Irwin and Rippe's
INTENSIVE CARE MEDICINE

EIGHTH EDITION

Irwin and Rippe's Intensive Care Medicine

EIGHTH EDITION

Editors

Richard S. Irwin, MD, Master FCCP
Professor of Medicine and Nursing
University of Massachusetts Medical School
Chair, Critical Care Operations
UMass Memorial Medical Center
Worcester, Massachusetts

Craig M. Lilly, MD, FCCP
Professor of Medicine, Anesthesiology, and Surgery
University of Massachusetts Medical School
Vice Chair, Critical Care Operations
Director, Tele-ICU Program
UMass Memorial Medical Center
Worcester, Massachusetts

Paul H. Mayo, MD, FCCP
Academic Director Critical Care
Division of Pulmonary, Critical Care, and Sleep Medicine
Department of Medicine
Northwell Health LIJ/NSUH Medical Center
Professor of Clinical Medicine
Zucker School of Medicine at Hofstra/Northwell
Hempstead, New York

James M. Rippe, MD
Founder and Director
Rippe Lifestyle Institute
Shrewsbury, Massachusetts

Wolters Kluwer

Philadelphia • Baltimore • New York • London
Buenos Aires • Hong Kong • Sydney • Tokyo

Acquisitions Editor: Brian Brown
Product Development Editor: Lauren Pecarich
Marketing Manager: Dan Dressler
Production Project Manager: David Saltzberg
Design Coordinator: Holly Reid McLaughlin
Manufacturing Coordinator: Beth Welsh
Prepress Vendor: S4Carlisle Publishing Services

Eighth edition

9 8 7 6 5 4 3

Printed in China

Library of Congress Cataloging-in-Publication Data

ISBN-13: 978-1-4963-0608-1
ISBN-10: 1-4963-0608-2

Cataloging-in-Publication data available on request from the Publisher.

LWW.com

CCS0521

To Our Families and Patients

Contributors List

Cynthia K. Aaron, MD, FACMT, FACEP
Program Director, Medical Toxicology
Regional Poison Center
Children's Hospital of Michigan
Detroit, Michigan

Gregory A. Abrahamian, MD
Surgical Director of Kidney Transplantation
University Transplant Center
University of Texas Health Science Center, San Antonio
San Antonio, Texas

Konstantin Abramov, MD, MHL
Assistant Professor of Medicine
Division of Renal Medicine
UMass Memorial Medical Center
Worcester, Massachusetts

Christopher D. Adams, PharmD
Clinical Assistant Professor
Department of Pharmacy
Robert Wood Johnson University at Somerset
Somerville, New Jersey

Sumera R. Ahmad, MD
Division of Pulmonary, Allergy and Critical Care
Department of Medicine
University of Massachusetts Medical School
Worcester, Massachusetts

Alfred Aleguas, Jr, BS Pharm, PharmD, DABAT, FAACT
Managing Director
Florida Poison Information Center-Trauma
Tampa General Hospital
Tampa, Florida

Gilman B. Allen, MD
Associate Professor
Department of Medicine
Division of Pulmonary Medicine and Critical Care
University of Vermont Medical Center
Burlington, Vermont

Jennifer E. Allen, MD
Palliative Medicine Consultant
Department of Oacis Services
Lehigh Valley Health Network
Allentown, Pennsylvania

Diana C. Anderson, MD, MArch
Founder, Dochitect
Physician, American Board of Internal Medicine (ABIM)
Architect, American College of Healthcare Architects (ACHA)
Montreal, Quebec, Canada

Gustavo Guillermo Angaramo, MD
Associate Professor of Anesthesiology and Critical Care
Director of Perianesthesia Unit
Department of Anesthesiology and Perioperative Medicine
University of Massachusetts Medical School
Worcester, Massachusetts

Luis F. Angel, MD
Professor, Department of Medicine
Professor, Department of Cardiothoracic Surgery
Medical Director, Lung Transplantation
NYU Langone Health
New York

Kevin E. Anger, PharmD
Pharmacy Supervisor
Department of Pharmacy
Brigham and Women's Hospital
Boston, Massachusetts

Derek C. Angus, MD
Distinguished Professor and Mitchell P. Fink Endowed Chair
Department of Critical Care Medicine
University of Pittsburg School of Medicine
Pittsburgh, Pennsylvania

Robert Arntfield, MD
Associate Professor of Critical Care
Western University
Department of Critical Care
London Health Sciences Centre
London, Ontario

Neil Aronin, MD
Chief, Division of Endocrinology
Professor, University of Massachusetts Medical School
UMass Memorial Medical Center
Worcester, Massachusetts

Seth M. Arum, MD
Clinical Associate Professor of Medicine
Department of Medicine/Endocrinology
UMass Memorial Medical Center
Worcester, Massachusetts

Samuel J. Asirvatham, MD
Consultant
Department of Cardiovascular Medicine
Division of Pediatric Cardiology
Department of Physiology and Biomedical Engineering
Professor of Medicine and Pediatrics
Medical Director, Electrophysiology Laboratory
Director of Strategic Collaborations
Center for Innovation, Program Director
Electrophysiology Fellowship Program
Mayo Clinic
Rochester, Minnesota

Philip J. Ayvazian, MD
Department of Urology
UMass Memorial Medical Center
Worcester, Massachusetts

Riad Azar, MD
Associate Professor of Medicine
Washington University School of Medicine
Gastroenterology Division
Department of Internal Medicine
Barnes-Jewish Hospital- North Campus
St. Louis, Missouri

Ednan K. Bajwa, MD, MPH
Assistant Professor of Medicine
Division of Pulmonary and Critical Care Medicine
Harvard Medical School
Massachusetts General Hospital
Boston, Massachusetts

Jerry P. Balikian, MD
Professor
Thoracic Imaging
UMass Memorial Medical Center
Worcester, Massachusetts

Ian M. Ball, MD, MSc(Epi), FACEP, FCCP, FRCPC
Assistant Professor
Department of Epidemiology and Biostatistics
Division of Critical Care Medicine
Western University
Critical Care Trauma Center
London Health Sciences Center
London, Ontario, Canada

Julia Baltz, MD
Chief Resident
Dermatology Residency Program
Department of Medicine
University of Massachusetts Medical School
Worcester, Massachusetts

Stephen L. Barnes, MD, FACS
Professor and Chief, Acute Care Surgery
Department of Surgery
University of Missouri Hospital and Clinics
Columbia, Missouri

Ribal Bassil, MD
Chief Resident
Department of Neurology
University of Massachusetts Medical School
Worcester, Massachusetts

David M. Bebinger, MD
Assistant Professor of Medicine
Department of Infectious Disease and Immunology
UMass Memorial Medical Center
Worcester, Massachusetts

Robert W. Belknap, MD
Director, Denver Metro TB Program
Department of Public Health and Infectious Diseases
Denver Health and Hospital Authority
Denver, Colorado

Isabelita R. Bella, MD
Associate Professor of Clinical Neurology
Department of Neurology
UMass Memorial Medical Center
Worcester, Massachusetts

Emanuelle A. Bellaguarda, MD
Assistant Professor
Department of Medicine Gastroenterology, Hepatology
Northwestern University Feinberg School of Medicine
Chicago, Illinois

Michael C. Bennett, MD
Instructor of Medicine
Department of Internal Medicine
Division of Gastroenterology
Washington University
Barnes-Jewish Hospital
St. Louis, Missouri

Hannah Bensimhon, MD
Chief Resident Physician
Department of Medicine
University of North Carolina
Chapel Hill, North Carolina

Andrew C. Bernard, MD
Professor, Chief of Trauma and Acute Care Surgery
Department of Surgery
University of Kentucky Healthcare
Lexington, Kentucky

Kristen Berrebi, MD
Division of Dermatology
University of Massachusetts Medical School
Worcester, Massachusetts

Mary T. Bessesen, MD
Associate Professor of Medicine
University of Colorado Denver
Chief, Infectious Diseases
Department of Internal Medicine
VA-Eastern Colorado Healthcare System
Denver, Colorado

Michael C. Beuhler, MD
Medical Director, Carolinas Poison Center
Department of Emergency Medicine
Carolinas Medical Center
Charlotte, North Carolina

Bonnie J. Bidinger, MD
Rheumatologist
Division of Rheumatology
Milford Regional Medical Center
Mendon, Massachusetts

Christine L. Bielick, MD
Assistant Professor
Department of Medicine
Division of Pulmonary, Allergy and Critical Care
University of Massachusetts Medical School
Worcester, Massachusetts

Steven B. Bird, MD
Professor
Department of Emergency Medicine
University of Massachusetts Medical School
Worcester, Massachusetts

Luke Bisoski, MD
Emergency Medicine Specialist
Sinai-Grace Hospital
Detroit, Michigan

Bruce R. Bistrian, MD
Professor of Medicine, Harvard Medical School
Chief, Clinical Nutrition
Department of Medicine
Beth Israel Deaconess Medical Center
Boston, Massachusetts

Robert M. Black, MD
Clinical Professor of Medicine
University of Massachusetts Medical School
Director, Division of Renal Medicine
Department of Renal Medicine
St. Vincent Hospital
Worcester, Massachusetts

Marc P. Bonaca, MD, MPH
Medical Director
Aortic Center
Assistant Professor
Department of Medicine
Division of Vascular Medicine and Cardiology
Brigham and Women's Hospital
Boston, Massachusetts

Naomi F. Botkin, MD
Associate Professor of Medicine
Department of Medicine
Division of Cardiology
University of Massachusetts Medical School
UMass Memorial Medical Center
55 Lake Avenue North
Worcester, Massachusetts

Adel Bozorgzadeh, MD, FACS
Professor of Surgery
Chief, Division of Organ Transplantation
Department of Surgery
UMass Memorial Medical Center
Worcester, Massachusetts

Suzanne F. Bradley, MD
Professor, Department of Internal Medicine
Medical Services, Division of Infectious Diseases
Veterans Affairs Ann Arbor Healthcare System
University of Michigan Medical School
Ann Arbor, Michigan

Brian Buchanan, BSc (Hon), MD, FRCPC
Clinical Lecturer
Department of Critical Care Medicine
University of Alberta
Edmonton, Alberta

Jennie A. Buchanan, MD
Denver Health & Hospital Authority Staff Physician
Rocky Mountain Poison & Drug Center Staff Physician
Associate Professor University of Colorado Department of Emergency Medicine
Denver, Colorado

Keith K. Burkhart, MD
Division of Applied Regulatory Science
Office of Clinical Pharmacology Office of Translational Science Center for Drug Evaluation and Research
United States Food and Drug Administration
Silver Spring, Maryland

Mitchell Cahan, MD, MBA, FACS
Associate Professor of Surgery
Director of Acute Care Surgery
University of Massachusetts Medical School
Worcester, Massachusetts

Brian T. Callahan, MD
Medical Director
Surgical Services
Emerson Hospital
Concord, Massachusetts

Alexis P. Calloway, MD
Physician, Digestive Healthcare of Georgia, PC
Department of Gastroenterology
Piedmont Atlanta Hospital
Atlanta, Georgia

Christine Campbell-Reardon, MD
Associate Professor of Medicine
Department of Pulmonary and Critical Care Medicine
Boston University School of Medicine
Boston Medical Center
Boston, Massachusetts

Jason P. Caplan, MD
Professor and Chair of Psychiatry
Department of Psychiatry
Creighton University School of Medicine, Phoenix
Phoenix, Arizona

Raphael A. Carandang, MD
Assistant Professor
Departments of Neurology, Anesthesiology and Surgery
University of Massachusetts Medical School
Vascular and Critical Care Neurology
UMass Memorial Medical Center
Worcester, Massachusetts

Paul A. Carpenter, MD
Professor of Pediatrics
Clinical Research Division
Fred Hutchinson Cancer Research Center
Seattle, Washington

James E. Carroll, Jr, MD, FACS
Assistant Professor of Surgery
Department of Surgery
Division of General and Laparoscopic Surgery
UMass Memorial Medical Center
University of Massachusetts Medical School
Worcester, Massachusetts

Karen C. Carroll, MD
Professor of Pathology
Department of Pathology
Division of Medical Microbiology
The Johns Hopkins University School of Medicine
John Hopkins Hospital
Baltimore, Maryland

Benjamin E. Cassell, MD
Fellow
Division of Gastroenterology
Washington University School of Medicine
St. Louis, Missouri

Richard Castriotta, MD
Professor and Director
Department of Internal Medicine
Division of Pulmonary and Sleep
McGovern Medical School
University of Texas Health Science Center at Houston
Houston, Texas

David R. Cave, MD, PhD
Professor of Medicine
Department of Internal Medicine
UMass Memorial Medical Center
Worcester, Massachusetts

Kelly L. Cervellione, MA, Mphil
Director, Department of Clinical Research
Jamaica Hospital Medical Center
Jamaica, New York

David A. Chad, MD
Associate Professor of Neurology
Department of Neurology
Massachusetts General Hospital
Neuromuscular Diagnostic Center
Boston, Massachusetts

Steven Y. Chang, MD, PhD
Associate Professor of Medicine
Department of Medicine
Division of Pulmonary and Critical Care
David Geffen School of Medicine at UCLA
Los Angeles, California

Sarah H. Cheeseman, MD
Professor of Medicine, Pediatrics and Microbiology, and Physiological Systems
Division of Infectious Diseases and Immunology
UMass Memorial Medical Center
Worcester, Massachusetts

Annabel A. Chen-Tournoux, MD
Assistant Professor
Department of Cardiology
Jewish General Hospital
Montreal, Quebec, Canada

Sonia Nagy Chimienti, MD
Vice Provost for Student Life and Campus Enrollment
Clinical Associate Professor, Medicine
Department of Medicine/Infectious Diseases
UMass Memorial Medical Center
Worcester, Massachusetts

William K.Chiang, MD
Associate Professor of Emergency Medicine
NYU School of Medicine
Bellevue Hospital Center
New York, New York

Eunpi Cho, MD
Hematology/Oncology Fellow
Department of Medicine
University of Washington
Fred Hutchinson Cancer Research Center
Seattle, Washington

Eric S. Christenson, MD
Medical Oncology Clinical Fellow
Department of Medical Oncology
Johns Hopkins Hospital
Baltimore, Maryland

Felicia C. Chu, MD
Assistant Professor
Department of Neurology
University of Massachusetts Medical School
Worcester, Massachusetts

Mary Dawn T. Co, MD
Assistant Professor of Medicine
Department of Medicine, Infectious Disease
University of Massachusetts Medical School
Worcester, Massachusetts

Christopher M. Coleman, MD
Post Doctoral Fellow
Microbiology and Immunology
University of Maryland School of Medicine
Baltimore, Maryland

Nancy A. Collop, MD
Emory Sleep Disorders Center
Wesley Woods Health Center
Emory University
Atlanta, Georgia

Brandon Colvin, MD
General Surgery Resident
University of Massachusetts Medical School
Worcester, Massachusetts

Laura S. Connelly-Smith, MBBCh, DM
Assistant Clinical Professor
Division of Hematology
School of Medicine
University of Washington
Assistant Medical Director of Apheresis and Cellular Therapy
Seattle Cancer Care Alliance
Seattle, Washington

Sara E. Cosgrove, MD
Professor of Medicine
Division of Infectious Disease
The Johns Hopkins University School of Medicine
Baltimore, Maryland

Filippo Cremonini, MD, PhD, MSc
Professor of Gastroenterology, Italian Ministry of University (MIUR)
Las Vegas Gastroenterology
Las Vegas, Nevada

Gerard Criner, MD, FACP, FACCP
Chairman, Department of Thoracic Medicine and Surgery
Temple University
Department of Thoracic Medicine and Surgery
Philadelphia, Pennsylvania

Ruy J. Cruz, Jr, MD, PhD
Associate Professor of Surgery
Surgical Director, Intestinal Rehabilitation and Transplant Center
Thomas E. Starzl Transplantation Institute
University of Pittsburgh
Pittsburgh, Pennsylvania

Hongyi Cui, MD, PhD, FACS
Clinical Associate Professor of Surgery
Department of Surgery
University of Massachusetts Medical School
Worcester, Massachusetts

Armagan Dagal, MD, FRCA
Associate Professor
Service Chief of Spine and Orthopaedic Anesthesia Services
Enhanced PeriOperative Care (EPOC)Program Co-Medical Director
Department of Anesthesiology and Pain Medicine
Department of Orthopedics and Sport Medicine
Department of Neurological Surgery (Adj.)
Harborview Medical Center
University of Washington
Seattle, Washington

Seth T. Dahlberg, MD
Associate Professor of Medicine and Radiology
University of Massachusetts Medical School
Department of Cardiology
UMass Memorial Medical Center
Worcester, Massachusetts

Jennifer S. Daly, MD
Professor of Medicine, Microbiology and Physiological Systems
Department of Medicine
University of Massachusetts Medical School
Worcester, Massachusetts

Lloyd E. Damon, MD
Professor of Clinical Medicine
Department of Medicine
Division of Hematology–Oncology
University of California
San Francisco, California

Raul E. Davaro, MD
Associate Professor of Clinical Medicine
Department of Internal Medicine
UMass Memorial Medical Center
Worcester, Massachusetts

Konrad L. Davis, MD, FCCP, FCCM
Associate Professor of Medicine
Department of Pulmonary and Critical Care Medicine
Uniformed Services University of Health Sciences
Naval Medical Center San Diego
San Diego, California

James A. de Lemos, MD
Professor
Department of Medicine
UT Southwestern Medical Center
Dallas, Texas

Gregory J. Della Rocca, MD, PhD, FACS
Associate Professor
Department of Orthopaedic Surgery
University of Missouri
Missouri Orthopaedic Institute
Columbia, Missouri

Mario De Pinto, MD
Associate Professor
Department of Anesthesiology
University of California
San Francisco, California

G. William Dec, MD
Roman W. DeSanctis Professor of Medicine
Division of Cardiology
Massachusetts General Hospital
Harvard Medical School
Boston, Massachusetts

Jeremy R. Degrado, PharmD
Clinical Pharmacist
Department of Pharmacy
Brigham and Women's Hospital
Boston, Massachusetts

Elizabeth R. DeGrush, DO
Resident Physician
Department of Neurology and Psychiatry
University of Massachusetts Medical School
Worcester, Massachusetts

Paul F. Dellaripa, MD
Associate Professor of Medicine
Harvard Medical School
Staff Physician
Department of Rheumatology
Brigham and Women's Hospital
Boston, Massachusetts

Thomas G. Deloughery, MD, MACP, FAWN
Professor of Medicine, Pathology, and Pediatrics
Department of Hematology
Oregon Health & Sciences University
Portland, Oregon

Deborah M. DeMarco, MD, FACP
Professor of Medicine
Department of Medicine
Senior Associate Dean of Clinical Affairs
University of Massachusetts Medical School
Worcester, Massachusetts

Mark Dershwitz, MD, PhD
Professor of Anesthesiology and Biochemistry & Molecular Pharmacology
Department of Anesthesiology
University of Massachusetts Medical School
Worcester, Massachusetts

Asha V. Devereaux, MD, MPH
Associate Professor of Clinical Medicine
UCSD-Pulmonary Division
San Diego, California
Clinical Pulmonologist
Department of Pulmonary/Critical Care Medicine
Disaster Medicine Consultant
Sharp Coronado Hospital
Coronado, California

Christopher R. DeWitt, MD
Associate Professor of Emergency Medicine and Consulting Medical Toxicologist
Department of Emergency Medicine and British Columbia Drug and Poison Centre
University of British Columbia
Saint Paul's Hospital
Vancouver, British Columbia, Canada

Abduljabbar Dheyab, MD
Fellow
Division of Pulmonary, Allergy, and Critical Care
Department of Medicine
University of Massachusetts Medical School
Worcester, Massachusetts

Kate H. Dinh, MD, MS
Resident
Department of Surgery
University of Massachusetts Medical School
Worcester, Massachusetts

Christian P. DiPaola, MD
Assistant Professor
Spine Surgery Division
Department of Orthopaedics and Rehabilitation
Department of Radiation Oncology
UMass Memorial Medical Center
Worcester, Massachusetts

Peter Doelken, MD
Pulmonary Critical Care Medicine
Pulmonary Medicine
Albany Medical Center
Albany, New York

Jon D. Dorfman, MD, FACS
Assistant Professor of Surgery
Department of Surgery
Division of Trauma and Surgical Critical Care
UMass Memorial Medical Center—University Campus
Worcester, Massachusetts

Robert P. Dowsett, BMBS, GDipClinEd, FACEM
Senior Lecturer (Assessment)
Department of Medical Education
Melbourne Medical School
Melbourne, Australia

David A. Drachman, MD
(deceased)
Professor of Neurology
Chairman Emeritus
Department of Neurology
University of Massachusetts Medical School
Worcester, Massachusetts

David F. Driscoll, PhD
Associate Professor of Medicine
Department of Medicine
University of Massachusetts Medical School
Worcester, Massachusetts

Dino Druda, MB, BCh, FACEM
Consultant Emergency Physician and Clinical Toxicologist
Monash Toxicology, Emergency Medicine Program, Monash Health
Dandenong Hospital
Dandenong, Victoria, Australia

David L. Dunn, MD
Vice President for Health Sciences
Professor of Surgery
Department of Microbiology and Immunology
University at Buffalo
Executive Vice President for Health Affairs
University of Louisville
Louisville, Kentucky

Angelina Edwards, MD
Nephrologist
Department of Nephrology
Memorial Hermann
Houston, Texas

Heather Elias, MD
Assistant Professor
Division of Endocrinology Metabolism and Diabetes
University of Massachusetts Medical School
Worcester, Massachusetts

Richard T. Ellison, III, MD
Hospital Epidemiologist
Professor of Medicine, Microbiology and Physiological Systems
University of Massachusetts Medical School
Department of Medicine
Division of Infectious Diseases
UMass Memorial Medical Center
Worcester, Massachusetts

Ashkan Emadi, MD, PhD
Associate Professor of Medicine, Pharmacology and Experimental Therapeutics
Director, Hematology & Medical Oncology Fellowship
Department of Medicine, Hematology/Medical Oncology
University of Maryland School of Medicine
Marlene & Stewart Greenebaum Comprehensive Cancer Center
Baltimore, Maryland

Charles H. Emerson, MD
Professor Emeritus of Medicine
Division of Endocrinology and Metabolism
University of Massachusetts Medical School
Worcester, Massachusetts

Timothy A. Emhoff, MD, FACS
Chief Trauma and Surgical Critical Care
Department of Surgery
UMass Memorial Medical Center
Worcester, Massachusetts

Jennifer L. Englund, MD
Emergency Medicine Physician
Maplewood, Minnesota

Robert M. Esterl, Jr, MD
Professor of Surgery
Department of Surgery
The University of Texas Health Science Center at San Antonio
San Antonio, Texas

Julien Fahed, MD
Resident
Department of Internal Medicine
UMass Memorial Medical Center
Worcester, Massachusetts

Pang-Yen Fan, MD
Professor of Medicine
Department of Medicine
University of Massachusetts Medical School
Worcester, Massachusetts

James C. Fang, MD
Adjunct Professor
Department of Medicine
Case Western Reserve University School of Medicine
Cleveland, Ohio

John Fanikos, BS, MBA
Director of Pharmacy
Department of Pharmacy
Brigham and Women's Hospital
Boston, Massachusetts

Harrison W. Farber, MD
Professor of Medicine
Director, Pulmonary Hypertension Center
Boston University
Boston Medical Center
Boston, Massachusetts

Khaldoun Faris, MD
Clinical Associate Professor
Director, Anesthesiology CCM
Department of Anesthesiology
University of Massachusetts Medical School
Worcester, Massachusetts

Alan P. Farwell, MD
Chief, Section of Endocrinology, Diabetes and Nutrition
Department of Medicine
Boston Medical Center/Boston University
Boston, Massachusetts

Alan M. Fein, MD
Clinical Professor of Medicine
Department of Pulmonary and Critical Care
Hofstra Northwell School of Medicine
Lake Success, New York

Stacey Feinstein, DO, MBA
Emergency Physician
Department of Emergency
Memorial Hospital Pembroke
Pembroke Pines, Florida

Sean Figy, MD
Resident Physician
Division of Plastics and Reconstructive Surgery
Department of Surgery
University of Massachusetts Medical School
Worcester, Massachusetts

Robert W. Finberg, MD
Richard M. Haidack Professor Medicine
Professor, Microbiology & Physiological Systems
Chair, Department of Medicine
University of Massachusetts Medical School
UMass Memorial Medical Center
Worcester, Massachusetts

Kimberly A. Fisher, MD
Assistant Professor
Department of Medicine
Division of Pulmonary and Critical Care
University of Massachusetts Medical Center
Worcester, Massachusetts

Christina Fitch, DO, MPH
Assistant Professor
Department of Palliative Care
University of Massachusetts Medical School
UMass Memorial Medical Center
Worcester, Massachusetts

Avegail G. Flores, MD
Assistant Professor, Hepatology Program
Division of Gastroenterology
Department of Medicine
Washington University
St. Louis, Missouri

Dee W. Ford, MD, MSCR
Associate Professor of Medicine
Department of Pulmonary and Critical
Care Medicine
Medical University of South Carolina
Charleston, South Carolina

Marsha D. Ford, MD
Emergency Medicine
Carolinas Medical Center
Charlotte, North Carolina

Kyle Fraielli, PharmD
Clinical Pharmacist
Department of Pharmacy
UMass Memorial Medical Center
Worcester, Massachusetts

Joseph J. Frassica, MD
Head, Phillips Research the Americas
Chief Medical Officer, Phillips North America
Professor, The Practice Institute for Medical Engineering and Science
Massachusetts Institute of Technology
Senior Consultant, Pediatric Critical Care
Massachusetts General Hospital for Children
Boston, Massachusetts

Ann-Kristin U. Friedrich, MD
Surgical Resident
Department of Surgery
University of Massachusetts Medical School
Worcester, Massachusetts
Saint Mary's Hospital
Waterbury, Connecticut

Matthew B. Frieman, MD
Associate Professor
Department of Microbiology and Immunology
University of Maryland, School of Maryland
Baltimore, Maryland

R. Brent Furbee, MD, FACMT
Professor Emeritus, Clinical Emergency Medicine
Department of Emergency Medicine
Division of Medical Toxicology
Indiana University School of Medicine
Indianapolis, Indiana

Brian S. Furukawa, MD
Assistant Professor
Department of Medicine
Division of Pulmonary and Critical Care Medicine
Loma Linda University
Loma Linda, California

Christos Galatas, MD
Cardiology Fellow
Department of Cardiology
McGill University
Montreal, Quebec, Canada

Sumanth Gandra, MD, MPH
Resident Scholar
The Center For Disease Dynamics, Economics & Policy
New Dehli, India

Javier Barreda Garcia, MD
Assistant Professor
Department of Internal Medicine
Division of Pulmonary and Critical Care Medicine
The University of Texas Health Science Center at Houston
Houston, Texas

Anne Garrison, MD
Director Obstetrics-Gynecology Clerkship
Assistant Professor
University of Massachusetts Medical School
UMass Memorial Medical Center - Memorial Campus
Worcester, Massachusetts

James Geiling, MD, MPH
Professor of Medicine, Geisel School of Medicine at Dartmouth
Veterans Affairs Medical Center
White River Junction, Vermont

Edith S. Geringer, MD
Boston, Massachusetts

Terry Gernsheimer, MD
Professor of Medicine
Division of Hematology
Medical Director of Transfusion
Seattle Cancer Care Alliance
University of Washington
Seattle, Washington

Hayley B. Gershengorn, MD
Assistant Professor
Department of Medicine
Albert Einstein College of Medicine
Montefiore Medical Center
Bronx, New York

Michael M. Givertz, MD
Medical Director, Heart Transplant and Mechanical Circulation Support
Brigham and Women's Hospital
Professor of Medicine
Harvard Medical School
Boston, Massachusetts

Richard H. Glew, MD
Professor of Medicine and Microbiology and Physiological Systems
Department of Medicine/Infectious Diseases
UMass Memorial Medical Center
Worcester, Massachusetts

Richard P. Goddeau, Jr, DO, FAHA
Associate Professor of Neurology
Department of Neurology
University of Massachusetts Medical School
UMass Memorial Medical Center
Worcester, Massachusetts

Dori Goldberg, MD
Assistant Professor
Division of Dermatology
University of Massachusetts Medical School
Worcester, Massachusetts

Andrew J. Goodwin, MD, MSCR
Assistant Professor
Division of Pulmonary, Critical Care, Allergy and Sleep Medicine
Medical University of South Carolina
Charleston, South Carolina

Susan E. Gorman, MD
Associate Director for Science
Division of Strategic National Stockpile
Centers for Disease Control and Prevention
Bethesda, Maryland

Andis Graudins, MBBS (Hons), PhD, FACEM, FCMT
Professor of Emergency Medicine and Toxicology Research
School of Clinical Sciences at Monash Health, Monash University
Director, Clinical Toxicology Services
Monash Toxicology, Emergency Medicine Program, Monash Health
Dandenong Hospital
Dandenong, Victoria, Australia

Gay Graves, MS, RD/LDN
Nutrition Support Dietitian
Department of Center for Human Nutrition
Vanderbilt University Hospital
Center for Human Nutrition
Nashville, Tennessee

Damian J. Green, MD
Assistant Member and Assistant Professor of Medicine
Clinical Research Division
Fred Hutchinson Cancer Research Center
University of Washington
Seattle, Washington

Bruce Greenberg, MD
Assistant Professor
Department of Medicine
Assistant Director
UMass Memorial Medical Center
Division of Pulmonary, Allergy and Critical Care
University of Massachusetts Medical School
Worcester, Massachusetts

Thomas C. Greenough, MD
Associate Professor
Department of Medicine
University of Massachusetts Medical School
Worcester, Massachusetts

Bonnie C. Greenwood, PharmD, BCPS
Clinical Program Director
Department of Clinical Pharmacy Services
University of Massachusetts Medical School
Shrewsbury, Massachusetts

Peeyush Grover, MD
Cardiology Fellow
Department of Cardiology
UMass Memorial Medical Center
Worcester, Massachusetts

Rainer W. G. Gruessner, MD, FACS, FICS
Professor of Surgery
Chief of Transplantation
Department of Surgery and Transplant Services
SUNY Upstate Medical University
Syracuse, New York

C. Prakash Gyawali, MD
Professor of Medicine
Division of Gastroenterology
Barnes Jewish Hospital
Washington University in St. Louis
St. Louis, Missouri

Michelle K. Haas, MD
Assistant Professor of Medicine
Division of Infectious Diseases
University of Colorado Health Science Center
Denver Public Health and Hospital Authority
Denver, Colorado

Shirin Haddady, MD, MPH
Clinical Assistant Professor
Department of Internal Medicine
Division of Endocrinology
Boston Medical Center
Boston University School of Medicine
Boston, Massachusetts

Wiley R. Hall, MD
Director of Neurocritical Care
UMass Memorial Medical Center
Worcester, Massachusetts

Hurst M. Hall, MD
Assistant Professor
Department of Medicine
Division of Cardiology
UT Southwestern Medical Center
Dallas, Texas

Neil A. Halpern, MD, MCCM, FACP, FCCP
Professor of Clinical Medicine
Professor of Medicine and Clinical Anesthesiology
Weill Cornell Medical College
Director, Critical Care Center
Chief, Critical Care Medicine Service
Department of Anesthesiology and Critical Care Medicine
Memorial Sloan Kettering Cancer Center
New York, New York

Tarek Abou Hamdan, MD
Gastroenterology and Interventional Endoscopy Consultant
Division of Gastroenterology
Clemenceau Medical Center Affiliated with Johns Hopkins International
Beirut, Lebanon

Samuel Y. Han, MD
Fellow
Department of Gastroenterology
University of Colorado
Aurora, Colorado

Stephen B. Hanauer, MD
Professor
Department of Medicine (Gastroenterology, Hepatology)
Northwestern University Feinberg School of Medicine
Chicago, Illinois

Sundaram Hariharan, MD
Professor of Medicine and Surgery
Robert J. Corry Chair of Surgery
Department of Medicine and Surgery
University of Pittsburgh Medical Center
Pittsburgh, Pennsylvania

David M. Harlan, MD
William and Doris Krupp Professor of Medicine
Co-Director, Diabetes Center of Excellence
Department of Medicine
Division of Diabetes
UMass Memorial Medical Center
Worcester, Massachusetts

Laura Harrell Raffals, MD, MS
Associate Professor of Medicine
Section of Gastroenterology and Hepatology
Mayo Clinic
Rochester, Minnesota

Steven Hatch, MD, MS
Associate Professor of Medicine
Division of Infectious Diseases
University of Massachusetts Medical School
Worcester, Massachusetts

Ashley Haynes, MD
Assistant Professor
Department of Emergency Medicine
Division of Medical Toxicology
University of Texas Southwestern
Parkland Health and Hospital System
Dallas, Texas

Lawrence J. Hayward, MD
Professor of Neurology
Department of Neurology
UMass Memorial Medical Center
University of Massachusetts Medical School
Worcester, Massachusetts

Stephen O. Heard, MD
Professor of Anesthesiology and Surgery
Department of Anesthesiology and Perioperative Medicine
UMass Memorial Medical Center
University of Massachusetts Medical School
Worcester, Massachusetts

Kennon Heard, MD
Professor of Emergency Medicine
Department of Emergency Medicine
University of Colorado School of Medicine
Aurora, Colorado

Benedikt H. Heidinger, MD
Research Fellow
Department of Radiology
Harvard Medical School
Beth Israel Deaconess Medical Center
330 Brookline Avenue
Boston, Massachusetts

Vitaly Herasevich, MD, PhD, FCCM
Associate Professor of Anesthesiology and Medicine
Department of Anesthesiology
Mayo Clinic
Rochester, Minnesota

Daniel Hetherman, MD
Resident
Department of Surgery
University of Massachusetts Medical School
Worcester, Massachusetts

Thomas L. Higgins, MD, MBA, FACP, MCCM
Chief Medical Officer and Interim President and CEO
Baystate Franklin Medical Center
Greenfield, Massachusetts
Professor of Medicine and Surgery and Anesthesiology
Tufts University School of Medicine
Boston, Massachusetts

Nicholas S. Hill, MD
Chief
Department of Pulmonary, Critical Care and Sleep Division
Tufts Medical Center
Boston, Massachusetts

John B. Holcomb, MD, FACS
Professor and Vice Chair
Department of Surgery
Memorial Hermann Hospital
Houston, Texas

Judd E. Hollander, MD
Associate Dean for Strategic Health Initiatives
Vice Chair for Finance and Healthcare Enterprises
Department of Emergency Medicine
Thomas Jefferson University Hospital
Philadelphia, Pennsylvania

Helen M. Hollingsworth, MD
Associate Professor of Medicine
Boston University School of Medicine
Boston Medical Center
Department of Pulmonary Allergy and Critical Care Medicine
UpToDate—Wolters Kluwer Health
Waltham, Massachusetts

Shelley A. Holmer, MD
Psychiatrist
Duke Health
Durham, North Carolina

Jonathan E. Holtz, MD
Clinical Instructor
Advanced Heart Failure Cardiologist
Department of Medicine
University of Pittsburgh Medical Center
Altoona, Pennsylvania

Donough Howard, MD
Consultant Rheumatologist
Hermitage Medical Clinic
Dublin, Ireland

Michael D. Howell, MD, MPH
Chief Quality Officer
Director, Center for Healthcare Delivery Science and Innovation
University of Chicago Medicine
Chicago, Illinois

Misha Huang, MD
Attending Physician
Denver Veterans Affairs Medical Center
Instructor
Department of Infectious Diseases
University of Colorado
Aurora, Colorado

Rolf D. Hubmayr, MD
Professor of Medicine and Physiology
Department of Pulmonary and Critical Care
Mayo Clinic
St. Louis Park, Minnesota

John Terrill Huggins, MD
Associate Professor
Department of Medicine
Division of Pulmonary and Critical Care
Medical University of South Carolina
Charleston, South Carolina

Abhinav Humar, MD
Thomas E. Starzl Professor in Transplantation Surgery
Clinical Director, Thomas E. Starzl Transplantation Institute
Chief, Division of Transplant Surgery
Department of Surgery
University of Pittsburgh
Pittsburgh, Pennsylvania

Benjamin Hyatt, MD
Assistant Professor of Medicine
Division of Gastroenterology
UMass Memorial Medical Center
Worcester, Massachusetts

Richard S. Irwin, MD, Master FCCP
Professor of Medicine and Nursing
University of Massachusetts Medical School
Chair, Critical Care Operations
UMass Memorial Medical Center
Worcester, Massachusetts

Margaret Isaac, MD
Adult Medicine Clinic and Palliative Care Service
Harborview Medical Center
Assistant Professor
University of Washington School of Medicine
Seattle, Washington

Janetta L. Iwanicki, MD
Assistant Professor, Emergency Medicine and Medical Toxicology
Department of Emergency Medicine
Denver Health and Hospital Authority
University of Colorado School of Medicine
Denver, Colorado

Colleen L. Jay, MD, MS
Assistant Professor of Surgery
University Transplant Center
University of Texas Health Science Center, San Antonio
San Antonio, Texas

Donald H. Jenkins, MD, FACS
Professor/Clinical
Division of Trauma and Emergency Surgery
Vice Chair for Quality
Department of Surgery
Betty and Bob Kelso Distinguished Chair in Burn and Trauma Surgery
Associate Deputy Director
Military Health Institute
University of Texas Health Science Center, San Antonio
San Antonio, Texas

Thanjira Jiranantakan, MD, MPH
Lecturer, Medical Toxicologist
Department of Preventive and Social Medicine
Division of Toxicology, Occupational & Environmental Medicine
Faculty of Medicine Siriraj Hospital
Mahidol University
Medical Toxicology
Attending Physician
Siriraj Poison Control Center
Bangkok Noi, Bangkok

Scott B. Johnson, MD
Chief of General Thoracic Surgery
Department of Cardiothoracic Surgery
University of Texas Health Science Center at San Antonio
San Antonio, Texas

Dejah R. Judelson, MD
Resident
Division of Vascular Surgery
UMass Memorial Medical Center
Worcester, Massachusetts

Bryan S. Judge, MD
Associate Professor
Department of Emergency Medicine
Spectrum Health
Grand Rapids Medical Education Partners/Michigan State University
College of Human Medicine Program in Emergency Medicine
Grand Rapids, Michigan

Firas Kaddouh, MD
Neurology Resident
Department of Neurology
UMass Memorial Medical Center
Worcester, Massachusetts

Marc J. Kahn, MD, MBA, FACP
Peterman-Prosser Professor
Senior Associate Dean
Departments of Medicine and Pharmacology
Division of Hematology/Medical Oncology
Tulane University School of Medicine
Office of Admissions and Student Affairs
New Orleans, Louisiana

Biren B. Kamdar, MD, MBA, MHS
Assistant Professor
Division of Pulmonary and Critical Care Medicine
David Geffen School of Medicine at
University of California
Los Angeles, California

Padmanaidu Karnam, MD
Rheumatology Fellow
Department of Rheumatology
UMass Memorial Medical Center
Worcester, Massachusetts

Sheetal Karne, MD
Hematology Oncology Fellow
Marlene and Stewart Greenebaum Cancer Center
University of Maryland
School of Medicine
Baltimore, Maryland

Jason N. Katz, MD, MHS
Associate Professor of Medicine
Department of Medicine
Division of Cardiology and Pulmonary & Critical Care Medicine
Medical Director, UNV Mechanical Heart Program
Medical Director, Cardiac Intensive Care Unit
Medical Director, Cardiothoracic Surgical Intensive Care Unit & Critical Care Service
Director, Cardiovascular Clinical Trials
University of North Carolina School of Medicine
Chapel Hill, North Carolina

Carol A. Kauffman, MD
Professor, Department of Internal Medicine
Chief, Division of Infectious Diseases
Veterans Affairs Ann Arbor Healthcare System
University of Michigan Medical School
Ann Arbor, Michigan

Andrew M. King, MD
Assistant Professor
Department of Emergency Medicine
Wayne State University School of Medicine
Detroit Medical Center
Detroit, Michigan

Mary A. King, MD, MPH
Pediatric Critical Care Medicine
Medical Director, PICU
Harborview Medical Center
Associate Professor
University of Washington
Seattle, Washington

Mark A. Kirk, MD
Associate Professor
Department, Emergency Medicine
UVA Health System
Charlottesville, Virginia

Karen M. Knops, MD
Medical Director, Palliative Care Program
Department of Palliative Care
Overlake Medical Center
Bellevue, Washington

Meghan S. Kolodziej, MD
Instructor in Psychiatry
Department of Psychiatry
Brigham and Women's Hospital
Boston, Massachusetts

Scott E. Kopec, MD
Associate Professor
Department of Medicine
Division of Pulmonary, Allergy and Critical Care
University of Massachusetts Medicine School
Worcester, Massachusetts

Pierre Kory, MD
Chief Critical Care Service
Medical Director, Trauma and Life Support Center
Department of Medicine
University of Wisconsin Hospital and Clinics
Madison, Wisconsin

Stephen J. Krinzman, MD
Clinical Associate Professor Medicine
University of Massachusetts Medical School
Division of Pulmonary and Critical Care
Department of Medicine
UMass Memorial Medical Center
Worcester, Massachusetts

Jason M. Kurland, MD
Assistant Professor of Medicine
Division of Renal Medicine
University of Massachusetts Medical School
Worcester, Massachusetts

Jennifer LaFemina, MD, FACS
Assistant Professor of Surgery
Department of Surgery
Division of Surgical Oncology
University of Massachusetts Medical School
Worcester, Massachusetts

Laura A. Lambert, MD
Associate Professor
Department of Surgery
Divisions of Surgical Oncology and Palliative Medicine
UMass Memorial Medical Center
Worcester, Massachusetts

Anthony J. Lembo, MD
Associate Professor of Medicine
Department of Medicine
Harvard Medical School
Beth Israel Deaconess Medical Center
Boston, Massachusetts

Adam B. Lerner, MD
Director, West Campus Clinical Operations
Department of Anesthesiology and Critical Care
Beth Isreael Deaconess Medical Center
Boston, Massachusetts

Stephanie M. Levine, MD
Professor of Medicine
Department of Medicine
Division of Pulmonary Diseases and Critical Care
University of Texas Health Center, San Antonio
San Antonio, Texas

William J. Lewander, MD
Vice Chair Pediatric Emergency Medicine
Department of Emergency
Hasbro Children's Hospital
Providence, Rhode Island

Daniel H. Libraty, MD
Professor of Medicine
Department of Medicine
University of Massachusetts Medical School
Worcester, Massachusetts

Craig M. Lilly, MD, FCCP
Professor of Medicine,
Anesthesiology, and Surgery
University of Massachusetts Medical School
Vice Chair, Critical Care Operations
Director, Tele-ICU Program
UMass Memorial Medical Center
Worcester, Massachusetts

Christopher H. Linden, MD
Professor
Division of Medical Toxicology
Department of Emergency Medicine
UMass Medical School
Department of Emergency Services
Milford Regional Medical Center
Milford, Massachusetts

Mark S. Link, MD
Professor of Medicine
Department of Cardiology
UT Southwestern Medical Center
Dallas, Texas

Carol F. Lippa, MD
Professor and Interim Chair
Department of Neurology
Drexel University College of Medicine
Philadelphia, Pennsylvania

Mauricio Lisker-Melman, MD
Professor of Medicine
Director of Hepatology
Department of Gastroenterology & Hepatology
Washington University School of Medicine
Barnes Jewish Hospital
St. Louis, Missouri

Diana E. Litmanovich, MD
Staff Radiologist, Cardiothoracic Imaging, BIDMC
Director, Cardiac Imaging
Director, Cardiothoracic Imaging Fellowship Program
Associate Professor of Radiology
Harvard Medical School
Boston, Massachusetts

Norman Scott Litofsky, MD
Professor and Chief, Director of Radiosurgery and
Neuro-Oncology
Division of Neurological Surgery
University of Missouri School of Medicine
Columbia, Missouri

Afroza Liton, MD
Attending Physician
Department of Internal Medicine
St. Peters Hospital
Albany, New York

Frederic F. Little, MD
Assistant Professor of Medicine
Program Director, Allergy/Immunology Fellowship
Medical Director, Pulmonary, Allergy and
Sleep Clinics
Department of Medicine
Boston University School of Medicine
Boston Medical Center
Boston, Massachusetts

Nancy Y. N. Liu, MD
Clinical Associate Professor
Department of Rheumatology
University of Massachusetts Medical School
UMass Memorial Medical Center-Memorial Campus
Worcester, Massachusetts

Melanie R. Loberman, MD
Instructor in Anaesthesia
Harvard Medical School
Department of Anesthesia, Critical Care & Pain Medicine
Beth Israel Deaconess Medical Center
Boston, Massachusetts

Dana Lustbader, MD
Professor of Medicine
Chair, Department of Palliative Care
Hofstra Northwell School of Medicine
ProHEALTH Care, an Optum Company
Lake Success, New York

Alice D. Ma, MD
Professor of Medicine
Department of Hematology/Oncology
University of North Carolina
Chapel Hill, North Carolina

J. Mark Madison, MD
Professor of Medicine and Microbiology
and Physiological Systems
Chief, Division of Pulmonary, Allergy and
Critical Care Medicine
Department of Medicine
UMass Memorial Medical Center
University of Massachusetts Medical School
Worcester, Massachusetts

Garbo Mak, MD
Assistant Professor
Division of Critical Care, Pulmonary and
Sleep Medicine
University of Texas Health Science Center at Houston,
Houston, Texas

Suzana K. E. Makowski, MD, MMM
Co-Chief, Division of Palliative Care
Department of Medicine
University of Massachusetts Medical School
UMass Memorial Medical Center
Worcester, Massachusetts

Atul Malhotra, MD
Professor
Department of Medicine
University of California San Diego
La Jolla, California

Samir Malkani, MD, MRCP (UK)
Clinical Professor of Medicine
University of Massachusetts Medical School
Diabetes Center of Excellence
Worcester, Massachusetts

Mary E. Maloney, MD
Chair, Division of Dermatology
University of Massachusetts Medical School
Worcester, Massachusetts

Max Mandelbaum, MD, PhD
Resident
Department of Neurology
UMass Memorial Medical Center
Worcester, Massachusetts

Paul E. Marik, MD, FCCM
Chief, Pulmonary and Critical Care Medicine
Department of Medicine
Eastern Virginia Medical School
Sentara Norfolk General Hospital
Norfolk, Virginia

William L. Marshall, MD
Associate Professor
Department of Medicine
Division of Infectious Diseases
University of Massachusetts Medical School
Worcester, Massachusetts

Carlos Martinez-Balzano, MD
Assistant Professor of Medicine
Division of Pulmonary, Critical Care and Sleep
SUNY Upstate Medical University
Syracuse, New York

Paulo Martins, MD, PhD
Assistant Professor
University of Massachusetts Medical School
UMass Memorial Medical Center
Worcester, Massachusetts

Christina Massey, MA
Predoctoral Intern
Department of Psychiatry
Massachusetts General Hospital
Boston, Massachusetts

Ryan C. Maves, MD, FACP, FIDSA
Attending Physician
Associate Professor of Medicine
Department of Infectious Disease and Critical Care Medicine
Uniformed Services University
San Diego, California

Paul H. Mayo, MD, FCCP
Academic Director Critical Care
Division of Pulmonary, Critical Care, and Sleep Medicine
Department of Medicine
Northwell Health LIJ/NSUH Medical Center
Professor of Clinical Medicine
Zucker School of Medicine at Hofstra/Northwell
Hempstead, New York

Guy Maytal, MD
Medical Director, Ambulatory Psychiatry
Department of Psychiatry
Massachusetts General Hospital
Boston, Massachusetts

Melanie Maytin, MD
Instructor in Medicine
Division of Cardiovascular Medicine
Brigham and Women's Hospital
Boston, Massachusetts

Joyce K. McIntyre, MD
Assistant Professor of Surgery, Pediatrics and Neurosurgery
Departments of Surgery, Pediatrics and Neurosurgery
Division of Plastics and Reconstructive Surgery
University of Massachusetts Medical School
UMass Memorial Medical Center
Worcester, Massachusetts

Brandy McKelvy, MD
Associate Professor
Department of Internal Medicine
Division of Pulmonary, Critical Care and Sleep Medicine
Memorial Herman Hospital Texas Medical Center
Lyndon B. Johnson General Hospital
University of Texas Health Science Center at Houston
Houston, Texas

Lloyd C. Meeks, MD
Intensivist, Regional Medical Director
Advanced ICU Care
St. Louis, Missouri

Brendan Merchant, MD
Fellow, Cardiovascular Medicine
Division of Cardiology
University of Massachusetts Medical School
UMass Memorial Medical Center
Worcester, Massachusetts

Marco Mielcarek, MD
Associate Professor of Medicine/Associate Member
Department of Medical Oncology
Clinical Research Division, FHCRC
University of Washington
Seattle, Washington

Abdul Mikati, MD
Neurology resident, Dept. of Neurology
University of Massachusetts Medical School
55 Lake Ave North
Worcester, Massachusetts

Ann L. Mitchell, MD
Clinical Associate Professor University of Massachusetts Medical School
UMass Memorial Medical Center
Worcester, Massachusetts

Lawrence C. Mohr, Jr, MD, ScD, FACP, FCCP
Professor of Medicine, Biometry and Epidemiology
Director, Environmental Biosciences Program
Medical University of South Carolina
Charleston, South Carolina

Jahan Montague, MD
Clinical Associate Professor of Medicine
Director, Nephrology Fellowship
Department of Medicine
Division of Renal Medicine
UMass Memorial Medical Center
Worcester, Massachusetts

Bruce Montgomery, MD
Professor
Department of Medicine
University of Washington and Seattle Cancer Alliance
Seattle, Washington

Majaz Moonis, MD, MRCP, DM, FRCP (I), FAAN, FAHA, FAASM
Professor of Neurology
Director of the Stroke Services
UMass Memorial Medical Center
Worcester, Massachusetts

Andrew H. Moraco, MD, MS
Fellow
Division of Pulmonary, Allergy and Critical Care
Department of Medicine
University of Massachusetts Medical School
Worcester, Massachusetts

John P. Mordes, MD
Professor of Medicine/Endocrinology
Department of Medicine
UMass Memorial Medical Center
Worcester, Massachusetts

David A. Morrow, MD, MPH
Professor of Medicine
Harvard Medical School
Directory, Levine Cardiac Intensive Care Unit
Division of Cardiovascular
Brigham and Women's Hospital
Boston, Massachusetts

Babak Movahedi, MD, PhD
Assistant Professor of Surgery
Department of Surgery
Division of Organ Transplantation
UMass Memorial Medical Center
Worcester, Massachusetts

James B. Mowry, PharmD, DABAT, FAACT
Director, Indiana Poison Center
Emergency Medicine and Trauma Center
Indiana University Health Methodist Hospital
Indianapolis, Illinois

Karol Mudy, MD
Cardiothoracic Clinics
Hennepin County Medical Center
Minneapolis, Minnesota

Susanne Muehlschlegel, MD, MPH, FNCS, FCCM
Associate Professor of Neurocritical Care
Department of Neurology, Anesthesia, Critical Care and Surgery
University of Massachusetts Medical School
Worcester, Massachusetts

Diana Wells Mulherin, PharmD, BCPS, BCNSP
Clinical Pharmacy Specialist, Nutrition Support
Department of Pharmacy Clinical Programs and Center for Human Nutrition
Vanderbilt University Medical Center
Nashville, Tennessee

Saori A. Murakami, MD
Attending Psychiatrist
Assistant Medical Director, McLean Franciscan Child and Adolescent Inpatient Program
Child and Adolescent Psychiatry
McLean Hospital
Brighton, Massachusetts

John G. Myers, MD
Professor and Chief
Division of Trauma and Emergency Surgery
University of Texas San Antonio
San Antonio, Texas

Nandita R. Nadig, MD, MSCR
Assistant Professor of Pulmonary and Critical Care
Department of Medicine
Medical University of South Carolina
Charleston, South Carolina

Ramana K. Naidu, MD
Assistant Professor
Department of Anesthesia and Perioperative Care
Division of Pain Medicine
University of California, San Francisco
San Francisco, California

Girish B. Nair, MD, FACP, FCCP
Associate Professor of Clinical Medicine
Division of Pulmonary and Critical Care Medicine
Oakland University William Beaumont School of Medicine
William Beaumont Hospital
Royal Oak, Michigan

Niyada Naksuk, MD
Division of Cardiovascular Diseases
Mayo Clinic
Rochester, Minnesota

Lena M. Napolitano, MD, FACS, FCCM, MCCM
Professor of Surgery
Division Chief, Acute Care Surgery
Department of Surgery
University of Michigan
Ann Arbor, Michigan

Reenu Nathan, PharmD, BCPS
Clinical Pharmacist
Department of Pharmacy
UMass Memorial Medical Center
Worcester, Massachusetts

Theresa A. Nester, MD
Medical Director of Integrated TSL
Bloodworks Northwest Medical Center
Associate Professor
Department of Laboratory Medicine
University of Washington
Seattle, Washington

Michael S. Niederman, MD, MACP, FCCP, FCCM, FERS
Clinical Director, Pulmonary and Critical Care Medicine
New York Presbyterian/Weill Cornell Medical Center
Professor of Clinical Medicine
Weill Cornell Medical College
New York, New York

Matthew A. Niemi, MD
Assistant Professor of Medicine
Division of Renal Medicine
Department of Medicine
UMass Memorial Medical Center
Worcester, Massachusetts

Anna Nolan, MD, MS
Assistant Professor of Medicine and Environmental Medicine
Department of Medicine and Environmental Medicine
Division of Pulmonary and Critical Care
New York University School of Medicine
New York, New York

Dominic J. Nompleggi, MD
Chief, Gastroenterology
Associate Professor
University of Massachusetts Medical School
Worcester, Massachusetts

Sean E. Nork, MD
Associate Professor of Orthopaedics and Sports Medicine
UW Medicine
Harborview Medical Center
Seattle, Washington

Gary O. Noroian, MD
Staff Nephrologist
Division of Nephrology
St. Vincent Hospital
Worcester, Massachusetts

Robert Lee Norris, MD
Professor of Surgery
Division of Emergency Medicine
Stanford University School of Medicine
Stanford, California

Patrick T. O'Gara, MD
Watkins Family Distinguished Chair in Cardiology
Division of Cardiovascular
Department of Medicine
Brigham and Women's Hospital
Boston, Massachusetts

Paulo J. Oliveira, MD, FCCP
Associate Professor of Medicine
Director of Interventional Pulmonary
Medical Director of Respiratory Care
Division of Pulmonary, Allergy and Critical Care Medicine
Department of Medicine
UMass Memorial Medical Center
Worcester, Massachusetts

Kent R. Olson, MD
Co-Medical Director
San Francisco Division California Poison Control System
Clinical Professor of Medicine & Pharmacy
University of California
San Francisco, California

Steven M. Opal, MD
Professor of Medicine
Department of Infectious Diseases
Alpert Medical School of Brown University
Rhode Island Hospital
Ocean State Clinical Coordinating Center
Providence, Rhode Island

Achikam Oren-Grinberg, MD
Director, Critical Care Echocardiography
Department of Anesthesia, Critical Care and Pain Management
Beth Israel Deaconess Medical Center
Boston, Massachusetts

David E. Ost, MD, MPH
Professor of Medicine
Department of Pulmonary Medicine
The University of Texas AD Anderson Cancer Center
Houston, Texas

John Scott Parrish, MD
Associate Program Director
Department of Pulmonary and Critical Care Medicine
Naval Medical Center San Diego
San Diego, California

Polly E. Parsons, MD
Professor of Medicine
Chair, Department of Medicine
University of Vermont Medical Center
Burlington, Vermont

Payal K. Patel, MD
Clinical Lecturer and Staff Infectious Diseases Physician
Division of Infectious Diseases
Department of Internal Medicine
Veterans Affairs Ann Arbor Healthcare System
University of Michigan Medical School
Ann Arbor, Michigan

Krunal Patel, MD
Fellow (Physician)
Division of Gastroenterology
University of Massachusetts Medical School
Worcester, Massachusetts

Marie T. Pavini, MD, FCCP
Intensivist
Department of Intensive Care Unit
Rutland Regional Medical Center
Rutland, Vermont

William D. Payne, MD
Professor
Department of Surgery
University of Minnesota
Minneapolis, Minnesota

Randall Pellish, MD
Assistant Professor of Medicine
Fellowship Program Director
Department of Medicine
Division of Gastroenterology
University of Massachusetts Medical School
UMass Memorial Medical Center
Worcester, Massachusetts

Catherine A. Phillips, MD
Associate Professor of Neurology
Department of Neurology
University of Massachusetts Medical School
UMass Memorial Medical Center
Worcester, Massachusetts

David J. Prezant, MD
Chief Medical Officer
Special Advisor to the Fire Commissioner for Health Policy
Co-Director WTC Medical Monitoring and Treatment Programs
New York City Fire Department
Professor of Medicine
Division of Pulmonary
Albert Einstein College of Medicine
Montefiore Medical Center
Bronx, New York

Timothy A. Pritts, MD, PhD, FACS
Professor of Surgery
Chief, Section of General Surgery
Department of Surgery
University of Cincinnati Medical Center
Cincinnati, Ohio

Juan Carlos Puyana, MD
Associate Professor of Surgery Department of Critical Care Medicine and Clinical Translational Science
The University of Pittsburgh
Pittsburgh, Pennsylviania

John Querques, MD
Chief, Inpatient Services
Department of Pyschology
Tufts Medical Center
Boston, Massachusetts

Jacob A. Quick, MD
Assistant Professor of Surgery
Department of Surgery
University of Missouri
Columbia, Missouri

Sunil Rajan, MD, FCCP
Pulmonary and Critical Care Physician
Department of Medicine
Centra Southside Community Hospital
Farmville, Virginia

Navitha Ramesh, MD
Associate
Geisinger Health
Wilkes Barre, Pennsylvania

Rajeev Ramgopal, MD
Chief Resident
Department of Internal Medicine
Barnes Jewish Hospital/Washington University
Saint Louis, Missouri

Britney M. Ramgopal, MD
Resident Physician
Department of Internal Medicine
Barnes Jewish Hospital/Washington University
Saint Louis, Missouri

Abbas A. Rana, MD
Assistant Professor of Surgery
Department of Surgery, Abdominal Transplantation
Baylor College of Medicine
Houston, Texas

Paula D. Ravin, MD
Department of Neurology
UCLA Health
Los Angeles, California

Daniel E. Ray, MD, MS, FAAHPM
Chief, Section of Palliative Medicine and Hospice
Department of Medicine
Lehigh Valley Health Network
Allentown, Pennsylvania

Mary Jane Reed, MD, FACS, FCCM, FCCP
Medical Director
Geisinger System Bio Containment Unit
Associate
Departments of Critical Care Medicine and Trauma Surgery
Geisinger Medical Center
Danville, Pennsylvania

Harvey S. Reich, MD, FACP, FCCP, FFSMB
Director, Critical Care Medicine
Department of Critical Care
Rutland Regional Medical Center
Rutland, Vermont

Jennifer E. Reidy, MD, MS, FAAHPM
Co-Chief, Division of Palliative Care
Department of Medicine and Family Medicine
UMass Memorial Medical Center
Assistant Professor
University of Massachusetts Medical School
Worcester, Massachusetts

Carole A. Ridge, MD
Consultant Radiologist
Mater Misericordiae University Hospital
Dublin

James M. Rippe, MD
Founder and Director
Rippe Lifestyle Institute
Shrewsbury, Massachusetts

Ray H. Ritz, BA, RRT, FAARC
Manager of Respiratory Care
Department of Respiratory Care
Beth Israel Deaconess Medical Center
Boston, Massachusetts

William P Robinson, III, MD
Associate Professor of Surgery
Program Director
Department of Vascular Surgery
University of Virginia School of Medicine
Charlottesville, Virginia

Kimberly A. Robinson, MD, MPH
Medical Director ICU
Department of Pulmonary and Critical Care Medicine
UMass Memorial Medical Center—Marlborough Campus
Marlborough, Massachusetts

Mark J. Rosen, MD
Division of Pulmonary, Critical Care and Sleep Medicine
North Shore University and Long Island Jewish Health System
Professor of Medicine
Hofstra North Shore-Long Island Jewish School of Medicine
New Hyde Park, New York

Marc S. Sabatine, MD
Professor of Medicine
Harvard Medical School
Physician
Chairman
TIMI Study Group
Cardiology Division
Brigham and Women's Hospital
Boston, Massachusetts

Marjorie S. Safran, MD, FACE
Clinical Professor Medicine
Division of Endocrinology
University of Massachusetts Medical School
Worcester, Massachusetts

Johnny S. Salameh
Associate Professor, Department of Neurology
Program Director, Neurology Residency
Chair, Quality Advisory Council
Director, ALS Clinic
American University of Beirut Medical Center
Beirut, Lebanon

Benkole Samuel, MD
General Surgery Resident
Department of Surgery
UMass Memorial Medical Center
Worcester, Massachusetts

Rolando Sanchez Sanchez, MD
Clinical Assistant Professor
Division of Pulmonary Diseases, Critical Care
University of Iowa
Iowa City, Iowa

Todd W. Sarge, MD
Director, Critical Care
Department of Anesthesia, Critical Care and Pain Medicine
Beth Israel Deaconess Medical Center
Boston, Massachusetts

Yaw Sarpong, MD, eMBA
Chief Resident
Division of Neurological Surgery
University of Missouri
Columbia, Missouri

Gregory A. Schmidt, MD
Professor
Division of Pulmonary Diseases, Critical Care, and Occupational Medicine
Associate Chief Medical Officer—Critical Care
University of Iowa Hospitals and Clinics
Iowa City, Iowa

Benjamin M. Scirica, MD, MPH
Senior Investigator
TIMI Study Group
Associate Professor of Medicine
Harvard Medical Group
Department of Medicine
Division of Cardiovascular
Brigham and Women's Hospital
Boston, Massachusetts

Joshua R. Scurlock, MD
Department of Surgery
UMass Memorial Medical Center
55 Lake Avenue
Worcester, Massachusetts

Douglas L. Seidner, MD, AGAF, FACG, FASPEN, CNSC
Associate Professor of Medicine
Director, Vanderbilt Center for Human Nutrition
Division of Gastroenterology
Vanderbilt University Medical Center
Nashville, Tennessee

Myron Michael Shabot, MD, FACS, FCCM, FACMI
Executive Vice President/System Chief Clinical Officer
Department of Executive Offices
Memorial Hermann Health System
Houston, Texas

Shahzad Shaefi, MD
Assistant Professor in Anesthesia
Harvard Medical School
Department of Anesthesia, Critical Care and Pain Medicine
Beth Israel Deaconess Medical Center
Boston, Massachusetts

Andrew W. Shaffer, MD
Fellow
Department of Cardiothoracic Surgery
University of Minnesota Medical Center
Minneapolis, Minnesota

Robert Sheiman, MD, BS, Ch. Eng
Professor of Abdominal and Interventional Radiology
University of Massachusetts Medical School
UMass Memorial Medical Center
Worcester, Massachusetts

Richard D. Shih, MD
Professor Clinical Biomedical Science
Department of Integrated Medical Science
Florida Atlanta University College of Medicine
Boynton Beach, Florida

Ryan G. Shipe, MD
Assistant Professor
Department of Medicine
Division of Pulmonary, Allergy and Critical Care Medicine
University of Massachusetts Medical School
Worcester, Massachusetts

Andrew F. Shorr, MD, MPH
Associate Director of Pulmonary and Critical Care Medicine
Chief
Pulmonary Clinic
MedStar Washington Hospital Center
Washington, DC

Bing Shue, MD
Resident Physician
Department of Vascular Surgery
University of Massachusetts Medical School
Worcester, Massachusetts

Sara J. Shumway, MD
Professor of Surgery
Vice Chief, Division of Cardiothoracic Surgery
University of Minnesota
Minneapolis, Minnesota

Michael G. Silverman, MD
Fellow
Department of Cardiovascular Medicine
Brigham and Women's Hospital
Boston, Massachusetts

Bruce J. Simon, MD
Associate Director, Trauma and Surgical Critical Care
Associate Professor, University of Massachusetts Medical School
UMass Memorial Medical Center
Worcester, Massachusetts

Marco L. A. Sivilotti, MD, MSc, FRCPC, FACEP, FACMT
Professor, Departments of Emergency Medicine and of Biomedical & Molecular Sciences
Queen's University at Kingston
Ontario, Canada

Craig S. Smith, MD
Assistant Professor
Medical Director, Coronary Care Unit
Department of Medicine and Cardiology
University of Massachusetts Medical School
UMass Memorial Medical Center
Worcester, Massachusetts

Heidi L. Smith, MD, PhD
Assistant Professor
Department of Medicine
University of Massachusetts Medical School
Mas Biologics of the University of Massachusetts Medical School, Clinical Affairs
Boston, Massachusetts

Brian S. Smith, PharmD
Vice President
Clinical Services and Quality
Department of Pharmacy
UMass Memorial Specialty Pharmacy
UMass Memorial Medical Center
Worcester, Massachusetts

Nicholas A. Smyrnios, MD, FACP, FCCP
Professor of Medicine
Associate Chief of Pulmonary, Allergy and Critical Care Medicine
University of Massachusetts Medical School
UMass Memorial Medical Center
Worcester, Massachusetts

Haley Snadecki, MD
Dermatology Resident
Division of Dermatology
University of Massachusetts Medical School
Worcester, Massachusetts

Rahul N. Sood, MD
Division of Pulmonary and Critical Care
Department of Medicine
University of Massachusetts Medical School
Worcester, Massachusetts

Andres F. Sosa, MD
Pulmonary and Critical Care Associate Physician
Department of Medicine
Baptist Hospital of Miami
South Florida Pulmonary and Critical Care
Miami, Florida

Judith A. Stebulis, MD
Assistant Professor of Medicine
Department of Medicine and Rheumatology
University of Massachusetts Medical School
UMass Memorial Medical Center
Worcester, Massachusetts

Mary Kathryn Steiner, MD
Instructor, Harvard Medical School
Pulmonary and Critical Care Attending
Division of Pulmonary, Critical Care
Department of Medicine
Deaconess Medical New England Baptist Hospital
Boston, Massachusetts

Jay S. Steingrub, MD, FACP, FCCP
Director, Medical Intensive Care Unit
Vice-chair of Research, Department of Medicine
Baystate Medical Center
Springfield, Massachusetts
Professor of Medicine
Tufts University School of Medicine
Boston, Massachusetts

Theodore A. Stern, MD
Chief, Avery D. Weisman Psychiatry Consultation Service, Massachusetts General Hospital
Director, Office for Clinical Careers, Massachusetts General Hospital
Ned H. Cassem Professor of Psychiatry in the Field of Psychosomatic Medicine/Consultation
Department of Psychiatry
Harvard Medical School
Massachusetts General Hospital
Boston, Massachusetts

Garrick C. Stewart, MD
Associate Physician
Department of Cardiovascular Medicine
Brigham and Women's Hospital
Boston, Massachusetts

Glenn Stokken, MD
Cardiology Fellow
Department of Cardiology
University of Massachusetts Medical School
Worcester, Massachusetts

Michael B. Streiff, MD, FACP
Associate Professor of Medicine and Pathology
Division of Hematology
Department of Medicine
Johns Hopkins University School of Medicine
Baltimore, Maryland

Shusen Sun, PharmD
Clinical Assistant Professor
Department of Pharmacy Practice
Western New England University College of Pharmacy
Springfield, Massachusetts

Banu Sundar, MD
Assistant Professor
Department of Neurology
UMass Memorial Medical Center
Worcester, Massachusetts

Arvind K. Sundaram, MD
Associate
Department of Critical Care Medicine and Pulmonary
Geisinger Commonwealth School of Medicine
Danville, Pennsylvania

Colin T. Swales, MD
Medical Director
Transplant Hepatology
Hartford Hospital
Hartford, Connecticut

Joan M. Swearer, PhD, ABPP
Professor of Clinical Neurology and Psychology
Department of Neurology
University of Massachusetts Medical School
Worcester, Massachusetts

Milton Tenenbein, MD, FRCPC, FAAP, FACCT, FACMT
Professor of Pediatrics and Child Health and Community Health Sciences
University of Manitoba
Children's Hospital
Winnipeg, Manitoba, Canada

Jeffrey J. Teuteberg, MD
Medical Director
Advanced Heart Failure
Department of Heart and Vascular Institute
University of Pittsburgh Medical Center
Pittsburgh, Pennsylvania

Jerry D. Thomas, MD
Assistant Professor
Emergency Medicine
Medical Toxicologist
Emory University Hospital Midtown
Atlanta, Georgia

John A. Thompson, MD
Fred Hutchinson Cancer Research Center
Seattle, Washington

Michael J. Thompson, MD
Clinical Research Chief, Adult Diabetes
Physician Unit Chief
Clinical Professor
University of Massachusetts Medical School
Worcester, Massachusetts

Robert M. Tighe, MD
Assistant Professor of Medicine
Department of Medicine
Division of Pulmonary, Allergy and Critical Care
Duke University Medical Center
Durham, North Carolina

Colleen Timlin, PharmD, BCOP
Clinical Pharmacy Specialist, Hematology/Oncology
Department of Pharmacy—Ground Rhoads
Hospital of the University of Pennsylvania
Philadelphia, Pennsylvania

Mira Sofia Torres, MD
Associate Professor and Fellowship Program Director
Department of Medicine
Division of Endocrinology
University of Massachusetts Medical School
Worcester, Massachusetts

Ulises Torres, MD
Assistant Professor of Surgery
Chief Quality Officer
Department of Surgery
Associate Program Director, General Surgery Residency
Program Director, Trauma Education and Outreach
UMass Memorial Medical Center
Worcester, Massachusetts

Matthew J. Trainor, MD
Assistant Professor of Medicine
Medical Director, University Dialysis Services
University of Massachusetts Medical School
Division of Renal Medicine
UMass Memorial Medical Center
Worcester, Massachusetts

Christoph Troppmann, MD
Professor of Surgery
Department of Surgery
University of California, Davis School of Medicine
Sacramento, California

Craigan T. Usher, MD
Associate Professor
Department of Psychiatry
Oregon Health & Science University
Portland, Oregon

Vaibhav R. Vaidya, MD
Instructor in Medicine
Department of Cardiovascular Diseases
Mayo Clinic
Rochester, Minnesota

John-Paul B. Velasco, MD
Vascular and Interventional Radiology
Department of Radiology
University of Massachusetts Medical School
Worcester, Massachusetts

Vivek Venugopal, MD
Orthopedic Surgery Resident
Baylor College of Medicine
Houston, Texas

Charles G. Volk, MD
Fellow
Department of Pulmonary
Naval Medical Center
San Diego, California

Javier C. Waksman, MD
Associate Clinical Professor Medicine-Clinical Pharmacology/Toxicology
Director
Medical Toxicology Practice
University of Colorado
Aurora, Colorado

J. Matthias Walz, MD, FCCP
Academic Vice Chair
Department of Anesthesiology and Perioperative Medicine
UMass Memorial Medical Center
Worcester, Massachusetts

Richard Y. Wang, DO
Senior Medical Officer
National Center for Environmental Health
Centers for Disease Control and Prevention
Atlanta, Georgia

Wahid Y. Wassef, MD
Director of Endoscopy
Professor of Medicine
Department of Medicine
UMass Memorial Medical Center
Worcester, Massachusetts

Paul M. Wax, MD, FACMT
Clinical Professor of Emergency Medicine (Medical Toxicology)
UT Southwestern Medical School
Executive Director, American College of Medical Toxicology
Dallas, Texas

Randy Wax, MD, MEd, FRCPC
Section Chief/Assistant Professor
Lakeridge Health/Queen's University
Department of Critical Care Medicine
Hospital Court
Oshawa, Ontario, Canada

John P. Weaver, MD
Associate Professor of Neurosurgery
Department of Neurosurgery
University of Massachusetts Medical School
Worcester, Massachusetts

Michael D. Weiden, MS, MD
Associate Professor of Medicine and Environmental Medicine
New York University School of Medicine
New York, New York

Mark Weir, MB, ChB, MRCP
Assistant Professor
Department of Thoracic Medicine and Surgery
Lewis Katz School of Medicine
Philadelphia, Pennsylvania

Vaughn E. Whittaker, MD, FACS
Assistant Professor of Surgery
Department of Surgery
Upstate Medical University
Syracuse, New York

Matthew J. Wieduwilt, MD, PhD
Assistant Clinical Professor of Medicine
Department of Medicine
Division of Blood and Marrow Transplantation
UC San Diego, Moores Cancer Center
La Jolla, California

Martin N. Wijkstrom, MD
Assistant Professor of Surgery
Department of Surgery/Transplant Division
University of Pittsburgh Medical Center
Pittsburgh, Pennsylvania

Mark M. Wilson, MD
Associate Professor of Medicine
Associate Director Medical Intensive
Care Units
Department of Medicine
University of Massachusetts Medical School
UMass Memorial Medical Center
Worcester, Massachusetts

John J. Wixted, MD
Assistant Professor of Clinical Orthopedics
Department of Orthopedic Surgery
Beth Israel Deaconess Medical Center
Boston, Massachusetts

Krysta S. Wolfe, MD
Fellow
Department of Pulmonary and Critical
Care Medicine
University of Chicago Medicine
Chicago, Illinois

Ann E. Woolfrey, MD
Member, Fred Hutchinson Cancer Research Center
Seattle, Washington

Peggy Wu, MD
Assistant Professor
Department of Rheumatology
UMass Memorial Medical Center
Worcester, Massachusetts

Omar Z. Yasin, MD, MS
Internal Medicine Resident
Division of Cardiovascular Medicine
Department of Internal Medicine
Mayo Clinic
Rochester, Minnesota

Shan Yin, MD, MPH
Assistant Professor of Pediatrics
Cincinnati Children's Hospital
Drug and Poison Information Center
Cincinnati, Ohio

Luke Yip, MD
Department of Medicine
Section of Medical Toxicology
Denver Health
Rocky Mountain Poison and Drug Center
Denver, Colorado

Hanbing Zhou, MD
Department of Orthopaedics and Rehabilitation
UMass Memorial Medical Center
Worcester, Massachusetts

Marya D. Zilberberg, MD, MPH, FCCP
Founder, President and CEO of EviMed
Research Group, LLC
Adjunct Associate Professor
The School of Public Health and Health Sciences at the
University of Massachusetts—Amherst
Senior Fellow
Jefferson School of Population Health
Thomas Jefferson University
Philadelphia
University of Massachusetts Amherst
Amherst, Massachusetts

Iva Zivna, MD
Assistant Professor
Division of Infectious Diseases
UMass Memorial Medical Center
Worcester, Massachusetts

Marc S. Zumberg, MD
Professor of Medicine
Section Chief, Benign Hematology
Department of Medicine
University of Florida
Gainesville, Florida

Section Editors

Neil Aronin, MD
Chief, Division of Endocrinology
Professor, University of Massachusetts Medical School
UMass Memorial Medical Center
Worcester, Massachusetts

Steven B. Bird, MD
Professor
Department of Emergency Medicine
University of Massachusetts Medical School
Worcester, Massachusetts

Mitchell Cahan, MD, MBA, FACS
Associate Professor of Surgery
Director of Acute Care Surgery
University of Massachusetts Medical School
Worcester, Massachusetts

Akshay S. Desai, MD, MPH
Associate Physician, Advanced Heart Disease Section
Cardiovascular Division,
Brigham and Women's Hospital
Instructor in Medicine, Harvard Medical School
Brigham and Women's Hospital
Boston, Massachusetts

David A. Drachman, MD
(deceased)
Professor of Neurology
Chairman Emeritus
Department of Neurology
University of Massachusetts Medical School
Worcester, Massachusetts

Timothy A. Emhoff, MD, FACS
Chief Trauma and Surgical Critical Care
Department of Surgery
UMass Memorial Medical Center
Worcester, Massachusetts

Pang-Yen Fan, MD
Professor of Medicine
Department of Medicine
University of Massachusetts Medical School
Worcester, Massachusetts

Robert W. Finberg, MD
Richard M. Haidack Professor Medicine
Professor, Microbiology & Physiological Systems
Chair, Department of Medicine
University of Massachusetts Medical School
UMass Memorial Medical Center
Worcester, Massachusetts

Patrick F. Fogarty, MD
Rare Disease, Global Product Development/
Medical Affairs
Pfizer, Inc
Collegeville, Pennsylvania

Joseph J. Frassica, MD
Head, Phillips Research the Americas
Chief Medical Officer, Phillips North America
Professor, The Practice Institute for Medical Engineering and Science
Massachusetts Institute of Technology
Senior Consultant, Pediatric Critical Care
Massachusetts General Hospital for Children
Boston, Massachusetts

Neil A. Halpern, MD, MCCM, FACP, FCCP
Professor of Clinical Medicine
Professor of Medicine in Clinical Anesthesiology
Weill Cornell Medical College
Director, Critical Care Center
Chief, Critical Care Medicine Service
Department of Anesthesiology and Critical Care Medicine
Memorial Sloan Kettering Cancer Center
New York, New York

David M. Harlan, MD
William and Doris Krupp Professor of Medicine
Co-Director, Diabetes Center of Excellence
Department of Internal Medicine
Division of Diabetes
UMass Memorial Medical Center
Worcester, Massachusetts

Kennon Heard, MD
Professor of Emergency Medicine
Department of Emergency Medicine
University of Colorado School of Medicine
Aurora, Colorado

Stephen O. Heard, MD
Professor of Anesthesiology and Surgery
Department of Anesthesiology and Perioperative Medicine
UMass Memorial Medical Center
University of Massachusetts Medical School
Worcester, Massachusetts

Richard S. Irwin, MD, Master FCCP
Professor of Medicine and Nursing
University of Massachusetts Medical School
Chair, Critical Care Operations
UMass Memorial Medical Center
Worcester, Massachusetts

Stephanie M. Levine, MD
Professor of Medicine
Department of Medicine
Division of Pulmonary Diseases and Critical Care
University of Texas Health Center, San Antonio
San Antonio, Texas

Nancy Y. N. Liu, MD
Clinical Associate Professor
University of Massachusetts Medical School
UMass Memorial Medical Center-Memorial Campus
Worcester, Massachusetts

J. Mark Madison, MD
Professor of Medicine and Microbiology
and Physiological Systems
Chief, Division of Pulmonary, Allergy and
Critical Care Medicine
Department of Medicine
UMass Memorial Medical Center
University of Massachusetts Medical School
Worcester, Massachusetts

Lawrence C. Mohr, Jr, MD, ScD, FACP, FCCP
Professor of Medicine, Biometry and Epidemiology
Director, Environmental Biosciences Program
Medical University of South Carolina
Charleston, South Carolina

David A. Morrow, MD, MPH
Professor of Medicine
Harvard Medical School
Directory, Levine Cardiac Intensive Care Unit
Division of Cardiovascular
Brigham and Women's Hospital
Boston, Massachusetts

Dominic J. Nompleggi, MD
Chief, Gastroenterology
Associate Professor
University of Massachusetts Medical School
Worcester, Massachusetts

Patrick T. O'Gara, MD
Watkins Family Distinguished Chair in Cardiology
Division of Cardiovascular
Department of Medicine
Brigham and Women's Hospital
Boston, Massachusetts

David Paydarfar, MD
Professor, Chair of Neurology
Interim Co-Director
Mulva Clinic for the Neurosciences
General Neurology
Dell Medical School at The University of Texas
Austin, Texas

John Querques, MD
Chief, Inpatient Services
Department of Pyschology
Tufts Medical Center
Boston, Massachusetts

Jennifer E. Reidy, MD, MS, FAAHPM
Co-Chief, Division of Palliative Care
Department of Medicine and Family Medicine
UMass Memorial Medical Center
Assistant Professor
University of Massachusetts Medical School
Worcester, Massachusetts

James M. Rippe, MD
Founder and Director
Rippe Lifestyle Institute
Shrewsbury, Massachusetts

Todd W. Sarge, MD
Director, Critical Care
Department of Anesthesia, Critical Care and Pain Medicine
Beth Israel Deaconess Medical Center
Boston, Massachusetts

Luke Yip, MD
Denver HealthRocky Mountain Poison and Drug Center
Department of Medicine, Section of Medical Toxicology
Denver, Colorado

Preface

It is with great pleasure that we present the eighth edition of *Irwin and Rippe's Intensive Care Medicine.* As with previous editions, the editorial challenge that we faced with this edition was to continue to ensure that the book remained at the cutting edge, evolving as the field has evolved. It also needed to continue to meet the varied and rigorous demands placed on it by the diverse group of specialty physicians and nonphysicians practicing in the adult intensive care environment without losing strengths that have made previous editions very useful and popular. We believe that the eighth edition of *Irwin and Rippe's Intensive Care Medicine* has met these challenges.

Over the past 32 years since the publication of the first edition of our book in 1985, dramatic changes have occurred in virtually every area of critical care, and these are reflected in the evolution of our book. Although our book initially focused primarily on medical intensive care medicine, it now provides an interprofessional emphasis on anesthesia, surgery, trauma, neuro and cardiovascular, as well as medical intensive care, with strong collaboration across all these disciplines. This reflects the reality that intensive care medicine has inevitably become more interprofessional and collaborative.

The eighth edition is approximately the same length as the previous edition. To update the text without expanding it, every section editor and author rose to the challenge and carefully balanced each chapter, emphasizing new evidence-based as well as state-of-the-art information and discarding outdated material. We take great pride in the quality of the section editors and chapter authors who have contributed to our eighth edition. All chapters in every section have been updated with recent references and other materials that reflect current information, techniques, and principles. New chapters have been added to reflect emerging areas of interest. An entirely new section has been added on "Palliative Care and Ethical Issues in the Critical Care Unit" that was ably edited by Jennifer E. Reidy.

Since publication of our last edition, point-of-care ultrasonography has become an important and arguably indispensable part of the bedside intensivist's tool kit. As such, its use is prominently featured in this edition. To reflect the rising importance of this diagnostic and therapeutic tool to the practice of modern intensive care medicine, a total of five hours video materials have been embedded into 23 chapters to aid and educate intensivists on the use of this tool. Each video has been personally selected, edited, and narrated by one of our senior editors, Paul H. Mayo, who is internationally known for his knowledge and expertise in ultrasonography.

Evidence-based medicine continues to play an ever-more prominent role in all branches of medicine including critical care. With this in mind, we have asked every chapter author, as in previous editions, to make recommendations that specifically reflect recent trials with a particular emphasis on prospective, randomized controlled trials. Authors have summarized such evidence when the data have allowed, with helpful tables.

In intensive care medicine, important changes and advances have occurred since the publication of the seventh edition. These include managing our ICUs according to the following guiding principles: (1) making our ICUs safer for our patients; (2) decreasing variability by following clinical practice guidelines based on the best available evidence to ensure better outcomes for our patients; and (3) doing more with less by choosing wisely to decrease the cost of caring for our patients. Although these principles have always been espoused, it has become clear that we must more consistently follow them. The appropriate uses of not only the electronic medical records, computer physician order entry, and clinical decision support tools, but also tele-ICU can help us operationalize these principles. All of these issues are covered in the section entitled "ICU Design, Organization, Operation, and Outcome Measures" edited by Neil A. Halpern.

With respect to managing cardiovascular problems and providing coronary care, it has been interesting to see how cardiovascular intensive care has dramatically changed since the publication of our first few editions as the advances in cardiology and cardiac surgery have become implemented. With respect to these problems, co-section editors Akshay S. Desai, David A. Morrow, and Patrick T. O'Gara have completely revamped their section to reflect the current state of their discipline.

Equally important advances have occurred in surgical critical care, shock, and trauma, including new therapies and techniques in a variety of conditions treated in this environment. These sections remain strengths of this book. We welcome new section editors, Mitchell Cahan for "Surgical Problems in the Intensive Care Unit" and Timothy A. Emhoff for "Shock, Trauma, and Sepsis Management." Both have done masterful jobs updating these sections.

Although our book has been updated and broadened to include new understandings, information, and techniques, our goal has been to maintain the practical, clinically oriented approach that readers have come to expect from previous editions. Our editorial focus remains on clinically relevant studies and information that readers have found very useful in the previous seven editions.

As in the past, our book opens with a detailed section on commonly performed procedures, techniques, and ultrasound in the intensive care unit, followed by a section covering minimally invasive monitoring. All chapters in these sections have been updated with new figures and descriptions of techniques that have been added to reflect changes since the seventh edition of the book. We are indebted to section editors Stephen O. Heard and Todd W. Sarge, who have done a superb job on these sections.

The Pharmacology, Overdoses, and Poisoning section, consisting of 30 chapters, remains a great strength of this book and essentially represents a textbook on the topics embedded into our larger book. For their tireless efforts on this outstanding and comprehensive section, we thank Luke Yip, Kennon Heard, and Steven B. Bird.

Our team of section editors continues to do a wonderful job coordinating large bodies of information that comprise the core of modern intensive care. Many of our section editors have been with us for one or more editions. Robert W. Finberg (Infectious Disease), Neil Aronin and David M. Harlan (Endocrinology), Stephanie M. Levine (Transplantation), Dominic J. Nompleggi (Gastroenterology and Metabolism/Nutrition), J. Mark Madison (Pulmonary), John Querques (Psychiatry), Nancy Y. N. Liu (Rheumatology), Pang-Yen Fan (Renal), Patrick F. Fogarty (Hematology and Oncology), Lawrence C. Mohr Jr. (Critical Care Consequences of Weapons [or Agents] of Mass Destruction), David A. Drachman and David Paydarfar (Neurology), and Joseph J. Frassica (Appendix, Calculations Commonly used in Critical Care) all fall into this category and have again made outstanding contributions.

As with previous editions, our emphasis remains on clinical management. Discussions of basic pathophysiology are also included and guided and supplemented by extensive references to help clinicians and researchers who wish to pursue more in-depth knowledge of these important areas. When therapies reflect institutional or individual bias or are considered controversial, we have attempted to indicate this.

We hope and believe that the outstanding efforts of many people over the past 5 years have continued to result in an evidence-based and state-of-the-art and comprehensive book that will elucidate the important principles in intensive care and will continue to guide and support the best efforts of practitioners in this challenging environment in their ongoing efforts to diagnose and treat complicated diseases and relieve human suffering.

Richard S. Irwin, MD, Master FCCP
Craig M. Lilly, MD, FCCP
Paul H. Mayo, MD, FCCP
James M. Rippe, MD

Acknowledgments

Numerous outstanding individuals have made significant contributions to all phases of writing and production of this book and deserve special recognition and thanks. First and foremost is our managing editor, Elizabeth Grady. Beth literally lives and breathes this book as it works its way through the production cycle every 4 to 5 years. She is the guiding and organizing force behind this book. It would simply not be possible without Beth's incredible organizational skills, good humor, and enormous energy. She has guided this book through eight editions—this book is as much hers as it is ours.

The major innovation of this edition is the focus on point-of-care ultrasonography. Assisting Paul H. Mayo with the task of developing the high-quality ultrasound videos was Yonathan Greenstein, while assisting in preparation of the utility of ultrasonography sections were Gisela Banauch, Ariel Shiloh, and Lewis Eisen. For their outstanding work, we owe them a large debt of gratitude.

Our administrative assistants, office assistants, and clinical coordinators, Sherry Jakubiak and Cynthia French, Linda Doherty, Debra Adamonis, and Carol Moreau have helped us continue to coordinate and manage our complex professional and personal lives and create room for the substantial amount of time required to write and edit. Our section editors have devoted enormous skill, time, and resources to every editions of this book. We have very much appreciated their deep commitment to this book and to advancing the field of intensive care medicine.

Our editors at Lippincott Williams & Wilkins including Brian Brown, Executive Editor, have been a source of great help and encouragement. As with the last edition, Nicole Dernoski continues to be extremely helpful and accommodating in supervising and coordinating all phases of production in an outstanding way. Lauren Pecarich handled the day-to-day details necessary with a book of this size. Last, we are grateful to Samson Premkumar and his staff for the outstanding job they have done copyediting the manuscript for this edition.

It is with great sadness that we report that David A. Drachman passed away before the publication of the edition of this book. David was a good friend and wonderful colleague who had been the neurology section editor or co-editor on every one of the eight editions of *Intensive Care Medicine*. He will be greatly missed.

Our families support our efforts with unfailing encouragement and love. To them, and the many others who have helped in ways too numerous to count, we are deeply grateful.

Richard S. Irwin, MD, Master FCCP
Craig M. Lilly, MD, FCCP
Paul H. Mayo, MD, FCCP
James M. Rippe, MD

Contents

Section 4 SHOCK AND TRAUMA AND SEPSIS MANAGEMENT

Section 5 SURGICAL PROBLEMS IN THE INTENSIVE CARE UNIT

Section 6 TRANSPLANTATION

Section 7 RHEUMATOLOGIC, IMMUNOLOGIC, AND DERMATOLOGIC DISEASES IN THE INTENSIVE CARE UNIT

Section 8 INFECTIOUS DISEASE PROBLEMS IN THE INTENSIVE CARE UNIT

Section 1 PROCEDURES, TECHNIQUES AND ULTRASONOGRAPHY

STEPHEN O. HEARD

Chapter 1 ■ Point-of-Care Critical Care Ultrasonography

PAUL H. MAYO

Critical care ultrasonography encompasses any application of ultrasonography that can be productively employed by the intensivist at the bedside for the diagnosis and management of the patient. In recognition of the importance of ultrasonography to intensive care medicine, the editors of this edition decided to incorporate the subject into the textbook insofar as possible. Where it is relevant, the reader will find within each chapter a section titled "Utility of Ultrasonography" that is written in cooperation with the chapter authors by a separate writing group, all of whom have been course leaders or senior faculty at American College of Chest Physicians national critical care ultrasonography courses and all of whom use ultrasonography in their daily critical care practice. Each ultrasonography section will connect to a video library coordinated with the subject matter of chapter that can be called out for review while reading the text. By design, the ultrasonography sections of the textbook do not emphasize technical aspects of machine design or ultrasound physics. These are well summarized in standard ultrasonography textbooks. Rather, the emphasis is on procedure- or disease-specific clinical applications of ultrasonography that are immediately relevant to the frontline intensivist, and that are well within their capability. The goal is to review those aspects of ultrasonography that a "typical" bedside intensivist would use on a routine basis. Complex aspects of ultrasonography are not part of the discussion, because they require expert level radiology and cardiology level capability.

COMPETENCE

By definition, the intensivist in charge of the case personally performs all aspects of the ultrasonography examination: image acquisition, image interpretation, and application of the results at point of care. This is very different from ultrasonography performed by the consultative service of radiology and cardiology, where the examination is delayed in its performance, and where the consultant is disassociated from the clinical reality of case. In using ultrasonography at point of care, the intensivist uses an imaging modality that is uniquely suited to the demands of intensive care medicine: immediately available, relatively inexpensive, flexible, and with multipurpose applications.

Competence in key parts of critical care ultrasonography are summarized in the ACCP/SRLF Statement on Competence in Critical Care Ultrasonography [1].This document lists the basic elements of the field that need to be mastered by the intensivist, and may be regarded as a minimum standard. This textbook reviews many other applications that are not listed in this Statement.

Competence in critical care ultrasonography requires mastery of image acquisition, image interpretation, and the cognitive elements of the field. Training in image acquisition may be accomplished initially on normal human subjects, but also requires scanning of patients under the direct supervision of a competent instructor. Training in image acquisition requires access to an image set that includes a large number of abnormal findings. The cognitive base is mastered by study of relevant material in a blended form comprising written material, lectures, or Internet-based information. Requirements for training relevant to the elements of the Competence Statement are summarized in the Statement on Training in Critical Care Ultrasonography that represents a multinational consensus on this subject [2].

At present, there is no national level certification process for critical care ultrasonography either in North America or any country in Europe. Competence is defined by local standards, so the intensivist has an important responsibility to seek out adequate training that focuses on achieving the standards defined in the Competence Statement. Some applications reviewed in this textbook are not mentioned in the Competence Statement, but have clinical utility. Competence in these is only assured by specific institutional standards. Critical care ultrasonography, once adopted by the active clinician, lends itself to an element of invention, local training effort, and adoption of techniques that are not initially widely used. One purpose of this textbook is to disseminate information on critical care ultrasonography that is not defined in the Competence Statement.

Machine Requirements

High-quality portable ultrasonography machines are widely available. Their cost is not prohibitive when compared to alternatives, such as computerized tomography (CT), and their operating costs are low. In addition, a team that uses ultrasonography as its primary imaging tool reduces utilization of other standard imaging methods [3]; this accrues cost savings, because more expensive imaging modalities are not used as often. Most recent generation machines have good image quality (with a few exceptions), so purchase decision should be predicated on other factors. Some key questions to consider include the following:

1. Is the machine durable? Can the machine be dropped, can the transducers be dropped, and is it impervious to fluid spills?
2. What is the service record of the company? Is the cost of the service contract included in the price of the machine, or is the machine a "loss leader" that requires an expensive service contract in addition? What is the turnaround time for service?
3. Is the machine easy to operate? What is the turn-on time? Is the control surface simple and easy to operate? Is there well-designed memory capability that uses a widely accepted video image format?
4. Is the machine truly portable? Can it be easily removed from the stand for situations that require a hand-carried device? What is the footprint of the stand?
5. Can the machine and probes be easily and safely cleaned with disinfecting fluids?

The intesive care unit (ICU) machine requires two probes. The linear vascular probe is high frequency, so that it has excellent resolution, but poor penetration. This makes it ideal for vascular access, examination of pleural morphology, and to characterize structures near the skin surface such as lymph nodes. The phased array cardiac transducer has less resolution, but better penetration, because it is designed for examination of deeper structures. Most machines allow the phased-array cardiac transducer to be configured for abdominal scanning. This results in cost savings, because the machine does not then need to be equipped with a curvilinear abdominal transducer which adds significantly to acquisition cost.

Machine Controls and Scanning Technique

Even with a simple-to-operate portable machine, a common failure point for the inexperienced scanner is poor gain, depth, frequency, and orientation control. This is remedied by effective hands-on training. Scanning technique is an important element of image acquisition. Excepting certain types of vascular access, the machine and the scanner are always placed on the same side as the patient. This permits the examiner to operate the machine controls with one hand while holding the probe with the other. This requires that the clinician be ambidextrous in terms of holding the probe, given that the patient may be surrounded by a variety of life support devices. Probe hold requires that some part of the hand rests on the patient while holding the probe in order to provide a stable image.

Scope of Practice

In considering the scope of practice of critical care ultrasonography, it is important to emphasize that not every intensivist needs to be competent in all aspects of the field. The consultative attending intensivist may not need any training, because their practice needs are not such that it is required. Other clinicians may wish to focus on procedural guidance with ultrasonography. For the active frontline intensivist, the Competence Statement is a good guide for the scope of practice, with additional skills added according to interest and practice requirements. This will require a higher level of training.

Competence should be defined by the scope of practice, but in some situations, there is an added layer of complexity. The hospital credentialing committee must grant the privilege to perform critical care ultrasonography. If the clinician has achieved competence during fellowship training as defined by their program director, hospital credentialing committees routinely grant privileges. This may not be the case for attending level intensivists, where other physician specialists perceive economic or political threat to granting the privilege to a physician who is not a radiologist or cardiologist. In this case, the intensivist may be competent, and yet be blocked from performing within their scope of practice. One solution to this problem is to provide strong evidence of training, such that the credentialing committee cannot but grant privileges. This evidence would include a comprehensive log of all scanning activity, cognitive training, image review, and course attendance. The American College of Chest Physicians has designed a training program to provide competence and to fulfil requirements to obtain hospital privileges.

Limitations of Critical Care Ultrasonography

Competence in critical care ultrasonography requires an understanding of its limitations. These include the following:

1. Related to patient factors: Obesity, heavy musculature, and edema may degrade the ultrasonography image to a major extent. The presence of subcutaneous air may block transmission of ultrasound, so that deeper structures cannot be visualized. Skin dressing and devices may block transmission of ultrasound. The critically ill patient often cannot be positioned for optimal image acquisition. For example, most critically ill patients are supine, so that posterior structures may be difficult to image.
2. Related to environmental factors: High ambient light levels degrade image quality. The patient may be surrounded by equipment that blocks access for scanning.
3. Related to the physics of ultrasonography: The physics of ultrasound limit the resolution and penetration of ultrasound in body tissues, and artifacts are common that may mimic abnormalities. Ultrasound is blocked by air owing to intense reflection such that the presence of air precludes any visualization of underlying structures. Bones markedly attenuate transmission of ultrasound, so that underlying structures are shadowed. Structures in the lung that are completely surrounded by air are invisible, ribs block visualization of the heart or brain, whereas gas-filled intestine blocks visualization of abdominal structures.
4. Related to the operator: The intensivist who performs critical care ultrasonography is responsible for all the aspects of image acquisition, interpretation, and application of the results to the clinical problem at hand. There is no expert radiologist or cardiologist to perform these critical functions. A limitation of critical care ultrasonography relates to the need for the intensivist to be fully trained and therefore competent in those aspects that are relevant to their practice needs.
5. Related to paradigm shift: The standard paradigm for imaging in the ICU is that the radiology or cardiology service is responsible for all aspects of image acquisition and interpretation. The intensivist is a passive participant in this process. The full integration of critical care ultrasonography into the daily function of the ICU requires a paradigm shift where the intensivists rely on their own skill at image acquisition and interpretation, and believe that ultrasonography often replaces standard imaging methods such as chest radiography and CT scan. As summarized by Oks et al.:

> "This approach to critical care ultrasonography requires several dedicated machines, a number of frontline intensivists who are skilled at critical care ultrasonography, the deployment of ultrasonography as a primary tool on work rounds, a team decision to rely on ultrasonography as a primary imaging tool as much as possible, and the decision that confirmatory imaging is not required for ultrasonography examinations performed by the MICU team." [3]

CONCLUSIONS

Critical care ultrasonography is an important aspect of intensive care medicine. Rather than having several stand-alone chapters summarizing various aspects of ultrasonography, the editors have embedded ultrasonography in a disease- or procedure-specific manner that is clinically relevant to the frontline intensivist. The accompanying video library serves to provide guidance for a wide variety of critical care ultrasonography applications.

References

1. Mayo PH, Beaulieu Y, Doelken P, et al: American College of Chest Physicians/ La Société de Réanimation de Langue Française statement on competence in critical care ultrasonography. *Chest* 135:1050–1060, 2009.
2. Cholley, B: International expert statement on training standards for critical care ultrasonography Expert Round Table on Ultrasound in ICU. *Intensive Care Med* 37:1077–1083, 2011.
3. Oks M, Cleven KL, Cardenas-Garcia J, et al: The effect of point-of-care ultrasonography on imaging studies in the medical ICU: a comparative study. *Chest* 146:1574–1577, 2014.

Chapter 2 ■ Anesthesia for Bedside Procedures

MARK DERSHWITZ

When a patient in an intensive care unit (ICU) requires a bedside procedure, it is usually the attending intensivist, as opposed to a consultant anesthesiologist, who directs the administration of the necessary hypnotic, analgesic, and/or paralytic drugs. Furthermore, unlike in the operating room, the ICU usually has no equipment for the administration of gaseous (e.g., nitrous oxide) or volatile (e.g., isoflurane) anesthetics. Anesthesia for bedside procedures in the ICU is thus accomplished via a technique involving total intravenous anesthesia (TIVA).

COMMON PAIN MANAGEMENT PROBLEMS IN ICU PATIENTS

Dosing of Agent

Selecting the proper dose of an analgesic to administer is problematic for several reasons, including difficulty in assessing the effectiveness of pain relief, pharmacokinetic (PK) differences between the critically ill and other patients, and normal physiologic changes associated with aging.

Assessing the Effectiveness of Pain Relief

Critically ill patients often are incapable of communicating their feelings because of delirium, obtundation, or endotracheal intubation. This makes psychological evaluation quite difficult, because surrogate markers of pain intensity (e.g., tachycardia, hypertension, and diaphoresis) are inherent in the host response to critical illness.

Pharmacokinetic Considerations

Most of the pressors and vasodilators administered in the ICU by continuous intravenous (IV) infusion have relatively straightforward PK behavior: They are water-soluble molecules that are minimally bound to plasma proteins. In contrast, the hypnotics and opioids used in TIVA have high lipid solubility, and most are extensively bound to plasma proteins, causing their PK behavior to be far more complex. After a single or a few bolus injections, these medications are typically short acting because of rapid redistribution out of the brain. However, following infusions of long duration (i.e., hours or days), the processes of metabolism and elimination become more important and drug effects can have a longer duration.

The PK behavior of the lipid-soluble hypnotics and analgesics given by infusion may be described by their context-sensitive half-times (CSHTs). This concept may be defined as follows: When a drug is given as an IV bolus followed by an IV infusion designed to maintain a constant plasma drug concentration, the time required for the plasma concentration to fall by 50% after termination of the infusion is the CSHT [1]. Figure 2.1 depicts the CSHT curves for the medications most likely to be used for TIVA in ICU patients. PK behavior in critically ill patients is unlike that in normal subjects for several reasons. Because ICU patients frequently have renal and/or hepatic dysfunction, drug metabolism or excretion is often significantly impaired. Hypoalbuminemia, common in critical illness, decreases protein binding and increases free-drug concentration. Because free drug is the only moiety available to tissue receptors, decreased protein binding increases the pharmacologic effect for a given plasma

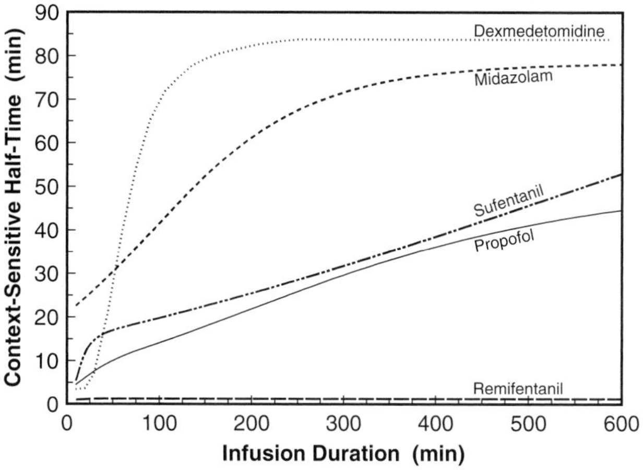

FIGURE 2.1 The context-sensitive half-times for propofol [26], midazolam [27], sufentanil [28], remifentanil [29], and dexmedetomidine [30] as a function of infusion duration.

concentration. It is therefore more important in the ICU patient that the doses of medications used for TIVA are individualized for a particular patient.

Physiologic Changes Associated with Aging

People 65 years of age and older comprise the fastest growing segment of the population and constitute the majority of patients in many ICUs. Aging leads to (1) a decrease in total body water and lean body mass; (2) an increase in body fat and, hence, an increase in the volume of distribution of lipid-soluble drugs; and (3) a decrease in drug clearance rates, because of reductions in liver mass, hepatic enzyme activity, liver blood flow, and renal excretory function. There is a progressive, age-dependent increase in pain relief and electroencephalographic suppression among elderly patients receiving the same dose of opioid as younger patients. There is also an increase in central nervous system (CNS) depression in elderly patients following administration of identical doses of benzodiazepines.

Selection of Agent

Procedures performed in ICUs today (Table 2.1) span a spectrum that extends from those associated with mild discomfort (e.g., esophagogastroscopy) to those that are quite painful (e.g., orthopedic manipulations, wound debridement, tracheostomy). Depending on their technical difficulty, these procedures can last from minutes to hours. To provide a proper anesthetic, medications should be selected according to the nature of the procedure and titrated according to the patient's response to surgical stimuli. In addition, specific disease states should be considered in order to maximize safety and effectiveness.

Head Trauma

Head-injured patients require a technique that provides effective yet brief anesthesia, so that the capacity to assess neurologic status is not lost for extended periods of time. In addition, the

TABLE 2.1

Bedside Procedures and Associated Levels of Discomfort

- Mild to moderately uncomfortable
  - Transesophageal echocardiography[a]
  - Transtracheal aspiration
  - Thoracentesis[a]
  - Paracentesis[a]
- Moderately to severely uncomfortable
  - Endotracheal intubation[a]
  - Flexible bronchoscopy[a]
  - Thoracostomy[a]
  - Bone marrow biopsy
  - Colonoscopy
  - Intraaortic balloon insertion[a]
  - Peritoneal dialysis catheter insertion[a]
  - Peritoneal lavage[a]
  - Percutaneous gastrostomy[a]
  - Percutaneous intraaortic balloon insertion[a]
- Extremely painful
  - Rigid bronchoscopy
  - Debridement of open wounds
  - Dressing changes
  - Orthopedic manipulations
  - Tracheostomy[a]
  - Pericardiocentesis/pericardial window[a]
  - Open lung biopsy
  - Ventriculostomy[a]

[a]Procedures in which the level of discomfort may be significantly mitigated by the use of local anesthesia.

technique must not adversely affect cerebral perfusion pressure. If the effects of the anesthetics dissipate too rapidly, episodes of agitation and increased intracranial pressure (ICP) may occur that jeopardize cerebral perfusion. In contrast, if the medications last too long, there may be difficulty in making an adequate neurologic assessment following the procedure.

Coronary Artery Disease

Postoperative myocardial ischemia following cardiac and noncardiac surgery strongly predicts adverse outcome [2]. Accordingly, sufficient analgesia should be provided during and after invasive procedures to reduce plasma catecholamine and stress hormone levels.

Renal and/or Hepatic Failure

The association between sepsis and acute renal failure has been recognized for many years. The risk of an adverse drug reaction is at least three times higher in azotemic patients than in those with normal renal function. This risk is magnified by excessive unbound drug or drug metabolite(s) in the circulation and changes in the target tissue(s) induced by the uremic state.

Liver failure alters the volumes of distribution of many drugs by impairing synthesis of the two major plasma-binding proteins, albumin and α_1-acid glycoprotein. In addition, reductions in hepatic blood flow and hepatic enzymatic activity decrease the clearance rates of many drugs.

CHARACTERISTICS OF SPECIFIC AGENTS USED FOR BEDSIDE PROCEDURES

Hypnotics

The characteristics of the hypnotics are listed in Table 2.2, and their recommended doses are listed in Table 2.3. When rapid awakening is desired, propofol or etomidate is the hypnotic agent of choice. Ketamine may be useful when a longer duration of anesthesia is needed. Midazolam is rarely used alone as a hypnotic; however, its profound anxiolytic and amnestic effects render it useful in combination with other agents. Dexmedetomidine does not reliably produce unconsciousness; however, its sedation is not accompanied by ventilatory depression and it potentiates opioid analgesia, thereby permitting lower opioid doses.

Propofol

Description

Propofol is a hypnotic agent associated with pleasant emergence and hangover characteristics. It is extremely popular because it is readily titratable and has more rapid onset and offset kinetics than midazolam. Thus, patients emerge from anesthesia more rapidly after propofol than after midazolam, a factor that may make propofol the preferred agent for sedation and hypnosis in general, and in particular for patients with altered level of consciousness.

The CSHT for propofol is about 10 minutes following a 1-hour infusion, and the CSHT increases about 5 minutes for each additional hour of infusion for the first several hours, as shown in Figure 2.1. Thus, the CSHT is about 20 minutes after a 3-hour infusion. The CSHT rises much more slowly for infusions longer than a day; a patient who is sedated (but not rendered unconscious) with propofol for 2 weeks will recover in approximately 3 hours [3]. This rapid recovery of neurologic status often makes propofol a desirable sedative in ICU patients, especially in those with head trauma, who may not tolerate mechanical ventilation without pharmacologic sedation.

Even though recovery following termination of a continuous infusion is faster with propofol than with midazolam, a comparative trial showed that the two drugs were roughly equivalent in effectiveness for overnight sedation of ICU patients [4]. For long-term sedation (e.g., more than 1 day), however, recovery is significantly faster in patients given propofol.

TABLE 2.2

Characteristics of Intravenous Hypnotic Agents

	Propofol	Etomidate	Ketamine	Midazolam	Dexmedetomidine
Onset	Fast	Fast	Fast	**Intermediate**	**Intermediate**
Duration	Short	Short	Intermediate	Intermediate	Intermediate
Cardiovascular effects	↓	**None**	↑	Minimal	↓
Ventilatory effects	↓	↓	**Minimal**	↓	**None**
Analgesia	None	None	**Profound**	None	**Moderate**
Amnesia	Mild	Mild	**Profound**	**Profound**	**None**

The listed doses should be reduced by 50% in elderly patients. Entries in bold type indicate noteworthy differences among the drugs.

TABLE 2.3

Usual Doses of Intravenous Anesthetic Agents Given by Continuous Infusion

	Propofol	Etomidate	Ketamine	Midazolam	Sufentanil	Remifentanil	Dexmedetomidine
Bolus dose (mg/kg)	1–2	0.2–0.3	1–2	0.05–0.15	0.5–1.5	0.5–1.5	0.5–1.0 (μg/kg)
Infusion rate (μg/kg/min)	100–200	NR[a]	25–100	0.25–1.5	0.01–0.03	0.05–0.5	0.003–0.012

The "usual doses" are for patients without preexisting tolerance and significant cardiovascular disease. The required doses will be higher in patients with tolerance, and should be reduced in elderly patients and in patients with decreased cardiovascular function. In all cases, the medications should be titrated to specific end points as described in the text.
[a]Not recommended because of the possibility of prolonged adrenal suppression.

In spontaneously breathing patients sedated with propofol, respiratory rate appears to be a more predictable sign of adequate sedation than hemodynamic changes. The ventilatory response to rebreathing carbon dioxide during a maintenance propofol infusion is similar to that induced by other sedative drugs (i.e., propofol significantly decreases the slope of the carbon dioxide response curve). Nevertheless, spontaneously breathing patients anesthetized with propofol are able to maintain normal end-tidal carbon dioxide values during most minor surgical procedures.

Bolus doses of propofol in the range of 1 to 2 mg per kg induce loss of consciousness within 30 seconds. Maintenance infusion rates of 100 to 200 μg/kg/min are adequate in younger subjects to maintain general anesthesia, whereas doses should be reduced by 20% to 50% in elderly individuals.

Adverse Effects

Cardiovascular. Propofol depresses ventricular systolic function and lowers afterload, but has no effect on diastolic function. Vasodilation results from calcium channel blockade. In patients undergoing coronary artery bypass surgery, propofol (2 mg per kg IV bolus) produced a 23% fall in mean arterial blood pressure, a 20% increase in heart rate, and a 26% decrease in stroke volume. In pigs, propofol caused a dose-related depression of sinus node and His-Purkinje system functions, but had no effect on atrioventricular node function or on the conduction properties of atrial and ventricular tissues. In patients with coronary artery disease, propofol administration may be associated with a reduction in coronary perfusion pressure and increased myocardial lactate production.

Neurologic. Propofol may improve neurologic outcome and reduce neuronal damage by depressing cerebral metabolism. Propofol decreases cerebral oxygen consumption, cerebral blood flow, and cerebral glucose utilization in humans and animals to the same degree as reported for thiopental and etomidate. Propofol frequently causes pain when injected into a peripheral vein. Injection pain is less likely if the injection site is located proximally on the arm or if the injection is made via a central venous catheter.

Metabolic. The emulsion used as the vehicle for propofol contains soybean oil and lecithin and supports bacterial growth; iatrogenic contamination leading to septic shock is possible. Currently available propofol preparations contain ethylenediamine tetraacetic acid (EDTA), metabisulfite, or benzyl alcohol as a bacteriostatic agent. Because EDTA chelates trace metals, particularly zinc, serum zinc levels should be measured daily during continuous propofol infusions. Hyperlipidemia may occur, particularly in infants and small children. Accordingly, triglyceride levels should be monitored daily in this population whenever propofol is administered continuously for more than 24 hours.

Etomidate

Description

Etomidate has onset and offset PK characteristics similar to propofol and an unrivaled cardiovascular profile, even in the setting of cardiomyopathy [5]. Not only does etomidate lack significant effects on myocardial contractility, but baseline sympathetic output and baroreflex regulation of sympathetic activity are well preserved. Etomidate depresses cerebral oxygen metabolism and blood flow in a dose-related manner without changing the intracranial volume–pressure relationship.

Etomidate is particularly useful (rather than thiopental or propofol) in certain patient subsets: Hypovolemic patients, multiple trauma victims with closed head injury, and those with low ejection fraction, severe aortic stenosis, left main coronary artery disease, or severe cerebral vascular disease. Etomidate may be relatively contraindicated in patients with established or evolving septic shock because of its inhibition of cortisol synthesis (see below).

Adverse Effects

Metabolic. Etomidate, when given by prolonged infusion, may increase mortality associated with low plasma cortisol levels [6]. Even single doses of etomidate can produce adrenal cortical suppression lasting 24 hours or more in normal patients undergoing elective surgery [7]. These effects are more pronounced as the dose is increased or if continuous infusions are used for sedation. Etomidate-induced adrenocortical suppression occurs because the drug blocks the 11β-hydroxylase that catalyzes the final step in the synthesis of cortisol. It is also noteworthy that etomidate causes the highest incidence of postoperative nausea and vomiting of any of the IV anesthetic agents.

In 2005, Jackson warned against the use of etomidate in patients with septic shock [8]. Since then, there have been several studies that have attempted to confirm or refute the safety of etomidate in critically ill patients, including those with sepsis. Unfortunately, some of these studies purportedly confirmed the danger of etomidate, whereas others support its continued use in patients with sepsis. Two recent meta-analyses of the available studies came to divergent conclusions [9,10]. Giving hydrocortisone to patients with septic shock may decrease overall mortality in patients who received etomidate for intubation as compared to other hypnotic agents [11].

Ketamine

Description

Ketamine induces a state of sedation, amnesia, and marked analgesia in which the patient experiences a strong feeling of dissociation from the environment. It is unique among the hypnotics in that it reliably induces unconsciousness by the intramuscular route. Ketamine is rapidly metabolized by the liver to norketamine that is pharmacologically active. Ketamine is both slower in onset and offset as compared with propofol or etomidate following IV administration.

Many clinicians consider ketamine to be the analgesic of choice in patients with a history of bronchospasm. In the usual dosage, it decreases airway resistance, probably by blocking norepinephrine uptake that in turn stimulates beta-adrenergic receptors in the lungs. In contrast to many beta-agonist bronchodilators, ketamine is not arrhythmogenic when given to asthmatic patients receiving aminophylline.

Ketamine may be safer than other hypnotics or opioids in unintubated patients because it depresses airway reflexes and ventilatory drive to a lesser degree. It may be particularly useful for procedures near the airway, where physical access and ability to secure an airway is limited (e.g., gunshot wounds to the face). Because ketamine increases salivary and tracheobronchial secretions, an anticholinergic (e.g., 0.2 mg glycopyrrolate) should be given prior to its administration. In patients with borderline hypoxemia despite maximal therapy, ketamine may be the drug of choice, because ketamine does not inhibit hypoxic pulmonary vasoconstriction.

Another major feature that distinguishes ketamine from most other IV anesthetics is that it stimulates the cardiovascular system (i.e., raises heart rate and blood pressure). This action appears to result both from direct stimulation of the CNS with increased sympathetic nervous system outflow and from blockade of norepinephrine reuptake in adrenergic nerves.

Because pulmonary hypertension is a characteristic feature of acute respiratory distress syndrome, drugs that increase right ventricular afterload should be avoided. In infants with either normal or elevated pulmonary vascular resistance, ketamine does not affect pulmonary vascular resistance as long as constant ventilation is maintained, a finding also confirmed in adults.

Cerebral blood flow does not change when ketamine is injected into cerebral vessels. In mechanically ventilated pigs with artificially produced intracranial hypertension in which ICP is on the shoulder of the compliance curve, 0.5 to 2.0 mg per kg IV ketamine does not raise ICP; likewise, in mechanically ventilated preterm infants, 2 mg per kg IV ketamine does not increase anterior fontanelle pressure, an indirect monitor of ICP. Unlike propofol and etomidate however, ketamine does not lower cerebral metabolic rate. It is relatively contraindicated in patients with an intracranial mass, with increased ICP, or who have suffered recent head trauma.

Adverse Effects

Psychological. Emergence phenomena following ketamine anesthesia have been described as floating sensations, vivid dreams (pleasant or unpleasant), hallucinations, and delirium. These effects are more common in patients older than 16 years, in females, after short operative procedures, after large doses (>2 mg per kg IV), and after rapid administration (>40 mg per minute). Pre- or concurrent treatment with benzodiazepines or propofol usually minimizes or prevents these phenomena [12].

Cardiovascular. Because ketamine increases myocardial oxygen consumption, there is risk of precipitating myocardial ischemia in patients with coronary artery disease if ketamine is used alone. On the other hand, combinations of ketamine plus diazepam, ketamine plus midazolam, or ketamine plus sufentanil are well tolerated for induction in patients undergoing coronary artery bypass surgery. Repeated bolus doses are often associated with tachycardia. This can be reduced by administering ketamine as a constant infusion.

Ketamine produces myocardial depression in the isolated animal heart. Hypotension has been reported following ketamine administration in hemodynamically compromised patients with chronic catecholamine depletion.

Neurologic. Ketamine does not lower the minimal electroshock seizure threshold in mice. When administered with aminophylline, however, a clinically apparent reduction in seizure threshold is observed.

Midazolam

Description

Although capable of inducing unconsciousness in high doses, midazolam is more commonly used as a sedative. Along with its sedating effects, midazolam produces anxiolysis, amnesia, and relaxation of skeletal muscle.

Anterograde amnesia following midazolam (5 mg IV) peaks 2 to 5 minutes after IV injection and lasts 20 to 40 minutes. Because midazolam is highly (95%) protein bound (to albumin), the drug effect is likely to be exaggerated in ICU patients. Recovery from midazolam is prolonged in obese and elderly patients and following continuous infusion because it accumulates to a significant degree. In patients with renal failure, active conjugated metabolites of midazolam may accumulate and delay recovery. Although flumazenil may be used to reverse excessive sedation or ventilatory depression from midazolam, its duration of action is only 15 to 20 minutes. In addition, flumazenil may precipitate acute anxiety reactions or seizures, particularly in patients receiving chronic benzodiazepine therapy.

Midazolam causes dose-dependent reductions in cerebral metabolic rate and cerebral blood flow, suggesting that it may be beneficial in patients with cerebral ischemia.

Because of its combined sedative, anxiolytic, and amnestic properties, midazolam is ideally suited both for brief, relatively painless procedures (e.g., endoscopy) and for prolonged sedation (e.g., during mechanical ventilation).

Adverse Effects

Respiratory. Midazolam (0.15 mg per kg IV) depresses the slope of the carbon dioxide response curve and increases the dead space–tidal volume ratio and arterial PCO_2. Ventilatory depression is even more marked and prolonged in patients with chronic obstructive pulmonary disease. Midazolam also blunts the ventilatory response to hypoxia.

Cardiovascular. Small (<10%) increases in heart rate and small decreases in systemic vascular resistance are frequently observed after administration of midazolam. It has no significant effects on coronary vascular resistance or autoregulation.

Neurologic. Because recovery of cognitive and psychomotor function may be delayed for up to 24 hours, midazolam as the sole hypnotic may not be appropriate in situations where rapid return of consciousness and psychomotor function are a high priority.

Dexmedetomidine

Description

Dexmedetomidine is the first α_2-adrenoceptor agonist specifically marketed as a sedative. It is considerably more selective for α_2-adrenoceptors than clonidine. The primary site of its action as a sedative is in the locus coeruleus, where its effect is to mimic physiologic sleep [13]. In rats, dexmedetomidine produces analgesia at the spinal cord level by activating descending inhibitory pathways originating in the midbrain, thereby reducing pain impulses that would otherwise ascend in the cord.

Dexmedetomidine produces intense sedation, although it cannot reliably produce amnesia, hypnosis, or general anesthesia [14]. It does not have anticonvulsant properties. As would be expected, dexmedetomidine lowers blood pressure and heart rate, and dramatic decreases have occasionally occurred in patients without preexisting cardiovascular disease. Higher doses of dexmedetomidine can produce an initial increase in blood pressure that is believed to result from stimulation of α_{2B}-adrenoceptors. Sympathetic stimulation is also responsible for the common side effect of dry mouth. Dexmedetomidine can markedly reduce the requirement for IV anesthetics and opioids. Sedative doses have very little effect on ventilation and do not appear to increase the ventilatory depressant effects of opioids [15].

Dexmedetomidine is approved for sedation of mechanically ventilated adult patients, but only for up to 24 hours, although longer trials have been published. The infusion typically is started near the end of an operative procedure before the patient is transported to the ICU or shortly after arrival. A bolus dose of 1 μg/kg is given over 10 minutes, followed by an infusion of 0.003 to 0.012 μg/kg/min. For infusions longer than an hour in duration, dexmedetomidine takes substantially longer to wear off than the other IV hypnotics as shown in Figure 2.1.

No ventilatory depression is associated with dexmedetomidine, and patients should require less opioid for management of postoperative pain. The heart rate usually is slow, although symptomatic bradycardia occasionally occurs, and dexmedetomidine should not be given to patients with preexisting heart block. Postoperative hypertension usually is well controlled; however, some patients experience hypotension and require pressor infusion, especially if they have preexisting ventricular dysfunction. Two multicenter studies showed that ventilated patients who were sedated with dexmedetomidine required a shorter period of mechanical ventilation compared with midazolam (5.1 vs. 6.8 days, $P = 0.03$), but not compared with propofol; the patients sedated with dexmedetomidine had more episodes of hypotension and bradycardia [16].

Dexmedetomidine is able to suppress postoperative shivering, probably via stimulation of α_{2B} receptors in the hypothalamus. An intriguing possibility is that perioperative administration of an α_2-adrenoceptor agonist decreases cardiovascular mortality. A meta-analysis concluded that such use decreases mortality and myocardial infarction after vascular surgery [17].

Opioids

Morphine

Description

Pain relief by morphine and its surrogates is relatively selective in that other sensory modalities (touch, vibration, vision, hearing) are not obtunded. Opioids blunt pain by (1) inhibiting pain processing by the dorsal horn of the spinal cord; (2) decreasing transmission of pain by activating descending inhibitory pathways in the brain stem; and (3) altering the emotional response to pain by actions on the limbic cortex.

Various types of opioid receptors (denoted by Greek letters) have been discovered in the CNS. The classical pharmacologic effects of morphine like analgesia and ventilatory depression are mediated by μ receptors. Other μ effects include sedation, euphoria, tolerance and physical dependence, decreased gastrointestinal motility, biliary spasm, and miosis. The κ receptor shares a number of effects with the μ receptor, including analgesia, sedation, and ventilatory depression. The δ receptor is responsible for mediating some of the analgesic effects of the endogenous opioid peptides, especially in the spinal cord. Few of the clinically used opioids have significant activity at δ receptors at the usual analgesic doses.

Morphine is a substrate for P-glycoprotein, a protein responsible for the transport of many molecules out of cells. The combination of slow CNS penetration due to lower lipid solubility and rapid efflux accounts for the slow onset of morphine's CNS effects. Peak analgesic effects may not occur for over an hour after IV injection; hence, the plasma profile of morphine does not parallel its clinical effects [18].

Morphine is unique among the opioids in causing significant histamine release after IV injection that occurs almost immediately. The beneficial effect of giving morphine to a patient with acute pulmonary edema is far more related to this hemodynamic effect rather than to its analgesic and sedating effects.

Adverse Effects

Gastrointestinal. Constipation, nausea, and/or vomiting are well-described side effects of morphine administration. Reduced gastric emptying and bowel motility (both small and large intestine), often leading to adynamic ileus, appear to be mediated both peripherally (by opioid receptors located in the gut) and centrally (by the vagus nerve). Fiber increasing agents, stool softeners, and mild cathartics are often prescribed for selected patients when a long duration of opioid analgesia requirement is expected.

Cardiovascular. Hypotension is not unusual following morphine administration, especially if it is given rapidly (i.e., 5 to 10 mg per minute). In patients pretreated with both H_1- and H_2-antagonists, the hypotensive response following morphine administration is significantly attenuated, despite comparable increases in plasma histamine concentrations. These data strongly implicate histamine as the mediator of these changes.

Respiratory. Morphine administration is followed by a dose-dependent reduction in responsiveness of brain stem ventilatory centers to carbon dioxide. Key features of this phenomenon include a reduction in the slope of the ventilatory and occlusion pressure responses to carbon dioxide, a rightward shift of the minute ventilatory response to hypercarbia, and an increase in resting end-tidal carbon dioxide and the apneic threshold (i.e., the PCO_2 value below which spontaneous ventilation is not initiated without hypoxemia). The duration of these effects often exceeds the time course of analgesia. In addition to blunting the carbon dioxide response, morphine decreases hypoxic ventilatory drive. Morphine administration in renal failure patients has been associated with prolonged ventilatory depression secondary to persistence of its active metabolite, morphine-6-glucuronide.

The administration of small doses of IV naloxone (40 μg) to patients in order to reverse the ventilatory depressant effect of morphine may produce adverse effects. Anecdotal reports describe the precipitation of vomiting, delirium, arrhythmias, pulmonary edema, cardiac arrest, and sudden death subsequent to naloxone administration in otherwise healthy patients after surgery. Furthermore, the duration of action of naloxone is shorter than any of the opioids it may be used to antagonize (except remifentanil). Recurring ventilatory depression therefore remains a distinct possibility, and in the spontaneously breathing patient, it is a source of potential morbidity.

Reversal with a mixed opioid agonist–antagonist, such as nalbuphine or butorphanol, appears to be safer than with naloxone. Mixed opioid agonist–antagonist agents may either increase or decrease the opioid effect, depending on the dose administered, the particular agonist already present, and the amount of agonist remaining.

For bedside procedures in the ICU, many of these problems can be obviated by using a shorter-acting opioid.

Neurologic. Morphine has little effect on cerebral metabolic rate or cerebral blood flow when ventilation is controlled. Morphine may affect cerebral perfusion pressure adversely by lowering mean arterial pressure.

Fentanyl and Its Congeners

Description

Fentanyl, sufentanil, and remifentanil enter and leave the CNS much more rapidly than morphine, thereby causing a much faster onset of effect after IV administration. The only significant difference among these agents is their PK behavior.

Fentanyl may be useful when given by intermittent bolus injection (50 to 100 μg), but when given by infusion, its duration becomes prolonged [19]. For TIVA in ICU patients in whom rapid emergence is desirable, sufentanil or remifentanil is the preferred choice for continuous infusion. When the procedure is expected to be followed by postoperative pain, sufentanil is preferred. Figure 2.1 shows that the CSHT of sufentanil is similar to that of propofol for infusions of up to 10 hours. When the procedure is expected to be followed by minimal postoperative pain (e.g., bronchoscopy), remifentanil is preferred. Its CSHT is about 4 minutes regardless of the duration of the infusion.

Remifentanil owes its extremely short duration to rapid metabolism by tissue esterases, primarily in skeletal muscle [20]. Its PK behavior is unchanged in the presence of severe hepatic [21] or renal [22] failure.

Sufentanil infusion for TIVA may be initiated with a 0.5 to 1.5 μg/kg bolus followed by an infusion at 0.01 to 0.03 μg/kg/min. If given with a propofol infusion, the two infusions may be stopped simultaneously as governed by the curves in Figure 2.1. Remifentanil infusion for TIVA may be initiated with a 0.5 to 1.5 μg/kg bolus followed by an infusion at 0.05 to 0.5 μg/kg/min. The remifentanil infusion should be continued until after the procedure is completed; if the patient is expected to have postoperative pain, another opioid should be given because the remifentanil effect will dissipate within a few minutes.

Adverse Effects

Cardiovascular. Although fentanyl, sufentanil, and remifentanil do not affect plasma histamine concentrations, bolus doses can be associated with hypotension, especially when infused rapidly (i.e., <1 minute). This action is related to medullary vasomotor center depression and vagal nucleus stimulation.

Neurologic. Fentanyl and sufentanil have been reported to increase ICP in ventilated patients following head trauma. Fentanyl and sufentanil may adversely affect cerebral perfusion pressure by lowering mean arterial pressure. All of the fentanyl derivatives may cause chest wall rigidity when a large bolus is given rapidly. This effect may be mitigated by neuromuscular blocking (NMB) agents as well as by coadministration of a hypnotic agent.

NEUROMUSCULAR BLOCKING AGENTS

There are two pharmacologic classes of NMB agents (see Chapter 4): Depolarizing agents (e.g., succinylcholine) and nondepolarizing agents (e.g., rocuronium, vecuronium, and cisatracurium). Succinylcholine is an agonist at the nicotinic acetylcholine receptor of the neuromuscular junction. Administration of succinylcholine causes an initial intense stimulation of skeletal muscle, manifested as fasciculations, followed by paralysis due to continuing depolarization. Nondepolarizing agents are competitive antagonists of acetylcholine at the neuromuscular junction; they prevent acetylcholine, released in response to motor nerve impulses, from binding to its receptor and initiating muscle contraction. Distinctions among the nondepolarizing agents are made on the basis of PK differences as well as by their cardiovascular effects.

NMB agents are used to facilitate endotracheal intubation and improve surgical conditions by decreasing skeletal muscle tone. Prior to intubation, the administration of an NMB agent results in paralysis of the vocal cords, increasing the ease with which the endotracheal tube may be inserted and decreasing the risk of vocal cord trauma. During surgery, the decrease in skeletal muscle tone may aid in surgical exposure (as during abdominal surgery), decrease the insufflation pressure needed during laparoscopic procedures, and make joint manipulation easier during orthopedic surgery. NMB agents should not be used to prevent patient movement that is indicative of inadequate anesthesia. Dosing of NMB agents should be based on monitoring evoked twitch response; ablation of two to three twitches of the train-of-four is sufficient for the majority of surgical procedures and permits easy reversal.

PRACTICAL CONSIDERATIONS FOR TIVA

Electing to perform common procedures (e.g., tracheostomy, percutaneous gastrostomy) in the ICU instead of the operating room represents a potential cost saving and increases access to these procedures. Not only does this strategy eradicate costly operating room time and support resources, it eliminates misadventures that sometimes occur in hallways and on elevators. Cost analyses estimate an average overall cost reduction of 50% or more compared with traditional operative procedures [23]. TIVA represents the most cost-effective method of facilitating this.

In most patients, safe and effective TIVA may be achieved via the infusions of propofol plus sufentanil or remifentanil. Premedication with midazolam decreases the required propofol doses and decreases the likelihood of recall for intraoperative events. Bolus doses should not be used in hemodynamically unstable patients, and lower bolus doses should be used in elderly individuals. NMB agents are also given if needed.

The opioid infusion rate is titrated to minimize signs of inadequate analgesia (e.g., tachycardia, tachypnea, hypertension, sweating, mydriasis), although differentiation of pain from the sympathetic responses to critical illness is difficult. The propofol infusion rate is titrated to the endpoint of loss of consciousness; the depth of anesthesia monitors that are based on analysis of the EEG waveform (bispectral index, patient state index, or spectral entropy) facilitates locating this endpoint more objectively. Loss of consciousness should be achieved prior to the initiation of muscle paralysis. It is possible for patients to be completely aware of intraoperative events at times when there is no change in hemodynamics or any manifestation of increased sympathetic activity [24,25]. Hence, administering an opioid to blunt incisional pain without inducing loss of consciousness with a hypnotic is inappropriate.

The following additional points deserve consideration in this context:

1. In subhypnotic doses, propofol is less effective than midazolam in producing amnesia. In the absence of coadministration of a benzodiazepine, propofol must cause unconsciousness in order to reliably prevent recall. Prompt treatment of patient responses (movement, tachycardia, hypertension) is important.
2. Medications infused for TIVA should be given via a carrier IV fluid running continuously at a rate of at least 50 mL per hour. This method not only helps deliver medication into the circulation, but also serves as another monitor of occlusion of the drug delivery system. Occlusion of the infusion line for more than a few minutes may lead to patient awareness.
3. In order to take advantage of the known CSHT values for the TIVA agents, communication with the surgeon during the procedure is important in order to anticipate the optimum time for stopping the infusions. Sufentanil and propofol infusions are stopped in advance of the end of the procedure, whereas remifentanil is infused until the procedure is completed.
4. To maintain reasonably constant propofol and sufentanil blood concentrations, the maintenance infusion rates should be decreased during the procedure because the plasma concentrations increase over time at constant infusion rates. An approximate guideline is to reduce the infusion rate by 10% every 30 minutes.
5. Strict aseptic technique is especially important during the handling of propofol.

References

1. Hughes MA, Glass PSA, Jacobs JR: Context-sensitive half-time in multicompartment pharmacokinetic models for intravenous anesthetic drugs. *Anesthesiology* 76:334–341, 1992.
2. Mangano DT, Browner WS, Hollenberg M: Association of perioperative myocardial ischemia with cardiac morbidity and mortality in men undergoing noncardiac surgery. *N Engl J Med* 323:1781–1788, 1990.
3. Barr J, Egan TD, Sandoval NF, et al: Propofol dosing regimens for ICU sedation based upon an integrated pharmacokinetic-pharmacodynamic model, *Anesthesiology* 95:324–333, 2001.
4. Ronan KP, Gallagher TH, Hamby BG: Comparison of propofol and midazolam for sedation in intensive care unit patients. *Crit Care Med* 23:286–293, 1995.
5. Erdoes G, Basciani RM, Eberle B: Etomidate—a review of robust evidence for its use in various clinical scenarios. *Acta Anaesthesiol Scand* 58:380–389, 2014.
6. Ledingham IM, Finlay WEI, Watt I, et al: Etomidate and adrenocortical function. *Lancet* 1:1434, 1983.
7. Fragen RJ, Shanks CA, Molteni A, et al: Effects of etomidate on hormonal responses to surgical stress. *Anesthesiology* 61:652–656, 1984.
8. Jackson WL: Should we use etomidate as an induction agent for endotracheal intubation in patients with septic shock? A critical appraisal. *Chest* 127:1031–1038, 2005.
9. Chan CM, Mitchell AL, Shorr AF: Etomidate is associated with mortality and adrenal insufficiency in sepsis: a meta-analysis. *Crit Care Med* 40:2945–2953, 2012.
10. Gu WJ, Wang F, Tang L, et al: Single-dose etomidate does not increase mortality in patients with sepsis: a systematic review and meta-analysis of randomized controlled trials and observational studies. *Chest* 147:335–346, 2015.
11. Jung B, Clavieras N, Nougaret S, et al: Effect of etomidate on complications related to intubation and on mortality in septic shock patients treated with hydrocortisone: a propensity score analysis. *Crit Care* 16:R224, 2012.
12. White PF: Pharmacologic interactions of midazolam and ketamine in surgical patients. *Clin Pharmacol Ther* 31:280, 1982.
13. Nelson LE, Lu J, Guo T, et al: The α2-adrenoceptor agonist dexmedetomidine converges on an endogenous sleep-promoting pathway to exert its sedative effects. *Anesthesiology* 98:428–436, 2003.
14. Coursin DB, Coursin DB, Maccioli GA: Dexmedetomidine. *Curr Opin Crit Care* 7:221–226, 2001.
15. Belleville JP, Ward DS, Bloor BC, et al: Effects of intravenous dexmedetomidine in humans. I. Sedation, ven-tilation, and metabolic rate. *Anesthesiology* 77:1125–1133, 1992.
16. Jakob SA, Ruokonen E, Grounds RM, et al: Dexmedetomidine vs midazolam or propofol for sedation during prolonged mechanical ventilation: two randomized controlled trials. *JAMA* 307:1151–1160, 2012.
17. Wijeysundera DN, Naik JS, Beattie WS: Alpha-2 adrenergic agonists to prevent perioperative cardiovascular complications: a meta-analysis. *Am J Med* 114:742–752, 2003.
18. Dershwitz M, Walsh JL, Morishige RJ, et al: Pharmacokinetics and pharmacodynamics of inhaled versus intravenous morphine in healthy volunteers. *Anesthesiology* 93:619–628, 2000.
19. Shafer SL, Varvel JR: Pharmacokinetics, pharmacodynamics, and rational opioid selection. *Anesthesiology* 74:53–63, 1991.
20. Dershwitz M, Rosow CE: Remifentanil: an opioid metabolized by esterases. *Exp Opin Invest Drugs* 5:1361–1376, 1996.
21. Dershwitz M, Hoke JF, Rosow CE, et al: Pharmacokinetics and pharmacodynamics of remifentanil in volunteer subjects with severe liver disease. *Anesthesiology* 84:812–820, 1996.
22. Hoke JF, Shlugman D, Dershwitz M, et al. Pharmacokinetics and pharmacodynamics of remifentanil in subjects with renal failure compared to healthy volunteers. *Anesthesiology* 87:533–541, 1997.
23. Barba CA, Angood PB, Kauder DR, et al: Bronchoscopic guidance makes percutaneous tracheostomy a safe, cost effective, and easy to teach procedure. *Surgery* 118:879–883, 1995.
24. Ausems ME, Hug CC Jr, Stanski DR, et al: Plasma concentrations of alfentanil required to supplement nitrous oxide anesthesia for general surgery. *Anesthesiology* 65:362–373, 1986.
25. Philbin DM, Rosow CE, Schneider RC, et al: Fentanyl and sufentanil anesthesia revisited: How much is enough? *Anesthesiology* 73:5–11, 1990.
26. Shafer A, Doze VA, Shafer SL: Pharmacokinetics and pharmacodynamics of propofol infusions during general anesthesia. *Anesthesiology* 69:348–356, 1988.
27. Persson P, Nilsson A, Hartvig P, et al: Pharmacokinetics of midazolam in total i.v. anaesthesia, *Br J Anaesth* 59:548–556, 1987.
28. Hudson RJ, Bergstrom RG, Thomson IR, et al: Pharmacokinetics of sufentanil in patients undergoing abdominal aortic surgery. *Anesthesiology* 70:426–431, 1989.
29. Egan TD, Lemmens HJM, Fiset P, et al: The pharmacokinetics of the new short acting opioid remifentanil (GI87084B) in healthy adult male volunteers. *Anesthesiology* 79:881–892, 1993.
30. Iirola T, Ihmsen H, LaitioR, et al: Population pharmacokinetics of dexmedetomidine during long-term sedation in intensive care patients. *Br J Anaesth* 108:460–468, 2012.

Chapter 3 ■ Management of Pain in the Critically Ill

MARIO DE PINTO • ARMAGAN DAGAL • RAMANA K. NAIDU

INTRODUCTION

In 2010, the International Association for the Study of Pain declared with the Declaration of Montreal that adequate pain management is a fundamental human right [1].

While goals of care in the intensive care unit (ICU) are mostly directed toward preventing mortality, it is equally, if not more important to consider the impact that morbidity may have on patients during the ICU phase of care; many decisions and interventions performed in the ICU can have a significant impact on the long-term well-being of patients.

In 2011, the Institute of Medicine estimated that 116 million Americans suffer from chronic pain, accounting for more health care costs than heart failure, diabetes, and cancer combined [2]. This report confirmed the significant impact pain has on our society.

We can look at the symptom pain as a dichotomy. On one hand, it is a signal of tissue damage and may offer protection from further insults. However, it can persist beyond the time of acute tissue damage, becoming a disease in its own right.

Pain may stem from acute medical or surgical illnesses as well as preexisting medical conditions. Mechanical ventilation, placement of indwelling tubes and catheters, procedures such as placement of chest tubes and intracranial pressure (ICP) monitors, turning and suctioning can all be causes of pain [3,4]. Exposure to high levels of pain can have negative psychological and physiological consequences, and its effective management is important in the maintenance of patient's dignity [5–7].

Critically ill patients should have their pain systematically observed and regularly assessed. All means of analgesic interventions should be evaluated in a coordinated, individualized, and goal-oriented interdisciplinary manner. Despite numerous improvement initiatives over the past two decades, pain is still a very common problem and often not treated appropriately for critically ill patients. It is estimated that as many as 70% of patients experience moderate-intensity procedure-related or postoperative pain during their stay in the ICU [8–11]. Pain is frequently treated inappropriately because of fears of depressing spontaneous ventilation, inducing opioid dependence, or precipitating cardiovascular instability. Moreover, many clinicians poorly understand the methods for assessing pain, the techniques for optimally treating it, and the benefits of its effective management. State-of-the-art pain management means not only decreasing pain intensity, but also reducing the side effects of anesthetics [12–14]. Studies also suggest that effective acute pain management may help reduce the development of chronic pain [15].

In 2005, the American Pain Society (APS) published guidelines for quality improvement in acute and cancer pain management [16]. In the guidelines, it is emphasized that it is important to

- recognize, identify, and treat pain promptly;
- involve patients and families in the pain management plan;
- reassess and adjust the pain management plan as needed; and
- monitor processes and outcomes of the pain management plan.

The primary goal of this structured approach to pain management is to prevent pain through the administration of analgesics at regular intervals and before performing potentially painful procedures. Implementation of the APS guidelines for 120 post–cardiac surgery patients over a 3-month period revealed that 95% had effective pain relief during every ICU staff shift for the first 6 days after surgery [17]. Analyses also revealed dramatically improved side-effect profile and reduced length of hospital stay. Implementation of a similar pain management protocol in a medical ICU resulted in a decrease in the number of days spent on the ventilator (from 10.3 to 8.9) and significant reductions of average hospital costs.

Pain management strategies for ICU patients should also incorporate the application of regional analgesia techniques (neuraxial and peripheral nerve blocks) whenever possible. While there are risks to the application and management of regional anesthesia and analgesia, these risks are generally low enough with knowledgeable and experienced practitioners to warrant its use. Regional anesthesia, when used appropriately, helps to reduce the total amount of opioid analgesics necessary to achieve adequate pain control without the development of potentially dangerous side effects.

PHYSIOLOGIC EFFECTS OF ACUTE PAIN

Pain leads to the development of increased catabolism, immunosuppression, and prolonged sympathetic responses as a result of the combination of tissue injury and pain that can contribute to increased rates of morbidity and mortality. These effects can be subclassified as follows:

Cardiovascular Effects

- Increased heart rate
- Increased blood pressure
- Increased stroke volume
- Increased myocardial O_2 demands and reduced supply leading to myocardial ischemia

Respiratory Effects

- Stimulation of respiration causing initial hypocapnia and respiratory alkalosis
- Diaphragmatic splinting and hypoventilation, atelectasis, hypoxia, and hypercapnia
- Impaired respiratory secretion clearance leading to chest infections

Endocrine Effects

- Catabolic and anabolic changes
- Decrease in insulin production and action
- Reduction in testosterone levels
- Fluid retention

Metabolic Effects

- Raised blood glucose levels and immune dysfunction

Gastrointestinal Effects

- Delayed gastric emptying
- Nausea and anorexia
- Reduced gastrointestinal (GI) motility and ileus

Coagulation

- Procoagulant effects of immobility
- Increased blood viscosity
- Hypercoagulability and deep vein thrombosis (DVT)

EVALUATION OF PAIN AND SEDATION IN THE ICU PATIENT

Appropriate assessment of pain for the adult ICU patient can be challenging. Structured approaches to pain assessment are mandatory for optimal patient outcomes and to understand the severity of pain from a population health perspective. Pain assessment tools are useful to monitor for deterioration or improvements over time, and evaluate and titrate analgesic therapy appropriately [7,18] (Fig. 3.1). There are several proposed methods available for pain assessment in the ICU. The chosen strategy should be adapted to the patient's capacity to interact with the practitioner in order to provide assessment of static (rest) and dynamic (while moving the affected part or while taking deep breaths or coughing) pain.

Assessment of pain should include determining its cause(s), type, intensity, duration, site, and prior responses to therapy. Categorization of pain into somatic, visceral, neuropathic in nature and identification of specific sites and characteristics, such as focal bone pain as opposed to allodynia, or diffuse bowel distention, is important because it helps determine the most effective type of intervention that improves the overall quality of pain care.

Subjective Pain Assessment

The **Visual Analog Scale** (VAS) is a 10-cm horizontal line, anchored by textual descriptors and/or pictures at each end. An end-point descriptor such as "no pain" (a score of 0) is marked at the left end and "worst pain imaginable" (a score of 10) is marked at the right end.

Five-Point Global Scale	None A little = 1 Some = 2 A lot = 3 The worst = 4
Verbal Quantitative Scale	0.......5.......10 None Worst imaginable
Visual Pain Analog Scale	No Worst .... Pain Pain Place a mark on the line

FIGURE 3.1 Several scales that can be useful for the evaluation of patient "self-reports" of pain before and after treatment. (From Stevens DS, Edwards WT: Management of pain in the critically ill. *J Intensive Care Med* 5:258, 1990, with permission.)

The **Numerical Rating Scale** (NRS) is a horizontal line with a scale from 0 to 10. Patients are asked to choose a number that relates to their pain intensity, where 0 represents no pain and 10 the worst imaginable pain. The NRS can be administered verbally or visually.

The **Faces Pain Scale** was first developed by Wong and Baker and is recommended for pediatric patients aged 3 and older. An explanation is given to the patient that each face is a person who feels happy because he or she has no pain or sad because he or she has some or a lot of pain. The patient is then asked to choose the face that best describes how they feel from six possible options.

NRSs have been reported to have the least variance and may be the preferred tool overall due to its rapid assessment. Mechanically ventilated and sedated patients will be unable to use the VAS ruler or other self-report pain assessment tools.

Objective Pain Assessment

When the patient is critically ill, sedated, and/or ventilated, pain severity can be estimated only by observing the behavioral and physiologic responses to pain:

- The **Behavioral Pain Scale** (BPS) is the earliest and most widely tested pain assessment tool for sedated patients.
  There are three component domains:
  "facial expression"
  "upper limb movement"
  "compliance with ventilation"
  Patients are scored from 1 to 4 on each section, giving a total score between 3 (no pain) and 12 (maximum pain) [19].
- The **Critical Care Pain Observation Tool** (CPOT)
  The CPOT has four domains:
  "facial expression"
  "body movement"
  "muscle tension"
  "compliance with ventilation"
  Patients are scored in each section between 0 and 2, giving an overall score of 0 (no pain) to 8 (maximum pain) [11,20].
- The **Non-Verbal Pain Scale** (NVPS)
  The NVPS incorporates three behavioral domains and two physiologic domains. The behavioral domains are "face," "activity (movement)," and "guarding." The first physiologic domain considers vital signs and the second incorporates other indicators including skin color and temperature, perspiration, and pupillary changes. Again, specific descriptors are given to enable the assessors to rate a patient's pain from 0 to 2 within each domain, giving a total pain score between 0 (no pain) and 10 (maximum pain) [21,22].

In general, none of these tools can be regarded as a gold standard and they require further evaluation and research to investigate the impact of their use on pain management in clinical practice. Nonetheless, they offer a consistent and systematic approach that might improve pain management in the ICU.

Analgesic trials can be another assessment tool if pain is suspected in ICU patients. They involve administration of a low dose of an analgesic followed by observation of the patient's pain-related behavior [7,23].

The **Pasero Opioid-Induced Sedation Scale** (POSS) [24] is a tool used for assessing opioid-induced sedation. It ranges from S (sleepy and easy to arouse) through four levels of sedation based on how drowsy the patient is. The utility of this scale is that it can forewarn the development of opioid-induced respiratory depression if used routinely and correctly.

The **Richmond Agitation Sedation Scale** (RASS) in contrast to POSS is used to assess sedation and agitation. When opioids are administered and the goal of therapy is analgesia, the POSS should be employed. If the goal of therapy is sedation, the RASS should be used. Both tools can be used in parallel, but it is important to know what the goals of care are when using these tools.

FORMULATION OF A TREATMENT PLAN

It is important to understand the characteristics of the pathologic process responsible for pain in order to establish the most effective therapy.

Character and Site

The location of current pain and any preexisting pain location(s) should always be documented.

Pain can be categorized as follows:

- **Nociceptive pain** occurs in response to a noxious stimulus and continues only in the presence of a persistent stimulus. It is transmitted through nonmyelinated C-sensory fibers and small myelinated A-delta (δ) fibers, propagating the noxious stimuli via the dorsal root ganglions (DRG) and spino-thalamic pathways to the spinal cord, thalamus, periaqueductal gray, and other centers in the brain [25]. Nociceptive pain is often dull, aching, sharp, or tender and can be categorized into somatic and visceral pain.
  - **Somatic pain** is due to nociceptive signals arising from the musculoskeletal system and is generally well localized.
  - **Visceral pain** is due to a disease process or abnormal function of an internal organ or its covering (parietal pleura, pericardium, and peritoneum). It can be frequently associated with nausea, vomiting, sweating, and changes in heart rate and blood pressure and is often described as diffuse and not well localized.
- **Inflammatory pain** occurs after tissue injury and the subsequent inflammatory response. In order to help healing of the injured body part, the sensory nervous system undergoes a profound change; normally innocuous stimuli now produce pain, and responses to noxious stimuli are both exaggerated and prolonged [26] due to plasticity in nociceptors and central nociceptive pathways [27,28]. Ablation of a specific set of nociceptor neurons, such as the one expressing the tetrodotoxin-resistant sodium channel Nav1.8, eliminates inflammatory pain, but leaves neuropathic pain intact, indicating a fundamental difference in the neuronal pathways responsible for these pain states [29,30].
- **Neuropathic pain** can be sharp, shooting, burning, tingling, or electric in character. Patients with neuropathic pain may describe positive or negative neurologic phenomena. Positive phenomena include spontaneous pain (arising without stimulus) and evoked pains (abnormal response to a stimulus). Negative phenomena include impaired sensation to touch or thermal stimuli. Neuropathic pain is initiated or caused by a primary lesion or dysfunction in the central or peripheral nervous system (CNS or PNS).

Central neuropathic pain most commonly results from spinal cord injury, stroke, or multiple sclerosis [31].

Peripheral neuropathic pain can be caused most commonly by [32]:

- Trauma (e.g., complex regional pain syndrome [CRPS], persistent postsurgical pain)
- Infection (e.g., postherpetic neuralgia, HIV-induced neuropathy)
- Ischemia (e.g., diabetic neuropathy, peripheral vascular disease)
- Metabolic (e.g., vitamin B_{12} deficiency)
- Cancer (e.g., invasion and compression of peripheral nerve structures)

- Chemically induced (e.g., chemotherapy-induced neuropathy)
- Radiation induced (e.g., medical radiation-induced neuropathy)

Damage to either the CNS or the PNS provokes maladaptive responses in nociceptive pathways that drive spontaneous pain and sensory amplification. This maladaptive plasticity leads to persistent changes and should be considered a disease state of the nervous system in its own right, independent of the etiologic factor(s) that trigger it. Studies suggest that peripheral and central sensitization mechanisms are also involved. In the PNS, they include altered gene expression and changes in ion channels that lead to ectopic activity. In the CNS, the expression of many genes is altered. In addition, synaptic facilitation and loss of inhibition at multiple levels of the neuraxis can produce central amplification. Neuronal cell death and aberrant synaptic connectivity provide the structural basis for persistently altered processing of both nociceptive and innocuous afferent inputs. Highly organized neuro-immunologic interactions as a result of neural damage play an important role in the development of persistent neuropathic pain. Genetically determined susceptibility is also likely to play a role in the development of neuropathic pain [30].

Hyperalgesia (an increased response to noxious stimuli), allodynia (the evocation of pain by non-noxious stimuli), hyperpathia (explosive pains evoked in areas with an increased sensory threshold when the stimulus exceeds the threshold), dysesthesia (spontaneous or evoked unpleasant abnormal sensation), and paresthesia (spontaneous or evoked abnormal sensation) are typical elements of neuropathic pain.

MEDICAL MANAGEMENT OF PAIN FOR THE ICU PATIENT

Consequences of inadequate sedation and analgesia in the ICU may result in excessive pain and anxiety, agitation, self-removal of tubes and catheters, violence toward caregivers, myocardial ischemia, patient–ventilator dysynchrony, hypoxemia, and pain-related immunosuppression. In contrast, excessive and/or prolonged sedation can lead to skin breakdown, nerve compression, delirium, unnecessary testing for altered mental status, prolonged mechanical ventilation, and associated problems such as ventilator-associated pneumonia, and perhaps posttraumatic stress disorder. A balanced treatment approach using both nonpharmacologic and pharmacologic methods is necessary for optimal pain management of the ICU patient [33,34]. Improvement in quality of pain care may result in reductions of the time spent on mechanical ventilation and length of stay in the ICU.

Nonpharmacologic Treatments

Nonpharmacologic interventions are easy to provide, safe, and effective. They may include attention to proper positioning of patients to avoid pressure points, stabilization of fractures, and elimination of irritating physical stimulation (e.g., avoiding traction on the endotracheal tube).

Several mechanisms have been proposed to explain how to inhibit or modulate the ascending transmission of a noxious stimulus from the periphery or, conversely, to stimulate descending inhibitory control from the brain [35]. They include the following:

- Gate control theory
- "Busy-line" effect
- Production of endogenous opioids at the periaqueductal gray, reticular activating system (RAS), and spinal gates
- Activation of monoaminergic neurons in the thalamus, hypothalamus, and brain stem
- Activation of second-order neurons in the dorsal horn, selective inhibition of abnormally hypersensitive neurons in the dorsal horn, and increased release of gamma (γ)-aminobutyric acid (GABA) from spinal neurons
- Descending inhibition from supraspinal centers via the pretectal zone and posterior columns

Stimulation-produced analgesia is a term that describes noninvasive or minimally invasive techniques such as acupuncture, electroacupuncture, acupressure, transcutaneous electric nerve stimulation (TENS), spinal cord stimulation, peripheral nerve stimulation, DRG stimulation, deep-brain stimulation, and motor cortex stimulation. Evidence suggests that these modalities are useful as a sole or supplementary analgesic technique for both acute and chronic painful conditions [35]. Peripherally applied heat causes local vasodilation that promotes circulatory removal of biomediators of pain from the site of injury, whereas cold application decreases the release of pain-inducing chemicals [36].

Given that pain is an unpleasant sensory and emotional experience, it is always important to address the emotional component as well. Pain psychologists have primarily been used on an outpatient basis in pain clinics, but their importance on the inpatient side is significant, especially in the ICU where patients have already or are undergoing a potentially "traumatic" experience. The ICU experience is associated with major life changes such as financial hardship from the cost of health care, loss of function, or potential death. Having family and friends in proximity can be very helpful for a patient, although at times, it can be a detriment depending on the relationship and circumstances. Some institutions have therapy animals, which can provide a positive distraction for specific patients.

Modifications of the ICU environment, such as creating units with single rooms, decreasing noise, setting a schedule for activity, providing music and windows or appropriate lighting that better reflect a day–night orientation [37], may help patients achieve normal sleep patterns and also improve pain control. For the cognitively intact ICU patients, provision of sensory and procedural information may improve their ability to cope with the discomfort.

Pharmacologic Treatments

The pharmacologic characteristics of the ideal analgesic medication include easy titration, rapid onset and offset of action without accumulation, and no side effects.

Cyclooxygenase Inhibitors—Nonsteroidal Anti-inflammatory Drugs

Cyclooxygenase (COX) is an enzyme located in all cells. It metabolizes arachidonic acid to generate prostaglandin H_2. A number of enzymes further modify this product to generate bioactive lipids (prostanoids) such as prostacyclin, thromboxane A_2, and prostaglandins D_2, E_2, F_2, and I_2. Isoforms COX-1 and COX-2 have been described. COX-1 is ubiquitous and constitutive. COX-2 is present in areas of inflammation and located in inflammatory cells. The COX-3 isoform was described in 2002 and was associated with a possible mechanism of action for acetaminophen but arguments exist as to why this is likely not so.

It is now recognized that COX-2 is expressed in normal endothelial cells in response to shear stress and its inhibition is associated with suppression of prostacyclin synthesis. Inhibition of COX-2 results in prothrombotic inclination on endothelial surfaces and an increase in sodium and water retention, leading to edema, as well as exacerbations of heart failure and hypertension. Loss of the protective effects of COX-2 upregulation in the setting of myocardial ischemia and infarction leads to a larger infarct size, greater thinning of the left ventricular wall in the infarct zone, and an increased tendency to myocardial rupture [38–40].

Blockade of the proinflammatory mediators by nonsteroidal anti-inflammatory drugs (NSAIDs) reduces the inflammatory response (and subsequent pain). Classically, their effect is anti-inflammatory, analgesic, and antipyretic because of the direct inhibition of prostaglandin production. Adding NSAIDs to intravenous (IV) opioid-based patient-controlled analgesia (PCA) reduces opioid consumption by 30% to 50% and results in a significant reduction in the incidence of nausea, vomiting, and sedation [41].

On the other hand, the nonspecific blockade of COX inhibits the physiologic role of COX-1 and results in clinically significant deterioration of renal function and risk of development of peptic ulcerations and upper GI hemorrhage, bronchospasm, and platelet dysfunction. A meta-analysis published in 2002 has shown that the risk of GI hemorrhage is related to the patient and drug-related factors and is irrespective of the type of NSAID used. Patients who smoke, those with history of GI hemorrhage, and those taking anticoagulants are at increased risk [42]. Prophylaxis with a proton-pump inhibitor, histamine-2 antagonist, misoprostol, or sucralfate, reduces the risk of COX-1-related gastritis.

Current evidence indicates that selective COX-2 inhibitors have important adverse cardiovascular effects that include increased risk for myocardial infarction, stroke, heart failure, and hypertension. The risk for these adverse effects is likely to be greatest in patients with a history of or at high risk for cardiovascular disease. These risks escalate with continued use after 30 days though it remains unclear if there is significant risk with short-term or "as needed" (PRN) use. In these patients, COX-2 inhibitors for pain relief should be used only if there are no alternatives and then only in the lowest dose and shortest duration necessary [43].

Opioid-sparing properties of NSAIDs have not been studied in critically ill patients, and so it is unclear if potential benefits outweigh potential risks such as GI bleeding or renal failure. Therefore, until more evidence for such agents becomes available, the clinician must carefully judge the risks and benefits on an individual basis.

Acetaminophen—Paracetamol

Acetaminophen is an analgesic and antipyretic. It may also have anti-inflammatory properties. The mechanism of action of acetaminophen remains unknown. Recent research indicates that acetaminophen inhibits prostaglandin synthesis in cells that have a low rate of synthesis and low levels of peroxide. When the levels of arachidonic acid are low, acetaminophen appears to be a selective COX-2 inhibitor. Acetaminophen has predominant effects on the CNS because the peroxide and arachidonic acid levels in the brain are lower than at peripheral sites of inflammation [44].

Acetaminophen is available in oral, rectal, and parenteral formulations. The parenteral formulation became available in the United States in 2010. It is an effective adjuvant to opioid analgesia, and a reduction in opioid requirement by 20% to 30% can be achieved when combined with a regular regimen of oral or rectal acetaminophen. One gram of acetaminophen significantly reduces postoperative morphine consumption over a 6-hour period. Doses greater than 1,000 mg have been reported to have a superior effect when compared with lower doses. IV acetaminophen has been shown to reduce PCA morphine requirements after spinal surgery [45] and hip arthroplasty. Its side-effect profile is comparable to placebo [46]; hypersensitivity reactions are rare. The major concerns with acetaminophen administration relate to the potential for hepatotoxicity, which is extremely rare following therapeutic dosing below 4 grams per day [47]. In patients with severe liver disease, the elimination half-life can be prolonged. A reduced dose of 1 gram two times a day with short duration of therapy is recommended. Prospective studies administering acetaminophen to patients consuming alcohol have found no increased evidence of liver injury [48]. Nonallergic hypotension has been reported in a cohort of ICU patients treated with therapeutic doses of acetaminophen. Brain injury and sepsis are potential risks for this type of hypotensive reaction [49].

Opioids

For the critically ill patient, opioids remain the main pharmacologic method for the treatment of pain. Despite their extensive side-effect profile, there are no alternatives currently available with the same therapeutic range (Table 3.1).

Opiates refer to the nonpeptide synthetic morphine-like drugs, while the term *opioid* is more generic, encompassing all substances that produce morphine-like actions.

Opioids can be loosely divided into four groups:

- Naturally occurring, endogenously produced opioid peptides (e.g., dynorphin and Met-enkephalin)
- Opium alkaloids, such as morphine or codeine, purified from the poppy (*Papaver somniferum*)
- Semisynthetic opioids (modifications to the natural morphine structure), such as diacetylmorphine (heroin), hydromorphone, oxycodone, and oxymorphone
- Synthetic derivatives with structure unrelated to morphine, which include the phenylpiperidine series (e.g., pethidine and fentanyl), methadone series (e.g., methadone and dextropropoxyphene), benzomorphan series (e.g., pentazocine), and semisynthetic thebaine derivatives (e.g., etorphine and buprenorphine)

Snyder et al. in 1973 reported on the presence of specific binding sites for opioids, providing the first evidence of the presence of distinct receptors for opioid medications. There are several types of opioid receptors. They differ in their potency, selective antagonism, and stereospecificity of opioid action. With a recent addition, the opioid receptor subtypes are listed as μ (MOR), κ (KOR), and δ (DOR), and nociceptin/orphanin FQ (N/OFQ) peptide receptor.

Opioids bind to the CNS and peripheral tissue receptors. μ_1-Receptors mediate analgesia, whereas μ_2-receptor binding produces respiratory depression, nausea, vomiting, constipation, and euphoria. κ-receptor activation causes sedation, miosis, and spinal analgesia. In addition to analgesia, opioid receptors may provide mild-to-moderate anxiolysis. Opioids have no reliable amnestic effect on patients. Opioid administration is associated with a dose-dependent, centrally mediated respiratory depression. The respiratory rate is reduced, whereas the tidal volume is initially preserved. The ventilatory response to hypoxia is eradicated, and the CO_2–response curve is shifted to the right. Opioids facilitate patients' compliance to the ventilator due to their cough-suppressant effects. Despite minimal cardiovascular effects in normovolemic patients, they may generate hypotension via decreased sympathetic tone and thus may decrease heart rate and systemic vascular resistance in critically ill patients. Additionally, some opiates can cause histaminergic vasodilation, which increases venous capacitance thereby decreasing venous return. Hypotension is more pronounced in hypovolemic patients.

Endogenous μ opioid receptors play a role in homeostatic peristalsis. Exogenous μ opioids can lead to opioid-induced ileus and constipation, a common problem in the critically ill patient. Some opioids are used for this particular effect (e.g., loperamide [Imodium] an enteric μ receptor agonist marketed as an antidiarrheal). Other methods to manage constipation and ileus secondary to the use of opioids include stool softeners, promotility agents, osmotic agents, and μ-receptor antagonists.

TABLE 3.1

Guidelines for Front-Loading Intravenous Analgesia

Drug	Total Front-Load Dose	Increments	Cautions
Morphine	0.08–0.12 mg/kg	0.03 mg/kg q 10 min	Bradycardia/hypotension (histamine) Nausea/vomiting Biliary colic Acute/chronic renal failure Elderly Bronchospasm
Methadone	0.08–0.12 mg/kg	0.03 mg/kg q 15 min	Accumulation/sedation Elderly
Hydromorphone	0.02 mg/kg	25–50 μg/kg q 10 min	Same as morphine Dosing errors
Fentanyl	1–3 μg/kg	0.5–2.00 μg/kg/h	Accumulation/sedation Elderly skeletal muscle rigidity
Remifentanil	0.25–1.00 μg/kg	0.05–2.00 μg/kg/min	Bradycardia/hypotension Pain on discontinuation Skeletal muscle rigidity
Ketamine	0.2–0.5 mg/kg	0.5–2.00 mg/kg/h	Delirium Increased ICP High myocardial O_2 requirement Hypotension Decreased CO

CO, cardiac output; ICP, intracranial pressure; q, every.

Morphine

Morphine has poor lipid solubility and thus has a relatively slow onset of action (5 to 10 minutes). The standard IV dose is 5 to 10 mg, and the approximate half-life is 3 hours. However, with repeated dosing or continuous infusions, half-life kinetics becomes unreliable. Morphine is conjugated by the liver to metabolites that include morphine-6-glucuronide, a potent metabolite with 20 times the activity of morphine. Both morphine and morphine-6-glucuronide are eliminated by the kidney; therefore, renal dysfunction results in a prolonged drug effect. Morphine-3-glucuronide is potentially neurotoxic and that can contribute to lowering the seizure threshold, the development of tremors, and, possibly, hyperalgesia. Morphine may also cause hypotension due to vasodilatation (secondary to the release of histamine).

Fentanyl

Fentanyl is highly lipid soluble with rapid onset of action (1 minute) and rapid redistribution into peripheral tissues, resulting in a short half-life (0.5 to 1.0 hour) after a single dose. The duration of action with small doses (50 to 100 μg) is short as a result of redistribution from the brain to other tissues. Larger or repeated doses, including those delivered via a continuous infusion, alter the context-sensitive half-time and result in drug accumulation and prolonged effects. The hepatic metabolism of fentanyl creates inactive metabolites that are renally excreted, making this drug a more attractive choice in patients with renal insufficiency. Fentanyl causes minor hemodynamic changes and does not affect inotropy.

Hydromorphone

Hydromorphone is a semisynthetic opioid that is five- to tenfold more potent than morphine, but with a similar duration of action. It has minimal hemodynamic effects and causes minor to no histamine release [50]. While the metabolite hydromorphone-3-glucoronide has been found to be neurotoxic in animal studies, there have been very few clinical reports of hydromorphone-related neurotoxicity, and therefore practitioners prefer it to morphine. Studies suggest that patients who received IV hydromorphone have a greater decrease in pain than those given an equianalgesic dose of IV morphine [51].

Methadone

Methadone is a synthetic opioid agent with unique properties. It can be given enterally and parenterally. The bioavailability of the drug is highly variable and can be altered by the administration of antibiotics, antipsychotics, and antidepressants because it is metabolized through multiple CYP450 pathways (3A4, 2B6, 2D6, 2C9, 2C19, 2C8) whose function is also affected by those classes of drugs [52]. Methadone does not follow a linear conversion in that with increasing doses, there is an exponential increase in opioid requirements.

Methadone is an attractive choice for opioid analgesia due to its long half-life and low cost. It produces *N*-methyl-D-aspartate (NMDA) antagonism, which makes it ideal for neuropathic pain. Although methadone is not the drug of choice for an acutely ill patient whose hospital course is rapidly changing, it is a good alternative for the patient who has preexisting opioid tolerance or may need prolonged ventilatory wean. It may help facilitate the tapering of opioid infusions [53]. Metabolized in the liver, 40% of the drug is eliminated from kidney and free from active metabolites. It does not accumulate in renal failure.

Oxycodone

Oxycodone is effective for management of postoperative pain. It has a higher bioavailability and a slightly longer half-life than oral morphine. When transferring patients from oral morphine to oral oxycodone, the dose should be based on a 1.5:1 ratio (i.e., 1 mg oral morphine = 0.5 to 0.7 mg oral oxycodone). Individual patient variability and incomplete cross-tolerance require careful titration [54].

The use of controlled-release oxycodone (OxyContin) is indicated for the treatment of moderate-to-severe pain when continuous analgesia is required for prolonged periods. Due to concerns about misuse, the Food and Drug Administration (FDA) has the ER/LA Risk Evaluation Mitigation Strategy program for the use of these drugs. Responding to concerns about misuse, the FDA approved an abuse-deterrent formulation of OxyContin in 2010 based on changes to the physical and chemical structure that makes it more difficult to inject or snort.

Remifentanil

Remifentanil (a derivative of fentanyl) is a powerful analgesic with an ultrashort duration of action. It is metabolized by nonspecific esterases to remifentanil acid, which has negligible activity in comparison. Its metabolism is independent from hepatorenal function. The context-sensitive half-time of remifentanil is consistently short (3.2 minutes), even after an infusion of long duration up to 72 hours [55].

In terms of safety, efficacy, and speed of onset and offset, remifentanil has been reported to have a better profile when compared with fentanyl [56]. When a morphine-based pain and sedation regimen was compared with another based on remifentanil, the mean duration of mechanical ventilation and extubation time were significantly shorter in the remifentanil group [57]. Breen et al. [58] compared a remifentanil-based analgesia–sedation regimen with another one based on midazolam and with the possible addition of fentanyl or morphine for analgesia, in a group of critically ill patients requiring prolonged mechanical ventilation for up to 10 days. The remifentanil-based sedation regimen was associated with significantly reduced duration of mechanical ventilation by more than 2 days.

Rozendaal et al. reported that in patients with anticipated short-term mechanical ventilation, a remifentanil–propofol analgesia–sedation regimen provides better control of sedation and agitation and reduces weaning time compared with conventional regimens. In addition, patients on a remifentanil–propofol–based regimen are almost twice as likely to be extubated and discharged from the ICU within the first 3 days of treatment than patients on conventional regimens [59]. In addition, remifentanil does not exert significantly prolonged clinical effects when administered to ICU patients with renal failure or chronic liver disease [55]. On the basis of these studies, it can be concluded that remifentanil is effective for providing both analgesia and sedation in critically ill patients, even those suffering from multiple organ failure. However, further data are needed to better guide clinicians on the use of this drug in ICU patients.

OPIOID SIDE EFFECTS

Opioid-related adverse effects occur commonly in the ICU [60].

Opioid-induced respiratory depression is generally dose related and is most deleterious for the spontaneously breathing ICU patient. The incidence of opioid-induced nausea and vomiting is low in the ICU. High-dose fentanyl may cause muscle rigidity. Opioid-induced hypotension occurs most commonly in patients who are hemodynamically unstable, volume depleted, or have a high sympathetic tone. The use of morphine is associated with histamine release; therefore, hypotension, urticaria, pruritus, flushing, and bronchospasm have been reported. Fentanyl can safely be used in patients with a suspected allergy to morphine. Excessive sedation from opioids is most often seen with the use of continuous infusions, particularly in patients with end-stage renal disease who are receiving fentanyl or morphine. Methadone may cause excessive sedation if the dose is not titrated downward after the first 5 days of therapy or if a human cytochrome P450 inhibitor is concomitantly administered. QTc-interval prolongation and the risk of development of torsades de pointes can occur with high doses of methadone because of its effects on the hERG channel, particularly if the chlorobutanol-containing IV formulation is used. Opioids may cause hallucinations, agitation, euphoria, sleep disturbances, and delirium [61]. Methadone may be the least likely drug to cause delirium because of its antagonistic activity at the NMDA receptor [62]. The effects of opioids on ICP in patients with traumatic brain injury remain unclear.

Ileus

Gastric retention and ileus are common in patients who are critically ill and receiving opioids. Prokinetic therapy and/or postpyloric access is often required in patients who are prescribed enteral nutrition. Prophylactic use of a stimulant laxative reduces the incidence of constipation. Methylnaltrexone, an opioid that does not cross an intact blood–brain barrier will only affect peripheral receptors and may have a role in treating opioid-induced constipation that fails to respond to laxative therapy [63]. Alvimopan has selectivity for peripheral μ receptors but is associated with an increased risk of myocardial infarction. Oral naloxone has been advocated for several years since it has very low bioavailability and can potentially antagonize enteric μ receptors without reversing analgesia. However, its use is not helpful when a patient already has impaired transit. Naloxegol, the most recent addition to the armamentarium, was approved in 2014. It adds polyethylene glycol to naloxol, a compound close in chemical structure to naloxone.

Addiction

The possibility of developing addiction with patients receiving long-term opioids related to transient ICU stay–related pain is extremely low. Addiction is defined by the American Society of Addiction Medicine as a primary, chronic disease, of brain reward, motivation, memory, and related circuitry. Dysfunction in these circuits leads to characteristic biologic, psychological, social, and spiritual manifestations. This is reflected in an individual pathologically pursuing reward and/or relief by substance use and other behaviors. Addiction is characterized by inability to consistently abstain, impairment in behavioral control, craving, diminished recognition of significant problems with one's behaviors and interpersonal relationships, and a dysfunctional emotional response. Like other chronic diseases, addiction often involves cycles of relapse and remission. Without treatment or engagement in recovery activities, addiction is progressive and can result in disability or premature death [64].

OPIOIDS ADMINISTRATION METHODS

Opioid analgesics can be administered by either continuous infusion or titration to provide better pain control and less drug-related adverse effects. "As needed" protocols make it difficult to achieve adequate analgesic plasma concentrations, with resultant poor pain control.

When a continuous infusion is used, a sedation vacation protocol allows more effective analgesic titration with a lower total dose of opioid used. Daily awakening may also be associated with a shorter duration of ventilation and ICU stay. For patients in whom a long recovery and a prolonged ventilatory wean are anticipated, the use of a long-acting medication (e.g., methadone) to achieve adequate background pain control in combination with bolus doses of a short-acting opioid for management of breakthrough pain may be an appropriate option.

Conventional Routes of Administration (Oral, Intramuscular, and Subcutaneous)

Because of first-pass metabolism in the liver, larger doses of medications are required when oral preparations are used. Immediate-release oral opioids (e.g., morphine, oxycodone, hydromorphone) are usually preferred. Onset of analgesia is obtained in 45 to 60 minutes with these medications. Fixed-interval dosing (e.g., every 4 hour) is preferable to a "when required" regimen to ensure adequate relief of moderate-to-severe pain. The rectal route is rarely used in the ICU, even though drugs absorbed from the lower half of the rectum bypass the portal vein and first-pass metabolism in the liver. Suppository formulations containing morphine, oxycodone, hydromorphone, and oxymorphone are available.

Intramuscular injections of opioids are useful if there is a lack of personnel trained to administer IV injections or if venous access is difficult. The intramuscular injection of morphine takes 30 to 60 minutes to be effective. Absorption of intramuscular opioids is variable and depends on the injection site, especially in critically ill patients. Subcutaneous injection via an indwelling cannula in the subcutaneous tissue of the upper outer aspect of the arm or thigh is a useful alternative route of administration. The rate of absorption of morphine after subcutaneous injection is similar to that of an intramuscular injection; therefore, the guidelines for titration are the same (Table 24.1)

Advanced Methods of Administration

The IV route is the preferred route of administration. There is less variability in blood levels when the IV route is used, making it easier to titrate the drug to an effective analgesia concentration. IV infusions are a commonly used method. An opioid infusion at a fixed rate takes five half-lives of the drug to reach 98% of a steady-state concentration. Therefore, a front-loading dose is needed to achieve adequate pain relief more rapidly before starting the infusion. If breakthrough pain occurs, more IV bolus doses may be needed to reestablish pain relief before the infusion rate is increased.

IV PCA devices allow the patient to self-administer a predetermined dose of opioid within the limits of a lockout period. This results in less variability in the blood levels of the drug, thereby enabling titration of the drug to effect [65].

The epidural and intrathecal routes of administration provide a more rapid analgesia due to the application of the drug directly within the CNS. Patient-controlled epidural analgesia (PCEA) regimens allow better titration of the medication. In general, the analgesic efficacy of neuraxial opioids is greater than that achieved with parenteral opioid administration, resulting in superior pain relief despite the smaller doses used in the subarachnoid or epidural space (e.g., subarachnoid morphine 0.1 mg = epidural morphine 1 mg = IV morphine 10 mg). Opioid solutions with preservative-free formulations should be used for neuraxial administration to avoid potential neurotoxicity.

Highly lipid-soluble opioids (e.g., fentanyl, buprenorphine) have been formulated as a skin patch for transdermal delivery, especially in the management of severe pain in chronic and palliative care. Fentanyl patches are usually not a recommended modality for acute analgesia because of their 12- to 24-hour delay to peak effect and similar lag time to complete offset once the patch is removed. However, it is appropriate to continue its use in the ICU if the patient has a known history of using this formulation of the medication before admission.

Given its peculiar pharmacologic characteristics (high affinity for the μ opioid receptor, antagonism at the κ opioid receptor, long half-life of approximately 24 hours), it is appropriate to discontinue the use of transdermal buprenorphine for patients who may require a long ICU stay. Because of the high affinity of buprenorphine for the μ receptor, high doses of other opioids with high affinity for the receptor (hydromorphone, fentanyl) may be necessary to achieve adequate pain control in these patients, especially during the initial phases of care.

ADJUVANT MEDICATIONS

Ketamine

Ketamine is a dissociative anesthetic that can be used for sedation and/or anti-hyperalgesia. It possesses strong analgesic properties at higher doses. It acts both centrally and peripherally by inhibition of glutamate activation via noncompetitive antagonism at the phencyclidine receptor of the NMDA channel. Nitric oxide (NO) synthase inhibition also contributes to its effects.

Water- and lipid-soluble characteristics of ketamine hydrochloride enable the IV, intramuscular, subcutaneous, epidural, oral, rectal, and transnasal routes of administration. Ketamine has a rapid onset and short duration of action [66]. Following metabolism in the liver, norketamine is produced, which is significantly less potent (20% to 30%) when compared with ketamine.

In subanesthetic or low doses (0.1 to 0.5 mg per kg IV or as an infusion at doses of 1 to 5 μg/kg/min), ketamine demonstrates significant anti-hyperalgesic efficacy without significant adverse pharmacologic effects. There is evidence that ketamine as an adjunct to a pain management plan reduces opioid consumption. Low-dose ketamine may play an important role in postoperative pain management when used as an adjunct to opioids, local anesthetics, and other analgesic agents [67–69]. Administration of regular benzodiazepines should be considered to minimize the risk of developing psychomimetic side effects associated with its use.

Ketamine infusions have been used for critically ill ICU patients who are very difficult to sedate with opioid and benzodiazepines. Because of the potential risk for developing hallucinations and vivid dreams, increased ICP, and myocardial depression, ketamine is not recommended for routine sedation and analgesia of the critically ill patient, but it can be useful for more difficult situations and/or when short surgical procedures with intense pain, such as placement of chest tubes, dressing changes, and/or wound debridement in burn patients, are necessary.

α_2-Adrenergic Agonists

α_2-Adrenergic activation represents an intrinsic mechanism of pain control at the level of the CNS. α_2-Adrenergic receptors exist in large numbers in the substantia gelatinosa of the dorsal horns of the spinal cord in humans. Agonists produce their pain control effect on those receptors.

Clonidine

Clonidine produces analgesia after systemic, epidural, or intrathecal administration. It has a short duration of action after a single dose and may produce sedation, bradycardia, and hypotension. Clonidine improves opioid analgesia and potentiates the effect of local anesthetic [70,71]. Its use for the ICU patient must be carefully considered, especially in patients with hemodynamic and cardiovascular instability.

Dexmedetomidine

Dexmedetomidine is a centrally acting α_2-agonist with sedative and analgesic properties. It has a much greater affinity for the α_2-receptors than clonidine. The sedative properties are facilitated through the locus coeruleus in the CNS. Analgesic effects occur via activation of the α_2-receptors and through potentiation of the action of opioids [72]. The drug causes no significant effect on the respiratory drive even when used with opioids. Dexmedetomidine has a biphasic effect on the cardiovascular system. The initial bolus injection is associated with vasoconstrictive effects, causing bradycardia and hypertension. Continuous infusion is associated with hypotension secondary to vasodilation caused by central sympatholysis. Studies conducted in postoperative ICU patients demonstrated successful short-term sedation and analgesic sparing effects [73]. There are a few studies examining long-term administration to critically ill, mechanically ventilated patients with encouraging results [74]. Suggested dosing recommendations would be a loading dose of 1 μg per kg over 10 minutes followed by an infusion at a rate of 0.2 to 0.7 μg/kg/h.

Lidocaine

Lidocaine has known analgesic, anti-hyperalgesic, and anti-inflammatory properties and some evidence to support the use of lidocaine infusions for pain management in selected group of patients has been reported.

Little is known about the incidence of risks associated with this type of intervention. However, in a recent review on the use of lidocaine infusions, its use was deemed safe when utilized in surgical patients at the appropriate dosing and when the appropriate contraindications are considered [75].

Lidocaine infusions are appropriate in patients undergoing major abdominal surgery, colorectal surgery in particular. Its use can reduce overall opioid requirements, ileus recovery time, and hospital length of stay [76,77]. However, one study comparing the use of IV lidocaine infusions with thoracic epidural analgesia (TEA) concluded that lidocaine does not reduce opioid consumption and pain scores when compared with TEA [78]. However, a lidocaine infusion may be considered for patients who may not be appropriate candidates for TEA (e.g., patient refusal, need for full-dose anticoagulation, presence of a localized or widespread infection).

The use of lidocaine infusions is contraindicated in patients with a known history of cardiac conditions such as atrio-ventricular conduction blockade and should be used with caution in patients with hepatic dysfunction. Serum levels should be obtained if one is concerned with systemic toxicity; the literature suggests that the threshold for lidocaine systemic toxicity is 5 μg per mL.

Antiepileptic Drugs—Calcium-Channel Membrane Stabilizers

Gabapentin and pregabalin (Gabapentinoids) are licensed for the management of neuropathic pain.

Despite its structural similarity to GABA, gabapentin does not bind to GABA receptors. It has a high affinity for α_2/δ-subunits of voltage-dependent calcium channels, resulting in postsynaptic inhibition of the calcium influx thereby reducing the presynaptic excitatory neurotransmitter release [79]. It markedly decreases postoperative opioid consumption when given at the time of anesthetic induction [80]. Several randomized controlled trials (RCTs) using different pain models have shown a positive effect of the gabapentinoids on postoperative pain in humans. Single doses of gabapentin up to 1,200 mg have been shown to reduce pain scores and/or morphine consumption after abdominal and vaginal hysterectomy, lower limb arthroplasty, and laparoscopic cholecystectomy. Different meta-analyses have confirmed these effects, which can persist for up to 24 hours after surgery [81]. Common side effects of these medications include dizziness and drowsiness. Gabapentin has minimal drug interactions.

Pregabalin has the same mechanism of action of gabapentin. It has higher efficacy due to its linear pharmacokinetics. In addition, it appears to have a faster onset of action, due in part to its smaller volume of distribution.

REGIONAL ANALGESIA TECHNIQUES

Neuraxial anesthesia and peripheral nerve blockade have the potential to reduce or eliminate the physiologic stress response to surgery and trauma, decreasing the risk of surgical complications and reducing the development of chronic pain. By optimizing pain control with regional anesthesia techniques, patient satisfaction scores and outcomes improve.

When used alone or in combination with other treatment modalities, regional analgesia techniques are an invaluable tool to address pain-related problems in critically ill patients, but the indications for their use must be established correctly. ICU patients are at risk for numerous complications, and the use of an inappropriate regional analgesia technique can cause a deterioration of the patient's clinical status, affecting potentially favorable outcomes.

The purpose of this section is to discuss risk and benefits of neuraxial and peripheral nerve blockade for the management of pain in the critically ill patient.

General Considerations

The use of ultrasound (US) technology in regional anesthesia allows an easier and more reliable identification of neural structures, the safe administration of lower doses of local anesthetic, and the insertion of nerve catheters even in the heavily sedated ICU patients. Ultrasound-guided (USG) techniques have reduced misplacement and failure rates in clinical practice. Effective identification of the needle allows for the reduction of the amount of administered drug volumes, which may be of importance in the critically ill, children, and patients who need more than one block, especially those who have undergone multisite surgery or sustained multiple injuries [82].

Regional analgesia techniques also effectively block sympathetic outflow. Many studies have shown that surgically related stress is reduced when regional anesthesia and analgesia techniques are used, neuraxial techniques in particular. The use of neuraxial analgesia has also been reported to decrease the rate of postoperative myocardial infarctions, shorten postoperative and posttraumatic ileus, improve the outcome, and shorten the length of ICU stay [83].

The use of such techniques may also reduce the incidence of chronic pain in patients undergoing surgical procedures, such as limb amputations and thoracotomies, two procedures in particular associated with the development of chronic persistent postsurgical pain [84].

Nerve Blocks for Thoracic and Abdominal Wall

Intercostal Nerve Blocks

Single and continuous intercostal nerve blocks are used to provide analgesia in patients with thoracic injuries and rib fractures and for the treatment of postoperative pain. Excellent pain relief and improvement in pulmonary mechanics have been reported [85]. Intercostal nerve blocks are associated with risk of pneumothorax and systemic local anesthetic toxicity. The patient's coagulation status must be checked to prevent the risk of bleeding and hematoma formation subsequent to the laceration of an intercostal vessel. Continuous intercostal nerve blockade after thoracotomy using an extrapleural catheter consistently results in better pain relief and preservation of pulmonary function than the use of systemic opioids and appears to be at least as effective as the relief provided by the epidural approach. The ease of the extrapleural approach and the low incidence of complications suggest that this technique should be used more frequently. Other methods of intercostal nerve blockade appear to be less effective. The use of a multifaceted approach to postthoracotomy analgesia that includes intercostal nerve blockade has been shown to be beneficial in the immediate postoperative period, as well as reduce the incidence of chronic pain.

Major pulmonary resections, which have been managed with a mini-thoracotomy and intrapleural intercostal nerve blockade, have been associated with reduced postoperative pain and improved outcomes. However, a recently published study in thoracotomy patients did not find a measurable difference in pain relief between intercostal catheters and epidural analgesia [86].

Although not frequently used, intercostal nerve blockade can be extremely useful for the ICU patient, especially when used as a single injection for painful procedures (e.g., placement of chest tubes), or as an infusion when the patient's hemodynamic conditions do not allow the use of TEA.

Paravertebral Block

Paravertebral nerve blocks (PVBs) provide analgesia for thoracic and upper abdominal pain. Paravertebral nerve blockade can be performed with a single injection or a continuous catheter technique [87]. Injection of contrast material into a paravertebral catheter shows flow of the dye laterally into the intercostal space, as well as up and down the ipsilateral paravertebral space, leading to the spreading of local anesthetics over several dermatomal levels.

The advantages of PVBs are similar to those of the intercostal nerve block technique. Analgesia can be obtained without the development of potentially deleterious widespread cardiovascular effects because only unilateral sympathetic blockade is produced.

Because the site of injection is medial to the scapula, this block is easier to perform at high thoracic levels than the intercostal nerve blocks. In contrast to routine intercostal blocks, the posterior primary ramus of the intercostal nerve is also covered with the paravertebral approach, providing analgesia of the posterior spinal muscles and the costovertebral ligaments.

Failure rate after PVB in adults varies from 6.1% to 10.7% and compares favorably with other regional procedures. In a prospective study of 319 adult patients, the incidence of complications after thoracic or lumbar PVB was reported to be as follows: hypotension 5%, vascular puncture 3.8%, pleural puncture 0.9%, and pneumothorax 0.3% [88,89].

Interpleural Analgesia

Interpleural blockade is a technique by which an amount of local anesthetic is injected into the thoracic cage between the parietal and visceral pleura to produce ipsilateral somatic block of multiple thoracic dermatomes. Local anesthetic solutions can be administered as single or intermittent boluses, or as continuous infusions via an indwelling interpleural catheter. It has been shown to provide safe, high-quality analgesia after cholecystectomy, thoracotomy, renal surgery, breast surgery, and some invasive radiologic procedures of the renal and hepatobiliary system. It has also been used successfully in the treatment of pain from multiple rib fractures, herpes zoster, CRPS, thoracic and abdominal cancer, and pancreatitis [85].

There are several methods proposed for the detection of the entry of the needle into the pleural space, and all of them involve the detection of the "negative pressure" when the needle has entered into the intrapleural space [90]. If a posterior approach is not possible, an anterior approach can be used. The catheter may also be positioned in the interpleural space under direct vision during surgery.

The risk of pneumothorax is 2%. The risk of systemic local anesthetic toxicity is 1.3%. Pleural inflammation increases the risk of toxicity.

It has been suggested that local anesthetic solution diffuses outward with the interpleural technique blocking multiple intercostal nerves, the sympathetic chain of the head, neck and upper extremity, the brachial plexus, splanchnic nerves, the phrenic nerve, the celiac plexus, and ganglia. As the injected local anesthetic diffuses out through both layers of the pleura, direct local effects on the diaphragm, lung, pericardium, and peritoneum may also contribute to some of its analgesic activity [86].

Transversus Abdominis Plane Block

Incisional pain represents a considerable portion of postoperative pain following abdominal operations. The abdominal wall consists of three muscle layers: external oblique, internal oblique, transversus abdominis, and their corresponding fascial sheaths. The skin, muscles, and parietal peritoneum of the anterior abdominal wall are innervated by the lower six thoracic nerves and the first lumbar nerve. The anterior primary rami of these nerves exit their respective intervertebral foramina and extend over the vertebral transverse process. They then pierce the musculature of the lateral abdominal wall to travel through a neurofascial plane between the internal oblique and transversus abdominis muscles. Deposition of local anesthetic dorsal to the midaxillary line blocks both the lateral cutaneous branch and the lateral cutaneous afferents, thus facilitating blockade of the entire anterior abdominal wall. The transversus abdominis plane thus provides a space into which local anesthetic can be deposited to achieve myo-cutaneous sensory blockade.

This regional anesthesia technique has been shown to provide good postoperative analgesia for a variety of procedures involving the abdominal wall [91]. The use of a fine-gauge, blunt-tipped, short-bevel needle, and USG have been proposed to reduce the incidence of possible complications (intraperitoneal injection with bowel injury/hematoma, liver laceration, transient femoral nerve palsy, accidental intravascular injection, infection, and catheter breakage). In addition, with US-guided techniques, upper and lower portions of the abdominal wall can be preferentially blocked [92].

Peripheral Nerve Blocks for the Upper Extremities

Severe trauma to the shoulders and arms is frequently present in acutely injured ICU patients. These injuries may be associated with blunt chest trauma requiring mechanical ventilation; they usually augment pain overall, especially during positioning [93]. If the orthopedic injury is part of complex trauma with closed-head injury causing alterations of mental status so that opioid-based analgesia regimens may mask the underlined neurologic condition, adequate analgesia can be provided with blocks of the brachial plexus. Continuous brachial plexus blocks consistently provide superior analgesia with minimal side effects, promoting earlier hospital discharge and possibly improving rehabilitation after major surgery [94].

Peripheral nerve injury is a rare complication of regional anesthesia for the upper extremities. A large study from France reported 0.04% overall risk of a serious adverse event after peripheral nerve blockade [95]. Several retrospective studies reported the incidence to be between 0.5% and 1.0%, whereas prospective studies published higher incidence rates between 10% and 15% [96].

Current evidence suggests that peripheral nerve blockade should not be routinely performed in most adults during general anesthesia (GA) or heavy sedation especially when using the interscalene approach. However, the risk-to-benefit ratio of performing a peripheral nerve block under these conditions versus using high doses of opioids to maintain adequate analgesia should be carefully considered in select ICU patients [97].

Furthermore, the advent of USG techniques, in combination with injection pressure monitoring and nerve stimulation, may help to significantly minimize possible serious complications in heavily sedated patients with increased success rate and potential benefits overall.

Peripheral Nerve Blockade for the Lower Extremities

Lower extremity injuries are also commonly present in critically ill ICU patients.

Reid et al. [98] recently conducted a study to compare the accuracy, success rates, and complications of USG femoral nerve blockade (FNBs) with the fascial pop technique in an emergency department. The result of this study favors the use of USG FNB. A similar study, conducted by Marhofer et al. [99] has demonstrated a clear benefit in the use of US over a peripheral nerve stimulator when performing a three-in-one nerve block. Use of both approaches (USG and peripheral nerve stimulation) may potentially improve the quality of the block, extend the duration, and provide better results with the use of smaller doses and less concentrated solutions of local anesthetic.

FNB is the preferred analgesic technique following injuries of the knee. Compared with epidural analgesia, it has a favorable morbidity profile, allows early mobilization, and there is no need for urinary catheterization. In addition, with USG, the technique is simple and easy to perform compared with the epidural blocks [100]. FNB and catheters are helpful in the management of acute pain following femoral fractures as well as after surgical stabilization [101].

Easy US-guided visualization of the sciatic nerve proximal to the popliteal fossa, before it divides into common peroneal nerve medially and tibial nerve laterally, makes the lateral approach to the sciatic nerve an ideal approach for management of pain secondary to distal tibia, ankle, and foot fractures [102]. This block can be conveniently performed in the supine position and enables more secure placement of a peripheral nerve catheter with high rates of success.

Epidural Analgesia

Epidural analgesia is the most frequently used regional anesthesia technique in the ICU [103] and has been reported to provide better pain relief than parenteral opioid administration [104]. However, there is conflicting evidence regarding a reduction of mortality with the use of epidural analgesia. The largest meta-analysis (CORTRA) to date and analysis of the Medicare claims database [105] associated a reduction in perioperative mortality with the use of perioperative neuraxial anesthesia. Procedure-specific meta-analyses and specific RCTs, however, have not demonstrated benefit from epidural anesthesia and analgesia regarding reduction in mortality. It is important to note that these specific meta-analyses and individual RCTs lack sufficient sample size due to the relatively low incidence of mortality (0.2% to 5%) overall [106].

A meta-analysis of more than 5,000 surgical patients [107] has shown that postoperative epidural analgesia reduces the time to extubation, length of ICU stay, incidence of renal failure, and morphine consumption during the first 24 hours after surgery, as well as maximal glucose and cortisol blood concentrations, and improves forced vital capacity. Many of these benefits may be relevant to ICU patients; they have been demonstrated to be beneficial in cardiac surgery [108] and thoracic trauma patients [109], as well as patients with severe acute pancreatitis [110].

Whether sepsis, with or without positive blood cultures, should be an absolute contraindication for the use of epidural analgesia is still a matter of debate [111]. In patients with ischemic heart disease, high TEA has been shown to improve systolic and diastolic myocardial function [112]. Data from a prospective randomized trial show that PCEA offers superior postoperative pain control after laparotomy for gynecologic surgery compared with traditional IV PCA [113].

TEA exerts a remarkable influence on the cardiovascular system. It reduces the risk of perioperative dysrhythmias except postoperative atrial fibrillation. In cardiac surgical patients, with decreased left ventricular function, the left ventricular global and regional wall motions are better preserved. TEA has also been associated with a reduction of cardiac oxygen consumption without jeopardizing coronary perfusion pressure by increasing the diameter of stenotic coronary segments. As a result, TEA reduces the overall incidence of myocardial infarction. It produces functional hypovolemia by inhibiting the vasoconstrictor sympathetic outflow; moreover, it interferes with the integrity of renin–angiotensin system and increases vasopressin plasma concentration. Despite causing hypotension, TEA has a beneficial outcome during hemorrhagic shock [114].

Issues of consent, coagulopathy, and infection can be addressed easily in elective conditions; they become a major problem in patients with multiple trauma or extremely painful conditions.

A study published in Sweden reports the risk of hematoma with neuraxial anesthesia to be 1.3 to 2.7 per 100,000 [115]. The current recommendations of the American Society of Regional Anesthesia should be followed [116].

Placing epidural catheters safely and confirming the presence of an adequate sensory block can be difficult in critically ill, sedated, and anesthetized patients. Awake and cooperative patients usually facilitate the placement of an epidural catheter, minimizing the possibility of undesirable complications. Current recommendations suggest that the possibility to miss systemic local anesthetic toxicity under GA or heavy sedation is not a valid reason not to perform a neuraxial block in this group of patients. However, the indications for neuraxial regional anesthesia should be carefully considered when the procedure is to be performed in patients whose sensorium is compromised by GA or heavy sedation [97]. The overall risk of neuraxial anesthesia should be weighed against its expected benefit.

Positioning the patient for the procedure may also represent a challenge depending on the underlying injury and the number and position of tubes, catheters, or external fixation devices present. Strict asepsis should always be maintained for neuraxial procedures. Bolus injections of long-acting local anesthetics, such as bupivacaine and ropivacaine, or the discontinuation of continuous infusions every morning can help neurologic and sensory assessment.

The most common side effects of TEA are bradycardia and hypotension related to sympathetic blockade; this can be more pronounced with intermittent bolus dosing in patients with hypovolemia or shock. Continuous low-rate local anesthetic and/or opioid (morphine) infusions can be safely used in this particular clinical setting. Currently, sepsis and bacteremia are considered contraindications to neuraxial blockade. Fever and increased white blood cell count alone in the absence of positive blood cultures do not provide a reliable diagnosis of bacteremia. High levels of the serum markers C-reactive protein, procalcitonin, and interleukin-6/8 have been shown to indicate bacterial sepsis with a high degree of sensitivity and specificity and can guide the decision as to whether or not to place an epidural catheter [117].

Because high-risk patients seem to profit most from epidural analgesia and the current literature does not address the specific problem of the critically ill patient with multiple comorbidities and organ failure, logic suggests that in carefully selected and closely monitored patients epidural analgesia may have significant benefits. Further research is needed before clear recommendations can be made.

INFLUENCE OF PAIN MANAGEMENT ON COMPLICATIONS, OUTCOMES, LENGTH OF HOSPITAL STAY, AND CHRONIC PAIN

A meta-analysis published in the year 2008 has concluded that epidural analgesia prevents postoperative major complications and may decrease postoperative mortality [77]. Other studies have reported that epidural anesthesia may selectively prevent the occurrence of respiratory and cardiovascular complications [118–120].

Conversely, other prospective trials have failed to confirm the beneficial effects of epidural anesthesia on postoperative morbidity and mortality after major abdominal or orthopedic surgery. Such a discrepancy is thought to be the result of overall improved postoperative medical care. As an example, a previously reported 50% reduction in DVT with epidural analgesia is no longer a valid criterion due to the recent introduction of low-molecular-weight heparin for management of DVT prophylaxis, which decreases the risk by more than 80%. Similarly, the use of prophylactic antibiotics and aggressive physiotherapy significantly reduces the postoperative pulmonary complications, and the preventive effect of epidural analgesia for chest infections has become less important. Consequently, there is no significant evidence to consider epidural analgesia beneficial for the prevention of morbidity, but as part of a multimodal pain management process, it may facilitate recovery after surgery and trauma. The superior quality of pain relief provided by epidural analgesia combined with parenteral analgesia does indeed have a positive impact on mobilization, bowel function, and early food intake with improvement in postoperative quality of life [121]. For orthopedic surgery patients, regional analgesia may provide functional benefits, allowing better patient involvement with physical therapy and shorter recovery time.

Improvements in perioperative outcomes following peripheral nerve block after major orthopedic surgery include significantly shorter hospital stay, earlier ambulation, improved joint range of motion, lower perioperative pain scores, and a reduction in postoperative nausea and vomiting. Patients treated with peripheral nerve blocks also had significantly lower opioid requirements when compared with controls, as well as significant reduction in urinary retention and postoperative ileus [122].

Although risk factors are difficult to identify, patients who experience severe pain and, above all, persistence of postoperative pain several days after the expected duration are prone to develop chronic pain. Postoperative chronic pain is defined as persisting pain, without relapse or pain-free interval, 2 months after the surgical intervention. Chronic pain syndromes have been described commonly after breast surgery, inguinal hernia repair, cholecystectomy, thoracic surgery, cardiac surgery, and limb or organ amputation. The incidence has been recorded to be up to 60% [123]. With such a high incidence, it is very important to provide good postoperative and posttrauma pain control to prevent the occurrence of chronic pain syndromes.

CONCLUSIONS

Pain control in critically ill patients is of paramount importance. Achieving adequate levels of analgesia in trauma and surgery patients decreases the stress response and improves morbidity and mortality. Individual units and acute pain teams should employ pain assessment techniques for patients with impaired cognition.

Lack of education, fear of possible side effects, and inappropriate use of medications contribute to the ineffective treatment of pain in critically ill ICU patients. The expertise of pain management specialists and anesthesiologists is often necessary for the management of these complex situations.

Choosing the treatment plan that best fits the patient's clinical conditions is mandatory. A potentially favorable outcome can be altered if inappropriate pain modalities are chosen and used.

A rational multimodal approach including the use of nonpharmacologic, pharmacologic, and regional analgesia techniques is desirable and often needed. The continued use of these techniques extended into the postoperative period may shorten recovery time and speed discharge.

Always assess and monitor the effects of a treatment modality on the patient's pain and clinical conditions as well. Be prepared to make changes in therapy as needed.

Regional analgesia techniques (epidural and peripheral nerve blockade), although proved to be safe and effective, are underused in the management of pain in critically ill patients. They allow a decrease in the overall use of opioid analgesics and sedatives and reduce the possibility of developing potentially dangerous side effects. A correct indication, as well as an appropriate timing for their use, is required in order to increase their beneficial effects.

The availability of new technologies (e.g., ultrasonography) improves the quality and safety of upper and lower extremity peripheral nerve blocks even in heavily sedated ICU patients.

References

1. International Association for the Study of Pain (IASP): Declaration of Montreal. Available at http://www.iasp-pain.org/DeclarationofMontreal.
2. Institute of Medicine (IOM): Relieving Pain in America: Report Brief. June 29, 2011. Available at https://iom.nationalacademies.org/Reports/2011/Relieving-Pain-in-America-A-Blueprint-for-Transforming-Prevention-Care-Education-Research/Report-Brief.aspx.
3. Sessler CN, Wilhelm W: Analgesia and sedation in the intensive care unit: an overview of the issues. *Crit Care* 12(Suppl 3):S1, 2008.
4. Sessler CN, Grap MJ, Brophy GM: Multidisciplinary management of sedation and analgesia in critical care. *Semin Respir Crit Care Med* 22(2):211–226, 2001.
5. Blakely WP, Page GG: Pathophysiology of pain in critically ill patients. *Crit Care Nurs Clin North Am* 13(2):167–179, 2001.
6. Summer GJ, Puntillo KA: Management of surgical and procedural pain in a critical care setting. *Crit Care Nurs Clin North Am* 13(2):233–242, 2001.
7. Herr K, Coyne PJ, Key T, et al: Pain assessment in the nonverbal patient: position statement with clinical practice recommendations. *Pain Manag Nurs* 7(2):44–52, 2006.
8. Dolin SJ, Cashman JN, Bland JM: Effectiveness of acute postoperative pain management: I. Evidence from published data. *Br J Anaesth* 89(3):409–423, 2002.
9. Apfelbaum JL, Chen C, Mehta SS, et al: Postoperative pain experience: results from a national survey suggest postoperative pain continues to be undermanaged. *Anesth Analg* 97(2):534–540, table of contents, 2003.
10. Puntillo KA, White C, Morris AB, et al: Patients' perceptions and responses to procedural pain: results from Thunder Project II. *Am J Crit Care* 10(4):238–251, 2001.
11. Gelinas C, Johnston C: Pain assessment in the critically ill ventilated adult: validation of the Critical-Care Pain Observation Tool and physiologic indicators. *Clin J Pain* 23(6):497–505, 2007.
12. Bonnet F, Marret E: Postoperative pain management and outcome after surgery. *Best Pract Res Clin Anaesthesiol* 21(1):99–107, 2007.
13. Basse L, Hjort Jakobsen D, Billesbolle P, et al: A clinical pathway to accelerate recovery after colonic resection. *Ann Surg* 232(1):51–57, 2000.
14. Kehlet H, Jensen TS, Woolf CJ: Persistent postsurgical pain: risk factors and prevention. *Lancet* 367(9522):1618–1625, 2006.
15. Kehlet H, Wilmore DW: Multimodal strategies to improve surgical outcome. *Am J Surg* 183(6):630–641, 2002.
16. Gordon DB, Dahl JL, Miaskowski C, et al: American Pain Society recommendations for improving the quality of acute and cancer pain management:

American Pain Society Quality of Care Task Force. *Arch Intern Med* 165(14):1574–1580, 2005.
17. Reimer-Kent J: From theory to practice: preventing pain after cardiac surgery. *Am J Crit Care* 12(2):136–143, 2003.
18. Gelinas C, Fortier M, Viens C, et al: Pain assessment and management in critically ill intubated patients: a retrospective study. *Am J Crit Care* 13(2):126–135, 2004.
19. Payen JF, Bru O, Bosson JL, et al: Assessing pain in critically ill sedated patients by using a behavioral pain scale. *Crit Care Med* 29(12):2258–2263, 2001.
20. Galinas C, Fillion L, Puntillo KA, et al: Validation of the Critical Care Pain Observation Tool in adult patients. *Am J Crit Care* 15(4):420–427, 2006.
21. Odhner M, Wegman D, Freeland N, et al: Assessing pain control in non-verbal critically ill adults. *Dimens Crit Care Nurs* 22(6):260–267, 2003.
22. Cade CH: Clinical tools for the assessment of pain in sedated critically ill adults. *Nurs Crit Care* 13(6):288–297, 2008.
23. Herr K: Pain assessment in cognitively impaired older adults. *Am J Nurs* 102(12):65–67, 2002.
24. Pasero C: Assessment of sedation during opioid administration for pain management. *J Perianesth Nurs* 24(3):186–190, 2009.
25. De Pinto M, Dunbar PJ, Edwards WT: Pain management. *Anesthesiol Clin* 24(1):19–37, vii, 2006.
26. Juhl GI, Jensen TS, Norholt SE, et al: Central sensitization phenomena after third molar surgery: a quantitative sensory testing study. *Eur J Pain* 12(1):116–127, 2008.
27. Huang J, Zhang X, McNaughton PA: Inflammatory pain: the cellular basis of heat hyperalgesia. *Curr Neuropharmacol* 4(3):197–206, 2006.
28. Hucho T, Levine JD: Signaling pathways in sensitization: toward a nociceptor cell biology. *Neuron* 55(3):365–376, 2007.
29. Abrahamsen B, Zhao J, Asante CO, et al: The cell and molecular basis of mechanical, cold, and inflammatory pain. *Science* 321(5889):702–705, 2008.
30. Costigan M, Scholz J, Woolf CJ: Neuropathic pain: a maladaptive response of the nervous system to damage. *Annu Rev Neurosci* 32:1–32, 2009.
31. Ducreux D, Attal N, Parker F, et al: Mechanisms of central neuropathic pain: a combined psychophysical and fMRI study in syringomyelia. *Brain* 129 (Pt 4):963–976, 2006.
32. Dworkin RH, Backonja M, Rowbotham MC, et al: Advances in neuropathic pain: diagnosis, mechanisms, and treatment recommendations. *Arch Neurol* 60(11):1524–1534, 2003.
33. Brush DR, Kress JP: Sedation and analgesia for the mechanically ventilated patient. *Clin Chest Med* 30(1):131–141, ix, 2009.
34. Sessler CN, Pedram S: Protocolized and target-based sedation and analgesia in the ICU. *Crit Care Clin* 25(3):489–513, viii, 2009.
35. Kotzé A, Simpson KH: Stimulation-produced analgesia: acupuncture, TENS and related techniques. *Anaesth Intensive Care Med* 9(1):29–32, 2008.
36. French SD, Cameron M, Walker BF, et al: Superficial heat or cold for low back pain. *Cochrane Database Syst Rev* (1):CD004750, 2006.
37. Cepeda MS, Carr DB, Lau J, et al: Music for pain relief. *Cochrane Database Syst Rev* (2):CD004843, 2006.
38. Hebbes C, Lambert D: Non-opioid analgesic drugs. *Anaesth Intensive Care Med* 9(2):79–83, 2008.
39. Timmers L, Sluijter JP, Verlaan CW, et al: Cyclooxygenase-2 inhibition increases mortality, enhances left ventricular remodeling, and impairs systolic function after myocardial infarction in the pig. *Circulation* 115(3):326–332, 2007.
40. Jugdutt BI: Cyclooxygenase inhibition and adverse remodeling during healing after myocardial infarction. *Circulation* 115(3):288–291, 2007.
41. Marret E, Kurdi O, Zufferey P, et al: Effects of nonsteroidal antiinflammatory drugs on patient-controlled analgesia morphine side effects: meta-analysis of randomized controlled trials. *Anesthesiology* 102(6):1249–1260, 2005.
42. Lewis SC, Langman MJ, Laporte JR, et al: Dose–response relationships between individual nonaspirin nonsteroidal anti-inflammatory drugs (NANSAIDs) and serious upper gastrointestinal bleeding: a meta-analysis based on individual patient data. *Br J Clin Pharmacol* 54(3):320–326, 2002.
43. Antman EM, Bennett JS, Daugherty A, et al: Use of nonsteroidal antiinflammatory drugs: an update for clinicians: a scientific statement from the American Heart Association. *Circulation* 115(12):1634–1642, 2007.
44. Kam P, So A: COX-3: uncertainties and controversies. *Curr Anaesth Crit Care* 20(1):50–53, 2009.
45. Hernandez-Palazon J, Tortosa JA, Martinez-Lage JF, et al: Intravenous administration of propacetamol reduces morphine consumption after spinal fusion surgery. *Anesth Analg* 92(6):1473–1476, 2001.
46. Barden J, Edwards J, Moore A, et al: Single dose oral paracetamol (acetaminophen) for postoperative pain. *Cochrane Database Syst Rev* (1):CD004602, 2004.
47. Benson GD, Koff RS, Tolman KG: The therapeutic use of acetaminophen in patients with liver disease. *Am J Ther* 12(2):133–141, 2005.
48. Kuffner EK, Green JL, Bogdan GM, et al: The effect of acetaminophen (four grams a day for three consecutive days) on hepatic tests in alcoholic patients—a multicenter randomized study. *BMC Med* 5:13, 2007.
49. Mrozek S, Constantin JM, Futier E, et al: Acetaminophen-induced hypotension in intensive care unit: a prospective study. *Ann Fr Anesth Reanim* 28(5):448–453, 2009.
50. Jacobi J, Fraser GL, Coursin DB, et al: Clinical practice guidelines for the sustained use of sedatives and analgesics in the critically ill adult. *Crit Care Med* 30(1):119–141, 2002.
51. Chang AK, Bijur PE, Meyer RH, et al: Safety and efficacy of hydromorphone as an analgesic alternative to morphine in acute pain: a randomized clinical trial. *Ann Emerg Med* 48(2):164–172, 2006.
52. Lugo RA, MacLaren R, Cash J, et al: Enteral methadone to expedite fentanyl discontinuation and prevent opioid abstinence syndrome in the PICU. *Pharmacotherapy* 21(12):1566–1573, 2001.
53. Fredheim OM, Moksnes K, Borchgrevink PC, et al: Clinical pharmacology of methadone for pain. *Acta Anaesthesiol Scand* 52(7):879–889, 2008.
54. Blumenthal S, Min K, Marquardt M, et al: Postoperative intravenous morphine consumption, pain scores, and side effects with perioperative oral controlled-release oxycodone after lumbar discectomy. *Anesth Analg* 105(1):233–237, 2007.
55. Breen D, Wilmer A, Bodenham A, et al: Offset of pharmacodynamic effects and safety of remifentanil in intensive care unit patients with various degrees of renal impairment. *Crit Care* 8(1):R21–R30, 2004.
56. Muellejans B, Lopez A, Cross MH, et al: Remifentanil versus fentanyl for analgesia based sedation to provide patient comfort in the intensive care unit: a randomized, double-blind controlled trial [ISRCTN43755713]. *Crit Care* 8(1):R1–R11, 2004.
57. Dahaba AA, Grabner T, Rehak PH, et al: Remifentanil versus morphine analgesia and sedation for mechanically ventilated critically ill patients: a randomized double blind study. *Anesthesiology* 101(3):640–646, 2004.
58. Breen D, Karabinis A, Malbrain M, et al: Decreased duration of mechanical ventilation when comparing analgesia-based sedation using remifentanil with standard hypnotic-based sedation for up to 10 days in intensive care unit patients: a randomised trial [ISRCTN47583497]. *Crit Care* 9(3):R200–R210, 2005.
59. Rozendaal FW, Spronk PE, Snellen FF, et al: Remifentanil-propofol analgo-sedation shortens duration of ventilation and length of ICU stay compared to a conventional regimen: a centre randomised, cross-over, open-label study in the Netherlands. *Intensive Care Med* 35(2):291–298, 2009.
60. Riker RR, Fraser GL: Adverse events associated with sedatives, analgesics, and other drugs that provide patient comfort in the intensive care unit. *Pharmacotherapy* 25(52):8S–18S, 2005.
61. Gaudreau JD, Gagnon P, Roy MA, et al: Opioid medications and longitudinal risk of delirium in hospitalized cancer patients. *Cancer* 109(11):2365–2373, 2007.
62. Benitez-Rosario MA, Feria M, Salinas-Martin A, et al: Opioid switching from transdermal fentanyl to oral methadone in patients with cancer pain. *Cancer* 101(12):2866–2873, 2004.
63. Thomas J, Karver S, Cooney GA, et al: Methylnaltrexone for opioid-induced constipation in advanced illness. *N Engl J Med* 358(22):2332–2343, 2008.
64. American Society of Addiction Medicine (ASAM): Definition of Addiction. Available at http://www.asam.org/for-the-public/definition-of-addiction.
65. Hudcova J, McNicol E, Quah C, et al: Patient controlled opioid analgesia versus conventional opioid analgesia for postoperative pain. *Cochrane Database Syst Rev* (4):CD003348, 2006.
66. Liu LL, Gropper MA: Postoperative analgesia and sedation in the adult intensive care unit: a guide to drug selection. *Drugs* 63(8):755–767, 2003.
67. Subramaniam K, Subramaniam B, Steinbrook RA: Ketamine as adjuvant analgesic to opioids: a quantitative and qualitative systematic review. *Anesth Analg* 99(2):482–495, table of contents, 2004.
68. Zakine J, Samarcq D, Lorne E, et al: Postoperative ketamine administration decreases morphine consumption in major abdominal surgery: a prospective, randomized, double-blind, controlled study. *Anesth Analg* 106(6):1856–1861, 2008.
69. Elia N, Tramer MR: Ketamine and postoperative pain—a quantitative systematic review of randomised trials. *Pain* 113(1–2):61–70, 2005.
70. Farmery AD, Wilson-MacDonald J: The analgesic effect of epidural clonidine after spinal surgery: a randomized placebo-controlled trial. *Anesth Analg* 108(2):631–634, 2009.
71. Andrieu G, Roth B, Ousmane L, et al: The efficacy of intrathecal morphine with or without clonidine for postoperative analgesia after radical prostatectomy. *Anesth Analg* 108(6):1954–1957, 2009.
72. Szumita PM, Baroletti SA, Anger KE, et al: Sedation and analgesia in the intensive care unit: evaluating the role of dexmedetomidine. *Am J Health Syst Pharm* 64(1):37–44, 2007.
73. Martin E, Ramsay G, Mantz J, et al: The role of the alpha2-adrenoceptor agonist dexmedetomidine in postsurgical sedation in the intensive care unit. *J Intensive Care Med* 18(1):29–41, 2003.
74. Venn M, Newman J, Grounds M: A phase II study to evaluate the efficacy of dexmedetomidine for sedation in the medical intensive care unit. *Intensive Care Med* 29(2):201–207, 2003.
75. McCarthy GC, Megalla SA, Habib AS. Impact of intravenous lidocaine on postoperative analgesia and recovery from surgery. *Drugs* 70(9):1149–1163, 2010.
76. Vigneault L, Turgeon AF, Cote D, et al: Perioperative intravenous lidocaine infusion for postoperative pain control: a meta-analysis of randomized controlled trials. *Can J Anesth* 58:22–37, 2011.
77. Marret E, Rolin M, Beaussier M, et al: Meta-analysis of intravenous lidocaine and postoperative recovery after abdominal surgery. *Br J Surg* 95:1331–1338, 2008.
78. Kuo CP, Jao SW, Chen M, et al: Comparison of the effects of thoracic epidural analgesia and i.v. infusion with lidocaine on cytokine response, postoperative pain and bowel function in patients undergoing colonic surgery. *Br J Anaesth* 97:640–646, 2006.
79. Bian F, Li Z, Offord J, et al: Calcium channel alpha2-delta type 1 subunit is the major binding protein for pregabalin in neocortex, hippocampus, amygdala, and spinal cord: an ex vivo autoradiographic study in alpha2-delta type 1 genetically modified mice. *Brain Res* 1075(1):68–80, 2006.
80. Hurley RW, Cohen SP, Williams KA, et al: The analgesic effects of perioperative gabapentin on postoperative pain: a meta-analysis. *Reg Anesth Pain Med* 31(3):237–247, 2006.

81. Seib RK, Paul JE: Preoperative gabapentin for postoperative analgesia: a meta-analysis. *Can J Anaesth* 53(5):461–469, 2006.
82. Wiebalck A, Grau T: Ultrasound imaging techniques for regional blocks in intensive care patients. *Crit Care Med* 35(5 Suppl):S268–S274, 2007.
83. Rodgers A, Walker N, Schug S, et al: Reduction of postoperative mortality and morbidity with epidural or spinal anaesthesia: results from overview of randomised trials. *BMJ* 321(7275):1493, 2000.
84. Jenewein J, Moergeli H, Wittmann L, et al: Development of chronic pain following severe accidental injury. Results of a 3-year follow-up study. *J Psychosom Res* 66(2):119–126, 2009.
85. Osinowo OA, Zahrani M, Softah A: Effect of intercostal nerve block with 0.5% bupivacaine on peak expiratory flow rate and arterial oxygen saturation in rib fractures. *J Trauma* 56(2):345–347, 2004.
86. Allen MS, Halgren L, Nichols FC III, et al: A randomized controlled trial of bupivacaine through intracostal catheters for pain management after thoracotomy. *Ann Thorac Surg* 88(3):903–910, 2009.
87. Eid HE: Paravertebral block: an overview. *Curr Anaesth Crit Care* 20(2):65–70, 2009.
88. Lonnqvist PA, MacKenzie J, Soni AK, et al: Paravertebral blockade. Failure rate and complications. *Anaesthesia* 50(9):813–815, 1995.
89. Dravid RM, Paul RE: Interpleural block—part 2. *Anaesthesia* 62(11):1143–1153, 2007.
90. Dravid RM, Paul RE: Interpleural block—part 1. *Anaesthesia* 62(10):1039–1049, 2007.
91. Belavy D, Cowlishaw PJ, Howes M, et al: Ultrasound-guided transversus abdominis plane block for analgesia after Caesarean delivery. *Br J Anaesth* 103(5):726–730, 2009.
92. Hebbard P: Subcostal transversus abdominis plane block under ultrasound guidance. *Anesth Analg* 106(2):674–675, 2008; author reply 675.
93. Schulz-Stübner S, Boezaart A, Hata JS: Regional analgesia in the critically ill. *Crit Care Med* 33(6):1400–1407, 2005.
94. Capdevila X, Ponrouch M, Choquet O: Continuous peripheral nerve blocks in clinical practice. *Curr Opin Anaesthesiol* 21(5):619–623, 2008.
95. Auroy Y, Benhamou D, Bargues L, et al: Major complications of regional anesthesia in France: The SOS Regional Anesthesia Hotline Service. *Anesthesiology* 97(5):1274–1280, 2002.
96. Sorenson EJ: Neurological injuries associated with regional anesthesia. *Reg Anesth Pain Med* 33(5):442–448, 2008.
97. Neal JM, Bernards CM, Hadzic A, et al: ASRA practice advisory on neurologic complications in regional anesthesia and pain medicine. *Reg Anesth Pain Med* 33(5):404–415, 2008.
98. Reid N, Stella J, Ryan M, et al: Use of ultrasound to facilitate accurate femoral nerve block in the emergency department. *Emerg Med Australas* 21(2):124–130, 2009.
99. Marhofer P, Schrogendorfer K, Koinig H, et al: Ultrasonographic guidance improves sensory block and onset time in three-in-one blocks. *Anesth Analg* 85(4):854–857; 1997.
100. Davies AF, Segar EP, Murdoch J, et al: Epidural infusion or combined femoral and sciatic nerve blocks as perioperative analgesia for knee arthroplasty. *Br J Anaesth* 93(3):368–374, 2004.
101. Chalmouki G, Lekka N, Lappas T, et al: Perioperative pain management in femoral shaft fractures. Continuous femoral nerve block vs systemic pain therapy. *Reg Anesth Pain Med* 33(5):e77, 2008.
102. Gray AT, Huczko EL, Schafhalter-Zoppoth I: Lateral popliteal nerve block with ultrasound guidance. *Reg Anesth Pain Med* 29(5):507–509, 2004.
103. Schulz-Stübner S: The critically ill patient and regional anesthesia. *Curr Opin Anaesthesiol* 19(5):538–544, 2006.
104. Werawatganon T, Charuluxanun S: Patient controlled intravenous opioid analgesia versus continuous epidural analgesia for pain after intra-abdominal surgery. *Cochrane Database Syst Rev* (1):CD004088, 2005.
105. Wu CL, Hurley RW, Anderson GF, et al: Effect of postoperative epidural analgesia on morbidity and mortality following surgery in medicare patients. *Reg Anesth Pain Med* 29(6):525–533, 2004; discussion 15–19.
106. Liu SS, Wu CL: Effect of postoperative analgesia on major postoperative complications: a systematic update of the evidence. *Anesth Analg* 104(3):689–702, 2007.
107. Guay J: The benefits of adding epidural analgesia to general anesthesia: a metaanalysis. *J Anesth* 20(4):335–340, 2006.
108. Liu SS, Block BM, Wu CL: Effects of perioperative central neuraxial analgesia on outcome after coronary artery bypass surgery: a meta-analysis. *Anesthesiology* 101(1):153–161, 2004.
109. Bulger EM, Edwards T, Klotz P, et al: Epidural analgesia improves outcome after multiple rib fractures. *Surgery* 136(2):426–430, 2004.
110. Bernhardt A, Kortgen A, Niesel H, et al: Using epidural anesthesia in patients with acute pancreatitis—prospective study of 121 patients. *Anaesthesiol Reanim* 27(1):16–22, 2002.
111. Low JH: Survey of epidural analgesia management in general intensive care units in England. *Acta Anaesthesiol Scand* 46(7):799–805, 2002.
112. Jakobsen CJ, Nygaard E, Norrild K, et al: High thoracic epidural analgesia improves left ventricular function in patients with ischemic heart. *Acta Anaesthesiol Scand* 53(5):559–564, 2009.
113. Ferguson SE, Malhotra T, Seshan VE, et al: A prospective randomized trial comparing patient-controlled epidural analgesia to patient-controlled intravenous analgesia on postoperative pain control and recovery after major open gynecologic cancer surgery. *Gynecol Oncol* 114(1):111–116, 2009.
114. Clemente A, Carli F: The physiological effects of thoracic epidural anesthesia and analgesia on the cardiovascular, respiratory and gastrointestinal systems. *Minerva Anestesiol* 74(10):549–563, 2008.
115. Moen V, Dahlgren N, Irestedt L: Severe neurological complications after central neuraxial blockades in Sweden 1990–1999. *Anesthesiology* 101(4):950–959, 2004.
116. Horlocker TT, Wedel DJ, Rowlingson JC, et al: Regional anesthesia in the patient receiving antithrombotic or thrombolytic therapy: American Society of Regional Anesthesia and Pain Medicine Evidence-Based Guidelines (Third Edition). *Reg Anesth Pain Med* 35(1):64–101, 2010.
117. Luzzani A, Polati E, Dorizzi R, et al: Comparison of procalcitonin and C-reactive protein as markers of sepsis. *Crit Care Med* 31(6):1737–1741, 2003.
118. Ballantyne JC, Carr DB, deFerranti S, et al: The comparative effects of postoperative analgesic therapies on pulmonary outcome: cumulative meta-analyses of randomized, controlled trials. *Anesth Analg* 86(3):598–612, 1998.
119. Beattie WS, Badner NH, Choi P: Epidural analgesia reduces postoperative myocardial infarction: a meta-analysis. *Anesth Analg* 93(4):853–858, 2001.
120. Meissner A, Rolf N, Van Aken H: Thoracic epidural anesthesia and the patient with heart disease: benefits, risks, and controversies. *Anesth Analg* 85(3):517–528, 1997.
121. Carli F, Mayo N, Klubien K, et al: Epidural analgesia enhances functional exercise capacity and health-related quality of life after colonic surgery: results of a randomized trial. *Anesthesiology* 97(3):540–549, 2002.
122. Hebl JR, Dilger JA, Byer DE, et al: A pre-emptive multimodal pathway featuring peripheral nerve block improves perioperative outcomes after major orthopedic surgery. *Reg Anesth Pain Med* 33(6):510–517, 2008.
123. Perttunen K, Tasmuth T, Kalso E: Chronic pain after thoracic surgery: a follow-up study. *Acta Anaesthesiol Scand* 43(5):563–567, 1999.

Chapter 4 ■ Therapeutic Paralysis

KHALDOUN FARIS

The most common indications for the use of neuromuscular blocking agents (NMBAs) in the intensive care unit (ICU) include emergency or elective intubations, optimization of patient–ventilator synchrony, management of increased intracranial pressure, reduction in oxygen consumption, and treatment of muscle spasms associated with tetanus. According to the American College of Critical Care Medicine and the Society of Critical Care Medicine clinical practice guidelines for sustained neuromuscular blockade in the adult critically ill patient, these medications should be used only when all other means of optimizing a patient's condition have been used. This recommendation is based on the concern that the administration of NMBAs may worsen patient outcome when administered during a course of critical illness, particularly if the patient is receiving systemic steroids at the same time [1]. However, this recommendation has recently been challenged. A prospective, multicenter, randomized study of 340 patients in the early stage of the acute respiratory distress syndrome (ARDS) demonstrated that use of cisatracurium for 48 hours was associated with improved survival without an increase in intensive care unit–acquired weakness (ICUAW) [2]. A retrospective cohort study examining several thousand mechanically ventilated patients with severe sepsis found that an early utilization of neuromuscular blockade was associated with lower mortality [3].

PHARMACOLOGY OF NMBAS

The neuromuscular junction (NMJ) consists of the motor nerve terminus, acetylcholine (ACh), and muscle end plate. In response to neuronal action potentials, ACh is released from presynaptic axonal storage vesicles into the synapse of the NMJ. Both the presynaptic membrane and the postsynaptic end plate contain specialized nicotinic ACh receptors (nAChRs). The chemical signal is converted into an electric signal by binding of two ACh molecules to the receptor ($\alpha\delta$- and $\alpha\varepsilon$-subunits), causing a transient influx of sodium and calcium, and efflux of potassium from muscle cells. This depolarization propagates an action potential that results in a muscle contraction. Unbound ACh is quickly hydrolyzed in the synapse by the enzyme acetylcholinesterase to acetic acid and choline, thus effectively controlling the duration of receptor activation. A repolarization of the motor end plate and muscle fiber then occurs.

THE NICOTINIC ACETYLCHOLINE RECEPTOR

The nAChR is built of five subunit proteins, forming an ion channel. This ionic channel mediates neurotransmission at the NMJ, autonomic ganglia, spinal cord, and brain. During early development, differentiation and maturation of the NMJ and transformation of the nAChR take place: fetal nAChRs gradually disappear with the rise of new, functionally distinct, mature nAChRs.

These mature nAChRs (also termed *adult*, *innervated*, *ε-containing*) have a subunit composition of two α, β, ε, *and* δ in the synaptic muscle membrane. The only structural difference from the fetal nAChR is in substitution of the γ for the ε-subunit, although functional, pharmacologic, and metabolic characteristics are quite distinct. Mature nAChRs have a shorter burst duration and a higher conductance to Na^+, K^+, and Ca^{2+}, and are metabolically stable with a half-life averaging about 2 weeks. The two α-, β-, δ-, and ε/γ-subunits interact to form a channel and an extracellular binding site for ACh and other mediators as well. As mentioned previously, simultaneous binding of two ACh molecules to $\alpha\delta$- and $\alpha\varepsilon$-subunits of an nAChR initiates opening of the channel and a flow of cations down their electrochemical gradient. In the absence of ACh or other mediators, the stable closed state (a major function of ε/γ-subunits) normally precludes channel opening [4].

Adult skeletal muscle retains the ability to synthesize not only adult, but also fetal (often called *immature* or *extrajunctional*)-type nAChRs. The synthesis of fetal nAChRs may be triggered in response to altered neuronal input, such as loss of nerve function or prolonged immobility, or in the presence of certain disease states. The major difference between fetal- and adult-type nAChRs is that fetal receptors migrate across the entire membrane surface and adult ones are mostly confined to the muscle end plate. In addition, these fetal nAChRs have a much shorter half-life, are more ionically active with prolonged open channel time that exaggerates the K^+ efflux, and are much more sensitive to depolarizing agents such as succinylcholine and resistant to nondepolarizing neuromuscular blockers.

The functional difference between depolarizing and nondepolarizing neuromuscular blockers lies in their interaction with AChRs. Depolarizing neuromuscular blockers are structurally similar to ACh and bind to and activate AChRs. Nondepolarizing neuromuscular blockers are competitive antagonists.

DEPOLARIZING NEUROMUSCULAR BLOCKERS

Succinylcholine is the only depolarizing neuromuscular blocker in clinical use. Its use is limited to facilitating rapid-sequence intubation in the emergency setting. Succinylcholine mimics the effects of ACh by binding to the ACh receptor and inducing a persistent depolarization of the muscle fiber. Muscle contraction remains inhibited until succinylcholine diffuses away from the motor end plate and is metabolized by serum (pseudo-) cholinesterase. The clinical effect of succinylcholine is a brief excitatory period, with muscular fasciculations followed by neuromuscular blockade and flaccid paralysis. The intravenous dose of succinylcholine is 1 to 1.5 mg per kg and offers the most rapid onset of action (60 to 90 seconds) of the NMBAs. Recovery to 90% muscle strength after an intravenous dose of 1 mg per kg takes from 9 to 13 minutes.

Potential adverse drug events associated with succinylcholine include hypertension, arrhythmias, increased intracranial and intraocular pressure, hyperkalemia, malignant hyperthermia, myalgias, and prolonged paralysis. Neuromuscular blockade can persist for hours in patients with genetic variants of pseudocholinesterase isoenzymes. Contraindications to succinylcholine use include major thermal burns, significant crush injuries, spinal cord transection, malignant hyperthermia, and upper or lower motor neuron lesions. Caution is also advised in patients with open-globe injuries, renal failure, serious infections, near-drowning victims, and immobilization beyond 2 weeks.

NONDEPOLARIZING NMBAS

Nondepolarizing NMBAs function as competitive antagonists and inhibit ACh binding to postsynaptic nAChRs on the motor end plate. They are categorized into two classes on the basis of chemical structure: benzylisoquinoliniums and aminosteroids. Within each of these classes, the therapeutic agents may further be categorized as short-acting, intermediate-acting, or long-acting agents. The benzylisoquinolinium agents commonly used in the critical care setting include atracurium, cisatracurium, and doxacurium, whereas the aminosteroid agents include vecuronium, rocuronium, pancuronium, and pipecuronium.

The nondepolarizing NMBAs are administered by the intravenous route and have volumes of distribution (V_ds) ranging from 0.2 to 0.3 L per kg in adults.

A clinical relationship exists between the time to onset of paralysis and neuromuscular blocker dosing, drug distribution, and ACh receptor sensitivity. An important factor to consider is V_d, which may change as a result of disease processes. Cirrhotic liver disease and chronic renal failure often result in an increased V_d and decreased plasma concentration for a given dose of water-soluble drugs. However, drugs dependent on renal or hepatic excretion may have a prolonged clinical effect. Therefore, a larger initial dose but smaller maintenance dose may be appropriate.

Alterations in V_d affect both peak neuromuscular blocker serum concentrations and time to paralysis. The pharmacokinetic and pharmacodynamic principles of commonly used NMBAs are summarized in Table 4.1.

Atracurium

Atracurium is an intermediate-acting nondepolarizing agent. Neuromuscular paralysis typically occurs between 3 and 5 minutes and lasts 25 to 35 minutes after an initial bolus dose. Atracurium undergoes ester hydrolysis as well as Hofmann degradation, a nonenzymatic breakdown process that occurs at physiologic pH and body temperature, independent of renal or hepatic function. Renal and hepatic dysfunction should not affect the duration of neuromuscular paralysis. The neuroexcitatory metabolite laudanosine is renally excreted. Laudanosine is epileptogenic in animals and may induce central nervous system excitation in patients with renal failure who are receiving prolonged atracurium infusions. Atracurium may induce histamine release after rapid administration.

TABLE 4.1

Pharmacokinetic and Pharmacodynamic Principles of Nondepolarizing Neuromuscular Blockers

	Benzylisoquinolinium Agents		
	Cisatracurium (Nimbex)	**Atracurium (Tracrium)**	**Doxacurium (Nuromax)**
Introduced	1996	1983	1991
95% Effective dose (mg/kg)	0.05	0.25	0.025–0.030
Initial dose (mg/kg)	0.1–0.2	0.4–0.5	Up to 0.1
Onset (min)	2–3	3–5	5–10
Duration (min)	45–60	25–35	120–150
Half-life (min)	22–31	20	70–100
Infusion dose (μg/kg/min)	2.5–3.0	4–12	0.3–0.5
Recovery (min)	90	40–60	120–180
% Renal excretion	Hofmann elimination	5–10 (Hofmann elimination)	70
Renal failure	No change	No change	↑o chan
% Biliary excretion	Hofmann elimination	Minimal	Unclear
Hepatic failure	Minimal to no change	Minimal to no change	?
Active metabolites	None, but laudanosine	None, but laudanosine	?
Histamine hypotension	No	Dose-dependent	No
Vagal block tachycardia	No	No	No
Ganglionic block hypotension	No	Minimal to none	No
Prolonged block reported	Rare	Rare	Yes

	Aminosteroidal Agents			
	Pancuronium (Pavulon)	**Vecuronium (Norcuron)**	**Pipecuronium (Arduan)**	**Rocuronium (Zemuron)**
Introduced	1972	1984	1991	1994
95% Effective dose (mg/kg)	0.07	0.05	0.05	0.30
Initial dose (mg/kg)	0.1	0.1	0.085–0.100	0.6–1.0
Onset (min)	2–3	3–4	5	1–2
Duration (min)	90–100	35–45	90–100	30
Half-life (min)	120	30–80	100	—
Infusion dose (μg/kg/min)	1–2	1–2	0.5–2.0	10–12
Recovery (min)	120–180	45–60	55–160	20–30
% Renal excretion	45–70	50	50+	33
Renal failure	↑Effect	↑Effect	↑Duration	Minimal
% Biliary excretion	10–15	35–50	Minimal	<75
Hepatic failure	Mild ↑ effect	Mild ↑ effect	Minimal	Moderate
Active metabolites	3-OH and 17-OH pancuronium	3-desacetyl vecuronium	None	None
Histamine hypotension	No	No	No	No
Vagal block tachycardia	Modest to marked	No	No	At high doses
Ganglionic block hypotension	No	No	No	No
Prolonged ICU block	Yes	Yes	No	No [-3pt]

↑, increased; ICU, intensive care unit.

Modified from Grenvik A, Ayres SM, Holbrook PR, et al: *Textbook of Critical Care*. 4th ed. Philadelphia, WB Saunders, 2000; Watling SM, Dasta JF: Prolonged paralysis in intensive care unit patients after the use of neuromuscular blocking agents: a review of the literature. *Crit Care Med* 22(5):884, 1994.

Cisatracurium

Cisatracurium and atracurium are similar intermediate-acting nondepolarizing agents. A bolus dose of 0.2 mg per kg of cisatracurium usually results in neuromuscular paralysis within 1.5 to 2.5 minutes and lasts 45 to 60 minutes. When compared with atracurium, cisatracurium is three times as potent and has a more desirable adverse drug event profile, including lack of histamine release, minimal cardiovascular effects, and less interaction with autonomic ganglia. It also undergoes ester hydrolysis as well as Hofmann degradation. However, plasma laudanosine concentrations after cisatracurium administration are 5 to 10 times lower than those detected after atracurium administration.

Rocuronium

Rocuronium is the fastest onset, shortest acting aminosteroidal NMBA. A bolus dose of 0.6 mg per kg usually results in neuromuscular paralysis within 60 to 90 seconds. It may be considered an alternative to succinylcholine for rapid-sequence intubation at a higher dose (1.2 mg per kg). Rocuronium is primarily eliminated in the liver and bile. Hepatic or renal dysfunction may reduce drug clearance and prolong recovery time.

Vecuronium

An initial intravenous bolus dose of 0.1 mg per kg of vecuronium typically results in neuromuscular paralysis within 3 to 4 minutes and lasts 35 to 45 minutes. Vecuronium lacks vagolytic effects, such as tachycardia and hypertension, and produces negligible histamine release. Hepatic metabolism produces three active metabolites, the most significant being 3-desacetyl vecuronium, with 50% to 70% activity of the parent drug. Both vecuronium and its active metabolites are renally excreted. There is potential for prolonged neuromuscular paralysis in patients with renal dysfunction receiving vecuronium by continuous infusion.

Pancuronium

Pancuronium is a long-acting nondepolarizing agent that is structurally similar to vecuronium. Unique features of pancuronium are its vagolytic and sympathomimetic activities and potential to induce tachycardia, hypertension, and increased cardiac output. Pancuronium is primarily excreted unchanged (60% to 70%) in the urine and bile, whereas the remaining 30% to 40% is hydroxylated by the liver to 3-hydroxy pancuronium. It has 50% activity of the parent drug and is renally eliminated. Renal dysfunction may result in the accumulation of pancuronium and its metabolites.

Doxacurium

Doxacurium is the most potent nondepolarizing agent available, but it has the slowest onset (as long as 10 minutes). It is practically devoid of histaminergic, vagolytic, or sympathomimetic effects. Doxacurium undergoes minimal hepatic metabolism, and excretion occurs unchanged in both the urine and the bile, with significantly prolonged effects seen in patients with renal dysfunction and, to a lesser extent, hepatic disease.

Pipecuronium

Pipecuronium is structurally related to pancuronium and its duration of action is 90 to 100 minutes, making it the longest acting NMBA. It is metabolized to 3-desacetyl pipecuronium by the liver, and both the parent compound and the metabolite are renally excreted. When compared with pancuronium, pipecuronium has a longer duration of action, less histamine release, and minimal cardiovascular effects.

REVERSAL AGENTS

The clinical effects of nondepolarizing neuromuscular blockers can be reversed by acetylcholinesterase inhibitors (anticholinesterases). These agents increase the synaptic concentration of ACh by preventing its synaptic degradation and allow it to competitively displace nondepolarizing NMBAs from postsynaptic nAChRs on the motor end plate. Because anticholinesterase drugs (e.g., neostigmine, edrophonium, and pyridostigmine) also inhibit acetylcholinesterase at muscarinic receptor sites, they are used in combination with the antimuscarinic agents (e.g., atropine or glycopyrrolate) to minimize adverse muscarinic effects (e.g., bradycardia, excessive secretions, and bronchospasm) while maximizing nicotinic effects. Typical combinations include neostigmine and glycopyrrolate (slower acting agents) and edrophonium and atropine (faster acting agents). The depth of neuromuscular blockade determines how rapidly neuromuscular activity returns [5].

Sugammadex is a new and novel agent (modified γ-cyclodextrin) that reverses rocuronium and other aminosteroid NMBAs by selectively binding and encapsulating the NMBA [6]. One of the advantages of sugammadex is the rapid reversal of the profound neuromuscular block, induced by the high dose of rocuronium needed for the rapid-sequence induction [7,8]—an effect that is equivalent to, if not better than, the spontaneous recovery from succinylcholine. Hence, rocuronium/sugammadex may prove to be an effective and safer alternative to succinylcholine in cases of the difficult airway and contraindications to the use of succinylcholine. Sugammadex is also useful as a reversal agent whenever the blockade is profound and there is an advantage for a timely reversal [8]. Sugammadex has been approved for use in Europe since 2008, but not in the United States. The initial nonapproval of the Food and Drug Administration (FDA) was based on concerns related to hypersensitivity and allergic reactions. However, a *Cochrane* systemic review concluded that sugammadex was not only effective but also equally safe when compared with placebo and neostigmine [9]. Sugammadex was finally approved for use in the United States in 2015. In addition to anaphylaxis, the FDA cautioned, in its approval statement, about marked bradycardia and cardiac arrest, observed within minutes of the administration of sugammadex.

DRUG INTERACTIONS

A substantial number of medications commonly used in clinical practice have the potential for interaction with NMBAs. These interactions typically influence the degree and duration of clinical effects through either potentiation of or resistance to neuromuscular blockade. The most clinically relevant drug interactions with NMBA are discussed here and summarized in Table 4.2.

Aminoglycosides and other antibiotics (e.g., tetracyclines, clindamycin, and vancomycin) have the ability to potentiate neuromuscular blockade and prolong the action of nondepolarizing agents through mechanisms including the inhibition of presynaptic ACh release, reduction in postsynaptic receptor sensitivity to ACh, blockade of cholinergic receptors, and impairment of ion channels. Penicillin and cephalosporin antibiotics do not interact with NMBAs and thus do not influence the degree of neuromuscular blockade.

Local, inhalational, and intravenous anesthetic and sedative agents may potentiate neuromuscular blockade. Local anesthetics reduce ACh release and decrease muscle contractions through direct membrane effects, whereas inhalational anesthetics desensitize the postsynaptic membrane and also depress muscle contractility.

Cardiovascular drugs such as furosemide, procainamide, quinidine, β-blockers, and calcium channel blockers have the ability to potentiate neuromuscular blocking effects. The role of the calcium ion in the release of ACh from vesicles into the synapse has been well established, although the exact interaction between calcium channel blockers and NMBAs remains to be determined. Verapamil, a calcium channel blocker, has local analgesic effects and direct skeletal muscle effects, but its significance in drug interaction with NMBAs remains to be defined.

TABLE 4.2

Drug Interactions with Neuromuscular Blocking Agents

Therapeutic Agent	Potential Interaction
Antibiotics	
Aminoglycosides	Potentiate blockade; decreased acetylcholine release
Tetracyclines	Potentiate blockade
Clindamycin and lincomycin	Potentiate blockade
Vancomycin	Potentiate blockade
Sedative/anesthetics	Potentiate blockade
Cardiovascular agents	
Furosemide	Low doses: potentiate blockade; high doses: antagonize blockade
β-Blockers	Potentiate blockade
Procainamide	Potentiate blockade
Quinidine	Potentiate blockade
Calcium channel blockers	Potentiate blockade
Methylxanthines	Antagonize blockade
Antiepileptic drugs	Acute: potentiate blockade; chronic: resistance to blockade
Phenytoin	
Carbamazepine	Resistance to blockade
Ranitidine	Antagonize blockade
Lithium	Potentiate blockade
Immunosuppressive agents	
Azathioprine	Mild antagonism; phosphodiesterase inhibition
Cyclosporin	Potentiate blockade
Corticosteroids	Potentiate steroid myopathy
Local anesthetics	Potentiate blockade

Adapted from Buck ML, Reed MD: Use of nondepolarizing neuromuscular blocking agents in mechanically ventilated patients. *Clin Pharm* 10(1):32, 1991.

Chronic antiepileptic therapy, specifically phenytoin and carbamazepine, can increase the resistance to neuromuscular blocking effects, whereas the acute administration of phenytoin potentiates neuromuscular blockade. Chronic phenytoin therapy appears to induce an upregulation of ACh receptors, resulting in decreased postsynaptic sensitivity. Carbamazepine has been shown to induce resistance and shorten recovery times in combination with both pancuronium and vecuronium, possibly resulting from competition at the NMJ.

MONITORING OF NMBAS

Current guidelines recommend the routine monitoring of depth of neuromuscular blockade in critically ill patients [1]. It is important to remember that NMBAs have no analgesic and sedative effect. Careful clinical monitoring of the patient for signs consistent with inadequate sedation or analgesia—such as tachycardia, hypertension, salivation, and lacrimation—while receiving NMBAs is important. A recommendation to use monitors such as the Bispectral Index or the Patient State Index to ensure adequate depth of sedation while receiving NMBAs seems plausible; however, more studies are needed to determine whether these monitors are reliable and cost-effective in the critical care setting and whether they contribute to improved outcomes [10–12]. The modality of choice to monitor the depth of nondepolarizing neuromuscular blockade at present is train-of-four (TOF) monitoring. To determine the depth of blockade, four supramaximal stimuli are applied to a peripheral nerve (ideally, the ulnar nerve to assess an evoked response of the adductor pollicis muscle) every 0.5 seconds (2 Hz). Each stimulus in the train causes the muscle to contract, and "fade" in the response provides the basis for evaluation. To obtain the TOF ratio, the amplitude of the fourth response is divided by the amplitude of the first response. Before administration of a nondepolarizing muscle relaxant, all four responses are ideally the same: the TOF ratio is 1:1. During a partial nondepolarizing block, the ratio decreases (fades) and is inversely proportional to the degree of blockade [13].

Three prospective clinical trials have examined the question whether the routine use of TOF monitoring in the ICU will increase the cost-effectiveness and decrease the incidence of prolonged neuromuscular weakness. TOF monitoring for vecuronium appears to improve the outcome and decrease the cost of therapy. However, these outcomes could not be demonstrated for the benzylisoquinolinium agents, atracurium, and cisatracurium [14–16].

ADVERSE EFFECTS OF DEPOLARIZING AND NONDEPOLARIZING NMBAS IN CRITICALLY ILL PATIENTS

Significant progress has been made in the recent past in our understanding of the changes in regulation and distribution of ACh receptors during a course of critical illness. The majority of patients hospitalized in an ICU will undergo postsynaptic upregulation of nAChRs due to immobility, upper and/or lower motor neuron lesions, and/or pharmacologic denervation (such as NMBAs and aminoglycoside antibiotics). As outlined previously, immature receptors are not confined to the NMJ proper, but can be found over the entire surface of skeletal muscle (Fig. 4.1). This will lead to increased sensitivity to depolarizing NMBAs and decreased sensitivity to nondepolarizing NMBAs. Furthermore, these changes in receptor distribution and physiology put the patient at a heightened risk of succinylcholine-induced hyperkalemia. This is based on the fact that immature (fetal) nAChRs are low conductance channels with prolonged opening times and significantly higher potassium efflux into the systemic circulation as compared to mature (adult) nAChRs. Furthermore, succinylcholine is metabolized more slowly as compared to ACh, thus prolonging the "open" state of the immature receptors. Although upregulation of receptors during periods of immobilization has been described as early as 6 to 12 hours into the disease process, clinical studies suggest that succinylcholine-induced hyperkalemia is unlikely to occur within 14 days of immobility [17]. In contrast, a reduction in the number of postsynaptic nAChRs will result in resistance to depolarizing and increased sensitivity to nondepolarizing NMBAs. For conditions associated with the potential for ACh receptor upregulation, see Table 4.3.

INTENSIVE CARE UNIT–ACQUIRED WEAKNESS

ICUAW is a term used to describe all weaknesses developed in critically ill patients after the onset of illness and in the absence of any identifiable causes. ICUAW is further classified into three entities: critical illness polyneuropathy (CIP), critical illness myopathy (CIM), and critical illness neuromyopathy [18,19] (see Chapter 154). These conditions occur in up to 50% to 70%

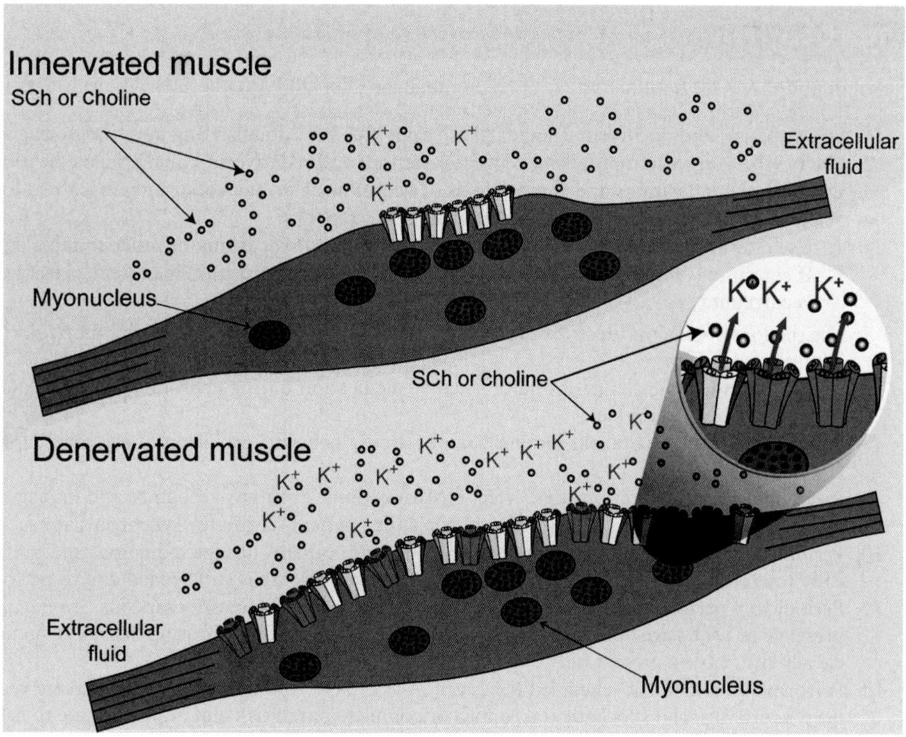

FIGURE 4.1 Schematic of the succinylcholine (SCh)-induced potassium release in an innervated (*top*) and denervated (*bottom*) muscle. In the innervated muscle, the systemically administered SCh reaches all of the muscle membrane, but depolarizes only the junctional ($\alpha1, \beta1, \delta, \varepsilon$) receptors because acetylcholine receptors (AChRs) are located only in this area. With denervation, the muscle (nuclei) expresses not only extrajunctional ($\alpha1, \beta1, \delta, \gamma$) AChRs, but also $\alpha7$AChRs throughout the muscle membrane. Systemic succinylcholine, in contrast to acetylcholine released locally, can depolarize all of the upregulated AChRs, leading to massive efflux of intracellular potassium into the circulation, resulting in hyperkalemia. The metabolite of SCh, choline, and possibly succinylmonocholine can maintain this depolarization via $\alpha7$AChRs, enhancing the potassium release and maintaining the hyperkalemia. (From Martyn JA, Richtsfeld M: Succinylcholine-induced hyperkalemia in acquired pathologic states: etiologic factors and molecular mechanisms. *Anesthesiology* 104:158, 2006, with permission.)

TABLE 4.3

Conditions Associated with the Potential for Nicotinic Acetylcholine Receptor Upregulation

Severe infection/SIRS
Muscle atrophy associated with prolonged immobility
Thermal injury
Upper and/or lower motor neuron defect
Prolonged pharmacologic or chemical denervation (e.g., NMBAs, magnesium, aminoglycoside antibiotics, and clostridial toxins)

NMBAs, neuromuscular blocking agents; SIRS, systemic inflammatory response syndrome.

of patients meeting diagnostic criteria for the systemic inflammatory response syndrome as well as in patients immobilized and on mechanical ventilation for more than a week [20]. They manifest as limb weakness and difficulty in weaning from the mechanical ventilator. Nondepolarizing muscle relaxants of both classes, aminosteroids and benzylisoquinoliniums, have been associated with the development of these neuromuscular disorders [21]; however, the etiology appears to be multifactorial and includes alterations in microvascular blood flow in conditions of sepsis/systemic inflammatory response syndrome and the concomitant administration of corticosteroids [20]. There is evidence suggesting that high-dose corticosteroids have direct physiologic effects on muscle fibers, resulting in a typical myopathy with loss of thick-filament proteins. Atrophy and weakness are observed primarily in muscles of trunk and extremities, and functional denervation of muscle with NMBAs in conjunction with corticosteroid therapy seems to heighten the risk of myopathy [21]. Furthermore, both methylprednisolone and hydrocortisone antagonize nAChRs, possibly potentiating the effects of NMBAs [22]. A differential diagnosis of weakness in ICU patients is presented in Table 4.4.

Critical Illness Polyneuropathy

Electrophysiologic findings of CIP are consistent with a primary, axonal degeneration, resulting in reduction in amplitudes of the compound muscle action potential and sensory nerve action potential. Although several case reports have suggested that NMBAs are causative agents in the etiology of this disorder, prospective studies of CIP have not confirmed a correlation between the use of NMBAs, steroids, and CIP [23] (see Chapter 180).

TABLE 4.4

Weakness in Intensive Care Unit Patients: Etiologies and Syndromes

Prolonged recovery from neuromuscular blocking agents (secondary to parent drug, drug metabolite, or drug–drug interaction)
Myasthenia gravis
Eaton–Lambert syndrome
Muscular dystrophy
Guillain–Barré syndrome
Central nervous system injury or lesion
Spinal cord injury
Steroid myopathy
Mitochondrial myopathy
Human immunodeficiency virus–related myopathy
Critical illness myopathy
Disuse atrophy
Critical illness polyneuropathy
Severe electrolyte toxicity (e.g., hypermagnesemia)
Severe electrolyte deficiency (e.g., hypophosphatemia)

Adapted from Murray MJ, Cowen J, DeBlock H, et al: Clinical practice guidelines for sustained neuromuscular blockade in the adult critically ill patient. *Crit Care Med* 30(1):142, 2002, with permission.

TABLE 4.5

Recommendations for Administration of Neuromuscular Blocking Agents (NMBAs) to ICU Patients

1. Develop, use, and document a standardized approach for administering and monitoring NMBA
2. Use NMBA only after optimizing ventilator settings and sedative and analgesic medication administration
3. Establish the indications and clinical goals of neuromuscular blockade, and evaluate at least daily
4. Select the best NMBA on the basis of patient characteristics:
   A. Use intermittent NMBA therapy with pancuronium, doxacurium, or other suitable agent if clinical goals can be met
   B. If continuous infusion is required and renal or hepatic dysfunction is present, select atracurium or cisatracurium, and avoid vecuronium
5. Use the lowest effective dose for the shortest possible time (<48 h if possible), particularly if corticosteroids are concomitantly administered
6. Administer adequate analgesic and/or sedative medication during neuromuscular blockade, and monitor clinically and by bispectral array EEG if available
7. Systematically anticipate and prevent complications, including provision of eye care, careful positioning, physical therapy, and DVT prophylaxis
8. Avoid the use of medications that affect NMBA actions. Promptly recognize and manage conditions that affect NMBA actions
9. Adjust NMBA dosage to achieve clinical goals (i.e., patient–ventilator synchrony, apnea, or complete paralysis)
10. Periodically (i.e., at least once or twice daily) perform NMBA dosage reduction, and preferably cessation (drug holiday) if clinically tolerated, to determine whether neuromuscular blockade is still needed and to perform physical and neurologic examination
11. Periodically perform and document a clinical assessment in which spontaneous respiration, as well as limb movement, and/or the presence of DTRs are observed during steady-state infusion and/or during dosage reduction/cessation. With deep blockade, muscle activity may be present only during dosage reduction/cessation
12. Perform and document scheduled (i.e., every 4–8 h) TOF testing for patients receiving vecuronium NMBA and/or undergoing deep neuromuscular blockade (i.e., apnea or complete paralysis), and adjust dosage to achieve one-fourth or more twitches. If clinical goals cannot be met when one-fourth or more twitches are present during steady-state infusion, demonstrate one-fourth or more twitches during dosage reduction/cessation. Consider TOF testing in all patients

DTR, deep tendon reflexes; DVT, deep venous thrombosis; EEG, electroencephalogram; TOF, train of four.
Modified from Gehr LC, Sessler CN: Neuromuscular blockade in the intensive care unit. *Semin Respir Crit Care Med* 22:175, 2001, with permission.

Critical Illness Myopathy

CIM can occur in association with, or independently of, CIP. A group of several myopathies of critical illness is now thought to be part of the same syndrome; these include acute quadriplegic myopathy, critical care myopathy, acute corticosteroid myopathy, acute hydrocortisone myopathy, acute myopathy in severe asthma, and acute corticosteroid and pancuronium-associated myopathy [24]. The major feature of this syndrome is flaccid, diffuse weakness, involving all limb muscles and neck flexors, and often the facial muscles and diaphragm. As with CIP, this can result in difficulty to wean from the mechanical ventilator. The syndrome is more difficult to diagnose than CIP, and diagnostic evaluations include electrophysiologic studies, muscle biopsy, and laboratory evaluations (plasma creatine kinase levels). Again, there is no definitive evidence suggesting that NMBAs are causative agents for this syndrome, but rather a component in a multifactorial etiology. However, the incidence of CIP and CIM appears to be higher in ICUs where these agents are more frequently used [25].

Although only limited data are available suggesting that CIP increases ICU and hospital mortality in critically ill patients, CIP and CIM appear to be important causes of increased morbidity during and after acute care hospital stay [26] (see Chapter 180).

SUMMARY AND RECOMMENDATIONS

Although there is currently insufficient evidence to demonstrate an unequivocal link between the use of NMBAs and an increase in morbidity and mortality in critically ill patients, it seems prudent to perform a careful risk–benefit analysis prior to the administration of this class of drugs in the ICU setting. Recent evidence suggests that the early utilization of neuromuscular blockade in ARDS and severe sepsis may improve survival [2,3]. However, more prospective data are needed to identify proper indications, selection of agents, and doses in the ICU setting. Concomitant use of drugs predisposing patients for the development of ICUAW, like steroids and aminoglycoside antibiotics, should alert the clinician for the increased risk in this setting. Succinylcholine can subject patients who are immobilized with upper and lower motor neuron lesions or with burns to a markedly increased risk of succinylcholine-induced hyperkalemia, and should be avoided in the ICU whenever possible. For recommendations for the administration of NMBAs to ICU patients, please see Table 4.5.

References

1. Murray MJ, Cowen J, DeBlock H, et al: Clinical practice guidelines for sustained neuromuscular blockade in the adult critically ill patient. *Crit Care Med* 30(1):142–156, 2002.
2. Papazian L, Forel J-M, Gacouin A, et al: Neuromuscular blockers in early acute respiratory distress syndrome. *N Engl J Med* 363(12):1107–1116, 2010.
3. Steingrub JS, Lagu T, Rothberg MB, et al: Treatment with neuromuscular blocking agents and the risk of in-hospital mortality among mechanically ventilated patients with severe sepsis. *Crit Care Med* 42(1):90–96, 2014.
4. Naguib M, Flood P, McArdle JJ, et al: Advances in neurobiology of the neuromuscular junction: implications for the anesthesiologist. *Anesthesiology* 96:202, 2002.
5. McManus MC: Neuromuscular blockers in surgery and intensive care, part 2. *Am J Health Syst Pharm* 58(24):2381–2395, 2001.
6. Naguib M: Sugammadex: another milestone in clinical neuromuscular pharmacology. *Anesth Analg* 104(3):575–581, 2007.
7. Lee C, Jahr JS, Candiotti KA, et al: Reversal of profound neuromuscular block by sugammadex administered three minutes after rocuronium: a comparison with spontaneous recovery from succinylcholine. *Anesthesiology* 110(5):1020–1025, 2009.
8. Rex C, Wagner S, Spies C, et al: Reversal of neuromuscular blockade by sugammadex after continuous infusion of rocuronium in patients randomized to sevoflurane or propofol maintenance anesthesia. *Anesthesiology* 111(1):30–35, 2009.

9. Abrishami A, Ho J, Wong J, et al: Sugammadex, a selective reversal medication for preventing postoperative residual neuromuscular blockade. *Cochrane Database Syst Rev* (4):CD007362, 2009.
10. Nasraway SS Jr, Wu EC, Kelleher RM, et al: How reliable is the Bispectral Index in critically ill patients? A prospective, comparative, single-blinded observer study. *Crit Care Med* 30(7):1483–1487, 2002.
11. Schneider G, Heglmeier S, Schneider J, et al: Patient State Index (PSI) measures depth of sedation in intensive care patients. *Intensive Care Med* 30(2):213–216, 2004.
12. Vivien B, Di Maria S, Ouattara A, et al: Overestimation of Bispectral Index in sedated intensive care unit patients revealed by administration of muscle relaxant. *Anesthesiology* 99(1):9–17, 2003.
13. Naguib M, Lien CA: Pharmacology of muscle relaxants and their antagonists, in Miller RD (ed): *Miller's Anesthesia*. 6th ed. New York, Churchill Livingstone: 518–522, 2005.
14. Baumann MH, McAlpin BW, Brown K, et al: A prospective randomized comparison of train-of-four monitoring and clinical assessment during continuous ICU cisatracurium paralysis. *Chest* 126(4):1267–1273, 2004.
15. Rudis MI, Sikora CA, Angus E, et al: A prospective, randomized, controlled evaluation of peripheral nerve stimulation versus standard clinical dosing of neuromuscular blocking agents in critically ill patients. *Crit Care Med* 25(4):575–583, 1997.
16. Strange C, Vaughan L, Franklin C, et al: Comparison of train-of-four and best clinical assessment during continuous paralysis. *Am J Respir Crit Care Med* 156(5):1556–1561, 1997.
17. Blanie A, Ract C, Leblanc PE, et al: The limits of succinylcholine for critically ill patients. *Anesth Analg* 115(4):873–879, 2012.
18. Stevens RD, Marshall SA, Cornblath DR, et al: A framework for diagnosing and classifying intensive care unit–acquired weakness. *Crit Care Med* 37(10, Suppl):S299–S308, 2009.
19. Vincent JL, Norrenberg M: Intensive care unit–acquired weakness: framing the topic. *Crit Care Med* 37(10, Suppl):S296–S298, 2009.
20. Bolton CF: Neuromuscular manifestations of critical illness. *Muscle Nerve* 32(2):140–163, 2005.
21. Larsson L, Li X, Edstrom L, et al: Acute quadriplegia and loss of muscle myosin in patients treated with nondepolarizing neuromuscular blocking agents and corticosteroids: mechanisms at the cellular and molecular levels. *Crit Care Med* 28(1):34–45, 2000.
22. Kindler CH, Verotta D, Gray AT, et al: Additive inhibition of nicotinic acetylcholine receptors by corticosteroids and the neuromuscular blocking drug vecuronium. *Anesthesiology* 92(3):821–832, 2000.
23. Berek K, Margreiter J, Willeit J, et al: Polyneuropathies in critically ill patients: a prospective evaluation. *Intensive Care Med* 22(9):849–855, 1996.
24. Lacomis D, Zochodne DW, Bird SJ: Critical illness myopathy. *Muscle Nerve* 23(12):1785–1788, 2000.
25. Lacomis D, Petrella JT, Giuliani MJ: Causes of neuromuscular weakness in the intensive care unit: a study of ninety-two patients. *Muscle Nerve* 21(5):610–617, 1998.
26. Latronico N, Shehu I, Seghelini E: Neuromuscular sequelae of critical illness. *Curr Opin Crit Care* 11(4):381–390, 2005.

Chapter 5 ■ Cerebrospinal Fluid Aspiration

FIRAS KADDOUH • SUSANNE MUEHLSCHLEGEL • JOHN P. WEAVER

This chapter presents guidelines for safe cerebrospinal fluid (CSF) aspiration for the emergency department or the intensive care physician. It also provides a basic understanding of the indications, techniques, and potential complications of these procedures.

Health care providers routinely and safely perform CSF aspiration procedures using equipment and sterile supplies readily accessible in most patient care areas. Most of those procedures are performed at the bedside using local anesthesia alone. Because it could be a painful and anxiety-provoking procedure, sedation may be required especially for children [1,2]. Radiographic imaging (fluoroscopy or ultrasound) can be helpful to provide adequate guidance for safe needle placement, particularly in the setting of anatomic variations, trauma, operative scars, congenital defects, body habitus, or degenerative changes. Fluoroscopy and myelography may be used for complicated lumbar and C1–C2 puncture. Computed tomography (CT) may be used for stereotactic placement of ventricular catheters. Although lumbar pucture is performed by many health care providers, clinicians should recognize the need for specialized equipment and training in selected cases of CSF aspiration.

CEREBROSPINAL FLUID ACCESS

Diagnostic Objectives

CSF analysis continues to be an important diagnostic tool in many diseases. The most common indication for CSF sampling is the suspicion of a cerebral nervous system (CNS) infection. CSF is also analyzed for the diagnosis of subarachnoid hemorrhage (SAH), demyelinating diseases, leptomeningeal spread of neoplasms, and neurodegenerative conditions. CSF access is necessary for some neurodiagnostic procedures that require injection of contrast agents, such as myelography, cisternography, or ventriculoperitoneal shunt patency. CSF access for pressure recording and monitoring is also important for the diagnosis of normal-pressure hydrocephalus, idiopathic intracranial hypertension, and some acute intracranial insults.

CSF is an ultrafiltrate of plasma in which the brain and the spinal cord float. It is normally clear and colorless. Abnormalities of color and clarity can reflect the presence of cells, protein, hemosiderin, or bilirubin that indicates pathologic processes. The diagnostic tests performed on the aspirated sample of CSF depend on the patient's age, history, and differential diagnosis. A basic profile includes glucose and protein values, a blood cell count with differential, Gram stain, and aerobic and anaerobic cultures.

CSF glucose depends on blood glucose levels and is equivalent to approximately 1/2 to 2/3 of the serum glucose, and slightly higher in neonates. Glucose is transported into the CSF via carrier-facilitated diffusion, and changes in spinal fluid glucose concentration lag blood levels by about 2 hours. Increased CSF glucose is nonspecific and usually reflects hyperglycemia. Hypoglycorrhachia (abnormally low CSF glucose) can result from infections, inflammatory, or neoplastic meningeal disorders; it reflects increased glucose use by nervous tissue, pathogens, or leukocytes and inhibited transport mechanisms. Elevated lactate levels caused by anaerobic glycolysis in bacterial and fungal meningitis usually accompany hypoglycorrhachia.

CSF protein content is usually less than 0.5% of that in plasma with an intact blood–brain barrier. Albumin constitutes appromixately 75% of CSF protein, and immunoglobulin G (IgG) is the major component of the γ-globulin fraction. IgG freely traverses a damaged blood–brain barrier. Although often nonspecific, elevated CSF protein is an indicator of CNS pathology. There is a gradient of total protein content in the spinal CSF column, with the highest level normally found in the lumbar subarachnoid space at 20 to 50 mg per dL, followed by the cisterna magna at 15 to 25 mg per dL and the ventricles at 6 to 12 mg per dL. A value exceeding 500 mg per dL is compatible with an intraspinal tumor or spinal compression, causing a complete subarachnoid block, meningitis, or blood in the CSF [3]. Low protein levels are seen in healthy children younger than

2 years, pseudotumor cerebri, recent lumbar pucture, chronic CSF leak, acute water intoxication, and leukemia.

A normal CSF cell count includes no erythrocytes and a maximum of five leukocytes per milliliter. A greater number of leukocytes is normally found in children (up to 10 per mL, mostly lymphocytes). Pathologically, increased white blood cells are present in infection, inflammation, leukemia, and hemorrhage.

Hemorrhage

A *nontraumatic* SAH in an adult may result from a ruptured aneurysm. A paroxysmal severe headache described as "the worst-headache-of-my-life" or a "thunderclap headache" is the classic symptom of aneurysmal rupture, but atypical headaches reminiscent of migraine are not uncommon. In one systematic review [4], De Falco reported that sentinel headache occurred in 10% to 43% of SAH patients in the 2 weeks preceeding the hemorrhage and seems to be caused by a minor leak of an aneurysm. Lumbar puncture can be helpful with such presenting headache when the head CT is normal.

SAH can cause acute obstructive hydrocephalus by intraventricular extension or obstruction to CSF resorptive mechanisms at the arachnoid granulations. The head CT demonstrates ventriculomegaly, which is best treated by CSF access and diversion using an external ventricular catheter.

A traumatic lumbar puncture presents a diagnostic dilemma, especially in the context of diagnosing suspected SAH. Differentiating characteristics include a decreasing red blood cell count in tubes collected serially during the procedure, the presence of a fibrinous clot in the sample, and a typical ratio of about 1 leukocyte per 500 to 1,000 red blood cells. Xanthochromia is more indicative of SAH and is quickly evaluated by spinning a fresh CSF sample and comparing the color of the supernatant to that of water, ideally using a spectrophotometer which significantly increases the sensitivity for xanthochromia detection. Spinal fluid accelerates red blood cell hemolysis, and hemoglobin products are released within 2 hours of the initial hemorrhage, creating the xanthochromia. Associated findings, such as a slightly depressed glucose level, increased protein, and an elevated opening pressure, are further suggestive of SAH.

Infection

CSF evaluation is the single most important aspect of the laboratory diagnosis of meningitis and encephalitis. The analysis usually includes a blood cell count with differential; protein and glucose levels; and Gram stain and cultures with antibiotic sensitivities. When tuberculosis or fungal meningitis is suspected, the fluid is analyzed by acid-fast stain, India ink preparation, cryptococcal antigen, and culture in appropriate media. More extensive cultures are helpful for evaluation of the immunocompromised patient.

Immunoprecipitation tests to identify bacterial antigens for *Streptococcus pneumoniae*, group B streptococcus, *Haemophilus influenzae*, and *Neisseria meningitidis* (meningococcus) allow rapid diagnosis and early specific treatment. Polymerase chain reaction (PCR) testing can be performed on CSF for rapid identification of several viruses. PCR testing exists for herpes viruses, including herpes simplex, varicella zoster, cytomegalovirus, and Epstein–Barr virus, as well as for toxoplasmosis and *Mycobacterium tuberculosis* [5].

Shunt Malfunction

A ventriculoperitoneal shunt is the most commonly implanted system for CSF diversion. It consists of a ventricular catheter connected to a reservoir and valve mechanism at the skull and a catheter that passes in the subcutaneous soft tissue in the neck and anterior chest wall to the peritoneum. The distal tubing can be alternatively inserted in the jugular vein, the pleura, or even the bladder. Failure of the ventricular catheter may occur because of choroid plexus obstruction or cellular debris from CSF infection. Valve or distal tubing obstruction also occurs from cellular debris, from disconnection, poor CSF absorption, or formation of an intra-abdominal pseudocyst.

The clinical presentation of an obstructed shunt is variable. It may be slowly progressive and intermittent, or a rapid decline in mentation progressing into a coma. A CT should be performed immediately to determine ventricular size. Ventriculomegaly is a reliable indicator of a malfunctioning shunt; however, the head CT should be compared with previous studies because the ventricular system in a shunted patient is often congenitally or chronically abnormal.

Aspiration from the reservoir or valve system of a shunt can be performed to determine patency and collect CSF to diagnose an infection. This invasive procedure itself carries a risk of contaminating the system with skin flora, and the resultant shunt infection requires a lengthy hospitalization for shunt externalization, antibiotic treatment, and replacement of all hardware. Therefore, the necessity of and procedure for a shunt tap is best left to a neurosurgeon and should be performed very selectively. When shunt failure is a result of distal obstruction, aspiration of CSF may temper neurologic impairment and even be lifesaving until surgical revision is performed.

Normal-Pressure Hydrocephalus

Serial lumbar punctures or continuous CSF drainage via a lumbar subarachnoid catheter can be used as diagnostic tests to select patients who would benefit from a shunt for CSF diversion. The results have a positive predictive value if the patient's gait improves. Lumbar CSF access may also be used for infusion tests, measurement of CSF production rate, pressure–volume index, and outflow resistance or absorption. Some studies suggest that these values are also predictive of therapeutic CSF diversion [6,7].

Idiopathic Intracranial Hypertension (Pseudotumor Cerebri)

Pseudotumor cerebri affects young persons, often obese young women. It produces nonlocalizing symptoms and could cause severe visual loss if left untreated [8]. Etiologic factors include dural sinus and internal jugular venous thrombosis, head injury, vitamin A overdosage, tetracycline, oral contraceptives, and pregnancy.

Intracranial pressure (ICP) is elevated (up to 40 cm H_2O) without ventriculomegaly or intracranial mass lesions. CSF dynamics demonstrates an increase in outflow resistance. Serial daily lumbar punctures can be therapeutic, with CSF aspirated until closing pressure is within normal limits ($<$20 cm H_2O), thus restoring the balance between CSF formation and absorption in some caes; other treatments include acetazolamide, diuretics, glycerol, steroids, and weight loss. If all these therapeutic interventions fail, placement of a permanent shunting system may be necessary.

Neoplasms

The subarachnoid space can be infiltrated by various primary or secondary tumors, giving rise to symptoms of meningeal irritation. CSF cytology can often but not always determine the presence of neoplastic cells. Systemic neoplasms, such as melanoma or breast cancer, have a greater propensity to metastasize into the CSF spaces than do primary CNS tumors and may even present primarily as meningeal carcinomatosis. Hematopoietic cancers such as acute leukemias and lymphoma also frequently infiltrate the subarachnoid spaces with little or no parenchymal involvement. Ependymoma, medulloblastoma, germinoma, and high-grade glioma are the most commonly disseminated primary tumors. CSF sampling is useful as an initial diagnostic and as a screening tool in the neurologically intact patient who harbors a tumor type with a high risk of CNS relapse. Lymphoma cells in primary CNS lymphoma are present in increased numbers, and pleocytosis correlates with positive cytology [9]. A generous amount of CSF or multiple samples may be required for diagnosis. Cisternal puncture may enhance the diagnosis if the lumbar CSF is nondiagnostic.

Myelography

Lumbar puncture is the most common access for lumbar and cervical myelography because the density of contrast material is higher than CSF and may be directed by gravity to the area of interest. Cervical C1–C2 puncture can be used for access; however, owing to its high risk and complications, it is often reserved for patients for whom a successful lumbar puncture is not possible.

Other Neurologic Disorders

There is extensive literature on CSF changes in demyelinating diseases, including mutiple sclerosis. Typical lumbar puncture findings are normal ICP, normal glucose levels, mononuclear pleocytosis, and elevated protein levels because of increased endothelial permeability. Immunoelectrophoresis reveals elevated IgG and oligoclonal bands that suggest inflammation in the CNS [10,11].

CSF findings described in other disease states include elevated τ protein and decreased β-amyloid precursor protein in Alzheimer disease and the presence of anti-GM1 antibodies and cytoalbumin dissociation in Guillain–Barré syndrome [12].

Therapeutic Interventions

Fistulas

CSF leaks occur because of a variety of traumatic and nontraumatic etiologies. Orthostatic headache is a characteristic symptom, and rhinorrhea may be evident. Postoperative CSF leaks may complicate surgery at the skull base. Fistulas following middle cranial fossa or cerebellopontine angle surgery occur infrequently, and CSF usually leaks through the eustachian tube to the nasopharynx. Following suboccipital craniectomy, a fistula can result in a pseudomeningocele, which manifests as subcutaneous swelling at the incision site because dural closure in the posterior fossa is often difficult and not watertight. Leaks following lumbar surgery are unusual, but may occur as a result of recent myelography, dural tear, or inadequate dural closure [13]. In children, repair of meningoceles or other spina bifida defects is more likely to present with a CSF leak because of dural or fascial defects.

The most common presentation of a CSF fistula follows trauma. Basilar skull fractures that traverse the ethmoid or frontal sinuses can cause CSF rhinorrhea. Fractures along the long axis of the petrous bone usually involve the middle ear, causing the hemotympanum or CSF otorrhea if the tympanic membrane is ruptured. Most CSF leaks present within 48 hours, but delayed leaks are not uncommon because the fistula can be temporarily occluded with adhesions, hematoma, or herniated brain tissue.

The diagnosis of a leak may be easily made on clinical examination; however, at times, the nature of a "drainage fluid" is uncertain, and laboratory characterization is necessary. Testing the fluid for glucose can be misleading because nasal secretions contain glucose. A chloride level often shows a higher value than in peripheral blood, but identification of β_2-transferrin is the most accurate diagnostic for CSF. This protein is produced by neuraminidase in the brain and is uniquely found in the spinal and perilymph fluids [14].

Elevation of the patient's head is the primary treatment of CSF leak. Placement of a lumbar drainage catheter or daily lumbar punctures should be considered when conservative therapy fails. The use of a continuous lumbar drainage by a catheter is somewhat controversial because of the potential for intracranial contamination from the sinuses if the ICP is lowered. To help prevent such complications, the lumbar drain collection bag can be maintained no lower than the patient's shoulder level and the duration of drainage should not exceed 5 days.

Intracranial Hypertension

Intracranial hypertension can cause significant neurologic morbidity or even death. There are mutiple etiologies which include cerebral edema that surrounds tumors, intracranial hematomas, stroke, traumatic contusions, following cranial surgery, or radiation therapy. Diffuse brain swelling also occurs in the setting of inflammatory and infectious disorders such as Reye syndrome or meningitis, or as a result of hyperthermia, carbon dioxide retention, or intravascular congestion. Access to the intracranial CSF space can be useful for diagnosis and treatment [15]. A ventriculostomy is commonly used as an ICP monitor and to treat by CSF drainage. An ICP-measuring device should be placed following traumatic brain injury for patients who exhibit a Glasgow Coma Scale score less than 8, a motor score less than 6 (for patients who are not aphasic), and have initial CT findings of diffuse brain edema, intercranial hematoma, cortical contusions, or absent or compressed basal cisterns [16]. Other indications for ICP monitoring include cerebrovascular diseases, including aneurysmal SAH; ischemic and hypoxic cerebral insults; and intraparenchymal and intraventricular hemorrhage. Obstructive hydrocephalus is another major indication for placement of a ventricular catheter.

Drug Therapy

CSF can be a route of administration for medications such as chemotherapeutic agents and antibiotics in disease processes such as lymphoma, leukemia, meningeal carcinomatosis, meningitis, and ventriculitis. Agents may be infused intrathecally through a lumbar route or an intraventricular injection via an implanted reservoir. Serial injections of small amounts are performed to minimize neurotoxicity. Careful selection of the agent, dose, and timing of administration is recommended, especially when the ventricular route is used, because many antibiotics can cause seizures or inflammatory ventriculitis when given intrathecally.

Thrombolytic Therapy in Intraventricular Hemorrhage

Intraventricular hemorrhage causing obstructive hydrocephalus in the setting of intracranial hemorrhage or aneurysmal SAH is indicative of poor outcome. External ventricular drain (EVD) placement is a standard procedure in such settings to monitor ICP and drain CSF. Therapy with low-dose recombinant tissue plasminogen activator given through the EVD has been shown to facilitate clot resolution in the ventricular system. Studies are being carried out to establish the relation of such treatment on longer term outcomes [17–19].

Lumbar Drainage in Thoracoabdominal Aortic Surgery

One of the most common and grave complications of thoracoabdominal aortic surgery is paraplegia. It usually results from spinal cord ischemia and spinal cord swelling in the setting of perioperative hypotension and compromise of segmental arteries supplying the spinal cord, the largest of which is the artery of Adamkiewicz. Many techniques have been developed to decrease the risk of such complication. Among those techniques is prophylatic lumbar CSF drainage which decreases the CSF pressure, thereby increasing the spinal cord perfusion pressure. There are growing data which demonstrate that this technique decreases the incidence of paraplegia in both open and endovascular aneurysm repairs [20,21].

TECHNIQUES OF CEREBROSPINAL FLUID ACCESS

There are several techniques for CSF aspiration. All procedures should be performed using sterile technique (including sterile gloves and a mask), and the skin is prepared with antiseptic solution and draped with sterile barriers.

Lumbar Puncture

Lumbar puncture is the common technique to aspirate CSF. Contraindications to lumbar puncture include skin infection at the entry site, anticoagulation or blood dyscrasias, papilledema in the presence of supratentorial masses, posterior fossa lesions, and known spinal subarachnoid block or spinal cord arteriovenous malformations. Hence, it should not be performed without prior CT if the patient has any focal neurologic deficit, or a depressed mental status, because this might indicate the presence of an intracranial mass lesion or brain edema, and lumbar puncture can increase the likelihood of downward transtentorial herniation.

In adults, lumbar puncture is often performed under local anesthesia using 1% lidocaine alone. In the pediatric population, however, sedation is often required and allows for a better-tolerated procedure. This is also true in the case of anxious, confused, or combative adult patients.

Oral or rectal chloral hydrate may be used in small children, and moderate sedation using intravenous midazolam, ketamine, fentanyl, or dexmedetomidine can be highly successful in appropriately monitored adults and children when performed by an experienced individual. The application of a topical anesthetic, such as lidocaine preceding injection, can also be useful. Conversely, it has been demonstrated in a controlled clinical trial that in the neonatal population, injection of a local anesthetic for lumbar puncture is probably not required and does not reduce perceived stress or discomfort [22].

Figures 5.1 and 5.2 depict some of the steps for lumbar puncture. The patient is placed in the lateral knee-chest position or with the patient sitting leaning forward over a bedside table. The sitting position may be preferred for obese patients in whom adipose tissue can obscure the midline or in elderly patients with significant lumbar degenerative disease. Following a time-out (correct patient, procedure, site, and equipment), the local anesthetic is injected subcutaneously using a 25- or 27-gauge needle. A 1.5-inch needle is then inserted through the skin wheal and additional local anesthetic is injected along the midline, thus anesthesizing the interspinous ligaments and muscles. This small anesthetic volume is usually adequate; however, a more extensive field block is accomplished by additional injections on each side of the interspinous space near the lamina [23].

The point of skin entry is midline at the level of the superior iliac crests, which is usually between the spinous processes of L3 to L4. Lower needle placement at L4 to L5 or L5 to S1 is required in children and neonates to avoid injury to the conus medullaris, which lies more caudal than in adults. The needle is advanced with the stylet in place to maintain needle patency and prevent iatrogenic intraspinal epidermoid tumors. The bevel of the needle should be parallel to the longitudinal fibers of the dura and spinal column. The needle should be oriented rostrally at an angle of about 30 degrees cephalad and virtually aimed toward the umbilicus. When properly oriented, the needle passes through the following structures before entering the subarachnoid space: skin, superficial fascia, supraspinous ligament, interspinous ligament, ligamentum flavum, epidural space with its fatty areolar tissue and internal vertebral plexus, dura, and arachnoid membrane (Fig. 5.3). The total depth varies from less than 1 inch in the very young patient to as deep

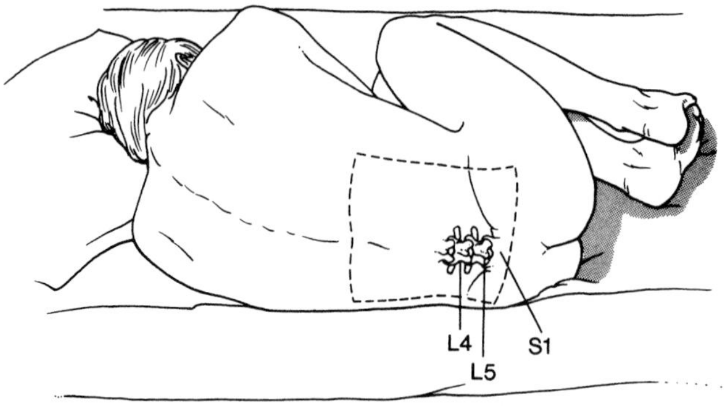

FIGURE 5.1 Patient in the lateral decubitus position with back on the edge of the bed and knees, hips, back, and neck flexed. (From Davidson RI: Lumbar puncture, in VanderSalm TJ (ed): *Atlas of Bedside Procedures*. 2nd ed. Boston, Little, Brown, 1988, with permission.)

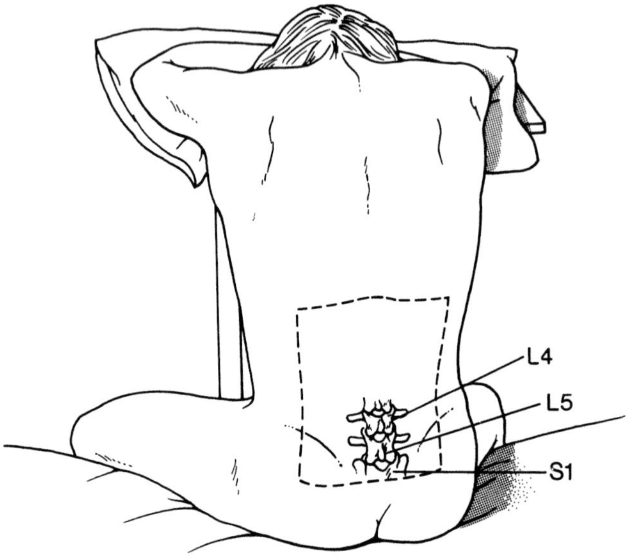

FIGURE 5.2 Patient sitting on the edge of the bed leaning on bedside stand. (From Davidson RI: Lumbar puncture, in VanderSalm TJ (ed): *Atlas of Bedside Procedures*. 2nd ed. Boston, Little, Brown, 1988, with permission.)

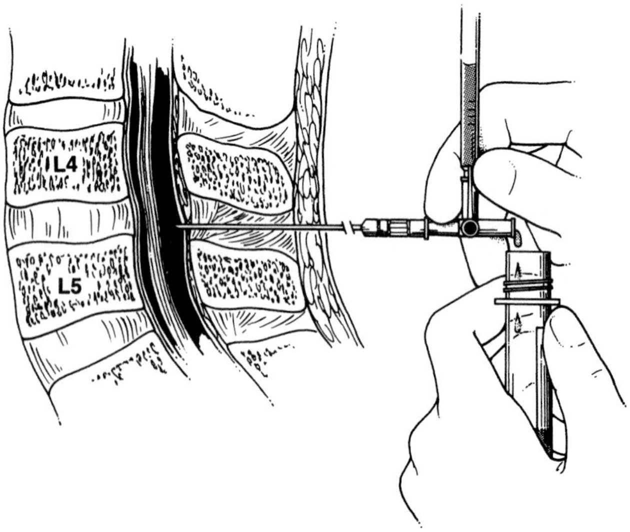

FIGURE 5.3 The spinal needle is advanced to the spinal subarachnoid space, and cerebrospinal fluid samples collected after opening pressure is measured. (From Davidson RI: Lumbar puncture, in VanderSalm TJ (ed): *Atlas of Bedside Procedures*. 2nd ed. Boston, Little, Brown, 1988, with permission.)

as 4 inches in the obese adult. The kinesthetic sensations of passing through the ligaments into the epidural space followed by dural puncture are quite consistent and recognized with practice. Once intradural, the bevel of the needle is redirected in a cephalad direction in order to improve CSF flow. A spinal needle no smaller than 22 gauge should be used for pressure measurement. The opening pressure is best measured with the patient's legs relaxed and extended from the knee-chest position. Pressure measurements may be difficult in children and may be estimated using CSF flow rate [24].

Once CSF is collected, the closing pressure is measured prior to needle withdrawal. It is best to replace the sterile stylet in the needle prior to exiting the subarachnoid space to prevent fistula formation. CSF pressure measurements are not accurate if performed in the sitting position because of the hydrostatic pressure of the CSF column above the entry point or if a significant amount of CSF was lost when the stylet is first withdrawn. If necessary, the pressure could be measured by reclining the patient to the lateral position once entry in the CSF space has been secured.

Although lumbar puncture is typically a safe procedure, there are a number of potential complications and risks involved. Among these complications, postural headache is the most common. Its reported frequency varies from 1% to 70% [25]. It is thought to be caused by excessive drainage of CSF or leakage into the paraspinous spaces, resulting in intracranial hypotension with stretching and expansion of the pain-sensitive intracerebral veins. Magnetic resonance imaging (MRI) has demonstrated a reduced CSF volume following lumbar puncture, but with no significant brain displacement and no correlation with headache [26]. Psychologic factors and previous history of headaches seem to strongly influence the patient's risk of and tolerance to headache [27]. A smaller needle size, parallel orientation to the dural fibers, a paramedian approach, and stylet reinsertion prior to withdrawal of the spinal needle have been reported to decrease the risk of headache after lumbar puncture [28]. The choice of needle type has been the subject of literature debate. Several needle tip designs are available, including the traditional Quincke needle with a beveled cutting tip, the Sprotte needle with a pencil point and side hole, and the Whitacre needle, which is similar to the Sprotte needle but with a smaller side hole. The use of an atraumatic needle seems to be adequate for the performance of a diagnostic lumbar puncture and is probably associated with a lower risk of a postpuncture headache [29]. Postdural puncture headache typically develops within 72 hours and lasts 3 to 5 days. Conservative treatment consists of bed rest, hydration, analgesics, and sometimes non-phenothiazine antiemetics if associated with nausea. If the symptoms are more severe, methylxanthines (caffeine or theophylline) are prescribed orally or parenterally. These agents are successful in up to 85% of patients [28,30]. If the headache persists, an epidural blood patch should be considered because it is one of the most effective treatments for this condition [31]. Epidural injection of other agents, such as saline, dextran, or adenocorticotropic hormone, has also been described and may be valuable under certain conditions (e.g., sepsis or immunodeficiencies).

Hemorrhage is uncommon but can be seen in association with bleeding disorders or anticoagulation therapy. Spinal SAH has been reported in such conditions, resulting in blockage of CSF outflow with subsequent back and radicular pain, sphincter disturbances, and even paraparesis [32]. Spinal subdural hematoma is likewise very infrequent, but it is associated with significant morbidity that may require prompt surgical intervention. Infection by introduction of the patient's skin flora or the operator's mouth or nose flora into the subarachnoid spaces, causing meningitis, is uncommon and preventable if aseptic techniques are used.

An uncommon sequela of lumbar puncture or continuous CSF drainage is hearing loss. Drainage decreases ICP, which is transmitted to the perilymph via the cochlear aqueduct and can cause hearing impairment [33]. The rate of occurrence of this complication is reported to be 0.4%, but is probably higher because it goes unrecognized and seems reversible. There are a few documented cases of irreversible hearing loss [34].

Transient sixth-nerve palsy has also been reported, probably beause of nerve traction following significant CSF removal. Neurovascular injury can occur uncommonly in the setting of a subarachnoid block as a result of spinal tumors. In this situation, CSF drainage leads to significant traction and spinal coning with subsequent neurologic impairment [35,36].

Utility of Ultrasonography for Performance of Lumbar Puncture

Ultrasonography has useful application for performance of lumbar puncture. In patients with standard anatomy, the use of ultrasonography does not offer advantage when compared with standard landmark technique [37]. However, ultrasonography has utility for guidance of lumbar puncture when patient-specific factors such as obesity or edema make it difficult to palpate the spinal processes or the midline of the lumbar region. In this case, the use of ultrasonography increases success rate and reduces the number of attempts required for otaining the CSF sample [38,39].

With the patient in standard position for lumbar puncture, the operator uses a high-frequency vascular probe to scan the lumbar area below the level of the superior iliac crests. With the probe perpendicular to the skin surface in longitudinal scanning plane, the sagittal section in midline allows identification of the adjacent spinous processes (Video 5.1). This allows visualization of the target interspace that is bounded by the spinal processs and the deeper interspinous ligament. The site is marked, the depth for needle penetration measured, and the angle of the transducer noted, because this defines the angle for needle penetration. If it is diffiult to locate the spinal processes in the sagittal scanning plane, a transverse scanning plane may be used for initial identification of the midline, followed by rotation of the probe to longitudinal orientation for verification of target site. The lumbar puncture is performed with standard technique and without real-time needle guidance. The main difficulty in using ultrasonography to aid in lumbar puncture relates to image quality. The patients in greatest need of ultrasonography guidance are the obese; and, yet, the greater the obesity, the more difficult it is to obtain adequate image quality, because of attenuation of the ultrasonography signal. Despite this, ultrasonography has value in this patient population.

Lateral Cervical (C1–C2) Puncture

The C1–C2, or lateral cervical, puncture was originally developed for percutaneous cordotomy. It may be used for myelography or aspiration of CSF if the lumbar route is inaccessible. It is most safely performed with fluoroscopic guidance with the patient supine, the head and neck flexed, and the lateral neck draped. The skin entry point is 1 cm caudal and 1 cm dorsal to the tip of the mastoid process. The site is infiltrated with a local anesthetic, and the spinal needle is introduced and directed toward the junction of the middle and posterior thirds of the bony canal to avoid an anomalous vertebral or posterior inferior cerebellar artery that may lie in the anterior half of the canal. The stylet should be removed frequently to check for CSF egress. When the procedure is performed under fluoroscopy, the needle is seen to be perpendicular to the neck and just under the posterior ring of C1. The same kinesthetic sensation is recognized when piercing the dura as in a lumbar puncture and the bevel is then directed cephalad in a similar manner. Complications of the lateral cervical puncture include injury to the spinal cord or the vertebral artery and irritation of a nerve root, causing local pain and headache.

Cisternal Puncture

A cisternal puncture provides CSF access via the cisterna magna when other routes are not possible. A preoperative lateral skull radiograph is performed to ensure normal anatomy. The patient is positioned sitting with the head slightly flexed. The hair is removed in the occipital region, and the area is prepared, draped, and infiltrated with lidocaine. The entry point is in the midline between the external occipital protuberance in the upper margin of the spinous process of C2 or via an imaginary line through both external auditory meati. The spinal needle is directed through a slightly cephalad course and usually strikes the occipital bone. It is then redirected more caudally in a stepwise manner until it passes through the atlanto-occipital membrane and dura, producing a "popping" sensation. The cisterna magna usually lies 4 to 6 cm deep to the skin; the needle should not be introduced beyond 7.0 to 7.5 cm from the skin to prevent injury to the medulla or the vertebral arteries. The procedure can be performed relatively safely in a cooperative patient because the cisterna magna is a large CSF space; however, it is rarely practiced owing to the greater potential morbidity.

Aspiration of Reservoirs and Shunts

An implanted reservoir or shunt system should not be accessed without prior consultation with a neurosurgeon, despite the apparent simplicity of the procedure itself. Violating implanted systems carries several risks, including infection, which can result in a lengthy hospitalization, prolonged antibiotic course, and several operative procedures for shunt externalization, hardware removal, and insertion of a new shunt system.

Subcutaneous reservoirs in ventriculoatrial or ventriculoperitoneal shunting systems are located proximal to the unidirectional valve and can be accessed percutaneously. The reservoirs are usually button sized, measuring approximately 7 to 10 mm in diameter and 2 mm in height. They can be located in the burr hole directly connected to the ventricular catheter (Fig. 5.4) or as an integral part of the valve system (Fig. 5.5). Indications for reservoir taps have been previously discussed.

The procedure can be performed in any hospital or outpatient setting using sterile techniques. The patient can be in any comfortable position that allows access to the reservoir. Sedation may be required for toddlers. Reference to a skull radiograph may be helpful in localization. The reservoir is palpated, overlying hair is removed with a clipper rather than a razor, and the skin cleansed. Local anesthesia is usually not required, and the use of topical anesthetic creams is occasionally considered. The needle is inserted perpendicular to the skin and into the reservoir, to a total depth of 3 to 5 mm. A manometer is then connected to the needle or butterfly tubing for pressure measurement. CSF collection or drug injection is performed only if CSF flow is demonstrated. A "dry tap" usually indicates faulty placement or catheter obstruction. Occasionally, an old reservoir may have retracted into the burr hole and not be palpable or may be too calcified for needle penetration, and some older shunting systems did not include a reservoir. Risks and complications of shunt aspiration include improper insertion, infection, introduction of blood in the shunt system, and choroid plexus hemorrhage caused by vigorous aspiration.

Lumboperitoneal Shunt

Lumboperitoneal shunts are placed via percutaneous insertion of a lumbar subarachnoid catheter or through a small skin incision. They are tunneled subcutaneously around the patient's flank to the abdomen, where the distal catheter enters the peritoneal

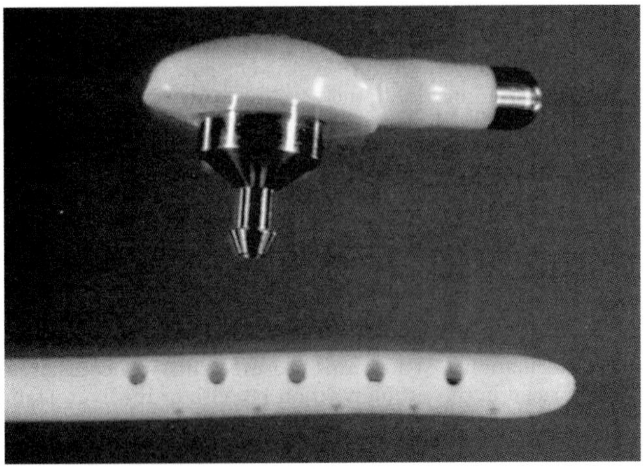

FIGURE 5.4 Close-up view of ventricular reservoir in the calvarial burr hole, with the funneled base connected directly to the proximal end of the ventricular catheter. The distal perforated end is shown.

cavity through a separate abdominal incision. A reservoir or valve or both may be used and are located on the lateral aspect of the flank. Careful palpation between the two incisions usually reveals the tubing path and reservoir placement in the nonobese patient. The patient is placed in lateral decubitus position, and a pillow under the dependent flank may be of assistance. The same technique as described for a ventricular shunt is then performed. Fluid aspiration should be particularly gentle because an additional risk of this procedure is nerve root irritation.

Ventricular Reservoirs

Ventricular reservoirs are inserted as part of a system consisting of a catheter located in a CSF space, usually the lateral ventricle, and without distal runoff. Such systems are placed for CSF access purposes, such as for instillation of antibiotics or chemotherapeutic agents, or CSF aspiration for treatment and monitoring. Ommaya reservoirs are dome-shaped structures (Fig. 5.6) with a diameter of 1 to 2 cm and have a connecting port placed at their base or side. They are placed subcutaneously and attached to a ventricular subarachnoid catheter (Fig. 5.7). Aspiration technique is essentially the same as from a shunt reservoir; however, the Ommaya reservoir is often larger and differs in shape from many shunt reservoirs. It is accessed, preferably, with a 25-gauge

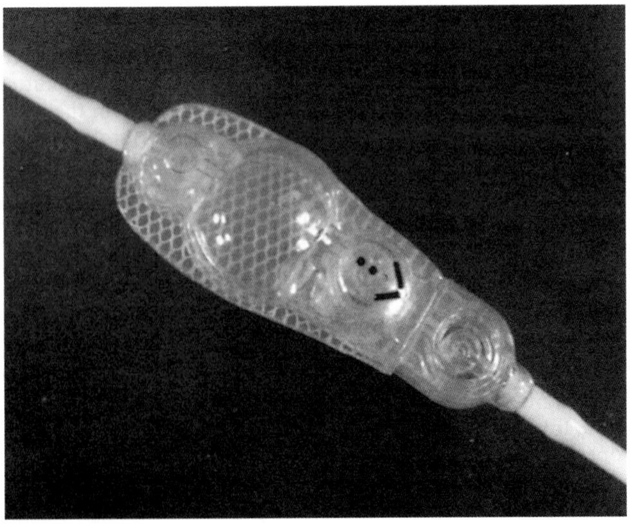

FIGURE 5.5 A domed reservoir in series in one type of shunt valve. The large, clear-domed area for puncture lies immediately proximal to the one-way valve.

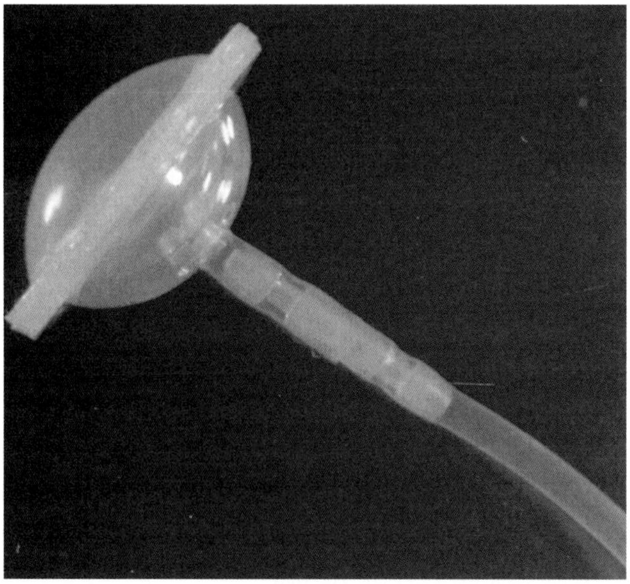

FIGURE 5.6 Close-up view of a ventricular (Ommaya) double-domed reservoir, the caudal half of which is designed to lie within the burr hole.

needle or butterfly. CSF is allowed to flow by gravity if possible; a volume equal to that to be instilled is removed and held for analysis or reinjection. The antibiotic or chemotherapeutic agent is injected; 1 mL of CSF or sterile saline can be used to flush the dose into the ventricle, or gentle barbotage of the reservoir may be performed. Risks and complications are essentially the same as in shunt aspirations (i.e., infection, bleeding, and improper insertion), with the addition of chemical ventriculitis or arachnoiditis.

Ventriculostomy

A ventriculostomy is a catheter placed in the lateral ventricle for CSF drainage or ICP monitoring and treatment. It is performed by a neurosurgeon in the operating room or at the bedside in the intensive care unit or emergency department. It is usually performed through the nondominant hemisphere and into the frontal horn of the lateral ventricle. An alternate approach is to cannulate the occipital horn or trigone through an occipital entry point located 6 cm superior to the inion and 4 cm from the midline. Premedication is not necessary unless the patient is very anxious or combative. Radiographic guidance is typically not required unless the procedure is being performed stereotactically. CT or MRI stereotaxy is needed if the ventricles are very small, as in diffuse brain swelling or slit ventricle syndrome. Complications of ventriculostomy placement include meningitis or ventriculitis, scalp wound infection, intracranial hematoma or cortical injury, and failure to cannulate the ventricle.

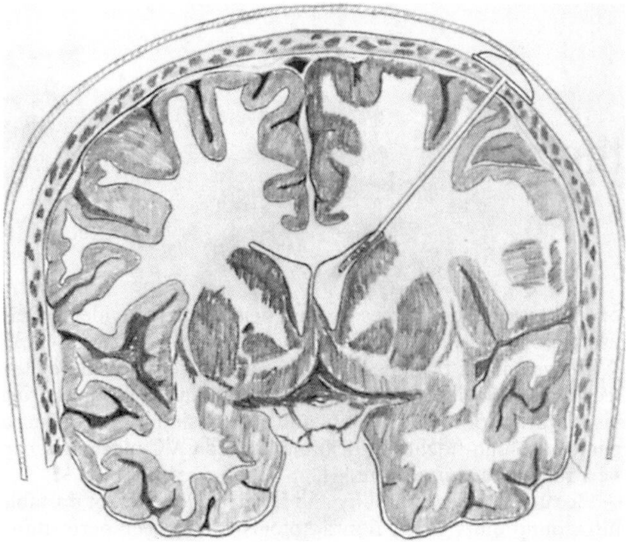

FIGURE 5.7 Coronal section through the brain at the level of the frontal horns, illustrating the subgaleal/epicalvarial location at the reservoir, with the distal perforated part of the catheter lying within the ventricle.

Lumbar Drainage

Continuous CSF drainage via a lumbar catheter is useful in the treatment of CSF fistulas and as a diagnostic test to demonstrate the potential benefit of shunting in normal-pressure hydrocephalus. Commercially available lumbar drainage kits are closed sterile systems that drain into a replaceable collection bag. Catheter placement is performed just as in lumbar puncture; however, a large-bore Tuohy needle is used, through which the catheter is threaded once CSF return has been confirmed. Needle orientation follows the same guidelines as for lumbar puncture and is even more important in the case of this large-gauge needle. Epidural catheter kits could also be used, although the catheters tend to be slightly stiffer and have a narrower diameter. Complications are essentially the same as in lumbar pucture, with the addition of supratentorial subdural hematoma secondary to overdrainage, which tends to be more common in elderly individuals. The potential for overdrainage is significant because of the large diameter of the catheter and because the amount of drainage depends on the cooperation of the patient and the nursing staff. In order to minmize the chances of such a complication, specialized kits are available that provide volume-limiting CSF drainage and monitoring (LimiTorr, Integra Lifescience Corporation, Plainsboro, NJ). These kits can be used in ventricular and lumbar drainge catheter systems and utilize a valve that halts drainage when the predetermined volume (usually 20 or 30 mL) is reached (Fig. 5.8).

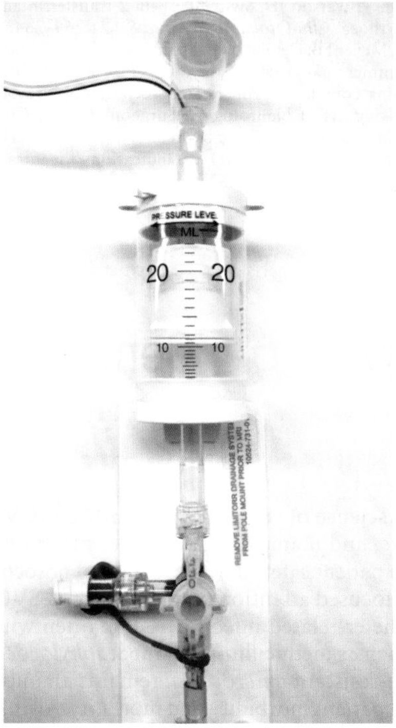

FIGURE 5.8 Volume-limiting CSF drainage system. It is attached to CSF collecting systems such as a lumbar drain to avoid overdrainage and subsequent complications, such as a supratentorial subdural hematoma. CSF, cerebrospinal fluid.

SUMMARY

CSF aspiration is a very improtant diagnostic and theraputic tool for many disease processes. Of the various techniques available for CSF access, lumbar puncture is the procedure most commonly and safely performed by the critical care practitioner. Other techniques are described that may require the assistance of a radiologist, neurologist, anesthesiologist, or neurosurgeon.

References

1. Hollman GA, Schultz MM, Eickhoff JC, et al: Propofol-fentanyl versus propofol alone for lumbar puncture sedation in children with acute hematologic malignancies: propofol dosing and adverse events. *Pediatr Crit Care Med* 9:616–622, 2008.
2. Dilli D, Dallar Y, Sorguc NH: Comparison of ketamine plus midazolam versus ketamine for sedation in children during lumbar puncture. *Clin J Pain* 25:349–350, 2009.
3. Wood J: Cerebrospinal fluid: techniques of access and analytical interpretation, in Wilkins RH, Rengachary SS: *Neurosurgery.* Vol 1. 2nd ed. New York, NY, McGraw-Hill, 1996.
4. de Falco FA: Sentinel headache. *Neurol Sci* 25[Suppl 3]:S215–S217, 2004.
5. d'Arminio Monforte A, Cinque P, Vago L, et al: A comparison of brain biopsy and CSF-PCR in the diagnosis of CNS lesions in AIDS patients. *J Neurol* 244:35–39, 1997.
6. Shprecher D, Schwalb J, Kurlan R: Normal pressure hydrocephalus: diagnosis and treatment. *Curr Neurol Neurosci Rep* 8:371–376, 2008.
7. Chotai S, Medel R, Herial NA, et al: External lumbar drain: a pragmatic test for prediction of shunt outcomes in idiopathic normal pressure hydrocephalus. *Surg Neurol Int* 5:51–59, 2014.
8. Thurtell MJ, Bruce BB, Newman NJ, et al: An update on idiopathic intracranial hypertension. *Rev Neurol Dis* 7:e56–e68, 2010.
9. Fischer L, Jahnke K, Martus P, et al: The diagnostic value of cerebrospinal fluid pleocytosis and protein in the detection of lymphomatous meningitis in primary central nervous system lymphomas. *Haematologica* 91:429–430, 2006.
10. Fishman RA: *Cerebrospinal Fluid in Diseases of the Nervous System.* 2nd ed. Philadelphia, PA, W.B. Saunders, 1992, pp 213–214.
11. Link H, Huang YM: Oligoclonal bands in multiple sclerosis cerebrospinal fluid: an update on methodology and clinical usefulness. *J Neuroimmunol* 180:17–28, 2006.
12. Fagan AM, Roe CM, Xiong C, et al: Cerebrospinal fluid tau/beta-amyloid(42) ratio as a prediction of cognitive decline in nondemented older adults. *Arch Neurol* 64:343–349, 2007.
13. Agrillo U, Simonetti G, Martino V: Postoperative CSF problems after spinal and lumbar surgery. General review. *J Neurosurg Sci* 35:93–95, 1991.
14. Nandapalan V, Watson ID, Swift AC: Beta-2-transferrin and cerebrospinal fluid rhinorrhoea. *Clin Otolaryngol Allied Sci* 21:259–264, 1996.
15. Lyons MK, Meyer FB: Cerebrospinal fluid physiology and the management of increased intracranial pressure. *Mayo Clin Proc* 65:684–707, 1990.
16. Brain Trauma Foundation, American Association of Neurological Surgeons (AANS), Congress of Neurological Surgeons (CNS): Guidelines for the management of severe traumatic brain injury. (AANS/CNS Joint Section on Neurotrauma and Critical Care) VI. Indications for intracranial pressure monitoring. *J Neurotrauma* 24:S37–S44, 2007.
17. Litrico S, Almairac F, Gaberel T, et al: Intraventricular fibrinolysis for severe aneurysmal intraventricular hemorrhage: a randomized controlled trial and meta-analysis. *Neurosurg Rev* 36:523–530, 2013.
18. Li Y, Zhang H, Wang X, et al: Neuroendoscopic surgery versus external ventricular drainage alone or with intraventricular fibrinolysis for intraventricular hemorrhage secondary to spontaneous supratentorial hemorrhage: a systematic review and meta-analysis. *PLoS One* 8:e80599, 2013.
19. Ziai WC, Tuhrim S, Lane K, et al: A multicenter, randomized, double-blinded, placebo-controlled phase III study of Clot Lysis Evaluation of Accelerated Resolution of Intraventricular Hemorrhage (CLEAR III). *Int J Stroke* 9:536–542, 2014.
20. Hnath JC, Mehta M, Taggert JB, et al: Strategies to improve spinal cord ischemia in endovascular thoracic aortic repair: outcomes of a prospective cerebrospinal fluid drainage protocol. *J Vasc Surg* 48:836–840, 2008.
21. Safi HJ, Miller CC 3rd, Huynh TT, et al: Distal aortic perfusion and cerebrospinal fluid drainage for thoracoabdominal and descending thoracic aortic repair: ten years of organ protection. *Ann Surg* 238:372–380, 2003.
22. Porter FL, Miller JP, Cole FS, et al: A controlled clinical trial of local anesthesia for lumbar punctures in newborns. *Pediatrics* 88:663–669, 1991.
23. Wilkinson HA: Field block anesthesia for lumbar puncture. *JAMA* 249:2177, 1983.
24. Ellis R 3rd: Lumbar cerebrospinal fluid opening pressure measured in a flexed lateral decubitus position in children. *Pediatrics* 93:622–623, 1994.
25. Strupp M, Brandt T: Should one reinsert the stylet during lumbar puncture? *N Engl J Med* 336:1190, 1997.
26. Grant R, Condon B, Hart I, et al: Changes in intracranial CSF volume after lumbar puncture and their relationship to post-LP headache. *J Neurol Neurosurg Psychiatry* 54:440–442, 1991.
27. Lee T, Maynard N, Anslow P, et al: Post-myelogram headache—physiological or psychological? *Neuroradiology* 33:155–158, 1991.
28. Ghaleb A, Khorasani A, Mangar D: Post-dural puncture headache. *Int J Gen Med* 5:45–51, 2012.
29. Vakharia VN, Lote H: Introduction of Sprotte needles to a single-centre acute neurology service: before and after study. *JRSM Short Rep* 3:82, 2012.
30. Basurto Ona X, Osorio D, Bonfill Cosp X: Drug therapy for treating post-dural puncture headache. *Cochrane Database Syst Rev* 7:CD007887:1–47, 2015.
31. van Kooten F, Oedit R, Bakker SL, et al: Epidural blood patch in post dural puncture headache: a randomised, observer-blind, controlled clinical trial. *J Neurol Neurosurg Psychiatry* 79:553–558, 2008.
32. Scott EW, Cazenave CR, Virapongse C: Spinal subarachnoid hematoma complicating lumbar puncture: diagnosis and management. *Neurosurgery* 25:287–292, 1989.
33. Walsted A, Salomon G, Thomsen J, et al: Hearing decrease after loss of cerebrospinal fluid. A new hydrops model? *Acta Otolaryngol* 111:468–476, 1991.
34. Michel O, Brusis T: Hearing loss as a sequel of lumbar puncture. *Ann Otol Rhinol Laryngol* 101:390–394, 1992.
35. Wong MC, Krol G, Rosenblum MK: Occult epidural chloroma complicated by acute paraplegia following lumbar puncture. *Ann Neurol* 31:110–112, 1992.
36. Mutoh S, Aikou I, Ueda S: Spinal coning after lumbar puncture in prostate cancer with asymptomatic vertebral metastasis: a case report. *J Urol* 145:834–835, 1991.
37. Peterson MA, Pisupati D, Heyming TW, et al: Ultrasound for routine lumbar puncture. *Acad Emerg Med* 21:130–136, 2014.
38. Strony R: Ultrasound-assisted lumbar puncture in obese patients. *Crit Care Clin* 26:661–664, 2010.
39. Nomura JT, Leech SJ, Shenbagamurthi S, et al: A randomized controlled trial of ultrasound-assisted lumbar puncture. *J Ultrasound Med* 26:1341–1348, 2007.

Chapter 6 ■ Central Venous Catheters

ANDREW H. MORACO • SCOTT E. KOPEC

The art and science of central venous catheter (CVC) insertion, maintenance, and management continues to evolve. Increased emphasis on patient safety and prevention of nosocomial complications has focused attention on the impact of CVCs on patient health. Catheter-related infection (CRI), often with a resistant organism such as methicillin-resistant *Staphylococcal aureus* or vancomycin-resistant *enterococci*, remains an important cause of increased patient morbidity and mortality. All institutions are encouraged to adopt evidence-based protocols and procedures designed to reduce CRI and other catheter complications [1]. Patient safety is also the main impetus for increased availability of simulation laboratories to train health care providers in the use of portable ultrasound to facilitate catheter insertion [2,3]. With systematic training, including a clear description of the technique with video examples, hands-on simulation emphasizing visualization of the needle tip, and supervision by experienced clinicians, high-fidelity ultrasound-guided CVC placement can be a reliably acquired skill [4].

Because of the availability and relatively low cost of portable ultrasound units, many nonradiologists have been performing bedside image-guided central venous cannulation. Ultrasound guidance allows visualization of the vessel, thus showing its precise location and patency in real time. It is especially useful for patients with suboptimal body habitus, volume depletion, shock, anatomic deformity, previous cannulation, underlying coagulopathy, or prior intravenous (IV) drug abuse. The use of ultrasound guidance has significantly decreased the failure rate, complication rate, and the number of attempts in obtaining central venous access. Experts agree that ultrasound guidance should be standard of care for all CVC insertions [4]. The Third Sonography Outcomes Assessment Program trial, a concealed, randomized, controlled multicenter study, demonstrated an odds ratio 53.5 times higher for success with ultrasound guidance compared with the landmark technique. It also demonstrated a significantly lower average number of attempts and average time of catheter placement [5,6].

In this chapter, we review the techniques and complications of the various routes available for central venous catheterization, and present a strategy for catheter management that incorporates all of the recent advances.

INDICATIONS AND SITE SELECTION

Like any medical procedure, CVC has specific indications and should be reserved for the patient who has potential to benefit from it. After determining that CVC is necessary, the health care provider should seek the most appropriate site and route for that particular patient. Table 6.1 lists general priorities in site selection for different indications of CVC; however, the final choice of site in a particular patient should, in part, be based on the operator experience. We recommend that all internal jugular and femoral vein (FV) cannulations be performed under ultrasound guidance, with consideration of using ultrasound guidance for the subclavian vein (SCV) approach depending on the operator experience.

Volume resuscitation alone is not an indication for CVC. A 2.5-inch, 16-gauge catheter used to cannulate a peripheral vein can infuse twice the amount of fluid as an 8-inch, 16-gauge CVC [7]. However, peripheral vein cannulation may be very difficult in the patient with shock, and, hence, CVC placement may be necessary. Long-term total parenteral nutrition is best administered through a peripherally inserted central catheter (PICC) because these lines are associated with fewer severe complications and significant cost savings [8]. The internal jugular vein (IJV) is the preferred site for acute hemodialysis: the SCV should be avoided because of the relatively high incidence of subclavian venous stenosis following temporary dialysis. This, in turn, may limit options for an arteriovenous fistula should long-term dialysis become necessary [9]. The FV is also suitable for acute short-term hemodialysis or plasmapheresis in the nonambulatory patient. However, FV catheters have a higher rate of infection and are not recommended unless absolutely necessary [10–12]. When used, FV catheters should be removed as soon as possible.

Emergent transvenous pacemakers and flow-directed pulmonary artery catheters are best inserted through the right IJV because of the direct path to the right ventricle. This route is associated with the fewest catheter tip malpositions. The SCV is an alternative second choice for pulmonary artery catheterization even in many patients with coagulopathy [13]. The left SCV is preferred to the right SCV because of a less torturous route to the heart. The reader is referred to Chapter 19 for additional information on the insertion and care of pulmonary artery catheters.

Preoperative CVC placement is desirable in a wide variety of clinical situations. One specific indication for preoperative right ventricular catheterization is the patient undergoing a posterior craniotomy or cervical laminectomy in the sitting position. These patients are at risk for air embolism, and the catheter can theoretically be used to aspirate air from the right ventricle, although data does not support the efficacy of this process [14]. Neurosurgical patients may benefit from the placement of an antecubital or a subclavian catheter, as opposed to IJV catheters. IJV catheters can theoretically obstruct blood

TABLE 6.1

Indications for Central Venous Catheterization (CVC)

Indication	Site selection: First	Second	Third
1. Pulmonary artery catheterization	RIJV	LSCV	LIJV
With coagulopathy	IJV	FV	
With pulmonary compromise or high-level positive end-expiratory pressure (PEEP)	RIJV	LIJV	FV
2. Total parenteral nutrition (TPN)	SCV	IJV (tunneled)	
Long term (surgically implanted)	SCV	PICC	
3. Acute hemodialysis/plasmapheresis	IJV	FV	SCV
4. Cardiopulmonary arrest	IO	FV	SCV
5. Emergency transvenous pacemaker	RIJV	SCV	
6. Hypovolemia, inability to perform peripheral IV	IJV	SCV	FV
7. Preoperative preparation	IJV	SCV	AV/PICC
8. General-purpose venous access, vasoactive agents, caustic medications, radiologic procedures	IJV	SCV	FV
With coagulopathy	IJV	EJV	FV
9. Emergency airway management	FV	SCV	IJV
10. Inability to lie supine	FV	EJV	AV/PICC
11. Central venous oxygen saturation monitoring	IJV	SCV	
12. Fluid management of ARDS (CVP monitoring)	IJV	EJV	SCV

IJV and FV assume ultrasound guidance (see text for details).

ARDS, acute respiratory distress syndrome; AV, antecubital vein; CVP, central venous pressure; EJV, external jugular vein; FV, femoral vein; IJV, internal jugular vein; IV, intravenous; L, left; PICC, peripherally inserted central venous catheter; R, right; SCV, subclavian vein.

return from the cranial vault potentially increasing intracranial pressure, although a small study suggests that venous return is not significantly reduced [15].

Venous access during cardiopulmonary resuscitation warrants special comment. Peripheral vein cannulation in circulatory arrest may prove impossible, and circulation times of drugs administered peripherally are prolonged when compared with central injection. Drugs injected through femoral catheters also have a prolonged circulation time, although the clinical significance is unclear [16]. Effective drug administration is a very important element of successful cardiopulmonary resuscitation, and all physicians should understand the appropriate techniques for establishing access. If venous access is not readily available, placement of an intraosseous device has been shown to be more efficient in establishing access, equivalent in pharmacokinetic studies and is considered the standard alternative to IV access [17].

The placement of CVC is common in patients with severe sepsis, septic shock, or acute respiratory distress syndrome. However, the necessity of CVC placement has been minimized in recent years, perhaps in part, to the ARISE, PROMISE, and ProCess trials, which showed no difference between early goal-directed therapy and what has become the standard of care. Thus, fewer central lines may be placed because of fewer indications for frequent monitoring of central venous oxygen saturations and central venous pressures [18,19].

GENERAL CONSIDERATIONS

General considerations for CVC independent of the site of insertion include the need for signed informed consent, ensuring patient comfort and safety, and ultrasound preparation. Determining the presence of coagulopathies, and preventions of complications such as vascular erosions, catheter-associated thrombosis, and air embolism, is also important.

Informed Consent

It seems intuitively obvious that a signed informed consent is mandatory before nonemergent CVC insertion, but, in clinical practice, many emergent insertions are required. CVC insertions in the ICU are extremely common, occur at all hours of the day, and may be crucial for early and appropriate resuscitation and commencement of care. Many critically ill patients have no immediately available family members or legal next of kin. Obtaining informed consent for these patients can prevent or delay the delivery of life-saving therapies. Because of these considerations, there is no uniform clinical or legal opinion regarding the necessity of individual informed consent prior to all CVC insertions or other ICU procedures [20]. Some institutions have dealt with this matter by developing a single general "consent form for critical care" that is signed one time for each individual ICU admission and covers all commonly performed bedside procedures. Up to 14% of all ICU included in a survey study used such a consent form, and overall consent practice varied widely. In general, health care providers in medical ICUs sought consent for CVC insertion more often than those in surgical ICUs [20]. Given the lack of agreement on this topic, it seems prudent to make a few recommendations: (1) Written informed consent should be obtained prior to all elective CVC insertion or other procedures. (2) Whenever possible, competent patients or legal next of kin of incompetent/incapacitated patients should be thoroughly informed of the indications, risks, and benefits of emergency CVC insertion prior to the performance of the procedure. If informed consent is not possible prior to CVC insertion, then consent should be obtained as soon as possible after completion of the procedure. A signed consent form is always preferable, but sometimes not feasible. Oral consent should be documented in the procedure note by the person obtaining assent. (3) Emergent CVC placement should not be delayed inappropriately by efforts to obtain consent—oral or written. Patients and family should be informed as soon as possible after insertion why the CVC was required. (4) A general consent form that is signed one time as close as possible to ICU admission is a reasonable way to try and inform patients of the benefits/risks of procedures without incurring unnecessary delays or consumption of clinical time. This form can also serve as a useful reference for patients and families of all the various common procedures that are performed in the ICU. (5) Finally, it is good practice to document the practice that is used in the institution's "Policies, Guidelines, and Procedures" along with the rationale for it [21].

Patient Comfort and Safety

Many patients requiring CVC have an unstable airway, are in respiratory distress, or are hemodynamically unstable. These patients may not tolerate lying flat for CVC placement. Patients with unstable airways or respiratory distress frequently require addressing their respiratory status prior to placing a CVC. These considerations should impact preparation and choice of site. In addition, many patients are claustrophobic and will not tolerate their face being covered. Every patient should be specifically assessed prior to CVC regarding their positioning, airway, and hemodynamic stability. Once the patient is stabilized, the appropriate site/catheter can then be inserted under less unstable/rigorous conditions.

Mobile Catheter Cart

Availability of a mobile catheter cart that contains all necessary supplies and that can be wheeled to each patient's bedside is good practice and likely reduces overall catheter infection rate by decreasing breaks in sterile technique [23]. The mobile cart is also an excellent way to standardize all catheter insertions, facilitate communication of procedural tasks (such as the use of a time-out), and allow for optimal documentation.

Catheter Tip Location

Catheter tip location is a very important consideration in CVC placement. The ideal location for the catheter tip is the distal innominate or proximal superior vena cava (SVC), 3 to 5 cm proximal to the cavotrial junction. Positioning of the catheter tip within the right atrium or right ventricle should be avoided. Cardiac tamponade secondary to catheter tip perforation of the cardiac wall is uncommon, with two-thirds of patients suffering this complication die [24]. Perforation likely results from vessel wall damage from infused solutions combined with catheter tip migration that occurs from the motion of the beating heart as well as patient arm and neck movements. Although not often considered, catheter tips can migrate up to 5 to 10 cm with antecubital catheters and 1 to 5 cm with IJV or SCV catheters [25]. Other complications from intracardiac catheter tip position include provocation of arrhythmias from mechanical irritation [26].

Correct placement of the catheter tip is relatively simple, beginning with an appreciation of anatomy. The cavoatrial junction is approximately 16 to 18 cm from right-sided skin punctures and 19 to 21 cm from left-sided insertions and is relatively independent of patient gender and body habitus [27]. A chest radiograph should be obtained following every initial CVC insertion to ascertain catheter tip location and to detect complications. The right tracheobronchial angle is the most reliable landmark on plain chest radiograph for the upper margin of the SVC, and is always at least 2.9 cm above the cavoatrial junction. The catheter tip should lie about 1 cm below this landmark, and above the right upper cardiac silhouette to ensure placement outside the pericardium [28].

Vascular Erosions

Large-vessel perforations secondary to CVCs are very rare, about 0.28 per 1,000 catheter days and occur on average between days 5 and 8 after insertion. Symptoms included dyspnea, chest pain, and palpitations. Radiographically, a pleural or pericardial effusion may be seen. This complication is more common in older patients and left-sided catheters and is considered to be related to the angle of the catheter tip adjacent to the superior vena cava [29]. Treatment should include removal of the catheter and symptomatic management of subsequent complications that arise, including possible thoracentesis, pericardiocentesis or chest tube placement. Additionally, given the significant morbidity and mortality associated with this complication, we would suggest consideration of a vascular surgery consultation [30].

Complications

Venous Air Embolism

Venous air embolism (VAE) is rare and preventable potentially life-threatening complication of CVC placement. As little as 200 mL of air has been theorized to cause a fatal embolism [31]. VAE often goes undiagnosed, leading to a fatal outcome. Potential mechanisms include air entry through the needle during placement, catheter disconnection resulting in the catheter being open to the atmosphere, and, more commonly, passage of air through a patent tract after catheter removal. Placing the patient in Trendelenburg (thereby increasing venous pressure) during catheter placement and removal will reduce this complication. VAE should be suspected in any patient with an indwelling or recently discontinued CVC who develops sudden unexplained hypoxemia or cardiovascular collapse. Often, VAE occurs after movement or when the patient is transferred out of bed. A characteristic mill wheel sound may be auscultated over the precordium. VAE can be confirmed with a bedside cardiac ultrasound. If VAE is found, the patient should be placed in the Trendelenburg and left lateral decubitus positions. This may trap the air in the apex of the right ventricle and prevent pulmonary artery outflow obstruction. Theoretically, a CVC can be used to aspirate the air from the right ventricle; this is rarely feasible [14]. The best treatment is prevention which can be effectively achieved through comprehensive nursing and physician-in-training educational modules and proper supervision of inexperienced operators [5,14,32].

Coagulopathy

Central venous access in the patient with a bleeding diathesis can be problematic. The SCV and IJV routes have increased risks in the presence of coagulopathy, but the true risk is frequently overestimated and it is not known at what degree of abnormality it becomes unacceptable. A coagulopathy is generally defined as an international normalized ratio greater than 1.5 or platelet count less than 50,000 per μL. Recently, studies have shown that we likely overestimate the increased risk of bleeding even with the subclavian approach and that ultrasound-guided IJV is safe even with significant coagulopathy. However, it is prudent to attempt to correct the coagulopathy and to favor a more compressible site, such as the IJV or FV, over the subclavian approach [33].

Thrombosis

Catheter-related thrombosis is common but usually of little clinical significance. The spectrum of thrombotic complications includes a fibrin sleeve surrounding the catheter from its point of entry into the vein distal to the tip; mural thrombus, a clot that forms on the wall of the vein secondary to mechanical or chemical irritation; or occlusive thrombus, which blocks flow and may result in collateral formation. All of these lesions are usually clinically silent; therefore, studies that do not use venography or color-flow Doppler imaging to confirm the diagnosis underestimate its incidence. However, the incidence may be as high as two-thirds of patients with CVC and underlying malignancy. In contrast, clinically overt symptoms of thrombosis occur between 5% and 25%. Infrequently, CVC-related upper extremity deep vein thromboses increase the risk of pulmonary embolism, with estimates ranging from 2% to 9% [34,35]. The presence of catheter-associated thrombosis is, however, associated with a higher incidence of infection [36]. If a CVC-associated thrombus is found, the catheter should be removed, and consideration for systemic anticoagulation should be entertained.

Infectious Complications

There are an estimated 18,000 cases of ICU central line–associated bloodstream infection annually in the United States [37]. Many factors impact the risk of developing these infections, including insertion technique, site, daily care, and type of catheter used. Table 6.2 summarizes current recommendations or interventions that have been shown to reduce the risk of CRI. A complete review of CRIs can be found in Chapter 79.

ROUTES OF CENTRAL VENOUS CANNULATION

In this section, the anatomy of the various approaches to achieving central venous access is described first, followed by how to achieve access using ultrasonography.

Antecubital Approach

The antecubital veins are used in the ICU for CVC with PICC and midline catheters. Specialized nursing teams are able to insert PICCs at beside with the use of real-time ultrasonography and sterile technique, thereby increasing safety and reducing the potential for infection. PICCs may be useful in ICU patients undergoing neurosurgery, with coagulopathy, or in the rehabilitative phase of critical illness for which general-purpose central venous access is required for parenteral nutrition or long-term medication access [38] (Table 6.1). Although many hospitals have a designated "PICC" insertion team, they may have significant work hour limitations that delay insertion of catheters and result in significant delays in delivery of care.

Anatomy

The basilic vein is preferred for CVC placement because it is almost always of substantial size and the anatomy is predictable. It provides an unimpeded path to the central venous circulation via the axillary vein and is formed at the ulnar aspect of the dorsal venous network of the hand. It may be found in the medial part of the antecubital fossa, where it is usually joined by the median basilic vein. It then ascends in the groove between the biceps brachii and pronator teres on the medial aspect of the arm to perforate the deep fascia distal to the midportion of the arm, where it joins the brachial vein to become the axillary vein.

TABLE 6.2

Steps to Minimize Central Venous Catheterization (CVC)–Related Infection

1. Institution-supported standardized education, with knowledge assessment, of all physicians involved in CVC insertion and care
2. Site preparation with approved chlorhexidine-based preparation
3. Maximal barrier precautions during catheter insertion
4. Use of mobile procedure carts, safety checklist, empowerment of staff
5. Strict protocols for catheter maintenance (including bandage and tubing changes), preferably by dedicated IV catheter team
6. Appropriate site selection, avoiding heavily colonized or anatomically abnormal areas; use of SCV for anticipated CVC of >4 d
7. For anticipated duration of catheterization exceeding 96 h, use of silver-impregnated cuff, sustained release chlorhexidine gluconate patch, and/or antibiotic/antiseptic-impregnated catheters
8. Prompt removal of any catheter which is no longer required
9. Remove pulmonary artery catheters and introducers after 5 d
10. Replace any catheter not placed with sterile precautions within 48 h (i.e., catheter placed in emergency)
11. Use multilumen catheters only when indicated; remove when no longer needed
12. Avoid "routine" guidewire exchanges
13. Use surgically implanted catheters or PICCs for long-term (i.e., >3 wk) or permanent CVC

IV, intravenous; PICC, peripherally inserted central catheter; SCV, subclavian vein.

Technique of Cannulation

Several kits are available for antecubital CVC. The PICC and midline catheters are made of silicone or polyurethane and, depending on catheter stiffness and size, are usually placed through an introducer. The method described below is for a PICC inserted through a tear-away introducer.

The success rates from either arm are comparable, although the catheter must traverse a greater distance from the left. With the patient's arm at his or her side, the antecubital fossa is prepared with chlorhexidine and draped using maximum barrier precautions (mask, cap and sterile gown, gloves and large drape covering the patient). A tourniquet is placed proximally by an assistant, and a portable ultrasound device is used to identify the basilic or its main branches. A vein can be distinguished from an artery by visualizing compressibility, color flow, and Doppler flow (Fig. 6.1). After a time-out and administration of local anesthesia subcutaneously, venipuncture is performed with the thin-wall entry needle a few centimeters proximal to the antecubital crease to avoid catheter breakage and embolism. When free backflow of venous blood is confirmed, the tourniquet is released and the guidewire carefully threaded into the vein for a distance of 15 to 20 cm. Leaving the guidewire in place, the thin-wall needle is withdrawn and the puncture site enlarged with a scalpel blade. The sheath introducer assembly is threaded over the guidewire with a twisting motion, and the guidewire removed. Next, leaving the sheath in place, the dilator is removed, and the introducer is now ready for PICC insertion. The length of insertion is estimated by measuring the distance along the predicted vein path from the venipuncture site to the manubriosternal junction, using the measuring tape provided in the kit. The PICC is typically supplied with an inner obturator that provides stiffness for insertion. The catheter is trimmed to the desired length and flushed with saline, and the obturator is inserted into the line upto the tip. The PICC/obturator assembly is inserted through the introducer to the appropriate distance, the introducer peeled away, and the obturator removed. The PICC is secured in place, and a chest X-ray is obtained to determine tip position.

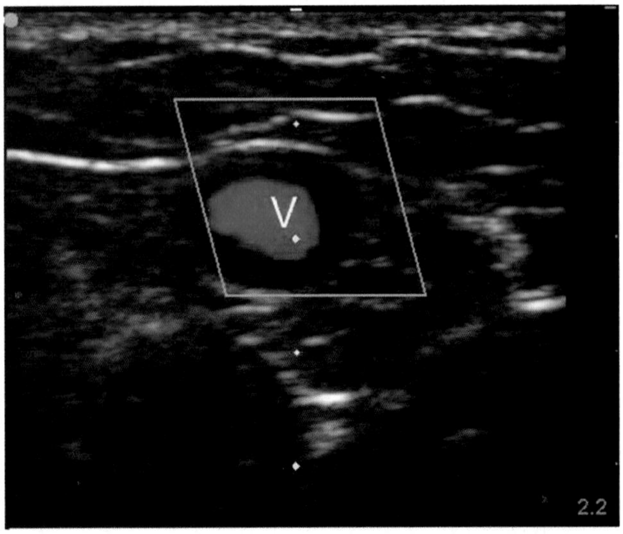

FIGURE 6.1 Ultrasound view of the basilica vein at the antecubital fossa.

If resistance to advancing the PICC is met, options are limited. Techniques such as abducting the arm are of limited value. If a catheter-through- or over-needle device has been used, the catheter must never be withdrawn without simultaneously retracting the needle to avoid catheter shearing and embolism. If the catheter cannot be advanced easily, another site should be chosen.

Success Rate and Complications

Using the abovementioned technique, PICC catheters have a 75% to 95% successful placement rate. Overall, PICCs appear to be at least as safe as CVCs, but important complications include sterile phlebitis, thrombosis (especially of the SCV and IJV), infection, limb edema, and pericardial tamponade. Phlebitis may be more common with antecubital CVCs, probably because of less blood flow in these veins as well as the proximity of the venipuncture site to the skin [39]. The risk of pericardial tamponade may also be increased if the catheter tip is inserted too far because of greater catheter tip migration occurring with arm movements [25]. Complications are minimized by strict adherence to recommended techniques for catheter placement and care.

Internal Jugular Approach

The IJV has been used for venous access in pediatric and adult patients for many years, and ultrasound has had its greatest impact by improving the efficiency of IJV cannulation because real-time direct visualization of the vein is easily obtained. This

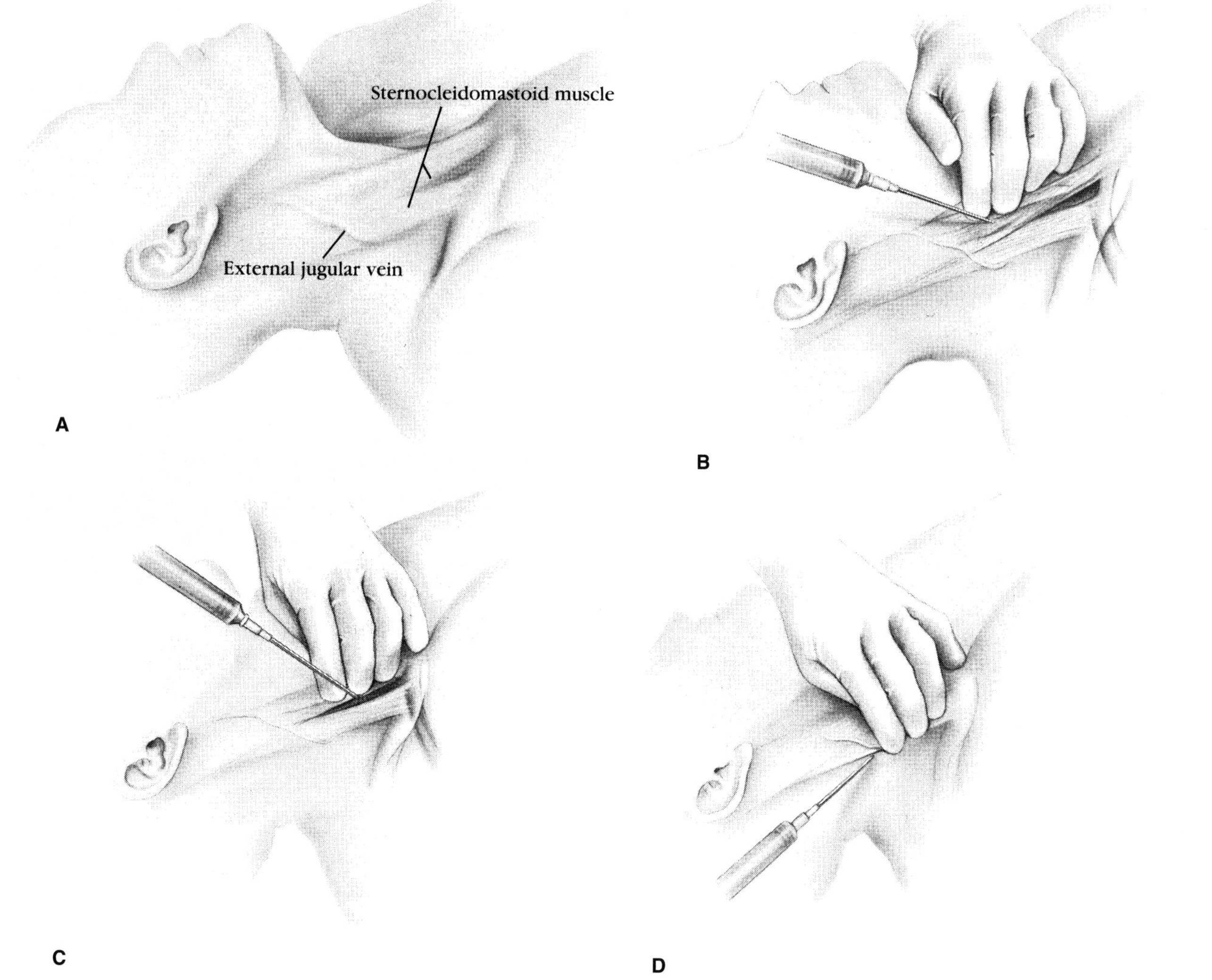

FIGURE 6.2 Surface anatomy and various approaches to cannulation of the internal jugular vein. A: Surface anatomy. B: Anterior approach. C: Central approach. D: Posterior approach. The external jugular vein is also shown.

minimizes the impact of hypovolemia or anatomic variations on overall success and has rendered ICU external jugular vein (EJV) catheterization extremely rare. Furthermore, under ultrasound guidance, the central approach is almost always used. Those interested in the anterior or posterior approaches, please refer to prior editions of this textbook. In general, these techniques differ mainly in the point of skin puncture (Fig. 6.2).

Anatomy

The IJV emerges from the base of the skull through the jugular foramen and enters the carotid sheath dorsally with the internal carotid artery (ICA). It then courses posterolaterally to the artery and runs beneath the sternocleidomastoid (SCM) muscle. The vein lies medial to the anterior portion of the SCM muscle superiorly and then runs beneath the triangle formed by the two heads of the muscle in its medial portion before entering the SCV near the medial border of the anterior scalene muscle at the sternal border of the clavicle. The junction of the right IJV (which averages 2 to 3 cm in diameter) with the right SCV forming the innominate vein follows a straight path to the SVC. As a result, catheter malposition and looping of the catheter inserted through the right IJV are unusual. In contrast, a catheter passed through the left IJV must negotiate a sharp turn at the left jugulosubclavian junction, which results in a greater percentage of catheter malpositions [40]. This sharp turn may also produce tension and torque at the catheter tip, which can result in a higher incidence of vessel erosion.

A knowledge of the structures neighboring the IJV is essential because they may be compromised by a misdirected needle. The ICA runs medial to the IJV but, rarely, may lie directly posterior or, rarely, anterior. Behind the ICA, just outside the sheath, lie the stellate ganglion and the cervical sympathetic trunk. The dome of the pleura, which is higher on the left, lies caudal to the junction of the IJV and SCV. Posteriorly, at the root of the neck, course the phrenic and vagus nerves. The thoracic duct lies posterior to the left IJV and enters the superior margin of the SCV near the jugulosubclavian junction. The right lymphatic duct has the same anatomic relationship but is much smaller, and chylous effusions typically occur only with left-sided IJV cannulations.

Technique of Cannulation

The *New England Journal of Medicine* has a step-by-step video showing the process of placing an internal jugular CVC (http://www.nejm.org/doi/full/10.1056/NEJMvcm0810156) [41]. With careful preparation of equipment and attention to patient comfort and safety as described earlier, the patient is placed in a 15-degree Trendelenburg position to distend the vein and minimize the risk of air embolism (Fig. 6.2). The use of ultrasonography to guide IJV catheter insertion is reviewed in Video 6.1. Using ultrasonography and a 7.5- to 10-MHz probe, the operator examines both sides of the neck to examine for an appropriate insertion site and factors that would contraindicate access. The IJV is examined in the transverse scanning plane along its length, and reexamined with compression in order to rule out isoechoic thrombus that would contraindicate venous access. It is recommended the operator holds the probe so that the probe marker is always oriented toward the left side of the operator. When the operator is standing at the patient's head and looking in caudal direction at the patient, the left side of the patient will project to the left side of the screen, given that the screen indicator is to the left on the screen. In this way, movement of the needle tip to the left or right will be seen as corresponding leftward and rightward movements on the screen.

While ipsilateral IJV thrombus is a strong contraindication to venous catheter insertion, the presence of a contralateral thrombus is a relative contraindication to ipsilateral IJV venous access out of concern for the possibility of formation of bilateral IJV thrombosis. Marked respiratory variation of IJV size may occur in the dyspneic patient that may contraindicate insertion attempt. Anatomic variation such as vessel size or position can also be identified with the preprocedure examination.

Before the procedure, the operator examines the anterior chest of the patient in order to rule out pneumothorax. The vascular probe is applied to the anterior chest bilaterally to observe for lung sliding (see Chapter 11 on Lung Ultrasonography). Its presence indicates that there is no pneumothorax before the start of the procedure.

Once an insertion site is identified, the ultrasound machine is positioned such that the operator can visualize the screen with minimal head movement; the line of sight along the needle insertion trajectory is as close as possible to that needed to see the screen. Bedside equipment may need to be moved in order to allow for proper machine positioning. For IJV access, the machine is best positioned contralateral to the planned insertion side with the screen angle adjusted for maximal clarity. The neck is then prepared with chlorhexidine and fully draped, using maximum barrier precautions, including a sterile probe cover with coupling gel. Before the procedure is begun, a time-out is performed. The operator holds the probe in the nondominant hand while examining the lower anterior neck in a transverse scanning plane. The IJV and adjacent carotid artery (CA) are identified, and the position and angle of the probe are adjusted such that the IJV is lateral to the CA, assuming normal anatomy (Fig. 6.3). If the CA is posterior to the IJV, needle insertion at this point into the IJV has high risk of unintentional CA puncture. The CA is usually medial to the IJV, but normal anatomic variants include a medial or posterior position that can only be identified with ultrasonography. Head rotation greater than 40 degrees increases the risk of overlap between the IJV and CA [42]. The most common site for insertion with ultrasonography guidance is toward the apex of the triangle formed by the sternal and clavicular heads of the SCM muscle (Fig. 6.2).

With the probe held over the target area, the target vessel is centered under the midpoint of the probe. Lidocaine is infiltrated with ultrasonography visualization to assure that the needle tract is well anesthetized. The access needle is held with the dominant hand and inserted through the skin at a 45-degree angle at a point corresponding to the center of the probe. The skin entry site is several millimeters from the probe face. As soon as the needle is through the skin, the scanning plane is angled toward the skin insertion site until the needle tip is identified as a hyperechoic structure that moves predictably with movement of the operator's hand. The operator moves the needle forward toward the IJV while angling the scanning plane in order to visualize the advance of the needle tip into the vessel. Blood return into the syringe confirms IV placement of the needle.

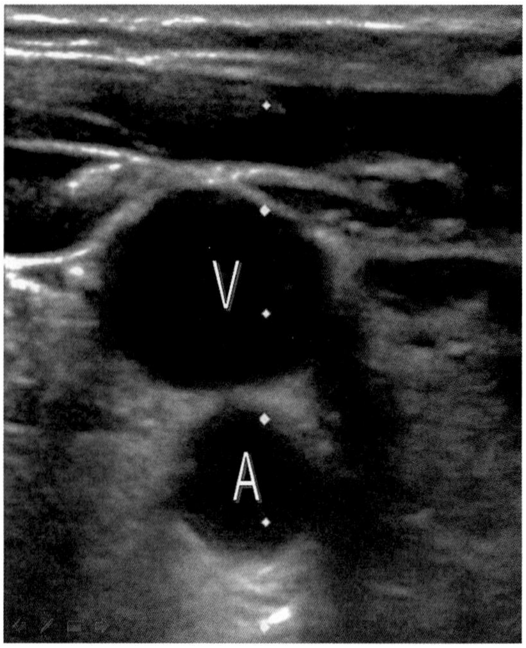

FIGURE 6.3 Ultrasound appearance of the right internal jugular vein and normal relationship with the internal carotid artery.

Some operators prefer to guide the needle using a longitudinal scanning plane while visualizing the needle in its long axis as it approaches and penetrates the IJV. This requires a high level of skill at needle control because the entire needle must be visualized during the insertion. There is no definitive evidence that supports the transverse or longitudinal approach to needle insertion. One problem with the longitudinal approach is that the CA and IJV are parallel to one another. The inexperienced operator may mistake one vessel for the other with risk of unintentional CA puncture. In our experience, the transverse scanning approach is favored by most operators.

Once venipuncture has occurred, the syringe is removed after ensuring that the backflow of blood is not pulsatile, and the hub is then occluded with a finger to prevent air embolism or excessive bleeding. The angle of the needle should be flattened to ensure smooth passage of the guidewire. The guidewire, with the J-tip oriented appropriately, is then inserted and should pass freely up to 20 cm, at which point the thin-wall needle or catheter is withdrawn. The tendency to insert the guidewire deeper than 15 to 20 cm should be avoided because it is the most common cause of ventricular arrhythmias during insertion and also poses a risk for cardiac perforation. Furthermore, if the patient has an inferior vena cava (IVC) filter in place, the guidewire can become entangled in the filter. Occasionally, the guidewire does not pass easily beyond the tip of the thin-wall needle. The guidewire should then be withdrawn, the syringe attached, and free backflow of blood reestablished and maintained, while the syringe and needle are brought to a more parallel plane with the vein. The guidewire should then pass easily. If resistance is still encountered, rotation of the guidewire during insertion often allows passage. If the wire still does not pass, the proceduralist should consider reaccessing the vessel in a different location. If there is concern that there are anatomic or mechanical obstructions (e.g., distal thrombus) preventing the wire from advancing, an alternative site for catheterization should be considered. Excessive force or manipulation leads only to complications.

The guidewire position is checked with ultrasonography before dilation of the insertion tract. This requires definitive identification of the wire in a long-axis view of the IJV. Unintentional passage of the wire into the CA, even when the needle insertion has been performed with ultrasonography guidance, is always a possibility, so checking wire position before dilation increases the safety of the procedure.

Next, a scalpel is used to make a stab incision at the skin entry site to facilitate passage of the vessel dilator. The dilator is inserted over the wire through the subcutaneous tissues and into the vein, ensuring that control and sterility of the guidewire is not compromised. The dilator is then withdrawn, and pressure is used at the puncture site to control bleeding and prevent VAE down the needle tract. Control of the guidewire with one hand while advancing guidewire with the other during dilation will help to minimize kinking of the wire. The catheter is then inserted over the guidewire, ensuring that the operator has control of the guidewire, either proximal or distal to the catheter, at all times to avoid intravascular loss of the wire. The catheter is then advanced 15 to 17 cm (17 to 19 cm for left IJV) into the vein, the guidewire withdrawn, and the distal lumen capped. Then, the proximal and middle lumens of a triple-lumen catheter are flushed with saline and capped. The catheter is sutured securely to limit tip migration and covered with a chlorhexidine-impregnated dressing.

At the end of the procedure, the operator checks for lung sliding in order to rule out pneumothorax. Loss of lung sliding when it was present before the procedure is strong evidence that there is a procedure-related pneumothorax. A chest radiograph should also be obtained to document tip location.

Ultrasonography may be used to confirm CVC position, as an alternative to chest radiography. Following insertion of the CVC, the operator uses the cardiac transducer to visualize the right atrium using the right ventricular inflow, subcostal long-axis, or a modified long-axis IVC view. Using a three-way stopcock and two 10 mL syringes, 10 mL of agitated saline contrast is injected into the distal port of the CVC while the operator is visualizing the right atrium.

The following four patterns result after the injection of the agitated contrast:

1. No contrast enters the atrium. This indicates malposition of the catheter, including the possibility of arterial cannulation.
2. Delayed (<2 seconds) contrast entry into the atrium. This indicates that the catheter is above the level of the SVC.
3. Immediate (>2 seconds) contrast entry into the atrium with laminar flow pattern of contrast into the atrium from the SVC. This indicates appropriate catheter position in the SVC.
4. Immediate contrast opacification of the atrium without laminar flow pattern. This indicates catheter position within the right atrium. This is often confirmed by visualization of the catheter tip in the right atrium.

If there is delayed contrast entry into the atrium, the operator may then examine the IJV and SCV veins to look for aberrant position of the catheter tip in the IJV or the SCV.

The use of agitated saline injection to confirm catheter tip position has been compared with chest radiography with excellent concordance of results. Vezzani et al. described the injection of agitated saline into the CVC in order to confirm appropriate position of the line tip [43]. They observed that appropriate catheter tip position was associated with a laminar inflow pattern of agitated saline contrast into the right atrium from the SVC that occurred within 2 seconds of the injection, whereas right atrial placement was identified by direct visualization of the catheter tip in the right atrium or by immediate opacification of the right atrium instead of a laminar flow pattern characteristic of SVC placement. No contrast entry into the right atrium or delayed entry of contrast indicated malposition of the catheter. Weekes et al. confirmed these results in two additional studies [44,45]. Both investigators also included examination for postprocedure pneumothorax using ultrasonography.

A major limitation of using ultrasonography is that not all patients have adequate cardiac views to permit visualization of the right atrium. In this case, chest radiography is required. Ultrasonography is useful if the results are unequivocal (i.e., if the catheter tip is visualized in the right atrium, if there is immediate nonlaminar opacification of the right atrium, or if there is immediate laminar flow of agitated saline contrast into the right atrium). With any other result, chest radiography is required. Other problems with using ultrasonography to check for the position of the central venous line tip include that the operator must have skill at cardiac ultrasonography and that it adds time to the procedure. Its advantage is that the skilled operator can promptly determine catheter tip position after insertion. Chest radiography has the advantage of simplicity, but the disadvantage of delay.

Success Rates and Complications

The use of direct ultrasound guidance clearly improves the success rate, decreases the number of attempts and complications, avoids unnecessary procedures by identifying unsuitable anatomy, and minimally impacts insertion time compared to the older anatomic techniques.

The overall incidence of complications in IJV catheterization with ultrasound guidance is quite rare; important complications include ICA puncture, pneumothorax, vessel erosion, thrombosis, and infection. In 2006, Karakitsos et al. randomized 900 patients to ultrasound-guided IJV placement versus the use of a landmark technique [46]. Complications with the ultrasound guidance were significantly lower and occurred very rarely with carotid puncture occurring in 1.1% of patients and hematoma in 0.4%. Hemothorax and pneumothorax did not occur in any of the ultrasound-guided IJV lines. In addition, the time and number of attempts was significantly reduced. This technique is an easily learned skill with proper teaching [46]. In the absence of a bleeding diathesis, arterial punctures are usually benign and are managed conservatively by applying local pressure for 10 minutes. Even in the absence of clotting abnormalities, a sizable hematoma may form, preventing further catheterization attempts [47]. Unrecognized arterial puncture can lead to catheterization of the ICA with a large-bore catheter or introducer. Options include pulling the catheter and applying pressure, percutaneous closure devices, internal stent grafting, or surgical repair [48,49]. For unintentional ICA catheters, it is safest to obtain vascular surgery consultation, although often removal of the catheter and holding pressure are the initial treatment of choice.

Pneumothorax, which may be complicated by hemothorax, infusion of IV fluid, or tension, is considered an unusual adverse consequence of IJV cannulation and is extraordinarily rare when the procedure is performed under direct ultrasound guidance [46]. Case reports indicate that any complication from IJV catheterization is possible, although in reality, the IJV route is reliable, with a low incidence of major complications. Operator experience is not as important a factor as in SCV catheterization; the incidence of catheter tip malposition is low, and patient acceptance is high. It is best suited for acute, short-term hemodialysis and for elective or urgent catheterizations, especially pulmonary artery catheterizations and insertion of temporary transvenous pacemakers. It is not the preferred site during airway emergencies, for parenteral nutrition, or for long-term catheterization.

External Jugular Vein Approach

With the advent of real-time ultrasound guidance, the EJV is now rarely used for CVC, but it remains an alternative. A description of the anatomy, the technique, and complications can be found elsewhere [50].

Femoral Vein Approach

The common femoral vein (CFV) has many practical advantages for CVC; it is directly compressible, it is remote from the airway and pleura, the technique is relatively simple, and the Trendelenburg position is not required during insertion. However, owing to increased risks for catheter-related infection compared to other sites, CFV catheters should be avoided wherever possible [10–12].

Anatomy

The FV (Fig. 6.4A) is a direct continuation of the popliteal vein and becomes the external iliac vein at the inguinal ligament. At the inguinal ligament, the CFV lies within the femoral sheath a few centimeters from the skin surface. The CFV lies medial to the femoral artery, which in turn lies medial to the femoral branch of the genitofemoral nerve. The medial compartment contains lymphatic channels and Cloquet node. The external iliac vein courses cephalad from the inguinal ligament along the anterior surface of the iliopsoas muscle to join its counterpart from the other leg and form the IVC anterior to and to the right of the fifth lumbar vertebra. Using ultrasound, the FV can be readily identified by placing the probe a few centimeters caudal to the inguinal ligament, just medial to the arterial pulsation (Fig. 6.4B).

Technique

FV cannulation is the easiest of all central venous procedures to learn and perform. The side chosen is based on the operator convenience. Ultrasound confirms the anatomy, identifies the depth needed for venipuncture, rules out preexisting thrombosis, and can directly guide venipuncture. The use of ultrasonography to guide CFV catheter insertion is reviewed in Video 6.2. The patient is placed in the supine position (if tolerated) with the leg extended and slightly abducted at the hip. Excessive hair should be clipped with scissors and the skin prepped with chlorhexidine. The CFV lies 1 to 1.5 cm medial to the arterial pulsation, and the overlying skin is infiltrated with 1% lidocaine.

The machine is positioned across the bed from the operator, and the screen is set at the appropriate angle. The right-handed operator is best positioned on the right side of the patient in order to be able to use their dominant hand for needle insertion while holding the probe with the left. The opposite applies to the left-handed operator.

Before sterile field preparation, the target area is scanned in its transverse axis to identify any contraindication to central venous access, such as thrombus. The CFV, which is the target vessel, is found medial to the common femoral artery; aberrant anatomy is very uncommon, unlike with the IJV.

Following application of maximum barrier precautions, the CFV is visualized in its transverse axis, and the needle is inserted at a 45-degree angle with constant ultrasonography visualization using the same technique as with IJV access. Needle penetration into the CFV should occur at the level of the inguinal crease. Slightly below this point, the CFV transitions to become the superficial FV that typically lies posterior to the superficial femoral artery. This position strongly contradicts any attempt at venous catheter insertion, out of concern for injury to the overlying artery.

When venous blood return is established, the syringe angle is depressed slightly and free aspiration of blood reconfirmed. The syringe is removed, ensuring that blood return is not pulsatile. The guidewire should pass easily and never forced, although rotation and minor manipulation are sometimes required. The

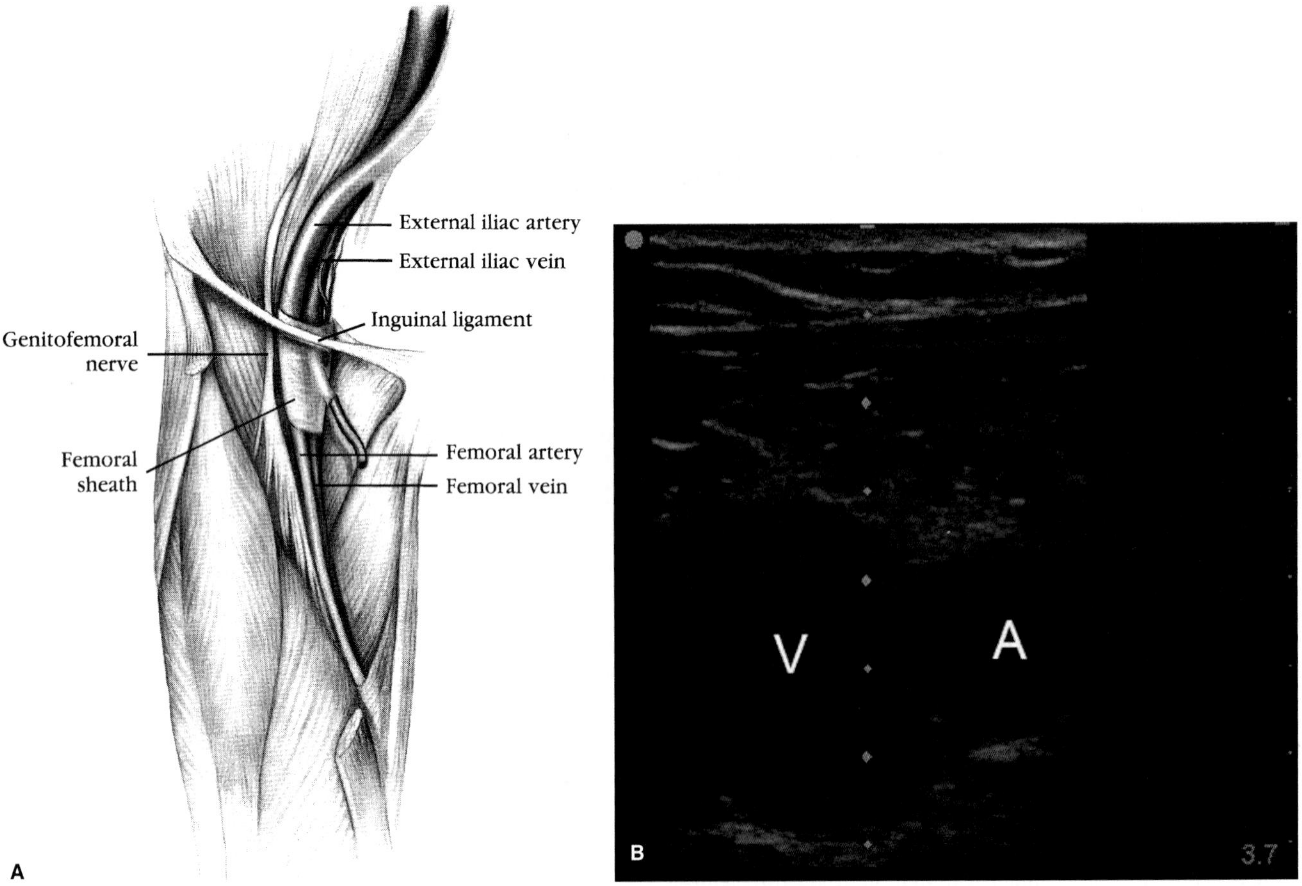

FIGURE 6.4 A: Anatomy of the femoral vein. B: Ultrasound appearance of femoral vein and artery.

needle is then withdrawn, and the wire is visualized with ultrasonography to be in the CFV before dilation and catheter insertion. Beyond direct visualization of the catheter in the vein, injection of agitated saline with rapid opacification of the right atrium using cardiac ultrasonography confirms an IV position of the catheter. The guidewire insertion site is enlarged with a scalpel and the vein dilator inserted over the wire. The dilator is then withdrawn and a catheter appropriate to clinical requirements inserted, taking care never to lose control of the guidewire. The guidewire is removed, the catheter is secured with a suture, and a chlorhexidine dressing is applied.

Success Rate and Complications

FV catheterization is successful in greater than 90% of patients, including those in shock or cardiopulmonary arrest, and has improved with the use of direct ultrasound guidance [51]. Unsuccessful catheterizations are usually a result of venipuncture failure, hematoma formation, or inability to advance the guidewire into the vein. Operator inexperience may increase the number of attempts and complication rate but does not appear to significantly decrease the overall success rate.

Three complications occur regularly with FV catheterization: arterial puncture with or without local bleeding, infection, and thromboembolic events. Other reported complications are rare and include scrotal hemorrhage, right lower quadrant bowel perforation, retroperitoneal hemorrhage, puncture of the kidney, and perforation of IVC tributaries. These complications occur when skin puncture sites are cephalad to the inguinal ligament or when long catheters are threaded into the FV.

Femoral artery puncture occurs in 5% to 10% of adults. Most arterial punctures are uncomplicated, but major hematomas may form in 1% of patients, especially in the presence of anticoagulants, fibrinolytics, or antithrombotic agents. As is the case with other routes, ultrasound significantly reduces the rate of these complications [52]. Even in the presence of coagulopathy, arterial puncture with the 18-gauge thin-wall needle is usually of minor consequence, but there is a potential for life-threatening thigh or retroperitoneal hemorrhage [53]. Arteriovenous fistula and pseudoaneurysm are rare chronic complications of arterial puncture; the former is more likely to occur when both femoral vessels on the same side are cannulated concurrently [54].

Infectious and thrombotic complications with FV catheters are more frequent than with other catheters. Specifically, there is a fourfold increased rate of colonization, and threefold increased risk of CRI [10,12]. As such, the Centers for Disease Control and Prevention guidelines recommend avoidance of the femoral site unless absolutely necessary [11].

Although catheter-associated thrombosis is a risk of all CVCs, regardless of the site of insertion, the risks associated with the femoral site are higher. Compared to the subclavian site, the FV was associated with a 14-fold increased odds ratio for thrombotic complications compared to a subclavian CVC [18]. In addition, lower extremity deep vein thromboses have a higher rate of symptomatic embolization compared to those in the upper extremity [35]. Although there are clearly increased risks associated with the FV approach, this site may be required in difficult clinical circumstances. In summary, available evidence supports the view that the FV may be cannulated safely in critically ill adults. FV catheterizations may be performed during airway emergencies and cardiopulmonary arrest, in patients with coagulopathy, in patients who are unable to lie flat, and for access during renal replacement therapy. The most common major complication during FV catheterization is arterial puncture, although this is minimized by direct ultrasound guidance. As stated earlier, infection is more common particularly when compared to the IJV and SCV and, as such, should be avoided if possible.

Subclavian Vein Approach

This route has been used for central venous access for many years and is associated with the most controversy, largely because of the relatively high incidence of pneumothorax and occasional-associated mortality. With the added safety of ultrasound-guided IJV catheterization, there has been some debate about abandonment of landmark-guided SCV catheterization. Ultrasound guidance is possible with the SCV, but it is more technically demanding and may require a different site for venipuncture [11]. The use of ultrasonography to guide SCV catheter insertion is reviewed in Video 6.3. Given these factors, we still believe the SCV is a valuable alternative in certain situations for experienced operators, who should have a pneumothorax rate well under 1%. Inexperienced operators have a far greater rate of pneumothorax; therefore, in settings where relatively inexperienced physicians perform the majority of CVC, the SCV should be used more selectively with close supervision. The advantages of this route include consistent identifiable landmarks, easier long-term catheter maintenance with a comparably lower rate of infection, and relatively high patient comfort. Assuming an experienced operator is available, the SCV is the preferred site for CVC in patients requiring long-term total parenteral nutrition and in patients with elevated intracranial pressure who require hemodynamic monitoring. It should not be considered the primary choice in the presence of thrombocytopenia (platelets $< 50{,}000$), for acute hemodialysis, or in patients with high PEEP (i.e., >12 cm H_2O).

Anatomy

The SCV is a direct continuation of the axillary vein, beginning at the lateral border of the first rib, extending 3 to 4 cm along the undersurface of the clavicle, and becoming the brachiocephalic vein where it joins the ipsilateral IJV at Pirogoff confluence behind the sternoclavicular articulation (Fig. 6.5). The vein is 1 to 2 cm in diameter, contains a single set of valves just distal to the EJV junction, and is fixed in position directly beneath the clavicle by its fibrous attachments. These attachments prevent collapse of the vein, even with severe volume depletion. Anterior to the vein throughout its course lie the subclavius muscle, clavicle, costoclavicular ligament, pectoralis muscles, and epidermis. Posteriorly, the SCV is separated from the subclavian artery and brachial plexus by the anterior scalenus muscle, which is 10 to 15 mm thick in the adult. Posterior to the medial portion of the SCV are the phrenic nerve and internal mammary artery as they pass into the thorax. Superiorly, the relationships are the skin, platysma, and superficial aponeurosis. Inferiorly, the vein rests on the first rib, Sibson fascia, the cupola of the pleura (0.5 cm behind the vein), and pulmonary apex [50]. The left thoracic duct and right lymphatic duct cross the anterior scalene muscle to join the superior aspect of the SV near its union with the IJV.

The clavicle presents a significant barrier for ultrasound visualization of the SCV, which may mandate using a different approach [11]. Typically, we identify the axillary vein–SCV junction by placing the probe inferior to the clavicle in the deltopectoral groove. We usually initially produce an axial view of the vein by placing the probe in the cranial–caudal direction. The probe is then rotated 90 degrees to produce a longitudinal view of the vein, which is maintained during venipuncture and guidewire insertion (Fig. 6.6). Although this method is often successful, it may be very difficult in patients with obesity, and tends to be more time consuming.

Landmark Technique

Although there are many variations, the SCV may be cannulated using surface landmarks by two basic techniques: infraclavicular [55] approach and supraclavicular approach (Fig. 6.7).

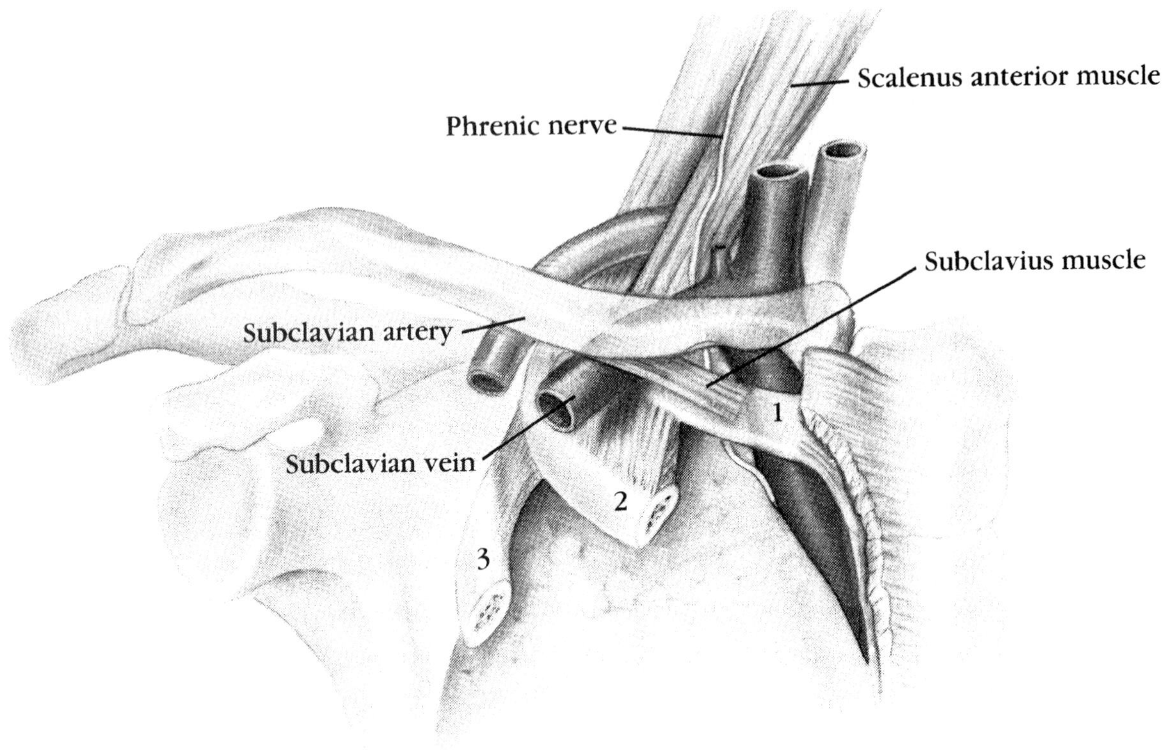

FIGURE 6.5 Anatomy of the subclavian vein and adjacent structures.

The differences in success rate, catheter tip malposition, and complications between the two approaches are negligible, although catheter tip malposition and pneumothorax may be less likely with supraclavicular cannulation [56]. In general, when discussing the success rate and incidence of complications of SV catheterization, there is no need to specify the approach used.

The 18-gauge thin-wall needle is preferable for SCV cannulation. The patient is placed in a 15- to 30-degree Trendelenburg position. Placement of a shoulder roll between the scapulas has been shown to reduce the cross-sectional area of the SCV with ultrasonography imaging. The head is turned slightly to the contralateral side, and the arms are kept to the side. The pertinent landmarks are the clavicle, the two muscle bellies of the SCM, the suprasternal notch, the deltopectoral groove, and the manubriosternal junction. For the infraclavicular approach (Fig. 6.7), the operator is positioned next to the patient's shoulder on the side to be cannulated. For reasons cited earlier, the left SCV should be chosen for pulmonary artery catheterization; otherwise, the success rate appears to be equivalent regardless of the side chosen. Skin puncture is 2 to 3 cm caudal to the clavicle at the deltopectoral groove, corresponding to the area where the clavicle turns from the shoulder to the manubrium. Skin puncture should be distant enough from the clavicle to avoid a downward angle of the needle in clearing the inferior surface of the clavicle, which also obviates any need to bend the needle. The path of the needle is toward the suprasternal notch. Using maximum barrier precautions, the skin is prepped with chlorhexidine. After skin infiltration and liberal injection of the clavicular periosteum with 1% lidocaine and a time-out, the 18-gauge thin-wall needle is mounted on a 10-mL syringe. Skin puncture is accomplished with the needle bevel up, and the needle is advanced in the plane until the tip abuts the clavicle. The needle is then "walked" down the clavicle until the inferior edge is cleared. To avoid pneumothorax, it is imperative the needle stay parallel to the floor and not angle down toward the chest. This is accomplished by using the operator's left thumb to provide downward displacement in the vertical plane after each attempt, until the needle advances under the clavicle.

As the needle is advanced further, the inferior surface of the clavicle should be felt hugging the needle. This ensures that the needle tip is as superior as possible to the pleura. The needle is advanced toward the suprasternal notch during breath holding or expiration, and venipuncture occurs when the needle tip lies beneath the medial end of the clavicle. This may require insertion of the needle to its hub. Blood return may not occur until slow withdrawal of the needle. If venipuncture is not accomplished on the initial attempt, the next attempt should be directed slightly more cephalad. If venipuncture does not occur by the third or fourth attempt, another site should be chosen or another operator should try, because additional attempts are unlikely to be successful and may result in complications.

When blood return is established, the bevel of the needle is rotated 90 degrees toward the heart. The needle is anchored firmly with the left hand, whereas the syringe is detached with the right. Blood return should not be pulsatile, and VAE prophylaxis is necessary at all times. The guidewire is then advanced through the needle to 15 cm and then the needle is withdrawn. To increase the success rate of proper placement of the catheter, the J-wire tip should point inferiorly [57]. The remainder of the procedure is as previously described. Triple-lumen catheters should be sutured at 15 to 16 cm on the right and 17 to 18 cm on the left to avoid intracardiac tip placement [27,58].

For the supraclavicular approach (Fig. 6.7), the important landmarks are the clavicular insertion of the SCM muscle and the sternoclavicular joint. The operator is positioned at the head of the patient on the side to be cannulated. The site of skin puncture is the claviculosternocleidomastoid angle, just above

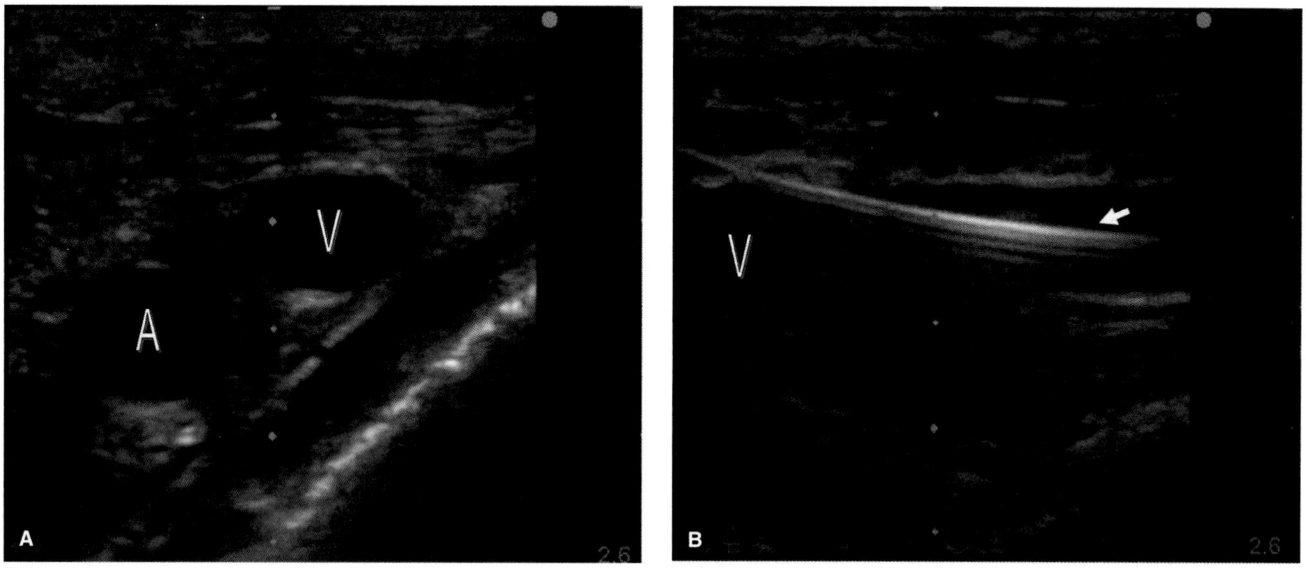

FIGURE 6.6 Ultrasound view of the subclavian vein. **A:** Axial view; **B:** longitudinal view. See text for details.

the clavicle and lateral to the insertion of the clavicular head of the SCM. The needle is advanced toward or just caudal to the contralateral nipple just under the clavicle. This corresponds to a 45-degree angle to the sagittal plane, bisecting a line between the sternoclavicular joint and clavicular insertion of the SCM. The depth of insertion is from just beneath the SCM clavicular head at a 10- to 15-degree angle below the coronal plane. The needle should enter the jugulosubclavian venous bulb after 1 to 4 cm, and the operator may then proceed with catheterization.

Ultrasound Technique

The patient is prepared as previously described. The ultrasound machine is positioned so that the operator can visualize the screen with minimal head movement, and the line of sight along the needle insertion trajectory is as close as possible to that required to see the screen. For SCV access, the machine is best positioned contralateral to the planned insertion directly across the patient with the screen angle adjusted for maximal clarity.

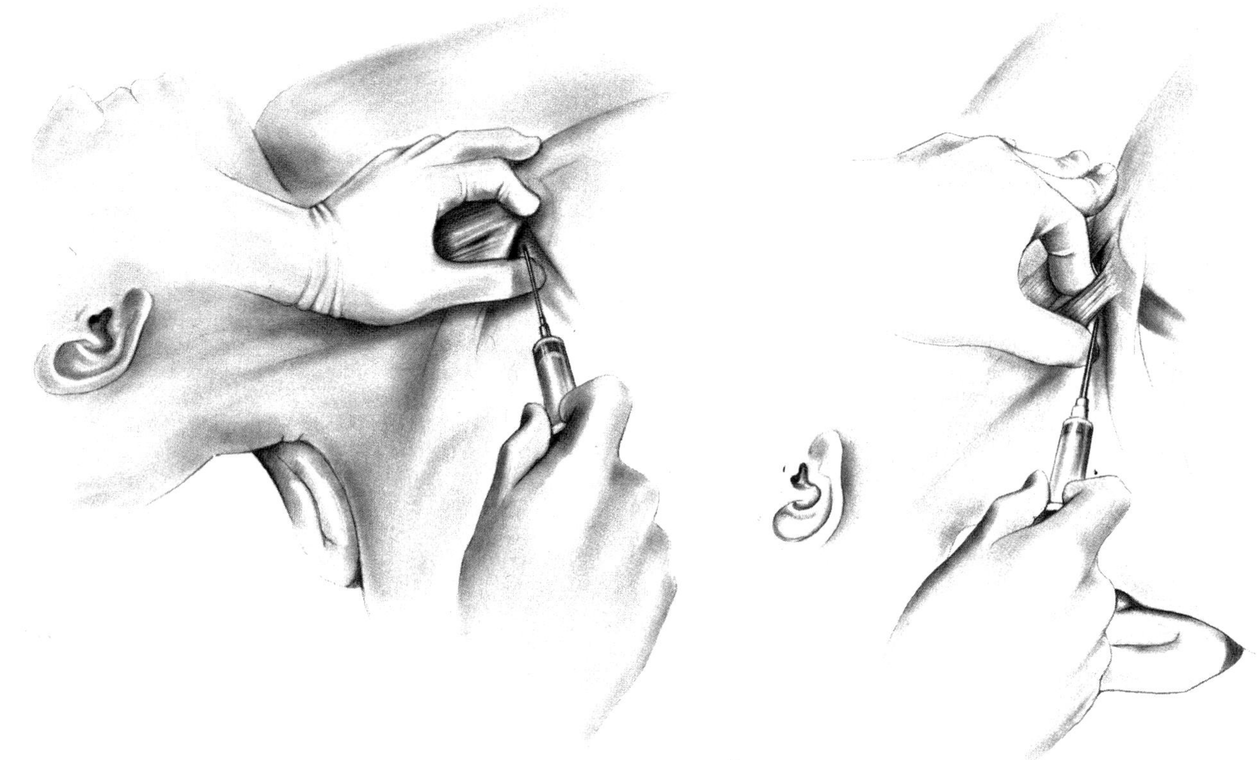

A B

FIGURE 6.7 **A:** Patient positioning for subclavian cannulation. **B:** Cannulation technique for supraclavicular approach.

The operator checks for lung sliding before the procedure to rule out pneumothorax.

Before sterile preparation, the target site is scanned to check for contraindications to IV access, such as thrombus, small size, or excessive respiratory variation. If using the subclavicular approach, the transducer is held in longitudinal orientation and placed on the clavicle using a sagittal scanning plane directed through the medial third of the clavicle. The transducer is then moved laterally on the clavicle until the SCV appears from underneath the clavicle. With further lateral movement of the probe, the target vessel and its paired artery are visualized in the subpectoral area away from the clavicle. The probe is then rotated 90 degrees in order to obtain a long-axis view of the vessel. If using the supraclavicular approach, the transducer is used to examine the supraclavicular area while angling medially. Once the SCV is identified, the transducer is rotated to obtain a view of the structure in longitudinal axis.

Because the SCV may not be as easily compressible as the IJV or FV, it may be difficult to distinguish the SCV from its paired artery. Respiratory variation or the presence of a venous valve is helpful in identifying the SCV. The use of spectral Doppler flow measurements is not recommended unless the operator has expert-level knowledge of Doppler ultrasonography. The use of color Doppler may be useful, because augmentation of color Doppler signal in the SCV occurs if the ipsilateral upper arm is manually compressed by the operator. Distinguishing the artery from the vein is a key element of performing safe SCV cannulation because the two structures are in close proximity.

Following the application of maximum barrier precautions, the vessel is visualized in its longitudinal axis, and the needle inserted with direct visualization of the entire needle throughout its insertion trajectory. Upon blood return into the syringe, the syringe is removed, and the wire is inserted. The operator holds the probe with their nondominant hand, whereas the needle and syringe are guided by the dominant hand. Some operators prefer to perform needle insertion using ultrasonography guidance with the vessel visualized in its transverse axis (longitudinal scanning plane). In this case, the needle tip is tracked real time, while it is moved forward into the vessel.

Before the dilation of the wire tract, the wire is confirmed to be in the SCV. It may be more difficult to image the wire in the SCV than with the IJV. Scanning from the supraclavicular approach may be helpful in checking for proper wire position. The remainder of the catheter insertion is as described previously. The operator checks for lung sliding in order to rule out procedure-related pneumothorax.

Although there is literature that supports the utility of ultrasonography for SCV venous access, there is consensus that it is difficult to master the technique. Unlike IJV and FV access, where the transverse axis approach is favored, SCV venous access requires that the operator be skilled at controlling the needle in its longitudinal axis. This requires precise insertion of the needle in the midpoint of the short axis of the probe. This may be challenging when the probe cover blocks clear view of the midpoint. In obese or edematous patients, the probe needs to be pressed into the chest tissue, with further difficulty in selecting the initial needle entry site. Even minimal deviation from the narrow tomographic plane of the probe may result in the operator losing control of the needle tip and mistaking the body of the needle for the tip, resulting in injury to the adjacent pleura or artery. Another challenge is maintaining a constant view of the target vessel in longitudinal axis while simultaneously keeping the entire needle in view while it is moved toward the target vessel. For the inexperienced operator, we recommend repeated deliberate practice on a vascular access model before the first closely supervised attempt on a patient. Subclavian venous access with landmark technique uses the clavicle as a definitive guide to successful cannulation, whereas ultrasonography does not. This requires the operator to rely totally on the ultrasonography image for guidance, and to discount the clavicle as a relevant landmark. When using ultrasonography for needle guidance into the SCV, the needle entry site is often more lateral and at a steeper angle than with the landmark technique. Initially, this may be disconcerting to the operator who is used to using landmark technique.

Success and Complication Rates

SCV catheterization is successful in 90% to 95% of cases, generally on the first attempt [59]. Unsuccessful catheterizations are a result of venipuncture failure or inability to advance the guidewire or catheter. Catheter tip malposition occurs in 5% to 20% of cases and tends to be more frequent with the infraclavicular approach. Malposition occurs most commonly to the ipsilateral IJV and contralateral SCV and is usually correctable without repeat venipuncture.

The overall incidence of noninfectious complications varies depending on the operator experience and the circumstances under which the catheter is inserted. Large series involving several thousand SCV catheters have reported an incidence of major complications of 1% to 3% [60]. Factors resulting in a higher complication rate are operator inexperience, multiple attempts at venipuncture, emergency conditions, variance from standardized technique, and body mass index. Major noninfectious complications include pneumothorax, arterial puncture, and thromboembolism. There are many case reports of isolated major complications involving neck structures or the brachial plexus; the reader is referred elsewhere for a complete listing of reported complications [60].

Pneumothorax accounts for one-fourth to one-half of reported complications, with an incidence of about 1.5%. The incidence varies inversely with the operator experience [60]. There is no magic figure whereby an operator matures from inexperienced to experienced. Fifty catheterizations are cited frequently as a cutoff number, but it is reasonable to expect an operator to be satisfactorily experienced after having performed fewer. For the experienced operator, a pneumothorax incidence of less than 1% is expected [61]. Most pneumothoraces are a result of lung puncture at the time of the procedure, but late-appearing pneumothoraces have been reported.

Approach to the treatment of pneumothoraces depends on the size of the defect. Many will require thoracostomy tube drainage with a small chest tube and a Heimlich valve, but some can be managed conservatively with 100% oxygen and serial radiographs or needle aspiration only [62]. Rarely, a pneumothorax is complicated by tension, hemothorax, infusion of IV fluid (immediately or days to weeks after catheter placement), chyle, or massive subcutaneous emphysema. Bilateral pneumothoraces can occur from unilateral attempts at venipuncture. Pneumothorax can result in death, especially when it goes unrecognized [63].

Subclavian artery puncture occurs in 0.5% to 1.0% of cases, constituting one-fourth to one-third of all complications. Arterial puncture is usually managed easily by applying pressure above and below the clavicle. Bleeding can be catastrophic in patients with coagulopathy, especially thrombocytopenia. As with other routes, arterial puncture may result in arteriovenous fistula or pseudoaneurysm [12,60].

Clinical evidence of central venous thrombosis, including SVC syndrome, development of collaterals around the shoulder girdle, and pulmonary embolism, is very rare occurring in 0% to 3% of SCV catheterizations, but routine phlebography performed at catheter removal reveals a much higher incidence of thrombotic phenomena. The importance of the discrepancy between clinical symptoms and radiologic findings is unknown, but upper extremity thrombosis, even if asymptomatic, is not a totally benign condition [61]. Duration of catheterization, catheter material, and patient condition probably impact the frequency of thrombosis, but to an uncertain degree.

In summary, the SCV is an extremely reliable and useful route for CVC, but because of the relatively high rate of pneumothorax and the increased success rate of ultrasound-guided IJV catheterization, its use should be limited to those operators skilled in the technique. Inexperienced operators should use an alternative site except with close supervision. Experienced operators should continue to use this route for certain indications (Table 6.1), but should scrupulously avoid it in patients who cannot tolerate a pneumothorax (severe lung disease, one lung), or in patients with severe coagulopathy, especially platelets <50,000.

ACKNOWLEDGMENTS

The authors thanked Michael G. Seneff, MD who contributed to previous editions of this chapter.

References

1. Pronovost P, Needham D, Berenholtz S, et al: An intervention to decrease catheter-related bloodstream infections in the ICU. *N Engl J Med* 355(26): 2725–2732, 2006. doi: 10.1056/NEJMoa061115.
2. Barsuk JH, McGaghie WC, Cohen ER, et al: Simulation-based mastery learning reduces complications during central venous catheter insertion in a medical intensive care unit. *Crit Care Med* 37(10):2697–2701, 2009.
3. Weiner MM, Geldard P, Mittnacht AJC: Ultrasound-guided vascular access: a comprehensive review. *J Cardiothorac Vasc Anesth* 27(2):345–360, 2013. doi: 10.1053/j.jvca.2012.07.007.
4. Airapetian N, Maizel J, Langelle F, et al: Ultrasound-guided central venous cannulation is superior to quick-look ultrasound and landmark methods among inexperienced operators: a prospective randomized study. *Intensive Care Med* 39(11):1938–1944, 2013. doi: 10.1007/s00134-013-3072-z.
5. Milling TJ, Rose J, Briggs WM, et al: Randomized, controlled clinical trial of point-of-care limited ultrasonography assistance of central venous cannulation: the Third Sonography Outcomes Assessment Program (SOAP-3) Trial. *Crit Care Med* 33(8):1764–1769, 2005.
6. Sandhu NS: Transpectoral ultrasound-guided catheterization of the axillary vein: an alternative to standard catheterization of the subclavian vein. *Anesth Analg* 99(1):183–187, 2004.
7. Graber D, Dailey RH: Catheter flow rates updated. *J Am Coll Emerg Physicians* 6:518, 1977.
8. Horattas MC, Trupiano J, Hopkins S, et al: Changing concepts in long-term central venous access: catheter selection and cost savings. *Am J Infect Control* 29(1):32–40, 2001. doi: 10.1067/mic.2001.111536.
9. Schwab SJ, Quarles LD, Middleton JP, et al: Hemodialysis-associated subclavian vein stenosis. *Kidney Int* 33(6):1156–1159, 1988.
10. Parienti J-J, Thirion M, Mégarbane B, et al: Femoral vs jugular venous catheterization and risk of nosocomial events in adults requiring acute renal replacement therapy: a randomized controlled trial. *JAMA* 299(20):2413–2422, 2008. doi: 10.1001/jama.299.20.2413.
11. O'Grady NP, Alexander M, Burns LA, et al: Summary of recommendations: guidelines for the Prevention of Intravascular Catheter-related Infections. *Clin Infect Dis Off Publ Infect Dis Soc Am* 52(9):1087–1099, 2011. doi: 10.1093/cid/cir138.
12. Merrer J, De Jonghe B, Golliot F, et al: Complications of femoral and subclavian venous catheterization in critically ill patients: a randomized controlled trial. *JAMA* 286(6):700–707, 2001.
13. Doerfler ME, Kaufman B, Goldenberg AS: Central venous catheter placement in patients with disorders of hemostasis. *Chest* 110(1):185–188, 1996.
14. Muth CM, Shank ES: Gas embolism. *N Engl J Med* 342(7):476–482, 2000. doi: 10.1056/NEJM200002173420706.
15. Vailati D, Lamperti M, Subert M, et al: An ultrasound study of cerebral venous drainage after internal jugular vein catheterization. *Crit Care Res Pract* 2012:685481, 2012. doi: 10.1155/2012/685481.
16. Emerman CL, Pinchak AC, Hancock D, et al: Effect of injection site on circulation times during cardiac arrest. *Crit Care Med* 16(11):1138–1141, 1988.
17. Reades R, Studnek JR, Vandeventer S, et al: Intraosseous versus intravenous vascular access during out-of-hospital cardiac arrest: a randomized controlled trial. *Ann Emerg Med* 58(6):509–516, 2011. doi: 10.1016/j.annemergmed.2011.07.020.
18. ARISE Investigators, ANZICS Clinical Trials Group; Peake SL, et al: Goal-directed resuscitation for patients with early septic shock. *N Engl J Med* 371(16):1496–1506, 2014. doi: 10.1056/NEJMoa1404380.
19. ProCESS Investigators; Yealy DM, Kellum JA, Huang DT, et al: A randomized trial of protocol-based care for early septic shock. *N Engl J Med* 370(18):1683–1693, 2014. doi: 10.1056/NEJMoa1401602.
20. Stuke L, Jennings A, Gunst M, et al: Universal consent practice in academic intensive care units (ICUs). *J Intensive Care Med* 25(1):46–52, 2010. doi: 10.1177/0885066609350982.
21. Schenker Y, Meisel A: Informed consent in clinical care: practical considerations in the effort to achieve ethical goals. *JAMA* 305(11):1130–1131, 2011. doi: 10.1001/jama.2011.333.
22. Stone MB, Nagdev A, Murphy MC, et al: Ultrasound detection of guidewire position during central venous catheterization. *Am J Emerg Med* 28(1):82–84, 2010. doi: 10.1016/j.ajem.2008.09.019.
23. Harting BP, Talbot TR, Dellit TH, et al: University HealthSystem Consortium quality performance benchmarking study of the insertion and care of central venous catheters. *Infect Control Hosp Epidemiol* 29(5):440–442, 2008. doi: 10.1086/587716.
24. Long R, Kassum D, Donen N, et al: Cardiac tamponade complicating central venous catheterization for total parenteral nutrition: a review. *J Crit Care* 2:39, 1987.
25. Curelaru I, Linder LE, Gustavsson B: Displacement of catheters inserted through internal jugular veins with neck flexion and extension. A preliminary study. *Intensive Care Med* 6:179, 1980.
26. Kusminsky RE: Complications of central venous catheterization. *J Am Coll Surg* 204(4):681–696, 2007. doi: 10.1016/j.jamcollsurg.2007.01.039.
27. Andrews RT, Bova DA, Venbrux AC: How much guidewire is too much? Direct measurement of the distance from subclavian and internal jugular vein access sites to the superior vena cava-atrial junction during central venous catheter placement. *Crit Care Med* 28(1):138–142, 2000.
28. Aslamy Z, Dewald CL, Heffner JE: MRI of central venous anatomy: implications for central venous catheter insertion. *Chest* 114(3):820–826, 1998.
29. Walshe C, Phelan D, Bourke J, et al: Vascular erosion by central venous catheters used for total parenteral nutrition. *Intensive Care Med* 33(3):534–537, 2007. doi: 10.1007/s00134-006-0507-9.
30. Duntley P, Siever J, Korwes ML, et al: Vascular erosion by central venous catheters. Clinical features and outcome. *Chest* 101(6):1633–1638, 1992.
31. Mirski MA, Lele AV, Fitzsimmons L, et al: Diagnosis and treatment of vascular air embolism. *Anesthesiology* 106(1):164–177, 2007.
32. Ely EW, Hite RD, Baker AM, et al: Venous air embolism from central venous catheterization: a need for increased physician awareness. *Crit Care Med* 27(10):2113–2117, 1999.
33. Kander T, Frigyesi A, Kjeldsen-Kragh J, et al: Bleeding complications after central line insertions: relevance of pre-procedure coagulation tests and institutional transfusion policy. *Acta Anaesthesiol Scand* 57(5):573–579, 2013. doi: 10.1111/aas.12075.
34. Muñoz FJ, Mismetti P, Poggio R, et al: Clinical outcome of patients with upper-extremity deep vein thrombosis: results from the RIETE Registry. *Chest* 133(1):143–148, 2008. doi: 10.1378/chest.07-1432.
35. Engelberger RP, Kucher N: Management of deep vein thrombosis of the upper extremity. *Circulation* 126(6):768–773, 2012. doi:10.1161/CIRCULATIONAHA.111.051276.
36. Timsit JF, Farkas JC, Boyer JM, et al: Central vein catheter-related thrombosis in intensive care patients: incidence, risks factors, and relationship with catheter-related sepsis. *Chest* 114(1):207–213, 1998.
37. Centers for Disease Control and Prevention (CDC): Vital signs: Central line—associated blood stream infections—United States, 2001, 2008, and 2009. *MMWR* 60(08):243–248.
38. Ng PK, Ault MJ, Maldonado LS: Peripherally inserted central catheters in the intensive care unit. *J Intensive Care Med* 11(1):49–54, 1996.
39. Duerksen DR, Papineau N, Siemens J, et al: Peripherally inserted central catheters for parenteral nutrition: a comparison with centrally inserted catheters. *JPEN J Parenter Enteral Nutr* 23(2):85–89, 1999.
40. Malatinský J, Faybík M, Griffith M, et al: Venepuncture, catheterization and failure to position correctly during central venous cannulation. *Resuscitation* 10(4):259–270, 1983.
41. Ortega R, Song M, Hansen CJ, et al: Ultrasound-guided internal jugular vein cannulation. *N Engl J Med* 362(16):e57, 2010. doi: 10.1056/NEJMvcm0810156.
42. Sulek CA, Gravenstein N, Bleackshear RH, et al: Head rotation during internal jugular cannulation and the risk of carotid artery puncture. *Anesth Analg* 82:125–128, 1996.
43. Vezzani A, Brusasco C, Palermo S, et al: Ultrasound localization of central vein catheter and detection of postprocedural pneumothorax: an alternative to chest radiography. *Crit Care Med* 38:533–538, 2010.
44. Weekes AJ, Johnson DA, Keller SM, et al: Central vascular catheter placement evaluation using saline flush and bedside echocardiography. *Acad Emerg Med* 21:65–72, 2014.
45. Weekes AJ, Keller SM, Efune B, et al: Prospective comparison of ultrasound and CXR for confirmation of central vascular catheter placement. *Emerg Med J* 33(3):176–180, 2016.
46. Karakitsos D, Labropoulos N, Groot ED, et al: Real-time ultrasound-guided catheterisation of the internal jugular vein: a prospective comparison with the landmark technique in critical care patients. *Crit Care* 10(6):R162, 2006. doi: 10.1186/cc5101.
47. Oliver WC, Nuttall GA, Beynen FM, et al: The incidence of artery puncture with central venous cannulation using a modified technique for detection and prevention of arterial cannulation. *J Cardiothorac Vasc Anesth* 11(7):851–855, 1997.
48. Nicholson T, Ettles D, Robinson G: Managing inadvertent arterial catheterization during central venous access procedures. *Cardiovasc Intervent Radiol* 27(1):21–25, 2004.

49. Shah PM, Babu SC, Goyal A, et al: Arterial misplacement of large-caliber cannulas during jugular vein catheterization: case for surgical management. *J Am Coll Surg* 198(6):939–944, 2004. doi: 10.1016/j.jamcollsurg.2004.02.015.
50. Irwin RS, Rippe JM (eds): Irwin and Rippe's intensive care medicine, in *External Jugular Vein Approach*. 7th ed. Lippincott Williams and Wilkins, 2012.
51. Deshpande KS, Hatem C, Ulrich HL, et al: The incidence of infectious complications of central venous catheters at the subclavian, internal jugular, and femoral sites in an intensive care unit population. *Crit Care Med* 33(1):13–20, 2005; discussion 234-235.
52. Prabhu MV, Juneja D, Gopal PB, et al: Ultrasound-guided femoral dialysis access placement: a single-center randomized trial. *Clin J Am Soc Nephrol* 5(2):235–239, 2010. doi: 10.2215/CJN.04920709.
53. Dailey RH: Femoral vein cannulation: a review. *J Emerg Med* 2(5):367–372, 1985.
54. Sharp KW, Spees EK, Selby LR, et al: Diagnosis and management of retroperitoneal hematomas after femoral vein cannulation for hemodialysis. *Surgery* 95(1):90–95, 1984.
55. Moosman DA: The anatomy of infraclavicular subclavian vein catheterization and its complications. *Surg Gynecol Obstet* 136(1):71–74, 1973.
56. Dronen S, Thompson B, Nowak R, et al: Subclavian vein catheterization during cardiopulmonary resuscitation. A prospective comparison of the supraclavicular and infraclavicular percutaneous approaches. *JAMA* 247(23):3227–3230, 1982.
57. Park H-P, Jeon Y, Hwang J-W, et al: Influence of orientations of guidewire tip on the placement of subclavian venous catheters. *Acta Anaesthesiol Scand* 49(10):1460–1463, 2005. doi: 10.1111/j.1399-6576.2005.00758.x.
58. McGee WT, Ackerman BL, Rouben LR, et al: Accurate placement of central venous catheters: a prospective, randomized, multicenter trial. *Crit Care Med* 21(8):1118–1123, 1993.
59. Seneff MG: Central venous catheterization: a comprehensive review. *J Intensive Care Med* 2:218, 1987.
60. Mansfield PF, Hohn DC, Fornage BD, et al: Complications and failures of subclavian-vein catheterization. *N Engl J Med* 331(26):1735–1738, 1994. doi: 10.1056/NEJM199412293312602.
61. Taylor RW, Palagiri AV: Central venous catheterization. *Crit Care Med* 35(5):1390–1396, 2007. doi: 10.1097/01.CCM.0000260241.80346.1B.
62. Laronga C, Meric F, Truong MT, et al: A treatment algorithm for pneumothoraces complicating central venous catheter insertion. *Am J Surg* 180(6):523–526, 2000; discussion 526-527.
63. Despars JA, Sassoon CS, Light RW: Significance of iatrogenic pneumothoraces. *Chest* 105(4):1147–1150, 1994.

Chapter 7 ▪ Arterial Line Placement and Care

CARLOS MARTINEZ-BALZANO • SCOTT E. KOPEC

Arterial catheterization remains an extremely important skill for the critical care physician. Arterial catheters are frequently required for close blood pressure monitoring of the hemodynamically unstable patient and for repeated arterial blood gas sampling for patients with respiratory failure or acid–base disorders. Newer technologies that necessitate arterial access continue to mature. In this sense, arterial pulse contour analysis can be used to predict fluid responsiveness and compute cardiac output (CO) reliably and less invasively for appropriately selected patients [1]. Although advancements of noninvasive technology, such as transcutaneous PCO_2 monitoring and pulse oximetry, may decrease the need for arterial catheter placement, intensivists need to be proficient with the insertion and interpretation of arterial catheter systems. In this chapter, we review the principles of hemodynamic monitoring and discuss the indications, insertion techniques, management, and complications of arterial cannulation.

INDICATIONS FOR ARTERIAL CANNULATION

Arterial catheters should be inserted only when they are specifically required and removed immediately when no longer needed. Too often they are left in place for convenience to allow easy access to blood sampling, which leads to increased laboratory testing and excessive diagnostic blood loss (DBL) [2,3], as well as an increased risk of infection. It should be noted that there are no large prospective clinical trials addressing the question of whether arterial cannulation influences mortality of intensive care unit (ICU) patients.

The indications for arterial cannulation can be grouped into three broad categories (Table 7.1): (1) hemodynamic monitoring (blood pressure and/or CO/pulse contour analysis); (2) frequent arterial blood gas sampling; (3) diagnostic or therapeutic interventions, including intra-aortic balloon pump (IABP) use and arterial administration of drugs, and procedures such as vascular stenting or embolization.

Noninvasive, indirect blood pressure measurements determined by auscultation of Korotkoff sounds distal to an occluding cuff (Riva–Rocci method) are generally accurate, although systolic readings are consistently lower compared to a simultaneous direct measurement. Although noninvasive blood pressure measurements are satisfactory for a majority of ICU patients, in very critically ill patients indirect techniques may provide grossly inaccurate blood pressure readings. Automated noninvasive oscillometric blood pressure measurement devices can also be inaccurate, providing discrepant readings of ≥10 mm Hg when compared to direct arterial measurements of critically ill patients [4,5]. The proprietary algorithms of these devices are in part to blame, and although their adjustment can result in higher accuracy, they still render imprecise measurements for an unacceptably high number of patients [6]. Based on these findings, and the fact that each automated device has a different proprietary algorithm that may not be validated for all ICU patients, the routine use of oscillometric devices cannot be recommended for all highest acuity critically ill patients, and for patients with severe hemodynamic instability.

Arterial catheterization allows monitoring of beat-to-beat changes and prompt initiation of appropriate therapeutic

TABLE 7.1

Indications for Arterial Cannulation

- Hemodynamic monitoring
  - Acutely hypertensive or hypotensive states
  - Assessment of the effects of vasoactive drugs (vasodilators or vasoconstrictors)
  - Continuous cardiac output monitoring
- Repeated blood sampling
  - Frequent blood gas sampling of patients with acute respiratory failure and/or receiving mechanical ventilation
  - Evaluation and management of acid–base disorders
  - Limited vascular access
- Diagnostic or therapeutic procedures
  - Administration of intra-arterial drugs
  - Vascular stenting
  - Intra-aortic balloon pump use
  - Arterial embolization

modalities; variations in individual pressure waveforms can also be diagnostic. Waveform inspection can rapidly diagnose electrocardiogram lead disconnection, indicate the presence of aortic valvular disease, help determine the effect of dysrhythmias on perfusion, and reveal the impact of the respiratory cycle on blood pressure (pulsus paradoxus). In addition, for mechanically ventilated patients, responsiveness to fluid boluses may be predicted by calculating the systolic pressure variation (SPV) or pulse pressure variation (PPV) from the arterial waveform, and stroke volume variation from the pulse contour analysis. For patients on mechanical ventilation, all of these techniques have been shown to predict, with a high degree of accuracy, the likelihood of responding (with an increase in stroke volume) to a fluid volume challenge [1]. It should be noted that all of these patients were well sedated, on a mechanical ventilation mode different from pressure support and receiving a tidal volume between 8 and 10 mL per kg of ideal body weight [1]. Lower tidal volumes, patient movement, and dysrhythmias could affect the accuracy of this diagnostic intervention.

CO can be monitored continuously using calibrated arterial pulse contour analysis. This method relies on the assumption that the contour of the arterial pressure waveform is proportional to the stroke volume [7,8]. This, however, does not take into consideration the differing impedances among the arteries of individuals under different disease states and, therefore, requires calibration with another method of CO determination [8]. This is usually done with the indicator dilution or transpulmonary thermodilution technique [8].

Uncalibrated pulse contour analysis devices, which do not use an additional method of determining CO, are available. They estimate impedance based upon a proprietary formula that uses waveform and patient demographic data [8,9]. This method has significant limitations (i.e., atrial fibrillation) and can provide inaccurate CO estimations for many critically ill patients [8,9].

Management of complicated patients in critical care units typically requires multiple laboratory and arterial blood gas determinations. In these situations, arterial cannulation facilitates obtaining laboratory tests without repeated needle sticks and vessel trauma. In our opinion, an arterial catheter for blood gas determination is justified when a patient requires two or more measurements daily.

EQUIPMENT, MONITORING, TECHNIQUES, AND SOURCES OF ERROR

The equipment necessary to display and measure an arterial waveform includes (a) an appropriate intra-arterial catheter, (b) fluid-filled tubing with stopcocks (ideally, it should be short and noncompliant), (c) a transducer, (d) a constant flush device with a fluid bag pressurized to 300 mm Hg, and (e) electronic monitoring equipment (signal processor, amplifier, and display). Using this equipment, intra-arterial pressure changes are transmitted through the hydraulic (fluid-filled) elements to the transducer, which converts mechanical displacement into a proportional electrical signal. This signal is amplified, processed, and displayed as a waveform by the monitor. Undistorted presentation of the arterial waveform depends on the performance of each component and an understanding of potential problems that can interfere with the overall fidelity of the system.

The major problems inherent to pressure monitoring with a catheter system are inadequate dynamic response, improper zeroing and leveling, zero drift, and improper transducer/monitor calibration. Most physicians are aware of zeroing and leveling techniques but do not appreciate the importance of dynamic response for ensuring system fidelity. Catheter-tubing-transducer systems used for pressure monitoring can best be characterized as underdamped second-order dynamic systems with mechanical parameters of elasticity, mass, and friction [10]. Overall, the dynamic response of such a system is determined by its natural frequency and damping coefficient.

Every system has a frequency at which it oscillates freely: the natural frequency. When an external force of similar frequency to the natural frequency is applied to a system, it will begin to oscillate at its maximum amplitude, a phenomenon called resonance. If the arterial pressure waveform approaches the natural frequency of the blood pressure measuring system, it will resonate causing progressive amplification of the output signal, and erroneously elevated blood pressure readings, particularly systolic, will result [11]. To ensure a flat frequency response (accurate recording across a spectrum of frequencies), the natural frequency of a monitoring system should be at least five times higher than the highest frequency in the input signal [10]. The natural frequency of a system may be increased by reducing its length, reducing its compliance, reducing its density, and increasing its diameter.

Physiologic peripheral arterial waveforms have a fundamental frequency of 3 to 5 Hz and therefore, the natural frequency of a system used to monitor arterial pressure should ideally be greater than 20 Hz to avoid resonance and systolic overshoot. The system component most likely to cause amplification of a pressure waveform is the hydraulic element. A good hydraulic system will have a natural frequency between 10 and 20 Hz, which may overlap with arterial pressure frequencies. Thus, amplification can occur, which may require damping to accurately reproduce the waveform [12].

The damping coefficient is a measure of how quickly an oscillating system dissipates energy and comes to rest. A system with a high damping coefficient dissipates mechanical energy well, causing a diminution in the transmitted waveform. Conversely, a system with a low damping coefficient results in underdamping and overestimation of systolic pressures. The damping coefficient of a system is increased by increasing its viscosity, increasing its density, decreasing its diameter, increasing its length, or decreasing its elasticity. Damping coefficient and natural frequency together determine the dynamic response of a recording system. If the natural frequency of a system is less than 7.5 Hz, the pressure waveform will be distorted no matter what the damping coefficient is. On the other hand, a natural frequency of 24 Hz allows a range in the damping coefficient of 0.15 to 1.1, without resultant distortion of the pressure waveform [10].

Although there are other techniques [13], the easiest method to test the damping coefficient and natural frequency of a monitoring system is the fast-flush test (also known as the square wave test). This is performed at the bedside by briefly opening and closing the continuous flush device, which exposes the system to a flush of fluid, with a pressure of 300 mm Hg producing a square wave displacement on the monitor followed by a few smaller oscillations and a return to baseline (Fig. 7.1). An optimal fast-flush test results in one undershoot followed by a small overshoot and then settles to the patient's waveform. The natural frequency is determined by dividing the paper or display speed by the interval between two successive oscillations. The damping coefficient can be calculated by measuring two successive peak amplitudes and determining their ratio. This ratio is then converted to the damping coefficient by equation or by matching it to published graphs and charts [10].

For peripheral pulse pressure monitoring, an adequate fast-flush test usually corresponds to a natural frequency of 10 to 20 Hz coupled with a damping coefficient of 0.5 to 0.7. To ensure the continuing fidelity of a monitoring system, dynamic response validation by fast-flush test should be performed frequently: at least every 8 hours, with every significant change in patient hemodynamic status, after each opening of the system (zeroing, blood sampling, tubing change), and whenever the waveform appears damped [10].

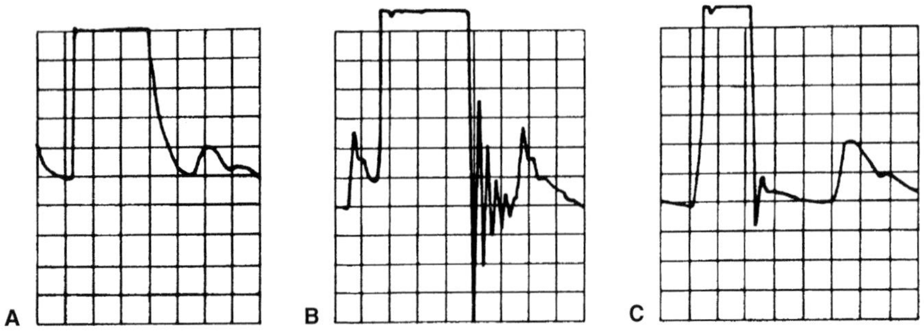

FIGURE 7.1 Fast-flush test. A: Overdamped system. B: Underdamped system. C: Optimal damping.

With consideration of the above concepts, the critical reader would note that many of the factors that increase the damping coefficient can decrease the natural frequency, and vice versa, producing effects that might be considered paradoxical. The interaction between damping coefficient and natural frequency is indeed complex and an exhaustive review of their physical characteristics is beyond the scope of this chapter. A more detailed discussion regarding hemodynamic waveforms can be found elsewhere [14]. However, we should emphasize that most components of the commercial monitoring systems are designed to optimize the frequency response of the entire system and that most clinically relevant effects of damping on the pressure waveform can be explained by the following examples.

Overdamped tracings (Fig. 7.1A) are usually caused by problems that are correctable, such as large air bubbles, tube or catheter kinks, clot formation, loose connections, a deflated pressure bag, or anatomic factors affecting the catheter (vasoconstriction). Catheter kinks can be fixed quickly by straightening the tubing, and thrombus occlusion can be rectified by flushing, usually. Air bubbles in the tubing and connecting stopcocks can be cleared by flushing through a stopcock. Loose connections and deflated pressure bags can be reconnected or replaced.

Underdamped tracings are common and have been seen in approximately 30% of selected patients admitted to the ICU [15]. An underdamped tracing results in resonance and systolic overshoot (Fig 7.1B) and is commonly secondary to excessive tubing length. Standard, noncompliant tubing is provided with most disposable transducer kits and should be as short as possible to minimize signal amplification [11]. The 18- and 20-gauge catheters used to gain arterial access were not considered to be a major source of distortion in the past, but a recent study showed that underdamping/resonance is associated with radial artery catheters with larger length and diameter (10 cm and 0.8 mm, respectively) and that the placement of a 20-gauge cannula (8 cm length and 0.6 mm diameter) decreases this phenomenon [15]. Other factors associated with underdamping are the presence of polydistrectual arteriopathy, chronic obstructive pulmonary disease, and arterial hypertension [15]. Increased sedation decreases underdamping [15].

Currently available disposable transducers incorporate microchip technology, are very reliable, and have relatively high resonant frequencies [16]. The transducer is attached to the electronic monitoring equipment by a cable. Modern monitors have internal calibration, filter artifacts, and print the display on request. The digital readout display is usually an average of values over time and therefore does not accurately represent beat-to-beat variability. Monitors provide the capability to freeze a display with on-screen calibration to measure beat-to-beat differences in amplitude precisely. This allows measurement of the effect of ectopic beats on blood pressure, PPV, SPV, or assessment of the presence and severity of pulsus paradoxus.

For the transducer to work accurately, atmospheric pressure and hydrostatic pressure (pressure exerted by the blood column) should be corrected for by zeroing and leveling the system. Improper zeroing and leveling, because of either a change in patient position or zero drift, is the single most important source of error. Zeroing can be performed by opening the transducer stopcock to room air, thus exposing it to atmospheric pressure. Leveling is done by aligning the transducer with the patient's heart, at the fourth or fifth intercostal space, in the midaxillary line, hence decreasing the effects of hydrostatic pressure on the system. Under these conditions, the pressure reading is calibrated to zero by the monitor. Zeroing and leveling should be repeated with every change of patient position (a transducer that is below the zero reference line will result in falsely high readings and vice versa), when significant changes of blood pressure occur, and routinely every 6 to 8 hours because of zero drift. Disposable pressure transducers incorporate semiconductor technology and are very small, yet rugged and reliable, and because of standardization, calibration of the system is not necessary [16]. Transducers are faulty on occasion, however, and calibration may be checked by attaching a mercury manometer to the stopcock and applying 100, 150, and/or 200 mm Hg pressure. A variation of ±5 mm Hg is acceptable. If calibration is questioned and the variation is out of range, or a manometer is not available for testing, the transducer should be replaced. When zero referencing and calibration are correct, a fast-flush test will assess the system's dynamic response.

Many monitors can be adjusted to filter out frequencies above a certain limit, which can eliminate frequencies in the input signal causing resonance. However, this may also cause inaccurate readings if clinically important frequencies are excluded. Ideally, an exhaustive search for potential causes of resonance and their solutions should be attempted before deciding to filter these frequencies.

TECHNIQUE OF ARTERIAL CANNULATION

Site Selection

Several factors are important when selecting the site for arterial cannulation. The ideal artery has extensive collateral circulation that will maintain the viability of distal tissues if thrombosis occurs. The site should be comfortable for the patient, accessible for insertion and nursing care, and close to the monitoring equipment. Sites involved by infection, disruption of the epidermal barrier, thrombosis, or ischemia need to be avoided. Certain procedures, such as coronary artery bypass grafting, may dictate preference for one site over another. Physicians should also be cognizant of differences of pulse contour recorded at different sites. Because the pressure pulse wave travels outward from the aorta, it encounters arteries of decreased caliber and elasticity, with multiple branch points, causing reflections of the pressure wave. This results in a peripheral pulse contour with increased slope and amplitude, causing artificially elevated pressure readings. As a result, distal extremity artery recordings yield higher systolic values than central aortic or femoral artery recordings.

Diastolic pressures tend to be less affected, and mean arterial pressures (MAPs) measured at the alternative sites are similar [17]. Therefore, MAP has been accepted as a more precise target, than systolic or diastolic pressures, for the titration of intravenous fluid and vasoconstrictor therapy in shock.

The most commonly used sites for arterial cannulation of adults are the radial, femoral, axillary, dorsalis pedis, and brachial arteries. Additional sites include the ulnar and superficial temporal arteries. Peripheral arteries are cannulated percutaneously with a 5-cm, 20-gauge, nontapered polytetrafluoroethylene (PTFE, Teflon) catheter-over-needle, whereas larger arteries are cannulated using the Seldinger technique with a prepackaged kit, typically containing a 15-cm, 18-gauge PTFE catheter, appropriate introducer needles, and guidewire.

Arterial catheterization is performed by physicians from many different specialties and usually the procedure to be performed dictates the site chosen. For example, insertion of an IABP is almost always performed through the femoral artery regardless of the specialty of the physician performing the procedure. Critical care physicians need to be facile with arterial cannulation at all sites, but the radial artery is used successfully for most arterial catheterizations performed for critically ill adults. Each site has unique complications, and they should be taken into account by the proceduralist [18–20]. Radial artery cannulation is usually attempted initially unless the patient is in severe shock, on high-dose vasopressors, and/or pulses are not palpable or adequately visualized with the use of the portable ultrasound. Traditional practice recommended femoral artery cannulation when the former failed, but it has been noted that femoral catheters may be associated with more frequent bloodstream infections [21]. Therefore, cannulation of alternative sites such as the dorsalis pedis, brachial, and axillary arteries should be considered first; however, data on the relative risk of infection of these sites are lacking [21]. Which of these is chosen depends on the exact clinical situation and the expertise of the operator.

Radial Artery Cannulation

A thorough understanding of normal arterial anatomy and common anatomic variants greatly facilitates insertion of catheters and management of unexpected findings at all sites. The radial artery is one of two final branches of the brachial artery. It courses over the flexor digitorum sublimis, flexor pollicis longus, and pronator quadratus muscles and lies just lateral to the flexor carpi radialis in the forearm. As the artery enters the floor of the palm, it ends in the deep volar arterial arch at the level of the metacarpal bones and communicates with the ulnar artery. A second site of collateral flow for the radial artery occurs via the dorsal arch running in the dorsum of the hand (Fig. 7.3).

The ulnar artery runs between the flexor carpi ulnaris and flexor digitorum sublimis in the forearm, with a short course over the ulnar nerve. In the hand, the artery runs over the transverse carpal ligament and becomes the superficial volar arch, which forms an anastomosis with a small branch of the radial artery. These three anastomoses provide excellent collateral flow to the hand [22]. A competent superficial or deep palmar arch must be present to ensure adequate collateral flow. At least one of these anastomoses may be absent in up to 20% of individuals.

Evaluation of Collateral Circulation of the Hand

Hand ischemia is a rare but potential devastating complication of radial artery catheterization that may require amputation [23]. Hand ischemia is rare because of the rich collateral circulation described earlier that ensures perfusion even if one of the main arteries thrombose. Historically, the modified Allen test [24] was used prior to radial catheterization to detect patients in whom the collateral circulation may not be intact and presumably at increased risk for hand ischemia. However, as a screening tool, the Allen test does not have a very good predictive value [25], and our institution, as well as many others, has abandoned its routine use. Doppler ultrasound has been used to screen selected patients for harvesting of the radial artery in elective coronary artery bypass grafting case series, and no ischemic complications were seen [26]. It is unclear if the patients that were excluded from these studies were indeed at increased risk of hand ischemia or not; ethical concerns may prevent the formulation of a clinical trial to answer that question. Based upon this study, we use Doppler ultrasound to evaluate collateral hand circulation with the caveat that it has not yet been validated for critically ill adults.

The best way to prevent hand ischemia is to avoid radial catheterization of patients perceived to be at increased risk (i.e., high-dose vasopressor therapy, scleroderma, vasculopathy) and to perform and document clinical evaluation of hand perfusion at frequent intervals. Any change of the hand distal to a radial artery catheter that suggests decreased perfusion (color or temperature change, paresthesias, or loss of capillary refill) should prompt immediate removal of the catheter and further investigation if the changes do not reverse.

Percutaneous Insertion

The hand is positioned in 30 to 60 degrees of dorsiflexion with the aid of a roll of gauze and armband, avoiding hyperabduction of the thumb. We next use ultrasound to determine the locations, depth, and size of the artery. The volar aspect of the wrist is prepared (alcoholic chlorhexidine) and draped using sterile technique, and approximately 0.5 mL of lidocaine is infiltrated on both sides of the artery through a 25-gauge or smaller needle. Lidocaine serves to decrease patient discomfort and may decrease the likelihood of arterial vasospasm [27]. The catheter over the needle approach necessitates cap, mask, sterile gloves, and a small fenestrated drape, whereas the Seldinger technique requires maximum barrier precautions. A time out confirming correct patient, correct site, correct equipment, and informed consent is necessary before the procedure begins.

A 20-gauge, nontapered, PTFE 5-cm catheter-over-needle apparatus is used for puncture. Entry is made at a 30- to 60-degree angle to the skin approximately 3 to 5 cm proximal to the distal wrist crease. An ultrasound image of the radial artery at this position is shown in Figure 7.2A. The needle and cannula are advanced until blood return is apparent in the hub, signifying intra-arterial placement of the tip of the needle. A small amount of additional advancement is necessary for the cannula tip to fully enter the artery lumen. With this accomplished, needle and cannula are brought flat to the skin and the cannula is advanced to its hub with a firm, steady rotary action. Correct positioning is confirmed by pulsatile blood return after removal of the needle. If the initial attempt is unsuccessful, subsequent attempts should be more proximal, rather than closer to the wrist crease, because the artery is of greater diameter [22], although this may increase the incidence of catheters becoming kinked or occluded [28].

If difficulty is encountered when attempting to pass the catheter, carefully replacing the needle and slightly advancing the whole apparatus may remedy the problem. Alternatively, a fixation technique can be attempted (Fig. 7.3). Advancing the needle and catheter through the far wall of the vessel purposely transfixes the artery. The cannula is then pulled back with the needle partially retracted within the catheter until vigorous arterial blood return is noted. The catheter can then be advanced up the arterial lumen, using the needle as a reinforcing stent.

Catheters with self-contained guidewires to facilitate passage of the cannula into the artery are available (Fig. 7.4). Percutaneous puncture is made in the same manner, but when blood return is

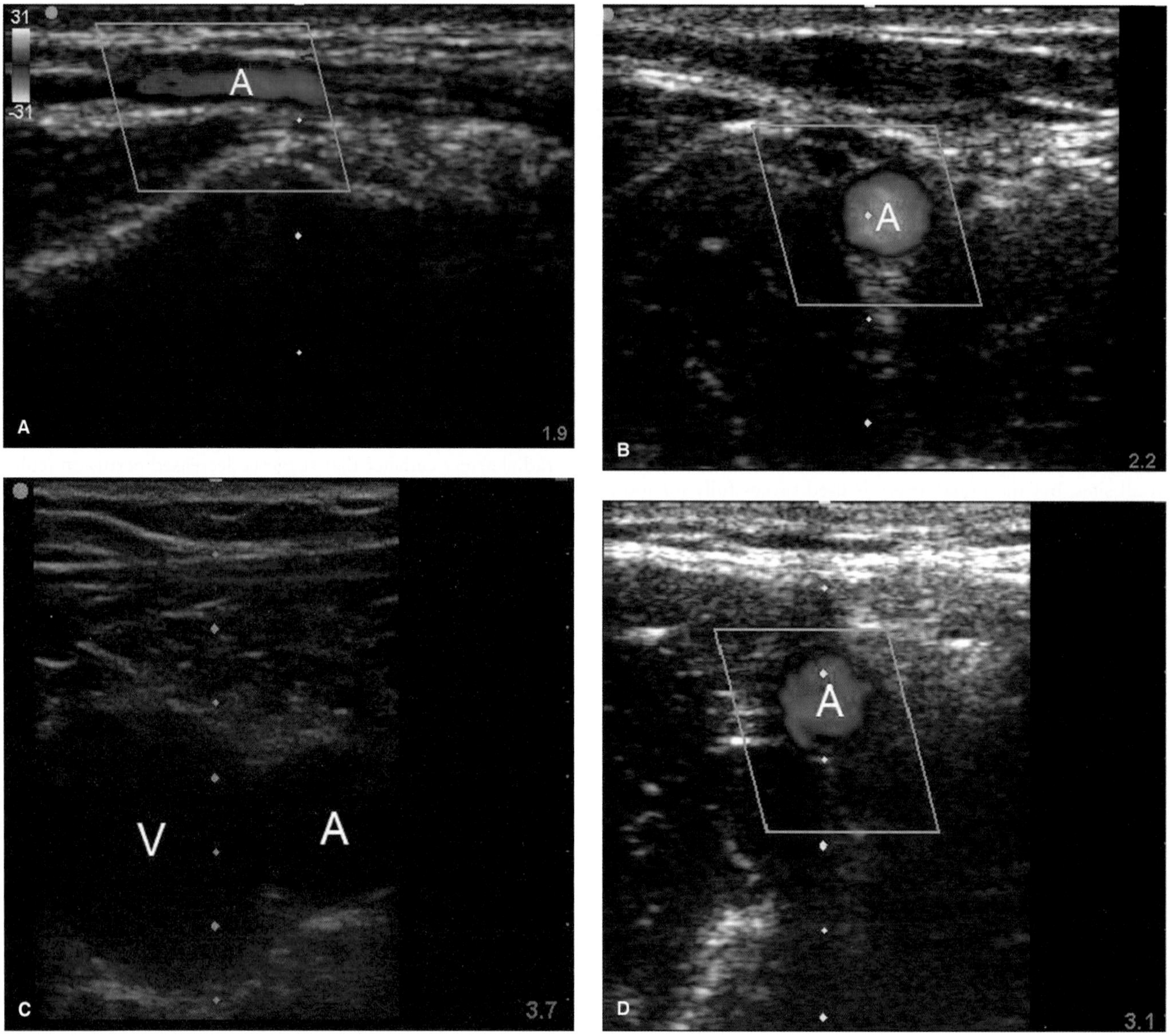

FIGURE 7.2 Portable ultrasound images. A: Radial artery longitudinal view. B: Brachial artery axial view. C: Femoral artery axial view. D: Axillary artery axial view. See text for details.

noted in the catheter hub the guidewire is passed through the needle into the artery, serving as a stent for subsequent catheter advancement. The guidewire and needle are then removed and placement confirmed by pulsatile blood return. The cannula is then secured firmly, attached to transducer tubing, and the site covered with a dressing. Video instruction for the insertion of a radial arterial catheter is available in Video 7.1 and on the Internet [29].

Dorsalis Pedis Artery Cannulation

Dorsalis pedis artery catheterization is uncommon in most critical care units; compared with the radial artery, the anatomy is less predictable and the success rate is lower [30]. The dorsalis pedis artery is the main blood supply of the dorsum of the foot. The artery runs from the ankle to the great toe. It lies very superficial and just lateral to the tendon of the extensor hallucis longus. The dorsalis pedis anastomoses with branches from the posterior tibial (lateral plantar artery) and, to a lesser extent, peroneal arteries, creating an arterial arch network analogous to the one in the hand.

The use of a catheter with a self-contained guidewire is recommended for dorsalis pedis catheterization. The foot is placed in plantar flexion and prepared in the usual fashion. Vessel entry is achieved approximately halfway up the dorsum of the foot where the palpable pulse is strongest; advancement is the same as with cannulation of the radial artery. Use of the ultrasound may increase the rate of successful insertion. Patients usually find catheterization here more painful but less physically limiting. Systolic pressure readings are usually 5 to 20 mm Hg higher with dorsalis pedis catheters than with radial artery catheters, but MAP values are generally similar.

Brachial Artery Cannulation

The brachial artery is cannulated in the bicipital groove proximal to the antecubital fossa at a point where there is no collateral circulation (Fig. 7.2B). In theory, clinical ischemia should be a greater risk, but in most series brachial artery catheters have complication rates comparable to other routes [20,22,31,32]. Even when diminution of distal pulses occurs, because of either proximal obstruction or distal embolization, clinical ischemia is

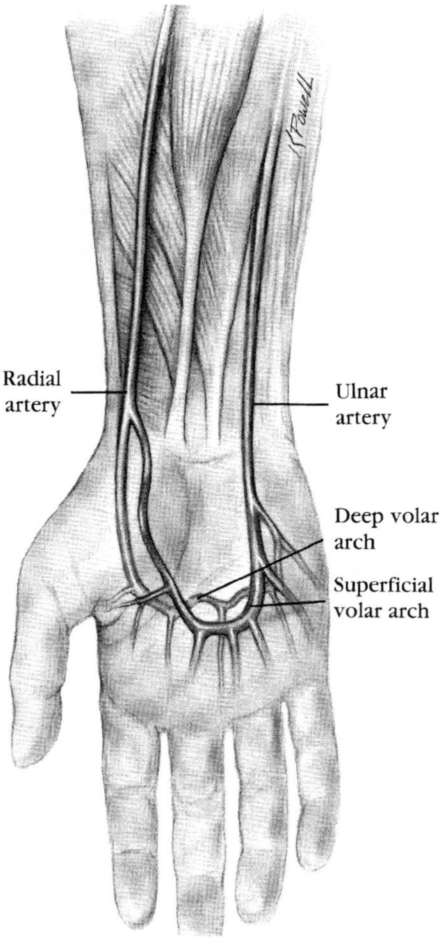

FIGURE 7.3 Anatomy of the radial artery. Note the collateral circulation to the ulnar artery through the deep volar arterial arch and dorsal arch.

unlikely. An important anatomic consideration is that the median nerve lies in close proximity to the brachial artery and may be punctured in 1% to 2% of cases [32]. This usually causes only transient paresthesias, but median nerve palsy has been reported. Median nerve palsy is a particular risk for patients with coagulopathy because even minor bleeding into the fascial planes can produce compression of the median nerve [33]. Coagulopathy may be considered a relative contraindication to brachial artery cannulation. Given all these considerations, brachial artery cannulation should be considered when the radial and dorsalis pedis sites are not available or appropriate. Ultrasound guidance for all brachial artery catheterizations is strongly recommended.

Cannulation of the brachial artery is best performed using a prepackaged kit designed for larger arteries. The brachial artery is punctured by extending the arm at the elbow and locating the pulsating vessel by palpation and ultrasound, a few centimeters proximal to the antecubital fossa, just medial to the bicipital tendon. Once catheterization is established, the elbow must be kept in full extension to avoid kinking or breaking the catheter. Clinical examination of the hand, and Doppler studies when indicated, should be performed and documented frequently while the brachial catheter is in place. The catheter should be promptly removed if diminution of any pulse occurs or there is evidence of embolism. An additional concern is air embolism because placement of a 15-cm catheter puts its tip in the axillary artery.

Femoral Artery Cannulation

Indwelling femoral artery catheters may be associated with a higher risk of health care–acquired infection [21] and should be placed only when insertion at others sites is not appropriate. The femoral artery is large and often palpable when other sites are not, easy to visualize with ultrasound and the technique of cannulation is simple to learn. The most common reason for failure to cannulate is severe atherosclerosis or stenosis from prior vascular procedures involving both femoral arteries. Complications unique to this site are rare but include retroperitoneal hemorrhage and intra-abdominal viscus perforation. These complications occur because of poor technique (puncture above the inguinal ligament) or in the presence of anatomic variations (i.e., large inguinal hernia). Ischemic complications from femoral artery catheters are very rare.

The external iliac artery becomes the common femoral artery at the inguinal ligament (Fig. 7.5). The artery courses under the inguinal ligament near the junction of the medial and the middle third of a straight line drawn between the pubis and the anterior superior iliac spine (Fig. 7.2C). The artery is cannulated using the Seldinger technique and any one of several available prepackaged kits. Kits contain the equivalent of a 19-gauge thin-wall needle, appropriate guidewire, and a 15-cm, 18-gauge PTFE catheter. The patient lies supine with the leg extended and slightly abducted. Skin puncture should be 3 to 5 cm caudal to the inguinal ligament to minimize the risk of retroperitoneal hematoma or bowel perforation, which can occur when needle puncture of the vessel is cephalad to the inguinal ligament. The thin-wall needle is directed, bevel up, cephalad at a 45-degree angle. When arterial blood return is confirmed, the needle and syringe may need to be brought down against the skin to facilitate guidewire passage. The guidewire should advance smoothly, but minor manipulation and rotation is sometimes required when the wire meets resistance at the needle tip or after it has advanced into the vessel. Inability to pass the guidewire may be because of an intimal flap over the needle bevel or atherosclerotic plaques in the vessel. In the latter instance, cannulation of that femoral artery may prove impossible. When the guidewire will not pass beyond the needle tip, it should be withdrawn and blood return reestablished by advancing the needle or repeat vascular puncture. The guidewire is then inserted, the needle withdrawn and the catheter threaded over the guidewire to its hub. The guidewire is withdrawn, the catheter sutured securely and connected to the transducer tubing.

Axillary Artery Cannulation

Axillary artery catheterization of critically ill adults occurs infrequently, but centers experiencing it report low rates of complications [18,20,34]. The axillary artery is large and frequently palpable when all other sites are not and has a rich collateral circulation. The tip of a 15-cm catheter inserted through an axillary approach lies in the subclavian artery, and thus central arterial pressures are effectively measured. The central location of the tip makes cerebral air embolism a greater risk; therefore, left axillary catheters are preferred for the initial attempt because air bubbles passing into the right subclavian artery are more likely to traverse the aortic arch. Caution should be exercised when flushing axillary catheters, which is best accomplished manually using low pressures and small volumes.

The axillary artery begins at the lateral border of the first rib as a continuation of the subclavian artery and ends at the inferior margin of the teres major muscle, where it becomes the brachial artery. The optimal site for catheterization is the junction of the middle and lower third of the vessel, which usually corresponds to its highest palpable point in the axilla. At this point, the artery is superficial and is located at the inferior border of the pectoralis major muscle (Fig. 7.2D). The artery is enclosed in a neurovascular bundle, the axillary sheath, with the medial, posterior, and lateral cords of the brachial plexus. Medial to the medial cord is the axillary vein. Not surprisingly, brachial plexus

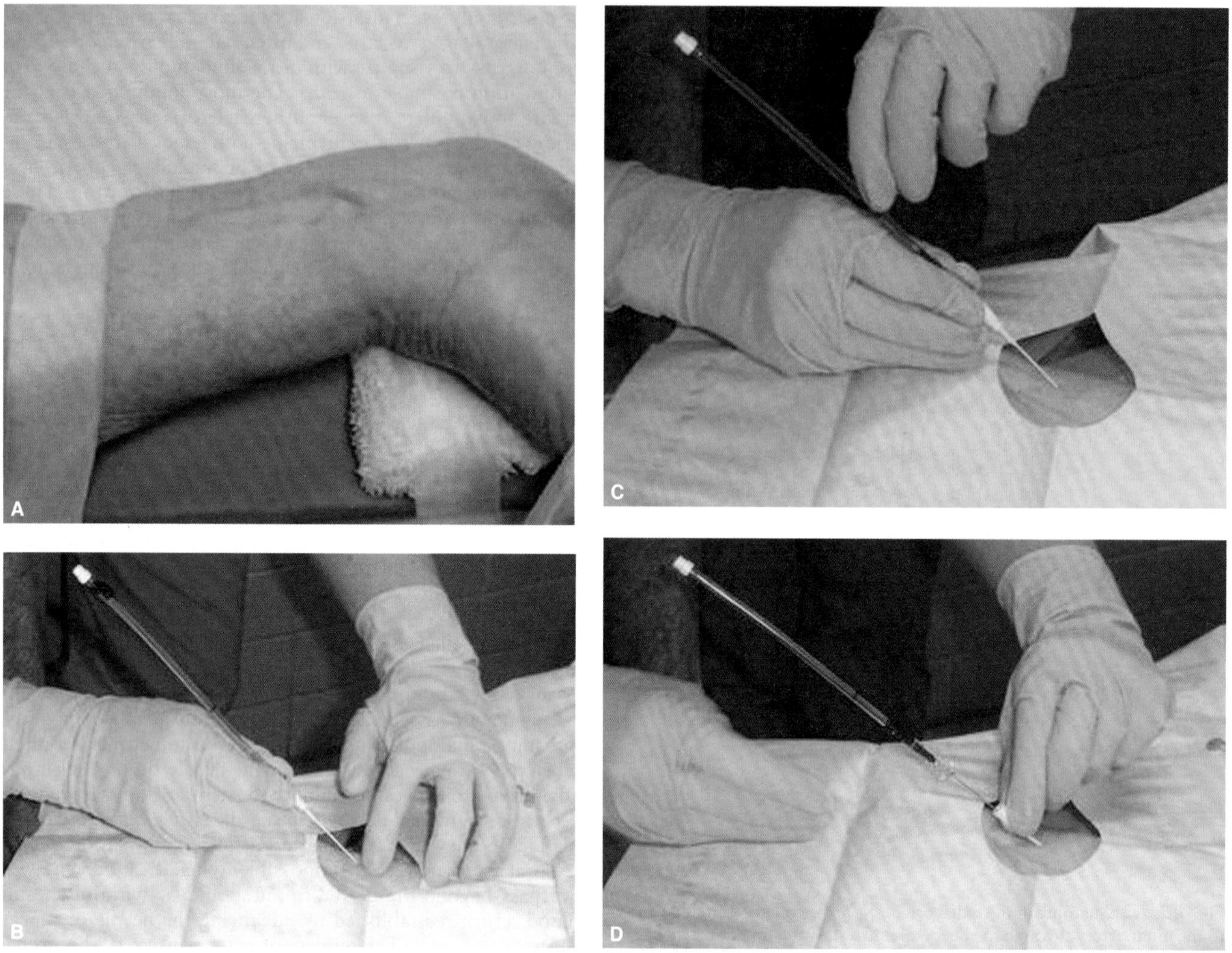

FIGURE 7.4 Cannulation of the radial artery. **A:** A towel is placed behind the wrist, and the hand is immobilized with tape. **B:** The catheter-needle-guidewire apparatus is inserted into the skin at a 30- to 60-degree angle. **C:** The guidewire is advanced into the artery after pulsatile blood flow is obtained. **D:** The catheter is advanced over the guidewire into the artery. (From Irwin RS, Rippe JM: *Manual of Intensive Care Medicine.* 4th ed. Philadelphia, PA, Lippincott Williams & Wilkins, 2006, p 17, with permission.)

neuropathies have been reported from axillary artery cannulation [35]. Coagulopathy is a relative contraindication, because the axillary sheath can rapidly fill with blood from an uncontrolled arterial puncture, resulting in a compressive neuropathy.

The axillary artery is cannulated using the Seldinger technique and a prepackaged kit. The arm is abducted, externally rotated, and flexed at the elbow by having the patient place the hand under his or her head. The artery is palpated at the lower border of the pectoralis major muscle and fixed against the shaft of the humerus. After site preparation and local infiltration with lidocaine, the thin-wall needle is introduced at a 30- to 45-degree angle to the vertical plane until return of arterial blood. The remainder of the catheterization proceeds as described for femoral artery cannulation.

An additional insertion technique, which is guided by ultrasound imaging, has been reported [36]. With this method, the arm is abducted to a 90-degree angle, the second portion of the axillary artery is identified by longitudinal sonographic views, the needle is then advanced under real-time imaging through the pectoral muscles and clavipectoral fascia until pulsatile blood return is seen. The artery is subsequently catheterized using the Seldinger technique. The potential benefits of this technique may include the ability to visualize and avoid puncturing the structures surrounding the axillary artery (i.e., brachial plexus) and an anterior insertion site that allows for easier care of the catheter.

Utility of Ultrasonography for Arterial Catheterization

Ultrasonography has useful application related to arterial catheterization. Although ultrasound guidance to decrease complication rates of central venous catheter insertion has become relatively commonplace, fewer clinicians are familiar with the use of ultrasound to guide arterial catheterization [37]. Traditional arterial palpation techniques for catheterization can be especially challenging for patients with obesity, edema, small vessel caliber, and shock states that obscure pulsatility. Additionally, repeated attempts after initial failure often result in arterial spasm, leading to further failed attempts with increased risk of complications. Multiple studies and meta-analyses have proven the benefits of real-time ultrasound-guided arterial catheterization by demonstrating increased success rates and overall reductions of rates of complications [38,39]. International, evidence-based recommendations advocate that ultrasound guidance as the method of choice for any kind of vascular cannulation, given its higher safety and efficacy [40]. The use of ultrasonography to guide radial artery catheter insertion is presented in Video 7.1.

Two-dimensional ultrasound and a high-frequency linear array transducer (5 to 10 MHz) are used for catheterization. Before sterile draping, potential access sites should be scanned for vessel depth, caliber, patency, tortuosity, atheromatous plaques, and adjacent vein and nerve location. Arteries are recognized

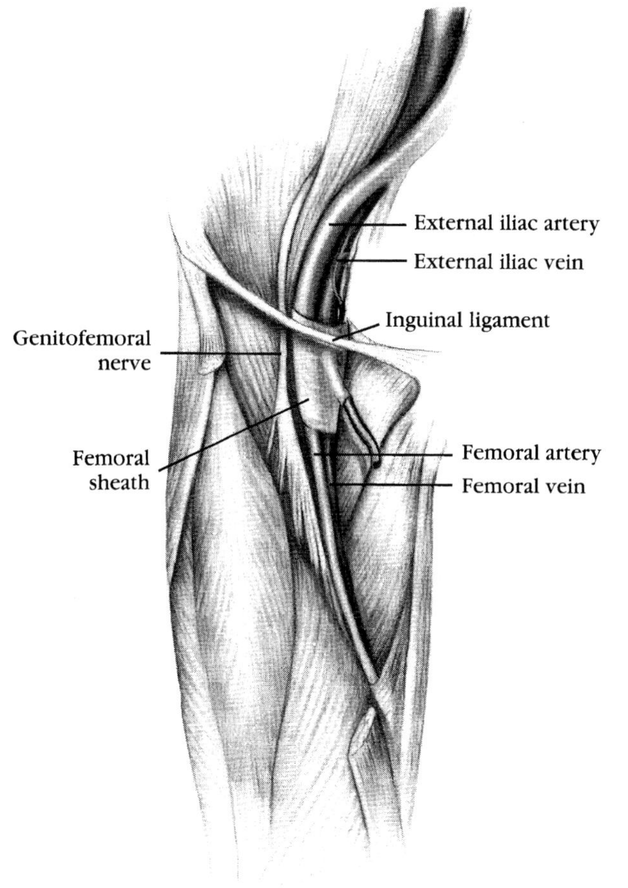

FIGURE 7.5 Anatomy of the femoral artery and adjacent structures. The artery is cannulated below the inguinal ligament.

and differentiated from veins and nerves by a discrete round shape, relatively thick walls, and above all pulsatility—which can be accentuated by partial compression of the artery. Color and pulsed-wave Doppler techniques can be used for vessel identification but are not required.

Sterile barrier precautions and a sterile probe cover should be used. The operator's dominant hand is used for needle control, whereas the nondominant hand is used to hold the transducer. The artery is centered on the screen. Both the transverse and the longitudinal views can be utilized as long as the operator maintains needle tip visualization throughout the procedure. Although the transverse approach allows for easier visualization and catheterization of smaller and tortuous arteries, the longitudinal approach may reduce perforation of the posterior arterial wall by direct visualization of the entire needle throughout the procedure [41]. A local anesthetic is injected under ultrasound guidance by visualizing an enlarging hypoechoic area in the subcutaneous tissue.

When using a transverse approach, the introducer needle is inserted through the skin at a 45-degree angle slightly distal to the transducer. Superficial arteries may require a shallower angle of insertion. Before any further advancement, the needle tip must be visualized under the skin surface, within the soft tissue, as a hyperechoic dot. The transducer is slowly angled back and forth to distinguish the needle tip from the shaft. Only when the tip is identified should the operator continue to slowly advance the needle toward the target artery. This can be achieved by advancing the needle and transducer simultaneously or by angulating the probe while advancing the needle. Both techniques require the needle tip to remain in view at all times. Once the artery is penetrated and blood flow obtained, the ultrasound probe is placed on the sterile field and catheterization is completed using the modified Seldinger technique. The wire should be visualized and confirmed within the artery before deploying the catheter. When the longitudinal approach is utilized, the needle must be advanced in-plane with the transducer at all times because any out-of-plane movement can potentially damage nonvisualized adjacent structures [41].

In addition to guidance, ultrasound can be used to identify the potential for complications. Before puncture of the radial artery, a Doppler ultrasound-guided Allen test can be performed to detect appropriate arterial blood flow to the hand [42]. The location of femoral artery puncture is directly related to post-procedural complications. "Low Stick" punctures below the bifurcation of the common femoral artery are associated with hematoma, pseudoaneurysm, arteriovenous fistula, and ischemic limb complications. Recognition and avoidance of the external iliac artery, superficial, and deep femoral arteries significantly reduces vascular complications. Retroperitoneal hemorrhage can be reduced by avoiding "high sticks" at or above the inferior epigastric artery. To reduce embolic complications, care should be taken to avoid catheterization through atheromas. Postprocedural complications, like hematomas, arteriovenous fistulas, and pseudoaneurysms, can be readily identified with ultrasound [43].

COMPLICATIONS OF ARTERIAL CANNULATION

Arterial cannulation is a relatively safe invasive procedure. Although estimates of the total complication rates range from 15% to 40%, clinically relevant complications occur in 5% or less of cannulations (Table 7.2). Risk factors for infectious and noninfectious complications have been identified and are listed in Table 7.3 [20,44,45].

Thrombosis

Thrombosis is the single most common complication of intra-arterial catheters. The incidence of thrombosis varies with

TABLE 7.2

Complications Associated with Arterial Cannulation

Site	Complication
All sites	Pain and swelling
	Thrombosis
	Embolization
	Hematoma
	Hemorrhage
	Limb ischemia
	Catheter-related infection including bacteremia
	Diagnostic blood loss
	Pseudoaneurysm
	Heparin-associated thrombocytopenia
Radial artery	Cerebral embolization
	Peripheral neuropathy
Femoral artery	Retroperitoneal hemorrhage
	Bowel perforation
	Arteriovenous fistula
	Higher risk of infection than radial insertion
Axillary artery	Cerebral embolization
	Brachial plexopathy
Brachial artery	Median nerve damage
	Cerebral embolization

TABLE 7.3

Factors Predisposing to Complications with Arterial Cannulation

Large tapered cannulas (>20 gauge except at the large artery sites)
Hypotension
Coagulopathy
Low cardiac output
Multiple puncture attempts
Use of vasoconstrictors
Atherosclerosis
Hypercoagulable state
Placement by surgical cutdown
Site inflammation
Intermittent flushing system
Bacteremia

the site, method of detection, size of the cannula, and duration of cannulation. Thrombosis is common with radial and dorsalis pedis catheters, but clinical sequelae are rare because of the collateral circulation [44,45]. When a 20-gauge nontapered PTFE catheter with a continuous 3 mL per hour heparinized-saline flush is used to cannulate the radial artery for 3 to 4 days, thrombosis of the vessel can be detected by Doppler study in 5% to 25% of cases [45]. Use of a flush solution containing heparin is no longer standard at our institution because of concern for heparin-induced thrombocytopenia (HIT); the incidence of thrombosis does not appear to be significantly higher using saline flush [46,47]. The risk of radial thrombosis seems to be proportionally associated with the diameter of the catheter used [20], and smaller catheters may be protective.

Thrombosis often occurs after catheter removal. Women have a preponderance of flow abnormalities following radial artery cannulation, likely explained by smaller arteries and a greater tendency to exhibit vasospasm [28]. Generally, thrombosed arteries recanalize by 3 weeks after removal of the catheter. Despite the high incidence of Doppler-detected thrombosis, clinical ischemia of the hand is rare and usually resolves following catheter removal. Symptomatic occlusion requiring surgical intervention occurs in fewer than 1% of cases, but can be catastrophic with tissue loss or amputation of the hand [23]. Most patients who develop clinical ischemia have an associated contributory cause, such as prolonged circulatory failure with high-dose vasopressor therapy requirements [44].

Regular inspection of the extremity for unexplained pain or signs of ischemia followed by immediate removal of the catheter, if indicated, minimize significant ischemic complications. When evidence of ischemia persists after catheter removal, anticoagulation, thrombolytic therapy, embolectomy, surgical bypass, or cervical sympathetic blockade are treatment options and should be pursued aggressively [23,44]. Early consultation of a vascular surgeon is recommended in this situation.

Cerebral Embolization

Continuous flush devices used with arterial catheters are designed to deliver 3 mL per hour of fluid from an infusion bag pressurized to 300 mm Hg. It was demonstrated that with rapid flushing of radial artery lines with relatively small volumes of radiolabeled solution, traces of the solution could be detected in the central arterial circulation in a time frame representative of retrograde flow [48]. Moreover, injection of greater than 2 mL of air into the radial artery of small primates results in retrograde passage of air into the vertebral circulation [35]. Factors that increase the risk of retrograde passage of air are patient size and position (air travels up in a sitting patient), injection site, and flush rate. Air embolism has been cited as a risk mainly for radial arterial catheters but logically could occur with all arterial catheters, especially axillary and brachial artery catheters. The risk is minimized by clearing all air from the tubing before flushing, opening the flush valve for no more than 2 to 3 seconds at a time, and avoiding overaggressive manual flushing of the line.

Diagnostic Blood Loss

DBL is blood loss that occurs in the patient because of frequent blood sampling obtained for laboratory testing. The significance of DBL is underappreciated. It is a particular problem for patients with standard arterial catheter setups that are used as the site for sampling, because 3 to 5 mL of blood are typically wasted (to avoid heparin/saline contamination) every time a sample is obtained. For patients with frequent arterial blood gas determinations, DBL can be substantial and results in a red cell transfusion [49]. There are several ways to minimize DBL, including tubing systems employing a reservoir for blood sampling, continuous intra-arterial blood gas monitoring, point of care microchemistry analysis, and the use of pediatric collection tubes. Given the expense and risks of blood transfusions, every ICU should have a blood conservation policy in place that includes minimizing DBL. Protocols that are designed to optimize laboratory utilization have resulted in significant cost savings and reduced transfusion requirements in our, as well as in other, institutions [50].

Other Mechanical and Technical Complications

Other noninfectious complications reported with arterial catheters are pseudoaneurysm formation, hematoma, local tenderness, hemorrhage, neuropathies, and catheter embolization [20]. Heparin use for flushing of vascular catheters may confer a small risk of HIT [51] and is associated with increased costs. The data supporting the use of heparin to maintain patency of arterial catheters is poor and does not provide sufficient proof for continuation of this practice [52]. Thus, it is our opinion that standard flushing of catheters should be done with saline solutions.

Infections

Infectious sequelae are the most important clinical complications caused by arterial cannulation. See Chapter 81 for a detailed review of catheter-related infections (CRIs). Catheter-associated infection is usually initiated when skin flora invades the intracutaneous tract, causing colonization of the catheter, and when not locally contained, bacteremia. An additional source of infection is contaminated infusate from the pressure monitoring system, which is at greater risk of infection than central venous catheters because (a) the transducer can become colonized as a consequence of stagnant flow, (b) the flush solution is infused at a slow rate (3 mL per hour) and may hang for several days, and (c) the stopcocks in the system can serve as entry sites for bacteria when they are accessed by several different personnel to obtain blood samples.

Appreciation of the mechanisms responsible for initiating arterial CRI is important for understanding how to minimize infection; thorough operator and site preparation is paramount. It should be noted that only one study evaluated the impact of maximum barrier precautions for the placement of radial and dorsalis pedis catheters [53] and that no studies have addressed this matter for larger arteries. With those considerations in mind, it is our practice to use full barrier precautions for all large artery insertions. Chlorhexidine should be used for skin preparation [54] and use of a chlorhexidine soaked dressing at the insertion site is an excellent practice. Breaks of sterile technique during insertion mandate termination of the procedure and replacement of compromised equipment. Nursing personnel should follow strict guidelines when drawing blood samples or manipulating connections. Blood withdrawn to clear the tubing prior to drawing samples should not be reinjected unless a specially designed system is in use [55]. Inspection of the site at the start of every nursing shift is mandatory, and the catheter should be evaluated and removed promptly when indicated. Routine change of the pressure monitoring system does not reduce infectious complications and may represent another opportunity to introduce colonization.

Arterial cannulation remains an underrecognized source of bloodstream infections. Historically, it was thought that arterial catheters had a lower risk for infection than central venous catheters, but research has proven this to be no longer true. Impressive reductions in overall CRI have occurred as a result of clinical research, better technology, and an emphasis on patient safety [21,56,57]. Using modern techniques, arterial catheter-related colonization may occur in up to 5% to 10% of catheters, but the incidence of catheter-related bacteremia is in the range of 0.5 to 2.0 per 1,000 catheter-days [18,19,21,56–58].

The site of insertion as an important factor impacting the incidence of infection has been a controversial issue. Previous research studies had conflicting reports about the risk of infection of femoral catheterizations, and the consensus among physicians was that they were generally safe [18–21,30]. A recent meta-analysis looked at this issue and found that CRI occurred in 1.5% of femoral catheterizations in contrast to 0.3% of radial cannulations [21]. The calculated relative risk of infection of the femoral site was 1.94 times greater than the radial site [21]. Rigorous data about the risk of infection of other insertion sites are not available. Based on these findings, placement of a catheter in the femoral artery should be avoided, when feasible, by cannulating another arterial site. In this regard, we have had a change of practice in our institution, where more brachial and axillary cannulations are done now.

Catheter duration is important and likely related to increased risk of infection [57]. We believe 5 to 7 days is an appropriate time to reassess the need for and the location of arterial catheterization [21,57], but each institution should determine its own catheter-associated infection rate so that rational policies can be formulated based on existing local infection rates.

When arterial catheter infection does occur, *Staphylococcus* species are commonly isolated. Gram-negative organisms are less frequent; they are predominantly contaminated infusate or equipment-related infections. Infection with *Candida* species is a greater risk for prolonged catheterization of the glucose-intolerant or immunocompromised patient but has been reported for all types of patients. PTFE catheters have a greater resistance to *Escherichia coli* and *Pseudomonas aeruginosa* [20]. Catheter-associated bacteremia should be treated with a 7- to 14-day course of appropriate antibiotics. For complicated cases, longer courses are sometimes necessary.

The optimal evaluation of febrile catheterized patients can be a challenging problem (see Chapter 79). If the site appears abnormal or the patient has sepsis of no other identified etiology, the catheter should be removed. More specific guidelines are difficult to recommend, and individual factors should always be considered. In general, arterial catheters in place less than 5 days are unlikely to be the source of fever unless insertion was contaminated. Catheters in place 5 days or longer should be changed to a different site, given the safety of arterial cannulation and the possibility of infection. Guidewire exchanges are not recommended in our institution because of the potential risk of infection.

RECOMMENDATIONS

The radial artery is an appropriate initial site for percutaneous arterial cannulation. When the radial artery is not appropriate for cannulation, other sites such as the brachial, axillary, dorsalis pedis, or femoral arteries can be safely cannulated. Most centers have more experience with femoral artery cannulation, but this site has been linked with a higher risk of infection and should be avoided as much as possible. Coagulopathy may be considered a relative contraindication for brachial and axillary arterial cannulation. Ultrasound guidance should be used for all catheterizations anticipated to be difficult and to avoid complications when a coagulopathy is present. Routine ultrasound use is also strongly advocated because it is associated with a higher first pass success rate and, potentially, less insertion time and fewer sites for successful placement. Arterial catheters should be removed as soon as clinically indicated, to decrease the risk of iatrogenic infection. Finally, arterial catheters are associated with overutilization of blood tests and iatrogenic anemia, and their prompt discontinuation may decrease these phenomena.

ACKNOWLEDGMENTS

The authors thanked Michael G. Seneff, MD who revised this chapter in previous editions of this textbook.

References

1. Marik PE, Cavallazzi R, Vasu T, et al: Dynamic changes in arterial waveform derived variables and fluid responsiveness in mechanically ventilated patients: a systematic review of the literature. *Crit Care Med* 37:2642–2647, 2009.
2. Low LL, Harrington GR, Stoltzfus DP: The effect of arterial lines on blood-drawing practices and costs in intensive care units. *Chest* 108:216, 1995.
3. Zimmerman JE, Seneff MG, Sun X, et al: Evaluating laboratory usage in the intensive care unit: patient and institutional characteristics that influence frequency of blood sampling. *Crit Care Med* 25:737, 1997.
4. Bur A, Hirschl MM, Herkner H, et al: Accuracy of oscillometric blood pressure measurement according to the relation between cuff size and upper-arm circumference in critically ill patients. *Crit Care Med* 28:371, 2000.
5. Ribezzo S, Spina E, Di Bartolomeo S, et al: Noninvasive techniques for blood pressure measurement are not a reliable alternative to direct measurement: a randomized crossover trial in ICU. *ScientificWorldJournal* 2014:353628, 2014.
6. Bur A, Herkner H, Vlcek M, et al: Factors influencing the accuracy of oscillometric blood pressure measurement in critically ill patients. *Crit Care Med* 31:793–799, 2003.
7. Hirschl MM, Kittler H, Woisetschlager C, et al: Simultaneous comparison of thoracic bioimpedance and arterial pulse waveform-derived cardiac output with thermodilution measurement. *Crit Care Med* 28:1798, 2000.
8. Thiele RH, Bartels K, Gan TJ: Cardiac output monitoring: a contemporary assessment and review. *Crit Care Med.* 43:177–185, 2015.
9. Mayer J, Boldt J, Poland R, et al: Continuous arterial pressure waveform-based cardiac output using the FloTrac/Vigileo: a review and meta-analysis. *J Cardiothorac Vasc Anesth* 23:401–406, 2009.
10. Gardner RM: Direct arterial pressure monitoring. *Curr Anaesth Crit Care* 1:239, 1990.
11. Boutros A, Albert S: Effect of the dynamic response of transducer-tubing system on accuracy of direct blood pressure measurement in patients. *Crit Care Med* 11:124, 1983.
12. Rothe CF, Kim KC: Measuring systolic arterial blood pressure. Possible errors from extension tubes or disposable transducer domes. *Crit Care Med* 8:683, 1980.
13. Billiet E, Colardyn F: Pressure measurement evaluation and accuracy validation: the Gabarith test. *Intensive Care Med* 24:1323, 1998.
14. Kleinman B: Understanding natural frequency and damping and how they relate to the measurement of blood pressure. *J Clin Monit* 5:137–147, 1989.
15. Romagnoli S, Ricci Z, Quattrone D, et al: Accuracy of invasive arterial pressure monitoring in cardiovascular patients: an observational study. *Crit Care* 18:644, 2014.
16. Gardner RM: Accuracy and reliability of disposable pressure transducers coupled with modern pressure monitors. *Crit Care Med* 24:879, 1996.
17. Pauca AL, Wallenhaupt SL, Kon ND, et al: Does radial artery pressure accurately reflect aortic pressure? *Chest* 102:1193, 1992.
18. Gurman GM, Kriemerman S: Cannulation of big arteries in critically ill patients. *Crit Care Med* 13:217, 1985.

19. Russell JA, Joel M, Hudson RJ, et al: Prospective evaluation of radial and femoral artery catheterization sites in critically ill adults. *Crit Care Med* 11:936, 1983.
20. Scheer BV, Perel A, Pfeiffer UJ: Clinical review: complications and risk factors of peripheral arterial catheters used for haemodynamic monitoring in anaesthesia and intensive care medicine. *Crit Care* 6:199–204, 2002.
21. O'Horo JC, Maki DG, Krupp AE, et al: Arterial catheters as a source of bloodstream infection: a systematic review and meta-analysis. *Crit Care Med* 426:1334–1339, 2014.
22. Mathers LH: Anatomical considerations in obtaining arterial access. *J Intensive Care Med* 5:110, 1990.
23. Valentine RJ, Modrall JG, Clagett GP: Hand ischemia after radial artery cannulation. *J Am Coll Surg* 201:18, 2005.
24. Allen EV: *Thromboangiitis obliterans*: method of diagnosis of chronic occlusive arterial lesions distal to the wrist with illustrative cases. *Am J Med Sci* 178:237, 1929.
25. Glavin RJ, Jones HM: Assessing collateral circulation in the hand—four methods compared. *Anaesthesia* 44:594, 1989.
26. Agrifoglio M, Dainese L, Pasotti S, et al: Preoperative assessment of the radial artery for coronary artery bypass grafting: is the clinical Allen test adequate? *Ann Thorac Surg* 79:570–572, 2005.
27. Giner J, Casan P, Belda J, et al: Pain during arterial puncture. *Chest* 110:1443, 1996.
28. Kaye J, Heald GR, Morton J, et al: Patency of radial arterial catheters. *Am J Crit Care* 10:104, 2001.
29. Tegtmeyer K, Brady G, Lai S, et al: Videos in clinical medicine. Placement of an arterial line. *N Engl J Med* 354:e13, 2006.
30. Martin C, Saux P, Papazian L, et al: Long-term arterial cannulation in ICU patients using the radial artery or dorsalis pedis artery. *Chest* 119:901, 2001.
31. Handlogten KS, Wilson GA, Clifford L, et al: Brachial artery catheterization: an assessment of use patterns and associated complications. *Anesth Analg* 118:288–295, 2014.
32. Mann S, Jones RI, Millar-Craig MW, et al: The safety of ambulatory intra-arterial pressure monitoring: a clinical audit of 1000 studies. *Int J Cardiol* 5:585, 1984.
33. Macon WL IV, Futrell JW: Median-nerve neuropathy after percutaneous puncture of the brachial artery in patients receiving anticoagulants. *N Engl J Med* 288:1396, 1973.
34. Brown M, Gordon LH, Brown OW, et al: Intravascular monitoring via the axillary artery. *Anesth Intensive Care* 13:38, 1984.
35. Sabik JF, Lytle BW, McCarthy PM, et al: Axillary artery: an alternative site of arterial cannulation for patients with extensive aortic and peripheral vascular disease. *J Thorac Cardiovasc Surg* 109:885–891, 1995.
36. Sandhu NS: The use of ultrasound for axillary artery catheterization through pectoral muscles: a new anterior approach. *Anesth Analg* 99:562–565, 2004.
37. Shiloh AL, Eisen LA: Ultrasound-guided arterial catheterization: a narrative review. *Intensive Care Med* 36:214–221, 2010.
38. Shiloh AL, Savel RH, Paulin LM, et al: Ultrasound-guided catheterization of the radial artery: a systematic review and meta-analysis of randomized controlled trials. *Chest* 139:524–529, 2011.
39. Sobolev M, Slovut DP, Lee Chang A, et al: Ultrasound-guided catheterization of the femoral artery: a systematic review and meta-analysis of randomized controlled trials. *J Invasive Cardiol* 27:318–323, 2015.
40. Lamperti M, Bodenham AR, Pittiruti M, et al: International evidence-based recommendations on ultrasound-guided vascular access. *Intensive Care Med* 38:1105–1117, 2012.
41. Sandhu NS, Patel B: Use of ultrasonography as a rescue technique for failed radial artery cannulation. *J Clin Anesth* 18:138–141, 2006.
42. Jarvis MA, Jarvis CL, Jones PR, et al: Reliability of Allen's test in selection of patients for radial artery harvest. *Ann Thorac Surg*70:1362–1365, 2000.
43. Davison BD, Polak JF: Arterial injuries: a sonographic approach. *Radiol Clin North Am* 42:383–396, 2004.
44. Wilkins RG: Radial artery cannulation and ischaemic damage: a review. *Anaesthesia* 40:896, 1985.
45. Weiss BM, Gattiker RI: Complications during and following radial artery cannulation: a prospective study. *Intensive Care Med* 12:424, 1986.
46. Clifton GD, Branson P, Kelly HJ, et al: Comparison of normal saline and heparin solutions for maintenance of arterial catheter patency. *Heart Lung* 20:115, 1990.
47. Hook ML, Reuling J, Luettgen ML, et al: Comparison of the patency of arterial lines maintained with heparinized and nonheparinized infusions. The Cardiovascular Intensive Care Unit Nursing Research Committee of St. Luke's Hospital. *Heart Lung* 16:693, 1987.
48. Lowenstein E, Little JW 3rd, Lo HH: Prevention of cerebral embolization from flushing radial-artery cannulas. *N Engl J Med* 285:1414, 1971.
49. Smoller BR, Kruskall MS: Phlebotomy for diagnostic laboratory tests in adults. Pattern of use and effect on transfusion requirements. *N Engl J Med* 314:1233, 1986.
50. Roberts DE, Bell DD, Ostryzniuk T, et al: Eliminating needless testing in intensive care–an information-based team management approach. *Crit Care Med* 21:1452, 1993.
51. Warkentin TE, Greinacher A, Koster A, et al; American College of Chest Physicians: Treatment and prevention of heparin-induced thrombocytopenia: American College of Chest Physicians Evidence-Based Clinical Practice Guidelines (8th Edition). *Chest* 133:340S–380S, 2008. Erratum in: *Chest* 139:1261, 2011.
52. Robertson-Malt S, Malt GN, Farquhar V, et al: Heparin versus normal saline for patency of arterial lines. *Cochrane Database Syst Rev* 5:CD007364, 2014.
53. Rijnders BJ, Van Wijngaerden E, Wilmer A, et al: Use of full sterile barrier precautions during insertion of arterial catheters: a randomized trial. *Clin Infect Dis* 36:743–748, 2003.
54. Mimoz O, Pieroni L, Lawrence C, et al: Prospective, randomized trial of two antiseptic solutions for prevention of central venous or arterial catheter colonization and infection in intensive care unit patients. *Crit Care Med* 24:1818, 1996.
55. Peruzzi WT, Noskin GA, Moen SG, et al: Microbial contamination of blood conservation devices during routine use in the critical care setting: results of a prospective, randomized trial. *Crit Care Med* 24:1157, 1996.
56. Maki DG, Kluger DM, Crnich CJ: The risk of bloodstream infection in adults with different intravascular devices: a systematic review of 200 published prospective studies. *Mayo Clin Proc* 81:1159–1171, 2006.
57. Lucet JC, Bouadma L, Zahar JR, et al: Infectious risk associated with arterial catheters compared with central venous catheters. *Crit Care Med* 38:1030–1035, 2010.
58. Traore O, Liotier J, Souweine B: Prospective study of arterial and central venous catheter colonization and of arterial- and central venous catheter-related bacteremia in intensive care units. *Crit Care Med* 33:1276, 2005.

Chapter 8 ■ Airway Management and Endotracheal Intubation

J. MATTHIAS WALZ • STEPHEN O. HEARD

In the emergency department and critical care environment, management of the airway to ensure optimal ventilation and oxygenation is of prime importance. Although initial efforts should be directed toward improving oxygenation and ventilation without intubating the patient (see Chapter 167), these interventions may fail and the placement of an endotracheal (ET) tube may be required. Although ET intubation is best left to the trained specialist, emergencies often require that the procedure be performed before a specialist arrives. Because intubated patients are commonly seen in the intensive care unit (ICU) and coronary care unit, all physicians who work in these environments should be skilled in the techniques of airway management, ET intubation, and management of intubated patients. For those intensivists who do not have the necessary training to become credentialed by their hospital for airway management, taking structured airway management courses, participating in simulation and intubating patients in the operating room or ICU under the watchful eye of a mentor should lead the way to the awarding of privileges.

ANATOMY

An understanding of the techniques of ET intubation and potential complications is based on knowledge of the anatomy of the respiratory passages [1]. Although a detailed anatomic description is beyond the scope of this book, an understanding of some features and relationships is essential to performing intubation.

Nose

The roof of the nose is partially formed by the cribriform plate. The anatomic proximity of the roof to intracranial structures dictates that special caution be exercised during nasotracheal intubations. This is particularly true in patients with significant maxillofacial injuries.

The mucosa of the nose is provided with a rich blood supply from branches of the ophthalmic and maxillary arteries, which allow air to be warmed and humidified. Because the conchae provide an irregular, highly vascularized surface, they are particularly susceptible to trauma and subsequent hemorrhage. The orifices from the paranasal sinuses and nasolacrimal duct open onto the lateral wall. Blockage of these orifices by prolonged nasotracheal intubation may result in sinusitis.

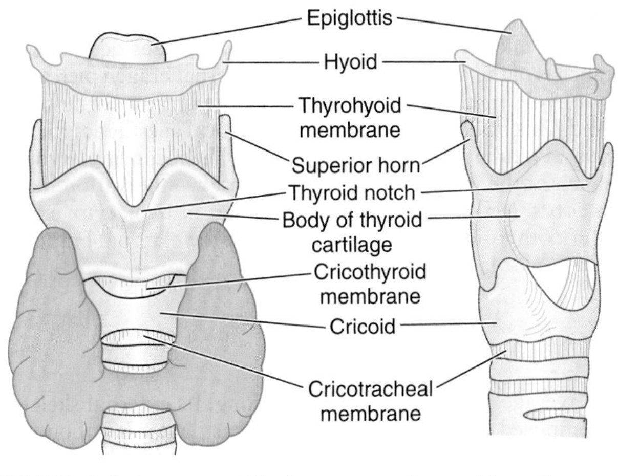

FIGURE 8.1 Anatomy of the larynx, anterior, and lateral aspects. (From Ellis H, Lawson AD: *Anatomy for Anaesthetists*. 9th ed. Oxford, Wiley-Blackwell, 2013, with permission.)

Mouth and Jaw

The mouth is formed inferiorly by the tongue, alveolar ridge, and mandible. The hard and soft palates compose the superior surface, and the oropharynx forms the posterior surface. Assessment of the anatomic features of the mouth and jaw is essential before orotracheal intubation. A clear understanding of the anatomy is also essential when dealing with a patient who has a difficult airway and when learning how to insert airway devices such as the laryngeal mask airway (LMA; discussed in "Management of the Difficult Airway" section).

Nasopharynx

The base of the skull forms the roof of the nasopharynx, and the soft palate forms the floor. The roof and the posterior walls of the nasopharynx contain lymphoid tissue (adenoids), which may become enlarged and compromise nasal airflow or become injured during nasal intubation, particularly in children. The Eustachian tubes enter the nasopharynx on the lateral walls and may become blocked secondary to swelling during prolonged nasotracheal intubation.

Oropharynx

The soft palate defines the beginning of the oropharynx, which extends inferiorly to the epiglottis. The palatine tonsils protrude from the lateral walls and, in children, occasionally become so enlarged that exposure of the larynx for intubation becomes difficult. A large tongue can also cause oropharyngeal obstruction. Contraction of the genioglossus muscle normally moves the tongue forward to open the oropharyngeal passage during inspiration. Decreased tone of this muscle (e.g., in the anesthetized state) can cause obstruction. The oropharynx connects the posterior portion of the oral cavity to the hypopharynx.

Hypopharynx

The epiglottis defines the superior border of the hypopharynx, and the beginning of the esophagus forms the inferior boundary (approximately 1 cm below the cricoid ring). The larynx is anterior to the hypopharynx. The pyriform sinuses that extend around both sides of the larynx are part of the hypopharynx.

Larynx

The larynx (Fig. 8.1) is bounded by the hypopharynx superiorly and is continuous with the trachea inferiorly. The thyroid, cricoid, epiglottic, cuneiform, corniculate, and arytenoid cartilages compose the laryngeal skeleton. The thyroid and cricoid cartilages are readily palpated in the anterior neck. The cricoid cartilage articulates with the thyroid cartilage and is joined to it by the cricothyroid ligament. When the patient's head is extended, the cricothyroid ligament can be pierced with a scalpel or large needle to provide an emergency airway (see Chapter 9). The cricoid cartilage completely encircles the airway. It is attached to the first cartilage ring of the trachea by the cricotracheal ligament. The anterior wall of the larynx is formed by the epiglottic cartilage, to which the arytenoid cartilages are attached. Fine muscles span the arytenoid and thyroid cartilages, as do the vocal cords. The true vocal cords and space between them are collectively termed the *glottis* (Fig. 8.2). The glottis is the narrowest space in the adult upper airway. In children, the cricoid cartilage defines the narrowest portion of the airway. Because normal phonation relies on the precise apposition of the true vocal cords, even a small lesion can cause hoarseness. Lymphatic drainage to the true vocal cords is sparse. Inflammation or swelling caused by tube irritation or trauma may take considerable time to resolve. The superior and recurrent laryngeal nerve branches of the vagus nerve innervate the structures of the larynx. The superior laryngeal nerve supplies sensory innervation from the inferior

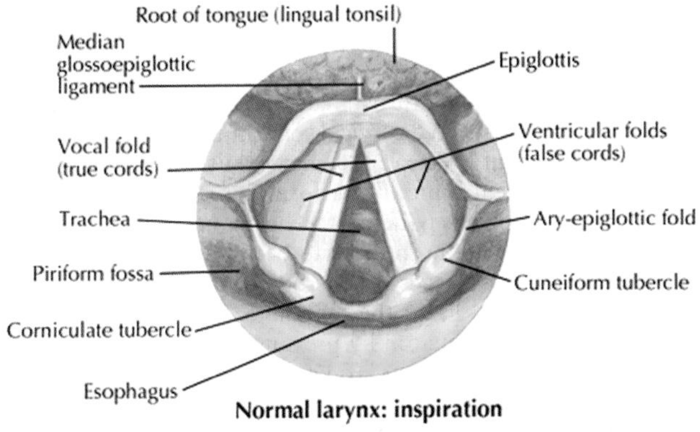

FIGURE 8.2 Superior view of the larynx (inspiration). (Netter FH: *Netter Atlas of Human Anatomy*. 6th ed. New York, NY, Saunders/Elsevier, 2014.)

surface of the epiglottis to the superior surface of the vocal cords. From its take-off from the vagus nerve, it passes deep to both branches of the carotid artery. A large internal branch pierces the thyrohyoid membrane just inferior to the greater cornu of the hyoid. This branch can be blocked with local anesthetics for oral or nasal intubations in awake patients. The recurrent laryngeal branch of the vagus nerve provides sensory innervation below the cords. It also supplies all the muscles of the larynx except the cricothyroid, which is innervated by the external branch of the superior laryngeal nerve.

Trachea

The average adult trachea is 15 cm long. Its external skeleton is composed of a series of C-shaped cartilages. It is bounded posteriorly by the esophagus and anteriorly for the first few cartilage rings by the thyroid gland. The trachea is lined with ciliated cells and has mucus glands; through the beating action of the cilia, foreign substances are propelled toward the larynx. The carina is located at the fourth thoracic vertebral level (of relevance when judging proper ET tube positioning on chest radiograph). The right main bronchus takes off at a less acute angle than the left, making right main bronchial intubation more common if the ET tube is in too far.

EMERGENCY AIRWAY MANAGEMENT

In an emergency situation, establishing adequate ventilation and oxygenation assumes primary importance. Too frequently, inexperienced personnel believe that this requires immediate intubation; however, attempts at intubation may delay establishment of an adequate airway. Such efforts are time consuming, can produce hypoxemia and arrhythmias, and may induce bleeding and regurgitation, making subsequent attempts to intubate significantly more difficult and contributing to significant patient morbidity and even mortality [2,3]. Some simple techniques and principles of emergency airway management can play an important role until the arrival of an individual who is skilled at intubation.

Airway Obstruction

Compromised ventilation often results from upper airway obstruction by the tongue, by substances retained in the mouth, or by laryngospasm. Relaxation of the tongue and jaw leading to a reduction in the space between the base of the tongue and the posterior pharyngeal wall is the most common cause of upper airway obstruction. Obstruction may be partial or complete. The latter is characterized by total lack of air exchange. The former is recognized by inspiratory stridor and retraction of neck and intercostal muscles. If respiration is inadequate, the head-tilt–chin-lift or jaw-thrust maneuver should be performed. In patients with suspected cervical spine injuries, the jaw-thrust maneuver (without the head tilt) may result in the least movement of the cervical spine. To perform the head-tilt maneuver, a palm is placed on the patient's forehead and applied pressure to extend the head about the atlanto-occipital joint. To perform the chin lift, several fingers of the other hand is placed in the submental area and lifted the mandible. Care must be taken to avoid airway obstruction by pressing too firmly on the soft tissues in the submental area. To perform the jaw thrust, lift up on the angles of the mandible (Fig. 8.3). Both of these maneuvers open the oropharyngeal passage. Laryngospasm can be treated by maintaining positive airway pressure using a face mask and bag valve device (see the following section). If the patient resumes spontaneous breathing, establishing this head position may constitute sufficient treatment. If obstruction persists, a check for foreign bodies, emesis, or secretions should be performed.

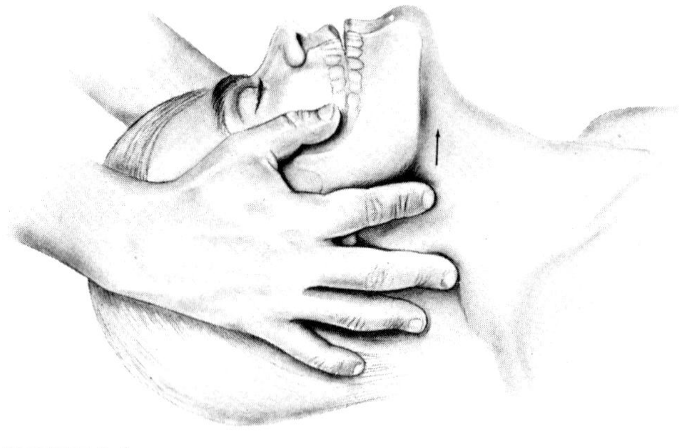

FIGURE 8.3 In an obtunded or comatose patient, the soft tissues of the oropharynx become relaxed and may obstruct the upper airway. Obstruction can be alleviated by placing the thumbs on the maxilla with the index fingers under the ramus of the mandible and rotating the mandible forward with pressure from the index fingers *(arrow)*. This maneuver brings the soft tissues forward and, therefore, frequently reduces the airway obstruction.

Use of Face Mask and Bag Valve Device

If an adequate airway has been established and the patient is not breathing spontaneously, oxygen can be delivered via face mask and a bag valve device. It is important to establish a tight fit with the face mask, covering the patient's mouth and nose. To perform this procedure, the mask is applied initially to the bridge of the nose and drawn it downward toward the mouth, using both hands. The operator stands at the patient's head and presses the mask onto the patient's face with the left hand. The thumb should be on the nasal portion of the mask, the index finger near the oral portion, and the rest of the fingers spread on the left side of the patient's mandible so as to pull it slightly forward (Fig. 8.4). The bag is then alternately compressed and released with the right hand. A good airway is indicated by the rise and fall of the chest; moreover, lung–chest wall compliance can be estimated from the amount of pressure required to compress the bag. The minimum effective insufflation pressure should be used to decrease the risk of insufflating the stomach with gas which increases the risk of aspiration.

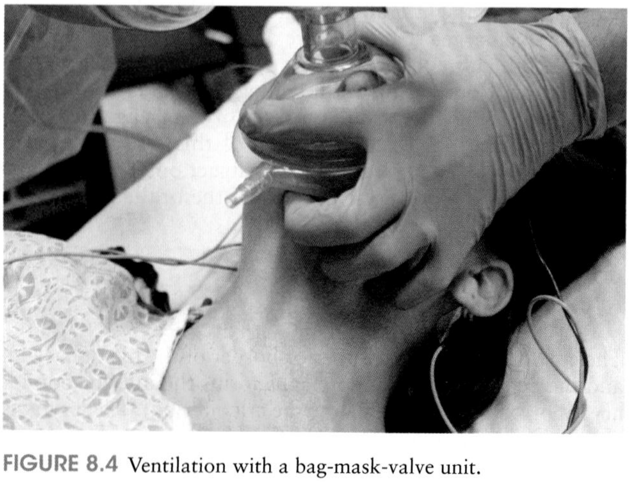

FIGURE 8.4 Ventilation with a bag-mask-valve unit.

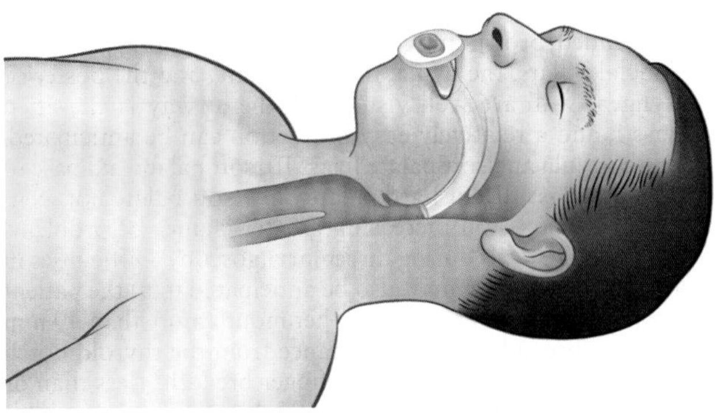

FIGURE 8.5 The proper position of the oropharyngeal airway. (Reproduced with permission from Janet Fong.)

Airway Adjuncts

If proper positioning of the head and neck or clearance of foreign bodies and secretions fails to establish an adequate airway, several airway adjuncts may be helpful if an individual who is skilled in intubation is not immediately available. An oropharyngeal or a nasopharyngeal airway occasionally helps to establish an adequate airway when proper head positioning alone is insufficient (Figs. 8.5 and 8.6). The oropharyngeal airway is semi-circular and made of plastic or hard rubber. The two types are the Guedel airway, with a hollow tubular design, and the Berman airway, with airway channels along the sides. Both types are most easily inserted by turning the curved portion toward the palate as it enters the mouth. It is then advanced beyond the posterior portion of the tongue and rotated downward into the proper position (Fig. 8.5). Often, depressing the tongue or moving it laterally with a tongue blade helps to position the oropharyngeal airway. Care must be exercised not to push the tongue into the posterior pharynx, causing or exacerbating obstruction. Because insertion of the oropharyngeal airway can cause gagging or vomiting or both, it should be used only in unconscious patients.

The nasopharyngeal airway is a soft tube approximately 15 cm long, which is made of rubber or plastic. It is inserted through the nostril into the posterior pharynx (Fig. 8.6). Before insertion, the airway should be lubricated with an anesthetic gel, and, preferably, a vasoconstrictor should be administered into the nostril. The nasopharyngeal airway should not be used in patients with extensive facial trauma or cerebrospinal rhinorrhea because it could be inserted through the cribriform plate into the brain.

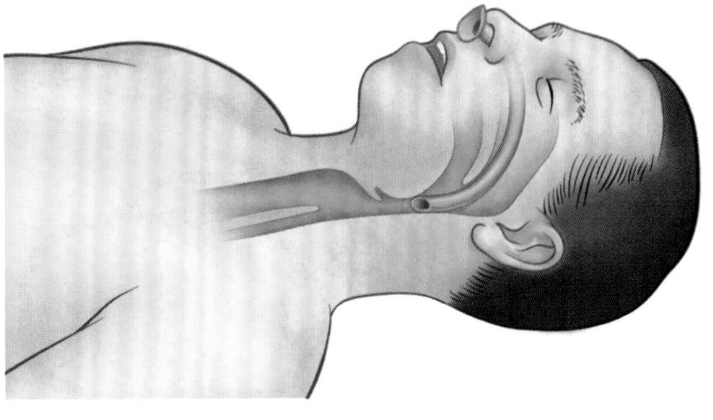

FIGURE 8.6 The proper position of the nasopharyngeal airway. (Reproduced with permission from Janet Fong.)

INDICATIONS FOR INTUBATION

The indications for ET intubation can be divided into four broad categories: (a) acute airway obstruction, (b) excessive pulmonary secretions or inability to clear secretions adequately, (c) loss of protective reflexes, and (d) respiratory failure (Table 8.1).

Preintubation Evaluation

Even in the most urgent situation, a rapid assessment of the patient's airway anatomy can expedite the choice of the proper route for intubation, the appropriate equipment, and the most useful precautions to be taken. In the less emergent situation, several moments of preintubation evaluation can decrease the likelihood of complications and increase the probability of successful intubation with minimal trauma.

Anatomic structures of the upper airway, head, and neck must be examined, with particular attention to abnormalities that might preclude a particular route of intubation. Evaluation of cervical spine mobility, temporomandibular joint function, and dentition is important. Any abnormalities that might

TABLE 8.1

Indications for Endotracheal Intubation

- Acute airway obstruction
  - Trauma
    - Mandible
    - Larynx (direct or indirect injury)
  - Inhalation
    - Smoke
    - Noxious chemicals
    - Foreign bodies
  - Infection
    - Acute epiglottitis
    - Croup
    - Retropharyngeal abscess
  - Hematoma
  - Tumor
  - Congenital anomalies
    - Laryngeal web
    - Supraglottic fusion
  - Laryngeal edema
  - Laryngeal spasm (anaphylactic response)
- Access for suctioning
  - Debilitated patients
  - Copious secretions
- Loss of protective reflexes
  - Head injury
  - Drug overdose
  - Cerebrovascular accident
- Respiratory failure
  - Hypoxemia
    - Acute respiratory distress syndrome
    - Hypoventilation
    - Atelectasis
    - Secretions
    - Pulmonary edema
  - Hypercapnia
    - Hypoventilation
    - Neuromuscular failure
    - Drug overdose

prohibit alignment of the oral, pharyngeal, and laryngeal axes should be noted.

Cervical spine mobility is assessed by flexion and extension of the neck (performed only after ascertaining that no cervical spine injury exists). The normal range of neck flexion–extension varies from 165 to 90 degrees, with the range decreasing approximately 20% by 75 years of age. Conditions associated with decreased range of motion include any cause of degenerative disk disease (e.g., rheumatoid arthritis, osteoarthritis, ankylosing spondylitis), previous trauma, or older than 70 years of age. Temporomandibular joint dysfunction can occur in any form of degenerative arthritis (particularly rheumatoid arthritis), in any condition that causes a receding mandible, and in rare conditions such as acromegaly.

Examination of the oral cavity is mandatory. Loose, missing, or chipped teeth and permanent bridgework are noted, and removable bridgework and dentures should be taken out. Mallampati et al. [4] (Fig. 8.7) developed a clinical indicator based on the size of the posterior aspect of the tongue relative to the size of the oral pharynx. The patient should be sitting, with the head fully extended, protruding the tongue and phonating [5]. When the faucial pillars, the uvula, the soft palate, and the posterior pharyngeal wall are well visualized, the airway is classified as class I, and a relatively easy intubation can be anticipated. When the uvula and soft palate (class II), soft palate and base of uvula only (class III), or hard palate only (soft palate not seen) are visible, there is an increasing greater chance of problems visualizing the glottis during direct laryngoscopy. Difficulties in orotracheal intubation may also be anticipated if (a) the patient is an adult and cannot open his or her mouth more than 40 mm (two-finger breadths), (b) the distance from the thyroid notch to the mandible is less than three-finger breadths (less than or equal to 7 cm), (c) the patient has a high arched palate, or (d) the normal range of flexion–extension of the neck is decreased (less than or equal to 80 degrees) [6]. The positive predictive values of these tests alone or in combination are not particularly high; however, a straightforward intubation can be anticipated if the test results are negative [7]. In the emergency setting, only

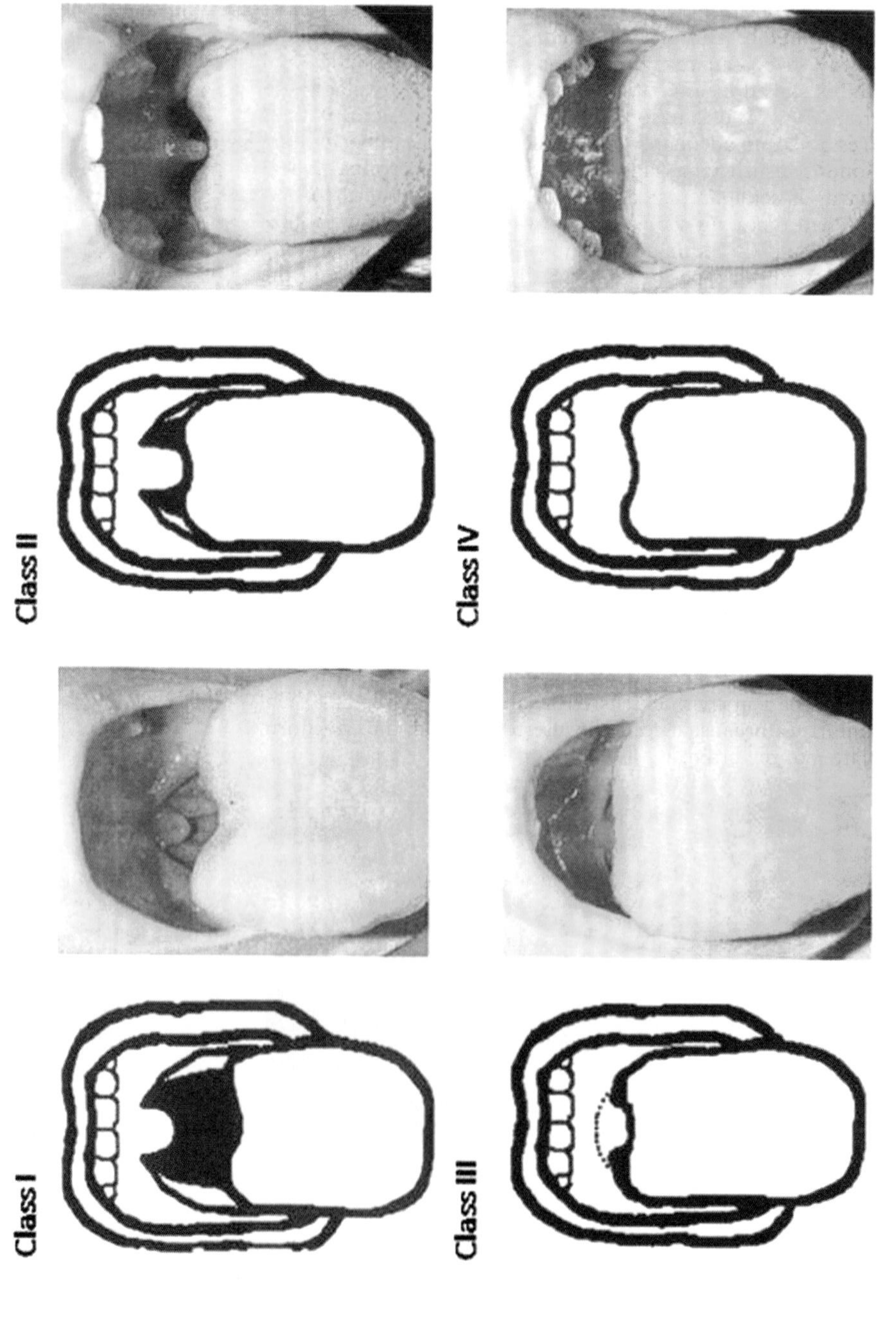

FIGURE 8.7 The modified Mallampati classification to predict difficult intubation. Class I: soft palate, uvula, fauces, and pillars are visible; Class II: soft palate and uvula are visible; Class III: soft palate and base of uvula visible; Class IV: only hard palate visible. (Reproduced from Huan H-H, Lee M-S, Shih Y-L, et al: Modified Mallampati classification as a clinical predictor of peroral esophagogastroduodenoscopy. *BMC Gastroenterol* 11:12, 2011.)

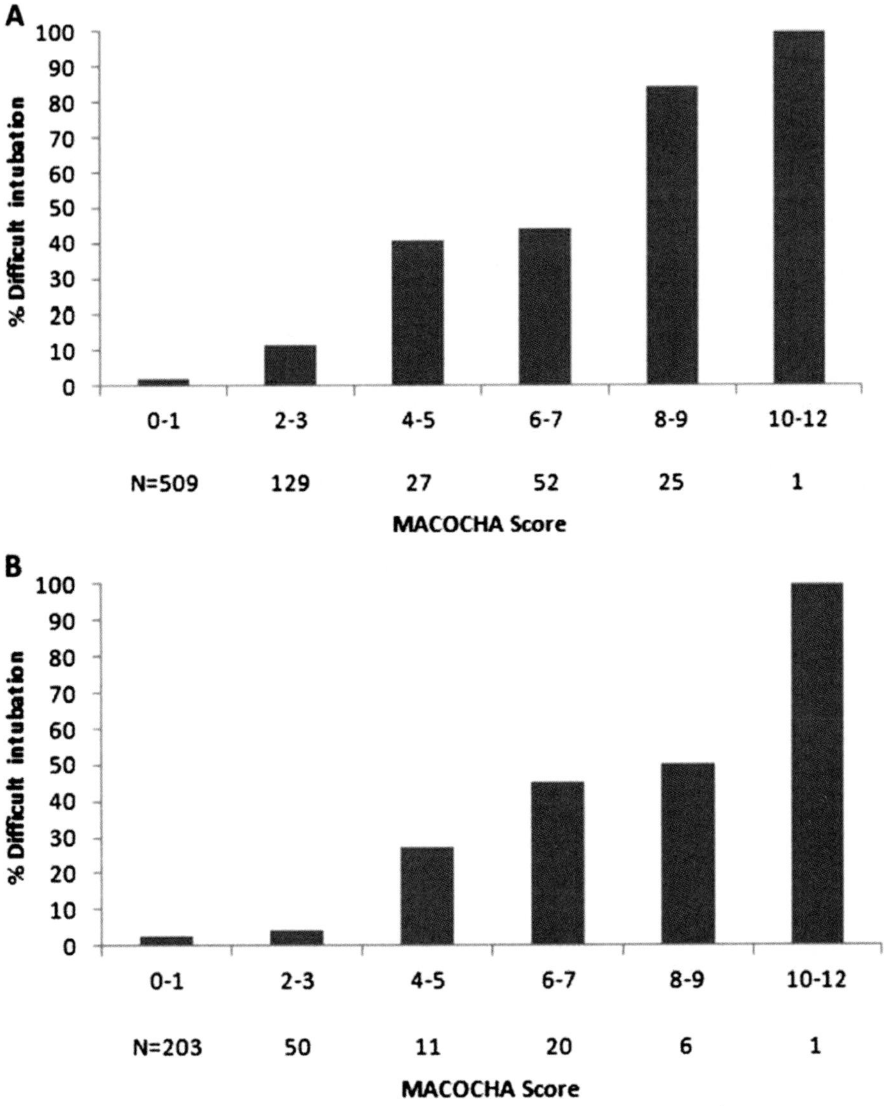

FIGURE 8.8 The MACOCHA score. (**A**) Original cohort and (**B**) is the validation cohort. An increasing score is associated with a higher degree of difficulty with intubation. Graphs A and B are the original and validation cohorts, respectively. (Reproduced with permission from De Jong A, Molinari N, Terzi, et al: Early identification of patients at risk for difficult intubation in the intensive care unit development and validation of the MACOCHA Score in a Multicenter Cohort Study. *Am J Respir Crit Care Med* 187:832–839, 2013.)

about 30% of airways can be assessed in this manner [8]. The MACOCHA (Mallampati, sleep Apnea syndrome, Cervical spine limitation, mouth Opening, Coma, Hypoxia, presence of an Anesthesiologist) score was developed by de Jong et al. (Fig. 8.8). Scores above 4 were associated with a greater than 20% incidence of difficult intubation [9]. Whenever possible, patients in need of elective and emergent airway management should be assessed for indicators of difficult mask ventilation because this may significantly influence the decision on the primary approach to airway management. In a large analysis, five independent predictors of impossible mask ventilation were identified by the authors: neck radiation changes, male sex, a diagnosis of sleep apnea, Mallampati class III or IV airway, and the presence of a beard [10]. Among these factors, neck radiation changes were the most significant predictor of impossible mask ventilation.

Education and Intubation Management

Emergent intubation in the acute care setting is associated with a high complication rate. It is, therefore, important to provide adequate training to practitioners working in this environment, and have an adequate number of trained personnel be available to assist the operator. Furthermore, a standardized approach to emergency airway management can improve patient outcomes. Although training on a mannequin is an important first step in acquiring competency in performing ET intubation, an investigation including nonanesthesia trainees has shown that approximately 50 supervised ET intubations in the clinical setting are needed to achieve a 90% probability of competent performance [11]. Whenever possible, residents and licensed independent practitioners should be supervised by an attending physician trained in emergency airway management during the procedure. This approach has led to a significant reduction in immediate complications from 21.7% to 6.1% in one pre- and postintervention analysis [12].

In addition, the use of a management bundle consisting of interventions that, in isolation have been shown to decrease complications during emergency airway management, can further improve patient outcomes. Elements that should be included in this approach are preoxygenation with noninvasive positive-pressure ventilation (NIPPV) if feasible, presence of two operators, rapid sequence intubation (RSI) with cricoid pressure, capnography, lung protective ventilation strategies, fluid loading prior to intubation unless contraindicated, and preparation and early administration of sedation and vasopressor use if needed [13].

EQUIPMENT FOR INTUBATION

Assembly of all appropriate equipment before attempted intubation can prevent potentially serious delays in the event of an unforeseen complication. Most equipment and supplies are readily available in the ICU but must be gathered so they are immediately at hand. To reduce the risk of having missing equipment during critical times, an intubation bag or cart with all necessary equipments and supplies should be developed. A supply of 100% oxygen and a well-fitting mask with attached bag valve device are mandatory, as is suctioning equipment, including a large-bore tonsil suction attachment (Yankauer) and suction catheters. Adequate lighting facilitates airway visualization. The bed should be at the proper height, with the headboard removed and the wheels locked. Other necessary supplies include gloves, Magill forceps, oral and nasal airways, laryngoscope handle and blades (straight and curved) and/or videolaryngoscope, ET tubes of various sizes, stylet, tongue depressors, a syringe for cuff inflation, and tape for securing the ET tube in position. Table 8.2 is a checklist of supplies needed.

TABLE 8.2

Equipment Needed for Intubation

Supply of 100% oxygen
Face mask
Bag valve device
Suction equipment
  Suction catheters
  Large-bore tonsil suction apparatus (Yankauer)
Stylet
Magill forceps
Oral airways
Nasal airways
Laryngoscope handle and blades (curved, straight; various sizes) or videolaryngoscope
Endotracheal tubes (various sizes)
Tongue depressors
Syringe for cuff inflation
Headrest
Supplies for vasoconstriction and local anesthesia
Tape
Tincture of benzoin

Laryngoscopes

The two-piece laryngoscope has a handle containing batteries that power the bulb in the blade. The blade snaps securely into the top of the handle, making the electrical connection. Failure of the bulb to illuminate suggests improper blade positioning, bulb failure, a loose bulb, or dead batteries. Modern laryngoscope blades with fiberoptic lights obviate the problem of bulb failure. Many blade shapes and sizes are available. The two most commonly used blades are the curved (MacIntosh) and straight (Miller) blades (Fig. 8.9). Although pediatric blades are available for use with the adult-sized handle, most anesthesiologists prefer a smaller handle for better control in the pediatric population. The choice of blade shape is a matter of personal preference and experience; however, one study has suggested that less force and head extension are required when performing direct laryngoscopy with a straight blade [14]. Video-assisted laryngoscopes (Fig. 8.10) are now widely available in many perioperative and acute care specialties and, in many institutions, have become the predominant method by which laryngoscopy and intubation are performed. The blades are equipped with antifogging technology and, distal angles of approximately 60 degrees to improve the view of the glottis and provide a view from near the tip of the scope. These devices have been shown to improve the success rate for difficult ET intubation performed by experienced physicians [15], as well as the rate of successful intubation by untrained individuals when performing normal

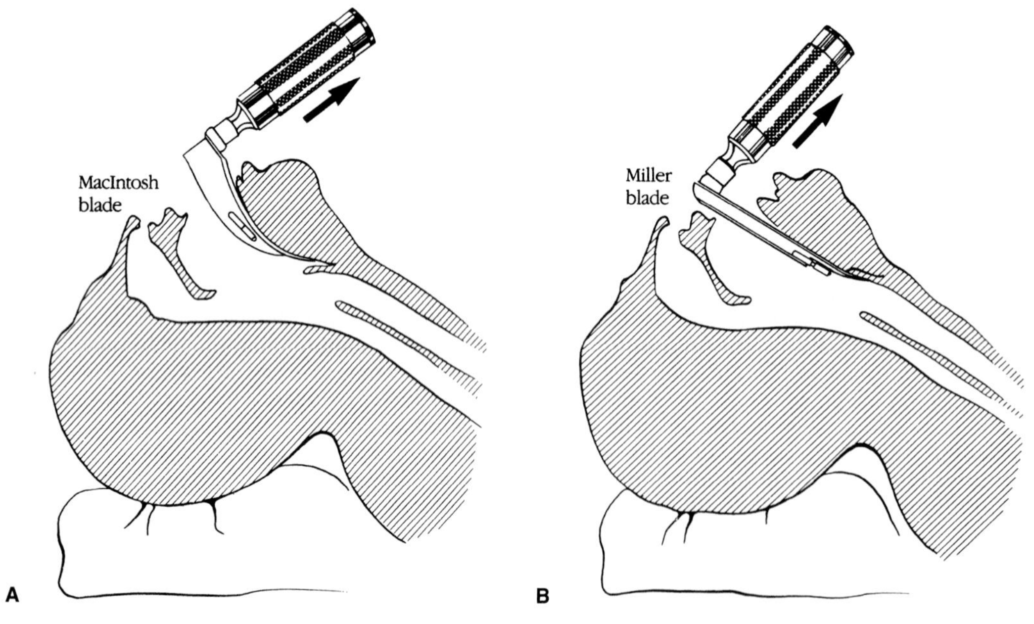

FIGURE 8.9 The two basic types of laryngoscope blades, MacIntosh (A) and Miller (B). The MacIntosh blade is curved. The blade tip is placed in the vallecula, and the handle of the laryngoscope pulled forward at a 45-degree angle. This allows visualization of the epiglottis. The Miller blade is straight. The tip is placed posterior to the epiglottis, pinning the epiglottis between the base of the tongue and the straight laryngoscope blade. The motion on the laryngoscope handle is the same as that used with the MacIntosh blade.

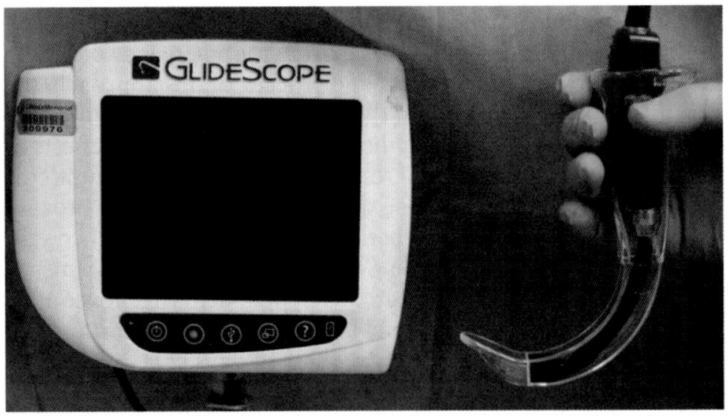

FIGURE 8.10 Videolaryngoscope with screen. Note the 60-degree angle of the blade.

intubations [16]. Hagberg has compiled an extensive list of commercially available videolaryngoscopes [17].

Endotracheal Tubes

The internal diameter of the ET tube is measured using both millimeters and French units. This number is stamped on the tube. Tubes are available in 0.5-mm increments, starting at 2.5 mm. Lengthwise dimensions are also marked on the tube in centimeters, beginning at the distal tracheal end. Selection of the proper tube diameter is of utmost importance and is a frequently underemphasized consideration. The resistance to airflow varies with the fourth power of the radius of the ET tube. Thus, selection of an inappropriately small tube can significantly increase the work of breathing. Moreover, certain diagnostic procedures (e.g., bronchoscopy) done through ET tubes require appropriately large tubes (see Chapter 10). In general, the larger the patient, the larger the ET tube that should be used. Approximate guidelines for tube sizes and lengths by age are summarized in Table 8.3. Most adults should be intubated with an ET tube that has an inner diameter of at least 8.0 mm, although occasionally nasal intubation in a small adult requires a 7.0-mm tube.

TABLE 8.3

Dimensions of Endotracheal Tubes Based on Patient Age

Age	Internal diameter (mm)	French unit	Distance between lips and location in midtrachea of distal end (cm)[a]
Premature	2.5	10–12	10
Full term	3.0	12–14	11
1–6 mo	3.5	16	11
6–12 mo	4.0	18	12
2 y	4.5	20	13
4 y	5.0	22	14
6 y	5.5	24	15–16
8 y	6.5	26	16–17
10 y	7.0	28	17–18
12 y	7.5	30	18–20
≥14 y	8.0–9.0	32–36	20–24

[a]Add 2 to 3 cm for nasal tubes.
Adapted from Stone DJ, Gal TJ, in Miller RD (ed): *Anesthesia*. 4th ed. New York, NY, Churchill Livingstone, 1994, with permission.

Endotracheal Tube Cuff

ET tubes have low-pressure, high-volume cuffs to reduce the incidence of ischemia-related complications. Tracheal ischemia can occur any time cuff pressure that exceeds capillary pressure (approximately 32 mm Hg), thereby causing inflammation, ulceration, infection, and dissolution of cartilaginous rings. Failure to recognize this progressive degeneration sometimes results in erosion through the tracheal wall (into the innominate artery if the erosion was anterior or the esophagus if the erosion was posterior) or long-term sequelae of tracheomalacia or tracheal stenosis. With cuff pressures of 15 to 30 mm Hg, the low-pressure, high-volume cuffs conform well to the tracheal wall and provide an adequate seal during positive-pressure ventilation. Although low cuff pressures can cause some damage (primarily ciliary denudation), major complications are rare. Nevertheless, it is important to realize that a low-pressure, high-volume cuff can be converted to a high-pressure cuff if sufficient quantities of air are injected into the cuff.

ANESTHESIA BEFORE INTUBATION

Because patients who require intubation often have a depressed level of consciousness, anesthesia is usually not required. If intubation must be performed on the alert, responsive patient, sedation or general anesthesia exposes the individual to potential pulmonary aspiration of gastric contents because protective reflexes are lost. This risk is a particularly important consideration if the patient has recently eaten and must be weighed against the risk of various hemodynamic derangements that might occur secondary to tracheal intubation and initiation of positive-pressure ventilation. Laryngoscopy in an inadequately anesthetized patient can result in tachycardia and an increase in blood pressure. This may be well tolerated in younger patients but may be detrimental in a patient with coronary artery disease or raised intracranial pressure. Sometimes laryngoscopy and intubation may result in a vasovagal response, leading to bradycardia and hypotension. Initiation of positive-pressure ventilation in a hypovolemic patient can lead to hypotension from diminished venous return.

Some of these responses can be attenuated by providing local anesthesia to the nares, mouth, and/or posterior pharynx before intubation. Topical lidocaine (1% to 4%) with phenylephrine (0.25%) or cocaine (4%, 200 mg total dose) can be used to anesthetize the nasal passages and provide local vasoconstriction. This allows the passage of a larger ET tube with less likelihood of bleeding. Aqueous lidocaine–phenylephrine or cocaine can be administered via atomizer, nose dropper, or long cotton-tipped swabs inserted into the nares. Alternatively, viscous 2% lidocaine can be applied via a 3.5-mm ET tube or small nasopharyngeal airway inserted into the nose. Anesthesia of the tongue and posterior pharynx can be accomplished with lidocaine spray (4% to 10%) administered via an atomizer or an eutectic mixture of two local anesthetics cream applied on a tongue blade and oral airway [18]. Alternatively, the glossopharyngeal nerve can be blocked bilaterally with an injection of a local anesthetic, but this should be performed by experienced personnel.

Anesthetizing the larynx below the vocal cords before intubation is controversial. The cough reflex can be compromised, increasing the risk of aspiration. However, tracheal anesthesia may decrease the incidence of arrhythmias or untoward circulatory responses to intubation and improve patient tolerance of the ET tube. Clinical judgment in this situation is necessary. Several methods can be used to anesthetize these structures. Transtracheal lidocaine (4%, 160 mg) is administered by cricothyroid membrane puncture with a small needle to anesthetize the trachea and larynx below the vocal cords. However, it may be difficult to identify the cricothyroid membrane by palpation in all patients [19]. Ultrasonography will reliably identify the cricothyroid membrane. Alternatively, after exposure of the vocal cords with the laryngoscope, the cords can be sprayed with lidocaine via an atomizer. Aerosolized lidocaine (4%, 6 mL) provides excellent anesthesia to the mouth, pharynx, larynx, and trachea. The superior laryngeal nerve can be blocked with 2 mL of 1.0% to 1.5% lidocaine injected just inferior to the greater cornu of the hyoid bone. The rate of absorption of lidocaine differs by method, being greater with the aerosol and transtracheal techniques. The patient should be observed for signs of lidocaine toxicity (circumoral paresthesia, agitation, and seizures).

If adequate topical anesthesia cannot be achieved or if the patient is not cooperative, general anesthesia may be required for intubation. Table 8.4 lists common drugs and doses that are used to facilitate intubation. Ketamine and etomidate are two drugs that are used commonly because cardiovascular stability is maintained. Caution should be exercised when using etomidate in patients with signs and symptoms consistent with severe sepsis or septic shock. Owing to inhibition of 11β-hydroxylase, even a single dose of etomidate can cause adrenal suppression for up to 72 hours. Studies examining its use as an induction agent for intubation have reported inconsistent effects on mortality. Administration of corticosteroids after etomidate use is likely unnecessary. Use of opioids such as morphine, fentanyl, sufentanil, alfentanil, or remifentanil allows the dose of the induction drugs to be reduced and may attenuate the hemodynamic response to laryngoscopy and intubation. Muscle relaxants can be used to facilitate intubation, but unless the practitioner has extensive experience with these drugs and airway management, alternative means of airway control and oxygenation should be used until an anesthesiologist or other expert in airway management arrives to administer the anesthetic and performs the intubation. Although the use of muscle relaxants is associated with improved laryngoscopy grade during intubation, their use may not be associated with a decrease in overall airway-related complications, hypotension or hypoxemia.

Reviews have extolled the virtue of RSI [20]: the process by which a drug such as etomidate, thiopental, ketamine, or propofol (Table 8.4) is administered to the patient to induce anesthesia and is followed immediately by a muscle relaxant to facilitate intubation. Although numerous studies exist in the emergency medicine literature attesting to the safety and efficacy of this approach, the practitioner who embarks on this route to intubation in the ICU must be knowledgeable about the pharmacology and side effects of the agents used, *and* the use of rescue methods should attempt(s) at intubation fail. Succinylcholine should be used cautiously because of its propensity to cause hyperkalemic cardiac arrest in certain critically ill populations, including burned and spinal injured patients. Prolonged bed rest can also lead to a hyperkalemic response after succinylcholine administration. This risk increases substantially if patients are in the ICU for more than 14 days [21]. Experience and an approached based on a validated algorithm will increase patient safety. In an analysis of 6,088 trauma patients undergoing emergency airway management in a single center over 10 years, intubation by anesthesiologists experienced in the management of trauma patients utilizing a modification of the American Society of Anesthesiologists difficult airway algorithm was very effective, resulting in a rate of surgical airway management in only 0.3% of patients included in the analysis [22].

TECHNIQUES OF INTUBATION

In a true emergency, some of the preintubation evaluation is necessarily neglected in favor of rapid control of the airway. Attempts at tracheal intubation should not cause or exacerbate hypoxia. Whenever possible, an oxygen saturation monitor should be used. Preoxygenation (denitrogenation), which replaces the nitrogen in the patient's functional residual capacity with oxygen, can maximize the time available for intubation. During laryngoscopy, apneic oxygenation can occur from this reservoir. Preoxygenation is achieved by providing 100% oxygen at a high flow rate via a tight-fitting face mask for 3.5 to 4.0 minutes. Extending the time of preoxygenation from 4 to 8 minutes does not seem to increase the PaO_2 to a clinically relevant extent and may actually reduce the PaO_2 in the interval from 6 to 8 minutes in some patients [23]. In patients who are being intubated for airway control, preoxygenation is usually efficacious, whereas the value of preoxygenation in patients with acute lung injury is

TABLE 8.4

Drugs Used to Facilitate Intubation

Drug	IV dose (mg/kg)	Onset of action	Other side effects	Effect on rate of ventilation	ICP	CBF	$CMRO_2$
Induction drugs							
Propofol	1.0–2.5	<60 s	Pain on injection	↓↓↓	↓↓↓	↓↓↓	↓↓↓
Midazolam	0.02–0.20	30–60 s		↓–↓↓	↓↓	↓↓	↓↓
Ketamine	0.5–2.0	30–60 s	Increase in secretions, Emergence reactions	0/↓	↑↑↑	↑↑↑	↑
Dexmedetomidine	1.0 μg/kg then 0.2—0.7 μg/kg/h	30 min	Bradycardia, Hypotension	0/↓	0	↓	0, ↓
Etomidate	0.2–0.3	20–50 s	Adrenal insufficiency, Pain on injection	0/↓	↓↓↓	↓↓↓	↓↓↓
Supplemental Drugs							
Fentanyl	50–100 μg	10–20 min	Chest wall rigidity	↓↓–↓↓↓	0/↑	0/↓	0/↓
Muscle relaxants							
Succinylcholine	1.0–2.0	45–60 s	Hyperkalemia	↓↓↓	0/↑	↑	?
Rocuronium	0.6–1.0	60–90 s		↓↓↓	0	a	a

Adapted from Heard SO and Watson NC. Airway Management and Upper Airway Obstruction. In: Roberts PR and Todd SR (eds), Comprehensive Critical Care : Adult. Society of Critical Care Medicine (Mount Prospect) 2012.
ICP, intracranial pressure; CBF, cerebral blood flow; CMRO2, cerebral metabolic rate of oxygen.

less certain [24]. Whenever possible, NIPPV or high flow nasal oxygen should be utilized as the mode of preoxygenation prior to intubation of hypoxemic patients. These approaches have been shown to be more effective than the standard approach in maintaining SpO_2 values before, during, and even after the intubation procedure [25–27]. In obese patients, the use of the 25-degree head-up position improves the effectiveness of preoxygenation.

Just before intubation, the physician should assess the likelihood of success for each route of intubation, the urgency of the clinical situation, the likelihood that intubation will be prolonged, and the prospect of whether diagnostic or therapeutic procedures such as bronchoscopy will eventually be required. Factors that can affect patient comfort should also be weighed. In the unconscious patient in whom a secure airway must be established immediately, orotracheal intubation with direct visualization of the vocal cords is generally the preferred technique. In the conscious patient, direct laryngoscopy or awake fiberoptic intubation may be performed after obtaining adequate anesthesia of the airway. Alternatively, blind nasotracheal intubation is an option but requires significant skill by the clinician. Nasotracheal intubation should be avoided in patients with coagulopathies or those who are anticoagulated for medical indications. In the obese patient, employing the ramped position, whereby blankets are place under the head, shoulders, and upper back to insure that the tragus is at the level of the suprasternal notch, will increase the probability of a successful intubation (Fig. 8.11A and B). In trauma victims with extensive maxillary and mandibular fractures and inadequate ventilation

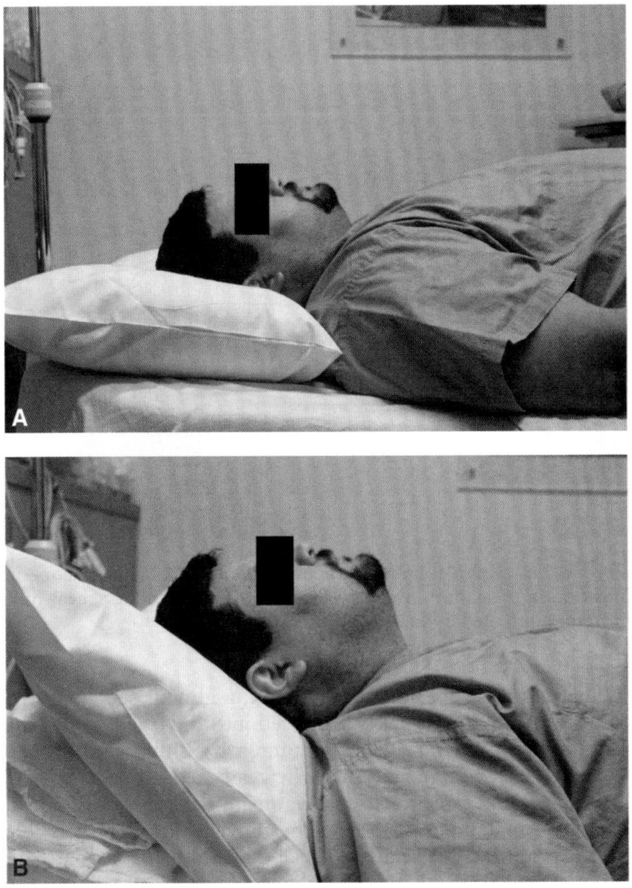

FIGURE 8.11 **A:** Obese subject with head placed on pillow. The tragus is below the level of the suprasternal notch. **B:** After "ramping" with blankets beneath upper back and head, the tragus is at the level of the suprasternal notch.

or oxygenation, cricothyrotomy may be mandatory (see Chapter 9). In patients with cervical spine injury or decreased neck mobility, intubation using the flexible bronchoscope may be necessary. Many of these techniques require considerable skill and should be performed only by those who are experienced in airway management.

Specific Techniques and Routes of Endotracheal Intubation

Orotracheal Intubation

Orotracheal intubation is the technique most easily learned and most often used for emergency intubations in the ICU. Traditional teaching dictates that successful orotracheal intubation requires alignment of the oral, pharyngeal, and laryngeal axes by putting the patient in the "sniffing position" in which the neck is flexed and the head is slightly extended about the atlanto-occipital joint. However, a magnetic resonance imaging (MRI) study has called this concept into question because the alignment of these three axes could not be achieved in any of the three positions tested: neutral, simple extension, and the "sniffing position" [28]. In addition, a randomized study in elective surgery patients examining the utility of the sniffing position as a means to facilitate orotracheal intubation failed to demonstrate that such positioning was superior to simple head extension [29,30].

In a patient with a full stomach, compressing the cricoid cartilage posteriorly against the vertebral body can reduce the diameter of the hypopharynx. This technique, known as *Sellick maneuver*, may prevent passive regurgitation of stomach contents into the trachea during intubation. However, an MRI study of awake volunteers demonstrated that the esophagus was lateral to the larynx in more than 50% of the subjects. Moreover, cricoid pressure *increased* the incidence of an unopposed esophagus by 50% and caused airway compression of greater than 1 mm in 81% of the volunteers [31]. These findings are in contrast to a more recent MRI study demonstrating that the location and movement of the esophagus is irrelevant to the efficacy of Sellick maneuver to prevent gastric regurgitation into the pharynx because the esophagus begins approximately 1 cm below the cricoid ring. In addition, the hypopharynx is attached to the cricoid ring by ligaments and muscles [32]. Consequently, compression of the alimentary tract was demonstrated with midline and lateral displacement of the cricoid cartilage relative to the underlying vertebral body [32]. Cadaver studies have demonstrated the efficacy of cricoid pressure [33], and clinical studies have shown that gastric insufflation with gas during mask ventilation is reduced when cricoid pressure is applied [34]. In aggregate, these data suggest that it is prudent to continue to use cricoid pressure in patients suspected of having full stomachs. In addition, placing the patient in the partial recumbent or reverse Trendelenburg position may reduce the risk of regurgitation and aspiration.

The laryngoscope handle is grasped in the left hand whereas the patient's mouth is opened with the gloved right hand. Often, when the head is extended in the unconscious patient, the mouth opens; if not, the thumb and index finger of the right hand are placed on the lower and upper incisors, respectively, and moved past each other in a scissor-like motion. The laryngoscope blade is inserted on the right side of the mouth and advanced to the base of the tongue, pushing it toward the left. If the straight blade is used, it should be extended below the epiglottis. If the curved blade is used, it is inserted in the vallecula.

With the blade in place, the operator should lift forward in a plane 45 degrees from the horizontal to expose the vocal cords (Figs. 8.2 and 8.9). This motion decreases the risk of the blade striking the upper incisors and either chipping or dislodging teeth. Both lips should be swept away from between the teeth and blade to avoid soft tissue damage. The ET tube is then held in the right hand and inserted at the right corner of the patient's mouth in a plane that intersects with the laryngoscope blade at the level of the glottis. This prevents the ET tube from obscuring the view of the vocal cords. The ET tube is advanced through the vocal cords until the cuff just disappears from sight. The cuff is inflated with enough air to prevent a leak during positive-pressure ventilation with a bag valve device. Videos 8.1 and 8.2 of the technique are available at https://video.search.yahoo.com/video/play?p=New+England+Journal+of+Medicine+Intubation&vid=3d7c0a1192ea871c2f64b8f9284b4ebb&turl=http%3A%2F%2Fts1.mm.bing.net%2Fth%3Fid%3DWN.Y0KiUOeOK9JsM7ZMbMzHVQ%26pid%3D15.1%26h%3D225%26w%3D300%26c%3D7%26rs%3D1&rurl=https%3A%2F%2Fwww.youtube.com%2Fwatch%3Fv%3D8SS_AhR-DUw&tit=Orotracheal+Intubation%2CPart-1&c=0&h=225&w=300&l=318&sigr=11btmomgp&sigt=10totfb9s&sigi=12kui7qjn&ct=p&age=1325589995&fr2=p%3As%2Cv%3Av&fr=yhs-mozilla-003&hsimp=yhs-003&hspart=mozilla&tt=b **AND** https://video.search.yahoo.com/video/play?p=New+England+Journal+of+Medicine+Intubation&vid=36d72b18a61e59101009ea1764b9eac3&turl=http%3A%2F%2Fts2.mm.bing.net%2Fth%3Fid%3DWN.ruA%252bnLZEzCLF3F0oXeASQA%26pid%3D15.1%26h%3D225%26w%3D300%26c%3D7%26rs%3D1&rurl=https%3A%2F%2Fwww.youtube.com%2Fwatch%3Fv%3Dt_8lNoaP6Oo&tit=Orotracheal+Intubation%2C+part-2&c=1&h=225&w=300&l=409&sigr=11bkvot9h&sigt=10utkvs4n&sigi=12msuh1g6&ct=p&age=1325760089&fr2=p%3As%2Cv%3Av&fr=yhs-mozilla-003&hsimp=yhs-003&hspart=mozilla&tt=b; both accessed June 25, 2015.

Intubation using a videolaryngoscope is accomplished by holding the handle with the left hand and inserting the blade into the mouth and advancing the tip to the vallecula (Fig. 8.12A, B and C). The view of the glottis is usually very good, but intubation can sometimes be problematic because the proprietary stylets are rigid and cannot be molded to the optimal curvature. Inserting the ET tube from the right at 90 degrees from the usual position may help if there is difficulty. Complications can include mucosal damage or perforation of the palatoglossal arch, palatopharyngeal arch, or the retromolar trigone. Direct visualization when inserting the tube into the mouth will reduce the risk of mucosal damage. (On-line tutorials are available: Turk M, Gravenstein D (2007): Storz DCI Video Laryngoscope, the University of Florida Department of Anesthesiology, Center for Simulation, Advanced Learning and Technology Web site: http://vam.anest.ufl.edu/airwaydevice/storz/index.html, accessed September 7, 2017 **AND** https://www.youtube.com/watch?v=4VAMBj2kc2Y, accessed September 7, 2017.)

A classification grading the view of the laryngeal aperture during direct laryngoscopy has been described [35] and is depicted in Figure 8.13. Occasionally, the vocal cords cannot be seen entirely; only the corniculate and cuneiform tubercles, interarytenoid incisure, and posterior portion of the vocal cords or only the epiglottis is visualized (grades II to IV view; Fig. 8.13). In this situation, it is helpful to insert the soft metal stylet into the ET tube and bend it into a hockey-stick configuration. The stylet should be bent or coiled at the proximal end to prevent the distal end from extending beyond the ET tube and causing tissue damage. The stylet should be lubricated to ensure easy removal. The BURP maneuver (*b*ackward–*u*pward–*r*ightward *p*ressure on the larynx) improves the view of the laryngeal aperture [36]. Alternatively, a control-tip ET tube can be used (Endotrol, Mallinckrodt, St. Louis, MO). This tube has a nylon cord running the length of the tube attached to a ring at the proximal end, which allows the operator to direct the tip of the tube anteriorly. Another aid is a stylet with a light (light wand). With the room lights dimmed, the ET tube containing the lighted stylet is inserted into the oropharynx and advanced in the midline.

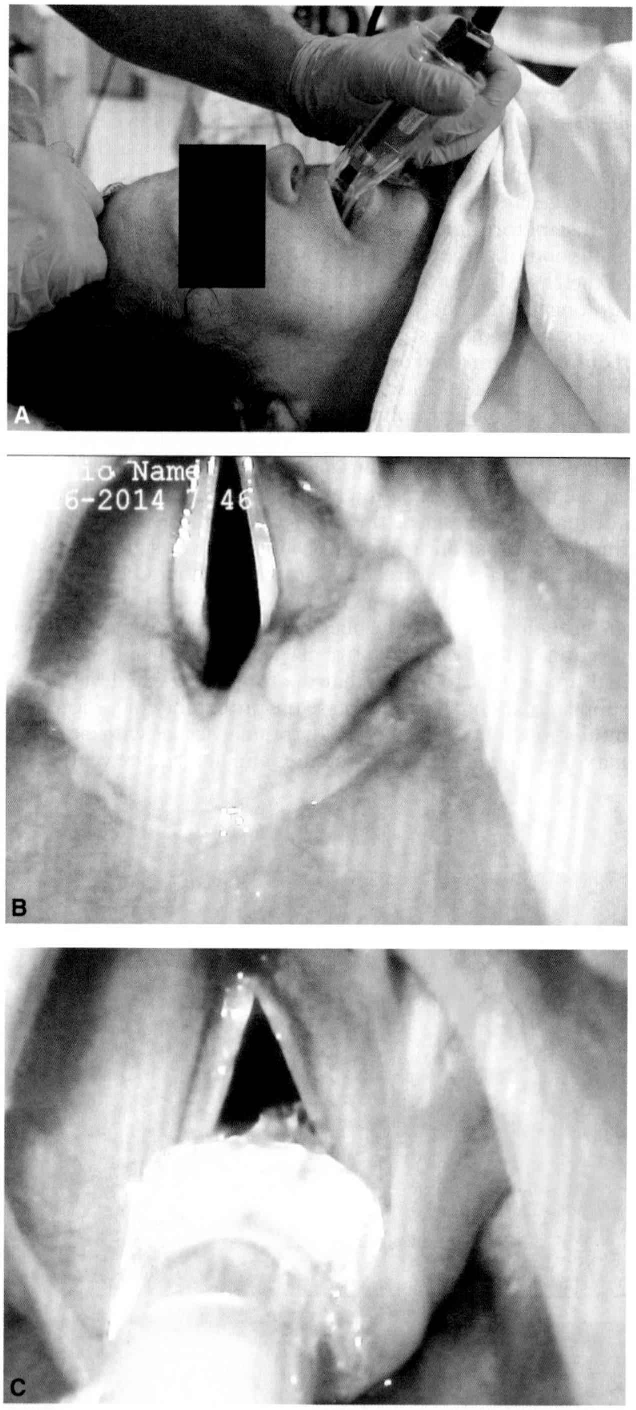

FIGURE 8.12 Videolaryngoscope intubation. **A:** Laryngoscope in position in the mouth. **B:** View of the glottis. **C:** Endotracheal tube insertion into the larynx.

When it is just superior to the larynx, a glow is seen over the anterior neck. The stylet is advanced into the trachea, and the tube is threaded over it. The light intensity is diminished if the wand enters the esophagus (http://www.wakehealth.edu/School/Anesthesiology/Tutorials/Lightwand-Intubation-Tutorial.htm [accessed September 7, 2017]). The gum elastic bougie (flexible stylet) is another alternative device that can be passed into the larynx; once in place, the ET tube is advanced over it and the stylet is removed. ET tubes and stylets are now available that have a fiberoptic bundle intrinsic to the tube or the stylet that can be attached to a video monitor. If the attempt to intubate

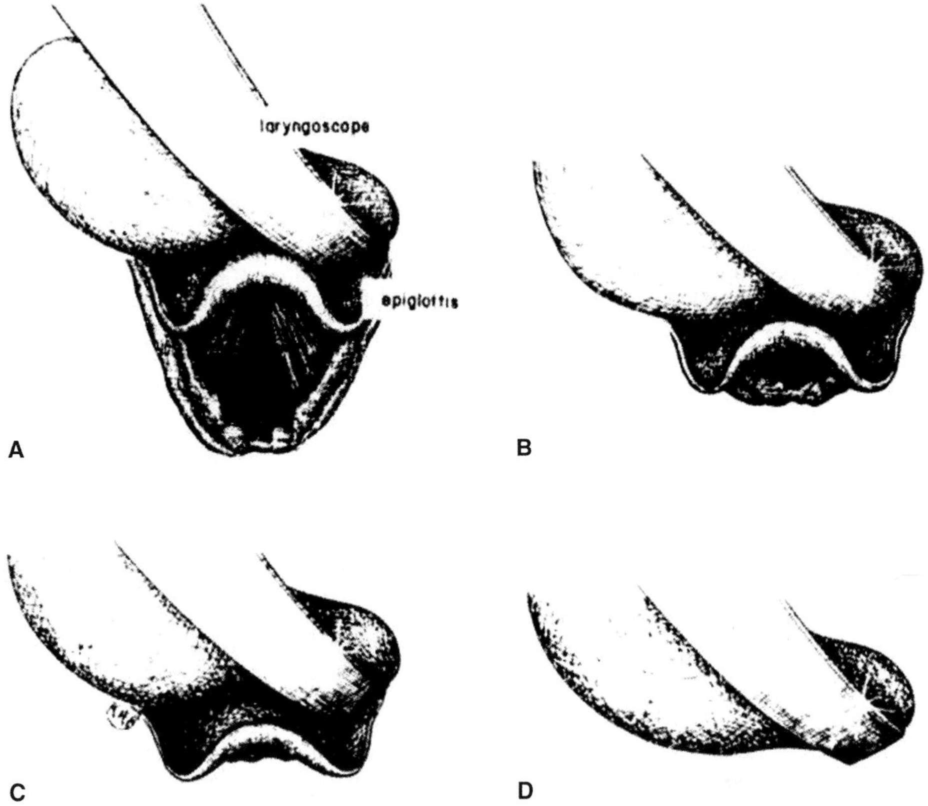

FIGURE 8.13 The four grades of laryngeal view during direct laryngoscopy. **A:** Grade I: the entire glottis is seen. **B:** Grade II: only the posterior aspect of the glottis is seen. **C:** Grade III: only the epiglottis is seen. **D:** Grade IV: the epiglottis is not visualized. (From Cormack RS, Lehane J: Difficult tracheal intubation in obstetrics. *Anaesthesia* 39:1105–1111, 1984, with permission.)

is still unsuccessful, the algorithm should be followed (see "Management of the Difficult Airway" section of this chapter).

Proper depth of tube placement is clinically ascertained by observing symmetric expansion of both sides of the chest and auscultating equal breath sounds in both lungs. The stomach should also be auscultated to ensure that the esophagus has not been entered. If the tube has been advanced too far, it will lodge in one of the main bronchi (particularly the right bronchus), and only one lung will be ventilated. If this error goes unnoticed, the nonventilated lung may collapse. A useful rule of thumb for tube placement in adults of average size is that the incisors should be at the 23-cm mark in men and the 21-cm mark in women. Alternatively, proper depth (5 cm above the carina) can be estimated using the following formula: (height in cm/5) − 13 [37]. Palpation of the anterior trachea in the neck may detect cuff inflation because air is injected into the pilot tube and can serve as a means to ascertain correct tube position. Measurement of end-tidal carbon dioxide by standard capnography if available or by means of a calorimetric chemical detector of end-tidal carbon dioxide (e.g., Easy Cap II, Nellcor, Inc., Pleasanton, CA) should be used to verify correct ET tube placement or detect esophageal intubation. The latter device is attached to the proximal end of the ET tube and changes color on exposure to carbon dioxide. An additional method to detect esophageal intubation uses a bulb that attaches to the proximal end of the ET tube (AMBU, Ballerup, Denmark). The bulb is squeezed. If the tube is in the trachea, the bulb reexpands, and if the tube is in the esophagus, the bulb remains collapsed. It must be remembered that none of these techniques is fool proof. Bronchoscopy is the only method to be absolutely sure the tube is in the trachea. After estimating proper tube placement clinically, it should be confirmed by chest radiograph or bronchoscopy because the tube may be malpositioned. The tip of the ET tube should be several centimeters above the carina (T-4 level). It must be remembered that flexion or extension of the head can advance or withdraw the tube 2 to 5 cm, respectively.

Nasotracheal Intubation

Many of the considerations concerning patient preparation and positioning outlined for orotracheal intubation apply to nasal intubation as well. Blind nasal intubation is more difficult to perform than oral intubation because the tube cannot be observed directly as it passes between the vocal cords. Nasal intubation should not be attempted in patients with abnormal bleeding parameters, nasal polyps, extensive facial trauma, cerebrospinal rhinorrhea, sinusitis, or any anatomic abnormality that would inhibit atraumatic passage of the tube. Nasal intubation is rarely performed because of the risk of maxillary sinusitis.

As previously discussed in "Airway Adjuncts" section, after the operator has alternately occluded each nostril to ascertain that both are patent, a topical vasoconstrictor and anesthetic are applied to the nostril that will be intubated. The nostril may be dilated with lubricated nasal airways of increasing size to facilitate atraumatic passage of the ET tube. The patient should be monitored with a pulse oximeter, and supplemental oxygen should be given as necessary. The patient may be either supine or sitting with the head extended in the sniffing position. The tube is guided slowly but firmly through the nostril to the posterior pharynx. Here the tube operator must continually monitor for the presence of air movement through the tube by listening for breath sounds with the ear near the open end of the tube. The tube must never be forced or pushed forward if breath sounds are lost, because damage to the retropharyngeal mucosa can result. If resistance is met, the tube should be withdrawn 1 to 2 cm and the patient's head repositioned (extended further or turned to either side). If the turn still cannot be negotiated, the other nostril or a smaller tube should be tried. Attempts at nasal intubation should be abandoned and oral intubation performed if these methods fail.

Once positioned in the oropharynx, the tube is advanced to the glottis while listening for breath sounds through the tube. If breath sounds cease, the tube is withdrawn several centimeters until breath sounds resume, and the plane of entry is adjusted slightly. Inflation of the cuff will facilitate alignment of the ET tube with the glottis. Passage through the vocal cords should be timed to coincide with inspiration. Entry of the tube into the larynx is signalled by an inability to speak. The cuff should be inflated and proper positioning of the tube ascertained as previously outlined.

Occasionally, blind nasal intubation cannot be accomplished. In this case, after adequate topical anesthesia, laryngoscopy can be used to visualize the vocal cords directly and Magill forceps used to grasp the distal end of the tube and guide it through the vocal cords. Assistance in pushing the tube forward is essential during this maneuver so that the operator merely guides the tube. The balloon on the tube should not be grasped with the Magill forceps.

Management of the Difficult Airway

A difficult airway may be recognized (anticipated) or unrecognized at the time of the initial preintubation airway evaluation. Difficulty managing the airway may be the result of abnormalities such as congenital hypoplasia, hyperplasia of the mandible or maxilla, or prominent incisors; injuries to the face or neck; acromegaly; tumors; and previous head and neck surgery. Difficulties ventilating the patient with a mask can be anticipated if two of the following factors are present: older than 55 years of age, body mass index greater than 26 kg per m^2, beard, lack of teeth, and a history of snoring [38]. When a difficult airway is encountered, the algorithm as detailed in Figure 8.14 should be followed. When a difficult airway is recognized before the patient is anesthetized, an awake tracheal intubation is usually the best option. Multiple techniques can be used and include (after adequate topical or local anesthesia) direct laryngoscopy, LMA (or variants), blind or bronchoscopic oral or nasal intubation, retrograde technique, rigid bronchoscopy, lighted stylet, or a surgical airway.

Flexible Bronchoscopic Intubation

Flexible bronchoscopy is an efficacious method of intubating the trachea in difficult cases. It may be particularly useful when the upper airway anatomy has been distorted by tumors, trauma, endocrinopathies, or congenital anomalies. This technique is sometimes valuable in accident victims in whom a question of cervical spine injury exists and the patient's neck cannot be manipulated. An analogous situation exists in patients with severe degenerative disk disease of the neck or rheumatoid arthritis with markedly impaired neck mobility. After adequate topical anesthesia is obtained (discussed in "Anesthesia before Intubation" section), the bronchoscope can be used to intubate the trachea via either the nasal or oral route. An appropriately sized warmed and lubricated ET tube that has been preloaded onto the bronchoscope is advanced through the vocal cords into the trachea and positioned above the carina under direct vision. The flexible bronchoscope has also been used as a stent over which ET tubes are exchanged and as a means to assess tracheal damage periodically during prolonged intubations. (A detailed discussion of bronchoscopy is found in Chapter 10.) Intubation by this technique requires skill and experience and is best performed by a fully trained operator.

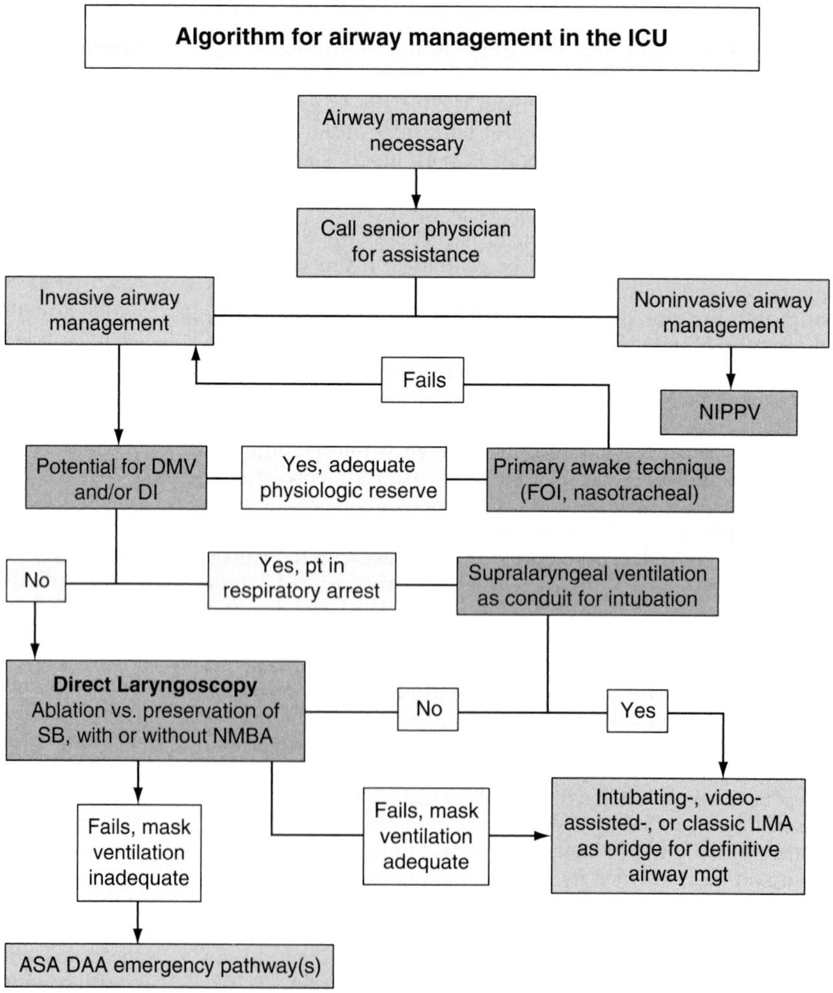

FIGURE 8.14 Modification of the difficult airway algorithm. ASA DAA, American Society of Anesthesiologists difficult airway algorithm; DMV, difficult mask ventilation; FOI, fiberoptic intubation; LMA, laryngeal mask airway; NIPPV, noninvasive positive-pressure ventilation; NMBA, neuromuscular blocking agents; SB, spontaneous breathing. (From Walz JM, Zayaruzny M, Heard SO: Airway management in critical illness. *Chest* 131(2):608–620, 2007, with permission.)

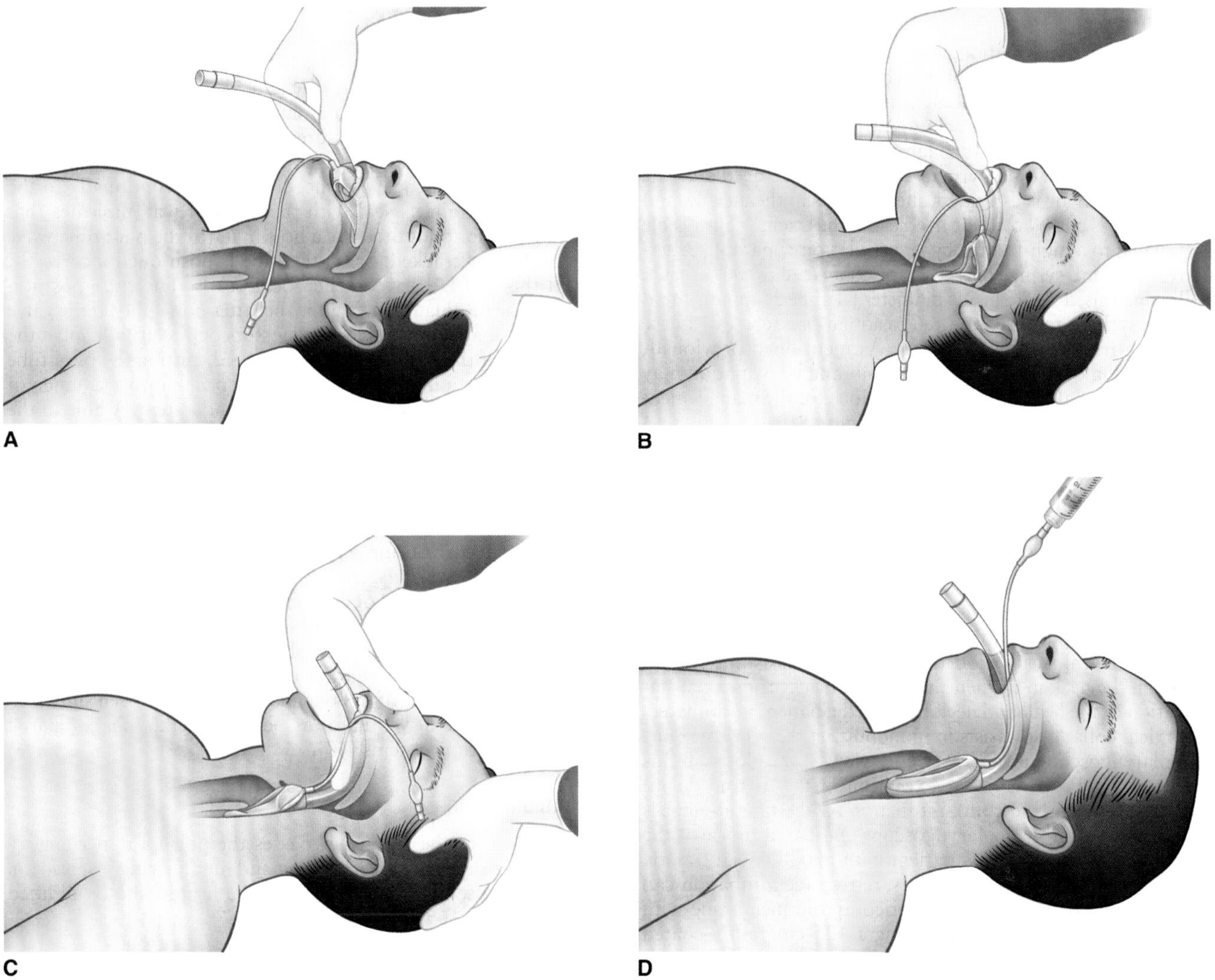

FIGURE 8.15 A–D: Technique for insertion of the laryngeal mask airway. (Reproduced with permission from Janet Fong.)

If the operator is able to maintain mask ventilation in a patient with an unrecognized difficult airway, a call for experienced help should be initiated (Fig. 8.14). If mask ventilation cannot be maintained, a cannot ventilate–cannot intubate situation exists and immediate lifesaving rescue maneuvers are required. Options include an emergency cricothyrotomy or insertion of a supraglottic ventilatory device, such as an LMA or a Combitube (Puritan Bennett, Pleasanton, CA).

Other Airway Adjuncts

The LMA is composed of a plastic tube attached to a shallow mask with an inflatable rim (Fig. 8.15A–D). When properly inserted, it fits over the laryngeal inlet and allows positive-pressure ventilation of the lungs. Although aspiration can occur around the mask, the LMA can be lifesaving in a cannot ventilate–cannot intubate situation. An intubating LMA (LMA-Fastrach; LMA North America, Inc., San Diego, CA) has a shorter plastic tube and can be used to provide ventilation as well as to intubate the trachea with or without the aid of a flexible bronchoscope (Fig. 8.16). The Combitube (Puritan Bennett) combines the features of an ET tube and an esophageal obturator airway and reduces the risk of aspiration. Personnel who are unskilled in airway management can easily learn how to use the LMA and the Combitube together.

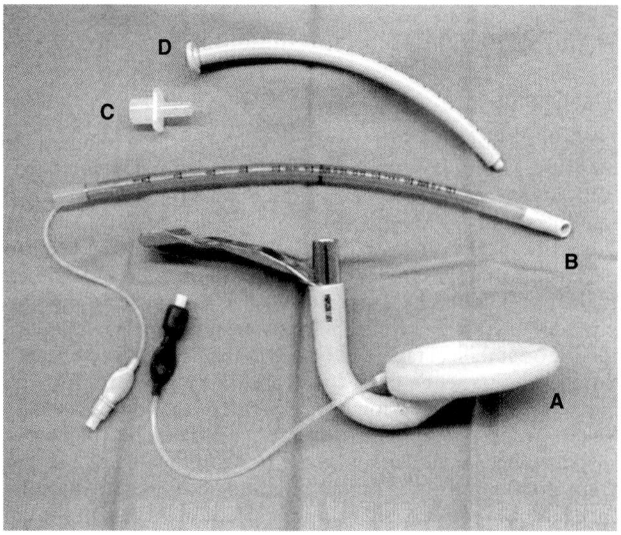

FIGURE 8.16 The laryngeal mask airway (LMA)-Fastrach (A) has a shorter tube than a conventional LMA. A special endotracheal tube (B) (without the adapter (C)) is advanced through the LMA-Fastrach into the trachea. The extender (D) is attached to the endotracheal tube, and the LMA-Fastrach is removed. After the extender is removed, the adapter is placed back on the tube.

Cricothyrotomy

In a truly emergent situation, when intubation is unsuccessful, a cricothyrotomy may be required. The technique is described in detail in Chapter 9. The quickest method, needle cricothyrotomy, is accomplished by introducing a large-bore (i.e., 14-gauge) catheter into the airway through the cricothyroid membrane while aspirating with a syringe attached to the needle of the catheter. When air is aspirated, the needle is in the airway, and the catheter is passed over the needle into the trachea. The needle is attached to a high-frequency jet ventilation apparatus. Alternatively, a 3-mL syringe barrel can be connected to the catheter. Following this, a 7-mm inside diameter ET tube adapter is fitted into the syringe and is connected to a high-pressure gas source or a high-frequency jet ventilator. As mentioned previously, identification of the cricothyroid membrane by palpation may be difficult. An algorithm with suggestions for the management of the difficult airway is provided in Figure 8.14.

Management of the Airway in Patients with Suspected Cervical Spine Injury

Any patient with multiple trauma who requires intubation should be treated as if cervical spine injury was present. In the absence of severe maxillofacial trauma or cerebrospinal rhinorrhea, nasal intubation can be considered. However, in the profoundly hypoxemic or apneic patient, the orotracheal approach should be used. If oral intubation is required, an assistant should maintain the neck in the neutral position by ensuring axial stabilization of the head and neck because the patient is intubated. A cervical collar also assists in immobilizing the cervical spine. Videolaryngoscopy provides a better view of the glottis in this situation. However, with the exception of the Airtraq device (Airtraq, www.airtraq.com), intubation on the first attempt is not improved with videolaryngoscopy compared to use of the MacIntosh blade [39]. In a patient with maxillofacial trauma and suspected cervical spine injury, retrograde intubation can be performed by puncturing the cricothyroid membrane with an 18-gauge catheter and threading a 125-cm Teflon-coated (0.025-cm diameter) guidewire through the catheter. The wire is advanced into the oral cavity, and the ET tube is then advanced over the wire into the trachea. Alternatively, the wire can be threaded through the suction port of a 3.9-mm bronchoscope.

Airway Management in the Intubated Patient

Securing the Tube

Properly securing the ET tube in the desired position is important for three reasons: (a) to prevent accidental extubation, (b) to prevent advancement into one of the main bronchi, and (c) to minimize damage to the upper airway, larynx, and trachea caused by patient motion. The ET tube is usually secured in place with adhesive tape wrapped around the tube and applied to the patient's cheeks. Tincture of benzoin sprayed on the skin provides greater fixation. Alternatively, tape, intravenous (IV) tubing, or umbilical tape, can be tied to the ET tube and brought around the patient's neck to secure the tube. Care must be taken to prevent occlusion of neck veins. Other products (e.g., Velcro straps) to secure the tube are available. A bite block can be positioned in patients who are orally intubated to prevent them from biting down on the tube and occluding it. Once the tube has been secured and its proper position verified, it should be plainly marked on the portion protruding from the patient's mouth or nose so that advancement can be noted.

Cuff Management

Although low-pressure cuffs have markedly reduced the incidence of complications related to tracheal ischemia, monitoring cuff pressures remains important. The cuff should be inflated just beyond the point where an audible air leak occurs. Maintenance of intracuff pressures between 17 and 23 mm Hg should allow an adequate seal to permit mechanical ventilation under most circumstances while not compromising blood flow to the tracheal mucosa. The intracuff pressure should be checked periodically by attaching a pressure gauge and syringe to the cuff port via a three-way stopcock. The need to add air continually to the cuff to maintain its seal with the tracheal wall indicates that (a) the cuff or pilot tube has a hole in it, (b) the pilot tube valve is broken or cracked, or (c) the tube is positioned incorrectly, and the cuff is between the vocal cords. The tube position should be revaluated to exclude the latter possibility. If the valve is broken, attaching a three-way stopcock to it will solve the problem. If the valve housing is cracked, cutting the pilot tube and inserting a blunt needle with a stopcock into the lumen of the pilot tube can maintain a competent system. A hole in the cuff necessitates a change of tube.

Tube Suctioning

A complete discussion of tube suctioning can be found in Chapter 169. Routine suctioning should not be performed in patients in whom secretions are not a problem. Suctioning can produce a variety of complications, including hypoxemia, elevations in intracranial pressure, and serious ventricular arrhythmias. Preoxygenation should reduce the likelihood of arrhythmias. Closed ventilation suction systems (Stericath) may reduce the risk of hypoxemia but have not been shown to reduce the rate of ventilator-associated pneumonia compared to open suction systems [40].

Humidification

Intubation of the trachea bypasses the normal upper airway structures responsible for heating and humidifying inspired air. It is thus essential that inspired air be heated and humidified (see Chapter 169).

Tube Replacement

At times, ET tubes may need to be replaced because of an air leak, obstruction, or other problems. Obstruction can be relieved with balloon-tipped catheters. The catheter is inserted into the tube and advanced to the tip, and the balloon is inflated. The catheter is pulled back, and the obstructing debris is dislodged from the tube. Before attempting to change an ET tube, one should assess how difficult it will be. After ensuring appropriate nil per os status, obtaining appropriate topical anesthesia or IV sedation and achieving muscle relaxation, direct laryngoscopy can be performed to ascertain whether there will be difficulties in visualizing the vocal cords. If the cords can be seen, the defective tube is removed under direct visualization and reintubation is performed using the new tube. If the cords cannot be seen on direct laryngoscopy, the tube can be changed over an airway exchange catheter (e.g., Cook Critical Care, Bloomington, IN) which allows insufflation of oxygen via either standard oxygen tubing or a bag valve device [41].

COMPLICATIONS OF ENDOTRACHEAL INTUBATION

Table 8.4 is a partial listing of the complications associated with ET intubation. Factors implicated in the etiology of complications include tube size, characteristics of the tube and cuff, trauma during intubation, duration and route of intubation, metabolic or nutritional status of the patient, tube motion, and laryngeal motor activity.

TABLE 8.5

Complications of Endotracheal Intubation

- Complications during intubation
  - Spinal cord injury
  - Excessive delay of cardiopulmonary resuscitation
  - Aspiration
  - Damage to teeth and dental work
  - Corneal abrasions
  - Perforation or laceration of
    - Pharynx
    - Larynx
    - Trachea
  - Dislocation of an arytenoid cartilage
  - Passage of endotracheal tube into cranial vault
  - Epistaxis
  - Cardiovascular problems
    - Ventricular premature contractions
    - Ventricular tachycardia
    - Bradyarrhythmias
    - Hypotension
    - Hypertension
    - Hypoxemia
  - Complications while tube is in place
    - Blockage or kinking of tube
    - Dislodgment of tube
    - Advancement of tube into a bronchus
    - Mechanical damage to any upper airway structure
    - Problems related to mechanical ventilation (see Chapter 166)
- Complications following extubation
  - Immediate complications
    - Laryngospasm
    - Aspiration
  - Intermediate- and long-term complications
    - Sore throat
    - Ulcerations of lips, mouth, pharynx, or vocal cords
    - Tongue numbness (hypoglossal nerve compression)
    - Laryngitis
    - Vocal cord paralysis (unilateral or bilateral)
    - Laryngeal edema
    - Laryngeal ulcerations
    - Laryngeal granuloma
    - Vocal cord synechiae
    - Tracheal stenosis

During ET intubation, traumatic injury can occur to any anatomic structure from the lips to the trachea. Possible complications include aspiration; damage to teeth and dental work; corneal abrasions; perforation or laceration of the pharynx, larynx, or trachea; dislocation of an arytenoid cartilage; retropharyngeal perforation; epistaxis; hypoxemia; myocardial ischemia; laryngospasm with noncardiogenic pulmonary edema; and death [2,3]. Many of these complications can be avoided by paying careful attention to technique and ensuring that personnel with the greatest skill and experience perform the intubation. Complications during ET intubation vary according to the location of the patient in need of emergency airway management. Although the complication rates on the regular hospital floor and in the ICU appear to be high at around 28% for both locations, they can be modified with standardized algorithms as outlined previously. The most frequent complications encountered in these two settings are multiple intubation attempts and esophageal intubation in the general hospital units, and severe hypoxemia and hemodynamic collapse in the ICU. The presence of acute respiratory failure and shock appears to be an independent risk factor for the occurrence of complications in the latter setting [42,43].

Complications during Intubation

A variety of cardiovascular complications can accompany intubation. Ventricular arrhythmias have been reported in 5% to 10% of intubations. Ventricular tachycardia and ventricular fibrillation are uncommon but have been reported. Patients with myocardial ischemia are susceptible to ventricular arrhythmias, and lidocaine prophylaxis (100 mg IV bolus) before intubation may be warranted in such individuals. Bradyarrhythmias can also be observed and are probably caused by stimulation of the laryngeal branches of the vagus nerve. They may not require therapy but usually respond to IV atropine (1 mg IV bolus). Hypotension or hypertension can occur during intubation. In the patient with myocardial ischemia, short-acting agents to control blood pressure (nitroprusside and nicardipine) and heart rate (esmolol) during intubation may be needed.

Complications While the Tube is in Place

Despite adherence to guidelines designed to minimize damage from ET intubation, the tube can damage local structures. Microscopic alterations to the surface of the vocal cords can occur within 2 hours after intubation. Evidence of macroscopic damage can occur within 6 hours. As might be expected, clinically significant damage typically occurs when intubation is prolonged. The sudden appearance of blood in tracheal secretions suggests anterior erosion into overlying vascular structures, and the appearance of gastric contents suggests posterior erosion into the esophagus. Both situations require urgent bronchoscopy, and it is imperative that the mucosa underlying the cuff be examined. Other complications include tracheomalacia and stenosis and damage to the larynx. Failure to secure the ET tube properly or patient agitation can contribute to mechanical damage.

Another complication is blockage or kinking of the tube, resulting in compromised ventilation. Placing a bite block in the patient's mouth can minimize occlusion of the tube caused by the patient biting down on it. Suctioning can usually solve blockage from secretions, although changing the tube may be necessary.

Unplanned extubation and endobronchial intubation are potentially life threatening. Judicious use of sedatives and analgesics and appropriately securing and marking the tube can minimize these problems. Other complications that occur while the tube is in position relate to mechanical ventilation (e.g., pneumothorax) and are discussed in detail in Chapter 58.

Complications after Extubation

Sore throat occurs after 40% to 100% of intubations. Using a smaller ET tube may decrease the incidence of postextubation sore throat and hoarseness. Ulcerations of the lips, mouth, or pharynx can occur and are more common if the initial intubation was traumatic. Pressure from the ET tube can traumatize the hypoglossal nerve, resulting in numbness of the tongue that can persist for 1 to 2 weeks. Irritation of the larynx appears to be caused by local mucosal damage and occurs in as many as 45% of individuals after extubation. Unilateral or bilateral vocal cord paralysis is an uncommon but serious complication following extubation.

Some degree of laryngeal edema accompanies almost all ET intubations. In adults, this is usually clinically insignificant. In children, however, even a small amount of edema can compromise the already small subglottic opening. In a newborn, 1 mm of laryngeal edema results in a 65% narrowing of the airway. Laryngeal ulcerations are commonly observed after extubation. They are more commonly located at the posterior portion of the vocal cords, where the ET tube tends to rub. Ulcerations become increasingly common the longer the tube is left in place. The incidence of ulceration is decreased by the use of ET tubes that conform to the anatomic shape of the larynx. Laryngeal granulomas and synechiae of the vocal cords are extremely rare, but these complications can seriously compromise airway patency. Surgical treatment is often required to treat these problems.

A feared late complication of ET intubation is tracheal stenosis. This occurs much less frequently now that high-volume, low-pressure cuffs are routinely used. Symptoms can occur weeks to months after extubation. In mild cases, the patient may experience dyspnea or ineffective cough. If the airway is narrowed to less than 5 mm, the patient presents with stridor. Dilation may provide effective treatment, but, in some instances, surgical intervention is necessary.

EXTUBATION

The decision to extubate a patient is based on (a) a favorable clinical response to a carefully planned regimen of weaning from mechanical ventilation (see Chapter 168), (b) recovery of consciousness following anesthesia, or (c) sufficient resolution of the initial indications for intubation.

Technique of Extubation

The patient should be alert, lying with the head of the bed elevated to at least a 45-degree angle. The posterior pharynx must be thoroughly suctioned. The procedure is explained to the patient. The cuff is deflated, and positive pressure is applied to expel any foreign material that has collected above the cuff as the tube is withdrawn. Supplemental oxygen is then provided.

In situations in which postextubation difficulties are anticipated, equipment for emergency reintubation should be assembled at the bedside. In addition, administration of pre-extubation steroids will reduce the risk of developing stridor [44]. Some clinicians have advocated the "leak test" as a means to predict the risk of stridor after extubation. The utility of this procedure is limited in routine practice, but for patients with certain risk factors (e.g., traumatic intubation, prolonged intubation, and previous accidental extubation), a leak volume of greater than 130 mL or 12% of the tidal volume has a sensitivity and specificity of 85% and 95%, respectively, for the development of postextubation stridor [45]. Probably, the safest way to extubate the patient if there are concerns about airway edema or the potential need to reintubate a patient with a difficult airway is to use an airway exchange catheter. This device is inserted through the ET tube and then the tube is removed over the catheter. Supplemental oxygen can be provided via the catheter to the patient, and the catheter can be used as a stent for reintubation if necessary.

One of the most serious complications of extubation is laryngospasm, and it is more likely to occur if the patient is not fully conscious. The application of positive pressure can sometimes relieve laryngospasm. If this maneuver is not successful, a small dose of succinylcholine (by the IV or intramuscular route) can be administered. Succinylcholine can cause severe hyperkalemia in a variety of clinical settings; therefore, only clinicians who are experienced with its use should administer it. Ventilation with a mask and bag unit is needed until the patient has recovered from the succinylcholine.

Tracheostomy

The optimal time of conversion from an ET tube to a tracheostomy remains controversial. The reader is referred to Chapter 9 for details on tracheostomy.

Utility of Ultrasonography for Airway Management

Ultrasonography has several useful applications related to airway management.

Identification of Gastric Fluid

Ultrasonography examination of the stomach is a useful means of identifying gastric contents [46]. Identification of a full stomach during setup for urgent ET intubation allows the team to avoid the catastrophic complication of massive aspiration during urgent ET intubation sequence. A proficient operator can scan for gastric contents in less than 1 minute, so the examination is feasible as a routine safety measure during urgent ET intubations. With the phased array probe configured for abdominal scanning, the examination is performed with longitudinal (coronal) scanning plane over the lower left lateral thorax in the midaxillary line. The tomographic ultrasonography plane is angled through the target area. The spleen maybe used as a sonographic window. An alternative method is to examine the left upper quadrant from the anterior approach, although gas artifact frequently blocks adequate imaging. If significant gastric fluid is present (Video 8.3), the team may elect to insert a gastric tube to empty the stomach. If the patient is so unstable that this is not possible, the team, alerted to the risk of massive aspiration, may take specific steps to reduce this risk, such as utilization of a paralytic agent, preparing extra suction devices, and assigning the intubation to the team member with highest skill level.

Identification of Endotracheal Tube Position

Ultrasonography may be used to verify the position of the ET tube [47,48]. The high-frequency vascular transducer is used to obtain a transverse-axis image of the trachea immediately above the suprasternal notch (Video 8.4). The anterior wall of the trachea appears as a curvilinear echogenic line often in association with a posterior comet tale artifact. With real-time scanning, the ET tube may be seen to pass through the image plane into the trachea or into the adjacent esophagus appearing as an echogenic line within the boundaries of the trachea. Alternatively, the operator may opt to identify ET tube position immediately following the insertion of the ET tube. The esophagus is usually immediately posterior and to the left of the trachea. Less commonly, it is to the right or posterior to the trachea. In case of unintentional esophageal intubation, the ET tube is visualized in transverse scanning plane posterior and usually to the left of the laryngeal structures. One limitation of ultrasonography of the trachea for ET tube placement is that, if there is air interposed between the anterior tracheal wall and the ET tube, the air will block visualization of the ET tube. For this reason, visualization of the ET tube within the trachea should only be used when other standard techniques of verification are not immediately available or deemed unreliable for clinical reasons.

Ultrasonography may be used to indirectly infer ET tube position using lung ultrasonography. Instead of directly identifying the position of the tube in the airway, successful ET intubation is verified by the presence of bilateral lung sliding, which may be rapidly ascertained by examination for lung sliding during bag valve breaths [49] (see Chapter 11 on Lung Ultrasonography). The combination of direct visualization methods described earlier with lung sliding has been reported to have very high predictive value for identification successful ET tube insertion [50].

Ultrasonography may be used to rapidly identify the presence of a right mainstem intubation [51]. In this case, the inflated ET tube cuff may block off the left mainstem bronchus with persistent hypoxemia and rapid resorptive atelectasis of the left lung. As a result, lung sliding will be present on the right side but absent on the left side. The ET tube may be pulled back under ultrasonography control until lung sliding is observed bilaterally.

References

1. Ellis H, Lawson AD: *Anatomy for Anaesthetists*. 9th ed. Oxford, UK, Wiley-Blackwell, 2014.
2. Mort TC: The incidence and risk factors for cardiac arrest during emergency tracheal intubation: a justification for incorporating the ASA Guidelines in the remote location. *J Clin Anesth* 16(7):508–516, 2004.
3. Mort TC: Emergency tracheal intubation: complications associated with repeated laryngoscopic attempts. *Anesth Analg* 99(2):607–613, 2004.
4. Mallampati SR, Gatt SP, Gugino LD, et al: A clinical sign to predict difficult tracheal intubation: a prospective study. *Can Anaesth Soc J* 32(4):429–434, 1985.
5. Lewis M, Keramati S, Benumof JL, et al: What is the best way to determine oropharyngeal classification and mandibular space length to predict difficult laryngoscopy? *Anesthesiology* 81(1):69–75, 1994.
6. Gal TJ: Airway management, in Miller RD (ed): *Anesthesia*. 6th ed. Philadelphia, PA, Churchill Livingstone, 2005, pp 1617–1652.
7. Tse JC, Rimm EB, Hussain A: Predicting difficult endotracheal intubation in surgical patients scheduled for general anesthesia: a prospective blind study. *Anesth Analg* 81(2):254–258, 1995.
8. Levitan RM, Everett WW, Ochroch EA: Limitations of difficult airway prediction in patients intubated in the emergency department. *Ann Emerg Med* 44(4):307–313, 2004.
9. De Jong A, Molinari N, Terzi N, et al: Early identification of patients at risk for difficult intubation in the intensive care unit: development and validation of the MACOCHA score in a multicenter cohort study. *Am J Respir Crit Care Med* 187(8):832–839, 2013.
10. Kheterpal S, Martin L, Shanks AM, et al: Prediction and outcomes of impossible mask ventilation: a review of 50,000 anesthetics. *Anesthesiology* 110(4):891–897, 2009.
11. Mulcaster JT, Mills J, Hung OR, et al: Laryngoscopic intubation: learning and performance. *Anesthesiology* 98(1):23–27, 2003.
12. Schmidt UH, Kumwilaisak K, Bittner E, et al: Effects of supervision by attending anesthesiologists on complications of emergency tracheal intubation. *Anesthesiology* 109(6):973–977, 2008.
13. Jaber S, Jung B, Corne P, et al: An intervention to decrease complications related to endotracheal intubation in the intensive care unit: a prospective, multiple-center study. *Intensive Care Med* 36(2):248–255, 2010.
14. Hastings RH, Hon ED, Nghiem C, et al: Force, torque, and stress relaxation with direct laryngoscopy. *Anesth Analg* 82(3):456–461, 1996.
15. Lim TJ, Lim Y, Liu EH: Evaluation of ease of intubation with the GlideScope or Macintosh laryngoscope by anaesthetists in simulated easy and difficult laryngoscopy. *Anaesthesia* 60(2):180–183, 2005.
16. Nouruzi-Sedeh P, Schumann M, Groeben H: Laryngoscopy via Macintosh blade versus GlideScope: success rate and time for endotracheal intubation in untrained medical personnel. *Anesthesiology* 110(1):32–37, 2009.
17. Hagberg CA: Current concepts in the management of the difficult airway. *Anesthesiol News* 1–28, 2014.
18. Larijani GE, Cypel D, Gratz I, et al: The efficacy and safety of EMLA cream for awake fiberoptic endotracheal intubation. *Anesth Analg* 91(4):1024–1026, 2000.
19. Aslani A, Ng SC, Hurley M, et al: Accuracy of identification of the cricothyroid membrane in female subjects using palpation: an observational study. *Anesth Analg* 114(5):987–992, 2012.
20. Reynolds SF, Heffner J: Airway management of the critically ill patient: rapid-sequence intubation. *Chest* 127(4):1397–1412, 2005.
21. Blanie A, Ract C, Leblanc PE, et al: The limits of succinylcholine for critically ill patients. *Anesth Analg* 115(4):873–879, 2012.
22. Stephens CT, Kahntroff S, Dutton RP: The success of emergency endotracheal intubation in trauma patients: a 10-year experience at a major adult trauma referral center. *Anesth Analg* 109(3):866–872, 2009.
23. Mort TC, Waberski BH, Clive J: Extending the preoxygenation period from 4 to 8 mins in critically ill patients undergoing emergency intubation. *Crit Care Med* 37(1):68–71, 2009.
24. Mort TC: Preoxygenation in critically ill patients requiring emergency tracheal intubation. *Crit Care Med* 33(11):2672–2675, 2005.
25. Baillard C, Fosse JP, Sebbane M, et al: Noninvasive ventilation improves preoxygenation before intubation of hypoxic patients. *Am J Respir Crit Care Med* 174(2):171–177, 2006.
26. Barjaktarevic I, Berlin D: Bronchoscopic intubation during continuous nasal positive pressure ventilation in the treatment of hypoxemic respiratory failure. *J Intensive Care Med* 30(3):161–166, 2015.
27. Miguel-Montanes R, Hajage D, Messika J, et al: Use of high-flow nasal cannula oxygen therapy to prevent desaturation during tracheal intubation of intensive care patients with mild-to-moderate hypoxemia. *Crit Care Med* 43(3):574–583, 2015.
28. Adnet F, Borron SW, Dumas JL, et al: Study of the "sniffing position" by magnetic resonance imaging. *Anesthesiology* 94(1):83–86, 2001.
29. Adnet F, Baillard C, Borron SW, et al: Randomized study comparing the "sniffing position" with simple head extension for laryngoscopic view in elective surgery patients. *Anesthesiology* 95(4):836–841, 2001.
30. Akihisa Y, Hoshijima H, Maruyama K, et al: Effects of sniffing position for tracheal intubation: a meta-analysis of randomized controlled trials. *Am J Emerg Med* 33:1606–1611, 2015.
31. Smith KJ, Dobranowski J, Yip G, et al: Cricoid pressure displaces the esophagus: an observational study using magnetic resonance imaging. *Anesthesiology* 99(1):60–64, 2003.
32. Rice MJ, Mancuso AA, Gibbs C, et al: Cricoid pressure results in compression of the postcricoid hypopharynx: the esophageal position is irrelevant. *Anesth Analg* 109(5):1546–1552, 2009.
33. Salem MR, Joseph NJ, Heyman HJ, et al: Cricoid compression is effective in obliterating the esophageal lumen in the presence of a nasogastric tube. *Anesthesiology* 63(4):443–446, 1985.
34. Lawes EG, Campbell I, Mercer D: Inflation pressure, gastric insufflation and rapid sequence induction. *Br J Anaesth* 59(3):315–318, 1987.
35. Cormack RS, Lehane J: Difficult tracheal intubation in obstetrics. *Anaesthesia* 39(11):1105–1111, 1984.
36. Ulrich B, Listyo R, Gerig HJ, et al: The difficult intubation. The value of BURP and 3 predictive tests of difficult intubation. *Anaesthesist* 47(1):45–50, 1998.
37. Cherng CH, Wong CS, Hsu CH, et al: Airway length in adults: estimation of the optimal endotracheal tube length for orotracheal intubation. *J Clin Anesth* 14(4):271–274, 2002.
38. Langeron O, Masso E, Huraux C, et al: Prediction of difficult mask ventilation. *Anesthesiology* 92(5):1229–1236, 2000.
39. Suppan L, Tramer MR, Niquille M, et al: Alternative intubation techniques vs Macintosh laryngoscopy in patients with cervical spine immobilization: systematic review and meta-analysis of randomized controlled trials. *Br J Anaesth* 116:27–36, 2016.
40. Subirana M, Sola I, Benito S: Closed tracheal suction systems versus open tracheal suction systems for mechanically ventilated adult patients. *Cochrane Database Syst Rev* (4):CD004581, 2007.
41. Loudermilk EP, Hartmannsgruber M, Stoltzfus DP, et al: A prospective study of the safety of tracheal extubation using a pediatric airway exchange catheter for patients with a known difficult airway. *Chest* 111(6):1660–1665, 1997.
42. Benedetto WJ, Hess DR, Gettings E, et al: Urgent tracheal intubation in general hospital units: an observational study. *J Clin Anesth* 19(1):20–24, 2007.
43. Jaber S, Amraoui J, Lefrant JY, et al: Clinical practice and risk factors for immediate complications of endotracheal intubation in the intensive care unit: a prospective, multiple-center study. *Crit Care Med* 34(9):2355–2361, 2006.
44. Khemani RG, Randolph A, Markovitz B: Corticosteroids for the prevention and treatment of post-extubation stridor in neonates, children and adults. *Cochrane Database Syst Rev* (3):CD001000, 2009.
45. Jaber S, Chanques G, Matecki S, et al: Post-extubation stridor in intensive care unit patients. Risk factors evaluation and importance of the cuff-leak test. *Intensive Care Med* 29(1):69–74, 2003.
46. Koenig S, Laktikoca V, Mayo PH: Utility of ultrasonography for detection of gastric fluid during emergency endotracheal intubation. *Intensive Care Med* 37:627–631, 2011.
47. Werner SL, Smith CE, Goldstein JR, et al: Pilot study to evaluate the accuracy of ultrasonography in confirming endotracheal tube placement. *Ann Emerg Med* 49:75–80, 2007.
48. Chou HC, Tseng WP, Wang CH, et al: Tracheal rapid ultrasound exam (T.R.U.E.). *Resuscitation* 82:1279–1284, 2011.
49. Sim SS, Lien WC, Chou HC, et al: Ultrasonographic lung sliding sign in confirming proper endotracheal intubation during emergency intubation. *Resuscitation* 83:307–312, 2012.
50. Park SC, Ryu JH, Yeom SR, et al: Confirmation of endotracheal intubation by combined ultrasonographic methods in the Emergency Department. *Emerg Med Australas* 21:293–297, 2009.
51. Blaivas M, Tsung JW: Point-of-care sonographic detection of left endobronchial main stem intubation and obstruction versus endotracheal intubation. *J Ultrasound Med* 27:785–789, 2008.

Chapter 9 ■ Tracheostomy

CHRISTINE L. BIELICK • SCOTT E. KOPEC • TIMOTHY A. EMHOFF

Tracheostomy first started to be performed regularly in the 1800s when used by Trousseau and Bretonneau in the management of diphtheria. In the early 1900s, this procedure was used to treat difficult cases of respiratory paralysis from poliomyelitis. Largely because of improvements in tubes and advances in clinical care, endotracheal intubation has become the treatment of choice for short-term airway management.

Although urgent tracheostomy or emergent cricothyrotomy is occasionally required in critically ill and injured patients who cannot be intubated for various reasons (e.g., cervical spine injury, upper airway obstruction, laryngeal injury, and anatomic considerations), the most common use of this procedure today is to provide long-term access to the airway in patients who are dependent on mechanical ventilation. With improvements in critical care medicine over the past 30 years, more patients are surviving their initial episodes of acute respiratory failure, trauma, and extensive surgeries, and require prolonged periods of mechanical ventilation. It is now common practice to convert these patients from translaryngeal intubation to tracheostomy. Tracheostomy is becoming a common procedure in the intensive care unit (ICU). The prevalence of tracheostomies in ICU patients ranges from 8% to more than 30% [1,2].

In this chapter, we review the indications, contraindications, complications, and techniques associated with tracheostomy. We also discuss the timing of converting from translaryngeal intubation to a tracheostomy.

TABLE 9.1

Indications for Tracheostomy [3,4]

- Upper airway obstruction
  - Laryngeal dysfunction: Vocal cord paralysis
  - Trauma: Upper airway obstruction caused by hemorrhage, edema, or crush injury; unstable mandibular fractures; injury to the larynx; cervical spine injuries
  - Burns and corrosives: Hot smoke, caustic gases, corrosives
  - Foreign bodies
  - Congenital anomalies: Stenosis of the glottic or subglottic area
  - Infections: Croup, epiglottitis, Ludwig's angina, deep neck space infections
  - Neoplasms: Laryngeal cancer
  - Postoperative: Surgeries of the base of the tongue and hypopharynx; rigid fixation of the mandibular
  - Obstructive sleep apnea
- Clearance of Secretions
  - Inability to clear secretions: Generalized weakness, altered mental status, and excess secretions
  - Neuromuscular disease
  - Ventilatory support: Prolonged or chronic

INDICATIONS

The indications for tracheostomy can be divided into three general categories: (1) to bypass obstruction of the upper airway, (2) to provide an avenue for removal of secretions retained in the airways, and (3) to provide a means for prolonged ventilatory support. These indications are summarized in Table 9.1 [3,4].

Anticipated prolonged ventilatory support, especially for patients receiving mechanical ventilation via translaryngeal intubation, is the most common indication for placing a tracheostomy in the ICU. There are several advantages and disadvantages of both translaryngeal intubation and tracheostomy in patients requiring prolonged ventilator support, and these are summarized in Table 9.2 [4–6]. Most authors feel that when the procedure is performed by a skilled specialist, the potential benefits of tracheostomy over translaryngeal intubation for most patients justify the application despite its potential risks. However, there are no detailed prospective clinical trials rigorously evaluating the advantages of tracheostomy in patients requiring prolonged mechanical ventilation. In a retrospective and a nonrandomized study, there were conflicting data on mortality in patients with respiratory failure of more than 1 week with regard to receiving a tracheostomy or continuing with an endotracheal tube [1,2].

CONTRAINDICATIONS

There are no absolute contraindications to tracheostomy. Relative complications include uncorrected coagulopathy, high levels of ventilator support (i.e., high levels of positive end-expiratory pressure [PEEP]), and abnormal anatomy of the upper airway. However, a prospective cohort study has demonstrated that percutaneous tracheostomy can be safely preformed in patients with refractory coagulopathy from liver disease [7]. Morbidly obese patients with body mass index greater than 30 kg per m^2 also appear to be at higher risk for complications with both open tracheostomy [8] and possibly percutaneous tracheostomy [9]. In patients with severe brain injury, percutaneous tracheostomy can be safely performed without significantly further increasing intracranial pressure [10].

Certain conditions warrant special attention. In patients undergoing conversion from translaryngeal intubation to a tracheostomy for prolonged ventilatory support, the procedure should be viewed as an elective or semielective procedure. Therefore, the patient should be optimally physiologically stabilized before the procedure, and all attempts should be made to correct coagulopathies, including uremia. The patient should tolerate submaximal ventilator settings because during the exchange positive pressure is lost temporarily. If not already on low levels (5 cm H_2O) of PEEP, placing the patient supine and using 5 or 7.5 cm H_2O of PEEP temporarily is a good test to decide if the patient will tolerate the exchange. Emergent tracheostomies for upper airway obstruction may need to be performed when the patient is unstable or has a coagulopathy.

TIMING OF TRACHEOSTOMY

Recommendations on when to perform a tracheostomy on an intubated, critically ill patient have varied over time. However, with the release of some consistent and recent studies, more sound recommendations can be made. Table 9.3 summarizes several studies comparing early versus late tracheostomy [11–21]. In 2003, Heffner recommended consideration of tracheostomy if a patient remains ventilator dependent after a week of translaryngeal intubation. If the patient has barriers to weaning and

TABLE 9.2

Advantages and Disadvantages of Intubation and Tracheostomy [5–7]

Advantages	Disadvantages
Translaryngeal intubation	
Reliable airway during urgent intubation	Bacterial airway colonization
Avoidance of surgical complications	Unintentional extubation
Lower initial cost	Laryngeal injury
	Tracheal stenosis
	Purulent sinusitis (nasotracheal intubations)
	Patient discomfort
Tracheostomies	
Avoids direct injury to the larynx	Complications (see Table 9.4)
Facilitates nursing care	Bacterial airway colonization
Enhances patient mobility	Cost
More secure airway	Surgical scar
Improved patient comfort	Tracheal and stomal stenosis
Permits speech	
Provides psychologic benefit	
More rapid weaning from mechanical ventilation	
Better oral hygiene	
Decreased risk of nosocomial pneumonia	

appears unlikely to be extubated within 7 days, a tracheostomy should be performed. Conversely, if the patient has minimal barriers to weaning and is likely to be extubated within 7 days, tracheostomy should be avoided. In those whose status is unclear, the need for tracheostomy should be readdressed daily [4].

Subsequently, a meta-analysis in 2005 [11] suggested advantages to "early tracheostomy" performed within 7 days of translarygneal intubation over a "late tracheostomy" (>7 days) in critically ill patients requiring mechanical ventilation. The meta-analysis combined five prospective studies and included

TABLE 9.3

Studies Evaluating Early (≤7 Days) Versus Late (>7 Days) Tracheostomy

Study	No. of patients	Study type	Patient type	Results
Rodriquez et al., 1990	106	Prospective Randomized	Surg	Decreased ICU LOS and MV days with early tracheostomy
Sugarman et al., 1997	127	Prospective Randomized	Surg, Trauma	No difference in mortality, VAP rate, or ICU LOS
Brook et al., 2000	90	Prospective Observational	Med, Surg	Decreased MV days and hospital costs
Rumbak et al., 2004	120	Prospective	Med	Decreased mortality, VAP 2004 rate, ICU LOS, and MV days with early trach
Griffiths et al., 2005		Meta-analysis	Med, Surg	Decreased MV days and ICU LOS with early trach, no difference in mortality or VAP rate
Scales et al., 2008	10,927	Retrospective Cohort	Med, Surg	Decreased mortality, MV days, ICU LOS with early trach
Blot et al., 2008	123	Prospective Randomized	Med, Surg	No difference in mortality, VAP rate, or ICU LOS
Durbin et al., 2010	641	Meta-analysis	Med, Surg	No difference in mortality, VAP rate, or MV days
Terragni et al., 2010	419	Prospective Randomized	Med, Surg	No difference in VAP rate ICU LOS or mortality, but decreased MV days
Wang et al., 2011	1,044	Meta-analysis	Med, Surg	No difference in VAP rate, mortality, LOS, MV days
Young et al., 2013	909	Prospective Randomized	Med, Surg	No difference in mortality, antibiotic usage, MV days, but decrease in sedation days

406 patients and suggested that early tracheostomy resulted in a decrease in length of ICU stay by an average of 15.3 days and a decrease in duration of mechanical ventilation by an average of 8.5 days [11]. Potential reasons for the decrease in duration of mechanical ventilation include easier weaning due to less dead space; lower airflow resistance; and less frequent episodes of obstruction due to mucus plugging in patients with tracheostomies. There was no significant increase in hospital mortality or risk of hospital-acquired pneumonia. However, there were limitations to the meta-analysis, including the inclusion of insufficiently randomized studies. Since this meta-analysis, multiple randomized controlled studies have been published which have consistently contradicted these results [20]. A subsequent 2011 meta-analysis of seven randomized controlled studies which included 1,044 patients showed no difference in mortality, mechanical ventilator days, or ICU length of stay [20]. More recently, in a study performed in the UK, 909 adult patients with respiratory failure not attributed to chronic neurologic disease were randomized to undergo "early" tracheostomy performed within 4 days of intubation, or "late" tracheostomy as defined by after 10 days if still indicated. Patients were identified by Intensive Care Day 4, as likely to require mechanical ventilation for at least an additional 7 days, and subsequently randomized to either group. There was no difference in 30-day, 1-year, or 2-year mortality between groups. Median critical care unit length of stay and need for antibiotics were similar in the groups, whereas the median days of intravenous sedation was lower in the early group: 5 versus 8 days, $p < 0.001$ [21]. Interestingly, tracheostomy was avoided in 53.7% in the late group, suggesting that identification of patients who will require long-term ventilation is not clear-cut [21].

In summary, despite previous research suggesting otherwise, the benefits of "early" tracheostomy are not sufficient to recommend tracheostomy prior to 7 to 10 days of translaryngeal intubation. Delayed tracheostomy likely leads to avoidance of trachoestomy in many patients, and correspondingly avoidance of potential complications associated with the procedure.

Early tracheostomy may be beneficial in some specific instances; however, the majority of the data is based on retrospective studies. Patients with blunt, multiple-organ trauma have a shorter duration of mechanical ventilation, fewer episodes of nosocomial pneumonia [22], and a significant reduction in hospital costs [23] when the tracheostomy is performed within 1 week of their injuries. Similar benefits have been reported in patients with head trauma and poor Glasgow Coma Score [24], acute spine trauma [25], and thermal injury [26] if a tracheostomy is performed within a week after the injury. Also, patients with facial injuries may require early tracheostomy to allow or facilitate facial fracture surgery, fixation, and immobilization.

PROCEDURES

Emergency Tracheostomy

Emergency tracheostomy is a moderately difficult procedure requiring training and skill, experience, adequate assistance, time, lighting, and proper equipment and instrumentation. When time is short, the patient is uncooperative, anatomy is distorted, and the aforementioned requirements are not met, then tracheostomy can be very hazardous. Emergency tracheostomy comprises significant risks to nearby neurovascular structures, particularly in small children in whom the trachea is small and not well defined. The risk of complications from emergency tracheostomy is two to five times higher than for elective tracheostomy [27,28]. Nonetheless, there are occasional indications for emergency tracheostomy [29], including transected trachea; anterior neck trauma with crushed larynx [30]; severe facial trauma; acute laryngeal obstruction or near-impending obstruction; and pediatric (younger than 12 years) patients requiring an emergency surgical airway in whom a cricothyrotomy is generally not advised. In emergency situations, when there is inadequate time or personnel to perform an emergency tracheostomy, a cricothyrotomy may be a more efficient and expedient manner to provide an airway.

Cricothyrotomy

Although initially condemned because of a high rate of complications, cricothyrotomy may have some potential advantages over tracheostomy. These include technical simplicity; speed of performance; low complication rate [31]; suitability as a bedside procedure; usefulness for isolation of the airway for median sternotomy and radical neck dissection [32]; lack of need to hyperextend the neck; and formation of a smaller scar. Also, because cricothyrotomy results in less encroachment on the mediastinum, there is less chance of esophageal injury and virtually no chance of pneumothorax or tracheal arterial fistula [33]. Despite these considerations, many authorities currently recommend that cricothyrotomy be used as an elective long-term method of airway access only in highly selected patients [34]. Use of cricothyrotomy in the emergency setting, particularly for managing trauma, is not controversial [35–37]. Emergency cricothyrotomy is useful because it requires a small number of instruments and less training than tracheostomy, and can be performed quickly as indicated as a means of controlling the airway in an emergency when oral or nasotracheal intubation is nonsuccessful or contraindicated. The cricothyroid membrane is higher in the neck than the tracheal rings and therefore closer to the surface and more accessible. In emergency situations, translaryngeal intubations fail because of massive oral or nasal hemorrhage or regurgitation; structural deformities of the upper airway; muscle spasm and clenched teeth; and obstruction by foreign body through the upper airway [35]. Cricothyrotomy finds its greatest use in trauma management, axial or suspected cervical spine injury, alone or in combination with severe facial trauma, where nasotracheal and orotracheal intubation is both difficult and hazardous. Thus, cricothyrotomy has an important role in emergency airway management [36].

Use and Contraindications

Cricothyrotomy should not be used to manage airway obstruction that occurred immediately after endotracheal extubation because the obstruction may be found below the larynx [36]; likewise, with primary laryngeal trauma or diseases such as a tumor or an infection, cricothyrotomy may prove to be useless. It is contraindicated in infants and children younger than 10 to 12 years under all circumstances because stenosis and even transection are possible [36]. In this age group, percutaneous needle catheter transtracheal ventilation may be a temporizing procedure until the tracheostomy can be performed.

Anatomy

The cricothyroid space is no larger than 7 to 9 mm in its vertical dimension, smaller than the outside diameter of most tracheostomy tubes (outside diameter 10 mm). The cricothyroid artery runs across the midline in the upper portion, and the membrane is vertically in the midline. The anterior superior edge of the thyroid cartilage is the laryngeal prominence. The cricothyroid membrane is approximately 2 to 3 cm below the laryngeal prominence and can be identified as an indentation immediately below the thyroid cartilage. The lower border of the cricothyroid membrane is the cricoid cartilage [33,35]. A description of the cricothyrotomy procedure is contained in standard surgical texts.

Complications

The report of incidents of short- and long-term complications of cricothyrotomy ranges from 6.1% for procedures performed in elective, well-controlled, carefully selected cases to greater than 50% for procedures performed under emergency or other suboptimal conditions [3,36]. The incidence of subglottic stenosis after cricothyrotomy is 2% to 3% [3,31]. This major complication occurs at the tracheostomy or cricothyrotomy site, but not at the cuff site [38]. Necrosis of cartilage due to iatrogenic injury to the cricoid cartilage or pressure from the tube on the cartilage may play a role [37]. Possible reasons that subglottic stenoses may occur more commonly with cricothyrotomy than with tracheostomy are as follows: the larynx is the narrowest part of the laryngotracheal airway; subglottic tissues, especially in children, are intolerant of contact; and division of the cricothyroid membrane and cricoid cartilage destroy the only complete rings supporting the airway. Furthermore, the range of tube sizes is limited because of the rigidity of the surrounding structures (cricoid and thyroid cartilages), and the curvature of the tracheostomy tube at this level may obstruct the airway because of posterior membrane impingement [39]. Prior laryngotracheal injury, as with prolonged translaryngeal intubation, is a major risk factor for the development of subglottic stenosis after cricothyrotomy [31].

The association of cricothyrotomy with these possible complications leads most authorities to consider replacing a cricothyrotomy within 48 to 72 hours with a standard tracheostomy procedure. This is commonly done by an open surgical tracheostomy (OST), which occurs between the second and third tracheal rings, as compared to a percutaneous dilational tracheostomy (PDT), which usually occurs between the cricoid cartilage and the first ring or the first and second rings [39].

TRACHEOSTOMY PROCEDURES IN THE INTENSIVE CARE UNIT

Tracheostomy is one of the most common surgical ICU procedures and is commonly performed for weaning from mechanical ventilation; clearance of secretions; and airway protection for patients requiring prolonged ventilation. There are two major techniques for tracheostomy, open and percutaneous, with various modifications of each. The different surgical tracheostomy techniques are well described in the references for this chapter [3,40].

Open Surgical Tracheostomy

In OST, the patient's neck is extended, and the surgical field is exposed from the chin to several inches below the clavicle. This area is prepped and draped, and prophylactic antibiotics are administered at the discretion of the surgeon. A vertical or horizontal incision may be used; however, a horizontal incision will provide a better cosmetic result. The platysma muscle is divided in line with the incision, and the strap muscles are separated in the midline. The thyroid isthmus is then mobilized superiorly or divided as needed to access the trachea. In the event of a low-lying cricoid cartilage, dissection on the anterior wall of the trachea helps to mobilize the trachea out of the mediastinum, and also the use of a cricoid hook will elevate the trachea to expose the second or third tracheal ring. Following identification of the second or third tracheal ring, a vertical tracheostomy is created, or a tracheal flap (Bjork flap) is fashioned to create a fistulous tract by suturing the tracheal mucosal flap to the skin in the incision.

Variations on this technique include the use of retention sutures through the lateral aspect of the tracheal walls for retraction purposes during tracheostomy tube insertion and for expeditious reinsertion of a tracheostomy tube in the event of accidental tube decannulation [40]. The tracheal "stoma" will, in most cases, mature after 7 to 10 days and will form a tract that will facilitate tube exchange or downsizing, thereby minimizing the risk of tube misplacement.

Percutaneous Dilational Techniques

The PDT are divided into several techniques; however, all are alike in that they depend on the basic technique of guidewire placement through the anterior tracheal wall, followed by dilation over this guidewire to create a tracheal stoma. The procedure is performed with monitoring of O_2 saturation, cardiac rhythm, and blood pressure. Successful cannulation of the trachea may be verified with $ETCO_2$ monitoring. There are several different modifications from the original technique that was described by Ciaglia et al. [41] in 1988. These modifications are described in detail elsewhere [3].

Both techniques, PDT and OST, can be performed in either the ICU or the operating room. There have been several meta-analyses comparing OST with PDT, most showing no significant difference in mortality or major complications between the two methods of performing the tracheostomy. Freeman et al. [42] reviewed multiple prospective controlled studies published between 1991 and 1999 totaling 236 patients and concluded that there is no difference in mortality between PDT and OST, and that PDT was associated with less bleeding and stomal infections and was performed more rapidly. Delancy et al. [43] reported that there was no significant difference in mortality and major complications between PDT and OST in a meta-analysis consisting of 17 randomized trials and a total of 1,212 patients. They also showed a decrease in stomal infections in the PDT group, but no difference in bleeding complications. Similar findings were demonstrated by meta-analysis studies by Higgins and Punthakee [44] and Oliver et al. [45]. However, Dulguerov et al. [46] reviewed 3,512 patients from 48 studies performed between 1960 and 1996 and concluded that OST was more favorable than PDT. Subsequent critiques of these papers indicate the inherent weakness of heterogeneous patient populations, and the use of case series and nonrandomized studies in meta-analyses [47–49]. It is likely that experience and technical modifications allow both the techniques to be performed in appropriate patients with the same degree of safety and efficiency (<1% procedure-related mortality) [50].

Other factors have been used to justify the use of one procedure over the other such as cost efficiency [51]; bleeding; infection; procedural time; and estimated time from the decision to proceed to successful completion of the procedure [50]. Each factor can be used to justify one procedure over another, but it is likely that institutional practice variations and operator experience are more important in the selection of one procedure over another. This is particularly relevant with respect to the target population where ICU daily expenses far outweigh the procedural costs of either technique [52], and the expected patient mortality can be as high as 35% [53].

It is probably more important to judiciously use the institutional resources and the operator experience in providing the "best" tracheal technique for these compromised patients. It is possible that the target population may vary from one institution to another (cardiac vs. trauma vs. neurosurgical vs. medical ICU patients), which may influence the decision to perform one technique over another. Patient body habitus also plays a large role in selection: difficulty palpating tracheal rings in a short, thick-necked patient makes percutaneous tracheostomy not only difficult but dangerous. This patient is better served in an operating room setting where optimum sedation/paralysis (if needed) and positioning can be accomplished while directly exposing the anterior trachea, mobilizing it if necessary to access the airway with an appropriately sized, sometimes custom-made, tube.

Nonetheless, there are certain distinct advantages of PDT that can be outlined as follows: (a) easier access for timing of the procedure; (b) reduced operating room and person power utilization; (c) PDT is less expensive than OST (even if both the procedures are performed in the ICU); (d) PDT has no requirement for transportation of critically ill patients to an operating room; (e) improved cosmetic results; and (f) possibly reduced rates of stomal infection, bleeding, and reduced tracheal secretions in the parastomal area owing to the tight fitting of the stoma around the tracheostomy tube.

We do recommend considering performing OST instead of PST in the following patients: (a) patients with severe respiratory failure ($FiO_2 > 0.60$, PEEP > 10, and complicated translaryngeal intubation or a nonpalpable cricoid cartilage or a cricoid cartilage <3 cm above the sternal notch [51]); (b) obese patients with abundant pretracheal subcutaneous fat; (c) patients with large goiters; (d) abnormal airways secondary to congenital or acquired conditions; (e) the need for constant attendance of a second physician to monitor ventilation or circulatory abnormalities; (f) abnormal bleeding diathesis that cannot be adequately corrected [54].

Utility of Ultrasonography for Percutaneous Tracheostomy

Ultrasonography has several useful applications related to PDT.

Identification of Aberrant Vascular Anatomy. A small proportion of patients have aberrant vascular anatomy that contraindicates PDT. Preprocedure ultrasonography examination of the anterior neck can identify dangerous vascular anatomy that precludes PDT [55–59]. The high frequency vascular transducer is used to obtain a transverse axis image of the anterior neck. Starting at the thyroid cartilage, the operator moves the probe down the anterior neck in order to identify anomalous midline vascular structures that would preclude bedside PDT (Chapter 9 Videos 9.1 and 9.2). Once at the suprasternal notch, the probe is angled downward to examine for any high riding mediastinal artery or vein. The examination takes a few minutes, and is an effective means of improving the safety of the procedure.

Aberrant position of the carotid, brachiocephalic, right subclavian, or thyroid artery, or aortic arch, though rare, has been associated with severe hemorrhage during PDT (Chapter 9 Video 9.2). Large midline veins are also an occasional finding that contraindicates PDT (Chapter 9 Video 9.2). If and when dangerous vascular anatomy has been identified, this situation requires that the procedure be performed with standard open surgical technique in the operating room.

Selection of Insertion Site. While examining for vascular structures, the operator identifies the thyroid cartilage, the cricoid membrane, and the prominent cricoid cartilage below which are the tracheal rings. The insertion site is targeted to be below the first tracheal ring (Chapter 9 Video 9.1). Ultrasonography is particularly useful for selection of insertion site when physical examination is challenging such as with obesity or in the elderly patient with a low position of the cricoid cartilage. Once a safe site is identified, the operator may mark it for subsequent needle insertion, or proceed with real-time guidance of needle insertion using ultrasonography.

Guidance of Needle Insertion. Real-time ultrasonography guidance of needle insertion into the trachea may be performed during PDT [60]. It improves first pass success rate and accuracy of needle insertion when compared to standard technique [61]. Should the operator choose the option of real-time guidance, the probe is held in the transverse axis, and the needle is inserted into the trachea while tracking its movement with ultrasonography. Some operators insert the needle before making the skin incision. Alternatively, the skin incision is made first, with subsequent needle insertion under ultrasonography control.

TUBES AND CANNULAS

Characteristics of a good tracheostomy tube are flexibility to accommodate varying patient anatomies; inert material; wide internal diameter; the smallest external diameter possible; a smooth surface to allow easy insertion and removal; and sufficient length to be secured once placed, but not so long as to impinge the carina or other tracheal parts. Until the late 1960s, when surgeons began to experiment with silicone and other synthetic materials, tracheostomy tubes and cannulas were made of metal. At present, almost all tracheostomy tubes are made of synthetic materials. One disadvantage of a silicone tube over a metal one is the increased thickness of the tube wall, resulting in a larger outer diameter. Silicone tubes are available with or without a cuff. The cuff allows occlusion of the airway around the tube, which is necessary for positive-pressure ventilation. It may also minimize aspiration. In the past, cuffs were associated with a high incidence of tracheal stenosis caused by ischemia and necrosis of the mucus membrane and subsequent cicatricial contracture at the cuff site. High-volume, low-pressure cuffs diminish pressure on the wall of the trachea, thereby minimizing (but not eliminating) problems caused by focal areas of pressure necrosis [62]. Cuff pressures should be maintained at 15 to 20 cm H_2O, because higher pressures impair mucosal capillary blood flow leading to ischemic injury to the trachea [63]. Cuff pressures should be checked with a manometer daily in critically ill patients. Once the patient is weaned from mechanical ventilation, the cuff should be deflated, or consideration should be given to placing an uncuffed tracheostomy tube until the patient can be decannulated. When the only purpose of the tube is to secure the airway (sleep apnea) or provide access for suctioning secretions, a tube without a cuff can be placed. A comprehensive review of tracheostomy tubes can be found elsewhere [64].

POSTOPERATIVE CARE

The care of a tracheostomy tube is important. Highlighted below are some specific issues that all intensivists need to know when caring for patients with tracheostomies.

Wound and Dressing Care

Daily examinations of the stoma are important in identifying infections or excoriations of the skin at the tracheostomy site [65]. In addition, keeping the wound clean and free of blood and secretions is important, especially in the immediate posttracheostomy period. Dressing changes should be performed at least twice a day and when the dressings are soiled. Some authors recommend cleaning the stoma with 1:1 mixture of hydrogen peroxide and sterile saline [65]. When changing dressings and tapes, special care is needed to avoid accidental dislodging of the tracheostomy tube. Sutures, placed either for fixation and/or through the rings themselves for exposure, should be removed as soon as practical, usually after 1 week when an adequate stoma has formed, to facilitate cleaning the stomal area. Malodorous tracheal "stomatitis" that can lead to an enlarging stoma around the tube should be treated with topical antimicrobial dressings such as 0.25% Dakin's solution to facilitate resolution. Significant induration and/or cellulitis should be managed with a systemic antibiotic such as clindamycin. Occasionally, the secretions become extremely malordorous, indicating a gram-negative or anaerobic infection or overgowth: this should be treated with topical and systemic antimicrobials.

Inner Cannulas

The inner cannulas should be used at all times in most tracheostomy tubes in the ICU. Bivona makes a tracheostomy tube that is lined with silicone and does not require an inner cannula. In other tracheotomy tubes, inner cannulas serve to extend the life of the tracheostomy tubes by preventing the buildup of secretions within the tracheostomy. The inner cannulas can be easily removed and either cleaned or replaced with a sterile, disposable one. Disposable inner cannulas have the advantage of quick and efficient changing; a decrease in nursing time; decreased risk of cross-contamination; and guaranteed sterility. The obturator should be kept at the bedside at all times in the event that reinsertion of the tracheostomy is necessary.

Humidification

One of the functions of the upper airway is to moisten and humidify inspired air. Because tracheostomies bypass the upper airway, it is vital to provide patients who have tracheostomies with warm, humidified air. Humidification of inspired gases prevents complications in patients with tracheostomies. Failure to humidify the inspired gases can result in obstruction of the tube by inspissated secretions, impaired mucociliary clearance, and decreased cough.

Suctioning

Patients with tracheostomies frequently have increased amounts of airway secretions coupled with decreased ability to clear them effectively. Keeping the airways clear of excess secretions is important for decreasing the risk of lung infection and airway plugging [65]. Suctioning is frequently required in patients with poor or ineffective cough. Suction techniques should remove the maximal amount of secretions while causing the least amount of airway trauma. Routine suctioning, however, is not recommended [66]. In the patient who requires frequent suctioning because of secretions, who otherwise appears well, without infection and without tracheitis, the tube itself may be the culprit. Downsizing the tube or even a short trial (while being monitored) with the tube removed may result in significantly less secretions, obviating the need for the tube.

Tracheostomy Tube Changes

Tracheostomy tubes do not require routine changing. In fact, there may be significant risks associated with routine tracheostomy tube changes, especially if this is performed within a week of the initial procedure and by inexperienced caregivers. A survey of accredited otolaryngology training programs suggested a significant incidence of loss of airway and deaths associated with routine changing of tracheostomy tubes within 7 days of initial placement, especially if they are changed by inexperienced physicians [67]. In general, the tube needs to be changed only under the following conditions: (a) there is a functional problem with it, such as an air leak in the balloon; (b) when the lumen is narrowed because of the buildup of dried secretions; (c) when switching to a new type of tube; or (d) when downsizing the tube prior to decannulation. Ideally, a tracheostomy tube should not be changed until 7 to 10 days after its initial placement. The reason for this is to allow the tracheal stoma and the tract to mature. Patients who have their tracheostomy tube changed before the tract is fully mature risk having the tube misplaced into the soft tissue of the neck. If the tracheostomy tube needs to be replaced before the tract has had time to mature, the tube should be changed over a guide, such as a suction catheter or tube changer with personnel and equipment readily available at the bedside to perform orotracheal intubation if needed.

Oral Feeding and Swallowing Dysfunction Associated with Tracheostomies

Caution should be exercised before initiating feedings by mouth in patients with tracheostomy, because numerous studies have demonstrated that patients are at a significantly increased risk for aspiration when a tracheostomy is in place. Physiologically, patients with tracheostomies are more likely to aspirate because the tracheostomy tube tethers the larynx, preventing its normal upward movement needed to assist in glottic closure and cricopharyngeal relaxation. Tracheostomy tubes also disrupt normal swallowing by compressing the esophagus and interfering with deglutition, decreasing duration of vocal cord closure and resulting in uncoordinated laryngeal closure [68,69]. In addition, prolonged translaryngeal intubation can result in swallowing disorders that persist even after the endotracheal tube is converted to a tracheostomy [70]. It is therefore not surprising that between 40% and 65% of patients with tracheostomies aspirate when swallowing [71]. It is felt that between 73% and 77% of the episodes are clinically silent [71].

Before attempting oral feedings in a patient with a tracheostomy, several objective criteria must be met. The patient must be consistently alert, and able to follow complex commands. The patient should have adequate cough and swallowing reflexes; adequate oral motor strength; and a significant respiratory reserve. These criteria are probably best assessed by a certified speech therapist. However, bedside clinical assessment may only identify 34% of the patients at high risk for aspiration [72]. Augmenting the bedside swallowing evaluation by coloring feedings or measuring the glucose in tracheal secretions does not appear to increase the sensitivity in detecting the risk of aspiration [73]. A video barium swallow may identify between 50% and 80% of patients with tracheostomies who are at a high risk to aspirate oral feeding [72]. A laryngoscopy to observe directly a patient's swallowing mechanics, coupled with a video barium swallow, may be more sensitive in predicting which patients are at risk for aspiration [72]. Scintigraphic studies may be the most sensitive test for identifying aspiration [74]. Plugging of the tracheostomy [67] or using a Passy–Muir valve may reduce aspiration in patients with tracheostomies who are taking oral feedings, but this is not a universal finding [75].

Because of the high risk for aspiration and the difficulty assessing which patients are at high risk to aspirate, we do not institute oral feedings in our patients with tracheostomy in the ICU. We believe that the potential risks of a percutaneous endoscopically placed gastrostomy feeding tube or maintaining a nasogastric feeding tube are much less than the risk of aspiration of oral feedings and its complications (i.e., recurrent pneumonia, acute respiratory distress syndrome, and prolonged weaning).

Discharging Patients with Tracheotomies from the ICU to the General Ward

Multiple studies have raised concern about the safety of patients who have been weaned from mechanical ventilation and who are transferred from the ICU to the general hospital ward with the tracheostomy in place [76,77]. Fernandez et al. retrospectively showed an increased mortality in patients with tracheostomy tubes versus those decannulated prior to transfer out of the ICU, especially among patients with a poorer overall prognosis [76]. Martinez et al. prospectively studied 73 patients who received tracheostomies, who were without neurologic injury, and who were transferred from the ICU to the general ward [77]. Thirty-five of these patients were decannulated prior to transfer to the wards. The decannulated group had a significantly lower mortality. Factors found to be associated with increased mortality in patients not decannulated prior to transfer include body mass index greater than 30 kg per m^2 and tenacious secretions.

Patients with tracheostomies who are transferred to the general medical wards need special attention. A multidisciplinary care model has been shown to significantly expedite the decannulation process while also reducing the complication rate in a small study in the UK [78]. We suggest that patients with tracheostomies can be safely cared for in the general ward, provided there is an interprofessional team approach between physicians, nurses, and respiratory therapists.

COMPLICATIONS

Tracheostomies, whether inserted by percutaneous dilatation or open surgical procedure, are associated with a variety of complications. These complications are best grouped by the time of occurrence after the placement and are divided into immediate, intermediate, and late complications (Table 9.4). The reported incidence of complications varies from 4% [79] to 39% [19], with reported mortality rates from 0.03% to 0.6% [46,80]. Complication rates decrease with increasing experience of the physician performing the procedure [81]. Posttracheostomy mortality and morbidity are usually caused by iatrogenic tracheal laceration, hemorrhage, tube dislodgment, infection, or obstruction [3]. Neurosurgical patients have a higher posttracheostomy complication rate than other patients [3]. Tracheostomy is more hazardous in children than in adults, and carries special risks in the very young, often related to the experience of the surgeon [82]. A comprehensive understanding of immediate, intermediate, and late complications of tracheostomy and their management is essential for the intensivist.

TABLE 9.4

Complications of Tracheostomies [3,7]

Immediate complications (0–24 h)
- Tube displacement
- Arrhythmia
- Hypotension
- Hypoxia/hypercapnia
- Loss of airway control
- Pneumothorax
- Pneumomediastinum
- Acute surgical emphysema
- Major hemorrhage
- Bacteremia
- Tracheal cartilage fracture
- Esophageal injury (*uncommon*)
- Cardiorespiratory arrest (*uncommon*)
- Tracheolaryngeal injury (*uncommon*)
- Crushed airway from dilational tracheostomy (*uncommon*)

Intermediate complications (from Day 1 to Day 7)
- Persistent bleeding
- Tube displacement
- Tube obstruction (mucus, blood)
- Major atelectasis
- Wound infection/cellulitis

Late complications (>Day 7)
- Tracheoinnominate artery fistula
- Tracheomalacia
- Tracheal stenosis
- Necrosis and loss of anterior tracheal cartilage
- Tracheoesophageal fistula
- Major aspiration
- Chronic speech and swallowing deficits
- Tracheocutaneous fistula

Multiple studies have suggested an increased complication rate of surgical tracheostomy in patients with a BMI > 30 [8,83]. There is conflicting evidence regarding the complication rate of percutaneous tracheostomy in these patients. Byhahn et al. found a complication rate of percutaneous tracheostomy of 43.8% in 32 patients with a BMI > 27, compared to 18.2% in 73 patients with a BMI < 27 ($p < 0.001$). Additionally, the rate of severe complication in the obese group was nearly five times that of those in the nonobese group [84]. However, a subsequent study by Romero et al. of 25 obese patients and 80 nonobese patients undergoing fiber-optic bronchoscopy-guided percutaneous tracheostomy with ultrasound support did not show any significant difference in complication rates (8% vs. 7.5%, $p = 1$) [85]. In the largest study to date, McCague et al. retrospectively reviewed 131 obese patients and 295 nonobese patients undergoing bronchoscopy-guided percutaneous tracheostomy and did not find a significant difference in complication rate [86]. Overall, these studies are limited by the small numbers; retrospective or observational nature; and lack of long-term follow-up.

Obstruction

Obstruction of the tracheostomy tube is a potentially life-threatening complication. The tube may become plugged with clotted blood or inspissated secretions. In this case, the inner cannula should be removed immediately and the patient suctioned. Should that fail, it may be necessary to remove the outer cannula also, a decision that must take into consideration the reason the tube was placed and the length of time it has been in place. Obstruction may also be caused by angulation of the distal end of the tube against the anterior or posterior tracheal wall. An undivided thyroid isthmus pressing against the angled tracheostomy tube can force the tip against the anterior tracheal wall, whereas a low superior transverse skin edge can force the tip of the tracheostomy tube against the posterior tracheal wall. An indication of this type of obstruction is an expiratory wheeze. Division of the thyroid isthmus, and proper placement of transverse skin incisions prevent anterior or posterior tube angulation and obstruction.

Tube Displacement/Dislodgment

Dislodgment of a tracheostomy tube that has been in place for 2 weeks or longer is managed by replacing the tube. If it cannot be immediately replaced or if it is replaced and the patient cannot be ventilated (indicating that the tube is not in the trachea), orotracheal intubation should be performed. Immediate postoperative displacement can be fatal, if the tube cannot be promptly replaced and the patient cannot be reintubated.

Dislodgment in the early postoperative period is usually caused by one of several technical problems. Failure to divide the thyroid isthmus may permit the intact isthmus to ride up against the tracheostomy tube and thus displace it. Excessively low placement of the stoma (i.e., below the second and third rings) can occur when the thoracic trachea is brought into the neck by overextending the neck or by excessive traction on the trachea. When the normal anatomic relationships are restored, the trachea recedes below the suprasternal notch, causing the tube to be dislodged from the trachea. The risk of dislodgment of the tracheostomy tube, a potentially lethal complication, can be minimized by (a) transection of the thyroid isthmus at surgery, if indicated; (b) proper placement of the stoma; (c) avoidance of excessive neck hyperextension and/or tracheal traction; (d) application of sufficiently tight tracheostomy tube retention tapes; (e) suture of the tracheostomy tube flange to the skin in patients with short necks; and (f) insertion of a tracheostomy tube of an appropriate length for the patient's anatomy. Some surgeons apply retaining sutures to the trachea for use in the early postoperative period in case the tube becomes dislodged, allowing the trachea to be pulled into the wound for reintubation. Making a Bjork flap involves suturing the inferior edge of the trachea stoma to the skin, thus allowing a sure pathway for tube placement. Bjork flaps, however, tend to interfere with swallowing and promote aspiration. Reintubation of a tracheostomy can be accomplished by using a smaller, beveled endotracheal tube and then applying a tracheostomy tube over the smaller tube, using the Seldinger technique [87].

If a tracheostomy becomes dislodged within 7 to 10 days of surgery, we recommend translaryngeal endotracheal intubation to establish a safe airway. The tracheostomy tube can then be replaced under less urgent conditions, with fiber-optic guidance if needed.

Subcutaneous Emphysema

Approximately 5% of patients develop subcutaneous emphysema after tracheostomy [87]. It is most likely to occur when dissection is extensive and/or the wound is closed tightly. Partial closure of the skin wound is appropriate, but the underlying tissues should be allowed to approximate naturally. Subcutaneous emphysema generally resolves over the 48 hours after tracheostomy, but when the wound is closed tightly and the patient is coughing or on positive-pressure ventilation, pneumomediastinum, pneumopericardium, and/or tension pneumothorax may occur [3].

Pneumothorax and Pneumomediastinum

The cupola of the pleura extends well into the neck, especially in patients with emphysema; thus, the pleura can be damaged during tracheostomy. This complication is more common in the pediatric age group because the pleural dome extends more cephalad in children. The incidence of pneumothorax after tracheostomy ranges from 0% to 5% [79,87]. Many surgeons routinely obtain a postoperative chest radiograph.

Hemorrhage

Minor postoperative fresh tracheostomy bleeding occurs in approximately 12.5% of cases and is the most common complication of this procedure [88]. Postoperative coughing and straining can cause venous bleeding by dislodging a clot or ligature. Elevating the head of the bed, packing the wound, and/or using homeostatic materials usually controls minor bleeding. Major bleeding can occur in up to 5% of tracheotomies and is caused by hemorrhage from the isthmus of the thyroid gland; loss of a ligature from one of the anterior jugular veins; or injury to the transverse jugular vein that crosses the midline just above the jugular notch. Persistent bleeding may require a return to the operating room for management. Techniques to decrease the likelihood of early posttracheostomy hemorrhage include (a) use of a vertical incision; (b) careful dissection in the midline, with care to pick up each layer of tissue with instruments rather than simply spread tissues apart; (c) liberal use of ligatures rather than electrocautery; and (d) careful division and suture ligation of the thyroid isthmus. Late hemorrhage after tracheostomy is usually because of bleeding granulation tissue or another relatively minor cause. However, in these late cases, a tracheoinnominate artery fistula needs to be ruled out.

Tracheoinnominate Artery Fistula

At one point, it had been reported that 50% of all tracheostomy bleeding occurring more than 48 hours after the procedure was because of an often fatal complication of rupture of the innominate artery caused by erosion of the tracheostomy tube at its tip or cuff into the vessel [87]. However, because of the advent of the low-pressure cuff, the incidence of this complication has decreased considerably and occurs less than 1% of the time [89].

Eighty-five percent of tracheoinnominate fistulas occur within the first month after tracheostomy [90], although they have been reported as late as 7 months after operation. Other sites of delayed exsanguinating posttracheostomy hemorrhage include the common carotid artery; superior and inferior thyroid arteries; aortic arch; and innominate vein [90]. Rupture and fistula formation are caused by erosion through the trachea into the artery because of excessive cuff pressure or by angulation of the tube tip against the anterior trachea. Infection and other factors that weaken local tissues, such as malnourishment and steroids, also seem to play a role [91]. The innominate artery rises to about the level of the sixth ring anterior to the trachea, and low placement of the stoma can also create close proximity of the tube tip or cuff to the innominate artery. Rarely, an anomaly of the innominate, occurring with an incidence of 1% to 2% [90], is responsible for this disastrous complication. Pulsation of the tracheostomy tube is an indication of potentially fatal positioning [90]. Initially, hemorrhage from a tracheoinnominate fistula is usually not exsanguinating. Herald bleeds must be investigated promptly using fiber-optic tracheoscopy. If a tracheoinnominate fistula seems probable (minimal tracheitis and anterior pulsating erosions), the patient should be taken to the operating room for evaluation. Historically, definitive management involves resection of the artery. However, there are several reported cases of successful treatment with endovascular stenting of the innominate artery [92,93]. The mortality rate approaches 100%, even with emergent surgical intervention [3]. Sudden exsanguinating hemorrhage may be managed by hyperinflation of the tracheostomy cuff tube or reintubation with an endotracheal tube through the stoma, attempting to place the cuff at the level of the fistula. A lower neck incision with blind digital compression on the artery may be part of a critical resuscitative effort. If a tracheoinnominate artery fistula is suspected, the patient should be evaluated in the operating room and preparations should be made for a possible sternotomy.

Misplacement of Tube

Misplacement of the tube can occur at the time of surgery or when the tube is changed or replaced through a fresh stoma. If not recognized, associated mediastinal emphysema and tension pneumothorax can occur, along with alveolar hypoventilation. Injury to neurovascular structures, including the recurrent laryngeal nerve, is possible [3]. The patient must be orally intubated or the tracheostoma recannulated. Some advise placing retaining sutures in the trachea at the time of surgery. The availability of a tracheostomy set at the bedside after tracheostomy facilitates emergency reintubation.

Tracheal Cartilage Fracture

Tracheal ring fracture is a common, though likely unrecognized, complication, with a rate of 9.6% in one series of 219 percutaneous tracheostomy procedures [94].These fractures likely are associated with the development of stenosis over time. Many preventative techniques have been suggested, including assuring bronchoscopic confirmation of placement; avoiding rotational torque at insertion site; perpendicular insertion; application of counterforce to the anterior tracheal wall with the endotracheal tube/bronchoscope; complete adequate skin incision and blunt soft tissue dissection to prevent excessive force on insertion; ensuring proper fit between tracheostomy and obturator; the use of tapered tracheostomies; and the smallest tracheostomy required by the patient.

Stomal Infections

A less than 2% incidence of local infection rate has been reported with tracheostomy [8]. The risk of serious infection is less than 0.5% [79]. Attention to the details of good stoma care and early use of antibiotics are advised. However, prophylactic antibiotics are not recommended [95].

Tracheoesophageal Fistula

Tracheoesophageal fistula caused by injury to the posterior tracheal wall and cervical esophagus occurs in less than 1% of patients, more commonly in the pediatric age group. Early postoperative fistula is a result of iatrogenic injury during the procedure [87]. The chances of creating a fistula can be minimized by entering the trachea initially with a horizontal incision between two tracheal rings (the second and third), thereby eliminating the initial cut into a hard cartilaginous ring [3]. A late tracheoesophageal fistula may be because of tracheal necrosis caused by tube movement or angulation, as in neck hyperflexion, or excessive cuff pressure [87]. A tracheoesophageal fistula should be suspected in patients with cuff leaks, abdominal distention, recurrent aspiration pneumonia, and reflux of gastric fluids through the tracheostomy site. It may be demonstrated on endoscopy and contrast studies. Tracheoesophageal fistulas require surgical repair. For patients who could not tolerate a major surgical procedure, placement of an esophageal and a tracheal stent may be used [96].

Tracheal Stenosis

Some degree of tracheal stenosis is seen in 40% to 60% of patients following tracheostomy [80,97]. However, only 3% to 12% of these stenoses are clinically significant enough to require intervention [98]. Stenosis most commonly occurs at the level of the stoma or just above the stoma, but distal to the vocal cords [3]. The stenosis typically results from bacterial infection or chondritis of the anterior and lateral tracheal walls. Granulation tissue usually develops first. Ultimately, the granulation tissue matures, becoming fibrous and covered with a layer of epithelium. The granulation tissue itself can also result in other complications, such as obstructing the airway at the level of the stoma, making changing the tracheostomy tube difficult, and occluding tube fenestrations. Identified risk factors for developing tracheal stenosis include sepsis; stomal infections; hypotension; advanced age; male gender; corticosteroid use; excess motion of the tracheostomy tube; oversized tube; prolonged placement; elevated cuff pressures; excessive excision of the anterior tracheal cartilage; and fracturing a tracheal ring during PDT [99]. Using properly sized tracheostomy tubes, inflating cuffs only when indicated, and maintaining intracuff pressures to less than 15 to 20 mm Hg may decrease the incidence of tracheal stenosis [100]. Tracheal stenosis, as well as other long-term complications, appears to be less frequent with the percutaneous procedure [101,102].

Treatment options for granulation tissue include topical strategies (such as topical antibiotic or steroids, silver nitrate, and polyurethane form dressings) or surgical strategies (laser excision, electrocautery, and surgical removal) [3]. Treatment options for symptomatic tracheal stenosis include dilatation with a rigid bronchoscopy with coring, intralumen laser excision, or surgical resection with end-to-end tracheal anastomosis.

Tracheomalacia

Tracheomalacia is a weakening of the tracheal wall resulting from ischemic injury to the trachea, followed by chondritis, then destruction, and necrosis of the tracheal cartilage. Consequently, there is collapse of the affected portion of the trachea with expiration, resulting in airflow limitation, air trapping, and retention of airway secretions. Tracheomalacia may ultimately result in the patient failing to wean from mechanical ventilation. A short-term therapeutic approach to tracheomalacia is to place a longer tracheostomy tube to bypass the area of malacia. Long-term treatment options include stenting, tracheal resection, or tracheoplasty.

Dysphagia and Aspiration

The major swallowing disorder associated with tracheostomy is aspiration (see the section Oral Feeding and Swallowing Dysfunction **Associated with Tracheostomies**). Because of the high risk for aspiration, we do not recommend oral feeding in ICU patients with tracheostomies.

Tracheocutaneous Fistula

Although the tracheostoma generally closes rapidly after decannulation, a persistent fistula may occasionally remain, particularly when the tracheostomy tube is present for a prolonged period. If this complication occurs, the fistula tract can be excised and the wound closed primarily under local anesthesia. More complicated or persistent fistulas required a more formal procedure under general anesthesia involving the use of a local muscle flap between the tracheal opening and the subcutaneous tissues.

CONCLUSIONS

Tracheostomy is one of the most common surgical procedures preformed in the ICU and appears to be the airway of choice for patients requiring mechanical ventilation for more than 10 to 14 days. In the majority of patients, there is unlikely a benefit to tracheostomy prior to 7 to 10 days of mechanical ventilation. The physician performing the tracheostomy procedure needs to assess each patient to determine the best technique (whether it be performed bedside percutaneously or open in the operating room) for that specific patient. The patient's medical condition; the physician's experience with the various techniques; and the hospital's resources all need to be considered in determining the type of procedure performed.

References

1. Clec'h C, Alberti C, Vincent F, et al: Tracheostomy does not improve the outcome of patients requiring mechanical ventilation: a propensity analysis. *Crit Care Med* 35:132, 2007.
2. Combes A, Luyt CE, Nieszkowska A, et al: Is tracheostomy associated with better outcomes for patients requiring long-term mechanical ventilation? *Crit Care Med* 25:802, 2007.
3. Kopec SE, Emhoff TA: Tracheostomy, in Irwin RS, Rippe JM (eds): *Intensive Care Medicine*. 7th ed. Lippincott, Williams, and Wilkins, Philadelphia, 2012, p 105.
4. Heffner JE: Tracheostomy application and timing. *Clin Chest Med* 24:389, 2003.
5. Durbin CG: Indications for and timing of tracheostomy. *Respir Care* 50:483, 2005.
6. Conlan AA, Kopec SE: Tracheostomy in the ICU. *J Intensive Care Med* 15:1, 2000.

7. Auzinger G, O'Callaghan GP, Bernal W, et al: Percutaneous tracheostomy in patients with severe liver disease and a high incidence of refractory coagulopathy: a prospective trial. *Crit Care* 11:R110, 2007.
8. El Solh AA, Jaafar W: A comparative study of the complications of surgical tracheostomy in morbidly obese critically ill patients. *Crit Care* 11:R3, 2007.
9. Aldawood AS, Arabi YM, Haddad S: Safety of percutaneous tracheostomy in obese critically ill patients: a prospective cohort study. *Anaesth Intensive Care* 36:69, 2008.
10. Milanchi S, Magner D, Wilson MT, et al: Percutaneous tracheostomy in neurosurgical patients with intracranial pressure monitoring is safe. *J Trauma Injury Infect Crit Care* 65:73, 2008.
11. Griffiths J, Barber VS, Morgan L, et al: Systematic review and meta-analysis of studies of the timing of tracheostomy in adult patients undergoing artificial ventilation. *BMJ* 330:1243, 2005.
12. Rodriguez JL, Steinberg SM, Luchetti FA, et al: Early tracheostomy for primary airway management in the surgical critical care setting. *Surgery* 108:655, 1990.
13. Sugerman HJ, Wolfe L, Pasquele MD, et al: Multicenter, randomized, prospective trial on early tracheostomy. *J Trauma* 43:741, 1997.
14. Brook AD, Sherman G, Malen J, et al: Early versus late tracheostomy in patients who require prolonged mechanical ventilation. *Am J Crit Care* 9:352, 2000.
15. Rumbak MJ, Newton M, Truncale T, et al: A prospective, randomized study comparing early percutaneous dilatational tracheostomy to prolonged translaryngeal intubation in critically ill medical patients. *Crit Care Med* 32:1689, 2004.
16. Scales DC, Thiruchelvam D, Kiss A, et al: The effect of tracheostomy timing during critical illness on long-term survival. *Crit Care Med* 36:2547, 2008.
17. Blot F, Similowski T, Trouillet JL, et al: Early tracheostomy versus prolonged endotracheal intubation in unselected severely ill ICU patients. *Intensive Care Med* 34:1779, 2008.
18. Durbin CG, Perkins MP, Moores LK: Should tracheostomy be performed as early as 72 hours in patients requiring prolonged mechanical ventilation? *Respir Care* 55:76, 2010.
19. Terragni PP, Antonelli M, Fumagalli R, et al: Early vs late tracheostomy for prevention of pneumonia in mechanically ventilated adult ICU patients. *JAMA* 303:1483, 2010.
20. Wang F, Wu Y, Bo L, et al: The timing of tracheotomy in critically ill patients undergoing mechanical ventilation: a systematic review and meta-analysis of rnadomized controlled trials. *Chest* 140(6):1456–1465, 2011.
21. Young D, Harrison DA, Cuthbertson BH, et al: Effect of early vs. late tracheostomy placement on survival in patients receiving mechanical ventilation; the TracMan randomized trial. *JAMA* 309:20, 2013.
22. Lesnik I, Rappaport W, Fulginiti J, et al: The role of early tracheostomy in blunt, multiple organ trauma. *Am Surg* 58:346, 1992.
23. Armstrong PA, McCarthy MC, Peoples JB: Reduced use of resources by early tracheostomy in ventilator-dependent patients with blunt trauma. *Surgery* 124:763, 1998.
24. Teoh WH, Goh KY, Chan C: The role of early tracheostomy in critically ill neurosurgical patients. *Ann Acad Med Singapore* 30:234, 2001.
25. Romero J, Vari A, Gambarrutta C, et al: Tracheostomy timing in traumatic spinal cord injury. *Eur Spine J* 18:1452, 2009.
26. Sellers BJ, Davis BL, Larkin PW, et al: Early predictors of prolonged ventilator dependence in thermally injured patients. *J Trauma* 43:899, 1997.
27. Stock CM, Woodward CG, Shapiro BA, et al: Perioperative complications of elective tracheostomy in critically ill patients. *Crit Care Med* 14:861, 1986.
28. Skaggs JA, Cogbill CL: Tracheostomy: management, mortality, complications. *Am Surg* 35:393, 1969.
29. American College of Surgeons Committee on Trauma: *Advanced Trauma Life Support Course for Physicians, Instructor Manual*. Chicago, American College of Surgeons, 1985, p 159.
30. Kline SN: Maxillofacial trauma, in Kreis DJ, Gomez GA (eds): *Trauma Management*. Boston, Little, Brown, 1989.
31. Cole RR, Aguilar EA: Cricothyroidotomy versus tracheotomy: an otolaryngologist's perspective. *Laryngoscope* 98:131, 1988.
32. Sise MJ, Shacksord SR, Cruickshank JC, et al: Cricothyroidotomy for long term tracheal access. *Ann Surg* 200:13, 1984.
33. O'Connor JV, Reddy K, Ergin MA, et al: Cricothyroidotomy for prolonged ventilatory support after cardiac operations. *Ann Thorac Surg* 39:353, 1985.
34. Kuriloff DB, Setzen M, Portnoy W, et al: Laryngotracheal injury following cricothyroidotomy. *Laryngoscope* 99:125, 1989.
35. Hawkins ML, Shapiro MB, Cue JI, et al: Emergency cricothyrotomy: a reassessment. *Am Surg* 61:52, 1995.
36. Mace SE: Cricothyrotomy. *J Emerg Med* 6:309, 1988.
37. Robinson RJS, Mulder DS: Airway control, in Mattox KL, Feliciano DV, Moore EE (eds): *Trauma*. New York, McGraw-Hill, 2000, p 171.
38. Brantigan CO, Grow JB: Subglottic stenosis after cricothyroidotomy. *Surgery* 91:217, 1982.
39. Epstein SK: Anatomy and physiology of tracheostomy. *Respir Care* 50:476, 2005.
40. Walts PA, Murthy SC, DeCamp MM: Techniques of surgical tracheostomy. *Clin Chest Med* 24:413, 2003.
41. Ciaglia P, Firsching R, Syniec C: Elective percutaneous dilatational tracheostomy: a new simple beside procedure. Preliminary report. *Chest* 87:715, 1985.
42. Freeman BD, Isabella K, Lin N, et al: A meta-analysis of prospective trials comparing percutaneous and surgical tracheostomy in critically ill patients. *Chest* 118:412, 2000.
43. Delancy A, Bagshaw SM, Nalos M: Percutaneous dilatational tracheostomy versus surgical tracheostomy in critically ill patients: a systemic review and meta-analysis. *Crit Care* 10:R55, 2006.
44. Higgins KM, Punthakee X: Meta-analysis comparison of open versus percutaneous tracheostomy. *Laryngoscope* 117:447, 2007.
45. Oliver ER, Gist A, Gillespie MB: Percutaneous versus surgical tracheostomy: an updated meta-analysis. *Laryngoscope* 117:1570, 2007.
46. Dulguerov P, Gysin C, Perneger TV, et al: Percutaneous or surgical tracheostomy: a meta-analysis. *Crit Care Med* 27:1617, 1999.
47. Anderson JD, Rabinovici R, Frankel HL: Percutaneous dilational tracheostomy vs open tracheostomy. *Chest* 120:1423, 2001.
48. Heffner JE: Percutaneous dilational vs standard tracheostomy: a meta-analysis but not the final analysis. *Chest* 118:1236, 2000.
49. Susanto I: Comparing percutaneous tracheostomy with open surgical tracheostomy. *BMJ* 324:3, 2002.
50. Angel LF, Simpson CB: Comparison of surgical and percutaneous dilational tracheostomy. *Clin Chest Med* 24:423, 2003.
51. Massick DD, Yao S, Powell DM, et al: Bedside tracheostomy in the intensive care unit: a perspective randomized trial comparing surgical tracheostomy with endoscopically guided percutaneous dilational tracheotomy. *Laryngoscope* 111:494, 2001.
52. Garland A: Improving the ICU: part 1. *Chest* 127:2151, 2005.
53. Combes A, Luyt CE, Trouillet JL, et al: Adverse effects on a referral intensive care unit's performance of accepting patients transferred from another intensive care unit. *Crit Care Med* 33:705, 2005.
54. Stocchetti N, Parma A, Lamperti M, et al: Neurophysiologic consequences of three tracheostomy techniques: a randomized study in neurosurgical patients. *J Neurosurg Anesthesiol* 12:307, 2000.
55. Shlugman D, Satya-Krishna R, Loh L: Acute fatal haemorrhage during percutaneous dilatational tracheostomy. *Br J Anaesth* 90:517, 2003.
56. Ayoub OM, Griffiths MV: Aortic arch laceration: a lethal complication after percutaneous tracheostomy. *Laryngoscope* 117:176, 2007.
57. Otchwemah R, Defosse J, Wappler F, et al: Percutaneous dilatation tracheostomy in the critically ill: use of ultrasound to detect an aberrant course of the brachiocephalic trunk. *J Cardiothorac Vasc Anesth* 26:e72, 2012.
58. Khan SM, Alzahrani T: Common carotid artery surprise during percutaneous dilatational tracheostomy—a near miss, confirmed with ultrasound. *Saudi J Anaesth* 5:353, 2011.
59. Gilbey P: Fatal complications of percutaneous dilatational tracheostomy. *Am J Otolaryngol* 33:770, 2012.
60. Yavuz A, Yılmaz M, Göya C, et al: Advantages of US in percutaneous dilatational tracheostomy: randomized controlled trial and review of the literature. *Radiology* 273:927, 2014.
61. Rudas M, Seppelt I, Herkes R, et al: Traditional landmark versus ultrasound guided tracheal puncture during percutaneous dilatational tracheostomy in adult intensive care patients: a randomised controlled trial. *Crit Care* 18:514, 2014.
62. Grillo HZ, Cooper JD, Geffin B, et al: A low pressured cuff for tracheostomy tubes to minimize tracheal inner injury. *J Thorac Cardiovasc Surg* 62:898, 1971.
63. Seegobin RD, van Hasselt GL: Endotracheal cuff pressure and tracheal mucosal blood flow, endoscopic study of effects of four large volume cuffs. *BMJ* 288:965, 1984.
64. Hess DR: Tracheostomy tubes and related appliances. *Respir Care* 50:497, 2005.
65. Wright SE, van Dahn K: Long-term care of the tracheostomy patient. *Clin Chest Med* 24:473, 2003.
66. Lewis RM: Airway clearance techniques for patients with artificial airways. *Respir Care* 47:808, 2002.
67. Tabaee A, Lando T, Rickert S, et al: Practice patterns, safety, and rationale for tracheostomy tube changes: a survey of otolaryngology training programs. *Laryngoscope* 117:573, 2007.
68. Shaker R, Dodds WJ, Dantas EO: Coordination of deglutitive glottic closure with oropharyngeal swallowing. *Gastroenterol* 98:1478, 1990.
69. Buckwater JA, Sasaki CT: Effect of tracheostomy on laryngeal function. *Otolaryngol Clin North Am* 21:701, 1988.
70. Devita MA, Spierer-Rundback MS: Swallowing disorders in patients with prolonged intubation or tracheostomy tubes. *Crit Care Med* 18:1328, 1990.
71. Romero CM, Marambio A, Larrondo J, et al: Swallowing dysfunction in nonneurologic critically ill patients who require percutaneous dilatational tracheostomy. *Chest* 137(6):1278–1282, 2010.
72. Tolep K, Getch CL, Criner GJ: Swallowing dysfunction in patients receiving prolonged mechanical ventilation. *Chest* 109:167, 1996.
73. Metheny NA, Clouse RE: Bedside methods for detecting aspiration in tube-fed patients. *Chest* 111:724, 1997.
74. Muz J, Hamlet S, Mathog R, et al: Scintigraphic assessment of aspiration in head and neck cancer patients with tracheostomy. *Head Neck* 16:17, 1994.
75. Leder SB, Tarro JM, Burell MI: Effect of occlusion of a tracheostomy tube on aspiration. *Dysphagia* 11:254, 1996.
76. Fernandez R, Bacelar N, Hernandez G, et al: Ward mortality in patients discharged from the ICU with tracheostomy may depend on patient's vulnerability. *Intensive Care Med* 34:1878, 2008.
77. Martinez GH, Fernandez R, Casado MS, et al: Tracheostomy tube in place at intensive care unit discharge is associated with increased ward mortality. *Respir Care* 54:1644, 2009.
78. Cetto R, Arora A, Hettige R, et al: Improving tracheostomy care: a prospective study of the multidisciplinary approach. *Clin. Otolaryngol* 36:482–488, 2011.
79. Goldenberg D, Ari EG, Golz A, et al: Tracheostomy complications: a retrospective study of 1130 cases. *Otolaryngol Head Neck Surg* 123:495, 2000.
80. Walz MK, Peitgen K, Thurauf N, et al: Percutaneous dilatational tracheostomy—early results and long-term outcome of 326 critically ill patients. *Intensive Care Med* 24:685, 1998.

81. Petros S, Engelmann L: Percutaneous dilatational tracheostomy in a medical ICU. *Intensive Care Med* 23:630, 1997.
82. Shinkwin CA, Gibbin KP: Tracheostomy in children. *J R Soc Med* 89:188, 1996.
83. Cordes SR, Best AR, Hiatt KK: The impact of obesity on adult tracheostomy complication rate. *Laryngoscope* 125:105–110, 2015.
84. Byhahn C, Lischke V, Meininger D, et al: Perio-operative complications during percutaneous tracheostomy in obese patients. *Anaesthesia* 60:12–15, 2005.
85. Romero CM, Cornejo RA, Ruiz MH, et al: Fiberoptic bronchoscopy-assisted percutaneous tracheostomy is safe in obese critically ill patients: a prospective and comparative study. *J Crit Care* 24:494–500, 2009.
86. McCague A, Aljanabi H, Wong D: Safety analysis of percutaneous dilational tracheostomies with bronchscopy in the obese patient. *Laryngoscope* 122:1031–1034, 2012.
87. Heffner JE, Miller KS, Sahn SA: Tracheostomy in the intensive care unit, 2: complications. *Chest* 90:430, 1986.
88. Glossop AJ, Meekings TC, Hutchinson SP, et al: Complications following tracheostomy insertion in critically ill patients-experience from a large teaching hospital. *JICS* 12:4:301–306, 2011.
89. Schaefer OP, Irwin RS: Tracheoarterial fistula: an unusual complication of tracheostomy. *J Intensive Care Med* 10:64, 1995.
90. Mamikunian C: Prevention of delayed hemorrhage after tracheotomy. *Ear Nose Throat J* 67:881, 1988.
91. Oshinsky AE, Rubin JS, Gwozdz CS: The anatomical basis for post-tracheotomy innominate artery rupture. *Laryngoscope* 98:1061, 1988.
92. Deguchi J, Furuya T, Tanaku N, et al: Successful management of trachea-innominate artery fistula with endobronchial stent graph repair. *J Vasc Surg* 33:1280, 2001.
93. Palchik E, Bakkan AM, Saad N, et al: Endobronchial treatment of tracheoinnominate artery fistula: a case report. *Vasc Endovasc Surg* 41:258, 2007.
94. Ferraro F, Marfella R, Esposito M, et al: Tracheal ring fracture secondary to percutaneous tracheostomy: is tracheal flaccidity a risk factor? *J Cardiothorac Vasc Anesth* 29(3):560–564, 2015.
95. Myers EN, Carrau RL: Early complications of tracheostomy. Incidence and management. *Clin Chest Med* 12:589, 1991.
96. Dartevelle P, Macchiarini P: Management of acquired tracheoesophageal fistula. *Chest Surg Clin North Am* 6:819, 1996.
97. Dollner R, Verch M, Schweiger P, et al: Laryngotracheoscopic findings in long-term follow-up after Griggs tracheostomy. *Chest* 122:206, 2002.
98. Streitz JM, Shapshay SM: Airway injury after tracheostomy and endotracheal intubation. *Surg Clin North Am* 71:1211, 1991.
99. Stauffer JL, Olsen DE, Petty TL: Complications and consequences of endotracheal intubation and tracheostomy: a prospective study of 150 critically ill adult patients. *Am J Med* 70:65, 1981.
100. Arola MK, Puhakka H, Makela P: Healing of lesions caused by cuffed tracheotomy tubes and their late sequelae: a follow-up study. *Acta Anaesthesiol Scand* 24:169, 1980.
101. Friedman Y, Franklin C: The technique of percutaneous tracheostomy: using serial dilation to secure an airway with minimal risk. *J Crit Illn* 8:289, 1993.
102. Crofts SL, Alzeer A, McGuire GP, et al: A comparison of percutaneous and operative tracheostomies in intensive care patients. *Can J Anaesth* 42:775, 1995.

Chapter 10 ■ Bronchoscopy

PAULO J. OLIVEIRA • RAHUL N. SOOD • RICHARD S. IRWIN

Flexible bronchoscopy (FB) was first introduced in 1968 by Dr. Shigeto Ikeda, the Japanese physician, who is regarded as the "father" of FB. Since then, further technological advances have facilitated its widespread utilization and it has evolved into an invaluable tool for diagnosis and therapy of a wide variety of respiratory diseases in the intensive care unit (ICU) [1]. Because of its safety and low complication rate [2], FB has largely replaced rigid bronchoscopy as the procedure of choice for most endoscopic evaluations of the airway and lung parenchyma. However, rigid bronchoscopy still plays a potential and pivotal role in the evaluation and management of (a) brisk, massive hemoptysis, defined broadly as 200 to 600 mL per 24 hours; (b) extraction of foreign bodies; (c) endobronchial resection of granulation tissue that can occur after traumatic and/or prolonged intubation; (d) biopsy of potentially vascular tumors (e.g., bronchial carcinoid), in which brisk and excessive bleeding can be controlled by packing and enhanced suction capabilities; (e) endoscopic-mechanical and laser-based debridement/destruction of airway tumors; and (f) dilation of tracheobronchial strictures and management of extrinsic airway constriction via placement of airway stents. In the last three decades, there has been renewed interest in the use of rigid bronchoscopy by pulmonologists, driven by the advent of dedicated endobronchial prostheses (airway stents) in the early 1990s for the management of both malignant and benign central airway obstruction [3,4]. These advances have fueled the growth of the established field of interventional pulmonology (IP); comprehensive guidelines have been published in the last decade by the American College of Chest Physicians and European Respiratory Society [3,5]. In this chapter, we discuss primarily the role of FB in the ICU but the reader is referred to Chapter 182 for the role of IP in the ICU.

GENERAL CONSIDERATIONS

Because FB can be performed easily even in intubated patients, the same general indications apply to critically ill patients on ventilators and non-critically ill patients; however, only the diagnostic and therapeutic indications most commonly encountered in the ICU are discussed here. Where relevant, the potential application of advanced bronchoscopic diagnostic and therapeutic interventions in the ICU setting are also discussed.

COMMON DIAGNOSTIC INDICATIONS

Hemoptysis

Hemoptysis is one of the most common clinical problems for which bronchoscopy is indicated [6]. Whether the patient complains of blood streaking or massive hemoptysis, bronchoscopy should be considered to localize/lateralize the site of bleeding and possibly diagnose the cause. Localization of the site of bleeding is crucial if temporizing or definitive therapy, such as surgery, becomes necessary, and it is also useful to guide angiographic procedures (bronchial or pulmonary artery embolization). Whenever patients have an endotracheal or tracheostomy tube in place, hemoptysis should always be evaluated, because it may indicate potentially life-threatening tracheal injury. Unless the bleeding is massive, a flexible bronchoscope, rather than a rigid bronchoscope, is the initial instrument of choice for evaluating hemoptysis. In the setting of massive hemoptysis, however, the patient is at risk of imminent decompensation and death due to asphyxiation. Stabilization of the patient, focusing on establishing a secure airway, and timely communication with pulmonology/IP, thoracic surgery, anesthesiology, and interventional radiology is of utmost importance. This coordinated, interprofessional effort should focus on rapid transfer to the operation room suite for rigid bronchoscopy. The rigid bronchoscope is ideal in this situation because it provides a secure route for ventilation, serves as a larger conduit for adequate suctioning, and can quickly isolate the lung in the case of a lateralized bleeding source. In most situations, once an adequate airway has been established and initial suctioning of excessive blood has been performed, the flexible bronchoscope can be used as a complementary modality inserted through the rigid bronchoscope to more accurately assess, localize, and temporize the source of bleeding within and beyond the main bronchi [7].

Diffuse Parenchymal Disease

The clinical setting influences the choice of procedure. When diffuse pulmonary infiltrates suggest sarcoidosis, lymphangitic carcinomatosis, or eosinophilic pneumonia, for example, transbronchial lung biopsy (TBLB) should be considered initially because it has an extremely high yield in these situations. However, TBLB has a low yield for the definitive diagnosis of most idiopathic interstitial pneumonias, inorganic pneumoconiosis, and pulmonary vasculitides [8]; when these disorders are suspected, surgical lung biopsy is the gold standard and procedure of choice. Although TBLB is usually not adequate for histologic diagnosis of pulmonary fibrosis and acute interstitial pneumonia, it may provide sufficient information to guide therapy in a critically ill patient by excluding infection.

Ventilator-Associated Pneumonia

The ability to determine the probability of ventilator-associated pneumonia (VAP) is very limited, with a sensitivity of only 50% and a specificity of 58% [9]. Quantitative cultures obtained via bronchoscopy may thus play an important role in the diagnostic strategy. Quantitative cultures of bronchoalveolar lavage (BAL) fluid and protected specimen brush (PSB), with thresholds of 10^4 colony-forming units (CFU) per mL and 10^3 CFU per mL, respectively, are most commonly employed prior to initiation of antimicrobial therapy when a semi-invasive approach is taken. Cultures of bronchial washings do not add to the diagnostic yield of quantitative BAL culture alone [10]. For a brief description of how to perform BAL and obtain PSB cultures, see the "Procedure" section, given later in the chapter.

For BAL, an evidence-based analysis of 23 prior investigations yielded a sensitivity of 73% and a specificity of 82%, indicating that BAL cultures fail to diagnose VAP in almost one-fourth of all cases [11]. A similar analysis of PSB cultures indicates a very wide range of results, with a sensitivity of 33% to greater than 95% and a median of 67%, and a specificity of 50% to 100% with a median of 95% [12]. PSB is thus more specific than it is sensitive, and negative results may not be sufficient to exclude the presence of VAP. Blind protected telescoping catheter specimens yield similar results to bronchoscopically directed PSB and BAL cultures [13]. Despite the greater accuracy of quantitative bronchoscopic cultures, prospective randomized trials of early invasive diagnostic strategies employing bronchoscopy and quantitative lower respiratory tract cultures for VAP have not demonstrated significant advantages in mortality or other major clinical end points over simpler methods [14]. A Cochrane database review combining five such randomized controlled trials showed no improvement in mortality, duration of mechanical ventilation, or length of ICU stay [15]. On the basis of these findings, routine use of bronchoscopy over semiquantitative endotracheal suctioning cultures in immunocompetent adults with suspected VAP cannot be recommended.

Pulmonary Infiltrates in Immunocompromised Patients

When an infectious process is suspected, the diagnostic yield depends on the organism and the immune status of the patient. Numerous recent investigations have examined the utility of bronchoscopy in immunocompromised patients. Most of these investigations have found that the diagnostic yield of BAL in such patients is approximately 50% and that the results of BAL lead to a change in treatment in 17% to 38% of patients. In one prospective multicenter trial [16], BAL was the only conclusive diagnostic study in 33% of patients. Although it is difficult to distinguish respiratory decompensation caused by bronchoscopy from the natural history of the patients' underlying disease, the same study found that 48% of patients developed deterioration in respiratory status after bronchoscopy and 27% of patients were intubated. Because of these concerns, novel approaches to FB have been used in such patients including the utilization of noninvasive positive pressure ventilation or high flow nasal cannula during the procedure [17]. Transbronchial biopsy may add only a little to the diagnostic yield of BAL in immunocompromised patients, with an incremental yield of 7% to 12% [18]. In some series, the major complication rate of transbronchial biopsy was greater than the diagnostic utility, including a 14% incidence of major bleeding requiring intubation [18]. However, in AIDS patients, the sensitivity of lavage and/or TBLB for identifying all opportunistic organisms can be as high as 87% [19]. Transbronchial biopsy adds significantly to the diagnostic yield in AIDS patients and may be the sole means of making a diagnosis in up to 24% of patients, including diagnoses of *Pneumocystis jirovecii*, *Cryptococcus neoformans*, *Mycobacterium tuberculosis*, and occasionally nonspecific interstitial pneumonitis [20]. Lavage alone may have a sensitivity of up to 97% for the diagnosis of *P. jirovecii* pneumonia [21]. However, because induced sputum samples can also be positive for *P. jirovecii* in up to 79% of cases [21], induced expectorated sputum, when available, should be evaluated first for this organism before resorting to bronchoscopy. More recently, the use of serum-based markers such as β-2 glucan and galactomannan have also been used in certain settings to guide diagnosis and therapy [22] when *P. jirovecii* and aspergillus infections are considered.

Acute Inhalation Injury

In patients suffering from smoke inhalation, flexible nasopharyngoscopy, laryngoscopy, and bronchoscopy are indicated to identify the anatomic level and severity of injury. Prophylactic intubation should be considered if considerable upper airway mucosal injury is noted early; acute respiratory failure is more likely in patients with mucosal changes seen at segmental or lower levels. Upper airway obstruction is a life-threatening problem that usually develops during the initial 24 hours after inhalation injury. It correlates significantly with increased size of cutaneous burns, burns of the face and neck, and rapid intravenous fluid administration, and also portends a greater mortality [23].

Blunt Chest Trauma

Patients may present with atelectasis, pulmonary contusion, hemothorax, pneumothorax, pneumomediastinum, or hemoptysis. Prompt bronchoscopic evaluation of such patients has a diagnostic yield of 53%; findings may include tracheal or bronchial laceration or transection (14%), aspirated material (6%), supraglottic tear with glottic obstruction (2%), mucus plugging (15%), and distal hemorrhage (13%) [24,25]. Many of these diagnoses may not be clinically evident and require surgical intervention.

Postresectional Surgery and Lung Transplantation

FB can identify a disrupted suture line causing bleeding and pneumothorax following surgery and an exposed endobronchial suture causing refractory cough. In these postpneumonectomy situations, the location of dehiscence and the subsequent bronchopleural fistula (BPF) can be identified visually via FB at the stump site. However, when the BPF occurs in the setting of acute respiratory distress syndrome (ARDS) or necrotizing pneumonia, localization at the segmental and subsegmental level (defects less than 2 to 5 mm in diameter) can be more challenging. FB also appears to be safe and effective in guiding clinical management in critically ill lung transplant recipients when considering infection or rejection [26].

Assessment of Intubation-Related Injury

When a nasotracheal or orotracheal tube of the proper size is in place, the balloon can be routinely deflated and the tube withdrawn over the bronchoscope to look for upper airway injury. The technique involves withdrawing the tube up through the vocal cords and over the flexible bronchoscope to assess glottic and supraglottic damage. This technique may be useful after reintubation for stridor, or when deflation of the endotracheal tube cuff does not produce a significant air leak, suggesting the potential for life-threatening upper airway obstruction when extubation takes place. The flexible bronchoscope may readily identify mechanical problems such as increased airway granulation tissue leading to airway obstruction, tracheal tears, tracheal stenosis at pressure points along the artificial airway–tracheal interface, and tracheobronchomalacia.

THERAPEUTIC INDICATIONS

Atelectasis

Bronchoscopy has a success rate of up to 89% in cases of lobar atelectasis, but only produced clinical improvement in 44% of patients when performed for retained secretions [27]. Two randomized trials found no advantage of bronchoscopy over a very aggressive regimen of frequent chest physiotherapy, recruitment maneuvers, saline nebulization, and postural drainage [28,29]. These studies also found that the presence of air bronchograms on the initial chest X-ray predicted relative failure of either intervention to resolve the atelectasis. Occasionally, the direct instillation of *N*-acetylcysteine through the bronchoscope may be necessary to liquefy the thick, tenacious inspissated mucus [30]. Because *N*-acetylcysteine may induce bronchospasm in patients with asthma, these patients should be pretreated with a bronchodilator. In cases of complete lobar collapse, a bronchoscope with the largest suction/working channel diameter available (3 to 3.2 mm working channel) should be used.

Foreign Bodies

Although the rigid bronchoscope is considered by many to be the instrument of choice for removing foreign bodies, especially in the pediatric population, devices with which to grasp objects have been created and are available for use with the flexible bronchoscope. A recent systematic review of the adult literature showed that FB has a high success rate (92%) in removal of inhaled foreign bodies [31]. The success of FB for foreign body removal can be enhanced by rigorous preprocedure preparation, assuring the availability of appropriate ancillary grasping equipment, practicing a "dry run," and ensuring that a bronchoscopist with experience in foreign body removal is involved. It is also important to have an appreciation for situations for which rigid bronchoscopy with added ancillary interventions, such as laser therapy or cryotherapy, might be useful (e.g., an embedded foreign body with significant granulation tissue reaction at risk of bleeding) [32].

Endotracheal Intubation

Intubation under endoscopic visualization may be planned in cases of a suspected difficult airway that cannot be easily intubated or properly ventilated using the flexible bronchoscope as an obturator for tube passage [33]. This is also useful for the intubation of patients with central airway stents, as blind intubation carries the risk of stent migration and malpositioning of the endotracheal tube [34]. The bronchoscope of choice should be one with an outer diameter of 5.7 mm or more because thinner more flexible scopes lack the stiffness and enhanced maneuverability needed for successful intubation.

Hemoptysis

On rare occasions where brisk bleeding threatens asphyxiation, endobronchial tamponade may stabilize the patient before definitive therapy is performed. With the use of the flexible bronchoscope, usually passed through a rigid bronchoscope or endotracheal tube, a Fogarty catheter with balloon is passed into the bleeding lobar orifice. When the balloon is inflated and wedged tightly, the patient may be transferred to surgery or angiography for bronchial arteriography and bronchial artery embolization [35]. Other bronchial blocking and lung separation techniques have been described and reviewed in the literature [36]. The Arndt blocker is a dedicated bronchial blocker that has a wire loop at its distal end, which when looped around the distal end of the flexible bronchoscope, can be guided to the bleeding airway and inflated. Its position can be adjusted under direct visualization and it can be fixed to the outer proximal portion of the endotracheal tube. More simple techniques that take advantage of the flexible bronchoscope's ability to act as a stylet for a single-lumen endotracheal tube can be used to isolate one lung. One can use the bronchoscope to preferentially intubate the right main or left main bronchus in an emergent situation. Hemostasis may also be achieved by using FB to apply oxidized regenerated cellulose mesh to the bleeding site, instill thrombin/thrombin–fibrinogen preparations, tranexamic acid and more traditionally, perform iced saline lavage or apply topical epinephrine (1:20,000) to decrease the bleeding [37]. In the case of a visibly bleeding endobronchial tumor, hemostasis can be attained with laser photocoagulation (Nd-YAG laser), electrocautery, or argon plasma coagulation.

Central Obstructing Airway Lesions

Some patients with cancer and others with benign lesions that obstruct the larynx, trachea, and major bronchi can be treated by electrocautery, laser photoresection, argon plasma coagulation, cryotherapy, or photodynamic therapy applied through the bronchoscope (rigid or flexible) [38,39]. FB can also be used to place catheters that facilitate endobronchial delivery of radiation (brachytherapy). Metallic or silicone endobronchial stents can be placed bronchoscopically to relieve stenosis of large central airways. Adequate insertion of stents and relief of stenosis (especially due to extrinsic compression) is typically accompanied by dilation of the airway via rigid bronchoscopy or with balloon dilation applied with the aid of FB. Several issues regarding airway stents should be noted: silicone stents can only be placed via rigid bronchoscopy and metallic stents should generally not be used in the setting of a nonmalignant central airway obstruction because they are associated with excessive growth of granulation tissue with subsequent worsening of airway obstruction and can be very challenging to remove once this complication occurs [40]. The primary goal of the interventions described earlier for the management of malignant central airway obstruction is palliative. In many instances, these procedures also facilitate liberation from mechanical ventilation and liberation from the ICU [41]. It appears that for intubated ICU patients, FB performed at the bedside with stent deployment and resective interventions, when necessary, is just as effective as rigid bronchoscopic interventions in the appropriately selected patient [42].

Closure of Bronchopleural Fistula

After placement of a chest tube, drainage of the pleural space, and stabilization of the patient (e.g., infection and cardiovascular and respiratory systems), bronchoscopy can be used to visualize a proximal BPF or localize a distal BPF; it can also be used in attempts to close the BPF [43]. Please see Chapter 176 that comprehensively covers this topic.

Percutaneous Dilatational Tracheostomy

Flexible bronchoscopic guidance is extremely helpful during bedside percutaneous tracheostomy [44,45]. Please see Chapter 9 that comprehensively covers this topic.

COMPLICATIONS

When performed by a trained specialist, *routine* FB is extremely safe [2]. The rare deaths have been due to excessive premedication or topical anesthesia, respiratory arrest from hemorrhage, laryngospasm or bronchospasm, and cardiac arrest from acute myocardial infarction [46]. Nonfatal complications occurring within 24 hours of the procedure include fever that is usually cytokine mediated (1.2% to 24%), pneumonia (0.6% to 6%), vasovagal reactions (2.4%), laryngospasm or bronchospasm (0.1% to 0.4%), cardiac arrhythmias (0.9% to 4%), pneumothorax, anesthesia-related problems (0.1%), and aphonia (0.1%) [47]. Most investigations have found that the incidence of bacteremia after transoral FB is very low (0.7%) [48]. Current guidelines by the American Heart Association for respiratory tract procedures recommend prophylactic antibiotics only when incision or biopsy of the respiratory tract mucosa is anticipated. Prophylaxis is further restricted to patients with high-risk cardiac conditions (prosthetic valves, prior history of infective endocarditis, congenital heart disease, and cardiac transplantation with valvulopathy) only and no distinction is made between rigid bronchoscopy and FB [49].

Although routine bronchoscopy is extremely safe, critically ill patients appear to be at higher risk for complications. Patients with asthma are prone to develop laryngospasm and bronchospasm. Bone marrow and stem cell transplant recipients are more likely to develop major bleeding during bronchoscopy (0% to 14%) [50], particularly if PSB or TBLB is performed (7% to 14% vs. 1.5% for BAL alone). One investigation found that aspirin use did not increase bleeding risk after transbronchial biopsy [51]. However, a prospective cohort study showed that clopidogrel use greatly increases the risk of bleeding after TBLB and therefore should be discontinued 7 days before bronchoscopy with biopsies [52]. In critically ill, mechanically ventilated patents, bronchoscopy causes a transient decrease in PaO_2 (partial arterial oxygen pressure) of approximately 25% [53], and TBLB is more likely to result in pneumothorax (7% to 23%), particularly in patients with ARDS (up to 36%) [54].

CONTRAINDICATIONS

Bronchoscopy should not be performed (a) unless an experienced bronchoscopist is available; (b) when the patient will not or cannot cooperate; (c) when adequate oxygenation cannot be maintained during the procedure; (d) in unstable cardiac patients [55]; and (e) in untreated symptomatic patients with asthma [56]. British Thoracic Society (BTS) guidelines recommend a platelet count of at least 20,000 per μL for FB with BAL, but to liaison with the hematology team if TBLB is considered [1]. Other considerations include patients with uremia and lung transplantation, who are also at a higher risk of bleeding with TBLB [1]. In patients with recent cardiac ischemia, the major complication rate is low (3% to 5%) and is similar to that of other critically ill populations [57]. The major contraindications to rigid bronchoscopy include inability to tolerate general anesthesia, an unstable cervical spine, limited range of motion of the spine, any condition that inhibits opening of the jaw, and an inexperienced operator and staff [3].

Consideration of bronchoscopy in neurologic and neurosurgical patients requires attention to the effects of bronchoscopy on intracranial pressure (ICP) and cerebral perfusion pressure (CPP). In patients with head trauma, bronchoscopy causes the ICP to increase by at least 50% in 88% of patients and by at least 100% in 69% of patients despite the use of deep sedation and paralysis [58]. Because mean arterial pressure tends to rise in parallel with ICP, there is often no change in CPP. A recent retrospective cohort study showed no increase in neurologic or sedation-specific complications in patients with malignant space occupying brain lesions undergoing flexible or rigid bronchoscopy [59]. In such patients, the procedure should be accompanied by deep sedation, paralysis, and medications for cerebral protection for which thiopental and lidocaine should be considered. Cerebral hemodynamics should be continuously monitored to ensure that ICP and CPP are within acceptable levels in high-risk patients whenever possible. Caution is warranted in patients with markedly elevated baseline ICP or with borderline CPP.

PROCEDURE

For nonintubated patients, FB can be performed by the transnasal or transoral route with a bite block. There has also been a recent interest in performing noninvasive ventilation-assisted FB via face mask, first described in eight immunocompromised patients with infiltrates and severe hypoxemia ($PaO_2/FiO_2 < 100$) [60]. The procedure was well tolerated with either maintenance of or an improvement in oxygenation noted throughout, and none of the patients required intubation. Since then, multiple small randomized controlled trials using similar applications of noninvasive ventilation during bronchoscopy in expanded patient populations with severe hypoxemia ($PaO_2/FiO_2 < 200$) have been described with similar outcomes [61]. Thus, it appears that this technique, augmented by BAL, appears to be a safe, effective, and viable option for obtaining an early and accurate diagnosis of pneumonia in nonintubated, otherwise marginally stable, patients with severe hypoxemia. In intubated and mechanically ventilated patients, the flexible bronchoscope can be passed into the tube through a swivel adapter with a rubber diaphragm that will prevent loss of the delivered respiratory gases. To prevent dramatic increases in airway resistance and an unacceptable loss of tidal volume, the lumen of the endotracheal tube should be at least 2 mm larger than the outer diameter of the bronchoscope [62]. Thus, FB with an average adult-sized instrument (outside diameter of scope 4.8 to 5.9 mm) can be performed in a ventilated patient if there is an endotracheal tube in place that is 8 mm or larger in internal diameter. If the endotracheal tube is smaller, a pediatric bronchoscope (outside diameter 3.5 mm) or intubation endoscope (outside diameter 3.8 mm) must be used to prevent damage to the bronchoscope. Both diagnostic and therapeutic interventions via FB have also been performed more frequently in the last decade through laryngeal mask airways used to secure the airway in spontaneously breathing under general anesthesia [63].

Premedication

Topical anesthesia may be achieved using nebulized lidocaine with lidocaine jelly as a lubricant and by instilling approximately 3 mL of 1% or 2% lidocaine at the main carina and, if needed, into the lower airways. Lidocaine is absorbed through the mucus membranes, producing peak serum concentrations that are nearly as high as that when the equivalent dose is administered intravenously, although toxicity is rare if the total dose does not exceed 6 to 7 mg per kg. In 2000, a study performed in otherwise healthy patients with asthma demonstrated the safety of topical lidocaine doses up to 8.2 mg per kg in this population [64] and subsequently led to this upper limit being recommended by the BTS in their guidelines for diagnostic FB [65]. A recent randomized control trial showed 1% lidocaine solution to be as effective as the 2% solution in achieving adequate topical anesthesia, at significantly lower cumulative doses [66]. In patients with hepatic or cardiac insufficiency, lidocaine clearance is reduced, and the dose should be decreased to a maximum of 4 to 5 mg per kg [67]. Administering nebulized lidocaine prior to the procedure substantially increases the total lidocaine dose without improving cough or patient comfort [68]. Moderate sedation with incremental doses of midazolam, titrated to produce light sleep, produces amnesia in more than 95% of patients, but adequate sedation may require a total of greater than 20 mg in some subjects [69]. Cough suppression is more effective when narcotics are added to benzodiazepine premedication regimens [70]. Premedication with intravenous anticholinergics has not been found to reduce secretions, decrease coughing, or prevent bradycardia, and has been associated with greater hemodynamic fluctuations when compared to placebo [71]. Propofol and fospropofol [72] have also been used with success during moderate sedation for bronchoscopy, and may have the advantage of more rapid onset and shorter recovery time. More recently, a double blinded prospective study showed that a sedative regimen of dexmedetomidine and propofol was associated with fewer episodes of desaturation when compared to remifentanil and propofol in patients undergoing FB, though it was associated with longer recovery times and slightly worse bronchoscopist satisfaction scores [73].

Mechanical Ventilation

Maintaining adequate oxygenation and ventilation while preventing breath stacking and positive end expiratory pressure (auto-PEEP) may be challenging when insertion of the bronchoscope reduces the effective lumen of the endotracheal tube by more than 50%. PEEP caused by standard scopes and tubes will approach 20 cm H_2O with the potential for volutrauma. The inspired oxygen concentration must be temporarily increased to 100% prior to starting the procedure. Expired volumes should be constantly monitored to ensure that they are adequate [62]. Meeting these ventilatory goals may require increasing the high-pressure limit in volume-cycled ventilation to near its maximal value, allowing the ventilator to overcome the added resistance caused by the bronchoscope. Although this increases the measured peak airway pressure, the alveolar pressure is not likely to change significantly because the lung is protected by the resistance of the bronchoscope [62]. Alternatively, decreasing the inspiratory flow rate in an attempt to decrease measured peak pressures may paradoxically increase alveolar pressures by decreasing expiratory time and thus increasing auto-PEEP. Suctioning should be kept to a minimum and for short periods of time because it will decrease the tidal volumes being delivered and may lead to derecruitment and associated hypoxemia [74].

Quantitative Cultures

BAL is performed by advancing the bronchoscope until the tip wedges tightly in a distal bronchus in the area of greatest clinical interest. If the disease process is diffuse, perform the procedure in the right middle lobe because this is the area from which the largest returns are most consistently obtained. Three aliquots of saline, typically 35 to 50 mL, are then instilled and withdrawn; in some protocols, the first aliquot is discarded to prevent contamination with more proximal secretions. A total instilled volume of 100 mL with at least 5% to 10% retrieved constitutes an adequate specimen [75]. PSB may be performed through a bronchoscope by advancing the plugged catheter assembly until it projects from the bronchoscope. When the area of interest is reached (e.g., purulent secretions can be seen), the distal plug is ejected and the brush is then fully advanced beyond the protective sheath. After the specimen is obtained, the brush is pulled back into the sheath and only then is the catheter assembly removed from the bronchoscope.

ACKNOWLEDGMENTS

Dr. Stephen Krinzman contributed to previous editions of this chapter.

References

1. Du Rand IA, Blaikley J, Booton R: BTS guideline for diagnostic flexible bronchoscopy in adults. *Thorax* 68:i1–i44, 2013.
2. Facciolongo N, Patelli M, Gasparini S: Incidence of complications in bronchoscopy: multi-centre prospective study of 20,986 bronchoscopies. *Monaldi Arch Chest Dis* 71:8–14, 2009.
3. Bolliger CT, Mathur PN, Beamis JF, et al: ERS/ATS statement on interventional pulmonology. *Eur Respir J* 19(2):356–373, 2002.
4. Wahidi MM, Ernst A: Role of the interventional pulmonologist in the intensive care unit. *J Intensive Care Med* 20(3):141–146, 2005.
5. Ernst A, Silvestri GA, Johnstone D: Interventional pulmonary procedures, guidelines from the American College of Chest Physicians. *Chest* 123:1693–1717, 2003.
6. Sakr L, Dutau H. Massive hemoptysis: an update on the role of bronchoscopy in diagnosis and management. *Respiration* 80(1):38–58, 2010.
7. Susanto I: Managing a patient with hemoptysis. *J Bronchol* 9:40–45, 2002.
8. Bradley B, Branley HM, Egan JJ, et al: Interstitial lung disease guideline: the British Thoracic Society in collaboration with the Thoracic Society of Australia and New Zealand and the Irish Thoracic Society. *Thorax* 63[Suppl 5]:v1–v58, 2008.
9. Fartoukh M, Maitre B, Honore S, et al: Diagnosing pneumonia during mechanical ventilation: the clinical infection score revisited. *Am J Respir Crit Care Med* 168:173, 2003.
10. Pinckard JK, Kollef M, Dunne WM: Culturing bronchial washings obtained during bronchoscopy fails to add diagnostic utility to culturing the bronchoalveolar lavage fluid alone. *Diagn Microbiol Infect Dis* 43:99, 2002.
11. Torres A, El-Ebiary M: Bronchoscopic BAL in the diagnosis of ventilator-associated pneumonia. *Chest* 117:198, 2000.
12. Baughman RP: Protected-specimen brush technique in the diagnosis of ventilator associated pneumonia. *Chest* 117:203S–206S, 2000.
13. Fujitani S, Yu VL: Diagnosis of ventilator-associated pneumonia: focus on nonbronchoscopic techniques (nonbronchoscopic bronchoalveolar lavage,

including mini-BAL, blinded protected specimen brush, and blinded bronchial sampling) and endotracheal aspirates. *J Intensive Care Med* 21:17–21, 2006.
14. Canadian Critical Care Trials Group: A randomized trial of diagnostic techniques for ventilator-associated pneumonia. *N Engl J Med* 355:2619, 2006.
15. Berton DC, Kalil AC, Teixeira PJZ: Quantitative versus qualitative cultures of respiratory secretions for clinical outcomes in patients with ventilator-associated pneumonia. *Cochrane Database Syst Rev* 10:CD006482, 2014.
16. Azoulay, E, Mokart, D, Rabbat A, et al: Diagnostic bronchoscopy in hematology and oncology patients with acute respiratory failure: prospective multicenter data. *Crit Care Med* 36:100, 2008.
17. Simon M, Braune S, Frings D, et al: High-flow nasal cannula oxygen versus non-invasive ventilation in patients with acute hypoxaemic respiratory failure undergoing flexible bronchoscopy—a prospective randomised trial. *Crit Care* 18(6):712, 2014.
18. Patel N, Lee P, Kim J, et al: The influence of diagnostic bronchoscopy on clinical outcomes comparing adult autologous and allogeneic bone marrow transplant recipients. *Chest* 127:1388, 2005.
19. Broaddus C, Dake MD, Stulbarg MS, et al: Bronchoalveolar lavage and transbronchial biopsy for the diagnosis of pulmonary infections in the acquired immunodeficiency syndrome. *Ann Intern Med* 102:747, 1985.
20. Raoof S, Rosen MJ, Khan FA: Role of bronchoscopy in AIDS. *Clin Chest Med* 20:63, 1999.
21. Hopewell PC: Pneumocystis carinii pneumonia: diagnosis. *J Infect Dis* 157:1115, 1988.
22. Desmet S, Van Wijngaerden E, Maertens J, et al: Serum (1–3)-beta-D-glucan as a tool for diagnosis of *Pneumocystis jirovecii* pneumonia in patients with human immunodeficiency virus infection or hematological malignancy. *J Clin Microbiol* 47:3871–3874, 2009.
23. Dries DJ, Endorf FW: Inhalation injury: epidemiology, pathology, treatment strategies. *Scand J Trauma Resusc Emerg Med*;21:31, 2013.
24. Barmada H, Gibbons JR: Tracheobronchial injury in blunt and penetrating chest trauma. *Chest* 9:74–78, 1994.
25. Hara KS, Prakash UBS: Fiberoptic bronchoscopy in the evaluation of acute chest and upper airway trauma. *Chest* 96:627, 1989.
26. Mohanka MR, Mehta AC, Budev MM, et al: Impact of bedside bronchoscopy in critically ill lung transplant recipients. *J Bronchology Interv Pulmonol* 21(3):199–207, 2014.
27. Kreider ME, Lipson DA: Bronchoscopy for atelectasis in the ICU: a case report and review of the literature. *Chest* 124:344, 2003.
28. Jaworski A, Goldberg SK, Walkenstein MD, et al: Utility of immediate postlobectomy fiberoptic bronchoscopy in preventing atelectasis. *Chest* 94(1):38–43, 1988.
29. Marini JJ, Pierson DJ, Hudson LD: Acute lobar atelectasis: a prospective comparison of fiberoptic bronchoscopy and respiratory therapy. *Am Rev Respir Dis* 119:971, 1979.
30. Lieberman J: The appropriate use of mucolytic agents. *Am J Med* 49:1, 1970.
31. Sehgal IS, Dhooria S, Ram B, et al: Foreign body inhalation in the adult population: experience of 25,998 bronchoscopies and systematic review of the literature. *Respir Care* 60(10):1438–1448, 2015.
32. Mehta AC, Rafanan AL: Extraction of airway foreign body in adults. *J Bronchol* 8:123–131, 2001.
33. Apfelbaum JL, Hagberg CA, Caplan RA, et al: American Society of Anesthesiologists Task Force on Management of the Difficult Airway. Practice guidelines for management of the difficult airway: an updated report by the American Society of Anesthesiologists Task Force on Management of the Difficult Airway. *Anesthesiology* 118(2):251–270, 2013.
34. Bonnet M, Monteiro MB: Fiberoptic bronchoscopy in intensive care—particular aspects. *Rev Port Med Int* 12:17–19, 2003.
35. Schramm R, Abugameh A, Tscholl D, et al: Managing pulmonary artery catheter-induced pulmonary hemorrhage by bronchial occlusion. *Ann Thorac Surg* 88:284–287, 2009.
36. Campos JH: An update on bronchial blockers during lung separation techniques in adults. *Anesth Analg* 97:1266–1274, 2003.
37. Valipour A, Kreuzer A, Koller H, et al: Bronchoscopy-guided topical hemostatic tamponade therapy for the management of life threatening hemoptysis. *Chest* 127:2113, 2005.
38. Beamis J: Interventional pulmonology techniques for treating malignant large airway obstruction: an update. *Curr Opin Pulm Med* 11:292, 2005.
39. Ernst A, Feller-Kopman D, Becker HD, et al: Central airway obstruction. *Am J Respir Crit Care Med* 169:1278–1297, 2004.
40. Swanson KL, Edell ES, Prakash UB, et al: Complications of metal stent therapy in benign airway obstruction. *J Bronchol* 14:90–94, 2007.
41. Colt HG, Harrell JH: Therapeutic rigid bronchoscopy allows level of care changes in patients with acute respiratory failure from central airways obstruction. *Chest* 112:202–206, 1997.
42. Saad CP, Murthy S, Krizmanich G, et al: Self-expandable metallic airway stents and flexible bronchoscopy. *Chest* 124:1993–1999, 2003.
43. Lois M, Noppen M: Bronchopleural fistulas, an overview of the problem with special focus on endoscopic management. *Chest* 128:3955–3965, 2005.
44. Madi JM, Trottier SJ: Percutaneous dilatational tracheostomy technique. *J Bronchol* 10:146–149, 2003.
45. Madsen KR, Guldager H, Rewers M, et al: Danish Guidelines 2015 for percutaneous dilatational tracheostomy in the intensive care unit. *Dan Med J* 61(3), 2015.
46. Suratt PM, Smiddy JF, Gruber B: Deaths and complications associated with fiberoptic bronchoscopy. *Chest* 69:747, 1976.
47. Stubbs SE, Brutinel WM: Complications of bronchoscopy, in Prakash USB (ed): *Bronchoscopy*. New York, Lippincott Williams & Wilkins, 1994, p 357.
48. Yigla M, Oren I, Solomonov A, et al: Incidence of bacteraemia following fiberoptic bronchoscopy. *Eur Respir J* 14:789, 1999.
49. Wilson M, Taubert KA, Gewitz M, et al: Prevention of endocarditis, guidelines from the American Heart Association. *Circulation* 116:1736–1754, 2007.
50. Dunagan DP, Baker AM, Hurd DD: Bronchoscopic evaluation of pulmonary infiltrates following bone marrow transplantation. *Chest* 111:135, 1997.
51. Herth FJ, Becker HD, Ernst A: Aspirin does not increase bleeding complications after transbronchial biopsy. *Chest* 122:1461, 2002.
52. Ernst A, Eberhardt R, Wahidi M, et al: Effect of routine clopidogrel use on bleeding complications after transbronchial biopsy in humans. *Chest* 129(3):734–737, 2006.
53. Antonelli M, Conti G, Rocco M, et al: Noninvasive positive-pressure ventilation vs. conventional oxygen supplementation in hypoxemic patients undergoing diagnostic bronchoscopy. *Chest* 121(4):1149–1154, 2002.
54. Bulpa PA, Dive AM, Mertens L, et al: Combined bronchoalveolar lavage and transbronchial lung biopsy: safety and yield in ventilated patients. *Eur Respir J* 21:489, 2003.
55. Luck JC, Messeder OH, Rubenstein MJ, et al: Arrhythmias from fiberoptic bronchoscopy. *Chest* 74:139, 1978.
56. Sahn SA, Scoggin C: Fiberoptic bronchoscopy in bronchial asthma: a word of caution. *Chest* 69:39, 1976.
57. Dweik RA, Mehta AC, Meeker DP, et al: Analysis of the safety of bronchoscopy after recent acute myocardial infarction. *Chest* 110:825, 1996.
58. Kerwin AJ, Croce MA, Timmons SD, et al: Effects of fiberoptic bronchoscopy on intracranial pressure in patients with brain injury; a prospective clinical study. *J Trauma* 48:878, 2000.
59. Grosu HB, Morice RC, Sarkiss M, et al: Safety of flexible bronchoscopy, rigid bronchoscopy, and endobronchial ultrasound-guided transbronchial needle aspiration in patients with malignant space-occupying brain lesions. *Chest* 147(6):1621–1628, 2015.
60. Antonelli M, Conti G, Riccioni L, et al: Noninvasive positive-pressure ventilation via face mask during bronchoscopy with BAL in high-risk hypoxemic patients. *Chest* 110:724–728, 1996.
61. Simon M, Braune S, Frings D, et al: High-flow nasal cannula oxygen versus non-invasive ventilation in patients with acute hypoxaemic respiratory failure undergoing flexible bronchoscopy—a prospective randomized trial. *Crit Care* 18(6):712, 2014.
62. Lawson RW, Peters JI, Shelledy DC: Effects of fiberoptic bronchoscopy during mechanical ventilation in a lung model. *Chest* 118:824, 2000.
63. Sung A, Kalstein A, Radhakrishnan P, et al: Laryngeal mask airway: use and clinical applications. *J Bronchol* 14:181–188, 2007.
64. Langmack EL, Martin RJ, Pak J, et al: Serum lidocaine concentration in asthmatics undergoing research bronchoscopy. *Chest* 117:1055–1060, 2000.
65. Honeybourne D, Jabb J, Bowie P, et al: British Thoracic Society guidelines on diagnostic flexible bronchoscopy. *Thorax* 56[Suppl I]:i1–i21, 2001.
66. Kaur H, Dhooria S, Aggarwal AN, et al: A randomized trial of 1% vs 2% lignocaine by the spray-as-you-go technique for topical anesthesia during flexible bronchoscopy. *Chest* 148(3):739–745, 2015.
67. Bose AA, Colt HG: Lidocaine in bronchoscopy: practical use and allergic reactions. *J Bronchology* 15:163–166, 2008.
68. Stolz D, Chhajed PN, Leuppi J, et al: Nebulized lidocaine for flexible bronchoscopy: a randomized, double-blind, placebo-controlled trial. *Chest* 128:1756, 2005.
69. Williams TJ, Bowie PE: Midazolam sedation to produce complete amnesia for bronchoscopy: 2 years' experience at a district hospital. *Respir Med* 93:361, 1999.
70. Cowl CT, Prakash UBS, Kruger BR: The role of anticholinergics in bronchoscopy: a randomized clinical trial. *Chest* 118:188, 2000.
71. Malik JA, Gupta D, Agarwal AN, et al: Anticholinergic premedication for flexible bronchoscopy—a randomized, double-blind, placebo-controlled study of atropine and glycopyrrolate. *Chest* 136(2):347–354, 2009.
72. Silvestri GA, Vincent BD, Wahidi MM, et al: A phase-3, randomized, double blind study to assess the efficacy and safety of fospropofol disodium injection for moderate sedation in patients undergoing flexible bronchoscopy. *Chest* 135:41–47, 2009.
73. Ryu JH, Lee SW, Lee JH, et al: Randomized double-blind study of remifentanil and dexmedetomidine for flexible bronchoscopy. *Br J Anaesth* 108(3):503–511, 2012.
74. Lindholm CE, Ollman B, Snyder JV, et al: Cardiorespiratory effects of flexible fiberoptic bronchoscopy in critically ill patients. *Chest* 74(4):362–368, 1978.
75. Meyer KC: The role of bronchoalveolar lavage in interstitial lung disease. *Clin Chest Med* 25:637, 2004.

Chapter 11 ■ Lung Ultrasonography

PIERRE KORY • NAVITHA RAMESH • PAUL H. MAYO

INTRODUCTION

Dr. Daniel Lichtenstein defined the key elements of lung ultrasonography (LUS) with the publication of a series of landmark articles that described the important features and the standard semiology of the field. Based on his original work, there have been numerous subsequent studies from other groups which have served to further validate and define the clinical applications of LUS. LUS is easy to learn, simple to perform, and has strong utility for the critical care that are well supported by the literature, in particular for the evaluation of respiratory failure.

BASIC PRINCIPLES OF LUS

Air-filled lung at the pleural surface prevents visualization of normal lung parenchyma owing to intense reflection of ultrasound that occurs at the interface of the aerated lung and overlying chest wall. The clinical utility of LUS in the critically ill is based on two factors: (1) in cases of respiratory distress or failure, over 90% of attributable lung pathology will contact the pleura at some point in the thorax, revealing identifiable pathologic patterns to the provider at the pleural surface and (2) these patterns can be correlated with discrete causes of respiratory dysfunction [1,2].

MACHINE REQUIREMENTS

LUS may be performed with a wide variety of ultrasound machines with two-dimensional (2D) scanning capability. A 3.5 to 5.0 MHz transducer similar to one used for cardiac applications is used for the entire spectrum of applications. Higher frequency (7.5 to 10 MHz) linear probes work well for identification of lung sliding and detailed characterization of pleural morphology.

PERFORMANCE OF LUS

By convention, the transducer is held in a longitudinal scanning plane. The transducer should be held like a pen, perpendicular to the chest wall with the transducer orientation marker pointing cephalad. The screen marker should be set to the left upper side of the screen. This being the case, cephalad structures will be projected to the left on the screen, whereas those that are caudad will be projected to the right on the screen. The scanning axis is perpendicular to the pleural surface. In areas of the thorax where the pleural surface is curvilinear, the probe is adjusted to obtain a perpendicular to the pleural surface, requiring the operator to tilt the transducer to ensure proper orientation of the ultrasonography beam. Proper probe orientation results in a horizontally orientated pleural line on the screen.

Unlike a chest radiograph, where an entire view of both hemithoraces is obtained in one image; thoracic ultrasonography relies on examining the pleural surfaces at multiple sites over each hemithorax, thus creating an image map of the lungs that is the summation of multiple tomographic cuts produced by movement of the ultrasonography scanning plane over the thorax. Many different scanning protocols have been proposed for LUS. Most divide the thorax into the anterior area, bordered by the sternum and the anterior axillary line; the lateral area, bordered by the anterior axillary and posterior axillary lines; and the posterior area, bordered by the posterior axillary line and the spine. Investigators designate specific points within these areas for examination and assign point values to the focal findings at each point. This is useful for research purposes, but impractical for clinical practice. The simplest protocol is that proposed by Lichtenstein that examines three defined points on each hemothorax in the anterior, lateral, and posterolateral area with characterization of LUS findings at each site [2]. An alternative approach is to perform a series of adjacent scan lines over the chest in order to define areas of abnormality that require more focused scanning (Chapter 11 Video 11.1).

The importance of examining the posterolateral chest is emphasized for the critically ill patient, given that the majority of pleural effusions and consolidations are found in the dependent hemithoraces. To adequately image this area, the transducer base is pressed into the mattress with the probe face angled anteriorly. Alternatively, the patient may be rolled to a lateral decubitus position to fully expose the posterior thorax.

IMAGING PATTERNS IN LUS

Pleural line artifacts and associated appearances of lung and pleural pathology described in the following sections are differentially produced according to the ratio of fluid and air produced by the various disease processes. These artifacts and patterns include analysis of the pleural line; the horizontal appearing reverberation artifacts seen in "dry" lung (A lines); the vertical appearing artifacts seen with interstitial fluid (B lines); the airless or fluid-filled lung seen in alveolar consolidation; and the accumulation of fluid seen with pleural effusions.

MAIN LUS PATTERNS

Novice lung ultrasonographers are often challenged by the lack of visually familiar anatomical correlates that are seen when scanning other organs such as the heart or kidney whose boundaries can be well delineated. Many lung images are not intuitively obvious to the novice, given that the condition of the lung is often abstracted from artifactual linear echogenic patterns deep to the pleural line. These patterns are few, discrete, and easy to master. The key findings of LUS for critical care applications are as follows:

NORMAL ANATOMY

On ultrasonography examination, the chest wall consists of skin overlying a layer of soft tissue and muscle covering the rib cage. Below the inner surface of the ribs lies the parietal pleura, against which the outer surface of lung, the visceral pleura, moves in respirophasic and cardiophasic synchrony. The rib edges form a distinctive hyperechoic curvilinear line. The pleural line is the first horizontal hyperechoic line just below the ribs and represents the interface between parietal and visceral pleura (Chapter 11 Video 11.2).

The interface of visceral and parietal pleura is readily visible with ultrasonography. Deep to the visceral pleura are the air-filled alveoli within lobules that are subtended by the interlobular septa. These septa insert into the visceral pleura, but cannot be seen under normal conditions, because their width is below the resolution of standard diagnostic ultrasonography transducers. With normally aerated lung, ultrasonography is intensely reflected from the pleural surface, so that the air-filled lung is not visible as an identifiable structure. It is only when the interlobular septae or the alveolar compartment underlying the visceral pleura are diseased that they become visible to the examiner. These resulting patterns allow ultrasonography to discriminate normal from abnormal lung.

FINDINGS OF LUS

Lung Sliding

With the transducer in a longitudinal orientation, perpendicular to the skin surface, and centered between two adjacent ribs; the pleural line is first located as detailed above, followed by identification of the dynamic movement of the pleural surfaces during the respiratory cycle. This movement, seen as a shimmering mobile pleural line that moves in synchrony with the respiratory cycle, is called lung sliding (Chapter 11 Video 11.3). A related finding is lung pulse, whereby the pleural line moves with cardiophasic movement caused by transmitted cardiac pulsations (Chapter 11 Video 11.4).

The identification of lung sliding or lung pulse excludes the presence of a pneumothorax at the site of transducer application with certainty [3]. Lung sliding and pulse can only be seen when the ultrasound waves propagate to the visceral pleura. When pleural air is interposed between the pleural surfaces, as that occurs with pneumothorax, the air acts as a barrier to ultrasound, so the movement of the underlying visceral pleura cannot be seen. In this case, lung sliding and lung pulse will be absent (Chapter 11 Video 11.5).

As air within the pleural space usually distributes to the anterior thorax in the supine patient, the critically ill patient is ideally positioned to examine for pneumothorax. Multiple rib interspaces sites may be rapidly examined for sliding lung over both hemithoraces, so that the intensivist can promptly and confidently rule out a clinically significant pneumothorax with superior accuracy to chest radiography [3–5].

Although the presence of lung sliding rules out the presence of pneumothorax at the site being examined, the absence of lung sliding is not diagnostic of pneumothorax. Loss of lung sliding may occur in other processes that reduce the movement of the visceral pleura such as pleural symphysis from inflammatory, neoplastic, or therapeutic pleurodesis. Mainstem bronchial intubation or occlusion (e.g., mucus plug, blood clot, foreign body, and tumor) will also ablate lung sliding on the side of the blockage.

In summary, the presence of lung sliding is a very useful sign, because it rules out the possibility of a pneumothorax being present. The absence of lung sliding is less useful, and always requires the clinician to consider whether there might be an alternative explanation for the lack of lung sliding.

Lung Point

When faced with the loss of lung sliding, identifying a lung point can confirm the presence of pneumothorax. The lung point represents the border of the pneumothorax, where the partially collapsed lung interfaces with the air-filled pneumothorax space. Some pneumothoraces are total, but most are partial with some remaining apposition of the visceral and parietal pleura at some point in the thorax, usually lateral or posterior depending on the size of the pneumothorax. A lung point is described as the intermittent respirophasic appearance of lung sliding from the edge of the screen (Chapter 11 Video 11.6). Although 100% specific for pneumothorax, lung point has only a 66% sensitivity for detection of pneumothorax [3].

A Lines

The normally aerated lung yields characteristic air artifacts called "A lines." An A line is a horizontally orientated line that is deep to the pleural line and separated by the same distance as the probe is to the pleural line (Chapter 11 Video 11.7). The A line is a reverberation of the pleural line, caused by echoes which reflect off of the visceral pleura owing to the inability of ultrasound to penetrate aerated lung tissue. The reflected pulse returns to the probe face and is reflected off of its surface to be in turn reflected back from the pleural line. When this pulse returns to transducer, it is interpreted by the ultrasound machine as arising from an identical, but more distant tissue plane. This is known as a reverberation artifact and occurs when there is an air–tissue interface deep to the probe. A lines can appear singly or multiply and are separated from each other by the same distance. When A lines appear with lung sliding, this represents a normal aeration pattern. When present without sliding lung, A lines represent either air between the visceral and parietal pleura (i.e., a pneumothorax) or aerated lung in association with lack of lung sliding as might occur with pleurodesis from inflammation or intervention.

B Lines

Using standard scanning technique with depth set to examine deeper structures, LUS may yield a characteristic pattern of artifact termed B lines. B lines have several distinct characteristics, as follows (Chapter 11 Video 11.8).

- B lines are vertical in orientation and may occur as one or more per field.
- They originate at the pleural interface.
- They extend ray-like to the bottom/far periphery of the screen.
- They move in synchrony with lung sliding (although mobility is not required, as in the case of B lines in the absence of lung sliding).
- They are hyperechoic.
- They efface A lines at their point of intersection.

B lines reflect the presence of a process that infiltrates or widens the interlobular septae of the lung, such as inflammation, neoplasm, or scarring; or that fills the alveolar space [6,7]. The presence of B lines is strongly correlated with alveolar or interstitial pattern abnormalities on computed tomography (CT) scan (ground-glass or reticular pattern abnormality) [8]. Depending on the disease process that is causing the B lines, they may be focal, scattered, or diffuse in distribution. Like any radiographic abnormality on standard chest radiograph or chest CT, clinical correlation is required to determine the cause of the B lines. More than two B lines in a single field are considered significant, with the exception that in normal individuals, several B lines may be present in the basilar-dependent rib interspaces. Pneumonia may manifest with focal B lines detected in the segment or lobe that is involved. Cardiogenic pulmonary edema (CPE) is associated with profuse, bilateral, and often anterior B lines, whereas idiopathic pulmonary fibrosis results in scattered, irregularly appearing B lines in association with pleural line irregularity (Chapter 11 Video 11.9).

The artifacts that are sometimes confused with B-lines include Z lines and E lines. Z-lines are artifacts arising from the pleural line, but attenuate before the periphery and are not as discrete B lines. Z lines have no pathologic significance. E Lines are vertical appearing artifacts that arise proximal to the pleural line from subcutaneous emphysema.

As B lines originate from the visceral pleural surface, their presence indicates that the lung is fully inflated at the site of the transducer application to the chest wall. The presence of B lines therefore rules out a pneumothorax [9]. Loss of lung sliding may occur in ARDS, because the lung is so diseased and the tidal volume so low that it could cause loss of pleural movement. Multiple B lines are characteristic of ARDS, so their presence assures the clinician that no pneumothorax is present, if this is a concern.

Consolidation

Consolidated lung yields a characteristic tissue density pattern on ultrasound examination (Chapter 11 Video 11.10) [10]. Consolidated lung has an echogenicity that is similar to liver (sonographic hepatization of the lung). If the bronchial structures that supply the affected consolidated lung are patent, the consolidated lung may have sonographic air bronchograms within it, appearing as small hyperechoic foci within the parenchyma. These represent small amounts of air in the bronchi. They may be mobile, reflecting movement of air within the bronchus owing to respiratory activity (Chapter 11 Video 11.11). Dynamic air bronchograms are highly suggestive of pneumonia as the cause of the consolidation [11]. The examiner may localize consolidation to a specific lobe or segment of the lung. The finding of consolidation with LUS is strongly correlated with results of chest CT [8]. The finding of consolidation on LUS is purely descriptive, and similar to the finding of consolidation on chest radiography or chest CT. Any process that renders the alveolar compartment airless will demonstrate consolidation on LUS or with other radiographic techniques. All causes of airless lung, such as atelectasis (compressive, resorptive, or cicatricial), infiltrative processes (tumor, purulent material as in pneumonia), or severe pulmonary edema with complete filling of the alveolar compartment will yield the ultrasonographic finding of lung consolidation. LUS identifies the consolidation; the clinician determines its cause.

PATTERN ANALYSIS OF LUS

Differentiating Causes of Acute Respiratory Failure and Dyspnea

Knowledge of LUS patterns allows the intensivist to improve the accuracy of diagnosis of acute respiratory failure when compared to use of standard clinical testing and assessment [12,13]. Given the utility of LUS to identify the cause of respiratory failure, the thoracic ultrasound examination may replace standard chest radiography as a more effective and efficient imaging modality [14–16]. When evaluating the patient with dyspnea and/or respiratory failure, the critical care clinician associates various profiles described below with the corresponding cause of respiratory failure compromise. This allows for early categorization of the disease process.

Generalized A Lines with Lung Sliding

This normal aeration pattern is seen among healthy patients; but when it is associated with dyspnea, the diagnostic possibilities include (1) the airway compartment (Chronic Obstructive Pulmonary Disease [COPD] or asthma), (2) the vascular compartment (pulmonary embolism), or (3) non-pulmonary causes such as neurologic, neuromuscular, metabolic, and toxic. This pattern rules out diseases that compromise the alveolar and/or interstitial compartment (pulmonary edema, pneumonia, fibrosis, etc.) or the pleural compartment. Identification of a normal aeration pattern of the dyspneic patient where pulmonary embolism is a concern requires the intensivist to perform a study for venous thromboembolism (see Chapter 92 on Venous Thromboembolism).

A Lines, Absence of Lung Sliding, Presence of Lung Point

When lung sliding is absent with A lines, pneumothorax is a possibility. For this situation, identification of a lung point confirms that there is a pneumothorax. If no lung point is identified, other methods are required to confirm if there is a pneumothorax, given the low sensitivity of lung point. The presence of lung pulse, B lines, or consolidation also rules out pneumothorax at the interspace being examined. Multiple interspaces are examined in a short period of time.

Alveolar/Interstitial Disease: B Line Patterns

Detection of profuse B lines at multiple symmetric points over the anterior chest indicates a high probability of an alveolar and/or interstitial process. CPE with profuse B line pattern is associated with a smooth pleural line morphology. This requires examination of the pleural line with the high frequency linear vascular probe. A rare cause of unilateral profuse B line pattern with smooth pleural morphology is unilateral CPE related to asymmetric mitral valve regurgitation.

Detection of multiple focal B lines with asymmetric distribution suggests primary lung injury pattern such as pneumonia, acute respiratory distress syndrome (ARDS), or other alveolar/interstitial process. For instance, when B lines are detected from subsegmental, segmental, lobar, or unilateral distribution, or involving one hemithorax with A line pattern for the rest of the lung, pneumonia is a prime consideration. Primary lung injury results in irregular pleural morphology. This requires examination of the pleural line with the high-frequency linear vascular probe. Thus, depending on the pattern of B profiles over the hemithorax (unilateral vs bilateral; irregular pleural line; sliding or non-sliding lung; sparing or uniform areas), the provider can differentiate CPE versus primary lung injury as the cause of respiratory failure.

Alveolar Consolidation Pattern

Alveolar consolidation is readily identified with LUS. It may appear as small multifocal areas of consolidation immediately below the pleural interface or in subsegmental, segmental, lobar, whole lung pattern with unifocal or multifocal distribution. As with chest radiography and chest CT, the finding of alveolar consolidation pattern with LUS is descriptive and not diagnostic, given that there are many causes for alveolar consolidation.

For pneumonia, the consolidation appears as tissue density without volume loss (Chapter 11 Video 11.10). The interface between the pleural surface and the consolidation is linear, whereas the interface between the consolidation and the adjacent aerated lung is irregular and often is associated with comet tail artifacts. This irregular interface is called the "shred sign" (Chapter 11 Video Clip 11.12). Pneumonias often contain dynamic air bronchograms, which appear as mobile, branching, and hyperechoic within the parenchyma (Chapter 11 Video 11.11). Although suggestive of pneumonia, mobile air bronchograms may be found in association with non-pneumonia consolidation; a hypoechoic area with well-defined borders within an area of alveolar consolidation is consistent with necrosis or abscess (Chapter 11 Video 11.13).

Atelectasis of lung results in an alveolar consolidation pattern that can be readily identified with LUS. The mechanism of the atelectasis may differ (compressive, resorptive, or cicatricial), but there is a characteristic loss of lung volume in association with the alveolar consolidation. Mobile air bronchograms are uncommon, although static air bronchograms are often present, unless the cause for the atelectasis is complete endobronchial occlusion [11].

A common cause of alveolar consolidation is that which occurs with pleural effusion. Compressive atelectasis from a pleural effusion causes the atelectatic lung to float within the effusion often in association with respirophasic or cardiophasic movement of the lung (Chapter 11 Video 11.14). Areas of posterior basilar alveolar consolidation commonly occur in patients on ventilatory support. The dual mechanism of compressive and resorptive atelectasis results in the airless lung that reinflates when the patient is successfully extubated. Differentiation from pneumonia may be challenging and requires clinical correlation. Endobronchial occlusion by mucus; tumor; foreign body aspiration; or block of the left mainstem bronchus with the endotracheal tube balloon (because of unintentional right mainstem bronchial intubation) results in resorptive atelectasis that is detected as alveolar consolidation with LUS. Bronchial occlusion results in absence of mobile air bronchograms. If the blockage is at the mainstem bronchial level, the affected lung undergoes major volume loss with associated marked ipsilateral shift of mediastinal and cardiac structures. This can occur rapidly if the patient is on a high FiO_2 as is the case immediately following endotracheal intubation.

CLINICAL APPLICATIONS OF LUS

Clarification of the Ambiguous Chest Radiograph

The technique of the intensive care unit (ICU) chest radiograph is often suboptimal. The anteroposterior projection combines with rotation, penetration, and density summation artifact to make interpretation difficult. Chest radiography results in a 2D representation of a complex structure, whereas thoracic ultrasonography yields a three-dimensional representation of the thoracic compartment by virtue of the multiple tomographic planes used in the examination. LUS may replace chest radiography for evaluation of the dyspneic patient; for identification of consolidation related to pneumonia; and for the evaluation of pleuritic chest pain [14–16]. The routine use of LUS was associated with reduced use of chest radiography and chest CT in a medical ICU [17]. An ambiguous chest radiograph requires clarification with LUS.

As performance of LUS is superior to the standard ICU chest radiograph for detection of normal aeration pattern, alveolar/interstial pattern, consolidation, pneumothorax, and pleural effusion [8]; the argument may be made that LUS could largely replace chest radiography in the ICU [18]. Although chest radiography does remain useful for determining the location of a variety of intrathoracic devices (see Chapter 179 Chest Radiographic Examination), the location of central venous catheters may, in many cases, be determined with ultrasonography (See Chapter 6 Central Venous Catheters).

Differentiation of ARDS from Cardiogenic Pulmonary Edema

Copetti et al. demonstrated the ability of LUS to discriminate between acute respiratory distress syndrome (ARDS) and CPE [19]. The most specific sign for ARDS was the finding of both an area of normal aeration within a single interspace co-existing with a focus on B lines/interstitial syndrome. Such a pattern was found in 100% of ARDS patients and 0% of CPE patients. Pleural line abnormalities such as thickening >2 mm, coarse irregular appearance, or subpleural consolidations were found in 100% of ARDS patients and 25% of CPE patients. Profuse B line pattern with a smooth pleural surface was highly suggestive of CPE. The finding of new onset B lines bilaterally during cardiac stress testing is indicative of inducible cardiac ischemia with increase in left-sided filling pressures [20]. An increase in extravascular lung water—as assessed independently by chest CT, chest X-ray, and thermodilution techniques—is associated with B lines [21].

Prediction of Extubation Failure

The amount of extravascular lung water and non-aerated lung can be accurately estimated using the LUS scoring system proposed by Rouby et al. [22]. In their scoring system, a value of 0 is assigned to any interspace examined which revealed A lines with sliding lung, a value of 1 to interspaces with regularly spaced B lines consistent with interlobular septal thickening, a value of 2 to interspaces with confluent B lines filling the visualized interspace, and a value of 3 was assigned to interspaces with consolidation. Assigning a score to 6 interspaces over each hemithorax led to a maximum LUS score of 36. When performing LUS scores before and after a 30-minute spontaneous breathing trial (SBT), an increase in the LUS score of more than 4 points predicted extubation failure. Additionally, any end-SBT LUS score >17 strongly predicted extubation failure.

Measurement of Lung Recruitment with PEEP

The above LUS score can also be used to predict the effects of positive end-expiratory pressure (PEEP) in ARDS patients [23]. When varying PEEP levels from 0 to 15, a decrease of 8 points in the LUS score described above using the higher PEEP, resulted in an average increase of lung volume >600 mL. If the LUS score increased by 4 or less, the volume increased by an average of 75 to 450 mL. The authors of this report caution that they could not distinguish whether the augmentation of lung volume resulted from lung recruitment or from overdistention of lung.

Diagnosis of Pneumonia

LUS is useful in establishing the diagnosis of pneumonia and following its evolution [24,25]. Of interest to the intensivist, the resolution of ventilator associated pneumonia (VAP) with antibiotic therapy can tracked with LUS [26], and the combination of LUS with sputum analysis is useful for the diagnosis of VAP [27].

Algorithmic Diagnosis of Respiratory Failure

Dr. Lichtenstein has developed a useful algorithm for the use of LUS in determining the cause of respiratory failure (the bedside lung ultrasound in emergency [BLUE] protocol) [2]. Using a simple three-point examination technique and simple LUS signs, the algorithm identified the etiology of respiratory failure in a high proportion of cases.

Estimates of Left Atrial Pressure

Patients with symptomatic CPE have a bilateral B line pattern. Conversely, if the patient has A line pattern with lung sliding, there is a high probability that the pulmonary occlusion pressure is below 18 mm Hg and probably less that 12 mm Hg [28]. Beyond its clinical utility in diagnosis of respiratory failure, this information has application during cardiac stress testing. EKG monitoring and serial segmental wall analysis with echocardiography are standard means of detecting ischemia during the stress test. The sudden appearance of B lines coincident with the onset of dyspnea while under exercise load is consistent with elevation of left atrial pressures with resultant CPE precipitated by cardiac ischemia [20].

Combination of LUS with Echocardiography

In evaluating patients with acute respiratory failure, Bataille et al. reported that the addition of echocardiography to LUS was superior to performing LUS alone [29]. Sekiguchi et al. confirmed that LUS is productively combined with echocardiography for the evaluation of respiratory failure [30].

Diagnosis of Pulmonary Embolism

Koenig et al. and Nazerian et al. both found that LUS combined with echocardiography and DVT study is a means of reducing unnecessary chest CT angiograms when pulmonary embolism is a diagnostic consideration. A definite alternative diagnosis of pulmonary embolism using ultrasonography excluded pulmonary embolism with a high level of certainty [31,32]. Mathis et al. reported that pulmonary emboli commonly result in small areas of consolidation immediately deep to the pleural interface with preferential distribution to the lower lobes of the lung [33]. This is a difficult area to image in the critically ill patient who is generally in supine position, so their results have uncertain application for the intensivist.

Timing of Chest Tube Removal

Maury et al. used LUS to document lung expansion following chest tube insertion for pneumothorax [34]. Once the lung is fully inflated by LUS criteria, the chest tube is clamped and LUS performed to observe for recurrence of the PTX. If there is no recurrence by LUS, the chest tube may be safely removed. The investigators found that this method was superior to standard chest radiography. From a practical point of view, this method offers a convenient, efficient, and cost-effective means of timing the removal of chest tube.

LUS for Guidance of Procedures

LUS may be used to guide transthoracic needles to biopsy peripheral lung lesions that abut the chest wall and thus are visible, given that no aerated lung is interposed [35]. Similarly, intraparenchymal lung abscess can be drained if clinically indicated [36].

Utility of LUS for Thoracic Trauma

The utility of LUS for thoracic trauma is reviewed in Chapter 43 on Thoracic and Cardiac Trauma.

Utility of LUS for Airway Management

The utility of LUS for airway management is reviewed in Chapter 8 on Airway Management.

References

1. Lichtenstein D: *Whole body ultrasonography in the critically ill*. Heidelberg: Springer, 2010.
2. Lichtenstein DA, Mezière GA: Relevance of lung ultrasound in the diagnosis of acute respiratory failure: the BLUE protocol. *Chest* 134:117–125, 2008.
3. Lichtenstein DA, Menu Y: A bedside ultrasound sign ruling out pneumothorax in the critically ill: lung sliding. *Chest* 108:1345–1348, 1995.
4. Soldati G, Testa A, Sher S, et al: Occult traumatic pneumothorax: diagnostic accuracy of lung ultrasonography in the emergency department. *Chest* 133:204–211, 2008.
5. Blaivas M, Lyon M, Duggal SA: Prospective comparison of supine chest radiography and bedside ultrasound for the diagnosis of traumatic pneumothorax. *Acad Emerg Med* 12:844–849, 2005.
6. Lichtenstein D, Meziére G: A lung ultrasound sign allowing bedside distinction between pulmonary edema and COPD: the comet-tail artifact. *Intensive Care Med* 2:1331–1334, 1998.
7. Agricola E, Bove T, Oppizzi M, et al: "Ultrasound comet-tail images": a marker of pulmonary edema. *Chest* 127:1690–1695, 2005.
8. Lichtenstein D, Goldstein I, Mourgeon E, et al: Comparative diagnostic performances of auscultation, chest radiography, and lung ultrasonography in acute respiratory distress syndrome. *Anesthesiology* 100:9–15, 2004.
9. Lichtenstein D, Mezière G, Biderman P, et al: The comet-tail artifact: an ultrasound sign ruling out pneumothorax. *Intensive Care Med* 25:383–388, 1999.
10. Lichtenstein DA, Lascols N, Mezière G, et al: Ultra-sound diagnosis of alveolar consolidation in the critically ill. *Intensive Care Med* 30:276–281, 2004.
11. Lichtenstein D, Meziere G, Seitz J: The dynamic air bronchogram. A Lung ultrasound sigh of alveolar consolidation ruling out atelectasis. *Chest* 135(6):1421–1425, 2009.
12. Laursen CB, Sloth E, Lambrechtsen J, et al: Focused sonography of the heart, lungs, and deep veins identifies missed life-threatening conditions in admitted patients with acute respiratory symptoms. *Chest* 144(6):1868–1875, 2013.
13. Silva S, Biendel C, Ruiz J, et al: Usefulness of cardiothoracic chest ultrasound in the management of acute respiratory failure in critical care practice. *Chest* 144(3):859–865, 2013.
14. Zanobetti M, Poggioni C, Pini R: Can chest ultrasonography replace standard chest radiography for evaluation of acute dyspnea in the ED? *Chest* 139(5):1140–1147, 2011.
15. Cortellaro F, Colombo S, Coen D, et al: Lung ultrasound is an accurate diagnostic tool for the diagnosis of pneumonia in the emergency department. *Emerg Med J* 29:19–23, 2012.
16. Volpicelli G, Caramello V, Cardinale L, et al: Diagnosis of radio-occult pulmonary conditions by real-time chest ultrasonography in patients with pleuritic pain. *Ultrasound Med Biol* 34(11):1717–1723, 2008.
17. Oks M, Cleven KL, Cardenas-Garcia J, et al: The effect of point-of-care ultrasonography on imaging studies in the medical ICU: a comparative study. *Chest* 146:1574–1577, 2014.
18. Xirouchaki N, Magkanas E, Vaporidi K, et al: Lung ultrasound in critically ill patients: comparison with bedside chest radiography. *Intensive Care Med* 37:1488–1493, 2011.
19. Copetti R, Soldati G, Copetti P: Chest sonography: a useful tool to differentiate acute cardiogenic pulmonary edema from acute respiratory distress syndrome. *Cardiovasc Ultrasound* 6:16, 2008.
20. Agricola E, Picano E, Oppizzi M, et al: Assessment of stress-induced pulmonary interstitial edema by chest ultrasound during exercise echocardiography and its correlation with left ventricular function. *J Am Soc Echocardiogr* 19:457–463, 2006.
21. Picano E, Frassi F, Agricola E, et al: Ultrasound lung comets: a clinically useful sign of extravascular lung water. *J Am Soc Echocardiogr* 19:356–363, 2006.
22. Soummer A, Perbet S, Brisson H, et al; the Lung Ultrasound Study Group: Ultrasound assessment of lung aeration loss during a successful spontaneous breathing trial predicts postextubation distress. *Crit Care Med* 40:2064–2072, 2012.
23. Bouhemad B, Bresson H, Le-Guen M, et al: Bedside ultrasound assessment of positive end-expiratory pressure-induced lung recruitment. *Am J Resp Crit Care Med* 183:341–347, 2011.
24. Ye X, Xiao H, Chen B, et al: Accuracy of lung ultrasonography versus chest radiography for the diagnosis of adult community-acquired pneumonia: review of the literature and meta-analysis. *PLoS One* 10(6):e0130066, 2015.
25. Reissig A, Copetti R, Mathis G, et al: Lung ultrasound in the diagnosis and follow-up of community-acquired pneumonia: a prospective, multicenter, diagnostic accuracy study. *Chest* 142:965–972, 2012.
26. Bouhemad B, Liu ZH, Arbelot C, et al: Ultrasound assessment of antibiotic-induced pulmonary reaeration in ventilator-associated pneumonia. *Crit Care Med* 38:84–92, 2010.
27. Mongodi S, Via G, Girard M, et al: Lung ultrasound for early diagnosis of ventilator-associated pneumonia. *Chest* 149:969–980, 2016.
28. Lichtenstein DA, Mezière GA, Lagoueyte JF, et al: A-lines and B-lines: lung ultrasound as a bedside tool for predicting pulmonary artery occlusion pressure in the critically ill. *Chest* 136:1014–1020, 2009.
29. Bataille B, Riu B, Ferre F, et al: Integrated use of bedside lung ultrasound and echocardiography in acute respiratory failure: a prospective observational study in ICU. *Chest* 146:1586–1593, 2014.
30. Sekiguchi H, Schenck LA, Horie R, et al: Critical care ultrasonography differentiates ARDS, pulmonary edema, and other causes in the early course of acute hypoxemic respiratory failure. *Chest* 148:912–918, 2015.

31. Koenig S, Chandra S, Alaverdian A, et al: Ultrasound assessment of pulmonary embolism in patients receiving CT pulmonary angiography. *Chest* 145:818–823, 2014.
32. Nazerian P, Vanni S, Volpicelli G, et al: Accuracy of point-of-care multiorgan ultrasonography for the diagnosis of pulmonary embolism. *Chest* 145:950–957, 2014.
33. Mathis G, Blank W, Reissig A, et al: Thoracic ultrasound for diagnosing pulmonary embolism: a prospective multicenter study of 352 patients. *Chest* 128:1531–1538, 2005.
34. Galbois A, Ait-Oufella H, Baudel JL, et al: Pleural ultrasound compared with chest radiographic detection of pneumothorax resolution after drainage. *Chest* 138:648–655, 2010.
35. Yang PC: Ultrasound-guided transthoracic biopsy of peripheral lung, pleural, and chest-wall lesions. *J Thorac Imaging* 12:272–284, 1997.
36. Yang PC, Luh KT, Lee YC, et al: Lung abscesses: US examination and US-guided transthoracic aspiration. *Radiology* 180:171–175, 1991.

Chapter 12 ■ Thoracentesis

MARK M. WILSON • RICHARD S. IRWIN

Thoracentesis is an invasive procedure that involves the introduction of a needle, cannula, or trocar into the pleural space to remove accumulated fluid or air. Although a few studies have critically evaluated the clinical value and complications associated with it [1–6], most studies concerning thoracentesis have dealt with the interpretation of the pleural fluid analyses [7–11].

INDICATIONS

Although history (cough, dyspnea, or pleuritic chest pain) and physical findings (dullness to percussion, decreased breath sounds, and decreased vocal fremitus) suggest that an effusion is present, chest radiography or ultrasonic examination is essential to confirm the clinical suspicion. Thoracentesis can be performed for diagnostic or therapeutic reasons. When done for diagnostic reasons, the procedure should be performed whenever possible before any treatment has been given to avoid confusion in interpretation. Analysis of pleural fluid has been shown to yield clinically useful information in more than 90% of cases. The four most common diagnoses for symptomatic and asymptomatic pleural effusions are malignancy, congestive heart failure (CHF), parapneumonia, and postoperative sympathetic effusions. A diagnostic algorithm for evaluation of a pleural effusion of unknown etiology is presented in Figure 12.1. In patients whose exudative pleural effusion remains undiagnosed after thoracentesis, closed pleural biopsy or thoracoscopy should be considered. Thoracoscopy provides for visualization of the pleura and directed biopsy, and yields a diagnosis in more than 80% of patients with recurrent pleural effusions that are not diagnosed by repeated thoracentesis, closed pleural biopsy, or bronchoscopy.

Therapeutic thoracentesis is indicated to remove fluid or air that is causing cardiopulmonary embarrassment, or for relief of severe symptoms. Definitive drainage of the pleural space with a thoracostomy tube must be done for a tension pneumothorax (PTX) and should be considered for: a PTX that is slowly enlarging; any size PTX in the mechanically ventilated patient; hemothorax; or the instillation of a sclerosing agent after drainage of a recurrent malignant pleural effusion.

CONTRAINDICATIONS

Absolute contraindications to performing a thoracentesis are an uncooperative patient; a lack of expertise in performing the procedure; and the presence of a coagulation abnormality that cannot be corrected. Relative contraindications to a thoracentesis include entry into an area where known bullous lung disease exists; a patient on positive end-expiratory pressure (PEEP); and a patient who has only one "functioning" lung (the other having been surgically removed or that has severe disease limiting its gas exchange function).

COMPLICATIONS

A number of prospective studies have documented that complications associated with the procedure are not infrequent [1–6,12]. The overall complication rate has been reported to be as high as 50% to 78% and can be further categorized as major (15% to 19%) or minor (31% to 63%) [12]. Complication rates appear to be inversely related to experience level of the operator; the more experienced the operator, the fewer the complications. Although death due to the procedure is infrequently reported, complications may be life threatening.

Major complications include PTX; bleeding (e.g., hemopneumothorax, hemoperitoneum, and hematoma); hypotension; soft tissue infection; empyema; spleen or liver puncture; and reexpansion pulmonary edema. The reported incidence of PTX is up to 30% (with most studies reporting rates of nearly 12%) and up to one-third to one-half of those with demonstrated PTX requiring subsequent intervention [2,12]. Tube thoracostomy should be considered for any PTX that is large or progressive and in any patient that is mechanically ventilated or symptomatic after the procedure. Several nonrandomized studies involving spontaneously breathing patients undergoing ultrasound-guided thoracentesis (USGT) performed by trained operators have demonstrated a reduction in the rate of PTX to less than 2% [5,6,13]. The risk of PTX for patients receiving positive-pressure mechanical ventilation is approximately 1% to 7% with the use of USGT [1,3]. The use of PEEP does not appear to increase the risk of PTX for USGT [11].

Various investigators have reported associations ("risk factors") between PTX and underlying lung disease (chronic obstructive pulmonary disease, prior thoracic radiation, prior thoracic surgery, and lung cancer); needle size and technique; number of passes required to obtain a sample; aspiration of air during the procedure; operator experience; use of a vacuum bottle; smaller size of the effusion; and mechanical ventilation versus spontaneously breathing patients [2,12]. Small sample sizes and observational study design limit the generalization of reported findings to allow for the delineation of a clear risk profile for the development of a PTX due to thoracentesis. The presence of baseline lung disease; low level of operator experience with the procedure; lack of use of ultrasound guidance; and the use of positive-pressure mechanical ventilation appear for now to be the best-established risk factors in the literature. Recognition and optimization of modifiable risk factors has been shown to improve the safety of thoracentesis [5,6,13]. Given the evidence of the value of ultrasound guidance in the performance of thoracentesis [1,3,5,6,13–16], the Accreditation Council for Graduate Medical Education (ACGME) has stated that effective July 2012 pulmonary/critical care fellows "must demonstrate competence in procedural and technical skills, including: use of ultrasound techniques to perform thoracentesis and place intravascular and intracavitary tubes and catheters." Thoracic ultrasound techniques for the sampling/removal of pleural fluid are described in more detail below.

Although PTX is most commonly caused by laceration of lung parenchyma, room air may enter the pleural space around or through a thoracentesis needle or catheter that is open to room air when a spontaneously breathing patient takes a deep breath (intrapleural pressure is subatmospheric). The PTX may be small and asymptomatic, resolving spontaneously, or large and associated with respiratory compromise, requiring chest tube drainage. Hemorrhage can occur from laceration of an intercostal artery or unintentional puncture of the liver or spleen, even if coagulation studies are normal. The risk of intercostal artery laceration is greatest in the elderly because of increased tortuosity of their vessels. This last complication is potentially lethal, and risk is minimized at sites 9 to 10 cm lateral to the spine (essentially the posterior axillary line, and this is the preferred puncture site, assuming accessibility of the fluid collection) [17,18].

Hypotension may occur during the procedure (as part of a vasovagal reaction or tension PTX) or hours after the procedure (uncommon, but most likely because of reaccumulation of fluid into the pleural space or the pulmonary parenchyma from the intravascular space). Hypotension in the latter settings responds to volume expansion; it can usually be prevented by limiting pleural fluid drainage to 1.5 L or less or alternatively by using serial measurements of pleural pressure (manometry) during large volume thoracentesis to determine a "safe" volume of fluid to be removed (described elsewhere) [19]. Other major complications are rare and may include implantation of tumor along the needle tract of a previously performed thoracentesis; venous and cerebral air embolism (the so-called

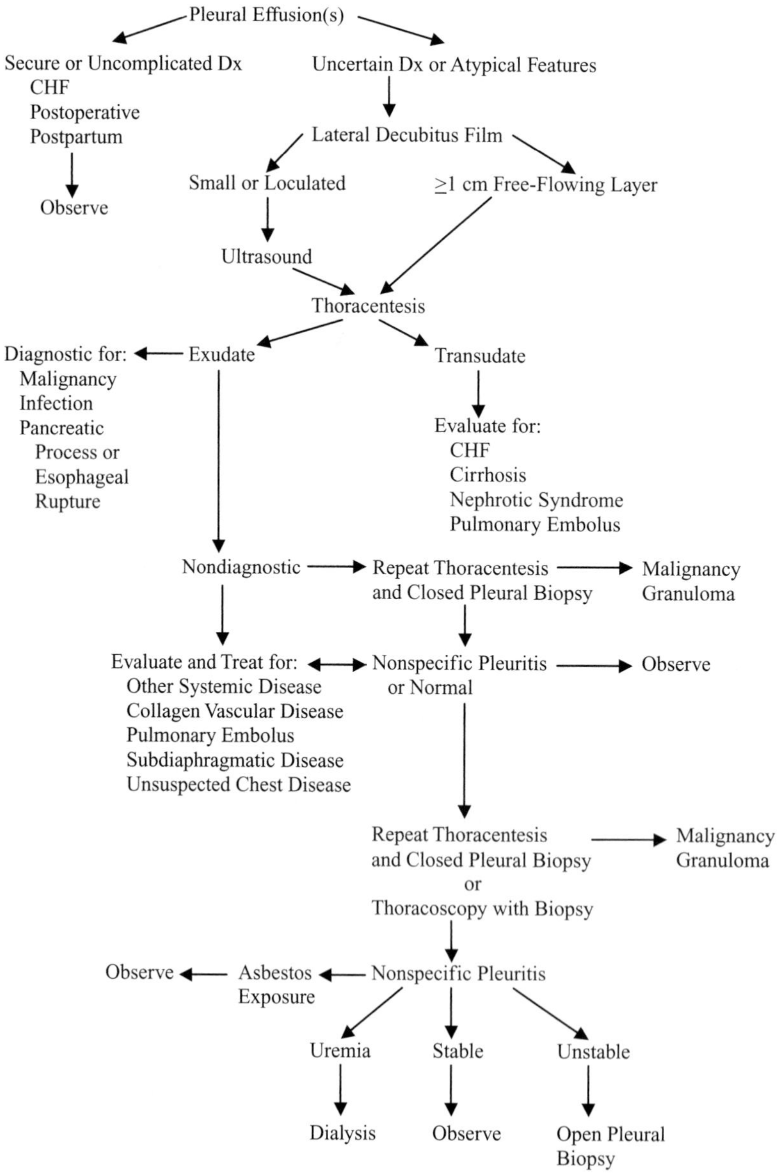

FIGURE 12.1 Diagnostic algorithm for evaluation of pleural effusion. CHF, congestive heart failure; Dx, diagnosis; USGT, ultrasound-guided thoracentesis; VATS, video-assisted thoracoscopic surgery; Bx, biopsy; TB, tuberculosis; Ca, cancer. (Adapted from Smyrnios NA, Jederlinic PJ, Irwin RS: Pleural effusion in an asymptomatic patient. Spectrum and frequency of causes and management considerations. *Chest* 97:192, 1990).

pleural shock); and accidental shearing of the catheter in the pleural space [12].

Minor complications include dry tap or insufficient fluid; pain; subcutaneous hematoma or seroma; anxiety; dyspnea; and cough. Reported rates for these minor complications range from 16% to 63% [12]. Dry tap and insufficient fluid are technical problems and expose the patient to increased risk of morbidity because of the need to perform multiple needle passes or repeated thoracentesis attempts at an alternate site. Pain may originate from parietal pleural nerve endings from inadequate local anesthesia; unintentional scraping of rib periosteum; or piercing an intercostal nerve during a misdirected needle thrust.

PROCEDURES

General Considerations

The most common techniques for performing thoracentesis are catheter-over-needle; needle only; and needle under direct sonographic guidance (multiple commercially available kits available). The catheter-through-needle technique has been used much less frequently over the past few decades. Performing thoracentesis without ultrasound guidance (using auscultation and percussion exam techniques to establish a fluid level) is suggested only in the presence of a large, free-flowing effusion and limited availability of ultrasound. Otherwise, USGT is the method of choice.

Technique for Diagnostic Sampling of a Large, Freely Flowing Pleural Effusion (Clinical Exam Guided)

1. Obtain a lateral decubitus chest radiograph to confirm a large, free-flowing pleural effusion. This is only required if ultrasonography is not available.
2. Describe the procedure to the patient and obtain written informed consent. Operators should be thoroughly familiar with the procedure that they will perform, and should receive appropriate supervision from an experienced operator before performing thoracentesis on their own.
3. With the patient sitting, arms at sides, mark the inferior tip of the scapula on the side to be tapped. This approximates the eighth intercostal space and should be the lowest interspace punctured, unless it has been previously determined by sonography that a lower interspace can be safely entered, or chest radiographs and sonography show the diaphragm to be higher than the eighth intercostal space.
4. Position the patient sitting at the edge of the bed, comfortably leaning forward over a pillow-draped, height-adjusted, bedside table (Fig. 12.2). The patient's arms should be crossed in front to elevate and spread the scapulae. An assistant should stand in front of the patient to prevent any unexpected movements.
5. Percuss the patient's posterior chest to determine the highest point of the effusion. The interspace below this point should be entered in the posterior axillary line, unless it is below the eighth intercostal space. Gently mark the superior aspect of the rib in the chosen interspace with your fingernail (The inferior portion of each rib contains an intercostal artery and should be avoided.).
6. Cleanse a wide area with 0.05% chlorhexidine or 10% povidone–iodine solution and allow it to dry. Using sterile technique, drape the area surrounding the puncture site.
7. Perform a time out and anesthetize the superficial skin with 2% lidocaine using a 25-gauge needle. Change to an 18- to 22-gauge needle, 2 inches long, and generously anesthetize the deeper soft tissues, aiming for the top of the rib. Always aspirate through the syringe as the needle is advanced and before instilling lidocaine to ensure that the needle is not in a vessel or the pleural space. Carefully aspirate through the syringe as the pleura is approached (the rib is 1 to 2 cm thick). Pleural fluid enters the syringe on reaching the pleural space. The patient may experience discomfort as the needle penetrates the well-innervated parietal pleura. Be careful not to instill anesthetic into the pleural space; it is bactericidal for most organisms, including *Mycobacterium tuberculosis*. Place a gloved finger at the point on the needle where it exits the skin (to estimate the required depth of insertion) and remove the needle.
8. Attach a three-way stopcock to a 20-gauge, 1.5-inch needle and to a 50-mL syringe. The valve on the stopcock should be open to the needle to allow aspiration of pleural fluid during needle insertion.
9. Insert the 20-gauge needle (or the catheter-over-needle apparatus) into the anesthetized tract with the bevel of the needle down and always aspirate through the syringe as the needle/catheter-over-needle is slowly advanced. When pleural fluid is obtained using the needle-only technique, stabilize the needle by attaching a clamp to the needle where it exits the skin to prevent further advancement of the needle into the pleural space. Once pleural fluid is obtained with the catheter-over-needle technique, direct the needle-catheter apparatus downward to ensure that the catheter descends to the most dependent area of the pleural space. Advance the catheter forward in a single smooth motion as the inner needle is simultaneously pulled back out of the chest.
10. Once you have reached a point when pleural fluid can easily be obtained, fill a heparinized blood gas syringe from the side port of the three-way stopcock for measurement of fluid pH. Express all air bubbles from the sample, cap it, and place it in a bag containing iced slush for immediate transport to the laboratory.
11. Fill the 50-mL syringe and transfer its contents into the appropriate collection tubes and containers. Always maintain a closed system during the procedure to prevent room air from entering the pleural space. For most diagnostic studies, 50 to 100 mL should be an ample volume [20,21]. Always ensure that the three-way stopcock has the valve closed toward the patient when changing syringes.
12. When the thoracentesis is completed, remove the needle (or catheter) from the patient's chest as they hum or perform a Valsalva maneuver. Apply pressure to the wound for several minutes, and then apply a sterile bandage.
13. A routine chest radiograph after thoracentesis is not generally indicated for most asymptomatic, nonventilated patients. Obtain a post-procedure upright end-expiratory chest radiograph if air was aspirated during the procedure; if PTX is suspected by developing signs or symptoms; or if multiple needle passes were required [1,12,22]. Whether a post-thoracentesis chest radiograph is necessary for patients who are mechanically ventilated is controversial [3,22]; however, it should be remembered that any PTX in a ventilated patient creates the risk that a tension PTX may occur rapidly.

Technique for Therapeutic Removal of Freely Flowing Fluid

To perform the technique for therapeutic removal of freely flowing fluid, steps 1 to 7 should be followed as described previously. Removal of more than 100 mL pleural fluid generally involves placement of a catheter into the pleural space to minimize the risk of PTX from a needle during this longer procedure. Commercially available kits generally use a catheter-over-needle system, although catheter-through-needle systems are still available in some locations. Each kit should have a specific set

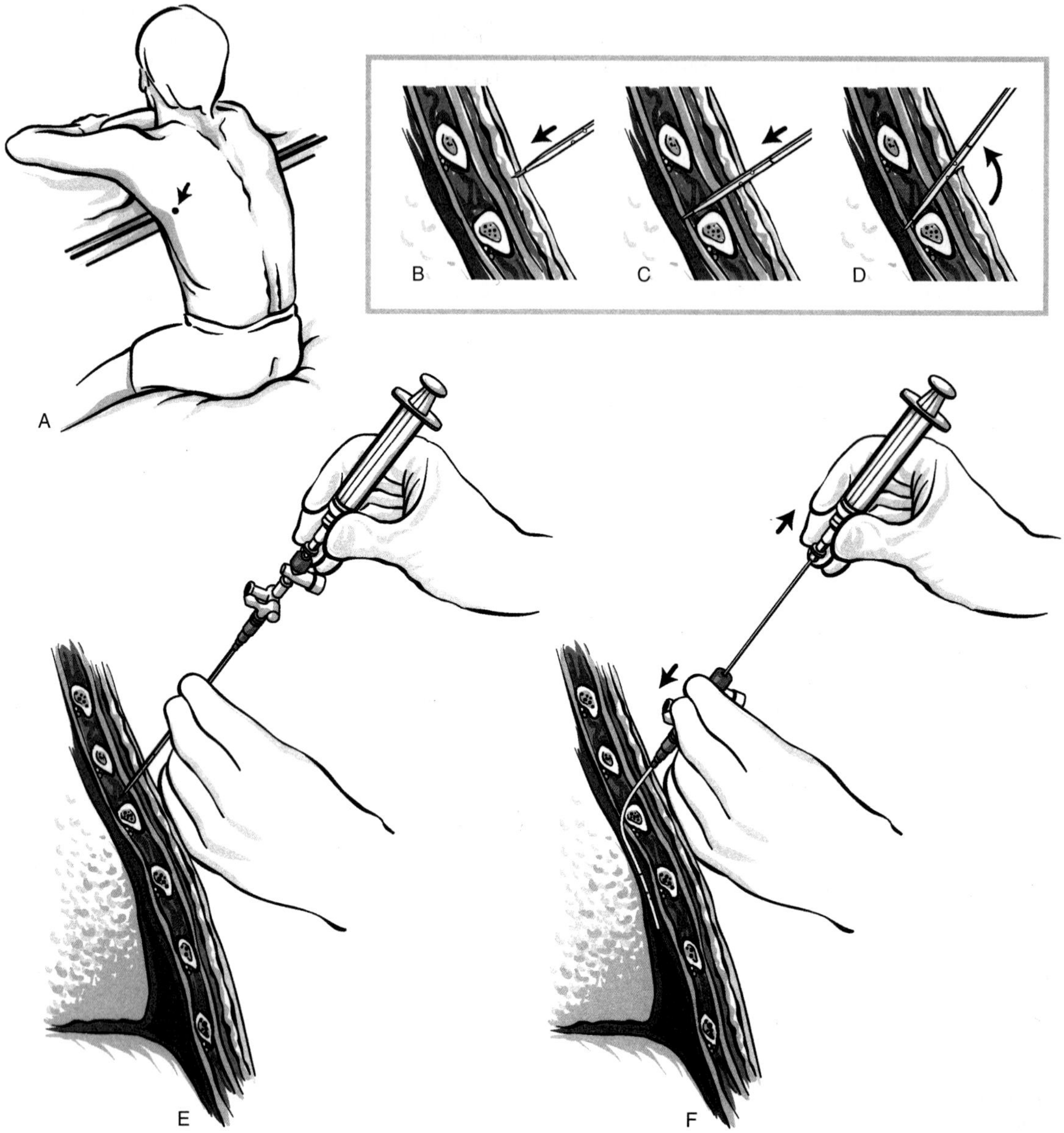

FIGURE 12.2 Catheter-over-needle technique for thoracentesis of freely flowing pleural field. **A:** The patient is comfortably positioned, sitting up and leaning forward over a pillow-draped, height-adjusted, bedside table. The arms are crossed in front of the patient to elevate and spread the scapulae. The preferred entry site is along the posterior axillary line. **B:** The catheter apparatus is gently advanced through the skin and across the upper surface of the rib. The needle is advanced several millimeters at a time while continuously aspirating through the syringe. **C:** As soon as the parietal pleura has been punctured, pleural fluid will appear in the syringe. **D:** Before the catheter is advanced any farther, the apparatus is directed downward. **E,F:** In rapid sequence, the catheter is advanced fully to the chest wall and the needle withdrawn from the apparatus. The one-way valve in the apparatus maintains a closed system until the operator manually changes the position of the stopcock to allow drainage of the pleural fluid.

of instructions for performing this procedure, and all will generally mirror the procedure described above. Operators should be thoroughly familiar with the recommended procedure for the catheter system that they will use and should receive appropriate supervision from an experienced operator before performing thoracentesis on their own.

Technique for Removal of Freely Moving Pneumothorax

The technique for removal of freely moving PTX is as follows:

1. Follow the same catheter-over-needle protocol described for removing freely moving fluid, but position the patient supine with the head of the bed elevated 30 to 45 degrees.
2. Prepare the second or third intercostal space in the anterior midclavicular line (this avoids hitting the more medial internal mammary artery) for the needle and catheter insertion.
3. Have the bevel of the needle facing up, and direct the needle upward so that the catheter can be guided toward the superior aspect of the hemithorax.
4. Air can be actively withdrawn by syringe or pushed out when intrapleural pressure is supraatmospheric (e.g., during a cough) as long as the catheter is intermittently open to the atmosphere. In the latter setting, air can leave but not reenter if the catheter is attached to a one-way check-valve apparatus (Heimlich valve) or if it is put to underwater seal.
5. When local anesthesia and skin cleansing are not possible because a tension PTX is life threatening, perform the procedure without them. If a tension PTX is known or suspected to be present and a chest tube is not readily available, quickly

insert a 14-gauge needle and 16-gauge catheter according to the above technique to avoid puncturing the lung. If a tension PTX is present, air escapes under pressure. When the situation has stabilized and the tension PTX has been diagnosed, leave the catheter in place until a sterile chest tube can be inserted.

Utility of Ultrasonography for Guidance of Thoracentesis

Whether to guide simple needle insertion for diagnostic thoracentesis or to perform more complex pleural procedures, the use of ultrasonography should be considered as a key feature of any pleural intervention. Ultrasonography guidance of thoracentesis reduces the rate of PTX [2,23]; facilitates the identification and targeting of the pleural effusion; and is more accurate in determining a safe site for needle insertion than physical examination [24]. It allows for performance of thoracentesis on patients who are on mechanical ventilator support [14] and for targeted insertion of drainage catheters into loculated pleural effusion.

Ultrasonography is effective for the identification of pleural fluid, because the fluid is either anechoic or hypoechoic compared to soft tissue; it also allows for characterization of the location, volume, and internal complexity of the effusion (Chapter 12 Videos 12.1–12.33). Although this information may provide details regarding the etiology of the effusion, sampling the fluid is often an important part of management, as is the need for pleural interventions that require catheter insertion. There are several considerations when using ultrasonography to guide thoracentesis.

Equipment

The ultrasonography examination is performed using a phased-array cardiac probe (3.5 to 5.0 MHz) whose small footprint allows for examination between rib interspaces. A curvilinear adominal probe may also be used. The linear high frequency probe lacks sufficient penetration to visualize deeper thoracic structures such as atelectatic lung underlying the pleural effusion.

Scanning Technique

A series of scan lines are performed over the chest in order to identify and characterize the pleural effusion, and to establish a safe site for needle insertion that avoids injury to adjacent organs.

Patient Position

The critically ill patient is generally in the supine position, which makes it difficult to identify a safe site for needle insertion unless the pleural effusion is large, because pleural fluid, unless loculated, assumes a dependent position in the thorax. In the case of a smaller effusion in a supine patient, the effusion will be posterior in location and readily identified by pressing the probe into the mattress with anterior angulation. However, this probe position cannot be duplicated by the needle–syringe assembly, which is a key requirement for safe needle insertion trajectory. In the case of a large effusion, the effusion will be visible with ultrasonography in a more anterior position, with a probe angulation that may be duplicated with the needle–syringe assembly. In the case of a small effusion, if no safe site can be identified with the patient in supine position, the head of the bed may be raised to semirecumbent position and the ipsilateral arm adducted in order to expose the posterolateral chest. The probe is used to scan the lower posterolateral chest to establish a safe site for needle insertion. The limitation of this method is that a team member must hold the patient in position for the entire duration of the procedure.

An alternative is to place the patient in a lateral decubitus position with the hemithorax contralateral to the effusion in the dependent position. The pleural effusion is identified by scanning over the posterior nondependent hemithorax. Both of these methods require significant movement of the patient who may be intubated with various life support devices in place. Care is taken to avoid accidental extubation or dislodgement of other life support equipment. This requires that several team members be involved with the procedure. For the patient who is able to sit up while leaning forward on an examination table, which is the standard position for thoracentesis performed by the intensivist, the effusion is identified by scanning over the posterior thorax.

Identification of Fluid

The examiner seeks three characteristic findings that are typical for a pleural effusion.

a. An anechoic or relatively hypoechoic space that is surrounded by typical anatomic boundaries. This space represents the pleural effusion.
b. Typical anatomic boundaries: This requires unequivocal identification of the chest wall, the surface of the lung, and the diaphragm. The heart may form an anatomic boundary on the left side. Identification of the diaphragm is a critical element of safe site selection as subdiaphragmatic device insertion may result in splenic or hepatic injury. Identification of the diaphragm requires definitive identification of the subdiaphragmatic organs (spleen or liver; and kidneys). The inexperienced scanner may misidentify the hepatorenal or splenorenal space as the diaphragm and consider the overlying liver or spleen to be an echo-dense effusion, because the spaces may appear as a curvilinear structure that may be mistaken for the diaphragm. This dangerous error is avoided by emphasizing the identification of the kidney as a discrete structure that is well below the diaphragm.
c. Dynamic changes: This requires identification of dynamic changes that are typical of a pleural effusion such as diaphragmatic movement; lung movement; and movement of internal echogenic elements within the pleural effusion.

Site Selection

Once the pleural effusion is identified, the transducer is moved over the target area in order to identify a safe site for needle insertion that maximizes the distance between the chest wall and the underlying lung while avoiding adjacent anatomic structures such as the diaphragm or heart (on the left side). As much as possible, the examiner holds the probe perpendicular to the chest wall, because this angle is easiest to duplicate with the needle–syringe assembly. Once a suitable site is identified, it is marked; the depth of needle penetration to access the fluid is measured; and the angle of the probe is determined. This angle will be duplicated by the operator during needle insertion.

A rare complication of thoracentesis is laceration of an intercostal wall vessel with subsequent hemothorax. This risk may be reduced by using the high-frequency vascular probe to scan the proposed needle trajectory. Using color Doppler, identification of a vessel may allow the operator to select an alternative site [25].

Performance of Needle Insertion

Once the site is selected, there can be no further patient movement, because this may shift the position of the pleural effusion within the chest cavity relative to the insertion site. The time between the ultrasonography examination and needle insertion is minimized. Immediately before the sterile preparation, the operator rechecks the site, angle, and depth for needle insertion. The thoracentesis is performed with free hand technique by inserting the needle–syringe assembly at the site mark, duplicating the angle at which the probe was held to determine a safe trajectory. Real-time guidance of needle insertion is not required for safe thoracentesis. If a wire is inserted through the needle for Seldinger technique device insertion, some operators identify the wire position before using the dilator. Likewise, final device position may be determined with ultrasonography.

As a routine, the patient should be checked for PTX before the procedure by examining for lung sliding, lung pulse, and/or B lines. Their presence reliably rules out PTX (see Chapter 11 on Lung Ultrasonography). Following the procedure, the examination is repeated. The continued presence of these three signs rules out PTX so reliably that chest radiography is not necessary, and may be misleading [26]. Their absence is strong evidence of a procedure-related PTX.

Pitfalls of Imaging

a. Skin compression: In the edematous or obese patient, skin compression artifact may cause an underestimation of the depth for successful needle insertion. In this case, the operator pushes the probe into the skin surface in order to improve image quality. This causes indentation of the skin surface at the target site that rebounds when the probe is removed. This is problematic at the time of needle insertion, because the operator must insert the needle to a depth greater than that measured with indentation of the skin.
b. Site mark movement: If lateral force is applied to the skin at the time of marking the insertion site, the skin mark may be moved to a substantial extent. This is of particular concern when accessing a smaller effusion. At the time of needle insertion, the operator takes care to not move the mark site when applying pressure to the skin surface.
c. Difficult scanning conditions: It may be difficult to achieve adequate image quality in the massively obese or edematous patient. The pleural effusion may be so echogenic that it could cause uncertainty as to its size or location.

INTERPRETATION OF PLEURAL FLUID ANALYSIS

To determine the etiology of a pleural effusion, a number of tests on pleural fluid are helpful. The initial determination should be to classify the effusion as a transudate or an exudate using the criteria discussed below. Additional studies can then be ordered to help establish a final diagnosis for the etiology of the pleural effusion, especially in the setting of an exudate.

Transudates versus Exudates

A transudate is biochemically defined by meeting all of the following classic (Light's) criteria [7]: pleural fluid–serum total protein ratio of less than 0.5; pleural fluid–serum lactate dehydrogenase (LDH) ratio of less than 0.6; and pleural fluid LDH of less than two-thirds the normal serum level. Transudates are generally caused by hydrostatic or oncotic pressure imbalances, or from the migration of pleural fluid from peritoneal or retroperitoneal spaces to the pleural space. An exudate is present when any of the foregoing criteria for transudates are not met. Exudates arise through a variety of mechanisms that result primarily from inflammation of the lung or pleura, impaired lymphatic drainage, or migration of fluid from the peritoneal space.

A wide variety of alternative diagnostic criteria have been studied since Light's original work was published. Abbreviated criteria with similar diagnostic accuracy, but without the need for concurrent serum measurements, have been proposed [8–10]. A meta-analysis of 8 studies (1,448 patients) indicates that a classic transudate can be identified with equal accuracy by the combination of both pleural fluid cholesterol of less than 45 mg per dL and a pleural fluid LDH less than 0.45 times the upper limit of normal for serum LDH [8]. Clinical judgment will be required when analyzing any borderline test results.

If a transudate is present, generally no further tests on pleural fluid are indicated (Table 12.1). If an exudate is identified, further laboratory evaluation is generally warranted (Fig. 12.1). If subsequent testing does not narrow the differential diagnosis and tuberculous pleuritis is a diagnostic consideration, a percutaneous pleural biopsy should be considered given the improved sensitivity over thoracentesis alone. If mesothelioma is considered a distinct possibility, consideration should be given to proceeding directly to thoracoscopic or open pleural biopsy to provide a large enough tissue sample to optimize diagnostic success. Thoracoscopy-guided pleural biopsy should be considered in patients with pleural effusion of unknown etiology while following the above-listed evaluation.

Selected Tests that are Potentially Helpful to Establish Etiology for a Pleural Effusion

pH

Pleural fluid pH determinations may have diagnostic and therapeutic implications [12]. For instance, the differential diagnosis associated with a pleural fluid pH of less than 7.2 is consistent with systemic acidemia; bacterially infected effusion (empyema); malignant effusion; rheumatoid pleuritis; tuberculous effusion; ruptured esophagus, noninfected parapneumonic effusion that needs drainage; paragonimiasis; and urinothorax. Pleural effusions with a pH of less than 7.2 are potentially sclerosis provoking and require consideration for chest tube drainage to aid resolution [12].

Glucose

All transudates and most exudates will have pleural glucose levels similar to blood glucose concentrations. Some exudates will have low pleural fluid glucose values (defined as less than 60 mg per dL) and in this situation, the differential diagnosis overlaps with those causes listed above for low pH effusions. Potentially important to note is that whereas pleural glucose levels are not significantly impacted by the duration of time the sample awaits analysis or the presence of air or lidocaine in the same sampling syringe, there can be clinically significant increases (time delay, air) or decreases (lidocaine) noted in the pleural fluid pH by these factors [27]. Therefore, glucose levels may serve as a surrogate for pleural fluid pH if there is any concern that the measured pH may be inaccurate.

Protein, LDH, and Protein Gradient

The main purpose for measuring pleural fluid protein and LDH levels is the separation of transudative from exudative effusions. An additional key point is that the pleural fluid LDH can serve as an indirect reflection of the degree of pleural inflammation, and any effusion classified as an exudate based on LDH criterion alone (and not by protein level as well) suggests the presence of pleural space infection or a malignant effusion. Also, importantly, the serum protein minus pleural fluid protein gradient may be of value in distinguishing a truly transudative effusion due to CHF in a patient who has undergone diuresis, from a truly exudative effusion. If in the setting of a patient who has undergone diuresis for CHF, the protein gradient is greater than 3.1 g per dL (or if greater than 1.2 g per dL when an albumin gradient is measured instead), that effusion is most likely transudative in nature and caused by CHF.

Amylase

A pleural fluid amylase level that is greater than the normal serum level may be seen in patients with acute and chronic pancreatitis;

TABLE 12.1

Causes of Pleural Effusions

Etiologies of Effusions That Are Virtually Always Transudates
Congestive heart failure
Nephrotic syndrome
Hypoalbuminemia
Urinothorax
Trapped lung
Cirrhosis
Atelectasis
Peritoneal dialysis
Constrictive pericarditis
Superior vena caval obstruction

Etiologies of Effusions That Are Typically Exudates

Infections
Parapneumonic
Tuberculous pleurisy
Parasites (amebiasis, paragonimiasis, and echinococcosis)
Fungal disease
Atypical pneumonias (virus, *Mycoplasma*, Q fever, and *Legionella*)
Nocardia, *Actinomyces*
Subphrenic abscess
Hepatic abscess
Splenic abscess
Hepatitis
Spontaneous esophageal rupture

Noninfectious Inflammations
Pancreatitis
Benign asbestos pleural effusion
Pulmonary embolism[a]
Radiation therapy
Uremic pleurisy
Sarcoidosis[c]
Postcardiac injury syndrome
Hemothorax
Acute respiratory distress syndrome

Malignancies[b]
Carcinoma
Lymphoma
Mesothelioma
Leukemia
Chylothorax[c]

Chronically Increased Negative Intrapleural Pressure
Atelectasis
Trapped lung[c]
Cholesterol effusion

Iatrogenic
Drug-induced (nitrofurantoin and methotrexate)
Esophageal perforation
Esophageal sclerotherapy
Central venous catheter misplacement or migration
Enteral feeding tube in space

Connective Tissue Disease
Lupus pleuritis
Rheumatoid pleurisy
Mixed connective tissue disease
Churg–Strauss syndrome
Wegener's granulomatosis
Familial Mediterranean fever

Endocrine Disorders
Hypothyroidism[c]
Ovarian hyperstimulation syndrome

Lymphatic Disorders
Malignancy
Yellow nail syndrome
Lymphangioleiomyomatosis

Movement of Fluid from Abdomen to Pleural Space
Pancreatitis
Pancreatic pseudocyst
Meigs' syndrome
Malignant ascites
Chylous ascites

[a] 10% to 20% may be transudates.
[b] 3% to 10% are transudates.
[c] Occasional transudates.
Adapted from Sahn SA: The pleura. *Am Rev Respir Dis* 138:184, 1988.

pancreatic pseudocyst that has dissected or ruptured into the pleural space; malignancy; and esophageal rupture. Salivary isoenzymes predominate with malignancy and esophageal rupture, whereas intrinsic pancreatic disease is characterized by the presence of pancreatic isoenzymes.

Triglyceride and Cholesterol

Chylous pleural effusions are biochemically defined by a triglyceride level greater than 110 mg per dL and the presence of chylomicrons on a pleural fluid lipoprotein electrophoresis [12]. The usual appearance of a chylous effusion is milky, but an effusion with elevated triglycerides may also appear serous. The measurement of a triglyceride level is therefore important. Chylous effusions occur when the thoracic duct has been disrupted somewhere along its course. The most common causes are trauma and malignancy (e.g., Non–Hodgkin lymphoma) as well as in 25% of patients with lymphangioleiomyomatosis. A pseudochylous effusion appears grossly milky because of an elevated cholesterol level (>220 mg per dL), but the triglyceride level is usually normal and no chylomicrons are present. Chronic effusions, especially those associated with rheumatoid and tuberculous pleuritis are characteristically pseudochylous.

Adenosine Deaminase

Adenosine deaminase (ADA) is abundant in lymphocytes and therefore is potentially a good marker for tuberculous pleural effusion, especially given its simpler testing methodology and lower cost as compared with measurement of pleural fluid interferon gamma level or nucleic acid polymerase chain amplification assessment [28]. Meta-analysis of ADA for the diagnosis of pleural TB has shown a sensitivity and specificity of 92% and 90%, respectively [29]. Whereas a pleural fluid ADA level <40 IU per L virtually excludes the diagnosis, levels >40 IU per L support the diagnosis and ADA levels >70 IU per L highly suggest pleural TB [24]. Because the predictive value of any test is dependent on the prevalence of disease in the specific population being tested, the use of a highly sensitive test such as the ADA in the majority of the USA (generally a low prevalence area for pleural TB) implies that the major strength of the ADA is in its negative predictive value. Multiple possible causes of false-positive ADA testing exist and include: infection, malignancy (especially lymphoma), and connective tissue diseases [29].

Cell Counts and Differential

Although pleural fluid white blood cell count and differential are never diagnostic of any disease, it would be distinctly unusual for an effusion other than one associated with bacterial pneumonia to have a white blood cell count exceeding 50,000 per μL. In an exudative pleural effusion of acute origin, polymorphonuclear leukocytes predominate early, whereas mononuclear cells predominate in chronic exudative effusions. Although pleural fluid lymphocytosis is nonspecific, severe lymphocytosis (greater than 80% of cells) is suggestive of tuberculosis or malignancy. Finally, pleural fluid eosinophilia ($\geq$10%) is nonspecific and is most commonly associated with either blood or air in the pleural space.

A red blood cell count of 5,000 to 10,000 cells per μL must be present for a fluid to appear pinkish. Grossly bloody effusions containing more than 100,000 red blood cells per μL are most consistent with trauma, malignancy, or pulmonary infarction. To distinguish a traumatic thoracentesis from a preexisting hemothorax, several observations are helpful. First, because a preexisting hemothorax has been defibrinated, it does not form a clot on standing. Second, a hemothorax is suggested when a pleural fluid hematocrit value is 50% or more of the serum hematocrit value.

Cultures and Stains

To maximize the yield from pleural fluid cultures, anaerobic and aerobic cultures should be obtained. Because acid-fast stains may be positive in up to 20% of tuberculous effusions, they should always be performed in addition to smears using Gram's stain. By submitting closed pleural biopsy pieces to pathology and microbiology laboratories, it is possible to diagnose up to 95% of tuberculous effusions with the combination of thoracentesis and percutaneous biopsy [7].

Cytology

Malignancies can produce pleural effusions by implantation of malignant cells on the pleura or impairment of lymphatic drainage secondary to tumor obstruction. The tumors that most commonly cause pleural effusions are lung, breast, and lymphoma. Pleural fluid cytology should be performed for an exudative effusion of unknown etiology, using at least 60 mL fluid [20,30]. If initial cytology results are negative and strong clinical suspicion exists, additional samples of fluid can increase the chance of a positive result to approximately 60% to 70%. The addition of a directed pleural biopsy (i.e., thoracoscopy) increases the yield to over 90%. In addition to malignancy, cytologic examination can definitively diagnose rheumatoid pleuritis, whose pathognomonic picture consists of slender, elongated macrophages and giant, round, multinucleated giant cells ("tadpole cells"), accompanied by an amorphous granular background material.

References

1. Ault MJ, Rosen BT, Scher J, et al: Thoracentesis outcomes: a 12 year experience. *Thorax* 70:127–132, 2015.
2. Gordon CE, Feller-Kopman D, Balk EM, et al: Pneumothorax following thoracentesis: a systematic review and meta-analysis. *Arch Intern Med* 170:332–339, 2010.
3. Goligher EC, Leis JA, Fowler RA, et al: Utility and safety of draining pleural effusions in mechanically ventilated patients: a systematic review and meta-analysis. *Crit Care* 15:R46, 2011.
4. Hibbert RM, Atwell TD, Lekah A, et al: Safety of ultrasound-guided thoracentesis in patients with abnormal preprocedural coagulation parameters. *Chest* 144:456–463, 2013.
5. Mercaldi CJ, Lanes SF: Ultrasound guidance decreases complications and improves the cost of care among patients undergoing thoracentesis and paracentesis. *Chest* 143:532–538, 2013.
6. Perazzo A, Gatto P, Barlascini C, et al: Can ultrasound guidance reduce the risk of pneumothorax following thoracentesis? *J Bras Pneumol* 40:6–12, 2014.
7. Light RW, MacGregor MI, Luchsinger PC, et al: Pleural effusions: the diagnostic separation of transudates and exudates. *Ann Intern Med* 77:507–513, 1972.
8. Heffner JE, Brown LK, Barbieri CA: Diagnostic value of tests that discriminate between exudative and transudative pleural effusions. *Chest* 111:970–980, 1997.
9. Gonlugur U, Gonlugur TE: The distinction between transudates and exudates. *J Biomed Sci* 12:985–990, 2005.
10. Kummerfeldt CE, Chiuzan CC, Huggins JT, et al: Improving the predictive accuracy of identifying exudative effusions. *Chest* 145:586–592, 2014.
11. Wilcox ME, Chong CA, Stanbrook MB, et al: Does this patient have an exudative pleural effusion? The Rational Clinical Examination systematic review. *JAMA* 311:2422–2431, 2014.
12. Wilson MM, Irwin RS: Thoracentesis, in Irwin RS, Rippe JM (eds): *Intensive Care Medicine*. 7th ed. Philadelphia, PA, Wolters Kluwer/Lippincott Williams & Wilkins, 2012, pp 95–101.
13. Daniels CE, Ryu JH: Improving the safety of thoracentesis. *Curr Opin Pulm Med* 17:232–236, 2011.
14. Mayo PH, Goltz HR, Tafreshi M, et al: Safety of ultrasound-guided thoracentesis in patients receiving mechanical ventilation. *Chest* 125:1059–1062, 2004.
15. Barnes TW, Morgenthaler TI, Olson EJ, et al: Sonographically guided thoracentesis and rate of pneumothorax. *J Clin Ultrasound* 33:442–446, 2005.
16. Duncan DR, Morganthaler TI, Ryu JH, et al: Reducing iatrogenic risk in thoracentesis: establishing best practice via experimental training in a zero-risk environment. *Chest* 135:1315–1320, 2009.
17. Salmonsen M, Ellis S, Paul E, et al: Thoracic ultrasound demonstrates variable location of the intercostal artery. *Respiration* 83:323–329, 2012.
18. Helm EJ, Rahman NM, Talakoub O, et al: Course and variation of the intercostal artery by CT scan. *Chest* 143:634–639, 2013.
19. Feller-Kopman D, Walkey A, Berkowitz D, et al: The relationship of pleural pressure to symptom development during therapeutic thoracentesis. *Chest* 129:1556–1560, 2006.
20. Abouzgheib W, Bartter T, Dagher H, et al: A prospective study of the volume of pleural fluid required for accurate diagnosis of malignant pleural effusion. *Chest* 135:999–1001, 2009.
21. Swiderek J, Morcos S, Donthireddy V, et al: Prospective study to determine the volume of pleural fluid required to diagnose malignancy. *Chest* 137:68–73, 2010.
22. Temes RT: Thoracentesis. *N Engl J Med* 356:641, 2007.
23. Cavanna L, Mordenti P, Bertè R, et al: Ultrasound guidance reduces pneumothorax rate and improves safety of thoracentesis in malignant pleural effusion: report on 445 consecutive patients with advanced cancer. *World J Surg Oncol* 12:139, 2014.
24. Diacon AH, Brutsche MH, Solèr M: Accuracy of pleural puncture sites: a prospective comparison of clinical examination with ultrasound. *Chest* 123:436–441, 2003.
25. Kanai M, Sekiguchi H: Avoiding vessel laceration in thoracentesis: a role of vascular ultrasound with color Doppler. *Chest* 147:e5–e7, 2015.
26. Reissig A, Kroegel C: Accuracy of transthoracic sonography in excluding post-interventional pneumothorax and hydropneumothorax. Comparison to chest radiography. *Eur J Radiol* 53:463–470, 2005.
27. Rahman NM, Mishra EK, Davies H, et al: Clinically important factors influencing the diagnostic measurement of pleural fluid pH and glucose. *Am J Respir Crit Care Med* 178:483–490, 2008.
28. Gopi A, Madhavan S, Sharma SK, et al: Diagnosis and treatment of tuberculous pleural effusion 2008. *Chest* 131:880–889, 2007.
29. Light RW: Update on tuberculous pleural effusion. *Respirology* 15:451–458, 2010.
30. Heffner JE, Klein JS: Recent advances in the diagnosis and management of malignant pleural effusions. *Mayo Clin Proc* 83:235–250, 2008.

Chapter 13 ■ Chest Tube Insertion and Care

ULISES TORRES • JOSHUA R. SCURLOCK

Chest tube insertion involves placement of a sterile tube into the pleural space to evacuate air or fluid into a closed collection system to restore negative intrathoracic pressure; promote lung expansion; and prevent potentially lethal levels of pressure from developing in the thorax. Most life-threatening thoracic injuries can be treated with airway control or an appropriately placed chest tube or needle [1].

PLEURAL ANATOMY AND PHYSIOLOGY

The pleural space is a potential space that separates the visceral and parietal pleura with a thin layer of lubricating fluid. Although up to 500 mL per day of fluid may enter the pleural space, 0.1 to 0.2 mL per kg surrounds each lung in the pleural space at any given time. These two layers are lined by an extensive lymphatic network that ultimately drains into the thoracic duct via the mediastinal and intercostal lymph nodes. These lymphatics prevent the accumulation of this pleural fluid. It is estimated that this mechanism allows clearance of up to 20 mL of pleural fluid per hour per hemithorax in a 70-kg human. The elastic coil of the chest wall and lung creates a subatmospheric pressure in the space, between −5 and −10 cm H_2O, which binds the lung to the chest wall [2,3].

Drainage of the pleural space is necessary when the normal physiologic processes are disrupted by increased fluid into the space owing to alterations in hydrostatic pressures (e.g., congestive heart failure) or oncotic pressures or by changes of the parietal pleura itself (e.g., inflammatory diseases that reduce the area available for fluid resorption). A derangement in lymphatic drainage—as with lymphatic obstruction; disruption of pleural anatomy; and/or lung parenchymal anatomy due to malignancy—may also result in excess fluid accumulation.

CHEST TUBE PLACEMENT

Indications

The indications for closed intercostal drainage include a variety of disease processes in the hospital setting (Table 13.1). The procedure may be performed to palliate a chronic disease process or to relieve an acute, life-threatening process. Chest tubes also may provide a vehicle for pharmacologic interventions, as when used with antibiotic therapy; tissue plasminogen activator/fibrinolytic agents; or instillation of sclerosing agents to prevent recurrence of malignant effusions.

TABLE 13.1

Indications for Chest Tube Insertion

- Pneumothorax
  - Primary or spontaneous
  - Secondary
    - Chronic obstructive pulmonary disease
    - Pneumonia
    - Abscess/empyema
    - Malignancy
  - Traumatic
  - Iatrogenic
    - Central line placement
    - Positive-pressure ventilation
    - Thoracentesis
    - Lung biopsy
- Hemothorax
  - Traumatic
    - Blunt
    - Penetrating (trauma or biopsy)
  - Iatrogenic
  - Malignancy
  - Pulmonary arteriovenous malformation
  - Blood dyscrasias
  - Ruptured thoracic aortic aneurysm
- Empyema
  - Parapneumonic
  - Posttraumatic
  - Postoperative
  - Septic emboli
  - Intra-abdominal infection
- Chylothorax
  - Traumatic
  - Surgical
  - Congenital
  - Malignancy
- Pleural effusion
  - Transudate
  - Exudate (malignancy, inflammatory)

Pneumothorax

Accumulation of air in the pleural space is the most common indication for chest tube placement. Symptoms include tachypnea, dyspnea, and pleuritic pain, although some patients (in particular, those with a small spontaneous pneumothorax) may be asymptomatic. Physical findings include increased work of breathing, diminished breath sounds, and hyperresonance to percussion on the affected side.

Diagnosis is often confirmed by chest radiography or ultrasound (US) (details of performing this examination can be found below). The size of a pneumothorax may be estimated, but this is at best a rough approximation of a three-dimensional space using a two-dimensional view. Although the gold standard for the identification of a pneumothorax (independent of location within the thorax) has been a computed tomography (CT) scan of the chest, US identification has been shown to have the same sensitivity as that of a CT scan. Furthermore, US estimates of the extension of the pneumothorax correlate well with CT scan [4]. The sensitivity of detecting a pneumothorax with US ranges from 86% to 89%, compared to a range of 28% to 75% with a supine chest X-ray [4–6].

Immediate tube decompression is indicated for patients who are symptomatic; those who have a large or expanding pneumothorax; or those who are being mechanically ventilated. The mechanically ventilated patient is of particular concern because of acute deteriorating oxygenation that occurs with a pneumothorax in the setting of increased pleural pressure. However, a small, stable, asymptomatic pneumothorax can be followed with serial chest radiographs. Reexpansion occurs at the rate of approximately 2.2% of lung volume per day [7].

Persistent leaking of air into the pleural space with no route of escape will ultimately collapse the affected lung, flatten the diaphragm, and eventually produce contralateral shift of the mediastinum. This is referred to as a tension pneumothorax. The combination of a collapsed lung on the affected side and the increasing pressure on the contralateral lung results in hypoxemia. The accompanying hypotension is a result of pressure on the inferior vena cava which compromises venous return. Emergency needle decompression with a 14- or 16-gauge catheter in the midclavicular line of the second intercostal space may be lifesaving while preparations for chest tube insertion are being made.

Hemothorax

Accumulation of blood in the pleural space can be classified as spontaneous, iatrogenic, or traumatic. Attempted thoracentesis or tube placement may result in injury to the intercostal arteries, internal mammary arteries or to the pulmonary parenchyma. Up to a third of patients with traumatic rib fractures may have an accompanying pneumothorax or hemothorax [8]. Pulmonary parenchymal bleeding from chest trauma is often self-limited owing to the low pressure of the pulmonary vascular system. However, systemic sources (intercostal, internal mammary, or subclavian arteries, aorta, or heart) may persist and become life threatening.

Indications for open thoracotomy in the setting of traumatic hemothorax include initial blood loss greater than 1,500 mL or continued blood loss exceeding 200 mL per hour for 2 to 4 hours. This decision is not based solely on the rate of continuing blood loss, but also on the patient's physiologic status. If a hemothorax is suspected, placement of large-bore (36 to 40 French [Fr]) drainage tubes encourages evacuation of blood and helps determine the need for immediate thoracotomy [1].

Empyema

The management principles for pleural infection have come a long way from employing antibiotic therapy and thoracentesis to the current availability of semi-invasive and invasive procedures like video assisted thoracostomy and fibrinolytics. Use of advanced imaging like US and CT scans widens the scope of diagnosing and for treating effusions seen on a routine posteroanterior chest radiograph. Observation is usually adequate for a small (<10 mm) unseptated, free flowing effusions. Any other effusions warrant a diagnostic thoracentesis. If the aspirated fluid fulfills the criteria for being infected (pH <7.2, glucose <40 mg per dL, culture positive), a prompt plan for its drainage is recommended. Currently, large bore tube thoracostomy is the treatment option of choice for patients with empyema, but data are accumulating for treating parapneumonic effusions with small-bore intercostal drains. Early thoracoscopy is an alternative to thrombolytics. Local expertise will dictate the choice between therapeutic thoracentesis, intrapleural fibrinolytics, and medical thoracoscopy as well as conversion to open drainage when thoracoscopy fails until randomized trials provide better evidence [9].

Chylothorax

Chylothorax is a rare condition with multiple etiologies. Pleural fluid analysis can identify this condition when clinical suspicion exists. Conservative management is generally recommended for most non-iatrogenic cases with surgery being reserved for those who have a large or persistent leak or in those who become immunologically challenged or malnourished. Conservative treatment initially involves replacing the nutrients lost in the chyle and draining large chylothoraces using chest tube insertion if necessary, to ensure complete lung expansion. Nothing by mouth or the administration of low-fat, medium-chain triglyceride enteral diet results in resolution of approximately 50% of congenital or traumatic chylothoraces. Other invasive treatments are available and are discussed in the respective sections of this book. Some of these treatments are pleurodesis; lymphangiography and embolization; and ligation of the thoracic duct thoracoscopically or by thoracotomy [10].

Pleural Effusion

Approximately 1.5 million people develop a pleural effusion in the USA each year. One of the main reasons to perform a thoracentesis (see Chapter 12) in a patient with an undiagnosed pleural effusion is to determine whether the patient has a transudative or an exudative pleural effusion. The reason to make this differentiation is that the existence of a transudative pleural effusion indicates that systemic factors such as heart failure or cirrhosis are responsible for the effusion, whereas the existence of an exudative effusion indicates that local factors are responsible for the effusion. If the patient has a transudative effusion, the systemic abnormality can be treated, and no attention needs to be diverted to the pleura. Alternatively, if an exudative effusion is present, investigations need to be directed toward the pleura to find out the cause of the local problem. Exudative effusion is present if one or more of the following conditions are met: (1) pleural fluid protein/serum protein level greater than 0.5, (2) pleural fluid lactic acid dehydrogenase (LDH)/serum LDH level greater than 0.6, or (3) pleural fluid LDH level greater than two-thirds the upper normal limit for serum LDH. The differential diagnosis list is extensive; please refer to Chapter 176 on pleural effusion for a more detailed discussion of this subject. Tube thoracostomy could be indicated to treat and/or diagnose the etiology of the pleural effusion, but there are a lot of other modalities, like thoracentesis, pleural biopsy, bronchoscopy, thoracoscopy, and/or imaging that could be useful for the diagnosis or treatment of effusions [11].

CONTRAINDICATIONS

Published guidelines state that there are no absolute contraindications for drainage via tube thoracostomy, except when a lung is completely adherent to the chest wall throughout the hemithorax, or upon patient refusal. Relative contraindications include risks of bleeding due to coagulopathies or anticoagulation medication, and infection overlying the insertion site. Whenever possible, coagulopathies and platelet defects should be corrected prior to the procedure. Overlying cellulitis or herpes zoster infection should be avoided by choosing another puncture site. Other relative contraindications include multiple pleural adhesions, emphysematous blebs, and scarring [12].

TECHNIQUE

Chest tube insertion requires knowledge not only of the anatomy of the chest wall and intrathoracic and intra-abdominal structures, but also of general aseptic technique. The procedure should be performed or supervised only by experienced personnel, because the complications of an improperly placed tube may have immediate life-threatening results. Before tube placement, the patient must be evaluated thoroughly by physical examination and chest films to avoid insertion of the tube into a bulla or lung abscess; into the abdomen; or even into the wrong side. Particular care must be taken before and during the procedure to avoid intubation of the pulmonary parenchyma.

The necessary equipment is listed in Table 13.2. Sterile technique is mandatory whether the procedure is performed in

TABLE 13.2

Chest Tube Insertion Equipment

Chlorhexidine or povidone–iodine solution
Sterile towels and drapes with full body cover
Sterile sponges
1% lidocaine without epinephrine (40 mL)
10-mL syringe
18-, 21-, and 25-gauge needles
Two Kelly clamps, one large and one medium
Mayo scissors
Standard tissue forceps
Towel forceps
Needle holder
0-Silk suture with cutting needle
Scalpel handle and no. 10 blade
Chest tubes (24, 28, 32, and 36 Fr)
Chest tube drainage system (filled appropriately)
Petrolatum gauze 2 inch nonelastic adhesive tape
Sterile gowns and gloves, masks, caps

the operating room; in the intensive care unit; in the emergency room; or on the ward. Detailed informed consent is obtained, and a time-out is performed to make sure that all the equipment is ready and available, and that the procedure is being done on the correct side and correct patient.

Careful titration of parenteral narcotics or benzodiazepines, and careful, generous administration of local anesthetic agents provide for a relatively painless procedure. Standard, large-bore drainage tubes are made from either Silastic or rubber. Silastic tubes are either right angled or straight; have multiple drainage holes; and contain a radiopaque stripe with a gap to mark the most proximal drainage hole. They are available in sizes ranging from 6 to 40 Fr, with size selection dependent on the patient population (6 to 24 Fr for infants and children) and the collection being drained (24 to 28 Fr for air; 32 to 36 Fr for pleural effusions; and 36 to 40 Fr for blood or pus). Small-caliber Silastic tubes have been increasingly employed for chest drainage, particularly after open-heart surgery, to decrease pain and allow earlier ambulation [13].

Before performing the procedure, it is important to review the steps to be taken and to ensure that all necessary equipment is available. Patient comfort and safety are paramount. There are three techniques for insertion of a thoracostomy tube. The first two direct techniques require a surgical incision and are (a) blunt dissection and (b) trocar puncture. Only the former technique is discussed here, because the latter is not commonly employed. The third technique is the percutaneous method, which can also be done at the bedside with US guidance.

1. With the patient supine and the head of the bed adjusted for comfort, the involved side is elevated slightly with the ipsilateral arm brought up over the head (Fig. 13.1). Supplemental oxygen is administered as needed. The triangle of safety is identified. This area is bordered by the anterior border of the latissimus dorsi; the lateral border of the pectoralis major muscle; a line superior to the horizontal level of the nipple; and the apex below the axilla [12].
2. The tube is usually inserted through the fourth or fifth intercostal space in the anterior axillary line. An alternative entry site (for decompression of a pneumothorax) is the second intercostal space in the midclavicular line, but for cosmetic reasons and to avoid the thick pectoral muscles, the former site is preferable in adults.
3. Under sterile conditions, the area is prepped in standard sterile fashion; and it is draped to include the nipple, which serves as a landmark, as well as the axilla. A 2- to 3-cm area is infiltrated with 1% lidocaine to raise a wheal two finger-breadths below the intercostal space to be penetrated. (This allows for a subcutaneous tunnel to be developed, through which the tube will travel, and discourages air entry into the chest following removal of the tube.)
4. A 2-cm transverse incision is made at the wheal, and additional lidocaine is administered to infiltrate the tissues through which the tube will pass, including a generous area in the intercostal space (especially the periosteum of the ribs above and below the targeted interspace). Care should be taken to anesthetize the parietal pleura fully, because it (unlike the visceral pleura) contains somatic pain fibers. Each injection of lidocaine should be preceded by aspiration of the syringe to prevent injection into the intercostal vessels. Up to 30 to 40 mL of 1% lidocaine may be needed to achieve adequate local anesthesia.
5. To confirm the location of air or fluid, a thoracentesis is then performed at the proposed site of tube insertion. If air or fluid is not aspirated, the anatomy should be reassessed, and chest radiographs and CT scans reexamined before proceeding.
6. A short tunnel is created to the chosen intercostal space using Kelly clamps, and the intercostal muscles are bluntly divided (Fig. 13.2).
7. The closed clamp is carefully inserted through the parietal pleura, hugging the superior portion of the lower rib to

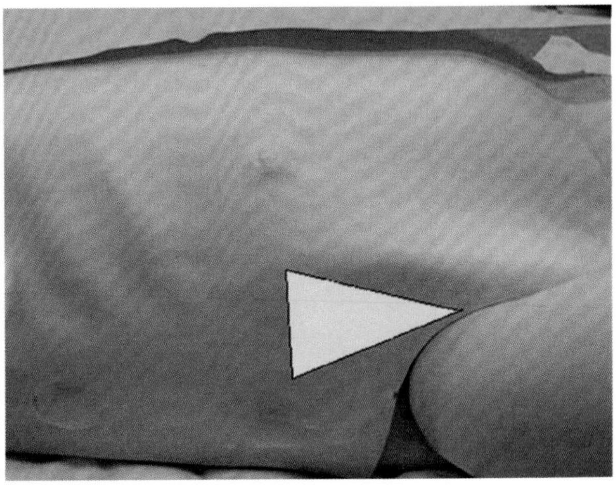

FIGURE 13.1 Positioning of the patient with the arm flexed over the head. Identification of the triangle of safety.

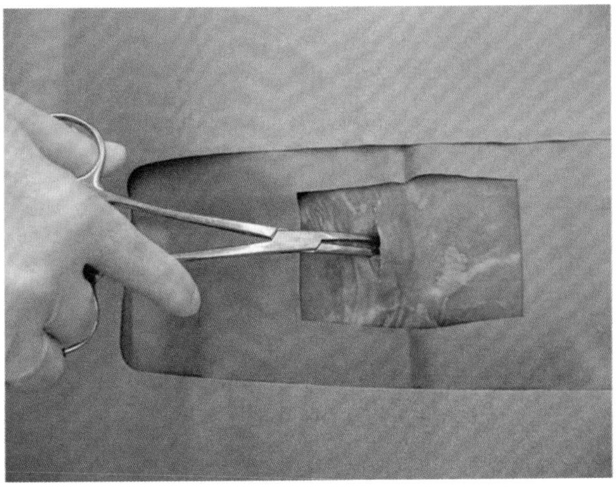

FIGURE 13.2 Dissection with Kelly clamp.

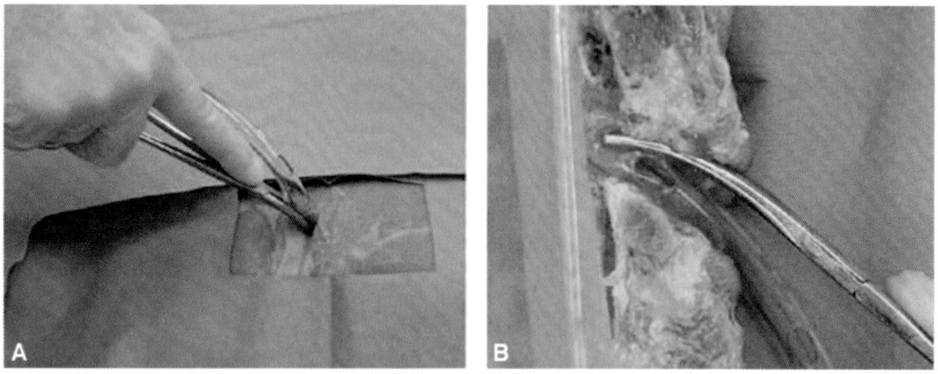

FIGURE 13.3 A, B: The clamp penetrates the intercostal muscle. The end of the chest tube is grasped with a Kelly clamp and guided with a finger through the chest incision. The clamp can be placed above or below the tube.

prevent injury to the intercostal bundle of the rib above. The clamp is placed to a depth of less than 1 cm to prevent injury to the intrathoracic structures, and is spread open approximately 2 cm.

8. A finger is inserted into the pleural space to explore the anatomy and confirm proper location and lack of pleural symphysis. Only easily disrupted adhesions should be broken. Bluntly dissecting strong adhesions may tear the lung and initiate bleeding.
9. The end of the chest tube is grasped with the clamp and guided with the finger through the tunnel into the pleural space. Once the tip of the tube is in the pleural space, the clamp is removed, and the chest tube is advanced and positioned apically for a pneumothorax and dependently for fluid removal (Fig. 13.3A, B). All holes must be confirmed to be within the pleural space. The use of undue pressure or force to insert the tube should be avoided (Fig. 13.4A, B).
10. The location of the tube should be confirmed by observing the flow of air (seen as condensation within the tube) or fluid from the tube. It is then sutured to the skin securely to prevent slippage (Fig. 13.5). A simple suture to anchor the tube can be used, or a horizontal mattress suture can be used to allow the hole to be tied closed when the tube is removed. An occlusive petrolatum gauze dressing is applied, and the tube is connected to a drainage apparatus and securely taped to the dressing and to the patient. All connections between the patient and the drainage apparatus must also be tight and securely taped.

COMPLICATIONS

Chest tube insertion may be accompanied by significant complications. In one series, insertion and management of pleural tubes in patients with blunt chest trauma carried a 9% incidence of complications. Major complications requiring surgical intervention, or administration of blood products or intravenous antibiotics occurred in only four (1.7%) patients [14] (Table 13.3). The use of small-caliber, less rigid, Silastic drains has been found to be as safe and efficacious as the more rigid, conventional chest tubes [15].

CHEST TUBE MANAGEMENT AND CARE

While a chest tube is in place, the tube and drainage system must be checked at least daily for adequate functioning. Most institutions use a three-chambered system that contains a calibrated collection trap for fluid; an underwater seal unit to allow escape of air while maintaining negative pleural pressure; and a suction regulator. Suction is routinely established at 15 to 20 cm water, controlled by the height of the column in the suction regulator unit, and maintained as long as an air leak is present. The drainage system is examined daily to ensure that appropriate levels are maintained in the underwater seal and suction regulator chambers. Connections between the chest tube and the drainage system should be tightly fitted and securely taped. For continuous drainage, the chest tube and the

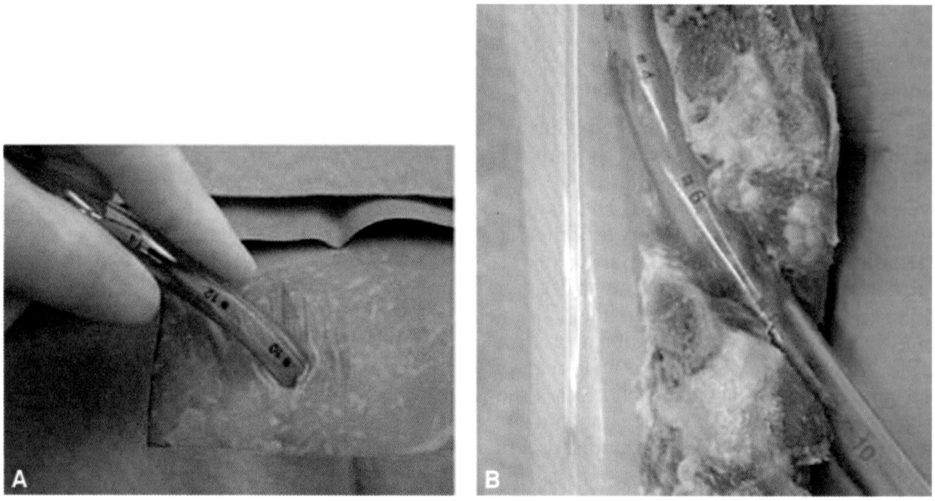

FIGURE 13.4 A, B: Advance the tube once the clamp has been removed.

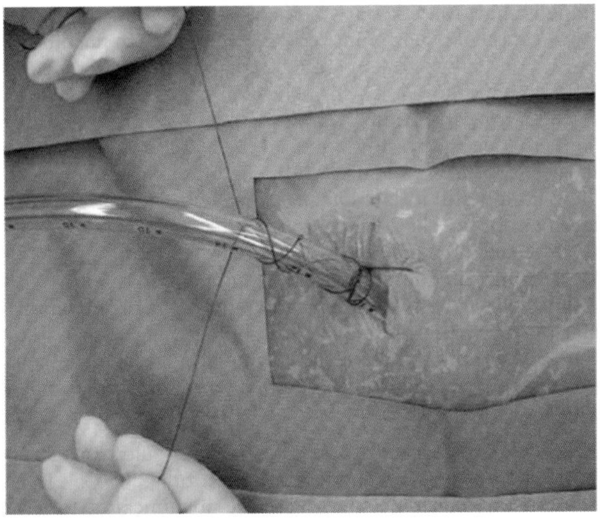

FIGURE 13.5 The tube is securely sutured to the skin with a 1-0 or 2-0 silk suture. This suture is left long, wrapped around the tube, and secured with tape. To seal the tunnel, the suture is tied when the tube is pulled out.

drainage system tubing should remain free of kinks; should not be left in a dependent position; and should never be clamped. Routine milking and stripping of chest tubes is discouraged primarily in postoperative cardiac surgical patients. The data do not support routine milking and stripping, unless there is a clot in the tubing [16]. Irrigation of the tube is discouraged. Dressing changes should be performed every 2 or 3 days and as needed, making sure that no dressing with high content of petroleum-based ointment is present, because this would macerate the skin around the chest tube insertion site. Adequate pain control is mandatory to encourage coughing and ambulation to facilitate lung reexpansion.

Daily chest radiographs rarely influence chest tube management or patient care decisions, and are no longer recommended. If the patient develops clinical symptoms including shortness of breath, decreasing oxygen saturation, or subcutaneous emphysema, then radiographic evaluation is indicated [17]. A tube should never be readvanced into the pleural space, and if a tube is to be replaced, it should always be at a different site. If a pneumothorax persists, increasing the suction level may be beneficial, but an additional tube may be required if no improvement results; other etiologies should be considered after this point and further evaluation with a CT scan of the chest. Proper positioning may also be confirmed by chest CT scanning [18].

TABLE 13.3

Complications of Chest Tube Insertion

- Unintentional tube placement into vital structures (lung, liver, spleen, etc.)
- Intercostal vessel laceration
- Retroperitoneal placement
- Misplacement
- Empyema
- Kinked tube
  - Advanced too deeply
  - Unresolved pneumothorax
  - Inadequately advanced
- Reaccumulation of pneumothorax
- Persistent pleural effusion

CHEST TUBE REMOVAL

Indications for removal of chest tubes include resolution of the pneumothorax or fluid accumulation in the pleural space, or both. For a pneumothorax, the drainage system is left on suction until the air leak stops. If an air leak persists, brief clamping of the chest tube can be performed to confirm that the leak is from the patient and not from the system. If, after several days, an air leak persists, placement of an additional tube may be indicated. When the leak has ceased for more than 24 to 48 hours (or if no fluctuation is seen in the underwater seal chamber), the drainage system is placed on water seal by disconnecting the wall suction, followed by a chest film several hours later. If no pneumothorax is present and no air leak appears in the system with coughing; deep breathing; and reestablishment of suction, the tube can be removed. For fluid collections, the tube can be removed when drainage is less than 200 mL per 24 hours [19], unless sclerotherapy is planned.

When the chest tube is removed, the lungs should be fully expanded, which minimizes the pleural space. This can only be achieved when the patient holds his/her breath while performing the Valsalva maneuver (i.e., trying to exhale against a closed glottis or bearing down) or at the end of expiration. US examination can confirm that lung reexpansion is complete, and chest X-ray is required only if the patient develops clinical symptoms that suggest the original problem has reoccurred [20].

RELATED SYSTEMS

Percutaneous aspiration of the pleural space to relieve a pneumothorax without an active air leak has been reported. Success rate for patients with nontraumatic PTX has ranged from 64% to 87% in adults, and 90% to 95% in children. Variation of success rates could be affected by a number of reasons including the underlying disease, the use of mechanical ventilation, or other factors [21]. Also, there have been reports of successful management of small and large pneumothoraces with small size (8.5 Fr) or pigtail catheters, connected to a portable one-way valve. Massongo et al. treated 60 patients in a prospective study, and 48 patients with large pneumothoraces were treated with small tubes and achieved a success rate of 83%. Thirty-six (60%) patients were discharged after 4 hours, and 30 patients (50%) were managed as outpatients. The 1-year recurrence rate was 17%. No severe complications were observed. The mean length of hospitalization was 2.3 ± 3.1 days. This change in management resulted in a 40% reduction in hospital stay–related costs [22].

Utility of Ultrasonography for Chest Tube Insertion and Care

Ultrasonography is superior to standard supine chest X-ray and is similar to chest CT radiography for detection of pneumothorax and pleural fluid [23,24]. Because evacuation of a pneumothorax and removal of pleural fluid are the main indications for chest tube insertion, ultrasonography has application for chest tube insertion and care.

Equipment

The ultrasonography examination is performed using a phased-array cardiac probe (3.5 to 5.0 MHz) with abdominal preset whose small footprint allows for examination between rib interspaces. A curvilinear abdominal probe may also be used. The linear high frequency probe lacks sufficient penetration to visualize deeper thoracic structures such as atelectatic lung underlying the pleural effusion, but is useful for identification of lung point while mapping out the extent of a pneumothorax.

Pleural Effusion Scanning Technique

A series of scan lines is performed over the chest in order to identify and characterize the pleural effusion, and to establish a safe site for needle insertion that avoids injury to adjacent organs. A free-flowing pleural effusion will assume a dependent position in the thorax owing to gravitational effect, so the operator examines for fluid over the lateral chest in the supine patient. A loculated pleural effusion may be located at any point in the thorax. The operator can readily locate a loculated effusion and insert a targeted chest tube for drainage of the pleural fluid [25].

Chest Tube Insertion and Care

Ultrasonography permits selection of a chest tube with the appropriate and safe angle and depth for insertion into a pleural effusion. The principles of site selection for chest tube insertion are the same as for thoracentesis (see Chapter 12 Thoracentesis). Site selection can be done rapidly in the emergency situation (thoracic trauma, tension pneumothorax on ventilatory support). Unintentional insertion of the chest tube in a subdiaphragmatic position with injury to the liver or spleen, cardiac perforation, or lung insertion are all recognized complications of chest tube insertion that can be avoided by the simple expedient of using ultrasonography for all chest tube insertions, if the capability is available [26].

Once the chest tube is in place, ultrasonography is useful for tracking adequacy of fluid drainage. Owing to the simplicity of the examination, ultrasonography is used to assess the amount of residual fluid. On occasion, a chest tube will not adequately drain the pleural effusion because of misplacement, tube blockage, or loculations. Ultrasonography can detect the adequacy of drainage; and, if the fluid is not being removed, guide decisions related to chest tube replacement or manipulation. Follow-up ultrasonography examinations take little time and are performed by the intensivist team at point of care as often as required in order to guide ongoing management of the chest tube. The decision to remove the tube may be determined with ultrasonography. At the appropriate time, the tube is clamped. Ultrasonography is used to determine if there is significant fluid reaccumulation. If not, the chest tube may be removed. It is feasible to use ultrasonography as the main imaging modality for management of pleural fluid removal.

Pneumothorax

Scanning Technique

A series of scan lines are performed over the chest in order to locate the pneumothorax and to establish a safe site for chest tube insertion that avoids injury to adjacent organs. In the supine patient, air in the pleural space will distribute anteriorly; so the examination for pneumothorax is concentrated over the anterior and lateral chest. Not all pneumothoraces assume a typical distribution. A loculated pneumothorax is always a possibility. This may occur with pleural adhesions that cannot be detected with ultrasonography. Excepting the emergency situation where an acute life-threatening tension pneumothorax is under consideration, ultrasonography is integrated with the review of the chest radiography and chest CT in order to rule out the presence of a loculated pneumothorax before targeted insertion of a chest tube.

Chest Tube Insertion and Care

The presence of lung sliding, lung pulse, or B lines rules out pneumothorax at the site of the examination (See Chapter 11 Lung Ultrasonography). Multiple intercostal spaces can be examined in a short period time in order to exclude pneumothorax with a high level of certainty in the patient. The absence of lung sliding is characteristic but not diagnostic for a pneumothorax. Identification of a lung point verifies the presence of pneumothorax [27] and allows the operator to map out the lateral extent of the pneumothorax. This is helpful in determining a safe site for chest tube insertion [28]. Most pneumothoraces are not complete (i.e., they result in partial lung atelectasis). The chest tube needs to be inserted into the pneumothorax space. Insertion where lung is still inflated against the chest wall may result in placement of the chest tube into the lung. The operator inserts the device into the area of the chest that lacks lung sliding and that is demarcated laterally by the lung point.

Once the tube is inserted, adequacy of lung inflation is determined by the return of lung sliding, lung pulse, and/or B lines. The timing of chest tube removal following chest tube insertion for pneumothorax is guided with ultrasonography as follows [29–31]:

1. The lung is determined to be fully inflated by ultrasonography, and there is no air leak from the chest tube.
2. The team determines that there are no clinical factors that require continued chest tube use.
3. The tube is clamped, and the chest is examined with ultrasonography immediately for evidence of reaccumulation of the pneumothorax.
4. Over the course of several hours, the chest is examined with ultrasonography for evidence of delayed pneumothorax accumulation.
5. If the lung remains inflated by ultrasonography criteria, the tube may be removed.

ACKNOWLEDGMENTS

Robert A. Lancey, M.D., contributed to previous revisions of this chapter.

References

1. American College of Surgeons. Committee on Trauma: *ATLS, Advanced Trauma Life Support for Doctors: Student Course Manual.* 9th ed. American College of Surgeons, 2012, p 96.
2. Brunelli A, Beretta E, Cassivi SD, et al: Consensus definitions to promote an evidence-based approach to management of the pleural space. A collaborative proposal by ESTS, AATS, STS, and GTSC. *Eur J Cardiothorac Surg* 40(2):291–297, 2011.
3. Finley DJ, Rusch VW: Anatomy of the pleura. *Thorac Surg Clin* 21(2):157–163, 2011.
4. Soldati G, Testa A, Sher S, et al: Occult traumatic pneumothorax: diagnostic accuracy of lung ultrasonography in the emergency department. *Chest* 133(1):204–211, 2008.
5. Wilkerson RG, Stone MB: Sensitivity of bedside ultrasound and supine anteroposterior chest radiographs for the identification of pneumothorax after blunt trauma. *Acad Emerg Med* 17(1):11–17, 2010.
6. Blasivas M, Lyon M, Duggal S: A prospective comparison of supine chest radiography and bedside ultrasound for the diagnosis of traumatic pneumothorax. *Acad Emerg Med* 12(9):844–849, 2005.
7. Kelly A-M, Loy J, Tsang AY, et al: Estimating the rate of re-expansion of spontaneous pneumothorax by a formula derived from computed tomography volumetry studies. *Emerg Med J* (23):780–782, 2006.
8. Ziegler DW, Agarwal NN: The morbidity and mortality of rib fractures. *J Trauma* 37:975, 1994.
9. Girdhar A, Shujaat A, Bajwa A: Management of infectious processes of the pleural space: a review. *Pulm Med* 2012:816502, 2012.
10. McGrath EE, Blades Z, Anderson PB: Chylothorax: aetiology, diagnosis and therapeutic options. *Respir Med* 104(1):1–8, 2010.
11. Light RW: Pleural effusions. *Med Clin North Am* 95(6):1055–1070, 2011.
12. Kuhajda I, Zarogoulidis K, Kougioumtzi I, et al: Tube thoracostomy; chest tube implantation and follow up. *J Thorac Dis* 6(4):S470, 2014.
13. Ishikura H, Kimura F: The use of flexible silastic drains after chest surgery: novel thoracic drainage. *Ann Thorac Surg* 81:231, 2006.
14. Sethuraman KN, Duong D, Mehta S, et al: Complications of tube thoracostomy placement in the emergency department. *J Emerg Med* 40(1):14–20, 2011.
15. Frankel TL, Hill PC, Stamou SB, et al: Silastic drains versus conventional chest tubes after coronary artery bypass. *Chest* 124:108, 2003.

16. Lotano VE. *Chest Tube Thoracostomy. Critical Care Medicine: Principles of Diagnosis and Management in the Adult (Expert Consult-Online and Print)*. Philadelphia, PA, Elsevier Saunders, 2013, p 219.
17. Cerfolio RJ, Bryant AS: The management of chest tubes after pulmonary resection. *Thorac Surg Clin* 20(3):399–405, 2010.
18. Cameron EW, Mirvis SE, Shanmuganathan K, et al: Computed tomography of malpositioned thoracostomy drains: a pictorial essay. *Clin Radiol* 52:187, 1997.
19. Younes RN, Gross JL, Aguiar S, et al: When to remove a chest tube? A randomized study with subsequent prospective consecutive validation. *J Am Coll Surg* 195:658–662, 2002.
20. Durai R, Hoque H, Davies TW: Managing a chest tube and drainage system. *AORN J* 91(2):275–283, 2010.
21. Kulvatunyou N, Vijayasekaran A, Hansen A, et al: Two-year experience of using pigtail catheters to treat traumatic pneumothorax: a changing trend. *J Trauma* 71(5):1104–1107, 2011.
22. Massongo M, Leroy S, Scherpereel A, et al: Outpatient management of primary spontaneous pneumothorax: a prospective study. *Eur Respir J* 43(2):582–590, 2014.
23. Lichtenstein D, Goldstein I, Mourgeon E, et al: Comparative diagnostic performances of auscultation, chest radiography, and lung ultrasonography in acute respiratory distress syndrome. *Anesthesiology* 100:9–15, 2004.
24. Xirouchaki N, Magkanas E, Vaporidi K, et al: Lung ultrasound in critically ill patients: comparison with bedside chest radiography. *Intensive Care Med* 37(9):1488–1493, 2011.
25. Moulton JS: Image-guided management of complicated pleural fluid collections. *Radiol Clin North Am* 38:345–374, 2000.
26. Havelick T, Teoh R, Laws D, et al; Pleural Disease Guideline Group: Pleural procedures and thoracic ultrasound. British Thoracic Society pleural disease guidelines 2010. *Thorax* 65:i61–i76, 2010.
27. Lichtenstein D, Mezière G, Biderman P, et al: The "lung point": an ultrasound sign specific to pneumothorax. *Intensive Care Med* 26(10):1434–1440, 2000.
28. Soldati G, Testa A, Sher S, et al: Occult traumatic pneumothorax: diagnostic accuracy of lung ultrasonography in the emergency department. *Chest* 133:204–211, 2008.
29. Galbois A, Ait-Oufella H, Baudel JL, et al: Pleural ultrasound compared with chest radiographic detection of pneumothorax resolution after drainage. *Chest* 138:648–655, 2010.
30. Soult MC, Collins JN, Novosel TJ, et al: Thoracic ultrasound can predict safe removal of thoracostomy tubes. *J Trauma Acute Care Surg* 77:256–261, 2014.
31. Lavingia KS, Soult MC, Collins JN, et al: Basic ultrasound training can replace chest radiography for safe tube thoracostomy removal. *Am Surg* 80:783–786, 2014.

Chapter 14 ■ Cardiopulmonary Resuscitation

BRUCE GREENBERG • ABDULJABBAR DHEYAB

INTRODUCTION

The era of modern resuscitation can be most directly traced to a report of electrical reversal of ventricular fibrillation (VF) by externally applied electrodes described in 1956 by Zoll et al. [1]. This ability to reverse a fatal arrhythmia without opening the chest challenged the medical community to develop a method of sustaining adequate ventilation and circulation long enough to bring the electric defibrillator to the patient's aid. By 1958, adequate rescue ventilation became possible with the development of the mouth-to-mouth technique described by Safar et al. [2] and Elam et al. [3]. In 1960, Kouwenhoven et al. [4] described "closed chest cardiac massage," thus introducing the modern era of cardiopulmonary resuscitation (CPR). The simplicity of this technique—"all that is needed are two hands"—has led to its widespread dissemination. The interaction of this technique of sternal compression with mouth-to-mouth ventilation was developed as basic CPR. The first national conference on CPR was sponsored by the National Academy of Sciences in 1966 [5]. Instructions in CPR for both professionals and the public soon followed through community programs in basic life support (BLS) and advanced cardiac life support (ACLS) [6] and have been updated periodically.

For individuals with adequately preserved cardiopulmonary and neurologic systems, the cessation of breathing and cardiac contraction may be reversed if CPR and definitive care are quickly available. The short period during which the loss of vital signs may be reversed is often referred to as *clinical death*. If ventilation and circulation are not restored before irreversible damage to vital structures occurs, then irreversible death occurs. This is referred to as *biologic death*. In difficult circumstances, the best single criterion (medical and legal) for the ultimate death of the functioning integrated human individual (i.e., the person) is brain death [7,8]. By this criterion, we can make decisions as to the appropriateness of continuing "life-sustaining" techniques.

EFFICACY

High quality CPR produces a cardiac output of 25% to 33% of normal [9,10].The benefit of rapid initiation of CPR has been demonstrated in numerous studies [11–14]. A large registry that recorded outcomes of over 70,000 cardiac arrest patients noted that survival from sudden cardiac arrest has slowly improved, with 8.3% of patients surviving to hospital discharge [15]. Survival with a good neurologic outcome, usually defined as being no worse than moderate disability, has also improved. In a large randomized controlled trial comparing different target temperatures after cardiac arrest of patients who survived to hospital admission and maintained a pulse for 20 minutes, survival at 6 months was approximately 50%, and the majority of survivors had good neurologic outcomes [16]. Data from prehospital care systems in Seattle showed that 43% of patients found in VF were discharged from the hospital if CPR (i.e., BLS) was applied within 4 minutes and defibrillation (i.e., ACLS) within 8 minutes. If the onset of CPR was delayed, or if the time to defibrillation was longer than 10 minutes, the probability was greater that the patient was in asystole or in *fine* VF that converted to asystole. Survival decreases as each minute passes without return of spontaneous circulation (ROSC), and a compression rate of 85 to 100 is associated with better survival than higher or lower rates [17]. Early access to defibrillation via the use of automated external defibrillators (AEDs) also improves survival [18].

Even though patients experiencing cardiac arrest in the hospital can be expected to receive CPR and definitive therapy well within the 4- and 8-minute time frames, the outcomes of in-hospital cardiac arrests are poor. The largest report of survival after in-hospital cardiac arrest recorded that 15% of victims survive to hospital discharge [19]. With the wide availability of AEDs in the community, two large registry studies have suggested that survival with intact neurologic function may be improving. In a study from Japan, survival with good neurologic function increased from 3.3% to 8.2% from 2005 to 2012 [20]. In a statewide study from North Carolina, survival with a favorable neurologic outcome increased from 7.1% to 9.7% from 2010 to 2013 [21]. In both of these studies bystander defibrillation was associated with a substantial increase in survival with intact neurologic function.

Researchers continue to evaluate new approaches and techniques, and further refinements in the delivery of CPR can be expected. Although research into improved CPR techniques and devices should be encouraged, research in this field is difficult. Animal models vary, and animal data may not be valid in humans. Before new CPR techniques can be adopted, they must have been demonstrated, ideally in humans, to improve either survival or neurologic outcomes.

Any significant improvement in CPR technique would seem to require an understanding of the mechanism by which blood flows during CPR. While there is no conclusive evidence as to the mechanism of blood flow during CPR, the two main theories are the cardiac compression (or pump) theory and the thoracic pump theory [22].

In 1960, when Kouwenhoven et al. [4] reported on the efficacy of closed chest cardiac massage, most researchers accepted the theory that blood is propelled by compressing the heart trapped between the sternum and the vertebral columns—the cardiac compression theory. According to this theory, during sternal compression, intraventricular pressures rise higher than the pressures elsewhere in the chest. With each sternal compression, semilunar valves would be expected to open and atrioventricular (AV) valves to close. With sternal release, pressure in the ventricles would be expected to fall and AV valves would open, allowing the heart to fill from the lungs and systemic veins.

In contrast to the cardiac compression theory, the thoracic pump theory proposes that the propulsion of blood during sternal compression is due to increased intrathoracic pressure [23,24]. According to this theory, the heart serves as a conduit only during CPR. Forward flow is generated by a pressure gradient between intrathoracic and extrathoracic vascular structures. Flow to the arterial side is favored by functional venous valves and greater compressibility of veins, compared to arteries, at their exit points from the thorax. Studies using pressure measurements [13] and angiography [23] support this hypothesis, as do most echocardiographic studies [25]. It is noteworthy that the dominating mechanism may vary among individual patients, with one large review suggesting that the cardiac pump predominates in children, whereas the thoracic pump is more important in adults [22].

EXPERIMENTAL AND ALTERNATIVE TECHNIQUES OF CPR

Several experimental and alternative techniques of CPR have been proposed, though none are recommended for general use according to the American Heart Association (AHA) 2010 guidelines [10]. High frequency chest compressions, such as at a rate >120 per minute, may improve hemodynamics, but have not improved clinical outcomes. Open chest CPR, in which the heart is manually compressed via a left thoracotomy incision, may have a role in select cases of penetrating trauma or in the early postoperative period after cardiothoracic surgery. This technique should not be attempted unless adequate facilities and trained personnel are available. Interposed abdominal compression CPR was developed by Ralston et al. [26] and Babbs et al. [27]. This technique includes manual compression of the abdomen by an extra rescuer during the relaxation phase of chest compression. The mid-abdomen is compressed at a point halfway between the xiphoid process and the umbilicus with a force of approximately 100 mm Hg of external pressure. This pressure is estimated to be equivalent to that required to palpate the aortic pulse in a subject with a normal pulse. Two randomized clinical trials have demonstrated a statistically significant improvement in outcome measures for in-hospital cardiac arrest [28,29] but no improvement has been shown for out-of-hospital arrest [30]. On the basis of these findings, interposed abdominal compression CPR is recommended as an option for in-hospital cardiac arrest when sufficient trained personnel are available [10]. However, the safety and efficacy of interposed abdominal compression CPR for patients with recent abdominal surgery, pregnancy, or aortic aneurysm has not been studied.

Several mechanical assist devices have been designed to provide or augment compressions (CPR vests, powered piston devices, active decompression devices using a suction cup applied to the anterior chest). However, none of these have been clearly shown to improve outcomes, and none are recommended by the AHA 2010 guidelines [10]. The use of an impedance threshold device is an option according to the AHA guidelines. These devices limit air entry into the lungs during decompression, allowing the resulting negative pressure to induce more effectively venous return. They are typically used with an advanced airway (supraglottic or endotracheal) [10]. One review identified an improvement in survival to hospital admission, but no improvement in survival to discharge or in neurologic outcome with the use of an impedance threshold device in out-of-hospital cardiac arrest [31].

INFECTIOUS DISEASES AND CPR

The fear provoked by the spread of human immunodeficiency virus (HIV) may lead to excessive caution when dealing with strangers. Fear of acquiring infection during the performance of CPR, specifically mouth-to-mouth ventilation, can best be counteracted by continued education.

Saliva has not been implicated in the transmission of HIV even after bites, percutaneous inoculation, or contamination of open wounds with saliva from HIV-infected patients [32–34]. In fact, neither hepatitis B or C nor HIV have been reported to have been acquired via CPR, excepting needle sticks and prolonged exposure of damaged skin to blood (not saliva). Infections thought to have been transmitted by CPR include *Mycobacterium tuberculosis*, meningococcus, herpes simplex, *Shigella*, *Streptococcus pyogenes*, *Salmonella*, and *Neisseria gonorrhoeae* [34].

Implications for Rescuers with Known or Potential Infection

Potential rescuers who know or are highly suspicious that they are infected with a serious pathogenic organism should not perform mouth-to-mouth ventilation if another rescuer is available who is less likely to be infectious or if the circumstances allow for any other immediate and effective method of ventilation, such as using mechanical ventilation devices. Compression-only CPR is a reasonable and safe alternative.

Health care professionals with known or potential infections should have ready access to mechanical ventilation devices. Bag–valve–mask devices should be available as initial ventilation equipment, and early endotracheal intubation should be encouraged when possible. Masks with one-way valves and plastic mouth and nose covers with filtered openings are available and provide some protection from transfer of oral fluids and aerosols. S-shaped mouthpieces, masks without one-way valves, and handkerchiefs provide little, if any, barrier protection and should not be considered for routine use. With these guidelines in mind, health care professionals are reminded that they have a special moral and ethical, and in some instances legal, obligation to provide CPR, especially in the setting of their occupational duties.

STANDARD PROCEDURES AND TEAM EFFORT

The distinctive function of the intensive care unit (ICU) is to serve as a locus of concentrated expertise in medical and nursing care, life-sustaining technologies, and treatment of complex multiorgan system derangements. Historically, it was the development of effective treatment for otherwise rapidly fatal arrhythmias during acute myocardial infarction that impelled the medical community to establish ICUs [35]. Rapid response by medical personnel has been facilitated by constant professional attendance and the development of widely accepted guidelines for resuscitation. Each member of the professional team is expected to respond in accordance with these guidelines.

Avoiding the need for CPR and ACLS by early intervention is a goal of rapid response teams (RRT). RRT, also called medical evaluation teams (MET), have been consistently shown to decrease hospital cardiorespiratory arrest rates [36]. Some studies have found a decrease in hospital mortality with the use of RRT, though this has not been found in all studies. How RRT can best be organized and implemented, as well as which hospitals benefit most, is yet to be determined [37].

The skills necessary to perform adequately during a cardiac or respiratory arrest and to interface smoothly with ACLS techniques cannot be mastered by reading texts and manuals alone. CPR courses taught according to AHA guidelines allow hands-on experience that approximates the real situation and tests the psychomotor skills needed in an emergency. All those who engage in patient care should be trained in BLS techniques. Those whose duties require a higher level of performance should be trained in ACLS as well. As these skills deteriorate with disuse, they need to be maintained. It is worth noting that there is no "certification" in BLS or ACLS. Issuance of a "card" is neither a license to perform these techniques nor a guarantee of skill, but simply an acknowledgment that an individual attended a specific course and passed the required tests. If employers or government agencies require such a card of their health workers, it is by their own mandate.

The ensuing discussion of BLS and ACLS techniques follows the recommendations and guidelines established by the AHA [38].

BASIC LIFE SUPPORT FOR ADULTS WITH AN UNOBSTRUCTED AIRWAY

BLS is meant to support the circulation and respiration of those who have experienced cardiac or respiratory arrest. After recognizing and ascertaining its need, definitive help is summoned without delay and CPR is initiated. A major focus of the 2010 guidelines is on the supremacy of effective compressions, with limited interruptions. The importance of early defibrillation is also stressed.

Respiratory Arrest

Respiratory arrest may result from airway obstruction, near-drowning, stroke, smoke inhalation, drug overdose, electrocution, or physical trauma. In the ICU, infections, pulmonary congestion, respiratory distress syndrome, and mucus plugs are frequent causes of primary respiratory arrests. The heart usually continues to circulate blood for several minutes, and the residual oxygen in the lungs and blood may keep the brain viable. Early intervention by opening the airway and providing ventilation may prevent cardiac arrest and may be all that is required to restore effective respiration. In the intubated patient, careful suctioning of the airway and attention to the ventilator settings are required. Lay rescuers should not check for a pulse, but if a health care professional ascertains that the patient does have a pulse, then rescue breaths should be performed at a rate of one breath every 5 to 6 seconds while arranging for more definitive airway management.

Cardiac Arrest

Cardiac arrest results in rapid depletion of oxygen in vital organs. After 6 minutes, brain damage is expected to occur, except in cases of hypothermia (e.g., near-drowning in cold water). Therefore, early bystander CPR (within 4 minutes) and rapid ACLS with attempted defibrillation (within 8 minutes) are essential in improving survival and neurologic recovery rates [39].

The sequence of steps in CPR may be summarized as the CABs of CPR: *c*irculation, *a*irway, and *b*reathing. This mnemonic is useful for teaching the public, but it should be remembered that each step is preceded by *assessment* of the need for intervention: before starting compressions, the rescuer determines unresponsiveness; before breathing, the rescuer determines breathlessness (Table 14.1).

Assessment and Determination of Unresponsiveness and Alerting of Emergency Medical Services

A person who has undergone cardiac arrest may be found in an apparently unconscious state (i.e., an unwitnessed arrest) or may be observed to suddenly lapse into apparent unconsciousness (i.e., a witnessed arrest). In either case, the rescuer must react promptly to assess the person's responsiveness by attempting to wake and communicate with the person by tapping or gently shaking and shouting. The rescuer should summon nearby staff for help. If no other person is immediately available, the rescuer should activate emergency medical services (EMS) or call the hospital emergency line for the resuscitation team to respond ("code blue").

In the ICU, nearly all arrests should be witnessed. Early recognition of cardiac and respiratory arrests is facilitated by electronic and video monitoring. Unfortunately, it is quite possible for a patient to become lost behind this profusion of electronic signals, the dependability of which varies widely. For several precious minutes, a heart with pulseless electric activity (PEA) continues to provide a comforting electronic signal, while the brain suffers hypoxic damage. A high frequency of false alarms and an overwhelming volume of alarms may dangerously raise the threshold of awareness and prolong the response time of the ICU team. [40]. The overall efficacy of the monitoring devices depends highly on meticulous skin preparation and care of electrodes, transducers, pressure cables, as well as caregiver response to alarms.

Sudden apparent loss of consciousness, occasionally with seizures, may be the first signal of arrest and requires prompt reaction. After determining unresponsiveness, the pulse is assessed by a health care provider for no more than 10 seconds. If the carotid pulse cannot definitely be palpated in 5 to 10 seconds and a defibrillator is not immediately available, CPR should be begun. Compressions should be performed at a rate of 100 per minute, compressing the chest 2 inches with each repetition and allowing the chest to recoil fully. Interruptions to compressions should only be allowed for essential interventions, such as intubation or defibrillation. Note that, in the 2010 guidelines, compressions should be started *before* assessing breathing.

Opening the Airway and Determining Breathlessness

After establishing unresponsiveness, activating EMS, and delivering 30 compressions and positioning the individual on his or her back, the next step is to open the airway and check for spontaneous breathing (see Chapter 8). In a monitored arrest with VF or tachycardia, this step is taken after initial attempts to defibrillate. Meticulous attention to establishing an airway and supplying adequate ventilation is essential to any further resuscitative effort. The team leader must carefully monitor the adequacy of ventilation, as well as direct the resuscitative effort. The leadership role is best accomplished if the leader does not directly perform procedures.

TABLE 14.1

Experimental and Alternate Techniques of Cardiopulmonary Resuscitation (CPR)

Researcher [Reference]	Technique	Notes
Taylor et al. [15]	Longer compression	Proposed use of longer duration to 40%–50% of the duration compression–relaxation cycle
Chandra et al. [14,16]	Simultaneous chest compression and lung inflation	High airway pressures of 60–110 mm Hg are used to augment carotid flow, requiring intubation and a mechanical ventilator. Its use has not met with universal success
Harris et al. [39]	Abdominal binding	Abdominal binding increases intrathoracic pressure by redistributing blood into the thorax during CPR. Studies have demonstrated adverse effects on coronary perfusion, cerebral oxygenation, and canine resuscitation
Redding [17] Koehler et al. [18] Chandra et al. [19] Ralston et al. [20]	Interposed abdominal	Abdominal compression is released when the sternum is compressed. Higher oxygen delivery and cerebral and myocardial blood flows are reported. One study suggests an improved survival and neurologic outcome
Barranco et al. [21]	Simultaneous chest	Simultaneous chest and abdominal compression provided higher intrathoracic pressures in compression in humans
Maier et al. [22]	High-impulse CPR	At compression rates of 150/min (with moderate force and brief duration), cardiac output in dogs increased as the coronary flow remained as high as 75% of prearrest values. High impulse and high compression rates can result in rescuer fatigue and increased injury
Cohen et al. [23]	Active compression	Forceful rebound using a plunger-like device resulted in improved hemodynamics. Clinical results are equivocal
Halperin et al. [24]	Vest inflation	Circumferential chest pressure with an inflatable vest showed improved hemodynamics and survival in dogs

The head tilt–chin lift maneuver is usually successful in opening the airway. The head is tilted backward by a hand placed on the forehead. The fingers of the other hand are positioned under the mandible and the chin is lifted upward. The teeth are almost approximated, but the mouth is not allowed to close. Because considerable cervical hyperextension occurs, this method should be avoided in patients with cervical injuries or suspected cervical injuries. The jaw-thrust maneuver provides the safest initial approach to opening the airway of a patient with a cervical spine injury; it usually allows excellent airway opening with a minimum of cervical extension. The angles of the mandible are grasped using both hands and lifting upward, thus tilting the head gently backward.

Rescue Breathing

If spontaneous breathing is absent, rescue breathing with an airway–mask–bag unit must be initiated (see Chapter 8). If equipment is immediately available and the rescuer is trained, intubation and ventilatory adjuncts should be used initially. Each breath should be delivered during 1 second, allowing the patient's lungs to deflate between breaths. A rate of 10 to 12 breaths per minute is maintained for as long as necessary, with tidal volumes of approximately 600 mL. Delivering the breath during 1 second helps to prevent gastric insufflation compared with faster delivery. Melker et al. [41] demonstrated airway pressures well in excess of those required to open the lower esophageal sphincter when quick breaths are used to ventilate patients. If the patient wears dentures, they are usually best left in place to assist in forming an adequate seal.

If air cannot be passed into the patient's lungs, another attempt at opening the airway should be made. The jaw-thrust maneuver may be necessary. If subsequent attempts at ventilation are still unsuccessful, the patient should be considered to have an obstructed airway and attempts should be made to dislodge a potential foreign body obstruction.

Chest Compressions

Artificial circulation depends on adequate chest compression through sternal depression. Recent recommendations for CPR are to push hard and push fast at a rate of 100 compressions per minute, allow full chest recoil, and minimize interruptions in chest compressions [42]. The safest manner of depressing the sternum is with the heel of the rescuer's hand at the nipple line, with the fingers kept off the rib cage. It is usually most effective to cover the heel of one hand with the heel of the other, the heels being parallel to the long axis of the sternum. If the rescuer's hands are placed either too high or too low on the sternum, or if the fingers are allowed to lie flat against the rib cage, broken ribs and organ laceration can result. Although it is important to allow the chest to recoil to its normal position after each compression, it is not advisable to lift the hands from the chest or change their position.

The rescuer's elbows should be kept locked and the arms straight, with the shoulders directly over the patient's sternum. This position allows the rescuer's upper body to provide a perpendicularly directed force for sternal depression. The sternum is depressed 2.0 inch (4 to 5 cm) at a rate of approximately 100 compressions per minute. In large patients, a slightly greater depth of sternal compression may be needed to generate a palpable carotid or femoral pulse. At the end of each compression, pressure is released and the sternum is allowed to return to its normal position. Equal time should be allotted to compression and relaxation with smooth movements, avoiding jerking or bouncing the sternum. Ventilation and sternal compression should not be interrupted except under special circumstances. Warranted interruptions include execution of ACLS procedures (e.g., endotracheal intubation and placement of central venous lines) or an absolute need to move the patient. Even in these limited circumstances, interruption of CPR should be minimized. In a retrospective analysis of VF patients, interruption of CPR was associated with a decreased probability of conversion of VF to another rhythm [43].

New data suggest that chest compression-only CPR is as effective as standard CPR (chest compression plus rescue breathing) for out-of-hospital arrest [44,45]. Subgroup analysis in one study suggested a trend for increased survival to hospital discharge for chest compression-only CPR if the cause of the arrest was cardiac in origin or the rhythm was shockable [44]. For lay persons, the 2010 AHA guideline supports compression-only CPR.

Two-Rescuer CPR

The combination of artificial ventilation and circulation can be delivered more efficiently and with less fatigue by two rescuers. One rescuer, positioned at the patient's side, performs sternal compressions, while the other, positioned at the patient's head, maintains an open airway and performs ventilation. This technique should be mastered by all health care workers called on to perform CPR. Lay people have not been routinely taught this method in the interest of improving retention of basic skills. The compression rate for two-rescuer CPR, as for one-rescuer CPR, is approximately 100 compressions per minute. The recommendation of the compression-to-ventilation ratio is 30 to 2. The only exception to this recommendation is when two health care workers are providing CPR to a child or infant (except newborns); in this instance, a 15 to 2 compression-to-ventilation ratio should be used [42]. When the rescuer performing compressions is tired, the two rescuers should switch responsibilities with the minimum possible delay.

Complications of BLS Procedures

Proper application of CPR should minimize serious complications, but serious risks are inherent in BLS procedures and should be accepted in the context of cardiac arrest. Awareness of these potential complications is important to the postresuscitative care of the arrest patient.

Gastric distention and regurgitation are common complications of artificial ventilation without endotracheal intubation. These complications are more likely to occur when ventilation pressures exceed the opening pressure of the lower esophageal sphincter. In mask ventilation, 1 second should be allowed for air delivery. Although an esophageal obturator airway may decrease the threat of distention and regurgitation during its use, the risk is increased at the time of its removal. To obviate this risk, the trachea should be intubated and protected with an inflated cuff before the esophageal cuff is deflated and the esophageal obturator removed.

Complications of sternal compression and manual thrusts include rib and sternal fractures, costochondral separation, flail chest, pneumothorax, hemothorax, hemopericardium, subcutaneous emphysema, mediastinal emphysema, pulmonary contusions, bone marrow and fat embolism, and lacerations of the esophagus, stomach, inferior vena cava, liver, or spleen [46]. Although rib fractures are common during CPR, especially in the elderly, no serious sequelae are likely unless tension pneumothorax occurs and is not recognized. The more serious complications are unlikely to occur if proper hand position is maintained and exaggerated depth of sternal compression is avoided. Overzealous or repeated abdominal or chest thrusts for relief of airway obstruction are more likely to cause fractures or lacerations. For this reason, abdominal thrust is not recommended for the infant younger than 1 year.

Monitoring the Effectiveness of Basic Life Support

The effectiveness of rescue effort is assessed regularly by the ventilating rescuer, who notes the chest motion and the escape of expired air. Unintentional hyperventilation is frequent during CPR, with studies in clinical situations showing that patients are commonly ventilated at a rate of 18 to 30, far faster than recommended [47]. The adequacy of circulation is assessed by noting an adequate carotid pulse with sternal compressions.

Pupillary response, if present, is a good indicator of cerebral circulation. However, fixed and dilated pupils should not be accepted as evidence of irreversible or biologic death. Ocular diseases, such as cataracts, and a variety of drugs (e.g., atropine and ganglion-blocking agents) interfere with the pupillary light reflex. The decision to cease BLS should be made only by the physician in charge of the resuscitation effort; this decision should not be made until it is obvious that the patient's cardiovascular system will not respond with ROSC to adequate administration of ACLS, including electric and pharmacologic interventions. Remediable problems such as airway obstruction, severe hypovolemia, and pericardial tamponade should also have been reasonably excluded by careful attention to ACLS protocols. Published guidelines suggest that BLS can be stopped if all of the following are present: the event was not witnessed by EMS personnel, no AED has been used, and there is no ROSC in the prehospital setting [48] (Table 14.2).

PEDIATRIC RESUSCITATION

The 2010 AHA guidelines for pediatric CPR are similar to the adult guidelines, with the exception that when performing two-person CPR, a ratio of 15 compressions to two breaths should be used. The rate of compressions remains 100 per minute, and the depth of compressions from 1.5 inches or infants to 2 inches for children; another way to gauge compression depth is to target one-third of the anteroposterior (AP) size of the patient [49].

OBSTRUCTED AIRWAY

An unconscious patient can experience airway obstruction when the tongue falls backward into the pharynx. Alternatively, the epiglottis may block the airway when the pharyngeal muscles are lax. In the sedated or ill patient, regurgitation of stomach contents into the pharynx is a frequent cause of respiratory arrest. Blood clots from head and facial injuries are another source of pharyngeal and upper airway obstruction. Even otherwise healthy people may have foreign body obstruction from poorly chewed food, large wads of gum, and so forth. The combination of attempting to swallow inadequately chewed food, drinking alcohol, and laughing is particularly conducive to pharyngeal obstruction. Children's smaller airways are likely to obstruct with small nuts or candies. Children are also prone to airway obstruction by placing toys or objects such as marbles or beads in their mouths.

Patients who experience partial obstruction with reasonable gas exchange should be encouraged to continue breathing efforts with attempts at coughing. A patient whose obstruction is so severe that air exchange is obviously markedly impaired (cyanosis with lapsing consciousness) should be treated as having complete obstruction.

Patients who experience complete obstruction may still be conscious, but are unable to cough or vocalize. A subdiaphragmatic

TABLE 14.2

Summary of Basic Life Support ABCD Maneuvers for Infants, Children, and Adults (Newborn Information Not Included)

Maneuver	Adult Lay Rescuer: 8 y HCP: adolescent and older	Child Lay Rescuers: 1–8 y HCP: 1 y–adolescent	Infant Younger than 1 y of age
Airway	Head tilt–chin lift (HCP: suspected trauma, use jaw thrust)		
Breathing: initial	Two breaths at 1 s/breath	Two effective breaths at 1 s/breath	
HCP: rescue breathing without chest compressions	10–12 breaths/min (approximate)	12–20 breaths/min (approximate)	
HCP: rescue breaths for CPR with advanced airway		8–10 breaths/min (approximate)	
Foreign body airway obstruction	Conscious: abdominal thrusts		Infant conscious: back slaps
	Unconscious: CPR		Infant unconscious: CPR
Circulation HCP: pulse check (≤10 s)	Carotid		Brachial or femoral
Compression landmarks	Lower half of the sternum, between nipples		Just below the nipple line (lower half of the sternum)
Compression method: Push hard and fast	Heel of one hand, other hand on top	Heel of one hand or as for adults	Two or three fingers
Allow complete recoil			HCP (two rescuers): two thumb–encircling hands
Compression depth	1½–2 in	Approximately one-third to one-half the depth of the chest	
Compression rate	Approximately 100/min		
Compression-to-ventilation ratio	30:2 (one or two rescuers)	30:2 (single rescuer)	
		HCP: 15:2 (two rescuers)	
Defibrillation: AED	Use adult pads Do not use child pads	Use AED after five cycles of CPR (out of hospital) Use pediatric system for children 1–8 y if available HCP: for sudden collapse (out of hospital) or in-hospital arrest use AED as soon as available	No recommendation for infants <1 y of age

Note: Maneuvers used by only health care providers are indicated by "HCP." CPR, cardiopulmonary resuscitation; AED, automatic external defibrillator. Adapted from ECC Committee, Subcommittees and Task Forces of the American Heart Association: 2005 American Heart Association Guidelines for Cardiopulmonary Resuscitation and Emergency Cardiovascular Care. *Circulation* 112[24, Suppl]:IV1–203, 2005.

abdominal thrust may force air from the lungs in sufficient quantity to expel a foreign body from the airway [50].

If the person is still standing, the rescuer stands behind the person and wraps his or her arms around the person's waist. The fist of one hand is placed with the thumb side against the person's abdomen in the midline, slightly above the umbilicus and well below the xiphoid process. The fist is grasped with the other hand and quickly thrust inward and upward. It may be necessary to repeat the thrust six to ten times to clear the airway. Each thrust should be a separate and distinct movement.

If the patient is responsive and lying down, he or she should be positioned face up in the supine position. The rescuer kneels beside or astride the person's thighs and places the heel of one hand against the person's abdomen, slightly above the umbilicus and well below the xiphoid process. The other hand is placed directly on top of the first and pressed inward and upward with a quick forceful thrust. If the patient is unresponsive, CPR should be initiated.

If attempted rescue breathing in an arrested patient fails to move air into the lungs, an obstructed airway must be presumed to be present. It may simply be due to the tongue or epiglottis, rather than a foreign body. If the airway remains closed after repositioning the head, other maneuvers to open the airway, including the jaw-thrust and tongue-jaw lift, must be used. Chest thrusts may be substituted for abdominal thrusts in patients in advanced stages of pregnancy, in patients with severe ascites, or in the markedly obese. The fist is placed in midsternum for the erect and conscious patient. For the supine patient, the hand is positioned on the lower sternum, as for external cardiac compression. Each thrust is delivered slowly and distinctly.

If attempts at dislodging a foreign body or relieving airway obstruction fail, special advanced procedures are necessary to provide oxygenation until direct visualization, intubation, or cricothyroidotomy is performed (Chapter 8).

ADVANCED CARDIAC LIFE SUPPORT IN ADULTS

The use of adjunctive equipment, more specialized techniques, and pharmacologic and electric therapy in the treatment of a person who has experienced cardiac or respiratory arrest is generally referred to as *ACLS*. As with any skill, excellence requires both training and practice. An improvement in survival after in-hospital cardiac arrest has been demonstrated after medical house officers were trained in ACLS [51]. An in-depth discussion is available in the ACLS text published by the AHA.

The focus of the following sections is on the techniques and medications used in the initial resuscitative efforts. The demarcation from therapies more commonly reserved for the ICU is often indistinct; indeed, it is expected to vary with the experience of the team and the degree of physician supervision. In general, most ACLS measures should be applied by trained personnel operating within an EMS system in the community, in transport, or in the hospital setting.

Airway and Ventilatory Support

Oxygenation and optimal ventilation are prerequisites for successful resuscitation. Supplemental oxygen should be administered as soon as it becomes available, beginning with 100%. In the postresuscitation period, the amount of administered oxygen may be decreased as guided by oxygen saturation.

Emergency ventilation commonly begins with the combined use of a mask and oral airway. The AHA guideline continues to recommend ventilation during CPR when performed by ACLS providers, but ventilation should neither interrupt early compressions nor delay defibrillation. Mouth-to-mask ventilation is very effective as long as an adequate seal is maintained between the mask and the face; this method is recommended for single-rescuer ACLS. Most masks are best fitted by flaring the top and molding it over the bridge of the nose. The inflated rim is then carefully molded to the cheeks as the mask is allowed to recoil. Relatively firm pressure is required to maintain the seal. Masks with one-way valves also provide a measure of isolation from the patient's saliva and breath aerosol. Bag–valve–mask ventilation requires strong hands and a self-inflating bag. The bag should be connected to a gas reservoir and to oxygen so that 100% oxygen delivery can be approximated. It cannot be overemphasized that the success of this method depends on airway patency and an adequate seal between the mask and the face. Equally important is adequate compression of the bag to deliver the required tidal volume of approximately 600 mL. It is advisable that everyone who uses this technique practice on a manikin to assess the adequacy of the method in his or her hands. Many people will discover that their hands are not large enough or strong enough to deliver 600 mL air. Some may have to squeeze the bag between their elbow and chest wall to supply adequate ventilation. If two people are available to ventilate, one should secure the mask while the other uses both hands to attend to the bag.

Cricoid pressure is not recommended during bag mask ventilation. Nasopharyngeal and oropharyngeal airways are both reasonable options to improve airway patency prior to an advanced airway. Nasopharyngeal airways may cause bleeding, and should be avoided in patients with basilar skull fractures.

The mask should include the following features:

- The use of transparent material, which allows the rescuer to assess lip color and to observe vomitus, mucus, or other obstructing material in the patient's airway.
- A cushioned rim around the mask's perimeter to conform to the patient's face and to facilitate a tight seal.
- A standard 15- to 22-mm connector, which allows the use of additional airway equipment.
- A comfortable fit to the rescuer's hand.
- An oxygen insufflation inlet, which allows oxygen supplementation during mouth-to-mask ventilation.
- A one-way valve, which allows some protection during mouth-to-mask ventilation.
- Availability in appropriate sizes and shapes, for various-sized faces. Most adults will be accommodated by a standard medium-sized (no. 4) oval-shaped mask.

Ventilating bags must be designed to include the following features:

- A self-refilling bag, which allows operation independent of a fresh gas source.
- A fresh gas inlet, which allows ambient air or supplemental oxygen to flow into the reservoir bag through a valve inlet.
- A nipple for oxygen connection, located near the gas inlet valve.
- An oxygen reservoir bag.
- Availability in pediatric and adult sizes.
- A nonrebreathing valve directing flow to the patient during inhalation and to the atmosphere during exhalation. The valve casing should be transparent to allow visual inspection of its function. A pop-off feature is often present to prevent high airway pressures; however, such valves should have provision to override the pop-off feature because higher airway pressures are sometimes required to ventilate lungs with unusually high resistances, especially in children.
- Reservoir tubing that can be attached to the fresh gas inlet valve which allows oxygen to refill the reservoir bag during exhalation. Such a reservoir allows delivered oxygen to approach 100%; without it, the self-refilling bag can deliver only 40% to 50% oxygen.

For patients undergoing prolonged arrest, or for whom mask ventilation is unsuccessful, placement of an advanced airway should be performed. Precisely when to perform airway placement during resuscitation is not well defined, but it should be delayed at least until the first round of CPR and defibrillation in arrests felt to be primarily cardiac (rather than respiratory) in origin. In view of minimizing interruptions to compressions, it should be noted that supraglottic airways can be placed without stopping compressions.

Selection of which advanced airway device to use depends on the situation and especially upon the skill of the providers present. Advanced airways include supraglottic devices and endotracheal devices. Supraglottic devices do not require visualization of the glottis and are technically less demanding to place. Esophageal tracheal tubes (Combitube) allow blind placement and effective ventilation at rates similar to those achieved with endotracheal tube placement by inexperienced providers [52]. The laryngeal tube, which is designed to be placed in the esophagus and is inflated via a single port, is also an option.

The laryngeal mask airway (LMA) has been effective for maintaining airway patency during anesthesia since 1988 and is an acceptable alternative to mask ventilation during ACLS. The LMA provides a more stable and consistent means of ventilation than bag mask ventilation. Current research concludes that regurgitation is less common with LMA than with the bag mask, and although it cannot provide complete protection from aspiration, it is less frequent when used as the first-line airway device [53,54]. Multiple studies have documented the advantages of LMA for its relative ease with insertion and ease of use by a variety of personnel: nurses, medical students, respiratory therapists, and EMS, many with little prior experience using the device. Studies have shown that inexperienced personnel achieved an 80% to 94% success rate on first placement attempts and achieved 98% and 94% on subsequent attempts of adult and pediatric cases, respectively [54]. The LMA provides adequate and effective ventilation when measured against endotracheal intubation [55]. Additionally, less equipment and training are needed to insert the device successfully. It may also have advantages over the endotracheal tube when patient airway access is obstructed, when the patient has an unstable neck injury, or when suitable positioning of the patient for endotracheal intubation is unattainable. LMA insertion has been successful when attempts at endotracheal intubation by experts were unsuccessful [55]. Endotracheal tubes can be fiberoptically inserted through an established LMA.

Relative contraindications for LMA use include the patient with an increased risk of aspiration pneumonitis. Examples of such situations include morbid obesity, pregnancy, recent food ingestion, gastrointestinal obstruction, and hiatal hernia. Despite these considerations, oxygenation and ventilation during cardiac arrest receive top priority and the LMA should be used if it is the fastest and most efficient means of providing airway patency.

When an endotracheal tube is chosen during ACLS, interruptions to compressions should be limited to not more than 10 seconds if possible. Once placed, correct endotracheal tube placement must be verified as unrecognized misplacement or displacement is common. One study of 108 patients found a 25% rate of misplaced endotracheal tubes on emergency room arrival [56]. Providers should confirm correct placement of the endotracheal tube by examination of the chest as well as capnography and ultrasonography. Continuous capnography is recommended as this allows rapid recognition of endotracheal tube displacement during transport. Alternatives to capnography include end-tidal CO_2 detectors and esophageal detector devices. When an end-tidal CO_2 detector is positive (CO_2 detected), the provider can be confident the tube is endotracheal. False-negative end-tidal CO_2 detectors (i.e., no color change but the tube is endotracheal) may occur, most commonly due to low blood flow during CPR. If CO_2 is not detected using an end-tidal CO_2 detector, laryngoscopy or an esophageal detection device (EDD) should be used to confirm placement, though the evidence supporting the use of EDDs is limited.

While not discussed in the AHA guidelines, if attempts at relieving an obstructed airway have failed, several advanced techniques may be used to secure the airway until intubation or tracheostomy is successfully performed. Transtracheal catheter ventilation is performed by inserting a catheter over a needle through the cricothyroid membrane. The needle is removed and intermittent jet ventilation initiated (see Chapter 8). In cricothyrotomy, an opening is made in the cricothyroid membrane with a scalpel (see Chapters 8, 9). Tracheostomy, if still necessary, is best performed in the operating room by a skilled surgeon after the airway has already been secured by one of the aforementioned techniques.

After placement of an advanced airway, compressions should not be interrupted and should be continued at a rate of 100 per minute with respirations delivered at a rate of 8 to 10 per minute. Hyperventilation should be consciously avoided as hyperventilation during resuscitation is common and may be detrimental [47].

Circulatory Support

Chest compression should not be unduly interrupted while adjunctive procedures are instituted. The rescuer coordinating the resuscitation effort must ensure that adequate pulses are generated by the compressor. The carotid or femoral pulse should be evaluated every few minutes, and while not well studied, the palpation of a carotid pulse during CPR is often used to help assess the adequacy of compressions. When available, quantitative end-tidal CO_2 monitoring is a reasonable adjunct to monitor the adequacy of CPR (goal: > 10 mm Hg). If an abrupt rise in end-tidal CO_2 is seen in the absence of a dose of bicarbonate, this may indicate ROSC.

ACLS: Defibrillation and Rhythm-Based Therapies

Electrocardiographic (ECG) monitoring is necessary during resuscitation to guide appropriate electric and pharmacologic therapy. Until ECG monitoring allows diagnosis of the rhythm, the patient should be assumed to be in VF (see the section "Ventricular Fibrillation and Pulseless Ventricular Tachycardia").

Most defibrillators currently marketed have built-in monitoring circuitry in the paddles or pads (quick look). On application of the defibrillator paddles, the patient's ECG is displayed on the monitor screen. This facilitates appropriate initial therapy. For continuous monitoring beyond the first few minutes, a standard ECG monitoring unit should be used.

ECG monitoring must never be relied on without frequent reference to the patient's pulse and clinical condition. What appears on the monitor screen to be VF or asystole must not be treated as such unless the patient is found to be without a pulse. An apparently satisfactory rhythm on the monitor must be accompanied by an adequate pulse and blood pressure.

Defibrillation

Electric defibrillation is the definitive treatment for most cardiac arrests. It should be delivered as early as possible and repeated frequently until VF or pulseless ventricular tachycardia (VT) has been terminated.

Electric defibrillation involves passing an electric current through the heart and causing synchronous depolarization of the myofibrils. As the myofibrils repolarize, the opportunity arises for the emergence of organized pacemaker activity.

Proper use of the defibrillator requires special attention to the following:

1. *Selection of proper energy levels.* This lessens myocardial damage and arrhythmias occasioned by unnecessarily high energies. For biphasic defibrillators, the energy should be 120 to 200 J. For monophasic defibrillators, the energy should be 360 J [57].
2. *Proper asynchronous mode.* The proper mode must be selected if the rhythm is VF. The synchronizing switch must be deactivated or the defibrillator will dutifully await the R wave that will never come. For rapid pulseless VT (approximately 150 to 200 beats per minute), it is best not to attempt synchronization with the R wave because this increases the likelihood of delivering the shock on the T wave. If the countershock should fall on the T wave and induce VF, another unsynchronized countershock must be delivered promptly after confirming pulselessness.
3. *Proper position of the paddles or pads.* This allows the major energy of the electric arc to traverse the myocardium. The anterolateral position requires that one paddle or pad be placed to the right of the upper sternum, just below the clavicle. The other paddle or pad is positioned to the left of the nipple in the left midaxillary line. In the anteroposterior position, one paddle or pad is positioned under the left scapula with the patient lying on it. The anterior paddle or pad is positioned just to the left of the lower sternal border.
4. *Adequate contact between paddles or pads and skin.* This should be ensured, using just enough electrode paste to cover the paddle face without spilling over the surrounding skin. The rescuer should hold the paddles with firm pressure (approximately 25 lb). The pressure should be delivered using the forearms; leaning into the paddles should be avoided for fear that the rescuer may slip. If defibrillator electrode paddles are used, the skin must be carefully prepared according to the manufacturer's directions.
5. *No contact with anyone other than the patient.* The rescuer must be sturdily balanced on both feet and not standing on a wet floor. CPR must be discontinued with no one remaining in contact with the patient. It is the responsibility of the person defibrillating to check the patient's surroundings, ensure the safety of all participants, loudly announce the intention to countershock, and provide the shock. The use of an automatic or semiautomatic defibrillator does not decrease the operator's need for diligence.
6. If no skeletal muscle twitch or spasm has occurred, the equipment, contacts, and synchronizer switch used for elective cardioversions should be rechecked.

Electric energy delivered in a biphasic waveform is clearly superior to monophasic waveforms for implantable defibrillators (see Chapters 15, 18), but there is a paucity of evidence to show that one waveform is superior over another with regard to ROSC or survival to hospital discharge. External defibrillators are now available with biphasic waveforms.

Excepting symptomatic bradycardia, pacing is no longer recommended during ACLS.

Ventricular Fibrillation and Pulseless Ventricular Tachycardia

The primary therapy for VF and VT without a pulse is defibrillation. If the initial shock, *followed by 2 minutes of CPR*, is unsuccessful, then epinephrine, vasopressin, and later amiodarone should be used. Although not included in the most recent 2010 ACLS guidelines, the use of *both* vasopressin 20 units *and* epinephrine 1 mg in place of epinephrine alone (for each dose where the below figures call for epinephrine) for the first five doses of epinephrine, along with a single dose of methylprednisolone 40 mg during the first cycle of CPR, improved outcomes in a single large multicenter trial [58]. Until further study, the combination of vasopressin and epinephrine with methylprednisolone should be considered as a reasonable substitute for epinephrine alone in all instances during ACLS. If steroids are given, hydrocortisone 300 mg per day should be given for up to 7 days and tapered in patients who achieve ROSC. Those who have experienced an acute myocardial infarction should only receive hydrocortisone for 3 days.

Particularly if the arrest has been unwitnessed and defibrillation is not immediately occurring, CPR should be started while placing defibrillator pads and powering on the machine. If amiodarone is unavailable, lidocaine may be given, though the benefit of lidocaine is unproven. Magnesium is only given for torsades de pointes.

PEA and Asystole

The algorithm for PEA and asystole is simple: epinephrine should be given every 3 to 5 minutes until a shockable rhythm or ROSC occurs, or until efforts are terminated. Treatment of the underlying causes, the "Hs and Ts" (discussed below) should be addressed. Atropine is no longer recommended as an agent for asystole or PEA.

Correction of Hypoxia

Hypoxia should be corrected early during CPR with administration of the highest possible oxygen concentration. Inadequate perfusion, decreased pulmonary blood flow, pulmonary edema, atelectasis, and ventilation–perfusion mismatch all contribute to the difficulty in maintaining adequate tissue oxygenation. Inadequate tissue oxygenation results in anaerobic metabolism, the generation of lactic acid, and the development of metabolic acidosis.

Correction of Acidosis

Correction of acidosis (increased H^+ concentration) must be considered when the arrest has lasted for more than several minutes. *Metabolic acidosis* develops because of tissue hypoxia and conversion to anaerobic metabolism. *Respiratory acidosis* occurs because of apnea or hypoventilation with intrapulmonary ventilation–perfusion abnormalities, and the marked decrease in pulmonary blood flow that exists even with well-performed CPR.

Sodium bicarbonate reacts with hydrogen ions to buffer metabolic acidosis by forming carbonic acid and then carbon dioxide and water. Each 50 mEq sodium bicarbonate generates 260 to 280 mL carbon dioxide, which can be eliminated only through expired air. Because carbon dioxide of exhaled gas during CPR is decreased, the carbonic acid generated by sodium bicarbonate cannot be effectively eliminated. Paradoxic intracellular acidosis is likely to result, and arterial blood gases may not correctly reflect the state of tissue acidosis. The sodium and osmolar load of bicarbonate is high; excessive administration results in hyperosmolarity, hypernatremia, and worsened cellular acidosis. Sodium bicarbonate is of questionable value in treating the metabolic acidosis during cardiac arrest; it has not been shown to facilitate ventricular defibrillation or survival in cardiac arrest [59–61]. In any case, bicarbonate should not be used during cardiac arrest until at least 10 minutes have passed, the patient is intubated, and the patient has not responded to initial defibrillation and drug intervention. An exception is the patient with known preexisting hyperkalemia in whom administration of bicarbonate is recommended. The use of bicarbonate may also be of value in patients who have a known preexisting bicarbonate-responsive acidosis or a tricyclic antidepressant overdosage, or to alkalinize the urine in drug overdosage. When bicarbonate is used, 1 mEq per kg may be given as the initial dose. When possible, further therapy should be guided by the calculated base deficit. To avoid iatrogenically induced alkalosis, complete correction of the calculated base deficit should be avoided.

Volume Replacement

Increased central volume is often required during CPR, especially if the initial attempts at defibrillation have failed. PEA is particularly likely to be caused either by acute severe hypovolemia (e.g., exsanguination) or by a cardiovascular process for which volume expansion may be a lifesaving temporizing measure (e.g., pericardial tamponade, pulmonary embolism, and septic shock). The usual clues for hypovolemia, such as collapsed jugular and peripheral veins and evidence of peripheral vasoconstriction, are unavailable during cardiac arrest; furthermore, dry mucus membranes and absence of normal secretions (tears and saliva) are unreliable in acute hypovolemia. Most physical findings of tamponade, pulmonary embolism, or septic shock are absent during arrest. Therefore, one must be guided by an appropriate clinical history and have a low threshold to administer volume during CPR.

Simple crystalloids, such as 5% dextrose in water (D_5W), are inappropriate for rapid expansion of the circulatory blood volume. Isotonic crystalloids (0.9% saline and Ringer's lactate), colloids, or blood is necessary for satisfactory volume expansion. Crystalloids are more readily available, easier to administer, and less expensive than colloids. They are also free of the potential to cause allergic reactions or infections.

If the patient has a weak pulse, simple elevation of the legs, or a passive leg raise, may help by promoting venous return to the central circulation. Volume challenges should be given as needed until pulse and blood pressure have been restored or until there is evidence of volume overload.

Venous Access

Although venous access with a reliable intravenous (IV) route must be established early in the course of the resuscitative effort to allow for the administration of necessary drugs and fluids, *initial defibrillation attempts and effective CPR* should not be delayed for the placement of an IV line. If skills allow, central venous access may be the most reliable, but intraosseous and peripheral IV access are also reasonable options. If medications are delivered via peripheral route, a 20-mL bolus should be used to flush the drug.

Although central lines may be associated with an increased incidence of complications for patients receiving fibrinolytic therapy, they are not an absolute contraindication to its use.

Drugs such as epinephrine, atropine, and lidocaine can be administered via the endotracheal tube if there is delay in achieving venous access. However, this route requires a higher dose to achieve an equivalent blood level, and a sustained duration of action (a "depot effect") can be expected if there is a return in spontaneous circulation [61]. It is suggested that 3 to 10 times the IV dose of epinephrine be administered when using the endotracheal route. Delivery of the drug to the circulation is facilitated by diluting the drug in 10 mL of sterile water and delivering it through a catheter positioned beyond the tip of the endotracheal tube. Stop chest compressions, spray the solution quickly down the endotracheal tube, and give several quick insufflations before reinitiating chest compressions. Intracardiac injection of epinephrine is to be avoided.

DRUG THERAPY

Sympathomimetic Drugs and Vasopressors

Sympathomimetic drugs act either directly on adrenergic receptors or indirectly by releasing catecholamines from nerve endings. Most useful during cardiac emergencies are the adrenergic agents, which include the endogenous biogenic amines epinephrine, norepinephrine, and dopamine, and the synthetic agent isoproterenol and its derivative dobutamine. Of note, none of the sympathomimetics can be administered in the same line as an alkaline infusion. Extravasation of any agent with α-adrenergic activity can result in tissue necrosis, so they should be infused via a central venous catheter when possible. If extravasation does occur, 5 to 10 mg phentolamine in 10 to 15 mL saline should be infiltrated as soon as possible into the area of extravasation.

Epinephrine

Epinephrine is a naturally occurring catecholamine that has both α- and β-activities. Although epinephrine is the pressor agent used most frequently during CPR, the evidence that it improves the outcome in humans is scant.

Indications for the use of epinephrine include all forms of cardiac arrest because its α-vasoconstrictive activity is important in raising the perfusion pressure of the myocardium and brain. The importance of α-adrenergic activity during resuscitation has been noted in several studies [62], whereas administration of pure β-agonists (e.g., isoproterenol or dobutamine) has been shown to be ineffective [63]. The β-action of epinephrine is theoretically useful in asystole and bradycardic arrests by increasing heart rate. The β-effect has also been touted to convert asystole to VF or to convert "fine" VF to "coarse." Coarse or wide-amplitude VF is easier to convert to a perfusing rhythm than fine or small-amplitude VF. However, this may be primarily due to the shorter time course of the arrest in patients still manifesting wide-amplitude rather than small-amplitude VF.

Epinephrine is best administered intravenously. As soon as possible after failed ventricular defibrillation attempts (or if defibrillation is not an option), an adult in cardiac arrest should be given a 1-mg dose at a 1 to 10,000 dilution (10 mL). It should be given in the upper extremity or centrally (see the earlier discussion in the section "Venous Access"), and may be repeated every 5 minutes. If a peripheral line is used, the drug should be administered rapidly and followed by a 20-mL bolus of IV fluid and elevation of the extremity. If an IV line has not been established, the endotracheal route may be used, but the intracardiac route should be avoided because it is prone to serious complications such as intramyocardial injection, coronary laceration, and pneumothorax. An IV infusion of 1 to 10 mcg per minute can also be given for inotropic and pressor support. Two multicenter trials evaluating the effectiveness of high-dose epinephrine in cardiac arrest failed to demonstrate an improvement in survival or neurologic outcome [64,65], and doses above 1 mg (excepting endotracheal administration) should not be used.

Risks in the use of epinephrine and other α-agonists include tissue necrosis from extravasation and inactivation from admixture with bicarbonate.

Norepinephrine

Norepinephrine is a potent α-agonist with β-activity. Its salutary α-effects during CPR are similar to those of epinephrine [66]. However, there are no data to support that it is superior to epinephrine during an arrest.

The major effect of norepinephrine is on the blood vessels. Initial coronary vasoconstriction usually gives way to coronary vasodilatation, probably as a result of increased myocardial metabolic activity. In a heart with compromised coronary reserve, this may cause further ischemia. During cardiac arrest, its usefulness, like that of epinephrine, is most likely due to peripheral vasoconstriction with an increase in perfusion pressure. In patients with spontaneous circulation who are in cardiogenic shock (when peripheral vasoconstriction is often already extreme), its effect is more difficult to predict.

Indications for the use of norepinephrine during cardiac arrest are similar to those for epinephrine, although there does not appear to be any reason to prefer it to epinephrine. Norepinephrine appears to be most useful in the treatment of shock caused by inappropriate decline in peripheral vascular resistance, such as septic shock and neurogenic shock. It is administered by IV infusion and titrated to an adequate perfusion pressure. Norepinephrine bitartrate, 4 to 8 mg (2 to 4 mg of the base), should be diluted in 500 mL D_5W or 5% dextrose in normal saline. A typical starting infusion rate is 0.5 mcg per minute and most adults respond to 2 to 12 mcg per minute, but some require rates up to 30 mcg per minute. Abrupt termination of the infusion (as may occur in transport) may lead to sudden severe hypotension.

Precautions to the use of norepinephrine include its inappropriate use in hypovolemic shock and in patients with already severe vasoconstriction. Intraarterial pressure monitoring is recommended when using norepinephrine because indirect blood pressure measurement is often incorrect in patients with severe vasoconstriction. In patients with myocardial ischemia or infarction, the myocardial oxygen requirements are increased by all catecholamines, but there is limited evidence to guide vasopressor selection in this population. Heart rate, rhythm, ECG evidence for ischemia, direct systemic and pulmonary pressures, urine output, and cardiac output should be closely monitored when using this drug in patients with myocardial ischemia or infarction.

Isoproterenol

This synthetic catecholamine has almost pure β-adrenergic activity. Its cardiac activity includes potent inotropic and chronotropic effects, both of which will increase the myocardium's oxygen demand. In addition to bronchodilatation, the arterial beds of the skeletal muscles, kidneys, and gut dilate, resulting in a marked drop in systemic vascular resistance. Cardiac output can be expected to increase markedly unless the increased myocardial oxygen demand results in substantial myocardial ischemia. Systolic blood pressure is usually maintained because of the rise in cardiac output, but the diastolic and mean pressures usually decrease. As a result, coronary perfusion pressure drops at the same time that the myocardial oxygen requirement is increased. This combination can be expected to have deleterious effects in patients with ischemic heart disease, especially during cardiac arrest. The main clinical usefulness of isoproterenol is in its ability to stimulate pacemakers within the heart.

Indications for isoproterenol are primarily in the setting of atropine-resistant, hemodynamically significant bradyarrhythmias, including profound sinus and junctional bradycardia, as well as various forms of high-degree AV block. It should be used only as an interim measure, until effective transcutaneous or IV pacing can be instituted. If the aortic diastolic pressure is already low, epinephrine is likely to be better tolerated as a stimulus to pacemakers. *Under no circumstances should isoproterenol be used during cardiac arrest.*

Isoproterenol is administered by titration of an IV solution. 1 mg isoproterenol (Isuprel) is diluted with either 250 mL D_5W (4 mg per mL) or 500 mL D_5W (2 mg per mL). The infusion rate should be only rapid enough to effect an adequate perfusing heart rate (2 to 20 mcg per minute, or 0.05 to 0.5 mcg per kg per minute). Depending on the adequacy of cardiac reserve, a target heart rate as low as 50 to 55 beats per minute may be satisfactory. Occasionally, more rapid rates are necessary.

Precautions in the use of isoproterenol are largely due to the increase in myocardial oxygen requirement, with its potential for provoking ischemia; *this effect, coupled with the possibility of dropping the coronary perfusion pressure, makes isoproterenol a dangerous selection in patients with myocardial ischemia.* The marked chronotropic effects may cause tachycardia and provoke serious ventricular arrhythmias, including VF. Isoproterenol is usually contraindicated if tachycardia is already present, especially if the arrhythmia may be secondary to digitalis toxicity. If significant hypotension develops with its use, it may be combined with another β-agonist with α-activity. However, switching to dopamine or epinephrine is usually preferable; better yet is the use of pacing for rate control.

Dopamine

This naturally occurring precursor of norepinephrine has α-, β-, and dopamine-receptor–stimulating activities. The dopamine-receptor activity theoretically dilates renal and mesenteric arterial beds at low doses (1 to 2 mcg per kg per minute), though the clinical relevance of this is unclear [67]. β-Adrenergic activity is more prominent with doses from 2 to 10 mcg per kg per minute, whereas α-adrenergic activity is predominant at doses greater than 10 mcg per kg per minute. It has not been shown that these dose ranges have relevance in the clinical setting. Indications for the use of dopamine are primarily significant hypotension and cardiogenic shock.

Dopamine is administered by IV titration in the range of 2 to 20 μg per kg per minute. Rarely, a patient may need in excess of 20 mcg per kg per minute. A 200-mg ampule is diluted to 250 or 500 mL in D_5W or 5% dextrose in normal saline for a concentration of 800 or 400 mg per mL. As with all catecholamine infusions, the lowest infusion rate that results in satisfactory perfusion should be the goal of therapy.

Precautions for dopamine are similar to those for other catecholamines. Tachycardia or ventricular arrhythmias may require reduction in dosage or discontinuation of the drug. If significant hypotension occurs from the dilating activity of dopaminergic or β-active doses, small amounts of an α-active drug may be added. Dopamine may increase myocardial ischemia.

Dobutamine

Dobutamine is a potent synthetic β-adrenergic agent that differs from isoproterenol in that tachycardia is less problematic. Unless ischemia supervenes, cardiac output will increase, as will renal and mesenteric blood flow.

Dobutamine is indicated primarily for the short-term enhancement of ventricular contractility in the patient with heart failure. It may be used for stabilization of the patient after resuscitation or for the patient with heart failure refractory to other drugs. It may also be used in combination with IV nitroprusside, which lowers peripheral vascular resistance and thereby left ventricular afterload. Although nitroprusside lowers peripheral resistance, dobutamine maintains perfusion by augmenting the cardiac output.

Dobutamine is administered by slow-titrated IV infusion. A dose as low as 0.5 mcg per kg per minute may prove to be effective, but the usual dose range is 2.5 to 10.0 mcg per kg per minute. A 250-mg vial is dissolved in 10 mL of sterile water and then to 250 or 500 mL D_5W for a concentration of 1.0 or 0.5 mcg per mL.

Precautions for dobutamine are similar to those for other β-agonists. Dobutamine may cause tachycardia, ventricular arrhythmias, myocardial ischemia, and extension of infarction.

Vasopressin

Vasopressin is not a catecholamine, but a naturally occurring antidiuretic hormone. In high doses, it is a powerful constrictor of smooth muscles and as such has been studied as an adjunctive therapy for cardiac arrest in an attempt to improve perfusion pressures and organ flows. Vasopressin may be especially useful in prolonged cardiac arrest as it remains effective as a vasopressor even in severe acidosis [68]. It may be used as a first-line agent in arrest in lieu of epinephrine or as the second-line agent if the first dose of epinephrine failed to cause a return in pulse. The dose of vasopressin is 40 units IV or intraosseously (IO). It may also be used in combination with epinephrine 1 mg and methylprednisolone 40 mg (once) at 20 units for each cycle of ACLS [58].

Antiarrhythmic Agents

Antiarrhythmic agents have been thought to play an important role in stabilizing the rhythm in many resuscitation situations; however, the data in support of their value are scant. Although lidocaine, bretylium, and procainamide had been considered useful in counteracting the tendency to ventricular arrhythmias, convincing evidence of benefit to their use for pulseless VT and VF is wanting. On the basis of available data, amiodarone is the agent of choice for the emergency treatment of refractory VT and VF [69].

Amiodarone

Amiodarone is a benzofuran derivative that is structurally similar to thyroxine and contains a considerable level of iodine. Gastrointestinal absorption is slow; therefore, when given orally, the onset of action is delayed while the drug slowly accumulates in adipose tissue. The mean elimination half-life is 64 days (range, 24 to 160 days). IV administration allows rapid onset of action, with therapeutic blood levels achieved with 600 mg given over 24 hours.

Amiodarone decreases myocardial contractility and also causes vasodilatation, which counterbalances the decrease in contractility. In general, it is well tolerated even by those with myocardial dysfunction.

Amiodarone given IV has been successful in terminating a variety of reentrant and other types of supraventricular and ventricular rhythms. In a major study of out-of-hospital cardiac arrest due to ventricular arrhythmias refractory to shock, patients were initially treated with either amiodarone (246 patients) or placebo (258 patients). Patients given amiodarone had a higher incidence of bradycardia (41% vs. 25%) and hypotension (59% vs. 48%), besides a higher rate of survival to hospital admission (44% vs. 34%) [69]. This study did not demonstrate an increase in survival to hospital discharge or in neurologic status. On the basis of this study, amiodarone has been given status as an option for use after defibrillation attempts and epinephrine therapy in refractory ventricular arrhythmias during cardiac arrest. It is also an option for ventricular rate control in rapid atrial arrhythmias in patients with impaired left ventricular function. Other optional uses are for control of hemodynamically stable VT, polymorphic VT, preexcited atrial arrhythmias, and wide-complex tachycardia of uncertain origin. It may also be useful for chemical cardioversion of atrial fibrillation or as an adjunct to electric cardioversion of refractory paroxysmal supraventricular tachycardia (PSVT) and atrial fibrillation or flutter.

Administration in cardiac arrest (pulseless VT or VF) is by rapid IV infusion of 300 mg diluted in 20 to 30 mL of saline or D_5W. Supplementary infusions of 150 mg may be used for recurrent or refractory VT or VF.

Administration for rhythms with a pulse is by IV infusion of 150 mg given for 10 minutes, followed by infusion of 1 mg per minute for 6 hours and then 0.5 mg per minute. Supplemental infusions of 150 mg may be given for recurrent or resistant arrhythmias to a total maximum dose of 2 g for 24 hours.

Lidocaine

This antiarrhythmic agent has been used for ventricular arrhythmias, such as premature ventricular complexes and VT. Premature ventricular complexes are not unusual in apparently healthy people and most often are benign. Even in the patient with chronic heart disease, premature ventricular complexes and nonsustained VT are usually asymptomatic, and controversy exists concerning the need to treat under these circumstances.

Administration of lidocaine begins with an IV bolus. The onset of action is rapid. Its duration of action is brief, but may be prolonged by continuous infusion. A solution of lidocaine, typically 20 mg per mL (2%), should be prepared for IV administration. If the patient has suffered an acute myocardial infarction and has had ventricular arrhythmias, the infusion is continued for hours to days and tapered slowly. If the cause of the arrhythmia has been corrected, the infusion may be tapered more rapidly.

Precautions should be taken against excessive accumulation of lidocaine. The dosage should be reduced in patients with low cardiac output, congestive failure, hepatic failure, and age older than 70 years because of the decreased liver metabolism of the drug. Toxic manifestations are usually neurologic, and can vary from slurred speech, tinnitus, sleepiness, and dysphoria to localizing neurologic symptoms. Frank seizures may occur with or without preceding neurologic symptoms and may be controlled with short-acting barbiturates or benzodiazepines. Conscious patients should be warned about possible symptoms of neurologic toxicity and asked to report them immediately if they occur. Excessive blood levels can significantly depress myocardial contractility.

Adenosine

Adenosine is an endogenous purine nucleoside that depresses AV nodal conduction and sinoatrial nodal activity. Because of the delay in AV nodal conduction, adenosine is effective for terminating arrhythmias that use the AV node in a reentrant circuit (e.g., PSVT) [70]. For supraventricular tachycardias, such as atrial flutter or atrial fibrillation, or atrial tachycardias that do not use the AV node in a reentrant circuit, blocking transmission through the AV node may prove helpful in clarifying the diagnosis [71,72]. In the 2010 ACLS guidelines, the use of adenosine in wide-complex tachycardia of uncertain origin to discriminate between VT and supraventricular tachycardia with aberrancy is encouraged. Adenosine may also be used in the diagnosis and treatment of stable and unstable narrow complex tachycardias. The half-life of adenosine is less than 5 seconds because it is rapidly metabolized.

Administration is by IV bolus of 6 mg given for 1 to 3 seconds, followed by a 20-mL saline flush. An additional dose of 12 mg may be given if no effect is seen within 1 to 2 minutes. Patients taking theophylline may need higher doses.

Side effects caused by adenosine are transient and may include flushing, dyspnea, bronchoconstriction, and angina-like chest pain (even in the absence of coronary disease). Sinus bradycardia and ventricular ectopy are common after terminating PSVT with adenosine, but the arrhythmias are typically short lived so as to be clinically unimportant. The reentrant tachycardia may recur after the effect of adenosine has dissipated and may require additional doses of adenosine or a longer acting drug, such as verapamil or diltiazem.

Theophylline and other methylxanthines, such as theobromine and caffeine, block the receptor responsible for adenosine's electrophysiologic effect; therefore, higher doses may be required in their presence. Dipyridamole and carbamazepine, on the other hand, potentiate and may prolong the effect of adenosine; therefore, other forms of therapy may be advisable. Be careful not to give to asthmatics.

Verapamil and Diltiazem

Unlike other calcium channel–blocking agents, verapamil and diltiazem increase refractoriness in the AV node and significantly slow conduction. This action may terminate reentrant tachycardias that use the AV node in the reentrant circuit (e.g., PSVT). These drugs may also slow the ventricular response of patients with atrial flutter or fibrillation and even for patients with multifocal atrial tachycardia. They should be used only for patients for whom the tachycardia is known to be supraventricular in origin.

Administration of verapamil is by IV bolus of 2.5 to 5.0 mg for 2 minutes. In the absence of a response, additional doses of 5 to 10 mg may be given at 15- to 30-minute intervals to a maximum of 20 mg. The maximum cumulative dose is 20 mg. Diltiazem may be given as an initial dose of 0.25 mg per kg with a follow-up dose of 0.35 mg per kg, if needed. A maintenance infusion of 5 to 15 mg per hour may be used to control the rate of ventricular response in atrial fibrillation.

Verapamil and diltiazem should be used for arrhythmias known to be supraventricular in origin and in the absence of preexcitation. Both verapamil and diltiazem may decrease myocardial contractility and worsen congestive heart failure or even provoke cardiogenic shock in patients with significant left ventricular dysfunction. They should, therefore, be used with caution in patients with known cardiac failure or suspected diminished cardiac reserve and in the elderly. If worsened failure or hypotension develops after the use of these agents, calcium should be administered, as described in the section "Other Agents."

Magnesium

Cardiac arrhythmias and even sudden cardiac death have been associated with magnesium deficiency [72]. Hypomagnesemia decreases the uptake of intracellular potassium and may precipitate VT or fibrillation. Routine use of magnesium in cardiac arrest or after myocardial infarction is not recommended. Magnesium may be of value for patients with torsades de pointes, even in the absence of hypomagnesemia.

Magnesium is administered IV. For rapid administration during VT or VF with suspected or documented hypomagnesemia, 1 to 2 g may be diluted in 100 mL of D_5W and given for 1 to 2 minutes. A 24-hour infusion of magnesium may be used for periinfarction patients with documented hypomagnesemia. A loading dose of 1 to 2 g is diluted in 100 mL D_5W and slowly given for 5 minutes to 1 hour, followed by an infusion of 0.5 to 1 g per hour during the ensuing 24 hours. Clinical circumstances and the serum magnesium level dictate the rate and duration of the infusion. Hypotension or asystole may occur with rapid administration.

Other Agents

Additional drugs occasionally found useful or necessary during resuscitation or in the immediate postresuscitation period include atropine, calcium, nitroprusside, and nitroglycerine; these agents are discussed in the following sections. Many other drugs may be required in particular circumstances and are discussed in other parts of this text. An incomplete list of these drugs includes beta-blockers, ibutilide, propafenone, flecainide, sotalol, digoxin, antibiotics, thiamine, thyroxine, morphine, naloxone, adrenocorticoids, fibrinolytic agents, anticoagulants, antiplatelet agents, and dextrose.

Atropine Sulfate

Atropine is an anticholinergic drug that increases heart rate by stimulating pacers and facilitating AV conduction that is suppressed by excessive vagal tone.

Atropine is indicated primarily for bradycardias causing hemodynamic difficulty or associated with ventricular arrhythmias. Atropine may be useful in AV block at the nodal level. It is no longer used in asystole and bradycardic arrests.

Atropine is administered by IV bolus. If a satisfactory response has not occurred within 3 to 5 minutes, additional 1-mg doses should be given in a bolus, to a maximum dose of 3 mg (0.04 mg per kg). For bradycardia with a pulse, the initial dose should be 0.5 mg repeated every 5 minutes until the desired effect is obtained, to a maximum dose of 3 mg (0.04 mg per kg). Atropine may be given by the endotracheal route at doses 2.5 times the IV dose.

Precautions for atropine include the requirement that an inordinately rapid heart rate not be produced. Patients with ischemic heart disease are likely to have worsened ischemia or ventricular arrhythmias if the rate is too rapid. Uncommonly, a patient will have a paradoxic slowing of rate with atropine; this is more likely to occur with smaller first doses and is caused by a central vagal effect. This effect is rapidly counteracted by additional atropine. In this situation, the next dose of atropine should be given immediately. If additional atropine does not correct the problem, the patient may require judicious use of isoproterenol or pacemaker therapy.

Calcium

The positive inotropic effect of calcium has led to its use in cardiac arrest. The contractile state of the myocardium depends in part on the intracellular concentration of the calcium ion. Transmembrane calcium flux serves an important regulatory function in both active contraction and active relaxation. The use of calcium in cardiac arrest is based on an early report by Kay and Blalock [73] in which several pediatric cardiac surgical patients were successfully resuscitated, apparently with the aid of calcium. However, several field studies have failed to demonstrate an improvement in survival or neurologic outcome with the use of calcium versus a control [74]. In addition, after standard doses of calcium administered during cardiac arrest, many patients are found to have very high calcium blood levels [75]. This is apparently due to the markedly contracted volume of distribution of the ion in the arrested organism. In addition, calcium has the theoretic disadvantage of facilitating postanoxic tissue damage, especially in the brain and heart. Digitalis toxicity may be exacerbated by the administration of calcium.

Calcium is indicated only in specific circumstances: calcium channel blocker toxicity, severe hyperkalemia, severe hypocalcemia, arrest after multiple transfusions with citrated blood, fluoride toxicity, and while coming off heart–lung bypass after cardioplegic arrest.

Calcium is available as calcium chloride, calcium gluceptate, and calcium gluconate. The gluconate salt is unstable and less frequently available. The chloride salt provides the most direct source of calcium ion and produces the most rapid effect. The gluceptate and gluconate salts require hepatic degradation to release the free calcium ion. Calcium chloride is, therefore, the best choice. It is highly irritating to tissues and must be injected into a large vein with precautions to avoid extravasation. Calcium chloride is available in a 10% solution. An initial dose of 250 to 500 mg may be administered slowly during several minutes. It may be repeated as necessary at 10-minute intervals if strong indications exist.

Precautions for calcium use include the need for slow injection without extravasation. If bicarbonate has been administered through the same line, it must be cleared before introducing the calcium. If the patient has a rhythm, rapid injection may result in bradycardia. Calcium salts must be used with caution in patients receiving digitalis.

CLINICAL SETTINGS

The procedures involved in the resuscitation of a person who has experienced cardiovascular or respiratory collapse are all part of a continuum progressing from the initial recognition of the problem and the institution of CPR to intervention with defibrillators, drugs, pacemakers, transport, and postresuscitative evaluation and care. The following sections focus on the pharmacologic and electric interventions appropriate to various clinical settings common in cardiac arrest.

Special Situations

Patients who have nearly drowned in cold water may recover after prolonged periods of submersion. Apparently, the hypothermia and bradycardia of the diving reflex may serve to protect against organ damage [76]. Successful resuscitation has been described after considerable periods of submersion [76]. Because it is often difficult for bystanders and rescuers to estimate the duration of submersion, in most cases it is warranted to initiate CPR at the scene, unless physical evidence exists of irreversible death, such as putrefaction or dependent rubor.

Hypothermia may occur with environmental exposures other than cold water drowning. The body's ability to maintain temperature is diminished by alcohol, sedation, antidepressants, neurologic problems, and advanced age. Because of the associated bradycardia and oxygen-sparing effects, prolonged hypothermia and arrest may be tolerated with complete recovery. A longer period may be needed to establish breathlessness and pulselessness because of profound bradycardia and slowed respiratory rate. Resuscitative efforts should not be abandoned until near-normal temperature has been reestablished.

Electric shock and lightning strike may lead to tetanic spasm of respiratory muscles or convulsion, causing respiratory arrest. VF or asystole may occur from the electric shock or after prolonged respiratory arrest. Before initiating assessment and CPR, the potential rescuer must ascertain whether the person who has been shocked is still in contact with the electric energy and that live wires are not in dangerous proximity. If the individual is located at the top of a utility pole, CPR is best instituted after the person is lowered to the ground [77].

Termination of ACLS and Post ACLS Care

Induced therapeutic hypothermia (32°C to 34°C) for 12 to 24 hours improves survival and neurologic outcome in comatose patients who have survived an out-of-hospital VF arrest [78,79]. More recent evidence suggests that targeting a temperature of 36°C rather than 33°C may offer the same benefit, and has the advantage of less infectious risks and easier use of existing literature to help determine prognosis

[16]. Hypothermia may also be beneficial for in-hospital arrests, though evidence is lacking. Lower cardiac index and hyperglycemia tend to occur more frequently in hypothermic patients, as do infections [80]. Shivering must be prevented to reduce the risk of increasing the metabolic rate. Please see Chapter 184 on hypothermia for an in-depth discussion of induced therapeutic hypothermia.

When to stop CPR or CLS is not always clearly defined. For emergency room patients with a rhythm of either PEA or asystole, there were no cases of ROSC when cardiac standstill was demonstrated by echocardiography [81]. Providers considering use of echo to assist in deciding to terminate resuscitative efforts should consider their own skill in performing echocardiography and the overall clinical situation. The ethics section of the ACLS guidelines suggests criteria for limiting resuscitation in several settings [48]. CPR should not begin in any setting when a valid do-not-resuscitate (DNR) order exists, when it is unsafe for the provider or rescuer, or when obvious signs of death are present such as rigor mortis, dependent livedo, decapitation, or decomposition. If CPR is begun, it is stopped when ROSC is achieved, the provider is too exhausted to continue, or when care is handed off to another provider team. Out-of-hospital arrest resuscitation (BLS and ALCS) may also be terminated if patients meet *all three* of the following criteria: (1) arrest not witnessed by EMS personnel; (2) no defibrillation attempted before transport; and (3) no ROSC before transport [48,82]. For most patients who undergo resuscitation but do not achieve ROSC, the decision to terminate resuscitation efforts is often based on the clinical situation, including factors such as whether a pulse was obtained at some point during the resuscitation, premorbid state, initial rhythm, arrest duration both before starting CPR and duration of the resuscitation. Prearrest functional status and duration of resuscitation impact survival [83,84]. Duration of CPR is often the simplest decision criterion, and while there is no well-defined threshold, after 10 to 30 minutes of CPR, survival is unlikely [84–86].

Arrests in the ICU are often felt to have a very poor prognosis. However, among ICU arrest patients for whom resuscitation is attempted, one 5-year series reported surprisingly good outcomes, with 1 and 5 year survivals of 24% and 16%, respectively [86]. Many ICU arrests can be anticipated and communication with patients and families with an emphasis on advanced care decision-making are often the most important aspects of resuscitation management in the ICU.

Utility of Ultrasonography for Cardiopulmonary Resuscitation

Ultrasonography has utility during the performance of CPR. Focused echocardiography can be performed during the pauses in CPR intended for checks of ROSC [87], and does not impair the quality of CPR when the no-flow period is not extended [88,89].

The operator is positioned such that a subcostal long axis view can be obtained during pulse checks. This requires that a portable ultrasonography machine be placed at the thigh level of the patient as close to the bed as possible with the screen adjusted for optimal image clarity. The operator faces the screen while pressing the probe into the subcostal area in anticipation of the pulse check. Machine setup and operator positioning are not permitted to interrupt chest compressions, as these take absolute priority. When the code team leader alerts the team that a pulse check is required, a team member assumes position contralateral to the ultrasonography machine to prepare to manually check for a pulse in the femoral area, while the ultrasonography operator pre-positions the probe in order to obtain an immediate subcostal long axis view of the heart during the pulse check. When the code leader orders that chest compressions stop for the 5-second pulse check, a skilled scanner can obtain a good quality view of the heart. During chest compressions, it is not possible to obtain any useful images due to the marked translational movement of the heart that occurs during chest compressions (Videos 14.1 and 14.2).

If the CPR team is so equipped, a transesophageal echocardiography probe can be easily inserted during CPR. This can only be performed if the patient has a well secured endotracheal tube in place. The probe is inserted with 0^0 transducer rotation to obtain the transgastric short axis view of the left ventricle. In this way, the CPR effort is monitored both during chest compressions and pulse checks (Videos 14.3 and 14.4).

Limited view transthoracic echocardiography is useful during CPR for three reasons:

1. Identification of potentially reversible causes of cardiac arrest such as a large pericardial effusion with tamponade, a severely dilated right ventricle with acute cor pulmonale related to a pulmonary embolism, or a heart that is profoundly hypovolemic. These findings are uncommon during CPR; however, when found, they may result in a lifesaving intervention (Videos 14.5–14.7).
2. Identification of cardiac contractile activity without palpable pulse (pseudo PEA). Echocardiographic imaging during CPR allows reclassification of some patients who are clinically classified as having pulseless electrical activity, because even very weak endogenous cardiac contractility can be observed sonographically (Videos 14.8 and 14.9). The prognosis for ROSC is improved when there is some echocardiographic evidence of endogenous myocardial contractility [90]. This finding is not uncommon, and leads to the consideration that resuscitation efforts should be continued if the clinical situation warrants this.
3. Identification of the absence of cardiac contractile activity. In the patient who is receiving CPR in the emergency department, complete absence of cardiac contractile activity is a strong indicator that the resuscitation effort will not be successful [91] (Videos 14.10 and 14.11). In ICU patients, the absence of endogenous myocardial contractility on echocardiography performed during CPR confers a significantly lower likelihood of ROSC and very low likelihood of survival to hospital discharge compared to finding the presence of cardiac contractile activity [92,93]. While the absence of cardiac contractile activity is not an absolute indicator that the CPR effort will fail, it may combine with other clinical indicators in the decision to terminate CPR attempts.

Ultrasonography is also useful for detecting correct endotracheal tube placement during CPR. Unintentional esophageal intubation may be difficult to detect during CPR because end-tidal CO_2 levels may not be detectable in full cardiac arrest, and chest auscultation may not be accurate. Laryngeal ultrasonography examination during endotracheal intubation allows detection of correct insertion of the endotracheal tube into the trachea in patients receiving CPR [94], and the presence of bilateral lung sliding with bag ventilation confirms correct tube position in the trachea [95] (Videos 14.12 and 14.13).

Interosseous needle insertion provides rapid access for drug delivery during CPR. Ultrasonography may be used to confirm intraosseous (I/O) needle placement [96,97]. At the tibial insertion site, the operator places the linear vascular probe next to the holding flange of the I/O needle while angling the scanning plane toward the needle tip. The periosteum of the anterior tibia appears as a distinct hyperechoic line. The color Doppler map is positioned below the periosteum and 5 cc of sterile saline is injected into the I/O needle. If the needle is well positioned, a color Doppler signal will result deep to the periosteum during the injection (Video 14.14). A color Doppler signal that is seen superficial to the periosteum indicates misplacement of the needle with the risk of extravasation of adrenergic medication into the subcutaneous compartment.

References

1. Zoll PM, Linenthal AJ, Gibson W, et al: Termination of ventricular fibrillation in man by externally applied electrical countershock. *N Engl J Med* 254:727, 1956.
2. Safar P, Escarraga L, Elam JO: A comparison of the mouth to mouth and mouth to airway methods of artificial respiration with the chest pressure arm-lift method. *N Engl J Med* 258:671, 1958.
3. Elam JO, Green DG, Brown ES, et al: Oxygen and carbon dioxide exchange and energy cost of expired air resuscitation. *JAMA* 167:328, 1958.
4. Kouwenhoven WB, Jude JR, Knickerbocker GG: Closed chest cardiac massage. *JAMA* 173:1064, 1960.
5. Cardiopulmonary resuscitation: statement by the Ad Hoc Committee on Cardiopulmonary Resuscitation of the Division of Medical Sciences, National Academy of Sciences—National Research Council. *JAMA* 198:372, 1966.
6. Standards for cardiopulmonary resuscitation (CPR) and emergency cardiac care (ECC). *JAMA* 227[Suppl]:833, 1974.
7. Guidelines for the determination of death: report of the medical consultants on the diagnosis of death to the President's Commission for the Study of Ethical Problems in Medicine and Biomedical and Behavioral Research. *JAMA* 246:2184, 1981.
8. Wijdicks EFM: The diagnosis of brain death. *N Engl J Med* 344:1215, 2001.
9. Del Guercio LR, Feins NR, Cohn JD, et al: Comparison of blood flow during external and internal cardiac massage in man. *Circulation* 31[Suppl 1]:171, 1965.
10. Cave DM, Gazmuri RJ, Otto CW, et al: Part 7: CPR techniques and devices: 2010 American Heart Association Guidelines for Cardiopulmonary Resuscitation and Emergency Cardiovascular Care. *Circulation* 122[18 Suppl 3]: S720–S728, 2010.
11. Copley DP, Mantle JA, Roger WJ, et al: Improved outcome for prehospital cardiopulmonary collapse with resuscitation by bystanders. *Circulation* 56:902, 1977.
12. Holmberg M, Holmberg S, Herlitz J: Effect of bystander cardiopulmonary resuscitation in out-of-hospital cardiac arrest patients in Sweden. *Resuscitation* 47:59, 2000.
13. Rudikoff MT, Maughan WL, Effron M, et al: Mechanisms of blood flow during cardiopulmonary resuscitation. *Circulation* 61:345, 1980.
14. Chandra N, Weisfeldt ML, Tsitlik J, et al: Augmentation of carotid flow during cardiopulmonary resuscitation by ventilation at high airway pressure simultaneous with chest compression. *Am J Cardiol* 48:1053, 1981.
15. Chan PS, McNally B, Tang F, et al. Recent trends in survival from out-of-hospital cardiac arrest in the United States. *Circulation* 130:1876–1882, 2014.
16. Nielsen N, Wetterslev J, Cronberg T, et al: Targeted temperature management at 33°C versus 36°C after cardiac arrest. *N Engl J Med* 369:2197–2206, 2013.
17. Wallace SK, Abella BS, Becker LB: Quantifying the effect of cardiopulmonary resuscitation quality on cardiac arrest outcome: a systematic review and meta-analysis. *Circ Cardiovasc Qual Outcomes* 6:148–156, 2013.
18. Valenzuela TD, Roe DJ, Nichol G, et al: Outcomes of rapid defibrillation by security officers after cardiac arrest in casinos. *N Engl J Med* 343:1206, 2000.
19. Goldberger ZD, Chan PS, Berg RA, et al: Duration of resuscitation efforts and survival after in-hospital cardiac arrest: an observational study. *Lancet* 27;380(9852):1473–1481, 2012.
20. Nakahara S, Tomio J, Ichikawa M, et al: Association of bystander interventions with neurologically intact survival among patients with bystander-witnessed out-of-hospital cardiac arrest in Japan. *JAMA* 314:247–254, 2015.
21. Hansen M, Kragholm K, Pearson DA, et al: Association of bystander and first-responder intervention with survival after out-of-hospital cardiac arrest in North Carolina, 2010–2013. *JAMA* 314(3):255–264, 2015.
22. Georgiou M, Papathanassoglou E, Xanthos T: Systematic review of the mechanisms driving effective blood flow during adult CPR. *Resuscitation* 85(11):1586–1593, 2014.
23. Niemann JT, Rosborough JP, Brown D, et al: Cough-CPR: documentation of systemic perfusion in man and in an experimental model—a "window" to the mechanism of blood flow in external CPR. *Crit Care Med* 8:141, 1980.
24. Niemann JT, Rosborough JP, Hausknecht M, et al: Pressure-synchronized cineangiography during experimental cardiopulmonary resuscitation. *Circulation* 64:985, 1981.
25. Werner JA, Greene HL, Janko CL, et al: Visualization of cardiac valve motion in man during external chest compression using two-dimensional echocardiography: implications regarding the mechanism of blood flow. *Circulation* 63:1417, 1981.
26. Ralston SH, Babbs CF, Niebauer MJ: Cardiopulmonary resuscitation with interposed abdominal compression in dogs. *Anesth Analg* 61:645, 1982.
27. Babbs CF, Ralston SH, Geddes LA: Theoretical advantages of abdominal counterpulsation in CPR as demonstrated in a simple electrical model of the circulation. *Ann Emerg Med* 13:660, 1984.
28. Sack JB, Kesselbrenner MB, Bregman D: Survival from in-hospital cardiac arrest with interposed abdominal counterpulsation during cardiopulmonary resuscitation. *JAMA* 267:379, 1992.
29. Ward KR, Sullivan RJ, Zelenak RR, et al: A comparison of interposed abdominal compression CPR and standard CPR by monitoring end-tidal PCO_2. *Ann Emerg Med* 18:831, 1989.
30. Mateer JR, Steuven HA, Thompson BM, et al: Pre-hospital IAC-CPR versus standard CPR: paramedic resuscitation of cardiac arrests. *Am J Emerg Med* 3:143, 1985.
31. Cabrini L, Beccaria P, Landoni G, et al: Impact of impedance threshold devices on cardiopulmonary resuscitation: a systematic review and meta-analysis of randomized controlled studies. *Crit Care Med* 36:1625–1632, 2008.
32. Fox PC, Wolff A, Yeh CK, et al: Saliva inhibits HIV-1 infectivity. *J Am Dent Assoc* 116:635, 1988.
33. Sande MH: Transmission of AIDS: the case against casual contagion. *N Engl J Med* 314:380–382, 1986.
34. Mejicano GC, Maki, DG: Infections acquired during cardiopulmonary resuscitation: estimating the risk and defining strategies for prevention. *Ann Intern Med* 129(10):813–828, 1998.
35. Adgey AA, Allen JD, Geddes JS, et al: Acute phase of myocardial infarction. *Lancet* 2:501–504, 1971.
36. Konrad D, Jaderling G, Bell M, et al: Reducing in-hospital cardiac arrests and hospital mortality by introducing a medical emergency team. *Intensive Care Med* 36:100–106, 2010.
37. Winters BD, Pham JC, Hunt EA, et al: Rapid responses systems: a systematic review. *Crit Care Med* 35:1238–1243, 2007.
38. AHA 2010 Guidelines for CPR & ECC. *Circulation* 122[18, Suppl 3]: S640–S656, 2010.
39. Thompson RG, Hallstrom AP, Cobb LA: Bystander-initiated cardiopulmonary resuscitation in the management of ventricular fibrillation. *Ann Intern Med* 90:737–740, 1979.
40. Drew BJ, Harris P, Zègre-Hemsey JK: Insights into the problem of alarm fatigue with physiologic monitor devices: a comprehensive observational study of consecutive intensive care unit patients *PLoS One* 9:e110274, 2014.
41. Melker R, Cavallaro D, Krischer J: One-rescuer CPR—a reappraisal of present recommendations for ventilation. *Crit Care Med* 9:423, 1981.
42. Travers AH, Rea TD, Bentley J, et al: CPR overview: 2010 American Heart Association Guidelines for cardiopulmonary resuscitation and emergency cardiovascular care. *Circulation* 122:S676–S684, 2010.
43. Eftestol T, Sunde K, Steen PA: Effects of interrupting precordial compressions on the calculated probability of defibrillation success during out-of-hospital cardiac arrest. *Circulation* 105:2270, 2002.
44. Rea TD, Fahrenbruch C, Culley L, et al: CPR with chest compression alone or with rescue breathing. *N Engl J Med* 363:423–433, 2010.
45. Svensson L, Bohm K, Castren M, et al: Compression-only CPR or standard CPR in out-of-hospital arrest. *N Engl J Med* 363:434–442, 2010.
46. Powner DJ, Holcombe PA, Mello LA: Cardiopulmonary resuscitation-related injuries. *Crit Care Med* 12:54–55, 1984.
47. Aufderheide TP, Lurie KG: Death by hyperventilation: a common and life-threatening problem during cardiopulmonary resuscitation. *Crit Care Med* 32[Suppl]:S345–S351, 2004.
48. Morrison LJ, Kierzek G, Diekema DS, et al: Ethics: 2010 American Heart Association Guidelines for cardiopulmonary resuscitation and emergency cardiovascular care. Circulation 122:S665–S675, 2010.
49. Berg MD, Schexnayder SM, Chameides L, et al: Pediatric basic life support: 2010 American Heart Association Guidelines for cardiopulmonary resuscitation and emergency cardiovascular care. *Circulation* 122:S862–S875, 2010.
50. Heimlich HJ, Uhtley MH: The Heimlich maneuver. *Clin Symp* 31:22–30, 1979.
51. Lowenstein SR, Sabyan EM, Lassen CF, et al: Benefits of training physicians in advanced cardiac life support. *Chest* 89:512–516, 1986.
52. Rumball C, Macdonald D, Barber P, et al: Endotracheal intubation and esophageal tracheal Combitube insertion by regular ambulance attendants: a comparative trial. *Prehosp Emerg Care* 8:15–22, 2004.
53. Stone BJ, Chantler PJ, Baskett PJ: The incidence of regurgitation during: cardiopulmonary resuscitation: a comparison between the bag valve mask and laryngeal mask airway. *Resuscitation* 38:3–6, 1998.
54. Kokkinis K: The use of the Laryngeal Mask Airway in CPR. *Resuscitation* 27:9–12, 1994.
55. Samarkandi AH, Seraj MA, Dawlatly A, et al: The role of laryngeal mask airway in cardiopulmonary resuscitation. *Resuscitation* 28:103–106, 1994.
56. Katz SH, Falk JL: Misplaced endotracheal tubes by paramedics in an urban emergency medical services system. *Ann Emerg Med* 37:32–37, 2001.
57. Link MA, Atkins DL, Passman RS, et al: Part 6: electrical therapies: automated external defibrillators, defibrillation, cardioversion, and pacing: 2010 American Heart Association Guidelines for Cardiopulmonary Resuscitation and Emergency Cardiovascular Care. Circulation 122:S706–S719, 2010.
58. Mentzelopoulos SD, Malachias S, Chamos C et al: Vasopressin, steroids, and epinephrine and neurologically favorable survival after in-hospital cardiac arrest. *JAMA* 310:270–279, 2013.
59. Guerci AD, Chandra N, Johnson E, et al: Failure of sodium bicarbonate to improve resuscitation from ventricular fibrillation in dogs. Circulation 74[6 Pt 2]:IV75–IV79, 1986.
60. Dybrik T, Strand T, Steen PA: Buffer therapy during out-of-hospital cardiopulmonary resuscitation. *Resuscitation* 29:89–95, 1995.
61. Hahnel J, Lindner KH, Ahnefeld FW: Endobronchial administration of emergency drugs. *Resuscitation* 17:261–272, 1989.
62. Otto CW, Yakaitis RW, Redding JS, et al: Comparison of dopamine, dobutamine, and epinephrine in CPR. *Crit Care Med* 9:640–643, 1981.
63. Niemann JT, Haynes KS, Garner D, et al: Postcountershock pulseless rhythms: response to CPR, artificial cardiac pacing, and adrenergic agonists. *Ann Emerg Med* 15:112–120, 1986.
64. Stiell IG, Hebert PC, Weitzman BN, et al: High-dose epinephrine in adult cardiac arrest. *N Engl J Med* 327:1045–1050, 1992.

65. Brown CG, Martin DR, Pepe PE, et al: A comparison of standard-dose and high-dose epinephrine in cardiac arrest outside the hospital. *N Engl J Med* 327:1051, 1992.
66. Robinson LA, Brown CG, Jenkins J, et al: The effect of norepinephrine versus epinephrine on myocardial hemodynamics during CPR. *Ann Emerg Med* 18:336, 1989.
67. De Backer D, Biston P, Devriendt J, et al: Comparison of dopamine and norepinephrine in the treatment of shock. *N Engl J Med* 362:779–789, 2010.
68. Lindner KH, Prengel AW, Brinkmann A, et al: Vasopressin administration in refractory cardiac arrest. *Ann Intern Med* 124:1061–1064, 1996.
69. Dorian P, Cass D, Schwartz B, et al: Amiodarone as compared with lidocaine for shock-resistant ventricular fibrillation. *N Engl J Med* 346:884–890, 2002.
70. MacMahon S, Collins R, Peto R, et al: Effects of prophylactic lidocaine in suspected acute myocardial infarction: an overview of results from the randomized controlled trials. *JAMA* 260:1910–1916, 1988.
71. DiMarco JP, Sellers TD, Berne RM, et al: Adenosine: electrophysiologic effects and therapeutic use for terminating paroxysmal supraventricular tachycardia. *Circulation* 68:1254–1263, 1983.
72. Teo KK, Yusuf S, Collins R, et al: Effects of intravenous magnesium in suspected acute myocardial infarction: overview of randomised trials. *BMJ* 303:1499–1503, 1991.
73. Kay JH, Blalock A: The use of calcium chloride in the treatment of cardiac arrest in patients. *Surg Gynecol Obstet* 93:97, 1951.
74. Stueven HA, Thompson BM, Aprahamian C, et al: Use of calcium in prehospital cardiac arrest. *Ann Emerg Med* 12:136–139, 1983.
75. Dembo DH: Calcium in advanced life support. *Crit Care Med* 9:358–359, 1981.
76. Southwick FS, Dalgish PH: Recovery after prolonged asystolic cardiac arrest in profound hypothermia. A case report and literature review. *JAMA* 243:1250–1253, 1980.
77. Gordon AS, Ridolpho PF, Cole JE: *Definitive Studies on Pole-Top Resuscitation*. Camarillo, CA, Research Resuscitation Laboratories, Electric Power Research Institute, 1983.
78. The Hypothermia After Cardiac Arrest Study Group: Mild therapeutic hypothermia to improve the neurologic outcome after cardiac arrest. *N Engl J Med* 346:549–556, 2002.
79. Benard SA, Gray TW, Buist MD, et al: Treatment of comatose survivors of out-of-hospital cardiac arrest with induced hypothermia. *N Engl J Med* 346:557–563, 2002.
80. Geurts M, Macleod MR, Kollmar R, et al: Therapeutic hypothermia and the risk of infection: a systematic review and meta-analysis. *Crit Care Med* 42:231–242, 2014.
81. Salen P, Melniker L, Chooljian C, et al: Does the presence or absence of sonographically identified cardiac activity predict resuscitation outcomes of cardiac arrest patients? *Am J Emerg Med* 23:459–462, 2005.
82. Ruygrok ML, Byyny RL, Haukoos JS: Validation of 3 termination of resuscitation criteria for good neurologic survival after out-of-hospital cardiac arrest. *Ann Emerg Med* 54:239–247, 2009.
83. Abbo ED, Yuen TC, Buhrmester L, et al: Cardiopulmonary resuscitation outcomes in hospitalized community-dwelling individuals and nursing home residents based on activities of daily living. *J Am Geriatr Soc* 61:34–39, 2013.
84. Kantamineni P, Emani V, Saini A, et al: Cardiopulmonary resuscitation in the hospitalized patient: impact of system-based variables on outcomes in cardiac arrest. *Am J Med Sci* 348:377–381, 2014.
85. Donaghue AJ, Abella BS, Merchant R, et al: Cardiopulmonary resuscitation for in-hospital events in the emergency department: a comparison of adult and pediatric outcomes and care processes. *Resuscitation* 92:94–100, 2015.
86. Kutsogiannis DJ, Bagshaw SM, Laing B, et al: Predictors of survival after cardiac or respiratory arrest in critical care units. *CMAJ*. 183:1589–1595, 2011.
87. Breitkreutz R, Price S, Steiger HV, et al: Focused echocardiographic evaluation in life support and peri-resuscitation of emergency patients: a prospective trial. *Resuscitation* 81:1527–1533, 2010.
88. Breitkreutz R, Walcher F, Seeger FH: Focused echocardiographic evaluation in resuscitation management: concept of an advanced life support-conformed algorithm. *Crit Care Med* 35[5 Suppl]:S150–S161, 2007.
89. Niendorff DF, Rassias AJ, Palac R, et al: Rapid cardiac ultrasound of inpatients suffering PEA arrest performed by nonexpert sonographers. *Resuscitation* 67:81–87, 2005.
90. Flato UA, Paiva EF, Carballo MT, et al: Echocardiography for prognostication during the resuscitation of intensive care unit patients with non-shockable rhythm cardiac arrest. *Resuscitation* 92:1–6, 2015.
91. Blaivas M, Fox JC: Outcome in cardiac arrest patients found to have cardiac standstill on the bedside emergency department echocardiogram. *Acad Emerg Med* 8:616–621, 2001.
92. Blyth L, Atkinson P, Gadd K, et al: Bedside focused echocardiography as predictor of survival in cardiac arrest patients: a systematic review. *Acad Emerg Med* 19:1119–1126, 2012.
93. Tomruk O, Erdur B, Cetin G, et al: Assessment of cardiac ultrasonography in predicting outcome in adult cardiac arrest. *J Int Med Res* 40:804–809, 2012.
94. Chou HC, Chong KM, Sim SS, et al: Real-time tracheal ultrasonography for confirmation of endotracheal tube placement during cardiopulmonary resuscitation. *Resuscitation* 84:1708–1712, 2013.
95. Sim SS, Lien WC, Chou HC, et al: Ultrasonographic lung sliding sign in confirming proper endotracheal intubation during emergency intubation. *Resuscitation* 83:307–312, 2012.
96. Stone MB, Teismann NA, Wang R: Ultrasonographic confirmation of intraosseous needle placement in an adult unembalmed cadaver model. *Ann Emerg Med* 49:515–519, 2007.
97. Tsung JW, Blaivas M, Stone MB: Feasibility of point-of-care colour Doppler ultrasound confirmation of intraosseous needle placement during resuscitation. *Resuscitation* 80:665–668, 2009.

Chapter 15 ■ Cardioversion and Defibrillation

GLENN STOKKEN • MARK S. LINK • NAOMI F. BOTKIN

The use of electric shock to terminate arrhythmia is one of the sentinel medical advances of the last century and underlies much of the modern treatment of arrhythmias. Thanks to the pioneering work of Zoll and Lown in the late 1950s and early 1960s, the use of electric shock gained widespread acceptance. Although incorporating the same mechanism and physics, *cardioversion* refers to the use of direct-current electric shock to terminate arrhythmias other than ventricular fibrillation (VF), whereas *defibrillation* refers to the termination of VF. Cardioversion shocks are delivered at the time of the electrical QRS complex (to avoid the initiation of VF which may result from shocks on the T-wave) while defibrillation occurs with an unsynchronized shock.

PHYSIOLOGY OF ARRHYTHMIA AND SHOCK

Arrhythmias require both a trigger for initiation and an appropriate substrate for maintenance. Arrhythmias may be due to reentry, increased automaticity, or triggered activity. Many of the commonly encountered arrhythmias are due to a fixed reentrant mechanism, including atrial flutter (AFL), atrioventricular nodal reentrant tachycardia (AVNRT), AV reentrant tachycardia (AVRT), and most ventricular tachycardias (VT). Atrial fibrillation (AF), once thought exclusively initiated by reentry, has also been shown to be initiated by automatic foci in the pulmonary veins in many individuals [1,2]. AF appears to be maintained by one of three mechanisms: functional reentry, one or more rapidly firing foci from an autonomic cardiac ganglion plexi, or "rotors" [2]. VF is also due to functional reentry. Cardioversion and defibrillation terminate these arrhythmias by simultaneously depolarizing all excitable tissue, disrupting the process of reentry.

Arrhythmias may also be due to disorders of impulse formation (increased automaticity or triggered activity). These include sinus tachycardia, focal atrial tachycardia (AT), and idiopathic VT (i.e., VT in a structurally normal heart). Sinus tachycardia is a physiologic response and not a pathologic tachycardia; thus sinus tachycardia will not respond to cardioversion, but AT and VT generally will terminate.

Insight into the effect of shock on fibrillating myocardial cells has grown in the past few decades. Although it was initially thought that all activation fronts had to be terminated simultaneously to stop AF and VF, it is now believed that if the vast majority of myocardium is silenced, the remaining mass is insufficient to perpetuate the arrhythmia. The effect of shock on the fibrillating myocardium is complex and is dependent on multiple factors including energy, waveform, and myocardial refractory state [3]. Electrical shocks at low energy levels may fail to terminate AF and VF. And finally, VF can be triggered in patients not already in this rhythm if shock occurs on a vulnerable portion of the T-wave. Thus, synchronization of shocks with the R-wave will minimize the risk of VF.

INDICATIONS AND CONTRAINDICATIONS

Cardioversion and defibrillation are performed for a variety of reasons in the intensive care setting. In the case of hemodynamic instability due to tachyarrhythmia of nearly any type, the urgent use of shock is strongly indicated. One must be careful, however, not to shock sinus tachycardia, which is commonly present in patients who are hypotensive for noncardiac reasons, as doing so may provoke arrhythmias. Acute congestive heart failure and angina that are secondary to an acute tachyarrhythmia are also indications for urgent cardioversion; however, there is usually sufficient time to provide some anesthesia. In the absence of hemodynamic instability or significant symptoms, cardioversion is usually considered elective and the risks and benefits of the procedure must be carefully weighed.

Extreme caution should be exercised in patients with digitalis toxicity or electrolyte imbalance because of their increased risk of VT or fibrillation after being shocked. Patients with severe sinus node disease may exhibit significant bradyarrhythmia after cardioversion from AF. In addition, patients who have been in AF for greater than 48 hours are at risk of thromboembolism after cardioversion; appropriate measures should be taken to minimize this risk (see below) [2].

CLINICAL COMPETENCE

A clinical competence statement by the American College of Cardiology and American Heart Association outlines the cognitive and technical skills required for the successful and safe performance of elective external cardioversion (Table 15.1). A minimum of eight cardioversions should be supervised before a physician is considered to be competent to perform the procedure independently. In addition, a minimum of four procedures should be performed annually to maintain competence [4].

TABLE 15.1

Cognitive and Technical Skills Necessary for Performing External Cardioversion

Physicians should have knowledge of the following:
- Electrophysiologic principles of cardioversion
- Indications for the procedure
- Anticoagulation management
- Proper use of antiarrhythmic therapy
- Use of sedation and the management of overdose
- Direct current cardioversion equipment, including the selection of appropriate energy and synchronization
- Treatment of possible complications, including ACLS, defibrillation, and pacing
- Proper placement of paddles or pads
- Appropriate monitor display and recognition of arrhythmias
- Ability to differentiate failure to convert atrial fibrillation from an immediate recurrence of atrial fibrillation
- Baseline 12-lead electrocardiogram reading, recognition of acute changes, drug toxicity, and contraindications

Physicians should have the following technical skills:
- Proper preparation of skin and electrode placement, including application of saline jelly or saline-soaked gauze
- Achievement of artifact-free monitored strips and synchronization signal/marker
- Technically acceptable 12-lead electrocardiograms before and after DCCV
- Temporary pacing and defibrillation capabilities
- Ability to perform advanced cardiac life support, including proper airway management

ACLS, advanced cardiovascular life support; DCCV, direct current cardioversion.
From Tracy CM, Akhtar M, DiMarco JP, et al. American College of Cardiology/American Heart Association 2006 Update of the Clinical Competence Statement on invasive electrophysiology studies, catheter ablation, and cardioversion: a report of the American College of Cardiology/American Heart Association/American College of Physicians-American Society of Internal Medicine Task Force on Clinical Competence. *Circulation* 114:1654–1668, 2006.

Methods

Patient Preparation

In the case of unconsciousness due to tachyarrhythmia, shock must be performed emergently. In more elective settings, patient safety and comfort become paramount. As with any procedure, informed consent should be obtained. In elective settings, patients should refrain from eating and drinking for several hours in order to decrease the risk of aspiration (6 hours for solids, 2 hours for clear liquids). Constant heart rhythm monitoring should be used throughout the procedure, and a 12-lead electrocardiogram should be obtained before and after the shock.

Medications with rapid onset and short half-life are favored for achieving analgesia, sedation, and amnesia. The combination of a benzodiazepine, such as midazolam, and a narcotic, such as fentanyl, is a common choice in the absence of anesthesiology assistance. Propofol is often used when an anesthesiologist is present to assist with airway management and sedation. Existing hospital policies for monitoring during conscious sedation should be followed, including frequent assessment of blood pressure and pulse oximetry. Supplemental oxygen is delivered via nasal cannula, face mask, or, in the case of heavier sedation, an Ambu bag. The goal of sedation should be minimal or no response to verbal stimulus.

Shock Waveforms

Defibrillators that employ biphasic waveforms have largely replaced those utilizing monophasic waveforms. Advantages of biphasic waveforms are lower defibrillation thresholds, meaning shocks using biphasic waveforms require less energy to achieve defibrillation, and they are less likely to cause skin burns and myocardial damage [3]. Biphasic truncated exponential waveform and biphasic rectilinear waveform are both commercially available, with the former being more common. Randomized trials comparing the two types of biphasic waveforms in the cardioversion of AF have failed to show any significant difference in efficacy [5–7].

The efficacy of biphasic shocks in the termination of VF has been well established [8]. Furthermore, clinical studies of AF cardioversion have established the superiority of biphasic over monophasic waveform shocks [9]. For instance, one study demonstrated the equivalent efficacy of a 120 to 200 J biphasic sequence with a 200 to 360 J monophasic sequence [9]. Biphasic waveforms allow fewer shocks to be given and a lower total energy delivery. Whether or not this translates into a significant clinical advantage remains to be demonstrated. However, there is evidence that biphasic shocks result in less dermal injury, and no significant difference in myocardial damage [10]. Although an animal model suggested better maintenance of cardiac function after biphasic shocks, human data on myocardial function are not yet available [11].

Electrodes

Self-adhesive pads and handheld paddles are employed for cardioversion and defibrillation. Limited data are available comparing the two modalities, but one study suggested the superiority of paddles over pads in cardioverting AF [12]. This phenomenon might be explained by the lower transthoracic impedance achieved with paddles. Whichever modality is used, impedance can be minimized by avoiding positioning over breast tissue, by clipping body hair when it is excessive, by delivering the shock during expiration, and by firm pressure on the pads or paddles. Burns secondary to self-adhesive pads are common and very rarely observed with paddles.

The optimal anatomic placement of pads and paddles is not clear; however, the general principal holds that the heart must lie between the two electrodes [3]. Anterior-lateral and anterior-posterior (AP) placements are both acceptable (Fig. 15.1). The anterior paddle is placed on the right infraclavicular chest. In anterior-lateral placement, the lateral paddle should be located lateral to the left breast and should have a longitudinal orientation, since this placement results in a lower transthoracic impedance than horizontal orientation. When AP positioning is used, the posterior pad is commonly located to the left of the spine at the level of the lower scapula, although some physicians favor placement to the right of, or directly over, the spine. There are data to suggest that AP placement is more successful in the cardioversion of AF than anterior-lateral positioning when monophasic waveforms are used [13,14]. It is thought that AP positioning directs more of the delivered energy to the atria than anterior-lateral placement. However, a study employing biphasic waveforms failed to show any difference of success with anterior-lateral compared to AP pad positions [15]. It should also be noted that if a patient has an internal ICD, AP positioning is recommended to minimize the potential for damage to the device.

Using the Defibrillator

External defibrillators are designed for easy operation. After the patient is adequately prepared and the electrodes are applied, attention may be turned to the device itself. If the QRS amplitude on the rhythm tracing is small and difficult to see, a different lead should be selected. If cardioversion—rather than defibrillation—is to be performed, the synchronization function should be selected. Many defibrillators require that external leads be applied for synchronization. The appropriate initial energy is selected. Finally, the capacitor is charged, the area is cleared, and the shock is delivered. One should be aware that the synchronization function is automatically deselected after each shock in most devices, meaning that it must be manually reselected prior to any further shock delivery if another synchronized shock is desired.

Table 15.2 provides a checklist for physicians involved in cardioversion. Table 15.3 gives recommendations for the initial energy selection for defibrillation and cardioversion of various arrhythmias. Recommendations specific to each device are available in the manufacturer manuals and should be consulted by physicians unfamiliar with their particular device.

Treatment of Ventricular Fibrillation and Pulseless Ventricular Tachycardia

The algorithm for the treatment of pulseless VT and VF in the most recently published American Heart Association guidelines included some minor changes from the prior 2005 guidelines. A change from A-B-C to C-A-B, emphasis on "high-quality CPR" along with postcardiac arrest care, and de-emphasis of drugs and mechanical compression devices were the major updates in the 2010 guidelines [16]. "High-quality CPR" refers to minimizing interruptions in cardiopulmonary resuscitation (CPR) (especially at the time of shock delivery), adequate compression depth, and allowing for adequate chest recoil. In the 2010 algorithm, vasopressors (epinephrine or vasopressin) may be given before or after the second shock, and antiarrhythmics such as amiodarone and lidocaine may be considered before or after the third shock (Table 15.4). Both VF and pulseless VT are treated

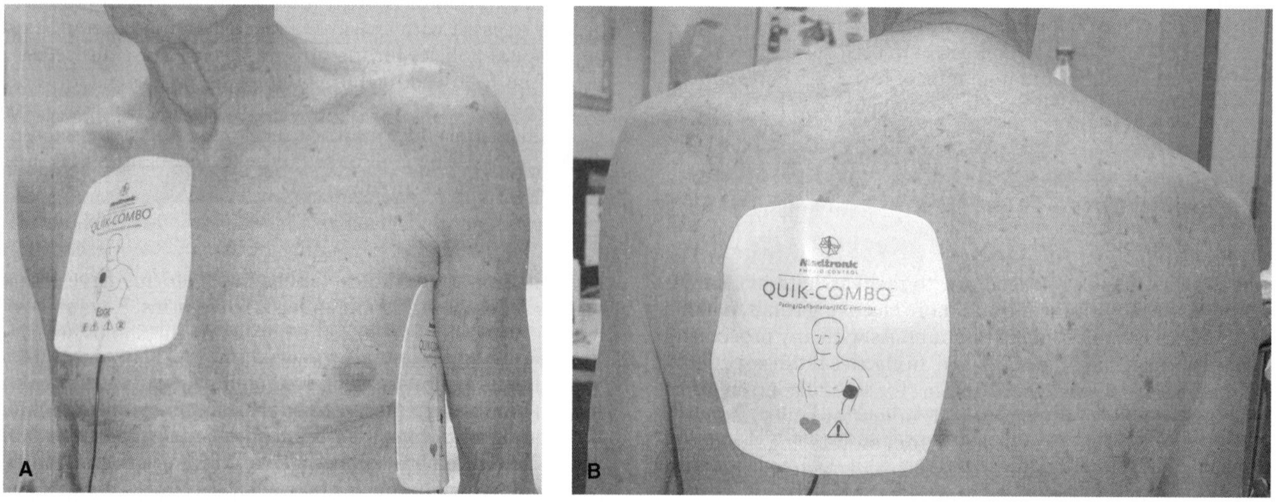

FIGURE 15.1 A: Self-adhesive defibrillator pads in the anterior and lateral positions. **B:** Self-adhesive defibrillator pad in the posterior position. When posterior positioning is used, the second pad is placed anteriorly.

TABLE 15.2

Checklist for Performing External Cardioversion

Preparing the patient:
1. Ensure NPO status (6 h for solids, 2 h for clear liquids)
2. Obtain informed consent
3. Apply self-adhesive pads (clip hair if needed)
4. Apply external lead
5. Achieve adequate sedation and analgesia
6. Monitor vital signs and cardiac rhythm throughout

Performing the cardioversion:
1. Select initial energy appropriate for specific device
2. Select the synchronization function
3. Confirm that arrhythmia is still present
4. Charge, clear, and deliver shock
5. If no change in rhythm, escalate energy as appropriate

NPO, nil per os (nothing by mouth).

TABLE 15.3

Suggested Initial Energy for Cardioversion and Defibrillation

Rhythm	Monophasic	Biphasic
Ventricular fibrillation, pulseless ventricular tachycardia	360 J	120–200 J
Ventricular tachycardia with pulse	100 J	50 J
Atrial fibrillation	100–200 J	200 J [2,4]
Atrial flutter	50–100 J	50 J

TABLE 15.4

Treatment of Ventricular Fibrillation and Pulseless Ventricular Tachycardia

Begin CPR (Emphasis of C-A-B)
Assess rhythm
Deliver 1 shock
- Monophasic: 360 J
- Biphasic: use device-specific energy; if unknown, 200 J

Resume compressions immediately and perform five cycles of CPR, consider advanced airway
Check rhythm—if still VT/VF, shock again
- Monophasic: 360 J
- Biphasic: same as first shock or higher dose

Resume compressions immediately and perform five cycles of CPR
Give a vasopressor during CPR, either before or after the second shock
- Epinephrine 1 mg IV/IO/IT, repeat every 3–5 min, OR
- Vasopressin 40 U IV/IO/IT may replace first or second dose of epinephrine

Check rhythm—if still VT/VF, shock again
Consider an antiarrhythmic before or after third shock:
- Amiodarone 300 mg IV/IO once, then consider additional 150 mg once OR
- Lidocaine 1–1.5 mg/kg first dose, then 0.5–0.75 mg/kg IV/IO, maximum three doses.

CPR, cardiopulmonary resuscitation; IO, intraosseous; IV, intravenous; IT, intratracheal, VF, ventricular fibrillation; VT, ventricular tachycardia.

with unsynchronized, high-energy shocks of 120 to 200 J with biphasic defibrillators (or 360 J in the case of devices that use monophasic waveforms). If there is any uncertainty regarding which energy should be used, it is best to shock with the highest available energy.

Treatment of Wide Complex Tachycardia with a Pulse

When a pulse is present, a regular, wide complex tachycardia may be VT, supraventricular tachycardia with aberrant conduction, or a supraventricular tachycardia with preexcitation. If signs of instability are present (such as chest pressure, altered mental status, hypotension, or heart failure) and are thought to be secondary to the tachycardia, urgent cardioversion is indicated. A starting energy of 100 J is recommended when a monophasic shock waveform is being used. With a biphasic device, the 2010 ACLS guidelines recommend 50 to 100 J. The energy should be escalated with each successive shock.

If the patient is stable, however, one might consider enlisting the assistance of an expert in distinguishing between ventricular and supraventricular arrhythmia. If this is not possible, it is generally safest to assume a ventricular etiology. Stable VT may be treated initially with antiarrhythmic agents such as amiodarone, lidocaine, or procainamide. Elective cardioversion can be performed if necessary, once anesthesia is assured. Adenosine may also be considered for a diagnostic and therapeutic option for a regular, monomorphic, wide complex tachycardia (a new addition to the 2010 guidelines).

Irregular, wide complex tachycardia in a stable patient is probably AF with aberrant conduction; alternatively, it may represent AFL with variable AV block or multifocal AT [10]. In the unstable patient, polymorphic VT or torsades de pointes is more likely. With preexcited AF (Wolff–Parkinson–White syndrome), AV nodal blocking agents are contraindicated and treatment options include procainamide, ibutilide, or amiodarone. If the patient exhibits signs or symptoms of hypoperfusion and instability mentioned above, immediate cardioversion is advised.

Treatment of Supraventricular Tachycardia

The most common narrow complex tachycardia is sinus tachycardia which is an appropriate cardiac response to some other physiologic condition. AF and AFL are the next most common, followed by AVNRT, AVRT, and AT. Supraventricular tachycardia—defined as a non-VT other than sinus tachycardia, AF, or AFL—should be suspected when the arrhythmia starts suddenly, when it is more rapid than maximal sinus rates (220-age), and when P-waves are absent or closely follow the QRS. Initial therapy involves vagal maneuvers and adenosine. If these fail, nondihydropyridine calcium channel antagonists or β-blockers may terminate the arrhythmia. Cardioversion is indicated only rarely for clinical instability, usually in patients with underlying heart disease in whom the initial therapies fail. The recommended initial biphasic energy is 50 to 100 J.

Treatment of Atrial Fibrillation and Flutter

Rate Control

Although the majority of patients with AF and AFL remain hemodynamically stable, many develop bothersome symptoms such as palpitations, chest pressure, and, occasionally, pulmonary edema. However, a rapid ventricular response is usually secondary to, rather than the cause of, heart failure and ischemia. β-blockers, nondihydropyridine calcium channel antagonists, digoxin, amiodarone, and intravenous magnesium sulfate are used to slow the ventricular response rate by slowing AV nodal conduction [17]. Many patients become asymptomatic or minimally symptomatic with adequate rate control, allowing the decision about cardioversion to be made electively.

Electrical Cardioversion

Cardioversion for AF or AFL is usually performed electively. The risk of thromboembolism dictates a thoughtful decision about treatment options. When cardioversion is performed, an appropriate initial starting dose is 100 to 360 J for monophasic waveform shock and 120 to 200 J for biphasic shock, and higher initial energies are recommended to reduce total energy delivered and duration of sedation, especially when the AF duration is >48 hours. AFL responds to lower energy, so a starting dose of 50 to 100 J is recommended with a monophasic waveform. The ideal starting energy for biphasic devices has not yet been defined, but should be lower than that of monophasic devices. If AF or AFL fails to terminate, shock energy should be escalated. For most defibrillators, the synchronization function must be reselected after each shock.

Anticoagulation

Patients with AF or AFL may develop thrombus in the left atrial appendage or left atrial cavity, leading to thromboembolism during or after cardioversion. One study demonstrated a risk of peri-cardioversion thromboembolism of 5.3% in patients who were not anticoagulated and 0.8% in those who were [18].

There is general agreement that cardioversion of patients who have been in AF for less than 24 to 48 hours is unlikely to cause thromboembolism, and as such, a transesophageal echocardiogram (TEE) is not required. Current guidelines indicate that peri-cardioversion anticoagulation with unfractionated heparin, low molecular weight heparin, direct thrombin inhibitor, or a factor Xa inhibitor are all acceptable options [2,19]. Individuals in AF or AFL for greater than 48 hours are at risk of thromboembolism. In these individuals, a TEE is necessary to exclude left atrial thrombus in all but the most emergent cases. Alternatively, one may anticoagulate for at least 3 weeks prior to cardioversion. It is recommended that anticoagulation continue for 3 weeks after cardioversion, as the risk of thromboembolism still exists during this period.

Pharmacologic Cardioversion

Cardioversion can be achieved not only electrically but also pharmacologically. Pharmacologic cardioversion is used mainly for AF and AFL of relatively short duration. Although electrical cardioversion is quicker and has a higher probability of success, pharmacologic cardioversion does not require sedation. The risk of thromboembolism with pharmacologic cardioversion has not been well established but is thought to be similar to that of electrical shock because it is the return of sinus rhythm rather than the shock itself that is believed to precipitate thromboembolism [5].

Dofetilide, flecainide, ibutilide, propafenone, amiodarone, and quinidine have been demonstrated to have some degree of efficacy in restoring sinus rhythm [19]. Each of these medications has potential toxicities including malignant arrhythmias and hypotension. The risks and benefits should be carefully weighed when selecting a pharmacologic agent. Although β-blockers and calcium channel antagonists are often believed to facilitate cardioversion, their efficacy has not been established in controlled trials.

Management of Resistant Atrial Fibrillation

Although electrical cardioversion is generally successful, up to 10% of AF and AFL patients have early recurrences of arrhythmia. The duration of AF is inversely related to the probability of successful cardioversion.

When cardioversion fails to even temporarily terminate the arrhythmia, the operator's technique should be reviewed and modified. Electrode position may be altered, from AP to anterior-lateral or vice versa. Firmer pressure may be employed via the paddles or pads. If a device that delivers monophasic waveform shocks is being employed, it may be exchanged for one that delivers biphasic waveform shocks. Sotalol, ibutilide, dofetilide, or amiodarone may be initiated prior to another attempt at cardioversion. Other antiarrhythmic agents may reduce the recurrence of arrhythmia. It is worthwhile mentioning that while digoxin is useful as a rate-controlling agent, it has pro-fibrillatory effects and therefore can precipitate AF.

Complications of Defibrillation and Cardioversion

Burns

Shock can cause first-degree burns and pain at the paddle or pad site. One study documented moderate to severe pain in nearly one quarter of patients undergoing cardioversion. Pain was directly related to total energy delivered and number of shocks [20]. Another study showed a lower rate of dermal injury with biphasic rather than monophasic shocks, and is associated with lower energy necessary with biphasic shocks. The lowest effective energy should be used to minimize skin injury; however, this must be balanced against a requirement for multiple shocks when a low energy shock fails to terminate an arrhythmia. In addition, burns are much more common with self-adhesive pads, so that for elective cardioversion, paddles may be preferable.

Thromboembolism

Cardioversion of AF and AFL carries a risk of thromboembolism. Please see "Anticoagulation" section above for recommendations about prevention of thromboembolism.

Arrhythmias

Bradyarrhythmias such as sinus arrest and sinus bradycardia are common immediately after shock and are almost always short-lived. Patients who have AF may have concomitant sinus node dysfunction that is masked by the AF and unmasked by cardioversion.

VT and VF can occasionally be precipitated by shock, particularly in patients with digitalis toxicity or hypokalemia [21,22]. Elective cardioversion should therefore be avoided in patients with these conditions. If cardioversion or defibrillation must be performed urgently, one should anticipate the ventricular arrhythmias to be more refractory to shock than usual.

Myocardial Damage

Occasionally, one may see transient ST elevations on post-shock electrocardiograms [23] This is unlikely to signify clinically relevant myocardial injury. Although a study of cardioversion using higher-than-usual energy levels demonstrated an increase in creatine kinase-MB levels above that expected from skeletal muscle damage in 10% of patients, there was no elevation in troponin-T or -I [24]. This observation suggests that clinically significant myocardial damage from cardioversion or defibrillation is unlikely. Nonetheless, it has been suggested that any two consecutive shocks be delivered no less than 1 minute apart to minimize the chance of myocardial damage. Of course, this recommendation applies only to nonemergent situations.

Miscellaneous Topics

Patients with Implanted Pacemakers and Defibrillators

Patients with implanted pacemakers and defibrillators may undergo external cardioversion and defibrillation safely. However, one must be aware of the possibility that external energy delivery may alter the programming of the internal device. Furthermore, energy may be conducted down an internal lead, causing local myocardial injury and a resultant change (typically an increase) in the pacing or defibrillation threshold. The paddles or pads used for external electric shock should never be placed over the device. In addition, interrogation of the device immediately after any external shock delivery is recommended.

Chest Thump

The use of a manual "thump" on the chest to successfully terminate VT was described in several patients in 1970. Unfortunately, this technique may inadvertently trigger VF if the blow happens to fall during the vulnerable period of the ventricle. A chest thump is extremely unlikely to terminate VF [25]. For these reasons, chest thump is considered a therapy of last resort, administered only to a pulseless patient when a defibrillator is unavailable and unlikely to become available soon. It should not be administered when a pulse is present.

Cardioversion and Defibrillation in Pregnancy

Cardioversion and defibrillation have been performed in all trimesters of pregnancy without obvious adverse fetal effects or premature labor [13]. It has been suggested that the fetal heart rhythm be monitored during cardioversion [26].

REFERENCES

1. Haissaguerre M, Jais P, Shah DC, et al: Spontaneous initiation of atrial fibrillation by ectopic beats originating in the pulmonary veins. *N Engl J Med* 339:659–666, 1998.
2. January CT, Wann LS, Alpert JS, et al: 2014 AHA/ACC/HRS guideline for the management of patients with atrial fibrillation: a report of the American College of Cardiology/American Heart Association Task Force on Practice Guidelines and the Heart Rhythm Society. *J Am Coll Cardiol* 64(21):e1–e76, 2014.
3. Part 5: Electrical Therapies: Automated External Defibrillators, Defibrillation, Cardioversion, and Pacing. *Circulation* 112:IV-35-IV-46, 2005.
4. Tracy CM, Akhtar M, DiMarco JP, et al: American College of Cardiology/American Heart Association 2006 Update of the Clinical Competence Statement on invasive electrophysiology studies, catheter ablation, and cardioversion: a report of the American College of Cardiology/American Heart Association/American College of Physicians-American Society of Internal Medicine Task Force on Clinical Competence. *Circulation* 114:1654–1668, 2006.
5. Neal S, Ngarmukos T, Lessard D, et al: Comparison of the efficacy and safety of two biphasic defibrillator waveforms for the conversion of atrial fibrillation to sinus rhythm. *Am J Cardiol* 2003;92:810–814.
6. Kim ML, Kim SG, Park DS, et al: Comparison of rectilinear biphasic waveform energy versus truncated exponential biphasic waveform energy for transthoracic cardioversion of atrial fibrillation. *Am J Cardiol* 2004;94:1438–1440.
7. Alatawi F, Gurevitz O, White RD, et al: Prospective, randomized comparison of two biphasic waveforms for the efficacy and safety of transthoracic biphasic cardioversion of atrial fibrillation. *Heart Rhythm* 2:382–387, 2005.
8. Schneider T, Martens PR, Paschen H, et al: Multicenter, randomized, controlled trial of 150-J biphasic shocks compared with 200- to 360-J monophasic shocks in the resuscitation of out-of-hospital cardiac arrest victims. Optimized Response to Cardiac Arrest (ORCA) Investigators. *Circulation* 2000;102:1780–1787.
9. Scholten M, Szili-Torok T, Klootwijk P, et al: Comparison of monophasic and biphasic shocks for transthoracic cardioversion of atrial fibrillation. *Heart* 89:1032–1034, 2003.
10. Winterhalter M, Piepenbrock T, Leyh RG, et al: Effectiveness and safety of internal rectilinear biphasic versus monophasic defibrillation in patients undergoing cardiac surgery. *J Cardiothorac Vasc Anesth* 19(6):739–745, 2005.
11. Tang W, Weil MH, Sun S, et al: The effects of biphasic and conventional monophasic defibrillation on postresuscitation myocardial function. *J Am Coll Cardiol* 34:815–822, 1999.
12. Kirchhof P, Monnig G, Wasmer K, et al: A trial of self-adhesive patch electrodes and hand-held paddle electrodes for external cardioversion of atrial fibrillation (MOBIPAPA). *Eur Heart J* 26:1292–1297, 2005.
13. Schroeder JS, Harrison DC: Repeated cardioversion during pregnancy. Treatment of refractory paroxysmal atrial tachycardia during 3 successive pregnancies. *Am J Cardiol* 27:445, 446, 1971.
14. Manning WJ, Leeman DE, Gotch PJ, et al: Pulsed Doppler evaluation of atrial mechanical function after electrical cardioversion of atrial fibrillation. *J Am Coll Cardiol* 13:617–623, 1989.
15. Walsh SJ, McCarty D, McClelland AJ, et al: Impedance compensated biphasic waveforms for transthoracic cardioversion of atrial fibrillation: a multi-centre comparison of antero-apical and antero-posterior pad positions. *Eur Heart J* 26:1298–302, 2005.
16. Neumar RW, Otto CW, Link MS, et al: American Heart Association guidelines for cardiopulmonary resuscitation and emergency cardiovascular care science part 8: adult advanced cardiovascular life support. *Circulation* 122:S729–S767, 2010.
17. Sleeswijk ME, Tulleken JE, Van Noord T, et al: Efficacy of magnesium-amiodarone step-up scheme in critically ill patients with new-onset atrial fibrillation: a prospective observational study. *J Intensive Care Med* 23(1):61–66, 2008.
18. Bjerkelund CJ, Orning OM: The efficacy of anticoagulant therapy in preventing embolism related to D.C. electrical conversion of atrial fibrillation. *Am J Cardiol* 23:208–216, 1969.
19. Fuster V, Ryden LE, Cannom DS, et al: ACC/AHA/ESC 2006 Guidelines for the Management of Patients with Atrial Fibrillation: a report of the American College of Cardiology/American Heart Association Task Force on Practice Guidelines and the European Society of Cardiology Committee for Practice Guidelines (Writing Committee to Revise the 2001 Guidelines for the Management of Patients With Atrial Fibrillation): developed in collaboration with the European Heart Rhythm Association and the Heart Rhythm Society. *Circulation* 114:e257–e354, 2006.
20. Ambler JJ, Sado DM, Zideman DA, et al: The incidence and severity of cutaneous burns following external DC cardioversion. *Resuscitation* 61:281–288, 2004.
21. Lown B, Kleiger R, Williams J: Cardioversion and digitalis drugs: changed threshold to electric shock in digitalized animals. *Circ Res* 17:519–531,
22. 1965.
23. Aberg H, Cullhed I: Direct current countershock complications. *Acta Med Scand* 183:415–421, 1968.
24. Van Gelder IC, Crijns HJ, Van der Laarse A, et al: Incidence and clinical significance of ST segment elevation after electrical cardioversion of atrial fibrillation and atrial flutter. *Am Heart J* 121:51–56, 1991.
25. Lund M, French JK, Johnson RN, et al: Serum troponins T and I after elective cardioversion. *Eur Heart J* 21:245–253, 2000.
26. Madias C, Maron BJ, Alsheikh-Ali AA, et al: Precordial thump for cardiac arrest is effective for asystole but not for ventricular fibrillation. *Heart Rhythm* 6:1495–1500, 2009.
27. Meitus ML: Fetal electrocardiography and cardioversion with direct current countershock. Report of a case. *Dis Chest* 48:324–325, 1965.

Chapter 16 ■ Critical Care Echocardiography

BRIAN BUCHANAN • ROBERT ARNTFIELD • PAUL H. MAYO

INTRODUCTION

Critical care echocardiography (CCE) enables the intensivist to identify and differentiate many distinct causes of hemodynamic failure, and to initiate targeted therapy at the point of care. CCE is an essential skill for frontline intensivists and is an important component of critical care training. There is no other bedside method of cardiac imaging that is as immediate and relevant for assessment of cardiopulmonary failure. When combined with other aspects of critical care ultrasonography, it is a key element of the whole-body ultrasonography approach to the critically ill patient, because, when combined with the history and physical examination, it affords the intensivist the ability to promptly diagnose and manage hemodynamic failure. In view of the central importance of CCE, consensus statements have been published with international collaboration among critical care societies regarding competencies, training standards, and scope of practice of CCE [1–3]. This chapter reviews key aspects of both basic and advanced CCE.

Unlike the standard workflow of conventional diagnostic echocardiography as performed by or under the direction of the cardiologist, the CCE examination may be limited in scope and goal-directed; or, depending on the clinical situation and skill of the operator, it may be as comprehensive as the consultative cardiology type examination. With CCE, the intensivist or an individual under their direction is responsible for all image acquisition and interpretation at the point of care and uses the information immediately to address specific hypotheses and to guide ongoing therapy; so the intensivist is required to have skill at image acquisition; image interpretation; and the cognitive elements required for immediate application of the results of the examination. The intensivist has full knowledge of the case, and is able to integrate the results of the CCE examination into the management plan more effectively than echocardiography performed within the constraints of the traditional echocardiography service model, where there are often delays of performance of the study; delays in interpretation; and delays of transmission of the results to the clinical team. In addition, the reader of the echocardiography service study may not be fully aware of the clinical facts of the case. Another difference with consultative echocardiography is that the CCE examination may be repeated as often as required in order to assess the effects of treatment; to follow evolution of the clinical condition; and to check for new diagnoses.

The ACCP/SRLF on Statement of Competence in Critical Care Ultrasonography was adopted as the foundation document for the International Statement on training in critical care ultrasonography that was developed and endorsed by 22 international societies [1,2]. The Competence Statement divides CCE into two parts: basic CCE and advanced CCE. These two categories require separate discussion.

BASIC CRITICAL CARE ECHOCARDIOGRAPHY

Equipment Requirements

Performance of basic CCE requires a portable machine capable of two-dimensional (2D) imaging that is equipped with a phased-array cardiac probe of frequency 2 to 5 MHz. Probes of this design have sufficient penetration for cardiac imaging, and their small footprint allows scanning between adjacent ribs. Modern portable ultrasonography machines have excellent image quality, and many have full Doppler capability, so that they are useful for both basic and advanced CCE. For basic CCE, color Doppler is recommended, but spectral Doppler (pulsed wave and continuous wave) is not mandatory, unless the machine is to be used for advanced CCE. Current generation devices that are designed to fit into pocket of the intensivist have serviceable image quality, but generally lack spectral Doppler capability. Devices available at the time of publication are suitable for basic CCE, but not for advanced CCE.

Technical Problems

Skill at transducer manipulation; optimization of machine settings; and knowledge of standard scanning planes are necessary for consistent, high-quality image acquisition. Patient positioning is an important component of image acquisition, but may be challenging in the intensive care unit (ICU). Although left arm abduction and left lateral decubitus positioning improve the quality of parasternal and apical cardiac views, optimal patient position may be difficult to achieve for all critically ill patients who may be supported with multiple life support devices; who require orthopedic immobilization; and/or who are obese. Mechanical ventilation and chronic obstructive pulmonary disease can block image acquisition owing to lung hyperinflation, and chest wall bandages and drains can limit transthoracic imaging windows. Respirophasic movement of the heart results in translational artifact, as the critically ill patient cannot suspend respiration. As a result, it may be difficult to obtain a stable tomographic plane in the dyspneic patient who has a high respiratory rate.

Training in Basic Critical Care Echocardiography

Competence for basic CCE requires mastery of three learning domains:

1. The cognitive base: The intensivist has a comprehensive knowledge of the cognitive elements of basic CCE. This includes machine operation; ultrasonography physics; cardiac anatomy; clinical applications; indications; and integration of results into other aspects of critical care ultrasonography. Resources include primary literature, review papers, textbooks, formal courses, and internet-based educational material that can be used in blended manner.
2. Image acquisition: The intensivist has definitive skill at image acquisition that includes the five standard views of basic echocardiography. Because there may be no echocardiography technician to perform the study, the quality of the images may be entirely dependent on the skill of the intensivist scanner. Competence at image acquisition is achieved by deliberate practice on normal models under the direct supervision of qualified faculty with transition to supervised scanning of critically ill patients. As the learner becomes more skilled, an autodidactic approach is effective while working with a mentor. Consensus holds that completion of a minimum of 30 acceptable quality studies is needed for competence in basic CCE [2].
3. Image interpretation: Access to a comprehensive video image collection that has a wide variety of abnormal cases provides the learner with skill at image interpretation. Image interpretation training sessions productively combine case-based learning with interpretation of the ultrasonography images. It is not reasonable to expect that the learner will, through personal scanning activity, collect sufficient examples of relevant cardiac dysfunction during their training period. This can be accomplished with a review of a well-designed image library.

Many noncardiologists have achieved competence in basic CCE. This extension of basic echocardiography competence has been supported by The American College of Echocardiography [4] and has been well documented [5–14].

The Basic Critical Echocardiography Examination

As described in the ACCP/SRLF consensus statement, the basic CCE examination consists of the parasternal long-axis (PSL) view, parasternal short-axis (PSS) view, apical four-chamber (AP4) view, subcostal long-axis view, and inferior cava long-axis (IVC) view. Color Doppler may be used to assess the mitral valve (MV) and the aortic valve (AV). Although desirable, a running ECG tracing is not required for every basic echocardiography examination. However, a running ECG tracing generally is required when performing an advanced CCE examination.

Parasternal Long-Axis View

The transducer is placed adjacent to the sternum perpendicular to the skin surface in the left third intercostal space, with the transducer index mark pointing to the right shoulder of the patient. Movement of the transducer in the caudal direction brings the parasternal long axis into view with the best image obtained in the third, fourth, or fifth intercostal space. The transducer is adjusted in small increments until the tomographic plane bisects the MV, the AV and includes the axis with the longest achievable left ventricular (LV) cavity. An optimal long-axis view displays the heart horizontally on the screen (Video of image acquisition). Patient positioning, abdominal obesity/distention, and examiner inexperience may result in a more vertical view of the heart.

Utility of the Parasternal Long-Axis View. The PSL view is used for qualitative assessment of ejection fraction (EF); right ventricular outflow tract (RVOT) and LV wall thickness and function; evaluation of AV/MV structure; evaluation of AV/MV function with screening color Doppler analysis; septal kinetics; LA chamber size; the descending aorta; and the pericardial space (Video Clips).

Pitfalls of the Parasternal Long-Axis view

1. Inability to assess RV size: The PSL view assesses the RVOT, so that it cannot be used to determine RV size. The AP4 and SCL are used for assessment of RV size.
2. Inaccurate LV size and function: Off-axis views of the LV due to rotation or angulation may lead to erroneous assessment of LV size and function. In particular, the LV may appear to be hyperdynamic with end-systolic effacement if the transducer is not orientated to identify the largest LV cavity and aligned through the midpoint of the AV and MV (Video Clips).
3. Inaccurate assessment of MV and AV function: The MV and AV may appear to be anatomically normal on 2D view, but can have substantial degrees of regurgitation, discernible only with color or spectral Doppler analysis. Proficiency in basic CCE does not allow the examiner to reliably exclude severe valvular regurgitation. Color Doppler has limitations not intuitively obvious to the inexperienced examiner. These include gain settings ("dial a jet"); wall jet effect (Coandă effect); angle effect (both of transducer and by Doppler interrogation angle relative to the jet); and shadowing by surrounding structures such as a prosthetic valve apparatus or a calcified annulus (Video Clips).
4. Inaccurate assessment of pericardial and pleural effusion: Identification of a pleural effusion requires that the depth setting on the ultrasound machine be increased such that the structures posterior to the heart are visualized. A pleural effusion will be seen as a relatively hypoechoic space posterior to the LV and posterior to the descending aorta. A pericardial effusion will track anterior to the descending aorta (Video Clips).

Parasternal Short-Axis Mid-Ventricular View

From the PSL long-axis view, the transducer is rotated 90° clockwise without angulation or tilting. This results in a cross-sectional view of the heart. Rotation of the transducer may be achieved using a two-handed approach accomplished by keeping the transducer steady with one hand while rotating it with the other hand. The transducer is rotated until the short axis of the heart is obtained with the transducer index mark pointing toward the left shoulder (Video of image acquisition). By angling the transducer along a right shoulder–left hip axis, multiple tomographic views of the heart may be obtained. For the basic CCE examination, the only view that is required is the mid-ventricular tomographic plane (papillary muscle level) (Video Clips).

Utility of the Parasternal Short-Axis View. The PSS view is used for qualitative assessment of EF; RV/LV wall thickness; LV segmental wall function; LV/RV chamber size and function; septal kinetics; and the pericardial space.

Pitfalls of the Parasternal Short-Axis View

1. Inaccurate assessment of LV configuration: The normal LV should be circular in short axis. An elliptical appearance results from an off-axis view related to a nonperpendicular tomographic plane or underrotation/overrotation of the transducer. An off-axis view may result in inaccurate diagnosis of systolic segmental wall abnormality or septal flattening (Video Clips). The supine position; ventilatory support with lack of diaphragmatic movement; obesity; and elevation of intra-abdominal pressures may all cause the heart to be rotated such that the short-axis view tends to assume a more vertical position in the critically ill. This results in an off-axis view of the LV in the transverse scanning plane. This cannot be corrected by transducer manipulation. An alternative method of obtaining a short-axis view of the LV may be realized with the subcostal approach.
2. Inability to visualize the RV free wall: Estimates of RV size require visualization of the RV wall, which may be difficult in the parasternal short-axis view of the LV. The AP4 and subcostal views are superior for assessment of RV size and function.

Apical Four-Chamber View

The transducer is placed at the anatomic apex of the LV with the probe marker pointing toward the 3 to 4 o'clock position. Ideally, the patient should be placed in the left lateral decubitus position, although this is often not possible in the critically ill patient. The window for the AP4 view is often small and difficult to locate (Video of image acquisition). The septum should be orientated vertically in the center of the screen, and the tomographic plane adjusted such that it bisects the apex, the ventricles, and the atria (Video Clips).

Utility of the Apical Four-Chamber View. The AP4 view is used for qualitative assessment of EF; RV/LV wall thickness, size and function; LV segmental wall function; septal kinetics; right atrium (RA) and LA chamber size; evaluation of tricuspid valve (TV) and MV anatomy with screening color Doppler analysis; and the pericardial space.

Pitfalls of the Apical Four-Chamber View

1. Off-axis image: The AP4 view is the most difficult for the basic-level echocardiographer to obtain. There are three goals for adequate image quality. First, the position of the septum should be in the center of the screen (Video Clip). Second, the tomographic plane should bisect the anatomical apex as well as bisecting the midpoint of the MV and TV annuli (Video Clip). Finally, the transducer rotation should be adjusted such that the RV size is maximal (Video Clip). Because LV-to-RV size ratio is important measurement of basic CCE, proper orientation is important. An off-axis view may result in an inability to visualize the RV free wall, and counterclockwise transducer rotation may result in underestimation of RV size. The subcostal view is the best alternative approach, in the case of suboptimal image quality in the AP4 view position.

Subcostal Long-Axis View

This view is best obtained with the patient lying supine. The transducer is placed just below the xiphoid process, pointing toward the left shoulder. The transducer index mark is orientated to the 3 to 4 o'clock position. This view requires the transducer to be held on its top surface, because some or most of its bottom surface will be contacting the patient (Video of image acquisition). This yields a four-chamber view with the tomographic plane sectioning the heart from the right side through to the left side (Video Clip). Often the subcostal view is the best quality image of the basic CCE examination. In the hyperinflated patient on ventilatory support it may be the only obtainable image. During a cardiopulmonary resuscitation sequence, it is the preferred image plane for rapid assessment of cardiac function during short pulse checks.

Utility of the Subcostal Long-Axis View. The subcostal long-axis view is used for qualitative assessment of EF; RV/LV wall thickness, size and function; LV segmental wall function; septal kinetics; evaluation of TV/MV anatomy with screening color Doppler analysis; and the pericardial space.

Pitfalls of the Subcostal Long-Axis View

1. Off-axis view: The tomographic plane should be orientated such that the RV and LV size are maximal in size and both atria are visible. The subcostal view is particularly susceptible to translational artifact that occurs with the respiratory cycle. The heart can be pushed out of plane in patients who are in respiratory distress or on mechanical ventilatory support (Video Clips)

Inferior Vena Cava (IVC) Longitudinal View

There are several methods of obtaining the IVC longitudinal view. From the subcostal four-chamber view, the transducer is rotated counterclockwise so the index marker is in the 12 o'clock position followed by angulation of the tomographic plane toward the right (Video Clip). Alternatively, the transducer can be moved directly to a right paramedian longitudinal plane, in either subcostal or transcostal position to locate the target structure (Video Clip). If bowel gas or surgical dressings block these anterior views, the transducer should be moved to the right mid-axillary line with the tomographic cut orientated in a coronal plane (Video Clip).

Utility of the IVC View. The IVC view is used for determination of volume responsiveness.

Pitfalls of the IVC View

1. Misidentification of the aorta as the IVC: The aorta is to the left of the midline and is posterior to the heart. The IVC is to the right of the midline, is closely associated with the liver, and passes through the diaphragm into the heart (Video Clip).
2. Off-axis view: Determination of preload sensitivity requires an accurate measurement of the IVC diameter. The scanning plane must be orientated along the longitudinal midline of the IVC to assure accurate diameter measurement (Video Clip).
3. Translational artifact: Volume responsiveness includes measurement of IVC diameter change when the patient is on ventilatory support and without spontaneous respiratory effort. When the ventilator cycles, the liver is displaced by the diaphragmatic movement. This may move the IVC out of the initial scanning plane, giving the impression of a change in diameter that actually is a translational artifact (Video Clip). This is an important consideration, because volume responsiveness may be determined by the IVC diameter change. Translational artifact may result in an inaccurate measurement of diameter change.

Clinical Applications of Goal-Directed Echocardiography

Basic CCE is a standard part of the evaluation of the patient with cardiopulmonary failure. Because image acquisition and interpretation is performed by or under the direction of the intensivist at the point of care, this allows the results to be immediately integrated with the history, the physical examination, and the laboratory assessment into the plan of care. By giving an immediate assessment of cardiac anatomy and function, the results influence management in a timely manner.

1. Identification of an immediately life-threatening cause for hemodynamic failure: The use of basic echocardiography allows for early identification of an imminently life-threatening process where early intervention may be lifesaving, such as pericardial tamponade; major valve failure; severe reduction in left ventricular function; or massive pulmonary embolism. Though it is uncommon, the possibility of an immediate diagnosis of a life-threatening process justifies early basic CCE for every patient in shock (Video Clips).
2. Categorization of shock state and initial management strategy: The five standard views of basic CCE allow the intensivist to rapidly categorize shock as cardiogenic, obstructive, hypovolemic, or distributive in pattern, thereby allowing for a targeted management strategy as well as guiding the search for treatable specific causes of the hemodynamic failure (Video Clips).
3. Evolution of disease and response to therapy: Critical illness is a dynamic process, as is, often, response to therapy, so a standard aspect of basic CCE is that it is repeated in serial fashion to follow the evolution of hemodynamic failure and response to treatments. The frontline intensivist uses serial basic CCE examinations on a routine basis, with the need determined by the clinical circumstances (Video Clips).
4. Identification of coexisting diagnoses: The critically ill patient may have more than one diagnosis that may preexist or modify the acute hemodynamic phenotype. These complicating factors can occur de novo or coexist at the time of a hemodynamic insult. The basic echocardiography examination is useful to identify both the primary hemodynamic insult and important coexisting diagnoses, and clarify the best comprehensive management plan (Video Clips).

Limitations of Basic Critical Care Echocardiography

It is important to recognize some of the limitations of goal-directed echocardiography (GDE). Recognition of these allows the ICU team to adjust their training and scanning strategy accordingly.

1. Limited Image Set: The basic CCE examination does not replace advanced level CCE, because it is limited to five views and does not include spectral Doppler. With Doppler measurements absent, it cannot include hemodynamic measurements such as stroke volume; pulmonary artery pressures; or quantitative measurement of valvular function. A key aspect of competence in basic CCE is knowledge of when to request a full echocardiography study.
2. Failure of Image Acquisition: A major limitation of both basic and advanced CCE is inadequate image quality related to patient-specific factors such as body habitus; difficulty with positioning the patient; and respirophasic translational artifacts. In this case, TEE may be indicated.
3. Inadequate Training: Failure of acquisition and interpretation of adequate quality images, or lack of knowledge of clinical applications of basic CCE can derive from inadequate training. Faculty have a special responsibility to provide rigorous training in all aspects of basic echocardiography and to develop effective means of quality assessment before the trainee or technician is considered competent in basic CCE.
4. Challenges of Documentation: The critical care team that uses basic CCE as a primary tool for initial and serial evaluation of hemodynamic failure faces the challenge of documenting a large number of studies that are performed on a daily basis in a busy ICU. Facing this reality, basic CCE comes to resemble

physical examination, where not every encounter is documented as a matter of practical necessity. This becomes problematic when trying to compare serial examinations. The solution to the challenge of documentation requires the development of methods of image storage and interpretation that can be used at the point of care. As wireless solutions become more widely available, the documentation issue will be less problematic. Integration of these data collection systems into ICU function requires training and buy-in by the intensivist staff.

Advanced Critical Care Echocardiography

Advanced CCE uses the same machine, the transducer, the image interpretation methods, and much of the same knowledge base and standard views as the cardiologist, but it differs in some ways from consultative cardiology echocardiography.

1. The examination may be as complete as the consultative cardiology examination or limited in scope. Because it is performed by the intensivist team at the point of care, the clinician decides what components of the examination are relevant given the clinical context.
2. The intensivist integrates the findings into a clinical management plan in ways that differ from consultative cardiology echocardiography, particularly when the intensivist uses advanced CCE as a hemodynamic monitoring tool. Advanced CCE is used to perform sequential examinations for patients to assess the effectiveness of changes in responses to therapy. The intensivist, in addition to having skill similar to the cardiologist in terms of diagnosis of cardiac dysfunction, also has skill at using echocardiography for sequential assessment of hemodynamics; evolution of disease; and responses to therapies.
3. The intensivist should have skill with all aspects of image acquisition related to advanced CCE, including the full image set that is typical of consultative cardiology echocardiography with comprehensive use of Doppler measurements. As with basic CCE, the intensivist can be personally responsible for image acquisition at the point of care. This is different from the standard echocardiography model in North America, where echocardiography technicians perform the examination for subsequent interpretation by the cardiologist. This is not the case in Europe, where echocardiography technicians are not the norm. This is an evolving field with increased use of off-site real-time interpretation of images obtained by bedside caregivers or technicians.
4. Unlike the cardiologist, the intensivist who performs advanced CCE is competent in general critical care ultrasonography (thoracic ultrasonography, including lung and pleura; screening abdominal ultrasonography; and vascular study for deep venous thrombosis), so the results of advanced CCE can be productively integrated into a whole-body ultrasonography approach to assessment of critical illness.

Training in advanced CCE is not required for the majority of intensivists. Competence in advanced CCE requires a substantial course of training, so the need for it is determined by the practice requirements of the intensivist. In a large ICU with a full-time team, all team members have skill at GDE, but only a small proportion need advanced CCE skill. Based on the experience in France, where there is a well-organized training sequence for advanced CCE, between 10% and 20% of the intensivist team have training in advanced CCE, whereas the others are competent in basic CCE.

Training Requirements

The training requirements for advanced CCE are summarized in a recent consensus statement that explicitly defines the process required to become competent in image acquisition; image interpretation; and the cognitive elements of the field [3]. The document forms the basis for the requirements for certification in advanced CCE that has been developed by the European Society of Critical Care Medicine. There is possibility that a similar certification process will be developed in North America under the aegis of the National Board of Echocardiography. Important elements of advanced CCE are reviewed in Chapter 29 of this textbook, and in relevant papers [15–17] and standard textbooks.

Transesophageal Echocardiography

TEE is part of advanced CCE. TEE can be performed with a high degree of safety for the intubated patient on mechanical ventilatory support, and it has strong clinical utility particularly for post–cardiac surgery ICU patients. Its main indication is in the situation where transthoracic echocardiography results in inadequate image quality to answer the clinical question at hand. This often occurs owing to patient-specific factors (e.g., obesity, heavy musculature, and cardiac surgery), or when TTE is known to be inadequate as a scanning method (e.g., intracardiac thrombus, and evaluation for endocarditis). The European certification process for advanced CCE includes TEE as a mandatory component of the training. This reflects the fact that TEE is widely used by intensivists in Europe. The situation is different than in North America, where it is still not common for intensivists to perform TEE. At present, the North American intensivist who decides to become competent in TEE is advised to follow the training requirements used in Europe [3]. TEE simulators are an effective means of accelerating skill at image acquisition [18].

Limitations of Advanced Echocardiography

Certain aspects of echocardiography remain under the purview of the cardiology echocardiographer. These include full assessment of artificial heart valves; stress echocardiography; complex congenital heart disease; decisions related to timing of valve replacement; intraoperative assessment of valve repair/replacement; and guidance of certain cardiac procedures. It is unlikely that an intensivist would have sufficient volume of service or interest to develop competence in these applications.

References

1. Mayo PH, Beaulieu Y, Doelken P, et al: American College of Chest Physicians/La Société de Réanimation de Langue Française statement on competence in critical care ultrasonography. *Chest* 135:1050–1060, 2009.
2. Cholley B: International expert statement on training standards for critical care ultrasonography Expert Round Table on Ultrasound in ICU. *Intensive Care Med* 37:1077–1083, 2011.
3. Expert Round Table on Echocardiography in ICU: International consensus statement on training standards for advanced critical care echocardiography. *Intensive Care Med* 40:654–666, 2014.
4. Labovitz AJ, Noble VE, Bierig M, et al: Focused cardiac ultrasound in the emergent setting: a consensus statement of the American Society of Echocardiography and American College of Emergency Physicians. *J Am Soc Echocardiogr* 23:1225–1230, 2010.
5. Mandavia DP, Hoffner RJ, Mahaney K, et al: Bedside echocardiography by emergency physicians. *Ann Emerg Med* 383:77–382, 2001.
6. Moore CL, Rose GA, Tayal VS, et al: Determination of left ventricular function by emergency physician echocardiography of hypotensive patients. *Acad Emerg Med* 9:186–193, 2002.
7. Vignon P, Chastagner C, François B, et al: Diagnostic ability of hand-held echocardiography in ventilated critically ill patients. *Crit Care* 7:R84–R91, 2003.
8. Randazzo MR, Snoey ER, Levitt MA, et al: Accuracy of emergency physician assessment of left ventricular ejection fraction and central venous pressure using echocardiography. *Acad Emerg Med* 10:973–977, 2003.
9. Lemola K, Yamada E, Jagasia D, et al: A hand-carried personal ultrasound device for rapid evaluation of left ventricular function: use after limited echo training. *Echocardiography* 20:309–312, 2003.

10. DeCara JM, Lang RM, Koch R, et al: The use of small personal ultrasound devices by internists without formal training in echocardiography. *Eur J Echocardiogr* 4:141–147, 2003.
11. Pershad J, Myers S, Plouman C, et al: Bedside limited echocardiography by the emergency physician is accurate during evaluation of the critically ill patient. *Pediatrics* 114:e667–e671, 2004.
12. Jones AE, Tayal VS, Sullivan DM, et al: Randomized, controlled trial of immediate versus delayed goal-directed ultrasound to identify the cause of nontraumatic hypotension in emergency department patients. *Crit Care Med* 32:1703–1708, 2004.
13. Royse CF, Seah JL, Donelan L, et al: Point of care ultrasound for basic haemodynamic assessment: novice compared with an expert operator. *Anaesthesia* 61:849–855, 2006.
14. Melamed R, Sprenkle MD, Ulstad VK, et al: Assessment of left ventricular function by intensivists using hand-held echocardiography. *Chest* 135:1416–1420, 2009.
15. Narasimhan M, Koenig SJ, Mayo PH: Advanced echocardiography for the critical care physician: part 1. *Chest* 145:129–134, 2014.
16. Narasimhan M, J Koenig S, Mayo PH: Advanced echocardiography for the critical care physician: part 2. *Chest* 145:135–142, 2014.
17. Mayo PH, Narasimhan M, Koenig S: Critical care transesophageal echocardiography. *Chest* 148:1323–1332, 2015.
18. Prat G, Charron C, Repesse X, et al: The use of computerized echocardiographic simulation improves the learning curve for transesophageal hemodynamic assessment in critically ill patients. *Ann Intensive Care* 6:27, 2016.

Chapter 17 ▪ Pericardiocentesis

PEEYUSH GROVER • CRAIG S. SMITH

Pericardial diseases are commonly encountered in the critical care setting. The diagnosis and management of these disorders is challenging for physicians owing to a paucity of randomized clinical data. Pericardiocentesis offers an excellent diagnostic and therapeutic tool for the treatment of potentially life-threatening pericardial diseases. This chapter reviews the indications for emergent and urgent pericardiocentesis; summarizes the pathobiology of pericardial effusions; and provides a step-by-step approach to pericardiocentesis, including management of patients following the procedure.

INDICATIONS FOR PERICARDIOCENTESIS

The initial management of patients with a known or suspected pericardial effusion is largely determined by clinical status. In the absence of hemodynamic instability or suspected purulent bacterial pericarditis, there is no need for emergent or urgent pericardiocentesis. Diagnostic pericardiocentesis may be performed to establish the etiology of an effusion, but should be considered only after a thorough noninvasive workup has been completed [1].

Despite an extensive differential diagnosis of a new pericardial effusion, a diagnosis based on initial history and physical examination is highly predictive [2,3]. The clinical context in which diagnostic pericardiocentesis is performed affects its predictive value, with greater diagnostic yield for large effusions than for acute pericarditis [4,5]. Primarily owing to the routine use of echocardiographic guidance, the major (1.2%) and minor (3.5%) complications of pericardiocentesis have significantly decreased over the past several decades, with successful single needle passage rates approaching 90% and relief of tamponade in over 97% [6]. As a result, current guidelines recommend pericardiocentesis as the method of choice for pericardial fluid removal/sampling [7]. Surgical intervention is recommended for recurring large effusions for which repeated pericardiocentesis has not been effective; loculated or posterior effusions of hemodynamic consequence; purulent pericarditis; traumatic hemopericardium; constrictive pericarditis; and effusions due to aortic dissection [7].

In contrast to diagnostic pericardiocentesis, the management of hemodynamically compromised patients requires emergent removal of pericardial fluid to restore adequate ventricular filling (preload) and hasten clinical stabilization. Fluid resuscitation and inotropic agents, although largely ineffective, are the mainstays of medical management that should be used only as a bridge to pericardial drainage. The method and timing of the procedure is determined by the patient's degree of stability [8]. Although echocardiographic and fluoroscopic guidance is preferred, unguided (or blind) pericardiocentesis may be required in patients with severe hypotension not responsive to temporizing measures. In this setting, there are no absolute contraindications to the procedure, and it should be performed without delay at the patient's bedside.

Urgent pericardiocentesis is indicated if patients are initially hypotensive but responsive to hemodynamic support. Unlike acute tamponade, subacute tamponade is more likely to present with protean symptoms such as dyspnea and fatigue. Patients with preexisting hypertension may not demonstrate severe hypotension due to a persistent sympathetic response. Echocardiographic assessment of effusion size; hemodynamic impact; and optimal percutaneous approach are of paramount importance [9]. The procedure should be performed within several hours of presentation while careful monitoring and support continue. As in elective circumstances, pericardiocentesis in these patients should be undertaken with appropriate visual guidance, the method of which depends on the physician's expertise and resources.

Three additional points must be stressed regarding patients undergoing expedited pericardiocentesis. First, coagulation parameters—prothrombin time, partial thromboplastin time, and platelet count ($>50,000/\mu L$)—should be checked and, when possible, quickly normalized prior to the procedure. If clinically feasible, the procedure should be postponed until the international normalized ratio (INR) is less than 1.4, and an anti-Xa level is recommended for patients receiving low–molecular weight heparin. For emergent pericardiocentesis performed on anticoagulant therapy, prolonged and continuous drainage is recommended. Second, many critical care specialists advocate performance of all pericardiocentesis procedures in the catheterization laboratory with concomitant right heart pressure monitoring to document efficacy of the procedure and to exclude a constrictive element of pericardial disease, although excessive delays must be avoided. Finally, efforts to ensure a cooperative and stationary patient during the procedure greatly facilitate the performance, safety, and success of pericardiocentesis.

ANATOMY

The clinical presentation of pericardial effusion is greatly influenced by pericardial anatomy and physiology. The pericardium is a membranous structure with two layers: the visceral and parietal pericardium. The visceral pericardium is a monolayer of mesothelial cells adherent to the epicardial surface by a loose collection of small blood vessels, lymphatics, and connective tissue. The parietal pericardium is a relatively inelastic 2 mm-dense outer network of collagen and elastin with an inner surface of mesothelial cells. It is invested around the great vessels and defines the shape of the pericardium, with attachments to the sternum, diaphragm, and anterior mediastinum while anchoring the heart in the thorax [10]. Posteriorly, the visceral epicardium is absent, with the parietal epicardium attached directly to the heart at the level of the vena cavae [11]. The potential space between the visceral and parietal mesothelial cell layers normally contains 15 to 50 mL of serous fluid in the AV and interventricular grooves, which is chemically similar to plasma ultrafiltrate [12]. The pericardium is relatively avascular, but is well innervated and may produce significant pain with vagal responses during procedural manipulation or inflammation [13].

Owing to the inelastic physical properties of the parietal pericardium, the major determinant of when and how pericardial effusions come to clinical attention is directly related to the speed of accumulation. Effusions that collect rapidly (over minutes to hours) may cause hemodynamic compromise with volumes of 250 mL or less. These effusions are usually located posteriorly and are often difficult to detect without echocardiography or other imaging modalities such as multislice computed tomography (CT) or cardiac magnetic resonance imaging (MRI). In contrast, effusions developing slowly (over days to weeks) allow for dilation of the fibrous parietal membrane. Volumes of 2,000 mL or greater may accumulate without significant hemodynamic compromise. As a result, chronic effusions may present with symptoms owing to compression of adjacent thoracic structures such as cough, dyspnea, dysphagia, or early satiety. Conversely, intravascular hypovolemia; impaired ventricular systolic function; and ventricular hypertrophy with decreased elasticity of the myocardium (diastolic dysfunction) may exacerbate hemodynamic compromise without significant effusions present evident by imaging methods.

Effusive-constrictive pericarditis (up to 7% of patients with tamponade) results from the accumulation of fluid between the visceral and parietal pericardium and may be transient (chemotherapy) or persistent. This diagnosis is important to make owing to its likelihood to evolve into a persistent constriction [14]. It is defined as failure of the right atrial pressure to decrease by more than 50% or to <10 mm Hg after pericardiocentesis as well as persistent signs of constriction on right heart catheter and on physical exam. Like most effusions, the clinical course is determined by the underlying etiology, but if symptoms of right heart failure persist, a visceral pericardectomy must be performed.

PROCEDURE

Since the first blind (or closed) pericardiocentesis performed in 1840 [15], numerous approaches to the pericardial space have been described. Marfan [16] performed the subcostal approach in 1911, which then became the standard approach for unguided pericardiocentesis, because it is extrapleural and avoids the coronary and internal mammary arteries.

The advent of clinically applicable ultrasonography has opened a new chapter in diagnostic and therapeutic approaches to pericardial disease, allowing clinicians to quantitate and localize pericardial effusions quickly and noninvasively [17–21]. Callahan et al. [22] at the Mayo Clinic established the efficacy and safety of two-dimensional (2D) echocardiography to guide pericardiocentesis. Although direct quantification of total fluid accumulation with echo is difficult, circumferential effusions >10 mm are considered large (500 mL), and guidelines recommend pericardiocentesis for effusions >20 mm, regardless of the presence of hemodynamic compromise [7]. Typically, at least 250 mL of fluid is required for safe pericardiocentesis. The routine use of echocardiography has resulted in two major trends in clinical practice: First, 2D echocardiography is commonly used to guide pericardiocentesis, with success rates comparable to traditionally fluoroscopic guided procedures [19,23–25]. Second, approaches other than the traditional subxiphoid method have been investigated owing to the ability to clearly define the anatomy (location and volume) of each patient's effusion [22]. In one series of postsurgical patients, the subxiphoid approach was the most direct route in only 12% of effusions [26]. With the use of echocardiographic guidance, apical and parasternal pericardiocentesis are increasingly performed with comparable success rates to the subxiphoid approach. In the apical approach, the needle is directed parallel to the long axis of the heart toward the aortic valve. Parasternal pericardiocentesis is performed with needle insertion 1 cm lateral to the sternal edge, to avoid internal mammary laceration. All approaches employ a Seldinger technique of over-the-wire catheter insertion. Because the subxiphoid approach remains the standard of practice and is the preferred approach for unguided emergent pericardiocentesis, it is described below.

Regardless of the approach used, confirmation of appropriate positioning is mandatory and preferably performed before a dilation catheter is advanced over the wire. Direct visualization of the needle with either echocardiography or fluoroscopy and injection of agitated saline (echo-guided) contrast (fluoroscopy-guided) should be performed to confirm the correct position [21].

In addition to two large-bore peripheral intravenous lines for aggressive resuscitative efforts, standard electrocardiographic monitoring is mandatory. Historically, an electrocardiogram (ECG) lead directly attached to the puncture needle has been used to detect contact with the myocardium via the appearance of a large "injury current" (ST elevation). Owing to the fact that a suboptimally grounded needle could fibrillate the heart (and the widespread availability of echocardiography), it is considered an inadequate safeguard [7].

The materials required for bedside pericardiocentesis are listed in Table 17.1. Table 17.2 lists the materials required for

TABLE 17.1

Materials for Percutaneous Pericardiocentesis

Site preparation
- Antiseptic
- Gauze
- Sterile drapes and towels
- Sterile gloves, masks, gowns, caps
- 5-mL or 10-mL syringe with 25-gauge needle
- 1% lidocaine (without epinephrine)
- Code cart
- Atropine (1-mg dose vial)

Procedure
- No. 11 blade
- 20-mL syringe with 10 mL of 1% lidocaine (without epinephrine)
- 18-gauge, 8-cm, thin-walled needle with blunt tip
- Multiple 20- and 40-mL syringes
- Hemostat
- Electrocardiogram machine
- Three red-top tubes
- Two purple-top (heparinized) tubes
- Culture bottles

Postprocedure
- Suture material
- Scissors
- Sterile gauze and bandage

TABLE 17.2

Materials for Intrapericardial Catheter

Catheter placement
Teflon-coated flexible J-curved guidewire
6 Fr dilator
8 Fr dilator
8 Fr, 35-cm flexible pigtail catheter with multiple fenestrations (end and side holes)
Drainage system[a]
Three-way stopcock
Sterile IV tubing
500-mL sterile collecting bag (or bottle)
Sterile gauze and adhesive bag (or bottle)
Suture material

simultaneous placement of an intrapericardial drainage catheter. The materials are available in prepackaged kits or individually (Figures 17.1 and 17.2).

The subxiphoid approach for pericardiocentesis is as follows:

1. Patient preparation: Assist the patient in assuming a comfortable supine position with the head of the bed elevated to approximately 45 degrees from the horizontal plane. Extremely dyspneic patients may need to be positioned fully upright, with a wedge if necessary. Elevation of the thorax allows free-flowing effusions to collect inferiorly and anteriorly, the sites that are safest and easiest to access using the subxiphoid approach.

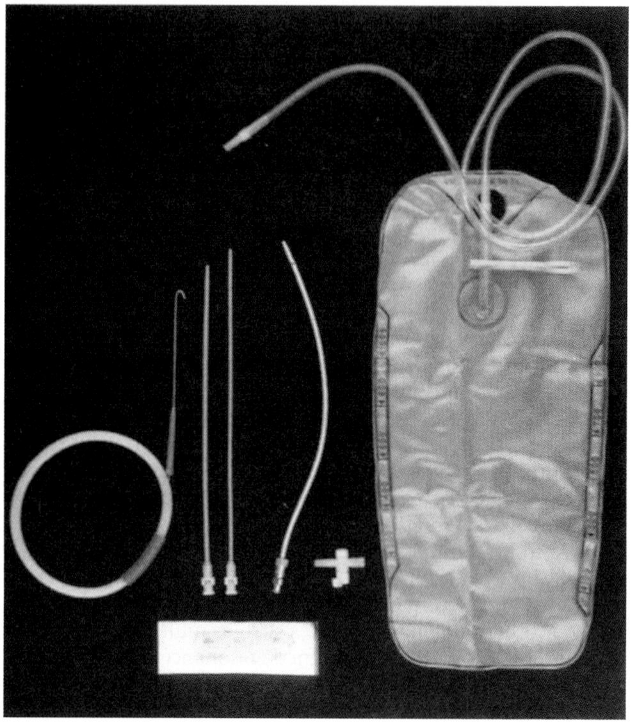

FIGURE 17.2 Materials required for intrapericardial catheter placement and drainage (*clockwise from lower left*): Teflon-coated flexible 0.035-inch J-curved guidewire, 8 Fr dilator, 6.3 Fr dilator, 8 Fr catheter with end and side holes (35-cm flexible pigtail catheter not shown), three-way stopcock, 500-mL sterile collecting bag and tubing, suture material.

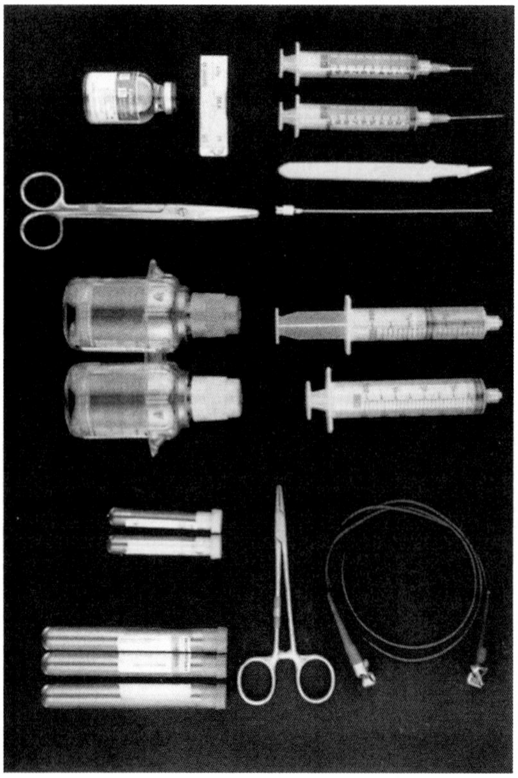

FIGURE 17.1 Materials required for pericardiocentesis (*clockwise from upper left*): 1% lidocaine solution; suture material; 10-mL syringe with 25-gauge needle; 10-mL syringe with 22-gauge needle; no. 11 blade; 18-gauge 8-cm thin-walled needle; 20-mL syringe; 30-mL syringe; alligator clip; hemostat; three red-top tubes; two purple-top tubes; culture bottles; and scissors.

2. Needle entry site selection: Locate the patient's xiphoid process and the border of the left costal margin using inspection and careful palpation. The needle entry site should be 0.5 cm to the (patient's) left of the xiphoid process and 0.5 to 1.0 cm inferior to the costal margin (Fig. 17.3). It is

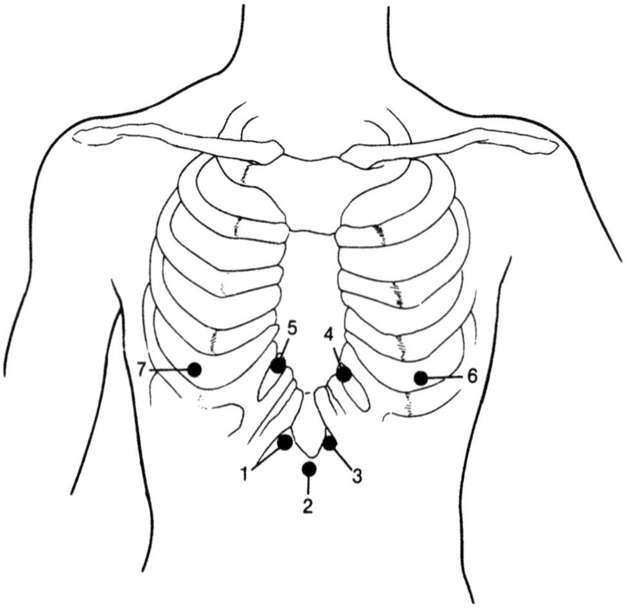

FIGURE 17.3 Selected locations for pericardiocentesis. In most cases, the subxiphoid approach (1 to 3) is preferred. (From Spodick DH: *Acute Pericarditis*. New York, Grune & Stratton, 1959, with permission.)

helpful to estimate (by palpation) the distance between the skin surface and the posterior margin of the bony thorax: This helps guide subsequent needle insertion. The usual distance is 1.0 to 2.5 cm, increasing with obesity or protuberance of the abdomen.

3. Site preparation: Strict sterile techniques must be maintained at all times in preparation of the needle entry site. Prepare a wide area in the subxiphoid region and lower thorax with a povidone–iodine or alcohol chlorhexidine solution and drape the field with sterile towels, leaving the subxiphoid region exposed. After a time-out, raise a 1- to 2-cm subcutaneous wheal by infiltrating the needle entry site with 1% lidocaine solution (without epinephrine). To facilitate needle entry, incise the skin with a No. 11 blade at the selected site after achieving adequate local anesthesia.
4. Insertion of the needle apparatus: The angle of entry with respect to the skin should be approximately 45 degrees in the subxiphoid area. Direct the needle tip superiorly, aiming for the patient's left shoulder. Continue to advance the needle posteriorly while alternating between aspiration and injection of lidocaine (with a half-filled 20 mL syringe of 1% lidocaine), until the tip has passed just beyond the posterior border of the bony thorax (Fig. 17.4). The posterior border usually lies within 2.5 cm of the skin surface. If the needle tip contacts the bony thorax, inject lidocaine after aspirating to clear the needle tip and anesthetize the periosteum. Then, walk the needle behind the posterior (costal) margin.
5. Needle direction: Once under the costal margin, reduce the angle of contact between the needle and skin to 15 degrees: This will be the angle of approach to the pericardium; the needle tip, however, should still be directed toward the patient's left shoulder. A 15-degree angle is used regardless of the height of the patient's thorax (whether at 45 degrees or sitting upright) (Fig.17.5).
6. Needle advancement: Advance the needle slowly while alternating between aspiration of the syringe and injection of 1% lidocaine solution. Obtain a baseline lead V tracing and monitor a continuous ECG tracing for the presence of ST-segment elevation or premature ventricular contractions (evidence of epicardial contact) as the needle is advanced. Advance the needle along this extrapleural path until either:
    a. A "give" is felt, and fluid is aspirated from the pericardial space (usually 6.0 to 7.5 cm from the skin) (Fig. 17.6). Some patients may experience a vasovagal response at this point and require atropine intravenously to increase their blood pressure and heart rate.

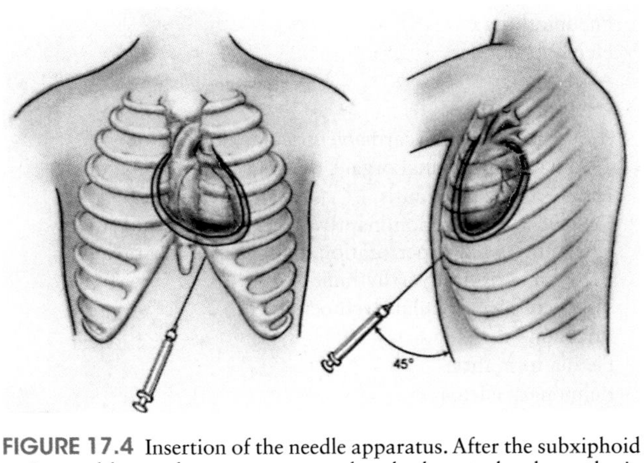

FIGURE 17.4 Insertion of the needle apparatus. After the subxiphoid region and lower thorax are prepared and adequate local anesthesia is given, the pericardiocentesis needle is inserted in the subxiphoid incision. The angle of entry (with the skin) should be approximately 45 degrees. The needle tip should be directed superiorly, toward the patient's left shoulder.

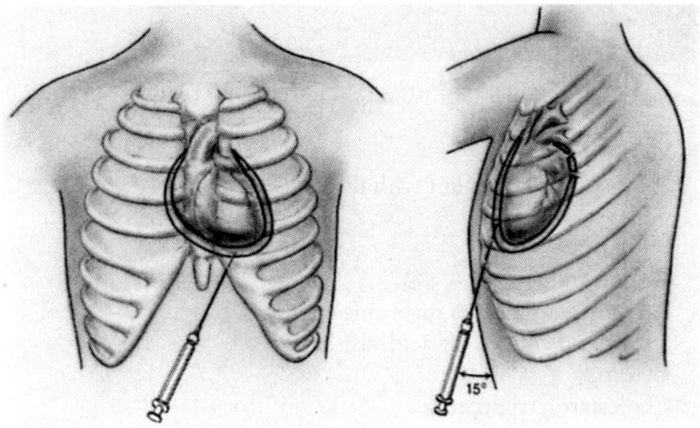

FIGURE 17.5 Needle direction. The needle tip should be reduced to 15 degrees once the posterior margin of the bony thorax has been passed. Needle advancement: The needle is advanced toward the left shoulder slowly while alternating between aspiration and injection. A "give" is felt, and fluid is aspirated when the pericardial space is entered.

    b. ST-segment elevation or premature ventricular contractions are observed on the electrocardiographic lead V tracing when the needle tip contacts the epicardium. If ST-segment elevation or premature ventricular complexes occur, immediately (and carefully) withdraw the needle toward the skin surface while aspirating. Avoid any lateral motion, which could damage the epicardial vessels. Completely withdraw the needle if no fluid is obtained during the initial repositioning.

    If a sanguineous fluid is aspirated, the differentiation between blood and effusion must be made immediately. In addition to confirming catheter position by saline, contrast, or pressure transduction, several milliliters of fluid can be kept and observed for clotting. Intrinsic fibrinolytic activity in the pericardium prevents subacute/

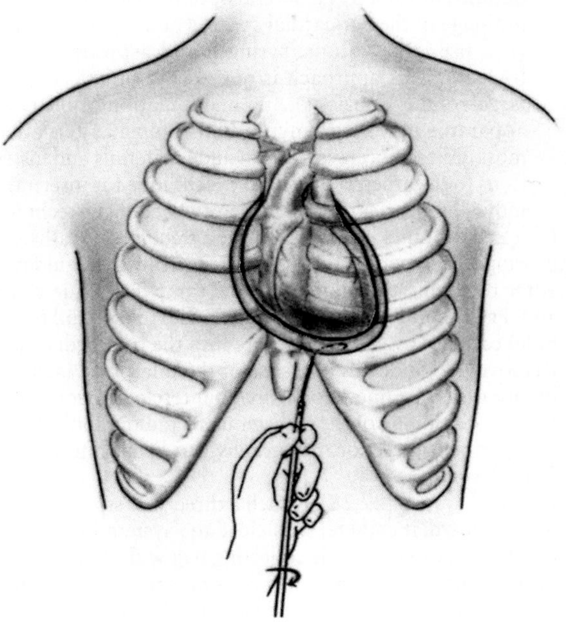

FIGURE 17.6 Placement technique. Holding the needle in place, a Teflon-coated, 0.035-inch guidewire is advanced into the pericardial space. The needle is then removed. After a series of skin dilations, an 8 Fr, 35-cm flexible pigtail catheter is placed over the guidewire into the pericardial space. Passage of dilators and the pigtail catheter is facilitated by a gentle clockwise/counterclockwise motion.

TABLE 17.3

Diagnostic Studies Performed on Pericardial Fluid

Hematocrit
White blood cell count with differential
Glucose
Protein
Gram's stain
Routine aerobic and anaerobic cultures
Smear and culture for acid-fast bacilli
Cytology
Cholesterol, triglyceride
Amylase
Lactate dehydrogenase
Special cultures (viral, parasite, and fungal)
Antinuclear antibody
Rheumatoid factor
Total complement, C3

chronic effusions from clotting, where frank hemorrhage or intraventricular blood will overwhelm fibrinolysis.

The patient's hemodynamic status should improve promptly with removal of sufficient fluid. Successful relief of tamponade is supported by (a) a fall of intrapericardial pressure to levels between −3 and +3 mm Hg, (b) a fall in right atrial pressure and a separation between right and left ventricular diastolic pressures, (c) augmentation of cardiac output, (d) increased systemic blood pressure, and (e) reduced pulsus paradoxus to physiologic levels (10 mm Hg or less). An improvement may be observed after removal of the first 50 to 100 mL of fluid. If the right atrial pressure remains elevated after fluid removal, an effusive-constrictive process should be considered. The diagnostic studies performed on pericardial fluid are outlined in Table 17.3. Several options exist for continued drainage of the pericardial space. The simplest approach is to use large-volume syringes and aspirate the fluid by hand. This approach is not always practical (i.e., in large-volume effusions), and manipulation of the needle apparatus may cause myocardial trauma. Alternatively, most pericardiocentesis kits include materials and instructions for a catheter-over-needle technique for inserting an indwelling pericardial drain via the Seldinger technique.

7. Pericardial Drain Placement: Create a tract for the catheter by passing a 6 French (Fr) dilator over a firmly held guidewire. After removing the dilator, use the same technique to pass an 8 Fr dilator. Then advance an 8 Fr flexible pigtail (or side hole) catheter over the guidewire into the pericardial space. Remove the guidewire. Passage of the dilators is facilitated by use of a torquing (clockwise/counterclockwise) motion. Proper positioning of the catheter using radiography, fluoroscopy, or bedside echocardiography can be used to facilitate fluid drainage.
8. Drainage system [27,28]: Attach a three-way stopcock to the intrapericardial catheter and close the system by attaching the stopcock to the sterile collecting bag with the connecting tubing. The catheter may also be connected to a transducer, allowing intrapericardial pressure monitoring. The system may be secured as follows:
   a. Suture the pigtail catheter to the skin, making sure that the lumen is not compressed. Cover the entry site with a sterile gauze and dressing.
   b. Secure the drainage bag (or bottle) using tape at a level approximately 35 to 50 cm below the level of the heart. Echocardiography or fluoroscopic guidance may be used to reposition the pigtail catheter, facilitating complete drainage of existing pericardial fluid.

It is recommended to drain fluid in sequential steps of <1,000 mL to avoid acute right-ventricular dilation—a rare but serious complication [7,29]. Drainage is recommended until pericardial pressure is subatmospheric with inspiration. The catheter should be flushed manually every 4 to 6 hours using 10 to 15 mL of normal saline solution until volume of aspiration falls to <25 mL per day [30].

SHORT-TERM AND LONG-TERM MANAGEMENT

After pericardiocentesis, close monitoring is required to detect evidence of recurrent tamponade and procedure-related complications. Table 17.4 lists the most common serious complications associated with pericardiocentesis [1,7,31,32]. Factors associated with an increased risk of complications include (a) small effusion (less than 250 mL), (b) posterior effusion, (c) loculated effusion, (d) maximum anterior clear space (by echocardiography) less than 10 mm, and (e) unguided percutaneous approach. All patients undergoing pericardiocentesis should have a portable chest radiograph after the procedure to exclude the presence of pneumothorax. A transthoracic 2D echocardiogram should be obtained within several hours to evaluate the adequacy of pericardial drainage and confirm catheter placement. Because pericardiocentesis typically does not remove all of the effusion (and active bleeding or secretion may occur), the pericardial catheter is typically left in place for 24 to 72 hours or until drainage subsides. Extended catheter drainage is safe, and is associated with a trend toward lower recurrence rates over a 4-year follow-up [30]. Catheter drainage of >100 mL per day after 3 days should prompt consideration of surgical intervention, sclerosing agents, or percutaneous balloon pericardotomy.

The long-term management of patients with significant pericardial fluid collections is beyond the scope of this chapter; however, the indications for surgical intervention are reviewed briefly above. The etiology of the pericardial effusion (Table 17.5),

TABLE 17.4

Complications of Pericardiocentesis

Cardiac puncture with hemopericardium
Coronary artery laceration (hemopericardium or myocardial infarction)
Pneumothorax
Hemothorax
Arrhythmias
Bradycardia
Ventricular tachycardia/ventricular fibrillation
Trauma to abdominal organs (liver, gastrointestinal tract)
Hemorrhagic peritonitis
Cardiac arrest (predominantly pulseless electrical activity from myocardial perforation, but occasionally tachyarrhythmia or bradyarrhythmia)[a]
Transient biventricular dysfunction
Infection
Fistula formation
Pulmonary edema

[a]Incidence has varied from 0% to 5% in studies and was less common in guided procedures, more common in "blind" procedures.

From Permayer-Miulda G, Sagrista-Savleda J, Soler-Soler J: Primary acute pericardial disease: a prospective study of 231 consecutive patients. *Am J Cardiol* 56:623,1985; Wong B, Murphy J, Chang CJ, et al: The risk of pericardiocentesis. *Am J Cardiol* 44:1110, 1979; Krikorian JG, Hancock EW: Pericardiocentesis. *Am J Med* 65:808, 1978.

TABLE 17.5

Common Causes of Pericardial Effusion

Idiopathic
Malignancy (primary, metastatic; solid tumors, hematologic)
Uremia
Graft-versus-host disease
Extramedullary hematopoiesis
Postpericardiotomy syndrome
Connective tissue disease
Trauma
Blunt
Penetrating
Infection
Viral (including HIV)
Bacterial
Fungal
Tuberculosis
Aortic dissection
Complication of cardiac catheterization, percutaneous coronary intervention or pacemaker insertion
Myxedema
Postirradiation

HIV, human immuno deficiency virus.

and the patient's functional status are of central importance for determining the preferred treatment. Aggressive attempts at nonsurgical management of chronically debilitated patients or those with metastatic disease involving the pericardium may be appropriate [33,34]. Percutaneous balloon pericardotomy or pericardial sclerosis with tetracycline, cisplatin, and other agents has benefited carefully selected patients with malignant pericardial disease [35–37]. Patients with a guarded prognosis who fail aggressive medical therapy should be offered the least invasive procedure.

Utility of Ultrasonography for Management of Pericardial Effusion

Ultrasonography has several useful applications related to the management of pericardial effusion.

1. Identification of Pericardial Fluid
   Pericardial fluid is readily identified by echocardiographic examination. The pericardial space is, in health, a virtual space that contains no fluid. Fluid accumulation in the pericardial space is hypoechoic and defined by the anatomic boundaries of the pericardium. Using the standard five-view basic echocardiography examination sequence (See Chapter 16 on Critical Care Echocardiography), pericardial fluid can be readily identified and characterized. Small pericardial effusions are visualized posterior to the heart in the parasternal long-axis and short-axis, and subcostal long-axis views of the heart. When moderate or large in volume, the effusion surrounds the heart, and is visible in the apical four-chamber view (Chapter 17 Video 17.1). Pericardial fluid is often hypoechoic, but infection or malignancy may result in increased echogenicity, stranding, septations, or masses within the fluid (Chapter 17 Video 17.2).

   Pericardial fluid is readily identified with transesophageal echocardiography (TEE) (Chapter 17 Video 17.3). With TEE, the pericardial space extends to the base of the heart in a series of complex reflections that are visible when distended with fluid. These may cause confusion, if misidentified by the inexperienced examiner. A specific application of TEE is for identification of loculated pericardial effusions post–cardiac surgery that may cause local pericardial tamponade due to chamber compression (Chapter 17 Video 17.3). These may not be visible with transthoracic echocardiography. Unexplained hypotension in the post–cardiac surgery patient requires TEE to rule out this potentially lethal complication.

   Anterior pericardial fat may be mistaken for pericardial fluid. Pericardial fat has hyperechoic elements within it that move with cardiac contraction. The absence of a coexisting posterior effusion favors anterior pericardial fat. In the parasternal long-axis view, pleural effusion may be confused with pericardial fluid. Pericardial fluid distributes anterior to the descending aorta on the parasternal long-axis view, whereas pleural fluid is posterior to the aorta (Chapter 17 Video 17.4).
2. Assessment for Pericardial Tamponade
   2D echocardiography is useful for identifying findings consistent with pericardial tamponade (Chapter 17 Video 17.5). Chamber collapse is suggestive, but not diagnostic of tamponade physiology. It is useful to have an ECG tracing on the ultrasonography screen in order to accurately time any chamber collapse. Right atrial (RA) collapse is best seen from the apical four-chamber and subcostal long-axis view. Normally, the right atrium should fill during systole, so the finding of a systolic RA collapse is abnormal. Early diastolic collapse of the right atrium is sensitive for tamponade. High RA pressures and severe tricuspid regurgitation may mask RA collapse.

   Right ventricular (RV) collapse is best seen from the parasternal short and subcostal long-axis views. The right ventricle fills during diastole, so a collapse of the right ventricle during diastole is abnormal. The collapse of the RV outflow track (RVOT) occurs before the RV free wall is involved, owing to the fact the RVOT is a thinner-walled structure. The RVOT is best imaged from the parasternal long-axis view, whereas the RV free wall is best imaged from the apical four-chamber and subcostal long-axis views. High right-sided pressures and RV wall hypertrophy may mask RV collapse. The presence of chamber compression does not in itself indicate that there is tamponade physiology, nor does its absence rule it out.

   The presence of a swinging heart within large pericardial effusion is suggestive of pericardial tamponade, as is respirophasic variation of chamber size on M-mode obtained with the sample line placed through the right ventricle and left ventricle from the parasternal long-axis view. Pericardial tamponade predictably results in distention of the inferior vena cave (IVC). The presence of a small IVC makes pericardial tamponade very unlikely. Doppler echocardiography has utility for assessment for pericardial tamponade. A characteristic feature of tamponade physiology is respirophasic variation of stroke volume (SV) owing to accentuation of ventricular interdependence. This is manifested with respirophasic variation of mitral valve and tricuspid valve diastolic inflow velocities. A greater than 30% respirophasic variation of mitral valve E wave velocity is characteristic of pericardial tamponade measured from the apical four-chamber view. Respirophasic variation of SV is measured in the LVOT from the apical five-chamber view and represents the echocardiographic equivalent of paradoxical pulse.

   Doppler analysis has limitations. It requires advanced level training and is time-consuming for the frontline intensivist. Major variation of intrathoracic pressure, such as that occurs with airway obstruction due to asthma or upper airway obstruction, causes respirophasic variation of SV. Translational artifact due to respirophasic movement of the heart may cause changes in Doppler signal that are unrelated to SV variation.

   Both 2D and Doppler echocardiography are helpful in identifying the patient with pericardial tamponade. Because there are sufficient confounders, echocardiographic findings, though helpful, should never be considered diagnostic.

Pericardial tamponade remains a clinical diagnosis that may or may not be supported by echocardiographic findings.

3. Guidance of Pericardiocentesis

Ultrasonography is the preferred method for safe performance of pericardiocentesis when compared to fluoroscopic guidance. Seward et al. described 1,127 serial pericardiocenteses performed with ultrasonographic guidance with a very low complication rate [25]. Guidance with fluoroscopy is performed using the subcostal approach. Because fluoroscopy is a 2D imaging technique, the position of the liver; the relationship of the needle to the myocardium; and the relationship of the lung to the needle trajectory is less certain than with ultrasonography imaging.

Pericardiocentesis performed with ultrasonographic guidance uses the same principles as those of thoracentesis and paracentesis. The fluid collection is identified, and the operator determines a safe site, angle, and depth for needle insertion while avoiding injury to adjacent anatomic structures. The operator needs to be skilled at image acquisition and interpretation, because an injury to the myocardium or coronary artery is a catastrophic complication of pericardiocentesis (Chapter 17 Video 17.6).

4. Site Selection and Preparation
   - Using ultrasonography, the best site is determined by where the most fluid is found. This may be at any point on the anterior or lateral chest or from the subcostal view. The best site is often found on the lateral chest using the apical four-chamber view (Chapter 17 Video 17.6). If the effusion is very large, the parasternal view may offer a good approach. When the effusion is predominately posterior in location, changing the patient's body position may distribute the fluid into a more favorable position. The left lateral decubitus position may shift the fluid for an improved apical view, whereas a semisupine position may improve the subcostal view.
   - The distance between the site of needle penetration into the pericardium and the heart is an important determinant of safety. The heart changes in size throughout the contractile cycle; cardiac "swinging" is a common phenomenon in severe tamponade, and the respirophasic translational movement of the heart is accentuated during the respiratory cycle. As a result, the thickness of the pericardial effusion may change a major extent during cardiac movement. A reasonable approach is to require at least 1 cm of fluid depth between the heart and the planned needle entry point into the pericardial fluid.
   - An important element in safe site selection is the avoidance of injury to adjacent structures. The lung is of concern. Fortunately, aerated or consolidated lung is easy to identify and therefore easy to avoid (see Chapter 11 on Lung Ultrasonography). The liver is readily identified, and therefore avoided when considering the subcostal approach. Color Doppler examination of the planned needle trajectory is mandatory when using the parasternal approach, in order to avoid the internal mammary vessels. A pleural effusion may occur concomitantly with the pericardial effusion, and may block access to the pericardial fluid. In this situation, it is best to drain the pleural effusion, and then to determine the best approach to the pericardial effusion. Occasionally, ascites may be mistaken for pericardial effusion in the subcostal long-axis view.
   - The best site and angle for needle insertion is determined, and the site is marked. Using the calipers function, the depth of needle penetration is measured from a frozen image on the ultrasound screen. Before obtaining a final confirmatory scan, equipment setup should be complete. This reduces the period between the final scan and needle insertion, thereby allowing the operator to maintain recent memory of the angle of approach during needle insertion. Following sterile skin preparation, the patient is covered with a full body drape. The transducer with sterile sleeve is part of the field setup, thereby allowing scanning during the procedure, because the operator may choose to reconfirm site, depth, and angle for needle insertion following sterile site preparation. The angle of needle insertion for device insertion duplicates the angle of probe angle that identified the safe trajectory for needle insertion.
   - The operator proceeds with needle–wire insertion, followed by catheter insertion. Confirmation of wire or catheter insertion may be accomplished by direct visualization using 2D ultrasonography. If there is a question of proper position, several milliliters of agitated saline may be injected through the catheter to document catheter position.
   - Similar to thoracentesis and paracentesis, pericardiocentesis does not require real-time guidance with ultrasonography. The largest published study [25] on the subject did not use real-time guidance. However, it is important to have the transducer with sterile cover in place for immediate use throughout the procedure, in case there is a need to rescan and document successful device insertion.

5. Pitfalls: Common and Uncommon
   - Skin compression artifact is a common problem, because it may cause an underestimation of the depth for needle insertion. This occurs in the obese or edematous patient when the operator pushes the probe into the skin while searching for a safe needle insertion site. Measurement of needle insertion distance is made while compressing the skin and underlying soft tissue. On removal of the probe pressure, the skin rebounds, such that the needle insertion is underestimated. During actual needle insertion, the operator is appropriately concerned, if there is no fluid obtained at the depth measured from the ultrasound machine screen. The solution to this problem is to rescan the patient, confirm the angle of insertion, and estimate the compression artifact more accurately. Another cause for difficulty is movement of the mark that designates the appropriate site for needle insertion. Skin is movable, so the injudicious application of force by the operator's hand may shift the skin mark. The needle should be inserted at the mark without any tension applied to the area that might shift the mark position. Similarly, a "dry tap" might result from inaccurate duplication of the angle at which the transducer was held, or an inaccurate skin mark. The solution remains to rescan the patient to recheck the angle and site. Generally, it is easier to duplicate a perpendicular transducer angle than one that is acutely angled. This favors an anterior or lateral chest wall approach (if fluid is accessible), because the transducer is often perpendicular to the chest wall when scanning in these areas. This is not the case in the subcostal approach.
   - An unusual cause of a "dry tap" is a blocked needle, resulting from an overly deep needle insertion. Clotted blood or skin plug may be the culprit. Overly vigorous probing of the anterior costal cartilage (if using a parasternal approach) may also block the needle with cartilage, causing the operator to insert the needle too deeply, with potential complications to the patient.
   - A large anterior pericardial fat pad may be mistaken for a pericardial effusion by the inexperienced ultrasonographer. Pericardial fat has some element of echogenicity and moves in synchrony with cardiac contraction. However, it is very uncommon for a consequential pericardial effusion to occur anterior to the heart without a significant posterior pericardial effusion also being present.
   - An uncommon pitfall of pericardiocentesis occurs when the anesthesia needle penetrates the pericardium after having traversed a pleural effusion. The pericardial effusion may then drain into the pleural space through the defect in the pericardium made by the anesthesia needle. This may occur if there is a delay before definitive pericardial device

insertion. The operator is unpleasantly surprised by the lack of pericardial effusion, and the presence of a new pleural effusion. To avoid this situation, device insertion should promptly follow infiltration of the local anesthesia.

SUMMARY

Ultrasonography permits safe pericardiocentesis. Ultrasonography allows the intensivist to select a safe site, angle, and depth for needle and device insertion. Careful attention to image acquisition and interpretation allows the operator to avoid the serious complication of myocardial or coronary artery laceration. The critical care ultrasonographer is strongly encouraged to develop proficiency in ultrasound guidance of pericardiocentesis, because it is superior to subcostal fluoroscopic guidance.

References

1. Permayer-Miulda G, Sagrista-Sauleda J, Soler-Soler J: Primary acute pericardial disease: a prospective study of 231 consecutive patients. *Am J Cardiol* 56:623, 1985.
2. Levy PY, Corey R, Berger P, et al: Etiologic diagnosis of 204 pericardial effusions. *Medicine (Baltimore)* 82:385, 2003.
3. Sagrista-Sauleda J, Merce J, Permanyer-Miralda G, et al: Clinical clues to the causes of large pericardial effusions. *Am J Med* 109:95, 2000.
4. Corey GR, Campbell PT, van Trigt P, et al: Etiology of large pericardial effusions. *Am J Med* 95:209, 1993.
5. Zayas R, Anguita M, Torres F, et al: Incidence of specific etiology and role of methods for specific etiologic diagnosis of primary acute pericarditis. *Am J Cardiol* 75:378, 1995.
6. Quinones M, Douglas P, Foster E, et al: ACC/AHA clinical competence statement on echocardiography. *JACC* 41 (4):687–708, 2003.
7. Maisch B, Seferovic P, Ristic AD, et al. Guidelines on the diagnosis and management of pericardial diseases. The task force on the diagnosis and management of pericardial diseases of the European Society of Cardiology. *Eur Heart J* 25(7):587–610, 2004.
8. Spodick DH: Medical treatment of cardiac tamponade, in Caturelli G, (ed). *Cura Intensive Cardiologica*. Rome, TIPAR Poligrafica, 1991, pp 265–268.
9. Cheitlin MD, Armstrong WF, Aurigemma GP et al: ACC/AHA/ASE 2003 guideline for the clinical application of echocardiography. *JACC* 42(5):954–970, 2003.
10. Spodick DH: Macrophysiology, microphysiology, and anatomy of the pericardium: a synopsis. *Am Heart J* 124:1046–1051, 1992.
11. Loukas M, Walter A, Boon JM, et al: Pericardiocentesis: a clinical anatomy review. *Clin Anat* 25:872, 2012.
12. Ellis H: The clinical anatomy of pericardiocentesis. *Br J Hosp Med* 71:M100, 2010.
13. Little W, Freeman G: Pericardial disease. *Circulation* 113:1622–1632, 2006.
14. Sagrista-Sauleda J, Angel J, Sanchez A, et al: Effusive-constrictive pericarditis. *N Engl J Med* 350:469, 2004.
15. Schuh R: Erfahrungen uber de Paracentese der Brust und des Herz Beutels. *Med JahrbOsterrStaates Wien* 33:388, 1841.
16. Marfan AB: Poncitian du pericarde par l espigahe. *Ann Med Chir Infarct* 15:529, 1911.
17. Tibbles CD, Porcaro W: Procedural applications of ultrasound. *Emerg Med Clin North Am* 22:797, 2004.
18. Rifkin RD, Mernoff DB: Noninvasive evaluation of pericardial effusion composition by computed tomography. *Am Heart J* 149:1120, 2005.
19. Degirmencioglu A, Karakus G, Guvenc TS, et al: Echocardiography-guided or "sided" pericardiocentesis. *Echocardiography* 30:997, 2013.
20. Nagdev A, Mantuani D: A novel in-plane technique for ultrasound-guided pericardiocentesis. *Am J Emerg Med* 31:1424.e5, 2013.
21. Ainsworth CD, Salehian O: Echo-guided pericardiocentesis: let the bubbles show the way. *Circulation* 123:e210, 2011.
22. Callahan JA, Seward JB, Nishimura RA: 2-dimensional echocardiography-guided pericardiocentesis: experience in 117 consecutive patients. *Am J Cardiol* 55:476, 1985.
23. Tsang TSM, Freeman WK, Sinak LJ, et al: Echocardiographically guided pericardiocentesis: evolution and state-of-the-art technique. *Mayo Clin Proc* 73:647, 1998.
24. Callahan JA, Seward JB, Tajik AJ: Cardiac tamponade: pericardiocentesis directed by two-dimensional echocardiography. *Mayo Clin Proc* 60:344, 1985.
25. Tsang TS, Enriquez-Sarano M, Freeman WK, et al: Consecutive 1127 therapeutic echocardiographically guided pericardiocentesis: clinical profile, practice patterns, and outcomes spanning 21 years. *Mayo Clin Proc* 77:429, 2002.
26. Fagan S, Chan KL: Pericardiocentesis. *Chest* 116:275–276, 1999.
27. Kapoor AS: Technique of pericardiocentesis and intrapericardial drainage, in Kapoor AS (ed): *International Cardiology*. New York, NY, Springer-Verlag, 1989, p 146.
28. Patel AK, Kogolcharoen PK, Nallasivan M, et al: Catheter drainage of the pericardium: practical method to maintain long-term patency. *Chest* 92:1018, 1987.
29. Armstrong WF, Feigenbaum H, Dillon JC: Acute right ventricular dilation and echocardiographic volume overload following pericardiocentesis for relief of cardiac tamponade. *Am Heart J* 107:1266–1270, 1984.
30. Tsang TS, Barnes ME, Gersh BJ, et al: Outcomes of clinically significant idiopathic pericardial effusion requiring intervention. *Am J Cardiol* 91(6):704–707, 2002.
31. Wong B, Murphy J, Chang CJ, et al: The risk of pericardiocentesis. *Am J Cardiol* 44:1110, 1979.
32. Krikorian JG, Hancock EW: Pericardiocentesis. *Am J Med* 65:808, 1978.
33. Shepherd FA, Morgan C, Evans WK, et al: Medical management of malignant pericardial effusion by tetracycline sclerosis. *Am J Cardiol* 60:1161, 1987.
34. Morm JE, Hallonby D, Gonda A, et al: Management of uremia pericarditis: a report of 11 patients with cardiac tamponade and a review of the literature. *Ann Thorac Surg* 22:588, 1976.
35. Reitknecht F, Regal AM, Antkowiak JG, et al: Management of cardiac tamponade in patients with malignancy. *J Surg Oncol* 30:19, 1985.
36. Maisch B, Ristic AD, Pankuweit S, et al: Neoplastic pericardial effusion. Efficacy and safety of intrapericardial treatment with cisplatin. *Eur Heart J* 23:1625, 2002.
37. Ziskind AA, Pearce AC, Lemon CC, et al: Percutaneous balloon pericardiotomy for the treatment of cardiac tamponade and large pericardial effusions: description of technique and report of the first 50 cases. *JACC* 21:1–5, 1993.

Chapter 18 ■ Temporary Cardiac Pacing

BRENDAN MERCHANT • SETH T. DAHLBERG

Temporary cardiac pacing may be urgently required for the treatment of cardiac conduction and rhythm disturbances seen in the intensive care unit (ICU). Therefore, ICU personnel should be familiar with the indications and techniques for initiating and maintaining temporary cardiac pacing, as well as the possible complications of this procedure. Recommendations for training in the performance of transvenous pacing have been published by a Task Force of the American College of Physicians (ACC), American Heart Association (AHA), and American College of Cardiology (ACC) [1]. Competence in the performance of transvenous pacing also requires the operator to have training in central venous access (Chapter 6) and hemodynamic monitoring (Chapter 28) [2].

INDICATIONS FOR TEMPORARY CARDIAC PACING

As outlined in Table 18.1, temporary pacing is indicated in the diagnosis and management of a number of serious rhythm and conduction disturbances.

Bradyarrhythmias

The most common indication for temporary pacing in the ICU setting is a hemodynamically significant or symptomatic

TABLE 18.1

Indications for Acute (Temporary) Cardiac Pacing

A. **Conduction disturbances**
   1. Symptomatic persistent third-degree AV block with inferior myocardial infarction
   2. Third-degree AV block, new bifascicular block (e.g., right bundle branch block and left anterior hemiblock, left bundle branch block, first-degree AV block), or alternating left and right bundle branch block complicating acute anterior myocardial infarction
   3. Symptomatic idiopathic third-degree AV block, or high-degree AV block

B. **Rate disturbances**
   1. Hemodynamically significant or symptomatic sinus bradycardia
   2. Bradycardia-dependent ventricular tachycardia
   3. AV dissociation with inadequate cardiac output
   4. Polymorphic ventricular tachycardia with long QT interval (torsades de pointes)
   5. Recurrent ventricular tachycardia unresponsive to medical therapy

AV, atrioventricular.

bradyarrhythmia such as sinus bradycardia or high-grade atrioventricular (AV) block.

Sinus bradycardia and AV block are commonly seen in patients with acute coronary syndromes, hyperkalemia, myxedema, or increased intracranial pressure. Infectious processes such as endocarditis or Lyme disease may impair AV conduction. Bradyarrhythmias also result from treatment or intoxication with digitalis, antiarrhythmic, β-blocker, or calcium channel blocker medications, and may also result from exaggerated vasovagal reactions to ICU procedures such as suctioning of the tracheobronchial tree in the intubated patient. Bradycardia-dependent ventricular tachycardia may occur in association with ischemic heart disease.

Tachyarrhythmias

Temporary cardiac pacing is used less often for the prevention and termination of supraventricular and ventricular tachyarrhythmias.

Atrial pacing in the ICU setting is often performed when temporary epicardial electrodes have been placed during cardiac surgery. Pacing termination of atrial flutter in cardiac surgery patients with epicardial leads may be preferable to synchronized cardioversion, which carries the risk associated with sedation. A critical pacing rate (usually 125% to 135% of the flutter rate) and pacing duration (usually about 10 seconds) are important in the successful conversion of atrial flutter to sinus rhythm [3].

Temporary pacing may be required for the prevention of paroxysmal polymorphic ventricular tachycardia in patients with prolonged QT intervals (torsades de pointes), particularly when secondary to drugs [4,5]. Temporary cardiac pacing with a mild tachycardia is the treatment of choice to stabilize the patient while a type I antiarrhythmic agent exacerbating ventricular irritability is metabolized. The effectiveness of cardiac pacing probably relates to decreasing the dispersion of refractoriness of the ventricular myocardium (shortening the QT interval).

Temporary ventricular pacing may be successful in terminating ventricular tachycardia. If ventricular tachycardia must be terminated urgently, cardioversion is mandated (Chapter 15). However, in less urgent situations, conversion of ventricular tachycardia via rapid ventricular pacing may be useful. "Overdrive" ventricular pacing is often effective in terminating monomorphic ventricular tachycardia in a patient with remote myocardial infarction or in the absence of heart disease. This technique is less effective when ventricular tachycardia complicates acute myocardial infarction or cardiomyopathy. Rapid ventricular pacing is most successful in terminating ventricular tachycardia when the ventricle can be "captured" (asynchronous pacing for 5 to 10 beats at a rate of 50 beats per minute greater than that of the underlying tachycardia). A cardiac defibrillator should be immediately available, because pacing may result in acceleration of ventricular tachycardia or degeneration to ventricular fibrillation.

DIAGNOSIS OF RAPID RHYTHMS

Temporary atrial pacing electrodes may be helpful for the diagnosis of tachyarrhythmias when the morphology of the P wave and its relation to the QRS complexes cannot be determined from the surface electrocardiogram (ECG) [6]. A recording of the atrial electrogram is helpful in a regular, narrow-complex tachycardia in which the differential diagnosis includes atrial flutter, AV node reentry, or other supraventricular rhythm. This technique may also assist in the diagnosis of wide-complex tachycardias in which the differential diagnosis includes supraventricular tachycardia with aberrant conduction; sinus tachycardia with bundle branch block; and ventricular tachycardia.

To record an atrial ECG, the ECG limb leads are connected in the standard fashion, and a precordial lead (usually V_1) is connected to the proximal electrode of the atrial pacing catheter or to an epicardial atrial electrode. A multichannel ECG rhythm strip is run at a rapid paper speed, simultaneously demonstrating surface ECG limb leads as well as the atrial electrogram obtained via lead V_1. This rhythm strip should reveal the conduction pattern between atria and ventricles as antegrade, simultaneous, retrograde, or dissociated.

ACUTE MYOCARDIAL INFARCTION

Sinus node dysfunction, disorders of AV conduction and disorders of intraventricular conduction may occur in the acute stages of an infarction [7]. Recommendations for temporary cardiac pacing have been provided by a Task Force of the ACC and the AHA (Table 18.2) [8]. Bradyarrhythmias unresponsive to medical treatment that result in hemodynamic compromise or symptoms require urgent treatment. Patients with anterior infarction and bifascicular block or Mobitz type II second-degree AV block, though hemodynamically stable, are at risk for development of complete heart block with an unstable escape rhythm and should be considered for a temporary pacemaker [9].

Prophylactic temporary cardiac pacing has aroused debate for its role in a complicated anterior wall myocardial infarction. The left anterior descending artery is the major blood supply to the His bundle and the bundle branches, and an anterior wall infarction with new bundle branch block represents extensive

TABLE 18.2

ACC/AHA American College of Cardiology/American Heart Association Recommendations for Treatment of Atrioventricular and Intraventricular Conduction Disturbances during STEMI

Intraventricular Conduction	AV Conduction													
			First-Degree AV Block				Mobitz I Second-Degree AV Block				Mobitz II Second-Degree AV Block			
	Normal		AMI		NonAMI		AMI		NonAMI		AMI		NonAMI	
	Action	Class	Action	Class	Action	Class	Action	Class	Action	Class	Action	Class	Action	Class
Normal	OB	1	OB	1	OB	1	OB	2B	OB	2A	OB	3	OB	3
	A	3	A	3	A	3	A*	3	A	3	A	3	A	3
	TC	3	TC	2B	TC	2B	TC	1	TC	1	TC	1	TC	1
	TV	3	TV	3	TV	3	TV	3	TV	3	TV	2A	TV	2A
Old or new Fascicular Block (LAFB or LPFB)	OB	1	OB	2B	OB	2B	OB	2B	OB	2B	OB	3	OB	3
	A	3	A	3	A	3	A*	3	A	3	A	3	A	3
	TC	2B	TC	1	TC	2A	TC	1	TC	1	TC	1	TC	1
	TV	3	TV	3	TV	3	TV	3	TV	3	TV	2A	TV	2B
Old BBB	OB	1	OB	3	OB	3	OB	3	OB	3	OB	3	OB	3
	A	3	A	3	A	3	A*	3	A	3	A	3	A	3
	TC	2B	TC	1	TC	1	TC	1	TC	1	TC	1	TC	1
	TV	3	TV	2B	TV	2B	TV	2B	TV	2B	TV	2A	TV	2A
New BBB	OB	3	OB	3	OB	3	OB	3	OB	3	OB	3	OB	3
	A	3	A	3	A	3	A*	3	A	3	A	3	A	3
	TC	1	TC	1	TC	1	TC	1	TC	1	TC	2B	TC	2B
	TV	2B	TV	2A	TV	2A	TV	2A	TV	2A	TV	1	TV	1

(*continued*)

TABLE 18.2

ACC/AHA American College of Cardiology/American Heart Association Recommendations for Treatment of Atrioventricular and Intraventricular Conduction Disturbances during STEMI (*continued*)

Fascicular block + RBBB	OB	3	OB	3	OB	3	OB	3	OB	3	OB	3	OB	3
	A	3	A	3	A	3	A*	3	A	3	A	3	A	3
	TC	1	TC	1	TC	1	TC	1	TC	1	TC	2B	TC	2B
	TV	2B	TV	2A	TV	2A	TV	2A	TV	2A	TV	1	TV	1
Alternating Left and Right BBB	OB	3	OB	3	OB	3	OB	3	OB	3	OB	3	OB	3
	A	3	A	3	A	3	A*	3	A	3	A	3	A	3
	TC	2B	TC	2B	TC	2B	TC	2B	TC	2B	TC	2B	TC	2B
	TV	1	TV	1	TV	1	TV	1	TV	1	TV	1	TV	1

This table is designed to summarize the AV (column headings) and intraventricular (row headings) conduction disturbances that may occur during acute anterior or nonanterior STEMI, the possible treatment options, and the indications for each possible therapeutic option.

ACC/AHA, American College of Cardiology/American Heart Association; LAFB, left anterior fascicular block; LPFB, left posterior fascicular block; RBBB, right bundle-branch block; BBB, bundle-branch block; OB, observe; A, atropine; TC, transcutaneous pacing; TV, temporary transvenous pacing; STEMI, ST elevation myocardial infarction; AV, atrioventricular; MI, myocardial infarction; AMI, anterior myocardial infarction; nonAMI, non-anterior myocardial infarction.

Action: There are four possible actions, or therapeutic options, listed and classified for each bradyarrhythmia or conduction problem:

1. Observe: continued ECG monitoring, no further action planned.
2. A, and A*: atropine administered at 0.6 to 1.0 mg IV every 5 minutes to up to 0.04 mg per kg. In general, because the increase in sinus rate with atropine is unpredictable, this is to be avoided unless there is symptomatic bradycardia that will likely respond to a vagolytic agent, such as sinus bradycardia or Mobitz I, as denoted by the asterisk, above.
3. TC: application of transcutaneous pads and standby transcutaneous pacing with no further progression to transvenous pacing imminently planned.
4. TV: temporary transvenous pacing. It is assumed, but not specified in the table, that at the discretion of the clinician, transcutaneous pads will be applied and standby transcutaneous pacing will be in effect as the patient is transferred to the fluoroscopy unit for temporary transvenous pacing.

Class: Each possible therapeutic option is further classified according to ACC/AHA criteria as Class 1: indicated, 2A: probably indicated, 2B: possibly indicated, and 3: not indicated.

Level of Evidence: This table was developed from published observational case reports and case series, published summaries, not meta-analyses, of these data; and expert opinion, largely from the prereperfusion era. There are no published randomized trials comparing different strategies of managing conduction disturbances after STEMI. Thus, the level of evidence for the recommendations in this table is C.

How to Use the Table: Example: A 54-year-old man is admitted with an anterior STEMI and a narrow QRS on admission. On day 1, he develops a right bundle-branch block (RBBB), with a PR interval of 0.28 seconds.

1. RBBB is an intraventricular conduction disturbance, so look at row 'New bundle-branch block.'
2. Find the column for "First-Degree AV Block."
3. Find the "Action" and "Class" cells at the convergence.
4. Note that "Observe" and "Atropine" are class 3, not indicated; transcutaneous pacing (TC) is class 1. Temporary transvenous pacing (TV) is class 2B.

From ref. [28] with permission.

myocardial damage and confers an increased risk of heart failure and mortality. Thrombolytic therapy or percutaneous coronary intervention takes precedence over placement of prophylactic cardiac pacing, because prophylactic pacing has not been shown to improve mortality. Transthoracic (transcutaneous) cardiac pacing is safe and usually effective [10], and would be a reasonable alternative to prophylactic transvenous cardiac pacing, particularly soon after the administration of thrombolytic therapy.

When right ventricular involvement complicates inferior myocardial infarction, cardiac output may be very sensitive to ventricular preload and AV synchrony. Therefore, AV sequential pacing is frequently the pacing modality of choice in patients with right ventricular infarction [11].

EQUIPMENT AVAILABLE FOR TEMPORARY PACING

Several methods of temporary pacing are currently available for use in the ICU. Transvenous pacing of the right ventricle or right atrium with a pacing catheter or modified pulmonary artery catheter is the most widely used technique; intraesophageal, transcutaneous, and epicardial pacing techniques are also available.

Transvenous Pacing Catheters

Some of the many transvenous pacing catheters available for use in the critical care setting are illustrated in Figure 18.1. Pacing catheters range in size from 4 Fr (1.2 mm) to 7 Fr (2.1 mm). In urgent situations, or where fluoroscopy is unavailable, a flow-directed flexible balloon-tipped catheter (Fig. 18.1, top) may be placed in the right ventricle using ECG guidance. After gaining access to the central venous circulation (Chapter 6), the catheter is passed into the vein and the balloon inflated. After advancing the catheter into the right ventricle, the balloon can be deflated and the catheter tip advanced to the right ventricular apex. Cardiac ultrasound can confirm placement of the catheter in the right ventricle [12]. Although the balloon-tipped catheter may avoid the need for fluoroscopy, placement may be ineffective in the setting of low blood flow during cardiac arrest or in the presence of severe tricuspid regurgitation. Stiff catheters (Fig. 18.1, middle) are easier to manipulate but require insertion under fluoroscopic or ultrasound guidance [13].

A flexible J-shaped catheter (Fig. 18.1, bottom), designed for temporary atrial pacing, is also available [14]. This lead is positioned by "hooking" it in the right atrial appendage under fluoroscopic guidance, providing stable contact with the atrial endocardium.

A multilumen pulmonary artery catheter is available with a right ventricular port. Placement of a small (2.4 Fr) bipolar pacing lead through the right ventricular lumen allows intracardiac pressure monitoring and pacing through a single catheter [15]. Details on its use and insertion are described in Chapter 19.

Utility of Ultrasonography for Transvenous Pacemaker Insertion

Ultrasonography has useful applications related to transvenous pacemaker insertion.

Real-time guidance of pacemaker insertion with ultrasonography is a safe, effective, and fast way to perform the procedure. It has advantage over fluoroscopic guidance, because it requires no patient transport or complex equipment and can be performed at the bedside of the critically patient. Ultrasonography guided

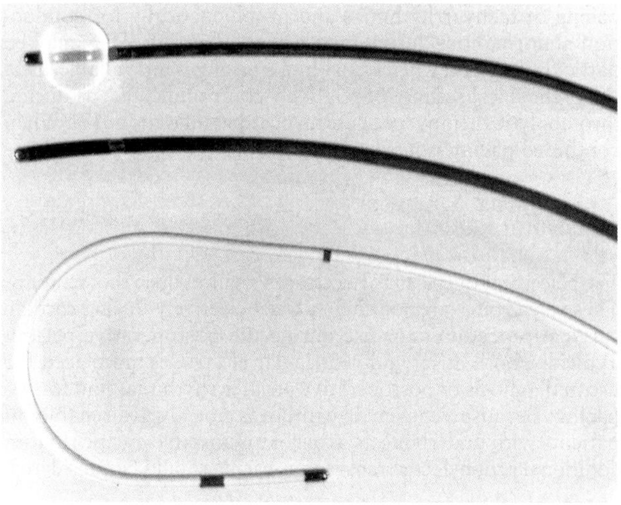

FIGURE 18.1 Cardiac pacing catheters. Several designs are available for temporary pacing in the critical care unit. **Top:** Balloon-tipped, flow-directed pacing wire. **Middle:** Standard 5 Fr pacing wire. **Bottom:** Atrial J-shaped wire.

insertion is performed more rapidly and with fewer complications than with fluoroscopic control [13,16].

The right atrium (RA), tricuspid valve (TV), and right ventricle (RV) are imaged from the subcostal views or the right ventricular inflow view according to operator preference. If a femoral approach is used, the longitudinal view of inferior vena cava permits visualization of the pacer wire (Chapter 18 Video 18.1). The catheter tip is visualized as it enters the RA. The operator manipulates the catheter under direct visualization through the TV. Once in the RV cavity, the balloon is deflated and the catheter advanced into the RV apex. Visualization of the catheter approach to the RV apex requires an apical four-chamber view. Because it may be difficult to image the wire during its final advance into the RV apex, the procedure is done with ECG monitoring from catheter tip, so as to confirm final position with detection of a current of injury pattern. In intubated patients with inadequate image quality from transthoracic images, transesophageal echocardiography is an effective alternative. In this case, the bicaval view allows initial visualization of the catheter, whereas the mid-esophageal four-chamber view permits assessment of catheter movement into the RV.

Esophageal Electrode

An esophageal "pill" electrode allows atrial pacing and recording of atrial depolarizations without requiring central venous cannulation. Because the electrode can be uncomfortable and may not give consistent, stable capture, the esophageal electrode is typically limited to short-term use for diagnosis of arrhythmias in pediatric patients.

Transcutaneous External Pacemakers

Transcutaneous external pacemakers have external patch electrodes that deliver a higher current (up to 200 mA) and longer pulse duration (20 to 40 ms) than transvenous pacemakers. External pacing can be implemented immediately and the risks of central venous access avoided. Some patients may require sedation for the discomfort of skeletal muscle stimulation. Transcutaneous external pacemakers have been used to treat bradyasystolic cardiac arrest, symptomatic bradyarrhythmias, and overdrive pacing of tachyarrhythmias and prophylactically for conduction abnormalities during myocardial infarction. They may be particularly useful when transvenous pacing is unavailable, as in the prehospital setting, or relatively contraindicated, as during thrombolytic therapy for acute myocardial infarction [17]. When continued pacing is needed, transvenous pacing is preferable.

Epicardial Pacing

The placement of epicardial electrodes requires open thoracotomy. These electrodes are routinely placed electively during cardiac surgical procedures for use during the postoperative period. Typically, both atrial and ventricular electrodes are placed for use in diagnosis of postoperative atrial arrhythmias and for AV pacing. Because ventricular capture is not always reliable, in patients with underlying asystole or an unstable escape rhythm additional prophylactic transvenous pacing should be considered.

Pulse Generators for Temporary Pacing

Temporary pulse generators are capable of ventricular, atrial, and dual chamber sequential pacing with adjustable ventricular and atrial parameters that include pacing modes (synchronous or asynchronous), rates, current outputs (mA), sensing thresholds (mV), and AV pacing interval/delay (ms). Because these generators have atrial sensing/inhibiting capability, they are also set with an upper rate limit (to avoid rapid ventricular pacing while "tracking" an atrial tachycardia); in addition, an atrial pacing refractory period may be programmed (to avoid pacemaker-mediated/endless loop tachyarrhythmias).

CHOICE OF PACING MODE

A pacing mode must be selected when temporary cardiac pacing is initiated. Common modes for cardiac pacing are outlined in Table 18.3. The mode most likely to provide the greatest hemodynamic benefit should be selected. In patients with hemodynamic instability, establishing ventricular pacing is of paramount importance prior to attempts at AV sequential pacing.

Ventricular pacing effectively counteracts bradycardia and is most frequently used in ICU patients; however, it cannot restore normal cardiac hemodynamics because it disrupts AV synchrony [18,19]. In patients with noncompliant ventricles (ischemic heart disease, left ventricular hypertrophy, aortic stenosis, and right ventricular infarction), loss of the atrial contribution to ventricular stroke volume (the atrial "kick") during ventricular pacing may result in increased atrial pressure;and intermittent mitral and tricuspid regurgitation with reduced cardiac output and blood pressure.

In addition to the hemodynamic benefit of atrial or AV sequential pacing, temporary atrial pacing after CABG has been shown to decrease the incidence of postoperative atrial fibrillation [20].

TABLE 18.3

Common Pacemaker Modes for Temporary Cardiac Pacing

AOO	Atrial pacing: pacing is asynchronous
AAI	Atrial pacing, atrial sensing: pacing is on demand to provide a minimum programmed atrial rate
VOO	Ventricular pacing: pacing is asynchronous
VVI	Ventricular pacing, ventricular sensing: pacing is on demand to provide a minimum programmed ventricular rate
DVI	Dual-chamber pacing, ventricular sensing: atrial pacing is asynchronous, ventricular pacing is on demand following a programmed A-V delay
DDD	Dual-chamber pacing and sensing: atrial and ventricular pacing is on demand to provide a minimum rate, ventricular pacing follows a programmed A-V delay, and upper-rate pacing limit should be programmed

PROCEDURE TO ESTABLISH TEMPORARY PACING

After achieving venous access, most often via the internal jugular or subclavian approach (Chapter 6), the pacing catheter is advanced to the central venous circulation and then positioned in the right heart using fluoroscopic or ECG guidance [21]. To position the electrode using ECG guidance, the patient is connected to the limb leads of the ECG machine, and the distal (negative) electrode of the balloon-tipped pacing catheter is connected to lead V_1 with an alligator clip or a special adaptor supplied with the lead. Lead V_1 is then used to continuously monitor a unipolar intracardiac electrogram. The morphology of the recorded electrogram indicates the position of the catheter tip (Fig. 18.2). The balloon is inflated in the superior vena cava, and the catheter is advanced while observing the recorded intracardiac electrogram. When the tip of the catheter reaches the right ventricle, the balloon is deflated and the catheter advanced to the right ventricular apex. ST segment elevation of the intracardiac electrogram owing to a current of injury indicates contact of the catheter tip with the ventricular endocardium.

After the tip of the pacing catheter is satisfactorily inserted in the right ventricular apex, the leads are connected to the ventricular output connectors of the pulse generator, with the pacemaker box in the off position. The pacemaker is then set to asynchronous mode (VOO) and the ventricular rate set to exceed the patient's intrinsic ventricular rate by 10 to 20 beats per minute. The threshold current for ventricular pacing is set

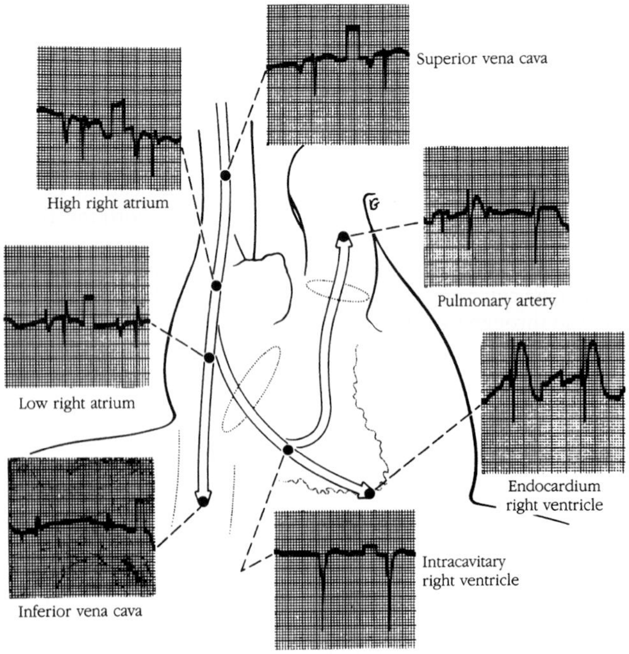

FIGURE 18.2 Pattern of recorded electrogram at various locations in the venous circulation. (From reference [21], with permission.)

at 5 to 10 mA. Then the pacemaker is switched on. Satisfactory ventricular pacing is evidenced by a wide QRS complex, with ST segment depression and T wave inversion immediately preceded by a pacemaker depolarization (spike). With pacing from the apex of the right ventricle, the paced rhythm usually demonstrates a pattern of left bundle branch block on the surface ECG [22].

Ventricular pacing is maintained as the output current for ventricular pacing is slowly reduced. The pacing threshold is defined as the lowest current at which consistent ventricular capture occurs. With the ventricular electrode appropriately positioned at or near the apex of the right ventricle, a pacing threshold of less than 0.5 to 1.0 mA should be achieved. If the output current for continuous ventricular pacing is consistently greater than 1 to 1.5 mA, the pacing threshold is too high. Possible causes of a high pacing threshold include relatively refractory endomyocardial tissue (fibrosis) or, most commonly, unsatisfactory positioning of the pacing electrode. The tip of the pacing electrode should be repositioned in the region of the ventricular apex until satisfactory ventricular capture at a current of less than 1.0 mA is consistently maintained. The ventricular output is set to exceed the threshold current at least threefold to guarantee uninterrupted ventricular capture despite any modest increase in the pacing threshold.

The pacemaker is now in VOO mode. However, the pacing generator generally should be set in the VVI ("demand") mode, because this prevents pacemaker discharge soon after any spontaneous activity in the paced chamber, while the heart lies in the electrically vulnerable period for induction of sustained ventricular arrhythmias. To set the pacemaker in VVI mode, the pacing rate is set at 10 beats per minute less than the intrinsic rate, and the sensitivity control is moved from asynchronous to the minimum sensitivity level. The sensitivity is gradually increased until pacing spikes appear. This level is the sensing threshold. The sensitivity is then set at a level slightly below the determined threshold and the pacing rate reset to the minimum desired ventricular rate.

If AV sequential pacing is desired, the atrial J-shaped pacing catheter should be advanced into the right atrium and rotated anteromedially to achieve a stable position in the right atrial appendage; however, positioning the atrial catheter usually requires fluoroscopy [23]. The leads are then connected to the atrial output of the pulse generator. The atrial current is set to 20 mA and the atrial pacing rate adjusted to at least 10 beats per minute greater than the intrinsic atrial rate. The AV interval is adjusted at 100 to 200 ms (shorter intervals usually provide better hemodynamics), and the surface ECG is inspected for evidence of atrial pacing (electrode depolarization and capture of the atrium at the pacing rate).

Atrial capture on ECG is indicated by atrial depolarization (P waves) immediately following the atrial pacing spikes. In patients with intact AV conduction, satisfactory atrial capture can be verified by shutting off the ventricular portion of the pacemaker and demonstrating AV synchrony during atrial pacing. As long as the atrial pacing rate continually exceeds the intrinsic sinus rate, the atrial P wave activity should track with the atrial pacing spike.

The DDD mode is the most commonly used setting in patients with atrial and ventricular leads. Although there is a risk of tracking atrial tachyarrhythmias in DDD mode, this risk can be mitigated by setting a maximum tracking rate or an upper rate limit on the temporary pulse generator [24].

COMPLICATIONS OF TEMPORARY PACING

Transvenous pacing in the ICU setting is most often performed via the internal jugular or subclavian approach. Appropriate selection of the optimal route requires an understanding of the results and complications of each technique.

Complications of temporary pacing from any venous access route include pericardial friction rub, arrhythmia, right ventricular perforation, cardiac tamponade, infection, unintentional arterial injury, diaphragmatic stimulation, phlebitis, and pneumothorax. The Mayo Clinic experience revealed that percutaneous cannulation of the right internal jugular vein provided the simplest, most direct route to the right-sided cardiac chambers [25].

Complications of internal jugular venous cannulation may include pneumothorax, carotid arterial injury, venous thrombosis, and pulmonary embolism (Chapter 6) [26]. These risks are minimized by use of ultrasound, knowledge of anatomic landmarks adherence to proved techniques, and use of a small-caliber needle to localize the vein before insertion of the large-caliber needle (for a full discussion, see Chapter 6). Full-dose systemic anticoagulation, thrombolytic therapy, and prior neck surgical procedures are relative contraindications to routine internal jugular vein cannulation.

Percutaneous subclavian venipuncture is also frequently used for insertion of temporary pacemakers [27]. This approach should be avoided in patients with severe obstructive lung disease or a bleeding diathesis (including thrombolytic therapy), in whom the risk of pneumothorax or bleeding is increased.

The femoral venous approach is used for electrophysiologic studies or during cardiac catheterization when the catheter is left in place for only a few hours. This approach is less desirable when long-term cardiac pacing is required, because there is a risk of deep venous thrombosis or infection. Central venous access by the subclavian or internal jugular route provides more stable long-term positioning of the pacing lead.

References

1. Francis GS, Williams SV, Achord JL, et al: Clinical competence in insertion of a temporary transvenous ventricular pacemaker: a statement for physicians from the ACP/ACC/AHA Task Force on Clinical Privileges in Cardiology. *Circulation* 89:1913–1916, 1994.
2. Birkhahn RH, Gaeta TJ, Tloczkowski J, et al: Emergency medicine-trained physicians are proficient in the insertion of transvenous pacemakers. *Ann Emerg Med* 43:469–474, 2004.
3. Deo R, Berger R: The clinical utility of entrainment pacing. *J Cardiovasc Electrophysiol* 20:466–470, 2009.
4. Khan IA: Long QT syndrome: diagnosis and management. *Am Heart J* 143:7–14, 2002.
5. Kossaify A: Temporary endocavitary pacemakers and their use and misuse: the least is better. *Clin Med Insights Cardiol* 8:9–11, 2014.
6. Reade MC: Temporary epicardial pacing after cardiac surgery: a practical review. Part 2: Selection of epicardial pacing modes and troubleshooting. [Review] [11 refs]. *Anaesthesia* 62:364–373, 2007.
7. Brady WJ Jr, Harrigan RA: Diagnosis and management of bradycardia and atrioventricular block associated with acute coronary ischemia. *Emerg Med Clin North Am* 19:371–384, xi–xii, 2001.
8. O'Gara PT, Kushner FG, Ascheim DD, et al: 2013 ACCF/AHA guideline for the management of ST-elevation myocardial infarction: a report of the American College of Cardiology Foundation/American Heart Association Task Force on Practice Guidelines. *Circulation* 127(4):e362–e425, 2013.
9. Singh SM, FitzGerald G, Yan AT, et al: High-grade atrioventricular block in acute coronary syndromes: insights from the Global Registry of Acute Coronary Events. *Eur Heart J* 36(16):976–983, 2015.
10. Falk RH, Ngai STA: External cardiac pacing: influence of electrode placement on pacing threshold. *Crit Care Med* 14:931–932, 1986.
11. Topol EJ, Goldschlager N, Ports TA, et al: Hemodynamic benefit of atrial pacing in right ventricular myocardial infarction. *Ann Intern Med* 96:594–597, 1982.
12. Labovitz AJ, Noble VE, Bierig M, et al: Focused cardiac ultrasound in the emergent setting: a consensus statement of the American Society of Echocardiography and American College of Emergency Physicians. *J Am Soc Echocardiogr* 23(12):1225–1230, 2010.
13. Pinneri F, Frea S, Najd K, et al: Echocardiography-guided versus fluoroscopy-guided temporary pacing in the emergency setting: an observational study. *J Cardiovasc Med (Hagerstown)* 14:242–246, 2013.
14. Littleford PO, Curry RC Jr, Schwartz KM, et al: Clinical evaluation of a new temporary atrial pacing catheter: results in 100 patients. *Am Heart J* 107:237–240, 1984.
15. Simoons ML, Demey HE, Bossaert LL, et al: The Paceport catheter: a new pacemaker system introduced through a Swan-Ganz catheter. *Cathet Cardiovasc Diagn* 15:66–70, 1988.
16. Ferri LA, Farina A, Lenatti L, et al: Emergent transvenous cardiac pacing using ultrasound guidance: a prospective study versus the standard

fluoroscopy-guided procedure. *Eur Heart J Acute Cardiovasc Care* 5:125–129, 2016. pii: 2048872615572598.
17. Hedges JR, Syverud SA, Dalsey WC, et al: Prehospital trial of emergency transcutaneous cardiac pacing. *Circulation* 76:1337–1343, 1987.
18. Romero LR, Haffajee CI, Doherty P, et al: Comparison of ventricular function and volume with A-V sequential and ventricular pacing. *Chest* 80:346–346, 1981.
19. Murphy P, Morton P, Murtaugh G, et al: Hemodynamic effects of different temporary pacing modes for the management of bradycardias complicating acute myocardial infarction. *Pacing Clin Electrophysiol* 15:391–396, 1992.
20. Neto VA, Costa R, Da Silva KR, et al: Temporary atrial pacing in the prevention of postoperative atrial fibrillation. *Pacing Clin Electrophysiol* 30 Suppl 1:S79–S83, 2007.
21. Harthorne JW, McDermott J, Poulin FK: Cardiac pacing, in Johnson RA, Haber E, Austen WG, (eds). *The Practice of Cardiology: The Medical and Surgical Cardiac Units at the Massachusetts General Hospital*. Boston, Little, Brown, 1980.
22. Morelli RL, Goldschlager N: Temporary transvenous pacing: resolving postinsertion problems. *J Crit Illness* 2:73, 1987.
23. Fitzpatrick A, Sutton R: A guide to temporary pacing. *BMJ* 304(6823):365–369, 1992.
24. Reade MC: Temporary epicardial pacing after cardiac surgery: a practical review: part 1: general considerations in the management of epicardial pacing. *Anaesthesia* 62(3):264–271, 2007.
25. Hynes JK, Holmes DR, Harrison CE: Five year experience with temporary pacemaker therapy in the coronary care unit. *Mayo Clin Proc* 58:122–126, 1983.
26. Gammage MD: Temporary cardiac pacing. *Heart* 83(6):715–720, 2000.
27. Donovan KD: Cardiac pacing in intensive care. *Anaesth Intensive Care* 13:41–62, 1984.
28. Antman EM, Anbe DT, Armstrong PW, et al: ACC/AHA guidelines for the management of patients with ST-elevation myocardial infarction--executive summary. A report of the American College of Cardiology/American Heart Association Task Force on Practice Guidelines (Writing Committee to revise the 1999 guidelines for the management of patients with acute myocardial infarction). *J Am Coll Cardiol* 44:671–719, 2004.

Chapter 19 ■ Pulmonary Artery Catheters

HARVEY S. REICH

Since their introduction into clinical practice in 1970 by Swan et al. [1], balloon-tipped, flow-directed pulmonary artery (PA) catheters (PACs) have found widespread use in the clinical management of critically ill patients. However, in recent years, both the safety and efficacy of these catheters have been brought into question. In this chapter, I review the physiologic basis for their use; some history regarding their development and use; the concerns raised about their use; and suggestions for appropriate use of the catheters and the information obtained from them.

PHYSIOLOGIC RATIONALE FOR USE OF PULMONARY ARTERY CATHETER

In unstable situations, during which hemodynamic changes often occur rapidly, clinical evaluation may be misleading. PACs allow for direct and indirect measurement of several major determinants and consequences of cardiac performance—preload, afterload, cardiac output (CO)—thereby supplying additional data to aid in clinical decision-making [2].

Cardiac function depends on the relationship between muscle length (preload); the load on the muscle (afterload); and the intrinsic property of contractility. Until the development of the flow-directed PA catheter, there was no way to assess all of these by using one instrument in a clinically useful way at bedside. The catheter allows the reflection of right ventricular (RV) preload (right atrial pressure); RV afterload (PA pressure); left ventricular preload—PA occlusion pressure (PAOP) or pulmonary capillary wedge pressure (PCWP)—and contractility (stroke volume or CO). Left ventricular afterload is reflected by the systemic arterial pressure. This information allows for the calculation of numerous parameters, including vascular resistances. However, monitors such as transthoracic or transesophageal echocardiography; esophageal Doppler; bioreactance; and pulse contour analysis have become increasingly popular, thereby diminishing the use of the PAC.

CONTROVERSIES REGARDING USE OF PULMONARY ARTERY CATHETER

Despite all of the advantages of the PA catheter, a number of clinical studies have been published in the past 20 years that have shown either no benefit or an increased risk of morbidity or mortality associated with its use (See Table 19.1 for a summary of the evidence for its utility.) Consequently, a number of clinicians have elected to minimize the use of this monitoring device.

Furthermore, the relationship of central venous (CV) pressure and PAOP to predict ventricular filling was studied in normal volunteers by Kumar et al. [43] who found that there was a poor correlation between initial CV pressure and PAOP, with both respective end diastolic ventricular volume and stroke volume indices. Their data call into question the basic tenet of the theoretical benefit of the PA catheter.

INDICATIONS FOR USE OF PULMONARY ARTERY CATHETER

Clinicians who use a PAC for monitoring should understand the fundamentals of the insertion technique; the equipment used; and the data that can be generated.

The use of PAC for monitoring has four central objectives: (a) to assess left or right ventricular function, or both; (b) to monitor changes in hemodynamic status; (c) to guide treatment with pharmacologic and nonpharmacologic agents; and (d) to provide prognostic information. The conditions under which PA catheterization may be useful are characterized by a clinically unclear or rapidly changing hemodynamic status. Table 19.2 is a partial listing of the indications. The use of PACs in specific disease entities is discussed in other chapters.

CATHETER FEATURES AND CONSTRUCTION

The catheter is constructed from polyvinylchloride and has a pliable shaft that softens further at body temperature. Because polyvinylchloride has a high thrombogenicity, the catheters are generally coated with heparin. Heparin bonding of catheters, introduced in 1981, has been shown to be effective in reducing catheter thrombogenicity [44] but can cause heparin-induced thrombocytopenia (HIT). The standard catheter length is 110 cm, and the most commonly used external diameter is 5 or 7 French (Fr) (1 Fr = 0.0335 mm). A balloon is fastened 1 to 2 mm from the tip (Fig. 19.1); when inflated, it guides the catheter (by virtue of fluid dynamic drag) from the greater intrathoracic veins through the right heart chambers into the PA. When fully inflated in a vessel of sufficiently large caliber, the balloon protrudes above

TABLE 19.1

Evidence Basis for the PA Catheter

Authors	Year	*N*	Design	Outcomes
Lower morbidity/mortality				
Rao et al. [3]	1983	733/364	Historical controls/ cohort	Lower mortality
Hesdorffer et al. [4]	1987	61/87	Historical controls/ cohort	Lower mortality
Shoemaker et al. [5]	1988	146	RCT	Lower mortality
Berlauk et al. [6]	1991	89	RCT	Lower morbidity
Fleming et al. [7]	1992	33/34	RCT	Lower morbidity
Tuchschmidt et al. [8]	1992	26/25	RCT	Decreased LOS; trend toward lower mortality
Boyd et al. [9]	1993	53/54	RCT	Lower mortality
Bishop et al. [10]	1995	50/65	RCT	Lower mortality
Schiller et al. [11]	1997	53/33/30	Retrospective cohort	Lower mortality
Wilson et al. [12]	1999	92/46	RCT	Lower mortality
Chang et al. [13]	2000	20/39	Prospective retrospective cohort	Lower morbidity
Polonen et al. [14]	2000	196/197	RCT	Decreased morbidity
Friese et al. [15]	2006	51,379 (no PAC) /1933 (PAC)	Retrospective analysis of National Trauma Data Bank	Improved survival in patients older than 60 or with ISS 25–75 and severe shock
No difference				
Pearson et al. [16]	1989	226	RCT	No difference
Isaacson et al. [17]	1990	102	RCT	No difference
Joyce et al. [18]	1990	40	RCT	No difference
Yu et al. [19]	1993	35/32	RCT	No difference
Gattinoni et al. [20]	1995	252/253/257	RCT	No difference
Yu et al. [21]	1995	89	RCT	No difference
Durham et al. [22]	1996	27/31	Prospective cohort	No difference
Afessa et al. [23]	2001	751	Prospective observational	No difference
Rhodes et al. [24]	2002	201	RCT	No difference
Richard [25]	2003	676	RCT	No difference
Yu et al. [26]	2003	1,010	Prospective cohort	No difference
Sandham et al. [27]	2003	997/997	RCT	No difference in mortality; increased risk of pulmonary embolism in PA group
Sakr et al. [28]	2005	3,147	Observational cohort	No difference
Harvey et al. [29]	2005	519/522	RCT	No difference in mortality
Binanay et al. [30]	2005	433	RCT	No difference in mortality
The National Heart, Lung and Blood Institute ARDS Clinical Trials Network [31]	2006	513/487	RCT	No difference in mortality or organ function
Higher or worse morbidity/mortality				
Tuman et al. [32]	1989	1,094	Controlled prospective cohort	Increased ICU stay with PAC
Guyatt [33]	1991	33/148	RCT	Higher morbidity
Hayes et al. [34]	1994	50	RCT	Higher mortality
Connors et al. [35]	1996	5,735	Prospective cohort	Higher mortality
Valentine et al. [36]	1998	60	RCT	Increased morbidity
Stewart et al. [37]	1998	133/61	Retrospective cohort	Increased morbidity
Ramsey et al. [38]	2000	8,064/5,843	Retrospective cohort	Higher mortality
Polanczyk et al. [39]	2001	215/215	Prospective cohort	Increased morbidity
Chittock et al. [40]	2004	7,310	Observational cohort	Increased mortality in low severity; decreased mortality in high severity
Peters et al. [41]	2003	360/690	Retrospective case control	Increased risk of death
Cohen et al. [42]	2005	26,437/735	Retrospective cohort	Increased mortality

ARDS, acute respiratory distress syndrome; ICU, intensive care unit; ISS, injury security score; LOS, length of stay; PA, pulmonary artery; PAC, pulmonary artery catheter; RCT, randomized control trial.

TABLE 19.2

General Indications for Pulmonary Artery Catheterization

Management of complicated myocardial infarction
- Hypovolemia versus cardiogenic shock
- Ventricular septal rupture versus acute mitral regurgitation
- Severe left ventricular failure
- Right ventricular infarction
- Unstable angina
- Refractory ventricular tachycardia

Assessment of respiratory distress
- Cardiogenic versus noncardiogenic (e.g., acute respiratory distress syndrome) pulmonary edema
- Primary versus secondary pulmonary hypertension

Assessment of shock
- Cardiogenic
- Hypovolemic
- Septic
- Pulmonary embolism

Assessment of therapy in selected individuals
- Afterload reduction in patients with severe left ventricular function
- Inotropic agent
- Vasopressors
- Beta-blockers
- Temporary pacing (ventricular vs. atrioventricular)
- Intra-aortic balloon counterpulsation
- Mechanical ventilation (e.g., with positive end-expiratory pressure)

Management of postoperative open-heart surgical patients

Assessment of cardiac tamponade/constriction

Assessment of valvular heart disease

Perioperative monitoring of patients with unstable cardiac status during noncardiac surgery

Assessment of fluid requirements in critically ill patients
- Gastrointestinal hemorrhage
- Sepsis
- Acute renal failure
- Burns
- Decompensated cirrhosis
- Advanced peritonitis

Management of severe preeclampsia

the catheter tip, thus distributing tip forces over a large area and minimizing the chances for endocardial damage or arrhythmia induction during catheter insertion (Fig. 19.2). Progression of the catheter is stopped when it impacts in a PA slightly smaller in diameter than the fully inflated balloon. From this position, the PAOP is obtained. Balloon capacity varies according to catheter size, and the operator must be aware of the individual balloon's maximal inflation volume, as recommended by the manufacturer. The balloon is usually inflated with air, but filtered carbon dioxide should be used in any situation in which balloon rupture might result in access of the inflation medium to the arterial system (e.g., if a right-to-left intracardiac shunt or a pulmonary arteriovenous fistula is suspected). If carbon dioxide is used, periodic deflation and reinflation may be necessary, because carbon dioxide diffuses through the latex balloon at a rate of approximately 0.5 cm^3 per

A variety of catheter constructions are available, each designed for particular clinical applications. Double-lumen catheters allow balloon inflation through one lumen, and a distal opening at the tip of the catheter is used to measure intravascular pressures and sample blood. Triple-lumen catheters have a proximal port terminating 30 cm from the tip of the catheter, allowing simultaneous measurement of right atrial and PA or occlusion pressures. The most commonly used PAC in the ICU setting is a quadruple-lumen catheter, which has a lumen containing electrical leads for a thermistor positioned at the catheter surface 4 cm proximal to its tip (Fig. 19.1) [45]. The thermistor measures PA blood temperature and allows for thermodilution CO measurements. A five-lumen catheter is also available, with the fifth lumen opening 40 cm from the tip of the catheter. The fifth lumen provides additional central venous access for fluid or medication infusions when peripheral access is limited or when drugs requiring infusion into a large vein (e.g., dopamine and epinephrine) are used. Figure 19.2 shows the balloon on the tip inflated.

Several special-purpose PAC designs are available. Pacing PACs incorporate two groups of electrodes on the catheter surface, enabling intracardiac electrocardiographic (ECG) recording or temporary cardiac pacing [46]. These catheters are used for emergency cardiac pacing, although it is often difficult to position the catheter for reliable simultaneous cardiac pacing and PA pressure measurements. A five-lumen catheter allows passage of a specially designed 2.4-Fr bipolar pacing electrode (probe) through the additional lumen (located 19 cm from the catheter tip) and allows emergency temporary intracardiac pacing without the need for a separate central venous puncture. The pacing probe is Teflon coated to allow easy introduction through the pacemaker port lumen; the intracavitary part of the probe is heparin impregnated to reduce the risk of thrombus formation. One report demonstrated satisfactory ventricular pacing in 19 of 23 patients using this catheter design (83% success rate) [47]. When a pacing probe is not in use, the fifth lumen may be used for additional central venous access or continuous RV pressure monitoring.

Continuous mixed venous oxygen saturation measurement is clinically available using a fiber-optic five-lumen PAC [48]. Catheters equipped with a fast-response (95 ms) thermistor and intracardiac ECG-monitoring electrodes are also available. These catheters allow for determination of the RV ejection fraction and RV systolic time intervals in critically ill patients [49]. Aside from the intermittent determination of CO by bolus administration of cold injectate, PACs have been adapted to determine near continuous CO by thermal pulses generated by a heating filament on the catheter to produce temperature changes [50]. The accuracy and reliability of CO determination by this heating–cooling cycle have been confirmed [51].

Pressure Transducers

Hemodynamic monitoring requires a system able to convert changes in intravascular pressure into electrical signals suitable for interpretation. The most commonly used hemodynamic monitoring system is a catheter–tubing–transducer system. A fluid-filled intravascular catheter is connected to a transducer by a fluid-filled tubing system (For more details, see the discussion in Chapters 7 and 28.)

INSERTION TECHNIQUES

General Considerations

Recommendations of manufacturers should be carefully followed. All catheter manufacturers have detailed insertion and training materials.

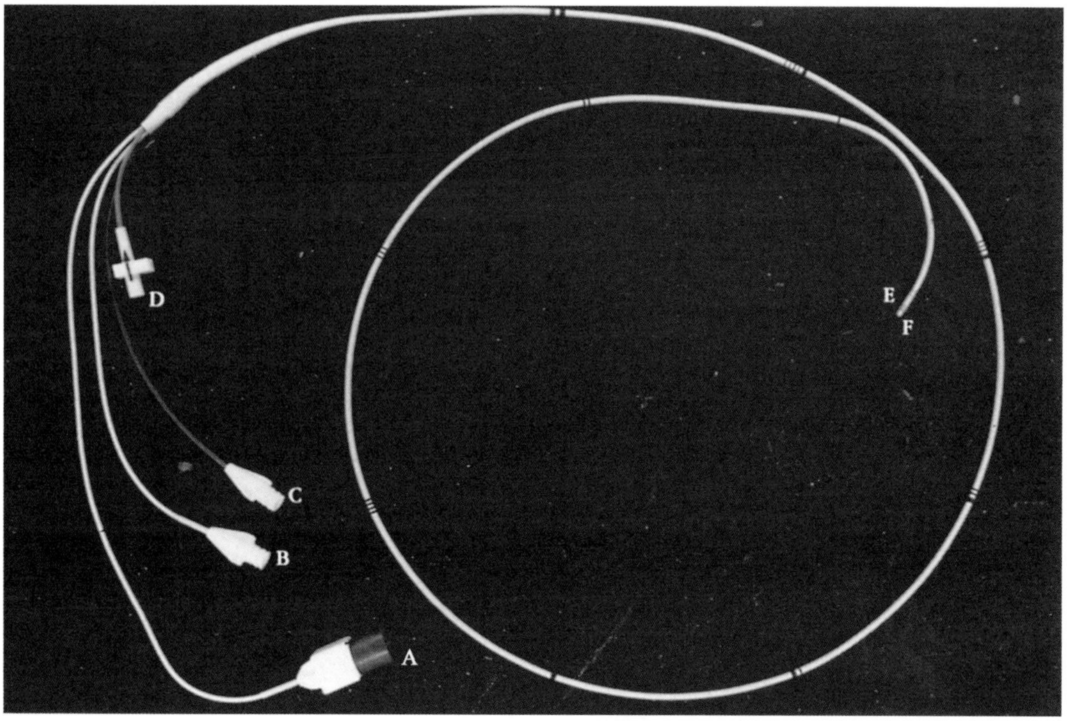

FIGURE 19.1 Quadruple-lumen pulmonary artery catheter. A: Connection to thermodilution cardiac output computer. B: Connection to distal lumen. C: Connection to proximal lumen. D: Stopcock connected to balloon at the catheter tip for balloon inflation. E: Thermistor. F: Balloon. Note that the catheter is marked in 10-cm increments.

PA catheterization can be performed in any hospital location where continuous ECG and hemodynamic monitoring are possible and where equipment and supplies needed for cardiopulmonary resuscitation are readily available. Fluoroscopy is not essential, but it can facilitate difficult placements. Properly constructed beds and protective aprons are mandatory for safe use of fluoroscopic equipment. Meticulous attention to sterile technique is of obvious importance; all involved personnel must wear sterile caps, gowns, masks, and gloves, and the patient must be fully covered by sterile drapes.

The catheter should be inserted percutaneously (not by cutdown) into the basilic, brachial, femoral, subclavian, or internal jugular veins by using techniques described in Chapter 6. Threading the catheter into the PA is more difficult from the basilic, brachial, or femoral vein.

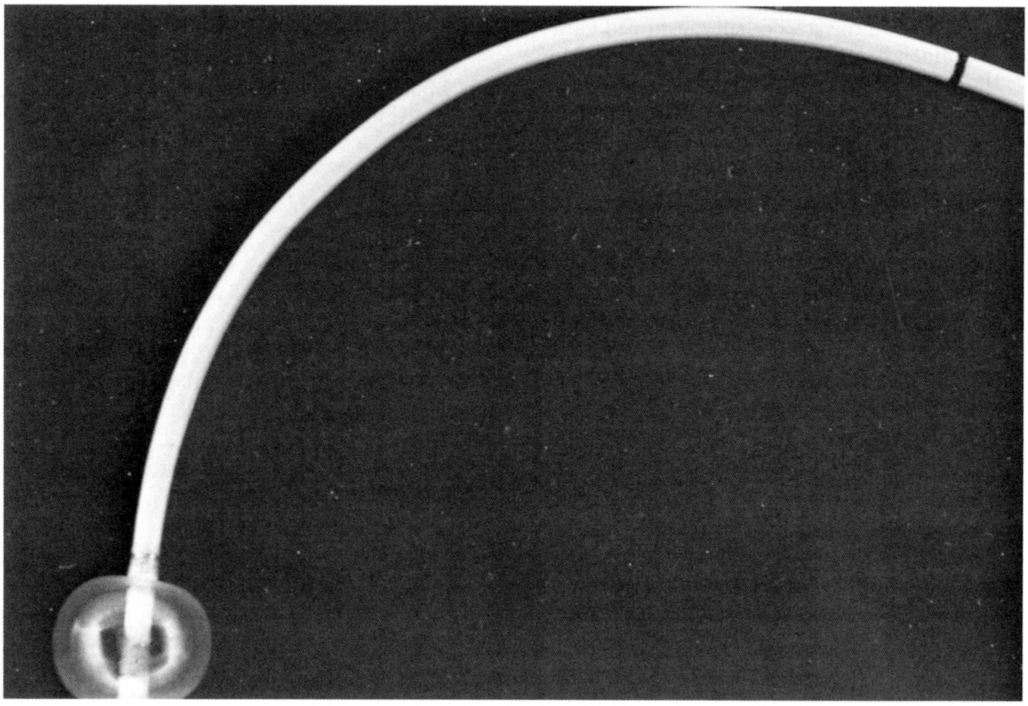

FIGURE 19.2 Balloon properly inflated at the tip of a pulmonary artery catheter. Note that the balloon shields the catheter tip and prevents it from irritating cardiac chambers on its passage to the pulmonary artery.

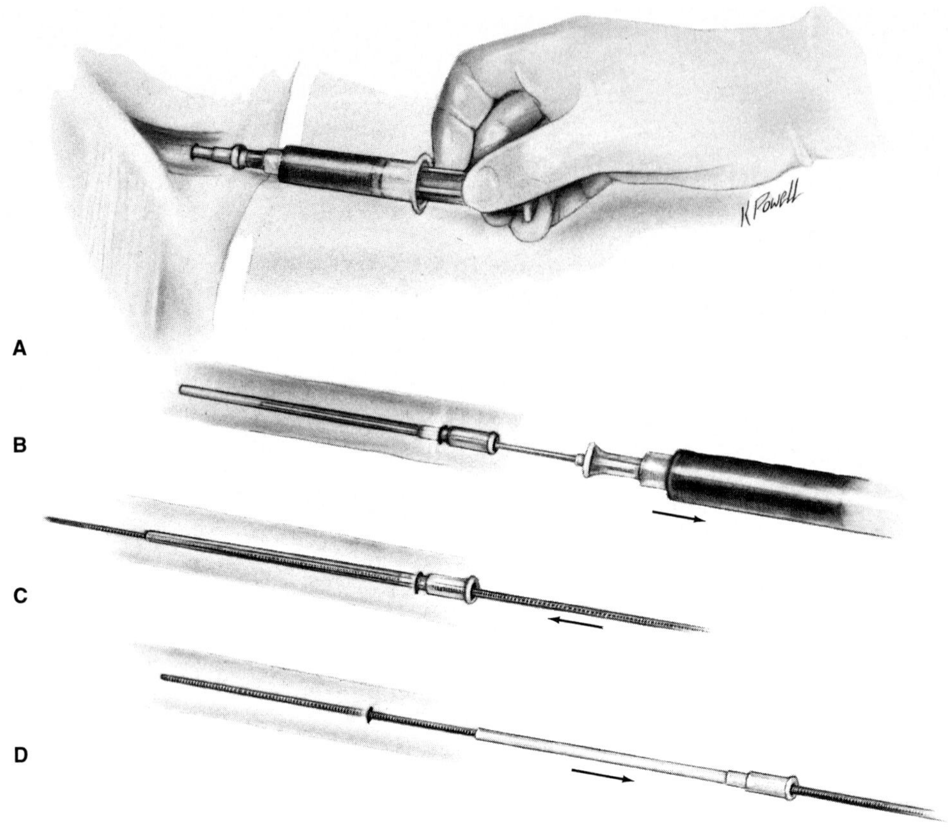

FIGURE 19.3 A: Easy blood aspiration has been demonstrated using the guidewire introducer needle. B: The inner needle is removed. C: The spring guidewire is advanced, soft end first, through the cannula into the vessel. D: With the guidewire held in place, the cannula is withdrawn from the vessel by being pulled over and off the length of the guidewire.

Typical Catheter Insertion Procedure

The procedures for typical catheter insertion are as follows:

1. Prepare and connect pressure tubing, manifolds, stopcocks, and transducers. Remove the sterile balloon-tipped catheter from its container. Balloon integrity may be tested by submerging the balloon in a small amount of fluid and checking for air leaks as the balloon is inflated (using the amount of air recommended by the manufacturer). Deflate the balloon.
2. After a time out, insert a central venous cannula or needle into the vein as described in Chapter 6. Using the Seldinger technique, thread the guidewire contained in the catheter kit into the vein and remove the catheter or needle (Figs. 19.3 and 19.4).
3. Make a small incision with a scalpel to enlarge the puncture site (Fig. 19.5). While holding the guidewire stationary,

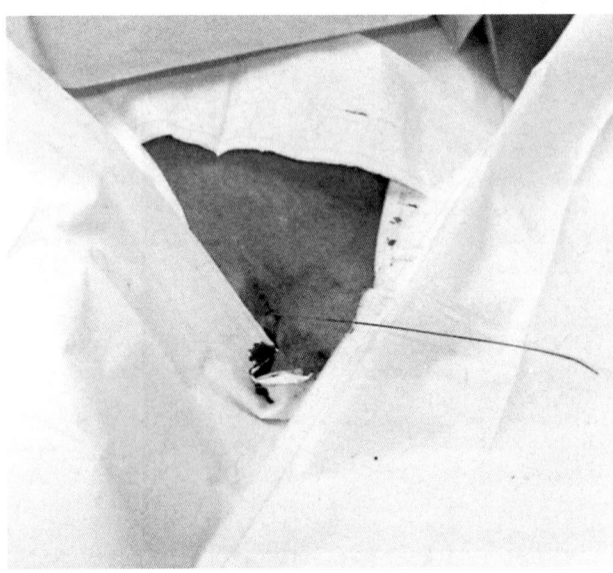

FIGURE 19.4 The spring guidewire, stiff end protruding, is now located in the subclavian vein.

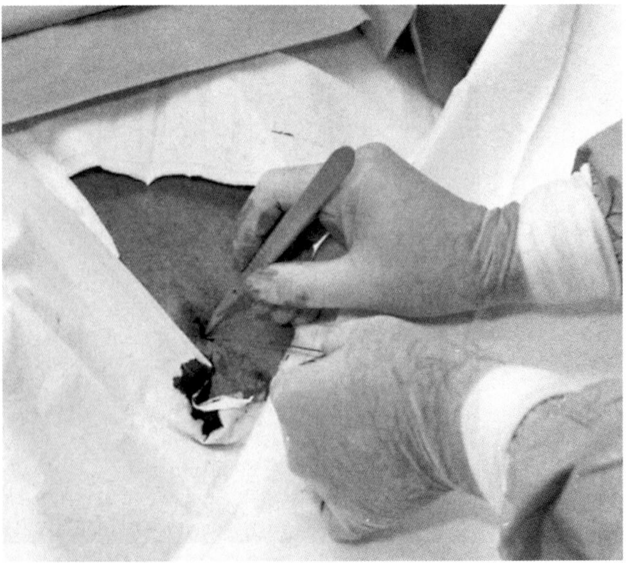

FIGURE 19.5 A small incision is made with a scalpel to enlarge the puncture site.

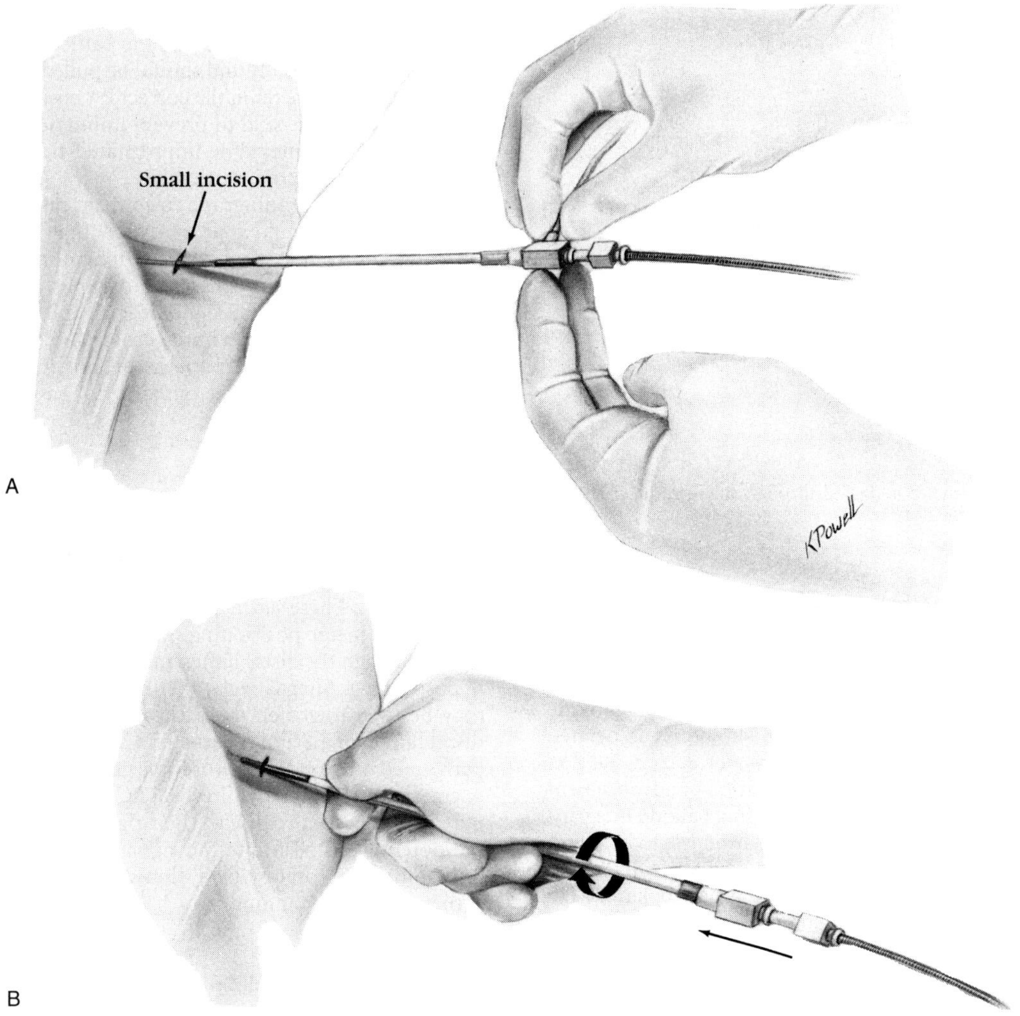

FIGURE 19.6 **A:** The vessel dilator-sheath apparatus is threaded over the guidewire and advanced into the vessel. **B:** A twisting motion is used to thread the apparatus into the vessel.

thread a vessel dilator-sheath apparatus (the size should be 8 Fr if a 7-Fr catheter is to be used) over the guidewire and advance it into the vessel, using a twisting motion to get through the puncture site (Fig. 19.6). The dilator and sheath should only be advanced until the tip of the sheath is in the vessel—estimated by the original depth of the cannula or needle required to access the vein. At that point, the dilator and guidewire are held stationary and the sheath is advanced off the dilator into the vessel. Advancing the dilator further may cause great vessel or cardiac damage.

4. Remove the guidewire and vessel dilator, leaving the introducer sheath in the vessel (Fig. 19.7). Suture the sheath in place.
5. Pass the proximal portion of the catheter to an assistant and have that person attach the stopcock-pressure tubing-transducer system to the right atrial and PA ports of the PA catheter. Flush the proximal and distal catheter lumens with normal saline.
6. If a sterile sleeve adapter is to be used, insert the catheter through it and pull the adapter proximally over the catheter to keep it out of the way. Once the catheter is advanced to its desired intravascular location, attach the distal end of the sleeve adapter to the introducer sheath hub.
7. Pass the catheter through the introducer sheath into the vein (Fig. 19.8). Advance it, using the marks on the catheter shaft indicating 10-cm distances from the tip, until the tip is in the right atrium. This requires advancement of approximately 35 to 40 cm from the left antecubital fossa, 10 to 15 cm from the internal jugular vein, 10 cm from the subclavian vein, and 35 to 40 cm from the femoral vein. A right atrial waveform on the monitor, with appropriate fluctuations accompanying respiratory changes or cough, confirms proper intrathoracic location (Fig. 19.9, center). If desired, obtain right atrial blood for oxygen saturation from the distal port. Flush the distal lumen with saline and record the

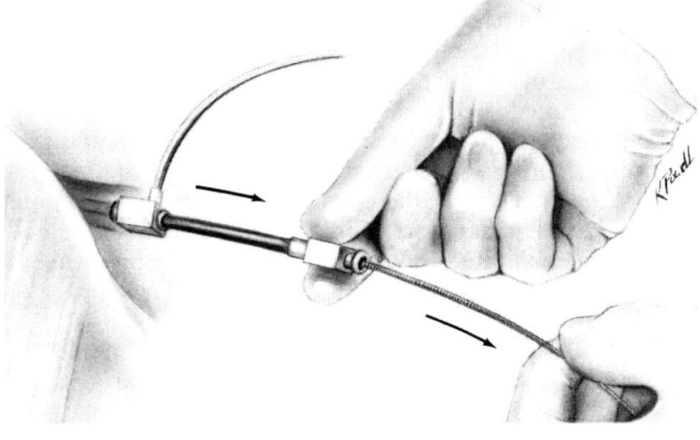

FIGURE 19.7 The guidewire and vessel dilator are removed, leaving the introducer sheath in the vessel.

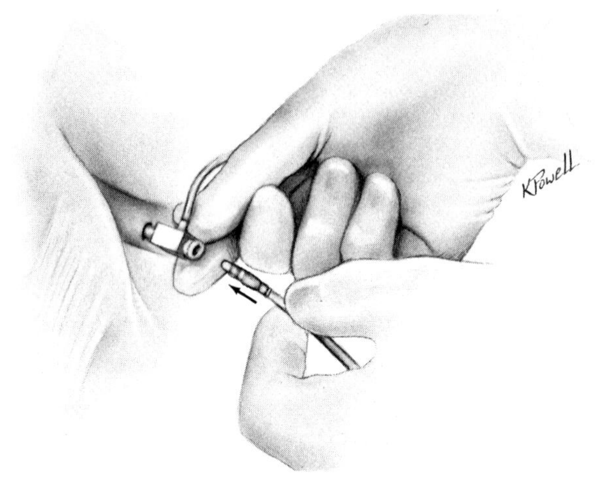

FIGURE 19.8 The catheter is passed through the introducer sheath into the vein.

right atrial pressures. (Occasionally, it is necessary to inflate the balloon to keep the tip from adhering to the atrial wall during blood aspiration.)

8. With the catheter tip in the right atrium, inflate the balloon with the recommended amount of air or carbon dioxide (Fig. 19.9A). Inflation of the balloon should be associated with a slight feeling of resistance—if it is not, suspect balloon rupture and do not attempt further inflation or advancement of the catheter before properly reevaluating balloon integrity. If significant resistance to balloon inflation is encountered, suspect malposition of the catheter in a small vessel; withdraw the catheter and readvance it to a new position. Do not use liquids to inflate the balloon, because they might be irretrievable and could prevent balloon deflation.
9. With the balloon inflated, advance the catheter until an RV pressure tracing is seen on the monitor (Fig. 19.9, center). Obtain and record RV pressures. Catheter passage into and through the RV is an especially risky time in terms of arrhythmias. Maintaining balloon inflation in the RV minimizes ventricular irritation (Fig. 19.9B), but it is important to monitor vital signs and ECG throughout the entire insertion procedure. Elevating the head of the bed to 5 degrees and a right tilt position will facilitate the passage of the catheter through the right ventricle and minimize the generation of arrhythmias.
10. Continue advancing the catheter until the diastolic pressure tracing rises above that in the RV (Fig. 19.9, center), indicating PA placement (Fig. 19.9C). If an RV trace still appears after the catheter has been advanced 15 cm beyond the original distance needed to reach the right atrium, suspect curling in the ventricle; deflate the balloon, withdraw it to the right atrium, then reinflate it and try again. Advancement beyond the PA position results in a fall on the pressure tracing from the levels of systolic pressure noted in the RV and PA. When this is noted, record the PAOP (Fig. 19.9, center, D) and deflate the balloon. Phasic PA pressure should reappear on the pressure tracing when the balloon is deflated. If it does not, pull back the catheter with the deflated balloon until the PA tracing appears. With the balloon deflated, blood may be aspirated for oxygen saturation measurement. Watch for intermittent RV tracings indicating slippage of the catheter backward into the ventricle.
11. Carefully record the balloon inflation volume needed to change the PA pressure tracing to the PAOP tracing. If PAOP is recorded with an inflation volume significantly lower than the manufacturer's recommended volume, or if subsequent PAOP determinations require decreasing amounts of balloon inflation volume as compared with an initial appropriate amount, the catheter tip has migrated too far peripherally and should be pulled back immediately.
12. Secure the catheter in the correct PA position by suturing or taping it to the skin to prevent unintetional advancement. Apply a chlorhexidine-impregnated transparent dressing at the introducre insertion site.
13. Order a chest radiograph to confirm catheter position; the catheter tip should appear no more than 3 to 5 cm from the midline. To assess whether peripheral catheter migration has occurred, daily chest radiographs are recommended to supplement pressure monitoring and checks on balloon inflation volumes. An initial cross-table lateral radiograph may be obtained in patients on positive end-expiratory pressure (PEEP) to rule out superior catheter placement.

Special Considerations

In certain disease states (right atrial or RV dilatation, severe pulmonary hypertension, severe tricuspid insufficiency, low CO syndromes), it may be difficult to position a flow-directed catheter properly. These settings may require fluoroscopic guidance to aid in catheter positioning. Infusion of 5 to 10 mL of cold saline through the distal lumen may stiffen the catheter and aid in positioning. Alternatively, a 0.025-cm guidewire 145 cm long may be used to stiffen the catheter when placed through the distal lumen of a 7-Fr PA catheter. This manipulation should be performed only under fluoroscopic guidance by an experienced operator. Rarely, nonflow-directed PACs (e.g., Cournand catheters) may be required. Because of their rigidity, these catheters have the potential to perforate the right heart and must be placed only under fluoroscopy by a physician experienced in cardiac catheterization techniques.

Utility of Ultrasonography for Pulmonary Artery Catheter Insertion

Ultrasonography has useful application related to PAC insertion. The PAC is usually inserted without difficulty using standard flow guided flotation technique in conjunction with real-time observation of the typical waveforms. Occasionally, the insertion may be difficult, particularly in patients with high right sided pressures, dilated right heart chambers, and/or severe tricuspid regurgitation. Real time guidance of PAC insertion with ultrasonography is a safe, effective, and fast method of insertion that has advantage over fluoroscopic guidance, given that it can be performed at the bedside of the critically patient and it requires no patient transport or complex equipment [52,53].

The right atrium (RA), tricuspid valve (TV), and right ventricle (RV) are imaged from the subcostal view or the right ventricular inflow view according to operator preference (See Chapter 18 Video 18.1 for an example of device insertion). The catheter tip is visualized as it enters the RA. The operator manipulates the catheter under direct visualization through the RV. The catheter is visualized as it enters the main PA from the short axis view of the base of the heart. Alternatively, it is visualized from the subcostal PA view where, imaging conditions permitting; it may be seen entering the right or left PA. In patients with inadequate image quality for transthoracic images, transesophageal echocardiography is an effective alternative [54] (Chapter 19 Video 19.1). In this case, the bicaval view allows initial visualization of the catheter, the mid-esophageal four chamber view permits assessment of catheter movement into the RV, the and final placement is visualized from the upper esophageal PA view.

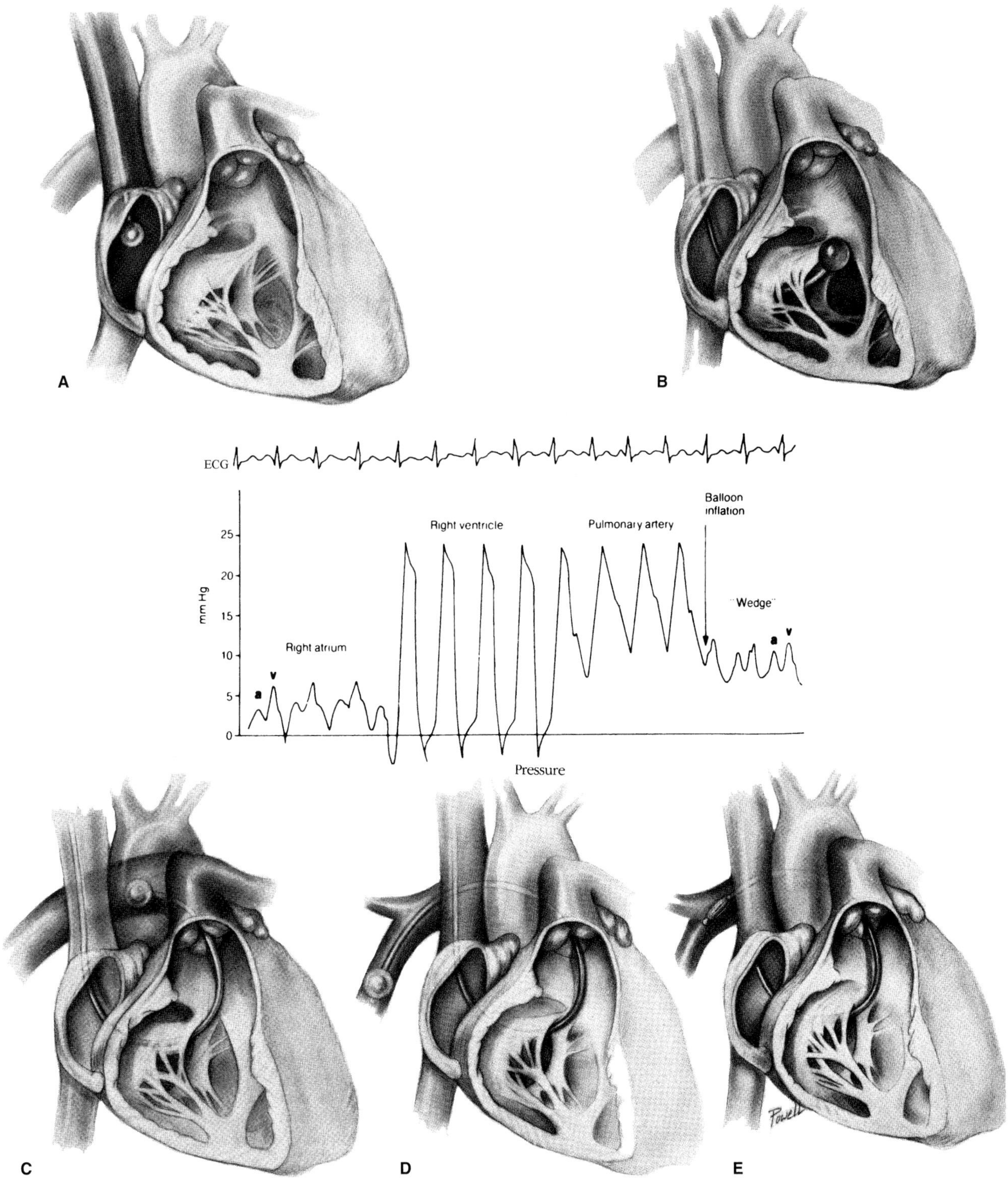

FIGURE 19.9 **A:** With the catheter tip in the right atrium, the balloon is inflated. **B:** The catheter is advanced into the right ventricle with the balloon inflated, and right ventricle pressure tracings are obtained. (*Center*): Waveform tracings generated as the balloon-tipped catheter is advanced through the right heart chambers into the pulmonary artery. (Adapted from Wiedmann HP, Matthay MA, Matthey RA: Cardiovascular pulmonary monitoring in the intensive care unit (Part 1) *Chest* 85:537;1984, with permission.) **C:** The catheter is advanced through the pulmonary valve into the pulmonary artery. A rise in diastolic pressure should be noted. **D:** The catheter is advanced to the pulmonary artery occlusion pressure position. A typical pulmonary artery occlusion pressure tracing should be noted with a and v waves. **E:** The balloon is deflated. Phasic pulmonary artery pressure should reappear on the monitor. (See text for details.)

PHYSIOLOGIC DATA

Measurement of a variety of hemodynamic parameters and oxygen saturations is possible using the PAC. A summary of normal values for these parameters is found in Tables 19.3 and 19.4.

Pressures

Right Atrium

With the tip of the PAC in the right atrium (Fig. 19.9A), the balloon is deflated and a right atrial waveform recorded (Fig. 19.10). Normal resting right atrial pressure is 0 to 6 mm Hg. Two major positive atrial pressure waves, the a wave and v wave, can usually be recorded. On occasion, a third positive wave, the c wave, can also be seen. The a wave is caused by atrial contraction and follows the simultaneously recorded ECG P wave [55]. The a wave peak generally follows the peak of the electrical P wave by approximately 80 ms. The v wave represents the pressure generated by venous filling of the right atrium while the tricuspid valve is closed. The peak of the v wave occurs at the end of ventricular systole when the atrium is maximally filled, corresponding to the point near the end of the T wave on the ECG. The c wave is caused by the sudden motion of the atrioventricular valve ring toward the right atrium at the onset of ventricular systole. The c wave follows the a wave by a time equal to the ECG P–R interval. The c wave is more readily visible in cases of P–R prolongation. The x descent follows the c wave and reflects atrial relaxation. The y descent is caused by rapid emptying of the atrium after opening of the tricuspid valve. The mean right atrial pressure decreases during inspiration with spontaneous respiration (secondary to a decrease in intrathoracic pressure), whereas the a and v waves and the x and y descents become more prominent. Once a multilumen PAC is in position, right atrial blood can be sampled and pressure monitored using the proximal lumen. It should be noted that the pressures obtained via the proximal lumen may not accurately reflect right atrial pressure owing to positioning of the lumen against the atrial wall or within the introducer sheath.

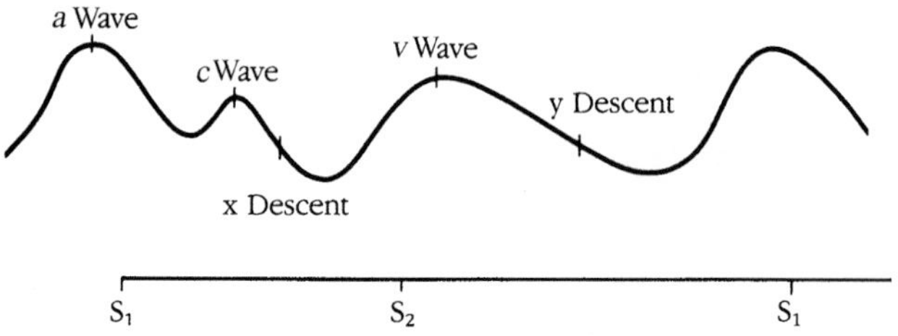

FIGURE 19.10 Stylized representation of a right atrial waveform in relation to heart sounds. (See text for discussion of a, c, and v waves and *x* and *y* descents.) S_1, first heart sound; S_2, second heart sound.

TABLE 19.3

Normal Resting Pressures Obtained during Right Heart Catheterization

Cardiac chamber	Pressure (mm Hg)
Right atrium	
Range	0–6
Mean	3
Right ventricle	
Systolic	17–30
Diastolic	0–6
Pulmonary artery	
Systolic	15–30
Diastolic	5–13
Mean	10–18
Pulmonary artery occlusion (mean)	2–12

Adapted from JM Gore, JS Alpert, JR Benotti, et al: *Handbook of Hemodynamic Monitoring*. Boston, MA, Little, Brown, 1984.

TABLE 19.4

Approximate Normal Oxygen Saturation and Content Values

Chamber sampled	Oxygen content (vol%)	Oxygen saturation (%)
Superior vena cava	14.0	70
Inferior vena cava	16.0	80
Right atrium	15.0	75
Right ventricle	15.0	75
Pulmonary artery	15.0	75
Pulmonary vein	20.0	98
Femoral artery	19.0	96
Atrioventricular oxygen content difference	3.5–5.5	—

Right Ventricle

The normal resting RV pressure is 17 to 30/0 to 6 mm Hg, recorded when the PAC crosses the tricuspid valve (Fig. 19.9B). The RV systolic pressure should equal the PA systolic pressure (except in cases of pulmonic stenosis or RV outflow tract obstruction). The RV diastolic pressure should equal the mean right atrial pressure during diastole when the tricuspid valve is open. Introduction of the catheter with a pacing lumen allows continuous monitoring of RV hemodynamics when the pacing wire is not in place. Using special catheters, RV end-diastolic volume index and RV ejection fraction can be accurately measured [56].

Pulmonary Artery

With the catheter in proper position and the balloon deflated, the distal lumen transmits PA pressure (Fig. 19.9E). Normal resting PA pressure is 15 to 30/5 to 13 mm Hg, with a mean pressure of 10 to 18 mm Hg. The PA waveform is characterized by a systolic peak and diastolic trough with a dicrotic notch due to closure of the pulmonic valve. The peak PA systolic pressure occurs in the T wave of a simultaneously recorded ECG.

Because the pulmonary vasculature is normally a low-resistance circuit, PA diastolic pressure (PADP) is closely related to mean PAOP (PADP is usually 1 to 3 mm Hg higher than mean PAOP) and thus can be used as an index of left ventricle filling pressure in patients in whom an occlusion pressure is unobtainable or in whom PADP and PAOP have been shown to correlate closely. However, if pulmonary vascular resistance is increased, as in pulmonary embolic disease, pulmonary fibrosis, or reactive pulmonary hypertension (see Chapter 174), PADP may markedly exceed mean PAOP and thus become an unreliable index of left heart function. Similar provisos apply when using PA mean pressure as an index of left ventricular function.

Pulmonary Artery Occlusion Pressure

An important application of the balloon flotation catheter is the recording of PAOP. This measurement is obtained when

TABLE 19.5

Checklist for Verifying Position of Pulmonary Artery Catheter

	Zone 3	Zone 1 or 2
PAOP contour	Cardiac ripple (A + V waves)	Unnaturally smooth
PAD versus PAOP	PAD > PAOP	PAD < PAOP
PEEP trial	ΔPAOP <½ ΔPEEP	ΔPAOP >½ ΔPEEP
Respiratory variation of PAOP	< ½ P_{ALV}	≥ ½ Δ P_{ALV}
Catheter-tip location	LA level or below	Above LA level

the inflated balloon impacts a slightly smaller branch of the PA (Fig. 19.9D). In this position, the balloon stops the flow, and the catheter tip senses pressure transmitted backward through the static column of blood from the next active circulatory bed—the pulmonary veins. Pulmonary venous pressure is a prime determinant of pulmonary congestion and thus of the tendency for fluid to shift from the pulmonary capillaries into the interstitial tissue and alveoli. Also, pulmonary venous pressure and PAOP closely reflect left atrial pressure (except in rare instances, such as pulmonary veno-occlusive disease, in which there is obstruction in the small pulmonary veins), and serve as indices of left ventricular filling pressure [57]. The PAOP is required to assess left ventricular filling pressure, because multiple studies have demonstrated that right atrial (e.g., central venous) pressure correlates poorly with PAOP [58].

The PAOP is a phase-delayed, amplitude-dampened version of the left atrial pressure. The normal resting PAOP is 2 to 12 mm Hg and averages 2 to 7 mm Hg below the mean PA pressure. The PAOP waveform is similar to that of the right atrium, with a, c, and v waves and x and y descents (Fig. 19.10). However, in contradistinction to the right atrial waveform, the PAOP waveform demonstrates a v wave that is slightly larger than the a wave [13]. Because of the time required for left atrial mechanical events to be transmitted through the pulmonary vasculature, PAOP waveforms are further delayed when recorded with a simultaneous ECG. The peak of the a wave follows the peak of the ECG P wave by approximately 240 ms, and the peak of the v wave occurs after the ECG T wave has been inscribed. Occlusion position is confirmed by withdrawing a blood specimen from the distal lumen and measuring oxygen saturation. Measured oxygen saturation of 95% or more is satisfactory [57]. The lung segment from which the sample is obtained will be well ventilated if the patient breathes slowly and deeply.

A valid PAOP measurement requires a patent vascular channel between the left atrium and catheter tip. Thus, the PAOP approximates pulmonary venous pressure (and therefore left atrial pressure) only if the catheter tip lies in Zone 3 of the lungs [55] (The lung is divided into three physiologic zones, dependent on the relationship of PA, pulmonary venous, and alveolar pressures. In Zone 3, the PA and pulmonary venous pressure exceed the alveolar pressure, ensuring an uninterrupted column of blood between the catheter tip and the pulmonary veins.). If, on portable lateral chest radiograph, the catheter tip is below the level of the left atrium (posterior position in supine patients), it can be assumed to be in Zone 3. This assumption holds if applied PEEP is less than 15 cm H_2O and the patient is not markedly volume depleted. Whether the catheter is positioned in Zone 3 may also be determined by certain physiologic characteristics (Table 19.5). A catheter occlusion outside Zone 3 shows marked respiratory variation, an unnaturally smooth vascular waveform, and misleading high pressures.

With a few exceptions [59], estimates of capillary hydrostatic filtration pressure from PAOP are acceptable. It should be noted that measurement of PAOP does not take into account capillary permeability, serum colloid osmotic pressure, interstitial pressure, or actual pulmonary capillary resistance. These factors all play roles in the formation of pulmonary edema, and the PAOP should be interpreted in the context of the specific clinical situation.

Mean PAOP correlates well with left ventricular end-diastolic pressure (LVEDP), provided the patient has a normal mitral valve and normal left ventricular function. In myocardial infarction, conditions with decreased left ventricular compliance (e.g., ischemia and left ventricular hypertrophy), and conditions with markedly increased left ventricular filling pressure (e.g., dilated cardiomyopathy), the contribution of atrial contraction to left ventricular filling is increased. Thus, the LVEDP may be significantly higher than the mean left atrial pressure or PAOP [55].

The position of the catheter can be misinterpreted in patients with the presence of giant v waves. The most common cause of these v waves is mitral regurgitation. During this condition, left ventricular blood floods a normal-sized, noncompliant left atrium during ventricular systole, causing giant v waves in the occlusion pressure tracing (Fig. 19.11). The giant v wave of mitral regurgitation may be transmitted to the PA tracing, yielding a bifid PA waveform composed of the PA systolic wave and the v wave. Because the catheter is occluded, the PA systolic wave is lost, but the v wave remains. It is important to note that the PA systolic wave occurs earlier in relation to the QRS complex of a simultaneously recorded ECG (between the QRS and T waves) than does the v wave (after the T wave).

Although a large v wave is not diagnostic of mitral regurgitation and is not always present in this circumstance, acute mitral regurgitation remains the most common cause of giant v waves in the PAOP tracing. Prominent v waves may occur whenever the left atrium is distended and noncompliant owing to left ventricular failure from any cause (e.g., ischemic heart

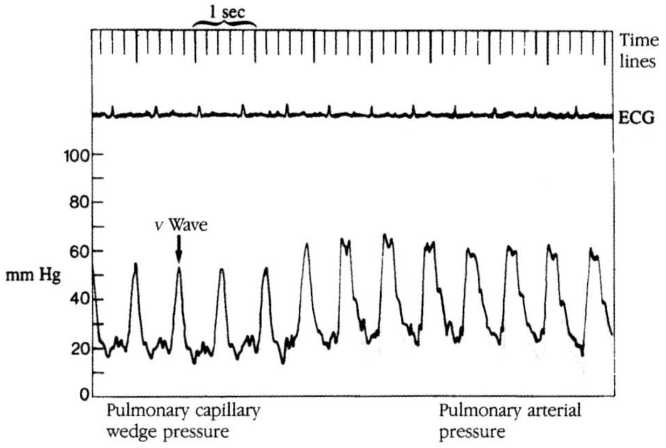

FIGURE 19.11 Pulmonary artery and pulmonary artery occlusion tracings with giant v waves distorting with pulmonary artery recording. ECG, electrocardiogram.

disease and dilated cardiomyopathy) [60], or secondary to the increased pulmonary blood flow in acute ventricular septal defect. Acute mitral regurgitation is the rare instance when the PA end-diastolic pressure may be lower than the computer-measured mean occlusion pressure.

End expiration provides a readily identifiable reference point for PAOP interpretation because pleural pressure returns to baseline at the end of passive deflation (approximately equal to atmospheric pressure). Pleural pressure can exceed the normal resting value with active expiratory muscle contraction or use of PEEP. How much PEEP is transmitted to the pleural space cannot be estimated easily, because it varies depending on lung compliance and other factors. When normal lungs deflate passively, end-expiratory pleural pressure increases by approximately one half of the applied PEEP. In patients with reduced lung compliance (e.g., patients with acute respiratory distress syndrome; ARDS), the transmitted fraction may be one-fourth or less of the PEEP value. In the past, PEEP levels greater than 10 mm Hg were thought to interrupt the column of blood between the left atrium and PAC tip, causing the PAOP to reflect alveolar pressure more accurately than left atrial pressure. However, two studies suggest that this may not hold true in all cases. Teboul et al. [61] could find no significant discrepancy between PAOP and simultaneously measured LVEDP at PEEP levels of 0, 10, and 16 to 20 cm H_2O in patients with ARDS. He hypothesized that (a) a large intrapulmonary right-to-left shunt may provide a number of microvessels shielded from alveolar pressure, allowing free communication from PA to pulmonary veins, or (b) in ARDS, both vascular and lung compliance may decrease, reducing transmission of alveolar pressure to the pulmonary microvasculature and maintaining an uninterrupted blood column from the catheter tip to the left atrium.

Although it is difficult to estimate precisely the true transmural vascular pressure in a patient on PEEP, temporarily disconnecting PEEP to measure PAOP is not recommended. Because the hemodynamics have been destabilized, these measurements will be of questionable value. Venous return increases acutely after discontinuation of PEEP [61], and abrupt removal of PEEP will cause hypoxia, which may not reverse quickly on reinstitution of PEEP [62].

Cardiac Output

Thermodilution Technique

A catheter equipped with a thermistor 4 cm from its tip allows calculation of CO by using the thermodilution principle [45,63]. The thermodilution principle holds that if a known quantity of cold solution is introduced into the circulation and adequately mixed (passage through two valves and a ventricle is adequate), the resultant cooling curve recorded at a downstream site allows for calculation of net blood flow. CO is inversely proportional to the integral of the time-versus-temperature curve.

In practice, a known amount of cold or room temperature solution (typically 10 mL of 0.9% saline in adults, and 5 mL of 0.9% saline in children) is injected into the right atrium via the catheter's proximal port. The thermistor allows recording of the baseline PA blood temperature and subsequent temperature change. The resulting curve is usually analyzed by computer, although it can be analyzed manually by simple planimetric methods. Correction factors are added by catheter manufacturers to account for the mixture of cold indicator with warm residual fluid in the catheter injection lumen and the heat transfer from the catheter walls to the cold indicator.

Reported coefficients of variation using triplicate determinations, using 10 mL of cold injectate and a bedside computer, are approximately 4% or less. Variations in the rate of injection can also introduce error into CO determinations, and it is thus important that the solution be injected as rapidly as possible. Careful attention must be paid to the details of this procedure; even then, changes of less than 10% to 15% above or below an initial value may not truly establish directional validity. Thermodilution CO is inaccurate in low-output states, tricuspid regurgitation, and in cases of atrial or ventricular septal defects [64].

Normal values for arterial–venous oxygen content difference, mixed venous oxygen saturation, and CO can be found in Table 19.6.

TABLE 19.6

Selected Hemodynamic Variables Derived from Right Heart Catheterization

Hemodynamic variable	Normal range
Arterial–venous content difference	3.5–5.5 mL/100 mL
Cardiac index	2.5–4.5 L/min/m^2
Cardiac output	3.0–7.0 L/min
Left ventricular stroke work index	45–60 g/beat/m^2
Mixed venous oxygen content	18.0 mL/100 mL
Mixed venous saturation	75% (approximately)
Oxygen consumption	200–250 mL/min
Pulmonary vascular resistance	120–250 dynes/sec/cm^{-5}
Stroke volume	70–130 mL/contraction
Stroke volume index	40–50 mL/contraction/m^2
Systemic vascular resistance	1,100–1,500 dynes/sec/cm^2

Adapted from JM Gore, JS Alpert, JR Benotti, et al: *Handbook of Hemodynamic Monitoring*. Boston, MA, Little, Brown, 1984.

Analysis of Mixed Venous Blood

CO can be approximated merely by examining mixed venous (PA) oxygen saturation. Theoretically, if CO rises, then the mixed venous oxygen partial pressure will rise, because peripheral tissues need to exact less oxygen per unit of blood. Conversely, if CO falls, peripheral extraction from each unit will increase to meet the needs of metabolizing tissues. Serial determinations of mixed venous oxygen saturation may display trends in CO. Normal mixed venous oxygen saturation is 70% to 75%; values of less than 60% are associated with heart failure and values of less than 40% with shock [65]. Potential sources of error in this determination include extreme low-flow states where poor mixing may occur, contamination of desaturated mixed venous blood by saturated pulmonary capillary blood when the sample is aspirated too quickly through the nonwedged catheter or in certain disease states (e.g., sepsis) where microcirculatory shunting may occur. Fiber-optic reflectance oximetry PACs can continuously measure and record mixed venous oxygen saturations in appropriate clinical situations [48].

Derived Parameters

Useful hemodynamic parameters that can be derived using data with PACs include the following:

1. Cardiac index = CO (L per minute)/BSA (m^2)
2. Stroke volume = CO (L per minute)/heart rate (beats per minute)
3. Stroke index = CO (L per minute)/(heart rate [beats per minute] × BSA [m^2])

4. Mean arterial pressure (mm Hg) = ([2 × diastolic] + systolic)/3
5. Systemic vascular resistance (dyne/s/cm^{-5}) = ([mean arterial pressure − mean right atrial pressure {mm Hg}] × 80)/CO (L per minute)
6. Pulmonary arteriolar resistance (dyne/s/cm^{-5}) = ([mean PA pressure − PAOP {mm Hg}] × 80)/CO (L per minute)
7. Total pulmonary resistance (dyne/s/cm^{-5}) = ([mean PA pressure {mm Hg}] × 80)/CO (L per minute)
8. Left ventricular stroke work index = 1.36 (mean arterial pressure − PAOP) × stroke index/100
9. Oxygen delivery (DO_2)(mL/min/m^2) = cardiac index × arterial O_2 content × 10

Normal values are listed in Table 19.6.

CLINICAL APPLICATIONS OF THE PULMONARY ARTERY CATHETER

Normal Resting Hemodynamic Profile

The finding of normal CO associated with normal left and right heart filling pressures is useful in establishing a noncardiovascular basis to explain abnormal symptoms or signs and as a baseline to gauge a patient's disease progression or response to therapy. Right atrial pressures of 0 to 6 mm Hg, PA systolic pressures of 15 to 30 mm Hg, PADPs of 5 to 12 mm Hg, PA mean pressures of 9 to 18 mm Hg, PAOP of 5 to 12 mm Hg, and a cardiac index exceeding 2.5 L/min/m^2 characterize a normal cardiovascular state at rest.

Table 19.7 summarizes specific hemodynamic patterns for a variety of disease entities in which PACs have been indicated and provide clinical information that can impact patient care.

COMPLICATIONS

Minor and major complications associated with bedside balloon flotation PA catheterization have been reported (Table 19.8). During the 1970s, in the first 10 years of clinical catheter use, a number of studies reported a relatively high incidence of certain complications. Consequent revision of guidelines for PAC use and improved insertion and maintenance techniques resulted in a decreased incidence of these complications in the 1980s [66]. The majority of complications are avoidable by scrupulous attention to detail in catheter placement and maintenance.

Complications Associated with Central Venous Access

The insertion techniques and complications of central venous cannulation are discussed in Chapter 6. Reported local vascular complications include local arterial or venous hematomas, unintentional entry of the catheter into the carotid system, atrioventricular fistulas, and pseudoaneurysm formation [67]. Adjacent structures, such as the thoracic duct, can be damaged, with resultant chylothorax formation. Pneumothorax can be a serious complication of insertion, although the incidence is relatively low (1% to 2%) [67]. The incidence of pneumothorax is higher with the subclavian approach than with the internal jugular approach in some reports [68], but other studies demonstrate no difference between the two sites [69]. The incidence of complications associated with catheter insertion is generally considered to be inversely proportional to the operator's experience.

Balloon Rupture

Balloon rupture occurred more frequently in the early 1970s than it does now and was generally related to exceeding recommended inflation volumes. The main problems posed by balloon rupture are air emboli gaining access to the arterial circulation and balloon fragments embolizing to the distal pulmonary circulation. If rupture occurs during catheter insertion, the loss of the balloon's protective cushioning function can predispose to endocardial damage and attendant thrombotic and arrhythmic complications.

TABLE 19.7

Hemodynamic Parameters in Commonly Encountered Clinical Situations (Idealized)

	RA	RV	PA	PAOP	AO	CI	SVR	PVR
Normal	0–6	25/0–6	25/6–12	6–12	130/80	≥2.5	1,500	≤250
Hypovolemic shock	0–2	15–20/0–2	15–20/2–6	2–6	≤90/60	<2.0	>1,500	≤250
Cardiogenic shock	8	50/8	50/35	35	≤90/60	<2.0	>1,500	≤250
Septic shock								
Early	0–2	20–25/0–2	20–25/0–6	0–6	≤90/60	≥2.5	<1,500	<250
Late[a]	0–4	25/4–10	25/4–10	4–10	≤90/60	<2.0	>1,500	>250
Acute massive pulmonary embolism	8–12	50/12	50/12–15	≤12	≤90/60	<2.0	>1,500	>450
Cardiac tamponade	12–18	25/12–18	25/12–18	12–18	≤90/60	<2.0	>1,500	≤250
AMI without LVF	0–6	25/0–6	25/12–18	≤18	140/90	≤2.5	>1,500	≤250
AMI with LVF	0–6	30–40/0–6	30–40/18–25	>18	140/90	>2.0	>1,500	>250
Biventricular failure secondary to LVF	>6	50–60/>6	50–60/25	18–25	120/80	~2.0	>1,500	>250
RVF secondary to RVI	12–20	30/12–20	30/12	<12	≤90/60	<2.0	>1,500	>250
Cor pulmonale	>6	80/>6	80/35	<12	120/80	~2.0	>1,500	>400
Idiopathic pulmonary hypertension	0–6	80–100/0–6	80–100/40	<12	100/60	<2.0	>1,500	>500
Acute ventricular septal rupture[b]	6	60/6–8	60/35	30	≤90/60	<2.0	>1,500	>250

TABLE 19.8

Complications of Pulmonary Artery Catheterization

Associated with central venous access
Balloon rupture
Knotting
Pulmonary infarction
Pulmonary artery perforation
Thrombosis, embolism
Arrhythmias
Intracardiac damage
Infections
Miscellaneous complications

Knotting

Knotting of a catheter around itself is most likely to occur when loops form in the cardiac chambers and the catheter is repeatedly withdrawn and readvanced [70]. Knotting is avoided if care is taken not to advance the catheter significantly beyond the distances at which entrance to the ventricle or PA would ordinarily be anticipated. Knotted catheters usually can be extricated transvenously; guidewire placement, venotomy, or more extensive surgical procedures are occasionally necessary.

Knotting of PACs around intracardiac structures [71] or other intravascular catheters has been reported. Rarely, entrapment of a PAC in cardiac sutures after open-heart surgery has been reported, requiring varying approaches for removal [72].

Pulmonary Infarction

Peripheral migration of the catheter tip (caused by catheter softening and loop tightening over time) with persistent, undetected wedging in small branches of the PA is the most common mechanism underlying pulmonary ischemic lesions attributable to PACs [73]. These lesions are usually small and asymptomatic, often diagnosed solely on the basis of changes in the chest radiograph that demonstrate an occlusion-shaped pleural-based density with a convex proximal contour.

Severe infarctions are usually produced if the balloon is left inflated in the occlusion position for an extended period, thus obstructing more central branches of the PA, or if solutions are injected at relatively high pressure through the catheter lumen in an attempt to restore an apparently damped pressure trace. Pulmonary embolic phenomena resulting from thrombus formation around the catheter or over areas of endothelial damage can also result in pulmonary infarction.

The reported incidence of pulmonary infarction secondary to PACs in 1974 was 7.2% [73], but subsequent studies reported much lower rates of pulmonary infarction. Boyd et al. [74] found a 1.3% incidence of pulmonary infarction in a prospective study of 528 PA catheterizations. Sise et al. [75] reported no pulmonary infarctions in a prospective study of 319 PAC insertions. Use of continuous saline flush solutions and careful monitoring of PA waveforms are important reasons for the decreased incidence of this complication.

Pulmonary Artery Perforation

A serious and feared complication of PA catheterization is rupture of the PA leading to hemorrhage, which can be massive and sometimes fatal [76,77]. Rupture may occur during insertion or may be delayed a number of days [77]. PA rupture or perforation has been reported in approximately 0.1% to 0.2% of patients [68,78]. Pathologic data suggest the true incidence of PA perforation is somewhat higher [79]. Proposed mechanisms by which PA rupture can occur include (a) an increased pressure gradient between PAOP and PA pressure brought about by balloon inflation and favoring distal catheter migration, where perforation is more likely to occur; (b) an occluded catheter tip position favoring eccentric or distended balloon inflation with a spearing of the tip laterally and through the vessel; (c) cardiac pulsation causing shearing forces and damage as the catheter tip repeatedly contacts the vessel wall; (d) presence of the catheter tip near a distal arterial bifurcation where the integrity of the vessel wall against which the balloon is inflated may be compromised; and (e) simple lateral pressure on vessel walls caused by balloon inflation (this tends to be greater if the catheter tip was occluded before inflation began). Patient risk factors for PA perforation include pulmonary hypertension, mitral valve disease, advanced age, hypothermia, and anticoagulant therapy. In patients with these risk factors and in whom PADP reflects PAOP reasonably well, avoidance of subsequent balloon inflation altogether constitutes prudent prophylaxis.

Another infrequent but life-threatening complication is false aneurysm formation associated with rupture or dissection of the PA [80]. Technique factors related to PA hemorrhage are distal placement or migration of the catheter; failure to remove large catheter loops placed in the cardiac chambers during insertion; excessive catheter manipulation; use of stiffer catheter designs; and multiple or prolonged balloon inflations. Adherence to strict technique may decrease the incidence of this complication. In a prospective study reported in 1986, no cases of PA rupture occurred in 1,400 patients undergoing PA catheterization for cardiac surgery [69].

PA perforation typically presents with massive hemoptysis. Emergency management includes immediate occlusion arteriogram and bronchoscopy; intubation of the unaffected lung; and consideration of emergency lobectomy or pneumonectomy. Application of PEEP to intubated patients may also tamponade hemorrhage caused by a PAC [81].

Thromboembolic Complications

Because PACs constitute foreign bodies in the cardiovascular system and can potentially damage the endocardium, they are associated with an increased incidence of thrombosis. Thrombi encasing the catheter tip and aseptic thrombotic vegetations forming at endocardial sites in contact with the catheter have been reported [74]. Extensive clotting around the catheter tip can occlude the pulmonary vasculature distal to the catheter, and thrombi anywhere in the venous system or right heart can serve as a source of pulmonary emboli. Subclavian venous thrombosis, presenting with unilateral neck vein distention and upper extremity edema, may occur in up to 2% of subclavian placements [82]. Venous thrombosis complicating percutaneous internal jugular vein catheterization is fairly commonly reported, although its clinical importance remains uncertain. Consistently damped pressure tracings without evidence of peripheral catheter migration or pulmonary vascular occlusion should arouse suspicion of thrombi at the catheter tip. A changing relationship of PADP to PAOP over time should raise concern about possible pulmonary emboli.

If an underlying hypercoagulable state is known to exist, if catheter insertion was particularly traumatic, or if prolonged monitoring becomes necessary, one should consider cautiously anticoagulating the patient.

Heparin-bonded catheters reduce thrombogenicity [44] and are commonly used. However, an important complication of heparin-bonded catheters is HIT [83]. Routine platelet counts are recommended for patients with heparin-bonded catheters in place. Because of the risk of HIT, some hospitals have abandoned the use of heparin-bonded catheters.

Rhythm Disturbances

Atrial and ventricular arrhythmias occur commonly during insertion of PACs [84]. Premature ventricular contractions occurred during 11% of the catheter insertions originally reported by Swan et al. [1].

Studies have reported advanced ventricular arrhythmias (three or more consecutive ventricular premature beats) in approximately 30% to 60% of patients undergoing right heart catheterization [68,85,86]. Most arrhythmias are self-limited and do not require treatment, but sustained ventricular arrhythmias requiring treatment occur in 0% to 3% of patients [74,85,86]. Risk factors associated with increased incidence of advanced ventricular arrhythmias are acute myocardial ischemia or infarction, hypoxia, acidosis, hypocalcemia, and hypokalemia [85]. A right lateral tilt position (5-degree angle) during PAC insertion is associated with a lower incidence of malignant ventricular arrhythmias than is the Trendelenburg position.

Although the majority of arrhythmias occur during catheter insertion, arrhythmias may develop at any time after the catheter has been correctly positioned. These arrhythmias are caused by mechanical irritation of the conducting system and may be persistent. Ventricular ectopy may also occur if the catheter tip falls back into the RV outflow tract. Evaluation of catheter-induced ectopy should include a portable chest radiograph to evaluate catheter position and assessment of the distal lumen pressure tracing to ensure that the catheter has not slipped into the RV. Lidocaine may be used but is unlikely to ablate the ectopy because the irritant is not removed. If the arrhythmia persists after lidocaine therapy or is associated with hemodynamic compromise, the catheter should be removed. Catheter removal should be performed by physicians under continuous ECG monitoring, because the ectopy occurs almost as frequently during catheter removal as during insertion [87].

Right bundle branch block (usually transient) can also complicate catheter insertion [88]. Patients undergoing anesthesia induction, those in the early stages of acute anteroseptal myocardial infarction, and those with acute pericarditis appear particularly susceptible to this complication. Patients with preexisting left bundle branch block are at risk for developing complete heart block during catheter insertion, and some have advocated the insertion of a temporary transvenous pacing wire, a PAC with a pacing lumen, or pacing PAC with the pacing leads on the external surface of the catheter. However, use of an external transthoracic pacing device should be sufficient to treat this complication.

Intracardiac Damage

Damage to the right heart chambers, tricuspid valve, pulmonic valve, and their supporting structures as a consequence of PA catheterization has been reported [89–91]. The reported incidence of catheter-induced endocardial disruption detected by pathologic examination varies from 3.4% to 75% [92], but most studies suggest a range of 20% to 30% [90,91]. These lesions consist of hemorrhage, sterile thrombus, intimal fibrin deposition, and nonbacterial thrombotic endocarditis. Their clinical significance is not clear, but there is concern that they may serve as a nidus for infectious endocarditis.

Direct damage to the cardiac valves and supporting chordae occurs primarily by withdrawal of the catheters while the balloon is inflated [1]. However, chordal rupture has been reported despite balloon deflation. The incidence of intracardiac and valvular damage discovered on postmortem examination is considerably higher than that of clinically significant valvular dysfunction.

Infections

Catheter-related septicemia (the same pathogen growing from blood and the catheter tip) was reported in up to 2% of patients undergoing bedside catheterization in the 1970s [93]. However, the incidence of septicemia related to the catheter appears to have declined in recent years, with a number of studies suggesting a septicemia rate of 0% to 1% [68,94]. In situ time of more than 72 to 96 hours significantly increases the risk of catheter-related sepsis. Right-sided septic endocarditis has been reported [95], but the true incidence of this complication is unknown. Becker et al. [89] noted two cases of left ventricular abscess formation in patients with PACs and *Staphylococcus aureus* septicemia. Incidence of catheter colonization or contamination varies from 5% to 20%, depending on the duration of catheter placement and the criteria used to define colonization [95,96]. In situ catheter-related bloodstream infection may be diagnosed by quantitative blood cultures.

Pressure transducers have also been identified as an occasional source of infection [97]. The chance of introducing infection into a previously sterile system is increased during injections for CO determinations and during blood withdrawal. Approaches to reduce the risk of catheter-related infection include use of a sterile protective sleeve and antibiotic bonding to the catheter [69,98]. Scheduled changes of catheters do not reduce the rate of infection [99].

Other Complications

Rare miscellaneous complications that have been reported include (a) hemodynamically significant decreases in pulmonary blood flow caused by balloon inflation in the central PA in postpneumonectomy patients with pulmonary hypertension in the remaining lung, (b) disruption of the catheter's intraluminal septum as a result of injecting contrast medium under pressure [100], (c) artifactual production of a midsystolic click caused by a slapping motion of the catheter against the interventricular septum in a patient with RV strain and paradoxic septal motion [101], (d) thrombocytopenia secondary to heparin-bonded catheters [83], and (e) dislodgment of pacing electrodes [102]. Multiple unusual placements of PACs have also been reported, including in the left pericardiophrenic vein, via the left superior intercostal vein into the abdominal vasculature, and from the superior vena cava through the left atrium and left ventricle into the aorta after open-heart surgery [103].

GUIDELINES FOR SAFE USE OF PULMONARY ARTERY CATHETERS

Multiple revisions and changes in emphasis to the original recommended techniques and guidelines have been published [66,104]. These precautions are summarized as follows:

1. Avoiding complications associated with catheter insertion.
   a. Inexperienced personnel performing insertions must be supervised. Many hospitals require that PACs be inserted by a fully trained intensivist, cardiologist, or anesthesiologist. Use of ultrasound guidance is recommended.
   b. Keep the patient as still as possible. Restraints or sedation may be required but the patient should be fully monitored with ECG and pulse oximetry.
   c. Strict sterile technique is mandatory. A chlorhexidine skin prep solution and maximum barrier precautions are recommended.
   d. Examine the postprocedure chest radiograph (or ultrasonography) for pneumothorax (especially after subclavian or internal jugular venipuncture) and for catheter tip position.

2. Avoiding balloon rupture.
   a. Always inflate the balloon gradually. Stop inflation if no resistance is felt.
   b. Do not exceed recommended inflation volume. At the recommended volume, excess air will automatically be expelled from a syringe with holes bored in it that is constantly attached to the balloon port. Maintaining recommended volume also helps prevent the accidental injection of liquids.
   c. Keep the number of inflation–deflation cycles to a minimum.
   d. Do not reuse catheters designed for single usage, and do not leave catheters in place for prolonged periods.
   e. Use carbon dioxide as the inflation medium if communication between the right and left sides of the circulation is suspected.
3. Avoiding knotting. Discontinue advancement of the catheter if entrance to right atrium, RV, or PA has not been achieved at distances anatomically anticipated from a given insertion site. If these distances have already been significantly exceeded, or if the catheter does not withdraw easily, use fluoroscopy before attempting catheter withdrawal. Never pull forcefully on a catheter that does not withdraw easily.
4. Avoiding damage to pulmonary vasculature and parenchyma.
   a. Keep recording time of PAOP to a minimum, particularly in patients with pulmonary hypertension and other risk factors for PA rupture. Be sure the balloon is deflated after each PAOP recording. There is never an indication for continuous PAOP monitoring.
   b. Constant pressure monitoring is required each time the balloon is inflated. It should be inflated slowly, in small increments, and must be stopped as soon as the pressure tracing changes to PAOP or damped.
   c. If an occlusion is recorded with balloon volumes significantly less than the inflation volume recommended on the catheter shaft, withdraw the catheter to a position where full (or nearly full) inflation volume produces the desired trace.
   d. Anticipate catheter tip migration. Softening of the catheter material with time, repeated manipulations, and cardiac motion make distal catheter migration almost inevitable.
      i. Continuous PA pressure monitoring is mandatory, and the trace must be closely watched for changes from characteristic PA pressures to those indicating a PAOP or damped tip position.
      ii. Decreases over time in the balloon inflation volumes necessary to attain occlusion tracings should raise suspicion regarding catheter migration.
      iii. Confirm satisfactory tip position with chest radiographs immediately after insertion and at least daily.
   e. Do not use liquids to inflate the balloon. They may prevent deflation, and their relative incompressibility may increase lateral forces and stress on the walls of pulmonary vessels.
   f. Hemoptysis is an ominous sign and should prompt an urgent diagnostic evaluation and rapid institution of appropriate therapy.
   g. Avoid injecting solutions at high pressure through the catheter lumen on the assumption that clotting is the cause of the damped pressure trace. First, aspirate from the catheter. Then consider problems related to catheter position, stopcock position, transducer dome, transducers, pressure bag, flush system, or trapped air bubbles. Never flush the catheter in the occlusion position.
5. Avoiding thromboembolic complications.
   a. Minimize trauma induced during insertion.
   b. Consider the judicious use of anticoagulants in patients with hypercoagulable states or other risk factors.
   c. Avoid flushing the catheter under high pressure.
   d. Watch for a changing PADP–PAOP relationship, as well as for other clinical indicators of pulmonary embolism.
6. Avoiding arrhythmias.
   a. Constant ECG monitoring during insertion and maintenance, as well as ready accessibility of all supplies for performing cardiopulmonary resuscitation, defibrillation, and temporary pacing, are mandatory.
   b. Use caution when catheterizing patients with an acutely ischemic myocardium or preexisting left bundle branch block.
   c. When the balloon is deflated, do not advance the catheter beyond the right atrium.
   d. Avoid over manipulation of the catheter.
   e. Secure the introducer in place at the insertion site.
   f. Watch for intermittent RV pressure tracings when the catheter is thought to be in the PA position. An unexplained ventricular arrhythmia in a patient with a PAC in place indicates the possibility of catheter-provoked ectopy.
7. Avoiding valvular damage.
   a. Avoid prolonged catheterization and excessive manipulation.
   b. Do not withdraw the catheter when the balloon is inflated.
8. Avoiding infections.
   a. Use meticulously sterile technique on insertion.
   b. Avoid excessive number of CO determinations and blood withdrawals.
   c. Avoid prolonged catheterization.
   d. Remove the catheter if signs of phlebitis develop. Culture the tip and use antibiotics as indicated.

SUMMARY

Hemodynamic monitoring enhances the understanding of cardiopulmonary pathophysiology in critically ill patients. Nonetheless, the risk-to-benefit profile of PA catheterization in various clinical circumstances remains uncertain [105]. Large trials have concluded that there may be no outcome benefit to patients with PACs used as part of clinical decision-making [106]. There is concern that data obtained during PA catheterization may not be optimally used, or perhaps in specific groups may increase morbidity and mortality. A meta-analysis of 13 randomized clinical trials concluded that the use of the PAC neither increased overall mortality or hospital days, nor conferred any benefit. The authors concluded that despite nearly 20 years of randomized clinical trials involving the PA catheter, there has not been a clear strategy in its use which has led to improved survival [107].

Until the results of future studies are available, clinicians using hemodynamic monitoring should carefully assess the risk-to-benefit ratio on an individual patient basis. The operator should understand the indications, insertion techniques, equipment, and data that can be generated before undertaking PAC insertion. PA catheterization must not delay or replace bedside clinical evaluation and treatment.

References

1. Swan HJC, Ganz W, Forrester J, et al: Catheterization of the heart in man with use of a flow-directed balloon-tipped catheter. *N Engl J Med* 283:447, 1970.
2. Gorlin R: Current concepts in cardiology: practical cardiac hemodynamics. *N Engl J Med* 296:203, 1977.
3. Rao TK, Jacobs KH, El-Etr AA: Reinfarction following anesthesia in patients with myocardial infarction. *Anesthesiology* 59:499, 1983.
4. Hesdorffer CS, Milne JF, Meyers AM, et al: The value of Swan-Ganz catheterization and volume loading in preventing renal failure in patients undergoing abdominal aneurysmectomy. *Clin Nephrol* 28:272, 1987.
5. Shoemaker WC, Appel PL, Kram HB, et al: Prospective trial of supranormal values of survivors as therapeutic goals in high-risk surgical patients. *Chest* 94:1176, 1988.
6. Berlauk JF, Abrams JH, Gilmour IL, et al: Preoperative optimization of cardiovascular hemodynamics improves outcome in peripheral vascular surgery: a prospective, randomized clinical trial. *Ann Surg* 214:289, 1991.
7. Fleming A, Bishop M, Shoemaker W, et al: Prospective trial of supernormal values as goals of resuscitation in severe trauma. *Arch Surg* 127:1175, 1992.

8. Tuchschmidt J, Fried J, Astiz M, et al: Elevation of cardiac output and oxygen delivery improves outcome in septic shock. *Chest* 102:216, 1992.
9. Boyd O, Grounds RM, Bennett ED: A randomized clinical trial or the effect of deliberate perioperative increase of oxygen delivery on mortality in high-risk surgical patients. *JAMA* 270:2699, 1993.
10. Bishop MH, Shoemaker WC, Appel PL, et al: Prospective randomized trial of survivor values of cardiac index, oxygen delivery, and oxygen consumption as resuscitation endpoints in severe trauma. *J Trauma* 38:780, 1995.
11. Schiller WR, Bay RC, Garren RL, et al: Hyperdynamic resuscitation improves in patients with life-threatening burns. *J Burn Care Rehabil* 18:10, 1997.
12. Wilson J, Woods I, Fawcett J, et al: Reducing the risk of major elective surgery: randomized controlled trial of preoperative optimization of oxygen delivery. *BMJ* 318:1099, 1999.
13. Chang MC, Meredith JW, Kincaid EH, et al: Maintaining survivors' of left ventricular power output during shock resuscitation: a prospective pilot study. *J Trauma* 49:26, 2000.
14. Polonen P, Ruokonen E, Hippelainen M, et al: A prospective, randomized study of goal-oriented hemodynamic therapy in cardiac surgical patients. *Anesth Analg* 90:1052, 2000.
15. Friese RS, Shafi S, Gentilello LM: Pulmonary artery catheter use is associated with reduced mortality in severely injured patients: a National Trauma Data Bank analysis of 53,312 patients. *Crit Care Med* 34:1597, 2006.
16. Pearson KS, Gomez MN, Moyers, JR, et al: A cost/benefit analysis of randomized invasive monitoring for patients undergoing cardiac surgery. *Anesth Analg* 69:336, 1989.
17. Isaacson IJ, Lowdon JD, Berry AJ, et al: The value of pulmonary artery and central venous monitoring in patients undergoing abdominal aortic reconstructive surgery: a comparative study of two selected, randomized groups. *J Vasc Surg* 12:754, 1990.
18. Joyce WP, Provan JL, Ameli FM, et al: The role of central hemodynamic monitoring in abdominal aortic surgery: a prospective randomized study. *Eur J Vasc Surg* 4:633, 1990.
19. Yu M, Levy M, Smith P: Effect of maximizing oxygen delivery on morbidity and mortality rates in critically ill patients. *Crit Care Med* 21:830, 1993.
20. Gattinoni L, Brazzi L, Pelosi P, et al: A trial of goal-oriented hemodynamic therapy in critically ill patients. *N Engl J Med* 333:1025, 1995.
21. Yu M, Takanishi D, Myers SA, et al: Frequency of mortality and myocardial infarction during maximizing oxygen delivery: a prospective, randomized trial. *Crit Care Med* 23:1025, 1995.
22. Durham RM, Neunaber K, Mazuski JE, et al: The use of oxygen consumption and delivery as endpoints for resuscitation in critically ill patients. *J Trauma* 41:32, 1996.
23. Afessa B, Spenser S, Khan W, et al: Association of pulmonary artery catheter use with in-hospital mortality. *Crit Care Med* 29:1145, 2001.
24. Rhodes A, Cusack RJ, Newman PJ, et al: A randomized, controlled trial of the pulmonary artery catheter in critically ill patients. *Intensive Care Med* 28:256, 2002.
25. Richard C: Early use of the pulmonary artery catheter and outcomes in patients with shock and acute respiratory distress syndrome: a randomized controlled trial. *JAMA* 290:2713, 2003.
26. Yu DT, Platt R, Lanken PN, et al: Relationship of pulmonary artery catheter use to mortality and resource utilization in patients with severe sepsis. *Crit Care Med* 31:2734, 2003.
27. Sandham JD, Hull RD, Brant RF, et al: A randomized, controlled trial of the use of pulmonary-artery catheters in high-risk surgical patients. *N Engl J Med* 348:5, 2003.
28. Sakr Y, Vincent JL, Reinhart K, et al: Use of the pulmonary artery catheter is not associated with worse outcome in the ICU. *Chest* 128:2722, 2005.
29. Harvey S, Harrison DA, Singer M, et al: Assessment of the clinical effectiveness of pulmonary-artery catheters in management of patients in intensive care (PAC-Man): a randomized controlled trial. *Lancet* 366:472, 2005.
30. Binanay C, Califf RM, Hasselblad V, et al: Evaluation study of congestive heart failure and pulmonary artery catheterization effectiveness: the ESCAPE trial. *JAMA* 294:1625, 2005.
31. The National Heart, Lung and Blood Institute ARDS Clinical Trials Network: Pulmonary artery versus central venous catheter to guide treatment of acute lung injury. *N Engl J Med* 354:2213, 2006.
32. Tuman KJ, McCarthy RJ, Spiess BD, et al: Effect of pulmonary artery catheterization on outcome in patients undergoing coronary artery surgery. *Anesthesiology* 70:199, 1989.
33. Guyatt G: A randomized control trial of right heart catheterization in critically ill patients. Ontario Intensive Care Study Group. *J Intensive Care Med* 6:91, 1991.
34. Hayes MA, Timmins AC, Yau H, et al: Elevation of systemic oxygen delivery in the treatment of critically ill patients. *N Eng J Med* 330:1717, 1994.
35. Connors AF, Speroff T, Dawson NV, et al: The effectiveness of right heart catheterization in the initial care of critically ill patients. *JAMA* 276:889, 1996.
36. Valentine RJ, Duke ML, Inman MH, et al: Effectiveness of pulmonary artery catheters in aortic surgery: a randomized trial. *J Vasc Surg* 27:203, 1998.
37. Stewart RD, Psyhojos T, Lahey SJ, et al: Central venous catheter use in low risk coronary artery bypass grafting. *Ann Thorac Surg* 66:1306, 1998.
38. Ramsey SD, Saint S, Sullivan SD, et al: Clinical and economic effects of pulmonary artery catheterization in nonemergent coronary artery bypass graft surgery. *J Cardiothorac Vasc Anesth* 14:113, 2000.
39. Polanczyk CA, Rohde LE, Goldman L, et al: Right heart catheterization and cardiac complications in patients undergoing noncardiac surgery: an observational study. *JAMA* 286:348, 2001.
40. Chittock DR, Dhingra VK, Ronco JJ, et al: Severity of illness and risk of death associated with pulmonary artery catheter use. *Crit Care Med* 32:911, 2004.
41. Peters SG, Afessa B, Decker PA, et al: Increased risk associated with pulmonary artery catheterization in the medical intensive care unit. *J Crit Care* 18:166, 2003.
42. Cohen MG, Kelley RV, Kong DF, et al: Pulmonary artery catheterization in acute coronary syndromes: insights from the GUSTO IIb and GUSTO III trials. *Am J Med* 118:482, 2005.
43. Kumar A, Anel R, Bunnell E: Pulmonary artery occlusion pressure and central venous pressure fail to predict ventricular filling volume, cardiac performance, or the response to volume infusion in normal subjects. *Crit Care Med* 32:691, 2004.
44. Hoar PF, Wilson RM, Mangano DT, et al: Heparin bonding reduces thrombogenicity of pulmonary-artery catheters. *N Engl J Med* 305:993, 1981.
45. Forrester JS, Ganz W, Diamond G, et al: Thermodilution cardiac output determination with a single flow-directed catheter. *Am Heart J* 83:306, 1972.
46. Chatterjee K, Swan JHC, Ganz W, et al: Use of a balloon-tipped flotation electrode catheter for cardiac monitoring. *Am J Cardiol* 36:56, 1975.
47. Simoons ML, Demey HE, Bossaert LL, et al: The Paceport catheter: a new pacemaker system introduced through a Swan–Ganz catheter. *Cathet Cardiovasc Diagn* 15:66, 1988.
48. Baele PL, McMechan JC, Marsh HM, et al: Continuous monitoring of mixed venous oxygen saturation in critically ill patients. *Anesth Analg* 61:513, 1982.
49. Vincent JL, Thirion M, Bumioulle S, et al: Thermodilution measurement of right ventricular ejection fraction with a modified pulmonary artery catheter. *Intensive Care Med* 12:33, 1986.
50. Nelson LD: The new pulmonary arterial catheters: right ventricular ejection fraction and continuous cardiac output. *Crit Care Clin* 12:795, 1996.
51. Haller M, Zollner C, Briegel J, et al: Evaluation of a new continuous thermodilution cardiac output monitor in critically ill patients: a prospective criterion standard study. *Crit Care Med* 23:860, 1995.
52. Tuggle DW, Pryor R, Ward K, et al: Real-time echocardiography: a new technique to facilitate Swan-Ganz catheter insertion. *J Pediatr Surg* 22:1169, 1987.
53. Alraies MC, Alraiyes AH, Salerno D: Pulmonary artery catheter placement guided by echocardiography. *QJM* 106:1149, 2013.
54. Rimensberger PC, Beghetti M: Pulmonary artery catheter placement under transoesophageal echocardiography guidance. *Paediatr Anaesth* 9:167, 1999.
55. Marini JJ: Hemodynamic monitoring with the pulmonary artery catheter. *Crit Care Clin* 2:551, 1986.
56. Huford WE, Zapol WM: The right ventricle and critical illness: a review of anatomy, physiology, and clinical evaluation of its function. *Intensive Care Med* 14:448, 1988.
57. Alpert JS: The lessons of history as reflected in the pulmonary capillary occlusion pressure. *J Am Coll Cardiol* 13:830, 1989.
58. Forrester JS, Diamond G, McHugh TJ, et al: Filling pressures in the right and left sides of the heart in acute myocardial infarction. *N Engl J Med* 285:190, 1971.
59. Timmis AD, Fowler MB, Burwood RJ, et al: Pulmonary edema without critical increase in left atrial pressure in acute myocardial infarction. *BMJ* 283:636, 1981.
60. Pichard AD, Kay R, Smith H, et al: Large V waves in the pulmonary occlusion pressure tracing in the absence of mitral regurgitation. *Am J Cardiol* 50:1044, 1982.
61. Teboul JL, Zapol WM, Brun-Buisson C, et al: A comparison of pulmonary artery occlusion pressure and left ventricular end diastolic pressure during mechanical ventilation with PEEP in patients with severe ARDS. *Anesthesiology* 70:261, 1989.
62. DeCampo T, Civetta JM: The effect of short-term discontinuation of high-level PEEP in patients with acute respiratory failure. *Crit Care Med* 7:47, 1979.
63. Ganz W, Swan HJC: Measurement of blood flow by thermodilution. *Am J Cardiol* 29:241, 1972.
64. Grossman W: Blood flow measurement: the cardiac output, in Grossman W (ed): *Cardiac Catheterization and Angiography*. Philadelphia, PA, Lea & Febiger, 1985, p 116.
65. Goldman RH, Klughaupt M, Metcalf T, et al: Measurement of central venous oxygen saturation in patients with myocardial infarction. *Circulation* 38:941, 1968.
66. Matthay MA, Chatterjee K: Bedside catheterization of the pulmonary artery: risks compared with benefits. *Ann Intern Med* 109:826, 1988.
67. McNabb TG, Green CH, Parket FL: A potentially serious complication with Swan-Ganz catheter placement by the percutaneous internal jugular route. *Br J Anaesth* 47:895, 1975.
68. Damen J, Bolton D: A prospective analysis of 1,400 pulmonary artery catheterizations in patients undergoing cardiac surgery. *Acta Anaesthesiol Scand* 14:1957, 1986.
69. Senagere A, Waller JD, Bonnell BW, et al: Pulmonary artery catheterization: a prospective study of internal jugular and subclavian approaches. *Crit Care Med* 15:35, 1987.
70. Lipp H, O'Donoghue K, Resnekov L: Intracardiac knotting of a flow-directed balloon catheter. *N Engl J Med* 284:220, 1971.
71. Meister SG, Furr CM, Engel TR, et al: Knotting of a flow-directed catheter about a cardiac structure. *Cathet Cardiovasc Diagn* 3:171, 1977.
72. Loggam C, Sanborn TA, Christian F: Ventricular entrapment of a Swan-Ganz catheter: a technique for nonsurgical removal. *J Am Coll Cardiol* 13:1422, 1989.
73. Foote GA, Schabel SI, Hodges M: Pulmonary complications of the flow-directed balloon-tipped catheter. *N Engl J Med* 290:927, 1974.
74. Boyd KD, Thomas SJ, Gold J, et al: A prospective study of complications of pulmonary artery catheterizations in 500 consecutive patients. *Chest* 84:245, 1983.

75. Sise MJ, Hollingsworth P, Bumm JE, et al: Complications of the flow directed pulmonary artery catheter: a prospective analysis of 219 patients. *Crit Care Med* 9:315, 1981.
76. Barash PG, Nardi D, Hammond G, et al: Catheter-induced pulmonary artery perforation: mechanisms, management and modifications. *J Thorac Cardiovasc Surg* 82:5, 1981.
77. Lapin ES, Murray JA: Hemoptysis with flow-directed cardiac catheterization. *JAMA* 220:1246, 1972.
78. Shah KB, Rao TL, Laughlin S, et al: A review of pulmonary artery catheterization in 6245 patients. *Anesthesiology* 61:271, 1984.
79. Fraser RS: Catheter-induced pulmonary artery perforation: pathologic and pathogenic features. *Hum Pathol* 18:1246, 1987.
80. Declen JD, Friloux LA, Renner JW: Pulmonary artery false-aneurysms secondary to Swan-Ganz pulmonary artery catheters. *AJR Am J Roentgenol* 149:901, 1987.
81. Scuderi PE, Prough DS, Price JD, et al: Cessation of pulmonary artery catheter-induced endobronchial hemorrhage associated with the use of PEEP. *Anesth Analg* 62:236, 1983.
82. Dye LE, Segall PH, Russell RO, et al: Deep venous thrombosis of the upper extremity associated with use of the Swan-Ganz catheter. *Chest* 73:673, 1978.
83. Laster JL, Nichols WK, Silver D: Thrombocytopenia associated with heparin-coated catheters in patients with heparin-associated antiplatelet antibodies. *Arch Intern Med* 149:2285, 1989.
84. Geha DG, Davis NJ, Lappas DG: Persistent atrial arrhythmias associated with placement of a Swan-Ganz catheter. *Anesthesiology* 39:651, 1973.
85. Sprung CL, Pozen PG, Rozanski JJ, et al: Advanced ventricular arrhythmias during bedside pulmonary artery catheterization. *Am J Med* 72:203, 1982.
86. Iberti TJ, Benjamin E, Grupzi L, et al: Ventricular arrhythmias during pulmonary artery catheterization in the intensive care unit. *Am J Med* 78:451, 1985.
87. Damen J: Ventricular arrhythmia during insertion and removal of pulmonary artery catheters. *Chest* 88:190, 1985.
88. Morris D, Mulvihill D, Lew WY: Risk of developing complete heart block during bedside pulmonary artery catheterization in patients with left bundle branch block. *Arch Intern Med* 147:2005, 1987.
89. Becker RC, Martin RG, Underwood DA: Right-sided endocardial lesions and flow-directed pulmonary artery catheters. *Cleve Clin J Med* 54:384, 1987.
90. Lange HW, Galliani CA, Edwards JE: Local complications associated with indwelling Swan-Ganz catheters. *Am J Cardiol* 52:1108, 1983.
91. Sage MD, Koelmeyer TD, Smeeton WMI: Evolution of Swan-Ganz catheter related pulmonary valve nonbacterial endocarditis. *Am J Forensic Med Pathol* 9:112, 1988.
92. Ford SE, Manley PN: Indwelling cardiac catheters: an autopsy study of associated endocardial lesions. *Arch Pathol Lab Med* 106:314, 1982.
93. Prochan H, Dittel M, Jobst C, et al: Bacterial contamination of pulmonary artery catheters. *Intensive Care Med* 4:79, 1978.
94. Pinella JC, Ross DF, Martin T, et al: Study of the incidence of intravascular catheter infection and associated septicemia in critically ill patients. *Crit Care Med* 11:21, 1983.
95. Greene JF, Fitzwater JE, Clemmer TP: Septic endocarditis and indwelling pulmonary artery catheters. *JAMA* 233:891, 1975.
96. Myers ML, Austin TW, Sibbald WJ: Pulmonary artery catheter infections: a prospective study. *Ann Surg* 201:237, 1985.
97. Weinstein RA, Stamm WE, Kramer L: Pressure monitoring devices: overlooked source of nosocomial infection. *JAMA* 236:936, 1976.
98. Heard SO, Davis RF, Sherertz RJ, et al: Influence of sterile protective sleeves on the sterility of pulmonary artery catheters. *Crit Care Med* 15:499, 1987.
99. Cobb DK, High KP, Sawyer RG, et al: A controlled trial of scheduled replacement of central venous and pulmonary artery catheters. *N Engl J Med* 327:1062, 1992.
100. Schluger J, Green J, Giustra FX, et al: Complication with use of flow-directed catheter. *Am J Cardiol* 32:125, 1973.
101. Isner JM, Horton J, Ronan JAS: Systolic click from a Swan-Ganz catheter: phonoechocardiographic depiction of the underlying mechanism. *Am J Cardiol* 42:1046, 1979.
102. Lawson D, Kushkins LG: A complication of multipurpose pacing pulmonary artery catheterization via the external jugular vein approach (letter). *Anesthesiology* 62:377, 1985.
103. Lazzam C, Sanborn TA, Christian F: Ventricular entrapment of a Swan-Ganz catheter: a technique for nonsurgical removal. *J Am Coll Cardiol* 13:1422, 1989.
104. Ginosar Y, Sprung CL: The Swan–Ganz catheter: twenty-five years of monitoring. *Crit Care Clin* 12:771, 1996.
105. Fleisher LA, Fleischmann KE, Aurbach AD, et al: 2014 ACC/AHA guideline on perioperative cardiovascular evaluation and management of patients undergoing noncardiac surgery: executive summary: a report of the American College of cardiology/American Heart Association Task Force on Practice Guidelines. *Circulation* 130(24):2215, 2014.
106. Rajram SS, Desani NK, Kaira A, et al: Pulmonary artery catheters for adult patients in critical care. *Cochrane Database Syst Rev* 2:CD003408, 2013.
107. Shah MR, Hasselblad V, Stevenson LW, et al: Impact of the pulmonary artery catheter in critically ill patients. *JAMA* 294:1664, 2005.

Chapter 20 ■ Gastrointestinal Endoscopy

SAMUEL Y. HAN • RANDALL PELLISH • DAVID R. CAVE • WAHID Y. WASSEF

Gastrointestinal (GI) endoscopy has evolved into an essential diagnostic and therapeutic tool for the treatment of patients in the intensive care unit (ICU). This chapter reviews general aspects of current indications and contraindications, provides an update of emerging technologies in the field, and concludes by discussing potential future directions.

PATIENT SELECTION

The indications for GI endoscopy in the ICU are summarized in Table 20.1. They are divided into those for (a) evaluation of the upper GI tract (esophagus, stomach, and duodenum); (b) evaluation of the pancreaticobiliary tract; (c) evaluation of the mid-GI tract (jejunum and ileum); and (d) evaluation of the lower GI tract (colon and rectum). In general, endoscopic interventions are contraindicated when the patient is hemodynamically unstable, when there is suspected perforation, or when adequate patient cooperation or consent cannot be obtained [1]. Other contraindications are listed in Table 20.2.

Evaluation of the Upper Gastrointestinal Tract

Common indications for evaluation of the upper GI tract in the ICU include, but are not limited to, upper GI bleeding (UGIB), caustic or foreign body ingestion (FBI), placement of gastroduodenal stents for gastric outlet obstruction (GOO), and placement of feeding tubes for nutrition.

Upper Gastrointestinal Bleeding

With an estimated 400,000 admissions annually, acute UGIB presents as a common medical emergency with mortality rates as high as 16% in the ICU [2]. This condition is suspected in patients who present with melena, hematemesis, or blood in the nasogastric (NG) aspirate, as studies have shown improved outcomes with urgent endoscopic management in critically ill patients with hemodynamic instability or continuing transfusion requirements [3,4]. Urgent evaluation allows differentiation between nonvariceal (peptic ulcer, esophagitis, Mallory–Weiss tear, and angiodysplasia) and variceal lesions (esophageal or gastric varices), thereby promoting targeted therapy [5]. Furthermore, urgent evaluation allows the identification and stratification of stigmata of bleeding, promoting appropriate triage and risk stratification. Finally, urgent evaluation allows the early identification of patients who may require surgical or invasive radiological intervention [3].

Foreign Body Ingestions

FBI can be divided into two groups: (i) food impaction and (ii) caustic ingestions. Food impactions constitute the majority of

TABLE 20.1

Indications for GI Endoscopy

Upper GI endoscopy
Upper GI bleeding (variceal or nonvariceal)
Caustic or foreign body ingestion
Placement of feeding or drainage tubes
Endoscopic retrograde cholangiopancreatography
Severe gallstone pancreatitis
Severe cholangitis
Bile leak
Lower GI endoscopy
Lower GI bleeding
Decompression of nontoxic megacolon or sigmoid volvulus
Unexplained diarrhea in the immunocompromised (graft vs. host disease and cytomegalovirus infection)

GI, gastrointestinal.

TABLE 20.2

Contraindications to Endoscopy

Absolute contraindications
Suspected or impending perforated viscus
Risks to the patient outweigh benefits of the procedure
Relative contraindications
Adequate patient cooperation or consent cannot be obtained
Hemodynamic instability or myocardial infarction
Inadequate airway protection or hypoxemia
Severe coagulopathy or thrombocytopenia
Inflammatory changes with increased risk of perforation (e.g., diverticulitis or severe inflammatory bowel disease)

FBI. Although most will pass spontaneously, endoscopic removal will be needed for 10% to 20% of cases, and 1% of patients will ultimately require surgery [6]. Evaluation is crucial to determine the underlying cause of the obstruction (strictures, rings, and carcinoma). Although caustic ingestions constitute only a small number of FBI, they are frequently life threatening, especially when they occur intentionally in adults, and warrant endoscopic evaluation to prognosticate and triage this group of patients [7].

Endoscopic Stenting for Gastric Outlet Obstruction

Although GOO is typically managed conservatively with receiving nothing by mouth, intravenous (IV) fluids, and decompression with a NG tube, GOO secondary to a malignancy can be treated with an endoscopically placed stent. Often used as a palliative measure, duodenal self-expandable metal stents (SEMS) have been found effective in providing relief from obstructive symptoms, allowing patients to resume eating, and improving quality of life [8].

Feeding Tubes

Enteral nutrition is associated with improved outcomes for critically ill patients and is preferred over parenteral nutrition in patients with a functional GI tract [9]. Although nasoenteric and oroenteric feeding tubes may be used for short-term enteral nutrition, these tubes are felt to carry a higher risk of aspiration, displacement, and sinus infections than endoscopically placed percutaneous tubes. Percutaneous endoscopic gastrostomy (PEG) [10] is appropriate for most patients in the ICU when there is a reversible disease process likely to require more than 4 weeks of enteral nutrition (e.g., neurologic injury, tracheostomy, and neoplasms of the upper aerodigestive tract) [21]. PEG with a jejunostomy tube and direct percutaneous endoscopic jejunostomy tubes are appropriate for selected patients in the ICU with high risk of aspiration. This includes patients with severe gastroesophageal reflux disease and those with gastroparesis. Enteral feeding beyond the ligament of Treitz with a nasojejunal tube or a jejunostomy tube has been demonstrated to be beneficial in patients with necrotizing pancreatitis, although a study demonstrated that there was no difference in mortality or infection rate between early, nasoenteric feeding and oral feeding 72 hours after admission in patients with acute pancreatitis [12]. Occasionally, endoscopic gastrostomies or jejunostomies may be indicated for decompression in patients with GI obstruction [13]. Although these procedures are technically simple and can be performed at the bedside under moderate sedation, the risks and benefits should always be weighed carefully in this critically ill group of patients.

Evaluation of the Pancreaticobiliary Tract

The indications for evaluation of the pancreaticobiliary tract by endoscopic retrograde cholangiopancreatography (ERCP) in critically ill patients are described in detail in Chapter 208 and only briefly discussed here. They include biliary tract obstruction by gallstones [14–16], pancreatic duct leaks, and bile duct leaks (generally a postoperative or traumatic complication) [17,18]. ERCP with sphincterotomy and/or stenting is the treatment of choice. When conventional ERCP is unsuccessful, the recent introduction of miniature endoscopes (cholangioscopes or pancreatic scopes) with direct endoscopic visualization into these ductal systems has proved to be beneficial through the use of advanced techniques such as electrohydraulic lithotripsy, laser lithotripsy, and topical glue [19]. Additionally, endoscopic necrosectomy for walled-off pancreatic necrosis via endoscopic ultrasound (EUS) has been validated as a viable alternative to surgical necrosectomy for this complication of pancreatitis [20].

Evaluation of the Mid-Gastrointestinal Tract (Jejunum and Ileum)

Persistent, GI bleeding without an identified site is the most common indication for mid-GI tract evaluation. Although this area of the GI tract had been difficult to evaluate in the past, this is no longer the case. The progression of video capsule endoscope (VCE), double-balloon enteroscopy (DBE), and spiral enteroscopy has made this area of the GI tract readily accessible. VCE is usually the first test performed to look for possible sites of bleeding in the jejunum and ileum (Fig. 20.1A and B). If bleeding or lesions are identified, DBE (Fig. 20.2) or the spiral endoscope (Fig. 20.3) can be used to implement therapy.

Evaluation of the Lower Gastrointestinal Tract

Lower GI tract evaluation is urgently needed in ICU patients in cases of severe lower GI bleeding (LGIB), acute colonic distention, and at times of refractory diarrhea for the evaluation of infection, such as *Clostridium difficile* [21].

Lower Gastrointestinal Bleeding

Severe LGIB is predominantly a disease of the elderly. It is defined as bleeding from a source distal to the ligament of Treitz for less than 3 days [22]. Common causes include, but are not

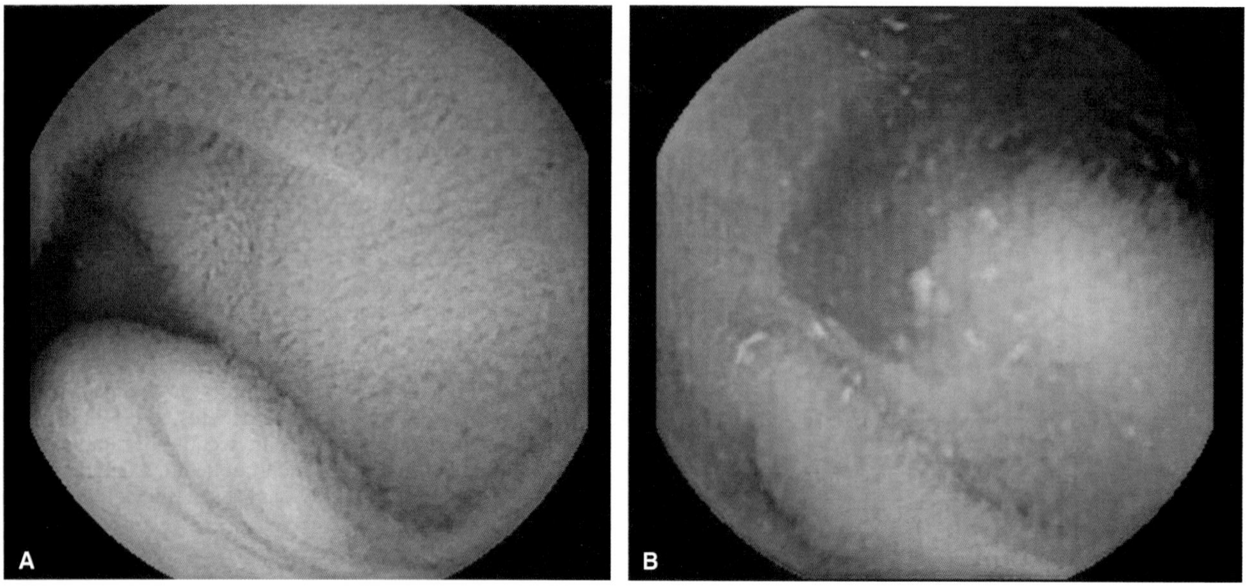

FIGURE 20.1 **A:** Normal jejunal image as seen by video capsule endoscope (VCE). **B:** Bleeding seen in jejunum on VCE. (Courtesy of David Cave, MD: Professor of Medicine, University of Massachusetts Medical School.)

limited to, diverticular bleeding, ischemic colitis, and vascular abnormalities (arteriovenous malformations, AVMs). The site of bleeding is not always identified easily; as many as 11% of patients initially suspected of having a LGIB are ultimately found to have an UGIB [23]. Therefore, UGIB sources should always be considered first in patients with LGIB, particularly in patients with unstable hemodynamics. Once an upper GI source has been excluded, colonoscopy should be performed to evaluate the lower GI tract and administer appropriate therapy. Although urgent colonoscopy within 24 to 48 hours has shown to decrease the length of hospital stay [24] and endoscopic intervention is often successful, 80% to 85% of LGIBs stop spontaneously [25]. If the bleeding is severe or a source cannot be identified at colonoscopy, a technetium (TC)-99m red blood cell scan with or without angiography should be considered [26].

Acute Colonic Distention

This condition can be caused by acute colonic obstruction or acute colonic pseudoobstruction. Acute colonic obstruction can be caused by neoplasms, diverticular disease, and volvulus [27]. Volvulus is a "closed-loop obstruction" and is considered an emergency because unlike the other causes of colonic obstruction, it can rapidly deteriorate from obstruction to ischemia, to perforation, and even result in death. However, if identified and treated early, it can be reversed. Acute colonic pseudoobstruction is a syndrome of massive dilation of the colon without mechanical obstruction that develops in hospitalized patients with serious underlying medical and surgical conditions due to impaired colonic motility. Increasing age, cecal diameter, delay in decompression, and status of the bowel significantly influence mortality, which is approximately 40% when ischemia or perforation is present. Evaluation of the markedly distended colon in the ICU setting involves excluding mechanical obstruction and other causes of toxic megacolon, such as *C. difficile* infection, and assessing for signs of ischemia and perforation. The risk of colonic perforation in acute colonic pseudoobstruction increases when cecal diameter exceeds 12 cm and when the distention has been present for greater than 6 days [28].

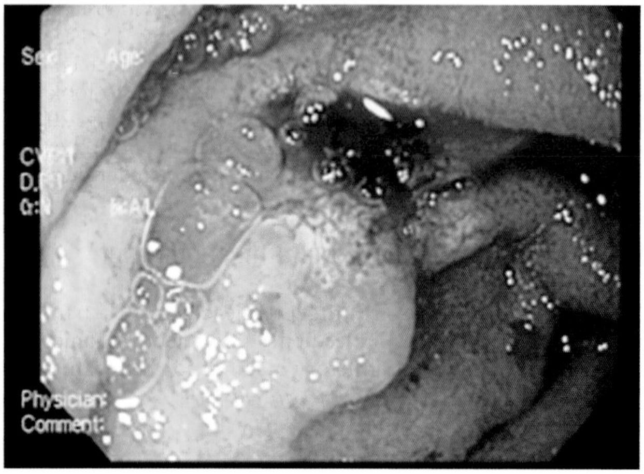

FIGURE 20.2 Bleeding in distal duodenum seen during double-balloon enteroscopy (DBE). (Courtesy of David Cave, MD: Professor of Medicine, University of Massachusetts Medical School.)

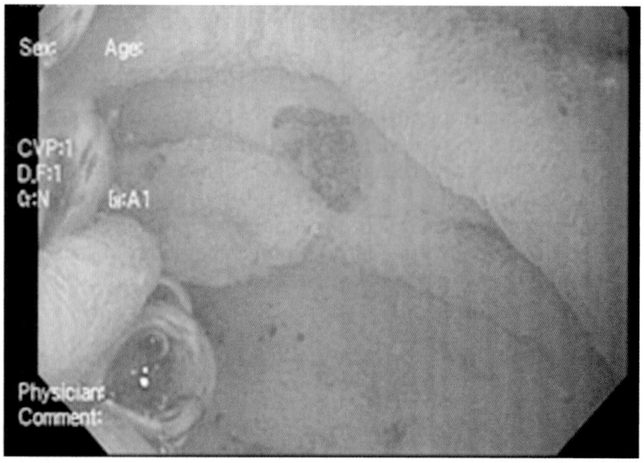

FIGURE 20.3 Bleeding seen in jejunum during spiral endoscopy. (Courtesy of David Cave, MD: Professor of Medicine, University of Massachusetts Medical School.)

PREPROCEDURAL CARE

When endoscopic interventions are contemplated, for any of the previously discussed indications, a number of issues need to be addressed: appropriate resuscitation, reversal of coagulopathies, adequate sedation, and antibiotics, especially in patients with ascites or endocarditis who present with GI bleeding [29,30]. In selected cases, proper sedation may simply involve light sedation [31]. In other cases, such as in uncooperative, confused, or hypoxemic patients, proper sedation may require deep sedation or endotracheal intubation with general anesthesia. Although this type of sedation does not significantly alter the risk of acquired pneumonia or cardiovascular events [32], it does generate controlled conditions during the procedure and may help prevent massive aspiration (especially in patients with variceal bleeding).

In all patients with UGIB, an empty stomach is crucial for thorough evaluation and identification of the bleeding lesion. Through proper identification and treatment, studies have shown a reduction in the risk of rebleeding and in the need for surgical intervention [33]. Gastric lavage with an NG tube or through use of the endoscope can clear the stomach of blood and clot. At times, the use of prokinetic agents such as erythromycin (250 mg in 50 mL of normal saline IV, 20 minutes prior to the procedure) may also be helpful. Studies have in fact shown that this approach may improve the endoscopic visualization, improve the outcome, and decrease the need for "second-look" endoscopy [34].

If a variceal hemorrhage is suspected, on the basis of a clinical history or physical examination that suggests portal hypertension, adjunctive therapy should be initiated immediately in the absence of contraindications. Both somatostatin analogues (octreotide) or vasopressin and its analogues have been used IV to reduce portal pressures and prevent recurrent bleeding [35]. Octreotide is usually given as a onetime bolus of 50 to 100 μg IV, followed by 25 to 50 μg IV per hour for 3 to 5 days. In addition, prophylactic antibiotics should be given to patients with active esophageal variceal bleeding for the prevention of bacterial infections [36]. In contrast to nonvariceal hemorrhage, volume resuscitation should be performed judiciously in variceal bleeding as volume repletion can theoretically increase portal pressures. Unlike the other types of endoscopies discussed previously, this is the only one requiring a preprocedure bowel preparation. In urgent situations, this can be done through a technique known as a rapid purge. This technique is usually achieved by drinking 4 L or more polyethylene glycol–based solutions over a 2- to 3-hour period. Approximately one-third of hospitalized patients require an NG tube for this type of preparation [37]. Metoclopramide (10 mg IV × 1), administered prior to starting the preparation, may help to control nausea and promote gastric emptying [34].

INTRAPROCEDURAL CARE

Upper Gastrointestinal Endoscopy

Upper Gastrointestinal Bleeding

If the bleeding source is found to be a peptic ulcer, the intervention will depend on the specific endoscopic findings [38]. If the ulcer has a clean base with no signs of active bleeding, endoscopic intervention is not indicated. If an actively bleeding or a nonbleeding visible vessel is identified in the crater of the ulcer, endoscopic hemostatic techniques are recommended. A number of endoscopic methods have been developed for hemostasis, including injection therapy, thermal cautery therapy, and mechanical hemostasis with clips (Table 20.3). The combination of injection therapy with thermal coaptive therapy is superior to either alone [36,39]. Although no single solution for endoscopic injection therapy appears superior to another, an epinephrine–saline solution is usually injected in four quadrants surrounding the lesion. Heater probe and multipolar electrocoagulation instruments are subsequently applied with firm pressure to achieve optimal coaptation. Mechanical hemostasis with hemoclips have the advantage of minimal tissue damage, leading to potentially faster ulcer healing and it has been found effective for ulcer bleeding alone or in conjunction with other therapies (Fig. 20.4) [40]. Argon plasma coagulation is a noncoaptive technique that provides cautery to tissues by means of ionized argon gas. This method appears to be most effective for shallow and broadly defined bleeding lesions such as vascular ectasias, but has been found to be as effective in ulcer management as other common modalities [38]. The yttrium-aluminum-garnet laser has fallen out of favor in the acute management of high-risk patients because of its poor portability and associated high cost. Hemospray is a hemostatic powder (Cook Medical, Winston-Salem, NC) recently introduced for the management of GI bleeding that is both a cohesive and adhesive substance that creates a mechanical barrier. Applied in short bursts with carbon dioxide propulsion directly to the bleeding site, Hemospray is given until hemostasis is seen. It has been studied as both primary therapy and salvage

TABLE 20.3

Endoscopic Methods for Hemostasis

- Thermal methods of hemostasis
  - Heater probe
  - Multipolar electrocoagulation (bicap)
  - Neodymium yttrium-aluminum-garnet laser
  - Argon plasma coagulation
- Injection therapy for hemostasis
  - Distilled water or saline
  - Epinephrine (adrenaline)
  - Sclerosants (cyanoacrylate, polidocanol, ethanol, ethanolamine oleate, sodium tetradecyl sulfate, sodium morrhuate)
  - Thrombin fibrin glue
- Mechanical methods
  - Clips
  - Band ligation
  - Detachable loops

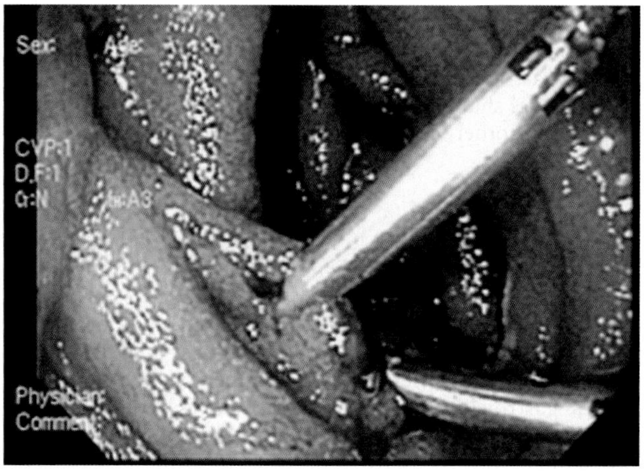

FIGURE 20.4 Hemostatic clip placed on a arteriovenous malformation in the proximal jejunum during a spiral enteroscopy. (Courtesy of David Cave, MD: Professor of Medicine, University of Massachusetts Medical School.)

therapy and has been shown to be effective in UGIB and LGIB [41,42]. Similarly, cryotherapy has gained wider recognition as it allows for tissue destruction via freezing by delivering a 25 to 30 mL per minute outflow of nitric monoxide at a temperature of −89.5°C and creating a 2 to 10 mm ice layer on the surface of the mucosa. It has found particular success in the management of angiodysplasia (AVM) [43].

In the last several years, several other modalities have emerged as effective treatment methods in UGIB. The over-the-scope-clip (OTSC) system, first developed in Germany, is a device that can be used to achieve hemostasis and close perforations, fistulas, or anastamotic leaks. Similar to the esophageal banding device, the OTSC cap can be loaded onto the tip of the scope, which can then be placed over the lesion, sucking the lesions in and allowing for the clip to be deployed. This device has now been studied in many different indications, and has enjoyed success in cases refractory to traditional hemostatic methods [44,45].

EUS has now been incorporated into the management of refractory GI bleeding. Under EUS visualization of a bleeding vessel with Doppler, the vessel is punctured with a 19-gauge needle and injected with a sclerosing agent such as cyanoacrylate (glue) or coils. Doppler monitoring then allows for viewing of the disappearance of the Doppler signal, signaling the cessation of bleeding. This method of EUS-guided angiotherapy has found success in a variety of bleeding etiologies, including gastric varices, ulcers, and malignancy [46].

In esophageal variceal bleeding, endoscopic variceal ligation (EVL) has become the procedure of choice [47,48]. With this technique, the varix is suctioned into a banding device attached to the tip of the endoscope and a rubber band is then deployed at its base to obliterate the varix. In contrast, endoscopic sclerotherapy (EST) causes obliteration by injection of a sclerosing agent (e.g., sodium morrhuate) in or around the bleeding varix. A meta-analysis by Laine and Cook [48] suggested that EVL was superior to EST in all major outcomes (recurrent bleeding, local complications such as ulcers or strictures, time to variceal obliteration, and survival). However, EST is effective in controlling active bleeding in more than 90% of cases and can be injected even with poor visualization during an active bleed.

Endoscopic methods (EST, EVL, and injection of fibrin glue) have also been used for the treatment of bleeding gastric varices. These methods, however, carry a considerable risk of rebleeding and mortality. Patients with bleeding gastric varices generally require urgent placement of a transjugular intrahepatic portosystemic shunt [49]. Balloon-occluded retrograde transvenous obliteration, a procedure first developed in Asia, has slowly been introduced in the United States, and consists of retrograde injection of sclerosing agents into gastric varices after balloon occlusion of the gastrorenal shunt, taking advantage of the tendency of gastric fundal varices to drain into the left renal vein via a gastrorenal shunt. Given its high success rate, this procedure represents another viable method to treat gastric varices [50].

Enteral Stents

The use of uncovered SEMS has been widely studied for use in GOO secondary to a malignancy. As long as a guidewire is able to be passed through the obstruction, the stent can be placed onto the guidewire and advanced under fluoroscopic guidance. A large systematic review demonstrated that there were no significant differences between the stent placement and surgical gastrojejunostomy in technical success, complications, or persistent of symptoms [51]. Stent placement, however, did have a higher rate of recurrent obstructive symptoms (18% vs. 1%) and decreased mean survival (105 vs. 164 days). Despite this, enteral stent placement does have a 90% initial clinical success rate, and should be pursued for palliative purposes in patients with a less than 6-month life expectancy.

Enteric Feeding Tubes

Please see Chapter 21 for more details on the placement of enteric feeding tubes.

Pancreaticobiliary Endoscopy

Refer to Chapter 208.

Small Bowel Endoscopy

The techniques are essentially the same as those for upper GI endoscopy (above).

Lower Gastrointestinal Endoscopy

Lower Gastrointestinal Bleeding

The endoscopic treatment options for LGIB are similar to those for UGIB (see earlier in the chapter) and should be based on the stigmata of bleeding that are identified. Hemostasis is usually approached through a combination approach of injection therapy with clipping or coagulation therapy.

Decompressive Endoscopy

A water-soluble contrast enema or computed tomography should be the initial procedure to perform in patients with acute colonic distention. This will establish the presence or absence of mechanical obstruction. Subsequently, the patient should undergo resuscitation with IV fluids, frequent repositioning, NG and rectal tube placements, correction of metabolic imbalances, and discontinuation of medications known to slow intestinal transit [52]. If conservative measures are unsuccessful, decompressive endoscopy with minimal inflation of air resolves acute obstruction of the colon in the majority of cases (81%) [53]. Despite a high recurrence rate (23% to 57%), colonoscopy is often considered the initial procedure of choice in the absence of intestinal ischemia [54]. This may be reduced with the placement of a decompression tube beyond the splenic flexure [55]. In patients with mechanical obstruction, SEMS can be placed with good outcome [56]. In patients with nonmechanical obstruction, medical therapy with the parasympathomimetic agent neostigmine should be considered. On the basis of a double-blind, placebo-controlled, randomized trial, the parasympathomimetic agent neostigmine has been shown to reduce colonic distention significantly, reduce recurrence, with minimal risk [57]. This agent should only be given in the absence of contraindications and under close cardiorespiratory monitoring with atropine at the bedside. Percutaneous, endoscopic, or surgical cecostomy presents another alternative if the aforementioned interventions are unsuccessful.

Fecal Microbiota Transplantation

The increase in prevalence of *Clostridium difficile* infection (CDI) and particularly recurrent CDI has brought fecal microbiota transplantation (FMT) to the forefront. Numerous studies have demonstrated its high success rate, but it remains poorly studied in cases of severe CDI, which will often require ICU care [58]. Nevertheless, the ability to perform FMT via upper endoscopy, colonoscopy, and rectal enema presents an alternative treatment option in patients with CDI who have failed conventional antibiotic therapy.

Perforations, Fistulas, and Anastamotic Leaks

Recently, the OverStitch (Apollo Endosurgery Inc., Austin, TX) has emerged as an endoscopic suturing device that can also be used to closing perforations and fistulas (Fig. 20.5). This system is attached to a standard endoscope and allows for a detachable needle to be used to suture lesions with a suture-cinching tool used to secure the deployed suture [59,60]. This may represent a method to close small perforations and fistulas without the need for surgical intervention.

POST-PROCEDURAL CARE

Although major complications of endoscopic procedures are infrequent, critically ill patients may be particularly sensitive to adverse outcomes due to multiple comorbidities. It is crucial to monitor patients for complications post procedures. These can be divided into two groups: (i) general complications and (ii) specific complications (Table 20.4).

In patients with UGIB, post procedure pharmacotherapy is also indicated. In patients with nonvariceal UGIB, for example, antisecretory therapy with a proton pump inhibitor (PPI) following endoscopic hemostasis is encouraged [40]. IV administration of a PPI is a faster way to achieve gastric acid suppression than is oral administration of the same agent. Peak suppression after IV administration occurs within hours, compared with several days later after oral administration. This is crucial because it can reduce the risk of rebleeding and the need for surgery [40]. The PPIs currently approved for IV use in the United States include pantoprazole, lansoprazole, and esomeprazole. In contrast, patients with variceal UGIB should receive daily nonselective β-blockers for secondary prevention in addition to repeat EVL every 3 to 4 weeks until obliteration of the varices is achieved [61].

FUTURE DIRECTIONS

The constantly evolving landscape of endoscopic technologies and methods will continue to expand the reach of endoscopic intervention. One area in particular is the developing role of endoscopic suturing in the GI tract, especially in the care and management of mucosal perforation, in the treatment of GI bleeding, and the closure of fistulas. Although case reports are in the literature, larger studies are needed before this technique can be recommended on a regular basis. Other areas of development are the evaluation and management of small bowel bleeding. With the advent of viewers linked in to video capsule and the development of the power spiral endoscopy, this may allow earlier recognition and treatment of small bowel disease than thought previously; however, studies are needed to determine the efficacy and benefits of these techniques.

TABLE 20.4

Complications of Endoscopy

- General complications
  - Complications of conscious sedation (cardiopulmonary, allergic, paradoxical reactions)
  - Bleeding (e.g., treatment of lesions, sphincterotomy)
  - Perforation (caused by endoscope, accessories, or air insufflation)
  - Aspiration
  - Myocardial ischemia
- Specific complications (examples)
  - Endoscopic retrograde cholangiopancreatography: pancreatitis, cholangitis, perforation
  - Sclerotherapy: ulceration, mediastinitis
  - Stenting procedures: stent migration

References

1. American Society for Gastrointestinal Endoscopy: Appropriate use of gastrointestinal endoscopy. *Gastrointest Endosc* 52:831–837, 2000.
2. Koch A, Buendgens L, Dückers H, et al: Bleeding origin, patient-related risk factors, and prognostic indicators in patients with acute gastrointestinal hemorrhages requiring intensive care treatment. A retrospective analysis from 1999 to 2010. *Med Klin Intensivmed Notfmed* 108(3):214–222, 2013.
3. Khamaysi I, Gralnek IM: Nonvariceal upper gastrointestinal bleeding: timing of endoscopy and ways to improve endoscopic visualization. *Gastrointest Endosc Clin N Am* 25(3):443–448, 2015.
4. Chak A, Cooper GS, Lloyd LE, et al: Effectiveness of endoscopy in patients admitted to the intensive care unit with upper GI hemorrhage. *Gastrointest Endosc* 53:6–13, 2001.
5. Beejay U, Wolfe MM: Acute gastrointestinal bleeding in the intensive care unit. The gastroenterologist's perspective. *Gastroenterol Clin North Am* 29:309–336, 2000.
6. Eisen GM, Baron TH, Dominitz JA, et al: Guideline for the management of ingested foreign bodies. *Gastrointest Endosc* 55:802–806, 2002.
7. Poley JW, Steyerberg EW, Kuipers EJ, et al: Ingestion of acid and alkaline agents: outcome and prognostic value of early upper endoscopy. *Gastrointest Endosc* 60:372–377, 2004.
8. van Hooft JE, Dijkgraaf MG, Timmer R, et al: Independent predictors of survival in patients with incurable malignant gastric outlet obstruction: a multicenter prospective observational study. *Scand J Gastroenterol* 45:1217–1222, 2010.
9. Eisen GM, Baron TH, Dominitz JA, et al: Role of endoscopy in enteral feeding. *Gastrointest Endosc* 55:699–701, 2002.
10. Fan AC, Baron TH, Rumalla A: Comparison of direct percutaneous endoscopic jejunostomy and PEG with jejunal extension. *Gastrointest Endosc* 56:890–894, 2002.
11. DeLegge MH, McClave SA, DiSario JA, et al: Ethical and medicolegal aspects of PEG-tube placement and provision of artificial nutritional therapy. *Gastrointest Endosc* 62:952–959, 2005.
12. Bakker OJ, van Brunschot S, van Santvoort HC: Early versus on-demand nasoenteric tube feeding in acute pancreatitis. *N Engl J Med* 371(21):1983–1993, 2014.
13. Herman LL, Hoskins WJ, Shike M: Percutaneous endoscopic gastrostomy for decompression of the stomach and small bowel. *Gastrointest Endosc* 38:314–318, 1992.
14. Sharma VK, Howden CW: Metaanalysis of randomized controlled trials of endoscopic retrograde cholangiography and endoscopic sphincterotomy for the treatment of acute biliary pancreatitis. *Am J Gastroenterol* 94:3211–3214, 1999.
15. Adler DG, Baron TH, Davila RE, et al: ASGE guideline: the role of ERCP in diseases of the biliary tract and the pancreas. *Gastrointest Endosc* 62:1–8, 2005.
16. Lai EC, Mok FP, Tan ES, et al: Endoscopic biliary drainage for severe acute cholangitis. *N Engl J Med* 326:1582–1586, 1992.
17. Kaffes AJ, Hourigan L, De Luca N, et al: Impact of endoscopic intervention in 100 patients with suspected postcholecystectomy bile leak. *Gastrointest Endosc* 61:269–275, 2005.
18. Sandha GS, Bourke MJ, Haber GB, et al: Endoscopic therapy of bile leak based on a new classification: results in 207 patients. *Gastrointest Endosc* 60:567–574, 2004.
19. Tringali A, Lemmers A, Meves V: Intraductal biliopancreatic imaging: European Society of Gastrointestinal Endoscopy (ESGE) technology review. *Endoscopy* 47(8):739–753, 2015.
20. Gardner TB, Coelho-Prabhu N, Gordon SR, et al: Direct endoscopic necrosectomy for the treatment of walled-off pancreatic necrosis: results from a multicenter U.S. series. *Gastrointest Endosc* 73(4):718–726, 2011.
21. Church J, Kao J: Bedside colonoscopy in intensive care units: indications, techniques, and outcomes. *Surg Endosc* 28(9):2679–2682, 2014.
22. Davila RE, Rajan E, Adler DG, et al: ASGE guideline: the role of endoscopy in the patient with lower GI-bleeding. *Gastrointest Endosc* 62:656–660, 2005.
23. Jensen DM, Machicado GA: Diagnosis and treatment of severe hematochezia. The role of urgent colonoscopy after purge. *Gastroenterology* 95:1569–1574, 1998.
24. Strate LL, Syngal S: Timing of colonoscopy: impact on length of hospital stay in patients with acute lower GI bleeding. *Am J Gastroenterol* 98:317–322, 2003.
25. Farrell JJ, Friedman LS: Review article: the management of lower gastrointestinal bleeding. *Aliment Pharmacol Ther* 21:1281–1298, 2005.
26. Strate LL, Syngal S: Predictors of utilization of early colonoscopy vs. radiography for severe lower intestinal bleeding. *Gastrointest Endosc* 61:46–52, 2005.
27. Frizelle FA, Wolff BG: Colonic volvulus. *Adv Surg* 29:131–139, 1996.
28. Saunders MD, Kimmey MB: Colonic pseudo-obstruction: the dilated colon in the ICU. *Semin Gastrointest Dis* 14(1):20–27, 2003.
29. Rajala MW, Ginsberg GG: Tips and tricks on how to optimally manage patients with upper gastrointestinal bleeding. *Gastrointest Endosc Clin N Am* 25(3):607–617, 2015.
30. Tang X, Gong W, Jiang B: Antibiotic prophylaxis for GI endoscopy. *Gastrointest Endosc* 81(6):1503–1504, 2015.
31. Lichenstein DR, Jagannath S, Baron TH, et al: ASGE Standards of Practice Committee: Sedation and anesthesia in GI endoscopy. *Gastrointest Endosc* 68(5):815–826, 2008.
32. Wassef W, Rullan R: Interventional endoscopy. *Curr Opin Gastroenterol* 21:644–652, 2005.
33. Meltzer AC, Klein JC: Upper gastrointestinal bleeding: patient presentation, risk stratification, and early management. *Gastroenterol Clin North Am* 43(4):665–675, 2014.

34. Frossard JL, Spahr L, Queneau PE, et al: Erythromycin intravenous bolus infusion in acute upper gastrointestinal bleeding: a randomized, controlled, double-blind trial. *Gastroenterology* 123:17–23, 2002.
35. Wells M, Chande N, Adams P, et al: Meta-analysis: vasoactive medications for the management of acute variceal bleeds. *Aliment Pharmacol Ther* 35(11):1267–1278, 2012.
36. Barkun AN, Bardou M, Kuipers EJ, et al: International consensus recommendations on the management of patients with nonvariceal upper gastrointestinal bleeding. *Ann Intern Med* 152(2):101–113, 2010.
37. Elta GH: Technological review. Urgent colonoscopy for acute lower-GI bleeding. *Gastrointest Endosc* 59:402–408, 2004.
38. Lu Y, Chen YI, Barkun A: Endoscopic management of acute peptic ulcer bleeding. *Gastroenterol Clin North Am* 43(4):677–705, 2014.
39. Calvet X, Vergara M, Brullet E, et al: Addition of a second endoscopic treatment following epinephrine injection improves outcome in high-risk bleeding ulcers. *Gastroenterology* 126(2):441–450, 2004.
40. Laine L, McQuaid KR: Endoscopic therapy for bleeding ulcers: an evidence-based approach based on meta-analyses of randomized controlled trials. *Clin Gastroenterol Hepatol* 7(1):33–47, 2009.
41. Sulz MC, Frei R, Meyenberger C, et al: Routine use of Hemospray for gastrointestinal bleeding: prospective two-center experience in Switzerland. *Endoscopy* 46(7):619–624, 2014.
42. Changela K, Papafragkakis H, Ofori E: Hemostatic powder spray: a new method for managing gastrointestinal bleeding. *Therap Adv Gastroenterol* 8(3):125–135, 2015.
43. Fujii-Lau LL, Wong Kee Song LM, Levy MJ: New technologies and approaches to endoscopic control of gastrointestinal bleeding. *Gastrointest Endosc Clin N Am* 25(3):553–567, 2015.
44. Sulz MC, Bertolini R, Frei R, et al: Multipurpose use of the over-the-scope-clip system ("Bear claw") in the gastrointestinal tract: Swiss experience in a tertiary center. *World J Gastroenterol* 20(43):16287–16292, 2014.
45. Mönkemüller K, Peter S, Toshniwal J, et al: Multipurpose use of the 'bear claw' (over-the-scope-clip system) to treat endoluminal gastrointestinal disorders. *Dig Endosc* 26(3):350–357, 2014.
46. Gavini H, Lee JH: Endoscopic ultrasound-guided endotherapy. *J Clin Gastroenterol* 49(3):185–193, 2015.
47. Baron TH, Wong Kee Song LM: Endoscopic variceal band ligation. *Am J Gastroenterol* 104:1083–1085, 2009.
48. Laine L, Cook D: Endoscopic ligation compared with sclerotherapy for treatment of esophageal variceal bleeding: a metaanalysis. *Ann Intern Med* 123:280–287, 1995.
49. Sharara AI, Rockey DC: Gastroesophageal variceal bleed. *N Engl J Med* 345:669–681, 2001.
50. Park J, Saab S, Kee S, et al: Balloon-occluded retrograde transvenous obliteration (BRTO) for treatment of gastric varices: review and meta-analysis. *Dig Dis Sci* 60(6):1543–1553, 2015.
51. Jeurnink SM, van Eijck CH, Steyerberg EW, et al: Stent versus gastrojejunostomy for the palliation of gastric outlet obstruction: a systematic review. *BMC Gastroenterol* 7:18, 2007.
52. Eisen GM, Baron TH, Dominitz JA, et al: Acute colonic pseudo-obstruction. *Gastrointest Endosc* 56:789–792, 2002.
53. Grossmann EM, Longo WE, Stratton MD, et al: Sigmoid volvulus in Department of Veterans Affairs Medical Centers. *Dis Colon Rectum* 43:414–418, 2000.
54. Saunders MD, Kimmey MB: Systematic review: acute colonic pseudo-obstruction. *Aliment Pharmacol Ther* 22:917–925, 2005.
55. Geller A, Petersen BT, Gostout CJ: Endoscopic decompression for acute colonic pseudo-obstruction. *Gastrointest Endosc* 44:144–150, 1996.
56. Dronamraju SS, Ramamurthy S, Kelly SB, et al: Role of self-expanding metallic stents in the management of malignant obstruction of the proximal colon. *Dis Colon Rectum* 52(9):1657–1661, 2009.
57. Ponec RJ, Saunders MD, Kimmey MB: Neostigmine for the treatment of acute colonic pseudo-obstruction. *N Engl J Med* 341:137–141, 1999.
58. Han S, Shannahan S, Pellish R: Fecal microbiota transplant: treatment options for *Clostridium difficile* infection in the intensive care unit. *J Intensive Care Med* 31(9):577–586, 2016.
59. Sharaiha RZ, Kumta NA, DeFilippis EM, et al: A large multicenter experience with endoscopic suturing for management of gastrointestinal defects and stent anchorage in 122 patients: a retrospective review. *J Clin Gastroenterol* 50(5):388–392, 2016.
60. Rieder E, Dunst CM, Martinec DV, et al: Endoscopic suture fixation of gastrointestinal stents: proof of biomechanical principles and early clinical experience. *Endoscopy* 44(12):1121–1126, 2012.
61. Garcia-Tsao G, Sanyal AJ, Grace ND, et al: Practice Guidelines Committee of the American Association for the Study of Liver Diseases; Practice Parameters Committee of the American College of Gastroenterology: Prevention and management of gastroesophageal varices and variceal hemorrhage in cirrhosis. *Hepatology* 46(3):922–938, 2007.

Chapter 21 ■ Endoscopic Placement of Feeding Tubes

LENA M. NAPOLITANO

INDICATIONS FOR ENTERAL FEEDING

Nutritional support is an essential component of intensive care medicine (see Chapters 212–214).

National and international guidelines [1–4] and comprehensive reviews [5] all strongly recommend that enteral nutrition be used in preference to parenteral nutrition when possible.

Provision of nutrition through the enteral route aids in prevention of gastrointestinal mucosal atrophy, thereby maintaining the integrity of the gastrointestinal mucosal barrier. Other advantages of enteral nutrition are preservation of immunologic gut functions and normal gut flora, improved use of nutrients, and reduced costs. Some studies suggest that clinical outcomes are improved and infectious complications are less frequent in patients who receive enteral nutrition compared with parenteral nutrition.

Although there are absolute or relative contraindications to enteral feeding in selected cases, most critically ill patients can receive some or all of their nutritional requirements via the gastrointestinal tract. Enteral feeding is even recommended in severe acute pancreatitis, and nasogastric or nasojejunal feedings are both well tolerated [6]. Even when some component of nutritional support must be provided by parenteral nutrition, feeding via the gut is desirable.

Several developments—including new techniques for placement of feeding tubes, availability of smaller caliber, minimally reactive tubes, and an increasing range of enteral formulas—have expanded the ability to provide enteral nutritional support to critically ill patients. Relative or absolute contraindications to enteral feeding include fistulas, intestinal obstruction, upper gastrointestinal hemorrhage, and severe inflammatory bowel disease or intestinal ischemia. Enteral feeding is not recommended in patients with severe malabsorption or early in the course of severe short-gut syndrome.

ACCESS TO THE GASTROINTESTINAL TRACT

After deciding to provide enteral nutrition, the clinician must decide whether to deliver the formula into the stomach, duodenum, or jejunum, and determine the optimal method for accessing the site, which is based on the function of the patient's gastrointestinal tract, duration of enteral nutritional support required, and risk of pulmonary aspiration. Gastric feeding provides the most normal route for enteral nutrition, but may not be tolerated in the critically ill patient because of gastric dysmotility with delayed emptying [7]. Enteral nutrition infusion into the duodenum or jejunum may decrease the incidence of aspiration because of the protection afforded by a competent pyloric sphincter; however, the risk of aspiration is not completely eliminated by feeding distal to the pylorus [8–10]. An advantage of this site of administration is that enteral feeding can be initiated early in the postoperative period, because postoperative ileus primarily affects the colon and stomach and only rarely involves the small intestine.

TECHNIQUES

Enteral feeding tubes can be placed via the transnasal, transoral, or percutaneous transgastric or transjejunal routes. If these procedures are contraindicated or unsuccessful, the tube may be placed by endoscopy, using endoscopic and laparoscopic technique, or surgically via a laparotomy [11].

Nasoenteric Route

Nasoenteric tubes are the most commonly used means of providing enteral nutritional support in critically ill patients. This route is preferred for short- to intermediate-term enteral support when eventual resumption of oral feeding is anticipated. It is possible to infuse enteral formulas into the stomach using a conventional 16- or 18-French (Fr) polyvinyl chloride nasogastric tube, but patients are usually much more comfortable if a small-diameter silicone or polyurethane feeding tube is used. Nasoenteric tubes vary in luminal diameter (6 to 14 Fr) and length, depending on the desired location of the distal orifice: stomach, 30 to 36 inches; duodenum, 43 inches; jejunum, at least 48 inches. Some tubes have tungsten-weighted tips designed to facilitate passage into the duodenum via normal peristalsis, whereas others have a stylet. Most are radiopaque. Some tubes permit gastric decompression while delivering formula into the jejunum.

Nasoenteric feeding tubes should be placed with the patient in a semi-Fowler's or sitting position. The tip of the tube should be lubricated, placed in the patient's nose, and advanced to the posterior pharynx. If the patient is alert and can follow instructions, the patient should be permitted to sip water as the tube is slowly advanced into the stomach. To avoid unintentional airway placement and serious complications, position of the tube should be ascertained after it has been inserted to 30 cm. Acceptable means of documenting intraesophageal location of the tube include a chest radiograph or lack of CO_2 detection through the lumen of the tube by capnography or colorimetry. If the tube is in the airway, CO_2 will be detected and the tube must be removed. Alternatively, commercial systems are now available to track tube progression from the esophagus through the stomach to the duodenum by electromagnetic means. Proper final placement of the tube in the stomach must be confirmed by chest or upper abdominal radiograph before tube feeding is begun. The following methods to assess final tube placement are unreliable and do not assess tube misdirection into the lower respiratory tract: auscultation over the left upper quadrant with air insufflation through the tube, assessment of pH with gastric content aspiration, and easy passage of the tube to its full length with the absence of gagging and coughing [12]. The tube should be securely taped to the nose, forehead, or cheek without tension. Nasal bridles are more effective at securing nasoenteric tubes than use of tape [13].

Delayed gastric emptying has been confirmed in critically ill patients and may contribute to gastric feeding intolerance. Spontaneous transpyloric passage of enteral feeding tubes in critically ill patients is commonly unsuccessful, secondary to the preponderance of gastric atony. The addition of a tungsten weight to the end of enteral feeding tubes and the development of wire or metal stylets in enteral feeding tubes are aimed at improving the success rate for spontaneous transpyloric passage. Once the tube is documented to be in the stomach, various bedside techniques, including air insufflation, pH-assisted, magnet-guided and spontaneous passage with or without motility agents, may help facilitate transpyloric feeding tube passage.

Intravenous (IV) metoclopramide and erythromycin have been recommended as prokinetic agents. But a Cochrane Database Systematic Review concluded that doses of 10 or 20 mg of IV metoclopramide were equally ineffective in facilitating transpyloric feeding tube placement [14]. No matter which techniques are used to facilitate transpyloric passage of enteral feeding tubes, these tubes must be inserted by skilled practitioners using defined techniques.

If the tube does not pass into the duodenum on the first attempt, placement can be attempted under endoscopic assistance or fluoroscopic or electromagnetic guidance. The latter method requires specialized equipment. Endoscopic placement of nasoenteral feeding tubes is easily accomplished in the critically ill patient and can be performed at the bedside using portable equipment [15]. Transnasal or transoral endoscopy can be used for placement of nasoenteral feeding tubes in critically ill patients. The patient is sedated appropriately (see Chapter 20), and topical anesthetic is applied to the posterior pharynx with lidocaine or benzocaine spray. A 43- to 48-inches-long nasoenteric feeding tube with an inner wire stylet is passed transnasally into the stomach. The endoscope is inserted and advanced through the esophagus into the gastric lumen. An endoscopy forceps is passed through the biopsy channel of the endoscope and used to grasp the tip of the enteral feeding tube. The endoscope, along with the enteral feeding tube, is advanced distally into the duodenum as far as possible (Fig. 21.1).

The endoscopy forceps and feeding tube remain in position in the distal duodenum as the endoscope is withdrawn back into the gastric lumen. The endoscopy forceps are opened, the feeding tube released, and the endoscopy forceps withdrawn carefully back into the stomach. On first pass, the feeding tube is usually lodged in the second portion of the duodenum. The portion of the feeding tube that is redundant in the stomach is advanced slowly into the duodenum using the endoscopy forceps to achieve a final position distal to the ligament of Treitz (Fig. 21.2). An abdominal radiograph is obtained at the completion of the procedure to document the final position of the nasoenteral feeding tube. Endoscopic placement of postpyloric enteral feeding tubes is highly successful, eliminates the risk of transporting the patient to the radiology department for fluoroscopic placement, and allows prompt achievement of nutritional goals, because enteral feeding can be initiated immediately after the procedure.

The recent development of ultrathin endoscopes (outer diameter 5.1 to 5.9 mm vs. 9.8 mm in standard gastroscope) has enabled nasoenteric feeding tube placement via transnasal endoscopy using an over-the-wire technique. A 90% success rate was documented with endoscopic procedure duration of approximately 13 minutes, shorter than fluoroscopic procedure

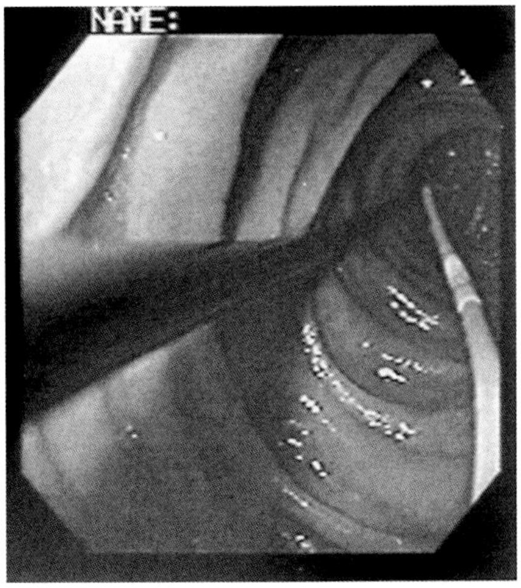

FIGURE 21.1 Endoscopic placement of nasoenteral feeding tube. Endoscopy forceps and gastroscope advance the feeding tube in the duodenum.

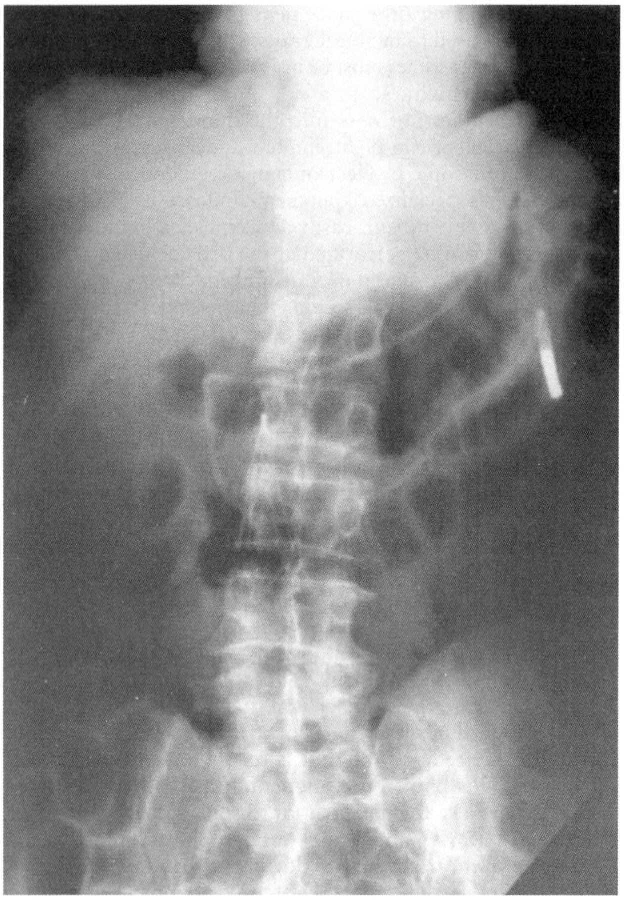

FIGURE 21.2 Abdominal radiograph documenting the optimal position of an endoscopically placed nasoenteral feeding tube, past the ligament of Treitz.

duration, and without the need for additional sedation [16]. Transnasal ultrathin endoscopy without the need for sedation can also be used for feeding tube or percutaneous endoscopic gastrostomy (PEG) placement in patients who are unable to undergo transoral endoscopy, that is, those who have partial or complete occlusion of the mouth [17].

Electromagnetic guidance employs a feeding tube with a guidewire that emits electromagnetic waves. A box with three receivers that is placed on the patient's xiphoid process triangulates the position of the tube. The clinician is able to "view" the tip on a monitor as it passes down the esophagus through the stomach and into the duodenum. An X-ray is still required to confirm and document tube placement.

Percutaneous Route

PEG tube placement, introduced by Ponsky et al. [18] in 1990, has become the procedure of choice for patients requiring prolonged enteral nutritional support. PEG tubes range in size from 20 to 28 Fr. PEG rapidly replaced open gastrostomy as the method of choice for enteral nutrition. Unlike surgical gastrostomy, PEG does not require general anesthesia and laparotomy and eliminates the discomfort associated with chronic nasoenteric tubes. This procedure can be considered for patients who have normal gastric emptying and low risk for pulmonary aspiration, and can be performed in the operating room, in an endoscopy unit, or at the bedside in the intensive care unit with portable endoscopy equipment.

PEG should not be performed in patients with near or total obstruction of the pharynx or esophagus, in the presence of coagulopathy, or when transillumination is inadequate. Relative contraindications are ascites, gastric cancer, and gastric ulcer. Previous abdominal surgery is not a contraindication. The original method for PEG was the pull technique; more recent modifications are the push and introducer techniques.

Pull Technique

The pull technique is performed with the patient in the supine position. After a time-out, the abdomen is prepared and draped. The posterior pharynx is anesthetized with a topical spray or solution (e.g., benzocaine spray or viscous lidocaine), and IV sedation (e.g., 1 to 2 mg of midazolam; see Chapter 20) is administered. A prophylactic antibiotic, usually a first-generation cephalosporin, is administered before the procedure. The fiberoptic gastroscope is inserted into the stomach, which is then insufflated with air. The lights are dimmed, and the assistant applies digital pressure to the anterior abdominal wall in the left subcostal area approximately 2 cm below the costal margin, looking for the brightest transillumination (light reflex). The endoscopist should be able to clearly identify the indentation in the stomach created by the assistant's digital pressure on the anterior abdominal wall (digital reflex); otherwise, another site should be chosen.

When the correct spot has been identified, the assistant anesthetizes the anterior abdominal wall. The endoscopist then introduces a polypectomy snare through the endoscope. A small incision is made in the skin, and the assistant introduces a large-bore catheter–needle stylet assembly into the stomach and through the snare. The snare is then tightened securely around the catheter. The inner stylet is removed, and a looped insertion wire is introduced through the catheter and into the stomach. The cannula is slowly withdrawn so that the snare grasps the wire. The gastroscope is then pulled out of the patient's mouth with the wire firmly grasped by the snare. The end of the transgastric wire exiting the patient's mouth is then tied to a prepared gastrostomy tube. The assistant pulls on the end of the wire exiting from the abdominal wall, whereas the endoscopist guides the lubricated gastrostomy tube into the posterior pharynx and the esophagus. With continued traction, the gastrostomy tube is pulled into the stomach so that it exits on the anterior abdominal wall. The gastroscope is reinserted into the stomach to confirm adequate placement of the gastrostomy tube against the gastric mucosa and to document that no bleeding has occurred. The intraluminal portion of the tube should contact the mucosa, but excessive tension on the tube should be avoided because this can lead to ischemic necrosis of the gastric wall. The tube is secured to the abdominal wall using sutures. Feedings may be initiated immediately after the procedure or 24 hours later.

Push Technique

The push technique is similar to the pull technique. The gastroscope is inserted and a point on the anterior abdominal wall localized, as for the pull technique. Rather than introducing a looped insertion wire, however, a straight guidewire is snared and brought out through the patient's mouth by withdrawing the endoscope and snare together. A commercially developed gastrostomy tube (Sachs–Vine) with a tapered end is then passed in an aboral direction over the wire, which is held taut. The tube is grasped and pulled out the rest of the way. The gastroscope is reinserted to check the position and tension on the tube.

Introducer Technique

The introducer technique uses a peel-away introducer technique originally developed for the placement of cardiac pacemakers and central venous catheters. The gastroscope is inserted into the stomach, and an appropriate position for placement of the tube is identified. After infiltration of the skin with local anesthetic, a 16- or 18-gauge needle is introduced into the stomach. A J-tipped guidewire is inserted through the needle into the stomach, and the needle is withdrawn. Using a twisting motion, a 16-Fr introducer with a peel-away sheath is passed over the guidewire into the gastric lumen [19,20]. The guidewire and introducer are removed, leaving in place the sheath that allows placement of a 14-Fr Foley catheter. The sheath is peeled away after the balloon is inflated with 10 mL of normal saline. Some advocate this as the optimal method for PEG in patients with head and neck cancer, related to an overall lower rate of complications in this patient population [21].

Percutaneous Endoscopic Gastrostomy/Jejunostomy

If postpyloric feeding is desired, a PEG/jejunostomy may be performed. The tube allows simultaneous gastric decompression and duodenal/jejunal enteral feeding [22]. A second, smaller feeding tube can be attached and passed through the gastrostomy tube and advanced endoscopically into the duodenum or jejunum. When the PEG is in position, a guidewire is passed through it and grasped using endoscopy forceps. The guidewire and endoscope are passed into the duodenum as distally as possible. The jejunal tube is then passed over the guidewire through the PEG into the distal duodenum, advanced into the jejunum, and the endoscope is withdrawn. An alternative method is to grasp a suture at the tip of the feeding tube or the distal tip of the tube itself and pass the tube into the duodenum, using forceps advanced through the biopsy channel of the endoscope. This obviates the need to pass the gastroscope into the duodenum, which may result in dislodgment of the tube when the endoscope is withdrawn.

Direct Percutaneous Endoscopic Jejunostomy

Jejunostomy tubes can be placed endoscopically by means of a PEG with jejunal extension (PEG-J) or by direct percutaneous jejunostomy (PEJ) [23]. Because the size of the jejunal extension of the PEG-J tube is significantly smaller than that of the direct PEJ, some have suggested that the PEJ provides more stable jejunal access for those who require long-term jejunal feeding. Unfortunately, a low success rate (68%) and a high adverse event rate (22.5%) have been documented in the largest series to date [24]. New methods using balloon-assisted enteroscopy with fluoroscopy have improved technical success rates to 96% [25].

Fluoroscopic Technique

Percutaneous gastrostomy and gastrojejunostomy can also be performed using fluoroscopy [26,27]. The stomach is insufflated with air using a nasogastric tube or a skinny needle if the patient is obstructed proximally. Once the stomach is distended and position is checked again with fluoroscopy, the stomach is punctured with an 18-gauge needle. T-fastener gastropexy may be used, deployed via the 18-gauge needle. A heavy-duty wire is passed, and the tract is dilated to accommodate a gastrostomy or gastrojejunostomy tube.

Complications

The most common complication after percutaneous placement of enteral feeding tubes is infection, usually involving the cutaneous exit site and surrounding tissue [28]. Gastrointestinal hemorrhage has been reported, but it is usually caused by excessive tension on the tube, leading to necrosis of the stomach wall. Gastrocolic fistulas, which develop if the colon is interposed between the anterior abdominal wall and the stomach when the needle is introduced, have been reported. Adequate transillumination aids in avoiding this complication. Separation of the stomach from the anterior abdominal wall can occur, resulting in peritonitis when enteral feeding is initiated. In most instances, this complication is caused by excessive tension on the gastrostomy tube. Another potential complication is pneumoperitoneum, secondary to air escaping after puncture of the stomach during the procedure, and is usually clinically insignificant. If the patient develops fever and abdominal tenderness, a Gastrografin study should be obtained to exclude the presence of a leak.

All percutaneous gastrostomy and jejunostomy procedures described here have been established as safe and effective. The method is selected on the basis of the endoscopist's experience and training and the patient's nutritional needs.

SURGICAL PROCEDURES

Since the advent of PEG, surgical placement of enteral feeding tubes is usually performed as a concomitant procedure as the last phase of a laparotomy performed for another indication. Occasionally, an operation solely for tube placement is performed in patients requiring permanent tube feedings when a percutaneous approach is contraindicated or unsuccessful. In these cases, the laparoscopic approach to enteral access should be considered. Laparoscopic gastrostomy was introduced in 2000, 10 years after the advent of PEG. Patients who are not candidates for PEG, as a result of head and neck cancer, esophageal obstruction, large hiatal hernia, gastric volvulus, or overlying intestine or liver, should be considered for laparoscopic gastrostomy or jejunostomy.

Gastrostomy

Gastrostomy is a simple procedure when performed as part of another intra-abdominal operation. It should be considered when prolonged enteral nutritional support is anticipated after surgery.

Complications are quite common after surgical gastrostomy. This may reflect the poor nutritional status and associated medical problems in many patients who undergo this procedure. Potential complications include wound infection, dehiscence, gastrostomy disruption, internal or external leakage, gastric hemorrhage, and tube migration.

Needle–Catheter Jejunostomy

The needle–catheter jejunostomy procedure consists of the insertion of a small (5-Fr) polyethylene catheter into the small intestine at the time of laparotomy for another indication. Kits containing the necessary equipment for the procedure are available from commercial suppliers. A needle is used to create a submucosal tunnel from the serosa to the mucosa on the antimesenteric border of the jejunum. A catheter is inserted through the needle and then the needle is removed. The catheter is brought out through the anterior abdominal wall, and the limb of the jejunum is secured to the anterior abdominal wall with sutures. The tube can be used for feeding immediately after the operation. The potential complications are similar to those associated with gastrostomy, but patients may have a higher incidence of diarrhea. Occlusion of the needle–catheter jejunostomy is common because of its small luminal diameter, and elemental nutritional formulas are preferentially used.

Transgastric Jejunostomy

Critically ill patients who undergo laparotomy commonly require gastric decompression and a surgically placed tube for enteral nutritional support. Routine placement of separate gastrostomy and jejunostomy tubes is common in this patient population and achieves the objective of chronic gastric decompression and early initiation of enteral nutritional support through the jejunostomy. Technical advances in surgically placed enteral feeding tubes led to the development of transgastric jejunostomy [29] and duodenostomy tubes, which allow simultaneous decompression of the stomach and distal feeding into the duodenum or the jejunum. The advantage of these tubes is that only one enterotomy into the stomach is needed, eliminating the possible complications associated with open jejunostomy tube placement. In addition, only one tube is necessary for gastric decompression and jejunal feeding, eliminating the potential complications of two separate tubes for this purpose.

The transgastric jejunostomy tube is placed surgically in the same manner as a gastrostomy tube, and the distal portion of the tube is advanced manually through the pylorus into the duodenum, with its final tip resting as far distally as possible in the duodenum or the jejunum (Fig. 21.3). The transgastric jejunostomy tube is preferred to transgastric duodenostomy tube because it is associated with less reflux of feedings into the stomach and a decreased risk of aspiration pneumonia. Surgical placement of transgastric jejunostomy tubes at the time of laparotomy is recommended for patients who likely require prolonged gastric decompression and enteral feeding.

DELIVERING THE TUBE-FEEDING FORMULA

The enteral formula can be delivered by intermittent bolus feeding, gravity infusion, or continuous pump infusion. In the intermittent bolus method, the patient receives 300 to 400 mL of formula every 4 to 6 hours. The bolus is usually delivered with the aid of a catheter-tipped, large-volume (60-mL) syringe. The main advantage of bolus feeding is simplicity. This approach is often used for patients requiring prolonged supplemental enteral nutritional support after discharge from the hospital. Bolus feeding can be associated with serious side effects, including gastric distention, nausea, cramping, and aspiration. The intermittent bolus method should not be used when feeding into the duodenum or the jejunum because boluses of formula can cause distention, cramping, and diarrhea.

Gravity-infusion systems allow the formula to drip continuously during 16 to 24 hours or intermittently during 20 to 30 minutes, four to six times per day. This method requires constant monitoring because the flow rate can be extremely irregular. The main advantages of this approach are simplicity, low cost, and close simulation of a normal feeding pattern.

Continuous pump infusion is the preferred method for the delivery of enteral nutrition in the critically ill patient. A peristaltic pump can be used to provide a continuous infusion of formula at a precisely controlled flow rate, which decreases problems with distention and diarrhea. Gastric residuals tend to be smaller with continuous pump-fed infusions, and the risk of aspiration may be decreased.

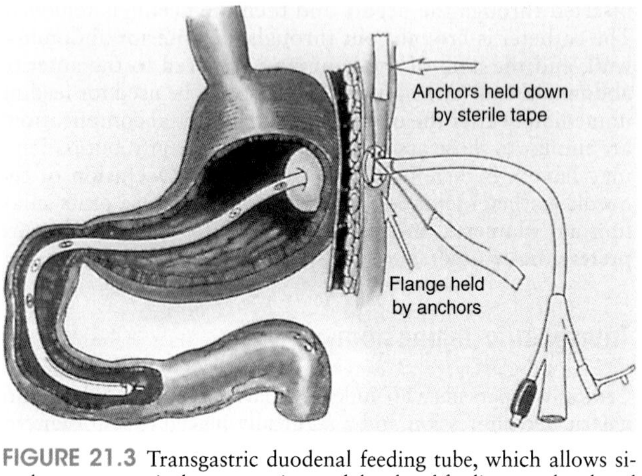

FIGURE 21.3 Transgastric duodenal feeding tube, which allows simultaneous gastric decompression and duodenal feeding, can be placed percutaneously (with endoscopic or fluoroscopic assistance) or surgically.

MEDICATIONS

When medications are administered via an enteric feeding tube, it is important to be certain that the drugs are compatible with each other and with the enteral formula. In general, medications should be delivered separately rather than as a combined bolus. For medications that are better absorbed in an empty stomach, tube feedings should be suspended for 30 to 60 minutes before administration.

Medications should be administered in an elixir formulation via enteral feeding tubes, whenever possible, to prevent occlusion of the tube. Enteral tubes should always be flushed with 20 mL of saline after medications are administered. To use an enteral feeding tube to administer medications dispensed in tablet form, often the pills must be crushed and delivered as slurry mixed with water. This is inappropriate for some medications, however, such as those absorbed sublingually or formulated as a sustained-released tablet or capsule.

COMPLICATIONS

Enteral tube placement is associated with few complications if practitioners adhere to appropriate protocols and pay close attention to the details of the procedures [30].

Nasopulmonary Intubation

Passage of an enteral feeding tube into the tracheobronchial tree most commonly occurs in patients with diminished cough or gag reflexes as a result of obtundation, altered mental status, or other causes such as the presence of endotracheal intubation. The presence of a tracheostomy or an endotracheal tube does not guarantee proper placement. A chest (or upper abdominal) radiograph should always be obtained before initiating tube feedings with a new tube to ensure that the tube is properly positioned. Endotracheal or transpulmonary placement of a feeding tube can be associated with pneumothorax, hydrothorax, pneumonia, pulmonary hemorrhage, abscess formation, or death [31]. A chest radiograph or a means of detecting CO_2 through the tube after it has been inserted 30 cm should be obtained to prevent unintentional placement of small-bore feeding tubes into the lungs. Alternatively, electromagnetic guidance can reduce the risk in intrapulmonary placement.

Aspiration

Pulmonary aspiration is a serious and potentially fatal complication of enteral nutritional support. The incidence of this complication varies and depends on the patient population studied. Traditional clinical monitors of aspiration with glucose oxidase strips and blue food coloring should no longer be used [32]. Nonrecumbent positioning is an evidence-based method for aspiration prevention that needs to be initiated in all patients receiving enteral nutrition.

Major risk factors for aspiration include obtundation or altered mental status, absence of cough or gag reflexes, delayed gastric emptying, gastroesophageal reflux, persistently high gastric residual volumes, and feeding in the supine position. The risk of pulmonary aspiration is minimized when the enteral feeding tube is positioned in the jejunum past the ligament of Treitz.

Gastrointestinal Intolerance

Delayed gastric emptying is sometimes improved by administering prokinetic agents. Combination therapy (metoclopramide 10 mg IV every 6 hours and erythromycin 200 mg IV every 12 hours) was highly effective compared to either agent alone for feeding intolerance in critical illness [33]. Dumping syndrome (i.e., diarrhea, distention, and abdominal cramping) can limit the use of enteral feeding. Dumping may be caused by delivering a hyperosmotic load into the small intestine.

Diarrhea in critically ill patients should not be attributed to intolerance of enteral feeding until other causes are excluded. Other possible etiologies for diarrhea include medications (e.g., magnesium-containing antacids and sorbitol-containing medications), alterations in gut microflora owing to prolonged antibiotic therapy, antibiotic-associated colitis, ischemic colitis, viral or bacterial enteric infection, electrolyte abnormalities, and excessive delivery of bile salts into the colon. Diarrhea can also be a manifestation of intestinal malabsorption because of enzyme deficiencies or villous atrophy [34].

Even if diarrhea is caused by enteral feeding, it can be controlled in nearly 50% of cases by instituting a continuous infusion of formula (if bolus feedings are used), slowing the rate of infusion, changing the formula (lower calorie, more elemental), adding fiber to the enteral formula, or adding antidiarrheal agents (e.g., loperamide, diphenoxylate/atropine, or tincture of opium).

Metabolic Complications

Prerenal azotemia and hypernatremia can develop in patients fed with hyperosmolar solutions. The administration of free water, either added to the formula or as separate boluses to replace obligatory losses, can avert this situation. Deficiencies of essential fatty acids and fat-soluble vitamins can develop after prolonged support with enteral solutions that contain minimal amounts of fat. Periodic enteral supplementation with linoleic acid or IV supplementation with emulsified fat can prevent this. The amount of linoleic acid necessary to prevent chemical and clinical fatty acid deficiency has been estimated to be 2.5 to 20.0 g per day.

Bacterial Contamination

Bacterial contamination of enteral solutions occurs when commercial packages are opened and mixed with other substances, and more commonly, it occurs with hospital-formulated and powdered feeds that require preparation compared to commercially prepared, ready-to-feed enteral formulas supplied in cans. The risk of contamination also depends on the duration of feeding. Contaminated formula may also play a significant role in the etiology of diarrhea in patients receiving enteral nutrition.

Occluded Feeding Tubes

Precipitation of certain proteins when exposed to an acid pH may be an important factor leading to the solidifying of formulas. Most premixed intact protein formulas solidify when acidified to a pH less than 5. To prevent occlusion of feeding tubes, the tube should be flushed with water before and after checking residuals. Small-caliber nasoenteric feeding tubes should be flushed with 20 mL of water every 4 to 6 hours to prevent tube occlusion, even when enteral feedings are administered by continuous infusion.

Medications are a frequent cause of clogging [35]. When administering medications enterally, liquid elixirs should be used, if available, because even tiny particles of crushed tablets can occlude the distal orifice of small-caliber feeding tubes. If tablets are used, it is important to crush them to a fine powder and solubilize them in liquid before administration. In addition, tubes should be flushed with water before and after the administration of any medications.

Several maneuvers are useful for clearing a clogged feeding tube. The tube can be irrigated with warm saline, a carbonated liquid, cranberry juice, or a pancreatic enzyme solution (e.g., Viokase). Commonly, a mixture of lipase, amylase, and protease (Pancrease) dissolved in sodium bicarbonate solution (for enzyme activation) is instilled into the tube with a syringe and the tube clamped for approximately 30 minutes to allow enzymatic degradation of precipitated enteral feedings. The tube is then vigorously flushed with saline. The pancreatic enzyme solution was successful in restoring tube patency in 96% of cases where formula clotting was the likely cause of occlusion and use of cola or water had failed [36,37]. Prevention of tube clogging with flushes and pancreatic enzyme are, therefore, the methods of choice in maintenance of chronic enteral feeding tubes.

Utility of Ultrasonography for Feeding Tube Insertion

Ultrasonography has useful application related to insertion of a feeding tube.

The insertion of a gastric tube may be facilitated with ultrasonography by identifying the nasogastric tube in the upper esophagus and confirming its placement in the stomach by direct visualization (Video 21.1) [38,39]. The tube may also be guided into a postpyloric position using real-time ultrasonography guidance (Video 21.1) [40,41]. For this application when compared to blind insertion technique, ultrasonography guidance has a higher success rate, takes less time, and reduces the need for postprocedure radiograph. Being a straightforward bedside technique, it has advantage over fluoroscopic, endoscopic, or electromagnetic guidance of postpyloric tube placement, given the simplicity of ultrasonography. The main disadvantage to ultrasonography guidance is that abdominal wounds and dressings can prevent its use, and patient specific factors such as obesity or intestinal gas may block visualization of the tube as it passes into the duodenum or the jejunem.

References

1. Taylor BE, McClave SA, Martindale RG, et al: Society of Critical Care Medicine; American Society of Parenteral and Enteral Nutrition. Guidelines for the Provision and Assessment of Nutrition Support Therapy in the Adult Critically Ill Patient: Society of Critical Care Medicine (SCCM) and American Society for Parenteral and Enteral Nutrition (A.S.P.E.N.). *Crit Care Med.* 44(2):390–438, 2016.
2. Dhaliwal R, Cahill N, Lemieux M, et al: The Canadian critical care nutrition guidelines in 2013: an update on current recommendations and implementation strategies. *Nutr Clin Pract* 29(1):29–43, 2014. http://www.criticalcarenutrition.com/docs/CPGs%202015/Summary%20CPGs%202015%20vs%202013.pdf.
3. Kreymann KG, Berger MM, Duetz NEP, et al: ESPEN guidelines on enteral nutrition: intensive care. *Clin Nutr* 25(2):210, 2006.
4. Jacobs DG, Jacobs DO, Kudsk KA, et al: Practice management guidelines for nutritional support of the trauma patient. *J Trauma* 57:660, 2004.
5. Casaer MP, Van den Berghe G: Nutrition in the acute phase of critical illness. *N Engl J Med* 370(13):1227–1236, 2014.
6. Chang YS, Fu HQ, Xiao YM, et al: Nasogastric or nasojejunal feeding in predicted severe acute pancreatitis: a meta-analysis. *Crit Care* 17(3):R118, 2013.
7. Ritz MA, Fraser R, Edwards N, et al: Delayed gastric emptying in ventilated critically ill patients: measurement by 13 C-octanoic acid breath test. *Crit Care Med* 29:1744, 2001.
8. Alkhawaja S, Martin C, Butler RJ, et al: Post-pyloric versus gastric tube feeding for preventing pneumonia and improving nutritional outcomes in critically ill adults. *Cochrane Database Syst Rev* 8:CD008875, 2015.
9. Alhazzani W, Almasoud A, Jaeschke R, et al: Small bowel feeding and risk of pneumonia in adult critically ill patients: a systematic review and meta-analysis of randomized trials. *Crit Care* 17(4):R127, 2013.
10. Deane AM, Dhaliwal R, Day AG, et al: Comparisons between intragastric and small intestinal delivery of enteral nutrition in the critically ill: a systematic review and meta-analysis. *Crit Care* 17(3):R125, 2013.

11. Haslam D, Fang J: Enteral access for nutrition in the intensive care unit. *Curr Opin Clin Nutr Metab Care* 9(2):155, 2006.
12. Burns SM, Carpenter R, Blevins C, et al: Detection of inadvertent airway intubation during gastric tube insertion: capnography versus a colorimetric carbon dioxide detector. *Am J Crit Care* 15:1, 2006.
13. Bechtold ML, Nguyen DL, Palmer LB, et al: Nasal bridles for securing nasoenteric tubes: a meta-analysis. *Nutr Clin Pract* 29(5):667–671, 2014.
14. Silva CC, Bennett C, Saconato H, et al: Metoclopramide for post-pyloric placement of naso-enteral feeding tubes. *Cochrane Database Syst Rev* 1:CD003353, 2015.
15. Foote JA, Kemmeter PR, Prichard PA, et al: A randomized trial of endoscopic and fluoroscopic placement of postpyloric feeding tubes in critically ill patients. *JPEN J Parenter Enteral Nutr* 28(3):154, 2004.
16. Fang JC, Hilden K, Holubkov R, et al: Transnasal endoscopy vs. fluoroscopy for the placement of nasoenteric feeding tubes in critically ill patients. *Gastrointest Endosc* 62(5):661, 2005.
17. Vitale MA, Villotti G, D'Alba L, et al: Unsedated transnasal percutaneous endoscopic gastrostomy placement in selected patients. *Endoscopy* 37(1):48, 2005.
18. Ponsky JL, Gauderer MWL, Stellato TA, et al: Percutaneous approaches to enteral alimentation. *Am J Surg* 149:102, 1985.
19. Dormann AJ, Glosemeyer R, Leistner U, et al: Modified percutaneous endoscopic gastrostomy (PEG) with gastropexy—early experience with a new introducer technique. *Z Gastroenterol* 38:933, 2000.
20. Maetani I, Tada T, Ukita T, et al: PEG with introducer or pull method: A prospective randomized comparison. *Gastrointest Endosc* 57(7):837, 2003.
21. Foster J, Filocarno P, Nava H, et al: The introducer technique is the optimal method for placing percutaneous endoscopic gastrostomy tubes in head and neck cancer patients. *Surg Endosc* 21(6):897–901, 2007.
22. Melvin W, Fernandez JD: Percutaneous endoscopic transgastric jejunostomy: a new approach. *Am Surg* 71(3):216, 2005.
23. Fan AC, Baron TH, Rumalla A, et al: Comparison of direct percutaneous endoscopic jejunostomy and PEG with jejunal extension. *Gastrointest Endosc* 56(6):890, 2002.
24. Maple JT, Petersen BT, Baron TH, et al: Direct percutaneous endoscopic jejunostomy: outcomes in 307 consecutive attempts. *Am J Gastroenterol* 100(12):2681, 2005.
25. Velázquez-Aviña J, Beyer R, Díaz-Tobar CP, et al: New method of direct percutaneous endoscopic jejunostomy tube placement using balloon-assisted enteroscopy with fluoroscopy. *Dig Endosc* 27(3):317–322, 2015.
26. Perona F, Castellazzi G, De Iuliis A, et al: Percutaneous radiologic gastrostomy: a 12-year series. *Gut Liver* 4 Suppl 1:S44–S49, 2010.
27. Covarrubias DA, O'Connor OJ, McDermott S, et al: Radiologic percutaneous gastrostomy: review of potential complications and approach to managing the unexpected outcome. *AJR Am J Roentgenol* 200(4):921–931, 2013.
28. Singh A, Gelrud A: Adverse events associated with percutaneous enteral access. *Gastrointest Endosc Clin N Am* 25(1):71–82, 2015.
29. Shapiro T, Minard G, Kudsk KA: Transgastric jejunal feeding tubes in critically ill patients. *Nutr Clin Pract* 12:164, 1997.
30. Baskin WN: Acute complications associated with bedside placement of feeding tubes. *Nutr Clin Pract* 21(1):40–55, 2006.
31. Sparks DA, Chase DM, Coughlin LM, et al: Pulmonary complications of 9931 narrow-bore nasoenteric tubes during blind placement: a critical review. *JPEN J Parenter Enteral Nutr* 35(5):625–629, 2011.
32. McClave SA, DeMeo MT, DeLegge MH, et al: North American Summit on Aspiration in the Critically Ill Patient: consensus statement. *JPEN J Parenter Enteral Nutr* 26[6 Suppl]:S80–S85, 2002.
33. Nguyen NQ, Chapman MJ, Fraser RJ, et al: Erythromycin is more effective than metoclopramide in the treatment of feed intolerance in critical illness. *Crit Care Med* 35(2):483–489, 2007.
34. Trabal J, Leyes P, Hervas S, et al: Factors associated with nosocomial diarrhea in patients with enteral tube feeding. *Nutr Hosp* 23(5):500–504, 2008.
35. Phillips NM, Nay R: A systematic review of nursing administration of medication via enteral tubes in adults. *J Clin Nurs* 17(17):2257–2265, 2008.
36. Williams TA, Leslie GD: A review of the nursing care of enteral feeding tubes in critically ill adults. *Intensive Crit Care Nurs* 21(1):5, 2005.
37. Bourgalt AM, Heyland DK, Drover JW, et al: Prophylactic pancreatic enzymes to reduce feeding tube occlusions. *Nutr Clin Pract* 18(5):398–401, 2003.
38. Chenaitia H, Brun PM, Querellou E, et al; WINFOCUS (World Interactive Network Focused On Critical Ultrasound) Group France: Ultrasound to confirm gastric tube placement in prehospital management. *Resuscitation* 83(4):447–451, 2012.
39. Brun PM, Chenaitia H, Lablanche C, et al: 2-Point ultrasonography to confirm correct position of the gastric tube in prehospital setting. *Mil Med* 179(9):959–963, 2014. doi: 10.7205/MILMED-D-14-00044.
40. Gok F, Kilicaslan A, Yosunkaya A: Ultrasound-guided nasogastric feeding tube placement in critical care patients. *Nutr Clin Pract* 30:257–260, 2015. doi: 10.1177/0884533614567714.
41. Hernández-Socorro CR, Marin J, Ruiz-Santana S, et al: Bedside sonographic-guided versus blind nasoenteric feeding tube placement in critically ill patients. *Crit Care Med* 24(10):1690–1694, 1996.

Chapter 22 ■ Gastroesophageal Balloon Tamponade for Acute Variceal Hemorrhage

MARIE T. PAVINI • JUAN CARLOS PUYANA

Gastroesophageal variceal hemorrhage is an acute and catastrophic condition that occurs in one-third to one-half of patients with portal pressures greater than 12 mm Hg or a portal–IVC pressure gradient of ≥5 [1]. Because proximal gastric varices and varices in the distal 5 cm of the esophagus lie in the superficial lamina propria, they are more likely to bleed and respond to endoscopic treatment [2]. Variceal rupture may be predicted by Child–Pugh class, red wale markings indicating epithelial thickness, and variceal size [1]. Although urgent endoscopy, sclerotherapy, and band ligations are considered first-line treatments, balloon tamponade remains a valuable intervention for the treatment of bleeding esophageal varices. Balloon tamponade is accomplished using a multilumen tube, approximately 1 m in length, with esophageal and gastric cuffs that can be inflated to compress esophageal varices and gastric submucosal veins, thereby providing hemostasis through tamponade, while incorporating aspiration ports for diagnostic and therapeutic usage.

HISTORICAL DEVELOPMENT

In 1930, Westphal described the use of an esophageal sound as a means of controlling variceal hemorrhage. In 1947, successful control of hemorrhage by balloon tamponade was achieved by attaching an inflatable latex bag to the end of a Miller–Abbot tube. In 1949, a two-balloon tube was described by Patton and Johnson. A triple-lumen tube with gastric and esophageal balloons, as well as a port for gastric aspiration, was described by Sengstaken and Blakemore in 1950. In 1955, Linton and Nachlas engineered a tube with a larger gastric balloon capable of compressing the submucosal veins in the cardia, thereby minimizing flow to the esophageal veins, with suction ports above and below the balloon. The Minnesota tube was described in 1968 as a modification of the Sengstaken–Blakemore tube, incorporating the esophageal suction port, which is described later. Several studies have published combined experience with tubes such as the Linton–Nachlas tube; however, the techniques described here are limited to the use of the Minnesota and Sengstaken–Blakemore tubes.

ROLE OF BALLOON TAMPONADE FOR THE MANAGEMENT OF BLEEDING ESOPHAGEAL VARICES

Treatment of portal hypertension to prevent variceal rupture includes primary and secondary prophylaxis. Primary prophylaxis consists of β-blockers, band ligation, and endoscopic surveillance, whereas secondary prophylaxis includes nitrates, transjugular intrahepatic portosystemic shunt (TIPS), and surgical shunts [3]. Management of acute variceal bleeding involves multiple simultaneous and sequential modalities. Balloon tamponade is considered a temporary bridge within these modalities. Self-expanding metal stents as an alternative to balloon tamponade are promising and currently under investigation [4,5].

Splanchnic vasoconstrictors such as somatostatin; octreotide; terlipressin (the only agent shown to decrease mortality); or vasopressin (with nitrates to reduce cardiac side effects) decrease portal blood flow and pressure, and should be administered as soon as possible [6–8]. In fact, Pourriat et al. [9] advocate administration of octreotide by emergency medical personnel before patient transfer to the hospital. Emergent therapeutic endoscopy in conjunction with pharmacotherapy is more effective than pharmacotherapy alone and is also performed as soon as possible. Band ligation has a lower rate of rebleeding and complications when compared with sclerotherapy, and should be performed preferentially, provided that visualization is adequate to ligate or sclerose varices successfully [3,10]. Tissue adhesives such as polidocanol and cyanoacrylate delivered through an endoscope are being used and studied outside the United States though glue embolization remains a concern [5].

Balloon tamponade is performed to control massive variceal hemorrhage, with the hope that band ligation or sclerotherapy and secondary prophylaxis will then be possible (Fig. 22.1). If bleeding continues beyond these measures, TIPS [11] is considered. Shunt surgery [12] may be considered when TIPS is contraindicated. Other alternatives include percutaneous transhepatic embolization; emergent esophageal transection with stapling [13]; esophagogastric devascularization with esophageal transection and

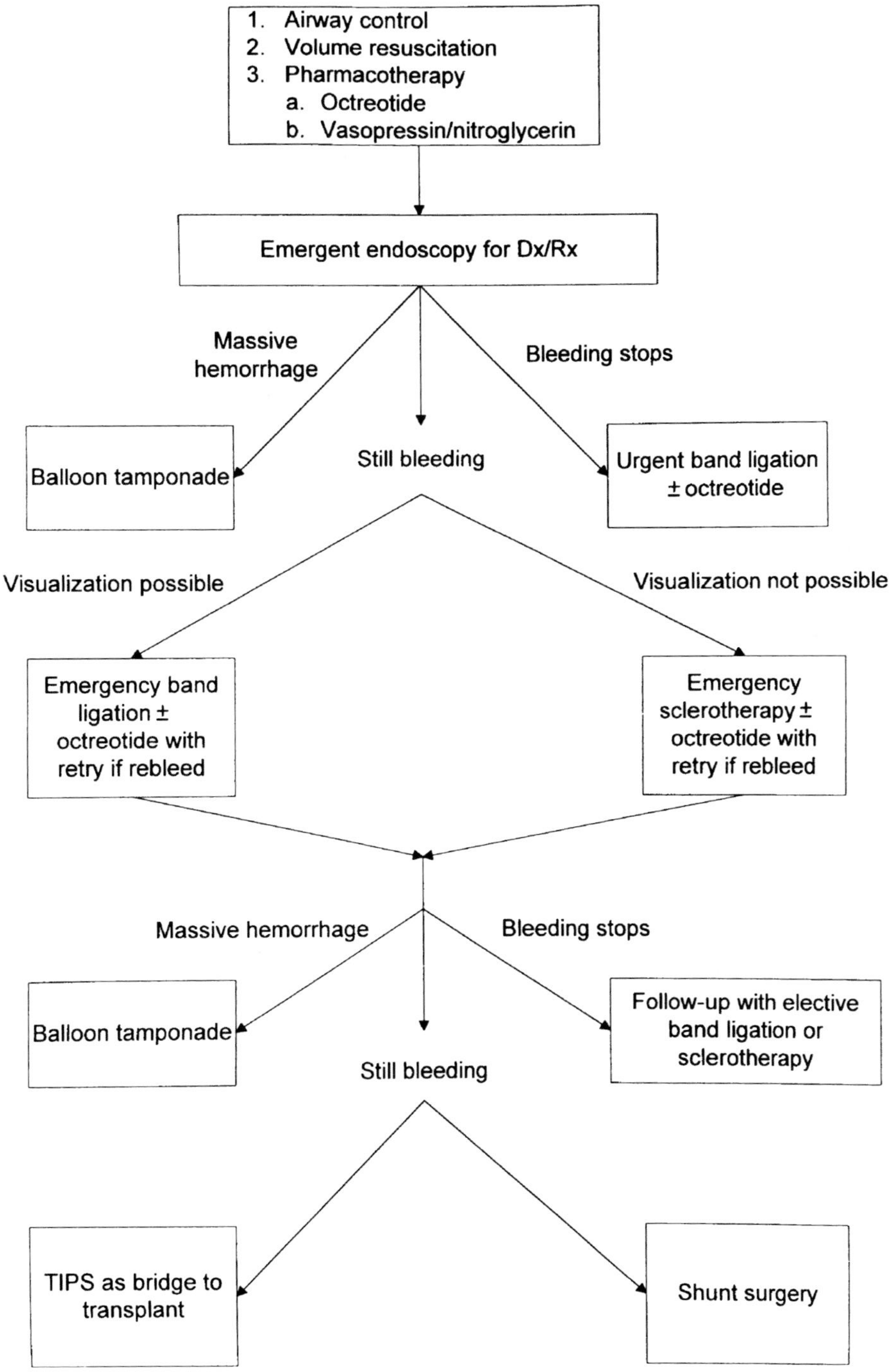

FIGURE 22.1 Management of esophageal variceal hemorrhage. Dx, diagnosis; Rx, therapy; TIPS, transjugular intrahepatic portosystemic shunt.

splenectomy; and hepatic transplantation. When gastric varices are noted, therapeutic options include endoscopic administration of the tissue adhesive cyanoacrylate; TIPS; balloon-occluded retrograde transvenous obliteration [14]; balloon-occluded endoscopic injection therapy [15]; and devascularization with splenectomy, shunt surgery, or liver transplantation.

INDICATIONS AND CONTRAINDICATIONS

A Minnesota or Sengstaken–Blakemore tube is indicated for patients with a diagnosis of esophageal variceal hemorrhage, in which neither band ligation nor sclerotherapy is technically possible, readily available, or has failed [16]. If at all possible, making an adequate anatomic diagnosis is critical before any of these balloon tubes are inserted. Severe upper gastrointestinal bleeding attributed to esophageal varices in patients with clinical evidence of chronic liver disease results from other causes in up to 40% of cases. The observation of a white nipple sign (platelet plug) during endoscopy is indicative of a recent variceal bleed. A balloon tube is contraindicated for patients with recent esophageal surgery or esophageal stricture [17]. Some authors do not recommend balloon tamponade when a hiatal hernia is present, but there are reports of successful hemorrhage control in some of these patients [18]. When there are no other options, it may be practical to titrate to the lowest effective balloon pressures especially when repeated endoscopic sclerotherapy has been performed, because there is increased risk of esophageal perforation [19].

TECHNICAL AND PRACTICAL CONSIDERATIONS

Airway Control

Endotracheal intubation (see Chapter 8) is imperative in patients with upper gastrointestinal bleeding and hemodynamic compromise; encephalopathy; or both. The incidence of aspiration pneumonia is directly related to the presence of impaired mental status [20]. Suctioning of pulmonary secretions and blood that accumulates in the hypopharynx is facilitated in patients who have been intubated. Sedatives and analgesics are more readily administered to intubated patients, and may be required when balloon tamponade is poorly tolerated, because retching or vomiting may lead to esophageal rupture [21]. The incidence of pulmonary complications is significantly lower when endotracheal intubation is routinely used [22].

Hypovolemia, Shock, and Coagulopathy

Adequate intravenous access should be obtained with large-bore venous catheters for blood product administration and fluid resuscitation with crystalloids and colloids. Packed red blood cells should be administered keeping four to six units available in case of severe recurrent bleeding, which commonly occurs among these patients. Coagulopathies, thrombocytopenia, or qualitative platelet disorders should be treated emergently. Octreotide and other vasoconstrictive therapies should be initiated as indicated.

Clots and Gastric Decompression

If time permits, placement of an Ewald tube and aggressive lavage and suctioning of the stomach and duodenum facilitates endoscopy, diminishes the risk of aspiration, and may help control hemorrhage from causes other than esophageal varices. It should be removed prior to balloon tamponade.

Infection, Ulceration, and Encephalopathy

Mortality is increased when infection is present in bleeding cirrhotic patients. The rate of early rebleeding is also increased in the presence of infection [23]. Prophylactic antibiotic use reduces the incidence of early rebleeding and increases survival [24]. Intravenous proton pump inhibitors are more efficacious than histamine-2-receptor antagonists for maintaining gastric pH at a goal of 7 or greater. Ulcers can form from sclerotherapy, banding, or direct cuff pressure during balloon tamponade. Shaheen et al. [25] found that the postbanding ulcers for patients receiving a proton pump inhibitor were two times smaller than those of patients who had not received a proton pump inhibitor. Rifaximin, lactulose, or lacitol may be useful, because blood and ammonia-forming bacteria in the gastrointestinal tract may contribute to encephalopathy.

Balloons, Ports, and Preparation

All lumens should be flushed to assure patency and the balloons inflated underwater to check for leaks. Two clean 100-mL (or larger) Foley-tip syringes and two to four rubber-shod hemostats should be readied for inflation of the balloons. To ensure that the gastric balloon will not be positioned in the esophagus, preinsertion compliance should be tested by placing 100-mL aliquots of air up to the listed maximum recommended volumes into the gastric inflation port while recording the corresponding pressures using a manometer attached to the gastric pressure port. In this way, postinsertion pressures can be compared. A portable handheld manometer allows for simpler continuous monitoring as well as patient transport and repositioning. When possible, a second manometer should be attached to the esophageal pressure port to facilitate inflation and continuous monitoring. Place a plug or hemostat on the other arm of the esophageal inflation port instead of a 100-mL syringe, because the manometer may also be used for inflation, rendering the syringe superfluous [26,27]. Both balloons are then completely deflated using suction and clamped with rubber hemostats or plugged before lubrication. The Minnesota tube (Fig. 22.2) includes a fourth lumen that allows for suctioning above the esophageal balloon [18], whereas the Sengstaken–Blakemore tube (Fig. 22.3) must have a 14 to 18 French nasogastric tube secured a few centimeters proximal to the esophageal balloon to be used for esophageal decompression. The nasogastric tube should be used even when the esophageal balloon is not inflated because inflation of the gastric balloon precludes proper drainage of esophageal secretions [28]. When the patient is to be placed in an aircraft (i.e., for evacuation), water should be instilled into balloon(s) instead of air [29].

Insertion and Placement of the Tube

The head of the bed should be elevated to reduce the risk of aspiration. Oral suction should be readied and the correct length of the tube to reach the patient's stomach should be selected (usually 45 to 60 cm orally). If the patient is not intubated, head down with left lateral positioning should be attained to minimize the risk of aspiration [17]. When using a Minnesota tube, the esophageal aspiration port should be set to continuous suction and the tube generously lubricated with lidocaine jelly prior to inserting it through the nose or mouth into the stomach. However, the nasal route is not recommended for patients with coagulopathy or thrombocytopenia. When insertion is difficult, the tube may be placed endoscopically [30] or with a guidewire [31]. Duarte described a technique of placing the tube in a longitudinally split Ewald tube [32]. Auscultation in the epigastrium while air is injected through the gastric lumen verifies the position of the tube, but the position of the gastric

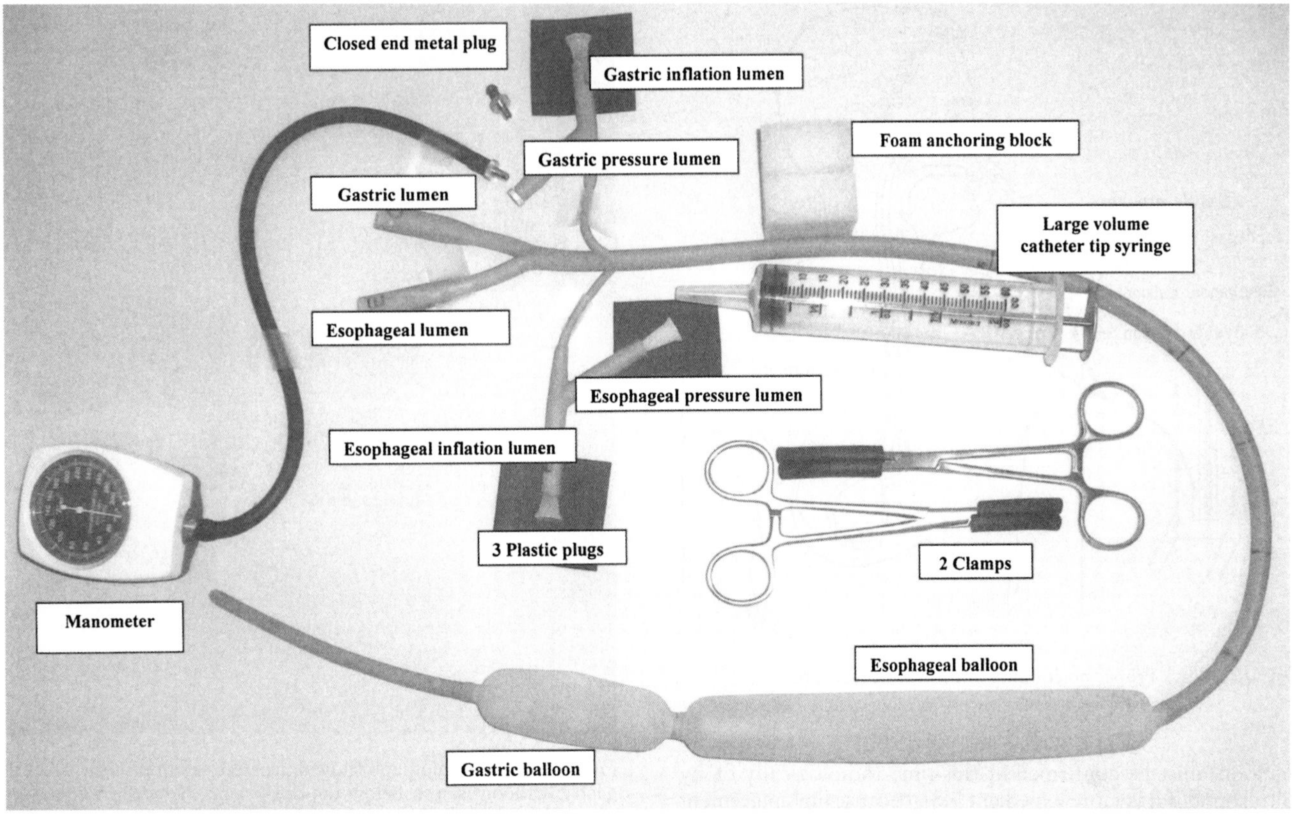

FIGURE 22.2 Minnesota tube.

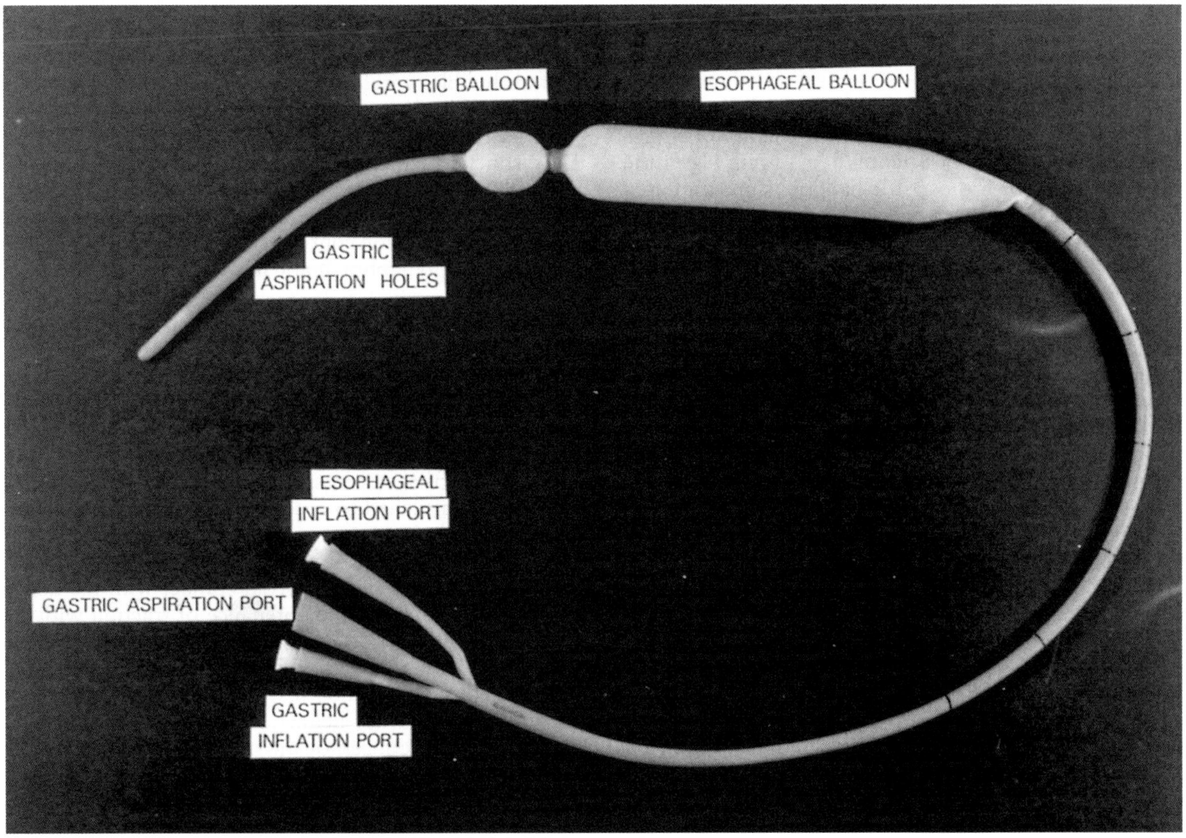

FIGURE 22.3 Sengstaken–Blakemore tube.

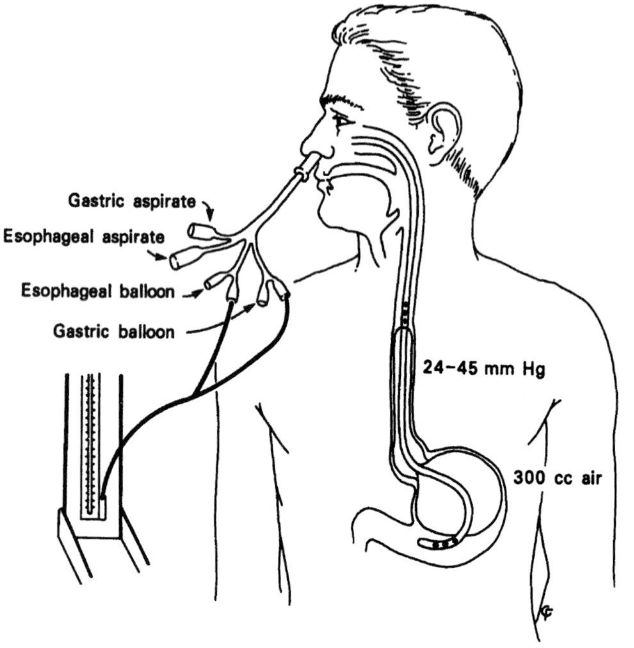

FIGURE 22.4 Proper positioning of the Minnesota tube.

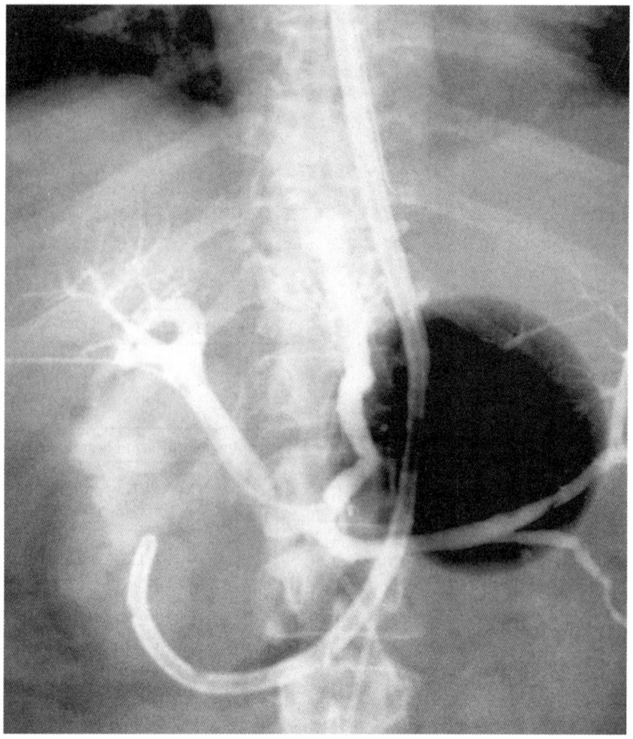

FIGURE 22.5 Radiograph showing correct position of the tube; the gastric balloon is seen below the diaphragm. Note the Salem sump above the gastric balloon and adjacent to the tube (Courtesy: Ashley Davidoff, MD.).

balloon must be confirmed at this time radiologically or by ultrasound if it is more expedient [33], because high placement can lead to esophageal rupture and low placement to duodenal rupture [34]. The manometer is then connected to the gastric pressure port and the gastric balloon is inflated with no more than 80 mL of air. A pressure of greater than 15 mm Hg at this stage suggests esophageal placement [27,35]. A (portable) radiograph or ultrasound must be obtained that includes the upper abdomen and lower chest (Figs. 22.4 and 22.5). When it is documented that the gastric balloon is below the diaphragm, it should be further inflated with air in 100 mL aliquots to a volume of 250 to 300 mL. The gastric balloon of the Minnesota tube can be inflated to 450 to 500 mL. If the change of manometric pressure for an aliquot is more than 15 mm Hg of the preinsertion pressure or if the gastric balloon is underinflated causing upward migration, erroneous esophageal placement should be considered. Record tube insertion depth (i.e., at the teeth). Tube balloon inlets should be clamped with rubber-shod hemostats after insufflation. Hemorrhage is frequently controlled with insufflation of the gastric balloon alone without applying traction, but for patients with torrential hemorrhage, it is necessary to apply traction (vide infra). If the bleeding continues, the manometer attached to the esophageal pressure port is used to inflate the esophageal balloon to a pressure of approximately 45 mm Hg. Some authors inflate the esophageal balloon for all patients immediately after insertion. When there is still bleeding, deflate the esophageal balloon, apply more traction, and reinflate in the event that it is a gastric variceal bleed. Pressures should be monitored and maintained.

Ultrasonography for Tube Insertion

Although a confirmatory radiograph is still warranted to document the final position of the inflated gastric balloon, an advantage to ultrasonography is that it can be used real time during insertion at the bedside of the patient [33,36]. The examiner uses the phased array probe in abdominal preset to locate the stomach. This may require several different tomographic views over the anterior and lateral upper quadrant. Frequently, the stomach is easy to locate because it is often filled with blood. The tube is visualized as a linear echogenic structure within the stomach. If the tube is not easily visible, injection of 50 mL of air into the gastric lumen of the tube will yield a characteristic pattern of air bubbles within the stomach. Once the tube is confirmed to be within the stomach, the operator slowly injects air into the gastric balloon. The inflated gastric balloon is visualized as a distinct structure within the stomach that has an echogenic curvilinear surface and that generates a strong acoustic shadow (Chapter 22 Video 22.1). The balloon enlarges in size within the stomach as inflation continues. The properly positioned gastric balloon is subdiaphragmatic in position.

Fixation and Traction Techniques

Fixation of the tube, and traction on the tube depend on the route of insertion. When the nasal route is used, attachment of a sponge rubber cuff around the tube at the nostril prevents skin and cartilage necrosis. When traction is required, the tube should be attached to a cord that is passed over a catcher's mask for maximum transportability [37] or a pulley in a bed with an overhead orthopedic frame and aligned directly as it comes out of the nose to avoid contact with the nostril. This type of system allows maintenance of traction with a known weight of 500 to 1,500 g either temporarily with IV fluid bags [17] or more permanently with block weights. When the tube is inserted through the mouth, traction is better applied by placing a football or hockey helmet on the patient and attaching the tube to the face mask of the helmet after a similar weight is applied for tension. Pressure sores can occur on the head and forehead if the helmet does not fit properly or if it is used for a prolonged period. Several authors recommend overhead traction for either oral or nasal insertion [38].

Maintenance, Monitoring, and Care

Periodically flush ports to ensure patency. To reduce encephalopathy, the gastric aspiration port should be used to thoroughly lavage the stomach before being set to low intermittent suction. It may be used later for medication administration. The esophageal port may be set to intermittent or continuous suction, depending on the extent of bleeding and drainage [35]. Tautness and inflation should be checked often and at least 1 hour after insertion, allowing for only transient fluctuations of as much as 30 mm Hg with respirations and esophageal spasm. Sedation or a pressure decrease may be necessary if large pressure fluctuations persist. If repositioning of the tube is required, assure that the esophageal balloon is deflated. Upper limb restraints should also be in use and the head of the bed elevated. The tube is left in place a minimum of 24 hours with gastric balloon tamponade maintained continuously for up to 48 hours. The esophageal balloon should be deflated for 5 minutes every 6 hours to help prevent mucosal ischemia and esophageal necrosis. Radiographic assurance of correct placement should be obtained every 24 hours and when dislodgement is suspected (Fig. 22.5). Watch for localized cervical edema, which may signal obstruction or malpositioning [39]. A pair of scissors should be kept with the apparatus in case rapid decompression becomes necessary, because balloon migration can acutely obstruct the airway or rupture the esophagus. It is advisable to take care not to utilize bare hemostats and to clamp at the thicker portion of the ports, because it is possible for the lumen to become obliterated and the tube thus impacted [40].

Removal of the Tube

Once hemorrhage is controlled, the esophageal balloon is deflated first. This may be done incrementally over time if desired. The gastric balloon is left inflated for an additional 24 to 48 hours and may be deflated when there is no evidence of bleeding. The tube is left in place 24 hours longer. If bleeding recurs, the balloon is reinflated. The tube is removed if no further bleeding occurs. Primary therapy and secondary prophylaxis, as described previously, should be considered because balloon tamponade is a bridge intervention and rebleeding occurs in up to two-thirds of patients within 3 months without therapy [3].

COMPLICATIONS

Rebleeding when the cuff(s) is deflated should be anticipated. The highest risk of rebleeding is in the first few days after balloon deflation. By 6 weeks, the risk of rebleeding returns to the premorbid risk level. Independent predictors of mortality of patients undergoing balloon tamponade, described by Lee et al. [41], include blood transfusion greater than 10 units; coagulopathy; presence of shock; abnormal Glasgow Coma Score; and high total volume of sclerosing agent (ethanolamine).

Aspiration pneumonia is the most common complication of balloon tamponade with incidence ranging from 0% to 12%. Acute laryngeal obstruction and tracheal rupture are the most severe of all complications, and the worst examples of tube migration or malpositioning. Migration of the tube occurs when the gastric balloon is not inflated properly after adequate positioning in the stomach or when excessive traction (>1.5 kg) is used, causing migration cephalad to the esophagus or hypopharynx. Mucosal ulceration of the gastroesophageal junction is common and is directly related to prolonged traction times (>36 hours). Perforation of the esophagus has been reported as a result of misplacing the gastric balloon above the diaphragm (Fig. 22.6). The incidence of complications that are a direct cause of death ranges from 0% to 20%.

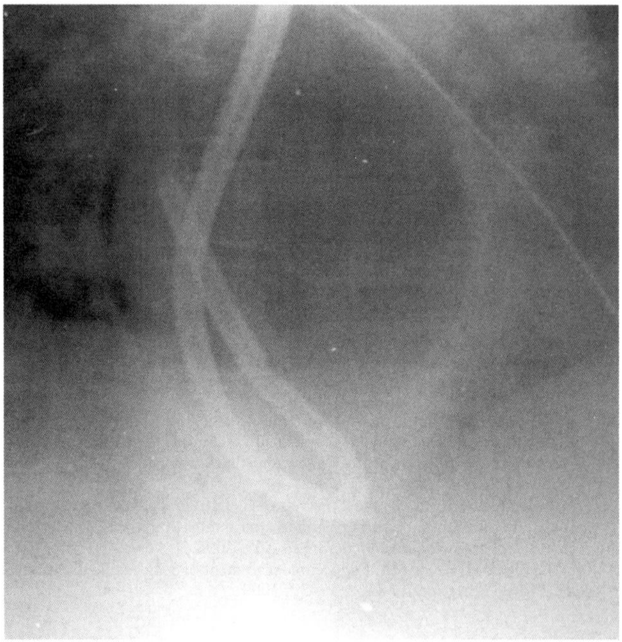

FIGURE 22.6 Chest radiograph showing distal segment of the tube coiled in the chest and the gastric balloon inflated above the diaphragm in the esophagus (Courtesy: Ashley Davidoff, MD.).

References

1. Rikkers LF: Surgical complications of cirrhosis and portal hypertension, in Townsend CM, Beauchamp RD, Evers BM, et al (eds): *Sabiston's Textbook of Surgery*. 17th ed. Philadelphia, PA, WB Saunders, 2004, p 1175.
2. Tsokos M, Turk EE: Esophageal variceal hemorrhage presenting as sudden death in outpatients. *Arch Pathol Lab Med* 126:1197, 2002.
3. Zaman A, Chalasani N: Bleeding caused by portal hypertension. *Gastroenterol Clin North Am* 34:623, 2005.
4. Zehetner J, Shamiyeh A, Wayand W, et al: Results of a new method to stop acute bleeding from esophageal varices; implantation of a self-expanding stent. *Surg Endosc* 22:2149–2152, 2008.
5. El Sayed G, Tarf S, O'Beirne J, et al: Endoscopy management algorithms: role of cyanoacrylate glue injection and self-expanding metal stents in acute variceal haemorrhage. *Frontline Gastroenterol* 6(3):208–216, 2015.
6. Sandford NL, Kerlin P: Current management of oesophageal varices. *Aust N Z J Med* 25:528, 1995.
7. Stein C, Korula J: Variceal bleeding: what are the options? *Postgrad Med* 98:143, 1995.
8. Erstad B: Octreotide for acute variceal bleeding. *Ann Pharmacother* 35:618, 2001.
9. Pourriat JL, Leyacher S, Letoumelin P, et al: Early administration of terlipressin plus glyceryl trinitrate to control active upper gastrointestinal bleeding in cirrhotic patients. *Lancet* 346:865, 1995.
10. Avgerinos A, Armonis A, Manolakpoulos S, et al: Endoscopic sclerotherapy versus variceal ligation in the long-term management of patients with cirrhosis after variceal bleeding: a prospective randomized study. *J Hepatol* 26:1034, 1997.
11. Banares R, Casado M, Rodriquez-Laiz JM, et al: Urgent transjugular intrahepatic portosystemic shunt for control of acute variceal bleeding. *Am J Gastroenterol* 93:75, 1998.
12. Lewis JJ, Basson MD, Modlin IM: Surgical therapy of acute esophageal variceal hemorrhage. *Dig Dis Sci* 10[Suppl 1]:46, 1992.
13. Mathur SK, Shah SR, Soonawala ZF, et al: Transabdominal extensive oesophagogastric devascularization with gastro-oesophageal stapling in the management of acute variceal bleeding. *Br J Surg* 84:413, 1997.
14. Kitamoto M, Imamura M, Kamada K, et al: Balloon-occluded retrograde transvenous obliteration of gastric fundal varices with hemorrhage. *AJR Am J Roentgenol* 178:1167, 2002.
15. Shiba M, Higuchi K, Nakamura K, et al: Efficacy and safety of balloon-occluded endoscopic injection sclerotherapy as a prophylactic treatment for high-risk gastric fundal varices: a prospective, randomized, comparative clinical trial. *Gastrointest Endosc* 56:522, 2002.
16. Burnett DA, Rikkers LF: Nonoperative emergency treatment of variceal hemorrhage. *Surg Clin North Am* 70:291, 1990.
17. McCormick PA, Burroughs AK, McIntyre N: How to insert a Sengstaken-Blakemore tube. *Br J Hosp Med* 43:274, 1990.
18. Minocha A, Richards RJ: Sengstaken-Blakemore tube for control of massive bleeding from gastric varices in hiatal hernia. *J Clin Gastroenterol* 14:36, 1992.

19. Chong CF: Esophageal rupture due to Sengstaken-Blakemore tube misplacement. *World J Gastroenterol* 11(41):6563–6565, 2005.
20. Pasquale MD, Cerra FB: Sengstaken-Blakemore tube placement. *Crit Care Clin* 8:743, 1992.
21. Zeid SS, Young PC, Reeves JT: Rupture of the esophagus after introduction of the Sengstaken-Blakemore tube. *Gastroenterology* 36:128–131, 1959.
22. Cello JP, Crass RA, Grendell JH, et al: Management of the patient with hemorrhaging esophageal varices. *JAMA* 256:1480, 1986.
23. Papatheodoridis GV, Patch D, Webster JM, et al: Infection and hemostasis in decompensated cirrhosis: a prospective study using thromboelastography. *Hepatology* 29:1085, 1999.
24. Pohl J, Pollmann K, Sauer P, et al: Antibiotic prophylaxis after variceal hemorrhage reduces incidence of early rebleeding. *Hepatogastroenterology* 51(56):541, 2004.
25. Shaheen NJ, Stuart E, Schmitz S, et al: Pantoprazole reduces the size of postbanding ulcers after variceal band ligation: a randomized control trial. *Hepatology* 41:588, 2005.
26. Greenwald B: Two devices that facilitate the use of the Minnesota tube. *Gastroenterol Nurs* 27:268–270, 2004.
27. Bard, Inc: Bard Minnesota four lumen esophagogastric tamponade tube for the control of bleeding from esophageal varices [package insert], 1997.
28. Boyce HW: Modification of the Sengstaken-Blackmore balloon tube. *Nord Hyg Tidskr* 267:195, 1962.
29. Pinto-Marques P, Romaozinho J, Ferreira M, et al: Esophageal perforation-associated risk with balloon tamponade after endoscopic therapy. Myth or reality? *Hepatogastroenterology* 53:536–539, 2006.
30. Lin TC, Bilir BM, Powis ME: Endoscopic placement of Sengstaken-Blakemore tube. *J Clin Gastroenterol* 31(1):29–32, 2000.
31. Wilcox G, Marlow J: A special maneuver for passage of the Sengstaken-Blakemore tube. *Gastrointest Endosc* 30(6):377, 1984.
32. Duarte B: Technique for the placement of the Sengstaken-Blakemore tube. *Surg Gynecol Obstet* 168(5):449–450, 1989.
33. Lock G, Reng M, Messman H, et al: Inflation and positioning of the gastric balloon of a Sengstaken-Blakemore tube under ultrasonographic control. *Gastrointest Endosc* 45(6):538, 1997.
34. Kandel G, Gray R, Mackenzie RL, et al: Duodenal perforation by a Linton-Nachlas balloon tube. *Am J Gastroenterol* 83(4):442–444, 1988.
35. Isaacs K, Levinson S: Insertion of the Minnesota tube, in Drossman D (ed): *Manual of Gastroenterologic Procedures*. 3rd ed. New York, NY, Raven Press, 1993, pp 27–35.
36. Lin A C-M, Hsu Y-H, Wang T-L, et al: Placement confirmation of Sengstaken-Blakemore tube by ultrasound. *Emerg Med J* 23:487, 2006.
37. Kashiwagi H, Shikano S, Yamamoto O, et al: Technique for positioning the Sengstaken-Blakemore tube as comfortably as possible. *Surg Gynecol Obstet* 172(1):63, 1991.
38. Hunt PS, Korman MG, Hansky J, et al: An 8-year prospective experience with balloon tamponade in emergency control of bleeding esophageal varices. *Dig Dis Sci* 27:413, 1982.
39. Juffe A, Tellez G, Eguaras M, et al: Unusual complication of the Sengstaken-Blakemore tube. *Gastroenterology* 72(4, Pt 1):724–725, 1977.
40. Bhasin DK, Zargar SA, Mandal M, et al: Endoscopic removal of impacted Sengstaken-Blakemore tube. *Surg Endosc* 3(1):54–55, 1989.
41. Lee H, Hawker FH, Selby W, et al: Intensive care treatment of patients with bleeding esophageal varices: results, predictors of mortality, and predictors of the adult respiratory distress syndrome. *Crit Care Med* 20:1555, 1992.

Chapter 23 ■ Paracentesis and Diagnostic Peritoneal Lavage

LENA M. NAPOLITANO

ABDOMINAL PARACENTESIS

Indications

Abdominal paracentesis is a simple procedure that can be easily performed at the bedside in the intensive care unit and may provide important diagnostic information or therapy for critically ill patients with ascites. As a *diagnostic* intervention, abdominal paracentesis with removal of 20 mL of peritoneal fluid is performed to determine the etiology of the ascites or to ascertain whether infection is present, as in spontaneous bacterial peritonitis [1]. It can also be used in any clinical situation in which the analysis of a sample of peritoneal fluid might be useful in ascertaining a diagnosis or guiding therapy. The evaluation of ascites should therefore include ascitic fluid analysis.

As a therapeutic intervention, abdominal paracentesis is usually performed to drain large volumes of abdominal ascites, termed large-volume paracentesis (LVP), sometimes with removal of more than 5 L of ascitic fluid [2]. Ascites is the most common presentation of decompensated cirrhosis, and its development heralds a poor prognosis, with a 50% 2-year survival rate. Effective first-line therapy for ascites includes sodium restriction (2 g per day), use of diuretics, and LVP. When tense or refractory ascites is present, LVP is safe and effective, and has the advantage of producing immediate relief from ascites and its associated symptoms [3]. LVP can be palliative by diminishing abdominal pain from distention or relieving respiratory symptoms by allowing better diaphragmatic excursion in patients who have ascites refractory to aggressive medical management.

Refractory ascites occurs in 10% of patients with cirrhosis and is associated with substantial morbidity and a 1-year survival of less than 50% [4,5]. For patients with refractory ascites, transjugular intrahepatic portosystemic shunt (TIPS) is superior to LVP for long-term control of ascites, but it is associated with greater encephalopathy risk and does not affect mortality [6,7].

Techniques

Before abdominal paracentesis is initiated, a catheter may be inserted to drain the urinary bladder, and correction of any underlying coagulopathy or thrombocytopenia should be considered. A consensus statement from the International Ascites Club states that "there are no data to support the correction of mild coagulopathy with blood products prior to therapeutic paracentesis, but caution is needed when severe thrombocytopenia is present" [3]. The practice guideline from the American Association for the Study of Liver Diseases (AASLD) states that routine correction of prolonged prothrombin time or thrombocytopenia is not required when experienced personnel perform paracentesis [2]. This has been confirmed in a study of 1,100 LVPs in 628 patients [8]. But in critically ill patients, there is still uncertainty as to the optimal platelet count and prothrombin time for the safe conduct of paracentesis.

The patient must next be positioned correctly. In critically ill patients, the procedure is performed in the supine position with the head of the bed elevated at 30 to 45 degrees. If the patient is clinically stable and therapeutic LVP is being performed, the patient can be placed in the sitting position, leaning slightly forward, to increase the total volume of ascites removed.

The site for paracentesis on the anterior abdominal wall is then chosen (Fig. 23.1). The preferred site is in the lower abdomen, lateral to the rectus abdominis muscle and inferior to the umbilicus. It is important to stay lateral to the rectus abdominis muscle to avoid injury to the inferior epigastric artery and vein. In patients with chronic cirrhosis and caput medusae (engorged

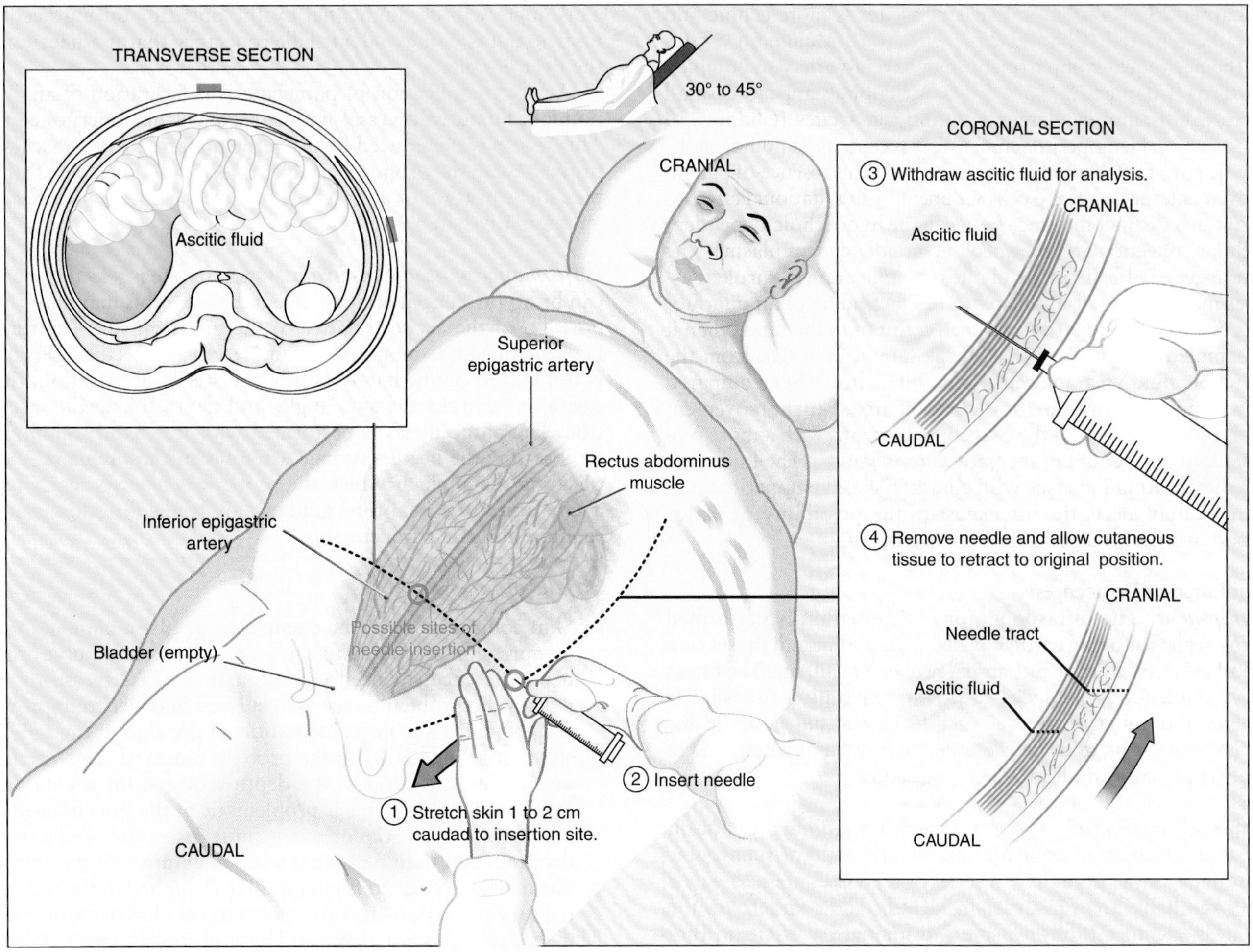

FIGURE 23.1 Recommended sites and appropriate technique for paracentesis.

anterior abdominal wall veins), these visible vascular structures must be avoided. Injury to these veins can cause significant bleeding because of the underlying portal hypertension and may result in hemoperitoneum. The left lower quadrant of the abdominal wall is preferred over the right lower quadrant for abdominal paracentesis because critically ill patients often have cecal distention. The ideal site is therefore in the left lower quadrant of the abdomen, lateral to the rectus abdominis muscle in the midclavicular line and inferior to the umbilicus. It has also been determined that the left lower quadrant is significantly thinner and the depth of ascites greater compared with the infraumbilical midline position, confirming the left lower quadrant as the preferred location for paracentesis [9].

If the patient had previous abdominal surgery limited to the lower abdomen, it may be difficult to perform a paracentesis in the lower abdomen and ultrasonic guidance is recommended for site selection. The point of entry, however, remains lateral to the rectus abdominis muscle in the midclavicular line. If there is concern that the ascites is loculated because of a previous abdominal surgery or peritonitis, abdominal paracentesis should be performed under ultrasound guidance to prevent iatrogenic complications.

Abdominal paracentesis can be performed by the needle technique, by the catheter technique, or with ultrasound guidance. Diagnostic paracentesis usually requires 20 to 50 mL peritoneal fluid and is commonly performed using the needle technique. However, if large volumes of peritoneal fluid are required, the catheter technique is used, because it is associated with a lower incidence of complications. LVP should always be performed with the catheter technique. Ultrasound guidance is recommended because it can be helpful both in diagnostic paracentesis using the needle technique and in LVP using the catheter technique.

Utility of Ultrasonography for Guidance of Paracentesis

Compared to standard landmark technique, guidance of paracentesis with ultrasonography is associated with a higher success rate and lower complication rate [10,11].

Identification of Ascites. Intra-abdominal fluid is readily identified with ultrasonography. In small amounts, it is identified in the hepatorenal recess, the splenorenal recess, and the pelvic area (Chapter 23 Video 23.1). In larger amounts, it accumulates in the prehepatic space, the presplenic space, the subphrenic area, in the pelvis; and the flanks bilaterally (Chapter 23 Video 23.2). Air-filled bowel will float on the ascitic fluid; so characteristically, ultrasonography examination of the anterior abdomen detects air artifact with the fluid distributing in dependent position.

Characterization of Ascites. Intra-abdominal fluid may have a variety of appearances. Uncomplicated ascites, as occurs with heart failure or portal hypertension, is typically anechoic

(Chapter 23 Video 23.3). Purulent ascites is more echoic and may be septated (Chapter 23 Video 23.4). Malignant ascites in the peritoneal compartment may have a variety of complex patterns (Chapter 23 Video 23.5). Air bubbles appear as small hyperechoic mobile elements within the ascites (Chapter 23 Video 23.6). Hemoperitoneum, if very recent, has a homogenous echoic pattern (Chapter 23 Video 23.7). In the absence of patient movement, the red blood cells sediment by gravitational effect to result in a distinct interface between the hypoechoic-dependent cellular collection and the anechoic-nondependent plasma. The interface may be distinct and linear in appearance. Purulent ascites may also result in this pattern. The finding of an interface has implications regarding the cell count of in the fluid when it is sampled with paracentesis. If the sample is drawn from the anechoic fluid area, the cell count will be low when compared to a sample drawn from the dependent area. Patient movement will result in mixing of the two compartments, with a more representative cell count of the paracentesis sample. The finding of a sedimentation interface with clinical risk of hemoperitoneum immediately alerts the intensivist to the possibility of major blood loss into the peritoneal compartment.

Guidance of Paracentesis

Equipment. The ultrasonography examination is performed using a phased-array cardiac probe with abdominal preset or a standard curved array abdominal probe, if available. The linear high frequency probe lacks sufficient penetration to visualize deeper abdominal structures such as bowel, but is useful for examining the planned needle trajectory for vascular structures that would contraindicate device insertion.

Scanning technique. The lower lateral abdominal quadrant areas are the preferred site for paracentesis with the suprapubic approach as an alternative. A series of scan lines are performed over the flank areas in order to identify and characterize the ascites; and to establish a safe site for needle insertion that avoids injury to adjacent organs.

The critically ill patient is generally in supine position, unlike thoracentesis; this in usually not a problem for paracentesis. Occasionally, the patient will need to be rolled into an ipsilateral decubitus position in order to distribute the fluid into a better target position.

Identification of fluid. The examiner seeks three characteristic findings that are typical for ascites.

a. An anechoic or relatively hypoechoic space that is surrounded by typical anatomic boundaries. This space represents the ascites.
b. Typical anatomic boundaries: This requires unequivocal identification of bowel structures, the liver, or the spleen.
c. Dynamic changes: This requires identification of dynamic changes that are typical of ascites such as movement of bowel within the fluid and shape change of the ascitic fluid with forward force application of the probe against the abdominal wall (Chapter 23 Video 23.8). This characteristic of shape change of the ascites does not occur with pleural fluid, because forward force application of the probe against the rigid chest wall does not alter the shape of the pleural effusion.

Site selection. The transducer is moved over the target area, in order to identify a safe site for needle insertion that maximizes the distance between the abdominal wall and underlying bowel and anatomic structures such as the liver or spleen. As much as possible, the examiner holds the probe perpendicular to the abdominal wall, because this angle is easiest to duplicate with the needle–syringe assembly. Once a suitable site is identified, it is marked; the depth of needle penetration to access the fluid is measured; and the angle of the probe is determined. This angle will be duplicated by the operator during needle insertion. It is best avoid a needle trajectory that is adjacent to the liver or spleen.

A rare complication of paracentesis is laceration of an abdominal blood wall vessel with subsequent hemoperitoneum. This risk may be reduced by using the high frequency vascular probe to scan the proposed needle trajectory. Using color Doppler, identification of a vessel may allow the operator to select an alternative site.

Performance of needle insertion. Once the site is selected, there can be no further patient movement, because this may shift the position of the ascites relative to the insertion site. The time between the ultrasonography examination and needle insertion is minimized. Immediately before the sterile preparation, the operator rechecks the site, angle, and depth for needle insertion. The paracentesis is performed with free-hand technique by inserting the needle–syringe assembly at the site mark, duplicating the angle at which the probe was held to determine a safe trajectory. Real-time guidance of needle insertion is not required for safe paracentesis.

Pitfalls of imaging

a. Skin compression: In the edematous or obese patient, skin compression artifact may cause an under estimation of the depth for successful needle insertion. In this case, the operator pushes the probe into the skin surface in order to improve image quality causing indentation of the skin at the target site that rebounds when the probe is removed. This results in a underestimation of the depth required for the needle to access the fluid. This is problematic at the time of needle insertion, because the operator must insert the needle to a depth greater than measured with indentation of the skin.
b. Site mark movement: If lateral force is applied to the skin at the time of marking the insertion site, the skin mark may be moved to a substantial extent. This is of special concern when accessing a smaller amount of ascites. At the time of needle insertion, the operator takes care to not move the mark site when applying pressure to the skin surface.
c. Difficult scanning conditions: It may be difficult to achieve adequate image quality in the obese or edematous patient.
d. Aberrant position of vascular structure: The epigastric artery is ordinarily positioned at the lateral border of the rectus muscle, so it is well away from the usual site of paracentesis which is lower in the flank area. However, the vessel may have an aberrant position, and dilated veins associated with portal hypertension may be positioned in the path of needle insertion [12]. Injury of an aberrant vessel may result in severe bleeding into the peritoneal cavity or formation of a pseudoaneurysm [13–15]. Hiroshi et al. have proposed examination of the needle trajectory before needle insertion using the high frequency vascular probe [16]. If a vessel is identified, the operator seeks an alternative site.

Needle Technique

With the patient in the appropriate position and the access site for paracentesis determined, the patient's abdomen is prepared with 2% chlorhexidine gluconate and 70% isopropyl alcohol and sterile aseptic technique is used. If necessary, intravenous sedation is administered to prevent the patient from moving excessively during the procedure (see Chapter 2). After a time out, local anesthesia, using 1% or 2% lidocaine with 1:200,000 epinephrine, is infiltrated into the site. A skin wheal is created with the local anesthetic, using a short 25- or 27-gauge needle. Then, using a 22-gauge, 1.5-inch needle, the local anesthetic is infiltrated into the subcutaneous tissues and anterior abdominal wall, with the needle perpendicular to the skin. Before the anterior abdominal wall and peritoneum are infiltrated, the skin is pulled taut inferiorly, allowing the peritoneal cavity to be entered at a different location than the skin entrance site, thereby decreasing the chance of ascitic leak (*Z-track technique*). While tension is maintained inferiorly on the abdominal skin the needle is advanced through the abdominal wall fascia and peritoneum, and local anesthetic is injected. Intermittent aspiration identifies when the peritoneal cavity is entered, with return of ascitic fluid into the syringe. The needle is held securely in this position with the left hand, and the right hand is used to withdraw approximately 20 to 50 mL ascitic fluid into the syringe for a diagnostic paracentesis.

Once adequate fluid is withdrawn, the needle and syringe are withdrawn from the anterior abdominal wall and the paracentesis site is covered with a sterile dressing. The needle is removed from the syringe, because it may be contaminated with skin organisms. A small amount of peritoneal fluid is sent in a sterile container for Gram stain and 10 mL or quantity sufficient to achieve the fill line is inoculated into blood culture bottles immediately at bedside for culture and sensitivity. The remainder of the fluid is sent for appropriate studies, which may include cytology; cell count and differential; protein; specific gravity; amylase; pH; lactate dehydrogenase; bilirubin; triglycerides; and albumin. A serum to ascites albumin gradient (SAAG) greater than 1.1 g per dL is indicative of portal hypertension and cirrhosis (Table 23.1) [17]. Peritoneal fluid can be sent for smear and culture for acid-fast bacilli if tuberculous peritonitis is in the differential diagnosis.

Catheter Technique

Positioning; use of aseptic technique; and local anesthetic infiltration are the same as for the needle technique. A 22-gauge, 1.5-inch needle attached to a 10-mL syringe is used to document the free return of peritoneal fluid into the syringe at the chosen site. This needle is removed from the peritoneal cavity and a catheter-over-needle assembly is used to gain access to the peritoneal cavity. If the anterior abdominal wall is thin, an 18- or 20-gauge Angiocath can be used as the catheter-over-needle assembly. If the anterior abdominal wall is quite thick, as in obese patients, it may be necessary to use a long (5.25-inch, 18- or 20-gauge) catheter-over-needle assembly or a percutaneous single- or multiple-lumen central venous catheter (18- or 20-gauge) and gain access to the peritoneal cavity using the Seldinger technique.

The peritoneal cavity is entered as for the needle technique. The catheter-over-needle assembly is inserted perpendicular to the anterior abdominal wall using the Z-track technique; once peritoneal fluid returns into the syringe barrel, the catheter is advanced over the needle, the needle is removed, and a 20- or 50-mL syringe is connected to the catheter. The tip of the catheter is now in the peritoneal cavity and can be left in place until the appropriate amount of peritoneal fluid is removed. This technique, rather than the needle technique, should be used when LVP is performed, because complications (e.g., intestinal perforation) may occur if a needle is left in the peritoneal space for an extended period.

When the Seldinger technique is used in patients with a large anterior abdominal wall, access to the peritoneal cavity is initially gained with a needle or catheter-over-needle assembly. A guidewire is then inserted through the needle and an 18- or 20-gauge single- or multiple-lumen central venous catheter is threaded over the guidewire. It is very important to use the Z-track method for the catheter technique to prevent development of an ascitic leak, which may be difficult to control and may predispose the patient to peritoneal infection. If continued drainage of a peritoneal fluid collection is desired, a radiologist or qualified proceduralist can place a chronic indwelling peritoneal catheter using a percutaneous guidewire technique. A video for the correct procedural technique for paracentesis is available for review [18].

TABLE 23.1

Etiologies of Ascites Based on Normal or Diseased Peritoneum and SAAG

Normal peritoneum
Portal hypertension (SAAG >1.1 g/dL)
Hepatic congestion
Congestive heart failure
Constrictive pericarditis
Tricuspid insufficiency
Budd–Chiari syndrome
Liver disease
Cirrhosis
Alcoholic hepatitis
Fulminant hepatic failure
Massive hepatic metastases
Hypoalbuminemia (SAAG < 1.1 g/dL)
Nephrotic syndrome
Protein-losing enteropathy
Severe malnutrition with anasarca
Miscellaneous conditions (SAAG < 1.1 g/dL)
Chylous ascites
Pancreatic ascites
Bile ascites
Nephrogenic ascites
Urine ascites
Ovarian disease
Diseased peritoneum infections (SAAG < 1.1 g/dL)
Bacterial peritonitis
Tuberculous peritonitis
Fungal peritonitis
HIV-associated peritonitis
Malignant conditions
Peritoneal carcinomatosis
Primary mesothelioma
Pseudomyxoma peritonei
Hepatocellular carcinoma
Other rare conditions
Familial Mediterranean fever
Vasculitis
Granulomatous peritonitis
Eosinophilic peritonitis

SAAG, serum to ascites albumin gradient; HIV, human immunodeficiency virus.

Complications

The most common complications related to abdominal paracentesis are bleeding and persistent ascitic leak. Because most patients in whom ascites has developed also have some component of chronic liver disease with associated coagulopathy and thrombocytopenia, it is very important to consider correction of any underlying coagulopathy before proceeding with abdominal paracentesis. In addition, it is very important to select an avascular access site on the anterior abdominal wall. The Z-track technique is very helpful in minimizing persistent ascitic leak and should always be used. Another complication associated with abdominal paracentesis is intestinal or urinary bladder perforation, with associated peritonitis and infection. Intestinal injury is more common when the needle technique is used than when the catheter technique is used. Because the needle is free in the peritoneal cavity, iatrogenic intestinal perforation may occur if the patient moves or if intra-abdominal pressure increases with Valsalva maneuver or coughing. Urinary bladder injury is less common and underscores the importance of draining the urinary bladder with a catheter before the procedure. This injury is more common when the abdominal access site is in the suprapubic location; therefore, this access site is not recommended when direct visualization is not available. Careful adherence to proper technique of paracentesis minimizes associated complications.

In patients who have large-volume chronic abdominal ascites, such as that secondary to hepatic cirrhosis or ovarian carcinoma; transient hypotension; and paracentesis-induced circulatory dysfunction (PICD) may develop during LVP. PICD is characterized by worsening hypotension and arterial vasodilation; hyponatremia; azotemia; and an increase in plasma renin activity. Evidence is accumulating that PICD is secondary to an accentuation of established arteriolar vasodilation with multiple etiologies, including the dynamics of paracentesis (the rate of ascitic fluid extraction); release of nitric oxide from the vascular endothelium; and mechanical modifications of flow dynamics due to abdominal decompression [19].

PICD is associated with increased mortality and may be prevented with the administration of plasma expanders. It is very important to obtain reliable peripheral or central venous access in these patients so that fluid resuscitation can be performed if PICD develops during the procedure. Systematic reviews and meta-analyses have found that albumin was associated with fewer complications of LVP (PICD, hyponatremia, and overall morbidity and mortality) compared to other treatments [20,21]. AASLD guidelines suggest that albumin (6 to 8 g per liter ascites removed) can be considered for LVP in which >5 L of ascites is removed.

Because PICD pathogenesis may be caused by accentuated splanchnic vasodilation, trials comparing terlipressin (a vasoconstrictor), midodrine, or octreotide with albumin have reported conflicting results for improving systemic and renal hemodynamics and renal function, including the prevention of PICD. Additional studies are warranted to establish their efficacy [22].

LVP is only transiently therapeutic; the underlying chronic disease induces reaccumulation of the ascites. Percutaneous placement of a tunneled catheter is a viable and safe technique to consider in patients who have symptomatic malignant ascites that require frequent therapeutic paracentesis for relief of symptoms [23]. An automated pump system for treatment of refractory ascites is undergoing investigation [24].

DIAGNOSTIC PERITONEAL LAVAGE

Before the introduction of diagnostic peritoneal lavage (DPL) by Root et al. [25] in 1965, nonoperative evaluation of the injured abdomen was limited to standard four-quadrant abdominal paracentesis. Abdominal paracentesis for the evaluation of hemoperitoneum was associated with a high false-negative rate. This clinical suspicion was confirmed by Giacobine and Siler [26] in an experimental animal model of hemoperitoneum documenting that a 500-mL blood volume in the peritoneal cavity yielded a positive paracentesis rate of only 78%. The initial study by Root et al. [25] reported 100% accuracy in the identification of hemoperitoneum using 1-L peritoneal lavage fluid. Many subsequent clinical studies confirmed these findings, with the largest series reported by Fischer et al. [27] in 1978. They reviewed 2,586 cases of DPL and reported a false-positive rate of 0.2%; false-negative rate of 1.2%; and overall accuracy of 98.5%. Following its introduction in 1965, DPL was a cornerstone in the evaluation of hemoperitoneum due to blunt and penetrating abdominal injuries. However, it is nonspecific for determination of the type or extent of organ injury.

Recent advances have led to the use of ultrasound (focused assessment with sonography in trauma [FAST]; Fig. 23.2) and rapid helical computed tomography (CT) in the emergent evaluation of abdominal trauma [28]. FAST has replaced DPL as the initial screening modality of choice for severe abdominal trauma, and FAST is now part of the Advanced Trauma Life Support course [29]. Practice management guidelines from the Eastern Association for the Surgery of Trauma recommend FAST as the initial diagnostic modality to exclude hemoperitoneum [30]. DPL remains a valuable adjunct to modern imaging techniques in early trauma assessment, particularly in hemodynamically unstable patients with initial FAST examination that is negative or equivocal and in the assessment of potential hollow visceral injury in blunt abdominal trauma [31]. Diagnostic peritoneal aspiration, without a full lavage, has also been utilized successfully in these circumstances [32].

Indications

The primary indication for DPL is evaluation of blunt abdominal trauma in patients with associated hypotension. If the initial FAST examination is positive for hemoperitoneum, surgical intervention (laparotomy) is required. If the FAST examination is negative or equivocal, DPL can be considered. If the patient is hemodynamically stable and can be transported safely, CT scan of the abdomen and pelvis is the diagnostic method of choice. If the patient is hemodynamically unstable or requires emergent surgical intervention for a craniotomy, thoracotomy, or vascular procedure, it is imperative to determine whether there is a coexisting intraperitoneal source of hemorrhage to prioritize treatment of life-threatening injuries. FAST or DPL can be used to diagnose hemoperitoneum in patients with multisystem injury, who require general anesthesia for the treatment of associated traumatic injuries. Patients with associated thoracic or pelvic injuries should also have definitive evaluation for abdominal trauma, and DPL can be used in these individuals. DPL can also be used to evaluate for traumatic hollow viscus injury, and a cell count ratio (defined as the ratio between white blood cell (WBC) and red blood cell (RBC) count in the lavage fluid divided by the ratio of the same parameters in the peripheral blood) less than or equal to 1 has a specificity of 97% and sensitivity of 100% [33].

DPL can also be used to evaluate penetrating abdominal trauma; however, its role differs from that in blunt abdominal trauma [34]. A hemodynamically unstable patient with abdominal penetrating injuries requires no further investigation and immediate laparotomy should be undertaken. Instead, the role of DPL in the hemodynamically stable patient with penetrating abdominal injury is to identify hemoperitoneum; and hollow viscus or diaphragmatic injury. DPL has also been recommended as the initial diagnostic study in stable patients with penetrating trauma to the back and flank, defining an RBC count greater than 1,000 per μL as a positive test [35]. Implementation of this protocol decreased the total celiotomy rate from 100% to 24%, and the therapeutic celiotomy rate increased from 15% to 80%.

DPL can also serve a therapeutic role. It is very effective in rewarming patients with significant hypothermia. DPL should not be performed for patients with clear signs of significant abdominal trauma and hemoperitoneum associated with hemodynamic instability or peritonitis. These patients should undergo emergent celiotomy. Pregnancy is a relative contraindication to DPL; it may be technically difficult to perform because of the gravid uterus and is associated with a higher risk of complications. Bedside

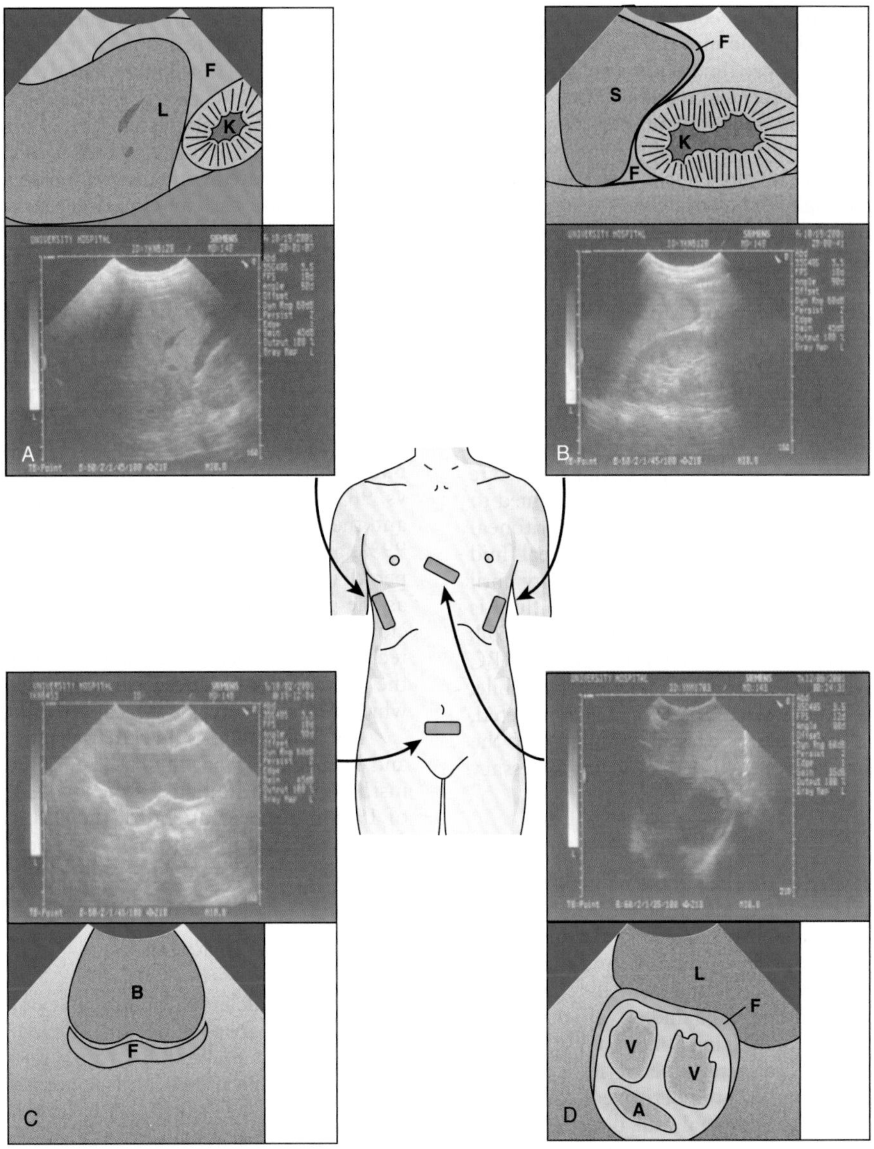

FIGURE 23.2 The FAST examination. FAST; focused assessment with sonography in trauma.

ultrasound evaluation of the abdomen in the pregnant trauma patient is associated with least risk to the woman and to the fetus. An additional relative contraindication to DPL is multiple previous abdominal surgeries due to abdominal adhesions, and difficulty in gaining access to the free peritoneal cavity. If DPL is indicated and ultrasound examination does not identify a safe pathway, it must be performed by the open technique to prevent iatrogenic complications such as intestinal injury.

Techniques

Three techniques can be used to perform DPL: (a) the closed percutaneous technique, (b) the semiclosed technique, and (c) the open technique. The closed percutaneous technique, introduced by Lazarus and Nelson [36] in 1979, is easy to perform, can be done rapidly, is associated with a low complication rate, and is as accurate as the open technique. It should not be used in patients who have had previous abdominal surgery or a history of abdominal adhesions. The open technique entails the placement of the peritoneal lavage catheter into the peritoneal cavity under direct visualization. It is more time-consuming than the closed percutaneous technique. The semiclosed technique requires a smaller incision than does the open technique and uses a peritoneal lavage catheter with a metal stylet to gain entrance into the peritoneal cavity. It has become less popular, because clinicians have become more familiar and skilled with the closed technique.

The patient is placed in the supine position for all three techniques. A catheter is placed into the urinary bladder and a nasogastric tube is inserted into the stomach to prevent iatrogenic bladder or gastric injury. The nasogastric tube is placed on continuous suction for gastric decompression. The skin of the anterior abdominal wall is prepared with 2% chlorhexidine solution and sterilely draped, leaving the periumbilical area exposed. Standard aseptic technique is used throughout the procedure. Local anesthesia with 1% or 2% lidocaine with 1:200,000 epinephrine is used as necessary throughout the procedure. The infraumbilical site is used unless there is clinical concern of possible pelvic fracture and retroperitoneal or pelvic hematoma, in which case the supraumbilical site is optimal.

Closed Percutaneous Technique

With the closed percutaneous technique, local anesthesia is infiltrated inferior to the umbilicus and a 5-mm skin incision is made just at the inferior umbilical edge. An 18-gauge needle is inserted through this incision and into the peritoneal cavity, angled toward the pelvis at approximately a 45-degree angle with the skin. The penetration through the linea alba and then through the peritoneum is felt as two separate "pops." A J-tipped guidewire is passed through the needle and into the peritoneal cavity, again directing the wire toward the pelvis by maintaining the needle at a 45-degree angle to the skin. The 18-gauge needle is then removed and the DPL catheter inserted over the guidewire into the peritoneal cavity, using a twisting motion and guided inferiorly toward the pelvis. The guidewire is then removed, and a 10-mL syringe is attached to the catheter for aspiration. If free blood returns from the DPL catheter before the syringe is attached or if gross blood returns in the syringe barrel, hemoperitoneum has been documented, the catheter is removed, and the patient is quickly transported to the operating room for emergent celiotomy. If no gross blood returns on aspiration through the catheter, peritoneal lavage is performed using 1 L Ringer's lactate solution or normal saline that has been previously warmed to prevent hypothermia. The fluid is instilled into the peritoneal cavity through the DPL catheter; afterward, the peritoneal fluid is allowed to drain out of the peritoneal cavity by gravity until the fluid return slows. A minimum of 250 mL lavage fluid is considered a representative sample of the peritoneal fluid [37]. A sample is sent to the laboratory for determination of RBC count; WBC count; amylase concentration; and presence of bile, bacteria, or particulate matter. When the lavage is completed, the catheter is removed and a sterile dressing applied over the site. Suture approximation of the skin edges is not necessary when the closed technique is used for DPL.

Semiclosed Technique

Local anesthetic is infiltrated in the area of the planned incision and a 2- to 3-cm vertical incision made in the infraumbilical or supraumbilical area. The incision is continued sharply down through the subcutaneous tissue and linea alba, and the peritoneum is then visualized. Forceps, hemostats, or Allis clamps are used to grasp the edges of the linea alba and elevate the fascial edges to prevent injury to the underlying abdominal structures. The DPL lavage catheter with a metal inner stylet is inserted through the closed peritoneum into the peritoneal cavity at a 45-degree angle to the anterior abdominal wall, directed toward the pelvis. When the catheter–metal stylet assembly is in the peritoneal cavity, the DPL catheter is advanced into the pelvis and the metal stylet removed. A 10-mL syringe is attached to the catheter, and aspiration is conducted as previously described. When the lavage is completed, the fascia must be reapproximated with sutures, the skin closed, and a sterile dressing applied.

Open Technique

After the administration of appropriate local anesthetic, a vertical midline incision approximately 3 to 5 cm long is made. This incision is commonly made in the infraumbilical location, but in patients with presumed pelvic fractures or retroperitoneal hematomas or in pregnant patients, a supraumbilical location is preferred. The vertical midline incision is carried down through the skin, subcutaneous tissue, and linea alba under direct vision. The linea alba is grasped on either side using forceps, hemostats, or Allis clamps; and the fascia is elevated to prevent injury to the underlying abdominal structures. The peritoneum is identified, and a small vertical peritoneal incision is made to gain entrance into the peritoneal cavity. The DPL catheter is then inserted into the peritoneal cavity under direct visualization and advanced inferiorly toward the pelvis. It is inserted without the stylet or metal trocar. When in position, a 10-mL syringe is attached for aspiration. If aspiration of the peritoneal cavity is negative (i.e., no gross blood returns), peritoneal lavage is performed, as described earlier in the chapter. As in the semiclosed technique, the fascia and skin must be reapproximated to prevent dehiscence or evisceration, or both.

A prospective randomized study documented that closed percutaneous DPL can be performed faster than the open procedure (1 to 3 minutes vs. 5 to 24 minutes) [38]. The closed percutaneous technique was as accurate as the open procedure and was associated with a lower incidence of wound infections and complications. The closed percutaneous technique, using the Seldinger technique, should therefore be used initially in all patients except those who have had previous abdominal surgery or in pregnant patients. This has been confirmed in a study of 2,501 DPLs performed over a 75-month period for blunt or penetrating abdominal trauma [39]. The majority (2,409, or 96%) were performed using the closed percutaneous technique, and 92 (4%) were done open because of pelvic fractures, previous scars, or pregnancy. Open DPL was less sensitive than closed DPL in patients who sustained blunt trauma (90% vs. 95%), but slightly more sensitive in determining penetration (100% vs. 96%). Overall, there were few (21, [0.8%]) complications, and the overall sensitivity, specificity, and accuracy were 95%, 99%, and 98%, respectively, using an RBC count of 100,000 per μL in blunt trauma and 10,000 per μL in penetrating trauma as the positive threshold. A meta-analysis concluded that the closed DPL technique is comparable to the standard open DPL technique in terms of accuracy and major complications, with the advantage of reduced performance time with closed DPL, which is offset by increased technical difficulties and failures [40].

A DPL modification [41] that resulted in more rapid infusion and drainage of lavage fluid used cystoscopy irrigation tubing for instillation and drainage of the lavage fluid, saving an average of 19 minutes per patient for the DPL completion. This modification can be applied to the closed percutaneous or open DPL technique to decrease the procedure time in critically ill patients.

Interpretation of Results

The current guidelines for interpretation of positive and negative results of DPL are provided in Table 23.2. A positive result can be estimated by the inability to read newsprint or typewritten print through the lavage fluid as it returns through clear plastic tubing. This test is not reliable, however, and a quantitative RBC count in a sample of the peritoneal lavage fluid must be performed [42]. For patients with nonpenetrating abdominal trauma, an RBC count greater than 100,000 per μL of lavage fluid is considered positive and requires emergent celiotomy. Fewer than 50,000 RBCs per μL is considered negative and RBC counts of 50,000 to 100,000 per μL are considered indeterminate. The guidelines for patients with penetrating abdominal trauma are much less clear with clinical studies using an RBC count of greater than 1,000 or 10,000 per μL to greater than 100,000 per μL as the criterion for a positive DPL in patients with penetrating thoracic or abdominal trauma. The lower the threshold, the more sensitive the test, but the higher the nontherapeutic laparotomy rate.

Determination of hollow viscus injury by DPL is much more difficult. A WBC count greater than 500 per μL of lavage fluid or an amylase concentration greater than 175 units per dL of lavage fluid is usually considered positive. These studies, however, are not as accurate as the use of RBC count in the lavage fluid to determine the presence of hemoperitoneum. One study in patients with blunt abdominal trauma determined that the WBC count in lavage fluid has a positive predictive value of only 23% and probably should not be used as an indicator of a positive DPL [43]. Other studies analyzed alkaline phosphatase levels in DPL fluid to determine if this assay is helpful in the diagnosis of hollow viscus injuries [44,45], but the results have been variable. A prospective study used a diagnostic algorithm of initial abdominal ultrasound, followed by helical CT and subsequent DPL (if CT

TABLE 23.2

Interpretation of Diagnostic Peritoneal Lavage Results

POSITIVE
Nonpenetrating abdominal trauma
Immediate gross blood return via catheter
Immediate return of intestinal contents or food particles
Aspiration of 10 mL blood via catheter
Return of lavage fluid via chest tube or urinary catheter
RBC count >100,000/mL
WBC count >500/μL
Cell count ratio (defined as the ratio between WBC and RBC count in the lavage fluid divided by the ratio of the same parameters in the peripheral blood) ≥1
Amylase >175 U/100 mL
Penetrating abdominal trauma
Immediate gross blood return via catheter
Immediate return of intestinal contents or food particles
Aspiration of 10 mL blood via catheter
Return of lavage fluid via chest tube or Foley catheter
RBC count used is variable, from >1,000/μL to >100,000/μL
WBC count >500/μL
Amylase >175 U/100 mL
NEGATIVE
Nonpenetrating abdominal trauma
RBC count <50,000/μL
WBC count <100/μL
Cell count ratio (defined as the ratio between WBC and RBC count in the lavage fluid divided zby the ratio of the same parameters in the peripheral blood) <1
Amylase <75 U/100 mL
Penetrating abdominal trauma
RBC count used is variable, from <1,000/μL to <50,000/μL
WBC count <100/μL
Amylase <75 U/100 mL

RBC, red blood cell; WBC, white blood cell.

was suggestive of blunt bowel or mesenteric injury) using a cell count ratio (defined as the ratio between WBC and RBC count in the lavage fluid divided by the ratio of the same parameters in the peripheral blood) greater than or equal to 1 to determine the need for laparotomy in patients with blunt abdominal injuries [46]. This proposed algorithm had a high accuracy (100%) while requiring the performance of DPL in only a few (2%) patients.

It must be stressed that DPL is not accurate for determination of retroperitoneal visceral injuries or diaphragmatic injuries [47]. The incidence of false-negative DPL results is approximately 30% in patients who sustained traumatic diaphragmatic rupture. In addition, DPL is insensitive in detecting subcapsular hematomas of the spleen or liver that are contained, without hemoperitoneum.

Complications

Complications of DPL by the techniques described here include malposition of the lavage catheter; injury to the intra-abdominal organs or vessels; iatrogenic hemoperitoneum; wound infection or dehiscence; evisceration; and possible unnecessary laparotomy. DPL is a very valuable technique, however, and if it is performed carefully, with attention to detail, these complications are minimized. In the largest series published to date, with more than 2,500 DPLs performed, the complications rate was 0.8% [39]. Wound infection, dehiscence, and evisceration are more common with the open technique; therefore, the closed percutaneous technique is recommended in all patients who do not have a contraindication to this technique. Knowledge of all techniques is necessary, however, because the choice of technique should be based on the individual patient's presentation.

References

1. Wong CL, Holroyd-Leduc J, Thorpe KE, et al: Does this patient have bacterial peritonitis or portal hypertension? How do I perform a paracentesis and analyze the results? *JAMA* 299(10):1166–1178, 2008.
2. Runyon BA; AASLD Practice Guidelines Committee: Management of adult patients with ascites due to cirrhosis: update 2012. *Hepatology* 57:1651–1653, 2013.
3. European Association for the Study of the Liver: EASL clinical practice guidelines on the management of ascites, spontaneous bacterial peritonitis, and hepatorenal syndrome in cirrhosis. *J Hepatol* 53(3):397–417, 2010.
4. Wong F: Management of ascites in cirrhosis. *J Gastroenterol Hepatol* 27(1):11–20, 2012.
5. Garcia-Tsao G, Lim JK, Members of Veterans Affairs Hepatitis C Resource Center Program: Management and treatment of patients with cirrhosis and portal hypertension: recommendations from the Department of Veterans Affairs Hepatitis C Resource Center Program and the National Hepatitis C Program. *Am J Gastroenterol* 104(7):1802–1829, 2009.
6. Saab S, Nieto JM, Lewis SK, et al: TIPS versus paracentesis for cirrhotic patients with refractory ascites. *Cochrane Database Syst Rev* (4):CD004889, 2006.
7. Salerno F, Camma C, Enea M, et al: Transjugular intrahepatic portosystemic shunt for refractory ascites: a meta-analysis of individual patient data. *Gastroenterology* 133(3):825–834, 2007.
8. Grabau CM, Crago SF, Hoff LK, et al: Performance standards for therapeutic abdominal paracentesis. *Hepatology* 40:484, 2004.
9. Sakai H, Sheer TA, Mendler MH, et al: Choosing the location for non-image guided abdominal paracentesis. *Liver Int* 25(5):984, 2005.
10. Nazeer SR, Dewbre H, Miller AH: Ultrasound-assisted paracentesis performed by emergency physicians vs the traditional technique: a prospective, randomized study. *Am J Emerg Med* 23:363, 2005.
11. Patel PA, Ernst FR, Gunnarsson CL: Evaluation of hospital complications and costs associated with using ultrasound guidance during abdominal paracentesis procedures. *J Med Econ* 15(1):1, 2012.
12. Pache I, Bilodeau M: Severe haemorrhage following abdominal paracentesis for ascites in patients with liver disease. *Aliment Pharmacol Ther* 21:525, 2005.
13. Seidler M, Sayegh K, Roy A, et al: A fatal complication of ultrasound-guided abdominal paracentesis. *J Clin Ultrasound* 41:457, 2013.
14. Arnold C, Haag K, Blum HE, et al: Acute hemoperitoneum after large-volume paracentesis. *Gastroenterology* 113:978, 1997.
15. Lam EY, McLafferty B, Taylor M Jr, et al: Inferior epigastric artery pseudoaneurysm: a complication of paracentesis. *J Vasc Surg* 28:566, 1998.
16. Sekiguchi H, Suzuki J, Daniels CE: Making paracentesis safer: a proposal for the use of bedside abdominal and vascular ultrasonography to prevent a fatal complication. *Chest* 143:1136, 2013.
17. McGibbon A, Chen GI, Peltekian KM, et al: An evidence-based manual for abdominal paracentesis. *Dig Dis Sci* 52(12):3307–3315, 2007.
18. Thomsen TW, Shaffer RW, White B, et al: Paracentesis. Videos in clinical medicine. *N Engl J Med* 355:e21, 2006. Available at: http://content.nejm.org/cgi/video/355/19/e21/. Accessed June 1, 2017.
19. Lindsay AJ, Burton J, Ray CE Jr: Paracentesis-induced circulatory dysfunction: a primer for the interventional radiologist. *Semin Intervent Radiol* 31(3):276–278, 2014.
20. Bernardi M, Caraceni P, Navickis RJ, et al: Albumin infusion in patients undergoing large-volume paracentesis: a meta-analysis of randomized trials. *Hepatology* 55:1172–1181, 2012.
21. Kwok CS, Krupa L, Mahtani A. et al: Albumin reduces paracentesis-induced circulatory dysfunction and reduces death and renal impairment among patients with cirrhosis and infection: a systematic review and meta-analysis. *Biomed Res Int* 2013:295153, 2013.
22. Singhal S, Baikati KK, Jabbour II, et al: Management of refractory ascites. *Am J Ther* 19(2):121–132, 2012.
23. Rosenberg SM: Palliation of malignant ascites. *Gastroenterol Clin North Am* 35(1):189, xi, 2006.
24. Bellot P, Welker MW, Soriano G, et al: Automated low flow pump system for the treatment of refractory ascites: a multi-center safety and efficacy study. *J Hepatol* 58(5):922–927, 2013.
25. Root H, Hauser C, McKinley C, et al: Diagnostic peritoneal lavage. *Surgery* 57:633, 1965.
26. Giacobine JW, Siler VE: Evaluation of diagnostic abdominal paracentesis with experimental and clinical studies. *Surg Gynecol Obstet* 110:676, 1960.
27. Fischer R, Beverlin B, Engrav L, et al: Diagnostic peritoneal lavage 14 years and 2586 patients later. *Am J Surg* 136:701, 1978.

28. Stengel D, Rademacher G, Ekkernkamp A, et al: Emergency ultrasound-based algorithms for diagnosing blunt abdominal trauma. *Cochrane Database Syst Rev* 9:CD004446, 2015.
29. American College of Surgeons Committee on Trauma: *Advanced Trauma Life Support for Doctors*. 9th ed. Chicago, American College of Surgeons, 2012.
30. Hoff WS, Holevar M, Nagy KK, et al: Practice management guidelines for the evaluation of blunt abdominal trauma: the EAST practice management guidelines work group. *J Trauma* 53:602–615, 2002.
31. Cha JY, Kashuk JL, Sarin EL, et al: Diagnostic peritoneal lavage remains a valuable adjunct to modern imaging techniques. *J Trauma* 67(2):330–334, 2009; discussion 334–336.
32. Kuncir EJ, Velmahos GC: Diagnostic peritoneal aspiration—the foster child of DPL: a prospective observational study. *Int J Surg* 5(3):167–171, 2007.
33. Fang JF, Chen RJ, Lin BC: Cell count ratio: new criterion of diagnostic peritoneal lavage for detection of hollow organ perforation. *J Trauma* 45(3):540, 1998.
34. Sriussadaporn S, Pak-art R, Pattaratiwanon M, et al: Clinical uses of diagnostic peritoneal lavage in stab wounds of the anterior abdomen: a prospective study. *Eur J Surg* 168(8–9):490, 2002.
35. Pham TN, Heinberg E, Cuschieri J, et al: The evaluation of the diagnostic work-up for stab wounds to the back and flank. *Injury* 40(1):48–53, 2009.
36. Lazarus HM, Nelson JA: A technique for peritoneal lavage without risk or complication. *Surg Gynecol Obstet* 149:889, 1979.
37. Sweeney JF, Albrink MH, Bischof E, et al: Diagnostic peritoneal lavage: volume of lavage effluent needed for accurate determination of a negative lavage. *Injury* 25:659, 1994.
38. Howdieshell TR, Osler RM, Demarest GB: Open versus closed peritoneal lavage with particular attention to time, accuracy and cost. *Am J Emerg Med* 7:367, 1989.
39. Nagy KK, Roberts RR, Joseph KT, et al: Experience with over 2500 diagnostic peritoneal lavages. *Injury* 31:479, 2000.
40. Hodgson NF, Stewart TC, Girotti MJ: Open or closed diagnostic peritoneal lavage for abdominal trauma? A metaanalysis. *J Trauma* 48(6):1091, 2000.
41. Cotter CP, Hawkins ML, Kent RB, et al: Ultrarapid diagnostic peritoneal lavage. *J Trauma* 29:615, 1989.
42. Gow KW, Haley LP, Phang PT: Validity of visual inspection of diagnostic peritoneal lavage fluid. *Can J Surg* 39:114, 1996.
43. Soyka J, Martin M, Sloan E, et al: Diagnostic peritoneal lavage: is an isolated WBC count greater than or equal to 500/mm^3 predictive of intra-abdominal trauma requiring celiotomy in blunt trauma patients? *J Trauma* 30:874, 1990.
44. Megison SM, Weigelt JA: The value of alkaline phosphatase in peritoneal lavage. *Ann Emerg Med* 19:5, 1990.
45. Jaffin JH, Ochsner G, Cole FJ, et al: Alkaline phosphatase levels in diagnostic peritoneal lavage as a predictor of hollow visceral injury. *J Trauma* 34:829, 1993.
46. Menegaux F, Tresallet C, Gosgnach M, et al: Diagnosis of bowel and mesenteric injuries in blunt abdominal trauma: a prospective study. *Am J Emerg Med* 24(1):19, 2006.
47. Fischer RP, Freeman T: The inadequacy of peritoneal lavage in diagnosing acute diaphragmatic rupture. *J Trauma* 16:538, 1976.

Chapter 24 ■ Interventional Radiology: Percutaneous Drainage Techniques

JOHN-PAUL B. VELASCO • BRIAN T. CALLAHAN • ROBERT SHEIMAN

Image-guided percutaneous drainage procedures have been established as safe and effective alternatives to surgery for the first-line treatment of clinically important fluid collections in the body. Image guidance typically provided by ultrasonography or computed tomography (CT) allows for precise localization of fluid collections and faster patient recovery times than open surgical techniques. Rapid image localization and percutaneous treatment has played a major role for avoiding the morbidity and mortality associated with surgical exploration [1–4].

GENERAL AIMS

The interventional radiologist should be part of the clinical team to help determine the clinical impact of a fluid collection and the expected outcome of percutaneous treatment. Close communication between interventional and critical care staff is, therefore, essential. Image-guided aspiration or drainage procedures can alleviate symptoms because of mass effect or infection, provide fluid samples for laboratory characterization to refine treatment, and cause reduction in sepsis [5]. A list of fluid collections amenable to image-guided procedures is provided in Table 24.1.

DIAGNOSTIC IMAGING

CT and ultrasound are the two main imaging modalities used for percutaneous image guidance. Magnetic resonance imaging (MRI)-guided drainage is available at some academic institutions, but has been limited by availability, cost, and paucity of MRI-compatible interventional devices. The choice between CT and ultrasound is ultimately determined by experienced operator, availability of equipment, and nature of the collection, such as size and location. Advantages of ultrasound include portability, lack of radiation, relatively low cost, and real-time visualization of needle placement into a collection (Fig. 24.1). Because ultrasound machines all currently have Doppler capability, arterial and venous structures along access routes to fluid are identified and avoided. Ultrasound is also not limited in its approach to a target as with CT which usually requires working in a fixed plane (axial). Limitations of ultrasound include poor visualization of deep collections secondary to large body habitus, bone, overlying bowel gas, or surgical dressings. CT, on the other hand, may provide better visualization of deep collections, such as those located in the pelvis or retroperitoneal space, [6] and a fluid collection's location relative to vital structures. The main limitations of CT include its lack of portability, radiation exposure, and cost. With the advent of faster parallel processors and reconstruction algorithms, CT fluoroscopy now exists that allows procedures to be performed faster and with less radiation to the patient [7,8].

TABLE 24.1

Fluid Collections Successfully Treated with Percutaneous Drainage

Sterile	Nonsterile
Ascites	
Hematoma	Enteric abscess
Lymphocele	Lung abscess and empyema
Pancreatic pseudocyst	Ruptured appendicitis
Postsurgical seroma	Pancreatic abscess
Urinoma	Tubo-ovarian abscess
Multilocular fluid collections	Cholecystitis

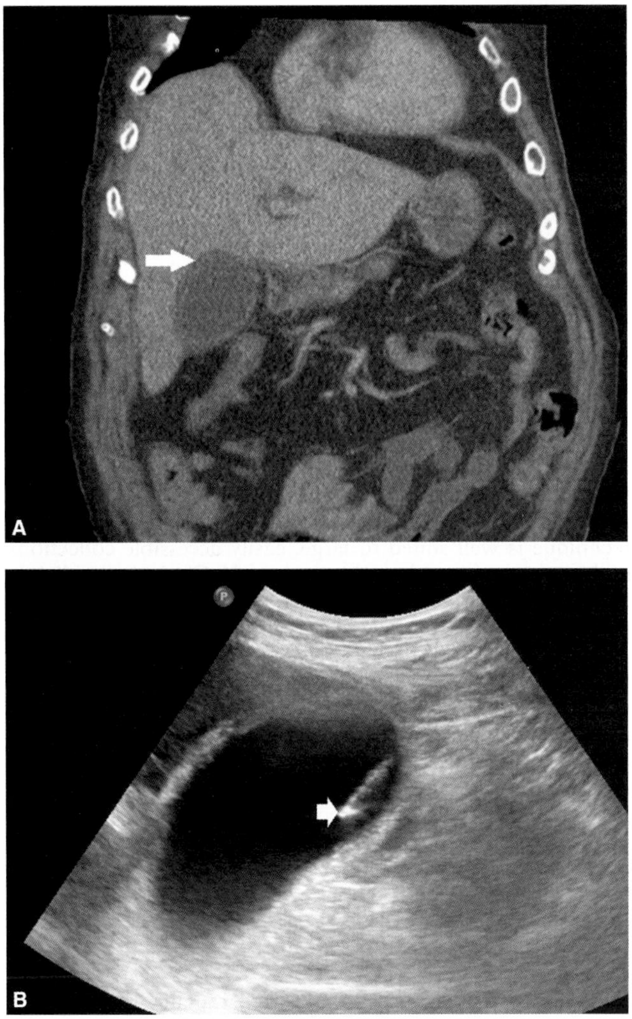

FIGURE 24.1 A 72-year-old male with a non–ST-elevation myocardial infarction presented with right upper quadrant pain and fever. **A:** Coronal computed tomography (CT) image demonstrating a thickened gallbladder wall with fluid in the gallbladder fossa (*arrow*). **B:** An ultrasound image demonstrating needle placement into the distended gallbladder (*arrowhead*) during ultrasound-guided cholecystostomy tube placement.

INDICATIONS

The indications for image-guided drainage and aspiration include, but are not limited to, fluid sampling to assess infected versus sterile collections, and abscess drainage. Sampling of a presumed infected collection for culture and antibiotic sensitivity, even after broad-spectrum antibiotics have been started, has been found to help tailor therapy in most patients [9]. Although fluid collections regardless of whether they are infected or benign (such as a seroma, lymphocele, or cyst of the kidney or liver) may cause issues for the patient, this is rare. Specific instances do exist and should be considered for critically ill patients, such as large volume ascites or pleural effusions causing continuous ventilator dependence or mass effect causing ureteral, biliary, or venous obstruction. For the critically ill patient, catheter drainage may stabilize the patient's condition so that a more definitive surgical procedure can be performed at a later time [10,11]. Abscess size and consistency are important determinants of the need for percutaneous drainage. Many patients with abscesses smaller than 4 cm in maximum diameter can be treated conservatively with broad-spectrum antibiotics [12]. When the interventional radiologist believes a collection represents an infected hematoma or a maturing infection, regardless of size, they may request initial conservative management and follow-up imaging to determine when catheter placement will lead to successful drainage.

CONTRAINDICATIONS

Absolute contraindications for percutaneous drainage historically have included the absence of a safe access route or uncorrectable coagulopathy, but these scenarios are now rare. A coagulopathy can usually be reversed (see Preprocedure Preparation below). Prior imaging may show a collection is inaccessible, but this is not absolute. In view of bowel motility and other options such as patient positioning, use of sterile fluid to displace structures temporarily (hydrodissection), inflation or deflation of the stomach or bladder for example, a safe route can often be found. The interventional radiologist should be able to think out of the box and offer a solution, especially in those cases where the only other alternative is surgery. For example, a transenteric (small bowel) route may allow for needle aspiration of a collection previously thought to be inaccessible [13]. If no direct route is available, the liver, kidney, and stomach may be safely transgressed during needle aspiration. Transgluteal, transvaginal, transrectal, or trans- inferior vena cava sampling provides more options for collections previously felt to be inaccessible [14–17].

When difficult to access or a coagulopathy does exist, risks and benefits have to be weighed, and this should be done in consensus with the intensive care unit (ICU) staff, and patient or health care proxy. Depending on the potential complication, the interventionalist may consider surgical backup. Patients or their health care proxy should be educated by both the clinical staff and radiologist to ensure that they are comfortable with their decision concerning a drainage procedure.

RISKS, BENEFITS, AND ALTERNATIVES

Overall complications associated with percutaneous drainage or aspiration are reported to be less than 15% [18]. These include damage to vital structures, bleeding, infection, among others. Mortality (ranging from 1% to 6%) is frequently secondary to sepsis or multiorgan failure rather than the procedure itself. Depending on the location and physical properties of an infected or a sterile collection, percutaneous drainage is curative in 75% to 90% of cases [6,18,19]. In approximately 10% of cases, percutaneous drainage can serve as a temporizing measure, allowing surgery to be postponed [12].

PREPROCEDURE PREPARATION

Regardless of the interventional procedure to be performed, certain basic principals apply to all patients. After review of the risks, benefits, and alternatives to the procedure, informed consent should be obtained from the patient or health care proxy [20]. The radiologist should have a firm understanding of the patient's clinical status which requires a comprehensive history and physical exam. A team approach is essential. Simply ordering a procedure without direct communication of concerns and goals with the interventional radiologist is suboptimal. Each case requires image review by the interventional radiologist and a discussion with the referring physicians to determine whether additional imaging is required, the procedure is technically possible, medically warranted, or if other treatment alternatives exist.

Once a collection has been identified and determined to be clinically relevant, the access route is planned with the basic rule that it should be the shortest and least invasive path. Prior to the procedure, the patient's primary caregivers should stop all anticoagulant medications, given that the benefits of the drainage procedure outweigh the risk to the patient from thrombosis. For example, clopidogrel (Plavix), an antiplatelet agent, should be held for 7 to 10 days before the procedure [21]. The role of a platelet transfusion just prior to a procedure in patients taking clopidogrel or other P2Y12 inhibitors is not well defined, although one unit of platelets may be prophylactically given. Rapid reversal of vitamin K agonists, such as Coumadin, can be achieved with fresh-frozen plasma and intravenous or oral vitamin K, and in extreme circumstances, a prothrombin complex concentrate. If time permits, holding Coumadin and bridging anticoagulation with low-molecular-weight heparin (given subcutaneously) or intravenous unfractionated heparin (given intravenously) [21,22] is another option. Newer target-specific anticoagulants, such as rivaoxaban and apixaban (target Factor Xa) and dabigatran (target Factor IIa), have gained traction because of predictable pharmacokinetics. A Food and Drug Administration–approved reversal agent is currently available for dabigatran, and other reversal agents for other drugs are in development [23]. It is believed that anticoagulants can be safely restarted 6 to 8 hours following the procedure. The goal is to achieve a the prothrombin time below 15 seconds, partial thromboplastin time less than 35 seconds, a platelet count greater than 50,000 per mL, and an international normalized ratio less than 1.5. However, the interventional radiologist should be flexible with these thresholds, depending on the urgency of the procedure.

The patient should have nothing to eat or drink for 4 to 6 hours prior to the study which includes tube feeds if applicable, to reduce the risk of aspiration during moderate sedation. Transient bacteremia associated with percutaneous drainage of an infected collection may require prophylactic treatment with antibiotics. The most common bacteria found in intra-abdominal abscesses are Gram-negative rods and anaerobes, particularly *Escherichia coli*, *Bacteroides fragilis*, and *Enterococcus* species. Thus, the current practice guidelines put forth by the Society of Interventional Radiology recommend the use of a third-generation cephalosporin [24]. Rarely, intravenous contrast is required to help identify a collection, so the patient's renal function (blood urea nitrogen and creatinine) should be evaluated. If abnormal (serum creatinine > 1.5 mg per dL, GFR < 30 mL/min/1.73 m^2), the patient may require hydration and pretreatment with sodium bicarbonate and oral or intravenous *N*-acetylcysteine (Mucomyst) [25]. For patients with a history of a prior contrast reaction, the incident should be discussed to determine whether symptoms were truly an anaphylactic reaction. In the setting of a validated contrast reaction, patients are usually pretreated with a combination of a steroid and an antihistamine. An acceptable approach is 50 mg of prednisone or 32 mg of methylprednisolone 12 hours prior to the procedure and then repeated at 2 hours prior to the procedure along with 50 mg diphenhydramine. Oral contrast may be given to patients prior to CT to better delineate bowel loops, keeping in mind the 6-hour window for nothing by mouth status to allow for sedation. Reports of unopacified bowel mistaken for an abscess collection are not uncommon.

ANESTHESIA AND MONITORING

Most image-guided drainage procedures are performed under local anesthesia in combination with moderate sedation. Typically, local anesthesia is achieved using 1% to 2% lidocaine, but longer acting agents, such as tetracaine gel or bupivacaine (lasting 4 to 8 hours), are available for procedures lasting more than a couple hours. For moderate sedation, the procedure is typically performed using a combination of intravenous fentanyl and midazolam or propofol. The interventional radiologist should be certified in the usage of conscious sedation and also be ACLS trained. Vital signs must be continuously monitored by an individual other than the radiologist and include pulse oximetry, blood pressure, and electrocardiography. For the infrequent event of cardiopulmonary resuscitation, a defibrillator, backboard, and code cart supplied with the necessary medications for advanced life support should always be available.

THERAPEUTIC CATHETER DRAINAGE

Catheter drainage systems can be introduced using the trocar or Seldinger technique. The trocar system consists of a 6.5- to 16-Fr pigtail catheter coaxially loaded over a hollow metal stiffener with a sharp inner stylet. Under image guidance, the trocar system is advanced together into the fluid collection. Next, the catheter is advanced off the cannula into the cavity, assuming its pigtail configuration. Advantages of the trocar technique include a single pass and less chance of access loss. The trocar technique is well suited to large, easily accessible collections and can be performed quickly and safely. Given the rigidity of the system, the trocar system is not recommended for drainage procedures where the collection is small or difficult to access.

An alternative to the trocar system for drain placement is the use of the Seldinger technique (Fig. 24.2). The Seldinger system involves two steps starting with insertion of an 18-gauge needle into a collection under image guidance through which a 0.035-inch guidewire is advanced into the cavity [26]. The guidewire is subsequently used for tract dilatation and catheter placement. This technique is best performed under continuous image guidance, such as CT fluoroscopy, because guidewire access can easily be lost in inexperienced hands.

Catheter Selection and Fixation

Catheter lengths are fairly standardized, ranging from 20 to 35 cm in length, and make use of a locking pigtail which must be released before catheter removal. A second type of locking device, a Malecot or "mushroom" catheter, can be deployed when the abscess cavity does not contain enough room for pigtail formation. Initial catheter size is chosen based on anticipated viscosity of the fluid being drained, but catheter upsizing using the same tract is straightforward when the current size is inadequate. For large collections or deep collections that cannot be reached by a standard 35 cm catheter, the interventional radiologist may become creative and use a biliary drainage catheter or nephroureteral stent, both of which contain numerous side holes and come in longer lengths. In addition to pigtail anchorage, skin adherent locking devices are used for catheter security. In some cases (disoriented patient, prior catheter dislodgement), suturing the catheter to the skin at its entrance site may be indicated. When the time comes, the universal approach to catheter removal is to cut the catheter at the distal end closest to the hub. This will release any type of anchoring mechanism. Because a pigtail is locked using a string, this must be accounted for and may come out with the catheter or be left after removal but clearly seen emerging from the catheter entrance site. This then is removed with gentle continuous traction.

One important side note must be taken into consideration. Cholecystitis has been reported in up to 1% of critically ill patients [27], and cholecystostomy tube placement is considered first-line treatment. Because the gallbladder may be in communication with the biliary tree through ducts of Luschka, or recannalization of an occluded cystic duct can occur, the tube needs to remain in place for at least 4 weeks to create a mature tract. This ensures that upon removal, there will be no bile leakage into the peritoneal cavity. This time aspect of cholecystostomy

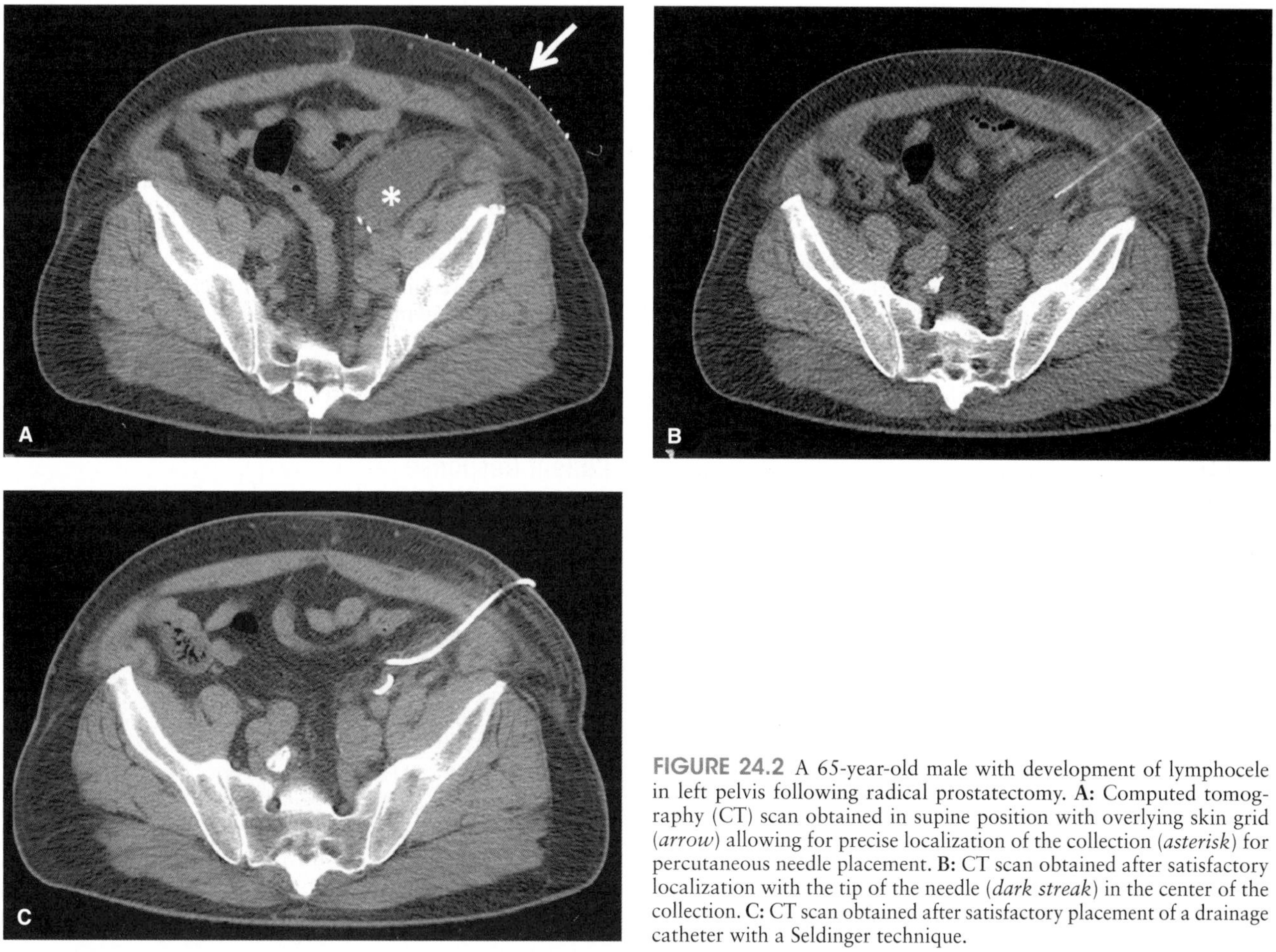

FIGURE 24.2 A 65-year-old male with development of lymphocele in left pelvis following radical prostatectomy. **A:** Computed tomography (CT) scan obtained in supine position with overlying skin grid (*arrow*) allowing for precise localization of the collection (*asterisk*) for percutaneous needle placement. **B:** CT scan obtained after satisfactory localization with the tip of the needle (*dark streak*) in the center of the collection. **C:** CT scan obtained after satisfactory placement of a drainage catheter with a Seldinger technique.

tube placement must be considered by the clinical team and also communicated to the patient or family.

Diagnostic or Therapeutic Aspiration

Usually, a 22- or 20-gauge needle is used for simple aspiration of a fluid collection. For a hematoma or more viscous collection, 16- or 18-gauge large-bore needles can be used [2,28]. Aspirated fluid can be sent for culture, Gram stain, and cytology when indicated. Additional laboratory tests can be added, such as in the case of evaluating fluid for amylase in a peripancreatic collection or creatinine in suspected urinomas. The relevance of collections felt to be clinically important solely because of their mass effect can be tested by large volume aspiration. In general, conversion from aspiration to catheter drainage can be done easily and is usually an anticipated possibility by the interventional radiologist.

PROCEDURE

General Considerations

With the advent of portable, high-resolution ultrasound machines, some diagnostic or therapeutic procedures may be performed at the bedside, the commonest being drainage of ascites, pleural effusions, and placement of cholecystostomy tubes. A variety of size needles, guidewires, and catheters should be available to the radiologist during the procedure. Given the variation in equipment on hand and the unanticipated need for other equipment not available in an ICU, such procedures should be solely reserved for subjects who are too unstable for transport.

All procedures are done adhering to sterile technique. In principle, a unilocular collection with a well-developed cavity wall is optimal but not required for percutaneous drainage. Loculated collections can often be handled by mechanical disruption using the guidewire placed while employing the Seldinger technique for catheter placement. Some authors advocate the use of thrombolytic agents, such as tissue plasminogen activator infused through the catheter once placed to aid in breaking down loculations [29]. For multiloculated or semisolid collections unresponsive to these measures, multiple drain placements may be required. If possible, drains should be inserted into the most dependent portion of the collection and as much of the collection drained at initial placement. The clinical success of catheter placement can be related to how well the collection responds to the reduction of its volume [30]. If the collection is felt to be the result of perforation of a hollow viscous (appendicitis, diverticulitis, and perforated ulcer), or leakage from the biliary tree or urinary tract for example, then after drain placement and immediate aspiration of contents, a catheter sinogram can be performed. Gentle injection of contrast or air under CT or fluoroscopic imaging (sonogram) can identify any communication which can be invaluable when developing a treatment plan for the patient (Fig. 24.3). The chance of creating sepsis or transient bacteremia from performing a sinogram at the time of drainage is a theoretical concern but rare in practice.

Catheter Management

Daily rounds by the interventional radiology team should be conducted to ensure the catheter is functioning correctly. It is useful to mark the level of the skin insertion on the catheter during initial placement to allow for easy assessment of catheter dislodgement. During rounds, the skin insertion site, catheter tubing, and amount of drainage should be evaluated. Most catheters are connected to a bag for passive external drainage. If dependent catheter position in the cavity undergoing drainage is not possible, Jackson–Pratt bulb suctioning can be used. Gentle irrigation of the abscess cavity with 10 to 20 mL of sterile saline is recommended three to four times daily to ensure patency [31]. Daily dressing changes should also be performed. In anticipation of the patient's discharge from the hospital, the patient and his or her family should be instructed in catheter care, and visiting nursing service is arranged. The patient is advised to return to the department in the event of abdominal pain, leakage from the catheter entry site, fever, or chills. When long-term drainage is anticipated, catheters should be exchanged approximately every 3 months to avoid blockage from encrustation or debris.

When to Remove a Catheter

Removal of a drainage catheter too early is one of the more common causes of postprocedural morbidity and mortality. The percutaneous drainage catheter should remain in place until the volume of drainage is less than 10 mL per day for 2 consecutive days, and the patient is showing clinical improvement. Reflux around the catheter during irrigation or new pain during irrigation are also signs of complete collection response and cavity collapse. Follow-up imaging on simple collections is typically not required prior to catheter removal. Continuous high drainage (>50 mL per day) should alert the radiologist for a possible fistulous tract to bowel, pancreas, or biliary tree, and the appropriate imaging modality should be used for further evaluation [10,32] if not already performed.

Patient Response

Depending on the location and makeup of an infected or sterile collection, image-guided percutaneous drainage is successful in

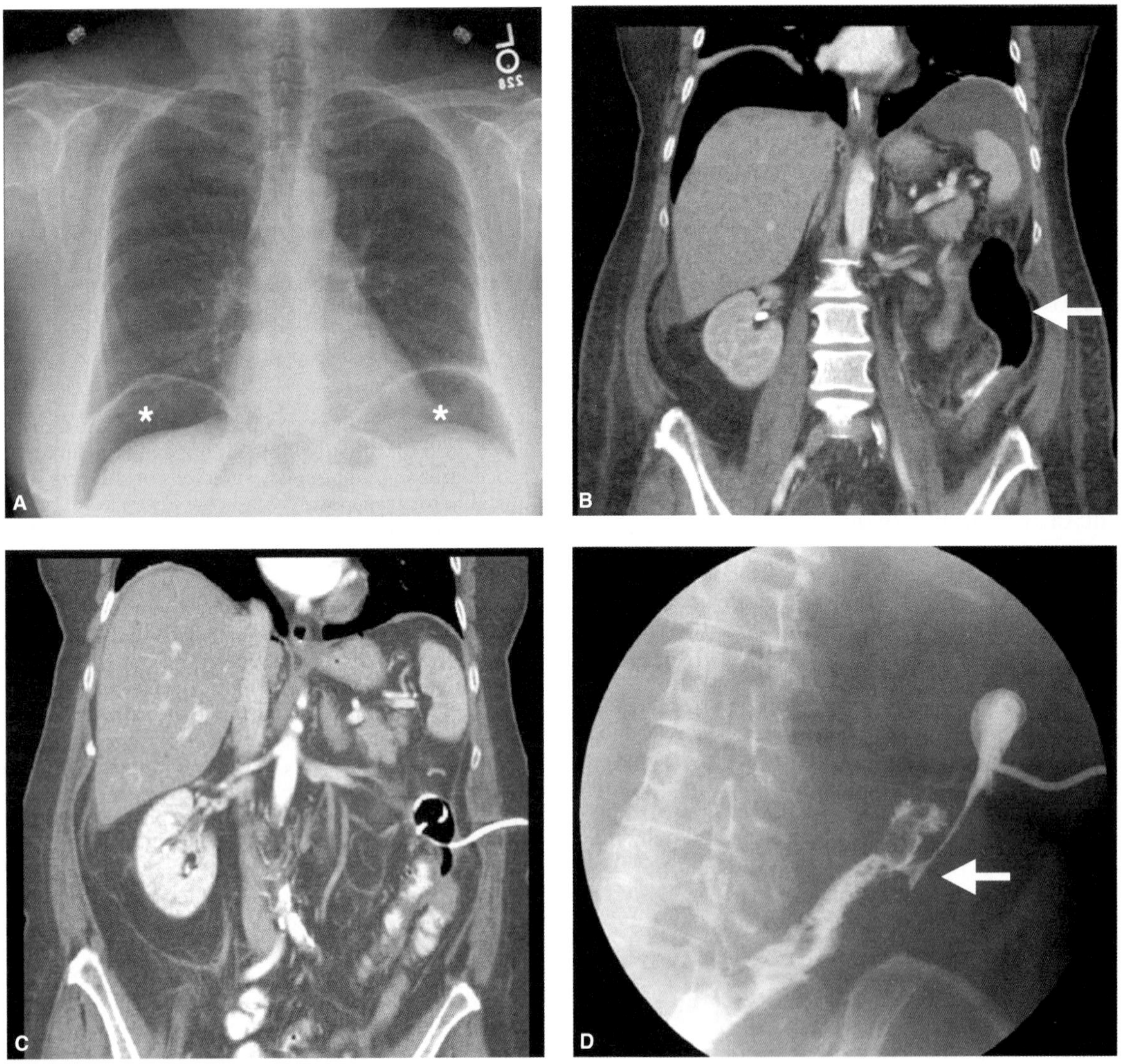

FIGURE 24.3 A 63-year-old female status post–recent sigmoid resection presenting with abdominal pain. **A:** Chest X-ray showing large amount of free intraperitoneal air (*asterisks*) concerning for bowel perforation. **B:** Computed tomography (CT) scan obtained with oral contrast showing large gas and fluid containing collection (*arrow*) from leak at the surgical anastomosis. **C:** CT scan performed after satisfactory position of drainage catheter into the collection. **D:** Owing to high drainage output (>50 mL per day), abscessogram was performed demonstrating a fistulous communication (*arrow*) with the descending colon.

70% to 90% of cases. Following complete evacuation of purulent material from an infected cavity, improved clinical response should be seen in a matter of hours to several days [10,13]. The parameters of improving clinical status include defervescence, reduction in pain, and resolution of leukocytosis. If there is no improvement after 2 to 3 days, suspicion should be raised for a separate, undrained collection, catheter dislodgement, or malfunction. In such cases, follow-up imaging using CT, ultrasound, or fluoroscopy with contrast injection into the collection is recommended. Semisolid collections, such as infected hematomas or pancreatic abscesses, are more resistant to drainage. In the case of a collection of necrotic debris from pancreatitis, one or more large-bore catheters (chest tubes) up to 24 Fr have been used with success, allowing a patient to avoid the morbidity of surgical debridement [33,34].

Complications

Overall complications of percutaneoue drainage are reported to be less than 15% [1–4], and most are minor. Major complications (under 5%) include infection, bleeding, septicemia, injury to adjacent structures such as bowel, and death. Mortality from the procedure usually related to sepsis or organ failure, compares favorably to the surgical literature rates of 10% to 20% [35]. Inadvertent contamination of a previously sterile collection is also a possibility with prolonged catheter drainage but only occurs among approximately 1% of cases [24]. Enteric transgression can usually be treated conservatively with delayed catheter removal to allow for a mature fistulous tract to develop. Minor complications include pain, infection at the skin insertion site, transient bacteremia, and malfunction of the catheter secondary to kinking, dislodgement, or clogging with debris, such as blood clots. Pain can be minimized by judicious use of analgesics. Daily catheter evaluation by the interventional staff can serve to reduce catheter malfunction. The recurrence rate following abscess drainage has been estimated to be between 5% and 10%. Recurrence may be caused by early catheter removal, failure to completely drain a loculated collection, or fistulous communication with the bowel, pancreatic duct, or biliary system. Repeat drainage of these cavities has been shown to be successful in 50% of patients with the need for surgical drainage reduced by half [3,36].

In conclusion, image-guided percutaneous aspiration and drainage has been established as the first-line treatment for sterile or infected fluid collections in the abdomen and pelvis. Awareness of the advantages and limitations of the procedure together with an integrated management approach between interventional and critical care staff will serve to benefit the patient and improve clinical outcomes.

References

1. Bufalari A, Giustozzi G, Moggi L: Postoperative intraabdominal abscesses: percutaneous versus surgical treatment. *Acta Chir Belg* 96:197, 1996.
2. vanSonnenberg E, Ferrucci JT, Mueller PR, et al: Percutaneous drainage of abscesses and fluid collections: technique, results and applications. *Radiology* 142:1, 1982.
3. Nakamoto DA, Haaga JR: Percutaneous drainage of postoperative intra-abdominal abscesses and collections, in Cope C (ed): *Current Techniques in Interventional Radiology*. Philadelphia, PA, Current Medicine, 1995.
4. vanWaes P, Feldberg M, Mali W, et al: Management of loculated abscesses that are difficult to drain: a new approach. *Radiology* 147:57, 1983.
5. Krebs TL, Daly B, Wong JJ, et al: Abdominal and pelvis therapeutic procedures using CT-fluoroscopic guidance. *Semin Intervent Radiol* 16:191, 1999.
6. Harisinghani MG, Gervais DA, Hahn PF, et al: CT-guided transgluteal drainage of deep pelvic abscesses: indications, technique, procedure-related complications, and clinical outcome. *RadioGraphics* 22:1353, 2002.
7. Daly B, Templeton P: Real-time CT floroscopy: evolution of an interventional tool. *Radiology* 211:309–315, 1999.
8. Carlson SK, Bender CE, Classic KL, et al: Benefits and safety of CT fluoroscopy in interventional radiologic procedures. Radiology 219(2):515–520, 2001.
9. McGillen KL, Boos J, Nathavitharana R, et al: Diagnostic yield and clinical impact of microbiologic diagnosis from CT-guided drainage in patients previously treated with empiric antibiotics. *Abdom Radiol* 42:298, 2017.
10. vanSonnenberg E, Wing VW, Casola G, et al: Temporizing effect of percutaneous drainage of complicated abscesses in critically ill patients. *AJR Am J Roentgenol* 142:821, 1984.
11. Bernini A, Spencer MP, Wong WD, et al: Computed tomography-guided percutaneous abscess drainage in intestinal disease. *Dis Colon Rectum* 40:1009, 1997.
12. Siewert B, Tye G, Kruskal J, et al: Impact of CT-guided drainage in the treatment of diverticular abscesses: size matters. *Am J Roentgenol* 186:680, 2006.
13. vanSonnenberg E, Gerhard R, Wittich MD, et al: Percutaneous abscess drainage: update. *World J Surg* 25:362, 2001.
14. Walser E, Raza S, Hernandez A, et al: Sonographically guided transgluteal drainage of pelvic abscesses. *Am J Roentgenol* 181:498, 2003.
15. Kuligowska E, Keller E, Ferrucci JT: Treatment of pelvic abscesses: value of one-step sonographically guided transrectal needle aspiration and lavage. *Am J Roentgenol* 164:201, 1995.
16. Sudakoff GS, Lundeen SJ, Otterson MF: Transrectal and transvaginal sonographic intervention of infected pelvic fluid collections: a complete approach. *Ultrasound Q* 21:175, 2005.
17. Gupta S, Ahrar K, Morello F, et al: Masses in or around the pancreatic head: CT-guided coaxial fine-needle aspiration biopsy with a posterior transcaval approach. *Radiology* 222(1):63–69, 2002.
18. vanSonnenberg E, Mueller PR, Ferrucci JT Jr: Percutaneous drainage of 250 abdominal abscesses and fluid collections. Part I. Results, failures, and complications. *Radiology* 151:337, 1984.
19. Lambiase RE, Deyoe L, Cronan JJ, et al: Percutaneous drainage of 335 consecutive abscesses: results of primary drainage with 1-year follow-up. *Radiology* 184:167, 1992.
20. Appelbaum PS, Grisso T: Assessing patients' capacities to consent to treatment. *N Engl J Med* 319(25):1635, 1988.
21. Kearon C, Hirsh MD: Management of Anticoagulation before and elective surgery. *N Engl J Med* 336(21):1506, 1997.
22. Douketis JD, Berger PB, Dunn AS, et al: The perioperative management of antithrombic therapy. *Chest* 133:299S, 2008.
23. Babilonia K, Trujillo T: The role of prothrombin complex concentrates in reversal of target specific anticoagulants. *Thromb J* 12:8, 2014.
24. Wallace JM, Chin KW, Fletcher TB et al: Quality improvement guidelines for percutaneous drainage/aspiration of abscess and fluid collections. *J Vasc Interv Radiol* 21:431–435, 2010.
25. Pannu N, Wiebe N, Tonelli M, et al: Prophylaxis strategies for contrast-induced neuropathy. *JAMA* 295(23):2765, 2006.
26. Harisinghani MG, Gervais DA, Maher MM, et al: Transgluteal approach for percutaneous drainage of deep pelvic abscesses: 154 cases. *Radiology* 228:701, 2003.
27. Laurila J, Syrjälä H, Laurila PA, et al: Acute acalculous cholecystitis in critically ill patients. *Acta Anaesthesiol Scand* 48(8):986–991, 2004.
28. vanSonnenberg E, Mueller PR, Ferrucci JT Jr: Percutaneous drainage of 250 abdominal abscesses and fluid collections. Part II Current procedural concepts. *Radiology* 151:343, 1984.
29. Shenoy-Bhangle AS, Gervais DA: Use of fibrinolytics in abdominal and pleural collections. *Semin Intervent Radiol* 29(4):264–269, 2012.
30. Kassi F, Dohan A, Soyer P, et al: Predictive factors for failure of percutaneous drainage of postoperative abscess after abdominal surgery. *Am J Surg* 207(6):915–921, 2014.
31. Hassinger SM, Harding G, Wongworawat D: High pressure pulsatile lavage propagates bacteria into soft tissue. *Clin Orthop Relat Res* 439:27, 2005.
32. Hui GC, Amaral J, Stephens D, et al: Gas distribution in intraabdominal and pelvic abscesses on CT is associated with drainability. *Am J Roentgenol* 184:915, 2005.
33. Freeny PC, Hauptmann E, Althaus SJ, et al: Percutaneous CT-guided catheter drainage of infected acute necrotizing pancreatitis: techniques and results. *Am J Roentgenol* 170(4):969–975, 1998.
34. Lee JK, Kwak KK, Park JK et al: The efficacy of nonsurgical treatment of infected pancreatic necrosis. *Pancreas* 34(4):399–404, 2007.
35. Deveney CW, Lurie K, Deveney KE: Improved treatment of intra-abdominal abscess: a result of improved localization, drainage, and patient care, not technique. *Arch Surg* 123:1126, 1988.
36. Gervais DA, Ho CH, O'Neill MJ, et al: Recurrent abdominal and pelvic abscesses: incidence, results of repeated percutaneous drainage, and underlying causes in 956 drainages. *Am J Roentgenol* 182:463, 2004.

Chapter 25 ■ Percutaneous Suprapubic Cystostomy

PHILIP J. AYVAZIAN

Percutaneous suprapubic cystostomy is used to divert urine from the bladder when standard urethral catheterization is impossible or undesirable [1–9]. The procedure for placement of a small diameter catheter is rapid, safe, and easily accomplished at the bedside under local anesthesia. This chapter will first address methods for urethral catheterization before discussing the percutaneous approach.

URETHRAL CATHETERIZATION

Urethral catheterization remains the principal method for bladder drainage. The indications for the catheter should be clarified, as they influence the type and size used. A history and physical examination with particular attention to the patient's genitourinary system is important.

Catheterization may be difficult with male patients in several instances. Patients with lower urinary tract symptoms (e.g., urinary urgency, frequency, nocturia, decreased stream, and hesitancy) may have benign prostatic hypertrophy. These patients may require a larger bore catheter, such as 20 or 22 French (Fr). Patients with a history of prior prostatic surgery such as transurethral resection of the prostate, open prostatectomy, or radical prostatectomy may have an irregular bladder neck as a result of contracture after surgery. The use of a coude tip catheter, which has an upper deflected tip, may help in negotiating the altered anatomy after prostate surgery. The presence of a high-riding prostate or blood at the urethral meatus suggests urethral trauma. In this situation, urethral integrity must be demonstrated by retrograde urethrogram before urethral catheterization is attempted.

Urethral catheterization for gross hematuria requires large catheters such as the 22 or 24 Fr, which have larger holes for irrigation and removal of clots. Alternatively, a three-way urethral catheter may be used to provide continuous bladder irrigation to prevent clotting. Large catheters impede excretion of urethral secretions, however, and can lead to urethritis or epididymitis if used for prolonged periods.

Technique

In males, after the patient is prepared and draped, 10 mL of a 2% lidocaine hydrochloride jelly is injected retrograde into the urethra. Anesthesia of the urethral mucosa requires 5 to 10 minutes after occluding the urethral meatus either with a penile clamp or manually to prevent loss of the jelly. The balloon of the catheter is tested, and the catheter tip is covered with a water-soluble lubricant. After stretching the penis upward perpendicular to the body, the catheter is inserted into the urethral meatus. The catheter is advanced up to the hub to ensure its entrance into the bladder. The balloon is not inflated until urine is observed in the drainage tubing to prevent urethral trauma. Irrigation of the catheter with normal saline helps verify the position. A common site of resistance to catheter passage is the external urinary sphincter within the membranous urethra, which may contract voluntarily. Any other resistance may represent a stricture necessitating urologic consultation. In patients with prior prostate surgery, an assistant's finger placed in the rectum may elevate the urethra and allow the catheter to pass into the bladder.

In females, short, straight catheters are preferred. Typically, a smaller amount of local anesthesia is used. Difficulties in catheter placement occur after urethral surgery, vulvectomy, vaginal atrophy, or with morbid obesity. In these cases, the meatus is not visible and may be retracted under the symphysis pubis. Blind catheter placement over a finger located in the vagina at the palpated site of the urethral meatus may be successful.

When urologic consultation is obtained, other techniques for urethral catheterization can be used. Flexible cystoscopy may be performed to ascertain the reason for difficult catheter placement and for insertion of a guidewire. A urethral catheter then can be placed over the guidewire by a Seldinger technique. Filiforms and followers are useful for urethral strictures.

Indications

On occasion, despite proper technique (as outlined previously), urethral catheterization is unsuccessful. These are the instances when percutaneous suprapubic cystostomy is necessary. Undoubtedly, the most common indication for percutaneous suprapubic cystostomy is for the management of acute urinary retention in men. Other indications for a percutaneous suprapubic cystostomy in the intensive care unit are listed in Table 25.1.

Contraindications

The contraindications to percutaneous suprapubic cystostomy are listed in Table 25.2. An inability to palpate the bladder or distortion of the pelvic anatomy from previous surgery or trauma makes percutaneous entry of the bladder difficult. In these situations, the risks of penetrating the peritoneal cavity become substantial. The bladder may not be palpable if the patient is in acute renal failure with oliguria or anuria, has a small contracted neurogenic bladder, or is incontinent. When the bladder is not palpable, it can be filled in a retrograde manner with saline to distend it. In men, a 14-Fr catheter is placed in the fossa navicularis just inside the urethral meatus, and the balloon is filled with 2 to 3 mL of sterile water to occlude the urethra. Saline is injected slowly into the catheter until the bladder is palpable; then, the suprapubic tube may be placed. In patients with a contracted neurogenic bladder, it is impossible to adequately distend the bladder by this approach. For these and most patients, ultrasonography is used to locate the bladder and allow the insertion of a 22-gauge spinal

TABLE 25.1

Indications for Percutaneous Cystostomy

- Unsuccessful urethral catheterization in the setting of acute urinary retention
- After prostatic surgery
- Presence of urethral trauma
- After anti-incontinence procedures
- Prostatic bilobar hyperplasia
- Urethral stricture
- Severe hypospadias
- Periurethral abscess
- Presence of severe urethral, epididymal, or prostate infection

TABLE 25.2

Contraindications to Percutaneous Cystostomy

Nonpalpable bladder
Previous lower abdominal surgery
Coagulopathy
Known bladder tumor
Clot retention

needle. Saline is instilled into the bladder via the needle to distend the bladder enough for suprapubic tube placement (Fig. 25.1).

In patients with previous lower abdominal surgery, ultrasonographic guidance is often necessary before a percutaneous cystostomy can be performed safely. Previous surgery can lead to adhesions that can hold a loop of intestine in the area of insertion. Other relative contraindications include patients with coagulopathy, a known history of bladder tumors, or active hematuria and retained clots. In patients with bladder tumors, percutaneous bladder access should be avoided because tumor cell seeding can occur along the percutaneous tract. Suprapubic cystostomy tubes are of small caliber and therefore do not function effectively with severe hematuria and retained clots. Instead, open surgical placement of a large caliber tube is necessary if urethral catheterization is impossible.

Technique

There are two general types of percutaneous cystostomy tubes that range in size from 8 to 14 Fr. The first type uses an obturator with a preloaded catheter. Examples include the Stamey catheter (Cook Urological, Spencer, IN) and the Bonanno catheter (Beckton Dickinson and Co., Franklin Lakes, NJ) [10]. The Stamey device is a polyethylene Malecot catheter with a luer lock hub that fits over a hollow needle obturator (Fig. 25.2A). When the obturator is locked to the hub of the catheter, the Malecot flanges are pulled inward (closed), and the system is ready for use. The Bonanno catheter uses a flexible 14-Fr Teflon tube, which is inserted over a hollow 18-gauge obturator (Fig. 25.2B). The obturator locks into the catheter hub and extends beyond the catheter tip. When the obturator is withdrawn, the tube pigtails in the bladder. One advantage of the Stamey catheter is that the flanges provide a secure retaining system. The Bonanno catheter generally induces fewer bladder spasms, however, and is better tolerated.

The second type of percutaneous cystostomy tube consists of a trocar and sheath, which are used to penetrate the abdominal wall and bladder. One of the most popular systems is the Lawrence suprapubic catheter (Rusch, Duluth, GA). This system allows a standard Foley catheter to be placed after removal of the trocar (Fig. 25.2C).

The patient is placed in the supine position; a towel roll may be placed under the hips to extend the pelvis. Trendelenburg may help to move the abdominal contents away from the bladder. The bladder is palpated to ensure that it is distended. The suprapubic region is clipped, prepared with 10% povidone-iodine solution, and draped with sterile towels. The insertion site is several centimeters above the symphysis pubis in the midline. This approach avoids the epigastric vessels. In obese patients with a large abdominal fat pad, the fold is elevated. The needle should be introduced into the suprapubic crease, where the fat thickness is minimal. After obtaining consent and performing a time-out, 1 % lidocaine is used to anesthetize the skin, subcutaneous tissues, rectus fascia, and retropubic space. A 22-gauge spinal needle with a 5-mL syringe is directed vertically and advanced until urine is aspirated. If the bladder is smaller or if the patient had previous pelvic surgery, the needle is directed

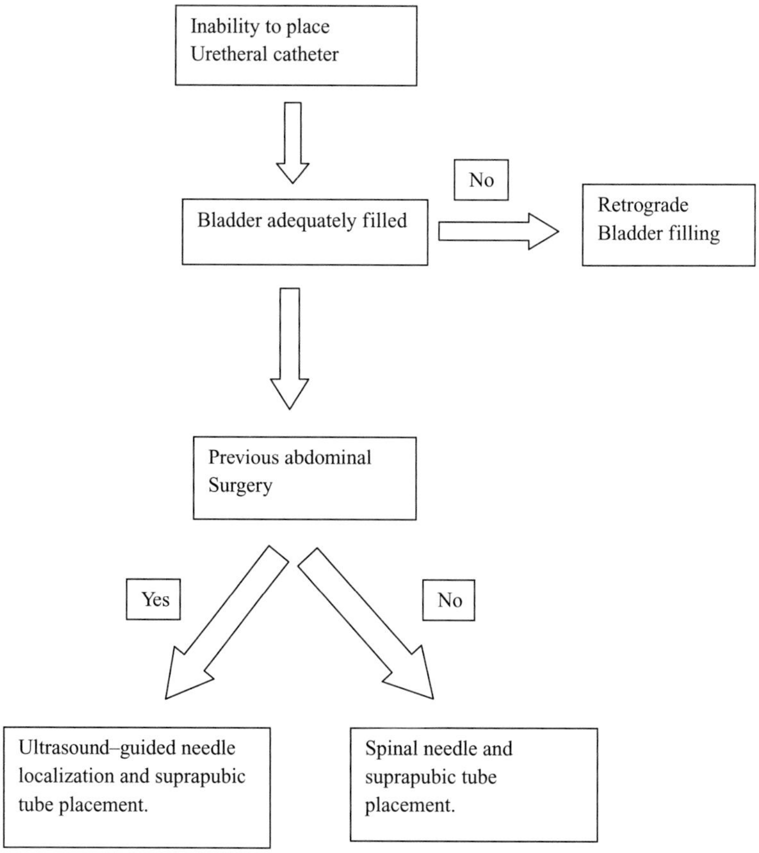

FIGURE 25.1 Algorithm for percutaneous suprapubic tube placement.

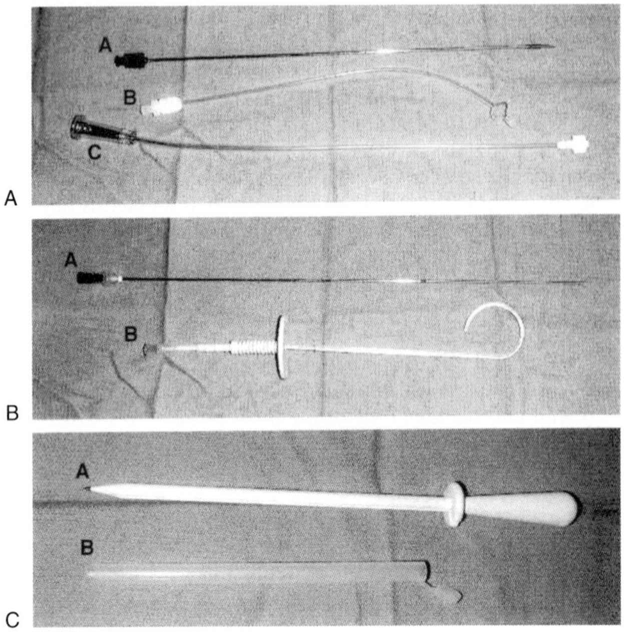

FIGURE 25.2 **A:** Stamey suprapubic cystostomy trocar set (A is the obturator, B is the Malecot catheter, and C is the drainage tube). **B:** Bonanno catheter set (A is the obturator and B is the catheter). **C:** Lawrence suprapubic catheter (A is the trocar and B is the sheath).

at a 60-degree caudal angle. Insertion of the cystostomy tube is predicated on the feasibility of bladder puncture and after the angle and depth of insertion is established with the spinal needle (Fig. 25.3).

At the site of bladder puncture, a small 2-mm incision is made with a No. 11 blade. The catheter mounted on the obturator is advanced toward the bladder. Two hands are used to grasp the system to provide a forceful, but controlled, thrust through the abdominal wall. One hand can be positioned on the obturator at a site marking the depth of the bladder. A syringe attached to the end of the obturator is used to aspirate urine and confirm obturator placement. Once the bladder is penetrated, the entire system is advanced 2 to 3 cm. This prevents the catheter tip from withdrawing into the retropubic space when the bladder decompresses. After unlocking the obturator from the catheter, the obturator acts as a guide while the catheter is advanced into the bladder. When using a Stamey catheter, the catheter can be gently withdrawn until the Malecot flanges meet resistance against the anterior bladder wall. The Stamey catheter is then advanced 2 cm back into the bladder to allow for movement. This maneuver pulls the catheter away from the bladder trigone and helps reduce bladder spasms. The same general technique applies to placement of the Lawrence suprapubic catheter system. After the bladder is penetrated, urine appears at the hub of the suprapubic catheter introducer (trocar plus sheath). The trocar is then removed, and a Foley catheter is inserted. The Foley catheter balloon is inflated to secure it in the bladder. Pulling the tab at the top of the peel-away sheath allows the remaining portion of the sheath to be removed away from the catheter.

The patency of the catheter is assessed by irrigating the bladder after decompression. The catheter can be fixed with a simple nylon suture and sterile dressing. The Bonanno catheter contains a suture disc. The Lawrence suprapubic catheter does not require extra fixation, because the balloon on the Foley catheter secures it in place.

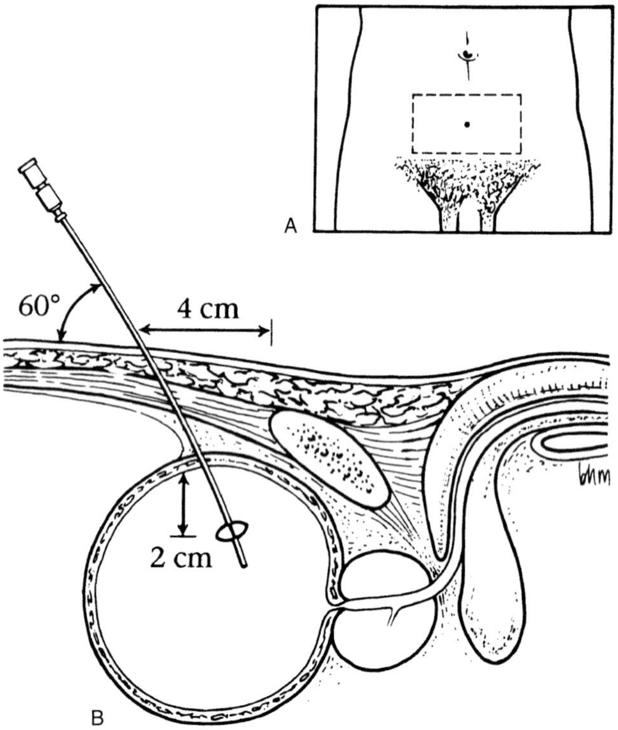

FIGURE 25.3 Technique of suprapubic trocar placement. **A:** Area to be shaved, prepared, and draped before trocar placement. **B:** Position of the Stamey trocar in the bladder. The angle, distance from the pubis, and position of the catheter in relation to the bladder wall are demonstrated.

SUPRAPUBIC CATHETER CARE

Bladder spasms occur commonly after suprapubic catheter placement. When using a Stamey catheter or a Foley catheter, bladder spasms can be prevented by withdrawing the tube until it meets the anterior bladder wall and then advancing 2 cm back into the bladder. Persistent bladder spasms can be treated with anticholinergic therapy (e.g., oxybutynin and hyoscyamine). This medication should be discontinued before removing the suprapubic tube to prevent urinary retention.

A suprapubic tube that ceases to drain is usually caused by kinking of the catheter or displacement of the catheter tip into the retropubic space. If necessary, suprapubic catheters may be replaced using either an exchange set (available for Stamey catheters) or by dilating the cystostomy tract. Closure of the percutaneous cystostomy tract is generally prompt after the tube is removed. Prolonged suprapubic tube use can lead to a mature tract, which may take several days to close. If the tract remains open, bladder decompression via a urethral catheter may be required.

COMPLICATIONS

Placement of suprapubic cystostomy tubes is generally safe with infrequent complications.

Possible complications are listed in Table 25.3. Bowel complications are severe but rare with this procedure [11,12]. Penetration of the peritoneal cavity or bowel perforation produces peritoneal or intestinal symptoms and signs. This complication can be avoided by attempting the procedure only on well-distended bladders and using a midline approach no more than 4 cm above the pubis.

In patients who have had previous lower abdominal or pelvic surgery, an ultrasound should be used to properly place the suprapubic tube and rule out entrapped bowel (Fig. 25.4).

TABLE 25.3

Complications of Percutaneous Cystostomy

Peritoneal and bowel perforation
Hematuria
Retained or calcified catheter
Bladder stones
Postobstructive diuresis
Hypotension
Bladder perforation

Patients who develop peritoneal symptoms and signs require a full evaluation of not only the location of the suprapubic tube (by a cystogram) but also of the cystostomy tract. A kidney-ureter-bladder X-ray and computed tomography scans may be required.

Hematuria is the most common complication after suprapubic tube placement. Rarely, it requires open cystostomy for placement of a large caliber tube for irrigation. Hematuria can occur secondary to laceration of a submucosal vessel or rapid decompression of a chemically distended bladder. It can be avoided by gradual bladder decompression.

Complications associated with the catheter include loss of a portion of the catheter in the bladder, calcification of the catheter, or bladder stone formation. These complications can be avoided by preventing prolonged catheter use. Beyond 4 weeks, evaluation and replacement or removal must be considered.

When chronically distended bladders are decompressed, patients are at risk of postobstructive diuresis. Patients who are at greatest risk include those with azotemia, peripheral edema, congestive heart failure, and mental status changes. Patients with postobstructive diuresis (i.e., urine outputs greater than 200 mL per hour) require frequent monitoring of vital signs and intravenous fluid replacement.

Hypotension rarely occurs after suprapubic tube placement. It may be caused by a vasovagal response or relief of pelvic veins compressed by bladder distention. Prompt fluid administration is the treatment for this complication.

Another rare complication is through-and-through bladder perforation. This is treated conservatively with bladder decompression.

UTILITY OF ULTRASONOGRAPHY FOR PERCUTANEOUS CYSTOSTOMY AND URETHRAL CATHETERIZATION

Ultrasonography has useful application for the performance of percutaneous cystostomy [13]. The experienced urologist will generally not use ultrasonography to perform percutaneous cystostomy; as, in their expert hands, the procedure can be performed with a high degree of safety [14]. The exception would be when there is history of lower abdominal surgery, where the risk of bowel injury is increased. It is unusual for an intensivist to perform percutaneous cystostomy, but, should the need arise, ultrasonography is particularly helpful to the less experienced operator, as the fluid-filled bladder can be readily identified with ultrasonography [7]. This allows for accurate identification of safe site, depth, and angle for device insertion into the bladder, similar in principle to that required for thoracentesis or paracentesis.

Using a transverse imaging plane, the phased array probe (or curvilinear abdominal probe if available) is placed immediately above the pubic bone in the midline. The fluid-filled bladder is identified as an anechoic space subtended by characteristic boundaries. When filled to moderate extent, the bladder has a square configuration; when distended, it becomes rounded in shape. By angling the probe from the transverse plane downward into the pelvis, the entire structure can be examined. The best site for device insertion that avoids interposed bowel is identified and marked. The risk that the bowel might be in the target area is of special concern, if there is history of lower abdominal surgery. The depth and best angle for device insertion is determined, followed by performance of the procedure. Ascites may be mistaken for a full bladder. This pitfall may be avoided by identifying bowel loops within the ascites, and by detection of ascites elsewhere in the abdomen. Ultrasonography also has useful application for the performance of difficult urethral catheterization. In the male patient with an enlarged prostate, passage of the urethral catheter may be difficult. The tip of the catheter may enter the bladder with drainage of urine, but with the catheter balloon remaining in the proximal urethra at the level of the prostate. Inflation of the balloon may injure the proximal urethra. When there is difficulty with catheter insertion and uncertainty concerning the position of the catheter balloon, real-time ultrasonography of the bladder during catheter insertion allows the intensivist to determine proper balloon position prior to its inflation. Ultrasonography guidance of catheter insertion is not required for routine urethral catheterization.

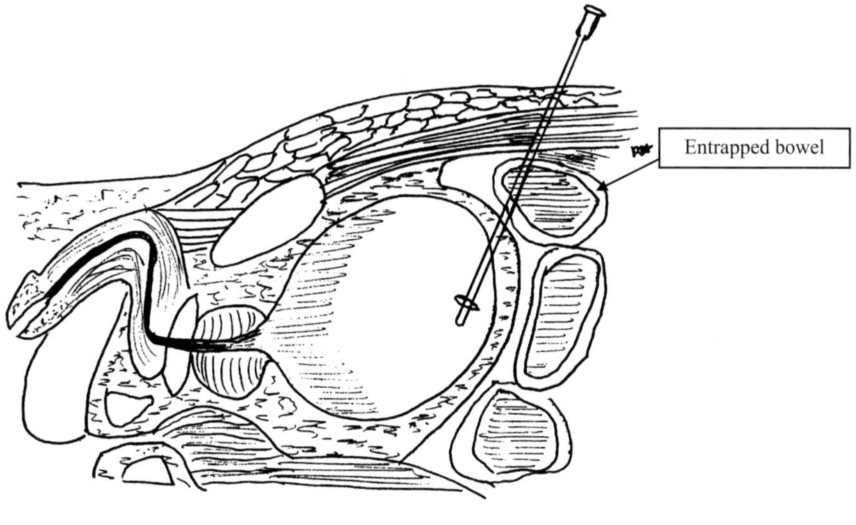

FIGURE 25.4 Placement of the suprapubic tube can perforate the entrapped bowel.

References

1. Sethia KK, Selkon JB, Berry AR, et al: Prospective randomized controlled trial of urethral versus suprapubic catheterization. *Br J Surg* 74:624–625, 1987.
2. Wein AJ, Kavocsi LR, Novick AC, et al: *Campbell-Walsh Urology*. 9th ed. Philadelphia, PA: Saunders/Elsener, 2007.
3. O'Brien WM: Percutaneous placement of a suprapubic tube with peel away sheath introducer. *J Urol* 145:1015–1016, 1991.
4. Chiou RK, Morton JJ, Engelsigjerd JS, et al: Placement of large suprapubic tube using peel-away sheath introducer. *J Urol* 153:1179–1181, 1995.
5. Meessen S, Bruhl P, Piechota HJ: A new suprapubic cystostomy trocar system. *Urology* 56:315–316, 2000.
6. Lee MJ, Papanicolaou N, Nocks BN, et al: Fluoroscopically guided percutaneous suprapubic cystostomy for long-term bladder drainage: an alternative to surgical cystostomy. *Radiology* 188:787–789, 1993.
7. Aguilera PA, Choi T, Durham BA: Ultrasound-guided suprapubic cystostomy catheter placement in the emergency department. *J Emerg Med* 26(3):319–321, 2004.
8. Irby PB, Stoller ML: Percutaneous suprapubic cystostomy. *J Endourol* 7(2):125–130, 1993.
9. Lawrentschuk N, Lee D, Marriott P, et al: Suprapubic stab cystostomy: a safer technique. *Urology* 62(5):932–934, 2003.
10. Bonanno PJ, Landers DE, Rock DE: Bladder drainage with the suprapubic catheter needle. *Obstet Gynecol* 35:807–812, 1970.
11. Drutz HP, Khosid HI: Complications with Bonanno suprapubic catheters. *Am J Obstet Gynecol* 149:685–686, 1984.
12. Dogra PN, Goel R: Complication of percutaneous suprapubic cystotomy. *Int Urol Nephrol* 36(3):343–344, 2004.
13. Harrison SC, Lawrence WT, Morley R, et al: British Association of Urological Surgeons' suprapubic catheter practice guidelines. *BJU Int* 107:77–85, 2011.
14. Johnson S, Fiscus G, Sudakoff GS, et al: The utility of abdominal ultrasound during percutaneous suprapubic catheter placement. *Can J Urol* 20:6840–6843, 2013.

Chapter 26 ■ Aspiration of the Knee and Synovial Fluid Analysis

PADMANAIDU KARNAM • BONNIE J. BIDINGER • DEBORAH M. DEMARCO

Arthrocentesis is a safe and relatively simple procedure that involves the introduction of a needle into a joint space to remove synovial fluid. It constitutes an essential part of the evaluation for arthritis of unknown cause, frequently with the intent to rule out a septic process [1–3].

Ropes and Bauer [4] first categorized synovial fluid as *inflammatory* or *noninflammatory* in 1953. In 1961, Hollander et al. [5] and Gatter and McCarty [6] coined the term *synovianalysis* to describe the process of joint fluid analysis and were instrumental in establishing its critical role in the diagnosis of certain forms of arthritis. Septic arthritis and crystalline arthritis can be diagnosed by synovial fluid analysis alone. They may present similarly but require markedly different treatments, thus necessitating early arthrocentesis and prompt synovial fluid analysis.

INDICATIONS

Arthrocentesis is performed for diagnostic and therapeutic purposes. The main indication for arthrocentesis is to assist in the evaluation of arthritis of unknown cause. In the intensive care unit, it is most commonly performed to rule out septic arthritis or crystalline arthritis. As many types of inflammatory arthritis mimic septic arthritis, synovial fluid analysis is essential in differentiating the various causes of inflammatory arthritis [4,7] (Table 26.1). Therefore, patients presenting with acute monoarthritis or oligoarthritis require prompt arthrocentesis with subsequent synovial fluid analysis, preferably before initiation of treatment.

Arthrocentesis is also used for therapeutic purposes. In a septic joint, serial joint aspirations are often required to remove accumulated inflammatory or purulent fluid. This accomplishes complete drainage of a closed space and allows serial monitoring of the total white blood cell count, Gram stain, and culture to assess treatment response. Inflammatory fluid contains many destructive enzymes that contribute to cartilage and bony degradation; removal of the fluid may slow this destructive process [8,9]. Additionally, arthrocentesis allows for injection of long-acting corticosteroid preparations into the joint space, which may be a useful treatment for various inflammatory and noninflammatory forms of arthritis [10].

TABLE 26.1

Common Causes of Noninflammatory and Inflammatory Arthritides

Noninflammatory	Inflammatory
Osteoarthritis	Rheumatoid arthritis
Trauma/internal derangement	Spondyloarthropathies
Avascular necrosis	Psoriatic arthritis
Hemarthrosis	Reiter's syndrome/reactive arthritis
Malignancy	Ankylosing spondylitis
Benign tumors	Ulcerative colitis/regional enteritis
Osteochondroma	Crystal-induced arthritis
Pigmented villonodular synovitis	Monosodium urate (gout)
	Calcium pyrophosphate deposition disease (pseudogout)
	Calcium pyrophosphate dihydrate (pseudogout)
	Hydroxyapatite
	Infectious arthritis
	Bacterial
	Mycobacterial
	Fungal
	Connective tissue diseases
	Systemic lupus erythematosus
	Vasculitis
	Scleroderma
	Polymyositis
	Hypersensitivity
	Serum sickness

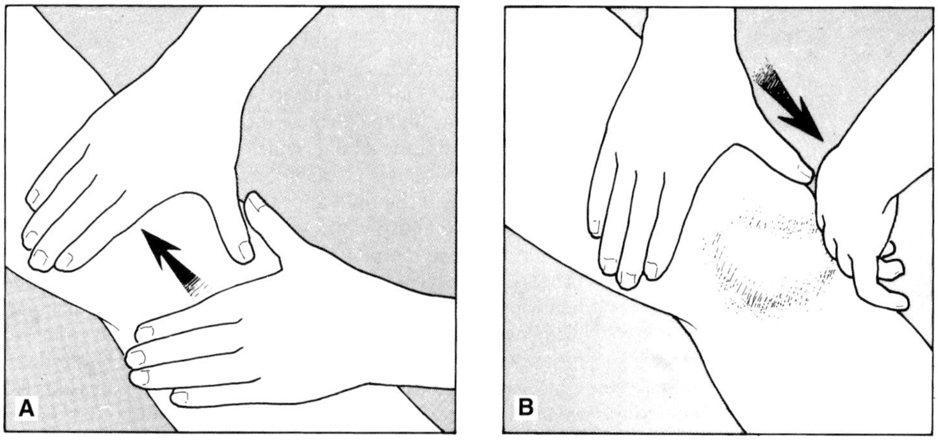

FIGURE 26.1 The bulge test. **A:** Milk fluid from the suprapatellar pouch into the joint. **B:** Slide the hand down the lateral aspect of the joint line and watch for a bulge medial to the joint.

Before performing arthrocentesis, it must be ascertained that the true joint is inflamed and an effusion is present. This requires a meticulous physical examination to differentiate arthritis from periarticular inflammation. Bursitis, tendinitis, and cellulitis all may mimic arthritis. In the knee, the examination begins with assessment of swelling. A true effusion may cause bulging of the parapatellar gutters and the suprapatellar pouch [11]. The swelling should be confined to the joint space. To check for small effusions, the bulge test is performed [12]. Fluid is stroked from the medial joint line into the suprapatellar pouch and then from the suprapatellar pouch down along the lateral joint line. If a bulge of fluid is noted at the medial joint line, a small effusion is present (Fig. 26.1). If a large effusion is present, one can detect a ballotable patella by pushing it against the femur with the right index finger while applying pressure to the suprapatellar pouch with the left hand [13]. Comparison with the opposite joint is helpful. Many texts describe joint examination and assessment for fluid in the knee and other joints [11–13].

CONTRAINDICATIONS

Absolute contraindications to arthrocentesis include local infection of the overlying skin or other periarticular structures and severe coagulopathy [1–3,10]. If coagulopathy is present and septic arthritis is suspected, every effort should be made to correct the coagulopathy (with fresh-frozen plasma or alternate factors; see Chapters 88 & 89 Disorders of Hemostasis) before joint aspiration. Therapeutic anticoagulation is not an absolute contraindication, but every effort should be made to avoid excessive trauma during aspiration, including using a smaller size needle. Known bacteremia is a relative contraindication because inserting a needle into the joint space disrupts capillary integrity, allowing joint space seeding [14]. However, if septic arthritis is strongly suspected, joint aspiration is indicated. The presence of articular instability (e.g., that seen with badly damaged joints) is a relative contraindication, although the presence of a large amount of presumed inflammatory fluid may still warrant joint aspiration.

COMPLICATIONS

The major complications of arthrocentesis are iatrogenically induced infection and bleeding, both of which are extremely rare [1]. The risk of infection after arthrocentesis has been estimated to be less than one in 10,000 [15]. Hollander [16] reported an incidence of less than 0.005% in 400,000 injections. Strict adherence to aseptic technique reduces the risk of postarthrocentesis infection. Significant hemorrhage is also extremely rare. Correction of prominent coagulopathy before arthrocentesis reduces this risk.

Another potential complication of arthrocentesis is direct injury to the articular cartilage by the needle. This is not quantifiable, but any injury to the cartilage could be associated with degenerative change over time. To avoid cartilaginous damage, the needle should be pushed in only as far as necessary to obtain fluid, and excessive movement of the needle during the procedure should be avoided.

Other complications include discomfort from the procedure itself, allergic reactions to the skin preparation or local anesthetic, and in the case of steroid injection, postinjection flare and local soft-tissue atrophy from the glucocorticoid [17].

TECHNIQUE

Joint aspiration is easily learned. A sound knowledge of the joint anatomy, including the bony and soft-tissue landmarks used for joint entry, is needed. Strict aseptic technique must be followed to minimize risk of infection, and relaxation of the muscles surrounding the joint should be encouraged because muscular contraction can impede the needle's entry into the joint.

Most physicians in the intensive care unit can aspirate the knee because it is one of the most accessible joints. Other joints should probably be aspirated by an appropriate specialist, such as a rheumatologist or an orthopedic surgeon. Certain joints are quite difficult to enter blindly and are more appropriately entered using guidance with ultrasonography, fluoroscopy, or computed tomography; these include the hip, sacroiliac, and temporomandibular joints. Many texts describe in detail the aspiration technique of other joints [3,16–18]. The technique for knee aspiration is as follows:

1. Describe the procedure to the patient, including the possible complications, and obtain written informed consent.
2. Collect all items needed for the procedure (Table 26.2).
3. With the patient supine and the knee fully extended, examine the knee to confirm the presence of an effusion, as described previously.
4. Identify landmarks for needle entry. The knee may be aspirated from a medial or lateral approach. The medial approach is more commonly used and is preferred when small effusions are present. Identify the superior and inferior borders of the patella. Entry should be halfway between the borders, just inferior to the undersurface of the patella (Fig. 26.2). The entry site may be marked with pressure from the needle cover with the needle removed. An indentation mark should be visible.
5. Cleanse the area with 10% povidone-iodine or 2% chlorhexidine in 70% isopropyl alcohol (if the patient is allergic to iodine) and allow the area to dry. Practice universal precautions: wear gloves at all times while handling any body fluid, although

TABLE 26.2

Arthrocentesis Equipment

Procedure	Equipment
Skin preparation and local anesthesia	10% povidone-iodine or 2% chlorhexidine in 70% isopropyl alcohol Ethyl chloride spray For local anesthesia—1% lidocaine; 25-gauge, 1.5-in needle; 22-gauge, 1.5-in needle; 5-mL syringe Sterile sponge/cloth
Arthrocentesis	Gloves 20- to 60-mL syringe (depending on size of effusion) 18- to 22-gauge, 1.5-in needle Sterile sponge/cloth Sterile clamp Sterile bandage
Collection	15-mL anticoagulated tube (with sodium heparin or ethylenediaminetetraacetic acid) Sterile tubes for routine cultures Slide, cover slip

they need not be sterile for routine knee aspiration. Do not touch the targeted area once it has been cleaned.

6. Apply local anesthesia. A local anesthetic (1% lidocaine) may be instilled subcutaneously with a 25-gauge, 1.5-in needle. Once numbing has occurred, deeper instillation of the local anesthetic to the joint capsule can be performed. Some physicians use ethyl chloride as an alternative anesthetic. However, this agent provides only superficial anesthesia of the skin. Spray ethyl chloride directly onto the designated area and stop when the first signs of freezing are evident in order to limit potential for skin damage.

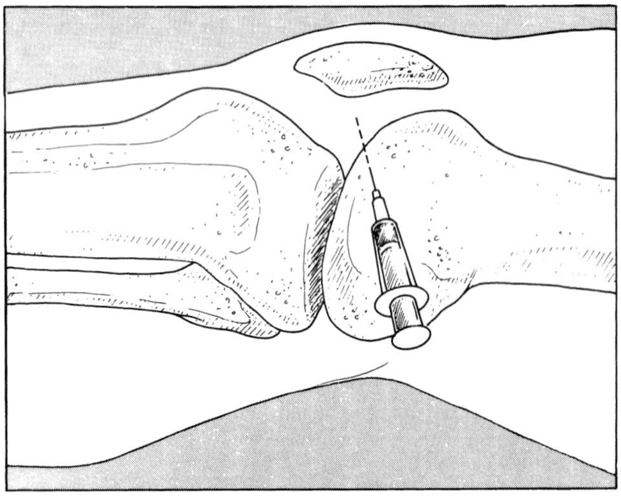

FIGURE 26.2 Technique of aspirating the knee joint. The needle enters halfway between the superior and inferior borders of the patella and is directed just inferior to the patella.

7. To enter the knee joint, use an 18- to 22-gauge, 1.5-in needle with a 20- to 60-mL syringe. Use a larger gauge needle particularly if septic arthritis is suspected as the aspirated fluid may be purulent and more difficult to aspirate. Use a quick thrust through the skin and on through the capsule to minimize pain. Avoid hitting periosteal bone, which causes significant pain, or cartilage, which causes cartilaginous damage. Aspirate fluid to fill the syringe. If the fluid appears purulent or hemorrhagic, try to tap the joint dry, which will remove mediators of inflammation that may perpetuate an inflammatory or destructive process. If the syringe is full and more fluid remains, a sterile hemostat may be used to clamp the needle, thus stabilizing it, while switching syringes. When the syringes have been switched, more fluid can be withdrawn. The syringes must be sterile.
8. On occasion, effusions can be difficult to aspirate. Reasons for this include increased fluid viscosity, fibrin and other debris impeding flow through the needle, loculated fluid, and use of a needle with an inappropriately small gauge. Additionally, the fluid may not be accessible by the approach being used [19]. At times, one can obtain a small drop of joint fluid by using continuous suction as the needle is withdrawn from the joint space [17]. This small specimen can then be sent for Gram stain, culture, and if possible, crystal analysis.
9. When fluid has been obtained, quickly remove the needle and apply pressure to the needle site with sterile gauze. When bleeding has stopped, remove the gauze, clean the area with alcohol, and apply an adhesive bandage. If the patient is receiving anticoagulation therapy or has a bleeding diathesis, apply prolonged pressure.
10. Document the amount of fluid obtained and perform a gross examination, noting the color and clarity. Send fluid for cell count with differential count, Gram stain, routine culture, specialized cultures for *Gonococcus*, *Mycobacterium*, and fungus, if indicated, and polarized microscopic examination for crystal analysis. Other tests, such as glucose and complement determinations, are generally not helpful. Use an anticoagulated tube to send fluid for cell count and crystal analysis. Sodium heparin or ethylenediaminetetraacetic acid are appropriate anticoagulants. Lithium heparin and calcium oxalate should be avoided because they can precipitate out of solution to form crystals, thus potentially giving a false-positive assessment for crystals [6,20]. Fluid may be sent for Gram stain and culture in the syringe capped with a blunt tip or in a sterile redtop tube. It is best to check with the institution's laboratory in advance as procedures vary regarding the handling of synovial fluid and the proper tubes in which to send it.

UTILITY OF ULTRASONOGRAPHY FOR KNEE JOINT ASPIRATION

Ultrasonography has several useful applications related to aspiration of the knee joint.

Identification of Knee Joint Effusion

Ultrasonography examination of the knee is a useful means of verifying whether there is a fluid collection in the knee joint. As indicated in this chapter, physical examination is an effective means of identifying a knee joint effusion. However, patient-specific factors such as obesity, edema, or anatomic abnormalities as well as lack of experience by the examiner may degrade the standard physical examination for knee effusion. In this case, ultrasonography is useful in identifying fluid [21]. This avoids errors that could lead to an attempt at arthrocentesis when no fluid is present or the converse, where fluid is present but not identified. The knee is examined with the leg in a straight and fully supported position. The linear vascular probe is preferred, as it has excellent resolution; and most knee joint effusions are within its depth range. The probe is placed over the medial or lateral knee joint in coronal scanning plane. The initial tomographic plane is anterior in order to identify the periosteum of the patella. The probe is moved posteriorly to move the scanning plane deep to the patella. The knee effusion is identified as an anechoic or hypoechoic space between the patella and the more posterior periosteum of the long bones of the leg. Stranding or loculations may be present suggesting a complex effusion. Other scanning planes may be utilized, but the medial or lateral approach is generally sufficient and has the added advantage that the follow through arthrocentesis is often performed at these scanning sites (Videos 26.1 and 26.2).

Guidance of Knee Aspiration

Ultrasonography may be used to guide needle insertion for aspiration of a knee effusion. Following identification of the fluid, the site is marked and, with sterile technique, the needle is inserted into the fluid collection with needle trajectory determined by the probe angle used to identify the fluid and depth for needle penetration measured from a frozen image using the caliper function of the machine. Real-time guidance of needle insertion is not required. Ultrasonography is superior to the landmark technique in terms of patient pain, volume of fluid aspirated, and overall success rate [22]. Ultrasonography is particularly useful for the patient with difficult anatomy [23]; and for the less experienced operator who performs only an occasional knee aspiration [24]; as may hold for the intensivist.

SYNOVIAL FLUID ANALYSIS

Synovial fluid analysis is identical for all joints and begins with bedside observation of the fluid. The color, clarity, and viscosity of the fluid are characterized. Synovial fluid is divided into noninflammatory and inflammatory types on the basis of the total nucleated cell count. A white blood cell count less than or equal to 2,000 per μL indicates a *noninflammatory fluid* and a count greater than 2,000 per μL indicates an *inflammatory fluid*. Table 26.3 shows how fluid is divided into major categories on the basis of appearance and cell count.

GROSS EXAMINATION

Color

Color and clarity should be tested using a clear glass tube. Translucent plastic, as used in most disposable syringes, interferes with proper assessment [1]. Normal synovial fluid is colorless. Noninflammatory and inflammatory synovial fluids appear yellow or straw colored. Septic effusions frequently appear purulent and whitish. Depending on the number of white blood cells present, pure pus may be extracted from a septic joint. Hemorrhagic effusions appear red or brown. If the fluid looks like pure blood, the tap may have aspirated venous blood. The needle is removed, pressure is applied, and the joint is reentered from an alternate site. If the same bloody appearance is noted, the fluid is a hemorrhagic effusion and probably not related to the trauma of the aspiration. If any question remains, the hematocrit of the effusion is compared with that of peripheral blood. The hematocrit in a hemorrhagic effusion is typically lower than that of peripheral blood. In the case of a traumatic tap, the hematocrit of the fluid should be equal to that of peripheral blood. For causes of a hemorrhagic effusion, refer to Table 26.4.

Clarity

The clarity of synovial fluid depends on the number and types of cells or particles present. Clarity is tested by reading black print on a white background through a glass tube filled with the synovial fluid. If the print is easily read, the fluid is transparent. This is typical of normal and noninflammatory synovial fluid. If the black print can be distinguished from the white background, but is not clear, the fluid is translucent. This is typical of inflammatory effusions. If nothing can be seen through the fluid, it is opaque. This occurs with grossly inflammatory, septic, and hemorrhagic fluids.

Viscosity

The viscosity of synovial fluid is a measure of the hyaluronic acid content. Degradative enzymes such as hyaluronidase are released in inflammatory conditions, thus destroying hyaluronic acid and other proteinaceous material, resulting in a thinner, less viscous fluid. Highly viscous fluid, on the other hand, can be seen in myxedematous or hypothyroid effusions.

Viscosity can be assessed at the bedside using the string sign [1]. A drop of fluid is allowed to fall from the end of the needle or syringe and the length of the continuous string that forms is estimated. Normal fluid typically forms at least a 6-cm continuous string. Inflammatory fluid does not form a string; instead, it drops off the end of the needle or syringe like water dropping from a faucet.

CELL COUNT AND DIFFERENTIAL

The cell count should be obtained as soon as possible after arthrocentesis, as a delay of even several hours may cause an artificially low white blood cell count [25]. The total white

TABLE 26.3

Joint Fluid Characteristics

Characteristic	Normal	Noninflammatory	Inflammatory	Septic
Color	Clear	Yellow	Yellow or opalescent	Variable—may be purulent
Clarity	Transparent	Transparent	Translucent	Opaque
Viscosity	Very high	High	Low	Typically low
White blood cell count per μL	200	200–2,000	2,000–100,000	>50,000, usually >100,000
Polymorphonuclear cells (%)	<25	<25	>50	>75
Culture	Negative	Negative	Negative	Usually positive

TABLE 26.4

Causes of a Hemorrhagic Effusion

Trauma (with or without fracture)
Hemophilia and other bleeding disorders
Anticoagulant therapy
Tumor (metastatic and local)
Hemangioma
Pigmented villonodular synovitis
Ehlers–Danlos syndrome
Scurvy

blood cell count of synovial fluid differentiates noninflammatory from inflammatory fluid, as noted previously. In general, the higher the total white blood cell count, the more likely the joint is to be infected. This is not absolute, however, and there is considerable overlap. For instance, a total white cell count greater than 100,000 per μL may be seen in conditions other than infection, whereas a total white blood cell count of 50,000 per μL may be due to infection, crystalline disease, or systemic inflammatory arthropathy [26].

The differential white blood cell count is also performed using the technique used for peripheral blood, typically using Wright's stain. The differential is calculated on the basis of direct visualization. The differential count includes cells typically seen in peripheral blood, such as polymorphonuclear cells, monocytes, and lymphocytes, as well as cells localized to the synovial space. In general, the total white blood cell count and the polymorphonuclear cell count increase with inflammation and infection. Septic fluid typically has a differential of greater than 75% polymorphonuclear cells (see Table 26.3).

CRYSTALS

All fluid should be assessed for the presence of crystals. As with cell count, crystal analysis should be performed as soon as possible after arthrocentesis. A delay is associated with a decreased yield [25]. One drop of fluid is placed on a slide and covered with a coverslip; this is examined for crystals using a compensated polarized light microscope. The presence of intracellular monosodium urate (MSU) or calcium pyrophosphate dihydrate (CPPD) crystals confirms a diagnosis of gout or pseudogout, respectively. MSU crystals are typically long and needle shaped: they may appear to pierce through a white blood cell. The crystals are strongly negatively birefringent, appearing yellow when parallel to the plane of reference. Typically, CPPD crystals are small and rhomboid. The crystals are weakly positively birefringent, appearing blue when oriented parallel to the plane of reference. Rotating the stage of the microscope by 90 degrees and thereby the orientation of the crystals (now perpendicular to the plane of reference) changes their color: MSU crystals turn blue and CPPD crystals turn yellow.

In addition to MSU and CPPD crystals, other less common crystals may induce an inflammatory arthropathy. Basic calcium crystals (e.g., hydroxyapatite) and oxalate crystals are two such types. Much like MSU crystals in gout, hydroxyapatite crystals can incite acute articular and periarticular inflammation, which can be difficult to distinguish clinically from septic arthritis and cellulitis, respectively [27]. On light microscopy, however, crystals appear as clumps of shiny nonbirefringent globules, and with alizarin red S stain, the clumps appear red-orange [28,29]. If hydroxyapatite is suspected, alizarin red S stain must be requested specifically from the laboratory as it is not a routine component of the crystal analysis. Calcium oxalate crystals can also induce an inflammatory arthritis. This is generally seen in patients on long-term hemodialysis [30,31], but may also be seen in young patients with primary oxalosis [27]. Synovial fluid typically reveals characteristic bipyramidal crystals as well as polymorphic forms [27].

It is important to note that even in the presence of crystals, infection must be considered because crystals can be seen concomitantly with a septic joint.

Other crystals include cryoimmunoglobulins in patients with multiple myeloma and essential cryoglobulinemia [32], and cholesterol crystals in patients with chronic inflammatory arthropathies, such as rheumatoid arthritis. Cholesterol crystals are a nonspecific finding and appear as platelike structures with a notched corner.

GRAM STAIN AND CULTURE

The Gram stain is performed as with other body fluids. It should be performed as soon as possible to screen for the presence of bacteria. It has been reported that the sensitivity of synovial fluid Gram stain in septic arthritis ranges between 50% and 75% for nongonococcal infection and less than 10% for gonococcal infection [26]. Specificity is much higher; this suggests that a positive Gram stain, despite a negative culture, should be considered evidence of infection. In fact, it is not uncommon for only the Gram stain to be positive in the setting of infection [26]. However, the absence of bacteria by the Gram stain does not rule out a septic process.

Synovial fluid in general should be cultured routinely for aerobic and anaerobic bacterial organisms. A positive culture confirms septic arthritis. In certain circumstances (e.g., in chronic monoarticular arthritis), fluid may be cultured for the presence of mycobacteria, fungus, and spirochetes. If disseminated gonorrhea is suspected, the laboratory must be notified because the fluid should be plated directly onto chocolate agar or Thayer–Martin medium. Just as Gram stain of synovial fluid in gonococcal infection is often negative, so too is synovial fluid culture. Synovial fluid culture is positive approximately 10% to 50% of the time, versus 75% to 95% of the time for nongonococcal infection [26]. However, cultures of genitourinary sites and mucosal sites in gonococcal infection are positive approximately 80% of the time [33]. Therefore, when suspicion of gonococcal arthritis is high (e.g., in a young, healthy, sexually active individual with a dermatitis-arthritis syndrome), the diagnosis must often be confirmed by a positive culture from the urethra, cervix, rectum, or pharynx.

In addition to documenting infection and identifying a specific organism, synovial fluid culture can be useful in determining antibiotic sensitivities and subsequent treatment. Furthermore, serial synovial fluid cultures can help in assessing response to therapy. For example, a negative follow-up culture associated with a decrease in synovial fluid polymorphonuclear cell count is highly suggestive of improvement.

Other studies on synovial fluid (e.g., glucose, protein, lactate dehydrogenase, complement, and immune complexes) are generally not helpful. Shmerling et al. [34] observed that synovial fluid glucose and protein were "highly inaccurate." The synovial fluid glucose and protein misclassified effusions as inflammatory versus noninflammatory 50% of the time. In contrast, synovial fluid cell count and differential were found to be reliable and complementary; sensitivity and specificity of cell count was 84% for both and for the differential was 75% and 92%, respectively [30]. Of note, there are special stains for synovial fluid that can be helpful as the clinical picture warrants; these include Congo red staining for amyloid arthropathy. Amyloid deposits display an apple-green birefringence with polarized light [35]. Prussian blue stain for iron deposition may reveal iron in synovial lining cells in hemochromatosis [19]. However, neither of these studies should be considered a routine component of synovial fluid analysis.

References

1. Gatter RA, Schumacher HR: *A Practical Handbook of Joint Fluid Analysis*. Philadelphia, Lea & Febiger, 1991.
2. Stein R: *Manual of Rheumatology and Outpatient Orthopedic Disorders*. Boston, Little, Brown, 1981.
3. Krey PR, Lazaro DM: *Analysis of Synovial Fluid*. Summit, NJ, CIBA-GEIGY, 1992.
4. Ropes MW, Bauer W: *Synovial Fluid Changes in Joint Disease*. Cambridge, MA, Harvard University Press, 1953.
5. Hollander JL, Jessar RA, McCarty DJ: Synovianalysis: an aid in arthritis diagnosis. *Bull Rheum Dis* 12:263, 1961.
6. Gatter RA, McCarty DJ: Synovianalysis: a rapid clinical diagnostic procedure. *Rheumatism* 20:2, 1964.
7. Schumacher HR: Synovial fluid analysis. *Orthop Rev* 13:85, 1984.
8. Greenwald RA: Oxygen radicals, inflammation, and arthritis: pathophysiological considerations and implications for treatment. *Semin Arthritis Rheum* 20:219, 1991.
9. Robinson DR, Tashjian AH, Levine L: Prostaglandin E2 induced bone resorption by rheumatoid synovia: a model for bone destruction in RA. *J Clin Invest* 56:1181, 1975.
10. Gray RG, Tenenbaum J, Gottlieb NL: Local corticosteroid injection treatment in rheumatic disorders. *Semin Arthritis Rheum* 10:231, 1981.
11. Polley HF, Hunder GG: *Rheumatologic Interviewing and Physical Examination of the Joints*. 2nd ed. Philadelphia, WB Saunders, 1978.
12. Doherty M, Hazelman BL, Hutton CW, et al: *Rheumatology Examination and Injection Techniques*. 2nd ed. London, WB Saunders, 1999.
13. Davis JM, Moder KG, Hunder GG: History and physical examination of the musculoskeletal system, in Firestein GS, Budd RC, Gabriel S, et al: (eds): *Kelley's Textbook of Rheumatology*. 9th ed. Philadelphia, Elsevier Saunders, 2013, p 559.
14. McCarty DJ Jr: A basic guide to arthrocentesis. *Hosp Med* 4:77, 1968.
15. Gottlieb NL, Riskin WG: Complications of local corticosteroid injections. *JAMA* 243:1547, 1980.
16. Hollander JL: Intrasynovial steroid injections, in Hollander JL, McCarty DL Jr (eds): *Arthritis and Allied Conditions*. 8th ed. Philadelphia, Lea & Febiger, 1972, p 517.
17. Wise C: Arthrocentesis and injection of joints and soft tissues, in Firestein GS, Budd RC, Gabriel S, et al: (eds): *Kelley's Textbook of Rheumatology*. 9th ed. Philadelphia, Elsevier Saunders, 2013, p 770.
18. Gerlag DM, Tak PP: Minimally invasive procedures, in Hochberg MC, Silman AJ, Smolen JS, et al: (eds): *Rheumatology*. 6th ed. Philadelphia, Elsevier Mosby, 2015, p 242.
19. Schumacher HR Jr: Synovial fluid analysis, in Katz WA (ed): *Diagnosis and Management of Rheumatic Diseases*. 2nd ed. Philadelphia, JB Lippincott, 1988, pp 248–255.
20. Tanphaichitr K, Spilberg I, Hahn B: Lithium heparin crystals simulating calcium pyrophosphate dihydrate crystals in synovial fluid [letter]. *Arthritis Rheum* 9:966, 1976.
21. Adhikari S, Blaivas M: Utility of bedside sonography to distinguish soft tissue abnormalities from joint effusions in the emergency department. *J Ultrasound Med* 29:519–526, 2010.
22. Sibbitt WL Jr, Kettwich LG, Band PA, et al: Does ultrasound guidance improve the outcomes of arthrocentesis and corticosteroid injection of the knee? *Scand J Rheumatol* 41:66–72, 2012.
23. Hurdle MF, Wisniewski SJ, Pingree MJ: Ultrasound-guided intra-articular knee injection in an obese patient. *Am J Phys Med Rehabil* 91:275–276, 2012.
24. Wiler JL, Costantino TG, Filippone L, et al: Comparison of ultrasound-guided and standard landmark techniques for knee arthrocentesis. *J Emerg Med* 39:76–82, 2010.
25. Kerolus G, Clayburne G, Schumacher HR Jr: Is it mandatory to examine synovial fluids promptly after arthrocentesis? *Arthritis Rheum* 32:271, 1989.
26. Shmerling RH: Synovial fluid analysis. A critical reappraisal. *Rheum Dis Clin North Am* 20(2):503, 1994.
27. Reginato AJ, Schumacher HR Jr: Crystal-associated arthropathies. *Clin Geriatr Med* 4(2):295, 1988.
28. Paul H, Reginato AJ, Schumacher HR: Alizarin red S staining as a screening test to detect calcium compounds in synovial fluid. *Arthritis Rheum* 26:191, 1983.
29. Hoffman G, Schumacher HR, Paul H, et al: Calcium oxalate microcrystalline associated arthritis in end stage renal disease. *Ann Intern Med* 97:36, 1982.
30. Reginato AJ, Feweiro JL, Barbazan AC, et al: Arthropathy and cutaneous calcinosis in hemodialysis oxalosis. *Arthritis Rheum* 29:1387, 1986.
31. Schumacher HR, Reginato AJ, Pullman S: Synovial fluid oxalate deposition complicating rheumatoid arthritis with amyloidosis and renal failure. Demonstration of intracellular oxalate crystals. *J Rheumatol* 14:361, 1987.
32. Dornan TL, Blundell JW, Morgan AG: Widespread crystallization of paraprotein in myelomatosis. *Q J Med* 57:659, 1985.
33. Balsa A, Martin-Mola E: Gonococcal arthritis, in Hochberg MC, Silman AJ, Smolen JS, et al: (eds): *Rheumatology*. 6th ed. Philadelphia, Elseveir Mosby, 2015, p 891.
34. Shmerling RH, Delbanco TL, Tosteson ANA, et al: Synovial fluid tests. What should be ordered? *JAMA* 264:1009, 1990.
35. Lakhanpal S, Li CY, Gertz MA, et al: Synovial fluid analysis for diagnosis of amyloid arthropathy. *Arthritis Rheum* 30(4):419, 1987.

Section 2
MINIMALLY INVASIVE MONITORING
TODD W. SARGE

Chapter 27 ■ Routine Monitoring of Critically Ill Patients
KRYSTA S. WOLFE • MICHAEL D. HOWELL

A key difference between intensive care units (ICUs) and other hospital units is the level of detail with which patients are routinely monitored. This careful monitoring alerts the health care team to changes in the patient's severity of illness—helping to both diagnose disease and assess prognosis. Careful monitoring also helps the health care team safely apply therapies such as volume resuscitation, vasoactive infusions, and mechanical ventilation.

This chapter deals with the routine, predominantly noninvasive monitoring that is often done for many patients in ICUs. It examines the indications for, the technology of, and problems encountered with the routine monitoring of temperature, blood pressure, electrocardiographic (ECG) rhythm, ST segments, respiratory rate, and oxygen and carbon dioxide levels. In addition, it reviews noninvasive monitoring of tissue perfusion, with particular attention to gastric tonometry, sublingual capnometry, and transcutaneous oxygen and carbon dioxide monitoring.

MONITORING SYSTEMS

When ICUs came into being in the late 1950s, nurses monitored patients' vital signs manually and intermittently. Continuous measurement was either unavailable or necessitated invasive procedures. However, nearly all routine vital signs can now be monitored accurately, noninvasively, and continuously. As a result, patients now are monitored more intensively and continuously in the ICU than in any other part of the hospital, with the possible exception of the operating room.

Over the past decades, the trend for monitoring systems has been toward multipurpose systems that integrate monitoring of a variety of parameters. Multipurpose systems eliminate the need for multiple, freestanding devices—reducing clutter and improving workflow ergonomics at the bedside. These systems also interface with critical care information systems to provide more efficient data management, quality improvement reporting, and in some cases prospective data-driven alerts.

TEMPERATURE MONITORING

Temperature abnormalities of the critically ill are associated with significant morbidity and mortality [1] (see Chapters 184 and 185)—making it clinically important to recognize an abnormal temperature. In one surgical ICU study, rectal temperatures on admission were normal in only 30% of patients, were above 37.6°C in 38%, and were below 36.8°C in 32% [2]. An abnormal temperature is frequently the earliest clinical sign of infection, inflammation, central nervous system dysfunction, or drug toxicity. Unfortunately, the type of thermometer and the site where the temperature is taken can affect the accuracy of this vital measurement. Clinicians should understand the impact of the thermometer type and the measurement site on how to interpret the patient's reported temperature.

Indications for Temperature Monitoring

The Society of Critical Care Medicine's Task Force on Guidelines' recommendations for care in a critical care setting grades temperature monitoring as an essential service for all critical care units [3]. Critically ill patients are at high risk of temperature dysregulation because of debility, impaired control of temperature, use of sedative drugs, and a high frequency of infection. All critically ill patients should have core temperature measured at least intermittently. Patients with marked temperature abnormalities should be considered for continuous monitoring; patients undergoing active interventions to alter temperature, such as breathing heated air or using a cooling–warming blanket, should have continuous monitoring to prevent overtreatment or undertreatment of temperature abnormalities.

Measurement Sites

The goal of temperature measurements is generally to estimate *core temperature*—the deep body temperature that is carefully regulated by the hypothalamus so as to be independent of transient small changes in ambient temperature. Core temperature exists more as a physiologic concept than as the temperature with an anatomic location. An ideal measurement site would be protected from heat loss, painless, convenient to use, and would not interfere with the patient's ability to move or communicate. No one location provides an accurate measurement of core temperature in all clinical circumstances.

Sublingual Temperature Measurements

Sublingual temperature measurements are convenient, but suffer numerous limitations. Although open-mouth versus closed-mouth breathing and use of nasogastric tubes do not alter temperature measurement [4], oral temperature is obviously altered if measured immediately after the patient has consumed hot or cold drinks. Falsely low oral temperatures may occur because of cooling from tachypnea. Sixty percent of sublingual temperatures are more than 1°F lower than simultaneously measured rectal temperatures; 53% differ by 1°F to 2°F, and 6% differ by more than 2°F. Continuous sublingual measurement is not generally practical. Sublingual measurement is best suited for intermittent monitoring when some inaccuracy can be tolerated.

Axillary Temperature Measurements

Axillary temperatures are commonly used as an index of core temperature. Although some studies indicate close approximation of the axillary site with pulmonary artery temperatures [5], temperatures average 1.5°C to 1.9°C lower than tympanic temperatures [6]. Positioning the sensor over the axillary artery may improve accuracy. The accuracy and precision of axillary temperature measurements are less than at other sites [6], perhaps due in part to the difficulty of maintaining a good probe position.

Rectal Temperature Measurements

Rectal temperature is the most widely accepted method for measuring core temperature in clinical use. Before a rectal thermometer is inserted, a digital rectal examination should be performed because feces can blunt temperature measurement. Readings are more accurate when the sensor is passed more than 10 cm (4 inches) into the rectum. Rectal temperature correlates well in most patients with distal esophageal, bladder, and tympanic temperatures [7]. Rectal temperatures typically respond to induced changes in temperature more slowly than other central measurement sites [8]. Many practitioners recommend against rectal manipulation in patients with neutropenia. Additionally, reusable, electronic, sheath-covered rectal thermometers have been associated with the transmission of *Clostridium difficile* and vancomycin-resistant *Enterococcus*, so disposable probes are generally preferred.

Esophageal Temperature Measurements

Esophageal temperature is usually measured with an electric, flexible temperature sensor. On average, esophageal temperatures are 0.6°C lower than rectal temperatures [9]. However, the measured temperature can vary greatly depending on the position of the sensor in the esophagus. In the proximal esophagus, temperature is influenced by ambient air [10]. During hypothermia, temperatures in different portions of the esophagus may differ by up to 6°C [10]. Because of the proximity of the distal esophagus to the great vessels and heart, the distal esophageal temperature responds rapidly to changes in core temperature [11]. Changes in esophageal temperature may inaccurately reflect changes in core temperature when induced temperature change occurs because of the inspiration of heated air, gastric lavage, or cardiac bypass or assist [11].

Tympanic Temperature Measurements

Health care providers can measure tympanic temperature with specifically designed thermometers that are commonly used in the ICU. However, several studies have demonstrated poor correlation with ICU patients' core temperatures [12,13]. Accuracy depends in part on operator experience—but even when trained, experienced ICU nurses use tympanic thermometers, the variability in repeated measurements was more than 0.5°F in 20% of patients [14]. Unlike temporal artery measurements, which are not known to have complications, tympanic temperature measurements come with some risk. Perforation of the tympanic membrane and bleeding from the external canal due to trauma from the probe have been reported.

Temporal Artery Measurements

Temporal artery measurements are not known to have complications. Their accuracy is reviewed later in this chapter.

Urinary Bladder Temperature Measurements

Providers can easily measure the urinary bladder temperature with a specially designed temperature probe embedded in a Foley catheter [6–8]. In patients undergoing induced hypothermia and rewarming, bladder temperatures correlate well with great vessel and rectal temperatures [7,8]. Bladder temperature under steady-state conditions is more reproducible than those taken at most other sites [7].

Central Circulation Temperature Measurements

ICU practitioners can measure the temperature of blood in the pulmonary artery using a thermistor-equipped pulmonary artery catheter. The temperature sensor is located at the distal tip and can record accurate great vessel temperatures once the catheter is in place in the pulmonary artery. Pulmonary artery temperatures have generally been accepted as the gold standard for accurate measures of core temperature, although readings might be expected to differ from core temperature when heated air was breathed or warm or cold intravenous fluids were infused. However, this understanding may not be true for neurosurgical patients. A study of patients undergoing neurosurgical procedures with induced hypothermic circulatory arrest found that pulmonary arterial temperature measurement was not effective in assessing core brain temperature with a correlation coefficient of 0.63. A greater degree of correlation was found in bladder temperature [15]. Inserting a central venous thermistor specifically to monitor temperature is probably warranted only when other sites are felt to be unreliable and accurate, and rapid continuous temperature measurements are critical to the patient's management.

Types of Thermometers

Mercury Thermometers

Although mercury thermometers were historically the most common type in clinical use, environmental and health concerns related to mercury have resulted in several state and local legislative efforts to phase out this type of thermometer. Mercury and other liquid–expansion-based thermometers can give a falsely low measurement when the thermometer is left in place for too short a period; falsely high temperatures result from failure to shake the mercury down.

Liquid Crystal Display Thermometers

Liquid crystal display (LCD) thermometers contain liquid crystals embedded in thin adhesive strips that are directly attached to the patient's skin. LCD thermometers are most commonly applied to the forehead for ease of use and steady perfusion, but can be applied to any area of the skin. Like all skin temperature measurements, they may poorly reflect core temperature when the skin is hypoperfused or for patients with vasomotor instability. Forehead skin temperature is typically lower than core temperatures by 2.2°C [16], and changes in LCD forehead temperature lag behind changes in core temperature by more than 12 minutes [17]. LCD skin thermometry is probably best used for patients with stable, normal hemodynamics who are not expected to experience major temperature shifts and in whom the trend of temperature change is more important than the accuracy of an individual measurement.

Standard Digital Thermometers: Thermocouples and Thermistors

Electric thermometers convert an electrical temperature signal into digital displays, frequently by use of thermocouples and thermistors as probes. Thermocouples and thermistors can be fashioned into thin wires and embedded in flexible probes that are suitable for placing in body cavities to measure deep temperature.

Thermocouples consist of a junction of two dissimilar metals. The voltage change across the junction can be precisely related to temperature. The measuring thermocouple must be calibrated against a second constant-temperature junction for absolute temperature measurements. In the range of 20°C to 50°C, thermocouples may have a linearity error of less than 0.1 [18].

Thermistors consist of semiconductor metal oxides in which the electrical resistance changes inversely with temperature. A linearity error of up to 4°C may occur over the temperature range of 20°C to 50°C, but this can be substantially reduced by mathematical adjustments and electrical engineering techniques [18]. Semiconductors measure temperature by taking advantage of the fact that the base-to-emitter voltage change is temperature dependent, whereas the collector current of the silicon resistor is constant. Thermistors are more sensitive, faster responding, and less linear than thermocouples or semiconductors [18].

Infrared Emission Detection Thermometers

Tympanic Thermometers. Commonly used in a hospital setting, infrared emission detection tympanic thermometers use a sensor that detects infrared energy emitted by the core temperature tissues behind the tympanic membrane. Infrared emissions through the tympanic membrane vary linearly with temperature. Operator technique is important: errors due to improper calibration, setup, or poor probe positioning can significantly alter temperatures [19]. Measurements are most accurate when the measuring probe blocks the entrance of ambient air into the ear canal and when the midposterior external ear is tugged posterosuperiorly so as to direct the probe to the anterior, inferior third of the tympanic membrane. Studies are mixed on whether tympanic thermometers provide accurate core temperature measurements, ranging from a 4% clinically meaningful error rate [14] to a finding that 21% of tympanic readings might result in delays in therapy for or evaluation of fever [20].

Temporal Artery Thermometers. Infrared technology can also measure temperature over the temporal artery. A probe is passed over the forehead and searches for the highest temperature; some systems also scan the area behind the ear. An algorithm estimates ambient heat loss and blood cooling to calculate core temperature. The device is convenient, painless, and provides a rapid reading. Although one small study of normothermic patients found good correlation with pulmonary artery temperatures [5], another study in patients with a broader temperature range found that 89% of measurements differed from pulmonary artery temperatures by more than 0.5°C, the amount the authors had specified a priori as clinically significant [21].

Selecting the Measurement Site

The site used to monitor temperature must be an individualized choice, but certain generalizations can be made. When intermittent temperature measurement is all that is clinically needed (e.g., in routine monitoring), or the consequences of inaccurate measurement are low, rectal or sublingual measurement may be preferred. If less accuracy is required, tympanic, temporal, or axillary sites may be chosen. When more accurate measurement is needed, bladder, esophageal, and rectal temperatures in general appear to be most accurate and reproducible—although rectal temperatures may lag behind other temperatures when the patient's status is changing quickly [7,13]. However, routine measurement of esophageal temperatures would necessitate inserting an esophageal probe in all patients. In addition, small changes in probe position can affect the accuracy of esophageal measurements, so this mode is probably best used in patients undergoing active, aggressive temperature management in centers with substantial experience with the modality. Meanwhile, rectal probes may be extruded or may be refused by patients. The third option, bladder temperature monitoring, is simplified by the fact that many critically ill patients have an indwelling Foley catheter. Monitoring the bladder temperature for these patients requires only a thermistor-equipped catheter. Patients with a thermistor-tipped pulmonary artery catheter already in place require no additional temperature monitoring.

Patient Safety and Temperature Monitoring

Therapeutic hypothermia is increasingly prevalent in ICU settings (Chapter 184). Some devices used to induce hypothermia are closed-looped systems. Since core temperature probes can fail (e.g., dislodgement of a rectal probe to a position outside the patient), practitioners should consider monitoring core temperature from two sites when temperature is being actively manipulated.

ARTERIAL BLOOD PRESSURE MONITORING

The first recorded blood pressure measurement occurred in 1733 and—somewhat surprisingly—was intraarterial pressure monitoring. The Reverend Stephen Hales placed a 9-foot brass tube in a horse's crural artery and found a blood pressure of about 8 feet 3 inches. This was obviously not clinically applicable. In the mid-1800s, Carl Ludwig recorded the first arterial pressure waveforms, but it was not until 1881 that the first noninvasive blood pressure recordings were made. In 1896, Riva-Rocci developed and popularized the mercury sphygmomanometer, which was then adopted and disseminated at least in part by Harvey Cushing. In 1905, Korotkoff developed techniques for detecting diastolic pressure by listening for what are now called Korotkoff sounds. More clinical techniques for direct blood pressure measurement by intraarterial cannula were developed in the 1930s and popularized in the 1950s [22]. These measurements were soon accepted as representing true systolic and diastolic pressures.

Since that time, a variety of invasive and alternative indirect methods have been developed that equal and even surpass auscultation in reproducibility and ease of measurement. This section examines the advantages and disadvantages of various methods of arterial pressure monitoring and provides recommendations for their use in the ICU.

Noninvasive (Indirect) Blood Pressure Measurement

Providers can indirectly monitor blood pressure using a number of techniques, most of which describe the external pressure applied to block blood flow to an artery distal to the occlusion. These methods therefore actually detect blood *flow*, not intraarterial pressure, although one method describes the pressure required to maintain a distal artery with a transmural pressure gradient of zero. These differences in what is actually measured are the major points of discrepancy between direct and indirect measurements.

Indirectly measured pressures vary depending on the size of the cuff used. Cuffs of inadequate width and length can provide falsely elevated readings. Bladder width should equal 40% and bladder length at least 60% of the circumference of the extremity measured [23]. Anyone who makes indirect pressure measurements must be aware of these factors and carefully select the cuff to be used.

Manual Methods

Auscultatory (Riva-Rocci) Pressures

The traditional way to measure blood pressure involves inflating a sphygmomanometer cuff around an extremity and auscultating over an artery distal to the occlusion. Sounds from the vibrations of the artery under pressure (Korotkoff sounds) indicate systolic and diastolic pressures. The level at which the sound first becomes audible is taken as the systolic pressure. The point at which there is an abrupt diminution in or disappearance of sounds is used as diastolic pressure. This method, still commonly used in the ICU, yields an acceptable value in most situations. Its advantages include low cost, time-honored reliability, and simplicity. Disadvantages include operator variability, susceptibility to environmental noise, and the absence of Korotkoff sounds when pressures are very low. Auscultatory pressures also correlate poorly with directly measured pressures at the extremes of pressure [24].

Manual Oscillation Method

When a cuff is slowly deflated and blood first begins to flow through the occluded artery, the artery's walls begin to vibrate. This vibration can be detected as an oscillation in pressure and has served as the basis for the development of several automated blood pressure monitoring devices. However, it also continues to be used in manual blood pressure measurement. The first discontinuity in the needle movement of an aneroid manometer indicates the presence of blood flow in the distal artery and is taken as systolic pressure [25]. The advantages of the oscillation method are its low cost and simplicity. The disadvantages include the inability to measure diastolic pressure, poor correlation with directly measured pressures [25], and lack of utility in situations in which Riva-Rocci measurements are also unobtainable. Aneroid manometers may also be inaccurate: in one study, 34% of all aneroid manometers in use in one large medical system gave inaccurate measurements, even when more lenient standards were used than those advocated by the National Bureau of Standards and the Association for the Advancement of Medical Instrumentation [26]. In the same survey, 36% of the devices were found to be mechanically defective—pointing out the need for regular maintenance. Although the manometers themselves can also be used for auscultatory measurements, oscillometric readings probably provide no advantage over auscultation in the ICU.

Palpation, Doppler, and Pulse Oximetric Methods

Systolic pressures can be measured via any method that detects flow in a distal artery as the blood pressure cuff is slowly deflated. Palpation of the radial artery is the most commonly used technique; it is most useful in emergency situations in which Korotkoff sounds cannot be heard and an arterial line is not in place. The inability to measure diastolic pressure makes the palpation method less valuable for ongoing monitoring. In addition, palpation obtains no better correlation with direct measurements than the previously described techniques. In one study, variation from simultaneously obtained direct pressure measurements was as high as 60 mm Hg [24]. Like other indirect methods, palpation tends to underestimate actual values to greater degrees at higher levels of arterial pressure. Any method which detects blood flow distal to a sphygmomanometer cuff may be used in this fashion. Doppler machines are commonly used and may be particularly useful in situations where the pulse is not palpable or environmental noise precludes auscultation. Pulse oximeters have been similarly used and correlate well with other methods; the point at which a plethysmographic trace appears is taken as the systolic pressure [27].

Automated Methods

Automated indirect blood pressure devices operate on one of several principles: Doppler flow, infrasound, oscillometry, volume clamp, arterial tonometry, and pulse wave arrival time.

Doppler Flow

Systems that operate on the Doppler principle take advantage of the change in frequency of an echo signal when there is movement between two objects. Doppler devices emit brief pulses of sound at a high frequency that are reflected back to the transducer [28]. The compressed artery exhibits a large amount of wall motion when flow first appears in the vessel distal to the inflated cuff. This causes a change in frequency of the echo signal, known as a *Doppler shift*. The first appearance of flow in the distal artery represents systolic pressure. In an uncompressed artery, the small amount of motion does not cause a change in frequency of the reflected signal. Therefore, the disappearance of the Doppler shift in the echo signal represents diastolic pressure [29].

Infrasound

Infrasound devices use a microphone to detect low-frequency (20 to 30 Hz) sound waves associated with the oscillation of the arterial wall. These sounds are processed by a minicomputer, and the processed signals are usually displayed in digital form [30].

Oscillometry

Oscillometric devices operate on the same principle as manual oscillometric measurements. The cuff senses pressure fluctuations caused by vessel wall oscillations in the presence of pulsatile blood flow [31]. Maximum oscillation is seen at mean pressure, whereas wall movement greatly decreases below diastolic pressure [32]. As with the other automated methods described, the signals produced by the system are processed electronically and displayed in numeric form.

Volume Clamp Technique

The volume clamp method avoids the use of an arm cuff. A finger cuff is applied to the proximal or middle phalanx to keep the artery at a constant size [33]. The pressure in the cuff is changed as necessary by a servocontrol unit strapped to the wrist. The feedback in this system is provided by a photoplethysmograph that estimates arterial size. The pressure needed to keep the artery at its *unloaded volume* can be used to estimate the intraarterial pressure [34]. There have been a number of studies examining this method in the past decade, mostly in the anesthesia literature. This method has been shown to be reliable in patients at risk of hypotensive episodes, but has variable results in critically ill patients [35]. Limitations include a lag time of 7.5 to 10 seconds and inaccuracies associated with peripheral vasoconstriction from vasopressors, hypothermia, or collagen vascular disorders.

Arterial Tonometry

Arterial tonometry provides continuous noninvasive measurement of arterial pressure, including pressure waveforms. It slightly compresses the superficial wall of an artery (usually the radial). Pressure tracings obtained in this manner are similar to intraarterial tracings. A generalized transfer function can convert these tracings to an estimate of aortic pressure [36]. This method has not yet achieved widespread clinical use. One available system studied in ICU patients had approximately one-third of mean arterial pressure (MAP) readings which differed by ≥10 mm Hg compared with intraarterial pressure measurements and was associated with significant drift during the course of the study [37]. However, more studies of a different system reported more accurate readings in patients undergoing anesthesia [38], including those with induced hypotension [39].

Utility of Noninvasive Blood Pressure Measurements

Only four of the methods described previously (infrasound, oscillometry, Doppler flow, volume clamp) are associated with significant clinical experience. Of these, methods that use infrasound technology correlate least well with direct measures of arterial blood pressure [31,40]. Therefore, infrasound is rarely used in systems designed for critical care.

Although they have not been consistently accurate, automated methods have the potential to yield pressures as accurate as values derived by auscultation. Commonly used oscillometric methods can correlate to within 1 mm Hg of the directly measured group average values [31] but may vary substantially from intraarterial pressures in individual subjects, particularly at the extremes of pressure. One study revealed as good a correlation with directly measured pressures as Riva-Rocci pressures have traditionally obtained [31]. Another study demonstrated that MAPs determined by auscultation were extremely close to those measured by automated devices [41].

When volume clamp methods using a finger cuff have been compared with standard methods [42,43], these devices have been found to respond rapidly to changes in blood pressure and give excellent correlation in group averages. In one study looking at a large number of measurements, 95% of all measurements using this method were within 10 mm Hg of the directly measured values [44]. Studies by Aitken et al. [43] and Hirschl et al. [42] demonstrated acceptable correlation of volume clamp technique with systolic pressures measured directly. However, other studies have shown clinically significant differences between the volume clamp technique and invasively measured pressures in patients undergoing anesthesia [45].

One of the proposed advantages of automated noninvasive monitoring is patient safety. Avoiding arterial lines eliminates the risk of vessel occlusion, hemorrhage, and infection. Automated methods, however, have complications of their own. Ulnar nerve palsies have been reported with frequent inflation and deflation of a cuff [46]. Decreased venous return from the limb and eventually reduced perfusion to that extremity can also be seen when the cuff is set to inflate and deflate every minute [46,47].

In summary, automated noninvasive blood pressure forms a major component of modern critical care monitoring. Oscillometric and Doppler-based devices are adequate for frequent blood pressure checks in patients without hemodynamic instability, in patient transport situations in which arterial lines cannot be easily used, and in the severely burned patient, in whom direct arterial pressure measurement may lead to an unacceptably high risk of infection [48]. Automated noninvasive blood pressure monitors have a role for following trends of pressure change [49] and when group averages, not individual measurements, are most important. In general, they have significant limitations for patients with rapidly fluctuating blood pressures and may diverge substantially from directly measured intraarterial pressures. Given these limitations, critical care practitioners should be wary of relying solely on these measurements for patients with rapidly changing hemodynamics or in whom very exact measurements of blood pressure are important.

Direct Invasive Blood Pressure Measurement

Direct blood pressure measurement is performed with an intraarterial catheter. Chapter 7 reviews insertion and maintenance of arterial catheters. Here, we discuss the advantages and disadvantages of invasive monitoring compared with noninvasive methods.

Arterial catheters contain a fluid column that transmits the pressure back through the tubing to a transducer. A low-compliance diaphragm in the transducer creates a reproducible volume change in response to the applied pressure change. The volume change alters the resistance of a Wheatstone bridge and is thus converted into an electrical signal. Most systems display the pressure in both wave and numeric forms.

Problems in Direct Pressure Monitoring

System-Related Problems. Several technical problems can affect the measurement of arterial pressure with intraarterial catheters. Transducers must be calibrated to zero at the level of the heart. Improper zeroing can lead to erroneous interpretation. Thrombus formation at the catheter tip can occlude the catheter, making accurate measurement impossible. This problem can be largely eliminated by using a 20-gauge polyurethane catheter, rather than a smaller one, with a slow, continuous heparin flush [50], although this can be associated with heparin-induced thrombocytopenia [51]. Because movement may interrupt the column of fluid and prevent accurate measurement, the patient's limb should be immobile during readings.

The frequency response of the transducer system is a phenomenon not only of transducer design but also of the tubing and the fluid in it. The length, width, and compliance of the tubing all affect the system's response to change. Small-bore catheters are preferable because they minimize the mass of fluid that can oscillate and amplify the pressure [52]. The compliance of the system (the change in volume of the tubing and the transducer for a given change in pressure) should be low [52]. In addition, bubbles in the tubing can affect measurements in two ways. Large amounts of air in the measurement system dampen the system response and cause the system to underestimate the pressure [53]. This is usually easily detectable. Small air bubbles cause an increase in the compliance of the system and can significantly amplify the reported pressure [52,53].

Arterial Catheter Infections. Recent data challenge the classical perception that arterial catheters are less likely to become infected [54] than central venous catheters. A prospective cohort study examined 321 arterial and 618 central venous catheters and found that arterial catheter colonization occurred with similar incidence to central venous catheter colonization [55]. Another recent study found similar results [56]. There is good evidence to support a link between the incidence of catheter colonization and catheter-related bloodstream infections [57]. Although one study suggested that full barrier precautions did not reduce the incidence of arterial line infection, interpretation of this trial is complex [58]. Taken together, the weight of evidence suggests that arterial catheters are an important potential source for infection of the critically ill patient and should be treated similar to central venous catheters in this setting. A recent study documented wide national variation in aseptic practices in arterial line insertion [59].

Finally, the location within the hospital where the procedure is performed is important as catheters placed in non-ICU locations may be associated with an increased risk of colonization versus those placed in the ICU [55].

Site Selection. The radial artery is the most common site of arterial cannulation for pressure measurement. This site is accessible and can be easily immobilized to protect both the catheter and the patient. The major alternative site is the femoral artery. Both sites are relatively safe for insertion [60,61]. The ulnar, brachial, dorsalis pedis, and axillary arteries are also used with some frequency [62]. Mechanical complications such as bleeding and nerve injury are discussed in Chapter 7. How should a provider choose a site? Although there are a number of theoretical considerations about comparing blood pressures from one site to another, there are little data from critically ill patients. A systematic review of 19,617 radial, 3,899 femoral, and 1,989 axillary cannulations found that serious complications occurred infrequently (<1% of cannulations) and were similar between all sites [62]. In 14 septic surgical patients on vasopressors, radial pressures were significantly lower than femoral arterial pressures. In 11 of the 14 patients, vasopressor dose was reduced based on the femoral pressure without untoward consequences; after vasopressors were discontinued, radial and femoral pressures equalized. The authors concluded that clinical management based on radial artery pressures may lead to excessive vasopressor administration [63]. Similar significant differences in systolic pressures between the radial and femoral sites were found in the reperfusion phase of liver transplantation, although MAPs did not differ [64]. However, another somewhat larger observational study of critically ill patients [65] found no clinically meaningful differences in blood pressures between the sites. Although data are sparse, MAP readings between the radial and femoral sites are probably interchangeable in many or most patients. There may be a preference toward using femoral arterial pressure readings in patients with vasopressor resistant shock, but this decision should be balanced by the risks of the femoral approach.

Should the risk of infection drive site selection? The data are mixed. Earlier work suggested that there was no difference in infection rates between the femoral and radial sites [62]. More recently, a prospective observational study of 2,949 catheters in the ICU found that the incidence of catheter-related bloodstream infection was significantly higher for femoral access (1.92/1,000 catheter-days) than for radial access (0.25/1,000 catheter-days) (odds ratio, 1.9; $p = 0.009$). Localized skin infections were also significantly increased in femoral versus radial arterial catheters. In addition, femoral arterial catheter bloodstream infections may have an increased association with gram-negative bacteria when compared to the radial site, similar to previous data from central venous catheters [66].

Advantages

Despite technical problems, direct arterial pressure measurement offers several advantages. Arterial lines actually measure the end-on pressure propagated by the arterial pulse. In contrast, indirect methods report the external pressure necessary to obstruct flow or to maintain a constant transmural vessel pressure. Arterial lines can also detect pressures at which Korotkoff sounds are either absent or inaccurate. Arterial lines provide a continuous measurement, with heartbeat-to-heartbeat blood pressures. In situations in which frequent blood drawing is necessary, indwelling arterial lines eliminate the need for multiple percutaneous punctures. Finally, analysis of the respiratory change in systolic or pulse pressure may provide important information on cardiac preload and fluid responsiveness.

Conclusions

Indirect methods of measuring the blood pressure estimate the arterial pressure by reporting the external pressure necessary to either obstruct flow or maintain a constant transmural vessel size. Arterial lines measure the end-on pressure propagated by the arterial pulse. Direct arterial pressure measurement offers several advantages for many, but not all, patients. Although an invasive line is required, the reported risk of complications is low [62]. Arterial lines provide heartbeat-to-heartbeat measurements, can detect pressures at which Korotkoff sounds are either absent or inaccurate, and do not require repeated inflation and deflation of a cuff. In addition, they provide easy access for phlebotomy and blood gas sampling, and they may provide additional information about cardiac status. However, particular care should be taken with aseptic insertion technique and line site maintenance, since the reported incidence of arterial line infection approaches that of central venous catheterization. Regardless of the method used, the MAP should generally be the value used for decision-making for most critically ill patients.

ELECTROCARDIOGRAPHIC MONITORING

Almost all ICUs in the United States routinely perform continuous ECG monitoring. Continuous ECG monitoring combines the principles of ECG, which have been known since 1903, with the principles of biotelemetry, which were first put into practical application in 1921 [67]. Here we review the principles of arrhythmia monitoring, automated arrhythmia detection, and the role of automated ST segment analysis.

ECG monitoring in most ICUs is done over hard-wired apparatus. Skin electrodes detect cardiac impulses and transform them into an electrical signal, which is transmitted over wires directly to the signal converter and display unit. This removes the problems of interference and frequency restrictions that can be seen with telemetry systems.

Arrhythmia Monitoring in the ICU

Continuous ECG is generally considered the standard of care for all critically ill patients in intensive care, regardless of whether the patient's primary admitting diagnosis is related to a cardiac problem [68]. Approximately 20% of patients in a general ICU have significant arrhythmias, mostly atrial fibrillation or ventricular tachycardia [69]. There is also a substantial incidence of arrhythmia following major surgery [70]. Although no studies address whether monitoring for arrhythmias in a general ICU population alters outcomes, this monitoring is generally accepted and considered standard care [68]. In postmyocardial infarction patients, on the other hand, the data are compelling. Arrhythmia monitoring was shown to improve the prognosis of patients admitted to the ICU for acute myocardial infarction (AMI) many years ago [71]. It has been a standard of care in the United States since that time. Although ventricular tachycardia and fibrillation after myocardial infarction have declined in frequency over the years, they still occur in about 7.5% of patients [72]. Monitoring enables the rapid detection of these potentially lethal rhythms.

Evolution of Arrhythmia Monitoring Systems for Clinical Use

After ICUs implemented continuous ECG monitoring, practitioners recognized some deficiencies with the systems. Initially, the responsibility for arrhythmia detection was assigned to specially trained coronary care nurses. Despite this, several studies documented that manual methods failed to identify arrhythmias, including salvos of VT, in up to 80% of cases [73]. This failure was probably due to an inadequate number of staff nurses to watch the monitors, inadequate staff education, and faulty monitors [74]. Subsequently, monitors equipped with built-in rate alarms that sounded when a preset maximum or minimum rate was detected proved inadequate because some runs of VT are too brief to exceed the rate limit for a given time interval [73,75]. Ultimately, computerized arrhythmia detection systems were incorporated into the monitors. The software in these systems is capable of diagnosing arrhythmias based on recognition of heart rate, variability, rhythm, intervals, segment lengths, complex width, and morphology [76]. These systems have been validated in coronary care and general medical ICUs [73,77]. Computerized arrhythmia detection systems are well accepted by nursing personnel, who must work most closely with them [78].

Ischemia Monitoring

Just as simple monitoring systems can miss episodes of VT and ventricular fibrillation, they can fail to detect significant episodes of myocardial ischemia. This is either because the episode is asymptomatic or because the patient's ability to communicate is impaired by intubation or altered mental status. ECG monitoring systems with automated ST segment analysis have been devised to attempt to deal with this problem.

In most ST segment monitoring systems, the computer initially creates a template of the patient's normal QRS complexes. It then recognizes the QRS complexes and the J points of subsequent beats and compares an isoelectric point just before the QRS with a portion of the ST segment 60 to 80 milliseconds after the J point [79]. It compares this relationship to that of the same points in the QRS complex template. The system must decide whether the QRS complex in question was generated and conducted in standard fashion or whether the beats are aberrant, which negates the validity of comparison. Therefore, an arrhythmia detection system must be included in all ischemia monitoring systems. Standard systems can monitor three leads simultaneously. These leads are usually chosen to represent the three major axes (anteroposterior, left-right, and craniocaudal). The machine can either display these axes individually or sum up the ST segment deviations and display them in a graph over time [79].

Automated ST segment analysis has gained widespread popularity among cardiologists. Since 1989, the American Heart Association has recommended that ischemia monitoring be included in new monitoring systems developed for use in the coronary care unit [80]. In patients admitted for suspected acute coronary syndromes, ischemia is both frequently silent and strongly associated with adverse events after discharge [68]. Although noting that no randomized clinical trials document improved patient outcomes when automated ST segment monitoring is used to detect ischemia, the American Heart Association recommends ST segment monitoring for patients with a number of primary cardiac issues (e.g., acute coronary syndromes), based on expert opinion. The guidelines make no statement regarding ST segment monitoring for ICU patients [68].

Newer Techniques

Because conventional three-lead monitoring detects only about one-third of transient ischemic events in patients with unstable coronary syndromes [81], some authors have advocated the use of continuous 12-lead ECG systems in the care of acute coronary syndromes. However, continuous 12-lead ECG monitoring can be impractical given the large number of leads required, patient discomfort, interference with medical procedures, and susceptibility to motion artifact. Some systems based on the dipole hypothesis of vectorcardiography allow the derivation of a 12-lead ECG from four recording electrodes and a reference electrode. Good correlation has been demonstrated between the EASI system and traditional 12-lead ECG in detection of ST segment deviation in acute myocardial ischemia and also in analyzing cardiac rhythm [82]. Other proposed enhancements to continuous ECG monitoring include signal-averaged ECG, QT dispersion, QT interval beat-to-beat variability, and heart rate variability [83]. Although associated with subsequent arrhythmic events, these have not yet reached common clinical use.

Technical Considerations

As with any other biomedical measurement, technical problems can arise when monitoring cardiac rhythms. Standards have been devised to guide manufacturers and purchasers of ECG monitoring systems [84].

The possibility of electrical shock exists whenever a patient is directly connected to an electrically operated piece of equipment by a low-resistance path. Electrical shocks would most commonly occur with improper grounding of equipment when a device such as a pacemaker is in place. Necessary precautions to avoid this potential catastrophe include (a) periodic checks to ensure that all equipment in contact with the patient is at the same ground potential as the power ground line; (b) insulating exposed lead connections; and (c) using appropriately grounded electrical outlets [85]. Each hospital's biomedical engineering department should have a documented preventive maintenance plan for all equipment in the unit.

The size of the ECG signal is important for accurate recognition of cardiac rate and rhythm. Several factors may affect signal size. The amplitude can be affected by a mismatch between the skin-electrode and preamplifier impedance. The combination of high skin-electrode impedance, usually the result of poor contact between the skin and electrode, with low-input impedance of the preamplifier can decrease the size of the ECG signal. Good skin preparation, site selection, and conducting gels can promote low skin-electrode impedance. A high preamplifier input impedance or the use of buffer amplifiers can also improve impedance matching and thereby improve the signal obtained. Another factor that affects complex size is critical damping, the system's ability to respond to changes in the input signal. An underdamped system responds to changes in input with displays that exaggerate the signal, called *overshoot*. An overdamped system responds slowly to a given change and may underestimate actual amplitude. The ECG signal can also be affected by the presence of inherent, unwanted voltages at the point of input. These include the common mode signal, a response to surrounding electromagnetic forces; the direct current skin potential produced by contact between the skin and the electrode; and a potential caused by internal body resistance. Finally, the ECG system must have a frequency response that is accurate for the signals being monitored. Modern, commercially available systems have incorporated features to deal with each of these problems.

Personnel

The staff's ability to interpret the information received is crucial to effective ECG monitoring [80]. Primary interpretation may be by nurses or technicians under the supervision of a physician. All personnel responsible for interpreting ECG monitoring should have formal training developed cooperatively by the hospital's medical and nursing staffs. At a minimum, this training should include basic skills for proper lead placement, ECG interpretation, and arrhythmia recognition. Hospitals should also establish and adhere to formal protocols for responding to and verifying alarms. Finally, a physician should be available in the hospital to assist with interpretation and make decisions regarding therapy.

Principles of Telemetry

Intensive care patients frequently continue to require ECG monitoring after they are released from the ICU, and many postoperative critical care patients begin mobilization while in the ICU. At this point, increased mobility is important to allow physical and occupational therapy as well as other rehabilitation services. Telemetry systems can facilitate this.

Telemetry means measurement at a distance and biomedical telemetry consists of measuring various vital signs, including heart rhythm, and transmitting them to a distant terminal [86]. Telemetry systems in the hospital consist of four major components [86]: (a) A signal transducer detects heart activity through skin electrodes and converts it into electrical signals; (b) a radio transmitter broadcasts the electrical signal; (c) a radio receiver detects the transmission and converts it back into an electrical signal; and (d) the signal converter and display unit present the signal in its most familiar format. Continuous telemetry requires an exclusive frequency so the signal can be transmitted without interruption from other signals, which means the hospital system must have multiple frequencies available to allow simultaneous monitoring of several patients. The telemetry signal may be received in one location or simultaneously in multiple locations, depending on staffing practices. The signal transducer and display unit should also be equipped with an automatic arrhythmia detection and alarm system to allow rapid detection and treatment of arrhythmias. Notably, telemetry systems may be subject to interference by cellular phones [87] or other radio equipment. Telemetry systems may also transmit over existing 802.11-type wireless networks.

Summary

Continuous ECG monitoring is usually considered the standard of care for all critically ill ICU patients [68]. Because ICU staff can miss a large percentage of arrhythmias when they use monitors without computerized arrhythmia detection systems, these computerized systems should be standard equipment for ICUs, especially those which care for patients with AMI. It appears that computerized monitoring devices can also detect a significant number of arrhythmias not detected manually in noncardiac patients and a concerning percentage of these lead to an alteration in patient care. Automated ST segment analysis facilitates the early detection of ischemic episodes. Telemetry provides close monitoring of recuperating patients while allowing them increased mobility.

RESPIRATORY MONITORING

Critical care personnel should monitor several primary respiratory parameters, including respiratory rate, tidal volume or minute ventilation, and oxygenation for critically ill patients. Routine monitoring of arterial carbon dioxide levels would be desirable, but the technology for monitoring these parameters is not yet developed enough to consider mandatory continuous monitoring. Among mechanically ventilated patients, many physiologic functions can be monitored routinely and continuously by the ventilator. This section does not discuss monitoring by the mechanical ventilator (see Chapter 30) but examines devices that might be routinely used to monitor the aforementioned parameters continuously and noninvasively.

Respiratory Rate, Tidal Volume, and Minute Ventilation

Clinical examination of the patient often fails to detect clinically important changes in respiratory rate and tidal volume [88]. Physicians, nurses, and hospital staff frequently report inaccurate respiratory rates, possibly because they underestimate the measurement's importance [89]. In another study, ICU staff had a greater than 20% error more than one-third of the time when the recorded respiratory rate was compared with objective tracings [90]. This is particularly surprising since the respiratory rate is an especially important predictor of outcomes for many severity of illness scores such as the APACHE prediction system [91]. In fact, respiratory rate has been called "the neglected vital sign" [92]. Providers' clinical assessment of tidal volume and minute ventilation is similarly inaccurate [93]. Therefore, objective monitoring must be used because clinical evaluation is inaccurate.

Impedance Monitors

ICUs commonly use impedance monitors to measure respiratory rates and approximate tidal volume. These devices typically use ECG leads and measure changes in impedance generated by the change in distance between leads as a result of the thoracoabdominal motions of breathing. Obtaining a quality signal requires placing the leads at points of maximal change in thoracoabdominal contour or using sophisticated computerized algorithms. Alarms can then be set for high and low rates or for a percentage drop in the signal that is thought to correlate with a decrease in tidal volume.

In clinical use, impedance monitors can suffer confounding problems. They have failed to detect obstructive apnea when it has occurred and falsely detected apnea when it has not [94,95]. About one-third of all apnea alarms from this technology are false-positives [96]. In situations with moving patients, they are even less accurate for the quantification of respiratory rate [97]. Impedance monitors alone are poor detectors of obstructive apnea because they may count persistent chest wall motion as breaths when the apneic patient struggles to overcome airway obstruction [94,95]. In general, respiratory rate monitoring in the ICU results in a very high fraction of clinically irrelevant alarms: in one study, only 4% of respiratory alarms were deemed clinically relevant [98]. Although impedance monitors offer the advantage of being very inexpensive when ECG monitoring is already in use, they lack accuracy when precise measurements of apnea, respiratory rate, airflow, or tidal volume are required.

Respiratory Inductive Plethysmography

Respiratory inductive plethysmography (RIP) measures changes in the cross-sectional area of the chest and abdomen that occur with respiration and processes these signals into respiratory rate and tidal volume. This technology may be familiar to providers and patients because it is often used in polysomnograms. Typically, two elastic bands with embedded wires are placed above the xiphoid and around the abdomen. As the cross-sectional area of the bands changes with respiration, the self-inductance of the coils changes the frequency of attached oscillators. These signals are generally calibrated to a known gas volume, or may be internally calibrated so that further measurements reflect a percentage change from baseline rather than an absolute volume. RIP can accurately measure respiratory rate and the percentage change in tidal volume, as well as detect obstructive apneas [99–101]. RIP has been used to follow lung volumes in patients undergoing high-frequency oscillatory ventilation [102]. These measurements are often more accurate than impedance measurements [95]. However, some studies have found problems with RIP's estimation of lung volumes. Notably, RIP must be calibrated against a known gas volume in order to provide tidal volume estimates. This calibration is not always accurate and may result in errors of >10% for 5% to 10% of patients even in highly controlled circumstances [99,103]. In mechanically ventilated patients, RIP had significant measurement drift (25 cm^3 per minute) and imprecise volume estimates. Only about two-thirds of tidal volume estimates were accurate to within 10% of the reference value [104].

In addition to displaying respiratory rate and percentage change in tidal volume, RIP can provide asynchronous and paradoxical breathing measurements and alarms, which are common during early weaning and may be helpful for predicting respiratory failure [105]. The noninvasive nature of the tidal volume measurement may be helpful for patients in whom technical problems or leaks make it difficult to directly measure expired volume (e.g., patients with bronchopleural fistulas). In addition, RIP can display changes in functional residual capacity, which permits health care providers to assess the effects of changing positive end-expiratory pressure (PEEP) or response to bronchodilator therapy. Providers can determine the presence and estimation of the amount of auto (intrinsic) PEEP by observing the effect of applied (extrinsic) PEEP on functional residual capacity [106], with the caveats noted earlier regarding possible inaccuracy of volume measurements.

RIP systems are available with central monitoring station configurations, which have been used in noninvasively monitored respiratory care units; these units have allowed ICU-level patients to be safely moved to a less labor-intensive level of care [107]. Compared with impedance methods, RIP is more accurate and offers a variety of other useful measurements but is less convenient and more expensive.

Other Methods

Although health care providers can also use pneumotachometers, capnographs, and electromyography to accurately measure respiratory rate, these methods are not commonly used in the ICU. A pneumotachometer requires complete collection of exhaled gas and, therefore, either intubation or use of a tight-fitting face mask is not practical simply for monitoring. A second alternative, capnography, works exceedingly well as a respiratory rate monitor. Because it does not require intubation or a face mask, it can be a useful tool in many circumstances. Capnography is discussed in more detail later in this chapter. A third option, surface electromyography of respiratory muscles, can be used to calculate respiratory rate accurately [108] but cannot detect obstructive apnea or provide a measure of tidal volume. Electromyography works well for infants but presents difficulties in adults, especially in obese adults and those with edema.

Recently, substantial research has focused on better ways to noninvasively monitor respiratory rate. All of these need clinical validation in a critical care setting, but examples of potentially emerging technologies include mechanical contact sensors placed in patient beds or pillows, acoustical respiratory monitoring, photoplethysmography, and monitoring based on the humidity of exhaled gas.

Measurements of Gas Exchange

Pulse Oximetry

Clinical estimation of hypoxemia is exceptionally unreliable [109,110]. Pulse oximeters measure the saturation of hemoglobin in the tissue during the arterial and venous phases of pulsation and mathematically derive arterial saturation. A meta-analysis of 74 oximeter studies suggests that these estimates are usually accurate within 5% of simultaneous gold standard measurements [111]. However, up to 97% of physicians and nurses who use pulse oximeters do not understand their underlying fundamental principles [112]. This section reviews the essential technology involved in pulse oximetry and practical problems that limit its use.

Theory. Oximeters distinguish between oxyhemoglobin and reduced hemoglobin on the basis of their differential absorption of light. Oxyhemoglobin absorbs much less red (±660 nm) and slightly more infrared (±910 to 940 nm) light than nonoxygenated hemoglobin. Oxygen saturation thereby determines the ratio of red to infrared absorption. When red and infrared light are directed from light-emitting diodes (LEDs) to a photodetector across a pulsatile tissue bed, the absorption of each wavelength by the tissue bed varies cyclically with pulse. During diastole, absorption is due to the nonvascular tissue components (e.g., bone, muscle, and interstitium) and venous blood. During systole, absorption is determined by all of these components and arterialized blood. The pulse amplitude accounts for only 1% to 5% of the total signal [113]. Thus, the difference between absorption in systole and diastole is in theory due to the presence of arterialized blood. The change in the ratio of absorption between systole and diastole can then be used to calculate an estimate of arterial oxygen saturation. Absorption is typically measured hundreds of times per second. Signals usually are averaged over several seconds and then displayed numerically. The algorithm used for each oximeter is determined by calibrations from human volunteers. Most oximeters under ideal circumstances measure the saturation indicated by the pulse oximeter (SpO_2) to within 2% of arterial oxygen saturation [114].

Cooximeters perform measurements on whole blood obtained from an artery or a vein. They frequently measure absorbance at multiple wavelengths and compute the percentage of oxyhemoglobin, deoxyhemoglobin, methemoglobin, and carboxyhemoglobin (COHb) in total hemoglobin based on different absorption spectra. They are mostly free of the artifacts that limit the accuracy of tissue oximeters and are regarded as a gold standard by which other methods of assessing saturation can be measured.

Technology. Many manufacturers market pulse oximeters. Because of the variety of manufacturers, the numerous algorithms used, and the diverse patient populations studied, it is difficult to generalize from studies performed with one particular instrument, with its specific version of software, in one defined group of patients, to critically ill patients in general. The reader should always check with an oximeter's manufacturer before generalizing the following discussion to his or her oximeter and patient population.

Problems Encountered in Use. Because pulse oximeters are ubiquitous, all ICU providers must understand their limitations. A meta-analysis of problems encountered in pulse oximetry trials identified severe hypoxemia, dyshemoglobinemia, low perfusion states, skin pigmentation, and hyperbilirubinemia as having the potential to affect the accuracy of pulse oximeter readings [111]. Any process that affects or interferes with the absorption of light between the LEDs and photodetector alters the quality of pulsatile flow, or changes the hemoglobin that may distort the oximeter's calculations. Pulse oximeters should be able to obtain valid readings in 98% of patients in an operating room or postanesthesia care unit [115]. Table 27.1 lists the problems that must be considered in clinical use.

Calibration. Manufacturers use normal volunteers to derive pulse oximeter calibration algorithms. This creates three problems. First, manufacturers use different calibration algorithms, which results in a difference in SpO_2 of up to 2.7% between different manufacturers' oximeters used to measure the same patient [116]. Second, the alternative manufacturers have defined SpO_2 differently for calibration purposes. Calibration may or may not account for the interference of small amounts of dyshemoglobinemia (e.g., methemoglobin or COHb). For

TABLE 27.1

Conditions Adversely Affecting Accuracy of Oximetry

May result in poor signal detection	
Probe malposition	No pulse
Motion	Vasoconstriction
Hypothermia	Hypotension
Falsely lowers SpO_2	**Falsely raises SpO_2**
Nail polish	Elevated carboxyhemoglobin
Dark skin	Elevated methemoglobin
Ambient light	Ambient light
Elevated serum lipids	Hypothermia
Methylene blue	
Indigo carmine	
Indocyanine green	

SpO_2, saturation indicated by the pulse oximeter.

example, if an oximeter is calibrated on the basis of a study of nonsmokers with a 2% COHb level, the measured SpO_2 percentage would differ depending on whether the value used to calibrate SpO_2 included or excluded the 2% COHb [116]. Third, it is difficult, for ethical reasons, for manufacturers to obtain an adequate number of validated readings in people with an SpO_2 of less than 70% to develop accurate calibration algorithms in this saturation range. Most oximeters give less precise readings in this saturation range [117]. Unless better calibration algorithms become available, oximeters should be considered unreliable when SpO_2 is less than 70%, although this may have little clinical impact since emergent intervention is usually required for all SpO_2 readings <70%.

Measurement sites. Careful sensor positioning is crucial for obtaining accurate results from a pulse oximeter [118]. Practitioners can obtain accurate measurements from fingers, forehead, and earlobes. The response time from a change in the partial pressure of arterial oxygen (PaO_2) to a change in displayed SpO_2 is delayed for finger and toe probes compared to ear, cheek, or glossal probes [119,120]. Forehead edema, wetness, and head motion may result in inaccurate forehead SpO_2 values [121]. Motion and perfusion artifacts are the greatest problems with finger or toe measurements. The earlobe is believed to be the site least affected by vasoconstriction artifact [122], but paradoxically the finger may give a better signal at times of hypoperfusion [111].

Fingernails. Long fingernails may prevent correct positioning of the finger pulp over the LEDs used in inflexible probes and therefore produce inaccurate SpO_2 readings without affecting the pulse rate [123]. Synthetic nails have also produced erroneous results [114]. Adhesive tape, even when placed over both sides of a finger, did not affect measured SpO_2 [124]. Since pulse oximetry depends fundamentally on color, nail polish may falsely lower SpO_2. In a 1988 study, blue, green, and black polish showed greater decreases than red or purple [125]. However, a 2002 study with a newer generation oximeter did not find this effect [126]. In addition, placing the probe sideways across the fingernail bed appeared to ameliorate any effect of fingernail polish in one study [127].

Skin color. The effect of skin color on SpO_2 was assessed in a study of 655 patients [128]. Although patients with the darkest skin had significantly less accurate SpO_2 readings, the mean inaccuracy in SpO_2 (compared with cooximetry) between subjects with light skin and those with the darkest skin was only 0.5%, a clinically insignificant difference. Pulse oximeters, however, encountered difficulties in obtaining readings in darker skinned patients; 18% of patients with darker skin triggered warning lights or messages versus 1% of lighter skinned patients. A study of 284 patients with a newer generation oximeter also found that skin color did not affect measurement accuracy. Poor-quality readings were found more often in darker skinned patients, although this was a rare event (<1% of all patients) [129]. Thus, dark skin may prevent a measurement from being obtained, but when the oximeter reports an error-free value, the value is generally accurate enough for clinical use [130].

Ambient light. Ambient light that affects absorption in the 660- or 910-nm wavelengths, or both, may affect calculations of saturation and pulse. Xenon arc surgical lights [131], fluorescent lights [132], and fiberoptic light sources [133] have caused falsely elevated saturation but typically are accompanied by obvious dramatic elevations in reported pulse. An infrared heating lamp [134] has produced falsely low saturations and a falsely low pulse, and a standard 15-W fluorescent bulb resulted in falsely low saturation without a change in heart rate [135]. Interference from surrounding lights should be suspected by the presence of pulse values discordant from the palpable pulse or ECG, or changes in the pulse-saturation display when the probe is transiently shielded from ambient light with an opaque object. Most manufacturers have now modified their probes to minimize this problem. Studies report that ambient lighting has little or no effect on newer generation oximeters [136], although this varies among manufacturers [137].

Hyperbilirubinemia. Bilirubin's absorbance peak is maximal in the 450-nm range but has tails extending in either direction [138]. Bilirubin, therefore, does not typically affect pulse oximeters that use the standard two-diode system [138,139]. However, it may greatly interfere with the measurement of saturation by cooximeters. Cooximeters typically use four to six wavelengths of light and measure absolute absorbance to quantify the percentage of all major hemoglobin variants. Serum bilirubin values as high as 44 mg per dL had no effect on the accuracy of pulse oximeters but led to falsely low levels of oxyhemoglobin measured by cooximetry [138].

Dyshemoglobinemias. Conventional (two-diode) pulse oximeters cannot detect the presence of methemoglobin, COHb, or fetal hemoglobin. Fetal hemoglobin may confound readings in neonates but is rarely a problem in adults. On the other hand, acquired methemoglobinemia—although uncommon—is seen in routine practice, largely due to the use of methemoglobinemia-inducing drugs such as topical anesthetics [140]. Because methemoglobin absorbs more light at 660 nm than at 990 nm, it affects pulse oximetry readings [141]. Moreover, higher levels of methemoglobin tend to bias the reading toward 85% to 90% [142]. COHb is typically read by a two-diode oximeter as 90% oxyhemoglobin and 10% reduced hemoglobin [143], resulting in false elevations of SpO_2. A gap between pulse oximetry and PO_2 or cooximetrically measured oxygen saturation may suggest elevated COHb levels, particularly in patients with smoke inhalation or potential carbon monoxide poisoning [144]. Because COHb may routinely be 10% among smokers, pulse oximetry may fail to detect significant desaturation in this group of patients. Oxygen saturation in smokers, when measured by cooximetry, was on average 5% lower than pulse oximetric values [145]. Hemolytic anemia may also elevate COHb up to 2.6% [146]. Because other etiologies of COHb are rare in the hospital and the half-life of COHb is short, this problem is unusual in the critical care setting except in newly admitted patients, patients with active hemolysis, or those on COHb-inducing drugs such as sodium nitroprusside [147]. More recently, some pulse oximeters that use multiwavelength technology have been able to successfully report methemoglobin and COHb levels [148].

Anemia. Few clear data are available on the effect of anemia on pulse oximetry. In dogs, there was no significant degradation in accuracy until the hematocrit was less than 10% [149]. In one study of humans who had hemorrhagic anemia, there appeared to be little effect on pulse oximetry accuracy [150].

Lipids. Patients with elevated chylomicrons and those receiving lipid infusions may have falsely low SpO_2 because of interference in absorption by the lipid [151]. This also affects cooximetry and may lead to spurious methemoglobin readings [152].

Glycohemoglobin A1C. A study of 261 patients with type 2 diabetes mellitus showed that a HbA1c greater than 7% leads to an overestimation of SpO_2 by an average of 2.3% when compared to those with a HbA1c less than 7% [153].

Hypothermia. Good-quality signals may be unobtainable in 10% of hypothermic patients [154]. The decrease in signal quality probably results from hypothermia-induced vasoconstriction. When good-quality signals could be obtained, SpO_2

differed from cooximetry-measured saturation by only 0.6% [154] in one series.

Intravascular dyes. Methylene blue, used to treat methemoglobinemia, has a maximal absorption at 670 nm and therefore falsely lowers measured SpO_2 [155]. Indocyanine green and indigo carmine also lower SpO_2, but the changes are minor and brief [156]. Fluorescein has no effect on SpO_2 [156]. Because of the rapid vascular redistribution of injected dyes, the effect on oximetry readings typically lasts only 5 to 10 minutes [157]. Patent V dye, which is used to visualize lymphatics in sentinel node mapping, confounds pulse oximetry, an effect which may persist for more than 90 minutes [158].

Motion artifact. Shivering and other motions that change the distance from diode to receiver may result in artifact. Oximeters account for motion by different algorithms. Some oximeters display a warning sign, others stop reporting data, and others display erroneous values. The display of a plethysmographic waveform rather than a signal strength bar helps to indicate to providers that artifact has distorted the pulse signal and lowered the quality of the SpO_2 reading. Newer generation oximeters appear to have significantly less susceptibility to motion artifact than earlier models [159].

Hypoperfusion. During a blood pressure cuff inflation model of hypoperfusion, most oximeters remained within 2% of control readings [160]. Increasing systemic vascular resistance and decreasing cardiac output can also make it harder to obtain a good-quality signal. In one series, the lowest cardiac index and highest systemic vascular resistance at which a signal could be detected were 2.4 L/min/m^2 and 2,930 dynes second/cm^5/m^2, respectively [161]. Warming the finger [162] or applying a vasodilating cream [161] tended to extend the range of signal detection in individual patients. The oximeter's ability to display a waveform and detect perfusion degradation of the signal was crucial for determining when the readings obtained were valid [160].

Pulsatile venous flow. In physiologic states in which venous and capillary flows become pulsatile, the systolic pulse detected by the oximeter may no longer reflect the presence of just arterial blood. In patients with severe tricuspid regurgitation, the measured saturation may be falsely low, especially with ear probes [163].

Indications. The Society of Critical Care Medicine considers pulse oximetry (or transcutaneous oxygen measurement) essential monitoring for all ICU patients receiving supplemental oxygen [164]. Unsuspected hypoxemia is common among critically ill patients. Sixteen percent of patients not receiving supplemental oxygen in the recovery room following general anesthesia have saturations of less than 90% [165]. In 35% of patients, saturations of less than 90% develop during transfer out of the operating room [166]. Because of the high frequency of hypoxemia among critically ill patients, the frequent need to adjust oxygen flow, and the unreliability of visual inspection to detect mild desaturation, oximeters should be used for most critically ill patients for routine, continuous monitoring. In one study that randomized more than 20,000 operative and perioperative patients to continuous or no oximetric monitoring, the authors concluded that oximetry permitted detection of more hypoxemic events, prompted increases in the fraction of oxygen in inspired gas, and significantly decreased the incidence of myocardial ischemia but did not significantly decrease mortality or complication rates [167].

Oximeters have been used in the ICU for reasons other than continuous monitoring. For example, oximeters may be helpful during difficult intubations. Once desaturation occurs, attempts to intubate should be postponed until manual ventilation restores saturation. Note, however, that oximetry is not helpful for promptly detecting inadvertent esophageal intubation because desaturation may lag significantly behind apnea in preoxygenated patients [168]. Oximeters can be useful for detecting systolic blood pressure (see arterial pressure monitoring earlier), and have been used in other clinical applications with varying degrees of success. Notably, a normal SpO_2 reading should *not* be used to exclude pulmonary embolism [169].

Capnography

Capnography involves the measurement and display of expired PCO_2 concentrations. This section reviews the technology, the sources of differences between end-tidal PCO_2 ($EtCO_2$) and $PaCO_2$, and the indications for capnography in the ICU.

Technology. The partial pressure of expired CO_2 is usually determined by infrared absorbance or mass spectrometry. The infrared technique relies on the fact that carbon dioxide has a characteristic absorbance of infrared light, with maximal absorbance near a wavelength of 4.28 mm. A heated wire with optical filters is used to generate an infrared light of appropriate wavelength. When carbon dioxide passes between a focused beam of light and a semiconductor photodetector, an electronic signal can be generated that, when calibrated, accurately reflects the partial pressure of the tested gas.

A mass spectrometer bombards gas with an electron stream. The ion fragments that are generated can be deflected by a magnetic field to detector plates located in precise positions to detect ions that are characteristic of the molecule being evaluated. The current generated at the detector can be calibrated to be proportional to the partial pressure of the molecule being evaluated.

The two techniques have different strengths. Mass spectrometers can detect the partial pressures of several gases simultaneously and can monitor several patients at once. Infrared techniques measure only PCO_2 and are usually used on only one patient at a time. The calibration and analysis time required for mass spectrometry is significantly longer than with infrared techniques. Infrared systems respond to changes in approximately 100 milliseconds, whereas mass spectrometers take 45 seconds to 5 minutes to respond [170]. Although costs vary widely, mass spectrometers are in general far more expensive and are most frequently purchased to be the central component of a carbon dioxide monitoring system. In the operating room, mass spectrometry has the advantage of being able to measure the partial pressure of anesthetic gases, and the need for a technical specialist to oversee its operation can be more easily justified. For these reasons, mass spectrometry has achieved much more popularity in the operating room than in the ICU.

Gases can be sampled by mainstream or sidestream techniques. Mainstream sampling involves placing the capnometer directly in line in the patient's respiratory circuit. All air leaving the patient passes through the capnometer. The sidestream sampling techniques pump 100 to 300 mL expired gas per minute through thin tubing to an adjacent analyzing chamber.

The mainstream method can be used only for patients who are intubated or wearing a tight-fitting laryngeal, face, or nose mask. Mainstream sampling offers the advantage of almost instantaneous analysis of sampled air, but it increases the patient's dead space and adds weight to the endotracheal tube. Sidestream sampling removes air from the expiratory circuit, altering measurement of tidal volume. Slower aspirating flow rates and longer tubing lengths significantly worsen the ability to detect a rapid rise in carbon dioxide and cause delay between physiologic changes in the patient and the display of changes on the monitor [171]. When the delay exceeds the respiratory cycle time, the generated data are inaccurate [171]. Located near the mouth or nose, sidestream sampling lines are also prone to clogging with secretions, saliva, or water condensation. Sidestream sampling can be used in nonintubated patients to detect cyclic changes in carbon dioxide concentrations. Because of these issues, accurate sidestream sampling requires short sampling tubes and attention to the possibility of clogged sample lines.

Differences Between End-Tidal and Arterial Carbon Dioxide. The PCO_2 of exhaled air measured at the mouth changes in a characteristic pattern for normal people that reflects the underlying physiologic changes in gas exchange (Fig. 27.1). During inspiration, the PCO_2 is negligible, but it rises abruptly with expiration. The rapid rise reflects mixing and the washout of dead space air with air from perfused alveoli, which contain higher levels of CO_2. A plateau concentration is reached after dead space air has been exhaled. The plateau level is determined by the mean alveolar PCO_2, which is in equilibration with pulmonary capillary PCO_2. The end-alveolar plateau level of PCO_2 measured during the last 20% of exhalation is the $EtCO_2$. In normal people at rest, the difference between $EtCO_2$ and $PaCO_2$ is ±1.5 mm Hg. A difference exists because of the presence of dead space and normal physiologic shunting. Changes in dead space or pulmonary perfusion alter ventilation–perfusion ratios and change the relationship between end-tidal and arterial PCO_2 values. As dead space increases, the $EtCO_2$ represents more the (lower) PCO_2 of nonperfused alveoli, thereby diverging from the $PaCO_2$ value. As perfusion decreases, fewer alveoli are perfused, creating a similar effect.

For most equipment, the $EtCO_2$ level is determined by a computerized algorithm. Because algorithms are imperfect, a waveform display is considered essential for accurate interpretation of derived values [171]. For slowly breathing patients, cardiac pulsations may cause the intermittent exhalation of small amounts of air at the end of the lungs' expiratory effort. This results in oscillations that may obscure the plateau phase. An irregular respiratory pattern or large increases in dead space can also cause distortion of the plateau phase. Visual inspection of traces can detect situations in which algorithms are prone to produce errors [170].

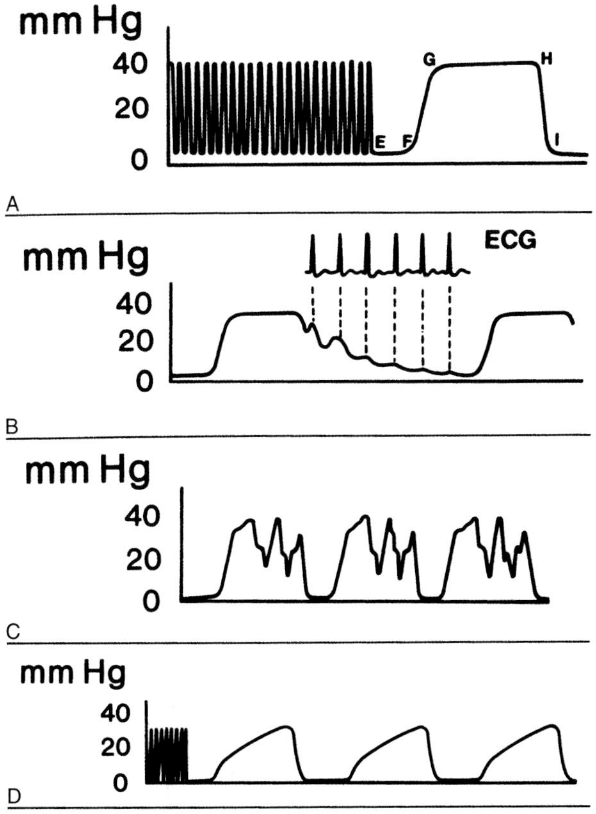

FIGURE 27.1 Normal and abnormal capnograms. In the normal capnogram (**A**), on the right of the trace, the paper speed has been increased. The *EF* segment is inspiration. The *FG* segment reflects the start of expiration with exhalation of dead space gas. The *GH* segment is the alveolar plateau. End-tidal values are taken at point *H*. *HI* is the beginning of inspiration. In the abnormal capnograms, the alveolar plateau is distorted and the end-tidal point cannot be clearly determined because of cardiac oscillations (**B**), erratic breathing (**C**), and obstructive airway disease (**D**). ECG, electrocardiogram. (Modified from Stock MC: Noninvasive carbon dioxide monitoring. *Crit Care Clin* 4:511, 1988.)

Indications. In the ICU, capnography is most useful for (1) detection of extubation, (2) determining the presence or absence of respiration, and (3) detecting return of spontaneous circulation after cardiac arrest. Such determinations do not require that $EtCO_2$ be measured accurately, only that changes be detected reliably. Alarms for apnea and tachypnea can be set and relied on, although capnography cannot discriminate between obstructive and central apnea. Capnography is a useful adjunct for detecting unintentional extubation, malposition of the endotracheal tube, or absence of perfusion. Cyclic variation of $EtCO_2$ is absent in esophageal intubation or disconnection from the ventilator [172], although pharyngeal intubation with adequate ventilation may produce a normal capnogram.

Capnography can demonstrate the return of circulation after cardiopulmonary arrest or bypass and is a useful indicator of endotracheal tube placement. In full cardiac arrest, $EtCO_2$ is low because of lack of perfusion; a rapid rise in $EtCO_2$ indicates return of circulation and successful delivery of CO_2 to the alveoli [173]. Capnography also detects esophageal intubation [174]. The American Heart Association 2015 Emergency Cardiovascular Care Guidelines include a Class I recommendation for using quantitative waveform capnography for verifying endotracheal tube placement after intubation for cardiac arrest. They also suggest consideration of using capnography to monitor CPR quality in real-time, titrate vasopressor therapy, and detect return of spontaneous circulation as a IIb recommendation. Finally, because $EtCO_2$ reflects cardiac output, the guidelines note that "failure to achieve an $EtCO_2$ of greater than 10 mm Hg by waveform capnography after 20 minutes of CPR may be considered as one component of a multimodal approach to decide when to end resuscitative efforts but should not be used in isolation" [175].

Can capnography be used as an approximation of arterial $PaCO_2$ for most critically ill patients? The answer is no. $EtCO_2$ measurements are unreliable indicators of $PaCO_2$ among critically ill patients. Since these patients undergo rapid changes in dead space fraction and pulmonary perfusion, the relationship of $EtCO_2$ to arterial $PaCO_2$ may change rapidly and unpredictably. In one study of anesthetized, stable, generally healthy adults, $PaCO_2$ could not be reliably determined from end-tidal values [176]. In patients undergoing weaning from mechanical ventilation, $EtCO_2$ was also shown to have no predictable relationship to $PaCO_2$ [177]. Although end-tidal and arterial values correlated well ($r = 0.78$) and rarely differed by more than 4 mm Hg, changes in $EtCO_2$ correlated poorly with changes in arterial PCO_2 ($r^2 = 0.58$). Because of changes in dead space and perfusion, arterial and end-tidal measurements at times moved unpredictably in opposite directions. $EtCO_2$ values can also be altered depending on the site of sampling as shown in a study comparing sidestream versus mainstream sampling among critically ill patients. In that study, $EtCO_2$ differed from $PaCO_2$ by 13 mm Hg on average for mainstream sampling and 9.7 mm Hg for sidestream sampling [178]. Although theoretically attractive, the use of end-tidal carbon dioxide measurements to evaluate changes in ventilation–perfusion mismatch in response to ventilator changes has failed to yield consistent clinical benefits [179].

Capnography has been helpful in the operating room for detecting air and pulmonary embolism as well as malignant hyperthermia [170]. In these situations, the capnograph does not provide a diagnosis; it records a change that, if limits are exceeded, signals an alarm. The responsibility for accurately interpreting the subtleties of changes of the capnogram remains the task of an experienced physician.

Conclusions. Capnography should be used after cardiac arrest to confirm endotracheal tube placement, and should be considered for monitoring the quality of CPR during an arrest. It is also an accurate monitor of respiratory rate (unlike many other technologies). In general, it should *not* be used as a substitute for $PaCO_2$ monitoring because the relationship of $PaCO_2$ and $EtCO_2$ varies for patients with changing cardiac output, fluctuating respiratory function, or chronic lung disease. This is important between patients, but also within the same patient over time. Capnography has an accepted role in the operating room, where its value is increased because of its ability to help detect endotracheal tube malposition, air embolism, pulmonary embolism, and malignant hyperthermia, and where there is a highly skilled anesthesiologist immediately available to interpret subtle changes in the capnogram.

NONINVASIVE TISSUE PERFUSION MONITORING

Bedside providers usually monitor tissue perfusion based on clinical signs such as skin temperature and capillary refill time. However, several noninvasive technologies provide quantitative data about overall or regional tissue perfusion. Unlike most of the other monitoring technologies described in this chapter, clinical adoption of these techniques has been relatively limited and heterogeneous [180]. This section reviews three such technologies that measure local PCO_2 or PO_2: gastric tonometry, sublingual capnometry, and transcutaneous oxygen and carbon dioxide monitoring. Measurements from each of these techniques correlate with meaningful clinical outcomes such as patient survival.

Physiology: Why Regional PO_2 and PCO_2 Reflect Tissue Perfusion and Not Just Global Gas Exchange

At first glance, it would appear that measurement of regional PO_2 or PCO_2 in the skin, stomach, or tongue would reflect global gas exchange and might be used for noninvasive blood gas estimation. In some cases, this is true. In healthy adults, for example, transcutaneously measured PO_2 and PCO_2 ($PtcO_2$ and $PtcCO_2$) accurately reflect PaO_2 and $PaCO_2$ [181]. The measured transcutaneous values of oxygen and carbon dioxide are typically 10 mm Hg lower [182] and 5 to 23 mm Hg higher [183] than arterial values, respectively.

However, local PO_2 and PCO_2 therefore depend not only on global gas exchange, cardiac output, and oxygen content, but also on regional blood flow and oxygen delivery to the site of measurement. Under normal circumstances, oxygen delivery far exceeds consumption. In critical illness, however, regional hypoperfusion or inadequate regional delivery of oxygen may occur for any number of reasons: hypotension, regional vasoconstriction, low cardiac output states, anemia, vascular occlusion, etc. If there is no flow to the region, there can be no delivery of oxygen and no elimination of carbon dioxide by the vasculature—thus creating lower local PO_2 and higher local PCO_2 than in the arterial circulation. When tissue is hypoperfused, local metabolism then further alters local PO_2 and PCO_2. As cellular processes use available oxygen for the production of adenosine triphosphate (ATP), local PO_2 falls. When these cells use ATP faster than they replenish it, they liberate hydrogen ions (H^+) and reduce local pH. (Alternatively, cells may produce lactic acid through the anaerobic metabolic pathway.) These additional hydrogen ions are then buffered by tissue bicarbonate, generating CO_2 by the reaction:

$$H^+ + HCO_3^- \rightarrow H_2O_3 \rightarrow H_2O + CO_2.$$

This increases the local PCO_2 above the corresponding global/arterial values [184]. For these reasons, local PO_2 and PCO_2 vary not only with global gas exchange, but also with local tissue perfusion and other factors.

Gastric Tonometry

Gastric tonometry, probably the most commonly used of the three perfusion monitoring techniques discussed in this section, assesses regional splanchnic perfusion based on the stomach's mucosal PCO_2. The splanchnic circulation has several properties which make this region particularly useful to assess in critically ill patients. Early in the development of shock states, the splanchnic circulation vasoconstricts, shunting cardiac output toward other core organs. Although this helps to prevent circulatory collapse, it may also result in intestinal mucosal ischemia—increasing the risk of gastric stress ulceration, mesenteric ischemia, and translocation of gut bacteria into the systemic circulation [185]. The gut is particularly sensitive to hypoperfusion and so may provide earlier warning of occult hypoperfusion than other vascular beds—leading some to liken it to a coal miner's canary [186]. Gastric tonometry measures gastric luminal PCO_2 and estimates gastric intramucosal PCO_2 and pH (pHi).

Technical Considerations

Development. Early measurements of visceral mucosal pH required operative implantation of monitors and focused on the gallbladder, urinary bladder, and small bowel [187,188]. Development of silastic tubing [189]—which is exceptionally permeable to O_2 and CO_2—and confirmation that gases in tissue equilibrate rapidly with fluid in the lumen of a hollow viscus [190] allowed development of the modern gastrointestinal tonometer.

Technique. The upper gastrointestinal catheter is inserted with a standard technique for nasogastric tube placement, and placement is confirmed radiographically. The stopcock is flushed with fluid to eliminate any trapped air, the balloon is filled to the manufacturer's specifications with fluid, and the tonometer lumen is closed to the outside environment. The fluid is allowed to equilibrate with the fluid in the lumen of the organ being monitored, a process believed to require approximately 90 minutes, although formulas are available to correct the values obtained with 30 to 90 minutes of equilibration [191]. After adequate time for equilibration, the dead space (usually 1.0 mL) is aspirated and discarded, and the fluid in the balloon is completely aspirated under anaerobic conditions. An ABG sample is taken simultaneously, and both samples are sent for analysis. The PCO_2 of the tonometer sample is measured directly. Providers can then calculate an arterial/mucosal PCO_2 gap or, using the HCO_3^- of arterial blood and the modified Henderson–Hasselbalch equation, pHi [192,193].

An air-based tonometer has also gained popularity. This device operates on the same principles as the saline-based tonometer, but automatically aspirates small amounts of air from a semipermeable balloon. This is substantially more convenient than the saline-based device, and allows semicontinuous measurement of gastric mucosal PCO_2. Results are generally similar to saline-based tonometry [194].

Technical Limitations. Several issues may confound the clinical use of gastric tonometry. Two of these apply only to saline-based tonometry. The fluid in the tonometer balloon requires 90 minutes for full equilibration with the fluid in the stomach. In a rapidly changing patient, this time window may not be appropriately timely. In addition, manufacturers calibrate blood gas analyzers to measure PCO_2 in blood, not saline. PCO_2 measurements in tonometer saline, therefore, may vary based on the blood gas analyzer used [195]. Other limitations apply to the general principle of measured gastric luminal PCO_2 to estimate mucosal perfusion. Tonometrically derived gastric pHi can be affected by the acid-secretory status of the stomach. In one study, mean gastric pHi was 7.30 in untreated normal volunteers but 7.39 in a similar group treated with ranitidine [196]. This was because the PCO_2 in the gastric fluid of the treated patients was 42 ± 4 mm Hg, compared with 52 ± 14 mm Hg in the untreated group. The difference in carbon dioxide content of the fluid is thought to be due to production of carbon dioxide by the conversion of secreted H^+ and HCO_3^- into water and carbon dioxide. Enteral feeding may also affect pHi reading. Tube feedings may lead to increased production of carbon dioxide through the interaction of secreted hydrogen ions and HCO_3^-. Some suggest temporarily discontinuing tube feeds before doing pHi measurements [197], although the PCO_2 effect appears to diminish after 24 hours of continuous feeding [198]. Finally, pHi is a calculated variable which uses the systemic arterial bicarbonate value; this probably does not reflect regional perfusion [193]. The present consensus favors the use of arterial-gastric PCO_2 gap rather than pHi [194,199].

Clinical Usefulness and Limitations. pHi correlates well with a number of clinically important end points. Changes in pHi during weaning from mechanical ventilation predict weaning failure [200]. Intraoperative and postoperative cardiac surgery patients have been particularly well studied, and in that group gastric pHi appears to predict complications well [201,202]. Most importantly, pHi predicts mortality of septic [203], acutely injured [204], and general ICU patients [205].

For a diagnostic tool to be *therapeutically* useful, however, we must be able to act on its results in a way that improves patient outcome [206]. Therapeutic protocols based on gastric tonometry have produced conflicting results. A randomized, controlled trial of 260 ICU patients, reported in 1992, found that gastric pHi-based therapy had no effect on mortality of patients with a low admission pHi but was associated with reduced mortality among patients with a normal admission pHi [207]. However, the interpretation of this finding is severely limited because the authors did not analyze the results in an intention-to-treat fashion, thus abandoning many of the benefits of randomization [208], and 21 patients were withdrawn from the study due to protocol noncompliance by treating physicians. A subsequent randomized, controlled trial of 210 general ICU patients, reported in 2000, found no difference between intervention and control arms [209]. For patients with a normal initial pHi, there was a nonsignificant trend toward increased 30-day mortality in the group treated based on pHi. A 2005 study randomized 151 trauma patients to pHi-driven therapy, splanchnic ischemia/reperfusion-based protocol, or usual care. The authors found no significant differences in mortality, organ dysfunction, ventilator days, or length of stay in an intention-to-treat analysis [210]. A recent meta-analysis of pHi-driven therapy showed no reduction in-hospital or ICU mortality, length of stay, or days of intubation. It did however show a decrease in overall mortality in patients who presented with a normal pHi [211].

Alternative Regional PCO_2 Measurement: Sublingual Capnometry. Sublingual capnometry operates on the same fundamental principles as gastric tonometry. A sensor is placed under the tongue and CO_2 diffuses across a semipermeable membrane into a dye, which fluoresces differently based on CO_2 concentration. A fiberoptic cable transmits light of the appropriate wavelength and detects the resulting fluorescence, which is proportional to CO_2 concentration in the sensor [180]. Results from this technique correlate with gastric tonometry [212] and patient outcomes [213]. No randomized intervention trials based on sublingual capnometry have yet been published.

Summary. Although gastric tonometry predicts many important clinical outcomes, high-quality data do not support gastric tonometry–based resuscitation. At this time, it remains largely a research tool. Researchers are continuing to investigate the use of sublingual capnometry, a similar technology, as a potential resuscitation end point.

Transcutaneous Oxygen and Carbon Dioxide Measurement in Adults

Transcutaneous measurements of the partial pressures of oxygen ($PtcO_2$) and carbon dioxide ($PtcCO_2$) are frequently used for neonatal blood gas monitoring but have not gained widespread clinical acceptance in adult ICUs [180]. In adults, similar to gastric tonometry, $PtcO_2$ and $PtcCO_2$ reflect *local* tissue oxygen and carbon dioxide levels and therefore blur the boundary between assessment of global gas exchange and regional tissue perfusion monitoring. More recently, measurements of transcutaneous hemoglobin oxygen saturation (StO_2) have entered the research and clinical realms.

This section refers only to transcutaneous monitoring in adults.

Technique

Oxygen and carbon dioxide diffuse out of the capillaries, into the interstitium, and through the skin. The skin usually resists O_2 and CO_2 diffusion, but heating the skin promotes diffusion by changing the structure of the stratum corneum, shifting the oxygen dissociation curve, and promoting arterialization of dermal capillaries [180]. Transcutaneous systems take advantage of these properties to measure partial pressures of oxygen ($PtcO_2$) and carbon dioxide ($PtcCO_2$). Typically, a unit less than 1 inch in diameter is attached with an airtight seal to the skin with an adhesive. An electrode heats the skin to improve gas exchange; a temperature sensor measures skin temperature at the skin surface and adjusts the heater to provide a constant temperature—typically about 44°C. Oxygen and carbon dioxide diffuse out of the capillaries into the interstitium and through the skin to measuring electrodes.

Technical Limitations

Because units use electrodes for partial pressure measurement, problems with calibration and electrode drift during prolonged monitoring can clearly alter measurements. Drift may alter readings by up to 12% over a 2-hour period [214]. Because of the heating requirement, probe sites must be changed at least every 4 hours to prevent burns [215]. Units must be recalibrated whenever the probe temperature is changed and every 4 to 6 hours to prevent artifact from electrode drift. Many units take 15 to 60 minutes to warm the skin and establish stable readings. Probes must be firmly attached to the skin, or leaks from the surrounding atmosphere lower $PtcCO_2$ and alter $PtcO_2$ values. Adhesion is a problem in diaphoretic patients.

Thick or edematous skin provides a diffusion barrier that amplifies differences between arterial and transcutaneous PO_2 and PCO_2. The longer the distance the gases must diffuse to be measured, the more important are the effects of temperature, perfusion, and local metabolism. This appears to be the fundamental reason why transcutaneous measurements are usually more closely related to arterial values in neonates than in adults. Edema, burns, abrasions, or scleroderma would all be expected to alter transcutaneous values.

Clinical Usefulness and Limitations

Because $PtcO_2$ and $PtcCO_2$ reflect local PO_2 and PCO_2, they change in response both to regional perfusion/oxygen delivery and to global derangements. In stable, healthy adults without hemodynamic or respiratory instability, $PtcO_2$ and $PtcCO_2$ accurately reflect PaO_2 and $PaCO_2$ [181,214]. The measured transcutaneous values of oxygen and carbon dioxide are typically 10 mm Hg lower [182] and 5 to 23 mm Hg higher [216] than arterial values, respectively. In stable patients, it may be reasonable to use transcutaneously measured values as surrogates for arterial PO_2 and PCO_2. However, systemic hypoperfusion due to low cardiac output, regional hypoperfusion due to sepsis or shock, and local hypoperfusion due to cutaneous vasoconstriction caused by medication or cold produces discrepancies. For these cases, transcutaneous measurements cease to reflect arterial values and better track oxygen delivery and tissue metabolism [217]. For these reasons, many authors have argued against relying on $PtcO_2$ and $PtcCO_2$ to estimate arterial PO_2 and PCO_2 for critically ill adults [217,218].

Several studies have demonstrated the value of transcutaneous oxygen measurements as indices of perfusion or oxygen delivery. When PaO_2 remains constant, a decrease in $PtcO_2$ is probably due to changes in perfusion. Changes in local perfusion and metabolism may cause $PtcO_2$ values to fall to zero and $PtcCO_2$ values to climb to more than 30 mm Hg above arterial values [216]. During cardiac decompensation and arrest, $PtcO_2$ correlates best with cardiac output [219]. In hemorrhagic shock, the ratio of $PtcO_2$ to PaO_2 decreases, even though PaO_2 may remain normal [220]. Because the measurements are very sensitive to changes in flow, they can be useful in predicting or warning of imminent change before a blood pressure response is seen. In a small series of high-risk perioperative patients, declines in the $PtcO_2/PaO_2$ ratio predicted subsequent hemodynamic collapse [221]. Transcutaneous $PtcO_2$ also correlates with mortality. Among emergency department patients with severe sepsis or septic shock, $PtcO_2$ was lower in nonsurvivors than in survivors [222]. Among trauma patients, $PtcO_2$ values were significantly higher in survivors than in nonsurvivors ($p < 0.001$) with an area under the receiver operating characteristics curve of 0.74 for predicting in-hospital mortality [223].

Ongoing Development

More recent work has focused on the use of near-infrared spectroscopy to measure tissue hemoglobin oxygen saturation. This technique, rather than quantifying partial pressures of oxygen, instead measures the percent of microvascular hemoglobin saturated with oxygen. It has shown clinical correlations with invasive hemodynamic measures for those with sepsis [224] and severity of shock for trauma victims [225]. Further research is required to define the role of StO_2 as a potential resuscitation end point.

Summary

Transcutaneous monitors have little role in the ICU as simple tools to replace other means of measuring arterial gases. They predictably reflect arterial PO_2 and PCO_2 values only in hemodynamically stable patients, who are least likely to demand intensive care or to benefit from ICU monitoring. As monitors of trends in PCO_2 and PO_2, they can be regarded as effective only in the sense that they typically do not produce false-negative alarms—that is, if the arterial values change, the transcutaneous values reflect the change. So many other factors, such as changes in tissue edema and perfusion, may result in alterations in transcutaneous trends that the supervising staff can initially determine only that *something* has changed. An accurate interpretation of the clinical event usually requires reassessment of either cardiac status or arterial gases.

Therefore, transcutaneous monitors are inadequate cardiac monitors and inadequate pulmonary monitors but are good cardiopulmonary monitors. When perfusion is stable, values reflect gas exchange. When gas exchange is stable, values reflect perfusion. When both are unstable, the results cannot be interpreted without additional information. The use of near-infrared spectroscopy to measure tissue hemoglobin oxygenation—StO_2—is a promising development, but one that requires further clinical study.

References

1. Peres Bota D, Lopes Ferreira F, Melot C, et al: Body temperature alterations in the critically ill. *Intensive Care Med* 30:811–816, 2004.
2. Kholoussy AM, Sufian S, Pavlides C: Central peripheral temperature gradient: its value and limitations in the management of critically ill surgical patients. *Am J Surg* 140(5):609–612, 1980.
3. Haupt MT, Bekes CE, Brilli RJ, et al: Guidelines on critical care services and personnel: recommendations based on a system of categorization of three levels of care. *Crit Care Med* 31:2677–2683, 2003.
4. Heinz J: Validation of sublingual temperatures in patients with nasogastric tubes. *Heart Lung* 14(2):128–130, 1985.
5. Myny D, De Waele J, Defloor T, et al: Temporal scanner thermometry: a new method of core temperature estimation in ICU patients. *Scott Med J* 50:15–18, 2005.
6. Cork RC, Vaughan RW, Humphrey LS: Precision and accuracy of intraoperative temperature monitoring. *Anesth Analg* 62(2):211–214, 1983.
7. Bone ME, Feneck RO: Bladder temperature as an estimate of body temperature during cardiopulmonary bypass. *Anaesthesia* 43(3):181–185, 1988.
8. Ramsay JG, Ralley FE, Whalley DG: Site of temperature monitoring and prediction of afterdrop after open heart surgery. *Can Anaesth Soc J* 32(6):607–612, 1985.
9. Crocker BD, Okumura F, McCuaig DI: Temperature monitoring during general anaesthesia. *Br J Anaesth* 52(12):1223–1229, 1980.
10. Severinghaus JW: Temperature gradients during hypothermia. *Ann N Y Acad Sci* 80:515–521, 1962.
11. Vale RJ: Monitoring of temperature during anesthesia. *Int Anesthesiol Clin* 19(1):61–84, 1981.
12. Giuliano KK, Scott SS, Elliot S, et al: Temperature measurement in critically ill orally intubated adults: a comparison of pulmonary artery core, tympanic, and oral methods. *Crit Care Med* 27:2188–2193, 1999.
13. Moran JL, Peter JV, Solomon PJ, et al: Tympanic temperature measurements: are they reliable in the critically ill? A clinical study of measures of agreement. *Crit Care Med* 35:155–164, 2007.
14. Amoateng-Adjepong Y, Del Mundo J, Manthous CA: Accuracy of infrared tympanic thermometer. *Chest* 115(4):1002–1005, 1999.
15. Camboni D, Philipp A, Schebesch KM, et al: Accuracy of core temperature measurement in deep hypothermic circulatory arrest. *Interact Cardiovasc Thorac Surg* 7:922–924, 2008.
16. Burgess GE III, Cooper JR, Marino RJ, et al: Continuous monitoring of skin temperature using a liquid-crystal thermometer during anesthesia. *South Med J* 71:516–518, 1978.
17. Roberts NH: The comparison of surface and core temperature devices. *J Am Assoc Nurse Anesth* 48:53, 1980.
18. Silverman RW, Lomax P: The measurement of temperature for thermoregulatory studies. *Pharmacol Ther* 27:233–242, 1985.
19. Terndrup TE, Rajk J: Impact of operator technique and device on infrared emission detection tympanic thermometry. *J Emerg Med* 10:683–687, 1992.
20. Farnell S, Maxwell L, Tan S, et al: Temperature measurement: comparison of non-invasive methods used in adult critical care. *J Clin Nurs* 14:632–639, 2005.
21. Suleman MI, Doufas AG, Akca O, et al: Insufficiency in a new temporal-artery thermometer for adult and pediatric patients. *Anesth Analg* 95:67–71, 2002; table of contents.
22. Pierce EC: Percutaneous arterial catheterization in man with special reference to aortography. *Surg Gynecol Obstet* 93:56–74, 1951.
23. Carrol GC: Blood pressure monitoring. *Crit Care Clin* 4:411–434, 1988.
24. Van Bergen FH, Weatherhead S, Treloar AE, et al: Comparison of direct and indirect methods of measuring arterial blood pressure. *Circulation* 10:481–490, 1954.
25. Bruner JM, Krenis LJ, Kunsman JM, et al: Comparison of direct and indirect methods of measuring arterial blood pressure: Part III. *Med Instrum* 15:182, 1981.
26. Bailey RH, Knaus VL, Bauer JH: Aneroid sphygmomanometers: an assessment of accuracy at a university hospital and clinics. *Arch Intern Med* 151:1409, 1991.
27. Talke P, Nichols RJ Jr, Traber DL: Does measurement of systolic blood pressure with a pulse oximeter correlate with conventional methods? *J Clin Monit* 6:5–9, 1990.
28. Zagzebski JA, ed: *Physics and Instrumentation in Doppler and B-Mode Ultrasonography*. Orlando, FL: Grune & Stratton, 1986.

29. Hochberg HM, Salomon H: Accuracy of automated ultrasound blood pressure monitor. *Curr Ther Res Clin Exp* 13:129, 1971.
30. Puritan BC: *Infrasonde Model D4000 Electronic Blood Pressure Monitor Operating Manual*. Los Angeles, CA: Puritan Bennett Corporation.
31. Nystrom E, Reid KH, Bennett R, et al: A comparison of two automated indirect arterial blood pressure meters: with recordings from a radial arterial catheter in anesthetized surgical patients. *Anesthesiology* 62:526, 1985.
32. Borow KM, Newberger JW: Non-invasive estimation of central aortic pressure using the oscillometric method for analyzing systemic artery pulsatile blood flow: comparative study of indirect systolic, diastolic, and mean brachial artery pressure with simultaneous direct ascending aortic pressure measurements. *Am Heart J* 103:879, 1982.
33. Van Egmond J, Hasenbros M, Crul JF: Invasive v. non-invasive measurement of arterial pressure. *Br J Anaesth* 57:434, 1985.
34. Bogert LW, van Lieshout JJ: Non-invasive pulsatile arterial pressure and stroke volume changes from the human finger. *Exp Physiol* 90:437–446, 2005.
35. Ilies C, Kiskalt H, Siedenhans D, et al: Detection of hypotension during caesarean section with continuous non-invasive arterial pressure device or intermittent oscillometric arterial pressure management. *Br J Anaesth* 109(3):413–419, 2012.
36. O'Rourke MF, Adji A: An updated clinical primer on large artery mechanics: implications of pulse waveform analysis and arterial tonometry. *Curr Opin Cardiol* 20:275–281, 2005.
37. Steiner LA, Johnston AJ, Salvador R, et al: Validation of a tonometric noninvasive arterial blood pressure monitor in the intensive care setting. *Anaesthesia* 58:448–454, 2003.
38. Janelle GM, Gravenstein N: An accuracy evaluation of the T-Line Tensymeter (continuous noninvasive blood pressure management device) versus conventional invasive radial artery monitoring in surgical patients. *Anesth Analg* 102:484–490, 2006.
39. Szmuk P, Pivalizza E, Warters RD, et al: An evaluation of the T-Line Tensymeter continuous noninvasive blood pressure device during induced hypotension. *Anaesthesia* 63:307–312, 2008.
40. Reder RF, Dimich I, Cohen ML: Evaluating indirect blood pressure measurement techniques: a comparison of three systems in infants and children. *Pediatrics* 62:326, 1978.
41. Yelderman M, Ream AK: Indirect measurement of mean blood pressure in the anesthetized patient. *Anesthesiology* 50:253, 1979.
42. Hirschl MM, Binder M, Herkner H, et al: Accuracy and reliability of noninvasive continuous finger blood pressure measurement in critically ill patients. *Crit Care Med* 24:1684, 1996.
43. Aitken HA, Todd JG, Kenny GN: Comparison of the Finapres and direct arterial pressure monitoring during profound hypotensive anesthesia. *Br J Anaesth* 67:36, 1991.
44. Rutten AJ, Isley AH, Skowronski GA, et al: A comparative study of the measurement of mean arterial blood pressure using automatic oscillometers, arterial cannulation and auscultation. *Anaesth Intensive Care* 14:58, 1986.
45. Stokes DN, Clutton-Brock T, Patil C, et al: Comparison of invasive and non-invasive measurements of continuous arterial pressure using the Finapres. *Br J Anaesth* 67:26–35, 1991.
46. Sy WP: Ulnar nerve palsy possibly related to use of automatically cycled blood pressure cuff. *Anesth Analg* 60:687–688, 1981.
47. Betts EK: Hazard of automated noninvasive blood pressure monitoring. *Anesthesiology* 55:717–718, 1981.
48. Bainbridge LC, Simmons HM, Elliot D: The use of automatic blood pressure monitors in the burned patient. *Br J Plast Surg* 43:322–324, 1990.
49. Hutton P, Prys-Roberts C: An assessment of the Dinamap 845. *Anaesthesia* 39:261–267, 1984.
50. Gardner RM, Schwarz R, Wong HC: Percutaneous indwelling radial-artery catheters for monitoring cardiovascular function. *N Engl J Med* 290:1227–1231, 1974.
51. McNulty I, Katz E, Kim KY: Thrombocytopenia following heparin flush. *Prog Cardiovasc Nurs* 20:143–147, 2005.
52. Rothe CF, Kim KC: Measuring systolic arterial blood pressure: possible errors from extension tubes or disposable transducer domes. *Crit Care Med* 8:683–689, 1980.
53. Shinozaki T, Deane RS, Mazuzan JE: The dynamic responses of liquid filled catheter systems for direct measurements of blood pressure. *Anesthesiology* 53:498–504, 1980.
54. Mermel LA, Farr BM, Sherertz RJ, et al: Guidelines for the management of intravascular catheter-related infections. *Clin Infect Dis* 32:1249–1272, 2001.
55. Koh DB, Gowardman JR, Rickard CM, et al: Prospective study of peripheral arterial catheter infection and comparison with concurrently sited central venous catheters. *Crit Care Med* 36:397–402, 2008.
56. Traore O, Liotier J, Souweine B: Prospective study of arterial and central venous catheter colonization and of arterial- and central venous catheter-related bacteremia in intensive care units. *Crit Care Med* 33:1276–1280, 2005.
57. Fraenkel DJ, Rickard C, Lipman J: Can we achieve consensus on central venous catheter-related infections? *Anaesth Intensive Care* 28:475–490, 2000.
58. Rijnders BJ, Van Wijngaerden E, Wilmer A, et al: Use of full sterile barrier precautions during insertion of arterial catheters: a randomized trial. *Clin Infect Dis* 36:743–748, 2003.
59. Cohen DM, Carino GP, Heffernan DS, et al: Arterial catheter use in the ICU: a national survey of antiseptic technique and perceived infectious risk. Crit Care Med 43:2346–2353.
60. Davis FM, Stewart JM: Radial artery cannulation. *Br J Anaesth* 52:41–47, 1980.
61. Russell JA, Joel M, Hudson RJ: Prospective evaluation of radial and femoral artery catheterization sites in critically ill adults. *Crit Care Med* 11:936–939, 1983.
62. Scheer B, Perel A, Pfeiffer UJ: Clinical review: complications and risk factors of peripheral arterial catheters used for haemodynamic monitoring in anaesthesia and intensive care medicine. *Crit Care* 6:199–204, 2002.
63. Dorman T, Breslow MJ, Lipsett PA, et al: Radial artery pressure monitoring underestimates central arterial pressure during vasopressor therapy in critically ill surgical patients. *Crit Care Med* 26:1646–1649, 1998.
64. Arnal D, Garutti I, Perez-Pena J, et al: Radial to femoral arterial blood pressure differences during liver transplantation. *Anaesthesia* 60:766–771, 2005.
65. Mignini MA, Piacentini E, Dubin A: Peripheral arterial blood pressure monitoring adequately tracks central arterial blood pressure in critically ill patients: an observational study. *Crit Care* 10:R43, 2006.
66. Lorente L, Santacreu R, Martin MM, et al: Arterial catheter-related infection of 2,949 catheters. *Crit Care* 10:R83, 2006.
67. Winters SR: Diagnosis by wireless. *Sci Am* 124:465, 1921.
68. Drew BJ, Califf RM, Funk M, et al: Practice standards for electrocardiographic monitoring in hospital settings: an American Heart Association scientific statement from the Councils on Cardiovascular Nursing, Clinical Cardiology, and Cardiovascular Disease in the Young: endorsed by the International Society of Computerized Electrocardiology and the American Association of Critical-Care Nurses. *Circulation* 110:2721–2746, 2004.
69. Reinelt P, Karth GD, Geppert A, et al: Incidence and type of cardiac arrhythmias in critically ill patients: a single center experience in a medical-cardiological ICU. *Intensive Care Med* 27:1466–1473, 2001.
70. Brathwaite D, Weissman C: The new onset of atrial arrhythmias following major noncardiothoracic surgery is associated with increased mortality. *Chest* 114:462–468, 1998.
71. Kimball JT, Killip T: Aggressive treatment of arrhythmias in acute myocardial infarction: procedures and results. *Prog Cardiovasc Dis* 10:483–504, 1968.
72. Henkel DM, Witt BJ, Gersh BJ, et al: Ventricular arrhythmias after acute myocardial infarction: a 20-year community study. *Am Heart J* 151:806–812, 2006.
73. Vetter NJ, Julian DG: Comparison of arrhythmia computer and conventional monitoring in coronary-care unit. *Lancet* 1:1151–1154, 1975.
74. Holmberg S, Ryden L, Waldenstrom A: Efficiency of arrhythmia detection by nurses in a coronary care unit using a decentralized monitoring system. *Br Heart J* 39:1019–1025, 1977.
75. Romhilt DW, Bloomfield SS, Chou TC, et al: Unreliability of conventional electrocardiographic monitoring for arrhythmia detection in coronary care units. *Am J Cardiol* 31:457–461, 1973.
76. Watkinson WP, Brice MA, Robinson KS: A computer-assisted electrocardiographic analysis system: methodology and potential application to cardiovascular toxicology. *J Toxicol Environ Health* 15:713–727, 1985.
77. Alcover IA, Henning RJ, Jackson DL: A computer-assisted monitoring system for arrhythmia detection in a medical intensive care unit. *Crit Care Med* 12:888–891, 1984.
78. Badura FK: Nurse acceptance of a computerized arrhythmia monitoring system. *Heart Lung* 9:1044–1048, 1980.
79. Clements FM, Bruijn NP: Noninvasive cardiac monitoring. *Crit Care Clin* 4:435–454, 1988.
80. Mirvis DM, Berson AS, Goldberger AL: Instrumentation and practice standards for electrocardiographic monitoring in special care units. *Circulation* 79:464–471, 1989.
81. Drew BJ, Pelter MM, Adams MG, et al: 12-lead ST-segment monitoring vs single-lead maximum ST-segment monitoring for detecting ongoing ischemia in patients with unstable coronary syndromes. *Am J Crit Care* 7:355–363, 1998.
82. Wehr G, Peters RJ, Khalife K, et al: A vector-based, 5-electrode, 12-lead monitoring ECG (EASI) is equivalent to conventional 12-lead ECG for diagnosis of acute coronary syndromes. *J Electrocardiol* 39:22–28, 2006.
83. Balaji S, Ellenby M, McNames J, et al: Update on intensive care ECG and cardiac event monitoring. *Card Electrophysiol Rev* 6:190–195, 2002.
84. Association for the Advancement of Medical I: *American National Standard for Cardiac Monitors, Heart Rate Meters, and Alarms (EC 13–1983)*. Arlington, VA: ANSI/AAMI, 1984.
85. Starmer CF, Whalen RE, McIntosh HD: Hazards of electric shock in cardiology. *Am J Cardiol* 14:537–546, 1964.
86. Pittman JV, Blum MS, Leonard MS: *Telemetry Utilization for Emergency Medical Services Systems*. Atlanta, GA: Georgia Institute of Technology, 1974.
87. Tri JL, Severson RP, Firl AR, et al: Cellular telephone interference with medical equipment. *Mayo Clin Proc* 80:1286–1290, 2005.
88. Mithoefer JC, Bossman OG, Thibeault DW, et al: The clinical estimation of alveolar ventilation. *Am Rev Respir Dis* 98:868–871, 1968.
89. McFadden JP, Price RC, Eastwood HD: Raised respiratory rate in elderly patients: a valuable physical sign. *Br J Med* 284:626–627, 1982.
90. Krieger B, Feinerman D, Zaron A: Continuous noninvasive monitoring of respiratory rate in critically ill patients. *Chest* 90:632–634, 1986.
91. Knaus WA, Wagner DP, Draper EA, et al: The APACHE III prognostic system. Risk prediction of hospital mortality for critically ill hospitalized adults. *Chest* 100:1619–1636, 1991.
92. Cretikos MA, Bellomo R, Hillman K, et al: Respiratory rate: the neglected vital sign. *Med J Aust* 188:657–659, 2008.
93. Semmes BJ, Tobin MJ, Snyder JV, et al: Subjective and objective measurement of tidal volume in critically ill patients. *Chest* 87:577–579, 1985.

94. Shelly MP, Park GR: Failure of a respiratory monitor to detect obstructive apnea. *Crit Care Med* 14:836–837, 1986.
95. Sackner MA, Bizousky F, Krieger BP: Performance of impedance pneumograph and respiratory inductive plethysmograph as monitors of respiratory frequency and apnea. *Am Rev Respir Dis* 135:A41, 1987.
96. Wiklund L, Hok B, Stahl K, et al: Postanesthesia monitoring revisited: frequency of true and false alarms from different monitoring devices. *J Clin Anesth* 6:182–188, 1994.
97. Lovett PB, Buchwald JM, Sturmann K, et al: The vexatious vital: neither clinical measurements by nurses nor an electronic monitor provides accurate measurements of respiratory rate in triage. *Ann Emerg Med* 45:68–76, 2005.
98. Tsien CL, Fackler JC: Poor prognosis for existing monitors in the intensive care unit. *Crit Care Med* 25:614–619, 1997.
99. Chadha TS, Watson H, Birch S, et al: Validation of respiratory inductive plethysmography using different calibration procedures. *Am Rev Respir Dis* 125:644–649, 1982.
100. Sackner MA, Watson H, Belsito AS, et al: Calibration of respiratory inductive plethysmograph during natural breathing. *J Appl Physiol* 66:410–420, 1989.
101. Tobin MJ, Jenouri G, Lind B, et al: Validation of respiratory inductive plethysmography in patients with pulmonary disease. *Chest* 83:615–620, 1983.
102. Wolf GK, Arnold JH: Noninvasive assessment of lung volume: respiratory inductance plethysmography and electrical impedance tomography. *Crit Care Med* 33:S163–S169, 2005.
103. Stradling JR, Chadwick GA, Quirk C, et al: Respiratory inductance plethysmography: calibration techniques, their validation and the effects of posture. *Bull Eur Physiopathol Respir* 21:317–324, 1985.
104. Neumann P, Zinserling J, Haase C, et al: Evaluation of respiratory inductive plethysmography in controlled ventilation: measurement of tidal volume and PEEP-induced changes of end-expiratory lung volume. *Chest* 113:443–451, 1998.
105. Tobin MJ, Guenther SM, Perez W: Konno-Mead analysis of ribcage-abdominal motion during successful and unsuccessful trials of weaning from mechanical ventilation. *Am Rev Respir Dis* 135:1320–1328, 1987.
106. Hoffman RA, Ershowsky P, Krieger BP: Determination of auto-PEEP during spontaneous and controlled ventilation by monitoring changes in end-expiratory thoracic gas volume. *Chest* 96:613–616, 1989.
107. Krieger BP, Ershowsky P, Spivack D: One year's experience with a noninvasively monitored intermediate care unit for pulmonary patients. *JAMA* 264:1143–1146, 1990.
108. O'Brien MJ, Van Eykern LA, Oetomo SB, et al: Transcutaneous respiratory electromyographic monitoring. *Crit Care Med* 15:294–299, 1987.
109. Mower WR, Sachs C, Nicklin EL: A comparison of pulse oximetry and respiratory rate in patient screening. *Respir Med* 90:593–599, 1996.
110. Brown LH, Manring EA, Korengay HB: Can prehospital personnel detect hypoxemia without the aid of pulse oximetry. *Am J Emerg Med* 14:43–44, 1996.
111. Jensen LA, Onyskiw JE, Prasad NG: Meta-analysis of arterial oxygen saturation monitoring by pulse oximetry in adults. *Heart Lung* 27:387–408, 1998.
112. Stoneham MD, Saville GM, Wilson IH: Knowledge about pulse oximetry among medical and nursing staff. *Lancet* 344:1339–1342, 1994.
113. Huch A, Huch R, Konig V: Limitations of pulse oximetry. *Lancet* 1:357–358, 1988.
114. New W: Pulse oximetry. *J Clin Monit* 1:126–129, 1985.
115. Moller JT, Pederen T, Rasmussen LS: Randomized evaluation of pulse oximetry in 20,802 patients: I. Design, demography, pulse oximeter failure rate, and overall complications rate. *Anesthesiology* 78:436–444, 1993.
116. Choe H, Tashiro C, Fukumitsu K: Comparison of recorded values from six pulse oximeters. *Crit Care Med* 17:678–681, 1989.
117. Severinghaus JW, Naifeh KH, Koh SO: Errors in 14 pulse oximeters during profound hypoxia. *J Clin Monit* 5:72–81, 1989.
118. Barker SJ, Hyatt J, Shah NK: The effect of sensor malpositioning on pulse oximetry accuracy during hypoxemia. *Anesthesiology* 79:248–254, 1993.
119. Severinghaus JW, Naifeh KH: Accuracy of responses of six pulse oximeters to profound hypoxia. *Anesthesiology* 67:551–558, 1987.
120. Reynolds LM, Nicolson SC, Steven JM: Influence of sensor site location on pulse oximetry kinetics in children. *Anesth Analg* 76:751–754, 1993.
121. Cheng EY, Hopwood MB, Kay J: Forehead pulse oximetry compared with finger pulse oximetry and arterial blood gas measurement. *J Clin Monit* 4:223–226, 1988.
122. Evans ML, Geddes LA: An assessment of blood vessel vasoactivity using photoplethysmography. *Med Instrum* 22:29–32, 1988.
123. Tweedie IE: Pulse oximeters and finger nails. *Anaesthesia* 44:268, 1989.
124. Read MS: Effect of transparent adhesive tape on pulse oximetry. *Anesth Analg* 68:701–702, 1989.
125. Cote CJ, Goldstein EA, Fuchsman WH: The effect of nail polish on pulse oximetry. *Anesth Analg* 67:683–686, 1988.
126. Brand TM, Brand ME, Jay GD: Enamel nail polish does not interfere with pulse oximetry among normoxic volunteers. *J Clin Monit Comput* 17:93–96, 2002.
127. Chan MM, Chan MM, Chan ED: What is the effect of fingernail polish on pulse oximetry? *Chest* 123:2163–2164, 2003.
128. Ries AL, Prewitt LM, Johnson JJ: Skin color and ear oximetry. *Chest* 96:287–290, 1989.
129. Adler JN, Hughes LA, Vivilecchia R, et al: Effect of skin pigmentation on pulse oximetry accuracy in the emergency department. *Acad Emerg Med* 5:965–970, 1998.
130. Bothma PA, Joynt GM, Lipman J: Accuracy of pulse oximetry in pigmented patients. *S Afr Med J* 86:594–596, 1996.
131. Costarino AT, Davis DA, Keon TP: Falsely normal saturation reading with the pulse oximeter. *Anesthesiology* 67:830–831, 1987.
132. Hanowell L, Eisele JH Jr, Downs D: Ambient light affects pulse oximeters. *Anesthesiology* 67:864–865, 1987.
133. Block FE Jr: Interference in a pulse oximeter from a fiberoptic light source. *J Clin Monit* 3:210–211, 1987.
134. Brooks TD, Paulus DA, Winkle WE: Infrared heat lamps interfere with pulse oximeters. *Anesthesiology* 61:630, 1984.
135. Amar D, Neidzwski J, Wald A: Fluorescent light interferes with pulse oximetry. *J Clin Monit* 5:135–136, 1989.
136. Fluck RR Jr, Schroeder C, Frani G, et al: Does ambient light affect the accuracy of pulse oximetry? *Respir Care* 48:677–680, 2003.
137. Gehring H, Hornberger C, Matz H, et al: The effects of motion artifact and low perfusion on the performance of a new generation of pulse oximeters in volunteers undergoing hypoxemia. *Respir Care* 47:48–60, 2002.
138. Beall SN, Moorthy SS: Jaundice, oximetry, and spurious hemoglobin desaturation. *Anesth Analg* 68:806–807, 1989.
139. Veyckemans F, Baele P, Guillaume JE: Hyperbilirubinemia does not interfere with hemoglobin saturation measured by pulse oximetry. *Anesthesiology* 70:118–122, 1989.
140. Moore TJ, Walsh CS, Cohen MR: Reported adverse event cases of methemoglobinemia associated with benzocaine products. *Arch Intern Med* 164:1192–1196, 2004.
141. Watcha MF, Connor MT, Hing AV: Pulse oximetry in methemoglobinemia. *Am J Dis Child* 143:845–847, 1989.
142. Reynolds KJ, Palayiwa E, Moyle JTB: The effect of dyshemoglobins on pulse oximetry: I. Theoretical approach. II. Experimental results using an in vitro system. *J Clin Monit* 9:81–90, 1993.
143. Barker SJ, Tremper KK: The effect of carbon monoxide inhalation on pulse oximetry and transcutaneous PO_2. *Anesthesiology* 66:677–679, 1987.
144. Buckley RG, Aks SE, Eshom JL: The pulse oximetry gap in carbon monoxide intoxication. *Ann Emerg Med* 24:252–255, 1994.
145. Glass KL, Dillard TA, Phillips YY: Pulse oximetry correction for smoking exposure. *Mil Med* 161:273–276, 1996.
146. Coburn RF, Williams WJ, Kahn SB: Endogenous carbon monoxide production in patients with hemolytic anemia. *J Clin Invest* 45:460–468, 1966.
147. Lopez-Herce J, Borrego R, Bustinza A, et al: Elevated carboxyhemoglobin associated with sodium nitroprusside treatment. *Intensive Care Med* 31:1235–1238, 2005.
148. Barker SJ, Badal JJ: The measurement of dyshemoglobins and total hemoglobin by pulse oximetry. *Curr Opin Anaesthesiol* 21:805–810, 2008.
149. Lee SE, Tremper KK, Barker SJ: Effects of anemia on pulse oximetry and continuous mixed venous oxygen saturation monitoring in dogs. *Anesth Analg* 67:S130, 1988.
150. Jay GD, Hughes L, Renzi FP: Pulse oximetry is accurate in acute anemia from hemorrhage. *Ann Emerg Med* 24:32–35, 1994.
151. Cane RD, Harrison RA, Shapiro BA: The spectrophotometric absorbance of intralipid. *Anesthesiology* 53:53–55, 1980.
152. Sehgal LR, Sehgal HL, Rosen AL, et al: Effect of Intralipid on measurements of total hemoglobin and oxyhemoglobin in whole blood. *Crit Care Med* 12:907–909, 1984.
153. Pu LJ, Shen Y, Lu L, et al: Increased blood glycohemoglobin A1c levels lead to overestimation of arterial oxygen saturation by pulse oximetry in patients with type 2 diabetes. *Cardiovasc Diabetol* 11:110, 2012.
154. Gabrielczyk MR, Buist RJ: Pulse oximetry and postoperative hypothermia: an evaluation of the Nellcor N-100 in a cardiac surgical intensive care unit. *Anaesthesia* 43:402–404, 1988.
155. Rieder HU, Frei FJ, Zbinden AM: Pulse oximetry in methemoglobinemia: failure to detect low oxygen saturation. *Anaesthesia* 44:326–327, 1989.
156. Scheller MS, Unger RJ, Kelner MJ: Effects of intravenously administered dyes on pulse oximetry readings. *Anesthesiology* 65:550–552, 1986.
157. Unger R, Scheller MS: More on dyes and pulse oximeters. *Anesthesiology* 67:148–149, 1987.
158. Koivusalo AM, Von Smitten K, Lindgren L: Sentinel node mapping affects intraoperative pulse oximetric recordings during breast cancer surgery. *Acta Anaesthesiol Scand* 46:411–414, 2002.
159. Barker SJ: "Motion-resistant" pulse oximetry: a comparison of new and old models. *Anesth Analg* 95:967–972, 2002; table of contents.
160. Morris RW, Nairn M, Torda TA: A comparison of fifteen pulse oximeters: I: a clinical comparison. II: a test of performance under conditions of poor perfusion. *Anaesth Intensive Care* 17:62–73, 1989.
161. Palve H, Vuori A: Pulse oximetry during low cardiac output and hypothermia states immediately after open heart surgery. *Crit Care Med* 17:66–69, 1989.
162. Paulus DA: Cool fingers and pulse oximetry. *Anesthesiology* 71:168–169, 1989.
163. Stewart KG, Rowbottom SJ: Inaccuracy of pulse oximetry in patients with severe tricuspid regurgitation. *Anaesthesia* 46:668–670, 1991.

164. Critical Care Services and Personnel: Recommendations based on a system of categorization into two levels of care. American College of Critical Care Medicine of the Society of Critical Care Medicine. *Crit Care Med* 27:422–426, 1999.
165. Smith DC, Canning JJ, Crul JF: Pulse oximetry in the recovery room. *Anaesthesia* 44:345–348, 1989.
166. Tyler IL, Tantisera B, Winter PM: Continuous monitoring of arterial oxygen saturation with pulse oximetry during transfer to the recovery room. *Anesth Analg* 64:1108–1112, 1985.
167. Moller JT, Johannenssen NW, Espersen K: Randomized evaluation of pulse oximetry in 20,802 patients: II. Perioperative events and postoperative complications. *Anesthesiology* 78:445–453, 1993.
168. Guggenberger H, Lenz G, Federle R: Early detection of inadvertent esophageal intubation: pulse oximetry vs. capnography. *Acta Anaesthesiol Scand* 33:112–115, 1989.
169. Stein PD, Goldhaber SZ, Henry JW, et al: Arterial blood gas analysis in the assessment of suspected acute pulmonary embolism. *Chest* 109:78–81, 1996.
170. Stock MC: Noninvasive carbon dioxide monitoring. *Crit Care Clin* 4:511–526, 1988.
171. Schena J, Thompson J, Crone R: Mechanical influences on the capnogram. *Crit Care Med* 12:672–674, 1984.
172. Murray IP, Modell JH: Early detection of endotracheal tube accidents by monitoring of carbon dioxide concentration in respiratory gas. *Anesthesiology* 59:344–346, 1983.
173. Garnett AR, Ornato JP, Gonzalez ER, et al: End-tidal carbon dioxide monitoring during cardiopulmonary resuscitation. *JAMA* 257:512–515, 1987.
174. Grmec S: Comparison of three different methods to confirm tracheal tube placement in emergency intubation. *Intensive Care Med* 28:701–704, 2002.
175. Link MS, Berkow LC, Kudenchuk PJ, et al: Part 7: Adult advanced cardiovascular life support: 2015 American Heart Association Guidelines Update for Cardiopulmonary Resuscitation and Emergency Cardiovascular Care. Circulation 2015;132:S444–S464.
176. Raemer DB, Francis D, Philip JH: Variation in PCO_2 between arterial blood and peak expired gas during anesthesia. *Anesth Analg* 62:1065–1069, 1983.
177. Morley TF, Giaimo J, Maroszan E: Use of capnography for assessment of the adequacy of alveolar ventilation during weaning from mechanical ventilation. *Am Rev Respir Dis* 148:339–344, 1993.
178. Pekdemir M, Cinar O, Yilmaz S, et al: Disparity between mainstream and sidestream end-tidal carbon dioxide values and arterial carbon dioxide levels. *Respir Care* 58:1152–1156, 2013.
179. Jardin F, Genevray B, Pazin M: Inability to titrate PEEP in patients with acute respiratory failure using end tidal carbon dioxide measurements. *Anesthesiology* 62530–533, 1985.
180. Lima A, Bakker J: Noninvasive monitoring of peripheral perfusion. *Intensive Care Med* 31:1316–1326, 2005.
181. Rooth G, Hedstrand U, Tyden H: The validity of the transcutaneous oxygen tension method in adults. *Crit Care Med* 4:162–165, 1976.
182. Gothgen I, Jacobsen E: Transcutaneous oxygen tension measurement: I. Age variation and reproducibility. *Acta Anaesthesiol Scand* 67:66–70, 1978.
183. Tremper KK, Waxman K, Shoemaker WC: Use of transcutaneous oxygen sensors to titrate PEEP. *Ann Surg* 193:206–209, 1981.
184. Cerny V, Cvachovec K: Gastric tonometry and intramucosal pH–theoretical principles and clinical application. *Physiol Res* 49:289–297, 2000.
185. Reilly PM, Wilkins KB, Fuh KC, et al: The mesenteric hemodynamic response to circulatory shock: an overview. *Shock* 15:329–343, 2001.
186. Dantzker DR: The gastrointestinal tract. The canary of the body? *JAMA* 270:1247–1248, 1993.
187. Bergofsky EM: Determination of tissue O_2 tensions by hollow visceral tonometers: effects of breathing enriched O_2 mixtures. *J Clin Invest* 43:193–200, 1964.
188. Dawson AM, Trenchard D, Guz A: Small bowel tonometry: assessment of small gut mucosal oxygen tension in dog and man. *Nature* 206:943–944, 1965.
189. Kivisaari J, Niinikoski J: Use of silastic tube and capillary sampling technic in the measurement of tissue pO_2 and pCO_2. *Am J Surg* 125:623–627, 1973.
190. Fiddian-Green RG, Pittenger G, Whitehouse WM: Back-diffusion of CO_2 and its influence on the intramural pH in gastric mucosa. *J Surg Res* 33:39–48, 1982.
191. Fiddian-Green RG: Tonometry: theory and applications. *Intensive Care World* 9:60–65, 1992.
192. Fiddian-Green RG: Gastric intramucosal pH, tissue oxygenation and acid–base balance. *Br J Anaesth* 74:591–606, 1995.
193. Schlichtig R, Mehta N, Gayowski TJ: Tissue-arterial PCO_2 difference is a better marker of ischemia than intramural pH (pHi) or arterial pH-pHi difference. *J Crit Care* 11:51–56, 1996.
194. Marshall AP, West SH: Gastric tonometry and monitoring gastrointestinal perfusion: using research to support nursing practice. *Nurs Crit Care* 9:123–133, 2004.
195. Riddington D, Venkatesh B, Clutton-Brock T, et al: Measuring carbon dioxide tension in saline and alternative solutions: quantification of bias and precision in two blood gas analyzers. *Crit Care Med* 22:96–100, 1994.
196. Heard SO, Helsmoortel CM, Kent JC: Gastric tonometry in healthy volunteers: effect of ranitidine on calculated intramural pH. *Crit Care Med* 19:271–274, 1991.
197. Marik PE, Lorenzana A: Effect of tube feedings on the measurement of gastric intramucosal pH. *Crit Care Med* 24:1498–1500, 1996.
198. Marshall AP, West SH: Gastric tonometry and enteral nutrition: a possible conflict in critical care nursing practice. *Am J Crit Care* 12:349–356, 2003.
199. Beale RJ, Hollenberg SM, Vincent JL, et al: Vasopressor and inotropic support in septic shock: an evidence-based review. *Crit Care Med* 32:S455–S465, 2004.
200. Mohsenifar Z, Hay A, Hay J, et al: Gastric intramural pH as a predictor of success or failure in weaning patients from mechanical ventilation. *Ann Intern Med* 119:794–798, 1993.
201. Fiddian-Green RG, Baker S: Predictive value of the stomach wall pH for complications after cardiac operations: comparison with other monitoring. *Crit Care Med* 15:153–156, 1987.
202. Landow L, Phillips DA, Heard SO: Gastric tonometry and venous oximetry in cardiac surgery patients. *Crit Care Med* 19:1226–1233, 1991.
203. Friedman G, Berlot G, Kahn RJ, et al: Combined measurements of blood lactate concentrations and gastric intramucosal pH in patients with severe sepsis. *Crit Care Med* 23:1184–1193, 1995.
204. Kirton OC, Windsor J, Wedderburn R, et al: Failure of splanchnic resuscitation in the acutely injured trauma patient correlates with multiple organ system failure and length of stay in the ICU. *Chest* 113:1064–1069, 1998.
205. Maynard N, Bihari D, Beale R, et al: Assessment of splanchnic oxygenation by gastric tonometry in patients with acute circulatory failure. *JAMA* 270:1203–1210, 1993.
206. Keenan SP, Guyatt GH, Sibbald WJ, et al: How to use articles about diagnostic technology: gastric tonometry. *Crit Care Med* 27:1726–1731, 1999.
207. Gutierrez G, Palizas F, Doglio G, et al: Gastric intramucosal pH as a therapeutic index of tissue oxygenation in critically ill patients. *Lancet* 339:195–199, 1992.
208. Heritier SR, Gebski VJ, Keech AC: Inclusion of patients in clinical trial analysis: the intention-to-treat principle. *Med J Aust* 179:438–440, 2003.
209. Gomersall CD, Joynt GM, Freebairn RC, et al: Resuscitation of critically ill patients based on the results of gastric tonometry: a prospective, randomized, controlled trial. *Crit Care Med* 28:607–614, 2000.
210. The Miami Trauma Clinical Trials Group: Splanchnic hypoperfusion-directed therapies in trauma: a prospective, randomized trial. *Am Surg* 71:252–260, 2005.
211. Zhang X, Xuan W, Ping Y, et al: Gastric tonometry guided therapy in critical care patients: a systematic review and meta-analysis. *Critical Care* 19:22, 2015.
212. Marik PE: Sublingual capnography: a clinical validation study. *Chest* 120:923–927, 2001.
213. Marik PE, Bankov A: Sublingual capnometry versus traditional markers of tissue oxygenation in critically ill patients. *Crit Care Med* 31:818–822, 2003.
214. Wimberley PD, Pedersen KG, Thode J: Transcutaneous and capillary pCO_2 and pO_2 measurements in healthy adults. *Clin Chem* 29:1471–1473, 1983.
215. Wimberley PD, Burnett RW, Covington AK, et al: Guidelines for transcutaneous pO_2 and pCO_2 measurement. *J Int Fed Clin Chem* 2:128–135, 1990.
216. Eletr S, Jimison H, Ream AK: Cutaneous monitoring of systemic PCO_2 on patients in the respiratory intensive care unit being weaned from the ventilator. *Acta Anaesthesiol Scand* 68:123–127, 1978.
217. Tremper KK, Shoemaker WC: Transcutaneous oxygen monitoring of critically ill adults, with and without low flow shock. *Crit Care Med* 9:706–709, 1981.
218. Hasibeder W, Haisjackl M, Sparr H, et al: Factors influencing transcutaneous oxygen and carbon dioxide measurements in adult intensive care patients. *Intensive Care Med* 17:272–275, 1991.
219. Tremper KK, Waxman K, Bowman R, et al: Continuous transcutaneous oxygen monitoring during respiratory failure, cardiac decompensation, cardiac arrest, and CPR. Transcutaneous oxygen monitoring during arrest and CPR. *Crit Care Med* 8:377–381, 1980.
220. Shoemaker WC, Fink S, Ray CW: Effect of hemorrhagic shock on conjunctival and transcutaneous oxygen tensions in relation to hemodynamic and oxygen transport changes. *Crit Care Med* 12:949–952, 1984.
221. Nolan LS, Shoemaker WC: Transcutaneous O_2 and CO_2 monitoring of high risk surgical patients during the perioperative period. *Crit Care Med* 10:762–764, 1982.
222. Shoemaker WC, Wo CC, Yu S, et al: Invasive and noninvasive haemodynamic monitoring of acutely ill sepsis and septic shock patients in the emergency department. *Eur J Emerg Med* 7:169–175, 2000.
223. Shoemaker WC, Wo CC, Lu K, et al: Outcome prediction by a mathematical model based on noninvasive hemodynamic monitoring. *J Trauma* 60:82–90, 2006.
224. Mesquida J, Masip J, Gili G, et al: Thenar oxygen saturation measured by near infrared spectroscopy as a noninvasive predictor of low central venous oxygen saturation in septic patients. *Intensive Care Med* 35:1106–1109, 2009.
225. Crookes BA, Cohn SM, Bloch S, et al: Can near-infrared spectroscopy identify the severity of shock in trauma patients? *J Trauma* 58:806–813; discussion 813–816, 2005.

Chapter 28 ■ Minimally Invasive Hemodynamic Monitoring

BRIAN S. FURUKAWA • EDNAN K. BAJWA • ATUL MALHOTRA • ANDREW J. GOODWIN

INTRODUCTION

The assessment and optimization of cardiac output (CO) has historically been considered important for the management of critically ill patients. The etiology of shock in a hypotensive patient may not be obvious clinically and is often multifactorial. In these circumstances, it is helpful to characterize what type of shock, i.e., distributive, cardiogenic, hypovolemic, is playing a role in a patient's presentation as well as monitor their response to interventions, such as volume loading. Determination of CO is thought to be a critical component of this process and thus has long been a matter of interest to clinicians.

The physical examination can be unreliable for assessing hemodynamics of systolic heart failure [1] and for critically ill patients without recent myocardial infarction [2]. As such, more dependable measurements may be required to treat such patients optimally. Since its introduction [3], the flow-directed pulmonary artery catheter (PAC) has been useful for obtaining measurements of CO and has been used both diagnostically as well as to gauge response to treatment. Indeed, for many years, the PAC thermodilution technique was considered to be the "gold standard" of intensive care unit (ICU) hemodynamic measurement. However, this philosophy has been called into question over the last several decades in light of mounting evidence that clinicians may be using the PAC ineffectively [4] and that morbidity and mortality in a variety of clinical situations are not improved with its use [5–7], and in some cases may be worsened [8,9].

As the paradigm of hemodynamic monitoring for the critically ill has steadily shifted away from PAC use, attention has turned to the study of alternative and less invasive methods of determining cardiac function. These methods can be divided into two broad categories: (1) direct measurement and optimization of CO and (2) indirect measurement of oxygen delivery and/or tissue perfusion as surrogates for CO. The goal of this research has been to develop feasible, minimally invasive techniques with accuracy for the ICU patient and in some cases, these studies have focused on adapting monitoring technology that is already routinely used in this patient population. In this chapter, we focus on several emerging technologies being used to determine CO and tissue perfusion in the ICU. We will conclude with a summary of practice recommendations and future directions.

CARDIAC OUTPUT

CO is the amount of blood flow through the cardiovascular system over a period of time. Conventionally, it is reported in liters per minute and can be normalized for a person's body surface area to provide the cardiac index. In the normal patient, CO is directly related to that subject's metabolic rate and oxygen consumption (VO_2). The fundamental principles of CO will be described in more detail elsewhere in this text. The therapies for a hypotensive patient with diminished CO (cardiogenic or obstructive shock) are fundamentally different from the therapies for a patient with diminished vascular tone (distributive shock). Therefore, accurate measurement of cardiac function can be a helpful guide for the effective treatment of hypotension.

Traditionally, a number of techniques have been used for the assessment of cardiac function. Jugular venous pulsations, S3 gallop, and skin temperature are physical examination findings that have all been used to estimate CO with mixed results [10–12]. Pulmonary artery occlusion pressure (PAOP) and central venous pressure (CVP) have also been used as surrogates for left and right ventricular end-diastolic volume, respectively. The PAOP is commonly used to establish the diagnosis of pulmonary venous hypertension or hypotension for the hypotensive patient and is often used to guide resuscitation, whereas Magder and colleagues [13,14] demonstrated that the CVP could provide useful information about the volume status of critically ill patients. Because the majority of the blood volume is in the systemic veins, and the right ventricle can be the major determinant of CO, some have argued that the CVP should receive more attention as the focus of hemodynamic resuscitation protocols [15]. Unfortunately, PAOP and CVP only represent the end-diastolic pressures of their respective chambers. These variables do not always reflect accurately end-diastolic volumes or equate with systolic function and CO. In addition, invasive assessment of PAOP [16,17] and clinical assessment of CVP [18] have been notoriously difficult to define accurately and reliably.

Over the last few decades, considerable research has been devoted to the accurate measurement of CO by minimally invasive means. At present, there exist several modalities, which are able to provide estimates of CO on a continuous or near-continuous basis. As described below, some have accumulated enough supporting data to warrant increasing use in clinical settings (esophageal Doppler [ED], pulse contour analysis [PCA], thoracic bioreactance) while the clinical usefulness of others is still unclear (partial carbon dioxide rebreathing) and will not be discussed further here.

Esophageal Doppler

Background

Ultrasound (US) creates images through the transmission of sound waves from a transducer and the subsequent measurement of sound waves which are reflected back. As the sound waves travel through the body, they are reflected back when they encounter adjacent structures or tissues which have different acoustic impedances. The degree of wave reflection is directly proportional to the magnitude of the difference in acoustic impedances between the adjacent structures such that interfaces between structures with highly different properties (i.e., blood and endocardium) will be reflected back to a greater degree. Image resolution and tissue penetration are dependent upon the frequency of the emitted sound wave such that higher frequency transducers provide superior image resolution at the expense of a reduced depth of penetration.

Motion-mode (M-mode), the most basic mode of US, represents the structures along the path of a single one-dimensional (1-D) vector. Sound waves reflected from this vector are displayed over time and its narrow scanning sector produces superior resolution for fast moving structures. Another clinically utilized mode of US is Doppler US that is used to calculate the velocity of a moving target, i.e., blood. This mode utilizes the Doppler shift principle, whereby a transmitted sound wave encountering a moving structure or fluid will reflect at a predictably different frequency based on the structure or fluid's properties. For example, in a fluid-filled tube such as a blood vessel, the magnitude of Doppler shift will vary in direct proportion to the velocity of blood flow in the vessel. Thus, Doppler US can provide information on both the velocity and the direction of intravascular blood flow.

The most commonly used mode is two-dimensional (2-D). Real-time 2-D images are created when the US beam is continuously swept to and fro in an arc and multiple 1-D images are aligned. This allows movement of cardiac structures such as the myocardial walls to be observed. In a landmark study in 1974, Griffith and Henry [19] were able to visualize the heart's structure and function in vivo using a handheld scanner that swept through a 30° arc at a speed of 30 cycles per second, along with real-time display and video recording. Although transthoracic echocardiography (TTE) was revolutionary in its ability to evaluate cardiac function noninvasively, it was often limited by body habitus and an inability to visualize posterior cardiac structures. To overcome these limitations, Schluter and colleagues [20] were among the first to revolutionize the clinical use of transesophageal echocardiography (TEE) by attaching miniaturized transducers to a gastroscope, allowing structures not normally visualized on TTE to be clearly visible. Over time, as the value of cardiac US as a diagnostic tool became apparent, efforts have been made to improve its technical capabilities and clarity. This has led to the increasing use of both TTE and TEE in the ICU as minimally invasive monitoring modalities. As a separate chapter in this text focuses primarily on TTE, this chapter will cover ED and its uses in critically ill patients.

Estimating Cardiac Output

Transesophageal assessment of hemodynamics in critical care has evolved over time in parallel with advancements in technology. The initial esophageal probes possessed only Doppler functionality giving rise to the commonly used nomenclature esophageal Doppler. Later iterations successfully added M-mode capability such that both blood flow and aortic diameter could simultaneously be measured. The first use of ED in humans was described by Side and Gosling [21] in 1971 when they used a Doppler probe to measure CO by analyzing stroke volume (SV) in the descending aorta. The ED system estimates SV by modeling the aorta as a cylinder (Fig. 28.1A). Using this geometric model, the SV is calculated by multiplying the cross-sectional area (CSA) of the aorta by the stroke distance which is the length of the aorta that a given SV travels:

$$SV = CSA \times \text{stroke distance}$$

As the aortic cross section closely approximates a circle, the CSA can be calculated by measuring the diameter (D) of the aorta using M-mode or by estimating the diameter from nomograms in the absence of M-mode capability:

$$CSA = \pi(D/2)^2$$

The length that a SV travels is then estimated by measuring the velocity time integral (VTI) of the aortic jet by Doppler (Fig. 28.1B).

$$\text{Stroke distance} = VTI$$

SV can then be estimated as follows:

$$SV = \pi(D/2)^2 \times VTI$$

As this measurement of aortic blood flow does not account for the component of total SV that travels to the coronary, carotid, and subclavian arteries, a correction factor must finally be applied to estimate the total SV. When using ED, important inaccuracies can occur if the aortic diameter measurement has even a small error as this value is ultimately squared during the calculation of SV [22]. Therefore, some operators will estimate a surrogate of SV using the VTI measurement alone. Additionally, SV can be underestimated if the Doppler signal is measured from a plane that is not parallel to that of blood flow [23].

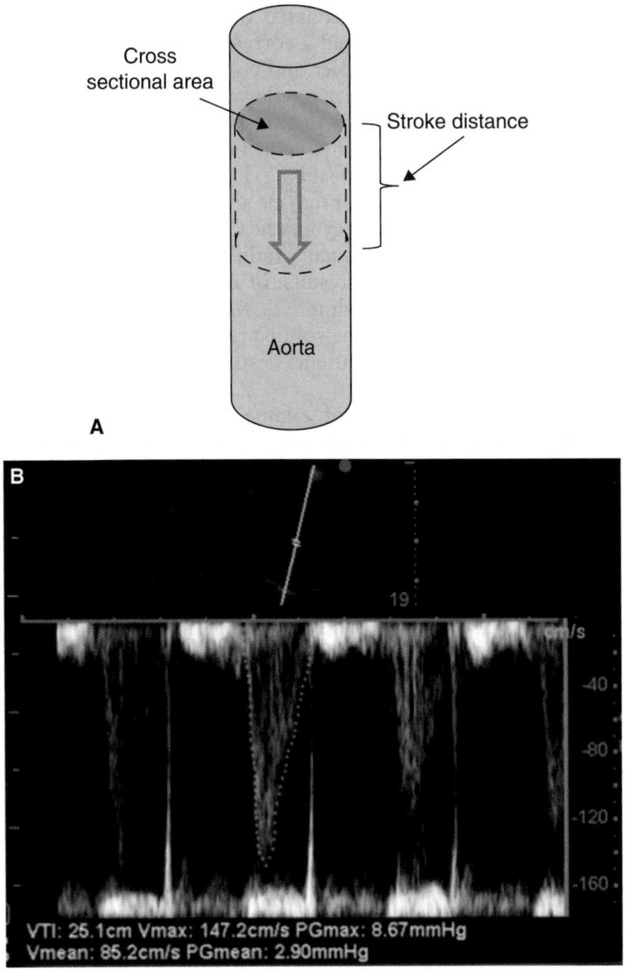

FIGURE 28.1 Esophageal Doppler measures stroke volume (SV) in the descending aorta. **A:** The aorta can be modeled as a cylinder. SV can be estimated by multiplying the cross-sectional area of the cylinder by the stroke distance. **B:** The velocity time integral (VTI) estimates stroke distance. The VTI is quantified as the area under the waveform and represents the stroke distance. SV is then calculated: SV = CSA × stroke distance.

The majority of recent studies that have compared ED-derived CO to the "gold standard" of thermodilution have been performed in either intraoperative or postoperative settings and have revealed mixed results. One single-center study of 35 patients during off-pump coronary artery bypass graft surgery showed very poor correlation between the two techniques [24]. Other studies, including a meta-analysis of 11 trials, have shown that ED systems are better at following changes in CO in response to fluid challenges than they are at measuring the absolute CO [25–27]. As the ability to monitor the response to interventions is arguably as important as measuring actual CO, these data suggest that ED may be a useful tool in the perioperative setting. The authors of the meta-analysis also highlight that the poor reproducibility inherent in the thermodilution technique will likely affect the limits of agreement between ED systems and thermodilution even if ED systems were accurate [25]. This concept was described by Bland and Altman [28] and has important implications when comparing the accuracy of absolute CO measured by any system when compared to thermodilution.

Optimizing Cardiac Output using Esophageal Doppler

Beyond providing an estimate of CO, ED systems can provide information about the preload and the contractility of the heart. Singer et al. [29,30] analyzed the flow velocity waveform derived from an ED system and discovered that the corrected flow time (FT_c) directly correlated with preload. Wallmeyer and colleagues [31] described a correlation between the peak velocity measured by Doppler and contractility measured by electromagnetic catheter measured flow. Singer et al. [32] further substantiated this finding by demonstrating that dobutamine infusions increased peak flow velocities measured by an ED system in a dose-dependent fashion. These observations suggest that an experienced operator may be able to extrapolate useful hemodynamic parameters, beyond the CO, through careful data synthesis. However, subsequent studies evaluating the utility of FT_c have shown mixed results. In a medically critically ill patient population, a baseline FT_c was poorly sensitive for discerning those who will be volume responsive and it significantly increased in some patients despite a lack of increase in CO [33,34].

Dynamic measurements of volume responsiveness have the best evidence supporting their utility for discriminating volume responsiveness. Monnet and colleagues [35] studied the utility of a passive leg raise (PLR) maneuver in a mechanically ventilated medically ill population and found that an increase in aortic blood flow ≥10% on ED could predict volume responsiveness with excellent accuracy. This study also showed that the change in aortic blood flow was a useful marker in those with arrhythmias and spontaneous ventilation, a population where other dynamic measurements of volume responsiveness have poor correlation [35–37].

Clinical Utility of Esophageal Doppler

The majority of studies which have examined the impact of ED on clinical outcomes focused on the perioperative setting. The transesophageal approach has distinct advantages over transthoracic in this setting including the ability to monitor continuously as well as to overcome limited access to the chest wall for TTE for most surgical patients. In 2006, a randomized double-blinded clinical trial of ED-guided intraoperative fluid resuscitation during colorectal surgery demonstrated that ED use was associated with earlier time to discharge, faster tolerance of a diet, and less need for inotropes [38]. Figus et al. [39] showed similar outcomes for patients undergoing reconstructive surgery and observed that although the total amount of fluid administered was not different between the two groups, the ED-guided group achieved a significantly lower net balance. Their findings were consistent with a recent meta-analysis which suggested that a balanced fluid approach (net zero) for patients undergoing colorectal surgery resulted in less perioperative complications and shorter lengths of stay [40]. These data challenge the prevailing paradigm of perioperative care which has historically resulted in positive fluid balances. Accordingly, judicious fluid use and a closer scrutiny on fluid balance has become a cornerstone of the modern enhanced recovery after surgery (ERAS) programs [41–43]. As such, a minimally invasive method of estimating fluid responsiveness intraoperatively may be of considerable value during larger surgeries. Interestingly, however, when ED was examined in the context of an ERAS approach, its use did not confer clinical benefit despite better optimization of SV [44]. While far from conclusive, these data suggest that (1) as long as CO is adequate, further optimization may be unnecessary and/or (2) a net zero fluid balance can be achieved without any monitoring of CO in many surgical patients.

There are few studies which examine the clinical impact of ED use among critically ill patients outside of standard perioperative management. A small, single-center study of trauma patients with hemorrhagic shock demonstrated that ED-guided resuscitation decreased the incidence of occult shock and was associated with fewer infectious complications and significantly reduced hospital length of stay [45]. Although further studies are needed to confirm the clinical utility, it does suggest that ED can be a meaningful diagnostic tool in the ICU.

Advantages and Disadvantages of Esophageal Doppler

There are several potential advantages to using ED for hemodynamic monitoring in the critically ill (Table 28.1). First, as outlined above, ED systems provide continuous data, which allows for earlier recognition of hemodynamic deterioration or improvement in response to a therapeutic intervention. Additionally, an ED probe can be placed in minutes and has been associated with a low incidence of major iatrogenic complications [46–48]. Some data also suggest that once inserted, an esophageal probe can be left in situ safely for more than 2 weeks [49]. Finally, as the esophagus is a non-sterile environment, it is logical to assume that the infectious risk of an ED probe is minimal.

ED monitoring has a few potential disadvantages as well. Transesophageal monitoring cannot be used from patient to patient as readily as the transthoracic approach and, therefore, multiple devices would be required if more than one examination is needed at a given time and has cost implications. Also, ED can only be utilized in intubated patients and are contraindicated in patients with esophageal perforation or stricture. Finally, while ED probes can be left in for extended periods of time for continuous hemodynamic monitoring, they have been noted to be frequently dislodged despite best efforts to keep patients adequately sedated [45].

Future Research

While the use of critical care echocardiography is expanding, and existing literature has shown its use affects management, there are little data to suggest it alters outcomes. The current management paradigm for septic shock with acute respiratory distress syndrome (ARDS) involves early and aggressive volume resuscitation [50] coupled with avoidance of unnecessary fluid that may exacerbate lung injury and lengthen ventilation time [51]. ED assessment of fluid responsiveness may better achieve optimal fluid status than CVP and could lead to more refined resuscitation protocols that affect patient outcomes. Similarly, a greater focus on fluid balance for surgical patients as part of ERAS programs may involve more incorporation of this modality. As these programs evolve and disseminate, more robust analyses of their clinical impact will likely follow.

Ongoing advancements in echocardiography technology will also impact its role in the future of intensive care. A 5.5 mm disposable monoplane TEE device has recently been developed and preliminary studies show that it is easy to place, can be safely left in for up to 72 hours, and can have a significant impact on management of medical ICU patients [52]. This technology may lead to more widespread adoption of using continuous 2-D TEE in the future.

TABLE 28.1

Advantages and Disadvantages of Esophageal Doppler for Cardiac Output Monitoring

Concept: Doppler probe measures stroke volume in the aorta

Advantages
- Continuous monitoring
- Proximity to the aorta
- Quick placement
- Estimates CO and predicts volume responsiveness
- Low infection risk
- Can remain in place for 2 weeks

Disadvantages
- Unable to use on > 1 patient
- Requires intubation
- Need for repositioning

CO, cardiac output.

The optimal training method to establish competence in ED use also requires further investigation. While cardiology-based certifications have traditionally relied upon volume-based metrics to establish competency [53], the American College of Chest Physicians has recently developed a competency-based training course for critical care US [54]. This novel and pragmatic approach combines online material with sequential didactic seminars that progress from basic to more advanced material. Learners are then instructed to return to their practices and assemble a portfolio of images which can be remotely reviewed by expert ultrasonographers to ensure competence in image acquisition in a real-world environment. Once competence has been confirmed, learners are able to complete a final examination to obtain certification. Rigorous assessment of the success of this model may lead to more effective training methods for both fellows and practicing intensivists.

Pulse Contour Analysis

Background

PCA is another modality for measuring CO noninvasively that has been extensively studied. This method relies on the theory, first described by Frank in the early part of the 20th century, that SV and CO can be derived from the characteristics of an aortic pressure waveform [55]. Wesseling and colleagues [56] published in 1983 an algorithm to link mathematically SV and the pressure waveform. This original approach calculated SV continuously by dividing the area under the curve of the aortic pressure waveform by the aortic impedance. As aortic impedance varies among patients, it had to be measured using another modality, usually arterial thermodilution, to calibrate the PCA system prior to obtaining SV data. Aortic impedance, however, is not a static property. It is based upon the complex interaction of the resistive and compliant elements of each vascular bed, which are often dynamic, especially among hemodynamically unstable patients. Since the first PCA algorithm was introduced, several unique algorithms have been created to model accurately the properties of the human vascular system for use in PCA systems.

PCA involves the use of an arterial placed catheter with a pressure transducer, which can measure pressure tracings on a beat-to-beat basis. Such catheters are now routinely used in operating rooms and ICUs as they provide a continuous measurement of blood pressure that is superior to intermittent noninvasive measurements in hemodynamically unstable patients. These catheters are interfaced with a PCA system, which uses its unique algorithm to provide a continuously displayed measurement of CO. Thus, the reliability of a PCA system depends upon the accuracy of the algorithm that it employs. Because each algorithm is unique in the weight that it ascribes to each element of vascular conductivity, it has been impossible to ensure that a system will be able to reproduce the results of another system under similar conditions [57]. Keeping this in mind, one cannot conclude that all systems are equally reliable.

PiCCO (Pulsion SG, Munich, Germany) is a PCA system that has received considerable attention in the literature. Numerous studies have demonstrated a strong correlation between this system and pulmonary thermodilution for both critically ill and surgical patients [58–62]. Notably, this system did not require recalibration during these study periods, which were performed under static ventricular loading conditions. The system involves the placement of a central arterial catheter equipped with a pressure transducer and a thermistor for arterial thermodilution. The system is calibrated by injecting cold saline via a central venous catheter at the right atrium in a manner similar to pulmonary arterial thermodilution. Instead of using a thermistor in the pulmonary artery, however, the thermistor on the central arterial catheter allows for a transpulmonary thermodilution and calculation of CO. This initial value of CO is then used to calibrate the PCA system that is coupled to the arterial catheter. When compared to pulmonary artery thermodilution, the transpulmonary thermodilution method was found to be accurate, implying that it is an acceptable method for calibration of a PCA system [58–60].

A competitor PCA system known as the Flotrac (Edwards Lifesciences, LLC, Irvine, CA) has also been widely used in the intensive care setting. It is designed to "autocalibrate" on a continuous basis. It calculates SV using a general equation: $SV = K \times \text{pulsatility}$, where K is a constant including arterial compliance and vascular resistance [63]. This constant is initially derived by patient variables such as height, weight, sex, and age using a method described by Langewouters and colleagues [64] and is subsequently adjusted once per minute using arterial waveform characteristics. Pulsatility is determined by analyzing the standard deviation of the arterial pressure waveform over preceding 20-second intervals. Thus, the variables used to calculate SV are updated at least once per minute. This algorithm offers the advantage of not needing an alternative method for calculating CO for calibration purposes. When compared to PAC thermodilution in a postcardiac surgery setting, this system showed good correlation over a wide range of COs. Additionally, it appears that a radial artery catheter is just as accurate as a femoral artery catheter in this setting, which is another advantage of this system [63]. However, autocalibrated CO measurements have been shown to be inaccurate in hyperdynamic and vasodilated states, such as sepsis or after liver transplantation [65,66]. Thus, Edwards has worked to upgrade its algorithm in order to improve its accuracy across a broader range of physiologic conditions [67]. Although these modifications have been shown to improve the technology's accuracy and ability to trend CO, they are met with mixed results, and the widespread applicability is still unsettled [68,69].

Clinical Utility

As mentioned above, the initial trials studying PCA systems used data from static ventricular loading conditions. Both the critically ill and intraoperative patients, however, often experience rapid changes in ventricular preload. The accuracy of the PiCCO system with dynamic changes of preload was addressed in a subsequent study, which used a modified algorithm. Felbinger and colleagues showed that changes in CO in response to preload could be accurately measured for a cardiac surgical ICU population when compared to pulmonary thermodilution [70].

While being able to monitor changes in CO during volume loading is important, being able to predict a priori when a patient would benefit from volume loading is perhaps more useful. Pulse pressures commonly vary throughout the respiratory cycle. Pulse pressure variation (PPV) is defined as the result of the minimum pulse pressure subtracted from the maximum pulse pressure divided by the mean of these two pressures.

$$PPV = \frac{\text{Pulse Pressure}_{max} - \text{Pulse Pressure}_{min}}{\text{Pulse Pressure}_{mean}} \qquad (1)$$

The magnitude of the PPV in a patient can predict preload responsiveness [71–73] and has been shown to be more accurate than traditional static measurements of preload such as CVP or PAOP [74,75]. Analogous to PPV, an additional piece of data that PCA systems can provide is the stroke volume variation (SVV). The SVV represents the percent change in SV over time due to fluctuations in preload caused by respiration and is calculated using the same equation format as PPV (Fig. 28.2). A meta-analysis of PPV and SVV measured by PCA found that a PPV of 12.5% and SVV of 11.6% had moderate sensitivity and specificity when predicting a response to volume [76].

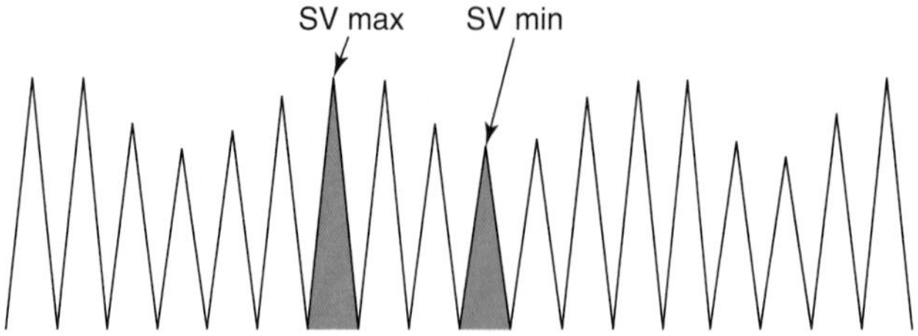

FIGURE 28.2 Stroke volume variation predicts volume responsiveness. The maximum and minimum stroke volumes during the respiratory cycle are calculated using a pulse contour analysis (PCA) system's algorithm. Larger variations in stroke volume predict volume responsiveness in the passively ventilated patient.

Due to these known limitations of the sensitivities and specificities of PPV and SVV to predict fluid responsiveness, some investigators have begun to examine the utility of using a range of PPV and SVV cutoffs. Cannesson and colleagues studied this approach in 413 elective surgical patients. They found that a PPV of 9% or less provided 90% accuracy that a patient would not respond to volume loading whereas a PPV of 13% or greater predicted with 90% accuracy that someone would respond. Up to 24% of the patient population studied fell into the "gray zone" where PPV was between 9% and 13%. In the gray zone, the predictive accuracy of PPV is limited and the authors argue that the decision to volume challenge should be made on a case-by-case basis after analyzing the relative risks and benefits [77]. This pragmatic approach to hemodynamic management has inherent appeal and could easily be applied to other modalities.

An important difference between PCA systems which have the ability to perform transpulmonary thermodilution (PiCCO, VolumeView) and those that do not (Flotrac) is the ability of the thermodilution systems to provide volumetric estimates of preload. Through analysis of the thermodilution curve and the application of known mathematical relationships between intrathoracic volumes, these systems provide estimates of global end-diastolic volumes (GEDV) and extravascular lung water (ELW) [78,79]. Indexed values of GEDV may be used as an assessment of preload and is preferred over traditional measures such as CVP by some clinicians [80]. Additionally, elevations of indexed ELW have been associated with higher mortality rates and, thus, may provide prognostic data in the critically ill population [81]. Despite the addition of these volumetric data, there are little data at present to suggest whether volumetric-based assessments of preload provide any clinical advantage to patient care compared with non-volumetric technology.

In fact, there are limited data to suggest that the use of PCA systems in the intensive care setting impacts clinically relevant outcomes [82]; however, their use in high-risk surgery has been associated with clinical benefit. In the OPTIMISE (Optimization of Cardiovascular Management to Improve Surgical Outcome) trial, 734 high-risk patients undergoing major gastrointestinal surgery were randomized to an uncalibrated PCA to guide CO optimization versus standard of care during surgery and up to 6 hours postoperatively. The trial showed a nonsignificant trend toward a reduction in a composite of postoperative complications including mortality. When the authors included the trial's data in a meta-analysis, they found a 23% reduction in the postoperative complications and a trend toward reduced mortality [83].

Advantages and Disadvantages

Overall, the PCA system offers several advantages over the traditional "gold standard" of pulmonary artery thermodilution (Table 28.2). Depending on the system, only an arterial catheter (Flotrac) or an arterial catheter and a central venous catheter (PiCCO) are required, both of which are commonly in place in critically ill and higher risk surgical patients. Thus, unlike PACs, no additional invasive procedures are required to use these systems. The PCA systems also provide a continuous measurement of CO as opposed to the intermittent nature of traditional thermodilution systems. This approach not only facilitates faster response times to hemodynamic derangements but also saves the clinician the time required to perform repeat CO or volume responsive assessments as would be required with TTE. Finally, PCA systems require minimal to no training to interpret and, therefore, may be an ideal modality to use in a busy clinical setting.

As with any noninvasive method of monitoring hemodynamics, there are disadvantages to the PCA systems as well. Regardless of the system employed, their accuracy and precision in vasodilated states are still questioned in situations with extremes of SVR such as septic shock, liver transplantation, or vasopressor titration [68,69,84–86]. Further, it is critical for clinicians to recall that the use of SVV to predict fluid responsiveness using PCA systems has only been validated in passively mechanically ventilated patients, usually at tidal volumes >8 mL per kg [76]. Thus, the reliability of using SVV in the spontaneous breathing patients is unknown and likely limited. Another known limitation to the PCA systems is their inability to reliably predict volume responsiveness when currently recommended lung protective strategies (<6 mL per kg) are used [87]. Fortunately, this limitation may be diminished at higher PEEP levels and may also be circumvented by transiently increasing tidal volumes at the time of SVV measurement [88]. In addition to tidal volume, respiratory rate (RR) has also recently been shown to impact the association between SVV or PPV and volume responsiveness. On average, the transit time of blood through the pulmonary circulation is approximately three to four beats resulting in a slight delay in the impact of a positive pressure breath on SV. In theory, if the RR is high enough such that the ventilator is cycling between inspiration and expiration faster than the pulmonary transit time, PPV variation may become challenging to quantify. Indeed, De Backer et al. [89] demonstrated that when the HR to RR ratio was decreased to <3.6 in hypovolemic patients, PPV could no longer be detected. These findings suggest that PCA systems may have limited efficacy in volume status assessment for patients with severe ARDS who require high RRs in the setting of lung protective ventilation and high dead space fractions. Finally, because pulse pressure and SV are dependent upon preload

TABLE 28.2

Advantages and Disadvantages of the Pulse Contour Analysis Method for Cardiac Output Monitoring

Concept: Arterial catheter used to determine stroke volume from aortic pressure waveforms

Advantages
- Continuous
- Utilizes catheters that are already commonly used in ICU patients
- Does not require calibration with pulmonary artery catheter
- Minimal training requirements

Disadvantages
- SVV inaccurate during low tidal volume ventilation and spontaneous breathing
- Questionable accuracy during low systemic vascular resistance states
- Questionable accuracy during vasoconstrictor use

ICU, intensive care unit; SVV, stroke volume variation

which is proportional to diastolic filling time, arrhythmias such as atrial fibrillation which result in variable R-R intervals will generate large PPV and SVV which are independent of volume status. This concept limits the ability to use PCA systems in the presence of these common arrhythmias, although newer algorithms are making improvements in this regard [67].

Future Research

Future studies that may help in defining the clinical role of PCA systems could focus on several points. First, a better understanding of how changes in vascular tone and vasopressor use affect the accuracy of a particular system's algorithm will help to determine if and when particular systems can be reliably used. Further exploration of the use of PCA systems to create clinical protocols akin to the previously described "gray zone" approach may help to reshape the ubiquitous clinical question, "Will this patient respond to fluids?" into the more patient-centered question, "Should I give this patient fluids?" Finally, examinations of how PCA systems could affect patient outcomes through tailored resuscitation protocols in sepsis and ARDS would further help to define their role in critical care.

Noninvasive Cardiac Output Monitoring (Bioreactance)

Background

The thoracic bioimpedance technique was first developed by Kubicek [90] as a means of noninvasively measuring the CO of astronauts. It involves the delivery of low amplitude, high frequency electrical current across the thorax. A series of sensing electrodes, which measure the change in voltage amplitude, are placed along the path of this current and can be used to calculate the electrical impedance intrinsic to the thorax. Because of the conductive properties of fluid, the thoracic bioimpedance is inversely proportional to the amount of fluid in the thorax at the time of measurement. Thus, as intrathoracic fluid volume increases during each cardiac cycle, the bioimpedance measured by the sensing electrodes decreases. This principle provides the basis for measuring the SV and, hence, CO using this technique. In order to estimate CO accurately, however, aortic blood flow must be distinguished from other sources of intrathoracic fluid movement. Simultaneously recording the electrocardiogram and using a computer algorithm to filter electrical noise caused by other fluid movement can accomplish this.

Investigations into the accuracy of bioimpedance have yielded mixed results. A large meta-analysis which compared CO measurement by thoracic bioimpedance and PAC thermodilution revealed a broad range of correlation ranging from 0.44 to 0.75 [91]. A potential limitation which may impact the device's accuracy is the electrical "noise" generated by extravascular fluid in the form of pulmonary edema and pleural effusions. Accordingly, a prior study in ventilated patients with acute lung injury demonstrated a poor correlation between CO measured by bioimpedance and PACs [92]. Further, data regarding the effects of obesity on the accuracy of bioimpedance measurements are inconsistent. Sageman and Amundson [93] found no correlation ($r^2 = 0.00$) between invasive cardiac index measurements and those measured by thoracic bioimpedance in a subset of obese patients post coronary bypass. In contrast, a retrospective review of a prospective database revealed that patients with a body mass index (BMI) greater than 30 kg per m^2 actually had equivalent correlation and less bias between thoracic bioimpedance and thermodilution when compared to patients with a BMI less than 30 kg per m^2 [94].

As suboptimal signal-to-noise ratios likely resulted in the substantial limitations of bioimpedance for these clinical scenarios, efforts have been made to improve the system's accuracy. A newer modality known as bioreactance was developed which appears to offer reduction in electrical noise. Unlike bioimpedance which monitors changes in the voltage amplitude imparted by intrathoracic blood flow, the noninvasive cardiac output monitoring (NICOM) bioreactance system monitors the phase shift of electrical waves which occurs due to this flow [95]. Similar to bioimpedance, a set of electrodes are placed upon the chest which transmit alternating electrical current at a known frequency to a set of receiving electrodes. Additional sensing electrodes are placed in the path of the electrical current and transmit information regarding the current back to the NICOM system. Specifically, the sensing electrodes measure the amount of time delay or phase shift that occurs as the current travels across the thorax. Because alternating current is delayed by traveling through fluid, the measured phase shift is directly proportional to the amount of intrathoracic fluid present at any given moment. Thus, small fluctuations in phase shift can be detected between systole and diastole (Fig. 28.3) and can be extrapolated into a SV using proprietary algorithms. Further, changes in SV in response to volume expansion can be detected by comparing the phase shift before and after volume challenge allowing for an assessment of fluid responsiveness using this system.

Clinical Utility

Since its inception, several studies have compared the accuracy of the CO measured by the NICOM bioreactance system to that measured by PACs or other minimally invasive modalities. Two early single-center studies demonstrated tight correlation between this system and PACs for both surgical and nonsurgical cardiac care unit patients [96,97]. This correlation was present during periods of stability and during periods of increasing or decreasing CO. Additionally, the bioreactance system detected changes in CO faster than traditional PAC monitoring. When compared to ED monitoring of an abdominal surgical population, there was substantial disagreement of absolute CO measurements; however, the modalities were concordant when assessing CO changes in response to volume loading [98].

As with other minimally invasive monitoring modalities, the ability of bioreactance to predict fluid responsiveness has also been examined. Unlike PCA or echocardiography assessment of inferior vena cava (IVC) diameter, bioreactance does not provide a respirophasic, dynamic measurement that can be determined without intervening on a patient. Instead, the phase shift is measured both before and after a fluid challenge and a ΔCO is calculated where any value $\geq$10% is considered fluid responsive. This approach requires that a fluid bolus be given and, therefore, may expose nonresponders to unnecessary volume before their status can be established. In order to circumvent this shortcoming, investigators have begun to examine whether a ΔCO measured during a PLR can offer predictive

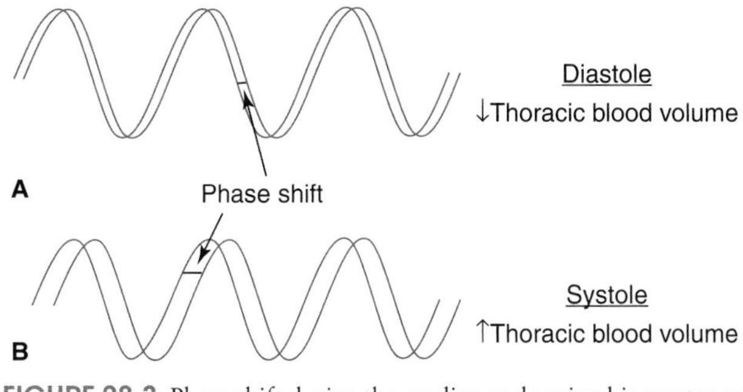

FIGURE 28.3 Phase shift during the cardiac cycle using bioreactance. Noninvasive cardiac output monitoring (NICOM) detects phase shifts in electrical current during (**A**) diastole and (**B**) systole that are elicited by changes in intrathoracic blood volume. The measured phase shifts can be used to estimate stroke volume (SV), CO, and response to volume loading.

capability without exposure to a fluid bolus. Benomar et al. [99] demonstrated that changes in CO during PLR correlated well with changes in CO after a 500-mL fluid challenge in a postcardiac surgery patient population using the bioreactance system. Tong and colleagues demonstrated similar findings in a small study examining bioreactance use in a septic population while simultaneously demonstrating that ΔCO during a PLR was a more accurate predictor of fluid responsiveness than SVV using a PCA system [100]. These same observations were also made for a heterogeneous critically ill population in which ΔCO during a PLR predicted fluid responsiveness with a 94% sensitivity and a 100% specificity [101].

The potential impact of thoracic bioreactance on clinical outcomes is still being determined. One early study examined the role of using the NICOM bioreactance system in trauma patients presenting to the ED. The authors report that CO derangements could be seen with a variety of clinical conditions including some in which hypotension was not present. Further, the length of stay during the study was significantly shorter in a subset of patients with injury severity scores ≥ 15 as compared to a similar cohort over two preceding years [102]. Lee et al. [103] also examined the impact of bioreactance monitoring on length of stay in a small cohort of patients undergoing valvular heart surgery. While they found no significant difference in length of stay with its use, they did discover that patients who received bioreactance monitoring experienced lower rates of both epinephrine use and prolonged mechanical ventilation. At present, additional studies examining the clinical benefits of this technology are lacking.

Advantages and Disadvantages

Perhaps the biggest advantage of the bioreactance monitoring system is its truly noninvasive nature (Table 28.3). Unlike PCA or ED, this system has no invasive components similar to TTE. Unlike TTE, however, bioreactance monitoring has the additional advantage of providing CO measurement on a near-continuous basis. The system displays the average CO over a preceding 1-minute interval which allows it to display accurate, real-time information without dramatic fluctuations from transient artifactual readings. Thus, the system allows for early detection of derangements akin to PCA and ED while remaining completely noninvasive. Another advantage of the bioreactance system is its compatibility with arrhythmias. Whereas minimally invasive modalities such as PCA are confounded by the impact that irregular diastolic filling times have on the beat-to-beat variation in SV, the bioreactance system has been shown to function reliably in the setting of atrial fibrillation [103]. Finally, patient positioning, and the need for frequent repositioning do not affect the accuracy of the bioreactance system offering a potential advantage over ED monitoring which can require adjustment each time a patient is moved [98].

As with all minimally invasive monitoring systems, there are potential disadvantages to the NICOM bioreactance system as well. First, as described above, the system is unable to predict fluid responsiveness without: (a) giving a fluid challenge or (b) performing a PLR maneuver. As 40% to 60% of patients in shock are not fluid responsive, the first approach may lead to frequent administration of unnecessary fluid [104,105]. Because the NICOM displays CO representative of an average value over the preceding minute, there is a brief delay before the response to a PLR would be observed. As data suggest that the effects of a PLR can disappear after 1 minute, it is possible that augmentations of CO from the PLR maneuver may be underestimated by bioreactance [35]. This may explain some of the mixed results about its efficacy at predicting volume responsiveness using this approach [101,106]. An additional disadvantage of the bioreactance system is its inability to accurately measure CO in certain clinical scenarios. Most notably, the system has been shown to perform poorly during upper abdominal surgery likely due to alterations in torso geometry, which can affect the derivation of SV from phase shift data [107]. This same limitation was again noted during liver transplantation but has not been seen in surgeries on the lower abdomen [107,108]. Finally, as the bioreactance system is based upon the measurement and analysis of electrical current, the introduction of extrinsic electrical signals may confound its accuracy. Accordingly, intraoperative electrical cautery has been shown to distort the signals of the bioreactance system and affect its accuracy [98]. The impact of implantable cardiac pacing devices on the system's accuracy is not fully known as interference has been reported but at least one study reports adequate performance during pacing [96,109].

TABLE 28.3

Advantages and Disadvantages of the NICOM Bioreactance Method for Cardiac Output Monitoring

Concept: External thoracic electrodes estimate stroke volume by monitoring the phase shift of current applied to the chest wall

Advantages
- Completely noninvasive
- Provides continuous measurements of CO
- Accurate with atrial fibrillation
- Not affected by patient positioning/repositioning

Disadvantages
- Ability to predict volume responsiveness without volume challenge is limited
- Limited accuracy during upper abdominal surgery
- Impact of electrical cardiac pacing not completely characterized

CO, cardiac output; NICOM, noninvasive cardiac output monitoring.

FUTURE DIRECTIONS

The thoracic bioreactance technology demonstrates considerable promise as a noninvasive means of monitoring CO and has supplanted bioimpedance due to its superior signal-to-noise capture. However, many questions regarding the clinical benefit of this technology remain. Although previous studies have investigated the accuracy of this system for hemodynamically unstable patients, the proportion of subjects who had pulmonary edema was either zero or not reported in these studies [96,101]. As pulmonary edema was a known confounder of the bioimpedance system, more data regarding its effect on the performance of the bioreactance system are necessary before this system can be broadly recommended. Further clarification of the system's ability to predict fluid responsiveness during a PLR maneuver is also important and should be performed with careful attention to the PLR protocol to avoid confounding [110]. Finally, as with most minimally invasive monitoring technologies, data regarding this technology's impact on clinical outcomes such as mortality, organ failure, length of stay, and cost are currently lacking. Only once these data are available can definitive practice recommendations be made.

OXYGEN DELIVERY AND TISSUE PERFUSION

While directly measuring CO can provide information vital to the management of critically ill patients, one can also argue that accurate knowledge of oxygen delivery and/or adequacy of tissue perfusion can be similarly useful. Proponents of this concept are less interested in the absolute CO as long as tissue oxygenation is adequate. Commonly used indirect measurements of oxygen delivery are central venous oxygen saturation ($S_{cv}O_2$) and lactate. Alternative modalities for measuring tissue perfusion are gastric tonometry and sublingual capnometry, which measure the concentration of CO_2 at the tissue level as a surrogate for tissue perfusion [111,112]. While some early studies found gastric tonometry-based protocolized resuscitation strategies to be of clinical benefit [113,114], others have not [115–117]. Although conceptually appealing, gastric tonometry and sublingual capnometry have failed to gain widespread popularity and, thus, will not be discussed further here.

$S_{cv}O_2$

Background

$S_{cv}O_2$ is an indirect measure of the oxygen content returning from the upper body through a properly placed central venous line in the superior vena cava (SVC). It is reflective of the balance between systemic oxygen delivery (DO_2) and systemic oxygen consumption ($\dot{V}O_2$). Conceptually, as CO (and DO_2) decrease, tissue extraction of oxygen will undergo a compensatory increase in order to sustain $\dot{V}O_2$ leading to a reduction in $S_{cv}O_2$. Thus, monitoring $S_{cv}O_2$ can provide useful information regarding the adequacy of CO over time.

The $S_{cv}O_2$ is analogous to the mixed venous oxygen saturation (S_vO_2), which is used less frequently in noncardiac ICUs as it requires a PAC. As S_vO_2 is considered to be a more exact measurement of global body oxygen delivery, several studies have examined the relationship of the two variables in order to determine the utility of $S_{cv}O_2$. An early study in healthy humans found that $S_{cv}O_2$ tended to be approximately 5% to 10% lower than S_vO_2 likely related to insufficient mixing of blood from the SVC, IVC, and coronary sinus in the right atrium [118]. However, more recent data suggest that in the setting of critical illness or surgery, the relationship between $S_{cv}O_2$ and S_vO_2 reverses with the former having larger values possibly caused by alterations in regional perfusion related to these conditions [119–121]. Regardless of the cause, these data have raised the question of whether $S_{cv}O_2$ is truly an appropriate surrogate marker of systemic oxygen delivery. In support of its adequacy, Reinhart et al. found a very good correlation ($r = 0.81$) between $S_{cv}O_2$ and S_vO_2 in a heterogeneous population of high-risk surgical and medically ill patients. In addition, the authors observed that changes in S_vO_2 led to proportionate changes in $S_{cv}O_2$ in both direction and magnitude over 90% of the time [119]. In contrast, numerous studies have demonstrated a relatively poor correlation between the two values in the setting of anesthesia or circulatory failure, particularly when S_vO_2 is <70% [121–124]. In these studies, the oxygen extraction ratio was repeatedly identified as a predictor of poor correlation. Intriguingly, one study demonstrated that a large discrepancy between S_vO_2 and $S_{cv}O_2$ was an independent risk factor for postoperative complications suggesting that the discrepancy is both real and may have clinical ramifications [125].

Despite the apparent controversy surrounding the accuracy of $S_{cv}O_2$ as a measure of oxygen delivery, much focus has been given to studying its use as a prognostic marker. As many as 60% of patients admitted with septic shock in the absence of preexisting heart disease experience myocardial dysfunction in the setting of their acute illness [126]. A prospective study of this population demonstrated that a $S_{cv}O_2$ cutoff of <64% predicted a reduced cardiac index with high positive and negative predictive values [127]. Supranormal $S_{cv}O_2$ levels, however, can also be associated with impaired oxygen delivery if the tissues have suffered significant damage and are unable to extract oxygen effectively in the setting of mitochondrial failure [128]. In fact, both low and elevated $S_{cv}O_2$ levels have been associated with increased mortality rates of patients admitted with sepsis [129,130].

Clinical Utility

Due to its minimally invasive nature and the development of catheters which allow for continuous measurement, $S_{cv}O_2$ has been used as a protocolized resuscitation target with mixed success. In an early landmark single-center trial, Rivers et al. demonstrated a significant reduction in mortality among patients with septic shock who were treated with an early and aggressive protocolized resuscitation which included interventions to target a $S_{cv}O_2 \geq 70\%$ [50]. These data were counter to an earlier study which had targeted normal S_vO_2 levels in a similar population [131] and were felt by many to be related to the early nature of the intervention. However, recent multicenter studies designed to validate the utility of early protocolized management of oxygen delivery using $S_{cv}O_2$ measurement have failed to demonstrate its benefit over the current standard of care [132–134]. The Protocolized Care for Early Septic Shock study (ProCESS) randomized patients into three arms: (1) an early goal-directed therapy (EGDT) arm whose care mimicked that of the original Rivers' study; (2) a protocolized resuscitation arm based on clinical assessment which did not require the use of a central venous catheter or the measurement of $S_{cv}O_2$; and (3) a usual care group in which all interventions were left to the clinical care team. Despite more dobutamine use and blood product administration in the EGDT arm, there was no mortality difference in the three treatment arms, while overall mortality was lower than predicted at 19% [132]. Similarly, the Australian Resuscitation in Sepsis Evaluation (ARISE) study enrolled 1,600 subjects to EGDT vs. usual care, and also found no difference in all-cause 90-day mortality (18%) despite a high level of adherence to the EGDT protocol [133]. Finally, the Protocolised Management in Sepsis (ProMISe) trial randomized 1,260 subjects with septic shock to EGDT versus usual care. Once again, resuscitation protocols incorporating $S_{cv}O_2$ as a surrogate end point provided no mortality benefit, however, did result in longer ICU stays and modest increases in cost [134].

At present, it is not clear why protocolized targeting of $S_{cv}O_2$ does not improve outcomes in septic shock. Possibilities include its known limitation for accurately reflecting oxygen delivery in those with circulatory failure as well as a heightened awareness that the standard of care for sepsis management should include early and aggressive resuscitation. Regardless, the utility of targeting $S_{cv}O_2$ in distributive shock appears to be limited at present. However, its use in guiding inotropic therapy for cardiogenic shock is still highly prevalent and may also have a role in perioperative care where it has been shown to be associated with reductions in length of stay and postoperative complications [135].

Lactate

Background

The physiologic basis for lactate production is a shift from mitochondrial oxidative phosphorylation to anaerobic glycolysis during times of circulatory failure or tissue hypoxia. Elevated lactate levels have been repeatedly associated with worse outcomes among critically ill patients [136–138]. This association is present even when clinical signs of macrocirculatory failure are absent and after adjustment for other confounding factors such as age and organ failure [139,140]. As such, investigators have been interested in exploring the prognostic capabilities of lactate as well as its utility as a resuscitation target.

Bakker et al. [136] noted that in addition to higher initial levels of lactate, non-survivors of septic shock also failed to clear lactate from their bloodstream. Subsequently, Nguyen and colleagues prospectively evaluated if early change in lactate levels, termed "lactate clearance," was a clinically useful indicator of survival in patients with suspected severe sepsis:

$$\text{Lactate Clearance} = [(\text{Lactate}^{\text{ED presentation}} - \text{Lactate}^{\text{Hour 6}})/\text{Lactate}^{\text{ED presentation}}] \times 100$$

They found that survivors had a significantly higher rate of lactate clearance (38.1% vs. 12%) at hour 6 and that for each 10% increase in lactate clearance, mortality decreased by 11% in a multivariate analysis [141]. A similar association between lactate clearance and survival has also been seen in trauma and burn populations [137,138], and lactate clearance has also been associated with improved neurologic outcomes after cardiac arrest [142].

Clinical Utility

When compared to targeting $S_{cv}O_2$ levels for septic shock, targeting lactate clearance appears to be more efficacious. This was suggested initially in retrospective studies which analyzed outcomes from a prospective trial of sepsis resuscitation in emergency departments. The authors observed that patients who did not successfully clear lactate had high mortality rates despite the fact that the majority of these patients had achieved a $S_{cv}O_2 \geq 70\%$ [143]. In a follow-up study, they demonstrated that achieving a lactate clearance of at least 10% in the absence of achieving a $S_{cv}O_2 \geq 70\%$ was associated with a fivefold reduction in mortality as compared to achieving a $S_{cv}O_2 \geq 70\%$ but failing to achieve lactate clearance [144]. These findings have been further substantiated by a recent meta-analysis which demonstrated that lactate clearance is associated with survival among critically ill patients [145].

In light of the association between lactate clearance and improved outcomes, Jansen et al. [146] investigated whether specific lactate-guided treatment protocols in the first 8 hours of ICU admission improves outcomes over standard of care for patients admitted with hyperlactemia. They prospectively randomized critically ill patients with a serum lactate ≥ 3 mEq per L on presentation to an intervention arm whose therapeutic goal was a 20% clearance in lactate every 2 hours or to a usual care arm. Although there was no significant difference in lactate levels between the two groups, the lactate-guided arm accomplished faster weaning from mechanical ventilation, shorter ICU stays, and reduced adjusted in-hospital mortality [146]. Finally, protocolized therapy targeting lactate clearance has also been compared head-to-head with protocolized targeting of $S_{cv}O_2$. In a multicenter non-inferiority randomized controlled trial, septic patients were randomized to receive early resuscitation using either $S_{cv}O_2$ or lactate clearance as an end point of oxygen delivery. In-hospital mortality rates were 17% in the lactate-guided group and 23% in the $S_{cv}O_2$ group and met the criteria for non-inferiority [147].

Advantages and Disadvantages

There are several theoretical advantages to blood markers of tissue perfusion such as $S_{cv}O_2$ and lactate (Table 28.4). Because they are indicators of the adequacy of tissue perfusion rather than a measurement of actual CO, they may be a more clinically appropriate method of guiding hemodynamic management. Although $S_{cv}O_2$ measurement requires a central venous catheter placed either in the internal jugular vein or in the subclavian vein, many patients who require close monitoring of oxygen delivery already have such central venous access. Thus, $S_{cv}O_2$ measurement does not increase the invasiveness of care in most patients. In addition, point of care measurement of $S_{cv}O_2$ is rapid and relatively inexpensive. The development of continuous $S_{cv}O_2$ monitoring catheters further improves the ability to monitor oxygen delivery in a convenient and real-time fashion [67], although it does represent an increase in the cost of care. Similarly, lactate measurement is also fast and affordable and has the added advantage of not requiring a central venous catheter. Finally, the accumulating evidence that lactate clearance is associated with clinical outcomes, including mortality, suggests that its monitoring may provide valuable clinical data [143–145].

There are limitations to the use of $S_{cv}O_2$ and lactate as well. First, while derangements in each value can identify the presence of inadequate oxygen delivery, neither will provide information regarding the underlying etiology of the derangement. Thus, their use may still require additional diagnostic testing in addition to clinical acumen. Additionally, the accuracy of $S_{cv}O_2$ measurements is dependent upon the position of the central venous catheter. Femoral catheters only provide evidence of oxygen delivery and extraction to the lower extremities and, thus, are not useful for assessment of vital organs. As outlined above, catheters placed in the internal jugular and subclavian veins may also provide inadequate representations of global oxygen delivery, particularly in the setting of circulatory failure [121–124]. The accuracy of $S_{cv}O_2$ levels may improve if the catheter tip is positioned in the right atrium [148]; however, the appropriateness and safety of such positioning is debated [149]. A further limitation is the fact that elevated levels of $S_{cv}O_2$ are not always indicative of adequate tissue oxygenation but, instead, may occur in the setting of mitochondrial failure when ischemic tissue loses the ability to extract oxygen effectively. As such, the clinician must not be falsely reassured by normal or supranormal values when other clinical clues suggest ongoing shock. Finally, and most importantly, accumulating evidence suggests that $S_{cv}O_2$-targeted therapy does not impact relevant clinical outcomes calling into question the appropriateness of its use in specific diagnoses such as septic shock [132–134].

The use of lactate and its clearance as surrogates for ongoing tissue hypoxia and anaerobic metabolism also have some limitations. There is evidence to suggest that hyperlactemia can result from aerobic glycolysis of well oxygenated tissues. One explanation for this finding is that epinephrine-induced

TABLE 28.4

Advantages and Disadvantages of Markers of Perfusion and Tissue Oxygenation Method for Cardiac Output Monitoring

Concept: Using lactate and $S_{cv}O_2$ as surrogate markers for adequate supply (CO) for a given metabolic demand

Advantages
- Utilizes catheters that are already commonly used in ICU
- No upfront capital investment
- Readily available, inexpensive tests
- Lactate clearance linked to clinical outcomes
- Representative of cellular function
- Potentially continuous

Disadvantages
- $S_{cv}O_2$
  - Not associated with clinical outcomes
  - Accuracy is position dependent
  - Levels above goal may represent ongoing tissue ischemia
- **Lactate**
  - Falsely elevated due to:
  - Aerobic production
  - Impaired clearance
  - Not continuous

CO, cardiac output; ICU, intensive care unit; $S_{cv}O_2$, central venous oxygen saturation.

activity of skeletal muscle Na^+–K^+ ATPase leads to hyperlactemia [150,151]. In times of stress, such as sepsis, endogenous and exogenous levels of epinephrine rise which can increase detectable levels of lactate despite adequate tissue perfusion [150]. Similarly, impairment of lactate clearance can also confound lactate levels in critically ill patients. Liver dysfunction and sepsis-related alterations in pyruvate dehydrogenase activity have both been associated with impaired lactate clearance and increased blood lactate levels [152,153], and higher baseline lactate levels have been associated with impaired clearance in a sepsis population [154].

Future Research

Although $S_{cv}O_2$-guided protocolized care does not appear to impact clinical outcomes from sepsis, the clinical utility of lactate-guided protocols is still being determined. Further examination of strategies using lactate clearance as a resuscitation end point will likely be forthcoming and informative of this measure's therapeutic potential. Alternatively, in light of the strong association between lactate clearance and survival, lactate levels may also find a role as a surrogate end point for other interventions over time. Finally, future research into the capabilities of markers of tissue perfusion to predict which patients are likely to experience complications early in the course of presentation may help to better triage patients and facilitate rapid interventions for patients with occult shock.

PRACTICE RECOMMENDATIONS

Independent of which hemodynamic monitoring technique is employed, a strategy that should be utilized for all patients with shock is early intervention aimed at restoring organ perfusion (Table 28.5). Mounting evidence suggests that mitochondrial failure may play a role in late shock [128] and efforts to correct hemodynamic derangements early in shock have shown promising results [50]. However, the accumulation of data suggesting that protocolized targeting of $S_{cv}O_2$ does not improve outcomes in sepsis argues that focus on oxygen delivery may not be a crucial component to an interventional approach so long as volume resuscitation and pressor support are supplied early [132–134].

The optimal method for hemodynamic monitoring is yet to be determined. Although pulmonary artery thermodilution remains the "gold standard" for measuring CO, its use continues to decline among noncardiac critically ill patients. ED offers the benefits of continuous monitoring, low infectious risk, and relative ease in placement. Its use during major surgery has been associated with earlier tolerance of oral nutrition and shorter lengths of stay; thus, its use can be recommended in this clinical setting. Similarly, PCA-guided optimization of CO during high-risk abdominal surgery has also been associated with reduced postoperative complications and its use is also recommended.

A common finding in nearly all studies of minimally invasive hemodynamic monitoring modalities is that dynamic measures of fluid responsiveness are superior to traditionally used static measurements such as CVP or PAOP. Accordingly, the authors recommend that regardless of which minimally invasive monitoring modality is used, clinical decision-making regarding volume resuscitation can be aided by dynamic measurements such as PPV, SVV, or ΔVTI. However, before clinical decisions are made based on these techniques, it is imperative that clinicians who use them understand the limitations of each measurement and the clinical situations in which they can and cannot be accurately used.

Finally, the role of lactate and its clearance for the management of shock is still to be determined. Although lactate clearance has been shown to be non-inferior to $S_{cv}O_2$ as a resuscitation end point, the utility of $S_{cv}O_2$ targeting is now in question [147]. Further studies may allow for more definitive recommendations regarding its use as a resuscitation guide in the future.

TABLE 28.5

Summary of Practice Recommendations based upon Randomized Controlled Clinical Trials

Early intervention in shock is beneficial [50]
$S_{cv}O_2$-targeted therapy in septic shock is not recommended [132–134]
Esophageal Doppler can be used to improve postoperative outcomes in high-risk patients [21,42,43]
Pulse contour analysis can be used to improve postoperative outcomes in high-risk patients [83]
Stroke volume variation cannot reliably be used to estimate preload responsiveness during low tidal volume ventilation [76,87,88]

$S_{cv}O_2$, central venous oxygen saturation.

FUTURE DIRECTIONS

As medical technology continues to advance at an explosive rate, it is easy to imagine that ICU practice will change in the not too distant future. The next generation of intensivists and likely younger members of this generation may find themselves looking back with awe at the "archaic" methods of current practice. In particular, the widespread application of high throughput proteomic and transcriptomic analyses to patients with shock has great potential to unlock new noninvasive biomarkers that may aid in both the prognosis and hemodynamic management of these patients.

Genome-wide association studies and predictive modeling have identified candidate genes and their associated proteins that have been associated with increased mortality in septic shock [155]. When tested in an adult population, a signature of five plasma proteins combined with age, lactate, and chronic illness burden were found to have superior predictive accuracy to the widely used APACHE II score [156]. The investigators went on to examine quantitative expression levels of messenger RNA in a larger previously identified group of 100 genes. They demonstrated that the expression patterns of this combinatorial signature could successfully classify children with sepsis into different subclasses, and that subclass designation was associated with organ failure, mortality [157], and the response to steroid therapy [158]. Importantly, using the investigators' methodology, patients could be subclassified within 12 hours raising the possibility of real-world clinical applicability. Thus, proteomic and genomic analyses may be finally approaching the era of rapid turnaround personalized medicine. Similar discoveries in the future could potentially influence a wide variety of hemodynamic management decisions including volume status management and pressor choice.

References

1. Thomas JT, Kelly RF, Thomas SJ, et al: Utility of history, physical examination, electrocardiogram, and chest radiograph for differentiating normal from decreased systolic function in patients with heart failure. *Am J Med* 112:437–445, 2002.
2. Connors AF Jr, McCaffree DR, Gray BA: Evaluation of right-heart catheterization in the critically ill patient without acute myocardial infarction. *N Engl J Med* 308:263–267, 1983.

3. Swan HJ, Ganz W, Forrester J, et al: Catheterization of the heart in man with use of a flow-directed balloon-tipped catheter. *N Engl J Med* 283:447–451, 1970.
4. Iberti TJ, Fischer EP, Leibowitz AB, et al: A multicenter study of physicians' knowledge of the pulmonary artery catheter. Pulmonary Artery Catheter Study Group. *JAMA* 264:2928–2932, 1990.
5. Gore JM, Goldberg RJ, Spodick DH, et al: A community-wide assessment of the use of pulmonary artery catheters in patients with acute myocardial infarction. *Chest* 92:721–727, 1987.
6. Richard C, Warszawski J, Anguel N, et al: Early use of the pulmonary artery catheter and outcomes in patients with shock and acute respiratory distress syndrome: a randomized controlled trial. *JAMA* 290:2713–2720, 2003.
7. Wheeler AP, Bernard GR, Thompson BT, et al: Pulmonary-artery versus central venous catheter to guide treatment of acute lung injury. *N Engl J Med* 354:2213–2224, 2006.
8. Binanay C, Califf RM, Hasselblad V, et al: Evaluation study of congestive heart failure and pulmonary artery catheterization effectiveness: the ESCAPE trial. *JAMA* 294:1625–1633, 2005.
9. Connors AF Jr, Speroff T, Dawson NV, et al: The effectiveness of right heart catheterization in the initial care of critically ill patients. SUPPORT Investigators. *JAMA* 276:889–897, 1996.
10. Rame JE, Dries DL, Drazner MH: The prognostic value of the physical examination in patients with chronic heart failure. *Congest Heart Fail* 9:170–175, 8, 2003.
11. Kaplan LJ, McPartland K, Santora TA, et al: Start with a subjective assessment of skin temperature to identify hypoperfusion in intensive care unit patients. *J Trauma* 50:620–627, 2001; discussion 7-8.
12. Joly HR, Weil MH: Temperature of the great toe as an indication of the severity of shock. *Circulation* 39:131–138, 1969.
13. Magder S, Lagonidis D, Erice F: The use of respiratory variations in right atrial pressure to predict the cardiac output response to PEEP. *J Crit Care* 16:108–114, 2001.
14. Magder S, Cheong G, Cheong T: Respiratory variations in right atrial pressure predict the response to fluid challenge. *J Crit Care* 7:76–85, 1992.
15. Magder S: More respect for the CVP. *Int Care Med* 24:651–653, 1998.
16. Morris AH, Chapman RH, Gardner RM: Frequency of technical problems encountered in the measurement of pulmonary artery wedge pressure. *Crit Care Med* 12:164–170, 1984.
17. Marik P, Heard SO, Varon J: Interpretation of the pulmonary artery occlusion (wedge) pressure: physician's knowledge versus the experts' knowledge. *Crit Care Med* 26:1761–1764, 1998.
18. Eisenberg PR, Jaffe AS, Schuster DP: Clinical evaluation compared to pulmonary artery catheterization in the hemodynamic assessment of critically ill patients. *Crit Care Med* 12:549–553, 1984.
19. Griffith JM, Henry WL: A sector scanner for real time two-dimensional echocardiography. *Circulation* 49:1147–1152, 1974.
20. Schluter M, Langenstein BA, Polster J, et al: Transoesophageal cross-sectional echocardiography with a phased array transducer system. Technique and initial clinical results. *Br Heart J* 48:67–72, 1982.
21. Side CD, Gosling RG: Non-surgical assessment of cardiac function. *Nature* 232:335–336, 1971.
22. Lewis JF, Kuo LC, Nelson JG, et al: Pulsed Doppler echocardiographic determination of stroke volume and cardiac output: clinical validation of two new methods using the apical window. *Circulation* 70:425–431, 1984.
23. Otto CM: *Textbook of Clinical Echocardiography*. 5th ed. Philadelphia, PA, Elsevier Saunders, 2013.
24. Sharma J, Bhise M, Singh A, et al: Hemodynamic measurements after cardiac surgery: transesophageal Doppler versus pulmonary artery catheter. *J Cardiothorac Vasc Anesth* 19:746–750, 2005.
25. Dark PM, Singer M: The validity of trans-esophageal Doppler ultrasonography as a measure of cardiac output in critically ill adults. *Int Care Med* 30:2060–2066, 2004.
26. Kim K, Kwok I, Chang H, et al: Comparison of cardiac outputs of major burn patients undergoing extensive early escharectomy: esophageal Doppler monitor versus thermodilution pulmonary artery catheter. *J Trauma* 57:1013–1017, 2004.
27. Roeck M, Jakob SM, Boehlen T, et al: Change in stroke volume in response to fluid challenge: assessment using esophageal Doppler. *Intensive Care Med* 29:1729–1735, 2003.
28. Bland JM, Altman DG: Statistical methods for assessing agreement between two methods of clinical measurement. *Lancet* 1:307–310, 1986.
29. Singer M, Clarke J, Bennett ED: Continuous hemodynamic monitoring by esophageal Doppler. *Crit Care Med* 17:447–452, 1989.
30. Singer M, Bennett ED: Noninvasive optimization of left ventricular filling using esophageal Doppler. *Crit Care Med* 19:1132–1137, 1991.
31. Wallmeyer K, Wann LS, Sagar KB, et al: The influence of preload and heart rate on Doppler echocardiographic indexes of left ventricular performance: comparison with invasive indexes in an experimental preparation. *Circulation* 74:181–186, 1986.
32. Singer M, Allen MJ, Webb AR, et al: Effects of alterations in left ventricular filling, contractility, and systemic vascular resistance on the ascending aortic blood velocity waveform of normal subjects. *Crit Care Med* 19:1138–1145, 1991.
33. Monnet X, Rienzo M, Osman D, et al: Esophageal Doppler monitoring predicts fluid responsiveness in critically ill ventilated patients. *Int Care Med* 31:1195–1201, 2005.
34. Lafanechere A, Pene F, Goulenok C, et al: Changes in aortic blood flow induced by passive leg raising predict fluid responsiveness in critically ill patients. *Crit Care* 10:R132, 2006.
35. Monnet X, Rienzo M, Osman D, et al: Passive leg raising predicts fluid responsiveness in the critically ill. *Crit Care Med* 34:1402–1407, 2006.
36. Heenen S, De Backer D, Vincent JL: How can the response to volume expansion in patients with spontaneous respiratory movements be predicted? *Crit Care* 10:R102, 2006.
37. Soubrier S, Saulnier F, Hubert H, et al: Can dynamic indicators help the prediction of fluid responsiveness in spontaneously breathing critically ill patients? *Int Care Med* 33:1117–1124, 2007.
38. Noblett SE, Snowden CP, Shenton BK, et al: Randomized clinical trial assessing the effect of Doppler-optimized fluid management on outcome after elective colorectal resection. *Br J Surg* 93:1069–1076, 2006.
39. Figus A, Wade RG, Oakey S, et al: Intraoperative esophageal Doppler hemodynamic monitoring in free perforator flap surgery. *Ann Plast Surg* 70:301–307, 2013.
40. Varadhan KK, Lobo DN: A meta-analysis of randomised controlled trials of intravenous fluid therapy in major elective open abdominal surgery: getting the balance right. *Proc Nutr Soc* 69:488–498, 2010.
41. Varadhan KK, Lobo DN, Ljungqvist O: Enhanced recovery after surgery: the future of improving surgical care. *Crit Care Clin* 26:527–547, x, 2010.
42. Tang J, Humes DJ, Gemmil E, et al: Reduction in length of stay for patients undergoing oesophageal and gastric resections with implementation of enhanced recovery packages. *Ann R Coll Surg Engl* 95:323–328, 2013.
43. Thiele RH, Rea KM, Turrentine FE, et al: Standardization of care: impact of an enhanced recovery protocol on length of stay, complications, and direct costs after colorectal surgery. *J Am Coll Surg* 220:430–443, 2015.
44. Phan TD, D'Souza B, Rattray MJ, et al: A randomised controlled trial of fluid restriction compared to oesophageal Doppler-guided goal-directed fluid therapy in elective major colorectal surgery within an Enhanced Recovery After Surgery program. *Anaesth Intensive Care* 42:752–760, 2014.
45. Chytra I, Pradl R, Bosman R, et al: Esophageal Doppler-guided fluid management decreases blood lactate levels in multiple-trauma patients: a randomized controlled trial. *Crit Care* 11:R24, 2007.
46. Daniel WG, Erbel R, Kasper W, et al: Safety of transesophageal echocardiography. A multicenter survey of 10,419 examinations. *Circulation* 83:817–821, 1991.
47. Singer M: Esophageal Doppler monitoring of aortic blood flow: beat-by-beat cardiac output monitoring. *Int Anesthesiol Clin* 31:99–125, 1993.
48. Valtier B, Cholley BP, Belot JP, et al: Noninvasive monitoring of cardiac output in critically ill patients using transesophageal Doppler. *Am J Respir Crit Care Med* 158:77–83, 1998.
49. Gan TJ, Arrowsmith JE: The oesophageal Doppler monitor. *BMJ* 315:893–894, 1997.
50. Rivers E, Nguyen B, Havstad S, et al: Early goal-directed therapy in the treatment of severe sepsis and septic shock. *N Engl J Med* 345:1368–1377, 2001.
51. National Heart L, Blood Institute Acute Respiratory Distress Syndrome Clinical Trials N, Wiedemann HP, et al: Comparison of two fluid-management strategies in acute lung injury. *N Engl J Med* 354:2564–2575, 2006.
52. Vieillard-Baron A, Slama M, Mayo P, et al: A pilot study on safety and clinical utility of a single-use 72-hour indwelling transesophageal echocardiography probe. *Intensive Care Med* 39:629–635, 2013.
53. Quinones MA, Douglas PS, Foster E, et al: ACC/AHA clinical competence statement on echocardiography: a report of the American College of Cardiology/American Heart Association/American College of Physicians-American Society of Internal Medicine Task Force on Clinical Competence. *J Am Col Cardiol* 41:687–708, 2003.
54. Critical Care Ultrasonography: http://www.chestnet.org/education/advanced-clinical-training/certificate-of-completion-program/critical-care-ultrasonography, Accessed January 27, 2017.
55. Frank O. Wellen- und windkesselthrorie Estimation of the strok volume of the human heart using the "windkessel" theory [in German]. *Zeitschr Biol* 90:405–409, 1930.
56. Wesseling K, de Wit Bd, Weber J, et al: A simple device for the continuous measurement of cardiac output. *Adv Cardiovasc Phys* 5:16–52, 1983.
57. Pinsky MR. Probing the limits of arterial pulse contour analysis to predict preload responsiveness. *Anesth Analg* 96:1245–1247, 2003.
58. Della Rocca G, Costa MG, Pompei L, et al: Continuous and intermittent cardiac output measurement: pulmonary artery catheter versus aortic transpulmonary technique. *Br J Anaesth* 88:350–356, 2002.
59. Della Rocca G, Costa MG, Coccia C, et al: Cardiac output monitoring: aortic transpulmonary thermodilution and pulse contour analysis agree with standard thermodilution methods in patients undergoing lung transplantation. *Can J Anaesth* 50:707–711, 2003.
60. Godje O, Hoke K, Goetz AE, et al: Reliability of a new algorithm for continuous cardiac output determination by pulse-contour analysis during hemodynamic instability. *Crit Care Med* 30:52–58, 2002.
61. Mielck F, Buhre W, Hanekop G, et al: Comparison of continuous cardiac output measurements in patients after cardiac surgery. *J Cardiothorac Vasc Anesth* 17:211–216, 2003.
62. Rauch H, Muller M, Fleischer F, et al: Pulse contour analysis versus thermodilution in cardiac surgery patients. *Acta Anaesthesiol Scand* 46:424–429, 2002.
63. Manecke GR Jr, Auger WR: Cardiac output determination from the arterial pressure wave: clinical testing of a novel algorithm that does not require calibration. *J Cardiothorac Vasc Anesth* 21:3–7, 2007.
64. Langewouters GJ, Wesseling KH, Goedhard WJ: The pressure dependent dynamic elasticity of 35 thoracic and 16 abdominal human aortas in vitro described by a five component model. *J Biomech* 18:613–620, 1985.

65. Sakka SG, Kozieras J, Thuemer O, et al: Measurement of cardiac output: a comparison between transpulmonary thermodilution and uncalibrated pulse contour analysis. *Br J Anaesth* 99:337–342, 2007.
66. Biancofiore G, Critchley LA, Lee A, et al: Evaluation of an uncalibrated arterial pulse contour cardiac output monitoring system in cirrhotic patients undergoing liver surgery. *Br J Anaesth* 102:47–54, 2009.
67. The FloTrac Sensor: http://www.edwards.com/products/mininvasive/Pages/FloTracSensor.aspx.
68. Biancofiore G, Critchley LA, Lee A, et al: Evaluation of a new software version of the FloTrac/Vigileo (version 3.02) and a comparison with previous data in cirrhotic patients undergoing liver transplant surgery. *Anesth Analg* 113:515–522, 2011.
69. De Backer D, Marx G, Tan A, et al: Arterial pressure-based cardiac output monitoring: a multicenter validation of the third-generation software in septic patients. *Intensive Care Med* 37:233–240, 2011.
70. Felbinger TW, Reuter DA, Eltzschig HK, et al: Cardiac index measurements during rapid preload changes: a comparison of pulmonary artery thermodilution with arterial pulse contour analysis. *J Clin Anesth* 17:241–248, 2005.
71. Gunn SR, Pinsky MR: Implications of arterial pressure variation in patients in the intensive care unit. *Curr Opin Crit Care* 7:212–217, 2001.
72. Michard F, Teboul JL: Using heart-lung interactions to assess fluid responsiveness during mechanical ventilation. *Crit Care* 4:282–289, 2000.
73. Michard F, Teboul JL: Predicting fluid responsiveness in ICU patients: a critical analysis of the evidence. *Chest* 121:2000–2008, 2002.
74. Osman D, Ridel C, Ray P, et al: Cardiac filling pressures are not appropriate to predict hemodynamic response to volume challenge. *Crit Care Med* 35:64–68, 2007.
75. Marik PE, Baram M, Vahid B: Does central venous pressure predict fluid responsiveness? A systematic review of the literature and the tale of seven mares. *Chest* 134:172–178, 2008.
76. Marik PE, Cavallazzi R, Vasu T, et al: Dynamic changes in arterial waveform derived variables and fluid responsiveness in mechanically ventilated patients: a systematic review of the literature. *Crit Care Med* 37:2642–2647, 2009.
77. Cannesson M, Le Manach Y, Hofer CK, et al: Assessing the diagnostic accuracy of pulse pressure variations for the prediction of fluid responsiveness: a "gray zone" approach. *Anesthesiology* 115:231–241, 2011.
78. PiCCO: http://www.pulsion.com/international-english/critical-care/parameter. Accessed January 27, 2017.
79. Volume View Set. http://www.edwards.com/gb/devices/Hemodynamic-Monitoring/VolumeView
80. Michard F, Alaya S, Zarka V, et al: Global end-diastolic volume as an indicator of cardiac preload in patients with septic shock. *Chest* 124:1900–1908, 2003.
81. Jozwiak M, Silva S, Persichini R, et al: Extravascular lung water is an independent prognostic factor in patients with acute respiratory distress syndrome. *Crit Care Med* 41:472–480, 2013.
82. Takala J, Ruokonen E, Tenhunen JJ, et al: Early non-invasive cardiac output monitoring in hemodynamically unstable intensive care patients: a multi-center randomized controlled trial. *Crit Care* 15:R148, 2011.
83. Pearse RM, Harrison DA, MacDonald N, et al: Effect of a perioperative, cardiac output-guided hemodynamic therapy algorithm on outcomes following major gastrointestinal surgery: a randomized clinical trial and systematic review. *JAMA* 311:2181–2190, 2014.
84. Krejci V, Vannucci A, Abbas A, et al: Comparison of calibrated and uncalibrated arterial pressure-based cardiac output monitors during orthotopic liver transplantation. *Liver Transpl* 16:773–782, 2010.
85. Meng L, Tran NP, Alexander BS, et al: The impact of phenylephrine, ephedrine, and increased preload on third-generation Vigileo-FloTrac and esophageal doppler cardiac output measurements. *Anesth Analg* 113:751–757, 2011.
86. Marque S, Gros A, Chimot L, et al: Cardiac output monitoring in septic shock: evaluation of the third-generation Flotrac-Vigileo. *J Clin Monit Comput* 27:273–279, 2013.
87. De Backer D, Heenen S, Piagnerelli M, et al: Pulse pressure variations to predict fluid responsiveness: influence of tidal volume. *Intensive Care Med* 31:517–523, 2005.
88. Freitas FG, Bafi AT, Nascente AP, et al: Predictive value of pulse pressure variation for fluid responsiveness in septic patients using lung-protective ventilation strategies. *Br J Anaesth* 110:402–408, 2013.
89. De Backer D, Taccone FS, Holsten R, et al: Influence of respiratory rate on stroke volume variation in mechanically ventilated patients. *Anesthesiology* 110:1092–1097, 2009.
90. Kubicek WG, Karnegis JN, Patterson RP, et al: Development and evaluation of an impedance cardiac output system. *Aerosp Med* 37:1208–1212, 1966.
91. Raaijmakers E, Faes TJ, Scholten RJ, et al: A meta-analysis of three decades of validating thoracic impedance cardiography. *Crit Care Med* 27:1203–1213, 1999.
92. Genoni M, Pelosi P, Romand JA, et al: Determination of cardiac output during mechanical ventilation by electrical bioimpedance or thermodilution in patients with acute lung injury: effects of positive end-expiratory pressure. *Crit Care Med* 26:1441–1445, 1998.
93. Sageman WS, Amundson DE: Thoracic electrical bioimpedance measurement of cardiac output in postaortocoronary bypass patients. *Crit Care Med* 21:1139–1142, 1993.
94. Brown CV, Martin MJ, Shoemaker WC, et al: The effect of obesity on bioimpedance cardiac index. *Am J Surg* 189:547–550, 2005; discussion 50-1.
95. Keren H, Burkhoff D, Squara P: Evaluation of a noninvasive continuous cardiac output monitoring system based on thoracic bioreactance. *Am J Physiol Heart Circ Physiol* 293:H583–H589, 2007.
96. Squara P, Denjean D, Estagnasie P, et al: Noninvasive cardiac output monitoring (NICOM): a clinical validation. *Intensive Care Med* 33:1191–1194, 2007.
97. Raval NY, Squara P, Cleman M, et al: Multicenter evaluation of noninvasive cardiac output measurement by bioreactance technique. *J Clin Monit Comput* 22:113–119, 2008.
98. Conway DH, Hussain OA, Gall I: A comparison of noninvasive bioreactance with oesophageal Doppler estimation of stroke volume during open abdominal surgery: an observational study. *Eur J Anaesthesiol* 30:501–508, 2013.
99. Benomar B, Ouattara A, Estagnasie P, et al: Fluid responsiveness predicted by noninvasive bioreactance-based passive leg raise test. *Intensive Care Med* 36:1875–1881, 2010.
100. Tong H, Hu C, Hao X, et al: The prediction value of noninvasive bioreactance-based passive leg raising test in assessing fluid responsiveness in elderly patients with sepsis[in Chinese]. *Zhonghua nei ke za zhi* 54:130–133, 2015.
101. Marik PE, Levitov A, Young A, et al: The use of bioreactance and carotid Doppler to determine volume responsiveness and blood flow redistribution following passive leg raising in hemodynamically unstable patients. *Chest* 143:364–370, 2013.
102. Dunham CM, Chirichella TJ, Gruber BS, et al: Emergency department noninvasive (NICOM) cardiac outputs are associated with trauma activation, patient injury severity and host conditions and mortality. *J Trauma Acute Care Surg* 73:479–485, 2012.
103. Lee S, Lee SH, Chang BC, et al: Efficacy of Goal-Directed Therapy Using Bioreactance Cardiac Output Monitoring after Valvular Heart Surgery. *Yonsei Med J* 56:913–920, 2015.
104. Charron C, Caille V, Jardin F, et al: Echocardiographic measurement of fluid responsiveness. *Curr Opin Crit Care* 12:249–254, 2006.
105. Maizel J, Airapetian N, Lorne E, et al: Diagnosis of central hypovolemia by using passive leg raising. *Intensive Care Med* 33:1133–1138, 2007.
106. Kupersztych-Hagege E, Teboul JL, Artigas A, et al: Bioreactance is not reliable for estimating cardiac output and the effects of passive leg raising in critically ill patients. *Br J Anaesth* 111:961–966, 2013.
107. Huang L, Critchley LA, Zhang J: Major upper abdominal surgery alters the calibration of bioreactance cardiac output readings, the NICOM, when comparisons are made against suprasternal and esophageal doppler intraoperatively. *Anesth Analg* 121:936–945, 2015.
108. Han S, Lee JH, Kim G, et al: Bioreactance is not interchangeable with thermodilution for measuring cardiac output during adult liver transplantation. *PLoS One* 10:e0127981, 2015.
109. Khan FZ, Virdee MS, Pugh PJ, et al: Non-invasive cardiac output measurements based on bioreactance for optimization of atrio- and interventricular delays. *Europace* 11:1666–1674, 2009.
110. Monnet X, Teboul JL: Passive leg raising: five rules, not a drop of fluid! *Crit Care* 19:18, 2015.
111. Krebs H, Woods HF, Alberti KGMM: Hyperlactataemia and lactic acidosis. *Essays Biochem* 1:81–103, 1970.
112. Neviere R, Chagnon JL, Teboul JL, et al: Small intestine intramucosal PCO(2) and microvascular blood flow during hypoxic and ischemic hypoxia. *Crit Care Med* 30:379–384, 2002.
113. Gutierrez G, Palizas F, Doglio G, et al: Gastric intramucosal pH as a therapeutic index of tissue oxygenation in critically ill patients. *Lancet* 339:195–199, 1992.
114. Barquist E, Kirton O, Windsor J, et al: The impact of antioxidant and splanchnic-directed therapy on persistent uncorrected gastric mucosal pH in the critically injured trauma patient. *J Trauma* 44:355–360, 1998.
115. Miami Trauma Clinical Trials Group: Splanchnic hypoperfusion-directed therapies in trauma: a prospective, randomized trial. *Am Surg* 71:252–260, 2005.
116. Ivatury RR, Simon RJ, Islam S, et al: A prospective randomized study of end points of resuscitation after major trauma: global oxygen transport indices versus organ-specific gastric mucosal pH. *J Am Coll Surg* 183:145–154, 1996.
117. Gomersall CD, Joynt GM, Freebairn RC, et al: Resuscitation of critically ill patients based on the results of gastric tonometry: a prospective, randomized, controlled trial. *Crit Care Med* 28:607–614, 2000.
118. Lee J, Wright F, Barber R, et al: Central venous oxygen saturation in shock: a study in man. *Anesthesiology* 36:472–478, 1972.
119. Reinhart K, Kuhn HJ, Hartog C, et al: Continuous central venous and pulmonary artery oxygen saturation monitoring in the critically ill. *Intensive Care Med* 30:1572–1578, 2004.
120. Chawla LS, Zia H, Gutierrez G, et al: Lack of equivalence between central and mixed venous oxygen saturation. *Chest* 126:1891–1896, 2004.
121. Varpula M, Karlsson S, Ruokonen E, et al: Mixed venous oxygen saturation cannot be estimated by central venous oxygen saturation in septic shock. *Intensive Care Med* 32:1336–1343, 2006.
122. Sander M, Spies CD, Foer A, et al: Agreement of central venous saturation and mixed venous saturation in cardiac surgery patients. *Intensive Care Med* 33:1719–1725, 2007.
123. Turnaoglu S, Tugrul M, Camci E, et al: Clinical applicability of the substitution of mixed venous oxygen saturation with central venous oxygen saturation. *J Cardiothorac Vasc Anesth* 15:574–579, 2001.
124. Ho KM, Harding R, Chamberlain J, et al: A comparison of central and mixed venous oxygen saturation in circulatory failure. *J Cardiothorac Vasc Anesth* 24:434–439, 2010.
125. Suehiro K, Tanaka K, Matsuura T, et al: Discrepancy between superior vena cava oxygen saturation and mixed venous oxygen saturation can predict postoperative complications in cardiac surgery patients. *J Cardiothorac Vasc Anesth* 28:528–533, 2014.
126. Vieillard-Baron A, Caille V, Charron C, et al: Actual incidence of global left ventricular hypokinesia in adult septic shock. *Crit Care Med* 36:1701–1706, 2008.

127. Perner A, Haase N, Wiis J, et al: Central venous oxygen saturation for the diagnosis of low cardiac output in septic shock patients. *Acta Anaesthesiol Scand* 54:98–102, 2010.
128. Levy RJ. Mitochondrial dysfunction, bioenergetic impairment, and metabolic down-regulation in sepsis. *Shock* 28:24–28, 2007.
129. Pope JV, Jones AE, Gaieski DF, et al: Multicenter study of central venous oxygen saturation (ScvO(2)) as a predictor of mortality in patients with sepsis. *Ann Emerg Med* 55:40.e1–46.e1, 2010.
130. Textoris J, Fouche L, Wiramus S, et al: High central venous oxygen saturation in the latter stages of septic shock is associated with increased mortality. *Crit Care* 15:R176, 2011.
131. Gattinoni L, Brazzi L, Pelosi P, et al: A trial of goal-oriented hemodynamic therapy in critically ill patients. SvO2 Collaborative Group. *N Engl J Med* 333:1025–1032, 1995.
132. Yealy DM, Kellum JA, Huang DT, et al: A randomized trial of protocol-based care for early septic shock. *N Engl J Med* 370:1683–1693, 2014.
133. Peake SL, Delaney A, Bailey M, et al: Goal-directed resuscitation for patients with early septic shock. *N Engl J Med* 371:1496–1506, 2014.
134. Mouncey PR, Osborn TM, Power GS, et al: Trial of early, goal-directed resuscitation for septic shock. *N Engl J Med* 372:1301–1311, 2015.
135. Donati A, Loggi S, Preiser JC, et al: Goal-directed intraoperative therapy reduces morbidity and length of hospital stay in high-risk surgical patients. *Chest* 132:1817–1824, 2007.
136. Bakker J, Coffernils M, Leon M, et al: Blood lactate levels are superior to oxygen-derived variables in predicting outcome in human septic shock. *Chest* 99:956–962, 1991.
137. Kamolz LP, Andel H, Schramm W, et al: Lactate: early predictor of morbidity and mortality in patients with severe burns. *Burns* 31:986–990, 2005.
138. Odom SR, Howell MD, Silva GS, et al: Lactate clearance as a predictor of mortality in trauma patients. *J Trauma Acute Care Surg* 74:999–1004, 2013.
139. Howell MD, Donnino M, Clardy P, et al: Occult hypoperfusion and mortality in patients with suspected infection. *Intensive Care Med* 33:1892–1899, 2007.
140. Mikkelsen ME, Miltiades AN, Gaieski DF, et al: Serum lactate is associated with mortality in severe sepsis independent of organ failure and shock. *Crit Care Med* 37:1670–1677, 2009.
141. Nguyen HB, Rivers EP, Knoblich BP, et al: Early lactate clearance is associated with improved outcome in severe sepsis and septic shock. *Crit Care Med* 32:1637–1642, 2004.
142. Lee TR, Kang MJ, Cha WC, et al: Better lactate clearance associated with good neurologic outcome in survivors who treated with therapeutic hypothermia after out-of-hospital cardiac arrest. *Crit Care* 17:R260, 2013.
143. Arnold RC, Shapiro NI, Jones AE, et al: Multicenter study of early lactate clearance as a determinant of survival in patients with presumed sepsis. *Shock* 32:35–39, 2009.
144. Puskarich MA, Trzeciak S, Shapiro NI, et al: Prognostic value and agreement of achieving lactate clearance or central venous oxygen saturation goals during early sepsis resuscitation. *Acad Emerg Med* 19:252–258, 2012.
145. Zhang Z, Xu X: Lactate clearance is a useful biomarker for the prediction of all-cause mortality in critically ill patients: a systematic review and meta-analysis. *Crit Care Med* 42:2118–2125, 2014.
146. Jansen TC, van Bommel J, Schoonderbeek FJ, et al: Early lactate-guided therapy in intensive care unit patients: a multicenter, open-label, randomized controlled trial. *Am J Respir Crit Care Med* 182:752–761, 2010.
147. Jones AE, Shapiro NI, Trzeciak S, et al: Lactate clearance vs central venous oxygen saturation as goals of early sepsis therapy: a randomized clinical trial. *JAMA* 303:739–746, 2010.
148. Kopterides P, Bonovas S, Mavrou I, et al: Venous oxygen saturation and lactate gradient from superior vena cava to pulmonary artery in patients with septic shock. *Shock* 31:561–567, 2009.
149. Vesely TM: Central venous catheter tip position: a continuing controversy. *J Vasc Interv Radiol* 14:527–534, 2003.
150. Luchette FA, Jenkins WA, Friend LA, et al: Hypoxia is not the sole cause of lactate production during shock. *J Trauma* 52:415–419, 2002.
151. McCarter FD, Nierman SR, James JH, et al: Role of skeletal muscle Na+-K+ ATPase activity in increased lactate production in sub-acute sepsis. *Life Sci* 70:1875–1888, 2002.
152. Pastor CM, Billiar TR, Losser MR, et al: Liver injury during sepsis. *J Crit Care* 10:183–197, 1995.
153. Vary TC: Sepsis-induced alterations in pyruvate dehydrogenase complex activity in rat skeletal muscle: effects on plasma lactate. *Shock* 6:89–94, 1996.
154. Levraut J, Ciebiera JP, Chave S, et al: Mild hyperlactatemia in stable septic patients is due to impaired lactate clearance rather than overproduction. *Am J Respir Crit Care Med* 157:1021–1026, 1998.
155. Wong HR: Clinical review: sepsis and septic shock--the potential of gene arrays. *Crit Care* 16:204, 2012.
156. Wong HR, Lindsell CJ, Pettila V, et al: A multibiomarker-based outcome risk stratification model for adult septic shock. *Crit Care Med* 42:781–789, 2014.
157. Wong HR, Cvijanovich N, Lin R, et al: Identification of pediatric septic shock subclasses based on genome-wide expression profiling. *BMC Med* 7:34, 2009.
158. Wong HR, Cvijanovich NZ, Anas N, et al: Developing a clinically feasible personalized medicine approach to pediatric septic shock. *Am J Respir Crit Care Med* 191:309–315, 2015.

Chapter 29 ■ Echocardiography as a Monitor in the ICU

ACHIKAM OREN-GRINBERG • TODD W. SARGE • ADAM B. LERNER

INTRODUCTION

The past decade of patient care can easily be described as the ultrasound revolution. Improvement of ultrasound technology allowed for miniaturization of equipment and reduced costs, allowing this technology to find its way into all corners of patient care. The concept of "point-of-care (POC) ultrasound" was born and has dominated the bedside patient evaluation in many areas. Today, clinicians all over the world depend on ultrasound machines to manage critically ill patients. Ultrasound is used for diagnosis (e.g., cardiac disease, lung pathology peritoneal fluid and bleeding, deep vein thrombosis [DVT], etc.) and for procedures (e.g., vascular access, thoracentesis, paracentesis, etc.).

Many clinicians quickly adopted echocardiography, and the more focused form of it—focused cardiac ultrasound—as a diagnostic tool for their patients. Echocardiography provides both anatomic and functional information about the heart. The relative ease of use, rapid retrieval of information along with low complication rates, has all led to adaptation of echocardiography to the critical care environment. Nevertheless, the revolution is still ongoing—graduated clinicians continue to pursue education about this new modality, and student doctors learn focused cardiac ultrasound as part of new POC ultrasound curricula at many medical schools.

With growing experience and knowledge managing patients with this new modality, echocardiography is now used by critical care physicians not only for initial diagnosis but also as a form of monitoring. This paradigm shift challenges the traditional way of "doing business" with regard to hemodynamic monitoring. Although there is still no clear-cut evidence of its benefits, echocardiography is well received by clinicians, maybe because "seeing is believing." Clinicians can now perform cardiac ultrasound at the bedside and quickly determine the cause of hemodynamic derangement. However, patient safety and optimal outcome depend heavily on a thorough understanding of both the strengths and limitations of the available technologies and their applications. This chapter concentrates on the use of echocardiography in the intensive care unit (ICU) with an emphasis on its role as a hemodynamic monitor.

LIMITATIONS OF HEMODYNAMIC MONITORS

Hemodynamic monitors play an essential role in the management of critically ill patients. The pulmonary artery catheter (PAC) that was introduced in the early 1970s [1] changed the care of critically ill patients by allowing clinicians to measure extensive hemodynamic variables, such as cardiac output (CO), cardiac filling pressures, and global oxygen transport, at the patient's bedside. For many years, the PAC was considered the standard of care in critical care. However, formal studies on the impact of the PAC have documented increased mortality and increased utilization of resources with the use of the PAC [2]. While several large randomized controlled trials could not confirm these findings, they also failed to demonstrate improved outcomes when patients were managed using the PAC [3–6]. These and other publications led to a significant decline in utilization of PAC over the ensuing years [7,8].

The void of hemodynamic monitoring was quickly filled with "new" hemodynamic monitors, usually less invasive and some considered completely noninvasive. Although most of these monitors were evaluated by both experimental and clinical studies, to-date, no specific monitoring device has been found to reduce mortality for critically ill patients [9]. The reality is that no hemodynamic monitoring technique can improve outcomes by itself. Rather, outcomes can only improve if the following three conditions are met: (1) the technique provides accurate data; (2) the data obtained is relevant to patient management; and (3) significant management changes are made based on the data obtained [10]. It is also important that the data is interpreted and applied correctly and that the applied therapies are not ineffective or harmful [10].

One major advantage echocardiography has over many other hemodynamic monitors is that it provides crucial diagnostic information during the vital moments of the first patient encounter and at the time of hemodynamic instability. It can then be used for monitoring key hemodynamic parameters (e.g., CO, PA pressure, etc.) after application of therapies or their adjustment in a paradigm that optimizes hemodynamic responses.

ECHOCARDIOGRAPHY AS A HEMODYNAMIC MONITOR

Until recently, echocardiography has been considered as a useful diagnostic modality and was not regarded as a hemodynamic monitoring technique. This concept is changing with the fast growing field of POC ultrasound [11]. POC ultrasound—ultrasonography performed and interpreted by the clinician at the bedside—allows clinicians to gain experience with using comprehensive echocardiography as well as focused cardiac ultrasound for the management of critically ill patients. The growing use of ultrasound and specifically cardiac ultrasound for the management of critically ill patients leads to a paradigm shift with regard to hemodynamic monitoring. Thus, it is not surprising that with this growing change of practice, current guidelines recommend using cardiac ultrasound to monitor therapeutic responses of critically ill patients [12,13].

Although echocardiography has many advantages, both as a diagnostic tool and as a monitoring technology, it is important to understand how its use differs from the more traditional hemodynamic monitoring. First, unlike most hemodynamic monitors that provide data continuously, echocardiography provides information only intermittently. The exception is when transesophageal echocardiography (TEE) is used in periods of hemodynamically instability, where it can provide continuous information for as long as the TEE probe is left in position and a qualified clinician is there for interpretation of the images. Despite this limitation, there is no proven advantage to continuous over intermittent monitoring. Second, echocardiography requires considerable initial and continuing education whereas, typically, there are no such requirements for the use of other hemodynamic monitors. Although this could be perceived as an advantage for traditional hemodynamic monitors, a relative lack of knowledge without continuing education may provide the clinician with an incorrect understanding of a patient's hemodynamic status. Lastly, echocardiography may be not useful for some patients owing to poor image quality. Reasons for poor image quality include body habitus (either high [14] or low body mass index [15]), patient's comorbidities (e.g., chronic obstructive pulmonary disease [COPD]), mechanical ventilation, high positive end-expiratory pressure, surgical dressings, chest tubes and drains, poor positioning, operator experience, and machine quality.

COMPARISON BETWEEN TRANSTHORACIC ECHOCARDIOGRAPHY AND TRANSESOPHAGEAL ECHOCARDIOGRAPHY IN THE ICU

Although both transthoracic echocardiography (TTE) and TEE are used by intensivists for the management of critically ill patients, TTE use is more widespread. Each modality has its advantages and disadvantages with regard to image quality, cardiac anatomy obtained, and logistics. Understanding the similarities, differences, and benefits of the two modalities can be useful for the intensivist.

Whereas TEE generally provides superior image quality compared to TTE, anterior structures such as the right ventricle (RV), right ventricular outflow tract (RVOT), pulmonic valve, and anterior pericardium can be better imaged by TTE. In addition, the apical TTE views provide better imaging of the left ventricular apex. Posterior structures such as the left atrium; mitral valve and subvalvular apparatus; and interatrial septum and left atrial (LA) appendage are best imaged with TEE [16]. TEE is also better than TTE for evaluating patients for a potential source of cerebral embolus [17].

TEE is somewhat invasive and, although rare, has been associated with complications, some of which may be significant [18–20]. TTE, on the other hand, is noninvasive and outside misinterpretation, is practically risk free. Logistically, TEE is more costly and challenging to maintain because it requires cleaning and disinfection after each use in a dedicated disinfecting apparatus. It also requires special storage and handling and is limited to use in one patient at a time with a few hours of cleaning time in between patients. This limits the number of patients that one TEE probe can service in a single day. In contrast, TTE can be rapidly disinfected and used repeatedly on the same or different patients and can be used anywhere in the hospital (e.g., during resuscitations on the wards) and even at prehospital settings. TEE performed by noncardiologists is usually limited to the perioperative environment, ICU [21], and the emergency department [22].

CARDIAC OUTPUT

Introduction

CO is a critical factor affecting global oxygen transport to tissues and organs. Although there are no absolute values that reflect adequate circulation for an individual patient, most clinicians agree that very low values (e.g., CI < 2.0 L per m^2) are associated with worse outcomes. Thus, it is reasonable to monitor CO in critical illness to assess for impairments of cardiac function with the goal of normalization as is feasible.

Current CO techniques include (1) thermodilution (either the transpulmonary technique or intracardiac technique using the PAC); (2) arterial pulse contour analysis; (3) noninvasive bioreactance; (4) Doppler technologies measuring blood flow in the ascending or descending aorta; (5) partial CO_2 rebreathing technique (using the modified Fick equation); and (6) arteriovenous oxygen content differences using the Fick equation (that also requires a PAC). Each of these techniques and methods has strengths and limitations that should be considered when choosing a method to evaluate an individual patient.

Echocardiographic Measurement Technique

CO can be measured relatively easily and quickly with echocardiography, and can be integrated into the clinician's assessment of critically ill patients [23]. In contrast to many hemodynamic monitors, CO measurement with echocardiography is not continuous and requires the clinician to be at the patient's bedside. It can be repeated as needed to monitor response to therapies (e.g., volume expansion therapy or initiation of inotropes).

Although there are several echocardiographic techniques that can be used to measure CO, most clinicians use a continuity-based assessment of flow in the left ventricular outflow tract (LVOT). In this technique, the LVOT is assumed to have a cylindrical shape and its cross section estimated by a circle. Because the volume of a cylinder is calculated by multiplying its cross-sectional area (CSA) with its height, one can see that the same calculations can be applied to the volume of the LVOT, resulting in calculation of a patient's stroke volume (SV).

The circular CSA of a cylinder is calculated by the formula πr^2. To calculate the CSA of the LVOT with TTE, the parasternal long-axis (PLAX) view (Video 29.1) is used to measure the LVOT diameter, from which the computer computes the radius. A key to success is optimizing the image quality and then zooming in on the LVOT before measuring its diameter (Video 29.1). This will improve accuracy and minimize measurement error because any error of the diameter/radius measurement will be squared. It is best to standardize the point of measurement of LVOT diameter, and many clinicians choose the point of aortic valve leaflet attachment to the LVOT (aortic valve annulus) as the measurement point.

To calculate the height of the cylinder, usually the apical 5-chamber (A5CH) view is used (Video 29.1), but if the quality of this view is suboptimal, the apical 3-chamber (A3CH) view can also be used, provided its angle of interrogation is less than 20 degrees off the flow of blood (Video 29.1). Blood flow velocity through the LVOT is measured with pulse wave Doppler, ideally at the same point where the diameter was measured (at the level of the aortic annulus). A characteristic spectral display is generated, where each wave represents velocity over time of one SV. By tracing one of these curves, the computer calculates the velocity time integral (VTI), which is the area under the curve. Conceptually, this is the average displacement (i.e., distance) of the column of blood that moved through the LVOT in the measured wave. This "stroke distance" is the height of the cylinder in centimeters that is used to complete the calculation of the LVOT cylinder SV.

Multiplying the LVOT cylinder's CSA (cm^2) with its height (cm) produces one SV (cm^3 or mL). The computer then calculates CO by multiplying SV with the heart rate.

If TEE is used, the midesophageal long-axis view is used to measure the LVOT diameter (Video 29.1), and the VTI is measured in the deep transgastric view (Video 29.1).

Stroke Volume Estimation

For critically ill patients, close attention should be made to SV because it can provide important information on the patient's hemodynamic state. For example, a patient with CO of 5 L per minute and heart rate of 60 beats per minute has normal SV of 83 mL per minute. In contrast, the SV of a different patient with the same CO and heart rate of 125 beats per minute is only 40 mL per minute, which is likely to be pathologic.

Therefore, SV can be monitored serially to assess improvement after initiation of therapy. Critically ill patients often have difficult windows yielding suboptimal image quality. For example, a patient with a difficult PLAX view may prohibit the accurate measurement of the LVOT diameter. In such patients, the velocity time index (VTI), which is a reflection of SV, can be followed serially. As the LVOT is an anatomic structure, its diameter and, thus, the CSA do not change significantly with therapies. Thus, in reality, it is the VTI and changes to the VTI that are more critical for monitoring a patient's CO and hemodynamic responses to therapies. On average, a normal VTI is greater than 18 cm that corresponds to an SV of roughly 60 mL (low normal SV). Serially following the VTI can help guide the clinician toward success for optimizing a hemodynamic therapeutic intervention [24].

Pitfalls and Limitations of Cardiac Output Measurement

Left Ventricular Outflow Tract Diameter Measurement

Because any error in the measurement of the LVOT diameter will be squared in the CO calculation, it is important to generate quality PLAX view, zoom on the LVOT, and measure it meticulously. Averaging several measurements of LVOT diameter will reduce the measurement error.

Doppler Measurement of Velocity Time Integral

The measured Doppler velocity is a function of the cosine of the angle between blood flow and the ultrasound beam. Therefore, accurate VTI measurement occurs when the Doppler beam is parallel to blood flow, and care should be taken to ensure that the Doppler beam is parallel to the LVOT when making this measurement. An angle of less than 20 degrees is desirable to maintain an error of less than 6%. Similar to LVOT measurement, averaging several VTI measurements will reduce its measurement error.

Arrhythmias

Arrhythmias (e.g., atrial fibrillation) often lead to beat-to-beat variation in SV and VTI. To improve accuracy, several VTIs should be measured and averaged to better gauge SV, particularly in the setting of irregular heart rhythms.

FLUID MANAGEMENT

Introduction

Early and adequate resuscitation is an important determinant of outcome for many critically ill patients. For example, among septic patients, early resuscitation is a part of the surviving sepsis bundle [25]. On the other hand, overly aggressive fluid administration has been linked to worsened outcomes and increased complications associated with lung physiology [26]. Therefore, determining an individual patient's volume status and response to fluids has been one of the most challenging tasks for critical care professionals. Hemodynamic optimization of the critically ill patient requires the fine balance between preload, afterload, and myocardial contractility. Although echocardiography can help to some degree with understanding preload and fluid responsiveness, there are many limitations that must be taken into account when assessing the patient's volume status. However, it should also be noted that this is true for all monitoring modalities with regard to fluid responsiveness. In this section, we discuss two aspects of volume status with case examples: (1) recognition of the patient with severe hypovolemia and (2) assessment of fluid responsiveness.

Severe Hypovolemia

Severe hypovolemia, the cause of hypovolemic shock, occurs with rapid and significant loss of blood volume or body fluid (e.g., diarrhea). If unrecognized and untreated, this life-threatening condition leads to inadequate organ perfusion and eventually death. Echocardiography can help for the diagnosis of severe hypovolemia and guide resuscitation.

The echocardiographic findings associated with severe hypovolemia include decreased dimensions of both the LV and RV cavities during systole and diastole, and a small inferior vena cava (IVC) diameter [13]. In addition, the IVC often collapses more than 50% with respiration. It is important to note that the IVC diameter is used not in isolation, but rather as part of a pattern to support a diagnosis of hypovolemia.

In the extreme situation of an "empty heart," echocardiography can be very useful for following the response to aggressive fluid resuscitation. With volume loading, ventricular size is expected to increase, and serial examinations can document such effect of therapy.

However, assessment of severe hypovolemia may be more complex for patients with chronic heart disease. In this population of patients, dilatation of cardiac chambers can obscure associations between chamber size and assessments of preload. Therefore, a thorough patient history is extremely important, and no monitoring technology can substitute for this valuable information. For example, in the setting of chronically dilated LV, LA, right atrial (RA), or RV as well as left ventricular hypertrophy and right ventricular hypertrophy, the ability of a single echocardiographic session to detect hypovolemia is severely limited [27].

Dynamic Parameters

In the past decade, dynamic parameters (e.g., SV variation, pulse pressure variation, etc.) have gained acceptance as more sensitive indices for assessing fluid responsiveness during mechanical ventilation [28]. Fluid responsiveness is defined as an increase of SV in response to fluid administration. These parameters take advantage of the heart–lung interaction during positive pressure ventilation, as long as the patient is in a regular rhythm. In short, positive pressure inspiration temporarily decreases right-sided venous return and RV SV. The same positive pressure inspiration initially leads to a temporary increase of the LV SV, because the increased intrathoracic pressure compresses the pulmonary veins, pushing blood forward to the LV. The end result is an increased LV SV via Starling forces and greater pulse pressure during the initial portion of inspiration. This is followed by a decrease in the SV effects of both the ventricles during exhalation. This normal phenomenon is exaggerated during hypovolemia. Modern hemodynamic monitors (including those with pulse contour analysis as well as pulse oximetry and discussed in Chapter 28) can quantify these changes using the stroke volume variation and pulse pressure variation to discriminate patients who are fluid responsive from those who are not. These respiratory effects on SV that occur as the result of heart–lung interaction can be assessed with echocardiography.

Aortic Flow Index

The aortic flow index (AFI) takes advantage of the heart–lung interaction that is the foundation of fluid responsiveness. This index uses pulse wave Doppler ultrasound to measure changes of the velocity of blood exiting the heart through the LVOT during positive pressure ventilation. In essence, this index is the ultrasound equivalent of the pulse pressure variation. As mentioned earlier, SV increases with initiation of positive pressure inspiration and decreases during exhalation. With ultrasound, higher left ventricular SV translates to higher velocities and VTIs of blood in the LVOT and ascending aorta. Measuring these flows is relatively easy with either TTE or TEE, and most modern ultrasound machines can be programmed to calculate this index automatically. The AFI is calculated as the difference between the highest and lowest peak velocities measured at the ascending aorta (or even more conveniently in the LVOT) divided by the mean of these two velocities, expressed as percentage (Fig. 29.1). An index of 12% allows discrimination between fluid responders and nonresponders with very high sensitivity and specificity [29].

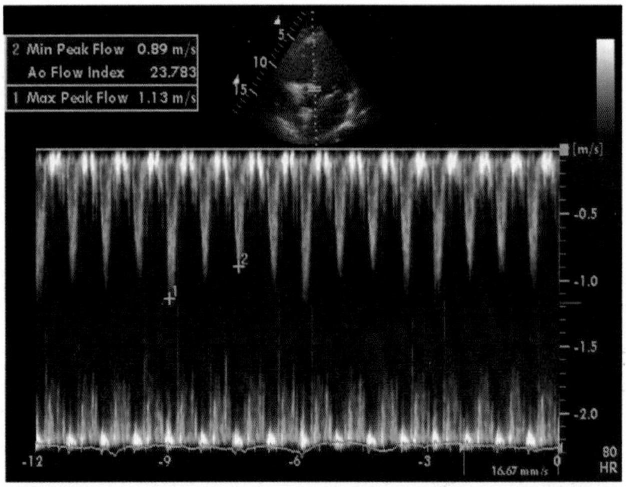

FIGURE 29.1 Aortic flow index is measured in the apical 5-chamber view (TTE) or deep trans-gastric view (TEE). The sweep speed is reduced to capture more stroke volume spectral display. While blood flow can be measured in the ascending aorta, it can be also very conveniently measured in the LVOT. Peak flow is measured at the highest and lowest stroke volumes, which represent flow during positive pressure inhalation and exhalation, respectively. Most modern ultrasound machines can be programmed to calculate equations, and, in this example, the aortic flow index is calculated to be almost 24%. LVOT, left ventricular outflow tract; TEE, transesophageal echocardiography; TTE, transthoracic echocardiography.

$$AFI = (V_{max} - V_{min})/[(V_{max} + V_{min})/2] \times 100\%$$

Inferior Vena Cava Distensibility Index

The IVC, as an extrathoracic structure, dilates during positive pressure inspiration because of increased intrathoracic pressure that resists venous return to the right heart. During exhalation, it decreases in size. Quantifying the degree of dimensional change of the IVC, defined as distensibility, can help predict fluid responsiveness in patients who are mechanically ventilated with positive pressure ventilation [30,31]. Two different distensibility indices have been described in the literature.

The first distensibility index (dIVC, where the "d" signifies "delta") is defined as the difference between the maximum IVC diameter at end-inspiration (D_{max}) and the minimum IVC diameter at end expiration (D_{min}) divided by D_{min} and expressed as percentage (Fig. 29.2) [30]. An index larger than 18% defines fluid responsiveness for this index.

$$dIVC = (D_{max} - D_{min})/D_{min} \times 100\%$$

The second index defines the distensibility as the difference between the maximum diameter at the end of inspiration (D_{max}) and the minimum IVC diameter at end expiration (D_{min}) divided by the mean of the two and expressed as percentage (Fig. 29.2) [31].

$$dIVC = (D_{max} - D_{min})/[(D_{max} + D_{min})/2] \times 100\%$$

Using this method, an index larger than 12% defines fluid responsiveness.

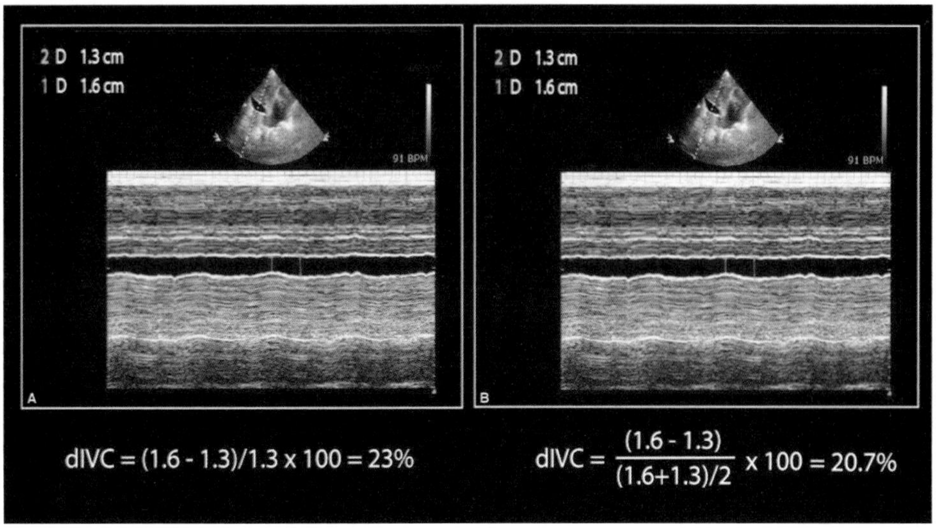

FIGURE 29.2 Two types of distensibility index. **A:** Calculation of the distensibility index using the minimum IVC diameter at end expiration in the denominator. **B:** Calculation of the distensibility index using the mean of IVC diameter in inspiration and expiration in the denominator. IVC, inferior vena cava.

Superior Vena Cava Collapsibility Index

Because the superior vena cava (SVC) is an intrathoracic structure hidden by the right lung, it cannot be viewed using TTE. TEE provides the ability to view this vessel relatively clearly. Although the concept is the same as for the IVC distensibility index, being an intrathoracic structure, the effect is reversed, and SVC diameter decreases (or "collapses") with positive pressure inspiration. The SVC collapsibility index (dSVC) is defined as the difference between the maximum SVC diameter at end expiration (D_{max}) and the minimum diameter at the end of inspiration (D_{min}) divided by the maximum diameter and expressed as a percentage (Fig. 29.3) [32].

$$\text{dIVC} = (D_{max} - D_{min})/D_{max} \times 100\%$$

For this index, a result larger than 36% indicates fluid responsiveness.

SVC collapsibility index appears to be more accurate than the IVC distensibility index for predicting fluid responsiveness [33]. This is likely because, physiologically, the SVC and IVC are exposed to significantly different pressures. For example, only 20% of the airway pressure is transmitted to the abdomen [34], and the relationship between venous transmural pressure and venous size is curvilinear [35].

Velocity Time Integral

As mentioned earlier, for monitoring CO response to inotropes or volume expansion, a simple approach to monitoring fluid resuscitation for critically ill patients is simply to serially measure the VTI. VTI is measured in the A5CH view and considred the Doppler surrogate of SV. Therefore, the VTI increases when SV increases as a result of fluid administration. For an average size patient, a normal VTI is larger than 18 cm that corresponds to SV of roughly 60 mL; however, it is the change in response to a fluid bolus that is desired to demonstrate fluid responsiveness.

Passive Leg Raise Test

The passive leg raise (PLR) test has been advocated in recent years as an excellent technique to assess fluid responsiveness for patients subjected to passive controlled ventilation [36] as well as those breathing spontaneously [37]. It is a simple reversible maneuver that mimics rapid fluid loading, thereby increasing the cardiac preload and SV of preload-dependent patients. The technique requires semicontinuous monitoring of CO that can detect short-term and transient changes of CO during the test. In theory, echocardiography may qualify as an approach for monitoring by investigating the change in LVOT by measuring VTI in the semi-recumbent, baseline position and the VTI in the supine position with the patient's legs elevated. However, technical challenges may limit its use for the PLR test. For example, in a study of the PLR test among healthy volunteers, only 65% of the patients had adequate Doppler images of the VTI for analysis [38]. The ability to obtain adequate Doppler images may be lower among critically patients as a result of obesity, comorbidities, mechanical ventilation, and other factors. Another limitation includes translation of displacement from the motion of the heart

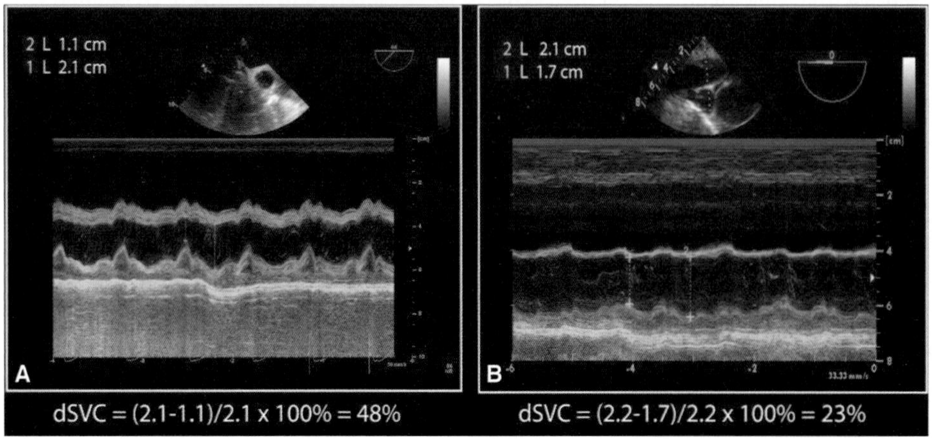

FIGURE 29.3 **A:** SVC collapsibility index of a patient who is fluid responsive. **B:** SVC collapsibility index of a patient who is fluid unresponsive. The SVC diameter is measured with TEE in the upper esophageal window. A cutoff of 36% discriminates between fluid responders and nonresponders; dSVC higher than 36% indicates fluid responders, and dSVC smaller than 36% indicates nonresponders. SVC, superior vena cava; TEE, transesophageal echocardiography.

when a semi-recumbent patient is moved to the supine position, preventing the sonographer from obtaining a timely recording of the VTI. Finally, with the PLR test, the CO should be measured for 3 to 5 minutes following transition to supine position with elevated legs [39,40], and the highest CO measurement used for the analysis. Therefore, echocardiography is likely to be less attractive for this purpose, because the sonographer is required to first record VTI loops for at least 3 minutes, choose the highest VTI out of these loops and then compare it to the baseline VTI and make the necessary calculations.

Limitations of Echocardiography Use for the Assessment of Fluid Responsiveness

Left Ventricular Preload

For over four decades, fluid optimization of critically ill patients was achieved by assessing right and left ventricular preload through measuring central venous pressure (CVP) and pulmonary artery occlusion pressure, respectively. It is now well accepted that filling pressures alone cannot be used to adequately assess ventricular preload [41]. A potentially attractive alternative is echocardiographic assessment of LV preload using direct visualization of left ventricular size and, more specifically, end-diastolic area (LVEDA). Unfortunately, because LV size is a highly variable parameter, LVEDA has a low sensitivity in detecting blood volume changes in critically ill patients [42,43]. In addition, LV size fails to predict fluid responsiveness among patients with shock [44]. Therefore, assessing fluid responsiveness by LVEDA is not recommended. However, in the extreme situation of pure hypovolemic shock, LEVDA may be useful and this is discussed later.

Static Inferior Vena Cava Diameter

The IVC is a very compliant vessel, and it is easily imaged from the subcostal view. Its size and collapsibility are affected by several factors, such as total blood volume, CVP, intrathoracic pressure (which in turn, can be affected by the patient's respiratory pattern), and intra-abdominal pressure. Despite the attractiveness of using the IVC to diagnose hypovolemia and predict fluid responsiveness using its size and respiratory variability for spontaneously breathing patients, this correlation appears to be poor and unpredictable [45–47]. Therefore, clinicians are discouraged from using the IVC in isolation from other parameters for diagnosing hypovolemia.

Case 1

A 35-year-old man was admitted to the ICU from the operating room after 12 hours of surgery for polytrauma. He underwent extensive vascular surgery of the pelvis, as well as an exploratory laparotomy and splenectomy. He lost a significant amount of blood and was aggressively resuscitated by the anesthesia team with blood products and fluids.

Upon arrival to the ICU, the patient was on low-dose phenylephrine infusion for hemodynamic support. Blood pressure (BP) was 110/55 mm Hg, and lactate was 7.2 mmol per L. Owing to the surgical dressing and body habitus, only the apical 4-chamber (A4CH) view was available for imaging. It demonstrated no evidence of chronic heart disease or severe hypovolemia. The RV was not well seen, but it appeared to be very small in size and with normal function. Severe hypovolemia was diagnosed based on the presence of LV end-systolic cavity obliteration (commonly known as "kissing walls"), and very small LVEDA using the eyeballing technique. In fact, the LV walls barely separated from each other in diastole (Video 29.2). Based on these findings, a liter of lactated ringer's solution was rapidly administered, and a follow-up examination showed that both ventricles enlarged in

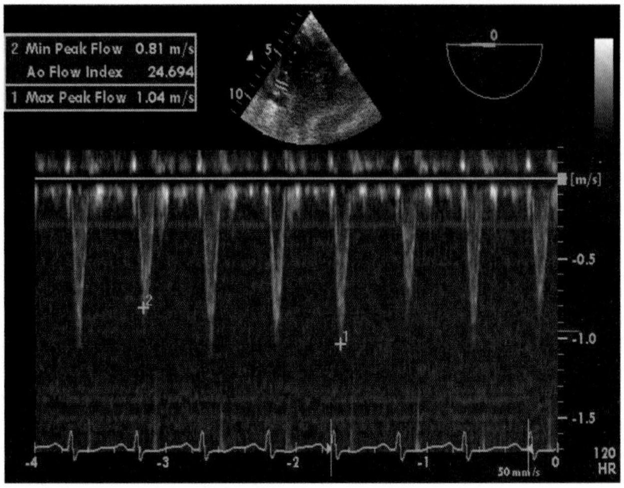

FIGURE 29.4 TEE deep transgastric view measuring flow of blood in the LVOT over several cardiac cycles. The spectral display waves with higher blood velocity occur during positive pressure inspiratory cycles and those with lower blood velocity occur during exhalation. The ultrasound machine has been programmed to automatically calculate the aortic flow index once the maximum and minimum peak velocities are measured. LVOT, left ventricular outflow tract; TEE, transesophageal echocardiography.

size and volume (Video 29.2). However, both appeared to still be significantly underfilled, as indicated by the small end-diastolic size. Another liter of lactate ringer's solution was rapidly administered, and the follow-up TTE examination demonstrates further increase in biventricular size that now appeared to be normal (Video 29.2).

Case 2

A 65-year-old woman was admitted to the ICU in septic shock, likely from a urologic source. During intubation in the emergency department, she vomited and aspirated and subsequently became hypotensive. Severe hypotension persisted in the ICU despite infusion of four pressors and inotropic agents. A TEE was performed to help with the management of shock and demonstrated hyperdynamic LV, normal RV function, and high AFI of 24% (Fig. 29.4). After administration of 500 mL of colloid solution, a repeat TEE examination showed that the AFI was reduced to 15% (Fig. 29.5). Further resuscitation with 250 mL bolus of colloid solution reduced the AFI to 11% (Fig. 29.6). Based on these findings, aggressive fluid resuscitation was held at that time. BP stabilized, and the dose of the vasopressor and inotropes was weaned successfully.

Pitfalls and Recommendations for Use of Echocardiography for Fluid Management

- **A.** Assessment of "fluid status" with echocardiography can only be done in the absence of chronic heart disease.
- **B.** Except for the extreme condition of severe hypovolemia, static measurements of LV preload by end-diastolic and end-systolic areas cannot predict fluid responsiveness.
- **C.** IVC size is affected by many factors and does not correlate with fluid responsiveness. Therefore, it should not be used in isolation to guide fluid management.
- **D.** In the absence of chronic heart disease, the pattern of severe hypovolemia includes very small right and left ventricular areas in both end diastole and end systole in the presence of a very small and collapsing IVC.
- **E.** The dynamic indices can be useful for predicting fluid responsiveness, but limited only for patients ventilated with positive pressure ventilation, sinus rhythm, and tidal volume of 8 to

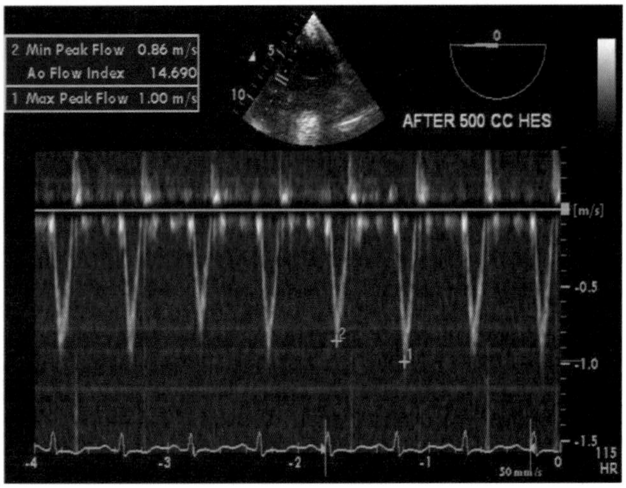

FIGURE 29.5 TEE deep transgastric view measuring flow of blood in the LVOT of several cardiac cycles after administration of 500 mL of colloid solution. Compared with the baseline examination, the maximum peak flow during positive pressure inspiration slightly decreased from 1.04 to 1.00 m per second and the maximum peak flow during exhalation increased from 0.81 to 0.86 m per second. This narrowing of the difference between the peak flows leads to a reduction of the aortic flow index from 24% to 15%. LVOT, left ventricular outflow tract; TEE, transesophageal echocardiography.

10 mL per kg. Cautious should be exercised in patients with RV failure who are passively ventilated because the presence of RV dysfunction may limit left chamber filling and results in a lack of the usual left-sided responsiveness predictors.

F. A simple and practical method to assess fluid responsiveness is by improved SV and thus VTI in the A5CH or A3CH views following administration of fluids.

PULMONARY EMBOLISM

Introduction

Venous thromboembolism (VTE) is a spectrum of disease ranging from DVT to pulmonary embolism (PE). In terms of prevalence, VTE is the third most frequent diagnosis among cardiovascular disorders [48]. Although the incidence of VTE is unclear, it is estimated to be approximately 100 to 400 cases per 100,000 people per year [49,50]. VTE is a frequent cause of hospitalization, morbidity, and mortality; it is estimated that 60,000 to 100,000 Americans die annually from VTE, and sudden death is the first symptom in about 25% of people who have PE. In addition, one-half of patients who have had DVT develop long-term complications [51]. This section analyzes the echocardiographic and ultrasonographic findings that are used to evaluate patients suspected of having a VTE. Specific emphasis is placed on the diagnosis of PE and the limitations of ultrasound for this purpose, particularly the issues with sensitivity and specificity for this diagnosis by ultrasound.

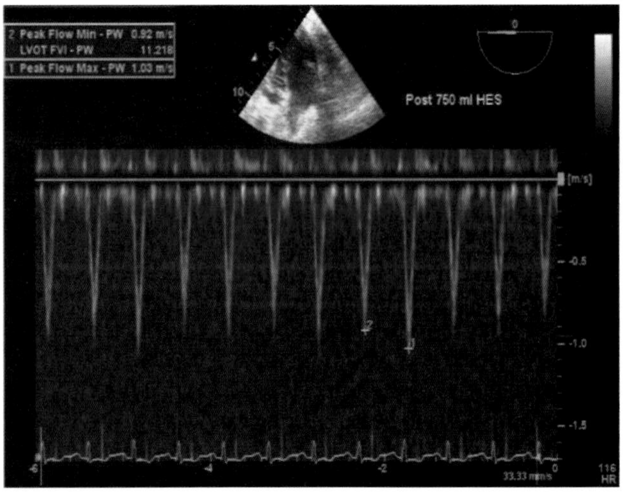

FIGURE 29.6 Same TEE view after resuscitation with a second bolus of 250 mL of colloid solution. This fluid bolus further reduced the aortic flow index to 11%, which changes the patient's physiology from fluid responsive to unresponsive by the defined limit for normal of 12%. TEE, transesophageal echocardiography.

Pathophysiology

Although acute PE can interfere with both gas exchange and circulation, the primary cause of death in PE is acute, right-sided heart failure caused by increased pulmonary vascular resistance (PVR) [52]. Right ventricular failure occurs when the RV experiences a sudden and profound increase in afterload from increased PVR. Under normal conditions, the PVR is low because of high compliance of the pulmonary vessels. This relationship changes when more than 30% of the pulmonary arterial vasculature is occluded by thromboemboli, at which point the PA pressure starts to increase [52].

In addition to anatomic obstruction of blood flow, the abrupt increase of PVR is explained by vasoconstriction caused by vasoactive mediators released mainly by activated platelets. Thromboxane A2 and serotonin are likely the two most important pulmonary vasoconstrictors in this context [53], and this hemodynamic effect can be reversed by vasodilators [54,55].

The effects of sudden and significant increases of PVR on the right heart can be devastating. Because the right ventricular free wall is a thin structure, the RV cannot withstand sudden pressure overload. It dilates when exposed to high-pressure conditions, thereby leading to increased wall tension and myocardial stretch. Both processes affect the contractile properties of the right ventricular myocardium, and while increased catecholamine levels may temporarily help compensate by increasing heart rate and contractility, the RV eventually fails. Its contraction time becomes prolonged into early diastole of the left ventricle (LV). This leads to interventricular septum shift toward the LV, further decreasing CO by reducing left ventricular preload [56] and contributing to hemodynamic instability [57].

RV infarction is uncommon in the setting of acute PE; yet, the presence of elevated levels of myocardial biomarkers (e.g., troponin) suggest RV ischemia as a result of imbalance between oxygen supply and demand [58,59]. This ischemia further exacerbates RV systolic function and contributes to hemodynamic instability.

To summarize the pathophysiology of PE, a large mechanical obstruction of the pulmonary vasculature prevents blood movement from the RV to the left heart. This leads to decreased CO and hypotension. In addition, the sudden and significant increase of RV afterload leads to RV dilatation and increased RV wall tension that frequently causes tricuspid insufficiency. RV pressure overload also leads to septal bowing to the LV, further decreasing CO. It also leads to neurohormonal activation as a compensatory mechanism (e.g., catecholamine release), tachycardia, and increased inotropy. These processes cause an increase of RV oxygen demand and ischemia, that eventually leads to decreased RV contractility, decreased RV CO, hemodynamic collapse, and death.

Role of Echocardiography for the Diagnosis of Pulmonary Embolism

Diagnostic Strategy

The diagnostic strategy for suspected PE might differ based on the hemodynamic status of the patient. In general, computed tomography angiography (CTA) is the gold standard imaging modality for the diagnosis of PE. It allows for adequate visualization of the pulmonary arteries down to the segmental level and potentially beyond [60,61]. Some patients, however, may not have access to CTA owing to either lack of a CT scanner in the treating facility or contraindications such as renal insufficiency, allergy to intravenous contrast, or profound hemodynamic instability, preventing transport of the patient out of the ICU to a remote CT scanner.

It is **only** in this setting of significant shock with high suspicion of acute PE that echocardiography can be recommended for the diagnosis or suggestion of acute PE [62]. It is important to realize, however, that despite widespread use of echocardiography during the initial management of acute PE, there is very little published data on its efficacy in this setting. This may explain the recommendation by several societies not to use echocardiography to establish the diagnosis of acute PE [63].

However, strategies that exclude bedside echocardiography from the diagnostic algorithm fail to provide guidance or useful information for patients with life-threatening shock. An alternative strategy recognizes that CTA should be done for all patients with suspicion of PE, unless CTA is not immediately available (such as the case of a patient with hemodynamic collapse who cannot to be transferred to the radiology suite). In this scenario, echocardiography can be used to look for direct and indirect signs of PE [62]. Also of note, TEE will likely provide better image quality than TTE and may allow for direct visualization of thrombi in the PA and its main branches, but is more invasive and, therefore, requires more training.

Adding lower body compression ultrasonography to the workup for PE may be valuable in this setting because up to 50% of patients with PE have also DVT [64–66]. When indicated, it is important to also investigate for upper extremity DVT in this setting. Although less frequent, upper extremity DVT accounts for 10% of all DVT cases [67], and its prevalence appears to be increasing, likely because of the increased use of indwelling central venous catheters as well as peripherally inserted central catheters [68,69]. Thus, echocardiography (TTE or TEE) along with a comprehensive ultrasound examination for DVT is a reasonable diagnostic alternative for patients with no access to CTA who have high probability of PE and shock.

Echocardiographic Findings

Direct Clot Visualization. Direct clot visualization confirms the diagnosis of acute PE for patients with shock and high suspicion of PE. TTE visualization of thrombi (usually in the right atrium or ventricle) occurs for about 5% of patients with acute PE [70]. TEE can visualize thrombi in the central pulmonary arteries (main, right, and occasionally proximal left PA) more readily than TTE.

Indirect Signs

RV strain and pressure/volume overload. Indirect signs of PE include RV dilatation, RV free wall hypokinesis (together referred to RV strain), and septal dyskinesia—an abnormal motion of the septum toward the LV. In pure RV pressure overload, the interventricular septum is pushed toward the LV in systole, leading to D-shaped LV during systole in cross-sectional views (Fig. 29.7). In pure RV volume overload, the interventricular septum is pushed toward the LV in diastole, leading to D-shaped LV in diastole (Fig. 29.8). When the LV is D-shaped during systole and diastole, there is pressure and volume overload.

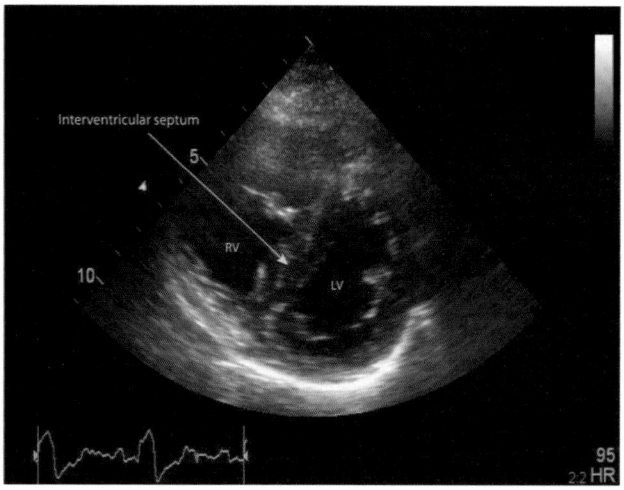

FIGURE 29.7 Parasternal short-axis view showing the left and right ventricles (LV and RV, respectively). The interventricluar septum is pushed toward the LV during systole (red bar on the ECG tracing), leading to a D-shaped LV. This is indicative of pressure overload. ECG, electrocardiogram.

McConnell sign. McConnell sign is a distinctive pattern of pathologic RV free wall regional motion that includes severe RV free wall hypokinesis (and sometimes akinesis) with sparing of the apical portion. That is, the RV apex is spared from hypokinesis/akinesis and contracts normally and may even behyperdynamic [71]. Originally, McConnell sign was regarded as a highly specific echocardiographic finding for acute PE [71]. However, it is now well accepted that it has poor positive predictive value for diagnosis of acute PE [72,73]. McConnell sign is also seen with other instances of acute cor pulmonale (e.g., RV infarction and acute respiratory distress syndrome [ARDS]) and, thus, should not be used in isolation for the diagnosis of acute PE.

Doppler signs of PE. Pulse wave Doppler interrogation of the RVOT and continuous wave Doppler interrogation of the tricuspid regurgitant (TR) jet are used to support the diagnosis of acute PE. Pulse wave Doppler of the RVOT creates a typical spectral display (Fig. 29.9). The acute development of high PA pressure can affect this pattern. Coexistence of short

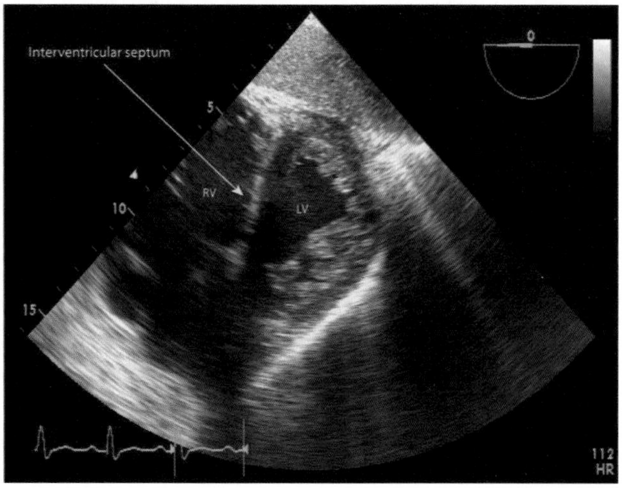

FIGURE 29.8 TEE transgastric short-axis view showing the left and right ventricles (LV and RV respectively). The interventricular septum is pushed toward the LV at the end of diastole (red bar on the ECG tracing), leading to a D-shaped LV. This is indicative of volume overload. TEE, transesophageal echocardiography.

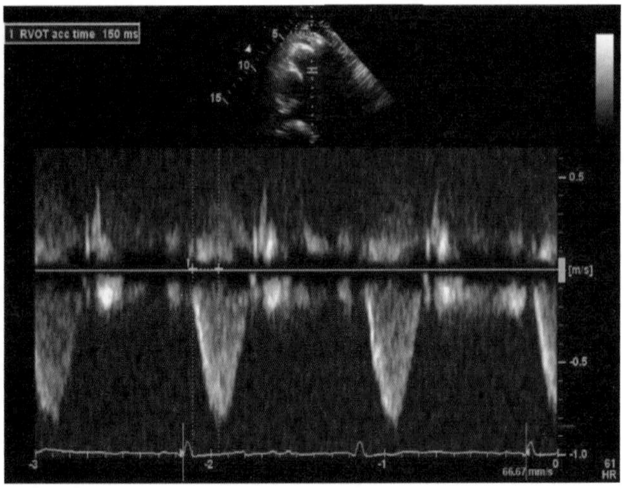

FIGURE 29.9 Parasternal short-axis view of the base of the heart with pulse wave interrogation of the right ventricular outflow tract (RVOT). A characteristic spectral display of laminar flow is displayed as strong signal at the periphery with the center clear of blood and thus seen as black.

acceleration time (the time from the beginning to peak RVOT flow) and midsystolic deceleration also known as midsystolic "notch"; Figure 29.10 is consistent with severe acute pulmonary hypertension [74]. With acute PE, RVOT acceleration time is much shorter (less than 60 ms) than other causes of pulmonary hypertension [74]. In addition, contrary to initial belief, a heart with baseline normal RV size, wall thickness, and function is unable to generate high PA pressures in the setting of an acute large PE. Echocardiography can be used to estimate PA pressure using the continuous wave Doppler modality and the Bernoulli equation. The simplified Bernoulli equation relates flow across a valve to the pressure difference between two chambers:

$$RVSP = 4(TR_{velocity})^2 + P_{RA}$$

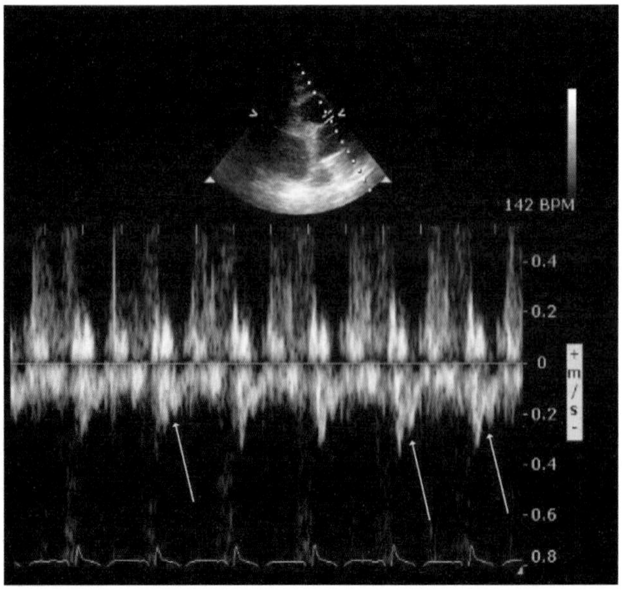

FIGURE 29.10 Parasternal short-axis view at the base of the heart with the pulse wave Doppler interrogation of the right ventricular outflow tract (RVOT). The normal spectral display of the RVOT is replaced with much reduced flow and with a midsystolic notch (*arrow*). This indicates acute RV pressure overload. RV, right ventricle.

where RVSP is the RV systolic pressure, $TR_{velocity}$ is the maximal velocity of the TR jet (in meters per second), and P_{RA} is an estimate (or measured, when the CVP is available) of the RA pressure [75]. In the absence of pulmonary stenosis, the RVSP equals PA systolic pressure, and as a result, this approach provides a simple and usually accurate estimation of the presence and severity of PA hypertension [75]. In comparison to patients with other causes of elevated PA pressure (chronic proximal PE, patients with COPD, and patients with primary pulmonary hypertension), patients with acute PE have only mild elevation in systolic PA pressure where the average TR peak gradient is only 48 mm Hg [76], indicating mild PA hypertension.

These two Doppler signs—RVOT acceleration time and TR peak jet gradient—have been described as the "60/60 sign"—an RVOT acceleration time of less than 60 milliseconds in the presence of TR pressure gradient of less than 60 mm Hg. Although the "60/60 sign" is not very sensitive, it is very specific (94%) for the diagnosis of acute PE [77].

Case 3

A 63-year-old diabetic man with severe peripheral arterial disease was admitted to the hospital with gangrenous right third and fourth digits for which he underwent toe amputation. The immediate perioperative course was uneventful, but, on the day of discharge, he collapsed in his room. He was found to be in pulseless electrical activity (PEA) arrest. Cardiopulmonary resuscitation and advanced cardiovascular life support were initiated, and, as part of the resuscitative efforts, echocardiography was used after return of spontaneous circulation. The parasternal short-axis view (PSAX) view demonstrated a large mass moving between the right atrium and ventricle (Video 29.3). In the setting of an acute event leading to hemodynamic collapse and PEA arrest, the large mass was considered "clot in transit," and heparin as well as tissue plasminogen activator (tPA) therapy was administered within 15 minutes of the arrest. Follow-up echocardiography 25 minutes after the initiation of therapy demonstrated absence of right-sided mass that was assumed to be a result of the tPA therapy (Video 29.3). Diagnostic angiography confirmed the diagnosis of significant PE with total occlusion of left main PA (Video 29.3).

Case 4

A 45-year-old woman underwent an uneventful laparoscopic esophagectomy for esophageal cancer. The postoperative course was uneventful, and, on the sixth postoperative day, she developed acute respiratory distress necessitating ICU admission. She required immediate intubation and developed profound shock; while on maximum doses of three vasopressors, her systolic BP remained less than 60 mm Hg. A TTE was performed, and the A4CH view demonstrated a massively enlarged RV, RV free wall akinesis with apical sparing (McConnell sign), and a very small and underfilled LV (Video 29.4). The PSAX view demonstrated a D-shaped LV through most of systole and throughout diastole, indicating RV pressure and volume overload (Video 29.4). These image findings are signs of cor pulmonale. Doppler interrogation demonstrated an RVOT pattern with a midsystolic notch and very short acceleration time of less than 60 milliseconds. The TR pressure gradient assessed in the A4CH view was 34 mm Hg, consistent with a positive "60/60 sign."

In the setting of acute respiratory failure and overwhelming shock without prior history of heart disease, these echocardiographic signs were highly suggestive of acute and massive PE as the etiology of this patient's shock. Because the patient was hemodynamically unstable, she could not be transported to the CT scanner. She was treated with heparin and tPA after discussion with cardiology and her thoracic surgeon. Roughly 30 minutes later, her hemodynamics stabilized, and a repeat echocardiogram showed an impressive decrease in the RV size, with improved free wall systolic function (Video 29.4). A repeated echocardiographic examination two days later demonstrated complete resolution of the cor pulmonale with normal RV size and function (Video 29.4).

Recommendations and Pitfalls of Using Echocardiography for the Diagnosis of Acute Pulmonary Embolism

A. CTA is the gold standard diagnostic modality for acute PE. Generally, echocardiography should be used cautiously in the diagnosis of acute PE.
B. Echocardiography may have a role **only** for patients with acute shock and high suspicion for a PE (i.e., high pretest probability) who do not have access to CTA.
C. Echocardiographic signs of acute PE include evidence of RV strain (RV dilatation, severe RV free wall hypokinesis, or akinesis) and septal flattening indicative of RV pressure and volume overload. These echocardiographic findings are consistent with acute cor pulmonale.
D. McConnell sign—severe hypokinesis of the RV free wall with apical sparing is a nonspecific sign for elevated pulmonary pressure (acute cor pulmonale). It is also seen in the settings of RV infarction and ARDS.
E. The "60/60 sign"—RVOT acceleration time shorter than 60 milliseconds in the presence of a TR pressure gradient of less than 60 mm Hg—is a nonsensitive but specific sign for the diagnosis of acute PE.
F. The decision on how to manage patients with suspected and echocardiographic evidence of PE (e.g., thrombolytic therapy) should be made only after multidisciplinary discussion with experts in managing patients with PE.

PERICARDIAL TAMPONADE

Introduction

Cardiac tamponade is a clinical syndrome that results from increased intrapericardial pressure and leads to impaired cardiocirculatory function and, ultimately, hemodynamic collapse. It is defined as significant compression of the heart chambers by accumulating pericardial contents, including fluid, blood, tumor, thrombus, pus, and gas—singly or in combination [78]. Rapid recognition of this life-threatening condition is essential for initiating life-saving treatment. Although tamponade is a clinical diagnosis, this section reviews the echocardiographic findings associated with tamponade as well as provides key limitations of using ultrasound for making this diagnosis.

Pathophysiology

The causes of pericardial disease and tamponade are diverse [79]. They include malignancy, infection (e.g., HIV), trauma, complications from myocardial infarction, surgery/procedures, uremia, collagen-vascular disease (e.g., systemic lupus erythematosus), drugs, idiopathic, and others.

The function of the normal volume of pericardial fluid (15 to 35 mL) is most likely lubrication of the pericardial sac in support of cardiac function. Although the pericardium has some degree of elasticity, at any instant, it is relatively inextensible. Because fluid starts to accumulate within the pericardial sac, it initially distends the parietal pericardium by filling the numerous sinuses and recesses of the pericardium. Once the elastic limit is reached, the heart and the pericardial content compete for the fixed intrapericardial volume [78]. Continued fluid accumulation eventually exceeds the pericardium's ability to stretch. At that point, the pressure within the pericardial sac increases and can quickly exceed the pressure within the heart chambers, eventually leading to their collapse.

Sequence of Chamber Collapse

A cardiac chamber will first show signs of collapse when its pressure is at its lowest during the cardiac cycle. For the ventricles, this time point is just at the beginning of diastole after the blood has been completely ejected. For the atria, this is also during diastole, which, with reference to the cardiac cycle, occurs during ventricular systole. As pressure builds up in the pericardial sac, it will first lead to right heart collapse because the right heart normally operates at much lower pressures than the left. Therefore, the sequence of chamber collapse, with reference to the cardiac cycle, is the right atrium during systole, right ventricle during diastole, left atrium during systole, and eventually left ventricle during diastole. It is important to keep in mind that some pericardial fluid accumulations may be confined to specific areas. This is most often seen after cardiac surgical procedures or among patients with pericardial septa that form in the setting of chronic pericardial fluid collections, especially when infectious in nature. For these cases, pressure may be exerted only on a specific chamber or chambers, sparing others. This can lead to deviation from the normal sequence of chamber collapse expected based on intracavitary pressures. As the chambers become progressively smaller, diastolic compliance is reduced, leading to reduced preload, low CO, and hypotension.

Reduced Venous Return

Venous return is normally bimodal with peaks during ventricular systole and early diastole. It is determined by the pressure difference between the pulmonary veins (which is affected by intrathoracic pressure) and the left atrium. As tamponade becomes more severe and chamber compression becomes more pronounced throughout the cardiac cycle, LA pressure increases. This, in turn, causes venous return to progressively occur during systole as diastolic flow diminishes. The end result is reduced venous return that leads to further reduction of CO and higher degrees of hypotension.

Ventricular Interdependence

Ventricular interdependence (Video 29.5) is the term used to describe the phenomenon of size, shape, and compliance of one ventricle that affects the size, shape, and pressure–volume relationship of the other ventricle through direct mechanical interactions [80]. During tamponade, ventricular interdependence affects hemodynamics to a much greater degree than during normal conditions.

Under normal physiology, there is respiratory variation of venous return to the heart. With normal negative pressure inspiration, the decline of thoracic pressure is transmitted through the pericardium to the right side of the heart, promoting venous return. The effect on the left heart is opposite; the decrease of the intrathoracic pressure decreases the pressure within the pulmonary veins, leading to a decreased pressure gradient to the left atrium and decreased venous return to the left heart.

During tamponade, the heart is isolated from the thorax, thus altering this normal physiology. The stiff pericardium prevents the right ventricular free wall from expanding during inspiration. As a result, the distension of the RV is limited. The structure that can best accommodate diastolic right ventricular filling is the interventricular septum that along with compromised left ventricular filling causes the septum to bulge to the left. The end result is further reduction of left ventricular size and compliance during diastole, contributing even further to decreased left ventricular filling during inspiration. This ventricular interdependence further contributed to lower CO and resulting hypotension.

To summarize, tamponade physiology consists of three processes that contribute to a significant decrease of CO. First, the mechanical compression of heart chambers decreases ventricular size and preload. Second, increased LA pressure results in decreased venous return to the left heart. Third, in the setting of a stiff pericardium, ventricular interdependence leads to diastolic bulging of the interventricular septum toward the LV, further decreasing its preload. These three processes lead to a reduction of CO, which can progress to hemodynamic collapse.

Role of Echocardiography for the Diagnosis of Tamponade

As mentioned previously, it is important to emphasize that tamponade is a clinical and not an echocardiographic diagnosis. Clinical findings of patients with tamponade include sinus tachycardia, tachypnea, distended neck veins, pulsus paradoxus, pericardial rub, muffled heart sounds, and electrical alternans on electrocardiogram. Echocardiography, however, plays a major role in the identification of a pericardial effusion and for assessing its hemodynamic significance [81].

Two-dimensional Evaluation

Although "size does not matter"—a small effusion can lead to tamponade (e.g., a young trauma patient with small hemopericardium)—in most cases of pericardial tamponade, a moderate-to-large effusion is present. On the other hand, the presence of a pericardial effusion does not necessarily secure the diagnosis of tamponade, and careful echocardiographic evaluation is required in order to make this diagnosis. Typically, cardiac chamber collapse occurs before clinical hemodynamic failure. When assessing for cardiac tamponade, it is important to identify abnormalities of the cardiac cycle where atrial diastole occurs during ventricular systole.

When intrapericardial pressure exceeds intracardiac pressure, collapse of any chamber can occur [82]. Following is a discussion of the individual chamber collapse.

Right Atrial Systolic Collapse. The right atrium is a thin, nonmuscular, and compliant structure, with the lowest pressure among all heart chambers (1 to 8 mm Hg) [83]. As a result, when intrapericardial pressure slightly exceeds intracavitary RA pressure, the RA will collapse [84]. Although brief RA collapse can occur in the absence of cardiac tamponade, when it persists for more than one-third of the cardiac cycle, it is highly sensitive and specific for cardiac tamponade [85].

Right Ventricular Diastolic Collapse. The RV is a thin muscular structure (up to 5-mm thickness), which like the RA is also susceptible to elevated intrapericardial pressure. The normal right ventricular diastolic pressure is 1 to 8 mm Hg, and the peak systolic pressure is 15 to 30 mm Hg [83]. RV diastolic collapse occurs in early diastole when the RV volume is still low [82]. RV diastolic collapse is less sensitive than RA systolic collapse for the presence of cardiac tamponade, but is very specific for the diagnosis of tamponade [86]. Caution should be exercised when investigating a patient with long-standing pulmonary hypertension because the hypertrophied RV may prevent RV free wall collapse [84].

Left Atrial Systolic Collapse. LA collapse is less common than right-sided collapse because the LA operates on a higher intracavitary pressure; the normal mean LA pressure is between 4 and 12 mm Hg [83]. It is seen in only 25% of patients with hemodynamic compromise [87], but it is very specific for cardiac tamponade [81,88,89].

Left Ventricular Collapse. Despite having similar diastolic pressure as the LA (LVEDP between 4 and 12 mm Hg) [83], the LV is less likely to collapse owing to its much higher and thicker muscle mass (wall thickness of 11 mm). It can collapse, however, at the end of the tamponade process when intrapericardial pressure becomes extremely high. LV collapse often precedes complete hemodynamic collapse and death.

Inferior Vena Cava Plethora. IVC plethora refers to IVC dilatation (>2.1 cm) and less than a 50% reduction in its diameter during inspiration. IVC plethora indicates marked elevation in CVP, as expected in tamponade. IVC plethora is expected in more than 90% of patients with tamponade [90], and, therefore, its absence should raise the suspicion for absence of tamponade physiology.

Doppler Evaluation

The ventricular interdependence discussed above can be evaluated using pulse wave Doppler. It is important to emphasize that this evaluation can be done only for spontaneously breathing patients because positive pressure ventilation can affect ventricular interdependence.

As discussed previously, ventricular interdependence is increased during tamponade, leading to reciprocal changes in left and right ventricular volumes with respiration. Pulse wave Doppler can be used to evaluate the respiratory variation of the tricuspid or mitral valve inflow by measuring blood flow velocities into the RV and LV, respectively. Under normal physiology, the respiratory change in tricuspid flow velocity is no more than 15%, and the change in mitral flow velocity is no more than 10% [91]. During tamponade, flow velocities are significantly increased with inspiration, thus reflecting increased ventricular interdependence (Video 29.5). Usually, changes of mitral flow velocities of more than 30% and tricuspid flow velocities greater than 60% are considered consistent with tamponade physiology [92]. However, in the absence of chamber collapse or abnormal IVC plethora, Doppler evaluation alone should not be used to diagnose tamponade.

Localized Tamponade

Presentation of cardiac tamponade among patients after cardiac surgery is often atypical [93] and can pose a serious diagnostic challenge. Effusions that contain clots can be challenging to identify by TTE and are often better evaluated with TEE or CT. A high level of suspicion should be maintained, and consultation with an expert echocardiographer should be solicited for this patient population.

Case 5

A 66-year-old man with extensive smoking history was diagnosed with squamous cell lung carcinoma and a medium-sized mass in the left upper lung lobe. He underwent chemoradiation and was treated for the year prior to admission with Coumadin as a result of left lower extremity DVT and bilateral lobar pulmonary emboli. The patient was readmitted 2 weeks after hospitalization for video-assisted thoracoscopic surgery (VATS) and left upper lobectomy. Following an uneventful surgery, he was discharged home but reported malaise following the VATS 2 weeks earlier with significant shortness of breath in the supine position and dyspnea on exertion, all of which has become progressively worse. The patient denied fever, chills, or chest pain. He was admitted to the ICU with significant shortness of breath and became acutely hypotensive.

Bedside TTE demonstrated a large pericardial effusion with RA systolic collapse and right ventricular diastolic collapse (Video 29.5) and mitral valve Doppler inflow pattern consistent with tamponade. The patient was transferred urgently to the cardiac catheterization lab where 1,150 mL of fluid was drained with resolution of his hypotension. The following day, an echocardiogram was repeated to verify resolution of the effusion (Video 29.5).

Case 6

A 35-year-old woman was admitted to the ICU from the emergency department with chest pain and severe shortness of breath when lying supine. The patient had history of aortic insufficiency and aortic stenosis, as well as end-stage renal disease requiring hemodialysis, which was complicated by recurrent episodes of endocarditis. She had undergone several cardiac surgeries for aortic valve replacements, most recently a month prior to this admission.

On physical examination, the patient was sitting in the upright position with significant shortness of breath and difficulty speaking full sentences. Her BP was 105/65 mm Hg, and heart rate was 100 beats per minute with an oxygen saturation of 97% on room air. The patient also suffered from lower back pain and asked for help to turn on her left side. Immediately after turning, her BP decreased to 50/30 mm Hg. She was immediately turned and positioned upright and her BP recovered. A TTE was performed demonstrating a large thrombus compressing the entire right atrium (Video 29.6). Based on this echocardiographic examination, she was urgently taken to the operating room where a large clot was removed.

Role of Echocardiography for the Diagnosis of Pericardial Tamponade

A. Tamponade is a clinical and not a radiographic diagnosis. However, echocardiography can be extremely helpful during the diagnostic process.
B. "Size does not matter." Tamponade can occur with even small amount of pericardial effusion (e.g., a young trauma patient with hemopericardium).
C. Not all effusions lead to tamponade. Very large effusions—as large as 2 L—can build up over a significant length of time and have insignificant hemodynamic effects (e.g., a cancer patient with slow fluid accumulation).
D. 2D echocardiographic evidence of tamponade in chronologic order: RA systolic collapse, RV diastolic collapse, LA systolic collapse, and LV collapse. In addition, IVC plethora is expected.
E. Patients with long-standing pulmonary hypertension and RV hypertrophy can have tamponade without RV collapse.
F. Doppler evidence of tamponade includes a respiratory change of the mitral valve inflow velocity of more than 30% and a respiratory change of the tricuspid valve inflow velocity of more than 60%. This reflects increased ventricular interdependence.
G. Localized tamponade can occur postcardiac surgery and may lead to diagnostic challenge. Help from expert echocardiographers should be solicited for this patient population.

PUMP FAILURE

Introduction

The term "pump failure" is commonly used to describe clinically relevant systolic dysfunction of either ventricle. Systolic dysfunction can be chronic, acute, or acute on chronic and can be either global or regional or both. Although there can be several causes that can lead to acute or acute on chronic ventricular dysfunction, this section focuses on the common etiologies that lead to shock and the associated echocardiographic findings of the critical care setting.

Septic Cardiomyopathy

Sepsis, a spectrum of disease ranging from systemic inflammatory response syndrome to septic shock, is a leading cause of death in the United States and the leading cause of death among critically ill patients [94–96]. Reversible myocardial dysfunction is a recognized manifestation of this syndrome [97–99], and coronary flow is often preserved or even supranormal [100]. Although cardiac function can be very depressed, death occurs principally because of multiorgan system failure [97,101,102].

Sepsis-induced cardiac dysfunction likely results from several simultaneous processes, including elevated circulating cytokines, mitochondrial dysfunction, high level of adrenergic stimulation, metabolic changes of cardiomyocytes, myocardial edema, elevated levels of nitric oxide (NO), myofibrillar dysfunction, and others [101]. Myocardial cell death, however, is a rare event during sepsis and likely does not contribute to the reversible functional cardiac depression. Finally, activation of endothelial cells and induction of the coagulation system also contribute to the pathophysiology of sepsis.

The circulatory abnormalities seen during early sepsis and septic shock are related to severe vasodilatation and intravascular volume depletion. This results in significantly reduced preload along with a reduction of CO, ultimately leading to an imbalance of oxygen supply and demand of different organ beds [103]. This process can be improved, however, with adequate fluid resuscitation [104]. The typical pattern of an adequately resuscitated patient with septic shock includes hyperdynamic cardiac function/output with warm extremities as a result of a low systemic vascular resistance (SVR) (i.e., "warm shock") [105,106]. Some of the initial reports suggested that patients surviving septic shock had significantly higher levels of CO and oxygen delivery content [107,108]. More recent evidence, however, suggests that 40% to 50% of patients with prolonged septic shock develop myocardial dysfunction, which is manifested as a decreased ejection fraction (EF) [109,110]. While EF is dependent on preload, afterload, and contractility, load-independent advanced techniques of assessing myocardial function among patients with sepsis has also demonstrated significant myocardial dysfunction [111]. This myocardial depression may be severe enough to mimic cardiogenic shock ("cold shock") [112], and it is often reversible with proper management [110,113]. In addition to systolic dysfunction, diastolic dysfunction has been also reported among patients with sepsis and septic shock [114,115]. Recent data suggest higher mortality rates among patients with grade I diastolic dysfunction than in those without dysfunction, which may suggest inadequate volume expansion at the time of ICU admission [116].

Echocardiographic Findings

Warm Shock. Echocardiographic findings in patients with septic shock depend on the shock state during the evaluation. In "warm shock" with low SVR and high CO, hypovolemia may coexist (the degree of which will depend on the amount of fluid administered by the time the exam is performed). Patients who have undergone adequate fluid resuscitation demonstrate a characteristic pattern of hyperdynamic ventricles (Video 29.7). Unfortunately, this pattern can be confused with the pattern of severe hypovolemia (Video 29.7) because the left ventricular end-systolic area is very small for both.

Additionally, ventricular walls may touch at the end systole (end-systolic cavity obliteration, commonly known also as "kissing walls"). The difference between severe hypovolemia and the pattern of septic shock is the diastolic area, which is a surrogate for end-diastolic volume. While end-diastolic area is very small during severe hypovolemia, it is normal or only slightly reduced for patients with septic shock [117].

Cold Shock. As noted earlier, up to 50% of patients with septic shock develop myocardial dysfunction. Often, both ventricles are affected simultaneously with a similar pattern of dysfunction [118]. However, for some cases, only left ventricular function is impacted. It is important to identify these patients with depressed myocardial function because the management may change significantly. For example, while aggressive fluid resuscitation is the main recommended therapy for the initial stage of sepsis, once myocardial dysfunction is recognized, therapy may be changed from fluid therapy to the addition of inotropic support. When using echocardiography for the management of septic patients, it is important to repeat the exam frequently. This allows the clinician to identify patients who transition from the initial presentation of a hyperdynamic cardiac function to the second stage of myocardial depression and systolic heart failure.

Case 7

A 72-year-old female with a history of renal cell carcinoma and nephrectomy and on chemotherapy was admitted to the emergency department (ED) with septic shock. She was diagnosed with perforated sigmoid diverticulitis and was waiting for urgent surgery. She was aggressively resuscitated with 5 L of crystalloid and was on a high-dose norepinephrine infusion. Initial lab work demonstrated pH of 7.15, base excess of −13 and lactate of 5.3 mmol per L. Echocardiography was performed and demonstrated normal right and left ventricular size with hyperdynamic systolic function of both ventricles (Video 29.7). She underwent sigmoid colectomy and Hartmann procedure and was transferred to the ICU after surgery. She had received about 12 L of fluid and blood products and remained on high-dose norepinephrine and vasopressin infusions to support her BP. Lab work on arrival to the ICU demonstrated a pH of 7.19, base excess of −10 and lactate of 4.6 mmol per L. Repeated echocardiogram demonstrated significant change from the baseline exam. Her repeat echocardiogram now demonstrated severe bi-ventricular systolic dysfunction, with an estimated left ventricular ejection fraction of ~10% (Video 29.7). This dramatic change of systolic function was attributed to rapidly developing septic cardiomyopathy. Based on this unexpected finding, fluid administration was stopped and inotropic support with dobutamine was started. The following morning, a third echocardiogram established resolution of the septic cardiomyopathy, and she now was noted to once again have hyperdynamic left-and-right ventricular systolic function (Video 29.7).

Stress Cardiomyopathy

Stress cardiomyopathy, also known as Takotsubo cardiomyopathy, apical-balloon syndrome or "broken heart syndrome," is a form of acute and usually reversible heart failure that occurs in the absence of obstructive coronary artery lesions. Patients may present with signs and symptoms mimicking myocardial infarction, but there is no angiographic evidence of obstructive coronary artery disease or acute plaque rupture [119,120]. It was first described in Japan in 1990 as Takotsubo cardiomyopathy [119] and, despite gaining worldwide awareness, current understanding of this syndrome is still lacking. It is characterized by transient systolic and diastolic left ventricular dysfunction with a variety of wall motion abnormalities [121,122], and affects mostly elderly women, with a female to male ratio of 9:1 [123]. While emotional stress was initially implicated as the main trigger for the development of stress cardiomyopathy [124], it appears that physical triggers, such as neurologic or psychiatric disorders, more frequently provoke it in up to 50% of patients [123]. It has been described in patients with subarachnoid hemorrhage [125], epilepsy [126], electroconvulsive therapy [127], traumatic brain injury [128], stroke [129], and anxiety or depression [130].

Excess catecholamine is suggested as having a potential role for the pathogenesis of stress cardiomyopathy [131]. While β-blockers have been proposed as a therapeutic strategy [132], no prospective trials evaluating therapies in stress cardiomyopathy have been performed to-date. Nevertheless, this may be very plausible given that the coronary microcirculation is innervated by neurons originating in the brain stem that mediate vasoconstriction that can potentially lead to microvascular dysfunction and reversible myocardial stunning [133]. In addition, histopathologic findings from cardiac tissue samples obtained from patients with sudden unexpected death during epilepsy or subarachnoid hemorrhage strongly resembled those of patients who died during an episode of Takotsubo cardiomyopathy [134,135].

Patients with stress cardiomyopathy commonly present with symptoms similar to those of an acute coronary syndrome [136], and, therefore, initial diagnosis and treatment of these patients remains challenging. Troponin levels and electrocardiographic changes on admission are not sufficient to differentiate between these two disorders [137]. Therefore, early coronary angiography may be necessary to rule out an acute coronary syndrome and consultation with cardiology is required.

Echocardiographic Findings

While the presentation of patients with stress cardiomyopathy varies (e.g., acute substernal chest pain, dyspnea, syncope, and others), in the ICU setting, it is often associated with shock. Stress cardiomyopathy has unique morphology of apical ballooning and relative compensatory hypercontractility of the basal segments. This initial description of left ventricular apical ballooning [119] is the most common form of stress cardiomyopathy (81.7%). However, it is now known that there are three other forms: midventricular type (14.6%), basal type (2.2%), and focal type (1.5%) [123].

Typically, LV function is impaired on hospital admission and resolves within days to weeks after initial presentation (mean 18 days) [138]. However, roughly 22% of patients have serious in-hospital complications. These rates are equal to or higher than those of patients with an acute coronary syndrome [123]. Patients with stress cardiomyopathy have lower mean left ventricular ejection fraction (40.7% vs. 51.5%) when compared to patients presenting with acute coronary syndrome [123]. In addition to low EF and CO, stress cardiomyopathy appears to predispose these patients to dynamic obstruction of the LVOT, with a high prevalence of 25% in this patient population [139]. With regard to pathophysiology, basal hypercontractility (possibly aggravated by inotropic agents) may accentuate the Venturi effect that draws the anterior mitral valve leaflet toward the interventricular septum during systole. This movement of the anterior mitral leaflet is known as systolic anterior motion (SAM). The end result can be a dynamic obstruction of blood flow through the LVOT and a further reduction in CO. Furthermore, mitral regurgitation may result from SAM and may contribute to the worsening hemodynamic status of the patient. The diagnosis is generally made with 2D echocardiography with the A5CH (Video 29.8) and A3CH views. Continuous wave Doppler is also useful, which can be used to follow the degree of gradient across the LVOT as well as its response to therapy.

There is no single test or imaging modality that can conclusively confirm the diagnosis of stress cardiomyopathy. Therefore, it remains a diagnosis of exclusion for patients with severe myocardial dysfunction in the proper setting. Suggested diagnostic criteria include the findings of transient left ventricular wall motion as described above, absence of obstructive coronary disease on angiogram, new electrocardiographic abnormalities (ST-segment elevation or T-wave inversion), and modest troponin elevation—all in the absence of myocarditis or pheochromocytoma [137]. Because stress cardiomyopathy can mimic an acute coronary syndrome, consultation with cardiology is warranted. Although echocardiography plays a significant role for the diagnosis and management of patients with stress cardiomyopathy, early angiography is still recommended for the initial diagnosis to exclude an acute coronary syndrome. Angiography, however, may not be feasible for some patients (e.g., patients with subarachnoid hemorrhage) because systemic anticoagulation and anti-platelet therapy is contraindicated for these patients. Therefore, management should be decided after multidisciplinary discussion with cardiology and other treating physicians and after carefully reviewing the patient's history and events leading to hospitalization.

Case 8

A 65-year-old woman was found unresponsive by her husband and she was transported to the hospital where a head CT showed subarachnoid hemorrhage. She underwent successful coiling of a ruptured aneurysm, but developed shock after the procedure. Echocardiography demonstrated severe LV systolic dysfunction and stress cardiomyopathy was presumed owing to the patient's history and LV apical ballooning (Video 29.8). Inotropic support was initiated and the patient underwent daily echocardiograms in the following days until resolution of shock. Two weeks after initial presentation a follow-up echocardiography confirmed resolution of apical ballooning and cardiomyopathy (Video 29.8).

CONCLUSION

The ongoing ultrasound revolution is changing the management of critically ill patients. Ultrasound machines have become ubiquitous in ICUs and have long been used for both diagnosis and procedural guidance. In recent years, many clinicians have undergone training in echocardiography and "focused cardiac ultrasound," leading to a paradigm shift where echocardiography is now becoming an important modality for the management of critically ill patients. Currently, echocardiography is a promising tool to provide the clinician at the bedside with valuable diagnostic information about the etiology of shock (or equally important—rule out common etiologies). However, focused echocardiography can also be used very effectively as a monitor—as demonstrated by the clinical examples of this chapter. It is also very important to understand the limitations of echocardiography and to maintain a high level of skill and knowledge to ensure that patients are not being harmed and to improve outcomes by the optimal use of this modality.

References

1. SwanHJ, Ganz W, Forrester J, et al: Catheterization of the heart in man with use of a flow-directed balloon-tipped catheter. *N Engl J Med* 283:447–451, 1970.
2. Connors AF, Speroff T, Dawson NV, et al: The effectiveness of right heart catheterization in the initial care of critically ill patients. SUPPORT Investigators. *JAMA* 276:889–897, 1996.
3. Richardv C, Warszawski J, Anguel N, et al: Early use of the pulmonary artery catheter and outcomes in patients with shock and acute respiratory distress syndrome: a randomized controlled trial. *JAMA* 290:2713–2720, 2003.
4. Sandham JD, Hull RD, Brant RF, et al: A randomized, controlled trial of the use of pulmonary-artery catheters in high-risk surgical patients. *N Engl J Med* 348:5–14, 2003.
5. Harvey S, Harrison DA, Singer M, et al: Assessment of the clinical effectiveness of pulmonary artery catheters in management of patients in intensive care (PAC-Man): a randomised controlled trial. *Lancet* 366:472–477, 2005.
6. Clinical Trials Network; Wheeler AP, Bernard GR, Thompson BT, et al: Pulmonary-artery versus central venous catheter to guide treatment of acute lung injury. National Heart, Lung, and Blood Institute Acute Respiratory Distress Syndrome (ARDS). *N Engl J Med* 354:2213–2224, 2006.
7. Vincent JL, Pinsky MR, Sprung CL, et al: The pulmonary artery catheter: in medio virtus. *Crit Care Med* 36:3093–3096, 2008.
8. Gershengorn HB, Wunsch H. Understanding changes in established practice: pulmonary artery catheter use in critically ill patients. *Crit Care Med* 41:2667–2676, 2013.
9. Ospina-Tascon GA, Cordioli RL, Vincent JL: What type of monitoring has been shown to improve outcomes in acutely ill patients? *Intensive Care Med* 34:800–820, 2008.
10. Vincent JL, Rhodes A, Perel A, et al: Clinical review: update on hemodynamic monitoring—a consensus of 16. *Crit Care* 15:229–236, 2011.
11. Moore CL, Copel JA: Point-of-care ultrasonography. *N Engl J Med* 364:749–757, 2011.
12. Labovitz AJ, NV, Bierig M, et al: American Society of Echocardiography consensus statement focused cardiac ultrasound in the emergent setting: a consensus statement of the American Society of Echocardiography and American College of Emergency Physicians. *J Am Soc Echocardiogr* 23:1225–1230, 2010.
13. Via A, Hussain A, Wells M, et al: International evidence-based recommendations for focused cardiac ultrasound. *J Am Soc Echocardiogr* 27:683.e1–683.e33, 2014.
14. Siadecki SD Frasure SE, Lewiss RE, et al: High body mass index is strongly correlated with decreased image quality in focused bedside echocardiography. *J Emerg Med* 50:295–301, 2016.
15. Personal comunication. Marylin Riley B, RDCS, Clinical Manger of the Cardiac Echo Lab, Beth Israel Deaconess Medical Center, Boston.
16. Shillcutt SK, Bick JS: Echo didactics: a comparison of basic transthoracic and transesophageal echocardiography views in the perioperative setting. *Anesth Analg* 116:1231–1236, 2013.
17. Blum A, Reisner S, Farbstein Y: Transesophageal echocardiography (TEE) vs. transthoracic echocardiography (TTE) in assessing cardio-vascular sources of emboli in patients with acute ischemic stroke. *Med Sci Monit* 9:CR521–CR523, 2004.
18. Colreavy FB, Donovan K, Lee KY, et al: Transesophageal echocardiography in critically ill patients. *Crit Care* 30:989–996, 2002.
19. Daniel WG, Erbel R, Kasper W, et al: Safety of transesophageal echocardiography. A multicenter survey of 10,419 examinations. *Circulation* 83:817–821, 1991.
20. Hüttemann E, Schelenz C, Kara F, et al: The use and safety of transoesophageal echocardiography in the general ICU—a minireview. *Acta Anaesthesiol Scand* 48:827–836, 2004.
21. Oren-Grinberg A, Talmor D, Brown S: Focused critical care echocardiography. *Crit Care Med* 41:2618–2626, 2013.
22. Blaivas M: Transesophageal echocardiography during cardiopulmonary arrest in the emergency department. *Resuscitation* 78:135–140, 2008.
23. Vieillard-Baron A, Slama M, Cholley B, et al: Echocardiography in the intensive care unit: from evolution to revolusion? *Intensive Care Med* 34:243–249, 2008.
24. Bergenzaun L, Gudmundsson P, Öhlin H: Assessing left ventricular systolic function in shock: evaluation of echocardiographic parameters in intensive care. *Crit Care* 15:R200, 2011.
25. Dellinger RP, Levy MM, Rhodes A, et al: Surviving sepsis campaign: international guidelines for management of severe sepsis and septic shock: 2012. *Crit Care Med* 41:580–637, 2013.
26. Wiedemann HP, Wheeler AP, Bernarg GR, et al: Comparison of two fluid-management strategies in acute lung injury. *N Engl J Med* 24:2564–2575, 2006.
27. Armstrong WE, Ryan T: ICU and operative/perioperative application, in DeStefano FR (ed): *Fingenbaum's Echocardiography*. 7th ed. Philadelphia, USA, Lippincott Williams & Wilkins, 2010, p 667.
28. Bendjelid K, Romand JA: Fluid responsiveness in mechanically ventilated patients: a review of indices used in intensive care. *Intensive Care Med* 29:352–360, 2003.
29. Feissel M, Michard F, Mangin I, et al: Respiratory changes in aortic blood velocity as an indicator of fluid responsiveness in ventilated patients with septic shock. *Chest* 119:867–873, 2001.

30. Barbier C, Loubieres Y, Schmit C, et al: Respiratory changes in inferior vena cava diameter are helpful in predicting fluid responsiveness in ventilated septic patients. *Intensive Care Med* 30:1740–1746, 2014.
31. Feissel M, Michard F, Faller JP, et al: The respiratory variation in inferior vena cava diameter as a guide to fluid therapy. *Intensive Care Med* 30:1834–1837, 2014.
32. Vieillard-Baron A, Chergui K, Rabiller A, et al: Superior vena caval collapsibility as a gauge of volume status in ventilated septic patients. *Intensive Care Med* 30:1734–1739, 2004.
33. Charbonneau H, Riu B, Faron M, et al: Predicting preload responsiveness using simultaneous recordings of inferior and superior vena cavae diameters. *Crit Care* 18:473–481, 2014.
34. van den Berg PCM, Jansen JR, Pinsky MR: Effect of positive pressure on venous return in volume-loaded cardiac surgical patients. *J Appl Physiol* 92:1223–1231, 2002.
35. Amoore JN, Santamore WP: Venous collapse and the respiratory variability in systemic venous return. *Cardiovasc Res* 28:472–479, 1994.
36. Boulain T, Achard JM, Teboul JL, et al: Changes in BP induced by passive leg raising predict response to fluid loading in critically ill patients. *Chest* 121:1245–1252, 2002.
37. Monnet X, Rienzo M, Ozman D, et al: Passive leg raising predicts fluid responsiveness in the critically ill. *Crit Care Med* 34:1402–1407, 2006.
38. Godfrey GEP, Dubrey SW, Handy JM: A prospective observational study of stroke volume responsiveness to a passive leg raise manoeuvre in healthy nonstarved volunteers as assessed by transthoracic echocardiography. *Anaesthesia* 69:306–313, 2014.
39. Marik PE, Levitov A, Young A: The use of bioreactance and carotid doppler to determine volume responsiveness and blood flow redistribution following passive leg raising in hemodynamically unstable patients. *Chest* 143:364–370, 2013.
40. Cavallaro F, Sandroni C, Marano C, et al: Diagnostic accuracy of passive leg raising for prediction of fluid responsiveness in adults: systematic review and meta-analysis of clinical studies. *Intensive Care Med* 36:1475–1483, 2010.
41. Michard F, Teboul JL: Predicting fluid responsiveness in ICU patients: a critical analysis of the evidence. *Chest* 121:2000–2008, 2002.
42. Lamia B, Ochagavia A, Monnet X: Echocardiographic prediction of volume responsiveness in critically ill patients with spontaneously breathing activity. *Intensive Care Med* 33:1125–1132, 2008.
43. Cheung AT, Savino JS, Weiss SJ: Echocardiographic and hemodynamic indexes of left ventricular preload in patients with normal and abnormal ventricular function. *Anesthesiology* 81:376–387, 1994.
44. Slama M, Teboul JL: Assessment of cardiac preload and volume responsiveness using echocardiography, in Vincent JL (ed): *Intensive Care Medicine*. New York, NY, Springer, 2003, pp 491–498.
45. Airapetian N, Maizel J, Alyamani O, et al: Does inferior vena cava respiratory variability predict fluid responsiveness in spontaneously breathing patients? *Crit Care* 19:400–407, 2015.
46. Bauman Z, Coba V, Gassner M, et al: Inferior vena cava collapsibility loses correlation with internal jugular vein collapsibility during increased thoracic or intra-abdominal pressure. *J Ultrasound* 18:343–348, 2015.
47. Juhl-Olsen P, Vistisen ST, Christiansen LK, et al: Ultrasound of the inferior vena cava does not predict hemodynamic response to early hemorrhage. *J Emerg Med* 45:592–597, 2013.
48. Huisman MV, Klok FA: Current challenges in diagnostic imaging of venous thromboembolism. *Blood* 126:2376–2382, 2015.
49. Bonderman D, Wilkens H, Wakounig S, et al: Risk factors for chronic thromboembolic pulmonary hypertension. *Eur Respir J* 33:325–331, 2009.
50. Deitelzweig SB, Johnson BH, Schulman KL, et al: Prevalence of clinical venous thromboembolism in the USA: current trends and future projections. *Am J Hematol* 86:217–220, 2011.
51. Venous Thromboembolism (Blood Clots). http://www.cdc.gov/ncbddd/dvt/data.html. Centers for Disease Control and Prevention, 2015.
52. McIntyre KM, Sasahara AA: The hemodynamic response to pulmonary embolism in patients without prior cardiopulmonary disease. *Am J Cardiol* 28:288–294, 1971.
53. Smulders Y: Pathophysiology and treatment of haemodynamic instability in acute pulmonary embolism: the pivotal role of pulmonary vasoconstriction. *Cardiovascular Res* 48:23–33, 2000.
54. Delcroix M, Mélot C, Lejeune P, et al: Effects of vasodilators on gas exchange in acute canine embolic pulmonary hypertension. *Anesthesiology* 72:77–84, 1990.
55. Huet Y, Brun-Buisson C, Lemaire F, et al: Cardiopulmonary effects of ketanserin infusion in human pulmonary embolism. *Am Rev Respir Dis* 135:114–117, 1987.
56. Marcus JT, Gan CT, Zwanenburg JJ, et al: Interventricular mechanical asynchrony in pulmonary arterial hypertension: left-to-right delay in peak shortening is related to right ventricular overload and left ventricular underfilling. *J Am Coll Cardiol* 51:750–757, 2008.
57. Mauritz GJ, Marcus JT, Westerhof N, et al: Prolonged right ventricular post-systolic isovolumic period in pulmonary arterial hypertension is not a reflection of diastolic dysfunction. *Heart* 97:473–478, 2011.
58. Lankeit M, Jiménez D, Kostrubiec M, et al: Predictive value of the high-sensitivity troponin T assay and the simplified pulmonary embolism severity index in hemodynamically stable patients with acute pulmonary embolism: a prospective validation study. *Circulation* 124:2716–2724, 2011.
59. Mehta NJ, Jani K, Khan IA: Clinical usefulness and prognostic value of elevated cardiac troponin I levels in acute pulmonary embolism. *Am Heart J* 145:821–825, 2003.
60. Ghaye B, Szapiro D, Mastora I, et al: Peripheral pulmonary arteries: how far in the lung does multi-detector row spiral CT allow analysis? *Radiology* 219:629–636, 2001.
61. Patel S, Kazerooni EA, Cascade PN: Pulmonary embolism: optimization of small pulmonary artery visualization at multi-detector row CT. *Radiology* 227:455–460, 2003.
62. Konstantinides SV, Torbicki A, Agnelli G, et al: 2014 ESC Guidelines on the diagnosis and management of acute pulmonary embolism. *Eur Heart J* 35:3033–3073, 2014.
63. Douglas PS, Garcia MJ, Haines DE, et al: ACCF/ASE/AHA/ASNC/HFSA/HRS/SCAI/SCCM/SCCT/SCMR 2011 appropriate use criteria for echocardiography. *J Am Soc Echocardiogr* 24:229–267, 2011.
64. Righini M, Le Gal G, Aujesky D, et al: Diagnosis of pulmonary embolism by multidetector CT alone or combined with venous ultrasonography of the leg: a randomised non-inferiority trial. *Lancet* 371:1343–1352, 2008.
65. Kearon C, Ginsberg JS, Hirsh J, et al: The role of venous ultrasonography in the diagnosis of suspected deep venous thrombosis and pulmonary embolism. *Ann Intern Med* 129:1044–1049, 1998.
66. Perrier A, Bounameaux H: Ultrasonography of leg veins in patients suspected of having pulmonary embolism. *Ann Intern Med* 3:243–245, 1998.
67. Engelberger RP, Kucher N: Management of deep vein thrombosis of the upper extremity. *Circulation* 126:768–773, 2012.
68. Munoz FJ, Mismetti P, Poggio R: Clinical outcome of patients with upper-extremity deep vein thrombosis: results from the RIETE Registry. *Chest* 133:143–148, 2008.
69. Joffe HV, Kucher N, Tapson VF, et al: Upper-extremity deep vein thrombosis: a prospective registry of 592 patients. *Circulation* 110:1605–1611, 2004.
70. Cohen R, Loarte P, Navarro V, et al: Echocardiographic findings in pulmonary embolism: an important guide for the management of the patient. *World J Cardiovasc Dis* 2:161–164, 2012.
71. McConnell MV, Solomon SD, Rayan MD, et al: Regional right ventricular dysfunction detected by echocardiography in acute pulmonary embolism. *Am J Cardiol* 78:469–473, 1996.
72. Casazza F, Bongarzoni A, Capozi A: Regional right ventricular dysfunction in acute pulmonary embolism and right ventricular infarction. *Eur J Echocardiogr* 6:11–14, 2005.
73. Vaid U, Singer E, Marhefka GD, et al: Poor positive predictive value of McConnell's sign on transthoracic echocardiography for the diagnosis of acute pulmonary embolism. *Hosp Pract* 41:23–27, 2013.
74. Kitabatake A, Inoue M, Asao M, et al: Non-invasive evaluation of pulmonary hypertension by a pulsed wave Doppler technique. *Circulation* 68:302–309, 1983.
75. Armstrong WE, Ryan T: Left and right atrium, and right ventricle, in DeStefano FR (ed): *Fingenbaum's Echocardiography*. 7th ed. Philadelphia, USA, Lippincott Williams & Wilkins, 2010, p 212.
76. Torbicki A, Kurzyna M, Ciurzynski M, et al: Proximal pulmonary emboli modify right ventricula ejection pattern. *Eur Respir J* 13:616–621, 1999.
77. Kurzyna M, Torbicki A, Pruszczyk P, et al: Disturbed right ventricular ejection pattern as a new doppler echocardiographic sign of acute pulmonary embolism. *Am J Cardiol* 90:507–511, 2002.
78. Spodick DH: Pathophysiology of cardiac tamponade. *Chest* 113:1372–1378, 1998.
79. Spodick DH: Pericardial diseases, in Braunwald E, Zipes D, Libby P (eds): *Heart Disease: A Textbook of Cardiovascular Medicine*. Philadelphia, PA, W.B. Saunders, 2001, pp 1823–1876.
80. Santamore WP, Dell'Italia LJ: Ventricular interdependence: significant left ventricular contributions to right ventricular systolic function. *Prog Cardiovasc Dis* 40:289–308, 1998.
81. Adler Y, Charron P, Imazio M, et al: 2015 ESC Guidelines for the diagnosis and management of pericardial diseases: The Task Force for the Diagnosis and Management of Pericardial Diseases of the European Society of Cardiology (ESC) Endorsed by: The European Association for Cardio-Thoracic Surgery (EACTS). *Eur Heart J* 36:2921–2964, 2015.
82. Reydel B, Spodick DH: Frequency and significance of chamber collapses during cardiac tamponade. *Am Heart J* 119:1160–1163, 1990.
83. Kem MJ: Cardiac catheterization techniques: normal hemodynamics, in Cutlip D (ed): *Cardiovascular Medicine*. UpToDate, 2015.
84. Leimgruber PP, Klopfenstein HS, Wann LS, et al: The hemodynamic derangement associated with right ventricular diastolic collapse in cardiac tamponade: an experimental echocardiographic study. *Circulation* 68:612–620, 1983.
85. Gillam LD, Guyer DE, Gibson TC, et al: Hydrodynamic compression of the right atrium: a new echocardiographic sign of cardiac tamponade. *Circulation* 68:294–301, 1983.
86. Kerber RE, Gascho JA, Litchfield R, et al: Hemodynamic effects of volume expansion and nitroprusside compared with pericardiocentesis in patients with acute cardiac tamponade. *N Engl J Med* 307:929–931, 1982.
87. Hoit BD: Cardiac tamponade, in Gersh BJ, Hoekstra J (ed): *Cardiovascular Medicine*. UpToDate, 2015.
88. Spodick DH: Acute cardiac tamponade. *N Engl J Med* 349:684–690, 2003.

89. Torelli J, Marwick TH, Salcedo EE: Left atrial tamponade: diagnosis by transesophageal echocardiography. *J Am Soc Echocardiogr* 4:413–414, 1991.
90. Himelman RB, Kircher B, Rockey DC, et al: Inferior vena cava plethora with blunted respiratory response: a sensitive echocardiography sign of cardiac tamponade. *J Am Coll Cardiol* 12:1470–1477, 1988.
91. Haddad F, Hunt SA, Rosenthal D, et al: Right ventricular function in cardiovascular disease, part I: anatomy, physiology, aging, and functional assessment of the right ventricle. *Circulation* 117:1436–1448, 2008.
92. Klein AL, Abbara S, Agler DA, et al: ASE Expert Consensus Statement American Society of Echocardiography clinical recommendations for multimodality cardiovascular imaging of patients with pericardial disease endorsed by the society for cardiovascular magnetic resonance and society of cardiovascular computed tomography. *J Am Soc Echocardiogr* 26:965–1012, 2013.
93. Chuttani K, Tischler MD, Pandian NG, et al: Diagnosis of cardiac tamponade after cardiac surgery: relative value of clinical, echocardiographic, and hemodynamic signs. *Am Heart J* 127:913–918, 1994.
94. Hotchkiss RS, Karl IE: The pathophysiology and treatment of sepsis. *N Engl J Med* 348:138–150, 2003.
95. Annane D, Bellissant E, Cavaillon J-M: Septic shock. *Lancet* 365:63–78, 2005.
96. Mayr FB, Yende S, Angus DC: Epidemiology of severe sepsis. *Virulence* 5:4–11, 2014.
97. Kumar A, Haery C, Parrillo JE: Myocardial dysfunction in septic shock. *Crit Care Clin* 16:251–287, 2000.
98. Court O, Kumar A, Parrillo JE, et al: Myocardial depression in sepsis and septic shock. *Crit Care* 6:500–507, 2002.
99. Levy RJ, Deutschman CS: Evaluating myocardial depression in sepsis. *Shock* 22:1–10, 2004.
100. Cunnion RE, Schaer GL, Parker MM, et al: The coronary circulation in human septic shock. *Circulation* 73:637–644, 1986.
101. Rudiger A, Singer M: Mechanisms of sepsis-induced cardiac dysfunction. *Crit Care Med* 35:1599–1608, 2007.
102. Torgersen C, Moser P, Luckner G, et al: Macroscopic postmortem findings in 235 surgical intensive care patients with sepsis. *Anesth Analg* 108:1841–1847, 2009.
103. Hotchkiss RS, Karl IE: Reevaluation of the role of cellular hypoxia and bioenergetic failure in sepsis. *JAMA* 267:1503–1510, 1992.
104. Rivers E, Nguyen B, Havstad S, et al: Earlygoal-directed therapy in the treatment of severe sepsis and septic shock. *N Engl J Med* 345:1368–1377, 2001.
105. Winslow E, Loeb HS, Rahimtoola S, et al: Hemodynamic studies and results of therapy in 50 patients with bacteremic shock. *Am J Med* 54:421, 1972.
106. Parrillo J: Pathogenetic mechanisms of septic shock. *N Engl J Med* 328:1471–1477, 1993.
107. Shoemaker WC, Montgomery ES, Kaplan E, et al: Physiologic pattern in surviving and nonsurviving shock patients. *Arch Surg* 106:630–636, 1973.
108. Bland RD, Shoemaker WC, Abraham E, et al: Hemodynamic and oxygen transport pattern in surviving and nonsurviving patients. *Crit Care Med* 13:85–90, 1985.
109. Vieillard-Baron A, Caille V, Charron C, et al: Actual incidence of global left ventricular hypokinesia in adult septic shock. *Crit Care Med* 36:1701–1706, 2008.
110. Jardin F, Fourme T, Page B, et al: Persistent preload defect in severe sepsis despite fluid loading: a longitudinal echocardiographic study in patients with septic shock. *Chest* 116:1354–1359, 1999.
111. Belcher E, Mitchell J, Evans T: Myocardial dysfunction in sepsis: no role for NO? *Heart* 87:507–509, 2002.
112. Jardin F, Brun-Ney D, Auvert B, et al: Sepsis related cardiogenic shock. *Crit Care Med* 18:1055–1060, 1990.
113. Parker MM, Shelhamer JH, Bacharach SL, et al: Profound but reversible myocardial depression in patients with septic shock. *Ann Intern Med* 100:483–490, 1984.
114. Jafri SM, Lavine S, Field BE, et al: Left ventricular diastolic function in sepsis. *Crit Care Med* 18:709–714, 1990.
115. Poelaert J, Declerck C, Vogelaers D, et al: Left ventricular systolic and diastolic function in septic shock. *Intensive Care Med* 23:553–560, 1997.
116. Brown SM, Pittman JE, Hirshberg EL, et al: Diastolic dysfunction and mortality in early severe sepsis and septic shock: a prospective, observational echocardiography study. *Crit Ultrasound J* 4:8, 2012.
117. Subramaniam B, Talmor D: Echocardiography for management of hypotension in the intensive care unit. *Crit Care Med* 35[Suppl]:S401–S407, 2007.
118. Parker MM, McCarthy KE, Ognibene FP, et al: Right ventricular dysfunction and dilatation, similar to left ventricular changes, characterize the cardiac depression of septic shock in humans. *Chest* 97:126–131, 1990.
119. Sato HTH, Uchida T, Dote K, et al: Tako-tsubo-like left ventricular dysfunction due to multivessel coronary spasm, in Kodama KHK, Hori M (eds): Clinical aspect of myocardial injury: from ischemia to heart failure. Tokyo, Kagakuhyoronsha Publishing, 1990, pp 56–64.
120. Bybee KA, Kara T, Prasad A, et al: Systematic review: transient left ventricular apical ballooning: a syndrome that mimics ST-segment elevation myocardial infarction. *Ann Intern Med* 141:858–865, 2004.
121. Hurst RT, Prasad A, Askew JW III, et al: Takotsubo cardiomyopathy: a unique cardiomyopathy with variable ventricular morphology. *JACC Cardiovasc Imaging* 3:641–649, 2010.
122. Medeiros K, O'Connor M, Baicu CF, et al: Systolic and diastolic mechanics in stress cardiomyopathy. *Circulation* 129:1659–1667, 2014.
123. Templin C, Ghadri JR, Diekmann J, et al: Clinical features and outcomes of takotsubo (stress) cardiomyopathy. *N Engl J Med* 373:929–938, 2015.
124. Tsuchihashi K, Ueshima K, Uchida T, et al: Transient left ventricular apical ballooning without coronary artery stenosis: a novel heart syndrome mimicking acute myocardial infarction: angina pectorismyocardial infarction investigations in Japan. *J Am Coll Cardiol* 38:11–18, 2001.
125. Lee VH, Connolly HM, Fulgham JR, et al: Tako-tsubo cardiomyopathy in aneurysmal subarachnoid hemorrhage: an underappreciated ventricular dysfunction. *J Neurosurg* 105:264–270, 2006.
126. Le Ven F, Pennec PY, Timsit S, et al: Takotsubo syndrome associated with seizures: an underestimated cause of sudden death in epilepsy? *Int J Cardiol* 146:475–479, 2011.
127. Sharp RP, Welch EB. Takotsubo cardiomyopathy as a complication of electroconvulsive therapy. *Ann Pharmacother* 45:1559–1565, 2011.
128. Riera M, Llompart-Pou JA, Carrillo A, et al: Head injury and inverted Takotsubo cardiomyopathy. *J Trauma* 68:E13–E15, 2010.
129. Yoshimura S, Toyoda K, Ohara T, et al: Takotsubo cardiomyopathy in acute ischemic stroke. *Ann Neurol* 64:547–554, 2008.
130. Summers MR, Lennon RJ, Prasad A: Pre-morbid psychiatric and cardiovascular diseases in apical ballooning syndrome (tako-tsubo/stress-induced cardiomyopathy): potential pre-disposing factors? *J Am Coll Cardiol* 55:700–701, 2010.
131. Wittstein IS, Thiemann DR, Lima JAC, et al: Neurohumoral Features of Myocardial Stunning Due to Sudden Emotional Stress. *N Engl J Med* 352:539–548, 2005.
132. Kyuma M, Tsuchihashi K, Shinshi Y, et al: Effect of intravenous propranolol on left ventricular apical ballooning without coronary artery stenosis (ampulla cardiomyopathy): three cases. *Circ J* 66:1181–1184, 2002.
133. Galiuto L, De Caterina AR, Porfidia A, et al: Reversible coronary microvascular dysfunction: a common pathogenetic mechanism in Apical Ballooning or Tako-Tsubo Syndrome. *Eur Heart J* 31:1319–1327, 2010.
134. Bybee KA, Prasad A: Stress-related cardiomyopathy syndromes. *Circulation* 118:397–409, 2008.
135. Samuels MA: The brain-heart connection. *Circulation* 116:77–84, 2007.
136. Prasad A, Lerman A, Rihal CS: Apical ballooning syndrome (Tako-Tsubo or stress cardiomyopathy): a mimic of acute myocardial infarction. *Am Heart J* 155:408–417, 2008.
137. Sharkey SW, Windenburg DC, Lesser JR, et al: Natural history and expansive clinical profile of stress (tako-tsubo) cardiomyopathy. *J Am Coll Cardiol* 55:333–341, 2010.
138. Nef HM, Möllmann H, Akashi YJ, et al: Mechanisms of stress (Takotsubo) cardiomyopathy. *Nat Rev Cardiol* 7:187–193, 2010.
139. El Mahmoud R, MN, Pilliére R, et al: Prevalence and characteristics of left ventricular outflow tract obstruction in Tako-Tsubo syndrome. *Am Heart J* 156:543–548, 2008.

Chapter 30 ■ Respiratory Monitoring during Mechanical Ventilation

MELANIE R. LOBERMAN • RAY H. RITZ • TODD W. SARGE

Respiratory function may be simply classified into ventilation and oxygenation, which are quantified by the ability of the respiratory system to eliminate carbon dioxide and form oxy-hemoglobin, respectively. The goal of respiratory monitoring in any setting is to allow the clinician to ascertain the status of the patient's ventilation and oxygenation. The data must then be used appropriately to correct the patient's abnormal respiratory physiology. As with all data, it is imperative to remember that interpretation and appropriate intervention are still the onus of the clinician, who must integrate these data with other pieces of information in order to make a final intervention. For the critically ill patient, the principal intervention with regard to respiratory function and monitoring usually involves the initiation, modification, or withdrawal of mechanical ventilatory support. This chapter will focus on respiratory monitoring for the mechanically ventilated patient.

Mechanical ventilation (MV) entails the unloading of the respiratory system via the application of positive pressure to achieve the goal of lung insufflation (i.e., inspiration) followed by the release of pressure to allow deflation (i.e., expiration). These simplified goals of mechanical ventilation are achieved in spite of complex and dynamic interactions of mechanical pressure with the physical properties of the respiratory system, namely, elastance (E_{rs}) and resistance (R_{rs}). Furthermore, the patient's overall clinical condition (e.g., neurological or muscular) often times affects the goals of respiration; thus, they need to be monitored and evaluated using an integrative approach. Therefore, this chapter will focus on three specific areas of monitoring for the mechanically ventilated patient: (a) the evaluation of gas exchange, (b) respiratory mechanics, and (c) respiratory neuromuscular function.

GAS EXCHANGE

Basic Physics of Gas Exchange

As mentioned, the primary function of the respiratory system is gas exchange (i.e., elimination of carbon dioxide while instilling oxygen to form oxy-hemoglobin). Inadequate ventilation and oxygenation within the intensive care setting are typically caused by hypoventilation, diffusion impairment, and ventilation–perfusion ($\dot{V}$–$\dot{Q}$) mismatch.

Hypoventilation is defined as inadequate alveolar ventilation and is commonly caused by drug side effects, neurological impairment, or muscle weakness/fatigue, which results in hypercarbia, according to the following equation:

$$PaCO_2 = (\dot{V}_{CO_2}/\dot{V}_A)\ k$$

where $PaCO_2$ is the arterial partial pressure of carbon dioxide, $\dot{V}_{CO_2}$ the production of carbon dioxide in the body, $\dot{V}_A$ is alveolar ventilation, and k is a constant. Fortunately, the institution of mechanical ventilatory support readily corrects hypoventilation while the underlying cause is determined and corrected.

Diffusion impairment is the result of inadequate exchange of oxygen across the capillary-alveolar membrane, resulting in hypoxemia. This may occur due to pathological thickening of the membrane or high cardiac output states such as sepsis. However, the relative clinical significance of diffusion impairment in the intensive care unit (ICU) is debatable. This is because the hypoxemia that results from the acute exacerbation of diffusion impairment is usually corrected by supplemental oxygen therapy. Of note, $PaCO_2$ is rarely affected by diffusion impairments because it is highly soluble and can be eliminated in multiple forms, e.g., as bicarbonate.

The most common cause of hypoxemia in the ICU is ventilation–perfusion ($\dot{V}$–$\dot{Q}$) mismatch. Ventilation–perfusion mismatch is the result of an inequality of the normal ventilation to perfusion ratio within the lung. $\dot{V}$–$\dot{Q}$ mismatch is a spectrum of abnormal ratios signifying inadequate gas exchange at the alveolar level. When ventilation is significantly decreased with respect to perfusion (i.e., a $\dot{V}$–$\dot{Q}$ ratio $<< 1$), hypoxemia ensues. In general, hypoxemia from $\dot{V}$–$\dot{Q}$ mismatch can be overcome with supplemental oxygen. However, in the extreme, as the $\dot{V}$–$\dot{Q}$ ratio in an alveolus approaches zero (i.e., no ventilation while the alveolus is still being perfused), it approaches "true shunt." At the other end of the spectrum, as the ratio in the alveolus approaches infinity (i.e., no perfusion in a ventilated alveolus), it becomes physiologic "dead space." Dead space will be described in greater detail later in this chapter.

As mentioned, true shunt is one extreme of $\dot{V}$–$\dot{Q}$ mismatch that occurs when ventilation in the alveolus approaches zero with ongoing perfusion. The true shunt fraction is the proportion of the cardiac output that results in venous blood mixing with end-arterial blood without participating in gas exchange. This has little effect on carbon dioxide tension; however, increases in shunt result in worsening hypoxemia. The true shunt fraction is expressed via the shunt equation as follows:

$$\dot{Q}_s/\dot{Q}_t = (C_c - C_a)/(C_c - C_v)$$

where $\dot{Q}_s$ and $\dot{Q}_t$ are the shunt and total blood flows, and C_c, C_a, and C_v represent the oxygen contents of pulmonary end-capillary, arterial, and mixed venous blood, respectively. The absolute oxygen content of arterial and mixed venous blood is calculated according to the oxygen content equation:

$$Cx = (1.34 \times Hb \times SxO_2) + (PxO_2 \times 0.003)$$

where Cx, SxO_2, and PxO_2 are the oxygen content, saturation, and partial pressure of oxygen within arterial and mixed venous blood, respectively. The oxygen content of end-capillary blood is estimated by the alveolar gas equation as follows:

$$C_c = (P_{atm} - P_{H_2O}) \times FiO_2 + PaCO_2/RQ$$

where P_{atm} and P_{H_2O} are the partial pressures of the atmosphere and water (typically 760 mm Hg and 47 mm Hg at sea level), respectively; while FiO_2 is the concentration of inspired oxygen, $PaCO_2$ is the arterial partial pressure of carbon dioxide and RQ is the respiratory quotient (approximately 0.8 at steady state, but varies depending on the utilization of carbohydrates, protein, and fat). The clinical significance of true shunt is the fact that it is not amenable to supplemental oxygen therapy. Shunted blood re-enters the circulation and dilutes oxygenated blood, resulting in a lower partial pressure of oxygen (PaO_2) in the arterial system. Increasing the FiO_2 will not improve oxygenation since the shunted fraction of blood does not meet alveolar gas.

Direct Blood Gas Analysis

Monitors of gas exchange for the mechanically ventilated patient are typically directed at measurements of gas content and their gradients from the ventilator circuit to the alveolus and from the alveolus to the end-artery. As with most monitors, sources of error abound at many points as gases flow according to their concentration gradients. The most accurate assessment of gas exchange is direct measurement from an arterial blood sample. This provides the partial pressures of carbon dioxide ($PaCO_2$) and oxygen (PaO_2) in the blood as well as the pH, base deficit, and co-oximetry of other substances such as carboxyhemoglobin and methemoglobin. Advantages of arterial blood gas (ABG) analysis include the fact that it is a fairly exact representation of the current state of the patient with regard to acid-base status, oxygenation, and ventilation. However, the limitations of blood gas analysis as a tool for monitoring gas exchange are numerous, including the fact that it is invasive, wasteful (blood), expensive, and intermittent (i.e., it is only a snapshot of the patient's condition at the time the ABG is drawn).

Central and peripheral venous blood gas sampling has been proposed as an acceptable surrogate to arterial blood for monitoring pH, $PaCO_2$, and base deficit [1]. The obvious advantage is that it is less invasive (i.e., patients are not required to have arterial access or punctures), while the disadvantages are the need for correlation and inability to assess oxygenation. With the exception of patients undergoing cardiopulmonary resuscitation [2], good correlation has been observed between arterial and venous pH and $PaCO_2$ among patients with acute respiratory diseases, with one author noting an average difference of 0.03 for pH and 5.8 for $PaCO_2$ [1]. Another study of mechanically ventilated trauma patients also demonstrated good correlation between arterial and central venous pH, $PaCO_2$, and base deficit; however, the authors concluded that the limits of agreement (−0.09 to 0.03 for pH and −2.2 to 10.9 for $PaCO_2$) represented clinically significant ranges that could affect management and therefore should not be used in initial resuscitation efforts of trauma patients [3].

Pulse Oximetry

Without question, pulse oximetry has been the most significant advance in respiratory monitoring in the past several decades. Based on the established oxy-hemoglobin dissociation curve (Fig. 30.1), pulse oximetry allows for the continuous, noninvasive estimate of a patient's oxy-hemoglobin and is expressed as a percentage of total hemoglobin. A detailed explanation of pulse oximetry including the physics and limitations is provided in the Chapter "Routine Monitoring of Critically Ill Patients" (Chapter 27).

Expired Carbon Dioxide Measurements

Capnometry is the quantification of the carbon dioxide concentration in a sample of gas. Quantitative waveform capnography is the continuous plotting of carbon dioxide values over time (Fig. 30.2). The inhaled and exhaled carbon dioxide is displayed on the monitor along with its corresponding numerical measurement. When capnography is performed on continuous samples of gas from the airway circuit, a waveform is created whereby the maximum value is expressed in millimeters Hg and termed end-tidal carbon dioxide or $P_{et}CO_2$.

Capnography can be very useful for assessing changes in a patient's cardiovascular status. For example, increases in $P_{et}CO_2$ can signify an increase in cardiac output as spontaneous circulation returns during cardiopulmonary resuscitation (CPR) as was shown in several experimental studies [4–6]. According to the

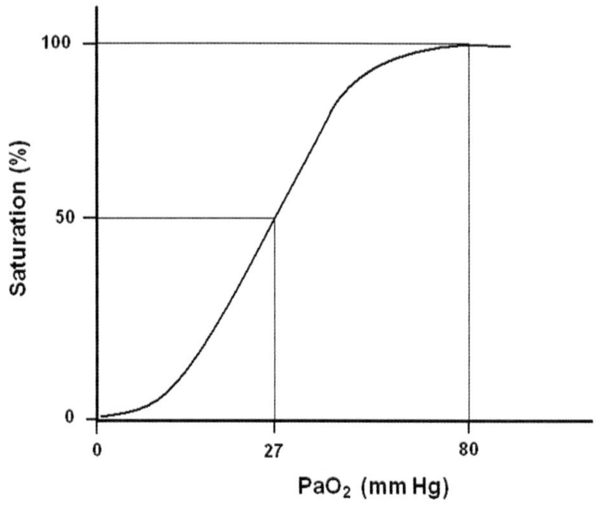

FIGURE 30.1 Schematic demonstrating a normal hemoglobin dissociation curve with 50% saturation at PaO_2 of 27 mm Hg and approaching 100% saturation at a PaO_2 of 80 mm Hg.

2010 to 2015 American Heart Association (AHA) guideline's for Advanced Cardiac Life Support (ACLS), continuous quantitative waveform capnography is recommended for confirmation and monitoring of endotracheal tube placement [7]. $P_{et}CO_2$ is also recommended during CPR since it allows providers to monitor CPR quality, optimize chest compressions, and detect return of spontaneous circulation (ROSC). That is, $P_{et}CO_2$ directly monitors ventilation and indirectly measures metabolism and cardiac output. Normal $P_{et}CO_2$ for an adult patient is 35 to 45mm Hg, and good quality chest compressions in a patient that is endotracheally intubated should result in $P_{et}CO_2$ levels of >10 mm Hg. Einav et al. postulated in their prospective cohort study that computerized $P_{et}CO_2$ carries potential as a tool for early, real-time decision-making during some resuscitations [8]. With return of spontaneous circulation, a significant increase in the $P_{et}CO_2$ to near normal levels can be observed [9]. For a detailed explanation of capnography and its uses, please refer to Chapter 27, "Routine Monitoring of Critically Ill Patients."

Dead Space Measurements

Dead space is defined as any space in the respiratory system that is ventilated but not perfused, thereby not participating in gas exchange. Measurement of dead space is a marker of respiratory efficiency with regard to carbon dioxide elimination. Dead space can be subdivided into alveolar and anatomic. Anatomic dead space is the sum of the inspiratory volume that does not reach the alveoli and therefore, does not participate in gas exchange. For mechanically ventilated patients, the anatomic dead space includes the proximal airways, trachea, endotracheal tube, and breathing circuit components from the Y-adapter to the endotracheal tube. In healthy human subjects, anatomic dead space in cubic centimeters is approximately 2 to 3 times the ideal body weight in kilograms, or 150 to 200 mL. Alveolar dead space is the conceptual sum of all alveoli that are ventilated but not participating in gas exchange, otherwise described as "West Zone 1" [10]. Physiologic dead space (V_d) is the sum of anatomic and alveolar dead space volumes and is usually expressed as a ratio of the total tidal volume (V_t) and can be calculated at the bedside using the modified Bohr equation:

$$V_d/V_t = PaCO_2 - P_{exp}CO_2/PaCO_2,$$

where $PaCO_2$ is the partial pressure of carbon dioxide and $P_{exp}CO_2$ is the partial pressure of carbon dioxide in the expired tidal

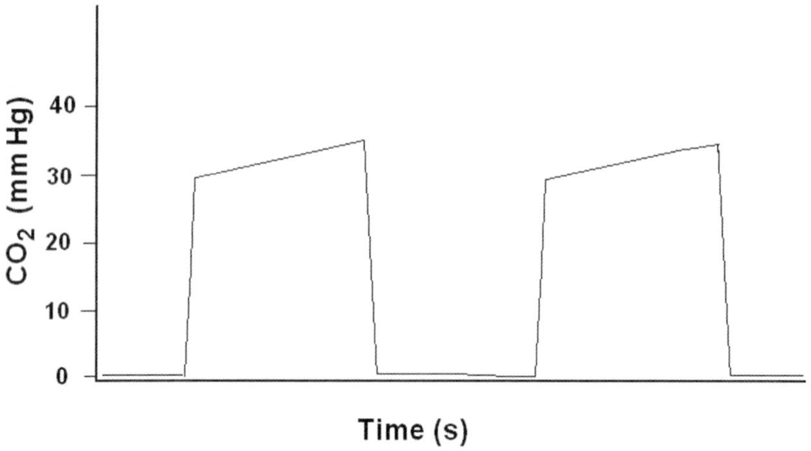

FIGURE 30.2 Schematic representation of a capnograph waveform with the expiratory plateau delineating the end-tidal CO_2 between 30 to 40 mm Hg.

volume of gas. The $P_{exp}CO_2$ is difficult to measure, often requiring metabolic monitoring systems. However, *volume capnography* is a relatively novel and simple approach to estimating $P_{exp}CO_2$, involving measurements of carbon dioxide at the Y-adapter, and has been shown to correlate with more complex methods of metabolic monitoring [11]. The $PaCO_2$ can be estimated as end-tidal carbon dioxide, $P_{et}CO_2$; however, this is known to be inaccurate in certain disease states. Therefore, determination of the $PaCO_2$ is most often measured directly via an ABG.

Physiologic dead space, V_d/V_t, is often increased in critical illnesses that cause respiratory failure, such as acute respiratory distress syndrome (ARDS) and chronic obstructive pulmonary disease (COPD). V_d/V_t can also increase with excessive Positive End Expiratory Pressure (PEEP) due to over-inflation of alveoli, which impedes pulmonary artery blood flow effectively increasing the "West Zone 1" volume. Serial measurements of V_d/V_t have been shown to correlate with outcomes of ARDS patients [12] and have been used to monitor the degree of respiratory insult and provide prognostic information for critically ill patients [13]. However, these data have not translated into changes in treatment. Furthermore, Mohr et al. [14] found no appreciable difference in V_d/V_t while studying a series of post-tracheostomy patients successfully weaned from mechanical ventilation versus those who had failed weaning.

RESPIRATORY MECHANICS

Basic Pulmonary Variables

Modern ventilators allow manipulation and measurement of the airway pressures (P_{aw}), including peak and plateau, in addition to mean and end-expiratory volumes (V) and flows ($\dot{V}$) It is also possible to measure the actual (or total) PEEP ($PEEP_t$) during static hold maneuvers on the ventilator to determine the extent of "air-trapping" or auto-PEEP. Auto-PEEP is also known as intrinsic PEEP ($PEEP_i$) and will be defined later in this chapter. Integration of these measurements allows assessment of the mechanical components of the respiratory system. The mechanical components are influenced by various disease states, and understanding these relationships could promote the delivery of more appropriate ventilator support as well as pharmacologic management.

The airway pressure (P_{aw}) is described by the equation of motion and must be equal to all opposing forces. For the relaxed respiratory system ventilating at normal frequencies, the major forces that oppose P_{aw} are the elastive and resistive properties of the respiratory system as they relate to the tidal volume (V_t) and flow ($\dot{V}$), respectively:

$$P_{aw} = E_{rs}V_t + R_{rs}(\dot{V})$$

where E_{rs} and R_{rs} are the elastance and resistance of the respiratory system, respectively. Constant flow inflation in a relaxed, ventilator-dependent patient produces a typical picture as depicted in Figure 30.3 [15]. The rapid airway occlusion method at end-inflation results in zero flow and a drop in P_{aw} from the peak value (PIP) to a lower initial value and then a gradual decrease over the rest of the inspiratory period until a plateau pressure (P_{plat}) is observed. The P_{plat} measured at the airway represents the static end-inspiratory recoil of the entire respiratory system [16]. It is important that the P_{plat} measurement is preformed when the patient is passive as any inspiratory or expiratory efforts will create an error in the obtained value.

Measurement of the pleural pressures would allow further partitioning of these pressures into the lung (i.e., transpulmonary pressure, P_L) and chest wall (i.e., pleural pressure, P_{pl}) components using the equation:

$$P_{aw} = P_L + P_{pl}$$

Unfortunately, direct measurements of pleural pressure are not practical in the intensive care setting. Therefore, pleural pressures have often been estimated via an esophageal balloon catheter measuring the pressure in the esophagus (P_{es}), which

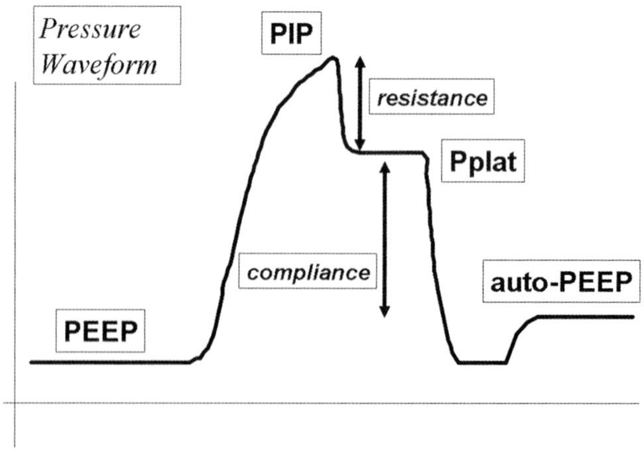

FIGURE 30.3 Schematic drawing of an airway pressure waveform delineating PEEP, auto-PEEP, Peak inspiratory pressure (PIP), plateau pressure (P_{plat}), resistance, and compliance.

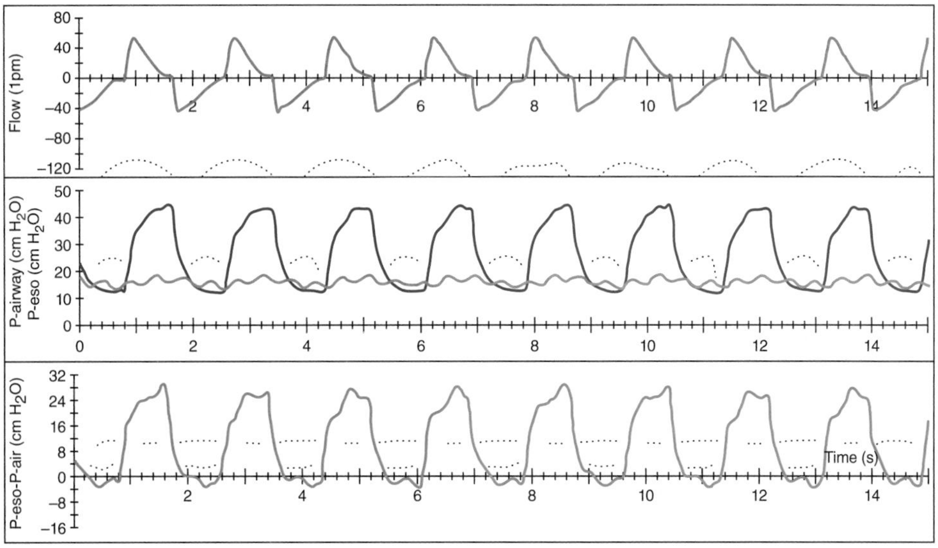

FIGURE 30.4 Esophageal pressure tracing (P-eso) can be seen superimposed on the airway pressure tracing (P-air) during pressure control ventilation (PCV). Transpulmonary pressure has been estimated as the difference between these pressures with specific assumptions.

lies in close proximity to the pleura at the mid-lung level. This alters the above equation as follows:

$$P_{aw} = P_L + P_{es}$$

These pressures are presented graphically in Figure 30.4.

Compliance and Elastance

The static compliance ($C_{st, rs}$) of the respiratory system and its reciprocal, elastance ($E_{st, rs}$), are easily measured at the bedside using the aforementioned end-inspiratory airway occlusion method to produce zero flow and thus negate the resistive forces within the system. The elastance of the respiratory system ($E_{st, rs}$) is simply the pressure gradient between the total PEEP ($PEEP_t$) and the plateau pressure (P_{plat}) divided by the tidal volume (V_t) to yield the following equation:

$$E_{st, rs} = (P_{plat} - PEEP_t)/V_t$$

$E_{st, rs}$ may also be separated into its lung (E_L) and chest wall (E_{cw}) components by applying this equation to the P_L and P_{es} tracings obtained using P_{es} tracings (see Fig. 30.4) and by the equation:

$$E_{st, rs} = E_L + E_{cw}$$

The relative contributions of the lung and chest wall to the total elastance may be dependent on the etiology of respiratory failure. By way of example, pulmonary edema, either cardiogenic or as a result of ARDS, will lead to an elevated lung elastance (E_{st}) and reduced compliance. ARDS of a nonpulmonary origin, sepsis as an example, may also lead to edema of the chest wall and abdominal distension. Both of these will lead to an additional increase in the elastance of the total respiratory system ($E_{st, rs}$) as a result of an increase in the elastance of the chest wall (E_{cw}).

Resistance

According to Ohm's law, resistance is a function of the airway pressure gradient (ΔP_{aw}) divided by flow ($\dot{V}$). Respiratory system resistance is a complex and dynamic construct that relates the difference of alveolar to airway opening pressures to airflow. Airway resistance can be measured for ventilator-dependent patients by using the technique of rapid airway occlusion during constant flow inflation. The resistance of the respiratory system (R_{RS}) can be estimated as:

$$R_{RS} = [P_{peak} - P_{plat}]/\dot{V}$$

R_{RS} reflects intrinsic resistance of the airways, dynamic tissue interactions based on respirophasic changes on airway geometry including the pendelluft effect, resistive effects of mucus, blood, cellular debris, and other airway contents, and the viscoelastic properties of the gasses moving through them. Recognizing that airway resistance is abnormally high suggests that airway tube position and patency should be verified, airway contents removed by suctioning or cleaning the tube, and that the bronchodilator administration may be indicated.

Intrinsic PEEP (Auto-PEEP)

The desired PEEP set by the clinician on the ventilator is the target pressure at end-exhalation. However, the actual pressure remaining in the alveoli and ventilator circuit at end-exhalation may be higher due to flow limitations or early closing capacity within a patient's lungs. The actual pressure at end-exhalation is called total PEEP ($PEEP_t$), and the difference between the set PEEP and $PEEP_t$ is referred to as the intrinsic PEEP ($PEEP_i$). $PEEP_i$ can be measured on most modern ventilators during a static breath hold maneuver during exhalation (Fig. 30.3), when the ventilator is able to measure the remaining pressure in the circuit and lungs to determine the $PEEP_t$ and thus the $PEEP_i$. As with P_{plat} measurements, care must be taken to ensure $PEEP_t$ measurements are made while the patient is passive to avoid errors due to muscle activity.

Especially among patients with severe obstructive pulmonary disease (e.g., asthma or COPD), $PEEP_i$ can impact the ability to trigger the mechanical ventilator. Such patients often have high resistance to both inhalation and exhalation and may not complete exhalation prior to the next inspiratory cycle. Dynamic hyperinflation is the result of increasing $PEEP_t$ in the airway circuit with each breath ("breath-stacking") due to the $PEEP_i$ and results in increasing dead space and over-distension. Respiratory rate, I:E ratio, and severity of obstructive pulmonary disease all influence the $PEEP_i$ and therefore may worsen dynamic hyperinflation. Care must be taken to set the high airway pressure ventilator alarms properly and to recognize significant increases in $PEEP_i$ to minimize the risk of dynamic hyperinflation, which can lead to decreased cardiac output and barotrauma (e.g., pneumothorax). For intubated patients breathing spontaneously, high $PEEP_i$ can result in ineffective triggering and increased WOB, which will be discussed later in this chapter. It is worth noting that manipulations of respiratory rate and tidal volume that do not reduce the patient's overall minute ventilation will rarely reduce the $PEEP_i$ level.

Driving Pressure

Driving pressure (ΔP) is the absolute pressure required to attain a given tidal volume and is proportional to the respiratory system compliance. It can be expressed by the equation:

$$(\Delta P = V_t/C_{st,\,rs})$$

where ΔP is the driving pressure, V_t is the tidal volume, and $C_{st,\,rs}$ is the static compliance of the respiratory system. In patients without spontaneous respiratory efforts, the driving pressure is simply the difference between plateau pressure and PEEP. In a retrospective study analyzing the variation and trends for a number of respiratory variables, Amato et al. demonstrated that changes in ΔP were most predictive of mortality [17]. Specifically, the authors found that a single standard deviation increment in ΔP (approximately 7 cm of water) was associated with a significant increase in mortality (relative risk, 1.41; 95% confidence interval [CI], 1.31 to 1.51; $p < 0.001$) [17]. The authors noted that this risk persisted even for those patients receiving "lung protective" tidal volumes and plateau pressures, whereas individual changes to tidal volume and PEEP were not independently associated with mortality [17]. Amato and co-authors have argued for a ventilator strategy in which PEEP and tidal volume are manipulated with the specific goal of minimizing ΔP. However, prospective trials are needed to determine whether ΔP can be manipulated to affect survival or it is merely a marker for disease severity and progression.

Pressure Volume Curves

Static Measurements of the Pressure–Volume Curve

The gold standard of pressure–volume (P–V) curve measurement is the super-syringe method. Using a calibrated syringe, in increments of 50 ± 100 mL, gas is used to inflate the lung up to a total volume of 1,000 ± 2,000 mL. After each increment, the static airway pressure is measured during a pause lasting a few seconds during which there is no flow and the pressure is the same in the entire system from the super-syringe to the alveoli. The lung is then deflated in the same manner and the pressure at each decrement of gas is recorded and the inspiratory and expiratory P–V curves are plotted. Continued oxygen uptake from the blood during this slow inflation-deflation cycle, coupled with equalization of the partial pressure of CO_2 in the blood and alveoli, will lead to a decrease in the deflation volume as compared to the inflation volume of gas. This artifact may appear to contribute to the phenomenon of hysteresis. The more important mechanical cause of hysteresis is based on the slow inflation of the lung during the P–V curve maneuver. This slow inflation recruits areas of the lung with slow time constants and collapsed alveoli. This again will lead to a decreased expiratory volume and hysteresis.

Semistatic Measurements of the Pressure–Volume Curve

There are two methods for obtaining semistatic measurements of the P–V curve. These methods do not require the specialized skill and equipment needed for the super-syringe technique. The *multiple occlusion technique* uses a sequence of different-sized volume-controlled inflations with end-inspiratory pauses [18,19]. Pressure and volume are plotted for each end-inspiratory pause to form a static P–V curve. If expiratory interruptions are done as well, the deflation limb of the P–V curve may also be plotted. This process may take several minutes to complete, but yields results close to those obtained by static measurements. The second method is the *low-flow inflation technique*. This technique uses a very small constant inspiratory flow to generate a large total volume. The slope (compliance) of the curve is parallel with a static P–V curve only if airway resistance is constant throughout the inspiration. This is likely not the case as the low flow lessens airway resistance. The low flow also causes a minimal but recognizable pressure decrease over the endotracheal tube, which means that the dynamic inspiratory pressure volume curve will be shifted to the right [20,21]. The long duration of the inspiration produces the same artifacts as the super-syringe technique, which is represented as hysteresis. Another drawback of static and semistatic methods is that they require stopping therapeutic ventilation while the maneuver is performed. Therefore, the question has been raised if these maneuvers are relevant in predicting the mechanical behavior of the lung under dynamic conditions, where resistance and compliance depend on volume, flow, and respiratory frequency.

Dynamic Measurements of the Pressure–Volume Curve

Dynamic measurement of the P–V curve allows continuous monitoring of the respiratory mechanics and in particular of the response to ventilator changes. These measurements are done with the patient on therapeutic ventilator settings whereby pressure is plotted against tidal volume to produce a dynamic P–V curve. However, the pressures are most commonly recorded proximal to the endotracheal tube and are thus heavily influenced by the resistance of the endotracheal tube. Neither the peak pressure nor the end-expiratory pressures are accurately recorded at this position, thus leading to an underestimation of compliance [19].

Clinical Use of the Pressure–Volume Curve

There is a characteristic shape to the static respiratory system P–V curve of patients with injured lungs. This shape includes an S-shaped inflation curve with an upper and lower inflection point (UIP and LIP respectively; Fig. 30.5), an increased recoil pressure at all lung volumes and reduced compliance (Fig. 30.6), which is seen in the slope of the inflation curve between LIP and UIP. The LIP has often been considered the critical opening pressure of collapsed lung units and has been used as a method of setting the optimal PEEP in patients with acute lung injury. The pressure at the UIP, in turn, was considered to indicate alveolar over-distension that should not be exceeded during mechanical ventilation [22]. These ideas have been challenged for multiple reasons. Accurate identification of the LIP and UIP is challenging even for experienced clinicians [23]. Additionally changes in the P–V curve are not specific for alveolar collapse and have been observed in saline-filled lungs, such as would be seen in patients with pulmonary edema [24,25]. When applied clinically to patients mechanically ventilated with ARDS, Amato et al. [26] demonstrated that use of the P–V curve and titration of PEEP to a level that exceeds the LIP may be part of a successful lung protective strategy. It is unclear from this study, however, what the relative importance of the higher levels of PEEP was in the context of the ventilatory strategy, which included delivery of low tidal volumes and the use of intermittent recruitment maneuvers.

Subsequent trials have confirmed the survival benefit for patients ventilated using low tidal volumes; however, studies with higher PEEP have been mixed. Although several early high PEEP trials were negative [27,28], these trials were criticized for not using a physiological basis to guide PEEP as Amato had done. In a randomized controlled trial involving 983 patients with

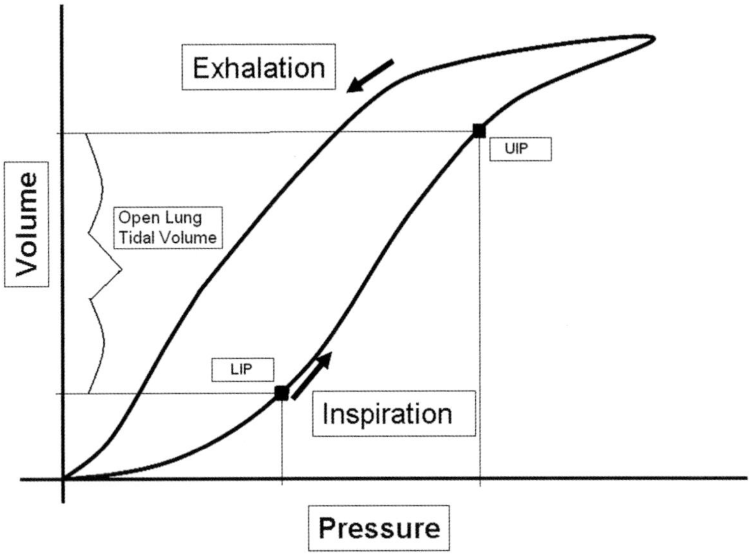

FIGURE 30.5 Schematic representation of normal pressure–volume curve (PV curve) with upper and lower inflection points (UIP and LIP, respectively) delineating the more compliant portion of the inspiratory limb and corresponding tidal volume that has been proposed as an "open lung" approach to ventilation in ARDS.

ARDS, Meade et al. compared an established low tidal volume ventilation strategy with an experimental strategy based on the original "open lung" approach (combining low tidal volume, lung recruitment maneuvers, and high PEEP) [29]. The authors found no significant difference in all-cause hospital mortality or barotrauma, but the "open lung" strategy appeared to improve secondary endpoints related to hypoxemia and use of rescue therapies [29]. Another trial by Mercat et al. was aimed to evaluate the optimal level of PEEP by assigning patients to a moderate PEEP strategy versus an increased recruitment strategy during which the level of PEEP was set to reach a plateau pressure of 28 to 30 cm H_2O [30]. While this study utilized a physiological variable for PEEP titration (based on plateau pressures), they did not find a significant reduction of mortality. However, the authors reported an improvement of lung function and reduced duration of mechanical ventilation as well as duration of organ failure [30]. In a secondary analysis of the aforementioned trials, Goligher et al. found that patients with ARDS who responded to increased PEEP by improved oxygenation had a lower risk of death and postulated that the response to PEEP might be used to predict whether patients would benefit from higher versus lower PEEP levels [31]. In summary, the optimum level of PEEP remains elusive and a matter of ongoing debate and subject for further trials.

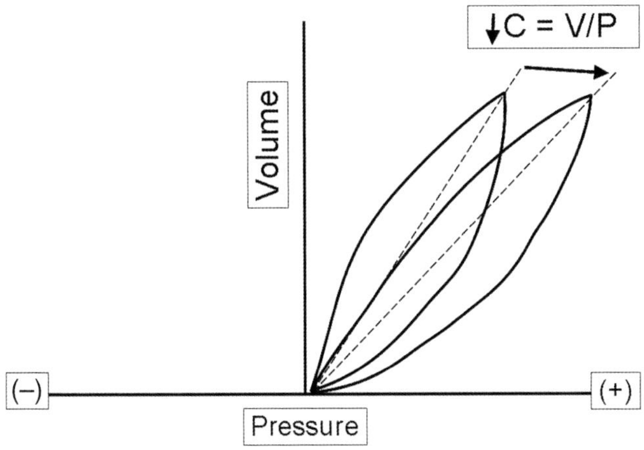

FIGURE 30.6 Schematic representation of altered compliance (C) and the effect on the volume-pressure (V/P) curve as occurs with pulmonary edema.

Stress Index

In recognition of the various difficulties encountered in determining the LIP and UIP of the P–V curve, the "stress index" was developed as a tool to determine optimal PEEP settings for injured lungs. The stress index is a dimensionless number, the coefficient b of the following power equation:

$$\Delta P_{aw} = a \times \Delta t^{b} + c$$

and describes the shape of the airway pressure–time curve during constant flow tidal inflation. In this equation, ΔP_{aw} is the change in airway pressure over time t; the coefficient a is the slope of the curve; and coefficient c is the value of P_{aw} at time 0. A stress index (SI) <1 (progressive increase in slope over tidal inflation) suggests tidal recruitment throughout tidal inflation, whereas a SI >1 (progressive decrease in the slope) suggests hyperinflation and a SI = 1 suggests adequate alveolar recruitment without over-distending the lungs [32].

Although large clinical trials on the use of Stress Index for PEEP titration are lacking, Grasso et al. showed that alveolar hyperinflation for patients with focal ARDS ventilated with the ARDSnet protocol is attenuated by a physiological approach to PEEP setting based on the stress index [32]. Several other experimental and small clinical studies have shown that when ventilatory parameters are adjusted to a noninjurious SI (0.95 to 1.05) [33], there is a decrease in lung inflammation and lung injury [33–35]. Ferrando et al. found in their experiment with a swine model that setting the tidal volume to a noninjurious stress index in an open lung condition improved alveolar ventilation and prevented over-distension without increasing lung injury [36]. However, large clinical trials with mortality benefit are lacking; therefore, the use of this measurement has not been incorporated into routine clinical practice.

Separating the Lung and Chest Wall Components of Respiratory Mechanics

Esophageal Pressure Monitoring

Ventilator-induced lung injury (VILI) arguably depends on the transpulmonary pressure ($P_{aw} - P_{pl}$), whereas current recommendations for management of ARDS specify limits for pressure applied across the whole respiratory system and are based on pressures measured at the airway. This approach could be seriously misleading if P_{pl} were to vary substantially among patients. In healthy subjects and upright spontaneously breathing patients, P_{pl} is often estimated by measuring esophageal pressure (P_{es}); however, this has rarely been done for critically ill patients with respiratory failure and ARDS, possibly because of a widespread, but untested, belief that artifacts make P_{es} unreliable as an estimate of P_{pl} [37]. However, in a lung-injured canine model, Pelosi et al. demonstrated good correlation at mid-lung height between an esophageal balloon catheter measuring the pressures in the esophagus (P_{es}) and the pleural pressures measured via pressure-transducing wafers inserted directly in the thorax [38]. Although the absolute values of the esophageal pressures were not identical with the pleural pressures, Pelosi noted the excursions of esophageal pressure were the same as those observed in the directly measured pleural pressures. The authors therefore concluded that the changes in esophageal pressures were accurate, but the absolute values were not [38]. Others have postulated the explicit assumption that absolute values of P_{es}, corrected for a positional artifact, may reliably reflect an effective P_{pl} in critically ill patients [39].

Variations of P_{pl} may have contributed to inconsistent outcomes among clinical trials of ventilation strategies in ARDS. Whereas one large-scale randomized trial demonstrated a survival benefit from use of low tidal volume ventilation, results from other studies have been equivocal [27,40,41]. It is possible that in some patients with high P_{pl}, low tidal volume ventilation coupled with inadequate levels of PEEP results in cyclic alveolar collapse at end-expiration. In such cases, resulting atelectrauma might negate the benefit of limiting tidal volume. Similarly, higher levels of PEEP have been shown to be lung-protective in numerous animal models of ARDS but have demonstrated inconsistent benefit in clinical investigations [26,28]. This too may reflect failure to account for P_{pl}, leading to under- or over-application of PEEP in some patients as well as misinterpretation of high plateau airway pressures as evidence of lung over-distension [42,43]. Measuring P_{es} to estimate transpulmonary pressure may allow ventilator settings to be individualized to accommodate variations in lung and chest wall mechanical characteristics. Such an individual approach may reduce the risk of further lung injury during ARDS [37,42,44]. This was the hypothesis of a single-center, randomized control trial (EPVENT Trial) of 61 patients by Talmor et al. in which ARDS and ALI patients with low-tidal lung protective ventilation were randomized to a high or low PEEP group. Uniquely when compared to prior trials, the intervention group received PEEP based on the contribution of the chest wall as measured by esophageal pressure manometry. The control group received PEEP based on the PEEP:FiO_2 tables from earlier trials that were created from expert opinion and without individualization based on physiologic measurements. The primary endpoint was oxygenation (PaO_2:FiO_2) with secondary endpoints of compliance, ventilator free days, and mortality. The authors demonstrated that ventilation with a strategy that utilized esophageal pressures measurements to determine PEEP settings was superior as evidenced by improved oxygenation, compliance, and a trend towards improved mortality [45]. A multicenter, prospective, randomized follow-up study is currently being conducted to examine the impact of mechanical ventilation directed at maintaining a positive transpulmonary pressure in patients with moderate-severe ARDS [46].

Gastric Pressure

Esophageal pressure monitoring is not a trivial task, requiring specialized equipment and experienced operators. Gastric pressure may provide a reasonable surrogate measure for P_{pl}. In a prior study, Talmor et al. [39] have demonstrated that there is a correlation between pressure measured in the esophagus and gastric pressures (Fig. 30.7). This relationship may be particularly important in patients suffering from ARDS, resulting from extrapulmonary causes, where abdominal distension and hypertension may contribute significantly to alveolar collapse.

Bladder Pressure

An alternative measurement of intraabdominal pressure may be obtained by measuring the pressure in the urinary bladder [47]. Instilling 50 to 100 mL of sterile water through a Foley catheter, clamping the catheter, and measuring the resulting bladder pressure have been shown to correlate well with intraabdominal pressure measured through a gastric tube [48]. These pressures have also been shown to correlate well with esophageal pressures [49]. Studies are still required to validate

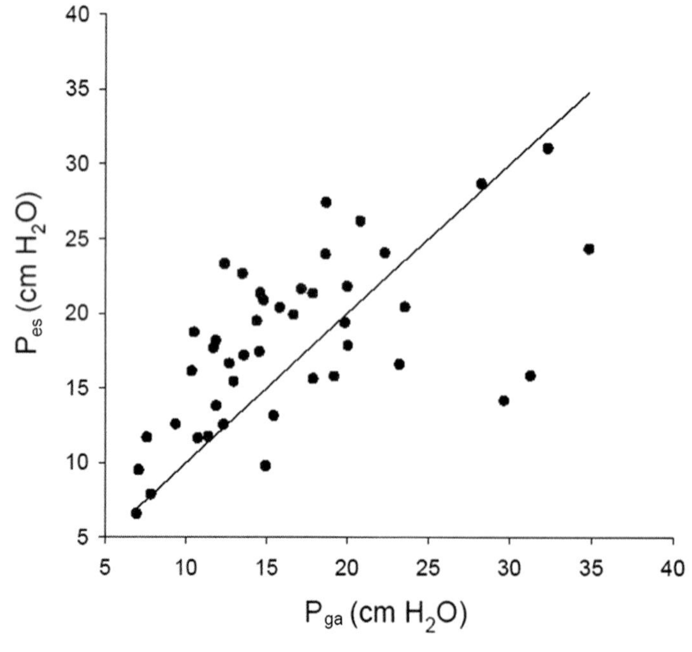

FIGURE 30.7 This graph demonstrates the correlation between pressures measured in the esophagus (P_{es}) and gastric pressure (P_{ga}).

the use of any of these measurements in the clinical care of patients with respiratory failure.

Respiratory Neuromuscular Function

During mechanical ventilation, the clinician aims to unload the patient's failing respiratory system and thereby reduce the work of breathing in the setting of respiratory failure [50]. Obviously, this goal is temporary with the later goal of weaning mechanical ventilation once the patient begins to recover from his or her disease process. To accomplish these goals, the clinician needs to have an understanding of the patient's respiratory function, which impacts each of these goals differently. For example, complete unloading of the respiratory system is common in the operating room with general anesthesia, muscle relaxants, and controlled mechanical ventilation. However, the use of deep sedation and muscle relaxants for prolonged periods in the ICU has deleterious effects on the latter goal of ultimately preparing critically ill patients for extubation with several studies demonstrating increases in ventilator days, hospital length of stay, and associated costs [51–53]. Furthermore, assisted modes of ventilation with partial unloading have been surmised as beneficial for maintaining the conditioning of the diaphragm and reducing sedation requirements in the critical care setting [50,54]. No one has defined the ideal degree of unloading [50], which would presumably vary by individual and disease state. Nevertheless, it is helpful to understand and quantify the patient's neuromuscular function in order to facilitate unloading of the respiratory system, minimize patient–ventilator dyssynchrony, and ultimately wean patients from ventilatory support. This requires an understanding of respiratory neuromuscular physiology and how it cooperates with the ventilator. This relationship has been termed *patient–ventilator interaction*.

Respiratory Neuromuscular Anatomy

The respiratory system is involuntarily controlled by specialized neurons in the pons and medulla oblongata that control both inspiration and expiration. These neurons in the brainstem coordinate many inputs and feedback loops to control respiration and ensure adequate gas exchange. The specific types of feedback can be mechanical, chemical, and behavioral, all of which directly affect the neurons' rate and intensity of neural firing [55]. Together these neurons and their feedback loops constitute the respiratory control center. Under normal resting conditions, neurons in the inspiratory center stimulate contraction of the diaphragm and intercostal muscles via the phrenic and spinal nerves, which creates a negative force in the chest cavity relative to the airway (i.e., a pressure gradient), thus allowing air to flow into the lungs (Fig. 30.8). Subsequent exhalation is typically passive and air is exhaled as a consequence of lung and chest wall elastance or recoil. However, when the respiratory center is stimulated in the presence of carbon dioxide, acidosis, or hypoxemia, exhalation can be made more active by contraction of abdominal and chest wall muscles. The cerebral cortex has the ability to take control of the respiratory system by overriding the brainstem to change the frequency, depth, and rhythm of respirations. This is of minimal concern in the mechanically ventilated patient, whose cerebral cortex is often sedated, either by medications or by illness, such that respiratory neuromuscular function is typically under the control of the brainstem as described above.

The muscular component of the respiratory system has been described as a pump that, when stimulated, creates a pressure, P_{mus} [55]. During assisted mechanical ventilation, this pressure can be added to a second pump, which is the airway pressure generated by the ventilator, P_{aw}. The sum of these two pressures, P_T provides the total driving pressure for inspiratory flow [55]. Although neglecting inertia, the equation for motion in the respiratory system states that P_T is dissipated while overcoming the elastive and resistive properties of the lungs as follows:

$$P_T = P_{mus} + P_{aw} = (E_{rs} \times V_t) + (R_{rs} \times \dot{V})$$

where the variables represent elastance (E_{rs}), tidal volume (V_t), resistance (R_{rs}), and flow ($\dot{V}$) in the respiratory system [55]. Since the ventilator generated pressure, P_{aw}, is intended to unload the patient's respiratory muscles, it should be synchronous with the neural impulses generated by the respiratory center and thus P_{mus}.

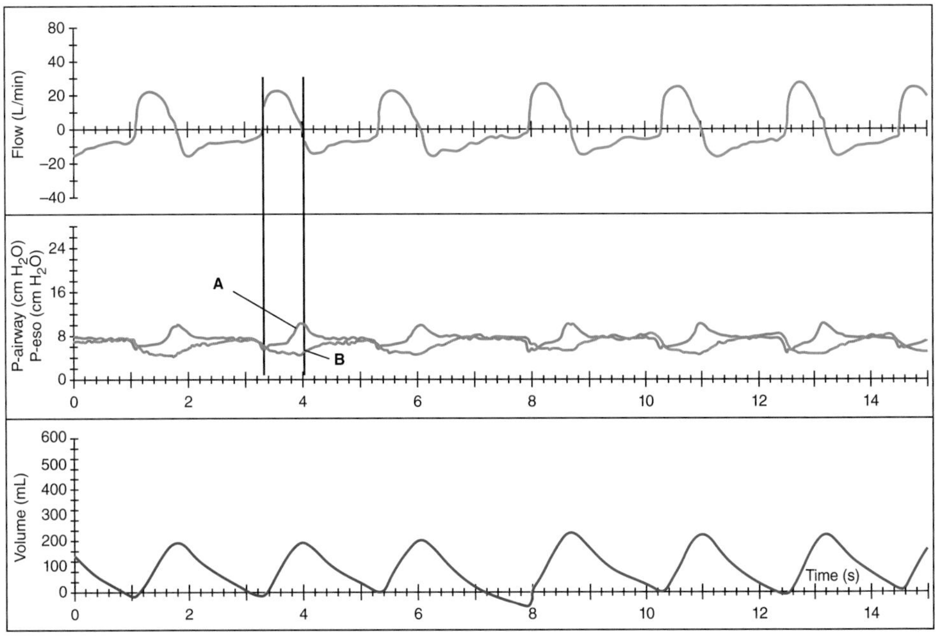

FIGURE 30.8 Spontaneous ventilation with continuous positive airway pressure (CPAP) at 7.5 mm Hg. Airway and esophageal pressure tracings are superimposed and marked as *A* and *B*, respectively. Note the onset of inspiration and flow, marked by the first vertical line, as esophageal (P-eso) and airway (P-air) pressures separate, creating a pressure gradient. Flow then ceases, as marked by the second vertical line, when the expiratory valve is opened on the ventilator and airway pressure quickly decreases.

To be synchronous with the patient driven inspiration, the ventilator would need to initiate support simultaneously with the patient's neural firing at the onset of inspiration, continue this support throughout the neural firing, and stop support at the end of neural firing. In reality, this goal is extremely difficult to achieve, though a newer mode of mechanical ventilation—Neuraly Adjusted Ventilator Assist (NAVA)—which will be described later in this chapter, delivers a pressure that is directly proportional to the integral of the electrical activity of the diaphragm. Rather than monitoring neural impulses, most modern ventilators sense changes in pressure and flow within the circuit in an effort to match the patient's respiratory cycle. The variables that we will discuss in regard to the patient–ventilator interaction include ventilator triggering, cycling-off, and delivery of gas between these two events (i.e., the post-trigger phase). However, it is essential to first define some of the measures of respiratory drive and effort that are commonly used to assess patient–ventilator interaction and weaning such as work of breathing, pressure–time product, airway occlusion pressure, maximal inspiratory force, vital capacity, and rapid shallow breathing index.

Work of Breathing

A patient's respiratory effort is typically discussed and quantified via some measure of the patient's "work of breathing." *Work* is defined as the force acting on an object to cause displacement of that object. Therefore, mechanical "work of breathing" includes the measurement of a force required to create a change in volume of gas and is expressed in Joules per liter. However, measurements that are based on volume frequently fail to account for the work done by the diaphragm and respiratory muscles during isometric contraction against a closed valve [56], as occurs prior to triggering in some assisted modes of ventilation. The pressure–time product (PTP), which measures swings in intrathoracic pressure via an esophageal pressure monitor and correlates with oxygen requirements of breathing, is considered superior for quantifying a patient's effort and degree of unloading [50]. This is a calculation of the difference in the time integrals between esophageal pressure, P_{es} during assisted breathing, and the recoil pressure of the chest wall during passive breathing at a similar tidal volume and flow [56].

Airway Occlusion Pressure

Airway occlusion pressure at 0.1 seconds ($P_{0.1}$) is an indicator of respiratory drive and is determined by measuring the pressure in the airway a tenth of a second after the onset of inspiration, beginning at functional residual capacity (FRC). This has been shown to correlate well with work of breathing during pressure support ventilation [56]. Therefore, several authors have advocated its use as a potential predictor for discontinuation of mechanical ventilation [57–60]. The threshold value for $P_{0.1}$ of 6 cm H_2O appeared to delineate success versus failure in one study. Although the utility of this measurement is still debated, it has been incorporated into several commercially available ventilators.

Maximal Inspiratory Force

Maximal inspiratory pressure (MIP), also known as negative inspiratory force (NIF), is another marker of respiratory muscle function and strength and is determined by measuring the maximum pressure that can be generated by the inspiratory muscles against an occluded airway beginning at FRC. A normal value is considered to be approximately 80 cm H_2O, with respiratory compromise typically observed at values less than 40% of normal. The major disadvantage and limitation of this measurement is the fact that it is extremely effort dependent, which can make its measurement as well as interpretation difficult in severely ill, sedated, and neurologically impaired patients.

Vital Capacity

Vital capacity (VC) is the sum of tidal volume, inspiratory reserve volume, and expiratory reserve volume. Forced vital capacity (FVC) is measured by instructing a patient to inspire maximally to total lung capacity (TLC), followed by forced expiration while measuring the expired volume as the integral of the flow rate. FVC has also been used as an indicator of respiratory muscle function. However, similar to MIP, FVC is also effort dependent and therefore can lead to variable results. With limited success, it has been used to monitor trends in respiratory muscle strength in patients with neurologic impairment and muscle disorders such as cervical spine injury, myasthenia gravis, and the Guillain–Barré syndrome [61–63].

Frequency/Tidal Volume Ratio

Respiratory distress is often marked by tachypnea and decreased tidal volumes, leading to inadequate ventilation and increases in $PaCO_2$ secondary to disproportionate ventilation of anatomic dead space and inadequate alveolar ventilation. Therefore, the ratio of frequency to tidal volume, also known as the rapid shallow breathing index (RSBI), has been used to gauge respiratory distress and facilitate weaning and readiness for extubation [59,64–66]. As a criterion for extubation, the RSBI has had mixed success. Values of 100 to 105 breaths/min/L are typically used as a cutoff to predict extubation success from failure. The RSBI is limited by the fact that rapid and shallow breathing, although sensitive indicators of respiratory distress are not specific. For example, pain and anxiety are also consistent with an abnormally high RSBI and are common among critically ill patients weaning from mechanical ventilation. In a clinical trial using a RSBI of <105 as a strict criteria for a spontaneous breathing trial (SBT), the authors found that a weaning protocol that required a favorable RSBI leads to more time on the ventilator without affecting extubation success [67]. Therefore, the RSBI should not automatically prevent the clinician from proceeding with an SBT unless there is just reason and it may be better as a monitor of progress rather than as a strict extubation criterion. For a more detailed explanation of RSBI and ventilator discontinuation, please see Chapter 168, "Discontinuation of Mechanical Ventilation."

PATIENT VENTILATOR INTERACTION

Ventilator Triggering Variable

During assisted modes of ventilation, the patient's inspiratory effort is sensed by the ventilator, which is then "triggered" to deliver support at a preset volume or pressure (Fig. 30.9). There are two distinct methods of triggering the ventilator-pressure and flow. *Pressure triggering* depends on patient's inspiratory effort, creating a change in pressure that exceeds a preset requirement (typically -2 cm H_2O) to open the inspiratory valve on the ventilator and initiate ventilator support. Likewise, *flow triggering* depends on a patient's inspiratory effort creating flow detected by a flow meter within the inspiratory limb that exceeds a preset threshold (typically 2 L per minute) for triggering the ventilator inspiratory support. The significant difference between these two triggering criteria is the presence of a closed demand

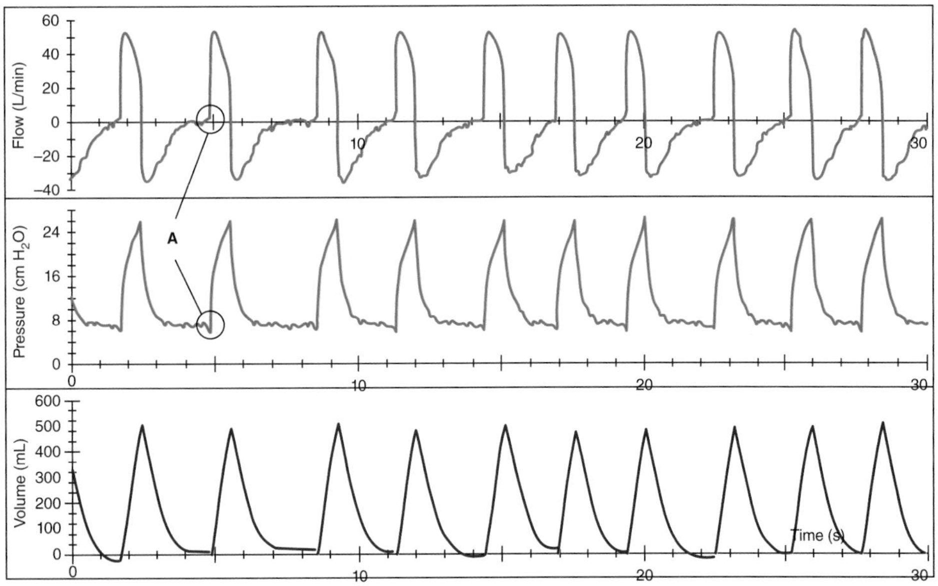

FIGURE 30.9 Normal triggering in assist-control ventilation. The *circles* marked *A* denote the pressure and flow that correspond to patient neural inspiration that is detected by the ventilator and leads to delivery of a mechanical breath.

valve in the inspiratory limb in pressure-triggered ventilators. In general, flow triggering has been considered superior to pressure-triggered algorithms in that it is believed that the work of breathing is less in a system that does not require an initial inspiratory effort against this closed valve. Many studies have compared flow triggering and pressure triggering with respect to work of breathing with most showing significant advantages in favor of flow-triggered systems [68–70]. This is partially explained by the fact that flow triggering results in improved responsiveness with shorter delay between onset of diaphragm contraction and ventilator triggering [70].

The main variable that can be controlled on the ventilator with regard to triggering is termed *sensitivity*. Typical values for pressure triggering are 1 to 2 cm H_2O, while those for flow triggering are 2 to 3 L per minute. The sensitivity threshold is important because it is required to strike a balance between two main problems associated with triggering. First, if the sensitivity is set too low, patients may experience *autotriggering*, in which pressure and flow changes that occur from sources of artifact such as cardiac oscillations, water in the circuit, patient movement or resonance within the system leading to irregular breathing patterns and dyssynchrony. Second, sensitivity settings that are too high will lead to *ineffective triggering*, which has the consequences of increased and wasted work and energy (Fig. 30.10). Ineffective triggering is also common in the setting of dynamic hyperinflation, as seen in obstructive disorders such as asthma and chronic obstructive pulmonary disease. In the setting of obstructive diseases, dynamic hyperinflation leads to elevations in the intrinsic PEEP ($PEEP_i$) above a critical threshold such that the patient's respiratory drive is insufficient to overcome the elastic recoil of the lung and chest wall and trigger the ventilator [50]. Clearly, this is also disadvantageous to the patient in terms of work of breathing and may contribute to ventilator dyssynchrony. Leung et al. [71] demonstrated that ineffective trigger attempts required 38% increases in patient effort as compared to successfully triggered breaths. Obviously, autotriggering and ineffective triggering can create a challenge to the clinician when attempting to optimize the ventilator settings. In general, it is helpful to reduce the trigger threshold to a point where the delay between neural firing and ventilator support is minimized without allowing autotriggering to occur.

Cycle-Off Variable

Neurons in the respiratory center continue firing beyond ventilator triggering and throughout inspiration. The cessation of firing is an important time point in the respiratory cycle and marks the beginning of expiration. The neural inspiratory time is often variable from breath to breath [50]. This can lead to considerable dyssynchrony in controlled modes of ventilation such as assisted-control, pressure-control, and intermittent mandatory ventilation, where the "cycle-off" variable for the ventilator into expiration is the inspiratory time (T_i) and is generally constant from one breath to the next. This can lead to increased sedation requirements, which are inconsistent with the goal of ventilator weaning, as mentioned earlier. Ideally, the ventilator should be able to detect the end of neural firing and react accordingly to halt the inspiratory pressure supplied. This is one of the goals and advantages of the "supportive" modes of ventilation such as pressure support ventilation.

Supportive modes of ventilation have the ability to detect patient expiration and stop ventilator inspiration such that the T_i is variable. This can be accomplished by measuring flow or pressure changes within the circuit. As neural firing ceases and P_{mus} decreases to baseline with muscle relaxation, total pressure and thus flow should decrease according to the elastive and resistive properties of the lung according to the equation of motion previously described. Typically, support modes have software that detects a preset decrement in flow, which in turn leads to cycling off the inspiratory support. This preset threshold can be an absolute value of flow or a percentage of maximum flow in the circuit, or both. Often, an increase in pressure that exceeds the programmed support level will also signal the ventilator to stop inspiration as well as open the expiratory valve.

Just as with triggering, the cycle-off variable can be a source of serious tribulations with the patient–ventilator interaction. For example, in the setting of decreased lung elastance, such as emphysematous lung disease, flow may not diminish enough to be detected properly despite a drop in P_{mus} at the end of neural inspiratory time. This can lead to patient discomfort and was studied by Jubran et al. [72], who noticed that 5 out of 12 patients with chronic obstructive pulmonary disease required active exhalation to cycle off the ventilator during pressure

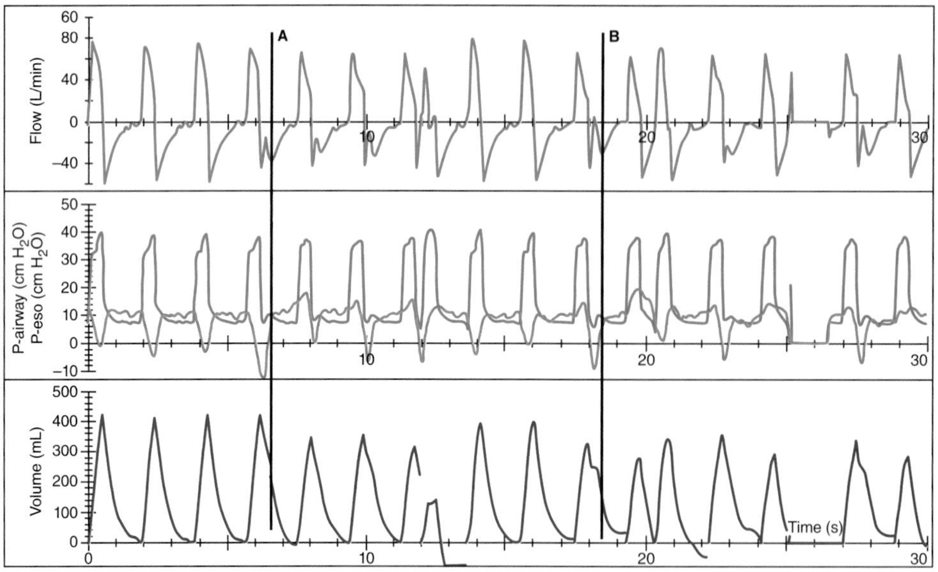

FIGURE 30.10 This pressure and flow tracing demonstrated failed trigger attempts that can be appreciated by the negative deflections in the expiratory limbs in the flow waveform and delineated by lines *A* and *B*.

support ventilation at 20 cm H_2O. Active exhalation is counterproductive to both the primary goal of respiratory muscle unloading and ventilator synchrony (Fig. 30.11). Furthermore, active exhalation will decrease transpulmonary pressure, which can lead to premature airway closure and increased intrinsic $PEEP_i$ as closing capacity increases.

Inspiratory Flow Variable

Inspiratory flow is now being recognized as an important parameter for assisted modes of ventilation. Critically ill patients in acute respiratory failure often have elevated respiratory drives that appear to demand greater flow to overcome the resistance of the failing respiratory system and ventilator breathing circuit [50]. Classically, this appears as a depression on the inspiratory limb of the airway pressure tracing and has been described by some practitioners as "flow hunger" (Fig. 30.12). Clinically, the response has been to increase flow, which typically ranges between 30 and 80 L per minute during assisted modes of mechanical ventilation in an effort to decrease the work of breathing and intrinsic PEEP in these situations. However, a recent series of studies has shown that this may in fact be counterproductive due to a phenomenon now recognized as "flow-associated tachypnea" [50]. Puddy and Younes [73] demonstrated this phenomenon by adjusting inspiratory flow in awake volunteers breathing on a volume-cycled ventilator in assist-control mode in which inspiratory T_i was variable. Laghi et al. [74] later delineated the contributions of flow, tidal volume, and inspiratory time in their study in which flow was increased from 60 to 90 L per minute and balanced with tidal volume settings of 1.0 and 1.5 L to maintain a constant inspiratory time, where frequency did not change. They were able to show that imposed ventilator inspiratory time during mechanical ventilation can determine

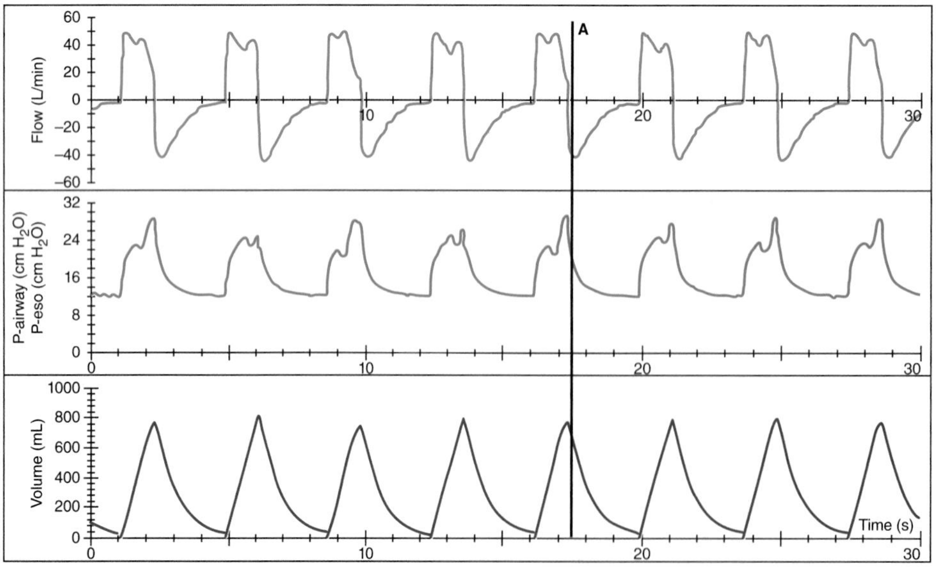

FIGURE 30.11 The pressure and flow waveforms demonstrate active recruitment of expiratory muscles to terminate ventilator inspiration. Note the time point marked by line *A* in which flow decreases rapidly corresponding to a sharp increase in the airway pressure due to active exhalation.

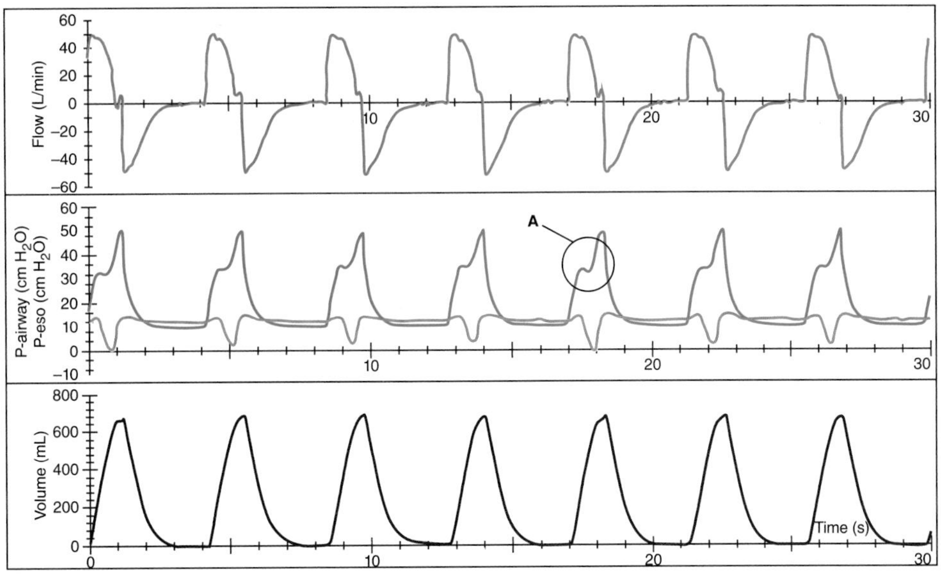

FIGURE 30.12 The pressure and flow waveforms above demonstrate the classic depressions on the inspiratory airway (P-air) pressure tracing in a patient with an elevated respiratory drive as highlighted by *circle A*. P-eso, esophageal pressure.

frequency independent of delivered inspiratory flow and tidal volume. Therefore, the clinician must consider the counteracting *variables* of flow, tidal volume, and inspiratory time when attempting to ventilate patients with elevated respiratory drive in acute respiratory failure and how one may negatively influence the other.

Neurally Adjusted Ventilator Assist (NAVA)

Thille et al. have shown that as many as 24% of intubated patients undergoing pressure support ventilation had severe asynchrony [75]. Asynchrony increases respiratory muscle load [55] and is associated with longer duration of mechanical ventilation [75,76]. Neurally Adjusted Ventilator Assist (NAVA) is a method of ventilation designed to improve patient comfort and ventilator synchrony. By improving the ventilator synchrony to better correlate with a patient's neuronal respiratory drive, one could decrease the work of breathing and possibly the duration of mechanical ventilation.

More specifically, NAVA is a pressure-assisted mode of MV, which delivers a pressure proportional to the integral of the electrical activity of the diaphragm (EAdi) recorded continuously through an esophageal probe and therefore is proportional to the neural output of the patient's central respiratory command [77]. As a result, it depends on the patient's respiratory center neural output how much pressure is delivered. Correct positioning of the esophageal probe is of paramount importance for obtaining representative EAdi signals from the diaphragm. Barwing et al. found that positioning the EAdi-catheter using a method of measurement from the nose, ear and xiphoid, gives a good approximation of the catheter position in most patients [78].

With NAVA, the ventilator is triggered and cycled-off based on the EAdi value, which directly reflects the activity of the neural respiratory command [79]. The inspiratory airway pressure applied by the ventilator is determined by the following equation:

$$P_{aw} = \text{NAVA level} \times \text{EAdi}$$

where P_{aw} is the instantaneous airway pressure (cm H_2O), EAdi is the instantaneous integral of the diaphragmatic electrical activity signal (μV), and the NAVA level (cm H_2O/μV or per arbitrary unit) is a proportionality constant set by the clinician [79]. NAVA thus has two important features: the delivered pressure is, in theory, synchronous with the diaphragmatic activity and the tidal volume is completely controlled by the output of the patient's respiratory control center [77]. Therefore, the level of pressure delivered is determined by the patient's respiratory-center neural output [79].

In a prospective interventional study of spontaneously breathing patients with respiratory failure, Piquilloud et al. compared the inspiratory trigger delay, the excess inspiratory time and the frequency of patient–ventilator asynchrony between 22 patients. Compared with standard pressure support ventilation (PSV), NAVA improved patient–ventilator synchrony by reducing the inspiratory trigger delay and the total number of asynchrony events and by improving expiratory cycling-off [80]. Furthermore, there is good evidence suggesting that NAVA—as compared to PSV—offers protection against excessive P_{aw} and tidal volume values because there is a downregulation of EAdi in response to increasing assistance levels [80–85].

SUMMARY

Respiratory monitoring is a complicated task for the critically ill patient who requires mechanical ventilation. The clinician must carefully balance a plethora of data acquired from studying variables of gas exchange, pulmonary mechanics, neuromuscular function, and patient–ventilator interactions. Skilled intensive care–trained personnel must then process these data so that a plan of respiratory support, often with mechanical ventilation, can be instituted. This plan must proceed in such a way that the patient is safely ventilated and oxygenated without imposing the undo harm that is associated with injurious modes of mechanical ventilation.

References

1. Kelly AM, Kyle E, McAlpine R: Venous pCO(2) and pH can be used to screen for significant hypercarbia in emergency patients with acute respiratory disease. *J Emerg Med* 22(1):15–19, 2002.
2. Weil MH, Rackow EC, Trevino R, et al: Difference in acid-base state between venous and arterial blood during cardiopulmonary resuscitation. *N Engl J Med* 315(3):153–156, 1986.

3. Malinoski DJ, Todd SR, Slone S, et al: Correlation of central venous and arterial blood gas measurements in mechanically ventilated trauma patients. *Arch Surg* 140(11):1122–1125, 2005.
4. Isserles SA, Breen PH: Can changes in end-tidal PCO_2 measure changes in cardiac output? *Anesth Analg* 73(6):808–814, 1991.
5. Jin X, Weil MH, Tang W, et al: End-tidal carbon dioxide as a noninvasive indicator of cardiac index during circulatory shock. *Crit Care Med* 28(7):2415–2419, 2000.
6. Pernat A, Weil MH, Sun S, et al: Stroke volumes and end-tidal carbon dioxide generated by precordial compression during ventricular fibrillation. *Crit Care Med* 31(6):1819–1823, 2003.
7. Callaway C, Soar J, Aibiki M, et al: Part 4: advanced life support: 2015 International Consensus on cardiopulmonary resuscitation and emergency cardiovascular care science with treatment recommendations. *Circulation* 132[16 Suppl 1]:S84–145, 2015.
8. Einav S, Bromiker R, Weiniger CF, et al: Mathematical modeling for prediction of survival from resuscitation based on computerized continuous capnography: proof of concept. *Acad Emerg Med* 18(5):468–475, 2011.
9. Meaney PA, Bobrow BJ, Mancini ME, et al: Cardiopulmonary resuscitation quality: [Corrected] improving cardiac resuscitation outcomes both inside and outside the hospital: a consensus statement from the American Heart Association. *Circulation* 128(4):417–435, 2013.
10. West JB, Dollery CT, Naimark A: Distribution of blood flow in isolated lung; relation to vascular and alveolar pressures. *J Appl Physiol* 19:713–724, 1964.
11. Kallet RH, Daniel BM, Garcia O, et al: Accuracy of physiologic dead space measurements in patients with acute respiratory distress syndrome using volumetric capnography: comparison with the metabolic monitor method. *Respir Care* 50(4):462–467, 2005.
12. Kallet RH, Alonso JA, Pittet JF, et al: Prognostic value of the pulmonary dead-space fraction during the first 6 days of acute respiratory distress syndrome. *Respir Care* 49(9):1008–1014, 2004.
13. Wathanasormsiri A, Preutthipan A, Chantarojanasiri T, et al: Dead space ventilation in volume controlled versus pressure controlled mode of mechanical ventilation. *J Med Assoc Thai* 85 Suppl 4:S1207–S1212, 2002.
14. Mohr AM, Rutherford EJ, Cairns BA, et al: The role of dead space ventilation in predicting outcome of successful weaning from mechanical ventilation. *J Trauma* 51(5):843–848, 2001.
15. Bates JH, Rossi A, Milic-Emili J: Analysis of the behavior of the respiratory system with constant inspiratory flow. *J Appl Physiol* 58(6):1840–1848, 1985.
16. Polese G, Rossi A, Appendini L, et al: Partitioning of respiratory mechanics in mechanically ventilated patients. *J Appl Physiol* 71(6):2425–2433, 1991.
17. Amato MBP, Meade MO, Slutsky AS, et al: Driving pressure and survival in the acute respiratory distress syndrome. *N Engl J Med* 372:747–755, 2015.
18. Iotti GA, Braschi A, Brunner JX, et al: Respiratory mechanics by least squares fitting in mechanically ventilated patients: applications during paralysis and during pressure support ventilation. *Intensive Care Med* 21(5):406–413, 1995.
19. Stenqvist O: Practical assessment of respiratory mechanics. *Br J Anaesth* 91(1):92–105, 2003.
20. Lu Q, Vieira SR, Richecoeur J, et al: A simple automated method for measuring pressure-volume curves during mechanical ventilation. *Am J Respir Crit Care Med* 159(1):275–282, 1999.
21. Servillo G, Coppola M, Blasi F, et al: The measurement of the pressure-volume curves with computerized methods. *Minerva Anestesiol* 66(5):381–385, 2000.
22. Roupie E, Dambrosio M, Servillo G, et al: Titration of tidal volume and induced hypercapnia in acute respiratory distress syndrome. *Am J Respir Crit Care Med* 152(1):121–128, 1995.
23. Harris RS, Hess DR, Venegas JG: An objective analysis of the pressure-volume curve in the acute respiratory distress syndrome. *Am J Respir Crit Care Med* 161(2 Pt 1):432–439, 2000.
24. Hubmayr RD: Perspective on lung injury and recruitment: a skeptical look at the opening and collapse story. *Am J Respir Crit Care Med* 165(12):1647–1653, 2002.
25. Martin-Lefevre L, Ricard JD, Roupie E, et al: Significance of the changes in the respiratory system pressure-volume curve during acute lung injury in rats. *Am J Respir Crit Care Med* 164(4):627–632, 2001.
26. Amato MB, Barbas CS, Medeiros DM, et al: Effect of a protective-ventilation strategy on mortality in the acute respiratory distress syndrome. *N Engl J Med* 338(6):347–354, 1998.
27. The Acute Respiratory Distress Syndrome Network: Ventilation with lower tidal volumes as compared with traditional tidal volumes for acute lung injury and the acute respiratory distress syndrome. *N Engl J Med* 342(18):1301–1308, 2000.
28. Brower RG, Lanken PN, MacIntyre N, et al: Higher versus lower positive end-expiratory pressures in patients with the acute respiratory distress syndrome. *N Engl J Med* 351(4):327–336, 2004.
29. Meade MO, Cook DJ, Guyatt GH, et al: Ventilation strategy using low tidal volumes, recruitment maneuvers, and high positive end-expiratory pressure for acute lung injury and acute respiratory distress syndrome: a randomized controlled trial. *JAMA* 299(6):637–645, 2008.
30. Mercat A, Richard J-CM, Vielle B, et al: Positive end-expiratory pressure setting in adults with acute lung injury and acute respiratory distress syndrome: a randomized controlled trial. *JAMA* 299(6):646–655, 2008.
31. Goligher EC, Kavanagh BP, Rubenfeld GD, et al: Oxygenation response to positive end-expiratory pressure predicts mortality in acute respiratory distress syndrome. A secondary analysis of the LOVS and ExPress trials. *Am J Respir Crit Care Med* 190(1):70–76, 2014.
32. Grasso S, Stripoli T, De Michele M, et al: ARDSnet ventilatory protocol and alveolar hyperinflation: role of positive end-expiratory pressure. *Am J Respir Crit Care Med* 176(8):761–767, 2007.
33. Terragni PP, Filippini C, Slutsky AS, et al: Accuracy of plateau pressure and stress index to identify injurious ventilation in patients with acute respiratory distress syndrome. *Anesthesiology* 119(4):880–889, 2013.
34. Grasso S, Terragni P, Mascia L, et al: Airway pressure-time curve profile (stress index) detects tidal recruitment/hyperinflation in experimental acute lung injury. *Crit Care Med* 32(4):1018–1027, 2004.
35. Ranieri VM, Zhang H, Mascia L, et al: Pressure-time curve predicts minimally injurious ventilatory strategy in an isolated rat lung model. *Anesthesiology* 93(5):1320–1328, 2000.
36. Ferrando C, Suárez-Sipmann F, Gutierrez A, et al: Adjusting tidal volume to stress index in an open lung condition optimizes ventilation and prevents overdistension in an experimental model of lung injury and reduced chest wall compliance. *Crit Care* 19(1):9, 2015.
37. de Chazal I, Hubmayr RD: Novel aspects of pulmonary mechanics in intensive care. *Br J Anaesth* 91(1):81–91, 2003.
38. Pelosi P, Goldner M, McKibben A, et al: Recruitment and derecruitment during acute respiratory failure: an experimental study. *Am J Respir Crit Care Med* 164(1):122–130, 2001.
39. Talmor D, Sarge T, O'Donnell CR, et al: Esophageal and transpulmonary pressures in acute respiratory failure. *Crit Care Med* 34(5):1389–1394, 2006.
40. Brochard L, Roudot-Thoraval F, Roupie E, et al: Tidal volume reduction for prevention of ventilator-induced lung injury in acute respiratory distress syndrome. The Multicenter Trail Group on Tidal Volume reduction in ARDS. *Am J Respir Crit Care Med* 158(6):1831–1838, 1998.
41. Stewart TE, Meade MO, Cook DJ, et al: Evaluation of a ventilation strategy to prevent barotrauma in patients at high risk for acute respiratory distress syndrome. Pressure- and Volume-Limited Ventilation Strategy Group. *N Engl J Med* 338(6):355–361, 1998.
42. Matthay MA, Bhattacharya S, Gaver D, et al: Ventilator-induced lung injury: in vivo and in vitro mechanisms. *Am J Physiol Lung Cell Mol Physiol* 283(4):L678–L682, 2002.
43. Terragni PP, Rosboch GL, Lisi A, et al: How respiratory system mechanics may help in minimising ventilator-induced lung injury in ARDS patients. *Eur Respir J Suppl* 42:15s–21s, 2003.
44. Milic-Emili J, Mead J, Turner JM, et al: Improved technique for estimating pleural pressure from esophageal baloons. *J Appl Physiol* 19(2):207–211, 1964.
45. Talmor D, Sarge T, Malhotra A, et al: Mechanical ventilation guided by esophageal pressure in acute lung injury. *N Engl J Med* 359(20):2095–2104, 2008.
46. Fish E, Novack V, Banner-Goodspeed VM, et al: The Esophageal Pressure-Guided Ventilation 2 (EPVent2) trial protocol: a multicentre, randomised clinical trial of mechanical ventilation guided by transpulmonary pressure. *BMJ Open* 4(9):e006356, 2014.
47. Malbrain ML: Abdominal pressure in the critically ill: measurement and clinical relevance. *Intensive Care Med* 25(12):1453–1458, 1999.
48. Collee GG, Lomax DM, Ferguson C, et al: Bedside measurement of intra-abdominal pressure (IAP) via an indwelling naso-gastric tube: clinical validation of the technique. *Intensive Care Med* 19(8):478–480, 1993.
49. Chieveley-Williams S, Dinner L, Puddicombe A, et al: Central venous and bladder pressure reflect transdiaphragmatic pressure during pressure support ventilation. *Chest* 121(2):533–538, 2002.
50. Tobin MJ, Jubran A, Laghi F: Patient-ventilator interaction. *Am J Respir Crit Care Med* 163(5):1059–1063, 2001.
51. Carson SS, Kress JP, Rodgers JE, et al: A randomized trial of intermittent lorazepam versus propofol with daily interruption in mechanically ventilated patients. *Crit Care Med* 34(5):1326–1332, 2006.
52. Kress JP, Pohlman AS, O'Connor MF, et al: Daily interruption of sedative infusions in critically ill patients undergoing mechanical ventilation. *N Engl J Med* 342(20):1471–1477, 2000.
53. Prielipp RC, Coursin DB, Wood KE, et al: Complications associated with sedative and neuromuscular blocking drugs in critically ill patients. *Crit Care Clin* 11(4):983–1003, 1995.
54. Le Bourdelles G, Viires N, Boczkowski J, et al: Effects of mechanical ventilation on diaphragmatic contractile properties in rats. *Am J Respir Crit Care Med* 149(6):1539–1544, 1994.
55. Kondili E, Prinianakis G, Georgopoulos D: Patient-ventilator interaction. *Br J Anaesth* 91(1):106–119, 2003.
56. Jubran A: Advances in respiratory monitoring during mechanical ventilation. *Chest* 116(5):1416–1425, 1999.
57. Capdevila X, Perrigault PF, Ramonatxo M, et al: Changes in breathing pattern and respiratory muscle performance parameters during difficult weaning. *Crit Care Med* 26(1):79–87, 1998.
58. Murciano D, Boczkowski J, Lecocguic Y, et al: Tracheal occlusion pressure: a simple index to monitor respiratory muscle fatigue during acute respiratory failure in patients with chronic obstructive pulmonary disease. *Ann Intern Med* 108(6):800–805, 1988.
59. Sassoon CS, Mahutte CK: Airway occlusion pressure and breathing pattern as predictors of weaning outcome. *Am Rev Respir Dis* 148(4 Pt 1):860–866, 1993.
60. Sassoon CS, Te TT, Mahutte CK, et al: Airway occlusion pressure. An important indicator for successful weaning in patients with chronic obstructive pulmonary disease. *Am Rev Respir Dis* 135(1):107–113, 1987.
61. Chevrolet JC, Deleamont P: Repeated vital capacity measurements as predictive parameters for mechanical ventilation need and weaning success in the Guillain-Barre syndrome. *Am Rev Respir Dis* 144(4):814–818, 1991.
62. Loveridge BM, Dubo HI: Breathing pattern in chronic quadriplegia. *Arch Phys Med Rehabil* 71(7):495–499, 1990.
63. Rieder P, Louis M, Jolliet P, et al: The repeated measurement of vital capacity is a poor predictor of the need for mechanical ventilation in myasthenia gravis. *Intensive Care Med* 21(8):663–668, 1995.

64. Krieger BP, Isber J, Breitenbucher A, et al: Serial measurements of the rapid-shallow-breathing index as a predictor of weaning outcome in elderly medical patients. *Chest* 112(4):1029–1034, 1997.
65. Vallverdu I, Calaf N, Subirana M, et al: Clinical characteristics, respiratory functional parameters, and outcome of a two-hour T-piece trial in patients weaning from mechanical ventilation. *Am J Respir Crit Care Med* 158(6):1855–1862, 1998.
66. Yang KL, Tobin MJ: A prospective study of indexes predicting the outcome of trials of weaning from mechanical ventilation. *N Engl J Med* 324(21):1445–1450, 1991.
67. Tanios M, Nevins M, Hendra K, et al: A randomized, controlled trial of the role of weaning predictors in clinical decision making. *Crit Care Med* 34(10):2530, 2006.
68. Aslanian P, El Atrous S, Isabey D, et al: Effects of flow triggering on breathing effort during partial ventilatory support. *Am J Respir Crit Care Med* 157(1):135–143, 1998.
69. Barrera R, Melendez J, Ahdoot M, et al: Flow triggering added to pressure support ventilation improves comfort and reduces work of breathing in mechanically ventilated patients. *J Crit Care* 14(4):172–176, 1999.
70. Branson RD, Campbell RS, Davis K Jr, et al: Comparison of pressure and flow triggering systems during continuous positive airway pressure. *Chest* 106(2):540–544, 1994.
71. Leung P, Jubran A, Tobin MJ: Comparison of assisted ventilator modes on triggering, patient effort, and dyspnea. *Am J Respir Crit Care Med* 155(6):1940–1948, 1997.
72. Jubran A, Van de Graaff WB, Tobin MJ: Variability of patient-ventilator interaction with pressure support ventilation in patients with chronic obstructive pulmonary disease. *Am J Respir Crit Care Med* 152(1):129–136, 1995.
73. Puddy A, Younes M: Effect of inspiratory flow rate on respiratory output in normal subjects. *Am Rev Respir Dis* 146(3):787–789, 1992.
74. Laghi F, Karamchandani K, Tobin MJ: Influence of ventilator settings in determining respiratory frequency during mechanical ventilation. *Am J Respir Crit Care Med* 160(5 Pt 1):1766–1770, 1999.
75. Thille AW, Rodriguez P, Cabello B, et al: Patient–ventilator asynchrony during assisted mechanical ventilation. *Intensive Care Med* 32:1515–1522, 2006.
76. Chao DC, Scheinhorn DJ, Stearn-Hassenpflug M: Patient-ventilator trigger asynchrony in prolonged mechanical ventilation. *Chest* 112:1592–1599, 1997.
77. Sinderby C, Navalesi P, Beck J, et al: Neural control of mechanical ventilation in respiratory failure. *Nat Med* 5:1433–1436, 1999.
78. Barwing J, Ambold M, Linden N, et al: Evaluation of the catheter positioning for neurally adjusted ventilatory assist. *Intensive Care Med* 35:1809–1814, 2009.
79. Terzi N, Piquilloud L, Rozé H, et al: Clinical review: update on neurally adjusted ventilatory assist—report of a round-table conference. *Crit Care* 16(3):225, 2012.
80. Piquilloud L, Vignaux L, Bialais E, et al: Neurally adjusted ventilatory assist improves patient–ventilator interaction. *Intensive Care Med* 37:263–271, 2011.
81. Brander L, Leong-Poi H, Beck J, et al: Titration and implementation of neurally adjusted ventilatory assist in critically ill patients. *Chest* 135:695–703, 2009.
82. Colombo D, Cammarota G, Bergamaschi V, et al: Physiologic response to varying levels of pressure support and neutrally adjusted ventilatory assist in patients with acute respiratory failure. *Intensive Care Med* 34:2010–2018, 2008.
83. Allo JC, Beck JC, Brander L, et al: Influence of neurally adjusted ventilatory assist and positive end-expiratory pressure on breathing pattern in rabbits with acute lung injury. *Crit Care Med* 34:2997–3004, 2006.
84. Brander L, Sinderby C, Lecomte F, et al: Neurally adjusted ventilatory assist decreases ventilator-induced lung injury and non-pulmonary organ dysfunction in rabbits with acute lung injury. *Intensive Care Med* 35:1979–1989, 2009.
85. Sinderby C, Beck J, Spahija J, et al: Inspiratory muscle unloading by neurally adjusted ventilatory assist during maximal inspiratory efforts in healthy subjects. *Chest* 131:711–717, 2007.

Chapter 31 ■ Neurologic Multimodal Monitoring

RAPHAEL A. CARANDANG • WILEY R. HALL

Neurologic function is a major determinant of quality of life. Injury or dysfunction can have profound effects on a patient's ability to be alert, communicate, and interact with his or her environment meaningfully, and function as an independent human being. The brain is a highly complex organ with specialized areas of function and is exquisitely sensitive to metabolic and physical insults such as hypoxemia, acidosis, trauma, and hypoperfusion. The goal of neurocritical care is to protect the brain and preserve neurologic functions for the critically ill patient. The impetus for multimodal monitoring of brain function arises from both its importance and vulnerability and also the difficulty in obtaining a satisfactory assessment of function in the setting of numerous insults and processes including toxic and metabolic encephalopathy, sedation and chemical restraints, and primary central nervous system (CNS) processes like stroke and traumatic brain injury (TBI).

There has been rapid growth and there continues to be much interest in the field as numerous devices and modalities are developed to monitor brain function and processes including intracranial pressure (ICP) monitoring, electroencephalography, corticography, global and regional brain tissue oxygen monitoring, cerebral blood flow (CBF) measurements, and neurochemical and cellular metabolism assessment by microdialysis.

As with any diagnostic or therapeutic tool, an understanding of the indications, limitations, risks and benefits of an intervention are essential in the effective utilization, interpretation, and application of the obtained information to the management of the individual patient. Important characteristics of monitoring devices include the ability to detect important abnormalities (sensitivity), to differentiate between dissimilar disease states (specificity), and to prompt changes in care that alter long-term outcomes (Table 31.1). Limitations of techniques include risks to patients (during placement, use, and removal), variability errors in generation of data (e.g., calibration and drift), and inherent trade-offs between specificity and sensitivity. Monitors with high specificity—values fall outside of threshold levels only when a disease state is unequivocally present—are unlikely to detect less profound levels of disease, while monitors with high sensitivity (will detect any value outside of the normal range) are likely to demonstrate small deviations from normal, which may be trivial in individual patients. The advantage of multimodal monitoring is it increases the sensitivity and accuracy of our detection of physiologic and cellular changes that signal further impending clinical deterioration by using different monitoring modalities in a complementary fashion. A legitimate concern raised by some is that the vast amounts of data generated by these devices require computer-supported data analyses that have been costly and time-consuming, may overwhelm the ill-prepared clinician, and could negate whatever benefits may be gained from the new technology [1]. Most agree that careful consideration should go into selecting the appropriate patient to monitor, the modalities to use, and that determining the most beneficial application of these technologies requires further prospective study.

The compelling theoretical importance of brain monitoring is based on the high vulnerability of the brain to hypoxic and ischemic injuries. The brain uses more oxygen and glucose per weight of tissue than any other organ, yet has no appreciable reserves of oxygen or glucose. The brain is thus completely dependent on uninterrupted CBF to supply metabolic substrates that are required for continued function and survival and to remove toxic by-products. Even transient interruptions of CBF, whether local or global, can injure or kill neural cells. These perturbations may not result in immediate cell death, but can initiate metabolic or cellular processes (e.g., gene transcription, secondary injury) that may lead to cell death days, months, or years after the insult. Therefore, clinical monitoring of neuronal well-being should emphasize early detection and reversal of potentially harmful conditions. Although there are limited conclusive data to demonstrate that

TABLE 31.1

Glossary of Neurologic Monitor Characteristics

Term	Definition
Bias	Average difference (positive or negative) between monitored values and "gold standard" values
Precision	Standard deviation of the differences (bias) between measurements
Sensitivity	Probability that the monitor will demonstrate cerebral ischemia when cerebral ischemia is present
Positive predictive value	Probability that cerebral ischemia is present when the monitor suggests cerebral ischemia
Specificity	Probability that the monitor will not demonstrate cerebral ischemia when cerebral ischemia is not present
Negative predictive value	Probability that cerebral ischemia is not present when the monitor reflects no cerebral ischemia
Threshold value	The value used to separate acceptable (i.e., no ischemia present) from unacceptable (i.e., ischemia present)
Speed	The time elapsed from the onset of actual ischemia or the risk of ischemia until the monitor provides evidence

morbidity and mortality are reduced by the information gathered from current neurologic monitoring techniques, most clinicians caring for patients with critical neurologic illness have confidence that their use improves management. In this chapter, we review currently available techniques with an emphasis on the current scientific literature and indications for utilization.

GOALS OF BRAIN MONITORING

Monitoring devices cannot independently improve outcomes. Instead, they contribute physiologic data that can be integrated into a care plan that, while frequently adding risks (associated with placement, use, and removal), may lead to an overall decrease in morbidity and mortality.

Neurologic monitoring can be categorized into three main groups: (1) monitors of neurologic function (e.g., neurologic examination, electroencephalogram [EEG], evoked potentials, functional magnetic resonance imaging [MRI]), (2) monitors of physiologic parameters (e.g., ICP, CBP, transcranial Doppler), and (3) monitors of cellular metabolism (e.g., jugular venous oxygen saturation [$SjvO_2$], near-infrared spectroscopy [NIRS], brain tissue oxygen tension, microdialysis, positron emission tomography [PET], magnetic resonance spectroscopy). Most categorizations are arbitrary and obviously overlaps and interrelationships between modalities (e.g., blood flow and electrical activity, oxygenation, and perfusion) blur the lines of distinction. All categories provide information that may be useful in assessing the current status of the brain and nervous system and in directing therapies as well as monitoring responses to interventions, but it cannot be overemphasized that the data obtained from these monitoring devices should always be interpreted in relation to the overall clinical picture of the individual patient.

CEREBRAL ISCHEMIA AND BLOOD FLOW

Given the brain's dependence and sensitivity to perturbations of oxygenation, many, if not all, monitors are concerned with the detection of cerebral ischemia defined as cerebral delivery of oxygen (CDO_2) insufficient to meet metabolic needs. Cerebral ischemia is traditionally characterized as global or focal, and complete or incomplete (Table 31.2). Systemic monitors readily detect most global cerebral insults, such as hypotension, hypoxemia, or cardiac arrest. Brain-specific monitors can provide additional information primarily for situations, such as stroke, subarachnoid hemorrhage (SAH) with vasospasm, and TBI, for which systemic oxygenation and perfusion can appear to be adequate when focal cerebral oxygenation is impaired.

The severity of ischemic brain damage has traditionally been thought to be proportional to the magnitude and duration of reduced CDO_2. For monitoring to influence long-term patient morbidity and mortality, prompt recognition of reversible cerebral hypoxia/ischemia is essential. Numerous animal studies and human studies using different imaging techniques such as PET, MRI, and single-photon emission computed tomography (SPECT) have concluded that the ischemic threshold for reversible injury or penumbra is a CBF of 20 mL/100 g/minute below which tissue is at risk of irreversible damage [2,3]. The tolerable duration of more profound ischemia is inversely proportional to the severity of CBF reduction (Fig. 31.1). Ischemia and hypoxemia initiate a cascade of cellular reactions that involve multiple pathways including energy failure from anaerobic glycolysis with accumulation of lactic acid and increase in lactate/pyruvate ratios, loss of ion homeostasis and failure of ATP-dependent ion pumps to maintain ion gradients. This leads to sodium and calcium influx into the cell and activation of enzymes such as phospholipases that result in further membrane and cytoskeletal damage, glutamate release and excitotoxicity, lipoperoxidases and free fatty acid breakdown, and free radical formation and inflammation with microvascular changes. Endonucleases which alter gene regulation and protein synthesis and activate the caspase pathways that trigger apoptosis are also released [4,5]. Other proteins synthesized in response to altered oxygen delivery, such as hypoxia-inducible factors, have been identified as adaptive mechanisms that respond to variations in oxygen partial pressure [6] and may be protective. These multiple pathways and cellular mediators and their interactions are potential areas for therapeutic intervention. By-products of these reactions provide potential biomarkers for secondary injury

TABLE 31.2

Characteristics of Types of Cerebral Ischemic Insults

Characteristics	Examples
Global, incomplete	Hypotension, hypoxemia, cardiopulmonary resuscitation
Global, complete	Cardiac arrest
Focal, incomplete	Stroke, subarachnoid hemorrhage with vasospasm

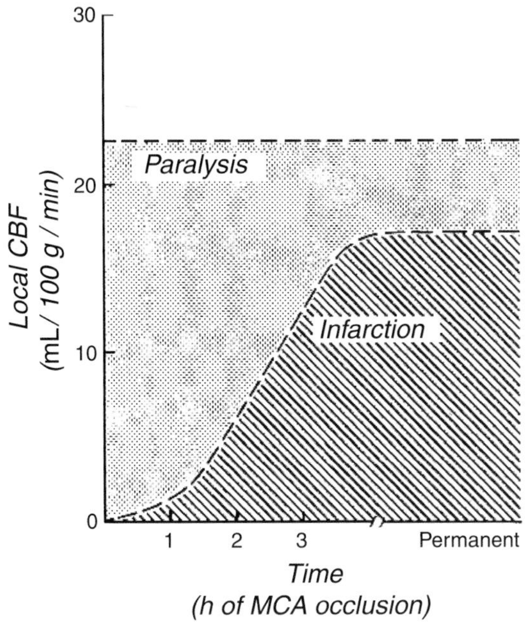

FIGURE 31.1 Schematic representation of ischemic thresholds in awake monkeys. The threshold for reversible paralysis occurs at local cerebral blood flow (local CBF) of approximately 23 mL/100 g/min. Irreversible injury (infarction) is a function of the magnitude of blood flow reduction and the duration of that reduction. Relatively severe ischemia is potentially reversible if the duration is sufficiently short. MCA, middle ceberal artery. (From Jones TH, Morawetz RB, Crowell RM, et al: Thresholds of focal cerebral ischemia in awake monkeys. *J Neurosurg* 54:773–782, 1981, with permission.)

that can be used for monitoring. Our current understanding of how the data is best used is still evolving; and currently, when a cerebral monitor detects ischemia, the results must be carefully interpreted. Often, all that is known is that cerebral oxygenation in the region of the brain that is assessed by that monitor has fallen below a critical threshold. Such information neither definitively implies that ischemia will necessarily progress to infarction nor does it clearly define what biochemical or genetic transcriptional changes may subsequently occur. Also, because more severe ischemia produces neurologic injury more quickly than less severe ischemia, time and dose effects must be considered. More importantly, if regional ischemia involves structures that are not components of the monitored variable, then infarction could develop without warning.

Among healthy persons, CBF is tightly regulated through multiple pathways such that CDO_2 is adjusted to meet the metabolic requirements of the brain. In the normal, "coupled" relationship, CBF is dependent on the cerebral metabolic rate for oxygen ($CMRO_2$), which varies directly with body temperature and with the level of brain activation (Fig. 31.2A). As $CMRO_2$ increases or decreases, CBF increases or decreases to match oxygen requirements with oxygen delivery. Pressure autoregulation maintains CBF at a constant rate (assuming unchanged metabolic needs) over a wide range of systemic blood pressures (Fig. 31.2B). When pressure autoregulation is intact, changes in cerebral perfusion pressure (CPP) do not alter CBF over a range of pressures of 50 to 130 mm Hg. CPP can be described by the equation CPP = MAP – ICP, where MAP equals mean arterial pressure. After neurologic insults (e.g., TBI), autoregulation of the cerebral vasculature may be impaired such that CBF may not increase sufficiently in response to decreasing CPP [7]. This failure to maintain adequate CDO_2 can lead to ischemia and add to preexisting brain injury, a process termed secondary injury, at blood pressures that would not normally be associated with cerebral ischemia/injury. Normally, arterial partial pressure of carbon dioxide ($PaCO_2$) significantly regulates cerebral vascular resistance (CVR) over a range of $PaCO_2$ of 20 to 80 mm Hg (Fig. 31.2C). CBF is acutely halved if $PaCO_2$ is halved, and doubled if $PaCO_2$ is doubled. This reduction in CBF (via arteriolar vasoconstriction) results in a decrease in cerebral blood volume and a decrease in ICP. Conceptually, decreasing $PaCO_2$ to decrease ICP may appear to be desirable. Hyperventilation as a clinical tool was described by Lundberg et al. [8] in 1959 as a treatment for increased ICP and was a mainstay of treatment for over 40 years. However, for the healthy brain, there are limits to maximal cerebral vasoconstriction with falling $PaCO_2$ (as well as vasodilation with increasing $PaCO_2$), such that, as CBF decreases to the point of producing inadequate CDO_2, local vasodilatory mechanisms tend to restore CBF and CDO_2. As a consequence, for the healthy brain, hyperventilation does not produce severe cerebral ischemia; however, after TBI, hypocapnia can generate cerebral ischemia as reflected by decreased partial pressure of brain tissue oxygen concentration ($PbtO_2$) and $SjvO_2$ [9,10]. For this reason, hyperventilation has fallen out of favor as a treatment modality for intracranial hypertension and is only used as an immediate intervention to bridge a patient to emergent definitive surgery such as decompressive craniectomy or removal of an offending mass lesion. If hyperventilation is required to acutely reduce ICP, administration of an increased inspired oxygen concentration can markedly increase $SjvO_2$ (Fig. 31.3). In response to decreasing arterial oxygen content (CaO_2), whether the reduction is secondary to

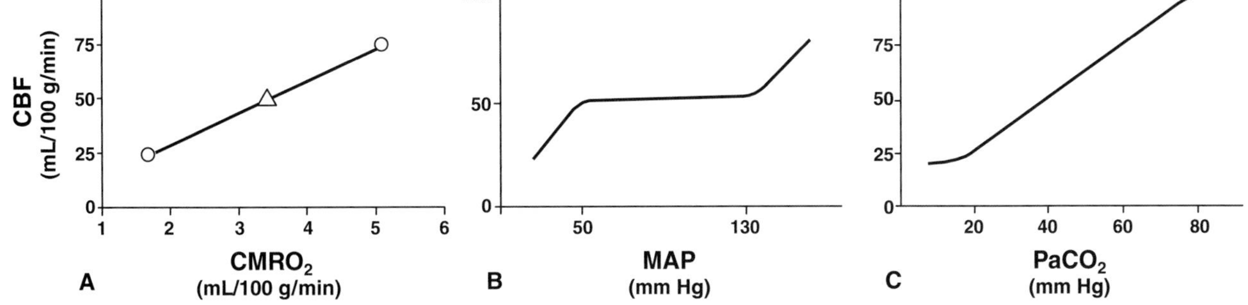

FIGURE 31.2 **A:** The normal relationship between the cerebral metabolic rate of oxygen consumption ($CMRO_2$) and cerebral blood flow (CBF) is characterized by closely coupled changes in both variables. Normally, CBF is 50 mL/100 g/min in adults (*open triangle*). As $CMRO_2$ increases or decreases, CBF changes in a parallel fashion (*solid line*). **B:** Effect of mean arterial pressure (MAP) on CBF. Note that changes in MAP produce little change in CBF over a broad range of pressures. If intracranial pressure (ICP) exceeds normal limits, substitute cerebral perfusion pressure on the horizontal axis. **C:** Effect of $PaCO_2$ on CBF. Changes in $PaCO_2$ exert powerful effects on cerebral vascular resistance across the entire clinically applicable range of values.

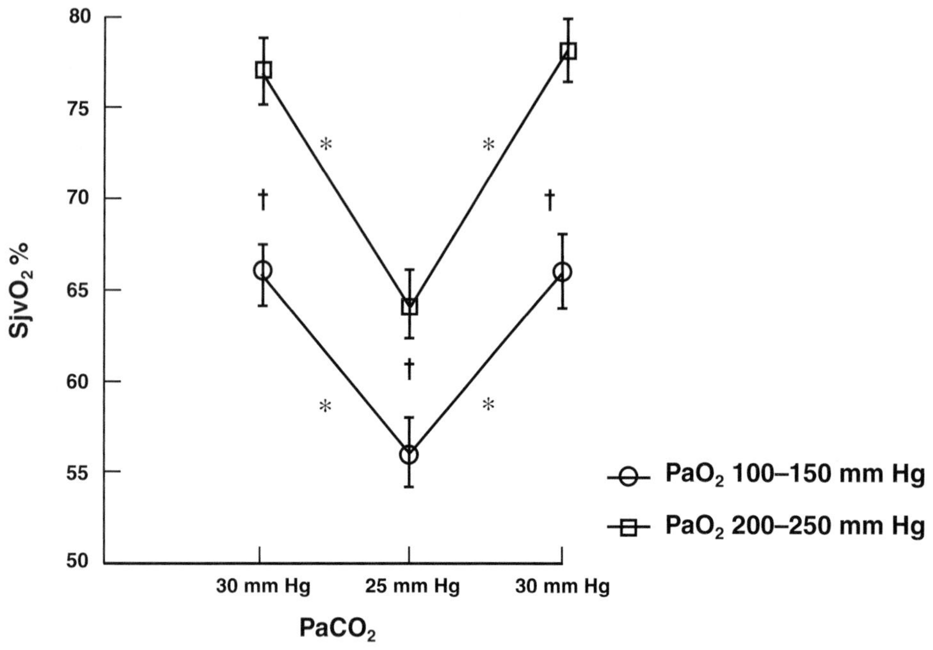

FIGURE 31.3 The effect of hyperoxia on percentage of oxygen saturation of jugular venous blood ($SjvO_2$) at two levels of $PaCO_2$. $^{*}p < 0.001$ for $SjvO_2$ at $PaCO_2$ 25 to 30 mm Hg at each PaO_2. $^{\dagger}p < 0.001$ for $SjvO_2$ between PaO_2 at each $PaCO_2$ level. (From Thiagarajan A, Goverdhan PD, Chari P, et al: The effect of hyperventilation and hyperoxia on cerebral venous oxygen saturation in patients with traumatic brain injury. *Anesth Analg* 87:850–853, 1998, with permission.)

a decrease in hemoglobin (Hgb) concentration or in arterial oxygen saturation (SaO_2), CBF normally increases, although injured brain tissue has impaired ability to increase CBF when it lacks autoregulation [11].

TECHNIQUES OF NEUROLOGIC MONITORING

Neurologic Examination

Frequent and accurately recorded neurologic examinations are an essential aspect of medical care, but are often limited among patients with moderate to severe neurologic compromise. Neurologic examination quantifies three key characteristics: level of consciousness, focal brain dysfunction, and trends in neurologic function. Recognition of changing consciousness or new focal deficits may warn of a variety of treatable conditions, such as progression of intracranial hypertension, new mass lesions such as expansion of intraparenchymal contusions or subdural hematoma and systemic complications of intracranial pathology, such as hyponatremia.

The Glasgow Coma Scale (GCS) score, originally developed as a tool for the assessment of impaired consciousness [12], has also been used as a prognostic tool for patients with TBI [13]. The GCS score at the time of initial hospitalization is used to characterize the severity of TBI, with severe TBI defined as a GCS score less than or equal to 8, moderate TBI as a GCS score of 9 to 12, and mild TBI as that associated with a GCS score greater than 12. Lower GCS scores are generally associated with poorer long-term outcomes, although correlation to individual patients with TBI is complicated by the significant variations of mortality rates and functional outcomes [14]. Significant concern has arisen regarding the validity of the initial GCS score on presentation given the aggressive prehospital management of these patients over the last decade or so, that includes sedation and intubation in the field or the administration of paralytics and sedatives in the emergency room. Some authors have reported a loss of predictive value of the GCS score from 1997 onward and call for a critical reconsideration of its use [15]. Other studies have looked at GCS in the field versus GCS upon arrival and have found good correlation and prognostic value for predicting outcomes and have even found the changes in scores from field GCS to arrival GCS to be highly predictive of outcomes for patients with moderate to severe TBI [16]. Many centers use the best GCS or postresuscitation GCS during the first 24 hours or just the motor component of the GCS instead of initial GCS given these issues. Nevertheless, the GCS score is popular as a quick, reproducible estimate of level of consciousness (Table 31.3). It

TABLE 31.3

Glasgow Coma Scale

Component	Response	Score
Eye opening	Spontaneously	4
	To verbal command	3
	To pain	2
	None	1
		Subtotal: 1–4
Motor response (best extremity)	Obeys verbal command	6
	Localizes pain	5
	Flexion-withdrawal	4
	Flexor (decorticate posturing)	3
	Extensor (decerebrate posturing)	2
	No response (flaccid)	1
		Subtotal: 1–6
Best verbal response	Oriented and converses	5
	Disoriented and converses	4
	Inappropriate words	3
	Incomprehensive sounds	2
	No verbal response	1
		Subtotal: 1–5
		Total: 3–15

is a common tool for the serial monitoring of consciousness, and has been incorporated into various outcome models, such as the Trauma score, Acute Physiology and Chronic Health Evaluation (APACHE), and the Trauma-Injury Severity score. The GCS score, which includes eye opening, motor responses in the best functioning limb, and verbal responses, is limited and by no means replaces a thoughtful and focused neurologic examination. It should be supplemented by recording pupillary size and reactivity, cranial nerve examination, and more detailed neurologic testing depending on the relevant neuroanatomy involved in the disease process. Given the limitations of assessing the GCS, particularly the verbal score in intubated patients, a mathematical model was developed to estimate the verbal score based on the eye and motor scores and is currently being utilized by some stroke trials but needs further validation [17]. A more comprehensive coma assessment score was formulated by Wijdicks and colleagues called the Full Outline of UnResponsiveness or FOUR Score. This removes the verbal score altogether, includes assessments of command following nonverbally, expands the eye assessment to include tracking, blinking to threat and blinking to command, incorporates brainstem function assessments of pupillary and corneal reflexes as well as breathing patterns, and has been validated in multiple populations of critically ill patients and been found to have good prognostic value [18] (Fig. 31.4).

Systemic Monitoring

Although not specific to neurologic monitoring, systemic parameters, including blood pressure, SaO_2, $PaCO_2$, serum glucose concentration, and temperature, have clinical relevance in the management of patients with neurologic dysfunction or injury. The relationships between these systemic variables and long-term outcome after neurologic insults are closely linked and are subject to continuing research.

Perhaps the most important systemic monitor is blood pressure, as CBF is dependent on the relationship between CPP and CVR, and can be modeled generally by the equation: CBF = CPP/CVR. As discussed previously, CBF is maintained relatively constant over a wide range of blood pressures (pressure autoregulation) through arteriolar changes in resistance (assuming no change in brain metabolism) in healthy individuals. After brain injury, autoregulation may become impaired, especially in traumatically brain-injured patients. Chesnut et al. [19,20] reported that even brief periods of hypotension (systolic blood pressure less than 90 mm Hg) worsened outcomes after TBI, and recommended that systolic blood pressure be maintained greater than 90 mm Hg (with possible benefit from higher pressures) [21]. These recommendations have also been promoted by the Brain Trauma Foundation for patients with severe TBI [22]. To achieve this goal, the use of vasoactive substances, such as norepinephrine, may be required [23]. Nevertheless, optimal blood pressure management for patients with TBI has yet to be defined. Some clinical data suggest that the influence of hypotension on outcomes after TBI is equivalent to the influence of hypotension on outcomes after non-neurologic trauma [24]. Current proposed treatment protocols often recommend CPP greater than 50 to 70 mm Hg [25]. The augmentation of CPP above 70 mm Hg with fluids and vasopressors has, however, been associated with increased risk of acute respiratory distress syndrome (ARDS) and is not universally recommended [25]. CPP goals need to be formulated with concomitant assessments of ICP, regional oxygenation and electrical-metabolic brain activity, and cerebral autoregulation.

Another essential step in insuring adequate CDO_2 is the maintenance of adequate CaO_2, which in turn is dependent on Hgb and SaO_2; therefore, anemia and hypoxemia can reduce CDO_2, which would normally result in compensatory increases in CBF. However, these compensatory mechanisms are limited.

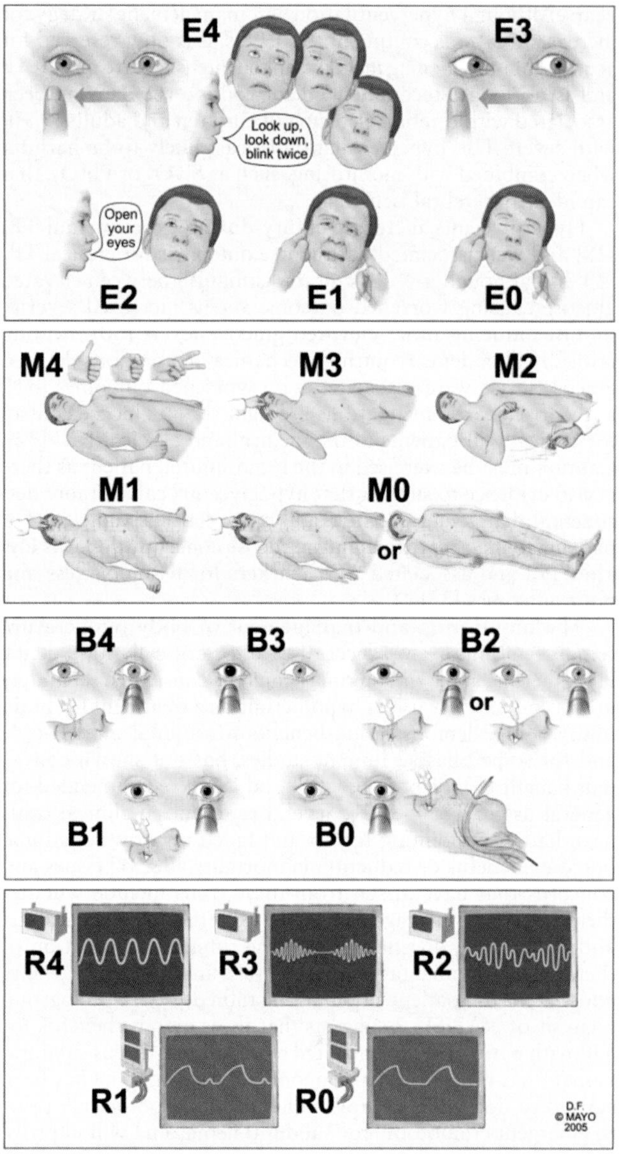

FIGURE 31.4 Description of Full Outline of UnResponsiveness (FOUR) Score. Eye response: E4, eyelids open or opened, tracking, or blinking to command; E3, eyelids open but not tracking; E2, eyelids closed but open to loud voice; E1, eyelids closed but open to pain; E0, eyelids remain closed with pain. Motor response: M4, thumbs-up, fist, or peace sign; M3, localizing to pain; M2, flexion response to pain; M1, extension response to pain; M0, no response to pain or generalized myoclonus status. Brainstem reflexes: B4, pupil and corneal reflexes present; B3, one pupil wide and fixed; B2, pupil or corneal reflexes absent; B1, pupil and corneal reflexes absent; B0, absent pupil, corneal, and cough reflex. Respiration pattern: R4, not intubated, regular breathing pattern; R3, not intubated, Cheyne–Stokes breathing pattern; R2, not intubated, irregular breathing; R1, breathes above ventilatory rate; R0, breathes at ventilator rate or apnea.

As SaO_2 (or PaO_2) decreases below the compensatory threshold, $SjvO_2$ and jugular venous oxygen content ($CjvO_2$), which reflect the ability of CDO_2 to supply $CMRO_2$, also decrease. The correlation is most evident below a PaO_2 of approximately 60 mm Hg, the PaO_2 at which SaO_2 is 90% and below which SaO_2 rapidly decreases. In contrast, as Hgb is reduced by normovolemic hemodilution, $SjvO_2$ remains relatively constant unless severe anemia is present [26].

The management of arterial CO_2 for patients with neurologic injury has changed dramatically during the past 10 years. Although hyperventilation as a management strategy for increased ICP was routine in the 1990s, it is now reserved for acute or life-threatening increases in the intensive care unit (ICU) and is no longer recommended for routine use. Having been associated with cerebral ischemia of children and adults [9,10] with severe TBI, hyperventilation is least likely to be harmful when combined with monitoring, such as $SjvO_2$ or $PbtO_2$, that can identify cerebral ischemia.

Hyperglycemia increased injury during experimental TBI [28] and was associated with worse outcomes for clinical TBI [29,30], although it is difficult to distinguish between elevated glucose causing worsened outcome versus increased severity of TBI inducing more elevated glucose levels [30]. Among critically ill patients requiring mechanical ventilation, elevated glucose levels were associated with worsened outcomes [31], and current recommendations are tight serum glucose control for critically ill patients in the medical and surgical ICU [32]. Caution must be exercised in the brain-injured patient as there is also evidence to suggest that hypoglycemia can be more detrimental than hyperglycemia, and microdialysis studies of TBI patients found that extracellular glucose concentration was low after TBI and associated with markers for tissue distress and poor outcomes [33].

The monitoring and management of body temperature remains an important aspect of care for critically ill patients. Hypothermia and hyperthermia should be considered separately in this context. The use of hypothermia as a treatment for brain injury, while demonstrating benefits for animal models [34] and for some phase 2 human studies, has not shown consistent benefit in larger studies [35] and is not recommended for general use in TBI [36,37]. Several randomized clinical trials have had disappointing results and failed to show functional outcome benefits or reduction in mortality. [38,39] Issues and concerns that have arisen from these trials include whether there was proper management of the side effects of hypothermia and rewarming, questions about the timing and duration of therapy, the optimal target temperature and the heterogeneity and size of the patient population studied [40,41]. Subgroup analysis of NABISH-2 suggests that there may be benefits for TBI with patients with evacuated mass lesions such as subdural hematomas [42,43] and an ongoing multicenter trial has been started to determine if rapid induction of hypothermia prior to emergent craniotomy for subdural hematoma will improve outcomes as measured by Glasgow Outcome Scale-Extended (GOSE) at 6 months [44]. In contrast, induced hypothermia after resuscitation from cardiac arrest (secondary to ventricular tachycardia or fibrillation) has improved outcomes of some trials [45,46].

Hyperthermia is common among critically ill patients, occurring in up to 90% of patients with neurologic disease, related to both diagnosis and length of stay [47,48]. Hyperthermia is generally associated with poorer outcomes when associated with neurologic injury of adults and children [49], but direct evidence for a causal link with adverse outcomes (as with serum glucose levels) is lacking. It is unclear whether increased temperatures result in worsened long-term neurologic outcomes, or whether a greater severity of brain injury is associated with more frequent or severe increases in systemic temperature.

The method of temperature monitoring is important. Thermal gradients exist throughout the body, and the site of measurement influences the diagnosis of hypothermia, normothermia, or hyperthermia. Measurements of systemic temperature may underestimate brain temperature. In studies of temperature monitoring by site, variations of up to 3°C have been identified between the brain and other routinely used monitoring sites, emphasizing the importance of monitoring site selection for patients with neurologic injury and the need to appreciate the difference between brain temperature and the active site of measurement used clinically for a given patient.

EEG/Electrocorticography

Electroencephalographic (EEG) monitoring has long been used in neurology for diagnosis and intraoperative monitoring, but has less frequently been used as a neurologic monitoring technique for critically ill patients. EEG is indicated in response to suspicion of a new or progressive abnormality such as cerebral ischemia or new onset of seizures. The cortical EEG or electrocorticography, which is altered by mild cerebral ischemia and abolished by profound cerebral ischemia, can be used to indicate potentially damaging cerebral hypoperfusion. More recent research has documented its utility for the detection of cortical spreading depression and peri-infarct and posttraumatic depolarizations which are thought to be early indicators of delayed ischemic injury of the acutely injured human cortex after TBI, SAH, malignant ischemic stroke, or intracerebral hemorrhage [50–53]. The EEG can document seizures, either convulsive or nonconvulsive, and provide information as to the efficacy of antiseizure therapy. Other functions include defining the depth or type of coma, documenting focal or lateralizing intracranial abnormalities, and supporting the diagnosis of brain death.

When the EEG is to be used for monitoring, care must be taken and weaknesses of the technique appreciated. In the ICU, electrical noise from other equipment may produce artifacts and interfere with technically adequate tracings. Continuous EEG recording was cumbersome in the past owing to the sheer volume of data (300 pages per hour of hard copy on as many as 16 channels), but techniques for digital recording and networking direct computer recording of EEG data are now available given adequate computer power and storage. Scalp fixation has also been a significant limiting factor, although newer fixation techniques are easier to apply and more stable. Techniques of mathematical data analysis, such as rapid Fourier analysis, can be used to determine the relative amplitude in each frequency band (σ—less than 4 Hz, θ—4 to 8 Hz, α—8 to 13 Hz, β—greater than 13 Hz), which can then be displayed graphically in formats such as the compressed spectral array or density spectral array [54]. Alpha variability and the delta to alpha ratio has been found to predict vasospasm/delayed cerebral ischemia in SAH patients [55], and the percentage of alpha variability was found to have prognostic value for TBI patients [56,57]. Analytical software has been developed that processes the raw EEG signal to provide single number interpretation of the "depth of sedation." These devices have been recommended for use during general anesthesia as a means to reduce the risk of awareness [58], although the scientific justification for this claim is not conclusive. The American Society of Anesthesiologists has developed a practice advisory on this issue [59]. Use of this type of monitoring has also been implemented by some for use in the ICU for monitoring sedation levels of the critically ill, the utility of which has yet to be proven [60,61]. All devices use proprietary analyses of an EEG signal (either spontaneous or evoked, with or without electromyogram monitoring), which is converted to a single number that is intended to correspond to an awareness level based on an arbitrary scale. The role and evidence of improved patient outcomes with this monitoring modality is undergoing further study and development as well as efforts to standardize reporting, facilitate multicenter collaborative research and improve applicability [62,63]. A more detailed discussion of the clinical indications, technical aspects, and limitations can be found in recent reviews [64,65].

Evoked Potentials

Sensory evoked potentials (EPs), which include somatosensory EPs (SSEPs), brainstem auditory EPs (BAEPs), and visual EPs (VEPs), can be used as qualitative threshold monitors to detect severe neural ischemia and injury and test the integrity of structures and connections between the CNS (e.g., brainstem and cortex) and the peripheral nervous system. Unlike EEG that records the continuous, spontaneous activity of the brain, EPs evaluate the responses of the brain to specific stimuli. To record SSEPs, stimuli are applied to a peripheral nerve, usually the median nerve at the wrist or posterior tibial nerve at the ankle, by a low-amplitude current of approximately 20 ms in duration. The resultant sensory (afferent) nerve stimulation and resultant cortical response to the stimulus are recorded at the scalp. Repeated identical stimuli are applied and signal averaging is used to remove the highly variable background EEG and other environmental electrical noise and thereby visualize reproducible evoked responses (Fig. 31.5).

EPs are described in terms of the amplitude of cortical response peaks and the conduction delay (latency) between the stimulus and the appearance of response waveform. Because peripheral nerve stimulation can be uncomfortable, SSEPs are usually obtained from sedated or anesthetized patients. SSEPs are unaffected by neuromuscular blocking agents but may be significantly influenced by sedative, analgesic, and anesthetic agents, often in a dose-dependent manner. In general, however, the doses of drugs required to influence EPs are sufficient to produce general anesthesia and are not usually clinically important in the ICU. If a patient is undergoing EP monitoring and requires large doses of analgesic or sedative agents, potential impairment of monitoring should be considered. Motor EPs represent a method of selectively evaluating descending motor tracts. Stimulation of proximal motor tracts (cortical or spinal) and evaluation of subsequent responses yield information that can be used for intraoperative and early postoperative neurosurgical management. Induction of motor EP and its interpretation is exquisitely sensitive to sedative, analgesic, and anesthetic drugs, making clinical use difficult when drugs are given concurrently. Despite these limitations, motor EP evaluation has been used successfully for the management of neuro-ICU patients and may become more common as techniques and equipment evolve [66,67].

Likewise, BAEPs and VEPs utilize auditory and visual sensory stimulation and record responses to them from the auditory and visual cortices and test the integrity of connections to and from them to the periphery.

The sensitivity of EP monitoring is similar to that of EEG monitoring. EPs, especially BAEPs, are relatively robust, although they can be modified by trauma, hypoxia, or ischemia. Because obliteration of EPs occurs only under conditions of profound cerebral ischemia or mechanical trauma, EP monitoring is one of the most specific ways in which to assess neurologic integrity of specific monitored pathways. However, as with the discussion of cerebral ischemia, there is a dose–time interaction that ultimately determines the magnitude of cerebral injury. As a result, neurologic deficits occur that have not been predicted by changes in EPs, and severe changes in EPs may not be followed by neurologic deficits. The most definitive indication for SSEPs is in the prognostication of anoxic brain injury after cardiac arrest. The absence of the N20 response on bilateral SSEPs of the median nerve within 3 days postarrest has been found to be a reliable predictor of negative outcome or recovery of consciousness for anoxic postarrest coma and is part of the American Academy of Neurology (AAN) practice parameter in the prognostication of postanoxic coma [68]. Different EPs have been studied after anoxia, TBI, coma as well as brain death, and have been found to have prognostic value to varying degrees. Various reviews and consensus statements have been published that provide specific indications and criteria [69,70].

Intracranial Pressure Monitoring

The symptoms and signs of intracranial hypertension are neither sensitive nor specific. Usually, the physical findings associated with increasing ICP (e.g., Cushing's response–hypertension and Cushing's triad–hypertension, reflex bradycardia, and alterations in respiratory function) become apparent only when intracranial hypertension has become sufficiently severe to injure the brain. Likewise, papilledema is a late development and is often difficult to identify clinically. Because ICP cannot otherwise be adequately assessed, direct measurement and monitoring of ICP has become a common intervention, especially in the management of TBI [71], and less commonly after critical illnesses such as SAH or stroke. Although there is no level 1 evidence that the use of this technique improves outcomes, there is a large body of clinical evidence supporting its use to guide therapeutic interventions after TBI that have potential risks (such as aggressive osmotherapy, induced hypothermia, and barbiturate coma), to aid with the detection of intracranial mass lesions and to provide prognostic data [72]. ICP monitoring has been found to improve outcome prediction after TBI and next to clinical parameters such as age, GCS motor score, and abnormal pupillary responses, the proportion of hourly ICP recordings greater than 20 mm Hg

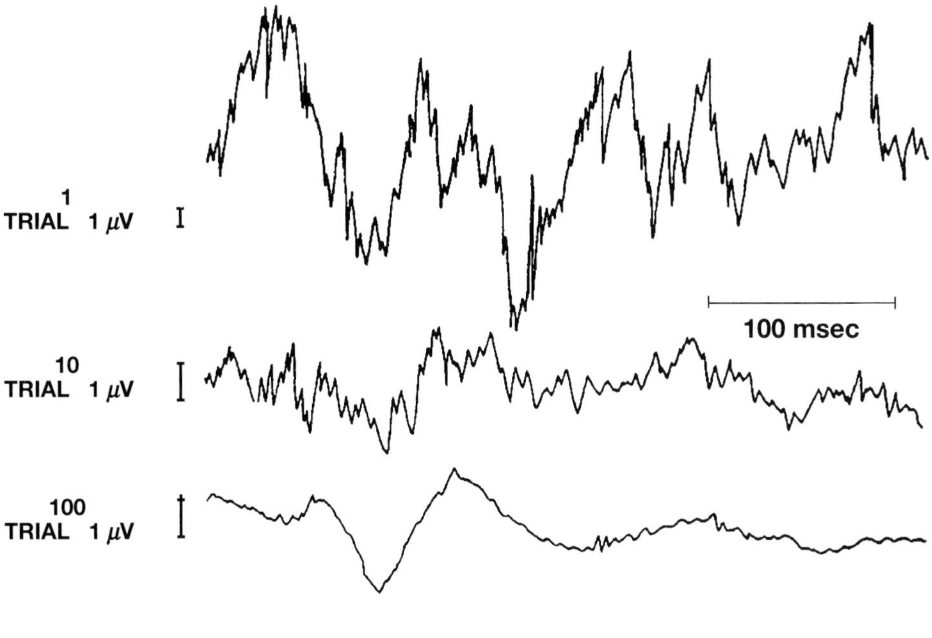

FIGURE 31.5 Averaging reduces background noise. After 100 trials, this visual evoked potential (EP) is relatively noise-free. The same EP is hard to distinguish after only 10 trials and would be impossible to find in the original unaveraged data. (From Nuwer MR: *Evoked Potential Monitoring in the Operating Room*. New York, Raven Press, 1986, p 29, with permission.)

was the next most robust predictor of outcomes in an analysis done of the National Traumatic Coma Data Bank [73]. Based on these data, the Brain Trauma Foundation/American Association of Neurosurgeons Guidelines recommend ICP monitoring for all patients with severe TBI (GCS < 8) and an abnormal CT scan or a normal scan with patients who are greater than 40 years old, have motor posturing, or a systolic BP <90 mm Hg [74,75]. This guideline is controversial however because it was not based on randomized trial data. Moreover, a recent multicenter randomized clinical trial comparing an ICP monitoring-driven treatment regimen to one without ICP monitoring performed in South America (because of the lack of clinical equipoise in the United States) demonstrated no benefits of monitoring and controlling ICP <20 mm Hg. This trial has only added to the controversy of ICP monitoring [76].

ICP functions as the outflow pressure apposing MAP (CPP = MAP – ICP) when ICP exceeds jugular venous pressure. Because the skull is not distensible, the brain, cerebrospinal fluid (CSF), and cerebral blood volume have little room to expand without increasing ICP. It is important to appreciate that some increase in intracranial volume is possible without much change in ICP, but when the compensatory mechanisms are exhausted, even small changes in volume can lead to significant increases in pressure. Although CBF cannot be directly inferred from knowledge of MAP and ICP, severe increases in ICP reduce CPP and CBF. ICP monitoring provides temporally relevant, quantitative information. The problems associated with ICP monitoring fall generally into three categories: direct morbidity due to monitor placement (e.g., intracranial hemorrhage, cortical damage, and infections), inaccurate measurement, and misinterpretation or inappropriate use of the data. Clinically, only two sites are used to measure ICP: a lateral ventricle with an external ventricular drain (EVD) or the surface of the brain with an intraparenchymal monitor. Ventricular catheterization, when performed using strict aseptic technique, is the method of choice for ICP monitoring and CSF drainage in patients with acute intracranial hypertension and excess CSF (i.e., acute hydrocephalus). In practice, intraventricular catheters may be difficult to place if cerebral edema or brain swelling has compressed the ventricular system. Intraventricular pressure monitoring can also be performed with fiberoptic catheters (instead of a hollow catheter) that use a variable reflectance pressure sensing system (transducer tip) to measure pressure (Camino Laboratories, San Diego, CA). These fiberoptic catheters are less susceptible to short-term malfunction than conventional, fluid-filled catheters but may slowly and unpredictably drift over days to weeks [77].

Previously used monitors include subdural ICP monitors such as a fluid-coupled bolt (simple transcranial conduit), fluid-coupled subdural catheters (or reservoirs), or fiberoptic transducer-tipped catheters have fallen out of use because of technical issues with fixation and reliability and complications such as the possibility of brain tissue herniating into the system, obstructing the system, distorting measurements, and potentially damaging the cerebral cortex including causing subdural hematomas.

Intraparenchymal placement of a fiberoptic catheter is also possible and is associated with complications similar to ventricular fiberoptic catheters. Complications are generally noted to be highest with ventriculostomies (when compared with fiberoptic catheter usage), and complications of ICP monitoring are associated with a worse GCS score.

The interpretation and utility of ICP readings from EVDs and intraparenchymal monitors are subject to numerous limitations. First, the monitors are often single monitors placed in a specific region of the brain parenchyma (often the right frontal lobe as it is non-eloquent cortex that will not result in neurologic dysfunction) usually in or adjacent to the most severely damaged hemisphere [78]. Because of this, however, it only reflects pressure in one region of the brain. There are pressure gradients that exist among various sites within the calvarium, and the pressure in the middle cranial fossa and posterior cranial fossa may not be reflected by ICP readings from the right frontal lobe and it is possible for patients to have middle cranial or inferior cranial fossa herniation without ICP elevations. For this reason, some have recommended bilateral or multiple ICP monitors be placed to circumvent this problem [79]. This is not practical and significantly increases the risk of the procedure and many neurosurgeons would oppose this. Even EVDs, although placed in the lateral ventricle and considered the gold standard for measuring ICP, can be misleading in the presence of posterior cranial fossa pressure. Shift and mass effect as well as hydrocephalus and significant clinical herniation can occur immediately prior to or without ICP elevations in certain situations. As with any monitoring device, clinical examination and interpretation in light of synthesis of all the other data is essential.

Management decisions based on ICP data continue to be the focus of ongoing debate and study. Previous clinical studies after TBI had demonstrated that increased ICP was associated with worse outcome [80]. Therefore, control of ICP had been considered by some clinicians to be the primary focus of treatment [22], while other clinicians considered restoration of CPP (by increasing MAP) to be the primary goal of medical management [81]. Although there was a possible suggestion of improved neurologic outcomes with cerebral perfusion-driven protocols, the problem was there were also more complications including ARDS [82].

All the data and trials investigating ICP and its effects on brain physiology after TBI had previously been non-randomized and II to III level of evidence. Given the lack of clinical equipoise, a clinical trial could not be done in the United States. Chesnut and colleagues conducted a multicenter controlled trial in Bolivia and Ecuador, of 324 severe TBI patients who were being treated in the ICU and randomly assigned them to either an ICP-driven treatment protocol which utilized ICP monitors and treated ICP greater than 20 mm Hg or a protocol of treatment based on clinical examination and serial imaging [76]. The primary outcome was a composite measure of survival time, impaired consciousness, functional outcome at 3 and 6 months, and neuropsychologic status at 6 months. There were no differences among the groups in terms of functional outcomes, mortality, or length of stay. The ICP monitoring group had fewer days of brain-specific treatments such as osmotherapy but did have more frequent administration of barbiturates or hypertonic saline. Given that there were no ICP measurements in the control group, a true comparison of the impact of the ICPs is difficult to conclude. This study did further emphasize that clinical assessments continue to be an important evaluation of brain function for which we have no current adequate substitute, as well as a conceptual problem of thinking that summated pressures as measured by ICP monitors will always be increased in the setting of mechanical tissue displacements that occur regionally in the brain and skull [83]. Rather than resulting in the abandonment of this monitoring modality, this study has reemphasized the need for clinical and imaging assessments and changed the way that ICP is utilized in that the cutoff value of 20 mm Hg is no longer an absolute goal. Many were not surprised with the results of this study given the now better understood complexity of the pathophysiology of TBI with multiple clinical and physiologic factors and numerous secondary injury pathways possibly influencing neurologic function and clinical outcomes. ICP monitoring continues to be utilized; but many intensivists have revised their protocols to include more nuanced assessments of pressure, including cerebral perfusion and assessments of autoregulation as well as other modalities such as regional and global oxygenation [84]. Figure 31.6 is an example.

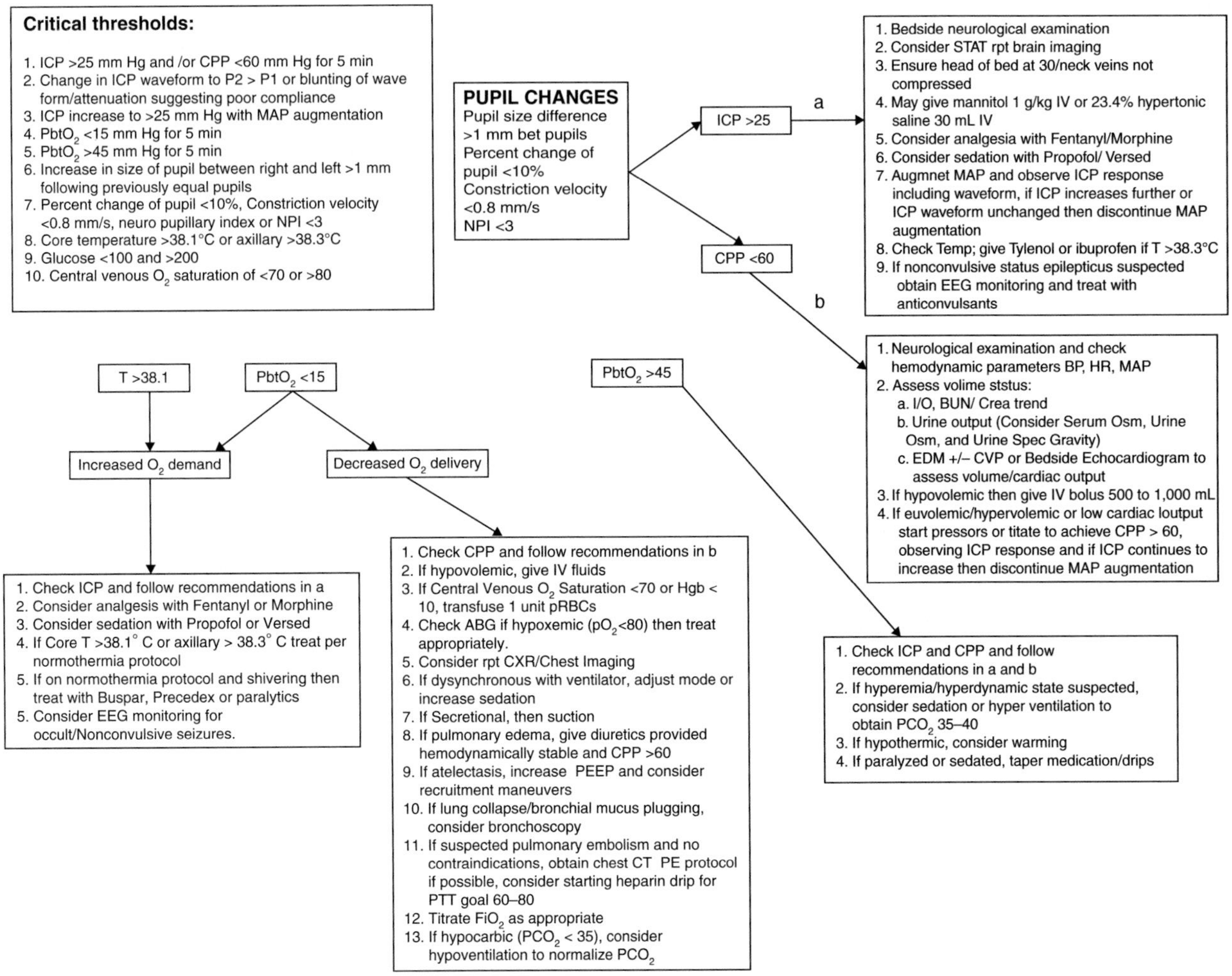

Critical thresholds:
1. ICP >25 mm Hg and /or CPP <60 mm Hg for 5 min
2. Change in ICP waveform to P2 > P1 or blunting of wave form/attenuation suggesting poor compliance
3. ICP increase to >25 mm Hg with MAP augmentation
4. PbtO2 <15 mm Hg for 5 min
5. PbtO2 >45 mm Hg for 5 min
6. Increase in size of pupil between right and left >1 mm following previously equal pupils
7. Percent change of pupil <10%, Constriction velocity <0.8 mm/s, neuro pupillary index or NPI <3
8. Core temperature >38.1°C or axillary >38.3°C
9. Glucose <100 and >200
10. Central venous O2 saturation of <70 or >80
PUPIL CHANGES
Pupil size difference >1 mm bet pupils
Percent change of pupil <10%
Constriction velocity <0.8 mm/s
NPI <3
ICP >25
CPP <60
a
b
1. Bedside neurological examination
2. Consider STAT rpt brain imaging
3. Ensure head of bed at 30/neck veins not compressed
4. May give mannitol 1 g/kg IV or 23.4% hypertonic saline 30 mL IV
5. Consider analgesia with Fentanyl/Morphine
6. Consider sedation with Propofol/ Versed
7. Augmnet MAP and observe ICP response including waveform, if ICP increases further or ICP waveform unchanged then discontinue MAP augmentation
8. Check Temp; give Tylenol or ibuprofen if T >38.3°C
9. If nonconvulsive status epilepticus suspected obtain EEG monitoring and treat with anticonvulsants
1. Neurological examination and check hemodynamic parameters BP, HR, MAP
2. Assess volime ststus:
a. I/O, BUN/ Crea trend
b. Urine output (Consider Serum Osm, Urine Osm, and Urine Spec Gravity)
c. EDM +/– CVP or Bedside Echocardiogram to assess volume/cardiac output
3. If hypovolemic then give IV bolus 500 to 1,000 mL
4. If euvolemic/hypervolemic or low cardiac loutput start pressors or titate to achieve CPP > 60, observing ICP response and if ICP continues to increase then discontinue MAP augmentation
T >38.1
PbtO2 <15
PbtO2 >45
Increased O2 demand
Decreased O2 delivery
1. Check ICP and follow recommendations in a
2. Consider analgesis with Fentanyl or Morphine
3. Consider sedation with Propofol or Versed
4. If Core T >38.1° C or axillary > 38.3° C treat per normothermia protocol
5. If on normothermia protocol and shivering then treat with Buspar, Precedex or paralytics
5. Consider EEG monitoring for occult/Nonconvulsive seizures.
1. Check CPP and follow recommendations in b
2. If hypovolemic, give IV fluids
3. If Central Venous O2 Saturation <70 or Hgb < 10, transfuse 1 unit pRBCs
4. Check ABG if hypoxemic (pO2<80) then treat appropriately.
5. Consider rpt CXR/Chest Imaging
6. If dysynchronous with ventilator, adjust mode or increase sedation
7. If Secretional, then suction
8. If pulmonary edema, give diuretics provided hemodynamically stable and CPP >60
9. If atelectasis, increase PEEP and consider recruitment maneuvers
10. If lung collapse/bronchial mucus plugging, consider bronchoscopy
11. If suspected pulmonary embolism and no contraindications, obtain chest CT PE protocol if possible, consider starting heparin drip for PTT goal 60–80
12. Titrate FiO2 as appropriate
13. If hypocarbic (PCO2 < 35), consider hypoventilation to normalize PCO2
1. Check ICP and CPP and follow recommendations in a and b
2. If hyperemia/hyperdynamic state suspected, consider sedation or hyper ventilation to obtain PCO2 35–40
3. If hypothermic, consider warming
4. If paralyzed or sedated, taper medication/drips

FIGURE 31.6 Example of a multimodal monitoring protocol in current use in a level 1 academic trauma center. (From Carandang R.A. The role of invasive monitoring in traumatic brain injury. *Current Trauma Reports* 1:125–132, 2015, with permission.)

Cerebral Blood Flow Monitoring

The first quantitative clinical method of measurement of CBF, the Kety–Schmidt technique, calculated global CBF from the difference between the arterial and jugular bulb concentration curves of an inhaled, inert gas as it equilibrated with blood and brain tissue. Later techniques used extracranial γ detectors to measure regional cortical CBF from washout curves after intracarotid injection of a radioisotope such as 133-xenon (Xe 133). Carotid puncture was avoided by techniques that measured cortical CBF after inhaled or intravenous administration of Xe 133, using γ counting of exhaled gas to correct clearance curves for recirculation of Xe 133. Because Xe is radiodense, saturation of brain tissue increases radiographic density in proportion to CBF. Imaging of the brain after equilibration with stable (nonradioactive) Xe provides a regional estimate of CBF that includes deep brain structures. Clinical studies of CBF after TBI performed using stable xenon computed tomography (CT) have prompted a radical revision of conventional understanding by demonstrating that one-third of patients had evidence of cerebral ischemia within 8 hours of trauma. Although slow in becoming a routine clinical tool, Xe CT is becoming a more common technique for monitoring CBF in patients. The use of helical and spiral CT scanners (with very short acquisition times) reduces radiation exposure to the patient and decreases the time needed for a scan, improving clinical utility [85]. A newer method of measuring CBF that provides continuous bedside quantitative measurements is the thermal diffusion technique. This consists of the insertion of a microprobe into the brain parenchyma with a thermistor at the tip and a temperature sensor proximal to it. The thermistor is heated to 2° above tissue temperature and CBF is calculated using the thermal gradient and provides a quantified regional CBF measurement in mL/100 g/minute. Some studies suggest a correlation with regional brain tissue oxygenation and a possible role for guiding management of ICP. Technical issues such as the invasive nature of the device, frequent calibration, and the limitations seen among febrile patients have kept this method from becoming more widely adopted [86]. Another CT-based technique, perfusion CT, uses iodinated contrast infusion with repeated images to calculate local CBF. This technique is limited to smaller regions and may not provide uniform results between brain regions [87]. Other techniques, such as SPECT and magnetic resonance perfusion imaging, also can provide information about CBF, but their clinical utility is still under study.

Transcranial Doppler Ultrasound

Transcranial Doppler ultrasonography can be used to estimate changes in CBF. For most patients, cerebral arterial flow velocity in intracranial vessels can be measured easily, especially the middle

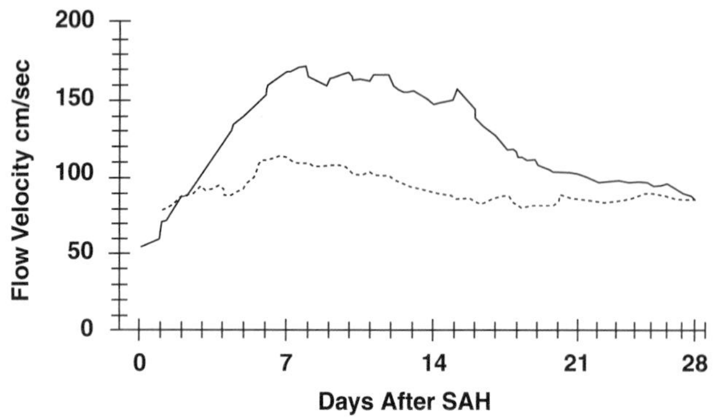

FIGURE 31.7 Mean flow velocity (FV, in cm/s) curves of 18 patients with laterally localized aneurysms (arising from the internal carotid and middle cerebral arteries). The side of the ruptured aneurysm (*continuous line*) shows a higher FV than the unaffected side (*dotted line*). SAH, subarachnoid hemorrhage. (From Seiler RW, Grolimund P, Aaslid R, et al: Cerebral vasospasm evaluated by transcranial ultrasound correlated with clinical grade and CT-visualized subarachnoid hemorrhage. *J Neurosurg* 64:594–600, 1986, with permission.)

cerebral artery, using transcranial Doppler ultrasonography. Doppler flow velocity uses the frequency shift, proportional to velocity, which is observed when sound waves are reflected from moving red blood cells. Blood moving toward the transducer shifts the transmitted frequency to higher frequencies; blood moving away, to lower frequencies. Velocity is a function of both blood flow rate and vessel diameter. When diameter remains constant, changes in velocity are proportional to changes in CBF; however, intersubject differences in flow velocity correlate poorly with intersubject differences in CBF. Entirely noninvasive, transcranial Doppler measurements can be repeated at frequent intervals or even applied continuously. The detection and monitoring of post-SAH vasospasm remains the most common use of transcranial Doppler (Fig. 31.7) [88]. However, further clinical research is necessary to define those situations for which the excellent capacity for rapid trend monitoring can be exploited, including assessment of vascular autoregulation, ancillary testing to detect intracranial hypertension, and brain death.

Jugular Venous Bulb Oxygen Saturation

Several measurements of cerebral oxygenation are clinically useful, including measurement of $SjvO_2$. To insert a retrograde jugular venous bulb catheter, the internal jugular vein can be located by ultrasound guidance or by external anatomic landmarks and use of a "seeker" needle, namely, the same technique used for antegrade placement of jugular venous catheters. Once the vessel is identified, the catheter is directed cephalad, toward the mastoid process, instead of centrally. A lateral cranial radiograph can confirm the position just superior to the base of the skull. The decision to place a jugular bulb catheter in the left or right jugular bulb is important. Simultaneous measurements of $SjvO_2$ in the right and left jugular bulb demonstrate differences in saturation [89], suggesting that one jugular bulb frequently is dominant, carrying the greater portion of cerebral venous blood. Differences in the cross-sectional areas of the vessels that form the torcula and the manner in which blood is distributed to the right and left lateral sinus contribute to differences between the two jugular bulbs. Ideally, a jugular bulb catheter should be placed on the dominant side, which can be identified as the jugular vein that, if compressed, produces the greater increase in ICP or as the vein on the side of the larger jugular foramen as detected by CT [90].

In general, $SjvO_2$ reflects the adequacy of CDO_2 to support $CMRO_2$, but mixed cerebral venous blood, like mixed systemic blood, represents a global average of cerebral venous blood from regions that are variably perfused and may not reflect marked regional hypoperfusion/ischemia of small regions. In contrast to ICP and CPP, which provide only indirect information concerning the adequacy of CDO_2 to support $CMRO_2$, $SjvO_2$ directly reflects the balance between these variables on a global or hemispheric level. CBF, $CMRO_2$, CaO_2, and $CjvO_2$ are modeled by the equation: $CMRO_2 = CBF\ (CaO_2 - CjvO_2)$. For a healthy brain, if $CMRO_2$ remains constant as CBF decreases, $SjvO_2$ and $CjvO_2$ decrease [25]. If flow-metabolism coupling is intact, decreases in $CMRO_2$ result in parallel decreases in CBF while $SjvO_2$ and $CjvO_2$ remain constant [25]. Abnormally low $SjvO_2$ (i.e., less than 50%, compared to a normal value of 65%) suggests the possibility of cerebral ischemia, but normal or elevated $SjvO_2$ does not prove the adequacy of cerebral perfusion because of possible saturation averaging between normal and abnormal areas of perfusion. This is especially true for focal areas of hypoperfusion. Therefore, the negative predictive value of a normal $SjvO_2$ is poor. After placement of a jugular catheter, monitoring of $SjvO_2$ can be achieved through repeated blood sampling. However, repeated blood sampling yields only "snapshots" of cerebral oxygenation and thus provides discontinuous data that may miss rapid changes in saturation. To achieve continuous monitoring of $SjvO_2$, indwelling fiberoptic oximetric catheters have been used. Because oxyhemoglobin and deoxyhemoglobin absorb light differently, $SjvO_2$ can be determined from differential absorbance. Oximetric jugular bulb catheters have proven somewhat challenging to maintain, requiring frequent recalibration, repositioning, and confirmation of measured saturation by analyzing blood samples in a CO-oximeter. The highest frequency of confirmed desaturation episodes occurs in patients with intracerebral hematomas, closely followed by those with SAH. For patients with TBI, the number of jugular desaturations is strongly associated with poor neurologic outcome; even a single desaturation episode is associated with a doubling of the mortality rate [91]. Clinical application of jugular venous bulb cannulation has been limited, perhaps in part because the technique is invasive, although the risks of cannulation injury, including hematoma and injury to the adjacent carotid, are low. Several modifications of jugular venous oxygen monitoring have been proposed. Cerebral extraction of oxygen, which is the difference between SaO_2 and $SjvO_2$ divided by SaO_2, is less confounded by anemia than the cerebral A-VDO_2 [92]. Another concept, termed cerebral hemodynamic reserve, is defined as the ratio of percentage of change in global cerebral extraction of oxygen (reflecting the balance between $CMRO_2$ and CBF) to percentage of change in CPP. This equation attempts to integrate cerebral hemodynamics and metabolism with intracranial compliance. Cruz et al. [92] found that cerebral hemodynamic reserve decreased as intracranial compliance decreased, even as a consequence of minor elevations in ICP. Theoretically, this variable may allow more precise management of cerebral hemodynamics in patients with decreased intracranial compliance.

Brain Tissue Oxygen Tension

Another promising technique for monitoring the adequacy of CDO_2 is direct assessment of brain tissue oxygen tension or $PbtO_2$. Monitoring of $PbtO_2$ overcomes one important limitation of $SjvO_2$ monitoring, which is that the global saturation measurements provide no information about regional or focal tissue oxygenation. Only relatively profound focal global ischemia causes $SjvO_2$ to decrease to less than the accepted critical threshold of 50%. Even severe regional ischemia may not result in desaturation if venous effluent from other regions is normally saturated, in part because the absolute flow of poorly saturated blood returning from ischemic regions is by definition less per volume of tissue than flow from well-perfused regions, resulting

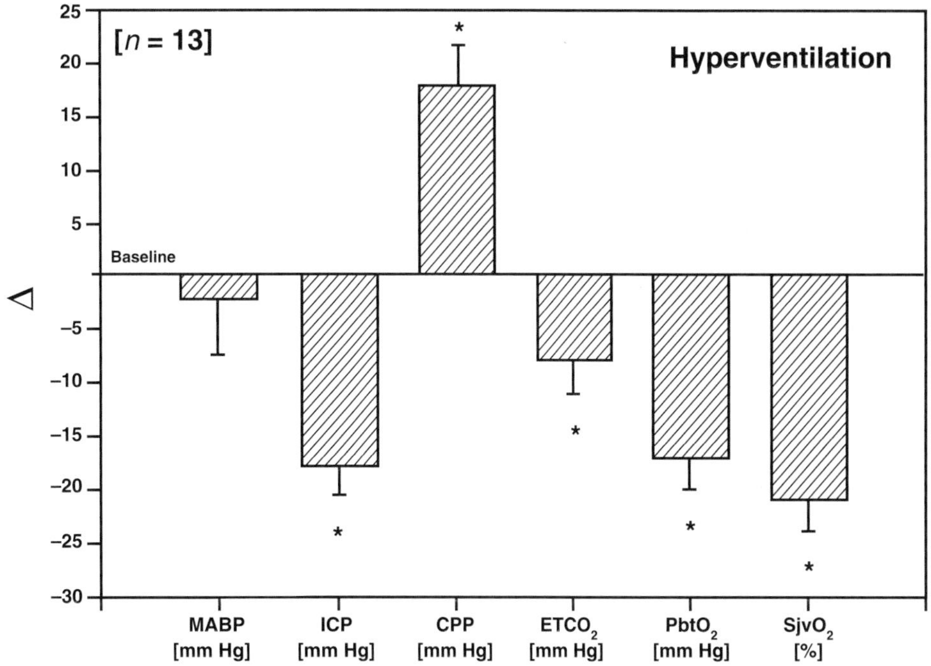

FIGURE 31.8 The effect of hyperventilation-induced hypocapnia on changes in mean arterial blood pressure (MABP), intracranial pressure (ICP), cerebral perfusion pressure (CPP), end-tidal CO_2 ($ETCO_2$), $PtiO_2$, and jugular bulb oximetry ($SjvO_2$). $*p < 0.05$; before hyperventilation versus 10 min later. (From Unterberg AW, Kiening KL, Härtl R, et al: Multimodal monitoring in patients with head injury: evaluation of the effects of treatment on cerebral oxygenation. *J Trauma* 42:S32–S37, 1997, with permission.)

in a smaller percentage of poorly oxygenated to well-oxygenated blood. Intracranial, intraparenchymal probes have been developed that monitor only $PbtO_2$ or that also monitor brain tissue PCO_2 and pH [93]. Modified from probes designed for continuous monitoring of arterial blood gases, intraparenchymal probes can be inserted through multiple-lumen ICP monitoring bolts. Although these probes provide no information about remote regions, they nevertheless provide continuous information about the region that is contiguous to the probe. They also carry the theoretical risks of hematoma formation, infection, and direct parenchymal injury. Evaluation of $PbtO_2$ after severe TBI has shown that low partial pressures ($PbtO_2$ less than 10 mm Hg for greater than 15 minutes) powerfully predict poor outcomes and that $PbtO_2$ probes are safe [94,95]. Both $PbtO_2$ and $SjvO_2$ may reflect changes in cerebral oxygenation secondary to alterations in CBF (Fig. 31.8) [96]. However, comparisons of simultaneous $PbtO_2$ and $SjvO_2$ monitoring suggest that each monitor detects cerebral ischemia that the other fails to detect. In 58 patients with severe TBI, the two monitors detected 52 episodes in which $SjvO_2$ decreased to less than 50% or $PbtO_2$ decreased to less than 8 mm Hg; of those 52 episodes, both monitored variables fell below the ischemic threshold in 17, only $SjvO_2$ reflected ischemia in 19, and only $PbtO_2$ reflected ischemia in 16 (Fig. 31.9) [97]. There have been eight completed studies comparing ICP/CPP-guided therapy to $PbtO_2$ + ICP/CPP-driven protocols, six retrospective studies, and two prospective studies in severe TBI patients, and results have been mixed. One study showed worse functional independence measures at discharge, three showed no benefit looking at GOS scores at 6 months and mortality at discharge, two showed reduced mortality at discharge and at 3 months, and two showed a trend toward better outcome or better outcome as measured by GOS at 3 and 6 months, respectively. The studies are nicely summarized and thoughtfully discussed in a review by DeGeorgia [98]. Preliminary results of the ongoing phase 2 randomized multicenter clinical trial investigating the safety and efficacy of brain tissue oxygen monitoring in severe

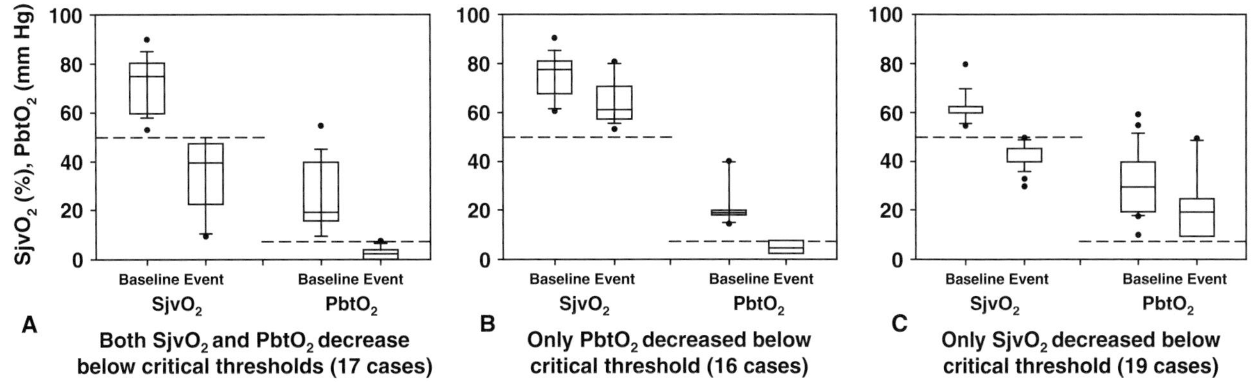

FIGURE 31.9 Changes in jugular venous oxygen saturation ($SjvO_2$) and brain tissue PO_2 ($PbtO_2$) during 52 episodes of cerebral hypoxia/ischemia. The horizontal line across the box plot represents the median, and the lower and upper ends of the box plot are the 25th percentile and 75th percentile, respectively. The error bars mark the 10th and 90th percentiles. The closed circles indicate any outlying points. **A:** Summary of the 17 cases in which both $SjvO_2$ and $PbtO_2$ decreased to less than their respective thresholds, as defined in the text. **B:** Summary of the 16 cases in which $PbtO_2$ decreased to less than the defined threshold; but $SjvO_2$, although decreased, did not decrease to less than 50%. **C:** Summary of the 19 cases in which $SjvO_2$ decreased to less than the threshold, but $PbtO_2$ remained at greater than 10 torr. (From Gopinath SP, Valadka AB, Uzura M, et al: Comparison of jugular venous oxygen saturation and brain tissue PO_2 as monitors of cerebral ischemia after head injury. *Crit Care Med* 27:2337–2345, 1999, with permission.)

TBI (BOOST-2) were presented at the Neurocritical Care Society meeting in October 2014. Patients aged 14 years and older with severe nonpenetrating TBI were randomized to treatment with ICP monitoring alone or with ICP and $PbtO_2$ monitoring which showed no differences in adverse events and safety but also met non-futility measures with lower overall mortality and lower poor outcome in the ICP and $PbtO_2$-monitored group. Initial conclusions were that a TBI treatment protocol guided by ICP and $PbtO_2$ reduced the duration of measured brain tissue hypoxia and was relatively safe [99]. The findings of this study will be used to determine the phase 3 study sample size [100].

Neurochemical Monitoring

Neuronal injury is associated with the release or production of chemical markers such as free radicals, inflammatory mediators, metabolic products, and excitatory amino acids [4]. Neurochemical monitoring via microdialysis allows assessment of the chemical milieu of cerebral extracellular fluid, provides valuable information about neurochemical processes in various neuropathologic states, and is used clinically in the management of severe TBI [101] and SAH [102,103]. There are data to suggest that chemical changes detected by microdialysis precede secondary neurologic injury and clinical worsening for intracranial hypertension, SAH, and ischemic stroke patients. Substances monitored via microdialysis include energy-related metabolites such as glucose, lactate, pyruvate, adenosine, and xanthine; neurotransmitters such as glutamate, aspartate, γ-amino butyric acid; markers of tissue damage such as glycerol and potassium [104], and alterations in membrane phospholipids by oxygen radicals [105]. Lactate levels and lactate/pyruvate ratios are reliable markers of ischemia and have been found to correlate well with PET, CPP, and jugular venous bulb oxygen saturation values, and associated with outcomes after TBI and SAH. Elevations of the excitatory neurotransmitter glutamate have been found after hypoxic-ischemic injury seen in low CBF, jugular venous bulb desaturation, seizures and low CPP, and correlated with poor outcomes following TBI. The magnitude of release of these substances correlates with the extent of ischemic damage. The time-dependent changes in these substances and the clinical implications are being evaluated, and their incorporation into standard practice is being studied. Certain issues related to quantification, bedside presentation of data, implantation strategies, and standardization of protocols need to be addressed. An excellent review of the current status, issues surrounding potential future developments, and methodological aspects of microdialysis are discussed in detail in an article by Hillered and colleagues [106].

Near-Infrared Spectroscopy

Theoretically, the best monitor of brain oxygenation would be a noninvasive device that characterizes brain oxygenation in real time: NIRS might eventually offer the opportunity to assess the adequacy of brain oxygenation continuously and noninvasively, although to date the use of the technique in adults has been limited.

Near-infrared light penetrates the skull and, during transmission through or reflection from brain tissue, undergoes changes in intensity that are proportional to the relative concentrations of oxygenated and deoxygenated hemoglobin in the arteries, capillaries, and veins within the field [107]. The absorption (A) of light by a chromophore (i.e., hemoglobin) is defined by Beer's law: $A = abc$, where a is the absorption constant, b is the path length of the light, and c is the concentration of the chromophore, namely, oxygenated and deoxygenated hemoglobin. Because it is impossible to measure the path length of NIRS light in tissue, approximations as to relative lengths and arterial versus venous contribution must be made.

Extensive preclinical and clinical data demonstrate that NIRS detects qualitative changes in brain oxygenation [108]. Studies have been done comparing NIRS to other technologies and assessing its correlation with EEG, transcranial Doppler, $PbtO_2$, and jugular venous O_2 saturation changes. NIRS was found to correlate with EEG, TCD, and PtO_2 during transient cerebral hypoxia, after SAH, and during intraoperative monitoring for carotid endarterectomy. It did not correlate well with $SjvO_2$ [109] values but was thought to provide complementary focal oxygenation data to $SjvO_2$'s global oxygenation assessment. Clinical applications include TBI where an rSO_2 of less than 55% was thought to suggest inadequate CPP and NIRS values were lower for the high ICP group of patients vasospasm detection in the setting of SAH, and the detection of intracranial hemorrhages such as subdural and epidural hematomas but studies are not definitive [110]. Despite the promise and enthusiasm generated by NIRS, many problems remain with the technology including tissue penetration, spatial and temporal resolution, artifacts from subcutaneous blood flow and methods of quantitative analysis which need to be resolved [111]. Therefore, validation studies suggest that NIRS may be more useful for qualitatively monitoring trends in brain tissue oxygenation than for actual quantification and its current clinical use is limited to a few centers and is adjunctive at best [108,112]. Some of the liabilities of NIRS may be overcome by optoacoustic monitoring of cerebral venous saturation. Optoacoustic monitoring of cerebral venous saturation depends on the generation by near-infrared light of ultrasonic signals in blood. The acoustic signals are then transmitted linearly through tissue and bone, and provide a focused, depth-resolved signal that reflects venous oxygenation [113].

Neuroimaging

MRI, PET scans, cerebral angiography, and radionuclide scans do not function as monitors per se. Rather, they are indicated in response to suspicion of a new or progressive anatomic lesion, such as a subdural or intracerebral hematoma or cerebral arterial vasospasm, that requires altered treatment. Most neuroimaging modalities provide static, discontinuous data and require moving a critically ill patient from the ICU to a remote location. Even so, these techniques play an important role in the overall management of patients with brain injury [114]. With the introduction of portable CT scanners and the development of ultrafast helical and spiral CT scanners, availability and acquisition time for evaluations have significantly decreased and can now be used for serial monitoring of ongoing neurologic processes and for evaluation of changes in CBF (see above).

CT scans obtained at the time of admission to the hospital can provide valuable prognostic information. Marshall et al. [115] predicted outcome of head-injured patients in relation to four grades of increasingly severe diffuse brain injury and the presence of evacuated or nonevacuated intracranial mass lesions (Table 31.4). Normal CT scans at admission in patients with GCS scores less than 8 are associated with a 10% to 15% incidence of ICP elevation [116,117]; however, the risk of ICP elevation increases for patients older than age 40 years, those with unilateral or bilateral motor posturing, or those with systolic blood pressure less than 90 mm Hg [116].

Although MRI often provides better resolution than CT scans, the powerful magnetic fields make the use of ferrous metals impractical (and dangerous), a ubiquitous component of life-support equipment. To address this issue, MRI-compatible ventilators, monitors, and infusion pumps have been developed, although the logistics of transport and the time required for scans continues to make this technique difficult for repeated

TABLE 31.4

Outcome at Discharge in Relation to Intracranial Diagnosis (% of Patients)

Outcome	DI I	DI II	DI III	DI IV	Evacuated Mass	Nonevacuated Mass
GR	27.0	8.5	3.3	3.1	5.1	2.8
MD	34.6	26.0	13.1	3.1	17.7	8.3
SD	19.2	40.7	26.8	18.8	26.0	19.4
PVS	9.6	11.2	22.9	18.8	12.3	16.7
Death	9.6	13.5	34.0	56.2	38.8	52.8
Total	100	100	100	100	100	100

DI, diffuse injury, DI categories I to IV represent increasingly severe classes of diffuse brain injury; GR, good recovery; MD, moderate disability; PVS, persistent vegetative state; SD, severe disability.
From Marshall LF, Marshall SB, Klauber MR, et al: A new classification of head injury based on computerized tomography. *J Neurosurg* 75:S14–S20, 1991, with permission.

monitoring. Recent advances in MRI technology, such as diffusion-weighted imaging, magnetic resonance spectroscopy (carbon labeled, phosphorus labeled, and nitrogen labeled), phase-contrast angiography, and functional MRI provide information about oxidative metabolic pathways, cerebral blood volume, functional CBF, and neuronal activation [114,118,119]. These techniques, while undergoing further evaluation and validation, may 1 day prove useful for evaluating brain injury and guiding its management. Recent clinical evidence of brain mitochondrial dysfunction after TBI, despite apparently adequate

TABLE 31.5

Summary of Modalities with Supporting Studies and Issues

Mode	Critical Thresholds	Data	Studies	Issues
ICP	>25	Pressure	[73, Cremer 2005]	RCT negative
			[Shafi 2009, 76]	Unclear threshold
CPP	<60 and >70	Perfusion	[Rosner 1995, 82]	Increased risk of ARDS
PRx	>0.2	Autoregulation	[Steiner 2002, Howells 2005]	Large data, calculations, and processing
$PbtO_2$	<10–25	Regional oxygen	[Narotam 2009, Spiotta 2010]	Unclear best location for placement
			[Steifel 2005]	Requires calibration
$SjvO_2$	<50%,	Global oxygen	Gopinath et al. [91]	Risk of venous thrombosis, durability
	>80%	Oxygen utilization	Cruz et al. [92]	Need for recalibration, gaps in data
MD	Glucose <2.0	Decreased perfusion	[Schulz 2000, 33]	Not widely available, logistical requirements
	L/P ratio >20–25	Metabolic crisis/ ischemia	[Hillered 1996, Robertson 1998, Valadka 1998]	Selection of biomarkers, quantification
			[93, Nordstrom 2003, Stahl 2001]	Computer interfacing, presentation of data
	Glut >15–20	Excitotoxicity	[Bullock 1995, Hutchinson 2000]	Implantation strategies
	Glycerol >100	Cell membrane degradation	[Marklund 1997, Hillered 1998, Reinstrup 2000]	Standardization of protocols
CBF	<18 mL/100 g/min	Ischemia	[Thome 2001, 86]	Needs validation, limited by temperature
	<15 mL/g/min	Vasospasm	[Vajkoczy 2003]	Frequent calibration
NIRS	rSO_2 <55%	Ischemia	Unterberg et al. [109]	Spatial resolution, needs validation
EEG	PAV <0.1	Electrical activity	Vespa et al. [56]	Large data, analytic software needed
	ADR >10% decrease	Vasospasm/DCI	[Claasen 2004, Finnigan 2007, Leon-Carrion 2009]	Scalp fixation, artifacts, cumbersome
ECoG	Depolarizations	Cortical spreading depression	[Hartings 2009, 53]	Cumbersome, analytic software, large data Needs further validation

ARDS, acute respiratory distress syndrome; ADR; DCI; CBF, cerebral blood flow; CPP, cerebral perfusion pressure; ICP, intracranial pressure; EEG, electroencephalogram; ECoG; L/P, lactate/pyruvate; MD, moderate disability; NIRS, near-infrared spectroscopy; PAV; PRx; $PbtO_2$, partial pressure of brain tissue oxygen concentration; RCT, randomized controlled trial; rSO_2; $SjvO_2$, jugular venous oxygen saturation.
From Carandang RA: The role of invasive monitoring in traumatic brain injury. *Curr Trauma Rep* 1:125–132, 2015, with permission.

CDO_2, suggests that functional cellular evaluation and associated therapy may someday be as important as maintaining CDO_2 [120]. In addition to providing information regarding ischemia and defining tissue at risk, MRI-based diffusion tensor imaging has been found to be helpful for further defining the anatomy of fiber tracts that have been damaged and has also been found to have prognostic value after severe TBI [121]. Functional MRI provides information regarding neural activity, localization, and the physiology of brain function but is currently in use only for neurosurgical planning, brain mapping, and in the investigation of neurobehavioral aspects and neuropsychologic sequelae of disorders such as Alzheimer's disease, stroke, multiple sclerosis, brain tumors, and TBI.

MULTIMODAL MONITORING STRATEGIES

With technological advances and active ongoing research, the field of neurologic monitoring is developing rapidly. Multimodal monitoring takes into account the limitations of each monitoring modality and compensates by combining different techniques into a generalized strategy that help to further elucidate the pathophysiology and underlying cellular mechanisms of disease and focuses care on the physiologic aspects of disease. This concept is not new (consider the operating room and the role of the anesthesiologist) and is becoming more common in the management of brain injury [122] as well as other neurologic diseases. There are multiple modalities with data to support their use but also issues with each modality (Table 31.5). Currently, there is multidisciplinary consensus on the use of multimodal monitoring strategies from various societies who endorse it as an important feature of neurocritical care but do raise concerns about the amount of data generated and emphasize the need for integration and synthesis of all relevant clinical data in the care of the individual patient. It is anticipated that further research and developments in technology, interfaces, database infrastructure, and bioinformatics as well as further elucidation of meaningful, normative, and validated data will improve the utility of monitoring devices and lead to improvements in therapeutics and patient outcomes [123,124].

References

1. Wright WL: Multimodal monitoring in the ICU: when could it be useful? *J Neurol Sci* 261:10–15, 2007.
2. Baron JC: Perfusion thresholds in human cerebral ischemia: historical perspective and therapeutic implications. *Cerebrovasc Dis* 11:2–8, 2001.
3. Cunningham AS, Salvador R, Coles JP, et al: Physiological thresholds for irreversible tissue damage in contusional regions following traumatic brain injury. *Brain* 128:1931–1942, 2005.
4. Carmichael ST: Gene expression changes after focal stroke, traumatic brain and spinal cord injuries. *Curr Opin Neurol* 16:699–704, 2003.
5. Enriquez P, Bullock R: Molecular and cellular mechanisms in the pathophysiology of severe head injury. *Curr Pharm Des* 10:2131–2143, 2004.
6. Acker T, Acker H: Cellular oxygen sensing need in CNS function: physiological and pathological implications. *J Exp Biol* 207:3171–3188, 2004.
7. Hlatky R, Furuya Y, Valadka AB, et al: Dynamic autoregulatory response after severe head injury. *J Neurosurg* 97:1054–1061, 2002.
8. Lundberg N, Kjällquist Å, Bien C: Reduction of increased intracranial pressure by hyperventilation. *Acta Psychiatr Neurol Scand Suppl* 34:5–57, 1959.
9. Marion DW, Puccio A, Wisniewski SR, et al: Effect of hyperventilation on extracellular concentrations of glutamate, lactate, pyruvate, and local cerebral blood flow in patients with severe traumatic brain injury. *Crit Care Med* 30:2619–2625, 2002.
10. Coles JP, Minhas PS, Fryer TD, et al: Effect of hyperventilation on cerebral blood flow in traumatic head injury: clinical relevance and monitoring correlates. *Crit Care Med* 30:1950–1959, 2002.
11. Tommasino C, Moore S, Todd MM: Cerebral effects of isovolemic hemodilution with crystalloid or colloid solutions. *Crit Care Med* 16:862–868, 1988.
12. Teasdale G, Jennett B: Assessment of coma and impaired consciousness: a practical scale. *Lancet* 2:81–84, 1974.
13. Langfitt TW: Measuring the outcome from head injuries. *J Neurosurg* 48:673–678, 1978.
14. Udekwu P, Kromhout-Schiro S, Vaslef S, et al: Glasgow Coma Scale score, mortality, and functional outcome in head-injured patients. *J Trauma* 56:1084–1089, 2004.
15. Balestreri M, Czosnyka M, Chatfield DA, et al: Predictive value of Glasgow Coma Scale after brain trauma: change in trend over the past ten years. *J Neurol Neurosurg Psychiatry* 75:161–162, 2004.
16. Davis DP, Serrano JA, Vilke GM, et al: The predictive value of field versus arrival GCS and TRISS calculations in moderate to severe TBI. *J Trauma* 60:985–990, 2006.
17. Meredith W, Rutledge R, Fakhry SM, et al: The conundrum of the Glasgow Coma Scale in intubated patients: a linear regression prediction of the Glasgow verbal score from the Glasgow eye and motor scores. *J Trauma* 44:839–844, 1998.
18. Wijdicks EF, Bamlet WR, Maramattom BV, et al: Validation of a new coma scale: the FOUR score. *Ann Neurol* 58(4):585–593, 2005.
19. Chesnut RM, Marshall SB, Piek J, et al: Early and late systemic hypotension as a frequent and fundamental source of cerebral ischemia following severe brain injury in the Traumatic Coma Data Bank. *Acta Neurochir* 59:121–125, 1993.
20. Chesnut RM, Ghajar J, Mass AIR, et al: Management and prognosis of severe traumatic brain injury. Part II. Early indications of prognosis in severe traumatic brain injury. *J Neurotrauma* 17:555–627, 2000.
21. Bullock RM, Chesnut RM, Clifton GL, et al: Resuscitation of blood pressure and oxygenation. *J Neurotrauma* 17:471–478, 2000.
22. Brain Trauma Foundation, American Association of Neurological Surgeons Congress of Neurological Surgeons Joint Section on Neurotrauma and Critical Care: Guidelines for the management of severe traumatic brain injury: cerebral perfusion pressure. Brain Trauma Foundation, Inc. Available from the Agency for Healthcare Research and Quality (AHRQ), http://www.guideline.gov/summary/summary.aspx?doc_id=3794. Retrieved December 5, 2006. Accessed January 25, 2017.
23. Johnston AJ, Steiner LA, Chatfield DA, et al: Effect of cerebral perfusion pressure augmentation with dopamine and norepinephrine on global and focal brain oxygenation after traumatic brain injury. *Intensive Care Med* 30:791–797, 2004.
24. Shafi S, Gentilello L: Hypotension does not increase mortality in brain-injured patients more than it does in non-brain-injured patients. *J Trauma* 59:830–834, 2005.
25. Bullock RM, Chesnut RM, Clifton GL, et al: Guidelines for cerebral perfusion pressure. *J Neurotrauma* 17:507–511, 2000.
26. Feldman Z, Robertson CS: Monitoring of cerebral hemodynamics with jugular bulb catheters. *Crit Care Clin* 13:51–77, 1997.
27. Kinoshita K, Kraydieh S, Alonso O, et al: Effect of posttraumatic hyperglycemia on contusion volume and neutrophil accumulation after moderate fluid-percussion brain injury in rats. *J Neurotrauma* 19:681–692, 2002.
28. Jeremitsky E, Omert LA, Dunham CM, et al: The impact of hyperglycemia on patients with severe brain injury. *J Trauma* 58:47–50, 2005.
29. Cochran A, Scaife ER, Hansen KW, et al: Hyperglycemia and outcomes from pediatric traumatic brain injury. *J Trauma* 55:1035–1038, 2003.
30. Rovlias A, Kotsou S: The influence of hyperglycemia on neurological outcome in patients with severe head injury. *Neurosurgery* 46:335–343, 2000.
31. Van den Berghe G, Wouters P, Weekers F, et al: Intensive insulin therapy in critically ill patients. *N Engl J Med* 345:1359–1367, 2001.
32. Van Den Berghe G, Wouters PJ, Bouillon R, et al: Outcome benefit of intensive insulin therapy in the critically ill: insulin dose versus glycemic control. *Crit Care Med* 31:359–366, 2003.
33. Vespa PM, McArthur D, O'Phelan K, et al: Persistently low ECF glucose correlates with poor outcome 6 months after human traumatic brain injury. *J Cereb Blood Flow Metab* 23:865–877, 2003.
34. Clifton GL, Jiang JY, Lyeth BG, et al: Marked protection by moderate hypothermia after experimental traumatic brain injury. *J Cereb Blood Flow Metab* 11:114–121, 1991.
35. Clifton G: Hypothermia and severe brain injury. *J Neurosurg* 93:718–719, 2000.
36. McIntyre LA, Fergusson DA, Hebert PC, et al: Prolonged therapeutic hypothermia after traumatic brain injury in adults: a systematic review. *JAMA* 289:2992–2999, 2003.
37. Henderson WR, Dhingra VK, Chittock DR, et al: Hypothermia in the management of traumatic brain injury. A systematic review and meta-analysis. *Intensive Care Med* 29:1637–1644, 2003.
38. Clifton Gl, Miller ER, Choi SC, et al: Lack of effect of induction of hypothermia after acute brain injury. *N Engl J Med* 344:556–563, 2001.
39. Hutchison JS, Ward RE, Lacroix J, et al: Hypothermia therapy after traumatic brain injury in children. *N Engl J Med* 358:2447–2456, 2008.
40. Polderman K, Ely EW, Badr AE, et al: Induced hypothermia for TBI: considering conflicting results of meta-analysis and moving forward. *Intensive Care Med* 30:1860–1864, 2004.
41. Peterson K, Carson S, Carney N: Hypothermia treatment for traumatic brain injury: a systematic review and meta-analysis. *J Trauma* 25:62–71, 2008.
42. Clifton G, Valadka A, Zygun D et al: Very early hypothermia induction in patients with severe brain injury (the National Acute Brain Injury Study: Hypothermia II): a randomised trial. *Lancet Neurol* 10(20):131–139, 2011.
43. Suehiro E, Kozuimi H, Fujisawa H, et al: Diverse effects of hypothermia therapy in patients with severe traumatic brain injury based on the computed tomography classification of the Traumatic Coma Data Bank. *J Neurotrauma* 32(5):353–358, 2015.
44. Yokobori S, Yokota H: Targeted Temperature management in traumatic brain injury. *J Intensive Care* 4(28):1–10. 2016

45. Hypothermia After Cardiac Arrest Study Group: Mild therapeutic hypothermia to improve the neurologic outcome after cardiac arrest. *N Engl J Med* 346:549–556, 2002.
46. Bernard SA, Gray TW, Buist MD, et al: Treatment of comatose survivors of out-of-hospital cardiac arrest with induced hypothermia. *N Engl J Med* 346:557–563, 2002.
47. Kilpatrick MM, Lowry DW, Firlik AD, et al: Hyperthermia in the neurosurgical intensive care unit. *Neurosurgery* 47:850–856, 2000.
48. Schwarz S, Hafner K, Aschoff A, et al: Incidence and prognostic significance of fever following intracerebral hemorrhage. *Neurology* 54:354–361, 2000.
49. Natale JE, Joseph JG, Helfaer MA, et al: Early hyperthermia after traumatic brain injury in children: risk factors, influence on length of stay, and effect on short-term neurologic status. *Crit Care Med* 28:2608–2615, 2000.
50. Fabricius M, Fuhr S, Bhatia R, et al: Cortical spreading depression and peri infarct depolarization in acutely injured human cerebral cortex. *Brain* 129:778–790, 2006.
51. Drier JP, Woitzik J, Fabricius M, et al: Delayed ischemic neurological deficits after subarachnoid hemorrhage are associated with clusters of spreading depolarizations. *Brain* 129:3224–3237, 2006.
52. Drier JP: The role of spreading depression, spreading depolarization and spreading ischemia in neurological disease. *Nat Med* 17:439–447, 2011.
53. Hartings JA, Watanabe T, Bullock MR et al: Spreading depolarizations have prolonged direct current shifts and are associated with poor outcome in brain trauma. *Brain* 134:1529–1540, 2011.
54. Nuwer M: Assessment of digital EEG, quantitative EEG, and EEG brain mapping: report of the American Academy of Neurology and the American Clinical Neurophysiology Society. *Neurology* 49:277–292, 1997.
55. Vespa PM, Nuwer MR, Juhasz C, et al: Early detection of vasospasm after acute subarachnoid hemorrhage using continuous EEG ICU monitoring. *Electroencephalogr Clin Neurophysiol* 103:607–615, 1997.
56. Vespa PM, Boscardin WJ, Becker DP, et al: Early persistent impaired percent alpha variability on continuous EEG monitoring as predictive of poor outcome after TBI. *J Neurosurgery* 97:84–92, 2002
57. Hebb MO, McArthur DL, Alger J, et al: Impaired percent alpha variability on continuous electroencephalography is associated with thalamic injury and predicts poor long-term outcome after human traumatic brain injury. *J Neurotrauma* 2007;24:579–590.
58. Preventing and managing the impact of anesthesia awareness. *JCAHO Sentinel Event Alert* 2004. Available from the Joint Commission on Accreditation of Healthcare Organizations, http://www.jointcommission.org/SentinelEvents/SentinelEventAlert/seq_32.htm Retrieved December 5, 2006. Accessed January 25, 2017.
59. American Society of Anesthesiologists practice advisory for intraoperative awareness and brain function monitoring: *House of Delegates*. Available from the American Society of Anesthesiologists, http://www.asahg.org/publicationsandServices/AwareAdvisoryFinalOct5.pdf. Retrieved December 5, 2006. Accessed January 25, 2017.
60. Nasraway SA Jr, Wu EC, Kelleher RM, et al: How reliable is the bispectral index in critically ill patients? A prospective, comparative, single-blinded observer study. *Crit Care Med* 30:1483–1487, 2002.
61. Bruhn J, Bouillon TW, Shafer SL: Electromyographic activity falsely elevates the bispectral index. *Anesthesiology* 92:1485–1487, 2000.
62. Beniczsky S, Aurlien H, Brogger JC, et al: Standardized computer based organization reporting of EEG: SCORE. *Epilepsia* 54(6):112–124, 2013.
63. Lee JW, LaRoche S, Choi H, et al: Development and feasibility testing of a critical care EEG monitoring database for standardized clinical reporting and multicenter collaborative research. *J Clin Neurophysiol* 33(2):133–140, 2016.
64. Friedman D, Claasen J, Hirsch LJ: Continuous EEG monitoring in the ICU. *Anesth Analg* 109:506–523, 2009.
65. Kurtz P, Hanafy KA, Claasen J: Continuous EEG monitoring: Is it ready for primetime? *Curr Opin Crit Care* 15(2):99–109, 2009.
66. Lotto ML, Banoub M, Schubert A: Effects of anesthetic agents and physiologic changes on intraoperative motor evoked potentials. *J Neurosurg Anesthesiol* 16:32–42, 2004.
67. Schwarz S, Hacke W, Schwab S: Magnetic evoked potentials in neurocritical care patients with acute brainstem lesions. *J Neurol Sci* 172:30–37, 2000.
68. Wijdicks EF, Hijdra A, Young GB, et al: Practice parameter: prediction of outcome in comatose survivors after cardiopulmonary resuscitation (an evidence-based review): report of the quality standards subcommittee of the American Academy of Neurology. *Neurology* 67:203–210, 2006.
69. Guérit JM, Amantini A, Amodio P, et al: Consensus on the use of neurophysiological tests in the intensive care unit (ICU): electroencephalogram (EEG), evoked potentials (EP), and electroneuromyography (ENMG). *Clin Neurophysiol* 39:71–83, 2009.
70. Koenig MA, Kaplan PW: Clinical applications for EPs in the ICU. *J Clin Neurophysiol* 32(6):472–480, 2015.
71. Marion DW, Spiegel TP: Changes in the management of severe traumatic brain injury: 1991–1997. *Crit Care Med* 28:16–18, 2000.
72. Smith M: Monitoring intracranial pressure in traumatic brain injury. *Anesth Analg* 106:240–248, 2008.
73. Marmarou A, Anderson RL, Ward JD, et al: Impact of ICP instability and hypotension on outcome in patients with severe head trauma. *J Neurosurg* 75:S59–S66, 1991.
74. Bullock RM, Chesnut RM, Clifton GL, et al: Management and prognosis of severe traumatic brain injury. Part I. Guidelines for the management of severe traumatic brain injury. *J Neurotrauma* 17:449–553, 2000.
75. Bullock RM, Chesnut RM, Clifton GL, et al: Indications for intracranial pressure monitoring. *J Neurotrauma* 17:479–491, 2000.
76. Chesnut RM, Temkin N, Carney N et al: A trial of intracranial pressure monitoring in traumatic brain injury. *N Eng J Med* 367:2471–2481, 2012.
77. Bullock RM, Chesnut RM, Clifton GL, et al: Recommendations for intracranial pressure monitoring technology. *J Neurotrauma* 17:497–506, 2000.
78. Martinez-Manas RM, Santamarta D, de Campos JM, et al: Camino intracranial pressure monitor: prospective study of accuracy and complications. *J Neurol Neurosurg Psychiatry* 69:82–86, 2000.
79. Chambers IR, Kane PJ, Signorini DF, et al: Bilateral ICP monitoring: its importance in detecting the severity of secondary insults. *Acta Neurochir Suppl* 71:42–43, 1998.
80. Juul N, Morris GF, Marshall SB, et al: Intracranial hypertension and cerebral perfusion pressure: influence on neurological deterioration and outcome in severe head injury. *J Neurosurg* 92:1–6, 2000.
81. Robertson CS: Management of cerebral perfusion pressure after traumatic brain injury. *Anesthesiology* 95:1513–1517, 2001.
82. Robertson CS, Valadka AB, Hannay HJ, et al: Prevention of secondary ischemic insults after severe head injury. *Crit Care Med* 27:2086–2095, 1999.
83. Ropper AH. Brain in a box. *N Eng J Med* 367:2539–2541, 2012.
84. Carandang RA: The role of invasive monitoring in traumatic brain injury. *Current Trauma Reports* 1:125–132, 2015.
85. Latchaw RE: Cerebral perfusion imaging in acute stroke. *J Vasc Interv Radiol* 15:S29–S46, 2004.
86. Jaeger M, Siehke M, Meixenberger J, et al: Correlation of continuously monitored regional cerebral blood flow and brain tissue oxygen. *Acta Neurochir* 147:51–56, 2005.
87. Sase S, Honda M, Machida K, et al: Comparison of cerebral blood flow between perfusion computed tomography and xenon-enhanced computed tomography for normal subjects: territorial analysis. *J Comput Assist Tomogr* 29:270–277, 2005.
88. Qureshi AI, Sung GY, Razumovsky AY, et al: Early identification of patients at risk for symptomatic vasospasm after aneurysmal subarachnoid hemorrhage. *Crit Care Med* 28:984–990, 2000.
89. Lam JM, Chan MS, Poon WS: Cerebral venous oxygen saturation monitoring: is dominant jugular bulb cannulation good enough? *Br J Neurosurg* 10:357–364, 1996.
90. Metz C, Holzschuh M, Bein T, et al: Monitoring of cerebral oxygen metabolism in the jugular bulb: reliability of unilateral measurements in severe head injury. *J Cereb Blood Flow Metab* 18:332–343, 1998.
91. Gopinath SP, Robertson CS, Contant CF, et al: Jugular venous desaturation and outcome after head injury. *J Neurol Neurosurg Psychiatry* 57:717–723, 1994.
92. Cruz J, Jaggi JL, Hoffstad OJ: Cerebral blood flow and oxygen consumption in acute brain injury with acute anemia: an alternative for the cerebral metabolic rate of oxygen consumption? *Crit Care Med* 21:1218–1224, 1993.
93. Zauner A, Doppenberg EM, Woodward JJ, et al: Continuous monitoring of cerebral substrate delivery and clearance: initial experience in 24 patients with severe acute brain injuries. *Neurosurgery* 41:1082–1093, 1997.
94. Maloney-Wilensky E, Gracias V, Itkin A, et al: Brain tissue oxygen and outcome after severe TBI: a systematic review. *Crit Care Med* 37:2057–2063, 2009.
95. van den Brink WA, van Santbrink H, Steyerberg EW, et al: Brain oxygen tension in severe head injury. *Neurosurgery* 46:868–878, 2000.
96. Unterberg AW, Kiening KL, Härtl R, et al: Multimodal monitoring in patients with head injury: evaluation of the effects of treatment on cerebral oxygenation. *J Trauma* 42:S32–S37, 1997.
97. Gopinath SP, Valadka AB, Uzura M, et al: Comparison of jugular venous oxygen saturation and brain tissue PO_2 as monitors of cerebral ischemia after head injury. *Crit Care Med* 27:2337–2345, 1999.
98. DeGeorgia MA: Brain tissue oxygen monitoring in neurocritical care. *J Intensive Care Med* 30(8):473–483, 2015
99. http://beta.neurocriticalcare.org/news/2014-annual-meeting-highlights
100. Brain Tissue Oxygen Monitoring in Traumatic Brain Injury, BOSST 2. NCT 00974259. Available at www.clinicaltrials.gov. Accessed January 25, 2017.
101. Mazzeo AT, Bullock R: Effect of bacterial meningitis complicating severe head trauma upon brain microdialysis and cerebral perfusion. *Neurocrit Care* 2:282–287, 2005.
102. Sarrafzadeh AS, Sakowitz OW, Kiening KL, et al: Bedside microdialysis: a tool to monitor cerebral metabolism in subarachnoid hemorrhage patients? *Crit Care Med* 30:1062–1070, 2002.
103. Bellander BM, Cantais E, Enblad P, et al: Consensus meeting on microdialysis in neurointensive care. *Intensive Care Med* 30:2166–2169, 2004.
104. Johnston AJ, Gupta AK: Advanced monitoring in the neurology intensive care unit: microdialysis. *Curr Opin Crit Care* 8:121–127, 2002.
105. Peerdeman SM, Girbes AR, Vandertop WP: Cerebral microdialysis as a new tool for neurometabolic monitoring. *Intensive Care Med* 26:662–669, 2000.
106. Hillered L, Vespa PM, Hovda DA: Translational neurochemical research in acute human brain injury: the current status and potential future of cerebral Microdialysis. *J Neurotrauma* 22:3–41, 2005.
107. Ferrari M, Mottola L, Quaresima V: Principles, techniques, and limitations of near infrared spectroscopy. *Can J Appl Physiol* 29:463–487, 2004.
108. Pollard V, Prough DS, DeMelo AE, et al: Validation in volunteers of a near-infrared spectroscope for monitoring brain oxygenation in vivo. *Anesth Analg* 82:269–277, 1996.
109. Unterberg A, Rosenthal A, Schneider GH, et al: Validation of monitoring of cerebral oxygenation by near-infrared spectroscopy in comatose patients, in Tasubokawa T, Marmarou A, Robertson C, et al (eds): *Neurochemical*

Monitoring in the Intensive Care Unit. New York, Springer-Verlag, 1995, pp 204–210.
110. Arnulphi MC, Alaraj A, Slavin KV: Near infrared technology in neuroscience: past, present and future. *Neurol Res* 31:605–614, 2009.
111. Nicklin SE, Hassan IA, Wickramasinghe YA, et al: The light still shines, but not that brightly? the current status of perinatal near infrared spectroscopy. *Arch Dis Child* 88:F263–F268, 2003.
112. Henson LC, Calalang C, Temp JA, et al: Accuracy of a cerebral oximeter in healthy volunteers under conditions of isocapnic hypoxia. *Anesthesiology* 88:58–65, 1998.
113. Petrov YY, Prough DS, Deyo DJ, et al: Optoacoustic, noninvasive, real-time, continuous monitoring of cerebral blood oxygenation: an in vivo study in sheep. *Anesthesiology* 102:69–75, 2005.
114. Newberg AB, Alavi A: Neuroimaging in patients with head injury. *Semin Nucl Med* 33:136–147, 2003.
115. Marshall LF, Marshall SB, Klauber MR, et al: A new classification of head injury based on computerized tomography. *J Neurosurg* 75:S14–S20, 1991.
116. Narayan RK, Kishore PRS, Becker DP, et al: Intracranial pressure: to monitor or not to monitor? A review of our experience with severe head injury. *J Neurosurg* 56:650–659, 1982.
117. Eisenberg HM, Gary HE Jr, Aldrich EF, et al: Initial CT findings in 753 patients with severe head injury. A report from the NIH Traumatic Coma Data Bank. *J Neurosurg* 73:688–698, 1990.
118. Kemp GJ: Non-invasive methods for studying brain energy metabolism: what they show and what it means. *Dev Neurosci* 22:418–428, 2000.
119. Watson NA, Beards SC, Altaf N, et al: The effect of hyperoxia on cerebral blood flow: a study in healthy volunteers using magnetic resonance phase-contrast angiography. *Eur J Anaesthesiol* 17:152–159, 2000.
120. Verweij BH, Muizelaar JP, Vinas FC, et al: Impaired cerebral mitochondrial function after traumatic brain injury in humans. *J Neurosurg* 93:815–820, 2000.
121. Tollard E, Galanaud D, Perlbarg V, et al: Experience of diffusion tensor imaging and H-spectroscopy for outcome prediction in severe TBI. *Crit Care Med* 37:1448–1455, 2009.
122. De Georgia MA, Deogaonkar A: Multimodal monitoring in the neurological intensive care unit. *Neurologist* 11:45–54, 2005.
123. Elf K, Nilsson P, Enblad P: Outcome after traumatic brain injury improved by an organized secondary insult program and standardized neurointensive care. *Crit Care Med* 30:2129–2134, 2003.
124. LeRoux P, Menon DK, Citerio G. et al: Consensus summary statement of the International Multidisciplinary Consensus Conference on Multimodality Monitoring in Neurocritical Care. A statement of healthcare professionals from the Neurocritical Care Society and the European Society of Intensive Care Medicine. *Intensive Care Med* 40(9):1189–1209, 2014.

Chapter 32 ▪ Telemedicine and Critical Care Delivery

LLOYD C. MEEKS • SHAHZAD SHAEFI • CRAIG M. LILLY

NEW FORMS OF ELECTRONIC SUPPORT FOR CRITICAL CARE PROFESSIONALS

The challenge of delivering critical care medicine in the 21st century has become increasingly clear, and there is broad consensus for making safe and effective care more available by controlling costs. This challenge is multifactorial and consists of several well-documented elements including a growing number of critically ill patients [1,2], an aging population [3], an unprecedented focus on accountable care and reducing healthcare spending [4], an inadequate number and maldistribution of qualified critical care providers [5–8], and public expectations for patient safety and the reduction of medical errors [9]. Ongoing efforts continue to center on finding evidence-based approaches to these complex and competing factors. One approach to solving the current challenges is "Telemedicine," defined as the application of communications and information technologies to allow specialty-trained physicians to care for patients remotely. This chapter will explore the rationale, advantages, and limitations associated with using telemedicine to care for critically ill patients under the current challenges facing healthcare.

Most proponents of healthcare improvement advocate ideas and solutions that can be encapsulated by the Institute for Healthcare Improvement's Triple Aim [10]. As health systems develop or transform, the Triple Aim provides a framework centered on three cornerstones that are simultaneously pursued—improving the quality and satisfaction of the patient care experience, improving the health of populations, and reducing the per capita cost of healthcare. The choices surrounding how to deliver critical care are important because both spending and mortality in the critical care setting are the highest for all of healthcare [11]. Annually, almost 6 million Americans are admitted to one of the 6,300 intensive care units (ICUs) located in 3,200 acute care hospitals, where 55,000 patients receive ICU care every day [12–14]. Recent evidence shows that from 2000 to 2009, the number of hospital beds did not grow substantially likely owing to the shift of healthcare to the outpatient setting. However, there was a substantial increase in the number of ICU beds, signifying a trend that a growing proportion of hospital operations are focused on the care of the critically ill [2]. Annually, these patients have required intensive care that contributes up to $100 billion of the over $3 trillion spent on all of US healthcare, corresponding to about 1% of the gross domestic product (GDP) [15]. In comparison, other countries spend as little as 0.1% of their GDP on critical care without appreciable differences in patient outcomes or life expectancy [16]. Further evidence shows that 25% of all US healthcare spending is in the final year of life and that approximately 20% of deaths occur in or soon after an ICU stay [17].

The combination of the post-World War II population expansion, known as the "baby boom," and the increase in life expectancy for US adults has led to large increases in older segments of our population that have required more critical care services [3,18]. By 2030, it is estimated that over 70 million US residents will be over 65, an age group that currently requires three times as much critical care resources as that of younger groups of patients. In addition, patients 85 years and older require six times as much critical care, and the size of this age group is projected to triple by 2030 compared with the 2006 population. The challenge associated with this expansion is compounded by the increasing focus on patient and family-centered care, which is the assurance that clinical care decisions are guided by the values and preferences of individual patients and their loved ones [19]. Healthcare information technology as a means to access healthcare is increasingly preferred by patients because it combines convenience with the ability to connect to specialists and other providers in ways that meet their expectations, which have traditionally been largely unmet [20]. These issues have spawned efforts by health policy experts and administrators to find solutions to increase the quality and efficiency of critical care delivery. The integration of telecommunications technologies and health information system data is allowing telemedicine to become an increasingly important part of the healthcare delivery system [21].

The increased need for critical care and the high costs associated with caring for critically ill adults have led to an intense interest in practical methods for increasing the efficiency of critical care delivery. A growing body of literature indicates that care delivered by intensive care–trained professionals can increase quality and improve important outcomes such as lowering mortality and length of stay (LOS) [22,23]. Healthcare payers, both governmental and private, are shifting payment models from traditional fee-for-service to value-based reimbursement systems [4]. Accordingly, hospitals and healthcare organizations are beginning to focus on quality standards and increased efficiency as the backbone of their delivery models as opposed to simply increasing the volume of services provided. One of the largest advocates in patient safety and quality has been The Leapfrog Group, a nonprofit organization and consortium of Fortune 500 companies that has established measures of improvement for all of healthcare [24]. Leapfrog compliance has continued to be a priority for hospitals and includes intensivist staffing as one of its key measures, or "leaps." The Leapfrog standard requires intensivists to be dedicated exclusively to providing care in the ICU during daytime hours [14]. If intensivists are unavailable, Leapfrog states that they must be reachable within 5 minutes and arrange for specifically trained nonintensivists, including nonphysicians, to reach the patient within 5 minutes. These initiatives are based on broadly accepted evidence that intensivist-led ICU teams can lower mortality, lower LOS, and increase quality [25]. However, less than one-quarter of ICUs in Leapfrog's recent surveys meet the intensivist staffing marker [26], a failure and an indicator of the broad difficulty of providing ICU patients healthcare by dedicated, specialty-trained, and certified providers. Interestingly, as telemedicine delivery models have grown, The Leapfrog Group has identified tele-intensivist programs as compliant with their standards [27], thus indicating strong support of ICU telemedicine programs as a leveraging technology that provides a practical way to deliver high-quality critical care.

Termed a "crisis," many critical care societies have publicly acknowledged the growing discrepancy between the supply of intensivists and the demand for critical care [28]. The etiology of this shortage is multifactorial and includes an inadequate growth of ICU fellowship and graduate medical education (GME) training programs [6], decreased interest in critical care as a career [29,30], and high rates of physicians leaving the field before retirement age [31]. In addition, not all qualified providers spend the majority of their time in the critical care setting because most ICU professionals trained in pulmonary medicine, anesthesiology, neurology, or surgery practice critical care as only part of their careers [32]. The simplest strategy to address this supply shortage is to produce more intensivists by increasing the number of GME training positions [7,33]. However, this strategy would increase costs by adding to the more than $15 billion currently spent on GME, which comes directly out of the US healthcare budget [34,35]. Furthermore, it could have unintended consequences on other areas of healthcare that are also thought to have an inadequate number of qualified providers [36]. The critical care physician shortage also has an element of maldistribution because there are a disproportionately larger number of critical care specialists in urban hospital ICUs than in rural areas [37]. Critical care is delivered throughout the United States in a variety of settings, but the majority of ICU beds are located in nonteaching community hospitals with fewer than 300 beds [14]. A critically ill patient with access to an ICU, unfortunately, does not uniformly indicate high quality and comprehensive care because wide variation exists in when and how critical care specialists, if available, provide care [38]. Furthermore, critical illnesses such as sepsis, acute respiratory distress syndrome, acute coronary syndrome, acute cerebrovascular accidents, and venous thromboembolism require timely standardized intervention delivered by healthcare teams comprised of individuals with adequate recent experience to maintain proficiency. Telemedicine support can increase the frequency of high-quality care at locations that would have otherwise delayed care in view of the need to transport patients to locations with qualified providers. ICU telemedicine programs have the potential to reduce mortality in diseases that require early goal-directed care, reduce costs associated with transport, and allow tertiary care hospitals to manage higher acuity cases that require services that are not available locally. ICU telemedicine programs also have the potential to improve access to high-quality care at community hospitals that are closer to the patient's home.

Importantly, simply increasing the number of intensivists might not solve the maldistribution issue because most qualified providers prefer to work in urban and suburban areas, whereas most ICUs without intensivists are in rural areas [39]. In addition, with limited numbers of providers at a particular location, it remains difficult for hospitals to retain intensivists owing in part to the increased workload and inadequate staffing and inadequate night and weekend coverage for their ICUs [40]. The US Health Resources and Services Administration (HRSA) recently projected a workforce gap of over 3,300 intensivist full-time equivalents by 2020 [6]. Well-intended strategies to solve this supply matrix crisis include increasing the training and distribution of advanced practice providers (APPs), either physician assistants (PA) or nurse practitioners (NP) [41]. More than 200,000 NPs and more than 90,000 PAs are currently practicing in the United States [42,43]. However, less than half of these providers are educated and trained in acute and critical care, including only 4,000 NPs who are actively working in critical care environments [44]. While intensivists often provide care in ratios of 1:12 and above, APPs often provide care in ratios of 1:4–5. To date, this approach has not provided an adequate supply of critical care providers to solve the workforce demand.

Government funding, through the creation of the Affordable Care Act [45], has recently initiated funding for healthcare innovation ideas across the full spectrum of healthcare delivery. One such example includes a financially successful initiative that integrates specific critical care training with APPs along with telemedicine oversight by intensivists to serve the high demand for ICU care professionals in underserved areas [46]. In addition to the federal government, state appropriations and foundation grants have similarly appropriated funds to technology-based innovation in telehealth with the common theme of improving access to high-quality care.

Telemedicine integration into ICU healthcare delivery helps solve the supply problem because it removes geographic barriers to high-quality care, thus increasing the number of ICU patients that can receive evaluation and management services from a critical care specialist–led team. Intensivist-led tele-ICU teams can serve a substantially larger population of patients than intensivists using traditional telephonic tools [47,48]. This is due in part to the use of dedicated workstations that run software designed to collect and display clinical information in a format that allows more efficient management of critically ill adults. These workstations include bidirectional audio/video, clinical decision support, population management software, and smart alarms and alerts that allow earlier detection of physiologic instability and abnormal laboratory values. They are also designed to support the efficient recording of provider orders and care protocols. These tools allow increased provider productivity based on the ability of the technology to collect real-time clinical data from the bedside and display electronic signatures of care need to off-site providers. The effectiveness of this approach depends on the timing and effectiveness of the delivery of evaluation and management services by the ICU telemedicine team [49]. Proactive critical care interventions coupled with provider documentation facilitated by technology such as alarms, alerts, and real-time reporting tools can create a more efficient and effective ICU delivery workflow than the traditional daily time-based rounding and documentation carried out by bedside providers. The optimal number of patients that one tele-intensivist should be responsible for is not well established and would vary widely depending on a variety of factors including local resources, ICU acuity, and telemedicine staffing and support structure [50]. In addition to increasing the number of patients who are able to receive care from a critical care specialist, more community-based ICUs can retain an intensivist because ICU telemedicine practice models reduce off-shift workload for bedside intensivists [51].

Some healthcare experts have not only proposed solutions to the issue with supply of ICU providers, but have emphasized potential measures to reduce the demand for ICU care [52]. Although standard ICU admission criteria exist, significant variability in ICU admission practices occurs that can lead to overutilization of resources, increased costs, increased LOS, and more frequent preventable complications [53]. It seems clear that admission to an ICU, either urban or rural, is currently based not on standardized criteria but rather on a variety of factors that often do not reflect the patient's potential for physiologic instability. Patients with borderline indications for ICU admission often get admitted to the ICU owing to the uncertainty regarding potential deterioration and thus receive more costly care that is unnecessary. An investigation of a large database of ICU admissions showed that only two-thirds of patients admitted to an ICU received an ICU-level intervention [54]. Similarly, less than 40% of patients in another ICU population received mechanical ventilation at any time during their ICU stay [55]. There is wide variation in the way ICUs are used in the United States, and hospitals that tend to use more critical care resources have not shown improved outcomes [56]. Telecommunications and health information technology including bidirectional audio/video, electronic monitoring, and clinical decision support can exist in acute care environments outside of the ICUs to augment in-hospital clinical teams and make better use of constrained resources with tools available to focus on best practices, sepsis management, pain management, readmission risk, and fall prevention. This electronic oversight captures physiologic data and alerts dedicated off-site clinical teams of potential patient deterioration and the need for escalation to ICU-level care through early detection, resulting in the ability to more appropriately utilize costly ICU resources.

Innovative critical care delivery models are gaining attention with the intention to provide safe, timely, consistent, and effective care with a limited number of qualified providers. In this chapter, we will focus on providing the evidence that supports the utilization of telemedicine support systems as a potential innovative technology solution by reengineering the flow of clinical information from the patient to their ICU provider (Fig. 32.1). These tools allow critical care specialists to obtain real-time actionable clinical information and provide evaluation and management services. Connecting to critically ill patients in this way can improve outcomes, lower complications, and increase patient and family satisfaction [57]. Utilizing remote workstations equipped with the necessary technology, tele-ICU teams consisting of intensivists, APPs, and critical care–certified nurses can provide high-quality critical care where and when it is needed.

TECHNOLOGIC SOLUTIONS

ICUs continue to evolve in parallel with the rapid maturation of health information technologies. In addition, major advances in the field of critical care medicine have produced meaningful improvements in patient survival. However, the penetration of these advances has been limited by inefficiencies of critical care delivery due to ineffective design or lack of qualified specialists [58]. Remote real-time support for acutely ill patients is a promising strategy that can improve the efficiency of critical care delivery by reengineering the interface between the patient and the ICU care delivery system [59]. Widespread acceptance of healthcare technology into certain healthcare delivery processes has been slow because a period of diffusion of innovation is followed by rapid expansion based on social acceptance [60]. Rapid expansion of technology and mobile communications has heightened societal expectations regarding the ability to access information anywhere, anytime, on personal electronic devices. Convenient access to healthcare is increasingly demanded, and delivery models have not fully integrated available technologies that can reduce inefficiencies, enhance the quality of care, and improve the patient experience. Telemedicine has the potential to provide an on-demand experience that can enhance the patient and family-centered care in ICUs by allowing easier access to desired providers. Interactions with families in ICUs are frequent and important because critically ill patients are often unable to directly participate in complex discussions of diagnosis, prognosis, treatment options, and end-of-life preferences [61]. Because families often rate communication with providers as being as important as clinical skill [62], telecommunication technologies can allow families access to these valuable discussions without being present at the bedside. Anywhere, anytime connectivity can enhance integration of families into the process of critical care delivery, provide an improved family experience during an often stressful time, and reduce overutilization of invasive treatments of little clinical benefit.

Over 100 years ago, attempts at electrocardiogram transmission over telephone lines allowed real-time off-site interpretation [63]. Telemedicine integration into ICU care occurred in the latter half of the past century [64], but the first comprehensive ICU telemedicine program was not implemented until 2000 in Virginia [65]. Wider acceptance did not occur until just over 10 years ago when investigators at Johns Hopkins showed acuity-adjusted improvements in both ICU and hospital mortality based on a continuous intensivist-led tele-ICU care model for two adult ICUs [66]. The tele-ICU platform used in this investigation has remained the dominant infrastructure and design of tele-ICU delivery to date, although expansion of technologic capabilities and alternative platforms has evolved. Most believe this initial model of continuous telemedicine delivery of intensivist care was the impetus for the growth of the field of ICU telemedicine.

Since the first program installation and the associated patient safety and efficiency of care benefits, there has been growth of programs with similar designs. Based on recent evidence attempting to quantify the expansion of tele-ICU programs in the United States, five integrated tele-ICU programs had been implemented in hospitals prior to 2003 [67]. Adoption of ICU telemedicine occurred in 218 hospitals between 2003 and 2010, an average annual increase of approximately 60%. Within this expansion, the number of ICU beds involved in tele-ICU delivery grew almost 50% per year from 598 to 5,799, while the number of dedicated support centers with tele-ICU professionals grew beyond 40 with wide geographic dispersion across the United States. With expanding technologies, increasing numbers of vendors, and a better understanding of the variation of designs that could potentially meet the needs of the full spectrum of urban and rural hospitals, further growth and saturation is anticipated. An estimated 15% of nonfederal hospital ICU beds in the United States are currently receiving support from a continuous ICU telemedicine model of care [38]. Recent expansion of alternative technology platforms, mobile telecommunications, and episodic care models suggests that the number of ICU patients receiving telemedicine support is larger than the number of closed model bedside intensivist-led ICUs [68].

With regard to design and infrastructure, ICU telemedicine capabilities have broadened in recent years (Table 32.1). Recent literature provides a detailed report of various ways to utilize telemedicine support systems for the care of critically ill patients [48,69,70]. Based on supportive literature, most new ICU telemedicine systems are based on a single design consisting of a centralized support center and provide a continuous model of care with a closed communication architecture. A centralized,

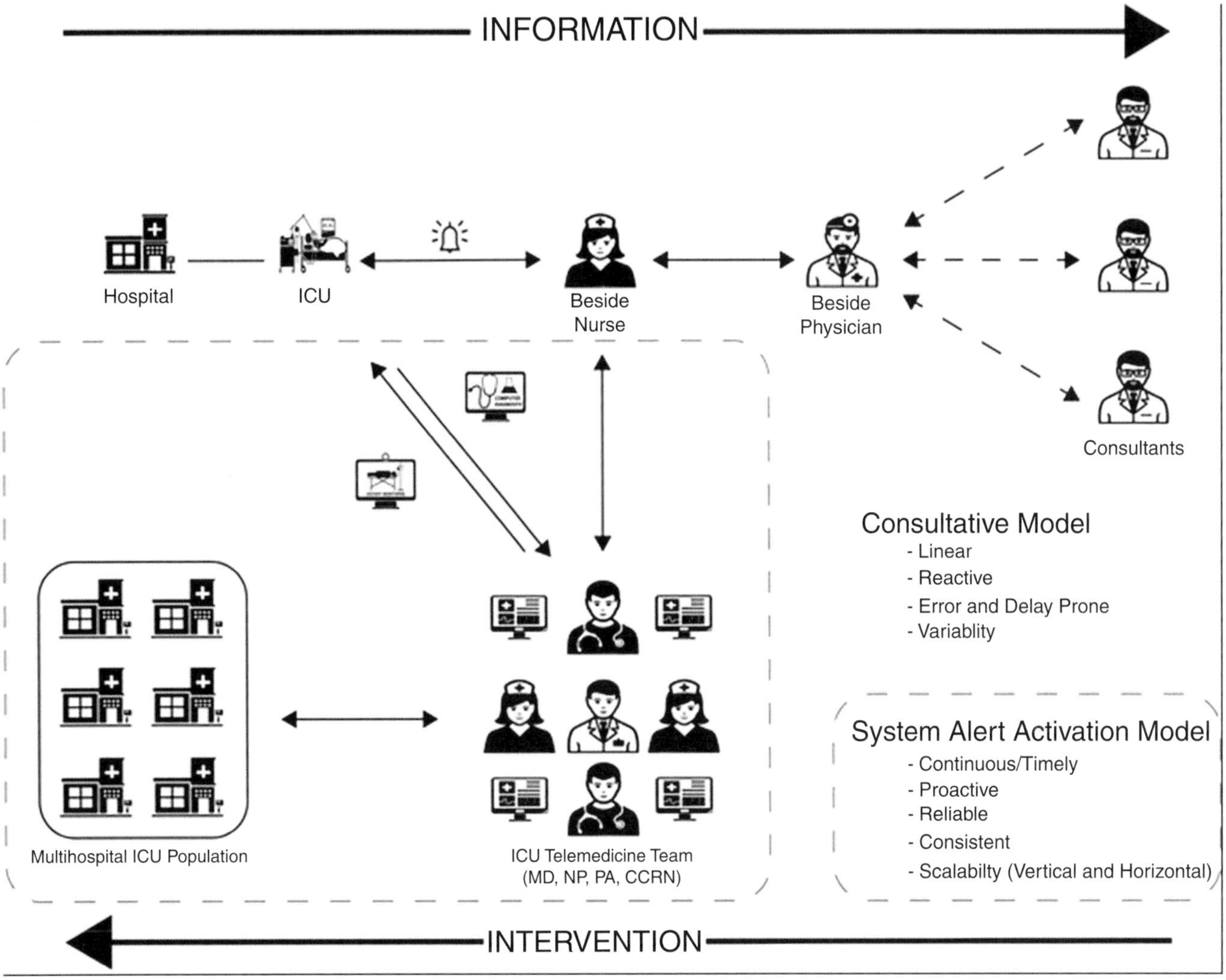

FIGURE 32.1 Contrasting traditional intensive care unit (ICU) flow of clinical information with a reengineered workflow utilizing electronic support tools to provide remote qualified ICU professionals with the ability to provide more timely care led by an intensive care physician specialist across a larger ICU population. NP, nurse practitioners; PA, physician assistants.

closed model consists of a monitoring center—housed by varying staffing models of intensivists, APPs, RNs, and support staff—with sophisticated computer workstations that utilize high-speed communication lines that securely and reliably link multiple hospitals to a central location. This platform provides bidirectional audio/visual capabilities, real-time interfacing and trending of physiologic data, connections to clinical information systems, and audio video connections to patients. A closed "hub and spoke" model generally indicates that providers outside of the monitoring center, such as subspecialists, would not have access to the tele-ICU system and could only provide patient care utilizing traditional modes of communication and data review. In contrast to a centralized closed architecture, a decentralized "virtual hub" offers open access to tele-ICU team members regardless of their geographic location. An open architecture generally indicates Internet connectivity linking multiple providers from multiple sites to multiple ICUs. In addition, open access allows the ICU telemedicine program to offer virtual subspecialty care to patients, with providers such as cardiologists and neurologists able to access the tele-ICU system from their secure personal devices. ICU telemedicine programs can be structured in ways to provide continuous or episodic care. Continuous care provides the tele-ICU team with the ability to deliver 24/7 critical care management using near real-time responses to electronic signatures of evolving physiologic instability. A discontinuous, or episodic, care model consists of a tele-ICU patient assessment only during designated times either scheduled or requested at the discretion of a bedside clinician. Incorporating various aspects

TABLE 32.1

ICU Telemedicine Delivery Models [128]

1. Continuous Care Model—Proactive care that occurs on a 24/7 continuous basis servicing an ICU population utilizing a centralized operational center staffed by a team of ICU professionals led by a qualified intensive care physician specialist.
2. Episodic Care Model—Proactive care that occurs intermittently connecting patient–provider or provider–provider on a predetermined basis (e.g., daily rounds) or at unscheduled times.
3. Responsive Care Model—Reactive care, when virtual consults are prompted by an alert (e.g., patient alarm, telephone call).

ICU, intensive care unit.

of all the elements of tele-ICU design can create hybrid systems that can facilitate high-quality multispecialty care to critically ill patients in a timely and effective manner [48]. Comparative trials of alternative systems have not been performed in part because systems that meet current telecommunications industry standards have sufficient speed and capacity to achieve nearly equivalent performance.

Since the introduction of the first tele-ICU system, technology and equipment have involved advanced workstations that allow the simultaneous display of data from multiple sources that can allow users to view information from more than one patient at a time. One key safety element is how the systems are designed to assure that a given intervention is prescribed to the patient for which it is intended. Tele-ICU monitoring centers often colocate workstations that include multiple computers, multiple monitor displays, microphones, speakers, and broadband capabilities for teams of providers. This creates efficiency because intensivists can leverage nurses and prescribing APP partners (NP or PA) to complete and document tasks. This tiered and shared strategy allows one intensivist to provide urgent evaluation and management services to as many as 150 critically ill adults.

ICU patient rooms include fixed high-resolution cameras with pan, tilt, and zoom capabilities along with speakers, a microphone, and a display monitor. In addition to the networking architecture, portable and mobile solutions have emerged for both ends of the system. Mobility implies Internet connectivity because intensivists and other involved providers can use an Internet-capable laptop or mobile device to gain access to a private viewing environment. Furthermore, mobile systems are often made available on carts equipped with audio/visual and networking equipment, including some robotic systems that do not require transportation or activation by bedside providers. As innovation continues, mobility and functionality are expected to expand.

The availability of sophisticated technology for the delivery of critical care alone does not improve performance [71]. Maximizing ICU telemedicine effectiveness requires a comprehensive understanding of the determinants of improved clinical and financial outcomes for its optimal application. More is now known about how ICU telemedicine reduces mortality and LOS. A multicenter trial that measured an alternative process of care identified several factors that are associated with greater reductions in mortality and LOS [72]. Early intensivist involvement in the form of workstation-assisted care plan reviews, more rapid responses to alerts and alarms for evolving physiologic instability, interdisciplinary collaboration, high rates of adherence to ICU best practices, and near real-time review of ICU performance data by a leadership team that takes action were associated with lower mortality and shorter LOS. Another study of the ability of off-site nurse reviews and communication to the bedside team reported significantly improved adherence to best practices [73]. Each of the elements that were associated with improved outcomes is concordant with the safety and clinical engineering literature. Studies to date have not identified a particular type or size of ICU that predicts improved outcomes. The approach to improving outcomes may depend less on the type or size of the ICU and more on the ability of a particular approach and system to impact these key processes in the environment in which it is deployed.

Telemedicine infrastructure can allow intensivist-led teams to provide critical care expertise across a large population of patients through workflow optimization and the efficient and effective use of near real-time analyses of trending clinical information. Without technology support systems, a bedside nurse or provider must recognize and interpret complex and dynamic physiologic and clinical data before action can occur. Relying upon human recognition and interpretation in an ICU environment can produce delay and error [59]. During critical illness, vital signs, laboratory data, imaging results, and medical equipment can produce hundreds of variables occurring simultaneously. Excessive and error-prone medical device alarms in the ICU environment can cause ICU staff mental fatigue (so-called "alarm fatigue"), often resulting in desensitization and delayed response with potential negative impacts on clinical outcomes and patient safety [74–76]. Based on current design, bedside nurses and providers are often multitasking and responding to unpredictable events elsewhere with the ability to interpret only a small fraction of the myriad of clinical information produced [77]. Further delay can occur if an ICU professional is not readily available to provide an intervention or has yet to become engaged in the patient's care. Current bedside delivery often involves provider rounding and a series of individual evaluations at single points in time. This evaluation includes assessment of current biosensor and clinical information but often does not include tools to detect concerning trends of these factors that can predict deviation from the intended trajectory [78]. ICU telemedicine can provide earlier intervention by ICU professionals along with integration into modern comprehensive patient monitoring systems that enable acquisition, storage, and pattern recognition of the large amounts of patient-specific data. Acquired, organized, and stored data with pattern recognition technology transmitted instantaneously to a tele-ICU can expedite care by enabling earlier recognition of often subtle changes in patient pathophysiology, transitioning from reactive care to proactive and predictive care. With additional connectivity and interoperability among multiple bedside medical devices, such as mechanical ventilators and infusion pumps, complex interactions between patients and therapies can be acquired and interpreted utilizing electronic support [79]. In addition, these systems allow qualified experts to interpret radiographic and ultrasonographic images in near real time. Real-time tele-ICU support for ultrasonography can also improve the quality of acquired images. Clinical decision support system integration further assists the ICU professional in tailoring interventions to the underlying disease process in near real time [80]. Ultimately, an integrated critical care informatics architecture can include real-time acquisition and storage of all raw clinical data that can be stored, processed, and translated into actionable information to be used by a remote ICU professional to provide management services in a more efficient manner across a larger population of patients [81].

DATA AND OUTCOMES

Clinical Outcomes and Process Measures

As evidence accrues (Table 32.2), it has become more established what particular aspects of critical care delivery are associated with meaningful improvements in outcomes. Significant effort has been placed on attempts to determine the impact of bedside intensivist staffing on patient outcomes. Access to intensivists in high intensity settings has been associated with reductions in both ICU and hospital mortality. This was most recently observed in a meta-analysis including 52 composite studies that showed high intensity staffing was associated with lower ICU mortality (risk ratio = 0.81; 95% confidence interval (CI), 0.68–0.96), lower hospital mortality (risk ratio = 0.83; 95% CI, 0.70–0.99), reduced ICU LOS (-0.38 days, 95% CI, -0.55 to -0.20 days), and reduced hospital LOS (-0.17 days, 95% CI, -0.31 to -0.03 days) [22]. The additional support of 24-hour in-hospital intensivist coverage did not improve ICU or hospital mortality, which is consistent with a majority of studies [82–84]. The inability of 24/7 intensivist models to provide incremental benefits is an important concept for the current paradigm of scarce critical care resources. Not only are nighttime intensivists costly to hospital systems, this model reduces the number of intensivists available for other ICUs competing for an already

TABLE 32.2

Effect of ICU Telemedicine on Clinical Outcomes

Source		n	Acuity[a]	ICU Mortality (%)	ICU LOS (d)	Hospital Mortality (%)	Hospital LOS (d)
Rosenfeld et al. [65]	Control	225	43	9.8	2.7	11.6	9.2
	Telemedicine	201	38	1.5	2.0	4.5	9.3
Breslow et al. [66]	Control	1,396	39	8.6	4.3	12.9	12.8
	Telemedicine	744	38	6.3	3.6	9.4	11.1
Marcin et al. [125]	Control	116	7.5	2.6	2.3	NR	NR
	Telemedicine	47	9.6	2.1	3.1	NR	NR
Thomas et al. [88]	Control	2,034	35	9.2	4.3	12	9.8
	Telemedicine	2,108	34	7.8	4.6	9.9	10.7
Zawada et al. [126]	Control	188	38	4.8	3.8	8.5	10.1
	Telemedicine	2,445	44	NR	2.1	NR	7.8
McCambridge et al. [127]	Control	954	57	15.8	4.1	21.4	9.1
	Telemedicine	959	58	11.5	3.8	14.7	9.2
Morrison et al. [89]	Control	1,371	49	6.6	2.6	9.9	7.7
	Telemedicine	1,430	47	7.4	3.2	10.1	7.9
Lilly et al. [92]	Control	1,529	45	10.7	6.4	13.6	13.3
	Telemedicine	4,761	58	8.6	4.5	11.8	9.8
Willmitch et al. [90]	Control	6,504	2.81	NR	4.2	12.3	11.4
	Telemedicine	18,152	2.95	NR	3.9	11.3	10.4
Kohl et al. [128]	Control	246	46	8	5	11	15.6
	Telemedicine	1,499	54	3	3.3	6	15.1
Lilly et al. [72]	Control	11,558	47	8	4.4	11	10.3
	Telemedicine	107,432	53	6	3.5	10	9.7

ICU, intensive care unit; LOS, length of stay; NR, not reported.

[a]APACHE III (Acute Physiology and Chronic Health Evaluation)—Rosenfield, Breslow, Morrison, Lilly 2011, Kohl; APACHE IV—Norman, McCambridge, Lilly 2014; PRISM III (Pediatric Risk of Mortality Score)—Marcin; SAPS II (Simplified Acute Physiology Score)—Thomas; APR-DRG (All Patient Refined—Diagnosis Related Groups)—Willmitch.

inadequate supply. Furthermore, findings from recent studies suggest that the presence of an intensivist at the bedside is not as important as when and how an intensivist is involved in patient care [85]. Engagement using telemedicine support tools that ensure earlier intensivist involvement, more timely response to physiologic instability, and improved adherence to best practices was shown to improve outcomes in both high- and low-intensity bedside staffing models similarly.

The ICU telemedicine evidence base has grown such that there are now two meta-analyses available [86,87] to determine the exact clinical and financial impact of telemedicine on critical care. Initially, most of the data revolving around tele-ICU implementation were reports in the non–peer-reviewed literature. However, two influential early studies [65,66] that are thought to have sparked the growth of the tele-ICU field were published in peer-reviewed critical care literature. In 2000, a tele-ICU program installed at a 10-bed community hospital ICU was shown to reduce the severity-adjusted ICU mortality by 45%, hospital mortality and LOS by 30%, and costs by 16% [65]. Subsequently, a 2004 study from two integrated ICUs showed significant improvement in outcomes, including a 26% reduction in overall hospital and ICU mortality, a 16% reduction in LOS, and a 25% reduction in variable costs generating a greater than $3 million financial benefit in the 6-month study period [66]. A common theme of the implementations of these ICU telemedicine programs was collaboration of bedside and tele-ICU intensivists to provide the same quality of care 24/7.

Tele-ICU implementations that use collaborative governance to standardize key processes of critical care delivery have been associated with lower LOS and improved financial performance. Implementations that do not address competitive tendencies of bedside and tele-ICU physicians or allow inexperienced trainees to staff the ICU telemedicine support center have not been associated with significant improvements in performance. In 2009, a large multicenter study of six ICUs did not detect significant associations between tele-ICU implementation and severity-adjusted ICU or hospital mortality, LOS, or rates of complications [88]. Similarly, in 2010, a study from four ICUs in two community hospitals including over 4,000 unit stays failed to detect a reduction in mortality, LOS, or costs after implementation of an ICU telemedicine program [89]. A recent meta-analysis of published data concluded that ICU telemedicine was associated with a reduced risk of ICU mortality (RR 0.79; 95% CI, 0.65–0.96), a reduced risk of hospital mortality (RR 0.83; 95% CI, 0.73–0.94), shorter ICU LOS (-0.62 days; 95% CI, -1.21 to -0.04 days), and shorter hospital LOS (-1.26 days; 95% CI, -2.49 to -0.03 days) [87]. Notably, there was wide variation and poor characterization of the intervention characteristics and processes, making it difficult to identify the aspects of the intervention that were associated with improved performance. Proactive care by tele-intensivists is thought to be one of the hallmarks of positive outcomes in more recent studies. Published in 2012, a retrospective observational study of over 24,000 patients observed significant reductions in both LOS and mortality over a 3-year postimplementation period [90]. Tele-intensivists were encouraged to be proactive in their participation with the patient care plan, and bedside providers were offered various levels of preferred tele-ICU involvement. Severity-adjusted hospital LOS was lowered from 11.86 days (95% CI, 11.52–12.21) to 10.16 days (95% CI, 9.80–10.53), ICU LOS was lowered from 4.35 days (95% CI, 4.22–4.49) to 3.80 days (95% CI, 3.65–3.94), and the relative risk of hospital mortality decreased to 0.77 (95% CI, 0.69–0.87). However, in 2014, contrary results were published with a US Department of Veterans Affairs healthcare system where no outcome benefit was shown regarding the impact of tele-ICU on hospital LOS or ICU, hospital, and 30-day mortality [91]. The authors did note significant variability among ICUs in their readiness to adopt and implement tele-ICU. Also, the extraordinary low baseline mortality rate reduced the statistical power, thus making it difficult to establish significance regarding the outcomes studied.

In 2011, a study provided more detailed descriptions of the intervention and included analyses that related changes in process to changes in outcomes [92]. A collaborative implementation model of an ICU telemedicine program that included over 6,000 unit stays from seven ICUs in a single academic medical center reported significant associations with improved outcomes. Implementation lowered hospital mortality from 13.6% to 11.8% with an odds ratio (OR) of 0.4 (95% CI, 0.31–0.52) and ICU mortality from 10.7% to 8.6% (OR = 0.37; 95% CI, 0.28–0.49). ICU LOS decreased from 6.4 to 4.5 days postintervention, consistent with increased quality and greater efficiency. Process-focused mechanistic analyses demonstrated that increased adherence to established critical care best practices and lower rates of complications were significantly associated with improved outcomes. Contrasting differences in care delivery process aspects with implementation of the ICU telemedicine program allowed identification of process changes that could account for lower mortality and LOS. Redundant processes for promoting ICU best practice adherence, less than 3 minute responses to alerts and alarms of physiologic instability, and initial care plan reviews by intensivists using dedicated workstations designed to track trends in physiologic parameters and laboratory values were identified as correlates of lower mortality and LOS.

The associations of these and other structural and process-based aspects of critical care delivery that were known to be impacted by some ICU telemedicine programs [93,94] were measured in a 2014 multicenter study [72]. This study analyzed 118,990 ICU stays among patients admitted to ICUs between 2003 and 2008 across 56 ICUs in 32 hospitals from 19 US healthcare systems in a pre/postassessment of implementing an ICU telemedicine program. This study was notable for its size, statistical power, and scope as it was the first study to look at the effect of tele-ICU across the United States. Tele-ICU implementation resulted in improved outcomes, including a 20% lower ICU LOS (95% CI, 19%–22%; $p < 0.001$) and lowering hospital LOS by 15% (95% CI, 14%–17%; $p < 0.001$). More importantly, using a validated standardized survey [93] that reliably characterizes ICUs and their telemedicine structure and processes, additional analysis identified six individual quality improvement constructs that were drivers of larger improvements in mortality and LOS (Table 32.3). Many of these processes revolve around early proactive involvement by an intensivist, technology-enhanced alerting and reminding systems, or the use of data to drive quality improvement. Notably, the effects of individual process elements appeared to be small, but the cumulative effects were clinically significant and financially important [72]. This study is important because it identifies factors that explain some of the differences in outcomes among published studies. These factors involve how clinicians use telemedicine technologies, and it is increasingly clear that how the technology is used is at least as important as the technology itself.

In addition to the important patient-related outcomes revolving around ICU and hospital mortality, multiple investigators have evaluated the effect of tele-ICU implementation on several other relevant outcomes to understand its relevancy, usefulness, impact, and cost-effectiveness. In a consensus statement on the state of tele-ICU research [94], the Critical Care Societies Collaborative recommended the development of a comprehensive outcome evaluation including elements from the perspective of the patients, the providers, the healthcare system, and healthcare payers.

Staff Perceptions and Satisfaction

It is important to understand the bedside provider perspective as acceptance and buy in have been identified as hallmarks of effective programs [95]. Bedside provider enthusiasm depends on several factors, including how they were included in the change process and how long after program implementation their opinions were solicited. A survey administered in 2015 with respondents from a wide variety of hospitals related generally positive responses regarding all facets of tele-ICU [96]. In this survey, responders at hospitals with more frequent use and longer implementation periods were significantly ($p < 0.05$) more positive in their responses on multiple survey items than other respondents. Evaluation of ICU staff satisfaction and perceptions involving tele-ICU implementation has occurred among numerous smaller studies [97]. A recent systematic review including 23 studies involving staff acceptance indicated favorable perceptions by physicians and nurses across a variety of settings [51]. Despite initial skepticism, bedside staff believed tele-ICU improved the quality of care and would likely achieve its highest efficacy in healthcare settings with reduced resources. Staff acceptance is poorly characterized in peer-reviewed literature, but is increasingly important because of its vital role in operational success and critical care cost-effectiveness. Preimplementation inclusion in program planning, establishing the understanding and expectations of bedside staff, investigating the perceived need, and assessing the availability of local resources have been shown as factors that improve acceptance [98].

Trainee Education

Nearly half of the comprehensive tele-ICU programs include participation of residents and trainees for the care of critically ill patients [68]. Little is known regarding the effects of ICU telemedicine on the critical care educational experience. There has been an increased effort to detail the effects of telemedicine integration into medical education and critical care training programs [51,99]. These investigations suggest that the addition of an ICU telemedicine program provides more resources to residents and fellows with documented educational support at times when their primary educator is not in the ICU [100]. Approximately 82% of residents surveyed responded that this technology improved patient care, 73% indicated that it enabled better care of their patients when they were on call, and 67% desired tele-ICU involvement in the care of their patients. The majority reported usefulness regarding ventilator management, supervision during arrests, blood gas interpretation, acute respiratory changes, and goal-directed therapy. Importantly, tele-ICU involvement was not perceived as having an overall negative impact on education and training.

Cost-Effectiveness and Reimbursement

The healthcare system's viewpoint of tele-ICU programs is a unique perspective that is now being better defined because intense public scrutiny on higher-quality healthcare at lower costs has resulted in increased focus on cost-effectiveness. Currently, one must consider the cost-effectiveness of tele-ICU in the setting of a substantial initial capital investment [101] in technology along with increased operating costs on account of the general failure of payers to integrate models of tele-ICU payment into existing reimbursement systems [102]. Direct reimbursement for tele-ICU evaluation and management services is not supported in the United States at the time of publication of this text [103,104]. Payment for telehealth services does exist, but is limited through federal, state, and private insurance

TABLE 32.3

Factors Associated with Improved Outcomes after ICU Telemedicine Implementation [72]

Workstation-assisted intensivist reviews of the care plan within 1 h of ICU admission
Frequent and collaborative review and use of ICU performance data
Near-perfect rates of adherence to ICU best practices
Shorter response times for abnormal laboratory and alarms for physiologic instability
Performance of interdisciplinary rounds
High levels of perceived effectiveness of the institution's ICU committee

ICU, intensive care unit.

restrictions. Medicare and Medicaid public programs have paid for telemedicine services dating back to the federal Balanced Budget Act in 1997 when Medicare initiated formal payment models for telehealth services in rural areas [105]. However, Medicare spending on telemedicine remains a small fraction as only $5 million was allocated to telemedicine in 2012 Medicare spending which totaled $466 billion. To date, 47 states have some form of payment for telemedicine services through Medicaid, and 28 states have active laws governing private payer telemedicine coverage [106]. However, ICU telemedicine services are not among those that are eligible for reimbursement. Accordingly, one must consider the indirect financial aspects of a system's ICU telemedicine program.

Until recently, the lack of transparent cost data along with the absence of a standardized methodology for assessing cost-effectiveness has limited the quality of literature surrounding the financial aspects of ICU telemedicine. In 2015, a comprehensive cost-effectiveness analyses of ICU telemedicine based on published literature suggested that ICU telemedicine was cost-effective when compared with ICU care without telemedicine [107]. Using simulation analyses, this study investigated the relationship of the cost of a tele-ICU intervention and its extension of quality-adjusted life years estimating that ICU telemedicine was cost saving 37.2% of the time and cost-effective 66.8% of the time. This included a wide variety of sensitivity analyses using a broad range of assumptions. In 2013, a systematic review identified 8 studies from 29 ICUs that reported costs associated with tele-ICU implementations [101]. Wide variation in cost and reporting detail existed because the estimated cost of implementing the tele-ICU program, including the technology, monitoring, operations, and staffing for 1 year, ranged from $50,000 to $100,000 per ICU bed. The majority of these studies attempted to identify the impact of tele-ICU on hospital variable direct costs. Importantly, studies with a vendor connection reported a cost saving of $2,600 to $3,000 per patient and suggested that some tele-ICUs have increased hospital per case margin by $1,000 to $4,000 per patient [65,66,108]. Alternatively, studies without a vendor connection did not impact LOS and reported no variable cost savings and suggested increased hospital costs after implementation. It seems clear that the most frequently reported method for assessing cost savings is by gauging reductions in LOS. In community hospitals, positive financial outcomes have been reported because of increases in volume and acuity of critically ill patients who are retained as opposed to transferred elsewhere [108]. High-quality research involving the costs of tele-ICU programs remains limited and is one of the important barriers to growth.

Quality Metrics and Evidence-Based Care

Important data exist outside the hallmark outcomes of risk-adjusted mortality and LOS within a continuous comprehensive model of tele-ICU. There are an increasing number of focused investigations pertaining to the potential impact of ICU telemedicine on specific disease processes and quality performance improvements commonly encountered in the ICU. A responsive, or episodic, telemedicine care model has been shown to provide safe, reliable, cost-effective care that improves timely response to neurologic ICU emergencies, decreases hospital LOS, and improves functional outcomes [109–112]. The utility of neurology consultation using telemedicine tools to assess neurologic symptoms, review neuroradiologic imaging, determine the National Institutes of Health Stroke Scale score, and provide recommendations regarding the administration of tissue plasminogen activator for patients suffering a stroke is now broadly accepted [113,114]. Similarly, cardiology consultation utilizing telemedicine can potentially expedite the care of patients with ST elevation myocardial infarction or enhance the management for those with chronic congestive heart failure [115]. Prehospital triage and thrombolysis utilizing remote interaction with paramedics and ECG have been shown to decrease the time to reperfusion in the setting of ST elevation myocardial infarction [116]. Additionally, telemedicine tools allowing home monitoring of patients with a diagnosis of congestive heart failure have been associated with a reduction in the rate of hospital admissions and an increase in quality of life [117]. The impact of telemedicine tools for both acute and chronic care delivery continues to evolve, and future investigations of the clinical and financial impact will help reduce the uncertainty for health system policy makers and payers.

Quality of healthcare has been defined by the Institute of Medicine as care that is safe, timely, effective, efficient, equitable, and patient centered [19]. Quality improvement involves activities that focus on process and outcome measures that often revolve around a particular disease entity or patient cohort [118]. There is an increasing belief that implementation of telemedicine in critical care delivery is uniquely capable of enhancing quality improvement programs by providing process-based metrics that are linked to outcomes [119]. Effective tele-ICU programs are well equipped to collect, assimilate, and analyze larger amounts of more granular data, invest dedicated human resources, and promote a culture of safety as the predominant force moving the program forward toward the desired result. Quality improvement programs often focus on "best practice" process measures such as adherence to the Surviving Sepsis Guidelines or procedures for the prevention of ventilator-associated pneumonia. Utilizing on-demand reports and smart alerts, telemedicine programs have increased compliance with early sepsis management protocols and ventilator bundle element [92,120]. In some instances, telemedicine integration for quality improvement has increased adherence to near 100% for preventative practices for pneumonia, stress ulcer prophylaxis, and deep vein thrombosis prophylaxis [121]. In 2014, the authors investigated the impact of tele-ICU–led ventilator rounds on protective lung ventilation compliance, ventilator duration ratio, and ICU mortality at multiple sites across 11 hospitals [122]. Despite wide variability in adherence rates to lung protective ventilation before the intervention across hospitals, there were statistically significant improvements in all measured outcomes. The effectiveness of telemedicine-directed ventilator rounds was attributed to the ability of the tele-ICU intervention to provide human support to encourage action based on data management and timely performance reporting [123].

Empirical research and clinical experience can provide a framework to optimize the effectiveness of ICU telemedicine. In 2014, guidelines were developed by the American Telemedicine Association (ATA) to assist critical care professionals in delivering safe, effective, and collaborative care through the tele-ICU, focusing on the unique aspects of utilizing audiovisual communications and computer systems for the delivery of critical care services [124]. The ATA generated and reviewed 66 consensus guidelines to be used both as operational guidance and as an educational tool to aid in the appropriate care for critically ill patients in the ICU telemedicine model. Standards and recommendations included administrative, clinical, operational, and technical guidelines including aspects of leadership structure, patient privacy and confidentiality, documentation and storage, tele-ICU delivery and staffing models, licensing and credentialing, workflows, quality performance reporting, audiovisual and networking protocols, and data security. A comprehensive evidence database consisting of high-quality research derived through a sound methodological framework will be necessary to meet the standards of creating evidence-based guidelines for ICU telemedicine.

SUMMARY

As the changing critical care delivery paradigm becomes more apparent, the role of ICU telemedicine for meeting patient-centered and system goals for critical care is evolving. ICU telemedicine programs have improved access to critical care professionals, identified patients with evolving physiologic instability that has not been addressed, and helped to control costs associated with wide variation of care through standardization of care delivery processes. Widespread acceptance of telecommunications technologies has fostered the ability of telemedicine to make critical care professionals continuously available to geographically dispersed ICUs. These electronic systems enable remotely delivered comprehensive care, including the ability to independently evaluate patient care plans and deliver evaluation and management services. Although meta-analyses report improved quality outcomes, it remains evident that there is wide variation in the practice of ICU telemedicine programs. The substantial implementation and operational costs of ICU telemedicine programs are best justified by increased efficiency of critical care delivery. As enabling technologies become less expensive and better integrated with commercially available electronic health records, the incremental costs of telemedicine technologies are expected to decrease.

More research is needed on operational, quality, staffing, and financial outcomes from the point of view of all stakeholders, including patients, providers, hospitals, healthcare systems, and society as a whole. Divergent forces including an aging population growth, increased focus on controlling costs, and a maldistribution of ICU professionals have increased the need for adult critical care services and created interest in exploring the application of telecommunications technologies to improve the efficiency of critical care delivery. The ability to support the effective process of critical care delivery and to provide timely and actionable performance reports are key elements that promote high-quality ICU outcomes. ICU telemedicine interventions can leverage electronic tools to assist in ensuring that every patient receives appropriate intervention in the correct time frame in a reliable and cost-effective manner. The great promise of ICU telemedicine is its potential to improve outcomes yet control critical care costs.

References

1. Vincent J-L: Critical care-where have we been and where are we going? *Crit Care* 17[Suppl 1]:S2, 2013.
2. Halpern NA, Pastores SM: Critical care medicine in the United States 2000-2005: an analysis of bed numbers, occupancy rates, payer mix, and costs. *Crit Care Med* 38(1):65–71, 2010.
3. Vincent GK, Velkoff VA: *The Next Four Decades: The Older Population in the United States: 2010 to 2050*. Washington, DC: U.S. Department of Commerce, Economics and Statistics Administration, U.S. Census Bureau, 2010.
4. Reineck LA, Kahn JM: Quality measurement in the Affordable Care Act: a reaffirmed commitment to value in healthcare. *Am J Respir Crit Care Med* 187(10):1038–1039, 2013.
5. Kelley MA, Angus D, Chalfin DB, et al: The critical care crisis in the United States: a report from the profession. *Chest* 125(4):1514–1517, 2004.
6. Health Resources and Services Administration Report to Congress: *The Critical Care Workforce: A Study of the Supply and Demand for Critical Care Physicians*. Requested by: Senate Report 108-81.
7. Krell K: Critical care workforce. *Crit Care Med* 36(4):1350–1353, 2008.
8. Grover A: Critical care workforce: a policy perspective. *Crit Care Med* 34 [3, Suppl]:S7–S11, 2006.
9. Leape LL, Berwick DM: Five years after to err is human: what have we learned? *JAMA* 293(19):2384–2390, 2005.
10. Berwick DM, Nolan TW, Whittington J: The triple aim: care, health, and cost. *Health Aff (Millwood)* 27(3):759–769, 2008.
11. Halpern NA, Pastores SM: Critical care medicine beds, use, occupancy, and costs in the United States: a methodological review. *Crit Care Med* 43(11):2452–2459, 2015.
12. Society of Critical Care Medicine: Critical Care Statistics. http://www.sccm.org/Communications/Pages/CriticalCareStats.aspx. Accessed September 1, 2015.
13. American Hospital Association: *AHA Hospital Statistics 2015 Edition*. Chicago, IL: Health Forum, 2015.
14. Angus DC, Shorr AF, White A, et al: Critical care delivery in the United States: distribution of services and compliance with Leapfrog recommendations. *Crit Care Med* 34(4):1016–1024, 2006.
15. National Center for Health Statistics: *Health, United States, 2014: With Special Feature on Adults Aged 55–64*. Hyattsville, MD: National Center for Health Statistics, 2015.
16. Wunsch H, Angus DC, Harrison DA, et al: Comparison of medical admissions to intensive care units in the United States and United Kingdom. *Am J Respir Crit Care Med* 183(12):1666–1673, 2011.
17. Angus DC, Barnato AE, Linde-Zwirble WT, et al: Use of intensive care at the end of life in the United States: an epidemiologic study. *Crit Care Med* 32(3):638–643, 2004.
18. Angus DC: Current and projected workforce requirements for care of the critically ill and patients with pulmonary disease - can we meet the requirements of an aging population? *JAMA* 284(21):2762, 2000.
19. Institute of Medicine: *Crossing the Quality Chasm: A New Health System for the 21st Century*. Washington, DC: National Academy Press, 2001.
20. Finkelstein J, Knight A, Marinopoulos S, et al: *Enabling Patient-Centered Care through Health Information Technology*. Agency for Healthcare Research and Quality (US); 2012.
21. Kvedar J, Coye MJ, Everett W: Connected health: a review of technologies and strategies to improve patient care with telemedicine and telehealth. *Health Aff (Millwood)* 33(2):194–199, 2014.
22. Wilcox ME, Chong CAKY, Niven DJ, et al: Do intensivist staffing patterns influence hospital mortality following ICU admission? A systematic review and meta-analyses. *Crit Care Med* 41(10):2253–2274, 2013.
23. Pronovost PJ, Angus DC, Dorman T, et al: Physician staffing patterns and clinical outcomes in critically ill patients: a systematic review. *JAMA* 288(17):2151–2162, 2002.
24. Milstein A, Galvin RS, Delbanco SF, et al: Improving the safety of healthcare: the leapfrog initiative. *Eff Clin Pract*. 3(6):313–316, 2000.
25. Kahn JM, Matthews FA, Angus DC, et al: Barriers to implementing the Leapfrog Group recommendations for intensivist physician staffing: a survey of intensive care unit directors. *J Crit Care* 22(2):97–103, 2007.
26. Moran J, Scanlon D: Slow progress on meeting hospital safety standards: learning from the Leapfrog Group's efforts. *Health Aff (Millwood)* 32(1):27–35, 2013.
27. The Leapfrog Group: Fact Sheet: ICU Physician Staffing. http://www.leapfroggroup.org/sites/default/files/Files/IPS%20Fact%20Sheet.pdf. Accessed September 1, 2015.
28. Ewart GW, Marcus L, Gaba MM, et al: The critical care medicine crisis: a call for federal action: a white paper from the critical care professional societies. *Chest* 125(4):1518–1521, 2004.
29. Lorin S, Heffner J, Carson S: Attitudes and perceptions of internal medicine residents regarding pulmonary and critical care subspecialty training. *Chest* 127(2):630–636, 2005.
30. Kovitz KL: Pulmonary and critical care: the unattractive specialty. *Chest* 127(4):1085–1087, 2005.
31. Shanafelt TD, Boone S, Tan L, et al: Burnout and satisfaction with work-life balance among US physicians relative to the general US population. *Arch Intern Med*, 72(18):1377–1385, 2012.
32. Pronovost PJ, Thompson DA, Holzmueller CG, et al: The organization of intensive care unit physician services. *Crit Care Med* 35(10):2256–2261, 2007.
33. Siegal EM, Dressler DD, Dichter JR, et al: Training a hospitalist workforce to address the intensivist shortage in American hospitals: a position paper from the Society of Hospital Medicine and the Society of Critical Care Medicine. *Crit Care Med* 40(6):1952–1956, 2012.
34. Institute of Medicine: *Graduate Medical Education That Meets the Nation's Health Needs*. Washington, DC: National Academies Press, 2014.
35. Wilensky GR, Berwick DM: Reforming the financing and governance of GME. *N Engl J Med* 371(9):792–793, 2014.
36. Center for Workforce Studies Association of American Medical Colleges: *Recent Studies and Reports on Physician Shortages in the US*, 2012.
37. Fordyce MA, Chen FM, Doescher MP, et al: *2005 Physician Supply and Distribution in Rural Areas of the United States*. WWAMI Rural Health

Research Center, University of Washington, School of Medicine, Department of Family Medicine, 2007.
38. Lilly CM, Zubrow MT, Kempner KM, et al: Critical care telemedicine: evolution and state of the art. *Crit Care Med* 42(11):2429–2436, 2014.
39. Rabinowitz HK, Diamond JJ, Markham FW, et al: The relationship between entering medical students' backgrounds and career plans and their rural practice outcomes three decades later. *Acad Med* 87(4):493–497, 2012.
40. Embriaco N, Azoulay E, Barrau K, et al: High level of burnout in intensivists: prevalence and associated factors. *Am J Respir Crit Care Med* 175(7):686–692, 2007.
41. Garland A, Gershengorn HB: Staffing in ICUs: physicians and alternative staffing models. *Chest* 143(1):214–221, 2013.
42. AANP: National Nurse Practitioner Database, 2014. https://www.aanp.org/all-about-nps/np-fact-sheet. Accessed September 7, 2015.
43. AAPA: PA Fact Sheet, 2013. https://www.aapa.org/workarea/downloadasset.aspx?id=670. Accessed September 7, 2015.
44. Kleinpell R, Ward NS, Kelso LA, et al: Provider to patient ratios for nurse practitioners and physician assistants in critical care units. *Am J Crit Care* 24(3):e16–e21, 2015.
45. Legislative Council: Compilation of Patient Protection and Affordable Care Act. http://housedocs.house.gov/energycommerce/ppacacon.pdf. Accessed October 1, 2015.
46. Centers for Medicare and Medicaid Services: Rapid Development and Deployment of Non-Physician Providers in Critical Care. *Healthc Innov Award*. https://innovation.cms.gov/initiatives/Health-Care-Innovation-Awards/Georgia.html. Accessed January 11, 2015.
47. Lilly CM, Thomas EJ: Tele-ICU: experience to date. *J Intensive Care Med* 25(1):16–22, 2010.
48. Reynolds HN, Bander J, McCarthy M: Different systems and formats for tele-ICU coverage. *Crit Care Nurs Q* 35(4):364–377, 2012.
49. Cummings J, Krsek C, Vermoch K, et al: Intensive care unit telemedicine: review and consensus recommendations. *Am J Med Qual* 22(4):239–250, 2007.
50. Venkataraman R, Ramakrishnan N: Outcomes related to telemedicine in the intensive care unit: what we know and would like to know. *Crit Care Clin* 31(2):225–237, 2015.
51. Young LB, Chan PS, Cram P: Staff acceptance of tele-ICU coverage: a systematic review. *Chest* 139(2):279–288, 2011.
52. Kahn JM, Rubenfeld GD: The myth of the workforce crisis. Why the United States does not need more intensivist physicians. *Am J Respir Crit Care Med* 191(2):128–134, 2015.
53. Gooch RA, Kahn JM: ICU bed supply, utilization, and healthcare spending: an example of demand elasticity. *JAMA* 311(6):567–568, 2014.
54. Zimmerman JE, Kramer AA: A model for identifying patients who may not need intensive care unit admission. *J Crit Care* 25(2):205–213, 2010.
55. Wunsch H, Wagner J, Herlim M, et al: ICU occupancy and mechanical ventilator use in the United States. *Crit Care Med* 41(12):2712–2719, 2013.
56. Seymour CW, Iwashyna TJ, Ehlenbach WJ, et al: Hospital-level variation in the use of intensive care. *Health Serv Res* 47(5):2060–2080, 2012.
57. Scurlock C, D'Ambrosio C: Telemedicine in the intensive care unit: state of the art. *Crit Care Clin* 31(2):187–195, 2015.
58. Kohn LT, Corrigan JM, Donaldson MS: *To Err is Human: Building a Safer Health System*. Washington, DC: National Academic Press, 2002.
59. Pickering BW, Litell JM, Herasevich V, et al: Clinical review: the hospital of the future-building intelligent environments to facilitate safe and effective acute care delivery. *Crit Care* 16(2):220, 2012.
60. Rogers EM: *Diffusion of Innovations*. New York: Simon and Schuster, 2010.
61. Curtis JR, Engelberg RA, Bensink ME, et al: End-of-life care in the intensive care unit: can we simultaneously increase quality and reduce costs? *Am J Respir Crit Care Med* 186(7):587–592, 2012.
62. Fox MY: Improving communication with patients and families in the intensive care unit: palliative care strategies for the intensive care unit nurse. *J Hosp Palliat Nurs* 16(2):93–98, 2014.
63. Einthoven LT: Le telecardiogramme. *Arch Int Physiol* 4:132–164, 1906.
64. Grundy BL, Jones PK, Lovitt A: Telemedicine in critical care: problems in design, implementation, and assessment. *Crit Care Med* 10(7):471–475, 1982.
65. Rosenfeld BA, Dorman T, Breslow MJ, et al: Intensive care unit telemedicine: alternate paradigm for providing continuous intensivist care. *Crit Care Med* 28(12):3925–3931, 2000.
66. Breslow MJ, Rosenfeld BA, Doerfler M, et al: Effect of a multiple-site intensive care unit telemedicine program on clinical and economic outcomes: an alternative paradigm for intensivist staffing. *Crit Care Med* 32(1):31–38, 2004.
67. Kahn JM, Cicero BD, Wallace DJ, et al: Adoption of ICU telemedicine in the United States. *Crit Care Med* 42(2):362–368, 2014.
68. Lilly CM, Zuckerman IH, Badawi O, et al: Benchmark data from more than 240,000 adults that reflect the current practice of critical care in the United States. *Chest* 140(5):1232–1242, 2011.
69. Reynolds HN, Rogove H, Bander J, et al: A working lexicon for the tele-intensive care unit: we need to define tele-intensive care unit to grow and understand it. *Telemed e-Health* 17(10):773–783, 2011.
70. Reynolds HN, Bander JJ: Options for tele-intensive care unit design: centralized versus decentralized and other considerations. *Crit Care Clin* 31(2):335–350, 2015.
71. Kellermann AL, Jones SS: What it will take to achieve the as-yet-unfulfilled promises of health information technology. *Health Aff (Millwood)*. 2013;32(1):63–68.
72. Lilly CM, McLaughlin JM, Zhao H, et al: A multicenter study of ICU telemedicine reengineering of adult critical care. *Chest* 145(3):500–507, 2014.
73. Kahn JM, Gunn SR, Lorenz HL, et al: Impact of nurse-led remote screening and prompting for evidence-based practices in the ICU*. *Crit Care Med* 42(4):896–904, 2014.
74. Donchin Y, Seagull FJ: The hostile environment of the intensive care unit. *Curr Opin Crit Care* 8(4):316–320, 2002.
75. Imhoff M, Kuhls S, Gather U, et al: Smart alarms from medical devices in the OR and ICU. *Best Pract Res Clin Anaesthesiol* 23(1):39–50, 2009.
76. Joint Commission: Medical device alarm safety in hospitals. *Sentin Event Alert* 50:1, 2013.
77. Patel VL, Zhang J, Yoskowitz NA, et al: Translational cognition for decision support in critical care environments: a review. *J Biomed Inform* 41(3):413–431, 2008.
78. Buchman TG: Novel representation of physiologic states during critical illness and recovery. *Crit Care* 14(2):127, 2010.
79. Halpern NA: Innovative designs for the smart ICU: Part 3: advanced ICU informatics. *Chest* 145(4):903–912, 2014.
80. Celi LA, Csete M, Stone D: Optimal data systems: the future of clinical predictions and decision support. *Curr Opin Crit Care* 20(5):573–580, 2014.
81. De Georgia MA, Kaffashi F, Jacono FJ, et al: Information technology in critical care: review of monitoring and data acquisition systems for patient care and research. *ScientificWorldJournal* 2015:727694, 2015.
82. Kerlin MP, Harhay MO, Kahn JM, et al: Nighttime intensivist staffing, mortality, and limits on life support: a retrospective cohort study. *Chest* 147(4):951–958, 2015.
83. Kerlin MP, Small DS, Cooney E, et al: A randomized trial of nighttime physician staffing in an intensive care unit. *N Engl J Med* 368(23):2201–2209, 2013.
84. Kerlin MP, Halpern SD: Nighttime physician staffing in an intensive care unit. *N Engl J Med* 369(11):1075, 2013.
85. Costa DK, Wallace DJ, Kahn JM: The association between daytime intensivist physician staffing and mortality in the context of other ICU organizational practices. *Crit Care Med* 43(11):2275–2282, 2015.
86. Young LB, Chan PS, Lu X, et al: Impact of telemedicine intensive care unit coverage on patient outcomes: a systematic review and meta-analysis. *Arch Intern Med* 171(6):498–506, 2011.
87. Wilcox ME, Adhikari NKJ: The effect of telemedicine in critically ill patients: systematic review and meta-analysis. *Crit Care* 16(4):R127, 2012.
88. Thomas EJ, Lucke JF, Wueste L, et al: Association of telemedicine for remote monitoring of intensive care patients with mortality, complications, and length of stay. *JAMA* 302(24):2671–2678, 2009.
89. Morrison JL, Cai Q, Davis N, et al: Clinical and economic outcomes of the electronic intensive care unit: results from two community hospitals*. *Crit Care Med* 38(1):2–8, 2010.
90. Willmitch B, Golembeski S, Kim SS, et al: Clinical outcomes after telemedicine intensive care unit implementation. *Crit Care Med* 40(2):450–454, 2012.
91. Nassar BS, Vaughan-Sarrazin MS, Jiang L, et al: Impact of an intensive care unit telemedicine program on patient outcomes in an integrated healthcare system. *JAMA Intern Med* 174(7):1160–1167, 2014.
92. Lilly CM, Cody S, Zhao H, et al: Hospital mortality, length of stay, and preventable complications among critically ill patients before and after tele-ICU reengineering of critical care processes. *JAMA* 305(21):2175–2183, 2011.
93. Lilly CM, Fisher KA, Ries M, et al: A national ICU telemedicine survey: validation and results. *Chest* 142(1):40–47, 2012.
94. Kahn JM, Hill NS, Lilly CM, et al: The research agenda in ICU telemedicine: a statement from the critical care societies collaborative. *Chest* 140(1):230–238, 2011.
95. Rogove H: How to develop a tele-ICU model? *Crit Care Nurs Q* 35(4):357–363, 2012.
96. Ward MM, Ullrich F, Potter AJ, et al: Factors affecting staff perceptions of tele-ICU service in rural hospitals. *Telemed J E Health* 21(6):459–466, 2015.
97. Ramnath VR, Ho L, Maggio LA, et al: Centralized monitoring and virtual consultant models of tele-ICU care: a systematic review. *Telemed J E Health* 20(10):936–961, 2014.
98. Moeckli J, Cram P, Cunningham C, et al: Staff acceptance of a telemedicine intensive care unit program: a qualitative study. *J Crit Care* 28(6):890–901, 2013.
99. Coletti C, Elliott DJ, Zubrow MT: Resident perceptions of a tele-intensive care unit implementation. *Telemed J E Health* 16(8):894–897, 2010.
100. Mora A, Faiz SA, Kelly T, et al: Resident perception of the educational and patient care value from remote telemonitoring in a medical intensive care unit [MeetingAbstracts]. *Chest J* 132(4):443a–443, 2007.
101. Kumar G, Falk DM, Bonello RS, et al: The costs of critical care telemedicine programs: a systematic review and analysis. *Chest* 143(1):19–29, 2013.
102. Rogove H, Stetina K: Practice challenges of intensive care unit telemedicine. *Crit Care Clin* 31(2):319–334, 2015.
103. McCambridge MM, Tracy JA, Sample GA: Point: should tele-ICU services be eligible for professional fee billing? Yes. Tele-ICUs and the triple aim. *Chest* 140(4):847–849, 2011; discussion 852-853.
104. Hoffmann S: Counterpoint: should tele-ICU services be eligible for professional fee billing? No. *Chest* 140(4):849–851, 2011; discussion 851-852.
105. Neufeld JD, Doarn CR: Telemedicine spending by medicare: a snapshot from 2012. *Telemed J E Health* 21(8):686–693, 2015.
106. Center for Connected Health Policy: State Telehealth Laws and Medicaid Program Policies: A Comprehensive Scan of the 50 states and District of Columbia. 2015. www.cchpca.org. Accessed October 15, 2015.
107. Yoo B-K, Kim M, Sasaki T, et al: Economic evaluation of telemedicine for patients in ICUs. *Crit Care Med,* 2015. doi:10.1097/CCM.0000000000001426.

108. Fifer S, Everett W, Adams M, et al: *Critical Care, Critical Choices: The Case for Tele-ICUs in Intensive Care*. Cambridge, MA: New England Healthcare Institute, 2010.
109. Audebert HJ, Schenkel J, Heuschmann PU, et al: Effects of the implementation of a telemedical stroke network: the Telemedic Pilot Project for Integrative Stroke Care (TEMPiS) in Bavaria, Germany. *Lancet Neurol* 5(9):742–748, 2006.
110. Audebert HJ, Schultes K, Tietz V, et al: Long-term effects of specialized stroke care with telemedicine support in community hospitals on behalf of the Telemedical Project for Integrative Stroke Care (TEMPiS). *Stroke* 40(3):902–908, 2009.
111. Vespa PM, Miller C, Hu X, et al: Intensive care unit robotic telepresence facilitates rapid physician response to unstable patients and decreased cost in neurointensive care. *Surg Neurol* 67(4):331–337, 2007.
112. Weber JE, Ebinger M, Rozanski M, et al: Prehospital thrombolysis in acute stroke: results of the PHANTOM-S pilot study. *Neurology* 80(2):163–168, 2013.
113. Audebert HJ, Schwamm L: Telestroke: scientific results. *Cerebrovasc Dis*. 2009;27[Suppl 4]:15–20.
114. Hubert GJ, Müller-Barna P, Audebert HJ: Recent advances in TeleStroke: a systematic review on applications in prehospital management and Stroke Unit treatment or TeleStroke networking in developing countries. *Int J Stroke* 9(8):968–973, 2014.
115. Raikhelkar JKJ, Raikhelkar JKJ: The impact of telemedicine in cardiac critical care. *Crit Care Clin*. 2015;31(2):305–317.
116. Brunetti ND, Di Pietro G, Aquilino A, et al: Pre-hospital electrocardiogram triage with tele-cardiology support is associated with shorter time-to-balloon and higher rates of timely reperfusion even in rural areas: data from the Bari- Barletta/Andria/Trani public emergency medical service 118 regist. *Eur Hear J Acute Cardiovasc Care* 3(3):204–213, 2014.
117. Conway A, Inglis SC, Clark RA: Effective technologies for noninvasive remote monitoring in heart failure. *Telemed J E Health*. 2014;20(6):531–538.
118. Curtis JR, Cook DJ, Wall RJ, et al: Intensive care unit quality improvement: a "how-to" guide for the interdisciplinary team*. *Crit Care Med* 34(1):211–218, 2006.
119. Weled BJ, Adzhigirey LA, Hodgman TM, et al: Critical care delivery. *Crit Care Med* 43(7):1520–1525, 2015.
120. Rincon TA, Bourke G, Seiver A: Standardizing sepsis screening and management via a tele-ICU program improves patient care. *Telemed J E Health* 17(7):560–564, 2011.
121. Sadaka F, Palagiri A, Trottier S, et al: Telemedicine intervention improves ICU outcomes. *Crit Care Res Pract* 2013:456389, 2013.
122. Kalb T, Raikhelkar J, Meyer S, et al: A multicenter population-based effectiveness study of teleintensive care unit-directed ventilator rounds demonstrating improved adherence to a protective lung strategy, decreased ventilator duration, and decreased intensive care unit mortality. *J Crit Care* 29(4):691.e7–691.e14, 2014.
123. Kalb TH: Increasing quality through telemedicine in the intensive care unit. *Crit Care Clin* 31(2):257–273, 2015.
124. American Telemedicine Association: Guidelines for TeleICU Operations. May 2014. http://www.learnicu.org/SiteCollectionDocuments/Guidelines-ATA-TeleICU.pdf. Accessed September 1, 2015.
125. Marcin JP, Nesbitt TS, Kallas HJ, et al: Use of telemedicine to provide pediatric critical care inpatient consultations to underserved rural Northern California. *J Pediatr* 144(3):375–380, 2004.
126. Zawada ET, Herr P, Larson D, et al: Impact of an intensive care unit telemedicine program on a rural healthcare system. *Postgrad Med* 121(3):160–170, 2009.
127. McCambridge M, Jones K, Paxton H, et al: Association of health information technology and teleintensivist coverage with decreased mortality and ventilator use in critically ill patients. *Arch Intern Med* 170(7):648–653, 2010.
128. Kohl BA, Fortino-Mullen M, Praestgaard A, et al: The effect of ICU telemedicine on mortality and length of stay. *J Telemed Telecare* 18(5):282–286, 2012.

Section 3 PALLIATIVE CARE AND ETHICAL ISSUES IN THE CRITICAL CARE UNIT

JENNIFER E. REIDY

Chapter 33 ■ Integrating Palliative Care in the Intensive Care Unit

NANDITA R. NADIG • DANA LUSTBADER • DEE W. FORD

The integration of high-quality palliative care is an essential part of comprehensive critical care medicine. Critical care providers are often required to provide pain and symptom relief to patients with serious illness; conduct family meetings to clarify goals of care; give bad news; or deliver end-of-life care to terminally ill patients while providing support to their loved ones. It is important that critical care clinicians acquire basic palliative care skills for the management of pain and suffering and learn the necessary skills for effective serious illness conversations. The Institute of Medicine (IOM), now renamed The National Academy of Medicine, conducted a comprehensive evaluation of end-of-life care in the USA and found numerous shortcomings, concluding with a call to action for systematic improvement in access to high-quality palliative care across all care settings [1]. This is especially true for the intensive care unit (ICU), where death is common and those who survive their ICU stay often experience significant morbidity and emotional suffering months and even years post–hospital discharge [2]. In the USA, a significant portion of health-care expenditure goes toward the care of critically ill patients more than for any other country in the world [3], and a significant amount of this spending is for patients who die in the ICU despite the use of advanced technologies and therapeutic interventions. A recent national assessment of end-of-life care among Medicare beneficiaries found that 30% of beneficiaries have an ICU admission in the last month of life [4]. What is concerning is that the use of life sustaining therapies, particularly in the final days or weeks of life, may in fact not be consistent with actual patient preferences [5]. Another study found that 20% of all deaths in the USA occur in the ICU or shortly thereafter. In an effort to address the discordance between what patients say they want and the care they actually get, the National Quality Forum developed a palliative care and hospice framework that advocates access for all eligible patients. This initiative also asserted that health-care providers in critical care require education and skills training in the practice of high-quality palliative care.

There are unique issues associated with providing palliative care in the ICU setting (see Table 33.1). Patients and families want both disease-modifying treatment and palliative care, and clinicians cannot always predict who will survive, who will die or who will remain chronically critically ill. For patients with terminal illness who are unlikely to benefit from life-sustaining treatments, an ICU admission can result in unnecessary suffering and treatment that may be discordant with their preferences for health care [6]. This often occurs from lack of prior conversations about patients' goals and preferences for care as well as the appropriate available palliative options to meet those goals as an illness progresses over time. An ICU admission for a terminally ill patient can be associated with inadequate treatment of pain, anxiety, dyspnea, thirst and other symptoms. In addition, family members of critically ill patients can suffer significant psychologic distress such as anxiety; posttraumatic stress; and depression [6] which has been associated with low-quality communication and the high burden of medical decision-making [7]. Critical care clinicians experience the emotional labor of providing end-of-life care in an ICU setting, and can suffer moral distress and burnout.

TABLE 33.1

Domains of ICU Palliative Care Quality as Defined by Critical Care/Palliative Care Professionals and by Adult ICU Patients/Families (The IPAL-ICU Project, Center to Advance Palliative Care, 2010)

A. Professionals' Definition (Experts in critical care and palliative care)	B. Patients' and Families' Definition (Recovered patients with ≥5-day ICU stay; and families of survivors and nonsurvivors)
Symptom management and comfort care	Clinical care of the patient: • Maintaining comfort, dignity, personhood, and privacy
Communication within team and with patients/families	Communication by clinicians: • Timely, ongoing, clear, complete, and compassionate • Addressing condition, prognosis, and treatment
Patient- and family-centered decision-making	Patient-focused medical decision-making: • Aligned with patient values, care goals, and treatment preferences
Emotional and practical support for patients and families	Care of the family: • Open access and proximity to patients • Interdisciplinary support in the ICU • Bereavement care for families of patients who died
Spiritual support for patients and families	
Continuity of care	
Emotional and organizational support for ICU clinicians	

ICU, intensive care unit.
Reprinted with permission from the Center to Advance Palliative Care (CAPC), The IPAL-ICU Project.

Hospice and palliative medicine emerged as a distinct medical subspecialty in 2006 when it was recognized by the American Board of Medical Specialties. Palliative care is a team-based model of care that focuses on the relief of pain and symptoms related to serious illness, regardless of prognosis. Palliative care teams include specially trained physicians, nurses, social workers, and chaplains who provide expert symptom management,

TABLE 33.2

Expected Benefits from an Initiative to Improve ICU Palliative Care

- Improved family satisfaction and comprehension
- Lower levels of family anxiety, depression, and posttraumatic stress disorder
- Less conflict in the ICU
- Timely implementation of care plans that are realistic, appropriate, and consistent with patients' preferences
- Reductions in the use of nonbeneficial treatments and lengths of stay in ICU/hospital—with stable ICU mortality
- Professional gratification for clinicians
- Significant cost savings for the hospital

ICU, intensive care unit.
Reprinted with permission from the Center to Advance Palliative Care (CAPC), IPAL-ICU Project.

clarify patients' goals and values, and reduce the stress of serious illness for patients and their loved ones. Palliative care teams collaborate and coordinate care with a patient's other clinicians while providing support to the patient and their family in the context of their lives, culture, faith, and community outside the hospital (see Table 33.2).

Ensuring access to high-quality palliative care across all settings from home to the ICU has become a national priority as patients and families begin to insist on better integration of goals and treatment plans. According to the National Palliative Care Registry, 90% of U.S. hospitals with more than 300 beds offered palliative care services in 2014 [8]. However, these inpatient teams were often understaffed and saw only 3.4% of annual hospital admissions on average. Based on national demographics and hospital data, the Center to Advance Palliative Care estimates that at least 8% of all hospital admissions require specialty palliative care, which results in a gap of 1 to 1.8 million patients with unmet needs. The field of palliative medicine is facing a serious workforce shortage, with only 7,000 board-certified physicians in 2014 among 10 primary specialties, and the current capacity of fellowship programs remains insufficient to meet the need [9]. As a result, the field is focused on training all providers who care for people with serious illness in "generalist palliative care" skills (see Table 33.3) in addition to building subspecialty programs. The current transformation of health care from a fee-for-service to a shared-risk model also incentivizes health systems and payers to develop palliative care services, especially in caring for the sickest patients who are often high health-care utilizers. Multiple studies have shown that palliative care improves quality, and can reduce harm by avoiding unwanted, nonbeneficial, and costly admissions, procedures, and treatments at the end of life [10]. There are also small studies demonstrating palliative care can prolong survival in metastatic lung cancer, COPD, and among hospice patients [11,12].

There is often confusion about the difference between hospice and palliative care (see Table 33.4). Hospice is specialized palliative care during the final 6 months of life. Patients generally must also forgo most disease-directed therapies like chemotherapy and dialysis to be eligible for hospice care. Hospice care is generally provided where the patient lives (e.g., nursing home, home) but can also be provided in an inpatient setting for a variety of reasons including refractory symptoms and family respite care. Hospice care is a benefit covered by Medicare, Medicaid and most commercial health plans. In contrast, palliative care can be provided at any point during serious illness—even over many years—and is usually delivered alongside disease-directed treatments.

In an effort to promote best practices, the National Consensus Project Clinical Practice Guidelines for Quality Palliative Care

TABLE 33.3

Knowledge and Skills for Generalist and Specialist Palliative Care

Generalist palliative care	Specialist palliative care
Management of pain and common symptoms	Management of refractory pain and symptoms
Management of depression and anxiety	Management of complex depression, anxiety, and emotional/existential suffering
First-line discussions about: • Prognosis • Goals of care • Code status • Patient/family distress	Conflict resolution over goals and treatment options: • Among family members • Between ICU team and families • Between ICU and specialist teams
	Help with navigating cases of medical futility

ICU, intensive care unit.

TABLE 33.4

Comparing Palliative Care and Hospice

	Palliative care	Hospice
Provides relief from pain and symptoms	Yes	Yes
Team based approach to care	Yes	Yes
Requires that death is likely within 6 months	No	Yes
Must forgo disease-directed therapies (chemotherapy and dialysis)	No	Yes
Reimbursed through Medicare, Medicaid, and other health plans	Variable	Yes

created an important theoretical framework and practical guide to improve care [13]. The report promotes the philosophies embedded in palliative care and outlines essential elements to ensure quality, including the structure and processes of care; the physical, psychosocial, spiritual, and cultural aspects of clinical care; caring for the imminently dying patient; and ethical and legal aspects of care. Guided by these principles, palliative care has been shown to reduce physical and psychologic suffering [14]; increase patient and family satisfaction; and decrease ICU admissions, ICU length of stay (LOS), and overall hospital costs [15]. This chapter discusses models for palliative care delivery in the ICU; clinical triggers for palliative care engagement; the barriers to palliative care; and quality improvement strategies.

EXPLORING MODELS OF PALLIATIVE CARE DELIVERY

An important feature of palliative care is that it can be offered simultaneously with medical treatments aimed at extending life, and does not require a distinct choice between treatment-focused critical care or comfort care. There are two approaches to palliative care delivery in the ICU: (1) the integrative model, which

TABLE 33.5

Consultative versus Integrated Model of ICU Palliative Care Delivery

Trigger/Initiative	Intervention	Outcome	Refs
Consultative model			
Provide a model of care for critically ill patients at the end of life a. ICU admission after hospital stay of > or =10 days b. Age >80 years in the presence of two or more life-threatening comorbidities (e.g., end-stage renal disease, severe congestive heart failure) c. Active Stage IV malignancy d. Status post cardiac arrest e. Intracerebral bleed requiring mechanical ventilation. To merge palliative and critical care cultures in the medical ICU.	Palliative care consult based on discussion between ICU team and palliative care team Proactive palliative care consultation Training nurses, educating house officers about palliative practices, Presence of a palliative care specialist during work rounds, Modeling of interdisciplinary teamwork.	Improved quality of life, higher rates of formalization of advance directives and utilization of hospice, as well as lower use of certain nonbeneficial life-prolonging treatments for critically ill patients who are at the end of life. Patients in the proactive palliative care group had significantly shorter lengths of stay in the ICU Identification of palliative care nurse champion program, Open visiting hours, Introduction of "Get to know me poster" of the patient.	[5,27,47]
Integrative model			
Initiative	**Intervention**	**Outcome**	**Refs**
Integration of palliative care in the surgical intensive care unit. Improve palliative care in a community hospital ICU Focus on palliative care quality improvement	Identify challenges, strategies and models, to promote effective integration of palliative care in surgical critical care. New palliative order sets, Extended visiting hours, Use of communication ambassadors. Palliative care clinician education; identifying local champions; feedback to clinicians; and system support.	Identified models to improve efficient work systems and practical tools to change attitudinal factors and bring about culture change. Significant reductions in ICU length of stay and decreased conflict over goals of care. Although not objectively measured, they showed improvement in the process and education interventions in the daily nature of discourse in the ICU among staff and between the staff, patients, and families. Significant improvement in nurse-assessed quality of dying and reduction in ICU length of stay with an intervention to integrate palliative care in the ICU No improvement in quality of dying and no change in ICU length of stay before death or time from ICU admission to withdrawal of life-sustaining measures.	[19,20,41,48]

ICU, intensive care unit.

integrates palliative care practices into everyday critical care routines for all ICU patients; and (2) the consultative model, which relies on consultants to provide care for selected ICU patients [16]. Table 33.5 provides a synopsis of studies that have investigated different strategies and outcomes associated with both models. The consultative model has generally shown greater improvement of outcomes compared to the integrative model. Ideally, ICUs would implement a combination of both models and be capable of providing basic, generalist palliative care by ICU clinicians and referring more complex cases to the palliative care consultation team [17].

Given the significant morbidity and mortality associated with critical illness, a large number of ICU patients and their family members will have palliative needs; therefore, integrating palliative care into the ICU routine and rounding protocols may be useful. Few ICU clinicians are fellowship-trained in palliative care, but formal training programs are becoming increasingly more common for clinicians at all stages of training. The Task Force from the Society of Critical Care Medicine, American College of Chest Physicians, American Thoracic Society, American Board of Internal Medicine, and the Association of Pulmonary and Critical Care Medicine Program Directors recommend palliative care training for ICU clinicians [18]. Based on this overwhelming consensus, educational efforts should be targeted for physicians, nurses, social workers, chaplains, and other members of the critical care team to strengthen the internal capacities for integrated ICU palliative care.

Integrative Models

Strategies to integrate palliative care into ICU practice have demonstrated variable results. A single center study showed significant improvement for nurse-assessed quality of dying and reduction of ICU LOS [19], but the same group assessed these outcomes in a multicenter study and found no improvement [20]. This suggests that it may be useful to focus on a narrow range of clearly defined goals that are achievable in individualized settings and culture given the locally available resources. One such example is the "care and communication bundle [21]" that addresses domains of palliative care quality that have been identified as important by ICU patients, families and professionals. Based on this bundle, there are preset ICU LOS triggers to identify medical decision-makers; investigate advance directives; address preferences for resuscitation; distribute information leaflets; offer social work and spiritual support; and conduct interdisciplinary family meetings. Pilot testing of this bundle in 19 ICUs showed feasibility and also revealed opportunities for improvement in clinician–patient–family serious illness communication [22]. A recent systematic review of factors associated with family satisfaction with end-of-life care in the ICU found recurring themes of higher satisfaction with good quality communication and expression of empathy by physicians, supporting the value of communication bundles [23].

An area of ICU practice for which evidence of palliative care integration is emerging is during rapid response team activations. An initial study by Jones et al. found that issues surrounding end-of-life care and limitations of medical therapy arose among approximately one-third of rapid response calls, suggesting an area for further integration [24]. A retrospective chart review at a Veterans Administration hospital in New York evaluated rapid response calls and found a 28% incidence of do not resuscitate (DNR) order placement after the call, suggesting that rapid response teams must frequently have an emergent goals-of-care conversation during a crisis [25]. Another study from Canada found that rapid response calls led to an increased incidence of patient and family conferences regarding treatment preferences within 48 hours [26]. This highlights the need for palliative care clinicians and other members of the rapid response team to be well skilled in having conversations about preferences for end-of-life care, particularly during a hospital admission or at times of hemodynamic instability. Strategies include clinician training for complex goals-of-care discussions and system initiatives to enhance awareness of opportunities to initiate goal-oriented conversations and avoid burdensome or unwanted ICU care (see Chapter 34).

Consultative Models

The consultative model for the ICU focuses on increasing the involvement and effectiveness of palliative care consultants for the care of ICU patients and their families, especially those at highest risk for poor outcomes. Typically, the consultative model can only accommodate a subset of the most challenging or symptomatic patients rather than all patients in the ICU, owing to the workforce shortage of palliative care providers and lack of round-the-clock, on-site coverage. The consultative model has helped to identify proactive clinical triggers for palliative care consultation. One study used five clinical triggers for automatic consultation: pre-ICU admission hospital LOS >10 days; age >80 years; terminal malignancy; status post–cardiac arrest; and intracerebral bleed requiring mechanical ventilation [27]. Other studies have used advanced dementia; multiorgan dysfunction syndrome; and the prior requirement for CPR as useful clinical triggers.

Consult teams may generate a halo effect resulting from their increased presence in the ICU, indirectly influencing care of other patients through modeling high-quality serious illness communication and symptom management. This may be especially true for conducting complex family meetings. Other providers may attend a specialist-led family meeting to discuss serious illness, observe skilled palliative care clinicians, and in turn apply some of the communication strategies to their own practices. An important advantage of the consultative model includes expert opinion from an interdisciplinary team of specially trained palliative care physicians, nurses, social workers, and others who can offer continuity of care before, during, and after an ICU admission, including transfer out of the ICU for end-of-life care when needed.

As a practical matter, many ICUs will function best with a hybrid model that offers the advantages of both the integrative and consultative models. A systematic review evaluated interventions in the ICU that improved end-of-life care and found that high-quality communication was the single most important factor for improving care, irrespective of the model [28]. Communication initiated by the palliative care consultants, along with family meetings and psychosocial support, improved quality in end-of-life care and family satisfaction. For the integrative model, trainees and interdisciplinary staff in an ICU showed higher rates of end-of-life discussions. Like any ICU procedure, conducting an effective family meeting requires training, skills practice, and feedback. The best model for any specific ICU depends on the locally available resources, particularly related to education, training, and commitment from all ICU clinicians to strengthen their knowledge and skills for palliative care practice. In addition, receptivity for collaboration with a multidisciplinary team is the key to efficient delivery of palliative care irrespective of the model.

TRIGGERING PALLIATIVE CARE IN THE ICU

Patients who are likely to benefit from palliative care consultative services should be identified early in their ICU stay. However, recognizing this population and initiating appropriate palliative care interventions are often at the discretion of the treating physician, potentially limiting the impact of consult teams. Over the last decade, a number of studies have investigated the use of standardized triggers to proactively initiate a palliative care consultation (Table 33.6). One medical ICU study proposed clinical parameters such as age greater than 80 years; LOS >10 days; prior cardiac arrest; terminal malignancy; and intracerebral bleed requiring mechanical ventilation as triggers initiating palliative care consultation and found that patients in the proactive palliative care group had significantly shorter ICU LOS [27]. Another study that used advanced dementia as a trigger to offer early assistance to the ICU staff found a decrease in hospital and medical ICU LOS. Notably, a proactive approach to palliative care intervention decreased the time between identification of the poor prognosis and the establishment of a DNR order and also reduced the use of nonbeneficial resources, which resulted in reduced patient and family burden and lower cost of care. In the severe brain injury cohort, the trigger-based approaches resulted in earlier and more systematic discussions with families about prognosis, patient values, and acceptable quality-of-life outcomes. In addition, there were higher rates of family satisfaction and a decrease in the number of tracheostomies for chronic respiratory failure [29].

Others have used prognostic triggers such as patients with a terminal condition as determined by the physician or a high risk of hospital death despite the continuation or escalation of medical therapies [30]. Patients with advanced cancer experience a complex web of these problems and evidence has demonstrated that specialist palliative care significantly improves patient outcomes in the domains of pain, symptom control, anxiety, and also reduces hospital admissions. In addition, patients with a palliative care consultation have higher rates of DNR orders before death suggesting they are protected more often from nonbeneficial cardiopulmonary resuscitation [31]. Evidence shows that families of patients who have a palliative care consultation during the last month of life are more satisfied with

TABLE 33.6

Triggers for Palliative Care in the ICU [27,34]

Clinical triggers
- Age >80 years
- Brain injury or global cerebral ischemia
- Status post–cardiac arrest
- Stage 4 malignancy
- Pre ICU admission length of stay >10 days
- Intracerebral hemorrhage requiring mechanical ventilation
- Multiorgan failure >3 organ systems
- Advanced stage dementia
- Death likely during this hospital admission

Complex communication triggers
- Goal-discordant care
- Disagreement regarding treatments among stakeholders (clinicians, patient, family members)
- Quality-of-life concerns

Surgical ICU triggers
- Greater than three admissions to the SICU during the index hospitalization
- Length of surgical ICU stay >1 month
- Multiorgan failure >3 organ systems in a patient over 60 years of age
- Transcranial gunshot wound
- Any disease with median survival < 4 months
- Family request
- GCS <8 for >1 week
- Carcinamatosis and unresectable malignancy

ICU, intensive care unit; SICU, surgical intensive care unit; GCS, Glasgow Coma Scale.

goals-of-care discussions and staff communication prior to their loved one's death [32].

The use of proactive clinical triggers for palliative care has demonstrated favorable outcomes in many settings. In the outpatient setting, patients are significantly more likely to have discussions about goals of care, improved quality of life (QOL) and lower depressive symptoms with trigger-initiated palliative care consultation. Specific to critical care, several studies showed that proactive approaches to palliative care consultation improve the concordance between the care provided and the care the patient actually wanted; increased use of advance directives; increased hospice referrals, and less use of nonbeneficial life-prolonging treatments for patients who are dying. A proactive palliative care approach has demonstrated a decreased ICU LOS; decreased hospital LOS; and less aggressive ICU interventions for patients that die in the ICU. Proactive palliative care has also shown to improve family satisfaction with the quality of care; understanding treatment options; and bereavement outcomes. Several outpatient studies have demonstrated that patients with serious illness who receive palliative care live longer, and proactive palliative care consultation has shown no increased mortality or discharge disposition [27].

One study looked at objective physiologic and medical parameters to predict palliative care need without consideration of communication or psychosocial factors. This study showed that about one in seven ICU patients could benefit from palliative care. There was no significant variation between the type of hospital (community vs. academic) or type of ICU (surgical, medical, neurologic, and mixed), and the prevalence of patients meeting certain palliative care triggers. Thus, the authors concluded that approximately one in seven ICU admissions met triggers for palliative care consultation using a single set of triggers, with an upper estimate of one in five patients using multiple sets of triggers. Notably, the triggers investigated by the authors were all objective, and clinical criteria and did not include issues such as ethical dilemmas, communication challenges, or symptom management; therefore, this is probably an underestimation of the number of ICU patients who would benefit from palliative care consultation [33]. Because palliative care needs are not unique to medical ICUs, various professional societies have their own specific guidelines. The American College of Surgeons convened a consensus panel of surgical palliative care specialists and surgical intensivists and developed "ten trigger" criteria for palliative care consultation, including multiorgan failure; expectation of death in the SICU; length of SICU stay >1 month; and more than three admissions to the SICU during the index hospitalization [34]. Several of these clinical criteria directly addressed terminal conditions, whereas others associated with a poor prognosis for neurologic recovery were also included (such as a Glasgow Coma Scale score <8 for more than 1 week in a patient older than 75 years). Triggers in the surgical literature can be used to proactively and systematically improve palliative care access for patients and families.

From the oncology literature, a concept known as "early palliative care" or "early integration" has been recommended by organizations such as the American Society of Clinical Oncology. The recommendation is that palliative care should be provided in all stages of advanced cancer in conjunction with disease-modifying treatments and is supported by randomized-controlled trials [35]. A recent study has also demonstrated that cancer patients receiving palliative care spend less time in the hospital or ICU; and have a better QOL, less depression, and longer survival [11]. Similarly, the American Thoracic Society instituted the End-of-Life Care Task Force whose primary purpose was to identify the core values and principles related to palliative care. Among the recommendations is that palliative care services be provided to all patients with chronic or advanced respiratory disease, regardless of age or social circumstances.

RECOGNIZING AND ADDRESSING BARRIERS TO PALLIATIVE CARE IN THE ICU

There are several important barriers to reliable high-quality palliative care delivery in the ICU, including educational gaps; time constraints; and local cultures of ICUs.

Physicians practice how they were trained. Most physicians practicing today did not receive formal training in communication; pain management; or spiritual assessment regarding the impact of serious illness on patients and their loved ones. Because all physicians received extensive training and supervision in the diagnosis and management of disease, it is often the default to offer and provide more medical treatments to patients regardless of their values and preferences, which often go unknown. Providers may lack the essential core skills to conduct an effective family meeting aimed at discussing serious illness; treatment options including palliative care; and patient or family preferences. Great efforts over the past few years to correct these knowledge and skill deficits are underway [36]. For example, an evidence-based conversation guide for providers regarding serious illness is available as a checklist to facilitate these difficult communication tasks [37]. The purpose of this script is to provide a framework for the clinician with phrases to use during a conversation about treatment preferences in the context of serious illness. This tool includes scripted sentences such as "What are you worried about most right now?" There are well-placed pauses intended to help the clinician be quiet and listen to the patient and family member, which allows them to process strong emotions; absorb medical information; and engage in important decisions. Such a tool models best practices and prompts clinicians to use, for example, periods of silence to more effectively listen and discern goals and values in order

TABLE 33.7

Internet-based Educational Resources for ICU Palliative Care

Resource	Description
C-3	Seven curriculum modules used in communication skills training program for intensive care fellows (free)
IPPC	Five curriculum modules on pediatric palliative care (free)
Palliative Care Fast Facts and Concepts (cross-published in the Journal of Palliative Medicine)	Concise, practical, peer-reviewed, evidence-based summaries on key topics (free; also available as an app)
EPEC	16 modules on core palliative care topics (available for purchase; CME credit)
ELNEC—Critical Care	Eight modules on critical care topics by expert faculty (available for purchase)
Center to Advance Palliative Care's Online Curriculum	Courses in pain and symptom management, and communication skills, among others (requires membership; CME credit)

ICU, intensive care unit; C-3, Communicating About Critical Care; IPPC, Initiative for Pediatric Palliative Care; EPEC, Education in Palliative and End-of-Life Care Project; CME, Continuing Medical Education; ELNEC, End-of-Life Nursing Education Consortium.

to make an appropriate treatment recommendation (e.g., to continue or discontinue the ventilator).

Knowledge gaps exist regarding pain and symptom assessment as well. Pain, dyspnea, and thirst are three of the most prevalent, intense, and distressing symptoms in ICU patients, but often underrecognized and undertreated. An interdisciplinary advisory board of the Improving Palliative Care in the ICU (IPAL-ICU) Project conducted a comprehensive review of literature in 2014 on the palliation of pain, dyspnea, and thirst. They identified evidence-based approaches for assessment and treatment, and recommended training of clinicians and well-designed work systems to implement best practices to ensure comfort and improve outcomes for the critically ill [38]. Pain management and palliative care are increasingly part of the core curricula in medical and nursing schools, and incorporated into academic milestones within residency and fellowship programs. A working group from the American College of Chest Physicians, the American Thoracic Society, the Association of Pulmonary and Critical Care Medicine Program Directors, and the Society for Critical Care Medicine designed entrustable professional activities that require pulmonary and critical care fellows to master the skills in facilitating effective family meetings and providing palliative care to patients and their families [39].

Another challenge is the fast pace and acuity of ICU care, which requires management of symptom crises and urgent decision-making about life-sustaining therapies without prior knowledge of patient preferences. This time pressure creates unique and additional stress on families and ICU staff. National leaders in critical care and palliative care have developed curricula for teaching and practicing urgent goals of care discussions during a medical crisis (see Table 33.7). In addition, the adoption of regular, brief family meetings from the beginning of an ICU stay about a patient's medical status, prognosis, and goals (before a new crisis) has been shown to reduce anxiety, depression, and posttraumatic stress in family members, as well as reduce nonbeneficial health-care utilization as a side effect [40]. As a further incentive, it is important these conversations are billed appropriately to compensate providers for this high-level work. In the USA, reimbursement for critical care professional services is time-based, and current Center for Medicare and Medicaid Services (CMS) guidelines allow physicians to include time spent communicating with family members when the following criteria are met: (1) the patient does not have decision-making capacity and cannot participate in the meeting; (2) the clinician is on the floor or unit while communicating with families (by telephone or in person); and (3) the discussion focuses on patient management and medical decision-making. More recently, CMS announced that they will reimburse "advance care planning" conversations in both inpatient and outpatient settings as of January 2015, and these discussions should be documented and billed separately, much like technical procedures.

Finally, assessment of local ICU culture is crucial for understanding potential barriers as well as opportunities of palliative care growth. Some ICUs embrace family meetings, include family members during rounds and encourage 24/7 visitation, whereas other ICUs are less forward facing to family members. As more data emerges regarding the negative impact of an ICU death on survivors, a trend is emerging toward family-centered ICU structures. The American College of Critical Care Medicine created evidence-based clinical practice guidelines for support of the family in the ICU [38] (see Table 33.8). Evidence and models from pediatric and neonatal ICUs suggest increased family satisfaction when loved ones are included in daily rounds, but highlight the need for careful design to maintain efficient workflows; patient privacy; and integration of teaching students, residents, and fellows. Some medical ICUs have incorporated "Get to Know Me" posters that encourage family to share personal information and photographs. ICUs that foster partnership with families and collaboration within their interdisciplinary teams may be better equipped to prevent or manage conflict, and help families and staff alike to cope with suffering. Much like central line infections, dying badly or in a manner discordant with patient preferences should become a "never event" within ICU culture.

1. Medical ICUs have increasingly adopted a closed model of care in which the intensivist is the primary provider; however, surgical ICUs often utilize an open model in which the surgeon retains primary care responsibility throughout the critical illness. Surgeons may have been trained to cure, and focus on mortality endpoints rather than patient-oriented endpoints. Death may be seen as a personal failure rather than the natural course of a terminal disease, which can lead to avoidance or poor communication with family about prognosis and end of life care. The surgical perspective is discussed in Chapter 55. In many of these ICUs, surgical intensivists may have less influence in discussing goals of care and shared decision-making. The Improving Palliative Care in the Intensive Care Unit (IPAL-ICU) [41] group recommended addressing attitudes and culture change through local champions and grassroots quality engagement to improve palliative care for the surgical and trauma professionals.

PALLIATIVE CARE QUALITY IMPROVEMENT

Quality improvement measures and related initiatives have swept through medical care at a rapid pace, especially with health-care reform. Landmark reports have demonstrated unacceptably high rates of medical errors and hospital-acquired complications, in addition to mandates around transparency and financial penalties for poor performance. Inevitably, the lack of palliative and end-of-life care has emerged as a major quality improvement issue, and this is particularly germane for ICUs owing to the morbidity and mortality associated with critical illness. Additionally, health systems are now being "graded" on their hospital mortality ratios as well as measures of patient–physician

TABLE 33.8

Selected Recommendations from the American College of Critical Care Medicine Clinical Practice Guidelines for Support of the Family in the Patient-Centered Intensive Care Unit [38]

- Practitioners fully disclose the patient's current status and prognosis to designated surrogates and clearly explain all reasonable management options.
- ICU caregivers strive to understand the level of life-sustaining therapies desired by patients, either directly from those patients or via their surrogates.
- Family meetings with the multiprofessional team begin within 24–48 hours after ICU admission and are repeated as dictated by the condition of the patient with input from all pertinent members of the multiprofessional team.
- Nurses and physicians assigned to each patient are as consistent as possible.
- Families are encouraged to provide as much care as the patient's condition will allow and they are comfortable providing.
- Family support is provided by the interprofessional team, including social workers, clergy, nursing, medicine, and parent support groups.
- The inter-professional team is kept informed of treatment goals so messages given to the family are consistent, thereby reducing friction within the team and between the team and family.
- A mechanism is created whereby all staff members may request a debriefing to voice concerns with the treatment plan; to decompress; to vent feelings; or to grieve.
- Spiritual needs of the patient are assessed by the health-care team, and findings that affect health and healing are incorporated into the plan of care.
- Physicians review reports of ancillary team members such as chaplains, social workers, and nurses to integrate their perspectives into patient care.
- Open visitation in the adult intensive care environment allows flexibility for patients and families, and is determined on a case-by-case basis.
- Whenever possible, adult patients or surrogate decision-makers are given the opportunity to participate in rounds.
- The family is educated about the signs and symptoms of approaching death in a developmentally and culturally appropriate manner.
- As appropriate, the family is informed about and offered referral to hospice, palliative care, or other community-based health-care resources.

ICU, intensive care unit.

communication and patient/family satisfaction, and palliative care can often impact these scores.

A useful lens for viewing palliative care as a quality improvement topic is the commonly applied Donabedian framework in which health-care quality outcomes are contingent upon the structures and processes of care within a health-care delivery system. The structure of palliative care services includes triggers; clinical models of care delivery; availability of palliative care expertise; and symptom management protocols. Examples of process measures include routine, structured family meetings; obtaining and documenting treatment preferences; and assessing and managing symptoms. Clinical outcomes such as mortality should be balanced with patient- and family-centered outcomes such as the QOL; quality of dying; decision-making processes at the end-of-life; and bereavement. Embedded in these clinical outcomes are issues of symptom management; communication; and adherence to patient goals and values. Other important quality outcomes include utilization of ICU resources and cost savings from nonbeneficial and unwanted care at end of life [5]. Ensuring that patients get the care they want and value may be the most powerful metric; however, this remains difficult to measure.

The National Quality Forum and the "Measuring What Matters" campaign [42] have studied and endorsed a variety of quality measures for palliative care. These measures could readily be applied to specific ICU-based quality improvement initiatives, such as improving pain control in the final 48 hours of life; assessing and treating dyspnea quickly; screening for spiritual distress; and triggering family conferences. Given the challenges intrinsic to outcome measures in palliative care, several consensus panels recommend indicators of structures and processes of care as proxies to reflect the quality of palliative care in the ICU. Process of care quality indicators for ICU palliative care include routine, structured family meetings; determining treatment preferences and surrogate decision-making roles; symptom management; and psychosocial support during and after end-of-life care. Quality indicators with respect to organizational structure include availability of palliative care consultative teams, religious/spiritual support services, protocols for withdrawing or withholding life support, and family-centered, open visitation spaces and policies.

An example of systematic palliative care integration through performance improvement is the "care and communication bundle," which was developed as part of the national Transformation of the ICU program by the Voluntary Hospital Association (VHA), Inc. This bundle of measures evaluates nine evidence-based care processes in established quality domains, using a denominator of patients in the ICU for at least 5 days (see Table 33.9). The program uses a time-triggered strategy to prompt critical palliative care processes by scheduling them into specific ICU days. On Day 1 of admission, the team identifies a medical decision-maker for a patient, followed by a serious illness conversation with documentation of advance directives and resuscitation status. On Days 2 through 5, there are daily family meetings to discuss ongoing goals of care or acute events. The program also included providing an informational brochure that introduced families to the ICU; the roles of each health-care providers, and logistics such as phone numbers and parking information. Before or by Day 3, patients and families were referred to social workers and/or chaplains for emotional, psychologic, and spiritual support as needed. Each day, the program required routine pain assessment, treatment and follow-up to ensure optimal care. The VHA "care and communication bundle" is posted on the National Quality Measures Clearinghouse website and maintained by the Agency for Healthcare Research and Quality [43]. The bundle formed the basis of a large-scale collaborative improvement project by multiple ICUs in the VHA TICU program, a major faith-based hospital system, and medical ICUs in the Veterans Integrated Service Network.

Other quality measures under scrutiny are hospital mortality rates, which are now publicly reported. The value and meaning of these ratings are debatable [44]. Some mortality rates are global and apply to an entire hospital or organization, whereas others are specific to an illness such as pneumonia or myocardial infarction. Within this reporting, it is important to delineate hospital deaths that are expected or unavoidable, especially when dying patients are admitted for terminal care. The reporting entities that construct mortality rates have grappled with this issue, using various strategies with proprietary statistical tools [45]. In order to better understand how palliative and hospice care codes impact hospital mortality rates, one study compared methodologies between four major vendors and found substantial variation [46]. Certain palliative care codes impact the inclusion or exclusion of decedents for some reporting entities and make this data difficult to compare in a meaningful way. As a result, some patients who receive end-of-life care in a hospital setting

TABLE 33.9

Voluntary Hospital Association's "Care and Communication Bundle" of Palliative Care Process Measures for Adult ICUs

Quality indicator	Numerator for quality measure
Medical Decision-Maker Documentation of efforts to identify a medical decision-maker (family member or other appropriate surrogate) for the patient on or before Day 1 in ICU	*Numerator*: Number of patients who have documentation of ICU efforts to identify a health-care proxy (or other appropriate surrogate decision-maker) on or before Day 1 of the ICU admission
Advance Directive Documentation of advance directive status on or before Day 1 in ICU	*Numerator*: Number of patients who have documentation of advance directive status on or before Day 1 in ICU
Resuscitation Status Documentation of resuscitation status on or before Day 1 in ICU	*Numerator*: Number of patients who have documentation of resuscitation status on or before Day 1 in ICU
Family Information Leaflet Documentation of information leaflet distribution to ICU family members on or before Day 1 in ICU	*Numerator*: Number of patients whose families were personally given a printed information leaflet by an ICU team member on or before Day 1 in ICU
Pain Assessment Regular pain assessment	*Numerator*: Total number of 4-hour intervals (on Day 0 and Day 1 in ICU) for which pain was assessed and documented *Denominator*: Total number of 4-hour intervals (on Day 0 and Day 1 in ICU) for patients with an ICU length of stay ≥5 days (this number cannot be greater than 12)
Pain Management Optimal pain management	*Numerator*: Total number of 4-hour intervals (on Day 0 and Day 1 in ICU) for which the documented pain score was ≤3 *Denominator*: Total number of 4-hour intervals (on Day 0 and Day 1 in ICU) with numerical pain values of 0 to 10, for patients with an ICU length of stay ≥5 days (this number cannot be greater than 12)
Social Work Support Social work support offered to ICU patients and/or families on or before Day 3 in ICU	*Numerator*: Number of patients who have documentation in the medical record that social work support was offered to the patient and/or family on or before Day 3 in the ICU
Spiritual Support Spiritual support offered to ICU patients and/or families on or before Day 3 in ICU	*Numerator*: Number of patients who have documentation in the medical record that spiritual support was offered to the patient and/or family on or before Day 3 in the ICU
Interdisciplinary Family Meeting Adequate clinician–patient/family communication on or before Day 5 in ICU	*Numerator*: Number of patients who have documentation in the medical record that an interdisciplinary meeting was conducted on or before Day 5 in the ICU

Unless otherwise indicated, the denominator for each of these measures is the number of patients with an ICU stay ≥5 days.
ICU, intensive care unit.
Reprinted with permission from the Center to Advance Palliative Care, The IPAL-ICU Project.

may indeed impact hospital-specific mortality data. The variations present among hospital mortality rate determinations in general and specifically with respect to palliative care offer a cautionary note, and ICU clinicians' efforts are probably best spent at this time on substantive strategies and assessment tools to improve the quality of bedside care for palliation in the ICU.

GUIDING SUCCESSFUL INTEGRATION OF PALLIATIVE CARE IN THE ICU

A new approach to better meeting the palliative needs of ICU patients begins with an organized initiative, including a working group, a needs assessment, and a focused action plan. A working group should include critical care clinicians (including the ICU medical and nursing directors), palliative care experts, nurses, social workers, chaplains, case managers, pharmacists, and administrators who demonstrate commitment and can serve as local champions and sponsors. Although palliative care has empirically demonstrated benefits, it is important for these stakeholders to adapt these lessons to their local ICU culture and resources. Initial planning should be based on a survey of existing clinical, educational, and financial resources to enhance feasibility and success without overwhelming the system. The working group should conduct a needs assessment to define problems; identify opportunities for improvement; and prioritize their agenda. This process also helps build support within the ICU and provides baseline data for evaluating results, which can be leveraged to strengthen a case for more resources from hospital leadership. Potential sources of data include patient mortality; LOS; readmissions; patient symptom ratings; family satisfaction surveys; presence of documentation of surrogate decision-makers in the medical record; proportion of patients seen by specialty palliative care; and surveys or focus groups of ICU staff.

Based on the needs assessment and inventory of resources, the working group should identify a specific and actionable opportunity for improvement relevant to their specific ICU. Examples include improving patients' symptoms through the regular use of assessment scales and analgesic equivalency charts, or improving communication with patients and families with structured family meetings (see Table 33.10).

Some of the most important aspects of successful integration of palliative care in the ICU include cultivating key stakeholders; designing effective and efficient systems for delivering palliative care; and promoting institutional culture change. The interdisciplinary leadership is crucial in elevating the importance of psychosocial, spiritual, and cultural factors that contextualize people's suffering and inform decision-making by patients and families [47].

TABLE 33.10

Example of an Abbreviated Action Plan

Overall goal	Improve communication between the clinical team and families of critically ill patients
Specific target	By Month 6, at least half of families of patients in the ICU for ≥5 days will have opportunity to meet with interdisciplinary ICU team for goal setting.
Clinical practice/system change actions	ICU social worker will track admissions and arrange meetings by scheduled day; new plan for coverage will free bedside RN to attend; meeting reminder to be included in Daily Goals Sheet; families to be given Meeting Guide on patient's admission.
Documentation actions	New family meeting documentation template to be placed in chart.
Measurement actions	Numerator and denominator for family meeting measure, including specifications defining participants to attend meetings and topics for discussion; measure will be collected by review of medical records by Quality RN.
Assignments	• Develop plan for nurse coverage: ICU Nursing Director • Develop new document templates: Dr. A and Nurse B • Develop Family Meeting Guide: Dr. C, Nurse D, and Social Worker • Plan program of educational support: Nurse Educator with Palliative Care Team members in workgroup; review of plan by ICU Director • Specify family meeting measure: ICU MD and RN Directors

ICU, intensive care unit; RN, registered nurse; MD, managing director.
Reprinted with permission from the Center to Advance Palliative Care (CAPC), The IPAL-ICU Project.

Education and training of clinicians, as described above, is critical to early success but also long-term sustainability of integrated palliative care. Clinicians must learn to manage multiple symptoms in patients with multiorgan failure and potential adverse effects from medications. They also should understand the legal and bioethical constructs for surrogate decision-making and limits on life-prolonging therapies, as well as strategies for dealing with uncertainty about prognosis and conflict resolution. This education should include skills practice, especially in advanced communication procedures such as sharing prognosis and discussing goals of care. These communication procedures can be especially challenging owing to the acuity of illness; incapacitated patients; reliance on surrogate decision-makers; and the lack of longitudinal relationships with patients and families. Whereas physicians provide information on diagnosis and prognosis, families provide expertise on patients' beliefs and values. The recommended framework is a shared decision-making model in which the physician and family jointly assume responsibility for decisions about end-of-life care.

In order for evidence-based education and training to translate into everyday clinical practice, structural and process factors that facilitate high-quality palliative care in the ICU are essential. These include the availability of specialists and multidisciplinary care teams, the feasibility of the consultative versus integrative models, and the creation and implementation of protocols. The protocols and order sets should address routine pain and symptom management; documentation of advanced directives; time-triggered family conferences; withdrawal of life support; and discharge for survivors to community-based palliative care or hospice.

Effective implementation of any program involves setting short- and long-term goals, and varies depending on the need of each ICU. For example, a working group might begin with a specific plan to improve communication between ICU clinicians and families (organizing regular family meetings; designing a meeting guide; and involving nurses in family meetings) that evolves into broader system changes over time (creating templated, retrievable electronic notes about goals and care preferences; hiring and incorporating chaplains, redesigning patient rooms and hospital spaces for more comfortable and effective family meetings.). Once integration of palliative care into the ICU environment is successful, focus should be directed to sustain it by creating a supportive ICU environment such that members of the interdisciplinary team feel responsible, empowered, and respected. This can be done by regular team huddles or debriefs that address ongoing challenges and quality concerns.

Nearly one in five Americans die during a hospitalization that involves ICU care, and nearly 100,000 ICU survivors continue with critical illness on a chronic basis [6]. Critical care providers play a key role for ensuring that high-quality palliative care is reliable and available to all patients with advanced illness in the ICU and their loved ones. This requires a commitment to ongoing palliative care education with training and feedback; regular assessment of quality measures such as symptom scores and numbers of structured family meetings; and measurement that care provided was concordant with patient preferences. This last measure, perhaps the most difficult to measure, is especially important as we strive to deliver the type of critical care that people want and value. The successful integration of palliative care is an essential to the delivery of high-quality critical care, especially the effective management of pain and symptoms of advanced illness and the mastery of skills required for serious illness communication.

Summary Table of Recommendations

Study/Organization	Consensus Statement/ Recommendations/ Conclusions	Refs
National Consensus Project Guidelines for Quality Palliative Care	The report promotes the philosophies embedded in palliative care and outlines essential elements to ensure quality, including the structure and processes of care; the physical, psychosocial, spiritual, and cultural aspects of clinical care; caring for the imminently dying patient, and ethical and legal aspects of care	[13]
A communication strategy and brochure for relatives of patients dying in the ICU	Providing families with a brochure on bereavement and using a proactive communication strategy may lessen the burden of bereavement	[40]

Task Force from the Society of Critical Care Medicine, American College of Chest Physicians, American Thoracic Society, American Board of Internal Medicine, and the Association of Pulmonary and Critical Care Medicine Program Directors	Recommend palliative care training for all ICU clinicians	[18]
National Quality Measures Clearinghouse of the Agency for Healthcare Research and Quality endorse the Voluntary Hospital Association "care and communication bundle"	Nine care process measures, which has served as the basis for ICU palliative care improvement efforts (see Table 33.9)	[22]
American Society of Clinical Oncology	Palliative care should be provided in all stages of advanced cancer in conjunction with disease-modifying treatments	[11]

References

1. Dying in America: *Improving Quality and Honoring Individual Preferences Near the End of Life. Committee on Approaching Death: Addressing Key End of Life Issues; Institute of Medicine*. Washington (DC), National Academies Press (US), 2015.
2. Hopkins RO, Girard TD: Medical and economic implications of cognitive and psychiatric disability of survivorship. *Semin Respir Crit Care Med* 33(4):348–356, 2012.
3. Pastores SM, Dakwar J, Halpern NA: Costs of critical care medicine. *Crit Care Clin* 28(1):1–10, 2012.
4. Teno JM, Gozalo PL, Bynum JP, et al: Change in end-of-life care for Medicare beneficiaries: site of death, place of care, and health care transitions in 2000, 2005, and 2009. *JAMA* 309(5):470–477, 2013.
5. O'Mahony S, McHenry J, Blank AE, et al: Preliminary report of the integration of a palliative care team into an intensive care unit. *Palliat Med* 24(2):154–165, 2010.
6. Davidson JE, Jones C, Bienvenu OJ: Family response to critical illness: postintensive care syndrome-family. *Crit Care Med* 40(2):618–624, 2012.
7. Zier LS, Sottile PD, Hong SY, et al: Surrogate decision makers' interpretation of prognostic information: a mixed-methods study. *Ann Intern Med* 156(5):360–366, 2012.
8. Morrison RS, Meier DE: America's care of serious illness: 2015 state-by-state report card on access to palliative care in our nation's hospitals. www.capc.org. Accessed May 30, 2017.
9. Lupu D: Estimate of current hospice and palliative medicine physician workforce shortage. *J Pain Symptom Manage* 40(6):899–911, 2010.
10. Morrison RS, Penrod JD, Cassel JB, et al: Cost savings associated with US hospital palliative care consultation programs. *Arch Intern Med* 168(16):1783–1790, 2008.
11. Temel JS, Greer JA, Muzikansky A, et al: Early palliative care for patients with metastatic non-small cell lung cancer. *N Engl J Med* 363(8)733–742, 2010.
12. Connor SR, Pyenson B, Fitch K, et al: Comparing hospice and non-hospice patient survival among patients who die within three-year window. *J Pain Symptom Manage* 33(3):238–236, 2007.
13. National Consensus Project for Quality Palliative Care: Clinical Practice Guidelines for quality palliative care, executive summary. *J Palliat Med* 7(5):611–627, 2004.
14. Enguidanos S, Housen P, Penido M, et al: Family members' perceptions of inpatient palliative care consult services: a qualitative study. *Palliat Med* 28(1):42–48, 2014.
15. Hsu-Kim C, Friedman T, Gracely E, et al: Integrating palliative care into critical care: a quality improvement study. *J Intensive Care Med* 30(6):358–364, 2015.
16. Nelson JE, Bassett R, Boss RD, et al: Models for structuring a clinical initiative to enhance palliative care in the intensive care unit: a report from the IPAL-ICU Project (Improving Palliative Care in the ICU). *Crit Care Med* 38(9):1765–1772, 2010.
17. Campbell ML, Weissman DE, Nelson JE: Palliative care consultation in the ICU #253. *J Palliat Med* 15(6):715–716, 2012.
18. Buckley JD, Addrizzo-Harris DJ, Clay AS, et al: Multi-society task force recommendations of competencies in Pulmonary and Critical Care Medicine. *Am J Respir Crit Care Med* 180(4):290–295, 2009.
19. Curtis JR, Treece PD, Nielsen EL, et al: Integrating palliative and critical care: evaluation of a quality-improvement intervention. *Am J Respir Crit Care Med* 178(3):269–275, 2008.
20. Curtis JR, Nielsen EL, Treece PD, et al: Effect of a quality-improvement intervention on end-of-life care in the intensive care unit: a randomized trial. *Am J Respir Crit Care Med* 183(3):348–355, 2011.
21. Black MD, Vigorito MC, Curtis JR, et al: A multifaceted intervention to improve compliance with process measures for ICU clinician communication with ICU patients and families. *Crit Care Med* 41(10):2275–2283, 2013.
22. Nelson JE, Mulkerin CM, Adams LL, et al: Improving comfort and communication in the ICU: a practical new tool for palliative care performance measurement and feedback. *Qual Saf Health Care* 15(4):264–271, 2006.
23. Hinkle LJ, Bosslet GT, Torke AM: Factors associated with family satisfaction with end-of-life care in the ICU: a systematic review. *Chest* 147(1):82–93, 2015.
24. Jones DA, Bagshaw SM, Barrett J, et al: The role of the medical emergency team in end-of-life care: a multicenter, prospective, observational study. *Crit Care Med* 40(1):98–103, 2012.
25. Smith RL, Hayashi VN, Lee YI, et al: The medical emergency team call: a sentinel event that triggers goals of care discussion. *Crit Care Med* 42(2):322–327, 2014.
26. Downar J, Rodin D, Barua R, et al: Rapid response teams, do not resuscitate orders, and potential opportunities to improve end-of-life care: a multicentre retrospective study. *J Crit Care* 28(4):498–503, 2013.
27. Norton SA, Hogan LA, Holloway RG, et al: Proactive palliative care in the medical intensive care unit: effects on length of stay for selected high-risk patients. *Crit Care Med* 35(6):1530–1535, 2007.
28. Scheunemann LP, McDevitt M, Carson SS, et al: Randomized, controlled trials of interventions to improve communication in intensive care: a systematic review. *Chest* 139(3):543–554, 2011.
29. Holloway RG, Quill TE: Treatment decisions after brain injury—tensions among quality, preference, and cost. *N Engl J Med* 362(19):1757–1759, 2010.
30. Sihra L, Harris M, O'Reardon C: Using the improving palliative care in the intensive care unit (IPAL-ICU) project to promote palliative care consultation. *J Pain Symptom Manage* 42(5):672–675, 2011.
31. Higginson IJ, Evans CJ: What is the evidence that palliative care teams improve outcomes for cancer patients and their families? *Cancer J* 16(5):423–435, 2010.
32. Casarett D, Johnson M, Smith D, et al: The optimal delivery of palliative care: a national comparison of the outcomes of consultation teams vs inpatient units. *Arch Intern Med* 171(7):649–655, 2011.
33. Hua MS, Li G, Blinderman CD, et al: Estimates of the need for palliative care consultation across united states intensive care units using a trigger-based model. *Am J Respir Crit Care Med* 189(4):428–436, 2014.
34. Bradley CT, Brasel KJ: Developing guidelines that identify patients who would benefit from palliative care services in the surgical intensive care unit. *Crit Care Med* 37(3):946–950, 2009.
35. Ford DW, Koch KA, Ray DE, et al: Palliative and end-of-life care in lung cancer: diagnosis and management of lung cancer, 3rd ed: American College of Chest Physicians evidence-based clinical practice guidelines. *Chest* 143(5 Suppl):e498S–e512S, 2013.
36. Nelson JE, Curtis JR, Mulkerin C, et al: Choosing and using screening criteria for palliative care consultation in the ICU: a report from the Improving Palliative Care in the ICU (IPAL-ICU) Advisory Board. *Crit Care Med* 41(10):2318–2327, 2013.
37. Bernacki RE, Block SD; American College of Physicians High Value Care Task Force: Communication about serious illness care goals: a review and synthesis of best practices. *JAMA Intern Med* 174(12):1994–2003, 2014.
38. Davidson JE, Powers K, Hedayat KM, et al: Clinical practice guidelines for support of the family in the patient-centered intensive care unit: American College of Critical Care Medicine Task Force 2004–2005. *Crit Care Med* 35(2):605–622, 2007.
39. Henry E, Fessler HE, Addrizzo-Harris D, et al: Entrustable professional activities and curricular milestones for fellowship training in pulmonary and critical care medicine: report of a Multi-Society Working Group. *Chest* 146:813–834, 2014.
40. Lautrette A, Darmon M, Megarbane B, et al: A communication strategy and brochure for relatives of patients dying in the ICU. *N Engl J Med* 356(5):469–478, 2007.
41. Mosenthal AC, Weissman DE, Curtis JR, et al: Integrating palliative care in the surgical and trauma intensive care unit: a report from the Improving Palliative Care in the Intensive Care Unit (IPAL-ICU) Project Advisory Board and the Center to Advance Palliative Care. *Crit Care Med* 40(4):1199–1206, 2012.
42. Dy SM, Kiley KB, Ast K, et al: Measuring what matters: top-ranked quality indicators for hospice and palliative care from the American Academy of Hospice and Palliative Medicine and Hospice and Palliative Nurses Association. *J Pain Symptom Manage* 49(4):773–781, 2015.
43. Care and Communication Quality Measures at the National Quality Measures Clearinghouse sponsored by the Agency for Healthcare Research and Quality. https://www.qualitymeasures.ahrq.gov/. Accessed May 30, 2017.
44. Shahian DM, Wolf RE, Iezzoni LI, et al: Variability in the measurement of hospital-wide mortality rates. *N Engl J Med* 363(26):2530–2539, 2010.
45. Chong CA, Nguyen GC, Wilcox ME: Trends in Canadian hospital standardised mortality ratios and palliative care coding 2004–2010: a retrospective database analysis. *BMJ Open* 2(6), 2012.
46. Cassel JB, Jones AB, Meier DE, et al: Hospital mortality rates: how is palliative care taken into account? *J Pain Symptom Manage* 40(6):914–925, 2010.
47. Billings JA, Keeley A, Bauman J, et al: Merging cultures: palliative care specialists in the medical intensive care unit. *Crit Care Med* 34[11 Suppl]:S388–S393, 2006.
48. Ray D, Fuhrman C, Stern G, et al: Integrating palliative medicine and critical care in a community hospital. *Crit Care Med* 34[11 Suppl]:S394–S398, 2006.

Chapter 34 ■ Effective Communication and Ethical Decision-Making in the ICU

DANIEL E. RAY • JENNIFER E. ALLEN • KAREN M. KNOPS

Timely, clear and compassionate communication is crucial to the care of critically ill patients and their families. Intensivists regularly share complex medical information, navigate prognosis and goals of care (GOC), and lead emotionally charged meetings with patients and families as part of their daily work. However, few clinicians receive formal training in communication skills and ethical decision-making. The costs of poor communication can result in increased patient and family psychological trauma, increased conflict, delayed or ineffective medical decision-making, moral distress among the ICU team, and the use of potentially inappropriate ICU resources. This chapter explores an approach to effective communication in the ICU, and the bioethical frameworks that guide shared decision-making between patients, families and clinicians.

FAMILY MEETINGS AND GOC DISCUSSIONS

Structured Family Meetings to Improve Communication

Communication presents one of the greatest challenges and therapeutic opportunities for medical care, regardless of clinical setting. Common barriers to communication include poor clinician training, time pressures, medical or legal concerns, and chasms of culture and health literacy [1,2]. Serious illness has potential to raise spiritual, existential, emotional, social, financial, and functional concerns for both the patient and his/her loved ones [3,4]. Patients and families meet numerous subspecialist physicians, specialized nurses and technicians and, in academic centers, trainees of every level, while patient care needs may change by the hour. Fragmented communication can create suffering and safety concerns, reducing satisfaction with care and increasing risk of malpractice claims [5–7].

The "family meeting" has been identified as a strategy to prevent miscommunication and directly address the emotional distress caused by the intensive care environment [8–10]. The term "family" will be used in this text to refer to a patient's loved ones, patient's legal guardian, health proxy, caregiver, next of kin, civil partner, clergy or friends that the patient has empowered to participate in his or her care. Such meetings save time and confusion by allowing a patient's loved ones to express feelings, hear each other's concerns, and ensure that the patient's individual goals and values are understood. This point has been evidenced by studies showing that an interdisciplinary communication intervention resulted in earlier consensus around goals and reduced length of stay in trauma ICU and liver transplant patients, without an increase of mortality [11,12].

Practitioners can promote quality care by using a consistent, evidence-based approach, planning ahead, and through skillful collaboration with the care team (Table 34.1). General discussion of clinical status, prognosis, patient-centered goals and options should be initiated by intensivists and the outpatient providers who have patient-valued relationships, such as oncologists, cardiologists and primary care clinicians. Such communication is considered to be "generalist" palliative care provided by many health professionals, while the expertise of the palliative care consultant is reserved for issues that remain unresolved in spite of the efforts of primary clinicians [13].

Interventions such as rounding tools and triggers have been used to ensure consistent communication practices. Triggers (see Chapter on Integrating Palliative Care in the ICU), including clinical factors, number of days in ICU, and staff assessments, can be used to prompt a structured family meeting with the ICU team and/or a referral to palliative care. Such triggers may be tailored to institutional goals, needs of a specific unit or patient population, and availability of ICU practitioners and palliative specialists. Structured approaches to communication are recommended to improve quality and timing of this important intervention [14] with extensive evidence for use in the ICU setting [15].

Evidenced-based curricula on communication training skills have been shown to be feasible and effective for clinicians [16]. The Vital Talk program [17] and the Critical Care Communication (C3) Course for intensive care fellows are high-quality examples. Such courses address knowledge, skills, and attitudes regarding serious illness communication. Because clear communication is so commonly needed following a resuscitation event, authors have also evaluated the need for skills in discussing bad news or goals of care linked with resuscitation exercises, which elicit a spectrum of emotional reactions within the clinician [18,19]. Clinicians can also "practice" by using skills in simpler, less emotionally charged interactions—ideally with feedback from mentors and inter-professional peers.

ICU-based initiatives and systematic literature reviews have identified key concepts in approaching family meetings, from vital preparatory steps to coherent documentation [8,20,21].

Anticipation: What to Discuss and Why

Determining the goal and content of the meeting sets the tone and guides subsequent steps. Failing to identify a shared goal can lead to confusion for the family and conflict for the care team. Through careful chart review, discussion with clinicians, and sharing one's intention with the patient or his/her proxy, one can refine the goals and create a shared agenda. Consensus about diagnosis, prognosis and treatment options should be reached during pre-meeting preparation. Patient/family distress will escalate if they perceive that physicians disagree or are not communicating effectively. The input of multiple specialists, (either in person, speaker phone or via relayed conversations) is helpful in situations where such information is vital for decision-making or for patient/family understanding.

When appropriate, advanced care planning documents are reviewed prior to the meeting for verification of patient proxy (for incapacitated patients) and values (if related to the clinical scenario). Discussions with outpatient physicians, social workers, nursing and spiritual care providers can reveal psychosocial and cultural influences on prognosis, treatment options and communication. Tensions among family members or between family and staff should be noted, but should not bias the perspective of the practitioner.

TABLE 34.1

The Goal-Setting Conference (Weissman)

Before the Meeting

Review chart—know all medical issues: history, prognosis, treatment options
- Coordinate medical opinions among consultant physicians
- Decide what tests/treatments are medically appropriate (i.e., likely to benefit the patient)
- Review Advance Care Planning documents
- Review/obtain family psychosocial information
- Decide who you want to be present from the medical team
- Clarify your goals for the meeting—What decisions are you hoping to achieve?

10-Step guide	Helpful language
1. Establish Proper Setting Private, comfortable; everyone seated, turn off/forward pager	
2. Introductions • Allow everyone to state name and relationship to patient • Build relationship: ask nonmedical question about patient	"Can you tell me something about your father? What kind of person is he?"
3. Assess Patient/Family Understanding • Encourage all present to respond • Ask for a description of changes in function over course of illness/hospitalization	"What have the doctors told you about your wife's condition at this point?" "What is your assessment of the current medical situation?"
4. Medical Review/Summary • Summarize "big picture" in few sentences—use "dying" if appropriate; avoid organ-by-organ medical review • Avoid jargon • Answer questions	"I'm afraid I have some bad news. I wish things were different. Based on what you have told me, and what I see, I believe your mother is dying."
5. Silence/Reactions • Respond to emotional reactions (have tissues available) • Prepare for common reactions: acceptance, conflict/denial, grief/despair, respond empathically	"This must be very hard" "I can only imagine how scary/difficult/overwhelming this must be." "You appear angry. Can you tell me what is upsetting you?"
6. Discuss Prognosis • Assess how much patient and family want to know • Provide prognostic data using a range • Respond to emotion	"Some people like to know every detail about their illness, others prefer a more general outline. What kind of person are you?" "Although I can't give you an exact time, given your illness and condition, I believe you have (hours to days) (weeks to months). This is an average, some live longer and some live shorter."
7. Assess Patient/Family Goals Possible Goals: • Prolong life • Improve function • Return home • See a family milestone • Relief of suffering • Staying in control	"What do you wish to accomplish?" "Are there any important goals or tasks left undone?" "What is most important to you at this time?" "Knowing that time is short, what goals do you have?" "How do you picture your death?" "Where do you want to be when you die?"
8. Present Broad Care Options • Stress priority of comfort, no matter the goal • Make a recommendation based on knowledge/experience	"Given what you have told me about your mother and her goals, I would recommend..." "These decisions are very hard; if (patients name) were sitting with us today, what do you think he/she would say?" "How will the decision affect you and other family members?"
9. Translate Goals into Care Plan • Review current and planned interventions—make recommendations to continue or stop based on goals • Discuss DNR, hospice/home care, artificial nutrition/hydration, future hospitalizations • Summarize all decisions made • Confirm your continued availability regardless of decisions	"You have told me your goals are _____. With this in mind, I do not recommend the use of artificial or heroic means to prolong your dying process. If you agree with this, I will write an order in the chart that when you die, no attempt to resuscitate you will be made, is this acceptable (ok)?" "All dying patients lose their interest in eating in the days to weeks leading up to death; this is the body's signal that death is coming." "I am recommending that the (tube feedings, IVF) be discontinued (or not started) as these will not improve her living and may only prolong her dying."

TABLE 34.1

The Goal-Setting Conference (Weissman) (*continued*)

10. Document and Discuss • Write a note: who was present, what decisions were made, follow-up plan • Discuss with team members (consultants, nurse, etc.) • Check your emotions	**Team Debriefing = Opportunity for Teaching and Reflection** Ask team members: "How do you think the meeting went?" "What went well?" What could have gone more smoothly? "What will you do differently in the future?"
Managing Conflict	
➢ Listen and make empathic statements ➢ Determine source of conflict: guilt, grief, culture, family, dysfunction, trust in med team, etc. ➢ Clarify misconceptions ➢ Explore values behind decisions ➢ Set time-limited goals with specific benchmarks (e.g., improved cognition, oxygenation, mobility) ➢ **When you need additional assistance or support, consider a palliative care consult.**	

Adapted from Weissman DE "The Family Goal Setting Conference" and "Communication Phrases Near the End of Life" pocket cards from Medical College of Wisconsin.

Anticipation: Whom to Include in the Family Meeting

After determining the goal of the meeting, consideration should be given to how the patient is represented. If doubt exists about patient capacity, an assessment should be performed (see section later in this chapter on "determining decision-making capacity"), as patients with the waxing and waning sensorium may lose or regain capacity quickly. Patients with dementia may also "cover" by giving vague answers and responding to social cues without real understanding. In general, encouraging a health care agent to attend the meeting is always advisable, especially if the patient has variable capacity or memory impairment, but also to prime the health care agent for future decision-making if and when the patient loses capacity.

Patients vary with regard to their desires to participate in decision making [22]. When explaining the goal of the discussion, inquire whether the patient prefers to be fully involved or if emotions or culture prompt him/her to defer. While a patient may be culturally expected to defer decision making, the patient should be asked what role her or she would like to play.

If the family request withholding information from the patient, understand the reason for the request. Common fears are often allayed with careful explanation and reassurance. Studies indicate that patients do not become more depressed when given a serious diagnosis [23]. Discussing the risks of non-disclosure—i.e., that the patient may already fear the worst, may make bad choices due to misinformation, or will eventually learn of the deception with devastating results—is important, as is explaining that disclosure will occur compassionately and only with patient consent to receive this information [23].

For a supportive presence, patients or surrogates may identify family, friends, or clergy. Many families have complex structure; it is helpful to ask open-ended questions to identify the necessary participants. Telephonic (including video) participation of those who cannot be present saves time and confusion. Encouraging the patient or surrogate to have a "second set of ears" (family member, friend, or staff member) can alleviate anxiety.

An interdisciplinary approach to the meeting will best meet the multifaceted needs of patients and families. For example, it is helpful to have a case manager present if the meeting will include discussion of complex discharge planning. Roles of members vary between institutions and even between care units, and may shift with the needs of a patient and family. A brief meeting of clinicians can clarify roles.

Anticipation: When and Where

Choosing a time and place that will not be interrupted can be a challenge but is vital for creating a sense of safety for patients and families. When possible, allow the patient or family to have a level of control over timing. If communication feels forced, trust may be damaged permanently. For cases with a great deal of clinical information or complex psychosocial barriers, begin conversations early, and choose a quiet, neutral setting where participants can sit comfortably.

Anticipation: How to Communicate

Communication aides such as telephonic or live interpreters, or an audio assistive device for a hearing-impaired participant, should be considered during the planning process, and techniques for use should be reviewed. For meetings that will address a new diagnosis, it may be beneficial to print information related to the patient's condition. For some types of illness, such as a precariously positioned tumor, allowing patient/family to view images with support from a clinical team member to assist in interpretation. Use available resources, such as white boards or electronic devices, which can help convey information or display images.

When multiple providers participate, a brief discussion of roles and goals is recommended. There is variability in the role of the physician in discussing end-of-life decisions in the ICU [24]. Depending on the level of certainty about medical options and prognosis and patient/family preferences, communication strategies for shared decision-making may emphasize paternalism or patient autonomy [8]. Mindfulness to one's own agenda and feelings is also helpful prior to entering a family meeting. Many providers are trained to have awareness of body language, eye contact, tone, and pacing of their speech. Just as clinicians must wash their hands to avoid bringing germs to the patient's bedside, they must take a moment to reflect on what emotions they carry. Such techniques have been shown to improve satisfaction with care [25]. Practitioners who enter the patient's or family's space carelessly or fail to maintain a professional appearance and countenance can inadvertently sabotage the clinical encounter before it even begins.

The Goal-Setting Conference

Step 1–Choose the Right Setting: While the team cannot always control availability of quiet conference areas, clinicians can inquire about the comfort level of patients and families and make every attempt to optimize it—offering a bathroom break, a warm blanket, or water before serious discussions. Chairs and tissues can be moved to a private space to prepare for discussion. Remove distractions from the setting, such as turning off televisions, silencing non-essential alarms and phones, and placing a sign on the door to request privacy, and warning if an interruption may occur. For meetings that include the patient, sit at eye level and encourage others to be seated. If the patient is incapacitated, determine with the family whether the meeting should be held with the patient present; if so, portray respect and acknowledge the patient's guiding "voice," even if s/he is unable to participate.

Step 2–Make Introductions and Share Intentions for the Meeting: While healthcare team members can prepare extensively for a family meeting, family members may have only moments to understand who is going to be speaking to them and why. Team members should be introduced and their roles explained. Terms like "resident" or "attending" may be meaningless to those without a medical background. Providing business cards of team members and offering materials to write down information can reduce distress. Some intensive care settings use brochures to explain the concept of family meetings [10].

Shaking hands, making good eye contact, offering a gentle smile, and bowing the head slightly can demonstrate respect, and sitting down sends a message of being willing to give time and attention [26]. Asking about proper pronunciation of patient's name or whether a nickname is preferred signals that the patient will be treated as a valued individual.

Step 3–Assess Patient/Family Understanding: It is easy to assume that patients or families "should" understand the diagnosis or prognosis based on prior conversations or the amount of time that a patient has been ill. Only by asking patients/families to share perspectives can the clinician gain insight into what the patient or family know. When traumatic events have occurred, the act of telling the story to an empathetic clinician helps the patient and family to accept what has occurred and improves satisfaction with care [27]. Ask about the patient as a person—goals, values, passions—in addition to the clinical summary.

Open-ended questions should be used to explore the patient or family's perception, resisting the urge to assume that broad comments such as "he's really sick" mean the same thing to everyone. For patients with chronic illness or frailty, inquire about baseline function. A technique called "ask-tell-ask" reminds clinicians to respond with questions rather than commentary. "Can you tell me more about that? I want to make sure I understand" is a simple yet empathic question. It is the feeling of being listened to that correlates with positive impressions of the clinician [27].

Allowing the patient or family to speak first allows the health professional to carefully assess factors such as emotional readiness to hear difficult information or make decisions, patient and family's health literacy, culture, any existing conflict within the family, and perspective on illness. Asking "Can you tell your biggest concern?" of all participants helps to focus the narrative and can elicit conflicts that may exist within the family. The attention of the clinician in lending a sympathetic ear is therapeutic [28]. If the topic of concern will not be covered in the meeting, the clinician can at least validate it and provide reassurance that the issue will be addressed in the future.

Step 4–Give a Concise Medical Review in Clear Language: A clinician summary can add recent events or details that inform the decision at hand and, by repeating back elements of the patient/family summary, events are placed in context. It can be helpful to ask what level of information is preferred: "Some families like a lot of detail about the clinical side, while others want to focus on the big picture—do you know what you prefer?" With highly sensitive information, it can be helpful to get permission to talk about the topic before proceeding, and this allows patient or family to prepare for difficult news: "I'm afraid some of the news about his current condition is concerning. May I tell you about my concerns?" The clinician should avoid jargon and use slow, even speech with frequent pauses to confirm understanding. Many people do not feel comfortable interrupting a clinician to ask for clarification. If a medical term is introduced, inquire about the patient/family's understanding of the term. Patients and families may also need explanations related to the nature of care in the ICU and common procedures.

Step 5–Allow Silence and Respond to Emotion: Response to emotion is critical at every point in the interaction. Discomfort with strong emotions is common, and failing to respond appropriately to emotions early in the interaction will limit the patient and family's trust in the clinician. Dire news is often difficult to accept and the perception that the clinician does not care provides a tempting reason to discount clinical opinions. For the medical caregiver, years of training emphasizing the importance of clinical knowledge and detail can create a reflexive desire to present more medical information than is valuable. Moments of silence often are vital to allow patients and families to process information. Well-intended efforts to reiterate clinical information may fall on deaf ears and hinder efforts by the patient or family to express themselves. "I feel like I should pause here for a moment—this can be a lot to take in" gives permission for patient/family to express emotion or their inability to continue the conversation. Family members who have suddenly lost eye contact or physically withdraw (leaning back, looking away, bowing the head, or crossing arms) may be indicating the need to pause. Asking if a break is needed, leaning in, or—if culturally appropriate and natural to the clinician—reaching gently forward to touch the other person are subtle ways to offer support.

Techniques for responding to emotion are summarized in the mnemonic NURSE (Naming, Understanding, Respecting, Supporting, and Empathizing). In the concept of naming emotion, the clinician begins by taking a step back to identify what emotion is being expressed. It is important to notice that anger may actually be rooted in another feeling, such as fear or shame. Rather than making a declarative, somewhat presumptive statement such as "you seem angry," normalize the emotion by saying "sometimes people begin to feel angry after talking about something like this." The same subtlety is important with Understanding. "I understand how you feel" may sound presumptuous, but saying "I can only imagine what this must be like for you" shows that you understand the complexity of the situation while trying to imagine what the other is going through.

Sadness and grief are common emotions in goals of care discussions. Tears may be a common response to difficult news and, while it may be uncomfortable to sit quietly, it is often the best response. Expressions of anger, frustration, or contempt can be unpleasant to hear. It is important to listen without defensiveness for areas where something can be done to allay the cause of the anger. Resist the urge to either make pacifying statements or become angry yourself, exhibit non-threatening body language, and speak calmly to prevent anger from overwhelming the interaction.

Anger is often secondary to other emotions, namely fear and guilt; gently identifying the sources of these underlying emotions can help defuse the anger. Families may fear that care at home was not adequate, that "signs" were missed, and fear future guilt and blame if the patient does not survive. Emphasizing that clinicians share in the lack of control over irreversible illness reduces guilt and builds the team's partnership with family members to care for their loved one—especially if they cannot collectively "fix" the situation [29].

Supporting people through times of strong emotion requires empathy and non-abandonment. Showing sadness when giving

TABLE 34.2

Ten Steps to Better Prognostication

Concept	10 steps to better prognostication			Action steps
Foresee				
Science	Disease	1.	Start with an Anchor Point	• Obtain details of known survival stats by stage of disease, SEER web, etc.; speak with expert about 1-, 5-, 10-y survival stats
	Function	2.	Assess changes in performance status (amount, rate of change)	• Use a functional status tool, which is part of prognosis (e.g., PPS, KPS, ECOG) to assess illness trajectory
	Tests	3.	Known physical signs and laboratory markers related to prognosis	• E.g., ↑ WBC, ↓ %lymphocytes, ↓ albumin • E.g., Delirium, dyspnea, anorexia, weight loss, dysphagia
	Tools	4.	Utilize palliative or end-stage prognostic tools	• PPS, PaP, PPI, SHFM, COORT, CHESS, nomograms, etc.
Skill	Judgment	5.	Clinician Prediction of Survival. Would I be Surprised?	• Use your clinical judgment to formulate • See if it fits with the above prognostic factors and adjust accordingly • Remember common optimistic bias and adjust further
Foretell				
Art	Centre	6.	What is important to my patient? To the family?	• Who/what do they want to know/not know? • Is it "how long" or "what will happen"? • What are their goals; what is hoped for?
	Frame it	7.	Use probabilistic planning and discussion	• Ball-park range; average survival; most will live...; outliers; talk in time-blocks; etc.
	Cautions	8.	Share limitations of your prognosis	• No one knows for sure; exceptions do occur • Changes can occur at any time
	Changes	9.	Review and Reassess Periodically	• "What is" will change • Especially if trigger's arise
	Follow-up	10.	Stay connected	• Discuss advance care planning as things may change further at anytime • Initiate effective symptom control • Involve interprofessional and home team; furthermore, patients want their physician to remain involved, even close to death, and will feel abandoned otherwise

The following table illustrates several aspects in the formulation (foresee) and communication (foretell) of prognosis. In utilizing these steps, the clinician begins with the primary illness including its current stage and complications. It is known that functional status is a significant factor affecting survival in advanced or terminal illnesses. There are also some symptoms and tests that are incorporated into prognostic models as noted. Furthermore, although there is variance in clinicians' ability to predict survival, it remains valuable as one incorporates the prior information into the experience and judgment of the physician to arrive at a reasonable prognosis. How this is shared with the patient and family depends a lot on what their goals and hopes are as well as how much/little they want to know. Rather than giving a specific estimated time of survival, it is prudent to frame the discussion within a range of possible times and their probabilities, given the fact that no one knows for sure and a wide variation in what could happen for this individual. That is, prognostic tools provide a population-based set of statistics but which cannot readily reflect the illness trajectory of any one patient. Finally, one needs to review and reassess the patient from time to time to revise the prognosis, as it is a process, not a proclamation. Ultimately, "staying connected" throughout the final trajectory is in general what is most appreciated.

PPS, Palliative Performance Scale; KPS, Kamofsky Performance Scale; PaP, Palliative Prognostic Score; PPI, Palliative Performance Index; ECOG, Eastern Cooperative Oncology Group performance status; SEER, surveillance epidemiology and end results; SHFM, Seattle Heart Failure Model; CCORT, Canadian Cardiovascular Outcomes Research Team; CHESS, changes in end-stage symptoms and signs.

Downing M: *10 Steps to Better Prognostication.* Victoria, DC, Victoria Hospice Society, 2009.

bad news with statements of emotion ("I am worried that your body is not improving with treatment") helps the patient and family to absorb the nature of the news. Clinicians who remain upbeat when giving bad news leave families thinking that the news was "mixed" due to incongruence of message and messenger, while those who withdraw without emotional expression add confusion and feelings of abandonment.

Patients and families faced with dire circumstances may still express hope, which requires a sensitive response from clinicians. Immediately discounting an outcome for which patients express hope can damage trust, yet it is imprudent to offer false hope in the form of non-beneficial treatments. An effective approach can be to simultaneously "hope for the best and prepare for the worst," which allows the team to acknowledge the patient and family's hopes while setting the stage for end-of-life planning. Family meetings allow everyone involved in a patient's care to process strong emotions, grasp medical realities, and find hope in shared and realistic goals.

Step 6–Discuss Prognosis: Prognosis is extremely important for guiding care decisions, yet is often not discussed explicitly due to clinical uncertainty, assumptions about awareness, and inclination to avoid uncomfortable topics. Keys to prognostication include formulating prognosis on the basis of medical facts and specialist input as needed; inquiring how much detail the patient and family desire; giving a range of times and probabilities, while acknowledging uncertainty; reassessing prognosis periodically with the patient and family; and responding empathically to emotion. Table 34.2 outlines a useful framework for formulating and communicating prognosis.

"Prognosis" or "recovery" can mean very different things to different people; such terms should be qualified in order to avoid confusion. For example, a patient with end-stage dementia may a

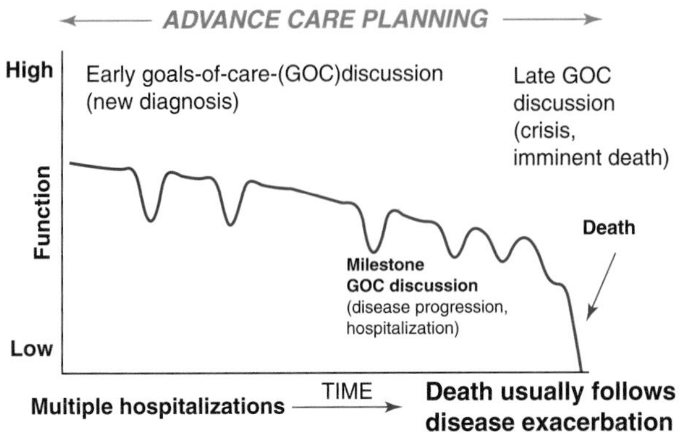

FIGURE 34.1 Trajectory of chronic illness with communication milestones.

good prognosis to survive to ICU discharge, while having a grim prognosis overall. Without qualifying statements, families may perceive being told conflicting information, halting their ability to make decisions and raising questions about the motives or competence of medical caregivers. It is important to understand that "prognosis" means more than survival to most people—that is, they hope to know if their loved one will be close to the same person they were prior to the recent illness. While uncertain, the team should estimate the likelihood of a patient's abilities to speak, walk, eat, recognize their families, etc., when discussing prognosis and treatment options with families.

Many patients with chronic critical illness have survived near-death experiences in the ICU; thus, family members may challenge the news of poor prognosis. In this situation, it can be helpful to reframe ("we're happy that your loved one has beaten the odds so far") and examine the "big picture" of the patient's illness trajectory (see Fig. 34.1). With compassionate and honest discussion of the illness trajectory, the team can "hope for the best and prepare for the worst" with the family as they face critical milestones of decision-making. The simultaneous acts of relationship-building and information-sharing build trust over time and allow the team to make medical recommendations to alleviate the burden of decision-making on grieving, stressed family members.

If a patient and family are aware of a grim prognosis but steadfastly choose to pursue aggressive treatment, simply reiterating the facts about prognosis may be unhelpful. Instead, compassionately exploring underlying factors such as family dynamics, cultural beliefs, and spiritual distress can be illuminating, and can lead the interdisciplinary team toward finding ways to partner with the family on a mutually acceptable outcome (see Tables 34.3 and 34.4).

Step 7–Explore Goals and Priorities: As discussed above, it is possible to express sincere hope for the patient to recover while also explaining the limitations and burdens of intensive care [30]. Understanding that surrogate's role as spokesperson for the patient's values and preferences (rather than "decider") not only ensures the appropriate ethical framework, but also reduces pressure on the surrogate. Questions such as "Given these circumstances, what would your loved one want to us focus on?"; "If he/she could hear the discussion and see our efforts, what concerns would be most important?"; or "What would he/she be hopeful for? What would be his/her greatest fear?" Because words like "recovery" and "improvement" are subjective, ask for clarification and explore the reasons behind preferences. This prevents miscommunication and also can prompt patients and families to more deeply explore feelings about illness and treatment. It may help to ask about the patient's approach to prior health or major life challenges. What core values were revealed? When has the patient been willing to make major changes in his or her life? If rapport and shared understanding exist, a clinician can not only present options, but make patient-centered recommendations.

Step 8–Present Broad Care Options: When the patient and family have fully understood the patient's current condition, existing treatments, and prognosis, it is possible to discuss broad options for care. Best, worst, and "most-likely" case scenarios may be discussed. Discussing specific care options without context can lead to contradictory, poorly designed care plans.

On the basis of the articulated values and the clinical condition of the patient, the care team may offer goals such as a trial of treatment to promote recovery to baseline function, improving quality of life, surviving to witness a significant family event, improving comfort, or creating a more peaceful environment for patient's death. Using techniques described in earlier steps, the clinical team can draw out patient/family perspective and respond to emotion during this process, in hope of prioritizing goals. Reassurance of the team's commitment to attend to the patient's comfort and dignity should be emphasized regardless of other goals.

Goals such as "hoping for a miracle" and "doing everything possible" should be further explored, examining the role of healthcare and the level of quality and quantity of life that is acceptable to the patient. Because feelings of guilt are common, it is helpful to emphasize that we only "choose" where to focus our efforts, we do not "choose" for a patient to die. While decision-making is shared, medical care in the ICU is ultimately the responsibility of the medical team.

Step 9–Translate Goals into a Care Plan: After reaching a shared understanding of clinical condition, prognosis, and patient-centered goals, the medical team makes recommendations for a care plan. Patients/families who have expressed desire for detail appreciate thorough descriptions of recommendations, while others prefer to feel that care is exclusively under the control of the medical team. Plan for management of physical, emotional, social, and spiritual needs of the patient and family. Rather than listing measures to be withdrawn or withheld, first emphasize the care that will be provided. Framing the withholding of a treatment as a means of protecting the patient from trauma emphasizes that the goal is not to "give up" but to honor the patient's condition and values.

Some patients or families request aggressive treatment in spite of a poor prognosis. If the patient/family will not follow medical advice, suggest planning for the most likely outcome (e.g., prolonged life support). Emphasize the resulting reduced ability to communicate preferences and that the treatment ultimately cannot prevent death. If there are repeated requests for non-beneficial care, the team should consider consulting palliative care and ethics for assistance (see Tables 34.3 and 34.4 on Managing Conflict and Case Example).

Concluding the interaction with a review of the next steps in care can help participants recall important points. Next steps should include plans to address any areas of uncertainty or conflict. Statements such as "we will always care for your loved one, no matter what happens" provide reassurance of the ICU team's treatment of the individual, not the disease [31]. Affirming the decisions of the family or patient and offering anticipatory guidance can address likely future scenarios [32]. Closing the discussion with a follow-up plan and ways to contact the care team reassures the family of ongoing support.

Step 10–Document and Debrief: Clinician documentation ensures patient safety and quality of care. A carefully crafted progress note, documenting not only time spent but the level of preparation, the participants, the role of the patient (i.e., patient capacity or desire to participate), the context of options discussed, broad goals, and next steps can provide vital information for members of the medical team. Good documentation protects the patient and family from "starting anew" with each caregiver. Documentation provides a medical/legal record of the quality of the care provided. In addition to the patient

TABLE 34.3

Principles of Managing Conflict [78,79]

Principle	Action steps
Convey professionalism and commitment to care of the patient in all interactions	Review facts and rule out misunderstanding as a source of conflict
Where might the team be wrong? Explore alternative views and perspectives	Take corrective action when appropriate
	Ensure that team members are using the same language; formalize processes for communication to prevent cross-talk
	Resist labeling—remain open to seeing the situation in a new way
Optimally address areas of uncertainty	Consider further input on clinical aspects from treating clinicians, second opinion, palliative care specialist, prognosis committee
	Identify additional sources of information about patient goals and values
	Review surrogate's understanding of his or her role; ensure all participants are focused on patient's values and interests
	Consider whether a patient may regain capacity—capacity and desire for participation may change
	Seek expert guidance for unfamiliar cultural, religious, legal, or psychosocial influence on conflict and educate staff
	Seek bioethics committee input on ethical questions
Offer a family meeting (see Fig. 34.1)	Perceived role of patient, illness, treatment, caregivers, family
	Future wants, needs, and fears of patient, family, and caregivers
	Spiritual, cultural, psychosocial, and cognitive influences
	Emotional responses
	Values and perceptions underlying positions, willingness to reframe meaning of past events and future options
Bridge differences in perception between patient/family and medical team	Praise efforts to work together and to put patient interests first
	Include family in hands-on care of the patient, increase transparency
	Provide care team with relevant details of patient/family perspective, education about unique cultural, spiritual, or psychosocial factors
	Encourage "I" statements to avoid laying blame; seek to understand why people feel and think what they do
Identify areas of persistent conflict	Name the conflict with a neutral statement, focusing on the issue and not on the participants
	Identify mutual concerns
	Include patient/family in brainstorming possible solutions that address mutual concerns
	Suggest strategies to minimize harm to the patient even if conflict cannot be resolved
	When possible, offer a follow-up meeting to allow emotions to subside and time for careful reflection
	If prognosis is in question, offer a trial of treatment [80]
	Consider whether another provider may be better aligned with patient/family wishes if there is direct conflict with your professional judgment
	Consider whether appointment of a guardian would be appropriate if family unit is being severely damaged by decision-making responsibility

medical record, the outcome of a family meeting—even if the outcome is a lack of consensus—ideally is discussed during a team meeting or hand-off with relevant health professionals. Caregivers may experience moral distress if the role of the care that they provide is not placed in context. Discussion among providers following a family meeting can also help staff to process the emotions of the event and to recognize opportunities for improvement.

Bioethical Principles

The ultimate irony of American health care: the growth of limitless technology coupled with resources that are limited [33].

The ever-evolving technologies available in the ICU allows medical teams to save and maintain lives in circumstances that would have been unthinkable years ago. These new technologies are exciting and hopeful, but often raise complex ethical issues. Decisions about when to use medical technology and resources can create moral dilemmas for clinicians as well as for patients and their families. These ethical debates can dramatically enter the public arena; for example, Americans witnessed intractable conflict within the family of Terri Schiavo regarding her prognosis and decisions about artificial nutrition, as well as the legal and political battles surrounding her case [34].

The American Medical Association first published a code of ethics in 1847. It wasn't until the mid-1900s that the concepts of autonomy and self-determination entered the discussion of medical ethics, stemming from historical disregard for patient rights and frank abuse of vulnerable populations, including discrimination of minorities and women, involuntary human experimentation during World War II under the Nazi regime, and the Tuskegee experiments [35].

The Patient Self-Determination Act, passed by the U.S. Congress in 1990, mandated patient autonomy as a guiding principle of medical decision-making. This law requires health care institutions to ask patients whether they have an advance directive. The institution must also record patient preferences

TABLE 34.4

Case—Managing Conflict

A 73-year-old Korean woman with metastatic gastric cancer is transferred to the ICU for management of sepsis. The hospitalist caring for the patient over the last week reports that the patient's son has "taken over" and has not been listening to staff attempts to discuss patient's poor prognosis. The physician feels the patient is dying and recommended against ICU transfer, but acquiesced to the son's wish. The patient requires pressor support and has multiple possible sources for infection. She is grossly edematous, with pressure ulcers and bruises from multiple needle sticks. She is pancytopenic as a result of recent chemotherapy, prolonged illness, and nutritional deficits. ICU caregivers report the patient is in pain. Although she speaks limited English, the patient tells staff at times that she wants to die. Her son, who continues to work full time, is listed as the primary contact in the medical record, and the patient and her husband defer all decision-making to their son. When the son visits with his pastor, he responds to information about her poor prognosis by suggesting the only option is to "pray for a miracle." The son insists that the patient's oncologist has said that his mother's cancer is "treatable." Nurses and other staff caring for the patient are feeling angry and uncomfortable about her care and interpret the son's behavior at the bedside as "cold" and "micromanaging."

Next steps and strategies:

1) ICU team huddle to clarify medical facts (including a conversation with the patient's oncologist); acknowledge staff emotion and distress; consult with social worker, chaplain, and medical interpreters who have worked with the patient and family to share insights on family dynamics and spiritual and culture issues.
2) Schedule a family meeting for a mutually convenient time. Negotiate who should be present (patient, her husband, son, pastor, medical interpreter, ICU team) and what to discuss ("we want to review her situation and figure out the best way to care for her going forward"). Use structured approach from Figure 34.1 to assess their understanding; respond to emotion; share difficult news about prognosis; explore hopes, fears, and goals; and create a plan on the basis of shared decision-making.
3) Offer spiritual and emotional support, and invite the patient's pastor to pray (including at the start or the end of family meetings). Ask the patient and family to teach the ICU team about their culture and faith traditions and how they may affect their coping and decision-making.
4) Allow time for the patient and family to absorb information and process emotion, and encourage them to spend meaningful time together as a family. If necessary, agree on a time-limited trial of interventions with specific goals (i.e., IV antibiotics for 5 days, with the goal of resolving the need for vasopressor support).

Outcome:

First meeting: At first, the patient's son appeared angry and suspicious and asked to meet with the ICU team outside his mother's room. He admitted to feeling overwhelmed by his mother's illness, as well as his own family and work responsibilities. As an only child, and as the most proficient English-speaker in his family, he felt protective of his elderly parents. They find hope and solace in their faith and lean on their pastor for guidance. The son worries what will become of his father, who faces his own health problems, after his mother dies someday. The son listens to the physician's assessment and news of poor prognosis, but says he still hopes for a miracle. The group negotiates to meet the next day at the patient's bedside, with the husband and pastor present to continue the discussion.

Second meeting: The pastor is invited to pray, which is comforting for the patient and family. The ICU team follows the same structured approach (Fig. 34.1), but this time assessing the patient and husband's understanding, and her goals and priorities. The patient acknowledges in front of her son that she is dying, and her faith in God supports her. The son says he doesn't want her to suffer, but can't believe "there isn't anything else to treat her cancer," despite the team's discussion with her primary oncologist who confirms this.

Third meeting: The ICU team arranges for the oncologist to call the son directly on the phone, and instead he is able to visit the patient and family the next day. The ICU team and oncologist express their caring and concern and reiterate that she is dying from progressive, incurable cancer. They stress how they will work to ensure excellent end-of-life care, introduce the concept of hospice, and give the family time to think. A few hours later, the son asks the team to arrange hospice care at his home and requests help in obtaining a family medical leave from work. The patient's oncologist remains as her attending physician under hospice care, and she is discharged the next day after equipment and medications are in place at the son's home.

in, and offer processes for completing advance directives if they have not yet been done [35]. There is controversy about whether this law is effective as advance directives do not address multiple specific medical situations and are difficult to use when prognosis is not clear.

The two types of advance directives are (1) "instructional directives," which provide guidance for caregivers, health care agents and representatives when making health care decisions for patients by way of substituted judgment and (2) "proxy directives", which name a patient's health care agent. Examples of instructional directives include living wills and the Five Wishes document. Proxy directive examples include health care durable power of attorney [35].

While autonomy is a cornerstone of medical decision-making, it is not the only ethical principle guiding complex care decisions in the ICU. Other bioethical principles include beneficence, nonmaleficence, and justice (see Table 34.5 for definitions and examples). These principles can help inform discussions among patients, families and the ICU team within the context of culture, faith, personal values and family dynamics. The Fifth International Consensus Conference in Critical Care issued a consensus statement on ethical principles in the ICU, and emphasized a patient-centered approach with the ultimate goal of acting within patients' best interests [36]. Ideally, this is accomplished through shared decision-making among the patient and family (who are experts in the patient's values and goals) and the ICU team (who are the medical experts on prognostication and viable therapeutic options).

Distributive justice is a core ethical principle, but is difficult and controversial to navigate at the bedside. While discussions about inappropriate use of resources and disproportionate care

TABLE 34.5

Bioethical Principles in the ICU

Ethical principle	Definition	ICU example
Autonomy	Respecting a person's right to determine a course of action/patient's right to make their own decisions regarding their health care	A patient chooses to forgo life-sustaining therapy despite the fact he will most certainly die without it but might recover with it (e.g., no mechanical ventilation for community-acquired pneumonia).
Beneficence	Desiring to benefit the patient	A clinician prescribes intravenous pain medication to control severe pain.
Nonmaleficence	Avoidance of harm	The team discontinues paralytics in patients undergoing terminal extubation.
Distributive Justice	Equal and fair distribution of resources	ICU care is costly and may significantly prolong the dying process in patients with irreversible conditions, which diverts resources from other patients.

occur in the ICU [37], the principle of justice should be utilized in policy decisions on the care of all patients in order to minimize partiality and bias. Some hospitals have already determined or are beginning to discuss how to allocate resources in the event of a natural disaster (e.g., Hurricane Katrina) or terrorist attack.

Decision-making Capacity and Substituted Judgment

In order to exercise autonomy, patients must have the capacity to make informed, reasoned medical decisions based on their values. Their capacity can be impaired by multiple factors, including acute illness, multiple medications, and chronic conditions [38]. Critically ill patients also suffer from varying degrees of hypoxia, hypotension, multi-organ dysfunction, and sepsis. Studies show that patients with compromised capacity to make medical decisions have an increased risk of mortality as well as increased cost of care [38]. In a review of 25 national studies using an array of assessment tools, the prevalence of incapacity among critically ill patients was significant: physicians missed 58% of patients who lacked decision-making capacity [39]. Physicians practicing critical care medicine need to understand how to assess a patient's capacity for medical decision-making. Although most physicians lack any formal training, a structured framework for assessing capacity can help guide a skilled evaluation at the bedside (see Table 34.6) [40].

Any physician—not necessarily a psychiatrist—can make a determination of a patient's decision-making capacity. Initially, capacity should be assessed when patients refuse a recommended procedure or treatment. If patients are amenable to proposed therapies, they are much less likely to have their capacity challenged. In situations where the benefits of an intervention outweigh the risks, a patient must meet a higher threshold for capacity in order to refuse the proposed procedure. If a patient is refusing a high-risk, low-benefit procedure, the threshold for capacity is lower [41].

The term "capacity" differs from competence. Only a judge can declare someone incompetent and legal standards for competence vary by state. A person deemed incompetent has more "general limitations" on his or her rights [41]. By comparison, capacity is both temporal and situational [39]. Capacity may vary, depending on the current medical condition of the patient. A patient may have capacity for simple, straightforward choices but not for complex decisions. In addition, cognitive impairment does not automatically imply a lack of capacity for all medical decisions. Assessment of capacity is warranted when patients have changes in their baseline mental status, are refusing recommended treatments, or have underlying conditions putting them at risk for impaired decision-making [42].

Of note, the dynamic and complex nature of the ICU also poses an increased risk of "pseudo-incapacity," which occurs when patients do not understand their situation due to poor communication, such as excessive use of medical jargon, primary language barriers and/or low health literacy. Decision-making capacity can be enhanced by treating underlying medical conditions, ensuring clear communication in the patient's primary language and educational level, and inviting a trusted confidant to help the patient cope with fear and anxiety when trying to process information.

Once a determination is made, it is important to document the assessment, including the use of any standardized evaluation tools. If a patient lacks capacity, the physician should invoke the patient's designated health care proxy. The proxy should use "substituted judgment" to make decisions on behalf of the patient, based on the patient's values and previously stated preferences. However, if a patient's preferences are unknown, the surrogate should work with the ICU team to understand the medical situation and act in the patient's best interests [43]. If the patient does not have a health care proxy, most states have established a hierarchy to determine a surrogate decision-maker; in general, the priority is the spouse, followed by adult children, parents, siblings and other relatives. If no surrogate decision-maker is available, the patient will require a court-appointed legal guardian for medical decision-making based on substituted judgment or, if substituted judgment is unknown, based on the best interests of the patient.

Withholding and Withdrawing Therapies

The decision to limit life-sustaining therapies (LST) prior to death in the ICU is difficult and complex. It is also a common practice, occurring in 74% to 90% of ICU deaths [44]. These decisions are influenced by many factors, including extent and severity of illness, prognosis, expected quality of life, perceived level of patient's suffering, prior health care experience, resource availability, family dynamics, and cultural and socioeconomic backgrounds [45].

From a bioethical perspective, there is no difference between withholding versus withdrawing a treatment. Patients, or their surrogate decision-makers, have the right to refuse treatments such as life support, cardiopulmonary resuscitation, and artificial nutrition/hydration before or after they have been started [46]. However, ICU clinicians report in surveys that withholding and withdrawing therapies "feel" different. This discomfort may arise from the perception that withholding a therapy is passive (by not interfering with a natural dying process), while withdrawing a therapy is active (by altering a course of

TABLE 34.6

Legally Relevant Criteria for Decision-Making Capacity and Approaches to Assessment of the Patient

Criterion	Patient's task	Physician's assessment approach	Questions for clinical assessment[a]	Comments
Communicate a choice	Clearly indicate preferred treatment option	Ask patient to indicate a treatment choice	Have you decided whether to follow your doctor's (or my) recommendation for treatment? Can you tell me what that decision is? (If no decision) What is making it hard for you to decide?	Frequent reversals of choice because of psychiatric or neurologic conditions may indicate lack of capacity.
Understand the relevant information	Grasp the fundamental meaning of information communicated by physician	Encourage patient to paraphrase disclosed information regarding medical condition and treatment	Please tell me in your own words what your doctor (or I) told you about: The problem with your health now The recommended treatment The possible benefits and risks (or discomforts) of the treatment Any alternative treatments and their risks and benefits The risks and benefits of no treatment	Information to be understood includes nature of patient's condition, nature and purpose of proposed treatment, possible benefits and risks of that treatment, and alternative approaches (including no treatment) and their benefits and risks
Appreciate the situation and its consequences	Acknowledge medical condition and likely consequences of treatment options	Ask patient to describe views of medical condition, proposed treatment, and likely outcomes	What do you believe is wrong with your health now? Do you believe that you need some kind of treatment? What is treatment likely to do for you? What makes you believe it will have that effect? What do you believe will happen if you are not treated? Why do you think your doctor has (or I have) recommended this treatment?	Courts have recognized that patients who do not acknowledge their illnesses (often referred to as "lack of insight") cannot make valid decisions about treatment. Delusions or pathologic levels of distortion or denial are the most common causes of impairment.
Reason about treatment options	Engage in a rational process of manipulating the relevant information	Ask patient to compare treatment options and consequences and to offer reasons for selection of option	How did you decide to accept or reject the recommended treatment? What makes (chosen option) better than (alternative option)?	This criterion focuses on the process by which a decision is reached, not the outcome of the patient's choice, since patients have the right to make "unreasonable" choices.

[a]Questions are adapted from Grisso and Appelbaum [31]. Patients' responses to these questions need not be verbal.

potentially life-prolonging treatment) [46]. These perceptions can provoke feelings of anxiety and moral distress. As a result, it is paramount that ICU clinicians gain knowledge and expertise in addressing patient, family, and ICU team distress over these bioethical decisions.

After skilled discussions about prognosis and goals of care, clinicians and family caregivers may decide to proceed with an acute withdrawal of LST for an imminently dying patient. In other cases, seriously ill patients may be gradually weaned from intensive care—sometimes referred to as "no escalation of care" [44,47]. Under this paradigm, the decision to continue or discontinue specific treatments is determined on an individual basis by the ICU team and the patient's decision makers. Based on a few observational studies, the "Do Not Resuscitate" (DNR) order is often the first step in limiting LST, preceding death by 1 to 2 days. Additional interventions including dialysis, vasopressors, laboratory and diagnostic studies, blood transfusions and antibiotics are also likely to be discontinued.

In contrast, artificial nutrition and hydration are initiated in some cases despite "no escalation of care," probably reflecting cultural beliefs by families or physicians that these therapies are more palliative than life-sustaining [44]. Decisions to withdraw this care can be controversial, and many families and caregivers view it as nurturing and vital for a dying patient. Families should be counseled on physiological changes during the dying process, including the loss of appetite and thirst, and the unintended consequences of fluid overload, including anasarca, pulmonary edema, ascites, secretions and incontinence with skin breakdown. In addition, there may be analgesic and anesthetic effects of dehydration, mediated by ketones and endogenous opioids [48]. It is important to reassure families that their loved ones are dying from their underlying disease and not from "starvation." As appropriate, families should be offered the opportunity to participate in other expressions of caregiving, such as providing mouth care, bed baths and hand or foot massages.

Mechanical ventilation is usually one of the last life-sustaining treatments to be withdrawn, and occurs among only half of the ventilated patients who die in the ICU. Factors influencing the decision to withdraw mechanical ventilation include physician prediction of a <10% likelihood of survival, physician prediction of severely impaired future cognitive function, and the physician's perception that the patient did not want life support [49,50].

It is important to emphasize that time to death after withdrawal of mechanical ventilation varies widely, and that some patients have survived to hospital discharge [49]. In one study, half of patients died within 1 hour, the majority died within 10 hours, and some patients survived 7 days until death [50].

There is no evidence supporting a specific approach to the withdrawal of mechanical ventilation, but clinicians should consider a patient's level of consciousness when managing symptoms [46]. It is important for families to know that brain-dead patients can exhibit dramatic movements (the "Lazarus sign") caused by the firing of spinal motor neurons in response to acute hypoxia. For patients who are comatose and unable to experience distress, clinicians can rapidly remove airway and ventilator support. If there is any concern that a patient may feel pain or anxiety, clinicians can pre-medicate the patient with analgesics and sedatives.

Patients who are conscious or semiconscious are more likely to experience distress during ventilation withdrawal. In these cases, a gradual decrease of supplemental oxygen may have an analgesic effect by creating hypoxia with normal carbon dioxide levels, followed by decreasing the ventilation rate [51]. During this "terminal weaning", the FiO_2 is reduced to room air and positive end-expiratory pressure is reduced to zero followed by assessment of patient comfort. Ventilator support is then reduced from baseline to zero, taking rarely more than 5 to 20 minutes [52]. There are limited data available to determine whether removing the artificial airway provides more patient comfort, but families are more satisfied if extubation occurs [47].

Another set of LST modalities include left ventricular assist devices and total artificial hearts (referred to as mechanical circulatory support [MCS]). The decision to deactivate these devices is controversial because deactivation can be a life-ending intervention. Recent guidelines state that discontinuation of MCS is equivalent to allowing a natural death when there is onset of irreversible medical problems. Examples include irreversible coma, circulatory shock, overwhelming infections, multi-organ failure, refractory hypoxia or catastrophic device failure. Under these circumstances, deactivation of the MCS is made in collaboration with the patient, family, ICU team, and the MCS team [53].

During and following withdrawal of LST, clinicians should be present to evaluate for signs and symptoms of distress that may require palliative interventions. The bedside clinicians should be capable of anticipating and addressing the needs of the patient and family [48]. Therapies should focus on comfort and symptom management, including antipyretics, anti-emetics, anti-epileptics, analgesics, sedatives, and/or anticholinergics to control secretions. If a patient has an automatic implantable cardiac defibrillator, it should be deactivated in order to prevent firing during the dying process. The benefits and burdens of routine ICU care (e.g., monitoring devices, wound debridement, and endotracheal suctioning) should be discussed and subsequently continued, limited, or eliminated as appropriate [48].

In order to foster a private and caring environment, the ICU team should remove visiting hour restrictions, remove patient restraints, lower the bedrails, and remove machines and monitors from the room as appropriate. Families also want to be assured of their loved one's comfort and have the opportunity to express emotions, stories, prayers and rituals.

The use of a standardized order set for the withdrawal of LST has been studied [54]. The order form includes four sections: (1) preparation for withdrawal of life support that included documentation for a family conference, discontinuation of labs, radiographs and prior medications, and completion of a DNR order; (2) a nurse-driven sedation and analgesia protocol; (3) protocol for withdrawing mechanical ventilation that focused on patient comfort; and (4) a set of principles to guide withdrawal of LST. The majority of physicians and nurses reported that the order form was helpful and that it resulted in an increased use of opioids and benzodiazepines for symptom management. Importantly, the intervention was not associated with any change in time from ventilator withdrawal to death, suggesting that the increased use of these medications did not hasten death.

Medical Futility

Advances in medicine have enabled critical care specialists to save lives. However, intensive care interventions can also prolong the dying process or, more often, sustain life under circumstances that would not be acceptable to the patient. Some of the most ethically challenging situations for ICU clinicians involve requests by patients and families for "futile" medical interventions.

Unfortunately, these conflicts are common. A study of ICUs in the United States revealed that roughly 20% of patients received at least 1 day of treatment that physicians defined as futile [55]. In a single-day, cross-sectional study performed in Europe, 27% of ICU clinicians believed they provided "inappropriate" (defined as excessive) care to at least one patient [56].

In the early 1990s, bioethicists and professional societies attempted to define the term "medical futility" and how to manage it [57–61]. Conceptually, futile care was divided into three categories: quantitative, qualitative, and physiological [62]. Quantitative futility occurs when the likelihood of an intervention benefiting a patient is exceedingly poor (i.e., $<1\%$ chance of success) [60,63]. Qualitative futility occurs when the benefit to quality of life produced by an intervention is exceedingly poor. Treatment that preserves permanent unconsciousness or dependence on intensive medical care may be considered qualitatively futile. Finally, physiological futility describes treatments that cannot attain physiologic goals [59]. For example, providing a fourth vasopressor for a patient in refractory shock will not achieve an improved blood pressure and thus would be considered physiologically futile.

Although futility policies have been developed across the United States, critics have argued that futility determinations are inherently value-laden [59,64]. There has been no clear consensus on the definition of futility due to the difficulty in establishing what defines "meaningful survival [65]." Recently, a multi-society statement recommended the term "potentially inappropriate" in describing treatments with only a small chance of benefit that are not justified on the basis clinician judgment and competing ethical considerations. The term "futile" should be used only in the rare circumstances in which an intervention simply cannot achieve the intended physiologic goal [58].

Recent qualitative research examined why ICU clinicians may provide inappropriate care. In one survey, physicians were uncomfortable with death, viewed death as avoidable and sought to delay it, or perceived a patient's death as a personal failure [66]. Other determinants included family demands, lack of timely or skilled communication, lack of consensus among the treatment team [66,67], cultural beliefs [68], legal pressures, and lack of prognostic certainty [66]. Inappropriate care has been associated with admission delays from the emergency department, delays in transfer of ICU patients from outside hospitals, and cancelation of patient transfers from other hospitals [69]. One study estimated the cost of inappropriate care as $2.6 million over a three-month period [55].

There is also the possibility that certain inappropriate medical interventions might pose risks to other patients [70]. For example, providing antibiotics to a patient who will not benefit may lead to increased risk for antibiotic-resistant organisms in other patients. In the era of pay-for-value, providing ventilator support to a patient who will not benefit increases the risk of ventilator-associated pneumonia. This "never event" might earn the hospital a reputation as a place with high infection rates, causing payers to withhold reimbursements, and limiting the hospital's resources to treat other patients [70].

Role of the Ethics Committee

The American Medical Association strongly recommends ethics committee consultations in situations where there is conflict over goals of care and end-of-life issues [71]. Often the disagreements between parties in these situations arise from differing morals and values. The central questions underlying these disputes often include:

- whether to pursue aggressive life-sustaining treatment in a seriously ill patient;
- whether to accede to family demands to provide life-sustaining treatment;
- how to deal with competing family members and companions wanting to make critical decisions on behalf of the patient; and
- what to do for a seriously ill, incapacitated patient who has no surrogate decision maker or advance directive [36].

Hospital ethics committees do not have a mandated composition and structure. Typically, the membership may include physicians, nurses, hospital administrators, social workers, allied health professionals, chaplains, lay community members, residents and medical students, hospital legal counsel and at times a bioethicist [72]. It has been recommended that the make-up of the committee reflect "the diversity of cultures, socioeconomic status and public opinion that exist in the community served by the institution [73]." Clinical ethicists "act as facilitators of communication and decision making about the goals for care, while directing attention to the ethical considerations underlying such decisions [74]." The American Society for Bioethics recommended core competencies for members of ethics committees in their report, "Core Competencies for Health Care Ethics Consultation [36]." It is important for all members of the committee to have some training and education in the field of bioethics. In reality, however, approximately 40% of those who perform ethics consultations in the U.S. have had no formal training, and only about 5% have had any graduate training in bioethics [75]. In fact, the vast majority of those who actually perform the consultations are clinicians rather than those lecturing and publishing about ethics in the academic world.

The primary role of ethics committees is offering critiques and suggestions for policy development and review. In this area, ethics committees can review policies and procedures related to end-of-life care, resource allocation, brain-death determination, advance directives, DNR policies, or anything else relating to patients' rights [72,73]. Final approval of hospital policy rests with the hospital administration in most cases, and the process of review is ongoing. As technology evolves and the health care system changes, there will be a continued need to update policies to help guide staffs and institutions.

Second, ethics committee members must not only address their own training but also educate other health care professionals and the lay community. This stakeholder education can take place in many forums: hospital grand rounds, ethics symposia, and lectures to students and staff [73].

The third most common function of ethics committees is clinical consultation. This has been defined as "a service provided by a committee, team, or individual to address the ethical issues involved in a specific, active clinical case [75]." The exact process varies by institution but primarily involves reviewing ethical dilemmas in patient care. Typically, there are three consultation models: full ethics committee evaluations, small-team models, or individual consultant models. Of these, research has shown that the most common model used in the U.S. is the small-team model [75]. In one large study of more than 500 U.S. hospital ethics committees, the committees recommended a "single best course of action for 46% of cases, described a range of acceptable actions for 41% of cases, and made no recommendation for 13% of cases [75]."

At most institutions, anyone, including patients and families, can request a consult—submitted anonymously, if desired. Unfortunately, there are limited available data on the effects and benefits of ethics consultations. One randomized controlled trial showed that ethics consultations in the ICU decreased length of stay and time spent in the ICU for patients who did not survive to discharge [36]. For patients who survived to discharge, there was no difference in ICU days or overall length of stay. In addition, the study found that an ethics consultation was associated with cost savings of $3,000 to $40,000 per patient, the bulk of which resulted from the care of patients remaining in the hospital for 10 days or longer after the consultation [36].

The decision to consult ethics versus palliative medicine can be framed in several different ways. Ethics consultation is often requested when there are questions or conflict related to values in order to help identify morally acceptable options. Palliative medicine consultants assist patients and families in synthesizing complex medical information, understanding prognosis, eliciting their priorities and goals, and facilitating shared decision-making. The American College of Critical Care Medicine recommends the availability of both ethics and palliative medicine consultations to improve end-of-life communication in the ICU [71]. Ethics consultants are often thought of as "outsiders" and viewed as a neutral party. The palliative care consultant serves the interest of the referring physician as well as the patient's interests and may be thought of as "clinical insiders," bringing a clinically oriented opinion to a particular case [76]. Both of these positions can be advantageous at different times depending on the situation and the emotions involved. As with any specialty consultation service, the culture of an institution, available resources and historical framework help in deciding which specific consultation may be most appropriate.

Treatment of Last Resort—Palliative Sedation

Palliative sedation (PS) is the intentional lowering of awareness towards, and including, unconsciousness for patients with severe and refractory symptoms, as defined by the American Academy of Hospice and Palliative Medicine (AAHPM). The following summary of the AAHPM's position statement [77] describes this procedure and its ethical implications:

PS is reserved for extreme situations, and should only be used after all available options have been exhausted to treat refractory symptoms. As with any procedure, PS must have a specific indication, a target outcome, and a benefit/risk ratio that is acceptable to the medical team, patient and family. The level of sedation should be proportionate to the patient's level of distress. Treatment of other symptoms must also be continued, since sedation may decrease the patient's ability to communicate or display discomfort.

Palliative sedation raises ethical concerns when it significantly reduces patient consciousness to the degree that the patient is unable to substantially interact with others, does not have the ability or opportunity to change his mind, and is unable to eat and drink (thus potentially shortening survival in particular circumstances). Palliative sedation is ethically defensible when used (1) after careful interdisciplinary evaluation and treatment of the patient, and (2) when palliative treatments that are not intended to affect consciousness have failed or, in the judgment of the clinician, are very likely to fail, (3) where its use is not expected to shorten the patient's time to death, and (4) only for the actual or expected duration of symptoms. Palliative sedation should not be considered irreversible in all circumstances. It may be appropriate, in some clinical situations when symptoms are deemed temporary, to decrease sedation after a predetermined time to assess efficacy, continued symptoms and need for ongoing sedation.

In clinical practice, palliative sedation usually does not alter the timing or mechanism of a patient's death, as refractory symptoms are most often associated with very advanced terminal illness. Practitioners who use palliative sedation should be clear in their intent to palliate symptoms and to not shorten survival. Because patients receiving palliative sedation are typically close to death, most patients will no longer have desire to eat or drink. Artificial nutrition and hydration are not generally expected to benefit the patient receiving palliative sedation, however questions about the use of artificial nutrition and hydration should be addressed before palliative sedation is undertaken.

There is no clear consensus or scientific evidence regarding the most appropriate medication(s) to effect palliative sedation. As elsewhere in medicine, the agent should be selected based on safety, efficacy, and availability [77].

Of note, opioids do not reliably achieve sedation. Palliative care clinicians often use benzodiazepines, sedating antipsychotics, barbiturates or propofol for palliative sedation, depending on the patient's co-morbid symptoms and clinical response [77].

References

1. Sharma RK, Dy SM: Cross-cultural communication and use of the family meeting in palliative care. *Am J Hosp Palliat Care* 28(6):437–444, 2011.
2. Haas LJ, Leiser JP, Magill MK, et al: Management of the difficult patient. *Am Fam Physician* 72(10):2063–2068, 2005.
3. King DA, Quill T: Working with families in palliative care: one size does not fit all. *J Palliat Med* 9(3):704–715, 2006.
4. Phelps AC, Maciejewski PK, Nilsson M, et al: Religious coping and use of intensive life-prolonging care near death in patients with advanced cancer. *JAMA* 301(11):1140–1147, 2009.
5. Hickson GB, Clayton EW, Githens PB, et al: Factors that prompted families to file medical malpractice claims following perinatal injuries. *JAMA* 267(10):1359–1363, 1992.
6. Levinson W: Doctor-patient communication and medical malpractice: implications for pediatricians. *Pediatr Ann* 26(3):186–193, 1997.
7. Denham CR, Dingman J, Foley ME, et al: Are you listening...are you really listening? *J Patient Saf* 4(3):148–161, 2008.
8. Curtis JR, White DB: Practical guidance for evidence-based ICU family conferences. *Chest* 134(4):835–843, 2008.
9. Powazki R, Walsh D, Hauser K, et al: Communication in palliative medicine: a clinical review of family conferences. *J Palliat Med* 17(10):1167–1177, 2014.
10. Lautrette A, Darmon M, Megarbane B, et al: A communication strategy and brochure for relatives of patients dying in the ICU. *N Engl J Med* 356(5):469–478, 2007.
11. Scheunemann LP, McDevitt M, Carson SS, et al: Randomized, controlled trials of interventions to improve communication in intensive care: a systematic review. *Chest* 139(3):543–554, 2011.
12. Lamba S, Murphy P, McVicker S, et al: Changing end-of-life care practice for liver transplant service patients: structured palliative care intervention in the surgical intensive care unit. *J Pain Symptom Manage* 44(4):508–519, 2012.
13. Weissman DE, Meier DE: Identifying patients in need of a palliative care assessment in the hospital setting: a consensus report from the Center to Advance Palliative Care. *J Palliat Med* 14(1):17–23, 2011.
14. Bernacki RE, Block SD: Communication about serious illness care goals: a review and synthesis of best practices. *JAMA Intern Med* 174(12):1994–2003, 2014.
15. Levin TT, Moreno B, Silvester W, et al: End-of-life communication in the intensive care unit. *Gen Hosp Psychiatry* 32(4):433–442, 2010.
16. Meyer EC, Sellers DE, Browning DM, et al: Difficult conversations: improving communication skills and relational abilities in health care. *Pediatr Crit Care Med* 10(3):352–359, 2009.
17. VitalTalk. www.vitaltalk.org. Accessed May 2, 2016.
18. Lamba S, Nagurka R, Offin M, et al: Structured communication: teaching delivery of difficult news with simulated resuscitations in an emergency medicine clerkship. *West J Emerg Med* 16(2):344–352, 2015.
19. Lamba S, Tyrie LS, Bryczkowski S, et al: Teaching surgery residents the skills to communicate difficult news to patient and family members: a literature review. *J Palliat Med* 19(1):101–107, 2016.
20. Billings JA, Keeley A, Bauman J, et al: Merging cultures: palliative care specialists in the medical intensive care unit. *Crit Care Med* 34(11 Suppl):S388–S393, 2006.
21. Nelson JE, Walker AS, Luhrs CA, et al: Family meetings made simpler: a toolkit for the intensive care unit. *J Crit Care* 24(4):626.e7–626.e14, 2009.
22. Levinson W, Kao A, Kuby A, et al: Not all patients want to participate in decision making. A national study of public preferences. *J Gen Intern Med* 20(6):531–535, 2005.
23. Hallenbeck J, Arnold R: A request for nondisclosure: don't tell mother. *J Clin Oncol* 25(31):5030–5034, 2007.
24. White DB, Malvar G, Karr J, et al: Expanding the paradigm of the physician's role in surrogate decision-making: an empirically derived framework. *Crit Care Med* 38(3):743–750, 2010.
25. Beach MC, Roter D, Korthuis PT, et al: A multicenter study of physician mindfulness and health care quality. *Ann Fam Med* 11(5):421–428, 2013.
26. Khan JS: Evaluation of the educational environment of postgraduate surgical teaching. *J Ayub Med Coll Abbottabad* 20(3):104–107, 2008.
27. McDonagh JR, Elliott TB, Engelberg RA, et al: Family satisfaction with family conferences about end-of-life care in the intensive care unit: increased proportion of family speech is associated with increased satisfaction. *Crit Care Med* 32(7):1484–1488, 2004.
28. Maisels MJ, Kring EA: A simple approach to improving patient satisfaction. *Clin Pediatr (Phila)* 44(9):797–800, 2005.
29. Selph RB, Shiang J, Engelberg R, et al: Empathy and life support decisions in intensive care units. *J Gen Intern Med* 23(9):1311–1317, 2008.
30. Back AL, Arnold RM, Quill TE: Hope for the best, and prepare for the worst. *Ann Intern Med* 138(5):439–443, 2003.
31. West HF, Engelberg RA, Wenrich MD, et al: Expressions of nonabandonment during the intensive care unit family conference. *J Palliat Med* 8(4):797–807, 2005.
32. Stapleton RD, Engelberg RA, Wenrich MD, et al: Clinician statements and family satisfaction with family conferences in the intensive care unit. *Crit Care Med* 34(6):1679–1685, 2006.
33. Benes R, Brobst K: Ethics in critical care: practitioners discuss collaborative approaches to decision making. *QRB Qual Rev Bull* 18(1):33–39, 1992.
34. Emanuel EJ: Legal aspects in palliative and end of life care. *UpToDate(R)* 2014. http://www.uptodate.com/contents/legal-aspects-in-palliative-and-end-of-life-care. Accessed April 8, 2015.
35. Luce JM, White DB: A history of ethics and law in the intensive care unit. *Crit Care Clin* 25(1):221–237, 2009.
36. Schneiderman LJ: Effect of ethics consultations in the intensive care unit. *Crit Care Med* 34(11 Suppl):S359–S363, 2006.
37. Kompanje EJ, Piers RD, Benoit DD: Causes and consequences of disproportionate care in intensive care medicine. *Curr Opin Crit Care* 19(6):630–635, 2013.
38. Chase J: A clinical decision algorithm for hospital inpatients with impaired decision-making capacity. *J Hosp Med* 9(8):527–532, 2014.
39. Sessums LL, Zembrzuska H, Jackson JL: Does this patient have medical decision-making capacity? *JAMA* 306(4):420–427, 2011.
40. Appelbaum PS: Clinical practice. Assessment of patients' competence to consent to treatment. *N Engl J Med* 357(18):1834–1840, 2007.
41. Carroll DW: Assessment of capacity for medical decision making. *J Gerontol Nurs* 36(5):47–52, 2010.
42. Tunzi M: Can the patient decide? Evaluating patient capacity in practice. *Am Fam Physician* 64(2):299–306, 2001.
43. Ilemona ER: An appraisal of ethical issues in end-of-life care. *Niger J Med* 23(4):358–364, 2014.
44. Morgan CK, Varas GM, Pedroza C, et al: Defining the practice of "no escalation of care" in the ICU. *Crit Care Med* 42(2):357–361, 2014.
45. Wiegand DL: Withdrawal of life-sustaining therapy after sudden, unexpected life-threatening illness or injury: interactions between patients' families, healthcare providers, and the healthcare system. *Am J Crit Care* 15(2):178–187, 2006.
46. Truog RD, Cist AF, Brackett SE, et al: Recommendations for end-of-life care in the intensive care unit: The Ethics Committee of the Society of Critical Care Medicine. *Crit Care Med* 29(12):2332–2348, 2001.
47. Gerstel E, Engelberg RA, Koepsell T, et al: Duration of withdrawal of life support in the intensive care unit and association with family satisfaction. *Am J Respir Crit Care Med* 178(8):798–804, 2008.
48. Cist AF, Truog RD, Brackett SE, et al: Practical guidelines on the withdrawal of life-sustaining therapies. *Int Anesthesiol Clin* 39(3):87–102, 2001.
49. Cook D, Rocker G, Marshall J, et al: Withdrawal of mechanical ventilation in anticipation of death in the intensive care unit. *N Engl J Med* 349(12):1123–1132, 2003.
50. Huynh TN, Walling AM, Le TX, et al: Factors associated with palliative withdrawal of mechanical ventilation and time to death after withdrawal. *J Palliat Med* 16(11):1368–1374, 2013.
51. Crippen D: Terminally weaning awake patients from life-sustaining mechanical ventilation: the critical care physician's role in comfort measures during the dying process. *Clin Intensive Care* 3:206–206, 1992.
52. Curtis JR: Interventions to improve care during withdrawal of life-sustaining treatments. *J Palliat Med* 8 Suppl 1:S116–S131, 2005.
53. Rady MY, Verheijde JL: Ethical challenges with deactivation of durable mechanical circulatory support at the end of life: left ventricular assist devices and total artificial hearts. *J Intensive Care Med* 29(1):3–12, 2014.
54. Treece PD, Engelberg RA, Crowley L, et al: Evaluation of a standardized order form for the withdrawal of life support in the intensive care unit. *Crit Care Med* 32(5):1141–1148, 2004.
55. Huynh TN, Kleerup EC, Wiley JF, et al: The frequency and cost of treatment perceived to be futile in critical care. *JAMA Intern Med* 173(20):1887–1894, 2013.
56. Piers RD, Azoulay E, Ricou B, et al: Perceptions of appropriateness of care among European and Israeli intensive care unit nurses and physicians. *JAMA* 306(24):2694–2703, 2011.
57. Valentin A, Druml W, Steltzer H, et al: Recommendations on therapy limitation and therapy discontinuation in intensive care units: Consensus Paper of the Austrian Associations of Intensive Care Medicine. *Intensive Care Med* 34(4):771–776, 2008.
58. Bosslet GT, Pope TM, Rubenfeld GD, et al: An official ATS/AACN/ACCP/ESICM/SCCM policy statement: responding to requests for potentially inappropriate treatments in intensive care units. *Am J Respir Crit Care Med* 191(11):1318–1330, 2015.
59. Truog RD, Brett AS, Frader J: The problem with futility. *N Engl J Med* 326(23):1560–1564, 1992.
60. Schneiderman LJ, Jecker NS, Jonsen AR: Medical futility: its meaning and ethical implications. *Ann Intern Med* 112(12):949–954, 1990.

61. Murphy DJ, Finucane TE: New do-not-resuscitate policies. A first step in cost control. *Arch Intern Med* 153(14):1641–1648, 1993.
62. Burns JP, Truog RD: Futility: a concept in evolution. *Chest* 132(6):1987–1993, 2007.
63. Schneiderman LJ, Jecker NS, Jonsen AR: Medical futility: response to critiques. *Ann Intern Med* 125(8):669–674, 1996.
64. Rubin SB. If we think it's futile, can't we just say no? *HEC Forum* 19(1):45–65, 2007.
65. Luce JM: A history of resolving conflicts over end-of-life care in intensive care units in the United States. *Crit Care Med* 38(8):1623–1629, 2010.
66. Palda VA, Bowman KW, McLean RF, et al: "Futile" care: do we provide it? Why? A semistructured, Canada-wide survey of intensive care unit doctors and nurses. *J Crit Care* 20(3):207–213, 2005.
67. Sibbald R, Downar J, Hawryluck L: Perceptions of "futile care" among caregivers in intensive care units. *CMAJ* 177(10):1201–1208, 2007.
68. Singal RK, Sibbald R, Morgan B, et al: A prospective determination of the incidence of perceived inappropriate care in critically ill patients. *Can Respir J* 21(3):165–170, 2014.
69. Huynh TN, Kleerup EC, Raj PP, et al: The opportunity cost of futile treatment in the ICU. *Crit Care Med* 42(9):1977–1982, 2014.
70. Niederman MS, Berger JT: The delivery of futile care is harmful to other patients. *Crit Care Med* 38(10 Suppl):S518–S522, 2010.
71. Truog RD, Campbell ML, Curtis JR, et al: Recommendations for end-of-life care in the intensive care unit: a consensus statement by the American College [corrected] of Critical Care Medicine. *Crit Care Med* 36(3):953–963, 2008.
72. Moeller JR, Albanese TH, Garchar K, et al: Functions and outcomes of a clinical medical ethics committee: a review of 100 consults. *HEC Forum* 24(2):99–114, 2012.
73. Gonsoulin TP, Taube JM: Hospital ethics committees: formation, function, and case consultation. *J La State Med Soc* 154(6):323–327, 2002.
74. Faith K, Chidwick P: Role of clinical ethicists in making decisions about levels of care in the intensive care unit. *Crit Care Nurse* 29(2):77–84, 2009.
75. Fox E, Myers S, Pearlman RA: Ethics consultation in United States hospitals: a national survey. *Am J Bioeth* 7(2):13–25, 2007.
76. Carter BS, Wocial LD: Ethics and palliative care: which consultant and when? *Am J Hosp Palliat Care* 29(2):146–150, 2012.
77. AAHPM palliative sedation position statement. 2014. http://aahpm.org/positions/palliative-sedation. Accessed February 23, 2016.
78. Wachs SR: Put conflict resolution skills to work. *J Oncol Pract* 4:37–40, 2008.
79. Back A, Arnold R, Tulsky J: *Mastering Communication with Seriously Ill Patients: Balancing Honesty with Empathy and Hope*. New York, NY, Cambridge University Press, 2009.
80. Quill TE, Holloway R: Time-limited trials near the end of life. *JAMA* 306(13):1483–1484, 2011.

Chapter 35 ■ Managing Symptoms in Critically Ill Patients

RICHARD CASTRIOTTA • JENNIFER E. REIDY • JAVIER BARREDA GARCIA • GARBO MAK • BRANDY MCKELVY

Patients in the intensive care unit (ICU) experience a variety of distressing symptoms caused by critical illness and/or its evaluation and treatment. Effective symptom management improves patients' abilities to heal from injuries, tolerate evaluation and treatment, cope with stress, and recover from severe illness or injury. This chapter reviews the management of common symptoms among ICU patients with severe illness or injury, including pain, dyspnea, nausea/vomiting, constipation, agitated delirium, anxiety, and depression.

PAIN MANAGEMENT IN PALLIATIVE CARE

Pain is a frequent and troubling symptom for patients with serious illness. ICU clinicians must have the knowledge and skills to effectively evaluate and treat the pain of critically ill patients. When pain is complicated and refractory, the ICU team should work with specialists from palliative care and pain anesthesia to formulate advanced approaches to complex pain. (For a complete and excellent discussion on pain assessment and treatment, see Chapter 3.) In addition, this section describes palliative care principles for the management of pain and offers pearls for clinical practice.

GENERAL PRINCIPLES

Pain is a multidimensional experience impacted by biologic, psychological, emotional, and social factors. Multiple studies show that pain perception does not always correlate with physical injury and that emotional pain or stress can activate the same brain structures as physical pain. Patients interpret sensations transmitted from nociceptors and peripheral and central nerves through their own personal mindset; in turn, these thoughts and emotions influence descending pathways from the brain to inhibit (or enhance) pain transmission through ascending neural pathways. When patients are faced with serious illness, physical pain inherently impacts multiple aspects of personhood (see Fig. 35.1). As a result, comprehensive pain assessment and management requires an interdisciplinary approach to address emotional, psychosocial, and existential/spiritual aspects of pain and suffering [1].

Table 35.1 outlines general principles for effective pain management, including whole-person assessment and care. Regular pain assessments with a consistent tool (selected after consideration of cultural, literacy, and personal factors) allows patients and staff to partner for managing pain. In addition to tools that quantify the pain intensity and/or observed behaviors, the interdisciplinary team should consider the following aspects of pain and suffering in patients with advanced illness:

- Understanding what the pain means to the patient;
- Inquiring about past experiences of pain;
- Exploring the patient's coping skills for pain and stress;
- Learning about the patient's knowledge, preferences, and expectations for pain management;
- Screening for any concerns about the use of controlled substances, especially opioids (which might include a history of addiction and/or fears of becoming addicted and refusing opioids);
- Assessing the impact of pain on the patient's mental health, quality of life, and functioning (including the ability to work on rehabilitation).

PEARLS FOR CLINICAL PRACTICE

Clinicians should always consider the pathophysiology of the pain and treat the underlying cause as possible (e.g., high-dose single-fraction palliative radiation for a painful bone metastasis). With pain medications, clinicians should understand and use pharmacologic principles to guide therapy, including (1) start low and go slow in frail, opioid-naïve patients; (2) use the intravenous route of administration for pain crises; (3) dose for breakthrough pain and procedures based on T_{Cmax} (time to maximum concentration in the blood); (4) scheduled dosing for continuous or chronic pain based on $T_{1/2}$ (half-life of the drug); and (5) prevent and manage side effects. Clinicians should always consider multimodal analgesia and/or interventional techniques depending on the pain pathophysiology (e.g., anticonvulsants

Domains of Issues Associated with Illness and Bereavement

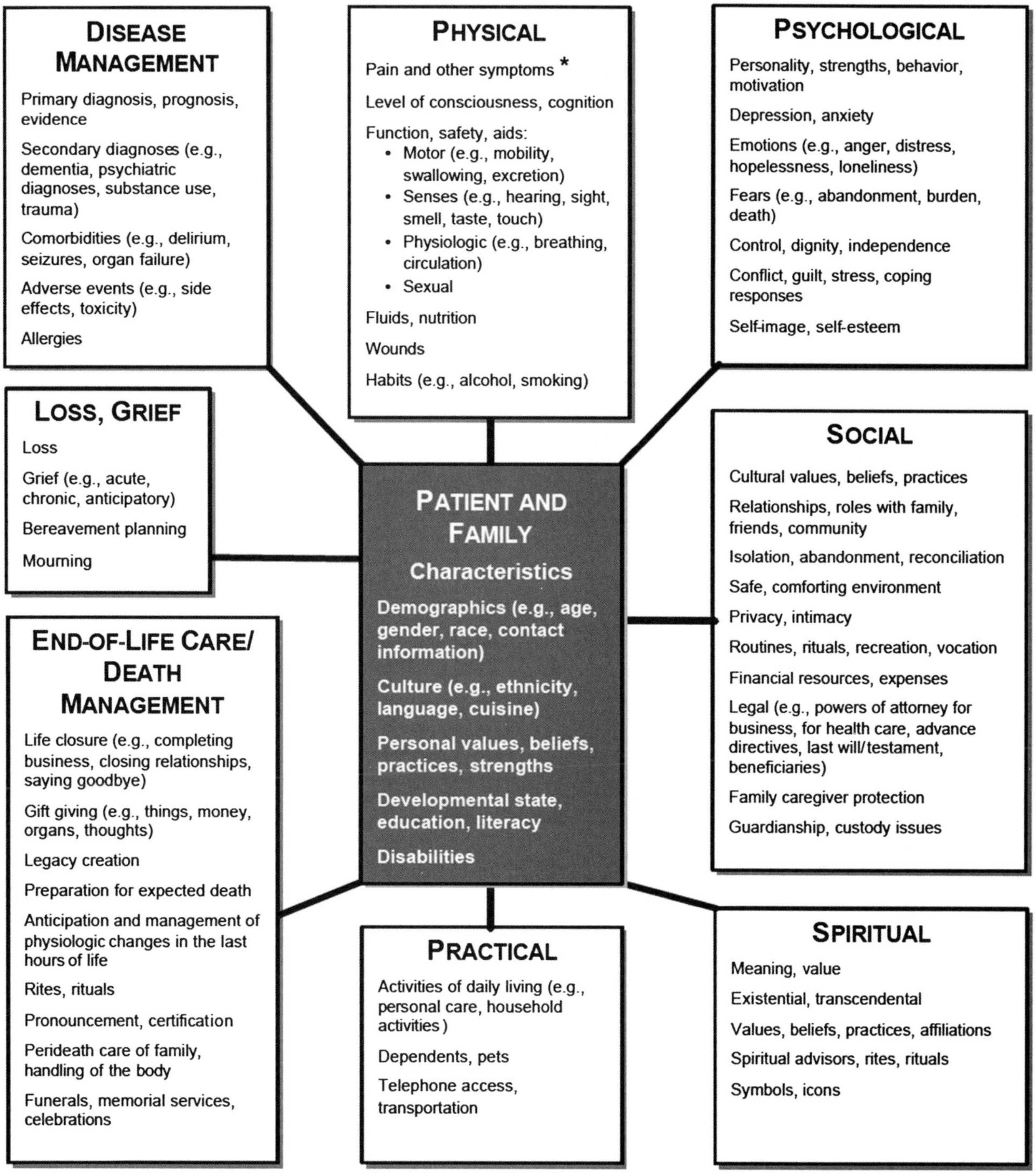

DISEASE MANAGEMENT
Primary diagnosis, prognosis, evidence
Secondary diagnoses (e.g., dementia, psychiatric diagnoses, substance use, trauma)
Comorbidities (e.g., delirium, seizures, organ failure)
Adverse events (e.g., side effects, toxicity)
Allergies
PHYSICAL
Pain and other symptoms *
Level of consciousness, cognition
Function, safety, aids:
• Motor (e.g., mobility, swallowing, excretion)
• Senses (e.g., hearing, sight, smell, taste, touch)
• Physiologic (e.g., breathing, circulation)
• Sexual
Fluids, nutrition
Wounds
Habits (e.g., alcohol, smoking)
PSYCHOLOGICAL
Personality, strengths, behavior, motivation
Depression, anxiety
Emotions (e.g., anger, distress, hopelessness, loneliness)
Fears (e.g., abandonment, burden, death)
Control, dignity, independence
Conflict, guilt, stress, coping responses
Self-image, self-esteem
LOSS, GRIEF
Loss
Grief (e.g., acute, chronic, anticipatory)
Bereavement planning
Mourning
PATIENT AND FAMILY
Characteristics
Demographics (e.g., age, gender, race, contact information)
Culture (e.g., ethnicity, language, cuisine)
Personal values, beliefs, practices, strengths
Developmental state, education, literacy
Disabilities
SOCIAL
Cultural values, beliefs, practices
Relationships, roles with family, friends, community
Isolation, abandonment, reconciliation
Safe, comforting environment
Privacy, intimacy
Routines, rituals, recreation, vocation
Financial resources, expenses
Legal (e.g., powers of attorney for business, for health care, advance directives, last will/testament, beneficiaries)
Family caregiver protection
Guardianship, custody issues
END-OF-LIFE CARE/ DEATH MANAGEMENT
Life closure (e.g., completing business, closing relationships, saying goodbye)
Gift giving (e.g., things, money, organs, thoughts)
Legacy creation
Preparation for expected death
Anticipation and management of physiologic changes in the last hours of life
Rites, rituals
Pronouncement, certification
Perideath care of family, handling of the body
Funerals, memorial services, celebrations
PRACTICAL
Activities of daily living (e.g., personal care, household activities)
Dependents, pets
Telephone access, transportation
SPIRITUAL
Meaning, value
Existential, transcendental
Values, beliefs, practices, affiliations
Spiritual advisors, rites, rituals
Symbols, icons

* Other common symptoms include, but are not limited to:

Cardio-respiratory: breathlessness, cough, edema, hiccups, apnea, agonal breathing patterns

Gastrointestinal: nausea, vomiting, constipation, obstipation, bowel obstruction, diarrhea, bloating, dysphagia, dyspepsia

Oral conditions: dry mouth, mucositis

Skin conditions: dry skin, nodules, pruritus, rashes

General: agitation, anorexia, cachexia, fatigue, weakness, bleeding, drowsiness, effusions (pleural, peritoneal), fever/chills, incontinence, insomnia, lymphoedema, myoclonus, odor, prolapse, sweats, syncope, vertigo

FIGURE 35.1 Whole person assessment and care.

TABLE 35.1

Pearls for Managing Pain in Palliative Care Patients

- Determine the underlying cause(s) and reverse what is treatable/modifiable;
- Perform structured pain assessments with a consistent tool;
- Work with interdisciplinary team to understand and treat the emotional, psychological, social, and existential/spiritual aspects of pain;
- Start low and go slow with medications in patients with altered absorption, metabolism, and excretion due to serious illness;
- Use IV route for pain crises, and premedicate before procedures;
- Understand pharmacokinetics of opioids and how to dose for continuous pain (based on half-life of drug) and breakthrough pain (based on time to maximum concentration in the serum);
- Utilize multimodal analgesia, including adjuvants, interventional modalities and nonpharmacologic approaches;
- Consider strategies to treat multiple symptoms simultaneously to minimize polypharmacy (i.e., corticosteroids for bone pain and nausea, antidepressants for neuropathic pain and mood);
- Monitor closely and adjust medications on the basis of analgesic response and side effects;
- Coordinate plan of care for pain management with outside providers if patient will be discharged out of the ICU.

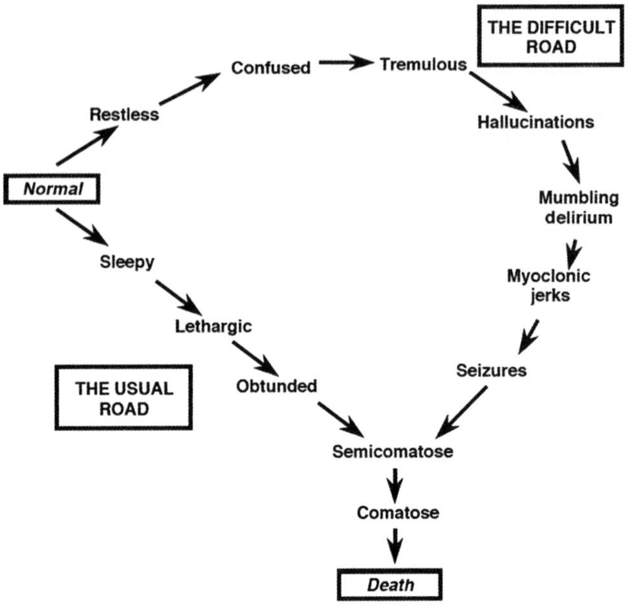

FIGURE 35.2 Two roads to death [49].

and/or antidepressants for peripheral neuropathy, or a celiac plexus block for epigastric pain related to pancreatic cancer). Studies show that opioids combined with adjuvants are more effective for neuropathic pain than opioids alone, and this approach reduces both the opioid dose and systemic side effects [2]. The ICU team should closely monitor and adjust the plan of care based on the patient's responses, and when the patient is close to discharge out of the ICU, coordinate closely with the next provider who will assume responsibility for ongoing pain management.

Finally, there are special considerations for patients who are dying in the ICU. The dying process itself is not recognized to be inherently painful; however, if a patient has a history of pain and/or clear causes of new pain, then pain should be effectively treated [3]. Agitated delirium (see Delirium section) can be misinterpreted as pain, and if incorrectly diagnosed and untreated, can lead to escalating opioid doses with worsening agitation and hyperalgesia [4]. In general, dying patients should never be started routinely on narcotic infusions in the absence of symptoms (i.e., "start morphine sulfate 1 mg per hour IV, titrate to comfort"), as sound pharmacologic principles always apply. Indiscriminate narcotic dosing can lead to build-up of active metabolites when renal failure occurs, resulting in agitated delirium from opioid neurotoxicity and/or hastened death (Fig. 35.2).

MANAGEMENT OF DYSPNEA

Dyspnea is defined as "a subjective experience of breathing discomfort that consists of qualitatively distinct sensations that vary in intensity [5]." More than 50% of patients report dyspnea during the months before death, and its prevalence increases as death becomes more imminent [6]. The underlying disease responsible for dyspnea seems to influence its prevalence and severity at the end of life. An observational study in Australia of 5,862 patients under hospice care showed that patients with a noncancer diagnosis experienced a higher prevalence and severity of dyspnea compared with cancer patients [7]. Patients with a primary respiratory disease were most affected. Surprisingly, even patients without an apparent cardiopulmonary condition reported a high frequency of shortness of breath (Table 35.2).

Mechanisms of Dyspnea

Currently, the mechanisms responsible for dyspnea are not fully characterized. Dyspnea is a result of the interplay between physiologic factors and psychological, social, and environmental elements [5]. Afferent impulses originate in, or are at least modified by, receptors located in the skin, chest wall, respiratory muscles and tendons, airways, lungs, pulmonary vessels, carotid and aortic bodies, and medulla. These impulses then activate the cortico-limbic region, which elicits a ventilation response. At any given moment, it is likely that multiple inputs are generated, transmitted through different pathways, and leading to a variety of uncomfortable respiratory sensations collectively described as dyspnea. Dyspnea occurs when a subject perceives an imbalance between respiratory demand and ventilatory response.

Treatment

As demonstrated by its high prevalence among patients under hospice care, alleviation of dyspnea at the end of life is often inadequate [7]. There is general agreement that the initial focus of management should be on treating the underlying disease process responsible for this symptom [8]. Nonspecific treatment of dyspnea should follow in situations of persistent shortness of breath. We have divided nonspecific therapies into the following categories: first-line therapies (recommended), second-line therapies (probably effective, considered for refractory situations), and interventions of unknown efficacy.

First-line Therapies

Systemic (oral or parenteral) opioids are effective for the treatment of dyspnea, and they are considered the primary therapies. Evidence for this therapy was derived from meta-analyses of randomized controlled trials (RCTs) of patients with cancer,

TABLE 35.2

Summary of Evidence-Based Recommendations in the Management of Dyspnea in Critically Ill Patients

Intervention	Year	Study	No. of patients	Findings	Reference
First-line therapy					
Any opioid	2002	Meta-analysis of RCTs	293	Improved dyspnea	[11]
Any opioid	2012	Meta-analysis of RCTs	130	Improved dyspnea	[10]
Any opioid	2015	Meta-analysis of RCTs	271	Improved dyspnea	[9]
Second-line therapies					
NIV	2013	RCT	200	Improved dyspnea	[12]
NIV	2013	RCT	30	Improved dyspnea compared with baseline	[13]
Handheld fan	2010	RCT	50	Improved dyspnea	[14]
Heliox	2004	RCT	12	Improved dyspnea	[15]
Inhaled furosemide	2013	RCT	100	Improved dyspnea	[16]
Oxygen	2010	RCT	239	No benefit	[18]
Oxygen	2011	RCT	143	No benefit	[17]

NIV, noninvasive ventilation; RCT, randomized controlled trial.

chronic obstructive pulmonary disease (COPD), and other dyspnea etiologies [9–11]. Their mechanism of action likely involves depression of the respiratory drive and changes at the cortical level [5]. Although effective, the magnitude of their benefit is unclear. They can be associated with a variety of side effects including nausea, vomiting, constipation, and drowsiness. Respiratory depression has been a particular concern of this therapy. However, it has not been reported with the opioid doses used for treating dyspnea, including in patients with advanced COPD [9]. Morphine is the best studied opioid therapy. In nonacute situations, it is reasonable to start with a low dose (oral, immediate-release formulation) and transition to a long-acting dose once a steady state has been reached [5].

Second-line Therapies

Dyspnea therapies in this group include interventions that have shown benefit from at least one RCT but for which positive effect was not consistently observed among other studies or when only small clinical trials were performed. They can be considered when dyspnea persists despite the use of opioids. These include noninvasive ventilation (NIV), fan, heliox, and inhaled furosemide.

Small clinical studies suggest that NIV might mitigate dyspnea for some patients. The best evidence is derived from an open-labeled RCT of 200 patients with end-stage solid cancer and acute respiratory failure who were randomized to NIV or oxygen groups for palliation of shortness of breath [12]. Patients of the NIV group demonstrated a faster improvement of dyspnea and used less morphine compared with the control group. In addition, one RCT showed an association between improved dyspnea and the use of NIV for cancer patients without acute respiratory failure [13].

Two other interventions that were shown to decrease dyspnea in single RCTs are the use of a fan directed to the face and heliox. The use of a handheld fan was associated with a reduction of dyspnea by an RCT of 50 patients with malignant and nonmalignant conditions [14]. A putative mechanism of action implicates stimulation of the trigeminal nerve by the cool air. It represents a low-cost and low-risk therapy that is widely available. Heliox was effective for reducing dyspnea and increasing walking distance in a phase II, double-blind, crossover RCT of 12 patients with lung cancer with dyspnea on exertion [15]. Its mechanism of action could involve a decrease in the work of breathing by increasing airflow at sites on airway narrowing by virtue of its lower density compared with air.

Inhaled furosemide is another second-line therapy for dyspnea. Several small RCTs of inhaled furosemide have shown improvement of dyspnea. These studies included healthy subjects with experimentally induced dyspnea and patients with COPD. The largest of these studies was a double-blinded study that included 100 patients with COPD exacerbations that were randomized to inhaled furosemide or normal saline [16]. Most of these trials used a 40-mg dose of furosemide as a single or daily dose. The mechanism of action of furosemide is unknown but could involve desensitization of the respiratory epithelium.

The use of oxygen with the intent to alleviate dyspnea should be considered for certain subgroups of patients. RCTs of patients with cancer, COPD, and other conditions suggest that oxygen does not relieve dyspnea compared with medical air [10,17,18]. However, most of the subjects from these studies were either outpatients or had no respiratory distress. Thus, it is unclear if the results from these trials can be extrapolated to patients in an ICU with severe dyspnea or at the end of life. It is also unknown if medical air, used as placebo in these studies, could have exerted a therapeutic effect by cooling the nasal mucosa, for example. Until new evidence is available, we suggest considering the use of oxygen in patients with respiratory distress because it is a low-risk intervention with potential benefits. Oxygen should be provided to breathless patients with hypoxemia [5,8].

INTERVENTIONS OF UNKNOWN EFFICACY

No definitive large-scale RCTs of inhaled opioids have been performed. Systematic reviews and meta-analyses that primarily included patients with COPD and cancer suggest that inhaled opioids provide little or no benefit for the treatment of dyspnea [9–11].

GASTROINTESTINAL SYMPTOMS: CONSTIPATION, NAUSEA, AND VOMITING

Gastrointestinal (GI) dysfunction, although a frequent and important determinant of ICU outcomes, currently lacks formal definition and classification [19]. Furthermore, treatment of GI symptoms during an ICU stay is often guided by experience and not evidence, with treatment strategies being extrapolated from non-ICU inpatients, outpatients, and palliative care settings.

Nausea, vomiting, and constipation can be associated with acute exacerbations of chronic illness, acute and rapid presentations of disease, or secondary to the interventions and medications prescribed during a hospitalization. The incidence of constipation in the ICU ranges from 69% to 83% and diarrhea occurs in as many as 36.1% of patients [20]. In fact, the incidence of critically ill patients, including mechanically ventilated patients who have at least one GI symptom, is 59% [21]. Development of two or more GI symptoms is associated with higher mortality and longer ICU stay [22].

GI symptoms frequently lead to discomfort for the patient and create obstacles to providing medical care. Constipation may lead to difficulty with ventilator weaning, enteral feeding intolerance, and a longer ICU stay [22]. Furthermore, nausea and vomiting may hinder reaching nutritional goals by delaying initiation of enteral feeding and complicate medication delivery and absorption. Providing palliative care for these symptoms during an ICU stay can be offered simultaneously with efforts to extend life and treat underlying medical issues with an overall goal to improve quality of life.

Constipation

Constipation is defined as infrequent or absent bowel movements that occur with difficulty of passing stool. In most ICU studies, the time period was at least 3 days [20]. The causes of constipation during an ICU stay include immobility, dehydration, and metabolic causes such as hypercalcemia and hypothyroidism. Medications are also a frequent cause of iatrogenic constipation during an ICU stay, including calcium-channel blockers and anticholinergic agents. Vasoactive drugs such as dopamine can cause constipation, and hemodynamic instability in the setting of hypoperfusion, shock, and endotoxin overproduction can decrease bowel motility. Opioids are regularly used for management of pain and sedation among critically ill patients and frequently cause constipation. The effect of opioids on the bowel includes reduced peristalsis throughout the GI tract, decreased intestinal fluid secretion, and increased intestinal fluid absorption resulting in constipation and the passage of hard stools [19].

Assessment

It is important to elicit a careful history, including the past medical history, the past abdominal surgical history, and prior bowel habits to establish whether chronic constipation was present or the patient has risk factors for constipation. Inpatient medications and medical interventions performed during the hospitalization must also be reviewed. The timing, quality, quantity, and frequency of stools since admission will characterize the degree of constipation. Some patients may present with unexplained nausea and vomiting. Abdominal pain may occur as the bowel attempts to evacuate hard stool. A physical exam, including abdominal and rectal examinations, is necessary. The abdominal examination may show firmness, distension, and the presence of hyperactive or hypoactive bowel sounds. Fecal impaction may be found on rectal examination. In some cases, fecal impaction may present as diarrhea with incontinence when fecal material higher in the colon is broken down into liquid form and flows past the mass. An empty rectal vault may suggest a proximal obstruction.

Patients with traumatic spinal cord injury often have neurogenic bowel, but clinicians may overlook it in nontraumatic etiologies such as multiple sclerosis, stroke, or cancer. In these patients, digital rectal and abdominal exams can help distinguish between upper motor neuron (a tight anal sphincter with peristalsis intact) and lower motor neuron lesions (a flaccid sphincter with no volitional contraction). In upper motor neuron injury, evacuation depends on stimulating the bowel wall digitally or with a suppository; by comparison, patients with lower motor neuron injury may need stool-bulking agents like fiber to control stool flow [23].

A plain abdominal radiograph can estimate the stool burden and differentiate between obstruction and constipation. In patients with continued symptoms and concern of alternative etiologies, computed tomography may aid in evaluation of small bowel obstruction, ileus, intra-abdominal abscess, bowel perforation or undiagnosed intraluminal or extraluminal abdominal masses.

Treatments

It can be effective to time medication use with a patient's normal toileting schedule and take advantage of the gastrocolonic response with meals to improve outcomes. In general, a greater volume of stool causes luminal stretch and triggers peristalsis. Hydration and high dietary fiber content are advantageous for healthy, active patients; however, additional dietary fiber such as psyllium may worsen constipation and should generally be avoided for critically ill patients who are not well hydrated.

If constipation due to secondary causes is suspected, interventions aimed at treating and reversing underlying etiologies should be attempted. Drugs that inhibit gastric motility should be withdrawn and avoided when possible. If impaction is suspected, a digital rectal examination and manual disimpaction is advised. Pharmacologic therapies that utilize different mechanisms and combine oral and rectal interventions may yield effective results.

The early use of supportive therapeutic agents is important and can be initiated independent of underlying pathology and bowel habits (see Table 35.3). Laxatives increase intestinal propulsion and secretion, and their use in the ICU is to improve intestinal fluid balance by promoting water secretion and preventing excessive water absorption. Stimulant laxatives such as senna and bisacodyl increase intestinal activity and secretion. Bisacodyl is activated in the small intestine by the hydrolytic activity of endogenous esterases. Senna is activated by colonic bacteria in the colon. Osmotic laxatives include magnesium salts, lactulose, and polyethylene glycol (PEG 3350), which are marginally reabsorbed and produce softer stool with larger volume by drawing in water during bowel transit. Magnesium salts must be used cautiously in renal insufficiency as this may lead to magnesium toxicity. Lactulose passes unabsorbed into the colon where bacteria break it down, thus possibly causing bloating and abdominal cramping. PEG 3350 is not metabolized by bacteria, resulting in no production of intestinal gas. It does not lead to a loss of fluids or electrolytes across the GI tract and is well tolerated with high effectiveness. PEG 3350 is also available without electrolytes (Miralax), which can be combined with a liquid.

Enemas and glycerol suppositories soften stool and generate peristalsis. Enemas are available as warm tap water, mineral oil, or sodium phosphate. Sodium phosphate enemas should be used with caution among elderly patients as they may cause hypotension, volume depletion, and electrolyte loss [24]. Metoclopramide is a prokinetic agent that antagonizes dopamine receptors, and it can be used in constipation that has not responded to other pharmacologic interventions.

Opioid receptor agonists are frequently used for sedation and pain in the ICU. The GI effect of opioids on the gut involves the enteric nervous system, and the agonism of enteric μ-opioid receptors of the GI tract inhibits gastric emptying, increases pyloric muscle tone, and delays transit through the small and large intestine. Methylnaltrexone is a peripheral opioid antagonist with limited ability to cross the blood–brain barrier and thus does not reverse centrally mediated analgesia. It is approved

TABLE 35.3

Medications for Managing Constipation

Medication	Class	Mechanism	Starting dose (max dose)	Side effects/ Precautions
Polyethylene glycol 3350	Osmotic laxative	Draws water into bowel to soften stool and trigger peristalsis	17 g PO daily (100 g daily in divided doses)	Take with 6–8 oz fluid; tasteless, with less gas or cramping
Lactulose	Osmotic laxative	Draws water into bowel to soften stool and trigger peristalsis	15–30 mL daily (tid)	Increased gas production, cramping
Magnesium citrate	Osmotic laxative	Draws water into bowel to soften stool and trigger peristalsis	150 mL PO daily (300 mL)	Systemic absorption of magnesium; avoid in renal failure
Sennosides	Stimulant laxative	Induces peristalsis; converted to active in colon	2 tabs at bedtime (4 tabs qid)	Cramping
Bisacodyl	Stimulant laxative	Induces peristalsis	Oral: 5–15 mg PO daily (30 mg) Rectal: 10 mg PR daily	Cramping
Docusate sodium	Stool softener	Facilitates mixing of aqueous and fatty substances to soften feces	100–200 mg PO daily (qid)	
Glycerin	Stool softener	Softens stool and stimulates peristalsis with insertion	1 suppository PR as needed	
Fleet's, tap water, mineral oil enemas	Enemas	Softens stool and stimulates peristalsis with insertion	1 enema PRN as needed	Avoid Fleet's in renal failure; avoid soap suds (damages mucosa)
Methylnaltrexone	Peripheral opioid receptor antagonist	Reverses opioid effect on bowel only	Weight-based (12 mg SC daily)	Caution if risk of bowel perforation

With chronic or opioid-induced constipation, best practice is to schedule daily laxatives for bowel maintenance (i.e., senna two tabs daily) and as-needed medications for rescue if no bowel movement in 48 hours (i.e., PEG 17 g daily or bisacodyl 10 mg PR PRN).

for treatment of opioid-induced constipation among patients with advanced illness and is effective for inducing laxation of palliative care patients with opioid-induced constipation where conventional laxatives have failed [25].

Nausea and Vomiting

Nausea, vomiting, and retching have distinct definitions. Nausea is a subjective sensation that precedes the need to vomit and may be associated with other symptoms including tachycardia, lightheadedness, diaphoresis, abdominal pain, and diarrhea. In contrast, vomiting and retching are objective. Vomiting involves expulsion of gastric contents after forceful contraction of abdominal musculature. Retching is contraction of the abdominal musculature in the presence of a closed glottis and no expulsion of gastric contents. Nausea may occur in isolation or precede vomiting and retching. Any of these symptoms in the most severe form may result in electrolytes imbalances, dehydration, and feeding intolerance with subsequent malnutrition.

Emesis is mediated by a complex interaction of afferent, humoral, and parasympathetic pathways. The vomiting center is located in the medulla oblongata and receives input from the chemoreceptor trigger zone (CTZ) located in the area postrema, the nucleus of the tractus solitarus, the GI tract, and the vestibular pathway. Dopamine, serotonin (5-HT), acetylcholine, histamine, and neurokinins are neurotransmitters involved in emetogenesis that bind to the receptors of the vomiting center, CTZ, and GI tract. The vomiting center additionally activates efferent pathways to the cranial nerves, diaphragm, and abdominal muscles [26,27]. Altogether, the activation of these various components triggers emesis (Fig. 35.3).

Primary causes of nausea and vomiting in the ICU include adynamic ileus, ketoacidosis, pancreatitis, liver dysfunction, Ogilvie syndrome and abdominal compartment syndrome. Secondary causes of symptoms are adverse effects from medications, shock, abnormal lab values, renal failure, intracranial lesions, increased intracranial pressure, heart failure, and non-abdominal surgery [19].

Assessment

Evaluation of nausea and vomiting in the critical care setting must involve patient assessment and corroboration of information from nursing staff. A thorough evaluation of the history, physical examination, laboratory, and radiographic data can frequently identify an etiology. Key components to assess are as follows:

- Symptoms of nausea, vomiting, retching, reflux, diarrhea, distension, abdominal pain, regurgitation, and constipation
- Timing, frequency, nature of the event (i.e., bloody or undigested food emesis), and the volume of gastric residuals if the patient is receiving enteral nutrition
- The inpatient medication list, especially opioids, antibiotics, and chemotherapeutic agents
- Physical examination including vital signs, fluid status assessment, abdominal distention, abdominal pain, and the presence of bowel sounds
- Review of laboratory values and looking for evidence of organ dysfunction
- Review of abdominal imaging

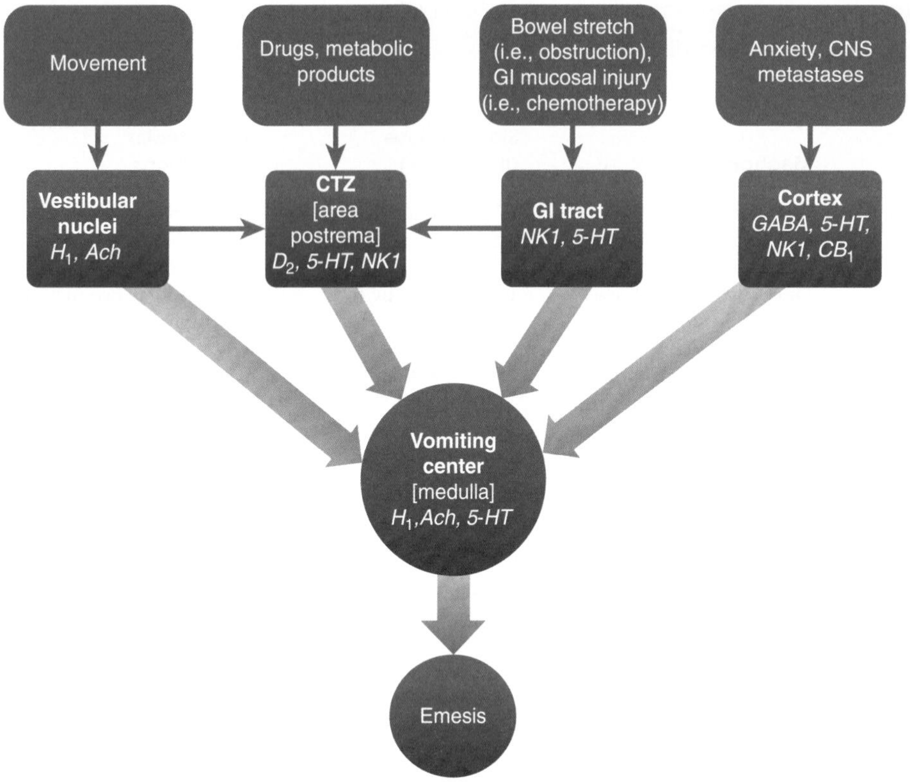

FIGURE 35.3 The emetic pathway. CTZ, chemoreceptor trigger zone; Ach, acetylcholine; D_2, dopamine; GABA, γ-aminobutyric acid; H_1, histamine; 5-HT, serotonin; NK1, neurokinin; CB_1, cannabinoid.

For example, the clinical assessment may reveal a pattern of delayed gastric emptying, which presents with intermittent nausea relieved by vomiting. Bilious or fecal emesis associated with abdominal discomfort and constipation or absence of bowel movements can suggest bowel obstruction. Constipation of the lower GI tract can precipitate nausea and is associated with use of opioids, sedatives, and intravenous catecholamines used for hemodynamic resuscitation. Ileus occurs after abdominal surgery, and general anesthesia also contributes to nausea among postoperative patients.

Treatment

A successful approach to managing the symptomatic patient incorporates thorough patient assessment, knowledge of the emetic pathophysiologic pathways, and a comprehensive treatment plan including pharmacologic and emotional support [26].

No guidelines exist for the pharmacologic treatment of nausea and vomiting for the critically ill. Published guidelines currently focus on chemotherapy-related and postoperative nausea management [27,28]. The occurrence of encephalopathy during critical illness may result in clinicians treating signs of emesis rather than symptoms. Although targeted antiemetic treatment blocks the neurotransmitters implicated in the underlying cause, empiric therapy may be necessary without a clear etiology, usually with a dopamine or serotonin antagonist [26]. (See Table 35.4 for an example of an order set with targeted pharmacologic and nonpharmacologic approaches.)

Metoclopramide and domperidone are dopamine (D_2) antagonists that work within the brain's CTZ, as well as increase gastric emptying and decrease small bowel transit time resulting in gut prokinesis. In addition to D_2 blockade, metoclopramide activates 5-HT_4 receptors that mediate acetylcholine release, thus increasing upper GI motility. Extrapyramidal adverse effects can occur, which may be treated with diphenhydramine. Dose adjustment must be made with renal insufficiency and in elderly patients. Domperidone is not available for use in the United States.

Phenothiazines are D_2 antagonists but have broader activity than do metoclopramide, as they additionally block cholinergic and histamine receptors. These drugs have potent antiemetic activity, but are frequently associated with adverse effects including hypotension, sedation, dry mouth, and extrapyramidal effects. Prochlorperazine, promethazine, chlorpromazine, and levomepromazine are several phenothiazines that are available. Haloperidol is a potent D_2 antagonist used for the treatment of delirium and agitation in ICUs. Among terminal cancer patients, it is commonly used for the management of nausea and vomiting, and it has also been used for postoperative nausea and vomiting [29]. However, data are lacking for its use as an antiemetic for the critically ill. Adverse effect monitoring should include electrocardiograms for QT prolongation and observation for extrapyramidal side effects.

More recently, there has been interest in the atypical antipsychotic olanzapine for chronic nausea and chemotherapy-induced nausea and vomiting. Olanzapine works through multiple neurotransmitters including D_2, 5-HT_2, 5-HT_3, acetylcholine, and histamine and thus may impact many areas of the emetic pathway in complex, refractory nausea. In addition, olanzapine has five times the affinity for 5-HT_2 over D_2 receptors, resulting in lower extrapyramidal side effects [30].

The 5-HT_3 receptors are found within the vagus nerve, brain, and gut enterochromaffin cells. Several 5-HT_3 antagonists are available, including dolasetron, granisetron, ondansetron, and palonosetron. Their use is established for the prevention and treatment of nausea with chemotherapy and also in the postoperative patient [27,31]. Although this drug class is commonly used for the critically ill, clinical trials are lacking. This class of drug is also associated with prolonged QT interval and can contribute to constipation.

Glucocorticoids are effective in chemotherapy-related and postoperative nausea, as well as in malignant bowel obstruction and elevated intracranial pressure from brain tumors. If nausea and vomiting is suspected due to corticosteroid insufficiency during acute illness, treatment with intravenous corticosteroids should be initiated.

TABLE 35.4

Example of an Order Set for Managing Nausea and Vomiting

Nausea/Vomiting	Circle antiemetic(s) below, based on etiology
Consider pathophysiology of patients' nausea to guide treatment.	**Corticosteroid** Dexamethasone 4 mg PO/IV daily in AM
Nonpharmacologic interventions	**Dopamine Antagonists (choose only one)** Haloperidol 1–2 mg PO q4h PRN nausea Prochlorperazine 10 mg PO q6h PRN nausea Promethazine 25 mg PR q6h PRN nausea Metoclopramide 10 mg PO/IV q6h PRN nausea Olanzapine (ODT) 5–10 mg SL q6h PRN nausea Olanzapine 2.5–5 PO mg q6h PRN nausea
Diet • Consider nutritionist consult • Encourage frequent small meals • Offer favorite foods and when patient wants it **Medications** • Give after meals when possible **Mouth care** • Provide good oral hygiene **Environment** • Limit unpleasant odors that worsen nausea • Adjust lighting in room as needed **Positioning** • Help patient find most comfortable positions **Relaxation Techniques** • Breathing, meditation, guided imagery **Distraction** • TV, videos, music **Company** • Volunteers as needed	**Serotonin Antagonists** Ondansetron 8 mg PO/IV q8h PRN nausea **Central Acting Agents** Dronabinol 2.5–10 mg PO t.i.d. PRN nausea Lorazepam 0.5–2 mg PO/IV q8h PRN nausea **Histamine Antagonists (choose only one)** Diphenhydramine 25 mg PO/IV q6h PRN nausea Meclizine 25–50 mg PO q6h PRN nausea Hydroxyzine 25–50 mg PO q6h PRN nausea **Acetylcholine Antagonists** Scopolamine 1.5–3 mg transdermal every 72 h **Antiacid Agents** Omeprazole 20 mg PO QD Calcium carbonate 1–2 tabs PO t.i.d. PRN nausea

PSYCHIATRIC SYMPTOMS: DELIRIUM, ANXIETY, AND DEPRESSION

Delirium

Delirium is a common and often devastating complication of advanced illness, occurring among nearly 85 percent of patients during their final weeks of life [32]. Delirium, which can be hyperactive, hypoactive, or mixed, is associated with increased morbidity and can be a sign of impending death of terminally ill patients. The symptoms of delirium can cause significant distress for patients, families, and staff. Delirium can also interfere with the assessment and management of other physical and psychological symptoms, such as pain. This section will focus on key management principles of palliative care patients, including

1. making a timely diagnosis,
2. determining reversibility versus irreversibility of the underlying cause(s),
3. understanding prognosis and goals of care to guide workup and management,
4. educating families and caregivers about delirium, and
5. using nonpharmacologic and pharmacologic measures to keep a patient comfortable and safe.

For a complete discussion of diagnosis, workup, and treatment of delirium, please see Chapter 157.

Assessment

Unfortunately, delirium (especially the hypoactive form) is often misdiagnosed and therefore untreated in terminally ill patients. Due to its high prevalence, ICU teams should use a consistent, evidence-based tool for diagnosis and screening, such as the Confusion Assessment Method for the ICU (CAM-ICU) and the Intensive Care Delirium Screening Checklist (ICDSC), which have been found to have a high degree of sensitivity and specificity in two meta-analyses [33]. Patients with advanced illness have multiple physiologic disturbances that can cause delirium, and many etiologies are irreversible in dying patients. However, there are common reversible etiologies as well, including constipation, urinary retention, and medication side effects for this population [34].

For determining reversibility of delirium, a clinician should review the patient's principal diagnosis, comorbidities, prognosis, and preadmission and current functional status. It is essential to hold a family meeting (including the patient if he or she is able to participate) in order to explain the nature of delirium, explore patient's goals and priorities, and weigh the benefits against burdens of further evaluation to elucidate the underlying causes (see Table 34.1 on structured family meetings of Chapter 34). Some patients, families, and ICU teams may agree on time-limited therapeutic trials and/or less invasive testing, especially if the results may allow an easy intervention that might reverse the delirium, reduce distress, or improve a patient's quality of life. Among other cases, the patient and family may decline a therapeutic trial or workup based on poor prognosis and/or need for burdensome testing, and delirium becomes effectively irreversible [34].

Prevention and Treatment

The most effective way of managing ICU delirium is to recognize the risk factors and attempt to prevent the development of delirium. These modifiable risk factors include polypharmacy, environmental factors (such as noise and sleep interruptions), and social interaction with visitors and the health care team. Windows may be associated with lower ICU delirium prevalence, but only if they allow enough light and a dark–light cycle [35]. In addition to light deprivation, noise levels can be lowered to reduce delirium in the ICU, but this may in fact be quite difficult to achieve [36]. The risk of delirium can be significantly lowered

TABLE 35.5

Changes during the Dying Process [49]

Change during the dying process	Manifest by/signs
Fatigue, weakness	Decreasing function, hygiene Inability to move around bed Inability to lift head off pillow
Cutaneous ischemia	Erythema over bony prominences Skin breakdown Wounds
Pain	Facial grimacing Tension in forehead; between eyebrows
Decreasing food intake, wasting	Anorexia Poor intake Aspiration, asphyxiation Weight loss, chiefly muscle and fat, notable in temples
Loss of ability to close eyes	Eyelids not closed Whites of eyes showing (with or without pupils visible)
Decreasing fluid intake, dehydration	Poor intake Aspiration Peripheral edema due to hypoalbuminemia Dehydration, dry mucous membranes/conjunctiva
Cardiac dysfunction, renal failure	Tachycardia Hypertension followed by hypotension Peripheral cooling Peripheral and central cyanosis (bluing of extremities) Mottling of the skin (livedo reticularis) Venous pooling along dependent skin surfaces Dark urine Oliguria, anuria
Neurologic dysfunction, including:	—
Decreasing level of consciousness	Increasing drowsiness Difficulty awakening Nonresponsive to verbal or tactile stimuli
Decreasing ability to communicate	Difficulty word finding Monosyllabic words, short sentences Delayed or inappropriate responses Not verbally responsive
Respiratory dysfunction	Change in ventilatory rate—increasing first, then slowing Decreasing tidal volume Abnormal breathing patterns—apnea, Cheyne-Stokes respirations, agonal breaths
Loss of ability to swallow	Dysphagia Coughing, choking Loss of gag reflex Buildup of oral and tracheal secretions Gurgling
Loss of sphincter control	Incontinence of urine or bowels Maceration of skin Perineal candidiasis
Terminal delirium	Early signs of cognitive failure, e.g., day-night reversal Agitation, restlessness Purposeless, repetitious movements Moaning, groaning
Rare, unexpected events	
Bursts of energy just before death occurs, the "golden glow"	
Aspiration, asphyxiation	

by utilizing ear plugs for patients [37]. Early mobilization has been utilized to reduce both the incidence and duration of delirium in the ICU [38]. There is no recommendation for using a pharmacologic delirium prevention protocol [39]. Numerous studies have found that the use of dexmedetomidine in place of benzodiazepines or propofol results in a lower risk of delirium, but none have compared it with placebo [40]. The best chance for reducing the incidence of ICU delirium may be the implementation of care bundles, which include early mobility, measures to improve sleep and circadian rhythm, and protocols for interruption of sedation, spontaneous breathing trials, and delirium monitoring [41].

Once an ICU patient develops delirium, it can be challenging to treat the symptoms, especially if the underlying cause is not reversible. The goals of symptom management are to keep a delirious patient safe and comfortable, while supporting and educating the family. The interdisciplinary team should provide intensive support to families holding vigil at the bedside, as they may perceive their loved one is "going crazy" and/or grieve the loss of the person they knew and loved before death arrives. Inadequate control of agitated symptoms can contribute to posttraumatic stress, anxiety, and depression in family members as well as the staff who witness these difficult deaths [32].

First-line treatment of symptoms should always be nonpharmacologic measures, including

- increasing supervision and companionship at the bedside;
- minimizing use of physical restraints;
- minimizing the number of invasive lines and catheters, as able;
- padding the bedrails and lowering the bed, as able;
- maximizing uninterrupted times for sleep at night; and
- ensuring the patient has access to glasses and hearing aids.

For the pharmacologic treatment of delirium, antipsychotics are the drugs of choice; however, there is no high-quality evidence for their use, and there are no FDA-approved medications for delirium [42]. One expert guideline in 2013 outlined a rapid and safe titration strategy for antipsychotics on the basis of their pharmacokinetics—much in the same way that opioids are titrated for a pain crisis [34]. For example, a sample order could read "haloperidol 1 mg IV q15 minutes PRN for agitated delirium; call provider if no improvement after three doses." This order is based on haloperidol's time to maximum concentration in the serum (15 minutes). The provider can then schedule the patient's total dose used in 24 hours in once-daily doses (not to exceed 100 mg per day) and continue the "as needed" doses that were previously effective for breakthrough agitation. For severe agitated delirium, chlorpromazine may be useful for its sedating, antihistamine properties as compared with haloperidol, which has stronger dopamine antagonism. Although benzodiazepines are generally avoided for treatment of delirium (and may cause delirium themselves), they can be effective for patients with a history of anxiety, alcohol use, previous benzodiazepine use, muscle spasm, and/or seizure risk [34].

For refractory agitated delirium of patients close to death, the ICU team can consider palliative sedation (PS) [32]. It is important to understand the differences in intent between aggressive symptom management of delirium and PS. PS is the intentional lowering of awareness toward, and including, unconsciousness for patients with severe and refractory symptoms, as defined by the American Academy of Hospice and Palliative Medicine. PS is reserved for extreme situations and should only be used after all available options have been exhausted to treat refractory symptoms (for full discussion on palliative sedation, see Chapter 34) [43].

Anxiety and Depression

Patients with serious illness confront daunting psychological challenges and emotional upheaval. In end-of-life situations, patients face what Byock calls "the last developmental stage of life," with opportunities for personal growth and enrichment of relationships [44]. This end-of-life work is difficult if physical and psychological symptoms, among other components of suffering, are not well managed. Although worry, sadness, and fear are normal responses to serious illness, ICU clinicians should be skilled in recognizing abnormal responses to stress, including anxiety disorders and depression. (For a comprehensive review of anxiety and depression, see Chapters 158 and 159 on Management of Anxiety and Depression.)

In one large study, nearly 50% of patients with advanced cancer met criteria for a psychiatric disorder, and among these patients, 68% had adjustment disorders with depressed or anxious mood, 13% had major depression, and 9% had organic mental disorders (delirium) [45]. Patients' psychological health fluctuates over the course of terminal illness, and so regular reassessment and treatment of symptoms is crucial. In general, clinicians should be mindful of their own biases ("Of course she's depressed—she's got metastatic cancer") that may impact their clinical judgment and ability to identify useful treatments and inadvertently convey a message of "giving up" on the patient.

Anxiety

It is common for patients to express anxiety and fear about the dying process and death. About 25% of patients with advanced illness suffer from debilitating anxiety symptoms and require treatment [46]. The ICU clinician should start with empathetically exploring a patient's anxiety ("can you tell me what you are worried about or afraid of?"). An effective strategy is to listen, acknowledge the patient's worries, provide empathetic support, and offer reassurance of ongoing care. If patients have persistently high levels of anxiety despite supportive-expressive therapy, a selective serotonin reuptake inhibitor (SSRI) and/or a low-dose benzodiazepine may be helpful (see Chapter 158 on Anxiety Management for specific medications and dosages). Mind–body treatments (e.g., meditation, cognitive-behavioral therapy, relaxation training) can be effective, especially when taught by a clinician trained in their use [47]. The ICU team should also diagnose and treat any contributors to a patient's anxiety, including poorly treated pain or dyspnea, unrecognized delirium, substance abuse (intoxication or withdrawal), or medication side effects (such as corticosteroids).

Depression

Depression is normal for patients with life-threatening illness, and it can be overlooked and thus untreated [45]. It is common for dying patients to experience poor appetite and energy, changes in sleep patterns, and difficulty with concentration; feelings of hopelessness, helplessness, worthlessness, and pervasive guilt are markers of depression in this population. Depression interferes with the patients' enjoyment of life, sense of purpose, and relationships with others. In addition, it can worsen pain and other physical symptoms and is associated with requests for hastened death. Risk factors include a previous history of depression, younger age, poor social supports, poor functional status, and pain [46]. In addition, certain medical conditions (hypo- or hyperthyroidism, anemia, and brain tumors) and medications (corticosteroids, interferon, tamoxifen, and other chemotherapeutic agents) can predispose patients to depression.

The single question, "Do you feel you are depressed?", is useful as a screening tool [48]. Among patients with end-stage disease, the ICU clinician must differentiate major depression from grief. People who are grieving experience waves of sadness related to loss (or anticipated loss), but retain the ability to feel joy and pleasure. They may have passive thoughts and desire for death at times, but continue to look forward to the future. Meanwhile, depressed patients have unrelenting, intense, persistent anhedonia; have no hope or optimism for the future; and may have active suicidal thoughts.

Depression is a treatable condition, even for patients with end-stage illness. Although no controlled clinical trials have evaluated the efficacy of combined interventions in this population, many experts recommend a combination of supportive psychotherapy, patient and family education, and antidepressants. (See Chapter 159 on Management of Depression for specific medications and dosing.) In particular, psychostimulants act rapidly, counteract opioid-induced sedation, and have analgesic activity. They can be the treatment of choice in patients facing a short prognosis, and they are often combined with an SSRI in severe depression (and while the SSRI is taking effect over weeks to a month). Serotonin-norepinephrine reuptake inhibitors can be good choices for patients with both depression and neuropathic pain, whereas the antidepressant mirtazapine also can improve appetite, anxiety, nausea, and insomnia at low doses.

The ICU team should consult specialists in palliative care and/or psychiatry for patients with refractory depression and anxiety, unusually intense grief, and/or persistent requests for hastened death.

Last Hours of Living and Syndrome of Imminent Death

ICU clinicians frequently witness patients dying of critical and chronic illness. These deaths can be sudden and unpredicted, or expected after a long decline; exhaustive after a lengthy medical "fight" to save or prolong a patient's life; calm with recognition and planning for end of life, or some combination of all of the above. Regardless of the path, the ways that patients die have profound ripple effects on families, loved ones, and ICU staff for years to come. It is paramount for ICU clinicians to have the knowledge and skills to expertly care for dying patients, and cultivate a calm, empathetic presence to counsel and reassure grieving families at the bedside [49].

Preparing for the Last Hours of Life

The ICU team should anticipate that actively dying patients require continuous skilled care and attempt to create an environment in the patient's room that supports privacy and intimacy. The patient and family should be reassessed regularly, and staff should be able to respond quickly to symptom crises and/or family concerns. Standardized order sets can help promote best practices, and utilization of the entire interdisciplinary team (including social work and chaplaincy) can address all aspects of suffering (see Fig. 35.1). If staff and family members feel confident in their caregiving abilities, the experience can be a meaningful time of life review, legacy creation, celebration, and healing. While the timing of death can be unpredictable, everyone should be aware of the potential time course, signs of the dying process, and how to manage any symptoms. The ICU team should also inquire about faith and cultural traditions (including after-death care and handling of the patient's body) and strive to honor any requests and rituals.

Physiological Changes and Symptoms

In order to effectively manage symptoms and counsel families, ICU clinicians need to understand the pathophysiology of the dying process and common associated issues [49] (see Fig. 35.1).

Medication use. As patients approach death, their absorption, metabolism, and excretion of drugs is highly impaired; therefore, clinicians should reassess the need for each medication and minimize polypharmacy and potential side effects as much as possible. Choosing the least invasive route of administration, medication should be used for relief of pain, dyspnea, excess secretions, agitated delirium, and seizure prophylaxis, depending on the clinical scenario. Patients should never be started routinely on morphine infusions ("start 1 mg per hour IV, titrate to comfort") in the absence of symptoms. Sound pharmacologic principles always apply, such as the use of morphine IV boluses as needed for intermittent pain, and calculation of basal infusions on the basis of the amount of as-needed dosing. Indiscriminate morphine dosing can lead to build-up of active metabolites [4] as renal failure occurs, resulting in agitated delirium from opioid neurotoxicity and/or hastened death (Fig. 35.1).

Fatigue and weakness. As a patient approaches death, providing sufficient cushioning on the bed will decrease the need for frequent turning and repositioning. Patients may have joint position fatigue and require passive range of motion of their joints every few hours.

Decreasing appetite, thirst, and intake. Families often worry that their loved one is "starving" and feel guilt that they are causing or contributing to death. Most patients lose their appetite and thirst, instead preferring bites and sips of favorite foods and fluids, and in the final hours prefer only mouth care. Studies show that parenteral or enteral feeding patients close to death neither prolongs life nor improves symptom control [50]. Instead, indiscriminate use of artificial nutrition and hydration can lead to anasarca, pulmonary edema, upper airway secretions, and increased incontinence, contributing to skin breakdown. Most experts agree that anorexia and dehydration as part of the dying process may be helpful as the resulting ketosis and endorphin release can promote a sense of well-being [51].

Mucosal and conjunctival care. Meticulous hydration of the lips, nose, and eyes can prevent discomfort from dry, cracked, and irritated mucous membranes. Moisten and clean the oral mucosa frequently, and treat oral candidiasis with topical nystatin. Coat the lips and anterior nasal mucosa with a thin layer of lubricant to reduce evaporation (which should be non-petroleum based if patient is using oxygen). If eyelids do not close, moisten conjunctiva with artificial tears or ophthalmic lubricating gel frequently.

Cardiac dysfunction and renal failure. Dying patients have diminishing peripheral blood perfusion, and families will notice mottling of their loved one's skin (livedo reticularis). Tachycardia, hypotension, peripheral cooling, and peripheral and central cyanosis are expected. Urine output drops as renal perfusion decreases, and eventually oliguria or anuria occurs.

Neurologic dysfunction. The neurologic changes associated with the dying process often follow two different patterns [49]—the "usual road" and the "difficult road" (see Fig. 35.1). Most patients follow the "usual road," which leads to decreasing levels of consciousness, coma, and death. In the "difficult road," patients experience increasing levels of confusion, restlessness, and agitated delirium (see management of delirium in this chapter). Despite patients' decreased abilities to communicate, families and clinicians should talk to the patient as if she or he were conscious because data from the operating room and "near death" experiences suggest patients may be more aware than caregivers perceive. Families and friends should also be encouraged to express their feelings to the patient to help with life closure ("I love you," "I forgive you," "Please forgive me," "Thank you," and "Goodbye") [52].

Respiratory dysfunction. As patients are close to death, their breathing patterns become shallow and rapid with periods of apnea (Cheyne–Stokes respirations), followed by agonal breaths in the moments before death. Families and clinicians often find these patterns distressing, and it is important to counsel them on these expected physiologic changes. If patients appear to have increased work of breathing (evidenced by accessory muscle use and grimacing), low doses of opioids can help reduce the perception of breathlessness [39].

Loss of ability to swallow. During the dying process, patients eventually use the ability to swallow due to weakness, impaired cognition, loss of gag reflex, and reflexive clearing of the oropharynx. As a result, oral secretions accumulate and may lead to gurgling or rattling sounds with each breath, which can be distressing to families. Repositioning and postural drainage can often resolve these sounds; if not, anticholinergic medications can be effective in drying these secretions. Glycopyrralate is the drug of choice because it does not cross the blood–brain barrier compared with other commonly used anticholinergic agents (atropine and scopolamine) and is likely less to induce or worsen delirium.

When death occurs. Even when death is expected, no one knows what it will feel like until it occurs. The interdisciplinary team is essential to supporting families in their acute grief, and following up on those with complicated grief. After a death, the ICU team should disconnect any lines or machines, remove catheters, and clean the patient to help create a peaceful vision of their loved one. Families should not feel rushed and encouraged to touch and hold the person's body (while maintaining universal body fluid precautions). The ICU team should take time to debrief their own sadness and distress, especially in challenging cases. Equally important is acknowledging the sense of satisfaction and meaning that comes with helping a patient die in comfort and dignity and supporting a family through this devastating time in their lives (see Chapter 36).

References

1. National Consensus Project for Quality Palliative Care: Clinical practice guidelines for quality palliative care. http://www.nationalconsensusproject.org. 2004. Accessed January 31, 2017.
2. Gilron I, Bailey JM, Tu D, et al: Morphine, gabapentin or their combination for neuropathic pain. *N Engl J Med* 352:1324–1334, 2005.
3. Moryl N, Coyle N, Foley K: Managing an acute pain crisis in a patient with advance cancer: "This is as much of a crisis as a code." *JAMA* 299(12):1457–1467, 2008.
4. Lee M, Silverman SM, Hansen H, et al: A comprehensive review of opioid-induced hyperalgesia. *Pain Physician* 14:145–161, 2011.
5. Parshall MB, Schwartzstein RM, Adams L, et al: An official American Thoracic Society statement: update on the mechanisms, assessment and management of dyspnea. *Am J Respir Crit Care Med* 185:435–452, 2012.
6. Singer AE, Meeker D, Teno JM, et al: Symptom trends in the last year of life from 1998 to 2010: a cohort study. *Ann Intern Med* 162:175–183, 2015.
7. Currow DC, Smith J, Davidson PM, et al: Do the trajectories of dyspnea differ in prevalence and intensity by diagnosis at the end of life? A consecutive cohort study. *J Pain Symptom Manage* 39:680–690, 2010.
8. Mahler DA, Selecky PA, Harrod CG, et al: American College of Chest Physicians consensus statement on the management of dyspnea in patients with advanced lung or heart disease. *Chest* 137:674–691, 2010.
9. Ekstrom M, Nilsson F, Abernethy A, et al: Effects of opioids on breathlessness and exercise capacity in chronic obstructive pulmonary disease: a systematic review. *Ann Am Thorac Soc* 12:1079–1092, 2015.
10. Ben-Aharon I, Gafter-Gvili A, Leibovici L, et al: Interventions for alleviating cancer-related dyspnea: a systematic review and meta-analysis. *Acta Oncol* 51:996–1008, 2012.
11. Jennings AL, Davies AN, Higgins JP, et al: A systematic review of the use of opioids in the management of dyspnea. *Thorax* 57:939–944, 2002.
12. Nava S, Ferrer M, Esquinas A, et al: Palliative use of non-invasive ventilation in end-of-life patients with solid tumors: a randomized feasibility trial. *Lancet Oncol* 14:219–227, 2013.
13. Hui D, Morgado M, Chisholm G, et al: High-flow oxygen and bilevel positive airway pressure for persistent dyspnea in patients with advanced cancer: a phase ii randomized trial. *J Pain Symptom Manage* 46:463–473, 2013.
14. Galbraith S, Fagan P, Perkins P, et al: Does the use of a handheld fan improve chronic dyspnea? A randomized, controlled, crossover trial. *J Pain Symptom Manage* 39:831–838, 2010.
15. Ahmedzai SH, Laude E, Robertson A, et al: A double-blind, randomized, controlled phase ii trial of heliox28 gas mixture in lung cancer patients with dyspnea on exertion. *Br J Cancer* 90:366–371, 2004.
16. Sheikh MVH, Mahshidfar B, Rabiee H, et al: The adjunctive effect of nebulized furosemide in COPD exacerbation: a randomized controlled clinical trial. *Respir Care* 58:1873–1877, 2013.
17. Moore RP, Berlowitz DJ, Denehy L, et al: A randomized trial of domiciliary, ambulatory oxygen in patients with COPD and dyspnea but without resting hypoxemia. *Thorax* 66:32–37, 2011.
18. Abernethy AP, McDonald CF, Frith PA, et al: Effect of palliative oxygen versus room air in relief of breathlessness in patients with refractory dyspnea: a double-blind, randomized controlled trial. *Lancet* 376:784–793, 2010.
19. Reintam Blaser A, Malbrain ML, Starkopf J, et al: Gastrointestinal function in ICU patients: terminology, definitions and management. Recommendations of the ESICM Working Group on Abdominal Problems. *Intensive Care Med* 38(3):384–394, 2012.
20. Guerra TL, Mendonca SS, Marshall NG: Incidence of constipation in an intensive care unit. *Rev Bras Ter Intensiva* 25(20):87–92, 2013.
21. Reintam A, Parm P, Kitus R, et al: Gastrointestinal symptoms in intensive care patients. *Acta Anaesthesiol Scand* 53(3):318–324, 2009.
22. Nguyen T, Frenette AJ, Johanson C, et al: Impaired gastrointestinal transit and its associated morbidity in the intensive care unit. *J Crit Care* 28(4):537.e11–537.e17, 2013.
23. Krassioukov A, Eng JJ, Claxton G, et al: Neurogenic bowel management after spinal cord injury: a systematic review of the evidence. *Spinal Cord* 48(10):718–733, 2010.
24. Mendoza J, Legido J, Rubio S, et al: Systematic review: the adverse effects of sodium phosphate enema. *Aliment Pharmacol Ther* 26(1):9–20, 2007.
25. Candy B, Jones L, Goodman ML, et al: Laxatives or methylnaltrexone for the management of constipation in palliative care patients. *Cochrane Database Syst Rev* (1):CD003448, 2011.
26. Wood GJ, Shega JW, Lynch B, et al: Management of intractable nausea and vomiting in patients at the end of life: "I was feeling nauseous all of the time. . . nothing was working". *JAMA* 298(10):1196–1207, 2007.
27. Rawlinson A, Kitchingham N, Hart C, et al: Mechanisms of reducing postoperative pain, nausea and vomiting: a systematic review of current techniques. *Evid Based Med* 17(3):75–80, 2012.
28. Basch E, Prestrud AA, Hesketh PJ, et al: Antiemetics: American Society of clinical oncology clinical practice guideline update. *J Clin Oncol* 29(31):4189–4198, 2011.
29. Buttner M, Walder B, von Elm E, et al: Is low-dose haloperidol a useful antiemetic? A meta-analysis of published and unpublished randomized trials. *Anesthesiology* 101(6):1454–1463, 2004.
30. Navari R: Olanzapine for the prevention and treatment of chronic nausea and chemotherapy-induced nausea and vomiting. *Eur J Pharm* 722:180–186, 2014.
31. Rojas C, Slusher BS: Pharmacological mechanisms of 5-HT_3 and tachykinin NK(1) receptor antagonism to prevent chemotherapy-induced nausea and vomiting. *Eur J Pharmcol* 684(1):1–7, 2012.
32. Breitbart W, Alici Y: Agitation and delirium at the end of life. . ."We couldn't manage him." *JAMA* 300(24):2898–2910, 2008.
33. Neto AS, Nassar AP, Cardoso SO, et al: Delirium screening in critically ill patients: a systematic review and meta-analysis. *Crit Care Med* 40:1946–1951, 2012.
34. Irwin SA, Pirrello RD, Hirst JM, et al: Clarifying delirium management: practical, evidence-based, expert recommendations for clinical practice. *J Pall Med* 16(4):1–13, 2013.
35. Zaal U, Spruyt CF, Peelen LM, et al: Intensive care unit environment may affect the course of delirium. *Intensive Care Med* 39:481–488, 2013.
36. Tainter CR, Levine AR, Quraishi SA, et al: Noise levels in surgical ICUs are consistently above recommended standards. *Crit Care Med* 44(1):147–152, 2016.
37. Litton E, Carnegie V, Elliott R, et al: The efficacy of earplugs as a sleep hygiene strategy for reducing delirium in the ICU: a systematic review and meta-analysis. *Crit Care Med* 44:992–999, 2016. PMID:26741578.
38. Schweickert WD, Pohlman MC, Pohlman AS, et al: Early physical and occupational therapy in mechanically ventilated, critically ill patients: a randomized controlled trial. *Lancet* 373:1874–1882, 2009.
39. Barr J, Fraser GL, Puntillo K, et al: Clinical practice guidelines for the management of pain, agitation, and delirium in adult patients in the intensive care unit. *Crit Care Med* 41(1):263–306, 2013.
40. Pasin L, Landoni G, Nardelli P, et al: Dexmedetomidine reduces the risk of delirium, agitation and confusion in critically ill patients: a meta-analysis of randomized controlled trials. *J Cardiothorac Vasc Anesth* 28(6):1459–1466, 2014.
41. Balas MC, Vasilevskis EE, Olsen KM, et al: Effectiveness and safety of awakening and breathing coordination, delirium monitoring/management, and early exercise/mobility bundle. *Crit Care Med* 42:1024–1036, 2014.
42. Lonergan E, Britton AM, Luxemberg J, et al: Antipsychotics for delirium. *Cochrane Database Syst Rev* (2):CD005594, 2007.
43. American Academy of Hospice and Palliative Medicine: AAHPM palliative sedation position statement 2014. Accessed at http://aahpm.org/positions/palliative-sedation. Accessed May, 2016.
44. Byock I: *The Best Care Possible: A Physician's Quest to Transform Care Through the End of Life*. Penguin Publishing Group, 2013.
45. Miovic M, Block S: Psychiatric disorders in advanced cancer. *Cancer* 110(8):1665–1667, 2007.
46. Kadan-Lottick NS, Vanderwerker LC, Block SD, et al: Psychiatric disorders and mental health service use in patients with advanced cancer: a report from the coping with cancer study. *Cancer* 104:2872–2881, 2005.
47. Peris A: Early intra-intensive care unit psychological intervention promotes recovery from post traumatic stress disorders, anxiety and depression symptoms in critically ill patients. *Crit Care* 15(1):R41, 2011.
48. Mitchell AJ: Are one or two simple questions sufficient to detect depression in cancer and palliative care? A Bayesian meta-analysis. *Br J Cancer* 98:1934–1943, 2008.
49. Ferris F: Last hours of living. *Clin Geriatr Med* 20:641–667, 2004.
50. Dev R, Dalal S, Bruera E: Is there a role for parenteral nutrition or hydration at the end of life? *Curr Opin Support Palliat Care* 6(3):365–370, 2012.
51. Ganzini L, Goy ER, Miller LL, et al: Nurses' experiences with hospice patients who refuse food and fluids to hasten death. *N Engl J Med* 349:359–365, 2003.
52. Byock I: *The Four Things that Matter Most*. Simon and Schuster, 2004.

Chapter 36 ■ Being with Suffering: Addressing Existential and Spiritual Distress

MARGARET ISAAC • SUZANA K. E. MAKOWSKI • CHRISTINA FITCH

INTRODUCTION

With modern medicine has come the ability to prolong the course of illnesses that previously caused rapid decline and death. Critical and life-threatening illness often brings existential and spiritual concerns to the fore. One consequence of our ability to delay death with modern medical treatments is the prolongation of existential suffering as patients cope with the knowledge that death is imminent. While clinicians may feel competent and knowledgeable in addressing physical symptoms and psychological distress, existential and spiritual concerns can be more intangible, complex, and challenging, falling outside of what most physicians consider to be their scope of practice [1].

Some data suggest that existential and spiritual concerns may cause more distress to patients than physical and psychological symptoms [2]. Despite this, a majority of patients do not feel that their spiritual needs are supported by medical providers [3]. Barriers identified by physicians include a lack of time, lack of experience, and the belief that addressing spiritual distress is not part of a physician's role [1]. Patients who feel that their spiritual needs are not addressed adequately by medical providers rate their care more poorly [4]. In contrast, patients and families who are satisfied with how their spiritual needs are met (and those for whom clergy have been involved at the end of life) are more satisfied overall with their care [5].

Starting a dialog about spiritual and existential concerns opens the door to a holistic model of care and healing. By developing an understanding of the types of existential and spiritual distress from which patients and their families can suffer, as well as specific approaches toward addressing this distress, clinicians can enhance their ability to provide compassionate and holistic care for patients at the end of life as well as their loved ones.

DEFINITIONS

Suffering was defined by Cassell [6] in his seminal work as "the state of severe distress associated with events that threaten the intactness of the person". Existential distress can be difficult to define—one review identified 56 different definitions in the literature [7]. In addition, there can be substantial overlap between the concepts of existential and spiritual distress. Kissane [8], building on the work of Yalom, describes eight main types of existential challenge: death anxiety, loss and change, freedom with choice or loss of control, dignity of the self, fundamental aloneness, altered quality of relationships, search for meaning, and mystery about what seems unknowable. Loss of control over one's life, loss of meaning, or the experience of being a burden (which relates to dignity of the self) are common symptoms that patients describe as being "unbearable" [9].

There are many definitions of spirituality described in the literature, though most include an exploration of meaning, transcendence, and relationships with self, others, and force(s) larger than oneself. An international group of experts has defined spirituality in specific terms: "Spirituality is a dynamic and intrinsic aspect of humanity through which persons seek ultimate meaning, purpose, and transcendence, and experience relationship to self, family, others, community, society, nature, and the significant or sacred. Spirituality is expressed through beliefs, values, traditions, and practices" [10]. Spirituality can be a key means through which patients cope with illness and mortality.

Religion can be defined as a particular system of faith and worship [11], and as a formal structure through which beliefs are practiced within a community.

RELIGIOUS TRADITIONS AT THE END OF LIFE

Religion and spirituality can impact medical decisions that are made at the end of life, though many differences across patients attributed to religion and spirituality are more accurately ascribed to cultural beliefs and values [12]. There are large and meaningful differences between spiritual and religious groups and, even more so, within them. Different religious traditions have heterogeneous views on the definition of death and on the withdrawal of life-sustaining interventions.

With the development of biomedical technologies and the medicalization of end-of-life care, spiritual and religious leaders are being increasingly called upon to speak to the appropriateness of end-of-life treatments and decisions. Specific formalized doctrines and proscriptions within individual traditions will be summarized below. These beliefs can shape the decisions of individuals around treatment decisions, though providers are cautioned to practice using a model of cultural humility rather than cultural competence [13]. In other words, physicians should avoid making assumptions about the beliefs of an individual, which may be very different than those expressed by the religious institution with whom they identify.

Christianity

Most Christian denominations support the withholding and withdrawal of life-sustaining treatments, though there is heterogeneity among Protestant denominations on physician aid in dying. The Greek Orthodox Church, in contrast, generally opposes the withholding and withdrawal of life-sustaining treatments and artificial nutrition, even for patients who wish to forego these treatments, maintaining in a statement from the Holy Synod that "the doctor has the moral obligation to assist the patient to consent to the effort being made to keep him alive" [14].

Catholicism

The Roman Catholic Church allows for the withholding and withdrawing of life-sustaining treatments if those treatments are deemed to be futile, burdensome, or disproportionate to the expected outcome. If treatment is deemed as such, the Church also supports the alleviation of suffering, even when consciousness is reduced and death hastened as unintentional side effects. However, the Church does not find it ethical to withhold or withdraw treatment based on patient's wishes if active treatment would be considered reasonable and life-prolonging [12,15].

Judaism

Jewish law (Halakha) dictates that death cannot be hastened, even when illness is terminal. A clear distinction is made between active and passive actions and between withdrawing and withholding life-sustaining interventions. Neither physician aid with dying nor withdrawal of *continuous* life-sustaining treatments that have already been initiated is allowed. Allowances can be made to first switch continuous treatments (such as mechanical ventilation) to intermittent settings (e.g., putting ventilators on timers), then discontinuing these treatments, given that continuing these interventions may cause suffering, the alleviation of which is a moral requirement [16]. Withholding life-prolonging treatments is considered permissible [12].

Islam

Islamic law (Shariah) dictates that all efforts should be made to prevent premature death, though withholding and withdrawing treatments at the end of life are permitted, provided that death is inevitable and that treatments are unlikely to improve outcomes or quality of life [12].

Hinduism and Buddhism

Buddhist and Hindu traditions share the belief that the body and the soul exist separately and that the body can be shed as the soul lives on or is reincarnated. In both traditions, it is believed that the time of physical death (e.g., death pronouncement) is only the beginning of the process of death for the soul [17]. Hinduism has many diverse interpretations and encompasses a myriad of traditions, though a "good death," late in life, peaceful, with one's affairs in order, is valued. The belief that this current life is a transition between the one before and the one after shapes views around end-of-life care and priorities [18].

Atheism

Little data exist describing the end-of-life preferences of patients who identify as atheist or agnostic. However, one small study found that atheists may have a conceptualization of a "good death" similar to other patients, but may have stronger preferences for evidence-based medical treatments at the end of life and physician aid when dying [19].

IMPACT OF RELIGIOSITY ON END-OF-LIFE DECISIONS

The literature evaluating the effect of religiosity on end-of-life care preferences is mixed. Some data suggest that other factors may have a bigger impact on resuscitation preferences than religiosity [20,21]. Other studies have demonstrated that patients and families who identify as religious or spiritual [3,22], who utilize spiritual coping strategies [23], and who express deference to God's will [24] are more likely to choose treatments to extend life. Patients who identify as religious may also be less likely to opt for a do-not-attempt-resuscitation order [25]. Additionally, those who feel that the length of life is determined by a higher power are less likely to engage in advance care planning [26].

DIAGNOSIS OF EXISTENTIAL SUFFERING AND LOSS OF PERSONHOOD

Existential suffering is poorly understood by many clinicians [7], which can make it difficult to recognize and treat. Because suffering is experienced by the whole person, and not limited to a specific part of the body or mind [27], developing an understanding of personhood is key to identifying and addressing suffering. Some existential distress is related to physical suffering and loss of dignity and personhood as patients struggle with life-limiting illness [28], and, conversely, loss of dignity and personhood is associated with an increase of physical, psychological [29], or existential suffering [30]. Personhood also has many definitions, though common themes include that persons are unique and rational, possessing of autonomy, intention, and purpose [31]. The notions of personhood and person-centered care are central to the provision of competent and holistic palliative and end-of-life care. Cassell highlights the wholeness of personhood, writing that "the understanding of the place of person during human illness requires a rejection of the historical dualism of mind and body" [6].

The Patient Dignity Question (PDQ) has been proposed by Harvey Chochinov and colleagues [32] as a means to evaluate personhood and is simple and straightforward to ask: "What do I need to know about you as a person to give you the best care possible?" Epstein and Back [33] have offered the question "What's the worst part of this for you?" as a means to recognize suffering, cultivate curiosity and empathy, and engage with patients in a deeper way—what they term "turning towards suffering".

Additionally, the Pictorial Representation of Illness and Self Measure (PRISM) tool was developed to aid with the assessment of suffering and the impact of illness and has been used specifically to assess spiritual and existential distress [34]. The PRISM tool consists of a white board and a fixed yellow circle representing the self. A smaller red circle represents their disease process, and patients are asked, "Where would you put the illness disk to represent its place in your life right now?" The distance between the middle of the self and the disease disk is termed the *self–illness separation*. This correlates inversely with suffering and positively with perceived control over illness and coping resources.

The Faith, Importance, Community, and Address (**FICA**) tool [35] is a useful guide to begin conversations between providers and patients about spirituality. The questions include:

- Faith, belief, and meaning
- Importance and influence
- Community
- Address/action in care

This tool can allow providers to open the door to further exploration and discussion around spiritual and existential distress and coping mechanisms. Another acronym, **HOPE**, provides a similarly useful framework for spiritual assessment [36]:

- H—sources of hope, meaning, connection, strength
- O—organized religion
- P—personal spirituality and practices
- E—effects on health care and end-of-life decision-making

Table 36.1 summarizes useful tools for spiritual assessment and sample questions.

ADDRESSING EXISTENTIAL AND SPIRITUAL DISTRESS: USE OF AN INTERDISCIPLINARY TEAM

The need to integrate the assessment and treatment of existential and spiritual distress is important for the care of the critically ill patient. This is particularly important given the acknowledgment, as outlined before, that increased sense of religiosity may impact preferences related to end-of-life care, and the fact that addressing spiritual and existential suffering improves quality of life even at the end of life [1]. Critical and palliative care teams commonly utilize an interdisciplinary approach involving psychologists and social workers to help address the emotional distress of patients. A similar model of interdisciplinary collaboration is

TABLE 36.1

Useful Tools for Spiritual/Existential Assessment

Framework	Domains	Sample questions
Single questions	Dignity and personhood (Patient dignity question)	"What do I need to know about you as a person to give you the best care possible?"[32]
	Suffering	"What's the worst part of this for you?"[33]
FICA[35]	Faith, belief, and meaning	"Do you consider yourself spiritual or religious?" "What gives your life meaning?"
	Importance and Influence	"What importance does your faith or belief have in your life?" "Do you have specific beliefs that might influence your health care decisions? If so, are you willing to share those with your health care team?"
	Community	"Are you a member of a spiritual or religious community?" "Is there a group of people you really love or who are important to you?" "Who matters the most to you?"
	Address/Action in Care	"How would you like me to address these issues in your health care?" "How can we honor these parts of your life while you are in the hospital?"
HOPE[36]	Sources of Hope, comfort, connection, strength, meaning	"What gives you hope?" "What sources of support do you have?" "What gives your life meaning?" "What gets you through difficult times?"
	Organized religion	"Do you belong to a religious community or tradition?" "What are the ways that this helpful to you (and not-so-helpful)?"
	Personal spirituality and practices	"Do you have any personal spiritual beliefs or practices?" "Do you have any spiritual beliefs outside of organized religion?" "What aspects of that practice are most helpful to you?"
	Effects on health care and end-of-life decision-making	"How do these beliefs and values shape your decisions about health care?" "Are there any ways in which you could imagine your religious beliefs coming into conflict with the care we are providing?" "Would you like for us to have our hospital chaplain explore this in more detail with you?" "How can we address these aspects of your care while you're in the hospital?"

needed to most effectively—and efficiently—meet the needs of our patients who experience spiritual suffering [37] (Fig. 36.1).

The hospital specialist in the spiritual domain is the chaplain. Within this specialty, there are two principal types of chaplains. This distinction should be recognized by clinicians to understand the nature of the relationship between patient and chaplain before hospitalization as well as the chaplain's familiarity with serious illness and the health care system:

1. The hospital or health-system–based chaplain (health care chaplain) is most often employed by the hospital. This type of chaplain serves the spiritual and religious needs of patients regardless of faith. They are often called to support patients and families whether or not they self-identify as religious or spiritual. The health care chaplain usually has a master's degree, and formal certification requires at least an additional 1,600 hours of training in clinical pastoral education or CPE. Just as with physicians, there is a tacit agreement to abide by a specific code of ethics and professional practice standards. These chaplains work closely with clinical teams, are integrated with the spiritual and faith communities of the patients they serve, and often collaborate with denominational chaplains (see the following paragraph).
2. The denominational chaplain is usually employed by a specific faith-based group, providing outreach to members

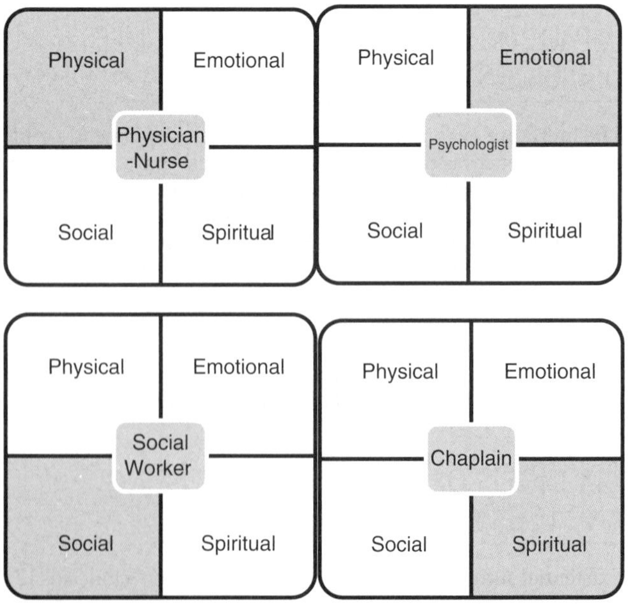

FIGURE 36.1 Interdisciplinary care of the critically ill patient [38]. Darkened box indicates primary focus of role.

BOX 36.1: CASE EXAMPLE

Addressing Spiritual Needs in the Intensive Care Unit

Ms. M is a 20 year-old young woman in a motor vehicle crash who sustained a severe traumatic brain injury and multiple fractures. Her hospital course has been complicated by multi-organ system failure. Due to the extent and nature of her injuries, the neurology consult service has communicated to the family that they do not think she will have any meaningful neurologic recovery, though she is not brain dead.

Her parents and two siblings have been involved in multiple family conferences over the course of her hospitalization. They identify as evangelical Christians and have been well supported by their church community during this time. They express a wish to continue life-sustaining treatments including mechanical intubation, and pressors indefinitely, stating that they have been praying for a miracle, and that Ms. M needs to be kept alive long enough to allow that miracle to occur.

The ICU team consulted both the hospital chaplain/spiritual care service, and the palliative care team. The chaplain first met with the family separately as well to explore their theology and their conceptualization of how a miracle might occur. Through these conversations, they came to feel that God would intervene with a miracle if He chose, independent of the artificial means of life support that were being provided by the medical team. They also felt strongly after these conversations that God would not want Ms. M to suffer. Over a series of family conferences that all began with prayer, the family agreed to make the patient DNAR, and later agreed to withdraw ventilator support and pressors.

of their religious community. These chaplains are not mandated to have the formal clinical training of their health care–based colleagues and can have a widely variable level of familiarity with critical illness and supporting those in medical crisis [38].

While the physician, nurse and social worker can assess and provide basic spiritual support for critically ill patients and their families, collaboration with chaplains, especially health care chaplains, is considered a best practice to address the spiritual needs of both patients and families [39].

Furthermore, as previously mentioned, data suggest that family members of patients who died in the intensive care unit (ICU) rate the overall experience better when chaplains were involved in the care of their critically ill loved ones during the final days of life [4]. Too often, chaplains are called in to see patients only in the final hours of their lives. Offering chaplaincy support to patients and families of critically ill patients earlier in their hospital stay may help address patient and family anxiety (see Box 36.1 for case example).

HOPE AND RESILIENCY—RESTORATION OF PERSONHOOD

Hopefulness is not merely an emotion, nor is it considered by psychologists to be something that is passively received. Rather, hope is a dynamic cognitive construct—both an emotion and a behavior. Hope not only has a role in life when looking forward to a bright or ambitious future, but also plays a critical role for helping people cope with and reframe serious life events, such as trauma, illness, and even death [40]. Redirection of what to hope for and supporting a means of hope may strengthen patient–clinician bonds and prevent feelings of abandonment [36].

When fighting a life-threatening illness, maintaining hope can help patients and families foster emotional resilience. Clinicians often hesitate to share prognostic information with patients and family members for fear of depriving them of hope. Research indicates that physicians avoid prognostication for fear of (1) causing anxiety and increased stress for patients and families, perhaps worsening their clinical outcomes; (2) influencing colleagues' attitudes about their effectiveness of care, potentially decreasing vigilance in the fight to cure; and (3) naming a possible negative outcome could make it more possible [41,42].

In contrast, many patients and families report that honest discussion about prognosis does not interfere with hope, and perhaps even helps support its maintenance. Despite this preference, family members of critically ill patients often demonstrate avoidant behaviors that suggest not wishing to "know all." This demonstrated ambivalence reflects the emotional struggle of not wanting to acknowledge their loved ones' serious prognosis. This difficulty can be mitigated by frequent clinician conversations to help patients and surrogate decision-makers process and prepare for the worst, while continuing to hold on to hope for the best realistically possible outcome [43,44] (e.g., "hope for the best, and prepare for the worst").

Furthermore, similar to suffering, a patient's individual notion of what hope is should be explored. Often, while the initial reflexive response is to survive or to return to good health, when examined further, the answers are more complex. Physicians often believe that when patients and their families ask whether something more can be done, they are referring to whether another procedure or intervention is possible. However, patients are often asking whether more can be done to help restore their personhood—some improvement in their physical well-being, an increased ability to return to performing in their identified roles, or simply to return home without suffering. They are also often asking for clarity in prognosis and support for themselves and their families to complete their life story with respect for the way they have always lived [45].

Life review and dignity therapy are psychotherapy methods specifically for patients with life-limiting illness. These approaches seek to support the dignity and resiliency of the person. Dignity therapy was developed by Dr. Harvey Chochinov to address sources of psychosocial and existential distress as well as provide a means of recording in a written legacy or "generativity document" thoughts they find valuable for their loved ones. The interview technique focuses on the events, roles, and accomplishments that were most important to the patient over their lifetime and also allows the dying person to share their hopes and dreams for those they will leave behind [46]. The meaning making that is created through dignity therapy has been shown to decrease patient suffering and increase a sense of both dignity and purpose [47].

IMPACT OF MEDICAL DECISIONS ON GRIEF AND BEREAVEMENT

Grief is a normal response to the loss of a family member or close friend. This can be a consequence not only of death itself, but also the loss of what constitutes the "personhood" of someone loved. For example, after 55 years of marriage, a wife can grieve the loss of her independent spouse who now needs to be placed in nursing home after a traumatic fall. A young athlete can grieve the loss of his sense of future and identity after having suffered a spinal cord injury. Grief also does not only occur after trauma, but also with protracted illness, or other intense loss.

Most people exhibit tremendous resiliency when grieving the death of a person loved. Resiliency can come from connection with sense of purpose, reflection on meaning of the relationship and life review, and both spiritual and religious factors. Respecting and infusing religious traditions and values at the end of life can further help add meaning to the loss. In many religions, ensuring a patient's honor and integrity at the end of life can support a family's bereavement. In Islamic tradition, for example, these efforts can reflect a family's acceptance of the Koranic teaching that there are times to let nature take its course (Al-Qur'an 39:42) and an assurance that their advocacy role as loving family members has been fulfilled [48].

However, approximately 10% of people who grieve develop protracted symptoms, what used to be called *complicated grief disorder*, but now is characterized as either depression or adjustment disorder of *DSM-5* [49]. Historically, a "bereavement exclusion" was made in the diagnosis of major depressive disorder—reflecting a belief that bereavement is a natural process and should not be pathologized. While it shares some symptomatology with major depression, grief has unique features as well, including the preservation of self-esteem, and positive memories and feelings related to the loved one combined with sadness. The bereavement exclusion was removed from *DSM-5* [49], though differentiating between major depression and grief remains complex [50].

Social isolation and underdeveloped coping mechanisms contribute to the risk of complex grief [51]. Perceived conflict between medical decisions and religious beliefs may contribute to increased suffering during bereavement [52,53]. In particular, this may be due to beliefs that the deceased may suffer consequences of decisions made during the final weeks of life. For example, in Buddhism, some believe that terminal delirium or confusion may cause the soul to become lost during the process of rebirth. It can be helpful for the medical team to seek guidance not only from the ethics committee, but also from religious leaders and experts to help inform how specific religious medical ethics and laws could influence decision-making. When appropriate, and with the help of chaplaincy, reassuring families that their decisions are consistent with their religious beliefs (especially around topics such as withholding or withdrawing life support, nutrition, or other interventions) can help mitigate grief responses that come out of spiritual distress or conflict.

SELF-CARE AND AVOIDING BURNOUT

Spirituality, as defined in this chapter, is broader than religion and religiosity. It is about resilience, hope, meaning making and purpose, and the ability to tend to suffering. As such, it is a concept that does not only apply to something assessed and offered to patients. Rather, in this broader sense, it can play a central role for preventing burnout among critical care physicians and nurses. Studies suggest that up to 50% of ICU physicians and 30% of ICU nurses meet criteria for severe burnout [54].

While for many, burnout is associated with long work hours and increased productivity pressures, for others, burnout is more causally related to end-of-life care conflicts, such as moral distress associated with poor interprofessional and provider–patient/family communication around end-of-life care issues [55]. Furthermore, burnout is linked with an individuals' level of motivation for excellence in their work and willingness to put aside self-awareness and self-care. Major characteristics of burnout include emotional (and physical) exhaustion, depersonalization, and a diminished sense of professional accomplishment or effectiveness. Physicians often correlate patient outcomes with their sense of personal effectiveness. In other words, for many, death of a patient—regardless of cause—equates with clinical failure. This makes care of patients at the end of life particularly high risk for clinician burnout. Unfortunately, research is demonstrating that patient outcomes may also be affected by clinician burnout [56].

In this way, the death of patients in the ICU adds not only to the emotional labor of the work, but also to the risk of burnout among clinicians.

Factors that help mitigate or prevent burnout include not only intrinsic personality characteristics such as hardiness, but also workplace factors such as perceived fairness and sense of support and control. Active spiritual practices such as mindfulness meditation, reflective writing, and cultivation of self-awareness have also demonstrated utility. The interdisciplinary team can play a role for supporting patient care providers' resiliency. Sharing the challenging experiences of caring for people with one's colleagues lends mutual support and counteracts the risk of burnout [57].

SUMMARY

In summary, spiritual and existential concerns are often at the forefront at the end of life (Table 36.2). Many physicians feel ill-equipped to address these issues, but engaging with patients around spiritual and existential distress is an essential part of holistic care. Religious theology and religiosity in general may influence decisions made at the end of life, though there is significant variability within religious and cultural traditions. Tools exist to help physicians assess spirituality and religiosity, as well as personhood and overall suffering. Interdisciplinary collaboration, particularly with chaplaincy, is critical in ensuring that the spiritual and existential needs of the person/patient have been fully addressed. Clinicians have an obligation to be truthful with patients and families about prognosis and also to help foster hope as a tool to build resiliency through critical

TABLE 36.2

Summary of Evidence-Based Recommendations

- Physicians should assess the spiritual and existential needs of patients at the end of life.
- Physicians should have an understanding of how religious and spiritual beliefs might affect decisions at the end of life.
- Loss of personhood and dignity are significant contributors to suffering at the end of life and screening for these is an important part of holistic palliative care.
- The FICA and HOPE tools and Patient Dignity Question can be used to better understand patients' religious/spiritual identities and personhood.
- Involving chaplaincy in the care of critically ill patients is considered a best practice and improves family satisfaction.
- Reframing hope within an honest discussion of prognosis can promote resiliency for patients and their families dealing with serious illness.
- Critical care physicians are at high risk for burnout and can take active steps to maintain their personal wellness as they care for patients at the end of life.

illness. Finally, clinicians who care for patients at the end of life and in the ICU are at high risk for burnout and are well served to use tools such as meditation and reflection, as well as the support of an interdisciplinary team to maintain their own personal wellness.

References

1. Ellis MR, Vinson DC, Ewigman B: Addressing spiritual concerns of patients: family physicians' attitudes and practices. *J Fam Pract* 48(2):105–109, 1999.
2. Puchalski CM, Lunsford B, Harris MH, et al: Interdisciplinary spiritual care for seriously ill and dying patients: a collaborative model. *Cancer J* 12(5):398–416, 2006.
3. Balboni TA, Vanderwerker LC, Block SD, et al: Religiousness and spiritual support among advanced cancer patients and associations with end-of-life treatment preferences and quality of life. *J Clin Oncol* 25(5):555–560, 2007.
4. Astrow AB, Wexler A, Texeira K, et al: Is failure to meet spiritual needs associated with cancer patients' perceptions of quality of care and their satisfaction with care? *J Clin Oncol* 25(36):5753–5757, 2007.
5. Wall RJ, Engelberg RA, Gries CJ, et al: Spiritual care of families in the intensive care unit. *Crit Care Med* 35(4):1084–1090, 2007.
6. Cassell E: *The Nature of Suffering and the Goals of Medicine*. 2nd ed. Oxford, Oxford University Press, 2004.
7. Boston P, Bruce A, Schreiber R: Existential suffering in the palliative care setting: an integrated literature review. *J Pain Symptom Manage* 41(3):604–618, 2011.
8. Kissane DW: The relief of existential suffering. *Arch Intern Med* 172:1501–1505, 2012.
9. Ruijs CD, Kerkhof AJ, van der Wal G, et al: Symptoms, unbearability and the nature of suffering in terminal cancer patients dying at home: a prospective primary care study. *BMC Fam Pract* 14:201, 2013.
10. Puchalski CM, Vitillo R, Hull SK, et al: Improving the spiritual dimension of whole person care: reaching national and international consensus. *J Palliat Med* 17(6):642–656, 2014.
11. Bowker, J: *The Oxford Dictionary of World Religions*, Oxford University Press, 1997.
12. Bülow HH, Sprung CL, Reinhart K, et al: The world's major religions' points of view on end-of-life decisions in the intensive care unit. *Intensive Care Med* 34(3):423–430, 2008.
13. Tervalon M, Murray-García J: Cultural humility versus cultural competence: a critical distinction in defining physician training outcomes in multicultural education. *J Health Care Poor Underserved* 9(2):117–125, 1998.
14. Hellenic Republic, The Holy Synod of the Church of Greece: Basic Positions on the Ethics of Euthanasia. Available from: http://bioethics.org.gr/en/10_frame_10.html. 2002. Accessed February 1, 2017.
15. Pius X: *Address to an International Group of Physicians*. AAS Congregation for the Doctrine of the Faith, Declaration on Euthanasia *Iura et Bona*, 24 February 1957. 49:547–548.
16. Ravitsky V: Timers on ventilators. *BMJ* 330(7488):415–417, 2005.
17. Setta SM, Shemie SD: An explanation and analysis of how world religions formulate their ethical decisions on withdrawing treatment and determining death. *Philos Ethics Humanit Med* 10:6, 2015.
18. Firth S: End-of-life: a Hindu view. *Lancet* 366(9486):682–686, 2005.
19. Smith-Stoner M: End-of-life preferences for atheists. *J Palliat Med* 10(4): 923–928, 2007.
20. Delgado-Guay MO, Chisholm G, Williams J, et al: The association between religiosity and resuscitation status preference among patients with advanced cancer. *Palliat Support Care* 13:1435–1439, 2015.
21. Karches KE, Chung GS, Arora V, et al: Religiosity, spirituality, and end-of-life planning: a single-site survey of medical inpatients. *J Pain Symptom Manage* 44(6):843–851, 2012.
22. True G, Phipps EJ, Braitman LE, et al: Treatment preferences and advance care planning at end of life: role of ethnicity and spiritual coping in cancer patients. *Ann Behav Med* 30(2):174–179, 2005.
23. Phelps AC, Maciejewski PK, Nilsson M, et al: Religious coping and use of intensive life-prolonging care near death in patients with advanced cancer. *JAMA* 301(11):1140–1147, 2009.
24. Winter L, Dennis MP, Parker B: Preferences for life-prolonging medical treatments and deference to the will of god. *J Relig Health* 48(4):418–430, 2009.
25. Jaul E, Zabari Y, Brodsky J: Spiritual background and its association with the medical decision of, DNR at terminal life stages. *Arch Gerontol Geriatr* 58(1):25–29, 2014.
26. Garrido MM, Idler EL, Leventhal H, et al: Pathways from religion to advance care planning: beliefs about control over length of life and end-of-life values. *Gerontologist* 53(5):801–816, 2013.
27. Sensky T: Suffering. *Int J Integr Care* 10 [Suppl]:e024, 2010.
28. Vehling S, Mehnert A: Symptom burden, loss of dignity, and demoralization in patients with cancer: a mediation model. *Psychooncology* 23(3):283–290, 2014.
29. Oechsle K, Wais MC, Vehling S, et al: Relationship between symptom burden, distress, and sense of dignity in terminally ill cancer patients. *J Pain Symptom Manage* 48(3):313–321, 2014.
30. Chochinov HM: Dying, dignity, and new horizons in palliative end-of-life care. *CA Cancer J Clin* 56(2):84–103, 2006; quiz 104-5.
31. Nelson G: Maintaining the integrity of personhood in palliative care. *Scott J Healthc Chaplaincy* 3(2):34–39, 2000.
32. Chochinov HM, McClement S, Hack T, et al: Eliciting personhood within clinical practice: effects on patients, families, and health care providers. *J Pain Symptom Manage* 49(6):974.e2–980.e2, 2015.
33. Epstein RM, Back AL: A PIECE OF MY MIND. Responding to suffering. *JAMA* 314(24):2623–2624, 2015.
34. Büchi S, Sensky T, Sharpe L, et al: Graphic representation of illness: a novel method of measuring patients' perceptions of the impact of illness. *Psychother Psychosom* 67(4–5):222–225, 1998.
35. Puchalski CM: The FICA spiritual history tool #274. *J Palliat Med* 17(1):105–106, 2014.
36. Anandarajah G, Hight E: Spirituality and medical practice: using the HOPE questions as a practical tool for spiritual assessment. *Am Fam Physician* 63(1):81–89, 2001.
37. Richardson P: Spirituality, religion and palliative care. *Ann Palliat Med* 3(3):150–159, 2014.
38. Sinclair S, Chochinov HM: The role of chaplains within oncology interdisciplinary teams. *Curr Opin Support Palliat Care* 6(2):259–268, 2012.
39. Davidson JE, Powers K, Hedayat KM, et al; American College of Critical Care Medicine Task Force 2004–2005: clinical practice guidelines for support of the family in the patient-centered intensive care unit: American College of Critical Care Medicine Task Force 2004–2005. *Crit Care Med* 35(2):605–622, 2007.
40. Fitzgerald Miller J: Hope: a construct central to nursing. *Nurs Forum* 42(1):12–19, 2007.
41. Christakis NA: Prognostication and bioethics. *Daedalus* 128(4):197–214, 1999.
42. Mack JW, Smith TJ: Reasons why physicians do not have discussions about poor prognosis, why it matters, and what can be improved. *J Clin Oncol* 30(22):2715–2717, 2012.
43. Apatira L, Boyd EA, Malvar G, et al: Hope, truth, and preparing for death: perspectives of surrogate decision makers. *Ann Intern Med* 149(12):861–868, 2008.
44. Schenker Y, White DB, Crowley-Matoka M, et al: "It hurts to know... and it helps": exploring how surrogates in the ICU cope with prognostic information. *J Palliat Med* 16(3):243–249, 2013.
45. Sulmasy DP: Spirituality, religion, and clinical care. *Chest* **135**(6):1634–1642, 2009.
46. Chochinov HM, Kristjanson LJ, Breitbart W, et al: Effect of dignity therapy on distress and end-of-life experience in terminally ill patients: a randomised controlled trial. *Lancet Oncol* 12(8):753–762, 2011.
47. Chochinov HM, Hack T, Hassard T, et al: Dignity therapy: a novel psychotherapeutic intervention for patients near the end of life. *J Clin Oncol* 23(24):5520–5525, 2005.
48. Kassim PN, Alias F: End-of-life decisions in Malaysia: Adequacies of ethical codes and developing legal standards. *J Law Med* 22(4):934–950, 2015.
49. American Psychiatric Association: *Diagnostic and Statistical Manual of Mental Disorders (DSM-5)*. 5th ed. American Psychiatric Publishing, 2013.
50. Pies RW: The bereavement exclusion and DSM-5: an update and commentary. *Innov Clin Neurosci* 11(7–8):19–22, 2014.
51. Thomas K, Hudson P, Trauer T, et al: Risk factors for developing prolonged grief during bereavement in family carers of cancer patients in palliative care: a longitudinal study. *J Pain Symptom Manage* 47(3):531–541, 2014.
52. Toscani F, Borreani C, Boeri P, et al: Life at the end of life: beliefs about individual life after death and "good death" models - a qualitative study. *Health Qual Life Outcomes* 1:65, 2003.
53. Anderson WG, Arnold RM, Angus DC, et al: Posttraumatic stress and complicated grief in family members of patients in the intensive care unit. *J Gen Intern Med* 23(11):1871–1876, 2008.
54. Embriaco N, Papazian L, Kentish-Barnes N, et al: Burnout syndrome among critical care healthcare workers. *Curr Opin Crit Care* 13(5):482–488, 2007.
55. Travado L, Grassi L, Gil F, et al: Physician-patient communication among Southern European cancer physicians: the influence of psychosocial orientation and burnout. *Psychooncology* 14(8):661–670, 2005.
56. Sansone RA, Sansone LA: Physician grief with patient death. *Innov Clin Neurosci* 9(4):22–26, 2012.
57. Kearney MK, Weininger RB, Vachon ML, et al: Self-care of physicians caring for patients at the end of life: "Being connected... a key to my survival". *JAMA* 301(11):1155–1164, E1, 2009.

Section 4 SHOCK AND TRAUMA AND SEPSIS MANAGEMENT

TIMOTHY A. EMHOFF

Chapter 37 ■ Resuscitation from Shock Following Hemorrhage

JACOB A. QUICK • DONALD H. JENKINS • JOHN B. HOLCOMB • STEPHEN L. BARNES

INTRODUCTION

Early recognition of exsanguinating hemorrhage is critical to the survivability of an acutely bleeding patient. Typical methods of in-hospital assessment, including blood pressure and hemoglobin levels, are often misleading, and reliance upon these methods frequently result in late recognition of hemorrhagic shock, giving rise to higher mortality rates. Advanced Trauma Life Support program teaches health care providers to incorporate basic physical examination skills (vital signs, pulse pressure, skin color, capillary refill, and mentation) to stratify injury severity, identify and treat immediate threats to life, and to quantify blood loss [1]. Rapid, focused assessment is necessary to expeditiously identify those patients who are either in hemorrhagic shock or at risk for developing it.

Surgical patients die from shock either abruptly via inadequate oxygen delivery or subacutely through development of multisystem organ dysfunction from late recognition or inadequate resuscitation. Unlike the typical nonsurgical critically ill patient, organ dysfunction is often resulted from the acute effects of exsanguination. Hemorrhage accounts for up to 40% of trauma deaths, second only to central nervous system injury [2–4]. Controlling hemorrhage is thus a priority for modern trauma patient care; however, the source of hemorrhage must first be identified, and identified early.

Prior to, during, and following surgical intervention, ongoing resuscitative efforts must proceed appropriately to avoid the sequelae of hypoperfusion. Although commonly utilized in nonbleeding patients, intravenous (IV) crystalloid infusion may only provide temporary volume repletion. Additionally, crystalloids increase acidosis, can contribute to coagulopathy, cause immunologic dysfunction, and impose pulmonary and renal risks, and, therefore, have limited use in the hemorrhaging patient [5]. Lost cellular components, coagulation factors, and oxygen-carrying capacity require directed replacement to achieve normal perfusion.

Trauma-induced and consumptive coagulopathy presents a unique challenge not present in other shock states. In addition to the quantitative loss of essential clotting components, hemorrhage results in hemostatic functional failure. Hyperfibrinolysis, progressive thrombocytopenia, acidosis, and hypothermia all contribute to worsening coagulopathy that mandates aggressive, early, and targeted management.

A variety of methods have been utilized to determine endpoints of resuscitation following significant hemorrhage. Failure to direct resuscitation to these specific goals may lead to over-or-under resuscitation and the multitude of deleterious effects of either. No single endpoint has proven adequate, further elucidating the importance of a keen understanding of the physiologic consequences of bleeding.

Following initial resuscitation, ongoing need for blood products and hemostatic adjuncts suggests the presence of a missed injury or ongoing surgical bleeding not yet controlled. Although not always clear, failing to recognize the need to return to the operating theatre or endoscopy or interventional suite will result in worsened physiology, often beyond recovery and repair.

The myriad of issues encompassing shock following hemorrhage require diligence, foresight, and intuition in order to orchestrate a successful resuscitative strategy, while minimizing the complications associated with the disease state, as well as complications of the resuscitation.

PHYSIOLOGIC RESPONSES TO HEMORRHAGE

Coagulopathy

Acute coagulopathy resulting from hemorrhage is not a new concept, but recent work has further elucidated causes and potential treatments for coagulation disturbances associated with acute, large-volume blood loss. When present, coagulopathy is associated with higher mortality, up to four times that of patients with normal coagulation profiles [6].

Dilutional coagulation dysfunction has long been at the forefront of arguments against the use of large-volume prehospital or in-hospital resuscitation with crystalloid volume. With continued hemorrhage, plasma constituents necessary for hemostasis are not repleted and diluted. Replacing only the lost *volume* with crystalloid not only fails to replenish plasma constituents but also dilutes those remaining coagulation elements, thereby worsening hemorrhage. Additionally, crystalloid dilutional resuscitation has also been linked with increased hyperfibrinolysis—a deadly combination. However, multiple studies have shown this to be only one component of coagulation disruption, because coagulopathy in the absence of crystalloid resuscitation remains a significant problem, most notably following injury [7].

Consumptive coagulopathy, originally thought to be the primary cause of clotting dysfunction seen in patients sustaining significant hemorrhage, is rooted in the concept of localized exhaustion of clotting factors, platelets, thrombin, and other hemostatic activators. In severe multisystem tissue damage, such as massive crush injury, this likely plays a key role in the basic view of hemorrhagic coagulation dysfunction. However, coagulopathy is often associated with major, single site hemorrhage where direct tissue damage is limited, such as intraoperative vascular injury or isolated organ trauma from a single gunshot wound, suggesting that systemic effects are at work [8].

Approximately 25% of traumatized patients will present with coagulopathy that differs from these classic interpretations of causative mechanisms [9]. Although dilutional and consumptive causes certainly play a role in the acute coagulopathy of hemorrhage, dysregulated systemic activation and deactivation of key hemostatic mediators, as well as hypoperfusion, significantly contribute to systemic hemostatic failure. This is evidenced by those patients who present with normal perfusion; and, despite massive tissue injury, the patients do not show signs of coagulopathy [10]. Direct tissue injury exposes tissue factor and type III collagen within the subendothelium of damaged vessels. Binding of von Willebrand factor, platelets, and factor VIIa leads to thrombin and fibrin formation. This process is then amplified by factor IX, propagating initial hemostatic response to hemorrhage. Because hemostasis is part of a coagulation continuum, whereby clot formation and lysis are principal components, the release of hemostatic factors is accompanied by concomitant increases in lytic factors. Endothelial exposure from injury and thrombin formation also result in release of tissue plasminogen activator (tPA). Additionally, plasminogen activator inhibitor 1 (PAI-1) is inhibited, leading to increased plasticity of forming clots [8,11].

These local responses to tissue damage do not, however, fully elucidate the widespread clotting malfunction seen with large-volume hemorrhage. Systemic activation in response to hypoperfusion and shock has been implicated as a fundamentally necessary component of the acute coagulopathy of hemorrhage. This is seen with the thrombin–thrombomodulin–protein C complex. Hemorrhagic shock leads to increased circulating thrombomodulin, resulting in whole-body activation of protein C. Activated protein C then exudes its anticoagulant effects through degradation of clotting factors, specifically factors V and VIII. Studies have shown those patients in shock, regardless of degree of tissue injury, and have universally demonstrated deficiency in factor V [7]. PAI-1 is consumed, and thrombin generation subsequently downregulated on a systemic level as a result of increased protein C and glycocalyx shedding. The endothelial glycocalyx is a key regulator of vascular permeability, cell adhesion, and inflammation. At least one of four key components, syndecan-1, is shed during hemorrhagic shock exposing the membrane to inflammatory molecule adhesion, increasing permeability, and hyperfibrinolysis. The glycocalyx has been shown, at least in an animal model, to be replenished in plasma-based resuscitation and not with crystalloids [12,13].

The presence of shock is associated with hyperfibrinolysis and worsened outcomes. When percentage of lysis at 30 minutes (LY30), as defined by thromboelastography (TEG), exceeded 3%, the associated mortality risk increased 10-fold [6]. Although fibrinolysis is a normal physiologic process, hypoperfusion-related dysregulation of mediating factors results in overactivation of the fibrinolytic process. Plasminogen activators (tPA) cleave plasminogen to plasmin and are systemically upregulated in response to hemorrhagic shock. Additionally, the downregulatory activities of PAI-1 are inhibited through depletion [11]. This sets the stage for unrestricted lysis, diffuse hemorrhage, and uncontrolled coagulopathy.

Often revered by clinicians as a key marker of a patient's hemostatic ability, thrombocytopenia is associated with worsened outcomes. However, a normal platelet count does not ameliorate the risk of mortality related to functional platelet abnormalities, especially when considering that thrombocytopenia on admission is a rare event. In a study examining 101 severely injured trauma patients with normal platelet counts, over 40% demonstrated a defect in platelet function on admission to the emergency department [14]. Again, the presence of shock is to blame. Hypoperfusion leading to organ dysfunction, specifically hepatic perturbations, leads to the release of substances, causing calcium channel disruption and platelet inhibition [15]. Impaired fibrinogen–platelet interactions, decreased platelet responsiveness to arachidonic acid, adenosine diphosphate, and thrombin receptor-activating peptide as well as the classic inhibitors of hemostasis—acidosis and hypothermia—resulting from hypoperfusion also contribute to decreased platelet function [16].

Hemodynamic

Hemodynamic physiologic changes occur as a result of the need to ensure adequate tissue perfusion to vital organs. This is accomplished at the outset of severe hemorrhage through a multitude of cardiovascular mechanisms, led by sympathetic upregulation. Sympathetic outflow resulting from atrial and carotid body baroreceptors and loss of vagal tonic inhibition as a function of hypovolemia, causes cardiac chronotropic and inotropic responses. Epinephrine increases heart rate, which in turn maintains cardiac output, despite falling stroke volume. This is first recognized clinically by an increase in diastolic pressure, and consequent narrowed pulse pressure. With worsening hypovolemia, respiratory variations in pulse pressure may develop, worsening mean perfusion pressures significantly. Sympathetic activation also increases contractility through cardiac β-receptor stimulation.

Decreased arterial and venous compliance secondary to epinephrine release improves venous return in the face of hypovolemia. Peripheral vasoconstriction is clinically identified by the presence of cool extremities. Blood is shunted away from the periphery to vital organs, such as the heart and brain. Splanchnic perfusion is compromised because endogenous vasopressin and other sympathetic substances, such as endothelin and angiotensin II, stimulate vasoconstrictive receptor systems. Consequently, renal blood flow is decreased to only a fraction of normal levels, leading to acute kidney injury and oliguria. Celiac vasoconstriction decreases hepatic and portal flow, resulting in release of proinflammatory mediators, such as interleukin 6 (IL-6) [15,17].

On a microvascular level, increases in cellular adhesion molecules cause neutrophils to adhere to the endothelial cells in the microcirculation, limiting the physical ability of red cells to navigate capillary beds. Inflammatory mediators induce endothelial cell swelling, further limiting the passage of blood constituents. Decreases of capillary flow provoke cellular ischemia and anaerobic metabolism with ensuing acidosis [18].

As hypovolemia progresses, hemodynamic compensation fails. Cardiac output falls despite increases in contractility and heart rate. Vasoconstriction is maximized through exponential quantities of endogenous catacholamines; however, without volume, it is to no avail. Acidosis rapidly follows, heart rate variability declines, and bradycardia emerges signifying irreversible shock.

Metabolic

In 1872, Gross called shock a "rude unhinging of the machinery of life." The machinery of cellular metabolism undergoes fundamental changes in the setting of hemorrhagic shock. Hypovolemic-induced depressions of cardiac output result in diminished perfusion to end organs. The remaining intravascular volume is deplete of hemoglobin *mass*, although *concentrations* may remain relatively stable in the initial phases. Limited hemoglobin mass correlates with decreasing levels of available oxygen. To counteract this, oxygen extraction increases, measured by declining mixed venous oxygen saturation, and the patient becomes dependent upon oxygen delivery to maintain aerobic metabolic pathways and stave off impending acidosis. As hemorrhage continues and the previously described hemodynamic changes occur, anaerobic metabolism begins to materialize. The resultant acidosis shifts the oxygen dissociation curve to the right, favoring oxygen offloading at the cellular level. Mild acidosis, therefore, executes a beneficial effect, curbing progressive anaerobic transformation temporarily. If hemorrhage control is not accomplished, the availability of cellular oxygen fades, and mitochondrial energy production is halted with accumulation of pyruvate. Reduction of the efficiency of the electron transport chain causes diversion of NADH that donates a proton to pyruvate with formation of lactate. Lactic acidosis then ensues until oxygen delivery restores the electron transport chain, at which time pyruvate may reenter the citric acid cycle and lactate production decreases.

Lactate clearance has been studied extensively as a marker of resuscitation effectiveness based on these basic physiologic mechanisms. For lactate formation rates to normalize, orderly aerobic cellular metabolism must be restored. This is evidenced through an understanding of the Cori cycle, which begins with glycolysis. Yielding two adenosine triphosphates (ATPs), glycolysis also produces two lactates, which are then transported to the liver. Lactate is then converted back to glucose through hepatic gluconeogenesis at the cost of six ATPs, resulting in a net negative energy balance. Glucose then participates in glycolysis again at the cellular level, and the process repeats itself. This large energy gap cannot be replenished without resumption of normal physiologic metabolism, which requires restoration of oxygen delivery through hemorrhage control and resuscitative efforts. Therefore, normalization of lactate levels signifies success from a resuscitation viewpoint.

Blood glucose and glucose utilization is intimately linked to the production of lactate and energy. In response to hypovolemia and acidosis, adrenal medullary and cortical hormones are released. Cortisol not only aids in vasoconstriction but also promotes glucose release in large quantities to combat essential cellular starvation as a result of hypoperfusion. Insulin is suppressed, favoring glucose utilization as opposed to storage. Insulin-independent GLUT membrane proteins allow for transport of glucose to vital organs such as the heart, kidneys, brain, and others, and thus provide an increased energy source. However, lactic acidosis will continue in the absence of adequate oxygen delivery. Hyperglycemic deleterious effects are far reaching, and include increased infection and elevated intracranial pressure. Regarding direct correlation to hemorrhagic shock, however, hyperglycemia may result in osmotic diuresis despite decreased renal blood flow and glomerular filtration rate augmented by renin–angiotensin–aldosterone system activation, thereby worsening the already depleted intravascular volume. Growth hormone and glucagon add to this process because they promote lipolysis and glycogenolysis.

Immunologic

Hemorrhagic shock results in a multitude of immune responses related to the upregulation of cellular signaling designed to protect, but often result in harm. Extensive research in the last decade has shown that hemorrhagic shock activates inflammatory cascades, resulting in profound abnormalities. The effect of immunologic dysregulation is often manifested by a spectrum of clinical problems, including acute respiratory distress syndrome (ARDS), systemic inflammatory response syndrome (SIRS), coagulation abnormalities, and multiple organ dysfunction syndrome (MODS). Cytokines such as IL-1, IL-6, tumor necrosis factor α, cellular signaling pathways involving toll-like receptors, and microRNA have all been implicated [19]. However, there have been no clear data regarding which of the many involved substances plays the key role in development and propagation of the overactive inflammatory response. One of the major areas of study involves the activated immune response that results in enhanced activation and adhesion of leukocytes. During this activated stage, neutrophils can release harmful reactive oxygen species, which are thought to play a major role in loss of capillary integrity. This leads to edema and the sequestration of fluid in the tissues and the interstitial space. Additionally, immunologic responses to therapy, specifically large-volume crystalloid infusion, may trigger the altered immune response to hemorrhage and has been a growing area of research [20].

SHOCK RECOGNITION

Early recognition of hemorrhagic shock is essential to prevent mortality. Aside from blatant exsanguination, hemorrhagic shock can be difficult to define in its early stages. A high index of suspicion is necessary for prompt, accurate diagnosis. Probable mechanisms of hemorrhagic shock must be thoroughly and rapidly examined and treated.

Every patient who is at risk for hemorrhage should be evaluated through methods delineated in the Advanced Trauma Life Support program. By quickly proceeding through the primary survey (evaluation), immediate life threats are recognized and can be treated [1]. This presents a departure from traditional methods of initial patient evaluation of taking a long, thorough history from the patient, discussing options, and planning a workup. A hemorrhaging patient does not have the luxury of time, and delayed recognition of shock often results in death. Immediate threats to life must be identified early, and minor injuries or findings must not derail the primary goal of addressing potentially lethal matters.

No one feature results in the diagnosis of hemorrhagic shock. Basic physical examination skills utilized in context often form a clinical impression that leads to the diagnosis. Heart rate and blood pressure, which are often used in the incorrect definition of shock, may be normal. β-Blockers, untreated hypertension, and physical fitness may confound interpretation of hemodynamic normalcy. A narrowed pulse pressure, however, is typically present, and often missed owing to a normal systolic value. Anxiety or belligerence may be a sign of shock, and can easily be confused for intoxication or isolated brain injury. Decreased mental status should be considered an ominous sign of impending decompensation. Cool, clammy extremities in a patient at risk for shock are clinical markers for peripheral vasoconstrictive compensation. Pallor may also be present, and in an otherwise healthy patient, should invoke a sense of urgency. Hypothermia, a key component of the lethal triad (hypothermia, coagulopathy, and acidosis) is an independent predictor of mortality in hemorrhaging patients.

Exhaustive laboratory studies are often unhelpful, especially in the early stages of shock. For example, hemoglobin and hematocrit levels are frequently normal, because the laboratory result is a measure of concentration—which remains unchanged until compensatory mechanisms and interstitial to intravascular fluid shifts have occurred. However, when a hemoglobin of less than 11 g per dL is present, it is associated with a mortality rate of nearly 40% [21]. Most patients with hemorrhagic shock were physiologically normal prior to the offending insult. This makes the arterial blood gas quite useful, because any acid–base abnormality can be presumed to be caused by the event that brought the patient to the hospital, and not underlying medical conditions. Patients with a base deficit (BD) greater than 6 are at higher risk of mortality and the need for massive transfusion. Severity of injury and mortality is linearly associated with the degree of the initial coagulopathy, and an international normalized ratio (INR) of greater than 1.5 reliably predicts the need for massive transfusion [10,22]. Tissue oxygen saturation continues to be investigated as a simple, reliable, and early marker of the presence of hemorrhagic shock [23].

Adjuncts to the clinical examination include very few imaging studies. For the injured patient, chest and pelvic radiographs may be of great utility because they can help identify major hemorrhage in two of the five key locations where deadly hemorrhage may occur. The Focused Assessment with Sonography for Trauma (FAST) may be utilized to identify tamponade, hemothorax, pneumothorax, and intraperitoneal hemorrhage. Long bone fractures are often readily identified. In nontrauma cases, a nasogastric tube may be inserted for suspected gastrointestinal hemorrhage to aid in localization. Endoscopy and interventional radiologic methods may also be employed emergently as conditions warrant.

Those patients who transiently respond to volume administration should undergo expeditious reevaluation to localize the cause of hemorrhage. Transient response conveys ongoing hemorrhage, and beseeches health care providers to act quickly to obtain hemorrhage control.

Shock scoring systems may aid in the clinical diagnosis of hemorrhagic shock when uncertainty exists. Many studies of hemorrhagic shock identification scoring systems use the necessity for transfusion as the outcome of interest. The Emergency Transfusion Score involves the use of nine markers, with a weighted coefficient assigned to each marker. For example, a systolic pressure of <90 mm Hg carries the most weight, at 2.5 times higher than mechanism of injury. The Trauma-Associated Severe Hemorrhage (TASH) system was developed in Germany and incorporates many of the clinical features described earlier, in addition to BD and hemoglobin. The TASH has been shown to reliably predict the need for massive transfusion [24]. A simplified method of identifying the probability of life-threatening hemorrhage was developed from military experience. Tachycardia, hypotension, acidosis, and acute anemia are all independent risk factors for the need of massive transfusion. When all four are present, approximately 80% of patients will require massive transfusion. The validity of this model, however, rests on a weighted evaluation, with pH carrying the most value, and thus is difficult to rapidly calculate. [25]. The ABC score was developed to eliminate the need for laboratory results to rapidly determine the presence of hemorrhagic shock and to predict the need for massive transfusion. Four components (penetrating mechanism, systolic pressure < 90 mm Hg, heart rate > 120 beats per minute, and positive FAST), each with equal weight make up the ABC score. Patients with all four variables present have a near 100% need for massive transfusion [26].

Utility of Ultrasonography for Diagnosis of Hemorrhagic Shock

As discussed earlier, early control of the site of bleeding is an essential part of the management of hemorrhagic shock. Source control requires identification of the source of bleeding. Ultrasonography has utility for this purpose, because it can be deployed at the point of care for urgent evaluation of the critically ill patient. Ultrasonography has the advantage of immediate application by the frontline clinical team who can integrate the results of the examination into the other key elements of emergency evaluation: the history, physical examination, and initial laboratory results. This is not to discount the importance of advanced imaging techniques, such as computerized tomography (CT) or angiography; yet, these suffer the disadvantage of some inevitable delay in their performance.

The ultrasonography examination is performed by a member of the trauma team while other key elements of initial resuscitation are ongoing. Modern bedside ultrasonography machines are small enough that they can be brought to the bedside without blocking access to the patient by other members of the trauma team. The machine has multiple uses beyond examination for life-threatening hemorrhage, such as vascular access, airway management, and assessment for alternative causes for shock.

Examination for Intra-abdominal Hemorrhage

The FAST examination utilizes ultrasonography to rapidly identify an intra-abdominal source of bleeding. It has replaced intra-abdominal lavage as the technique of choice for management of abdominal trauma and is standard practice for evaluation for intra-abdominal bleeding in trauma [39].

Scanning Technique

A phased array cardiac probe on abdominal preset gives serviceable images. If available, a curvilinear abdominal probe is used. The hepatorenal and splenorenal spaces are imaged in longitudinal axis to look for fluid collection. On the right side, the probe is placed in the midaxillary line on the lower chest wall in order to obtain a transcostal view of the liver in a coronal imaging plane (see Chapter 44 Critical Care of the Patient with Abdominal Trauma). Once the appropriate intercostal space is found, the probe is angled and tilted to achieve a clear image of the hepatorenal space. The presence of fluid is taken as an indication of intra-abdominal bleeding (Video 37.1). The examiner also checks for prehepatic fluid, and, using the liver as an acoustic window, examines the subdiaphragmatic space for fluid (Video 37.1). The scan is repeated on the left with examination of the splenorenal, presplenic, and subdiaphragmatic spaces (Video 37.1). The operator then checks for pelvic fluid. The probe is placed just above the level of the iliac crest in the midline using a transverse scanning plane and angled downward through the bladder to search for fluid in the pelvis (Video 37.1). Pelvic fluid indicates an intra-abdominal source of bleeding in the patient with hemorrhagic shock. Some examiners include examination of the right and left lower lateral abdominal quadrants to the FAST examination. The FAST examination may include the subxiphoid view of the heart (subcostal long-axis view) in order to exclude a hemoperidium with pericardial tamponade and to look for severe hypovolemia manifested with a small hyperdynamic left ventricle (Video 37.1). The subxiphoid view of the inferior vena cava (IVC) is included to examine for IVC size and respiratory variation. The presence of a small diameter IVC or respirophasic variation of IVC size suggests hypovolemia.

The FAST examination can be performed rapidly. If initially negative, it can be repeated as clinically indicated. In the presence of hemorrhagic shock, a positive examination indicates intra-abdominal bleeding and the need for urgent source control.

Examination for Hemothorax

The extended FAST examination uses elements of thoracic ultrasonography to evaluate the patient with hemorrhagic shock for hemothorax. In addition, the examination has utility to examine for pneumothorax and pericardial effusion on an emergency basis.

Scanning Technique

With the patient is supine position, fluid will distribute in the dependent thorax owing to gravitational effect. On both the right and left sides, the probe is placed in the midaxillary to posterior axillary line on the chest in a coronal imaging plane and moved over adjacent interspaces to examine for pleural effusion. The examination for pleural fluid may be performed by extending the scan performed for intra-abdominal fluid to the area above the diaphragm. The finding of significant pleural fluid in a patient with hemorrhagic shock indicates hemothorax and the need for consideration of urgent source control (Video 37.1).

Examination for Retroperitoneal Bleed

Retroperitoneal bleeding is a potentital cause of hemorrhagic shock that may be difficult to identify by physical examination. Ultrasound examination of the retroperitoneum is also limited, and has a high false negative rate. For this reason, in patients who present in hemorrhagic shock with no identifiable cause, a retroperitoneal source should be considered, and expedient operative intervention should proceed in instances where a high index of suspicion exists.

Scanning Technique

The probe is used to examine the flank area bilaterally. Using a coronal scanning plane, the probe is moved over the flank. Identification of retroperitoneal fluid collection indicates retroperitoneal bleeding and the urgent need for consideration of source control (Video 37.1).

Limitations of Ultrasonography

Ultrasonography readily identifies fluid collections. In hemorrhagic shock, the trauma team may reasonably assume that the fluid represents hemorrhage and takes action based upon this supposition. If the patient is unstable, this may result in early surgical intervention. If time permits, the finding may lead to further imaging with CT scan or angiography; if an interventional radiology approach seems appropriate.

Patient-specific characteristics such as obesity and edema may degrade the ultrasonography image. This is most likely to occur when imaging the retroperitoneum. Competence in scanning during emergency situations, such as for the evaluation of hemorrhagic shock, requires effective training for competence [40] because inaccurate results may have severe consequence in the unstable patient.

Perhaps the greatest limitation of using ultrasonography to identify sources of hemorrhagic shock, is misinterpretation of a negative result. Patients who exhibit signs of hemodynamic compromise related to hemorrhage may have a completely normal ultrasound examination. [41] When this occurs, providers should resist being lulled into complacency based upon the negative imaging examination, and must remain vigilant to ensure rapid hemorrhage control is obtained.

Despite these limitations, ultrasonography is an effective tool for the initial and ongoing evaluation of the patient with hemorrhagic shock. It can be fully integrated into the team effort at the bedside, and it gives immediate and valuable clinical information. As such, it is an essential component of the imaging strategy for the evaluation and management of hemorrhagic shock.

HEMORRHAGE CONTROL

Obvious external hemorrhage is controlled first by manual pressure. Pressure is the force applied per unit area. To effectively control hemorrhage with direct pressure, one must limit the area over which it is applied. For example, a finger placed deliberately is often more efficacious than two hands placed over a large surface.

Tourniquets have seen increasing use in both civilian and military populations in recent years. Commercially available tourniquets are simple to apply with minimal training, are lightweight, and effective at controlling extremity hemorrhage. Tourniquets should be utilized in manner in which they were designed, to occlude arterial hemorrhage. Isolated venous occlusion, without arterial cessation of hemorrhage, will worsen blood loss [27]. Junctional hemorrhage, occurring high in the groin, for example, is often difficult to control with pressure or tourniquets alone and, typically, requires emergent surgical intervention. However, adjuncts such as the junctional emergency tourniquet system may be useful for some patients [28].

Local hemostatic agents are widely available and have shown promise in controlling both external hemorrhage, and organ bleeding encountered in the operating suite. Topical hemostats are typically constructed of bioabsorbable material with the addition of thrombin and/or fibrin, and are available in a variety of application constructs. Polymerized sprays, injectable foam, and biologic sheets are among the many methods available. Cost and local availability often dictate which product may be utilized. It is important to avoid intravascular injection or placement of these products, because embolization is a risk.

Noncompressible torso hemorrhage has been identified as a major cause of death both in military and civilian studies [29]. Few techniques other than surgery are available to address noncompressible hemorrhage, such as bleeding in the abdomen, retroperitoneum, or chest. It is important to recognize that these techniques are temporizing measures in lieu of definitive hemorrhage control. Resuscitative thoracotomy, although effective for ceasing torso hemorrhage, is associated with high mortality rates, and is frequently impractical for the general physician to successfully accomplish. Resuscitative endovascular balloon occlusion of the aorta was first described over 50 years ago, and has seen increased use recently. It involves advancing and inflating an endovascular balloon into the aorta via percutaneous femoral artery access. This can be accomplished in the emergency department with minimal equipment and has been shown to be effective at controlling torso hemorrhage [30]. Self-expanding polyurethane foam, injected through percutaneous techniques intraperitoneally, has shown promise and efficacy. The liquid polymer rapidly expands, conforming to intra-abdominal anatomy and stopping hemorrhage. The foam is then removed at the time of surgery. Studies are currently underway to further characterize this technique [31].

Surgical control of hemorrhage is beyond the scope of this chapter; however, it warrants mention. Once hemorrhagic shock is identified, immediate control of hemorrhage must be undertaken. Delaying definitive care with exhaustive radiologic or laboratory studies is unwise. At centers without surgical capabilities, rapid transport to a tertiary facility, when hemorrhage is suspected, is safer than definitively identifying the source of that hemorrhage. Control in the operating room or angiography suite is crucial to avoid death, and initial evaluation and management should effectively move toward that goal.

Systemic adjuncts for controlling hemorrhage in the presence of coagulopathy may be utilized to help normalize coagulation disturbances, and avoid ongoing bleeding. Many of these pharmacologic adjuncts are utilized off-label; however, significant data exists to support their use in certain situations. Prothrombin complex concentrates, initially developed to treat isolated congenital factor deficiencies, provide rapid, effective correction of factor-based coagulation disruptions. Three-factor (factors II, IX, and X) and four-factor (factors II, IX, X, and VII) varieties are available and are associated with minimal adverse events [32]. Recombinant factor VIIa has been associated with normalization of conventional coagulation tests, and decreased transfusion requirements [33]. Anti-inhibitor binders have also been utilized in specific circumstances, such as coagulopathy in the presence of novel anticoagulants. Recently, a dabigatran-specific antibody fragment has been released. Prior to the inception of idarucizumab, no method of therapeutic reversal was available for patients anticoagulated with dabigatran [34]. Currently, several agents are being developed to target coagulopathy resultant from factor Xa inhibitors, direct thrombin inhibitors, and other novel mechanistic medications.

Tranexamic acid, an antifibrinolytic, arose to the forefront of pharmaceutic hemorrhage control after the release of the CRASH-2 trial [35]. This study showed significant reductions in mortality. Subsequent studies confirmed its efficacy, and it is now frequently utilized as an adjunct during resuscitation of hemorrhagic shock [36–38]. Its efficacy, low cost, and wide availability make tranexamic acid an attractive adjunct to hemostatic control.

HISTORY OF HEMORRHAGIC SHOCK RESUSCITATION

The modern-day trauma system owes a large debt to combat casualty care. Techniques from system development to operating room procedures have their roots in battlefield medicine. Resuscitation is no stranger to advancement during wartime as well. To understand the advancements made and differences that exist with modern combat resuscitation strategies, it is important to understand the history of combat resuscitation.

Empiric crystalloid administration owes its roots to strategies developed in the Vietnam War. Based on research by Shires [42,43], Dillon [44], and others, the need for volume resuscitation was brought to the forefront to replace an interstitial volume debt, secondary to intravascular movement in hemorrhagic shock. High-volume crystalloid resuscitation strategies were used to replace volume loss encountered by the bleeding soldier in ratios of 3:1 to as high as 8:1. The physiology was sound, but outcomes were disappointing, as survival rates did not improve. In fact, the adopted strategy of large-volume IV fluid administration spawned its own set of complications, most notably the emergence of Da Nang lung, known now as ARDS. Reports linking ARDS to crystalloid resuscitation and subsequent immunologic effects appeared as early as 1967 [45].

Despite this, massive volume resuscitation strategies prevailed for more than 30 years. In the early 1990s, Rotondo and colleagues published the first major data on damage control surgery, employing early, rapid hemorrhage control, and temporizing measures to avoid the effects of ongoing massive resuscitation related to prolonged operative escapades [46]. This sparked a fury among traditionalists, but led to a series of manuscripts debunking the idea of benefit associated with large-volume resuscitation.

A report by the Institute of Medicine in 1999, as well as two consensus conferences held by Office of Naval Research, the US Army Medical Research and Material Command and the Uniformed Services University of Health Sciences, in 2001 and 2002, addressed concerns of resuscitation techniques, further delineating the adverse effects of large-volume resuscitation and giving recommendations for alternative strategies. First noted was the paucity of Level I and II data to support the then standard of care. Second, the immunologic activity of common IV fluids and deleterious effects of high-volume resuscitation were best defined by complications related to their use. Third, the reports supported the initial battlefield use of low-volume hypertonic saline (HTS) resuscitation [47]. A 250-mL bolus of HTS was chosen based on research showing decreased neutrophil activation as well as increased oncotic properties. Fourth, triggers for fluid resuscitation were defined as systolic blood pressure < 80 mm Hg or the absence of palpable radial pulse, decreasing blood pressure, or altered mental status with no confounding brain injury [48]. This protocol allowed for "permissive hypotension" during resuscitation until definitive hemorrhage control. The goal was not to return blood pressure to normal, but rather to target clinical goals of mentation and palpable pulse. These protocols were developed with several civilian trauma studies in mind, showing survival benefit to limited initial resuscitation [49]. The combination of a large number of studies near the turn of the millennium ultimately culminated in a complete 180-degree shift from the high-volume crystalloid resuscitation seen in the Vietnam War. Currently, an injured soldier with a palpable pulse and is awake and alert will have an IV placed, but no volume will be infused. Oral hydration is encouraged, and rapid evacuation is undertaken. If fluids are given, they are in low volume and hypertonic in nature.

The concept is simple—without effective hemostasis, no amount of resuscitation will effect a mortality benefit. In the Iraq and Afghanistan Wars, the goal of resuscitation changed—from early volume resuscitation to early hemorrhage control. With this objective highlighted, tourniquets were reintroduced, and pharmaceutic adjuncts like recombinant factor VIIa and tranexamic acid were added to the armamentarium to aid cessation of hemorrhage [37].

Rural, marine, or mountainous areas typically require longer transport times and represent some the civilian austere environments. In these scenarios, much of the same wisdom gained from combat research should be utilized, with minimal prehospital resuscitation prior to arrival at definitive care. Once arriving at the tertiary facility, however, resuscitation may begin with the same tenant—crystalloid resuscitation is a thing of the past. Blood component therapy is now utilized early, rather than after several liters of lactated Ringers or saline. Higher ratios of plasma to red blood cells (RBCs) have been a point of study in recent years, with ratio of 1:1 showing improved outcomes [50]. Highlighting the value of replenishing specific blood components early in hemorrhagic shock resuscitation.

INITIAL RESUSCITATION

Previously, initial resuscitation of hemorrhagic shock involved large-volume fluid resuscitation and maintenance of normothermia. Although these methods aimed to address two of the three components of the lethal triad, coagulopathy was largely ignored. Today's resuscitation techniques specifically target the coagulopathy of hemorrhage through the concept of damage control resuscitation.

Damage control resuscitation focuses on several key goals, and begins immediately upon arrival to the emergency department. The first of which is to maintain a slightly lower-than-normal systolic blood pressure of approximately 90 mm Hg. This serves to limit clot disruption by allowing some degree of stasis to occur, increasing the chance for clot development, and strengthening. Peripheral vasoconstriction is preserved, and perfusion to vital organs is increased with permissive hypotension. Conversely, large amounts of IV fluids will reverse peripheral vasoconstriction and, without hemorrhage control, will ultimately worsen blood loss. Excessive or misdirected fluid resuscitation to achieve normal hemodynamics will lead to dilution of existing clotting factors, aggravating coagulopathy and exacerbating hemorrhage. The benefits of permissive hypotension were first recognized, and eloquently described, over 100 years ago by W.B. Cannon. His observations of the deleterious effects of copious volume resuscitation prior to hemorrhage control persist today. The current evolving hypotensive resuscitation literature continues to show improved mortality and morbidity in both traumatic and nontraumatic bleeding events [51].

Second, damage control resuscitation directly addresses the coagulopathy of hemorrhage. Fluid resuscitation commences with blood component therapy. As described earlier, crystalloids lack the essential elements necessary to combat the coagulopathy of hemorrhage, and are evidenced to exacerbate inflammatory dysregulation. Coagulopathy and inflammation are suppressed through administration of early plasma and platelets. These components also provide volume resuscitation, thus achieving both the first and second goals of the initial resuscitation. For patients in hemorrhagic shock, directly addressing hyperfibrinolysis is accomplished with tranexamic acid, which is most efficacious within 3 hours of injury. It acts to compete with plasmin, blocking fibrinolysis. Other antifibrinolytic pharmaceuticals are available, such as ε-aminocaproic acid. Concentrated clotting factors, such as prothrombin complex concentrates and recombinant factor VIIa, have the benefit of rapid repletion of essential clotting elements, with the effects within minutes of infusion, and should be considered in severely injured or hemorrhaging patients.

Third, blood component therapy serves not only to maintain the above state of permissive hypotension while replenishing the stores of circulating procoagulants but also to optimize oxygen delivery in the interlude prior to, and during surgical, endoscopic or interventional hemorrhage control. Increasing oxygen delivery through augmentation of the blood's oxygen-carrying capacity with red cells minimizes tissue oxygen debt in the setting of compromised circulation more so than crystalloid preparations. By relieving oxygen debt through increased oxygen delivery, acidosis is quelled because aerobic metabolism is supported and lactate production is limited. Decreased acidosis is crucial for normal global cellular and enzyme function.

Although there are clear benefits to blood component resuscitation, the optimal ratio of blood component therapy continues to be studied. A variety of ratios (fresh frozen plasma (FFP):PLT:RBC) exist to closely mimic the constituents of whole blood transfusion, which, in civilian centers, is rarely available. Early platelet and plasma administration have been associated with decreased mortality. In the PROMMTT study, investigators noted a three to fourfold increase in mortality in patients who received a 1:2 (FFP:RBC) transfusion ratio in the first 6 hours, as compared to those who received a 1:1 transfusion ratio [52]. This large, multicenter study showed clear benefit of early plasma initiation in the setting of hemorrhagic shock. More recently, Holcomb and colleagues tested the differences between 1:1:1 and 1:1:2 (FFP:PLT:RBC) ratios, and found equivocal mortality rates at both 24 hours and 30 days between the two. However, fewer deaths from exsanguination were noted in the 1:1:1 group [50]. Early, high-ratio transfusion of plasma and platelets aids not only in correction of coagulation dysfunction, but restores volume with necessary coagulation components shed during hemorrhagic shock.

Massive transfusion protocols have been widely adopted at both major centers and smaller hospitals. Development of these protocols has been associated with lower mortality rates. Although the term "massive," implies a greater volume of products, multiple studies have shown decreased overall product usage when these protocols are effectively utilized early in the resuscitation. Several reasons exist to explain this somewhat paradoxic finding. First, by limiting crystalloid resuscitation, blood loss is lessened and dilutional coagulopathy is curbed, which ultimately will result in less product transfusion. Second, early activation allows for efficient optimization of the tenets of damage control resuscitation, resulting in less acidosis, improved organ function, and less blood loss while hemorrhage is controlled. Third, for a patient presenting with hemorrhagic shock, predetermined massive transfusion protocols offer a streamlined method of delivering product to the patient while assuring that appropriate component ratios are maintained. Some published indicators for massive transfusion include (1) INR > 1.5, (2) BD > 6, (3) systolic blood pressure < 90 mm Hg, (4) hemoglobin < 11 g per dL, (5) heart rate > 120, and (6) positive FAST scan. The more of these factors that are present, the more likely the patient should undergo massive transfusion, with early plasma administration in a fixed-ratio paradigm.

Damage control resuscitation strives to reach a balance between achieving optimal physiologic function, while limiting the unwanted effects of the resuscitation itself, and is most useful from the time of presentation through the period of definitive surgical, endoscopic, or interventional hemorrhage control. It must expeditiously be initiated upon arrival in the emergency department, often with limited information. Prolonged resuscitation should not delay definitive hemorrhage control in order to achieve distant hemodynamic or physiologic goals. Time spent in the emergency department equates to lost time in the operating room, endoscopy, or interventional suites where damage control resuscitation may be continued and decisive hemorrhage control obtained. The initial phase continues through the operative intervention, and damage control principles are upheld by targeting the above physiologic goals. To this end, damage control *surgery* is often performed, which consists of surgical hemorrhage control, limitation of contamination and temporary closure, deferring definitive repair of non–life-threatening injuries until physiologic correction is achieved in the intensive care unit (ICU) in the second resuscitative phase.

ONGOING RESUSCITATION

While initial resuscitation of hemorrhagic shock is to serve as a bridge to operative, interventional, or endoscopic hemorrhage control, ongoing resuscitation following hemorrhage aims to restore normal physiologic parameters to ensure adequate oxygen delivery to resume normal bodily functions once hemorrhage has ceased. Despite effective damage control resuscitative measures, patients often exhibit varying degrees of physiologic instability in the ICU. Similar principles exist in the ongoing resuscitative phase, which is typically undertaken in the ICU. Patients arriving from the operating theater may remain hypovolemic, coagulopathic, hypothermic, and acidotic, necessitating further intensive management to achieve a successful resuscitation. Endpoints of resuscitation should be aggressively targeted in this phase to ensure rapid resolution of metabolic derangements that may have occurred during the preceding interventions.

Endpoints of Resuscitation

Traditional endpoints of resuscitation, such as heart rate, blood pressure, and urine output, are grossly inadequate as sole markers of physiologic normalization. Although these common methods provide insights into the overall clinical picture, they fail to accurately demonstrate resuscitation success. Confounding variables abound when considering these easily attainable, yet simplistic determinations. For example, heart rate is altered by a variety of mechanisms that may be unrelated to the adequacy of resuscitation. Pain and anxiety commonly cause tachycardia, whereas the widespread use of β-blockers and other cardiac medications may prevent it—rendering heart rate less useful. Urine output has long been utilized as an endpoint signifying the adequate restoration of perfusion to an end organ. However, oliguria may be present despite completion of resuscitation. CT evaluation is ubiquitous, and often utilizes IV contrast which commonly results in acute tubular necrosis despite aggressive resuscitation. Medications, specifically antibiotics, are known to cause acute interstitial nephritis. Additionally, the initial hypoperfusion event may have caused direct tubular injury resulting in oliguria, despite adequate resuscitation. Managing oliguria with large volumes of resuscitation fluid will inevitably result in the undesirable consequences of overresuscitation. Conversely, entities such as diabetes insipidus and cerebral salt wasting cause polyuria and may falsely reassure the clinician.

Hemorrhagic shock occurs as the result of hypoperfusion, and thus markers of hypoperfusion should be sought as valid endpoints. An arterial blood gas is commonly touted as the most beneficial laboratory test in the resuscitation of a patient in hemorrhagic shock because of the rapid, comprehensive information gained, including BD. The BD assumes a normal pCO_2, which is a crucial point to consider, because it allows for the true metabolic derangement to be elucidated. Clinicians typically examine the pH, and may miss significant acidosis, especially if the patient is compensating with tachypnea. For this reason, the BD is a test that requires virtually no analysis, and provides a simple number that, in hemorrhagic shock, is an accurate marker of perfusion. Through the mechanisms described earlier in this chapter, acidosis results as a function of hypoperfusion and anaerobic metabolism at the cellular level. As this acidosis worsens, BD becomes more negative. An initial BD less than -6 is associated with the need for massive transfusion and damage control resuscitation practice implementation. Similarly, a persistent BD following hemorrhage control suggests the need for further resuscitation. Multiple studies have shown benefits of using the BD as an endpoint of resuscitation [53,54]. The goal should be a rapid normalization of the BD. Decreased mortality is associated with normalization of the BD within the first 24 hours of hospitalization. Some issues with BD warrant mention however. If sodium bicarbonate is employed in the initial resuscitation phase, the BD becomes useless, secondary to the addition of exogenous base to the equation. Only in the most severe acidosis cases should bicarbonate even be considered. Another relative indication for bicarbonate administration is to increase the effectiveness of resuscitation adjuncts, such as prothrombin complex concentrate or recombinant factor VIIa, which have decreased efficacy below a pH of 7.2. The BD may be confounded by other acidotic states, such as hyperchloremia, which is typically iatrogenic in nature. Additionally, BD often lags behind the resuscitation, and its continued pursuit may lead to overresuscitation. When the BD persists, the presence of a missed injury or ongoing causes for hypoperfusion should be reviewed.

To counter the issues associated with BD, serum lactate is employed. In the setting of acute hemorrhagic shock, increases in lactate are the result of tissue and cellular mitochondrial dysfunction, and thus lactate provides insights into tissue perfusion. Parallel physiologic hypoperfusion mechanisms will cause the level of lactate to increase, secondary to anaerobic metabolism. Similar to BD, lactate clearance within 24 hours has been shown in many studies to be associated with lower mortality rates [55,56]. Several societies have incorporated lactate into their resuscitation guidelines, including the Society of Critical Care Medicine and the Eastern Association for the Surgery of Trauma; and an internal consensus conference on hemodynamic monitoring has recommended utilization of lactate clearance as an endpoint of resuscitation. Lactate clearance is affected by hepatic function, and, for those patients with either underlying or acute hepatic insufficiency, elevated lactate concentrations may persist secondary to decreased clearance by the liver and may be misleading in these circumstances. Some have further criticized the ability of lactate levels to determine perfusion adequacy by citing the multiple *aerobic* processes, including glucose utilization in the setting of hyperglycemia, as potential nonperfusion-related causes for hyperlactatemia. However, many consider lactate one of the most useful endpoints in the resuscitation of hemorrhagic shock.

Adequate tissue perfusion depends upon both oxygen delivery and tissue oxygen demand. This supply–demand relationship can be determined by examining central venous oxygen saturation ($ScvO_2$) measurement from a central venous catheter. Normal physiologic conditions incur approximately 25% oxygen extraction at the tissue level, resulting in a $ScvO_2$ of 75%, given an arterial saturation of 100%. When tissue demand increases, or oxygen delivery decreases, as in hemorrhagic shock, more oxygen is extracted, decreasing $ScvO_2$. $ScvO_2$ has been shown to be a marker of both fluid responsiveness and reinstatement of normal perfusion [57]. By restoring normal cardiac output with volume administration, preload and afterload optimization, and inotropic support; the delivery component of $ScvO_2$ is corrected. Complexity arises, however, in addressing the demand component of $ScvO_2$. Peripheral vasoconstriction, as described earlier, is a compensatory mechanism in the face of hypovolemia. This vasoconstriction ultimately leads to decreased tissue oxygen extraction and a rising $ScvO_2$. Conversely, in hemorrhagic shock tissue, oxygen demand and concomitant extraction are typically increased secondary to tissue-level hypoxia, resulting from acute hypovolemia and hypoperfusion. Increased oxygen extraction in response to hemorrhage leads to a delivery-dependent state and declining $ScvO_2$. These two competing forces have resulted in an argument against the efficacy of $ScvO_2$ as a resuscitation marker and work to confuse the interpretation of $ScvO_2$. Despite these intricacies, $ScvO_2$ remains an endpoint of interest, and abnormal elevations or decreases in $ScvO_2$ should prompt the clinician to adjust resuscitation based on results.

In hemorrhagic shock, restoration of normal oxygen delivery (DO_2) is the ultimate goal, making this calculated value extremely useful for determining sufficiency of resuscitation. The equation is defined as the product of arterial oxygen content and blood flow, and involves three main components: cardiac output, hemoglobin, and oxygen saturation (SaO_2). The contribution of partial pressure of oxygen is negligible and is often omitted in bedside calculations of DO_2. With the equation, we simplify the concept of perfusion, by separating it into two main determinants—flow and content. To address arterial oxygen content, first the SaO_2 is optimized through oxygen administration, increased FiO_2, or through ventilator methods to increase oxygenation. Hemoglobin is then optimized, keeping in mind the clear benefit of restrictive transfusion strategies shown in virtually all patient populations. Next, flow is maximized via optimization of cardiac output, which typically equates to targeting stroke volume through ongoing resuscitation or application of inotropic agents. Through these methods, normalizing oxygen delivery represents a valid and complete endpoint of resuscitation for hemorrhagic shock. Like the endpoints described earlier, DO_2 is not without limitation. In states of decreased tissue oxygen extraction, DO_2 may not coincide with cellular perfusion. Additionally, advanced monitoring is required to obtain stroke volume measurement, and depending upon the device used, significant error may be introduced into the equation.

Coagulation Endpoints

Many damage control resuscitation measures are directed at controlling the early coagulopathy of hemorrhage. The ongoing phase of resuscitation continues this focus. Conventional coagulation tests are helpful, and provide insight into ongoing coagulopathy. Considering the above endpoints, the clinician should consider normalizing coagulation function with plasma, platelets, cryoprecipitate, or pharmacologic means. Understanding each of the blood components and when to utilize them is crucial in the resuscitation of hemorrhagic shock. TEG and rotational thromboelastometry (ROTEM) have gained wide acceptance over the last decade owing to the ability to help guide resuscitation, and serve as a set of endpoints specifically relating to the coagulopathy associated with hemorrhage. Developed in 1948 to detect congenital factor deficiencies, this technology has broadened its use to hemorrhage of all types. TEG is a dynamic test that measures both the formation and lysis of the clot. Results are presented graphically and numerically and allow for a global assessment of clotting function, by illuminating abnormalities at specific sites in the clotting cascade and offering detailed information regarding coagulation function.

TEG and ROTEM share many similarities; however, the nomenclature differs between the two. Abnormalities in clot initiation are measured by R (TEG) or CT (ROTEM). Clot initiation is dependent upon clotting factors. Therefore, a prolonged R or CT value corresponds to a deficiency in clotting factors. Prolongations are commonly seen with anticoagulant use and in the presence of factor inhibitors. Therapies include plasma transfusion, prothrombin complex concentrates, and recombinant factor VII. As the clot develops, the tracing diverges and becomes parabolic in shape. The initial angle of this divergence is known as alpha (α). The α corresponds to the rapidity of clot development, and is mainly dependent upon fibrinogen, with a minor role played by platelets. A steep angle indicates overly rapid clot development, whereas a gradual angle indicates a slowly developing clot. Hypofibrinogenemia and hyperfibrinolysis often result in a low α value. Therapies include plasma, which has the greatest *amount* of fibrinogen, and cryoprecipitate, which has the highest *concentration* of fibrinogen. As the clot strengthens, the parabolic curve peaks, resulting in the maximal amplitude (MA) (TEG) or maximum clot firmness (MCF) (ROTEM) of the clot. This is largely dependent upon platelets, with fibrinogen and platelet–fibrinogen interactions contributing to a lesser extent. Low MA/MCF values are seen with thrombocytopenia and in the presence of antiplatelet agents, such as aspirin or clopidogrel. Treating low MA/MCF values is limited to platelet transfusion only. The down-sloping TEG tracing represents the time for clot lysis. Normal lysis at 30 minutes, LY30 (TEG) or CL30 (ROTEM), is 0%. Minor increases in lysis (3% to 8%) are associated with increased mortality and should be rapidly addressed. Therapy includes antifibrinolytic medications, such as tranexamic acid and ε-aminocaproic acid. Plasma and cryoprecipitate may also be employed to replace lost fibrinogen, but the mainstay of treatment is to cease hyperfibrinolysis with pharmacologic means [58].

Employing targeted pharmacologic and transfusion strategies based on TEG measurements allows for normalization of coagulopathy, while limiting untoward effects of overresuscitation or underresuscitation. Additionally, it may result in fewer transfusions, which in turn will decrease complications related to transfusion.

Monitoring

Today's ICUs utilize advanced technologies to determine volume status and resuscitation parameters. The Swan–Ganz pulmonary artery catheter (PAC), since its introduction in 1970, has provided a wealth of information regarding hemodynamics to a large variety of patient populations. However, multiple, large randomized trials have failed to show a mortality benefit when PAC parameters were used to guide resuscitation [59,60]. And, in some trials, higher mortality, increased morbidity, and larger volume fluid resuscitation were seen with PAC use. Additionally, with less-invasive monitors becoming more and more available, the PAC has fallen out of favor. The benefits of the PAC, however, should not be understated in certain instances. Patients with significant arrhythmias or those with pulmonary hypertension may benefit from PAC catheterization, because noninvasive methods frequently fail to demonstrate accurate hemodynamic results. Furthermore, perioperative use of PACs to guide resuscitation has shown in multiple studies to show a mortality and morbidity benefit [61]. For hemorrhagic shock, the PAC may provide information not available from noninvasive methods and, therefore, should be considered in select patient populations.

In addition to PACs, a variety of minimally invasive and noninvasive techniques are available to rapidly determine endpoints of resuscitation. Arterial waveform analysis methodologies have seen widespread use in recent years. Continuous pulse contour cardiac output monitors (PiCCO; Phillips) utilize proprietary thermodilution arterial catheters, typically inserted in the femoral artery, to determine cardiac output through pulse contour analysis. Frequent calibration is necessary, and a learning curve exists both from a physician and nursing point of view [62]. Lithium dilution cardiac output (LiDCO; LiDCO Limited) is measured through the injection of lithium via a central venous access line. The concentration changes of lithium are then measured with a lithium-sensitive sensor attached to an existing arterial line. Again, multiple daily calibrations are necessary; however, a variety of derived variables, including cardiac output, are readily calculated and have been shown to be equivalent to thermodilutional techniques [63]. Arterial waveform monitors (Vigileo; Edwards Lifesciences) provide cardiac output measurement through existing arterial lines, and do not require injection-based calibration. By measuring the pulse pressure variations, stroke volume is calculated and cardiac output is derived. Although typically less precise than the above dilutional methods, arterial waveform monitors provide information using existing catheters with minimal training [64].

Noninvasive methods of cardiac output determination continue to be developed. Ultrasonic cardiac output monitoring (USCOM; Uscom Ltd.) utilizes an ultrasound probe placed at the sternal notch to measure beat-to-beat variability, cardiac output, and systemic vascular resistance. It requires minimal training and has been validated against thermodilution. Obesity may be a barrier to utilizing this method, and may increase error rates in measurements [65]. Another noninvasive device (NICOM; Cheetah Medical) uses bioreactance to measure phase shifts and amplitude after passing a current between electrodes placed on the chest. The phase change correlates well with changes in stroke volume and aortic blood volume. This noninvasive monitor has shown good correlation and reliability both with Doppler ultrasound and thermodilutional methods [66]. It is important to note that reliable monitoring is crucial to determining adequacy of resuscitation. Blind resuscitation invariably misses the mark, resulting in either overresuscitation or underresuscitation and worsened outcomes.

Fluids and Component Therapy

Historically, crystalloid solutions were almost exclusively utilized in resuscitation following hemorrhage. Traditional regimens called for infusing crystalloids while awaiting blood products from the blood bank, with repeated bolus doses as necessary. Following at least 2 L of crystalloid infusion, PRBC were considered. Unfortunately, this approach led to worsened coagulopathy, worsened organ failure, and overall outcomes. Recent evidence has shown improved mortality and morbidity with earlier use of blood products, including plasma transfusion. As stated previously, a key component to both early damage control resuscitation and ongoing resuscitation in the ICU is that crystalloids offer little benefit for hemorrhagic shock. Unlike patients in septic shock, hypotension and hemodynamic collapse are secondary to blood loss. This simple idea of *replacing what was lost* is at the cornerstone of hemorrhagic shock management. Crystalloid preparations inevitably are used to some extent, either as medication carriers or transfusion flushes. However, their use should be limited as much as possible—especially in the early phases of resuscitation, before hemorrhage control is gained. Once in the ICU, targeted and thoughtful use of crystalloid may be employed, but again holding true to damage control tenants. Fluid shifts occurring as the result of hemorrhage are often profound and worsened by large-volume IV fluid administration. Control of coagulopathy and acidosis also falls victim to isotonic and hypotonic crystalloid volume use.

HTS is one crystalloid formula that has proven beneficial. Solutions of 3%, 5%, and 7.5% are commercially available. High concentrations of sodium chloride delivered to the vascular system favor the flux of water from the interstitial space and from the cells to augment the blood volume. This results in a rapid restoration of intravascular volume. Infusions of small amounts of these solutions lead to hemodynamic responses equivalent to much larger volumes of crystalloid solutions. This is advantageous because of both the rapidity of the response and the limited volume necessary to achieve the same goals. Recent work suggests these fluids decrease the activation of neutrophils, modulate cytokine and adhesion molecule expression, and suppress the production of reactive oxygen species. These immunomodulatory effects have been shown to decrease the risk of multiple organ dysfunction syndrome [67]. Proponents believe that the smaller volumes lead to less tissue edema and associated potential complications. Once fluid is drawn into the vascular space, sodium chloride is diluted and equilibrates across the fluid spaces of the body. As this happens, the effect of the HTS is gradually lost. Increases in mean arterial pressure are short-lived, with hemodynamic effects lasting only 15 to 75 minutes [68]. The largest potential danger with hypertonic solutions is hypernatremia. This may be accentuated in the previously dehydrated patient without additional extravascular fluid to donate to the vascular system. Although some rapid and transient hypernatremia seems to be tolerated, caution in administration and careful monitoring of sodium levels are important in the safe use of these solutions.

Whole blood contains all of the factors lost by the bleeding patient, including plasma proteins, clotting factors, platelets, and white blood cells, as well as erythrocytes. Although fresh whole blood is a superb resuscitation fluid, it has a short storage life and, therefore, has limited use in the typical civilian setting. Additionally, infectious disease testing and blood banking inventory management issues have made whole blood largely unavailable. However, whole blood is used in many centers, and clinical studies on whole blood are underway for civilian trauma patients. Prospective data collected in these studies may present an impetus for change in blood banking and provide access to this useful and efficacious resuscitative fluid.

RBC transfusion is common for the resuscitation from hemorrhage, and should be utilized early in the process. Initial resuscitation practices often employ uncrossed blood products with O-negative; however, packed red blood cells (PRBCs) should be typed and cross-matched as early as feasible to avoid transfusion reactions. PRBCs can be stored for 42 days according to current Food and Drug Administration standards. However, detrimental effects of stored PRBCs can be related to their age. Hyperkalemia is a well-known problem with red cell storage, because potassium is lost into the PRBC supernatant over time. Increased risk of cardiac events, infection, multisystem organ failure, and mortality are also associated with older RBCs [69,70]. Despite safeguards, clerical errors lead to mismatched blood administrations, with a rate of fatal major ABO blood group reactions of between 1 in 500,000 and 1 in 2 million. Currently, the risk of infection from a transfused unit is 1 in 30,000 to 1 in 150,000 for hepatitis C, and 1 in 200,000 to 1 in 2,000,000 for human immunodeficiency virus [71].

The benefits of early plasma administration continue to be realized through multiple randomized trials. Plasma should be considered an initial resuscitation fluid in hemorrhagic shock, along with PRBCs. Thawed plasma is plasma that is stored for up to 5 days at 1°C to 6°C. This storage timeline is based on similar RBC storage guidelines and preservation of factors V and VIII; however, clinical data is lacking [72,73]. Because more centers are using earlier and increased amounts of plasma, thawed plasma is now routinely available at many trauma centers, and increasingly stored in emergency departments. Type AB plasma, the universal donor for plasma, is chosen initially before cross-matched product is available. Group A plasma has been shown to be a safe alternative to Type AB, and empiric utilization of Group A plasma may expand the use of massive transfusion protocols, and help encourage the use of early plasma transfusion where AB availability is limited [74]. Having thawed plasma available in the emergency department allows for the initiation of a protocol driven high ratio of FFP to PRBCs. Plasma transfusion risks of TRALI, infection, and multisystem organ failure increase at the rate of approximately 2% with each unit transfused [75]. However, these observations have been made in the context of higher survival among patients who received high ratios of FFP, suggesting that those patients survived despite the potential cost of sepsis and multisystem organ failure development.

Platelets are transfused in two different formulations. Pooled whole blood–derived platelets are generally transfused in six-unit increments from five to six different blood donors. Apheresis platelet units are derived from a single donor and are transfused in volumes approximately equal to 5 to 6 units of pooled whole blood–derived platelets. Because evidence continues to emerge, it is becoming clear that platelets, once an afterthought during traditional resuscitation practices, should be transfused at higher ratios. Many massive transfusion protocols include platelets in the first or second tier of the transfusion guideline. Improved outcomes have been seen when fixed-ratio transfusion strategies include platelets early in the schema. Platelet counts of less than 20,000 per μL should always be corrected in any bleeding patient, whether or not a life-threatening injury has been identified. If the patient has a known history of antiplatelet use within the preceding 7 days, it may be necessary to transfuse platelets despite a platelet count greater than 50,000 per μL, particularly in those patients with head injury or those being managed nonoperatively for significant solid organ injury. Platelet counts of less than 100,000 per μL are a relative indication for platelet transfusion in the head-injured patient with evidence of intracranial hemorrhage, whether as a single-system injury or as part of multisystem injuries. It is possible that we have been overly restrictive in the use of platelet transfusions, because recent data suggests that increased and early use improves survival [52]. Both pooled and apheresis platelets are stored at room temperature for up to 5 days. Bacterial contamination remains the greatest risk of platelet transfusion; however, apheresis platelet units have been shown to have lower risk of infection because they are derived from a single donor.

Cryoprecipitate is a product of FFP that contains factor VIII, von Willebrand factor, fibrinogen, fibronectin, factor XIII, and platelet microparticles. The benefits of including cryoprecipitate in massive transfusion protocols have yet to be confirmed [76]. As a product of plasma, cryoprecipitate contains many of the constituents of plasma, only in concentrated, less voluminous form. For this reason, unless a specific coagulation defect is targeted, cryoprecipitate likely offers little benefit over FFP in the early resuscitation of hemorrhagic shock. Cryoprecipitate is made after centrifuging thawed plasma and removing the supernatant. It has a shelf life of 1 year when frozen at −20°C. Cryoprecipitate is customarily transfused in 10 unit bags, although this is highly variable. As a result of this practice, patients generally receive 2.5 g of cryoprecipitate per transfusion.

Vasopressor and Inotropic Support

Despite adequate volume resuscitation, some patients require additional pharmacologic means to attain hemodynamic goals. In these patients, selective use of vasopressor agents may be necessary. A keen understanding of each agent's receptor targets and their resultant effects is required to effectively make use of vasopressors in the resuscitation of hemorrhagic shock. Norepinephrine is widely used, and is at the forefront of many algorithms aimed to treat critically ill patients. Acting weakly on β_1 receptors, norepinephrine mildly increases contractility, while it acts to strongly activate α_1 receptors, affording potent vasoconstriction. Bradycardia is commonly seen and is, therefore, not recommended for those with bradyarrhythmias. Dopamine acts on multiple receptors and is strongly associated with tachycardia and the development of tachyarrhythmia. At lower doses, it acts as a dopamine (D_1) receptor agonist, and may produce vasodilation through action on β_2 receptors. The so-called "renal dose" dopamine, at low doses, has not been shown to improve renal perfusion or treat renal insufficiency, and although theoretical advantages exist, clinically it has no benefit. At somewhat higher doses, dopamine triggers β_1 receptors and increases contractility and heart rate. With increasing doses, α_1 receptors are activated and vasoconstriction results. Dopamine is typically a second-line agent for most situations relevant to hemorrhagic shock, because of the risk of tachyarrhythmia is increased in patients who are already tachycardic.

Epinephrine is a powerful agent acting strongly on both α and β receptors. In the case of cardiac arrest, 1 mg bolus doses remain a mainstay of treatment. When higher doses are used, tissue ischemia becomes more likely. High-dose epinephrine infusions worsen acidosis and ultimately may result in cardiac ischemia, and therefore are not recommended. Lower doses, however, may be beneficial as either intermittent boluses or infusions. Particular benefits may be seen prior to anesthetic induction for procedural hemorrhage control.

Phenylephrine is a pure α-agent, effecting potent vasoconstriction. Care should be taken when beginning a phenylephrine infusion in patients with hemorrhagic shock. These patients are typically maximally vasoconstricted via endogenous catecholamine release, and cardiac output is being sustained by the patient's tachycardia. Further vasoconstriction, without stimulation of β receptors, will worsen cardiac output by causing a reflex bradycardia, and reduced cardiac output. Additionally, phenylephrine infusions in elderly patients may increase afterload beyond that which the aging heart can function, causing acute heart failure and precipitous drop in cardiac output.

Vasopressin has been increasingly utilized in the resuscitation of patients following hemorrhage. Evidence suggests endogenous vasopressin stores are rapidly depleted in response to hemorrhage, and replacement with a low-dose infusion is warranted when hemodynamic profiles are not optimized. The greatest benefit appears to be when vasopressin is used in conjunction with other vasoactive medications, such as norepinephrine. When norepinephrine doses are greater than 12 μg per minute, concomitant vasopressin infusion has been shown to allow norepinephrine to be titrated down, while maintaining desirable hemodynamics. High-dose infusions (>0.04 units per minute) are strongly associated with coronary ischemia and are not recommended.

Dobutamine and milrinone are two inotropic agents that typically have limited use in hemorrhagic shock. Dobutamine, a pure β-agonist, has a strong effect on contractility and heart rate. It is also associated with vasodilation, and may result in up to a 10% drop in systemic vascular resistance. Milrinone, a phosphodiesterase inhibitor, increases contractility by increasing cyclic adenosine monophosphate. It too, acts as a vasodilator, and preferentially vasodilates the pulmonary vascular bed. Owing to their vasodilating properties, both of these pharmaceuticals offer limited benefit in the resuscitation following hemorrhage. In selected circumstances, principally preexisting heart failure, they may be utilized, but invasive monitoring is necessary to fully appreciate these benefits.

Additional Therapies

Coagulopathy may persist despite aggressive initial treatment. It is important to reevaluate coagulopathy within the first 48 hours of the ICU stay. Preexisting conditions, such as cirrhosis, may prevent adequate coagulopathic control without repeated dosing of medications, such as vitamin K, prothrombin complex concentrates, or plasma (if volume is necessary). Similarly, hyperfibrinolysis may still be present, and require dosing of tranexamic acid. If renal failure is present, the presence of uremic platelet dysfunction should be considered and treated with high-dose DDAVP.

Steroids have been studied in many shock states; however, they have shown little benefit in hemorrhagic shock. One area of interest where steroids may have benefit is in the realm of acute acquired adrenal insufficiency. In patients with persistent hypotension, despite adequate volume resuscitation, a random cortisol level and empiric dosing of either hydrocortisone or dexamethasone should be considered. Many clinicians use clinical judgment to guide administration of steroids in the face of a "relatively" low serum random cortisol. The cortisol stimulation test is controversial, but when used, the patient's cortisol level should increase a minimum of 9 μg per dL above baseline upon administration of cosyntropin.

Glycemic control should be initiated upon arrival to the ICU. Hyperglycemia encourages a proinflammatory state, and results in worsened outcomes. Targets should be reasonable, because iatrogenic hypoglycemia is associated with worsened outcomes as well. Nutritional support should be initiated as early as prudent, depending upon the patient's physiologic state. Intra-abdominal hemorrhage and subsequent operations often preclude early enteral feeding, as do the necessity of vasopressor agents. Most vasoactive medications decrease splanchnic circulation, which increases the risk of tube feed necrosis and other nutritionally related enteric disasters.

Evidence continues to emerge regarding the use of thromboembolic prophylaxis in the setting of hemorrhage. As directed treatment of coagulopathy is associated with improved outcomes, so is thromboembolic prevention. Hemorrhaging patients often are in a prothrombotic and paradoxically coagulopathic state. Overactivation of the clotting cascade combined with stasis from hypotension and vascular damage from the inciting event complete Virchow's triad, and therefore put patients at increased risk for thrombotic events. Once hemorrhage control has been demonstrated, thromboembolic prophylaxis should be initiated. In most cases, waiting more than 24 hours is unnecessary, and leads to higher rates of thromboembolic events.

Home medications should be reviewed and begun as necessary. Preinjury statin use is associated with increased rates of myocardial ischemia when these medications are not restarted upon admission. Withholding β-blocker medications may result in rebound tachycardia and tachyarrhythmias, and increase risk of cardiac ischemia. Diuretics are typically detrimental until the patient is beyond the resuscitative phases, and are generally withheld until stability is demonstrated. In those patients who take diuretics regularly, however, special attention is warranted in regard to volume overloaded states, and the development of pulmonary edema. Anticoagulants should be restarted with caution. Certain conditions, such as patients with mechanical heart valves or recent percutaneous coronary stents, may require anticoagulant or antiplatelet agents to be restarted as soon as possible. An accurate and thorough history is essential to obtain, especially in the aging population.

SUMMARY

Shock following hemorrhage represents a significant, multifaceted process impacting a significant number of patients. Early recognition is crucial to improve outcomes. Once recognized, hemorrhage control must rapidly be obtained to prevent further physiologic derangements, for without it, any resuscitation strategy is futile. Hemostatic adjuncts, both topical and IV, may be utilized to reach this goal. Damage control principles, with targeted treatment of coagulopathy, early use of plasma, and limited crystalloid volume, should be employed in patients at risk for exsanguination. Before, during, and after hemorrhage has ceased, resuscitation efforts must proceed with goals to normalize hemodynamic, coagulation, and perfusion parameters. Resuscitation endpoints should be targeted, with the combined use of advanced monitoring techniques, laboratory results, and clinical judgment.

References

1. Committee on Trauma: *Advanced Trauma Life Support Program*. Chicago, American College of Surgeons, 2012.
2. Sauaia A, Moore FA, Moore EE, et al: Epidemiology of trauma deaths: a reassessment. *J Trauma* 38:185, 1995.
3. Kauvar DS, Lefering R, Wade CE: Impact of hemorrhage on trauma outcome: an overview of epidemiology, clinical presentations, and therapeutic considerations. *J Trauma* 60:S3–S11, 2006.
4. Gunning AC, Lansink KW, van Wessem KJ, et al: Demographic patterns and outcomes of patients in Level I Trauma Centers in three international trauma systems. *World J Surg* 39:2677–2684, 2015.
5. Holcomb JB, Jenkins D, Rhee P, et al: Damage control resuscitation: directly addressing the early coagulopathy of trauma. *J Trauma* 62:307–310, 2007.
6. Cotton BA, Harvin JA, Kostousouv V, et al: Hyperfibrinolysis at admission is an uncommon but highly lethal event associated with shock and prehospital fluid administration. *J Trauma Acute Care Surg* 73:365–370, 2012.
7. Rizoli SB, Scarpelini S, Callum J, et al: Clotting factor deficiency in early trauma-associated coagulopathy. *J Trauma* 71:S427–S434, 2011.
8. Hess JR, Brohi K, Dutton RP, et al: The coagulopathy of trauma: a review of mechanisms. *J Trauma* 65:748–754, 2008.
9. Cohen MJ, Call M, Nelson M, et al: Critical role of activated Protein C in early coagulopathy and later organ failure, infection and death in trauma patients. *Ann Surg* 255:379–385, 2012.
10. Floccard B, Rugeria L, Faure A, et al: Early coagulopathy in trauma patients: an on-scene and hospital admission study. *Injury* 43:26–32, 2012.
11. Cardenas JC, Matijevic N, Baer LA, et al: Elevated tissue plasminogen activator and reduced plasminogen activator inhibitor promote hyperfibrinolysis in trauma patients. *Shock* 41:514–521, 2014.

12. Rahbar E, Cardenas JC, Baimukanova G, et al: Endothelial glycocalyx shedding and vascular permeability in severely injured trauma patients. *J Transl Med* 13:117, 2015.
13. Kozar RA, Peng Z, Zhang R, et al: Plasma restoration of endothelial glycocalyx in rodent model of hemorrhagic shock. *Anesth Analg* 112:1289–1295, 2011.
14. Kutcher ME, Redick BJ, McCreery RC, et al: Characterization of platelet dysfunction after trauma. *J Trauma Acute Care Surg* 73:13–19, 2012.
15. Wiener G, Moore HB, Moore EE, et al: Shock releases bile acid inducing platelet inhibition and fibrinolysis. *J Surg Res* 195:390–395, 2015.
16. Cardenas JC, Wade CE, Holcomb JB: Mechanisms of trauma-induced coagulopathy. *Curr Opin Hematol* 21:404–409, 2014.
17. Toung T, Reilly PM, Fu KC, et al: Mesenteric vasoconstriction in response to hemorrhagic shock. *Shock* 13:267–273, 2000.
18. Parillo JE, Dellinger RP (eds): *Critical Care Medicine*. 3rd ed. Philadelphia PA, Mosby, 2008.
19. Uhlich RM, Konie JA, Davis JW, et al: Novel microRNA correlations in the severely injured. *Surgery* 156:834–841, 2014.
20. Alam HB, Sun L, Ruff P, et al: E-and P-selectin expression depends on the resuscitation fluids used in hemorrhaged rats. *J Surg Res* 94:145, 2000.
21. Schreiber MA, Perkins JP, Kiraly L, et al: Early predictors of massive transfusion in combat casualties. *J Trauma* 205(4):541–545, 2006.
22. MacLeod J, Lynn M, McKenney MG, et al: Predictors of mortality in trauma patients. *Am Surg* 70:805, 2004.
23. Khasawneh MA, Zielinski MD, Jenkins DH, et al: Low tissue oxygen saturation is associated with requirements for transfusion in the rural trauma population. *World J Surg* 38:1892–1897, 2014.
24. Yucel N, Lefering R, Maegele M, et al: Trauma associated severe hemorrhage (TASH)-Score: probability of mass transfusion as surrogate for life threatening hemorrhage after multiple trauma. *J Trauma* 60:1228–1237, 2006.
25. McLaughlin DF, Niles SE, Salinas J, et al: A predictive model for massive transfusion in combat casualty patients. *J Trauma* 64:S57–S63, 2008.
26. Nunez TC, Voskresensky IV, Dossett LA, et al: Early prediction of massive transfusion in trauma: simple as ABC (Assessment of Blood Consumption)? *J Trauma* 66:346–352, 2009.
27. MacIntyre, AD, Quick JA, Barnes SL: Hemostatic dressings reduce tourniquet time while maintaining hemorrhage control. *Am Surg* 77:162–165, 2011.
28. Gates KS, Baer L, Holcomb JB: Prehospital emergency care: evaluation of the junctional emergency tourniquet tool with a perfused cadaver model. *J Spec Oper Med* 14:40–44, 2014.
29. Kisat M, Morrison JJ, Hasmi ZG, et al: Epidemiology and outcomes of non-compressible torso hemorrhage. *J Surg Res* 184:414–421, 2013.
30. Qasim Z, Brenner M, Menaker J, et al: Resuscitative endovascular balloon occlusion of the aorta. *Resuscitation* 96:275–279, 2015.
31. Chang JC, Holloway BC, Amisch M, et al: ResQFoam for the treatment of non-compressible hemorrhage on the front line. *Mil Med* 180:932–933, 2015.
32. Quick JA, Barnes SL: Correct coagulopathy quickly, effectively. *Lancet* 385:2024–2026, 2015.
33. Duchesne JC, McSwain NE, Cotton BA, et al: Damage control resuscitation: the new face of damage control. *J Trauma* 69:976–990, 2010.
34. Pollack CV, Reilly PA, Eikelboom J, et al: Idarucizumab for dabigatran reversal. *N Engl J Med* 373:511–520, 2015.
35. Shakur H, Roberts I, Bautista R, et al: Effects of tranexamic acid on death, vascular occlusive events, and blood transfusion in trauma patients with significant haemorrhage (CRASH-2): a randomized, placebo-controlled trial. *Lancet* 376:23–32, 2010.
36. Harvin JA, Peirce CA, Mims MM, et al: The impact of tranexamic acid on mortality in injured patients with hyperfibrinolysis. *J Trauma Acute Care Surg* 78:905–911, 2015.
37. Morrison JJ, Dubose JJ, Rasmussen TE, et al: Military application of tranexamic acid in trauma emergency resuscitation (MATTERs) study. *Arch Surg* 147:113–119, 2012.
38. *ACS TQIP Massive Transfusion in Trauma Guidelines*. Chicago, IL, American College of Surgeons Committee on Trauma, 2015.
39. Kirkpatrick AW: Clinician-performed focused sonography for the resuscitation of trauma. *Crit Care Med* 35[5 Suppl]:S162–S172, 2007.
40. Jang T, Kryder G, Sineff S, et al: The technical errors of physicians learning to perform focused assessment with sonography in trauma. *Acad Emerg Med* 19:98–101, 2012.
41. Gaarder C, Kroepelien CF, Loekke R, et al: Ultrasound performed by radiologists—confirming the truth about FAST in trauma. *J Trauma* 67:323–327, 2009.
42. Shires GT, Carrico CJ, Baxter CR, et al: Principles in treatment of severely injured patients. *Adv Surg* 4:255–324, 1970.
43. Shires GT, Coln D, Carrico J, et al: Fluid therapy in hemorrhagic shock. *Arch Surg* 88:688–693, 1964.
44. Dillon J, Lunch LJ, Meyers R, et al: A bioassay of treatment of hemorrhagic shock. *Arch Surg* 93:537–555, 1966.
45. Ashbaugh DG, Bigelow DB, Petty TL, et al: Acute respiratory distress in adults. *Lancet* 12:319–323, 1967.
46. Rotondo MF, Schwab CW, McGonigal MD, et al. 'Damage control': an approach for improved survival in exsanguinating penetrating abdominal injury. *J Trauma* 35:375–383, 1993.
47. Longnecker DE, French G: *Fluid Resuscitation: State of the Science for Treating Combat Casualties and Civilian Injuries*. Washington DC, Institute of Medicine, 1999.
48. Fluid Resuscitation in pre-hospital trauma care: a consensus view. *J R Army Med Corps* 147:147–152, 2001.
49. Bickel WH, Wall MJ, Pepe PE, et al: Immediate versus delayed fluid resuscitation for hypotensive patient with penetrating torso injuries. *N Engl J Med* 331:1105–1109, 1994.
50. Holcomb JB, Tilley BC, Baraniuk S, et al: Transfusion of plasma, platelets, and red blood cells in a 1:1:1 vs a 1:1:2 ratio and mortality in patients with severe trauma (PROPPR). *JAMA* 313:471–482, 2015.
51. Smith JB, Pittet JF, Pierce A: Hypotensive resuscitation. *Curr Anesthesiol Rep* 4:209–215, 2014.
52. Holcomb JB, del Junco DJ, Fox EE, et al: The Prospective, Observational, Multicenter, Major Trauma Transfusion (PROMMTT) Study: comparative effectiveness of a time-varying treatment with competing risks. *JAMA* Surg 148:127–136, 2013.
53. Mutschler M, Nienaber U, Brockamp T, et al: Renaissance of base deficit for the initial assessment of trauma patients: a base deficit-based classification for hypovolemic shock developed on data from 16,305 patients derived from the TraumaRegister DGU. *Crit Care* 17:R42, 2013.
54. Hodgman EI, Morse BC, Dente CJ, et al: Base deficit as a marker of survival after traumatic injury: consistent across changing patient populations and resuscitation paradigms. *J Trauma* 72:844–851, 2012.
55. Jones AE, Shapiro NI, Trzeciak S, et al: Lactate clearance vs central venous oxygen saturation as goals of early sepsis therapy. *JAMA* 303:739–746, 2010.
56. Regnier MA, Rauz M, Le Manach Y, et al: Prognostic significance of blood lactate and lactate clearance in trauma patients. *Anesthesiology* 117:1276–1288, 2012.
57. Giraud R, Siegenthaler N, Gayet-Ageron A, et al: $ScvO_2$ as a marker to define fluid responsiveness. *J Trauma* 70:802–807, 2011.
58. Sankarankutty A, Nascimento B, Teodoro da Luz L, et al: TEG and ROTEM in trauma: similar test but different results. *World J Emerg Surg* 7:S1, 2012.
59. Sandham JD, Hull RD, Brant RF, et al: A randomized, controlled trial of the use of pulmonary-artery catheters in high-risk surgical patients. *N Engl J Med* 348:5–14, 2003.
60. Stevenson LW, Binanay C, Califf RM, et al: Evaluation study of congestive heart failure and pulmonary artery catheterization effectiveness. *JAMA* 294:1625–1633, 2005.
61. Hamilton MA, Cecconi M, Rhodes A: A systematic review and meta-analysis on the use of preemptive hemodynamic intervention to improve postoperative outcomes in moderate and high-risk surgical patients. *Anesth Analg* 112:1392–1402, 2011.
62. Litton E, Morgan M: The PiCCO monitor: a review. *Anaesth Intensive Care* 40:393–409, 2012.
63. Mora B, Ince I, Birkenberg B, et al: Validation of cardiac output measurement with the LiDCO™ pulse contour system in patients with impaired left ventricular function after cardiac surgery. *Anaesthesia* 66:675–681, 2011.
64. Biancofore G, Critchley LAH, Lee A, et al: Evaluation of a new software version of the FloTrac/Vigileo (Version 3.02) and a comparison with previous data in cirrhotic patients undergoing liver transplant surgery. *Anesth Analg* 113:515–522, 2011.
65. Beltramo F, Menteer J, Razavi A, et al: Validation of an ultrasound cardiac output monitor as a bedside tool for pediatric patients. *Pediatr Cardiol* 37:177–183, 2016.
66. Cheung H, Dong Q, Dong R, et al: Correlation of cardiac output measured by non-invasive continuous cardiac output monitoring (NICOM) and thermodilution in patients undergoing off-pump coronary artery bypass surgery. *J Anesth* 29:416–420, 2015.
67. Motaharinia J, Etezadi F, Moghaddas A, et al: Immunomodulatory effect of hypertonic saline in hemorrhagic shock. *Daru* 23:47, 2015.
68. Tyagi R, Donaldson K, Loftus CM, et al: Hypertonic saline: a clinical review. *Neurosurg Rev* 30:277–290, 2007.
69. Sadjadi J, Cureton EL, Twomey P, et al: Transfusion, not just injury severity, leads to posttrauma infection: a matched cohort study. *Am Surg* 75:307–312, 2009.
70. Murrell Z, Haukoos JS, Putnam B, et al: The effect of older blood on mortality, need for ICU care, and length of ICU stay after major trauma. *Am Surg* 71:781–785, 2005.
71. Goodnough LT, Brecher ME, Kanter MH, et al: Transfusion medicine: first of two parts—blood transfusion. *N Engl J Med* 340:438, 1999.
72. Spinella PC, Holcomb JB: Resuscitation and transfusion principles for traumatic hemorrhagic shock. *Blood Rev* 23:231–240, 2009.
73. Lamboo M, Poland DC, Eikenboom JC, et al: Coagulation parameters of thawed fresh-frozen plasma during storage at different temperatures. *Transfus Med* 17:182–186, 2007.
74. Zielinski MD, Johnson PM, Jenkins D, et al: Emergency use of prethawed Group A plasma in trauma patients. *J Trauma Acute Care Surg* 74:69–75, 2013.
75. Watson GA, Sperry JL, Rosengart MR, et al: Fresh frozen plasma is independently associated with a higher risk of multiple organ failure and acute respiratory distress syndrome. *J Trauma* 67:221–227, 2009.
76. Holcomb JB, Fox EE, Zhang X, et al: Cryoprecipitate use in the Prospective Observational Multicenter Major Trauma Transfusion study (PROMMTT). *J Trauma Acute Care Surg* 75:S31–S39, 2013.

Chapter 38 ■ Trauma Systems

DANIEL HETHERMAN • TIMOTHY A. EMHOFF

INTRODUCTION

The number of preventable deaths from traumatic injuries worldwide is unfortunate, numbering in the millions annually. In the United States, trauma constitutes a public health crisis and is responsible for over 130,000 lives lost annually. Trauma is now the fourth leading cause of death in the United States based on 2013 statistics published by the Centers for Disease Control and Prevention (CDC). It also remains the leading cause of death among those aged 1 to 44 years. Trauma represents the second highest potential years of life lost, behind only malignant neoplasms. The impact of trauma goes beyond the number of deaths. For every death from trauma, there are 20 individuals who are admitted to the hospital and over 200 Emergency Department visits. The cost of injuries in terms of lost wages, and direct and indirect medical expenses, is estimated to exceed $400 billion annually [1–3].

BACKGROUND

Trauma is a time-sensitive disease. Classically trauma-related deaths were described in a trimodal fashion. Based on this early model, nearly half of all deaths occur immediately at the time of trauma before any medical intervention. The second group of patients reflects those who have ongoing bleeding and injuries that require critical care and may need operative intervention. This group best demonstrates the time-sensitive nature of trauma and is best described by the "Golden Hour" concept. Badly injured trauma patients have a "golden hour" during which time they should be transported to a trauma center and their injuries addressed. The last group of patients reflects those with late mortality related to complications from this initial traumatic insult and resulting medical care.

Today, trauma systems are focused on the rapid transport of injured patients to the most appropriate level of care. This means transportation to a verified trauma center rather than simply the closest hospital with an emergency department. The goal of trauma systems is to get the right patient to the right facility at the right time for the best outcomes.

DEFINITIONS

Typically, trauma patients are individuals suffering from penetrating, blunt, or thermal trauma. Combinations of mechanisms may occur, as well as special circumstances such as blast, near drowning, or electrical injuries. Trauma patients need to be triaged to the most appropriate facility for care. Triage is based both on severity of injuries identified and on the risk of severe injury. The potential severity of injuries is important because the total sum of injuries is not known until the patient has been fully evaluated at the appropriate trauma center. Hemodynamic normalcy at a given point in time does not assure that the patient will remain that way.

Trauma centers are hospitals that have been designated by the state or other designating authority as qualified to care for injured patients. The American College of Surgeons (ACS) maintains a Verification Review Committee that recommends designation for hospitals at certain levels of care using criteria in their document "Optimal Care of the Injured Patient," the sixth edition of which was published in 2015. There are usually a small number of trauma centers in a certain geographic area assuring that each receives an adequate volume of patients required to maintain clinical expertise. Most frequently, trauma centers are designated as Level I through Level IV (some states have also designated Level V trauma centers). Level I trauma centers provide the highest level of care, plus have research, teaching, and serve as a regional resource. Level II trauma centers are intended to also provide for the full spectrum of trauma care, but do not have the research and teaching requirements. Level III facilities do not provide the full spectrum of trauma care; they usually do not provide neurosurgical services. Level IV trauma centers provide trauma care commensurate with their existing resources and usually function as "points of entry" into the system.

HISTORY

The ACS in the 1920s established a committee to attempt to improve in-hospital management of traumatic injuries. This committee attempted to set standards for emergency room treatments and practices. There was some initial push for more involvement of prehospital first responders, but it was not until 1966, when the National Academy of Sciences and the National Research Council published "Accidental Death and Disability: The Neglected Disease of Modern Society," that progress was made with prehospital care. This paper highlighted trauma as a major public health problem and made specific recommendations to reduce accidental death and disability. Subsequent national and state legislation included the Highway Safety Act and the National Traffic and Motor Vehicle Safety Act, which was the first effort to regulate traffic safety and reduce automobile-related death and injuries. Then in 1973, the EMS Systems Act identified trauma systems as one of 15 essential components of an EMS system and appropriated federal funds [4].

VERIFICATION AND DESIGNATION

The trauma system encompasses the complete care of the injured patient from the point of injury prehospital to the completion of the rehabilitative process. Important activities of that system include injury prevention, education, research, and financial viability. For this, there needs to be a lead agency established by each state that has the authority to create and execute policy for the injured patients, as well as designate the trauma centers to manage the injured patients. In order to receive a designation, a hospital or medical center has to demonstrate the standards of care established by the designating authority to achieve their level of trauma center, I, II, III, or IV. The trauma center is then evaluated and verified by either an internal team or an external reviewer, such as the ACS, as meeting the necessary criteria to be a trauma center in the system. This verification is then recommended to the lead agency of the state for designation of a trauma center. The lead agency regulates the quality of trauma systems components and establishes trauma triage guidelines.

The ACS Committee on Trauma (COT) wrote the "Optimal Hospital Resources for Care of the Seriously Injured" in 1976 and is presently on its sixth edition, now called the "Resources for

Optimal Care of the Injured Patient." Since the ACS established this document, it has served as the standard by which trauma systems function and the quality of care is provided. The ACS verification process consists of hospital site reviews to determine a given center's quality of care and ability to manage seriously injured patients. This verification process is then often used by the state as the designating authority to either designate or maintain designation as a trauma center. Verification is currently for 3 years: the rationale being that hospital systems are usually in a constant state of flux and must be verified on an ongoing review process. The ACS–COT also reviews statewide trauma systems to make recommendations to the system as a whole for regional improvements [5,6].

QUALITY OF CARE

Early studies of trauma systems in California introduced the concept of preventable mortality. These studies were able to clearly identify a group of trauma patients, in nonregionalized trauma system areas, that died from inadequate care—preventable mortalities. This concept provided a tool that could be used to examine quality of trauma care in any region or system. It became increasingly clear that analyses of data were important for determining quality of care, trends, and preventable mortality. Trauma registries emerged as a required part of all ACS-verified trauma centers. Aggregations of these hospital-based trauma registries then developed as a result of state-sponsored trauma registries and research-oriented databases. With the ability to examine populations of trauma patients came the development of mathematical formulas calculating the probability of survival of an individual trauma patient and comparing quality of care at trauma centers based on patient survival [7].

Trauma registries continue to support the advancement of trauma care on a national scale. The National Trauma Data Bank (NTDB) is the largest aggregation of trauma patient data. It produces yearly reports and establishes benchmarks for patient care. The development of the ACS TQIP (Trauma Quality Improvement Program) has allowed individual centers to assess their own outcomes compared to national standards. These individualized reports allow institutions to understand areas in which they excel at or need improvement in. This focused feedback, compared to national standards, gives trauma centers specific information necessary to make targeted quality improvements. National aggregation of trauma patient data has allowed for several organizations to emerge and set guidelines for trauma care. AAST (American Association for the Surgery of Trauma), WEST (Western Trauma Association), and EAST (Eastern Association for the Surgery of Trauma) each publish practice guidelines for trauma centers. They use the wide breadth of available data to provide trauma centers with best practice guidelines based on available published evidence.

The ability to implement best practices at trauma centers requires education of both prehospital and hospital providers. The ACS–COT develops the prototype Advanced Trauma Life Support Course (ATLS) in 1978 [8]. The course has been adopted and managed by the American College as one of the most successful educational programs for doctors worldwide. ATLS lays out the framework for the management of trauma patients. Every trauma evaluation begins with a primary survey. The primary survey consists of an ABCDE assessment. In the primary survey, A is for airway, B is for breathing, C is for circulation, D is for disability, and E is for exposure. A secondary survey follows, during which a head-to-toe physical exam is performed and pertinent history obtained. The concept of the primary survey is to identify the most life-threatening problems first and begin treatment immediately. The remainder of the ATLS teaches diagnostic and life-saving interventions, as well as emphasizing the need to transfer a seriously injured patient to a trauma center. ATLS has been introduced in over 50 countries worldwide and is available in numerous different languages.

As one examines the challenges and successes of trauma systems, it remains clear that all phases of care are equally important for the successful outcome desired. These phases are:

A. *Identification/recognition of incident*: The first step in any system is to identify that an injury has occurred or the patient may succumb before medical care can be started. This happens not infrequently in rural and remote parts of our country. Even if the patient is found and transported to an appropriate trauma center, the delay in care may result in sepsis from open fractures not cared for in a timely manner or organ failure from delays or inadequate resuscitation. Some locations in our nation are so remote that even when the injured patient is recognized immediately, it can take more than 24 hours for him or her to arrive in a definitive care facility. The risk for poor outcomes is the same in either case.

B. *Prehospital care and transport*: Prehospital care systems are extremely variable across the United States. These systems range from volunteer to government-employed professionals or contracted professionals. As the first responders to any accident, these individuals often are the first to provide life-saving treatment. Quality EMS providers provide intensive care in the prehospital setting. Pre-Hospital Trauma Life Support (PHTLS) has been developed as a teaching tool for EMS and other prehospital providers to provide education and teaching about care of trauma patients. Inadequate or delayed care can have profound effects on outcomes. Many trauma systems set up regionalized trauma triage criteria that allow the more critically injured patients to bypass closer facilities in favor of higher-level trauma centers capable of providing more definitive care. This regionalization allows more critically injured patients to reach definitive care more quickly. This triage process is enabled by the national trauma field triage guidelines. These guidelines set up protocols for first responders to assist in the decision-making of when to bypass a closer hospital for a designated trauma center. The 2006 national field triage guidelines were reviewed again in 2011 against published data and published as *Guidelines for Field Triage of Injured Patients: Recommendations of the National Expert Panel on Field Triage, 2011* [9].

C. *Emergency department (ED) care*: The Emergency Department represents the advanced practioners first chance to evaluate trauma patients. Even in the ED, inadequate or delayed resuscitation may contribute to a worse outcome. This may happen many ways: too slow a resuscitation may result in prolonged hypotension with potential for organ damage—the brain being particularly susceptible. Conversely, over aggressive resuscitation in the face of some injuries such as brain injury or pulmonary contusion may also cause problems. In these cases, too much resuscitation fluid may result in unnecessary tissue edema. This will cause increased intracranial pressure and poor perfusion in the closed space of the skull. With the lungs, the leaky capillaries associated with pulmonary contusion will cause the contusion to worsen, with difficulty in ventilating and weaning the patient. Too aggressive crystalloid resuscitation in the severely burned puts the patient at increased risk of abdominal compartment syndrome. Inappropriate use of strictly crystalloid resuscitation, when blood/blood products are indicated, can lead to increased mortality.

Systems at individual centers are critical for the timely and effective assessment of the trauma patient. At higher-level trauma centers, these systems are often resource-heavy with large teams of staff prepared to quickly evaluate and treat trauma patients. However, at smaller or more rural centers, there may be only a small team or an individual practitioner who is charged with this patient's care. At these smaller facilities, prompt stabilization and transfer of critically injured patients to a higher-level center is essential.

D. *Operating room (OR) care*: Prior to intensive care unit (ICU) admission, many trauma patients will have required operative intervention. In the operating room, the trauma surgeon remains the principal manager of resuscitation. Although the surgeon is operating, other staff and resources are essential for effective patient care. Operating rooms must be capable and prepared with equipment and staff to explore any part of the body necessary. Inappropriate or inadequate resuscitation during operative intervention may worsen outcomes. As a result, anesthesia plays a critical role in the management of trauma patients in the operating room. Many centers have moved to a massive transfusion protocol both in the emergency department and in the operating room to help guide patient fluid management. These protocols focus on giving blood and blood products in predetermined ratios to optimize outcomes and trauma patient resuscitation.

E. *ICU care*: ICU critical care is essential for the management of the sickest trauma patients. Any and all organ systems can be adversely affected by trauma, and the ICU is critical in supporting and managing these diverse set of injuries. Patients who arrive from the operating room may still be cold, acidotic, or coagulopathic; and it is incumbent on the trauma system to have effective ICU care to manage the significant burden of disease. The ICU provides an opportunity to review and compile the data that has been collected to date and continue to evaluate the trauma patient for additional injuries: a so-called "tertiary survey." Central lines placed urgently in less than sterile conditions are removed and replaced with new sterile lines; blood work and physiologic monitoring are used to provide focused care and to direct care guided by end points of resuscitation. Other chapters in this section give details for the care of shock, resuscitation, management of sepsis, multiple organ dysfunction syndrome, traumatic brain injury, spinal cord injury, thoracic and cardiac trauma, abdominal trauma, burn management, and orthopedic injuries.

F. *Ward care after leaving the ICU:* Critical care trauma patients will need close follow-up on the trauma center wards. Sepsis may occur on the floor with MOD syndrome as well. The physicians following these patients must be capable of early recognition of these problems and institute immediate therapy when such problems are recognized. High-functioning trauma systems are not devoid of complications, but they do have systems and processes in place to "rescue" patients when they occur.

G. *Rehabilitation*: Though many think the rehabilitative process begins after leaving the hospital, it should begin on the first full hospital day. Patients need to be mobilized early, and physical and occupational therapy consults should be on the admission orders. All patients with even minor head injuries need cognitive testing and evaluation by speech and occupational therapists. Even patients on ventilators in the ICU should be part of an early mobilization program. Data suggest that these early mobilization programs significantly improve long-term outcomes for trauma patients [10]. Any patient with head or spinal cord injuries or with a cluster of serious injuries needs a physical medicine and rehabilitation physician involved with their care early in their hospitalization. The discharge plan needs to be formulated early and the resources of the patient and families need to be understood so the maximum benefit of rehabilitation and recovery can be realized. Many trauma patients are injured while using drugs or alcohol or owing to suicidal or depressive motives. These patients benefit significantly from directed psychiatric or social work interventions regarding their substance abuse issues. All seriously injured patients may suffer from posttraumatic stress. It is the obligation of the trauma service to address these issues and have social services, counselors, and psychiatric services as part of the team so that the patient has the opportunity for the best possible outcome.

H. *Performance improvement*: Providing evidence-based care and striving to provide the best care possible is the mission of every trauma service. Research, education, and injury prevention are all components of that mission. Opportunities for improvement in patient care from specific events or trends in complications must be recognized, dissected, and acted upon to promote quality medical care. Trauma registries serve as a central database for data collection and allow for the evaluation of trends and recognition of areas of improvement. As part of a verified trauma center, this information is shared with the National Trauma Data Bank at the ACS. The information obtained from the trauma center registry feeds an effective PI program. Using the information in the NTDB can identify areas of research and areas where injury prevention can be targeted to reduce traumatic injuries. The knowledge of which injuries are prevalent in that region will direct the focus of the injury prevention program; from helmet or seat belt use to preventing childhood or elderly falls. The wide research activity is encouraged at all trauma centers but is a requirement for Level I centers. Finally, ongoing educational programs of all care givers involved with trauma care, including prehospital and rehabilitative services, is ensured as an essential duty of a trauma center and the trauma system.

DISASTER MANAGEMENT

Most disasters are major incidents such as plane crashes, explosions in chemical factories, natural disasters such as hurricanes, or results of war, and terrorist activities such as the events of September 11, 2001 or at the Boston Marathon. An effective trauma system should be primed to manage these disasters. To successfully manage a disaster with many victims, there needs to be preplanning and organization of resources. There needs to be training done within the trauma system, stockpiling of supplies, an effective communication and triage system, and a clear understanding of the resources of each hospital and trauma center in the area. Without a trauma system, the wrong facilities would end up with the wrong patients (i.e., a seriously injured patient to a small hospital) or one hospital being overwhelmed while others close by go underused. The trauma system needs to predefine the triage of patients of a disaster according to severity of injury and volume of patients. The most important principle is triage of the most seriously injured to the higher level of care in the fastest amount of time, and to avoid overtriage of minor injuries to the major trauma center. Events such as the Boston Marathon Bombing highlight how an effective regional system allowed for effective care of over 250 injured patients with no in-hospital mortality for the 127 severely injured patients who were cared for at the area's trauma centers. These unfortunate events highlight the need for disaster planning within trauma systems to be prepared both prehospital and within the hospital in order to deal with the large volume of patients and prevent in-hospital mortality [11,12].

RURAL TRAUMA

The establishment of a trauma system in a rural environment is a unique challenge but important nonetheless to improve outcomes of the injured patients. Most of the problems with rural trauma relate to the time to definitive care at a trauma center. Studies have shown that rural trauma has a higher rate or mortality than urban trauma, but that those who reach definitive care often have similar outcomes. However, because of the rural environment, there is increased discovery time, time for the prehospital personnel to get to the patient, transportation over great distances, and hard terrain. Transfer to the highest level of medical center may take hours or even days depending on how remote an area may be. To decrease the mortality and morbidity of these patients, the trauma system needs to be firmly established; as also, there is a need to designate and train lower-level trauma centers in areas of sparse population, provide consistent training of the volunteer prehospital personnel, and establish effective communication and transport systems between the prehospital care givers and major trauma centers. The American College of Surgeons sponsors specific courses for training in both rural trauma and disaster management—the Rural Trauma Team Development Course (RTTDC) and the Disaster Management and Emergency Preparedness course (DMEP).

In summary, trauma systems provide for early recognition, prehospital care, resuscitation, and operative care critical care management, long-term care, and rehabilitation. Performance improvement remains an essential trauma system function.

References

1. Ten Leading Causes of Death by Age Group, United States 2013 (Chart): Center for Disease Control and Prevention.
2. Johnson NB, Hayes, LD, Brown K, et al: CDC National Health Report: leading causes of morbidity and mortality and associated behavior risk and protective factors—United States, 2005-2013. *MMWR Surveill Summ.* 63[Suppl 4]:3–27, 2014.
3. Injury Prevention & Control: Data & Statistics (WISQARS™): Cost of Injuries Report 2010. Center for Disease Control and Prevention.
4. Simpson AT: Transporting Lazarus: physicians, the State and the creation of the Modern Paramedic and Ambulance, 1955-73. *J His Med Allied Sci* 68(2):163–197, 2013.
5. Committee on Trauma, American College of Surgeons: *Resources for Optimal Care of the Injured Patient 2014.* Chicago: American College of Surgeons, 2014.
6. Celso B, Tepas J, Langland-Orban B, et al: A systematic review and meta-analysis comparing outcome of severely injured patients treated in trauma centers following the establishment of trauma systems. *J Trauma* 60(2):371–378, 2006.
7. Cales RH, Trunkey DD: Preventable trauma deaths. *JAMA* 254(8):1049–1053, 1985.
8. American College of Surgeons. *Advanced Trauma Life Support for Doctors.* 9th ed. Chicago: American College of Surgeons, 2012.
9. Centers for Disease Control and Prevention: Guidelines for field triage of injured patients: recommendations of the national expert panel on field triage, 2011. *MMWR Morb Mortal Wkly Rep* 61(1):1–21, 2012.
10. Adler J, Malone D: Early mobilization in the intensive care unit: a systematic review. *Cardiopulm Physi Ther J* 23(1):5–13, 2012.
11. Lennquist S: Management of major accidents and disasters: an important responsibility for the trauma surgeons. *J Trauma* 62(6):1321–1329, 2007.
12. Gates JD, Arabian S, Biddinger P, et al: The initial response to the Boston Marathon Bombings: lessons learned to prepare for the next disaster. *Ann Surg* 260(6):960–966, 2014.
13. Fatovich DM, Phillips M, Langford SA, et al: A comparison of metropolitan vs rural major trauma in Western Australia. *Resuscitation* 82(7):886–890, 2011.

Chapter 39 ■ The Management of Sepsis

PAUL E. MARIK

Sepsis is among the most common reasons for admission to ICUs throughout the world. An epidemiologic study in European ICUs demonstrated a prevalence of 37% for sepsis and 30% for severe sepsis [1]. The incidence of severe sepsis in the United States is estimated to be about 300 cases per 100,000 population [2–4]. Sepsis is reported to be more common in men and among non-White persons [3]. Surgical patients account for nearly one-third of sepsis cases in the United States; this is important as the management of "surgical" and "medical sepsis" differs somewhat. Patients who have had a septic episode are at an increased risk of death for up to 5 years following the acute event [5]. Data from 2004 to 2009 demonstrate a 13% average annual increase in the incidence of severe sepsis with a decrease in in-hospital mortality from 35% to 26% [2]. This study estimated that there were 229,044 deaths from severe sepsis in 2009, which would place severe sepsis as the third most common cause of death in the United States, after heart disease and malignant neoplasms [2]. However, several factors including international classification of disease (ICD) coding rules, the use of administrative data sets, and increased awareness and surveillance confound the interpretation of these epidemiologic data [6,7]. In 1987, the Australian and New Zealand Intensive Care Society (ANZICS) developed a high-quality database that prospectively collects data from all patients admitted to 171 ICUs in Australia and New Zealand [8]. An analysis of this database demonstrates a linear decrease in absolute mortality for severe sepsis and septic shock from 35% in 2000 to 16.7% in 2012, with an annual rate of absolute decrease of 1.3% [9]. It should be noted that the Surviving Sepsis Campaign was not endorsed by ANZICS and was poorly adopted in these two countries [10]. While it has been claimed that the Surviving Sepsis Campaign has contributed to the decline in mortality from sepsis around the world [11,12], this is clearly not the case for Australia and New Zealand. Furthermore, the decline in mortally from severe sepsis and septic shock in the United States was evident long before the "adoption" of the Surviving Sepsis Campaign [3]. It is likely that the earlier recognition and treatment of sepsis as well as advances in ICU care (lung-protective ventilation, conservative blood strategy, etc) are largely responsible for the improved outcomes of patients with sepsis. This chapter will provide an overview of sepsis with particular emphasis on the diagnosis and management of severe sepsis and septic shock.

DEFINITIONS

The word "sepsis" is derived from the ancient Greek word for rotten flesh and putrefaction. Since then, a wide variety of definitions have been applied to sepsis, including sepsis syndrome, severe sepsis, bacteremia, septicemia, and septic shock. In 1991, the American College of Chest Physicians (ACCP) and the Society of Critical Care Medicine (SCCM) developed a new set of terms and definitions to define sepsis in a more "precise manner" [13]. These definitions took into account the findings that sepsis may result from a multitude of infectious agents and microbial mediators and may not be associated with detectable bloodstream infection. The term "systemic inflammatory response syndrome" (SIRS) was coined to describe the common systemic response to a wide variety of insults. Four SIRS criteria were defined, namely tachycardia (heart rate >90 beats per minute), tachypnea (respiratory rate >20 breaths per minute), fever or hypothermia (temperature >38°C or less than 36°C), and leukocytosis, leukopenia, or bandemia (WBC >1,200 per μL, <4,000 per μL or bandemia ≥10%). Patients who met two or more of these criteria fulfilled the definition of SIRS. When SIRS was the result of a suspected or confirmed infectious process, patients were defined as having "sepsis." Severe sepsis was defined as sepsis plus organ dysfunction. Septic shock was a subset of severe sepsis and was defined as "sepsis-induced hypotension persisting despite adequate fluid resuscitation." However, it became evident that the use of the SIRS criteria to define sepsis was problematic, as it lacked both sensitivity and specificity [14]. Kaukonen et al. [15] evaluated the presence of the SIRS criteria in 109,603 patients with infection and organ failure. In this study, 12% of patients were classified as SIRS-negative sepsis (i.e., had <2 SIRS criteria). Conversely, when the SIRS criteria are applied to an unselected cohort of patients, many patients who do not have an infection are diagnosed as having sepsis [16]. In order to "improve" on these definitions, updated definitions for sepsis and septic shock were released in 2016 by the Third International Consensus Taskforce (Sepsis-3) [17–19]. Sepsis was defined as life-threatening organ dysfunction caused by a dysregulated host response to infection. For clinical operationalization, organ dysfunction was defined as an increase in the Sequential Sepsis Organ Assessment (SOFA) score of 2 or more points for patients in the ICU. A new bedside score termed *quickSOFA* (qSOFA) was developed to describe organ dysfunction in non-ICU patients. Patients required at least two of the following qSOFA criteria to be diagnosed as having sepsis: respiratory rate of 22 per minute or greater, altered mentation, or a systolic blood pressure of 100 mm Hg or less. Septic shock was defined as a subset of sepsis with "profound circulatory, cellular, and metabolic abnormalities." Patients with septic shock are identified by the requirement for vasopressors to maintain a mean arterial pressure of 65 mm Hg or greater and a serum lactate greater than 2 mmol per L in the "absence of hypovolemia." With the new definitions, the "SIRS criteria" are no longer used to screen for or diagnose sepsis and the term "severe sepsis" was removed. Only time will tell how much of an advance these new criteria provide our patients.

PATHOGENS AND SITES OF INFECTION

Sepsis studies conducted over the past two decades indicate that the lung (pneumonia) is the commonest site of infection, accounting for about 50% of cases, followed by abdominal/pelvic infection (25%), primary bacteremia (15%), urosepsis (10%), and blood stream infections related to vascular access devices (5%). Approximately 25% of patients with severe sepsis are infected with a gram-positive organism, 25% gram-negative organisms, 20% a mixed infection (gram-positive and gram-negative), with anaerobic and fungal infections occurring in less than 5% of cases. Viral pathogens are rare causes of sepsis (Ebola and H1N1 influenzae infections). Despite exhaustive microbiologic tests, a pathogen is not isolated in about 25% of patients. A recent study in patients with community-acquired pneumonia isolated a bacterial pathogen in only 14% of patients [20]. The spectrum of pathogens depends upon the site of infection and whether the patient is at risk of infection with drug-resistant pathogen (see below).

PATHOPHYSIOLOGY OF SEPSIS

Sepsis is probably the most complex disease known to man. The pathogenetic mechanisms and physiologic changes associated with sepsis are exceedingly complex, with our understanding of this topic rapidly evolving; the reader is referred to excellent reviews on this topic [21–26]. Exposure of human macrophages to bacterial antigens has been demonstrated to result in a significant change in the expression of over 950 genes [27]. These include genes for pro- and anti-inflammatory cytokines, chemokines, adhesion molecules, transcription factors, enzymes, clotting factors, stress proteins, and antiapoptotic molecules. These gene products alter the function of nearly every cell and tissue in the body. Furthermore, these mediators interact in complex positive and negative feedback loops and result in epigenetic modifications that further alter the expression of this network of mediators [25]. The early phase of sepsis is generally believed to result from the uncontrolled production of proinflammatory mediators, the so-called cytokine storm [21,22]. Sir William Osler was the first to recognize that "except on few occasions, the patient appears to die from the body's response to infection rather than from the infection" [28]. However, recent data suggest that both a proinflammatory and an opposing anti-inflammatory response occur concurrently in patients with sepsis [23,24,29]. In general, following a variable time course, patients transition from a predominantly proinflammatory to an anti-inflammatory immunosuppressive state [23,25,30]. Among elderly patients, particularly those with significant comorbidities, the anti-inflammatory response may predominate [23]. Similarly, surgical and trauma patients who become infected transition rapidly to a predominantly anti-inflammatory response [31].

The cardiovascular changes associated with severe sepsis play a central role in the early management of sepsis and will be briefly reviewed. The major cardiovascular changes in patients with severe sepsis and septic shock include vasoplegic shock, myocardial dysfunction, altered microvascular flow, and a diffuse endothelial injury [32,33]. Sepsis is characterized by increased expression and activation of endothelial adhesion molecules with adhesion and activation of platelets, leukocytes, and mononuclear cells and activation of the coagulation cascade [34]. This results in a diffuse endothelial injury, microvascular thrombosis, gaps between the endothelial cells (paracellular leak), and shedding of the endothelial glycocalyx [35,36]. The combination of these mechanisms contributes to a reduction of functional capillary density, heterogenous abnormalities in microcirculatory blood flow, and increased capillary permeability [37,38].

Asoplegic shock, due to failure of the vascular smooth muscle to constrict, results in arterial and veno-dilatation [32]. Vasoplegic shock is believed to result from increased expression of inducible nitric oxide synthetase with increased production of nitric oxide (NO), activation of K_{ATP} channels resulting in hyperpolarization of the muscle cell membrane, increased production of natriuretic peptides (which act synergistically with NO), and a relative vasopressin deficiency [32]. Veno-dilatation increases the size of the nonstressed blood volume decreasing venous return which compounds the intravascular volume deficit caused by the vascular leak.

Myocardial depression of patients with septic shock was first described in 1984 by Parker et al. [39] using radionuclide cineangiography. In a series of 20 patients, these investigators reported a 50% incidence of left ventricular (LV) systolic dysfunction. Notably, in this study, the initial ejection fraction and ventricular volumes were normal among nonsurvivors, and these indices did not change during serial studies; it is likely that these patients had significant diastolic dysfunction. The initial studies evaluating cardiac function for sepsis focused on LV systolic function. However, LV diastolic dysfunction has emerged as a common finding among patients with severe sepsis and septic shock [40]. Adequate filling during diastole is a crucial component of effective ventricular pump function. Diastolic dysfunction refers to the presence of an abnormal left ventricular diastolic distensibility, filling, or relaxation, regardless of LV ejection fraction. Predominant diastolic dysfunction appears to be at least twice as common as systolic dysfunction in patients with sepsis [40]. The largest study to date (n = 262), by Landesberg et al. [41], reported diastolic dysfunction for 40% of patients with sepsis, whereas 9.1% of patients had isolated systolic dysfunction. Unlike systolic LV dysfunction, diastolic dysfunction is an important prognostic marker for patients with sepsis [40–42]. Patients with diastolic dysfunction respond very poorly to fluid loading [41]. For these patients, fluid loading will increase cardiac filling pressures and increase venous and pulmonary hydrostatic pressures with the increased release of natriuretic peptides with minimal (if any) increase in SV [43].

COMPLICATIONS ASSOCIATED WITH SEPSIS

Complications associated with severe sepsis and septic shock include acute respiratory distress syndrome (ARDS), acute kidney injury (AKI), disseminated intravascular coagulation (DIC), critical illness polyneuropathy, critical illness myopathy, and septic encephalopathy. The risk of ARDS (and outcome) may be critically dependent on the fluid resuscitation strategy (see below). Sepsis is the leading cause of AKI in critically ill patients and is associated with a hospital mortality exceeding 50% [44,45]. Contrary to classic teaching, animal models and human studies have shown that the sepsis-induced AKI occurs in the setting of preserved or increased renal blood flow [46]. A "unifying theory" has been proposed to explain the development of sepsis-induced AKI, which includes the interplay between inflammation and oxidative stress, microvascular dysfunction, and the adaptive response of the tubular epithelial cell to the septic insult [46]. In addition, a high central venous pressure (CVP) caused by overzealous fluid resuscitation can be transmitted retrograde increasing venous pressures. The kidney is particularly affected by increased venous pressure, which leads to increased renal subcapsular pressure and lowered renal blood flow and glomerular filtration rate [47]. Legrand and colleagues demonstrated a linear relationship between increasing CVP and AKI, with a high CVP being the only hemodynamic variable independently associated with AKI [48]. A CVP >8 mm Hg (as proposed by Early Goal Directed Therapy-EGDT and the Surviving Sepsis Campaign) [49,50] can increase the risk of developing AKI [48,51].

Coagulopathy is a common feature of acute sepsis and comprises a wide spectrum of hemostatic changes ranging from thrombocytopenia and/or subclinical activation of blood coagulation to uncontrolled, systemic clotting activation with massive thrombin formation and fibrin deposition in the microcirculation, eventually leading to consumption of platelets and proteins of the hemostatic system (acute DIC) [26]. The widespread microvascular thrombosis is believed to play a major role in the pathogenesis of the multiorgan dysfunction syndrome (MODS) that is characteristic of severe sepsis and septic shock [52]. The key event underlying the development of DIC is the overwhelming inflammatory host response to the pathogen leading to the overexpression of inflammatory mediators. The latter, along with the microorganism and its derivatives, drive the major changes responsible for massive thrombin formation and fibrin deposition mediated by aberrant expression of tissue factor mainly by monocytes-macrophages. In addition, impairment of anticoagulant pathways, orchestrated by dysfunctional endothelial cells and suppression of fibrinolysis due to the overproduction of plasminogen activator inhibitor-1 by endothelial cells and thrombin-mediated activation of thrombin-activatable fibrinolysis inhibitor compounds the thrombotic dysfunction [26].

CLINICAL FEATURES AND DIAGNOSIS OF SEPSIS

Sepsis is a systemic disease with a variety of clinical manifestations. The initial symptoms of sepsis are nonspecific and include malaise, tachycardia, tachypnea, fever, and sometimes hypothermia. Although most patients with sepsis have an elevated white blood cell count, some patients present with low white blood cell counts, which in general is a poor prognostic sign. A band count in excess of 5% has been reported to have a high specificity (92%) but low sensitivity for the diagnosis of sepsis (43%) [53]. Other clinical manifestations include altered mental status, hypotension, respiratory alkalosis, metabolic acidosis, hypoxemia with acute lung injury, thrombocytopenia, consumptive coagulopathy, proteinuria, acute tubular necrosis, intra-hepatic cholestasis, elevated transaminases, hyperglycemia, and hypoglycemia. Patients may present with clinical features of a localized site of infection, such as cough, tachypnea, or sputum production resulting from pneumonia; flank pain and dysuria with urinary tract infection, or abdominal pain with intra-abdominal infection.

The manifestations of sepsis can sometimes be quite subtle, particularly in the very young, the elderly, and those patients with chronic debilitating or immunosuppressing conditions. These patients may present with normothermia or hypothermia. The failure to generate a temperature greater than 99.6°F (37.5°C) in the first 24 hours of clinical illness has been associated with an increased mortality rate. An altered mental state or an otherwise unexplained respiratory alkalosis may be the presenting feature of sepsis. The signs and symptoms of systemic inflammation are not useful in distinguishing infectious from noninfectious causes of SIRS.

Blood cultures are considered to provide a clinical gold standard for the diagnosis of bacterial infections. However, blood cultures are only positive in between 20% and 30% of patients with sepsis; moreover, it takes 2 to 3 days before the results become available. Despite exhaustive microbiologic tests, a pathogen is not isolated in between 25% and 50% of patients [54]. The use of antibiotics prior to microbiologic testing contributes to the low diagnostic yield of these tests. Molecular diagnostic techniques that do not depend on the growth of organisms in culture may offer distinct advantages over current microbiologic methods. Most of the early molecular methods relied upon culture amplification, which did not resolve the issue of the significant proportion of false-negative cultures. Furthermore, these techniques used targeted pathogen detection with limited pathogen coverage. SeptiFast (Roche Diagnostics, Germany) was the first real-time polymerase chain reaction (PCR)–based system approved for clinical use. A meta-analysis from 41 phase III diagnostic accuracy studies reported a sensitivity and specificity for SeptiFast compared with blood culture of 0.68 and 0.86, respectively [55]. Similarly, Chang and colleagues performed a meta-analysis evaluating multiplex PCR for the detection of pathogens in patients with presumed sepsis [56]. This meta-analysis, which included 34 studies and 6,012 patients, reported an overall sensitivity and specificity of 0.75 and 0.92, respectively. More recently, advanced PCR followed by electrospray ionization mass spectrometry (PCR/ESI-MS) has been described which can detect more than 800 relevant pathogens in a single assay and which can be completed in approximately 6 hours [57]. The Rapid Diagnosis of Infection in the Critically ill (RADICAL) study was a prospective observational multicenter study that evaluated 529 patients with suspected infection using the PCR/ESI-MS technology [58]. PCR/ESI-MS detected a pathogen in 35% of blood samples compared with 11% for conventional blood culture. This technique holds great promise for the early detection of blood stream infection, allowing for early targeted antibiotic therapy. The major limitation of this technology is that it cannot provide detailed antimicrobial susceptibility data and as such complements standard culture techniques. It is therefore important to emphasize that appropriate samples for culture be obtained prior to initiation of antibiotics to increase the diagnostic yield of these tests. Venipuncture is the preferred method for blood culture collection. Arterial blood samples do not increase diagnostic yield, and blood specimens obtained from intravascular lines have been associated with higher rates of contamination [59]. The Clinical and Laboratory Standards Institute (CLSI) recommends that if one must collect a blood culture from an intravenous line, it should be paired with a culture that is obtained via venipuncture to assist in the interpretation of positive results [60]. The total volume of blood cultured from adult patients is directly proportional to the yield of microorganisms recovered [59,61]. The timing of blood culture collection does not appear to significantly affect the recovery of clinically relevant microorganisms, and most authorities therefore recommend collecting multiple sets simultaneously or over a short period of time [59–61]. Classic teaching suggests that sets of blood cultures be separated in time (20 minutes to an hour); there is, however, no evidence to support this approach, which is logistically problematic and can delay the initiation of antibiotic therapy [61]. Optimally, two to three sets of blood specimens should be collected from independent venipuncture sites, and each set should consist of at least 20 mL of blood [59]. Therefore, the best strategy when performing blood culture is to obtain blood for 4 to 6 bottles (for a total volume of 40 to 60 mL), preferably at the same time [62]. Such a strategy increases the likelihood of obtaining positive blood cultures results yet minimizes the risk of contaminants and reduces the delay in the administration of antibiotics.

A number of biomarkers have been evaluated as adjunctive methods to improve the diagnosis of sepsis. Procalcitonin (PCT) has to date been the most useful biomarker to aid in the diagnosis of sepsis. PCT, a propeptide of calcitonin, is normally produced in the C-cells of the thyroid. In healthy individuals, PCT levels are very low (<0.01 ng per mL). In patients with sepsis, however, PCT levels increase dramatically, sometimes to more than several hundred nanograms per milliliter. The use of PCT for the diagnosis of sepsis and in determining the duration of antibiotics is controversial. The test is not perfect and should always be interpreted in the clinical context together with other diagnostic tests. Wacker et al. [63] performed a meta-analysis to evaluate the diagnostic accuracy of PCT. In this meta-analysis, the sensitivity was 0.77 (95% CI 0.72 to 0.81), the specificity was 0.79 (95% CI 0.74 to 0.84), and the area under the ROC curve was 0.85 (95% CI 0.81 to 0.88). This diagnostic accuracy is better than any other single test to diagnose sepsis. A PCT >0.5 ng per mL is highly suggestive of a bacterial infection, whereas a level <0.1 ng per mL makes this diagnosis less likely [64]. However, the optimal diagnostic threshold is unclear and has been reported to vary from 0.25 to 1.4 ng per mL [64,65] .This variation of diagnostic threshold may partly be explained by the case-mix of each study and the fact that patients with gram-negative infection have significantly higher PCT levels than those with gram-positive infections [66–68]. Infection with a gram-negative pathogen is highly likely in a patient with a PCT level >5 ng per mL. It should be noted that patients with fungal infections usually have much lower or "normal" PCT levels [66]. In hematologic patients, an elevated PCT level within 24 hours after the onset of neutropenic fever is highly predictive of gram-negative bacteremia [69]. In addition to being a very useful test to diagnose bacterial sepsis, the trend in the PCT level is useful for deciding when to discontinue antibiotics [70,71]. Furthermore, the trend in the PCT is strongly predictive of outcomes, with a persistently high level being associated with a poor outcome [72].

Presepsin is a "newer" biomarker that appears to have a diagnostic accuracy that is similar to PCT [73]. Presepsin, also named soluble cluster-differentiation 14 subtype (sCD14-ST), is a 13 kDa protein that is a truncated N-terminal fragment of CD14 [73]. CD14 is a high-affinity receptor for complexes of lipopolysaccharide (LPS) and LPS-binding proteins (LPB). Presepsin increases significantly in the blood of septic patients, and it has been studied as a marker to differentiate sepsis from other noninfectious causes of SIRS [74–76]. Similarly, soluble triggering receptor expressed on myeloid cells-1 (sTREM-1) levels has been demonstrated to have moderate diagnostic performance in differentiating sepsis from SIRS [77]. The "classic" proinflammatory mediators (IL1, IL-6, and TNF-α) are unable to distinguish between infectious and noninfectious causes of SIRS. IL-27 is produced by antigen-presenting cells on exposure to microbial derived molecules and inflammatory stimuli and has been shown to have a modest ability to predict bacterial infections, especially bloodstream infections [78,79]. It is likely that a decision tree using a number of biomarkers may improve the diagnostic accuracy as compared with a single biomarker alone [79].

Owing to the lack of specific criteria to diagnose sepsis, this diagnosis is often delayed. The early detection and treatment of sepsis are the most important factors for improving the outcome from this condition. However, for many patients admitted to hospital, there is frequently a long delay before the diagnosis of sepsis. Furthermore, it is not uncommon for febrile patients to be sent home from the Emergency Department or the physician's office with the diagnosis of "flu" only to return hours or days later in overt septic shock. The diagnosis of sepsis therefore requires a high index of suspicion, a comprehensive clinical evaluation together with supportive laboratory tests including appropriate microbiologic cultures, a complete blood count with differential, lactate and when rapidly available PCT levels [80]. It is important to emphasize that unlike PCT, lactate is not a specific "sepsis test." An elevated lactate is a useful marker of disease severity in patients with sepsis, and sepsis should be considered in the differential diagnosis of patients with an elevated lactate level.

Any one of the following features alone or in combination is suggestive of bacterial sepsis [80]:

- Fever >38.3°C or hypothermia (<36°C)
- Heart rate >120 per minute (sinus tachycardia)
- Systolic BP <90 mm Hg
- PCT >0.5 ng per mL
- Bandemia >5%
- Lymphocytopenia <0.5 × 10^3 μL
- Thrombocytopenia <150 × 10^3 μL
- Lactate >2.0 meq per L
- Increased neutrophil/lymphocyte ratio (>10:1)

MANAGEMENT OF SEPSIS

The optimal management of patients with severe sepsis and septic shock is highly controversial. It is important to emphasize that there is no Level 1 evidence (data from two or more adequately powered randomized controlled trials (RCTs) or a meta-analysis of RCTs) that demonstrates that any intervention reduces the mortality of patients with severe sepsis or septic shock. Multiple large RCTs have attempted to modulate the immune response or coagulation cascade in patients with severe sepsis and septic shock; these studies have universally met with failure. Although the timely administration of appropriate antibiotics and adequate source control are considered the cornerstones of the management of patients with severe sepsis and septic shock, no RCTs have been performed (or are likely to be performed) that demonstrate the benefit of these interventions. Furthermore, the narrow time window for the administration of antibiotics as advocated by the Surviving Sepsis Campaign Guidelines (administration within 3 hours of Emergency Department triage and within 1 hour of severe sepsis/septic shock recognition) is not supported by a meta-analysis of cohort studies that investigated this issue [81]. This section will focus on appropriate antibiotic therapy, hemodynamic management, source control, and adjunctive therapies that may be of potential benefit in patients with severe sepsis and septic shock.

Antimicrobial Therapy

Empiric intravenous antibiotic therapy should be started as soon as possible after appropriate cultures have been obtained. Although the tight window as suggested by the Surviving Sepsis Campaign is not supported by scientific evidence, common sense would dictate that delaying the administration of antibiotics serves no useful purpose. The choice of antibiotics is largely determined by the source or focus of infection, the patient's immunologic status, whether the patient has risk factors for a drug-resistant pathogen (DRP) as well as knowledge of the local microbiology and sensitivity patterns. Initial empiric anti-infective therapy should include one or more drugs that have activity against the likely pathogens and that penetrate into the presumed source of sepsis site. Because the identity of the infecting pathogen(s) and its sensitivity pattern(s) are unknown at the time of initiation of antibiotics, for patients with severe sepsis and septic shock the initial regimen should include two or more antibiotics or an extended spectrum β-lactam antibiotic. A number of studies have demonstrated that appropriate initial antimicrobial therapy, defined as the use of at least one antibiotic active in vitro against the causative bacteria, is associated with a lower mortality when compared with patients receiving initial inappropriate therapy [82,83]. Once a pathogen is isolated, monotherapy is adequate for most infections; this strategy of initiating broad-spectrum cover with two or more antibiotics and then narrowing the spectrum to a single agent when a pathogen is identified is known as "antimicrobial de-escalation" [84]. Antimicrobial de-escalation has been demonstrated to be associated with lower rates of hospital mortality [85]. The indications for continuation of double-antimicrobial therapy include enterococcal infections and severe intra-abdominal infections. In order to rapidly achieve adequate blood and tissue concentrations, antibiotics should be given intravenously, at least initially.

Inappropriate initial antibiotic therapy is usually associated with infection with a DRP. The following factors have been shown to increase the risk of infection with a DRP, with this risk increasing with the number of risk factors: hospitalization >2 days in the previous 90 days, antibiotics during the previous 90 days, nonambulatory status, patients receiving tube feeds, immunocompromised status, acid suppressive therapy, chronic hemodialysis in the preceding 30 days, infection or colonization with methicillin-resistant Staphylococcus Aureus (MRSA) in the previous 90 days, and current hospitalization >2 days [86]. With the widespread use of antibiotics, a group of pathogens have emerged that are resistant to multiple antibiotics. These pathogens, referred to as the "ESKAPE bugs," have emerged in hospitals in both the developing and the developed world and are the most important DRPs encountered in clinical practice [87,88]. The ESKAPE pathogens include *Enterococcus faecium, Staphylococcus aureus, Klebsiella pneumonia, Acinetobacter baumannii, Pseudomonas aeruginosa,* and *Enterobacter* species. Antimicrobial classes for which resistance has become a major problem for the ESKAPE pathogens include β-lactams, the glycopeptides (vancomycin), and fluoroquinolones [89].

The appropriate length of antibiotic treatment for patients with sepsis has not been well established, with marked variation between and within different countries and healthcare settings, independent of factors such as disease severity [90]. Christ-Crain and colleagues randomized 302 patients with community-acquired pneumonia to usual care or antibiotic therapy guided by PCT [91]. In the PCT group, antibiotics were discontinued when the PCT fell to less than 0.25 μg per mL or if the PCT fell by more than 10% in patients with high PCT values on admission (PCT > 10 μg per mL). The median duration of antibiotics use was 5 days in the PCT group as compared with 12 days in the usual care group ($p < 0.001$). There were no differences of outcomes between the two groups. A meta-analysis by the Cochrane group compared a short 7- to 8-day course of antibiotics with a prolonged 10- to 15-day course in patients with ventilator-associated pneumonia (VAP) [92]. This meta-analysis, which included eight studies, demonstrated a reduced recurrence of VAP caused by multi-resistant organisms for the short-course group (OR 0.44; 95% CI 0.21 to 0.95) without adversely affecting other outcomes. Sawyer et al. [93] randomized 518 patients with complicated intra-abdominal infection and adequate source control to receive antibiotics until 2 days after resolution of fever, leukocytosis, and ileus with a maximum of 10 days or to receive a fixed course of antibiotics for 4 ± 1 days. In this study, there were no differences for any of the outcomes studied between the two dosing strategies.

These data suggest that a 5- to 8-day course of antibiotics is adequate for most patients with sepsis who received initial appropriate therapy and have had a good clinical response, with no evidence of infection with a DRP. Patients infected with a DRP generally require 10 to 14 days of treatment. The trend in the PCT level may further aid in determining when it is safe to discontinue antibiotics.

Hemodynamic Support

On November 8, 2001, Emanuel Rivers and collaborators published a study entitled "Early Goal Directed Therapy in the treatment of severe sepsis and septic shock," in which they compared two protocols for the early resuscitation of patients with severe sepsis and septic shock (for 6 hours in the Emergency Department) [49]. Both protocols used the CVP to guide fluid therapy (target CVP > 8 mm Hg). The "treatment arm" (EGDT) required placement of an oximetric central venous catheter with protocolized interventions to maintain the saturation of the central venous oxygen ($ScvO_2$) >70%. The study, which enrolled 288 patients (25 were excluded after the fact), reported a 28-day mortality of 49.2% in the control group and 33.3% in the EGDT group ($p = 0.01$, with an absolute reduction of the risk of death of 16%). Within a short time, this small (severely underpowered), unblinded, single-center study came to be considered the standard of care around the world and formed the basis of the 6-hour resuscitation bundle of the 2004, 2008, and 2012 Surviving Sepsis Campaign Bundles [50,94,95]. However, soon after publication of the EGDT study, concerns were raised regarding the validity of the protocol as well as the conduct and reporting of the study [96–101]. The basic premise of EGDT was to optimize tissue oxygen transport to reverse tissue hypoxia with the use of continuous monitoring to prespecified physiologic targets. This premise is flawed as bioenergetic failure and cellular hypoxia are likely only preterminal events in patients with septic shock [102,103]. Most importantly, none of the elements of the protocol were supported by strong scientific evidence [96–101]; notably, the CVP is a poor reflection of volume status and fluid responsiveness, patients with sepsis usually have a high rather than a low $ScvO_2$, with a high rather than a low $ScvO_2$ being predictive of a poor outcome, that transfusing patients with a hemoglobin >7 g per dL is likely to be harmful and that driving up oxygen delivery (DO_2) without regard to cardiac function is potentially harmful.

In 2014, 13 years after the publication of the EGDT study, the ProCESS and ARISE studies were published [104,105], with PROMISE the final of the *Trilogy* of large multicenter RCTs being published in 2015 [106]. ProCESS, ARISE, and PROMISE demonstrated that EGDT did not improve outcomes for patients with severe sepsis and septic shock. Patients in the EGDT arm of PROMISE had worse organ-failure scores, a longer stay in the ICU with increased use of resources, and increased costs [106]. A meta-analysis of EGDT, which included the ProCESS, ARISE, and PROMISE studies, concluded that "EGDT is not superior to usual care for Emergency Department patients with septic shock but is associated with increased utilization of ICU resources" [107]. ProCESS, ARISE, and PROMISE together with this meta-analysis have now clearly established that we should move beyond EGDT. This does not mean that the approach to the management of sepsis does not matter! Patients with sepsis should be managed by a thoughtful individualized approach based on an understanding of human physiology, the pathophysiologic changes that occur with sepsis, the patients' comorbidities, and the best clinical evidence.

Fluid Therapy

Beyond the early administration of antibiotics, aggressive "supportive measures" may be harmful, and the "less is more" paradigm appears applicable for the management of patients with severe sepsis. In these highly vulnerable patients, more intensive treatment may promote the chances of unwanted adverse effects and hence iatrogenic injury [108]. Current teaching suggests that *aggressive fluid resuscitation* is the best initial approach for the cardiovascular instability of sepsis. Consequently, large volumes of fluid (10 to 15 L) are often infused in the early stages of sepsis. There is, however, no human data that large fluid boluses (>30 mL per kg) reliably improves blood pressure, urine output, or end-organ perfusion [109,110]. This approach is likely to lead to "iatrogenic salt water drowning" with severe ARDS, AKI, and death [111].

The only reason to give a patient a fluid bolus is to increase stroke volume (SV). If the fluid bolus does not increase SV, the fluid bolus serves the patient no useful purpose and may be harmful. This concept is referred to as "fluid responsiveness" [112,113]. By definition, a patient is considered to be fluid responsive if his or her SV increases by ≥10% following a fluid challenge (usually 500 mL crystalloid). The chest radiograph, CVP, central venous oxygen saturation ($ScvO_2$), and ultrasonography, including the vena-caval collapsibility index, have limited value in guiding fluid management and should not be used for this purpose [114–119]. The passive leg raising maneuver (PLR) or a fluid challenge coupled with real-time SV monitoring are accurate methods for determining fluid responsiveness [112,120,121].

Multiple studies of diverse populations of patients have demonstrated that only about 50% of hemodynamically unstable patients are fluid responsive [112,113]. This implies that for about 50% of hemodynamically unstable patients, fluid boluses may be harmful [111]. This challenges the "well established" notion in critical care medicine, anesthesiology, and emergency medicine that fluid boluses are the "cornerstone of resuscitation." Owing to increased diastolic compliance and an increase in the unstressed blood volume of septic patients, it is likely that less than 50% of patients with severe sepsis and septic shock are fluid responsive [122]. Large fluid boluses further decrease diastolic compliance of the ventricles, causing the CVP to increase more than the mean circulating filling pressure (MCFP), paradoxically decreasing the gradient for venous return [122,123]. Furthermore, the increased CVP is transmitted backward, increasing venous pressure, which can impair organ function and microcirculatory flow, particularly for encapsulated organs such as the kidney and liver [111]. To make matters worse, the hemodynamic response to fluids in patients with circulatory shock is small and short lived (less than an hour) because most (about 90% to 95%) of the fluid leaks into the tissues [124–127]. Glassford and colleagues performed a systematic review that examined the hemodynamic response of fluid boluses in patients with sepsis [128]. These authors reported that while the mean arterial pressure (MAP) increased by 7.8 ± 3.8 mm Hg immediately following the fluid bolus, the MAP had returned close to baseline at 1 hour with no increase in urine output. Although having a minimal effect on blood pressure, fluid boluses may cause a fall in effective arterial elastance and systemic vascular resistance, potentiating arterial vasodilatation and the hyperdynamic state characteristic of septic shock [129,130]. These data suggest that the majority of patients with severe sepsis and septic shock are not fluid responders. The hemodynamic changes of the fluid responders are small, short lived, and likely to be clinically insignificant. Furthermore, overaggressive fluid resuscitation will likely have adverse hemodynamic consequences including an increase in cardiac filling pressures, damage to the endothelial glycocalyx, arterial vasodilation, and tissue edema. Consequently, the concept that aggressive fluid resuscitation is the "cornerstone of resuscitation" of patients with severe sepsis and septic shock should be reconsidered [50,94,95,131].

The harmful effects of overaggressive fluid resuscitation on the outcome of sepsis are supported by experimental studies as well as data accumulated from clinical trials [132,133]. Multiple clinical studies have demonstrated an independent association between an increasingly positive fluid balance and increased mortality in patients with sepsis [1,45,134–141]. In a secondary analysis of the *Vasopressin in Septic Shock Trial* (VASST), Boyd and colleagues demonstrated that a greater positive fluid balance at both 12 hours and 4 days were independent predictors of death [141]. Kelm and colleagues [142] evaluated the fluid status and outcome of 405 patients with severe sepsis and septic shock who were admitted to the Mayo clinic and treated with EGDT. In this study, 67% of patients had clinical evidence of fluid overload at 24 hours with 48% having evidence of fluid overload at 72 hours. Fluid overload was an independent predictor of mortality (odds ratio of 1.92; 95% confidence interval of 1.16 to 3.22). The most compelling data that fluid loading for sepsis is harmful comes from the landmark "Fluid Expansion as Supportive Therapy (FEAST)" study performed in 3,141 sub-Saharan children with severe sepsis [143]. In this randomized study, aggressive fluid loading was associated with a significantly increased risk of death. Nevertheless, despite data suggesting that "aggressive fluid resuscitation" is associated with adverse outcomes and no randomized trials to indicate that this approach improves patient outcomes, the updated Surviving Sepsis Campaign Guidelines, published in April of 2015, mandates the administration of "30 mL/kg crystalloid for hypotension or lactate ≥4 mmol/L" within 3 hours of presentation to hospital [114].

In summary, these data support a "conservative" hemodynamically guided fluid resuscitation strategy in patients with severe sepsis and septic shock. From an evolutionary point of view, humans have evolved to deal with hypovolemia and not hypervolemia. Large fluid boluses may counter the live preserving homeostatic mechanisms of unstable critically ill patients, increasing the risk of death [144]. For some patients, hypotension and tachycardia do resolve with limited fluid resuscitation. It is likely that many of these patients have super-added dehydration owing to poor oral intake and a delay in seeking medical attention. However, fluids alone will not reverse the hemodynamic instability of patients with more severe sepsis; for these patients, fluids alone are likely to exacerbate the vasodilatory shock and increase the capillary leak and tissue edema. On the basis of these data, the initial resuscitation of patients with septic shock should logically include 500 mL boluses of crystalloid (Ringers Lactate) to a maximum of about 20 mL per kg [145]. Ideally, fluid resuscitation should be guided by the determination of fluid responsiveness [112,146]. Norepinephrine should be initiated in those patients who remain hypotensive (MAP < 65 mm Hg) despite this initial limited fluid strategy (see below) [145,147].

The septic patient with an intra-abdominal catastrophe who requires urgent surgical intervention represents one subgroup of patients that may require more aggressive fluid resuscitation. However, overly aggressive fluid resuscitation can result in intra-abdominal hypertension, which is associated with a high risk of complications and death [148,149]. For these patients, continuous SV monitoring is helpful, and ongoing fluid requirements should be guided by the trend in the SV as well as the hemodynamic response to small volume fluid boluses. In addition, perioperative intra-abdominal pressure monitoring is required in these patients [148].

The choice of fluid in patients with severe sepsis and septic shock is controversial. Normal saline (0.9% NaCl) is the most widely used crystalloid around the world. However, normal saline is an unphysiologic solution that is associated with a number of adverse effects. Normal saline causes a hyperchloremic metabolic acidosis [150–153]; it decreases renal blood flow [154] and increases the risk of renal failure [155]. In patients with sepsis, the use of normal saline as compared with physiologic salt solutions has been associated with an increased risk of death [156]. The SPLIT trial was a randomized double-blind, cluster randomized, double-crossover trial conducted in four ICUs in New Zealand that compared 0.9% Saline with Plasma-Lyte 148 for ICU fluid therapy [157]. The risk of AKI (primary outcome) as well as of all secondary outcomes did not differ between the two fluid groups. This study, however, has a number of significant limitations that preclude widespread generalizability of the results; most notably, 71% of patients were postoperative patients, only 4% were diagnosed with sepsis, and the volume of fluid administered was small (about 2.7 L in the first 4 days). Nevertheless, despite the findings of the SPLIT study, 0.9% Saline has no advantages over balanced salt solutions (except in patients with acute necrologic insults) and is best avoided.

Synthetic starch solutions increase the risk of renal failure and death in patients with sepsis and should be avoided [158,159]. The role of albumin for patients with sepsis is widely debated [160]. Nevertheless, the use of 4% albumin in patients with sepsis was associated with a survival benefit in the SAFE study [161]. In the ALBIOS study, hyperoncotic albumin (20%) was associated with a survival benefit in patients with septic shock [162]. It should be noted that exogenous albumin is one of the few therapies that can restore the endothelial glycocalyx in experimental systems [163]. We recommend the use of hyperoncotic albumin (20% or 25%) in patients with "resuscitated" septic shock who have a serum albumin of less than 3 g per L. Hyperoncotic albumin should not be given as a bolus because this form of administration will paradoxically dehydrate the glycocalyx. If a 20/25% albumin is used to stabilize the glycocalyx, it may be preferable to give this as a continuous infusion at a rate of 10 to 20 mL per hour.

Vasopressors and Inotropic Agents

A low MAP is a reliable predictor for the development of organ dysfunction. When the MAP falls below an organ's autoregulatory threshold, organ blood flow decreases in an almost linear fashion [164]. Because the autoregulatory ranges of the heart, brain, and kidney are above 60 mm Hg [164], an MAP below this level will likely result in organ ischemia and death [165]. Varpula and colleagues studied the hemodynamic variables associated with mortality of patients with septic shock [166]. These authors calculated the area under the curve (AUC) for various MAP thresholds over a 48-hour time period. The highest AUC values were found for an MAP < 65 mm Hg (AUC 0.83, 95% CI 0.772 to 0.934). Owing to the shift of the autoregulatory range (to the right) in patients with chronic hypertension, a higher MAP may be required in these patients. In the SEPSISPAM study (The *Assessment of Two Levels of Arterial Pressure on Survival in Patients with Septic Shock*), patients with septic shock were randomized to achieve a target MAP of 65 to 70 or 80 to 85 mm Hg. The primary outcome was 28-day mortality. Secondary outcomes included 90-day mortality and organ failure. *A priori* a secondary analysis was planned in patients with and without a history of hypertension. Overall, there was no difference in either primary or secondary end-point between the two treatment groups. However, the incidence of organ failure (particularly renal dysfunction) was higher in the subgroup of patients with chronic hypertension in the lower MAP group. Furthermore, much like the Varpula study, the time below the 65 mm Hg (but not 80 mm Hg) threshold was an independent predictor of death. On the basis of these data, we suggest targeting an initial MAP of 65 to 70 mm Hg for patients with septic shock. Among those patients with a history of chronic hypertension, it may be preferable to target a slightly higher MAP (80 to 85 mm Hg) [167].

Norepinephrine is the vasopressor of choice for patients with septic shock [145,168]. Dopamine increases the risk of arrhythmias and death and should be avoided [168–170]. Similarly, phenylephrine is not recommended as the first-line vasopressor because in experimental models it decreases cardiac output as well as renal and splanchnic blood flow [171]. Furthermore, phenylephrine has not been as well studied in patients with sepsis. In patients with septic shock, norepinephrine restores the stressed blood volume, increasing the MCFP, venous return, and cardiac output. Norepinephrine increases arterial vascular tone, further increasing blood pressure and organ blood flow [145]. Venous capacitance vessels are much more sensitive to sympathetic stimulation than are arterial resistance vessels, and consequently, low-dose $\alpha 1$ agonists cause greater veno- than vasoconstriction [172]. The increase in the stressed blood volume following the use of norepinephrine is caused by the mobilization of blood rather than a short-lived volume expander (crystalloid) [173]. Therefore, unlike fluids, the effect of $\alpha 1$ agonists on venous return is enduring and not associated with tissue edema. The early use of norepinephrine in patients with septic shock can increase preload, rendering the fluid-responsive patient fluid unresponsive [172]. This may allow the target blood pressure to be achieved and a significant reduction in the amount of fluid administered. Hamzaoui et al. [174] have demonstrated that the early administration of norepinephrine increased preload, cardiac output, and MAP, largely reversing the hemodynamic abnormalities of severe vasodilatory shock. Abid and colleagues demonstrated that the early use of norepinephrine in patients with septic shock was a strong predictor of survival [175]. It is noteworthy that norepinephrine may be safely given through a well-functioning peripheral venous catheter [176], precluding the requirement for emergent central venous catheterization, which is generally regarded as an obstacle to the early use of norepinephrine.

For patients with "refractory septic shock" who remain hypotensive despite an adequate dose of norepinephrine (approximately 0.1 to 0.2 μg/kg/min), we recommend further hemodynamic assessment to exclude severe systolic ventricular dysfunction, which between 10% and 20% of patients experience. Ventricular function is best assessed by bedside echocardiography and confirmed by minimally invasive cardiac output monitoring. Dobutamine at a starting dose of 2.5 μg/kg/min is recommended for patients with significant systolic ventricular dysfunction (milrinone is an alternative agent) [177]. The dose of dobutamine should be titrated to hemodynamic response as determined by minimally invasive cardiac output monitoring [177,178]. For patients with persistent hypotension and hyperdynamic ventricular function (who have severe failure of vasomotor tone), fixed-dose vasopressin (0.03 units per minute) should be initiated. Vasopressin reverses the "relative vasopressin deficiency" seen among patients with septic shock and increases adrenergic sensitivity [32,179]. Terlipressin is an alternative (although not FDA approved in the United States) [180,181]. The VASST trial randomized patients with septic shock to norepinephrine alone or norepinephrine plus vasopressin at 0.03 units per minute [182]. By intention-to-treat analysis, there was no difference in outcome between the groups. However, an *a priori* defined subgroup analysis demonstrated that survival among patients receiving <0.2 μg/kg/min norepinephrine at the time of randomization was better with the addition of vasopressin than those receiving norepinephrine at a dose >0.2 μg/kg/min. We therefore suggest the addition of vasopressin at a dose of norepinephrine between 0.1 and 0.2 μg/kg/min. Thereafter, the dose of norepinephrine should be titrated to achieve an MAP of at least 65 mm Hg.

β-Blockers and Phenylephrine for Septic Shock

As part of the stress response of patients with sepsis and septic shock, there is massive sympathetic activation with very high levels of circulating catecholamines [183]. Septic patients often have an elevated heart rate, even after excluding common causes of tachycardia such as hypovolemia, fever, pain, and agitation. The volume-depleted patient's tachycardia constitutes the main mechanism that compensates for the decrease in SV. However, persistence of tachycardia after fluid resuscitation (patients who are no longer fluid responsive) may indicate an inappropriate degree of sympathetic activation. Persistent tachycardia has been demonstrated to be a poor prognostic sign in patients with sepsis [184]. In 1987, Parker and colleagues reported that an initial heart rate of <106 beats per minute and a heart rate at 24 hours of <95 beats per minute were strong predictors of survival [185]. These factors have led investigators to consider the use of β-blockers for the management of "fully resuscitated" septic patients with persistent tachycardia [186,187]. However, reducing heart rate with β-blockers in the early phase of septic shock may potentially lead to an inappropriately low cardiac output with a consequent decrease in organ blood flow, increasing the risk of organ failure.

Morelli et al. [188] randomized 154 patients with "resuscitated septic shock" receiving norepinephrine to maintain an MAP >65 mm Hg and who had a persistent heart rate > 95 beats per minute to an infusion of esmolol (short-acting β1-selective β blocker) or placebo. The esmolol was titrated to achieve a heart rate between 80 and 94 beats per minute. Twenty-eight-day mortality was 49.4% in the esmolol group versus 80.5% in the control group (HR 0.39; CI 0.26 to 0.59; $p < 0.001$). For the patients receiving esmolol, there was a significant increase in the Left Ventricular Stroke Work Index (LVSWI) and Stroke Volume Index (SVI). It is important to emphasize that a highly select group of patients were enrolled into this study; these patients may represent only a small fraction of patients presenting with sepsis. The mortality in the control group was higher than that of any study published in the last two decades. Echocardiography was not performed, and it is therefore unclear how many patients had severe isolated diastolic dysfunction. In addition to attenuating the stress response, β-blockers modulate cytokine production, decrease energy expenditure, and modulate protein, fat, and carbohydrate metabolism.

β-blockers should be avoided during the initial resuscitation of patients with severe sepsis/septic shock, patients who are fluid responsive, and patients with predominant systolic LV dysfunction. β-blockers may have a role in the tachycardic septic patient with significant LV diastolic dysfunction. It would appear to be counterintuitive to simultaneously use an infusion of norepinephrine (β1, β2, α1 agonist) and esmolol. In this situation, it would appear more rational to use phenylephrine (α1 agonist) to achieve arterial and venoconstriction together with esmolol (for improvement of diastolic dysfunction). Only a short-acting β-blocker should be used (esmolol), its dose closely titrated and the effects of this combination on cardiac output, blood pressure, and SV closely monitored. β-blockers should be used only for patients who are fluid nonresponsive, for patients undergoing continuous SV monitoring, and after echocardiography has excluded systolic dysfunction.

Resuscitation End Points

A large number of hemodynamic, perfusion, oxygenation, and echocardiographic targets have been proposed as resuscitation goals in patients with severe sepsis and septic shock [50,189,190]. Most of these targets, however, are controversial and not supported by outcomes data. The 2012 and updated 2015 Surviving Sepsis Campaign Guidelines recommend a CVP of 8 to 12 mm Hg (12 to 15 mm Hg if mechanically ventilated), a central venous oxygen saturation ($ScvO_2$) > 70%, and a urine output > 0.5 mL/kg/h as targets for resuscitation [50,114]. As already discussed, targeting a CVP >8 mm Hg may be harmful and, as demonstrated by the ProCESS, ARISE, and PROMISE trials, targeting a $ScvO_2$ >70% does not improve patient outcomes [104–106]. Although urine output may be a valuable marker of renal perfusion in hypovolemic states, this clinical sign becomes problematic for sepsis-associated AKI, where experimental models suggest that oliguria occurs in the presence of marked global renal hyperemia [191–193]. Titration of fluids to urine output may therefore result in fluid overload. Furthermore, the Surviving Sepsis Campaign guideline recommends "targeting resuscitation to normalize lactate in patients with elevated lactate levels as a marker of tissue hypoperfusion" [50]. This recommendation is based on the notion that an elevated lactate is a consequence of tissue hypoxia and inadequate oxygen delivery [194] and is "supported" by two studies that used "lactate clearance" as the target of resuscitation [195,196]. However, the concept that sepsis is associated with tissue hypoxia is unproven and possibly incorrect [103,197,198]. Increasing oxygen delivery for patients with sepsis is often not associated with increased oxygen consumption [197,199,200]. Previous studies have demonstrated that targeting supramaximal oxygen delivery does not improve outcome and may be harmful [201,202]. Furthermore, in the study by Morelli et al. [188], oxygen delivery was reduced in the esmolol arm as compared with control patients, yet the lactate concentration decreased among esmolol arm subjects, whereas it increased for control arm patients. Although the lactate concentration is an important marker of severity of illness and the trend in lactate may be useful in prognostication, attempts to titrate treatment modalities to a lactate concentration may not be grounded on sound physiologic concepts [197,198].

The updated Surviving Sepsis Campaign Guidelines [114], which are now mandated by law in the United States (National Quality Forum Measure #0500 [203], Center for Medicare and Medicaid Services SEP-1 Quality measure), require reassessment of volume status and tissue perfusion (after a 30 mL per kg fluid bolus) with either: "repeat focused exam by a licensed independent practitioner including vital signs, cardiopulmonary refill, pulse and skin findings" (all these clinical findings) or two of the following: CVP, $ScvO_2$, bedside cardiovascular ultrasound, or dynamic assessment of fluid responsiveness with passive leg raise or fluid challenge. However, it has been well established that the chest radiograph, CVP, $ScvO_2$, and ultrasonography, including the vena-caval collapsibility index, have very limited value for guiding fluid management and should not be used for this purpose [115–119,204]. Furthermore, it has been well established that physical examination cannot be used to predict fluid responsiveness and that physical examination is unreliable for estimating intravascular volume status [205].

These data suggest that achieving an MAP of at least 65 mm Hg should be the primary target for the resuscitation of patients with septic shock. Furthermore, while attempts to achieve a supranormal cardiac index may be potentially harmful, we would suggest targeting a normal cardiac index (> 2.5 L/min/m^2) [201]. Although a falling arterial lactate concentration is a sign that the patient is responding to therapy (attenuation of the stress response), titrating therapy to a lactate concentration may not be grounded on sound physiologic principles [197,200]. Additional end points of resuscitation remain unproven at this time.

Source Control

It has been known for centuries that unless the source of the infection is controlled, the patient is often not cured of his/her infective process and that death will eventually ensue. It is important that specific diagnoses of infection that require emergent source control be made in a timely manner (e.g., necrotizing soft-tissue infection, peritonitis, cholangitis, intestinal infarction) and surgical consultation be immediately obtained [50,206]. When source control is required for a severely septic patient, the effective intervention associated with the least physiologic insult should be used (e.g., percutaneous rather than surgical drainage of an abscess) [50,207]. In patients with "urosepsis," an emergent renal ultrasound or abdominal CT scan should be obtained to exclude urinary tract obstruction, because urgent decompression of the urinary system is required for patients with evidence of obstruction. If intravascular access devices are a possible source of severe sepsis or septic shock, they should be removed promptly after other vascular access has been established [83].

Adjunctive Therapies

A myriad of adjunctive novel pharmacologic agents and interventions have been investigated in patients with severe sepsis and septic shock. To date, none of these therapies have consistently been demonstrated to improve patient outcomes. Ongoing issues that remain controversial include the use of corticosteroids, glycemic control, and nutritional interventions.

Corticosteroids

The use of low-dose corticosteroids in patients with severe sepsis remains controversial [208]. It has been proposed that inadequate cellular glucocorticoid activity (Critical Illness Related Corticosteroid Insufficiency) caused by either adrenal suppression or glucocorticoid tissue resistance results in an exaggerated and protracted proinflammatory response [209]. In addition to downregulating the proinflammatory response and modulating the anti-inflammatory response, corticosteroids may have additional beneficial effects including increasing adrenergic responsiveness [210] and preserving the endothelial glycocalyx [211]. Although there are divergent recommendations and large geographic variations in the prescription of glucocorticoids, up to 50% of patients with severe sepsis and septic shock receive such therapy [212]. A recent comprehensive meta-analysis that included a trial sequential analysis found no "evidence to support or negate the use of steroids in any dose in sepsis patients" [213]. Consequently, the use of glucocorticoids for patients with sepsis remains unclear. Currently, the Australian and New Zealand Intensive Care Society Clinical Trials Group are performing the ADRENAL study, in which 3,800 patients with septic shock will be randomized to receive hydrocortisone (200 mg per day as a continuous infusion) versus placebo [214]. The outcome of this study will, hopefully, resolve this ongoing therapeutic dilemma.

Nutritional Support

Current Clinical Practice Guidelines (CPG) emphasize early (within 24 to 48 hours of ICU admission) normocaloric enteral nutrition (daily caloric intake estimated to match 80% to 100% of energy expenditure) [215–218] However, a number of recent RCTs have failed to demonstrate an improvement in the outcomes for critically ill patients receiving a normocaloric feeding protocol as opposed to a strategy of intentional hypocaloric feeding. Indeed, a meta-analysis that compared trophic and permissive underfeeding with normocaloric nutrition (included six RCTs) reported no difference in the risk of secondary infections, ventilator-free days, hospital mortality, or ICU length of stay [219].

Early feeding may be particularly harmful for patients with sepsis. Anorexia is an evolutionary preserved acute host response to infection and is likely beneficial to the host. Complex and redundant pathways have evolved to ensure that the host develops anorexia during acute septic insults. Folklore that dates back to the 16th century suggests that "fasting is a great remedy for fever" [220]. The mechanisms whereby decreased nutrient intake is protective and promotes survival during acute illness are not entirely clear. The acute phase response is associated with a dramatic fall in serum iron concentrations [221]. Iron is an essential element required for the survival of many pathogens, and iron deprivation retards bacterial growth [222]. Food restriction results in a dramatic reduction of iron in the liver and serum of a variety of organisms [223]. It has been postulated that fever and iron deprivation act synergistically to inhibit bacterial growth [224]. Starvation promotes autophagy, and this may play a key role in promoting host defenses [225,226]. Autophagy is a component of innate immunity and is involved in host defense elimination of pathogens [226]. Autophagy contributes to immune response against intracellular bacteria, parasites, and viruses [227]. Autophagy plays a role in the degradation of both extracellular bacterial pathogens that invade the cell (e.g., group A Streptococcus) and true intracellular bacterial pathogens (e.g., *Mycobacterium tuberculosis* and *Shigella flexneri*) [228]. These data suggest that it may be beneficial to withhold enteral nutrition for the first 24 to 48 hours in patients with severe sepsis.

Randomized controlled trials proving that starvation is detrimental to critically ill and injured patients have until recently not been performed. This is likely because of the lack of equipoise by researchers and the notion that such an experiment would be unethical. However, recently, the Dutch Pancreatitis Study Group reported the results of the "Early versus On-Demand Nasoenteric Tube Feeding in Acute Pancreatitis study (PYTHON trial)" [229]; this study comes close to an RCT comparing initial starvation followed by an *ad libitum* diet with early enteral nutrition administered via a feeding tube. In this study, patients with acute severe pancreatitis were randomly assigned to nasoenteric tube feeding within 24 hours after randomization or to an oral diet initiated 72 hours after presentation with tube feeding provided the oral diet was not tolerated. There was no difference in any of the outcome variables between the two groups. Furthermore, there was no difference between the levels of CRP or the SIRS score between the groups over the 1st week, suggesting that early enteral nutrition did not attenuate the inflammatory response.

It should be recognized that in all the RCTs that failed to demonstrate a benefit from early aggressive enteral nutrition, patients received continuous rather than intermittent enteral nutrition [230]. No species eats continuously (day and night), and such an evolutionary design would seem absurd. The alimentary tract and metabolic pathways of humans appear designed for intermittent ingestion of nutrients a few times a day. Humans have evolved as intermittent meal eaters and are not adapted to a continuous inflow of nutrients; normal physiology appears to be altered when this approach is adopted. Continuous as opposed to intermittent enteral feeding likely limits protein synthesis, and this may be an important factor in promoting critical illness–acquired muscle weakness [230]. In addition to adversely affecting protein synthesis, continuous enteral feeding can have other adverse consequences including uncontrolled hyperglycemia, hepatic steatosis, functional changes of the small intestine, and diminished gall bladder contraction [230].

These data suggest that anorexia with limited nutrient intake is an evolutionary preserved response that may be beneficial during the first 24 to 48 hours of acute illness. In those patients who are unable to resume an oral diet after this time period, enteral nutrition via orogastric tube is recommended. Continuous tube feeding targeting normocaloric goals has not been proven to improve outcome; such a mode of feeding may be unphysiologic.

CONCLUSIONS

Sepsis is a complex and dynamic disease that is difficult to manage by simple treatment algorithms and checklists [231]. Each patient is unique, with a unique set of genes and comorbidities, and responds to illness and its treatment in a unique and often unpredictable manner. This dictates that patients with sepsis be treated with an appropriate physiologic approach that promotes healing and limits the potential for intragenic harm.

References

1. Vincent JL, Sakr Y, Sprung CL, et al: Sepsis in European intensive care units: results of the SOAP study. *Crit Care Med* 34:344–353, 2006.
2. Gaieski DF, Edwards JM, Kallan MJ, et al: Benchmarking the incidence and mortality of severe sepsis in the United States. *Crit Care Med* 41:1167–1174, 2013.
3. Martin GS, Mannino DM, Eaton S, et al: The epidemiology of sepsis in the United States from 1979 through 2000. *N Engl J Med* 348:1546–1554, 2003.
4. Angus DC, Linde-Zwirble WT, Lidicker J, et al: Epidemiology of severe sepsis in the United States: analysis of incidence, outcome and associated costs of care. *Crit Care Med* 29:1303–1310, 2001.
5. Wang HE, Szychowski JM, Griffin R, et al: Long term mortality after sepsis. *Chest* 21(12):E762–E769, 2013.
6. Jolley RJ, Sawka KJ, Yergens DW, et al: Validity of administrative data in recording sepsis: a systematic review. *Crit Care* 19:139, 2015.
7. Whittaker SA, Mikkelsen ME, Gaieski DF, et al: Severe sepsis cohorts derived from claims-based strategies appear to be biased toward a more severely ill patient population. *Crit Care Med* 41:945–953, 2013.
8. Stow PJ: Development and implementation of a high-quality clinical database: the Australian and New Zealand Intensive Care Society Adult Patient Database. *J Crit Care* 21:133–141, 2006.
9. Kaukonen KM, Bailey M, Suzuki S, et al: Mortality related to severe sepsis and septic shock among critically ill patients in Australia and New Zealand, 2000–2012. *JAMA* 311:1308–1316, 2014.
10. Hicks P, Cooper DJ, Webb S, et al: The surviving sepsis campaign: international guidelines for management of severe sepsis and septic shock: 2008. An assessment by the Australian and New Zealand Intensive Care Society. *Anaesth Intensive Care* 36:149–151, 2008.
11. Levy MM, Dellinger RP, Townsend SR, et al: The surviving sepsis campaign: results of an international guideline-based performance improvement program targeting severe sepsis. *Crit Care Med* 38:367–374, 2010.
12. Levy MM, Artigas A, Phillips GS, et al: Outcomes of the surviving sepsis campaign in intensive care units in the USA and Europe: a prospective cohort study. *Lancet Infect Dis* 2012;12:919–924.
13. Bone RC, Balk RA, Cerra FB, et al: Definitions for sepsis and organ failure and guidelines for the use of innovative therapies in sepsis. The ACCP/SCCM Consensus Conference Committee. American College of Chest Physicians/ Society of Critical Care Medicine. *Chest* 101:1644–1655, 1992.
14. Vincent JL, Opal SM, Marshall JC, et al: Sepsis definitions: time for change. *Lancet* 381:774–775, 2013.
15. Kaukonen KM, Baily M, Pilcher D, et al: Systemic inflammatory response syndrome criteria criteria in defining severe sepsis. *N Engl J Med* 372:1629–1638, 2015.
16. Whippy A, Skeath M, Crawford B, et al: Kaiser Permanente's performance improvement system, part 3: multisite improvements in care for patients with sepsis. *Jt Comm J Qual Patient Saf* 37:483–493, 2011.
17. Singer M, Deutschman CS, Seymour CW, et al: The third international consensus definitions for sepsis and septic shock (Sepsis-3). *JAMA* 315:801–810, 2016.
18. Shankar-Hari M, Phillips GS, Levy ML, et al: Developing a new definition and assessing new cliical criteria for septic shock. For the third international consensus definitions for sepsis and septic shock (Sepsis-3). *JAMA* 315:775–787, 2016.
19. Seymour CW, Liu VX, Iwashyna TJ, et al: Assessment of the clinical criteria for sepsis. For the third international consensus definitions for sepsis and septic shock (Sepsis-3). *JAMA*; 315:762–774, 2016.
20. Jain S, Self WH, Wunderink RG, et al: Community-acquired pneumonia requiring hospitalization among U.S. adults. *N Engl J Med* 373:415–427, 2015.
21. Rittirsch D, Flierl MA, Ward PA: Harmful molecular mechanisms in sepsis. *Nat Rev Immunol* 8:776–787, 2008.
22. Parrish WR, Gallowitsch-Puerta M, Czura CJ, et al: Experimental therapeutic strategies for severe sepsis: mediators and mechanisms. *Ann N Y Acad Sci* 1144:210–236, 2008.
23. Skrupky LP, Kerby PW, Hotchkiss RS: Advances in the management of sepsis and the understanding of key immunologic defects. *Anesthesiol* 115:1349–1362, 2011.
24. Stearns-Kurosawa DJ, Osuchowski MF, Valentine C, et al: The pathogenesis of sepsis. *Ann Rev Pathol* 6:19–48, 2011.
25. Leentjens J, Kox M, van der Hoeven JG, et al: Immunotherapy for the adjunctive treatment of sepsis: from immunosupression to immunostimulation. Time for a paradigm change? *Am J Respir Crit Care Med* 187:1287–1293, 2013.
26. Semeraro N, Ammollo CT, Semeraro F, et al: Coagulopathy of acute sepsis. *Semin Thromb Hemost* 41:650–658, 2015.
27. Nau GJ, Richmond JF, Schlesinger A, et al: Human macrophage activation programs induced by bacterial pathogens. *Proc Natl Acad Sci U S A* 99:1503–1508, 2002.
28. Osler W: *The Evolution of Modern Medicine*. New Haven, CT: Yale University Press, 1921.
29. Hotchkiss RS, Karl IE: The pathophysiology and treatment of sepsis. *N Engl J Med* 348:138–150, 2003.
30. Boomer JS, To K, Chang KC, et al: Immunosuppression in patients who die of sepsis and multiple organ failure. *JAMA* 306:2594–2605, 2011.
31. Marik PE, Flemmer MC: The immune response to surgery and trauma: implications for treatment. *J Trauma* 73:801–808, 2012.
32. Landry DW, Oliver JA: Pathogenesis of vasodilatory shock. *N Engl J Med* 345:588–595, 2001.
33. Lee WL, Slutsky AS: Sepsis and endothelial permeability. *N Engl J Med* 363:689–691, 2010.
34. Ait-Oufella H, Maury E, Lehoux S et al: The endothelium: physiological functions and role in microcirculatory failure during severe sepsis. *Intensive Care Med* 36:1286–1298, 2010.
35. Goldenberg NM, Steinberg BE, Slutsky AS, et al: Broken barriers: a new take on sepsis pathogenesis. *Sci Translation Med* 3:88ps25, 2011.
36. Hernandez G, Bruhn A, Ince C: Microcirculation in sepsis: new perspectives. *Curr Vasc Pharm* 11:161–169, 2013.
37. De Backer D, Creteur J, Preiser JC, et al: Microvascular blood flow is altered in patients with sepsis. *Am J Respir Crit Care Med* 166:98–104, 2002.
38. Trzeciak S, Rivers E: Clinical manifestations of disordered microcirculatory perfusion in severe sepsis. *Crit Care* 9 [Suppl 4]:S20–S26, 2005.
39. Parker MM, Shelhamer JH, Bacharach SL, et al: Profound but reversible myocardial depression in patients with septic shock. *Ann Intern Med* 100:483–490, 1984.
40. Sanfilippo F, Corredor C, Fletcher N, et al: Diastolic dysfunction and mortality in septic patients: a systematic review and meta-analysis. *Intensive Care Med* 41:1004–1013, 2015.
41. Landesberg G, Gilon D, Meroz Y, et al: Diastolic dysfunction and mortality in severe sepsis and septic shock. *Eur Heart J* 33:895–903, 2012.
42. Brown SM, Pittman JE, Hirshberg EL, et al: Diastolic dysfunction and mortality in early severe sepsis and septic shock: a prospective, observational echocardiography study. *Crit Ultrasound J* 4:8, 2012.
43. Ognibene FP, Parker MM, Natanson C, et al: Depressed left ventricular performance: response to volume infusion in patients with sepsis and septic shock. *Chest* 93:903–910, 1988.
44. Uchino S, Kellum JA, Bellomo R, et al: Acute renal failure in critically ill patients: a multinational, multicenter study. *JAMA* 294:813–818, 2005.
45. Payen D, de Pont AC, Sakr Y, et al: A positive fluid balance is associated with a worse outcome in patients with acute renal failure. *Crit Care* 12:R74, 2008.
46. Gomez H, Ince C, De Backer D, et al: A unified theory of sepsis-induced acute kidney injury: inflammation, microcirculatory dysfunction, bioenergetics, and the tubular cell adaption to injury. *Shock* 41:3–11, 2014.
47. Prowle JR, Kirwan CJ, Bellomo R: Fluid management for the prevention and attenuation of acute kidney injury. *Nat Rev Nephrol* 10:37–47, 2014.
48. Legrand M, Dupuis C, Simon C, et al: Association between systemic hemodynamics and septic kidney injury in critically ill patietns: a retrospective observational study. *Crit Care* 17:R278, 2013.
49. Rivers E, Nguyen B, Havstad S, et al: Early goal-directed therapy in the treatment of severe sepsis and septic shock. *N Engl J Med* 345:1368–1377, 2001.
50. Dellinger RP, Levy MM, Rhodes A, et al: Surviving sepsis campaign: international guidelines for management of severe sepsis and septic shock: 2012. *Crit Care Med* 41:580–637, 2013.
51. Mullens W, Abrahams Z, Francis GS, et al: Importance of venous congestion for worsening of renal function in advanced decompensated heart failure. *J Am Coll Cardiol*; 53:589–596, 2009.
52. Levi M, Schultz M, van der Poll T: Sepsis and thrombosis. *Semin Thromb Hemost* 39:559–566, 2013.
53. Cavallazzi R, Bennin CL, Hirani A, et al: Is the band count useful in the diagnosis of infection? An accuracy study in critically ill patients. *J Intensive Care Med* 25:353–357, 2010.
54. Ranieri VM, Thompson BT, Barie PS, et al: Drotrecogin Alfa (activated) in adults with septic shcok. *N Engl J Med* 366:2055–2064, 2012.
55. Dark P, Blackwood B, Gates S, et al: Accuracy of LightCycler SeptiFast for the detection and identification of pathogens in the blood of patients with suspected sepsis: a systematic review and meta-analysis. *Intensive Care Med* 41:21–33, 2015.
56. Chang SS, Hsieh WH, Liu TS, et al: Multiplex PCR system for rapid detection of pathogens in patients with presumed sepsis - a systemic review and meta-analysis. *PloS One* 8:e62323, 2013.

57. Bacconi A, Richmond GS, Baroldi MA, et al: Improved sensitivity for molecular detection of bacterial and Candida infections in blood. *J Clin Microbiol* 52:3164–3174, 2014.
58. Vincent JL, Brealey D, Abidi NE, et al: Rapid diagnosis of infection in the critically ill, a multicenter study of molecular detection in bloodstream infections, pneumonia, and sterile site infections. *Crit Care Med* 43:2283–2291, 2015.
59. Kirn TJ, Weinstein MP: Update on blood cultures: how to obtain, process, report, and interpret. *Clin Microbiol Infect* 19:513–520, 2013.
60. Clinical and Laboratory Standars Institute: *Principles and Procedures for Blood Cultures: Approved Guideleine*. Wayne, PA: Clinical and Laboratlry Standards Institute, 2007.
61. Li J, Plorde JJ, Carlson LG: Effects of volume and periodicity on blood cultures. *J Clin Microbiol* 32:2829–2831, 1994.
62. Lamy B, Roy P, Carret G, et al: What is the relevance of obtaining multiple blood samples for culture? A comprehensive model to optimize the strategy for diagnosing bacteremia. *Clin Infect Dis* 35:842–850, 2002.
63. Wacker C, Prkno A, Brunkhorst FM, et al: Procalcitonin as a diagnostic marker for sepsis: a systematic review and meta-analysis. *Lancet Infect Dis* 13:426–435, 2013.
64. Schuetz P, Chiappa V, Briel M, et al: Procalcitonin algorithms for antibiotic therapy desisions. A systematic review of randomized controlled trials and recommendations for clinical algorithms. *Arch Intern Med* 171:1322–1331, 2011.
65. Tromp M, Lansdorp B, Bleeker-Rovers CP, et al: Serial and panel analyses of biomarkers do not improve the prediction of bacteremia compared to one procalcitonin measurement. *J Infect* 65:292–301, 2012.
66. Brodska H, Malickova K, Adamkova V, et al: Significantly higher procalcitonin levles could differentiate Gram-negative sepsis from Gram-positive and fungal sepsis. *Clin Exp Med* 13:165–170, 2014.
67. Feezor RJ, Oberholzer C, Baker HV, et al: Molecular characterization of the acute inflammatory response to infections with gram-negative versus gram-positive bacteria. *Infect Immun* 71:5803–5813, 2003.
68. Charles PE, Ladoire S, Aho S, et al: Serum procalcitonin elevation in critically ill patients at the onset of bacteremia caused by either Gram negative or Gram positive bacteria. *BMC Infect Dis* 8:38, 2008.
69. Koivula I, Hamalainen S, Jantunen E, et al: Elevated procalcitonin predicts Gram-negative sepsis in haematological patients with febrile neutropenia. *Scand J Infect Dis* 43:471–478, 2011.
70. Matthaiou DK, Ntani G, Kontogiorgi M, et al: An ESICM systematic review and meta-analysis of procalcitonin-guided antibiotic therapy algorithm in adult critically ill patients. *Intensive Care Med* 38:940–949, 2012.
71. Kopterides P, Siempos IL, Tsangaris I, et al: Procalcitonin-guided algorithms of antibiotic therapy in the intensive care unit: a systematic review and meta-analysis of randomized controlled trials. *Crit Care Med* 38:2229–2241, 2010.
72. Schuetz P, Maurer P, Punjabi V, et al: Procalcitonin decrease over 72 hours in US critical care units predicts fatal outcome in sepsis patients. *Crit Care* 17:R115, 2013.
73. Faix JD: Presepsin - the new kid on the sepsis block. *Clin Biochem* 47:503–504, 2014.
74. Rabensteiner J: Diagnostic and prognostic potential of presepsin in Emergency Department patients presenting with systemic inflammatory response syndrome [Letter]. *J Infect* 69:627–630, 2014.
75. Shirakawa K, Naitou K, Hirose J, et al: Presepsin (sCD14-ST): development and evaluation of one-step ELISA with a new standard that is similar to the form of presepsin in septic patients. *Clin Chem Lab Med* 49:937–939, 2011.
76. Masson S: Circulating presepsin (soluble CD14 subtype) as a marker of host response in patients with severe sepsis or septic shock: data from the multicenter, randomized ALBIOS trial. *Intensive Care Med* 41:12–20, 2015.
77. Wu Y, Wang F, Fan X, et al: Accuracy of plasma sTREM-1 for sepsis diagnosis in systemic inflammatory patients: a systematic review and meta-analysis. [Review]. *Crit Care* 16:R229, 2012.
78. Hanna WJ, Berrens Z, Langer T, et al: Interleukin-27: a novel biomarker in predicting bacterial infection among the critically ill. *Crit Care* 19:378, 2015.
79. Wong HR, Lindsell CJ, Lahni P, et al: Interleukin 27 as a sepsis diagnostic biomarker in critically ill adults. Shock 40:382–386, 2013.
80. Marik PE: Don't miss the diagnosis of sepsis! *Crit Care* 18:529, 2014.
81. Sterling SA, Miller WR, Pryor J, et al: The impact of timing of antibiotics on outcomes in Severe Sepsis and Septic Shock: a systematic review and meta-analysis. *Crit Care Med* 43:1907–1915, 2015.
82. Kollef MH, Napolitano LM, Solomkin JS, et al: Health care-associated infection (HAI): a critical appraisal of the emerging threat-proceedings of the HAI Summit. *Clin Infect Dis* 47[Suppl 2]:S55–S99, 2008.
83. Mermel LA, Farr BM, Sherertz RJ, et al: Guidelines for the management of intravascular catheter-related infections. *Clin Infect Dis* 32:1249–1272, 2001.
84. Joung MK, Lee JA, Moon SY, et al: Impact of de-escalation therapy on clinical outcomes for intensive care unit-acquired pneumonia. *Crit Care* 15:R79, 2011.
85. Garnacho-Montero J, Gutierrez-Pizarraya A, Escoresca-Ortega A, et al: De-escalation of emperical therapy is associated with lower mortality in patients with severe sepsis and septic shock. *Intensive Care Med* 40:32–40, 2014.
86. Shindo Y, Ito R, Kobayashi D, et al: Risk factors for drug-resistant pathogens in community-acquired and healthcare-associated pneumonia. *Am J Respir Crit Care Med* 188:985–995, 2013.
87. Boucher HW, Talbot GH, Bradley JS, et al: Bad bugs, no drugs: no ESKAPE! An update from the Infectious Diseases Society of America. *Clin Infect Dis* 48:1–12, 2009.
88. Rice LB: Federal funding for the study of antimicrobial resistance in nosocomial pathogens: no ESKAPE. *J Infect Dis* 197:1079–1081, 2008.
89. Rice LB: Mechanisms of resistance and clinical relevance of resistance to beta-lactams, glycopeptides, and fluoroquinolones. *Mayo Clin Proc* 87:198–208, 2012.
90. Aliberti S, Blasi F, Zanaboni AM, et al: Duration of antibiotic therapy in hospitalised patients with community-acquired pneumonia. *Eur Respir J* 36:128–134, 2010.
91. Christ-Crain M, Stolz D, Bingisser R, et al: Procalcitonin guidance of antibiotic therapy in community-acquired pneumonia: a randomized trial. *Am J Respir Crit Care Med* 174:84–93, 2006.
92. Pugh R, Grant C, Cooke RP, et al: Short-course versus prolonged-course antibiotic therapy for hospital-acquired pneumonia in critically ill adults. *Cochrane Database Syst Rev* CD007577, 2011. doi:10.1002/14651858. CD007577.pub3.
93. Sawyer RG, Claridge JA, Nathens AB, et al: Trial of short-course antimicrobial therapy for intraabdominal infection. *N Engl J Med* 372:1996–2005, 2015.
94. Dellinger RP, Carlet JM, Masur H, et al: Surviving Sepsis Campaign guidelines for management of severe sepsis and septic shock. *Crit Care Med* 32:858–873, 2004.
95. Dellinger RP, Levy MM, Carlet JM, et al: Surviving sepsis Campaign: international guidelines for management of severe sepsis and septic shock: 2008. *Crit Care Med* 36:296–327, 2008.
96. Burton TM: New therapy for sepsis infection raises hope but many questions (lead article). *Wall Street J* 4:1, 2008.
97. Marik PE, Varon J: Goal-directed therapy in sepsis. *N Engl J Med* 346:1025, 2002.
98. Bellomo R, Warrillow SJ, Reade MC: Why we should be wary of single-center trials. *Crit Care Med* 37:3114–3119, 2009.
99. Marik PE, Varon J: Early Goal Directed Therapy (EGDT): On terminal lIfe support? *Am J Emerg Med* 28:243–245, 2010.
100. Marik PE: Surviving sepsis guidelines and scientific evidence? *J Intensive Care Med* 26:201–202, 2011.
101. Marik PE: Surviving sepsis: going beyond the guidelines. *Ann Intensive Care* 1:17, 2011.
102. Marik PE: The demise of early goal-directed therapy for severe sepsis and septic shock. *Acta Anaesthesiol Scand* 59:561–567, 2015.
103. Hotchkiss RS, Karl IE: Reevaluation of the role of cellular hypoxia and bioenergetics failure in sepsis. *JAMA* 267:1503–1510, 1992.
104. ProCESS Investigators, Yealy DM, Kellum JA, et al: A randomized trial of protocol-based care for early septic shock. *N Engl J Med* 370:1683–1693, 2014.
105. ARISE Investigators, ANZICS Clinical Trials Group, Peake SL, et al: Goal-directed resuscitation for patients with Early Septic Shock. *N Engl J Med* 371:1496–506, 2014.
106. Mouncey PR, Osborn TM, Power S, et al: Trial of early, goal-directed resuscitation for septic shock. *N Engl J Med* 372:1301–1311, 2015.
107. Angus DC, Barnato AE, Bell D, et al: A systematic review and meta-analysis of early goal-directed therapy for septic shock: the ARISE, ProCESS and ProMISe investigators. *Intensive Care Med* 41:1549–1560, 2015.
108. Knox M, Pickkers P: "Less is More" in Critically ill patients. Not too intensive. *JAMA Intern Med* 173:1369–1372, 2013.
109. Hilton AK, Bellomo R: A critique of fluid bolus resuscitation in severe sepsis. *Crit Care* 16:302, 2012.
110. Hilton AK, Bellomo R: Totem and taboo: fluids in sepsis. *Crit Care* 15:164, 2011.
111. Marik PE: Iatrogenic salt water drowning and the hazards of a high central venous pressure. *Ann Intensive Care* 4:21, 2014.
112. Marik PE, Monnet X, Teboul JL: Hemodynamic parameters to guide fluid therapy. *Ann Crit Care* 1:1, 2011.
113. Marik PE: Fluid responsiveness and the six guiding principles of fluid resuscitation. *Crit Care Med* 44:1920–1922, 2016.
114. Surviving Sepsis Campaign six hour bundle revised. Available at: http://www.survivingsepsis.org/News/Pages/SSC-Six-Hour-Bundle-Revised.aspx. Acessed January 28, 2017.
115. Marik PE, Cavallazzi R: Does the Central Venous Pressure (CVP) predict fluid responsiveness: An update meta-analysis and a plea for some common sense. *Crit Care Med* 41:1774–1781, 2013.
116. Wetterslev M, Haase N, Johansen RR, et al: Predicting fluid responsiveness with transthoracic echocardiography is not yet evidence based. *Acta Anaesthesiol Scand* 57:692–697, 2013.
117. Muller L, Bobbia X, Toumi M, et al: Respiratory variations of inferior vena cava diameter predict fluid responsiveness in spontaneously breathing patients with acute circulatory failure: need for a cautious use. *Crit Care* 16:R188, 2012.
118. Juhl-Olsen P, Vistisen ST, Christiansen LK, et al: Ultrasound of the inferior vena cava does not predict hemodynamic response to early hemorrhage. *J Emerg Med* 45:592–597, 2013.
119. Corl K, Napoli AM, Gardiner F: Bedside sonographic measurement of the inferior vena cava caval index is a poor predictor of fluid responsiveness in emergency department patients. *Emerg Med Australas* 24:534–539, 2012.
120. Monnet X, Teboul JL: Passive leg raising: five rules, not a drop of fluid! *Crit Care* 19:18, 2015.
121. Monnet X, Marik P, Teboul JL: Passive leg raising for predicting fluid responsiveness: a systematic review and meta-analysis. *Intensive Care Med* 42:1935–1922, 2016.

122. Marik P, Bellomo R: A rational apprach to fluid therapy in sepsis. *Br J Anaesth* 116(3):339–349, 2016.
123. Marik PE: The physiology of volume resuscitation. *Curr Anesthesiol Rep* 4:353–359, 2014.
124. Nunes T, Ladeira R, Bafi A, et al: Duration of hemodynamic effects of crystalloids in patients with circulatory shock after initial resuscitation. *Ann Intensive Care* 4:25, 2014.
125. Lammi MR, Aiello B, Burg GT, et al: Response to fluid boluses in the fluid and catheter treatment trial. *Chest* 148:919–926, 2015.
126. Sanchez M, Jimenez-Lendinez M, Cidoncha M, et al: Comparison of fluid compartments and fluid responsiveness in septic and non-septic patients. *Anaesth Intensive Care* 39:1022–1029, 2011.
127. Bark BP, Oberg CM, Grande PO: Plasma volume expansion by 0.9% NaCl during sepsis/systemic inflammatory response syndrome, after hemorrhage, and during a normal state. *Shock* 40:59–64, 2013.
128. Glassford NJ, Eastwood GM, Bellomo R: Physiological changes after fluid bolus therapy in sepsis: a systematic review of contemporary data. *Crit Care* 18:2557, 2014.
129. Monge-Garcia MI, Gonzalez PG, Romero MG, et al: Effects of fluid administration on arterial load in septic shock patients. *Intensive Care Med* 41:1247–1255, 2015.
130. Pierrakos C, Velissaris D, Scolletta S, et al: Can changes in arterial pressure be used to detect changes in cardiac index during fluid challenge in patients with septic shock? *Intensive Care Med* 38:422–428, 2012.
131. Hollenberg SM, Ahrens TS, Annane D, et al: Practice parameters for hemodynamic support of sepsis in adult patients: 2004 update. *Crit Care Med* 32:1928–1948, 2004.
132. Brandt S, Regueira T, Bracht H, et al: Effect of fluid resuscitation on mortality and organ function in experimental sepsis models. *Crit Care* 13:R186, 2009.
133. Rehberg S, Yamamoto Y, Sousse L, et al: Selective V(1a) agonism attenuates vascular dysfunction and fluid accumulation in ovine severe sepsis. *Am J Physiol Heart Circ Physiol* 303:H1245–H1254, 2012.
134. Rosenberg AL, Dechert RE, Park PK, et al: Review of a large clinical series: association of cumulative fluid balance on outcome in acute lung injury: a retrospective review of the ARDSnet tidal volume study cohort. *J Intensive Care Med* 24:35–46, 2009.
135. Alsous F, Khamiees M, DeGirolamo A, et al: Negative fluid balance predicts survival in patients with septic shock: a retrospective pilot study. *Chest* 117:1749–1754, 2000.
136. Murphy CV, Schramm GE, Doherty JA, et al: The importance of fluid management in acute lung injury secondary to septic shock. *Chest* 136:102–109, 2009.
137. Chung FT, Lin SM, Lin SY, et al: Impact of extravascular lung water index on outcomes of severe sepsis patients in a medical intensive care unit. *Respir Med* 102:956–961, 2008.
138. Bouchard J, Soroko SB, Chertow GM, et al: Fluid accumulation, survival and recovery of kidney function in critically ill patients with acute kidney injury. *Kidney Int* 76:422–427, 2009.
139. Micek SC, McEnvoy C, McKenzie M, et al: Fluid balance and cardiac function in septic shock as predictors of hospital mortality. *Crit Care* 17:R246, 2013.
140. Zhang Z, Zhang Z, Xue Y, et al: Prognostic value of B-type natriuretic peptide (BNP) and its potential role in guiding fluid therapy in critically ill septic patients. *Scand J Trauma Resus Emerg Med* 20:86, 2012.
141. Boyd JH, Forbes J, Nakada T, et al: Fluid resuscitation in septic shock: a positive fluid balance and elevated central venous pressure increase mortality. *Crit Care Med* 39:259–265, 2011.
142. Kelm DJ, Perrin JT, Cartin-Cebra R, et al: Fluid overload in patients with severe sepsis and septic shock treated with Early-Goal Directed Therapy is associated with increaed acute need for fluid-related medical interventions and hospital death. *Shock* 43:68–73, 2015.
143. Maitland K, Kiguli S, Opoka RO, et al: Mortality after fluid bolus in african children with severe infection. *N Engl J Med* 364:2483–2495, 2011.
144. Maitland K, George EC, Evans JA, et al: Exploring mechanisms of excess mortality with early fluid resuscitation: insights from the FEAST trial. *BMC Med* 11:68, 2013.
145. Marik PE: Early management of severe sepsis: current concepts and controversies. *Chest* 145:1407–1418, 2014.
146. Marik PE, Lemson J: Fluid responsiveness: an evolution of our understanding. *Br J Anaesth* 112:620–622, 2014.
147. Asfar P, Meziani F, Hamel JF, et al: High versus low blood-pressure target in patients with septic shock. *N Engl J Med* 370:1583–1593, 2014.
148. Kirkpatrick AW, Roberts DJ, De WJ, et al: Intra-abdominal hypertension and the abdominal compartment syndrome: updated consensus definitions and clinical practice guidelines from the World Society of the Abdominal Compartment Syndrome. *Intensive Care Med* 39:1190–1206, 2013.
149. Malbrain ML, Marik PE, Witters I, et al: De-resuscitation in the critically ill: what, why, when and how? Results of a meta-analysis and systematic review on the impact of fluid overload on morbidity and mortality. *Anesthesiol Intensive Ther* 46:361–380, 2014.
150. Scheingraber S, Rehm M, Sehmisch C, et al: Rapid saline infusion produces hyperchloremic acidosis in patients undergoing gynecologic surgery. Anesthesiology 90:1265–1270, 1999.
151. Kellum JA, Bellomo R, Kramer DJ, et al: Etiology of metabolic acidosis during saline resuscitation in endotoxemia. *Shock* 9:364–368, 1998.
152. Waters JH, Gottlieb A, Schoenwald P, et al: Normal saline versus lactated Ringer's solution for intraoperative fluid management in patients undergoing abdominal aortic aneurysm repair: an outcome study. *Anesth Analg* 93:817–822, 2001.
153. Reid F, Lobo DN, Williams RN, et al: (Ab)normal saline and physiological Hartmann's solution: a randomized double-blind crossover study. *Clin Sci* 104:17–24, 2003.
154. Chowdhury AH, Cox EF, Francis S, et al: A randomized, controlled, double-blind crossover study on the effects of 2-L infusions of 0.9% saline and plasma-lyte 148 on renal blood flow velocity and renal cortical tissue perfusion in healthy volunteers. *Ann Surg* 256:18–24, 2012.
155. Mohd Yunos N, Bellomo R, Hegarty C, et al: Association between a chloride-liberal vs chloride-restrictive intravenous fluid administration strategy and kidney injury in critically ill adults. *JAMA* 308:1566–1572, 2012.
156. Raghunathan K, Shaw A, Nathanson B, et al: Association between the choice of IV crystalloid and in-hospital mortality among critically ill adults with sepsis. *Crit Care Med* 42:1585–1591, 2014.
157. Young P, Bailey M, Beasley R, et al: Effect of a buffered crystalloid solution vs saline on acute kidney injury among patients in the intensive care unit. The SPLIT randomized clinical trial. *JAMA* 314:1701–1710, 2015.
158. Perner A, Haase N, Guttormsen AB, et al: Hydroxyethyl starch 130/0.4 versus Ringers Acetate in severe sepsis. *N Engl J Med* 367:124–134, 2012.
159. Haase N, Perner A, Hennings LI, et al: Hydroxyethyl starch 130/0.38-0.45 versus crystalloid or albumin in patients with sepsis: systematic review with meta-analysis and trial sequential analysis. *BMJ* 346:f839, 2013.
160. Patel A, Laffan MA, Waheed U, et al: Randomised trials of human albumin for adults with sepsis: systematic review and meta-analysis with trial sequential analysis of all-cause mortality. *BMJ* 349:g4561, 2014.
161. SAFE Study Investigators, Finfer S, McEvoy S, et al: Impact of albumin compared to saline on organ function and mortality of patients with severe sepsis. *Intensive Care Med* 37:86–96, 2011.
162. Caironi P, Tognoni G, Masson S, et al: Albumin replacement in patients with severe sepsis or septic shock. *N Engl J Med* 370:1412–1421, 2014.
163. Kremer H, Baron-Menguy C, Tesse A, et al: Human serum albumin improves endothelial dysfunction and survival during experimental endotoxemia: concentration-dependent properties. *Crit Care Med* 39:1414–1422, 2011.
164. Bellomo R, Di Giantomasso D: Noradrenaline and the kidney: friends or foes? *Crit Care* 5:294–298, 2001.
165. Lehman LW, Saeed M, Talmor D, et al: Methods of blood pressure measurement in the ICU. *Crit Care Med* 41:34–40, 2013.
166. Varpula M, Tallgren M, Saukkonen K, et al: Hemodynamic variables related to outcome in septic shock. *Intensive Care Med* 31:1066–1071, 2005.
167. Panwar R, Lanyon N, Davies AR, et al: Mean perfusion pressure deficit during the initial management of shock-an observational cohort study. *J Crit Care* 28:816–824, 2013.
168. Avni T, Lador A, Lev S, et al: Vasopressors for the treatment of septic shock: systematic review and meta-analysis. *PloS One* 10(8):e0129305, 2015.
169. Fawzy A, Evans SR, Walkey AJ: Practice patterns and outcomes associated with choice of initial vasopressor therapy for septic shock. *Crit Care Med* 43:2141–2146, 2015.
170. De Baker D, Aldecoa C, Njimi H, et al: Dopamine versus norepinephrine in the treatment of septic shock: a meta-analysis. *Crit Care Med* 40:725–730, 2011.
171. Malay MB, Ashton JL, Dahl K, et al: Heterogeneity of the vasoconstrictor effect of vasopressin in septic shock. *Crit Care Med* 32:1327–1331, 2004.
172. Monnet X, Jabot J, Maizel J, et al: Norepinephrine increases cardiac preload and reduces preload dependency assessed by passive leg raising in septic shock patients. *Crit Care Med* 39:689–694, 2011.
173. Persichini R, Silva S, Teboul JL, et al: Effects of norepinephrine on mean systemic pressure and venous return in human septic shock. *Crit Care Med* 40:3146–3153, 2012.
174. Hamzaoui O, Georger JF, Monnet X, et al: Early administration of norepinephrine increases cardiac preload and cardiac output in septic patients with life-threatening hypotension. *Crit Care* 14:R142, 2010.
175. Abid O, Akca S, Haji-Michael P, et al: Strong vasopressor support may be futile in the intensive care unit patient with multiple organ failure. *Crit Care Med* 28:947–949, 2000.
176. Cardenas-Garcia J, Schaub KF, Belchikov YG, et al: Safety of peripheral intravenous administration of vasoactive medication. *J Hosp Med,* 2015. doi:10.1002/jhm.2394.
177. Vieillard-Baron A, Caille V, Charron C, et al: Actual incidence of global left ventricular hypokinesia in adult septic shock. *Crit Care Med* 36:1701–1706, 2008.
178. Jellema WT, Groeneveld AB, Wesseling KH, et al: Heterogeneity and prediction of hemodynamic responses to dobutamine in patients with septic shock. *Crit Care Med* 34:2392–2398, 2006.
179. Landry DW, Levin HR, Gallant EM, et al: Vasopressin deficiency contributes to the vasodilation of septic shock. *Circulation* 95:1122–1125, 1997.
180. Morelli A, Ertmer C, Lange M, et al: Effects of short-term simultaneous infusion of dobutamine and terlipressin in patients with septic shock: the DOBUPRESS study. *Br J Anaesth* 100:494–503, 2008.
181. Morelli A, Ertmer C, Rehberg S, et al: Continuous terlipressin versus vasopressin infusion in septic shock (TERLIVAP): a randomized, controlled pilot study. *Crit Care* 13:R130, 2009.
182. Russell JA, Walley KR, Singer J, et al: Vasopressin versus norepinephrine infusion in patients with septic shock. *N Engl J Med* 358:877–887, 2008.
183. Chernow B, Alexander HR, Smallridge RC, et al: Hormonal responses to graded surgical stress. *Arch Intern Med* 147:1273–1278, 1987.

184. Jardin F, Fourme T, Page B, et al: Persistent preload defect in severe sepsis despite fluid loading: a longitudinal echocardiographic study in patients with septic shock. *Chest* 116:1354–1359, 1999.
185. Parker MM, Shelhamer JH, Natanson C, et al: Serial cardiovascular variables in survivors and nonsurvivors of septic shock: heart rate as an early predictor of prognosis. *Crit Care Med* 15:923–929, 1987.
186. Ackland GL, Yao ST, Rudiger A, et al: Cardioprotection, attenuated systemic inflammation, and survival benefit of beta1-adrenoceptor blockade in severe sepsis in rats. *Crit Care Med* 38:388–394, 2010.
187. Rudiger A: Beta-block the septic heart. *Crit Care Med* 38:S608–S612, 2010.
188. Morelli A, Ertmer C, Westphal M, et al: Effect of heat rate control with esmolol on hemodynamic and clinical outcomes in patients with septic shock. A randomized clinical trial. *JAMA* 310:1683–1691, 2013.
189. da Silva Ramos FJ, Azevedo LC: Hemodynamic and perfusion end points for volemic resuscitation in sepsis. *Shock* 34[Suppl 1]:34–39, 2010.
190. Bouferrache K, Amiel JB, Chimot L, et al: Initial resuscitation guided by the Surviving Sepsis Campaign recommendations and early echocardiographic assessment of hemodynamics in intensive care unit septic patients: a pilot study. *Crit Care Med* 40:2821–2827, 2012.
191. Langenberg C, Wan L, Egi M, et al: Renal blood flow and function during recovery from experimental septic acute kidney injury. *Intensive Care Med* 33:1614–1618, 2007.
192. Langenberg C, Wan L, Egi M, et al: Renal blood flow in experimental septic acute renal failure. *Kidney Int* 69:1996–2002, 2006.
193. Wan L, Bagshaw SM, Langenberg C, et al: Pathophysiology of septic acute kidney injury: what do we really know? *Crit Care Med* 36:S198–S203, 2008.
194. Angus DC, van der Poll T: Severe sepsis and septic shock. *N Engl J Med* 369:840–851, 2013.
195. Jansen TC, van BJ, Schoonderbeek FJ, et al: Early lactate-guided therapy in intensive care unit patients: a multicenter, open-label, randomized controlled trial. *Am J Respir Crit Care Med* 182:752–761, 2010.
196. Jones AE, Shapiro NI, Trzeciak S, et al: Lactate clearance vs central venous oxygen saturation as goals of early sepsis therapy: a randomized clinical trial. *JAMA* 303:739–746, 2010.
197. Marik PE, Bellomo R: Lactate clearance as a target of therapy in sepsis: a flawed paradigm. *OA Crit Care* 1:3, 2013.
198. Garcia-Alvarez M, Marik P, Bellomo R: Sepsis-associated hyperlactatemia. *Crit Care* 18:503, 2014.
199. Marik PE, Sibbald WJ: Effect of stored-blood transfusion on oxygen delivery in patients with sepsis. *JAMA* 269:3024–3029, 1993.
200. Garcia-Alvarez M, Marik PE, Bellomo R: Stress Hyperlactemia. *Lancet Endo Diab* 2:339–347, 2014.
201. Hayes MA, Timmins AC, Yau E, et al: Elevation of systemic oxygen delivery in the treatment of critically ill patients. *N Engl J Med* 330:1717–1722, 1994.
202. Gattinoni L, Brazzi L, Pelosi P, et al: A trial of goal-oriented hemodynamic therapy in critically ill patients. *N Engl J Med* 333:1025–1032, 1995.
203. National Quality Forum: Severe sepsis and septic shock: managment bundle, update. 2015. Available at: www.qualityforum.org. Accessed January 28, 2017.
204. Ibarra-Estrada MA, Lopez-Pulgarin JA, Mijangos-Mendez JC, et al: Variation in carotid peak systolic velocity predicts volume responsiveness in mechanically ventilated patients with septic shock: a prospective cohort study. *Crit Ultrasound J* 7:12, 2015.
205. Saugel B, Ringmaier S, Holzapfel K, et al: Physical examination, central venous pressure, and chest radiography for the prediction of transpulmonary thermodilution-derived hemodynamic parameters in critically ill patients: a prospective trial. *J Crit Care* 26:402–410, 2011.
206. Boyer A, Vargas F, Coste F, et al: Influence of surgical treatment timing on mortality from necrotizing soft tissue infections requiring intensive care management. *Intensive Care Med* 35:847–853, 2009.
207. Bufalari A, Giustozzi G, Moggi L: Postoperative intraabdominal abscesses: percutaneous versus surgical treatment. *Acta Chir Belg* 96:197–200, 1996.
208. Marik PE: Glucocorticoids in sepsis: disectiong facts from fiction. *Crit Care* 15:158, 2011.
209. Marik PE, Pastores SM, Annane D, et al: Recommendations for the diagnosis and management of corticosteroid insufficiency in critically ill adult patients: consensus statements from an international task force by the American College of Critical Care Medicine. *Crit Care Med* 36:1937–1949, 2008.
210. Annane D, Bellissant E, Sebille V, et al: Impaired pressor sensitivity to noradrenaline in septic shock patients with and without impaired adrenal function reserve. *Br J Clin Pharmacol* 46:589–597, 1998.
211. Chappell D, Jacob M, Hofmann-Kiefer K, et al: Hydrocortisone preserves the vascular barrier by protecting the endothelial glycocalyx. *Anesthesiology* 107:776–784, 2007.
212. Beale R, Janes JM, Brunkhorst FM, et al: Global utilization of low-dose corticosteroids in severe sepsis and septic shock: a report from the PROGRESS registry. *Crit Care* 14:R102, 2010.
213. Volbeda M, Wetterslev J, Gluud C, et al: Glucocorticosteroids for sepsis: systematic review with meta-analysis and trial sequential analysis. *Intensive Care Med* 41:1220–1234, 2015.
214. Venkatesh B, Myburgh J, Finfer S, et al: The ADRENAL study protocol: adjunctive corticosteroid treatment in critically ill patients with septic shock. *Crit Care Resus* 15:83–88, 2013.
215. Heyland DK, Dhaliwal R, Drover JW, et al: Canadian clinical practice guidelines for nutrition support in mechanically ventilated, critically ill adult patients. *JPEN* 27:355–373, 2003.
216. McClave SA, Martindale RG, Vanek VW, et al: Guidelines for the provision and assessment of nutrition support therapy in the adult critically ill patient: society of Critical Care Medicine (SCCM) and American Society for Parenteral and Enteral Nutrition (A.S.P.E.N.). *JPEN* 33:277–316, 2009.
217. Heyland DK, Dhaliwal R, Lemieux M, et al: 2015 Canadian Clinical Practice Guidelinee. Available at: http://www.criticalcarenutrition.com/. Retrieved September 9, 2015. Accessed January 28, 2017
218. Kreymann KG, Berger MM, Deutz NE, et al: ESPEN Guidelines on Enteral Nutrition: Intensive care. *Clin Nutr* 25:210–223, 2006.
219. Marik PE, Hooper MH: Normocaloric versus hypocaloric feeding on the outcomes of ICU patients: a systematic review and meta-analysis. *Intensive Care Med* 42:316–323, 2016.
220. Feed a cold, starve a fever. Available at: https://en.wiktionary.org/wiki/feed_a_cold,_starve_a_fever. Accessed January 28, 2017.
221. Wessling-Resnick M: Iron homeostasis and the inflammatory response. *Annu Rev Nutr* 30:105–122, 2010.
222. Sherman AR: Influence of iron on immunity and disease resistance. *Ann N Y Acad Sci* 587:140–146, 1990.
223. Conn CA, Kozak WE, Tooten PC, et al: Effect of voluntary exercise and food restriction in response to lipopolysaccharide in hamsters. *J Appl Physiol* 78:466–477, 1995.
224. Kluger MJ, Rothenburg BA: Fever and reduced iron: their interaction as a host defense response to bacterial infection. *Science* 203:374–376, 1979.
225. Choi AM, Ryter SW, Levine B: Autophagy in human health and disease. *N Engl J Med* 368:651–662, 2013.
226. Levine B, Mizushima N, Virgin HN: Autophagy in immunity and inflammation. *Nature* 469:323–335, 2011.
227. Rich KA, Burkett C, Webster P: Cytoplasmic bacteria can be targets for autophagy. *Cell Microbiol* 5:455–468, 2003.
228. Xu Y, Eissa NT: Autophagy in innate and adaptive immunity. *Proc Am Thorac Soc* 7:22–28, 2010.
229. Bakker OJ, van Goor H, Bosscha K, et al: Early versus on-demand nasoenteric tube feeding in acute pancreatitis. *N Engl J Med* 371:1983–1993, 2014.
230. Marik PE: Feeding critically ill patients the right "whey":thinking outside the box. A personal view. *Ann Intensive Care* 5:11, 2015.
231. Girbes AR, Robert R, Marik PE: More protocols: beware of regression to the mean and mediocrity. *Intensive Care Med* 41:2218–2220, 2015.

Chapter 40 ■ Multiple Organ Dysfunction Syndrome

TIMOTHY A. PRITTS • ANDREW C. BERNARD

Care of the critically ill has advanced substantially in the past 50 years to the point that patients who previously succumbed to illness or injury may now survive their initial insult. Unfortunately, this places them at risk for multiple organ dysfunction syndrome (MODS), with subsequent failure of organ systems and late mortality [1]. A thorough understanding of the pathophysiology and treatment of MODS is necessary to attempt to mitigate associated secondary morbidity and mortality.

MODS can be defined as "the inability of one or more organs to support its activities spontaneously without intervention" [2]. Initial recognition of MODS came during World War II as advances in resuscitation strategies allowed casualties to survive the initial hemorrhagic shock insult, but rendered them vulnerable to subsequent acute renal failure [3]. Improved intensive care and resuscitation strategies subsequently led to the recognition of pulmonary failure in the form of acute respiratory distress syndrome (ARDS) during the Vietnam conflict [4]. Although advances in support for failing organs, including continuous dialysis and advanced ventilator care, have potentially increased survival, MODS remains a common cause of death in the intensive care unit (ICU).

DIAGNOSTIC CRITERIA AND SCORING SYSTEMS

The severity of MODS determines mortality [5]. Organ failure severity scoring was initially described by Knaus in 1985 [6]. Modern scoring systems consider grade and severity and are intended to serve as predictors of outcome. Among the most commonly used scoring systems are the multiple organ dysfunction syndrome (MODS), sequential organ failure assessment (SOFA), and logistic organ dysfunction score (LODS) [7–9]. All include clinical and laboratory data for six organs: respiratory, cardiovascular, hematologic, hepatic, renal, and central nervous system (Table 40.1) [10]. The Denver Multiple Organ Failure (MOF) score is a straightforward 4-point scale that has similar or superior specificity to the SOFA score [11]. The Simplified Acute Physiology Score (SAPS) is easy to calculate with available clinical and laboratory data and may in fact be superior to acute physiology and chronic health evaluation (APACHE) in geriatric ICU patients [12]. A "cellular injury score" based on measures of cellular dysfunction has also been described [13]. Specialized scoring systems have been developed for unique populations. For example, the cardiac surgery score (CASUS) outperformed APACHE and SAPS in that special population [14]. No single scoring system has been proven superior, but all predict mortality more accurately than they predict health care resource utilization [11,15].

All scoring systems are intended to improve upon clinical judgment. The Denver Emergency Department Trauma Organ Failure Score uses six simple criteria available in the trauma room to predict MODS at 7 days more effectively than unaided emergency department attending judgment [16]. Such predictive

TABLE 40.1

Criteria Used in Common Organ Dysfunction Scoring Systems

Organ	Variable	Denver MOF [11]	SOFA [8]	LODS [9]	MODS [7]
Respiratory	PaO_2/FIO_2	Yes	Yes	Yes	Yes
	MV		Yes		
Hematology	Platelets	Yes	Yes	Yes	
	WBC			Yes	
Hepatic	Bilirubin	Yes	Yes	Yes	Yes
	Prothrombin time			Yes	
Cardiovascular	MAP		Yes		
	SBP			Yes	
	Heart rate			Yes	
	PAR [(HR × CVP)/MAP]				Yes
	Dopamine			Yes	
	Dobutamine			Yes	
	Epinephrine			Yes	
	Norepinephrine			Yes	
	Any inotrope	Yes			
CNS	GCS		Yes	Yes	Yes
Renal	Creatinine	Yes	Yes	Yes	Yes
	BUN			Yes	
	Urine output		Yes	Yes	

Denver MOF, Denver multiple organ failure score; SOFA, sequential organ failure assessment; LODS, logistic organ dysfunction score; MODS, multiple organ dysfunction syndrome; PaO_2, blood partial pressure of oxygen; FIO_2, fraction of inspired gas which is oxygen; MV, mechanical ventilation requirement; WBC, elevated white blood count; PAR, pressure-adjusted heart rate; HR, heart rate; CVP, central venous pressure; MAP, mean arterial pressure; SBP, systolic blood pressure; CNS, central nervous system; GCS, Glasgow Coma Scale score; BUN, blood urea nitrogen.
Modified from Mizock BA: The multiple organ dysfunction syndrome. *Dis Mon* 55(8):476–526, 2009.

models permit resource allocation and can be used to guide patient transfers. The APACHE, originally described by Knaus in 1985 [17], is a scoring system that considers patient factors unrelated to the acute illness as well as acute illness severity. APACHE considers many variables and is therefore not as easily calculable at the bedside as MODS, SOFA, LODS, or Denver, but it reliably predicts both outcome and resource utilization, has been refined to its current version, APACHE IVa, and may be useful for benchmarking ICU performance [18].

EPIDEMIOLOGY

Incidence of MODS varies on the basis of primary diagnosis and the scoring system used to determine organ dysfunction. Seventy-one percent of ICU patients have some organ dysfunction [19] and about half have MODS [20], depending on the criteria used. For example, in one adult trauma ICU 47% had MODS, defined by SOFA ≤3 in two or more systems [21]. Septic patients are more likely to have organ dysfunction and more organ failures than nonseptic patients, and mortality is higher in MODS when sepsis is present (31% vs. 21%) [19].

ETIOLOGY

MODS is most often the result of shock, sepsis, and trauma, but there are many causes (Table 40.2) [22]. Forty-one percent of those patients with organ dysfunction have sepsis [19]. Sepsis most commonly originates in the lung (68%) and abdomen (22%), but there are many causes of sepsis-induced MODS [19].

MECHANISMS OF MULTIORGAN DYSFUNCTION SYNDROME

The systemic inflammatory response syndrome (SIRS) is frequently viewed as a predecessor and lies on a continuum of dysfunction with MODS. Components of the SIRS response are seen in virtually all patients following an operation, febrile illness, or injury. SIRS frequently resolves without progression to MODS. MODS may be viewed as a result of an ongoing, dysregulated, or treatment refractory SIRS response with progressive organ system derangement.

Despite extensive efforts, the pathophysiology of MODS is not fully understood and remains an area of intensive investigation [23]. Several mechanisms for the onset and propagation of MODS have been proposed, including an initial insult in which ischemia, oxidative stress, mitochondrial dysfunction, and activation of apoptotic pathways lead immediately to organ failure, and a "two hit" model, where an initial stimulus primes the immune system to respond to a subsequent insult or stimulus with an exuberant reaction, and the concept that dysregulated immune responses lead to MODS [23].

A common theme in the onset and propagation of MODS is the presence of a disordered immune response. It is likely that ongoing tissue hypoxia leads to activation of the acute inflammatory response, oxidative imbalance, structural rearrangement of cellular proteins, dysregulation of the immune system, activation of apoptotic pathways, cell death, and organ dysfunction [24]. Although the inflammatory response is an important component of normal recovery from injury and illness, organ failure appears to result from a loss of the balance between the pro- and anti-inflammatory cascades [25]. The proinflammatory response to a stimulus predominates initially, with increased release of proinflammatory mediators, increased capillary permeability, macrophage and neutrophil activation with tissue invasion and damage, disordered apoptosis, and microvascular thrombosis [26]. This initial response is normally tempered by the anti-inflammatory response, but immune regulation may become dysfunctional. Widespread activation of proinflammatory pathways and impaired balanced resolution by anti-inflammatory pathways can lead to early onset of MODS. If the organism survives the initial insult and onset of MODS, a period of immunosuppression can follow. During this period, the patient becomes susceptible to nosocomial pathogens, with a normally survivable event such as pneumonia representing a life-threatening "second hit" [27].

As research into the pathophysiology of MODS has advanced, another phase of the process has been recognized. Termed PICS (persistent inflammation, immunosuppression, and catabolism syndrome), this syndrome consists of loss of lean body mass, recurrent sepsis, and increased debility [28]. PICS is associated with functionally irreversible immune system paralysis and may be a significant cause of late death after recovery from the acute phase of MODS [29].

TABLE 40.2

Risk Factors for MODS

- Infection
  - Peritonitis and intra-abdominal infection
  - Pneumonia
  - Necrotizing soft tissue infections
  - Tropical infections (e.g., falciparum malaria, typhoid fever, dengue fever)
- Inflammation
  - Pancreatitis
- Ischemia
  - Ruptured aortic aneurysm
  - Hemorrhagic shock
  - Mesenteric ischemia
- Immune reactions
  - Autoimmune disease
  - Reactive hemophagocytic syndrome
  - Antiphospholipid antibody syndrome
  - Transplant rejection
  - Graft-versus-host disease
- Iatrogenic causes
  - Delayed or missed injury
  - Blood transfusion
  - Injurious mechanical ventilation
  - Treatment associated increased intra-abdominal pressure
- Intoxication
  - Drug reactions (anticonvulsants, carboplatin, antiretrovirals, colchicines, propofol, amiodarone, monoclonal antibodies)
  - Arsenic
  - Drug intoxication (ecstasy, cocaine, salicylates, acetaminophen)
- Endocrine
  - Adrenal crisis
  - Pheochromocytoma
  - Thyroid storm
  - Myxedema coma

Reproduced from Mizock BA: The multiple organ dysfunction syndrome. *Dis Mon* 55(8):476–526, 2009.

CURRENT MANAGEMENT STRATEGIES

Course of MODS

Outcome for MODS partly depends upon host factors including genetics. Some patients are genetically predisposed to enhanced immune reactivity [30]. For most patients, MODS progression follows a typical sequence first described by Don Fry in 1980 [31], beginning with lung failure, followed by the liver, gastric mucosa, and kidney. Lung dysfunction has since been reaffirmed as the initial manifestation of MODS in the majority of patients [32]. MODS follows a bimodal onset with early and late MODS characterized by different patient characteristics and mechanisms of death [33]. An important distinction must also be made with early organ dysfunction during resuscitation, which is often reversible, and not necessarily the same as early MODS [34].

Respiratory organ dysfunction is the most common early manifestation of MODS but is often not associated with death [35]. Renal, central nervous, and hematologic system impairments characterize MODS progression and are more strongly associated with mortality. Treatment of MODS, therefore, is focused on early recognition of those at risk, removing the proinflammatory pathway trigger, and preventing MODS progression [36]. Clinicians should move briskly to optimize cardiorespiratory function, remove catabolic stressors, and provide nutrition while using antimicrobials selectively and avoiding blood product transfusion. Key advances in the treatment of patients with severe critical illness and MODS that is based on randomized controlled trials are summarized in Table 40.3.

Resuscitation

The Surviving Sepsis Guidelines summarize current best practice regarding resuscitation as of 2013 [37]. One major strategy to reduce MODS is to ensure optimal initial resuscitation. Resuscitation should target adequate oxygen delivery and normalization of physiology. Oxygen saturation in mixed venous blood has historically been an important, if not vital, resuscitation target (SvO_2-saturation in mixed venous blood obtained from a pulmonary artery catheter or $ScvO_2$-saturation in central venous blood obtained from a central venous catheter in superior vena cava). Rivers et al. [38] showed that by using oxygen delivery as a target for resuscitation with fluid, blood, and inotropes, lactic acidemia was less severe and outcomes were improved. Subsequent studies of such "goal-directed therapy" have failed to show similar benefit but those investigations have been conducted in an era when the norm in resuscitation is much more advanced monitoring [39]. There is no question that inadequate initial resuscitation contributes to MODS risk [40]. For a comprehensive discussion of this topic, see Chapter 39.

Preventing MODS Progression

Source control is critical to terminate the trigger of the proinflammatory response [36]. Antimicrobials should be used early and be targeted at a broad spectrum of likely organism, then tailored and de-escalated [15]. On the basis of the possible role of the gut and enteric bacteria as a "motor" for MODS, several groups have proposed cleansing the bowel of bacteria to disrupt this relationship, but studies have yielded conflicting results and this practice remains controversial [41]. Although some European studies support parenteral and topical oropharyngeal antibiotics in reducing mortality, this is not widely accepted in the United States [42]. Transfusion is a risk factor for MODS, suggesting that a conservative approach to blood transfusion is appropriate [43].

Mechanical ventilation may contribute to distant organ dysfunction in acute lung injury (ALI) and ARDS [44]. In the ARDSNet trial, the "lung protective strategy" of plateau $\leq$30 cm H_2O and tidal volumes $\leq$6 mL per kg body weight was associated with a reduction in all-cause mortality of 9% compared with conventional ventilation with plateau pressures $\leq$50 cm H_2O and tidal volumes $\leq$12 mL per kg body weight [45]. A European study affirmed that use of a ventilation strategy with volumes greater than ARDSNet (>7.4 mL tidal volume per kg body weight) increased mortality [46]. For a comprehensive discussion of this topic, see Chapters 163 and 166.

Although Van den Berghe et al. [47] initially reported reduced mortality with intensive insulin therapy and the mortality reduction was in septic MODS, unacceptably high rates of hypoglycemia have since been reported [48] without a mortality benefit.

Steroid therapy in patients with sepsis and MODS may be used for select indications. For a comprehensive discussion of this topic, see Chapter 39.

Nutrition

Early initiation of enteral nutrition is associated with improved outcome for patients with severe trauma, surgery, sepsis, and MODS. MODS may be attenuated among patients receiving enteral nutrition within 24 hours as opposed to initiation later [49,50]. Recent retrospective data support early enteral feeding to reduce ICU and hospital mortality [51]. Both the American and European Societies of Parenteral and Enteral Nutrition (ASPEN and ESPEN) recommend enteral nutrition for ventilated patients when hemodynamics are adequate and gastrointestinal function is sufficient [52,53]. Feeding patients at their full nutritional requirements does not, appear to be necessary early in their ICU course, however [54]. Arginine has been shown to be beneficial for surgical and trauma patients, but cannot be recommended for septic medical patients because of immunoinflammatory characteristics [53]. However, omega fatty acids do appear

TABLE 40.3

Advances in Management of Multiple Organ Dysfunction Syndrome Based on Randomized Controlled Clinical Trials

Advance	Reference	Remarks
Digestive tract or oropharynx decontamination with antimicrobials reduces 28-day mortality in ICU patients	[42]	Not widely practiced in the United States, as it conflicts with principles of antimicrobial stewardship
Lung protective ventilation strategies are associated with reduced mortality and increased ventilator-free days	[45]	Lung protective strategies are commonly utilized in ICU settings
Aggressive enteral nutrition is associated with improved immune function and less mortality in burned children	[50]	Landmark study suggested that protein repletion is essential for critically ill patients

beneficial for shortening length of stay, ventilator days, and mortality among septic patients in some studies. Serum selenium is depleted in trauma and surgical patients, and some evidence suggests that depletion may contribute to MODS. Selenium repletion reduced MODS in a multi-institutional prospective randomized trial in 2007, but subsequent prospective trials questions its efficacy [55,56]. For a comprehensive discussion of this topic, see Chapters 39, 212, 213, and 214.

Continuous renal replacement therapy has been associated with reduction of MODS severity, theoretically due to alteration of the balance of pro- and anti-inflammatory circulating cytokines [57], but no large studies currently support its use for this purpose. Renal replacement appears to reduce outcome and length of hospital stay when initiated early but only based upon meta-analyses of smaller heterogeneous studies [58]. Intense interest in renal replacement is reflected in the numerous studies published on the topic to date but well-designed, appropriately powered studies defining the optimal method, risks, and benefits have yet to be performed. Other novel therapies include pharmacologic manipulation of the microcirculation or augmentation of mitochondrial oxidative metabolism to enhance oxygen delivery or utilization [15].

PROGNOSIS AND ICU LENGTH OF STAY

Up to 20% of patients admitted to an ICU develop aspects of MODS, with significantly increased morbidity and mortality [59]. MODS severity is decreasing but ICU mortality remains stable, perhaps because overall acuity is increasing [60]. In an epidemiologic study of sepsis in 2001, Angus et al. [22] determined that dysfunction of one, two, or three organ systems conveys 1%, 4.7%, and 20.7% mortality, respectively. Four-organ dysfunction was associated with 65% to 74% mortality [19,22]. A more recent study examining the outcomes of critically ill patients reported ICU mortality of 10% for failure of three systems or less, increasing to 25% and 50% for four- and five-organ system failure, respectively. Mortality of seven-system failure was 100% [61]. In addition to mortality, MODS can also affect long-term functional outcomes [21].

MODS is the most common reason for prolonged stays in the ICU, exceeding single organ system failure and simply the need for ventilatory support [59]. Determining prognosis for individual patients with MODS remains challenging. Severity of organ dysfunction at the time of ICU admission or during the ICU stay correlates well with mortality, with the highest scores suggestive of a nonsurvivable injury or illness, but does not allow clinically actionable bedside prediction of an individual patient's outcome [7]. The strongest independent risk factors for death appear to be central nervous system failure (RR = 16.06) and cardiovascular failure (RR = 11.83) [61].

CONCLUSIONS

MODS is largely a result of medical progress and modern ICU care. A common denominator for the pathogenesis of MODS appears to be cellular hypoperfusion, leading to an imbalanced immune response, with resultant organ damage and failure. Treatment of patients at risk for MODS is supportive, ensuring adequate resuscitation, nutritional support, infection or tissue injury source control, and support of individual organ system functions. Despite modern critical care, MODS remains a common cause of death among critically ill patients.

References

1. Levine JH, Durham RM, Moran J, et al: Multiple organ failure: is it disappearing? *World J Surg* 20(4):471–473, 1996.
2. Baue AE: Multiple organ failure—the discrepancy between our scientific knowledge and understanding and the management of our patients. *Langenbecks Arch Surg* 385(7):441–453, 2000.
3. Churchill ED: *Surgeon to Soldiers: Diary and Records of the Surgical Consultant, Allied Force Headquarters, World War 2*. Philadelphia, PA, Lippincott, 1972.
4. Ashbaugh DG, Bigelow DB, Petty TL, et al: Acute respiratory distress in adults. *Lancet* 2(7511):319–323, 1967.
5. Barie PS, Hydo LJ: Influence of multiple organ dysfunction syndrome on duration of critical illness and hospitalization. *Arch Surg* 131(12):1318–1323, 1996; discussion 1324.
6. Knaus WA, Draper EA, Wagner DP, et al: Prognosis in acute organ-system failure. *Ann Surg* 202(6):685–693, 1985.
7. Marshall JC, Cook DJ, Christou NV, et al: Multiple organ dysfunction score: a reliable descriptor of a complex clinical outcome. *Crit Care Med* 23(10):1638–1652, 1995.
8. Vincent JL, Moreno R, Takala J, et al: The SOFA (sepsis-related organ failure assessment) score to describe organ dysfunction/failure. On behalf of the Working Group on Sepsis-Related Problems of the European Society of Intensive Care Medicine. *Intensive Care Med* 22(7):707–710, 1996.
9. Le Gall JR, Klar J, Lemeshow S, et al: The logistic organ dysfunction system. A new way to assess organ dysfunction in the intensive care unit. ICU Scoring Group. *JAMA* 276(10):802–810, 1996.
10. Afessa B, Gajic O, Keegan MT: Severity of illness and organ failure assessment in adult intensive care units. *Crit Care Clin* 23(3):639–658, 2007.
11. Sauaia A, Moore EE, Johnson JL, et al: Validation of postinjury multiple organ failure scores. *Shock* 31(5):438–447, 2009.
12. Haq A, Patil S, Parcells AL, et al: The simplified acute physiology score III is superior to the simplified acute physiology score II and acute physiology and chronic health evaluation II in predicting surgical and ICU mortality in the "Oldest Old". *Curr Gerontol Geriatr Res* 2014:934852, 2014.
13. Oda S, Hirasawa H, Sugai T, et al: Cellular injury score for multiple organ failure severity scoring system. *J Trauma* 45(2):304–310, 1998; discussion 310–311.
14. Exarchopoulos T, Charitidou E, Dedeilias P, et al: Scoring systems for outcome prediction in a cardiac surgical intensive care unit: a comparative study. *Am J Crit Care* 24(4):327–334, 2015.
15. Mizock BA: The multiple organ dysfunction syndrome. *Dis Mon* 55(8):476–526, 2009.
16. Vogel JA, Newgard CD, Holmes JF, et al: Validation of the Denver Emergency Department Trauma Organ Failure Score to predict post-injury multiple organ failure. *J Am Coll Surg* 222(1):73–82, 2016.
17. Knaus WA, Draper EA, Wagner DP, et al: APACHE II: a severity of disease classification system. *Crit Care Med* 13(10):818–829, 1985.
18. Zimmerman JE, Kramer AA, McNair DS, et al: Acute Physiology and Chronic Health Evaluation (APACHE) IV: hospital mortality assessment for today's critically ill patients. *Crit Care Med* 34(5):1297–1310, 2006.
19. Vincent JL, Sakr Y, Sprung CL, et al: Sepsis in European intensive care units: results of the SOAP study. *Crit Care Med* 34(2):344–353, 2006.
20. Barie PS, Hydo LJ: Epidemiology of multiple organ dysfunction syndrome in critical surgical illness. *Surg Infect (Larchmt)* 1(3):173–185, 2000; discussion 185–186.
21. Ulvik A, Kvale R, Wentzel-Larsen T, et al: Multiple organ failure after trauma affects even long-term survival and functional status. *Crit Care* 11(5):R95, 2007.
22. Angus DC, Linde-Zwirble WT, Lidicker J, et al: Epidemiology of severe sepsis in the United States: analysis of incidence, outcome, and associated costs of care. *Crit Care Med* 29(7):1303–1310, 2001.
23. Barie PS, Hydo LJ, Pieracci FM, et al: Multiple organ dysfunction syndrome in critical surgical illness. *Surg Infect (Larchmt)* 10(5):369–377, 2009.
24. Rittirsch D, Flierl MA, Ward PA: Harmful molecular mechanisms in sepsis. *Nat Rev Immunol* 8(10):776–787, 2008.
25. Ward NS, Casserly B, Ayala A: The compensatory anti-inflammatory response syndrome (CARS) in critically ill patients. *Clin Chest Med* 29(4):617–625, viii, 2008.
26. Lenz A, Franklin GA, Cheadle WG: Systemic inflammation after trauma. *Injury* 38(12):1336–1345, 2007.
27. Tschoeke SK, Hellmuth M, Hostmann A, et al: The early second hit in trauma management augments the proinflammatory immune response to multiple injuries. *J Trauma* 62(6):1396–1403, 2007; discussion 1403–1404.
28. Rosenthal MD, Moore FA: Persistent inflammation, immunosuppression, and catabolism: evolution of multiple organ dysfunction. *Surg Infect (Larchmt)* 17(2):167–172, 2016.
29. Gentile LF, Cuenca AG, Efron PA: Persistent inflammation and immunosuppression: a common syndrome and new horizon for surgical intensive care. *J Trauma Acute Care Surg* 72(6):1491–1501, 2012.
30. Villar J, Maca-Meyer N, Perez-Mendez L, et al: Bench-to-bedside review: understanding genetic predisposition to sepsis. *Crit Care* 8(3):180–189, 2004.
31. Fry DE, Pearlstein L, Fulton RL, et al: Multiple system organ failure. The role of uncontrolled infection. *Arch Surg* 115(2):136–140, 1980.
32. Ciesla DJ, Moore EE, Johnson JL, et al: The role of the lung in postinjury multiple organ failure. *Surgery* 138(4):749–757, 2005; discussion 757–758.
33. Moore FA, Sauaia A, Moore EE, et al: Postinjury multiple organ failure: a bimodal phenomenon. *J Trauma* 40(4):501–510, 1996; discussion 510–512.
34. Ciesla DJ, Moore EE, Johnson JL, et al: Multiple organ dysfunction during resuscitation is not postinjury multiple organ failure. *Arch Surg* 139(6):590–594, 2004; discussion 594–595.
35. Russell JA, Singer J, Bernard GR, et al: Changing pattern of organ dysfunction in early human sepsis is related to mortality. *Crit Care Med* 28(10):3405–3411, 2000.

36. Barie PS, Hydo LJ, Shou J, et al: Decreasing magnitude of multiple organ dysfunction syndrome despite increasingly severe critical surgical illness: a 17-year longitudinal study. *J Trauma* 65(6):1227–1235, 2008.
37. Dellinger RP, Levy MM, Rhodes A, et al: Surviving sepsis campaign: international guidelines for management of severe sepsis and septic shock: 2012. *Crit Care Med* 41(2):580–637, 2013.
38. Rivers E, Nguyen B, Havstad S, et al: Early goal-directed therapy in the treatment of severe sepsis and septic shock. *N Engl J Med* 345(19):1368–1377, 2001.
39. Pope JV, Jones AE, Gaieski DF, et al: Emergency Medicine Shock Research Network (EMShockNet) Investigators. Multicenter study of central venous oxygen saturation ($ScvO_2$) as a predictor of mortality in patients with sepsis. *Ann Emerg Med* 55(1):40–46, 2010.
40. Levy B, Sadoune LO, Gelot AM, et al: Evolution of lactate/pyruvate and arterial ketone body ratios in the early course of catecholamine-treated septic shock. *Crit Care Med* 28(1):114–119, 2000.
41. Marshall JC, Christou NV, Meakins JL: The gastrointestinal tract. The "undrained abscess" of multiple organ failure. *Ann Surg* 218(2):111–119, 1993.
42. Silvestri L, van Saene HK, Zandstra DF et al: Impact of selective decontamination of the digestive tract on multiple organ dysfunction syndrome: systematic review of randomized controlled trials. *Crit Care Med* 38(5):1370–1376, 2010.
43. Napolitano LM, Kurek S, Luchette FA, et al: Clinical practice guideline: red blood cell transfusion in adult trauma and critical care. *Crit Care Med* 37(12):3124–3157, 2009.
44. Slutsky AS, Tremblay LN: Multiple system organ failure. Is mechanical ventilation a contributing factor? *Am J Respir Crit Care Med* 157(6 Pt 1):1721–1725, 1998.
45. Ventilation with lower tidal volumes as compared with traditional tidal volumes for acute lung injury and the acute respiratory distress syndrome. The acute respiratory distress syndrome network. *N Engl J Med* 342(18):1301–1308, 2000.
46. Sakr Y, Vincent JL, Reinhart K, et al: High tidal volume and positive fluid balance are associated with worse outcome in acute lung injury. *Chest* 128(5):3098–3108, 2005.
47. van den Berghe G, Wouters P, Weekers F, et al: Intensive insulin therapy in the critically ill patients. *N Engl J Med* 345(19):1359–1367, 2001.
48. Mesotten D, Van den Berghe G: Glycemic targets and approaches to management of the patient with critical illness. *Curr Diab Rep* 12(1):101–107, 2012.
49. Moore FA, Moore EE: The evolving rationale for early enteral nutrition based on paradigms of multiple organ failure: a personal journey. *Nutr Clin Pract* 24(3):297–304, 2009.
50. Alexander JW, MacMillan BG, Stinnett JD, et al: Beneficial effects of aggressive protein feeding in severely burned children. *Ann Surg* 192(4):505–517, 1980.
51. Artinian V, Krayem H, DiGiovine B: Effects of early enteral feeding on the outcome of critically ill mechanically ventilated medical patients. *Chest* 129(4):960–967, 2006.
52. Kreymann KG, Berger MM, Deutz NE, et al: ESPEN Guidelines on enteral nutrition: Intensive care. *Clin Nutr* 25(2):210–223, 2006.
53. Taylor BE, McClave SA, Martindale RG, et al: Guidelines for the provision and assessment of nutrition support therapy in the adult critically ill patient: Society of Critical Care Medicine (SCCM) and American Society for Parenteral and Enteral Nutrition (A.S.P.E.N.). *Crit Care Med* 44(2): 390–438, 2016.
54. Arabi YM, Aldawood AS, Haddad SH, et al: Permissive underfeeding or standard enteral feeding in critically ill adults. *N Engl J Med* 372(25):2398–2408, 2015.
55. Angstwurm MW, Engelmann L, Zimmermann T, et al: Selenium in Intensive Care (SIC): results of a prospective randomized, placebo-controlled, multiple-center study in patients with severe systemic inflammatory response syndrome, sepsis, and septic shock. *Crit Care Med* 35(1):118–126, 2007.
56. Chelkeba L, Ahmadi A, Abdollahi M, et al: The effect of parenteral selenium on outcomes of mechanically ventilated patients following sepsis: a prospective randomized clinical trial. *Ann Intensive Care* 5(1):29, 2015.
57. Ratanarat R, Brendolan A, Piccinni P, et al: Pulse high-volume haemofiltration for treatment of severe sepsis: effects on hemodynamics and survival. *Crit Care* 9(4):R294–R302, 2005.
58. Liu Y, Davari-Farid S, Arora P, et al: Early versus late initiation of renal replacement therapy in critically ill patients with acute kidney injury after cardiac surgery: a systematic review and meta-analysis. *J Cardiothorac Vasc Anesth* 28(3):557–563, 2014.
59. Martin CM, Hill AD, Burns K, et al: Characteristics and outcomes for critically ill patients with prolonged intensive care unit stays. *Crit Care Med* 33(9):1922–1927, 2005.
60. Ciesla DJ, Moore EE, Johnson JL, et al: A 12-year prospective study of postinjury multiple organ failure: has anything changed? *Arch Surg* 140(5):432–438, 2005; discussion 438–440.
61. Mayr VD, Dunser MW, Greil V, et al: Causes of death and determinants of outcome in critically ill patients. *Crit Care* 10(6):R154, 2006.

Chapter 41 ■ Traumatic Brain Injury

WILEY R. HALL • RAPHAEL A. CARANDANG

The CDC estimates that traumatic brain injury (TBI) results in over 2.5 million ER visits, nearly 300,000 hospitalizations, and over 50,000 deaths annually in the US. Up to 3 million people are living in the US with disabilities related to TBI [1]. Falls are the most common of the causes overall, often seen among the pediatric and elderly populations. Motor vehicle accidents follow and are the most common cause among those aged 14 to 35. The estimated annual financial burden is 3 billion dollars for initial hospitalization costs to 60 billion dollars overall [2–4].

TRAUMA BAY AND INITIAL CRITICAL CARE

Care of the TBI patient involves early stabilization and longitudinal care to halt deterioration and maximize recovery. Injury from TBI is commonly divided into two subtypes. Primary injury is dealt directly to the brain by the initial insult and can be modified only by prevention. Much of prehospital, emergency department, and ICU care has long been targeted at reducing secondary injury, which affects up to 91% of TBI patients [5]. Hypotension, hypoxia, hemorrhage, intracranial hypertension, cerebral edema, seizures, and metabolic derangements all contribute to secondary injury [6]. Studies of permissive hypotension, a strategy for hemorrhagic trauma, have excluded patients with TBI owing to the concerns over cerebral perfusion pressure [7]. Systolic blood pressure is maintained over 90 mmHg, and management to maintain adequate cerebral perfusion pressure (CPP) improves outcomes [8,9]. Corticosteroids are contraindicated for the management of brain edema related to TBI because they are associated with worse outcomes [10].

The mainstay of urgent neuroimaging remains computed tomography (CT). Although MRI is more sensitive for axonal injury, small hemorrhage, and ischemia, CT is rapid, readily available, and more sensitive for acute SAH [11].

Isotonic fluids remain the primary vehicle for volume resuscitation. Studies of hypertonic saline as resuscitation fluid have been equivocal; 7.5% saline solution and 500m Osm per L sodium lactate showed improved outcome, while a study using 7% saline solution revealed no benefit [11–13]. Hyponatremic or hypoosmotic fluids induce and exacerbate cerebral edema and are avoided during resuscitation and throughout the critical care phase of TBI, even in the presence of hypernatremia. 5% dextrose as a resuscitation fluid for non-brain injured children has been associated with the evolution of cerebral edema [14]. A rat model of TBI comparing ringers lactate and 5% dextrose infusions reported significantly increased mortality for animals treated with 5% dextrose [15].

Mannitol 1gm per kg IV is the first choice for measured or when elevated ICP is presumed. Preoperative high-dose mannitol, 1.4gm per kg IV, benefits patients requiring emergent surgery for subdural and temporal lobe hematomas [16,17]. Mannitol is infused through a 5-micron filter and must not be infused through a cooled catheter such as those used for targeted temperature management, owing to the risk of precipitation of mannitol out of solution. Hypertonic saline solutions including 23.4% saline may be used in place of mannitol during trauma resuscitation and may improve outcomes [18]. An advantage favoring hypertonic saline is that it acts as a volume expander, whereas mannitol acts as an osmotic diuretic, possibly reducing the effectiveness of volume resuscitation. However, 23.4% saline solution must be infused through a central venous catheter, and issues surrounding the storage of concentrated electrolytes in Emergency Departments raised by the Joint Commission have prevented 23.4% saline from competing effectively with mannitol for this role in many centers [19].

Seizures may increase intracranial pressure and may lead to secondary injury. Prophylaxis during the first 7 days after severe injury is standard of care, though this has not been shown to alter long-term mortality, or even the incidence of long-term epilepsy. Phenytoin is a common choice as it is available in enteral and IV formulations, and levetiracetam is popular because of its low incidence of interactions. Neither has been shown to be superior to the other [20].

Reversal of Anticoagulation

Reversal of anticoagulation must be performed promptly for TBI patients with ICH [21]. Among patients receiving vitamin K antagonists with International Normalized ratio (INR) over 1.4, vitamin K 10 mg IV should be given, conventionally followed on days 2 and 3 by 5 to 10 mg enterally [22]. Reversal of anticoagulation with four-factor prothrombin complex concentrate (PCC), dosed by weight, and INR is faster than and superior to plasma transfusion [23–25]. KCentra is a PCC FDA approved for warfarin reversal among patients with major bleeding or requiring urgent surgery. For patients with a history of heparin-induced thrombocytopenia in the past 90 days, plasma transfusion or factor VIIa dosing may be considered because KCentra contains a small amount of heparin.

The anticoagulant effects of the direct thrombin inhibitor dabigatran (Pradaxa) can be reversed by the FDA approved reversal agent idarucizumab, which binds and inactivates dabigatran. If idarucizumab is not available, KCentra, hemodialysis, and hemofiltration have been attempted [26].

Factor Xa inhibitors currently lack a reversal agent, though andexanet alfa is moving through the approval process and is expected to be available. KCentra has been reported as a possible reversal agent [26].

For patients receiving aspirin, platelet transfusions may be considered for patients requiring urgent neurosurgery [27]. Transfusion is not as useful for patients receiving GPIIB/IIIa inhibitors as the transfused platelets are inactivated [26], though salvage transfusion is often considered.

Surgical Therapies for TBI

Surgical hematoma evacuation is commonly performed acutely for subdural hematomas over 1 cm in width and epidural hematomas with significant mass effect or progression. Routine evacuation of parenchymal hemorrhages is not indicated, as violation of otherwise healthy or recoverable tissue may be required to access the hematoma. However, intracranial hypertension refractory to medical management may be an indication for resection of parenchymal hematomas [28,29].

Decompressive craniectomy has historically been viewed as a last resort for management of TBI with intracranial hypertension [29,30]. One complication of decompressive craniectomy is injury to the brain tissue and blood vessels, especially veins, at the edges of the craniotomy defect. Authors recommend removal of at least a 12-cm-diameter bone flap, and extension of the craniectomy to the temporal bone is also sometimes recommended [31,32]. A retrospective review of TBI patients treated with decompressive craniectomy found no outcome benefits compared to historical controls. For many patients, surgery was performed late in the ICU course, and the subgroup of patients who had earlier surgery did have better outcomes at 6 months compared to controls [28]. Analysis of a non-randomized series of patients with GCS ≤9 and a midline shift greater than the width of an extra axial hematoma who were considered for decompressive surgery revealed that the treated patients had worse GCS on admission, but more survived to discharge and more were discharged to home or skilled nursing than those of the non-surgical group [29]. The often cited DECRA study randomized patients prospectively to decompressive surgery or medical therapy. This study demonstrated harm in the treatment group, however was plagued by problems with randomization in that the treatment group had significantly more patients with unreactive pupils than the medical group, and the study had intended to exclude patients with unreactive pupils altogether [33].

Neurological Critical Care

Multimodality Monitoring

Neurological monitoring relevant to TBI is covered in depth in Chapter 31. Although the physical examination remains the gold standard for neurological monitoring, many patients with severe TBI require sedation and other therapies, which make surrogate monitoring mandatory. Although important for the reduction of the duration of mechanical ventilation and the prevention of VAP [34], interruption of sedation is contraindicated for patients with elevated ICP [35]. Elevated ICP, particularly when not responsive to therapy, is associated with worse outcomes [36]. The recent BEST-TRIP trial demonstrated no improvement of outcomes with a protocol driven by ICP over one guided by clinical observations [37,38]. However, ICP monitoring remains the standard of care where available and is supported by consensus statements including one to which BEST-TRIPs lead investigator was a contributor. Although brain edema may preclude the selection of an external ventricular drain (EVD) over a parenchymal ICP monitor, EVDs have the advantage of offering the ability to decrease ICP by draining CSF and are thus favored when feasible, especially when hydrocephalus is present [35]. EEG is indicated when the mental status is worse than anticipated given the known injuries, and continuous EEG is favored [35]. Poor brain tissue oxygen tension is a predictor of poor outcome, and treatment guided by brain tissue oximetry has been shown to improve outcomes [39,40], and even with the use of brain oximetry or metabolic monitoring, ICP monitoring is still required [35]. See Chapter 31 for more detail.

Treatment of Elevated Intracranial Pressure

For all patients with elevated intracranial pressure, maintenance of intravascular volume is important because it improves cerebral perfusion pressure. For patients with significant acidosis or those requiring high volumes of crystalloid, the substitution of isonatremic sodium acetate for sodium chloride may limit the development of hyperchloremic metabolic acidosis [41]. Adequate analgesia and anxiolysis can help maintain adequate ICP. Head elevation to 30 degrees above horizontal decreases intracranial pressure without sacrificing cerebral perfusion or oxygenation [42].

Mannitol

Mannitol has long been known to lower intracranial pressure [43,44]. Doses of 0.25 to 1.4 g per kg IV are commonly used every 3 to 8 hours [16,45–47]. Our center favors 1gm per kg, rounded to the nearest 25gms, every 6 hours, to allow approximately 5 half-lives between doses and to avoid the development of idiogenic osmoles, which may lead to tolerance of osmotherapy [48,49]. Acutely with rapid infusion, mannitol increases circulating volume, blood pressure, and cardiac output and decreases blood viscosity [50,51]. This may lead to decreased ICP via an increase in CBF and autoregulatory decrease of cerebral blood volume (CBV) [45]. Mannitol also acts as an osmotic diuretic, recruiting water from the interstitial space through the blood brain barrier, which is nearly impervious to mannitol. Mannitol has been shown to preferentially shrink brain tissue where the blood–brain barrier is intact, though it has been shown that midline shift does not increase with mannitol's use [52,53].

Mannitol may leak into damaged brain tissue, but has been shown to leave that tissue once it clears the bloodstream. Additionally, it does not accumulate in concentrations higher than those of plasma; thus, no reverse gradient exists to exacerbate cerebral edema [49,54,55]. Mannitol clearance from the bloodstream can be monitored my measuring the osmotic gap [56,57].

Hypertonic Saline

Hypertonic saline (HS) may be used to decrease intracranial pressure, and like mannitol, HS has hemodynamic effects in addition to its osmotic effects on cerebral edema [48,58–60]. The use of HS at concentrations varying from 3% infusions to 29.2% boluses has been shown to improve ICP both as a primary measure and when mannitol fails [41,58,61–63]. At our center, we use 15 to 30 mL boluses of 23.4% sodium chloride every 4 to 6 hours when mannitol fails to control ICP or when renal failure precludes the use of mannitol. Randomized trials comparing serial doses of mannitol to hypertonic saline are not conclusive. Loss of efficacy of ICP control when HS is used over several days time may be due to the formation of osmolytes, as persistent hypernatremia frequently develops.

The relationship between hypernatremia, renal function, and outcomes is a complex one. Only one study has directly examined the relationship between varying levels of hypernatremia and outcomes [64]. Though patients with more severe injuries were more likely to be hypernatremic, likely owing to more aggressive osmotherapy, there was an independent association between a finding of serum sodium over 160 mEq per L and mortality. Although it is well known that hypernatremia in the setting of hypovolemia is associated with renal failure [65], the safety of euvolemic hypernatremia is not known. It is also known that a rapid decrease of serum sodium may lead to cerebral edema among healthy patients, and the dangers of hypotonic fluid administration for patients and experimental models with cerebral edema have been described above. When significant hypernatremia develops among patients with cerebral edema, it may be safer to limit treatments which raise sodium while resisting treatments which directly lower it. Diabetes insipidis is an ominous sign among those with TBI [66]. Treatment with vasopressin or DDVAP to limit free water diuresis may be a safer way to combat hypernatremia in this setting than parenteral-free water administration.

Cerebral Perfusion Pressure and the Lund Concept

In contrast to purely ICP based management, the "Lund Concept" describes a strategy for lowering ICP based partially on decreasing CPP [67,68]. In this strategy, it is postulated that increases of MAP may exacerbate cerebral edema, especially when large amounts of crystalloid solutions are administered. MAP is lowered to decrease hydrostatic capillary pressure and ameliorate cerebral edema. Mannitol and vasopressors are generally avoided. CPP is tolerated as low as 50 mmHg. Multimodality monitoring, often including bedside microdialysis, is required to monitor the metabolic reaction of vulnerable tissue to decreased CPP.

Temperature Management

Hyperthermia increases the body's metabolic demand, worsens cognitive impairment, and has been associated with worse outcomes among multiple models of neurological insults [69]. Induced hypothermia has been shown to improve neurological outcomes after witnessed cardiac arrest [70,71]. Recent studies suggest a target temperature of 36°C is as effective as a target of 33degrees; however, this has not been studied for TBI [72]. Induced hypothermia has been shown to improve outcomes using animal models [71,73,74]. The first hour after injury was found to be critical. A series of large, multicenter trials, however, failed to show a benefit of prophylactic-induced hypothermia after TBI [75–77].

Still, Class I evidence shows that induced hypothermia lowers ICP [78]. Side effects include hyperglycemia, immunosuppression, hypovolemia, and electrolyte imbalances largely due to "cold diuresis" [71]. Rapid rewarming or overshoot may lead to rebound intracranial hypertension and impaired cerebral vasoreactivity [79]. Patients presenting with mild hypothermia after TBI should not be aggressively rewarmed [71]. Fever, defined as core body temperature over 38°C, affects up to 68% of TBI patients within 72 hours of admission and is associated with worse outcome [69]. Although much effort is spent in ICUs to reduce fever, and induction of hypothermia remains a hot topic in critical care literature, neither effort has been conclusively shown to improve outcomes after TBI.

Induced Coma

Pharmacologically induced coma may be an appropriate step taken when ICP and CPP cannot be managed by the above means [80,81]. Prophylactic administration of barbiturates does not improve outcomes [8]. Pentobarbital is the most common agent reported for this purpose and is postulated to lower ICP by reducing the cerebral metabolic rate of oxygen ($CMRO_2$). Pentobarbital has numerous side effects, including hypotension, cardiac depression, immune system suppression, and hypothermia. Close attention must be paid to the maintenance of adequate hemodynamics [81,82]. Coma is induced with a slow bolus 5 to 10 mg per kg of pentobarbital, followed by an infusion of 1 to 3 mg/kg/h. Although many centers check pentobarbital levels, continuous EEG monitoring provides a more useful measure of dose effect, with the goal being a reduction of ICP to acceptable levels and the induction of burst suppression on EEG [80]. Serum drug levels are of value when evaluating for CNS function, for example, when brain death is contemplated and the clearance of drug from the bloodstream must be confirmed. Propofol has also been described as an agent for ICP control. When used to achieve burst suppression, a 2mg per kg loading dose followed by an infusion of up to 200g/kg/h is required. Severe hypotension and propofol infusion syndrome are concerns when using high-dose propofol.

Systemic Critical Care

Mechanical Ventilator Management

Hypoxia and hypercarbia may exacerbate secondary injury and complicate ICP and CPP management [83]. The Brain Trauma Foundation recommends maintaining SpO_2 over 90% and PO_2 over 60 for TBI patients [8]. Advanced modes of mechanical ventilation and inotropic and/or vasopressor are frequently required to maintain CPP and adequate gas exchange. For some patients, hypoxia may be resistant to conventional ventilator settings, and increases in PEEP and FIO_2 may be required.

Concern has been raised over the effect of PEEP on ICP. Published data, however, reveal varying effects of PEEP on ICP. One theory posits that PEEP raises intrathoracic pressure, thus decreasing venous return to the chest and thus increasing the volume of venous blood inside the cranial vault, leading to a rise in ICP [84]. In reality, it is unclear to what extent changes of PEEP are transmitted into the thoracic cavity, much less into the vascular system where venous return could be affected, especially among patients with ARDS where the stiffness of the diseased lung may not transmit PEEP efficiently [85]. A series of TBI patients with ALI/ARDS reported that ICP was more tightly associated with PCO_2 than levels of PEEP [86]. For refractory hypoxia, prone positioning has been reported in several series. Although in some neurocritical care series raised ICP has been reported, in a dedicated series on TBI patients with ARDS prone positioning was associated with improved oxygenation without detrimental effects on ICP or CPP [87,88].

Ventilation of the TBI patient demands attention to systemic acid base balance and to secondary effects on cerebral blood flow. Therapeutic hyperventilation (HV) is the fastest way to lower ICP, causing rapid vasoconstriction of the cerebral arterial supply. Animal experiments and human observations reveal that HV causes a decrease in the partial pressure of oxygen in brain tissue ($PbtO_2$) [89,90], is now contraindicated during the acute phase of TBI, and is discouraged by most authorities [8,89]. Even for normal brain tissue, decreases of PCO_2 below 30mmHg resulted in decreased CBF and evidence of anaerobic metabolism [89]. Although evidence of harm with less aggressive HV is lacking, evidence for its benefit is absent. This intervention cannot be recommended with enthusiasm. If used when other measures fail, HV should be monitored with one of the markers for tissue stress, such as brain tissue oximetry or microdialysis [91].

Glucose Management

A 2001 multicenter trial revealed that tight glycemic control improves outcome in critical care populations [92]. This finding leads to a revolution of ICU glucose management, with many hospitals implementing ICU-based protocols targeting maximum serum glucoses levels from 110 to 140 mg per dL. More recent trials have questioned this result, prominently the NICE SUGAR trial, which revealed increased mortality of patients treated with a tight control protocol targeting serum glucose under108 mg per dL compared to a protocol targeting glucose under 180 mg per dL [93]. For the TBI and neurocritical care population, concerns have been raised over glucose delivery to regions of vulnerable brain tissue, which may already be at risk of poor perfusion owing to cerebral edema. A study using microdialysis to examine glucose delivery revealed significantly low brain glucose levels associated with signs of metabolic stress among patients treated with a tight glycemic control strategy [94]. A meta-analysis concluded while blood sugars over 200 mg per dL were likely harmful, overly tight glycemic control was also harmful and a blood sugar target of under 180mg per dL was suggested [95].

Nutrition and Metabolism

A thorough review of the literature regarding energy expenditure of TBI patients found that historically held beliefs regarding brain injured patients' elevated metabolic rates and nutritional needs are valid [96]. Moderate to severely injured TBI patients exhibited metabolic rates 96% to 132% of predicted baseline when sedated and 105% to 160% over base when awake. Another review documented some findings where hypermetabolism reached 200% of predicted baseline [97]. TBI patients are also catabolic, exhibiting a −3 to −16gm per day nitrogen balance. The resultant decrease of muscle mass and related immune function deficits may worsen outcomes [96]. Although the common practice is to prescribe nutrition targeted to exceed baseline predicted needs by 40%, these authors favored the use of indirect calorimetry to better target each patient's individual needs. Although upper GI intolerance is common early among those with TBI, placing patients at risk for aspiration pneumonia, some studies do show a trend to improved outcomes with the institution of early feeding [96]. No conclusive data exist to suggest favoring post-pyloric feeding to gastric feeding.

Prevention of Venous Thromboembolism

Pulmonary embolism is the 3rd leasing cause of death among patients surviving past day one of TBI [98]. Trials comparing early to late chemoprophylaxis are lacking. Low molecular weight heparin (LMWH) is superior to unfractionated heparin (UFH) for preventing venous thromboembolism among patients with polytrauma and spinal cord injury, but data regarding TBI patients are limited. Consensus guidelines support therapy with intermittent pneumatic compression systems within 24 hours of admission and chemoprophylaxis with LMWH or UFH starting 24 to 48 hours after admission or completion of surgery as long as there is no evidence of continued bleeding [99].

Specialty Injury Subtypes

Penetrating Brain Injury

High-energy missile trauma produces brain injury through multiple mechanisms. Brain tissue along the tract of the missile is injured directly. With high-energy projectiles, a wave of energy precedes the missile, and significant damage is delivered by a wave of cavitation, which follows in the wake of the projectile. This cavitation may reverberate through the cranium, reflecting off the inside surface of the dura and skull [100,101]. Contusions, intracranial hemorrhage, and subdural and epidural hemorrhage may result. Vascular injury is common when the path of injury crosses near vascular structures, and arterio-venous fistulas and pseudoaneurysms may develop [101]. Vasospasm may develop early or late in the ICU course. Critical care focuses on control of intracranial pressure using methods similar to those used for closed head injury. Surgical debridement is indicated for missile and bone fragments in non-eloquent areas of the brain only [102]. Historically, from 15% to 50% of wounds become infected and antibiotic prophylaxis is standard practice. There is no consensus on which antimicrobials are more appropriate; most surgeons favor cephalosporins, whereas some centers use combinations including cephalosporins, metronidazole, and vancomycin. Invasion of an open-air sinus by the injury raises the risk of infection and may warrant broader coverage [101].

Blast Related Trauma

Experience in Iraq, Afghanistan, and to an extent Lebanon has revealed a previously poorly recognized variant of TBI: that delivered by blast injury [103–105]. With current protective armor, many warfighters survive previously fatal battlefield injuries [104,106]. Combatants and civilians exposed to high-energy blast trauma suffer brain injuries, which may have features seen in both closed and penetrating TBI [104]. Pseudoaneurysms and vasospasm were commonly detected among a cohort of [103] patients imaged either because of injury known to be near or involving cerebral vasculature or because of unexplained deterioration of neurological function. The prevalence of vasospasm and pseudoaneurysm in the general blast TBI population was not investigated. Vasospasm was been recognized as early as 48 hours after blast TBI and may occur as late as 10 to 14 days after injury. Warfighters returning to rehabilitation hospitals with severe injuries did demonstrate recoverability even in the worst cases; up to 50% of patients presenting to stateside rehabilitation with GCS score 3 to 5 eventually recovered to a Glasgow Outcome Scale (GOS) score ≥3 at 1- to 2-year follow-up [107].

Associated Vascular Injuries

Both blunt and penetrating trauma to the head and neck may induce the formation of aneurysms. Intervention is indicated when aneurysms are accessible to surgical or endovascular repair [108,109]. Dissections of the carotid and vertebral arteries may occur among TBI patients, especially when trauma also includes the cervical spine. Dissections may lead to ischemic strokes by either leading to occlusion of the involved vessel or by serving as an embolic source [108,110]. Treatment for dissections includes avoidance of hypertension and mitigation of embolic risk. Both antiplatelet drugs and heparin have significant hemorrhagic risks for patients with concomitant brain injury [111]. In extreme cases, surgical or endovascular occlusion of the affected vessel may be the safest choice to limit embolic risk [108,112].

Long-Term Outcomes

Prediction of outcomes after TBI is difficult due to the heterogeneity of the different injury subtypes, varying levels of concomitant non-neurological injuries, and medical complications of critical care. Bedside physician estimates of prognosis are often either overly pessimistic or unrealistically optimistic. When studied, physicians have reported that they feel their predictions are often inaccurate [113]. The need for better prognostication tools, as well as aids for shared decision making, has been noted by the CDC as recently as 2015 and is the subject of ongoing research [114,115]. Treatment by a specialized neurocritical care team is associated with decreased hospital costs, decreased length of stay, and improved outcomes at 6 months [116,117].

Findings of bilaterally fixed pupils confer a 70% to 90% likelihood of death or persistent vegetative state as the final outcome [11]. Absent bilateral Somatosensory Evoked Potentials (SEP) early in the ICU course predict death, whereas initially normal bilateral readings predict good outcome. SEPs may fluctuate over the course of each day; thus, single recordings are less informative than serial examinations, and improvement within the first 10 days predicts recovery [118,119]. Serial physical examinations combined with aggressive resuscitation for 72 hours are recommended by consensus guidelines [120,121].

References

1. Centers for Disease Control and Prevention. Report to Congress on Traumatic Brain Injury in the United States: Epidemiology and Rehabilitation. National Center for Injury Prevention and Control; Division of Unintentional Injury Prevention. Atlanta, GA, 2015.
2. McGarry LJ, Thompson D, Millham FH, et al: Outcomes and costs of acute treatment of traumatic brain injury. *J Trauma* 53(6):1152–1159, 2002.
3. Maas AI, Stocchetti N, Bullock R: Moderate and severe traumatic brain injury in adults. *Lancet Neurol* 7(8):728–741, 2008.
4. Maas AI, Marmarou A, Murray GD, et al: Prognosis and clinical trial design in traumatic brain injury: the IMPACT study. *J Neurotrauma* 24(2):232–238, 2007.
5. Jones PA, Andrews PJ, Midgley S, et al: Measuring the burden of secondary insults in head-injured patients during intensive care. *J Neurosurg Anesthesiol* 6(1):4–14, 1994.
6. Tisdall MM, Smith M: Multimodal monitoring in traumatic brain injury: current status and future directions. *Br J Anaesth* 99(1):61–67, 2007.
7. Alsawadi A: The clinical effectiveness of permissive hypotension in blunt abdominal trauma with hemorrhagic shock but without head or spine injuries or burns: a systematic review. *Open Access Emerg Med* 4:21–29, 2012.
8. Brain Trauma Foundation, American Association of Neurological Surgeons, Congress of Neurological Surgeons. Guidelines for the management of severe traumatic brain injury. *J Neurotrauma* 24(Suppl 1):S1–106, 2007.
9. Hammell CL, Henning JD: Prehospital management of severe traumatic brain injury. *BMJ* 338:b1683, 2009. Available from: http://dx.doi.org/10.1136/bmj.b1683.
10. Roberts I, Yates D, Sandercock P, et al: Effect of intravenous corticosteroids on death within 14 days in 10008 adults with clinically significant head injury (MRC CRASH trial): randomised placebo-controlled trial. *Lancet* 364(9442):1321–1328, 2004.
11. Moppett IK: Traumatic brain injury: assessment, resuscitation and early management. *Br J Anaesth* 99(1):18–31, 2007.
12. Vassar MJ, Fischer RP, O'Brien PE, et al: A multicenter trial for resuscitation of injured patients with 7.5% sodium chloride. The effect of added dextran 70. The multicenter group for the study of hypertonic saline in trauma patients. *Arch Surg* 128(9):1003–1011; discussion 1011–1013, 1993.
13. Shackford SR, Zhuang J, Schmoker J: Intravenous fluid tonicity: effect on intracranial pressure, cerebral blood flow, and cerebral oxygen delivery in focal brain injury. *J Neurosurg* 76(1):91–98, 1992.
14. Jackson J, Bolte RG: Risks of intravenous administration of hypotonic fluids for pediatric patients in ED and prehospital settings: let's remove the handle from the pump. *Am J Emerg Med* 18(3):269–270, 2000.
15. Feldman Z, Zachari S, Reichenthal E, et al: Brain edema and neurological status with rapid infusion of lactated ringer's or 5% dextrose solution following head trauma. *J Neurosurg* 83(6):1060–1066, 1995.
16. Cruz J, Minoja G, Okuchi K: Major clinical and physiological benefits of early high doses of mannitol for intraparenchymal temporal lobe hemorrhages with abnormal pupillary widening: a randomized trial. *Neurosurgery* 51(3):628–637; discussion 637–638, 2002.
17. Cruz J: Current international trends in severe acute brain trauma. *Arq Neuropsiquiatr* 58(3A):642–647, 2000.
18. Pascual JL, Maloney-Wilensky E, Reilly PM, et al: Resuscitation of hypotensive head-injured patients: is hypertonic saline the answer? *Am Surg* 74(3):253–259, 2008.
19. Wanzer LJ: Implementing national patient safety goal 3. *AORN J* 82(3):471, 473–474, 2005.
20. Jones KE, Puccio AM, Harshman KJ, et al: Levetiracetam versus phenytoin for seizure prophylaxis in severe traumatic brain injury. *Neurosurg Focus* 25(4):E3, 2008.
21. Veshchev I, Elran H, Salame K: Recombinant coagulation factor VIIa for rapid preoperative correction of warfarin-related coagulopathy in patients with acute subdural hematoma. *Med Sci Monit* 8(12):CS98–CS100, 2002.
22. Hung A, Singh S, Tait RC: A prospective randomized study to determine the optimal dose of intravenous vitamin K in reversal of over-warfarinization. *Br J Haematol* 109:537–539, 2000.
23. Frontera JA, Gordon E, Zach V, et al: Reversal of coagulopathy using prothrombin complex concentrates is associated with improved outcome compared to fresh frozen plasma in warfarin-associated intracranial hemorrhage. *Neurocrit Care* 21:397–406, 2014.
24. Woo CH, Patel N, Conell C, et al: Rapid warfarin reversal in the setting of intracranial hemorrhage: a comparison of plasma, recombinant activated factor VII, and prothrombin complex concentrate. *World Neurosurg* 81:110–115, 2014.
25. Sarode R, Milling TJ Jr, Refaai MA, et al: Efficacy and safety of a 4-factor prothrombin complex concentrate in patients on vitamin K antagonists presenting with major bleeding: a randomized, plasma controlled, phase IIIb study. *Circulation* 128:1234–1243, 2013.
26. Frontera JA, Lewin JJ 3rd, Rabinstein AA, et al: Guideline for Reversal of Antithrombotics in Intracranial Hemorrhage: A Statement for Healthcare Professionals from the Neurocritical Care Society and Society of Critical Care Medicine. *Neurocrit Care* 24(1):6–46, 2016.
27. Li X, Sun Z, Zhao W, et al: Effect of acetylsalicylic acid usage and platelet transfusion on postoperative hemorrhage and activities of daily living in patients with acute intracerebral hemorrhage. *J Neurosurg* 118:94–103, 2013.
28. Munch E, Horn P, Schurer L, et al: Management of severe traumatic brain injury by decompressive craniectomy. *Neurosurgery* 47(2):315–322; discussion 322–323, 2000.
29. Coplin WM, Cullen NK, Policherla PN, et al: Safety and feasibility of craniectomy with duraplasty as the initial surgical intervention for severe traumatic brain injury. *J Trauma* 50(6):1050–1059, 2001.
30. Gunnarsson T, Fehlings MG: Acute neurosurgical management of traumatic brain injury and spinal cord injury. *Curr Opin Neurol* 16(6):717–723, 2003.
31. Cooper DJ, Rosenfeld JV, Murray L, et al: Early decompressive craniectomy for patients with severe traumatic brain injury and refractory intracranial hypertension – a pilot randomized trial. *J Crit Care* 23(3):387–393, 2008.
32. Wagner S, Schnippering H, Aschoff A, et al: Suboptimum hemicraniectomy as a cause of additional cerebral lesions in patients with malignant infarction of the middle cerebral artery. *J Neurosurg* 94(5):693–696, 2001.
33. Cooper DJ, Rosenfeld JV, Murray L, et al: Decompressive craniectomy in diffuse traumatic brain injury. *N Engl J Med* 364:1493–1502, 2011.
34. Girard TD, Kress JP, Fuchs BD, et al: Efficacy and safety of a paired sedation and ventilator weaning protocol for mechanically ventilated patients in intensive care (Awakening and breathing controlled trial): a randomised controlled trial. *Lancet* 371:126–134, 2008.
35. Le Roux P, Menon DK, Citerio G, et al: Consensus Summary Statement of the international Multidisciplinary Consensus conference on Multimodality Monitoring in Neurocritical Care. A statement of healthcare professionals from the Neurocritical Care Society and the European Society of Intensive Care Medicine. *Neurocrit Care* 21(Suppl 2):S297–S361, 2014.
36. Badri S, Chen J, Barber J, et al: Mortality and long-term functional outcome associated with intracranial pressure after traumatic brain injury. *Intensive Care Med* 38(11):1800–1809, 2012.
37. Chesnut RM, Temkin N, Carney N, et al: A trial of intracranial-pressure monitoring in traumatic brain injury. *N Engl J Med* 367(26):2471–2481, 2012.
38. Chesnut RM: Intracranial pressure monitoring: headstone or a new head start. The BEST TRIP trial in perspective. *Intensive Care Med* 39(4):771–774, 2013.
39. Oddo M, Levine J, Mackenzie L, et al: brain hypoxia is associated with short-tem outcome after severe traumatic brain injury independently of intracranial hypertension and low cerebral perfusion pressure. *Neurosurgery* 69(5):1037–1045, 2011.
40. Brain Tissue Oxygen Monitoring in Traumatic Brain Injury, BOSST 2. NCT 00974259. www.clinicaltrials.gov.
41. Qureshi AI, Suarez JI, Bhardwaj A, et al: Use of hypertonic (3%) saline/acetate infusion in the treatment of cerebral edema: effect on intracranial pressure and lateral displacement of the brain. *Crit Care Med* 26(3):440–446, 1998.
42. Ng I, Lim J, Wong HB: Effects of head posture on cerebral hemodynamics: its influences on intracranial pressure, cerebral perfusion pressure, and cerebral oxygenation. *Neurosurgery* 54(3):593–597; discussion 598, 2004.

43. Allen CH, Ward JD: An evidence-based approach to management of increased intracranial pressure. *Crit Care Clin* 14(3):485–495, 1998.
44. McGraw CP, Howard G: Effect of mannitol on increased intracranial pressure. *Neurosurgery* 13(3):269–271, 1983.
45. Diringer MN, Zazulia AR: Osmotic therapy: fact and fiction. *Neurocrit Care* 1(2):219–233, 2004.
46. Wakai A, Roberts I, Schierhout G: Mannitol for acute traumatic brain injury [see comment][update of cochrane database syst rev. 2005;(4):CD001049; PMID: 16235278]. *Cochrane Database Syst Rev* (1):001049, 2007.
47. Wakai A, Roberts I, Schierhout G: Mannitol for acute traumatic brain injury [update in cochrane database syst rev. 2007;(1):CD001049; PMID: 17253453] [update of cochrane database syst rev. 2003;(2):CD001049; PMID: 12804397]. *Cochrane Database Syst Rev* (4):001049, 2005.
48. Doyle JA, Davis DP, Hoyt DB: The use of hypertonic saline in the treatment of traumatic brain injury. *J Trauma* 50(2):367–383, 2001.
49. Rudehill A, Gordon E, Ohman G, et al: Pharmacokinetics and effects of mannitol on hemodynamics, blood and cerebrospinal fluid electrolytes, and osmolality during intracranial surgery. *J Neurosurg Anesthesiol* 5(1):4–12, 1993.
50. Wallasch TM: The value of transcranial doppler sonography in neurosurgery. *Neurochirurgia (Stuttg)* 33(Suppl 1):58–60, 1990.
51. Burke AM, Quest DO, Chien S, et al: The effects of mannitol on blood viscosity. *J Neurosurg* 55(4):550–553, 1981.
52. Manno EM, Adams RE, Derdeyn CP, et al: The effects of mannitol on cerebral edema after large hemispheric cerebral infarct. *Neurology* 52(3):583–587, 1999.
53. Videen TO, Zazulia AR, Manno EM, et al: Mannitol bolus preferentially shrinks non-infarcted brain in patients with ischemic stroke. *Neurology* 57(11):2120–2122, 2001.
54. Maioriello AV, Chaljub G, Nauta HJ, et al: Chemical shift imaging of mannitol in acute cerebral ischemia. Case report. *J Neurosurg* 97(3):687–691, 2002.
55. Wise BL, Perkins RK, Stevenson E, et al: Penetration of C14-Labeled mannitol from serum into cerebrospinal fluid and brain. *Exp Neurol* 10:264–270, 1964.
56. Garcia-Morales EJ, Cariappa R, Parvin CA, et al: Osmole gap in neurologic-neurosurgical intensive care unit: its normal value, calculation, and relationship with mannitol serum concentrations. *Crit Care Med* 32(4):986–991, 2004.
57. Worthley LI, Guerin M, Pain RW: For calculating osmolality, the simplest formula is the best. *Anaesth Intensive Care* 15(2):199–202, 1987.
58. Hartl R, Ghajar J, Hochleuthner H, et al: Hypertonic/hyperoncotic saline reliably reduces ICP in severely head-injured patients with intracranial hypertension. *Acta Neurochir Suppl* 70:126–129, 1997.
59. Hijiya N, Horiuchi K, Asakura T: Morphology of sickle cells produced in solutions of varying osmolarities. *J Lab Clin Med* 117(1):60–66, 1991.
60. Shackford SR, Schmoker JD, Zhuang J: The effect of hypertonic resuscitation on pial arteriolar tone after brain injury and shock. *J Trauma* 37(6):899–908, 1994.
61. Horn P, Munch E, Vajkoczy P, et al: Hypertonic saline solution for control of elevated intracranial pressure in patients with exhausted response to mannitol and barbiturates. *Neurol Res* 21(8):758–764, 1999.
62. Worthley LI, Cooper DJ, Jones N: Treatment of resistant intracranial hypertension with hypertonic saline. Report of two cases. *J Neurosurg* 68(3):478–481, 1988.
63. Oddo M, Levine J, Frangos S, et al: Effect of Mannitol and hypertonic saline on cerebral oxygenation in patients with severe traumatic brain injury and refractory intracranial hypertension. *J Neurol Neurosurg Psychiatry* 80(8):916–920, 2009.
64. Aiyagari V, Deibert E, Diringer MN: Hypernatremia in the neurologic intensive care unit: How high is too high? *J Crit Care* 21(2):163–172, 2006.
65. Lima EQ, Aguiar FC, Barbosa DM, et al: Severe hypernatraemia (221 mEq/l), rhabdomyolysis and acute renal failure after cerebral aneurysm surgery. *Nephrol Dial Transplant* 19(8):2126–2129.
66. Bahloul M, Chelly H, Ben Hmida M, et al: Prognosis of traumatic head injury in south tunisia: a multivariate analysis of 437 cases. *J Trauma* 57(2):255–261, 2004.
67. Grande PO: The "lund concept" for the treatment of severe head trauma – physiological principles and clinical application. *Intensive Care Med* 32(10):1475–1484, 2006.
68. Nordstrom CH: Assessment of critical thresholds for cerebral perfusion pressure by performing bedside monitoring of cerebral energy metabolism. *Neurosurg Focus* 15(6):E5, 2003.
69. Aiyagari V, Diringer MN: Fever control and its impact on outcomes: what is the evidence? *J Neurol Sci* 261(1–2):39–46, 2007.
70. Hypothermia after Cardiac Arrest Study Group: Mild therapeutic hypothermia to improve the neurologic outcome after cardiac arrest. *N Engl J Med* 346(8):549–556.
71. Polderman KH: Induced hypothermia and fever control for prevention and treatment of neurological injuries.[see comment]. *Lancet* 371(9628):1955–1969, 2008.
72. Nielsen N, Wetterslev J, Cronberg T, et al: Targeted temperature management at 33°C versus 36°C after cardiac arrest. *N Engl J Med* 369:2192–2206, 2013.
73. Mcilvoy LH: The effect of hypothermia and hyperthermia on acute brain injury. *AACN Clin Issues* 16(4):488–500, 2005.
74. Povlishock JT: Pathophysiology of neural injury: therapeutic opportunities and challenges. *Clin Neurosurg* 46:113–126, 2000.
75. Clifton GL, Miller ER, Choi SC, et al: Lack of effect of induction of hypothermia after acute brain injury. *N Engl J Med* 344(8):556–563, 2001.
76. Clifton GL, Choi SC, Miller ER, et al: Intercenter variance in clinical trials of head trauma – experience of the national acute brain injury study: hypothermia. *J Neurosurg* 95(5):751–755, 2001.
77. Clifton GL, Drever P, Valadka A, et al: Multicenter trial of early hypothermia in severe brain injury. *J Neurotrauma* 26(3):393–397, 2009.
78. Marion D, Bullock MR: Current and future role of therapeutic hypothermia. *J Neurotrauma* 26(3):455–467, 2009.
79. Povlishock JT, Wei EP: Posthypothermic rewarming considerations following traumatic brain injury. *J Neurotrauma* 26(3):333–340, 2009.
80. Ling GS, Marshall SA: Management of traumatic brain injury in the intensive care unit. *Neurol Clin* 26(2):409–426, 2008.
81. Tang ME, Lobel DA: Severe traumatic brain injury: maximizing outcomes. *Mt Sinai J Med* 76(2):119–128, 2009.
82. Pickard JD, Czosnyka M: Management of raised intracranial pressure. *J Neurol Neurosurg Psychiatry* 56(8):845–858, 1993.
83. Oddo M, Nduom E, Frangos S, et al: Acute lung injury is an independent risk factor for brain hypoxia after severe traumatic brain injury. *Neurosurgery* 67(2):338–344, 2010.
84. Stevens RD, Lazaridis C, Chalela JA: The role of mechanical ventilation in acute brain injury. *Neurol Clin* 26(2):543–563, 2008.
85. Luecke T, Pelosi P: Clinical review: positive end-expiratory pressure and cardiac output. *Crit Care* 9(6):607–621, 2005.
86. Mascia L, Grasso S, Fiore T, et al: Cerebro-pulmonary interactions during the application of low levels of positive end-expiratory pressure. *Intensive Care Med* 31(3):373–379, 2005.
87. Thelandersson A, Cider A, Nellgard B: Prone position in mechanically ventilated patients with reduced intracranial compliance. *Acta Anaesthesiol Scand* 50(8):937–941, 2006.
88. Reinprecht A, Greher M, Wolfsberger S, et al: Prone position in subarachnoid hemorrhage patients with acute respiratory distress syndrome: effects on cerebral tissue oxygenation and intracranial pressure. *Crit Care Med* 31(6):1831–1838, 2003.
89. Clausen T, Scharf A, Menzel M, et al: Influence of moderate and profound hyperventilation on cerebral blood flow, oxygenation and metabolism. *Brain Res* 1019(1–2):113–123, 2004.
90. Manley GT, Pitts LH, Morabito D, et al: Brain tissue oxygenation during hemorrhagic shock, resuscitation, and alterations in ventilation. *J Trauma* 46(2):261–267, 1999.
91. Stocchetti N, Maas AI, Chieregato A, et al: Hyperventilation in head injury: a review. *Chest* 127(5):1812–1827, 2005.
92. van den Berghe G, Wouters P, Weekers F, et al: Intensive insulin therapy in the critically ill patients. *N Engl J Med* 345(19):1359–1367, 2001.
93. NICE-SUGAR Study Investigators, Finfer S, Chittock DR, Su SY, et al: Intensive versus conventional glucose control in critically ill patients. *N Engl J Med* 360(13):1283–1297, 2009.
94. Vespa P, Boonyaputthikul R, McArthur DL, et al: Intensive insulin therapy reduces microdialysis glucose values without altering glucose utilization or improving the lactate/pyruvate ratio after traumatic brain injury. *Crit Care Med* 34(3):850–856, 2006.
95. Kramer AH, Roberts DJ, Zygun DA: Optimal glycemic control in neurocritical care patients: a systematic review and meta-analysis. *Crit Care* 16(5):R203, 2012.
96. Krakau K, Omne-Ponten M, Karlsson T, et al: Metabolism and nutrition in patients with moderate and severe traumatic brain injury: a systematic review. *Brain Inj* 20(4):345–367, 2006.
97. Foley N, Marshall S, Pikul J, et al: Hypermetabolism following moderate to severe traumatic acute brain injury: a systematic review. *J Neurotrauma* 25(12):1415–1431, 2008.
98. Geerts WH, Bergqvist D, Pineo GF, et al: Prevention of venous thromboembolism: American College of Chest Physicians evidence-based clinical practice guidelines (8th Edition). *Chest* 133(6 Suppl):381S–453S, 2008.
99. Nyquist P, Bautista C, Jichici D, et al: Prophylaxis of venous thrombosis in neurocritical care patients: an evidence-based guideline: a statement for healthcare professionals from the neurocritical care society. *Neurocrit Care* 24(1):47–60, 2016.
100. Oehmichen M, Meissner C, Konig HG, et al: Gunshot injuries to the head and brain caused by low-velocity handguns and rifles. a review. *Forensic Sci Int* 146(2–3):111–120, 2004.
101. Esposito DP, Walker JB: Contemporary management of penetrating brain injury. *Neurosurg Q* 19(4):249–254, 2009.
102. Aarabi B, Alden TD, Chesnut RM: Guidelines for the management of penetrating brain injury. *J Trauma* 51:s1–s86, 2001.
103. Armonda RA, Bell RS, Vo AH, et al: Wartime traumatic cerebral vasospasm: recent review of combat casualties. *Neurosurgery* 59(6):1215–1225; discussion 1225, 2006.
104. Ling G, Bandak F, Armonda R, et al: Explosive blast neurotrauma. *J Neurotrauma* 26(6):815–825, 2009.
105. Levi L, Borovich B, Guilburd JN, et al: Wartime neurosurgical experience in lebanon, 1982-85. II: closed craniocerebral injuries. *Isr J Med Sci* 26(10):555–558, 1990.
106. Champion HR, Holcomb JB, Young LA: Injuries from explosions: physics, biophysics, pathology, and required research focus. *J Trauma* 66(5):1468–1477; discussion 1477, 2009.
107. Bell RS, Vo AH, Neal CJ, et al: Military traumatic brain and spinal column injury: a 5-year study of the impact blast and other military grade weaponry on the central nervous system. *J Trauma* 66(4):S104–S111, 2009.
108. Guyot LL, Kazmierczak CD, Diaz FG: Vascular injury in neurotrauma. *Neurol Res* 23(2–3):291–296, 2001.
109. Halbach VV, Higashida RT, Dowd CF, et al: Endovascular treatment of vertebral artery dissections and pseudoaneurysms. *J Neurosurg* 79(2):183–191, 1993.

110. Detante O, Colle F, Vu P, et al: Pontine infarct after fracture of the skull base. *Rev Neurol (Paris)* 159(3):326–328, 2003.
111. Marion DW: Complications of head injury and their therapy. *Neurosurg Clin N Am* 2(2):411–424, 1991.
112. Matsuura D, Inatomi Y, Saeda H, et al: Traumatic extracranial vertebral artery dissection treated with coil embolization – a case report. *Rinsho Shinkeigaku* 45(4):298–303, 2005.
113. Perel P, Edwards P, Wentz R, et al: Systematic review of prognostic models in traumatic brain injury. *BMC Med Inform Decis Mak* 6:38, 2006.
114. Cai X, Robinson J, Muehlschlegel S, et al: Patient preferences and surrogate decision making in neuroscience intensive care units. *Neurocrit Care* 23(1):131–141, 2015.
115. Muehlschlegel S, Shutter L, Col N, et al: Decision aids and shared decision-making in neurocritical care: an unmet need in our NeuroICUs. *Neurocrit Care* 23(1):127–130, 2015.
116. Patel HC, Menon DK, Tebbs S, et al: Specialist neurocritical care and outcome from head injury. *Intensive Care Med* 28(5):547–553, 2002.
117. Suarez JI, Zaidat OO, Suri MF, et al: Length of stay and mortality in neurocritically ill patients: impact of a specialized neurocritical care team. *Crit Care Med* 32(11):2311–2317, 2004.
118. Amantini A, Amadori A, Fossi S: Evoked potentials in the ICU. *Eur J Anaesthesiol Suppl* 42:196–202, 2008.
119. Claassen J, Hansen HC: Early recovery after closed traumatic head injury: somatosensory evoked potentials and clinical findings. *Crit Care Med* 29(3):494–502, 2001.
120. Izzy S, Compton R, Carandang R, et al: Self-fulfilling prophecies through withdrawal of care: do they exist in traumatic brain injury, too? *Neurocrit Care* 19(3):347–363, 2013.
121. Souter MJ, Blissitt PA, Blosser S, et al: Recommendations for the critical care management of devastating brain injury: prognostication, psychological, and ethical management. *Neurocrit Care* 23(1):4–13, 2015.

Chapter 42 ■ Spinal Cord Trauma

HANBING ZHOU • CHRISTIAN P. DIPAOLA

INTRODUCTION

The incidence of traumatic spinal cord injury (SCI) is approximately 40 SCIs per million persons per year in the United States [1]. Most traumatic spinal cord trauma (80.6%) occurs in males and most cases are among Whites (66%), followed by African Americans (26.2%) and Hispanics (8.3%). There has been an increase in the average age of injury since the 1970s from 28.7 years to 41 years. This is owing to an increase in people older than 65 years in the general population and a decrease in childhood trauma [1]. Traumatic SCI in the United States is reported to occur by motor vehicle accidents (47%), falls (23%), personal violence (14%), sports injuries (9%), and other sources of trauma (7%) [1].

Cervical injuries (C1–C7) account for approximately 55% of all traumatic SCIs. In the thoracolumbar spine, the most common location of fractures is between T12 and L2, with SCI in 10% to 25% of these fractures [2]. Thoracic fracture patients with less severe neurologic deficits have more favorable prognosis in the recovery of overall general health status compared to those with more significant neurologic deficits [3].

The trauma surgeon works as a part of a multidisciplinary team. A high degree of suspicion for spinal column injury with neurologic impairment must be maintained upon evaluation of most trauma patients. As the trauma team leader, he or she must be able to appropriately identify the pertinent history, examine the patient, provisionally stabilize the patient and the spine, and order appropriate imaging to identify or rule out injuries that may require orthopedic or neurosurgical consultation.

In order to execute these key fundamentals, a surgeon must understand the relevant anatomy, injury mechanisms, injury patterns, pathophysiology, and associated physical findings. Familiarity with "first responder" and in-hospital provisional spinal stabilization methods, patient resuscitation measures, and monitoring is the key to proper treatment.

ANATOMY

Spinal Column

The normal spinal column consists of 33 vertebrae, including 7 cervical, 12 thoracic, 5 lumbar, 5 fused sacral, and 4 fused coccygeal vertebrae. When anatomy is normal, the cervical and lumbar spines are lordotic, and the thoracic and sacral spines are kyphotic. These curvatures help to balance the spine and evenly distribute forces.

C1, which is also called the atlas, has neither a vertebral body nor a spinous process (Fig. 42.1). It is a ring-like structure with anterior and posterior arches separated by lateral masses on each side. It has two superior concave facets that articulate with the occipital condyles, accounting for approximately 50% of the neck flexion and extension [4].

C2, which is also called the axis, has an odontoid process (dens) and vertebral body (Fig. 42.1). It articulates with C1 (atlanto-axial) and accounts for 50% of cervical rotation. There is a vascular watershed area between the apex and base of the C2, and this limited blood supply is thought to affect healing in Type II odontoid fractures. The dens articulates with the posterior aspect of the anterior ring of C1 and is stabilized by the transverse ligament. There is no intervertebral disc at either the atlanto-occipital or the C1–C2 joints.

C1–C7 vertebrae typically have a transverse foramen, and the vertebral artery travels through the transverse foramen of C1–C6 in the majority of individuals. C7 has a prominent spinous process and is a useful landmark during physical examination.

In the thoracic spine, the articulations with the ribs lead to increased rigidity. Therefore, more force is required to produce a fracture in the thoracic region than the cervical or lumbar region.

The cervicothoracic junction represents a region that transitions from the fairly mobile cervical spine to the fairly rigid thoracic spine. Furthermore, it represents a transition from the lordotic cervical spine to the kyphotic thoracic spine. Biomechanically, this construct creates significant stress on the cervicothoracic junction. Disruptions of this anatomical region by trauma or tumor can lead to significant instability. Similarly, at the thoracolumbar junction, the vertebral column transitions from a relatively stiff construct in the thoracic spine to a more flexible construct. This transition point, especially T11–L2, acts as a zone of stress concentration and is more susceptible to injury than other adjacent portions of the spine.

Spinal Cord

The spinal cord is a tubular nervous tissue that extends from the brainstem and typically terminates as the conus medullaris

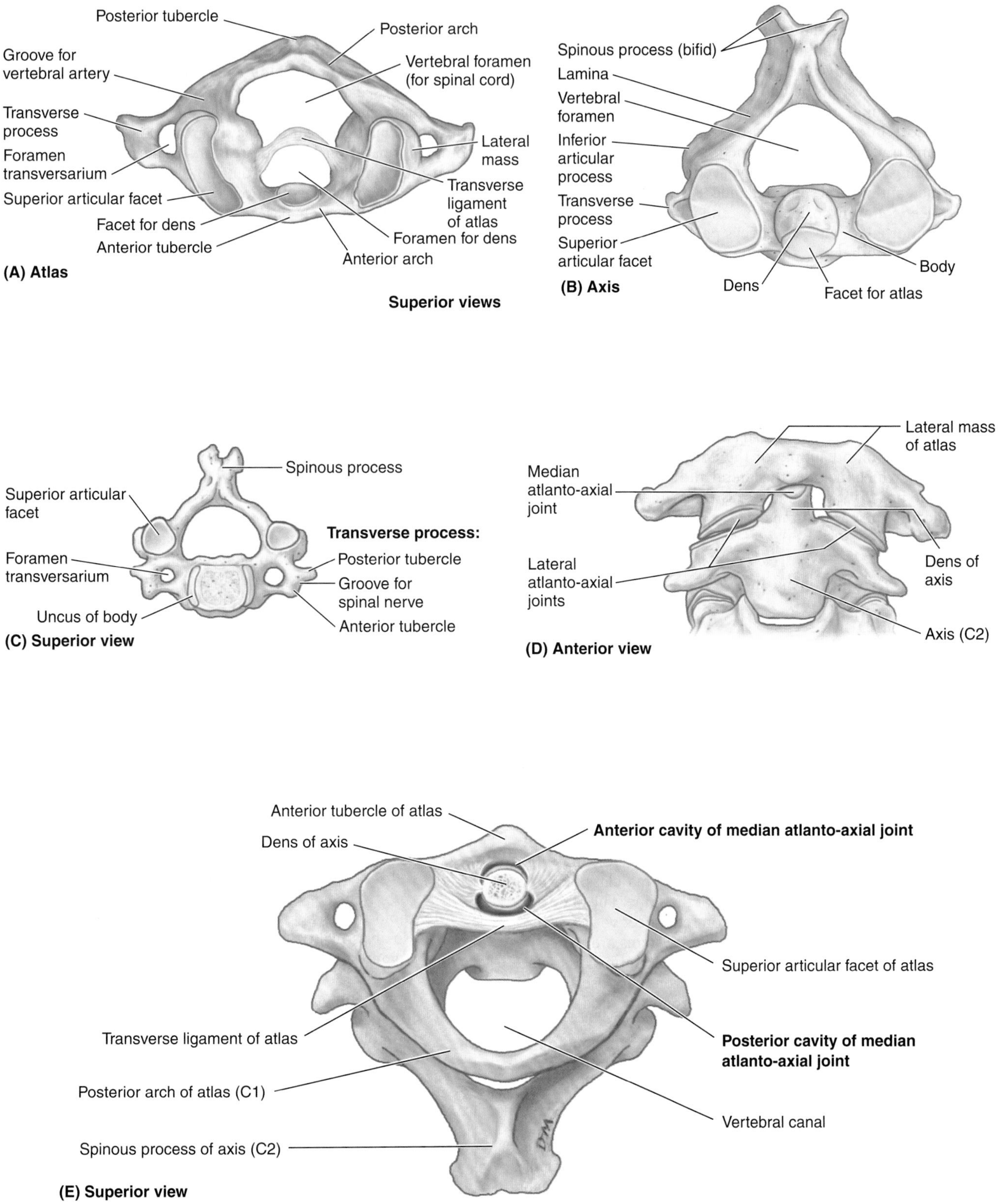
Posterior tubercle
Posterior arch
Groove for vertebral artery
Vertebral foramen (for spinal cord)
Transverse process
Foramen transversarium
Lateral mass
Superior articular facet
Transverse ligament of atlas
Facet for dens
Anterior tubercle
Foramen for dens
Anterior arch
(A) Atlas
Superior views
Spinous process (bifid)
Lamina
Vertebral foramen
Inferior articular process
Transverse process
Superior articular facet
Body
(B) Axis
Dens
Facet for atlas
Spinous process
Superior articular facet
Transverse process:
Foramen transversarium
Posterior tubercle
Groove for spinal nerve
Uncus of body
Anterior tubercle
(C) Superior view
Lateral mass of atlas
Median atlanto-axial joint
Lateral atlanto-axial joints
Dens of axis
Axis (C2)
(D) Anterior view
Anterior tubercle of atlas
Dens of axis
Anterior cavity of median atlanto-axial joint
Superior articular facet of atlas
Transverse ligament of atlas
Posterior cavity of median atlanto-axial joint
Posterior arch of atlas (C1)
Vertebral canal
Spinous process of axis (C2)
(E) Superior view

FIGURE 42.1 Anatomy of C1 (Atlas) and C2 (Axis) [40].

at the inferior border of L1. Extending from the distal tip of the conus medullaris, the cauda equina consists of the lumbar and sacral nerve roots and filum terminale surrounded by dura. The spinal cord acts as a shuttle that relays neuronal signals from the brain to the rest of the body and vice versa. Specific neural fibers with similar function form "tracts." Ascending tracts relay sensory information from the body to the brain and the descending tracts relay motor function to the body.

Ascending tracts include the dorsal columns, lateral spinothalamic tract, and ventral spinothalamic tract. The dorsal columns convey deep touch, proprioception, and vibratory sensation. The lateral spinothalamic tract conveys pain and temperature and the ventral spinothalamic tract conveys light touch. Descending tracts are comprised of lateral and ventral corticospinal tracts, which carry voluntary motor signals to the body.

The blood supply to the spinal cord originates from the segmental vessels, which are branches of the great vessels at the neck, thorax, and abdomen. These segmental vessels divide into anterior and posterior radicular arteries, which transverse the neuroforamen along with the segmental nerve root. The anterior and posterior radicular arteries finally terminate as the anterior and posterior spinal artery. The anterior spinal artery is the primary blood supply of the anterior two-thirds of the spinal cord, which includes the lateral and ventral corticospinal tracts. The posterior spinal artery is the primary blood supply to the dorsal sensory columns [5].

CLASSIFICATION OF INJURY AND ASSESSMENT OF SPINAL STABILITY

The vertebral column serves to transmit loads, permit motion, and protect the spinal cord. Spinal stability is one of the most important considerations in the management of spinal trauma. White and Panjabi defined spinal stability as the "ability of the spine under physiologic loads to limit patterns of displacement so as not to damage or irritate the spinal cord or nerve roots and, in addition, to prevent incapacitating deformity or pain due to structural changes [6]."

An ideal spinal column injury classification should be both descriptive and prognostic. The system should have consistent radiographic measures and guide clinical decision-making. There are a number of historical spinal trauma classification schemes utilized to assess the stability of the spine. The majority of them are not validated and based on retrospective views and experiences of individual surgeons. These systems are typically based on either mechanistic or anatomic description of spinal column injuries. Although there are numerous proposed injury classifications, many of them are not prognostic and do not guide clinical decision-making [7].

The Denis classification is an example of a three-column theory based on anatomic description of thoracolumbar fractures. This system divides the spine into anterior, middle, and posterior columns. The anterior column consists of the anterior half of the vertebral body, the anterior half of the intervertebral disk, and the anterior longitudinal ligament. The middle column consists of the posterior half of the vertebral body, the posterior half of the intervertebral disk, and the posterior longitudinal ligament. The posterior column consists of the posterior arch, the facet joint complex, the interspinous ligament, the supraspinous ligament, and the ligamentum flavum. The spine is considered unstable if two or more columns are disrupted. The Denis classification system does provide for an anatomic description of the zones of injury for thoracolumbar trauma but unfortunately does not account for neurologic status and guide clinical treatment decision.

Holdsworth described the first mechanistic classification of spinal injuries based on experiences of over 1,000 patients by categorizing fractures as simple wedge, dislocation, rotational fracture–dislocation, extension, burst, and shear [7]. This was the first classification to highlight the importance of posterior ligamentous complex (PLC). Allen and Ferguson [8], later in 1982, proposed a classification of subaxial spine fractures based on radiographic appearance and the inferred mechanism of disruptions. This classification has six groups including (1) flexion compression, (2) vertical compression, (3) flexion distraction, (4) extension compression, (5) extension distraction, and (6) lateral flexion. Mechanistic classifications have limited clinical application because they are mainly based on inferred mechanisms of injury rather than objective injury morphology. Furthermore, similar to anatomic descriptive classifications, neurologic status of the patient is not included, which is essential in treatment decision-making [7].

Because of the lack of clinical relevance of the previously established classification systems and an overall "gold standard" system, Vaccaro et al. [9] proposed the Subaxial Cervical Spine Injury Classification System (SLIC) and Thoracolumbar Injury Classification and Severity Score (TLICS) [10] system that is based on injury morphology, integrity of the disco-ligamentous complex (SLIC) (Fig. 42.2) or posterior ligamentous complex (TLICS) (Fig. 42.3) and neurologic status. These two systems were designed to incorporate key anatomic and clinical predictors of stability and severity of injury. The goal of these systems is to simplify communication, help guide treatment, and provide a common language upon which further study can be performed.

The three components of the SLIC system include: morphology, disco-ligamentous complex, and neurologic status. Each component is assigned a weighted score. The overall injury score is the sum of the weighted score of each component. Nonoperative treatment may be considered for a score <4, and operative treatment may be considered for score >4. If the score = 4, then either nonoperative or operative treatment may be considered.

The three components of the TLICS system include: morphology, posterior ligamentous complex, and neurologic involvement. Similar to SLIC system, each component has a weighted score and the overall injury score is the sum of the three components. Nonoperative treatment may be considered for score <4, and operative treatment may be considered for score >4. If score = 4 then, either nonoperative or operative treatment may be considered.

	Points
Morphology	
No abnormality	0
Compression	1
Burst	+1=2
Distraction (e.g., facet perch, hyperextension)	3
Rotation/Translation (e.g., facet dislocation, unstable teardrop or advanced staged flexion compression injury)	4
Disco-ligamentous complex	
Intact	0
Indeterminate (e.g., isolated interspinous widening, MRI signal change only)	1
Disrupted (e.g., widening of disc space, facet perch or dislocation)	2
Neurological status	
Intact	0
Root injury	1
Complete cord injury	2
Incomplete cord injury	3
Continuous cord compression in setting of neuro deficit (neuro modifier)	+1

FIGURE 42.2 Subaxial Cervical Spine Injury Classification System (SLIC) [9].

	Points
Morphology	
Compression Fracture	1
Burst Fracture	2
Translational/rotational	3
Distraction	4
Neurological involvement	
Intact	0
Nerve root	2
Cord, conus medullaris	
Incomplete	3
Complete	2
Cauda Equina	3
Posterior ligamentous complex	
Intact	0
Injury suspected/indeterminate	2
Injured	3

FIGURE 42.3 Thoracolumbar Injury Classification and Severity Score (TLICS) [10].

SLIC and TLICS systems are built on three components that are independent determinants of prognosis and optimal treatment. They are the first comprehensive spinal trauma classification systems that account for the neurologic status of the patient. Most importantly, SLIC and TLICS systems overcame the shortcomings of the previous classification systems by demonstrating good interobserver reliability and validity [10]. Furthermore, Patel et al. demonstrated that these systems can be easily incorporated into large clinical practice with physicians of different levels of experience from attending surgeons to fellows and residents [11].

Neurologic Injury

Assessing neurologic injury is the key in determining the level of injury and the severity of injury to the spinal cord. The extent of the injury can determine the treatment options and overall prognosis. Motor examination includes strength measurement (Grade 0–5) of five key upper- and lower-extremity myotomes. The upper extremity myotomes include C5, elbow flexion; C6, wrist extension; C7, elbow extension; C8, long finger flexion; T1, finger abductions. The lower-extremity myotomes include L2, hip flexion; L3, knee extension; L4, ankle dorsiflexion; L5, great toe extension; S1, ankle plantar flexion. Sensory examination is comprised of light touch and pinprick sensation along the dermatomes [12].

The ASIA (American Spinal Injury Association) scoring system [13,14] was proposed to allow for easy classification of neurologic impairment. The scoring system is based on motor, sensory, reflex, and rectal function (Fig. 42.4). For a complete neurologic examination, it is important to consider if the patient is in spinal shock by checking the bulbocavernosus reflex. This reflex is characterized by anal sphincter contraction in response to squeezing the glans penis. Tugging on an indwelling Foley catheter can also elicit the reflex.

It is also important to determine the neurologic level of injury. This is defined as the lowest segment with intact sensation and antigravity (grade 3 or more) motor function. In the regions where there is no myotome to test, motor level is presumed to be the same as sensory level. Another key component of the neurologic assessment is to determine whether the injury is complete or incomplete. Complete injury is defined as no anal contraction, 0/5 distal motor score, 0/2 distal sensory score, and present bulbocavernosus reflex. Incomplete is defined as voluntary anal contraction or present perianal sensation, or palpable/visible muscle contraction below the neurologic level.

The ASIA scoring system yields an ASIA Impairment Score (AIS), which groups each injury into five categories (A–E) based on severity (Fig. 42.5). Grade A is a complete neurologic injury with no motor or sensory preserved in the sacral segments (S4–S5). Grade B, C, D are incomplete neurologic injures. Grade B is defined as preserved sensory function but not motor function below the neurologic level and includes the sacral segments (S4–S5). Grade C has preserved motor function below the neurologic level and more than half of key muscles below the neurologic level have a muscle grade less than 3. Grade D has preserved motor function below the neurologic level with at least half of the key muscles below the neurologic level have a muscle grade of 3 or more. Grade E has normal neurologic function.

The AIS has prognostic value for determination. Fisher et al. found that patients with ASIA A (complete) spinal cord injury had no distal lower extremity functional recovery 2 years after the injury. Approximately half of AISA B patients will achieve ambulatory status, compared to ¾ of ASIA C patients and almost all patients with ASIA D injuries. Younger patients tend to have a better prognosis as well. Burns et al. found 91% of patients younger than 50 years with ASIA C were ambulatory at discharge compared to 42% in patients older than 50 years [12,15].

Patients with no motor or sensory function preserved in the lowest sacral segments (S4–S5) are AIS A. Those with sensory sparing in the lowest sacral segments but no motor functions are AIS B. Those with preserved motor function below the neurologic level but the majority of myotomes having a muscle grade of 2 or less are AIS C. Those with preserved motor function below the neurologic level with majority of myotomes having a muscle grade of 3 or more are AIS D. Patients with normal motor and sensory function are AIS E.

There are several incomplete neurologic injuries based on specific locations of the spinal cord that have predictable patterns of neurologic findings.

Anterior cord syndrome is characterized by loss of motor and loss of pain and temperature sensation below the level of the injury. Vibratory sense and proprioception are preserved. This is usually a result of flexion/compression injury that lead to either direct compression of the anterior spinal cord or disruption of anterior spinal artery (supplies anterior two-thirds spinal cord). This injury carries the worst prognosis of incomplete SCI.

Central cord syndrome is the most common incomplete cord injury. It often occurs in the elderly with extension type injury mechanisms. It is believed to be caused by spinal cord compression and central cord edema with injury/destruction of lateral corticospinal tract white matter. The classical finding on physical examination is more pronounced motor deficits in the upper extremities compared to the lower extremities. Hands typically have more pronounced motor deficits than arms. This is owing to the fact that hands are more "centrally" located in the corticospinal tract. Patients with central cord syndrome have good prognosis but full functional recovery is rare. Lower-extremities function typically recovers first and hand function is last to recover [16].

Posterior cord syndrome is very rare and examination findings include loss of proprioception with preserved motor, pain and light touch. It is a result of direct injury to the dorsal columns. Stabbing injuries to the back commonly cause this injury pattern.

Brown–Sequard syndrome is a complete cord hemitransection as a result of penetrating trauma or direct lateral injuries to the spinal cord. Patients on examination have ipsilateral deficit in motor, vibratory sense and proprioception below the level of the injury and contralateral loss of pain and temperature sensation. These patients have excellent overall prognosis with the majority of patients able to ambulate at final follow-up.

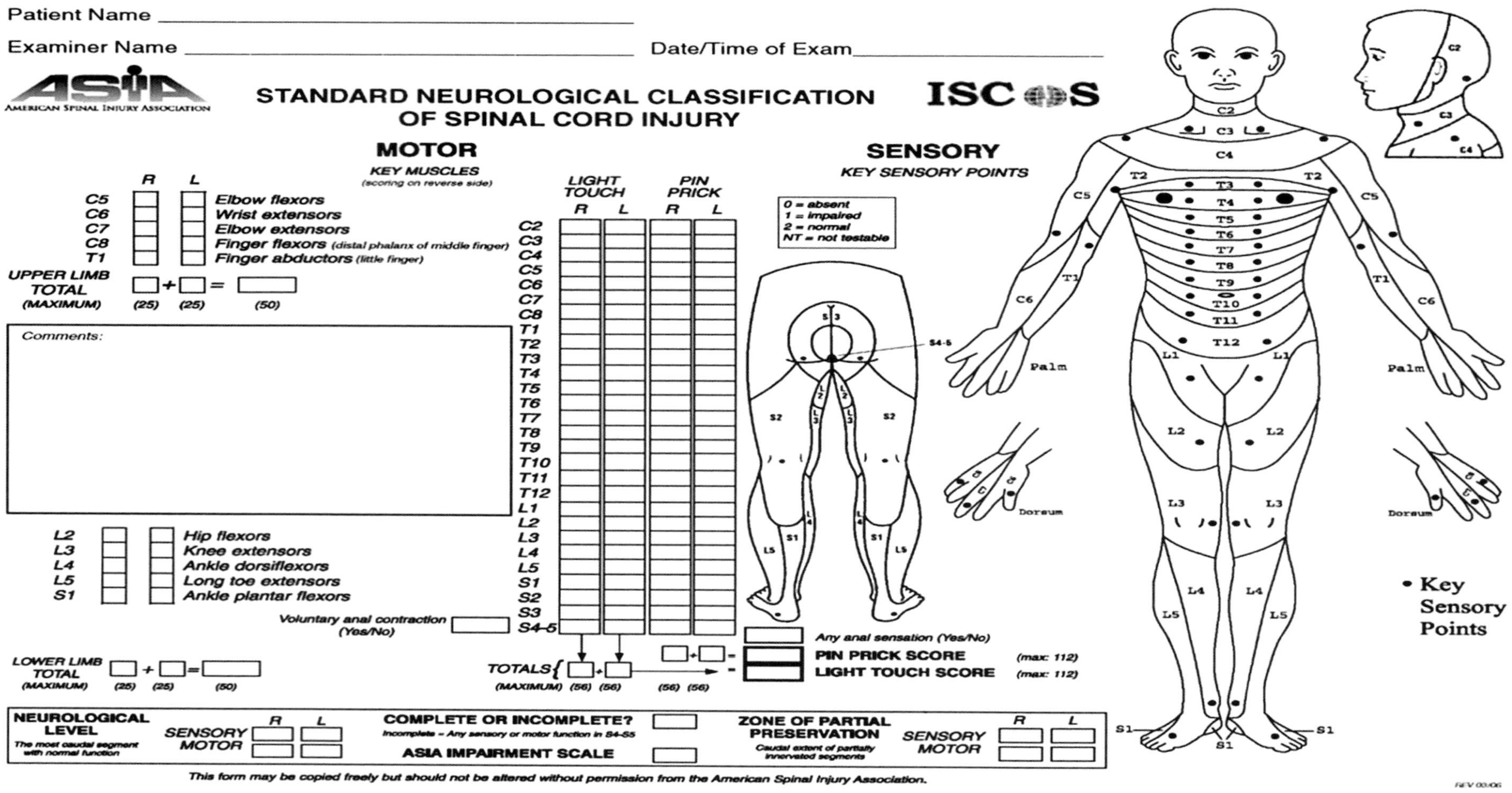
Patient Name ______________________

Examiner Name ______________________ Date/Time of Exam ______________________

ASIA — American Spinal Injury Association

ISCoS

STANDARD NEUROLOGICAL CLASSIFICATION OF SPINAL CORD INJURY

MOTOR

KEY MUSCLES (scoring on reverse side)

	R	L	
C5			Elbow flexors
C6			Wrist extensors
C7			Elbow extensors
C8			Finger flexors (distal phalanx of middle finger)
T1			Finger abductors (little finger)

UPPER LIMB TOTAL (MAXIMUM) ☐ + ☐ = ☐ (25) (25) (50)

Comments:

	R	L	
L2			Hip flexors
L3			Knee extensors
L4			Ankle dorsiflexors
L5			Long toe extensors
S1			Ankle plantar flexors

Voluntary anal contraction (Yes/No) ☐

LOWER LIMB TOTAL (MAXIMUM) ☐ + ☐ = ☐ (25) (25) (50)

SENSORY

KEY SENSORY POINTS

	LIGHT TOUCH R	LIGHT TOUCH L	PIN PRICK R	PIN PRICK L
C2				
C3				
C4				
C5				
C6				
C7				
C8				
T1				
T2				
T3				
T4				
T5				
T6				
T7				
T8				
T9				
T10				
T11				
T12				
L1				
L2				
L3				
L4				
L5				
S1				
S2				
S3				
S4-5				

TOTALS { ☐ + ☐ (MAXIMUM) (56) (56) ☐ + ☐ (56) (56)

0 = absent
1 = impaired
2 = normal
NT = not testable

Any anal sensation (Yes/No) ☐

PIN PRICK SCORE (max: 112)

LIGHT TOUCH SCORE (max: 112)

NEUROLOGICAL LEVEL — The most caudal segment with normal function — SENSORY R ☐ L ☐; MOTOR R ☐ L ☐

COMPLETE OR INCOMPLETE? ☐ Incomplete = Any sensory or motor function in S4-S5

ASIA IMPAIRMENT SCALE ☐

ZONE OF PARTIAL PRESERVATION — Caudal extent of partially innervated segments — SENSORY R ☐ L ☐; MOTOR R ☐ L ☐

REV 03/06

FIGURE 42.4 American Spinal Injury Association (ASIA) scoring system [13] documents the motor and sensory function to determine the severity of the neurologic injury. The motor score is comprised of 10 key muscles groups as seen on the left column of the figure. The sensory score for light touch and pinprick is comprised of sensation within 28 dermatomes. Perianal sensation and anal contraction assessment is critical to determine the functional preservation in the lowest sacral segments, S4–S5. An AIS (ASIA impairment score) grade is determined based on these neurologic findings.

A=Complete	No motor or sensory function is preserved in the sacral segments S4–S5
B=Incomplete	Sensory but no motor function is preserved below the neurological level and includes the sacral segments S4–S5
C=Incomplete	Motor function is preserved below the neurological level, and at least half of key muscles below the neurological level have a muscle grade of 3 or more
D=Incomplete	Motor function is preserved below the neurological level, and at least half of key muscles below the neurological level have a muscle grade of 3 or more
E=Normal	Motor and sensory function are normal

FIGURE 42.5 ASIA Impairment Score (AIS) neurologic severity grading scale, A through E. [13].

Conus medullaris syndrome presents with symmetric lower-extremity motor deficits and bowel and bladder dysfunction. Patients typically have symmetric perineal or "saddle" loss of sensation. This is a result of injuries to the conus medullaris at the thoracolumbar junction. Because of the significant amount of nerve roots emerging from this area of the spinal cord, patients are less likely to recover neurologically compared to nerve root injury.

Cauda equina syndrome is defined by symptoms that result from nerve root compression in the lumbosacral region. This is most commonly caused by disc herniation but in trauma patients this nerve root compression can result from retropulsion of fracture fragments or fracture dislocation of the vertebrae. Key features of cauda equina syndrome include bilateral leg pain, blower and bladder dysfunction, saddle anesthesia, and lower-extremity motor and sensory deficits. Certain lesions may affect the transition level between the conus medullaris and cauda equina, and symptoms may overlap. Cauda equina is predominantly lower motor neuron dysfunction, and deep tendon reflexes will be intact in the levels cranial to the level of injury. Patients with conus medullaris syndrome have predominantly upper motor neuron dysfunction, and patients will have absent deep tendon reflexes in the lower extremities.

Pathophysiology

Blunt Trauma

Damage to the spinal cord from blunt trauma injury occurs in two stages. The primary injury phase includes a combination of mechanical factors that cause direct injury to the spinal cord. This leads to direct neurologic dysfunction at and below the level of the injury. This direct mechanical disruption and persistent pressure on the spinal cord leads to secondary events that worsen the initial damage [17].

Within seconds to minutes after the injury (immediate phase), there is disruption of microvasculature that leads to possible hemorrhage in the gray matter, and edema in the white matter of the spinal cord [17,18]. This increases the extracellular fluid and pressure, which leads to decreased perfusion in the spinal cord. This decrease in perfusion ultimately results in ischemia owing to thrombosis and vasospasm [19].

After the immediate phase is the early acute phase, which occurs from 2 hours to 2 days after the initial injury. There is further damage from ionic dysregulation and excitotoxicity. Intracellular sodium concentration increases as a result of trauma-induced activation of voltage-sensitive sodium channels [19]. This increase in sodium is accompanied by influx of calcium through the sodium–calcium exchanger, which leads to intracellular acidosis and cytotoxic edema. Furthermore, this influx of sodium and calcium triggers release of excitatory neurotransmitter glutamate in the presynaptic neurons. This excessive accumulation of glutamate leads to amplification and propagation of depolarization, which eventually leads to postsynaptic neuron edema and death. Furthermore, there is increased infiltration of neutrophils, free radicals, and inflammatory mediators in this phase that contribute to neuronal damage [20].

In the subacute phase, which is from 2 days to 2 weeks postinjury, there is increased phagocytosis and apoptosis of the neuronal cells, and demyelination is followed by cyst formation [20].

Penetrating Trauma

Penetrating SCI comprises a distinct mechanism of spinal injury that deserves special consideration. Gunshot wounds and stabbings account for the greatest proportion of penetrating SCI followed by injuries from falls onto sharp objects and industrial type accidents [21].

Gunshot missiles impart damage in three ways: (1) Direct tissue destruction; (2) Pressure or shockwave effect; and (3) Temporary cavitation. The extent of tissue damage from a gunshot missile is related to the energy imparted by the projectile. Kinetic energy (KE) is calculated based on the equation $KE = 1/2\ mv^2$ (m = mass and v = velocity). Based on this principle, increases in velocity impart an exponential increase in kinetic energy, which transfers into a greater degree of tissue destruction. In general, guns with muzzle velocity below 2,000 feet/sec are considered "low velocity" (civilian pistols) and those over 2,000 feet/sec are considered "high velocity" (military rifles or assault weapons). Shotguns impart a low velocity but high energy owing to the large mass of the pellets or slug that is delivered. It is important to identify the type of weapons used as it will dictate the extent of soft-tissue damage and help guide treatment. Furthermore, the path which the bullet passes through or comes to a complete stop within the patient can also affect the extent of the damage. Bullets that are jacketed tend to pass through targets, whereas bullets that yaw (wobble) often enter the target at an angle thus resulting in a great cross-sectional area or tissue cavity.

SCI from stabbings involve cervical and thoracic locations in 80% of the cases, and are split equally in prevalence [22]. "Cord hemisection" injury is more commonly seen in stabbing injuries owing to the spinal column bony anatomy. The penetrating object typically finds the path of least resistance in the gutter between the transverse process and spinal process. Because of the orientation of the spinous process (caudal and sagittal), the knife typically is blocked from crossing the midline. This results in Brown–Sequard syndrome with loss of ipsilateral motor and proprioception and contralateral pain and temperature.

Acute Management

Early management of a patient with potential spinal cord/spinal column injury should begin immediately at the scene of the accident. Pathologic motion of the injured vertebrae can lead to worsening neurologic injury. It is estimated that 3% to 25% of spinal cord injuries deteriorate neurologically after the initial trauma owing to transit or early management of the patient [12,23]. There has been dramatic improvement in the neurologic status of trauma patients since the establishment of spinal immobilization protocols that stabilize patients from the scene of the accident to the hospital. Current recommendations for spinal immobilization consist of a rigid cervical collar, lateral supports, and tape and body straps to secure the patient to a backboard to immobilize the entire spine. Unwanted motion can still occur during transport or logrolling the patient, resulting in neurologic deterioration [12,23]. It also should be emphasized that a rigid cervical orthosis does not eliminate all cervical motion [24].

Physicians should review the details of the accident, the energy and mechanism of injury, and the general condition of the patient at the scene. Patients with closed head injuries and facial trauma should raise suspicion for a cervical spine injury owing to transmission of force. Patients with a "seat belt sign" may have a thoracolumbar spine injury consistent with flexion distraction of the spine about the fulcrum of the seatbelt. Patients who have fallen from height may have lumbar burst fractures with other distracting injuries such as open calcaneus or tibial plafond fractures. Physicians must be aware of certain patient populations such as pediatric patients or adults with preexisting kyphotic deformities that require special attention during prehospital management. In pediatric patients, the head size is disproportionally larger than the body. Anterior translation/flexion injury may occur if the patient is positioned on a flat surface. An occipital recess or a mattress placed under the torso is needed to maintain neutral spinal alignment. In patients with suspected neurologic injury without radiographic (plain radiograph or CT scan) abnormality (SCIWORA), MRI imaging is recommended. In adult patients suspected to have ankylosing spondylitis or diffuse idiopathic skeletal hyperostosis (DISH), physicians must be aware of a preexisting kyphotic deformity as well as the very rigid mechanical nature of their spines [12]. Placing a cervical collar and taping the head to a flat backboard can worsen an extension–distraction injury, resulting in further neurologic damage. Patients with AS and advanced kyphosis may require their heads to be propped up to maintain the preexisting deformities rather than cause an iatrogenic deformity that may lead to neurologic impairment [12].

Initial evaluation of a patient should follow the Advanced Trauma Life Support protocols (ATLS), including Airway (A), Breathing (B), Circulation (C), Disability (D), and Exposure (E). Airway management is essential in the trauma patient. In case of emergent intubation, in-line immobilization and neutral cervical position should be maintained at all times. Patients with neurologic injury at or above C3 often experience acute respiratory arrest and require mechanical ventilation [12]. Lower-level cervical or thoracic injuries may also lead to difficulty with breathing owing to impaired intercostal muscle function. Maintaining oxygenation and perfusion should be a priority in trauma patients. Hypotension should be treated aggressively and the etiology of suspected hemorrhage should be investigated thoroughly. Patients with seatbelt injures often have intra-abdominal pathologies along with thoracolumbar flexion–distraction injury [12]. Furthermore, one should suspect neurogenic shock in the setting of a hypotensive and bradycardic patient. Neurogenic shock occurs in approximately 20% of cervical spinal cord injuries and is a result of loss of sympathetic tone on the peripheral vasculature [25,26]. Neurogenic shock often occurs with injuries above the T4 level, and hypotension should be aggressively treated to prevent further ischemic cord damage. Pharmacologic interventions should be used in case of hypotension not responsive to fluid resuscitation. Alpha-agonists such as dopamine and norepinephrine can increase peripheral vascular resistance [12].

Radiographic Assessment

The goal of cervical spine clearance is to safely and efficiently rule out an injury that might, if missed, lead to neurologic injury or late instability [12]. Patients with neck pain, tenderness, and neurologic deficits and obtunded patients require radiologic evaluation. Patients who are temporarily cognitively impaired should be protected with spinal precautious until a definitive clinical examination is completed.

Diagnostic imaging modalities utilized to assess spinal column/spinal cord pathologies include plain radiographic films, computed tomography (CT) scans, and magnetic resonance imaging (MRI) scans. Two decision guidelines have previously been established to minimize use of unnecessary imaging in trauma patients. NEXUS Low Rick Criteria [27] (National Emergency X-radiography Use Study) was designed to identify patients who do not need diagnostic imaging to exclude a clinically significant cervical spine injury. Cervical spine radiographs are indicated unless the patients fit all of the following criteria: alert and not intoxicated, no posterior midline tenderness, no neurologic indications of injury, and have no distracting injuries. CCR [28] (Canadian C-Spine Rule) guidance states, "the patients who meet the following criteria do not require radiographic study: fully alert and oriented, involved in low-energy trauma, no neurologic symptoms, no midline tenderness, can actively rotate head 45 degrees in both directions, and have no distracting injuries" (Fig. 42.6).

Plain radiographs provide information on bony integrity and overall alignment. Upright plain radiographs including flexion/extension films are often used to assess spinal column alignment under physiologic load. CT scans provide a more sensitive and specific modality for evaluation of bony pathology. It has enhanced resolution compared to plain radiographs and it allows visualization of the occipitocervical and cervicothoracic junctions.

Patients with a known diagnosis of ankylosing spondylitis or diffuse idiopathic skeletal hyperostosis (DISH) should be treated with extra caution [12]. Owing to fusion of multiple spinal segments (especially in patients with ankylosing spondylitis), nondisplaced fractures behave like diaphyseal long-bone fractures and are potentially highly unstable. Previously mentioned scoring systems to assess stability do not apply to these patients and missed diagnosis can have catastrophic results. Patients with AS who have been in even a minor trauma that have back/neck pain should have CT/MRI to rule out fracture. Negative plain radiographs are not sufficient to make a definite diagnosis [12]. A prior study demonstrated a high rate of neurologic deterioration if fractures are missed in this patient population [29].

Magnetic resonance imaging (MRI) has become the gold standard for imaging neurologic tissues including the spinal cord. When a patient's neurologic examination does not match the fracture pattern seen on CT scan, MRI should be the utilized in the evaluation process. MRI allows better visualization of the spinal cord, ligaments, discs, vessels, and other soft tissues. Patients with cervical spine injuries have high rate of disc herniation (36%) on MRI, along with posterior ligamentous injuries (64%) [30]. Furthermore, MRI allows the surgeon to plan surgically and prognosticate in the setting of spinal cord injuries.

Four MRI imaging patterns of spinal cord injuries have been described, and include normal cord, single-level edema, multi-level edema, and mixed hemorrhage and edema. Patients with single-level edema had overall improvement of two grades in ASIA score compared to an improvement of one for patients with diffuse edema. Single-level edema patients had higher chance of returning to ASIA E grade compared to those with diffuse edema. Patients with edema and hemorrhage have the worst prognosis, with 95% classified as ASIA A at the time of initial presentation. These patients improved one ASIA grade only 5% of the time [30].

TREATMENT

Nonoperative

Patients with SCI often benefit from multidisciplinary nonoperative ICU care. Previous studies have shown improved management

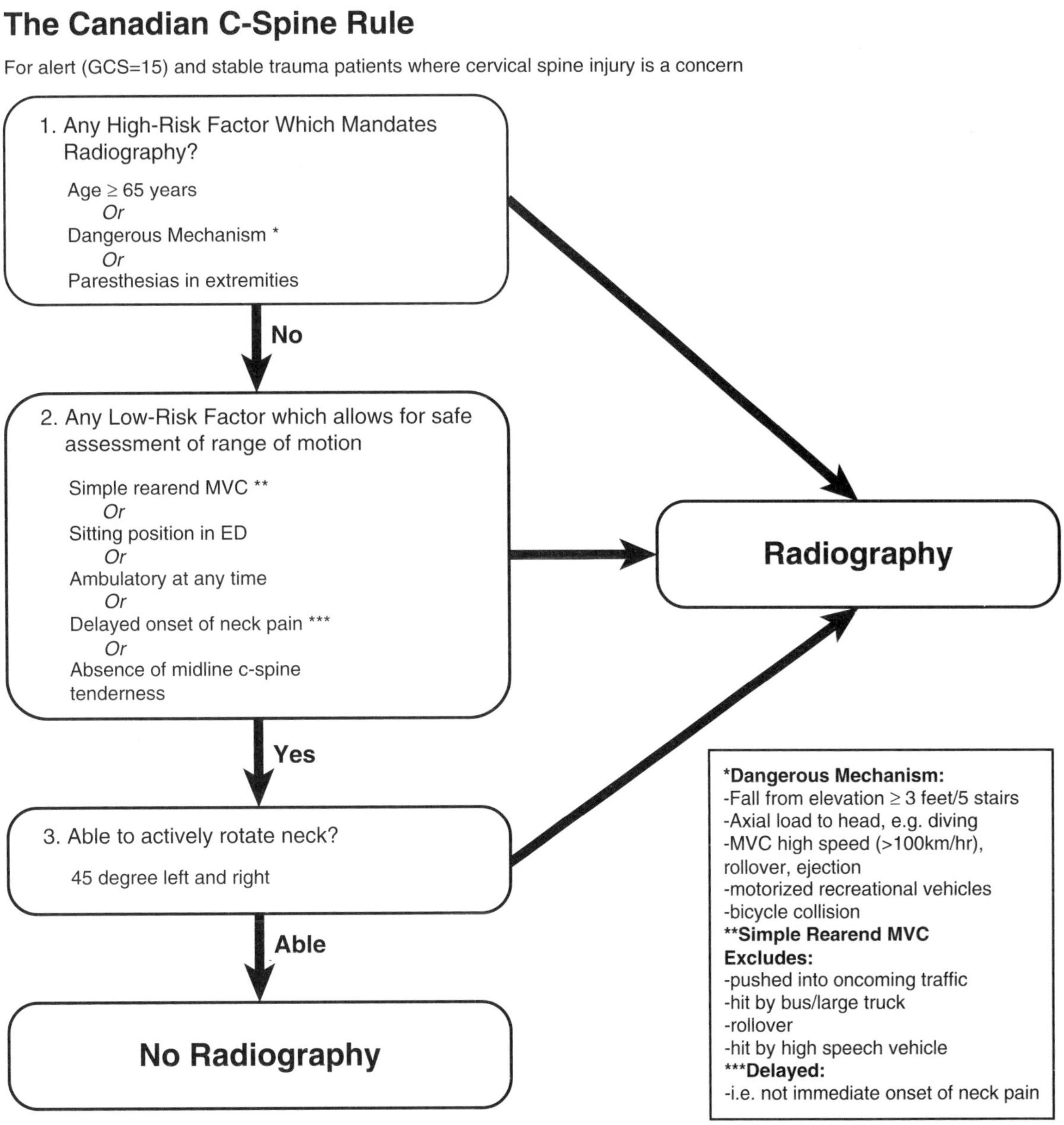

The Canadian C-Spine Rule
For alert (GCS=15) and stable trauma patients where cervical spine injury is a concern
1. Any High-Risk Factor Which Mandates Radiography?
Age ≥ 65 years
Or
Dangerous Mechanism *
Or
Paresthesias in extremities
No
2. Any Low-Risk Factor which allows for safe assessment of range of motion
Simple rearend MVC **
Or
Sitting position in ED
Or
Ambulatory at any time
Or
Delayed onset of neck pain ***
Or
Absence of midline c-spine tenderness
Yes
3. Able to actively rotate neck?
45 degree left and right
Able
No Radiography
Radiography
*Dangerous Mechanism:
-Fall from elevation ≥ 3 feet/5 stairs
-Axial load to head, e.g. diving
-MVC high speed (>100km/hr), rollover, ejection
-motorized recreational vehicles
-bicycle collision
**Simple Rearend MVC Excludes:
-pushed into oncoming traffic
-hit by bus/large truck
-rollover
-hit by high speech vehicle
***Delayed:
-i.e. not immediate onset of neck pain

FIGURE 42.6 The Canadian C-Spine Rule [28].

and lower morbidity and mortality following acute SCI with ICU monitoring and aggressive medical management [31,32]. Nonoperative SCI care can be categorized into two categories [41]: neuroprotective measures and indirect reduction with immobilization.

1. Neuroprotective measures
   Maintenance of adequate oxygenation and perfusion to the spinal cord may be neuroprotective against secondary SCI. Hypotension in animal models of SCI results in worse neurologic outcome [31]. No prospective controlled assessment of hypotension on human SCI patients has been performed, but previous observational or retrospective studies set a goal for MAP at a minimum of 85 to 90 mmHg based on evidence in the traumatic brain injury (TBI) patient population. Studies of TBI suggest that MAP less than 90 mmHg has been associated with increased morbidity and mortality. Current standard of care management includes support of arterial oxygenation and spinal cord perfusion pressure, and maintenance of MAP above 85 to 90 mmHg for the first 7 days following spinal cord injury is recommended [31].

   Pharmacologic intervention for spinal cord injury aims to minimize the secondary zone of injury [33]. The most publicized intervention was the use of high-dose methylprednisolone for spinal cord injury. NASCIS [34–36] (National Acute Spinal Cord Injury Studies) II and III studies found extremely modest yet inconsistent neurologic improvement with high-dose methylprednisolone. However, the complication rates were significant and include wound infection, hyperglycemia, GI hemorrhage, sepsis, steroid induced myopathy, and death. High-dose methylprednisolone can also significantly alter immune response with decreased T-cell count, and patients who received treatment are associated with higher rate of pneumonia and longer hospital stays [37]. The authors do not recommend the use of corticosteroid in the setting of traumatic SCI.

   GM-1 Ganglioside (Sygen) is another drug with promising results in early studies. This compound is found indigenously in cell membranes of mammalian central nervous system tissue and thought to have antiexcitotoxic activity, potentiate the effects of nerve growth factor, and prevent apoptosis. A multicenter study randomized 797 patients within 72 hours of injury to receive either GM-1 ganglioside or placebo. Although patients with ASIA grade C and D SCI treated with GM-1 ganglioside demonstrated significant neurologic improvement compared to placebo-treated patients at 4 and 8 weeks after injury, the advantage was lost at subsequent follow-up visits. No difference was noted in any of the outcome measures at 1 year [37].

A number of promising pharmacologic therapies are currently under investigation for neuroprotective effect in animal models. These include the sodium (Na^+) channel blocker riluzole, the tetracycline derivative minocycline, the fusogen copolymer polyethylene glycol (PEG), and the tissue-protective hormone erythropoietin (EPO) [17,38].

2. Indirect reduction and spinal immobilization

The goals of SCI treatment are to prevent neurologic deterioration, reestablish spinal column stability, and regain neurologic function. Neurologic deterioration is a real risk once the patient has come under the care of medical personal. Understanding the functions and limitations of spine orthoses is critical to limit those occurrences. SCI patients should first be immobilized with bed rest and "spine precautious." All cervical fracture patients should be protected by cervical orthosis. Previous cadaver studies have shown that specimens with cervical collar had similar cervical spine motion compared to those who did not during bed-to-bed transfer. For this reason, extra caution must be used during patient transfer despite the presence of cervical orthosis.

In patients with high cervical injuries including occipitocervical dissociation, rigid cervical collars may not adequately immobilize those spinal segments. The halo vest remains the orthosis of choice for these patients. A halo vest is the most rigid cervical external immobilizer. It restricts up to 75% of flexion/extension at C1–C2 level and has superior control of lateral bending and rotation compared to other cervical orthoses. Halo vest should not be used in patients with advanced age, chest trauma, cranial fractures, infection, or soft-tissue damage around the proposed pin sites [39].

Certain fracture/dislocations of the cervical spine may require in-line cervical traction with Gardner–Wells tongs to achieve fracture reduction. The patient should be awake/alert and positioned in reverse Trendelenburg position with shoulder straps attached to the end of the bed. Gardner–Wells tongs are typically applied 1 cm superior to the pinna of the ears. Traction weight should be applied and increased gradually and incrementally. At every step, a neurologic examination and lateral cervical X-ray must be performed. If reduction is successful, a postreduction CT or MRI scan should be done [39].

KTT (kinetic therapy treatment) is a laterally rotating bed created to substitute frequent patient positioning in order to minimize the complications of long-term bed rest. Previous cadaver studies have shown that KTT generated significantly less cervical and thoracolumbar spine motion in comparison to logroll [40]. The author recommends that KTT should be used for initial immobilization for patients with cervical, thoracic, or lumbar instability.

Medical Management of Spinal Cord–Injured Patients

Spinal cord injury may cause dysfunctions in multiple organ systems, leading to increased mortality and decreased quality of life [41]. SCI above T6 vertebra disrupts the descending pathways to the sympathetic neurons in the intermediolateral column of the spinal cord from T1–L2. Loss of sympathetic control results in increased sympathetic activity below the injury and loss of inhibition of parasympathetic nervous system above the level of injury [41].

Sympathetic neurons in the upper thoracic spinal cord (T1–T5) innervate the vessels of the upper body and heart [41]. Neurogenic shock, which is characterized by hypotension and bradycardia, is a result of intact parasympathetic influence via vagal nerve with a loss of sympathetic tone. Treatments of neurogenic shock include fluid resuscitation for hypotension, atropine in the setting of bradycardia, and vasopressors such as dopamine or norepinephrine in the setting of severe hemodynamic instability [31]. Owing to decreased transmission of cardiac pain (T4), patients with SCI above that level may have impaired perception of chest pain in case of ischemic cardiac events [41]. During the acute phase of SCI, vagal nerve disturbance can last 2 to 3 weeks; in certain cases, pacemakers are required to maintain a functional cardiac rhythm [41].

Autonomic dysreflexia is a sudden uncontrolled sympathetic response resulting in uncontrolled arterial blood pressure. This typically occurs in patients with SCI above T6. This is a life-threatening event, with blood pressures above 250 mmHg reported [42]. The incidence of AD was found to be 10% to 11% during the first 3 years postinjury [42]. The most common offending trigger is bladder distention owing to urinary retention or catheter blockage. Other triggers include constipation, urinary tract infection, and traumatic/painful stimuli. The mainstay of treatment for AD is prevention and avoidance of common triggers. Pharmacologic interventions should include drugs that are rapid-onset with short duration; that is, nifedipine, hydralazine, or sodium nitroprusside [43].

Respiratory insufficiency and pulmonary dysfunction are common after spinal cord injury, especially in the high cervical level owing to phrenic nerve innervation (C3–C5) [31]. Early initiation of vigorous pulmonary therapy after acute SCI is associated with increased survival, reduced incidence of pulmonary complications, and decreased need for ventilator support [31]. Aggressive secretion clearance, pulmonary toilet, and chest physiotherapy are highly recommended to lower the rate of pulmonary complications. In the thoracic spinal cord injury population, the location of injury is a predictor of the incidence of pulmonary complications. Maung et al. found a higher rate of pneumonia in high thoracic injury patients (T1–T6) compared to low thoracic injury patients (T7–T12), 43.3% versus 25.4%, respectively [44,45].

Spinal cord injury often leads to bladder dysfunction. This dysfunction can be classified as either an upper motor neuron or lower motor neuron syndrome [41]. Upper motor neuron syndrome leads to detrusor hyperactivity, where the bladder wall contracts in response to minor stretch without any voluntary external urethral sphincter control. This results in frequent, involuntary voiding. Lower motor neuron syndrome leads to decreased or absent detrusor contractility (flaccidity) with a distended bladder. Bladder management in SCI patients include sterile intermittent catheterization (SIC) in the hospital and clean intermittent self-catheterization outside the hospital [41]. Anticholinergic medications may be helpful with spastic bladder.

The incidence of thromboembolic events in the untreated patients with spinal cord injury is high, ranging from 7% to 100% [46,47]. There is a high rate of morbidity and mortality associated with occurrence of DVT and PEs in this population. Thromboembolic events are responsible for 9.7% of all deaths in the first year following SCI. Furthermore, SCI patients have 500-fold increased risk of PE-related death in the first month following the injury [47]. Previous systematic review has suggested that low-molecular-weight heparin (LMWH) is more effective than unfractionated heparin in preventing DVT in the SCI population [47]. IVC filters are not recommended as a routine prophylactic measure, but are recommended in patients who failed or are not candidates for anticoagulation therapy.

Operative

Operative treatment in patients with spine fractures has typically been for unstable fractures, progressive neurologic deficits, and patients unable to tolerate bracing (i.e., obesity, skin lesions, visceral injury, multi-extremity injuries).

The goal of surgical intervention in patients with spinal cord injury is to achieve spinal stability, deformity correction, neurologic recovery, and pain control, and allow for rehabilitation [48]. Surgical decompression and stabilization of the spine can be performed via an anterior, posterior, or combined approach. The anterior approach is indicated when neurologic deficits are caused by anterior compression such as bony retropulsion or disc herniation. This procedure may include corpectomy (removal of a portion of the vertebra and the adjacent intervertebral discs) and strut grafting using allograft, autograft, metal cages, or a combination of these. Corpectomy is usually supplemented with additional posterior instrumentation for increased spinal column stability. The posterior approach can achieve spinal cord decompression by either directly removing retropulsed vertebra through a transpedicular approach or via ligamentotaxis by restoring the vertebral height and alignment with posterior instrumentation.

Optimal timing of surgical intervention to achieve maximum neurologic recovery remains a controversial topic. Most of the studies performed on the timing of surgical decompression is usually classified as early (<72 hours) or late (>72 hours). This time delineation is likely based on preclinical studies that showed that early decompression of acute spinal cord injury could lead to improved neurologic function [49]. Previous data suggest that white matter is more resilient and damage is reversible up to 72 hours after injury, compared to irreversible damage to the gray matter [48]. Unfortunately, in clinical trials, there is no clear evidence to support early surgical decompression in improving neurologic outcomes. Dimar et al. showed no benefit with early surgery compared with late surgery in a randomized controlled trial of cervical spine injury [49]. Cengiz et al. [50] performed a prospective randomized clinical trial on thoracic fractures, which demonstrated a nonsignificant trend toward improved neurologic recovery in the early surgery group.

If the goal of surgery is for spine stabilization only, retrospective studies have shown early surgical stabilization (<72 hours) leading to improved outcome. A review by Bellabarba et al. [51] found seven studies reporting decreased hospital LOS with early stabilization, and decreased ICU stay with thoracic spine stabilization. A literature review by Dimar et al. [49] concluded that when neurologic recovery is not considered an outcome of interest, previous studies have consistently shown shorter hospital LOS, ICU LOS, fewer days on mechanical ventilation, and lower pulmonary complications in patients who had undergone early stabilization. Early stabilization leads to lower overall cost compared to late stabilization cohorts. Unfortunately, these retrospective studies have many confounding factors including significant associated injuries and baseline patient comorbidities [49].

References

1. Zhang S, Wadhwa R, Haydel J, et al: Spine and spinal cord trauma: diagnosis and management. *Neurol Clin* 31(1):183–206, 2013.
2. Furlan JC, Sakakibara BM, Miller WC, et al: Global incidence and prevalence of traumatic spinal cord injury. *Can J Neurol Sci* 40(4):456–464, 2013.
3. Schouten R, Lewkonia P, Noonan VK, et al: Expectations of recovery and functional outcomes following thoracolumbar trauma: an evidence-based medicine process to determine what surgeons should be telling their patients. *J Neurosurg Spine* 22(1):101–111, 2015.
4. Pimentel L, Diegelmann L: Evaluation and management of acute cervical spine trauma. *Emerg Med Clin North Am* 28(4):719–738, 2015.
5. Colman MW, Hornicek FJ, Schwab JH: Spinal cord blood supply and its surgical implications. *J Am Acad Orthop Surg* 23(10):581–591, 2015.
6. Kwon BK, Vaccaro AR, Grauer JN, et al: Subaxial cervical spine trauma. *J Am Acad Orthop Surg* 14(2):78–89, 2006.
7. Patel AA, Vaccaro AR: Thoracolumbar spine trauma classification. *J Am Acad Orthop Surg* 18(2):63–71, 2010.
8. Allen BL Jr, Ferguson RL, Lehmann TR, et al: A mechanistic classification of closed, indirect fractures and dislocations of the lower cervical spine. *Spine (Phila Pa 1976)* 7(1):1–27, 1982.
9. Vaccaro AR, Hulbert RJ, Patel AA, et al: The subaxial cervical spine injury classification system: a novel approach to recognize the importance of morphology, neurology, and integrity of the disco-ligamentous complex. *Spine (Phila Pa 1976)* 32(21):2365–2374, 2007.
10. Patel AA, Vaccaro AR, Albert TJ, et al: The adoption of a new classification system: time-dependent variation in interobserver reliability of the thoracolumbar injury severity score classification system. *Spine (Phila Pa 1976)* 32(3):E105–E110, 2007.
11. Joaquim AF, Fernandes YB, Cavalcante RA, et al: Evaluation of the thoracolumbar injury classification system in thoracic and lumbar spinal trauma. *Spine (Phila Pa 1976)* 36(1):33–36, 2011.
12. Schouten R, Albert T, Kwon BK: The spine-injured patient: initial assessment and emergency treatment. *J Am Acad Orthop Surg* 20(6):336–346, 2012.
13. Kirshblum SC, Burns SP, Biering-Sorensen F, et al: International standards for neurological classification of spinal cord injury (revised 2011). *J Spinal Cord Med* 34(6):535–546, 2011.
14. Kirshblum S, Waring W 3rd: Updates for the International standards for neurological classification of spinal cord injury. *Phys Med Rehabil Clin N Am* 25(3):505–517, vii, 2014.
15. Krishna V, Andrews H, Varma A, et al: Spinal cord injury: how can we improve the classification and quantification of its severity and prognosis? *J Neurotrauma* 31(3):215–227, 2014.
16. Aarabi B, Hadley MN, Dhall SS, et al: Management of acute traumatic central cord syndrome (ATCCS). *Neurosurgery* 72 (Suppl 2):195–204, 2013.
17. Nagoshi N, Nakashima H, Fehlings MG: Riluzole as a neuroprotective drug for spinal cord injury: from bench to bedside. *Molecules* 20(5):7775–7789, 2015.
18. Kwon BK, Sekhon LH, Fehlings MG: Emerging repair, regeneration, and translational research advances for spinal cord injury. *Spine (Phila Pa 1976)* 35(Suppl 21):S263–S270, 2010.
19. Fehlings MG, Wilson JR, Frankowski RF, et al: Riluzole for the treatment of acute traumatic spinal cord injury: rationale for and design of the NACTN Phase I clinical trial. *J Neurosurg Spine* 17(Suppl 1):151–156, 2012.
20. Yilmaz T, Kaptanoglu E: Current and future medical therapeutic strategies for the functional repair of spinal cord injury. *World J Orthop* 6(1):4–255, 2015.
21. Stuke LE, Pons PT, Guy JS, et al: Prehospital spine immobilization for penetrating trauma – review and recommendations from the Prehospital Trauma Life Support Executive Committee. *J Trauma* 71(3):763–769, 2011; discussion 769–770.
22. Saeidiborojeni HR, Moradinazar M, Saeidiborojeni S, et al: A survey on spinal cord injuries resulting from stabbings: a case series study of 12 years' experience. *J Inj Violence Res* 5(1):70–74, 2013.
23. Theodore N, Hadley MN, Aarabi B, et al: Prehospital cervical spinal immobilization after trauma. *Neurosurgery* 72(Suppl 2):22–34, 2013.
24. Sundstrom T, Asbjørnsen H, Habiba S, et al: Prehospital use of cervical collars in trauma patients: a critical review. *J Neurotrauma* 31(6):531–540, 2014.
25. Guly HR, Bouamra O, Lecky FE; Trauma Audit and Research Network: The incidence of neurogenic shock in patients with isolated spinal cord injury in the emergency department. *Resuscitation* 76(1):57–62, 2008.
26. Mallek JT, Inaba K, Branco BC, et al: The incidence of neurogenic shock after spinal cord injury in patients admitted to a high-volume level I trauma center. *Am Surg* 78(5):623–626, 2012.
27. Hoffman JR, Mower WR, Wolfson AB, et al: Validity of a set of clinical criteria to rule out injury to the cervical spine in patients with blunt trauma. National Emergency X-Radiography Utilization Study Group. *N Engl J Med* 343(2):94–99, 2000.
28. Stiell IG, Wells GA, Vandemheen KL, et al: The Canadian C-spine rule for radiography in alert and stable trauma patients. *JAMA* 286(15):1841–1848, 2001.
29. Caron T, Bransford R, Nguyen Q, et al: Spine fractures in patients with ankylosing spinal disorders. *Spine (Phila Pa 1976)* 35(11):E458–E464, 2010.
30. Bozzo A, Marcoux J, Radhakrishna M, et al: The role of magnetic resonance imaging in the management of acute spinal cord injury. *J Neurotrauma* 28(8):1401–1411, 2011.
31. Ryken TC, Hurlbert RJ, Hadley MN, et al: The acute cardiopulmonary management of patients with cervical spinal cord injuries. *Neurosurgery* 72(Suppl 2):84–92, 2013.
32. Casha S, Christie S: A systematic review of intensive cardiopulmonary management after spinal cord injury. *J Neurotrauma* 28(8):1479–1495, 2011.
33. Gupta R, Bathen ME, Smith JS, et al: Advances in the management of spinal cord injury. *J Am Acad Orthop Surg* 18(4):210–222, 2010.
34. Bracken MB, Shepard MJ, Collins WF Jr, et al: Methylprednisolone or naloxone treatment after acute spinal cord injury: 1-year follow-up data.

Results of the second National Acute Spinal Cord Injury Study. *J Neurosurg* 76(1):23–31, 1992.
35. Bracken MB, Holford TR: Effects of timing of methylprednisolone or naloxone administration on recovery of segmental and long-tract neurological function in NASCIS 2. *J Neurosurg* 79(4):500–507, 1993.
36. Bracken MB, Shepard MJ, Collins WF, et al: A randomized, controlled trial of methylprednisolone or naloxone in the treatment of acute spinal-cord injury. Results of the Second National Acute Spinal Cord Injury Study. *N Engl J Med* 322(20):1405–1411, 1990.
37. Hurlbert RJ, Hadley MN, Walters BC, et al: Pharmacological therapy for acute spinal cord injury. *Neurosurgery* 76(Suppl 1):S71–S83, 2015.
38. Pavlica S, Milosevic J, Keller M, et al: Erythropoietin enhances cell proliferation and survival of human fetal neuronal progenitors in normoxia. *Brain Res* 1452:18–28, 2012.
39. Lauweryns P: Role of conservative treatment of cervical spine injuries. *Eur Spine J* 19(Suppl 1):S23–S26, 2010.
40. Rechtine GR, Conrad BP, Bearden BG, et al: Biomechanical analysis of cervical and thoracolumbar spine motion in intact and partially and completely unstable cadaver spine models with kinetic bed therapy or traditional log roll. *J Trauma* 62(2):383–388, 2007; discussion 388.
41. Hagen EM, Faerestrand S, Hoff JM, et al: Cardiovascular and urological dysfunction in spinal cord injury. *Acta Neurol Scand Suppl* (191):71–78, 2011.
42. Hagen EM: Acute complications of spinal cord injuries. *World J Orthop* 6(1):17–23, 2015.
43. Milligan J, Lee J, McMillan C, et al: Autonomic dysreflexia: recognizing a common serious condition in patients with spinal cord injury. *Can Fam Physician* 58(8):831–835, 2012.
44. Maung AA, Schuster KM, Kaplan LJ, et al. Risk of venous thromboembolism after spinal cord injury: not all levels are the same. *J Trauma* 71(5):1241–1245, 2011.
45. Bransford RJ, Chapman JR, Skelly AC, et al: What do we currently know about thoracic spinal cord injury recovery and outcomes? A systematic review. *J Neurosurg Spine* 17(Suppl 1):52–64, 2012.
46. Dhall SS, Hadley MN, Aarabi B, et al: Deep venous thrombosis and thromboembolism in patients with cervical spinal cord injuries. *Neurosurgery* 72(Suppl 2):244–254, 2013.
47. Christie S, Thibault-Halman G, Casha S: Acute pharmacological DVT prophylaxis after spinal cord injury. *J Neurotrauma* 28(8):1509–1514, 2011.
48. O'Boynick CP, Kurd MF, Darden BV 2nd, et al: Timing of surgery in thoracolumbar trauma: is early intervention safe? *Neurosurg Focus* 37(1):E7, 2014.
49. Dimar JR, Carreon LY, Riina J, et al: Early versus late stabilization of the spine in the polytrauma patient. *Spine (Phila Pa 1976)* 35(Suppl 21):S187–S192, 2010.
50. Cengiz SL, Kalkan E, Bayir A, et al: Timing of thoracolomber spine stabilization in trauma patients; impact on neurological outcome and clinical course. A real prospective (rct) randomized controlled study. *Arch Orthop Trauma Surg* 128(9):959–966, 2008.
51. Bellabarba C, Fisher C, Chapman JR, et al: Does early fracture fixation of thoracolumbar spine fractures decrease morbidity or mortality? *Spine (Phila Pa 1976)* 35(Suppl 9):S138–S145, 2010.

Chapter 43 ■ Thoracic and Cardiac Trauma

BRUCE J. SIMON • SCOTT B. JOHNSON • JOHN G. MYERS

INTRODUCTION

Trauma continues to be the leading cause of death in the first four decades of life in the US; 130,000–150,000 deaths per year are trauma associated. Thoracic trauma is responsible for 20% to 25% of these deaths. Two-thirds of thoracic-related deaths occur in the prehospital setting, usually due to significant cardiac, great vessel, or tracheobronchial injuries. In a study of over 1,300 patients presenting to a level I trauma center with thoracic trauma, Kulshrestha and colleagues reported an overall mortality rate of 9.4%, with 56% of these occurring within the initial 24 hours. While the two strongest predictors of mortality were a low GCS and increased age, other factors including penetrating injury, liver or spleen injury, long bone fracture, and more than five rib fractures also predicted in hospital mortality [1]. In a study of trauma-related hospital deaths at an urban level I trauma center, Demetriades and colleagues found that penetrating mechanism, age more than 60, and chest AIS >3 to be significant variables were associated with patients who had no vital signs on admission [2].

Overall, motor vehicle collisions account for 70% to 80% of all thoracic injuries. The incidence of penetrating injuries varies widely but is usually more prevalent in urban centers. The majority of thoracic injuries can be treated with careful observation or tube thoracostomy. It is historically reported that 12% to 15% of patients with thoracic injury will require a thoracotomy. In a Western Trauma Association multicenter review, only 1% of all trauma patients required nonresuscitative thoracotomy [3]. With the improvements in prehospital care and transport, more severely injured patients, who would have previously died at the scene, are arriving at the hospital alive. Success of the management for these injuries rests in having a high index of suspicion for the life-threatening thoracic trauma and prompt recognition and treatment of associated injuries.

INDICATIONS FOR URGENT SURGICAL INTERVENTION

Bleeding

Hemothorax is second only to rib fractures as the most common associated finding of thoracic trauma, being present in approximately 25% of patients with thoracic trauma. Bleeding can arise from the chest wall, lung parenchyma, major thoracic vessels, heart, or diaphragm. A small or moderate-size hemothorax that stops bleeding immediately after placement of a tube thoracostomy and full lung inflation can usually be managed conservatively. However, if the patient continues to bleed at a rate of more than 200 cc per hour, exploration is indicated. In addition, the accumulation of more than 1,500 cc of blood within a pleural space is considered a massive hemothorax that is likely due to larger thoracic vessel injury and is an indication for exploration. If the patient becomes hemodynamically unstable at anytime and an intrathoracic source is suspected, emergent thoracotomy should be performed irrespective of chest tube drainage. A chest radiograph should always be obtained after placing a tube thoracostomy to ensure proper positioning of the tube and complete drainage of the pleural space. Video-assisted thoracoscopic surgery (VATS) can be considered in the stable patient with retained hemothorax or in a stable patient who continues to bleed at a slow but steady rate; however, the surgeon should not hesitate to convert to open thoracotomy if visualization is inadequate or drainage and evacuation of the pleural space is incomplete.

Cardiovascular Collapse

The indications for resuscitative emergency department thoracotomy (EDT) continue to be debated. Penetrating thoracic injuries, specifically stab wounds, have the highest rate of survival. Data for blunt trauma are much less encouraging but should not be used as a deterrent, as there are several functional survivors in most reported series. A retrospective study of 959 patients undergoing resuscitative thoracotomy concluded that EDT in blunt trauma with more than 5 minutes or penetrating trauma with more than 15 minutes of prehospital CPR is futile [4]. A wide range of institutional protocols have been developed. However, evidence indicates that almost all survivors are among the group of patients with penetrating thoracic trauma who have signs of life on arrival [5,6]. These patients generally have not exsanguinated but have a penetrating cardiac injury with tamponade, which can often be treated effectively by drainage of the pericardium and repair of the injury. In general, EDT is not indicated in any patients who have no signs of life or in blunt trauma patients who have only cardiac rhythm without pulses, as these patients have likely exsanguinated. When performed, resuscitative thoracotomy should be done early. Discovered tamponade should be released; massive pulmonary bleeding should be quickly controlled with staplers, clamping, or manual compression, and hemorrhage from cardiac wounds should be controlled. With no intrathoracic source, the aorta should be clamped and internal cardiac massage continued.

Massive Air Leak

Findings on initial presentation of significant subcutaneous emphysema, persistent pneumothorax after chest tube placement, a subsequent large or persistent air leak, or pneumomediastinum should alert the clinician to the presence of major tracheobronchial injury. This injury is potentially lethal but relatively rare, which was found in only 2% to 5% of patients with thoracic trauma. Significant tracheobronchial injuries may result in a massive air leak, leading to hypoventilation. In this situation, maneuvers to stabilize the patient should include decreasing airway pressures to minimize leak. Contralateral mainstem intubation can also be attempted. Major tracheobronchial injuries generally should be repaired as early as the patient's condition allows. For patients who are too unstable for surgery, temporizing measures for ventilator support include high frequency oscillator ventilation and independent lung ventilation [7].

Tamponade

Cardiac tamponade results when fluid or air collects within an intact pericardial sac, resulting in compression of the right heart with subsequent obstruction of venous return and cardiovascular collapse. Potential findings upon presentation include tachycardia and hypotension, cervical cyanosis, jugular venous distension, muffled heart sounds, and pulsus paradoxus. The diagnosis is confirmed with beside ultrasound, pericardial window, or at the time of emergent thoracotomy. Treatment requires prompt resuscitation and decompression of the pericardium, followed by repair of the bleeding source.

DIAGNOSTICS

Diagnostic imaging plays a key role in the management of patients after chest trauma and has a considerable impact on therapeutic decision-making. The chest radiograph (CXR) has traditionally been and remains the initial imaging study of choice to be obtained in patients with suspected chest injury. In many trauma centers, the thoracic component of the bedside ultrasound (extended FAST exam) is preceding the conventional X-ray as an immediate method of identifying pneumothorax and massive hemothorax [8,9]. Computed Tomography (CT) of the chest, however, is commonly used to more accurately identify the nature and severity of chest trauma. CT can be useful in assessing suspected traumatic aortic, pulmonary, airway, skeletal, and diaphragmatic injuries [10,11]. Magnetic resonance imaging (MRI) on the other hand has a limited role in the initial evaluation of any patient with suspected chest trauma. To undergo an MRI, the patient must be stable, and many trauma patients cannot be scanned because of bulky, mechanical supportive equipment. However, in selected patients who are hemodynamically stable, MRI may be particularly useful for the evaluation of vertebral ligamentous injury and spinal cord injury. Other imaging modalities available to the clinician include echocardiography, angiography, and VATS, which can be both diagnostic and therapeutic when appropriately indicated.

Plain Chest Radiograph

The frontal chest radiograph has traditionally been the initial radiographic study to obtain for the evaluation of patients with suspected chest injury. This study is particularly useful for helping to rule out major injury. Ideally, the radiograph should be obtained with the patient in the upright position because of mediastinal widening that is typically seen in the supine position. Chest radiography has a 98% negative predictive value and is therefore quite useful when normal. However, abnormal findings may be subtle and quite nonspecific. Radiographic findings that may indicate mediastinal injury, such as major aortic disruption, include abnormal contour or indistinctness of the aortic knob, apical pleural cap, rightward deviation of the nasogastric tube, thickening of the right paratracheal stripe, downward displacement of the left mainstem bronchus, rightward deviation of the trachea, and, not uncommonly, nonspecific mediastinal widening. Most life-threatening injuries can be screened by the plain chest radiograph and a careful physical exam. Blunt thoracic injuries detected by CT alone infrequently require immediate therapy. Rather, if immediate therapy is needed, findings will usually be visible on plain radiographs or obvious on clinical exam. Although a plain upright chest radiograph remains one of the basic imaging studies routinely performed on initial screening, it may be over-utilized. A recent study suggests that in the presence of a normal physical exam in the hemodynamically stable patient, obtaining a routine chest radiograph is actually unnecessary, since it rarely, if ever, changes clinical care [12].

Chest Computed Tomography

CT is highly sensitive in detecting thoracic injuries after blunt chest trauma and is superior to routine CXR for visualizing lung contusions, pneumothorax, and hemothorax, and it can often alter initial therapeutic management for a significant number of patients with suspected chest trauma. It has also been shown to detect unexpected injuries and abnormalities, resulting in altered management in a substantial number of patients when applied appropriately [13]. It can be particularly useful in screening for major intrathoracic aortic injury. In one study, contrast-enhanced CT scanning ("CT angiogram") was 100% sensitive in detecting major thoracic aortic injury based on clinical follow-up and was 99.7% specific, with 89% positive and 100% negative predictive values for an overall diagnostic accuracy of 99.7% [14]. An unequivocally normal mediastinum at CT, with no hematoma and a regular aorta surrounded by a normal fat pad, has essentially a 100% negative predictive value for aortic injury [14–17]. It has also been shown that CT scanning detects 11% of thoracic aortic injuries that are not detected by routine, plain chest radiography alone [18].

CT scanning can also be useful for detecting hemopericardium and/or hemothorax from any cause, injury to the brachiocephalic vessels, pneumothorax, rib fractures, pulmonary parenchymal contusion, and sternal fractures. It can also be useful for detecting pneumomediastinum caused by interstitial lung injury, bronchial or tracheal rupture (commonly associated with pneumothorax), esophageal rupture, iatrogenic barotrauma from mechanical ventilation, or traumatic intubation. In addition, CT scanning can detect injuries otherwise missed by routine plain radiograph. In one study comparing CT scanning with plain radiography, CT scanning detected serious injuries among 65% of those patients not found to have injury by plain film. These injuries included (in decreasing order of frequency) lung contusions, pneumothoraces, hemothoraces, diaphragmatic ruptures, and myocardial rupture [19]. Even for patients without suspected chest trauma, CT scanning of the abdomen, which commonly includes the lower portion of the thorax, often yields important information when intrathoracic injury is present. In one study, hematoma surrounding the intrathoracic aorta near the level of the diaphragmatic crura seen on intra-abdominal CT scanning was found to be a relatively insensitive but highly specific sign for thoracic aortic injury after blunt trauma. Therefore, the presence of this sign seen on abdominal CT imaging should prompt more specific imaging of the thoracic aorta to evaluate potential thoracic aortic injury [20]. CT scanning has also been shown to be useful to help define the extent of pulmonary contusion and identify patients at high risk for acute respiratory failure among patients with PaO_2/FiO_2 lower than 300. Digitally processed 3-D reconstruction views from CT scans have also been shown to be useful for diagnosing and determining the severity of sternal fractures [21]. With the advent of high resolution CT scanners that can reconstruct axial, coronal, and sagittal images, even penetrating diaphragmatic injuries, which are difficult to image preoperatively, can be diagnosed with a relatively high sensitivity and specificity [22]. Despite its usefulness, thoracic CT scanning is not routinely indicated for all patients with chest wall trauma. In addition, although there has been a dramatic increase in the utilization of CT scanning in the last decade, its usefulness for detecting clinically relevant injury has recently come into question, especially for patients with a normal screening plain chest radiograph [23].

Ultrasonography (Extended FAST Exam and TEE)

Over the last 10 years, the traditional Focused Abdominal Sonogram for Trauma or "FAST" exam has evolved to include bedside assessment for thoracic injuries and is now referred to as the extended FAST exam or "eFAST." This modality can provide immediate real-time assessment for pneumothorax by looking for secondary signs of lung inflation such as "sliding" of pleural surfaces and "comet tails" artifacts at the visceral pleura [8,9]. In some situations, the eFAST lung exam obviates the need for a screening chest X-ray, particularly when the patient is to have a chest CT scan. eFAST can also identify large hemothoraces and can assess the pericardium, identifying hemopericardium and tamponade. The results from eFAST are operator dependent with a significant learning curve. However, the results are reproduceable among those trained to use the modality and this has become part of the trauma armamentarium at most centers.

Transesophageal echocardiography (TEE) is rapidly gaining acceptance as an important diagnostic tool available to the trauma surgeon and is showing particular promise in diagnosing traumatic intrathoracic aortic injuries. Although somewhat invasive, its portability makes it a diagnostic procedure of choice in looking at the heart and great vessels in multiply injured trauma patients particularly in the operating room setting. In one study of 58 patients with thoracic trauma, TEE demonstrated its usefulness in diagnosing thoracic aortic injury and permitted the identification of small lesions not detectable by CT scanning or angiography [24]. TEE has shown to be an important diagnostic tool for examining the thoracic aorta and is valuable for identifying aortic injury among high-risk trauma patients who are too unstable to undergo transport to the aortography suite. When an aortic injury is present, typical findings on the TEE can include aortic wall hematomas, intimal flaps, or disruptions. Several groups have shown TEE to be accurate for identifying aortic pathology after trauma, with its diagnostic efficacy mainly limited by the experience of the person performing the exam [25–27]. In addition, it has been shown to be useful for diagnosing blunt cardiac rupture, when other diagnostic modalities have failed, as well as in diagnosing severe valvular regurgitation intraoperatively following foreign body removal [28,29].

Angiography

Thoracic aortography historically has been the gold standard for diagnosing thoracic aortic injury and for defining the extent of the injury and involvement of branch disease, when it is present. Aortography has largely been supplanted by dynamic thin-cut contrast CT scaning or CT angiography [11]. This modality involves a rapid high-resolution CT scan with timed contrast injection and subsequent computerized processing of the study. The accuracy of this study and its specificity in defining the anatomy of the aortic injury has made it more than adequate for planning surgical or endovascular interventions. Aortography is occasionally required for the rare situation when CT scan is equivocal. Diagnosis of aortic injury angiographically is usually made by finding one or more of the following: an irregular or discontinued contour of the aortic lumen, an intimal flap, an aortic dissection, and/or a luminal outpouching (i.e., pseudoaneurysm). Thoracic aortography can detect blunt traumatic aortic injuries with 96% sensitivity and 98% specificity. Angiography is invasive and can have associated complications. The complications associated with arteriography include allergic reactions, renal failure, local puncture site problems, stroke, and even death. Radiographic contrast media cause severe anaphylactic reactions in less than 2% of cases.

Video-Assisted Thoracoscopic Surgery (VATS)

The role of thoracoscopy in trauma has been explored by a number of investigators. Prior to the modern video era, Jones et al. described management of 36 patients with thoracoscopy under local anesthesia as a diagnostic tool to define intrathoracic injuries and to visualize ongoing hemorrhage [30]. Four patients in their series were spared abdominal exploration when the diaphragm was found devoid of injury. More recently, Ochsner et al. [31] and Mealy et al. have demonstrated the usefulness of VATS as a diagnostic tool for the assessment of diaphragmatic integrity among cases of penetrating and blunt thoracic injuries, respectively [32]. VATS has become an acceptable surgical modality in the diagnostic evaluation of suspected diaphragmatic injury and has been shown to have therapeutic benefit when evacuation of clotted hemothoraces is able to be performed in stable patients with penetrating chest injures [33]. Main indications for VATS include diagnosis of and treatment for diaphragmatic injuries, diagnosis of persistent hemorrhage, management of retained thoracic collections, assessment of cardiac and mediastinal structures, diagnosis of bronchopleural fistulas, and diagnosis of and treatment for persistent posttraumatic pneumothorax. In these situations, VATS has been shown to be a useful alternative to an open thoracotomy for selected patients. In select situations, VATS has been used as the primarily modality of treatment for acute traumatic thoracic hemorrhage meeting the criteria for thoracotomy among hemodynamically stable patients [34]. Because lung deflation with single-lung ventilation is a critical component of the technique, VATS is relatively contraindicated in patients unable to tolerate this. Caution should be used in patients with suspected obliteration to their pleural cavity secondary to previous infection ("pleurisy") or surgery. VATS should have no role in the management of unstable patients and is relatively contraindicated in those patients unable to tolerate formal thoracotomy for any reason. Whether VATS should be considered as the initial approach in the evaluation of all stable chest trauma patients when an intrathoracic injury is suspected is still debated, and appropriate patient selection remains important.

SPECIFIC INJURIES

Chest Wall

Rib Fractures

Rib fractures are the most common injury to the thorax occurring from blunt trauma and are often associated with other injuries. Rib fractures themselves may cause only minor problems in the young and otherwise healthy; however, they may be a marker of more severe injury, and it may be the underlying pulmonary contusion that often accompanies the rib fracture that may be more clinically relevant. A study by Flagel et al. showed that 13% of those patients in the National Trauma Data Bank who had one or more rib fractures ($n = 64{,}750$) developed complications including pneumonia, acute respiratory distress syndrome, pulmonary embolus, pneumothorax, aspiration pneumonia, empyema, and the need for mechanical ventilation. They also showed that increasing number of rib fractures correlated directly with increasing pulmonary morbidity and mortality. The overall mortality rate for patients with rib fractures was 10%. The mortality rates were higher ($p < 0.02$) with each additional rib fracture, independent of patient age. This ranged from 5.8% for a single rib fracture to 10% in the case of five fractured ribs. The mortality rates were dramatically higher for the groups with 6, 7, and 8 or more fractured ribs to 11.4%, 15.0%, and 34.4%, respectively [35]. It has been shown that rib fractures occurring in the very young should alert the clinician to possible nonaccidental trauma (NAT). In one study by Barsness et al., rib fractures in children under 3 years of age had a positive predictive value of NAT of 95%, and rib fracture was the only skeletal manifestation of NAT in 29% of the children [36]. With regards to the elderly, it has been shown that there is a linear relationship between age and complications, including mortality. It has been shown that elderly patients with rib fractures have up to twice the mortality of younger patients with similar injuries [37]. In addition, this increase in mortality may begin to be seen in patients as early as 45 years of age when more than four ribs are involved [38]. The location of the rib fracture(s) is also important, as it has been shown that left-sided rib fractures are associated with splenic injuries and right-sided rib fractures are associated with liver injuries. While isolated rib fractures have an associated incidence of vascular injury of only 3%, first rib fractures in association with multiple rib fractures have a 24% incidence of associated vascular injury. A first rib fracture along with findings of a widened mediastinum, upper extremity pulse deficit, brachial plexus injury, and/or expanding hematoma should prompt work-up for a possible subclavian arterial injury.

Pain control and effective respiratory secretion clearance remain the mainstays of therapy for rib fractures. Adequacy of pain control can be monitored by the ability to perform incentive spirometry. Regional analgesia by epidural or paraspinal catheter is appropriate when narcotics are inadequate to allow adequate lung volumes or are accompanied by unacceptable levels of sedation, particularly among the elderly [39–41]. In Flagel's study noted above, epidural analgesia was associated with a reduction in mortality for all patients sustaining rib fractures, particularly those with more than four fractures [35]. Since this was not a prospective randomized study, it is difficult to tell if there was a correlation between patients that received epidural catheters having an overall lower injury severity score. However, in one prospective randomized trial by Bulger et al., trauma patients with rib fractures were randomized to either receive epidural anesthesia or intravenous opioids for pain relief, and it was shown that those patients with epidural anesthesia had a lower incidence of nosocomial pneumonia and shorter duration of mechanical ventilation [42]. The number of patients that could receive epidural anesthesia was limited, however, due to strict inclusion criteria. The age of the patient sustaining rib fractures should be taken into account, as well as the location of the fractures. In many protocols, patients with multiple rib fractures and a certain age threshold, anywhere from 55 to 65 years, receive an epidural analgesia proactively as their preferred modality of pain control [39–41].

Flail Chest

Flail chest occurs when multiple adjacent ribs are broken in two locations, thereby allowing that portion of the chest wall to move independently of respiration. The anatomic definition of flail chest is the fracture of at least three consecutive ribs in two or more places; however, the clinical or functional definition requires a disjointed, "free-floating" segment of chest wall, which does not contribute to normal ventilatory excursion. This gives rise to the classical "paradoxical respiration" whereby the flail segment is "sucked inward" by the negative pressure of inspiration as the rest of the rib cage moves upward and outward. This is a mechanical problem in which negative pressure generated during inspiration within the thorax is dissipated by movement of the flail segment inward. This movement equalizes the intrathoracic pressure, which would normally be accomplished by the movement of air into the lungs. Despite this mechanical impairment, the major mortality and morbidity of flail chest can be attributed to the usual underlying pulmonary contusion, which leads to a ventilation perfusion mismatch, contributing to the hypoxia; the pain associated with multiple rib fractures can lead to splinting and contribute to lack of deep breathing, atelectasis, compromised secretion clearance, and further hypoxemia. Fortunately, large segment flail chest occurs relatively infrequently. Flagel et al. showed an overall incidence of flail chest of 3.95% in patients with six rib fractures, 4.84% in those with seven rib fractures, and 6.42% in those with eight or more rib fractures [35].

As for simple rib fracture, pain control remains the main therapy for flail chest so as to allow optimal ventilatory excursion and self-clearance of respiratory secretions" by deep breathing and coughing. Obligatory ventilatory support "internal pneumatic stabilization" of the fractures, first described in 1956, has given a way to selective ventilatory support as needed, with subsequent improved outcomes [42–45]. Surgical stabilization of the chest wall has been shown to be of some benefit with regard to shorter length of ventilator dependency, lower rates of pneumonia, and shorter intensive care unit stays, although this form of therapy is not yet widely practiced [46,47]. A number of proprietary systems for rib fracture fixation have been developed after biomechanical studies of the stresses on ribs *en vivo* (i.e., Rib-Loc, Acute Innovations, Hillsboro, OR, USA; Biomet System, Jacksonville FLa., USA). The benefits and appropriate indications for rib fracture repair remain to be fully defined. Pain control continues to be an important adjunct in any treatment regimen.

Sternal Fracture

Sternal fractures have been shown to decrease the stability of the thorax in cadavers [48]. They usually occur as a deceleration force during traffic accidents together with blunt force trauma from foreign objects, such as steering wheels, although they have been reported as a complication of CPR, which interestingly was found in 14% of medical autopsy cases that had received chest compressions prior to death [49]. Traffic accidents are the cause of sternal fractures in almost 90% of cases, with approximately 25% of fractures graded as moderately to severely displaced. Approximately 30% of patients will have associated injuries, with craniocerebral trauma and rib fractures being the most commonly associated injuries [50]. Displaced fractures are more likely to have associated thoracic and cardiac injuries and are more likely to require surgical fixation.

However, the majority of patients can be safely observed and even discharged home as long as the following criteria are met: (1) the injury is not one of the high-velocity impacts, (2) the fracture is not severely displaced, (3) there are no clinically significant associated injuries, and (4) complex analgesia is not required. Most serious complications and deaths that occur among patients with sternal fractures are not due to the fracture itself but rather are related to the associated injuries, such as flail chest, head injury, or pulmonary or cardiac contusion. Although approximately 22% of patients will exhibit electrocardiographic changes, elevated cardiac injury enzymes, or echocardiographic abnormalities, only approximately 6% of patients will exhibit a clinically significant myocardial contusion. In addition to myocardial contusion, other complications of sternal fracture such as mediastinal abscess, mediastinitis, and acute tamponade have all been reported. Indications for operative sternal fixation are certainly not absolute and should be judged individually. Generally accepted criteria include severe pain, sternal instability causing respiratory compromise, and severe displacement. Only a small percentage of patients (2% in one series) actually require sternal fixation [51]. A lack of consensus among surgeons on how to treat these injuries, in addition to a lack of randomized trials concerning their optimal approach, have led to this variability of practice.

Scapular Fracture

Scapular fractures are relatively rare and were once presumed to be an indicator of severe underlying trauma and subsequent higher mortality. They occur in only approximately 1% to 4% of blunt trauma patients who present to a level I trauma center and are associated with a higher incidence of thoracic injury compared to those patients who sustain blunt trauma without a scapular fracture. However, more recent studies have indicated that although patients with scapular fractures tend to have more severe chest injuries and a higher overall injury severity score, their length of intensive care unit stay, length of hospital stay, and overall mortality are not necessarily increased [52,53]. Treatment is usually conservative and, most of the time, aimed at the associated injuries that are commonly present.

Scapulothoracic Dissociation

Scapulothoracic dissociation is an infrequent injury with a potentially devastating outcome. Scapulothoracic dissociation results from massive traction injury to the anterolateral shoulder girdle with disruption of the scapulothoracic articulation. Identification of this injury requires a degree of clinical suspicion, based upon the injury mechanism and physical findings. Assessment of the degree of trauma to the musculoskeletal, neurologic, and vascular structures should be made. Based upon clinical findings, a rational diagnostic approach can be navigated and appropriate surgical intervention planned. Scapulothoracic dissociation is frequently associated with acromioclavicular separation, a displaced clavicular fracture, subclavian or axillary vascular disruption, and a sternoclavicular disruption. Clinically, patients usually present with a laterally displaced scapula, a flail extremity, an absent brachial pulse, and massive swelling of the shoulder. Vascular injury occurs in 88% of patients and severe neurologic injuries occur in 94% of patients. Many of these patients have poor outcomes and present with a flail, flaccid extremity that usually results in early amputation and have an overall mortality of 10%. One of the most devastating aspects of scapulothoracic dissociation is the brachial plexus injuries that occur, which are typically proximal, involving the roots and cords—brachial plexus avulsions are not unusual. Attempts at repair of complete brachial plexus injuries with grafts or nerve transfers have generally been unsuccessful [54]. Treatment includes arterial and venous ligation to stop exsanguination if present, orthopedic stabilization and consideration for elective above elbow amputation to allow for a more useful extremity if brachial plexus avulsion is present. Overall prognosis for limb recovery is poor.

Pleural Space

Pneumothorax

This section will only focus on pneumothoraces associated with trauma. For further general discussion of pneumothorax in the critically ill, readers are referred to Chapter 176. For in depth discussion of imaging studies on the topic of pneumothorax, readers are referred to Chapters 11 and 179. A traumatic pneumothorax occurs from either blunt or penetrating trauma, with resultant direct injury to the pleura. Rib fractures may or may not be present. Mechanical ventilation can also be considered a traumatic cause of pneumothorax and has an overall associated incidence of 5%. This incidence increases dramatically in patients with underlying lung diseases, such as COPD or acute respiratory distress syndrome (ARDS). Iatrogenic causes of pneumothorax also occur in the hospital setting. Central-line insertions are associated with a 3% to 6% incidence of pneumothorax.

All types of pneumothorax may progress to tension pneumothorax, which occurs in 1% to 3% of spontaneous pneumothoraces and can occur at any stage of treatment. As tension pneumothorax is a rapidly progressive condition, early identification is essential and immediate decompression should be performed when the clinical suspicion is high.

Tension pneumothorax is a clinical diagnosis, and treatment should never be delayed to obtain a confirmatory X-ray. Open pneumothorax is caused when a penetrating chest injury opens the pleural space to the atmosphere. Negative pressure cannot be generated to inflate the lung on inspiration, leading to a collapsed lung and a "sucking" chest wound. Open pneumothorax is an injury commonly seen on the battlefield. In civilian life, impalement by an object is a common cause. For injuries in which the chest wall wound diameter approaches two-thirds of the diameter of the trachea, air will preferentially enter the pleural space through the wound during inspiration, thereby inhibiting normal ventilation through the upper airway, leading to profound hypoventilation and subsequent hypoxia. Changes in venous return can occur similar to that seen in a tension pneumothorax because the injured side is now at atmospheric pressure, while the normal side has negative pressure, creating a mediastinal shift. This in turn can lead to hemodynamic instability. The presence of a "sucking" chest wound makes the diagnosis obvious. External wound size may not correlate with the degree of compromise, as it is the size of the atmospheric-pleural connection that correlates best.

Treatment includes appropriate resuscitative maneuvers, starting with the placement of a sterile occlusive dressing over the wound to allow effective negative pressure ventilation to resume. If this does not suffice, intubation and positive pressure mechanical ventilation may be necessary to correct the ventilatory and hemodynamic dysfunction. A standard method of coverage involves placing a nonporous dressing over the wound and taping it on three sides, allowing it to act as a one-way valve, allowing air to escape during expiration but occlusive during negative pressure inspiration. A chest tube is routinely inserted at a separate site away from the injury to treat any ongoing air leak that might arise from concurrent lung injury. The wound should be treated with local measures and associated injuries should be sought and treated appropriately.

Hemothorax

After rib fractures, hemothorax is the second most common complication of chest trauma. It can be caused by bleeding from anywhere in the chest cavity, including the chest wall, lung parenchyma, major thoracic vessels, heart, or diaphragm. It presents in approximately 25% of patients with chest trauma. Patients with hemothorax typically have decreased breath sounds and dullness to percussion over the affected side with associated dyspnea and tachypnea. Depending on the amount of blood loss, they may have hemodynamic changes. The major cause of significant hemothorax is usually due to a laceration to the lung or bleeding from an injured intercostal vessel or internal mammary artery. Radiographic films may not reveal a fluid collection of less than 300 mL. Small hemothoraces usually resolve within few days. Accumulation of more than 1,500 mL of blood within a pleural space is considered massive, is more commonly seen on the left side, and is usually due to aortic rupture (blunt trauma) or pulmonary hilar or major vessel injury (penetrating trauma). Severe blunt trauma where highly displaced rib fracture fragments puncture deep into the lung parenchyma may also lead to a massive hemothorax. Massive hemothorax can lead to hemodynamic instability including hypotension and circulatory collapse. Neck veins may be flat or distended, depending on whether or not blood loss or increased intrathoracic pressure predominates. A mediastinal shift with tracheal deviation is typically opposite from the side of blood accumulation.

Treatment for acute hemothorax includes supplemental oxygen therapy and, in most cases, the insertion of a large bore (i.e., 32 to 36 French) tube thoracostomy anterior to the midaxillary line at the fifth or sixth intercostal space. A moderate-size hemothorax (500 to 1,500 mL) that stops bleeding immediately after a tube thoracostomy can usually be managed conservatively with a closed drainage system. Bleeding from pulmonary parenchymal injuries that do not involve the hilum usually will stop spontaneously because of the low pulmonary pressures and high concentrations of tissue thromboplastin within the lung [55]. If, however, the patient continues to bleed at a rate of 100 to 200 mL per hour, then exploration is indicated. Likewise, if the patient bleeds out more than 1,500 mL initially through the chest tube, exploration is indicated. VATS exploration has been successfully utilized to control acute thoracic bleeding in patients who are stable [34]. If the patient is hemodynamically unstable at any time, and intrathoracic bleeding is suspected as the cause, emergent thoracotomy should be done regardless of chest tube output. A chest radiograph should always be obtained after placing a tube thoracostomy to check position of the tube and to make sure that the pleural space is adequately drained.

Once the patient is stable and acute bleeding has ceased, retained hemothorax may still be a problem when a large amount of retained blood and clot remains within the pleural space for 24 to 48 hours after tube thoracostomy, semielective exploration with open evacuation should be considered. VATS is an option for the stable patient with retained hemothorax. However, the surgeon should not hesitate to convert to an open thoracotomy if visualization is inadequate or drainage and evacuation of the pleural space is incomplete. If the retained hemothorax is not massive, nonoperative therapy can be considered as these may lyse with time. Alternatively, it has been shown that a retained hemothorax can be successfully treated with instillation of thrombolytics into the pleural space. This has been deemed safe even for patients who have sustained multiple trauma [56]. However, the use of thrombolytics for trauma patients remains debated with some reports of reactivation of thoracic bleeding after instillation of thrombolytics into the pleural space.

Lung

Pulmonary Contusion

Pulmonary contusion is a common injury found among patients sustaining blunt chest trauma, with an approximate incidence of 30% to 75%. Mortality is between 10% and 25%. Hemorrhage and interstitial edema result from injury to the lung. This can lead to alveolar collapse and the typical parenchymal consolidation seen on the radiograph. Injury to the parenchyma from blunt force trauma is thought to be caused by a combination of events that includes alveolar stretching, parenchymal tearing, and concussive forces. Lung injury in the absence of identifiable rib fractures typically exhibits diffuse injury, whereas rib fractures and flail chest are associated with more localized injuries. The extravasation of blood into the alveolar space causes subsequent consolidation, which can then lead to an intrapulmonary shunt. A flail chest may be associated with pulmonary contusion(s) approximately three-fourths of the time, which more than doubles the morbidity and mortality. Hypoxemia, although nonspecific, is the most common clinical finding associated with pulmonary contusions. Typical chest radiographic findings in the appropriate clinical setting remain the mainstay of diagnosis. Typical findings usually demonstrate a focal or diffuse consolidative process that does not typically follow anatomical segments or lobes. Rib fractures are the most common bony injuries seen and should raise suspicion for the diagnosis of pulmonary contusion, even if other clinical signs are absent at the time. While the respiratory effects of pulmonary contusion may occur soon after injury, they may not become radiographically apparent for up to 48 hours postinjury, with an average delay of 6 hours. On the other hand, CT scanning of the chest has been shown to be able to demonstrate the presence of pulmonary contusion almost immediately postinjury [57–60]. In addition, it can help estimate the total volume of injured lung present. This can be helpful for predicting the need for eventual ventilatory support. It has been shown that when pulmonary contusion involves 28% or more of the total lung volume, essentially all patients eventually require mechanical ventilation, whereas when 18% or less of the lung volume is involved, the need for mechanical ventilatory support is unlikely [61]. Treatment for pulmonary contusion is generally supportive. Close respiratory monitoring and frequent clinical examination is important, as approximately half of all respiratory failures secondary to pulmonary contusion occur within the first few hours postinjury. Once coexistent injuries are treated, and the need for emergent surgery is ruled out or performed as required, the patient with pulmonary contusion should be transferred to a monitored bed. Optimal respiratory secretion clearance should be employed and may be achieved through several mechanisms, including airway suctioning, chest physiotherapy, and postural drainage. This helps to minimize atelectasis and clear respiratory secretions. If patients are still unable to clear their secretions adequately, bronchoscopy can be helpful. Adequate analgesia for associated chest wall injuries is also important for maintaining adequate secretion clearance as the effects of the contusions and chest wall injuries are additive. Pain control can be achieved through systemic opioids or regional analgesia. Preferred methods of regional analgesia include nerve blocks, and epidural or paravertebral catheters. Inadequate analgesia as determined by low vital capacity (<15 mL per kg in otherwise healthy individual) or oversedation from opipods are indications for regional analgesia [39–41] (see section "Rib Fractures" above). Mechanical ventilation can minimize edema and increase functional residual capacity, which in turn can decrease shunt and reduce hypoxemia. Positioning patients with the injured lung in the nondependent position may also improve oxygenation, especially in those patients refractory to other measures. Fluid administration should be done judiciously, as hypervolemia may worsen fluid extravasation into the alveolar spaces and increase parenchymal consolidation, because capillary permeability is already compromised. However, under-resuscitation should also be avoided, as this may lead to thickened secretions and possible systemic effects if hypovolemia occurs. Obviously, fluid administration in these patients can be a difficult balancing act, and good clinical judgment is important. Positive end expiratory pressure (PEEP) should be maintained at the minimum value necessary to ensure adequate oxygenation, because excessive PEEP may actually worsen gas exchange and can actually extend the area of injury. Atelectasis can allow to bacterial growth that can lead to pneumonia, which typically develops several days after the injury. Pulmonary infections may develop in up to 50% of patients with pulmonary contusions. While used by some, diuresis has not been shown to decrease hypoxia or ventilator days in pulmonary contusion when cardiogenic pulmonary edema is not concurrent. Acute respiratory distress syndrome (ARDS) can complicate pulmonary contusion in 5% to 20% of cases, and respiratory dysfunction is a common sequela. Dyspnea may affect as many as 90% of patients during the first 6 months postinjury. In addition, functional reserve capacity has been found to be diminished as late as 4 years after injury, with the majority of patients demonstrating subtle changes on CT [62].

Tracheobronchial Injury/Lung Laceration

Tracheobronchial injury can be a challenge to diagnose, manage, and definitively treat. The true incidence of tracheobronchial injury is difficult to establish, as a large proportion (30% to 80%) of these patients will die before reaching the hospital. It is estimated on the basis of autopsy reports that 2.5% to 3.2% of patients who die as a result of trauma may have associated tracheobronchial injury [63,64]. More than 80% of tracheobronchial injury due to blunt trauma is located within 2.5 cm of the carina. Resuscitation of a patient with tracheobronchial injury can be difficult, since obtaining adequate ventilation may require novel approaches to securing the airway. Patients with tracheal or bronchial injuries make this initial assessment particularly challenging. The majority of patients with tracheobronchial injury seen in the emergency department have some degree of respiratory difficulty and require emergent measures to secure and control the airway, but some may have an initially innocuous presentation with subtle signs. However, several abnormalities can alert the physician to the diagnosis. Tachypnea and subcutaneous emphysema are common. Pneumothorax may or may not be seen on a plain radiograph. The liberal use of bronchoscopy is mandatory for identifying tracheobronchial injuries and constitutes the gold standard in diagnosis. Findings that can typically be seen on bronchoscopy include obstruction of the airway with blood and inability to visualize the more distal lobar bronchi because of collapsed proximal bronchi. Visualization of a bronchial tear is confirmatory.

Orotracheal intubation is the most common method used for airway control. If possible, the intubation should be done over a fiber optic bronchoscope so that the injury can be identified, avoided, and clearly bypassed with the endotracheal tube. It should be noted that merely identifying the glottic opening and vocal cords does not ensure proper placement of the endotracheal tube as there may be complete discontinuity distally. Patients with cervical injuries and open neck wounds can be intubated through the open wound to secure the airway if necessary.

Associated injuries are common and are usually related to the mechanism and location of the tracheobronchial injury. The injury most commonly associated with penetrating tracheobronchial injury is esophageal perforation. Most repairs of cervical tracheal injuries are approached through a collar incision. For patients with injuries high in the mediastinal trachea or with suspected great-vessel injury, a median sternotomy may be necessary. When the injury is associated with a unilateral pneumothorax or a bronchial injury is diagnosed preoperatively, an ipsilateral posterolateral thoracotomy is the incision of choice. For injuries to the mediastinal trachea, an approach by a right posterolateral thoracotomy (usually high through the fourth intercostal space) is reasonable. Since the initial report by Shaw and colleagues, primary repair of the injured tracheobronchial tree has been encouraged [63,65–69]. Most patients can undergo primary repair of their tracheobronchial injury using tailored surgical techniques specific to the injury. When a major bronchus is disrupted, lobectomy is the preferred method of treatment, with closure of the bronchial stump debrided back to healthy tissue. With injuries to the mainstem bronchi, primary repair is preferred over pneumonectomy whenever possible, due to the higher mortality associated with pneumonectomy, especially in the trauma setting. Injury to the trachea can be either primarily repaired or converted to a tracheostomy if necessary for airway control. Nonoperative management of tracheobronchial injury has been reported to be successful in selected cases. Those patients that seem most appropriate for this approach are those with membranous injuries. Patients that have cartilaginous injuries are more likely to require operative repair. Tracheobronchial injury encompasses a heterogeneous group of injuries that requires skillful airway management, careful diagnostic evaluation, and operative repairs that are often creative and necessarily unique to the given injury.

Heart

Blunt Cardiac Injury

Blunt cardiac injury, formerly referred to as myocardial contusion, is now recognized as a continuum of injury from minor contusion through fatal cardiac rupture [70–73]. Most blunt cardiac injuries are not serious. However, moderately severe cardiac injuries may cause arrhythmias or result in low-output cardiac failure. The clinical significance of myocardial contusion following blunt thoracic trauma is still largely unknown. In one study by Lindstaedt et al., approximately 20% of patients who were admitted to a surgical intensive care unit because of their injuries met the criteria for diagnosis of myocardial contusion [74]. Their criteria include exclusion of pathologic findings on ECG known to be present prior to injury; echocardiographic evidence of a kinetic wall motion abnormalities; combination of regional wall motion abnormality, significant isoenzyme elevation (CK-MB > 7%), and ECG abnormality; regional wall motion abnormality in the baseline echocardiogram and in the control echocardiogram at follow-up; or confirmation of myocardial contusion at autopsy or intraoperatively. Even though the prevalence of the injury was significant in their population, the overall prognosis was excellent, and the authors recommend that specific diagnostic and therapeutic measures should be limited to cases where cardiac complications develop. The combination of a normal ECG and normal serum troponin levels, drawn at the time of presentation and 8 hours later, essentially rules out significant myocardial contusion and is sufficient, in the absence of other reasons for hospitalization, to discharge such patients safely home [75]. However, patients with an abnormal ECG and elevated troponin should be monitored for at least 24 hours. Cardiac contusion may lead to cardiogenic shock resistant to inotropic support. The use of intra-aortic balloon counterpulsation as a mechanical means of augmenting cardiac function following cardiac contusion is rarely indicated but has been reported with success even in elderly patients [76].

At the other end of the severity spectrum, high energy injuries to the heart can result in cardiac rupture. Atrial and/or ventricular rupture can occur, leading to profound hemodynamic compromise. Rapid recognition of such injuries is necessary for successful treatment. Associated injuries are common and include closed head injury, pulmonary contusion and/or laceration, multiple rib fractures, liver and spleen injury, and traumatic aortic injury; these account for approximately 25% of fatalities seen in patients after blunt cardiac injury. The usual clinical presentation of cardiac rupture is cardiac tamponade secondary to hemopericardium, although less than 15% of these patients actually manifest physiological evidence of tamponade. Associated pericardial tears may allow for decompression of intrapericardial hemorrhage through the pleural space, preventing the development of cardiac tamponade but leading to exsanguinating hemothorax. Pericardial rupture is rare, but can occur in isolation or with associated injuries such as blunt cardiac or diaphragmatic rupture, which has a high mortality. Hypotension is usually present, and the diagnosis of cardiac rupture should be considered in any patient who has hypotension in the absence of overt blood loss. The chest radiograph may not show evidence of cardiac injury, even in the face of tamponade and hemodynamic compromise, since a rapid accumulation of blood into the pericardial space can occur without significantly altering the cardiac silhouette. The Extended FAST ultrasound exam can be useful in diagnosing pericardial tamponade. Diagnosis of blunt cardiac rupture should be strongly suspected when hemopericardium is seen by ultrasound in the setting of blunt trauma. The diagnostic dependability of pericardiocentesis is limited in the assessment of traumatic hemopericardium and potential cardiac rupture because of significant false-negative and false-positive results. Performing a pericardial window in the operating room, however, can be both diagnostic and therapeutic, and it can confirm hemopericardium and allow for rapid decompression and median sternotomy. Nevertheless, the diagnosis of blunt cardiac rupture requires a fair degree of clinical suspicion, particularly in the setting of hypotension that does not respond to adequate volume resuscitation. Perchinsky et al. reviewed a consecutive series of 27 patients seen between 1984 and 1993 with blunt cardiac rupture. Overall survival rate was 41%. Of note was that three out of nine (33%) patients presenting to the emergency department with no identifiable blood pressure or viable electrical heart rhythm survived resuscitation, surgery, and initial hospital care. No patient survived rupture of two or more cardiac chambers in their series, however [77]. Although cardiac exploration should be performed with cardiopulmonary bypass support nearby, repair of cardiac rupture does not necessarily require its use.

Cardiac Valvular Injuries

Blunt cardiac injury may rarely result in valvular insufficiency. The right ventricle is immediately behind the sternum, which makes it particularly vulnerable to injury. Acute severe elevation of right intraventricular pressures has been shown to result in injury of the tricuspid valvular apparatus [71,78]. The most common injury is chordal rupture, followed by rupture of the anterior papillary muscle and leaflet tears. Posttraumatic aortic valve regurgitation has also been reported and affects all ages and is often found in association with sternal or multiple rib fractures [79]. Traumatic mitral valve insufficiency has been shown to present with either complete papillary muscle avulsion from its ventricular attachment or with chordal tears and/or leaflet damage. Those with papillary muscle avulsion typically present with severe regurgitation. Those patients with less severe injuries to the mitral valve, such as chordal tears and/or leaflet damage, usually present with less severe symptoms and may even be asymptomatic. Not only can blunt cardiac injury cause acute valvular incompetence, but it can also predispose patients to delayed valvular dysfunction. In a study performed by Ismailov et al. looking at hospital patient discharges, patients who sustained blunt cardiac injury had an associated 12-fold increased risk for developing tricuspid valve insufficiency and a 3.4-fold increased risk of developing aortic valvular insufficiency later in life, which appeared to be independent of age, race, sex, and injury severity score [80]. There was no correlation found with increased risk for mitral valve insufficiency, however. Traumatic valve insufficiency, depending on severity and valve involved, may necessitate surgical treatment.

Penetrating Cardiac Injury

The clinical presentation of penetrating cardiac injury ranges from one of hemodynamic stability to complete cardiopulmonary arrest. Beck's Triad represents the classical presentation of the patient arriving in the emergency department in pericardial tamponade and includes venous hypertension with distended neck veins, arterial hypotension, and muffled heart sounds. Kussmaul's sign: jugular venous distention seen with expiration is another classic sign attributed to pericardial tamponade, though it may not necessarily be appreciated in the acute trauma setting. The physiology of pericardial tamponade is related to the relative inelastic and noncompliant pericardium. Sudden acute loss of intracardiac blood volume into the pericardial sac leads to an acute pressure rise and compression of the thin-walled right ventricle and atria. This decreases the heart's ability to fill, resulting in decreased left ventricular filling and ejection fraction, thus decreasing cardiac output. Subxiphoid pericardial window remains the gold standard for the diagnosis of cardiac injury, though today more cases are being diagnosed almost immediately upon patient arrival by the Extended FAST ultrasound examination. Jimenez et al. showed that echocaradiography had 90% accuracy, 97% specificity, and 90% sensitivity in detecting penetrating cardiac injuries [81]. The usefulness of the FAST cardiac echo may be in its ability to identify obvious hemopericardium, thereby allowing the trauma surgeon to proceed directly to median sternotomy and thus eliminating the need for a subxiphoid pericardial window in many cases.

Pericardial window can also be therapeutic and can be done under local anesthesia in the operating room to allow release of tamponade prior to the induction of general anesthesia. If blood is found, then the surgeon can proceed immediately to median sternotomy and cardiorrhaphy. For relatively stable patients who do not require emergency room thoracotomy, median sternotomy is the incision of choice to repair penetrating cardiac wounds [82,83]. TTE has clearly emerged as the technique of choice for the diagnosis of penetrating cardiac injuries.

Suspected or proven pericardial tamponade with loss of vital signs due to penetrating thoracic trauma is the major indications to perform EDT [6]. An anterolateral thoracotomy is typically performed in between chest compressions and should be extended through all of the subcutaneous tissues, as well as the anterior chest wall muscles, until the intercostal space is identified. Typically, the patient's vital signs quickly return to acceptable levels. Internal defibrillation may be necessary, as the heart is often found to be in ventricular fibrillation. Epinephrine and similar drugs should specifically be avoided, as release of the tamponade is usually more than sufficient to allow the patient's vital signs to return. Epinephrine can increase chronotropy, inotropy, and intraventricular pressures, which can potentially extend ventricular injuries and make repair difficult and unnecessarily challenging. If sinus rhythm cannot be restored despite all attempts, the prognosis is grave and the outcome is invariably poor. Once vital signs are reestablished, attention can then be given to repairing the cardiac injury. Definitive cardiac repair does not necessarily have to be done immediately, however, and in some cases may be ill-advised when performing an emergency room thoracotomy, since it is the tamponade and not the blood loss per se that causes hemodynamic collapse. Once the tamponade is released, digital pressure can be directly applied to the cardiac wound which is often all that is needed once vital signs are restored to maintain relative hemostasis until definitive repair can be done in an operating room. In the authors' opinion, the use of adjunct measures, such as balloon tamponade with a Foley catheter, can be fraught with creating more injuries or extending existing myocardial lacerations and should be avoided if possible. Vascular clamps can be placed on bleeding right atrial wounds but usually are not necessary and may cause more harm than not, extending small injuries into larger ones. In addition, cross-clamping of the thoracic aorta is generally not necessary and ill-advised with isolated penetrating cardiac wounds. If necessary, it can be temporarily occluded digitally against the bodies of the thoracic vertebrae until adequate resuscitation has taken place. An attempt should be made to trace the trajectory of the wounding agent, as missiles often enter into one thorax and then enter the contralateral hemithorax. Once the tamponade has been released, the patient has regained a rhythm and a blood pressure, and the bleeding sites are identified and digitally controlled, the experienced surgeon can then attempt closure of the cardiac wound in an appropriate equipped operating room. Total inflow occlusion of the heart can be done if the blood loss is substantial through the wound and proper placement of sutures difficult in the face of ongoing blood loss without the aid of cardiopulmonary bypass. This maneuver is performed by placing caval tapes around both the superior and inferior vena cavae within the pericardium, which, when tethered, results in immediate emptying of the heart. The tolerance of the injured heart to this maneuver is limited, however, and should be used only for short periods if found to be necessary. This procedure can result in cardiopulmonary arrest and ventricular fibrillation, and appropriate plans should be made prior to caval occlusion should this happen. Atrial injuries can be repaired with running 2-0 Prolene. Ventricular wounds may be repaired while digitally occluding the laceration while placing a horizontal mattress stitch with a pledget surrounding the wound, usually with 2-0 Prolene. Repairing cardiac injuries resulting from gunshot wounds can be more challenging when compared with stab wounds, since they tend to have associated blast effects, which can make repair difficult. The repair of ventricular wounds adjacent to or involving coronary arteries can be challenging. If the coronary artery is injured itself but is quite distal (e.g., distal 1/3 of the left anterior descending artery), simple ligation can be done without serious consequences. However, if the injury is more proximal than this, ligation of the injury with distal bypass using a segment of saphenous vein or mammary artery is recommended. This can be done on or off cardiopulmonary bypass but usually requires the expertise of an experienced cardiac surgeon to perform. If the injury does not involve the coronary artery but is in close proximity, suturing of the injury may require placement of a horizontal U-stitch underneath the bed of the coronary artery, thereby closing the injury without compromising coronary blood flow. Patients who have sustained injury to their coronary artery who has already sustained irreversible myocardial damage may require intra-aortic balloon counterpulsation as part of their resuscitation.

Recently, some cases of hemopericardium due to penetrating trauma have been managed by urgent, rather than emergent surgery for stable patients [84].

Esophagus

Iatrogenic injuries to the esophagus are the most common, particularly those of iatrogenic esophageal perforation. Traumatic injury and Boerhaave's syndrome account for most of the rest.

Patients who present with esophageal perforation usually complain of pain. Findings may include fever and subcutaneous or mediastinal air. Crepitus in the neck is relatively common following perforations of the cervical esophagus and can be detected on physical exam in approximately 60% of patients. Pleural effusions are present in more than 50% of patients with perforations of their thoracic esophagus. Radiologic studies are important for diagnosing patients with esophageal perforation. A plain chest radiograph may show subcutaneous emphysema, pneumomediastinum, pleural effusion, pneumothorax, or mediastinal air–fluid levels (hydropneumothorax). Radiographic abnormalities can be found in as many as 90% of patients on plain film. Contrast studies are performed to confirm the diagnosis of perforation and to define the exact site. The appropriate type of contrast agent to use for this study remains controversial. Water-soluble contrast agents such as Gastrografin have been the preferred agents of choice since if leakage through the perforation occurs, they will not seed the mediatinum with particulate matter that serves as a nidus for infection. However, Gastrografin can cause severe pneumonitis if aspirated into the lungs, and its use may not demonstrate small leaks. Because of this, some prefer to use thin barium, as it is more inert in the lungs and is better at detecting smaller leaks. CT scanning can be particularly helpful for showing mediastinal findings such as air, inflammation, and fluid collections when the perforation has already sealed.

The optimal management of esophageal perforation is patient specific and should take into account the clinical setting [85]. This includes consideration of the patient's underlying disease process, the degree of sepsis, if any, the location of the perforation, and whether or not the perforation is contained. A nonoperative approach may be considered for patients with minimal symptoms and physical findings who do not appear septic and have a small, contained leak. Nonoperative management should include the use of broad-spectrum intravenous antibiotics and nothing to eat or drink by mouth (NPO). A nasogastric tube should be specifically avoided. There is no clear consensus as to generally how long a patient with a contained leak should be left NPO or how long intravenous antibiotics should be continued. However, clear liquids can usually be safely started within a few days and the diet advanced cautiously, especially when no further extravasation is seen on repeat contrast study.

Surgery should be performed if the patient appears septic, the leak freely communicates with either the peritoneal or thoracic cavities, or there is an associated mediastinal abscess. Primary repair can be done regardless of the timing of the injury, as long as the tissues appear healthy at the time of surgery. Drainage alone can be done for cervical perforations, especially if the perforation cannot be found at the time of operation, which is not infrequent. Primary repair with drainage is the preferred method when possible; however, if the esophageal tissues do not appear viable to hold sutures, drainage alone, with or without proximal diversion may be necessary. It is important when primarily repairing the esophagus that the mucosal edges are defined, as the injury seen in the muscle layer is often only the "tip of the iceberg," and closure of the entire mucosal defect is necessary if adequate healing is to occur.

Esophagectomy is rarely necessary or safe in the acute trauma setting. If resection must be done, diversion should be done and esophageal reconstruction deferred until sepsis and the acute catabolic state have resolved. In these cases, it is better to create an end cervical esophagostomy and oversew the gastric stump with the placement of and enteral feeding catheter. Esophageal injuries due to penetrating trauma are rare, with most series averaging only a handful [86–88]. They result most commonly from transmediastinal gunshot wounds. Asensio et al. reported their experience consisting of 43 penetrating esophageal injuries managed over a period of 6 years. Overall, 28 of their 32 survivors (88%) were managed by primary repair alone [89]. The overall mortality for their series was 26%. The authors also reported that these mortality figures were consistent with others reported in the literature, which have remained high and relatively stable for the last 20 years, thus attesting to the critical nature of these injuries. Only Symbas et al. (48 cases) and Defore et al. (77 cases) have reported larger experiences but over much longer spans of time, 15 and 22 years, respectively [86,87]. Penetrating esophageal injuries are not easily detected and require a high index of suspicion. Delay in diagnosis is associated with higher mortality. However, mortality can exceed 20% even for patients who are promptly diagnosed. Esophagoduodenoscopy (EGD) is a sensitive and safe diagnostic test for the detection of esophageal injury. A study by Flowers et al. showed that EGD had a sensitivity of 100%, a specificity of 96%, and an accuracy of 97% in detecting penetrating esophageal injuries [90]. There was no morbidity related to the examination, and, most importantly, no esophageal injuries were missed. The authors commented that the most significant potential weakness of flexible EGD for esophageal trauma is that it actually may be too sensitive. EGD is most helpful in excluding esophageal injury in patients who require a surgical procedure for another injury. When found, prompt primary repair is the treatment of choice.

Caustic Injuries of the Esophagus

Caustic injuries of the esophagus can be very challenging to manage. They are most frequently due to suicide attempts in adults and accidental ingestion in children. The degree of injury to the esophagus is directly proportional to the amount of caustic substance ingested. Lye causes transmural liquefaction necrosis of the esophagus and therefore is most injurious. Diagnosis is usually from history, although patients attempting suicide may present with no history at all or, even worse, an inaccurate one. Examination of the buccal mucosa, mouth, tongue, and gums can often show chemical burns suggestive of the diagnosis. Endoscopy should be performed to document the proximal extent of the injury only; there is no need to pass the endoscope further, since it may actually be harmful and potentially lead to perforation. Passage of an NGT is controversial, although it may actually help to "stent" the esophagus open and be associated with lower rates of stricture formation. Arterial blood gases should be obtained with particular attention paid to the base deficit, as this can be a marker for severity of injury. Signs and symptoms of perforation and sepsis should be carefully monitored. The patient should be made NPO, and broad spectrum intravenous antibiotics should be given. Steroids are controversial but have been associated with lower rates of stricture formation in some series [91,92]. Intravenous fluids should be given and consideration given to performing esophagectomy, if signs of perforation and mediastinal sepsis are present. Intra-abdominal perforations can also occur, as well as injury to surrounding structures (e.g., spleen, colon). If esophageal resection becomes clinically indicated due to sepsis, immediate reconstruction is ill-advised. Esophagectomy can be performed either transhiatally or transthoracically, with creation of an end cervical esophagostomy. Intra-abdominal feeding tubes should be placed for enteral access. Delayed reconstruction can then be performed electively once the sepsis clears and the patient heals, usually several months later. Late stricture formation is common and can be difficult to manage. In addition, the pharyngeal phase of swallowing can be affected, leading to debilitating problems with speech and swallowing. It is not uncommon to require serial dilations or even late esophagectomy if stricture formation develops. It typically involves long segments of the esophagus and is panmural in depth, often making dilation impossible or at best marginally effective. Overall prognosis is variable depending on the degree of injury.

Thoracic Aortic Injury

Traumatic disruption of the thoracic aorta immediately leads to death in majority of the patients and is a common finding of autopsy series from high-speed motor vehicle accidents. These horizontal acceleration/deceleration injuries usually result from a disruption of the integrity of the aortic wall just distal to the ligamentum arteriosum. Patients fortunate enough to survive initial injury usually do so because the aortic adventitial tissues are able to tamponade the tear, thereby creating an expanding pseudoaneurysm and thus preventing or delaying fatal intrathoracic exsanguination. The risk of rupture is dependent on multiple factors, including the ability of the adventitial tissues to contain the leak, the patient's systemic blood pressure, and the size of the contained pseudoaneurysm.

While emergent operative repair of thoracic aortic tears has long been the standard of care, after 1997 there has been emerging evidence that not all thoracic aortic tears should be treated equally. In addition, associated injuries such as pulmonary contusions, intracranial hemorrhage, and/or intra-abdominal hemorrhage (which are common in these patients) may take precedence and may render major aortic surgery particularly hazardous. For these cases, the aortic injury can be acutely managed medically and definitive treatment delayed, so long as certain criteria are met. With careful medical management (strict blood pressure control, minimization of dP/dT), it has been shown that many thoracic aortic injuries can undergo delayed repair, perhaps resulting in superior outcomes when compared with those patients undergoing emergent repair [93,94]. A recent prospective, observational study sponsored by the American Association for the Surgery of Trauma (AAST) looked at the subgroup of patients that underwent immediate repair versus those that underwent delayed repair [95]. Those patients that underwent delayed repair of stable thoracic aortic injury actually had improved survival regardless of the presence of major associated injuries, although their length of ICU stay was longer. It should be noted that patients with no major associated injuries who underwent delayed repair had a significantly higher complication rates when compared to those patients undergoing immediate repair. Although there has not been a randomized, controlled trial of early versus delayed repair, these results probably are affected by selection bias. However, selection bias, which reflects the "art" of clinical treatment planning, should not be underscored when making decisions regarding these often multiply injured patients. In addition, successful nonoperative therapy of descending thoracic aortic injury has been reported [96]. Justification for nonoperative therapy includes favorable anatomy of the injury (contained, small injury, hemodynamic stability) as well as the presence of coexisting injuries, which would render the operative risk prohibitively high. These include patients with spinal cord injury that might make lateral decubitus positioning dangerous, patients with pulmonary contusions that may make single lung ventilation difficult, and patients with closed head injury, solid abdominal organ injury, or major fractures in which systemic heparinization would be ill-advised. One accepted method of operative repair is the "clamp-and-sew" technique, in which the proximal and distal aorta are simply clamped, thereby isolating the injury so that either primary repair or interposition grafting can be performed. Operative mortality is generally reported to be 10% to 20% in most series, with major morbidity including renal failure and paraplegia, which appears to increase with prolonged (i.e., >30 minutes) clamp times [97]. Another accepted method of operative repair utilizes bypass of the injured segment during repair, either with partial left heart bypass or with proximal to distal aortic shunt placement (i.e., Gott shunt). Partial left heart bypass (with cannulae in the left atrium and distal aorta) allows controlled off-loading of the left heart in addition to maintaining distal aortic perfusion, especially to the kidneys, that may decrease (but not negate) the incidence of paraplegia, especially when prolonged clamp times are anticipated. Since there has not been a randomized controlled trial comparing the two techniques, and there is no conclusive evidence that one technique is superior over the other in terms of outcome, both methods are acceptable, and their performance is usually based on surgeon preference.

The need for operative repair, however, which was once considered the gold standard, is now coming into question. There have been many reports showing that "TEVAR" (Thoracic Endovasclar Aneurysmal Repair) endovascular stent grafting of selected patients may actually be superior to that of "mandatory" operative repair [98–100]. A prospective, multicenter study sponsored by the AAST was recently published that clearly shows the early efficacy and safety of endovascular stent grafting in selected patients with traumatic thoracic aortic injuries [100]. The patients who underwent stent grafting had a significantly lower mortality (adjusted odds ratio: 8.42; 95% CI: [2.76 to 25.69]; adjusted p value <0.001) and fewer blood transfusions (adjusted mean difference: 4.98; 95% CI [0.14 to 9.82]; adjusted p value <0.046) compared to those patients that underwent operative repair. In addition, among the patients with major extrathoracic injuries, a significantly higher mortality and pneumonia rate were found in the operative group (adjusted p values 0.04 and 0.03, respectively). The major drawback seen for patients undergoing stent grafting were device-related complications, which developed among 20% of the patients. Their conclusion was that stent grafting of thoracic aortic injuries is now more commonly chosen by surgeons as the preferred method of repair and is associated with significantly lower mortality but that there is a considerable risk of serious device-related complications. The rate of device related complications is continually decreasing in recent literature. Additionally, the rate of paraplegia has ranged between 1% and 3%, significantly less than any open surgical method [98]. Also, systemic heparinization, a major risk in trauma patients, is not required. TEVAR has now become the method of choice in many centers for repair of thoracic aortic transection for the high risk or multi-injured patient who would not tolerate open surgery. As more experience is gained, it is conceivable that this method will supplant open surgical repair for all thoracic aortic injuries.

Traumatic Asphyxia

Traumatic asphyxia occurs as a result of a sudden or severe compression injury of the thorax or upper abdomen. It is most often associated with blunt trauma secondary to a crush injury. Entrapment of children under automatic garage doors is a prime example, as reported by Kriel et al. [101]. The true incidence of traumatic asphyxia is unknown, but it is considered to be a relatively rare event. The diagnosis is usually made based on the mechanism of injury and physical examination. Associated injuries are common and therefore should be investigated. The usual physical findings consist of facial edema, cyanosis, and petechial hemorrhages of the upper torso, neck, and face. The petechiae usually occur within the conjunctiva and oral mucosa and become most prominent a few hours after the initial injury. Neurologic findings are not rare and are thought to be secondary to anoxic injury, as well as possible cerebral edema and hemorrhage. The exact pathophysiology is thought to relate to prolonged elevation of central venous pressure (CVP). Prolonged application of high pressure to the mediastinum causes the heart to force blood out of the right atrium retrograde into the valveless innominate and jugular venous system. In addition, a sudden reflexive inspiration is thought to occur against a closed glottis, which may elevate the intrathoracic pressures to high levels. This results in a sudden and rapid increase in the pressure of the small veins of the face and neck, resulting in the typical petechial hemorrhages that are observed.

Treatment is generally supportive. Specific therapy for traumatic asphyxia is based on physiologic techniques to decrease intracranial pressure, including elevation of the head of the bed and oxygen therapy. If there is altered mental status, CT scanning of the head should be done. If there is evidence of increased intracranial pressure, ICP monitoring and treatment of intracranial hypertension may be needed. Laryngeal edema may occur necessitating airway control by endotracheal intubation or emergent cricothyroidotomy. The need to concurrently treat associated injuries is also likely. Commonly associated injuries include rib fractures, pulmonary contusions, extremity fractures, pneumothorax, hemothorax, flail chest, and blunt pelvic and intra-abdominal injuries (i.e., splenic and/or liver lacerations). The prognosis for patients with traumatic asphyxia is generally good, as long as the patient did not sustain prolonged apnea or hypoxia. The majority of fatalities are usually from associated injuries and their complications. When death does occur, it usually occurs in patients who have sustained a prolonged compression, causing massive irreversible neurologic insult from the resultant apnea and hypoxia.

Respiratory Complications

As a result of either primary lung contusion or from the treatment necessary to treat generalized traumatic injury (e.g., massive transfusions, mechanical ventilation, etc.), the lungs are susceptible to acute injury. Complications, which can develop, include transfusion related lung injury (TRALI), ventilator associated pneumonia (VAP), or ARDS. For an in depth discussion of these three complications, readers are referred to Chapters 89, 163, and 181.

UTILITY OF ULTRASONOGRAPHY FOR EVALUATION OF THORACIC AND CARDIAC TRAUMA

Ultrasonography is valuable for the immediate assessment of the critically ill patient with thoracic and cardiac trauma in the form of the extended FAST examination [102]. Chest CT and angiography are useful for definitive imaging of thoracic and cardiac trauma but cannot be used on an emergency basis. For some applications, ultrasonography is superior to standard supine chest radiography.

The ultrasonography examination is performed by a single member of the trauma team, while other key elements of initial resuscitation are ongoing. Modern bedside ultrasonography machines are small enough that they can be brought to the bedside without blocking access to the patient by other members of the trauma team. The machine has multiple uses beyond examination for life threatening complications of thoracic trauma such as vascular access, airway management, and assessment for alternative causes for shock.

Equipment Requirements

The extended FAST examination is performed using a phased array cardiac probe (2.0 to 5.0 MHz). For the thoracic assessment, the probe is configured with abdominal preset. The machine is switched back to cardiac preset when examining the heart. Many portable ultrasound machines have full TEE capability, so it is feasible to use TEE as an immediate imaging modality at point of care.

Scanning Technique

With the patient in supine position, the operator examines the anterior and lateral chest with the probe held perpendicular to the chest wall and adjusted to scan through the intercostal spaces. A series of scan lines are performed over the anterior and lateral chest, while the probe is moved over adjacent rib interspaces. Generally, it suffices to perform one scan line in the anterior midclavicular line, the anterior axillary line, and the posterior axillary line. In each intercostal space, the operator checks for lung sliding/pulse, A lines, B lines, consolidation, and pleural fluid (see Chapter 11 Lung Ultrasonography and Chapter 12 Thoracentesis). Following the thoracic examination, the operator obtains a subcostal long axis view of the heart in order to evaluate for the presence of pericardial fluid (see Chapter 17 Pericardiocentesis). If indicated, the examination can be extended to include the abdomen (see Chapter 37 Shock Following Hemorrhage).

Examination for Pneumothorax

The presence of lung sliding, lung pulse, or B lines rules out pneumothorax at the site of the examination (see Chapter 11 Lung Ultrasonography). Multiple intercostal spaces can be examined in a short period time in order to exclude pneumothorax with a high level of certainty in the patient with thoracic trauma. If lung sliding is absent with the presence of A line pattern, there is a high probability of a pneumothorax. Identification of a lung point verifies the presence of pneumothorax (see Chapter 11 Lung Ultrasonography). However, lung point requires a skilled operator. It is highly specific for pneumothorax, but its sensitivity depends on the skill of the examiner [103]. Ultrasonography is similar or superior to standard supine chest radiography for evaluation for pneumothorax [104,105]. Its performance characteristics are such that it may replace chest radiography for this purpose [8]. CT scan remains the gold standard, but, in comparison, ultrasonography gives similar results and offers the advantage of being a point of care technique.

Examination for Hemothorax

Hemothorax is readily detected with ultrasonography [106,107]. The hemothorax will accumulate in the dependent thorax, so the examination is focused on the lateral and posterolateral intercostal spaces. A very recent hemothorax has a swirling characteristic and significant echogenicity (see Chapter 12 Thoracentesis). Within a short period of time, blood becomes progressively more hypoechoic. The cellular elements within the blood collection undergo gravitational sedimentation; so it is common to see a clear sedimentation effect with an anechoic space clearly demarcated from a dependent more echoic area. This has been termed "hematocrit" sign. The blood may eventually form a mobile thrombus that is visualized as a distinct structure floating in the anechoic fluid collection. If a hemothorax is present, ultrasonography allows identification of a safe site for chest tube insertion.

Examination for Lung Contusion

Ultrasonography can detect lung contusion related to thoracic trauma. Contused lung appears as B lines or areas of areas of alveolar consolidation, depending on the severity of the injury. It may be focal, multifocal, unilateral, or bilateral in distribution (see Chapter 11 Lung Ultrasonography). The injury may appear rapidly following the trauma and may evolve in severity over time. The finding of B lines and alveolar consolidation is not diagnostic of lung contusion. Their presence is a nonspecific finding indicating lung injury of some type (e.g., aspiration, pneumonia, ARDS); the diagnosis of lung contusion remains a clinical diagnosis that may be supported by the ultrasonography findings. The severity of lung contusion detected by ultrasonography is predictive of the need for mechanical ventilatory support [108].

Examination for Cardiac Injury

The extended FAST examination includes the subcostal long axis view of the heart. This view is designed to detect a pericardial effusion. The finding of a pericardial effusion in the thoracic trauma patient with hemodynamic compromise requires consideration of pericardial tamponade requiring immediate decompression. An acute hemopericardium is relatively echogenic (See Chapter 17 Pericardiocantesis). The operator who is competent at goal directed echocardiography is able to recognize pericardial fluid, but, lacking skill at advanced critical care echocardiography, cannot make more advanced measurements that indicate the presence of tamponade physiology. These are not relevant to the patient who is near death from thoracic trauma with a pericardial effusion. In this situation, the finding of the pericardial effusion is sufficient to take definitive action to drain the fluid either percutaneously or with surgical intervention. Examination for cardiac contusion, valvular injury, and/or penetrating cardiac injury requires training in advanced critical care echocardiography. As goal directed echocardiography is not designed to reliably detect this type of injury, the management team obtains immediate consultative echocardiography, if there is clinical indication to do so.

TEE for Examination for Thoracic Aortic Injury

Transoesophageal echocardiography has utility in identifying thoracic aortic injury [109]. While CT and angiography are standard means to make the diagnosis, TEE has the advantage of immediate feasibility, safety, and utility in identification of thoracic aortic injury. Assuming that the trauma team has TEE capability, it is appropriate to use TEE as the primary imaging modality and reserve CT scan and angiography for cases where TEE is nondiagnostic or contraindicated. This approach is predicated on immediate availability of TEE to the trauma team and a team member who is competent in the procedure. As critical care echocardiography becomes more widespread, trauma specialists will develop capability with TEE, as the procedure is feasible, has low risk, and has strong clinical utility. However, its use requires an understanding of the limitations of TEE for evaluation of thoracic aortic injury.

1. TEE has contraindications that apply to all patients. Two of these are of special concern in the thoracic trauma patient. An absolute contraindication to TEE is esophageal injury, and cervical spine injury is a relative contraindication.
2. The aortic arch is often difficult to image with TEE due to the presence of the air-filled trachea that may block visualization of this area. The aortic arch includes the take-off of the brachiocephalic, left carotid, and subclavian arteries. Unless the TEE examination is definitive in this area, it may be necessary to proceed with alternative imaging technique such as CT or angiography [110].
3. While TEE has excellent sensitivity for detection of acute thoracic aortic injury, its specificity is reduced due to the

TABLE 43.1

Use of TEE Diagnostic Criteria to Distinguish Linear Artifacts from True Intra-aortic Flaps for the Diagnosis of Spontaneous AD and TDA

Variables (n = 121)	Sensitivity (%)	Specificity (%)	Positive predictive value (%)	Negative predictive value (%)
Ascending aorta				
At least one criterion[a]	92.9	68.2	65.0	93.8
At least two criteria	92.9	95.5	92.9	95.5
At least three criteria	92.9	100.0	100.0	95.7
All four criteria	42.9	100.0	100.0	73.3
Descending thoracic aorta				
At least one criterion[b]	97.1	100.0	100.0	87.5
At least two criteria	82.4	100.0	100.0	53.8
All three criteria	64.7	100.0	100.0	36.8

[a]Any of the following: (1) displacement of the linear image parallel to aortic walls, (2) similar blood flow velocities on both sides of the linear image, (3) thickness of the linear image > 2.5 mm, and (4) angle between the linear image and the aortic wall >85 degrees.
[b]Any of the following: (1) displacement of the linear image parallel to the aortic walls, (2) over position of blood flow on the linear image, and (3) similar blood flow velocities on both sides of the linear image.
Adapted from Vignon P, Martaillé JF, François B, et al: Transesophageal echocardiography and therapeutic management of patients sustaining blunt aortic injuries. *J Trauma* 58:1150–1158, 2005.).

problem of intraluminal linear artifacts that are often observed in the ascending aorta and less commonly in the descending aorta. These are classified as multiple-path artifacts that are the result of reverberations between strongly reflective surfaces. When the ultrasound beam strikes an interface with large impedance mismatch between media, multiple reflections occur, especially if the interface is perpendicular to the direction of sound propagation. In the case of the ascending aorta, these commonly occur when the left atrium or right pulmonary artery are smaller in diameter than the ascending aorta. The source of the reverberation artifact is the interface between the posterior wall of the ascending aorta and the anterior wall of the left atrium or right pulmonary artery. Reverberations between this interface and the esophageal transducer may occur with the resultant linear reverberation artifact occurring in the aorta. The resulting linear artifacts do not correspond to anatomic structures, as they derive from reverberation between an interface and the ultrasonography transducer in esophageal position. These linear artifacts may be misidentified as intraluminal dissection flaps and lead to surgical intervention for a false positive result [110]. The trauma specialist who is responsible for the examination has special skill at distinguishing linear artifacts within the thoracic aorta from true aortic dissection, as well as having mastery of the standard components of critical TEE that include other findings of thoracic trauma: cardiac injury, mediastinal hematoma, and aortic disruption (intimal vs. subadventitial) [111,112]. Table 43.1 and its accompanying reference 110 summarize useful TEE findings that allow the operator to identify linear artifacts within the thoracic aorta.

SUMMARY

In summary, most thoracic trauma can be managed without surgery or, at most, with minimally invasive interventions. Multiply injured patients with thoracic injuries need to be comprehensively evaluated and their injuries prioritized and as a result, their successful care often requires a multidisciplinary approach. The treatment for thoracic injuries is evolving and requires a working knowledge of a number of both diagnostic and therapeutic modalities. As with almost all other traumatic injuries, the key to optimal treatment and outcomes is dependent upon having a high index of suspicion for the injury and to identify it early. The ability to competently manage all aspects of a critically injured patient is also important in effecting a successful overall outcome.

References

1. Kulshrestha P, Munshi I, Wait R: Profile of chest trauma in a level I trauma center. *J Trauma* 57(3):576–581, 2004.
2. Demetriades D, Murray J, Charalambides K, et al: Trauma fatalities time and location of hospital deaths. *J Am Coll Surg* 198(1):20–26, 2004.
3. Karmy-Jones R, Jurkovich GJ, Shatz DV, et al: Management of traumatic lung injury: a Western Trauma Association multicenter review. *J Trauma* 51(6):1049–1053, 2001.
4. Martin SK, Shatney CH, Sherck JP, et al: Blunt trauma patients with prehospital pulseless electrical activity (PEA): poor ending assured. *J Trauma* 53(5):876–881, 2002.
5. Hunt PA, Greaves I, Owens WA: Emergency thoracotomy in thoracic trauma—a review. *Injury* 37:1–19, 2006.
6. Johannesdottir BK, Mogensen B, Gudbjartsson T: Emergency thoracotomy as a rescue treatment for trauma patients in Iceland. *Injury* 44:1186–1190, 2013.
7. Soni KD, Aggarwal R, Gupta A, et al: Is the use of high frequency oscillatory ventilator beneficial in managing severe chest injury with massive air leak? *BMJ Case Rep*, 2014.
8. Soult MC, Weireter LJ, Britt RC, et al: Can routine trauma bay chest x-ray be bypassed with an extended focused assessment with sonography for trauma examination. *Am Surg* 81(4):336–340, 2015.
9. Abdulrahman Y, Musthafa S, Haim S, et al: Utility of extended FAST in blunt chest trauma: is it the time to be used in the ATLS algorithm? *World J Surg* 39:172–178, 2015.
10. Blasinska-Przerwa K, Pacho R, Bestry I: The applicationof MDCT in the diagnosis of chest trauma. *Pneumonol Alergol Pol* 81(6):518–526, 2013.
11. de Mestral C, Dueck A, Sharma SS, et al: Evolution of the incidence, management and mortality of blunt thoracic aortic injury: A population-based analysis. *J Am Coll Surg* 216:1110–1115, 2013.
12. Wisbach GG, Sise MJ, Sack DI, et al: What is the role of chest x-ray in the initial assessment of stable trauma patients? *J Trauma* 62(1):74–79, 2007.
13. Deunk J, Dekker HM, Brink M, et al: The value of indicated computed tomography scan of the chest and abdomen in addition to the conventional radiologic work-up for blunt trauma patients. *J Trauma* 63(4):757–763, 2007.
14. Mirvis SE, Shanmuganathan K, Buell J, et al: Use of spiral computed tomography for the assessment of blunt trauma patients with potential aortic injury. *J Trauma* 45(5):922–930, 1998.
15. Wicky S, Wintermark M, Schnyder P, et al: Imaging of blunt chest trauma. *Eur Radiol* 10:1524–1538, 2000.
16. Patel NH, Stephens KE Jr, Mirvis SE, et al: Imaging of acute thoracic aortic injury due to blunt trauma: a review. *Radiology* 209:335–348, 1998.
17. Gavant ML: Helical CT grading of traumatic aortic injuries: impact on clinical guidelines for medical and surgical management. *Radiol Clin North Am* 37:553–574, 1999.

18. Ekeh AP, Peterson W, Woods RJ, et al: Is chest X-ray an adequate screening tool for the diagnosis of blunt thoracic aortic injury? *J Trauma* 65(5):1088–1092, 2008.
19. Chen MY, Miller PR, McLaughlin CA, et al: The trend of using computed tomography in the detection of acute thoracic aortic and branch vessel injury after blunt thoracic trauma: single-center experience over 13 years. *J Trauma* 56(4):783–785, 2004.
20. Wong H, Gotway MB, Sasson AD, et al: Periaortic hematoma at diaphragmatic crura at helical CT: sign of blunt aortic injury in patients with mediastinal hematoma. *Radiology* 231(13):185–189, 2004.
21. Kehdy F, Richardson JD: The utility of 3-D CT scan in the diagnosis and evaluation of sternal fractures. *J Trauma* 60(3):635–636, 2006.
22. Stein DM, Gregory B, York GB, et al: Accuracy of computed tomography (CT) scan in the detection of penetrating diaphragm injury. *J Trauma* 63(3):538–543, 2007.
23. Plurad D, Green D, Demetriades D, et al: The increasing use of chest computed tomography for trauma: is it being overutilized? *J Trauma* 62(3):631–635, 2007.
24. Goarin JP, Catoire P, Jacquens Y, et al: Use of transesophageal echocardiography for diagnosis of traumatic aortic injury. *Chest* 112:71–80, 1997.
25. Brooks SW, Young JC, Cmolik B, et al: The use of transesophageal echocardiography in the evaluation of chest trauma. *J Trauma* 32:761, 1992.
26. Goarin JP, Le Bret F, Riou B, et al: Early diagnosis of traumatic thoracic aortic rupture by transesophageal echocardiography. *Chest* 103:618, 1993.
27. Wolfenden H, Newman DC: Transesophageal echocardiography: an increasing role in the diagnosis of traumatic aortic rupture. *J Thorac Cardiovasc Surg* 106:757, 1993.
28. Yoon D, Hoftman N, Ren W, et al: Intraoperative transesophageal echocardiography in chest trauma. *J Trauma* 65(4):924–926, 2008.
29. Wong SSF: Penetrating thoracic injuries: the use of transesophageal echocardiography to monitor for complications after intracardiac nail removal. *J Trauma* 64(5):E69–E70, 2008.
30. Jones JW, Kitahama A, Webb WR, et al: Emergency thoracoscopy: a logical approach to chest trauma management. *J Trauma* 21:280–284, 1981.
31. Ochsner MG, Rozycki CS, Lucente F, et al: Prospective evaluation of thoracoscopy for diagnosing diaphragmatic injury in thoracoabdominal trauma: a preliminary report. *J Trauma* 34:704–709, 1993.
32. Mealy K, Murphy M, Broe P: Diagnosis of traumatic rupture of the right hemidiaphragm by thoracoscopy. *Br J Surg* 80:210–211, 1993.
33. Abolhoda A, Livingston DH, Donahoo JS, et al: Diagnostic and therapeutic video assisted thoracic surgery (VATS) following chest trauma. *Eur J Card Thor Surg* 12:356–360, 1997.
34. Wu N, Wu L, Qiu C, et al: A comparison of video-assisted thoracoscopic surgery with open thoractomy for the management of chest trauma: a systematic review and meta-analysis. *World J Surg* 29(4):940–952, 2015.
35. Flagel BT, Luchette FA, Reed RL, et al: Half-a-dozen ribs: the breakpoint for mortality. *Surgery* 138:717–725, 2005.
36. Katherine BA, Cha ES, Bensard DD, et al: The positive predictive value of rib fractures as an indicator of nonaccidental trauma in children. *J Trauma* 54:1107–1110, 2003.
37. Bulger EM, Arneson MA, Mock CN, et al: Rib fractures in the elderly. *J Trauma* 48:1040–1047, 2000.
38. Holcomb JB, McMullin NR, Kozar RA: Morbidity from rib fractures increases after age 45. *J Am Coll Surg* 196:549–555, 2003.
39. Gage A, Rivera F, Wang J, et al: The effect of epidural placement in patients after blunt thoracic trauma. *J Trauma Acute Care Surg* 76(1):39–46, 2014.
40. Yeh DD, Kutcher ME, Knudson MM, et al: Epidural analgesia for blunt thoracic injury—which patients benefit most? *Injury* 43:1667–1671, 2012.
41. Carrier FM, Turgeon Af, Nicole PC, et al: Effect of epidural analgesia i patients with traumatic rib fractures: a systematic review and meta-analysis of randomized controlled trials. *Can J Anaesth* 56(3):230–242, 2009.
42. Bulger EM, Edwards T, Klotz P, et al: Epidural analgesia improves outcome after multiple rib fractures. *Surgery* 136:426–430, 2004.
43. Simon B, Ebert J, Bokhari F, et al: Management of pulmonary contusion and flail chest: an Eastern Association for the Surgery of Trauma practice management guideline. *J Trauma Acute Care Surg* 73(5 Suppl 4):S351–S361, 2012.
44. Kilic D, Findikcioglu A, Akin S, et al: Factors affecting morbidity and mortality in flail chest: comparison of anterior and lateral location. *Thorac Cardioasc Surg* 59(1):45–48, 2011.
45. Athanassiadi K, Theakos N, Kalantzi, N, et al: Prognostic factors in flail chest patients. *Eur J Cardiothorac Surg* 38(4):466–471, 2012.
46. Zhang Y, Tang X, Xie H, et al: Comparison of surgical fixation and nonsurgical management of flail chest and pulmonary contusion. *Am J Emerg Med* 33(7):937–940, 2015.
47. Tanaka H, Yukioka T, Yamaguti Y, et al: Surgical stabilization of internal pneumatic stabilization? A prospective randomized study of management of severe flail chest patients. *J Trauma* 52:727–732, 2002.
48. Watkins R IV, Watkins R III, Williams L, et al: Stability provided by the sternum and rib cage in the thoracic spine. *Spine* 30(11):1283–1286, 2005.
49. Black CJ, Busuttil A, Robertson C: Chest wall injuries following cardiopulmonary resuscitation. *Resuscitation* 63:339–343, 2004.
50. Garrel TV, Ince A, Junge A, et al: The sternal fracture: radiographic analysis of 200 fractures with special reference to concomitant injuries. *J Trauma* 57:837–844, 2004.
51. Athanassiadi K, Gerazounis M, Moustardas M, et al: Sternal fractures: retrospective analysis of 100 cases. *World J Surg* 26:1243–1246, 2002.
52. Weening B, Walton C, Cole PA, et al: Lower mortality in patients with scapular fractures. *J Trauma* 59:1477–1481, 2005.
53. Veysi VT, Mittal R, Agarwal S, et al: Multiple trauma and scapula fractures: so what? *J Trauma* 55:1145–1147, 2003.
54. Sedel L: The results of surgical repair of brachial plexus lesions. *J Bone Joint Surg Br* 64:54–66, 1982.
55. Sherwood SF, Hartsock RL: Thoracic injuries, in McQuillian KA, Von Rueden KT, Hartstock RL, et al (eds): *Trauma Nursing From Resuscitation Through Rehabilitation*. 3rd ed. Philadelphia, PA, Saunders, 2002 pp 543–590.
56. Kimbrell BJ, Yamzon J, Petrone P, et al: Intrapleural thrombolysis for the management of undrained traumatic hemothorax: a prospective observational study. *J Trauma* 62(5):1175–1179, 2007.
57. Toombs BD, Sandlet SV, Lester RG: Computed tomography of chest trauma. *Radiology* 140:733–738, 1981.
58. Shin B, McAlslan TC, Hankins JR: Management of lung contusion. *Am Surg* 45:168–179, 1979.
59. Schild HH, Strunk H, Weber W: Pulmonary contusion: CT vs plain radiograms. *J Comput Assist Tomogr* 13:417–420, 1989.
60. Hankins JR, Attar S, Turney SZ: Differential diagnosis of pulmonary parenchymal changes in thoracic trauma. *Am Surg* 39:309–318, 1973.
61. Wagner RB, Jamieson PM: Pulmonary contusion: evaluation and classification by computed tomography. *Surg Clin N Am* 69:211–224, 1989.
62. Kishikawa M, Yoshioka T, Shimazu T: Pulmonary contusion causes long-term respiratory dysfunction with decreased functional residual capacity. *J Trauma* 31:1203–1210, 1991.
63. Roxburgh JC: Rupture of the tracheobronchial tree. *Thorax* 42:681–688, 1987.
64. Lynn RB, Iyengar K: Traumatic rupture of the bronchus. *Chest* 61:81–83, 1972.
65. Kiser AC, O'Brien SM, Detterbeck FC: Blunt tracheobronchial injuries: treatment and outcomes. *Ann Thorac Surg* 71:2059–2065, 2001.
66. Juvekar N, Deshpande S, Nadkarni A, et al: Perioperative management of tracheobronchial injury following blunt trauma. *Ann Cardiac Anaesth* 16(2):140, 2013.
67. Flynn AE, Thomas AN, Schecter WP: Acute tracheobronchial injury. *J Trauma* 29:1326–1330, 1989.
68. Baumgartner F, Sheppard B, de Virgilio C, et al: Tracheal and main bronchial disruptions after blunt chest trauma: presentation and management. *Ann Thorac Surg* 50:569–574, 1990.
69. Shaw RR, Paulson DL, Kee KL Jr: Traumatic tracheal rupture. *J Thorac Cardiovasc Surg* 42:281–297, 1961.
70. Marcolini EG, Keegan J: Blunt cardiac injury. *Emerg Med Clin North Am* 33(3):19-27, 2015-11-24
71. Mehotra, D, Dalley P, Mahon B: Tricuspid valve avulsion after blunt chest trauma. *Texas Heart Inst J* 39(5):668–670, 2012.
72. Ismailov RM, Ness RB, Redmond CK, et al: Trauma associated with cardiac dysrhythmias: results from a large matched case-control study. *J Trauma* 62(5):1186–1191, 2007.
73. Lin YC, Chang YS, Chen MS, et al: Effective myocardial salvage with percutaneous coronary intervention in late diagnosed acute post-traumatic ST-elevation myocardial infarction. *J Emerg Med* 42(1):28–35, 2012.
74. Lindstaedt M, Germing A, Lawo T, et al: Acute and long-term clinical significance of myocardial contusion following blunt thoracic trauma: results of a prospective study. *J Trauma* 52(3):479–485, 2002.
75. Clancy K, Velopulos C, Bilaniuk JW, et al: Screeing for blunt cardiac injury: an Eastern Association for the Surgery of Trauma practice management guideline. *J Trauma Acute Care Surg* 73(5 Suppl 4):S301–S306, 2012.
76. Penney DJ, Bannon PG, Parr MJ: Intra-aortic balloon counterpulsation for cardiogenic shock due to cardiac contusion in an elderly trauma patient. *Resuscitation* 55:337–340, 2002.
77. Perchinsky MJ, Long WB, Hill JG: Blunt cardiac rupture. The Emanuel Trauma Center experience. *Arch Surg* 130(8):852–856; discussion 856–857, 1995.
78. Perlroth MG, Hazan E, Lecompte Y, et al: Chronic tricuspid regurgitation and bifascicular block due to blunt chest trauma. *Am J Med Sci* 291(2):119–125, 1986.
79. Lundevall J: Traumatic rupture of the aorta, with special reference to road accidents. *Acta Pathol Microbiol Scand* 62:29–33, 1964.
80. Ismailov RM, Weiss HB, Ness RB, et al: Blunt cardiac injury associated with cardiac valve insufficiency: trauma links to chronic disease. *Injury* 36(9):1022–1028, 2005.
81. Nicol AJ, Navsaria PH, Beningfield S, et al: Screening for occult penetrating cardiac injuries. *Ann Surg* 261:573–578, 2015.
82. Asensio JA, Stewart BM, Murray J, et al: Penetrating cardiac injuries. *Surg Clin North Am* 76:685–725, 1996.
83. Duval P: Le incision median thoraco-laparotomy: Bull Et Mem Soc De Chir De Paris, xxxiii: 15. As quoted by Ballana C (1920) Bradshaw lecture. The surgery of the heart. *Lancet* CXCVIII:73–79, 1907.
84. Kremer H, Wilson J: Penetrating cardiac injury with urgent not emergent thoracotomy. *Missouri Med* 107(5):328–330, 2010.
85. Makhani M, Midani D, Goldberg A, et al: Pathogenesis and outcomes of traumatic injuries of the esophagus. *Dis Esophagus* 27(7):630–636, 2014.
86. Symbas PN, Hatcher CR, Vlasis SE: Esophageal gunshot injuries. *Ann Surg* 191:703, 1980.
87. Defore WW, Mattox KL, Hansen HA, et al: Surgical management of penetrating injuries of the esophagus. *Am J Surg* 134:734, 1977.
88. Cheadle W, Richardson JD: Options in management of trauma to the esophagus. *Surg Gynecol Obstet* 155:380, 1982.

89. Asensio JA, Berne J, Demetriades D, et al: Penetrating esophageal injuries: time interval of safety for preoperative evaluation-how long is safe? *J Trauma* 43(2):319–324, 1997.
90. Flowers JL, Graham SM, Ugarte MA, et al: Flexible endoscopy for the diagnosis of esophageal trauma. *J Trauma* 40(2):261–265; discussion 265–266, 1996.
91. Mamede RC, De Mello Filho FV: Treatment of caustic ingestion: an analysis of 239 cases. *Dis Esophagus* 15(3):210–213, 2002.
92. Bautista A, Varela R, Villanueva A, et al: Effects of prednisolone and dexamethasone in children with alkali burns of the esophagus. *Eur J Pediatr Surg* 6:198–203, 1996.
93. Pacini D, Angeli E, Fattor R, et al: Traumatic rupture of the thoracic aorta: ten years of delayed management. *J Thorac Cardiovasc Surg* 129:880–884, 2005.
94. Kwon CC, Gill IS, Fallon WF, et al: Delayed operative intervention in the management of traumatic descending thoracic aortic rupture. *Ann Thorac Surg* 74:S1888–S1891, 2002.
95. Demetriades D, Velmahos GC, Scalea TM, et al: Blunt traumatic thoracic aortic injuries: early or delayed repair—results of an American association for the surgery of trauma prospective study. *J Trauma* 66(4):967–973, 2009.
96. Hirose H, Gill IS, Malangoni MA: Nonoperative management of traumatic aortic injury. *J Trauma* 60(3):597–601, 2006.
97. Von Oppell UO, Dunne TT, De Groot MK, et al: Traumatic aortic rupture: twenty-year meta-analysis of mortality and risk for paraplegia. *Ann Thorac Surg* 58:585–593, 1994.
98. Spiliotopoulos K, Kokotsakis J, Argiriou M, et al: Endovascular repair for blunt thoracic aortic injury: 11-year outcomes and postoperative surveillance experience. *J Thorac Cardiovasc Surg* 148(6):2956–2961, 2014.
99. Piffaretti G, Benedetto F, Menegolo M: Outcomes of endovascular repair for blunt thoracic aortic injury. *J Vasc Surg* 58(6):1483–1489, 2013.
100. Demetriades D, Velmahos GC, Scalea TM, et al: Operative repair or endovascular stent graft in blunt traumatic thoracic aortic injuries: results of an American Association for the Surgery of Trauma Multicenter Study. *J Trauma* 64(3):561–571, 2008.
101. Kriel RL, Gormley ME, Krach LE, et al: Automatic garage door openers: hazards for children. *Pediatrics* 98:770–773, 1996.
102. Zanobetti M, Coppa A, Nazerian P, et al: Chest Abdominal-Focused Assessment Sonography for Trauma during the primary survey in the Emergency Department: the CA-FAST protocol. *Eur J Trauma Emerg Surg*, 2015.
103. Lichtenstein D, Mezière G, Biderman P, et al: The "lung point": an ultrasound sign specific to pneumothorax. *Intensive Care Med* 26:1434–1440, 2000.
104. Wilkerson RG, Stone MB: Sensitivity of bedside ultrasound and supine anteroposterior chest radiographs for the identification of pneumothorax after blunt trauma. *Acad Emerg Med* 17:11–17, 2010.
105. Kirkpatrick AW, Sirois M, Laupland KB, et al: Hand-held thoracic sonography for detecting post-traumatic pneumothoraces: the Extended Focused Assessment with Sonography for Trauma (EFAST). *J Trauma* 57:288–295, 2004.
106. Ojaghi Haghighi SH, Adimi I, Shams Vahdati S, et al: Ultrasonographic diagnosis of suspected hemopneumothorax in trauma patients. *Trauma Mon* 19:e17498, 2014. doi: 10.5812/traumamon.17498.
107. Hyacinthe AC, Broux C, Francony G, et al: Diagnostic accuracy of ultrasonography in the acute assessment of common thoracic lesions after trauma. *Chest* 141:1177–1183, 2012.
108. Leblanc D, Bouvet C, Degiovanni F, et al: Early lung ultrasonography predicts the occurrence of acute respiratory distress syndrome in blunt trauma patients. *Intensive Care Med* 40:1468–1474, 2014.
109. Vignon P, Lang RM: Use of transesophageal echocardiography for the assessment of traumatic aortic injuries. *Echocardiography* 16:207–219, 1999.
110. Vignon P, Spencer KT, Rambaud G, et al: Differential transesophageal echocardiographic diagnosis between linear artifacts and intraluminal flap of aortic dissection or disruption. *Chest* 119:1778–1190, 2001.
111. Vignon P, Martaillé JF, François B, et al: Transesophageal echocardiography and therapeutic management of patients sustaining blunt aortic injuries. *J Trauma* 58:1150–1158, 2005.
112. Vignon P, Guéret P, Vedrinne JM, et al: Role of transesophageal echocardiography in the diagnosis and management of traumatic aortic disruption. *Circulation* 92:2959–2968, 1995.

Chapter 44 ■ Critical Care of the Patient with Abdominal Trauma

JON D. DORFMAN

The success of nonoperative treatments and the ubiquitous availability of high-resolution CT scans have changed the management and possible complications from traumatic injuries. This chapter will focus on complications of abdominal trauma that an intensivist should recognize.

One possible origin of the word abdomen is the Latin *abdere*, meaning to conceal. Few areas of the human body are as difficult to assess following injury or to monitor subsequently as is the abdomen, particularly in the obtunded or intubated patient. Much of the morbidity and mortality due to abdominal injury results from delay in recognizing conditions that can be corrected once identified. Once the patient is admitted to the intensive care unit (ICU), the ability to follow changes occurring within the abdomen deteriorates.

ICU ADMISSION

In previous years, trauma patients arriving in the ICU were assumed to have had their injuries identified and definitively treated, frequently in the operating room. Today, the ICU plays a different role in the care of blunt trauma patients, commonly continuing the initial resuscitation to specified endpoints to allow the patient to return to the operating room for definitive care. In the majority of blunt trauma patients, who frequently are managed nonoperatively, the ICU must carefully follow the patients for signs of bleeding or failure of nonoperative management and monitor for the potential complications of "missed" injuries. In patients, who do have operations, they may undergo "damage control" surgery; these patients have staged operations with resuscitation in the ICU between operations. Furthermore, the resuscitation for traumatic abdominal injuries is now known to have systemic physiologic effects.

Trauma surgeons have traditionally separated injured patients into those injured by blunt mechanisms such as car crashes and falls and those injured by penetrating mechanisms, which are subdivided into gunshot wounds or stabbings. Blunt trauma patients are more frequently managed nonoperatively, whereas penetrating trauma, particularly gunshots wounds, more often require operative exploration.

Operative trauma patients will have had a laparotomy, and their injuries should have been defined. However, there still exists a rate of missed injuries of up to 10% [1]. There will be a tendency for the intensivist to consider these patients identical to the elective general surgical patient who has undergone a comparable operation. Although there are certainly areas of commonality, there are critical differences that must be considered. The general surgical patient will usually have only a single acute problem unlike the trauma patient who may have sustained injuries to multiple body regions and possibly more than one organ in the abdomen. These differences often lead to management problems and complications that would not be expected of the general surgical patient.

Many blunt injury patients and selective penetrating injury patients are now managed with the intention of not operating on them. This approach has grown out of the recognition that many trauma laparotomies are nontherapeutic as opposed to negative. For example, a laparotomy for hemoperitoneum that identifies a small liver laceration and a minor tear in the mesentery is certainly not a "negative" laparotomy, but if both injuries have stopped bleeding spontaneously, it is difficult to argue that the surgery was therapeutic. Nontherapeutic laparotomies are not without consequences. Operations are painful; they expose the patient to complications rates in older series of up to 41% [2] and in more recent studies of 14% [3]. Complications include wound infections, pneumonia, urinary tract infections, deep venous thrombosis as well as ileus, bowel obstruction, and incisional hernias. Thus, the risks and benefits of operating must be balanced by trauma surgeons.

NONOPERATIVE MANAGEMENT

Nonoperative management of intra-abdominal injury is so widely practiced that trauma surgeons often feel they have to attempt nonoperative management or justify why they want to operate on a splenic or liver laceration. Nonoperative management of abdominal solid organ injury is appropriate only for hemodynamically stable patients whose injuries are identified by imaging. Hemodynamic stability is not as easy to define as it would appear. Advance Trauma Life Support for Doctors defines hypotension as a systolic blood pressure of 90 mm Hg. However, there are exceptions to this rule. The elderly, in particular, have an increase in mortality with blood pressures lower that 110 to 120 mm Hg [4]. Certainly, patients who require ongoing resuscitation with blood and blood products or pressors to maintain normotension are not considered stable. Other factors to consider include tachycardia or metabolic acidosis, and if present, would also preclude a state of physiologic stability. Additional factors should be considered before a decision to attempt nonoperative management is made. Are there medical conditions such as portal hypertension or the use of anticoagulants? Patients with severe head injuries or ischemic heart disease are often considered to be at high operative risk, but a failure of nonoperative management also poses a high risk of mortality [5,6].

As imaging has improved, trauma surgeons have been given a more precise determination of the anatomic location and severity of the injury prior to deciding whether or not an operation is indicated. This information has allowed the construction of a number of models intended to predict the success of nonoperative management [7]. CT-based injury grading systems have been shown to correlate with clinical outcomes, but, as with most scoring systems, work better for analyzing populations than for predicting the outcome of an individual patient [8,9].

One of the most useful CT findings is the presence of extravasated vascular contrast. This contrast blush usually represents either active bleeding or a pseudoaneurysm of a parenchymal artery. Such patients have a higher probability of failing nonoperative management. Angiographic embolization of the injured vessel may help to restore them to the nonoperative pathway [10].

BLUNT TRAUMA

Spleen

The current practice of managing splenic injury nonoperatively comes from recognition of the immunologic importance of the spleen and the risk of overwhelming postsplenectomy sepsis. Furthermore, realization grew that many splenic injuries required no intervention. The practice of nonoperative management began in pediatrics and has gradually extended into the adult population, for whom nonoperative management is not as successful. Nonoperative failure rates range from 2% to 13% [11]. Predictors of failure of nonoperative management include grade of injury [12], active contrast extravasation, and in some studies, age over 55 years old [13]. Isolated lower grade injuries are unlikely to be admitted to the ICU as the risk of failure of nonoperative management and the risk of mortality are low. If low grade injury patients are admitted to the ICU, it is most likely due to concomitant injuries or significant patient comorbidities. The intensivist should remember that even low grade injuries have a small chance of bleeding that would require intervention. For injuries grade III and higher, the rate of failure of nonoperative management increases and is particularly significant in grade IV (60%) and grade V (75%) injuries [14].

Nonoperative management fails in up to 15% of all patients with splenic injury. In prior studies, 75% of these failures occur within 2 days, and almost 95% of the failures occurred within one week [13].

The nonoperative management of a ruptured spleen must be a joint effort between the surgical and the ICU teams. Parameters that change the management strategy should be agreed upon in advance. In general, any sign of ongoing hemorrhage should lead to immediate surgery and splenectomy. If the patient experiences a steadily falling hemoglobin level but never manifests any change in vital signs, there should be prior agreement regarding the number of units of packed red blood cells (PRBCs) to be transfused before intervening. The absolute number will vary with the estimated operative risk, and other factors predicting success or failure.

Splenic embolization may be an option in some facilities for those patients whose CT demonstrates a contrast blush within the spleen. Patients admitted to the ICU for nonoperative management of a higher grade (III to IV) isolated splenic injury should receive their planned immunizations, including pneumococcal, meningococcal, and Hemophilus influenza vaccine, since there is evidence that these vaccines are more effective with the spleen *in situ* [15].

Other elements of the patient's care are determined in conjunction with the trauma surgeon, or institution. Many centers have protocols that determine the frequency of hemoglobin blood draws, the advancement of activity, when to change the diet, and when to start venothromboembolism (VTE) chemoprophylaxis. Although many studies have been performed, the data have not been conclusive enough to guide the institution of these measures [16]. Most centers start VTE prophylaxis within 48 hours of injury, assuming hemodynamic stability and significant bleeding has ceased.

Another major complication is an infection involving the injured splenic parenchyma or the perisplenic hematoma resulting in either splenic or subphrenic abscess [17]. Unexplained fever, leukocytosis, or pleural effusion should lead to consideration for an abdominal CT scan looking for evidence of infection. Most infections can be effectively treated with antibiotics and percutaneous drainage, but failure to respond promptly should result in exploration, evacuation of the infected hematoma, and splenectomy.

Liver

The other commonly injured abdominal organ from blunt trauma is the liver. As in splenic injuries, nonoperative management of liver injuries has a high success rate (>80%). Although the surgical options differ from the spleen, the decision to operate should be based on similar considerations. The first criterion for successful nonoperative management is hemodynamic stability. A patient who does not meet this condition should be taken to the operating room and explored; surgically, the options include cauterization and placement of sutures. Formal liver resection has a high mortality rate. Treatment can be also be staged with placement of perihepatic packing with or without interventional radiology angiography and embolization with later reexploration after resuscitation, or transfer to a center with additional capabilities.

Patients who remain normotensive or who are successfully resuscitated in the trauma bay will likely have had a CT scan with intravenous contrast. In prior studies, contrast extravasation into the peritoneum on CT scan is likely to require an intervention (operative or angiographic), because these patients are likely to become hemodynamically unstable [18]. Contrast blush or high grade injury may be considered an indication for angiogembolization. Angioembolization is not without risks. Risks include hepatic necrosis requiring surgical debridment and, more commonly, gallbladder ischemia requiring cholecystectomy [19,20]. Liver injuries in the setting of cirrhosis, portal hypertension, or coagulopathy are much more likely to fail nonoperative management than comparable injured patients lacking these comorbidities.

Complications of nonoperative management include intraperitoneal hemorrhage, hemobilia, bile leak or biloma, biliary ascites, hepatic necrosis, and abdominal compartment syndrome [21]. Higher grades of liver injury are associated with higher rates of complications. Delayed bleeding from a liver laceration is uncommon, and if it were to happen, usually occurs within 24 hours postinjury.

Biliary complications occur later than delayed bleeding. Rising liver function tests, fevers, tachycardia, and worsening abdominal pain are an indication for repeat CT scan, or hepatobiliary iminodiacetic acid (HIDA) scan to evaluate for a bile leak. Management of biliary complications include percutaneous drainage of symptomatic bilomas, endoscopic retrograde cholangiopancreatography with biliary stenting, and laparoscopy or laparotomy. Frequently, multimodality treatment is necessary.

Hemobilia is an uncommon complication. Most cases are associated with penetrating rather than blunt hepatic trauma. The classic triad of gastrointestinal hemorrhage, jaundice, and right upper quadrant pain may suggest the diagnosis, although all three signs and symptoms are infrequently present. It may occur within days of the injury to years later. Diagnosis is often difficult and delayed. The bleeding may be intermittent so that diagnostic endoscopy may demonstrate no source for the bleeding. Hepatic angiogram and embolization is considered the first-line therapy, although rarely operative intervention is required [22].

Kidney

Renal injury is most often the result of blunt trauma and and rarely occurs in isolation. Right renal injury most frequently occurs in conjunction with hepatic injury, and left renal injury in conjunction with splenic injury. Renal injury management is usually determined by hemodynamic status. Hemodynamic instability due to a renal injury, typically a high grade renovascular injury (Grade V on the American College of Surgeons Scale of I to V), usually results in nephrectomy. The literature on attempting surgical repair shows that this is usually unsuccessful but should be considered if the trauma patient had only a single functional kidney to begin with [23]. However, in hemodynamically stable high grade IV and V injuries, nonoperative management is still possible and highly successful [24].

The complications of renal injury include hemorrhage and urine leak. Hemorrhage can present as hematuria, but the severity of the hematuria and the degree of the renal injury are often discordant. Gross hematuria may appear dramatic, but most renal bleeding diminishes spontaneously. In some persistent cases, angioembolization may be necessary. Microscopic hematuria is common after blunt abdominal trauma and is of little consequence. Hemorrhage requiring an operation can occur up to 4 days postinjury in some series [24].

Urine leak from an injured kidney can also occur but may resolve spontaneously. Extravasated contrast that is confined within Gerota's fascia does not mandate intervention. Leakage of urine as demonstrated by delayed contrast extravasation outside of Gerota's fascia may still resolve but is more likely to require intervention. Persistent urine leakage or urinoma may need treatment, which can include a combination of ureteral stents, a nephrostomy tube, or percutaneous drainage.

Pancreas

Blunt pancreatic injury is typically the result of high-energy impact to the epigastrium from such mechanisms as handle bar injury in bicyclists or steering wheel injury in a motor vehicle crash. Physical findings are usually minimal. Pancreatic injury rarely occurs by itself and is usually associated with injury to adjacent organs or structures such as the liver, kidneys, or spleen. Injury to these organs should heighten your vigilance. The challenge in detection is that laboratory and imaging studies are often nondiagnostic. Mortality rates of up to 40% are reported from high grade injuries. Injury to the pancreas is one of the classic "missed injuries" that may not become apparent until days later.

Serum amylase and lipase may be monitored after blunt abdominal trauma. Amylasemia is not specific to pancreatic injuries, and therefore the sensitivity and specificity is low. For example, traumatic brain injury and salivary gland injury can lead to a rise in amylase levels. Lipase is also not predictive of injury. Futhermore, serum amylase drawn within 3 hours of the injury is inaccurate. Finally, the extent of amylasemia elevation does not correlate with extent of injury [25].

Imaging of the pancreas also has limitations. Abdominal CT scans with intravenous contrast are commonly performed and are normal in up to 40% of patients with a pancreatic injury. The findings may be nonspecific and may not appear for 12 hours or more after injury. These findings include signs of inflammation or "stranding" around the pancreas. Other signs may include lacerations, contusions, or hematoma.

The critical factor that determines the management strategy of pancreatic injuries is whether or not the main pancreatic duct is injured. AAST low grade injuries (I and II) do not involve the duct, whereas high grade injuries (III to V) have main ductal injury. If pancreatic ductal disruption is present, distal resection or internal drainage produces much less morbidity than simple drainage or noninvasive management [26]. If no definitive reason for surgical exploration exists but there is reason to suspect or diagnose a pancreatic injury, it is imperative to evaluate the ductal integrity. If there is any suggestion of instability or peritoneal signs, this should be performed at the time of abdominal exploration. Otherwise, the patient may be a candidate for magnetic resonance cholangiopancreatography (MRCP) or ERCP. Delay in diagnosing and providing definitive therapy for a ductal injury may have devastating consequences.

Pelvic Fracture

Pelvic fractures may be the result of low-energy falls in the osteoporotic elderly or high-energy trauma in a young motorcyclist. In each case, pelvic fractures can lead to life-threatening hemorrhage and complications. There are multiple classification systems for pelvic fractures. One of the more commonly used systems is Young and Burgess, which classifies the fracture on the basis of four impact patterns—anterior posterior compression (APC), lateral compression (LC), vertical shear, and complex—for pelvic fractures that do not fit simply into one of the previous categories. APC and LC have 3 subtypes. The Young and Burgess system aids in understanding the stability of the fracture and the potential complications.

Hemorrhage can be significant; the source of the hemorrhage and hypotension may not initially be certain given the association of pelvic fractures with intra-abdominal solid organ injuries and long bone fractures. Other sources of bleeding must be considered, identified, and dealt with accordingly. Pelvic fracture–associated bleeding can be from injured pelvic arteries, disrupted veins, particularly of the sacral plexus, and even the fractured pelvic bones themselves. The fracture pattern has some association with potential blood loss; APC2 and APC3 fractures as well as LC3 and vertical shear are higher blood loss fracture patterns; APC3 fractures can require 10 units or more of PRBCs for resuscitation [27]. Management options include closing the pelvic ring in APC2 and APC3 fracture patients who are hemodynamically unstable. Wrapping the pelvis at the greater trochanters can achieve temporary closure of the pelvic ring and effectively reduce the pelvic volume. External fixation by orthopedic surgery can be performed in the operating room. Embolization of arterial extravasation is also an option; however, not all patients who have active extravasation on CT scan necessarily require embolization. Hemodynamic instability and ongoing blood transfusion requirements due to a pelvic fracture are indications for angiography [28]. Performing embolization, however, is not without potential complications. Gluteal muscle and skin necrosis have been reported along with soft tissue infection requiring debridement [29]. For uncontrolled venous hemorrhage, prepelvic packing is advocated at some trauma centers [30]. Even with this armamentarium, the mortality rate from pelvic injury can be quite high.

With large retroperitoneal hematomas, abdominal distension can lead to abdominal compartment syndrome. Ventilation, in particular, can be impaired as the abdominal contents reduce the thoracic volume. Respiratory failure leading to intubation can occur.

Associated injuries with pelvic fracture include long bone fractures and intra-abdominal injury. Intra-abdominal solid and hollow viscous organ injury will be addressed separately. Here it is important to discuss genitourinary and rectal injury, which are more commonly associated with "open book" fractures, APC2 and APC3. Urethral injuries are relatively uncommon (2%). Men are more likely to sustain a urethral injury than women. Suspicion for this injury should be elevated if blood is noted at the urethral meatus or there is a high-riding prostate on rectal examination. A retrograde urethrogram can confirm the injury; if found, this injury is treated with placement of a urinary catheter or temporized with a suprapubic tube. Bladder injury can occur as well and should be considered if gross hematuria is noted. CT cystogram can confirm the diagnosis and determine whether the injury to the bladder leads to intraperitoneal or extraperitoneal urine leakage. Intraperitoneal leakage requires operative repair via a laparotomy and with prolonged bladder decompression with a urinary catheter. Extraperitoneal leakage may be managed with only a urinary catheter for 2 weeks [31]. Rectal injury should also be considered for all pelvic fractures but is most commonly associated with APC2 and APC3. Blood on rectal examination should prompt rigid sigmoidoscopy and consideration for diverting colostomy. Untreated rectal injuries may lead to abscess formation and pelvic sepsis.

Other

Nonoperative management of abdominal injuries is the treatment strategy for the solid organs, including the liver and spleen, as previously discussed. Hollow viscous injuries are usually managed with an intervention except in two particular circumstances. These two exceptions are intramural hematoma of the duodenum and extraperitoneal rupture of the bladder.

Blunt duodenal injuries are primarily the result of a blunt force to the epigastrium such as from the steering wheel or seat belt in a motor vehicle crash and handle bars in a bicycle crash. In the AAST grading system, duodenal hematomas are either Grade I or II injuries, depending on the length of the duodenum involved [32]. Symptoms, when present, will usually be those of gastric outlet obstruction. Diagnosis is made from a CT scan with oral contrast or an upper gastrointestinal study. The patient should be carefully evaluated for any evidence of a concomitant pancreatic injury. If there are no associated injuries, nonoperative management is recommended. Gastric decompression with a nasogastric tube and nutritional support with total parenteral nutririon should be prescribed. Periodic radiographic reevaluation should occur to determine whether the obstruction has resolved. If it has not resolved within several weeks, evaluation for possible stricture should be considered.

Approximately 80% of bladder injuries occur in the setting of pelvic fracture, although only about 5% of pelvic fractures are associated with bladder injuries [33]. Bladder injuries are often extraperitoneal and result from perforation of the bladder by bone fragments from fractures of the parasymphyseal pelvis. This may occur even though the final position of the bone fragments as demonstrated on radiographs does not appear near the bladder. Bladder injury is also suggested by the inability to void, incomplete return of catheter irrigation into the bladder, and gross hematuria. Any pelvic fracture associated with gross hematuria requires a cystogram. Diagnosis requires retrograde contrast injection into the bladder with images taken in both the anteroposterior (AP) and lateral views and postvoiding. CT scan with contrast can also give a high-quality image of the bladder by clamping the Foley catheter to distend the bladder. Extraperitoneal injuries typically will heal with bladder decompression by a urinary catheter for 7 to 14 days. Prior to removal of the catheter, a repeat cystogram should be obtained to confirm resolution of the injury. Persistent extravasation may require surgical repair of the bladder.

PENETRATING INJURY

In some institutions, patients with penetrating trauma may be selected for nonoperative management and admitted to the ICU for close monitoring. As with blunt trauma, the fundamental requirement for nonoperative management is hemodynamic stability and the absence of peritonitis. Any hemodynamic instability or the development of peritoneal signs mandates exploration.

Stab wounds are much more likely to be monitored nonoperatively than gunshot wounds. This type of penetrating abdominal injury has a lower incidence of penetrating the posterior abdominal fascia, and even if penetration occurs, only a fraction of stabbings cause an injury that requires repair. The ICU team will monitor for hemodynamic changes, a change in abdominal examination, and signs of abdominal sepsis [34].

Gunshot wounds are infrequently managed nonoperatively if the bullet enters the peritoneal cavity because of the higher probability of visceral, particularly hollow viscus, injury. However, CT imaging is now allowing the nonoperative management of highly selected abdominal gunshot wounds. These cases are primarily patients who are hemodynamically stable, have no peritoneal signs on examination, or for whom the entire tract of the missile appears to lie within a solid organ (liver, spleen, kidney, retroperitoneum). Such patients should be monitored in a manner similar to blunt trauma patients with the exception that hollow viscus injury is still a concern [35].

MISSED INJURIES

Missed injuries may be a misnomer because the injury may not have been apparent or detectable at the time of arrival at the hospital. Furthermore, no matter how careful the initial evaluation of the trauma patient, almost all series report an approximately 10% incidence of missed injuries that are discovered in a delayed fashion [36]. Most of these are minor extremity fractures discovered as the patient begins to increase activity and reports pain. The delay in diagnosis is generally inconsequential. However, a delay of the diagnosis of a hollow viscus injury may have serious consequences. Avoiding delays in diagnosis requires the cooperation of the entire team providing care to the patient. The initial assessment should be thorough and take into account the mechanism of injury, external signs of trauma, patient complaints, and laboratory and radiographic findings. In spite of such a detailed and comprehensive evaluation, additional information will often become available over the first 24 to 48 hours. Bruises, abrasions, seat belt marks, will often be more apparent the next day. Laboratory and even imaging studies are less sensitive when the patient arrives at the trauma center within a few hours of injury. These facts have led many trauma centers to institute a formal tertiary survey within 24 hours of admission [37]. During the tertiary survey, the patient should be carefully reexamined from head to toe for new evidence of traumatic injury. Radiographs should be reexamined and compared with the now dictated radiology interpretation. Tertiary surveys are even more important when the patient is initially unstable, and examiners may be distracted by the urgency of the situation. Furthermore, patients who had altered mental status from traumatic brain injury or intoxication may now relay new symptoms. Patients who were intubated and unable to communicate may provide important subjective complaints once extubated. Repeat focused assessment sonography in trauma (FAST) or computed tomography (CT) scan should be considered if there is any change in status. Injuries such as pancreatic, or small bowel injuries may be more apparent on a CT scan performed at 24 hours postinjury than on the initial scan.

Bowel

One of the major concerns is the possibility of a missed bowel injury. Direct bowel rupture from blunt trauma is uncommon. Typically, injury occurs to the mesentery, and therefore the blood supply to a segment of small intestine is compromised. The segment of intestine supplied by injured mesentery becomes ischemic over time and may then become necrotic. A patient who has a bowel injury will likely not have peritoneal signs initially. Peritoneal signs develop over time but may not be apparent in a patient who has a traumatuc brain injury, intoxication, intubated on sedation, or has a distracting injury. On examination, a "seat belt" sign or abdominal wall injury from the seat belt has been associated with blunt bowel injury and should increase the index of suspicion.

Injuries can also be missed at the time of surgical exploration. Although the mesenteric injury to the small intestine may be apparent, the retroperitoneal colon injury from a seat belt would not be obvious in the operating room. The intensive care team must be cognizant of the possibility of missed injury and have a heightened vigilance for the signs and symptoms in patients who are not progressing or improving as would be expected. Patients arriving with "negative" abdominal CT scans and the patient admitted following abdominal exploration must be reevaluated for bowel injury if they show signs of unexplained sepsis, prolonged ileus, rising white blood cell (WBC) count, or failure to clear their acidosis.

Patients admitted to the ICU for planned nonoperative management are at particular risk. The sensitivity and specificity of CT scanning is low for hollow viscus injury [38]. Trauma CT scan protocols use intravenous contrast without oral contrast. Even with oral contrast, the free leak of oral contrast into the peritoneal cavity is a relatively infrequent finding. Free air may be demonstrated, but its absence certainly cannot exclude bowel injury. An area of localized thickening of the bowel wall is suggestive of injury, whereas a diffuse thickening is more compatible with either excess fluid administration or poor perfusion. CT findings that cause concern are intraperitoneal hemorrhage without evidence of a solid organ injury to account for the bleeding and signs of mesenteric injury. There is a debate about how much free fluid (hemorrhage) is enough to create concern for bowel injury. Some consider this sufficient evidence for exploration, whereas others disagree [39]. Recent studies attempted to devise scoring systems based on CT imaging, physical examination, and laboratory findings; however, nearly 16% of patients still required a delayed laparotomy [40].

Any mesenteric injury that is not explored surgically must be monitored carefully in the postinjury period to allow the recognition of ischemic bowel prior to perforation. Even with penetrating trauma, there is a missed injury rate. Urgency of hemorrhage control may lead to oversight. An apparently straight missile tract may not have been so straight. Bowel may have been in a different configuration at the time of penetration. Tangential injuries to the intestine on the mesenteric border that appeared not to have injured the intestine are a classic location of missed injury. Areas of bowel injury that did not appear transmural may have been deeper than was realized. Areas that did not appear injured such as the retroperitoneum may not have been explored. It is incumbent on the operating surgeon to explore the abdomen thoroughly, but in spite of this, injuries will at times be missed. Neither the operating surgeon nor the intensivist caring for the patient in the ICU should dismiss the possibility if the patient is not recovering as anticipated.

Pancreas

Signs and symptoms of pancreatic injury may not manifest immediately. As previously explained, serum amylase and serum lipase will not be elevated if checked within 3 hours of the injury. CT scan findings may be minimal or completely lacking within 12 to 24 hours of the injury. Fluid collections (pseudocysts), pancreatic ascites, pancreatitis, and sepsis may develop days after the injury.

Renal Collecting System

Injuries to the renal collecting system, including the renal pelvis, ureters, and bladder, may present as a rising blood urea nitrogen (BUN) without obvious explanation, as new onset nonhemorrhagic ascites without evidence of cirrhosis, as drainage of serosanguineous fluid from the incision, or as a mass in the flank or pelvis. The diagnosis is usually not difficult as long as a urine leak is considered. CT with intravenous contrast with appropriately timed delayed images will usually establish the diagnosis. Any unexplained fluid collection in the abdomen that is aspirated should be analyzed for creatinine and compared to the serum level. Most injuries that are diagnosed late can be managed with decompression or stenting, although complete transection of a ureter will require operative repair.

Solid Organs

The probability of missing a solid organ injury if the patient has received a CT scan with intravenous contrast is low. CT scans with intravenous contrast identify approximately 98%

of solid organ injuries. The probability of missing a significant solid organ injury is even lower. However, solid organ injuries can be missed if the patient does not receive a CT scan on the basis of what is perceived to be a normal physical examination with a false negative FAST examination. As previously discussed, many reasons exist for an erroneous physical examination. Blood in the peritoneal cavity may not cause peritoneal irritation immediately. Intoxication, traumatic brain injury, or distracting injuries can alter the abdominal examination. FAST examinations are intended to assess the presence or absence of free fluid in the abdomen, not injury to solid organs. Some liver, spleen, or kidney lacerations produce little or no free fluid on initial examination. Patients admitted to the ICU without abdominal CT scanning or with a noncontrast CT should be monitored closely. Any unexplained deterioration in vital signs or change in hemoglobin should prompt an immediate FAST examination or a CT scan if the patient is sufficiently stable to be transported to radiology.

ABDOMINAL COMPARTMENT SYNDROME

Abdominal compartment syndrome (ACS) is a recognized complication of traumatic injury and resuscitation, but the diagnosis may be delayed or missed all together. Recogntion of ACS began in the 1800s with reports of the deleterious results of intra-abdominal hypertension, but the clinical diagnosis was imprecise, unreliable, and infrequently made. With the publication by Kron et al. [41] of the indirect measurement of intra-abdominal pressure (IAP) by bladder pressure, diagnosis of ACS became feasible and quantifiable. ACS assumed even greater importance with the widespread use of damage control surgical resuscitation as patients at high risk for ACS should be considered for staged closure. A complete review of ACS is presented in its own chapter 52, including current definitions, pathophysiology, systemic consequences, measuring techniques, and management. We discuss it briefly here as it relates specifically to abdominal trauma.

Pathophysiology

The fundamental physiology of ACS does not differ from any other compartment syndrome. It may occur as a result of bleeding, edema, or packing within the abdomen, referred to as primary compartment syndrome, or as a result of ischemia-reperfusion and capillary leak associated with other disease processes such as major burns or systemic sepsis. This is referred to as secondary compartment syndrome. Pressure within the abdominal compartment increases until the perfusion pressure is inadequate to meet the oxygen and nutrient needs of the tissues within the abdomen or extra-abdominal organ failure results.

As IAP increases, the abdomen distends until it can expand no further. The increased intra-abominal pressure is transmitted to the surrounding structures. Although the most direct technique involves the insertion of catheter directly into the peritoneal cavity, this is not practical or necessary for injured patients. The accepted clinical technique is an indirect assessment by the bladder pressure measurement.

When IAP rises to a critical level, not only does it compromise blood flow to intra-abdominal organs, it also negatively impacts the respiratory, cardiovascular, and central nervous systems. ACS is defined as an abdominal pressure of more than 20 mm Hg with one or more organs showing signs of dysfunction [42].

Clinical Manifestations

Increases in IAP impact virtually every organ system. Often, the first measurable finding involves the respiratory system, where increased IAP is often the cause of hypercarbia due to decreased minute ventilation. In a pressure control mode, the tidal volumes will decrease. In a volume control setting, peak inspiratory pressures will rise. These changes may be subtle initially, but then dramatic changes will occur rapidly [43,44]. Other possible causes are frequently considered first, such as pulmonary edema and acute lung injury; however, ACS should not be forgotten on the differential diagnosis, or it will be missed and the consequences will be dire.

Increased IAP increases renal vein pressure with elevations in plasma renin and aldosterone as well as decreased renal blood flow, glomerular filtration, and urine output [45]. The result is oliguria and then anuria. In the midst of a trauma resuscitation, oliguria could easily be misinterpreted as hypovolemia and the need for additional resuscitation, which could exacerbate the problem.

The increase in IAP results in an elevated central venous pressure and pulmonary capillary wedge pressure. In spite of this, actual venous return declines, leading to decreased cardiac output and increased systemic and pulmonary vascular resistance. This compromise in venous return is transmitted to the central nervous system, resulting in increased intracranial pressure and decreased cerebral perfusion pressure.

Management of Intra-abdominal Hypertension

In patients judged to be at high risk for the development of ACS, the risk may be reduced by leaving the abdomen open at the time of surgery. Similarly, a patient whose abdominal wall is difficult to close because of edematous bowel or a large retroperitoneal hematoma may be better managed as an open abdomen from the beginning. Anytime there is a suspicion of ACS, the initial diagnostic step should be the measurement of IAP. If IAP is elevated, the therapeutic choices are to either reduce the volume of the abdominal contents by removing space occupying lesions or to enlarge the abdominal compartment. Bedside ultrasound allows the determination of whether there is a significant quantity of free fluid in the abdomen. If so, either a paracentesis or the insertion of a drain may remove enough simple fluid to reduce the abdominal pressure. Large quantities of fluid or gas within distended bowel loops may be removed with a nasogastric tube. IAP may also be reduced in some patients with the use of improved analgesia and even neuromuscular blockade. Although these few special cases should not be overlooked, many cases of ACS will require surgical decompression with some form of temporary abdominal closure.

Open Abdomen

Patients whose abdomen is opened to prevent or treat ACS will require some alternative method of closure to prevent evisceration, to manage fluid loss, and to prevent loss of domain of the abdominal viscera. One of the simplest forms of temporary abdominal wall closure that allows expansion of the abdominal cavity is the towel clip closure. This technique is based on the rapid closure of the skin only with multiple surgical towel clips [46]. Although it is inexpensive and fast, towel clip closure has largely been abandoned in recent years because it has been recognized that a significant number of patients developed a recurrent compartment syndrome. Other methods of temporary closure that allow expansion of the abdominal cavity include placing absorbable mesh or gauze packing [47]. Additional techniques have been based on the silo idea similar to that used for newborns with gastroschisis [46]. Several materials have been utilized for the silo, from 3 L bags of fluid to adhesive drapes to sterile silastic sheets.

Currently, the most popular management of the open abdomen is negative pressure wound therapy [48]. The fundamental principle is the application of a nonadherent barrier over the bowel, followed by negative pressure connection, and then a closed, sealed covering over the abdomen. The benefits of such a negative pressure dressing include reduced wound care, removal of fluid from the peritoneal cavity, and the collapse of any free space in the abdomen. The negative pressure may also minimize the retraction of the abdominal wall muscles. A number of homemade devices have been described, and several commercial systems are now also available.

Once the patient has been resuscitated and abdominal injuries addressed, the next priority is abdominal closure. The longer the abdomen remains open, the greater will be the difficulty in achieving closure as well as the greater the risk of enteroatmospheric fistula formation. To achieve closure of the adbominal wall will require coordination between the surgical and ICU teams, the patient should have a negative fluid balance, and diuretics should be administered as needed. Reapproximation of the midline fascia may require the use of pharmacologic muscle relaxants, multiple trips to the operating room to partially close the abdominal wall each time, or more complex surgical techniques such as component separation [49]. In some cases, fascial closure cannot be obtained, and coverage by closing skin only or placement of a split thickness will be required. This method is not ideal because it will lead to a ventral hernia that will require repair months to years later once the patient has recovered.

Prolonged exposure of the bowel by any of these techniques results in a substantial risk of enteroatmospheric fistula formation. Fistula formation greatly complicates the wound management as well as fluid and nutritional management. The primary goal of this phase of open abdominal management is to achieve some form of wound closure before enteroatmospheric fistula formation occurs.

DAMAGE CONTROL RESUSCITATION

Damage Control Surgery

Historically, trauma surgeons attempted a single definitive operation. In patients with large injury burdens or serious physiologic derangements, recognition of the benefits of staging the operation has occurred. In these carefully selected patients, hemorrhage control and then control of enteric spillage is prioritized. The reconstruction to obtain gastrointestinal continuity and closure of the abdominal wall is left to later procedures once the patient's physiologic condition improves. This damage control philosophy attempts to abort the cycle of the "triad of death" [50] in which hypothermia, acidosis, and coagulopathy worsen until the patient expires. This technique has become widely used and applied for traumatic and nontraumatic abdominal catastrophes. Damage control has been advocated in the following circumstances: if more than 10 units of blood has been transfused, base excess of −18 mmol per L or less if patient is less than 55 years old; base excess of −8 mmol per L or less if patient is greater than 55 years old; lactic acidosis greater than 5 mmol per L; hypothermia of less than 35°C [51]. Damage control surgery, as generally practiced, consists of three phases:

- **I.** Limited operative intervention aimed at controlling hemorrhage, usually by ligation, shunting, or packing, and at controlling contamination, usually by ligation or stapling. Little or no repair or reconstruction is performed at this stage. Abdominal closure is rapid and temporary.
- **II.** Resuscitation in the ICU to correct hypovolemia with blood products, hypothermia by active warming, and coagulopathy by replacement of coagulation factors.
- **III.** Planned return to the operating room to look for additional injuries, perform definite surgical procedure, remove packs, and to close the abdominal wall. This phase should take place only when the physiologic derrangements described above have been corrected.

Inability to resuscitate the patient and correct the physiologic deficits of acidosis, hypovolemia, hypothermia, and coagulopathy may reflect continued bleeding or an injury that needs to be addressed. It is not difficult to overlook a surgical bleeding site when it is obscured by diffuse nonsurgical bleeding. Furthermore, vessels may spasm and once hypotension is corrected in the ICU, may hemorrhage again. Making the decision to return to the OR before correction of the deficits is a difficult one. Various criteria have been described for emergent return to the OR [52], but in practice, the decision is often based on progress or the lack thereof. If the temperature, the pH, the coagulation studies, and the vital signs are getting better, it is usually worth continuing with resuscitation in the ICU. If there are signs of ongoing bleeding and physiologic parameters are worsening, it may be worth the risk of transporting the patient back to the OR for another look or considering angioembolization if the surgical team feels that an operative intervention will not be of benefit, for example, a liver injury that has been packed already.

Acidosis

Hypovolemic shock of the severely injured patient produces a metabolic derangement that will not have disappeared with the restoration of normal vital signs. One manifestation of this metabolic failure is a lactic acidosis. A variety of endpoints for resuscitation have been proposed, but none have been shown to be more reliable than resolution of the lactic acidosis. The role of crystalloid as a resuscitative fluid has changed over the past decades. Intravenous fluid is acidotic, and only a fraction remains intravascular. Crystalloid causes cellular swelling, organ edema, and dysfunction and is proinflammatory [53]. The resuscitative volume expander of choice in patients with hemorrhagic shock has become blood and blood products with limited crystalloid administration. Recent data suggest that more of the resuscitation should be based on blood and blood products with lower ratios with a proven benefit to patient outcomes [54,55].

Severe acidosis increases the risk of cardiac arrhythmias, reduces the effectiveness of endogenous and exogenous catecholamines, and worsens coagulopathy. The enzymes of the coagulation cascade do not function as well in pH ranges outside of homeostasis; furthermore, platelet dysfunction occurs. Thus, it may be appropriate to use alkalinizing agents such as sodium bicarbonate or THAM (trishydroxymethylaminomethane) to raise the pH above 7.2 [56]. There is no clinical proof of mortality benefit, however, from this practice of correcting the acidosis with alkalinizing agents.

Hypothermia

Hypothermia and traumatic injury are a lethal combination. Hypothermia in trauma begins at 36°C as opposed to isolated hypothermia from environmental exposure, which begins at 35°C. Mortality rates are as high as 40% in trauma patients with temperatures of 34°C and approach 100% when the patient's temperature is less than 32°C [51]. Hypothermia of the abdominal trauma patient is usually multifactorial. Patients may arrive hypothermic from exposure and shock. Further exposure to cold environments in the emergency department (ED) or the operating room (OR) worsens this problem; other factors include the infusion of cold fluids and blood products, and an open peritoneal cavity in the operating room. Inadequate oxygen delivery leads to a failure of heat production. Vasodilation from either intoxicants or anesthetic agents and loss of shivering ability from muscle relaxants also aggravate the situation. It is critical to prevent the development of hypothermia because it is difficult to correct once present.

However, despite efforts in the ED and the OR, many damage control patients will be delivered to the ICU already hypothermic. In this circumstance, aggressive efforts must be employed, including raising the room temperature, ensuring the patient is covered with blankets, warming blankets, and warming all intravenous fluids and blood products administered. Lavage of the stomach via the nasogastric tube or lavage of the pleural cavity via the chest tube with warm saline solution may be considered. In severe cases of hypothermia, it may be appropriate to utilize continuous arteriovenous rewarming as described by Gentilello et al. [57]. The inability to correct hypothermia if these measures have been employed usually indicates a failure of adequate resuscitation.

Coagulopathy

The cause of coagulopathy of trauma, as with many other conditions, is multifactoral. The attributed etiologies include consumption of coagulation factors from hemorrhage as well as dilution from infusion of crystalloids. Hypothermia and acidosis play an important part in the coagulation cascade because enzymatic processes function poorly outside of the homeostatic normal, as was discussed in previous sections. Hypothermia and acidosis should be corrected to reduce the coagulopathy.

However, blunt trauma, and, in particular, crush injury, is associated with coagulopathy from tissue injury. These patients may arrive at the hospital already coagulopathic. In fact, up to 25% of patients arrive coagulopathic; this coagulopathy is associated with higher injury severity scores and predicts worse outcomes [58].

On arrival in the ICU from the initial phase of damage control surgery, blood should immediately be sent to the laboratory for prothrombin time, activated partial thromboplastin time, platelet count, and fibrinogen level. Thromboelastography has become more widely used and is advocated by some centers as a better and more rapid assessment of coagulopathy and a way to determine which components of the coagulation cascade to replace.

SUMMARY

This chapter focuses on the unique aspects of critically ill abdominal trauma patients. With the increased use of nonoperative management and damage control resuscitation, the role of the intensivist has changed. The ICU must monitor closely for hemorrhage, signaling the failure of nonoperative management of solid organ injuries. All injuries may not have been identified prior to admission to the ICU, and a high index of suspicion must be maintained for missed injuries that are not readily apparent at presentation and are not easily found on the initial CT scan. For damage control resuscitation, the correction of hypovolemia, hypothermia, acidosis, and coagulopathy occurs as the patient transitions between the ED, the OR, and the ICU.

References

1. Lawson CM, Daley BJ, Ormsby CB, et al: Missed injuries in the era of the trauma scan. *J Trauma* 70:452–458, 2011.
2. Renz BM, Feliciano DV: Unnecessary laparotomies for trauma: a prospective study of morbidity. *J Trauma* 38(3):350–356, 1995.
3. Schnuriger B, Lam L, Inaba K, et al: Negative laparotomy in trauma: are we getting better? *Am Surg* 78(11):1219–1223, 2012.
4. Oyetunji TA, Chang DC, Crompton JG, et al: Redefining hypotension in the elderly: normotension is not reassuring. *Arch Surg* 146(7):865–869, 2011.
5. Peitzman AB, Heil B, Rivera L, et al: Blunt splenic rupture in adults: multi-institutional study of the eastern association for the surgery of trauma. *J Trauma* 49:177–87, 2000.
6. Godley CD, Warren RL, Sheridan RL, et al: Non-operative management of blunt splenic injury in adults: age over 55 years as a powerful indicator for failure. *J Am Coll Surg* 183:133–139, 1996.
7. Malhotra AK, Fabian TC, Croce MA, et al: Blunt hepatic injury: a paradigm shift from operative to non-operative management in the 1990s. *Ann Surg* 231:804–813, 2000.
8. Cohn SM, Arango JI, Myers JG, et al: Computed tomography grading systems poorly predict the need for intervention after spleen and liver injury. *Am Surg* 75:133–139, 2009.
9. MacLean AA, Durso A, Cohn SM, et al: A clinically relevant liver injury grading system by CT, preliminary report. *Emerg Radiol* 12:34–37, 2005.
10. Davis KA, Fabian TC, Croce MA, et al: Improved success in nonoperative management of blunt splenic injuries: embolization of splenic artery pseudoaneurysms. *J Trauma* 44:1008–1013, 1998.
11. Moore FA, Davis JW, Moore EE, et al: Western Trauma Association (WTA) critical decisions in trauma: management of adult blunt splenic trauma. *J Trauma* 65:1007–1011, 2008.
12. Tinkoff G, Esposito TJ, Reed J, et al: American association for the surgery of trauma organ injury scale I: spleen, liver, and kidney validation based on the national trauma data bank. *J Am Coll Surg* 207:646–655, 2008.
13. McIntyre LK, Schiff M, Jurkovich GJ: Failure of nonoperative management of splenic injuries. *Arch Surg* 40:563–569, 2005.
14. Vlahos GC, Zacharias N, Emhoff TA, et al: Management of the most severely injured spleen. *Arch Surg* 145(5):456–460, 2010.
15. Howdieshell TR, Heffernan D, Dipiro JT, et al: Surgical infection society guidelines for vaccination after traumatic injury. *Surg Infect (Larchmt)* 7:275–303, 2006.
16. Stassen NA, Bhullar I, Cheng JD, et al: Selective nonoperative management of blunt splenic injury: an eastern association for the surgery of trauma practice management guideline. *J Trauma Acute Care Surg* 73:S294–S300, 2012.
17. Sekikawa T, Shatney CH: Septic sequelae after splenectomy for trauma in adults. *Am J Surg* 145:667–673, 1983.
18. Fang JF, Wong YC, Lin BC, et al: The CT risk factors for the need of operative treatment in initially hemodynamically stable patients after blunt hepatic trauma. *J Trauma* 61:547–554, 2006.
19. Dabbs DN, Stein DM, Scalea TM: Major hepatic necrosis: a common complication after angioembolization for treatment of high-grade liver injuries. *J Trauma* 66:621–629, 2009.
20. Misselbeck TS, Teicher EJ, Cipolle MD, et al: Hepatic angioembolization in trauma patients: indications and complications. *J Trauma* 67:769–773, 2009.
21. Kozar RA, Moore FA, Cothren CC, et al: Risk factors for hepatic morbidity following nonoperative management. *Arch Surg* 141:451–459, 2006.
22. Forleea MV, Krigea JE, Welman CJ, et al: Haemobilia after penetrating and blunt liver injury: treatment with selective hepatic artery embolisation. *Injury* 35:23–28, 2004.
23. Santucci RA, Fisher MB: The literature increasingly supports expectant (Conservative) management of renal trauma—a systematic review. *J Trauma* 59:491–501, 2005.
24. van der Wilden GM, Velmahos GC, Joseph DK, et al: Successful nonoperative management of the most severe blunt renal injuries a multicenter study of the research consortium of New England centers for trauma. *JAMA Surg* 148(10):924–931, 2013.
25. Subramanian A, Dente CJ, Feliciano DV: The management of pancreatic trauma in the modern era. *Surg Clin N Am* 87:1515–1532, 2007.
26. Olah A, Issekutz A, Haulik L, et al: Pancreatic transaction from blunt abdominal trauma: early versus delayed diagnosis and surgical management. *Dig Surg* 20:408–414, 2003.
27. Dyer GS, Vrahas MS: Review of the pathophysiology and acute management of haemorrhage in pelvic fracture. *Injury* 37(7):602–613, 2006.
28. Cullinane DC, Schiller HJ, Zielinskiv MD, et al: Eastern association for the surgery of trauma practice management guidelines for hemorrhage in pelvic fracture—update and systematic review. *J Trauma* 71:1850–1868, 2011.
29. Yasumura K, Ikegami K, Kamohara T, et al: High incidence of ischemic necrosis of the gluteal muscle after transcatheter angiographic embolization for severe pelvic fracture. *J Trauma* 58:985–990, 2005.
30. Cothren CC, Osborn PM, Moore EE, et al: Preperitoneal pelvic packing for hemodynamically unstable pelvic fractures: a paradigm shift. *J Trauma* 62:834–842, 2007.
31. Flint L, Cryer HG: Pelvic fracture: the last 50 years. *J Trauma* 69:483–488, 2010.
32. Moore EE, Cogbill T, Malangoni M, et al: Organ injury scaling II: pancreas, duodenum, small bowel, colon and rectum. *J Trauma* 30:1427–1429, 1990.
33. Cass AS: The multiple injured patient with bladder trauma: *J Trauma* 24:731–734, 1984.
34. Biffl WL, Kaups KL, Cothren CC, et al: Management of patients with anterior abdominal stab wounds: a western trauma association multicenter trial. *J Trauma* 66:1294–1301, 2009.
35. Velmahos GC, Constantinou C, Tillou A, et al: Abdominal computed tomographic scan for patients with gunshot wounds to the abdomen selected for nonoperative management. *J Trauma* 59:1155–1161, 2005.
36. Chena CW, Chub CM, Yuc WY, et al: Incidence rate and risk factors of missed injuries in major trauma patients. *Accid Anal Prev* 43:823–828, 2011.
37. Biffl WL, Harrington DT, Cioffi WG: Implementation of a tertiary trauma survey decreases missed injuries. *J Trauma* 54:38–43, 2003.
38. Malhotra AK, Fabian TC, Katsis SB, et al: Blunt bowel and mesenteric injuries: the role of screening computed tomography. *J Trauma* 48:991–998, 2000.
39. Livingston DH, Lavery RF, Passannante MR, et al: Free fluid on abdominal computed tomography without solid organ injury after blunt abdominal does not mandate celiotomy. *Am J Surg* 182:6–9, 2001.
40. McNutt MK, Chinapuvvula NR, Beckmann NM, et al: Early surgical intervention for blunt bowel injury. *J Trauma Acute Care Surg* 78:105–111, 2015.
41. Kron IL, Harman PK, Nolan SP: The measurement of intra-abdominal pressure as a criterion for re-exploration. *Ann Surg* 199:28–30, 1984.

42. Kirkpatrick AW, Roberts DJ, De Waele J, et al: Intra-abdominal hypertension and the abdominal compartment syndrome: updated consensus definitions and clinical practice guidelines from the world society of the abdominal compartment syndrome. *Intensive Care Med* 39:1190–1206, 2013.
43. Meldrum DR, Moore FA, Moore EE, et al: Prospective characterization and selective management of the abdominal compartment syndrome. *Am J Surg* 174:667–672, 1997.
44. Cullen DJ, Coyle JP, Teplich R, et al: Cardiovascular, pulmonary, and renal effects of massively increased intra-abdominal pressure in critically ill patients. *Crit Care Med* 17:118–121, 1989.
45. Harman PK, Kron IL, McLachlan HD, et al: Elevated intra-abdominal pressure and renal function. *Ann Surg* 196:594–597, 1982.
46. Feliciano DV, Burch JM: Towel clips, silos, and heroic forms of wound closure, in Maull KI, Cleveland HC, Feliciano DV, et al (eds): *Advances in Trauma and Critical Care*. Vol 6. Chicago, IL, Year Book, 1991, p 231–250.
47. Saxe JM, Ledgerwood AM, Lucas CE: Management of the difficult abdominal closure. *Surg Clin North Am* 73:243–251, 1993.
48. Barker DE, Kaufman HJ, Smith LA, et al: Vacuum pack technique of temporary abdominal closure: a 7 year experience with 112 patients. *J Trauma* 48:201–206, 2000.
49. Ramirez OM, Ruas E, Dellon AL: "Components separation" method for closure of abdominal wall defects: an anatomic and clinical study. *Plast Reconst Surg* 86:519–526, 1990.
50. Rotondo MF, Schwab CW, McGonigal MD, et al: "Damage control": an approach for improved survival in exsanguinating penetrating abdominal injury. *J Trauma* 35:375–382, 1993.
51. Sagraves SG, Toschlog EA, Rotondo MF, et al: Damage control surgery—the intensivist's role. *J Intensive Care Med* 21(1):5–16, 2006.
52. Morris JA Jr, Eddy VA, Rutherford EF: The trauma celiotomy: the evolving concepts of damage control. *Curr Prob Surg* 33:611–700, 1996.
53. Santry HP, Alam HB: Fluid resuscitation: past, present, and the future. *Shock* 33(3):229–241, 2010.
54. Borgman BA, Spinella PC, Perkins JG, et al: The ratio of blood products transfused affects mortality in patients receiving massive transfusions at a combat support hospital. *J Trauma* 63:805–813, 207.
55. Holcomb JB, Tilley BC, Baraniuk S, et al: Transfusion of plasma, platelets, and red blood cells in a 1:1:1 vs a 1:1:2 ratio and mortality in patients with severe trauma the PROPPR randomized clinical trial. *JAMA* 313(5):471–482, 2015.
56. Pohlman TH, Walsh M, Aversa J, et al: Damage control resuscitation. *Blood Rev* 29(4):251–261, 2015.
57. Gentilello LM, Cobean RA, Offner PJ, et al: Continuous arteriovenous rewarming: rapid reversal of hypothermia in critically ill patients. *J Trauma* 32:316–325, 1992.
58. Brohi K, Singh J, Heron M, et al: Acute traumatic coagulopathy. *J Trauma* 54:1127–1130, 2003.

Chapter 45 ■ Orthopedic Injury

GREGORY J. DELLA ROCCA • SEAN E. NORK • VIVEK VENUGOPAL • JOHN J. WIXTED

EPIDEMIOLOGY

With an annual attributable mortality of more than 100,000 people in the United States, blunt and penetrating trauma is a leading cause of death for Americans younger than 45 years of age and results in staggering losses of health among surviving trauma patients [1]. Trauma evacuation systems have improved dramatically over the past few decades, and patients are much more likely to survive injuries that would have previously resulted in early mortality. Many polytraumatized patients sustain significant orthopedic injuries. These need to be recognized and addressed appropriately to minimize consequent morbidity and mortality. A dedicated orthopedic trauma service, specifically constructed to manage patients with complex fractures and dislocations in the setting of other systemic injuries, may be associated with improved outcomes for trauma patients [2]. The orthopedic traumatologist is not only trained in the surgical management of the individual orthopedic injuries, but is also comfortable functioning as a member of a multidisciplinary team that may include emergency physicians, anesthesiologists, general surgeons, neurosurgeons, urologists, and plastic surgeons.

Musculoskeletal injuries of trauma patients come in many varieties. Long-bone fractures can have direct impact upon a patient's early mortality and late morbidity. Pelvic fractures are associated with early mortality, and their recognition and acute management is vital as part of the life-saving efforts of the trauma team. Open fractures are associated with the development of sepsis if not properly managed. Articular (joint) fractures represent complex injuries requiring prolonged reconstruction; although they routinely occur among polytraumatized patients, their management is beyond the scope of this discussion. Compartment syndrome, a sequela of severe extremity trauma, is a soft tissue condition that can result in early morbidity, associated with the impact of myonecrosis on renal function, as well as late disability, associated with fibrosis of one or more muscles important for activities of daily living. Venous thromboembolism (VTE) is a danger for all trauma patients, and the risk of VTE has been shown to be increased significantly among patients with pelvic and hip fractures. Finally, lesser fractures can have dramatic implications on future function for trauma patients; it has been shown that failure to identify and/or address complex injuries of the foot, for example, is associated with poor long-term outcomes among patients who survive major trauma [3].

In this chapter, we will introduce challenges and share knowledge associated with multiple problems that affect trauma patients: Open fractures, pelvic fractures, long-bone fractures, knee dislocations, compartment syndrome, deep venous thrombosis (DVT), and neurological injury. It is our goal to discuss orthopedic treatment considerations for all of these trauma sequelae such that they can be integrated into the management of the patient who is the victim of polytrauma.

OPEN FRACTURES

Open fractures, or fractures with associated skin wounds allowing communication of the external environment with the fractured bone surfaces, are present in a high percentage of polytraumatized patients. These wounds are at high risk for infection without adequate and early treatment of the open wound. The basic treatment protocol for open fractures includes antibiotic administration, wound debridement, wound irrigation, fracture stabilization, and wound closure.

Initially published in 1976 [4], the Gustilo–Anderson classification scheme is an imperfect but widely utilized classification for open fractures. Type I open fractures are fractures with a clean wound measuring less than 1 cm in length. Type II open fractures are fractures with a laceration measuring more than 1 cm in length and without extensive soft tissue damage. Type III open fractures are fractures with extensive soft tissue damage or an open segmental fracture (a two-level fracture of the same long bone). Type III fractures, therefore, represented a highly heterogeneous group of severe open fractures; a modification of the classification scheme for type III open fractures was therefore developed and published in 1981 [5]. Type IIIA open fractures have extensive soft tissue damage but adequate soft tissue coverage, or are the result of high-energy trauma irrespective of laceration size. Type IIIB open fractures entail extensive soft tissue loss, periosteal stripping, bone exposure, and massive contamination. No mention of requirement for muscle flap fracture coverage is made by the authors (despite the fact that many of these wounds indeed do require flap coverage); this is a modification of the classification that has been propagated over the years [6], although it was suggested by Gustilo himself in a subsequent letter to the editors of the *Journal of Bone and Joint Surgery* [7]. Type IIIC open fractures are those associated with a vascular injury that requires repair. An important point must be made about this classification scheme: It is best utilized during operative debridement of the open fracture. The presence of a small open wound in the skin may belie the extensive soft tissue injury underneath, leading to a misclassification of the open fracture. The reliability of this classification scheme has hence been questioned [8–10]. Regardless, this system continues to be used at many institutions.

As infection is a feared complication of open fractures, antibiotic administration is crucial for decreasing rates of infection after open fractures [11]. Short courses of first-generation cephalosporins (typically, cefazolin), initiated as soon as possible after injury, are beneficial for limiting infections after open fracture [12]. Aminoglycosides and penicillins are often utilized in the treatment of type III open fractures and highly contaminated open fractures [13], respectively. Older studies have demonstrated that administration of broad-spectrum antibiotics lead to decreased infection rates [14]. However, the scientific evidence for this practice is limited [12]. Administration of aminoglycosides for the treatment of open fractures must be accomplished judiciously to minimize risk of oto- and nephrotoxicity. Quinolone antibiotics, effective against gram-negative bacteria, have been shown to be effective for reducing infection rates for type I and type II open fractures [15], but they may have an adverse effect on fracture healing, an effect suggested by animal studies [16,17]. Duration of antibiotic administration is a matter of debate. Older recommendations included 72 hours of antibiotic treatment for type I and type II open fractures and 120 hours for type III open fractures [18]; however, newer studies have demonstrated potentially equivalent outcomes in patients who have 24 hours of antibiotic therapy [19].

Surgical debridement of open fracture wounds in a complete and expeditious manner is an important additional factor for successful management. Sharp debridement should be meticulous, and all foreign material removed. Bone ends should be delivered into the wound, and complete exploration of the injury zone is necessary. Long longitudinal extensions of the traumatic wound are often necessary for adequate exploration. All tissue which is completely devitalized, including bone fragments devoid of soft tissue attachments, should be removed [20,21]. Judgments related to the removal of large articular (i.e., joint surface) fragments may be required to balance the risk of severe disability from the loss of said fragments versus the risk of infection with their retention. Devitalized extra-articular fragments can be cleaned and used as a reduction aid intraoperatively when fixation is proceeding immediately, or they may be stored and utilized later when fixation is delayed [22]. In general, therefore, it is better not to discard bone fragments from open fractures until the patient has arrived in the operating room for definitive management.

An ongoing source of debate for the management of open fractures relates to the timing of debridement. The previous benchmark that had been followed internationally is for open fractures to undergo urgent irrigation and debridement procedures within 6 hours. However, this has recently been questioned, as it appears to have little scientific evidence supporting it. In a seminal article on treatment of open fractures, Patzakis and Wilkins [14] demonstrated no relationship between the time from injury to surgical debridement of open fractures and subsequent development of infection. Another more recent prospective observational study of open fracture patients across eight trauma centers in the United States also failed to show a correlation between time to surgical debridement and the risk of infection of open fracture wounds [23]. Although urgency of treatment for open fractures associated with massive contamination, vascular injury, and/or limb crush is self-evident, routine emergent management does not appear to be required for open fractures, and after-hours surgery done in a hurried fashion by underexperienced practitioners and teams may result in increased rates of minor complications [24]. However, it is generally accepted among the international community that treatment of an open fracture is not an elective procedure [25].

Wound irrigation follows sharp debridement. Irrigation solutions generally are based upon normal saline (0.9% NaCl). Additives historically have included bacitracin, cefazolin, neomycin, soaps, bleach, Betadine, and other antiseptics (such as benzalkonium chloride). Some of these, such as antiseptics, have been shown to be detrimental to wound viability [26]. Antibiotics appear to offer no benefit over normal saline alone [27]. High- versus low-pressure lavage for open fracture wounds has also been a source of debate. However, much of the debate on additives to irrigant solutions and the role of high-pressure saline have been put to rest, as a recent randomized control trial that failed to demonstrate any benefit to soap additives, and showed similar outcomes with high- or low-pressure washing. No consensus exists on the volume of irrigant. Protocols vary between institutions and even within institutions, based on surgeon preference. Up to 9 L of irrigant are utilized in some centers, but there is no scientific evidence upon which a recommendation can be based. Ultimately, it is the opinion of most surgeons that wound debridement is the most critical aspect of treating open fracture wounds, and that the irrigation component of this treatment is of relatively less importance.

Methods of fixation for open fractures are variable. Historically, acute open reduction and internal fixation of open fractures was contraindicated, without good scientific evidence. However, the Harborview group in Seattle demonstrated that acute open reduction and internal fixation of open ankle fractures is a safe and effective method of treatment [28]. External fixation is relatively rapid and fixation points can be kept out of the zone of injury. Mobilization of fracture ends can be accomplished at the time of future debridement, if necessary, and staged open reduction and internal fixation with external fixator removal is safe and effective [29–31]. Plate or nail fixation at the time of irrigation and debridement is also safe and effective [28,32], but limits the surgeon's ability to redisplace bone ends for wound exploration if repeat debridement is indicated.

Early wound closure or coverage is preferred, as this appears to limit rates of infection of open fracture wounds [33]. Acute primary closure of open fracture wounds after debridement and fixation, if possible, has been shown to be a safe method of treatment [34]. Early coverage of open fracture wounds that are unable to be closed primarily has also been shown to be safe and effective [35]. Adjuncts to wound closure, especially in the setting of skin tension, include "pie-crusting" of skin about the wound(s) [36] or performing open wound management with a vessel loop closure technique to reapproximate wound edges [37] and/or use of negative-pressure wound dressings [38,39]. Also, if doubts about the safety of closure at the time of initial debridement and fixation persist, then open wound management and repeat debridement are appropriate until closure or coverage is considered safe. Negative-pressure wound dressings can be utilized successfully for open fracture wounds as a bridge to delayed closure with successful reduction of infection rates in some series [40], or as a bridge to delayed free tissue transfer with reduction of infection rates as compared to traditional dressings [41], perhaps allowing for a possible reduction of the

TABLE 45.1

Mangled Extremity Severity Score

Type	Characteristics	Injuries	Points
Skeletal/soft tissue group			
1	Low energy	Stab wound, simple closed fracture, small-caliber GSW	1
2	Medium energy	Open or multilevel fractures, dislocations, moderate crush injury	2
3	High energy	Shotgun blast, high-velocity GSW	3
4	Massive crush	Logging, railroad, oil rig accidents	4
Shock group			
1	Normotensive	BP stable in field and OR	0
2	Transiently hypotensive	BP unstable in field, responsive to IV fluids	1
3	Prolonged hypotension	Systolic BP <90 mm Hg in field and unresponsive to IV fluids	2
Ischemia group			
1	None	Pulsatile limb, no sign of ischemia	0[a]
2	Mild	Diminished pulses, no sign of ischemia	1[a]
3	Moderate	No pulse via U/S, sluggish CR, paresthesia, diminished motor	2[a]
4	Advanced	Pulseless, cool, paralyzed, numb limb without CR	3[a]
Age group			
1	<30 years		0
2	30–50 years		1
3	>50 years		2

MESS equals sum of scores for each of the group types; minimum score is 1, maximum score is 14.

[a]Points × 2 if ischemic time >6 h.

BP, blood pressure; CR, capillary refill; GSW, gunshot wound; IV, intravenous; MESS, mangled extremity severity score; OR, operating room.

Adapted from Helfet DL, Howey T, Sanders R, et al: Limb salvage versus amputation: preliminary results of the Mangled Extremity Severity Score. *Clin Orthop* 256:80–86, 1990.

need for free tissue transfer [42]. However, this may be a limited process, and earlier wound closure or flap coverage may reduce infection rates over late wound closure or coverage, despite utilization of the negative-pressure dressing [43].

Occasionally, the polytraumatized patient who sustains high-energy open fractures may not be a candidate for fixation, instead requiring amputation. Properly indicated, a well-executed amputation can be a life-saving procedure that can shorten rehabilitation times associated with prolonged reconstruction of a mangled extremity. The debate often centers on whether a limb might be amenable to salvage versus amputation at the time of the patient's arrival to the hospital. Errors in judgment regarding this can have devastating effects to the patient's outcome, both physiologically and psychologically. Multiple assessment tools have been developed to assist surgeons with making decisions regarding limb salvage versus amputation, including the Mangled Extremity Severity Score (MESS) [44,45] (Table 45.1). However, many of these tools are mediocre at best with regard to their predictive value. One example is the Lower Extremity Assessment Project (LEAP) [46,47]. A historically held indication for acute amputation in the setting of a mangled extremity, the lack of plantar foot sensation, has been refuted by the LEAP study team; many patients presenting with absent plantar foot sensation recovered it completely over time, indicating that the most tibial nerve injuries are neurapraxias (as opposed to complete disruptions) [48]. Ultimately, each injured patient must be carefully scrutinized, and no particular physical examination finding or trauma scale has been shown to be absolutely predictive of the success or failure of attempts at limb salvage. Therefore, thoughtful interpretation of trauma scores combined with assessment of the patient's functional goals is imperative prior to making the choice between salvage and amputation.

PELVIC FRACTURES

Evaluation

The pelvis contains the acetabulae, which represent the articulations with the lower extremities, and the lumbosacral junction, representing the articulation with the spine. Comprised of three bones (two hipbones and the sacrum) with three articulations (two sacroiliac joints and the pubic symphysis), the pelvic ring is designed to distribute the weight of the upper body onto the legs for bipedal ambulation. The sacroiliac joints and pubic symphysis are thought to have minimal motion, and are connected by stout ligaments. Incompetence of these joints can lead to laxity and chronic pain. This may occur after trauma, complicated vaginal birth in females, or idiopathically [49,50]. Further ligamentous connection between the posterior and anterior pelvis is provided by the sacrospinous and sacrotuberous ligaments. The transverse processes of the fifth lumbar vertebra are attached to the posterior iliac crests by the iliolumbar ligaments.

Disruption of the pelvic ring of young patients requires a high-energy mechanism, such as a motor vehicle crash or fall from a significant height. As the pelvis is functionally a single rigid ring, the discovery of a single break is a harbinger for others. For example, pubic ramus fractures, in the anterior aspect of the pelvic ring, may be obvious on plain radiographs, but associated sacral fractures may not be readily apparent on plain radiographs due to the overlying bowel gas, radio-opaque contrast agents in the bowel or bladder, or bony anatomy. A high index of suspicion must be maintained, and further injury may be visible on computed tomography (CT) scanning. It should also be emphasized that transverse acetabular fractures often

TABLE 45.2

Young and Burgess Classification System

Type	APC	LC	VS
I	APC I – Symphysis widening < 2.5 cm	LC I – Pubic ramus fracture and ipsilateral anterior sacral ala compression fracture	VS – Posterior and superior directed force
II	APC II – Symphysis widening > 2.5 cm. anterior SI joint diastasis. Disruption of sacrotuberous and sacrospinous ligament	LC II – Rami fracture and ipsilateral posterior ilium fracture–dislocation	
III	APC III – SI dislocation with associated vascular injury	LC III – Ipsilateral lateral compression and contralateral APC	

APC, anterior posterior compression; LC, lateral compression; SI, sacroiliac; VS, vertical shear.

represent a component of a pelvic ring disruption, and suspicion that such disruption has occurred should be maintained with these fracture patterns.

Multiple classification schemes exist that describe various aspects of pelvic ring injuries. The Young and Burgess [51] classification (Table 45.2) is the most commonly utilized descriptive scheme for pelvic ring injuries, in which they are classified as anteroposterior compression (APC) injuries, lateral compression (LC) injuries, vertical shear (VS) injuries, and "complex patterns". This classification can be helpful for identification of other problems that can be associated with the pelvic ring injury, such as increased incidence of head trauma with LC injuries and of abdominal and chest trauma with APC injuries [52], and it can be somewhat predictive of transfusion requirements in trauma patients [53]. Other commonly utilized classification schemes include the Tile classification [54] and the American Orthopedic (AO)/Orthopedic Trauma Association classification [55]. No pelvic fracture classification scheme, however, possesses all seven of the following requisites for universally applicable schemes: Ease of use, prognostic value (outcomes), descriptive value (describe the injury), therapeutic value (direct treatment), research value (allows direct comparison between groups), intraobserver reliability, and interobserver reliability.

Orthopedic examination of the pelvic fracture patient is similar to the orthopedic examination of all polytraumatized patients, covering the entire musculoskeletal system in a methodical manner. Focused examination of the pelvis includes observation of limb deformity; abnormal limb rotation or shortening in the setting of pelvis injury may be secondary either to pelvic deformity or to hip dislocation (with or without associated acetabular fracture), or to extrapelvic lower extremity fracture. Skin about the pelvis, including about the perineum, must be carefully examined for lacerations that can be associated with open pelvic fractures. Open wounds may be present within folds of skin, and a thorough examination is necessary. Lacerations may lurk within the fold of skin inferior to the scrotum in males, and examination of this area cannot be neglected. Extensive ecchymosis should be noted; these may be indicative of degloving injuries. Blood emanating from the anus or vagina can be an indicator of open pelvic fracture. Digital rectal examination is therefore required to detect occult open fractures into the rectum, and vaginal examination should be performed in a safe manner to detect open fractures violating the vaginal vault. Speculum examination is not generally performed in the trauma bay. Urethral disruptions can also occur with pelvic fracture, and blood at the urethral meatus can be indicative of such an injury. Manual palpation of the pelvis and gentle compression of the iliac crests may detect abnormal motion or crepitus associated with an unstable disruption of the pelvic ring, although this manipulation lacks sensitivity and specificity [56]. Pelvic manipulations must be undertaken judiciously; unstable pelvic ring disruptions can cause life-threatening hemorrhage, which can be exacerbated by repeated examinations. Repeated examinations also can induce severe patient discomfort. A neurovascular examination of both legs, as well as examination of anal sphincter tone and of the bulbocavernosus reflex, is routine.

Standard radiography of the pelvis begins with the anteroposterior view. The inlet radiograph, with the beam tilted approximately 40° caudal, can detect anteroposterior translation of the hemipelvis and rotational hemipelvic deformities. The outlet radiographs, with the beam tilted approximately 40° cephalad, can detect "vertical" translation (more often, a flexion deformity) of the hemipelvis and is useful for visualizing sacral fractures. Judet radiographs, with the patient or X-ray beam tilted approximately 45° to either side, are reserved for patients with acetabular fractures detected on anteroposterior radiographs. CT has become routine for polytraumatized patients, and provides extensive information regarding the bony anatomy of a pelvic fracture and/or dislocation. In the setting of pelvic and acetabular fractures, CT scanning is also invaluable for planning of the surgical reconstruction. The CT scan is of limited utility, however, for acetabular fractures if the hip remains dislocated during the scan. Therefore, it is desirable to reduce fracture–dislocations of the hip (acetabulum) prior to CT scanning of the pelvis for adequate delineation of fracture anatomy and for preoperative planning.

Acute Management

Pelvic fracture patients often have multiple associated injuries, all of which may contribute to the overall physiological condition of the patient. Early mortality of patients with pelvic fractures may be related to patient age and occurs as a result of catastrophic hemorrhage, head injury, or multiple organ system failure [57,58]. As the pelvic fracture may contribute directly to morbidity and mortality, early stabilization is preferred. This stabilization may be performed at the scene of the injury by emergency medical personnel, by the application of a circumferential sheet, pelvic binder, or other compressive garment. Sheets are readily available, inexpensive, and easy to apply [59]. The personnel applying the sheet should do their best to avoid wrinkling of the sheet, which may cause skin compromise [60]. Overcompression of the pelvic ring must be avoided, as the exact nature of the pelvic injury is unknown; overcompression of certain types of unstable fracture patterns may lead to laceration of the bladder, rectum, vagina, or other intrapelvic structures. Although circumferential pelvic wraps may assist with patient transport and comfort and can successfully reduce some types of pelvic ring disruptions [61], some studies fail to demonstrate decreases of mortality, transfusion requirements, or the need for pelvic angiography by their use [62].

Upon arrival at the trauma center, all circumferential clothing (including pelvic wraps/binders) is removed to allow for examination of the lower abdomen and pelvis. Binders can be reapplied after examination, and an effort should be made to keep patients warm to avoid coagulopathy. Although pelvic fractures may be associated with catastrophic hemorrhage, ongoing hemodynamic instability can arise from a number of causes unrelated to the specific pelvic injury. Grossly unstable pelvic injuries can be treated provisionally with the application of skeletal traction, on the same side(s) of the pelvic injury(ies), through either the distal femur or the proximal tibia as the side of pelvic instability. Skeletal traction is also used routinely for the provisional stabilization of acetabular fractures prior to definitive treatment in the operating room; traction can minimize contact of the femoral head with rough acetabular fracture edges.

Patients with pelvic ring disruptions may demonstrate hemodynamic instability that is refractory to volume resuscitation. An ongoing search for sources of blood loss is vital. One publication demonstrated that, at a single trauma center, 21% of patients with pelvic fractures and hemodynamic instability (systolic blood pressure < 90 mm Hg) refractory to a 2 L bolus of saline ultimately expired, and 75% of those patients expired as a result of exsanguination [63]. Unstable pelvic fractures are more highly associated with pelvic hemorrhage than are stable pelvic fractures. Therefore, investigation of other potential sources of hemorrhage is vital, especially for the hemodynamically unstable trauma patient with a stable pelvic fracture pattern [64]. Patients with unstable APC injuries have been demonstrated to require massive transfusions, followed by those patients with VS or complex mechanism pelvic ring disruptions, and lastly by those with LC injuries [53,65]. However, fracture pattern may not always be indicative of transfusion requirements or the need for angiographic arterial embolization [66].

Pelvic fracture-associated bleeding comes from three sources: Fracture surfaces, lacerated or ruptured veins, or lacerated or ruptured arteries. Fracture surfaces may not be a source of ongoing massive blood loss, and therefore may contribute negligibly to hemodynamic instability [67]. Distinguishing between major sources of pelvic hemorrhage—arterial or venous—represents a challenging but important task, and prior studies have examined multiple factors that may be associated with successful angiographic embolization, used for arterial hemorrhage, including patient age, trauma scores, shock on arrival to the trauma center, and fracture pattern [68]. Venous hemorrhage after pelvic fracture can be adequately treated with pelvic stabilization, either by circumferential pelvic wrap or by external fixation, while arterial hemorrhage can be addressed with angiographic embolization [69]. Transient response to initial resuscitation, lack of response to provisional pelvic stabilization, and presence of a contrast blush on pelvic CT scanning are all thought to be indicative of arterial hemorrhage that may be amenable to angiographic embolization [70,71].

Pelvic packing has been used for control of severe hemorrhage in hemodynamically unstable patients. It has been proposed that packing may be a more reliable method of treating severe pelvic fracture-associated hemorrhage than angiographic embolization with regard to controlling continued hemorrhage and limiting patient death due to exsanguination [72]. Angiography may also be delayed, and emergency stabilization of the fracture along with or without pelvic packing may be more reliable at controlling severe fracture-associated hemorrhage [73]. Another series documented a 30-day survival rate for pelvic fracture patients treated with extraperitoneal pelvic packing of 72%, and subsequent angiography was successful in detecting arterial hemorrhage in 80% of the patients after packing. Immediate increases in systolic blood pressure after packing were also noted [74]. Importantly, both angiography and pelvic packing must be used in a judicious fashion; this will help minimize complications related to both (such as gluteal necrosis).

Genitourinary injuries occur in a small subset of patients with pelvic fracture. This frequency has been shown to approximate 4.6% in a study of the U.S.A. National Trauma Data Bank [75]. Another recent study estimated a genitourinary injury rate of 6.8% in pelvic fractures; importantly, 23% of these injuries were missed at the time of initial evaluation [76]. Urological injuries most commonly take the form of urethral disruption, extraperitoneal bladder rupture, or intraperitoneal bladder rupture. Diagnosis is often by retrograde cystourethrogram, with careful attention to postdrainage images to detect bladder ruptures not detectable when the bladder is filled with contrast [77]. Urethral disruption appears to occur distal to the urogenital diaphragm, contrary to classical teaching [78]. Primary realignment, when possible, is accomplished endoscopically followed by threading of the urinary catheter by the Seldinger technique [79]. This repair may be accomplished at the time of pelvic fracture repair, using a team approach [80]. Routine use of suprapubic catheters for the management of urethral disruptions is discouraged, as it may increase the rate of infection, especially in the setting of open reduction and internal fixation of anterior pelvic ring injuries [81]. Bladder injuries are more commonly extraperitoneal. Nearly all present with gross hematuria. Intraperitoneal bladder ruptures are generally treated with surgical exploration, to delineate the extent of injury fully, and with Foley (preferred if open reduction and internal fixation of the pelvic ring fractures will be accomplished) or suprapubic catheters. Extraperitoneal ruptures may be managed with Foley catheters; the bulk of these require no formal repair [82]. However, if open reduction and internal fixation of the pelvic fracture is planned, then primary repair of the extraperitoneal rupture is also accomplished at the same time, with low rates of infection [80].

Open pelvic fractures represent a subset of severe injuries with a historically high mortality rates. A recent systematic review calculated the total mortality rate in open pelvic fracture patients across multiple published series prior to 1991 as 30%, and since 1991 as 18%, with the decrease likely owing to aggressive management of the pelvic fracture, selective diversion of the fecal stream, and advances in critical care medicine [83]. These open fractures may be occult, localized within the rectum or vagina. Visual as well as digital exploration is mandatory in these patients. Examination of bowel contents for gross or occult blood is also necessary. While selective fecal diversion does appear beneficial for open pelvic fracture patients with perineal wounds or for patients with extensive or posterior wounds, routine use of fecal diversion does not appear to reduce infection rates among patients with open pelvic fractures [84,85].

LONG-BONE FRACTURES

Femoral Shaft Fractures

Femoral shaft fractures often occur in conjunction with other injuries after high-velocity blunt or penetrating trauma. Fracture of the femur is associated with significant morbidity of the polytraumatized patient; significant hemorrhage can occur, even in the absence of open wounds. Bilateral femoral shaft fractures are associated with higher mortality rates than are seen in patients with unilateral femoral shaft fractures [86]. Open femoral shaft fractures are unusual and require significant energy to create the situation where the fracture fragments travel through the robust soft tissue envelope of the thigh.

Initial management of femoral shaft fractures often entails placement of traction devices in the field. These devices are meant to be portable, and they rest against the ischial tuberosity, against which they provide traction through the ankle or the foot. Splinting of femoral shaft fractures is marginally effective at best, as it requires a splint to include the trunk for effective immobilization. Portable traction devices should be removed as quickly as possible to prevent sciatic nerve pressure injury or skin ulceration. Skin or, more commonly, skeletal traction is routinely applied in the emergency department, as a temporizing measure prior to transport to the operating room and to allow for continued evaluation of the patient for other injuries. This traction provides patient comfort, provides immobilization for the fracture, and limits fracture shortening. It can also function as a temporary treatment modality in the setting of operating room unavailability. Evaluation of the patient prior to transport to the operating room should include an investigation of the ipsilateral femoral neck with thorough radiographic imaging. A high percentage of femoral neck fractures are missed in the setting of ipsilateral femoral shaft fractures, and CT scans do not appear to be 100% sensitive for their diagnosis [88].

Operative management is the mainstay of therapy for fractures of the femoral shaft. In the United States, definitive treatment of the femoral shaft fracture patient in skeletal traction is of historical interest only. A distinct advantage of femur fracture stabilization includes the ability to mobilize the patient, thereby avoiding complications associated with prolonged bed rest in critically injured patients, such as pneumonia, pressure ulcers, and deep vein thrombosis. The gold standard for treatment of closed fractures of the femoral shaft is reamed, statically locked, antegrade (from the hip region) medullary nailing. This method of treatment has been demonstrated to be highly effective in numerous studies [88–90], and it can allow for early unprotected weight-bearing [91]. Reaming prior to nailing appears to improve healing rates of femoral shaft fractures [92,93], although this may come at the expense of increased pulmonary injury in the setting of chest-injured patients [94].

Other methods of fixation for femoral shaft fractures include open reduction and internal fixation with a plate-and-screw construct and external fixation. Plate fixation is often reserved for extremely proximal or extremely distal femoral shaft fractures and for fractures in which intramedullary fixation is contraindicated (e.g., the presence of device, such as a total hip arthroplasty stem, within the femoral canal). Plate fixation has been employed successfully for polytraumatized patients with femoral shaft fractures [95].

Early femoral shaft stabilization is associated with improved outcomes among polytraumatized patients [96]. The method of stabilization is unimportant for these early outcomes; medullary nailing, plate-and-screw fixation, or external fixation provides benefit. Controversy remains regarding the optimal method of early femur fracture stabilization for the polytraumatized patient, including chest- and head-injured patients. The Hannover group has published extensively regarding the second-hit phenomenon of femoral nailing in polytraumatized patients, and has made recommendations that pulmonary- and head-injured patients perhaps undergo acute "damage-control orthopedic surgery" with external fixation of a femoral shaft fracture, followed by staged conversion from external fixation to medullary nailing when the patient's condition has improved and resuscitation has been completed [97–99]. However, some recent studies have demonstrated that reduced rates of acute respiratory distress syndrome (ARDS) can be achieved with acute nailing of femoral shaft fractures, instead of with damage-control orthopedics, for polytraumatized patients [100–102]. The utilization of reaming has been shown not to create increased rates of ARDS among polytraumatized patients undergoing medullary nailing of femur fractures, as compared to patients undergoing nailing without reaming [100]. Adequate resuscitation has been shown to be important prior to nailing [100].

Tibial Shaft Fractures

Fractures of the tibial shaft are common among polytraumatized individuals. Tibial fractures have a higher likelihood of being open [103,104], perhaps secondary to the thin soft tissue envelope surrounding the human tibia. This soft tissue envelope may also play a role for the increased likelihood of infection and nonunion for tibial fractures; infected nonunion is more common after tibial fracture than after any other fracture of a long bone [105]. Compartment syndrome is also common after high-energy fractures of the tibia, even when the fractures are open [10].

Principles of treatment for tibial shaft fractures are similar to those of femoral shaft fractures: Provide comfort, restore length, alignment, and rotation, and allow for early mobilization. Tibial fractures are commonly treated with medullary nailing techniques, unless there is intra-articular involvement. Nailing of tibial fractures can provide sufficient stability to allow for full weight-bearing after surgery [106]. Plating of tibial fractures is often done for those fractures that involve the articular surfaces of the tibia. External fixation is most often utilized in a temporary fashion, especially with large open wounds requiring repeat debridement, of complex fractures involving the tibial plateau or tibial plafond, or for patients with significant physiological instability. Conversion of external fixation to nailing is safe, when the patient's condition permits [30,31].

Tibial fractures in patients sustaining multisystem trauma can be stabilized in a delayed fashion, after the physiological condition of the patient has improved. Unlike femoral shaft fractures, tibial fractures can be effectively treated temporarily with long-leg splints. However, splinted tibial fractures must be carefully monitored for skin breakdown from the splinting material, compartment syndrome, and impending skin compromise from unstable fracture ends.

Humeral Shaft Fractures

Fractures of the humeral shaft are a source of morbidity among polytraumatized patients. They have implications for early rehabilitation as well as for future function. Humeral shaft fractures can be complicated by brachial artery and nerve injuries; the radial nerve is particularly susceptible to concomitant injury with humeral shaft fracture. Management of humeral shaft fractures and their sequelae are based upon the overall condition of the patient and on nature of the injury.

Isolated humeral shaft fractures are particularly amenable to closed management. Splinting, casting, and fracture bracing have all been noted to be highly successful in achieving union of humerus fractures [107,108], and long-term outcomes (at a minimum of 1 year) are thought to be as good as those after surgical repair [109]. Considerations for the management of humerus fractures of polytraumatized patients, however, likely are different.

Polytraumatized patients often require the use of both arms for effective mobilization and rehabilitation. They are subjected to prolonged bed rest, and may be incapable of the frequent fracture brace adjustment that is advocated by Sarmiento and colleagues [107]. As fracture braces are not generally utilized during the acute phase after fracture (delay of 1 to 3 weeks prior to application is common), early splints can be cumbersome and unwieldy for patients and caregivers and are not generally removable for the purposes of skin monitoring and vascular access. Obtunded patients also cannot complain about pressure points beneath a nonremovable splint, and they do not routinely change position in an effort to alleviate pressure points. Skin necrosis can be a danger in this setting. For all of these reasons, management of humeral shaft fractures for polytraumatized patients is typically operative.

Humerus fractures can be treated either with open reduction and internal fixation, utilizing a plate-and-screw construct, or with medullary nailing. Advocates of plate-and-screw fixation cite the ability of humeral shaft fracture patients to utilize their arms for assistance with ambulation (i.e., weight-bearing on crutches or a walker) after fixation [110]. Advocates of medullary nailing for humeral shaft fractures have demonstrated good outcomes [111], although no literature exists that provides evidence regarding immediate weight-bearing after nailing of humerus fractures. Some literature exists that appears to favor plating versus nailing for humeral shaft fractures, as shoulder impingement and reoperation risk appear to be lower with plating [112–114], although there is no definitive answer regarding optimal surgical treatment of humeral shaft fractures. In the setting of radial nerve palsy, present between 8% and 11% of the time [115,116], nerve exploration can also occur at the time of surgery. However, radial nerve palsy is not an indication for operative exploration of the nerve [117]; the bulk of radial nerve palsies appear to be neurapraxias, and one study reported that 89% recover normal distal neurological function after closed humeral shaft fracture management [118].

Forearm Fractures

Forearm fractures, while not often a contributing factor to mortality of the polytraumatized patient, are a source of long-term morbidity if not properly addressed. The forearm functions as a mobile unit that is dependent upon the anatomy of the radius and the ulna. The radius and ulna are "parallel" but curved bones, and this anatomy is vital for the maintenance of proper forearm pronation and supination. The maximal radial bow has been shown, in anatomical studies, to be approximately 16 mm and located near the junction between the middle and distal one-thirds of the forearm length [119]. Encroachment of either bone or of foreign material into this region may have adverse consequences on forearm rotation, and may create limitations of pronation, supination, or both.

Fracture of one bone of the adult forearm often leads to injury associated with the other bone, whether it is fracture or dislocation of the other bone. Dislocation, when it occurs, is either at the elbow (radius) or wrist (ulna). The anatomical connections between the radius and ulna include the proximal and distal radioulnar joints and the interosseous ligaments; deformation of one bone, due to fracture, that is not "compensated" by fracture of the other bone will cause the other bone to be drawn in the direction of the deformation, causing dislocation. Typical patterns include displaced proximal ulnar shaft fractures associated with dislocations of the radial head from the capitellum (the "Monteggia" fracture–dislocation) and displaced distal radial shaft fractures associated with dislocations of the ulnar head from the distal radioulnar joint (the "Galeazzi" fracture–dislocation).

Careful scrutiny of the elbow, forearm, and wrist is vital for the detection of these injuries, which may be overlooked in the setting of multiple traumas. Failure to recognize these injuries acutely can result in increased difficulty with surgical reconstruction (if accomplished late) or significant disability (if reconstruction is never accomplished). Forearm fractures tend to shorten, due to the powerful investing musculature of the forearm, and surgical repair is often more straightforward when it can be undertaken within a few days of injury. The repaired forearm is often protected and weight-bearing is restricted for a number of weeks. However, "platform" walkers or crutches may be utilized for assistance with ambulation for many cases; the weight of assisted ambulation is borne through the elbow (as opposed to the wrist and forearm) with these devices.

COMPARTMENT SYNDROMES

Muscle groups are divided into compartments by layers of noncompliant fascia. Injury to a particular muscular compartment can induce edema and/or hemorrhage within the compartment, leading to increased intracompartmental pressures. Increased intracompartmental pressure can lead to venous congestion and resultant muscle ischemia within the involved compartment(s). This scenario is termed "compartment syndrome." The number of muscle compartments is variable based on location in the body. The brachium has two muscular compartments (anterior and posterior), the forearm has three muscular compartments (dorsal, volar, and mobile wad), the thigh has three muscular compartments (anterior, posterior, and adductor), and the leg has four muscular compartments (anterior, lateral, superficial posterior, and deep posterior) (Table 45.3). The exact number of muscular compartments in the hand and the foot are a matter of debate. Hand compartments include the interosseous compartments as well as the thenar and hypothenar compartments, and foot compartments include the interosseous compartments as well as the abductor and adductor compartments.

The absolute intracompartmental pressure at which a compartment syndrome exists continues to be a matter of debate. Some authors have previously advocated threshold intracompartmental pressures, such as absolute values of 30 mm Hg or 40 mm Hg, as diagnostic of compartment syndrome. However, a differential between intracompartmental pressure and diastolic blood pressure is thought to be a more reliable indicator of evolving compartment syndrome. The pressure differential thought to be diagnostic of compartment syndrome is commonly accepted to be 30 mm Hg [120]. The improved reliability of ΔP measurements, as opposed to absolute measurements of intracompartmental pressures alone, was recently illustrated in a series of 101 tibial fracture patients. In this series, 41 patients had continuous leg intramuscular compartment pressures more than 30 mm Hg for over 6 hours in the setting of a satisfactory ΔP. No difference in outcome regarding return to function and muscle strength was noted, as compared to a control group of 60 patients without elevated intramuscular pressures [121].

Compartment syndrome is a problem that can arise among patients who have sustained high-energy injuries. Typical injuries associated with development of compartment syndrome include fractures, dislocations, crush injuries, and prolonged episodes of limb ischemia. The syndrome can also develop after reperfusion of a dysvascular limb that occurs after a revascularization procedure or after a manipulative reduction of a fracture that reduces kinking and occlusion of vessels. Penetrating injuries, such as gunshot and stab wounds, can lacerate arteries within a single compartment or multiple compartments, leading to hemorrhage under pressure into a confined environment and creating a compartment syndrome. The presence of a penetrating injury or open fracture (which results in fascial disruption) should *not* create a false sense that compartment syndrome will not develop; compartment syndromes have been documented to occur in the setting of penetrating injury or open fracture [122].

Compartment syndrome can also develop after stabilization of a fracture, such as after nailing a tibial fracture, once the compartment has been returned to its preinjury length and its available volume is thereby diminished. This "finger-trap" phenomenon was initially described in the literature by Matsen and Clawson [123]. Tibial traction or fracture reduction in the setting of tibial shaft fractures raises compartment pressures [124]. A fracture situation in which excessive shortening is corrected, or vigorous traction is required to maintain reduction, should perhaps prompt increased vigilance for the development of compartment syndrome. This risk must be balanced, however, during staged management of severe fractures, as the consequence of initial inadequate limb-length restoration may be increased difficulty of the definitive reconstructive procedure at the time of formal open reduction and internal fixation. Also, a recent report revealed that among tibial plateau fractures, application of an external fixator device that spans the knee and fracture may lead to transient elevations of intracompartmental pressure, but does not appear to cause a compartment syndrome [125].

TABLE 45.3

Muscle Compartments

Region	Compartment	Muscles	Nerves	Vasculature
Lower leg	Anterior	Extensor digitorum longus, extensor hallucis longus, tibialis anterior	Deep peroneal nerve	Anterior tibial artery
	Lower leg: Lateral	Peroneus longus, Peroneus brevis	Superficial peroneal nerve, prox portion of deep peroneal nerve	Peroneal artery
	Posterior deep	Popliteus, tibialis posterior, flexor hallicus longus, flexor digitorum longus	Tibial nerve	Posterior tibial artery, peroneal artery
	Posterior superficial	Gastrocnemius, soleus, plantaris	Branches tibial nerve branches	Posterior tibial artery, popliteal artery, peroneal artery, sural arteries
Upper leg	Anterior	Sartorius, rectus femoris, vastus lateralis, vastus intermedius, vastus medialis, articularis genus	Femoral nerve	Femoral artery
	Medial	Pectineus, external obturator, gracilis adductor longus, adductor brevis, adductor magnus	Obturator nerve	Deep femoral artery, obturator artery
	Posterior	Biceps femoris, semitendinosus, semimembranosus	Sciatic/tibial nerve. Short head of biceps femoris innervated by common peroneal nerve	Deep femoral artery
Arm	Anterior	Biceps brachii, brachialis, coracobrachialis	Musculocutaneous nerve	Brachial artery
	Posterior	Triceps brachii, anconeus	Radial nerve	Deep brachial artery
Forearm	Volar	Flexor carpi radialis, pronator teres, policis longus, flexor digitorum superficialis, flexor carpi ulnaris, flexor digitorum profundus	Median nerve, ulnar nerve	Ulnar artery
	Dorsal	Extensor carpi ulnaris, extensor digiti minimi, extensor digitorum, Supinator	Radial nerve	Radial artery
	Mobile wad	Brachioradialis, extensor carpi radialis longus, extensor carpi radialis brevis	Branches of radial nerve	Radial artery

Missed compartment syndromes can lead to significant morbidity. Frank muscle necrosis is a normal sequela of compartment syndrome, and associated joint contractures have been extensively described in the literature. Elevated levels of serum creatine phosphokinase (CPK) or the appearance of myoglobinuria (which can be misinterpreted as hematuria) are associated with muscle necrosis, and have been utilized in the past as diagnostic tools for evolving compartment syndromes [126,127]. Delayed treatment of compartment syndrome is fraught with complications [128]. Infection rates are dramatically increased when fasciotomy for compartment syndrome is delayed [129]. Fasciotomy revision, performed in a delayed fashion for inadequate index fasciotomy (and failure to relieve compartment syndrome), has been associated with increased rates of mortality and major amputation [130]. Often, it is not possible to determine the exact time of onset for a compartment syndrome. Therefore, the recommendation is that fasciotomy be undertaken as expeditiously as possible after diagnosis of compartment syndrome, and that a high index of suspicion for the development of compartment syndrome should be maintained in patients with high-energy trauma or trauma patients who are obtunded.

Compartment syndromes should be diagnosed during the evolution phase. A high clinical suspicion should be maintained for any patient who has sustained a high-energy injury. Pain out of proportion to the injury should alert the examiner to the possibility of impending compartment syndrome. Orthopedic injuries are very painful by their nature, and patients often have differing pain tolerances (sometimes affected by chronic narcotic use/abuse), so the examiner should be sensitive to *changes* in pain level as reported by the injured patient. Traditionally, the "five P's" have been utilized in the awake, responsive patient for examination of the leg and ruling out compartment syndrome: Pain with palpation of the compartment, pallor, paresthesia, pain with passive stretch, and pulselessness are commonly quoted as signs of compartment syndrome. Pulselessness, however, is an extreme late finding as it requires excessive pressures, in excess of systolic pressure, to occlude arteries and likely associated with complete myonecrosis within compartments involved. Excessive pain with passive stretch of muscles within each compartment should alert the examiner to evolving compartment syndrome. Awareness of the patient's injuries and their direct contribution to pain with the motion of a joint (e.g., intra-articular fracture) should be considered. All compartments of a traumatized extremity should be examined. Muscle compartments tend to be very firm in the setting of evolving compartment syndrome.

Direct monitoring of intracompartmental pressure is possible utilizing the wick catheter technique, an arterial pressure line setup, or a variety of commercially available devices. These methods provide direct measurements of intracompartmental pressures in mm Hg. It should be emphasized, however, that compartment syndrome is primarily a clinical diagnosis. Physical examination findings consistent with evolving compartment syndrome should prompt surgical intervention, even in the setting of compartment pressure measurements that indicate normal ΔP, as the consequences of missed compartment syndrome include myonecrosis and irreversible neurological injury. Complete reliance upon direct intracompartmental measurements may result in undertreatment or overtreatment of compartment syndrome. Intracompartmental pressure measurements have been shown to be highest within 5 cm of the fracture, and measurements taken outside of this zone may be spuriously low and lead to undertreatment [131]. Also, there is a documented decrease in diastolic blood pressure after induction of general anesthesia; intracompartmental pressure measurements obtained in a patient under anesthetic must be interpreted cautiously as the ΔP value may be spuriously low and lead to overtreatment [132]. Diagnosis of compartment syndrome is variably difficult, even at large trauma centers [133], and high indices of suspicion need to be maintained in order to correctly identify and treat patients.

For obtunded patients, serial exams should be vigilantly completed. The examiner should note compartment firmness and proceed appropriately. Significant degrees of subcutaneous edema can mask tense compartments. Compartment pressure monitoring with commercially available devices or with an arterial pressure line setup may be utilized for diagnosis in the obtunded patient, especially if the patient exhibits no response to painful stimuli and if physical examination of compartment tightness is impeded by extensive surrounding edema (e.g., with anasarca).

Techniques of fasciotomy have been described extensively. Adequate decompression of all compartments in the affected portion of the extremity is the goal. During fasciotomy, nonviable muscle is debrided. Following fasciotomy, closure of the fascia is not indicated and skin closure should be undertaken cautiously. It is imperative to verify that all compartments of the affected extremity have been released, regardless of the surgical approach utilized. Anatomy may be distorted due to fracture deformity, excessive hematoma, or soft tissue avulsion, and it occasionally can be difficult to discern fascial planes. Negative-pressure wound therapy devices may also be beneficial for promoting growth of granulation tissue within a fasciotomy bed, in anticipation of skin grafting, or in maintaining smaller wound dimensions, in anticipation of delayed primary closure [134,135].

Fasciotomy can be associated with both acute and long-term morbidity. Multiple neurovascular structures can be injured during fasciotomy. Risk can be minimized by careful and meticulous dissection technique, maintaining nerves and vessels within a cutaneous flap (if possible), and assuring that neither is directly exposed to the environment (dressing) at the conclusion of the case. At least one case of profound hemorrhage after erosion of an artery beneath a negative-pressure wound therapy device has been reported [136]. Analysis of long-term outcomes related to fasciotomy is difficult in the trauma setting due to the concomitant injuries that have invariably occurred and which can have an effect upon function. Nevertheless, a retrospective analysis of 40 patients undergoing leg fasciotomy for a variety of reasons has been published [137]. Complications of leg fasciotomy were common, and included neurological injury, hemorrhage, and infection. Only 45% of legs healed with a good functional result, and 27.5% had a severely disabled leg at the time of final healing. Another report indicated frequent patient complaints related to fasciotomy wounds, including decreased sensation, tethering of tendons, and recurrent ulceration [138]. Other known side effects of compartment release include pruritus, reflex sympathetic dystrophy, temperature sensitivity, venous stasis, and chronic edema. Despite these concerns, the morbidity and potential mortality of an untreated compartment syndrome is likely to be much higher. Also, a number of published reports, reviewed by Bong et al. [139], indicate that outcomes of fasciotomy for chronic exertional compartment syndrome (in the absence of trauma) are reliably good. These reports, however, require cautious interpretation for their application to trauma, as they did not include patients who required fasciotomy for trauma-related compartment syndrome.

OTHER SEQUELAE OF ORTHOPEDIC TRAUMA

Deep Venous Thrombosis

Polytraumatized patients with lower extremity or pelvic fractures often are subjected to prolonged periods of immobilization or reduced mobility. They are at risk for development of DVT and subsequent pulmonary thromboembolism (PE). Management of the orthopedic trauma patient must take into account the increased propensity for these patients to develop VTE disease.

There has been much debate in the literature about appropriate methods of DVT prophylaxis for orthopedic trauma patients. The Eastern Association for the Surgery of Trauma (EAST) states that the greatest risk factors in trauma patients for development of VTE are spinal fractures and spinal cord injury. EAST also states that insufficient evidence exists regarding risk of VTE in trauma patients as it relates directly to long-bone fracture or pelvic fracture [139]. Trauma patients with pelvic and acetabular fractures are thought to have an increased risk of VTE [140]. However, there is limited high-quality evidence in the literature, regarding the best method of DVT prophylaxis [141].

Prophylaxis of trauma patients, especially those with pelvic and acetabular fractures, is important to reduce the risk of DVT. Trauma patients have been shown to have lower rates of DVT when both chemical and mechanical means of prophylaxis are utilized [142]. Mechanical DVT prophylaxis can consist of foot pumps or pneumatic compression devices. Chemical DVT prophylaxis often consists of low-molecular-weight heparin (LMWH) for hospital inpatients; for patients thought to be at higher risk of VTE and who are awaiting surgical intervention for fracture repair, chemical prophylaxis does not need to be halted in anticipation of surgery [143]. Despite adequate prophylaxis, however, patients are still at risk for development of DVT [144].

As there are not any high-quality studies that dictate practice guidelines, the Orthopedic Trauma Association put together the recommendations based on expert opinion [145]. These recommendations include the following:

1. Initiation of LMWH in patients with musculoskeletal injury, who do not have contraindications within 24 hours.
2. LMWH should be held for 12 hours prior and subsequent to surgery.
3. Patients should be started on both pharmacological and pneumatic compression devices if able.
4. If pharmacological prophylaxis is contraindicated, pneumatic compression devices should be used.
5. For patients at high risk for VTE, the panel recommended four weeks of prophylaxis.
6. Routine screening for DVT is not recommended for asymptomatic patients with musculoskeletal injuries.
7. Low-risk patients do not require routine inferior **vena cava** (IVC) filter placement.
8. Though patients with closed head injuries with stable neurological exams and stable head CT can be anticoagulated in 24 to 48 hours, a neurosurgical consultation is recommended.

While these are current expert recommendations, the panel recommended that further high-quality studies are required [145].

Peripheral Nerve Injury

The bulk of peripheral nerve injuries that occur as a consequence of trauma are neurapraxias, which often will recover with time. Typical neurological injuries include radial nerve palsies in association with humeral shaft fractures, sciatic nerve palsies (peroneal branch, in particular) in association with pelvic and acetabular fractures, and brachial plexopathies in association with scapulothoracic dissociation.

Radial nerve palsies occur after approximately 12% of humeral shaft fractures [118]. An early description of radial nerve palsy in association with humeral shaft fracture was published by Holstein and Lewis, and describes the association with a spiral fracture of the humeral shaft located at the junction between the middle and distal one-thirds of the diaphysis [147]. The radial nerve supplies motor innervation to the extensors of the hand and wrist; patients with radial nerve motor palsies will lack the ability to extend the wrist or hyperextend the interphalangeal joint of the thumb, which is mediated by the extensor pollicis longus. The extensor digitorum communis (EDC), also supplied by the radial nerve, extends the metacarpophalangeal joints of the hand, but patients may recruit other muscles or perform other functions (such as wrist flexion) that will serve to extend the digits, even though the EDC is not functional. The interphalangeal joints of the fingers (index, long, ring, and small) are extended by the intrinsic muscles of the hand, which are innervated by the median and ulnar nerves, and therefore are not affected by radial nerve palsy. Radial nerve–mediated sensation includes the dorsal surfaces of the forearm and hand; the most specific location for radial nerve sensation is the dorsum of the first web space on the hand.

Most radial nerve palsies are thought to be traction injuries (neurapraxias), as opposed to complete disruptions (neurotmesis) or impalings on bone edges [146]. Rarely, the radial nerve may become entrapped within the humeral fracture site, creating neurological deficits [118]. In the setting of high-velocity penetrating injury (gunshot wounds), a radial nerve palsy may be secondary to blast effect of the projectile (as opposed to nerve transaction). Radial nerve palsy at presentation of a patient with a humeral shaft fracture is not considered an indication for surgery, either for nerve exploration or humeral shaft fracture fixation. In the past, humeral shaft fracture patients presenting with intact radial nerve function which then is lost after manipulation of the fracture (e.g., for reduction) was considered an indication for operative nerve exploration; it has been shown, however, that the bulk of these "iatrogenic" radial nerve palsies resolve on their own, with no residual deficit, and that fracture fixation or nerve exploration is not indicated in these patients either [118]. Humeral shaft fracture fixation should be undertaken for patients who would benefit (or who specifically request fixation), after thorough risk and benefit discussions with the patients and/or their families, and should not be prompted by the presence of a radial nerve deficit. Electromyography and nerve conduction studies are not helpful in the acute setting, and have low sensitivity and specificity regarding the etiology of radial nerve palsy immediately after injury. Ultrasonic examination, however, can be beneficial to detect nerve laceration or entrapment, when utilized by experienced practitioners [148].

Although radial nerve palsies are most often transient, their recovery can take many weeks to months. During this time, flexion contractures of the wrist and digits can occur. Splinting and occupational therapy, with daily manual stretching exercises, are beneficial to minimize this problem. Electromyography and nerve conduction studies may be performed between 6 and 12 weeks following the onset of the radial nerve palsy if there has been absolutely no recovery of function after the injury [146]. Functional recovery is slow; rapid recovery should not be expected. A good rule of thumb is that nerve recovery progresses at approximately 1 mm per day [149]. Therefore, an injury to the radial nerve at the midshaft of the humerus should be expected to result in dorsal hand sensory deficits for many weeks.

Sciatic nerve palsies can occur in conjunction with pelvic or acetabular fractures. Acetabular fractures with posterior dislocation of the hip have an association with the development of sciatic nerve palsy [150]. Pelvic or acetabular fractures, with extensions of fracture lines into the sciatic buttress at the greater sciatic notch, can result in direct laceration of the sciatic nerve; this pattern of fracture can also result in catastrophic hemorrhage due to laceration of the superior and/or inferior gluteal arteries. Pelvic ring disruptions, with wide displacement of the hemipelvis, can also cause sciatic nerve palsies or lumbosacral plexopathies [151], perhaps due either to avulsion of nerve roots or to neurapraxia [152,153]. Nerve roots may be lacerated in association with sacral fractures [154]. The peroneal division of the sciatic nerve is more commonly affected than the tibial division [155]; it has been postulated that this has to do with more points at which the peroneal nerves are tethered down the lower extremity than the tibial nerves.

The bulk of sciatic nerve palsies are also neurapraxias [152]. Prognosis of these, however, is poorer than that for radial nerve palsy, perhaps secondary to the long distance across which recovery must occur (the nerve bud must travel from the pelvis to at least the superior leg, where innervation of the peroneal muscles and ankle and toe dorsiflexors occurs) [155]. Electromyography and nerve conduction studies are useful for characterizing the injury, and many patients with mild injuries regain good function [156].

Scapulothoracic dissociation, likened to a closed forequarter amputation [157], occurs when the shoulder girdle and upper extremity are pulled away from the midline [158]. Prompt recognition of this injury complex is vital. Significant degrees of scapulothoracic dissociation can result in the rupture of subclavian or axillary vessels [157,159]. The injury complex can have devastating effects upon the neurological function of the upper extremity, due to the stretch of nerves or brachial plexus, or due to the avulsion of nerve roots from the cervical spine [157]. Degree of neurological injury and prognosis for recovery correlates with the location of vascular injury; more proximal vascular injury correlates with more severe neurological compromise and poorer prognosis [160]. Evidence of expanding hematoma within the axilla of a patient with such an injury should prompt emergent vascular surgical consultation. Careful attention to the vascular status of the distal upper extremity must be paid to any patient with a distracted clavicular fracture, a significantly displaced scapular fracture, or a clear increase in distance on anteroposterior chest radiograph between the thoracic spine and the medial border of the scapula, known as the scapular index [161]. CT is of questionable benefit for initial diagnosis, as the axis of the beam may not be perfectly perpendicular to the axial skeleton, and therefore determination of scapular index may be unreliable. Recovery of brachial plexus function after scapulothoracic dissociation is unreliable at best, especially after nerve root avulsion [159,160,162].

References

1. Anderson RN, Smith BL: Deaths: leading causes for 2001. *Natl Vital Stat Rep* 52:1–85, 2003.
2. Wixted JJ, Reed M, Eskander MS, et al: The effect of an orthopedic trauma room on after-hours surgery at a level one trauma center. *J Orthop Trauma* 22(4):234–236, 2008.
3. Stiegelmar R, McKee MD, Waddell JP, et al: Outcome of foot injuries in multiply injured patients. *Orthop Clin North Am* 32:193–204, 2001.
4. Gustilo RB, Anderson JT: Prevention of infection in the treatment of one thousand and twenty-five open fractures of long bones. *J Bone Joint Surg [Am]* 58:453–458, 1976.

5. Gustilo RB, Mendoza RM, Williams DN: Problems in the management of type III (severe) open fractures: a new classification of type III open fractures. *J Trauma* 24:742–746, 1981.
6. Anglen J: Letter to the editor. *J Orthop Trauma* 21:422, 2007.
7. Gustilo RB: Letter to the editor. *J Bone Joint Surg [Am]* 77:1291–1292, 1995.
8. Horn BD, Rettig ME: Interobserver reliability in the Gustilo and Anderson classification of open fractures. *J Orthop Trauma* 7:357–360, 1993.
9. Brumback RJ, Jones AL: Interobserver agreement in the classification of open fractures of the tibia: the results of a survey of two hundred and forty-five orthopedic surgeons. *J Bone Joint Surg [Am]* 76:1162–1166, 1994.
10. Giannoudis PV, Papakostidis C, Roberts C: A review of the management of open fractures of the tibia and femur. *J Bone Joint Surg [Br]* 88:281–289, 2006.
11. Gosselin RA, Roberts I, Gillespie WJ: Antibiotics for preventing infection in open limb fractures. *Cochrane Database Syst Rev* (1):CD003764, 2004.
12. Hauser CJ, Adams CA Jr, Eachempati SR, et al: Surgical Infection Society guideline: prophylactic antibiotic use in open fractures: an evidence-based guideline. *Surg Infect (Larchmt)* 7:379–405, 2006.
13. Zalavras CG, Patzakis MJ: Open fractures: evaluation and management. *J Am Acad Orthop Surg* 11:212–219, 2003.
14. Patzakis MJ, Wilkins J: Factors influencing infection rate in open fracture wounds. *Clin Orthop* 243:36–40, 1989.
15. Patzakis M, Bains RS, Lee J, et al: Prospective, randomized, double-blind study comparing single-agent antibiotic therapy, ciprofloxacin, to combination antibiotic therapy in open fracture wounds. *J Orthop Trauma* 14:529–533, 2000.
16. Huddleston PM, Steckelberg JM, Hanssen AD, et al: Ciprofloxacin inhibition of experimental fracture healing. *J Bone Joint Surg [Am]* 82:161–173, 2000.
17. Perry AC, Prpa B, Rouse MS, et al: Levofloxacin and trovafloxacin inhibition of experimental fracture-healing. *Clin Orthop* 414:95–100, 2003.
18. Wilkins J, Patzakis M: Choice and duration of antibiotics in open fractures. *Orthop Clin North Am* 22:433–437, 1991.
19. Hoff WS, Bonadies JA, Cachecho R, et al: East Practice Management Guidelines Work Group: update to practice management guidelines for prophylactic antibiotic use in open fractures. *J Trauma* 70(3):751–754, 2011.
20. Templeman DC, Gulli B, Tsukayama DT, et al: Update on the management of open fractures of the tibial shaft. *Clin Orthop* 350:18–25, 1998.
21. Ficke JR, Pollak AN: Extremity war injuries: development of clinical treatment principles. *J Am Acad Orthop Surg* 15:590–595, 2007.
22. Barei DP, Taitsman LA, Beingessner D, et al: Open diaphyseal long bone fractures: a reduction method using devitalized or extruded osseous fragments. *J Orthop Trauma* 21:574–578, 2007.
23. Pollak AN, Jones AL, Castillo RC, et al: The relationship between time to surgical debridement and incidence of infection after open high-energy lower extremity trauma. *J Bone Joint Surg [Am]* 92:7–15, 2010.
24. Ricci WM, Gallagher B, Brandt A, et al: Is after-hours orthopedic surgery associated with adverse outcomes? A prospective comparative study. *J Bone Joint Surg [Am]* 91:2067–2072, 2009.
25. Schmidt AH: Commentary & perspective on "The relationship between time to surgical débridement and incidence of infection after open high-energy lower extremity trauma" by Andrew N. Pollak, MD, et al: *J Bone Joint Surg [Am]* 92, 2010.
26. Conroy BP, Anglen JO, Simpson WA, et al: Comparison of castile soap, benzalkonium chloride, and bacitracin as irrigation solutions for complex contaminated orthopedic wounds. *J Orthop Trauma* 13:332–337, 1999.
27. Anglen JO: Wound irrigation in musculoskeletal injury. *J Am Acad Orthop Surg* 9:219–226, 2001.
28. Franklin JL, Johnson KD, Hansen ST Jr: Immediate internal fixation of open ankle fractures: report of thirty-eight cases treated with a standard protocol. *J Bone Joint Surg [Am]* 66:1349–1356, 1984.
29. Nowotarski PJ, Turen CH, Brumback RJ, et al: Conversion of external fixation to intramedullary nailing for fractures of the shaft of the femur in multiply injured patients. *J Bone Joint Surg [Am]* 82:781–788, 2000.
30. Bhandari M, Zlowodzki M, Tornetta P III, et al: Intramedullary nailing following external fixation in femoral and tibial shaft fractures. *J Orthop Trauma* 19:140–144, 2005.
31. Della Rocca GJ, Crist BD: External fixation versus conversion to intramedullary nailing for definitive management of closed fractures of the femoral and tibial shaft. *J Am Acad Orthop Surg* 14:S131–S135, 2006.
32. Henley MB, Chapman JR, Agel J, et al: Treatment of type II, IIIA, and IIIB open fractures of the tibial shaft: a prospective comparison of unreamed interlocking intramedullary nails and half-pin external fixators. *J Orthop Trauma* 12:1–7, 1998.
33. Okike K, Bhattacharyya T: Trends in the management of open fractures: a critical analysis. *J Bone Joint Surg [Am]* 88:2739–2748, 2006.
34. DeLong WG Jr, Born CT, Wei SY, et al: Aggressive treatment of 119 open fracture wounds. *J Trauma* 46:1049–1054, 1999.
35. Gopal S, Majumder S, Batchelor AG, et al: Fix and flap: the radical orthopedic and plastic treatment of severe open fractures of the tibia. *J Bone Joint Surg [Br]* 82:959–966, 2000.
36. Dunbar RP, Taitsman LA, Sangeorzan BJ, et al: Technique tip: use of "pie crusting" of the dorsal skin in severe foot injury. *Foot Ankle Int* 28:851–853, 2007.
37. Schnirring-Judge MA, Anderson EC: Vessel loop closure technique in open fractures and other complex wounds in the foot and ankle. *J Foot Ankle Surg* 48:692–699, 2009.
38. DeFranzo AJ, Argenta LC, Marks MW, et al: The use of vacuum-assisted closure therapy for the treatment of lower-extremity wounds with exposed bone. *Plast Reconstr Surg* 108:1184–1191, 2001.
39. Herscovici D Jr, Sanders RW, Scaduto JM, et al: Vacuum assisted wound closure (VAC therapy) for the management of patients with high energy soft tissue injuries. *J Orthop Trauma* 17:683–688, 2003.
40. Stannard JP, Volgas DA, Stewart R, et al: Negative pressure wound therapy after severe open fractures: a prospective randomized study. *J Orthop Trauma* 23:552–557, 2009.
41. Rinker B, Amspacher JC, Wilson PC, et al: Subatmospheric pressure dressing as a bridge to free tissue transfer in the treatment of open tibia fractures. *Plast Reconstr Surg* 121:1664–1673, 2008.
42. Dedmond BT, Kortesis B, Punger K, et al: The use of negative-pressure wound therapy (NPWT) in the temporary treatment of soft-tissue injuries associated with high-energy open tibial shaft fractures. *J Orthop Trauma* 21:11–17, 2007.
43. Bhattacharyya T, Mehta P, Smith M, et al: Routine use of wound vacuum-assisted closure does not allow coverage delay for open tibia fractures. *Plast Reconstr Surg* 121:1263–1266, 2008.
44. Johansen K, Daines M, Howey T, et al: Objective criteria accurately predict amputation following lower extremity trauma. *J Trauma* 30:568–572, 1990.
45. Helfet DL, Howey T, Sanders R, et al: Limb salvage versus amputation: preliminary results of the Mangled Extremity Severity Score. *Clin Orthop* 256:80–86, 1990.
46. Bosse MJ, MacKenzie EJ, Kellam JF, et al: A prospective evaluation of the clinical utility of the lower-extremity injury-severity scores. *J Bone Joint Surg [Am]* 83:3–14, 2001.
47. Ly TV, Travison TG, Castillo RC, et al: Ability of lower-extremity injury severity scores to predict functional outcome after limb salvage. *J Bone Joint Surg [Am]* 90:1738–1743, 2008.
48. Bosse MJ, McCarthy ML, Jones AL, et al: The insensate foot following severe lower extremity trauma: an indication for amputation? *J Bone Joint Surg [Am]* 87:2601–2608, 2005.
49. Garras DN, Carothers JT, Olson SA: Single-leg-stance (flamingo) radiographs to assess pelvic instability: how much motion is normal? *J Bone Joint Surg [Am]* 90:2114–2118, 2008.
50. Siegel J, Templeman DC, Tornetta P 3rd: Single-leg-stance radiographs in the diagnosis of pelvic instability. *J Bone Joint Surg [Am]* 90:2119–2125, 2008.
51. Young JW, Burgess AR, Brumback RJ, et al: Pelvic fractures: value of plain radiography in early assessment and management. *Radiology* 160:445–451, 1986.
52. Dalal SA, Burgess AR, Siegel JH, et al: Pelvic fracture in multiple trauma: classification by mechanism is key to pattern of organ injury, resuscitative requirements, and outcome. *J Trauma* 29:981–1000, 1989.
53. Magnussen RA, Tressler MA, Obremskey WT, et al: Predicting blood loss in isolated pelvic and acetabular high-energy trauma. *J Orthop Trauma* 21:603–607, 2007.
54. Tile M: Pelvic fractures: operative versus nonoperative treatment. *Orthop Clin North Am* 11:423–464, 1980.
55. Marsh JL, Slongo TF, Agel J, et al: Fracture and dislocation classification compendium–2007: Orthopedic Trauma Association classification, database and outcomes committee. *J Orthop Trauma* 21:S1–S133, 2007.
56. Hak DJ, Smith WR, Suzuki T: Management of hemorrhage in life-threatening pelvic fracture. *J Am Acad Orthop Surg* 17:447–457, 2009.
57. Kregor PJ, Routt MLC Jr: Unstable pelvic ring disruptions in unstable patients. *Injury* 30:SB19–SB28, 1999.
58. Sathy AK, Starr AJ, Smith WR, et al: The effect of pelvic fracture on mortality after trauma: an analysis of 63,000 trauma patients. *J Bone Joint Surg [Am]* 91:2803–2810, 2009.
59. Routt ML Jr, Falicov A, Woodhouse E, et al: Circumferential pelvic antishock sheeting: a temporary resuscitation aid. *J Orthop Trauma* 16:45–48, 2002.
60. Schaller TM, Sims S, Maxian T: Skin breakdown following circumferential pelvic antishock sheeting: a case report. *J Orthop Trauma* 19:661–665, 2005.
61. Krieg JC, Mohr M, Ellis TJ, et al: Emergent stabilization of pelvic ring injuries by controlled circumferential compression: a clinical trial. *J Trauma* 59:659–664, 2005.
62. Ghaemmaghami V, Sperry J, Gunst M, et al: Effects of early use of external pelvic compression on transfusion requirements and mortality in pelvic fractures. *Am J Surg* 194:720–723, 2007.
63. Smith W, Williams A, Agudelo J, et al: Early predictors of mortality in hemodynamically unstable pelvis fractures. *J Orthop Trauma* 21:31–37, 2007.
64. Eastridge BJ, Starr A, Minei JP, et al: The importance of fracture pattern in guiding therapeutic decision-making in patients with hemorrhagic shock and pelvic ring disruptions. *J Trauma* 53:446–450, 2002.
65. Burgess AR, Eastridge BJ, Young JW, et al: Pelvic ring disruptions: effective classification system and treatment protocols. *J Trauma* 30:848–856, 1990.
66. Sarin EL, Moore JB, Moore EE, et al: Pelvic fracture pattern does not always predict the need for urgent embolization. *J Trauma* 58:973–977, 2005.
67. Elzik ME, Dirschl DR, Dahners LE: Hemorrhage in pelvic fractures does not correlate with fracture length. *J Trauma* 65:436–441, 2008.
68. Starr AJ, Griffin DR, Reinert CM, et al: Pelvic ring disruptions: prediction of associated injuries, transfusion requirement, pelvic arteriography, complications, and mortality. *J Orthop Trauma* 16:553–561, 2002.
69. Miller PR, Moore PS, Mansell E, et al: External fixation or arteriogram in bleeding pelvic fracture: initial therapy guided by markers of arterial hemorrhage. *J Trauma* 54:437–443, 2003.
70. Stein DM, O'Toole RV, Scalea TM: Multidisciplinary approach for patients with pelvic fractures and hemodynamic instability. *Scand J Surg* 96:272–280, 2007.
71. Stephen DJ, Kreder HJ, Day AC, et al: Early detection of arterial bleeding in acute pelvic trauma. *J Trauma* 47:638–642, 1999.

72. Osborn PM, Smith WR, Moore EE, et al: Direct retroperitoneal pelvic packing versus pelvic angiography: a comparison of two management protocols for haemodynamically unstable pelvic fractures. *Injury* 40:54–60, 2009.
73. Gansslen A, Giannoudis P, Pape HC: Hemorrhage in pelvic fracture: who needs angiography? *Curr Opin Crit Care* 9:515–523, 2003.
74. Totterman A, Madsen JE, Skaga NO, et al: Extraperitoneal pelvic packing: a salvage procedure to control massive traumatic pelvic hemorrhage. *J Trauma* 62:843–852, 2007.
75. Bjurlin MA, Fantus RJ, Mellett MM, et al: Genitourinary injuries in pelvic fracture morbidity and mortality using the National Trauma Data Bank. *J Trauma* 67:1033–1039, 2009.
76. Ziran BH, Chamberlin E, Shuler FH, et al: Delays and difficulties in the diagnosis of lower urologic injuries in the context of pelvic fractures. *J Trauma* 58:533–537, 2005.
77. Porter SE, Schroeder AC, Dzugan SS, et al: Acetabular fracture patterns and their associated injuries. *J Orthop Trauma* 22:165–170, 2008.
78. Carroll PR, McAninch JW: Major bladder trauma: the accuracy of cystography. *J Urol* 130:887–888, 1983.
79. Mouraviev BV, Santucci RA: Cadaveric anatomy of pelvic fracture urethral distraction injury: most injuries are distal to the external urinary sphincter. *J Urol* 173:869–872, 2005.
80. Londergan TA, Gundersen LH, van Every MJ: Early fluoroscopic realignment for traumatic urethral injuries. *Urology* 49:101–103, 1997.
81. Routt ML, Simonian PT, Defalco AJ, et al: Internal fixation in pelvic fractures and primary repairs of associated genitourinary disruptions: a team approach. *J Trauma* 40:784–790, 1996.
82. Brandes S, Borrelli J Jr: Pelvic fracture and associated urologic injuries. *World J Surg* 25:1578–1587, 2001.
83. Kotkin L, Koch MO: Morbidity associated with nonoperative management of extraperitoneal bladder injuries. *J Trauma* 38:895–898, 1995.
84. Grotz MR, Allami MK, Harwood P, et al: Open pelvic fractures: epidemiology, current concepts of management and outcome. *Injury* 36:1–13, 2005.
85. Woods RK, O'Keefe G, Rhee P, et al: Open pelvic fracture and fecal diversion. *Arch Surg* 133:281–286, 1998.
86. Pell M, Flynn WJ, Seibel RW: Is colostomy always necessary in the treatment of open pelvic fractures? *J Trauma* 45:371–373, 1998.
87. Nork SE, Agel J, Russell GV, et al: Mortality after reamed intramedullary nailing of bilateral femur fractures. *Clin Orthop* 415:272–278, 2003.
88. Cannada LK, Viehe T, Cates CA, et al: A retrospective review of high-energy femoral neck-shaft fractures. *J Orthop Trauma* 23:254–260, 2009.
89. Winquist RA, Hansen SV, Clawson DK: Closed intramedullary nailing of femoral fractures: a report of 520 cases. *J Bone Joint Surg [Am]* 66:529–539, 1984.
90. Wolinsky PR, McCarty E, Shyr Y, et al: Reamed intramedullary nailing of the femur: 551 cases. *J Trauma* 46:392–399, 1999.
91. Brumback RJ, Uwagie-Ero S, Lakatos RP, et al: Intramedullary nailing of femoral shaft fractures. Part II: fracture-healing with static interlocking fixation. *J Bone Joint Surg [Am]* 70:1453–1462, 1988.
92. Brumback RJ, Reilly JP, Poka A, et al: Intramedullary nailing of femoral shaft fractures. Part I: decision-making errors with interlocking fixation. *J Bone Joint Surg [Am]* 70:1441–1452, 1988.
93. Tornetta P III, Tiburzi D: Reamed versus nonreamed anterograde femoral nailing. *J Orthop Trauma* 14:15–19, 2000.
94. Bhandari M, Guyatt GH, Tong D, et al: Reamed versus nonreamed intramedullary nailing of lower extremity long bone fractures: a systematic overview and meta-analysis. *J Orthop Trauma* 14:2–9, 2000.
95. Pape HC, Regel G, Dwenger A, et al: Influences of different methods of intramedullary femoral nailing on lung function in patients with multiple trauma. *J Trauma* 35:709–716, 1983.
96. Bosse MJ, MacKenzie EJ, Riemer BL, et al: Adult respiratory distress syndrome, pneumonia, and mortality following thoracic injury and a femoral fracture treated either with intramedullary nailing with reaming or with a plate: a comparative study. *J Bone Joint Surg [Am]* 79:799–809, 1997.
97. Bone LB, Johnson KD, Weigelt J, et al: Early versus delayed stabilization of femoral fractures: a prospective randomized study. *J Bone Joint Surg [Am]* 71:336–340, 1989.
98. Pape HC, Hildebrand F, Pertschy S, et al: Changes in the management of femoral shaft fractures in polytrauma patients: from early total care to damage control orthopedic surgery. *J Trauma* 53:452–461, 2002.
99. Harwood PJ, Giannoudis PV, van Griensven M, et al: Alterations in the systemic inflammatory response after early total care and damage control procedures for femoral shaft fracture in severely injured patients. *J Trauma* 58:446–452, 2005.
100. Pape HC, Rixen D, Morley J, et al: Impact of the method of initial stabilization for femoral shaft fractures in patients with multiple injuries at risk for complications (borderline patients). *Ann Surg* 246:491–499, 2007.
101. Anwar IA, Battistella FD, Neiman R, et al: Femur fractures and lung complications: a prospective randomized study of reaming. *Clin Orthop* 422:71–76, 2004.
102. Canadian Orthopaedic Trauma Society: Reamed versus unreamed intramedullary nailing of the femur: comparison of the rate of ARDS in multiple injured patients. *J Orthop Trauma* 20:384–387, 2006.
103. O'Toole RV, O'Brien M, Scalea TM, et al: Resuscitation before stabilization of femoral fractures limits acute respiratory distress syndrome in patients with multiple traumatic injuries despite low use of damage control orthopedics. *J Trauma* 67:1013–1021, 2009.
104. Howard M, Court-Brown CM: Epidemiology and management of open fractures of the lower limb. *Br J Hosp Med* 57:582–587, 1997.
105. Khatod M, Botte MJ, Hoyt DB, et al: Outcomes in open tibia fractures: relationship between delay in treatment and infection. *J Trauma* 55:949–954, 2003.
106. Patzakis MJ, Zalavras CG: Chronic posttraumatic osteomyelitis and infected nonunion of the tibia: current management concepts. *J Am Acad Orthop Surg* 13:417–427, 2005.
107. Finkemeier CG, Schmidt AH, Kyle RF, et al: A prospective, randomized study of intramedullary nails inserted with and without reaming for the treatment of open and closed fractures of the tibial shaft. *J Orthop Trauma* 14:187–193, 2000.
108. Sarmiento A, Zagorski JB, Zych GA, et al: Functional bracing for the treatment of fractures of the humeral diaphysis. *J Bone Joint Surg [Am]* 82:478–486, 2000.
109. Koch PP, Gross DF, Gerber C: The results of functional (Sarmiento) bracing of humeral shaft fractures. *J Shoulder Elbow Surg* 11:143–150, 2002.
110. Ekholm R, Tidermark J, Tornkvist H, et al: Outcome after closed functional treatment of humeral shaft fractures. *J Orthop Trauma* 20:591–596, 2006.
111. Tingstad EM, Wolinsky PR, Shyr Y, et al: Effect of immediate weightbearing on plated fractures of the humeral shaft. *J Trauma* 49:278–280, 2000.
112. Rommens PM, Kuechle R, Bord T, et al: Humeral nailing revisited. *Injury* 39:1319–1328, 2008.
113. McCormack RG, Brien D, Buckley RE, et al: Fixation of fractures of the shaft of the humerus by dynamic compression plate or intramedullary nail. *J Bone Joint Surg [Br]* 82:336–339, 2000.
114. Chapman JR, Henley MB, Agel J, et al: Randomized prospective study of humeral shaft fracture fixation: intramedullary nails versus plates. *J Orthop Trauma* 14:162–166, 2000.
115. Bhandari M, Devereaux PJ, McKee MD, et al: Compression plating versus intramedullary nailing of humeral shaft fractures–a meta-analysis. *Acta Orthop* 77:279–284, 2006.
116. Ekholm R, Adami J, Tidermark J, et al: Fractures of the shaft of the humerus: an epidemiological study of 401 fractures. *J Bone Joint Surg [Br]* 88:1469–1473, 2006.
117. Shao YC, Harwood P, Grotz MR, et al: Radial nerve palsy associated with fractures of the shaft of the humerus: a systematic review. *J Bone Joint Surg [Br]* 87:1647–1652, 2005.
118. Hak DJ: Radial nerve palsy associated with humeral shaft fractures. *Orthopedics* 32:111, 2009.
119. Schemitsch EH, Richards RR: The effect of malunion on functional outcome after plate fixation of fractures of both bones of the forearm in adults. *J Bone Joint Surg [Am]* 74:1068–1078, 1992.
120. McQueen MM, Gaston P, Court-Brown CM: Acute compartment syndrome: who is at risk? *J Bone Joint Surg [Br]* 82:200–203, 2000.
121. Park S, Ahn J, Gee AO, et al: Compartment syndrome in tibial fractures. *J Orthop Trauma* 23:514–518, 2009.
122. Blick SS, Brumback RJ, Poka A, et al: Compartment syndrome in open tibial fractures. *J Bone Joint Surg [Am]* 68:1348–1353, 1986.
123. Matsen FA III, Clawson DK: The deep posterior compartmental syndrome of the leg. *J Bone Joint Surg [Am]* 57:34–39, 1975.
124. Egol KA, Bazzi J, McLaurin TM, et al: The effect of knee-spanning external fixation on compartment pressures in the leg. *J Orthop Trauma* 22:680–685, 2008.
125. Velmahos GC, Toutouzas KG: Vascular trauma and compartment syndromes. *Surg Clin North Am* 82:125–141, 2002.
126. Olson SA, Glasgow RR: Acute compartment syndrome in lower extremity musculoskeletal trauma. *J Am Acad Orthop Surg* 13:436–444, 2005.
127. Sheridan GW, Matsen FA III: Fasciotomy in the treatment of the acute compartment syndrome. *J Bone Joint Surg [Am]* 58:112–115, 1976.
128. Williams AB, Luchette FA, Papaconstantinou HT, et al: The effect of early versus late fasciotomy in the management of extremity trauma. *Surgery* 122:861–866, 1997.
129. Ritenour AE, Dorlac WC, Fang R, et al: Complications after fasciotomy revision and delayed compartment release in combat patients. *J Trauma* 64[Suppl 2]:S153–S162, 2008.
130. Heckman MM, Whitesides TE Jr, Grewe SR, et al: Compartment pressure in association with closed tibial fractures. The relationship between tissue pressure, compartment, and the distance from the site of the fracture. *J Bone Joint Surg* 76:1285–1292, 1994.
131. Kakar S, Firoozabadi R, McKean J, et al: Diastolic blood pressure in patients with tibia fractures under anaesthesia: implications for the diagnosis of compartment syndrome. *J Orthop Trauma* 21:99–103, 2007.
132. O'Toole RV, Whitney A, Merchant N, et al: Variation in diagnosis of compartment syndrome by surgeons treating tibial shaft fractures. *J Trauma* 67:735–741, 2009.
133. Asgari MM, Spinelli HM: The vessel loop shoelace technique for closure of fasciotomy wounds. *Ann Plast Surg* 44:225–229, 2000.
134. Yang CC, Chang DS, Webb LX: Vacuum-assisted closure for fasciotomy wounds following compartment syndrome of the leg. *J Surg Orthop Adv* 15:19–23, 2006.
135. White RA, Miki RA, Kazmier P, et al: Vacuum-assisted closure complicated by erosion and hemorrhage of the anterior tibial artery. *J Orthop Trauma* 19:56–59, 2005.

136. Heemskerk J, Kitslaar P: Acute compartment syndrome of the lower leg: retrospective study on prevalence, technique, and outcome of fasciotomies. *World J Surg* 67:744–747, 2003.
137. Fitzgerald AM, Gaston P, Wilson Y, et al: Long-term sequelae of fasciotomy wounds. *Br J Plast Surg* 53:690–693, 2000.
138. Bong MR, Polatsch DB, Jazrawi LM, et al: Chronic exertional compartment syndrome: diagnosis and management. *Bull Hosp Jt Dis* 62:77–84, 2005.
139. Buerger PM, Peoples JB, Lemmon GW, et al: Risk of pulmonary emboli in patients with pelvic fractures. *Am Surg* 59:505–508, 1993.
140. Slobogean GP, Lefaivre KA, Nicolaou S, et al: A systematic review of thromboprophylaxis for pelvic and acetabular fractures. *J Orthop Trauma* 23:379–384, 2009.
141. Stannard JP, Lopez-Ben RR, Volgas DA, et al: Prophylaxis against deep-vein thrombosis following trauma: a prospective, randomized comparison of mechanical and pharmacological prophylaxis. *J Bone Joint Surg [Am]* 88:261–266, 2006.
142. Fuchs S, Heyse T, Rudofsky G, et al: Continuous passive motion in the prevention of deep-vein thrombosis: a randomized comparison in trauma patients. *J Bone Joint Surg [Br]* 87:1117–1122, 2005.
143. Stannard JP, Singhania AK, Lopez-Ben RR, et al: Deep-vein thrombosis in high-energy skeletal trauma despite prophylaxis. *J Bone Joint Surg [Br]* 87:965–968, 2005.
144. Sagi HC, Ahn J, Ciesla D, et al: Venous thromboembolism prophylaxis in orthopaedic trauma patients: a survey of OTA member practice patterns and OTA expert panel recommendations. *J Orthop Trauma* 29(10):e355–e362, 2015.
145. Patil S, Gandhi J, Curzon I, et al: Incidence of deep-vein thrombosis in patients with fractures of the ankle treated in a plaster cast. *J Bone Joint Surg [Br]* 89:1340–1343, 2007.
146. Bodner G, Buchberger W, Schocke M, et al: Radial nerve palsy associated with humeral shaft fracture: evaluation with US–initial experience. *Radiology* 219:811–816, 2001.
147. Lowe JB III, Sen SK, MacKinnon SE: Current approach to radial nerve paralysis. *Plast Reconstr Surg* 110:1099–1113, 2002.
148. Seddon HG: Nerve grafting. *J Bone Joint Surg [Br]* 45:447–461, 1963.
149. Cornwall R, Radomisli TE: Nerve injury in traumatic dislocation of the hip. *Clin Orthop* 377:84–91, 2000.
150. Helfet DL, Koval KJ, Hissa EA, et al: Intraoperative somatosensory evoked potential monitoring during acute pelvic fracture surgery. *J Orthop Trauma* 9:28–34, 1995.
151. Huittinen VM, Slatis P: Nerve injury in double vertical pelvic fractures. *Acta Chir Scand* 138:571–575, 1971.
152. Harris WR, Rathbun JB, Wortzman G, et al: Avulsion of lumbar roots complicating fracture of the pelvis. *J Bone Joint Surg [Am]* 55:1436–1442, 1973.
153. Denis F, Davis S, Comfort T: Sacral fractures: an important problem. *Clin Orthop* 227:67–81, 1988.
154. Schmeling GJ, Perlewitz TJ, Helfet DL: Chapter 39: Early complications of acetabular fractures, in Tile M, Helfet DL, Kellam JF (eds): *Fractures of the Pelvis and Acetabulum*. 3rd ed. Philadelphia, PA, Lippincott Williams & Wilkins, 2003, p 734.
155. Fassler PR, Swiontkowski MF, Kilroy AW, et al: Injury of the sciatic nerve associated with acetabular fracture. *J Bone Joint Surg [Am]* 75:1157–1166, 1993.
156. Brucker PU, Gruen GS, Kaufmann RA: Scapulothoracic dissociation: evaluation and management. *Injury* 36:1147–1155, 2005.
157. Ebraheim NA, An HS, Jackson WT, et al: Scapulothoracic dissociation. *J Bone Joint Surg [Am]* 70:428–432, 1988.
158. Althausen PL, Lee MA, Finkemeier CG: Scapulothoracic dissociation: diagnosis and treatment. *Clin Orthop* 416:237–244, 2003.
159. Sen RK, Prasad G, Aggarwal S: Scapulothoracic dissociation: level of vascular insult, an indirect prognostic indicator for the final outcome? *Acta Orthop Belg* 75:14–18, 2009.
160. Oreck SL, Burgess A, Levine AM: Traumatic lateral displacement of the scapula: a radiographic sign of neurovascular disruption. *J Bone Joint Surg [Am]* 66:758–763, 1984.
161. Zelle BA, Pape HC, Gerich TG, et al: Functional outcome following scapulothoracic dissociation. *J Bone Joint Surg [Am]* 86:2–8, 2004.
162. Mauser N, Gissel H, Henderson C, et al: Acute lower-leg compartment syndrome. *Orthopedics* 36(8):619–624, 2013.

Suggested Readings

Anglen JO: Comparison of soap and antibiotic solutions for irrigation of lower-limb open fracture wounds: a prospective, randomized study. *J Bone Joint Surg [Am]* 87:1415–1422, 2005.

Borer DS, Starr AJ, Reinert CM, et al: The effect of screening for deep vein thrombosis on the prevalence of pulmonary embolism in patients with fractures of the pelvis and acetabulum: a review of 973 patients. *J Orthop Trauma* 19:92–95, 2005.

Bosse MJ, MacKenzie EJ, Kellam JF, et al: An analysis of outcomes of reconstruction or amputation after leg-threatening injuries. *N Engl J Med* 347:1927–1931, 2002.

Cothren CC, Smith WR, Moore EE, et al: Utility of once-daily dose of low-molecular-weight heparin to prevent venous thromboembolism in multisystem trauma patients. *World J Surg* 31:98–104, 2007.

Draeger RW, Dirschl DR, Dahners LE: Debridement of cancellous bone: a comparison of irrigation methods. *J Orthop Trauma* 20:692–698, 2006.

Ekholm R, Ponzer S, Tornkvist H, et al: Primary radial nerve palsy in patients with acute humeral shaft fractures. *J Orthop Trauma* 22:408–414, 2008.

Goel DP, Buckley R, de Vries G, et al: Prophylaxis of deep-vein thrombosis in fractures below the knee: a prospective randomized controlled trial. *J Bone Joint Surg [Br]* 91:388–394, 2009.

Heini PF, Witt J, Ganz R: The pelvic C-clamp for the emergency treatment of unstable pelvic ring injuries: a report on clinical experience of 30 cases. *Injury* 27:SA38–SA45, 1996.

Henson JT, Roberts CS, Giannoudis PV: Gluteal compartment syndrome. *Acta Orthop Belg* 75:147–152, 2009.

Holstein A, Lewis GB: Fractures of the humerus with radial-nerve paralysis. *J Bone Joint Surg [Am]* 45:1382–1388, 1963.

Hope MJ, McQueen MM: Acute compartment syndrome in the absence of fracture. *J Orthop Trauma* 18:220–224, 2004.

Kenny C: Compartment pressures, limb length changes and the ideal spherical shape: a case report and in vitro study. *J Trauma* 61:909–912, 2006.

Kutty S, Laing AJ, Prasad CV, et al: The effect of traction on compartment pressures during intramedullary nailing of tibial-shaft fractures. A prospective randomised trial. *Int Orthop* 29:186–190, 2005.

Lindahl J, Hirvensalo E, Bostman O, et al: Failure of reduction with an external fixator in the management of injuries of the pelvic ring: long-term evaluation of 110 patients. *J Bone Joint Surg [Br]* 81:955–962, 1999.

MacKenzie EJ, Bosse MJ, Pollak AN, et al: Long-term persistence of disability following severe lower-limb trauma: results of a seven-year follow-up. *J Bone Joint Surg [Am]* 87:1801–1809, 2005.

McQueen MM, Court-Brown CM: Compartment monitoring in tibial fractures: the pressure threshold for decompression. *J Bone Joint Surg [Br]* 78:99–104, 1996.

Palmer S, Fairbank AC, Bircher M: Surgical complications and implications of external fixation of pelvic fractures. *Injury* 28:649–653, 1997.

Petrisor B, Jeray K, Schemitsch E, et al: Fluid lavage in patients with open fracture wounds (FLOW): an international survey of 984 surgeons. *BMC Musculoskelet Disord* 9:7, 2008.

Pohlemann T, Braune C, Gansslen A, et al: Pelvic emergency clamps: anatomic landmarks for a safe primary application. *J Orthop Trauma* 18:102–105, 2004.

Ricci WM, Schwappach J, Tucker M, et al: Trochanteric versus piriformis entry portal for the treatment of femoral shaft fractures. *J Orthop Trauma* 20:663–667, 2006.

Richard MJ, Tornetta P III: Emergent management of APC-2 pelvic ring injuries with an anteriorly placed C-clamp. *J Orthop Trauma* 23:322–326, 2009.

Rogers FB, Cipolle MD, Velmahos G, et al: Practice management guidelines for the prevention of venous thromboembolism in trauma patients: the EAST practice management guidelines work group. *J Trauma* 53:142–164, 2002.

Stover MD, Morgan SJ, Bosse MJ, et al: Prospective comparison of contrast-enhanced computed tomography versus magnetic resonance imaging veno-graphy in the detection of occult deep pelvic vein thrombosis in patients with pelvic and acetabular fractures. *J Orthop Trauma* 16:613–621, 2002.

White TO, Howell GE, Will EM, et al: Elevated intramuscular compartment pressures do not influence outcome after tibial fracture. *J Trauma* 55:1133–1138, 2003.

Zannis J, Angobaldo J, Marks M, et al: Comparison of fasciotomy wound closures using traditional dressing changes and the vacuum-assisted closure device. *Ann Plast Surg* 62:407–409, 2009.

Chapter 46 ■ Burn Management

SEAN FIGY • JOYCE K. McINTYRE

DEFINITION AND GENERAL CONSIDERATIONS

Patients with inappropriate or excessive exposure to thermal, chemical, electrical, or radioactive agents are burned. The degree of injury and depth of burn are proportional to the amount of energy delivered to the tissue and duration of exposure to the offending agent.

In 2015, approximately 450,000 burn-related injuries were reported in the United States, necessitating approximately 40,000 hospitalizations. The 2013 National Burn Repository Report from the American Burn Association found 3.3% of burn-related injuries were greater than 40% total body surface area (TBSA) [1].

All human tissue is susceptible to burn injury, although skin and aerodigestive tissues are commonly involved. The embryologically distinct epidermal and dermal layers of skin behave differently when burned. Ectodermally derived epidermis is vital for fluid management, pigmentation, and protective immunologic functions, but the epidermis has little structural integrity at seven cells thick. What the epidermis lacks in thickness it makes up for with its regenerative properties; the layer's abundant stem cells heal isolated injury of this layer without scar. The dermis, in contrast, is derived from mesenchymal cells and forms abundant scar while healing. The dermis gives skin its strong mechanical integrity and as such is the focus of much of acute burn care [2].

Burn thickness may range from superficial epidermal involvement to char of the deepest bone. Accurate burn depth assessment is critical in the patient's clinical management but remains a qualitative appraisal. Significant "bench to bedside" work has been performed using both laser Doppler and hyperspectral imaging to quantify tissue injury; however, clinical judgment remains the gold standard [3].

Burn depth occurs on a spectrum: superficial burns involve the thin epidermis only; partial-thickness or second-degree burns disrupt the epidermis' basement membrane and encroach into the dermis, resulting in blisters; the dermis is burned in full-thickness or third-degree burns, which often look pale, ashen, and leathery. Fourth-degree burns involve the underlying fat, fascia, or bone. Third- and fourth-degree burns typically outstrip the body's regenerative capacity and require operative excision of damaged tissues and restoration of skin integrity.

Because of the body's inflammatory response to the initial traumatic insult, burn depth may change over time, colloquially described as "deepening." Pink burned tissue with wheepy blisters on the day of presentation may progress to appear white and dry—a full-thickness injury—and much of acute burn care is directed toward preventing this conversion.

A burned patient is a trauma patient and should initially be evaluated in accordance with the systematic techniques of Advanced Trauma Life Support (ATLS) principles. Airway should be evaluated and secured when appropriate to facilitate breathing and ongoing oxygenation, followed by an evaluation of the patient's circulation. Primary traumatic survey should encompass evidence of head injury, long bone trauma, and acute hemorrhage. Evaluation of the burned tissue is part of a prompt secondary survey.

Accurate information around the mechanism of burn and location (closed or open space) inform the clinician's suspicion about concomitant injuries such as inhalational injury, deep muscle injury from electrocution or fractures from a high fall, and the like. The initial depth of the burn and TBSA affected should be documented in the medical record. Please see the section Inhalational Injury for further management of the burned airway.

TBSA can be calculated with the "rule of nines" and the Lund–Browder scales (useful for contiguous injury), whereas the palmar surface of the patient's hand, representing 1% TBSA, is used as a guide in noncontiguous injuries [4]. TBSA should include only partial and full-thickness burns; superficial burns confined to the epidermis are not included in this calculation [5].

Overall morbidity and mortality are influenced by TBSA, patient's age, medical comorbidities, and presence of inhalational injury. Burn patients with greater than 20% TBSA and those with inhalational injury are at risk for development of burn shock (see Burn Shock section). Age of the burned patient is of vital importance when predicting a patient's mortality; with increasing age, risk of death is greater with lower total body burn surface area. The Baux Score is a combination of TBSA and age and is predictive of burn mortality for burns greater than 15% [6].

The patient's predicted mortality rate rises to over 90% when the patient is older than 60 years, TBSA burned is more than 40%, and the patient has an inhalational injury; when two factors are present, calculated mortality is roughly 33%. Death is usually caused in such cases by multisystem organ failure as a result of sepsis. Burn care before the 1980s focused on topical antibiotics and delayed excision and grafting. The clinical paradigm has shifted in the past 35 years to early surgery (within 5 days), and survival rates of major burns—in conjunction with advances in critical care—have dramatically improved [7]. Because of the interdisciplinary care required to take care of the burned patient, prompt transfer to certified burn centers in accordance with American Burn Association guidelines has been shown to have the best outcomes, especially in cases of inhalational burns [8].

BURN SHOCK

Burn shock is a form of vasodilatory shock, akin to the general term "systemic inflammatory response," and creates a significant initial fluid volume resuscitation requirement for the burned patient. Large volume repletion is usually necessary only for patients with burns exceeding 20% TBSA and is essentially universal in larger surface area burns [9].

This fluid need comes from the body's systemic response to burned tissue. Kinins, serotonin, histamine, prostaglandins, and oxygen radicals are the vasoactive mediators released in response to the burn injury and stimulate systemic vascular permeability. These mediators increases vascular permeability, with resultant decreased capillary oncotic pressure and subsequent severe total body edema, even in nonburned tissues. Albumin is functionally lost into the interstitium, thereby increasing extravascular oncotic pressure, compounding the edema [10].

The burned patient's fluid "requirement" should be thought of as that volume needed to optimize organ function and tissue perfusion. Classically, this has been calculated with the Parkland formula using the patient's TBSA burn and weight, times the coefficient of 4, with half the isotonic fluid given in the first 8 hours from injury and the second half given in the subsequent 16 hours. However, goal-directed therapy is the gold standard of care, aiming for a urine output of 0.5 to 1 mL/kg/h, and the calculated fluid requirements should serve only as a general guide for meeting this goal. If the patient's urine output is greater than 1 mL/kg/h, the infusion rate should be decreased and titrated appropriately. If urine output remains high, urine electrolytes and glucose should be evaluated with specific attention to glycosuria secondary to the burn hypermetabolism.

Albumin is an increasingly popular component of the resuscitation of a burned elderly patient or in those whose fluid requirements in practice are significantly higher than their calculated needs [11]. Central venous access may be necessary to deliver the appropriate resuscitation in a timely manner and is ideally, but not essentially, placed through nonburned tissue [12].

The use of pressors requires clinical judgment and should be employed only in settings of persistent hypotension despite adequate fluid resuscitation with both crystalloid and colloid rescue therapy. For patients with persistent oliguria, preexisting renal failure, or congestive heart failure, a pulmonary artery catheter or the equivalent measuring tool to quantify hemodynamics is advised [13].

Adrenal insufficiency should be suspected when hypotension persists despite solid volume repletion and adequate vasopressor therapy and is further suggested by concurrent hyponatremia and hyperkalemia. Although somewhat unusual, a high mortality exists when disturbances of the hypothalamic–pituitary–adrenal axis are found early in a patient's burn shock course. A single blood cortisol of less than 15 μg per dL in a stressed patient is suggestive of adrenal insufficiency, although results of a corticotrophin stimulation test should not delay implementation of glucocorticoid replacement therapy in the face of circulatory collapse. In questionable cases, a corticotrophin stimulation test is confirmatory and not skewed by dexamethasone, which enhances vascular tone but does not have the mineral corticoid activity seen with hydrocortisone administration [14]. Glucocorticoids are known to unfavorably affect skin engraftment, although vitamin A supplementation seems to limit the wound-healing delay [15].

The pathophysiologic similarities between septic shock, systemic inflammatory response, and burn shock may have a common pathway that could be interrupted to improve outcomes. β-blockade, antihistamines, FFP, generous narcosis, nonsteroidal anti-inflammatory agents, and glucocorticosteroids are among the many approaches investigated to mitigate this cellular "hysteria." None of these approaches have proven superiority in multicenter prospective trials to date [16].

In the acutely burned patient, central shunting of blood compensates for anhydremia, yet deprives peripherally injured tissue of vital perfusion. This low blood flow to skin keeps essential nutrients and gas exchange from partly burned tissue, resulting in conversion of partial-thickness injury to full-thickness tissue loss. Excessive fluid resuscitation, however, has the same result by compounding extravascular tissue edema [10].

The biologic basis of burn wound conversion, also called *secondary burn progression*, has not been fully elucidated. Direct cellular damage, inflammation, and ischemia are significant contributing factors. Investigations into erythropoietin derivatives and resolvins have shown preservation of microvascular network in animal models. This may allow prevention of secondary burn progression [17].

The gastrointestinal tract is an underutilized resuscitative venue. Enteral nutrition and resuscitation may begin on the day of injury with the caveat that patients in shock or requiring vasopressors can develop bowel ischemia and enteral feeds may increase the metabolic needs of the gut, contributing to bowel ischemia and necrosis. This risk can be minimized by initiating enteral rehydration and nutrition within 24 hours of the initial burn [18]. Patient's not tolerating enteral feeds or those with abdominal hypertension (see Chapter 52) should be given total parenteral nutrition.

Typically, by the third postburn day, the patient's systemic inflammatory response has dampened and vascular integrity is returning, with decreased fluid requirements. After this point, it is reasonable to limit fluid replacement to maintenance levels and allow the patient to autodiurese or judiciously use diuretics in the elderly or cardiac-compromised patient [9].

CARDIOVASCULAR RESPONSE

Unresuscitated burn victims die of hypovolemic shock. An untreated victim would show progressively decreasing preload and cardiac output. Unfortunately, during the initial 4-to-24-hour postinjury period, even "adequate" volume repletion will not maintain baseline cardiac output, and decreased cardiac contractility and diastolic dysfunction prevail. This decrease in contractility is more pronounced among those with an inhalational injury and is related to both increased pulmonary vascular resistance and increased systemic nitric oxide production. This temporary and seemingly maladaptive cardiac dysfunction improves as time elapses from the initial injury and is followed by tachycardia, which is often maintained for weeks after burn [19,20].

Given this hyperdynamic response, the elderly and patients with preinjury cardiac compromise are more susceptible to heart failure in this period. Laboratory workup may reveal elevations in cardiac enzymes, including both creatine phosphokinase (CPK) and troponin-I, and although myocardium may be at risk, the evaluation of elevated cardiac labs in burn shock patients goes beyond a single lab value. Elevated troponins should not be used as an indication for emergent cardiac catheterization without other signs or symptoms of acute cardiac ischemia, such as electrocardiogram changes [19].

INHALATIONAL INJURY

An inhalational injury occurs when toxic combustants have been inhaled, causing a systemic inflammatory response and local injury in the bronchial pulmonary tree. History of fire or explosion in a closed space and findings of singed facial structures, carbonaceous sputum, and respiratory distress often corroborate the diagnosis. Approximately 3.5% of adult burn admissions have inhalational injury, which increases mortality rate for like burn size; however, larger burns have an incidence of inhalational injury closer to 15% [1]. Concurrent inhalational injury intensifies burn shock and may require up to 50% more fluid for adequate resuscitation. This component of the inhalational injury cascade appears to be driven by the sensory neuronal pathway, because the response can be truncated by sympathetic blockade in experimental animal models [21].

Clinically, in the acutely burned patient with an inhalational injury, airway management is paramount. The clinician should look for signs of upper airway obstruction secondary to edema, which often develops hours after initial injury. Stridorous patients should be intubated urgently; preferably with an 8-Fr endotracheal tube to allow for bronchoscopy and removal of respiratory tract secretions. Currently, no scale of severity for inhalational injury is used clinically. Bronchoscopy is most useful to characterize the presence or absence of tracheobronchial inflammation and provide therapeutic pulmonary lavage [22].

Immediate threats include carbon monoxide (CO) poisoning and cyanide (CN^-) toxicity. Generally, the lethal level is >60% COHgb. Breathing 100% oxygen by mask or endotracheal tubes should bring the half-life of COHgb to about 60 minutes [23]. CN^- poisoning causes cytochrome oxidase inhibition and loss of hypoxic pulmonary vasoconstriction, increasing lung dead space. CN^- is lethal in levels over 1 μg per mL, while 0.02 μg per mL occurs in healthy nonsmokers. For practical purposes, a normal COHgb rules out CN^- toxicity [23].

Inhalational injury has multiple sequelae, including endobronchial and interstitial edema, alveolar damage, mucociliary dysfunction, endobronchial slough with cast formation, functional pulmonary shunting, and decreased lung compliance. Increased bronchial blood flow causes increased interstitial edema. Bronchial epithelium sloughs and combines with exudates and fibrin to form "plugs" that nurture bacterial growth and create mechanical airway obstructions. Aerosolized heparin in conjunction with *N*-acetyl-cysteine may prevent cast formation and has been shown to decrease lung injury scores and ventilator days and has been especially helpful for pediatric patients where narrow airways easily obstruct [24,25].

Although burn patients are at increased risk for pneumonia because of their immunocompromised state, immobility, and inability to clear secretions, prophylactic antibiotics are not recommended. Pneumonia and tracheobronchitis should be treated by culture-directed therapy, using Gram stain, culture of sputum, or bronchoscopy specimens and incorporate a hospital's known bacterial sensitivities [26]. Aspiration risks should be minimized, and lung protective ventilator settings should be used. Patients' overall condition and pulmonary performance by way of usual weaning parameters dictate extubation time [27]. The risk of upper airway obstruction before extubation should be assessed by deflating the balloon and audible appreciation of air leak. If no air leak is present, extubation should not be performed.

METABOLIC AND NUTRITIONAL CONSIDERATIONS

The insensible fluid and protein losses from burn wounds are extraordinary. Protein catabolism, compounded by losses through the wound bed and the interstitium, results in severe hypoproteinemia, and the hypermetabolic response that occurs after a thermal injury is more than that observed after most other forms of trauma or sepsis. The loss of regulated vasomotor tone, possibly in an effort to provide maximal nutrient delivery and gas exchange to the wounded tissues, results in significant evaporative heat loss. Hypothermia from weeping wounds and dwindling energy supplies from the catabolic, muscle-wasting condition of burn shock is easily avoided with external warming. The ambient temperature in the patient's room should be kept warm, 90°F to 100°F, in an effort to shunt calories away from being used in thermostasis.

Muscle wasting, a difficult complication of the hypermetabolism associated with burn wounds, can be ameliorated through anabolic enhancement. The two most common approaches are recombinant human growth hormone (HGH) and oxandrolone. HGH is associated with hyperglycemia requiring insulin support and has largely been supplanted by oxandrolone, which must be given enterally at 0.2 mg/kg/d (max dose 20 mg) divided twice daily, thereby limiting its use in patients with ileus [28,29].

The patient with a major thermal injury has a metabolism characterized by increased muscle proteolysis, lipolysis, and gluconeogenesis. Burn wounds use glucose in greatly increased quantities. Hyperglycemia is common with burn catabolism, may exacerbate muscle wasting, and should be tightly controlled with insulin. Nitrogen loss should also be supplemented to combat muscle wasting and to enhance the immune system [30].

Burn patients need two to three times their basal energy expenditure in calories [30]. Significant burn injuries require 2 g per kg protein, glucose should contribute 50% to 60% of the calories, and the calorie-to-nitrogen ratio should approach 150:1. All attempts should be made to feed the patient enterally, and, ideally, enteral nutrition should be initiated within 24 hours of admission. Prompt enteral feeding has been shown to decrease patient's length of hospital stay as well as burn wound infection and is thought to maintain the integrity of the gastrointestinal track [14]. In addition to early enteral nutrition, supplementation with trace elements such as copper, zinc, and selenium is also important for helping decrease infectious complications [31].

BURN WOUND SEPSIS

Burn victims develop multiple defects in their immune system both mechanical and immunologic that predispose them to an increased risk of infection. Topical antimicrobials (e.g., silver sulfadiazine or mafenide acetate) in the context of good overall wound care help decrease the incidence of frank burn wound infections. However, primary treatment of infected burns remains surgical excision and tissue coverage with autograph or skin substitute (see "Early Excision and Grafting").

The signs of burn wound sepsis typically present as a greenish gray discoloration of the burn, purulent fluid from the wound, and eschar separation along with cellulitis in the surrounding unburned skin. If not treated at the earliest possible time, systemic sepsis will ensue. Diagnosis can be confirmed by biopsy of the wound with quantitative culture but should not preclude total and urgent excision [32]. Systemic antibiotics are started if florid infection is suspected and tailored or stopped once burn biopsies for quantitative bacterial counts and blood culture results are obtained.

The overall hypermetabolic state associated with severe burns can have significant effects on the pharmacokinetics and pharmacodynamics of many medications including anti-infectives. As one example, Mafenide acetate penetrates eschar and is most effective against Gram-negative organisms; however, Mafenide acetate is known to cause metabolic acidosis as a carbonic anhydrase inhibitor and may select for fungal overgrowth [26].

Immunity and Infection

Significant burn injury that induces a systemic inflammatory response may also induce a compensatory anti-inflammatory response syndrome. This combination can lead to persistent inflammation-immunosuppression catabolism syndrome. As such, large surface area burn patients are at high risk for infection, which is often the precipitating cause of late deaths [33]. The pulmonary tree and the burn wound beds themselves are the most common sites and foci for fatal infection. Early wound infections, within 10 days of injury, are typically Gram-positive organisms. Later, pseudomonas is a common and potentially lethal organism, although fungal infections may occur in the subacute period and are often ominous. Central lines and urinary catheters should also be evaluated as possible infectious nidi. A growing and considerable body of evidence links bacterial translocation from the gut as a source of unexplained bacteremia [26]. Presence of gut bacteria and endotoxin in the lymphatic system supports this theory [20]. This risk may be decreased by enteral feedings and supplementation with glutamine. Immunoenhancing regimens are an area of intense study [34].

SURGICAL CONSIDERATIONS

Early Excision and Grafting

By the 1980s, the operative paradigm had shifted toward early (within 5 days) excision of full-thickness burns to limit the inflammatory forces driving "burn shock." In the operating room, excision of full-thickness burns is performed to the level of healthy bleeding tissue. Blood loss of 0.5 mL of blood per kilogram of patient weight for every percentage of TBSA excised is routine.

Once an area has been grafted with autologous tissue, shear forces must be minimized because the grafted skin initially lives by diffusion of nutrients from the underlying wound bed and imbibition until inosculation and neovascularization can take place. The use of negative pressure wound therapy devices (NPWT) as protective dressings from graft-killing shear has become the standard of care [35].

In areas of mixed partial- and full-thickness burns, excision of partial-thickness burns in addition to full-thickness burns may be necessary in order to facilitate practical skin grafting. Using a combination of autografts on completely excised burns and xenografts on partial-thickness burns is also a means to facilitate timely healing. Xenografts will function as a biologic dressing, decrease insensible fluid loss, and do not need frequent dressing changes, allowing the newly applied autografts to inosculate and neovascularize unmolested.

Escharotomies

Burned tissue has significantly less compliance than normal unburned tissue and may acutely restrict breathing as well as blood flow to the extremities. In the initial evaluation period, it is important to evaluate respiratory status as well as peripheral perfusion. Poor oxygenation can be a sign of frankly restrictive respiratory physiology secondary to a burned torso, and acute limb ischemia can also develop from a badly burned limb. The treatment for both of these conditions is immediate escharotomy at the affected site. Torso escharatomies will improve excursion of the chest wall, and limb escharatomies alleviate the functional venous tourniquet of a significant burn, equivalent to a fasciotomy for acute compartment syndrome. On the torso, escharotomy incisions are made along the anterior axillary line and connect at the level of the second rib and the xyphoid. In the extremities, incisions are made along the medial and lateral aspects of the appendage. In rare situations, orbital pressures can be elevated secondary to retro-orbital edema, necessitating lateral canthotomies.

Abdominal Compartment Syndrome

The inflammatory cascade and changing oncotic pressures in a patient with an acute burn undergoing resuscitation can lead to abdominal compartment syndrome. Abdominal hypertension is typically first identified by decreased urine output and restrictive airway dynamics. Transurethral bladder pressures in a chemically paralyzed patient greater than 20 cm H_2O are considered diagnostic for abdominal hypertension. Failure to identify and treat abdominal compartment syndrome can have devastating consequences including renal and respiratory failure as well as abdominal organ ischemia secondary to abdominal vasculature compression. Definitive treatment is decompressive laparotomy [36]. Please see Chapter 52 for a detailed discussion of abdominal compartment syndrome.

SPECIFIC INJURIES

Electrical Injury

The magnitude of electrical injuries varies depending on the voltage of current delivered to human tissue. Low-voltage (less than 1,000 V) injuries create thermal burns, injuring tissue from the outside in, whereas high voltage (greater than 1,000 V) can initially be deceiving in their devastation because a significant portion of the injury is not cutaneous but rather to the underlying muscle and bone. Very high-voltage injuries will have both extensive deep tissue injury and obvious cutaneous injury [37].

Immediate life-threatening conditions related to electrical injuries include cardiac dysrhythmias and spinal cord injury, either from direct injury, fall, or because of tetany resulting in spinal column fracture and cord injury.

Exit and entry wounds should be identified when possible, because this will help identify potentially affected tissue. Compartment syndrome from myonecrosis is common, especially in the upper extremity, and patients should be monitored closely for this complication in the first 24 hours. Limbs injured by electricity with resultant compartment syndrome require fasciotomies rather than simple escharotomies [38].

Aggressive fluid resuscitation should be initiated quickly to limit the renal effects of myonecrosis and myoglobinuria. Maintaining high urine output can help prevent kidney injury associated with myoglobin crystallization in the renal tubules. Daily monitoring of CPK may be beneficial in identifying potential or ongoing muscle necrosis. Persistently high levels may indicate muscle necrosis and need for surgical debridement [39].

Chemical Injury

Acids and alkali bases injure tissues by different mechanisms. Alkali bases burn tissue by liquefactive necrosis of subcutaneous fat, thrombosing perfusing vessels. Acids in turn burn by coagulation necrosis and as such are typically more superficial in their penetration of tissue [40]. Hydrofluoric acid (HF) burns are unique, however, because HF is a strong calcium and magnesium chelator. This can lead to devastating cardiac dysrhythmias and cardiac arrest owing to severe hypocalcemia. Topical calcium gluconate slurries are a mainstay of treatment for HF burns. Systemically, intravenous calcium gluconate is frequently necessary, and intra-arterial infusions have been effective for pain relief and preservation of tissue in extremity burns caused by HF [41].

PSYCHIATRIC AND ANALGESIC CONSIDERATIONS

Beyond the physiologic stress induced by burns, the burned patient undergoes significant psychological stress. Posttraumatic stress disorder (PTSD) has been reported in up to 45% of burn patients [42], and previous psychiatric history has been shown to be a risk factor for PTSD in the broadly studied burn population. Self-immolation accounts for only 4% of burn admission; however, these patients present complex patient care problems, because there is typically significant psychopathology that may hinder recovery [43].

Adequate pain control during their hospitalizations and during dressing changes has been shown to limit the long-term psychiatric effects of burn trauma [44]. Opiates, benzodiazepines, and the full range of dissociative medications are indicated. Unlike other critically ill patients, "sedation holidays" are not commonly used because these breaks in regular analgesia can create undue physiologic and psychological stress for the patient, increase catabolism, cardiovascular stress, and risk for development of PTSD [45]. Once the burn has been treated, wounds closed, and shock resolved, tapering of sedatives and narcotics can be initiated such that the patient may be weaned from the ventilator and avoid withdrawal symptoms. Among patients with extremity burns, long-acting regional anesthetics may be beneficial for pain control and permit better burn care and therapy.

References

1. American Burn Association: 2015 National Burn Repository, 2015.
2. Hussain SH, Limthongkul B, Humphreys TR: The biomechanical properties of the skin. *Dermatol Surg* 39(2):193–203, 2013.

3. Khatib M, Jabir S, Fitzgerald O'Connor E, et al: A systematic review of the evolution of laser Doppler techniques in burn depth assessment. *Plast Surg Int* 2014:621792, 2014. doi:10.1155/2014/621792.
4. Lund C, Browder N: The estimation of areas of burns. *Surg Gynecol Obstet* 79:352–358, 1944.
5. Veeravagu A, Yoon BC, Jiang B, et al: National trends in burn and inhalation injury in burn patients: results of analysis of the nationwide inpatient sample database. *J Burn Care Res* 36(2):258–265, 2015.
6. Heng JS, Clancy O, Atkins J, et al: Revised baux score and updated Charlson comorbidity index are independently associated with mortality in burns intensive care patients. *Burns* 41(7):1420–1427, 2015.
7. Jackson PC, Hardwicke J, Bamford A, et al: Revised estimates of mortality from the Birmingham Burn Center, 2001-2010: a continuing analysis over 65 years. *Ann Surg* 259(5):979–984, 2014.
8. Cassidy TJ, Edgar DW, Phillips M, et al: Transfer time to a specialist burn service and influence on burn mortality in Australia and New Zealand: A multi-center, hospital based retrospective cohort study. *Burns* 41(4):735–741, 2015.
9. Peeters Y, Vandervelden S, Wise R, et al: An overview on fluid resuscitation and resuscitations endpoints in burns: past, present and future. Part 1-Historical background, resuscitation fluid and adjunctive treatment. *Anaesthesiol Intensive Ther* 47(5):s6–14, 2015. doi:10.5603/AIT.a2015.0063.
10. Edgar DW, Fish JS, Gomez M, et al: Local and systemic treatments for acute edema after burn injury: a systematic review of the literature. *J Burn Care Res* 32(2):334–347, 2011.
11. Lawrence A, Faraklas I, Watkins H, et al: Colloid administration normalizes resuscitation ratio and ameliorates "fluid creep." *J Burn Care Res* 31(1):40–47, 2010.
12. Tao L, Zhou J, Gong Y, et al: Risk factors for central line-associated bloodstream infection in patients with major burns and efficacy of the topical application of mupirocin at the Central Venous Catheter Exit Site. *Burns* 31(8):1831–1838, 2015.
13. Peeters Y, Lebeer M, Wise R, et al: An overview on fluid resuscitation and resuscitation endpoints in burns; past, present and future. Part 2-avoiding complications by using the right endpoints with a new personalized protocolized approach. *Anaesthesiol Intensive Ther* 47(5):s15–26, 2015. doi:10.5603/AIT.a2015.0064.
14. Mosier MJ, Lasinski AM, Gamelli RL: Suspected adrenal insufficiency in critically ill burned patients: etomidate-induced or critical illness-related corticosteroid insufficiency? A review of the literature. *J Burn Care Res* 36(2):272–278, 2015.
15. Wicke C, Halliday B, Allen D: Effects of steroids and retinoids on wound healing. *Arch Surg* 135(11):1265–1270, 2000.
16. Jeschke MG: Postburn hypermetabolism: past, present, and future. *J Burn Care Res* 37(2):86–96, 2015. doi:10.1097/BCR.0000000000000265.
17. Schmauss D, Rezaeian F, Finck T, et al: Treatment of secondary burn wound progression in contact burns-a systematic review of experimental approaches. *J Burn Care Res* 36(3):e176–e189, 2015.
18. Hu S, Liu W-W, Zhao Y, et al: Pyruvate-enriched oral rehydration solution improved intestinal absorption of water and sodium during enteral resuscitation in burns. *Burns* 40(4):693–701, 2014.
19. Abu-Sittah GS, Sarhane KA, Dibo SA, et al: Cardiovascular dysfunction in burns: review of the literature. *Ann Burns Fire Disasters* 25(1):26–32, 2012.
20. Sambol J, Deitch EA, Takimoto K, et al: Cellular basis of burn-induced cardiac dysfunction and prevention by mesenteric lymph duct ligation. *J Surg Res* 183(2):678–685, 2013.
21. Nunez-Villaveiran T, Sanchez M, Millan P, et al: Systematic review of the effect of propanolol on hypermetabolism in burn injuries. *Med Intensiva* 39(2):101–113, 2015.
22. You K, Yang HT, Kym D, et al: Inhalation injury in burn patients: establishing the link between diagnosis and prognosis. *Burns* 40(8):1470–1475, 2014.
23. Huzar TF, George T, Cross JM: Carbon monoxide and cyanide toxicity: etiology, pathophysiology and treatment in inhalation injury. *Expert Rev Respir Med* 7(2):159–170, 2013.
24. Desai MH, Mlcak RP, Richardson J, et al: Reduction in mortality in pediatric patients with inhalational injury with aerosolized heparin/acetylcystine therapy. *J Burn Care Rehabil* 19(3):210–212, 1998.
25. Elsharnouby NM, Eid HE, Abou Elezz NF, et al: Heparin/N-acetylcysteine: an adjuvant in the management of burn inhalation injury: a study of different doses. *J Crit Care* 29(1):182.e181–182.e 184, 2014.
26. Ravat F, Le-Floch R, Vinsonneau C, et al: Antibiotics and the burn patient. *Burns* 37(1):16–26, 2011.
27. Smailes ST, McVicar AJ, Martin R: Cough strength, secretions and extubation outcome in burn patients who have passed a spontaneous breathing trial. *Burns* 39(2):236–242, 2013.
28. Breederveld R, Tuinebreijer W: Recombinant human growth hormone for treating burns and donor sites (Review). *Cochrane Database Syst Rev* (9):CD008990, 2014. doi:10.1002/14651858.CD008990.pub3.
29. Li H, Guo Y, Yang Z, et al: The efficacy and safety of oxandrolone treatment for patients with severe burns: a systematic review and meta-analysis. *Burns* 42(4):717–727, 2015. doi:10.1016/j.burns.2015.08.023.
30. Rousseau AF, Losser MR, Ichai C, et al: ESPEN endorsed recommendations: nutritional therapy in major burns. *Clin Nutr* 32(4):497–502, 2013.
31. Kurmis R, Greenwood J, Aromataris E: Trace element supplementation following severe burn injury: a systematic review and meta-analysis. *J Burn Care Res* 37(3):143–159, 2016. doi:10.1097/BCR.0000000000000259.
32. Rafla K, Tredget EE: Infection control in the burn unit. *Burns* 37(1), 5–15, 2011.
33. Linden K, Scaravilli V, Kreyer SF, et al: Evaluation of the cytosorb hemoadsorptive column in a PIG model of severe smoke and burn injury. *Shock* 44(5):487–495, 2015.
34. Williams FN, Branski LK, Jeschke MG, et al: What, how, and how much should patients with burns be fed? *Surg Clin North Am* 91(3):609–629, 2011.
35. Kamolz LP, Lumenta DB, Parvizi D, et al: Skin graft fixation in severe burns: use of topical negative pressure. *Ann Burns Fire Disasters* 27(3):141–145, 2014.
36. Wise R, Jacobs J, Pilate S, et al: Incidence and prognosis of intra-abdominal hypertension and abdominal compartment syndrome in severely burned patients: pilot study and review of the literature. *Anaesthesiol Intensive Ther* 48(2):95–109, 2014.
37. Salehi SH, Fatemi MJ, Asadi K, et al: Electrical injury in construction workers: a special focus on injury with electrical power. *Burns* 40(2):300–304, 2014.
38. Aghakhani K, Heidari M, Tabatabaee SM, et al: Effect of current pathway on mortality and morbidity in electrical burn patients. *Burns* 41(1):172–176, 2015.
39. Saracoglu A, Kuzucuoglu T, Yakupoglu S, et al: Prognostic factors in electrical burns: a review of 101 patients. *Burns* 40(4):702–707, 2014.
40. Tan T, Wong DS: Chemical burns revisited: what is the most appropriate method of decontamination? *Burns* 41(4):761–763, 2015.
41. Wang X, Zhang Y, Ni L, et al: A review of treatment strategies for hydrofluoric acid burns: current status and future prospects. *Burns* 40(8):1447–1457, 2014.
42. Sveen J, Ekselius L, Gerdin B, et al: A prospective longitudinal study of post-traumatic stress disorder symptom trajectories after burn injury. *J Trauma* 71(6):1808–1815, 2011.
43. Caine PL, Tan A, Barnes D, et al: Self-inflicted burns: 10 year review and comparison to national guidelines. *Burns* 42(1):215–221, 2016.
44. Sheridan RL, Stoddard FJ, Kazis LE, et al: Long-term posttraumatic stress symptoms vary inversely with early opiate dosing in children recovering from serious burns: effects durable at 4 years. *J Trauma Acute Care Surg* 76(3):828–832, 2014.
45. Giannoni-Pastor A, Eiroa-Orosa FJ, Fidel Kinori SG, et al: Prevalence and predictors of posttraumatic stress symptomatology among burn survivors: a systematic review and meta-analysis. *J Burn Care Res* 37(1):e79–e89, 2016.

Section 5
SURGICAL PROBLEMS IN THE INTENSIVE CARE UNIT

MITCHELL CAHAN

Chapter 47 ■ Surgeon and Intensivist Collaboration in the Care of the ICU Patient

GUSTAVO GUILLERMO ANGARAMO • CRAIG M. LILLY

The modern intensive care unit (ICU) is teeming with technology; however, it is probably the most stressful place in the hospital [1]. Advanced technology has brought sophisticated instrumentation and databases to the bedside [2]. Entirely new therapies are possible for grave diseases, such as low tidal volume strategies for acute lung injury or early antimicrobial therapy for sepsis [3–5]. Increasing sophistication of care leads invariably to increased complexity. This complexity poses opportunities and potential hazards [2]. Patient turnover is rapid and survival rates continue to improve. Many caregivers are involved, and all of them expect some input into the process of care. Meanwhile, a designated credentialed provider always must be responsible for the overall care plan and occasionally adjudicate differences of opinion regarding difficult decisions, or reconcile conflicting recommendations from key team members. The conflicts arise not only from uncertainties about outcomes but also about what is understood as success. In the clinical world, success is defined as survival to leave the ICU; however, in the moral world of families and friends, success often means a patient returning to an independent life with resumption of normal activities. Effective care of patients requires that all parties involved understand each other's point of view.

DEFINITION OF ICU MODELS AND LEVELS OF CARE

The open ICU model is an ICU in which patients are admitted under the care of an internist, family physician, surgeon, or other primary attending of record, with intensivists often available providing expertise via elective consultation [6].

Intensivist co-management is an open ICU model in which all patients receive mandatory consultation from an intensivist. The internist, family physician, or surgeon is the co-attending of record with intensivists collaborating in the management of all ICU patients.

In a closed ICU model, patients admitted to the unit are transferred to the care of an intensivist assigned to the ICU on a full-time basis. Patients are accepted to the ICU only after approval by the intensivist. For periods ranging from 1 week to 1 month at a time, the intensivist's clinical duties consist of caring for patients in the ICU, with no other clinical responsibilities.

A mixed ICU model may consist of directorship and daily ICU rounds by the intensivist (closed unit and/or co-management), or simply the presence of a full-time intensivist in the ICU (including examples of all three models).

The American College of Critical Care Medicine has described three levels of hospital-based critical care centers to optimally match services and personnel with community needs [7]:

1. Level I critical care centers have ICUs that provide comprehensive care for a wide range of disorders requiring intensive care. They require the continuous availability of sophisticated equipment, specialized nurses, and physicians with critical care training.
2. Level II critical care centers have the capability to provide comprehensive critical care, but may not have resources to care for specific populations (e.g., cardiothoracic surgery, neurosurgery, trauma).
3. Level III critical care centers may provide initial stabilization of critically ill patients but are limited in their ability to provide comprehensive critical care.

COMMUNICATION AMONG ICU TEAM MEMBERS

Interprofessional tensions can threaten the delivery of quality health care in the hospital setting. Such tensions have been documented at several clinical locations including the ICU [8]. The ICU in particular is a nexus for interspeciality tensions because of its unique role in the care of the hospital's most critically ill patients and associated management of critical care resources [9]. Conflict in the ICU is frequent; more than 70% of ICU clinicians report experiencing conflict weekly [10,11]. The combination of caring for acutely ill patients, end-of-life decision-making, and coordination of large interprofessional teams can lead to frustration, communication breakdown, and discord among members of the health care team. The epidemiology of this conflict has been very well described in the Conflicus study [10]. Conflict has been associated with lower quality patient care [12,13], higher rates of serious medical errors [14], staff burn out [15,16], and greater direct and indirect costs of care [17]. ICU conflict can occur between the health care team and patients' families, among members of the ICU team, and among different groups of clinicians caring for the same patient, most notably between surgeons and intensivists.

Lingard et al. [9] studied the forces governing the interactions among professions (nurses and physicians) and specialties (ICU team and consultants). This group found out that the level of collaboration or conflict within the ICU team and between ICU and other specialties fluctuated on the basis of six important catalysts: authority, education, patient needs, knowledge, resources, and time. Two dominant mechanisms were also described and categorized in their analysis as "the perception of ownership" and the "process of trade."

Ownership was perceived as both collective (ICU team) and individual [9]. It promoted collaboration between members of the ICU team and was often established by contrast with those outside of the core team such as surgeons, internists, or nurses from the wards. Individual ownership is also a dominant issue and includes instances where members recognized their own or other's skill; this recognition is part of the smooth collaborative functioning of the team.

Within the process of trade, team members traded valued commodities including equipment, resources, respect, goodwill, and knowledge as they negotiated their collaborative work [9].

The forces of ownership and trade have a central role in the daily negotiations that constitute teamwork in the ICU setting. When ownership is not attended to, or one commodity is not offered in trade for another, tensions accumulate and collaboration is compromised [9].

The Surgeon's Perspective

The qualities that define a surgical personality have been described by anthropologist Joan Cassell [18] as decisiveness, control, confidence, and certitude. The surgeon often views his or her relationship with the patient as a covenant to cure. Actions that threaten this covenant as relinquishing responsibility for the care of a patient to another practitioner, losing control over key decisions, and proposals toward comfort with the expectation of death can be strongly rejected by the admitting surgeon [44]. This ownership searching for an ideal outcome is valuable in that the patient has a strong advocate to facilitate recovery; however, surgical obstinacy with respect to sharing responsibility for care and resulting reluctance to direct efforts toward comfort can deny the dying patient both dignity and control [19]. Surgeons are affected by the increasing demands of clinical practice, spending more time in the office and in the operating room, at the cost of less available time to see and manage patients in the ICU.

Olson et al. reported in a study on conflict of postoperative goals of care that 40% of surgeons who routinely perform high-risk operations reported conflict with critical care physicians and nurses regarding the goals of care for their patients with poor postoperative outcomes [20]. Surgeons who reported higher rates of conflict had fewer years in practice and worked in an academic setting. Surgeons with more experience may be more accepting and may have developed coping strategies for unwanted outcomes. Additionally, surgeons who practice in a closed ICU reported higher rates of conflict about goals of care.

The Intensivist's Perspective

In contrast to the surgeon's perspective, the intensivist's point of view is often more focused on symptom relief and comfort. This different perspective does not mean that intensivists are any less goal oriented than surgeons; intensivists actually embrace goal-directed care [19].

From the surgeon's perspective, persistence in the face of overwhelming odds is seen as a noble obligation. From the intensivist's perspective, persistence in the face of overwhelming odds can be costly, painful, and disrespectful if the patient has expressed any wish to avoid heroic measures.

The effectiveness of a dedicated intensivist caring for ICU patients has been shown in multiple reviews [21]. The presence and participation of an intensivist-directed team can identify and treat problems before catastrophic complications occur. Understanding of sepsis, mechanical ventilatory support for acute respiratory distress syndrome (ARDS), and description and treatment of endocrine dysfunction among the critically ill have led to protocol-driven care and improved survival [22,23].

Young and Birkmeyer [24] have provided estimates of the relative reduction of annual ICU mortality resulting from conversion of all urban ICUs to an intensivist model of management. Assuming an ICU mortality of 12% and estimating that 85% of urban ICUs are not currently intensivist managed, they calculated that there are approximately 360,000 preventable deaths annually in U.S. urban ICUs that lack intensivists. A conservative projection of a 15% relative reduction in mortality resulting from intensivist-managed ICUs yields a predicted annual saving of nearly 54,000 lives.

The ICU Nurse's Perspective

The ICU nurse has a fundamental role for supporting and comforting ICU patients and their families. Nurses spend the most time with ICU patients and family members and thus are a valuable resource for identifying the patient and family understanding and evaluating the effectiveness of communication. Moreover, nurses act as the medical intermediary for families, as well as the link between health care providers, particularly when surgeons and ICU physicians disagree [18,25,26].

METHODS FOR ACHIEVING AND MAINTAINING ICU TEAM CONSENSUS

Consensus is a process-based concept that is a core element of high-performing teams. It allows essential communication that enables teams to effectively perform high-fidelity tasks. Consensus is founded on assent of the team members and sometimes requires vetting, discussion, and even negotiation. Establishing a process by which consensus is consistently achieved is an important skill for ICU team leaders. Consensus is a state of acquiescence to team-based decisions that does not require that all team members are in full agreement with all of the details of a decision, rather that all key members assent to the critical concepts of the decision [27]. In the context of patient care, it is better to maintain a state of consensus than to attempt to build it after disagreement has festered [28]. A summary of helpful communication strategies is presented in Table 47.1.

One effective approach to build and maintain consensus is including key team members in an interprofessional rounding process [29]. In this context, "including" means listening and valuing input from all stakeholders and on occasion soliciting the opinions of those who may not be in consensus with the plan of care. Including key personnel like the surgeon [30] on

TABLE 47.1

Strategies for Achieving and Maintaining Team Consensus

Include the surgeon in all decision-making sessions with the patient and family
Include the surgeon on interprofessional rounds
Before all decision-making sessions: *Value* the surgical opinion and identify points of agreement
Before all decision-making sessions: Leverage consultants and diagnostic studies to resolve differences of opinion with regard to the medical facts
Have the patient or his or her medical decision maker participate in interprofessional rounds
Share medical images with the patient or medical decision maker in the presence of the surgeon
When the surgeon believes that continued aggressive care will lead to healing, agree on a time-limited trial of continued aggressive care
Discuss the functional outcome in the context of the patient's goals and values
Discuss whether continued aggressive care or a comfort-oriented plan is more consistent with the patient's values
Carefully assess how much unfavorable information the patient and the surgeon are ready to accept. Allow adequate time for processing difficult information

interdisciplinary rounds is one of the best methods for managing the consensus-building process [31,32]. An increasing number of ICU teams have found that including the patient and family members on bedside rounds [33–35] is helpful for preventing and resolving differences of opinion regarding the patient's goals for minimal functional outcomes [36,37]. This approach has the advantage of removing the nurse or intensivist from the messenger role and allowing a more balanced discussion of the merits of alternative goals for the care plan. Establishing clear patient-centered goals is often helpful for achieving consensus on specific care plan elements and increasing the comfort of reluctant team members to assent to a comfort-oriented care plan [38].

The process of avoiding confrontational and emotion-laden open or hidden disagreements involves active listening skills and the thoughtful inclusion of consultants, review of medical advanced testing and imaging, and inclusion of the patient or their medical decision maker in team discussions. The most important consensus-building skill for an ICU team leader is to value the dissenting opinions of team members, particularly those of the operating surgeon and nursing staff. Adaptation of the patient-focused V.A.L.U.E. system that was developed at the University of Washington for difficult communication can also be helpful in the context of team communication [39]. In this context, "V" is for valuing comments made by dissenting team members, "A" is for acknowledging the emotions associated with their point of view, "L" is for actively listening, "U" is for understanding the dissenters as individuals, and "E" is for eliciting their comments by creating safe space for their expression. This approach can be highly effective when routinely employed, and team members learn to present their opinions efficiently. One key concept is a proactive ICU team approach that prepares for managing potential compromised critical care functional outcomes before they have occurred.

Proactive management starts by identifying gaps between the patient or surgeon's goals for functional outcomes and those that are likely to be achieved. The identification of the gap in expectations can be managed in several ways and all start with achieving agreement on the medical facts [38,39]. When the medical facts are not clear, consultants, pathologic evaluation of tissue specimens, advanced laboratory studies, and radiologic testing can be helpful for achieving consensus regarding the diagnosis and for defining practically achievable alternative therapeutic approaches. Establishing the medical facts and options allows the team to discuss alternative care plans and the metrics by which their success or failure can be judged.

Team consensus, including that of the operating surgeon, on a specific approach allows implementation of a time-limited plan of aggressive care. Including "clinical milestones" or objective metrics by which the success or failure of the plan will be judged allows presentation of the plan to the patient and medical decision-makers with a date for a "difficult discussion" should the care plan not achieve the clinical milestones [38]. This approach has been shown to improve outcomes and support patient-defined values because it encourages team members that favor a comfort-only approach to contribute fully to an aggressive care trial and those who favor aggressive care to transition to a comfort-oriented approach [40]. Time-limited trials of aggressive care that use clinical milestones that medical decision-makers can easily identify have the advantage that ICU team members spend less time explaining unpleasant information and are better able to advocate for comfort and dignity at the end of life. This approach also supports physiologically improving patients because prescheduled communication events can be used to discuss preparation for the process of physical and emotional rehabilitation after severe critical illness when continued aggressive care leads to improvement.

The adoption of collaborative interprofessional teams that are led by critical care professionals who adopt a proactive approach that is supported by V.A.L.U.E.-based communication will only rarely require the services of an ethics consultant [41] or a palliative care specialist [42] to heal broken-down communication or to work on resolving refractory value-based differences among interprofessional team members or between the ICU team and the patient or medical decision maker.

SUMMARY

The structure of the ICU can pose a barrier to the continuity of the surgeon–patient relationship and contributes to conflict when the surgeon is replaced as the primary decision maker for his or her patients by an intensivist [12,19,20,43]. Clearly, some of the ICU models described earlier can promote conflict with juxtaposition of clinicians with unmanaged competing interests. This is where valuing the input of the surgeon can have the greatest impact by ensuring that his or her patients receive an adequate trial of aggressive care. The surgeon who communicates his or her wishes and participates in patient-focused discussions of alternative approaches is a valued ICU team member and patient advocate [19].

Conflict is a significant public health problem that diminishes quality of care for critically ill patients. Consequences of conflict underscores the importance of surgeon–patient preoperative discussion of goals and values to guide postoperative decisions in the event of an undesired outcome [20,44–46]. In the absence of cooperation, conflict can affect patients and families, leading to decreased satisfaction with care and increased stress [10,13,47].

It is time to move from the rhetoric of team collaboration, toward a more clear understanding of the skills required to function in the competitive setting of the interprofessional health care team. These findings have educational implications for both trainees and practicing intensivists. As a result, medical schools have adapted by requiring competence in domains such as communication and collaboration within the medical team [48].

Communication is the most important factor for the intensivist who ensures that adverse events are reported in a timely fashion, that important decisions are discussed, and that the surgeon is included in the process. The surgeon should be willing to discuss rather than dictate and consider different approaches [19]. Clinicians from all backgrounds should focus on streamlining communication to allow energies to be spent more productively on better care for our critically ill postoperative patients [20].

Further research, particularly into ideal communication among surgeons, intensivists, and ICU nurses, is needed.

References

1. Barie PS: Advances in critical care monitoring. *Arch Surg* 132:734–739, 1997.
2. Barie PS, Bacchetta MD, Eachempati SR: The contemporary surgical intensive care unit. *Surg Clin North Am* 80(3):791–804, 2000.
3. Fanelli V, Vlachou A, Ghannadian S, et al: Acute respiratory distress syndrome: new definition, current and future therapeutic options. *J Thorac Dis* 5(3):326–334, 2013.
4. Rivers E, Nguyen B, Havstad S, et al: Early goal-directed therapy in the treatment of severe sepsis and septic shock. *N Engl J Med* 345(19):1368–1377, 2001.
5. Monnet X, Teboul JL: Assessment of volume responsiveness during mechanical ventilation: recent advances. *Crit Care* 17(2):217, 2013.
6. Rothschild JM: "Closed" intensive care units and other models of care for critically ill patients. A critical analysis of patient safety practices. Agency for Healthcare Research and Quality. Chapter 36: 413–414, Available at: http://archive.ahrq.gov/clinic/ptsafety/. Accessed January 31, 2017.
7. Haupt MT, Bekes CE, Carl LC, et al: Guidelines on critical care services and personnel: recommendations based on a system of categorization of three levels of care. *Crit Care Med* 31(11):2677–2683, 2003.
8. Hawryluck LA, Espin S, Lingard L: Pulling together and pushing apart: tides of tension in the ICU team. *Acad Med* 77:S73–S76, 2002.
9. Lingard L, Espin S, Evans C, et al: The rules of the game: interprofessional collaboration on the intensive care unit team. *Crit Care* 8:R403–R408, 2004.
10. Azoulay E, Timsit JF, Sprung CL, et al: Prevalence and factors of intensive care unit conflicts: the Conflicus study. *Am J Respir Crit Care Med* 180(9):853–860, 2009.

11. Fassier T, Azoulay E: Conflicts and communication gaps in the intensive care unit. *Curr Opin Crit Care* 16(6):654–665, 2010.
12. Danjoux Meth N, Lawless B, Hawryluck L: Conflicts in the ICU: perspectives of administrators and clinicians. *Intensive Care Med* 35(12):2068–2077, 2009.
13. Studdert DM, Mello MM, Burns JP, et al: Conflict in the care of patients with prolonged stay in the ICU: types, sources, and predictors. *Intensive Care Med* 29(9):1489–1497, 2003.
14. Baldwin DC Jr, Daugherty SR: Interprofessional conflict and medical errors: results of a national multi-specialty survey of hospital residents in the US. *J Interprof Care* 22(6):573–586, 2008.
15. Embriaco N, Azoulay E, Barrau K, et al: High level of burnout in intensivists: prevalence and associated factors. *Am J Respir Crit Care Med* 175(7):686–692, 2007.
16. Poncet MC, Toullic P, Papazian L, et al: Burnout syndrome in critical care nursing staff. *Am J Respir Crit Care Med* 175(7):698–704, 2007.
17. Brinkert R: A literature review of conflict communication causes, costs, benefits and interventions in nursing. *J Nurs Manag* 18(2):145–156, 2010.
18. Cassell J: *Life and Death in the Intensive Care Unit*. Philadelphia: Temple University Press, 2005.
19. Penkoske P, Buchman T: The relationship between the surgeon and the intensivist in the surgical intensive care unit. *Surg Clin North Am* 86:1351–1357, 2006.
20. Olson TJ, Brasel KJ, Redmann AJ, et al: Surgeon reported conflict with intensivists about postoperative goals of care. *JAMA Surg* 148(1): 29–35, 2013.
21. Gasperino J: The Leapfrog initiative for intensive care unit physician staffing and its impact on intensive care unit performance: a narrative review. *Health Policy* 102:223–228, 2011.
22. Van Den Berghe G, Wouters P, Weekers F, et al: Intensive insulin therapy in critically ill patients. *N Engl J Med* 345(19):1359–1367, 2001.
23. The Acute Respiratory Distress Syndrome Network: Ventilation with lower tidal volumes as compared with traditional tidal volumes for acute lung injury and the acute respiratory distress syndrome. *N Engl J Med* 342:1301–1308, 2000.
24. Young MP, Birkmeyer JD: Potential reduction in mortality rates using an intensivist model to manage intensive care units. *Eff Clin Pract* 3:284–289, 2000.
25. Aslakson RA, Wyskiel R, Shaeffer D, et al: Surgical intensive care unit clinician estimates of the adequacy of communication regarding patient prognosis. *Crit Care* 14:R218, 2010.
26. Asch DA, Shea JA, Jedrziewski MK, et al: The limits of suffering: critical care nurses' views of hospital care at the end of life. *Soc Sci Med* 45:1661–1668, 1997.
27. Collins SA, Bakken S, Vawdrey DK, et al: Agreement between common goals discussed and documented in the ICU. *J Am Med Inform Assoc* 18(1):45–50, 2011.
28. Davidson JE, Powers K, Hedayat KM, et al: Clinical practice guidelines for support of the family in the patient-centered intensive care unit: American College of Critical Care Medicine Task Force 2004-2005. *Crit Care Med* 35(2):605–622, 2007.
29. Mosenthal AC, Murphy PA, Barker LK, et al: Changing the culture around end-of-life care in the trauma intensive care unit. *J Trauma* 64(6):1587–1593, 2008.
30. Pronovost PJ, Jenckes MW, Dorman T, et al: Organizational characteristics of intensive care units related to outcomes of abdominal aortic surgery. *JAMA* 281(14):1310–1317, 1999.
31. Puntillo KA, McAdam JL: Communication between physicians and nurses as a target for improving end-of-life care in the intensive care unit: challenges and opportunities for moving forward. *Crit Care Med* 34[11, Suppl]:S332–S340, 2006.
32. DeKeyser Ganz F, Engelberg R, Torres N, et al: Development of a model of interprofessional shared clinical decision making in the ICU: a mixed-methods study. *Crit Care Med* 44(4):680–689, 2016.
33. Cypress BS: Family presence on rounds: a systematic review of literature. *Dimens Crit Care Nurs* 31(1):53–64, 2012.
34. McPherson G, Jefferson R, Kissoon N, et al: Toward the inclusion of parents on pediatric critical care unit rounds. *Pediatr Crit Care Med* 12(6):e255–e261, 2011.
35. Mangram AJ, McCauley T, Villarreal D, et al: Families' perception of the value of timed daily "family rounds" in a trauma ICU. *Am Surg* 71(10):886–891, 2005.
36. Harris GM: Family-centered rounds in the neonatal intensive care unit. *Nurs Women's Health* 18(1):18–27, 2014.
37. Stickney CA, Ziniel SI, Brett MS, et al: Family participation during intensive care unit rounds: goals and expectations of parents and health care providers in a tertiary pediatric intensive care unit. *J Pediatr* 165(6):1245–1251 e1, 2014.
38. Lilly CM, De Meo DL, Sonna LA, et al: An intensive communication intervention for the critically ill. *Am J Med* 109(6):469–475, 2000.
39. Lautrette A, Darmon M, Megarbane B, et al: A communication strategy and brochure for relatives of patients dying in the ICU. *N Engl J Med* 356(5):469–478, 2007.
40. Lilly CM, Sonna LA, Haley KJ, et al: Intensive communication: four-year follow-up from a clinical practice study. *Crit Care Med* 31[5, Suppl]:S394–S399, 2003.
41. Luce JM: A history of resolving conflicts over end-of-life care in intensive care units in the United States. *Crit Care Med* 38(8):1623–1629, 2010.
42. Villarreal D, Restrepo MI, Healy J, et al: A model for increasing palliative care in the intensive care unit: enhancing interprofessional consultation rates and communication. *J Pain Symptom Manage* 42(5):676–679, 2011.
43. Buchman TG, Cassell J, Ray SE, et al: Who should manage the dying patient?: Rescue, shame, and the surgical ICU dilemma. *J Am Coll Surg* 194(5):665–673, 2002.
44. Schwarze ML, Bradley CT, Brasel KJ: Surgical "buy-in": the contractual relationship between surgeons and patients that influences decisions regarding life-supporting therapy. *Crit Care Med* 38(3):843–848, 2010.
45. Redmann AJ, Brasel KJ, Alexander GC, et al: Use of advance directives for high-risk operations: a national survey of surgeons. *Ann Surg* 255(3):418–423, 2012.
46. Sudore RL, Fried TR: Redefining the "planning" in advance care planning: preparing for end-of-life decision making. *Ann Intern Med* 153(4):256–261, 2010.
47. Breen CM, Abernathy AP, Abbott KH, et al: Conflict associated with decisions to limit life sustaining treatment in intensive care units. *J Gen Intern Med* 16(5):283–289, 2001.
48. CanMEDS Roles (Canadian Medical Education Directions for Specialists), Royal College of Physicians and Surgeons of Canada: Accreditation and postgraduate training guidelines. Available at: http://www.royalcollege.ca/rcsite/canmeds-e.

Chapter 48 ■ Surgical Infections in the Intensive Care Unit

ANN-KRISTIN U. FRIEDRICH • MITCHELL CAHAN

INTRODUCTION

Surgical infections present challenges of diagnosis and management in the intensive care setting. Manifestations may vary from simple superficial surgical site infection to complex generalized infections of the abdominal cavity. Abdominal infections are the third most common cause of sepsis in the intensive care unit (ICU) [1] and have been associated with high morbidity and mortality rates [2]. Rarely do surgical infections present as the sole reason for admission to ICUs. Patients who develop surgical site infections may have multiple comorbidities, be hemodynamically unstable, or even septic with concurrent failure of one or more organ systems, and are at high risk of treatment failure [3]. Early recognition and appropriate treatment is crucial in order to mitigate and control a potentially lethal infection.

PATHOGENESIS

Etiology of Surgical Infections

Surgical infections in the ICU population represent a complex clinical entity with a number of etiologic and contributory factors. This can be seen as a result of an inability of the host to adequately respond to a high number of pathogens of varying virulence. Patient-associated factors therefore play a significant role, including: malnutrition, as manifested by a low serum albumin concentration; older age; obesity; smoking; diabetes mellitus; localized malperfusion caused by vascular disease or a history of radiation to the site; and generalized malperfusion caused by peri- or intraoperative shock [4,5]. In addition, inadequate surgical technique, prolonged procedure time, or breaks in sterile technique may cause or contribute to the development of a surgical infection. Foreign body presence in the surgical field may help organisms to fester, as the number of bacteria required to cause a clinically significant infection may be lower in the presence of such a nidus [4]. In addition to skin flora as the source of causative organisms, surgical infections can be caused by spillage of enteric content or anastomotic leaks. Blunt abdominal trauma can also lead to perforation of the intestine or simple translocation of bacteria into the peritoneal cavity in the setting of intestinal wall hematoma or ischemia [6]. In an immunocompromised patient, this abdominal seeding may lead to peritonitis and infection, similar to a deep-organ space surgical site infection.

Abscess Formation

Abscess formation may occur when the patient's immune systems attempts to locally control a certain disease process, such as free entry of pathogenic organisms into the abdominal cavity via perforation, surgical intervention, or trauma. Intraabdominal abscesses are confined to a part of the abdomen without free access to the peritoneal cavity. Especially in sizable abscesses, free diffusion of antibiotics and host immune cells into its center is usually not possible. This makes it almost impossible to control a sizable lesion with antiinfective therapy alone. Drainage via either the radiologic or open surgical technique is usually required to prevent hematogenous spreading of pathogens or rupture of the abscess into the peritoneal cavity. Abscess formation may occur at any location of the body, including sites of venipunctures, chronic wounds or ulcers, and around indwelling catheters, and is a frequently observed intraabdominal process in postoperative critical care patients.

Peritonitis

Peritonitis is a generalized inflammatory reaction that may involve the partial or entire peritoneal cavity. It can be classified as primary, secondary, or tertiary peritonitis. The extent of peritoneal reaction may be dependent on the exact intestinal origin of the causative organism [7].

Primary Peritonitis

Infection of the peritoneum without obvious source or localized infection within the abdominal cavity is classified as primary peritonitis [8]. Obvious disruption of the gastrointestinal (GI) tract's anatomic barrier is absent. Primary peritonitis tends to be a community-acquired disease of patients with previously existing ascites due to cirrhotic liver disease. A single causative organism can usually be isolated. GI flora such as enterococci and gram-negative bacilli tend to be responsible [9]. Other causes of primary peritonitis include infection of an indwelling peritoneal dialysis catheter, as well as rare cases of primary peritonitis in otherwise healthy patients, primarily caused by group A streptococcus [10,11]. The latter presentation can be associated with toxic shock syndrome [12]. In postoperative patients in an intensive care setting, primary peritonitis is a very rare occurrence.

Secondary Peritonitis

Peritonitis in the setting of perforation of a hollow viscus is called secondary peritonitis. Gross spillage of GI flora into the peritoneal cavity follows this disruption of the anatomic barrier. Causes include inflammation, malignancy, anastomotic leak, necrosis, fistula, and blunt and/or penetrating trauma. Secondary peritonitis is a frequently encountered problem in surgical intensive care patients. Reported mortality rates associated with secondary peritonitis range from 15% to 23%; however, this may increase in the setting of simultaneous sepsis or shock, as well as comorbid disease processes [13–15]. When isolation of microbial pathogens is successful, cultures are usually polymicrobial [16]. Outcomes from secondary peritonitis are dependent on adequate and timely treatment, source control, and the patient's immune system [17].

Tertiary Peritonitis

Persistent peritonitis in the setting of exhaustive medical and interventional management is conventionally referred to as tertiary peritonitis [18]. The range of patients who progress from secondary to tertiary peritonitis can be as high as 20% [19]. It is however important to differentiate tertiary peritonitis from ongoing secondary peritonitis in the setting of inadequate source control, in the sense of failure to drain or evacuate existing abscesses or nidi of infection.

Tertiary peritonitis has been associated with a high incidence of nosocomial, multidrug-resistant organisms as well as immunologic dysfunction and altered endocrine stress response [20]. Different disease processes seem to be more or less prone to progress to tertiary peritonitis; for example, necrotizing pancreatitis has been associated with a high progression rate [19]. Tertiary peritonitis is linked to higher mortality, longer ICU stay, and more severe stage of end-organ impairment [21,22]. In a retrospective observational study with 92 cases of tertiary peritonitis, Evans et al. [23] could not correlate tertiary peritonitis as a sole prognostic factor of death after adjusting for other variables. Rather than being the cause of a patient's death, tertiary peritonitis may in fact be a symptom of a highly dysfunctional host response to inflammatory stress.

PATHOGENS

The spectrum of causative pathogens in surgical infections is broad and depends on the underlying site of the primary disease as well as the clinical course of the patient. Community-acquired diseases that lead to surgical postoperative infections often start with an obstructive disease pattern and eventually become superinfected by GI flora; classic examples include acute calculous cholecystitis or appendicitis. The causative pathogens vary depending on the area of perforation. De Ruiter et al. [7] analyzed peritoneal fluid of 221 patients with abdominal sepsis due to perforated viscus at the time of the primary operation. They most commonly observed aerobic and gram-negative bacteria in appendiceal and colonic perforations; gram-positive bacteria were encountered with colorectal disease. Gastroduodenal perforations were associated with Candida species, most commonly *Candida albicans*.

Nosocomial infections are different for a variety of reasons. Pathogens tend to be less susceptible to antibiotic regimens and may be multiresistant [24]. In addition to this, the patient's host response may be impaired or their GI flora may have been altered in the setting of prior antibiotic treatments, including potential overpopulation of virulent, ICU-acquired organisms. An increased risk of infection and subsequent multiorgan failure is observed among patients who are colonized with pathogens such as Candida species, *Staphylococcus epidermidis*, *Pseudomonas aeruginosa*, and *Enterococcus faecalis* [24,25].

Enterococcus is frequently isolated from patients with nonappendiceal peritonitis and is associated with the pathogenesis of many surgical abdominal infections [26,27]. Its involvement has been directly correlated with the severity of disease in the setting of anastomotic leakage [28]. However, antibiotic coverage of Enterococcus is not always indicated. Increasingly drug-resistant strains of Enterococci have emerged over the recent past and presented an increasingly difficult challenge. In particular, a growing population of vancomycin-resistant enterococci is feared, as this may lead to subsequent evolvement of vancomycin-resistant *Staphylococcus aureus* through genetic exchange among species.

Another challenge of surgical site infections is that caused by fungal pathogens. Fungal organisms benefit from decreased selection pressure from bacteria, especially after multiple courses of broad-spectrum antibiotics, and have been associated with the development of tertiary peritonitis [29,30]. High mortality has been associated with intraabdominal candidiasis infection, especially in an ICU setting [31]. Unfortunately, even adequate treatment of Candida species has not always been associated with improved outcomes [32]. It is not clear whether Candida spp. isolated from abdominal sources are true causative pathogens or rather a symptom of poor host immune response and severity of underlying disease.

DIAGNOSIS

Clinical Examination

Suspicion for a surgical site infection can be raised by clinical examination. Erythema, drainage, or dehiscence are the first signs of a superficial infection, and may necessitate opening the incision at least partially in order to ensure adequate drainage. Gentle probing of the underlying fascia can help for assessment of the depth of infection and differentiating fascial dehiscence due to an infectious process from a possible enterocutaneous fistula.

Deep-organ space infections can also become clinically apparent. Rebound and guarding on exam, as well as inappropriate tenderness to palpation, can be signs of peritonitis or intraabdominal abscesses. It is important to realize that clinical examination findings can however be obscured by coexisting diseases, altered level of consciousness, the patient's overall clinical deterioration, and the presence of sedating or paralyzing agents. Significant infections can also cause a change in vital signs, such as repeated febrile episodes as well as tachycardia, hypotension and tachypnea, and if not recognized and treated can lead to septic shock. In an ICU patient, these vital sign derangements may be the only reliable indication of an infection.

Laboratory Analysis

Persistent or increasing leukocytosis, often associated with an increased count of segmented neutrophils, should also raise suspicion of an infection of surgical and postoperative ICU patients. Other valuable parameters especially for monitoring the clinical course of the infectious disease process include acute phase proteins such as C-reactive protein and procalcitonin, a precursor of the hormone calcitonin [33]. Organ-specific parameters may prove helpful in potentially locating an abscess, such as altered liver function parameters in the setting of an intrahepatic abscess.

Cultures are an important tool for tailoring antibiotic regimens and assessing the course of disease. Blood cultures should be drawn in the setting of presumed sepsis and unexplained febrile episodes. Fluid draining from seromas and hematomas can be cultured, as well as aspirate from superficial and deep abscesses. The use of aspiration and analysis of peritoneal fluid in the setting of peritonitis remains controversial, especially as these cultures are often sterile in the setting of persistent secondary or tertiary peritonitis [16]. However, when possible, the isolation of a target organism and subsequent susceptibility testing are invaluable tools for the diagnosis and treatment of surgical infections.

Radiology

Different imaging modalities play a vital role in the setting of a surgical site infection. Radiographs can reveal free air, pneumatosis of the bowel wall, which indicates ischemia or necrosis, or gas in the soft tissue as potential signs of a localized infection. Ultrasound can be a helpful mobile bedside tool for evaluating the presence of an abscess. It is dependent upon the ability of the ultrasonographer and the patient's body habitus, and can be seriously limited in deep-organ spaces, when air-filled bowel loops may obstruct the view of a potential collection.

Computed tomography (CT) can be a very useful tool for evaluating deep surgical site infections, especially as image quality can be optimized by the application of intravenous, oral, or rectal contrast. This can be limited by the fact that many hemodynamically unstable patients may not be suitable for transport to the CT suite, and use of intravenous contrast can also contribute to impaired renal function.

Magnetic resonance imaging may be a helpful modality for evaluating compartments for patients whose radiation exposure should be minimized, such as pregnant or pediatric patients. Its use to assess surgical infections in intensive care patients is nonetheless limited due to the relatively long duration of the examination, and due to limited image quality of the thoracic and abdominal cavity due to motion artifacts from peristalsis of the bowel wall, as well as respiration and movement of the diaphragm.

THERAPY

Antiinfective Treatment

The general principles of antibiotic therapy apply in the setting of surgical site infections as well. Antibiotic treatment should commence as early as possible. Initially, a broad-spectrum empiric agent should be chosen, tailored to the likely site(s) of infection, local bacterial epidemiology, and known resistance patterns. Coverage is dependent on location, type, and severity of the surgical infection [34]. Usually, initial coverage includes gram negatives, gram positives, and anaerobes. One may also consider covering Candida in a high-risk setting. As a second step, antibiotic coverage is tailored to culture and susceptibility results in order to prevent the emergence of multiresistant bacterial strains [35]. Antibiotic coverage should not be prolonged unless necessary, such as in the setting of failed source control or superinfection.

Source Control

Despite adequate antiinfectious coverage, patient's mortality rates in the setting of surgical infection may be high without proper source control [31]. Source control is defined as "all physical measures undertaken to eliminate a source of infection, control ongoing contamination, and restore premorbid anatomy and function" [36]. In order to optimize outcomes, controlling the source of bacterial contamination and the removal of infectious foci should be performed in a timely fashion [37]. Ideally, the patient should be medically optimized before source control measures; necessary medical treatment may include fluid resuscitation, establishment of adequate intravenous access, transfusion of blood products, and optimization of coagulation. However, adequate source control should not be postponed for lengthy diagnostic or radiologic studies. Depending on the underlying extent of infection, source control measures may include drainage via either the open surgical or percutaneous technique, debridement of infected and necrotic tissue, decompression, diversion, or restoration of anatomy and organ function. Clinical judgment and experience of the intensivist and surgeon are warranted for timely intervention to ensure control of the ongoing cause of infection without causing further harm to the patient.

The ideal treatment approach to surgical infections is thus multimodal. Early adequate antibiotic coverage and source control ensure optimal control over pathogens, while the patient needs to be appropriately resuscitated and nutritionally supported.

PROGNOSIS

Prognosis of surgical infection is dependent on the extent of infection, resulting organ dysfunction, adequacy of source control and antibiotic treatment, and on basic patient factors such as age and immunologic competence. Origin of surgical infection may also influence outcomes; for example, appendiceal perforation as origin of infection has been found to be associated with better outcome when compared with other perforations within the abdomen [15]. Increased knowledge about appropriate resuscitation and improved antibiotic use have also contributed to improving overall mortality rates [38]. Surgical infections in an intensive care setting remain a challenge, but timely diagnosis and appropriate management will minimize complications and enhance rates of survival.

References

1. Moss M: Epidemiology of sepsis: race, sex, and chronic alcohol abuse. *Clin Infect Dis* 41[Suppl 7]:S490–S497, 2005.
2. Dohmen PM: Influence of skin flora and preventive measures on surgical site infection during cardiac surgery. *Surg Infect (Larchmt)* 7[Suppl 1]:13–17, 2006.
3. Friedrich AK, Cahan M: Intraabdominal infections in the intensive care unit. *J Intensive Care Med* 5:S247–S254, 2014.
4. Mangram AJ, Horan TC, Pearson ML, et al: Guideline for prevention of surgical site infection, 1999. Hospital Infection Control Practice Advisory Committee. *Infect Control Hosp Epidemiol* 20:247–278, 1999.
5. Cheadle WG: Risk factors for surgical site infection. *Surg Infect (Larchmt)* 7[Suppl 1]:S7–S11, 2006.
6. Barras JP, Gilg M, Regli B, et al: Secondary peritonitis after negative computerized tomography in blunt abdominal trauma. *Helv Chir Acta* 60(4):S513–S516, 1994.
7. de Ruiter J, Weel J, Manusama E, et al: The epidemiology of intra-abdominal flora in critically ill patients with secondary and tertiary abdominal sepsis. *Infection* 37(6):522–527, 2009.
8. Sheer TA, Runyon BA: Spontaneous bacterial peritonitis. *Dig Dis* 23(1):39–46, 2005.
9. Wiest R, Krag A, Gerbes A: Spontaneous bacterial peritonitis: recent guidelines and beyond. *Gut* 61(2):297–310, 2012.
10. Elkassem S, Dixon E, Conly J, et al: Primary peritonitis in a young healthy woman: an unusual case. *Can J Surg* 51(2):E40–E41, 2008.
11. Park JY, Moon SY, Son JS, et al: Unusual primary peritonitis due to Streptococcus pyogenes in a young healthy woman. *J Korean Med Sci* 27(5):553–555, 2012.
12. Saha P, Morewood T, Naftalin J, et al: Acute abdomen in a healthy woman: primary peritonitis due to group A streptococcus. *J Obstet Gynaecol* 26(7):700–701, 2006.
13. Hynninen M, Wennervirta J, Leppäniemi A, et al: Organ dysfunction and long term outcome in secondary peritonitis. *Langenbecks Arch Surg* 393(1):81–86, 2008.
14. Riché FC, Dray X, Laisné MJ, et al: Factors associated with septic shock and mortality in generalized peritonitis: comparison between community-acquired and postoperative peritonitis. *Crit Care* 13(3):R99, 2009.
15. Gauzit R, Péan Y, Barth X, et al: Epidemiology, management, and prognosis of secondary non-postoperative peritonitis: a French prospective observational multicenter study. *Surg Infect (Larchmt)* 10(2):119–127, 2009.
16. Berger D, Buttenschoen K: Management of abdominal sepsis. *Langenbecks Arch Surg* 383(1):35–43, 1998.
17. van Till JW, van Veen SQ, van Ruler O, et al: The innate immune response to secondary peritonitis. *Shock* 28(5):504–517, 2007.
18. Malangoni MA: Evaluation and management of tertiary peritonitis. *Am Surg* 66(2):157–161, 2000.
19. Weiss G, Meyer F, Lippert H: Infectiological diagnostic problems in tertiary peritonitis. *Langenbecks Arch Surg* 391(5):473–482, 2006.
20. Buijk SE, Bruining HA: Future directions in the management of tertiary peritonitis. *Intensive Care Med* 28(8):1024–1029, 2002.
21. Chromik AM, Meiser A, Hölling J, et al: Identification of patients at risk for development of tertiary peritonitis on a surgical intensive care unit. *J Gastrointest Surg* 13(7):1358–1367, 2009.
22. Nathens AB, Rotstein OD, Marshall JC: Tertiary peritonitis: clinical features of a complex nosocomial infection. *World J Surg* 22(2):158–163, 1998.
23. Evans HL, Raymond DP, Pelletier SJ, et al: Tertiary peritonitis (recurrent diffuse or localized disease) is not an independent predictor of mortality in surgical patients with intraabdominal infection. *Surg Infect (Larchmt)* 2(4):255–263; discussion 264–265, 2001.
24. De Waele JJ, Hoste EA, Blot SI: Blood stream infections of abdominal origin in the intensive care unit: characteristics and determinants of death. *Surg Infect (Larchmt)* 9(2):171–177, 2008.
25. Montravers P, Gauzit R, Muller C, et al: Emergence of antibiotic-resistant bacteria in cases of peritonitis after intraabdominal surgery affects the efficacy of empirical antimicrobial therapy. *Clin Infect Dis* 23(3):486–494, 1996.
26. Sitges-Serra A, Lopez MJ, Girvent M, et al: Postoperative enterococcal infection after treatment of complicated intra-abdominal sepsis. *Br J Surg* 89(3):361–367, 2002.
27. Swenson BR, Metzger R, Hedrick TL, et al: Choosing antibiotics for intra-abdominal infections: what do we mean by high-risk? *Surg Infect (Larchmt)* 10(1):29–39, 2009.
28. Kaffarnik MF, Urban M, Hopt UT, et al: Impact of enterococcus on immunocompetent and immunosuppressed patients with perforation of the small or large bowel. *Technol Health Care* 20(1):37–48, 2012.
29. Panhofer P, Izay B, Riedl M, et al: Age, microbiology and prognostic scores help to differentiate between secondary and tertiary peritonitis. *Langenbecks Arch Surg* 394(2):265–271, 2009.
30. Hughes MG, Chong TW, Smith RL, et al: Comparison of fungal and nonfungal infections in a broadbased surgical patient population. *Surg Infect (Larchmt)* 6(1):55–64, 2005.
31. Bassetti M, Right E, Ansaldi T, et al: A multicenter multinational study of abdominal candidiasis: epidemiology, outcomes and predictors of mortality. *Intensive Care Med* 41(9):1601–1610, 2015.
32. Sandven P, Qvist H, Skovlund E, et al: Significance of Candida recovered from intraoperative specimens in patients with intra-abdominal perforations. *Crit Care Med* 30(3):541–547, 2002.
33. Rau BM, Frigerio I, Büchler MW, et al: Evaluation of procalcitonin for predicting septic multiorgan failure and overall prognosis in secondary peritonitis: a prospective, international multicenter study. *Arch Surg* 142(2):134–142, 2007.
34. Herzog T, Chromik AM, Uhl W: Treatment of complicated intraabdominal infections in the era of multi-drug resistant bacteria. *Eur J Med Res* 15(12):525–532, 2010.
35. Augustin P, Kermarrec N, Muller-Serieys C, et al: Risk factors for multidrug resistant bacteria and optimization of empirical antibiotic therapy in postoperative peritonitis. *Crit Care* 14(1):R20, 2010.
36. Schein M, Marshall J: Source control for surgical infections. *World J Surg* 28(7):638–645, 2004.
37. De Waele JJ: Early source control in sepsis. *Langenbecks Arch Surg* 395(5):489–494, 2010.
38. Schneider CP, Seyboth C, Vilsmaier M, et al: Prognostic factors in critically ill patients suffering from secondary peritonitis: a retrospective, observational, survival time analysis. *World J Surg* 33(1):34–43, 2009.

Chapter 49 ■ Care of the Patient with Necrotizing Fasciitis

BRANDON COLVIN • BENKOLE SAMUEL • HONGYI CUI

INTRODUCTION

Necrotizing fasciitis (NF) originates from the Greek word *nekroun,* to make dead and from the Latin word *fascis* meaning bundle. NF is an aggressive disease commonly known as a condition involving flesh-eating bacteria. NF is on the broader spectrum of necrotizing soft tissue infections (NSTI) which all share common signs, symptoms, etiologies, pathophysiology, and treatments. All NSTI occur in the soft tissue compartment from the dermis down to and including the muscular layer. NF specifically spreads along the fascial planes at an aggressive rate. In addition, administration of antibiotics alone does not cure this disease making it a true surgical emergency. Mortality increases significantly if wide surgical debridement is delayed, thereby placing high importance on accurate and rapid diagnosis of this devastating disease.

NF has been identified for over two millennia; the first account is ascribed to Hippocrates. Hippocrates referred to a case of complicated erysipelas disease *ca.* 500 BCE, and the specific disease manifestations he described were similar to current descriptions of NF. In the 1700s, the chief surgeon at a hospital in France, Claude Colles, described a condition that he had seen that was consistent with NF. It was not until the American Civil War when Joseph Jones, a confederate physician whose notes are one of the mainstays of medical documentation of this war, identified an organism, specifically a bacillus, as the cause of multiple cases of gangrene. After the war, Jones published documentation of over 2,600 cases of gangrene. Weaponry and physical site (e.g., farmland) of battle were thought to have contributed to numerous accounts of gas gangrene, which led to one of the largest contemporaneous retrospective studies on gas gangrene. In his paper, he gave the first description of what we currently call NF, with a mortality rate nearing 50%. A variant of NF is Fournier gangrene and is attributed to Jean Alfred Fournier, a French dermatologist. Fournier gangrene is NF of the perianal, perineal, or genital area, which will be discussed later. He documented five cases of tissue necrosis of the perineum in the 1880s. NF became known as Meleney gangrene after Dr. Frank L Meleney discovered an association with the disease and β-hemolytic Streptococcus in the 1920s. In the 1950s, Dr. Ben Wilson coined the term NF as a more appropriate term [6].

Throughout history, despite our advances in medicine, mortality rates remain high in NSTI: reports range in the literature from 25% to 60%. One of the contributing factors to this high mortality rate is the non-specificity of symptoms. This non-specificity can make early diagnosis difficult and delay lifesaving surgical intervention, emphasizing the importance of accurate and early diagnosis. Many approaches have been developed to predict the risk of an infection truly being NF. The most commonly utilized is the LRINF (Laboratory Risk Indicator for Necrotizing Fasciitis) score described by Wong [1–6].

EPIDEMIOLOGY AND RISK FACTORS

The number of cases of adult NSTI in the United States ranges from 500 to 1,500 annually with an incidence rate 0.04/1,000 person-years [1,7,8].

Comorbidities are a major risk factor for the development of NF; one study showed that greater than 80% of patients had preexisting medical conditions. The most common risk factors include diabetes mellitus, age greater than 50, obesity, malnutrition, chronic renal disease, chronic liver disease, human immunodeficiency virus, immunosuppression, hypertension, peripheral vascular disease, cancer, pulmonary disease, and intravenous drug abuse (IVDA). Some studies even suggest use of nonsteroidal antiinflammatory drugs as a risk factor [9].

The literature has repeatedly demonstrated that delayed surgical intervention, generally considered greater than 24 hours after diagnosis, is the main risk factor for mortality. Other significant mortality factors recognized are *Clostridium* spp. infection, development of sepsis, chronic renal disease, cardiac or pulmonary disease, IVDA, and malignancy [1,9–11].

ETIOLOGIES

Most cases of NF are associated with a particular trauma or inciting event, allowing the pathogen to be inoculated through a break in the epidermal or mucosal surfaces into the subcutaneous tissue. NF is most commonly reported in the lower extremities, perineum, and the genitalia but can occur anywhere on the body. Documented sources of NF include skin infections (abscess), trauma, infected foot ulcers, surgical wound, perforated viscus, animal and insect bites, needle sticks (IVDA or subcutaneous insulin injection), percutaneous procedures, infected grafts, pressure ulcers (sacral decubitus ulcers), burns, or incarcerated hernias. While most cases of NF are trauma related, anywhere from 15% to 52% are idiopathic [1,2,4,6,9,10,12,13].

PATHOPHYSIOLOGY

Layers of skin from superficial to deep are epidermis, dermis, subcutaneous layer (hypodermis or superficial fascia), and deep fascia. The superficial fascial layer is termed dartos fascia in the genitalia, which is a continuance of the Colles fascia in the perineum, and the Scarpa fascia of the abdominal wall.

The disease course is similar regardless of the etiology or location. Once the pathogen has been inoculated into the subcutaneous tissue, it begins to replicate. The severity of infection is also determined by other factors including the size of the inoculum, virulence of the pathogen, blood flow to the tissue, presence of foreign bodies, as well as host response. Pathogens that are more virulent, if polymicrobial, work synergistically allowing for rapid reproduction in an anaerobic environment. Enzymes begin to necrose the hypodermis and cause vascular thrombosis of the nutrient vessels located in the hypodermis, leading to ischemia and edema (Fig. 49.1). Ischemia of the nerves causes hypoesthesia, anesthesia, and hyperesthesia (pain out of proportion to physical examination). Crepitus on physical examination and subcutaneous air seen on imaging is caused by the gas-forming anaerobic pathogens. The hypodermis is more likely to develop necrosis leading to the expected later finding of overlying epidermal and dermal changes, once the cutaneous circulation has thrombosed. This leads to erythema, edema, both serous and hemorrhagic bullae, and frank necrosis [1,2,7–9].

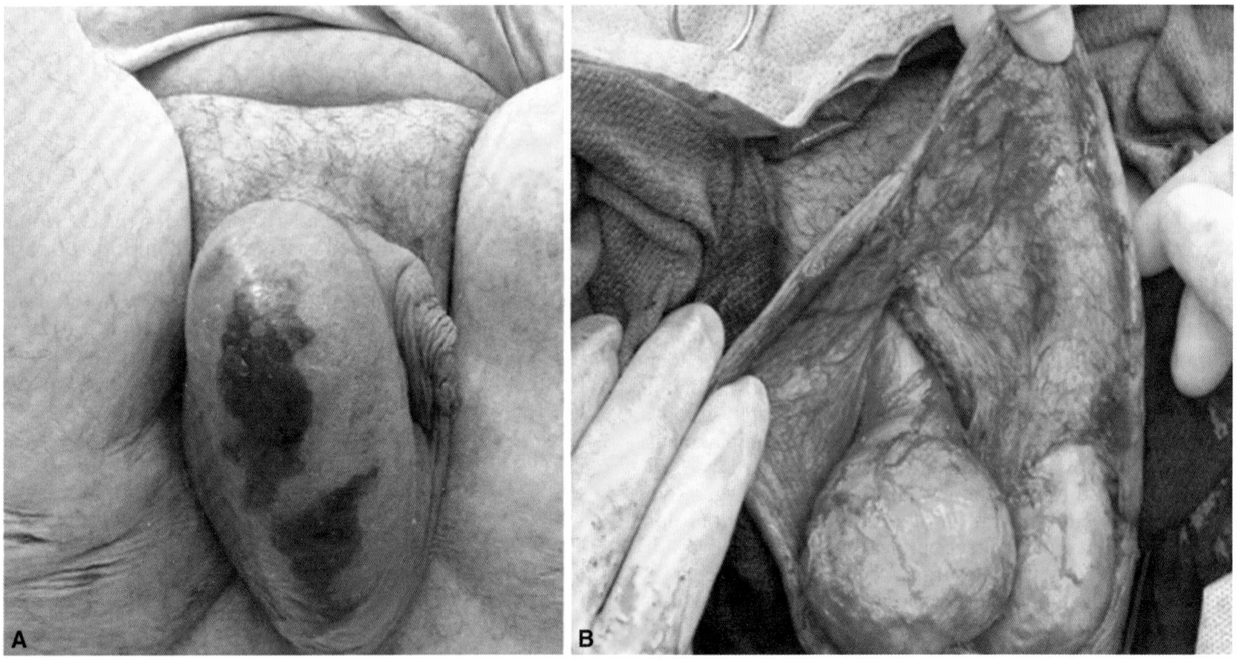

FIGURE 49.1 **A:** Patient with left lower extremity tissue necrosis, erythema, and edema consistent with necrotizing fasciitis. **B:** The same patient after wide surgical debridement.

CLASSIFICATIONS

Originally two types of NF were proposed. However, due to increased research and documentation, that classification has been expanded to a third and fourth type of NF as described by Misiakos et al. [8] These classifications are based on the bacteria as well as the number of bacteria causing NF. These classifications are also important for directing treatment which will be discussed in a later section.

Type I: Polymicrobial

This is by far the most common type of NF, accounting for upward of 70% of NF. Type I is generally seen in the elderly population and those with multiple comorbidities. Most of these infections are located in the trunk or perineum. At least two pathogens are detected in the surgical specimen culture, with an average of over four species identified. In historical terms, *Clostridium* spp. played a large role in type I NF. In more recent years, the incidence of *Clostridium* has declined significantly and is rare. This is thought to be due to improved sanitation, hygiene, and sterilization techniques. *Clostridium* is commonly found in soil in endemic areas of the United States and the world with rates around 10%. For further discussion of *Clostridium*, please refer to our discussion below of type 3 NF [1–3,7–9,13].

Fournier gangrene (Fig. 49.2) is considered a subtype of type I NF because it is a polymicrobial infection. Fournier was first described as a necrotizing infection of the penis and scrotum. Today's definition is a little broader, and now includes the genitalia of both male and females, perineal, and perianal areas. Particular considerations with this type of NF are that Scarpa fascia is continuous with Colles fascia and dartos fascia. This allows for the disease to spread easily from the groin superiorly

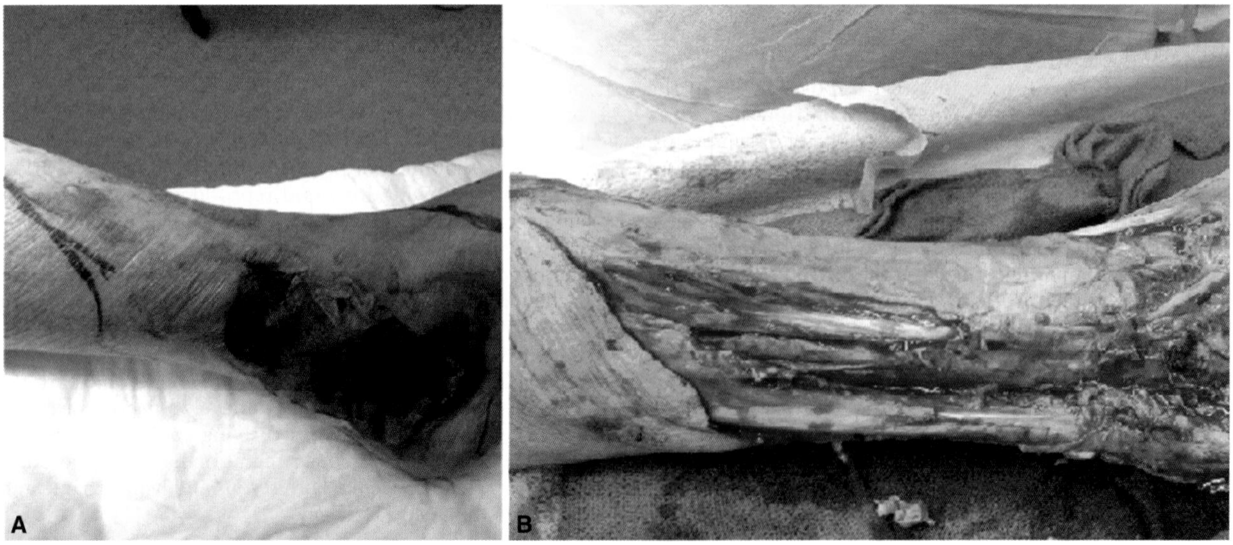

FIGURE 49.2 **A:** Neutrophils infiltrating the subcuatenous tissues **B:** Coagulation necrosis that can be seen in necrotizing fasciitis (NF).

to the anterior abdominal wall, making control of this disease more difficult [1–3,7–9,13–15].

Type II: Monomicrobial Gram Positive (β-hemolytic Streptococcus A alone or with MSSA or MRSA)

Group-A β-hemolytic streptococcus (gram-positive catalase-negative cocci in pairs or chains), also referred to as GAS, is the hallmark of type II NF. It can either occur by itself or in conjunction with *Staphylococcus aureus* (gram-positive cocci catalase-positive in clusters), and both methicillin sensitive (MSSA) and methicillin resistant (MRSA). GAS (*Streptococcus pyogenes*) has evolved to include several mechanisms to increase its toxicity; most importantly for the discussion of pathophysiology is the M protein. The M protein allows GAS to bind and activate T-cell receptors in a much larger number than would normally be activated. This causes an extremely large inflammatory response, by releasing inflammatory cytokines including interleukin-1, interleukin-6, and tumor necrosis factor-α. The M protein also leads to decreased phagocytosis by neutrophils. In addition, GAS has exotoxins that lead to neutrophil damage, decreased phagocytosis, and breakdown of connective tissue. Panton–Valentine leukocidin gene is a virulent factor seen with some *S. aureus* that is currently being studied and is thought to contribute to the severity of disease as well as resistance to certain antibiotic therapies [4]. With *Staphylococcus* spp., infection can lead to toxic shock syndrome, both by tissue necrosis and leukocyte destruction. This type of NF is more common in the extremities in young healthy patients and is commonly caused by trauma such as surgery and IVDA. Mortality rates of types I and II are comparable [2,8,9].

Type III: Monomicrobial Infection Caused by Clostridium or Gram-Negative Bacteria

Overall, type III NF is comparatively rare. The most common pathogen of type III is *Clostridium* spp. (gram-positive anaerobic spore-forming bacilli), with the most commonly isolated organism being *Clostridium perfringens*. This pathogen is associated with obstetrical and intestinal surgery, significant trauma, and IVDA. Other strains of *Clostridium* that have been implicated include *C. septicum* in patients with certain types of cancer without a traumatic injury and *C. sordellii* in subcutaneous injections of a particular type of heroin. *Clostridium* species are thought to produce two main toxins responsible for their virulence: α and θ toxins. α toxin causes damage locally by impairing neutrophil function, platelet function, and diapedesis. θ toxin damage is systemically active and is thought to cause hemolysis, decreased systemic vascular resistance through decreasing peripheral tone, and impaired phagocytosis. Gram-negative bacteria include both *Vibrio* spp. and *Aeromonas* spp. *Vibrio vulnificus* (gram-negative motile bacilli) are the most common *Vibrio* spp. seen in NF and are normally found with upper extremity trauma in patients with hepatic, renal, or adrenal failure. These bacteria are observed in warmer marine water, hence an increase in incidence during the summer months. *Aeromonas hydrophila* and *A. veronii* bv. sobria (gram-negative rod or bacilli) are also aquatic, usually fresh or brackish water, but can also be normal flora in human. Usually infection with *Aeromonas* spp. leads to gastroenteritis but it can also cause NF [1,8,9,15,16].

Type IV: Fungal

This type is very unusual, but is often seen in immunocompromised patients with a traumatic inoculation. Type IV NF has a very rapid course that is often attributed to the comorbidities of this patient population. Fungi seen are usually *Candida* species, more specifically *C. parapsilosis* [17], *C. albicans* [18], and *C. tropicalis* [14], as well as *Zygomycetes* [8].

SIGNS AND SYMPTOMS

Physical examination is of utmost importance for patients with NF. Attention to detail, especially with change or worsening conditions within a short time period, is extremely important. Pertinent signs and symptoms are listed below. These are not specific to NF but can be suggestive of this disease.

Symptoms

- Pain out of proportion to exam
- Nausea and vomiting
- Diarrhea
- Chills

Signs

- Skin erythema, which is common in many skin conditions and is more sensitive than specific (Fig. 49.3)
- Skin discoloration, necrosis
- Bullae or blistering

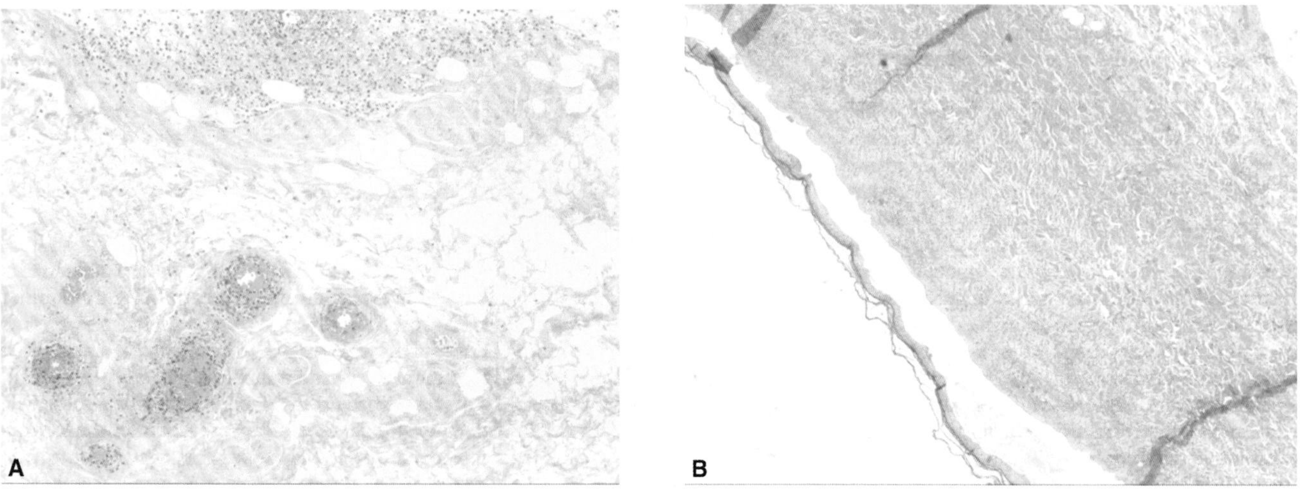

FIGURE 49.3 **A:** A case of scrotal necrotizing fasciitis (Fournier gangrene), requiring extensive wide debridement of affected tissue (**B**). Cultures demonstrated a polymicrobial infection.

- Warm to palpation
- Crepitus (more common with Clostridium or other gas-forming bacteria)
- Wound discharge, classically dishwater in character but can vary
- Induration, edema
- Laboratory anomalies (which will be discussed later)
- Fever
- Tachycardia
- Mental status changes

As the disease progresses, patients develop systemic inflammatory response syndrome (SIRS). SIRS criteria include heart rate greater than 90, white blood cell count $\leq$4,000, $\geq$12,000, or bands $\geq$10%, temperature greater than 38 or less than 36°C, respiratory rate greater than 20 breaths per minute or $PaCO_2$ less than 32. Despite adequate treatment, a number of patients develop septic shock with multiorgan dysfunction syndrome.

DIAGNOSTICS

Once again, physical examination is most important for the diagnosis of NF. The aforementioned symptoms can be detected on examination but there are other tools to assist in making the diagnosis.

Microbiology

Drainage from the wound can be sent for gram stain and culture. The culture takes 24 to 72 hours to identify the pathogen, but if gram stain is positive for gram-positive cocci or bacilli, this will aid in making the diagnosis, especially in conjunction with other signs and symptoms exhibited by the patient.

Surgical Biopsy

This can be done at the bedside or in the operating room if clinical suspicion is high. The main objective is to evaluate the fascia. Discoloration and peeling of unhealthy fascia is pathognomonic for NF. Surgery is the only definitive method of diagnosis for NF. This is the only way to truly evaluate fascial involvement.

X-rays

This may show air within subcutaneous tissue and musculature with edema (Fig. 49.4). Radiography tends to be more useful with *Clostridium* or gas-forming bacterium due to the subcutaneous emphysema.

Commuted Tomography (CT) Scan

CT scans can be helpful in making a diagnosis, especially with patient history and an examination. Stranding on CT is suggestive of inflammation. Air within fascial planes can also be better visualized on CT scans than X-rays.

Magnetic Resonance Imaging

This can also be useful in making the diagnosis, and is the most sensitive imaging. However, CT scan is often more efficient. If the diagnosis is still uncertain, including both laboratory values and physical examination, a CT scan can be obtained, saving both cost and time compared to magnetic resonance imaging (MRI).

Ultrasound

There is some evidence showing efficacy with the use of ultrasound in NF. A retrospective study evaluating the role of ultrasound in proven cases of NF revealed changes in muscle, fascia, and fat that would support evidence of an infection, but are nonspecific and are user dependent [19].

Despite the availability of these diagnostic modalities, it is still difficult to definitely differentiate NF from other soft tissue infections. In 2004, there was a retrospective study published

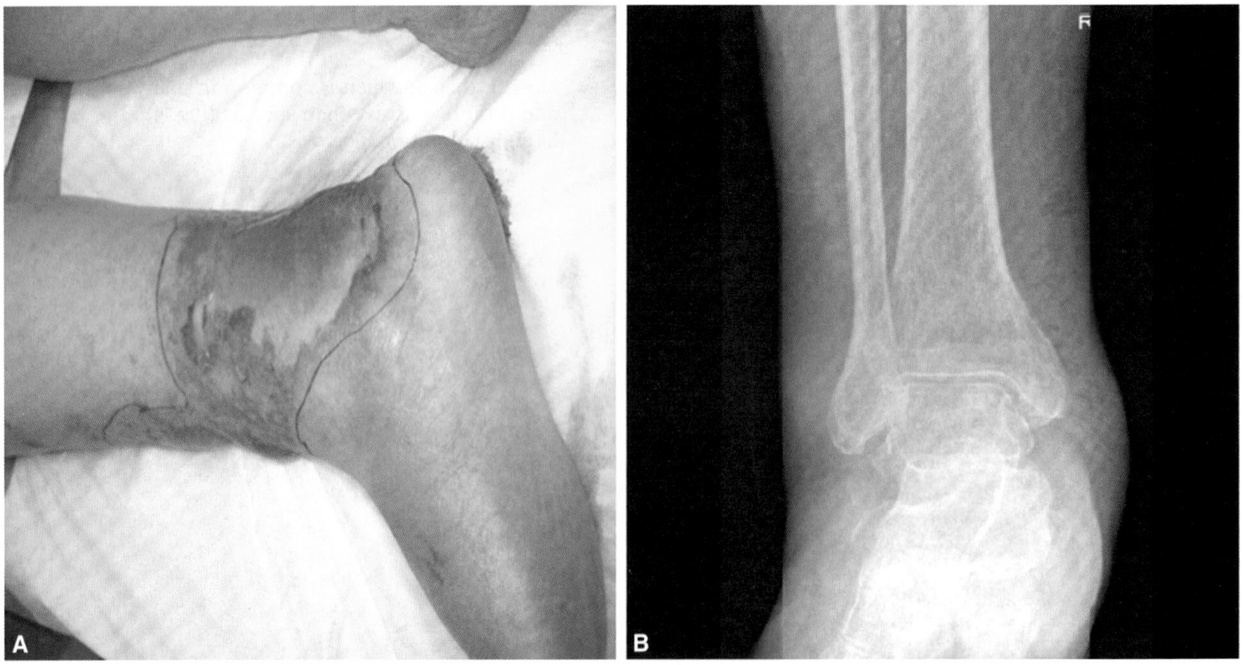

FIGURE 49.4 **A:** The patient is an 80-year-old diabetic immunosuppressed male with right ankle/foot erythema, ecchymosis, bullae, discharge, and edema. **B:** X-ray of the ankle shows soft tissue swelling and gas. Serous discharge was sent for gram stain, and culture demonstrated a polymicrobial infection. He was diagnosed with necrotizing fasciitis (NF) [15].

in the *Journal of Critical Care Medicine* on the subject of NF. The goal was to establish criteria to help differentiate NF from other soft tissue infections with a certain degree of reliability. A scoring system was developed that was very suggestive of NF if the patient scored above 6. However, about 10% of patients with scores below 6 were also found to have NF. Components of the laboratory risk factors are listed in Table 49.1. Laboratory values such as basic metabolic panel and complete blood count are routinely obtained in patients presenting to the emergency department. The C-reactive protein level is the only additional value that is required for the calculation [6].

LABORATORIES

Delay in diagnosis and time to the operating room increase mortality in patients with NF, as well as the lack of a fast and accurate imaging modality. Scoring scales based upon signs to help clinicians diagnose NF earlier have also been developed. The currently accepted scoring system is the LRINF.

TREATMENT

Surgery

The main goal when treating NF is removal of the involved tissues. Wide surgical excision is the mainstay of therapy. Patients usually require multiple returns to the operating room to evaluate the wound and to ensure all involved tissue is excised. Wounds may be left open and allowed to heal by secondary intention. Often multiple wet to dry dressing changes are required to adequately debride the tissue. Iodine, Dakin solution, as well as other chemicals can be added to the early wet to dry dressings to help decrease the bacterial load in the wound. Patients may ultimately require skin grafts if the area of debridement is extensive (Fig. 49.5).

TABLE 49.1

The Currently Accepted Scoring System, the LRINF [6]

Variable, Units	β	Score
C-reactive protein, mg/L		
<150	0	0
≥150	3.5	4
Total white cell count, per mm^3		
<15	0	0
15–25	0.5	1
>25	2.1	2
Hemoglobin, g/dL		
>13.5	0	0
11–13.5	0.6	1
<11	1.8	2
Sodium, mmol/L		
≥135	0	0
<135	1.8	2
Creatinine, μmol/L		
≤141	0	0
>141	1.8	2
Glucose, mmol/L		
≤10	0	0
>10	1.2	1

Final model constructed using factors found to be independently predictive of necrotizing fasciitis (NF) on multivariate analysis. β values are the regression coefficients of our model after adjusting for a shrinkage factor of .89. The maximum score is 13: a score of ≥6 should raise the suspicion of NF and a score of ≥8 is strongly predictive of this disease. To convert the values of glucose to mg per dL, multiply by 18.015. To convert the values of creatinine to mg per dL, multiply by 0.01131.

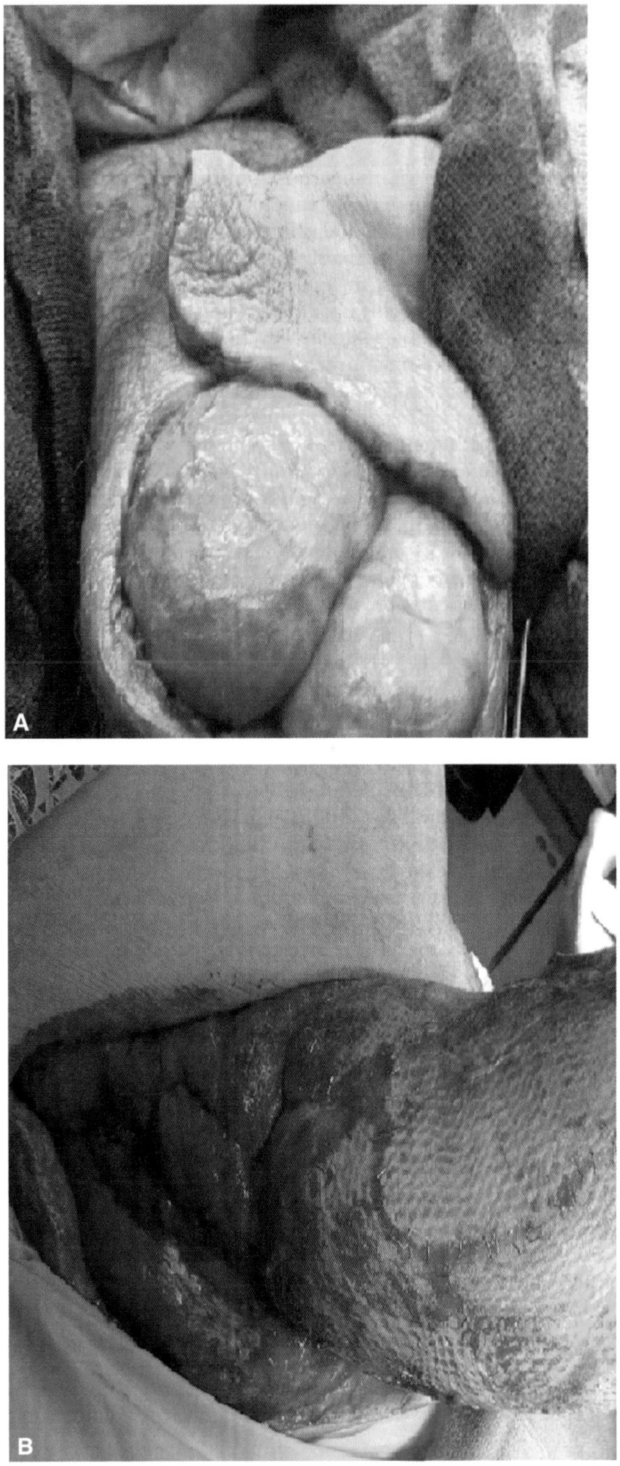

FIGURE 49.5 **A:** The patient who was previously discussed with Fournier gangrene after surgical debridement of the scrotum. **B:** The application of a split thickness skin graft to cover part of a large defect.

Antibiotics

Once diagnosis is made, antibiotics are started to help control the spread of the infection. Since the bacteria commonly found in this disease are gram-positive cocci, rods or anaerobes, broad-spectrum antibiotic coverage should be started initially. Once surgical cultures have resulted, the type of NF can be identified and antibiotic therapy can be targeted. The recommended regimen consists of a β-lactam inhibitor +/− β-lactamase inhibitor (penicillin, pipercillin/tazobactam), anaerobic coverage with clindamycin/metronidazole, and MRSA coverage with vancomycin. Other studies recommend use of meropenem plus clindamycin or ciprofloxacin, or clindamycin and metronidazole combination for broad-spectrum coverage. Clindamycin is also used frequently because it has been shown to decrease the release of *Clostridium* α-toxin as well as the *Streptococcal* M protein [9,13,20].

Intravenous Immune Globulin (IVIG)

The use of IVIG for NF is supported by some case reports and mainly as an adjunct in cases of GAS infections. It is not a widely accepted option for treatment and requires more research to evaluate its efficacy [9,21].

Hyperbaric Oxygen Therapy

The role of hyperbaric oxygen in NF appears to be as an adjunct. Some retrospective studies have shown an additional benefit in patients treated primarily with surgical debridement and antibiotics. At the current time, there is no randomized prospective trial evaluating the benefit of hyperbaric oxygen in these patients. Use of hyperbaric oxygen still remains controversial [9].

Negative Pressure Wound Therapy

Negative pressure wound therapy (NPWT) has become more popular for the treatment of large wounds. In cases of NF, NPWT is placed after surgical debridement has taken place. It has been shown that NPWT decreases cost of therapy in the long term and decreases time to complete wound healing [22]. More recently, there are case reports of adding a pure hypochlorous acid solution 0.01% (NeutroPhase, NovaBay Pharmaceuticals Inc, Emeryville, CA) for the treatment of NF. Hypochlorous acid inactivates *S. aureus* and *S. pyogenes* toxins [14]. Silver is another adjunct to NPWT described by Pour et al. in a case report that decreased hospital length of stay. Silver is thought to be antimicrobial by disabling growth enzymes [23].

CONCLUSIONS

NF is a true surgical emergency. The earlier diagnosis and intervention occur, the better the potential outcome for the patient. Surgery, which involves excision of all involved tissue, is the only known cure for all types of NF that have been discussed (types I-IV and Fournier). Antibiotics, IVIG, and other adjuncts can aid in the treatment. The difficulty is in early recognition and diagnosis. Retrospective studies have shown mortality to be between 25% and 60% [6,13]. Many factors are involved in predicting mortality, including time of diagnosis, time to surgery, patient's comorbidities and operative risk, and level of illness (SIRS, severe sepsis, septic shock, etc.). NF can easily be confused with other soft tissue infections but a good physical examination, attention to details, and potential use of imaging studies is the preferred approach for making the diagnosis.

References

1. Gamelli RL, Posluszny JA: Necrotizing soft tissue infections, in Irwin R, Rippe J (eds): *Irwin and Rippe's Intensive Care Medicine*. 7th ed. Philadelphia: Lippincott Williams & Wilkins, 2011, pp 1619–1626.
2. Lancerotto L, Tocco I, Salmaso R, et al: Necrotizing fasciitis: classification, diagnosis, and management. *J Trauma Acute Care Surg* 72(3):560–566, 2012.
3. McHenry CR, Piotrowski JJ, Petrinic D, et al: Determinants of mortality for necrotizing soft-tissue infections. *Ann Surg* 221(5):558–563; discussion 563–565, 1995.
4. Su YC, Chen HW, Hong YC, et al: Laboratory risk indicator for necrotizing fasciitis score and the outcomes. *ANZ J Surg* 78(11):968–972, 2008.
5. Taviloglu K, Yanar H: Necrotizing fasciitis: strategies for diagnosis and management. *World J Emerg Surg* 2:19, 2007.
6. Wong, CH, Khin LW, Heng KS, et al: The LRINEC (Laboratory Risk Indicator for Necrotizing Fasciitis) score: a tool for distinguishing necrotizing fasciitis from other soft tissue infections. *Crit Care Med* 32(7):1535–1541, 2004.
7. Hussein QA, Anaya DA: Necrotizing soft tissue infections. *Crit Care Clin* 29(4):795–806, 2013.
8. Misiakos EP, Bagias G, Patapis P, et al: Current concepts in the management of necrotizing fasciitis. *Front Surg* 1:36, 2014.
9. Hakkarainen TW, Kopari NM, Pham TN, et al: Necrotizing soft tissue infections: review and current concepts in treatment, systems of care, and outcomes. *Curr Probl Surg* 51(8):344–362, 2014.
10. Goh T, Goh LG, Ang CH, et al: Early diagnosis of necrotizing fasciitis. *Br J Surg* 101(1):e119–e125, 2014.
11. Thapaliya D, O'Brien AM, Wardyn SE, et al: Epidemiology of necrotizing infection caused by Staphylococcus aureus and Streptococcus pyogenes at an Iowa hospital. *J Infection Public Health* 8(6):634–641, 2015.
12. Khamnuan P, Chongruksut W, Jearwattanakanok K, et al: Necrotizing fasciitis: risk factors of mortality. *Risk Manag Healthc Policy* 8:1–7, 2015.
13. Machado NO: Necrotizing fasciitis: the importance of early diagnosis, prompt surgical debridement and adjuvant therapy. *North Am J Med Sci* 3:107–118, 2011.
14. Crew JR, Varilla R, Allandale Rocas Iii T, et al: Treatment of acute necrotizing fasciitis using negative pressure wound therapy and adjunctive neutrophase irrigation under the foam. *Wounds* 25(10):272–277, 2013.
15. Cui H, Hao S, Arous E: A distinct cause of necrotizing fasciitis: aeromonas veronii biovar sobria. *Surg Infect* 8(5):523–528, 2007.
16. Kuo YL, Shieh SJ, Chiu HY, et al: Necrotizing fasciitis caused by vibrio vulnificus: epidemiology, clinical findings, treatment and prevention. *Eur J Clin Microbiol Infect Dis* 26(11):785–792, 2007.
17. Zhang M, Chelnis J, Mawn LA: Periorbital necrotizing fasciitis secondary to candida parapsilosis and streptococcus pyogenes. *Ophthal Plast Reconstr Surg*, 2015. doi:10.1097/IOP.0000000000000476.
18. Chandawarkar RY, Jessie TA, Pennington GA, et al: Necrotizing fasciitis: diagnosis and management of an occult infective focus. *Can J Plast Surg* 12(3):149–153, 2004.
19. Parenti GC, Marri C, Calandra G, et al: Necrotizing fasciitis of soft tissues: role of diagnostic imaging and review of the literature. *Radiol Med* 99(5):334–339, 2000.
20. Buchanan, PJ, Mast BA, Lottenberg L, et al: Candida albicans necrotizing soft tissue infection: a case report and literature review of fungal necrotizing soft tissue infections. *Ann Plast Surg* 70(6):739–741, 2013.
21. Yong, JM: Rationale for the use of intravenous immunoglobulin in streptococcal necrotizing fasciitis. *Clin Immunother* 4(1):61–71, 1995.
22. Ye J, Xie T, Wu M, et al: Negative pressure wound therapy applied before and after split-thickness skin graft helps healing of Fournier Gangrene: a case report (CARE-Compliant). *Medicine* 94(5):e426, 2015.
23. Pour SM: Use of negative pressure wound therapy with silver base dressing for necrotizing fasciitis. *J Wound Ostomy Continence Nurs* 38(4):449–452, 2011.
24. Antimicrobial guidelines: Necrotizing fasciitis including Fournier's. East Kent Hospital University, NHS.Web. Available at: http://www.ekhuft.nhs.uk/staff/clinical/antimicrobial-guidelines/skin-and-soft-tissue-guidelines/necrotising-fasciitis/. Updated January 29, 2015.
25. Majeski J, Majeski E: Necrotizing fasciitis: improved survival with early recognition by tissue biopsy and aggressive surgical treatment. *South Med J* 90(11):1065–1068, 1997.
26. Morgan, MS: Diagnosis and management of necrotising fasciitis: a multiparametric approach. *J Hosp Infect* 75(4):249–157, 2010.

Chapter 50 ■ The ICU Management of Patients Undergoing Major Surgery for Gastrointestinal Cancers

KATE H. DINH • JENNIFER LAFEMINA

Major surgical procedures are now routine. However, high-risk, noncardiac populations, including those who are at high risk due to the presence of cancer, are a subgroup that requires special consideration. This chapter highlights operations for common gastrointestinal (GI) cancer requiring perioperative intensive care. As morbidity and mortality after major oncologic surgery for cancer can be substantial, herein we focus on the complications specific to these operations, which can have significant implications on perioperative management and outcomes.

PANCREATIC RESECTION

Pancreatic cancer is currently the fourth leading cause of cancer death in the United States; incidence and mortality rates are currently increasing. While survival remains dismal with little improvement in recent decades, surgical resection currently offers the best option for long-term survival and cure. The type of resection is largely dependent upon tumor characteristics such as size, location, and vascular involvement. Common standard segmental resections for pancreatic cancer include pancreaticoduodenectomy (PD; also known as the Whipple procedure) and distal pancreatectomy (DP). Total pancreatectomy for neoplastic purposes may be considered for selected cases, particularly in the setting of main duct intraductal papillary mucinous neoplasm.

Perioperative management remains largely surgeon- and institution-dependent. Early ambulation, pulmonary secretion clearance, and pain control (particularly with epidural analgesia) are paramount during the early postoperative period. Following PD, nasogastric decompression may be helpful. Once gastric decompression is discontinued, there is slow advancement of the diet. Attention should be paid to clinical signs of perioperative complications that warrant additional workup and management. Patients are at risk of postoperative diabetes and thromboembolic events and, therefore, generally receive close glucose monitoring and insulin supplementation and venous thromboembolism prevention. Feeding jejunostomies and parenteral nutrition are generally unnecessary unless a complication that would result in nutritional deficiency warrants their use.

Contemporary series of complications following PD report an overall complication rate of 31% to 38% and mortality rate ranging from 1% to 4% [1–7]. The most commonly reported complications include pancreatic fistula, hemorrhage related to pseudoaneurysm, delayed gastric emptying (DGE), and exocrine and endocrine insufficiency. Additional complications include, but are not limited to, wound infections, need for reoperation, other anastomotic leakage (biliary, gastric, or duodenal), cholangitis, pancreatitis, and complications of other organ systems reported with other operations (including deep venous thrombosis, pulmonary embolus, cardiopulmonary complications, cerebral complications including stroke, and urinary tract infection).

This discussion will focus on the common complications specific to pancreatic resection, including pancreatic fistula, hemorrhage related to pseudoaneurysm, DGE, and endocrine and exocrine insufficiency.

Postoperative Pancreatic Fistula

Postoperative pancreatic fistula (POPF; also known as pancreatic leak) remains a difficult management dilemma, which contributes significantly to postoperative morbidity and mortality. Numerous reports have been published exploring the incidence of this complications as well as means by which to prevent and treat this issue. The reported incidence of POPF is highly variable, ranging from 2% to 12% [1–6]. Many groups have proposed definitions based on surgical drain output quantity and quality, but the most commonly adopted terminology arises from the International Study Group on Pancreatic Fistula (ISGPF). This group defines POPF as "failure of healing/sealing of the pancreatic-enteric anastomosis or a parenchymal leak not directly related to the anastomosis" [7]. More specifically, the ISGPF consensus defines POPF as drain fluid output on postoperative day 3 with a fluid amylase level more than three times greater than a concurrent serum amylase value.

Within this system, POPFs are graded A through C based on the degree of severity and impact on the patient's clinical condition and management (Table 50.1). Grade A POPFs are generally short-lived and of little clinical significance. As the patients are clinically well with without signs of infection, these do not result in changes in management. Grade B fistulas are characterized by patients who are generally well, but may have a change in management: alteration in diet (i.e., nothing by mouth), use of parenteral nutrition, use of antibiotics if an infection is present, and/or use of octreotide. A postoperative collection, which preferably is drained via a percutaneous or endoscopic approach, may be identified on imaging and addressed. Grade C POPFs are considered the most severe and are defined by a clinically unwell patient who may be septic. These POPFs require major changes in management, including reoperation and delay in discharge, and may be associated with severe complications including death.

TABLE 50.1

Summary of Postoperative Pancreatic Fistula Grades

Postoperative Pancreatic Fistula Grade	A	B	C
Clinical condition	Well	Often well	Unwell
Management alteration[a]	No	Possible	Yes
Imaging findings	No	Possible	Yes
Prolonged drainage	No	Possible	Yes
Reoperation	No	No	Yes
Mortality	No	No	Possible
Readmission	No	Possible	Possible
Infection/Sepsis	No/No	Yes/No	Yes/Yes

[a]Includes change in diet, use of parenteral nutrition, antibiotics, somatostatin analogs, minimal invasive drainage. Amended from [7].

Conservative management of POPF is the mainstay of treatment. As noted previously, clinically insignificant Grade A POPFs do not require alterations in diet or additional medications. However, for more severe Grade B-C POPFs, bowel/pancreatic rest (i.e., nothing by mouth) and the use of parenteral nutrition (i.e., total parenteral nutrition [TPN]) may be necessary. Routine use of postoperative TPN is generally not necessary and has been associated with a higher risk of major complications [8]. When collections are present, drains (whether placed surgically or postoperatively via a percutaneous approach) allow for control of contamination. Antibiotics should be introduced for signs of infection or sepsis. Reoperation is uncommon, but should be considered in the setting of an unstable patient or in one who fails conservative management.

Extensive reports have discussed, and continue to lead to a debate about, the role of octreotide in the prevention and treatment of POPF [9–14]. Octreotide is a somatostatin analog and inhibits pancreatic secretion. Initial work reported a decrease in the postoperative complication rate, including POPF, with routine octreotide administration. However, two studies performed in the United States evaluated the role of octreotide following PD and failed to demonstrate a significant impact on postoperative complications, including POPF [11,14]. Pasireotide, a somatostatin analog with a longer half-life than octreotide and a broader binding profile, was recently reported to decrease the rate of clinically significant POPF following both PD and DP [15].

Similar to the role of octreotide, there is an extensive body of literature on proposed technical means to decrease the incidence of POPF. It is generally accepted that careful handling of the pancreas and preservation of the blood supply are critical to minimize morbidity. Variations in the technical construction of the pancreatic anastomosis have been explored. Multiple studies, including a recent multicenter randomized controlled trial, have failed to demonstrate that there are differences in the rate of fistula, irrespective of whether a pancreaticojejunostomy or pancreaticogastrostomy is performed [16–19]. Variations in reconstruction, with "binding" techniques, "invagination" techniques, and duct obliteration have been met with different levels of success [20–24] To date, a single method of pancreatic reconstruction has not been accepted as superior to others. At least with DP, there appears to be no difference in POPF or mortality whether the pancreatic stump is hand sewn or stapled [25].

The role of surgically placed drains for the prevention of POPF remains controversial. In a single-institution, prospective, randomized trial, intraoperative drain placement was associated with no overall increase in complications, but placement was associated with a significantly greater incidence of intraabdominal abscesses/collections [26]. The authors evaluated their more recent experience and again demonstrated that operatively placed drains were associated with a longer hospital stay, increased morbidity (including fistula rates), and increased readmission rates [27]. A multicenter, prospective randomized trial recently demonstrated that subjects who did not have routine intraoperative drainage had a higher incidence of gastroparesis, intraabdominal fluid collection and abscess, severe diarrhea, need for additional drainage, and prolonged length of stay [28]. Therefore, whether surgical placed drains should be routinely placed, particularly after PD, remains unclear.

Hemorrhage Related to Pseudoaneurysm

Pseudoaneurysm, particularly pseudoaneurysm of the gastroduodenal artery (GDA) following a PD, is a life-threatening surgical emergency. Patients with GDA pseudoaneurysms most commonly present with abdominal pain, massive GI hemorrhage (presenting as hematemesis, melena, or hematochezia) and hemoperitoneum. Computed tomography (CT) angiogram may confirm the diagnosis, and embolization by interventional radiology can control the hemorrhage. However, if embolization fails or the patient remains unstable, exploration and control of hemorrhage is warranted. It is critically important to have a high level of suspicion for this complication: if recognized and treated expeditiously, mortality is up to 15%. If untreated, mortality approaches 90% [29].

Delayed Gastric Emptying

The definition of DGE is variable. The International Study Group of Pancreatic Surgery (ISGPS) defines DGE as "the inability to return to a standard diet by the end of the first postoperative week" and includes prolonged nasogastric tube (NGT) use [30]. The pathologic mechanisms are poorly understood, though it has been proposed that duodenal resection, remnant duodenal length, disrupted innervation (i.e., the duodenal intestinal pacemaker), changes in motilin levels, and mechanical narrowing at the anastomosis may contribute to DGE. If DGE occurs, it is important to rule out additional etiologies, such as a POPF or collection, which might be contributing. The reported incidence of this common complication, particularly after PD, ranges from 7% to 16% [1–6].

It was thought that the risk of DGE would be decreased with pylorus-preserving pancreaticoduodenectomy (PPPD), compared to a standard PD in which the pylorus is resected en bloc. However, multiple trials have failed to demonstrate a difference in this complication based on the preservation or resection of the pylorus [31–33]. Several studies have, in fact, suggested a higher incidence of DGE after PPPD [30].

Gastric decompression with a NGT is an important component of management, particularly for a vomiting patient who is at risk of aspiration. Motility agents such as metoclopramide and erythromycin are first-line agents. The latter has been shown to significantly reduce the incidence of DGE from 30% to 19% following resection [34]. If DGE is prolonged, enteral nutrition via a nasojejunostomy or gastrostomy tube, or parenteral nutrition should be considered to optimize nutritional status. If a mechanical obstruction is identified, endoscopic dilation should be considered.

Endocrine and Exocrine Pancreatic Insufficiency

The incidence of postpancreatectomy endocrine and exocrine insufficiency has been most commonly reported among studies focusing on the chronic pancreatitis population. The risk for this population is perhaps greater than for the non-pancreatitis (i.e., neoplastic) population as pancreatic resection entails removal of at least some of the little remaining functional parenchyma. The estimated incidence of new onset diabetes following PD ranges from 11% to 54%. The risk of exocrine insufficiency followed PD has been reported as 24% to 78% [35–41]. The reported incidence from a similar population may be as high as 50% for endocrine and exocrine insufficiency, respectively, following DP [42,43]. Postoperative endocrine insufficiency is management with oral hypoglycemic or insulin. Postoperative exocrine insufficiency may be detected by continued postoperative weight loss or steatorrhea, and may be treated with enzyme supplementation.

ESOPHAGEAL RESECTION

Esophageal and gastroesophageal junction (GEJ) cancers remain therapeutic challenges with 5-year survivals of approximately 18% [44]. Due to substantial morbidity and mortality of esophagectomy as well as the large number of patients with advanced disease in whom surgery in unlikely to be curative, there has been an increasing interest in non-surgical options, including endomucosal resection, endoscopic ablation with techniques such as photodynamic therapy, and definitive chemoradiotherapy [45]. However, esophagectomy currently remains the best option for long-term survival and cure in early stage disease and to achieve local control (e.g., reduction in the risk of tracheal or bronchial obstruction) of locally advanced disease.

Common operative approaches include the Ivor Lewis esophagectomy, McKeown esophagectomy, Sweet procedure (left-sided thoracotomy), left thoracoabdominal approach, and the transhiatal esophagectomy. A number of factors determine the operative approach, including tumor location and stage, extent of lymphadenectomy, conduit options (e.g., stomach, colon, and small intestine), patient characteristics, and surgeon preference. There is ongoing debate about a number of issues, including the role of minimally invasive surgery, the extent of lymphadenectomy, and the location of the anastomosis (cervical versus thoracic). A more thorough analysis of these ongoing debates is beyond the scope of this chapter.

Chest physiotherapy, optimization of pain control (for instance with epidural analgesia), early ambulation incentive spirometry, careful fluid management, and early extubation, when possible, are paramount to try to minimize perioperative morbidity. Chest tubes and nasogastric decompression to prevent dilation are commonly employed, the latter to reduce distension which can lead to regurgitation and aspiration. The role of feeding jejunostomy or nasoduodenal tube placement for perioperative enteral feeding is variable among surgeons. Some advocate placement to allow for nutritional optimization, particularly if inadequate or delayed diet advancement is anticipated. While some surgeons will proceed with diet advancement based on the patient's clinical picture, a swallow study with Gastrografin contrast is the gold standard for diagnosis of complications, such as esophageal leak, and may be pursued prior to diet advancement.

Commonly reported complications include those named elsewhere in this chapter (such as cardiopulmonary complications including arrhythmias, pneumonia, and thromboembolic events), but specific to esophagectomy, morbidity can arise from esophageal anastomotic leak, DGE, dumping syndrome, anastomotic stricture, regurgitation and reflux, chylothorax, and hemi-vocal cord dysfunction from damage to the recurrent laryngeal nerve injury.

Esophageal Anastomotic Leak

Series from large volume centers have reported leak rates of approximately 10% [46–49], though an incidence of greater than 30% has been reported for low volume centers [50]. However, differences in operative techniques, such as stapled or hand-sewn anastomosis, have not necessarily shown to reduce this complication rate [51].

Within the first 48 hours of surgery, if a patient develops shock, one must consider hemorrhage or a fulminant leak due to anastomotic necrosis or gangrene. A chest X-ray (CXR) or CT, when patient stability allows, may help differentiate between etiologies and with the latter, localize blood, when present. Exploration is generally indicated for unstable patients. Should the anastomosis be the culprit, anastomotic resection with preservation of maximal esophageal length, cervical esophagostomy, and wide drainage is performed.

More commonly, esophageal leaks may be incidentally detected on radiologic studies (such as the planned Gastrografin swallow) or may be clinically apparent about a week after surgery. One should suspect an esophageal leak in a patient with fevers, tachycardia, tachypnea, shortness of breath, and shoulder pain. In the setting of a cervical anastomosis, neck pain or cellulitis may be present. The diagnosis may be confirmed on Gastrografin swallow or CT of the chest and/or neck with oral contrast, which may show a pleural effusion or pooling of oral contrast. If a chest tube is in place, drainage may be foul-smelling or turbid.

If the patient is hemodynamically stable, the patient may be managed conservatively with drainage, nutrition optimization, and antibiotics based on culture data. Proton pump inhibitors that reduce gastric acid secretion may be helpful. However, if these maneuvers fail or if the patient is unstable, re-exploration with drainage should be considered. Primary repair may not be possible in this setting. For cervical anastomotic leaks in a stable patient, the leak may be drained by opening the wound. When a leak is believed to be healed, a repeat Gastrografin swallow study can confirm healing prior to diet initiation. Upon diet advancement, instillation of methylene blue dye in clear liquids will also allow for determination of an active leak.

Delayed Gastric Emptying

DGE following esophagectomy is a common complication and can occur due a number of proposed mechanisms, including the presence of vagotomy, reduced volume, inadequate emptying after gastric conduit creation, spiraling of the gastric tube, narrowing at the diaphragmatic hiatus, and inadequate pyloromyotomy or pyloroplasty. The Pittsburgh group demonstrated that the risk of DGE is about 2%, and it is believed that using a pyloroplasty, rather than pyloromyotomy, may contribute to a lower rate [47]. Similar to DGE associated with pancreatic resection, medications such as metoclopramide and erythromycin may be used to alleviate symptoms. Endoscopic pyloric balloon dilation may be useful for cases in which an intact pylorus is contributing to the symptoms.

Chylothorax

Chylothorax will occur in approximately 3% of cases [47] and arises from leakage of chyle from the thoracic duct or its branches with subsequent accumulation in the pleural space. While uncommon, it can lead to significant morbidity and mortality, related to sepsis, acute respiratory distress syndrome, pneumonia, and need for reintubation.

Signs of this complication include drainage of an excessive amount of straw or cream-colored fluid, a contralateral pleural effusion, or milky fluid when enteral nutrition is given. The fluid has a characteristic lymphocytic predominance and high triglyceride levels (>110 mg per dL). If the triglyceride level is <110 mg per dL, the presence of chylomicrons can confirm the diagnosis. Lymphangiography may be used to diagnose and assess the degree of thoracic duct leak.

First-line management is conservative, including control of the initiating cause (if not related to the operation), adequate pleural drainage, and lung re-expansion, such as with a chest tube, and nutrition modification. Medications such as octreotide and somatostatin are rarely used. A reduced fat diet (<10 g per day) with avoidance of long-chain triglycerides and substitution with medium-chain triglycerides, and consideration of parenteral nutrition is recommended. If nonoperative measures fail, one may consider chemical pleurodesis or operative ligation of the thoracic duct (thoracoscopically, via thoracotomy, or via laparotomy). There are increasing reports about the role of percutaneous embolization via the cisterna chyli as an effective treatment, with up to a 70% success rates at some centers [52]. When these surgical maneuvers fail, pleuroperitoneal or pleurovenous shunts may prove beneficial.

Anastomotic Stricture

Postoperative dysphagia may be functional or mechanical, the latter due to anastomotic stricture. Dysphagia after esophagectomy is one of the more commonly reported complications, in part because of its subjective nature. The diagnosis may be suspected from clinical history and from upper endoscopy or upper GI radiography. Early strictures are generally benign, due to etiologies, such as scar tissue. If symptoms require, esophageal dilation can ameliorate symptoms. One should suspect recurrent cancer in the setting of late strictures. In these situations, upper endoscopy and staging studies may help elucidate the cause.

Dumping Syndrome

Following both esophagectomy and gastrectomy, dumping syndrome can be a common complication, associated with a spectrum of disease severity. Causes are similar to that of DGE. Symptoms result when hypertonic enteral feeds result in the translocation of fluid into the intestine, resulting in hypovolemic symptoms and/or GI symptoms such as diarrhea and bloating.

First-line management involves dietary modification, including a postgastrectomy diet of six small meals per day, limitation of foods high in monosaccharides, substitution of monosaccharides with polysaccharides, avoidance of dairy products, and limitation of excessive fluid intake after meals.

Recurrent Laryngeal Nerve Injury

Recurrent laryngeal nerve injury is an uncommon complication following cervical anastomoses, with an incidence reported to be as low as approximately 3% in high volume centers [47]. Due to the risk of pulmonary complications, it is a complication that should be diagnosed and treated early. The diagnosis may be made with bedside laryngoscopy, which allows for vocal cord visualization. Treatment initially is supportive and includes assessment by speech pathology. However, if necessary, vocal cord injection may improve glottic closure. If this fails, surgical intervention can accomplish vocal cord medialization.

GASTRIC RESECTION

Gastric cancer is the second leading cause of cancer deaths worldwide. In the United States, surgical resection with a total or subtotal gastrectomy with chemotherapy or chemoradiotherapy provides the best option for long-term survival and cure [53]. Postoperative morbidity risk is vaguely described. Particularly after total gastrectomy (TG), which is used for high-risk patients (i.e., those with a *CDH1* mutation), GEJ tumor, tumors of the proximal and middle stomach, and diffuse tumors, morbidity can approach 40% and mortality up to approximately 11% [53]. Complications include wound issues, anemia, cardiopulmonary complications, thromboembolic events, and anastomotic stricture. However, complications specific to gastrectomy, and particularly TG, including duodenal stump leak (DSL) and anastomotic leak, will be discussed here.

Similar to other cancers, the extent of resection is based upon the site and extent of the primary tumor. While TG may be used in specific cases noted above, a more limited resection, involving a proximal or subtotal resection, may be employed if margins are adequate and oncologic outcome is not compromised. The extent of lymphadenectomy and its impact on oncologic outcome remains debatable. However, an extended, D2 lymph node dissection, with a minimum of 15 nodes harvested, is the standard at this time.

Perioperatively, early ambulation, pulmonary secretion clearance measures, judicious fluid management, and pain control are paramount. Postoperative control with epidural analgesia should be considered. There is variability regarding the use of NGTs based on the extent of resection, though NGTs are generally employed after TG. Similar to esophagectomy, Gastrografin swallow study remains the gold standard to rule out postoperative anastomotic leaks. Some clinicians elect to forgo such a study for asymptomatic patients, as a leak in an asymptomatic patient is unlikely to be clinically significant. Diet is generally advanced to a postgastrectomy diet (see "Dumping Syndrome" section). The use of a surgically placed feeding jejunostomy tube is variable. When used, enteral feeding may be initiated and advanced slowly until the patient's oral intake is sufficient.

Esophagojejunal Anastomotic Leak

A substantial contribution of morbidity and mortality after TG arises from leakage from the esophagojejunal (EJ) anastomosis following TG with Roux-en-Y EJ. Reported EJ leak rates range from 0.5% to 13%. EJ leaks can be associated with significant morality, reported as high as 18%. Many groups have evaluated variations of surgical techniques to reduce the risk of EJ leakage (i.e., open versus laparoscopic, circular versus linear staplers), and all techniques appear largely comparable [54].

If an EJ leak is suspected in a stable patient, for instance when an otherwise clinically well patient develops tachycardia, tachypnea, abdominal pain, or an increasing left effusion, a Gastrografin upper GI swallow study may confirm the leak as an area of extravasation. A CT scan of the chest and abdomen with Gastrografin oral contrast may confirm pooling or leakage of contrast from the anastomotic site. If a small, contained leak is identified, patients may be managed conservatively with nothing by mouth and parenteral nutrition. Antibiotics should be considered with a suspected infection. Once healing is confirmed, often with a Gastrografin swallow study, oral diet may be resumed.

Reoperation may be necessary for an unstable patient, or for a patient with peritonitis or failure to resolve nonoperatively. In some circumstances, wide drainage with enteral feeding access (jejunostomy tube versus nasojejunal tube) may be sufficient. However, if a complete EJ dehiscence is identified, it might be necessary to take down the EJ and create a cervical esophagostomy with a feeding jejunostomy tube.

There are an increasing number of recent reports discussing the role of esophageal stents, particularly as an alternative to reoperation in high-risk patients. Theoretical benefits are that placement of a stent might allow for early enteral nutrition and be associated with a lower morbidity than reoperation. In comparison with non-stent endoscopic therapies (such as fibrin glue and endoscopically placed clips), esophageal stents had a greater sealing rate. Complications of stenting can include stent migration and non-sealing [55].

Duodenal Stump Leak

DSL is an uncommon complication (up to 3%) but can be severe and result in substantial morbidity and mortality [56,57]. Proposed risk factors include increasing age, inadequate closure of the stump, devascularization, duodenal distension (i.e., afferent loop syndrome), and local irritation from inflammation (i.e., pancreatitis), or hematoma [56,58]. Recently, reports on DSL are becoming less common, particularly with fewer resections (and therefore complications) in the setting of peptic ulcer disease. First-line therapy is conservative management. As with other complications, nutritional optimization may improve healing. If an intraabdominal abscess is identified, percutaneous drainage should be considered. If feasible, percutaneous biliary decompression may reduce the fistula output.

If unsuccessful, if the patient is unstable (such as with hemorrhage or sepsis), or if peritonitis is present, exploration, washout, and drainage is indicated [56]. Tube duodenostomy or Roux-en-Y duodenojejunostomy (particularly if a disrupted stump that cannot be closed or if a tube duodenostomy cannot be placed) may be considered based on the degree of contamination and inflammation. The former option converts a DSL to a controlled fistula and should be considered if primary closure of the duodenal stump is tenuous or not feasible. In the setting of hostile abdomen, these complex operations, such as PD, are generally avoided.

COLORECTAL RESECTION

Colorectal cancer is the third leading cause of cancer death in the United States. The risk of death has been declining in recent years, in part due to screening colonoscopy and precancerous polyp removal. The overall lifetime risk of developing colorectal cancer is 5%.

Surgical resection, chemotherapy (including targeted treatments), and radiotherapy may be used in various combinations based on the tumor location (colon versus rectum), tumor stage, and patient characteristics. Colectomy, which may be partial (segmental) or total, can be performed for colonic cancers. Increasingly, minimally invasive techniques, such as laparoscopic, laparoscopic-assisted, or robotic approaches, may be used in addition to the traditional open operations. Low anterior resection and abdominoperineal resections may be used for more distal colon and rectal cancers not amenable to local resection. The focus of this chapter will be related to complications of these latter two operations.

Typically, due to the high bacterial load in the colon, preoperative bowel preparation is indicated. There is controversy on what constitutes a bowel preparation and specifically, the role of a mechanical bowel preparation, preoperative oral antibiotics, and perioperative parenteral antibiotics. However, most would agree that a bowel preparation, of some type, is indicated [59].

The complications of surgery for colorectal cancer are similar to those noted above. However, some complications, such as anastomotic leaks as well as sexual and urinary dysfunction, deserve specific note.

Anastomotic Leak

Anastomotic leakage will occur in up to 20% of cases, usually within the first 7 days after surgery. Signs and symptoms may include fevers, tachycardia, increasing abdominal pain including peritonitis, or the presence of a fistula. If suspected, the diagnosis may be confirmed on an upright CXR, which can show free air. A CT scan of the abdomen and pelvis might demonstrate a postoperative fluid collection with air bubbles, possibly with accumulation of passed oral contrast. While awaiting confirmation, patients should be made nothing by mouth, and broad-spectrum parenteral antibiotics may be initiated.

Anastomotic leaks may be managed conservatively with bowel rest, intravenous antibiotics, and percutaneous drainage for a clinically stable patient without peritonitis. However, for a patient who is unstable, who has peritonitis, or who fails nonoperative management, exploration, abdominal washout, wide drainage, and diverting ileostomy or colostomy should be considered.

Genitourinary Dysfunction

Inadvertent injury to the sacral splanchnic and hypogastric nerves during rectal mobilization may lead to urinary and sexual dysfunction following rectal surgery. Radiation may further compound sexual dysfunction. More than 50% of patients will have a reduced sexual function and about one-third will have alterations in urinary function. In men, sexual dysfunction may manifest as impotence and difficulties with ejaculation; women may experience dyspareunia and vaginal dryness. These known complications carry with them a significant reduction in psychosocial well-being and quality of life [60]. It remains unclear if laparoscopic resection offers any benefits compared to open surgery regarding these complications.

If urinary dysfunction is a concern, particularly if there is involvement of the membranous urethra, Foley catheterization should be continued for an extended duration in the perioperative period. Patients may be discharged with a Foley catheter in place, to be discontinued later in the postoperative period. For sexual dysfunction in men, once recovered, a penile prosthetic device can be considered.

References

1. Balcom JH, Rattner DW, Warshaw AL, et al: Ten-year experience with 733 pancreatic resections: changing indications, older patients, and decreasing length of hospitalization. *Arch Surg* 136(4):391–398, 2001.
2. Buchler MW, Friess H, Wagner M, et al: Pancreatic fistula after pancreatic head resection. *Br J Surg* 87(7):883–889, 2000.
3. Kazanjian KK, Hines OJ, Eibl G, et al: Management of pancreatic fistulas after pancreaticoduodenectomy: results in 437 consecutive patients. *Arch Surg* 140(9):849–854, 2005.
4. Mullen JT, Lee JH, Gomez HF, et al: Pancreaticoduodenectomy after placement of endobiliary metal stents. *J Gastrointest Surg* 9(8):1094–1104, 2005.
5. Schmidt CM, Powell ES, Yiannoutsos CT, et al: Pancreaticoduodenectomy: a 20-year experience in 516 patients. *Arch Surg* 139(7):718–725, 2004.
6. Sohn TA, Yeo CJ, Cameron JL, et al: Resected adenocarcinoma of the pancreas-616 patients: results, outcomes, and prognostic indicators. *J Gastrointest Surg* 4(6):567–579, 2000.
7. Bassi C, Dervenis C, Butturini G, et al: Postoperative pancreatic fistula: an international study group (ISGPF) definition. *Surgery* 138(1):8–13, 2005.
8. Brennan MF, Pisters PW, Posner M, et al: A prospective randomized trial of total parenteral nutrition after major pancreatic resection for malignancy. *Ann Surg* 220(4):436–441, 1994.
9. Buchler M, Friess H, Klempa I, et al: Role of octreotide in the prevention of postoperative complications following pancreatic resection. *Am J Surg* 163(1):125–130, 1992.
10. Friess H, Beger HG, Sulkowski U, et al: Randomized controlled multicentre study of the prevention of complications by octreotide in patients undergoing surgery for chronic pancreatitis. *Br J Surg* 82(9):1270–1273, 1995.
11. Lowy AM, Lee JE, Pisters PW, et al: Prospective, randomized trial of octreotide to prevent pancreatic fistula after pancreaticoduodenectomy for malignant disease. *Ann Surg* 226(5):632–641, 1997.
12. Montorsi M, Zago M, Mosca F, et al: Efficacy of octreotide in the prevention of pancreatic fistula after elective pancreatic resections: a prospective, controlled, randomized clinical trial. *Surgery* 117(1):26–31, 1995.
13. Pederzoli P, Bassi C, Falconi M, et al: Efficacy of octreotide in the prevention of complications of elective pancreatic surgery. Italian Study Group. *Br J Surg* 81(2):265–269, 1994.
14. Yeo CJ, Cameron JL, Lillemoe KD, et al: Does prophylactic octreotide decrease the rates of pancreatic fistula and other complications after pancreaticoduodenectomy? Results of a prospective randomized placebo-controlled trial. *Ann Surg* 232(3):419–429, 2000.
15. Allen PJ, Gonen M, Brennan MF, et al: Pasireotide for postoperative pancreatic fistula. *N Eng J Med* 370(21):2014–2022, 2014.
16. Bassi C, Falconi M, Molinari E, et al: Reconstruction by pancreaticojejunostomy versus pancreaticogastrostomy following pancreatectomy: results of a comparative study. *Ann Surg* 242(6):767–771, 2005.
17. Duffas JP, Suc B, Msika S, et al: A controlled randomized multicenter trial of pancreatogastrostomy or pancreatojejunostomy after pancreatoduodenectomy. *Am J Surg* 189(6):720–729, 2005.
18. Keck T, Wellner UF, Bahra M, et al: Pancreatogastrostomy versus pancreatojejunostomy for RECOnstruction after PANCreatoduodenectomy (RECOPANC, DRKS 00000767): perioperative and long-term results of a multicenter randomized controlled trial. *Ann Surg* 263(3):440–449, 2015.
19. Yeo CJ, Cameron JL, Maher MM, et al: A prospective randomized trial of pancreaticogastrostomy versus pancreaticojejunostomy after pancreaticoduodenectomy. *Ann Surg* 222(4):580–588, 1995.
20. Berger AC, Howard TJ, Kennedy EP, et al: Does type of pancreaticojejunostomy after pancreaticoduodenectomy decrease rate of pancreatic fistula? A randomized, prospective, dual-institution trial. *J Am Coll Surg* 208(5):738–747, 2009.
21. Peng SY, Wang JW, Lau WY, et al: Conventional versus binding pancreaticojejunostomy after pancreaticoduodenectomy: a prospective randomized trial. *Ann Surg* 245(5):692–698, 2007.
22. Suc B, Msika S, Fingerhut A, et al: Temporary fibrin glue occlusion of the main pancreatic duct in the prevention of intra-abdominal complications after pancreatic resection: prospective randomized trial. *Ann Surg* 237(1):57–65, 2003.

23. Tran K, Van Eijck C, Di Carlo V, et al: Occlusion of the pancreatic duct versus pancreaticojejunostomy: a prospective randomized trial. *Ann Surg* 236(4):422–428, 2002.
24. Chou FF, Sheen-Chen SM, Chen YS, et al: Postoperative morbidity and mortality of pancreaticoduodenectomy for periampullary cancer. *Eur J Surg* 162(6):477–481, 1996.
25. Diener MK, Seiler CM, Rossion I, et al: Efficacy of stapler versus hand-sewn closure after distal pancreatectomy (DISPACT): a randomised, controlled multicentre trial. *Lancet* 377(9776):1514–1522, 2011.
26. Conlon KC, Labow D, Leung D, et al: Prospective randomized clinical trial of the value of intraperitoneal drainage after pancreatic resection. *Ann Surg* 234(4):487–493, 2001.
27. Correa-Gallego C, Brennan MF, D'angelica M, et al: Operative drainage following pancreatic resection: analysis of 1122 patients resected over 5 years at a single institution. *Ann Surg* 258(6):1051–1058, 2013.
28. Van Buren G, Bloomston M, Hughes SJ, et al: A randomized prospective multicenter trial of pancreaticoduodenectomy with and without routine intraperitoneal drainage. *Ann Surg* 259(4):605–612, 2014.
29. Lu M, Weiss C, Fishman EK, et al: Review of visceral aneurysms and pseudoaneurysms. *J Comput Assist Tomogr* 39(1):1–6, 2015.
30. Wente MN, Bassi C, Dervenis C, et al: Delayed gastric emptying (DGE) after pancreatic surgery: a suggested definition by the International Study Group of Pancreatic Surgery (ISGPS). *Surgery* 142(5):761–768, 2007.
31. Seiler CA, Wagner M, Bachmann T, et al: Randomized clinical trial of pylorus-preserving duodenopancreatectomy versus classical Whipple resection-long term results. *Br J Surg* 92(5):547–556, 2005.
32. Lin PW, Shan YS, Lin YJ, et al: Pancreaticoduodenectomy for pancreatic head cancer: PPPD versus Whipple procedure. *Hepatogastroenterology* 52(65):1601–1604, 2005.
33. Tran KT, Smeenk HG, van Eijck CH, et al: Pylorus preserving pancreaticoduodenectomy versus standard Whipple procedure: a prospective, randomized, multicenter analysis of 170 patients with pancreatic and periampullary tumors. *Ann Surg* 240(5):738–745, 2004.
34. Yeo CJ, Barry MK, Sauter PK, et al: Erythromycin accelerates gastric emptying after pancreaticoduodenectomy. A prospective, randomized, placebo-controlled trial. *Ann Surg* 218(3):229–237, 1993.
35. Jimenez RE, Fernandez-del Castillo C, Rattner DW, et al: Outcome of pancreaticoduodenectomy with pylorus preservation or with antrectomy in the treatment of chronic pancreatitis. *Ann Surg* 231(3):293–300, 2000.
36. Martin RF, Rossi RL, Leslie KA: Long-term results of pylorus-preserving pancreatoduodenectomy for chronic pancreatitis. *Arch Surg* 131(3):247–252, 1996.
37. Riediger H, Adam U, Fischer E, et al: Long-term outcome after resection for chronic pancreatitis in 224 patients. *J Gastrointest Surg* 11(8):949–959, 2007.
38. Rumstadt B, Forssmann K, Singer MV, et al: The Whipple partial duodenopancreatectomy for the treatment of chronic pancreatitis. *Hepatogastroenterology* 44(18):1554–1559, 1997.
39. Sakorafas GH, Farnell MB, Nagorney DM, et al: Pancreatoduodenectomy for chronic pancreatitis: long-term results in 105 patients. *Arch Surg* 135(5):517–523, 2000.
40. Sohn TA, Campbell KA, Pitt HA, et al: Quality of life and long-term survival after surgery for chronic pancreatitis. *J Gastrointest Surg* 4(4):355–364, 2000.
41. Traverso LW, Kozarek RA: Pancreatoduodenectomy for chronic pancreatitis: anatomic selection criteria and subsequent long-term outcome analysis. *Ann Surg* 226(4):429–435, 1997.
42. Howard TJ, Maiden CL, Smith HG, et al: Surgical treatment of obstructive pancreatitis. *Surgery* 118(4):727–734, 1995.
43. Sakorafas GH, Sarr MG, Rowland CM, et al: Postobstructive chronic pancreatitis: results with distal resection. *Arch Surg* 136(6):643–648, 2001.
44. National Cancer Institute: Cancer stat fact sheets: esophageal cancer. 2015. Available at: http://seer.cancer.gov/statfacts/html/esoph.html. Accessed February 1, 2017.
45. Luketich JD, Pennathur A, Awais O, et al: Outcomes after minimally invasive esophagectomy: review of over 1000 patients. *Ann Surg* 256(1):95–103, 2012.
46. Bailey SH, Bull DA, Harpole DH, et al: Outcomes after esophagectomy: a ten-year prospective cohort. *Ann Thorac Surg* 75(1):217–222, 2003.
47. Luketich JD, Alvelo-Rivera M, Buenaventura PO, et al: Minimally invasive esophagectomy: outcomes in 222 patients. *Ann Surg* 238(4):486–494, 2003.
48. Orringer MB, Marshall B, Iannettoni MD: Transhiatal esophagectomy for treatment of benign and malignant esophageal disease. *World J Surg* 25(2):196–203, 2001.
49. Swanson SJ, Batirel HF, Bueno R, et al: Transthoracic esophagectomy with radical mediastinal and abdominal lymph node dissection and cervical esophagogastrostomy for esophageal carcinoma. *Ann Thoracic Surg* 72(6):1918–1924, 2001.
50. Birkmeyer JD, Sun Y, Wong SL, et al: Hospital volume and late survival after cancer surgery. *Ann Surg* 245(5):777–783, 2007.
51. Law SYK, Wong J: Esophagogastrectomy for carcinoma of the esophagus and gastric cardia and the esophageal anastomosis, Chapter 63, in Fischer JE (ed): *Mastery of Surgery*. 5th ed. Philadelphia, PA: Lippincott, Williams & WIlkins, 2001. pp 752–771.
52. Itkin M, Kucharczuk JC, Kwak A, et al: Nonoperative thoracic duct embolization for traumatic thoracic duct leak: experience in 109 patients. *J Thoracic Cardiovasc Surg* 139(3):584–589, 2010.
53. Selby LV, Vertosick EA, Sjoberg DD, et al: Morbidity after total gastrectomy: analysis of 238 patients. *J Am Coll Surg* 220(5):863–871 e2, 2015.
54. LaFemina J, Vinuela EF, Schattner MA, et al: Esophagojejunal reconstruction after total gastrectomy for gastric cancer using a transorally inserted anvil delivery system. *Ann Surg Oncol* 20(9):2975–2983, 2013.
55. Shim C, Kim HI, Hyung WJ, et al: Self-expanding metal stents or nonstent endoscopic therapy: which is better for anastomotic leaks after total gastrectomy? *Surg Endosc* 28(3):833–840, 2014.
56. Aurello P, Sirimarco D, Magistri P, et al: Management of duodenal stump fistula after gastrectomy for gastric cancer: systematic review. *World J Gastroenterol* 21(24):7571–7576, 2015.
57. Cozzaglio L, Coladonato M, Biffi R, et al: Duodenal fistula after elective gastrectomy for malignant disease: an italian retrospective multicenter study. *J Gastrointest Surg* 14(5):805–811, 2010.
58. Kim KH, Kim MC, Jung GJ: Risk factors for duodenal stump leakage after gastrectomy for gastric cancer and management technique of stump leakage. *Hepatogastroenterology* 61(133):1446–1453, 2014.
59. Dellinger EP: Should a scheduled colorectal operation have a mechanical bowel prep, preoperative oral antibiotics, both, or neither? *Ann Surg* 261(6):1041–1043, 2015.
60. Lange MM, van de Velde CJ: Urinary and sexual dysfunction after rectal cancer treatment. *Nat Rev Urol* 8(1):51–57, 2011.

Chapter 51 ■ The ICU Approach to the Acute Abdomen

JAMES E. CARROLL, JR

While definitions of the "acute abdomen" differ, most clinicians will use this term to describe the sudden onset of severe abdominal pain of unclear etiology that frequently indicates the presence of a surgical pathology. Under ideal circumstances, a detailed history (including comorbid illness and prior surgeries), a thorough physical examination, ordering appropriate laboratories, and targeted imaging would reveal the source of the symptoms. The challenge for the intensive care physician begins with the many potential obstacles to early diagnosis, including altered patient sensorium, limited ability to communicate due to mechanical ventilation, concurrent antibiotic therapy, and the masking of reliable physical examination signs.

Abdominal catastrophes for intensive care unit (ICU) patients occur frequently among patients admitted for nonsurgical problems, and other systemic comorbidities, such as pulmonary, cardiovascular, renal, or multisystem disorders [1]. An acute abdomen of an already critically ill patient portends high mortality, especially for patients meeting criteria of severe sepsis, often with derangements of more than one organ system associated with widespread cellular dysfunction. Successful management of the acute abdomen of a critically ill adult has traditionally relied upon clinician-dependent factors such as sharp clinical acumen, early collaborative efforts, and diagnostic expediency, as much as evidence-based algorithms. Despite improvements in data collection and the integration of dedicated specialists into patient care plans, high-quality evidence and specific clinical guidelines are still inadequate [2].

EPIDEMIOLOGY

In a 5-year retrospective cohort study of 6,000 medical ICU admissions, 77 patients were identified with acute abdominal syndromes requiring surgical intervention, suggesting it may be a rare occurrence among critically ill patients [3]. Mortality of this group peaked at 63%, more than doubling APACHE III-predicted mortality (31%). In contrast, a 2-month prospective, observation cohort of 484 ICU patients from mainland China with severe sepsis demonstrated abdominal sources (18%) to be the second most common source of infection (behind lung) and carried a high mortality (~25%) [4]. Mesenteric ischemia was associated with both early and late mortality in a single-center, retrospective study of 543 patients over 6 years, causing 6.4% of early ICU deaths and 16.6% of late ICU deaths [5]. An observational study of 3,665 patients in 10 Chinese surgical ICUs found the abdomen to be the most common source of severe sepsis among critically ill patients (72.3%). Diagnoses included severe acute pancreatitis, intestinal or gastric perforation, bowel obstruction, and biliary infection, all of which were associated with high hospital mortality (33.2% to 65.4%) [6]. The 75-country EPIC II (Extended Prevalence of Infection in the ICU) study established that 19.6% of more than 7,000 patients were found to have an abdominal source of infection using International Sepsis Forum criteria, and also showed a higher mortality rate for abdominal infections than for infections of other systems (29.4% vs. 24.4%) [7].

HISTORY

When clinical parameters permit (e.g., hemodynamic stability), a focused history should be obtained from the patient. Beyond typical historical elements (onset, quality, severity, location, radiation, exacerbating and alleviating symptoms), additional information about constitutional symptoms, gastrointestinal, and gynecologic symptoms should be obtained. Special attention should be paid to prior medical and surgery history, medications, and social history. Overall, the sensitivity and specificity of a history for the diagnosis of abdominal pain is poor. However, the information obtained from the patient may be used to identify risk factors for particular intraabdominal processes (see Table 51.1).

PHYSICAL

The traditional abdominal examination begins with inspection, which may reveal prior surgical scars, ecchymosis, areas of discoloration, and visible hernias. Long regarded an essential part of the abdominal examination, auscultation is neither specific nor sensitive [8]. Percussion may elicit tympany, suggesting ileus or obstruction. Tenderness is elicited through palpation, with rebound and guarding indicating peritonitis. Frequently, multiple signs occur simultaneously; in one study, 95% of patients with abdominal complications in a medical ICU had findings of abdominal pain, while 73% had abdominal distention and 38% had documented peritoneal signs [3]. Patients with focal pain or obstructive symptoms should be carefully examined for evidence of inguinal or incisional hernias. Rectal and pelvic examination should be performed as indicated by the symptoms and findings. Comorbid conditions such as diabetes and chronic immunosuppression may blunt examination findings associated with intraabdominal pathologies.

TABLE 51.1

Representative Historical Elements and Associated Abdominal Pathology

ROS	Increases suspicion for:
Fevers and/or chills	Infectious processes (e.g., appendicitis, cholecystitis, diverticulitis, intraabdominal abscess)
Unintentional weight loss, change in stool caliber, night sweats	Malignancy (e.g., colon, esophageal or gastric CA)
Hematochezia	AVM, diverticular disease, malignancy, mesenteric ischemic
Vaginal discharge, multiple sexual partners	Pelvic inflammatory disease, tubo-ovarian abscess
Prior medical history	
Atrial fibrillation	Mesenteric ischemia, infarct
Venous thromboembolism	Mesenteric or portal vein thrombosis
Diabetes mellitus	Any intraabdominal infection
Clostridium difficile infection	Toxic megacolon
Prior surgeries	
Gastric bypass	Closed loop obstruction, internal hernia
Any intraabdominal procedure	Adhesions, small bowel obstruction
Social history	
Chronic alcohol use	Pancreatitis, esophageal/gastric cancer
Intravenous drug use	Hepatitis, intraabdominal abscess
Medications	
Anticoagulation (warfarin, dabigatran, apixaban, rivaroxaban)	Intraabdominal hemorrhage, rectus sheath hematoma, retroperitoneal hematoma
Corticosteroids	Peptic ulcer disease, perforated viscus, intraabdominal abscess
Immunosuppression	Any intraabdominal infection, certain agents associated with increased risk of perforation (e.g., bevacizumab)
Digoxin	Mesenteric ischemia

ROS, review of systems; CA, cancer; AVM, arteriovenous malformations.

IMAGING

Physical examination findings may fail to provide clinical clues regarding abdominal pathologies of the critically ill patient. Diagnostic imaging provides critical clinical data during the evaluation, particularly when physical examination findings are unreliable secondary to sedation, obtundation, delirium, or immunosuppression.

Plain Radiographs

Abdominal radiographs are rapidly and widely available, inexpensive studies that are frequently obtained for patients with abdominal pain. However, the utility of abdominal radiography is highest when applied for specific indications. The American College of Radiology (ACR) recommends that abdominal radiography be used to evaluate for the following conditions in adults: pneumoperitoneum, bowel obstruction or ileus, intraabdominal foreign bodies, urinary tract calculi, and medical device placement. The ACR identifies no absolute contraindications to abdominal X-rays, with pregnancy being the only relative contraindication [9]. After an intraabdominal exploration or procedure, free air should not persist for more than 48 to 72 hours. Contrast-enhanced X-rays can be used to confirm the placement of gastrostomy and jejunostomy tubes, or to evaluate bowel motility.

Abdominal Pelvic Computed Tomography

Computed tomography (CT) is the preferred imaging modality for the diagnosis of intraabdominal catastrophes. Moreover, CT plays an essential role in limiting the number of unnecessary exploratory laparotomies performed among critically ill patients; unnecessary laparotomy is associated with morbidity for 22% of these patients [10]. Intraabdominal processes like free air, pancreatitis, diverticulitis, infections (e.g., abscesses), inflammation (e.g., colitis), acute mesenteric ischemia, and bowel obstructions are all readily identified by abdominal pelvic CT [11]. Improvements in CT technology have obviated the need for oral contrast for most patients; oral contrast should be considered for patients with a history of gastric bypass, evaluation of anastomotic leaks, and in patients with inflammatory bowel disease. When not contraindicated by allergy or renal insufficiency, intravenous contrast should be administered to optimally evaluate vascular structures (such as the superior mesenteric artery [SMA]) and abscesses. While CT does frequently identify signs of cholecystitis, ultrasound remains superior for biliary tract (specifically common bile duct) imaging. Hemodynamic instability may preclude transport of patients to CT scan, while patients with morbid obesity may be unable to undergo a CT study due to mechanical limits.

Ultrasound

Ultrasound offers distinct advantages for evaluating abdominal pathologies of the critically ill care. Bedside ultrasonography is immediately available at most centers. Bedside ultrasound can be used to assess a variety of acute findings, including free fluid, pneumothorax, pericardial effusions, gallbladder disease, aortic aneurysm, intrauterine pregnancy, hydronephrosis, bladder volume, and inferior vena cava diameter (as a marker of volume resuscitation). Ultrasonography remains the test of choice for biliary tract pathologies. There are several settings in which technical limitations to ultrasound arise, including morbid obesity and the presence of bowel gas.

SPECIFIC CAUSES OF ABDOMINAL PAIN

The differential diagnosis for abdominal pain is extensive. Acute mesenteric ischemia and acalculous cholecystitis are discussed in detail here, as these are common reasons for surgical consultation for critically ill adults. Abdominal compartment syndrome, surgical infections, and necrotizing fasciitis (Fournier's gangrene) are separately covered within this section.

Acute Mesenteric Ischemia

Acute mesenteric ischemia can be a difficult diagnosis to make, and clinicians must maintain a high degree of suspicion particularly for elderly patients with severe abdominal pain. There are several etiologies for mesenteric ischemia, including SMA embolism, SMA thrombus, superior mesenteric vein (SMV) thrombosis, and nonocclusive mesenteric ischemia (frequently associated with low-flow states). The risk factors are different for each process. Atrial fibrillation, valvular heart disease, congestive heart failure (CHF), myocardial infarction (MI), and recent vascular surgery increase the risk of SMA embolism. In these cases, the embolus is nearly always generated in the heart, then lodges in the SMA due to its angle of takeoff from the aorta [12]. Cases of SMA thrombosis are frequently associated with smoking, peripheral vascular disease, and coronary artery disease. Risk factors for SMV thrombosis include recent abdominal surgery, hypercoagulable states, oral contraceptive use, and prior history of venous thromboembolism. Nonocclusive mesenteric ischemia risk factors include low-flow states (e.g., hypotension), CHF, end-stage renal disease, and digoxin or vasopressor use [13].

Regardless of the etiology, the diagnosis and treatment of acute mesenteric ischemia are challenging. With bacterial translocation occurring 6 hours after disruption of ischemic mucosal barrier, correcting the subsequent physiologic insults is challenging, because the diagnosis takes an average of 8 hours and treatment can take another 2.5 hours [14]. Even with prompt initiation of anticoagulation for thromboembolic events with intravenous heparin (5,000 International Units bolus followed by 20,000 International Units over 24 hours), morbidity and mortality are substantial. Among patients for whom the diagnosis is delayed by 24 hours, mortality nearly doubles from 36% to 69% [13].

Cholecystitis

Acalculous cholecystitis is more frequent among the critically ill than typical stone-based disease. Acalculous cholecystitis reflects ischemic or inflammatory changes to the gallbladder secondary to obstruction of the cystic duct, bile stasis, or distention [15]. Risk factors include older age, male gender, diabetes mellitus, hemodialysis, CHF, cardiac arrest, or cardiopulmonary resuscitation [1]. Acute acalculous cholecystitis is frequently diagnosed among patients with an admission diagnosis of sepsis [16]. Acalculous cholecystitis should be considered for any ICU patient with right upper quadrant pain, fevers, and worsening leukocytosis. The most common modality for the evaluation of acalculous cholecystitis is ultrasound; however, the absence of stones can decrease the sensitivity of this test [17]. Once the diagnosis is made, treatment alternatives can be considered. Definitive therapy with open or laparoscopic cholecystectomy is associated with increased perioperative mortality among critically ill patients, leading to alternatives (percutaneous cholecystostomy tube placement) [1]. A retrospective observational study of 56 patients treated for acalculous cholecystitis with percutaneous cholecystostomy demonstrated an efficacy of over 80%, with low rates of associated complications, mortality, or need for subsequent cholecystectomy [18]. Often representing a further progression of multisystem organ failure, acute acalculous cholecystitis requires prompt intervention with low-risk surgical interventions available that can accommodate patients unfit for anesthesia or transport [19].

Extraabdominal Causes of Abdominal Pain

Several extraabdominal medical emergencies can present with abdominal pain, including MI, pneumonia, and diabetic ketoacidosis. Clinicians must remain vigilant for extraabdominal sources of pain, particularly when abdominal imaging is unremarkable or equivocal.

SPECIAL POPULATIONS

Abdominal emergencies impact the elderly with particular resonance. Impaired or dwindling physiologic reserves exacerbate failing organ systems and potentiate comorbidities [20]. Multidisciplinary approaches involving palliative care teams, geriatricians, primary care physicians, as well as the surgeon and intensivist, enable the identification of cases where a comfort-oriented care plan is appropriate.

MANAGEMENT

Given the possible uncertainty amid a wide spectrum of differential diagnoses for abdominal sources of sepsis of the critically ill patient, early administration of broad-spectrum antibiotics, volume resuscitation, and rapid source control must occur immediately to prevent mortality related to delay of treatments. The Surviving Sepsis Campaign: International Guidelines for Management of Severe Sepsis and Septic Shock, 2012, summarizes evidence-supported early interventions for the septic patient by international consensus and are appropriate for the critically ill patient with abdominal sepsis. Recommendations include quantitative resuscitation with appropriate reevaluation of end points, acquisition of blood cultures prior to initiation of broad-spectrum antibiotics, prompt acquirement of ancillary imaging, and source control by appropriate modality (with consideration of risks and benefits) within 12 hours.

Hemodynamic lability in such circumstances may prevent patient transport, increasing the burden on the clinician to work with physical examination, and available laboratory, and ancillary bedside diagnostics. High clinical suspicion of intraabdominal sepsis in these circumstances warrants exploratory laparotomy and its associated high mortality and morbidity [11]. When associated with hypothermia, acidosis, and coagulopathy, the mortality risk becomes nearly prohibitive. Wide surgical source control of devitalized tissues, perforated viscus, or anastomotic failures remain a priority to reduce both bacterial load and source [21]. Bowel edema secondary to resuscitation, ongoing or unresolved contamination from perforated or compromises viscous, and clear anticipation of abdominal compartment syndrome may warrant leaving the abdomen open with placement of a negative pressure wound therapy device [22]. Open abdomens in the non-trauma patient have become more widely described in recent years with concerns noted for high mortality and enterocutaneous fistula formation, but with the caveat that many of these scenarios are predisposed to both outcomes as expected sequelae of inflamed, swollen bowel and severe sepsis [23,24]. There exists substantial heterogeneity regarding the indications for the open abdomen among critically ill patients, whether deliberate or unavoidable. While initial maneuvers performed during source control (damage control) surgery require debridement of devitalized tissues, removal of infected foreign bodies, irrigation and drainage of contaminated surfaces, and abdominal decompression, the subsequent restoration of anatomic function is less of an immediate priority [25]. An emerging literature has embraced delayed reconstruction of bowel continuity, with some indication that resuscitation and optimization of anastomosis creation may lead to improved survival and fewer complications [26].

CONCLUSIONS

Intraabdominal source control, prompt administration of antibiotics, and the application of due diligence to fluid resuscitation and correction of physiologic derangements represent the cornerstones of an ICU approach to the acute abdomen. Impediments to the pragmatic approach and treatment of the acute abdomen include patient complexity, poor clinical correlates, and delays in diagnosis secondary to confounding from coexisting ailments. A multidisciplinary approach designed to maximize utilization of physical examination findings, laboratory results, imaging modalities, and collaborative clinical judgment results in the best opportunity for early intervention and improved outcomes.

References

1. Rezende-Neto JB, Rotstein OD: Abdominal catastrophes in the intensive care unit setting. *Crit Care Clin* 29:1017–1044, 2013.
2. Mayumi T, Yoshida M, Tazuma S, et al: The practice guidelines for primary care of acute abdomen 2015. *Jpn J Radiol* 34:80–115, 2016.
3. Gajic O, Urrutia LE, Sewani H, et al: Acute abdomen in the medical intensive care unit. *Crit Care Med* 30:1187–1190, 2002.
4. Zhou J, Qian C, Zhao M, et al: Epidemiology and outcome of severe sepsis and septic shock in intensive care units in mainland China. *PLoS One* 9:e107181, 2014.
5. Daviaud F, Grimaldi D, Dechartres A, et al: Timing and causes of death in septic shock. *Ann Intensive Care* 5:16, 2015.
6. Cheng B, Xie G, Yao S, et al: Epidemiology of severe sepsis in critically ill surgical patients in ten university hospitals in China. *Crit Care Med* 35:2538–2546, 2007.
7. De Waele J, Lipman J, Sakr Y, et al: Abdominal infections in the intensive care unit: characteristics, treatment and determinants of outcome. *BMC Infect Dis* 14:420, 2014.
8. Felder S, Margel D, Murrell Z, et al: Usefulness of bowel sound auscultation: a prospective evaluation. *J Surg Educ* 71:768–773, 2014.
9. American College of Radiology and the Society for Pediatric Radiology. ACR-SPR Practice parameter for the performance of abdominal radiography, 2014.
10. Memon MA, Fitztgibbons RJ Jr: The role of minimal access surgery in the acute abdomen. *Surg Clin North Am* 77:1333–1353, 1997.
11. Crandall M, West MA: Evaluation of the abdomen in the critically ill patient: opening the black box. *Curr Opin Crit Care* 12:333–339, 2006.
12. Wyers MC: Acute mesenteric ischemia: diagnostic approach and surgical treatment. *Semin Vasc Surg* 23:9–20, 2010.
13. Carver TW, Vora RS, Taneja A: Mesenteric ischemia. *Crit Care Clin* 32:155–171, 2016.
14. Klar E, Rahmanian PB, Bucker A, et al: Acute mesenteric ischemia: a vascular emergency. *Dtsch Arztebl Int* 109:249–256, 2012.
15. Rehman T, Deboisblanc BP: Persistent fever in the ICU. *Chest* 145:158–165, 2014.
16. Laurila J, Syrjala H, Laurila PA, et al: Acute acalculous cholecystitis in critically ill patients. *Acta Anaesthesiol Scand* 48:986–991, 2004.
17. Trowbridge RL, Rutkowski NK, Shojania KG: Does this patient have acute cholecystitis? *JAMA* 289:80–86, 2003.
18. Kirkegard J, Horn T, Christensen SD, et al: Percutaneous cholecystostomy is an effective definitive treatment option for acute acalculous cholecystitis. *Scand J Surg* 104:238–243, 2015.
19. Treinen C, Lomelin D, Krause C, et al: Acute acalculous cholecystitis in the critically ill: risk factors and surgical strategies. *Langenbecks Arch Surg* 400:421–427, 2015.
20. Tridente A, Clarke GM, Walden A, et al: Association between trends in clinical variables and outcome in intensive care patients with faecal peritonitis: analysis of the GenOSept cohort. *Crit Care* 19:210, 2015.
21. Chromik AM, Meiser A, Holling J, et al: Identification of patients at risk for development of tertiary peritonitis on a surgical intensive care unit. *J Gastrointest Surg* 13:1358–1367, 2009.
22. Beckman M, Paul J, Neideen T, et al: Role of the open abdomen in critically ill patients. *Crit Care Clin* 32:255–264, 2016.
23. Atema JJ, Gans SL, Boermeester MA: Systematic review and meta-analysis of the open abdomen and temporary abdominal closure techniques in non-trauma patients. *World J Surg* 39:912–925, 2015.
24. Bruns BR, Ahmad SA, O'Meara L, et al: Nontrauma open abdomens: a prospective observational study. *J Trauma Acute Care Surg* 80:631–636, 2016.
25. Hecker A, Uhle F, Schwandner T, et al: Diagnostics, therapy and outcome prediction in abdominal sepsis: current standards and future perspectives. *Langenbecks Arch Surg* 399:11–22, 2014.
26. Sartelli M, Abu-Zidan FM, Ansaloni L, et al: The role of the open abdomen procedure in managing severe abdominal sepsis: WSES position paper. *World J Emerg Surg* 10:35, 2015.

Chapter 52 ■ Abdominal Compartment Syndrome

JON D. DORFMAN

INTRODUCTION

Since intraabdominal hypertension (IAH) and abdominal compartment syndrome (ACS) were first recognized, the incidence and importance has resulted in an increasing body of research and the formation of the World Society of Abdominal Compartment Syndrome. Normal abdominal pressure is typically less than 7 mm Hg. Once pressures are greater than 12 mm Hg, the patient is considered to have IAH. As pressures increase further, organ failure can develop. Pressures greater than 20 mm Hg with new onset organ failure is considered ACS and pressures greater than 25 mm Hg are considered significant enough to consider intervening [1].

ACS can be termed primary or secondary. Primary ACS occurs from an intraabdominal process, for example pancreatitis, liver failure, or abdominal trauma. Secondary ACS is the result of illness not directly related to the abdomen or pelvis. This secondary form is caused by severe systemic illness and the resultant capillary leak and typically is related to large volume resuscitation [2].

INCIDENCE

Many factors determine intraabdominal pressures. These factors include patient-related issues such as body mass index (BMI), severity of illness such as acute lung injury requiring increased positive end expiratory pressure (PEEP) as well as the technique by which the pressure was measured. The technique will be discussed in detail below. Increased BMI correlates with increased intraabdominal pressure in multiple studies [3]. In particular, a patient population with BMI 52 ± 1 kg per m^2 had measured intraabdominal pressures of 13.2 ± 0.5 mm Hg as compared with patients with a BMI 24 kg ± 2 kg per m^2 whose measured pressures were 5.1 ± 1.2 mm Hg [4]. PEEP has a variable effect on intraabdominal pressure. The effects of PEEP may be greater with higher intraabdominal pressures [3].

Setting an upper limit of 15 mm Hg, the incidence of IAH exceeding this cutoff was 28% for published cohorts [5,6]. If a lower threshold of 12 mm Hg was used, nearly 50% of critically ill patients had IAH [5,7]. It is important to note that intraabdominal pressures vary during the day when serially measured and one elevated pressure may or may not be significant. How studies define IAH also varies with some studies using the maximum daily measured intravesicular pressure; other studies calculate a mean daily pressure. Using the maximum daily pressure versus the mean pressure more than doubled the incidence of IAH [5]. The World Society of Abdominal Compartment Syndrome recommends pressures greater than 12 mm Hg on more than one occasion to diagnose IAH [1].

The risk factors for development of IAH/ACS vary among studies. Fluid resuscitation impacts the development of elevated intraabdominal pressures, with positive fluid balances in the first days of intensive care unit (ICU) admission being significantly different both statistically and clinically between patients with elevated intravesicular pressures and those patients with normal measured pressures [5,7]. The administered volume associated with IAH/ACS varies widely between studies from 3.5 L to greater than 15 L [5,8]. Other factors associated with elevated intraabdominal pressure include mechanical ventilation, acute respiratory distress syndrome (ARDS) [7], abdominal surgery, ileus, and liver failure [6]. Systemic diseases such as severe trauma, major burn injury. as well as sepsis and multiorgan failure (as determined by the Sepsis-related Organ Failure Assessment score [SOFA]) also place patients at risk of IAH/ACS [1].

Overall, 20% to 40% of surgical and medical ICU patients develop IAH. Patients may arrive to the ICU already with IAH or it can develop during their ICU stay. ACS occurs in up to 10% of these patients. Numerous risk factors are described and many case reports have been published. Many of these patient and disease factors are nonspecific making patient selection for intraabdominal pressure monitoring difficult. No clear recommendations have been published. Of the highest risk populations for IAH, severe trauma, major burn, severe pancreatitis, and liver failure patients should be considered for monitoring [9].

MEASUREMENT OF INTRAABDOMINAL PRESSURE

Many techniques have been developed to monitor intraabdominal pressure. Clinical examination has been assessed to determine its ability to detect IAH/ACS. A prospective study of 128 consecutive surgical patients admitted to the ICU compared the clinician's examination (scored as normal, moderately tense, markedly tense abdominal examination) with intravesicular pressure which was classified unremarkable if <18 mm Hg, elevated if between 18 and 25 mm Hg, and markedly elevated if >25 mm Hg. In this population of patients with 20% having elevated intravesicular pressures, and 1% having markedly elevated pressures, the clinical examiner impression had a sensitivity of 61%, specificity of 81%, and positive predictive value of only 45% [10]. Other series confirm the finding that physical examination poorly predicts IAH/ACS [11].

Quantitative techniques have been developed and include gastric, bladder, rectal, femoral vein, inferior vena cava (IVC), and direct intraperitoneal pressure monitoring [12]. Intravascular monitoring via the femoral vein or the IVC has been reported in animal models [13]. However, the invasiveness of the intravascular approach as well as the infectious and thrombotic risks make placement of these catheters impractical. Intraperitoneal pressure monitors have been compared with intravesicular pressure monitors in 40 postsurgical patients. The peritoneal catheters used were 14 French polyvinylchloride. Five patients had postoperative IAH and only one had ACS, which required surgical intervention. The correlation between the intraperitoneal catheter with the intravesicular monitor was excellent with $r = 0.96$ and most measurements had a less than 1 mm Hg difference between the methods [14].

Intravesicular pressure monitoring as a surrogate for intraabdominal pressure is now the standard. The technique involves instilling saline into a urinary catheter; the catheter is clamped between the culture aspiration port and the urometer. After waiting for 30 to 60 seconds, the culture aspiration port is connected to a pressure monitor. There have been many concerns over the validity of this technique and it has been widely studied. In particular, the proper volume to infuse has been examined and varied from 10 mL to as much as 250 mL; one study examined the effects of 10, 50, and 100 mL instillation volumes on the measured bladder pressure. The higher instillation instillation volumes of 50 mL and 100 mL increased the measured bladder pressures by 20% and 40% as compared to 10 mL instillation[15]. The current recommendation is the instillation of 25 mL [1].

The correct zero point has been investigated as has been the effects of different patient positions. Patient positions with the head of bed between 0 degrees (supine) and 45 degrees elevated have been shown to increase the intraabdominal pressure with increased elevation [16,17]. The most common zero point is set at the midaxillary line and iliac crest. Due to feasibility and expense, the current guidelines recommend bladder pressure assessment in a supine patient at end expiration with the zero point set at the midaxillary line [1].

PHYSIOLOGY

The classic compartment syndrome occurs in the cranium. The cranium is a rigid enclosed space whose bounds are the cranial bones; the intracranial volume is fixed. Within the cranium lies cerebral spinal fluid, blood within the arterial and venous systems, and brain parenchyma. If any of these components increase in volume, for example the amount of intracranial blood from a subdural hematoma, then intracranial pressure increases.

The abdominal compartment has a different structure. The volume is not fixed and can expand. This difference plays an important role in treatment options. Inferiorly and posteriorly the pelvis and the spine create a rigid barrier; however, the anterior and superior bounds are not rigid. The diaphragmatic muscles contract and relax with inspiration and expiration. The anterior abdominal wall musculature which lies between the anterior axillary lines is composed of the paired rectii muscles medially and the external obliques, internal obliques, and the transversus abdominus; these muscles also can contract or relax changing the intraabdominal volume [12].

Within the abdomen there are the solid organs and the arterial–venous systems; there is also the intraperitoneal space or third space where ascites can develop. Within the lumen of the gastrointestinal tract, air and succuss can take up a significant volume, for example from an ileus or Ogilvie syndrome. An increase in the volume of any of these components can increase the intraabdominal pressure.

ABDOMINAL COMPARTMENT SYNDROME

Increased intraabdominal pressure can have systemic effects for patients. Once new organ failure results from IAH, the patient is considered to have ACS. The pressure at which IAH causes ACS varies from patient to patient. Pressures below 20 mm Hg are unlikely to cause organ failure; organ failure is much more likely to occur once pressures exceed 25 mm Hg [2]. We will individually examine each organ system that may be affected.

Respiratory Failure

Pulmonary failure from ACS can result in hypoxia and hypercarbia. As intraabdominal volume and pressure increase, the diaphragm is elevated into the thorax. This upward pressure leads to compression and atelectasis of the lungs. Due to the ventilation and perfusion mismatch, hypoxia occurs.

Lung volumes can decrease, and among intubated patients, plateau pressures and peak inspiratory pressures can increase. In a swine animal mode of IAH, 50% of the IAH was transmitted to the plateau pressure under conditions of PEEP of 1 or 10 cm H_2O [18]. When a pressure control mode of ventilation is used, tidal volumes may insidiously decrease as abdominal pressures increase. When minute ventilation decreases, hypercarbia will occur and hypoxemia can result from perfusion of the collapsed lung. These signs, hypoxia, hypercarbia, and increased plateau pressure, are nonspecific and their relation to increased intraabdominal pressure may not be appreciated [19]. Among patients with ARDS, elevated peak inspiratory pressures and plateau pressures can be misinterpreted as being caused by worsening ARDS rather than evolving ACS.

Renal Failure

Renal dysfunction commonly occurs in ACS. The challenge in diagnosis is that acute renal failure is also common in the critical illnesses associated with ACS including sepsis, pancreatitis, and burns. Therefore, oliguria from ACS can easily be attributed to other factors.

Increased abdominal pressure leads to decreased renal venous flow. Ultimately, this decreased renal venous flow causes ischemia, tubular dysfunction, and oliguria. Decreased cardiac output from ACS may also contribute to acute renal failure. In a study of healthy volunteers, IAH, as measured by gastric pressure, was generated by an external binder, positive pressure ventilation, or by both methods. Ultrasound was used to assess renal arterial resistance and it significantly increased with IAH [20]. Dalfino et al. [21] measured intravesicular pressure in consecutive critically ill patients, and found that IAH greater than 12 mm Hg was predictive of acute renal failure, although other studies in postoperative patients have found a higher intraabdominal pressure (mean 27 mm Hg) is associated with acute renal failure [22].

Further compounding the problem is the kidney's physiologic responses to decreased perfusion. Antidiuretic hormone (ADH) is released and the renin–angiotensin pathway is activated leading to reabsorption of sodium and water. The increase in serum ADH has been confirmed in human studies. Among patients undergoing laparoscopic donor nephrectomy with a pneumoperitoneum of 12 mm Hg, serum ADH levels were increased from the patient's preinsufflation baseline as well as from open nephrectomy controls [23]. Increased water and sodium reabsorption may lead to further third space fluid volume and edema, and further increase IAH.

Cardiovascular

The cardiovascular effects of increased intraabdominal pressure are numerous. Thoracic and intraabdominal volumes are interrelated. As the abdominal pressure and abdominal volume increase, the diaphragm pushes cranially. The thoracic volume is subsequently decreased and this leads to increased intrathoracic pressure. In experimental models, the transmission of IAH to the thoracic cavity has been estimated to be around 50% [24]. Cardiac dysfunction and decreased output occur because of the effects on preload, contractility, and afterload.

Increased intrathoracic pressure leads to decreased inflow from the IVC and subsequently decreased cardiac preload. The elevation of the diaphragm also reduces the size of its caval opening and can constrict the IVC that further decreases venous return [25]. Parameters that have been commonly used to assess cardiac function and volume status for the critically ill may be unreliable in patients with IAH/ACS. For example, bedside ultrasound to assess the IVC size and collapsibility has been used to determine volume responsiveness [26]. This parameter may no longer be useful to assess volume responsiveness as inferior venal caval dimensions can be altered by IAH [20].

Pulse pressure variability and stroke volume variation have been used to predict patient responsiveness to volume loading. However, limited evidence suggests that the predictive ability of these parameters may be reduced in the presence of IAH/

ACS. In an IAH animal model, stroke volume variation was no longer found to be predictive of responsiveness. Pulse pressure variability remained predictive if >20.5% rather than the conventional cutoff of >11.5% [27].

Contractility of both the right and left ventricles can be impaired by IAH as well. With increased thoracic pressure and decreased thoracic volume, pulmonary arterial pressures can increase. The rise in pulmonary pressures can be large enough to cause significant increases in right ventricular afterload. The combination of reduced venous return and increased pulmonary vascular resistance can cause right ventricular failure. Due to ventricular interdependence, compromised right ventricle function can impair left ventricular function [28]. In humans, decreased left ventricular function has been noted on transesophageal echocardiography when IAH is caused by intraabdominal insufflation during laparoscopic surgery [29].

Not only can preload and contractility decrease, but an increase in afterload can occur, further impairing blood flow. Afterload increases result from two mechanisms. First, vascular resistance increases directly from increased thoracic pressure on the aorta and pulmonary vessels as well as direct pressure on the intraabdominal organs from IAH. Second, due to decreased cardiac output, there is the resultant increase in systemic vascular resistance.

Neurologic

The systemic effects of IAH are not just limited to the abdomen and chest, but also affect the central nervous system. As discussed previously, the intracranial compartment is a fixed space in adults. Inside this enclosed space are the brain parenchyma, cerebral spinal fluid, as well as the venous and arterial blood supply. Any increase in one of these components increases intracranial pressure. IAH appears to cause increased intrathoracic venous pressure that leads to elevated jugular venous pressure. The higher jugular venous pressure leads to decreased venous outflow and a rise in intracranial pressure.

Animal model data support this hypothesis. In a swine model, Bloomfield et al. measured intraabdominal, intrapleural, external jugular venous, and intracranial pressures as an abdominal balloon was inflated with saline. As IAH occurred, pleural pressure increased along with external jugular venous and intracranial pressure. Intracranial pressure was decreased with either desufflation of the intraabdominal balloon or via median sternotomy [30].

This relationship is also borne out in humans. An observational trial in trauma patients with intracranial monitors measured intraabdominal, central venous, and internal jugular venous pressures. Placement of a 15-L fluid-filled bag externally on the abdominal wall simulated increased IAH and resulted in statistically increased intracranial pressures. Temporally, pressures increased with the placement of a 15-L bag on the abdominal wall; however, the increase did not have a linear correlation between intrathoracic and intracranial pressures [31]. These findings have been confirmed in nontraumatic neurologically impaired patient populations [32] as well as in case reports of decompressive laparotomy for relieving ACS with concomitant reduction in measured intracranial pressure [33].

TREATMENT OPTIONS

Medical Management

Management strategies for ACS depend on the etiology and vary with the clinical scenario. While many recommendations exist, the clinical context is important and should be individualized to the patient.

To reduce intraabdominal pressure, the patient should have a functional nasogastric tube to decompress the stomach. A nasogastric tube is particularly important when small bowel ileus is the primary cause of IAH. If the patient has Ogilvie syndrome, or a paralytic ileus of the colon, a rectal tube, colonoscopic decompression, or neostigmine should be considered. A urinary indwelling catheter should also be in place, not only for monitoring of intraabdominal pressures and urine output, but also to decompress the bladder and to reduce the abdominal volume.

Negative fluid balance has been proposed as a useful method to reduce intraabdominal pressures. Diuresis has become an important part of the armamentarium. This treatment has not been specifically assessed in any clinical trial. Continuous venovenous hemodialysis and slow extended daily dialysis has been studied in a small series. In a study of nine patients with heterogeneous cause of critical illness, intraarterial pressure (IAP) decreased by a statistically significant difference but only from 12 to 10 mm Hg with volume removal [34]. With such limited data, no recommendation regarding hemodialysis was made by the World Society of Abdominal Compartment Syndrome [1].

Drainage of intraabdominal fluid collections is also an important adjunct in selected patients. Ascites can develop from liver failure, severe pancreatitis, or massive volume resuscitation. Hemorrhage and resultant clot formation is difficult to percutaneously drain. A study of nine patients with greater than 40% total body surface area burns who developed IAH/ACS from large volume resuscitation examined the efficacy of percutaneous drainage. Five required percutaneous drainage only and four failed percutaneous drainage and underwent decompressive laparotomy. In the percutaneous drainage-only group, 38 ± 28 mL per kg of fluid were drained by the catheter and 45 ± 20 mL per kg were removed initially in the percutaneous/decompressive laparotomy group. The author's conclusions were that drainage is a viable technique as no patient experienced any complications directly related to the percutaneous drainage [35]. In an observational matched case–control trial, 31 surgical ICU patients who had percutaneous treatment of IAH were compared with patients who had decompressive laparotomy. Bedside ultrasound was used to identify IAH/ACS patients with free fluid and to place a 14 French catheter under visualization. The IAH/ACS etiology was heterogeneous and included trauma (23%), burns (29%), postoperative (36%), and sepsis (12%) patients. Percutaneous drainage was successful for 81% of the patients with the remaining 19% of the patients requiring a decompressive laparotomy. Important predictors of failure of percutaneous drainage were drainage of less than 1,000 mL via the catheter and failure to reduce measured intraabdominal pressure by 9 mm Hg. It is important to note that during the study time period, decompressive laparotomy was performed for ACS in 265 patients. Therefore, percutaneous drainage was appropriate for a minority of patients [36].

Given that the abdominal cavity is not completely rigid, another medical management technique may include increasing the abdominal volume by relaxing the abdominal musculature with heavy sedation and neuromuscular blockade. De laet et al. performed a prospective cohort study, assessing the effect of neuromuscular blockade on nine patients with IAH. A single dose of cisatracurium reduced IAH from 18 to 14 mm Hg at 15 and 30 minutes, respectively [37].

Surgical Management

Decompressive laparotomy remains the standard of care when medical therapies fail. However, the mortality remains as high as 50% despite surgical decompression [38]. The mortality remains elevated as ACS is usually not the primary cause of the patient's critical illness. Furthermore, abdominal pressure remains elevated when measured after decompression [38]. Pulmonary and cardiac parameters improve but do not normalize. Additionally, ACS has been described in spite of the abdomen remaining open [39]. Vigilance is therefore still required after surgical decompression and it would seem prudent to continue to monitor abdominal pressures. Decompressive laparotomy is not without risks. Enterocutaneous fistula, intraabdominal abscesses, and organ failure are associated with an open abdomen [40]. The inability to close the abdominal wall may lead to a large ventral hernia.

After laparotomy, a variety of techniques have been employed for coverage of the abdominal viscera to prevent the development of entero-atmospheric fistulae, control fluid losses, and allow re-exploration. One of the easiest methods is to close the skin while leaving the fascia open beneath. Towel clips have been previously used as well as suturing the skin close. These techniques are quick and inexpensive but do not expand the abdomen volume well enough. Recurrent ACS is frequent.

Other techniques include repurposing sterile equipment as a temporary cover of the abdominal viscera. Sterile 3-L infusion bags or the Bogata bag are used by some centers. The use of sterile plastics covers for radiology cassettes has been described [41]. The drawback to these techniques is that peritoneal fluid loss is not well controlled.

Negative pressure wound therapy is now commonly employed. While there are commercially available products and suction devices, standard operating room equipment can be fashioned into a system. The benefit of this technique is that it (1) prevents the intraabdominal viscera from becoming adherent to the abdominal wall; (2) the negative pressure controls and removes fluid; (3) the negative pressure may prevent fascial retraction allowing for easier delayed abdominal wall closure; (4) dressing changes can be performed every 3 to 4 days simplifying wound management. However, cost remains a major drawback. Reported delayed closure rates vary widely in the literature.

Abdominal closure can be facilitated by placing tension on the fascia to prevent fascial retraction [42]. Protocols that specify scheduled re-exploration and partial closure with each trip to operating room has been advocated and their use has been associated with abdominal wall closure rates up to 100% [43]. Sequential closure, however, typically requires a week or more and multiple operations. Other techniques to obtain closure include acute component separation, or planned hernia with delayed component separation. Component separation closure is considered an important technique to electively repair hernias. This technique has not been studied for acutely ill patients who are not medically optimized and likely malnourished. The failure of component separation in the acute setting makes this method unavailable in the future for that patient when it would likely be successful. Current recommendations are to reserve component separation for elective repairs for medically optimized patients [44]. If the decision is to allow the patient to have a large abdominal wall hernia, coverage of the abdominal viscera with a split thickness skin graft or skin-only closure will usually be required.

PREVENTION

Prevention of ACS is an important strategy. Damage control resuscitation has been advocated for trauma patients. Among these patients, low normal blood pressure is permitted and over-resuscitation avoided. This concept emphasizes early control of hemorrhage, transfusion of blood and blood products, and reduced administration of crystalloids [45].

The type of fluid as well as the volume infused may prove consequential in secondary compartment syndrome. The use of albumin has been examined for burn patients. While a single-center study showed no change in the occurrence of ACS by including albumin along with crystalloids in burn resuscitation [46], another prospective study showed decreased intraabdominal pressures [47]. A meta-analysis suggested albumin use decreased the occurrence of all compartment syndromes but this study did not differentiate between the types of compartment syndromes [48]. The use of fluid types other than crystalloids as well as other patient populations and fluid effects on the development of ACS is unclear.

Damage control surgery and deciding not to close the abdomen at the index operation is also an important part of prevention. Data here is sparse. For trauma patients, major liver injury or any other injury requiring packing for hemostasis is one consideration. The occurrence of ACS was reduced from 80% to less than 24% in a retrospective cohort trial of severely injured trauma patients [49]. A small series examined the outcomes of 27 patients with a ruptured abdominal aortic aneurysm who were repaired by the open technique. In a retrospective analysis of patients who remained intubated postoperatively and had shock, colonic ischemia and ACS occurred only those patients with IAP of 21 mm Hg or higher [50]. The limitation of course is that the IAP was monitored postoperatively. Current societal recommendations for trauma and emergency surgery patients suggest the following intraoperative markers to consider leaving the abdomen open: large volume resuscitation defined as transfusion of greater than 10 units of packed red blood cells or the administration of greater than 15 L of crystalloid. Other factors to consider include hypothermia (temperature less than 35°C) and acidosis with a pH <7.2 [51].

CONCLUSIONS

Abdominal hypertension and ACS are common among surgical and medical patients, have significant detrimental physiologic effects, and are associated with an increase in mortality. Many risk factors for the development of IAH and ACS have been described. Selection of particular patients for intravesicular pressure monitoring remains unclear. The accuracy, feasibility, and low cost of intravesicular pressure monitoring should make unrecognized IAH/ACS uncommon. The many medical and surgical treatments available should be tailored to the individual patient. Decompressive laparotomy, however, remains the most common treatment option for ACS with organ dysfunction.

References

1. Kirkpatrick AW, Roberts DJ, De Waele J, et al: Intra-abdominal hypertension and the abdominal compartment syndrome: updated consensus definitions and clinical practice guidelines from the World Society of the Abdominal Compartment Syndrome. *Intensive Care Med* 39:1190–1206, 2013.
2. Carr JA: Abdominal compartment syndrome. *J Am Coll Surg* 216(1):135–146, 2013.
3. De Keulenaer BL, De Waele JJ, Powell B, et al: What is normal intra-abdominal pressure and how is it affected by positioning, body mass and positive end expiratory pressure. *Intensive Care Med* 35:969–976, 2009.
4. Sugarman H, Windsor A, Bessos M, et al: Intra-abdominal pressure, sagital abdominal diameter, obesity comorbidity. *J Intern Med* 241:71–79, 1997.
5. Malbrain ML, Chiumello D, Pelosi P, et al: Prevalence of intra-abdominal hypertension in critically ill patients: a Multicentre Epidemiological Study. *Intensive Care Med* 30:822–829, 2004.
6. Malbrain ML, Chiumello D, Pelosi P, et al: Incidence and prognosis of intra-abdominal hypertension in a mixed population of critically ill patients: a multiple-center epidemiological study. *Crit Care Med* 33:315–322, 2005.
7. Vidal MG, Ruiz Weisser J, Gonzalez F, et al: Incidence and clinical effects of intra-abdominal hypertension in critically ill patients. *Crit Care Med* 36:1823–1831, 2008.
8. Diaz JJ, Cullinane DC, Dutton WD: The management of the open abdomen in trauma and emergency general surgery: part 1-damage control. *J Trauma* 68(6):1425–1438, 2010.
9. Starkopf J, Tamme K, Blaser A: Should we measure intra-abdominal pressures in every intensive care patient. *Ann Intensive Care* 2[Suppl 1]:S9, 2012.
10. Sugrue MJ, Bauman A, Jones F, et al: Clinical examination is an inaccurate predictor of intraabdominal pressure. *World J Surg* 26:1428–1431, 2002.

11. Kirkpatrick AW, Brenneman FD, McLean RF, et al: Is clinical examination an accurate indicator of raised intra-abdominal pressure in critically injured patients. *Can J Surg* 43(3):207–211, 2000.
12. Malbrain ML, Roberts DJ, De laet I, et al: The role of abdominal compliance, the neglected parameter in critically ill patients—a consensus review of 16. Part 1: definitions and pathophysiology. *Anaesthesiol Intensive Ther* 46(5):392–405, 2014.
13. Gudmundsson FF, Viste A, Gislason H, et al: Comparison of different methods for measuring intra-abdominal pressure. *Intensive Care Med* 28(4):509–514, 2002.
14. Risin E, Kessel B, Ashkenazi I, et al: A new technique of direct intra-abdominal pressure measurement: a preliminary study. *Am J of Surg* 191:235–237, 2006.
15. De Waele j, Pletinckx P, Blot S, et al: Saline volume in transvesical intra-abdominal pressure measurement: enough is enough. *Intensive Care Med* 32:455–459, 2006.
16. Cheatham ML, De Waele JJ, De Laet I, et al: The impact of body position on intra-abdominal pressure measurement: a multicenter analysis. *Crit Care Med* 37:2187–2190, 2009.
17. McBeth PB, Zygun DA, Widder S, et al: Effect of patient positioning on intra-abdominal pressure monitoring. *Am J Surg* 193:644–647, 2007.
18. Cortes-Puentes GA, Cortes-Puentes LA, Adams AB, et al: Experimental intra-abdominal hypertension influences airway pressure limits for lung protective mechanical ventilation. *J Trauma Acute Care Surg* 24:1468–1473, 2013.
19. Lui F, Sangosanya A, Kaplan LJ: Abdominal compartment syndrome: clinical aspects and monitoring. *Crit Care Clin* 23(3):415–433, 2007.
20. Cavaliere F, Cina A, Biasucci D, et al: Sonographic assessment of abdominal vein dimensional and hemodynamic changes induced in human volunteers by a model of abdominal hypertension. *Crit Care Med* 39(2):344–348, 2011.
21. Dalfino L, Tullo L, Donadio I, et al: Intra-abdominal hypertension and acute renal failure in critically ill patients. *Intensive Care Med* 34:707–713, 2008.
22. Biancofiore G, Bindi ML, Romanelli AM, et al: Post-operative intra-abdominal pressure and renal function after liver transplantation. *Arch Surg* 138:703–706, 2003.
23. Hazebroek EJ, de Vos tot Nederveen Cappel R, Gommers D, et al: Antidiuretic hormone release during laparoscopic donor nephrectomy. *Arch Surg* 137(5):600–605, 2002.
24. Wauters J, Claus P, Brosens N, et al: Relationship between abdominal pressure, pulmonary compliance, and cardiac preload in a porcine model. *Crit Care Res Pract* 2012:763–781, 2012.
25. Malbrain ML, De Waele JJ, De Keulenaer BL: What every ICU clinician needs to know about the cardiovascular effects caused by abdominal hypertension. *Anaesthesiol Intensive Ther* 47(4):388–399, 2015.
26. Gunst M, Ghaemmaghami V, Sperry J, et al: Accuracy of cardiac function and volume status estimates using the bedside echocardiographic assessment in trauma/critical care. *J Trauma* 65:509–516, 2008.
27. Renner J, Gruenewald M, Quaden R, et al: Influence of increased intra-abdominal pressure on fluid responsiveness predicted by pulse pressure variation and stroke volume variation in a porcine model. *Crit Care Med* 37:650–658, 2009.
28. Pinsky M: Heart lung interactions. *Curr Opin Crit Care* 13:528–531, 2007.
29. Sakka SG, Huettemann E, Petrat G, et al: Transesophageal echocardiographic assessment of haemodynamic changes during laparoscopic herniorrhaphy in small children. *Br J Anaesth* 84(3):330–334, 2000.
30. Bloomfield GL, Ridings PC, Blocher CR, et al: A proposed relationship between increased intra-abdominal, intrathoracic, and intracranial pressure. *Crit Care Med* 25(3):496–503, 1997.
31. Citerio G, Vascotto E, Villa F, et al: Induced abdominal compartment syndrome increases intracranial pressure in neurotrauma patients: a prospective study. *Crit Care Med* 29:1466–1471, 2001.
32. Dereen DH, Dits H, Malbrain ML: Correlation between intra-abdominal and intracranial pressure in nontraumatic brain injury. *Intensive Care Med* 31:1577–1581, 2005.
33. Dorfman JD, Burns JD, Green DM, et al: Decompressive laparotomy for refractory intracranial hypertension after traumatic brain injury. *Neurocrit Care*15:516–518, 2011.
34. De Laet I, Deeren D, Schoonheydt K, et al: Renal replacement therapy with net fluid removal lowers intra-abdominal pressure and volumetric indices in critically ill patients. *Ann Intensive Care* 2[Suppl 1]: S20, 2012.
35. Latenser BA, Kowal-Vern A, Kimball D, et al: A pilot study comparing percutaneous decompression with decompressive laparotomy for acute abdominal compartment syndrome in thermal injury. *J Burn Care Rehabil* 23:190–195, 2002.
36. Cheatham ML, Safcsak K: Percutaneous catheter decompression in the treatment of elevated intraabdominal pressure. *Chest* 140(6):1428–1435, 2011.
37. De lae I, Hoste E, Verholen E, et al: The effect of neuromuscular blockade in patients with intra-abdominal hypertension. *Intensive Care Med* 33:1811–1814, 2007.
38. De Waele JJ, Hoste EA, Malbrain ML: Decompressive laparotomy for abdominal compartment syndrome—a critical analysis. *Crit Care* 10(2):R51, 2006.
39. Gracias VH, Braslow B, Johnson J, et al: Abdominal compartment syndrome in the open abdomen. *Arch Surg* 137(11):1298–1300, 2002.
40. Losanoff JE, Richman BW, Jones JW: Temporary abdominal coverage and reclosure of the open abdomen: frequently asked questions. *J Am Coll Surg* 195(1):105–115, 2002.
41. Tremblay LN, Feliciano DV, Schmidt J, et al: Skin only or silo closure in the critically ill patient with an open abdomen. *Am J Surg* 182(6):670–675, 2001.
42. Dennis A, Vizinas TA, Joseph K, et al: Not so fast to skin graft: transabdominal wall traction closes most "domain loss" abdomens in the acute setting. *J Trauma Acute Care Surg* 74:1486–1492, 2013.
43. Burlew CC, Moore EE, Biffl WL, et al: One hundred percent fascial approximation can be achieved in the postinjury open abdomen with a sequential closure protocol. *J Trauma Acute Care Surg* 72:235–241, 2012.
44. Diaz JJ Jr, Dutton WD, Ott MM, et al: Eastern association for the surgery of trauma: a review of the management of the open abdomen-part 2 "Management of the open abdomen". *J Trauma* 71(2):502–512, 2011.
45. Cotton BA, Reddy N, Hatch QM: Damage control resuscitation is associated with a reduction in resuscitation volumes and improvement in survival in 390 damage control laparotomy patients. *Ann Surg* 254(4):598–605, 2011.
46. Park SH, Hemmila MR, Wahl W: Early albumin use improves mortality in difficult to resuscitate burn patients. *J Trauma Acute Care Surg* 73(5):1294–1297, 2012.
47. O'Mara MS, Slater H, Goldfarb IW, et al: A prospective, randomized evaluation of intra-abdominal pressures with crystalloid and colloid resuscitation in burn patients. *J Trauma* 58(5):1011–1018, 2005.
48. Navickis RJ, Greenhalgh DG, Wilkes MM: Albumin in burn shock resuscitation: a meta-analysis of controlled clinical studies. *J Burn Care Res* 37(3):e268–e278, 2016.
49. Offner PJ, de Souza AL, Moore, EE: Avoidance of abdominal compartment syndrome in damage-control laparotomy after trauma. *Arch Surg* 136:676–680, 2001.
50. Djavani K, Wanhainen A, Bjorck M: Intra-abdominal hypertension and abdominal compartment syndrome following surgery for ruptured abdominal aortic aneurysm. *Eur J Vasc Endovasc Surg* 31:581–584, 2006.
51. Diaz JJ Jr, Cullinane DC, Dutton WD, et al: The management of the open abdomen in trauma and emergency general surgery: part 1-damage control. *J Trauma* 68(6):1425–1438, 2010.

Chapter 53 ■ Management of the Obstetrical Patient in the Intensive Care Setting

ANNE GARRISON

Up to 300,000 women died worldwide in 2015 as a result of pregnancy-related conditions [1]. Maternal mortality has been decreasing each year since 1990, with the greatest reductions in these deaths coming in developed countries. However, the overall rate in the United States has increased [2]. In 2013, the maternal mortality ratio was 18.5 per 100,000 live births, an increase of 1.7 percent from the rate of 1990 [3]. It is unknown if this difference is due to an improvement of identifying and coding for pregnancy-related deaths [4], or if it should be attributed to increases in maternal age, body mass index, and comorbidities. The leading cause of maternal mortality in the United States is cardiovascular disease and cardiomyopathy. Other common causes of mortality include thromboembolic events, hemorrhage, infections, and amniotic fluid embolism [5]. It is not surprising that, because the intensive care unit (ICU) is a common setting for care of these patients, both maternal and fetal mortality are high when a pregnant patient is admitted to the ICU [6].

This chapter will review the maternal anatomic and physiologic adaptations to pregnancy, considerations of potential fetal harm from diagnostic studies or medication administration, and specific pregnancy disease states that may complicate the care of the critically ill pregnant patient such as preeclampsia, eclampsia, obstetric hemorrhage, and trauma. Specifics related to the diagnosis and treatment of respiratory failure and other common medical problems in pregnancy is discussed elsewhere in the text (Chapter 164).

MATERNAL PHYSIOLOGIC ADAPTATIONS TO PREGNANCY

Cardiovascular System

The cardiovascular system undergoes significant alteration during pregnancy. The major changes seen include an increase in cardiac output, blood volume expansion, and reductions in systemic vascular resistance and blood pressure (BP). These changes start early in the first trimester, peak in the second trimester, and remain constant until delivery [7]. Hemodynamic changes surrounding labor and delivery are also significant.

Cardiac output rises up to 50% above baseline during pregnancy, with half of this rise coming in the first trimester. Cardiac output increases by several mechanisms including: (1) increasing preload (rise in blood volume), (2) decreasing afterload (decrease in vascular resistance) and (3) a rise in heart rate [8]. Initially, the increase in cardiac output comes from the rise in stroke volume, and later in pregnancy, heart rate is the major factor. Ejection fraction stays constant throughout pregnancy. This increase in workload can cause heart disease in women to decompensate during the later part of pregnancy. Both plasma volume and red blood cell mass expand during pregnancy; however, there is greater plasma expansion than red blood cell production, resulting in a physiologic anemia of pregnancy [9]. Both systolic and diastolic BPs fall early in pregnancy and average 5 to 10 mm Hg below baseline. In the third trimester, BP normalizes [10]. The drop in BP is induced by a reduction in systemic vascular resistance, the mechanism of which is not completely understood, though both are likely to be hormonally and placentally mediated.

Respiratory Adaptations

The respiratory tract undergoes profound changes during pregnancy. Progesterone is a known stimulant of both respiration and respiratory drive [11]. A relevant hyperventilation therefore occurs in pregnancy. Minute ventilation rises almost 50% by term, largely secondary to an increase in tidal volume [12]. Functional residual capacity decreases by 20% due to an upward shift of the diaphragm. Expiratory reserve volume and residual volume also decrease. However, inspiratory capacity increases, resulting in only minimally decreased total lung capacity [13]. There is an increase in PaO_2 and a decrease in $PaCO_2$ levels. This respiratory alkalosis leads to a compensatory excretion of bicarbonate by the kidneys, resulting in a relatively normal pH (7.4 to 7.45) [14]. Measurements of pulmonary function and disease should be interpreted in the context of the above changes [15].

Hematologic Adaptations

As stated previously, plasma volume during pregnancy increases by 50% from prepregnancy levels. The red cell mass will increase to a lesser degree. This phenomenon has been termed the physiologic anemia of pregnancy [16,17].

Increased catecholamine and steroid levels during pregnancy cause a demargination of mature leukocytes from the endothelium. This leads to a physiologic leukocytosis of pregnancy, with the white blood cell count increasing by 5,000 to 10,000 cells per mL [16,17].

Pregnancy is associated with changes in several clotting factors (resistance to activated protein C, decreases in protein S, increase in factors I, II, V, VII, X, and XII). This results in a reduction in prothrombin and partial thromboplastin times [18,19]. The net effect is the production of a hypercoagulable state. Venous thromboembolism occurs more frequently during pregnancy and presents a three to fourfold higher risk in the peripartum period than during pregnancy [20].

TABLE 53.1

Physiologic Maternal Adaptation to Pregnancy

System	Alternations
Cardiovascular	Cardiac output increased 20%–30%
Blood pressure	Decreased
Peripheral vascular resistance	Decreased
Pulmonary system	Tidal volume increased Respiratory rate increased Functional residual capacity reduced
Renal system	Renal artery perfusion increased Glomerular filtration rate increased Creatinine clearance increased BUN, serum creatinine, serum uric acid decreased Urinary stasis increased Dilated renal pelvises and ureters
Hematologic system	Plasma volume increased >RBC volume increase Leukocytosis Increased liver-produced clotting factors Increased fibrinogen Hypercoagulable state

BUN, blood urea nitrogen; RBC, red blood cell.

Renal Adaptations

Normal pregnancy provides both anatomic and functional changes to the renal system. The kidneys increase in size by 1 to 1.5 cm. The renal pelvises and calyces may be dilated and hydronephrosis and hydroureter may be seen in up to 80% of women [21]. Glomerular filtration rate (GFR) rises markedly during pregnancy, due to increases in cardiac output and renal blood flow. This results in a decrease in serum creatinine concentration. Among pregnant women with a normal serum creatinine at baseline, the creatinine may remain within the normal range despite a significantly reduced GFR. A small rise in serum creatinine usually reflects a marked reduction in renal function. Hence, careful attention to small fluctuations of serum creatinine is required to detect renal injury during pregnancy (Table 53.1).

DIAGNOSTIC RADIATION EXPOSURE

When caring for any critically ill patient, diagnostic imaging is critically important. When the patient is pregnant, care must be taken to weigh the risk of the imaging study with the potential change in management given the outcome of that study.

It is important to remember that there are no studies of humans to evaluate the risk of radiation. Most evidence is case reports and data from survivors of nuclear bombings/accidents [22,23].

There are four areas of potential harm when assessing radiation exposure: pregnancy loss, fetal malformations, disturbances of growth/development, and carcinogenic effects. The effect radiation will have on a fetus depends on the gestational age at the time of exposure and the dose of radiation that the fetus is exposed to.

The majority of diagnostic procedures expose the fetus to less than 0.05 Gy of radiation. There is no evidence that this level of exposure increases the risk of fetal anomalies, disability, growth restriction, or pregnancy loss at these levels; however, these low levels may increase the risk of childhood leukemia [24,25]. The threshold at which a fetus sustains risk is not completely known, though evidence suggests that the risk of malformations increases at doses greater than 0.1 Gy.

The timing of exposure is also important. The fetus is most sensitive to radiation exposure early in pregnancy. In early pregnancy, the "all or none" phenomenon applies, which means that the fetus either survives intact or is resorbed. This is true for the first 14 days after conception [26]. After the first 14 days, an embryo can be damaged. In the first trimester, the most common abnormalities seen are growth restriction or central nervous system abnormalities [27]. Radiation levels needed for these mutations are 0.1 to 0.2 Gy prior to 16 weeks and 0.5 to 0.7 Gy after 16 weeks of gestation [28]. Growth restriction usually is not seen until >1 Gy. After 20 weeks, the fetus is resistant to the teratogenic effects of radiation [29].

There are no known fetal effects from exposure to ultrasound or magnetic resonance imaging (MRI). MRI examinations are used as an adjunct to ultrasound in the second and third trimesters to aid in the diagnosis of certain fetal anomalies. Contrast agents should be avoided during the first trimester [30,31].

If a significant alteration in management is to be undertaken as a result of the information obtained from the procedure, the potential fetal risk should be considered. If excessive radiation doses to the pelvis are administered inadvertently, it is important to calculate the fetal isodose radiation exposure. An excess of 10 cGy delivered to the fetus may lead to significant fetal effects. Table 53.2 outlines both the amount of radiation of common imaging studies and the potential fetal effects of radiation exposure.

TABLE 53.2

Radiation Dose and Fetal Effects

Radiation dose to fetus (cGy)	Theoretical or actual fetal effect
0–5	No reported malformation; potential for oncogenesis, and increased cancer risk
5–10	Potential for oncogenesis; potential for IUGR
10–20	Microcephaly, IUGR, 2.4% mental retardation
20–50	Microcephaly, IUGR, fetal death, mental retardation
50–100	Microcephaly, IUGR, 18% mental retardation, fetal death

IUGR, intrauterine growth retardation.
From Gianopoulos JG: Breast disease in pregnancy, in Isaccs JH (ed): *Textbook of Breast Disease*. Philadelphia, PA, Mosby-Year Book, 1992, p 131, with permission.

MEDICATIONS AND PREGNANCY

Analgesic Agents

Opiate narcotic agents administered for short periods of time have been shown to be safe during pregnancy. They have shown no adverse fetal effects. Chronic opiate use during pregnancy has been associated with intrauterine growth restriction and neonatal abstinence syndrome [32].

Nonsteroidal antiinflammatory agents may decrease fetal renal blood flow, leading to oligohydramnios. They also will lead to the in utero closure of the ductus arteriosus, producing fetal pulmonary hypertension after 32 weeks of gestation. Short courses of indomethacin may be used with caution prior to 32 weeks of gestation.

Antibiotics

Penicillins, cephalosporins, erythromycin, clindamycin, and vancomycin are considered safe during pregnancy. There is some concern regarding renal toxicity with vancomycin. Aminoglycosides have been implicated in fetal ototoxicity [33]. However, only streptomycin and kanamycin have been implicated. Gentamicin has not been reported to have significant ototoxicity and is used commonly during pregnancy. Sulfonamides compete with bilirubin-binding sites and may lead to neonatal kernicterus if administered during the third trimester. Tetracycline is teratogenic, leading to brown teeth and abnormal long bone development [33–35] (Table 53.3).

Anticoagulants

Unfractionated heparin, because of its molecular size and ionic negative charge, has been shown not to cross the placental membrane [36]. Therefore, it is the anticoagulant of choice in all trimesters of pregnancy and may be used with relative fetal safety. Fractionated heparins also have been shown not to cross the placental membrane. They may be used throughout

TABLE 53.3

Antibiotics during Pregnancy

Safe in pregnancy
Penicillins/cephalosporins
Fosfomycin
Nitrofurantoin
Vancomycin
Clindamycin
Azithromycin, erythromycin
Risks in pregnancy
Aminoglycosides: renal and ototoxic, OK in life-threatening conditions
Tetracycline: bone demineralization and teeth staining
Sulfa drugs: OK in second trimester, risk of birth defects in first trimester, and kernicterus in third trimester
Fluoroquinolones: toxic to cartilage development

pregnancy as well. If fractionated heparins are used during pregnancy, it is advised to change to unfractionated heparin late in the third trimester because when surgical intervention is needed, unfractionated heparin may be reversed with protamine sulfate and because regional anesthesia can be used after reversal [37]. Warfarin and its derivatives are contraindicated during the first trimester as these agents are teratogenic, producing midline defects such as clefts, cardiac septal defect, and limb bud abnormalities. In all trimesters, warfarin crosses the placenta and may lead to spontaneous fetal bleeding [38–40]. In some selected cardiac patients (particularly those with mechanical valves), warfarin may be used during the second and early third trimesters. Fetal intracranial bleeding has been observed with warfarin use during the late third trimester.

Antihypertensives

Pregnant patients will require acute antihypertensive intervention when the systolic BP exceeds 160 mm Hg or the diastolic BP exceeds 110 mm Hg. Preservation of the fetal circulation must be kept in mind when treating these conditions. For the acute management of hypertensive crisis in pregnancy, labetolol or hydralazine are recommended [41,42]. Hydralazine is dosed as 10 mg IV push. Labetolol is given as a 10-mg dose IV, followed by a 20-mg dose at 10 minutes if no response is observed. If still no response in BP is observed, the dose may be increased to 40 mg in 10 minutes and followed by 80 mg in 10 minutes. The 80 mg dose may be repeated one time. The total dose should not exceed 220 mg [43,44].

Angiotensin-converting enzyme inhibitors and angiotensin receptor blocker agents are contraindicated during pregnancy. They have been associated with fetal anomalies and intrauterine fetal death secondary to fetal cardiovascular collapse.

SPECIFIC PREGNANCY DISORDERS

Hypertensive Disorders of Pregnancy

Preeclampsia is most commonly defined as hypertension (>140/90) in combination with proteinuria (>300 mg per day) beginning after the 20th week of pregnancy in a previously normotensive person. Eclampsia is defined as meeting the criteria for preeclampsia with the addition of seizures. Preeclampsia and eclampsia are multisystem diseases that develop only during pregnancy or, more rarely, during the postpartum period. Previously, preeclampsia was defined as mild or severe. In 2013, the American Congress of Obstetrics and Gynecology changed the categories; preeclampsia is now defined as being "with" or "without" severe features. Severe features are defined as BP >160/110 mmHg, or evidence of end organ disease. They also removed proteinuria as an essential criterion for diagnosis of preeclampsia with severe features and removed massive proteinuria (5 g per 24 hours) and fetal growth restriction as possible features of severe disease [45].

The underlying cause of preeclampsia is not fully understood, but likely involves maternal, fetal, and placental factors. Abnormalities of blood vessel development can result in placental underperfusion, hypoxia, and ischemia [46]. The severity of disease is influenced not only by maternal and placental factors but also likely by paternal and environmental factors [47].

It is the complications of preeclampsia that usually indicate ICU admission. Sequelae include refractory hypertension, neurologic manifestations (seizure, intercranial hemorrhage, and elevated intracranial pressure), renal failure, liver failure or rupture, pulmonary edema, HELLP syndrome, or disseminated intravascular coagulation (DIC) [6].

Management

Though all of the complications of preeclampsia can be treated, the ultimate treatment for preeclampsia is delivery. If a patient who develops preeclampsia is near term, prompt delivery is the recommendation. Patients who are preterm without evidence of severe features can be managed expectantly with close monitoring until term gestation is reached (37 weeks) or severe features develop. For selected patients remote from term with severe features, expectant management can be undertaken at a tertiary care center [45]. Patients remote from term should be given steroids to enhance fetal pulmonary maturity. Patients with severe features should be treated with IV magnesium. It has been shown to be superior to other antiepileptics for the prevention of seizure activity [48,49]. Magnesium is given as a 4-g bolus IV over the first hour, then at 2 g per hour until 24 hours post delivery with monitoring of reflexes and magnesium levels.

ICU care involves managing the complications of preeclampsia:

1. **Severe hypertension:** BP greater than 160/110 mmHg is generally treated with IV antihypertensives. Labetolol and hydralazine are the drugs of choice [50]. Exact dosing is the same as the algorithm above.
2. **Seizures:** Eclamptic seizures are treated with IV magnesium. In cases unresponsive to magnesium, benzodiazepines may be used. When the seizure activity persists, the next agent of choice is phenytoin. In severe refractory cases, muscle paralysis with general anesthesia and ventilatory support may be needed [48].
3. **DIC:** Treatment of DIC involves identifying the underlying cause. Placental abruption is a common cause among those with preeclampsia. Aggressive resuscitation with blood products to reverse coagulopathy is sometimes needed.
4. **Pulmonary edema:** Pulmonary edema may present with dyspnea or acute respiratory failure. Supportive management includes supplemental oxygen and fluid restriction. Diuresis is indicated when there is fluid overload, although this is rare because most patients are volume depleted.

Obstetrical Hemorrhage

Vaginal bleeding during pregnancy is a common event. The source of the bleeding is almost always maternal. The evaluation, differential diagnosis, and management of bleeding differ by trimester and volume. Vaginal bleeding during the third trimester can be a medical emergency. When significant hemorrhage occurs, prompt medical or surgical intervention is needed.

Antepartum Hemorrhage

The most common cause of bleeding during the first trimester is miscarriage. Miscarriage is common (up to 25% of pregnancies), and significant bleeding requiring transfusion, while rare, does occur [51]. Another less prevalent (~2% of pregnancies) cause of hemorrhage during the first trimester is ectopic pregnancy. Rupture of an ectopic pregnancy can be a life-threatening emergency and aggressive monitoring of hemodynamic status, fluid resuscitation, and administration of blood products may be required. Vaginal bleeding in the second and third trimester is less common but may be a medical emergency dependent on etiology; the possibilities are described below.

Placenta Previa

Placenta previa is defined as the placental tissue extending to or covering the cervical os. This diagnosis is uncommon, occurring in ~4/1,000 births [52], but the sequelae of this condition has the potential for severe bleeding. Classically, the patient with placenta previa will resent with painless vaginal bleeding; however, some women will present with pain or contractions in association with bleeding [53,54]. Any woman without an ultrasound documenting placental location who presents with bleeding should undergo ultrasound evaluation for placental location. Ultrasound should be performed prior to digital examination of the cervix to avoid palpation of the placenta and severe hemorrhage.

Women with placenta previa are at increased risk of hemorrhage during the antepartum, intrapartum, and postpartum periods [55]. They are therefore more likely to undergo blood transfusion, peripartum hysterectomy, uterine artery embolization to have a placenta accreta [56]. Maternal mortality secondary to previa is low in resource-rich countries; however, in the third world, this remains a high risk of maternal mortality [56]. Because the risk of severe bleeding and emergent, unscheduled delivery outweigh the risks of late preterm birth, delivery of patients with known previa is recommended by cesarean section between 36 and 37 weeks of gestation [57,58].

Though an actively bleeding placenta previa is a potential emergency, most cases of acute bleeding are self-limited. Patients should be admitted, a complete blood count and Type and Screen should be sent. Fetal monitoring should be employed. If the bleeding is active, both the mother and fetus should be closely monitored and supportive care provided. Indications for emergent cesarean delivery include refractory, life-threatening hemorrhage, non-reassuring fetal status or a significant bleed after 34 weeks of gestation. If the bleeding episode is self-limited, the patient can be monitored in the hospital. A course of antenatal corticosteroids should be given for fetal benefit given the potential for preterm delivery. If the patient is Rh negative, Rhogam should be given. When delivery is undertaken, close coordination and planning with anesthesia should be undertaken as the presence of previa increases the risk of hemorrhage and placenta accreta and percreta.

Abruption Placenta

Placental abruption is the premature separation of the placenta from the uterus (prior to the delivery of the infant). Abruption occurs in up to 1% of pregnancies and may be small and not clinically significant or may lead to severe life-threatening bleeding and DIC.

The clinical presentation of abruption is vaginal bleeding with associated uterine pain or contractions. There may or may not be associated fetal distress. In severe cases, DIC and coagulopathy occur. The bleeding may be vaginal or confined to the uterus, so the amount of vaginal bleeding is not a reliable indicator of severity. Ultrasound is not a reliable indicator of abruption (only 2% of abruption can be visualized on ultrasound). If coagulopathy occurs, resuscitation with blood-replacement products such as fresh-frozen plasma or cryoprecipitate should occur [59]. The definitive management is delivery and resuscitation. If the patient is preterm and the abruption is limited and fetal status is not affected, potential inpatient surveillance can be undertaken. Antenatal corticosteroids are given for fetal lung maturity.

Postpartum Hemorrhage

Significant hemorrhage postpartum occurs among 2% to 5% of deliveries. The most common cause is uterine atony. Other causes include retained products of conception, lacerations of the cervix and vagina, and unrecognized coagulopathies [60]. Blood loss of more than 500 mL at vaginal delivery or 1,000 mL at cesarean section is classified as postpartum hemorrhage. Delayed hemorrhage, 3 to 7 days postpartum, most often is due to retained placental fragments or unrecognized congenital coagulopathies [60].

The initial assessment should include a determination of the cause of hemorrhage. Careful examination of the cervix and vagina to assess for unrecognized lacerations is warranted. Manual exploration of the uterus is performed both to assess tone and to apply uterine massage if atony is noted. If uterine atony is encountered, uterotonics are given. Pitocin (oxytocin) is usually first line and is given IV with 20 to 40 units mixed in IV fluids [60–62].

If uterine atony persists, several other uterotonics may be given. Methergine, misoprostol and Hemabate may all be used and the order in which they are used does not appear to be important. Methergine is an ergot derivative. It is given as 0.2 mg IM and is contraindicated for patients with hypertension, as significant elevations in BP may occur. Hemabate and misoprostol are prostaglandins. Hemabate is given as 250 μg IM [63]. Misoprostol is given rectally at 400 to 800 μg. Hemabate may cause significant bronchospasm and is contraindicated for patients with asthma.

If medical management of postpartum hemorrhage is unsuccessful, surgical intervention is needed. An intrauterine examination under anesthesia for retained products and dilatation and uterine curettage may be performed. If still unresponsive, uterine artery embolization may be attempted. In cases of unresponsive atony, laparotomy and uterine-constricting b-lynch suture may be performed. If all measures have failed to resolve the bleeding, hysterectomy may be employed as a last resort [64–66].

Amniotic Fluid Embolism

Amniotic fluid embolism is an extremely rare event. Incidence is 1 to 12 cases per 100,000 deliveries [67]. Clinically, patients present with sudden onset of cardiovascular and respiratory collapse at or around the time of delivery [68]. When amniotic fluid enters the intervascular space, vasoactive and fibrinolytic components precipitate cardiovascular collapse and respiratory failure. Immediate identification and aggressive treatment is required. Despite this, mortality rates are still as high as 50% [69].

Intubation and mechanical ventilation with positive end-expiratory pressure is employed. Inotropic and vasoconstrictor agents are needed for cardiac and vascular support. Invasive right-sided cardiac monitoring is also indicated. These patients will often experience a rapid and fulminant DIC, requiring resuscitation with fresh-frozen plasma and cryoprecipitate. These patients require intensive monitoring and support. Extra corporeal membrane oxygenation has been used to rescue patients with refractory cardiorespiratory collapse. If the patient survives the initial insult, most will survive [70,71].

Trauma Complicating Pregnancy

Trauma is the most common cause of death during pregnancy not related to obstetric factors. Motor vehicle accidents and domestic violence make up the majority of cases; however, there are many other potential causes of trauma. Though trauma is a common occurrence during pregnancy, less than 1% will require hospitalization [72].

The physiologic alterations of pregnancy are discussed in detail above. Because of these, particularly the increased blood volume, the pregnant trauma patient is less likely to immediately manifest signs of shock. The abdominal position of the uterus in the third trimester makes this organ more susceptible to both blunt and penetrating trauma. As the uterus grows, the bladder is pulled superior and rendered more susceptible to traumatic injury in pregnancy.

Motor vehicle accidents account for 60% of injuries in pregnancy. The pregnancy outcome is directly related to the severity of maternal injuries. The most common cause of fetal death is maternal death [73,74].

Following blunt injury secondary to a motor vehicle accident, placental abruption is the most common complication associated with the pregnancy. Placental abruption occurs among 2% to 4% of patients with these injuries. Ultrasound to detect placental abruption is not sensitive, as stated above [74–76]. Contraction monitoring with a tocometer has a high negative predictive value for abruption and most abruptions will occur during the first 4 to 8 hours postinjury. No consensus exists as to the length of the post-trauma monitoring interval, but at least 4 hours is recommended [77,78]. Rarely, a delayed abruption up to 48 hours postinjury may occur. There is no sensitive test to predict delayed abruption. However, if fetal–maternal hemorrhage is observed, the incidence is higher. Patients can be screened with a Kleihauer–Betke assay to assess for fetal–maternal bleeding [79]. If positive, a longer period of observation may be indicated. As small amounts of fetal blood may enter the maternal circulation, all patients require blood type and screen, and Rh-negative patients should receive Rhogam. Continuous fetal monitoring should occur. The usual markers of severity of maternal illness—BP, heart rate, hematocrit, and arterial partial pressure of carbon dioxide—are not predictive of fetal outcomes. Imaging studies with ultrasound are the first line for assessment. In the second and third trimesters, computed tomography scans of the abdomen and pelvis may be undertaken when indicated. In severe cases, cesarean section may improve maternal outcomes, by removing the placental arteriovenous shunt [80]. Potential maternal lifesaving cesarean delivery can be performed at ~4 to 5 minutes into maternal code to attempt to remove placental blood flow.

Penetrating Trauma

Penetrating injuries of pregnant patients most commonly are gunshot wounds or knife wounds. Pregnant patients have a better prognosis after penetrating abdominal trauma as the large muscular uterus protects maternal vital organs. Maternal visceral injuries complicate 19% of penetrating abdominal trauma with a 3.9% maternal mortality rate [81]. The anterior and central location of the uterus subjects the fetus to significant risk from penetrating wounds. The fetus is injured in 66% of these cases, with a high 40% to 70% fetal mortality rate [82]. The management of these injuries remains controversial. Many experts advocate surgical exploration. Conservative management with imagining and observation may also be considered. A coordinated effort between the trauma surgeon and obstetrician is important for achieving the best outcomes for both mother and fetus [81–83].

References

1. Alkema L, Chou D, Hogan D, et al: Global, regional, and national levels and trends in maternal mortality between 1990 and 2015, with scenario-based projections to 2030: a systematic analysis by the UN Maternal Mortality Estimation Inter-Agency Group. *Lancet* 387:462–474, 2016.
2. Hogan MC, Foreman KJ, Naghavi M, et al: Maternal mortality for 181 countries, 1980–2008: a systematic analysis of progress towards Millennium Development Goal 5. *Lancet* 375:1609–1623, 2010.
3. Kassebaum NJ, Bertozzi-Villa A, Coggeshall MS, et al: Global, regional, and national levels and causes of maternal mortality during 1990–2013: a systematic analysis for the Global Burden of Disease Study 2013. *Lancet* 384:980–1004, 2014.
4. Berg CJ, Chang J, Callaghan WM, et al: Pregnancy-related mortality in the United States, 1991–1997. *Obstet Gynecol* 101:289, 2003.
5. Clark SL, Belfort MA, Dildy GA, et al: Maternal death in the 21st century: causes, prevention, and relationship to cesarean delivery. *Am J Obstet Gynecol* 199:36.e1–36.e5, 2008.
6. Pollock W, Rose L, Dennis CL: Pregnant and postpartum admissions to the intensive care unit: a systematic review. *Intensive Care Med* 36:1465–1474, 2010.
7. Chapman AB, Abraham WT, Zamudio S, et al: Temporal relationships between hormonal and hemodynamic changes in early human pregnancy. *Kidney Int* 54:2056–2063, 1998.
8. Robson SC, Hunter S, Boys RJ, et al: Serial study of factors influencing changes in cardiac output during human pregnancy. *Am J Physiol* 256:H1060–H1065, 1989.
9. Metcalfe J, Ueland K: Maternal cardiovascular adjustments to pregnancy. *Prog Cardiovasc Dis* 16:363–374, 1974.
10. Grindheim G, Estensen ME, Langesaeter E, et al: Changes in blood pressure during healthy pregnancy: a longitudinal cohort study. *J Hypertens* 30:342–350, 2012.
11. Liberatore SM, Pistelli R, Patalano F, et al: Respiratory function during pregnancy. *Respiration* 46:145–150, 1984.
12. Milne JA: The respiratory response to pregnancy. *Postgrad Med J* 55:318–324, 1979.
13. Bonica JJ: Maternal respiratory changes during pregnancy and parturition. *Clin Anesth* 10:1–19, 1974.
14. Lim VS, Katz AI, Lindheimer MD: Acid-base regulation in pregnancy. *Am J Physiol* 231:1764–1769, 1976.
15. Hernandez E, Angell CS, Johnson JW: Asthma in pregnancy: current concepts. *Obstet Gynecol* 55:739–743, 1980.
16. Lund CS, Donovan JC: Blood volume during pregnancy. *Am J Obstet Gynecol* 98:393–403, 1967.
17. Pritchard JA, Rowland RC: Blood volume changes in pregnancy and the puerperium. *Am J Obstet Gynecol* 88:391–395, 1964.
18. Talbert LM, Langdell RD: Normal values of certain factors in the blood clotting mechanism in pregnancy. *Am J Obstet Gynecol* 90:44–50, 1964.
19. Walker MC, Garner PR, Keely EJ, et al: Changes in activated protein C resistance during normal pregnancy. *Am J Obstet Gynecol* 177:162–169, 1997.
20. McColl MD, Ramsay JE, Tait RC, et al: Risk factors for pregnancy associated venous thromboembolism. *Thromb Haemost* 78:1183–1188, 1997.
21. Rasmussen PE, Nielsen FR: Hydronephrosis during pregnancy: a literature survey. *Eur J Obstet Gynecol Reprod Biol* 27:249–259, 1988.
22. Castronovo FP Jr: Teratogen update: radiation and Chernobyl. *Teratology* 60:100–106, 1999.
23. United Nations Scientific Committee on the Effects of Atomic Radiation: *Sources and Effects of Ionizing Radiation, UN Publication E.94.IX.2*. UN Publications, United Nations, New York, 1993.
24. Brent RL: The effect of embryonic and fetal exposure to x-ray, microwaves, and ultrasound: counseling the pregnant and nonpregnant patient about these risks. *Semin Oncol* 16:347–368, 1989.
25. Stewart A, Kneale GW: Radiation dose effects in relation to obstetric x-rays and childhood cancers. *Lancet* 1:1185–1188, 1970.
26. De Santis M, Cesari E, Nobili E, et al: Radiation effects on development. *Birth Defects Res C Embryo Today* 81:177–182, 2007.
27. Bentur, Y: Ionizing and nonionizing radiation in pregnancy, in Koren G (ed): *Maternal-fetal Toxicology*. 2nd ed. New York, NY, Marcel Dekker, 1994.
28. www.bt.cdc.gov/radiation/prenatalphysician.asp. Accessed March, 2016.
29. De Santis M, Di Gianantonio E, Straface G, et al: Ionizing radiations in pregnancy and teratogenesis: a review of literature. *Reprod Toxicol* 20:323–329, 2005.
30. Shellock FG, Kanal E: Bioeffects and safety of MRI procedures, in Edelman RR, Hesselink JR, Zlatkin MB (eds): *Clinical Magnetic Resonance Imaging*. 4th ed. Philadelphia, PA, WB Saunders, 2000, p 935.
31. Wienreb JC, Lowe TW, Santos-Ramos R, et al: Magnetic resonance imaging in obstetric diagnosis. *Radiology* 154:157–161, 1985.
32. Kandall SR, Albin S, Gartner LM, et al: The narcotic-dependent mother: fetal and neonatal consequences. *Early Hum Dev* 1:159–169, 1977.
33. Briggs GG, Bodendoter TW, Freeman RK, et al: *Drugs in Pregnancy and Lactation: A Reference Guide to Fetal and Neonatal Risk*. Baltimore, Williams & Wilkins, 1994.
34. Shepard TF: Human teratogenicity. *Adv Pediatr* 33:225–268, 1986.
35. Chow AW, Jewesson RJ: Pharmacokinetics and safety of antimicrobial agents in pregnancy. *Rev Infect Dis* 7:287–313, 1985.
36. Flessa HC, Klapstrom AB, Glueck MJ, et al: Placental transport of heparin. *Am J Obstet Gynecol* 93:570–573, 1965.
37. Sanson BJ, Lensing AW, Prins ML, et al: Safety of low molecular weight heparin in pregnancy: a systematic review. *Thromb Haemost* 81:668–672, 1999.
38. Forestier F, Daffos F, Capella-Pavlousky M: Low molecular weight heparin (PK 10169) does not cross the placenta during the second trimester of pregnancy: study by direct fetal blood sampling under ultrasound. *Thromb Res* 34:557–560, 1984.
39. Ginsberg B, Hirsch J, Turner C, et al: Risks to the fetus of anticoagulant therapy during pregnancy. *Thromb Haemost* 61:197–203, 1989.
40. Hall JG, Pavi RM, Wilson KM: Maternal and fetal sequelae of anticoagulants during pregnancy. *Am J Med* 68:122–140, 1978.
41. Magee LA, Cham C, Waterman ES, et al: Hydralazine for the treatment of severe hypertension in pregnancy: meta-analysis. *BMJ* 327:955–960, 2003.
42. Magee LA, Ornstein MP, Von Dadelszen P: Fortnightly review: management of hypertension in pregnancy. *BMJ* 318:1332–1336, 1999.
43. National High Blood Pressure Education Program: *Working Group Report on High Blood Pressure in Pregnancy*. Washington, DC, National Institutes of Health, 2000.
44. Duley L, Henderson-Smart DJ: Drugs for treatment of very high blood pressure during pregnancy. *Cochrane Database Syst Rev* 4:CD001449, 2002.

45. American College of Obstetricians and Gynecologists; Task Force on Hypertension in Pregnancy: Hypertension in pregnancy. Report of the American College of Obstetricians and Gynecologists' Task Force on Hypertension in Pregnancy. *Obstet Gynecol* 122:1122–1131, 2013.
46. Meekins JW, Pijnenborg R, Hanssens M, et al: A study of placental bed spiral arteries and trophoblast invasion in normal and severe pre-eclamptic pregnancies. *Br J Obstet Gynaecol* 101:669–674, 1994.
47. Trogstad L, Magnus P, Stoltenberg C: Pre-eclampsia: risk factors and causal models. *Best Pract Res Clin Obstet Gynaecol* 25:329–342, 2011.
48. Witlin AG, Sibai B: Magnesium sulfate therapy in preeclampsia and eclampsia. *Obstet Gynecol* 92:883–889, 1998.
49. Altman D, Carroli G, Duley L, et al; The Magpie Trial Collaborative Group: Do women with pre-eclampsia, and their babies, benefit from magnesium sulfate? The Magpie Trial: a randomized placebo controlled trial. *Lancet* 359:1877–1890, 2002.
50. Committee on Obstetric Practice: Committee opinion no. 623: emergent therapy for acute-onset, severe hypertension during pregnancy and the postpartum period. *Obstet Gynecol* 125:521–525, 2015.
51. Nanda K, Lopez LM, Grimes DA, et al: Expectant care versus surgical treatment for miscarriage. *Cochrane Database Syst Rev* 3:CD003518, 2012.
52. Faiz AS, Ananth CV: Etiology and risk factors for placenta previa: an overview and meta-analysis of observational studies. *J Matern Fetal Neonatal Med* 13:175–190, 2003.
53. Cotton DB, Read JA, Paul RH, et al: The conservative aggressive management of placenta previa. *Am J Obstet Gynecol* 137:687–695, 1980.
54. Silver R, Depp R, Sabbagha RE, et al: Placenta previa: aggressive expectant management. *Am J Obstet Gynecol* 150:15–22, 1984.
55. Crane JM, Van den Hof MC, Dodds L, et al: Maternal complications with placenta previa. *Am J Perinatol* 17:101–105, 2000.
56. Olive EC, Roberts CL, Algert CS, et al: Placenta praevia: maternal morbidity and place of birth. *Aust N Z J Obstet Gynaecol* 45:499–504, 2005.
57. Spong CY, Mercer BM, D'alton M, et al: Timing of indicated late-preterm and early-term birth. *Obstet Gynecol* 118:323–333, 2011.
58. American College of Obstetricians and Gynecologists: ACOG committee opinion no. 560: medically indicated late-preterm and early-term deliveries. *Obstet Gynecol* 121:908–910, 2013.
59. Hurd WW, Meodornik M, Hertzberg V, et al: Selective management of abruptio placentae: a prospective study. *Obstet Gynecol* 61:467–473, 1983.
60. Luea WE: Post partum hemorrhage. *Clin Obstet Gynecol* 23:637, 1980.
61. Cassidy GN, Moore DL, Bridenbaugh D: Postpartum hypertension after use of vasoconstrictor and oxytocin drugs: etiology incidences, complications and treatment. *JAMA* 172:1011–1015, 1960.
62. Hayashi RH, Castello MS, Noah ML: Management of severe postpartum hemorrhage due to uterine atony using an analogue of prostaglandin F_2. *Obstet Gynecol* 58:426–429, 1981.
63. Leary AM: Severe bronchospasm and hypotension after 15 methyl prostaglandin F_2 & in atonic postpartum hemorrhage. *J Obstet Anesth* 3:42–44, 1994.
64. Schwartz PE: The surgical approach to severe postpartum hemorrhage, in Bereowitz RL (ed): *Critical Care of the Obstetric Patient.* New York, NY, Churchill Livingstone, 1983, p 285.
65. Pais SO, Glickman M, Schwartz P, et al: Embolization of pelvic arteries for control of postpartum hemorrhage. *Obstet Gynecol* 53:754–758, 1980.
66. Ferguson JE II, Bourgesis FJ, Underwood P: B-Lynch suture for postpartum hemorrhage. *Obstet Gynecol* 95:1020–1022, 2000.
67. Abenhaim HA, Azoulay L, Kramer MS, et al: Incidence and risk factors of amniotic fluid embolisms: a population-based study on 3 million births in the United States. *Am J Obstet Gynecol* 199:49.e1–49.e8, 2008.
68. Gist RS, Stafford IP, Leibowitz AB, et al: Amniotic fluid embolism. *Anesth Analg* 108:1599–1602, 2009.
69. Gilbert W, Danielsen B: Amniotic fluid embolism: decreased mortality in a population based study. *Obstet Gynecol* 93:973–977, 1999.
70. Davies S: Amniotic fluid embolism and isolated disseminated intravascular coagulation. *Can J Anaesth* 46:456–459, 1999.
71. Gilmore DA, Wakins J, Secrest J, et al: Anaphylactoid syndrome of pregnancy: a review of the literature with latest management and outcome data. *AANA J* 71:120–126, 2003.
72. Lavery J, Staton-McCormick M: Management of moderate to severe trauma in pregnancy. *Obstet Gynecol Clin North Am* 22:69–90, 1995.
73. Peckham AF, King RA: A study of intercurrent conditions observed during pregnancy. *Am J Obstet Gynecol* 87:609–624, 1963.
74. Drost RF, Rosemary AS, Sherman HF, et al: Major trauma in pregnant women: maternal/fetal outcome. *J Trauma* 30:574–578, 1990.
75. Rothenberger D, Quattlebaum F, Perry J, et al: Blunt maternal trauma, a review of 103 cases. *J Trauma* 18:173–179, 1978.
76. Goodwin T, Breen M: Pregnancy outcome and fetal maternal hemorrhage after non-catastrophic trauma. *Am J Obstet Gynecol* 162:665–671, 1990.
77. Dahmus M, Sebai B: Blunt abdominal trauma, are there any predictive factors for abruptio placentae or maternal fetal distress? *Am J Obstet Gynecol* 169:1054–1059, 1993.
78. Connolly A, Katz V, Bash K, et al: Trauma and pregnancy. *Am J Perinatol* 14:331–336, 1997.
79. Pearlman M, Tintinalli J, Lorenz R: A prospective controlled study of outcome after trauma during pregnancy. *Am J Obstet Gynecol* 162:1502–1507, 1990.
80. Pearlman M, Tintinalli J, Lorenz R: Blunt trauma during pregnancy. *N Engl J Med* 323:1609–1613, 1990.
81. Committee on Trauma, American College of Surgeons: *Advanced Trauma Life Support Program for Physicians.* Chicago, American College of Surgeons, 1997.
82. Buchsbaum H (ed): *Penetrating Injury of the Abdomen. Trauma in Pregnancy.* Philadelphia, PA, Saunders, 1979, p 82.
83. Awwad J, Azar G, Seoud M, et al: High velocity penetrating wounds of the gravid uterus: review of 16 years of civil war. *Obstet Gynecol* 83:259–264, 1994.

Chapter 54 ■ Acute Limb Ischemia in the ICU Population

DEJAH R. JUDELSON[1] • BING SHUE[1] • WILLIAM P. ROBINSON, III

INTRODUCTION

Acute limb ischemia (ALI) occurs as a result of sudden inadequate arterial perfusion to an extremity. This state of hypoperfusion can result in a number of both local and systemic manifestations. These include loss of sensory and motor function of the affected extremity, gangrene leading to sepsis, as well as systemic acid–base disturbances and increased cardiopulmonary stress. Unfortunately, ALI also commonly develops in the setting of systemic illness and multiple other medical comorbidities. This is especially true in the intensive care unit (ICU) setting in which concomitant conditions such as myocardial infarction, hypercoagulable states, or hypotension requiring pharmacologic support play a role in both the etiology and disease progression [1]. Furthermore, revascularization can lead to ischemia–reperfusion injury impacting multiple organ systems and rhabdomyolysis as toxic by-products are reintroduced into the system circulation.

ALI is a devastating condition with 30-day mortality rates of 15%, and 5-year mortality rates of up to 50%. In addition, amputation rates range from 10% to 30% [2]. Due to its high rate of complications, ALI is a vascular surgery emergency necessitating expedient evaluation and treatment when indicated. This chapter reviews the etiology, evaluation, and management of both upper and lower extremity ALI of the critically ill patient.

ETIOLOGY

The most common causes of ALI are embolism and thrombosis. These two etiologies account for more than 90% of ALI cases [3,4]. Less common etiologies include aortic dissection and low flow states secondary to poor cardiac output. Embolic events typically originate from a cardiac source. The most common condition associated with cardiac emboli is atrial fibrillation but other cardiac sources include myocardial infarction leading to mural thrombus, valvular heart disease, and endocarditis [5,6].

[1] These authors contributed equally to the content in this chapter.

Myocardial infarction and endocarditis are especially dreadful causes of ALI as these patients are extremely high-risk surgical candidates due to the coexisting medical comorbidities.

Less common causes of peripheral emboli include paradoxical emboli, aortic mural thrombus, and arterial atheroemboli. The presence of a patent foramen ovale allows the thrombus to traverse from the deep venous to arterial circulation leading to an ALI event. Paradoxical emboli should be suspected among patients with concomitant deep vein thrombosis and ALI without other cardioembolic risk factors [7]. Aortic mural thrombus typically presents as an asymptomatic finding and is commonly seen in the setting of hypercoagulable states such as malignancy or underlying aortic pathology. Atheroembolic events occur as a result of disruption of cholesterol plaque. This can be related to vessel manipulation from recent interventions such as cardiac or cerebral catheterizations, or peripheral vascular interventions. It can also be spontaneous in the setting of significant aortic atherosclerotic disease. Atheroemboli typically migrate to the distal vasculature, resulting in distal vessel thrombosis or blue toe syndrome [8]. This is in contrast to cardiac sources of emboli which typically lodge at arterial bifurcations due to the change in vessel caliber at these locations. Over half of cardioemboli occur in the iliofemoral arteries; the popliteal and brachial arteries are less common areas of embolization [9].

Thrombosis of native arteries or previously placed stents or grafts is an increasingly common cause of ALI. In situ thrombosis of native arteries occurs among patients with significant preexisting atherosclerotic disease burden. Most patients will have risk factors for peripheral arterial disease (PAD) and a portion will have a discernible history of claudication, rest pain, or nonhealing ulcers prior to their acute thrombotic event. Common sites of thrombosis correlate with the location of preexisting lesions; these typically include the iliac or superficial femoral arteries [10]. Low flow states, hypercoagulability, and endothelial injury lead to disruption of atherosclerotic plaques and thrombus formation. This pathophysiology is exacerbated for the critically ill patient who suffers from cardiac compromise, sepsis, and vasopressor dependence. Critically ill patients exhibit elevated levels of inflammatory markers such as TNFα which has been shown to affect atherosclerotic plaque stability and increase the risk of thrombosis [11]. Critically ill patients also exhibit increased levels of procoagulant activity, especially in the setting of sepsis, heparin-induced thrombocytopenia, and disseminated intravascular coagulation [12]. These risk factors also have a significant impact on the patency of previously placed arterial stents or bypasses. Therefore, a detailed history of both endovascular and surgical revascularizations should be taken, as the presence of prior interventions will influence both the diagnosis and subsequent management.

Less common causes of ALI include arterial dissection, non-thrombotic limb ischemia secondary to low flow state, and traumatic arterial injury. Arterial dissection can occur spontaneously or as a result of iatrogenic injury secondary to arterial catheterization. Non-thrombotic limb ischemia often occurs in the setting of low cardiac output or vasopressor dependence. In these instances, the vessels remain patent; however, perfusion is limited by severe vasoconstriction at the arteriole and capillary level [13]. Blunt limb distraction injuries such as fractures and dislocations, or penetrating trauma from stabs or gunshot wounds, can lead to arterial injury. These can have a delayed presentation, so high-risk patients should be monitored with serial vascular examinations [14].

The etiology of an ALI event is critical for determining the subsequent evaluation and management. Patients who suffer embolic events typically do not have robust collateral peripheral circulation and can quickly develop permanent deficits if left untreated. On the other hand, thrombosis of native vessels is better tolerated due to the preexisting presence of collateral circulation in the setting of PAD. However, these patients often require more extensive revascularizations due to a heavier burden of underlying disease. Finally patients with non-thrombotic ALI secondary to low cardiac output or vasopressor dependence often improve with treatment of the underlying condition.

EVALUATION AND DIAGNOSIS OF ACUTE LIMB ISCHEMIA IN THE ICU POPULATION

A careful, detailed history and physical examination to elicit the etiology of ALI can have a tremendous impact on the overall management and prognosis for a patient. Assessment of the etiology, determining the extent of ischemia and neuromuscular damage, and establishing an appropriate treatment plan must be performed rapidly to minimize the time of ischemia. Patients in the ICU are often unable to provide necessary history and participate in a thorough examination; therefore, a thorough examination of their documented history and interviewing the family and critical care staff is often necessary to ascertain a complete picture. Medical records should be reviewed for key comorbidities including history of atrial arrhythmias, coagulation disorders, recent percutaneous interventions (i.e., cardiac catheterizations), history of claudication or rest pain, and previously lower extremity interventions should be investigated. Examining previous imaging including echocardiograms, computed tomography (CT) scans demonstrating aneurysmal disease or mural thrombus, and prior angiograms should be performed to understand possible etiologies or baseline disease.

A comprehensive physical examination is compulsory in order to determine the duration and extent of lower extremity ischemia; this will assist in deciding the appropriate management. To determine the diagnosis and duration of ALI, the six "Ps" of acute ischemia need to be evaluated—pain, paresthesias, pulselessness, pallor, poikilothermia, and paralysis. Bilateral lower extremities should be evaluated to determine if there are signs of underlying chronic PAD such as dependent rubor with elevation pallor, sparse hair growth, dystrophic nail growth, ulceration or nonhealing lesions, and lack of palpable pulses The extent of pallor, coolness, sensory and/or motor deficits, and mottling often indicates the level of arterial obstruction. Ischemic symptoms tend to occur one vascular bed distal to the level of obstruction—for example, mottling in the foot and calf implies an obstruction in the superficial femoral artery.

A careful pulse examination is a reliable method to determine the level of arterial obstruction. Bilateral pulse examination should be performed including the femoral, popliteal, dorsalis pedis, and posterior tibial arteries. When pulses are nonpalpable, continuous wave Doppler examination should be performed at the bedside. Assessing the quality of the pulse and the phasicity of the signal is important in assessing the severity of the occlusion; comparing the affected to the unaffected side is also important. Bedside ankle-brachial indices should be performed and compared to the contralateral limb and to any baselines values on the affected limb. Additional signs can indicate the pathophysiology. A "water hammer" pulse will indicate pulsation against an obstruction such as a recent embolus or thrombus. Evaluating for pulsatility, a palpable thrill, or an audible bruit can indicate an iatrogenic pseudoaneurysm or arteriovenous fistula in the setting of recent percutaneous intervention such as central line, arterial stick, cardiac catheterization, or angiogram.

Whether or not additional imaging is obtained will depend on the severity and acuity of the ischemia. Often a physical examination alone is enough to determine location of disease. If the patient is stable and the limb is not immediately threatened, additional imaging such as a CT angiogram can precisely identify the location of disease and define the arterial lesions in the affected limb. Duplex ultrasound can also be utilized, including at the bedside, to define suspected lesions. Such imaging should be readily available within a short timeframe and can be extremely helpful for operative planning. In cases where emergent revascularization is indicated and the burden of disease is not clear from clinical evaluation, a formal on-table angiogram in the operating room is a rapid way to define the pathophysiology and plan revascularization.

TREATMENT OF ACUTE LIMB ISCHEMIA IN THE ICU POPULATION

Treatment of ALI in the critical care population requires understanding of the etiology of the ischemia, the viability of the affected limb, and evaluation of the patient's overall medical status.

The main treatment modalities of ALI can be divided into medical and operative management. Medical management includes systemic anticoagulation and supportive care. A heparin infusion, with a goal partial thromboplastin time (PTT) of 60 to 80, is the usual form of systemic anticoagulation that should be initiated immediately to prevent thrombus propagation. However, in the cases of heparin-induced thrombocytopenia or heparin allergy, a direct thrombin inhibitor, such as argatroban, can be used. In many instances of ALI in a critical care setting, these patients require multiple pressors for blood pressure support. Weaning pressors as tolerated, supporting intravascular volume, and placing the patient in a reverse Trendelenburg position to allow for the benefits of gravity, and utilizing a Bair hugger are all supportive measures that can be an effective adjuncts to systemic anticoagulation.

Treatment of ALI can be guided by the revised Rutherford Criteria proposed by The Society for Vascular Surgery and International Society for Cardiovascular Surgery (SVS/ISCVS) which stratifies levels of severity of ALI (Table 54.1). Category I, or viable, limbs have no sensory or motor deficits. These patients are appropriate for observation or systemic anticoagulation, possible angiogram and thrombolysis if appropriate. Category II limbs are the most difficult to differentiate, and are separated into two categories, IIa and IIb. Category IIa limbs are marginally threatened; they have minimal sensory loss and revascularization can be directed by expeditious angiography after systemic anticoagulation. Diagnostic imaging should be performed to guide treatment. Duplex ultrasonography, CT angiogram, or magnetic resonance angiogram are all excellent modalities to precisely identify the location and extent of the lesion and help plan intervention. Category IIb limbs are immediately threatened with both motor and sensory loss; if these patients do not undergo immediate operative revascularization, they are at a high risk of limb loss. The additional time needed to get additional imaging can put them at higher risk of limb loss and often they are taken directly to the operating room without additional studies. Category III limbs have sustained irreversible damage; these patients are often insensate with profound paralysis of the limb; primary amputation for pain control and avoidance of sepsis is the mainstay of therapy. Attempts at revascularization will not only fail to result in limb salvage, but can be hazardous and precipitate multiorgan system dysfunction due to severe ischemia–reperfusion injury.

For critically ill patients, their overall medical status is a guiding factor to determine if they are appropriate for revascularization. If the patient is hemodynamically unstable or experiencing profound cardiopulmonary or multisystem organ dysfunction, surgical revascularization or even aggressive endovascular revascularization might precipitate the patient's demise. In these instances, revascularization should be delayed or deferred altogether to save "life over limb." Systemic anticoagulation, ongoing observation, and conservative measures become the mainstays of treatment. In rare instances of category III limb ischemia, primary amputation of a densely ischemic or secondarily infected limb is necessary to prevent failure of other organs.

OPEN SURGICAL REVASCULARIZATION

Open surgical revascularization offers the advantage of immediate reperfusion to the affected extremity. Surgical options are dictated by the level of arterial obstruction but generally include a combination of open surgical exploration with Fogarty balloon thromboembolectomy, thromboendarterectomy with patch angioplasty, and bypass.

The standard open operation for ALI secondary to embolism is surgical exploration with Fogarty balloon thromboembolectomy [15]. Successful embolectomy occurs when the arterial intima is not damaged and the distal arterial tree was patent prior to embolization. Typically a femoral exploration is performed for suspected aortic, iliac, or femoral thromboemboli while a

TABLE 54.1

Clinical Categories of Acute Limb Ischemia

Category	Description/ prognosis	Sensory loss	Muscle weakness	Doppler signal (arterial)	Doppler signal (venous)
I. Viable	Not immediately threatened	None	None	Audible	Audible
II. Threatened					
a. Marginally	Salvageable if promptly treated	Minimal (toes) or None	None	Inaudible	Audible
b. Immediately	Salvageable with immediate revascularization	More than toes, associated with rest pain	Mild, moderate	Inaudible	Audible
III. Irreversible	Major tissue loss or permanent nerve damage inevitable	Profound, anesthetic	Profound paralysis (rigor)	Inaudible	Inaudible

Modified from reporting criteria recommended by the Society for Vascular Surgery and the International Society for Cardiovascular Surgery [11], Vascular Surgery, and the North American Chapter.

below the knee popliteal exploration is performed for suspected popliteal or tibial thromboemboli.

If there is significant preexisting atherosclerotic occlusive disease, an endarterectomy with patch angioplasty may be a necessary adjunct to an embolectomy. This is seen commonly with in situ thrombosis of a diseased common femoral artery. When thrombosis of significant arterial segment occurs such that flow cannot be adequately restored by a focal thromboendarterectomy, a surgical bypass is generally necessary. In these instances, definition of a distal target for bypass with preoperative or on-table angiography is exceedingly helpful. The type of bypass is dictated by the clinical scenario. For example, when there is bilateral ALI, an aortic occlusion or saddle emboli is suspected. If bilateral femoral thromboembolectomy does not adequately restore perfusion, an axillobifemoral bypass may be undertaken.

ENDOVASCULAR ANGIOGRAPHY AND THROMBOLYSIS

Catheter-directed thrombolysis (CDT) for ALI was first introduced in the 1990s [16]. The goal of thrombolytic therapy is to restore flow through the occluded arterial segment and, in doing so, to "uncover" the underlying culprit lesion which can then be definitively addressed via standard open surgical or endovascular methods. The major advantages of using CDT to restore blood flow in the critical care population is the avoidance of a major open surgical operation and the gradual reestablishment of blood flow to the affected extremity avoiding ischemia–reperfusion injury. The most appropriate candidates for thrombolysis are patients with category I or IIa disease, or those with in situ thrombosis. Patients with imminently threatened limbs that may lose neurologic function without immediate revascularization are not appropriate candidates as thrombolysis may take 2 to 3 days to restore blood flow.

The general procedure is as follows:

1. Endovascular access is gained utilizing the Seldinger technique under ultrasound guidance.
2. Angiogram is accomplished to elucidate the location and extent of disease.
3. The occluded arterial segment is traversed with a guidewire.
4. A lysis catheter is placed across the occluded segment.
5. A thrombolytic agent is administered as a bolus and a continuous infusion is started.
6. Serial laboratory testing as well as neurovascular examinations are done.
7. Reimaging is done in 24 hours to ascertain the success of the thrombolysis and angioplasty/stenting can be performed at the conclusion of thrombolytic therapy.

Monitoring of patients undergoing thrombolysis is critical. After the initiation of thrombolysis, patients are returned to the ICU. Serial laboratory studies are performed to reduce the risk of a systemic thrombolytic state which would increase the risk of intracerebral hemorrhage (ICH) or other spontaneous bleeding. During fibrinolysis, thrombus dissolves and the body recruits coagulation factors to reform the thrombus; therefore coagulation factors and fibrinogen are consumed. Laboratory values monitored include fibrinogen, complete blood count, prothrombin time (PT)/international normalized ratio (INR), PTT. A decrease in fibrinogen by more than 50% or below 100 mg per dL implies an excessive consumption of coagulation factors leading to an increased risk of ICH. Serial PT/INR and PTTs should be assessed to reduce the risk of systemic anticoagulation.

In the United States, the most commonly used drugs are urokinase and recombinant tissue plasminogen activator usually marketed as alteplase.

TABLE 54.2

Absolute and Relative Contraindications to Treatment with Thrombolytic Therapy

Contraindications to thrombolytic therapy
Absolute
1. Established cerebrovascular event (including TIAs within last 2 mo)
2. Active bleeding diathesis
3. Recent gastrointestinal bleeding (<10 d)
4. Neurosurgery (intracranial, spinal) within last 3 mo
5. Intracranial trauma within last 3 mo
Relative major
1. Cardiopulmonary resuscitation within last 10 d
2. Major nonvascular surgery or trauma within last 10 d
3. Uncontrolled hypertension: >180 mm Hg systolic or >110 mm Hg diastolic
4. Puncture of noncompressible vessel
5. Intracranial tumor
6. Recent eye surgery
Relative minor
1. Hepatic failure, particularly those with coagulopathy
2. Bacterial endocarditis
3. Pregnancy
4. Diabetic hemorrhagic retinopathy

TIA, transient ischemic attack.
Modified from Working Party on Thrombolysis in the Management of Limb Ischemia: Thrombolysis in the management of lower limb peripheral arterial occlusion—consensus document. *J Vasc Interv Radiol* 7:S337–S349, 2003.

There are two multicenter randomized clinical trials that established the efficacy of CDT [17,18]. It should be noted that thrombolytic therapy is most effective for freshly formed thrombus and that the trials demonstrated poor efficacy for patients who had limb ischemia of the duration greater than 14 days.

Several professional societies have published consensus guidelines on the surgical management of ALI. The CHEST guidelines published in 2012 recommend open surgery as compared to CDT (Level 1B evidence), yet CDT is a recommended modality for appropriate patients [19]. In 2005, the American College of Cardiology/American Heart Association (ACC/AHA) guidelines on Peripheral Artery Disease (PAD) were published in collaboration with cardiologists, vascular surgeons, vascular medicine, and interventional radiology; their conclusion was CDT is effective and indicated for patients with ALI of fewer than 14 days' duration [20].

There are several adjunctive measures to improve the success of thrombolysis, notably mechanical thrombectomy and aspiration thrombectomy. There are two FDA-approved mechanical thrombectomy devices, the AngioJet and the Trellis Thrombectomy system, which can supplement thrombosis by reducing clot burden and more rapidly restoring perfusion. While CDT is an attractive option for a select patient group, it is contraindicated for patients at high risk of hemorrhagic complications. There are several contraindications to treatment with thrombolytic therapy (Table 54.2). When patients are selected appropriately, approximately 1% of patients will have a life-threatening hemorrhage, most ominously an ICH.

POSTOPERATIVE CARE

Postoperative management of the revascularized acute limb ICU patient focuses on resuscitation and anticoagulation. These patients must be aggressively resuscitated to prevent systemic complications of ischemia–reperfusion injury. Additionally, systemic anticoagulation must be continued as rethrombosis or recurrent embolism occurs among 6% to 46% of patients [21,22].

MANAGEMENT OF ISCHEMIA–REPERFUSION INJURY AND RHABDOMYOLSIS

Ischemia–reperfusion injury may result in limb and multisystem organ dysfunction. As ischemic muscle is reperfused, cellular edema and interstitial fluid shifts may occur. Symptoms include pain, hypoesthesia, and weakness of the involved limb. Rhabdomyolysis may occur; as the muscle groups are reperfused, the ischemic muscle is broken down and by-products are released into the bloodstream—notably myoglobin and potassium. The elevated potassium can lead to cardiac arrhythmias and the myoglobin can cause acute kidney injury. Treatment is mainly supportive, aggressive fluid resuscitation with an isotonic fluid; occasionally, a bicarbonate drip is indicated to alkalinize the urine. In cases of severe hyperkalemia, calcium carbonate may help to stabilize the cardiac myocyte membrane while IV insulin and an ampule of D50W can help to redistribute potassium into cells. Patients can become profoundly acidotic and in rare cases require hemodialysis [23].

COMPARTMENT SYNDROME

Compartment syndrome occurs when the reperfused muscle swells inside fixed factual compartments. When compartment pressures exceed 25 to 30 mm Hg, the extravascular pressure then exceeds capillary pressure and blood flow is restricted leading to tissue infarction. The first signs are pain, numbness, and paresthesias. Of the four compartments to the distal lower extremity, the anterior compartment is the most susceptible to compartment syndrome. Symptoms are focused around deep peroneal nerve injury and include numbness to the first web space and decreased foot dorsiflexion. Management is operative; immediate four-compartment fasciotomies are necessary to prevent any further nerve or muscle damage.

UPPER EXTREMITY ACUTE LIMB ISCHEMIA

Upper extremity ALI is far less commonly encountered than lower extremity ALI and typically results from cardioembolic events. In situ thrombosis is uncommon since atherosclerotic disease is rare in the upper extremities. Emboli typically lodge at the brachial or axillary artery. The clinical presentation can be similar to lower extremity ALI; however, more commonly, patients report decreased sensation and strength without pain. Upper extremity ALI can be diagnosed with history and physical examination alone, although duplex imaging can confirm the diagnosis. CT angiogram of the chest and upper extremities is a useful adjunct for determining the anatomic location of the occlusion and to assist with operative planning [24,25].

First-line treatment for upper extremity ALI is anticoagulation. Most patients report a significant improvement in symptoms with anticoagulation alone. The upper extremities have robust collateral circulation compared to the lower extremities, so the risk for tissue loss is lower. However, patients who develop upper extremity ALI are at risk of developing chronic arm claudication or even severe neuromuscular dysfunction with incidence rates of 50%. Therefore, patients who are medically able to tolerate surgery or at risk of loss of upper extremity function should undergo revascularization [26].

Surgical treatment of upper extremity ALI is generally performed through a brachial artery exploration and Fogarty balloon thromboembolectomy. The procedure can be performed under local or regional anesthesia with sedation if the patient is unable to tolerate general anesthesia. Postoperatively, the patient should remain anticoagulated and undergo serial neurovascular examinations. Upper extremity compartment syndrome is less common, so prophylactic fasciotomies are rarely performed. However, careful neurologic monitoring is indicated to identify a developing compartment syndrome. In addition, a full workup including cardiac echocardiogram and CT angiography of the chest should be performed to determine the etiology of the ALI event. Patency rates for upper extremity revascularizations are high and amputation rates are negligible. However, studies have shown overall mortality rates of patients with upper extremity ALI to be as high as 50% over 5 years due to the incidence of multiple medical comorbidities in the population.

RECOMMENDATIONS

In general, recommendations are as follows:

1. Systemic anticoagulation is a mainstay in the management of ALI in all patients to minimize propagation of thrombosis and prevent recurrent events after revascularization.
2. Immediate surgical revascularization is indicated for patients with an immediate threatened limb, Rutherford classification IIb, to avoid an unacceptable delay in reperfusion.
3. In patients with a marginally threatened limb, CDT is an appropriate treatment modality.
4. Primary amputation is indicated for patients with an irreversibly ischemic limb.
5. In hemodynamically unstable patients or those with severe multisystem dysfunction, the mortality risk of revascularization may be prohibitive. In these patients, conservative medical management with a "life over limb" approach may be appropriate.

References

1. Dormandy J, Heeck L, Vig S: Acute limb ischemia. *Semin Vasc Surg* 12: 148–153, 1999.
2. Genovese EA, Baril DT, Taha AG, et al: Risk factors for long-term mortality and amputation after open and endovascular treatment of acute limb ischemia. *Ann Vasc Surg* 30:82–92, 2016.
3. Abbott WM, Maloney RD, McCabe CC, et al: Arterial embolism: a 44 year perspective. *Am J Surg* 143:460–464, 1982.
4. Elliot JP Jr, Hageman J, Szilagyi D, et al: Arterial embolization: problems of source, multiplicity, recurrence, and delayed treatment. *Surgery* 88:833–845, 1980.
5. Menke J, Luthje L, Kastrup A, et al: Thromboembolism in atrial fibrillation. *Am J Cardiol* 105:502–510, 2010.
6. Asinger RW, Mikell FL, Elsperger J, et al: Incidence of left-ventricular thrombosis after acute transmural myocardial infarction. Serial evaluation by two-dimensional echocardiography. *N Engl J Med* 305(6):297–302, 1991.
7. Ward R, Jones D, Haponik E: Paradoxical embolism: an under-recognized problem. *Chest* 108:549–558, 1995.
8. Rhodes JM: Cholesterol crystal embolism: an important "new" diagnosis for the general physician. *Lancet* 347:1641, 1996.
9. Cambria RP, Abbott WM: Acute arterial thrombosis of the lower extremity. Its natural history contrasted with arterial embolism. *Arch Surg* 119:784–787, 1984.
10. Bentzon JF, Otsuka F, Virmani R, et al: Mechanisms of plaque formation and rupture. *Circ Res* 114:1852–1866, 2014.
11. Gopalakrishnan M, Silva-Palacios F, Taytawat P, et al: Role of inflammatory mediators in the pathogenesis of plaque rupture. *J Invasive Cardiol* 9;26(9): 484–492, 2014.
12. Boldt J, Papsordf M, Rothe A, et al: Changes of the hemostatic network in critically ill patients—is there a difference between sepsis, trauma, and neurosurgery patients? *Crit Care Med* 28(2):445–450, 2000.
13. Ljungman C, Adami HO, Bergqvist D, et al: Time trends in incidence rates of acute, non-traumatic extremity ischaemia: a population-based study during a 19-year period. *Br J Surg* 78:857–860, 1991.
14. Engelmann DT, Gabram SGA, Allen L, et al: Hypercoagulability following multiple trauma. *World J Surg* 20:5–10, 1996.
15. Fogarty TJ, Cranley JJ, Krause RJ, et al: A method for extraction of arterial emboli and thrombi. *Surg Gynecol Obstet* 116:241–244, 1963.
16. Ouriel K, Shortell CK, DeWeese JA, et al: A comparison of thrombolytic therapy with operative revascularization in the initial treatment of acuteperipheral arterial ischemia. *J Vasc Surg* 19(6):1021–1030, 1994.

17. STILE investigators: Results of a prospective randomized trial evaluating surgery versus thrombolysis for ischemia of the lower extremity. The STILE trial. *Ann Surg* 220(3):251–266, 1994; discussion 266-8.
18. Ouriel K, Veith FJ, Sasahara AA: A comparison of recombinant urokinase with vascular surgery as initial treatment for acute arterial occlusion of the legs. Thrombolysis or Peripheral Arterial Surgery (TOPAS) Investigators. *N Engl J Med* 16;338(16):1105–1111, 1998.
19. Alonso-Coello P, Bellmunt S, McGorrian C, et al; American College of Chest Physicians: Antithrombotic therapy in peripheral artery disease: Antithrombotic Therapy and Prevention of Thrombosis, 9th ed: American College of Chest Physicians Evidence-Based Clinical Practice Guidelines. *Chest* 141[2, Suppl]:e669S–e690S, 2012.
20. Hirsch AT, Haskal ZJ, Hertzer NR, et al: ACC/AHA 2005 Practice Guidelines for the management of patients with peripheral arterial disease (lower extremity, renal, mesenteric, and abdominal aortic): a collaborative report from the American Association for Vascular Surgery/Society for Vascular Surgery, Society for Cardiovascular Angiography and Interventions, Society for Vascular Medicine and Biology, Society of Interventional Radiology, and the ACC/AHA Task Force on Practice Guidelines (Writing Committee to Develop Guidelines for the Management of Patients With Peripheral Arterial Disease): endorsed by the American Association of Cardiovascular and Pulmonary Rehabilitation; National Heart, Lung, and Blood Institute; Society for Vascular Nursing; TransAtlantic Inter-Society Consensus; and Vascular Disease Foundation. *Circulation* 21;113(11):e463–e654, 2006.
21. Henke PK: Contemporary management of acute limb ischemia: factors associated with amputation and in-hospital mortality. *Semin Vasc Surg* 22:34–40, 2009.
22. Fukuda I, Chiyoya M, Taniquchi S, et al: Acute limb ischemia: contemporary approach. *Gen Thorac Cardiovasc Surg* 63:540–548, 2015.
23. Creager M, Kaufman JA, Conte MS: Clinical practice. Acute limb ischemia. *N Engl J Med* 366:2198–2206, 2012.
24. Eyers P, Earnshaw JJ: Acute non-traumatic arm ischaemia. *Br J Surg* 85:1340–1346, 1998.
25. Joshi V, Harding GE, Bottoni DA, et al: Determination of functional outcome following upper extremity arterial trauma. *Vasc Endovasc Surg* 41:111–114, 2007.
26. Hernandez-Richter T, Angele MK, Helmberger T, et al: Acute ischemia of the upper extremity: long-term results following thrombembolectomy with the Fogarty catheter. *Langenbecks Arch Surg* 386:261–266, 2001.

Chapter 55 ■ Palliative Surgery in the Intensive Care Unit

LAURA A. LAMBERT

Surgeons play an essential role in providing optimal palliative care for patients and families. Palliative surgery is best defined as the deliberate use of a procedure in the setting of incurable disease for the intention of relieving symptoms, minimizing patient distress and improving quality of life [1]. Because the goal of the surgery is not curative but rather the alleviation of suffering, the decision to proceed requires not only technical judgment, but also a sincere understanding of the patient's symptoms, the clinical, emotional, psychological, and social situation and the goals of care of both the patient and family. Typically, surgical outcomes are measured in terms of morbidity and mortality. However, given the stated goals of palliative surgery, morbidity and mortality are not necessarily the most effective measures of success. Rather outcomes such as the presence and duration of patient-acknowledged symptom relief may be much more salient [2,3]. Treatment plans which effectively achieve these goals must balance the potential benefit of durable symptom relief with the risk of treatment toxicity, while considering the patient's medical condition, performance status, prognosis and life expectancy, other medical treatment options and cost-effectiveness. The complex decisions required to manage these patients can challenge even the most experienced surgeons.

For patients with an incurable disease who are in the intensive care unit (ICU), the role of surgery in the management of their care may be even less clear than for patients whose clinical condition does not require intensive care. This lack of clarity is often multifactorial and includes a potentially more limited survival time, the patient's ability to undergo anesthesia safely, the magnitude of the surgery required to address the problem, whether or not the surgical problem is the cause or effect of the patient's critical condition, the likelihood of success of the surgery, the risk of complications, the availability of other treatment options, and the overall goals and wishes of the patient and family. Furthermore, the fact that most surgical procedures tend to inflict some pain initially adds an additional element of complexity to this equation. This chapter reviews the current status of, and evolving approach to, palliative surgery, as well as the management of some of the more common indications for palliative surgery consults in the ICU. It will also address ways to improve communication and decrease moral distress among surgeons related to interactions with patients and families in the end of life setting.

CURRENT STATUS OF PALLIATIVE SURGERY

The greatest experience with palliative surgery revolves largely around its use in patients with advanced malignancies. Palliative surgical consultations have been reported to represent up to 40% of all inpatient surgical consultations at major cancer cancers [4]. In fact, studies from two stand-alone cancer centers, the Memorial Sloan Kettering Cancer Center (MSKCC) in New York, New York, and the City of Hope Cancer Center in Duarte, California, showed that 6% and 12.5% of all surgical procedures were performed for palliation, respectively [5,6]. In the largest study ever looking at outcomes for palliative surgery from the MSKCC, Miner et al. [6] reported on the results of 1,022 palliative surgeries performed over the course of 1 year from July 2002 to June 2003. During that time, palliative interventions exceeded the combined number of esophagogastrectomies, gastrectomies, pancreatectomies, and hepatectomies performed. The most common indications for palliative surgery consults included gastrointestinal obstruction (34%), neurological symptoms (23%), pain (12%), dyspnea (9%), and jaundice (7%). Symptom improvement or resolution was achieved in 80% of patients by 30 days with a median duration of symptom control of 135 days. The primary symptom recurred in 25% of patients and treatment of additional symptoms was required in 29%. The 30-day morbidity and mortality associated with the palliative procedures was 29% and 11%, respectively. Not unexpectedly, postoperative complications had a negative impact and reduced the likelihood of symptom improvement to 17%. Median survival from the time of the palliative procedure was 194 days. The authors concluded that there is an opportunity for a significant number of patients to achieve durable improvement in quality of life given the median symptom-free survival of 135 days and a median survival of 194 days. Others have shown similar findings including an improved overall survival associated with symptom improvement in one study [1,6–8] (Table 55.1).

Because the primary goal of palliative surgery is to improve quality of life or relieve symptoms, it has been argued that traditional surgical outcome measures such as morbidity, mortality, disease recurrence, and survival are not sufficient to determine the success or failure of a palliative intervention. While understanding the risks (morbidity and mortality) of a procedure is important, it is equally important to assess the potential benefits.

TABLE 55.1

Outcomes in Palliative Surgery

Author/Year	Consultations	Surgical procedure (%)	Surgical morbidity %	Surgical mortality %	Symptom improvement %	Note
Krouse et al. [5]	240	170 (71) 70 (29)	25.9 10	12.2	NR	5 patients (2%) died within 5 d of surgery
Miner et al. [6]	1,022	713 (70) 309 (30)	29	11	80	Major complication reduced symptom improvement to 17%
Podnos et al. [8]	106	35 (33)	17	0	NR	Significant improvement in QOL and distress from primary symptom. Worsening overall QOL at 3 mo
Miner et al. [12]	227	106 (46.7)	16.7[a]	3.9	90.7	Use of palliative triangle
Badgwell et al. [7]	202	86(43) 35 (17)	43	9	67	Symptom improvement associated with improved overall survival

[a]Grade 3/4 major surgical morbidity only.
NR, not reported; QOL, quality of life

Because the impact of different specific palliative interventions can vary significantly—i.e., the impact of an indwelling catheter for a refractory pleural effusion may be significantly greater than that of a venting gastrostomy—it is difficult to quantify and compare the benefit of different procedures. One approach to addressing this issue is the use of patient-reported outcomes [2]. Patient-reported outcomes are surveys used to assess a patient's well-being from the patient's perspective. These surveys often include health-related quality of life or symptom assessment and are appropriate for assessing a surgical intervention intended to improve quality of life or relieve symptoms. However, currently, there are no validated quality of life instruments solely focused on palliative surgical outcomes, making it difficult to identify patients who benefit from these interventions, and the use of patient-reported outcomes in palliative surgery is limited [1,9]. One prospective pilot study using standardized, validated instruments demonstrated the challenges of interpreting outcomes after palliative interventions due to the continued loss of global health status during the end of life [1]. In a second study, the authors found that the death rate of 40% prior to study completion at 90 days post-procedure had a significant impact on the questionnaire response, clearly demonstrating the challenge of measuring the success of interventions in actively dying patients [10]. However, validating these interventions is essential given the high proportion of interventions that are palliative and the relatively high mortality rate which can significantly impact the overall operative mortality of an institution. In this age of quality-based reimbursement, this impact cannot be ignored and a means of incorporating palliative intent as a specific data element for comparing surgical outcomes needs to be devised.

As with any treatment—surgical or medical—another opportunity for improving the outcomes of palliative surgery is through optimal patient selection. The end of life setting presents a unique set of circumstances requiring difficult decisions with limited data. Using an open-ended questionnaire, Collins et al. [11] investigated the patient reasoning behind treatment choices after palliative surgical consultation. Of 98 patient enrolled in this prospective study, 54 were treated nonoperatively and 44 were treated with surgery. Symptom relief and/or quality of life was the reason for the treatment choice in only 46% of patients, and 40% said that they made their choice based on the doctor's recommendation. Twenty percent opted for care in hopes of prolonging their lives. This study demonstrates the powerful influence of the physician in the decision-making of patients at this stage of life, and the need for clear communication about goals and expectations between all parties.

Another critical party in these decisions is the patient's family. To help surgeons navigate this intriguing and often challenging dynamic, Miner et al. [1] have previously proposed and studied the use of the "palliative triangle" as an approach to improving patient selection and patient-acknowledged outcomes for palliative surgery (Fig. 55.1). Through the dynamics of the triangle, the patient's complaints, values, and emotional support are taken into account while weighing the medical and surgical alternatives. In addition, the triangle offers an opportunity to learn about and address a patient's and/or family's expectations regarding the intent of the proposed procedure helping to moderate any incongruent expectations between surgeon, patient, and family members. Miner et al. [12] prospectively investigated the use of the palliative triangle technique during palliative surgery consultation in 227 patients with symptomatic, advanced, incurable cancer. This is one of the few studies that included both patients who did and did not undergo a palliative procedure. More than half (53.3%) of the patients did not undergo a procedure. Reasons cited included low symptom severity, decision for nonoperative palliation, patient preference, and concerns about complications. Of the patients who did undergo a palliative procedure, 90.7% reported symptom resolution or improvement. The morbidity and mortality associated with these procedures was 20.1% and 3.9%, respectively. The median survival was 212 days. The authors concluded that use of the palliative triangle can help improve patient selection which is associated with significantly better symptom resolution and few postoperative complications compared with previously published results. The authors have also postulated that building this strong relationship may explain the observation of high patient satisfaction toward surgeons after palliative operation—even if there is no demonstrable benefit [1].

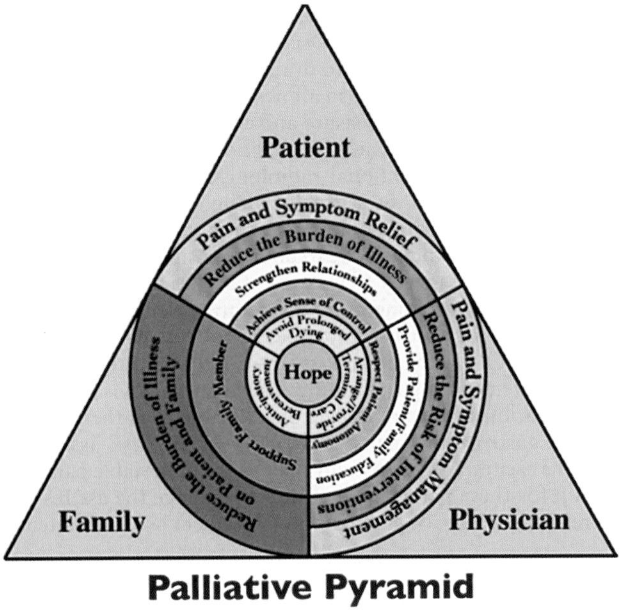

FIGURE 55.1 The palliative triangle. The palliative triangle facilitates interactions between patients, families, and surgeons, and helps guide patients to the best decisions regarding palliative surgery. (From Thomay AA, Jaques DP, Miner, TJ: Surgical palliation: getting back to our roots. *Surg Clin North Am* 89:33, 2009; permission requested.)

MANAGEMENT OF COMMON PALLIATIVE SURGERY CONSULTATIONS

This section reviews management options for some common palliative surgery consults in ICU patients. While this list is not comprehensive, it does offer a framework for approaching any palliative surgery situation. Management of other specific surgical problems encountered in the ICU is discussed elsewhere in the text. When surgery is not an option, it is important to know how to palliate common symptoms in patients with advanced illness (see Chapter 35).

Bowel Obstructions

One of the most common palliative surgical consults is for bowel obstruction. Bowel obstructions can occur at any level of the gastrointestinal tract from the stomach to the rectum. Depending upon the etiology (adhesions, cancer, stricture), the management can vary from nonoperative nasogastric decompression and bowel rest to bowel resection and/or intestinal diversion. In the setting of advanced illness such as cancer, and for patients who are in the ICU, management can be complicated and multimodal. Regardless of the etiology, initial management of a patient with a bowel obstruction should include appropriate intravenous fluid resuscitation based upon the degree of dehydration and the site of the obstruction and correction of any metabolic abnormalities. The bowel should be decompressed with a nasogastric tube if the patient is vomiting, and the patient should not be allowed to eat or drink to decrease gastrointestinal stimulation and secretions. Serial abdominal examinations for signs or symptoms of peritonitis are essential. Imaging studies, such as an abdominal series and/or a computed tomography scan of the abdomen and pelvis, are helpful to determine the level and nature of the obstruction. They can also demonstrate the presence of extraluminal air suggesting a perforation, and the presence or absence of ascites.

Patients who are hemodynamically stable, who do not have peritonitis and have a normal or only mildly elevated white blood count (especially in the setting of dehydration), can initially be monitored closely (with the measures mentioned above) and given a chance for the obstruction to resolve without surgery. Signs and symptoms of peritonitis or an imaging study suggesting a "closed loop" obstruction (a loop of intestine twisted around its mesentery) are indications for a more urgent surgical intervention. Often the exact nature of that intervention cannot be determined until the time of surgery—adding an additional element of cognitive and emotional uncertainty that must be borne by the patient, family, and surgeon. Surgery may include resecting the section of obstructed intestine if it appears to be an isolated site, performing an intestinal bypass if the site cannot be resected, performing a diverting ostomy (either small or large bowel depending on the location of the obstruction), or placing a decompression gastrostomy tube for venting the stomach if the obstruction cannot otherwise be relieved. In the setting of a malignancy, these operations can be challenging, both technically as well as with regard to the decision-making, and they pose a high risk for perioperative morbidity and mortality [13].

If the obstruction is located in the rectum or rectosigmoid colon or duodenum, it is reasonable to consider an endoscopic stent placement rather than surgery as the initial intervention. While the presence of carcinomatosis has been shown to increase the risk of failure of endoscopic stent placement for colonic obstruction, there is a 77% to 85% success rate [14–17]. For patients with a limited prognosis, an opportunity to avoid an operation that could involve either an intestinal diversion and ostomy or venting gastrostomy tube is an important consideration. For patients in whom it is felt that surgical or endoscopic relief of the bowel obstruction is not feasible, it is reasonable to evaluate them for a percutaneous endoscopic gastrostomy tube placement for gastric drainage.

Surgical decision-making becomes more challenging for end of life patients who are not stable and require a decision regarding an emergent operation. It may be argued that this is not a purely palliative surgery consult as the surgical intervention has the potential to rescue the patient from a life-threatening complication of their life-limiting illness. On the other hand, it may also be considered palliative as it will not cure the patient of the underlying disease process. Needless to say, this is often an emotionally charged time, even for patients with long-standing illness such as advanced cancer, because they are now faced with the imminent risk of dying. A recent study by Cauley et al. [18] reported the results of a retrospective cohort study of 875 disseminated cancer patients undergoing emergency surgery for obstruction (n = 376) or perforation (n = 499). Of the 376 patients who underwent emergency surgery for obstruction, the 30-day mortality rate was 18% with a 41% morbidity rate and 60% were discharged to an institution. Dependent functional status and ascites were independent preoperative predictors of death at 30 days. Postoperative predictors of mortality included respiratory and cardiac complications. Only 4% of patients had "do not resuscitate" orders in place prior to surgery. Further underscoring the dismal prognosis in this particular situation, a study by Pameijer et al. [19] showed that patients with metastatic cancer who presented with obstructive symptoms had a median survival of 3 months regardless of operative or no-operative management.

While most patients will survive the initial operation, a substantial number will die soon after the surgery and many experience postoperative complications, reoperations, stays in nursing homes, or hospital readmissions. Such events clearly impact the patient's quality of life. While these data are helpful for surgeons and caregivers to advise patients of the risks of surgery, set expectations for the postoperative experience, discharge location and overall survival, both at the time when the decisions is made for surgery and if complications occur, important data regarding whether the goals of the patients and families were met and whether or not they would make the same choice again are still severely lacking at this time.

Gastric Outlet and Duodenal Obstruction

Obstruction of the gastric outlet and/or duodenum is another common indication for palliative surgical consultation. Most patients present with nausea and vomiting of undigested food. Physical examination usually demonstrates upper abdominal distension and tympani. Imaging studies often reveal a distended stomach with retained enteric contents. As with a lower intestinal obstruction, acute symptoms should be initially managed with nasogastric decompression, bowel rest, and intravenous resuscitation, including aggressive electrolyte repletion. (For patients with chronic gastric outlet obstruction, special attention should be paid to chloride replacement which is lost in large quantities with emesis of gastric secretions.) If significant weight loss is present or if there may be a delay in definitive treatment, it may be reasonable to consider parenteral nutrition while planning additional palliative measures.

Options for managing upper gastrointestinal obstructions include intraluminal stenting, surgical bypass, and decompression gastrostomy with possible feeding jejunostomy. Similar to colonic stenting, the potential benefits of duodenal stenting include immediate palliation of nausea and vomiting with a less invasive procedure than surgical bypass and earlier return to oral nutrition [20,21]. (Restoring a person's ability to eat and drink is one of the most rewarding palliative interventions.) Stents may be particularly useful for patients with advanced malignancy, who are at increased risk of surgical complication or who are technically inoperable. Flexible self-expanding metal stents can be placed using endoscopic or fluoroscopic techniques. Stenting has been shown to provide a comparable survival outcome and equivalent morbidity and mortality to surgical bypass [22]. In a systematic review of the literature from 1990 to 2008 comparing endoscopic stenting with open surgical bypass, Ly et al. [22] found that endoscopic stenting was more likely to result in tolerance of oral intake (OR 2.6; $p = 0.002$) in a shorter period of time (mean difference of 6.9 days, $p < 0.001$) with a shorter hospital stay (mean difference 11.8 days, $p < 0.001$) as compared with open surgical bypass. Similar findings were reported by Zheng et al. [23] Based upon these findings, it is also likely that stenting is less expensive than surgical bypass. The major limiting factor for the endoscopic approach is being unable to pass the scope through the obstruction. The major complications reported are gastric ulceration, bowel perforation, biliary obstruction, stent dysfunction, and stent migration. Stent placement would be contraindicated in patients with multiple levels of intestinal obstruction and should be considered carefully for patients with peritoneal carcinomatosis who are at risk of more distal obstructions.

For patients in whom stenting is not an option, surgical bypass can relieve both the symptoms of the obstruction and allow the patient to resume enteral nutrition. Surgical bypass, most commonly in the form of a gastrojejunostomy, can either be performed laparoscopically or through a relatively small upper midline incision. The estimated risk of morbidity and mortality from these procedures is 25% to 60% and 0% to 25%, respectively [22,23]. While surgical bypass is usually technically successful, patient selection with regard to preoperative nutritional status and life expectancy is imperative to the palliative success of this approach. For example, in addition to general surgical risks such as bleeding or infection, a patient with chronic gastric outlet or duodenal obstruction who is malnourished is at increased risk of a leak from the intestinal anastomosis. Other potential complications specific to gastric bypass include dumping syndrome, alkaline reflux gastritis, and delayed gastric emptying.

Placement of a gastrostomy tube for decompression is another option for palliation of gastric outlet, duodenal and nonoperable small bowel obstruction or profound gastrointestinal dysmotility from carcinomatosis. Gastrostomy tubes can be placed either endoscopically, fluoroscopically, or surgically (either laparoscopic or open). Decompression gastrostomy tubes provide patients the ability to drain the stomach as for nausea and to avoid vomiting. It also allows them to drink liquids and eat some soft foods for pleasure and comfort. It does not allow for the enteric maintenance of nutrition. Many endoscopists, surgeons, and interventional radiologists are leery of placing gastrostomy tubes in the setting of malignant ascites. They are concerned about the risk of infecting the ascites, intraperitoneal leakage from the stomach due to poor apposition to the anterior abdominal wall, as well as leakage of ascites from around the tube. There is a growing body of literature demonstrating the safety of placing gastrostomy tubes in patients with malignant ascites from a variety of tumors [24–26]. Paracentesis prior to or concurrent with gastrostomy placement is advisable. Also, consideration of placing a peritoneal drainage catheter at the time of gastrostomy may also help lower any risk associated with the ascites. As gastrostomy may be the only viable palliative option for these patients, all efforts to manage the ascites and increase the safety of gastrostomy placement are warranted.

Ascites and Pleural Effusions

Two other common palliative surgical consultations for the ICU patient are for management of peritoneal ascites and pleural effusions. Unfortunately, while the symptom relief from a paracentesis or thoracentesis is immediately helpful, it is usually temporary. For patients requiring frequent drainage of either the peritoneal or pleural cavity, a tunneled intraperitoneal catheter that can be intermittently connected to a self-contained vacuum drainage system is a helpful option [27]. These catheters can be placed under local anesthesia either by interventional radiology or surgery. Another option for the treatment of malignant ascites is hyperthermic intraperitoneal chemotherapy (HIPEC). A number of studies have demonstrated the efficacy of HIPEC in the treatment of malignant ascites [28,29]. As there is often no cytoreductive surgery involved, this can be done laparoscopically, which, although less invasive, still does require general anesthesia. This option may be less appropriate for patients who are in the ICU and should typically be reserved for patients with a longer life expectancy and higher performance status.

Similarly, an alternative treatment option for patients with recurrent malignant pleural effusion is pleurodesis. Pleurodesis can be performed using a number of different agents including talc, chemotherapy, or abrasion. The intent is to create an inflammatory reaction within the pleural cavity resulting in fusion of the visceral and parietal pleura, thereby obliterating the peritoneal space and the opportunity for fluid re-accumulation. Talc has been shown to be the most effective pleurodesis agent in randomized clinical trials with reported success rates of 60% to 90% [30]. However, although these procedures can be done at the bedside, they do require the placement of a larger bore chest tube and can be rather painful [31].

Intestinal Perforation

Intestinal perforation due to a complication of a life-limiting illness can be one of the most challenging consults at the end of life in the ICU setting. Unlike patients with a bowel obstruction, patients with a perforated viscus are more likely to have pain from peritonitis, adding another element of consideration to both the decision-making process and the emotional charge of the situation. Currently, there is a small, but growing body of literature supporting the use of nonsurgical management for bowel perforation in select (hemodynamically stable, non-peritonitic) patients. Some studies have reported a greater than 90% success rate in nonsurgical management of patients with perforated diverticulitis [32]. Unfortunately, for patients with advanced cancer, who are not stable or who have peritonitis, and who undergo emergent surgery, the outcomes are even worse than for those with a bowel obstruction. In the study by Cauley et al. [18], among the 499 patients who underwent surgery for perforation, the 30-day mortality was 34% with a morbidity rate of 67%, and 52% of patients were discharged to an institution. Independent preoperative predictors of death at 30 days included renal failure, septic shock, ascites, dyspnea at rest, and dependent functional status. Postoperative respiratory complications and advanced age (greater than 75 years) were also predictors of mortality. Similar to the patients who presented with a bowel obstruction, only 4% had a "do not resuscitate" order in place prior to surgery despite the advanced nature of their cancer. Again, while data from studies like this may help surgeons answer questions about the risks associated with surgical interventions and guide some patients in their decisions, in a society in which people are not prepared for dying, these data can often make things harder for the surgeon who is asked to operate in the face of such overwhelming odds.

Avoiding Moral Distress

Caught between patients who are suddenly facing their own mortality and families who are not ready to let go, the smallest amount of hope that surgery offers makes even the most daunting risks seem worth taking. This is a setting in which surgeons, and other affiliated providers, experience moral distress. Professionalism demands that the surgeon make a sincere effort to understand and be understanding of the perspective of the patient and family—without realistic expectation of the same in return. This can be particularly challenging when the surgeon is busy or when these events occur in the middle of the night. In the name of "full disclosure and informed consent," some surgeons paint as bleak a picture as possible for the patient and family, in an effort to dissuade the patient from choosing surgery. When, despite these efforts, the patient and family ask for surgery, some surgeons expect a tacit agreement that the patient will endure to the end, including any additional procedures or maneuvers that may be required—surgery, feeding tubes, tracheotomy, dialysis, rehabilitation, etc. There is often a sense of frustration and betrayal on the part of the surgeon when within a few days after the index surgery, the family decides to stop any further life-prolonging care. It is for this reason that understanding the perspective of the patient and family is critical to both outcome of the encounter and the surgeon's well-being (see Chapter 36).

It is for challenging situations like this that the palliative triangle can be most helpful. As described above, use of the palliative triangle can help create a space in which all three parties are given a chance to express their concerns and be heard. It is also significant in that it helps the surgeon separate the patient's goals and understanding from that of the family's and vice versa. It also gives the surgeon's goals and understanding equal weight in the decision-making. However, success of the palliative triangle approach is predicated on the surgeon's mind-set. If the surgeon truly hopes to influence the behavior of the patient and the family in an efficient and professional manner, an outward mind-set, in which the patient's and family's objectives matter like the surgeon's objectives matter, is essential. The Arbinger Influence Pyramid is a proven leadership approach to influencing behavior which is readily applicable to patient–family–physician interactions [33] (Fig. 55.2). Starting at the base of the pyramid, the surgeon must adjust his or her mind-set to an outward mind-set in which the goals and objectives of the patient and family matter equally with his or hers. The outward mind-set will then facilitate building a relationship with the patient and those who have influence on the patient—namely the family. Building this relationship can happen simply through introductions and a sincere

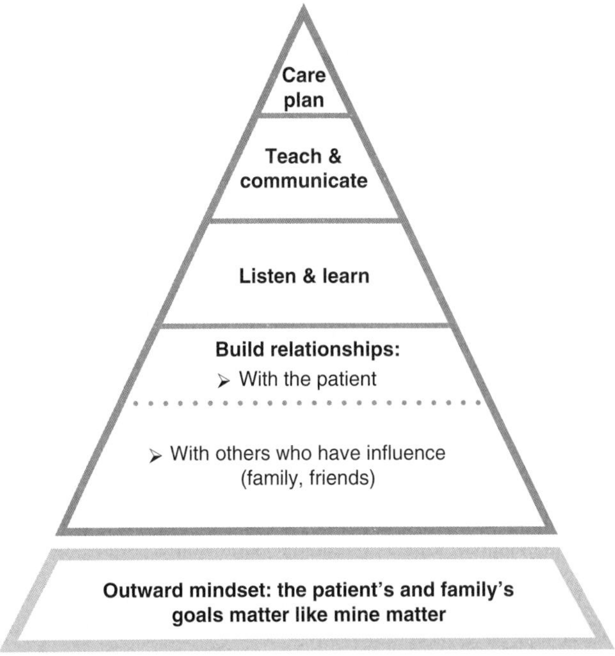

FIGURE 55.2 The Arbinger Influence Pyramid. The Influence Pyramid is a proven framework designed to help influence behavior and improve results beginning with a shift in mind-set. (Adapted from The Arbinger Institute: *The Anatomy of Peace—Resolving the Heart of Conflict*. Oakland, CA: Berrett-Koehler Publishers, Inc, 2015, with permission.)

expression of empathy for the challenging situation which the patient and family are facing. Next, the surgeon needs to listen and learn what the patient and family know about the situation and what their hopes, goals, and objectives are. Afterward, the surgeon can teach the patient and family what they need to know, correct any misconceptions, answer questions, review the risks, benefits, and indications for surgery and the alternative options, and make an engaged recommendation based upon the goals of all three parties. From there, the surgeon, patient, and family can usually come to a mutually agreed upon goal and care plan (see "structured family meetings" in Chapter 34). There are a few key points about using the Influence Pyramid. First, time and effort spent at the lower levels of the pyramid is what ensures effectiveness at the higher levels. Second, the solution to a problem at one level of the pyramid will be found in spending more time at a lower level of the pyramid. Third, the effectiveness at each level of the pyramid depends on the effectiveness of the level below and ultimately on the deepest level of the pyramid—the mind-set.

BENEFITS OF EARLY PALLIATIVE CARE CONSULTS

Initiation of a palliative surgery consultation is an appropriate time for initiating a palliative care consultation as well, if one has not already been obtained. While some physicians and patients view a palliative care consult as "giving up," this could not be further from the truth. Unlike hospice (which is a medical insurance benefit that requires a life expectancy of less than 6 months if the life-threatening disease is untreated and the patient forgoes disease-directed treatment), all patients with symptoms from an illness or its treatment benefit from palliative care. While most patients' symptoms can be adequately palliated by their primary physician (either their primary care provider or primary specialist), advanced, life-threatening illnesses, such as cancer, can pose additional challenges in terms of physical, emotional, psychological, spiritual, and social symptomatology. It is preferable to initiate a palliative care consultation before these symptoms become unmanageable, as this will make it seem less like "giving up" when there is an acute need for the expertise of a palliative care provider.

One way to overcome the inertia of referring patients to palliative care early is to normalize it. Many institutions have made it part of their cancer center's protocols to refer all patients with advanced cancer to palliative care from the initial cancer center visit. This allows the palliative care team to tell patients and their families that all patients with advanced cancer are seen by palliative care and that it is simply part of the multidisciplinary team effort to care for the patient and family. Similar efforts can also be made in the ICU for selected patients (see Chapter 33). Palliative care consultation can help take some of the burden off the primary specialist for conducting the harder conversations around goals of care and advanced directives and allowing them to focus on the plan of treatment. Having these difficult conversations early is essential for the comprehensive management of life-threatening illness and should not be avoided due to provider unease.

Earlier palliative care involvement can also help with the transition to hospice when appropriate. Recognition of that time may come first to the primary specialist when further illness-directed treatment is likely to do more harm than good to the patient and family when they decide that the burden of treatment is not worth the limited potential for more time. Unfortunately, it is not infrequent that both parties do not arrive at this recognition at the same time. The treating physician may find it easier to continue to treat the patient who insists on continuing to "fight" even knowing that "fighting" may take time away from the patient. Similarly, the patient may find it easier to keep doing treatment rather than "disappoint" the treating physician by stopping. With an early palliative care intervention, conversations about hospice as a potential option can be started early leaving plenty of time to correct any misconceptions. Patients and families can learn that the mission of hospice is neither to prolong life nor hasten death but to provide comfort and dignity and optimize the quality of life that is left. It can help dispel other concerns such as losing contact with the primary care provider, not being allowed to go to the hospital if necessary, not being allowed to come off hospice if a new treatment becomes available, etc. They will also learn that hospice provides support to both the patient and the family through an interdisciplinary team of providers including physicians, nurses, social workers, chaplains, and volunteers. Hospice also helps families prepare for their loss and provides bereavement programs after the death. It has also been shown that patients who understand their poorer prognosis near the end of life are unlikely to choose invasive treatments that can prolong suffering and time away from home [34–36]. A palliative care consultant who is an expert in communication can be a huge help with this aspect of the patient's care (see Chapter 34).

CONCLUSIONS

Surgery and surgeons are an essential component of comprehensive palliative care. Surgical decision-making for palliation in the end of life setting is complex and challenging. These situations often demand the highest level of surgical judgment. In addition to consideration of the risks in terms of the traditional surgical outcomes measures such as morbidity and mortality, decisions must also include end points such as the probability and duration of symptom resolution, the impact on overall quality of life, pain control, and cost-effectiveness. Regardless of the indication for a palliative surgery consultation, deliberations over surgical palliation must consider the clinical condition and performance status of the patient, the prognosis of the disease process, the availability and success of nonoperative management, and the individual patient's quality of life, life expectancy, and goals of care. Clinicians must remain flexible to meet the ever-changing needs of the patient and family. Use of a tool such as the palliative care triangle and the Influence Pyramid can facilitate the difficult conversations that often accompany these consults and help guide the patient, family, and surgeon to make the optimal choice for the patient. Early palliative care consultation has also been shown to improve outcomes in terms of quality of life, overall survival and cost-effectiveness, as well as mitigating some of the moral distress that can arise in these emotionally charged situations.

References

1. Miner TJ, Jaques DP, Shriver CD: A prospective evaluation of patients undergoing surgery for the palliation of an advanced malignancy. *Ann Surg Oncol* 9(7):696–703, 2002.
2. Badgwell B, Bruera E, Klimberg SV: Can patient reported outcomes help identify the optimal outcome in palliative surgery? *J Surg Oncol* 109(2):145–150, 2014.
3. Blakely AM, Heffernan DS, McPhillips J, et al: Elevated C-reactive protein as a predictor of patient outcomes following palliative surgery. *J Surg Oncol* 110(6):651–655, 2014.
4. Badgwell BD, Smith K, Liu P, et al: Indicators of surgery and survival in oncology inpatients requiring surgical evaluation for palliation. *Support Care Cancer* 17(6):727–734, 2009.
5. Krouse RS, Nelson RA, Farrell BR, et al: Surgical palliation at a cancer center: incidence and outcomes. *Arch Surg* 136(7):773–778, 2001.
6. Miner TJ, Brennan MF, Jaques DP: A prospective, symptom related, outcomes analysis of 1022 palliative procedures for advanced cancer. *Ann Surg* 240(4):719–726; discussion 726–717, 2004.
7. Badgwell BD, Aloia TA, Garrett J, et al: Indicators of symptom improvement and survival in inpatients with advanced cancer undergoing palliative surgical consultation. *J Surg Oncol* 107(4):367–371, 2013.
8. Podnos YD, Juarez G, Pameijer C, et al: Impact of surgical palliation on quality of life in patients with advanced malignancy: results of the decisions and outcomes in palliative surgery (DOPS) trial. *Ann Surg Oncol* 14(2):922–928, 2007.
9. Podnos YD, Juarez G, Pameijer C, et al: Surgical palliation of advanced gastrointestinal tumors. *J Palliat Med* 10(4):871–876, 2007.
10. Badgwell B, Krouse R, Cormier J, et al: Frequent and early death limits quality of life assessment in patients with advanced malignancies evaluated for palliative surgical intervention. *Ann Surg Oncol* 19(12):3651–3658, 2012.
11. Collins LK, Goodwin JA, Spencer HJ, et al: Patient reasoning in palliative surgical oncology. *J Surg Oncol* 107(4):372–375, 2013.
12. Miner TJ, Cohen J, Charpentier K, et al: The palliative triangle: improved patient selection and outcomes associated with palliative operations. *Arch Surg* 146(5):517–522, 2011.
13. Paul Olson TJ, Pinkerton C, Brasel KJ, et al: Palliative surgery for malignant bowel obstruction from carcinomatosis: a systematic review. *JAMA Surg* 149(4):383–392, 2014.
14. Yoon JY, Jung YS, Hong SP, et al: Clinical outcomes and risk factors for technical and clinical failures of self-expandable metal stent insertion for malignant colorectal obstruction. *Gastrointest Endosc* 74(4):858–868, 2011.
15. Sagar J: Colorectal stents for the management of malignant colonic obstructions. *Cochrane Database Syst Rev* (11):CD007378, 2011. doi:10.1002/14651858.CD007378.pub2.
16. Kim JH, Ku YS, Jeon TJ, et al: The efficacy of self-expanding metal stents for malignant colorectal obstruction by noncolonic malignancy with peritoneal carcinomatosis. *Dis Colon Rectum* 56(11):1228–1232, 2013.
17. Caceres A, Zhou Q, Iasonos A, et al: Colorectal stents for palliation of large-bowel obstructions in recurrent gynecologic cancer: an updated series. *Gynecol Oncol* 108(3):482–485, 2008.
18. Cauley CE, Panizales MT, Reznor G, et al: Outcomes after emergency abdominal surgery in patients with advanced cancer: Opportunities to reduce complications and improve palliative care. *J Trauma Acute Care Surg* 79(3):399–406, 2015.
19. Pameijer CR, Mahvi DM, Stewart JA, et al: Bowel obstruction in patients with metastatic cancer: does intervention influence outcome? *Int J Gastrointest Cancer* 35(2):127–133, 2005.
20. Mosler P, Mergener KD, Brandabur JJ, et al: Palliation of gastric outlet obstruction and proximal small bowel obstruction with self-expandable metal stents: a single center series. *J Clin Gastroenterol* 39(2):124–128, 2005.
21. Holt AP, Patel M, Ahmed MM: Palliation of patients with malignant gastroduodenal obstruction with self-expanding metallic stents: the treatment of choice? *Gastrointest Endosc* 60(6):1010–1017, 2004.
22. Ly J, O'Grady G, Mittal A, et al: A systematic review of methods to palliate malignant gastric outlet obstruction. *Surg Endosc* 24(2):290–297, 2010.
23. Zheng B, Wang X, Ma B, et al: Endoscopic stenting versus gastrojejunostomy for palliation of malignant gastric outlet obstruction. *Dig Endosc* 24(2):71–78, 2012.

24. Pothuri B, Montemarano M, Gerardi M, et al: Percutaneous endoscopic gastrostomy tube placement in patients with malignant bowel obstruction due to ovarian carcinoma. *Gynecol Oncol* 96(2):330–334, 2005.
25. Ryan JM, Hahn PF, Mueller PR: Performing radiologic gastrostomy or gastrojejunostomy in patients with malignant ascites. *AJR Am J Roentgenol* 171(4):1003–1006, 1998.
26. Shaw C, Bassett RL, Fox PS, et al: Palliative venting gastrostomy in patients with malignant bowel obstruction and ascites. *Ann Surg Oncol* 20(2):497–505, 2013.
27. Fleming ND, Alvarez-Secord A, Von Gruenigen V, et al: Indwelling catheters for the management of refractory malignant ascites: a systematic literature overview and retrospective chart review. *J Pain Symptom Manage* 38(3):341–349, 2009.
28. Facchiano E, Risio D, Kianmanesh R, et al: Laparoscopic hyperthermic intraperitoneal chemotherapy: indications, aims, and results: a systematic review of the literature. *Ann Surg Oncol* 19(9):2946–2950, 2012.
29. Randle RW, Swett KR, Swords DS, et al: Efficacy of cytoreductive surgery with hyperthermic intraperitoneal chemotherapy in the management of malignant ascites. *Ann Surg Oncol* 21(5):1474–1479, 2014.
30. Shaw P, Agarwal R: Pleurodesis for malignant pleural effusions. *Cochrane Database Syst Rev* (1):CD002916, 2004. doi: 10.1002/14651858.CD002916.pub2.
31. Rahman NM, Pepperell J, Rehal S, et al: Effect of opioids vs NSAIDs and larger vs smaller chest tube size on pain control and pleurodesis efficacy among patients with malignant pleural effusion: the TIME1 randomized clinicalt. *JAMA* 314(24):2641–2653, 2015.
32. Dharmarajan S, Hunt SR, Birnbaum EH, et al: The efficacy of nonoperative management of acute complicated diverticulitis. *Dis Colon Rectum* 54(6):663–671, 2011.
33. The Arbinger Institute: *The Anatomy of Peace—Resolving the Heart of Conflict.* Oakland, CA: Berrett-Koehler Publishers, 2015.
34. Mack JW, Weeks JC, Wright AA, et al: End-of-life discussions, goal attainment, and distress at the end of life: predictors and outcomes of receipt of care consistent with preferences. *J Clin Oncol* 28(7):1203–1208, 2010.
35. Weeks JC, Cook EF, O'Day SJ, et al: Relationship between cancer patients' predictions of prognosis and their treatment preferences. *JAMA* 279(21):1709–1714, 1998.
36. Zhang B, Nilsson ME, Prigerson HG: Factors important to patients' quality of life at the end of life. *Arch Intern Med* 172(15):1133–1142, 2012.

Chapter 56 ■ Management of the Organ Donor

CHRISTOPH TROPPMANN

In 2016, over 13,000 patients on the national organ transplant waiting list in the United States died or were delisted because they had become too ill before a suitable donor organ became available [1]. Almost assuredly, this number underestimates the actual magnitude of the problem. Many patients with end-stage organ failure are currently not even considered for transplantation (and consequently are not listed) because of the strict recipient selection criteria that are being applied—in part as a result of the severe, ongoing organ shortage. The widening gap between available deceased donor organs and the number of patients waiting is a result of the explosive, increased use of organ transplantation therapy over the past 40 years (Tables 56.1 and 56.2), with which the deceased donor pool has not kept pace (Fig. 56.1) [1,2].

The single most important factor that has been identified in this equation is the failure to maximize the conversion of potential deceased donors to actual donors, primarily because of the inability to obtain consent for organ recovery. The rates of consent granted by families of potential deceased donors range only from 0% to 75% and appear to vary widely among geographic regions and ethnic groups [10–12]. Lack of dissemination and poor presentation of information to the public, misperceptions in the general population regarding the beneficial nature of organ transplantation, and the necessity of organ recovery from deceased donors, as well as inappropriate coordination of the approach to families of potential donors contribute to the stagnation of the organ supply [11–13].

TABLE 56.1

Number of Solid Organ Transplants from Deceased Donors per Year in the United States: 1982 versus 2014

Organ	1982	2016
Kidney	3,681	13,431
Liver	62	7,496
Pancreas	38	1,031
Heart	103	3,190
Heart–lung	8	18
Lung	—[a]	2,327
Intestine	—[a]	147

[a]No lung or intestinal transplants were performed in 1982.
Data from references [1–4].

TABLE 56.2

One-Year Graft Survival Rates (Deceased Donors): 1982 versus 2013

Organ	1982 (%)[a]	2015 (%)
Kidney	80	94
Liver	35	89
Pancreas	23	86
Heart	65	90
Lung	—[b]	85
Intestine	—[b]	75

[a]Results without cyclosporin A–based immunosuppression.
[b]No lung or intestinal transplants were performed in 1982.
Data from references [4–8] (1982) and [1,2] (2015).

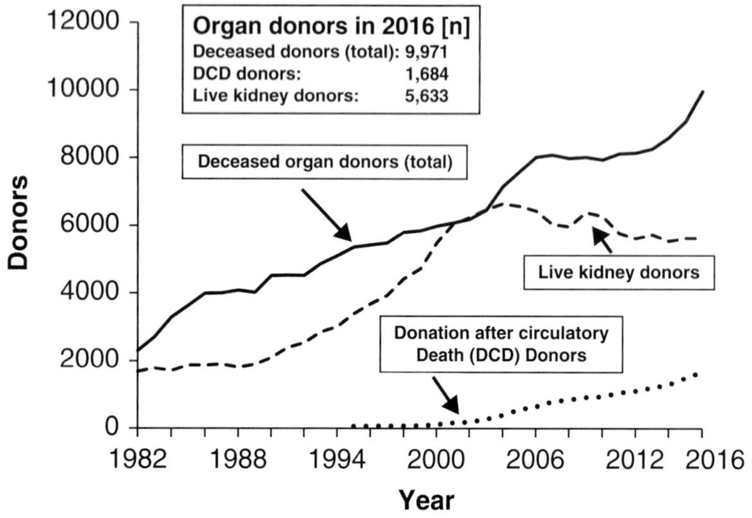

FIGURE 56.1 Evolution of the number of overall deceased organ donors, of donors after circulatory death, and of living kidney donors between 1982 and 2016 in the United States. (Data from references [1–4,9])

TABLE 56.3

Identification of Potential Organ Donors: Guidelines for Referral to the Local Organ Procurement Organization

Clinical triggers	All patients with a severe nonrecoverable neurologic injury on a ventilator with any of the following conditions: Head trauma Cerebral hemorrhage Primary brain tumor Hypoxic insult (including prolonged cardiopulmonary resuscitation, near-drowning, drug overdose, poisoning, cerebral edema, seizures, and asphyxiation injuries)
Referral guidelines	Refer patients within 1 hour of meeting one or more clinical triggers Refer all patients who meet clinical triggers regardless of age and underlying/associated diagnosis Refer all patients who meet clinical triggers prior to approaching the family regarding end-of-life decisions Refer patients prior to brain death evaluation Refer patients if the family raises the subject of donation Coroner case status does not constitute an exclusion criterion

The role of physicians who care for critically ill patients in altering this current situation is crucial [14]. It is their responsibility to minimize deceleration of the critical care provided to patients that have suffered a catastrophic brain injury, to identify potential donors, to seek their early referral to an organ procurement organization (OPO), and to ensure that families are adequately approached. This will maximize families' opportunities to donate a family member's organs and allow the families to experience the beneficial effects of donation for the bereavement process (Table 56.3) [15].

It is estimated that in the United States alone, approximately 250,000 additional life years could be saved annually if consent rates for potential deceased donors could be increased to 100% [16]. Intensive care and emergency medicine physicians are obligated ethically and morally to provide the best possible outcome for a very ill patient. However, after a potential donor has been identified, they are also obligated to seek the best possible outcome for patients with end-stage failure of a vital organ waiting for a transplant by attempting to ensure that organ donation occurs. It is becoming increasingly evident that implementation of critical pathways and standardized donor management protocols play an important role in this context [17–25].

DONOR CLASSIFICATION BASED ON THE CRITERIA USED FOR DETERMINATION OF DEATH

Brain-Dead Deceased Donors

Death is determined based on neurologic criteria. Donation after brain death is the most common type of organ donation (currently over 80% of all donors belong in this category) [2]. In most Western developed countries, brain death is legally equated with death. The diagnosis of brain death rests on the irreversibility of the neurologic insult and the absence of clinical evidence of cerebral *and* brain stem function. The details of the clinical examination that is required to unequivocally establish brain death are described in this chapter. Organ procurement proceeds only after brain death has been diagnosed and death has been declared.

Donation After Circulatory Death Donors (Formerly Known as Donation After Cardiac Death or Non–Heart-Beating Donors)

Death is determined based on circulatory and respiratory criteria. Further increases of the number of donors in this category are to be expected (Fig. 56.1) [1,2,24,26,27]. Most commonly, families of unconscious patients with severe irreversible traumatic or cerebrovascular brain injury, who do not fulfill the formal criteria of brain death, decide to forgo any further care and wish to donate the organs of their family member. Under this scenario, time and place of death are controlled. Circulatory and respiratory support technologies are discontinued in the critical care unit or the operating room and organ recovery is initiated once death has been pronounced by a physician not belonging to the organ recovery and transplant team [26].

An alternative, by far less common donation after circulatory death (DCD) scenario—uncontrolled death—involves a patient who expires, for example, in the emergency room following massive trauma or a sudden cardiovascular event. In the interest of minimizing warm ischemia time, flushing cannulas may be inserted and possibly even perfusion of internal organs with cold preservation solution might already be started while consent to proceed with organ donation is obtained from the patient's family. The discussion that surrounds this category of DCD donors includes concerns centered on when to stop the resuscitation effort and whether it is appropriate to perform a procedure (i.e., insertion of flushing cannulas) that presumes consent before actually obtaining it from the family. In light of the severe organ donor shortage, there is renewed public debate about more systematically considering uncontrolled DCD at a larger scale [28].

Other considerations that pertain to both controlled and uncontrolled DCD donors include: uncertainty regarding the exact definition of death after discontinuing circulatory and respiratory support (there is no standardized definition of, e.g., the minimal duration of asystole after the patient expires following withdrawal of support before death can be pronounced; this is currently subject to considerable interinstitutional variation), and the possibility of the patient at least temporarily surviving the withdrawal of support technologies (backup plans must be clearly defined by each individual institutional DCD donor protocol). Nevertheless, these considerations must be balanced with the right of self-determination based on an individual's previously documented preferences and the final wishes of a competent patient family. Further debate by the medical community and general public is crucial to address these complex ethical issues and to maximize acceptance of organ donation [28,29]. Without such thorough consideration, the deceased donor concept and the donation system that is currently in place might be harmed or discredited.

CURRENT STATUS OF SOLID ORGAN TRANSPLANTATION

The increased number of solid organ transplant procedures performed during the last 40 years has been paralleled by significant improvements in outcomes including rates of patient and graft survival (Table 56.2). This phenomenon has been attributed to a variety of factors that include (a) the introduction in the early

1980s of the powerful immunosuppressive agent cyclosporin A, followed a decade later by tacrolimus, mycophenolate mofetil, and other new immunosuppressants; (b) the availability of antilymphocyte antibody preparations to prevent and treat rejection episodes (e.g., antilymphocyte and antithymocyte globulin); (c) improvements in organ preservation (e.g., use of University of Wisconsin solution, *ex vivo* machine perfusion of donor organs); (d) thorough preoperative transplant candidate screening for the presence of comorbid disease processes; and (e) increasing sophistication in the postoperative intensive care of regular and high-risk recipients. In addition, the availability of potent, yet nontoxic, antibacterial, antifungal, and antiviral agents has allowed opportunistic infections in immunocompromised transplant patients to be treated more effectively. In combination with refinement of surgical techniques, these factors have led to increasing success of solid organ replacement therapy.

Thus, transplantation has become the treatment of choice for many patients with end-stage failure of the kidneys, liver, endocrine pancreas, heart, lungs, and small bowel. Successful hand, arm, larynx, and face transplants from deceased donors have also been reported [30–33]. Currently, the only patients who are excluded from undergoing transplantation are those with malignancies (metastatic or at high risk for recurrence) and uncontrolled infections, those who are unable to withstand transplant surgery, or those who have a significantly shortened life expectancy due to disease processes unrelated to their target organ dysfunction or failure.

Kidney

Currently, patients undergoing kidney transplants from deceased donors exhibit excellent graft survival rates (Table 56.2). Renal transplantation dramatically improves life expectancy and quality of life, decreases cardiovascular morbidity and mortality, and rehabilitates the recipients from a social perspective. Kidney transplants are also less expensive from a socioeconomic standpoint than is chronic hemodialysis. For pediatric patients with chronic renal failure, a functioning renal allograft is the only way to preserve normal growth and ensure adequate central nervous, mental, and motor development.

Liver

Patients with end-stage liver failure die unless they receive a transplant. Liver transplants are an effective treatment for many patients, pediatric and adult, regardless of the cause of liver failure: congenital (i.e., structural or metabolic defects), acquired (i.e., due to infection, trauma, or toxins), or idiopathic (e.g., cryptogenic cirrhosis, autoimmune hepatitis). A dramatic improvement in graft survival occurred after the introduction of cyclosporin A (Table 56.2). Currently, there are no reliable means to substitute, even temporarily, for a failing liver other than with a transplantation. Extracorporeal perfusion, using either animal livers or bioartificial liver devices (e.g., hepatocytes suspended in bioreactors), may someday bridge the gap between complete liver failure and liver transplantation, but these therapeutic modalities are still investigational and are far from becoming standard clinical tools. Hepatocyte and stem cell transplants to treat fulminant liver failure and to correct congenital enzyme deficiencies are being studied but are presently not a clinical reality.

Intestine

Small bowel transplants are performed in patients with congenital or acquired short gut, especially if liver dysfunction occurs because of long-term administration of total parenteral nutrition and when difficulty in establishing or maintaining central venous access is limiting. If liver disease is advanced, a combined liver–small bowel or, in highly selected cases, a multivisceral transplant (liver, stomach, small bowel, with or without pancreas) can be performed [34].

Pancreas and Islet

Primary prevention of type 1 insulin-dependent diabetes mellitus is not possible, but transplantation of the entire pancreas or isolated pancreatic islets can correct the endocrine insufficiency once it occurs. Glucose sensor systems that *continuously* monitor blood sugar levels coupled with real-time command of an insulin delivery system (implantable pump) and bioartificial and hybrid biomechanical insulin-secreting devices are not yet universally available for routine clinical use. The only effective current option to *consistently* restore continuous near-physiologic normoglycemia, however, is a pancreas transplant [35–37]. Good metabolic glycemic control decreases the incidence and severity of secondary diabetic complications (neuropathy, retinopathy, gastropathy and enteropathy, and nephropathy). Most pancreas transplants are performed simultaneously with a kidney transplant in preuremic patients with significant renal dysfunction or in uremic patients with end-stage diabetic nephropathy. Selected nonuremic patients with brittle type 1 diabetes mellitus (with progression of the autonomic neuropathy or recurrent severe hypoglycemic episodes, and with repetitive episodes of diabetic ketoacidosis) can benefit from a solitary pancreas transplant (without a concomitant kidney transplant) to improve their quality of life and to prevent the manifestation and progression of secondary diabetic complications. Evidence suggests that a successful pancreas transplant can achieve these goals in uremic and in nonuremic recipients and decrease mortality [35]. Islet transplants are undergoing intensive clinical investigation. Results of transplanting alloislets from deceased donors are encouraging in the short term [36]; however, long-term results are less favorable [37].

Heart

Heart transplantation is the treatment of choice for patients with end-stage congenital and acquired parenchymal and vascular diseases and is recommended generally after all conventional medical or surgical options have been exhausted. After a widely publicized start in 1967, poor results were observed over the ensuing decade. In the 1980s, however, the field of cardiac transplantation experienced dramatic growth (Table 56.1) because of significant improvements in outcome, probably most directly related to immunosuppressive therapy and to refinements in diagnosis and treatment of rejection episodes [38]. Mechanical pumps, such as implantable ventricular assist devices or the bioartificial heart, have contributed to this success because they can also serve as a bridge during the time between end-stage cardiac failure and a transplantation.

Heart–Lung and Lung

Heart–lung and lung transplants are an effective treatment for patients with advanced pulmonary parenchymal or vascular disease, with or without primary or secondary cardiac involvement. This field has evolved rapidly since the first single-lung transplant with long-term success was performed in 1983 (Table 56.1). The significant increase in lung transplantations is mainly due to technical improvements resulting in fewer surgical complications, as well as to the extremely limited availability of heart–lung donors. Previously, many patients with end-stage pulmonary failure would have waited for an appropriate heart–lung donor. Now, they undergo a single or a bilateral single-lung transplant instead [39]. Bilateral single-lung transplants are specifically indicated in patients with septic lung diseases (e.g., cystic fibrosis, α_1-antitrypsin deficiency) in which the remaining native contralateral lung could cross-contaminate a single transplanted lung. Double *en bloc* lung transplants have been abandoned because of technical difficulties related to the bronchial anastomotic blood supply. Mechanical ventilation or extracorporeal membrane oxygenation (ECMO) can be used as a temporary bridge to this type of transplant, but none of these modalities obviates the need for organ replacement therapy.

CURRENT STATUS OF ORGAN DONATION

Current organ supply does not meet demand.This is due to an insufficient augmentation of the donor pool (Tables 56.1 and 56.2; Fig. 56.1). The 55-mile-per-hour speed limit, stricter seat belt and helmet laws, advances in critical care, as well as the trend toward a deceleration of care in patients that have suffered a catastrophic brain injury have all had significant impacts on the number of brain-dead organ donors [1]. In 2016, the three leading causes of death among deceased donors in the United States were cerebral anoxia (e.g., due to a cardiac arrest), a cerebrovascular accident (e.g., due to a stroke or an intracranial aneurysmal bleed), and traumatic brain injury [1,2].

A positive trend is the increasing number of DCD donors (Fig. 56.1) [2,24]. These donors constitute currently nearly 20% of the overall deceased donor pool [2]. In DCD donors, refined surgical techniques allow for fast insertion of cannulas and perfusion of vital organs while these are rapidly excised. Innovative approaches, such as withdrawal of support technologies in the ICU (rather than in the operating room), in the presence of the donor's family, may further increase acceptance of DCD donation among potential donors' families and health care professionals [26,29]. Moreover, ongoing refinements of organ perfusion and preservation techniques, including maintenance of the DCD donor on ECMO until organ recovery can occur, and placement of the recovered organs on hypothermic or normothermic perfusion using a pump during the transport and preservation phase, all result in less ischemic organ injury and also allow for better organ preservation and increased utilization of DCD donor organs [24,40–43]. Currently, kidneys and livers are the organs most commonly recovered and transplanted from DCD donors [2].

According to estimates, there are at least 10,500 to 13,800 *potential* brain-dead donors in the United States per year [12]. In 2016, however, there were only 9,971 *actual* deceased organ donors in the United States [1]. According to a study, the overall consent rate (the number of families agreeing to donate divided by the number of families asked to donate) was 54% in the United States, and the overall conversion rate (the number of actual donors divided by the number of potential donors) was 42% [12]. The single most important reason for lack of organ recovery from 45% to 60% of the potential donor pool is the inability to obtain consent [12,24]. Several studies have shown that family refusal to provide consent and the inability to identify, locate, or contact family members to obtain consent within an appropriate time frame are the leading causes for the nonuse of many organs from potential donors [10–13,24]. A public opinion survey showed that 69% of respondents would be very or somewhat willing to donate their organs, and 93% would honor the expressed wishes of a family member [44]. However, only 52% of these individuals had communicated their wishes to their family. Moreover, 37% of respondents did not comprehend that a brain-dead person should be considered dead and unable to recover, and 59% either believed or were unsure whether or not organs can be bought and sold on the "black market." Also, 42% did not realize that organ donation does not cause any financial cost to the family of the deceased in the United States [44]. Finally, racial differences which are likely based on historical distrust in the health care system may adversely impact donation rates as well. For instance, African American families have been consistently found to be less willing to consent to organ donation than White families [45].

Correcting these misperceptions and attempting to increase awareness of the importance of organ transplantation must remain the focus of public educational campaigns [24,29]. The family's knowledge of the patient's previous wishes is central to decision-making [10,11,13]. Such efforts can be successful, especially among minorities, in whom mistrust and the perception of inequitable access to medical care and organ transplant therapy have led to disappointingly low organ donation and recovery rates [24,45]. It is very important that adequate communication, empathy, and an informative, humane approach to the family of the deceased occur to ensure reasonable consideration of donation. Families are more likely to donate if they are approached by an OPO coordinator, view the requestor as sensitive to their needs, and experience an optimal request pattern [11,13,22]. Educational efforts to enhance organ donation must therefore also be directed at health care professionals and medical students, whose views and knowledge of these issues are often inconsistent and limited [29,46]. Physicians, too, need to be better trained to recognize and refer potential organ donors and to not discuss organ donation until a member of the local OPO has approached their families [11,13,22]. As a result, since 1998, Conditions of Participation of the Centers for Medicare and Medicaid Services (CMS) require hospitals to use "designated requestors" to obtain family authorization. Finally, the potential for financial compensation or other rewards for deceased donor families (e.g., compensation for funeral expenses) has been considered as a means to increase donation rates [46]. But the potential effects of such an intervention on donation rates remain unclear.

OTHER OPTIONS TO INCREASE ORGAN AVAILABILITY

Additional mechanisms that might help to increase the number of available organs for transplantation include (a) optimization and maximal use of the current actual donor pool; (b) increasing the number of living donor transplants, including the provision of incentives for live donation; (c) enacting presumed consent laws; (d) allowing the use of organs from executed prisoners; and (e) xenotransplants (e.g., use of animal organs as a potentially unlimited supply for transplantation into humans, particularly after genetic engineering). Only the first two options are, however, of practical interest at this time.

Optimal Use of the Current Donor Pool

As a result of the ongoing organ shortage, transplant surgeons have attempted to refine procurement techniques so that maximal use of the available donor pool occurs (Fig. 56.2) [47]. On average, more than three organs are recovered and transplanted from each deceased donor (Fig. 56.2) [1,2].

Marginal donors—elderly patients, patients with a history of hypertension, poisoning victims, patients with significant organ injury (e.g., liver laceration due to blunt injury) or complications of brain death (e.g., hypotension, acute kidney injury with oliguria or anuria, disseminated intravascular coagulation)—are routinely used for recovery of kidneys and extrarenal organs [1,2,24]. Organ recovery techniques also have been adapted to facilitate use of older donors with significant aortic atherosclerosis [48]. The increased use of hypothermic machine perfusion of kidney grafts allows to assess the quality of grafts from marginal donors and facilitates—by improving preservation quality—organ allocation to geographically more distant transplant centers [42].

Organs with anatomic abnormalities (e.g., multiple renal arteries or ureters, horseshoe kidney, annular pancreas) also are

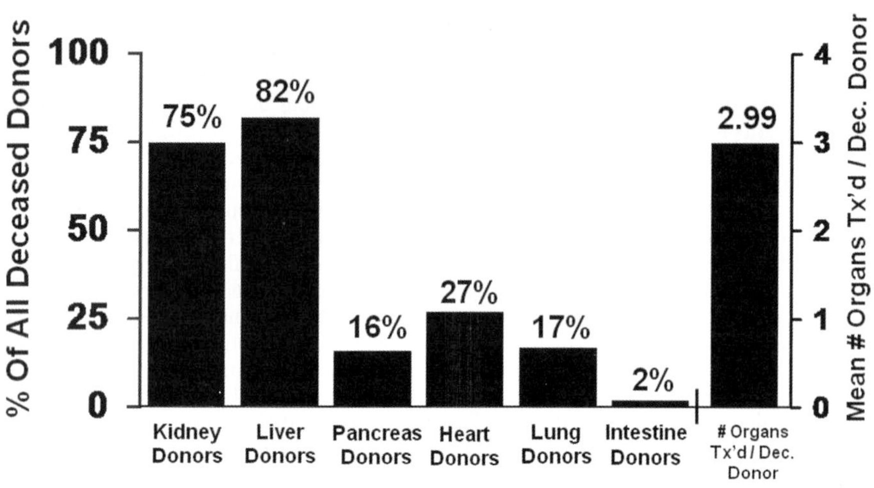

FIGURE 56.2 Transplant rates (by organ) from 8,085 deceased donors (100%; 2007) in the United States. The last bar represents the mean number of organs transplanted per deceased donor for the year 2013. Tx'd, transplanted; Dec., deceased. (Based on data from references [1,2])

being used routinely. Improvements in operative technique permit the *en bloc* transplantation of two kidneys from very young (e.g., infant) donors that would have been too small to be used separately in one recipient [49–51]. Similarly, transplantation of both kidneys from an *adult* donor into one recipient is, on occasion, done to avoid discarding suboptimal kidneys with an insufficient individual nephron mass. To maximize the use of livers, adult donor livers can be split and the two size-reduced grafts transplanted into two recipients (e.g., a pediatric and an adult recipient). A similar principle has also been proposed for the pancreas and has been reported on at least one occasion [52].

Explanted livers from patients undergoing liver transplantation for hepatic metabolic disorders that cause systemic disease without affecting other liver functions (e.g., familial amyloidotic polyneuropathy, hereditary oxalosis) can be used for transplanting other patients ("domino transplant") who are not candidates for deceased livers because of graft shortage (e.g., cirrhotic patients with hepatocellular carcinoma confined to the liver who are not in the group with good expected survival) [53]. The combination of split-liver and domino transplantation can even result in transplantation of three adult patients with one deceased donor graft [54].

The advent of single-lung transplants has made it possible to distribute the heart and lungs of one donor to three recipients. Formerly, transplanting a heart–lung bloc into one recipient was the treatment of choice for end-stage pulmonary disease. If the native heart of a heart–lung recipient is healthy, a domino transplant can be performed: The heart–lung recipient donates his or her heart to another patient in need of a heart transplant.

In an attempt to optimize use of scarce donor resources, the reuse of previously transplanted hearts, kidneys, and livers has also been reported. However, all these methods allow only for better use of organs from the existing donor pool. The cornerstone for an effective increase in the number of organ donors remains heightened awareness and education of the public, physicians, and other health care professionals to improve consent and conversion rates [11–13,24,29].

Living Donors

The use of organs from living donors, traditionally limited to kidney transplants, has been expanded to the liver, small bowel, pancreas, and lung [1,2]. In the more distant past, most living donors were genetically related to the recipient—siblings, parents, and adult children. As a result of the organ shortage, the use of living unrelated kidney donors, who are emotionally, but not genetically, related to the recipient (e.g., spouses, close friends), or are emotionally and genetically unrelated to the recipient (i.e., nondirected, "Good Samaritan" donors), has considerably increased over the past 25 years (Fig. 56.1) [1,2,55]. In order to increase the number of live donor transplants even further, paired-kidney-exchange programs and living donor chain transplants have been implemented [56,57]. In that setting, the supply of organs is increased for instance by exchanging kidneys from living donors who are ABO or crossmatch incompatible with their intended recipients, but ABO or crossmatch compatible with another donor–recipient pair (donor A would provide a kidney to [ABO or crossmatch compatible] recipient B, and donor B would provide a kidney to [ABO or crossmatch compatible] recipient A) [56,57]. In cases when paired-kidney-exchange or donor chain transplants are not available or feasible, it is alternatively possible to precondition (desensitize) the intended recipient of an ABO or crossmatch incompatible kidney (by use of plasmapheresis and/or intravenous immunoglobulin and pharmacologic intervention) to still facilitate a successful living donor kidney transplant.

Currently, there is considerable public debate on providing incentives for living kidney donation [58–61]. The debate centers on concerns that reimbursement might lead to the commercialization of organ donation, with the inherent risk of turning potential donors and transplantable organs into a commodity [59,60]. In the United States, those in support of compensating live donors stress that an Organ Procurement and Transplantation Network–run transparent system of paid living donation would ensure that donors are compensated fairly, eliminate transplant tourism to other countries, greatly diminish the currently existing black market for organs in those countries, and emphasize any potentially interested donor's autonomy—while at the same time increasing the organ supply [58,61]. In any case, paid living donation, while a reality in certain regions of the world, remains currently unlawful in the United States and most Western countries. Even when assuming that (i) public attitudes toward living donation will continue to evolve favorably (Fig. 56.1), (ii) innovative approaches as described above will be increasingly used, and (iii) other alternative means for finding living donors, such as donor solicitation via social media, would ultimately prove to be successful, only modest increases of the absolute number of living kidney donors could be expected [58–63]. Finally, compared with renal transplantation, the proportion of living donor transplants for extrarenal organs is much smaller (less than 5% for liver and less than 0.5% for pancreas, lung, and small bowel) [1]. Thus, living donor transplants will continue to help alleviate the organ shortage for certain organs (kidney, liver) to some extent, but will never be able to completely compensate—even under the best circumstances—for the severe lack of deceased donors.

Presumed Consent Laws

Presumed consent laws have been implemented in many areas of the world, most notably in several countries in Europe. These laws permit organ procurement unless the potential donor has objected explicitly. A permanently and easily accessible registry of objectors is a prerequisite for such a system. In the United States, proposals for presumed consent legislation have not had broad support. Moreover, presumed consent would not alleviate the problem of insufficient donor identification and referral [12].

The beneficial impact that such laws can have became evident in Spain. In that country, presumed consent laws coupled with the creation of a decentralized network of mostly hospital-based, specifically trained transplant coordinators (most of them physicians in intensive care units) in the early 1990s led not only to more efficient identification of eligible deceased donors but also to higher consent rates. Accordingly, the annual donation rate in Spain rose from 14.3 donors per million population (pmp) in 1989 to 34.2 pmp in 2008 (United States, 2008: 26.3 pmp) [64–66]. Interestingly, a similar approach (without the presumed consent component) using in-house coordinators at some hospitals in the United States did yield greater consent and conversion rates, too, and underscored the advantages that such a system could have, if implemented at a larger scale [67].

Organs from Executed Prisoners

Certain countries (e.g., China) routinely use organs from executed prisoners. This practice has been strongly rejected by the national and international transplant community [68]. Moreover, proposals to use organs from executed prisoners would engender a very passionate, emotional debate that would have a negative impact on public opinion and thereby decrease overall organ availability.

Xenotransplantation

Xenotransplantation of organs and tissues from animals into humans offers a potentially unlimited supply of donors [68,69]. Past attempts have received significant public attention [69], but numerous practical problems remain before this procedure could become a clinical reality. Ethical concerns regarding the use of animal organs for transplantation have also been raised. Immunologic concerns include hyperacute rejection (mediated by circulating, preformed natural antibodies), which occurs in vascularized solid organ transplantation between virtually all discordant species. Also, the biocompatibility of protein synthesized by an animal liver and the human organism is not fully established, and infectious diseases (e.g., caused by porcine endogenous retroviruses) could be transmitted when using nonhuman primates or pigs as donors. Genetic engineering of animals before their use as donors to overcome the immunologic barriers is an area of intensive investigation. Significant experimental progress in this area could fundamentally change the field of organ transplantation.

REGULATION AND ORGANIZATION OF ORGAN PROCUREMENT AND ALLOCATION

In the early 1980s, the introduction of new immunosuppressive agents engendered a rise in organ transplant activity. Tissue matching (e.g., by use of living related donor–recipient combinations) became less important, and the use of brain-dead donors increased (Fig. 56.1). In the wake of these developments, consolidation and national regulation of the organ sharing and allocation organizations, which had previously functioned mainly at a local and regional level, became necessary.

In the United States, the National Organ Transplant Act of 1984 called for a national system to ensure equitable access to transplant therapy for all patients, a major component of which was fair organ allocation. The federal government commissioned a task force on organ transplantation to define such an allocation system. This task force, whose members were appointed by the U.S. Department of Health and Human Services, resolved that human organs are a "national resource to be used for public good" and recommended the creation of a national Organ Procurement and Transplantation Network (OPTN) [3]. In 1986, the U.S. Department of Health and Human Services awarded the OPTN contract to the United Network for Organ Sharing (UNOS). Pursuant to the contract, UNOS was asked to design a network to achieve balance in the goals of equity in organ access and distribution and in optimal medical outcome [70]. In 1986, the Omnibus Budget Reconciliation Act mandated that only hospital members of the OPTN could perform Medicare- and Medicaid-reimbursed transplant procedures. In 1988, the Organ Transplant Amendments reaffirmed the federal interest in equitable organ allocation by locating authority in UNOS as opposed to local transplant organizations.

The national OPTN is currently operated under contract by UNOS, which is accountable to the U.S. Department of Health and Human Services. All patients on waiting lists of a transplant program are registered with UNOS, which maintains

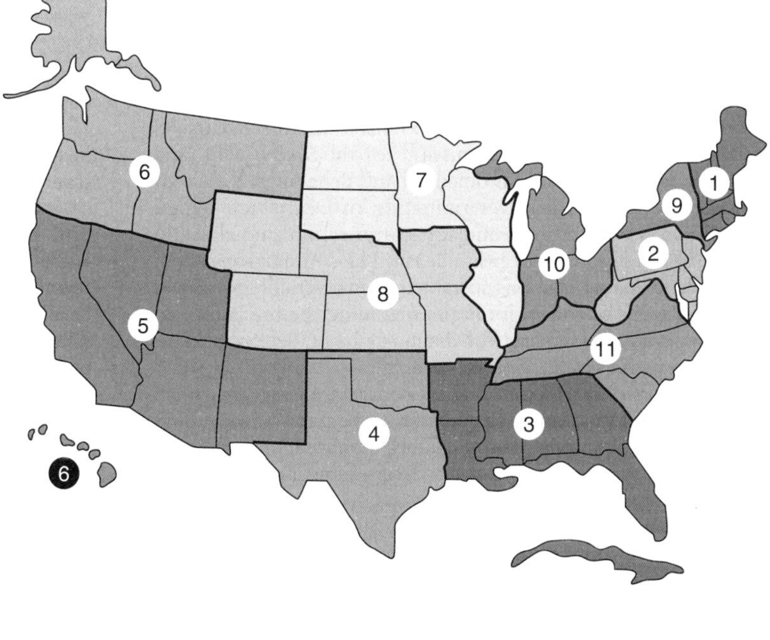

FIGURE 56.3 United Network for Organ Sharing (UNOS) regions in the United States (24-hour access number: 1-800-292-9537). The United States has been divided into 11 regions for organ procurement, allocation, and sharing purposes.

a centralized computer system linking all OPOs and transplant centers. The United States has been divided into 11 regions for organ procurement, allocation, and sharing purposes (Fig. 56.3). Organs are registered, shared, and allocated through use of the central UNOS computer, which generates a list of recipients for each available organ. Patients awaiting deceased donor transplantation are ranked according to UNOS policies, based on medical and scientific criteria that—depending on the organ—may include blood type, tissue type, length of time waiting on the list, age (pediatric vs. adult), level of presensitization (percentage of panel reactive antibody), and medical status. For kidneys, national sharing of virtual crossmatch compatible, very highly sensitized recipients is mandated. For the vast majority of all of the other organs, though, allocation first takes place locally and then regionally. If no suitable recipients are available, organs are then allocated nationally.

LEGAL ASPECTS OF ORGAN DONATION AND BRAIN DEATH

Uniform Anatomical Gift Act

The Uniform Anatomical Gift Act, adopted in 1968 and in force throughout the United States, allows any adult individual (over age 18 years) to donate all or part of their body for transplantation, research, or education. This act also provides the legal basis for recovery of organs from both DCD and brain-dead (*vide infra*) donors. Explicit consent is required. The act also specifies who may give consent (e.g., legal next of kin) for donation [71].

The 2006 Revised Uniform Anatomical Give Act honors the choice of an individual to be or not to be a donor and strengthens the language barring others from overriding a donor's first-person authorization to make an anatomical gift. The revised act also empowers minors that apply for a driver's license to become donors and encourages and establishes standards for donor registries [72].

Uniform Determination of Death Act

Over the past five decades, brain death has legally become equated with death in most Western developed countries. *Brain death* means that all brain and brain stem function has irreversibly ceased. The recognition of brain death became possible only after substantial advances in intensive care medicine (e.g., provision of cardiovascular support, prolonged mechanical ventilation). The first classic description of brain death was published in 1959 in France and termed *coma dépassé* (beyond coma). An *ad hoc* commission of the Harvard Medical School defined brain death criteria in the United States in 1968 [73]. These criteria were judged by some as being too extensive and too exclusive. In 1981, the President's Commission for the Study of Ethical Problems in Medicine and Biomedical and Behavioral Research formulated the Uniform Determination of Death Act, which established a common ground for statutory and judicial law related to the diagnosis of brain death. The commission stated that "an individual who has sustained . . . irreversible cessation of all functions of the entire brain, including the brainstem, is dead," and left the criteria for diagnosis to be determined by "accepted medical standards."

Those standards were defined in a related report to the President's Commission on the diagnosis of death by 56 medical consultants in 1981 [74]. The guidelines in that report have now been accepted as the standard for determining brain death in the United States. They are as follows: "Cessation is recognized when: (1) all cerebral functions and (2) all brainstem functions are absent. The irreversibility is recognized when: (1) the cause of the coma is established and is sufficient to account for the loss of brain functions, (2) the possibility of the recovery of any brain functions is excluded, and (3) the cessation of cerebral and brainstem function persists for an appropriate period of observation and/or trial of therapy" [74]. Confusion regarding this well-founded and accepted medicolegal concept of the equivalence of brain death and death of a human persists to this date among physicians, other health care professionals, and the general public [11,13]. Specifically, in the field of transplantation, it should be unequivocally clear to the potential donor's family and anyone involved in the patient's care that the time of death is the time at which the diagnosis of brain death is established and not the time of cardiac arrest during the organ recovery. Providing education targeted specifically at these groups and society at large is of paramount importance to optimize consent rates [11,13].

Required Request

Required request laws have now been enacted in all states in the United States. They obligate hospitals to notify an OPO of potential donors and to offer the option of donation to the families of potential donors (brain-dead and DCD donors). In order to optimize this process, the CMS' Conditions of Participation have been requiring hospitals since 1998 to use "designated requestors" to obtain authorization from legal next of kin for donation [75].

Clinical Diagnosis of Brain Death

The clinical diagnosis of brain death rests on three criteria: (a) irreversibility of the neurologic insult, (b) absence of clinical evidence of cerebral function, and, most important, (c) absence of clinical evidence of brain stem function (Table 56.4) [76–79]. Irreversibility is established if structural disease (e.g., trauma, intracranial hemorrhage) or an irreversible metabolic cause is known to have occurred. Hypothermia, medication side effects, drug overdose, and alcohol ingestion and intoxication must be ruled out when testing for brain death. Plasma concentrations of sedative or analgesic drugs sometimes correlate poorly with cerebral effects. Therefore, residual effects of those drugs can be excluded only by passage of time, if any doubts exist. As no evidence-based recommendations for a minimal waiting time prior to the first brain death examination can be made, good—individualized—clinical judgment is paramount. The observation period between two sequential brain death examinations should be at least 6 hours for structural causes and preferably 12 to 24 hours for metabolic causes, drug overdose, or intoxication [76–79]. Even with potentially reversible metabolic alterations (e.g., hepatic or uremic encephalopathy), recovery has not been described after duration of the brain death state for more than 12 hours and as long as all criteria in Table 56.4 (which are based on the 1995 American Academy of Neurology medical standards for death determination using neurologic criteria and on its 2010 update) are met [77,78]. Clinical testing of cerebral and brain stem function is detailed in Table 56.4 [76–81]. Although pediatric donors are not the focus of this chapter, it should be noted that brain death criteria are more stringent for very young pediatric patients, particularly newborns, in whom criteria for brain death also include demonstration of the absence of blood flow on cerebral flow studies.

After brain death, the pupils become fixed in midposition because sympathetic and parasympathetic input is lost. Decerebrate (abnormal extension) and decorticate (abnormal flexion) responses to painful stimuli imply the presence of some brain stem function and are incompatible with the diagnosis of brain death. In contrast, spinal cord–mediated tendon reflexes, automatic stepping, and other complex motor activities (which

TABLE 56.4

Brain Death Criteria and Clinical Diagnosis of Brain Death

Irreversible, well-defined etiology of coma

Structural disease or metabolic cause (requires documentation by neuroimaging)

Exclusion of: significant hypothermia (defined as core temperature <33°C); hypotension (systolic blood pressure must be >100 mm Hg); severe electrolyte, endocrine, or acid–base disturbance; and drug, alcohol or substance intoxication (may require toxicology screen; barbiturates, if present, serum level must be <10 μg/mL)

No spontaneous respirations

Absence of residual paralyzing agents

Sufficient observation period (at least 6 h) between two brain death examinations

No clinical evidence of cerebral function

No spontaneous movement, eye opening, or movement or response after auditory, verbal, or visual commands

No movement elicited by painful stimuli to the face and trunk (e.g., sternal rub, pinching of a nipple or fingernail bed) other than spinal cord reflex movements

No clinical evidence of brain stem function

No pupillary reflex: pupils are fixed and midposition; no change of pupil size in either eye after shining a strong light source in each eye sequentially in a darkened room

No corneal reflex: no eyelid movement after touching the cornea (not the conjunctiva) with a sterile cotton swab or tissue

No gag reflex: no retching or movement of the uvula after touching the back of the pharynx with a tongue depressor or after moving the endotracheal tube

No cough reflex: no coughing with deep tracheal irrigation and suctioning

No oculocephalic reflex (doll's eyes reflex): no eye movement in response to brisk turning of the head from side to side with the head of the supine patient elevated 30 degrees

No oculovestibular reflex (caloric reflex): no eye movements within 3 min after removing earwax and irrigating each tympanic membrane (if intact) sequentially with 50 mL ice water for 30 to 45 seconds while the head of the supine patient is elevated 30 degrees

No integrated motor response to pain: no localizing or withdrawal response (face; all four limbs), no extensor or flexor posturing

No respiratory efforts on apnea testing ($PaCO_2$ >60 mm Hg or 20 mm Hg higher than the normal baseline value): The patient is preoxygenated with an FiO_2 of 1.0 for 10–15 minutes to reach a PaO_2 >100 mm Hg (preferably with an arterial line in place for rapid blood gas measurements) while adjusting ventilatory rate and volume such that the $PaCO_2$ reaches ~40–45 mm Hg. After a baseline arterial blood gas value is obtained and the patient is disconnected from the ventilator, O_2 at 6–8 L/min is delivered through a cannula advanced 20–30 cm into the endotracheal tube (cannula tip at the level of the carina). Continuous pulse oximetry is used for early detection of desaturation, which does not usually occur when using this protocol. In most cases, a $PaCO_2$ >60 mm Hg is achieved within 3–5 minutes after withdrawal of ventilatory support; at this point, the patient should be reconnected to the ventilator (or earlier, should hemodynamic instability, desaturation, or spontaneous breathing movements occur). Obtaining an arterial blood gas sample immediately before reinstitution of mechanical ventilation is mandatory. If there is no evidence of spontaneous respirations before reinstitution of mechanical ventilation in the presence of a $PaCO_2$ >60 mm Hg or an increase of >20 mm Hg from the normal baseline value, the criteria for a positive apnea test are met.

Other points

- Spinal reflexes, such as deep tendon reflexes and triple flexion responses, can be preserved and do not exclude the diagnosis of brain death
- Shivering, piloerection, arm movements, reaching of the hands toward the neck, forced exhalation, and thoracic respiratory-like movements are possible after brain death and are likely to release phenomena of the spinal cord, including the upper cervical cord. All these findings are compatible with the diagnosis of brain death.
- Confirmatory tests should be used in cases in which the observation period needs to be shortened (e.g., unstable donors), if the apnea test had to be aborted in equivocal situations in children younger than 1 year old, or if one of the potential pitfalls (Table 56.6) cannot be ruled out (demonstration of absence of intracranial circulation by conventional cerebral angiogram, Tc-99m hexamethylpropyleneamine oxime single photon-emission computed tomography, transcranial Doppler ultrasonography, or electrocerebral silence documented by an electroencephalogram).

$PaCO_2$, partial arterial carbon dioxide pressure; FiO_2, fraction of inspired oxygen.
References [76–80].

can also occur during apnea testing) are compatible with brain death [78,79,82]. The occurrence of these movements can be quite distressing if observed by the next of kin; therefore, it is advisable that they not be present during the apnea test. Very rarely, ascending acute reversible inflammatory polyneuropathy (Guillain–Barré syndrome) can simulate brain death and inhibit all motor functions, including pupillary reactions and brain stem reflexes. The typical clinical history, coupled with evidence of progressive weakness, should yield the correct diagnosis and preclude a diagnosis of brain death from being established [76–79].

The American Academy of Neurology has stated that special confirmatory tests are not necessary to diagnose brain death in the vast majority of cases. Only in equivocal or questionable circumstances does a study demonstrating the absence of intracranial blood flow need to be performed [76–78]. The most sensitive and specific test for assessing intracranial blood flow is four-vessel catheter cerebral arteriography. Alternatively, Tc-99m hexamethylpropyleneamine oxime single photon-emission computed tomography may be used [78,80]. Other ancillary tests are either less sensitive (e.g., digital subtraction angiography, transcranial Doppler ultrasonography), less specific (e.g., brain stem acoustic evoked potentials), or measure only hemispheric flow.

Four-vessel cerebral catheter arteriography is indicated in all conditions that can temporarily cause an isoelectric

TABLE 56.5

Pitfalls in Clinical Brain Death Testing and Potential Remedial Measures[a]

Pitfalls	Remedial Measure(s)
Hypotension, shock	Institute fluid resuscitation, use pressor agents
Current hypothermia	Use warmed fluids, ventilatory warmer
Recent treatment with therapeutic hypothermia	Increase time under normothermic conditions until performance of first brain death exam (several days may be necessary to clear all previously administered muscle relaxants and mood or consciousness-altering drugs)
Intoxication, alcohol ingestion or drug overdose	Check drug and alcohol levels and toxicology screens or increase waiting time between brain death examinations
Presence of neuromuscular-inhibiting agents and sedative drugs, which can interfere with elicitation of motor responses	Discontinue muscle relaxants and mood- or consciousness-altering medications, increase waiting time between brain death examinations
Pupillary fixation, which may be caused by anticholinergic drugs (e.g., atropine given during a cardiac arrest), neuromuscular blocking agents, or preexisting disease	Discontinue anticholinergic medications and muscle relaxants, increase waiting time between brain death examinations, obtain careful patient history
Corneal reflexes absent due to overlooked contact lenses	Remove contact lenses before brain death examination
Oculovestibular reflexes diminished or abolished after prior use of ototoxic drugs (e.g., aminoglycosides, loop diuretics, vancomycin) or agents with suppressive side effects on the vestibular system (e.g., tricyclic antidepressants, anticonvulsants, and barbiturates) or due to preexisting disease	Obtain careful medication history and patient history

[a]If one of the listed conditions cannot be ruled out, confirmatory testing (cerebral flow studies or electroencephalography) is necessary before brain death is declared.

electroencephalogram (e.g., extreme intoxication). If the indication for cerebral arteriography is unclear, the benefits must be weighed against the potential risks of transporting an unstable patient. Confirmatory tests may serve to shorten the waiting period between the two brain death examinations, should donor hemodynamic instability occur. Certain potential pitfalls exist in clinical brain death testing, and the diagnosis should not be considered to have been established until these all have been excluded (Table 56.5) [79]. If these cannot be excluded, confirmatory testing is mandatory [79,80].

In summary, the diagnosis of brain death can be established by performance of routine neurologic examinations, including cold caloric and apnea testing on two separate occasions, coupled with prior establishment of the underlying diagnosis and prognosis in most cases [76–80]. More sophisticated tests are required in cases in which the diagnosis cannot be unequivocally established [78,80]. However, brain death must be diagnosed in accordance with local regulations and state laws. Details on the locally prevailing regulations are available through the state medical board and the local OPO.

ORGAN DONATION PROCESS

The three key elements leading to successful organ donation are (a) early referral of potential donors, (b) a well-coordinated approach in informing and dealing with the potential donor's family to request and obtain consent, and (c) appropriate critical care therapy of the donor [11,13]. The optimal course of events for both brain-dead and DCD donors is summarized in Table 56.6.

Early Donor Referral

Early referral of any potential donor to the local OPO minimizes the loss of transplantable organs due to unexpected cardiac arrest and death, hemodynamic instability, serious nosocomial infection, or complications related to intensive care [83,84]. For example, an inverse correlation exists between the duration of mechanical ventilation and the suitability of the donor for lung donation.

The evidence is substantial that brain death eventually leads to cardiac arrest, even when cardiorespiratory support is maintained [83,84]. Cardiac arrest occurs in 4% to 28% of potential donors in the maintenance phase, and as many as 50% of all potential donors die within 24 hours without appropriate support [83,84].

The previously outlined clinical triggers for early referral to the local OPO should therefore be applied to any neurologically severely injured patient after admission to the hospital or intensive care unit (Table 56.3). Early contact with the OPO is essential as the latter will provide assistance with further screening and the evaluation of any patient who might potentially become a donor.

DONOR EVALUATION

General Guidelines. During the initial contact with the OPO, the physician should provide the potential donor's name, age, sex, height, weight, and blood type. Also needed are the date of admission and diagnosis, the nature and extent of any trauma, a concise medical and social history, and the time of brain death (if applicable). Whether local investigative agencies (e.g., medical examiner, coroner) need to be notified also should be specified. The current medical status, including vital signs, urine output, cardiorespiratory status, medications, and culture results, must be communicated. Basic laboratory results should be obtained: arterial blood gas determinations; blood urea nitrogen, creatinine, and electrolyte values; hemoglobin, hematocrit, white blood cell and platelet counts, and tests for serum amylase, total bilirubin, alkaline phosphatase, alanine aminotransferase, and aspartate aminotransferase; coagulation profile (including prothrombin time or International Normalized Ratio); and urinalysis and urine culture, along with electrocardiogram and chest radiograph results. In the case of potential lung donors, chest circumference and radiographic thoracic measurements, as well as the results

TABLE 56.6

Organ Donation Algorithm

1. Early identification of the potential donor by the critical care physician or health care professional (Table 56.3).
2. Early contact with the local or regional OPO for medical, legal, and logistic assistance. If the local OPO's address or phone number is unknown, a 24-h access number to UNOS is available: 1-800-292-9537.
3. Completion of the preliminary screening by the OPO if necessary in consultation with the transplant surgeon for decisions regarding marginal donors.

4a. For potential DCD donors: await family decision regarding withdrawal of care. Proceed only if family decides to do so.
4b. For potential brain-dead donors: brain death diagnosis and confirmation (Tables 56.4 and 56.5), certification of death. Family notification and explanation of brain death with its legal and medical implications. Sufficient time for acceptance must be allowed.

5. Request for organ donation. Must be made after, and in clear temporal separation, from step 4a or 4b.
6. After consent for organ donation is obtained, the focus switches from treatment of elevated intracranial pressure and cerebral protection to preservation of organ function and optimization of peripheral oxygen delivery (Table 56.8).
7. All remaining laboratory and serologic studies as well as any further studies and tests required in equivocal situations are performed at this point.
8. Final organ allocation by the OPO and UNOS, coordination of the organ recovery operation, notification of the abdominal and thoracic surgical teams. Modification of the final steps may become necessary under special circumstances, for example, in hemodynamically unstable donors.
9. For controlled DCD donors: Support is withdrawn and death is certified (in the ICU or in the operating room).
10. Organ recovery operation (brain-dead and DCD donors).

OPO, organ procurement organization; UNOS, United Network for Organ Sharing; DCD, donation after circulatory death.
Steps 4, 5, and 9 should not involve physicians who are part of the transplantation team.

of an oxygenation challenge (partial arterial oxygen pressure [PaO_2] measurement after ventilation for 10 minutes with a fraction of inspired oxygen [FiO_2] of 1.0), are helpful.

The OPO provides further procedural, administrative, legal, and logistic help. Most importantly, the OPO coordinates how the family is approached. All further testing (including human leukocyte antigen tissue typing; serologic screening for cytomegalovirus [CMV], for hepatitis A, B, and C viruses [HAV, HBV, HCV], for human immunodeficiency virus [HIV], and syphilis; and blood, sputum, and urine cultures) is then coordinated through the OPO if the donor passes the preliminary screening tests. The organ allocation process begins only after the family has decided to withdraw support technologies (DCD donors) or brain death has been declared and consent has been obtained. If prospective tissue typing is to be done, it may occasionally be necessary to perform a bedside surgical inguinal lymph node biopsy at the donor hospital—after consent for organ donation has been obtained, but before proceeding with the actual organ recovery several hours later.

The medical status and the life expectancy of the potential recipient without the organ transplant are taken into account when considering the risks associated with a specific donor's medical characteristics and the final decision about transplantation of a specific donor organ is made. The ultimate decision regarding the use of a donor organ is made by the transplant surgeon. At this stage, the transplant center may need to obtain further tests to assess the functional status of one or more organ systems. For example, if the heart is to be recovered, an echocardiogram is usually obtained. In selected donors, coronary angiography is performed. Pulmonary status can be further assessed by bronchoscopy after considering the results of the chest radiograph, oxygenation challenge, and sputum cultures. For potential liver donors who might have fatty liver disease, a percutaneous bedside liver biopsy can be performed. If concern over the suitability of organs arises, direct inspection by the transplant surgeon is necessary at the time of the organ procurement operation. In some cases, an open biopsy (e.g., for kidney or liver) and frozen section pathologic analysis obtained at the time of organ recovery also help in the final decision-making. Direct inspection also is important in organ donors who suffered a blunt injury to the head and trunk (e.g., motor vehicle accident). Under these circumstances, intraabdominal organs have been used successfully despite the presence of parenchymal tears or subcapsular hematomas in either the liver or the kidney. Significant injuries to the pancreas preclude its use.

In summary, *each* patient with a severe nonrecoverable neurologic injury should be referred to the local OPO as a potential donor, regardless of the type of brain injury (e.g., trauma, stroke), history, age, or medical condition (Table 56.3). With few exceptions (*vide infra*), organ donation should never be excluded a priori because of the clinical situation, the results of imaging studies, or the magnitude of an injury, without first having contacted the local OPO (24-hour access number: 1-800-292-9537).

Organ-Specific Considerations. The use of kidneys from older donors, donors dying of cardiovascular disease, or donors requiring large doses of inotropic drugs for cardiovascular support entails a higher rate of delayed graft function and is associated with decreased graft survival [85,86]. Nevertheless, organs from these marginal donors are routinely used given the current prolonged periods (which can be longer than 8 to 10 years in some areas) that some recipients may wait for available organs, during which their medical condition may deteriorate. Marginal donor kidneys benefit from preservation on a pulsatile perfusion pump, which was shown to improve preservation quality, quality of early graft function, and long-term outcomes [42]. In equivocal cases (e.g., donors with elevated baseline serum creatinine levels or a history of hypertension), renal biopsies at the time of organ recovery may quantify the amount of preexisting donor arteriosclerosis or glomerulosclerosis. The critical shortage of organs has led to increasing relaxation of exclusion criteria, with satisfactory long-term results in many recipients.

Livers from donors with an abnormal liver enzyme or coagulation profile can frequently still be transplanted. Elevated hepatic enzyme levels may reflect transient hepatic ischemia at the time of resuscitation. The trends observed in the results of serial hepatic enzyme levels can be more informative than absolute values. Abnormal coagulation test results may be due to disseminated intravascular coagulation (commonly a result of brain injury, not primary hepatic dysfunction). Significant donor hypernatremia (e.g., >155 mg per dL), as commonly observed in under-resuscitated brain-dead donors with significant diabetes insipidus, may be a risk factor for primary liver graft nonfunction posttransplant. Aggressive intervention prior to procurement is warranted and will ultimately allow for safe transplantation of liver grafts from these hypernatremic donors. The decision to use a liver from a marginal donor has to be made on the basis of relatively limited information. Often, only direct inspection, with or without a biopsy of the liver, at the time of organ recovery provides a final answer and may be the only way to assess a donor with a history of significant ethanol intake. Severe macrovesicular hepatic steatosis is one of the most significant factors predictive of early posttransplant hepatic dysfunction or failure.

In general, donors older than 60 years of age are not considered for pancreas donation. However, donors with hyperglycemia [caused by peripheral insulin resistance, particularly after brain death (see the section "Endocrine Therapy") or with hyperamylasemia (which can be a consequence of severe head injury without actual pancreatitis)] are not to be excluded a priori from pancreas donation, because these factors do not necessarily influence posttransplant outcome [87,88]. A pancreas transplant registry analysis suggested a slightly higher incidence of graft thrombosis for pancreata that had been procured from donors treated with desmopressin (vs. those that did not) [89]. Clearly, further study is necessary to confirm or refute these findings and determine their clinical significance. Currently, the only absolute contraindications to pancreas donation are a history of impaired glucose tolerance or insulin-dependent diabetes mellitus, direct blunt or penetrating trauma to the pancreas, or the finding of acute or chronic pancreatitis at the time of the donor operation.

Regarding heart donation, an important criterion is good donor heart ventricular function immediately before retrieval, as judged by the cardiac surgeon at visual inspection during organ recovery. Ideally, no potential heart donor should be excluded solely on the basis of echocardiographic wall motion abnormalities, a borderline or abnormal ejection fraction, inotropic medication requirements, or heart murmurs, arrhythmias, or other electrocardiographic changes (which often occur in brain-dead individuals in whom no cardiac disease is present).

Risk factors associated with poorer outcomes after lung transplantation include a history of smoking, aspiration, purulent secretions observed during bronchoscopy, an abnormal chest radiograph, or an unsatisfactory oxygenation challenge (PaO_2 less than 300 mm Hg after 10 minutes of ventilation with FiO_2 of 1.0 and low positive end-expiratory pressure [PEEP] of 5 cm H_2O) alone or in combination in lung donors. However, even lungs with these characteristics have been successfully transplanted [90]. Bronchoscopy often is performed as a final preoperative confirmatory test in the operating room by the lung recovery surgeon. Direct intraoperative inspection of the lungs determines whether significant contusions are present, which could preclude use of the organs.

In conclusion, the traditional donor criteria have been considerably expanded over recent years, for both thoracic and abdominal organs, due to the ongoing, severe donor shortage.

Transmission of Infectious Diseases. Transmission of bacterial or fungal infection through organ transplantation can potentially be due to an infection of the donor or contamination of the organ itself during organ procurement or storage. Published evidence suggests that organs transplanted from bacteremic donors and from donors with bacterial meningitis do not transmit bacterial infection or result in poorer recipient outcomes provided that donor and recipient(s) are adequately treated with antibiotics [91]. Similarly, positive urine cultures do not preclude renal donation and transplantation. Organs from donors with serologic evidence of syphilis can be used as long as the recipients are given adequate antibiotic prophylaxis.

Seropositivity for HIV no longer constitutes an absolute contraindication to organ donation, as the federal ban on transplantation of organs from HIV-positive individuals has been lifted [92]. As of late 2015, transplant hospitals that meet specific criteria set forth by the OPTN can consider HIV-positive organs for HIV-positive kidney and liver candidates.

Organs from donors that fulfill the Public Health Service's behavioral criteria for being at increased risk for having acquired HBV, HCV, or HIV infection are frequently transplanted following careful case-by-case consideration and after obtaining specific recipient consent [93]. Decision-making by the OPOs and transplant centers regarding the use of organs from these high-risk donors has been greatly facilitated by the now widespread use of nucleic acid testing for those viral pathogens [94].

Potential donors that test positive for the HBV surface antigen, the HBe antigen, or for HBV-DNA are usually precluded from donating. Serologic positivity for the hepatitis B core antigen antibody, however, does not constitute an absolute contraindication to proceed with donation [95]. Acceptable organs from donors with serologic evidence of HBV are usually only transplanted into recipients that have demonstrated immunity against HBV (i.e., HBsAb positivity) [95]. Selected recipients may also receive HBV immunoglobulin or an antiviral agent (e.g., entecavir) or both, beginning at the time of transplant [95]. Ideally, however, all potential organ transplant recipients should have received HBV immunization prior to their pretransplant evaluation.

The use of HCV seropositive donors for selected recipients has become routine [96]. For adequate identification of HCV-positive donors, OPOs routinely perform besides HCV antibody testing and nucleic acid testing for HCV-RNA. HCV-infected livers and kidneys transplanted into HCV-infected recipients do not convey a worse outcome than HCV-negative grafts [96]. The final decision regarding the use of an HCV serology–positive donor must be made on an individual basis by each transplant surgeon. Factors that are taken into account in such circumstances include the likelihood of disease transmission, the recipient's current medical and serologic status, and the availability of modern drugs for the treatment and eradication of HCV [96].

CMV can also be transmitted by donor tissue, particularly to CMV-seronegative patients. Effective prophylaxis against, and treatment of, CMV disease has become routine because of the availability of highly effective antiviral agents such as ganciclovir and valganciclovir. Positive CMV serologies do therefore not preclude organ donation but have been used to identify high-risk donor–recipient combinations (i.e., CMV-seropositive donor to CMV-seronegative recipient) where enhanced prophylaxis should be used and careful surveillance for CMV disease is important.

However, organ donation is contraindicated if potential donors exhibit or develop active bacterial or fungal sepsis that is unresponsive to adequate source control and antibiotic therapy. Similarly, active tuberculosis is a contraindication to organ donation. Absolute contraindications to donation also include evidence of significant *acute* viral infections (e.g., viral encephalitis, systemic herpes simplex virus infections, acute viral HAV, HBV, or HCV). For similar reasons, donation should not proceed in patients in whom a definitive etiology for their febrile illness, encephalitis, meningitis, or flaccid paralysis is not ascertainable.

Transmission of Malignancy. The risk for transmission of a donor malignancy to a solid organ recipient is low overall [97]. In that regard, appropriate selection of donors with a current or past history of cancer is paramount. If a potential donor has had successful cancer treatment in the past, the transplant surgeon must weigh the small potential risk of transmitting micrometastases against discarding a potentially life-saving organ. In general, patients with a history of malignancy with little propensity to recur after therapy (e.g., small, noninvasive lesions treated by complete surgical excision) are considered as organ donors, particularly if they have remained without evidence of recurrence for more than 5 years. Patients who have experienced invasive cancer in which a substantial risk of late recurrence exists (e.g., breast cancer, malignant melanoma, lung cancer), particularly if a large lesion was initially present and chemotherapy or radiation therapy was used, should not be considered for donation. Similarly, patients with a history of leukemia or lymphoma should not be considered as donors.

Individuals with low-grade skin malignancies such as basal cell carcinoma and most squamous cell carcinomas, and with an in situ carcinoma of the uterine cervix are routinely used as donors.

Patients with tumors of the central nervous system (CNS) can be considered for donation on a case-by-case basis [97,98]. It is important to ensure that a CNS tumor does not represent a focus of metastatic disease from an extracerebral primary site. Metastases from choriocarcinomas, bronchial or renal malignancies, and malignant melanomas may present as what appears to be a primary brain tumor or may bleed and be mistaken for an intracranial hemorrhage. Previous treatment of a neoplasm, menstrual irregularities after a pregnancy or a spontaneous abortion in women of childbearing age (suggestive of a choriocarcinoma), or evidence of suspicious lesions at other sites in the patient with a purported primary CNS malignancy should preclude organ donation. Donors with primary CNS tumors should not be used if they have undergone radiotherapy, chemotherapy, ventriculoperitoneal or ventriculoatrial shunting, or craniotomies, because these treatments either are associated with high-grade malignancies or create potential pathways for the systemic dissemination of tumor cells [97,98].

Patients with low-grade CNS tumors (grades I to II) should be considered as acceptable donors as long as they were not subjected to any of the aforementioned interventions [18,97,98]. Those with a high-grade (grades III to IV) CNS malignancy and/or one of the aforementioned interventions are at a higher risk for malignancy transmission. In those cases, the transplant surgeon must therefore carefully assess the risk of malignancy transmission versus the risk to the potential recipient of not receiving the organ [18,96,97].

Required Request for Organ Donation and Consent

After the OPO determines the suitability of a potential donor, the next important steps are the brain death examination (when applicable) and the legally required request for organ donation (Table 56.6). Those steps should *not* involve any of the physicians associated with the transplant team, as this would represent a potential conflict of interest. In 1987, federal required request legislation became effective and has since been adopted by every state in the United States. This requirement has been further strengthened by the CMS's 1998 Conditions of Participation (*vide supra*) [75]. Required request laws mandate that the family of a potential organ donor be offered the option of organ donation. The hospital must notify the local OPO of the presence of a potential organ donor. Several studies have shown that consent rates are highest when an OPO coordinator—rather than a member of the patient's ICU team such as a physician or a nurse—approaches the family about organ donation [11–13,71].

Brain-Dead Donors

For brain-dead donors, it is of utmost importance to ensure that (a) the family understands and accepts the concept of brain death, including its legal and medical equivalence with death; (b) the request for organ donation *not* be made at the same time that brain death is explained (unless the family voiced the wish to consider donation earlier during the hospitalization); and (c) the approach and request be made by an OPO representative (rather than a member of the potential donor's care team). Sufficient time must be given to the next of kin to begin coping with this information and to accept the loss of the family member. Only then, in clear temporal separation from the explanation of death, should the subject of organ donation be broached and an appropriate request be made [11,13]. Also, the family must be informed that, after declaration of brain death and consenting to organ donation, all hospital costs relating to donation will be paid by the OPO.

DCD Donors

Families of patients with severe, irreversible brain injuries who do not fulfill the formal criteria of brain death might decide to forgo any further life-sustaining treatment. Only then can the subject of organ donation be broached with the family. As discussed earlier, it is paramount that the approach to the family and the request for organ donation be made by an OPO representative [18,26,27,99,100].

Consent

For those individuals that have not expressed in a legally binding form their desire to become an organ donor ("first-person authorization"), the Uniform Anatomical Gift Act of 1968 specifies the legal next-of-kin priority for donors over age 18 years in the following order: (a) spouse, (b) adult son or daughter, (c) either parent, (d) adult brother or sister, and (d) legal guardian [78]. Similarly, the order of priority for donors under age 18 years is as follows: (a) both parents, (b) one parent (if both parents are not available and no wishes to the contrary of the absent parent are known), (c) the custodial parent (if the parents are divorced or legally separated), and (d) the legal guardian (if there are no parents) [71]. The Revised Anatomical Gift Act of 2006 provides stipulations that bar others from overriding a donor's first-person authorization and empowers minors that apply for a driver's license to become donors (*vide supra*) [72,101]. First-person authorization may be provided by signing up with a donor registry (which is now possible online in all 50 States), notation on the driver's license, a donor card, or documentation of preferences (i) with a primary care provider, (ii) in a durable power of attorney, or (iii) in an advance directive [18]. In part as a result of these now available options, an increasing proportion of patients will have previously expressed preference for organ donation (i.e., will have provided first-person authorization). In 2015, for instance, 46% of all organ recovery operations were authorized through the donor's consent that he/she had previously registered with a state donor registry (first-person authorization) [101]. Critical care specialists must be aware that occasionally conflicts may arise from discrepancies between a donor's wishes expressed in a first-person authorization and the views of their family members or other surrogates. These sensitive situations require resolution through collaboration involving OPO representatives, ICU physicians, hospital representatives, and the patient's surrogates [18].

PERIOPERATIVE CRITICAL CARE OF THE BRAIN-DEAD ORGAN DONOR

There is an overall lack of randomized, controlled studies that could lead to a more evidence-based approach to the care of these patients. The levels of evidence provided by these studies are generally low. It is therefore important to acknowledge that some of the following recommendations may undergo substantial revision as additional, new evidence emerges (Table 56.7).

TABLE 56.7

Management of the Deceased Organ Donor: Selected Evidence Published 1993–2015

Study design	Study	Outcome	No. of cases	Reference
Effect of medical (primarily nonpharmacologic) interventions and of donor management protocols				
Case–control study	Effect of critical donor pathway (including hormonal resuscitation protocol component)	Significant increase of organs procured, organ quality unchanged	270	Rosendale et al. [19]
Case–control study	Impact of hospital-based OPO coordinators on conversion rates	Higher donor conversion rate in hospitals with hospital-based OPO coordinators	NA	Shafer et al. [67]
Prospective case series with historical controls	Impact of aggressive lung management strategies (incl. recruitment maneuvers, fluid restriction, diuresis, aspiration precautions) on lung recovery rates and transplant outcomes	Significant increase of lungs recovered without adverse effect on transplant outcomes	711	Angel et al. [102]
RCT	Effect of multipronged lung-protective strategy (incl. low tidal volume, higher PEEP) vs. conventional strategy on lung recovery rate	Lung-protective strategy nearly doubled the lung recovery rate	118	Mascia et al. [103]
RCT	Impact of mild hypothermia (target: 34°C–35°C) in brain-dead donors on early function of kidney grafts	Significant reduction of delayed graft function in recipients of kidney from the hypothermia donor group	370	Niemann et al. [104]
Effect of donor pretreatment—Single pharmacologic agents				
Retrospective cohort study	Effect of catecholamine administration to brain-dead donors on graft survival	Catecholamine use associated in dose-dependent manner with significantly better kidney graft survival	3,890	Schnuelle et al. [105]
Retrospective cohort study	Effect of dopamine administration on quality of early graft function in the recipients	Lower recipient delayed graft function rates and faster creatinine decrease in the dopamine group	254	Schnuelle et al. [106]
RCT	Effect of continuous low-dose dopamine infusion in stable donors with normal renal function on early recipient graft outcomes	Decreased posttransplant need for >1 dialysis session; no effect on rejection and short-term graft survival	265	Schnuelle et al. [107]
Case–control study	High-dose steroids and aggressive management for marginal lung donors	No graft survival differences for lungs from marginal vs. standard donors	194	Straznicka et al. [108]
RCT	Effect of high-dose continuous steroid infusion in liver donors on posttransplant outcomes	Improved posttransplant clinical reperfusion parameters (liver enzymes, bilirubin) and less early liver rejection for grafts from the steroid group	100	Kotsch et al. [109]
RCT	Effect of intensive lung donor management protocol + (steroids or T3 or [steroids + T3] or placebo) on prerecovery lung quality and lung yield	No effect of single-agent pharmacologic prerecovery interventions on lung yield; significantly less extravascular lung water accumulation in steroid groups	60	Venkateswaran et al. [23]
Retrospective cohort study	Effect of donor desmopressin use on pancreas graft thrombosis rates (UNOS recipient database)	Higher thrombosis rates in pancreas grafts from donors that had received desmopressin	2,804	Marques et al. [89]
Retrospective cohort study	Effect of use of individual drugs on organ yield (UNOS donor database)	Favorable impact of steroids or desmopressin, but not T4, on organ yield	15,601	Selck et al. [110]

TABLE 56.7 (*continued*)

Management of the Deceased Organ Donor: Selected Evidence Published 1993–2015

Study design	Study	Outcome	No. of cases	Reference
RCT	Effect of low-dose vasopressin vs. saline on donor hemodynamics and inotrope use	Increase in blood pressure and decrease in inotrope use in vasopressin group	24	Pennefather et al. [111]
RCT	Effect of T3 infusion (limited to the duration of the organ procurement operation) vs. no T3	No differences for posttransplant liver graft function	25	Randell et al. [112]
RCT	Effect of T3 infusion (within <5 h of organ recovery) vs. none on donor hemodynamics and adenine nucleotide concentration measured in graft biopsy tissue	No differences in hemodynamics and adenine nucleotide levels	52	Perez-Blanco et al. [113]
Effect of donor pretreatment—Combination hormonal replacement therapy				
Retrospective cohort study	Effect of T3 + steroids + insulin on need for inotropic support and organ yield in unstable donors	Hormonal treatment improved hemodynamics of unstable donors and resulted in similar organ yield as in stable donors	47	Roels et al. [114]
Retrospective cohort study	Impact on organ yield of (T3 or thyroxin) + steroids + vasopressin vs. none	Increased kidney, liver, pancreas, heart, and lung yield rates in donors that received hormonal replacement therapy	10,292	Rosendale et al. [20]
Retrospective cohort study	Impact of (T3 or thyroxin) + steroids + vasopressin vs. all other (<3 hormones) hormonal replacement regimens on heart yield and early heart graft function	Increased number of transplanted hearts and improved early heart graft function	4,543	Rosendale et al. [19]
RCT	Effect of intensive lung donor management protocol and (steroids or T3 or [steroids + T3] or placebo) on lung quality and yield	No effect of steroids + T3 on donor lung quality and yield	60	Venkateswaran et al. [23]
Retrospective cohort study	Effect of steroids + T4 on organ yield (UNOS donor database)	No effect of steroids + T4 on organ yield	15,601	Selck et al. [110]
RCT	Effect of T3 vs. steroids vs. (T3 + steroids) vs. placebo on donor cardiac function and heart yield	T3 and steroids (alone and in combination) did not affect donor cardiovascular function or heart yield	80	Venkateswaran et al. [115]

Levels of evidence that apply to this table based on current guidelines published by the Oxford Centre for Evidence-Based Medicine (www.cebm.net) (highest to lowest): Level 2: RCT(s); Level 3: nonrandomized controlled cohort studies; Level 4: case series, case–control studies (incl. historical controls).
OPO, organ procurement organization; NA, not applicable; RCT, randomized controlled trial; UNOS, United Network for Organ Sharing; T3, triiodothyronine; T4, thyroxin.

Pathophysiology of Brain Death

The majority of our knowledge of the pathophysiologic changes during and after brain death has been derived from experiments performed using animal models. Hemodynamic instability during the phase of impending brain herniation is the result of autonomic dysregulation secondary to the progressive loss of central neurohumoral regulatory control of vital functions. The continuous increase of intracranial pressure with worsening brain ischemia leads to severe systemic hypertension (Cushing's response) and frequently is associated with tachyarrhythmias. This process is mediated by an increase in sympathetic activity and an excess of circulating catecholamines ("autonomic storm") [116–118]. A brief period of transient bradycardia associated with the hypertensive response can be seen in the early phase of brain herniation (Cushing's reflex).

During the phase of increased sympathetic activity, there is evidence that coronary blood flow is significantly impaired, resulting in cardiac microinfarctions. Furthermore, decreased hepatic perfusion due to increased intrahepatic shunting has been demonstrated as a result of the excessive sympathetic activity. Neurogenic pulmonary edema is thought to develop during the autonomic storm phase secondary to the temporary elevation of pulmonary venous pressures over the level of pulmonary arterial and alveolar capillary pressures. This causes massive transudation of fluid from the microvasculature into the alveoli and hemorrhage [116–118]. Within approximately 15 minutes after brain herniation and brain death, catecholamines decrease to below baseline values.

The resting vagal tone is abolished because of destruction of the nucleus ambiguus, eliminating all chronotropic effects of atropine administered after brain death. The total carbon dioxide production after brain death is low, because of the absence of cerebral metabolism and the presence of hypothermia and decreased muscle tone. The subsequent chronic maintenance phase of brain-dead donors is frequently characterized by hypotension, resulting mainly from complete arterial and venous vasomotor collapse with significant peripheral venous pooling.

Experimental and clinical evidence also shows that brain death leads to activation of proinflammatory and immunoregulatory pathways [106,118–122]. Messenger ribonucleic acid and protein expression within peripheral solid organs of brain-dead donors is significantly increased for cytokines (e.g., interleukin-1β, interleukin-6, tumor necrosis factor-α, interferon gamma, tumor growth factor-β), adhesion molecules (e.g., P- and E-selectin), and vasoconstrictors (e.g., endothelin) [106,118–122]. Importantly, brain death has also been associated with enhanced expression of immunoregulatory molecules such as major histocompatibility complex class I and II proteins. Consistent with these findings, increased immunogenicity and accelerated rejection were noted in kidneys and hearts transplanted from brain-dead rodents [118,119].

Routine Care and Monitoring

Regular nursing care must be continued after brain death. Frequent turning to prevent decubitus ulcers, skin care, dressing changes, urinary and intravascular catheter care, and catheter site care must be meticulous to minimize the risk of infection. Other indwelling devices should be removed, if possible (e.g., ventriculostomies and ventriculoatrial or ventriculoperitoneal shunts, which may have been inserted in certain patients for monitoring or treating of elevated intracranial pressure). Any urinary and intravascular catheters that may have been inserted under suboptimal, emergent conditions without appropriate aseptic technique at the time of original injury should be replaced. A nasogastric tube should always be inserted for gastric decompression and prevention of aspiration.

Arterial lines should be inserted preferentially into peripheral arteries of the upper extremities because femoral arterial line readings can become inaccurate from surgical manipulation of the abdominal aorta during organ procurement. Similarly, central venous catheters should not be inserted through the femoral vein because dissection and manipulation of the interior vena cava occur during organ procurement. In addition, venous catheters inserted through the femoral vein can cause iliac vein thrombosis. This increases the risk of pulmonary embolization, particularly during surgical venous dissection. Thrombosis can also render the iliac veins unsuitable for use in vascular reconstruction, which may be necessary for some types of abdominal or thoracic organ transplants.

The following parameters must be determined routinely and frequently for all organ donors using various monitoring devices: core temperature (esophageal, rectal, or indwelling bladder catheter temperature probes), heart rate (continuous electrocardiographic monitoring), systemic blood pressure (arterial catheter), central venous blood pressure (subclavian or internal jugular central venous catheter), arterial oxygen saturation (pulse oximetry), and hourly urine output (Foley catheter). Use of a pulmonary artery catheter for measurement of cardiac output, cardiac index, pulmonary arterial and pulmonary arterial occlusion (wedge) pressure, and central venous oximetry is not routinely necessary; their use is typically reserved for selected unstable donors whose volume status is uncertain or who exhibit persistent acidosis with evidence of tissue hypoperfusion. Laboratory parameters also must be checked regularly, including arterial blood gas, serum electrolytes, blood urea nitrogen, creatinine, lactate, and liver enzyme values; total bilirubin; and hemoglobin, hematocrit, platelet count, and coagulation tests. Testing is adapted to the individual clinical situation—e.g., frequent electrolyte determinations if diabetes insipidus has been diagnosed, lactate monitoring in acidotic donors, and repeated coagulation profiles in the presence of disseminated intravascular coagulation.

If infection is suspected, blood, urine, sputum, cerebrospinal fluid, and wound drainage cultures must be obtained. Routine surveillance cultures (usually blood and urine cultures) may be required, depending on the protocol of the local OPO and the organ type. Blood cultures should be obtained using peripheral venipuncture, rather than arterial or central venous catheters, to avoid contamination. Prophylactic antibiotics should only be administered immediately before the retrieval procedure. Any source of infection should be identified, characterized from a microbiologic standpoint, and treated with pathogen-specific agents.

General Management Goals

The most important overall goal in the management of brain-dead multiple-organ donors is to optimize organ perfusion and tissue oxygen delivery. Organ viability and function after transplantation are closely correlated with adequacy of resuscitation and hemodynamic stability during the organ donor maintenance phase.

The events associated with the cause of brain death (e.g., hemorrhagic shock, cardiac arrest) can lead to significant physiologic abnormalities. Head injury preceding brain death is known to induce a hypermetabolic response, equivalent to that observed after a second- or third-degree burn involving approximately 40% of the total body surface area. Significant metabolic stress and impairment of organ perfusion occur during brain herniation, and both events are related to excessive catecholamine release. Any additional circulatory compromise in the time period afterward potentiates the deleterious consequences of these previous adverse events. Posttransplant organ function can be negatively affected by such episodes of cardiovascular dysregulation, particularly in such ischemia-sensitive organs as the heart and liver. For example, even with optimal heart donor management, the recipient often needs inotropic support and may exhibit subendocardial myocyte necrosis on biopsy specimens obtained during the early posttransplant period [21,119]. Anticipating these changes associated with brain death and providing optimal management should they occur during the organ donor maintenance phase, as well as optimizing organ function, are of utmost importance [21].

Parameters associated with adequate tissue perfusion in stable donors in the absence of lactic acidosis are listed in Table 56.7. They include a mean arterial pressure of >60 and/or a systolic blood pressure of 100 to 120 mm Hg, central venous pressure of 6 to 8 mm Hg, oxygen saturation of the arterial blood ≥95%, core temperature ≥35°C, and hemoglobin of 8 to 10 g per dL [19,25], the latter balancing the slightly decreased oxygen transport capacity of the red blood cell mass with the beneficial effects of low viscosity on blood flow. Maintaining adequate hemoglobin concentration is also essential in preparation for organ recovery, in which hemodynamic stability throughout the operation is crucial, especially if blood loss occurs.

Measurement of urine output alone as a means of assessing adequacy of fluid resuscitation is notoriously unreliable in brain-dead donors. A mean arterial pressure >60 mm Hg and the absence of metabolic acidosis (with or without infusion of a small amount of dopamine) with concurrent adequate urine output (at least 1 to 2 mL/kg/h) are usually better indirect indicators of donor stability and sufficient oxygen delivery to organs and tissues (Table 56.8). It is important to remember, however, that the use of vasoconstrictor or inotropic agents is not a substitute for adequate fluid resuscitation. Thus, proper

TABLE 56.8

Maintenance Therapy Endpoints for Brain-Dead Organ Donors

Variable	Therapeutic endpoint
Systolic blood pressure	100–120 mm Hg or mean arterial pressure ≥60 mm Hg
Central venous pressure	6–8 mm Hg
Urine output	>1 mL/kg/h
Core temperature	>35°C
Partial arterial oxygen pressure	80–100 mm Hg
Systemic arterial oxygen saturation	95%
pH	7.37–7.45
Hemoglobin	8–10 g/dL

fluid management remains the cornerstone of successful donor management.

The use of vasopressors should be minimized if at all possible because of their splanchnic vasoconstrictive effects. Efforts to elevate blood pressure beyond the normal range can adversely affect outcome and should be avoided: high doses of vasopressors can cause arrhythmias and increase myocardial oxygen consumption, and pulmonary edema after excessive fluid administration can render lungs unsuitable for transplantation. After the lung, the pancreas is the organ most prone to tissue edema. Normal central venous pressure and PEEP help maintain an adequate perfusion gradient across the hepatic microcirculatory bed (i.e., that between the portal vein and hepatic artery on one side and the inferior vena cava and right atrium on the other).

Selective use of pulmonary artery catheterization must be considered in donors who do not respond to routine management and continue to exhibit hypotension or persistent lactic acidosis after adequate volume loading, particularly in those in whom this occurs despite use of moderate doses of dopamine. Determining pulmonary artery and pulmonary artery occlusion pressures, cardiac output and index, pulmonary and systemic vascular resistive indices, oxygen availability and consumption, and other parameters helps to differentiate the cause of instability. In selected patients, echocardiographic assessment of the left ventricular ejection fraction may prove useful. Appropriate therapy can then be administered (e.g., fluid balance correction or PEEP adjustments, additional inotropic support, preload or afterload reduction). Once the hemodynamic instability has resolved, pulmonary artery catheters should be removed to eliminate the inherent risks of infection, induction of arrhythmias, and mechanical endomyocardial damage.

Cardiovascular Support

Hypotension is the most common hemodynamic abnormality seen in brain-dead organ donors. The usual cause is hypovolemia, because of a combination of vasomotor collapse after brain death and the effects of treatment protocols to decrease intracranial pressure, which require minimization of hydration and use of osmotic diuretics (Tables 56.9 and 56.10). After brain death is declared, adequate volume resuscitation of the donor can require several liters of fluid. Until a euvolemic state is achieved, dopamine (greater than 3 μg per kg per minute) can be used temporarily; the dose should be titrated to maintain an adequate systolic blood pressure [18]. Infusion rates greater than 10 μg/kg/min have been associated with increased rates of acute tubular necrosis and decreased renal allograft survival.

TABLE 56.9

Differential Diagnosis of Hypotension in the Brain-Dead Organ Donor

Diagnosis	Common Underlying Cause(s)
Hypovolemia	see Table 56.10
Hypothermia	Loss of central temperature control, administration of room-temperature intravenous fluids and blood products, heat loss during laparotomies and thoracotomies
Cardiac dysfunction	Arrhythmia (ischemia, catecholamines, hypokalemia, hypomagnesemia)
	Acidosis
	Hypooxygenation
	Excessive positive end-expiratory ventilatory pressure
	Congestive heart failure due to excessive fluid administration
	Hypophosphatemia
	Causes related to the injury leading to brain death (cardiac tamponade, myocardial contusion)
	Myocardial sequelae of autonomic storm
	Preexisting cardiac disease
Drug side effect or overdose	Long-acting β-blocker, calcium channel antagonist, antihypertensive agent
Hypocalcemia	Transfusions, hypomagnesemia (e.g., secondary to osmotic diuresis), acute renal failure

TABLE 56.10

Differential Diagnosis of Hypovolemia in the Brain-Dead Organ Donor

- Arterial and venous vasomotor collapse due to loss of central neurohumoral control
- Dehydration (fluid restriction to treat head injury)
- Insufficient resuscitation after the injury leading to brain death (e.g., ongoing hemorrhagic shock with coagulopathy after trauma)
- Polyuria
- Osmotic diuresis (mannitol, hyperglycemia)
- Diabetes insipidus
- Hypothermia
- Administration of other diuretics
- Massive third spacing in response to the original injury
- Decreased intravascular oncotic pressure after excessive resuscitation with crystalloid fluids

High infusion rates also lead to decreased perfusion of other organs because of splanchnic vasoconstriction.

Dopamine is also the drug of choice if hemodynamic instability persists after fluid resuscitation and adequate volume loading. Use of isoproterenol and dobutamine should be avoided in this context because of their vasodilatory effects. Drugs with α-adrenergic agonist effects such as phenylephrine (IV infusion 0.15 to 0.75 μg/kg/min) and norepinephrine (IV infusion up to 0.05 μg/kg/min) should be added only if hypotension persists in the face of euvolemia and titration of the dopamine infusion up to 15 μg/kg/min. α-Adrenergic agonists can cause severe peripheral vasoconstriction, reduce renal and hepatic perfusion, and may predispose to increased pulmonary capillary permeability. For these reasons, they must be used judiciously. Once these drugs are used, the need for their continued use must be frequently reassessed [18,25]. For the majority (>80%) of donors, adequate hemodynamic goals can be achieved with volume resuscitation and low to moderate doses of a single vasopressor agent (dopamine).

Several studies have suggested that administration of catecholamines, and in particular of dopamine, to brain-dead patients may exert a beneficial impact on early kidney graft function and graft survival [105–107,123]. Several potential mechanisms have been invoked to explain these observations, including favorable modulatory effects on ischemia–reperfusion and on upregulation of adhesion molecules that results from the inflammatory state induced by brain death [105–107].

Low-dose arginine vasopressin can serve as an alternative first-line or as an additional vasopressor. It enhances vascular sensitivity to catecholamines and causes vasoconstriction through multiple effector pathways; it may thus allow minimizing catecholamine dose and side effects [111,124,125]. Effective arginine vasopressin doses for improving hemodynamic stability range from 0.01 to 0.1 International Units per minute (starting dose: 0.01 to 0.04 International Units per minute) given as continuous intravenous infusion [18,111,124]. The use of arginine vasopressin in brain-dead organ donors has been associated with improvement of cardiac performance and increased rates of organ recovery [125].

When attempting to determine the etiology of hypotension in an organ donor, underlying cardiac disease (e.g., coronary artery disease, valve defects) and factors related to the cause of brain death (e.g., myocardial infarction, cardiac tamponade, or myocardial contusion) must be included in the differential diagnosis. Electrolyte abnormalities such as hypophosphatemia, hypocalcemia, hypokalemia, and hypomagnesemia are common in brain-dead organ donors. The presence of these entities must also be considered when hemodynamic instability is encountered, and frequent testing and correction of these significant electrolyte imbalances are important. Hypophosphatemia and hypocalcemia can decrease myocardial contractility and provoke hypotension [126]; hypokalemia and hypomagnesemia can also impair hemodynamics by causing arrhythmias.

For the treatment of arrhythmias or hypertension, medications that possess rapid reversibility and a short half-life are preferred. Hemodynamic instability can be pronounced after brain death, with wide swings between the extremes of hypotension and hypertension, rendering the brain-dead donor more susceptible to cardiovascular drug effects. Hypertension can be treated with short-acting vasodilatory agents (e.g., nitroprusside) or a rapidly reversible β-adrenergic antagonist (e.g., esmolol hydrochloride), because hypertension is usually associated with increased circulating catecholamines. Other drugs, such as calcium channel blockers (e.g., verapamil) or longer-acting β-blockers (e.g., labetalol, propranolol), should be avoided because of their negative inotropic effects and the inability to titrate them precisely. Bradyarrhythmias during the early phase of brain herniation are part of Cushing's reflex and do not usually require any treatment, unless they are associated with hypotension and asystole. Because of the lack of chronotropic effects by atropine after brain death, use of either isoproterenol or epinephrine is required to treat hemodynamically significant bradyarrhythmias.

Tachyarrhythmias are associated with the increased catecholamine release that occurs during and immediately after brain herniation. Administration of short-acting β-blockers (e.g., esmolol hydrochloride) serves not only to treat arrhythmias but also to mitigate hypertension during the autonomic storm. Use of additional short-acting IV antiarrhythmics (e.g., lidocaine) may become necessary if tachyarrhythmias do not resolve after β-blocker therapy. Calcium channel blockers (e.g., verapamil) must be avoided under these circumstances because of their negative inotropic effects. Cardiac glycosides (e.g., digoxin) also should not be used because they can induce and potentiate bradyarrhythmias and tachyarrhythmias, and they also have splanchnic vasoconstrictive side effects.

Cardiac arrest can occur in up to 25% of all donors during the maintenance phase after brain death and should be treated by routine measures, with the exception that isoproterenol or epinephrine must be substituted for atropine [83,84]. If these measures fail to result in the return of a cardiac rhythm, external (transcutaneous) pacing may be considered. However, the efficacy of external pacing for asystole associated with brain death is unknown. No intracardiac injections should be given during cardiopulmonary resuscitation because they can render the heart unsuitable for transplantation.

Respiratory and Acid–Base Maintenance

Use of endotracheal suctioning is usually minimized during the treatment of cerebral edema to avoid any unnecessary stimulation that would increase intracranial pressure. In contrast, after brain death is declared, vigorous tracheobronchial toilet is important, with frequent suctioning using sterile precautions. Percussion and turning for postural drainage are instituted as well. Even if the lungs are unsuitable for donation, it is important to minimize the risk of atelectasis and infection. Preventing atelectasis facilitates oxygenation and may obviate the need for detrimental high levels of PEEP. Steroids administered to some patients as part of the treatment for increased intracranial pressure predispose to pulmonary infectious complications. The presence of pneumonia can preclude donation of the lungs as well as other organs, depending on its severity and association with systemic sepsis. Routine respiratory care of all donors also includes the use of 5 cm H_2O PEEP to increase alveolar recruitment and prevent microatelectasis [18,19,25].

The etiology of pulmonary edema in organ donors can be cardiogenic, neurogenic, aspiration induced, a result of trauma or fluid overload, or a combination of these factors. Neurogenic pulmonary edema can preclude lung or combined heart–lung donation, but not donation of other organs (e.g., heart, kidney, liver, pancreas). The treatment for pulmonary edema is supportive and should be directed at maintaining adequate arterial oxygenation without using very high levels of PEEP. Fluids must be administered carefully to maintain organ perfusion while avoiding exacerbation of the edema.

In potential lung donors, the endotracheal tube should not be advanced more than several centimeters into the trachea, to prevent damage to areas that may become part of an anastomosis. A sample of sputum should be obtained for Gram's stain and cultures to exclude the presence of infection. The samples can be obtained using bronchoscopy, a procedure that is often routinely performed before lung donation.

Traditionally, tidal volumes of 10 to 12 mL per kg and relatively low PEEP target ranges (3 to 5 cm H_2O) have been recommended. However, there is now evidence that lung-protective ventilatory strategies that have become standard of care for regular ICU patients—i.e., tidal volumes of 6 to 8 mL per kg and PEEP of 8 to 10 cm H_2O—are also beneficial for the management of the often injured lungs of brain-dead donors [18,25,127,128]. In a randomized trial, the number of transplanted lungs doubled when a lung-protective strategy was pursued [102]. Aggressive living donor management protocols aimed at improving alveolar recruitment and oxygenation have proven successful with high rates of conversion from unacceptable to acceptable PaO_2/FiO_2 ratios [102]. For potential lung donors, the lowest FiO_2 that is capable of maintaining a PaO_2 of greater than 100 mm Hg should be selected. If oxygenation is insufficient, PEEP should be increased rather than increasing the FiO_2. Very high levels of PEEP may negatively affect cardiac output, which should be carefully monitored in this setting. If hypotension occurs, PEEP should be reduced. Under these circumstances, use of pulmonary artery catheterization should be considered to balance PEEP requirements against those of organ perfusion. In contrast, to correct insufficient arterial oxygenation in nonlung donors, an increase in FiO_2 is preferred over high levels of PEEP [25].

There is no direct evidence stemming from controlled trials that would support a specific fluid management strategy in prospective lung donors. Indirect evidence from studies that involved ICU patients with acute respiratory distress syndrome, as well as prospective lung donors, supports a conservative fluid management approach with prospective donors [102,129]. To date, there is no evidence that such a conservative fluid management approach in donors adversely impacts the function of kidney grafts obtained from the same donor [130]. Excessive use of crystalloid fluids during the initial resuscitation after brain death is declared can render the lungs unsuitable for transplantation. If relatively large amounts of fluid are required for resuscitation and hemodynamic stabilization, colloids (i.e., albumin solutions) or blood transfusions (if the hemoglobin is less than 8 g per dL) should be considered in addition to the infusion of crystalloid solutions [18].

Respiratory alkalosis can develop in brain-dead organ donors secondary to mechanical hyperventilation as part of the treatment protocol for elevated intracranial pressure. After brain death, the arterial pH should be adjusted to normal values because alkalosis has many undesirable side effects, such as increased cardiac output, systemic vasoconstriction, bronchospasm, and a shift to the left of the oxyhemoglobin dissociation curve. The latter decreases oxygen unloading in the tissues and impairs oxygen delivery, thereby diminishing tissue oxygenation and metabolism. Lactic metabolic acidosis is frequent in brain-dead donors; it should be treated by compensation with a slight respiratory alkalosis until the underlying abnormality has been corrected (e.g., dehydration, tissue ischemia). Administration of sodium bicarbonate should be contemplated only if the increased minute ventilation necessary to induce respiratory alkalosis leads to a decrease in cardiac output. In either situation, the most important aspect of managing metabolic acidosis is to treat the underlying cause. In selected patients this may require pulmonary artery catheterization to assess the adequacy of hydration, cardiac output, and tissue oxygen delivery.

Renal Function and Fluid and Electrolyte Management

Maintaining adequate systemic perfusion pressure while minimizing the use of vasopressors contributes to good renal allograft function and reduces the rate of acute tubular necrosis after transplantation. If the urine production is insufficient (e.g., less than 0.5 mL/kg/h) after adequate volume loading, loop diuretics (furosemide, ethacrynic acid, bumetanide) or osmotic diuretics (mannitol) can be considered to initiate diuresis. Nephrotoxic drugs (e.g., aminoglycosides) and agents that may exert adverse effects on renal perfusion (e.g., nonsteroidal anti-inflammatory drugs) are contraindicated. Cephalosporins, monobactams, carbapenems, and quinolones are examples of less nephrotoxic but effective antibiotics that can be used if infection occurs.

Polyuria in brain-dead donors is a frequent finding. It can be due to diabetes insipidus, osmotic diuresis (induced by mannitol administered to decrease elevated intracranial pressures or hyperglycemia), physiologic diuresis due to previous massive fluid administration during resuscitation after the original injury with return of third-space fluid into the intravascular space, or hypothermia. Diabetes insipidus often heralds brain death in head-injured patients. It is the most frequent cause of polyuria during the organ donor maintenance phase. Found in up to 80% of all brain-dead bodies [81], it is related to insufficient blood levels of antidiuretic hormone (vasopressin), resulting in the production of large quantities of dilute urine.

Diabetes insipidus should be suspected when urine volumes exceed 300 mL per hour (or 7 mL/kg/h) in conjunction with hypernatremia (serum sodium greater than 150 mEq per dL), elevated serum osmolality (greater than 310 mOsm per L) and a low urinary sodium concentration. In addition to hypernatremia, other electrolyte abnormalities frequently observed during diabetes insipidus include hypokalemia, hypocalcemia, and hypomagnesemia. The appropriate replacement of these electrolyte losses can be guided by urinary electrolyte determinations, which easily allow calculation of the amount of the electrolyte to be replaced. Because diabetes insipidus is so common, mannitol administration should be discontinued after brain death is declared. Other supportive care of patients with diabetes insipidus includes replacing urine output milliliter for milliliter with free water (e.g., 5% solution of dextrose in water IV).

Once urine output due to diabetes insipidus exceeds 300 mL per hour, desmopressin (desamino-8-D-arginine vasopressin), a synthetic analog of vasopressin (or arginine vasopressin), should be administered. Desmopressin has a long duration of action (6 to 20 hours) and a high antidiuretic-to-pressor ratio, without any undesirable splanchnic vasoconstrictive effects that can occur with administration of normal- and high-dose arginine vasopressin [18,25,131]. For example, doses of 1 to 2 μg desmopressin are administered intravenously every 8 to 12 hours to achieve a urine output less than 300 mL per hour [18,25,131]. Desmopressin can also be effectively administered subcutaneously, intramuscularly, and intranasally. Alternatively, in donors with diabetes insipidus that are also hypotensive due to a low systemic vascular resistance (SVR), an arginine vasopressin IV infusion can be started at 0.5 International Units per hour and titrated up to 6 International Units per hour, targeting a urine output of 0.5 to 3 mL/kg/h and a serum sodium of 135 to 145 mEq per L [18,25]. Compared to desmopressin, arginine vasopressin is easily titrated and adds beneficial hemodynamic effects.

The choice of the *resuscitation* fluid depends on the clinical circumstances and the donor's electrolyte, osmolar, and acid–base state. Generally, for intravascular volume replacement, an isotonic crystalloid is preferred (i.e., 0.9% saline solution [in hypoosmolar patients] or lactated Ringer's solution [in the setting of hyperchloremic metabolic acidosis]). For correction of hypernatremia in euvolemic or near-euvolemic patients, hypotonic fluids (e.g., D5W or 0.45% saline solution) can be administered (e.g., during the initial resuscitation phase after brain death is declared) [18]. For intravascular volume expansion to address acute hypotension, albumin 5% is the preferred colloid. Use of low- or high-molecular-weight hydroxyethyl starch (HES) is contraindicated as it is associated with acute kidney injury and coagulopathy because it is trapped within the hepatic reticuloendothelial system. Consistent with these concerns, HES use in donors was shown to result in higher delayed kidney graft function and failure rates [132].

Subsequently, *maintenance* fluid should consist of 5% dextrose in 0.45% sodium chloride with 20 mEq potassium added to each liter, administered at a rate of 2 mL/kg/h during the maintenance phase if urine output is adequate (greater than 1 to 2 mL/kg/h). If the urine output is greater than 2 mL/kg/h, IV fluids should be administered at a rate equal to the urine output during the previous hour (IV intake = urine output). If the serum sodium concentration exceeds 150 mEq per dL, the maintenance fluid should consist of 5% dextrose solution with 20 mEq potassium added to each liter. Should the hourly fluid administration rate exceed 500 mL per hour, the dextrose concentration of the maintenance fluid should be decreased to 1% to avoid excessive hyperglycemia. IV maintenance fluids administered to brain-dead organ donors should contain glucose, which is important to maintain intrahepatic glycogen stores that appear to be associated with normal liver allograft function in the early posttransplant period. In hypernatremic patients, the sodium content of certain IV fluids and plasma expanders (e.g., albumin solutions) must also be taken into consideration.

Endocrine Therapy

According to prior studies, pituitary hormone blood levels do not uniformly decrease after brain death. Diabetes insipidus develops in approximately 80% of brain-dead donors as a result of low or absent blood levels of vasopressin [80]. These findings are a direct consequence of brain death, which abolishes vasopressin production in the hypothalamic nuclei (supraoptic and paraventricular nuclei) and vasopressin storage and release in the posterior pituitary. In contrast, near-normal levels of anterior pituitary hormones, such as thyroid-stimulating hormone, adrenocorticotropic hormone, and growth hormone, have been documented after brain death in some studies [133–136]. Their persistence is probably due to the preservation of small subcapsular areas in the anterior pituitary, the blood supply of which is derived from small branches of the inferior hypophyseal artery. The latter arises from the extradural internal carotid artery, which is relatively protected from increases in intracranial pressure [137]. Clinical evidence, however, suggests deficient adrenal cortisol secretion after dynamic stimulation in brain-dead donors, irrespective of the level of pituitary dysfunction [138].

The principle of pharmacologic replacement therapy for deficient posterior pituitary vasopressin after brain death is well established [18,19,25,111]. A retrospective UNOS database analysis demonstrated a significant association between desmopressin use in donors and organ yield (Table 56.7) [110]. Low-dose vasopressin has been shown to exert beneficial hemodynamic effect in brain-dead donors (Table 56.7) [111,125].

In contrast, controversy still exists regarding the benefits of supplementation with triiodothyronine [T3] and thyroxine [T4], which are synthesized under anterior pituitary control (Table 56.7) [18,19,25,110,112,114,139–148]. Initially, the presence of low T3 blood levels was demonstrated after brain death in animal experiments [149]. Administration of exogenous T3 to donor animals improved a variety of metabolic parameters before and after organ preservation [150–152], as well as organ function after transplantation [153]. These findings suggested possibly positive effects of T3 also in human donors. A limited number of uncontrolled clinical trials suggested favorable influences of donor pretreatment with thyroid hormone on hemodynamic and metabolic parameters during the donor maintenance phase [84,154,155] and on outcome after heart transplantation [156–158]. But a number of other investigators failed to observe a significant benefit of thyroid hormone administration on biochemical and hemodynamic donor parameters and on posttransplant outcomes (Table 56.7) [112,113,159,160].

The latter outcomes could be explained at least in part by the findings of some studies which have suggested that the low T3 levels in human donors do not correlate with the presence of hemodynamic stability [161,162] or outcome after transplantation [163–166] to begin with. The typical thyroidal hormonal pattern after brain death consists of decreased T3, normal or decreased thyroxine, and normal thyroid-stimulating hormone. This pattern is not consistent with acute insufficiency of the hypothalamic–pituitary–thyroid axis or clinically overt hypothyroidism, but is similar to changes (sick euthyroid syndrome) observed in other groups of critically ill individuals. Thyroid hormone administration to such patients may not only be ineffective but may theoretically even be detrimental in some cases [145,146]. In summary, there is no conclusive evidence to date that supplementation of organ donors with thyroid hormone *alone* yields a significant clinical benefit. As per a consensus recommendation by leading North American critical care medicine societies and the U.S. Association of OPOs, thyroid hormone replacement therapy—either alone or as part of a combination protocol—should at present be considered for hemodynamically unstable donors with abnormal (<45%) left ventricular ejection fraction (*vide infra* for thyroid hormone dosing guidelines) [18].

By contrast, evidence for the potential benefits of routine administration of corticosteroids *alone* has emerged [18,108–110]. Normal human serum adrenocorticotropic hormone and cortisol levels have been demonstrated after brain death in some studies, whereas others have observed dysfunction of the hypothalamic–pituitary–adrenal axis in patients with traumatic brain injury [133–136]. Clinically, however, administration of high-dose steroids was noted to stabilize and improve lung function, leading to higher probability of lung recovery from brain-dead patients that had previously not been considered for lung donation, to increase organ yield, and to lead to improved outcomes after liver transplantation [19,108–110,167,168].

Published retrospective evidence suggests that institution of empiric donor management protocols that incorporate *combination* treatment with arginine vasopressin, high-dose corticosteroids, thyroid hormone, and insulin may stabilize and improve cardiac function in brain-dead donors and may result in increased probability of kidney, heart, liver, lung, and pancreas recovery and transplantation and may improve posttransplant outcomes (Table 56.7) [114,139,140,142–144]. These and other findings have served as the basis for recommendations from a national U.S. consensus conference held in 2001 that include: T3: 4 μg bolus, 3 μg per hour continuous infusion; arginine vasopressin: IU bolus, 0.5 to 4.0 International Units per hour continuous infusion (titrate SVR to 800 to 1,200 using a pulmonary artery catheter); methylprednisolone 15 mg per kg intravenous bolus, repeat every 24 hours; and insulin continuous intravenous infusion at a minimum rate of 1 unit per hour (titrate blood glucose to 120 to 180 mg per dL) [20,21]. However, given the uncertainty regarding potentially adverse side effects and the absence of high-level evidence, large prospective randomized trials are necessary before routine administration of hormonal combination therapy can be recommended for all donors—particularly because, for example, excellent lung procurement rates from marginal donors and good posttransplant outcomes have also been described in the current era without hormonal supplementation (Table 56.7) [169]. Moreover, the optimal dose and combination, as well as the contribution of each individual hormone to the observed overall outcome remain yet to be studied and elucidated. For now, it appears prudent to reserve routine *combination* hormone replacement therapy for hemodynamically unstable donors that require substantial catecholamine doses (e.g., dopamine >10 μg/kg/min) or have an ejection fraction of less than 45% [18,20,21,25].

Although brain death is not associated with primary pancreatic endocrine dysfunction, hyperglycemia is frequent in brain-dead donors. Hyperglycemia can be caused by increased catecholamine release, altered carbohydrate metabolism, steroid administration for treatment of cerebral edema, infusion of large amounts of dextrose-containing IV fluids, or peripheral insulin resistance. Treating hyperglycemia in brain-dead donors appears to be important with regard to pancreatic islet cell function. Experimental evidence suggests that high glucose levels may produce transient or irreversible damage to beta cells in the pancreatic islets, in vitro and in vivo [170,171]. This glucose toxicity was attenuated during in vivo experiments by correcting hyperglycemia [172]. Clinical studies in pancreas transplant recipients have demonstrated that donor hyperglycemia is a risk factor for decreased graft survival [88]. It was not established in these studies, however, whether donor hyperglycemia was indicative of marginal or insufficient beta-cell mass or whether impaired pancreatic graft function was related to islet cell dysfunction as a result of hyperglycemia.

Hyperglycemia in and of itself is known to cause insulin resistance [173]. Studies in brain-dead donors have suggested that a state of hyperinsulinemia coupled with peripheral insulin resistance exists, as evidenced by elevated C-peptide–glucose molar ratios [174]. For all the above reasons, it is prudent to maintain blood glucose levels in donors between 120 and 180 mg per dL [175]. Insulin should be administered as needed according to the blood glucose values to mitigate any potential adverse effects of hyperglycemia on pancreatic islets, which could impair glucose homeostasis after transplantation [175]. If hyperglycemia persists despite initial bolus insulin therapy, continuous IV insulin infusion should be instituted to facilitate titration of glucose levels. As in many other critical care patients, good glycemic control is also good standard practice for brain-dead donors, because it acts to prevent ketoacidosis and osmotic diuresis, both of which can be significant problems in the management of brain-dead donors, and because it may contribute to improved overall organ recovery and transplantation rates [176].

Hypothermia

After brain death, the body becomes poikilothermic because of the loss of thalamic and hypothalamic central temperature control mechanisms, and hypothermia usually ensues [177]. Systemic vasodilation causes additional heat loss. Hypothermia can be aggravated by administering room-temperature IV fluids and cold blood products. Adverse effects of significant hypothermia include decreased myocardial contractility, hypotension, cardiac arrhythmias, cardiac arrest, hepatic and renal dysfunction, and acidosis and coagulopathy [178–180]. Therefore, donor core temperature should be maintained at or above 35°C. It is usually sufficient to use humidified, heated ventilator gases; warmed IV fluids and blood products; and warming blankets to achieve rewarming and to maintain an adequate body temperature. Rewarming with peritoneal dialysis or bladder irrigations generally should not be performed in organ donors.

In a randomized trial, a mildly hypothermic target temperature range of 34°C to 35°C in brain-dead patients was associated with significantly decreased delayed graft function rates in the recipients of kidneys from these donors [104]. The effect of mild hypothermia on extrarenal donor organs, however, remains unknown for now. It is therefore premature to recommend a mildly hypothermic core temperature target range for all brain-dead donors.

Coagulation System

Coagulopathy and disseminated intravascular coagulation are common findings in brain-dead donors, particularly after head injuries. Pathologic activation of the coagulation cascade occurs when brain tissue, which is very rich in tissue thromboplastin, comes in contact with blood after trauma. Massive blood transfusions can produce dilutional thrombocytopenia, and subsequent ongoing hemorrhage, hypothermia, and acidosis are all able to trigger or further aggravate coagulopathy. Clinical findings can include pathologic bleeding, abnormal prothrombin time, thrombocytopenia, hypofibrinogenemia, and increased levels of fibrin/fibrinogen degradation products. Treatment of coagulopathy entails use of blood components such as platelets, fresh-frozen plasma, or cryoprecipitate and correction of the underlying pathophysiology (e.g., hypothermia, acidosis, surgical hemorrhage). ε-Aminocaproic acid and tranexamic acid should not be used because of their potential for inducing microvascular thrombosis, thereby rendering organs potentially unsuitable for transplantation [181].

Other Aspects

Brain death may also adversely affect the donor's nutritional status. Experimental studies have suggested a hypercatabolic state and decreased hepatic intracellular ATP levels [182]. Moreover, a suboptimal organ energy and redox status along with the inflammatory changes that result from the chemokine and cytokine release associated with brain death may exert a deleterious influence on the magnitude of, and recovery from, ischemia–reperfusion injury and on posttransplant organ function in the recipient. Appropriate nutritional support of the donor may be able to prevent depletion of micro- and macronutrients and may attenuate oxidative stress and ischemia–reperfusion injury. However, currently, there are no clinical data available that would directly support routine nutritional supplementation of brain-dead donors. For potential small bowel donors, it may be justified to continue any already instituted tube feedings given the beneficial effects of the latter for the maintenance of the intestinal mucosa's integrity [18,34].

Various pharmacologic donor pretreatment protocols to optimize donor and transplant outcomes have been reported. The potential clinical effects of administration of catecholamines, vasopressin (or its analog desmopressin), and of steroids on both donor and posttransplant outcomes have already been discussed in detail (Table 56.7). In other studies, verapamil mitigated the adverse impact of elevated cytosolic calcium levels on renal allograft function [183] after donor hemodynamic instability. Finally, donor pretreatment with immunosuppressants (other than steroids) may have a favorable impact by preventing upregulation of proinflammatory pathways and increased expression of major histocompatibility complex molecules that have been demonstrated to occur after brain death [120–122]. The latter pretreatment modalities, however, must be investigated more extensively before they can be routinely applied.

Multiple-Organ Donor Operation

After consent is obtained, the OPO schedules and organizes the organ recovery operation. Often, several surgical teams from different locations participate; their transportation and the preparation of the recipients in the various hospitals must be meticulously coordinated. After certification of death according to the state laws occurs, the brain-dead donor is brought to the operating room. Full cardiovascular and ventilatory support is maintained throughout the operation, until the organs are flushed and cooled. The principles of brain-dead donor management should be reviewed with the anesthesiologist, unless he or she is familiar with the specific clinical aspects of cardiovascular and ventilatory support for brain-dead organ donors. Hemodynamic stability must be maintained during the surgical organ retrieval, which is the equivalent of a combined major abdominal and thoracic operation and can last up to several hours. Transient tachycardia and hypertension may occur while the surgical incision is being made; they most likely reflect spinal reflexes causing vasoconstrictive responses and adrenal stimulation. Subsequently, consideration must be given to the increased heat loss caused by the wide abdominal and thoracic incisions and the duration of the surgery. Neuromuscular blocking agents (e.g., vecuronium, cisatracurium, or rocuronium) should be used to inhibit reflex muscular contractions [82]. Tubocurarine (which is not available anymore in many countries) should also not be used in brain-dead donors because of its association with hypotension as a consequence of histamine release and ganglionic blockade. Maintenance fluid administration throughout the operation must take into account the significant intraoperative fluid losses resulting from extensive dissection with evaporation and blood loss, transection of lymphatic channels, and massive third-space fluid loss.

All organs to be recovered are completely mobilized, and their vascular pedicles are dissected free. At the end of the operation, systemic heparinization occurs and cannulas are inserted (depending on the organs to be procured) into the abdominal aorta, inferior vena cava, portal vein, aortic arch, and pulmonary artery. Only then is circulatory and respiratory support terminated. The organs are flushed in situ with preservation solution to remove blood and to cool the organs to a temperature of 4°C to 7°C. Simultaneously, topical external cooling is provided by the application of sterile ice slush. The organs are then individually removed, by dividing the remaining attachments and vascular pedicles, and then packaged [47]. Storage in preservation solution at 4°C to 7°C in a cooler surrounded by crushed ice allows maximal preservation times of 4 to 6 hours for heart and lungs, approximately 30 hours for livers and pancreata, and about 40 hours for kidneys. These preservation constraints are taken into consideration as organs are allocated. Critical care of the donor ends when controlled cardiac arrest occurs at the completion of the surgical organ recovery. This finality is ephemeral, however, because it results in the start of new lives for the recipients after a successful organ transplant.

PERIOPERATIVE CRITICAL CARE OF THE DCD ORGAN DONOR

Preoperative Care of the Potential DCD Donor (Prior to Obtaining Consent for Organ Donation)

Therapy in those patients must remain primarily aimed at treating the underlying pathology (e.g., head trauma, cerebrovascular accident). Any premature (i.e., prior to the family having made the decision to withdraw care and prior to obtaining consent) change of therapeutic objectives would be unethical and may ultimately lead to overall lower consent rates, thereby further exacerbating the current donor organ shortage [26,27,97].

Preoperative Care of the Actual DCD Donor (After Having Obtained Consent for Organ Donation)

Once consent to proceed with organ donation has been obtained, the focus switches from cerebral protection to preservation of organ function and optimization of peripheral oxygen delivery [26,27,97]. Maintenance therapy endpoints in DCD donors are identical to those that apply for brain-dead organ donors (Table 56.8). Because DCD donors do not exhibit the same pathophysiologic characteristics as brain-dead donors, general management principles for DCD donors are more akin to those that apply to non–brain-dead patients in the ICU that are described elsewhere in this book. Organ-specific considerations (e.g., use of catecholamines) are the same as those described earlier for brain-dead donors.

Preterminal and Intraoperative Care of DCD Donors

Maintenance therapy as outlined earlier is continued until technologic support is withdrawn and the patient is extubated (either in the ICU or in the operating room). Any additional premortem interventions (e.g., surgical: insertion of femoral cannulas in preparation of organ recovery; pharmacologic: administration of intravenous heparin, opioids, and phentolamine) must occur in strict accordance with local OPO/hospital DCD protocols and policies [26,27,97,184,185]. Death is then pronounced by a physician (usually the patient's intensive care physician) not belonging to the organ recovery and transplant team, according to criteria that are specified by the local OPO/hospital DCD protocol.

Next, after an additional 2- to 5-minute waiting time, surgical organ recovery begins [26,184,185]. For DCD donors, the use of a rapid procurement technique is mandatory in order to minimize warm ischemia time, particularly when highly ischemia-sensitive organs such as the liver, pancreas, or lungs are to be recovered as well [48].

Disposition of the patient, if death does not occur within the specified waiting time (which typically ranges between 30 and 90 minutes) after withdrawal of support, is determined by the local protocol (e.g., return of patient to a non–intensive care hospital floor for comfort care only). This aspect is particularly important because as a result of the global efforts to maximize DCD, an increase in the numbers of "unsuccessful" withdrawals of support is to be expected (and must be acceptable to the providers that care for these patients during their terminal hospital admission).

References

1. https://optn.transplant.hrsa.gov/data/. Accessed July 14, 2017.
2. Organ Procurement and Transplantation Network (OPTN) and Scientific Registry of Transplant Recipients (SRTR): *OPTN/SRTR 2015 Annual Data Report*. Rockville, MD, Department of Health and Human Services, Health Resources and Services Administration, 2016. https://www.srtr.org/reports-tools/srtroptn-annual-data-report/. Accessed July 14, 2017.
3. Report of the Task Force on Organ Transplantation: *Organ Transplantation: Issues and Recommendation*. Washington, DC, US Department of Health and Human Services, 1986, p 36.
4. Heffron TG: Organ procurement and management of the multiorgan donor, in Hall JB, Schmidt GA, Wood LDH (eds): *Principles of Critical Care*. New York, NY, McGraw-Hill, 1992, p 891.
5. Najarian JS, Strand M, Fryd DS, et al: Comparison of cyclosporine versus azathioprine-antilymphocyte globulin in renal transplantation. *Transplant Proc* 15[Suppl 1]:2463, 1983.
6. Starzl TE, Iwatsuki S, Van Thiel DH, et al: Report of Colorado-Pittsburgh liver transplantation studies. *Transplant Proc* 15[Suppl 1]:2582–2585, 1983.
7. Sutherland DER: Pancreas transplantation: overview and current status of cases reported to the registry through 1982. *Transplant Proc* 15[Suppl 1]:2597, 1983.
8. Oyer PE, Stinson EB, Jamieson SW, et al: Cyclosporine in cardiac transplantation: a 2½-year follow-up. *Transplant Proc* 15[Suppl 1]:2546, 1983.
9. Evans RW, Orians CE, Ascher NL: The potential supply of organ donors: an assessment of the efficiency of organ procurement efforts in the United States. *JAMA* 267:239–246, 1992.
10. Siminoff LA, Arnold RM, Caplan AL, et al: Public policy governing organ and tissue procurement in the United States. *Ann Intern Med* 123:10–17, 1995.
11. Siminoff LA, Gordon N, Hewlett J, et al: Factors influencing families' consent for donation of solid organs for transplantation. *JAMA* 286:71–77, 2001.
12. Sheehy E, Conrad SL, Brigham LE, et al: Estimating the number of potential organ donors in the United States. *N Engl J Med* 349:667–674, 2003.
13. Rodrigue JR, Cornell DL, Howard RJ: Organ donation decision: comparison of donor and nondonor families. *Am J Transplant* 6:190–198, 2006.
14. Singbartl K, Murugan R, Kaynar AM, et al: Intensivist-led management of brain-dead donors is associated with an increase in organ recovery for transplantation. *Am J Transplant* 11:1517–1521, 2011.
15. Merchant SJ, Yoshida EM, Lee TK, et al: Exploring the psychological effects of deceased organ donation on the families of the organ donors. *Clin Transplant* 22:341–347, 2008.
16. Schnitzler MA, Whiting JF, Brennan DC, et al: The life-years saved by a deceased organ donor. *Am J Transplant* 5:2289–2296, 2005.
17. Patel M, Zatarain J, De La Cruz S, et al: The impact of meeting donor management goals on the number of organs transplanted per expanded criteria donor: a prospective study from the UNOS Region 5 Donor Management Goals workgroup. *JAMA Surg* 149:969–975, 2014.
18. Kotloff RM, Blosser S, Fulda GJ, et al: Management of the potential organ donor in the ICU: Society of Critical Care Medicine/American College of Chest Physicians/Association of Organ Procurement Organizations consensus statement. *Crit Care Med* 43:1291–1325, 2015.
19. Rosendale JD, Chabalewski FL, McBride MA, et al: Increased transplanted organs from the use of a standardized donor management protocol. *Am J Transplant* 2:761–768, 2002.
20. Rosengard BR, Feng S, Alfrey EJ, et al: Report of the Crystal City meeting to maximize the use of organs recovered from the cadaver donor. *Am J Transplant* 2:701–711, 2002.
21. Zaroff JG, Rosengard BR, Armstrong WF, et al: Consensus conference report: maximizing use of organs recovered from the cadaver donor: cardiac recommendations. *Circulation* 106:836–841, 2002.
22. Salim A, Martin M, Brown C, et al: The effect of a protocol of aggressive donor management: implications for the national organ donor shortage. *J Trauma* 61:429–433, 2006.

23. Venkateswaran RV, Patchell VB, Wilson IC, et al: Early donor management increases the retrieval rate of lungs for transplantation. *Ann Thorac Surg* 85:278–286, 2008.
24. Sung RS, Galloway J, Tuttle-Newhall JE, et al: Organ donation and utilization in the United States, 1997–2006. *Am J Transplant* 8:922–934, 2008.
25. Wood KE, Becker BN, McCartney JG, et al: Care of the potential organ donor. *N Engl J Med* 351:2730–2739, 2004.
26. Reich DJ, Mulligan DC, Abt PL, et al: ASTS recommended practice guidelines for controlled donation after cardiac death organ procurement and transplantation. *Am J Transplant* 9:2004–2011, 2009.
27. Gries CJ, White DB, Truog, R, et al; on behalf of the American Thoracic Society Health Policy Committee: An official American Thoracic Society/International Society for Heart and Lung Transplantation/Society of Critical Care Medicine/Association of Organ and Procurement Organizations/United Network of Organ Sharing statement: ethical and policy considerations in organ donation after circulatory determination of death. *Am J Respir Crit Care Med* 188:103–109, 2013.
28. Wall S, Plunkett C, Caplan A: A potential solution to the shortage of solid organs for transplantation. *JAMA*, 2015. doi:10.1001/jama.2015.5328.
29. D'Alessandro AM, Peltier JW, Phelps JE: Understanding the antecedents of the acceptance of donation after cardiac death by healthcare professionals. *Crit Care Med* 36:1075–1081, 2008.
30. Jones JW, Gruber SA, Barker JH, et al: Successful hand transplantation. One year follow-up. *N Engl J Med* 343:468–473, 2000.
31. Landin L, Cavadas PC, Nthumba P, et al: Preliminary results of bilateral arm transplantation. *Transplantation* 88:749–751, 2009.
32. Strome M, Stein J, Esclamado R, et al: Laryngeal transplantation and 40-month follow-up. *N Engl J Med* 344:1676–1679, 2001.
33. Smith CR: Dire wounds, a new face, a glimpse in a mirror. *N Y Times Web*:1A, 2005.
34. Sudan D: The current state of intestine transplantation: indications, techniques, outcomes and challenges. *Am J Transplant* 14:1976–1984, 2014
35. Gruessner RWG, Sutherland DER, Gruessner AC: Mortality assessment for pancreas transplants. *Am J Transplant* 4:2018–2026, 2004.
36. Shapiro J, Lakey J, Edmond R, et al: Islet transplantation in seven patients with type 1 diabetes mellitus using a glucocorticoid-free immunosuppressive regimen. *N Engl J Med* 343:230–238, 2000.
37. Ryan EA, Paty BW, Senior PA, et al: Five-year follow-up after clinical islet transplantation. *Diabetes* 54:2060–2069, 2005.
38. Kay MP: The Registry of the International Society for Heart and Lung Transplantation: tenth official report—1993. *J Heart Lung Transplant* 12:541–548, 1993.
39. Bolman RM III, Shumway SJ, Estrin JA, et al: Lung and heart-lung transplantation: evolution and new applications. *Ann Surg* 214:456–468, 1991.
40. Gravel MT, Arenas JD, Chenault R 2nd, et al: Kidney transplantation from organ donors following cardiopulmonary death using extracorporeal membrane oxygenation support. *Ann Transplant* 9:57–58, 2004.
41. Wang C-C, Wang S-H, Lin C-C, et al: Liver transplantation from an uncontrolled non-heart-beating donor maintained on extracorporeal membrane oxygenation. *Transplant Proc* 37:4331–4333, 2005.
42. Moers C, Smits JM, Maathuis M, et al: Machine perfusion or cold storage in deceased-donor kidney transplantation. *N Engl J Med* 360:7, 2009.
43. Gallup poll surveys views on organ donation. *Nephrol News Issues* 5:16, 1993.
44. Callender CO, Hall LE, Yeager CL, et al: Organ donation and blacks: a critical frontier. *N Engl J Med* 325:442–444, 1991.
45. Siminoff L, Arnold, R: Increasing organ donation in the african-american community: altruism in the face of an untrustworthy system. *Ann Intern Med* 130:607–609, 1999.
46. Rodrigue JR, Crist K, Roberts JP, et al: Stimulus for organ donation: a survey of the American Society of Transplant Surgeons membership. *Am J Transplant* 9:2172–2176, 2009.
47. Brockmann JG, Vaidya A, Reddy S, et al: Retrieval of abdominal organs for transplantation. *Br J Surg* 93:133–146, 2006.
48. Fukuzawa K, Schwartz ME, Katz E, et al: An alternative technique for in situ arterial flushing in elderly liver donors with atherosclerotic occlusive disease. *Transplantation* 55:445–447, 1993.
49. Troppmann C, Daily MF, McVicar JP, et al: Hypothermic pulsatile perfusion of small pediatric en bloc kidneys: technical aspects and outcomes. *Transplantation* 88:289–290, 2009.
50. Troppmann C: Procurement of pediatric en bloc kidneys, in: Englesbe MJ, Mulholland MW (eds): *Operative Techniques in Transplantation Surgery*. New York, NY, Wolters Kluwer Health, 2015, pp 9–14.
51. Troppmann C, Perez RV: Transplantation of pediatric en bloc kidneys, in: Englesbe MJ, Mulholland MW (eds): *Operative Techniques in Transplantation Surgery*. New York, NY: Wolters Kluwer Health, 2015, pp 65–80.
52. Sutherland DER, Morel P, Gruessner RWG: Transplantation of two diabetic patients with one divided cadaver donor pancreas. *Transplant Proc* 22:585, 1990.
53. Azoulay D, Didier S, Castaing D, et al: Domino liver transplants for metabolic disorders: experience with familial amyloidotic polyneuropathy. *J Am Coll Surg* 189:584–593, 1999.
54. Azoulay D, Castaing D, Adam R, et al: Transplantation of three adult patients with one cadaveric graft: wait or innovate. *Liver Transpl* 6:239–240, 2000.
55. Jacobs CL, Roman D, Garvey C, et al: Twenty-two nondirected kidney donors: an update on a single center's experience. *Am J Transplant* 4:1110–1116, 2004.
56. Ross LF, Rubin DT, Seigler M, et al: Ethics of a paired-kidney-exchange program. *N Engl J Med* 336:1752–1755, 1997.
57. Rees MA, Kopke JE, Pelletier RP, et al: A nonsimultaneous, extended, altruistic-donor chain. *N Engl J Med* 360:1096–1101, 2009.
58. Matas AJ, Hippen B, Satel S: In defense of a regulated system of compensation for living donation. *Curr Opin Organ Transplant* 13:379–385, 2008.
59. Radcliffe-Richards J, Daar AS, Guttmann RD, et al: The case for allowing kidney sales. *Lancet* 351:1950–1952, 1998.
60. Scheper-Hughes N: The global traffic in human organs. *Curr Anthropol* 41:191–224, 2000.
61. Starzl T, Teperman L, Sutherland D, et al: Transplant tourism and unregulated black-market trafficking of organs. *Am J Transplant* 9:1484, 2009.
62. Wright L, Campbell M: Soliciting kidneys on Web sites: Is it fair? *Semin Dial* 19:5–7, 2006.
63. Steinbrook R: Public solicitation of organ donors. *N Engl J Med* 353:441–444, 2005.
64. Matesanz R, Miranda B, Felipe C, et al: Continuous improvement in organ donation. *Transplantation* 61:1119–1121, 1996.
65. Matesanz R, Marazuela R, Domínguez-Gil B, et al: The 40 donors per million population plan: an action plan for improvement of organ donation and transplantation in Spain. *Transplant Proc* 41:3453–3456, 2009.
66. Council of Europe: International figures on donation and transplantation—2008. Newsletter Transplant 2009; Vol. 14, No 1. http://www.edqm.eu/medias/fichiers/Newsletter_Transplant_Vol_14_No_1_Sept_2009.pdf. Accessed February 3, 2017.
67. Shafer TJ, David KD, Holtzman SM, et al: Location of in-house organ procurement organization staff in level I trauma centers increases conversion of potential donors to actual donors. *Transplantation* 75:1330–1335, 2003.
68. Sharif A, Singh MF, Trey T, et al: Organ procurement from executed prisoners in China. *Am J Transplant* 14:2246–2252, 2014.
69. Starzl TE, Fung J, Tzakis A, et al: Baboon-to-human liver transplantation. *Lancet* 341:65–71, 1993.
70. Dennis JM: A review of centralized rule-making in American transplantation. *Transplant Rev* 6:130–137, 1992.
71. Sadler AM Jr, Sadler BL, Stason EB: The uniform anatomical gift act: a model for reform. *JAMA* 206:2505–2506, 1968.
72. National Conference of Commissioners on Uniform State Laws. http://www.uniformlaws.org/shared/docs/anatomical_gift/uaga_final_aug09.pdf. Accessed September 15, 2015.
73. Beecher HK, Adams RD, Barger AC, et al: A definition of irreversible coma: report of the ad hoc committee of the Harvard Medical School to examine the definition of brain death. *JAMA* 205:337–340, 1968.
74. Guidelines for the determination of death: Report of the medical consultants on the diagnosis of death to the President's Commission for the Study of Ethical Problems in Medicine and Biomedical and Behavioral Research. *JAMA* 246:2184–2186, 1981.
75. Department of Health and Human Services, Office of the Inspector General: Medicare Conditions of Participation for organ donation: An early assessment of the new donation rule. August 2000. http://oig.hhs.gov/oei/reports/oei-01-99-00020.pdf. Accessed September 15, 2015.
76. Wijdicks EFM: The diagnosis of brain death. *N Engl J Med* 344:1215–1221, 2001.
77. The Quality Standards Subcommittee of the American Academy of Neurology: Practice parameters for determining brain death in adults. *Neurology* 45:1012–1014, 1995.
78. Wijdicks EF, Varelas PN, Gronseth GS, et al; American Academy of Neurology: Evidence-based guideline update: determining brain death in adults. Report of the Quality of Standards Subcommittee of the American Academy of Neurology. *Neurology* 74:1911–1918, 2010.
79. Wijdicks E: Pitfalls and slip-ups in brain death determination. *Neurol Res* 35:169–173, 2013.
80. Heran MK, Heran NS, Shemie SD: A review of ancillary tests in evaluating brain death. *Can J Neurol Sci* 35:409–419, 2008.
81. Darby JM, Stein K, Grenvik A, et al: Approach to management of the heart-beating "brain dead" organ donor. *JAMA* 261:2222–2228, 1989.
82. Saposnik G, Bueri JA, Maurino J, et al: Spontaneous and reflex movements in brain death. *Neurology* 54:221–223, 2000.
83. Lytle FT, Afessa B, Keegan MT: Progression of organ failure in patients approaching brain stem death. *Am J Transplant* 9:1446–1450, 2009.
84. Taniguchi S, Kitamura S, Kawachi K, et al: Effects of hormonal supplements on the maintenance of cardiac function in potential donor patients after cerebral death. *Eur J Cardiothorac Surg* 6:96–101, 1992.
85. Troppmann C, Gillingham KJ, Benedetti E, et al: Delayed graft function, acute rejection, and outcome after cadaver renal transplantation. *Transplantation* 59:962–968, 1995.
86. Whelchel JD, Diethelm AG, Phillips MG, et al: The effect of high-dose dopamine in cadaver donor management on delayed graft function and graft survival following renal transplantation. *Transplant Proc* 18:523–527, 1986.
87. Bouwman DL, Altshuler J, Weaver DW: Hyperamylasemia: a result of intracranial bleeding. *Surgery* 94:318–323, 1983.
88. Gores PF, Gillingham KJ, Dunn DL, et al: Donor hyperglycemia as a minor risk factor and immunologic variables as major risk factors for pancreas allograft loss in a multivariate analysis of a single institution's experience. *Ann Surg* 215:217–230, 1992.
89. Marques RG, Rogers J, Chavin KD, et al: Does treatment of cadaveric organ donors with desmopressin increase the likelihood of pancreas graft thrombosis? Results of a preliminary study. *Transplant Proc* 36:1048–1049, 2004.
90. Bohrade SM, Vignaswaran W, McCabe MA, et al: Liberalization of donor criteria may expand the donor pool without adverse consequence in lung transplantation. *J Heart Lung Transplant* 19:1199–1204, 2000.

91. Freeman RB, Giatras I, Falagas ME, et al: Outcome of transplantation of organs procured from bacteremic donors. *Transplantation* 68:1107–1111, 1999.
92. The White House: HIV Organ Policy Equity (HOPE) Act is now law. https://www.whitehouse.gov/blog/2013/11/21/hiv-organ-policy-equity-hope-act-now-law. Accessed September 15, 2015.
93. Seem DL, Lee I, Umscheid CA, et al: PHS guideline for reducing human immunodeficiency virus, Hepatitis B Virus, and Hepatitis C Virus transmission through organ transplantation. *Public Health Rep* 128:247–343, 2013.
94. Theodoropoulos N, Jaramillo A, Ladner DP, et al: Deceased organ donor screening for HIV, Hepatitis B, and Hepatitis C viruses: a survey of organ procurement organization practices. *Am J Transplant* 13:2186–2190, 2013.
95. Dodson SF, Bonham CA, Geller DA, et al: Prevention of de novo hepatitis B infection in recipients of hepatic allografts from anti-HBc positive donors. *Transplantation* 68:1058–1061, 1999.
96. Reese P, Abt P, Blumberg E, et al: Transplanting Hepatitis C-positive kidneys. *N Engl J Med* 373:303–305, 2015.
97. Kauffman HM, Cherikh WS, McBride MA, et al: Deceased donors with a past history of malignancy: an organ procurement and transplantation network/United Network for Organ Sharing update. *Transplantation* 84:272–274, 2007.
98. Colquhoun SD, Robert ME, Shaked A, et al: Transmission of CNS malignancy by organ transplantation. *Transplantation* 57:970–974, 1994.
99. Bernat JL, D'Alessandro AM, Port FK, et al: Report of a national conference on donation after cardiac death. *Am J Transplant* 6:281–291, 2006.
100. Steinbrook R: Organ donation after cardiac death. *N Engl J Med* 357: 209–213, 2007.
101. Donate Life America: 2016 Annual Update. https://www.donatelife.net/wp-content/uploads/2016/06/DLA_AnnualReport_2016-low-res.pdf. Accessed July 14, 2017.
102. Angel LF, Levine DJ, Restrepo MI, et al: Impact of a lung transplantation donor-management protocol on lung donation and recipient outcomes. *Am J Respir Crit Care Med* 174:710–716, 2006.
103. Mascia L, Pasero D, Slutsky AS, et al: Effect of a lung protective strategy for organ donors on eligibility and availability of lungs for transplantation: a randomized controlled trial. *JAMA* 304:2620–2627, 2010.
104. Niemann, C, Feiner J, Swain S, et al: Therapeutic hypothermia in deceased organ donors and kidney-graft function. *N Engl J Med* 373:405, 2015.
105. Schnuelle P, Berger S, De Boer J, et al: Effects of catecholamine application to brain-dead donors on graft survival in solid organ transplantation. *Transplantation* 72:455–463, 2001.
106. Schnuelle P, Yard BA, Braun C, et al: Impact of donor dopamine on immediate graft function after kidney transplantation. *Am J Transplant* 4:419–426, 2004.
107. Schnuelle P, Gottmann U, Hoeger S, et al: Effects of donor pretreatment with dopamine on graft function after kidney transplantation. *JAMA* 302:1067–1075, 2009.
108. Straznicka M, Follette DM, Eisner MD, et al: Aggressive management of lung donors classified as unacceptable: Excellent recipient survival one year after transplantation. *J Thorac Cardiovasc Surg* 124:250–258, 2002.
109. Kotsch K, Ulrich F, Reutzel-Selke A, et al: Methylprednisolone therapy in deceased donors reduces inflammation in the donor liver and improves outcome after liver transplantation. *Ann Surg* 248:1042–1050, 2008.
110. Selck FW, Deb P, Grossman EB: Deceased organ donor characteristics and clinical interventions associated with organ yield. *Am J Transplant* 8:965–974, 2008.
111. Pennefather SH, Bullock RE, Mantle D, et al: Use of low dose arginine vasopressin to support brain-dead organ donors. *Transplantation* 59:58–62, 1995.
112. Randell TT, Höckerstedt KAV: Triiodothyronine treatment in brain-dead multiorgan donors: a controlled study. *Transplantation* 54:736–738, 1992.
113. Perez-Blanco A, Caturla-Such J, Canovas-Robles J, et al: Efficiency of triiodothyronine treatment on organ donor hemodynamic management and adenine nucleotide concentration. *Intensive Care Med* 31:943–948, 2005.
114. Roels L, Pirenne J, Delooz H, et al: Effect of triiodothyronine replacement therapy on maintenance characteristics and organ availability in hemodynamically unstable donors. *Transplant Proc* 32:1564–1566, 2000.
115. Venkateswaran RV, Steeds RP, Quinn DW, et al: The haemodynamic effects of adjunctive hormone therapy in potential heart donors: A prospective randomized double-blind factorially designed controlled trial. *Eur Heart J* 30:1771–1780, 2009.
116. Cooper DKC, Novitzky D, Witcomb WN: The pathophysiological effects of brain death on potential donor organs, with particular reference to the heart. *Ann R Coll Surg Engl* 71:261–266, 1989.
117. Smith M: Physiologic changes during brain stem death—lessons for management of the organ donor. *J Heart Lung Transplant* 23:S217–S222, 2004.
118. Bos EM, Leuvenink HG, van Goor H, et al: Kidney grafts from brain dead donors: inferior quality or opportunity for improvement? *Kidney Int* 72:797–805, 2007.
119. Takada M, Nadeau KC, Hancock WW, et al: Effects of explosive brain death on cytokine activation of peripheral organs in the rat. *Transplantation* 65:1533–1542, 1998.
120. Bouma HR, Ploeg RJ, Schuurs TA: Signal transduction pathways involved in brain death-induced renal injury. *Am J Transplant* 9:989–997, 2009.
121. Venkateswaran RV, Dronavalli V, Lambert PA, et al: The proinflammatory environment in potential heart and lung donors: prevalence and impact of donor management and hormonal therapy. *Transplantation* 88:582–588, 2009.
122. Powner DJ: Effects of gene induction and cytokine production in donor care. *Prog Transplant* 13:9–14, 2003.
123. Schnuelle P, Schmitt WH, Weiss C, et al: Effects of dopamine donor pretreatment on graft survival after kidney transplantation: a randomized trial. Clin J Am Soc Nephrol 12:493-501, 2017.
124. Russell JA, Walley KR, Singer J, et al: Vasopressin versus norepinephrine infusion in patients with septic shock. *N Engl J Med* 358:877–887, 2008.
125. Plurad DS, Bricker S, Neville A, et al: Arginine vasopressin significantly increases the rate of successful organ procurement in potential donors. *Am J Surg* 204:856–860, 2012.
126. Davis SV, Olichwier KK, Chakko SC: Reversible depression of myocardial performance to hypophosphatemia. *Am J Med Sci* 295:183–187, 1988.
127. Ventilation with lower tidal volumes as compared with traditional tidal volumes for acute lung injury and the acute respiratory distress syndrome. The Acute Respiratory Distress Syndrome Network. *N Engl J Med* 342:1301–1308, 2000.
128. Avlonitis VS, Fisher AJ, Kirby JA, et al: Pulmonary transplantation: the role of brain death in donor lung injury. *Transplantation* 75:1928–1933, 2003.
129. National Heart, Lung, and Blood Institute Acute Respiratory Distress Syndrome (ARDS) Clinical Trials Network, Wiedemann H, Wheeler A, et al: Comparison of two fluid-management strategies in acute lung injury. *N Engl J Med* 354:2564–2575, 2006.
130. Miñambres E, Rodrigo E, Ballesteros MA, et al: Impact of restrictive fluid balance focused to increase lung procurement on renal function after kidney transplantation. *Nephrol Dial Transplant* 25:2352–2356, 2010.
131. Richardson DW, Robinson AG: Desmopressin. *Ann Intern Med* 103:228–239, 1985.
132. Cittanova ML, Leblanc I, Legendre C, et al: Effect of Hydroxyethylstarch in brain-dead kidney donors on renal function in kidney-transplant recipients. *Lancet* 348:1620–1622, 1996.
133. Hall GM, Mashiter K, Lumley J, et al: Hypothalamic-pituitary function in the "brain-dead" patient. *Lancet* 2:1259, 1980.
134. Gramm H-J, Meinhold H, Bickel U, et al: Acute endocrine failure after brain death. *Transplantation* 54:851–857, 1992.
135. Howlett TA, Keogh AM, Perry L, et al: Anterior and posterior pituitary function in brain-stem-dead donors: a possible role for hormonal replacement therapy. *Transplantation* 47:828–834, 1989.
136. Powner DJ, Hendrich A, Lagler RG, et al: Hormonal changes in brain dead patients. *Crit Care Med* 18:702–708, 1990.
137. Seeger W (ed): *Atlas of Topographical Anatomy of the Brain and Surrounding Structures*. New York, NY, Springer-Verlag, 1978.
138. Dimopoulou I, Tsagarakis S, Anthi A, et al: High prevalence of decreased cortisol reserve in brain-dead potential organ donors. *Crit Care Med* 31:1113–1117, 2003.
139. Rosendale JD, Kauffman HM, McBride MA: Hormonal resuscitation yields more transplanted hearts with improved early function. *Transplantation* 75:1336–1341, 2003.
140. Rosendale JD, Kauffman HM, McBride MA, et al: Aggressive pharmacologic donor management results in more transplanted organs. *Transplantation* 75:482–487, 2003.
141. Novitzky D, Cooper DKC, Muchmore JS, et al: Pituitary function in brain-dead patients. *Transplantation* 48:1078–1079, 1989.
142. Macdonald PS, Aneman A, Bhonagiri D, et al: A systematic review and meta-analysis of of clinical trials of thyroid hormone administration to brain dead potential organ donors. Crit Care Med 40:1635-1644, 2012.
143. Salim A, Vassiliu P, Velmahos GC, et al: The role of thyroid hormone administration in potential organ donors. *Arch Surg* 136:1377–1380, 2001.
144. Reutzel-Selke A, Tullius SG, Zschockelt T, et al: Donor pretreatment of grafts from marginal donors improves long-term graft outcome. *Transplant Proc* 33:970–971, 2001.
145. Hershman JM: Free thyroxine in nonthyroidal illness. *Ann Intern Med* 98:947, 1983.
146. Hess ML: Letters to the Editor. *J Heart Transplant* 5:486, 1986.
147. Pennefather SH, Bullock RE: Triiodothyronine treatment in brain-dead multiorgan donors: a controlled study. *Transplantation* 55:1443, 1993.
148. Novitzky D, Cooper DKC, Rosendale JD, et al: Hormonal therapy of the brain-dead organ donor: experimental and clinical studies. *Transplantation* 82: 1396–1401, 2006.
149. Novitzky D, Wicomb WN, Cooper DKC, et al: Electrocardiographic, hemodynamic and endocrine changes occurring during experimental brain death in the chacma baboon. *J Heart Transplant* 4:63, 1984.
150. Novitzky D, Cooper DKC, Morrell D, et al: Change from aerobic to anaerobic metabolism after brain death, and reversal following triiodothyronine therapy. *Transplantation* 45:32–36, 1988.
151. Novitzky D, Wicomb WN, Cooper DKC, et al: Improved cardiac function following hormonal therapy in brain dead pigs: relevance to organ donation. *Cryobiology* 24:1–10, 1987.
152. Wicomb WN, Cooper DKC, Novitzky D: Impairment of renal slice function following brain death, with reversibility of injury by hormonal therapy. *Transplantation* 41:29–33, 1986.
153. Pienaar H, Schwartz I, Roncone A, et al: Function of kidney grafts from brain-dead donor pigs: the influence of dopamine and triiodothyronine. *Transplantation* 50:580–582, 1990.
154. Washida M, Okamoto R, Manaka D, et al: Beneficial effect of combined 3,5,3-triiodothyronine and vasopressin administration on hepatic energy status and systemic hemodynamics after brain death. *Transplantation* 54:44–49, 1992.
155. García-Fages LC, Antolín M, Cabrer C, et al: Effects of substitutive triiodothyronine therapy on intracellular nucleotide levels in donor organs. *Transplant Proc* 23:2495–2496, 1991.
156. Orlowski JP, Spees EK: Improved cardiac transplant survival with thyroxine treatment of hemodynamically unstable donors: 95.2% graft survival at 6 and 30 months. *Transplant Proc* 25:1535, 1993.

157. Novitzky D, Cooper DKC, Reichart B: Hemodynamic and metabolic responses to hormonal therapy in brain-dead potential organ donors. *Transplantation* 43:852–854, 1987.
158. Novitzky D, Cooper DKC, Chaffin JS, et al: Improved cardiac allograft function following triiodothyronine therapy to both donor and recipient. *Transplantation* 49:311–316, 1990.
159. Goarin J-P, Cohen S, Riou P, et al: The effects of triiodothyronine on hemodynamic status and cardiac function in potential heart donors. *Anesth Analg* 83:41–47, 1996.
160. Schwartz I, Bird S, Lotz Z, et al: The influence of thyroid hormone replacement in a porcine brain death model. *Transplantation* 55:474–476, 1993.
161. Robertson KM, Hramiak IM, Gelb AW: Endocrine changes and haemodynamic stability after brain death. *Transplant Proc* 21:1197–1198, 1989.
162. Koller J, Wieser C, Gottardis M, et al: Thyroid hormones and their impact on the hemodynamic and metabolic stability of organ donors and on kidney graft function after transplantation. *Transplant Proc* 22:355–357, 1990.
163. Wahlers T, Fieguth HG, Jurmann M, et al: Does hormone depletion of organ donors impair myocardial function after cardiac transplantation? *Transplant Proc* 20:792, 1988.
164. Macoviak JA, McDougall IR, Bayer MG, et al: Significance of thyroid dysfunction in human cardiac allograft procurement. *Transplantation* 43:824–826, 1987.
165. Gifford RRM, Weaver AS, Burg JE, et al: Thyroid hormone levels in heart and kidney cadaver donors. *J Heart Transplant* 5:249–253, 1986.
166. Mariot J, Sadoune L-O, Jacob F, et al: Hormone levels, hemodynamics, and metabolism in brain dead organ donors. *Transplant Proc* 27:793–794, 1995.
167. Follette D, Rudich S, Bonacci R, et al: Importance of an aggressive multidisciplinary management approach to optimize lung donor procurement. *Transplant Proc* 31:169–170, 1999.
168. Milano CA, Buchan K, Perreas K, et al: Thoracic organ transplantation at Papworth Hospital, in Terasaki PI, Cecka JM (eds): *Clinical Transplants 1999*. Los Angeles, UCLA Tissue Typing Laboratory, 1999.
169. Gabbay E, Williams TJ, Griffiths AP, et al: Maximizing the utilization of donor organs offered for lung transplantation. *Am J Respir Crit Care Med* 160:265–271, 1999.
170. Dohan FC, Lukens FDW: Lesions of the pancreatic islets produced in cats by administration of glucose. *Science* 105:183, 1947.
171. Collier SA, Mandel TE, Carter WM: Detrimental effect of high medium glucose concentration on subsequent endocrine function of transplanted organ-cultured fetal mouse pancreas. *Aust J Exp Biol Med Sci* 60:437–445, 1982.
172. Clark A, Bown E, King T, et al: Islet changes induced by hyperglycemia in rats: effects of insulin or chlorpropamide therapy. *Diabetes* 31:319–325, 1982.
173. Unger RH, Grundy S: Hyperglycemia as an inducer as well as a consequence of impaired islet cell function and insulin resistance: implications for the management of diabetes. *Diabetologia* 28:119–121, 1985.
174. Massen F, Thicoipe M, Gin H, et al: The endocrine pancreas in brain-dead donors. A prospective study in 25 patients. *Transplantation* 56:363–367, 1993.
175. Powner DJ: Donor care before pancreatic tissue transplantation. *Prog Transplant* 15:129–136, 2005.
176. Van den Berghe G, Wouters P, Weekers F, et al: Intensive insulin therapy in critically ill patients. *N Engl J Med* 345:1359–1367, 2001.
177. Powner DJ, Jastremski M, Lagler RG: Continuing care of multiorgan donor patients. *J Intensive Care Med* 4:75, 1989.
178. Swain JA: Hypothermia and blood pH. *Arch Intern Med* 148:1643–1646, 1988.
179. Koncke GM, Nichols RRD, Mendenhall JT, et al: Ectothermic philosophy of acid-base balance to prevent fibrillation during hypothermia. *Arch Surg* 121:303–304, 1986.
180. Reuler JB: Hypothermia: pathophysiology, clinical settings, and management. *Ann Intern Med* 89:519–527, 1978.
181. Revollo J, Cuffy M, Witte D, et al: Case report: hemolytic anemia following deceased donor renal transplantation associated with tranexamic acid administration for disseminated intravascular coagulation. *Transplant Proc* 47:2239–2242, 2015.
182. Singer P, Shapiro H, Cohen J: Brain death and organ damage: the modulating effects of nutrition. *Transplantation* 80:1363–1368, 2005.
183. Korb S, Albornoz G, Brems W, et al: Verapamil pretreatment of hemodynamically unstable donors prevents delayed graft function post-transplant. *Transplant Proc* 21:1236–1238, 1989.
184. Institute of Medicine (IOM): Report: Non-heart-beating organ transplantation: practice and protocols. Washington, DC, National Academy Press, 2000.
185. Institute of Medicine (IOM): Report: Non-heart-beating organ transplantation: medical and ethical issues in procurement. Washington, DC, National Academy Press, 1997.

Chapter 57 ■ Critical Care Problems in Kidney Recipients

ABBAS A. RANA • RAINER W.G. GRUESSNER

INTRODUCTION

Kidney transplantation is more than a life-enhancing endeavor; it is life-saving. A recent study estimated that more than 1.3 million life-years have been saved from over 300,000 kidney transplantations in the United States over the past 25 years [1]. Other studies have calculated a projected 10-year survival benefit for an average cadaveric kidney transplantation [2]. More than just survival benefit, a successful transplantation can free a patient from the demands of dialysis and provide a higher quality of life at a fraction of the overall cost compared to those not transplanted [3]. In the United States, the cumulative 1-year graft survival rate was 91.3% for deceased donor recipients and 96.4% for living donor recipients; and 5-year graft survival rate of 68.9% for deceased donor recipients and 81.5% for living donor recipients. The half-life graft survival is projected for deceased donor recipients to be 10 years; for living-related donor recipients, almost 18 years [4,5]. Enthusiasm for kidney transplantation is undoubtedly fueled by these promising outcomes; however, a donor shortage crisis remains. Over 100,000 patients are waitlisted for kidney transplantation on an ever-growing list. This waitlist is in the context of just 17,000 annual kidney transplants in the United States. In 2008, the median waiting time was 4.2 years, increased from 2.7 years in 1998 [6]. These protracted waiting times subject our patients to a great deal of harm from the ill effects of uremia and dialysis. Critical care providers, therefore, are facing a cohort of patients awaiting kidney transplantation who are sick and getting sicker. This chapter discusses the salient points of critical care to optimize outcomes after kidney transplantation.

PRETRANSPLANT EVALUATION

In addition to the aforementioned ill effects of prolonged dialysis, kidney transplant candidates are commonly plagued with significant comorbidities, often the etiology of their renal failure; including hypertension, diabetes, and cardiovascular disease. It is therefore imperative that the pretransplant evaluation should be exhaustive (covering cardiovascular, gastrointestinal, pulmonary, neurologic, genitourinary, and infection disease concerns). The goal is not only that the patient should survive the operation and hospitalization, but also survive in the long term so that there is a realization of the potential graft life of the donor allograft.

The cardiovascular examination is the most important because cardiac events constitute the most common cause of death in the perioperative and postoperative periods [7]. Ironically, our preoperative screening with noninvasive cardiac stress testing is notoriously unreliable. In a meta-analysis, the sensitivity of the pretransplant cardiac perfusion study for myocardial infarction was only 0.7; and for cardiac death, only 0.8 [8,9]. The onus remains on the transplant clinician to be highly suspicious of potential cardiac morbidity, even in younger patients with prolonged renal failure. Abnormalities detected by stress testing require coronary angiography to investigate the need for coronary stenting or even coronary artery bypass. It may also be reasonable to perform coronary angiography on high-risk patients with significant comorbidities or a pronounced history of cardiac problems with unremarkable stress testing.

Carotid duplex ultrasound should be used to screen candidates with a history of stroke or transient ischemic attacks (TIAs) for critical carotid stenosis. Pulmonary function testing should be used to screen patients with any history of pulmonary disease including COPD and asthma. Since hepatitis C exposure is so common in the hemodialysis (HD) population, screening with liver function test and hepatitis C (HCV) testing should be conducted [10]. Abnormal results should prompt consultation with a hepatologist and further testing. Since gastrointestinal diseases are more common in patients with end-stage renal disease, any upper GI symptoms should elicit an EGD. Screening with colonoscopy is mandatory for candidates older than 50 years. Recurrent urinary tract infections or bladder dysfunction requires urodynamic testing and urology consultation. Candidates with any history of hypercoagulability should undergo a complete thrombophilia evaluation. Abnormal results require hematology consultation and a plan for therapeutic measures in the perioperative period.

PERIOPERATIVE CARE

Pretransplant Preparation

Careful preparation in the days and hours before transplantation is essential to achieve ideal outcomes. For HD-dependent patients, a routine HD session on the day prior to transplant would be acceptable. If this is not the case, HD should be performed in the hours prior to surgery. An electrolyte panel should be checked within hours of anesthetic induction. Dialysis catheter sites should be inspected for infection for patients on HD. Peritoneal fluid should be obtained for culture and Gram stain for patients on peritoneal dialysis (PD). In addition to electrolyte screening, a complete history and physical examination, electrocardiogram, chest X-ray, and laboratory examination should be performed just prior to the operation to uncover any possible health derangements since the last physician visit. The history should include a comprehensive review of the medication list. Anticoagulants should be held including warfarin and Plavix. β-blockade should be continued through the perioperative period.

Intraoperative Care

The degree of invasive monitoring during the operation should reflect the extent of the recipient's comorbidities. Central venous catheters are commonly introduced to guide intraoperative and postoperative fluid management. This access is also essential to administer the most commonly used induction agent, thymoglobulin. Continuous arterial blood pressure monitoring is also quite common and facilitates blood pressure management during the case. It can also be instrumental to optimize the recipient's blood pressure just prior to reperfusion. Pulmonary artery pressure monitoring is used much more selectively. It is justified when recipients have significant cardiac dysfunction, valvular abnormalities, or significant pulmonary artery hypertension. A 20-F three-way Foley catheter is useful to inflate the bladder with saline that greatly facilitates the ureteroneocystostomy. After completion of this anastomosis, urine output is checked frequently to guide fluid resuscitation. Compression stockings and sequential compression devices provide deep venous thrombosis prophylaxis.

Optimizing the immediate perfusion of the allograft is vital to maximize graft function. This is achieved by maintaining adequate intravascular volume with a central venous pressure (CVP) between 10 and 15 mm Hg. The goal is a systolic blood pressure of greater than 120 mm Hg at the time of reperfusion. If this is not achieved with appropriate volume loading, then low-dose dopamine can be used. Other vasopressors should be avoided since they can effectively reduce perfusion of the allograft. Another strategy, shown to decrease the incidence of acute tubular necrosis (ATN), is to give Mannitol (1 g per kg) with furosemide prior to reperfusion to increase urine flow [11]. Optimizing the chance of immediate graft function requires careful communication and coordination between anesthesia and surgical teams. Immediate graft function is important because both ATN and delayed graft function (DGF) have been found to increase patient mortality [12].

Immediate Postoperative Care

Recipients with significant comorbidities may require admission to the intensive care unit (ICU) for optimal monitoring and fluid resuscitation. Most patients, however, can receive appropriate care on a solid-organ transplant ward provided there is mechanism for proper fluid resuscitation. This can be challenging, with the voluminous urine output often encountered with immediate graft function. The basis of the resuscitation is the equivalent replacement of urine output milliliter for milliliter, which is measured hourly. A 5% dextrose and 0.45 normal saline solution should be administered; potassium replacement may also be necessary, but should not exceed 0.3 mEq/kg/h. For recipients with cardiac dysfunction, replacement should be lower at 0.5 mL of replacements for 1 mL of urine. After 24 hours, the fluid replacements are converted to a continuous rate between 100 and 150 mL per hour based on the recipient weight and kidney function.

Serial blood counts, coagulation profiles, and chemistries should be obtained in the postoperative period. Electrolyte abnormalities, especially hyperkalemia, hypokalemia, hypomagnesaemia, and hypocalcaemia are common and should be corrected. Serial troponins should be obtained to exclude myocardial ischemia with select recipients with significant cardiac comorbidity. Chest X-ray and electrocardiograms are obtained in the immediate postoperative period.

ICU monitoring can become necessary at any time if complications should develop. Kidney transplant recipients are prone to complications owing to their significant comorbidities, intense immunosuppression, and variable graft function. It is estimated that between 15% and 30% of high-risk transplant candidates will require specific critical care.

CRITICAL EVALUATION OF DYSFUNCTIONAL GRAFTS

Immediate graft function is reliably indicated with the combination of brisk diuresis (>100 to 200 mL per hour) and a consistent downward trend in serum creatinine. Diuresis on its own may be a result of the urine produced by the recipient's native kidneys or the residual effect of diuretics infused during the operation. DGF is affected by a multitude of factors including prolonged cold ischemia time, advanced donor age, and donor diabetes among a host of others. [13] While rare with living donor transplants, the incidence of DGF in cadaveric donors is about 25% [14]. Most allografts with DGF start to recover by 10 days. Doppler ultrasound plays a vital role in the surveillance of the allograft in DGF or for allografts with immediate function that abruptly changes. Intensivists must be aware that ultrasound can rule out surgical complications that require immediate therapeutic maneuvers to salvage the graft including clearing of arterial or venous thromboses.

Medical Complications Leading to Early Graft Dysfunction

Acute Tubular Necrosis

There are a variety of medical and surgical causes of impaired kidney function after transplantation. The most common culprit is ATN, which fortunately has the best prognosis. It is estimated that up to 35% of deceased donor recipients have ATN, but is rare in living donor recipients. About 95% of recipients with ATN will eventually recover kidney function, in some cases requiring HD for several weeks. The causes of ATN are many and often multifactorial, with the most common cause being prolonged ischemia times. Other indicators of poor donor quality such as advanced donor age and donor diabetes mellitus (DM) are also common culprits. Donor and recipient instability requiring the use of vasopressors also contribute. There is a host of immunologic risk factors that are factors causing ATN, as well, including poor human leukocyte antigen (HLA) matching and donor-specific antibodies.

Although most recipients with ATN recover, ATN has a detrimental effect on graft function and graft survival. ATN leads to a higher incidence of rejection and chronic allograft nephropathy [15].

ATN is a diagnosis of exclusion. Most importantly, surgical complications need to be ruled out, most notably, thrombosis with a Doppler ultrasound. Next, the clinician is obligated to rule out urologic complications and rejection.

Acute Rejection

Acute rejection in kidney transplantation is of great significance, but a comprehensive review is beyond the scope of this chapter. There are two types of acute rejection, cellular rejection and antibody-mediated rejection; both can diminish graft function and survival [16]. At present, this diagnosis is secured with a kidney biopsy, although there are efforts underway for noninvasive diagnostics. After vascular thrombosis and urologic complications are ruled out, the next step is often a biopsy to rule out rejection. Acute cellular rejection, which is a lymphocytic attack against donor tissue, is most often treated with a course of steroids or thymoglobulin. Antibody-mediated rejection that may occur in conjunction with acute cellular rejection or occur on its own is most often treated with a course of plasmapheresis and IVIG and in some cases Rituximab. In antibody-mediated rejection, preformed or de novo alloantibodies target capillary endothelium and by activating the complement system can result in rapid destruction of the allograft.

Recurrence of Kidney Disease

Most types of kidney diseases rarely recur in the acute setting; the exception, however, are *focal segmental glomerulosclerosis* (FSGS) and *hemolytic uremic syndrome* (HUS) that can cause early and profound graft dysfunction. Nephrotic range proteinuria (i.e., >3.5 g per day) in a transplant recipient with known FSGS should prompt an immediate biopsy. Diffuse foot process effacement on biopsy is diagnostic. Early graft dysfunction with laboratory evidence of microvascular trauma including low haptoglobin levels, elevated lactate dehydrogenase levels, and the presence of schistocytes on blood smear should elicit suspicion of HUS and prompt a biopsy as well. It may be recurrent or de novo, with the patient's calcineurin inhibitor being a well-known causative agent [17].

Surgical Complications Leading to Early Graft Dysfunction

Hemorrhage after surgery is always a possibility but is rare in kidney transplantation because the surgical field is confined to the retroperitoneal space, so bleeding usually tamponades. Reexploration is uncommon. Bleeding is suspected if the patient is tachycardic, hypotensive, oliguric, and requiring blood transfusions. Subscapular bleeding in the allograft is an entirely different matter, as it can lead to compression and quick deterioration of allograft function. If this is recognized on Doppler ultrasound with evidence of compression, immediate reexploration is imperative to release the hematoma.

Arterial thrombosis is a devastating complication in kidney transplantation, as the renal arteries are end arteries without collateralization. Therefore, arterial thrombosis almost invariably results in graft loss; however, fortunately it is rare (0.7% to 5%) [18]. As mentioned earlier in the chapter, impaired graft function or a sudden change in urine output should elicit a Doppler ultrasound, which is usually diagnostic when thrombosis is present. If discovered early, within hours, graft salvage is possible although most cases result in irreparable damage necessitating transplant nephrectomy. Unidentified intimal flaps, allograft damage in the procurement, donor–recipient size discrepancy, hypotension, and technical difficulty with multiple arteries in the donor or diseased iliac vessels in the recipient are all identified causative factors [18].

Renal vein thrombosis is equally devastating and uncommon and occurs in 0.3% to 4.2% of recipients. It is most often diagnosed within a few days after the transplant and is characterized by sudden onset of pain and graft swelling, hematuria, and, in the case of iliofemoral thrombosis, an edematous leg. In addition to the vein thrombosis, the Doppler ultrasound often shows reversal of the diastolic flow in the arterial system and an enlarged kidney possibly surrounded by hematoma. Urgent allograft nephrectomy is necessary in complete thrombosis to prevent kidney rupture and devastating hemorrhage. Partial thrombosis is an indication for urgent surgical thrombectomy or thrombolytic therapy. It is most often caused by kinking of the anastomosis, intimal injury during organ procurement, pressure on the vein secondary to a fluid collection (i.e., lymphocele, urinoma, or hematoma), compartment syndrome, and extension of an iliofemoral thrombosis [19].

Other vascular complications include aneurysms and renal artery stenosis. Aneurysms can be anastomotic (pseudoaneurysm) or infected (mycotic) and require surgical repair. Recipients with renal artery stenosis require percutaneous balloon dilation, or if unsuccessful, surgical repair.

Urologic complications are much more common than vascular complications, but if addressed systematically, rarely threaten the viability of the allograft. Urologic complications, including hematuria, urine leaks, and ureteral stenosis, range from 5% to 14% [20].

Hematuria is not uncommon from operating on the distal ureter and bladder and often resolves within 24 hours; however, clot formation leading to obstructive uropathy can occur, especially with poor initial urine flow. Close monitoring of the urine output is necessary and any changes can indicate obstruction. Large clots can cause suprapubic pain and bladder spasms. Catheter irrigation can often remedy the situation. If unsuccessful, manual evacuation using a 20-F Six-eye Foley catheter can be used. Occasionally, hematuria can be caused by posttransplant biopsies with blot clots forming in the renal pelvis. In these situations, a percutaneously placed nephrostomy tube may be necessary.

Urine leaks are caused by technical error with the ureteroneocystostomy, presenting in the first few postoperative days, or from ureteral ischemia and necrosis, presenting in the first few weeks. The presentation can be quite varied, including wound drainage, persistent tenderness, fevers, or general swelling. They are also commonly diagnosed on surveillance Doppler ultrasound where a large perinephric fluid collection is aspirated and found to have a high creatinine content. Nephroscintigraphy or retrograde cystography can confirm the diagnosis. Minor leaks can spontaneously resolve with bladder decompression over several weeks. More significant leaks are approached with immediate exploration and reimplantation of the ureter or with percutaneous maneuvers to maximize drainage for 4 to 8 weeks. Both strategies have their advocates. Proponents of the percutaneous approach report success rates of 90%, avoiding significant morbidity from a reoperation [21].

Ureteral stenosis usually becomes evident months after transplantation when an elevated creatinine leads to a Doppler ultrasound that reveals hydronephrosis. Percutaneous nephrostomy elucidates the location and degree of stenosis as well the opportunity for therapeutic maneuvers including balloon dilatation with a temporary tent tube. If this approach fails, reoperation with operative repair is necessary. Extensive adhesions and lack of graft mobility make this operation quite difficult. On some occasions, reimplanting the distal ureter is possible, but in most cases a ureteroureterostomy (to native ureter) or a ureteropyelostomy (native ureter to the graft's renal pelvis) is necessary [21].

Perinephric fluid collections after transplantation are common and often innocuous. However, on occasion, they can cause compression of the iliac veins leading to leg edema or compression of the ureter leading to hydronephrosis. In these cases, percutaneous decompression is imperative. Most collections are residual hematomas or seromas and are self-limited. Lymphoceles, caused from disruption of lymphatic vessels along the external iliac artery, are the exception and can be quite persistent. In these cases, a surgically created peritoneal window must be created to drain the leakage and can often be approached laparoscopically.

NONRENAL POSTTRANSPLANTATION COMPLICATIONS

Cardiovascular Complications

Cardiac complications are the most common cause of death posttransplantation [22]. For this reason, clinicians are often very particular with the cardiac clearance prior to transplant, but despite careful preoperative evaluation, cardiac complications are not uncommon following transplantation. The immediate function of the transplanted kidney has a very influential effect on the incidence of cardiac complications. Immediate function corrects uremia which in turn improves cardiac index, stroke volume, and ejection fraction. On the other hand, DGF can exacerbate fluid shifts and fluid overload, as well as electrolyte derangements which can tip the patients into congestive heart failure (CHF) [23]. In these cases, expedient HD is essential. Patients who are at high risk for cardiac complications need careful ICU monitoring in the perioperative setting, especially for cases of DGF. This includes patients with long standing diabetes, hypertension, coronary artery disease, and impaired ventricular function. Further monitoring with a pulmonary artery catheter for optimal fluid management may be prudent for the highest-risk patients with diabetes and significant history of cardiac morbidity.

Although somewhat uncommon in the perioperative period, myocardial infarction is one of the major causes of death in the long term. Perioperative myocardial infarctions are more common among patients with diabetes and a history of coronary artery disease. Clinicians should maintain a high index of suspicion with this subgroup, monitoring continuous hemodynamic parameters and serial troponins in an ICU setting. Studies suggest that maintaining the hematocrit above 30% in diabetic patients reduces cardiac morbidity by 24% in the initial 6 months postoperatively [24]. High-risk patients with DGF should have HD initiated expeditiously.

Pericarditis following kidney transplantation occurs in 1% to 3% of patients [25]. The most common culprit is uremia but there are other possible etiologies including: infections (e.g., cytomegalovirus), fluid overload, and medications (minoxidil). Less frequently, bacterial pericarditis develops in recipients with advanced septic complications. In addition to antibiotics, bacterial pericarditis causing cardiac failure, hypotension, or tamponade requires urgent surgical or percutaneous decompression. Any symptoms of pericarditis require ICU monitoring.

Exacerbation of underlying hypertension can be an issue in the postoperative period. Fluid overload and calcineurin (CNI)-induced hypertension can lead to considerable hypertension. Systolic blood pressures above 180 mm Hg or diastolic pressures above 100 mm Hg require intensive monitoring which often includes ICU monitoring with IV antihypertensive infusions (sodium nitroprusside). The patient's home regimen should be restarted, and abrupt cessation of antihypertensives should be avoided with the exception of angiotensin-converting enzyme inhibitors. Calcium-channel blockers appear to be the best at obviating the renal vasoconstriction induced by CNIs [26]. The mechanism of CNI-induced hypertension is multifactorial, including vascular constriction by reducing prostacyclin and nitric oxide production while increasing serum levels of endothelin-1. Vasoconstriction of the kidney enhances sodium retention and exacerbates hypertension [27].

Hypotension can be catastrophic to the newly transplanted allograft and can lead to graft loss or severe dysfunction. More than just ATN, significant hypotension can perpetuate vascular thrombosis. In the operating room (OR), hypotension can be related to volume depletion or anesthetic agents and should be avoided with appropriate fluid loading using central venous pressure (CVP) monitoring. Induction immunosuppression with thymoglobulin can also lead to hypotension, which should be reversed by slowing the infusion rate. In the postoperative period, brisk diuresis with immediate graft function can lead to inadequate fluid replacement. Cardiac dysfunction and bleeding can also be contributing causes of hypotension.

Uremic patients have a greater incidence of deep venous thrombosis (DVT) compared to the general population, ranging from 1% to 4%. This risk is linked to high-dose corticosteroid therapy in the perioperative period and a hypercoagulable state secondary to decreased fibrinolytic activity and increase in plasminogen activation inhibitors [28]. Other factors for the development of DVT are postoperative immobilization, increased blood viscosity from posttransplant erythrocytosis, cyclosporine, and perinephric fluid collections that can diminish the venous return from the leg. Two-thirds of the time, DVT occurs on the side of the graft. Since the kidney allograft is a high-flow organ, DVT usually terminates at the level of or just distal to the renal vein anastomosis. Elevated hemoglobin levels in conjunction with other risk factors such as old recipient age or diabetes are thought to predispose to DVT and aggressive therapeutic phlebotomy should be used to maintain the hematocrit level at less than 55%.

Once the diagnosis of DVT is established, just as with any other patient, systemic heparin is administered followed by 3 to 6 months of anticoagulation with warfarin. If there is a contraindication to anticoagulation, an inferior vena cava filter can be inserted. In the very rare instance that phelgmasia cerulea dolens develops, venous thrombectomy and fasciotomy must be performed.

Pulmonary embolism is rare (<1%), but there is an increased risk after kidney transplantation. This is because the coagulation system is activated in the uremic patient after transplantation. After 1 week posttransplantation, the rate of pulmonary embolism is near pretransplant rates. Although rare, if a recipient develops a pulmonary embolism, the mortality rate is about 40%.

Pulmonary Complications

It is not common for kidney transplant recipients to require postoperative ventilator support. Those who do often have pulmonary dysfunction secondary to fluid overload, cardiac dysfunction, or underlying lung disease.

Over-resuscitation in the OR in conjunction with a poorly functioning graft can lead to pulmonary edema. Inadequate pretransplant HD may also contribute. As discussed previously, poor early graft function requires much more precise fluid management to optimize volume status for the graft, without placing the recipient at unacceptable risk for cardiopulmonary complications. Chest radiography in the recovery room to assess pulmonary status should be routine, and may help guide fluid resuscitation. A patient with pulmonary edema and DGF should prompt consideration for HD. Recurrent pulmonary edema may be an atypical manifestation of a kidney graft renal artery stenosis.

Pulmonary hypertension (PHT), although a profound risk factor for death in liver transplant recipients, has not been found to be an independent risk factor for mortality after kidney transplant. Nevertheless, kidney transplant recipients with known PHT may require ICU care postoperatively, guided by PAC monitoring [29].

Acute respiratory distress syndrome (ARDS) in kidney transplant recipients is very rare, affecting 0.2% of all patients. A precipitating factor can be induction immunosuppression with antithymocyte globulin. The mortality rate of KTx recipients with ARDS is prohibitive at well over 50% [30].

Metabolic Complications

Hyperkalemia is frequently encountered and can be quite dangerous in the perioperative setting making serial serum potassium levels and appropriate treatment indispensable. In the OR, surgical trauma and transfusion of banked blood can cause hyperkalemia. Postoperatively, hyperkalemia can develop quickly in the setting of DGF. In addition to impaired GFR and decreased plasma aldosterone levels, ATN damage to the distal tubules can contribute to hyperkalemia since the distal tubules are a major site of potassium secretion. Medications are also common culprits. CNIs cause vasoconstriction of the afferent arterioles and damage to the distal tubules leading to hyperkalemia. Other medications that decrease potassium excretion include: trimethoprim-sulfamethoxazole, ACE inhibitors, angiotensin-2 receptor-antagonists, and nonsteroidal anti-inflammatory agents. β-blockers cause hyperkalemia by impeding intracellular potassium entry. The standard therapy is to give IV glucose, insulin, and bicarbonate to rapidly decrease serum potassium, but this does not change the total body potassium content. A potassium-binding resin actual removes potassium from the body but is slow acting. Recipients with hyperkalemia from poor graft function often require HD.

The brisk diuresis from immediate graft function can lead to hypokalemia. Recipients requiring more than 0.3 mEq/kg/h should be placed on a cardiac monitor. Hypomagnesaemia and hypophosphatemia can also result from high-output diuresis. Other causes of hypomagnesaemia include drug-related renal wasting (e.g., cyclosporine, tacrolimus, diuretics, aminoglycosides, and amphotericin B), poor dietary intake, and malabsorption from the gastrointestinal tract. Other causes of hypophosphatemia include secondary hyperparathyroidism, glucocorticoids (inhibit the tubular reabsorption of phosphate), and antacids (which bind phosphate in the gastrointestinal tract).

Infectious Complications

Infectious diseases can be very complex in solid-organ transplant recipients. A comprehensive review is beyond the scope of this chapter, but we will try to cover the germane points for the immediate posttransplantation period. The earliest infections are caused by bacterial infection of breached anatomic sites, including the lungs, blood (indwelling catheters), superficial wounds, and the perinephric space. Viral and fungal infections can occur in the immediate postoperative course but are more common in later periods [31].

The most common infection posttransplant is, not surprisingly, a urinary tract infection, with an incidence of more than 30%. UTIs progress to the more sinister pyelonephritis and bacteremia in about 10% of recipients. Gram-negative bacilli are the cause 70% of the time, but Enterococcus, Staphylococcus, and Candida are other causative pathogens. Risk factors include prolonged bladder catheterization, neurogenic bladder, ureteral stent placement, and ureteral complications. It is paramount to initiate antibiotic therapy, even in cases of asymptomatic bacteruria. If the infection persists, the ureteral stent should be removed and further diagnostic tests ordered, including voiding cystourethrogram and CT scan [32].

Kidney transplant recipients have a wound infection rate of 1% to 6%. Every effort should be made to prevent wound infections including thorough skin preparation with chlorhexidine, prophylactic antibiotics, and irrigation of the urinary bladder with an antibiotic solution. Wound infections should be treated according to the standard surgical principles of drainage and antimicrobial therapy [33].

Pneumonia is a formidable problem in the posttransplant period, developing in 16% of kidney transplant recipients and carrying a mortality rate of 10% to 13%. In this period, 90% of these infections are bacterial, usually caused by Staphylococcus or nosocomial gram-negative species. Fungal pneumonias are less likely but occur, most commonly in patients with a more intensive immunosuppressive regimen or who had a prolonged prior course of antibiotics [34,35].

The diagnosis of bacterial pneumonia is not always clear-cut. There are many noninfectious causes of fever including atelectasis and medications. If a CXR reveals an infiltrate, a chest CT may delineate the pneumonia. Although there is no consensus on the role of bronchoalveolar lavage (BAL), it may be prudent to obtain a BAL in recipients with pneumonia who do not respond to antibiotic therapy in 48 to 72 hours. If a patient has suspected pneumonia, broad-spectrum antibiotics need to be initiated immediately; antimicrobial therapy cannot wait for culture results in solid-organ transplant recipients. Antifungal therapy should be initiated in appropriate situations. Surveillance cultures should be reviewed to exclude the presence of multidrug-resistant (MDR) bacteria. Antibiotics should later be tailored to culture results [35].

Since kidney transplant recipients have indwelling catheter, arteriovenous fistula, or arteriovenous grafts, they are at risk for bloodstream infections. Catheters should be removed as soon as possible. Staphylococcal species and gram-negative bacilli are the most likely pathogens and should be treated aggressively with IV antibiotics. Persistent bacteremia should prompt suspicions for infective endocarditis. Echocardiogram should reveal cardiac valve vegetation. Treatment is with prolonged antibiotics.

Viral infections can play a sinister role in the later posttransplant period. The predominant offenders are from the herpesvirus genus, including cytomegalovirus (CMV), Epstein–Barr virus, herpes simplex virus (HSV), and varicella-zoster virus (herpes zoster virus, HZV).

Primary infections by HSV are rare but reactivations are common with an incidence as high as 30% for adults and 8% for pediatric recipients. Diagnosis is confirmed by tissue culture or direct immunofluorescent antibody staining using the Tzanck preparation. A PCR test is now available which is thought to be up to two times more sensitive than tissue cultures. Symptomatic HSV infections are common with orofacial and genital lesions. Although much less common, conjunctivitis or corneal ulcerations may develop. Topical 5% acyclovir ointment shortens the duration of viral shedding. Oral acyclovir (200 mg five times per day) is also effective. IV acyclivor (5.0 mg per kg every 8 hours for 7 to 14 days) is used in cases of disseminated disease [36].

CMV infections are rare in the first month posttransplantation but can infect up to as many as 60% of recipients and by some estimates, cause invasive disease in up to 25%. Most infections occur within the first year and are of serious concern. Studies have shown that CMV infections decrease graft and patient survival. We risk-stratify patients based on seropositivity. Donor-seropositive (D+) and recipient-seronegative (R–) is the highest-risk group with an incidence of up to 60%. D+R+ and D–R+ groups have a lower risk profile with an incidence between 20% and 40%. CMV infections are possible in the D–R– group when they occur as primary infections or reactivations [37,38]. Prophylaxis with parental 9-[(1,3-dihydroxy-2-propoxy) methyl] guanine (DHPG) (ganciclovir) or enteral (valganciclovir) forms have successfully reduced rates of infection. Recipients with D+R– (high-risk) group should receive prophylactic oral DHPG for at least 6 months posttransplantation.

In addition to generalized symptoms of fever, malaise, myalgia, and headache, 70% of infected patients have leukopenia. CMV infections can manifest in many different sites, including: neuritis, gastritis, colitis, retinitis, hepatitis, pancreatitis, and nephritis. Most infections occur within the first 6 months. The gold standard for diagnosis is growth in tissue culture; however, PCR quantification techniques are becoming much more common. PCR techniques can detect viremia within 48 hours, allowing for prompt initiation of treatment. The treatment for an established infection is IV DHPG (5 mg per kg every 12 hours if creatinine <1.5 mg per dL with dose adjustment according to graft function). Treatment can be limited by leukopenia (white blood cell count $< 3,000$ cells per μL) or thrombocytopenia (platelet count $< 100,000$ per μL), requiring dose reduction or temporary cessation. The treatment course is 14 days of IV DHPG with the addition of CMV hyperimmune globulin for severe cases. Oral DHPG is then continued for 6 months.

EBV infections are often associated with mononucleosis-like symptoms: malaise, fevers, headaches, and sore throat. At its worst manifestation, it can present as widespread posttransplant lymphoproliferative disease (PTLD), a form of B-cell lymphoma. This usually occurs months to years posttransplantation. Immunosuppression impairs the ability of virus-specific cytotoxic T lymphocytes to control the expression of EBV-infected transformed B cells, leading to polyclonal and monoclonal proliferation of lymphocytes (which constitutes PTLD). Treatment entails cessation of immunosuppression accompanied by anti-CD-20 antibodies (rituximab), and antiviral therapy (e.g., ganciclovir, acyclovir, or anti-CMV immune globulin). Suboptimal responses necessitate conventional lymphoma treatment.

Varicella-zoster virus usually presents as dermatomal skin lesions. Therapy is a 7-day course of acyclovir. Varicella-zoster immune globulin is indicated for seronegative recipients. Recipients are at risk for other viruses as well, including adenoviruses and influenza, papovaviruses, and hepatitis. Human papillomavirus infections are also increased leading to higher incidence of cervical cancer.

Fungal infections are quite frequent and occur in 14% of kidney transplant recipients. Translocation of Candida from the gastrointestinal tract is a common source. *Aspergillus* species infections are common and can be serious. The most common infection is oropharyngeal candidiasis that can be treated with oral nystatin. Systemic fungal infections are usually quite serious and occur in significantly ill patients. Often, recipients are on broad-spectrum antibacterials and have poor graft function. Superinfections have a dismal prognosis. Patients with cerebral, pulmonary, or visceral involvement require significant reduction or cessation of immunosuppression [39].

Azole antifungals (e.g., fluconazole) are the first-line therapy given their safety profile. For life-threatening fungemia, stronger agents such as an echinocandin-like caspofungin, or amphotericin B should be used, especially for non-albicans Candida [40]. Liposomal form of amphotericin B can mitigate some of the agent's notorious nephrotoxicity. Specific fungal complications include: mycotic pseudoaneurysm from Candida, which often requires graft nephrectomy and IV amphotericin B. *Cryptococcus* and Asperillus can cause severe pulmonary and cerebral infections requiring systemic or intrathecal amphotericin B. *Pneumocystis jiroveci* (formerly known as *Pneumocystis carinii*) can manifest as interstitial pneumonia. Pneumocystic pneumonia (PCP) is rare now that TMP-SMX prophylaxis is the standard of care, but it can be seen with heavily immunosuppressed patients, presenting with fever, dyspnea, and nonproductive cough. Therapy consists of IV TMP-SMX with pentamidine or dapsone serving as alternatives. Reduction of immunosuppression or temporary cessation may also be necessary.

Mycobacterium tuberculosis infection is uncommon, infecting about 1% of kidney transplant recipients and is often a result of reactivation of a prior infection. Symptoms include fevers, malaise, night sweats, and weight loss. Sputum and blood samples should be used to identify acid-fast bacilli. Treatment should be aggressive since mortality rates are high; 6 months of a two- to three-drug regimen or a longer regimen is often required. Treatment agents include isoniazid, rifampin, pyrazinamide, ethambutol, and ciprofloxacin.

Gastrointestinal and Pancreaticobiliary Complications

Gastrointestinal tract complications are a major cause of morbidity and mortality for the kidney transplant population.

Peptic ulcer disease (PUD) with its associated complications (perforation, bleeding) is the most common gastrointestinal tract complication. There is some evidence to suggest that the prevalence of PUD is more common among renal failure patients compared to the general population. Historically, it was not uncommon for kidney transplant recipients to have suffered from severe upper GI bleeding; up to 10% of recipients had significant bleeding [41]. These problems declined considerably with the use of H_2 blockers and proton-pump inhibitors. If severe upper gastrointestinal tract bleeding does occur, the standard treatment algorithm should apply. ICU monitoring and resuscitation should be instituted immediately to stabilize the patient followed by conservative treatments with endoscopy with mucosal control measure including submucosal injection of epinephrine when indicated. If the patient is still bleeding, angiographic embolization should be performed which often requires embolization of two arteries. If all of these measures are unsuccessful, as a last resort, emergency gastric surgery should be performed with resection and vagotomy. Immunosuppression should be minimized during the perioperative period. A high incidence of CMV infection has been observed in peptic ulcers from kidney transplant recipients. Tissue samples should be tested for CMV and if positive, IV DHPG and anti-CMV immune globulin treatments initiated.

Small-bowel obstruction can occur following intra-abdominal placement of organs as is done with pediatric kidney transplantation or simultaneous pancreas–kidney transplantation in adults. The vast majority of adult kidney transplantations are placed in the retroperitoneum so small-bowel obstructions are usually not related to the operation; however, small bowel can incarcerate through an inadvertent tear in the peritoneum made during the dissection. More likely, obstruction is related to previous intra-abdominal procedures, infections, or PTLD in the small bowel or mesentery.

Colonic perforation and lower gastrointestinal tract hemorrhage are the most common lower gastrointestinal tract complications encountered, but have a very low incidence overall. Colonic perforation occurs in 1% to 2% of KTx recipients and is most commonly owing to diverticulitis, ischemic colitis, CMV colitis, and occasionally, stercoral ulceration. Colonic perforation in KTx recipients carries a very high mortality rate—20% to 38%. Immunosuppression complicates the diagnostic picture and is associated with high mortality rates. Peritoneal signs are usually absent in immunosuppressed kidney transplant recipients. The progression to septic shock can be very rapid. A successful outcome depends on maintaining a high index of suspicion, liberal use of imaging studies, and a low threshold for exploration. Diverting colostomies have been associated with better outcomes than other approaches [42–45].

Kidney transplant recipients, especially patients with polycystic kidney disease, have a greater incidence of colonic diverticulitis with higher rates of perforation. Steroids are thought to be responsible for this difference since they not only mask the symptoms but impair the patient's ability to localize and contain the infection. Historically, diverticular perforations had a disastrous prognosis, but recent experience suggests decreasing mortality rates. This is likely owing to the widespread acceptance of the principle that immunosuppressed patients need prompt surgical intervention. It may be prudent to perform sigmoid resections with a Hartmann pouch and diverting colostomy compared to the general population where primary anastomosis is often advocated. Given the significant morbidity from diverticulitis in this population, some surgeons advocate sigmoidectomy prior to transplantation for candidates with a single episode of diverticulitis [46,47].

Ischemic colitis is associated with significant arterial disease, immunosuppression, antibiotic therapy, and hypotension—so it is no surprise that there is a higher incidence in the kidney transplant population. On rare occasions, even young transplant recipients without significant risk factors can have ischemic colitis, with no apparent explanation. Ischemic colitis may be segmental or pancolic [48,49].

Pseudomembranous colitis caused by *Clostridium difficile* is being increasingly recognized. Due to immunosuppression, it can rapidly progress to toxic megacolon and perforation with a grim prognosis. Stool assays in conjunction with the clinical picture confirm the diagnosis. On occasion, visualization of the pseudomembranes on colonoscopy is necessary. Patients can be treated conservatively with metronidazole (250 mg four times daily for 10 days) or oral vancomycin (125 mg every 6 hours for 10 days), but there should be a low threshold for colonic resection when a patient's clinical condition deteriorates.

Neutropenic enterocolitis is associated with profound neutropenia and invasion by clostridial organisms; most commonly, *Clostridium septicum*. Treatment is with metronidazole and again, low threshold for surgical intervention. Infectious colitis is frequently owing to CMV infections but can also be due to bacterial, viral (e.g., herpes), or fungal pathogens. Diagnosis is confirmed by stool cultures, and if necessary, endoscopic biopsies. Empiric antibiotics should be started quickly with later tailoring of the regimen based on culture results. In most cases of infectious colitis, surgical intervention should be avoided [50].

Ogilvie syndrome or acute colonic pseudo-obstruction has an incidence of 1.5% among kidney transplant recipients. It is a paralytic colonic ileus that can cause pronounced cecal dilation and eventual rupture. The first line of therapy is conservative with nasogastric decompression, and neostigmine. If this fails, endoscopic colonic decompression can be tried. The last line of therapy is surgical resection. Again, the principle of prompt surgical intervention holds. Immunosuppression should be reduced. Rejection is very uncommon in patients with severe infections or extremis [51].

In addition to the common causes of lower gastrointestinal tract bleeding, transplant-specific pathologies are common in this population, including CMV colitis and fungal ulcerations. H_2 blockers and antacids that promote fungal overgrowth owing to achlorhydria can promote fungal ulceration. Steroids can also promote ulcers and impair the reparative mechanisms of the bowel wall. Additionally, uremia and diabetes result in colonic distention and impaction promoting colonic ulcers. Prompt diagnostic colonoscopy and treatment is essential [52].

Pancreatitis is also more common in the kidney transplant population compared to the general population. One to six percent suffer from an episode of pancreatitis. There are numerous transplant-specific risk factors, including: (1) immunosuppressants (e.g., corticosteroids, azathioprine, cyclosporine) and diuretics (e.g., furosemide, thiazide diuretics); (2) hypercalcemia with or without hyperparathyroidism [53]; (3) infections (e.g., CMV, HSV) [54]; (4) previous episodes of pancreatitis (uremia); and (5) cholelithiasis (i.e., related to cyclosporine). There is also speculation of a phenomenon called rejection pancreatitis where host antibodies react not only to the graft (vascular rejection) but also with antigens on the surface of the pancreas cells (vascular pancreatitis). The most frequent causes of pancreatitis in the general population, biliary tract disease and alcoholism, are not as common in the kidney transplant population [55,56].

Since hyperamylasemia is not uncommon in uremic patients, owing to reduced amylase clearance from the kidneys, the amylase/creatinine clearance ratio is a more sensitive index of pancreatitis. The degree of hyperamylasemia in not thought to be a prognostic factor. A contrast-enhanced CT scan is important for staging. Conservative therapy should be initiated. Any evidence of hemorrhagic or necrotizing pancreatitis requires ICU monitoring and careful fluid resuscitation with cardiac monitoring. Additionally, immunosuppression should be reduced and broad-spectrum antibiotics initiated when infection is suggested by imaging studies. Percutaneous drainage or aggressive surgical therapy should be pursued if there is any evidence of infected necrosis, including removal of all necrotic material in multiple trips to the OR that is sometimes necessary to achieve sufficient drainage by irrigation of the abdominal cavity. Overwhelming sepsis is the common cause of death. Furthermore, the mortality rate for posttransplant pancreatitis is higher than for other forms of pancreatitis. It is therefore essential to promptly initiate broad-spectrum antibiotics and reduce immunosuppression.

There is no clear evidence for prophylactic cholecystectomy for asymptomatic cholelithiasis in the pretransplant screening. In the posttransplant period, acute choleystitis should always be considered in patients with abdominal pain and sepsis. Acalculous cholecystitis should be considered with complicated posttransplant courses and prolonged hospital stays. Biliary scintigraphy is often necessary to establish the diagnosis. If a patient is not clinically stable enough for a formal operation, image-guided cholecystectomy drainage should be pursued.

Neurologic Complications

The incidence of life-threatening central nervous system (CNS)–related complications in the immediate posttransplant period is 1% to 5% [57–59]. The patient population is prone to comorbidities that are a setup for cerebrovascular events, including: diabetes, hypertension, hyperlipidemia, hypercoagulability, uremia, and advanced age. The most common cerebrovascular events, infarct, TIA, and hemorrhage, peak during the first few months postoperatively. The prognosis of hemorrhage is grim. Patients with strokes and TIAs should be treated immediately with heparin and aspirin. If there is an ulcerated carotid lesion or a stenosis that is severe but accessible, a carotid endarterectomy should be pursued.

CNS infections have a wide spectrum of severity, but all are considered serious. Infections are caused by bacteria (e.g., *Listeria monocytogenes*, *Pseudomonas* species), viruses (e.g., CMV, HSV), fungi (e.g., *Cryptococcus*, *Aspergillus*, *Mucor*), and parasites (*Toxoplasma*). *L. monocytogenes* is the most common infectious organism and usually causes meningitis. *Aspergillus* species can cause brain abscesses. Rhinocerebral mucormycosis infection can cause cavernous sinus thrombosis and rapid death. Dissemination of CMV may include the CNS, although the overall incidence is low [60]. Acute polyradiculoneuritis has also been associated with CMV infections. Similarly, dissemination of the VZV can involve the CNS or facial nerve (Ramsay–Hunt syndrome). It is crucial to diagnose and treat these infections early and aggressively. Intrathecal administration of antimicrobial drugs or drainage for recipients with brain abscesses may be necessary.

Seizures are most commonly associated with excessively high CNI serum levels. Hypertension and hypomagnesaemia may predispose recipients to seizure activity. Diagnosis can be confirmed with a brain MRI showing PRES (posterior reversible encephalopathy syndrome). PRES occurs in about 0.35% of kidney transplant recipients [61]. Treatment includes a reduction in CNI dosing or switching to a non-CNI immunosuppressant, in addition to anticonvulsants. ICU monitoring is mandatory. Tacrolimus more frequently causes neurologic problems than cyclosporine. Other forms of CNI neurotoxicity include tremor, headaches, paralysis, quadriplegia, and coma.

CURRENT CHALLENGES IN KIDNEY TRANSPLANTATION

Despite the many advances in kidney transplantation, several challenges remain (Table 57.1). During the past decade, the proportion of candidates on the active kidney transplantation waiting list >50 years of age has increased from 44% to 58% and those with diabetes and hypertension have increased from 24% to 28% and 17% to 22%, respectively. To maintain excellent short-term outcomes, an exhaustive pretransplantation cardiovascular evaluation followed by intense posttransplantation critical care has become mandatory for this high-acuity cohort of patients [8,9].

Mortality on the waiting list continues to stimulate the adoption of innovative desensitization protocols to allow high-risk recipients a transplantation opportunity. This, in turn, must be met with equally innovative therapies when antibody-mediated rejection occurs in the early postoperative period. Attempts at modulating the complement system are underway to mitigate early posttransplant injury in the allograft [62].

TABLE 57.1

Current Challenges in Kidney Transplantation

Clinical dilemma	Management
Higher-acuity KTx waiting list	Exhaustive pretransplant evaluation
Age > 50: 58%	Intense posttransplant critical care and subspecialty consultation
Diabetic: 28%	Desensitization protocols
Hypertensive: 22%	Innovative recipient immunomodulation
Waiting list mortality	Complement modulation
Organ scarcity	Live donor paired kidney exchange
Sensitized recipients	National live donor registries

KTx, kidney transplantation.

References

1. Rana A, Gruessner A, Agopian VG, et al: Survival benefit of solid-organ transplant in the United States. *JAMA Surg* 150(3):252–259, 2015.
2. Wolfe RA, Ashby VB, Milford EL, et al: Comparison of mortality in all patients on dialysis, patients on dialysis awaiting transplantation, and recipients of a first cadaveric transplant. *N Engl J Med* 341(23):1725–1730, 1999.
3. Laupacis A, Keown P, Pus N, et al: A study of the quality of life and cost-utility of renal transplantation. *Kidney Int* 50(1):235–242, 1996.
4. Hariharan S, Johnson CP, Bresnahan BA, et al: Improved graft survival after renal transplantation in the United States, 1988 to 1996. *N Engl J Med* 342(9):605–612, 2000.
5. Ishikawa N, Tanabe K, Tokumoto T, et al: Long-term results of living unrelated renal transplantation. *Transplant Proc* 31(7):2856–2857, 1999.
6. Matas AJ, Smith JM, Skeans MA, et al: OPTN/SRTR 2012 Annual Data Report: kidney. *Am J Transplant* 14[Suppl 1]:11–44, 2014.
7. Briggs JD: Causes of death after renal transplantation. *Nephrol Dial Transplant* 16(8):1545–1549, 2001.
8. Humar A, Kerr SR, Ramcharan T, et al: Peri-operative cardiac morbidity in kidney transplant recipients: incidence and risk factors. *Clin Transplant* 15(3):154–158, 2001.
9. Rabbat CG, Treleaven DJ, Russell JD, et al: Prognostic value of myocardial perfusion studies in patients with end-stage renal disease assessed for kidney or kidney-pancreas transplantation: a meta-analysis. *J Am Soc Nephrol* 14(2):431–439, 2003.
10. Fissell RB, Bragg-Gresham JL, Woods JD, et al: Patterns of hepatitis C prevalence and seroconversion in hemodialysis units from three continents: the DOPPS. *Kidney Int* 65(6):2335–2342, 2004.
11. van Valenberg PL, Hoitsma AJ, Tiggeler RG, et al: Mannitol as an indispensable constituent of an intraoperative hydration protocol for the prevention of acute renal failure after renal cadaveric transplantation. *Transplantation* 44(6):784–788, 1987.
12. Dawidson IJ, Sandor ZF, Coorpender L, et al: Intraoperative albumin administration affects the outcome of cadaver renal transplantation. *Transplantation* 53(4):774–782, 1992.
13. Perico N, Cattaneo D, Sayegh MH, et al: Delayed graft function in kidney transplantation. *Lancet* 364(9447):1814–1827, 2004.
14. Ojo AO, Wolfe RA, Held PJ, et al: Delayed graft function: risk factors and implications for renal allograft survival. *Transplantation* 63(7):968–974, 1997.
15. Humar A, Ramcharan T, Kandaswamy R, et al: Risk factors for slow graft function after kidney transplants: a multivariate analysis. *Clin Transplant* 16(6):425–429, 2002.
16. Matas AJ, Gillingham KJ, Payne WD, et al: The impact of an acute rejection episode on long-term renal allograft survival (t1/2). *Transplantation* 57(6):857–859, 1994.
17. Ducloux D, Rebibou JM, Semhoun-Ducloux S, et al: Recurrence of hemolytic-uremic syndrome in renal transplant recipients: a meta-analysis. *Transplantation* 65(10):1405–1407, 1998.
18. Benedetti E, Troppmann C, Gillingham K, et al: Short- and long-term outcomes of kidney transplants with multiple renal arteries. *Ann Surg* 221(4):406–414, 1995.
19. Englesbe MJ, Punch JD, Armstrong DR, et al: Single-center study of technical graft loss in 714 consecutive renal transplants. *Transplantation* 78(4):623–626, 2004.
20. Streeter EH, Little DM, Cranston DW, et al: The urological complications of renal transplantation: a series of 1535 patients. *BJU Int* 90(7):627–634, 2002.
21. Bassiri A, Simforoosh N, Gholamrezaie HR: Ureteral complications in 1100 consecutive renal transplants. *Transplant Proc* 32(3):578–579, 2000.
22. Matas AJ, Humar A, Gillingham KJ, et al: Five preventable causes of kidney graft loss in the 1990s: a single-center analysis. *Kidney Int* 62(2):704–714, 2002.
23. Debska-Slizien A, Dudziak M, Kubasik A, et al: Echocardiographic changes in left ventricular morphology and function after successful renal transplantation. *Transplant Proc* 32(6):1365–1366, 2000.
24. Djamali A, Becker YT, Simmons WD, et al: Increasing hematocrit reduces early posttransplant cardiovascular risk in diabetic transplant recipients. *Transplantation* 76(5):816–820, 2003.
25. Sever MS, Steinmuller DR, Hayes JM, et al: Pericarditis following renal transplantation. *Transplantation* 51(6):1229–1232, 1991.
26. Barbari A: Posttransplant hypertension: multipathogenic disease process. *Exp Clin Transplant* 11(2):99–108, 2013.
27. Cauduro RL, Costa C, Lhulier F, et al: Cyclosporine increases endothelin-1 plasma levels in renal transplant recipients. *Transplant Proc* 36(4):880–881, 2004.
28. Ozsoylu S, Strauss HS, Diamond LK: Effects of corticosteroids on coagulation of the blood. *Nature* 195:1214–1215, 1962.
29. Issa N, Krowka MJ, Griffin MD, et al: Pulmonary hypertension is associated with reduced patient survival after kidney transplantation. *Transplantation* 86(10):1384–1388, 2008.
30. Shorr AF, Abbott KC, Agadoa LY: Acute respiratory distress syndrome after kidney transplantation: epidemiology, risk factors, and outcomes. *Crit Care Med* 31(5):1325–1330, 2003.
31. Fishman JA: Infection in solid-organ transplant recipients. *N Engl J Med* 357(25):2601–2614, 2007.
32. Tolkoff-Rubin NE, Rubin RH: Urinary tract infection in the immunocompromised host. Lessons from kidney transplantation and the AIDS epidemic. *Infect Dis Clin North Am* 11(3):707–717, 1997.
33. Patel R, Paya CV: Infections in solid-organ transplant recipients. *Clin Microbiol Rev* 10(1):86–124, 1997.

34. Chang GC, Wu CL, Pan SH, et al: The diagnosis of pneumonia in renal transplant recipients using invasive and noninvasive procedures. *Chest* 125(2):541–547, 2004.
35. Linden PK: Approach to the immunocompromised host with infection in the intensive care unit. *Infect Dis Clin North Am* 23(3):535–556, 2009.
36. Slomka MJ, Emery L, Munday PE, et al: A comparison of PCR with virus isolation and direct antigen detection for diagnosis and typing of genital herpes. *J Med Virol* 55(2):177–183, 1998.
37. Sagedal S, Nordal KP, Hartmann A, et al: A prospective study of the natural course of cytomegalovirus infection and disease in renal allograft recipients. *Transplantation* 70(8):1166–1174, 2000.
38. Mengelle C, Pasquier C, Rostaing L, et al: Quantitation of human cytomegalovirus in recipients of solid organ transplants by real-time quantitative PCR and pp65 antigenemia. *J Med Virol* 69(2):225–231, 2003.
39. Hibberd PL, Rubin RH: Clinical aspects of fungal infection in organ transplant recipients. *Clin Infect Dis* 19[Suppl 1]:S33–S40, 1994.
40. Mora-Duarte J, Betts R, Rotstein C, et al: Comparison of caspofungin and amphotericin B for invasive candidiasis. *N Engl J Med* 347(25):2020–2029, 2002.
41. Sarosdy MF, Saylor R, Dittman W, et al: Upper gastrointestinal bleeding following renal transplantation. *Urology* 26(4):347–350, 1985.
42. Gautam A: Gastrointestinal complications following transplantation. *Surg Clin North Am* 86(5):1195–1206, vii, 2006.
43. Coccolini F, Catena F, Di Saverio S, et al: Colonic perforation after renal transplantation: risk factor analysis. *Transplant Proc* 41(4):1189–1190, 2009.
44. Flanigan RC, Reckard CR, Lucas BA: Colonic complications of renal transplantation. *J Urol* 139(3):503–506, 1988.
45. Lao A, Bach D: Colonic complications in renal transplant recipients. *Dis Colon Rectum* 31(2):130–133, 1988.
46. Scheff RT, Zuckerman G, Harter H, et al: Diverticular disease in patients with chronic renal failure due to polycystic kidney disease. *Ann Intern Med* 92(2, pt 1):202–204, 1980.
47. Pirenne J, Lledo-Garcia E, Benedetti E, et al: Colon perforation after renal transplantation: a single-institution review. *Clin Transplant* 11(2):88–93, 1997.
48. Indudhara R, Kochhar R, Mehta SK, et al: Acute colitis in renal transplant recipients. *Am J Gastroenterol* 85(8):964–968, 1990.
49. Hellstrom PM, Rubio C, Odar-Cederlof I, et al: Ischemic colitis of the cecum after renal transplantation masquerading as malignant disease. *Dig Dis Sci* 36(11):1644–1648, 1991.
50. Frankel AH, Barker F, Williams G, et al: Neutropenic enterocolitis in a renal transplant patient. *Transplantation* 52(5):913–914, 1991.
51. Love R, Starling JR, Sollinger HW, et al: Colonoscopic decompression for acute colonic pseudo-obstruction (Ogilvie's syndrome) in transplant recipients. *Gastrointest Endosc* 34(5):426–429, 1988.
52. Stylianos S, Forde KA, Benvenisty AI, et al: Lower gastrointestinal hemorrhage in renal transplant recipients. *Arch Surg* 123(6):739–744, 1988.
53. Frick TW, Fryd DS, Sutherland DE, et al: Hypercalcemia associated with pancreatitis and hyperamylasemia in renal transplant recipients. Data from the Minnesota randomized trial of cyclosporine versus antilymphoblast azathioprine. *Am J Surg* 154(5):487–489, 1987.
54. Kamalkumar BS, Agarwal SK, Garg P, et al: Acute pancreatitis with CMV papillitis and cholangiopathy in a renal transplant recipient. *Clin Exp Nephrol* 13(4):389–391, 2009.
55. Fernandez-Cruz L, Targarona EM, Cugat E, et al: Acute pancreatitis after renal transplantation. *Br J Surg* 76(11):1132–1135, 1989.
56. Johnson WC, Nabseth DC: Pancreatitis in renal transplantation. *Ann Surg* 171(2):309–314, 1970.
57. Adams HP Jr, Dawson G, Coffman TJ, et al: Stroke in renal transplant recipients. *Arch Neurol* 43(2):113–115, 1986.
58. Bruno A, Adams HP Jr: Neurologic problems in renal transplant recipients. *Neurol Clin* 6(2):305–325, 1988.
59. Lee JM, Raps EC: Neurologic complications of transplantation. *Neurol Clin* 16(1):21–33, 1998.
60. Simmons RL, Matas AJ, Rattazzi LC, et al: Clinical characteristics of the lethal cytomegalovirus infection following renal transplantation. *Surgery* 82(5):537–546, 1977.
61. Bartynski WS, Tan HP, Boardman JF, et al: Posterior reversible encephalopathy syndrome after solid organ transplantation. *Am J Neuroradiol* 29(5):924–930, 2008.
62. Colvin RB, Smith RN: Antibody-mediated organ-allograft rejection. *Nat Rev Immunol* 5(10):807–817, 2005.

Chapter 58 ■ Critical Care of Liver Transplant Recipients and Live Liver Donors

BABAK MOVAHEDI • PAULO MARTINS • SONIA NAGY CHIMIENTI • ADEL BOZORGZADEH

INTRODUCTION

From early experimental animal model implantations conducted in the 1950s, to the first successful liver transplant performed by Dr. Starzl in 1963, liver transplantation has evolved to become a safe and widely accepted treatment for patients with end-stage liver disease (ESLD) [1]. The current 1-year survival rate in recipients of deceased donor organs is approximately 91%, owing in part to improvements in surgical procurement and transplantation techniques, more effective immunosuppressive regimens, individualized approaches to immunosuppression, improved perioperative and postoperative critical care, and improvements in the management of rejection and infection (Source: OPTN data as of November 27, 2015. http://optn.transplant.hrsa.gov. Accessed December 1, 2015).

Despite these substantial improvements, liver transplantation is a major abdominal surgical procedure that confers significant risk for a variety of postsurgical and medical complications. The content of this chapter addresses the critical care of these complex, often critically ill patients, from the intraoperative through the immediate postoperative period, reviewing the management of selected posttransplant complications. Care of the live donor is also described. Detailed discussions regarding care of the patient with ESLD, approaches to immunosuppression management, and the diagnosis and management of rejection, infection, and malignancy for transplant recipients are found in other sections of this textbook.

ORGAN ALLOCATION AND DISPARITY

Expanding the Donor Pool

As liver transplant outcomes have improved, the indications for liver transplantation have expanded, and the number of individuals waitlisted for liver transplant has increased dramatically. According to Organ Procurement and Transplantation Network (OPTN) data, 15,064 patients were listed for liver transplant as of November 27, 2015. In the United States, 6,729 liver transplants were performed in 2014. Approximately 4% of liver transplants performed each year are from live donors (Source: OPTN data as of November 27, 2015; http://optn.transplant.hrsa.gov. Accessed December 1, 2015).

Given the growing problem of disparity between the number of liver transplant candidates and available donor organs, expansion of the donor pool has attracted increased interest. Donors with livers that are considered marginal are now allocated to carefully selected recipients, whereas they may not have been deemed acceptable for transplantation in the past. Although these so-called extended criteria donors have created opportunities for candidates who may not otherwise have received an organ, they are associated with an increased rate of primary nonfunction (PNF). In 2006, a retrospective study of more than 20,000 donors identified a number of factors associated with an increased risk of graft loss. This work contributed to the development of a "donor risk index," which is used to predict the rate of graft survival. Characteristics associated with a relative risk of at least 1.5 for liver graft loss include donor age over 60 years, donation after cardiac death, and use of partial/split grafts. Other donor factors, such as age between 40 and 60 years, African American race, and cerebrovascular accident, are also associated with an increased risk for graft loss, though to a lesser extent. Use of the donor risk index may help to optimize donor–recipient matching. Innovative surgical procedures have also been used to increase the donor pool, including living donor liver transplantation and split-liver transplantation. These procedures are each associated with unique problems, as will be discussed below.

DCD Organs

In recent years, the use of organs from donors after cardiac death (DCD) has emerged as an important source of grafts [2]. DCD donors have severe neurologic injury without meeting criteria for brain death [3–5]. In the United States in 2009, 4.6% of liver transplants performed were from DCD donors, up from 3% in 2004 [2–5]. Kidneys from DCD donors, despite their higher rate of delayed graft function, provide similar graft survival as do kidneys from brain death donors [6]. Results for liver transplantation with grafts from DCD donors have been mixed, and individual centers have reported outcomes ranging from excellent to very poor. An SRTR review of over 1500 DCD liver transplants between 2001 and 2009 revealed a 3-year patient survival of 64.9%. Furthermore, 13.6% required retransplantation [7]. The principal problem with the use of DCD livers is the risk of biliary complications and the development of ischemic cholangiopathy, which has been reported to occur in 16% to 29% of cases, often requiring retransplantation [8].

Reduced-Size and Split-Liver Transplantation

In reduced-size liver transplantation (RSLT), a whole deceased donor graft is tailored to fit the recipient. A portion of the liver, such as the right lobe, is resected and discarded, and the remaining left lateral segment is used for the transplantation. In split-liver transplantation (SLT), an adult deceased donor liver is divided into two grafts: the left lateral segment and the remaining right trisegment (right lobe plus segment 4). Both segments can then be utilized for transplantation. For most adult recipients with ESLD, the small graft size with this approach would not be sufficient. Thus, while this approach may be beneficial for pediatric transplantation, it does not serve to significantly increase the adult donor pool [9]. With appropriate donor and recipient selection criteria, however, SLT may be considered for two adult recipients.

Living Donor Liver Transplantation

Living donor liver transplant (LDLT) involves removing a segment of the liver from an adult donor and transplanting the segment into a carefully selected recipient. This approach typically provides sufficient liver tissue for a recipient. With LDLT, the transplant is optimally performed before the recipient's health deteriorates significantly, thereby shortening the wait time. In LDLTs for pediatric recipients, the left lateral segment is used; for adult recipients, however, depending on the donor and recipient size and the liver volume, either right or left lobe could be considered. In 2001, 524 LDLTs were performed in the United States, of the 5,195 liver transplants performed that year (10.1%) (OPTN data as of November 27, 2015, source http://optn.transplant.hrsa.gov). Since that all-time high, approximately 250 liver transplants each year have been LDLTs; in 2014, 280 of the 6,729 (4.2%) liver transplants performed were from live donors (OPTN data as of November 27, 2015, source http://optn.transplant.hrsa.gov).

The main disadvantage of LDLT is the peri- and postoperative risk to an otherwise healthy donor. All potential live liver donors are carefully evaluated through a detailed screening process, including assessment by a hepatologist, donor surgeon, independent donor advocate, social worker, psychiatrist, and other providers as indicated during the evaluation. Standardized radiologic and laboratory evaluation is performed in order to detect the presence of any underlying medical issues. This detailed screening process is conducted in order to ensure that the donor is medically healthy and able from both a physical and a psychosocial perspective to undergo liver donation. The decision to proceed with live liver donation occurs following this extensive evaluation, after careful consideration and discussion of the risks and potential complications of liver donation.

Hepatitis B–Positive Donors

Careful allocation of organs from donors with hepatitis B virus (HBV) infection may safely expand the donor pool. The risk of transmission of HBV varies depending on the serologic status of both donor and recipient, with the highest risk observed in transplantation of grafts from donors with active HBV (HBsAg+ or HBV DNA+ donors) to naïve recipients. Liver graft recipients are at highest risk for acquisition of de novo HBV, as compared with recipients of other grafts. Prevention of transmission includes use of universal prophylaxis with newer generation antivirals such as entecavir, and occasionally the targeted use of hepatitis B immune globulin (HBIg) intra- and postoperatively, for a specified duration. These strategies significantly lower the risk of transmission of HBV, and make this a reasonable approach, particularly for patients who may not otherwise receive a standard graft in a timely manner. With the use of antiviral prophylaxis, with or without HBIg, excellent outcomes have been demonstrated with transplantation of HBV core antibody-positive donor grafts to immune (vaccinated or natural immunity) recipients. The risks of transmission of HBV must be discussed with the transplant candidate in advance of transplantation, and the candidate must provide informed consent for the transplantation of organs from donors with past or active HBV infection. A comprehensive consensus guideline was recently published that provides guidance with regard to the management of recipients of grafts from donors with active or prior HBV infection [10].

Hepatitis C–Positive Donors

Historically, transplantation of grafts from donors with a past history of hepatitis C virus (HCV) infection was reserved for recipients with active genotype 1 HCV infection. Outcomes in this setting were demonstrated to be equivalent to those in HCV-positive recipients of HCV-negative grafts [11]. For optimal outcomes, grafts from HCV-positive donors should be from younger donors with no significant liver fibrosis or inflammation. Grafts from older donors may be associated with more rapidly progressive fibrosis related to HCV posttransplant. In the new era of effective treatment of HCV-infected recipients with direct acting antivirals, the approach to the use of HCV-positive grafts for HCV-positive recipients will likely change. Data and guidelines in this area are rapidly evolving.

PHS Increased Risk Donors

Some donors engage in behaviors that may put them at increased risk for infections that can be transmitted by blood or body

TABLE 58.1

Behaviors Associated with Increased Risk of Transmission of HIV, HBV, and HCV Infection [12]

Method of exposure	Risk behavior
Sexual (*vaginal, anal, oral*) (*prior 12 mo*)	Individuals who have had sex with a person known/suspected to have HIV, HBV, or HCV infection Men who have had sex with men (MSM) Women who have had sex with a man with a history of MSM Individuals who have exchanged sex for money or drugs Individuals who have had sex with a person who had sex in exchange for money or drugs Individuals who have had sex with a person who injected drugs (intravenous, intramuscular, or subcutaneous) for nonmedical reasons
Maternal/child	A child who is ≤18 mo of age and born to a mother known to be infected with, or at increased risk for, HIV, HBV, or HCV infection A child who has been breastfed within the preceding 12 mo and whose mother is known to be infected with, or at increased risk for, HIV infection
Injection drugs (*prior 12 mo*)	Individuals who have injected drugs (intravenous, intramuscular, subcutaneous) for nonmedical reasons Individuals who have been in jail/prison/correctional facility for >72 consecutive hours
History of sexually transmitted infections (*prior 12 mo*)	New diagnosis of or treatment for syphilis, gonorrhea, *Chlamydia,* or genital ulcers

fluids. These infections include human immunodeficiency virus (HIV), HBV, and HCV. Donors with these risk behaviors are referred to as Public Health Service (PHS) Increased Risk Donors (Table 58.1). Revised guidelines for the assessment of PHS Increased Risk Donors, and for the monitoring of recipients of grafts from these donors, were published in 2013 [12]. Prior to organ procurement, potential donors are tested for all of these viruses using both serologic tests and nucleic acid tests (NAT). Even in the setting of negative serologic and NAT testing, PHS Increased Risk Donors, who constitute up to 9% of the donor pool, may harbor low levels of these viruses, and may pose a risk for transmission of viral infection from donor to recipient. This typically occurs during a "window period" of infection, when a donor has recently been exposed to one or more of these viruses and has not yet developed a measurable antibody response to the virus(es). The advent of NAT testing has decreased this window period dramatically, but a small risk of transmission still exists. With the active antiviral treatments that are now available for HIV, HBV, and HCV, utilization of organs from PHS Increased Risk Donors is a very reasonable option for carefully selected recipients who may not otherwise receive an organ in a reasonable time frame, and for whom the risk of death from end-stage organ disease is more significant than the risk of transmission of infection from a PHS Increased Risk Donor. The risks of transmission must be discussed with the transplant candidate in advance of transplantation, and the candidate must provide informed consent for the transplantation of PHS Increased Risk organs.

CAUSES OF LIVER FAILURE AND LIVER TRANSPLANT CANDIDATE SELECTION

Indications for Liver Transplant

Within the array of available options for the management of patients with chronic liver disease, liver transplantation is the most definitive one. However, not every patient may benefit from a transplant, and risks and benefits of either option should be carefully evaluated for each individual patient. Typically, well-compensated cirrhotics have a low mortality risk secondary to their underlying liver diseases and may be managed medically. However, patients with signs of hepatic decompensation have a poor prognosis without a transplant and should be considered for transplantation. Furthermore, well-selected patients with certain malignancies confined to the liver may benefit from liver transplantation. In particular, patients with hepatocellular carcinoma may have excellent long-term disease-free outcome after liver transplantation.

As hepatic fibrosis progresses and liver function deteriorates, signs and symptoms of decompensated liver disease appear. Decompensated cirrhosis is defined as the presence of *any* one of the following, which leads to an acute care hospitalization: (1) portosystemic encephalopathy, (2) variceal hemorrhage, (3) spontaneous bacterial peritonitis, (4) hepatorenal syndrome or acute kidney injury in the setting of cirrhosis, or (5) hepatic hydrothorax. Critical care of patients with decompensated cirrhosis and fulminant hepatic failure is addressed in Chapters 206 and 207. Portal hypertension can lead to the development of esophageal varices and portal hypertensive gastropathy and eventually hemorrhage. Ascites may require large volume paracentesis and can be further complicated by spontaneous bacterial peritonitis (SBP) [13]. As portal blood is shunted away from the liver and ammonia is insufficiently cleared from the circulation, hepatic encephalopathy develops. Other complications of ESLD include hepatorenal syndrome (HRS), hepatopulmonary syndrome, portopulmonary syndrome, protein malnutrition and muscle wasting, and severe weakness and fatigue. Identifying and managing patients with decompensated cirrhosis or fulminant hepatic failure who may be candidates for orthotopic liver transplant (OLT) is a complex process, with interprofessional collaboration between medical and surgical services. For patients who are hospitalized with decompensated cirrhosis and who undergo a transplantation evaluation while in the hospital, coordinated care involving the transplant and critical care teams is crucial to facilitate candidate evaluation and selection, and to optimize care in the pretransplantation period.

Causes of Chronic Liver Disease

A variety of chronic liver diseases account for the majority of indications for liver transplantation, as compared with transplants for acute liver disease. The most common causes of chronic liver disease in North America include alcohol use, hepatitis C virus (HCV) infection, and nonalcoholic steatohepatitis (NASH). Autoimmune hepatitis may also lead to cirrhosis, primarily in women, and may develop either acutely or over a period of years [14]. Cholestatic disorders are also an important cause of chronic liver disease. In adults, the most common cholestatic causes of chronic liver disease are primary biliary cirrhosis (PBC) and primary sclerosing cholangitis (PSC). In children, biliary atresia is the most common cause of cholestatic liver disease. Metabolic diseases that can cause chronic liver injury and cirrhosis include hereditary hemochromatosis, α_1-antitrypsin deficiency, and Wilson disease [15].

Hepatocellular carcinoma (HCC) may develop as a complication of cirrhosis from any cause, but is most commonly seen in patients with hepatitis B virus (HBV) infection, HCV infection, hemochromatosis, and tyrosinemia. The best transplantation candidates are those with a single lesion less than 5 cm in size or with no more than three lesions, the largest no greater than 3 cm in size (known as the Milan criteria). Transplantation of patients with HCC lesions outside of these criteria is usually associated with higher recurrence rates, although some centers have shown acceptable 5-year survival in patients that have tumors that slightly exceed the Milan criteria [16,17]. Other diseases that may lead to chronic liver failure that are potentially amenable to treatment with a transplant include Budd–Chiari and polycystic liver disease.

In order to determine the cause of ESLD, if not already known, and to begin the liver transplant evaluation process, a comprehensive laboratory evaluation is performed, to identify the etiology of cirrhosis, to determine the presence of comorbid conditions, to rule out active infectious processes requiring treatment before transplantation, and to guide vaccination strategies.

Causes of Fulminant Hepatic Failure

Fulminant hepatic failure (FHF) is defined as the development of hepatic encephalopathy and profound coagulopathy rapidly after the onset of initial symptoms, such as jaundice, in patients without preexisting liver disease. UNOS criteria for FHF (OPTN Policy 9.1.A) include *all* of the following:

1. age at least 18 years old at the time of registration for transplant, *and*
2. life expectancy without a liver transplant of less than 7 days *and at least one of the following conditions*:
   a. acute decompensated Wilson Disease *or*
   b. fulminant liver failure, without preexisting liver disease and currently in the ICU, defined as the onset of hepatic encephalopathy within 8 weeks of the first symptoms of liver disease, and has *at least one of the following* criteria:
      i. ventilator dependency
      ii. requiring dialysis, continuous venovenous hemofiltration (CVVH), or continuous venovenous hemodialysis (CVVHD)
      iii. has an international normalized ratio (INR) greater than 2.0

Alternative criteria for FHF include the King's College Criteria, which are listed in Table 58.2.

The most common causes of FHF in the Western world include acetaminophen overdose, acute viral hepatitis, various drugs and hepatotoxins, and Wilson disease; often, however, no cause is identified [18]. Treatment consists of appropriate critical care support and providing patients with time for spontaneous recovery. The prognosis for spontaneous recovery depends on the patients' age (those younger than 10 and older than 40 years have a poor prognosis), the underlying cause, and the severity of liver injury (as indicated by degree of hepatic encephalopathy, coagulopathy, and kidney dysfunction) [19,20]. A subset of patients may have delayed onset of hepatic decompensation that occurs 8 weeks to 6 months after the onset of symptoms. This condition is often referred to as subacute hepatic failure; these patients rarely recover without a transplant.

TABLE 58.2

King's College Criteria for ALF [20]

Acetaminophen-induced ALF

1. Strongly consider OLT listing if arterial lactate >3.5 mmol/L after early fluid resuscitation
2. List for OLT if pH <7.3 or arterial lactate >3 mmol/L after adequate fluid resuscitation
3. List for OLT if, within a 24-h period, all of the following are present: presence of grade 3 or 4 hepatic encephalopathy and INR >6.5 and creatinine >3.4 mg/dL

Non-acetaminophen-induced ALF

1. List for OLT if INR >6.5 (with encephalopathy present, irrespective of grade)
2. List for OLT if any three of the following (with encephalopathy present, irrespective of grade):
   - Age <10 or >40 y
   - Jaundice for >7 d before development of encephalopathy
   - INR > 3.5
   - Serum bilirubin > 17.6 mg/dL
   - Unfavorable etiology (Wilson Disease, idiosyncratic drug reaction, seronegative hepatitis)

ALF, acute liver failure; OLT, orthotopic liver transplant; INR, international normalized ratio.

MELD and PELD

The severity of illness and prognosis of patients with chronic liver disease can be estimated by a variety of scoring models, including the Childs–Pugh–Turcotte score and the MELD score. The latter is now widely used in the United States for the allocation of organs. It is based on a predicted 3-month mortality for patients awaiting a liver transplant and uses three laboratory values to generate a score that determines priority for liver transplantation. The three laboratory values used are serum bilirubin, serum creatinine, and INR.

For pediatric patients, the scoring system is somewhat different. The PELD (pediatric ESLD) score is calculated on the basis of the following factors: serum bilirubin, albumin, and INR, the age of the patient (additional points if the patient is <1 year old), and growth trajectory (additional points if the patient has growth failure) [21]. MELD and PELD calculators can be readily found online, including on the OPTN website (http://optn.transplant.hrsa.gov/converge/resources/MeldPeldCalculator.asp?index=98).

Contraindications for Transplant

Absolute contraindications to liver transplantation are few and have decreased with time. There are no specific age or weight limits for recipients. Contraindications include irreversible cardiac or pulmonary disease, uncontrolled active systemic infection and active extra-hepatic malignancy. HCC patients with metastatic disease, obvious vascular invasion, or significant tumor burden are not good transplant candidates. Patients with other types of extra-hepatic malignancy should be deferred for at least 5 years after completing curative therapy before a transplant is attempted.

Currently in the United States, the most common contraindication to a liver transplant is ongoing, active substance abuse. Before considering patients for a transplant, most centers require a documented period of abstinence, demonstration of compliant behavior, and willingness to pursue a chemical dependency program.

Unique to patients with chronic liver disease, a transplant may be contraindicated in the presence of severe treatment-resistant porto-pulmonary syndrome or pulmonary hypertension. Hepatopulmonary syndrome is characterized by impaired gas exchange, resulting from intrapulmonary arteriovenous shunts. These shunts may lead to severe hypoxemia, especially when patients are in the upright position (orthodeoxia). A transplant may be contraindicated if intrapulmonary shunting is severe, as manifested by hypoxemia that is only partially improved with high inspired oxygen concentrations. Pulmonary hypertension (mean pulmonary artery pressure >25 mm Hg in the setting of portal hypertension) is seen in a small proportion of patients with established cirrhosis. Its exact cause is unknown [22]. Diagnosing pulmonary hypertension pretransplant is critical, because major surgical procedures in the presence of irreversible pulmonary hypertension are associated with a very high risk of mortality. The initial screening is usually performed with transthoracic Doppler echocardiography (TTE), which can estimate pulmonary arterial systolic pressure when tricuspid regurgitation is present. TTE presents a sensitivity of 97% and a specificity of 77% in diagnosing pulmonary hypertension in the setting of liver failure. In patients with elevated pulmonary arterial systolic pressure (>50 mm Hg), a more invasive assessment (right heart catheterization) is recommended. It has been shown that perioperative mortality is directly proportional to the mean pulmonary artery pressure (mPAP) and pulmonary vascular resistance. For these reasons, most transplant centers consider a mPAP greater than 35 mm Hg to be an absolute contraindication for transplant. If the mPAP can be lowered below that value using medications (epoprostenol, sildenafil), the patient can still be considered for transplant [22].

Another absolute contraindication for liver transplantation, in case of acute liver failure, is the presence of unresponsive cerebral edema with sustained elevation of intracranial pressure (>50 mm Hg) and a persistent decrease in cerebral perfusion pressure (<40 mm Hg).

INTRAOPERATIVE MANAGEMENT

The liver transplant operation itself may be divided into three phases: recipient hepatectomy, anhepatic phase, and reperfusion. The recipient hepatectomy phase involves mobilizing of the recipient's diseased liver in preparation for its removal. Adequate exposure is crucial for the safety of the procedure. The most commonly used incision is a bi-subcostal incision with upper midline extension. This allows for sufficient exposure of the liver hilum, inferior vena cava (IVC), and most of the abdominal aorta, in case access is needed during the procedure. The initial step in hepatectomy includes dissection of the hepatoduodenal ligament. Branches of hepatic artery and the common bile duct are ligated and transected close to the liver. The portal vein is then isolated. There are two major approaches to recipient hepatectomy; the conventional technique entails removal of the hepatic portion of the native IVC and replacing it with the donor IVC. This requires temporary interruption of portal and inferior caval flow, causing decreased venous return to the heart. Many centers routinely employ a venovenous bypass (VVB) system during this time: blood is drawn from the lower body and bowels via a cannula in the common femoral vein and portal vein, and returned through a central venous cannula in the upper body. Potential advantages of bypass include improved hemodynamic stability, reduction of bleeding and bowel edema from an engorged portal system, and avoidance of elevated venous pressures in the renal veins. However, many centers selectively use VVB for patients without portal hypertension or for those patients who demonstrate hemodynamic instability with a trial of caval clamping. The added complexity of VVB combined with its potential complications, which include air embolism, thromboembolism, hypothermia, hemodilution, cannula and incision-related morbidity, trauma to vessels, and incremental costs, has led to the development of the cava preserving technique. Here, the liver is dissected off the IVC, and all the short hepatic veins entering the IVC are individually ligated and transected. The main hepatic veins (right, middle, and left) are then isolated and transected after placement of a vascular clamp. Although use of either technique is mainly dictated by the preference of individual surgeon, a recent randomized study did demonstrate increased risk of posttransplant renal dysfunction using the conventional technique [23].

Given the presence of existing coagulopathy and portal hypertension associated intra- and retroperitoneal varices within the recipient, the hepatectomy may be very challenging and provoke excessive blood loss. Rapid infusion devices and use of intraoperative cell salvage machines are therefore extremely helpful. Liver transplantation is, by necessity, a team effort. Good communication between the surgeons and the anesthesia team is imperative throughout the case.

Once the in- and outflow of the liver are obstructed, the recipient liver is removed and the patient is considered anhepatic. At this time, the majority of the bleeding has subsided and the induction immunosuppression is administered. Next, the donor liver is anastomosed to the appropriate structures, to place the new liver in an orthotopic position. The suprahepatic caval anastomosis is performed first, followed by the infrahepatic cava. In the case of the piggyback technique, the donor's suprahepatic cava is anastomosed to the recipient's confluence of the hepatic veins. Once the portal vein anastomosis is performed, the caval and portal clamps are removed, allowing reperfusion of the new liver. The hepatic artery is then anastomosed.

The reperfusion phase may be associated with dramatic changes in the patient's hemodynamics, with hypotension and the potential for serious cardiac arrhythmia. Many centers routinely rinse the graft through the portal vein prior to reperfusion to remove excessive potassium and accumulated metabolites from the graft, in order to reduce the risk of postreperfusion syndrome. Although there are no standard rinsing protocols [24], we routinely use cold lactated Ringer solution. Furthermore, severe coagulopathy may also develop because of the release of natural anticoagulants from the ischemic liver or active fibrinolysis. Clot firmness, measured by thromboelastometry, is an excellent tool in the assessment of intraoperative coagulopathy and helps to guide treatment. Fresh frozen plasma, platelet concentrate, and fibrinogen are often needed to correct the postreperfusion coagulopathy [25].

For pediatric patients (particularly infants and small children), the chance of finding a size-matched cadaver graft may be very small; the vast majority of cadaver donors are adults. Reduced-size liver transplants, living related liver transplants, and split-liver transplants are used to size-adjust the donor liver to the recipient body.

For living donor (LD) liver transplantation, the recipient operation is not greatly different from whole-organ deceased donor liver transplants. The recipient hepatectomy is performed in cava preserving fashion. The LD graft typically has a single hepatic vein that is anastomosed to the recipient's right hepatic vein orifice or directly anastomosed to the IVC. Furthermore, the graft often has segmental veins (segments 5 and 8 in case of right lobe graft) that may require reconstruction to ensure adequate outflow and avoid venous congestion. Many centers perform porto-systemic shunts in all or selected patients, in order to protect the partial graft against high portal flow and pressure, which can increase the risk of hepatic artery thrombosis. Inflow to the graft can be reestablished by anastomosing the donor's portal vein and hepatic artery branch to the corresponding structures in the recipient. Bile duct anastomosis is performed between the graft's hepatic duct(s) and the patient's common bile duct or hepatic duct branches. Alternatively, a Roux-en-Y hepaticojejunostomy can be used for biliary drainage.

POSTOPERATIVE MANAGEMENT

The postoperative course after liver transplant can range from very straightforward to extremely challenging. Several factors influence the pace and progression of recovery; among the most important ones are the preoperative status of the patient (MELD score, presence of hepatorenal syndrome, hepatopulmonary syndrome, and malnutrition), graft quality (graft size, degree of steatosis, ischemic insult and ischemia–reperfusion injury), and development of postoperative complications. Early postoperative care for all liver recipients includes: (1) initial resuscitation and supportive care for the recovery of major organ systems; (2) assessment of the graft function and institution of immunosuppression; and (3) monitoring and treatment of postoperative complications.

Initial Resuscitation and Recovery of Major Organ Systems

Transplant surgery typically provokes a major physiologic stress to otherwise very sick patients. Patients with ESLD often have portal hypertension, coagulopathy, thrombocytopenia, and dysfunction involving organ systems other than the liver. The surgery itself causes rapid hemodynamic changes, massive fluid shifts, and alterations in electrolyte and acid–base balances. Hence, patients are usually kept under sedation, mechanically ventilated, and closely monitored in an intensive care setting for several hours following transplantation. This delay in extubation is intended to achieve and maintain adequate equilibrium in all organ systems in a highly controlled setting, while the newly grafted liver supersedes the previously dysfunctional cirrhotic liver.

When the patient is hemodynamically stable and sufficient liver function has been established, sedation is discontinued and the patient is allowed to regain consciousness. Once the patient demonstrates ability to protect his/her airway and maintain sufficient ventilation and oxygenation, the endotracheal tube is removed. Adequate fluid management, respiratory physiotherapy, incentive spirometry, and early ambulation will help to reduce the risk of respiratory complications.

The functions of the heart and liver are closely related. Chronic heart failure can cause liver dysfunction owing to congestion; similarly, certain conditions that lead to cirrhosis, such as chronic alcohol abuse and hemochromatosis, can also affect the heart. The state of cirrhosis itself impacts the heart as well [26]. A study of a cohort of 403 liver transplant recipients revealed 7% risk of myocardial infarction within the first 30 days posttransplant [27]. To minimize this risk, continuous hemodynamic surveillance is recommended; ECG and blood pressure monitoring through an arterial line, volume monitoring by use of a pulmonary artery catheter, transesophageal echocardiography or pulse dye densitometry should be considered. Information obtained should be used to ensure adequate perfusion of the graft and other vital organs. The preoperative hyperdynamic circulatory state will often persist into the postoperative period. Later, as hepatic function improves, the cardiac index progressively declines, and the SVR increases toward normal values. However, the myocardial dysfunction that is often seen early in the reperfusion phase may persist, with decreased compliance and contractility of the ventricles. The cause of this myocardial depression is unclear, but may be related to the release of vasoactive substances after reperfusion of the ischemic liver and decompression of the portal circulation. The usual treatment is to optimize preload and afterload, and use inotropic agents such as dopamine or dobutamine, as indicated.

To assess for possible bleeding, serial hematocrit measurements should be taken, initially every 4 to 6 hours. Coagulation parameters (prothrombin time, partial thromboplastin time, thrombin time) need to be carefully monitored because of frequent coagulopathy, most likely related to intraoperative blood loss and temporary ischemic damage of the revascularized new liver. Other laboratory values that must be monitored include serum transaminases and serum bilirubin. Normalization of these values, along with improvement in mental status and renal function, are valuable indicators of good graft function.

Fluid management, electrolyte status, and renal function require frequent evaluation after surgery. Most liver transplant recipients have a reduced intravascular volume as a result of insufficient correction of intraoperative bleeding, ongoing postoperative hemorrhage and/or fluid shifts through third spacing. Hypovolemia should be corrected using volume resuscitation. In contrast to nontransplant critical care patients, liver transplant recipients may benefit more from blood transfusions and albumin [28]. The osmotic effect of blood and colloids promotes the shift of fluids from the extravascular space into the circulation, thereby improving organ perfusion while reducing graft congestion. Attention should be given to potassium, calcium, magnesium, phosphate, and glucose levels. Potassium may be elevated because of poor renal function, residual reperfusion effect, or immunosuppressive medications. Diuretics may be required to remove excess fluid acquired intraoperatively, but may result in hypokalemia and may not be effective in patients with acute kidney injury or for those with a history of hepatorenal syndrome. Magnesium levels should be kept above 2 mg per dL to prevent seizures, particularly in the presence of tacrolimus, which may lower the seizure threshold. Normal phosphate levels are needed for proper support of the respiratory and alimentary tracts. Patients with a partial graft, such as LD recipients, often have low phosphate levels. Marked hyperglycemia may be seen secondary to steroids and should be treated with an insulin drip. Hypoglycemia is often an indication of poor hepatic function.

Nasogastric suction can usually be discontinued during the first postoperative day; patients with a choledochojejunostomy may need more time. Some form of prophylaxis for gastrointestinal (GI) bleeding should be maintained, because the physiologic stress after a liver transplant may lead to gastric erosions and ulcerations. The GI tract can be used for nutrition early on after liver transplant, often by the second postoperative day. Patients with ESLD are frequently protein malnourished; hence, there should be a low threshold for placing a Dobbhoff tube for supplemental enteral nutrition.

As soon as the patient enters the ICU, prevention, prophylaxis, and close monitoring for possible infections should begin. Given the magnitude of the operation, the often poor pretransplant medical status, and the need for immunosuppression, it is not surprising that more than 50% of liver recipients develop some type of infection. Close attention must be given to all invasive monitoring lines, which should be removed or changed every 5 to 7 days. Aggressive clearance of respiratory secretions is needed, because the lung is a common site of postoperative infection.

Graft Function and Immunosuppression

A crucial aspect of postoperative care is the repeated evaluation of graft function, which in fact begins intraoperatively, soon after the liver is reperfused. Signs of hepatic function include good texture and color of the graft, evidence of bile production, and restoration of hemodynamic stability. Once the patient arrives in the ICU, evaluation of hepatic function is continued on the basis of clinical signs and laboratory values. The patient who rapidly awakens from anesthesia and whose mental status progressively improves likely has a well-functioning graft. Laboratory values that corroborate good function include normalization of the coagulation profile, resolution of hypoglycemia, and clearance of serum lactate. Bilirubin levels may rise for a few days before trending down. Hemolysis of transfused and recycled blood, and ischemia–reperfusion injury may lead to postoperative hyperbilirubinemia in the presence of a functioning graft. Adequate urine production and good output of bile through the biliary tube (if present) are also indicators of good graft function. Serum transaminase levels will usually rise during the first 48 to 72 hours following transplant secondary to preservation injury, and then should fall rapidly over the subsequent 24 to 48 hours.

Induction immunosuppression posttransplant varies from center to center. Many programs use a triple immunosuppressive regimen based on a calcineurin inhibitor (cyclosporine or tacrolimus), antimetabolite (mycophenolate mofetil or azathioprine), and prednisone. Some centers also use antibody induction such as antilymphocyte antibody or Rituximab [29], either for all recipients or only for those with renal dysfunction. Other humanized monoclonal antibodies such as basiliximab and daclizumab are also being used as part of steroid sparing protocols or to reduce calcineurin inhibitors dose [30]. A detailed discussion of immunosuppression for transplant recipients can be found in Chapter 63.

POSTTRANSPLANT SURGICAL COMPLICATIONS

Posttransplant surgical complications are common, given the magnitude of the surgical procedure. Surgical complications related directly to the operation include postoperative hemorrhage, problems with any of the anastomoses (five vascular and one biliary), and wound complications.

Biliary Complications

Biliary complications are considered the technical "Achilles heel" of liver transplantation because of their morbidity and frequent occurrence. They include leakage, anastomotic strictures, nonanastomotic strictures, and ampullary dysfunction. In early reports, morbidity rates of up to 50% and related mortality rates of up to 25% to 30% were reported [31,32]. Recent improvements in organ selection, preservation, immunosuppression, and standardization of the methods of biliary reconstruction have all contributed to reduce the incidence of these complications. A recent meta-analysis showed that the overall incidence of biliary stricture is 13% (12% among deceased donor liver transplant (DDLT) recipients and 19% among LDLT recipients), and the overall incidence of biliary leakage is 8.2% (7.8% among DDLT and 9.5% among LDLT). The main risk factors for biliary complications include: small size of bile ducts, hepatic artery thrombosis, older donor age, prolonged ischemic times, and immunologic response (e.g., ABO incompatibility) [33]. The incidence of strictures in DCD transplants is particularly high (20% to 40% compared with 5% in grafts from brain-dead donors), possibly owing to significant ischemic damage to the biliary ducts before transplantation [34–36].

The management of biliary complications consists of: (1) endoscopic retrograde cholangiogram (ERCP) stenting, (2) percutaneous transhepatic biliary drainage (PTBD), (3) surgical revision, and (4) retransplantation. An endoscopic strategy is the first choice for biliary complications; treatment of biliary stricture with endoscopic modalities has a success rate of 57% [33].

Biliary Leaks

Biliary leaks typically occur early and are diagnosed by the presence of a biliary fistula or on a routine cholangiography. Increased inflammatory markers or fever might occur in the case of a biloma. The majority of bile leaks are seen either in the first month after liver transplant or after T-tube removal. Late onset of bile leaks up to 6 months after transplant occasionally occurs. Risk factors for biliary leak include small size of bile ducts, discrepancy between donor and recipient ducts size, ischemic injury, and devascularization of the bile duct.

T-tube removal is a common cause of biliary leak and is reported to occur in 5% to 33% of cases [33]. Because of this concern, many transplant centers have stopped using T-tubes, although this change in practice has not been demonstrated to decrease the incidence of biliary leakage (4.7% vs. 6.3% with and without a T-tube, respectively) [33].

The management of biliary leaks varies according to the location and the severity. Conservative treatment can be attempted in selected cases when there is a small leak at the cut surface of split-liver grafts or grafts from LDs. Most biliary leaks can be treated by ERCP papillotomy and biliary stenting. In some cases, a primary surgical revision is indicated, particularly with early leaks (<1 to 2 weeks after liver transplant), large defects, or if bile duct necrosis is suspected. Surgical intervention is also indicated after failure of endoscopic therapy. Duct-to-duct repairs are not always feasible and a bilioenteric anastomosis is often required, especially in the case of periductal infection and/or bile duct necrosis [37].

Biliary Strictures

Biliary strictures can be anastomotic and nonanastomotic. Anastomotic strictures are much more common and are associated with technical failure. Biliary stenoses often result in jaundice, increased cholestatic enzymes, and fever. Ultrasound examination is less sensitive after liver transplantation, since severe dilatation of the intrahepatic bile ducts is absent in >60% of patients with anastomotic stenosis, whereas an ERCP is able to detect the cause of biliary obstruction in 95% and the site of bile leaks in 90% of cases [37]. The use of a T-tube to prevent anastomotic biliary strictures is controversial. However, a recent meta-analysis indicated that the incidence of biliary stricture was 9.7% with a T-tube and 12.5% without a T-tube [33].

Nonanastomotic strictures, also called ischemic-type biliary lesions (ITBL), or ischemic cholangiopathy, are the most troublesome biliary complication after liver transplant. ITBL is a radiologic diagnosis, characterized by intrahepatic strictures and dilatations on a cholangiogram, in the absence of hepatic artery thrombosis. The exact mechanisms are not known, but are most likely multifactorial [38,39]. The risk of ischemic cholangiopathy in grafts from DCD donors is 10 times higher than for brain-dead donors [36]. Although the risk of ITBL is directly correlated with the degree of ischemia, currently there is no way to predict which grafts will display ITBL, and no pharmacologic approaches to prevent the development of ITBL. Available therapeutic approaches (endoscopic dilation/stenting, hepatico-jejuno anastomosis, liver resection, or retransplantation) are performed only when complications are already present. Eventually, up to 50% of patients with ITBL will die or require retransplantation [40].

The treatment of anastomotic stenosis is easier and typically achieved by ERCP repetitive balloon dilatation (every 2 to 3 months) and stenting. Severe and long anastomotic strictures are usually not amenable to endoscopic treatment, requiring surgical correction instead. For patients with bilioenteric anastomotic strictures, balloon dilatation is performed percutaneously (PTC).

ERCP and balloon dilation with or without stenting is the first choice of treatment for biliary stricture in the majority of centers (58%) and is indicated for 83% of patients. The success rate is approximately 57%.

Sphincter of Oddi Dysfunction/Papillary Stenosis

Outflow obstruction at the papillary region occurs in 2% to 7% of patients after liver transplantation and is thought to be associated with manipulation, denervation of the recipient bile duct, and inflammation or scarring of the sphincter of Oddi [41]. Clinical manifestations include increased cholestatic parameters and biliary dilatation. Endoscopic sphincterotomy is the treatment of choice and is effective in the vast majority of patients [42,43].

Vascular Complications

Vascular complications following liver transplantation include bleeding, thromboembolic events, and anastomotic failures (stenosis and thrombosis). Patients with ESLD are concurrently coagulopathic, hypercoagulable, and hyperfibrinolitic [44].

Bleeding

Despite advances in surgical technique and anesthetic management, extensive bleeding is still very common during and after liver transplantation. Bleeding negatively affects outcomes and the cost-effectiveness of liver transplantation [45–48]. Because of changes in procoagulant and anticoagulant pathways with cirrhosis, cirrhotic patients are at increased risk both of bleeding and of thromboembolic events. The most common source of bleeding after liver transplantation is from the vascular anastomosis, but it can also arise from varices, the retroperitoneum, or the liver anastomoses. The incidence of posttransplantation abdominal bleeding, defined as any hemorrhage requiring radiologic intervention or laparotomy within the first month, is 9%, occurring at a mean of 6.1 days (range, 1 to 21 days) posttransplantation. Active bleeding is controlled by endovascular interventional techniques for 39%, by surgical ligation or vascular reconstruction for 46%, or by sequential combinations of endovascular intervention and surgery for 15% [49].

Important risk factors for bleeding include SLT, retransplantation, previous abdominal operations, severe portal hypertension, and thrombocytopenia. The risk of bleeding can be minimized by meticulous surgical dissection and bleeding control. The use of procoagulants remains controversial [50–52].

Thromboembolic Events

Despite prolonged coagulation times and thrombocytopenia associated with ESLD, formation of thrombi in the circulation occurs more frequently during liver transplantation than during any other type of major surgery. For a long time, there has been a dogma that cirrhosis is associated with bleeding tendency. Recent literature has challenged this dogma, showing that the coagulation system of cirrhotic patients is dysfunctional and also associated with hypercoagulability tendency [53–55]. The incidence of deep vein thrombosis (DVT) or pulmonary embolism (PE) in cirrhotic patients is 0.5%, despite 21% of patients receiving some form of DVT prophylaxis [55]. In ESLD, the low number of platelets and reduced synthesis of procoagulant factors are compensated by deficient hepatic clearance of activated procoagulants and reduced hepatic synthesis of anticoagulant proteins (protein S and C, antithrombin III, heparin cofactor II, and α_2-macroglobulin), low levels of plasminogen, and elevated levels of von Willebrand factor and factor VIII [44,53,55].

In addition to the inherent hypercoagulability associated with ESLD, thromboembolism is more common during liver transplantation owing to surgical factors associated with this procedure, including the excessive activation of the coagulation system secondary to injury to a large capillary bed during hepatectomy, venous stasis during clamping of the portal vein and IVC, ischemic injury to the intestines, release of coagulation activators from the graft, and massive blood transfusion or administration of blood products [56]. Other factors that may contribute to thromboembolic complications include concomitant cancer (HCC), venovenous bypass, and use of vascular catheters [44].The overall incidence of massive embolism associated with liver transplantation ranges from 1.5% to 6.2% [44]. Although the estimated incidence of significant pulmonary embolism (PE) or intracardiac thrombosis among liver transplant recipients is low, these complications are potentially fatal, and therefore of great clinical relevance [44,56]. Thromboembolic events can occur during any phase of the transplantation (37% during reperfusion vs. 30% pre-anhepatic vs. 33% anhepatic) [57].

Vascular Anastomosis Failures

Although bleeding, stenosis, and thrombosis can arise at any of the vascular anastomoses, hepatic artery thrombosis (HAT) and portal vein thrombosis (PVT) are the most common.

HAT. The consequences of HAT are often life threatening, causing interruption of the graft blood supply, leading to early graft loss, long-term dysfunction, or patient death. Early HAT (within the first 3 weeks) commonly causes graft failure. Even if the graft is not lost, there will be long-term graft dysfunction. The biliary ducts are exclusively supplied by arterial blood [58], and interruption of arterial blood leads to ischemic cholangiopathy, which leads to biliary strictures, abscesses, biliary cast formation, and potentially sepsis [36]. HAT is reported to complicate 4% to 15% of OLTs and is generally more frequent after pediatric liver transplantation and LD liver transplantation [59].

Factors associated with HAT include small diameter (pediatric and LD graft), dissection of the hepatic arterial wall, anastomotic technical failures (leading to kinking, stenosis, or intima exposure), atherosclerosis (older donor age), and celiac stenosis or compression by the median arcuate ligament. Aberrant donor or recipient arterial anatomy, complex backtable arterial reconstruction of the allograft, and nonsurgical causes, such as transarterial chemoembolization, and high-resistance microvascular arterial outflow caused by severe ischemia–reperfusion injury, CMV infection, hypotension, hypercoagulable disorder, rejection are also important considerations [59–63].

Treatment of these complications has traditionally involved reexploration, surgical thrombectomy, and anastomotic revision. Failure of anastomotic revision usually requires retransplantation as a life-saving procedure. Early HAT should be treated with surgical exploration and thrombectomy. More recently, catheter-based and medical anticoagulant or thrombolytic interventions are available, but the results are inferior. However, up to 50% graft salvage rates using catheter-based treatment of HAT have been reported [64]. A single center experience with 4,200 liver transplants showed that graft salvage after early HAT requiring surgical revision, thrombectomy, and re-anastomosis was only 10.5%. Among all patients experiencing HAT, retransplantation was required in 75% of patients [59].

PVT. This complicates 3% to 7% of liver transplantations and, similar to HAT, significantly reduces both graft and patient survival [65,66]. Factors associated with posttransplant PVT include technical issues, preexisting PVT requiring thromboendovenectomy at the time of transplantation, small portal vein size (<5 mm), previous splenectomy, and the use of venous conduits for portal vein reconstruction. Presentation of PVT can include portal hypertension with gastrointestinal bleeding, ascites, elevated transaminases, and acute graft failure [59,67,68]. PVT occurs early for 65% of patients, and late for 35% [59]. Retransplantation for PVT is not always technically possible because it requires patent mesenteric graft inflow to provide hepatotrophic factors to the graft. In patients with extensive and organized PVT, this is not always possible, even with construction of a venous conduit [59,69,70].

Wound Complications

Wound complications are common following liver transplantation and may contribute to significant morbidity in the liver transplant recipient. Wound complications include infections and hematomas. Conventional risk factors for wound infections are all present in liver transplant recipients, including longer operative times, contamination with bowel or biliary contents, need for transfusion of blood products, poor nutritional status prior to transplantation, and steroid administration for immunosuppression to prevent rejection. Wound infections typically develop after the first week following liver transplantation, often presenting with fever, chills, erythema, and purulent drainage from the wound. Given the presence of immunosuppression, signs and symptoms of infection may be subtle, with the absence of typical features of inflammation. Management includes opening the wound to allow appropriate drainage of collections, frequent dressing changes, and allowing healing by secondary intention. Intravenous antibiotics may be necessary in the presence of significant cellulitis, deeper involvement, or systemic symptoms. Complicated skin and soft tissue infections, including necrotizing fasciitis, have been reported and require rapid, aggressive debridement together with appropriate selection of intravenous antibiotics.

POSTTRANSPLANT MEDICAL COMPLICATIONS

Medical complications following liver transplantation are quite common, considering the comorbidities and often poor functional status of transplant candidates at the time of transplantation, together with the impact of significant immunosuppression. Medical complications in the early posttransplant period may involve almost any organ system (Table 58.3).

Nontechnical Graft Dysfunction

In addition to the surgical complications listed earlier, hepatic graft dysfunction may occur early following transplant, unrelated to technical factors. Causes of nontechnical liver dysfunction after transplant include primary nonfunction (PNF) or primary dysfunction (PDF) of the graft, acute rejection, and infection.

Primary Nonfunction and Primary Dysfunction

Hepatic PNF/PDF is one of the most serious complications in the immediate postoperative period, and is defined as a severe form of reperfusion injury that results in irreversible graft failure without underlying surgical complication or rejection [71]. Early detection is key to improving outcomes. PNF is the most common reason for early retransplantation, occurring in up to 5.8% of DDLTs, and conferring a mortality rate of approximately 80% in the absence of retransplantation. Unrecognized PNF may result in recipient death within a week of transplantation. Several factors have been described in association with PNF, including donor gender (female donors), advanced donor age (>50 years), donor hospital length of stay in the ICU before organ procurement (>3 days), macrosteatosis (>30%), prolonged cold ischemia time (CIT) (>12 hours), DCD donor status, the duration in the operating room, and retransplantation [72]. PNF should be considered in recipients who have signs of continued poor hepatic function after admission to the ICU,

TABLE 58.3

Posttransplant Medical Complications

Nontechnical graft dysfunction
Primary nonfunction/dysfunction
Acute rejection
Infection
Neurologic complications
Altered levels of consciousness
Seizures
Cerebrovascular accidents
CNS infections (meningitis, meningoencephalitis, brain abscess)
CPM
Sepsis
Medications (opioids, sedatives)
Posterior reversible encephalopathy syndrome (PRES)
Uremia owing to renal failure
Hypoxic–ischemic encephalopathy
Ischemic or hemorrhagic CVAs
Sequelae of pretransplant comorbidities (hepatic encephalopathy, substance abuse, multiorgan failure)
Cardiovascular complications
PRS with malignant cardiac arrhythmias
Postoperative myocardial ischemia
Pulmonary complications
Infectious
Pneumonia (ventilator associated and/or healthcare-associated)
Noninfectious
Fluid overload/pulmonary edema
Decreased respiratory drive (sedatives, narcotics), atelectasis
Complications associated with mechanical ventilation
ARDS
Phrenic nerve injury
Persistent HPS
Renal complications
Hepatorenal syndrome
Acute tubular necrosis (secondary to hemodynamic compromise during surgery)
CNI toxicity
Sepsis, multiorgan dysfunction
Drug-related nephrotoxicity owing to drugs other than CNIs
Gastrointestinal complications
Technical complications
Upper GI bleeding
Peptic ulcer disease
Bleeding from esophageal varices
Stress gastritis
Hemobilia after liver biopsy
Bleeding from Roux-en-Y anastomosis
Lower GI bleeding
Colitis (cytomegalovirus, *Clostridium difficile*)
Noninfectious ulcers (steroids)
Bowel perforation or unrecognized injury to the bowel wall during transplantation

(*continued*)

TABLE 58.3

Posttransplant Medical Complications (*continued*)

Infectious complications (vary depending upon period posttransplant) [86]
First 30 d posttransplant
Nosocomial infections (bacterial and fungal)
Wound infections, including superficial, deep, and organ space infections
Urinary tract infections
Pneumonia
Biliary tract infections including infected bilomas
Sepsis
Invasive fungal infections (*Candida* spp.)
Previously undiagnosed pretransplant infections
C. difficile colitis
Donor-derived infections (LCMV, rabies, West Nile Virus, *Trypanosoma cruzi*, HIV)
Between 1 and 6 mo posttransplant (incidence varies depending on use of prophylaxis)
Biliary tract complications (infected bilomas, cholangitis, hepatic abscess)
Reactivation of latent viral infections (CMV, HBV, HCV, HSV, VZV)
Reactivation or acquisition of opportunistic infections (including fungal pathogens)
Community-acquired infections (including respiratory viral infections)
C. difficile colitis
Reactivation of latent infections (tuberculosis, strongyloides, schistosomiasis)
Later than 6 mo posttransplant
Community-acquired infections
Late-onset viral infections
Reactivation or acquisition of opportunistic infections (including fungal pathogens)

ARDS, acute respiratory distress syndrome; CNI, Calcineurin inhibitor; CNS, central nervous system; CPM, central pontine myelinolysis; CVA, cerebrovascular accidents; HPS, hepatopulmonary syndrome; PRS, postreperfusion syndrome

including persistent hemodynamic instability, worsening acidosis, persistent coagulopathy, poor bile production, worsening renal function, persistent hypoglycemia, or persistent altered mental status. There is no effective medical treatment for PNF other than supportive care; ultimately, retransplantation may be required for survival. Outcomes are typically better if retransplantation is performed as early as possible, before the development of significant multiorgan dysfunction [73].

Rejection

Graft rejection affects up to 30% of liver transplant recipients at some point posttransplantation. A detailed discussion of the diagnosis and management of graft rejection is addressed in Chapter 65. Rejection typically manifests as elevation of serum bilirubin and/or transaminase levels, occasionally with mild fever and malaise. The differential diagnosis of rejection includes vascular thrombosis, bile leaks, and underlying infection. Biopsy is required to confirm a diagnosis of rejection. Mild episodes may be managed by increasing the baseline level of immunosuppression, whereas moderate or severe rejection episodes usually require treatment with a pulse of high-dose intravenous corticosteroids.

Neurologic Complications

Neurologic complications are relatively common posttransplant, affecting 15% to 30% of liver transplant recipients. Neurologic issues may develop at any time in the posttransplant period, and include alterations in level of consciousness, seizures, cerebrovascular accidents, central nervous system (CNS) infections, and central pontine myelinolysis (CPM). Pretransplant conditions, such as hepatic encephalopathy, sepsis, multiorgan failure, and substance abuse, may also have an impact on posttransplant recovery [74].

Alterations of the level of consciousness may result from medications administered for pain control or sedation, with reduced clearance due to impaired liver and/or renal function. Immunosuppressants may also contribute, particularly the calcineurin inhibitors (CNIs), such as tacrolimus and cyclosporine. The CNIs, and rarely the mTor inhibitors (sirolimus, everolimus), may cause posterior reversible encephalopathy syndrome (PRES), which develops in <1% of solid-organ transplant recipients and can manifest with headaches, alterations in consciousness, and/or seizures. Brain magnetic resonance imaging (MRI) often has typical findings, specifically, increased T2-signal in the posterior white matter. PRES most commonly develops in the first 2 months after transplant and is managed by switching immunosuppressive medications and providing supportive care [75].

Metabolic encephalopathy may persist following transplantation owing to primary graft dysfunction or nonfunction (PDF/PNF), pretransplant metabolic derangements that are slow to resolve, medications (as described above), CNS infections, evolving sepsis, or uremia due to renal failure. Significant perioperative hypotension may cause hypoxic–ischemic encephalopathy, or even ischemic cerebrovascular accidents (CVAs). The latter are not common after liver transplantation, occurring in 2% to 4% of transplant recipients. Older recipients or those with diabetes mellitus may be at increased risk for CVAs [74].

Central pontine myelinolysis (CPM) or extrapontine myelinolysis (EPM) may develop among 1% to 2% of liver transplant recipients, in the setting of significant fluid shifts and excessively rapid correction of hyponatremia [74]. Factors that may confer increased risk include pretransplant hyponatremia or severe hepatic dysfunction prior to transplant. Manifestations include decreased levels of consciousness and spasticity. MRI of the brain may reveal characteristic T2 hyperintensity in the central pons.

Acute changes in mental status or development of focal neurologic findings should prompt urgent imaging to rule out a CNS hemorrhage or infection. Coagulopathy due to hepatic dysfunction pretransplantation may occasionally result in intracranial bleeding. Immunosuppressive medications confer an increased risk for meningitis, meningoencephalitis, or brain abscess. Early posttransplant, donor-derived infections must be considered (including lymphocytic choriomeningitis, a viral infection transmitted from rodents), as well as reactivation of infections in the recipient, including viruses such as herpes simplex virus (HSV), cytomegalovirus (CMV), and varicella zoster virus (VZV). The risk of CNS infection increases after the first month following transplantation, with etiologies reflecting both new exposures and reactivation of latent infections acquired via travel or endemic exposures. Potential etiologies include cryptococcal meningitis or other endemic mycoses, nocardiosis, and listeriosis. A detailed discussion of infections following transplantation is included below and in Chapter 65.

Posttransplant seizures have variable etiologies, depending on the timing of onset following transplantation. In the first few weeks posttransplant, seizures are typically the result of metabolic derangements or adverse effects from medications. However, it is crucial to also consider and rule out other causes, including a cerebrovascular accident, CNS bleeding, or infectious processes (meningitis, encephalitis, or an intracranial abscess). CNS imaging should be obtained routinely in patients with new-onset seizures, to rule out a mass lesion or bleed.

Cardiovascular Complications

Cardiovascular (CV) complications may develop among liver recipients with previously diagnosed cardiac disease, but may also occur among those not known to have preexisting cardiac comorbidities. As the mean age of liver transplant recipients increases, strategies to reduce the risk of cardiac events and optimization of medical management prior to liver transplant are essential, in order to minimize the risk of CV complications in the posttransplantation period. The hemodynamic and metabolic profiles associated with liver disease differ from those seen among other transplant candidates, and alter the risk and manifestations of CV events following transplantation. These differences include lower systemic blood pressure, lower peripheral vascular resistance, lower serum cholesterol levels, and relatively less atherosclerotic vascular disease [76]. Despite this lowered overall risk, CV events are reported to be a significant cause of morbidity and mortality among liver transplant recipients, contributing to 12% to 16% of deaths posttransplantation in the United States. CV-attributable mortality is usually late onset, beyond the first year posttransplantation [77].

The period after liver reperfusion is a time when the majority of intraoperative cardiac complications develop. Transient hypotension during liver reperfusion may cause a postreperfusion syndrome (PRS), which is defined as a decrease in mean arterial pressure (MAP) of at least 30% for 1 minute, during the first 5 minutes following reperfusion. The drop in MAP is accompanied by a decrease in myocardial contractility (decreased heart rate, increased CVP and PCWP) and a drop in SVR. PRS occurs in up to 30% of liver transplant recipients, and is likely because of multiple factors, including hyperkalemia and acidosis. In addition, factors released from the ischemic graft upon reperfusion, may effectively depress myocardial function. Although this phenomenon is usually transient, resolving within 5 minutes, it may have a significant and lasting impact, particularly for patients with preexisting cardiac disease. The bradycardia and hypotension may lead to cardiac arrest and malignant cardiac arrhythmias, such as ventricular tachycardia or fibrillation.

Postoperative myocardial ischemia may occur among as many as 13% of liver transplant recipients. To minimize the risk for cardiac complications, liver transplantation candidates with previously diagnosed coronary artery disease (CAD), or those with risk factors for CAD identified during the pretransplant evaluation, should be evaluated by a cardiologist prior to transplantation, so as to maximize medical management of cardiovascular risk factors. Pharmacologic cardiac stress testing is now the standard of care in the pretransplant evaluation of liver transplantation candidates who have risk factors for CAD. Transplantation candidates with positive results on pharmacologic stress testing should be referred to a cardiologist for consideration of diagnostic coronary angiography, so as to determine whether further intervention is indicated prior to transplantation.

Pulmonary Complications

Pulmonary complications in the setting of liver transplantation are quite common, reported in 40% to 47% of liver transplant recipients, and may be attributable to both infectious and noninfectious etiologies [78]. Noninfectious causes predominate during the first week posttransplant, owing to fluid shifts, fluid overload, decreased respiratory drive due to the use of sedative and narcotic medications to manage pain, and as a result of complications associated with mechanical ventilation. With increasing time following the transplant procedure, infectious pulmonary complications become more prevalent. In one study, causes of pulmonary infiltrates included pulmonary edema in 40%, pneumonia in 38%, atelectasis in 10%, and ARDS in 8% [79]. In this study, 87% of cases of pneumonia identified in the ICU setting occurred among patients who had been mechanically ventilated.

The majority of liver transplant recipients are extubated within the first 48 hours following transplantation. Recipients with prolonged hospitalizations prior to transplantation or preexisting pulmonary disease, those who are significantly malnourished at the time of transplantation, and those with significant infectious or hepatic complications posttransplant may require a prolonged course of mechanical ventilation following liver transplantation. A recent review of early respiratory complications following liver transplantation highlighted the most common preoperative risk factors for post–liver transplant pulmonary complications, including recipient age, female gender, history of tobacco use, severity of liver dysfunction, presence of pretransplantation hepatic encephalopathy, mental status changes, acute renal failure, preexisting pulmonary disease, preoperative ventilatory support, and pretransplant diabetes mellitus [78]. Preoperative mechanical ventilation is a significant risk factor owing in part to the increased risk of lower respiratory tract infection, and reflective of the severity of liver disease in the transplantation candidate, in the immediate pretransplantation period. Intraoperative risk factors for pulmonary complications are primarily related to fluid shifts and fluid overload related to resuscitation during surgery, and the abdominal surgical procedure itself, decreasing respiratory compliance and making extubation more difficult [78].

Postoperative factors associated with an increased risk for complications include the residual effects of anesthetics used during the transplantation, decreased hepatic and renal clearance of narcotic medications used to control pain, and continued fluid overload. Persistent large volume abdominal ascites may contribute to atelectasis and a 50% to 60% decrease in vital capacity. This may result in difficulty with weaning from ventilatory support and extubation [80]. While phrenic nerve recovery does occur, it can often be a prolonged process. Hepatic dysfunction, the need for reoperation/abdominal exploration for various issues, and continued poor nutritional status can all lead to a delay in weaning from mechanical ventilation.

Posttransplant pneumonia, classified as either healthcare associated and/or ventilator associated, may develop in up to 38% of liver transplant recipients. The incidence is highest between 7 and 10 days after transplantation, declining thereafter, unless additional risk factors remain. These include prolonged ventilatory support, poor nutritional status, severity of liver disease, pretransplant hospitalization, and medical comorbidities such as diabetes mellitus and preexisting pulmonary disease. Each of these factors will contribute to an increased risk of pneumonia in the posttransplantation period. If a healthcare-associated pneumonia is suspected, it is imperative to identify the causative organism, in order to tailor antimicrobial coverage appropriately. Liver transplantation candidates may be colonized with resistant nosocomial gram-negative organisms, by virtue of the frequency of their interactions with the healthcare environment, exposure to antimicrobial agents, the duration of pretransplantation hospitalization, as well as the presence of prolonged mechanical ventilatory support. Adequate sputum samples should be obtained and sent for Gram stain and culture to identify bacterial pathogens. Bronchoscopy with bronchoalveolar lavage may be necessary in order to identify a causative organism. Empiric antimicrobials should be chosen on the basis of the antibiogram of the local ICU, because the microbiology and sensitivity patterns can vary significantly between different hospitals and even between different units within a hospital.

Hepatopulmonary syndrome (HPS) is characterized by severe hypoxemia, significantly increased alveolar arterial oxygen gradient, and intrapulmonary vascular dilatations in the setting of chronic liver disease. HPS may be reversible in up to 90% of patients after liver transplantation, usually within a year following transplantation [81].

Renal Complications

The majority of liver transplantation recipients have some degree of renal dysfunction in the posttransplantation period. Renal dysfunction may be acute or chronic, with up to 10% of liver transplantation recipients requiring dialysis posttransplantation. Abnormalities may be attributable to complications from the surgical procedure itself or from the effects of transplant immunosuppression, specifically, the CNIs. Renal dysfunction may also be present prior to transplantation, for example, owing to preexisting hepatorenal syndrome, and may persist or progress after transplantation. Renal complications posttransplantation, whether new or progressive, increase transplantation-associated morbidity and may have a significant negative impact on both patient and graft survival [82].

Preexisting kidney disease owing to HRS or ATN may improve after restoration of normal hepatic function, but they may also confer a greater risk for the development of chronic kidney disease (CKD) after transplantation. Factors associated with a greater risk of progression to CKD include need for renal replacement therapy (RRT) before transplant, hemodynamic compromise during the transplant surgery, and CNI toxicity posttransplantation. Sepsis and multiorgan dysfunction during the posttransplant setting may also contribute to an increased risk for progressive renal disease. Drug-related nephrotoxicity is most commonly attributable to the CNIs (cyclosporine or tacrolimus) but may also result from other agents, including antimicrobials such as vancomycin, aminoglycosides, and amphotericin B. Individuals who were dependent on dialysis before transplant are unlikely to regain significant renal function after liver transplantation, and may be candidates for a combined liver–kidney transplant.

Management of renal dysfunction following liver transplantation, with the goal of preserving residual renal function, can be achieved with appropriate hemodynamic monitoring, maintenance of normal blood pressure through the use of resuscitation with fluids and/or blood products as indicated, and administration of antihypertensive agents as required. In addition, the use of nephrotoxic agents should be minimized.

Gastrointestinal Complications

Gastrointestinal (GI) complications are common after liver transplantation, and may result from technical complications, stress related to the postsurgical state, bleeding, or infections. Upper GI bleeding following liver transplantation may result from peptic ulcer disease, persistent bleeding from esophageal varices, or stress gastritis. Diffuse gastritis secondary to surgical stress is uncommon in the current era owing to the use of routine prophylaxis with proton pump inhibitors. Peptic ulcer disease remains a potential cause of upper GI bleeding, occurring most commonly in the first month posttransplantation, perhaps related to relatively higher doses of steroids. More unusual causes of GI bleeding include hemobilia after liver biopsy (incidence of 0.03%) and bleeding from the Roux-en-Y anastomosis in those patients who required choledochojejunostomy.

Lower GI bleeding following liver transplant is often secondary to colitis, typically owing to an infection such as CMV or *Clostridium difficile*. Noninfectious ulcers may also cause colonic bleeding, perhaps related to the effects of high-dose steroids used in induction therapy.

Bowel perforation is a devastating complication and is associated with a high mortality rate. The signs and symptoms that are typically associated with acute peritonitis, including high fever and severe abdominal pain, may be attenuated by the effects of immunosuppressive agents. Perforation may occur in the small or large bowel, the latter being associated with a higher mortality rate owing to the high risk of infection from heavy bacterial colonization of the large bowel. Unrecognized injury to the bowel wall during the transplant is uncommon, but when it occurs, it may later present as a perforation with peritonitis. Perforations may also be spontaneous; these occur more commonly in children, generally 1 to 2 weeks posttransplantation, and may be related to the effects of high-dose steroids. As with perforation in patients who have not undergone transplantation, early diagnosis with prompt reexploration and copious irrigation to decrease the degree of bacterial contamination is the best option.

Infectious Complications

Although infectious complications are common in all organ transplants, in liver transplant recipients the incidence is reported as high as 50% in some studies [86, 87]. The higher relative rates of infection in liver transplant recipients is due in part to operative factors (duration and type of surgery), the risk of biliary and enteric contamination during surgery, and the poor nutritional status and presence of medical comorbidities among patients with ESLD. Infectious complications following transplantation in general are discussed in detail in Chapter 65.

Despite the relatively higher risk of infection for liver transplant recipients, mortality rates attributable to infections have improved in recent years and are now reported as low as 10% in some series [86, 87]. Reasons for the decrease include improved posttransplant critical care, reduced use of venovenous bypass, thoughtful selection of appropriate antimicrobials, and careful titration of immunosuppression. Even with these improvements, infectious complications continue to impact patient and graft survival, hospital length of stay, and cost of care following transplantation.

Pretransplant identification of risk factors for infectious diseases, and modification of these risks when possible, can have a positive impact on outcomes. Effective prophylaxis to prevent reactivation or transmission of infection and a prompt response to the diagnosis and treatment of infections when they occur is crucial to decrease posttransplant morbidity and mortality related to infectious diseases.

Pretransplant Evaluation

The purpose of the pretransplant evaluation is to determine the risk for or presence of active or latent infectious diseases. Pretransplant serologic testing includes laboratory assessment of prior exposure to cytomegalovirus (CMV), Epstein–Barr virus (EBV), varicella zoster virus (VZV), syphilis, human immunodeficiency virus (HIV), and hepatitis viruses (A, B, and C). Latent infections that may reactivate during transplantation immunosuppression must be identified and are most optimally treated before transplantation. Pretransplant infectious disease screening should be tailored, with consideration of the travel history of the transplant candidate, and may include assessment for prior exposure to tuberculosis, strongyloides, and schistosomiasis [87].

Transplantation in the setting of untreated latent tuberculosis infection (LTBI) is reasonable; treatment of LTBI may be delayed until after transplantation if significant liver dysfunction precludes administration of medications for the treatment of LTBI or if delaying transplantation until LTBI treatment can be completed carries too high a risk of mortality for the liver transplant candidate. Vaccines for preventable infections should be administered at the time of the pretransplant evaluation, in accordance with current guidelines [87]. Active infections that require treatment before transplantation or that might delay transplantation should optimally be identified and addressed before candidate listing. Patients with ESLD have increased susceptibility to infectious complications even before transplantation, by virtue of their relative immune compromise due to cirrhosis and splenomegaly, when present. Infections that are frequently identified in patients with ESLD include spontaneous bacterial peritonitis, cholangitis, recurrent sinupulmonary infections, and more rarely, cryptococcal infection (cryptococcemia and meningitis). In cases where delaying transplant may increase the risk of mortality, it may in some cases be prudent to begin treatment of the underlying infection and then to proceed with transplantation while continuing antimicrobial treatment of the infection. Decisions such as this should be individualized, with a collaborative team approach involving the transplant team, the critical care team, and experts in infectious disease care of transplant candidates and recipients.

Perioperative Prevention of Infection

Perioperative antibiotics with activity against biliary tract pathogens are administered before surgical incision and are typically continued for up to 24 hours following transplant. The choice of agent varies by center but may include ceftriaxone, ampicillin-sulbactam, or piperacillin-tazobactam. Perioperative prophylactic strategies should be guided by the local flora that are commonly identified within the hospital, and protocols should be developed in consultation with infection control experts at the transplant center, recognizing the increasing complexity of these decisions in the setting of emerging multidrug-resistant pathogens [87]. Fluconazole may be added for 28 days to prevent the development of invasive fungal infection (IFI) for patients at increased risk for this complication [83]. Risk factors for IFI include preexisting renal dysfunction, duration of operative procedure, transfusion of significant volume of blood products during the transplantation procedure, retransplantation, abdominal or intrathoracic reoperations, cytomegalovirus infection, Roux-en-Y hepaticojejunostomy, and colonization with yeast at the time of transplantation [83,84].

Transplant recipients typically receive trimethoprim–sulfamethoxazole for 1 year or more to prevent infection due to *Pneumocystis jirovecci* (patients with sulfa allergy may receive dapsone or atovaquone as alternatives) and either valganciclovir (if donor or recipient is CMV IgG positive) or acyclovir (if both donor and recipient are CMV IgG negative) to prevent infection due to herpesviruses. Nystatin is provided for a short period, usually 1 to 3 months posttransplant, for those recipients who do not meet criteria for systemic antifungal prophylaxis.

Postoperative Assessment for Infection

The development of fever following liver transplantation should be thoroughly investigated to rule out infection, given the morbidity and mortality associated with a delay in treatment. The evaluation includes a comprehensive physical examination, with particular attention to the surgical wound, entry sites for indwelling catheters, and respiratory status. Liver transplant recipients, as with all solid-organ transplant recipients, develop typical postoperative complications such as line infections, pneumonias, urinary tract infections, and wound infections. The most common infections following liver transplantation are pulmonary infections, superficial incisional wound infections, and deeper, organ space intra-abdominal infections [85, 87].

As part of the initial evaluation, cultures should be obtained from blood, urine, sputum, ascitic fluid when present, and any other fluid collections identified through the clinical exam, laboratory testing, or imaging. A good-quality chest radiograph should be obtained in order to rule out a pulmonary source of the fever, understanding that plain radiography may not be sensitive enough to reveal an etiology in some patients and that chest CT may be required to more adequately assess any infiltrates present on a plain chest radiograph.

If physical examination combined with initial laboratory and radiographic evaluation does not reveal a source of infection, abdominal imaging with a CT scan may be necessary to identify fluid collections that could be a source of infection. If present, fluid collections should be sampled for Gram stain and culture. Initiation of broad-spectrum empiric antimicrobials should be considered if the recipient is febrile or has hemodynamic instability, even before a source is identified, because of the significant risk of rapid clinical decline in the setting of infection in transplant recipients. Reasonable initial coverage should include broad-spectrum antimicrobials that have activity against biliary pathogens. Coverage of multidrug-resistant organisms should be considered if there is an increased prevalence of these organisms at the transplant center. Consultation with infectious diseases physicians with expertise in transplant care and infection control is recommended to determine the optimal empiric regimen.

A detailed description of infectious complications after solid-organ transplantation is provided in Chapter 65. Infectious complications following solid-organ transplantation have been categorized as occurring early (within 1 month), between 1 and 6 months after transplant, and more than 6 months posttransplant and are dependent on the "net state of immunosuppression" of the recipient [86]. This phrase, described by Fishman, Rubin, and colleagues, refers to the intensity and duration of immunosuppression, together with host factors, that may impact risk of infection at different points in time following transplant [86].

Among liver transplant recipients, bacterial and fungal organisms are the most common causes of infection during the first month following transplant and are typically related to surgical complications, initial graft function, and recipient pretransplant comorbidities. Risk factors for early posttransplant infections include increasing duration of the transplantation surgical procedure, blood transfusions in the perioperative period, retransplantation, and surgical reexploration. Following the first month after transplant, the "net state of immunosuppression" becomes an important factor contributing to the ongoing risk for infection [86]. Opportunistic pathogens, including viral, fungal, and parasitic pathogens, are more commonly seen during this period. Administration of augmented immunosuppression to treat acute rejection episodes with either bolus high-dose steroids or antilymphocyte agents will increase the risk of infection due to opportunistic pathogens.

Bacterial infections following liver transplantation are most commonly related to the surgical wound, and may be superficial, deep, or organ-space infections. The bacterial pathogens commonly associated with surgical-site infections are from a biliary or bowel source and may complicate a biliary leak. The risk of infection from a biliary source is higher with choledochojejunostomy (CDJ) than with duct-to-duct biliary anastomosis. Wound infections may present with typical signs of infection, such as increased drainage, erythema, or fluctuance, or they may be subtle, with only minimal findings (fever, elevated white blood cell count, or hemodynamic instability) due to the effects of induction immunosuppression. Patients will usually present with signs of focal intra-abdominal infection or sepsis, often with evidence of cholangitis, discrete abscesses, or peritonitis. Abdominal CT scanning may help to identify the presence of a focal collection, which should be aspirated and cultured whenever feasible.

Management of wound infections may require opening of the wound, irrigation and drainage as indicated, serial dressing changes, healing by secondary intention, and administration of systemic antibiotics, depending on the severity and depth of the infection. Treatment of infected collections requires drainage of the collection, irrigation, and correction of biliary complications. Drainage may be open or percutaneous, depending on the size, location, and complications related to the collection. Broad-spectrum intravenous antibiotics should be chosen to cover the most likely pathogens, which include aerobic and anaerobic enteric gram-negative bacilli and gram-positive cocci. Local transplant center flora and the presence of multidrug-resistant pathogens should be considered when selecting empiric antibiotics. Antibiotic coverage can be tailored on the basis of culture results, to focus the antimicrobial treatment [87].

Liver transplant recipients have the highest incidence of fungal infection, although the incidence has been decreasing due to effective prophylactic approaches and improved perioperative techniques and care [87]. Risk factors and management have been well described elsewhere and are discussed in another chapter in this book [83, 87]. Candida species are the most commonly isolated pathogens and often develop early posttransplant, usually within the first 1 to 2 months. Opportunistic fungal infections usually occur later, as a result of a longer duration of immunosuppression or more intense/augmented immunosuppression.

Viral infections typically develop more than 1 month after transplant, as a result of the cumulative effects of immunosuppression [86]. Viral pathogens that reactivate in the setting of immunosuppression include CMV, EBV, HSV, and hepatitis viruses (B and C). Occasionally, primary infection due to these viruses can occur. Viral infections in transplant recipient result in both significant morbidity and increased cost of care. CMV is the most common viral infection diagnosed following liver transplantation. Infection with CMV is typically evident within 1 to 6 months after liver transplant and can be due to either reactivation (recipient seropositive pretransplant) or transmitted infection from the donor (donor seropositive/recipient seronegative) [87]. Manifestations of CMV infection include asymptomatic viremia or CMV disease [90]. Asymptomatic viremia may be detected through routine posttransplant surveillance. CMV disease is diagnosed by the presence of viremia together with clinical signs and symptoms such as fever, malaise, and leukopenia, with or without specific end-organ involvement. The diagnosis of tissue-invasive CMV disease requires biopsy with demonstrated presence of viral inclusions on histopathology. Tissue-invasive disease most commonly involves the liver, gut, or lungs, although encephalitis and retinitis are rarely described in this population [87, 90]. Strategies to prevent reactivation or transmission of primary CMV infection include universal prophylaxis with valganciclovir and preemptive treatment, with close monitoring to detect viremia and initiate antiviral treatment before significant end-organ disease due to CMV develops. Both strategies are effective; the reasons for choosing one approach over another include risk of CMV infection, feasibility of preemptive monitoring, the ability of the transplant center/staff to receive laboratory test results in a timely manner, cost, and adverse effects of valganciclovir prophylaxis. For patients at high risk for primary CMV disease (donor CMV IgG positive, recipient CMV IgG negative), universal prophylaxis is most commonly chosen for a duration of 3 to 6 months after transplantation [87, 90].

CARE OF THE LIVING LIVER DONOR

Living liver donation surgery is a partial hepatectomy, involving surgical removal of up to 60% to 70% of the liver. If at any point the surgical team believes that the donor is at risk or that the segment of the donor's liver is not appropriate for transplantation, the surgery is stopped. This happens in the United States at least 5% of the time. Following surgery, the donor is admitted to the intensive care unit for at least 1 day for observation. Live liver donors may be discharged approximately 5 to 7 days after surgery. The postoperative recovery period is from 4 to 6 weeks. Most donors return to their usual activities within 12 weeks, and may begin more demanding activities 6 months after their surgery.

Surgical Risks for LDs

Although living liver donation is highly successful, complications for the donor and the recipient may arise. The overall incidence of donor complications after LD liver donation ranges from 5% to 10%. There is also a small risk (<0.5%) of death [88,89]. Of note, mortality is higher for adult-to-adult donation (0.24% to 0.4%) compared with adult-to-child donation (0.09% to 0.2%). This is explained by the fact that adult-to-child donation usually involves removal of a smaller portion of the liver.

Adverse reactions may occur as a result of anesthesia or other medications administered at the time of surgery. Bleeding may occur postoperatively, possibly requiring blood transfusion(s). Other complications include infections (wound, urinary tract, pneumonia), blood clots in the legs, PE, gastrointestinal problems (bowel obstruction, nausea/vomiting, constipation), incisional pain, numbness around the incision, and abnormal sensation of the upper extremities. Other complications after donor surgery may include incisional problems such as hernias. The risks of DVT and PE are the same as for other major abdominal procedures. A rare but serious complication is liver failure that may require a liver transplant to correct (this occurs in about 2 transplants per 1,000 living liver donor surgeries), or death. The mortality rate of a living liver donor is 5 in 1,000.

Bile duct problems are the most worrisome complication after donor surgery. The rate of this happening across the country ranges from 5% to 15%. At our center, 5% of patients undergoing operations similar to live donor liver surgeries have had bile leaks. Bile may leak from the cut surface of the liver or from the site where the bile duct is divided. That site may later become strictured. Generally, bile leaks resolve spontaneously with simple drainage. Strictures and occasionally bile leaks may require an ERCP and stenting. If the above measures fail, a reoperation may be required. Intra-abdominal infections developing among donors are usually related to a biliary problem.

Biliary strictures (narrowing of the large ducts that drain the liver) can also occur after live donor partial hepatectomy. These strictures confer potential long-term complications. Current data suggest that these strictures are rare and that some of them can be fixed without additional surgery. Another rare event that may happen is injury to the spleen during the surgery. If this complication occurs, the spleen may be removed.

Postoperative ICU Care

Once stability is achieved, the patient is positioned on his or her left side with right side up during the first 48 hours postoperatively whenever the patient is in bed. Jackson Pratt drains are placed intraoperatively and monitored for the presence of normal (serosanguinous) versus abnormal (bilious, bloody, purulent) drainage. The donor typically has a nasogastric tube to low continuous suction, with the duration of placement determined by the donor transplant surgeon. Worsening abdominal pain warrants a thorough abdominal assessment for possible signs of bleeding, gastric dilatation, or pleuritic symptoms. As with the transplant recipient, the donor receives medications for stress ulcer prophylaxis. In addition, anticoagulation and venodyne boots are provided for DVT prophylaxis in accordance with published guidelines.

Complications following live donor partial hepatectomy include but are not limited to acute hemorrhage (manifest as hypotension, mental status changes, decreased hematocrit, tachycardia, and increasing abdominal pain), infection (wound infection or pneumonia most commonly), gastric dilatation (often developing by postoperative day 3 or 4, and manifest as bloating with nausea), hypophosphatemia (commonly developing around postoperative days 3 to 4), CNS abnormalities, and rarely renal, hepatic, cardiac, or respiratory dysfunction.

In order to decrease the risk of complications, donors should receive continued education regarding hospital expectations throughout their inpatient stay. Donors should be instructed on the correct use of an incentive spirometer and encouraged to cough and deep-breathe frequently with a therapeutic cough pillow. The donor's diet is advanced as his or her condition allows. The team will optimize the donor's nutrition to meet the latter's needs for wound healing. Donors may typically be assisted out of bed to chair on postoperative day 1 and advanced to ambulation as tolerated.

Expected ICU Course

Patients are managed with isotonic crystalloid (normal saline) with close monitoring. A low CVP is preferred, to minimize intra- and postoperative bleeding. Volume expansion in the postoperative period is expected to be associated with modest declines in the Hb levels. Urine flows of 0.5 mL/kg/hr. are desired, and additional boluses and rates of 125 mL per hour are not unexpected. The postoperative INR is expected to be in the 1-to-1.5 range, and may rise to as high as 2.5 in the early postoperative period. This is managed with vitamin K in some cases. FFP transfusions are not given. The platelet count is not expected to fall significantly. Transfusion is not expected, and the hematocrit rarely falls below 25. Postoperative pain is managed with a narcotic patient-controlled analgesia (PCA) pump. Additional small intravenous doses (50 mcg fentanyl, 1 mg morphine, 0.5 mg dilaudid) of narcotic are sometimes required. Patients are treated with a first-generation cephalosporin for 24 hours beginning at the time of incision, but are generally not needed after the initial 24 hours.

Postdonation Care

Live liver donors are followed by the transplant program for follow-up care, including evaluations such as blood pressure, lab studies, and other routine tests. Transplant centers are required to report follow-up information on all LDs for 2 years after donation.

SUMMARY

Care of liver transplant recipients before, during, and after surgery is a significant challenge, given the comorbidities and complications associated with ESLD. These patients are typically quite debilitated and deconditioned going into transplantation, and a variety of medical and surgical complications can occur following transplantation. Despite dramatic advances in the field, liver transplantation remains a major undertaking with the possibility of complications affecting every major organ system. A systematic approach is necessary to prevent, minimize, and manage these complications. Intensive medical care in an ICU setting may be necessary even pretransplantation, particularly for patients with FHF or severely decompensated chronic liver disease. Optimizing the overall medical status of transplant candidates with chronic liver failure is essential to decrease the likelihood of postoperative problems. Immediately posttransplantation, intensive monitoring in a critical care setting by providers with experience in the care of liver transplant recipients is necessary to ensure an optimal outcome. A thorough knowledge of potential complications is required to allow for rapid diagnosis and appropriate treatment.

ACKNOWLEDGMENT

The authors would like to acknowledge the authors of previous edition, Ruy J. Cruz Jr, William D. Payne and Abhinav Humar, for their work in writing this chapter, from which the current version is adapted.

References

1. Moore FD, Wheele HB, Demissianos HV, et al: Experimental whole-organ transplantation of the liver and of the spleen. *Ann Surg* 152:374–387, 1960.
2. Monbaliu D, Pirenne J, Talbot D: Liver transplantation using donation after cardiac death donors. *J Hepatol* 56:474–485, 2012.
3. Selck FW, Grossman EB, Ratner LE, et al: Utilization, outcomes, and retransplantation of liver allografts from donation after cardiac death: implications for further expansion of the deceased-donor pool. *Ann Surg* 248:599–607, 2008.
4. Reich DJ, Mulligan DC, Abt PL, et al: ASTS recommended practice guidelines for controlled donation after cardiac death organ procurement and transplantation. *Am J Transplant* 9:2004–2011, 2009.
5. de Vera ME, Lopez-Solis R, Dvorchik I, et al: Liver transplantation using donation after cardiac death donors: long-term follow-up from a single center. *Am J Transplant* 9:773–781, 2009.
6. Locke JE, Segev DL, Warren DS, et al. Outcomes of kidneys from donors after cardiac death: implications for allocation and preservation. *Am J Transplant* 7:1797–1807, 2007.
7. Mathur AK, Heimbach J, Steffick DE, et al: Donation after cardiac death liver transplantation: predictors of outcome. *Am J Transplant* 10:2512–2519, 2010.
8. Mourad MM, Algarni A, Liossis C, et al: Aetiology and risk factors of ischaemic cholangiopathy after liver transplantation. *World J Gastroenterol* 20:6159–6169, 2014.
9. Renz JF, Emond JC, Yersiz H, et al: Split-liver transplantation in the United States: outcomes of a national survey. *Ann Surg* 239:172–181, 2004.
10. Huprikar S, Danziger-Isakov L, Ahn J, et al: Solid organ transplantation from hepatitis B virus-positive donors: consensus guidelines for recipient management. *Am J Transplant* 15:1162–1172, 2015.
11. Northup PG, Argo CK, Nguyen DT, et al: Liver allografts from hepatitis C positive donors can offer good outcomes in hepatitis C positive recipients: a US National Transplant Registry analysis. *Transpl Int* 23:1038–1044, 2010.
12. Seem DL, Lee I, Umscheid CA, et al: PHS guideline for reducing human immunodeficiency virus, hepatitis B virus, and hepatitis C virus transmission through organ transplantation. *Public Health Rep* 128, 247–343, 2013.
13. Koulaouzidis A, Bhat S, Saeed AA: Spontaneous bacterial peritonitis. *World J Gastroenterol* 15:1042–1049, 2009.
14. Obermayer-Straub P, Strassburg CP, Manns MP: Autoimmune hepatitis. *J Hepatol* 32:181–197, 2000.
15. Brewer GJ: Recognition, diagnosis, and management of Wilson's disease. *Proc Soc Exp Biol Med* 223:39–46, 2000.
16. Mazzaferro V, Regalia E, Doci R, et al: Liver transplantation for the treatment of small hepatocellular carcinomas in patients with cirrhosis. *N Engl J Med* 334:693–699, 1996.
17. Yao FY, Ferrell L, Bass NM, et al: Liver transplantation for hepatocellular carcinoma: comparison of the proposed UCSF criteria with the Milan criteria and the Pittsburgh modified TNM criteria. *Liver Transpl* 8:765–774, 2002.
18. Ostapowicz G, Lee WM: Acute hepatic failure: a Western perspective. *J Gastroenterol Hepatol* 15:480–488, 2000.
19. Williams R: Classification, etiology, and considerations of outcome in acute liver failure. *Semin Liver Dis* 16:343–348, 1996.
20. O'Grady JG, Alexander GJ, Hayllar KM, et al: Early indicators of prognosis in fulminant hepatic failure. *Gastroenterology* 97:439–445, 1989.
21. McDiarmid SV, Merion RM, Dykstra DM, et al: Selection of pediatric candidates under the PELD system. *Liver Transpl* 10:S23–S30, 2004.
22. Singh C, Sager JS: Pulmonary complications of cirrhosis. *Med Clin North Am* 93:871–883, viii, 2009.
23. Brescia MD, Massarollo PC, Imakuma ES, et al: Prospective randomized trial comparing hepatic venous outflow and renal function after conventional versus piggyback liver transplantation. *PLoS One* 10:e0129923, 2015.
24. Houben P, Manzini G, Kremer M, et al: Graft rinse prior to reperfusion in liver transplantation: literature review and online survey within the Eurotransplant community. *Transpl Int* 28(11):1291–1298, 2015.
25. Sabate A, Dalmau A, Koo M, et al: Contreras, coagulopathy management in liver transplantation. *Transplant Proc* 44:1523–1525, 2012.
26. Ripoll C, Yotti R, Bermejo J, et al: The heart in liver transplantation. *J Hepatol* 54:810–822, 2011.
27. Safadi A, Homsi M, Maskoun W, et al: Perioperative risk predictors of cardiac outcomes in patients undergoing liver transplantation surgery. *Circulation* 120:1189–1194, 2009.
28. Rozga J, Piatek T, Malkowski P: Human albumin: old, new, and emerging applications. *Ann Transplant* 18:205–217, 2013.
29. Mangus RS, Fridell JA, Vianna RM, et al: Immunosuppression induction with rabbit anti-thymocyte globulin with or without rituximab in 1000 liver transplant patients with long-term follow-up. *Liver Transpl* 18:786–795, 2012.

30. Lupo L, Panzera P, Tandoi F, et al: Basiliximab versus steroids in double therapy immunosuppression in liver transplantation: a prospective randomized clinical trial. *Transplantation* 86:925–931, 2008.
31. Calne RY, McMaster P, Portmann B, et al: Observations on preservation, bile drainage and rejection in 64 human orthotopic liver allografts. *Ann Surg* 186:282–290, 1977.
32. Starzl TE, Putnam CW, Hansbrough JF, et al: Biliary complications after liver transplantation: with special reference to the biliary cast syndrome and techniques of secondary duct repair. *Surgery* 81:212–221, 1977.
33. Akamatsu N, Sugawara Y, Hashimoto D: Biliary reconstruction, its complications and management of biliary complications after adult liver transplantation: a systematic review of the incidence, risk factors and outcome. *Transpl Int* 24:379–392, 2011.
34. op den Dries S, Westerkamp AC, Karimian N, et al: Injury to peribiliary glands and vascular plexus before liver transplantation predicts formation of non-anastomotic biliary strictures. *J Hepatol* 60:1172–1179, 2014.
35. Martins PN: Normothermic machine preservation as an approach to decrease biliary complications of DCD liver grafts. *Am J Transplant* 13:3287–3288, 2013.
36. Jay CL, Lyuksemburg V, Ladner DP, et al: Ischemic cholangiopathy after controlled donation after cardiac death liver transplantation: a meta-analysis. *Ann Surg* 253:259–264, 2011.
37. Seehofer D, Eurich D, Veltzke-Schlieker W, et al: Biliary complications after liver transplantation: old problems and new challenges. *Am J Transplant* 13:253–265, 2013.
38. Op den Dries S, Sutton ME, Lisman T, et al: Protection of bile ducts in liver transplantation: looking beyond ischemia. *Transplantation* 92:373–379, 2011.
39. Buis CI, Hoekstra H, Verdonk RC, et al: Causes and consequences of ischemic-type biliary lesions after liver transplantation. *J Hepatobiliary Pancreat Surg* 13:517–524, 2006.
40. Verdonk RC, Buis CI, Porte RJ, et al: Biliary complications after liver transplantation: a review. *Scand J Gastroenterol Suppl* 243:89–101, 2006.
41. Gholson CF, Zibari G, McDonald JC: Endoscopic diagnosis and management of biliary complications following orthotopic liver transplantation. *Dig Dis Sci* 41:1045–1053, 1996.
42. Pfau PR, Kochman ML, Lewis JD, et al: Endoscopic management of postoperative biliary complications in orthotopic liver transplantation. *Gastrointest Endosc* 52:55–63, 2000.
43. Thuluvath PJ, Pfau PR, Kimmey MB, et al: Biliary complications after liver transplantation: the role of endoscopy. *Endoscopy* 37:857–863, 2005.
44. Warnaar N, Molenaar IQ, Colquhoun SD, et al: Intraoperative pulmonary embolism and intracardiac thrombosis complicating liver transplantation: a systematic review. *J Thromb Haemost* 6:297–302, 2008.
45. Feltracco P, Brezzi M, Barbieri S, et al: Blood loss, predictors of bleeding, transfusion practice and strategies of blood cell salvaging during liver transplantation. *World J Hepatol* 5:1–15, 2013.
46. Esmat Gamil M, Pirenne J, Van Malenstein H, et al: Risk factors for bleeding and clinical implications in patients undergoing liver transplantation. *Transplant Proc* 44:2857–2860, 2012.
47. Testa G, Malago M, Broelsch CE: Bleeding problems in patients undergoing segmental liver transplantation. *Blood Coagul Fibrinolysis* 11[Suppl 1]:S81–S85, 2000.
48. Roullet S, Biais M, Millas E, et al: Risk factors for bleeding and transfusion during orthotopic liver transplantation. *Ann Fr Anesth Reanim* 30:349–352, 2011.
49. Jung SW, Hwang S, Namgoong JM, et al: Incidence and management of postoperative abdominal bleeding after liver transplantation. *Transplant Proc* 44:765–768, 2012.
50. Bechstein WO, Neuhaus P: Bleeding problems in liver surgery and liver transplantation [in German]. *Chirurg* 71:363–368, 2000.
51. Neuhaus P, Bechstein WO, Lefebre B, et al: Effect of aprotinin on intraoperative bleeding and fibrinolysis in liver transplantation. *Lancet* 2:924–925, 1989.
52. Gurusamy KS, Pissanou T, Pikhart H, et al: Methods to decrease blood loss and transfusion requirements for liver transplantation. *Cochrane Database Syst Rev* CD009052 (12), 2011. doi: 10.1002/14651858.CD009052.pub2.
53. Lisman T, Porte RJ: Antiplatelet medication after liver transplantation: does it affect outcome? *Liver Transpl* 13:644–646, 2007.
54. Porte RJ: Coagulation and fibrinolysis in orthotopic liver transplantation: current views and insights. *Semin Thromb Hemost* 19:191–196, 1993.
55. Northup PG, McMahon MM, Ruhl AP, et al: Coagulopathy does not fully protect hospitalized cirrhosis patients from peripheral venous thromboembolism. *Am J Gastroenterol* 101:1524–1528, 2006; quiz 1680.
56. Gologorsky E, De Wolf AM, Scott V, et al: Intracardiac thrombus formation and pulmonary thromboembolism immediately after graft reperfusion in 7 patients undergoing liver transplantation. *Liver Transpl* 7:783–789, 2001.
57. Lerner AB, Sundar E, Mahmood F, et al: Four cases of cardiopulmonary thromboembolism during liver transplantation without the use of antifibrinolytic drugs. *Anesth Analg* 101:1608–1612, 2005.
58. Stapleton GN, Hickman R, Terblanche J: Blood supply of the right and left hepatic ducts. *Br J Surg* 85:202–207, 1998.
59. Duffy JP, Hong JC, Farmer DG, et al: Vascular complications of orthotopic liver transplantation: experience in more than 4,200 patients. *J Am Coll Surg* 208:896–903, 2009; discussion 903–895.
60. Mourad MM, Liossis C, Gunson BK, et al: Etiology and management of hepatic artery thrombosis after adult liver transplantation. *Liver Transpl* 20:713–723, 2014.
61. Pastacaldi S, Teixeira R, Montalto P, et al: Hepatic artery thrombosis after orthotopic liver transplantation: a review of nonsurgical causes. *Liver Transpl* 7:75–81, 2001.
62. Stringer MD, Marshall MM, Muiesan P, et al: Survival and outcome after hepatic artery thrombosis complicating pediatric liver transplantation. *J Pediatr Surg* 36:888–891, 2001.
63. Yao FY, Kinkhabwala M, LaBerge JM, et al: The impact of pre-operative loco-regional therapy on outcome after liver transplantation for hepatocellular carcinoma. *Am J Transplant* 5:795–804, 2005.
64. Boyvat F, Aytekin C, Harman A, et al: Endovascular stent placement in patients with hepatic artery stenoses or thromboses after liver transplant. *Transplant Proc* 40:22–26, 2008.
65. Englesbe MJ, Schaubel DE, Cai S, et al: Portal vein thrombosis and liver transplant survival benefit. *Liver Transpl* 16:999–1005, 2010.
66. Qi X, Dai J, Jia J, et al: Association between portal vein thrombosis and survival of liver transplant recipients: a systematic review and meta-analysis of observational studies. *J Gastrointestin Liver Dis* 24:51–59, 54 p following 59, 2015.
67. Charco R, Fuster J, Fondevila C, et al: Portal vein thrombosis in liver transplantation. *Transplant Proc* 37:3904–3905, 2005.
68. Wang JT, Zhao HY, Liu YL: Portal vein thrombosis. *Hepatobiliary Pancreat Dis Int* 4:515–518, 2005.
69. Llado L, Fabregat J, Castellote J, et al: Management of portal vein thrombosis in liver transplantation: influence on morbidity and mortality. *Clin Transplant* 21:716–721, 2007.
70. Kishi Y, Sugawara Y, Matsui Y, et al: Late onset portal vein thrombosis and its risk factors. *Hepatogastroenterology* 55:1008–1009, 2008.
71. Lock JF, Schwabauer E, Martus P, et al: Early diagnosis of primary nonfunction and indication for reoperation after liver transplantation. *Liver Transpl* 16:172–180, 2010.
72. Uemura T, Randall HB, Sanchez EQ, et al: Liver retransplantation for primary nonfunction: analysis of a 20-year single-center experience. *Liver Transpl* 13:227–233, 2007.
73. Kamath GS, Plevak DJ, Wiesner RH, et al: Primary nonfunction of the liver graft: when should we retransplant? *Transplant Proc* 23:1954, 1991.
74. Zivkovic SA: Neurologic complications after liver transplantation. *World J Hepatol* 5:409–416, 2013.
75. Bartynski WS, Tan HP, Boardman JF, et al: Posterior reversible encephalopathy syndrome after solid organ transplantation. *Am J Neuroradiol* 29:924–930, 2008.
76. Luca L, Westbrook R, Tsochatzis EA: Metabolic and cardiovascular complications in the liver transplant recipient. *Ann Gastroenterol* 28:183–192, 2015.
77. Watt KD, Pedersen RA, Kremers WK, et al: Evolution of causes and risk factors for mortality post-liver transplant: results of the NIDDK long-term follow-up study. *Am J Transplant* 10:1420–1427, 2010.
78. Feltracco P, Carollo C, Barbieri S, et al: Early respiratory complications after liver transplantation. *World J Gastroenterol* 19:9271–9281, 2013.
79. Singh N, Gayowski T, Wagener MM, et al: Pulmonary infiltrates in liver transplant recipients in the intensive care unit. *Transplantation* 67:1138–1144, 1999.
80. McAlister VC, Grant DR, Roy A, et al: Right phrenic nerve injury in orthotopic liver transplantation. *Transplantation* 55:826–830, 1993.
81. Krowka MJ, Cortese DA: Hepatopulmonary syndrome. Current concepts in diagnostic and therapeutic considerations. *Chest* 105:1528–1537, 1994.
82. Bahirwani R, Reddy KR: Outcomes after liver transplantation: chronic kidney disease. *Liver Transpl* 15[Suppl 2]:S70–S74, 2009.
83. Collins LA, Samore MH, Roberts MS, et al: Risk factors for invasive fungal infections complicating orthotopic liver transplantation. *J Infect Dis* 170:644–652, 1994.
84. Patel R, Portela D, Badley AD, et al: Risk factors of invasive Candida and non-Candida fungal infections after liver transplantation. *Transplantation* 62:926–934, 1996.
85. Kusne S, Dummer JS, Singh N, et al: Infections after liver transplantation. An analysis of 101 consecutive cases. *Medicine (Baltimore)* 67:132–143, 1988.
86. Fishman JA: Infection in solid-organ transplant recipients. *N Engl J Med* 357:2601–2614, 2007.
87. Hernandez MDP, Martin P, Simkins J: Infectious complications after liver transplantation. *Gastroenterol Hepatol* 11:741–753, 2015.
88. Trotter JF, Wachs M, Everson GT, et al: Adult-to-adult transplantation of the right hepatic lobe from a living donor. *N Engl J Med* 346:1074–1082, 2002.
89. Brown RS Jr, Russo MW, Lai M, et al: A survey of liver transplantation from living adult donors in the United States. *N Engl J Med* 348:818–825, 2003.
90. Razonable RR, Humar A, AST infectious diseases community of practice: cytomegalovirus in solid organ transplantation. *Am J Transplantation* 13:93–106, 2013.

Chapter 59 ■ Critical Care of the Lung Transplant Recipient

LUIS F. ANGEL • STEPHANIE M. LEVINE

Over the past three-plus decades, lung transplantation (LT) has become a successful therapeutic option for patients with end-stage pulmonary parenchymal or vascular disease. In the early era of LT, the primary complications associated with the procedure were dehiscence and impaired healing of the bronchial anastomosis, and early graft failure; these complications occurred in most patients who survived for more than 1 week. Improvements in donor and recipient selection, organ allocation and availability, and surgical techniques, the development of new immunosuppressive drugs, and better management of complications, such as primary graft dysfunction (PGD), rejection, and infections have all contributed to advancing the field (Table 59.1). Despite these advances, LT is still associated with numerous complications, often requiring intensive care management.

According to the 2015 report of the International Society for Heart and Lung Transplantation (ISHLT), more than 3,893 adult lung transplants were performed in 2013. The ISHLT Registry reports that the 1-year survival rate for lung transplant recipients is 80%, the 3-year rate is 65%, and the 5-year rate is 54% [1]. The median survival rate for the recent years was 5.7 years. However, there is a marked difference in survival rates according to the type of transplant procedure, with a median survival of 7.1 years for the bilateral lung transplantation (BLT) recipients compared with 4.5 years in those who underwent a single-lung transplantation (SLT) procedure. The recipients who survived to 1 year after primary transplantation had a conditional median survival of 7.9 years (9.7 years for bilateral recipients and 6.4 for single-lung recipients). It is important to mention that there is also high variability of survival rates among different LT programs; if one examines US-specific data from the Scientific Registry of Transplant Recipients (SRTR), survival rates at 1 year are higher than 88%, with experienced centers achieving 1-year survival rates >90% and 3-year survival rates over 75%. These higher survival rates may in part reflect advances in critical care management of lung transplant recipients [2].

The most common cause of mortality is PGD for the first 30 days following transplantation, non-cytomegalovirus (CMV) infection in the 1st year following transplantation, and chronic rejection for all subsequent time intervals [1].

INDICATIONS

The most frequent indications for SLT are obstructive nonsuppurative lung disease, such as emphysema resulting from tobacco use (42% of all SLT procedures reported to the ISHLT Registry) or α_1-antitrypsin deficiency (5%). It is also indicated for diffuse parenchymal lung diseases (39%) such as interstitial lung disease including idiopathic pulmonary fibrosis, familial pulmonary fibrosis, drug- or toxin-induced lung disease, and occupational lung disease, as well as sarcoidosis, limited scleroderma, lymphangioleiomyomatosis, eosinophilic granuloma, and other disorders resulting in end-stage fibrotic lung disease [1].

The steady increase in the overall number of lung transplants over the past 10 years has been due to a significant increase in the number of BLT procedures, now representing over 75% of the total number of LTs. The most frequent indications for BLT are suppurative pulmonary lung disease, cystic fibrosis (24%) and bronchiectasis, severe chronic obstructive pulmonary disease (COPD) resulting from tobacco use (27%), or α_1-antitrypsin deficiency (6%) and diffuse parenchymal lung diseases (22%). In addition, more than 95% of transplants for pulmonary hypertension (PH) are BLT procedures [1].

Heart–lung transplantation (HLT) is performed at only a few transplantation centers and should be reserved for patients who cannot be treated by LT alone. The most frequent indications for HLT are Eisenmenger syndrome with a cardiac anomaly that cannot be corrected surgically and severe end-stage lung disease with concurrent severe heart disease. HLT is discussed in more detail in Chapter 60.

TABLE 59.1

Major Advances or Changes in Lung Transplantation Over the Past 5 Years

Topic	Change	Reference
Selection of lung transplant candidates	A new consensus document for the selection of transplant candidates	[3]
Increased donor pool with protocols for donor management	Increasing the use of extended donors and the use of low tidal volume ventilator strategies in potential lung donors	[28,29]
DCD donors	Increased use of DCD donors with comparable outcomes	[20,21]
Ex vivo lung perfusion	Increasing the use of marginal/extended donor lungs	[31–33]
ECMO as bridge to lung transplantation	Considered as a viable option for end-stage pulmonary patients awaiting lung transplantation	[5,9]
Improved short-term survival and decreasing waiting time for lung transplant recipients	Experienced centers now with over 90% survival at 1 y and waiting time under 4 mo	[2,18]
Acute antibody-mediated rejection after lung transplantation	Establishes the role of antibodies in acute rejection and proposes criteria for diagnosis	[70,72]
Description of CLAD	Defines both phenotypes of the obstructive pattern as BOS and the RAS	[75,111]

BOS, bronchiolitis obliterans syndrome; CLAD, chronic lung allograft dysfunction; DCD, donation after circulatory death; RAS, restrictive allograft syndrome.

GUIDELINES FOR RECIPIENT SELECTION

An ISHLT consensus document recently updated the previous consensus-based guidelines (1998 and 2006) for the selection of lung transplant candidates [3]. LT should be considered for any patient with chronic, end-stage lung disease who meet all the following criteria: high (>50%) risk of death from lung disease within 2 years if LT is not performed, high (>80%) likelihood of surviving at least 90 days after transplantation, and a high (80%) likelihood of 5-year posttransplant survival from a general medical perspective provided that there is adequate graft function.

Age

The 2014 ISHLT consensus document for the selection of transplant candidates [3] suggest an age >65 years in association with low physiologic reserve as a relative contraindication regardless of procedure type, and 75 years as an absolute contraindication to LT.

Relative Contraindications

Transplantation is relatively contraindicated in patients with systemic diseases that have extrapulmonary involvement such as scleroderma, systemic lupus erythematous, polymyositis, and rheumatoid arthritis. Advanced atherosclerotic disease is also considered a relative contraindication unless this can be corrected before, or in very selected cases concurrently, with transplantation. Osteoporosis is a significant problem after LT, and preexisting symptomatic osteoporosis is also a relative contraindication.

Patients with active sites of infection are not considered to be good transplantation candidates. Treated tuberculosis and fungal disease pose a particular problem but are not contraindications for LT. Many centers will not consider performing a transplant in a patient who is chronically colonized with a resistant organism (e.g., *Burkholderia cenocepacia*, atypical mycobacterium such as *abscesses*), and it is recommended to try to eradicate these organisms in the pretransplant period and to consider each patient on an individual basis. However, if considered, these patients are candidates only for BLT procedures since the remaining colonized lung could pose a serious threat to the new graft in the case of an SLT. This issue is of particular concern in cystic fibrosis patients who are often infected with drug-resistant organisms. Both *Burkholderia cenocepacia* (specific strains) and *Burkholderia gladioli* are of concern due to poor posttransplantation outcomes [4].

As patients are now allocated lungs for transplantation according to the severity of their disease, requirements for invasive mechanical ventilation and extracorporeal life support are now more frequently seen. During this critical period, patients usually have multiple acute changes that pose a relative or absolute contraindication to transplantation, and the candidacy for this procedure should be assessed on a continuous basis [5–7]. In one small series of mechanically ventilated patients, there was a longer time on postoperative mechanical ventilation and a longer intensive care unit (ICU) stay following LT. Rates of PGD, survival, and total hospital stay were similar to those in patients undergoing LT not on mechanical ventilation [6]. Recently venovenous and/or venoarterial extracorporeal membrane oxygenation (ECMO) has been used as a bridge to transplantation for end-stage lung disease patients with good short-term function and survival rates [5,7]. In a large review of the United Network of Organ Sharing (UNOS) database of patients undergoing LT on mechanical respiratory support (586 on mechanical ventilation and 51 on ECMO as a bridge to LT), the authors found that patients on mechanical ventilation or ECMO have lower survival rates following LT compared with those not requiring support [8]. A small study of 25 patients receiving ECMO as a bridge to transplant showed that the duration of ECMO was related to mortality (which increased steadily with time on ECMO) and morbidity (ICU length of stay, days on mechanical ventilation, and hospital stay) following LT [9]. Noninvasive ventilatory support is not considered a relative contraindication to transplantation.

To be considered for transplantation, patients should have an ideal body weight of >70% or ≤130% predicted (BMI, 18 to 30 kg per m^2). Those patients with poor nutritional status may be too weak to withstand the surgical procedure; those patients who are obese (BMI, 30–35 kg per m^2) make more difficult surgical candidates and may have higher mortality rates than nonobese patients.

Prior thoracotomy or pleurodesis was once considered to be a relative contraindication to transplantation due to increased difficulty with the transplant pneumonectomy as well as with an increased risk of bleeding. Extensive prior chest surgery with lung resection remains a relative contraindication to LT. Despite this, transplantation can be successfully performed for these patients and for many of them SLT may be the best option. Other relative contraindications include well-controlled human immunodeficiency (HIV) disease, and hepatitis B or C without active cirrhosis.

Absolute Contraindications

The 2014 international guidelines identified several absolute contraindications to LT including untreatable major organ dysfunction, uncorrectable atherosclerotic disease, acute medical instability, and uncorrectable bleeding diatheses [3]. Active malignancy within the prior 2 years is also a contraindication to transplantation. For patients with a history of breast cancer greater than stage 2, colon cancer greater than Duke A stage, renal carcinoma, or melanoma greater than or equal to level 2, the waiting period should be at least 5 years. Restaging is suggested before transplant listing.

Severe non-osteoporotic skeletal disease, such as kyphoscoliosis, is often an absolute contraindication to transplantation, primarily because of the technical difficulties encountered during surgery, and residual restrictive lung disease after transplantation.

Drug abuse and alcoholism are considered to be contraindications to transplantation because patients with these conditions are associated with a high risk for noncompliance. Patients who continue to smoke despite having end-stage pulmonary disease are not candidates for LT. Transplant centers require patients to abstain from cigarette smoking, alcohol use, or narcotics use for 6 months to 2 years before being considered for lung transplant evaluation.

The patient must be well motivated and emotionally stable to withstand the extreme stress of the pretransplantation and perioperative periods. A history of nonadherence, significant psychiatric illness, or lack of an adequate support system are absolute contraindications. In addition, lack of potential for rehabilitation or extreme obesity ≥35.0 kg per m^2, are also absolute contraindications to LT. Chronic infection with pan-resistant organisms or active *Mycobacterium tuberculosis* infection also preclude LT.

DONOR ALLOCATION AND SELECTION

Until the spring of 2005, as established by the United Network of Organ Sharing, lungs were allocated primarily by time on the waiting list and not by necessity. In the spring of 2005, the system for donor allocation for lungs was revised and priority was assigned for lung offers on the basis of a benefit or need-based Lung Allocation Score (LAS) [10,11]. The LAS is calculated using the following measures: (1) waitlist urgency measure (i.e., the expected number of days lived without a transplant during an additional year on the waitlist); (2) posttransplant survival measure (i.e., the expected number of days lived during the 1st year after transplant); and (3) the transplant benefit measure (i.e., the posttransplant survival measure minus waitlist urgency measure) [12]. Now 10 years later, many of the goals of the system (decreased waiting list deaths and times, and prioritizing patients by urgency rather than time on the list) are being accomplished, with comparable survival rates except for those with the very high LAS scores (>46 in one study and >60 in another) [13–15]. In a large single-center study, patients with high LAS scores of ≥50 had lower survival rates at 30 days, 90 days, 1 year, and 3 years (92.6%, 87.8%, 71.5%, 52% vs. 96.9%, 93.5%, 83.2%, and 73.9%, respectively) and increased morbidity compared with those with LAS < 50 including prolonged need for ventilator support, need for tracheotomy, and longer ICU stays [16]. There also appears to be a stepwise decline in posttransplantation survival as the LAS score increases. In another study, patients with high LAS scores had higher morbidity including requirements for dialysis, infections, and longer lengths of stay [17]. Since the implementation of the LAS, the distribution of patient diagnoses on the list, and those transplanted, has also shifted from a majority of COPD patients to an increasing number of patients with pulmonary fibrosis. In addition, sicker patients are being transplanted.

In the United States, donor lungs are first distributed locally, then regionally, and finally nationally. Currently, the median time to transplant for waitlist patients is approximately 4.3 months (range 0.2 to 52 months) [18] and therefore close management of the listed transplant patient is required. Despite this close attention, a small percentage of patients die while awaiting transplantation.

A shortage of donor organs remains the primary factor limiting the number of LTs performed. Contributing to this shortage is the estimate that lungs for transplantation are procured from only 21% of multiorgan donors [19]. The vast majority of transplanted lungs are from brain-dead donors. A small number of LT procedures involving living related donors and an increasing number of lung donors from donation after circulatory death (DCD), previously referred as non–heart-beating donors, have been performed at institutions specializing in these procedures [20,21]. In a recent meta-analysis of DCD donation in LT involving 271 DCD and 2,369 donation after brain death (DBD) donors, no differences were found in 1-year survival, incidence of PGD, or acute rejection [20]. In the DCD Registry of the ISHLT, 306 DBD transplantations were compared to 3,992 DCD transplantations. The study found that 30-day, 1-year, and 3-year survival rates were comparable between the two groups. The DCD recipients had a slightly longer hospital stay following transplantation 18 days versus 16 days ($p = 0.016$) [21]. Ethical issues regarding DCD donation were recently reviewed in a multisociety policy statement [22].

The usual donor selection criteria are age younger than 60 to 65 years, no history of clinically significant lung disease, normal results from a sputum Gram stain, and a limited history of smoking (less than 20 pack-years). In addition, the lung fields should be clear as demonstrated by chest radiograph, and gas exchange should be adequate as demonstrated by a partial pressure of arterial oxygen (PaO_2) > 300 mm Hg, while receiving fractional inspired oxygen (FIO_2) equal to 1, or a PaO_2/FIO_2 ratio of more than 300, with a positive end-expiratory pressure (PEEP) of 5 cm H_2O. Bronchoscopy is also part of the evaluation of the donor. The main goal of the endobronchial evaluation is to rule out gross aspiration or purulent secretions in the distal airways. Lungs from extended donors (i.e., those who do not meet all of the criteria listed earlier) are now more frequently being transplanted in an attempt to expand the donor pool. Commonly extended criteria include the use of lungs from older donors and those from smokers [23,24]. In the Euro transplant community, lungs from extended donors are used for rescue offers with comparable outcomes [25]. Some centers are actively engaged in developing protocols for optimizing marginal donor lungs, thereby rendering them transplantable [26–29]. By instituting a protocol including educational and donor management interventions, and changing donor classification and selection criteria, a single-organ procurement organization was able to increase the percentage of lungs procured from 11.5% to 22.5% with an increase in the number of procedures performed, without adverse recipient outcomes [29]. A similar study using a protocol of protective ventilation including ventilator recruitment maneuvers, high levels of PEEP, fluid restriction, and hormonal resuscitation therapy also showed increased procurement rates from 20% to 50% without compromised survival or incidence of PGD [26]. The use of lung protective ventilation strategies such as low tidal volume ventilation to limit lung injury is now recommended when managing the potential lung donor, resulting in adequate functioning lungs [26–28,30]. A multicenter randomized controlled trial of potential organ donors managed with conventional versus protective ventilator strategies revealed that the latter resulted in a significant increase in the number of eligible (54% vs. 95%) and harvested (27% vs. 54%) lungs for LT. There were no differences in 6-month survival among recipients receiving lungs from donors ventilated by either strategy [28].

A new development in lung donation has been the use of ex vivo lung perfusion(EVLP), which in essence "reconditions" lungs that have previously not been acceptable for transplantation. In a prospective nonrandomized clinical trial from Toronto examining high-risk donor lungs transplanted after 4 hours of EVLP, the investigators found results similar to those obtained with conventionally selected lungs, including incidence of PGD, 30-day mortality and 1-year mortality, bronchial complications, duration of mechanical ventilation, and hospital and ICU length of stay [31,32]. Other studies using EVLP found similar results in addition to similar incidences of acute rejection and infection [33,34].

Donors are excluded from potential lung donation if there is evidence of active infection, human immunodeficiency virus, hepatitis, or malignancy. Donor and recipient compatibility is assessed by matching A, B, and O blood types and chest wall size. Human leukocyte antigen (HLA) matching is not routinely performed in LT except in patients with history of preformed donor-specific antibodies.

SURGICAL TECHNIQUES

Initially, double-lung transplantation was the procedure of choice with the anastomosis placed at the level of the trachea. However, the rate of ischemic airway complications was prohibitive. Now, SLT or BLT (essentially sequential SLT) with anastomoses at the level of the main stem bronchi is the preferred surgical technique. At the time of donor harvest, the donor lung is usually removed through a median sternotomy. The pulmonary veins are detached from the heart with a residual 5-mm cuff of left atrium. Each pulmonary artery and the main stem bronchus are transected between two staple lines. During transportation to the recipient site, the partially inflated donor lung graft is placed into preservation solution, usually a low-potassium dextran solution with extracellular electrolyte composition or a modified Euro-Collins solution with an intracellular electrolyte composition at 4°C.

For SLT, the recipient surgery is performed more commonly through a posterolateral thoracotomy or on occasion through a midsternotomy, or vertical axillary muscle-sparing minithoracotomy. Most centers start with the bronchial anastomosis, without a vascular anastomosis of the bronchial circulation of the recipient and donor lungs. Initially, most transplant procedures involved an end-to-end anastomosis, which was wrapped with a piece of omentum or pericardial fat with an intact vascular pedicle for assistance in bronchial revascularization. Subsequently, a telescoping technique was recommended, with the recipient and donor bronchi overlapping by approximately one cartilaginous ring. This procedure allowed the recipient's intact bronchial circulation to supply the donor bronchus. More recently, most anastomoses are performed with an end-to-end single suture in the membranous portion and a single or continuous suture in the cartilaginous portion, without omental wrap, and telescoping is performed when the donor and recipient bronchi differ in size and there is a natural, unforced telescoping of both bronchi [35].

After the bronchial anastomosis has been performed, the donor pulmonary veins are anastomosed end-to-end to the recipient's left atrium, and the pulmonary arteries are attached with an end-to-end anastomosis.

BLT is usually performed through a transverse thoracosternotomy (clamshell incision) or less frequently with median sternotomy followed by sequential single-lung procedures. Cardiopulmonary bypass may be required for patients with pulmonary hypertension or those who cannot tolerate single-lung ventilation or perfusion and who experience marked hypoxemia or hemodynamic instability. Although center specific, an increasing number of cases (nearly 50% of LT procedures at some institutions) are performed with the use of cardiopulmonary bypass.

GENERAL POSTOPERATIVE MANAGEMENT

After LT, patients remain intubated, require mechanical ventilation, and are transferred to the ICU. Most patients are ventilated in a volume-control mode, although in recent years some transplant centers have changed to pressure-control ventilation, or airway pressure release ventilation. In general, low tidal volume ventilation strategies are used. Airway pressures are kept as low as possible so that barotrauma and anastomotic dehiscence can be avoided. Many institutions use routine pharmacologic sedation. Patients are generally maintained with tidal volumes of 6 to 8 mL per kg postoperatively. At most institutions, a low level of PEEP (5.0 to 7.5 cm H_2O) is applied immediately after lung expansion in the operating room and is continued after transplantation. Early extubation is one of the main goals after LT, and lung transplant recipients who do not experience complications are extubated within the first 12 to 24 hours postoperatively if they meet the commonly accepted weaning criteria. Both postural drainage and chest physiotherapy can be routinely employed without concern for mechanical complications at the anastomosis, and patients should perform incentive spirometry soon after extubation.

A recent international survey, with 58% response rate, on mechanical ventilation practices after LT revealed that pressure assist control was used by 37% of respondents and volume assist control by 35%. Tidal volumes were based on recipient, not donor, characteristics, and most respondents selected 6 mL per kg of recipient ideal body weight as a target. Twenty-one percent selected 10 mL per kg, and none selected 15 mL per kg. Most respondents favored limiting FIO_2 over PEEP 69% versus 31% ($p = 0.006$), and the median minimum PEEP used was 5 cm H_2O and median maximum was 11.5 cm H_2O. In the setting of PGD, the plateau pressure limit for adjusting tidal volume was 30 cm H_2O [36].

Certain patient populations require special ventilator management. Most patients with idiopathic pulmonary hypertension undergo BLT; however, at a few centers some patients undergo SLT for pulmonary hypertension with an increased risk of reperfusion pulmonary edema because nearly all of the perfusion is going to the newly implanted lung.

Patients with obstructive lung disease can encounter problems if the delivered tidal volume or the required levels of PEEP are high. Occasionally, clinically significant acute native lung hyperinflation can occur and can compromise the newly transplanted lung and lead to hypotension and hemodynamic instability. To reduce this problem, some transplant centers avoid PEEP for patients undergoing SLT for obstructive disease. However, the problem is magnified when patients experience reperfusion injury or pneumonia after transplantation; in such cases, the compliance of the transplanted lung is decreased and higher PEEP is required for maintaining oxygenation. As a consequence, the more compliant emphysematous lung becomes overexpanded and can herniate toward the contralateral hemithorax [37]. Attempts to prevent this possible complication by using selective independent ventilation with a double-lumen endotracheal tube have been tried. Lung hyperinflation is associated with a significantly longer stay in the ICU, a longer duration of mechanical ventilation, and a trend toward higher mortality [38].

Pain control is usually provided by opiates, usually fentanyl, administered intravenously, or morphine sulfate via an epidural catheter with a patient-regulated pain-control system.

Because many patients are nutritionally depleted before transplantation as a result of their underlying disease, postoperative nutrition is important. Ideally, enteral nutrition should be provided as soon as tolerated.

Antibiotics are routinely administered for the first 48 to 72 hours after transplantation. Antibiotic regimens include broad-spectrum antibiotic coverage for both gram-negative and gram-positive bacteria. Most centers advocate empiric anaerobic coverage. Gram stains and cultures of sputum from the donor and the recipient may be used when available to guide the choice of appropriate antibiotics. Many centers routinely use antifungal agents such as inhaled amphotericin B, voriconazole, or itraconazole postoperatively. Most transplantation programs administer valganciclovir for CMV prophylaxis if either the patient or the donor IgG serology is CMV-positive before surgery.

Immunosuppression is begun preoperatively with tacrolimus or cyclosporine and corticosteroids. Corticosteroids are administered in the operating room as intravenous methylprednisolone 0.5 to 1 g (usually administered at the time of reperfusion) and then at doses of 1 to 3 mg per kg daily for the next 3 days, followed by 0.8 mg per kg daily and then conversion to an equivalent oral dose. Many centers currently use interleukin (IL)-2 receptor blockers (e.g., basiliximab) for induction immunosuppression. A retrospective registry analysis of the impact of induction therapy on survival following LT showed a survival advantage with the use of interleukin-2-receptor antagonists in both SLT and BLT recipients and in BLT recipients treated with anti-thymocyte globulin (ATG) [39]. After the transplantation procedure, most patients begin a triple immunosuppression protocol with a combination of prednisone, a calcineurin agent, tacrolimus or cyclosporine, and a cell-cycle–inhibiting agent, mycophenolate mofetil or azathioprine [40].

POSTOPERATIVE PROBLEMS

Primary Graft Dysfunction

Perhaps the most serious problem in the postoperative period after LT is PGD [41]. A 2005 consensus conference attempted to standardize the grading of PGD on the basis of gas exchange and the presence of radiographic infiltrates (Table 59.2) [42]. When the acute lung injury definition of acute respiratory distress syndrome (ARDS)—a PaO_2/FiO_2 ratio of less than 200—is used to define the most severe form of PGD (grade 3), it is estimated that as many as 5% to 25% of transplant recipients can develop PGD (grade 3) [42, 43]. PGD is a diagnosis of

TABLE 59.2

Grading of the Severity of Primary Graft Dysfunction

Grade	PaO_2/FiO_2	Radiographic infiltrates consistent with pulmonary edema
0	>300	No
1	>300	Yes
2	200–300	Yes
3	<200	Yes

Adapted from Christie JD, Carby M, Bag R, et al: Report of the ISHLT Working Group on Primary Lung Graft Dysfunction part II: definition. A consensus statement of the International Society for Heart and Lung Transplantation. *J Heart Lung Transplant* 24(10):1454–1459, 2005, with permission [42].

exclusion; the condition usually occurs hours to 3 days after LT, whereas rejection and infection are more common after the first 24 hours. A stenosis at the venous anastomosis presents with similar signs and symptoms, but this diagnosis can be excluded by transesophageal echocardiography. However, because the timing of these disorders may vary, differentiation may be difficult.

PGD can persist to various degrees for hours to days after LT. Clinically, PGD is characterized by the appearance of new alveolar or interstitial infiltrates on radiographs, a decrease in pulmonary compliance, an increase in pulmonary vascular resistance, and a disruption in gas exchange. The radiographic findings of these patients include a perihilar haze, patchy alveolar consolidations, and, in the most severe form, dense perihilar and basilar alveolar consolidations with air bronchograms (Fig. 59.1). Pathology reports from biopsy specimens, autopsies, or lung explants removed during retransplantation indicate diffuse alveolar damage. PGD usually stabilizes over the next 2 to 4 days and then begins to resolve, although PGD is the single most common cause of mortality in the first 30 days following transplantation.

PGD is managed supportively with diuretics and mechanical ventilation, often with protective ventilatory strategies [41]. Because

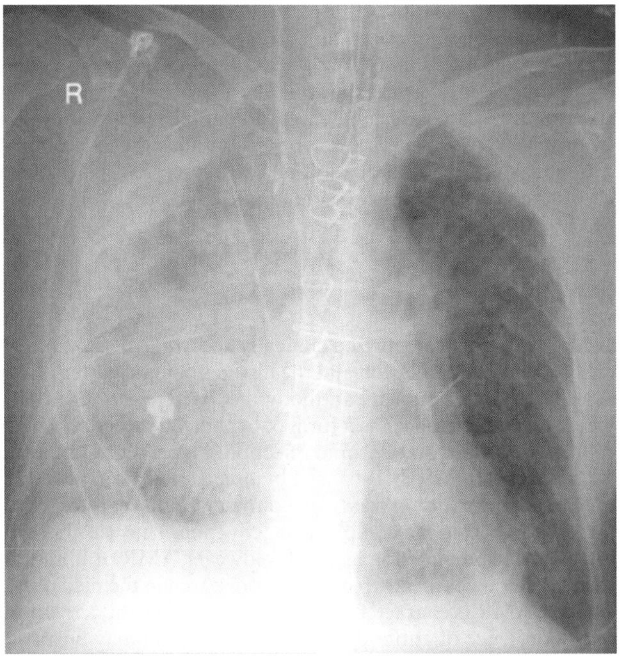

FIGURE 59.1 Severe primary graft dysfunction in the transplanted lung following a right single-lung transplant for idiopathic pulmonary fibrosis.

endogenous nitric oxide (NO) activity decreases after LT, there are several reports of the use of inhaled NO for hypoxemia and for pulmonary hypertension as a consequence of graft dysfunction after transplantation [44,45]. However, in one randomized, placebo-controlled trial (84 patients), the prophylactic inhalation of NO 10 minutes after reperfusion and for a minimum of 6 hours, was not shown to be beneficial for hemodynamic variables, reperfusion injury, oxygenation, time to extubation, length of intensive care or hospital stay, or 30-day mortality [46]. The use of artificial surfactant replacement has also been examined [47,48]. An open randomized prospective trial studying the use of instilled bovine surfactant immediately after establishment of the bronchial anastomosis, showed improved oxygenation and decreased PGD, shortened intubation time, and enhanced early post-LT recovery in the treatment group, although an unusually high incidence of PGD was found in the control group [47]. ECMO is also used for severe PGD unresponsive to protective lung ventilation with a hospital survival rate of 42% in an analysis of the Extracorporeal Life Support Organization registry study [49]. When used in this setting, ECMO should be initiated early to minimize the complications associated with prolonged mechanical ventilation. Veno-venous ECMO is the most commonly used ECMO for PGD, particularly since PGD usually resolves in a relatively short period of time. Retransplantation has also been performed, but the outcomes for patients undergoing retransplantation for PGD has been very poor.

Severe PGD usually leads to compromised short-term outcomes, including increase in the duration of mechanical ventilation and lengths of stay, poor 1-year survival rates, and compromised function among survivors. Long-term outcomes, such as pulmonary function and the incidence of bronchiolitis obliterans, are also impacted, and more severe PGD and longer duration of PGD are associated with the development of bronchiolitis obliterans syndrome (BOS) [50–52].

Although the mechanisms of PGD have not been completely delineated, several contributing factors have been postulated, including the disruption of lymphatics, bronchial vasculature, or nerves, and lung injury occurring either during preservation of the graft or after reperfusion [53]. Most likely, PGD is due to ischemia-reperfusion injury leading to increased capillary permeability and noncardiogenic pulmonary edema.

Multiple risk factors may be associated with the development of PGD [41,43,54–56]. Risk factors for severe PGD include some donor characteristics such as smoking history and hemodynamic instability following brain death; some events during the surgical procedure such as increased FIO_2 during allograft reperfusion, single-lung transplant, use of cardiopulmonary bypass, prolonged ischemic times, and blood product transfusions; and finally some recipient characteristics such as obesity, a preoperative diagnosis of sarcoidosis, and pre- and postoperative pulmonary arterial hypertension. Antibody-mediated rejection has also recently been postulated to be a risk factor for PGD [57].

ICU Outcomes

Few data are available for predicting outcomes and length of ICU stay after LT. It is known that the duration of mechanical ventilation is prolonged and the ICU mortality increased for patients who experience PGD. One study found that an immediate postoperative PaO_2/FIO_2 ratio of less than 200 predicted an ICU stay of 5 days or more [58]. Another study examined the value of intravascular volume status and central venous pressure (CVP) for predicting ICU outcomes; the results indicated that a CVP higher than 7 mm Hg after transplantation was associated with a longer duration of mechanical ventilation, longer ICU and hospital stays, and higher 2-month mortality rates [59].

Among patients requiring prolonged ICU stays, those who underwent tracheostomy were more likely to have undergone

BLT, required cardiopulmonary bypass during the procedure, experienced postoperative pneumonia, had more significant PGD at 48 hours, had longer initial periods of mechanical ventilation, and required reintubation more often [60].

Late Complications Requiring Admission to the ICU

The number of lung transplant recipients who are admitted to the ICU is expected to increase as the number of long-term survivors increases. The postoperative mortality rate has decreased because of improved surgical techniques and perioperative care, and approximately 97% of patients are discharged alive after transplantation [2]. However, after this immediate posttransplantation period, lung transplant recipients are more likely than some other solid-organ transplant recipients to experience infection or rejection that often require readmission to the ICU.

Nearly 25% of lung transplant recipients require an ICU admission after the initial hospital discharge. The most common admission diagnoses are respiratory failure and sepsis. These patients frequently require mechanical ventilation (53%), and the mortality rate is generally close to 40%. Prognostic factors for mortality include higher acute physiology and chronic health evaluation (APACHE) scores, a forced expiratory volume in one second (FEV_1) lower than the patient's best posttransplantation FEV_1, nonpulmonary organ dysfunction, low-serum albumin level, and longer duration of mechanical ventilation [61]. Patients admitted with a diagnosis of BOS who require mechanical ventilation are at the highest risk of mortality. In a large single-center study examining all admissions to the MICU in patients >30 days following LT, reasons for admission included respiratory failure in 50.5% and acute rejection in 16%. One quarter of patients required hemodialysis, and 53.5% required mechanical ventilation. In the study cohort, hospital survival was 88/101, but 6-month survival was 56.4%. Predictors of hospital survival were APACHE score on admission and SLT. Functional status at discharge was an independent predictor of 6-month survival [62]. In another study, again examining ICU admissions at >30 days post-LT in patients with diagnoses of idiopathic pulmonary fibrosis and COPD, 93% of patients required mechanical ventilation. Septic shock was the reason for admission in 55% of patients. ICU mortality was 62.5%. Mortality was associated with more frequent hospital admissions, a high severity score (SOFA), a diagnosis of sepsis, and requirement for mechanical ventilation. There was a higher incidence of BOS in nonsurvivors [63].

The long-term survival of patients who recover from the ICU stay is also compromised; however, a high percentage of patients (50%) can still enjoy long-term survival after an ICU admission.

A recent study supports the use of high-flow nasal cannula (HFNC) as supportive therapy for patients readmitted to the ICU for acute respiratory failure and was associated with a decreased risk of mechanical ventilation (absolute risk reduction of 29.8%). The number needed to treat to prevent one intubation was three [64]. In addition, those supported with HFNC had increased survival rates and did not experience adverse events.

Airway Complications

Because of the lack of revascularization of the bronchial circulation, anastomotic complications, such as bronchial dehiscence, bronchial stenosis, and bronchial infection, are the main airway complications reported in the first few weeks to months after LT [65,66]. The incidence of anastomotic complications has decreased as surgical techniques have improved and surgeons have gained experience with the procedure. The reported incidence of this complication ranges widely: some studies report it to be as high as 33%; others, as low as 1.6%. However, in reality, most recent series suggest a range of 7% to 18% [67], with a related mortality rate of 2% to 4%. Risk factors for airway complications include ischemia of the donor bronchus during the posttransplantation period, due to loss of bronchial blood flow (only the pulmonary vessels are revascularized during LT surgery), surgical techniques for the anastomosis, length of the donor bronchi, acute rejection, and bronchial infections.

Airway complications can be classified as early or late. Early airway complications usually occur during the first 4 to 12 weeks after transplantation and manifest themselves as a partial or complete anastomotic dehiscence or a fungal (usually *Aspergillus* or *Candida* species) or bacterial (usually *Staphylococcus* or *Pseudomonas* species) anastomotic infection. These conditions can subsequently result in anastomotic strictures or bronchomalacia. Clinically, bronchial dehiscence may cause prolonged air leaks in the early posttransplantation period. In some cases, the dehiscence may also lead to infection or the formation of peribronchial abscesses or fistulas. The results of chest radiographs and computed tomography (CT) scans are usually nonspecific; however, the appearance of extraluminal air on chest CT scans is very sensitive and specific for the diagnosis of anastomotic dehiscence.

Bronchoscopy is the preferred diagnostic method for evaluating the bronchial anastomosis. The initial bronchoscopies are done usually before extubation and again before discharge. In addition, the anastomosis is also evaluated carefully during surveillance or clinically indicated bronchoscopy particularly during the 1st year. The integrity of the mucosa should be assessed, and specimens from a bronchial wash or brush should be sent for cultures and cytologic examination. If there is any evidence of infection, antibiotics and antifungals (usually inhaled amphotericin with or without itraconazole or voriconazole) should be administered on the basis of culture results.

Late bronchial anastomotic complications, including stenosis (most common), bronchomalacia, and development of exophytic granulation tissue are often the result of ischemia, infection, or dehiscence during the early weeks after transplantation. These complications manifest themselves as cough, shortness of breath, wheezing, dyspnea on exertion, and worsening obstruction as documented by pulmonary function testing. The characteristic flow volume loop demonstrates a concave appearance in both the inspiratory loop and the expiratory loop. Bronchial strictures or stenosis may also be seen on chest radiographs or CT scans, or by bronchoscopy. Therapeutic options for anastomotic complications include balloon dilation of a stricture, stent placement, cryotherapy, argon beam coagulation, laser procedures, and, rarely, surgery.

Rejection

Graft rejection is categorized clinically according to the time of onset after transplantation and the histopathologic pattern. The three types of rejection are antibody-mediated rejection (AMR) which can rarely appear as a form of hyperacute rejection, acute cellular rejection, and chronic rejection. Hyperacute rejection is an acute form of AMR caused by preexisting alloantibodies that bind to the donor vascular epithelium and lead to vessel thrombosis because of complement activation. This was thought to be a rare complication after LT. However, AMR or humoral rejection is currently an area of active research in the field of LT [68,69]. AMR is characterized by local complement activation or the presence of antibody to donor HLAs and may be a risk factor for BOS [70]. Treatment of AMR includes plasmapheresis, intravenous immunoglobulin and/or rituximab, a monoclonal antibody against the CD-20 antigen.

Acute Rejection

As many as 50% to 55% of patients experience acute rejection during the first postoperative month, and as many as 90% will experience at least one episode of acute rejection within the 1st year [69]. Acute rejection usually occurs between 10 and 90 days after LT. It is not uncommon (20% of lung transplant recipients) for a single patient to experience either recurrent (more than two episodes) and/or persistent (failure to resolve with standard therapy) rejection. Acute rejection usually does not occur as frequently after the first postoperative year. Risk factors for acute rejection are poorly defined, but HLA mismatches may be correlated with its occurrence [71,72].

Clinically, acute rejection manifests itself as cough, shortness of breath, malaise, and fever. Occasionally, the presentation is asymptomatic. The majority of transplantation centers advocate surveillance bronchoscopy for the detection of this condition, although outcome data are not available [40]. Physical examination may detect rales or wheezing. The usefulness of chest radiography depends on the time since transplantation. Typically, during the 1st month the results of chest radiography can be abnormal in as many as 75% of rejection episodes; however, the results of radiography are abnormal in only 25% of rejection episodes that occur more than 1 month after transplantation. The most common radiographic patterns associated with acute rejection are a perihilar flare, and alveolar or interstitial localized or diffuse infiltrates with or without associated pleural effusion. In addition, CT may show ground-glass opacities, septal thickening, and volume loss. New pleural fluid or increases in the amount of pleural fluid produced during the 2nd to 6th week after LT is common among patients with acute lung rejection. The characteristics of the fluid are consistent with those of an exudate: the total lymphocyte count is often more than 80% of the total number of white blood cells.

Physiologic findings during periods of acute rejection include hypoxemia and deterioration in pulmonary function. Pulmonary function abnormalities are characterized by at least a 10% to 15% decline in FEV_1 from baseline and/or at least a 20% decline in forced expiratory flow (FEF) over 25% to 75% of expired vital capacity. Once again, these changes are nonspecific and can also be seen with infectious processes and graft complications.

Because clinical criteria alone cannot differentiate acute rejection from infection and less common graft complications, transbronchial biopsy (TBBx) with bronchoalveolar lavage (BAL) has become the primary diagnostic procedure. The sensitivity of diagnosing acute rejection by TBBx ranges from 61% to 94%, and the specificity ranges from 90% to 100%. A histologic grading system for acute pulmonary rejection was proposed in 1990 and revised in 1996 and 2007 [73]. Pathologically, acute rejection is characterized by perivascular, mononuclear lymphocytic infiltrates with or without airway inflammation; histologically, it is graded from A_0 to A_4 on the basis of the degree of perivascular inflammation. In addition, the airway can be involved by lymphocytic bronchitis or bronchiolitis, which is graded from B_0 to B_x. As rejection progresses, the perivascular lymphocytic infiltrates surrounding the venules and arterioles become dense and extend into the perivascular and peribronchiolar alveolar septa. Severe rejection may involve the alveolar space; parenchymal necrosis, hyaline membranes, and necrotizing vasculitis have been described; and respiratory failure requiring mechanical ventilation can occur.

Once acute rejection has been diagnosed, treatment consists of augmenting the level of immunosuppression. Intravenous methylprednisolone (10 to 15 mg per kg daily for 3 days) followed by an increase in the maintenance regimen of prednisone regimen to 0.5 to 1 mg per kg daily, with tapering over the next several weeks, is a standard treatment regimen. Maintenance immunosuppression should also be augmented. Typically, symptoms resolve in days, and histologic follow-up 3 to 4 weeks later should demonstrate resolution. Recurrent or persistent acute rejection may require alteration of the baseline immunosuppressive regimen. Lympholytic therapy, methotrexate, photophoresis, total lymphoid irradiation, and aerosolized cyclosporine have been used with varied success [74].

Chronic Lung Allograft Dysfunction

Chronic lung allograft dysfunction (CLAD) encompasses varied presentations of progressive allograft dysfunction with obstructive and restrictive physiology [75]. The most common form of CLAD has been equated with the histologic finding of obliterative bronchiolitis (OB); this form of chronic rejection is a primary cause of morbidity and mortality after LT and the leading single cause of death more than 1 year after transplantation [1]. The incidence of OB ranges from 35% to 50%. OB has been defined clinically by an obstructive functional defect and histologically by obliteration of terminal bronchioles. OB generally occurs at a mean of 16 to 20 months after LT, but it has been reported as early as 3 months after transplantation. More than 50% of recipients will experience some degree of OB by 5 years after transplantation [1]. A less common form of CLAD, the restrictive allograft syndrome (RAS), contributes to approximately 25% to 35% of the reported cases and carries a worse prognosis than BOS. It is characterized by various stages of diffuse alveolar damage and extensive fibrosis in the alveolar interstitium, visceral pleura, and interlobular septae. RAS presents radiologically as upper lobe–dominant fibrosis and/or interstitial opacities sometimes often with associated pleural thickening and with a restrictive pattern in the lung function tests (Total lung capacity [TLC] below 90% of the best baseline posttransplant) [75,76].

The causes of and risk factors for OB remain unclear. Several possible risk factors have been proposed, including uncontrolled acute rejection, lymphocytic bronchiolitis, CMV pneumonitis, CMV infection without pneumonitis, community-acquired respiratory viruses, gastroesophageal reflux disease, PGD, AMR, HLA-A mismatches, total HLA mismatches, absence of donor antigen-specific hyporeactivity, non-CMV infection, older donor age, and bronchiolitis obliterans with organizing pneumonia [50,51,77–79]. The most consistently identified risk factor is acute rejection, particularly in those patients who experience recurrent, high-grade episodes of acute rejection.

Clinically, OB can manifest itself as an upper respiratory tract infection and can be mistakenly treated as such. Other patients exhibit no clinical symptoms, but pulmonary function testing demonstrates gradual obstructive dysfunction. FEV_1 has been the standard spirometric parameter used for diagnosis, but midexpiratory flow rates may be a more sensitive parameter for early detection.

Typically, chest radiographs are not helpful in the diagnosis of OB because their results are unchanged from the results of baseline posttransplantation radiographs. High-resolution CT scans may show peripheral bronchiectasis, patchy consolidation, decreased peripheral vascular markings, air trapping, mosaicism, tree-in-bud changes, and bronchial dilation; these findings may aid in the diagnosis of OB [80]. Air trapping on end-expiratory high-resolution CT scans has been shown to be a sensitive (91%) and accurate (86%) radiologic indicator of OB, but it may not be able to provide an early diagnosis of this disorder. As with acute rejection, TBBx is used to diagnose OB, but primarily to exclude other diagnoses. The classic pathologic finding is constrictive bronchiolitis. Unfortunately, the sensitivity of TBBx for diagnosing OB is low (range: 15% to 87%), and the diagnosis of OB is often made by exclusion. OB is graded physiologically on the basis of the degree of change in pulmonary function (FEV_1) from baseline [78]. Because of the variability in obtaining bronchioles by TBBx, the ISHLT has established a staging system for BOS. This staging is based on a reduction in FEV_1 of more than 20% from baseline after transplantation and is associated with a decrease in the FEF 25% to 75%, with or without the pathologic documentation of OB [78].

Once OB has been diagnosed histologically or clinically by excluding alternative diagnoses, treatment involves administering high-dose methylprednisolone followed by a tapering course of oral corticosteroids. Therapy may stabilize pulmonary function, but it only rarely results in substantial improvement. Alternative immunosuppressants such as sirolimus have also been associated with stabilization of pulmonary function when used as rescue treatment for BOS. Lympholytic depleting agents such as ATG are the most commonly used rescue medications if there is no clinical response to corticosteroids. Several studies have shown prevention, stabilization, and/or improvement in BOS when azithromycin is added to the regimen or used prophylactically, likely due to the immunomodulating effects and is now a widespread practice [81,82]. Other alternatives with limited clinical success include alemtuzumab, basiliximab, methotrexate, total lymphoid radiation, and photophoresis.

Infection, including bronchiectasis, frequently complicates intensive immunosuppression for OB and may result in death. Pseudomonas is a common offender, and aerosolized aminoglycoside antibiotics or suppressive quinolone treatment may be considered. Because most cases of OB can only be stabilized, strategies directed at prevention, early diagnosis, and treatments are necessary for the preservation of lung function. Retransplantation has been performed with varied results. Survival rates are somewhat lower than those after the initial transplantation and are superior when performed for the indication of BOS, performed more than 1 year following the initial transplant and when a bilateral transplant is performed (1 year, 71%; 3 years, 46%; and 5 years, 34%) [1,83].

Infectious Complications

Infections are an important cause of early and late morbidity and mortality after transplantation and are the leading single specific cause of death during the 1st year following the transplantation procedure [1,84]. The incidence of infection is significantly higher among recipients of lung transplants than among recipients of most other solid-organ transplants; this higher incidence may be related to the continuous exposure of the allograft to the environment. Other predisposing factors include a diminished cough reflex because of denervation, poor lymphatic drainage, decreased mucociliary clearance, recipient-harbored infection, and, occasionally, transfer of infection from the donor organ. Nosocomial infections, such as urinary tract infections, ventilator-assisted pneumonia, and infections at the site of the surgical wound or the vascular access, also occur during the early postoperative period. However, in most circumstances the allograft(s) is/are the primary site of infection.

Bacterial Infections

Bacterial pneumonia is the most common life-threatening infection that develops during the early postoperative period. Its incidence during the first two postoperative weeks is reported to be as high as 35% [84–87], and in a single-center retrospective cohort study, 68% of patients developed at least one episode of pneumonia [88]. In another single-center study, 12% of patients suffered a ventilator-associated pneumonia, resulting in increases in hospital length of stay, increase in duration of mechanical ventilation, and an increase in hospital mortality. Pseudomonas and Enterobacteracie were the most common pathogens. Gastroperesis was associated with the development of pneumonia in this study [89]. Common organisms include *Pseudomonas aeruginosa* and *Staphylococcus* species. The incidence of perioperative bacterial pneumonia has been reduced to as low as 10% by prophylaxis with broad-spectrum antibiotics, usually an antipseudomonal cephalosporin and clindamycin, and by routine culture of the trachea of both the donor and the recipient at the time of transplantation. Prophylactic antibiotics are usually discontinued after 3 days if the results of cultures are negative; the antibiotics are tailored to the cultured organisms if the results are positive. For transplant recipients with bronchiectasis, postoperative bacterial prophylaxis is usually continued for 14 days. The incidence of bacterial pneumonia is high during the first 6 months after transplantation but decreases thereafter, although a second late peak of incidence often occurs when immunosuppression is augmented for the treatment of chronic rejection. During the early posttransplantation period, bacterial infection due to *Staphylococcus* or, less commonly, *Pseudomonas* can develop at or distal to the site of the anastomosis.

It is often difficult to distinguish pneumonia from other early graft complications, such as reperfusion injury, pulmonary edema, rejection, and other causes of infection. In addition, differentiating between colonization and invasion may be difficult and often requires invasive procedures such as bronchoscopy with BAL, quantitative sterile brush sampling, or TBBx.

Other Infections

Atypical pneumonias, including those due to Legionella, Mycobacteria, and Nocardia, are uncommon during the first month after transplantation but occur among 2% to 9% of recipients of lung or heart–lung transplants. At transplantation centers that routinely administer prophylaxis with trimethoprim–sulfamethoxazole during the 1st year after transplantation and continue or reinitiate it when immunosuppression is augmented, the incidence of pneumocystis pneumonia is less than 1%.

Most opportunistic infections occur within 6 months after transplantation. Sustained immunosuppression leading to a decrease in cell-mediated immunity predisposes the patient to infection with opportunistic organisms such as Aspergillus, Mycobacterium, Nocardia, and geographically endemic fungi.

Viral Infections

Viral infections are a primary cause of morbidity and mortality among lung transplant recipients. During the first 6 months after transplantation, CMV accounts for most of the viral infections among these patients [84,87,90]. The typical time period for the development of CMV infection is 30 to 150 days postoperatively; the incidence of illness (i.e., infection and disease) is approximately 50%. Risk factors for CMV disease depend on the serology of the donor and the recipient and on the use of high-intensity immunosuppressive therapy, including cytolytic therapy. Approximately 15% to 35% of CMV-positive patients who receive grafts from either CMV-positive or CMV-negative donors experience CMV disease, whereas approximately 55% of CMV-negative patients who receive a graft from a CMV-positive donor may experience CMV disease. Most studies indicate that CMV pneumonitis contributes to the development of chronic rejection [78].

CMV can cause a wide spectrum of disease, ranging from asymptomatic infection, such as shedding of the virus in the urine or BAL, to widespread dissemination. The most common presentation of CMV among lung transplant recipients is pneumonitis, but the infection may also present as gastroenteritis, hepatitis, or colitis. CMV pneumonitis can often be confused with acute rejection. Clinical findings of CMV pneumonitis include fever, cough, flu-like illness, hypoxemia, an interstitial or alveolar infiltrate, and leukopenia. A definitive diagnosis of invasive disease requires cytologic or histologic changes in a cell preparation or in tissue. Therefore, diagnosis often requires flexible bronchoscopy with TBBx and BAL; this combination can detect 60% to 90% of CMV pneumonias. Currently, plasma-based polymerase chain reaction (PCR) assays are used to screen patients and to detect CMV infection [91]. The risk of CMV pneumonitis after LT is usually related to the serum concentration of CMV DNA, and this measure is used in many programs for the preemptive management of CMV.

The pathologic hallmark of CMV infection is a cytomegalic 250-nm cell containing a large central basophilic intranuclear inclusion. This inclusion is referred to as an "owl's eye" because it is separated from the nuclear membrane by a halo. Identifying CMV cytologically is very specific (98%) but lacks sensitivity (21%) for detecting the presence of infection. Other pathologic findings in the lung parenchyma of patients with CMV pneumonia include a lymphocytic and mononuclear-cell interstitial pneumonitis.

Ganciclovir intravenous and oral valganciclovir are currently the mainstays of therapy for invasive CMV disease [90]. Bone marrow toxicity is one of the primary limiting side effects of ganciclovir therapy and may necessitate conversion to an alternative agent such as foscarnet. Most centers also use CMV-specific hyperimmunoglobulin to treat CMV disease.

Prophylaxis against CMV infections has become an important strategy at most transplantation centers. Initially, some centers attempted to match CMV-negative recipients with CMV-negative donors; however, the limited donor supply did not allow the continuation of this practice. The use of CMV-negative blood products is advocated. Prophylaxis with ganciclovir or valganciclovir seems to be effective in delaying the onset of CMV infection. Most centers give prophylaxis to all patients except CMV-negative recipients who receive grafts from CMV-negative donors. Prophylaxis is usually recommended for at least 90 days, but the majority of centers, particularly for CMV-negative recipients of grafts from CMV-positive donors, will continue prophylaxis for at least 1 year. A randomized, controlled, multicenter study examined the efficacy of extending valganciclovir prophylaxis from the standard 3 months to 12 months in at-risk (either donor or recipient CMV-positive) patients. The investigators found a significant reduction in CMV infection, disease, and disease severity without increased ganciclovir resistance or toxicity among those patients receiving the longer course of therapy [92]. For patients at highest risk of infection, CMV hyperimmunoglobulin may be added to the regimen. Preemptive strategies, such as initiating treatment when a high level of CMV DNA is detected by PCR, may also delay and decrease the severity of CMV infection and has become the standard of care at many centers.

Other viruses that affect lung transplant recipients include herpes simplex virus (early after transplantation), community-acquired respiratory viruses, such as respiratory syncytial virus, other paramyxoviruses (such as parainfluenza), influenza virus, metapneumovirus, and adenovirus [93]. Some transplantation programs initiate prophylaxis with acyclovir for herpes infection after the discontinuation of ganciclovir. Ribavirin has been used to treat respiratory syncytial virus infection in both nebulized and oral form, although the former is associated with bronchospasm and potential teratogenicity to health care workers.

Fungal Infections

Fungal infections are more common among recipients of LTs than among recipients of some other solid-organ transplantations [94,95]. The overall incidence of invasive fungal infection after LT ranges from 15% to 35%. Such infections usually develop during the first few months after transplantation. Fungal infections carry the highest morbidity and mortality rates of all infections after transplantation; mortality rates can range from 40% to 70%.

Aspergillus species such as *A. fumigatus*, *A. flavus*, *A. terreus*, and *A. niger* can be colonizing organisms; can cause an infection that suggests an indolent, progressive pneumonia; or can cause an acute fulminant infection that disseminates rapidly. *Aspergillus* can invade blood vessels and may appear as an infarct on chest imaging or present with hemoptysis. The radiographic findings of pulmonary aspergillosis include focal lower-lobe infiltrates, patchy bronchopneumonic infiltrates, single or multiple nodules with or without cavitation, thin-wall cavities, and opacification of the entire lung graft. High-resolution CT scans may reveal a halo sign that is believed to be pathognomonic for angioinvasive fungal infections such as aspergillosis. Other manifestations of *Aspergillus* infection include pseudomembranous tracheobronchitis, often at and distal to the site of the anastomosis. Diagnosing invasive aspergillosis requires identifying organisms within tissues. These organisms can appear as septate hyphae that branch at acute angles and can be detected on hematoxylin-eosin and methenamine silver stains.

Survival rates for patients with Aspergillus infection have been improved by the early initiation of broad-spectrum azoles (such as voriconazole or itraconazole, and more recently posaconazole), sometimes with the addition of an echinocandin, and a reduction in immunosuppressive therapy [96]. In patients with airway involvement with *Aspergillus* and for short-term prophylaxis following transplantation, inhaled amphotericin may be used. It is now rare to require systemic amphotericin or the less nephrotoxic liposomal formulation of amphotericin B. Prophylaxis with the azoles (voriconazole or itraconazole) for 3 to 6 months, and/or with aerosolized amphotericin, has shown promise for decreasing the incidence of *Aspergillus* infection after transplantation.

Candidal infections may occur during the early postoperative period but usually do not cause invasive disease. *Candida* species can cause a variety of syndromes among LT recipients; these syndromes include mucocutaneous disease, line sepsis, wound infection, and, rarely, pulmonary involvement. Fluconazole and caspofungin have emerged as effective alternatives for treating infections caused by *Candida albicans*. Fluconazole appears to be less active against other *Candida* species such as *C. glabrata* and *C. krusei*.

Less common causes of fungal infections among lung transplant recipients include *Cryptococcus neoformans* and the dimorphic fungi (*Coccidioides*, *Histoplasma*, and *Blastomyces*). The broad-spectrum azole agents are the initial therapeutic choices for treating serious infections with the invasive mycoses. Amphotericin B can be used for disseminated disease. The dose, duration of therapy, and alternative therapies differ depending on the organism.

Immunosuppression

After LT, a typical regimen for the maintenance of immunosuppression consists of tacrolimus at a dose of approximately 0.1 mg per kg orally every day in two divided doses (adjusted to maintain a serum concentration of 8 to 15 ng per mL), or cyclosporine 5 mg per kg orally every day in two divided doses (with dose adjusted to maintain serum concentrations of 250 to 350 ng per mL), and mycophenolate mofetil at a dose of 1 to 3 g daily, or azathioprine 1 to 2 mg per kg daily (adjusted to maintain a leukocyte count higher than 4,000 to 4,500 per mL), and prednisone approximately 0.5 mg per kg daily for the 1st month and then tapered by 5 mg per week over the next few months to a final maintenance dose of 5 mg per day. A minority of transplantation programs completely discontinue the administration of prednisone approximately 1 year after transplantation. The role of sirolimus after LT remains to be established. It is recommended that sirolimus not be used in the early perioperative period (<10 to 12 weeks) due to impaired wound healing.

Physicians caring for transplant recipients must be aware of the numerous drugs that can interact with tacrolimus and cyclosporine. For example, the azoles cause a significant increase in the serum concentrations of tacrolimus and cyclosporine. Likewise, discontinuing azole agents without increasing the dose of tacrolimus or cyclosporine can cause an acute and life-threatening decrease in the therapeutic concentrations of these drugs. Interactions with macrolide antibiotics, calcium-channel blockers, and gastric motility drugs have also been reported. The concentrations of tacrolimus or cyclosporine are decreased by rifampin and anticonvulsants.

All immunosuppressants are associated with toxicity and drug interactions [97,98]. The details of these complications are discussed in chapter 63. A unique toxicity of the calcineuerin agents particularly when used with sirolimus include thrombotic microangiopathy [99].

Miscellaneous Complications

Another possible complication of LT is postoperative hemorrhage, requiring reexploration. One of the early clues to this diagnosis is radiographic evidence of a hemothorax or what appears to be a retained clot, or a large volume of blood draining from the thoracostomy tubes. This complication may occur more frequently among patients who require cardiopulmonary bypass with its attendant requirement for anticoagulation or among patients with pleural adhesions from previous procedures such as pleurodesis or diagnostic or therapeutic lung surgery. Persistent air leaks can occasionally occur but are unlikely unless the bronchial anastomosis loses its integrity because the lung parenchyma is normally not entered during a routine LT procedure.

In addition to the bronchial anastomotic complications discussed earlier, vascular anastomotic complications can occur. A stenosis at the venous anastomosis is indicated by radiographic evidence of pulmonary edema and infiltrates; this condition can be confused with PGD and is usually diagnosed by transesophageal echocardiography. A stenosis at the arterial anastomosis is suggested by unexplained gas exchange abnormalities and pulmonary hypertension [100]. Phrenic nerve dysfunction and diaphragmatic paralysis, which occur in conjunction with other types of cardiothoracic surgery, occur after LT with an incidence of 3% to 9.3% and are associated with a prolongation in the number of days for which mechanical ventilation is required, an increase in the length of stay in the ICU, an increase in the use of ICU resources, and an increase in the need for tracheostomy [101]. An inability to wean the patient from mechanical ventilation may indicate phrenic nerve dysfunction; the diagnosis can be confirmed by phrenic nerve conduction studies. For patients who do not require ventilation, the diagnosis of phrenic nerve dysfunction can be made with a fluoroscopic "sniff test," and more recently with the use of bedside ultrasound. If the injury is the result of stretching of the phrenic nerve or trauma to the nerve during the surgical procedure but the nerve is not completely transected, a slow recovery can be anticipated. Complete transection is rare, but the damage is permanent. Diaphragmatic plication or pacing can be performed in some cases.

Pleural effusions can develop and/or persist following LT. The characteristics of these effusions are usually lymphocyte-predominant exudates and can be associated early on with severing of the lymphatics (i.e., chylous effusion) or with rejection. A single-center study of a large number of lung transplant patients found that 27% of pleural effusions in these patients required drainage. Of the effusions, 96% was exudates, and 27% of patient had infected pleural effusions with organisms such as fungal pathogens (specifically Candida most commonly), followed by bacterial etiologies. These infected effusions were characterized by high lactate dehydrogenase levels and neutrophilia [102]. Other causes of pleural effusions include heart failure, pulmonary embolism, and trapped lung. Rarely pleurodesis or decortication may be required.

Lung transplant recipients also experience gastroparesis, severe gastroesophageal reflux resulting in aspiration pneumonia, and an increased incidence of gastrointestinal emergencies. These conditions include colonic perforation, small-bowel obstruction, diverticulitis, CMV colitis, megacolon, prolonged ileus, ischemic bowel, and pancreatitis [103]. Gastroesophageal reflux may be more severe among transplant recipients with cystic fibrosis.

Renal insufficiency is also a frequent complication among lung transplant recipients. This complication results from a combination of infections leading to sepsis and acute tubular necrosis, or from medication-related renal toxicity. Another study reported an incidence of acute renal failure postoperatively in 39% of patients and identified the use of aprotinin and bilateral lung procedures as risk factors. Acute renal failure was not predictive of late renal dysfunction or decreased long-term survival [104].

Cardiac arrhythmias, especially atrial arrhythmias such as atrial fibrillation, commonly develop in the perioperative period with an incidence of 25% in one study with resulting increase in length of hospital stay and increased 1-year mortality. Risk factors for their development included older age, diagnosis of pulmonary fibrosis, right ventricular dysfunction, right ventricle enlargement and elevated right atrial pressure, left atrial enlargement diastolic dysfunction, and history of coronary artery disease [105]. Another study found an incidence of atrial fibrillation of 35%, which was associated with older age and cardiopulmonary bypass, with resulting increase in hospital length of stay but no increase in mortality, ICU length of stay, or days on mechanical ventilation [106].

In one series of lung transplant recipients, the incidence of deep venous thrombosis and pulmonary embolism was reported to be 8.6%. This complication was believed to be related to alterations in coagulability leading to a hypercoagulable state or hypercoagulability due to their underlying disease [107,108].

Posttransplant lymphoproliferative disease (PTLD) and other malignancies can occur among lung transplant recipients. The incidence of PTLD after LT reportedly ranges from 1.8% to 9.4% [109,110]. PTLD comprises a heterogeneous group of lymphoid proliferations, usually of the B-cell form, that are strongly associated with the Epstein–Barr virus (EBV). Patients for whom the results of pretransplantation serologic studies are negative for EBV but who receive an organ from an EBV-positive donor and experience seroconversion are at a higher risk of PTLD. Clinically, PTLD usually occurs during the first year after transplantation; it involves the allograft and manifests itself as radiographic findings of solitary or multiple pulmonary nodules. Treatment includes reducing the level of immunosuppression, institution of antiviral therapy, and administering the anti-CD20 monoclonal antibody rituximab. In some cases, chemotherapy or surgery may be indicated.

Significant advances have been made in the field of LT since its inception more than 30 years ago, allowing this procedure to be a successful therapeutic option for patients with end-stage parenchymal or vascular lung disease. However, despite these improvements, numerous complications, many of which are managed by critical care professionals, can arise in this group of patients, and the unique aspects of their care are important.

References

1. Yusen RD, Edwards LB, Kucheryavaya AY, et al: The Registry of the International Society for Heart and Lung Transplantation: thirty-second official adult lung and heart-lung transplantation report-2015; focus theme: early graft failure. *J Heart Lung Transplant* 34(10):1264–1277, 2015.
2. Scientific Registry of Transplant Recipients. Patient survival after lung transplantation. Available from: http://www.srtr.org. Accessed December 14, 2015.
3. Weill D, Benden C, Corris PA, et al: A consensus document for the selection of lung transplant candidates: 2014–an update from the Pulmonary Transplantation Council of the International Society for Heart and Lung Transplantation. *J Heart Lung Transplant* 34(1):1–15, 2015.

4. Stephenson AL, Sykes J, Berthiaume Y, et al: Clinical and demographic factors associated with post-lung transplantation survival in individuals with cystic fibrosis. *J Heart Lung Transplant* 34(9):1139–1145, 2015.
5. Chiumello D, Coppola S, Froio S, et al: Extracorporeal life support as bridge to lung transplantation: a systematic review. *Crit Care* 19:19, 2015.
6. Vermeijden JW, Zijlstra JG, Erasmus ME, et al: Lung transplantation for ventilator-dependent respiratory failure. *J Heart Lung Transplant* 28(4):347–351, 2009.
7. Javidfar J, Brodie D, Iribarne A, et al: Extracorporeal membrane oxygenation as a bridge to lung transplantation and recovery. *J Thorac Cardiovasc Surg* 144(3):716–721, 2012.
8. Mason DP, Thuita L, Nowicki ER, et al: Should lung transplantation be performed for patients on mechanical respiratory support? The US experience. *J Thorac Cardiovasc Surg* 139(3):765.e1–773.e1, 2010.
9. Crotti S, Iotti GA, Lissoni A, et al: Organ allocation waiting time during extracorporeal bridge to lung transplant affects outcomes. *Chest* 144(3):1018–1025, 2013.
10. Organ Procurement and Transplant Network. Lung Allocation Score (LAS) Calculator. Available from: http://optn.transplant.hrsa.gov/resources/allocation-calculators/las-calculator/. 2015. Accessed December 14, 2015.
11. Eberlein M, Garrity ER, Orens JB: Lung allocation in the United States. *Clin Chest Med* 32(2):213–222, 2011.
12. McShane PJ, Garrity ER Jr: Impact of the lung allocation score. *Semin Respir Crit Care Med* 34(3):275–280, 2013.
13. Takahashi SM, Garrity ER: The impact of the lung allocation score. *Semin Respir Crit Care Med* 31(2):108–114, 2010.
14. Liu V, Zamora MR, Dhillon GS, et al: Increasing lung allocation scores predict worsened survival among lung transplant recipients. *Am J Transplant* 10(4):915–920, 2010.
15. Merlo CA, Weiss ES, Orens JB, et al: Impact of U.S. Lung Allocation Score on survival after lung transplantation. *J Heart Lung Transplant* 28(8):769–775, 2009.
16. Horai T, Shigemura N, Gries C, et al: Lung transplantation for patients with high lung allocation score: single-center experience. *Ann Thorac Surg* 93(5):1592–1597, 2012; discussion 1597.
17. Russo MJ, Iribarne A, Hong KN, et al: High lung allocation score is associated with increased morbidity and mortality following transplantation. *Chest* 137(3):651–657, 2010.
18. Scientific Registry of Transplant Recipients. Time to transplant and waitlist for lung transplant patients. Available from: http://www.srtr.org. 2015. Accessed December 14, 2015.
19. Organ Procurement and Transplant Network. Donors Recovered in the U.S by Donor Type. Available from: http://optn.transplant.hrsa.gov.2015. Accessed December 15, 2015.
20. Krutsinger D, Reed RM, Blevins A, et al: Lung transplantation from donation after cardiocirculatory death: a systematic review and meta-analysis. *J Heart Lung Transplant* 34(5):675–684, 2015.
21. Cypel M, Levvey B, Raemdon DV, et al: International Society for heart and lung transplantation donation after circulatory death registry report. *J Heart Lung Transplant* 34(10):1278–1282, 2015.
22. Gries CJ, White DB, Truog RD, et al: An official American Thoracic Society/International Society for Heart and Lung Transplantation/Society of Critical Care Medicine/Association of Organ and Procurement Organizations/United Network of Organ Sharing Statement: ethical and policy considerations in organ donation after circulatory determination of death. *Am J Respir Crit Care Med* 188(1):103–109, 2013.
23. Taghavi S, Jayarajan SN, Komaroff E, et al: Single-lung transplantation can be performed with acceptable outcomes using selected donors with heavy smoking history. *J Heart Lung Transplant* 32(10):1005–1012, 2013.
24. Baldwin MR, Peterson ER, Easthausen I, et al: Donor age and early graft failure after lung transplantation: a cohort study. *Am J Transplant* 13(10):2685–2695, 2013.
25. Sommer W, Kuhn C, Tudorache I, et al: Extended criteria donor lungs and clinical outcome: results of an alternative allocation algorithm. *J Heart Lung Transplant* 32(11):1065–1072, 2013.
26. Minambres E, Coll E, Duerto J, et al: Effect of an intensive lung donor-management protocol on lung transplantation outcomes. *J Heart Lung Transplant* 33(2):178–184, 2014.
27. Bansal R, Esan A, Hess D, et al: Mechanical ventilatory support in potential lung donor patients. *Chest* 146(1):220–227, 2014.
28. Mascia L, Pasero D, Slutsky AS, et al: Effect of a lung protective strategy for organ donors on eligibility and availability of lungs for transplantation: a randomized controlled trial. *JAMA* 304(23):2620–2627, 2010.
29. Angel LF, Levine DJ, Restrepo MI, et al: Impact of a lung transplantation donor-management protocol on lung donation and recipient outcomes. *Am J Respir Crit Care Med* 174(6):710–716, 2006.
30. Kotloff RM, Blosser S, Fulda GJ, et al: Management of the potential organ donor in the ICU: Society of Critical Care Medicine/American College of Chest Physicians/Association of Organ Procurement Organizations Consensus Statement. *Crit Care Med* 43(6):1291–1325, 2015.
31. Cypel M, Yeung JC, Machuca T, et al: Experience with the first 50 ex vivo lung perfusions in clinical transplantation. *J Thorac Cardiovasc Surg* 144(5):1200–1206, 2012.
32. Cypel M, Yeung JC, Liu M, et al: Normothermic ex vivo lung perfusion in clinical lung transplantation. *N Engl J Med* 364(15):1431–1440, 2011.
33. Fildes JE, Archer LD, Blaikley J, et al: Clinical outcome of patients transplanted with marginal donor lungs via ex vivo lung perfusion compared to standard lung transplantation. *Transplantation* 99(5):1078–1083, 2015.
34. Boffini M, Ricci D, Bonato R, et al: Incidence and severity of primary graft dysfunction after lung transplantation using rejected grafts reconditioned with ex vivo lung perfusion. *Eur J Cardiothorac Surg* 46(5):789–793, 2014.
35. Boasquevisque CH, Yildirim E, Waddel TK, et al: Surgical techniques: lung transplant and lung volume reduction. *Proc Am Thorac Soc* 6(1):66–78, 2009.
36. Beer A, Reed RM, Bolukbas S, et al: Mechanical ventilation after lung transplantation. An international survey of practices and preferences. *Ann Am Thorac Soc* 11(4):546–553, 2014.
37. Ahya VN, Kawut SM: Noninfectious pulmonary complications after lung transplantation. *Clin Chest Med* 26(4):613–622, vi, 2005.
38. Angles R, Tenorio L, Roman A, et al: Lung transplantation for emphysema. Lung hyperinflation: incidence and outcome. *Transpl Int* 17(12):810–814, 2005.
39. Hachem RR, Edwards LB, Yusen RD, et al: The impact of induction on survival after lung transplantation: an analysis of the International Society for Heart and Lung Transplantation Registry. *Clin Transplant* 22(5):603–608, 2008.
40. Levine SM; Transplant/Immunology Network of the American College of Chest Physicians: A survey of clinical practice of lung transplantation in North America. *Chest* 125(4):1224–1238, 2004.
41. Lee JC, Christie JD: Primary graft dysfunction. *Clin Chest Med* 32(2):279–293, 2011.
42. Christie JD, Carby M, Bag R, et al: Report of the ISHLT Working Group on Primary Lung Graft Dysfunction part II: definition. A consensus statement of the International Society for Heart and Lung Transplantation. *J Heart Lung Transplant* 24(10):1454–1459, 2005.
43. Shah RJ, Diamond JM, Cantu E, et al: Objective estimates improve risk stratification for primary graft dysfunction after lung transplantation. *Am J Transplant* 15(8):2188–2196, 2015.
44. Perrin G, Roch A, Michelet P, et al: Inhaled nitric oxide does not prevent pulmonary edema after lung transplantation measured by lung water content: a randomized clinical study. *Chest* 129(4):1024–1030, 2006.
45. Ardehali A, Laks H, Levine M, et al: A prospective trial of inhaled nitric oxide in clinical lung transplantation. *Transplantation* 72(1):112–115, 2001.
46. Meade MO, Granton JT, Matte-Martyn A, et al: A randomized trial of inhaled nitric oxide to prevent ischemia-reperfusion injury after lung transplantation. *Am J Respir Crit Care Med* 167(11):1483–1489, 2003.
47. Amital A, Shitrit D, Raviv Y, et al: The use of surfactant in lung transplantation. *Transplantation* 86(11):1554–1559, 2008.
48. Struber M, Fischer S, Niedermeyer J, et al: Effects of exogenous surfactant instillation in clinical lung transplantation: a prospective, randomized trial. *J Thorac Cardiovasc Surg* 133(6):1620–1625, 2007.
49. Fischer S, Bohn D, Rycus P, et al: Extracorporeal membrane oxygenation for primary graft dysfunction after lung transplantation: analysis of the Extracorporeal Life Support Organization (ELSO) registry. *J Heart Lung Transplant* 26(5):472–477, 2007.
50. Huang HJ, Yusen RD, Meyers BF, et al: Late primary graft dysfunction after lung transplantation and bronchiolitis obliterans syndrome. *Am J Transplant* 8(11):2454–2462, 2008.
51. Daud SA, Yusen RD, Meyers BF, et al: Impact of immediate primary lung allograft dysfunction on bronchiolitis obliterans syndrome. *Am J Respir Crit Care Med* 175(5):507–513, 2007.
52. Arcasoy SM, Fisher A, Hachem RR, et al: Report of the ISHLT Working Group on Primary Lung Graft Dysfunction part V: predictors and outcomes. *J Heart Lung Transplant* 24(10):1483–1488, 2005.
53. Schnickel GT, Ross DJ, Beygui R, et al: Modified reperfusion in clinical lung transplantation: the results of 100 consecutive cases. *J Thorac Cardiovasc Surg* 131(1):218–223, 2006.
54. Diamond JM, Lee JC, Kawut SM, et al: Clinical risk factors for primary graft dysfunction after lung transplantation. *Am J Respir Crit Care Med* 187(5):527–534, 2013.
55. Barr ML, Kawut SM, Whelan TP, et al: Report of the ISHLT Working Group on Primary Lung Graft Dysfunction part IV: recipient-related risk factors and markers. *J Heart Lung Transplant* 24(10):1468–1482, 2005.
56. de Perrot M, Bonser RS, Dark J, et al: Report of the ISHLT Working Group on Primary Lung Graft Dysfunction part III: donor-related risk factors and markers. *J Heart Lung Transplant* 24(10):1460–1467, 2005.
57. Westall GP, Snell GI, McLean C, et al: C3d and C4d deposition early after lung transplantation. *J Heart Lung Transplant* 27(7):722–728, 2008.
58. Guillen RV, Briones FR, Marin PM, et al: Lung graft dysfunction in the early postoperative period after lung and heart lung transplantation. *Transplant Proc* 37(9):3994–3995, 2005.
59. Pilcher DV, Scheinkestel CD, Snell GI, et al: High central venous pressure is associated with prolonged mechanical ventilation and increased mortality after lung transplantation. *J Thorac Cardiovasc Surg* 129(4):912–918, 2005.
60. Padia SA, Borja MC, Orens JB, et al: Tracheostomy following lung transplantation predictors and outcomes. *Am J Transplant* 3(7):891–895, 2003.
61. Hadjiliadis D, Steele MP, Govert JA, et al: Outcome of lung transplant patients admitted to the medical ICU. *Chest* 125(3):1040–1045, 2004.
62. Banga A, Sahoo D, Lane CR, et al: Characteristics and outcomes of patients with lung transplantation requiring admission to the medical ICU. *Chest* 146(3):590–599, 2014.
63. Cohen J, Singer P, Raviv Y, et al: Outcome of lung transplant recipients requiring readmission to the intensive care unit. *J Heart Lung Transplant* 30(1):54–58, 2011.

64. Roca O, de Acilu MG, Caralt B, et al: Humidified high flow nasal cannula supportive therapy improves outcomes in lung transplant recipients readmitted to the intensive care unit because of acute respiratory failure. *Transplantation* 99(5):1092–1098, 2015.
65. Machuzak M, Santacruz JF, Gildea T, et al: Airway complications after lung transplantation. *Thorac Surg Clin* 25(1):55–75, 2015.
66. Puchalski J, Lee HJ, Sterman DH: Airway complications following lung transplantation. *Clin Chest Med* 32(2):357–366, 2011.
67. Santacruz JF, Mehta AC: Airway complications and management after lung transplantation: ischemia, dehiscence, and stenosis. *Proc Am Thorac Soc* 6(1):79–93, 2009.
68. Hachem R: Antibody-mediated lung transplant rejection. *Curr Respir Care Rep* 1(3):157–161, 2012.
69. Martinu T, Howell DN, Palmer SM: Acute cellular rejection and humoral sensitization in lung transplant recipients. *Semin Respir Crit Care Med* 31(2):179–188, 2010.
70. Witt CA, Gaut JP, Yusen RD, et al: Acute antibody-mediated rejection after lung transplantation. *J Heart Lung Transplant* 32(10):1034–1040, 2013.
71. Martinu T, Pavlisko EN, Chen DF, et al: Acute allograft rejection: cellular and humoral processes. *Clin Chest Med* 32(2):295–310, 2011.
72. McManigle W, Pavlisko EN, Martinu T: Acute cellular and antibody-mediated allograft rejection. *Semin Respir Crit Care Med* 34(3):320–335, 2013.
73. Stewart S, Fishbein MC, Snell GI, et al: Revision of the 1996 working formulation for the standardization of nomenclature in the diagnosis of lung rejection. *J Heart Lung Transplant* 26(12):1229–1242, 2007.
74. Iacono AT, Johnson BA, Grgurich WF, et al: A randomized trial of inhaled cyclosporine in lung-transplant recipients. *N Engl J Med* 354(2):141–150, 2006.
75. Verleden GM, Raghu G, Meyer KC, et al: A new classification system for chronic lung allograft dysfunction. *J Heart Lung Transplant* 33(2):127–133, 2014.
76. Sato M, Waddell TK, Wagnetz U, et al: Restrictive allograft syndrome (RAS): a novel form of chronic lung allograft dysfunction. *J Heart Lung Transplant* 30(7):735–742, 2011.
77. Glanville AR, Aboyoun CL, Havryk A, et al: Severity of lymphocytic bronchiolitis predicts long-term outcome after lung transplantation. *Am J Respir Crit Care Med* 177(9):1033–1040, 2008.
78. Meyer KC, Raghu G, Verleden GM, et al: An international ISHLT/ATS/ERS clinical practice guideline: diagnosis and management of bronchiolitis obliterans syndrome. *Eur Respir J* 44(6):1479–1503, 2014.
79. Weigt SS, Wallace WD, Derhovanessian A, et al: Chronic allograft rejection: epidemiology, diagnosis, pathogenesis, and treatment. *Semin Respir Crit Care Med* 31(2):189–207, 2010.
80. de Jong PA, Dodd JD, Coxson HO, et al: Bronchiolitis obliterans following lung transplantation: early detection using computed tomographic scanning. *Thorax* 61(9):799–804, 2006.
81. Corris PA, Ryan VA, Small T, et al: A randomised controlled trial of azithromycin therapy in bronchiolitis obliterans syndrome (BOS) post lung transplantation. *Thorax* 70(5):442–450, 2015.
82. Ruttens D, Verleden SE, Vandermeulen E, et al: Prophylactic azithromycin therapy after lung transplantation: post hoc analysis of a randomized controlled trial. *Am J Transplant* 16:254–261, 2016.
83. Thomas M, Belli EV, Rawal B, et al: Survival after lung retransplantation in the United States in the Current Era (2004 to 2013): better or worse? *Ann Thorac Surg* 100(2):452–457, 2015.
84. Burguete SR, Maselli DJ, Fernandez JF, et al: Lung transplant infection. *Respirology* 18(1):22–38, 2013.
85. Fishman JA: Infection in solid-organ transplant recipients. *N Engl J Med* 357(25):2601–2614, 2007.
86. Lease ED, Zaas DW: Complex bacterial infections pre- and posttransplant. *Semin Respir Crit Care Med* 31(2):234–242, 2010.
87. Remund KF, Best M, Egan JJ: Infections relevant to lung transplantation. *Proc Am Thorac Soc* 6(1):94–100, 2009.
88. Palacio F, Reyes LF, Levine DJ, et al: Understanding the concept of health care-associated pneumonia in lung transplant recipients. *Chest* 148(2):516–522, 2015.
89. Riera J, Baldirà J, Ramirez S, et al: Gastroparesis following lung transplantation: risk factor for pneumonia. *Eur Respir J* 46[Suppl 59], 2015.
90. Zamora MR, Davis RD, Leonard C; CMV Advisory Board Expert Committee: Management of cytomegalovirus infection in lung transplant recipients: evidence-based recommendations. *Transplantation* 80(2):157–163, 2005.
91. Hadaya K, Wunderli W, Deffernez C, et al: Monitoring of cytomegalovirus infection in solid-organ transplant recipients by an ultrasensitive plasma PCR assay. *J Clin Microbiol* 41(8):3757–3764, 2003.
92. Palmer SM, Limaye AP, Banks M, et al: Extended valganciclovir prophylaxis to prevent cytomegalovirus after lung transplantation: a randomized, controlled trial. *Ann Intern Med* 152(12):761–769, 2010.
93. Kumar D, Erdman D, Keshavjee S, et al., Clinical impact of community-acquired respiratory viruses on bronchiolitis obliterans after lung transplant. *Am J Transplant* 5(8):2031–2036, 2005.
94. Hosseini-Moghaddam SM, Husain S: Fungi and molds following lung transplantation. *Semin Respir Crit Care Med* 31(2):222–233, 2010.
95. Sole A, Salavert M: Fungal infections after lung transplantation. *Curr Opin Pulm Med* 15(3):243–253, 2009.
96. Limper AH, Knox KS, Sarosi GA, et al: An official American Thoracic Society statement: treatment of fungal infections in adult pulmonary and critical care patients. *Am J Respir Crit Care Med* 183(1):96–128, 2011.
97. Baughman RP, Meyer KC, Nathanson I, et al: Monitoring of nonsteroidal immunosuppressive drugs in patients with lung disease and lung transplant recipients: American College of Chest Physicians evidence-based clinical practice guidelines. *Chest* 142(5):e1S–e111S, 2012.
98. Taylor JL, Palmer SM: Critical care perspective on immunotherapy in lung transplantation. *J Intensive Care Med* 21(6):327–344, 2006.
99. Hachem RR, Yusen RD, Chakinala MM, et al: Thrombotic microangiopathy after lung transplantation. *Transplantation* 81(1):57–63, 2006.
100. Siddique A, Bose AK, Ozalp F, et al: Vascular anastomotic complications in lung transplantation: a single institution's experience. *Interact Cardiovasc Thorac Surg* 17(4):625–631, 2013.
101. Ferdinande P, Bruyninckx F, Van Raemdonck D, et al; Leuven Lung Transplant Group: Phrenic nerve dysfunction after heart–lung and lung transplantation. *J Heart Lung Transplant* 23(1):105–109, 2004.
102. Wahidi MM, Willner DA, Snyder LD, et al: Diagnosis and outcome of early pleural space infection following lung transplantation. *Chest* 135(2):484–491, 2009.
103. Lyu DM, Zamora MR: Medical complications of lung transplantation. *Proc Am Thorac Soc* 6(1):101–107, 2009.
104. Jacques F, El-Hamamsy I, Fortier A, et al: Acute renal failure following lung transplantation: risk factors, mortality, and long-term consequences. *Eur J Cardiothorac Surg* 41(1):193–199, 2012.
105. Orrego CM, Cordero-Reyes AM, Estep JD, et al: Atrial arrhythmias after lung transplant: underlying mechanisms, risk factors, and prognosis. *J Heart Lung Transplant* 33(7):734–740, 2014.
106. Raghavan D, Gao A, Ahn C, et al: Contemporary analysis of incidence of post-operative atrial fibrillation, its predictors, and association with clinical outcomes in lung transplantation. *J Heart Lung Transplant* 34(4):563–570, 2015.
107. Izbicki G, Bairey O, Shitrit D, et al: Increased thromboembolic events after lung transplantation. *Chest* 129(2):412–416, 2006.
108. Yegen HA, Lederer DJ, Barr RG, et al: Risk factors for venous thromboembolism after lung transplantation. *Chest* 132(2):547–553, 2007.
109. Neuringer IP: Posttransplant lymphoproliferative disease after lung transplantation. *Clin Dev Immunol* 2013:430209, 2013.
110. Reams BD, McAdams HP, Howell DN, et al: Posttransplant lymphoproliferative disorder: incidence, presentation, and response to treatment in lung transplant recipients. *Chest* 124(4):1242–1249, 2003.
111. Todd JL, Christie JD, Palmer SM: Update in lung transplantation 2013. *Am J Respir Crit Care Med* 190(1):19–24, 2014.

Chapter 60 ■ Specific Critical Care Problems in Heart and Heart–Lung Transplant Recipients

ANDREW W. SHAFFER • KAROL MUDY • SARA J. SHUMWAY

The advent of thoracic organ transplantation has brought new hope to patients who were previously afflicted by end-stage cardiac, pulmonary, or combined cardiopulmonary disease. The first heart transplant was performed on December 3, 1967. Fourteen years passed before the first successful heart–lung transplant was performed on March 9, 1981. Heart–lung transplantation established the potential for lung transplantation as a viable therapeutic option, and the first successful single-lung transplant was performed in 1983 [1].

HEART TRANSPLANTATION

The United Network for Organ Sharing (UNOS) is a nonprofit organization that maintains the nation's organ transplant waiting list. Patients awaiting cardiac transplantation are listed according to severity of illness. Organs are then allocated to those individuals who are most ill and have waited the longest. The waiting list for heart transplant has steadily grown because more patients are added than removed every year. The most current UNOS summary was published in 2012. The UNOS wait-list has approximately 3,000 patients awaiting transplant. Subsequently, the number of heart transplants has been increasing since 2004, with roughly 2,500 performed annually in the United States. Wait-list times peaked in 2007 and since then have decreased. The average wait-list time for status 1A candidates is 2.4 months, status 1B candidates is 6.9 months, and status 2 candidates is 20 months [2]. Status 1 heart candidates have the highest medical urgency. These are patients who have support either via a total artificial heart, ventricular assist device (VAD), intra-aortic balloon pump, or extracorporeal membrane oxygenation. It could also be an individual who has a mechanical assist device in place and either right or left ventricular support that is beginning to malfunction. It also includes individuals who are on continuous mechanical ventilation or on high-dose inotropic support that cannot be weaned. Status 2 candidates are individuals who need heart transplantation but have not been defined as being in the most urgent status. These patients typically are at home, still active, and taking heart-failure medications while awaiting transplantation.

The annual mortality rate on the waiting list has continued to decline over the last 10 years. In general, pretransplant mortality declined from 15.8 deaths per 100 wait-list years in 2002 to 12.4 in 2012 [2]. This slow decrease is related to the evolution of left ventricular assist devices (LVADs) and their acceptance as a bridge to heart transplantation.

In 2012, 54.0% of transplants were performed for cardiomyopathy, 32.8% in patients with coronary artery disease, and 9.9% in patients with congenital heart disease. The number of transplantations increased for patients with cardiomyopathy and congenital heart disease, 34% and 28%, respectively. The number of transplantations in patients with valvular heart disease decreased 44%. In 2012, 41.3% of patients had prior VAD support. Cardiac retransplantation represents approximately 4% of the adult heart transplant population annually. Most patients who received a transplant had private insurance; however, the proportion of insured versus those on Medicare decreased between 2002 and 2012 [2].

Patient Selection

Many of the specific critical care problems seen in thoracic organ recipients can be reduced by careful patient selection. In well-compensated patients, a week-long outpatient evaluation is performed. This applies to approximately 80% to 90% of patients seen at a cardiac transplant center. The other 10% to 20% are individuals who are critically ill and undergo an urgent transplant evaluation.

The recipient assessment consists of a general evaluation, an assessment of the functional and hemodynamic status, and a psychosocial evaluation. All parts are equally crucial. One of the first assessments is an oxygen-consumption treadmill test. For those patients who are capable of performing this test, there are excellent data which demonstrate that a peak oxygen consumption of less than 12 mL/kg/min is associated with a very poor 1-year survival rate without transplant. Individuals with a peak oxygen consumption of less than 15 mL/kg/min should be considered for listing [3,4]. The assessment then proceeds with a general evaluation. The patient's medical history is examined to try to determine the cause of the patient's heart disease. General laboratory tests are performed, including a creatinine clearance. Individuals who have a creatinine clearance of less than 50 mL per minute do have a significant increase in the need for postcardiac transplantation dialysis and have lower rates of survival than those with near-normal renal function. Individuals with severely abnormal creatinine clearance would be excluded from heart transplant or considered for heart-and-kidney transplantations. Individuals with diabetes need further end-organ evaluation prior to listing to understand the full scope of their risk.

Nutritional status is also crucial. Those individuals with a body mass index (BMI) less than 20 kg per m^2 or greater than 35 kg per m^2 would be asked to either gain or lose weight, respectively. Again, individuals at the extremes of the body mass index have higher rates of mortality in the postoperative period than those with normal BMI [5,6].

The hemodynamic evaluation consists of an echocardiogram to evaluate function and anatomy, and a cardiac catheterization. The cardiac catheterization includes evaluation of heart function by a right heart catheterization as well as a coronary angiogram. In this assessment, the patient's coronary anatomy is examined for potential intervention, and any abnormalities in the filling pressures, pulmonary capillary occlusion pressure, or pulmonary vascular resistance are identified.

Patients with heart failure and secondary pulmonary hypertension are a group who are of special interest. Pulmonary arterial and capillary wedge pressures are measured to determine the degree to which a patient has secondary pulmonary hypertension and whether or not it is reversible. The patient's hemodynamics should be optimized in the catheterization laboratory in an attempt to decrease the pulmonary arterial pressures to normal levels, and 100% oxygen, nitric oxide, and other pulmonary vasodilators can be used to test the reactivity of the pulmonary vasculature. The absolute exclusion criteria for heart transplantation are a pulmonary vascular resistance greater than 4 Wood units (WU) and, more importantly, a transpulmonary gradient greater than 15 mm Hg. Individuals with values outside these values would then be listed for heart–lung transplant, or be given a trial of pulmonary vasodilators.

The patient's ABO blood type and panel-reactive antibody (PRA) level are determined to quantitate the patient's preexisting antibodies and sensitization to the general population. If class II (locus D) is greater than 20%, it is recommended that a preoperative crossmatch be performed. The patient's HLA typing is also done at that time, and if the PRAs are significantly elevated, the laboratory should be able to identify the particular human leukocyte antigen to which the individual is reacting. Sensitization can occur in many situations. It may occur because of pregnancy, between sexual partners, from prior transplantation, or with transfusions often associated with the placement of a VAD. Individuals who carry a high PRA level have been treated in the past with plasmapheresis, intravenous immunoglobulin, cyclophosphamide, and mycophenolate mofetil (MMF). There have been inconclusive results with each of these. Recent studies from a nationwide sample of the UNOS database demonstrated that ABO-compatible versus ABO-identical transplantation recipients did not have significant differences in survival rates [7].

The psychosocial evaluation should be centered on evaluating not only the transplant recipient, but also the family support for the patient. This needs to be performed by a qualified professional experienced in social work and, when indicated, other mental health professionals who have a keen understanding of the demands made on a postoperative cardiac transplantation patient. Patients need to be medically compliant, have adequate neurocognitive function for the postoperative regimen, and adequate social support.

Once the evaluation has been completed, the patient is evaluated for any relative or absolute contraindication for heart transplantation. Those relative contraindications include: age greater than 70 years, previous chronic substance abuse, limited social support, limited adaptive ability, mild renal dysfunction, active peptic ulcer disease, cachexia, obesity, and cigarette smoking. It should be noted that to receive a heart transplantation, individuals who smoke are required to go through a smoking-cessation program, and many transplant programs require them to sign a contract stating that they will not resume smoking prior to or after the transplantation. They also are evaluated for chemical evidence of smoking during their waiting time [8].

Absolute contraindications to cardiac transplantation include: ongoing substance abuse, refractory psychiatric conditions, suicidal behavior, severe personality disorder, issues with ongoing medical noncompliance, inadequate neurocognitive ability, irreversible hepatic or renal dysfunction, severe peripheral or cerebral vascular disease, systemic disease that limits rehabilitation, insulin-dependent diabetes with severe end-organ damage, or evidence of severe, fixed, secondary pulmonary hypertension [8–10].

Implantable Cardiac Assist Devices

VADs represent the greatest advance in the treatment of end-stage heart failure and the field of heart transplantation in the past 10 years (Table 60.1). With an assist device implanted, patients who would otherwise not survive long enough to receive a heart transplantation are now living independently at home with reasonably good quality of life until a suitable organ becomes available. As of 2012, 35.6% of transplant recipients were using an LVAD at the time of operation. This has impacted the number of patients reliant on inotropes at the time of transplant, with a decrease from 43.4% in 2007 to 36.2% in 2012 [2,11].

From their increased use, a corpus of terminology has evolved to categorize and describe the devices themselves, their use, and technical aspects of their function and performance. Most devices are designed to assist the left ventricle and hence are called LVADs. However, some models are made to be implanted in either ventricle and when implanted on the right side are referred to as a right ventricular assist device (RVAD). When both ventricles are mechanically assisted, each with its own pump, the whole system together is referred to as a biventricular assist device, or BIVAD.

There are two broad categories of devices in use based on pump mechanism: pulsatile devices that employ some type of pneumatic pump, and continuous, or axial flow devices that involve a spinning propeller. The cycles of the pulsatile device are measured in beats per minute (bpm) and that of the continuous-flow pumps in revolutions per minute (rpm). Each device has an inflow cannula through which the patient's blood is drawn from the heart and into the pump and an outflow cannula that directs the blood back into the patient's circulation.

For both pulsatile pumps and continuous-flow pumps, there are two more classifications that can be described on the basis of the location of the pump when implanted: intracorporeal, wherein the entire pump is implanted inside the body with the exception of the drive-line that powers the device and passes through an exit site on the abdomen; the other is paracorporeal, or extracorporeal, wherein the pump sits outside the body and the inflow and outflow cannulae enter and exit the skin on the upper abdomen just below the costal margin. Most LVADs usually involve an inflow cannula placed in the apex of left ventricle and the outflow cannula in the ascending aorta.

The only permanent RVAD approved for use in the United States is the Thoratec Paracorporeal VAD and its inflow cannula is placed in the right ventricular free wall and the outflow cannula is anastomosed to the pulmonary artery. The Levitronix CentriMag (now owned by Thoratec) is approved for temporary right ventricular assistance up to 30 days and its inflow cannula may be placed in either the right atrium or the right ventricle.

Devices are categorized based upon the intended therapeutic goal for each particular patient. Bridge to transplant (BTT) indicates that the patient is or will become a heart transplant candidate and the device is intended to improve survival and other physiologic parameters until an organ is available. Destination therapy (DT) indicates that the patient is not a transplant candidate but the device is implanted to improve survival and quality of life for the remainder of the patient's life. Bridge to recovery refers to the patient who is expected to recover from heart failure and the device is used to sustain life until the time when it can be weaned off and explanted. Bridge to decision (BTD) refers to

TABLE 60.1

Advances of Ventricular Assist Devices in Heart-Failure Treatment

Topic	Finding	Reference
Destination therapy trial with pulsatile pumps	Improved survival at 1 y with mechanical assist device vs. medical management for Class III and IV heart failure	[11]
Bridge to transplant trial with continuous-flow pumps	HeartMate II provides effective support to transplant for at least 6 mo with 75% survival	[12]
Improved survival with continuous-flow pumps	Effective support, improved functional status, and quality of life with 72% survival at 18 mo	[48–50]

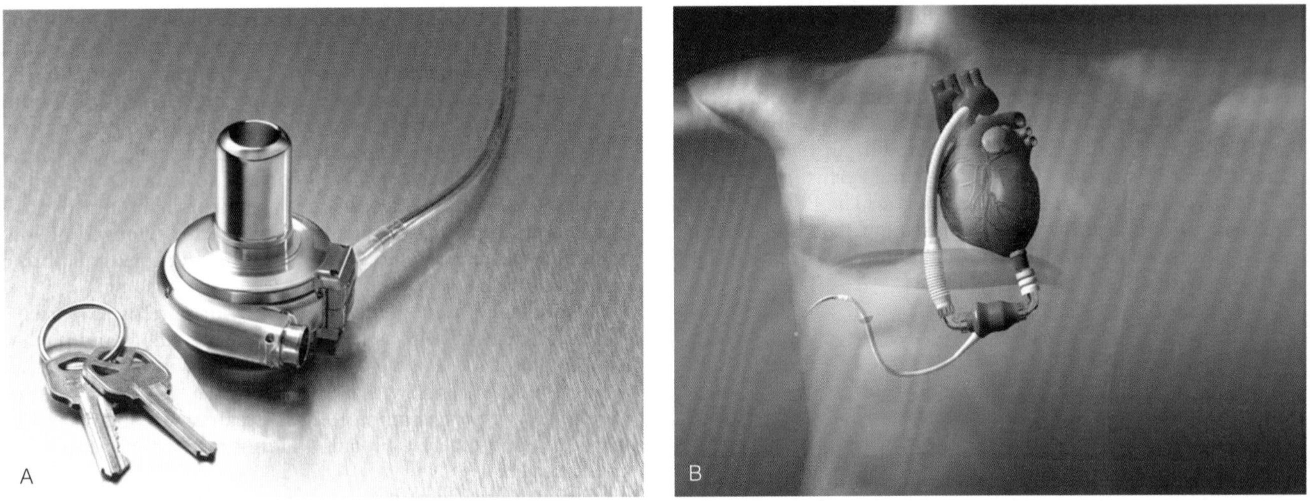

FIGURE 60.1 Continuous-flow ventricular assist devices. **A:** HeartWare ventricular assist device. **B:** HeartMate II ventricular assist device. (A, Reprinted with permission from HeartWare. B, Reprinted with permission from Thoratec.)

those patients for whom survival is not certain and a temporary assist device, such as the AbioMed BVS5000 or the Levitronix CentriMag, is used in the critical care setting to prolong life until it can be determined whether the patient ought to be implanted with a long-term device as those used in BTT or DT patients or be disconnected from the BTD device and allowed to expire.

The superior efficacy of VADs over optimal medical management in improving survival in end-stage, New York Heart Association Class 3 or 4 heart-failure patients was proven in the REMATCH trial: patients implanted with the Thoratec HeartMate VE had a 52% survival at 1 year compared to 25% in the medically managed group [12]. Subsequently, the Food and Drug Administration (FDA) approved the HeartMate XVE for DT. The Thoratec HeartMate II continuous-flow pump demonstrated efficacy in bridge to transplantation with 75% survival at 6 months postimplantation and 68% survival at 1 year [13]. It received approval by the FDA in April 2008 for bridge to transplantation and was subsequently approved for DT in January 2010. Smaller devices such as the Jarvik 2000 Flowmaker and the HeartWare VAD are currently under investigation in the United States with more than two dozen other devices presently in development (Fig. 60.1).

Knowing how these devices work and how these patients are managed will be an important part of the pretransplantation care of the recipient. Almost all of these patients will present anticoagulated on warfarin. It will be important not to begin administration of plasma and cryoprecipitate until the plan to proceed with the transplant is certain. Administration of blood products without completing the transplantation will only sensitize the recipient and increase the PRAs for any subsequent transplant offers [14]. The postoperative course is often complicated by bleeding. Drains for the VAD pocket are necessary and pericardial effusions are common.

Several studies have examined posttransplant survival and recent studies have shown that recipients of VADs have had equivalent or better posttransplant outcomes [15,16]. One exception is the patient who had VAD-related sepsis prior to transplantation, as these patients had a trend to slightly poorer posttransplantation rates of survival than those patients who did not have an infection [17].

Donor Criteria

The donor evaluation begins with the pronouncement of brain death. The local organ-procurement agency will obtain consent for donation from the family and proceed with the donor evaluation and support. The donor evaluation consists of taking a general history of any illnesses or risk factors such as heart disease, hypertension, diabetes, or cigarette smoking. Specifics are gathered surrounding the time and mode of death to determine whether there is any potential cardiac injury, down time, cardiopulmonary resuscitation, or cardioversion. The organ-procurement professionals will proceed with a hemodynamic evaluation of the patient. This consists of measuring central venous pressures and, potentially, full hemodynamic profiles if pulmonary artery catheter measurement capability exists at the hospital caring for the donor. Once the donor is stabilized hemodynamically, further studies are performed. The initial stabilization phase should include endocrine support with the administration of levothyroxine and corticosteroids, reduction of inotropic support if it is appropriate, and, potentially, diuresis or transfusion when indicated. A surface echocardiogram is then performed to make sure the heart is structurally normal and that function is normal. A 12-lead electrocardiogram is also obtained. It is not uncommon to find subtle ST changes in individuals who are brain-dead. It is generally accepted that a cardiac catheterization will be necessary in male donors more than 40 years old and female donors more than 45 years old, but catheterization should also be performed in younger donors when the donor has a significant history of hypertension, cigarette smoking, diabetes, or alcohol abuse. Cardiac enzymes need to be carefully evaluated and correlated to any severe hemodynamic instability, the use of cardiopulmonary resuscitation, as well as the time of herniation [18].

A number of studies have demonstrated correlations between elevations of troponin and early graft failure [19,20]. In one study, a cardiac troponin I value greater than 1.6 μg per L was a predictor of early graft failure, with a sensitivity of 73% and a specificity of 94% [19]. These data should be analyzed closely with the patient's hemodynamic function and echocardiographic findings.

A transplant center may request that a second echocardiogram be performed if the first echocardiogram was performed shortly after herniation. Catecholamine-induced left ventricular dysfunction can improve significantly in a short period of time and not preclude excellent short-and long-term outcomes. One must also take into consideration the ischemic time that will be incurred with procurement and travel time. The majority of transplant centers are willing to accept an ischemic time up to 4 hours for adult donors but no more than 6 hours.

The advent of ex vivo perfusion offers the possibility of warm perfused preservation of thoracic organ grafts. The technology is currently commercially available in Europe and is under FDA investigation in the United States. Ex vivo perfusion uses warm oxygenated blood and an extracorporeal pump to perfuse organs during transport and preservation. This technology offers the potential for longer extracorporeal periods and possibly altering the paradigm of cold preservation. The Organ Care System designed by TransMedics (Boston, MA) and Perfusix (Toronto, CA) are two examples of ex vivo perfusion. The PROCEED II trial was a noninferiority study confirming that OCS warm perfusion versus cold-storage in heart allografts was comparable in 30-day patient and graft survival [21].

Operative Techniques

Donor Operation

Once the donor has been prepared and the abdominal team has started their procedure, the median sternotomy incision is performed. If lungs are being harvested, both pleural spaces are also opened for inspection of both lungs. During this inspection, one should palpate the coronary arteries to discern any calcifications and also palpate the aortic root for calcifications. External evaluation of the heart is not a reliable evaluation of function unless there is something grossly abnormal, such as severe bruising from a myocardial contusion or a dilated right ventricle. Once it is determined that the heart is appropriate for transplantation and all of the other organ teams are ready, the donor is heparinized and cannulated. The heart is cannulated with a cardioplegia cannula in the ascending aorta. If the lungs are being harvested, a pulmonary artery cannula will be placed in the main pulmonary artery. Once all teams are ready, the aorta is cross-clamped and the flush solution is given. Between 1 and 2 L of cold cardioplegic solution is administered. The heart is vented via the left atrial appendage, excised, and is then submerged in ice slush saline, packaged sterilely, and placed in a cooler for rapid transport to the center caring for the recipient.

Recipient Operation

Once the recipient is prepared and draped, the median sternotomy incision is made and the heart is dissected free of any adhesions, and then cardiopulmonary bypass is established.

The recipient is placed on total cardiopulmonary bypass, before the cross-clamp is applied to the aorta, and the heart is excised along the atrioventricular groove. The great vessels are divided just above their respective semilunar valves. The anastomoses are performed in the following order: left atrial, inferior vena caval, pulmonary arterial, aortic, and superior vena caval [22]. Temporary pacing wires are left on the donor right atrium and right ventricle. The organ is reperfused and, once it has recovered, is separated from bypass. On separation from bypass, appropriate inotropic support is administered. Typically, the patient may require dopamine or epinephrine and milrinone for postoperative support. Isoproterenol is used to maintain an appropriate heart rate if bradycardia is a problem or the heart is paced. The pulmonary artery catheter should be floated through the new heart so that pulmonary artery pressures can be monitored closely and any signs of right heart failure can be detected early.

Postoperative Care

The immediate postoperative management of a heart transplant recipient is by and large not unlike that of other cardiac surgery patients. Drips and temporary pacing leads are modified to optimize cardiac index and end-organ perfusion. Typical inotropes used are epinephrine, dopamine, dobutamine, and milrinone. A pulmonary artery catheter is used with continuous mixed venous oximetry and preload is optimized with either volume or diuretic. Usually patients come out of the operating room on Isuprel (isoproterenol) to stimulate the heart rate and/or the temporary pacemaker set to a back-up rate of 90 to 100 bpm or higher. The ideal heart rate for these patients in the first few days postoperatively is 100 to 120 bpm. After the first several days, the heart rate is allowed to drift to its baseline as the cardiac index allows. Occasionally, patients exhibit a distributive shock immediately postoperatively characterized by low systemic vascular resistance and vasopressin or neosynephrine is used to treat it.

Ventilatory management varies from patient to patient. The ideal patient who is hemodynamically stable and has no signs of surgical bleeding can be extubated within a few hours. Sometimes, patients with right ventricular failure owing to pulmonary hypertension need to be treated with inhaled nitric oxide or epoprostenol (Flolan) and thus mechanical ventilation is continued.

Patients who have had a VAD placed as a bridge to transplantation frequently have had two or more prior sternotomies and arrive at the hospital on Coumadin. These patients have a tendency to bleed more postoperatively and one should keep a low threshold to return to the operating room for exploration if bleeding persists.

Serious ventricular failure after cardiac transplantation is unusual and can be related to poor donor-organ selection, poor graft preservation, a long ischemia time, or rejection owing to the presence of preformed antibodies. Early rejection is often heralded by atrial fibrillation and the manifestation of arrhythmias should prompt an immediate workup and treatment. Plasmapheresis can be very effective in removing preformed antibodies responsible for humoral rejection. Inotropes and pulmonary vasodilators are also often used to manage the right heart failure that frequently accompanies rejection, with the addition of an intra-aortic balloon pump if necessary. In cases of severe graft dysfunction, VADs can support the patient until either the donor heart recovers or retransplantation takes place.

Immunosuppression

Balanced triple-drug immunosuppression is still the most commonly used protocol, consisting of calcineurin inhibitors, an antimetabolite, and corticosteroids (Table 60.2). The calcineurin inhibitors include cyclosporine and tacrolimus. Cyclosporine is largely recognized as the agent that moved cardiac transplant from a feasible medical option to an acceptable medical treatment. The physicians at Stanford University performed a randomized controlled trial in cardiac transplant patients that demonstrated that cyclosporine immunosuppression improved 1-year survival to 80% from the mid-50% range [23]. Patients receiving either cyclosporine or tacrolimus have similar survival rates in heart transplantation, both long and short term [24–26]. However, in a controlled clinical trial by Kobashigawa et al. in 2006, studying 343 de novo cardiac transplant patients, tacrolimus in combination with either mycophenolate or sirolimus had fewer occurrences of grade 3 A or greater rejection or hemodynamic compromise rejection at 1 year when compared to cyclosporine and mycophenolate [27]. In addition, median serum creatinine and triglyceride levels were lowest in the tacrolimus and mycophenolate group. Cyclosporine is well known to also cause postoperative hypertension, nephrotoxicity, hepatotoxicity, gingival hyperplasia, hypertrichosis, and tremor. Tacrolimus also causes nephrotoxicity and many of the other side effects of cyclosporine but to a lesser extent, in particular, posttransplant hypertension and gingival hyperplasia. A review article from Stanford confirmed improved survival with the use of tacrolimus and improved postoperative infection prophylaxis [28].

TABLE 60.2

Balanced Triple-Drug Immunosuppression Protocol

Drug	Perioperative	Maintenance	Taper	Maintenance	Withdrawal
Corticosteroids					
Methylprednisolone	10 mg/kg intraoperatively or perioperatively; 125 mg IV q8 h three doses postoperatively				
Prednisone	0.5 mg/kg IV/PO qd in 2 divided doses	0.5 mg/kg IV/PO qd in 2 divided doses	Decrease dose by 5 mg/d until total daily dose is 0.3 mg/kg/d	1st mo: 0.3 mg/kg/d 2nd mo: 0.2 mg/kg/d 3rd mo: 0.1 mg/kg/d 4th mo: 0.05 mg/kg/d (or 2.5 mg PO qd)	5th mo: total steroid withdrawal (if no rejection for the past 3 mo)
Calcineurin inhibitors					
Tacrolimus	0.05 mg/kg PO preoperatively; 0.1 mg/kg PO qd in 2 divided doses; dose target levels 0–1 mo, 10–15	Dose target levels 2–6 mo, 10–12 7–12 mo, 10–12 12+ mo, 8–12			
Cyclosporine	2 mg/kg PO preoperatively; 1 mg/kg IV over 24 h, then 3–5 mg/kg PO qd in 2 divided doses (based on renal function); dose target levels 0–1 mo, 200–250	Dose target levels 2–6 mo, 150–225 7–12 mo, 125–175 12+ mo, 100–125			
Antimetabolite					
Mycophenolate mofetil	1,000 mg PO preoperatively; 2–3 g IV/PO qd in 2 divided doses; dosage to keep white blood cell count >4.0	2–3 g PO qd in 2 divided doses			
Azathioprine	34 mg/kg PO preoperatively; 3 mg/kg IV/PO qd postoperatively	1–3 mg/kg PO qd			

Data from Refs. [21–25].
IV, intravenously; PO, orally.

The antimetabolites include MMF and azathioprine. These inhibit purine synthesis and thus block the proliferation of both T and B cells. They are complementary to the calcineurin inhibitors. Kobashigawa et al. [29] demonstrated considerable benefits to MMF over azathioprine when coupled with cyclosporine in transplants performed in 1998. MMF is currently the most widely used antimetabolite in heart transplantation [26].

Corticosteroids remain a cornerstone of therapy. There are multiple regimens for early corticosteroid reduction to avoid the serious associated side effects including systemic hypertension, obesity, osteoporosis, and glucose intolerance. In spite of the negative side effects, in 2004, approximately 75% of patients were still taking corticosteroids 1 year following their transplants [30]. Monotherapy consisting of tacrolimus is currently being studied in heart transplant recipients. In one study, 75% of recipients were successfully converted to monotherapy [31]. Results from the group at Stanford confirm that therapy with tacrolimus and limited corticosteroid are linked to improved recipient and graft survival [28].

The use of IL-2 receptor blockade has become more prevalent during the last 4 to 5 years. These proliferation signal inhibitors, sirolimus and everolimus, block the activation of the T cell by binding the IL-2 receptor. They have shown promise in significantly reducing the severity of cardiac allograft vasculopathy, the main threat of long-term graft survival. But they remain only an adjunct to the calcineurin inhibitors that are still more effective in preventing acute rejection.

Outcomes

The Registry of the International Society for Heart and Lung Transplantation (ISHLT) has reported on survival after cardiac transplantation in adult patients. Survival rates have increased from 89% in 2008 to 94% in 2014 at 1 year [32]. The UNOS/OPTN (Organ Procurement and Transplantation Network) database also reported survival rates for the years 2005 to 2007 of 88% at 1 year, 81% at 3 years, and 75% at 5 years. UNOS notes that survival rates are lowest among the patients 18 to 34 years of age [2].

Over the years, the average survival rate for cardiac transplant patients improves. The median survival in patients who were transplanted between 1982 and 1988 was 8.1 years, and that has increased to 9.8 years for individuals transplanted between 1994 and 1998. A significant improvement that has occurred during the current era is the 1-year survival for cardiac retransplantation, which is markedly better than that reported in past eras. The 1-year survival for these patients is 82.4% [2].

General Complications of Heart Transplantation

Right Heart Failure and Pulmonary Hypertension

Frequently acute right heart failure in the postoperative heart transplant patient is secondary to pulmonary hypertension. As mentioned, patient selection is crucial in identifying those recipients with fixed pulmonary hypertension. Those with a pulmonary vascular resistance ≥4 WU, a systolic pulmonary artery pressure ≥60 mm Hg or a transpulmonary gradient ≥15 mm Hg that does not reverse with vasodilator therapy such as inhaled nitric oxide or a prostacyclin analogue such as epoprostenol should not receive a heart transplant. Despite this, there are still recipients who will have some degree of pulmonary hypertension that will cause right heart strain posttransplantation.

Though right heart failure is frequently accompanied by pulmonary hypertension, other causes include donor selection, poor preservation, or prolonged ischemia time. The main principles of management in all cases of right heart failure are to preserve coronary perfusion, optimize RV preload, and reduce afterload by using high inspired oxygen concentrations, inhaled nitric oxide, and/or prostacyclin [33]. Intravenous milrinone or dobutamine followed later by oral sildenafil are also mainstays of therapy. Finally, in severe cases of right heart failure in the acute postoperative setting, a temporary right VAD is used to bridge the heart to recovery. The need for mechanical assistance typically lasts only a few days to a week and a low threshold should be kept for implanting a device.

Rejection

Surveillance for rejection of the transplanted heart by evaluating endomyocardial biopsies of the right ventricle obtained via the right internal jugular vein is performed frequently during the first year and eventually lessens to two to three times per year. There are four types of rejection: hyperacute, acute cellular, acute humoral, and chronic. The grading scale for rejection was recently revised to simplify it and also because there appeared to be little clinical difference between grade 1A and 1B rejection in the old classification. There was evidence of a benign clinical course for grade 2 rejection in the old classification as well [34]. The new grading system is shown in Table 60.3.

The mainstay of treatment is pulse corticosteroids administered intravenously for 3 days, with or without a subsequent taper. In the case of hemodynamically significant rejection or suspected acute humoral rejection, ultrafiltration, and intravenous immunoglobulin are administered to lower circulating antibodies. The addition of methotrexate or cyclophosphamide also should be considered. Photopheresis has been used to treat patients who have preexistent high levels of PRAs [35]. Late chronic rejection manifests as cardiac allograft vasculopathy. It is thought to be owing to a combination of humoral and cellular rejection, and is the greatest threat to long-term survival. When a patient has no other options to treat chronic, unrelenting rejection, the last resort is retransplantation.

TABLE 60.3

ISHLT Cardiac Biopsy Grading for Acute Cellular Rejection

Grade	
0R	No rejection
1R, mild	Interstitial and/or perivascular infiltrate with up to one focus of myocyte damage
2R, moderate	Two or more foci of infiltrate with associated myocyte damage
3R	Diffuse infiltrate with multifocal myocyte damage ± edema, ± hemorrhage, ± vasculitis

ISHLT, International Society for Heart and Lung Transplantation.
Data from Stewart S, Winters GL, Fishbein MC, et al: Revision of the 1990 working formulation for the standardization of nomenclature in the diagnosis of heart rejection. *J Heart Lung Transplant* 24:1710, 2005.

Infection and Pneumonia

Patients who have undergone thoracic organ transplantation are susceptible to bacterial, fungal, and viral infections. The most morbid viral infection that occurs in thoracic organ transplant recipients is caused by cytomegalovirus (CMV) [36]. Transmission of CMV by a donor organ is very common and hence prophylaxis with ganciclovir is used in CMV-mismatched thoracic transplant recipients. Patients who are seronegative at the time of transplantation and receive a graft from a seropositive donor sustain the highest rate of infection and exhibit the most severe form of CMV disease. Ganciclovir is the treatment of choice.

Pulmonary complications occur in approximately a third of heart transplant recipients [36,37] and is the most common infectious complication in heart transplant recipients. In the first 6 months, hospital-acquired bacterial pneumonia is the most common pulmonary complication followed by Aspergillus pneumonia. The overall mortality associated with pneumonia is 35% to 55% and accounts for 40% of all-cause mortality. A heightened vigilance for pulmonary infection is critical and the presence of yeast or mold-positive sputum should be aggressively treated. Risk factors for pulmonary complications are older recipient age, moderate-to-severe rejection, and development of CMV antigenemia in a previously CMV-seronegative recipient [36].

Coronary Allograft Vasculopathy

The development of coronary allograft vasculopathy can lead to myocardial infarction and sudden death in the cardiac transplant recipient. Routine annual coronary angiography with intravascular ultrasound is performed to permit an accurate assessment of the time of onset and rate of progression of coronary artery disease. Graft atherosclerosis occurs in 30% to 40% of transplant recipients after 3 years and in 40% to 60% of patients by 5 years after transplantation [38]. It remains the major obstacle to long-term survival in cardiac transplant recipients. A correlation between CMV infection and accelerated allograft atherosclerosis has also been identified [39]. Immunologically-mediated endothelial damage has been proposed as a stimulus for the development of graft atherosclerosis. Treatment can be temporizing in the form of angioplasty for focal lesions; however, when the disease involves tapering of the distal vessels, only cardiac retransplantation can treat the problem.

Renal Failure

Renal failure in the perioperative period is often transient, and it may be the direct result of nephrotoxic immunosuppressive drugs. Mild impairment of renal function preoperatively is acceptable as long as the risk of severe renal impairment during the postoperative period is recognized as a possible complication. The lowest acceptable level for creatinine clearance in a potential thoracic organ transplant recipient is 50 mL per minute. For suitable patients, combined heart-and-kidney transplant can be considered. It is also possible for a patient to be listed for a kidney transplant following thoracic organ transplantation.

Posttransplant Lymphoproliferative Disease

Posttransplant lymphoproliferative disease is a common cause of late death following solid-organ transplantation. It is more commonly seen in the pediatric population and is associated with exposure to the Epstein–Barr virus (EBV). Those at greatest risk for posttransplant lymphoproliferative disease are individuals who are EBV-seronegative before transplant who convert after their transplant. Those individuals who are EBV-seropositive before transplant are at a lower risk, but are not risk free. Management includes vigilant monitoring of the patient's EBV status, EBV polymerase chain reaction testing, and regular examinations of lymph node beds for enlargement. Therapy once this problem occurs has not been standardized and includes the use of antiviral agents, reduction of immunosuppression, anti-CD20 antibodies (such as rituximab), chemotherapy, and radiation therapy. Many of these have been used in combination.

Gastrointestinal Problems

Approximately 40% of patients experience gastrointestinal complications posttransplantation. The majority are related to drug side effects, most notably MMF that can cause nausea, vomiting, and diarrhea [40]. These are most often managed with dose adjustments. Serious complications of the alimentary tract following heart and heart–lung transplantation have been well documented and remain a major source of morbidity and mortality [41]. For that reason, patients with active peptic ulcer disease or diverticular disease are not considered for thoracic organ transplantation, at least until these problems have resolved. Mild liver dysfunction as evidenced by elevation of serum transaminase values and hyperbilirubinemia may occur in patients receiving high doses of cyclosporine. This is a chemical hepatitis that usually responds to a decrease in the dosage. Other immunosuppressants such as azathioprine have been implicated in a similar process. Hepatitis may also be secondary to hepatitis B, CMV, herpes simplex virus, hepatitis A, or hepatitis C.

Biliary tract disease is common in the thoracic organ transplant population. In a series of heart transplant recipients, the incidence of cholelithiasis ranged from 30% to 39%, which is more than twice that expected for age- and gender-matched controls [42]. The primary cause of this problem is thought to be gallbladder stasis and the side effects of specific immunosuppressants [43].

Cardiac Retransplantation

Cardiac retransplantation represents a small fraction of the transplants that are performed annually (the UNOS/OPTN database: 3% to 5% annual retransplant rate) [2]. According to the ISHLT database, approximately 2% of all adult heart transplantations internationally are retransplants. In the pediatric heart transplant population, this rate is approximately 6% of all transplantations. Current 1-year survival for heart retransplant is 82%, closely approaching the 1-year survival of the original transplantation [44]. The primary indications for retransplantation appear to be early graft failure, and in later time periods, chronic rejection or graft atherosclerosis.

HEART–LUNG TRANSPLANTATION

Heart–lung transplants are performed almost exclusively in patients with surgically uncorrectable congenital heart disease and Eisenmenger physiology. Patients with unrelated severe cardiomyopathy and pulmonary disease may also be candidates for heart–lung transplantation. With the difficulty of obtaining a heart–lung block and the outcomes of these procedures, many surgeons repair the congenital heart defect and transplant only the lungs [45,46]. Increasing numbers of patients with primary pulmonary hypertension are being treated with bilateral single-lung transplant rather than with heart–lung transplantation.

There has been a constant decline in the number of heart–lung transplants performed since the mid-1990s, both nationally and internationally, with fewer than 90 heart–lung transplants being performed annually in the current era [2].

Donor Criteria and Organ Procurement

The donor criteria are similar to the criteria used for heart (as listed previously) and lung transplantation (see Chapter 59). The procurement of the heart–lung block entails simultaneous use of techniques that are otherwise used to procure these same organs separately.

Operative Technique

From the outset, the recipient is placed on cardiopulmonary bypass. The recipient heart is excised first, and then each lung is removed. The phrenic neurovascular bundles are protected bilaterally. The left recurrent laryngeal nerve is also at risk for damage in the region of the ligamentum arteriosum. For that reason, some surgeons leave a portion of the main and left pulmonary artery in situ. The tracheal anastomosis is performed first. Although it can be wrapped with omentum, it does not need to be, because the coronary–bronchial collateral circulation is generally excellent. Performance of the right atrial anastomosis or bicaval anastomoses is followed by the aortic anastomosis. Large aortopulmonary collaterals and bronchial vessels can develop in patients with chronic cyanosis and Eisenmenger physiology. Extreme care must be taken during the operative procedure in these patients to avoid postoperative bleeding.

Postoperative Care

Postoperative care of patients who have had heart–lung transplantation can be quite complex. Potential complications from the heart or the lungs can arise. The standard postoperative care most closely resembles that of a lung transplantation patient, and is discussed in Chapter 59. Postoperative bleeding can be quite profound in this subset of patients, even with careful operative control of collateral vessels.

Outcomes

As of 2009, the current registry reports from ISHLT demonstrate a 1-year survival rate of only 75% for individuals undergoing a heart–lung transplantation. The average survival for this group of patients who were transplanted between 1982 and 2003 was 3.2 years. Because of the significant mortality rate that occurred within the first year after the transplantation, the conditional half-life was higher at 9 years [30]. Early mortalities were owing to technical complications, graft failure, and non-CMV infections accounting for 73% of the deaths. Mortality that occurred beyond the first year was attributed to chronic lung rejection with bronchiolitis obliterans, whereas cardiac rejection or coronary vasculopathy played a minimal role.

In the field of heart–lung transplantation, it was initially thought that endomyocardial biopsy would be the appropriate diagnostic test to detect rejection [47,48]. However, with two organ systems involved, the lungs often reject despite normal findings on endomyocardial biopsy [45]. Transbronchial biopsy reveals what is occurring in the lungs during the perioperative period and, later, complications in the lung grafts may be suggested when there are changes on chest radiograph or in pulmonary function studies, and should be evaluated with transbronchial biopsy [49]. Treatment of recurrent lung rejection consists of pulse corticosteroids with or without a taper. Alternate therapies including lympholytic agents, photopheresis, methotrexate, or cyclophosphamide may be used for refractory cases of rejection [50].

CONCLUSION

The discipline of heart transplantation has recently passed its 40th anniversary, and many major advances have been made. In spite of the changes that have occurred in recipient criteria, the greater number of potential recipients coming to transplant who are more than 60 years of age, on inotropic support, or using mechanical assist, the outcomes of heart transplantation have improved with each passing year. The field has also enjoyed seeing a decrease in candidate waiting times on the list and the evolution of cardiac assist devices to improve candidates for heart transplant. Clearly, knowledge of cardiac transplantation is directly related to the duration of experimental and clinical experience. It is expected that, as understanding continues to expand, long-term survival of transplant recipients will increase.

References

1. Toronto Lung Transplant Group: Unilateral lung transplantation for pulmonary fibrosis. *N Engl J Med* 314(18):1140–1145, 1986.
2. United Network for Organ Sharing Statistics. Available at: http://optn.transplant.hrsa.gov/latestData/step2.asp. Accessed August 15, 2015.
3. Mancini DM, Eisen H, Kussmaul W, et al: Value of peak exercise oxygen consumption for optimal timing of cardiac transplantation in ambulatory patients with heart failure. *Circulation* 83(3):778–786, 1991.
4. Kao W, Jessup M: Exercise testing and exercise training in patients with congestive heart failure. *J Heart Lung Transplant* 13(4):S117–S121, 1994.
5. Jimenez J, Edwards L, Jara J, et al: Impact of body mass index on survival following heart transplantation. *J Heart Lung Transplant* 23:S119, 2004.
6. Grady KL, White-Williams C, Naftel D, et al: Are preoperative obesity and cachexia risk factors for post heart transplant morbidity and mortality: a multi-institutional study of preoperative weight-height indices. Cardiac Transplant Research Database (CTRD) Group. *J Heart Lung Transplant* 18(8):750–763, 1999.
7. Jawitz OK, Jawitz NG, Yuh DD, et al: Impact of ABO compatibility on outcomes after heart transplantation in a national cohort during the past decade. *J Thoracic Cardiovasc Surg* 146(5):1239–1246, 2013.
8. Kasper E, Achuff SC: Clinical evaluation of potential heart transplant recipients, in Baumgartner WA, Reitz BA, Kasper EK, et al (eds): *Heart and Lung Transplantation*. 2nd ed. Philadelphia: WB Saunders Company, 2002, pp 57–63.
9. Boyle A, Colvin-Adams M: Recipient selection and management. *Semin Thoracic Cardiovasc Surg* 16:358, 2004.
10. Miller LW: Listing criteria for cardiac transplantation: results of an American Society of Transplant Physicians-National Institutes of Health conference. *Transplantation* 66(7):947–951, 1998.
11. Mancini D, Colombo PC: Left ventricular assist devices: a rapidly evolving alternative to transplant. *J Am Coll Cardiol* 65(23):2542–2555, 2015.
12. Rose EA, Gelijns AC, Moskowitz AJ, et al: Long-term use of a left ventricular assist device for end-stage heart failure. *N Eng J Med* 345(20):1435–1443, 2001.
13. Miller LW, Pagani FD, Russell SD, et al: Use of a continuous-flow device in patients awaiting heart transplantation. *N Eng J Med* 357(9):885–896, 2007.
14. John R, Lietz K, Schuster M, et al: Immunologic sensitization in recipients of left ventricular assist devices. *J Thoracic Cardiovasc Surg* 125(3):578–591, 2003.
15. Jaski BE, Kim JC, Naftel DC, et al: Cardiac transplant outcome of patients supported on left ventricular assist device vs intravenous inotropic therapy. *J Heart Lung Transplant* 20(4):449–456, 2001.
16. Radovancevic B, Golino A, Vrtovec B, et al: Is bridging to transplantation with a left ventricular assist device a risk factor for transplant coronary artery disease? *J Heart Lung Transplant* 24(6):703–707, 2005.
17. Gordon RJ, Quagliarello B, Lowy FD: Ventricular assist device-related infections. *Lancet Infect Dis* 6(7):426–437, 2006.
18. John R: Donor management and selection for heart transplantation. *Semin Thorac Cardiovasc Surg* 16(4):364–369, 2005.
19. Potapov EV, Ivanitskaia EA, Loebe M, et al: Value of cardiac troponin I and T for selection of heart donors and as predictors of early graft failure. *Transplantation* 71(10):1394–1400, 2001.
20. Potapov EV, Wagner FD, Loebe M, et al: Elevated donor cardiac troponin T and procalcitonin indicate two independent mechanisms of early graft failure after heart transplantation. *Int J Cardiol* 92(2):163–167, 2003.
21. Ardehali A, Esmailian F, Deng M, et al: Ex-vivo perfusion of donor hearts for human heart transplantation (PROCEED II): a prospective, open-label, multicentre, randomised non-inferiority trial. *Lancet* 385(9987):2577–2584, 2015.
22. Smith CR: Techniques in cardiac transplantation. *Prog Cardiovasc Dis* 32(6):383–404, 1990.
23. Oyer P, Stinson E, Jamieson S, et al: Cyclosporine in cardiac transplantation: a 2 1/2 year follow-up. *Transplant Proc* 15[Suppl 1]:2546, 1983.
24. Taylor DO, Barr ML, Radovancevic B, et al: A randomized, multicenter comparison of tacrolimus and cyclosporine immunosuppressive regimens in cardiac transplantation: decreased hyperlipidemia and hypertension with tacrolimus. *J Heart Lung Transplant* 18(4):336–345, 1999.
25. Reichart B, Meiser B, Vigano M, et al: European multicenter tacrolimus heart pilot study: three year follow-up. *J Heart Lung Transplant* 20(2):249–250, 2001.
26. Kobashigawa JA, Patel J, Furukawa H, et al: Five-year results of a randomized, single-center study of tacrolimus vs microemulsion cyclosporine in heart transplant patients. *J Heart Lung Transplant* 25(4):434–439, 2006.
27. Kobashigawa JA, Miller LW, Russell SD, et al: Tacrolimus with mycophenolate mofetil (MMF) or sirolimus vs. cyclosporine with MMF in cardiac transplant patients: 1-year report. *Am J Transplant* 6(6):1377–1386, 2006.
28. Deuse T, Sista R, Weill D, et al: Review of heart–lung transplantation at Stanford. *Ann Thorac Surg* 90(1):329–337, 2010.
29. Kobashigawa J, Miller L, Renlund D, et al: A randomized active-controlled trial of mycophenolate mofetil in heart transplant recipients. Mycophenolate mofetil investigators. *Transplantation* 66(4):507–515, 1998.
30. Taylor DO, Edwards LB, Boucek MM, et al: Registry of the International Society for Heart and Lung Transplantation: twenty-second official adult heart transplant report—2005. *J Heart Lung Transplant* 24(8):945–955, 2005.
31. Baran DA, Zucker MJ, Arroyo LH, et al: Randomized trial of tacrolimus monotherapy: tacrolimus in combination, tacrolimus alone compared (the TICTAC trial). *J Heart Lung Transplant* 26(10):992–997, 2007.
32. ISHLT Database for North America. Available at: http://www.ishlt.org/registries/quarterlyDataReportResults.asp?organ=HR&rptType=recip_p_surv&continent=4. Accessed September 22, 2015.
33. Stobierska-Dzierzek B, Awad H, Michler RE: The evolving management of acute right-sided heart failure in cardiac transplant recipients. *J Am Coll Cardiol* 38(4):923–931, 2001.
34. Stewart S, Fishbein MC, Snell GI, et al: Revision of the 1996 working formulation for the standardization of nomenclature in the diagnosis of lung rejection. *J Heart Lung Transplant* 26(12):1229–1242, 2007.
35. Sulemanjee NZ, Merla R, Lick SD, et al: The first year post-heart transplantation: use of immunosuppressive drugs and warly complications. *J Cardiovascular Pharmacol Ther* 13(1):13–31, 2008.
36. Atasever A, Bacakoglu F, Uysal F, et al: Pulmonary complications in heart transplant recipients. *Transplantation Proc* 38:1530, 2006.
37. Lenner R, Padilla ML, Teirstein AS, et al: Pulmonary complications in cardiac transplant recipients. *Chest* 120(2):508–513, 2001.
38. Hunt SA, Haddad F: The changing face of heart transplantation. *J Am Coll Cardiol* 52(8):587–598, 2008.
39. Wang SS: Treatment and prophylaxis of cardiac allograft vasculopathy. *Transplant Proc* 40(8):2609, 2008.
40. Diaz B, Vilchez FG, Almenar L, et al: Gastrointestinal complications in heart transplant patients: MITOS study. *Transplant Proc* 39(7):2397, 2007.
41. Kirklin J, Holm A, Aldrete J, et al: Gastrointestinal complications after cardiac transplantation. Potential benefit of early diagnoses and prompt surgical intervention. *Ann Surg* 211(5):538, 1990.
42. Steck TB, Costanzo-Nordin MR, Keshavarzian A: Prevalence and management of cholelithiasis in heart transplant patients. *J Heart Lung Transplant* 10(6):1029–1032, 1990.
43. Stief J, Stempfle H, Götzberger M, et al: Biliary diseases in heart transplanted patients: a comparison between cyclosporine a versus tacrolimus-based immunosuppression. *Eur J Med Res* 14(5):206, 2009.
44. Everly MJ: Cardiac transplantation in the United States: an analysis of the UNOS registry. *Clin Transpl* 35–43, 2008.
45. Starnes V, Theodore J, Oyer P, et al: Evaluation of heart–lung transplant recipients with prospective, serial transbronchial biopsies and pulmonary function studies. *J Thorac Cardiovasc Surg* 98(5, pt 1):683–690, 1989.
46. Starnes VA: Heart–lung transplantation: an overview. *Cardiol Clin* 8(1):159–168, 1990.
47. Glanville AR, Imoto E, Baldwin JC, et al: The role of right ventricular endomyocardial biopsy in the long-term management of heart–lung transplant recipients. *J Heart Transplant* 6(6):357–361, 1986.
48. Griffith BP, Hardesty RL, Trento A, et al: Heart–lung transplantation: lessons learned and future hopes. *Ann Thoracic Surg* 43(1):6–16, 1987.
49. Barr ML, Meiser BM, Eisen HJ, et al: Photopheresis for the prevention of rejection in cardiac transplantation. *N Eng J Med* 339(24):1744–1751, 1998.
50. Glanville AR, Baldwin JC, Burke CM, et al: Obliterative bronchiolitis after heart–lung transplantation: apparent arrest by augmented immunosuppression. *Ann Intern Med* 107(3):300–304, 1987.

Chapter 61 ■ Care of the Pancreas Transplant Recipient

COLLEEN L. JAY • GREGORY A. ABRAHAMIAN • ANGELINA EDWARDS

Type 1 diabetes mellitus has two primary treatment options: (a) exogenous insulin administration or (b) β cell replacement by pancreas or islet transplantation. Despite the introduction of many new and improved modalities for insulin administration, exogenous administration requires complex and frequent monitoring and responsiveness from the patient, making it burdensome. Often, patients face a choice between imperfect glycemic control, predisposing them to secondary complications including retinopathy, neuropathy, and nephropathy, or too tight control possibly precipitating hypoglycemic unawareness, which can dramatically impact quality of life.

Pancreas and islet transplantation when successful produces a more physiologic euglycemic state and effectively treats hypoglycemia episodes. However, pancreas transplantation requires major surgery in which perioperative risks are often compounded by the comorbidities frequently seen in patients with long-standing diabetes. Additionally, the long-term effectiveness of islet transplantation continues to be a challenging goal. Moreover, both require long-term immunosuppression to prevent rejection, resulting in increased risks of infection and cancer.

In 1993, The Diabetes Control and Complications Trial [1] showed that intensive insulin therapy (multiple injections per day with doses adjusted by frequent blood sugar determinations) resulted in a 60% reduction in the risk of secondary complications despite typically failing to achieve normalization of glucose [2]. Current American Diabetes Association (ADA) guidelines recommend multiple-dose insulin injections (three to four injections daily of basal and prandial insulin) or continuous subcutaneous insulin pump with the goal of achieving an HbA1C <7% and <6.5% when risks of hypoglycemia or other adverse effects are low [3]. National Health and Nutrition Examination Survey (NHANES) data show that almost half (45%) of patients failed to achieve glycemic targets (HbA1C < 7%) [4].

Pancreas transplantation can produce insulin independence in diabetic recipients, decrease risks of life-disabling hypoglycemia, and slow progression and even reverse secondary complications including retinopathy, nephropathy, and neuropathy [5]. With major advances in technical aspects and management of pancreas transplantation, the success rate has progressively increased since its introduction. Currently, 1-year patient survival is 95% after pancreas transplantation [6]. One- and five-year pancreas graft survival was 74% to 78% and 51%, respectively, for pancreas transplant alone; 86% and 74%, respectively, for simultaneous pancreas–kidney transplantation; and 79% to 80% and 62%, respectively, for pancreas after kidney transplantation [6,7]. Today's recipients have a high probability of achieving insulin independence for years with pancreas transplantation, if not indefinitely.

Historically, islet transplantation has had lower rates of insulin independence than pancreas transplantation. In the late 1990s at the University of Alberta, insulin independence was achieved by sequential transplantation of islets from multiple donors and the use of a steroid-free, nondiabetogenic, immunosuppressive regimen [8]. In another series from the University of Minnesota with a similar immunosuppressive regimen, single-donor islet transplantation induced insulin independence [9]. In this series, the donors had a high body mass index (BMI) and the recipients had a low BMI so that the net number of islets transplanted per unit weight was similar in the Alberta and Minnesota series. In subsequent follow-up under the Edmonton protocol, 68% (44/65) of patients who received one to three islet transplants achieved insulin independence [10]. However, at 5-year follow-up, only 10% maintained insulin independence with a median duration of insulin independence of 15 months (interquartile range 6.2 to 25.5) [11]. Although outcomes with islet transplantation have improved, pancreas transplantation continues to provide higher rate of more durable success.

The main trade-off for recipients of β-cell allografts is the need for immunosuppression. A successful graft makes the recipient euglycemic and normalizes glycosylated hemoglobin levels, but the combined risks of immunosuppression and a major pancreas transplant surgery must be weighed against the long-term risks of imperfect glycemic control with exogenous insulin injection and of development of secondary complications. A randomized prospective trial has not been done to weigh these risks. The burden of daily management of diabetes with the need for multiple sticks to monitor blood sugar levels and to inject insulin tilts the balance in favor of a pancreas or islet transplant for many diabetic patients. Furthermore, antirejection strategies are continually being modified to decrease the complications of immunosuppression. Nevertheless, pancreas transplantation is more frequently performed later in the course of disease often after the recipient has become uremic and needs a kidney transplant. Currently, only 12% of pancreas transplantations are performed alone before the onset of end-stage renal disease [7].

The main indications for pancreas transplantation in patients with normal kidney function are progressive diabetic complications, glycemic lability, and hypoglycemic unawareness, the latter of which may emerge years after the onset of diabetes, particularly in patients with autonomic neuropathy. However, even for nonlabile diabetic patients who attempt tight control by intensive glucose monitoring, the diabetes literature shows a high rate of secondary complications that are just as morbid, balancing out the risks associated with chronic immunosuppression in pancreas transplantation recipients [12].

Given that most pancreas transplantation candidates have advanced diabetic nephropathy and require a kidney transplant also, the risks of immunosuppression are already assumed because of the kidney transplant, and so a simultaneous or sequential pancreas transplant does not pose significant additional risks other than those associated with surgery [13]. Although most pancreas transplantations are performed in type 1 diabetics with impending or chronic renal failure, some pancreas transplantations are performed in patients categorized as having type 2 diabetes [14]. Currently, approximately 7% of pancreas transplantations annually in the United States are performed in type 2 diabetics [7]. Many reports have shown successful outcomes with comparable survival rates as seen in type 1 diabetics [15,16]. There has been much controversy surrounding the increasing use of pancreas transplantation for type 2 diabetes and wide variability in the definitions used to categorize patients as type 1 versus type 2 diabetics and as such United Network of Organ Sharing (UNOS) has set strict guidelines regarding recipient BMI criteria in patients with detectable C-peptide levels (>2 ng per mL) in order to accrue waiting time [17].

While β-cell replacement therapies are ideal for type 1 diabetes management, this approach suffers from a lack of available suitable donors. Thus, stem cell–based therapies have the potential to make β-cell restoration possible, for both forms of diabetes. In addition to β-cell replacement, the use of mesenchymal stromal cells may modulate autoimmunity and promote regeneration of the recipient's islet cells [18]. Previous attempts at in vitro stem cell therapy for insulin production lacked uniformity in the generation, maintenance, and differentiation of βcells [19]. Recent advances in understanding pancreatic development in the mouse have led to considerable progress of in vitro development of functional islets and in vivo use in diabetic animal models [20]. Scientists have now generated stem cell–derived β cells that express cell markers found on mature β cells and exhibit calcium influx, membrane depolarization, and insulin exocytosis in response to a glucose challenge. These cells display the same activity once transplanted under the kidney capsule of immunosuppressed mice. These cells secrete human insulin in a glucose-related manner and ameliorate hyperglycemia for diabetic mice [21]. Although still in its infancy, this exciting discovery has brought scientists one step closer to realizing the potential that cell therapy may play in clinical transplantation.

PANCREAS TRANSPLANT RECIPIENT CATEGORIES

Pancreas transplantation candidates are divided into three categories: uremic (need a kidney transplant), posturemic (have a functioning kidney transplant), and nonuremic (do not need a kidney transplant, at least yet). For candidates who are uremic, the options are to receive kidney and pancreas transplantations either simultaneously in the same operation or sequentially in separate operations. Which option to take is usually based on the availability and suitability of living and deceased donors for one or both organs at that particular time.

Accordingly, there are three broad categories of pancreas transplantation procedures: simultaneous pancreas kidney (SPK) transplantation, pancreas after kidney (PAK) transplantation, and pancreas transplantation alone (PTA).

1. SPK transplantations: Most SPK transplantations are performed with both organs from the same deceased donor. Because a large number of patients wait on the UNOS list for a kidney organ, unless priority is given to SPK candidates, waiting times tend to be long (years). To avoid two operations and long waiting times, a simultaneous kidney and segmental pancreas transplantations from a living donor can be done, but historically only a few centers offered this, and this option has largely fallen out of favor as outcomes with deceased donor pancreas transplantations have improved [22,23]. A simultaneous living donor islet–kidney transplantations have been utilized anecdotally with some success [23,24]. If a living kidney donor is available, another option is a simultaneous living donor kidney and deceased donor pancreas transplantation [25]. However, due to logistical challenges associated with this approach, more commonly if a patient has an available living kidney donor and is thought to benefit from avoiding prolonged wait times and the morbidity and mortality risks associated with increased duration of dialysis, many center will proceed with living donor kidney transplant and subsequent PAK.
2. PAK transplantation: For diabetic patients who have already received a kidney transplantation from a living or deceased donor, a PAK transplantation can be performed. Most PAK transplantations today are performed from a deceased donor in a patient who previously received a living kidney transplantation. Although a PAK transplantation requires that a uremic diabetic patient undergoes two operations to achieve both a dialysis-free and insulin-independent state, the two transplantations done separately are "smaller" procedures than combined transplantations. The time interval between the living donor kidney transplantation and the deceased donor pancreas transplantation depends on several factors, including recipient recovery from the kidney transplantation and donor availability. Initial popularity of the PAK peaked at 28% of pancreas transplants performed in the United States in 2004 has now declined to around 12% [7]. Under the new kidney allocation system implemented in December 2014, equal prioritization was given to SPK and PAK recipients, obviating the advantage of shorter wait times with PAK versus SPK. Historically, PAK has been associated with inferior pancreas graft survival and higher rates of rejection compared with SPK transplantation, which has the immunologic advantage of a single donor [7,26]. More recently, some authors have argued for the increasing reconsideration of PAK especially in the era of modern immunosuppression regimens and improved pancreas transplantation outcomes since this could be performed after a patient receives a living donor kidney transplantation [26]. Improved patient and graft survival has been demonstrated after living donor compared with deceased donor kidney transplantation. Moreover, this approach could enable preemptive kidney transplantation, which is also associated with well-established survival benefits as well as decreased complications and costs.
3. PTA: For recipients with adequate kidney function, a solitary pancreas transplantation can be performed from either a living or deceased donor. With improved outcomes following deceased donor pancreas transplantation, living donor solitary pancreas transplantation is done infrequently, but is typically indicated if a candidate has a high panel-reactive antibody and a negative cross-match to a living donor. PTA candidates have problems with glycemic control, hypoglycemic unawareness, and frequent insulin reactions but as yet fairly normal renal function. A successful PTA not only obviates these problems, but also probably improves the quality of life and may ameliorate secondary diabetic complications, thus increasing the applicability of PTA [27–29].

Although the numbers of pancreas transplantations have declined over the past decade from a high of more than 1,400 annually in 2004 to 2005 to a little over 1,000 in 2013 and 2014, the most common category of pancreas transplantation is still SPK (76%). Approximately, 12% of pancreas transplantations were PAK or PTA each, respectively [7]. Although rare, pancreas transplants can also occur as multiorgan transplants in patients with unique medical problems.

HISTORICAL PERSPECTIVES, EVOLUTION, AND IMPROVEMENTS IN PANCREAS TRANSPLANTS

The first clinical pancreas transplantation was performed at the University of Minnesota in 1966 [30]. The number of transplants remained low during the 1970s, but progressively increased in the 1980s, due to the introduction of cyclosporine. By the end of 2010, more than 36,000 pancreas transplants were reported to the International Pancreas Transplant Registry (IPTR) from more than 1,000 centers worldwide, including more than 24,000 in the United States and more than 12,000 outside the United States [6]. More than 3,000 patients wait for a pancreas transplantation on the basis of OPTN data in June 2015, and more than 1,000 pancreas transplantations are performed annually in the United States [7].

The early history of pancreas transplantation was largely performed at the University of Minnesota and involved various surgical techniques, many of which were developed to manage pancreatic exocrine drainage [22]. The first clinical pancreas transplant was performed by Kelly et al. as a duct-ligated, segmental graft at the University of Minnesota in December 1966 [30,31]. In 1973, Lillehei described a series of 13 pancreas transplants at the University of Minnesota, first via a cutaneous duodenostomy and subsequently where he used enteric drainage (ED) of pancreatic secretions via a Roux-en-Y duodenojejunostomy [31,32]. In the 1970s, Gliedman reported a series of 11 segmental

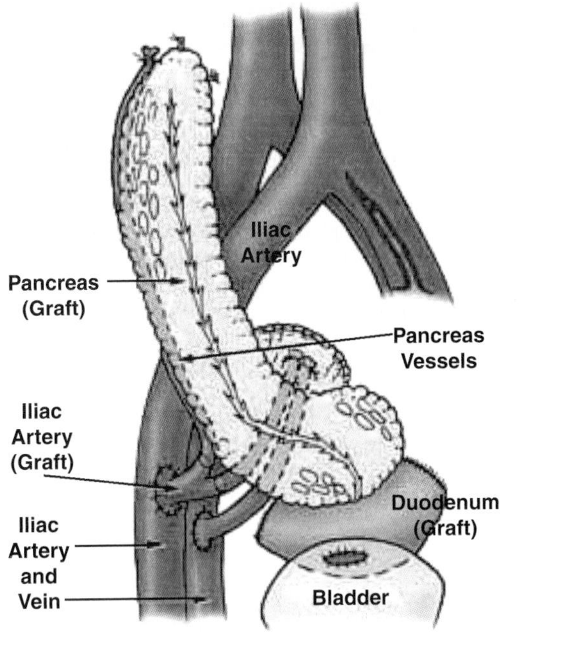

FIGURE 61.1 Bladder-drained pancreaticoduodenal transplant alone from a cadaveric donor.

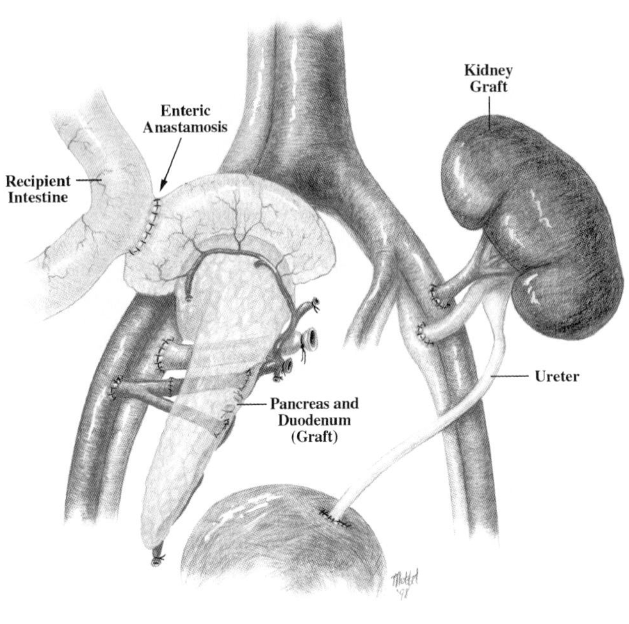

FIGURE 61.2 Enteric-drained simultaneous pancreas and kidney transplant from a cadaveric donor with systemic venous drainage.

pancreas transplants with a pancreatic duct–ureter anastomosis for exocrine drainage [31–34]. This technique did not develop widespread popularity because of leakage from the pancreatic duct–ureter anastomosis and the cut surface of the pancreas [31].

From the mid-1970s to mid-1980s, segmental pancreas transplantations predominated due to a historical belief that the pancreatic organ was less antigenic than the duodenal stump [31,32]. It was during this time that islet transplantation was viewed with increasing promise and the hope that it would replace pancreas transplantation. With segmental pancreas transplantations, two techniques were popularized to manage pancreatic exocrine secretion, including open intraperitoneal drainage by Bewick in 1976 and the University of Minnesota in 1978 [31,35] and synthetic polymer pancreatic duct injection by Dubernard in 1978 [31,36]. In 1983, Sollinger [37] reported the use of direct bladder drainage (BD) to manage pancreatic exocrine secretions in a segmental pancreas graft , and the next year he described a series of 10 segmental pancreas transplantations with BD that had very few surgical complications, and so BD became the predominant technique (Fig. 61.1) [31,37]. Additionally, the ease of measuring urinary amylase activity as a marker for rejection episodes contributed to the popularity of this technique over the next decade [22,31,38].

In mid-1980s, Starzl revived ED of the whole-organ pancreas transplantation described by Lellehei 20 years earlier (Fig. 61.2) [31,39]. In the mid-1980s to the mid-1990s, although BD had continued popularity, urinary complications including cystitis, urethritis, hematuria, metabolic acidosis, and dehydration led to enteric conversion of many whole-organ pancreas transplants in a technique first described by Tom in 1987 [31,40]. For SPK, monitoring of urinary amylase was less important as serum creatinine elevation typically preceded urinary amylase decline when rejection episode affected both organs [22]. As such, ED became the more common technique much earlier for SPK. Since 2010, enteric drainage was used in approximately 90% of pancreas transplantations [6].

Venous drainage of the pancreas has also evolved over the years. Portal drainage was used with segmental grafts in the 1980s [41–44]. In 1989, Mühlbacher [45] described the first case of whole-organ pancreas transplantation with portal venous drainage and exocrine BD. Until 1990s, systemic venous drainage had been the norm until portal drainage gained increased popularity with ED [46,47] as opposed to BD [45]. Most commonly, drainage of the portal vein was to the recipient superior mesenteric vein (Fig. 61.3). However, by 2010, the popularity of portal drainage was waning, with only portal drainage utilized in 18% of SPK and PAK and 10% of PTA [6].

Before standard techniques were developed to procure liver and pancreas grafts with intact blood supplies, segmental

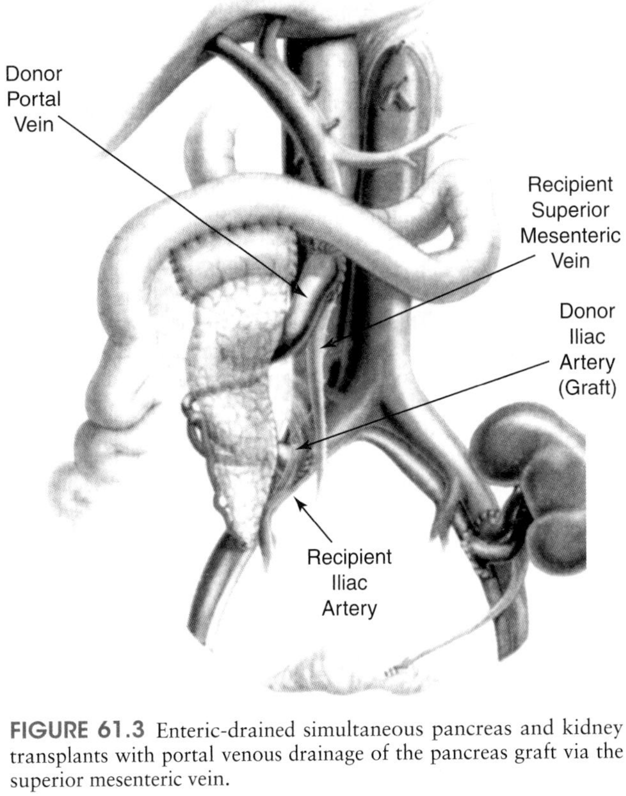

FIGURE 61.3 Enteric-drained simultaneous pancreas and kidney transplants with portal venous drainage of the pancreas graft via the superior mesenteric vein.

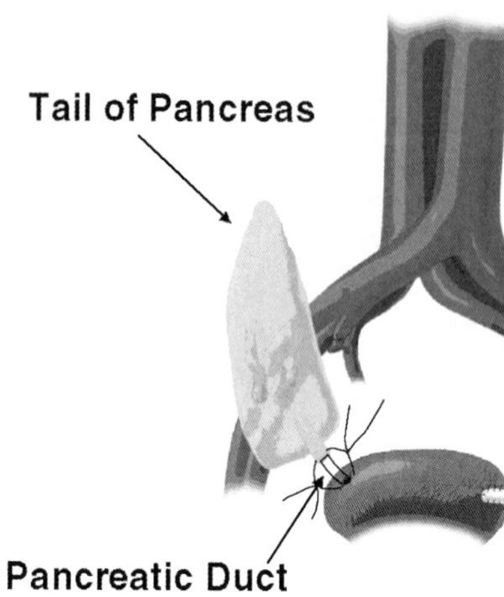

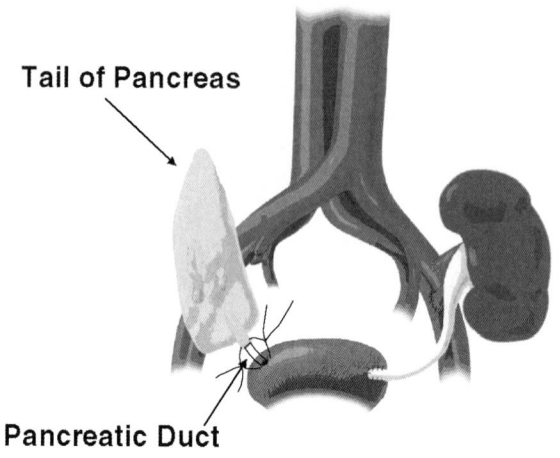

FIGURE 61.4 Simultaneous segmental pancreas and kidney transplant from a living donor. Either bladder- or enteric-drained technique can be used, but the bladder-drained technique has a lower complication rate and is illustrated.

TABLE 61.1

Summary of American Diabetes Association Recommendations for Indications for Pancreas Transplants

Indication for pancreas transplants
1. Imminent or established end-stage renal disease in patients who have had, or plan to have, a kidney transplantation
2. History of frequent, acute, and severe metabolic complications (e.g., hypoglycemia, hyperglycemia, ketoacidosis)
3. Incapacitating clinical and emotional problems with exogenous insulin therapy
4. Consistent failure of insulin-based management to prevent acute complications
5. Islet cell transplantation is experimental and should be performed only within the setting of controlled research studies

pancreas grafts were commonly used. Currently, whole-organ pancreaticoduodenal grafts predominate, although segmental grafts are still used for living donor pancreas transplantations. The first living donor pancreas transplantation was performed at the University of Minnesota in 1979 [48]. The early series of living donor pancreas transplantations consisted of solitary pancreata because the technical failure and rejection rates for deceased donor pancreata were so high [22,49]. In the 1990s, living donor pancreas transplantations were predominantly performed in combination with a kidney from the same donor (Fig. 61.4) [50–52]. Another approach, as previously mentioned, is to perform a living donor kidney transplantation simultaneously with a deceased donor pancreas transplantation [25].

Immunosuppressive regimens have made great strides over the years. Most immunosuppressive protocols use antibody induction, followed by maintenance therapy with tacrolimus in combination with mycophenolate mofetil [53]. Typically, patients received T-cell–depleting induction with either antithymocyte globulin or aletuzemab. Despite initial interest in nondepleting agents, utilization for pancreas transplant had declined to less than 10% according to the IPTR registry [6]. In the late 1990s and early 2000s, some centers including Northwestern University pushed for steroid-free regimens for pancreas transplantations [31]. In fact, according to the IPTR, a third of SPK and up to 45% of PTA/PAK transplantations were discharged on a steroid-free maintenance regimen [6,31,53].

In 2012, there were more than 100 pancreas transplant centers and 12 active allogeneic islet cell transplant centers in the United States [54]. Some centers have reported extensive experience, including more than 1,000 SPK transplantations at the University of Wisconsin and more than 1,900 pancreas transplantations of all categories at the University of Minnesota. Since 1980, the IPTR has collected data from all centers in the world [6,55] and remains an excellent resource for outcome analysis. In addition, the US Transplant Scientific Registry of Transplant Recipients (SRTR) provides detailed scientific analysis of national, regional, state, and center-specific pancreas graft and patient survival [7].

INDICATIONS AND CONTRAINDICATIONS FOR PANCREAS TRANSPLANTS

The indications for a pancreas transplantation have evolved and expanded over the years as the results have improved. The position statement of the American Diabetes Association [3] on indications for a pancreas transplant (Table 61.1) include patients with impending or existing end-stage renal failure, frequent and severe metabolic complications such as hypoglycemia especially hypoglycemic unawareness, incapacitating clinical or emotional problems with insulin therapy, and failure of insulin therapy to prevent acute complications. Pancreas transplantation also benefits patients who have developed secondary complications of diabetes including retinopathy, cardiovascular disease, nephropathy, and neuropathy. The progression of many of these complications is halted and potentially reversed by a functioning pancreas graft.

With a functioning pancreas transplant, improvements with sensory, motor, and autonomic neuropathy and paresthesias have been reported [56–61]. Patients with abnormal cardiorespiratory neurologic reflexes have reduced death rates after a functioning pancreas transplantation [61,62]. There is increased nerve conduction velocity in SPK recipients with functioning pancreas transplantation versus those with failed pancreas grafts [56,63–65]. Uremic patients who undergo SPK transplantation have improved symptoms of gastroparesis than do patients who have a kidney transplantation alone [57,66].

Similarly, a successful pancreas transplantation halts the progression of diabetic changes in the new kidney transplant, and several studies have demonstrated improvement of nephropathy after PTA [56,57,61]. One study showed that long-term normoglycemia due to a functioning pancreas transplant led to reversal of characteristic diabetic glomerular lesions that occurred in nonuremic PTA recipients who had established nephropathy [57,67]. In addition to improvement in glomerular architecture, this group also showed a reversibility of cortical interstitial expansion and reabsorption of atrophic renal tubules 10 years after PTA [57,68]. These changes in renal architecture may explain the reduction in blood pressure, albuminuria, and nephrotic range proteinuria that some PTA recipients demonstrate [57,69,70], but creatinine clearance can still deteriorate.

Several recent reports have shown stabilization or amelioration of diabetic retinopathy with a functioning pancreas transplant [56,57,61]. Ramsey et al. reported reduced deterioration in advanced retinopathy with a functioning pancreas transplant at 3 years [57,71]. Wang et al. reported regression of diabetic retinopathy in 43% of SPK recipients versus 23% of kidney-transplantation-alone recipients, although nearly 50% of both groups showed no benefit but follow-up was short at 1 year [61,72]. Giannarelli et al. examined 33 type 1 patients who received a pancreas transplantation versus 36 type 1 patients who had medical therapy only and noted that stabilization or amelioration of diabetic retinopathy was 91% versus 43%, respectively [56,73].

Several studies have examined the effects of pancreas transplantation on vasculopathy and cardiovascular risk factors. Severe and advanced vascular disease may be unaffected by a functioning pancreas transplant [56,61]. One series documented improvement in conjunctival microcirculation in 12 SPK patients when compared with five kidney-transplant-alone recipients [57,74], and other series reported improvement in carotid artery intima-media thickness (which correlates with decreased cardiovascular events) within 2 years of pancreas transplantation [57,61,75,76]. SPK transplants have also shown to improve cardiovascular risk factor profiles, left ventricular systolic and diastolic function, and endothelial function and slow progression of coronary atherosclerotic lesions [56,57,61,77–82]. Atherosclerosis regresses in nearly 40% of recipients with a functioning pancreas transplant, and this fact may explain improved quality of life and patient survival benefit after pancreas transplantation [56,61,82]. Fiorina et al. demonstrated normalization of left ventricular diastolic function at 4 years after a functioning pancreas graft [56,61,83], which leads to reduction in cardiovascular events [79]. Rates of myocardial infarction and pulmonary edema were lower in SPK recipients than in kidney-transplant-alone patients, although the kidney-alone patients tended to be quite older and the follow-up period was short [61,84–86]. Echocardiographic findings 2 years after pancreatic transplantation showed improvement in left ventricular shape and function when compared with kidney transplantation alone. Stabilization [61,62] and even improvement [61,87] in cardiac autonomic dysfunction can occur after pancreas transplantation. A pancreas transplantation preferably can be offered early, before the onset of these complications of diabetes, to interested patients who understand the risks of a significant operation and immunosuppression versus the benefit of insulin independence and freedom from diabetic complications.

Potentially, the most subjective outcome after pancreas transplantation, improved quality of life, may be the most important [57]. One study compared the quality of life of diabetic patients who underwent SPK transplants with a kidney transplants alone and noted that SPK recipients reported improved quality of life in regard to chronic symptoms, effects of kidney disease, cognitive function, pain, physical activity, and overall health [88]. Clear evidence regarding improvement in quality of life after PTA recipients is lacking.

Relative and absolute contraindications include those for any other transplantation, such as extremes of age, prohibitive cardiovascular and pulmonary risk, severe hepatic disease, malignancy, active acute and chronic infections, AIDS, severe persistent coagulation disorder, noncompliance, and serious psychosocial problems. Candidates with advanced vascular disease have increased risks of surgical complications, yet those patients who do well after pancreas transplantation greatly benefit from stabilization of their cardiovascular risk.

PRETRANSPLANTATION EVALUATION

The pretransplantation workup should include a detailed medical, surgical, and psychosocial evaluation. Cardiac risk assessment is mandatory because diabetes is a major risk factor for coronary artery disease (CAD). Cardiologists vary on the type of test to screen for CAD in pretransplantation diabetic patients. Coronary angiograms are performed in many candidates, especially those over 45 years of age. Noninvasive tests are not very sensitive for CAD and are poorly predictive for subsequent postoperative events in long-standing diabetic patients. Risks of contrast-induced nephropathy in patients with residual renal function must be balanced against the potential benefits of accurate cardiac risk stratification and potential intervention when evaluating patients for transplant. Revascularization by angioplasty, stenting, or bypass surgery may be needed when possible to address reversible ischemic and unstable cardiac disease. Revascularized transplantation candidates have significantly fewer postoperative cardiac events, as compared with those who received medical therapy alone. The minimum cardiac evaluation for consideration of pancreas transplant candidacy should include an electrocardiogram, chest radiograph, echocardiogram, and cardiac stress test [61].

A detailed physical examination must be done to rule out vascular insufficiency in the lower extremities. If such vascular insufficiency is found, it too may need pretransplant correction with angioplasty, endarterectomy, or revascularization because the transplant operation, often involving an anastomosis to the iliac artery, may further diminish lower extremity blood flow.

Pulmonary function tests are indicated in chronic smokers and patients with a history of chronic pulmonary disease. Postoperative intensive care unit monitoring and perioperative bronchodilator therapy may be indicated in some patients. Some transplant centers require smoking cessation for consideration for listing. Liver function tests should be done to rule out hepatic insufficiency and viral hepatitis. The diagnosis of viral hepatitis (especially hepatitis C) is associated with worse long-term outcome after extrahepatic transplantation. The presence of cirrhosis is a contraindication for pancreas transplant (unless the patient is a candidate for a multiorgan transplant). Autonomic dysfunction in terms of autonomic neuropathy and gastroparesis are frequent complications of long-standing diabetes. In some cases, symptoms of these can be unmasked or more severe during the early postoperative period. Some immunosuppressive medications also may worsen gastrointestinal dysfunction (mycophenolate mofetil can have significant gastrointestinal side effects). Prokinetic agents may be indicated to treat gastroparesis. A urologic evaluation is especially important for bladder-drained recipients because bladder dysfunction predisposes to graft pancreatitis and for SPK recipients because it may impact long-term kidney graft function.

CADAVERIC DONOR SELECTION

Pancreas donor selection criteria are not standardized and vary from center to center. Absolute contraindications are the obvious ones applied to most solid organs: active hepatitis B, hepatitis C (unless the recipient has hepatitis C), human immunodeficiency virus, most viral encephalitis, non-CNS malignancy, surgical or traumatic damage to the graft, history of diabetes mellitus, pancreatitis, and extremes of age (less than 10 or more than 60 years). Prolonged intensive care unit stay and duration of brain death have been associated with an increased risk of pancreas graft failure [89]. Many studies have shown that donor age is important. Even middle-aged donors (>45 years old) are associated with pancreas graft failure and increased complications [90–92]. Small donors (<28 kg) have been used for pancreas transplantation with good outcomes [93]. Obesity in the deceased donor is a common cause for refusal of solid-organ pancreas donation, and donors with a BMI > 35 kg per m^2 are virtually never used for solid-organ pancreas transplantation [61]. According to International Pancreas Transplant Registry data, the following variables are associated with an increased risk of pancreas allograft thrombosis: (1) donor age > 40 years; (2) nontraumatic cause of brain death; and (3) pancreas preservation time >24 hours [53,94]. Other reports have suggested that donor BMI > 30 and fatty infiltration of the pancreas gland on visual inspection increase risks of graft thrombosis [95,96]. Older and obese donors (>50 years old and >30 kg per m^2) are probably more suitable for islet cell than for solid-organ pancreas transplantation [61]. Elevated donor sodium levels (Na > 160 mg per dL) is considered a relative contraindication by some centers due to concerns for pancreatic edema and risks of graft pancreatitis and thrombosis. It is one of the factors along with donor age, BMI, duration of cardiac arrest and ICU stay, vasopressor use, and elevated serum amylase and lipase levels that make up the preprocurement pancreas allocation suitability score (P-PASS), which had been associated with differences in pancreatic graft survival rates [97]. Elevated amylase and lipase levels are considered contraindications by many centers, but care must be taken in interpreting amylase levels as these are frequently elevated in donors with head injury. More recently, a pancreas donor risk index (PDRI) score developed by Axelrod et al. [98] on the basis of multivariate regression predicts pancreas graft survival after transplantation on the basis of donor age, gender, race, BMI, height, cause of death, donation after cardiac death status, and elevated serum creatinine .

Still, donors after cardiac death are being used increasingly and successfully to expand the donor pool. One survey showed equivalent patient and graft survival at 1, 3, and 5 years in SPK transplant recipients from donors after cardiac death compared with ideal donors after brain death [64]. In general, a pancreas from a so-called marginal donor is associated with good outcome if the pancreas is found to be normal on gross inspection [64,99].

In nearly 3,200 consecutive pancreas donors procured between 2000 and 2005, Vinkers et al. [100] determined the influence of a "preprocurement pancreas suitability" score on the acceptance or refusal of deceased pancreatic organs . The investigators assigned a weight for several preprocurement factors including age, BMI, length of ICU stay, cardiac arrest as cause of death, serum sodium, amylase and lipase levels, and need for vasopressor support to develop a donor score. When the donor score was ≥17, pancreata from these deceased donors were three times more likely to be refused by transplant centers. Donor scoring systems such as this one may provide more objective information about the quality of a deceased pancreatic organ to promote wider pancreas donor acceptance.

Pancreas Preservation

University of Wisconsin solution was first used for pancreas preservation in a preclinical model in 1987 [101]. As with most solid organs, in vivo flush followed by simple storage in cold University of Wisconsin solution is still the gold standard for pancreas preservation. In the original canine model, pancreata were preserved for up to 96 hours [102], but in clinical transplantation, pancreas cold preservation exceeding 24 hours has been associated with increased graft dysfunction. Even for less than 24 hours, it is evident that the longer the cold ischemia time, the greater the technical complication rate. Therefore, every effort should be made to minimize the cold ischemia time to optimize graft function and to minimize complication rates. A general trend toward shorter preservation time has been noted over time with over 50% of pancreas transplants having a preservation time under 12 hours since 2005 [6].

The two-layer method (TLM) using University of Wisconsin solution and perfluorochemical has been used in clinical whole pancreas transplantation but more commonly for islet preservation [103]. This method improves pancreas oxygenation, allowing for longer preservation time while providing a mechanism for repair of ischemic damage due to cold storage [104–106]. Some studies show that TLM improves islet yields, islet viability, islet morphology, rates of successful islet isolations and transplants, and islet yields from marginal donors [105,107–113]. Other studies report that TLM has no effect or is even detrimental for pancreas preservation and show no difference in islet yields, islet viability, or islet transplant outcomes when pancreatic organs were preserved with the TLM versus University of Wisconsin solution [54,105,108,114]. More prospective, randomized, controlled trials are needed before the TLM becomes routine procedure.

Three main preservation solutions for pancreas transplantation are available today, including University of Wisconsin solution, Celsior, and histidine–tryptophan–ketoglutarate solution (HTK) [105,108]. HTK has been increasingly used in pancreas transplantation, and its advantages include lower viscosity, less potassium, lower cost, and no need for "on-shelf" cold storage, but it requires more solution to flush organs in the multiorgan donor (8 to 12 L of HTK solution vs. 4 to 6 L of Celsior vs. 4 to 6 L of University of Wisconsin solution) [105]. In pancreas transplantation, there have been only one retrospective study [107] and two prospective randomized studies [115,116], which compare University of Wisconsin solution with Celsior, and both solutions give similar results. Several reports have compared HTK with University of Wisconsin solution and most reports have described equal suitability for perfusion and organ preservation in clinical pancreas transplantation [117–121]. In an analysis of the UNOS pancreas transplant database from 2004 to 2008, Stewart et al. [122] noted that HTK preservation was associated with a 1.5-fold higher odds of early (<30 days) pancreas graft loss when compared with University of Wisconsin solution and was independently associated with increased pancreas graft loss in SPK and PTA recipients, especially when cold ischemia times were ≥12 hours. Further prospective, randomized studies will be necessary to determine which perfusion and preservation solution provides the best short-term and long-term pancreas graft survival.

Human Leucocyte Antigen (HCA) Matching

The impact of HLA matching on outcomes varies. HLA matching appears to have minor effect on patient, kidney, or pancreas graft survival after SPK transplantation [123,124], although increased acute rejection rates have been reported with poorer matches [125–127]. For PAK and PTA transplants the data are mixed, ranging from studies showing little impact [128] to registry data showing that higher HLA A and B mismatches are associated with increased immunologic graft loss [124]. A few centers offer desensitization to highly sensitized pancreas transplant candidates on the basis of the utilization of Intravenous Immune Globulin (IVIG) administration and plasma exchange [129]; however, this is not a routine practice or considered at most transplant centers. In general, pancreas transplantation is performed after confirmation of a negative cross-match that can now be accurately predicted on the basis of solid-phase assays, which can identify preformed HLA antibodies.

Anesthetic Considerations in Recipient

A patient with brittle diabetes and secondary complications (e.g., CAD, autonomic neuropathy) can pose special problems for the anesthesiologist. Dysautonomic response to drugs or hypoxia can lead to significant morbidity and even death. It is well documented that long-standing diabetes poses a challenge to the anesthesiologist during intubation. Awareness of these risks and use of an experienced anesthesiology team might help decrease the morbidity and mortality. A major operation such as a pancreas transplantation or combined kidney–pancreas transplantation is often prolonged and can be associated with significant blood loss. Prompt replacement with blood or colloid solutions should be instituted to avoid hypoperfusion after significant blood loss because pancreas hypoperfusion can lead to thrombosis. In the intra- and perioperative period, careful blood glucose monitoring is essential and insulin therapy may be necessary to maintain tight control of blood glucose levels. Blood glucose levels may be affected in the immediate postoperative period due to high-dose steroids, and so supplemental insulin therapy may be required to control hyperglycemia even in the setting of a functioning graft. Perioperative β-blockade should be considered for long-standing diabetic patients with a cardiac history.

BACK-TABLE PREPARATION OF THE DONOR PANCREAS

Back-table preparation of the pancreas organ is necessary before implantation, including these steps:

1. Donor splenectomy (taking care to avoid injury to the pancreatic tail)
2. Shortening the donor duodenum without damage to the main or accessory pancreatic duct (especially important with BD to minimize bicarbonate loss)
3. Ligation of the mesocolic and mesenteric stumps on the anterior aspect of the pancreas
4. Excision of excessive lymphatic and ganglionic tissue in the periportal area
5. Reconstruction of the splenic and superior mesenteric arteries with a donor Y graft including the iliac artery bifurcation (to provide for a single-arterial anastomosis in the recipient)
6. Some mobilization of the portal vein
7. Ligation of the bile duct stump

RECIPIENT OPERATION

Several techniques have been described for the recipient operation [130]. The techniques vary on the basis of whether a solitary pancreas transplant (PTA, PAK) or a combined transplant (SPK) is done. Most SPK transplants are performed through a midline intra-abdominal approach, although some are performed through bilateral iliac retroperitoneal incisions.

The major surgical considerations for pancreas transplants include the following:

1. Choice of exocrine secretion of the pancreas, ED versus BD: The 2004 IPTR noted that 81% of SPK, 67% of PAK, and 56% of PTA transplants had ED of pancreatic exocrine secretions [53]. Bladder drainage accounted for 10% to 20% of all pancreas transplants reported to the IPTR from 2004 through 2008 [131]. ED is much more physiologic and eliminates the complications of BD (e.g., acidosis, pancreatitis, urinary tract infections, hematuria, urethritis, urinary stricture, urinary disruption). Between 10% and 20% of BD recipients ultimately undergo enteric conversion at 6 to 12 months because of such complications. BD, however, allows for direct measurement of urinary amylase as a marker of exocrine function. A decrease in urinary amylase is sensitive, but not very specific, for acute rejection of the pancreas [53]. Hyperglycemia is a late event in rejection, and a decrease in urinary amylase occurs early in rejection. Thus, rejection episodes may be detected earlier with BD than with ED.
   In clinical practice, the choice of exocrine drainage varies. Some groups always use ED, some always use BD, and others determine the choice of exocrine drainage on the basis of the individual recipient's anatomic constraints and the risk of bowel/urologic complications. Patient and graft survival are similar with both techniques [91,132], but BD is associated with higher rates of urinary tract infections, in addition to urologic and metabolic complications [133,134]. ED is likely to predominate as the major technique in the future, as immunologic strategies to eliminate rejection are further refined. ED usually occurs as an anastomosis between the donor duodenal stump and the recipient proximal jejunum, but graft placement behind the right colon can allow for direct duodenostomy [133,135].
2. Choice of venous drainage, portal or systemic: The 2004 IPTR reported that in enteric-drained pancreas transplants, 20% of SPK, 23% of PAK, and 35% of PTA cases had venous drainage to the portal vein [53]. Portal drainage is more physiologic than systemic drainage. Theoretically, portal drainage preserves the first-pass metabolism of insulin in the liver. Therefore, pancreas recipients with portal venous drainage will have lower systemic insulin levels than recipients with systemic venous drainage. In one study [136] that compared portal with systemic venous drainage in SPK recipients, there were no significant differences in patient, kidney or pancreas allograft survival rates, or early graft loss by pancreatitis or thrombosis. There were no significant differences in early endocrine function, although HbA1C was lower at 6 and 12 months in the portal-drained group.
   Portal venous drainage is difficult to perform with BD unless there is a venous extension graft [45]. However, portal venous drainage is likely to increase in popularity, given some reports that rejection rates are lower in this category [132,137]. Recent modifications include a retroperitoneal portal-enteric drainage technique behind the right colon [138].
3. Choice of graft, whole-organ or segmental: Almost all deceased donor pancreas transplantations performed today are whole-organ grafts. Segmental grafts have little role to play in this group, except when a rare anatomic abnormality is noted such that the head of the pancreas cannot be used. A rare instance of a split deceased donor pancreas organ transplanted into two different recipients has been described [139]. All living donor pancreas transplants use segmental grafts (body and tail), which are still capable of maintaining normoglycemia in the recipient.

POSTOPERATIVE CARE

After an uncomplicated pancreas transplantation, the recipient is transferred to the postanesthesia care unit or the surgical intensive care unit. Centers that have a specialized monitored transplant unit (with central venous and arterial monitoring capabilities) transition the postoperative recipients through the postanesthesia care unit to the transplant unit. Other centers transfer patients directly to the surgical intensive care unit for the first 24 to 48 hours. Care during the first few hours after transplant is similar to care after any major operative procedure. Careful monitoring of vital signs, central venous pressure, oxygen saturation, urine output, and laboratory parameters is crucial. The following factors are unique to pancreas recipients and should be attended to:

1. Blood glucose levels: Any sudden, unexplained increase in blood glucose levels should raise the suspicion of graft thrombosis. An urgent ultrasound must be done to assess blood flow to the graft. Some centers believe that maintenance of tight glucose control (<150 mg per dL) using an IV insulin drip is important to "rest" the pancreas in the early postoperative period.
2. Intravascular volume: Because the pancreas is a "low-flow" organ, intravascular volume must be maintained to provide adequate perfusion to the graft. Central venous pressure monitoring is used to monitor intravascular volume status. In some cases, such as patients with depressed cardiac function, pulmonary artery catheter monitoring may be required during the first 24 to 48 hours. If the hypovolemia is associated with low hemoglobin levels, then packed red cell transfusions should be given; otherwise, crystalloid (and sometimes colloid) replacement should be used to treat hypovolemia.
3. Maintenance IV fluid therapy: The choice of IV fluid therapy can be 5% dextrose in 0.45% normal saline, as long as IV insulin is used to maintain tight blood glucose control, or 0.45% normal saline to maintain acceptable urine output. In SPK recipients, whose IV fluid rate is based on urine output, dextrose should be eliminated if the urine output is high (>500 mL per hour) because hyperglycemia may cause an osmotic diuresis, leading to worsening hypovolemia.

Maintenance IV fluid for BD recipients should also include HCO_3 10 mEq per L to account for the excess HCO_3 loss, or sodium lactate can be used as an alternative.

4. Antibiotic therapy: Broad-spectrum antibiotic therapy and antifungal therapy are instituted in the perioperative period. Antiviral prophylaxis is similar to that for other solid organs and is driven by cytomegalovirus (CMV) status.
5. Anticoagulation: At the University of Texas Health Science Center at San Antonio, all pancreas recipients receive enteric-coated aspirin 325 mg started on the first postoperative day and continued indefinitely. Recipients of solitary pancreas transplants or "high-risk" SPK transplants also receive an intraoperative dose of heparin (3,000 units), followed by a postoperative regimen of low-dose, continuous IV heparin at 500 units per hour for 24 hours. The partial thromboplastin time for heparin is not measured. Our experience is that therapeutic doses of heparin lead to excessive postoperative hemorrhage that requires reduction in heparin dose, and sometimes red cell transfusion or reoperation.

Immunosuppression

Immunosuppression is essential to thwart rejection in all allotransplant recipients. Before the advent of cyclosporine in the early 1980s, dual therapy with azathioprine and prednisone was the mainstay of immunosuppression for pancreas transplants. From the early 1980s to the mid-1990s, cyclosporine was introduced for maintenance therapy and resulted in significant improvement in immunologic outcomes. Since the mid-1990s, tacrolimus and mycophenolate mofetil have replaced cyclosporine and azathioprine as the primary maintenance immunosuppressive medications. In a prospective, randomized, multicenter study of tacrolimus versus cyclosporine in SPK recipients, Saudek et al. [140] noted that 3-year patient and kidney graft survival were comparable, but pancreas graft survival was superior in the tacrolimus-treated cohort (89% tacrolimus vs. 74% cyclosporine) . In addition, with antibody induction steroids have been successfully withdrawn or even avoided in some cases [141]. However, a 2014 review of several randomized controlled trials involving steroid avoidance or withdrawal concluded that there was insufficient evidence to support the benefits or harm of steroid withdrawal in pancreas transplantation [142]. Specific immunosuppressive regimens vary among different transplant programs.

Antibody induction has become the mainstay protocol for pancreas recipients. The debate continues as to which antibody preparations are best in pancreas transplant recipients [143]. The administration of depleting agents such as rabbit antithymocyte globulin (rATG) or alemtuzumab has increased over the years, while the use of IL-2 inhibitors has decreased, with the rationale that depleting antibodies provide good immunosuppressive coverage for innovative immunosuppressive strategies including steroid withdrawal or avoidance and minimization of calcineurin inhibitors.

Results

Outcomes after pancreas transplants have consistently improved over the years. The 2012 SRTR report [144] described pancreas transplant graft survival for patients transplanted in 2007. Adult unadjusted graft survival rates at 5 years for SPK, PAK, and PTA recipients were 73%, 65%, and 53%, respectively, at 60 months. The report does highlight the lack of uniformity by transplant centers in their definition of graft failure.

The latest report from the IPTR [131] focused on pancreas transplants in the United States from 2004 to 2008 and included 4,200 SPK, 1,136 PAK, and 491 PTA cases. One-year patient survival rates for all three categories were more than 95%. One-year pancreas graft survival rates were higher for SPK (84.9%) than for PAK (78.6%) and PTA (78.9%) recipients. Graft loss from rejection at 1 year was low in all three categories (2.1% SPK, 5.5% PAK, 6.6% PTA). In the majority of all transplants, ED was used for duct management (80% to 90%), and of the ED transplants, portal venous drainage use declined (15% to 21% of cases). Although overall graft function did not vary with ED or BD, the technical failure rate was higher in ED transplant recipients.

Donor and Recipient Causes of Pancreas Complications

Donor and recipient factors can influence the postoperative course after pancreas transplantation. In a study of 210 SPK transplants between 1995 and 2007, donor-specific risk factors correlating with postoperative pancreas-related complications included donor age, need for vasopressor support, need for preprocurement blood transfusions, and asystolic events >10 minutes [145]. Increasing donor age and BMI were associated with greater need for postoperative interventions. Graft preservation with HTK solution was associated with significantly higher postoperative complications, as was preexisting cardiac disease in the recipient. The choice of immunosuppression had a significant effect on pancreas-related complications, which were greater after induction therapy with rATG versus daclizumab, and maintenance immunosuppression with tacrolimus/rapamycin or cyclosporine/mycophenolate mofetil versus tacrolimus/mycophenolate mofetil. The duration of the pancreas transplant operation and the presence of elevated C reactive protein were associated with significantly more postoperative complications that required interventions. In another study, donor obesity (BMI > 30 kg per m^2) was associated with greater risk of graft thrombosis and deep wound infections [146]. Another trial [94] noted that technical failure of the pancreas graft occurred more commonly when (1) the donor BMI was >30 kg per m^2, (2) the cause of donor death was other than trauma, (3) the preservation time was >24 hours, (4) the duct management was ED versus BD, and (5) recipient BMI was >30 kg per m^2. In another study, multivariate analysis showed that technical failure of a pancreas transplant appeared to be the most significant risk factor for kidney graft loss [147]. This evidence underscores that careful donor and recipient selection in addition to improved preservation and surgical techniques play important roles to minimize complications after pancreas transplantation [148].

Surgical Complications

Prevention of surgical complications has critical implications not only on pancreas graft and patient survival, but also on financial impact associated with postoperative care. Early diagnosis and management of surgical complications can limit morbidity; delayed diagnosis and treatment of pancreas complications can lead not only to pancreas graft loss but also to kidney graft loss [148,149]. Common surgical complications of pancreas transplantation will now be addressed:

1. Hemorrhage: Postoperative hemorrhage is a frequent reason for early re-laparotomy in pancreas transplant recipients. Hemorrhage can occur from the pancreatic parenchyma, from poorly ligated mesenteric or splenic vascular stumps or from the anastomosis in an enteric-drained or bladder-drained pancreas transplant. The incidence of hemorrhage ranges from 6% to 7% [91], and this risk increases with the use of anticoagulation in the immediate postoperative period. Frequent physical examination and monitoring of hemoglobin

help to detect early hemorrhage. Heparin may be temporarily suspended to stabilize the patient. Packed cells should be administered if the recipient has symptomatic anemia. If hemorrhage continues, early operative intervention is indicated. If hemorrhage slows down or ceases, heparin should be resumed at a lower rate and judiciously increased as tolerated.

2. Thrombosis: Thrombosis after transplant ranges from 5% to 6% [91], and remains the most common cause of early pancreas graft failure. The risk increases after segmental pancreas transplantation because of the small caliber of vessels [51]. Most pancreas transplant thromboses are due to technical causes. Diagnosis is suspected by sudden hyperglycemia and confirmed by sonogram, computed tomography (CT) angiogram, formal angiogram, or MRI, which reveals an absence of arterial or venous flow to the graft. Aggressive anticoagulation will not prevent pancreas transplant thrombosis due to technical reasons. A short portal vein requiring an extension graft or atherosclerotic arteries in the pancreas graft increases the risk for thrombosis. A recipient narrow pelvic inlet with a deeply placed, poorly mobilized iliac vein, atherosclerotic disease of the iliac artery, a technically difficult vascular anastomosis, kinking of the vein by the pancreas graft, significant hematoma formation around the vascular anastomosis, hypovolemia, and a hypercoagulable state are some of the factors that increase the risk for thrombosis. The most common form of hypercoagulable state in the Western population is factor V Leiden mutation. Its incidence ranges from 2% to 5% but may be as high as 50% to 60% in patients with a history (self or family) of vascular thrombosis [150]. Other causes of hypercoagulable state include antithrombin III deficiency, protein C or S deficiency, activated protein C resistance, and anticardiolipin antibodies [151]. The transplant surgeon must have a high incidence of suspicion of these hypercoagulable states and treat them aggressively to prevent pancreas graft thrombosis. If thrombosis is suspected in the early postoperative period, operative exploration of the graft is warranted and findings of a thrombosed graft usually necessitates removal of the pancreas.
3. Duodenal stump leaks: The incidence of duodenal stump leaks ranges from 6% to 7% [91]. A leak from the anastomosis of the duodenum stump to the bowel almost always leads to re-laparotomy. Gross peritoneal contamination due to an enteric leak usually necessitates a graft pancreatectomy. The diagnosis is made by elevated pancreatic enzymes in a patient who has clinical signs of acute abdomen. A plain abdominal radiograph may show free air, and an abdominal CT scan may show free air and extravasation of contrast into the free peritoneal cavity. The differential diagnosis is pancreatitis, abdominal infection, or acute severe rejection. A Roux-en-Y anastomosis to the duodenal stump may be a preferred technique if the risk of leak is thought to be increased during the initial pancreas operation. Other novel techniques such as a venting Roux-en-Y pancreatic duodenojejunostomy have been used in selected recipients [152].
   Small duodenal stump leaks in bladder-drained recipients are usually managed nonoperatively with prolonged catheter decompression of the urinary bladder. The diagnosis of duodenal stump leak is made using plain or CT cystography. Large leaks may require operative intervention, including primary repair, enteric conversion, or even transplant pancreatectomy if there is significant compromise of the duodenal stump.
4. Major intra-abdominal infections: The incidence of significant intra-abdominal infections requiring reoperation ranges from 3% to 4% [91]. Performance of the enteric anastomosis with associated contamination predisposes to this higher rate of intra-abdominal infection, where fungal and gram-negative organisms predominate. With the advent of percutaneous procedures to drain intra-abdominal abscesses, the incidence of reoperations is fast decreasing. If the infection is uncontrolled or widespread, then graft pancreatectomy followed by frequent washouts may be necessary.
5. Renal pedicle torsion: Torsion of the kidney has been reported after SPK transplantation [153,154]. The intraperitoneal location of the kidney (allowing for more mobility) predisposes to this complication. Additional risk factors are a long renal pedicle and a marked discrepancy between the length of artery and vein. Prophylactic nephropexy to the anterior or lateral abdominal wall is recommended with intraperitoneal transplantations to avoid this problem. The colon can be mobilized and reapproximated over a kidney transplant in order to prevent torsion.
6. Others: Other surgical complications that may require re-laparotomy include wound dehiscence, incisional hernia, severe pancreatitis (sometimes hemorrhagic or necrotic), pseudocysts, pseudoaneurysms, arteriovenous (AV) fistula in the graft, severe painful rejection, and bowel obstruction [155]. The overall incidence of re-laparotomy for these complications decreased from 32% in the 1980s to 19% in the 1990s, and the mortality rate in recipients requiring re-laparotomy decreased from 9% to 1% over that same period. Improved antibiotic prophylaxis, surgical techniques, immunosuppression, and advances in interventional radiology have all contributed to this decrease [91].

Nonsurgical Complications

1. Pancreatitis: The incidence of posttransplant pancreatitis varies based on the type of exocrine drainage. Bladder-drained recipients with abnormal bladder function are at increased risk of pancreatitis secondary to incomplete bladder emptying and urinary retention causing resistance to flow of pancreatic exocrine secretions. Other causes of pancreatitis include drugs (corticosteroids, azathioprine, cyclosporine), hypercalcemia, viral infections (CMV or hepatitis C), and reperfusion injury after prolonged ischemia. Pancreatitis is usually manifested by an increase in serum amylase and lipase with or without local signs of inflammation. An abdominal ultrasound or CT scan may identify an enlarged, edematous, hypoechoic graft. The treatment usually consists of catheter decompression of the bladder for a period of 2 to 6 weeks, depending on the severity of pancreatitis. In addition, octreotide therapy may be used to decrease pancreatic secretions. The underlying urologic problem, if any, should be treated. The patient should be placed on NPO status and total parenteral nutrition should be administered if the pancreatitis is severe. If repeated episodes of pancreatitis occur, enteric conversion of a bladder-drained pancreas transplant may be indicated.
2. Rejection: The incidence of acute rejection ranges from 15% to 30% and immunologic graft loss from 2% to 15% for all types of pancreas transplants at 1 year [156]. The diagnosis is usually based on increased serum amylase and lipase levels in all pancreas transplant patients, and decreased urinary amylase levels in bladder-drained recipients. A sustained drop in urinary amylase levels from baseline should prompt a pancreas biopsy to rule out rejection. For enteric-drained recipients, one has to rely on serum amylase and lipase levels only. A rise in serum lipase levels has shown to correlate well with acute rejection in the pancreas transplant. Other signs and symptoms include tenderness over the graft, unexplained fever, and hyperglycemia (which is usually a late finding). Diagnosis of rejection can be suspected by a hypoechoic, enlarged graft by ultrasound or an enlarged, edematous graft by abdominal CT scan. Diagnosis of rejection can be confirmed by a percutaneous pancreas biopsy [157]. In cases for which percutaneous biopsy is not possible due to technical reasons, empiric therapy for rejection may be started. Rarely, open biopsy is indicated, and transcystoscopic biopsy of a

bladder-drained pancreas graft, which was used in the past, has been largely abandoned. Finally, in SPK recipients, isolated pancreas transplant rejection portends a worse renal allograft survival than in patients who experience no rejection [158].

3. Others: Other findings include infectious complications such as CMV, extra-abdominal bacterial or fungal infections, posttransplant malignancy such as posttransplant lymphoproliferative disorder, and other rare complications such as graft-versus-host disease. Many catheter infections are due to gram-positive organisms, with methicillin-resistant coagulase-negative isolates being quite common [159]. The diagnosis and management of these complications is similar to those of other solid-organ transplantations.

Radiologic Studies

1. Ultrasonography: This is the most frequent study used in pancreas recipients. Noninvasive, portable, and relatively inexpensive, it provides prompt information regarding blood flow to the pancreas, the presence of arterial or venous stenosis or occlusion, thrombosis, pseudoaneurysms, AV fistulae, resistance to blood flow within the pancreas (suggestive of either rejection or pancreatitis), and peripancreatic fluid collections.
2. CT scan: A CT scan provides more detail of pancreatic and surrounding anatomy. Use of oral, IV, and bladder contrast (in bladder-drained recipients) is recommended. Thus, a CT cystogram can be combined with an abdominal CT scan. A CT scan is frequently used as a guide in pancreatic biopsies or in placement of percutaneous drains for intra-abdominal infection.
3. Fluoroscopy: A contrast cystogram can be performed under fluoroscopy and can be used instead of, or in addition to, a CT cystogram to look for a bladder leak. The combination of the tests increases the sensitivity for detecting bladder leaks.
4. Magnetic resonance angiogram (MRA): An MRA is done if vascular abnormalities are suspected on the ultrasound. MRA provides accurate information about pancreatic vascular patency, but it is inferior to standard angiography in providing fine vascular detail.
5. Angiography: This is the gold standard test for evaluating arterial anatomy in and around the pancreas. However, it is rarely employed, except in cases in which angiographic intervention (such as angioplasty, stenting of a stenotic segment, or coiling of an AV fistula or pseudoaneurysm) is planned. Contrast nephropathy is feared in a solitary pancreas recipient with renal dysfunction, and reasonable alternatives (such as ultrasound) are available.

FUTURE DIRECTIONS

For type 1 diabetic patients with kidney dysfunction, an SPK or PAK transplant is the standard of care. A PTA, however, is less common because the long-term risks of diabetes are weighed against the long-term risks of immunosuppression. A successful pancreas transplantation can improve existing neuropathy and nephropathy in diabetic recipients, and the survival after a solitary pancreas transplant is better than remaining on the waiting list [160]. As the risks of immunosuppression decrease with novel methods of tolerance and immunomodulation, the balance will tilt in favor of an early transplantation. The limiting factor will then be the organ shortage, which could be alleviated if xenotransplantation is able to overcome its current barrier of hyperacute rejection.

The application of islet transplantation is rapidly growing. Recent successes suggest that islet transplants can provide all the benefits of pancreas transplants without the risks of major operation. Improvements in islet isolation, islet viability, islet functionality, islet implantation, and immunotherapy will improve islet outcomes so that only one donor will be necessary to achieve insulin independence [161]. Xenotransplantation of islets may be more readily achievable using encapsulation than with other organs. Prolonged diabetes reversal after intraportal xenotransplant in primates has been documented [162] and may pave the way for human xenotransplant trials. Also, stem cells from numerous sources (e.g., bone marrow, adipose, or cord blood) may be manipulated to differentiate into islets in order to provide a rich supply for transplantation, and islet transplants can be combined with immunomodulation and tolerogenic strategies to minimize or eliminate immunosuppression [161]. This combination would provide for minimally invasive islet cell transplantations for all type 1 diabetic patients without the need for long-term immunosuppression. The only scenario that would be better would be the thwarting of autoimmunity before the onset of isletitis, thereby preventing type 1 diabetes mellitus in the first place.

References

1. The effect of intensive treatment of diabetes on the development and progression of long-term complications in insulin-dependent diabetes mellitus. The Diabetes Control and Complications Trial Research Group. *N Engl J Med* 329(14):977–986, 1993.
2. Lifetime benefits and costs of intensive therapy as practiced in the diabetes control and complications trial. The Diabetes Control and Complications Trial Research Group. *JAMA* 276(17):1409–1415, 1996.
3. American Diabetes Association: Standards of medical care in diabetes-2015 abridged for primary care providers. *Clin Diabetes* 33(2):97–111, 2015.
4. Ali MK, Bullard KM, Gregg EW: Achievement of goals in U.S. Diabetes Care, 1999–2010. *N Engl J Med* 369(3):287–288, 2013.
5. Boggi U, Vistoli F, Amorese G, et al: Results of pancreas transplantation alone with special attention to native kidney function and proteinuria in type 1 diabetes patients. *Rev Diabet Stud* 8(2):259–267, 2011.
6. Gruessner AC: 2011 update on pancreas transplantation: comprehensive trend analysis of 25,000 cases followed up over the course of twenty-four years at the International Pancreas Transplant Registry (IPTR). *Rev Diabet Stud* 8(1):6–16, 2011.
7. Kandaswamy R, Skeans MA, Gustafson SK, et al: OPTN/SRTR 2013 Annual Data Report: pancreas. *Am J Transplant* 15[Suppl 2]:1–20, 2015.
8. Shapiro AM, Lakey JR, Ryan EA, et al: Islet transplantation in seven patients with type 1 diabetes mellitus using a glucocorticoid-free immunosuppressive regimen. *N Engl J Med* 343(4):230–238, 2000.
9. Hering BJ, Kandaswamy R, Harmon JV, et al: Transplantation of cultured islets from two-layer preserved pancreases in type 1 diabetes with anti-CD3 antibody. *Am J Transplant* 4(3):390–401, 2004.
10. Hering BJ, Kandaswamy R, Ansite JD, et al: Single-donor, marginal-dose islet transplantation in patients with type 1 diabetes. *JAMA* 293(7):830–835, 2005.
11. Ryan EA, Paty BW, Senior PA, et al: Five-year follow-up after clinical islet transplantation. *Diabetes* 54(7):2060–2069, 2005.
12. Krolewski AS, Warram JH, Freire MB: Epidemiology of late diabetic complications. A basis for the development and evaluation of preventive programs. *Endocrinol Metab Clin North Am* 25(2):217–242, 1996.
13. Gruessner A, Gruessner R, Moudry-Munns K, et al: Influence of multiple factors (age, transplant number, recipient category, donor source) on outcome of pancreas transplantation at one institution. *Transplant Proc* 25(1, Pt 2):1303–1305, 1993.
14. Light JA, Sasaki TM, Currier CB, et al: Successful long-term kidney-pancreas transplants regardless of C-peptide status or race. *Transplantation* 71(1):152–154, 2001.
15. Weems P, Cooper M: Pancreas transplantation in type II diabetes mellitus. *World J Transplant* 4(4):216–221, 2014.
16. Sener A, Cooper M, Bartlett ST: Is there a role for pancreas transplantation in type 2 diabetes mellitus? *Transplantation* 90(2):121–123, 2010.
17. UNOS/OPTN. Organ Procurement and Transplantation Network. Available from: http://optn.transplant.hrsa.gov/governance/policies/. 2015. Accessed February 7, 2017.
18. Weir GC, Cavelti-Weder C, Bonner-Weir S: Stem cell approaches for diabetes: towards beta cell replacement. *Genome Med* 3(9):61, 2011.
19. Li M, Ikehara S: Stem cell treatment for type 1 diabetes. *Front Cell Dev Biol* 2:9, 2014.
20. Muir KR, Lima MJ, Dochetry HM, et al: Cell therapy for type 1 diabetes. *QJM* 107(4):253–259, 2014.
21. Pagliuca FW, Millman JR, Gürtler M, et al: Generation of functional human pancreatic beta cells in vitro. *Cell* 159(2):428–439, 2014.
22. Sutherland DE, Gruessner RW, Dunn DL, et al: Lessons learned from more than 1,000 pancreas transplants at a single institution. *Ann Surg* 233(4):463–501, 2001.
23. Sutherland DE, Radosevich D, Gruessner R, et al: Pushing the envelope: living donor pancreas transplantation. *Curr Opin Organ Transplant* 17(1):106–115, 2012.

24. Matsumoto S, Okitsu T, Iwanaga Y, et al: Insulin independence of unstable diabetic patient after single living donor islet transplantation. *Transplant Proc* 37(8):3427–3429, 2005.
25. Farney AC, Cho E, Schweitzer EJ, et al: Simultaneous cadaver pancreas living-donor kidney transplantation: a new approach for the type 1 diabetic uremic patient. *Ann Surg* 232(5):696–703, 2000.
26. Fridell JA, Powelson JA: Pancreas after kidney transplantation: why is the most logical option the least popular? *Curr Opin Organ Transplant* 20(1):108–114, 2015.
27. Gruessner AC, Sutherland DE, Dunn DL, et al: Pancreas after kidney transplants in posturemic patients with type I diabetes mellitus. *J Am Soc Nephrol* 12(11):2490–2499, 2001.
28. Humar A, Ramcharan T, Kandaswamy R, et al: Pancreas after kidney transplants. *Am J Surg* 182(2):155–161, 2001.
29. Sutherland DE, Gruessner RG, Humar A, et al: Pretransplant immunosuppression for pancreas transplants alone in nonuremic diabetic recipients. *Transplant Proc* 33(1/2):1656–1658, 2001.
30. Kelly WD, Lillehei RC, Merkel FK, et al: Allotransplantation of the pancreas and duodenum along with the kidney in diabetic nephropathy. *Surgery* 61(6):827–837, 1967.
31. Squifflet JP, Gruessner RW, Sutherland DE: The history of pancreas transplantation: past, present and future. *Acta Chir Belg* 108(3):367–378, 2008.
32. Lillehei RC, Ruix JO, Aquino C, et al: Transplantation of the pancreas. *Acta Endocrinol Suppl (Copenh)* 205:303–320, 1976.
33. Gliedman ML, Gold M, Whittaker J, et al: Clinical segmental pancreatic transplantation with ureter-pancreatic duct anastomosis for exocrine drainage. *Surgery* 74(2):171–180, 1973.
34. Gold M, Whittaker JR, Veith FJ, et al: Evaluation of ureteral drainage for pancreatic exocrine secretion. *Surg Forum* 23:375–377, 1972.
35. Sutherland DE, Goetz FC, Najarian JS: Intraperitoneal transplantation of immediately vascularized segmental pancreatic grafts without duct ligation. A clinical trial. *Transplantation* 28(6):485–491, 1979.
36. Dubernard JM, Traeger J, Neyra P, et al: A new method of preparation of segmental pancreatic grafts for transplantation: trials in dogs and in man. *Surgery* 84(5):633–639, 1978.
37. Cook K, Sollinger HW, Warner T, et al: Pancreaticocystostomy: an alternative method for exocrine drainage of segmental pancreatic allografts. *Transplantation* 35(6):634–636, 1983.
38. Nghiem DD, Corry RJ: Technique of simultaneous renal pancreatoduodenal transplantation with urinary drainage of pancreatic secretion. *Am J Surg* 153(4):405–406, 1987.
39. Starzl TE, Iwatsuki S, Shaw BW Jr, et al: Pancreaticoduodenal transplantation in humans. *Surg Gynecol Obstet* 159(3):265–272, 1984.
40. Tom WW, Munda R, First MR, et al: Autodigestion of the glans penis and urethra by activated transplant pancreatic exocrine enzymes. *Surgery* 102(1):99–101, 1987.
41. Gil-Vernet JM, Fernández-Cruz L, Caralps A, et al: Whole organ and pancreaticoureterostomy in clinical pancreas transplantation. *Transplant Proc* 17(4):2019–2022, 1985.
42. Calne RY: Paratopic segmental pancreas grafting: a technique with portal venous drainage. *Lancet* 1(8377):595–597, 1984.
43. Sutherland DE, Goetz FC, Moudry KC, et al: Use of recipient mesenteric vessels for revascularization of segmental pancreas grafts: technical and metabolic considerations. *Transplant Proc* 19(1, pt 3):2300–2304, 1987.
44. Tyden G, Tibell A, Sandberg J, et al: Improved results with a simplified technique for pancreaticoduodenal transplantation with enteric exocrine drainage. *Clin Transplant* 10(3):306–309, 1996.
45. Muhlbacher F, Gnant MF, Auinger M, et al: Pancreatic venous drainage to the portal vein: a new method in human pancreas transplantation. *Transplant Proc* 22(2):636–637, 1990.
46. Rosenlof LK, Earnhardt RC, Pruett TL, et al: Pancreas transplantation. An initial experience with systemic and portal drainage of pancreatic allografts. *Ann Surg* 215(6):586–595, 1992; discussion 596–597.
47. Shokouh-Amiri MH, Gaber AO, Gaber LW, et al: Pancreas transplantation with portal venous drainage and enteric exocrine diversion: a new technique. *Transplant Proc* 24(3):776–777, 1992.
48. Sutherland DE, Goetz FC, Najarian JS: Living-related donor segmental pancreatectomy for transplantation. *Transplant Proc* 12[4, Suppl 2]:19–25, 1980.
49. Sutherland DE, Gores PF, Farney AC, et al: Evolution of kidney, pancreas, and islet transplantation for patients with diabetes at the University of Minnesota. *Am J Surg* 166(5):456–491, 1993.
50. Sutherland DE, Najarian JS, Gruessner R: Living versus cadaver donor pancreas transplants. *Transplant Proc* 30(5):2264–2266, 1998.
51. Gruessner RW, Sutherland DE: Simultaneous kidney and segmental pancreas transplants from living related donors—the first two successful cases. *Transplantation* 61(8):1265–1268, 1996.
52. Gruessner RW, Sutherland DE, Drangstveit MB, et al: Pancreas transplants from living donors: short- and long-term outcome. *Transplant Proc* 33(1/2):819–820, 2001.
53. Gruessner AC, Sutherland DE: Pancreas transplant outcomes for United States (US) and non-US cases as reported to the United Network for Organ Sharing (UNOS) and the International Pancreas Transplant Registry (IPTR) as of June 2004. *Clin Transplant* 19(4):433–455, 2005.
54. The CITR Coordinating Center and Investigators: The Collaborative Islet Transplant Registry 2010 Annual Report. NIDDK, 2010. www.citregistry.org
55. Sutherland DE: International human pancreas and islet transplant registry. *Transplant Proc* 12[4, Suppl 2]:229–236, 1980.
56. Gremizzi C, Vergani A, Paloschi V, et al: Impact of pancreas transplantation on type 1 diabetes-related complications. *Curr Opin Organ Transplant* 15(1):119–123, 2010.
57. Dean PG, Kudva YC, Stegall MD: Long-term benefits of pancreas transplantation. *Curr Opin Organ Transplant* 13(1):85–90, 2008.
58. Allen RD, Al-Harbi IS, Morris JG, et al: Diabetic neuropathy after pancreas transplantation: determinants of recovery. *Transplantation* 63(6):830–838, 1997.
59. Kennedy WR, et al: Effects of pancreatic transplantation on diabetic neuropathy. *N Engl J Med* 322(15):1031–1037, 1990.
60. Navarro X, Sutherland DE, Kennedy WR: Long-term effects of pancreatic transplantation on diabetic neuropathy. *Ann Neurol* 42(5):727–736, 1997.
61. White SA, Shaw JA, Sutherland DE: Pancreas transplantation. *Lancet* 373(9677):1808–1817, 2009.
62. Navarro X, Kennedy WR, Loewenson RB, et al: Influence of pancreas transplantation on cardiorespiratory reflexes, nerve conduction, and mortality in diabetes mellitus. *Diabetes* 39(7):802–806, 1990.
63. Solders G, Tydén G, Persson A, et al: Improvement of nerve conduction in diabetic neuropathy. A follow-up study 4 yr after combined pancreatic and renal transplantation. *Diabetes* 41(8):946–951, 1992.
64. Salvalaggio PR, Davies DB, Fernandez LA, et al: Outcomes of pancreas transplantation in the United States using cardiac-death donors. *Am J Transplant* 6(5, pt 1):1059–1065, 2006.
65. Martinenghi S, Comi G, Galardi G, et al: Amelioration of nerve conduction velocity following simultaneous kidney/pancreas transplantation is due to the glycaemic control provided by the pancreas. *Diabetologia* 40(9):1110–1112, 1997.
66. Hathaway DK, Abell T, Cardoso S, et al: Improvement in autonomic and gastric function following pancreas-kidney versus kidney-alone transplantation and the correlation with quality of life. *Transplantation* 57(6):816–822, 1994.
67. Fioretto P, Steffes MW, Sutherland DE, et al: Reversal of lesions of diabetic nephropathy after pancreas transplantation. *N Engl J Med* 339(2):69–75, 1998.
68. Fioretto P, Sutherland DE, Najafian B, et al: Remodeling of renal interstitial and tubular lesions in pancreas transplant recipients. *Kidney Int* 69(5):907–912, 2006.
69. Coppelli A, Giannarelli R, Boggi U, et al: Disappearance of nephrotic syndrome in type 1 diabetic patients following pancreas transplant alone. *Transplantation* 81(7):1067–1068, 2006.
70. Coppelli A, Giannarelli R, Vistoli F, et al: The beneficial effects of pancreas transplant alone on diabetic nephropathy. *Diabetes Care* 28(6):1366–1370, 2005.
71. Ramsay RC, Goetz FC, Sutherland DE, et al: Progression of diabetic retinopathy after pancreas transplantation for insulin-dependent diabetes mellitus. *N Engl J Med* 318(4):208–214, 1988.
72. Wang Q, Klein R, Moss SE, et al: The influence of combined kidney-pancreas transplantation on the progression of diabetic retinopathy. A case series. *Ophthalmology* 101(6):1071–1076, 1994.
73. Giannarelli R, Coppelli A, Sartini M, et al: Effects of pancreas-kidney transplantation on diabetic retinopathy. *Transpl Int* 18(5):619–622, 2005.
74. Cheung AT, Perez RV, Chen PC: Improvements in diabetic microangiopathy after successful simultaneous pancreas-kidney transplantation: a computer-assisted intravital microscopy study on the conjunctival microcirculation. *Transplantation* 68(7):927–932, 1999.
75. Larsen JL, Colling CW, Ratanasuwan T, et al: Pancreas transplantation improves vascular disease in patients with type 1 diabetes. *Diabetes Care* 27(7):1706–1711, 2004.
76. Larsen JL, Ratanasuwan T, Burkman T, et al: Carotid intima media thickness decreases after pancreas transplantation. *Transplantation* 73(6):936–940, 2002.
77. Fiorina P, La Rocca E, Venturini M, et al: Effects of kidney-pancreas transplantation on atherosclerotic risk factors and endothelial function in patients with uremia and type 1 diabetes. *Diabetes* 50(3):496–501, 2001.
78. Coppelli A, Giannarelli R, Mariotti R, et al: Pancreas transplant alone determines early improvement of cardiovascular risk factors and cardiac function in type 1 diabetic patients. *Transplantation* 76(6):974–976, 2003.
79. La Rocca E, Fiorina P, di Carlo V, et al: Cardiovascular outcomes after kidney-pancreas and kidney-alone transplantation. *Kidney Int* 60(5):1964–1971, 2001.
80. Luan FL, Miles CD, Cibrik DM, et al: Impact of simultaneous pancreas and kidney transplantation on cardiovascular risk factors in patients with type 1 diabetes mellitus. *Transplantation* 84(4):541–544, 2007.
81. Davenport C, Hamid N, O'Sullivan EP, et al: The impact of pancreas and kidney transplant on cardiovascular risk factors (analyzed by mode of immunosuppression and exocrine drainage). *Clin Transplant* 23(5):616–620, 2009.
82. Jukema JW, Smets YF, van der Pijl JW, et al: Impact of simultaneous pancreas and kidney transplantation on progression of coronary atherosclerosis in patients with end-stage renal failure due to type 1 diabetes. *Diabetes Care* 25(5):906–911, 2002.
83. Fiorina P, La Rocca E, Astorri E, et al: Reversal of left ventricular diastolic dysfunction after kidney-pancreas transplantation in type 1 diabetic uremic patients. *Diabetes Care* 23(12):1804–1810, 2000.
84. La Rocca E, Fiorina P, Astorri E, et al: Patient survival and cardiovascular events after kidney-pancreas transplantation: comparison with kidney transplantation alone in uremic IDDM patients. *Cell Transplant* 9(6):929–932, 2000.
85. Biesenbach G, Königsrainer A, Gross C, et al: Progression of macrovascular diseases is reduced in type 1 diabetic patients after more than 5 years successful combined pancreas-kidney transplantation in comparison to kidney transplantation alone. *Transpl Int* 18(9):1054–1060, 2005.

86. Gaber AO, Wicks MN, Hathaway DK, et al: Sustained improvements in cardiac geometry and function following kidney-pancreas transplantation. *Cell Transplant* 9(6):913–918, 2000.
87. Cashion AK, Hathaway DK, Milstead EJ, et al: Changes in patterns of 24-hr heart rate variability after kidney and kidney-pancreas transplant. *Transplantation* 68(12):1846–1850, 1999.
88. Ziaja J, Bozek-Pajak D, Kowalik A, et al: Impact of pancreas transplantation on the quality of life of diabetic renal transplant recipients. *Transplant Proc* 41(8):3156–3158, 2009.
89. Douzdjian V, Gugliuzza KG, Fish JC: Multivariate analysis of donor risk factors for pancreas allograft failure after simultaneous pancreas-kidney transplantation. *Surgery* 118(1):73–81, 1995.
90. Humar A, Harmon J, Gruessner A, et al: Surgical complications requiring early relaparotomy after pancreas transplantation: comparison of the cyclosporine and FK 506 eras. *Transplant Proc* 31(1/2):606–607, 1999.
91. Humar A, Kandaswamy R, Granger D, et al: Decreased surgical risks of pancreas transplantation in the modern era. *Ann Surg* 231(2):269–275, 2000.
92. Kapur S, Bonham CA, Dodson SF, et al: Strategies to expand the donor pool for pancreas transplantation. *Transplantation* 67(2):284–290, 1999.
93. Illanes HG, Quarin CM, Maurette R, et al: Use of small donors (<28 kg) for pancreas transplantation. *Transplant Proc* 41(6):2199–2201, 2009.
94. Humar A, Ramcharan T, Kandaswamy R, et al: Technical failures after pancreas transplants: why grafts fail and the risk factors—a multivariate analysis. *Transplantation* 78(8):1188–1192, 2004.
95. Stratta RJ: Donor age, organ import, and cold ischemia: effect on early outcomes after simultaneous kidney-pancreas transplantation. *Transplant Proc* 29(8):3291–3292, 1997.
96. Odorico JS, Heisey DM, Voss BJ, et al: Donor factors affecting outcome after pancreas transplantation. *Transplant Proc* 30(2):276–277, 1998.
97. Vinkers MT, Rahmel AO, Slot MC, et al: How to recognize a suitable pancreas donor: a Eurotransplant study of preprocurement factors. *Transplant Proc* 40(5):1275–1278, 2008.
98. Axelrod DA, Sung RS, Meyer KH, et al: Systematic evaluation of pancreas allograft quality, outcomes and geographic variation in utilization. *Am J Transplant* 10(4):837–845, 2010.
99. Bonham CA, Kapur S, Dodson SF, et al: Potential use of marginal donors for pancreas transplantation. *Transplant Proc* 31(1/2):612–613, 1999.
100. Vinkers MT, Rahmel AO, Slot MC, et al: Influence of a donor quality score on pancreas transplant survival in the Eurotransplant area. *Transplant Proc* 40(10):3606–3608, 2008.
101. Wahlberg JA, Love R, Landegaard L, et al: 72-hour preservation of the canine pancreas. *Transplantation* 43(1):5–8, 1987.
102. Kin S, Stephanian E, Gores P, et al: Successful 96-Hr cold-storage preservation of canine pancreas with UW solution containing the thromboxane A2 synthesis inhibitor OKY046. *J Surg Res* 52(6):577–582, 1992.
103. Kuroda Y, Kawamura T, Suzuki Y, et al: A new, simple method for cold storage of the pancreas using perfluorochemical. *Transplantation* 46(3):457–460, 1988.
104. Fujita H, Kuroda Y, Saitoh Y: The mechanism of action of the two-layer cold storage method in canine pancreas preservation–protection of pancreatic microvascular endothelium. *Kobe J Med Sci* 41(3):47–61, 1995.
105. Baertschiger RM, Berney T, Morel P: Organ preservation in pancreas and islet transplantation. *Curr Opin Organ Transplant* 13(1):59–66, 2008.
106. Tanioka Y, Kuroda Y, Saitoh Y: Amelioration of rewarming ischemic injury of the pancreas graft during vascular anastomosis by increasing tissue ATP contents during preservation by the two-layer cold storage method. *Kobe J Med Sci* 40(5/6):175–189, 1994.
107. Fraker CA, Alejandro R, Ricordi C: Use of oxygenated perfluorocarbon toward making every pancreas count. *Transplantation* 74(12):1811–1812, 2002.
108. Iwanaga Y, Sutherland DE, Harmon JV, et al: Pancreas preservation for pancreas and islet transplantation. *Curr Opin Organ Transplant* 13(2):135–141, 2008.
109. Matsumoto S, Qualley SA, Goel S, et al: Effect of the two-layer (University of Wisconsin solution-perfluorochemical plus O_2) method of pancreas preservation on human islet isolation, as assessed by the Edmonton Isolation Protocol. *Transplantation* 74(10):1414–1419, 2002.
110. Ramachandran S, Desai NM, Goers TA, et al: Improved islet yields from pancreas preserved in perflurocarbon is via inhibition of apoptosis mediated by mitochondrial pathway. *Am J Transplant* 6(7):1696–1703, 2006.
111. Salehi P, Mirbolooki M, Kin T, et al: Ameliorating injury during preservation and isolation of human islets using the two-layer method with perfluorocarbon and UW solution. *Cell Transplant* 15(2):187–194, 2006.
112. Tsujimura T, Kuroda Y, Avila JG, et al: Influence of pancreas preservation on human islet isolation outcomes: impact of the two-layer method. *Transplantation* 78(1):96–100, 2004.
113. Zhang G, Matsumoto S, Newman H, et al: Improve islet yields and quality when clinical grade pancreata are preserved by the two-layer method. *Cell Tissue Bank* 7(3):195–201, 2006.
114. Kin T, Mirbolooki M, Salehi P, et al: Islet isolation and transplantation outcomes of pancreas preserved with University of Wisconsin solution versus two-layer method using preoxygenated perfluorocarbon. *Transplantation* 82(10):1286–1290, 2006.
115. Boggi U, Vistoli F, Del Chiaro M, et al: Pancreas preservation with University of Wisconsin and Celsior solutions: a single-center, prospective, randomized pilot study. *Transplantation* 77(8):1186–1190, 2004.
116. Nicoluzzi J, Macri M, Fukushima J, et al: Celsior versus Wisconsin solution in pancreas transplantation. *Transplant Proc* 40(10):3305–3307, 2008.
117. Agarwal A, Murdock P, Pescovitz MD, et al: Follow-up experience using histidine-tryptophan ketoglutarate solution in clinical pancreas transplantation. *Transplant Proc* 37(8):3523–3526, 2005.
118. Englesbe MJ, Moyer A, Kim DY, et al: Early pancreas transplant outcomes with histidine-tryptophan-ketoglutarate preservation: a multicenter study. *Transplantation* 82(1):136–139, 2006.
119. Potdar S, Malek S, Eghtesad B, et al: Initial experience using histidine-tryptophan-ketoglutarate solution in clinical pancreas transplantation. *Clin Transplant* 18(6):661–665, 2004.
120. Becker T, Ringe B, Nyibata M, et al: Pancreas transplantation with histidine-tryptophan-ketoglutarate (HTK) solution and University of Wisconsin (UW) solution: is there a difference? *JOP* 8(3):304–311, 2007.
121. Schneeberger S, Biebl M, Steurer W, et al: A prospective randomized multicenter trial comparing histidine-tryptophane-ketoglutarate versus University of Wisconsin perfusion solution in clinical pancreas transplantation. *Transpl Int* 22(2):217–224, 2009.
122. Stewart ZA, Lonze BE, Warren DS, et al: Histidine-tryptophan-ketoglutarate (HTK) is associated with reduced graft survival of deceased donor kidney transplants. *Am J Transplant* 9(5):1048–1054, 2009.
123. Mancini MJ, Connors AF Jr, Wang XQ, et al: HLA matching for simultaneous pancreas-kidney transplantation in the United States: a multivariable analysis of the UNOS data. *Clin Nephrol* 57(1):27–37, 2002.
124. Gruessner AC, Sutherland DE, Gruessner RW: Matching in pancreas transplantation–a registry analysis. *Transplant Proc* 33(1/2):1665–1666, 2001.
125. Lo A, Stratta RJ, Alloway RR, et al: A multicenter analysis of the significance of HLA matching on outcomes after kidney-pancreas transplantation. *Transplant Proc* 37(2):1289–1290, 2005.
126. Malaise J, Berney T, Morel P, et al: Effect of HLA matching in simultaneous pancreas-kidney transplantation. *Transplant Proc* 37(6):2846–2847, 2005.
127. Berney T, Malaise J, Morel P, et al: Impact of HLA matching on the outcome of simultaneous pancreas-kidney transplantation. *Nephrol Dial Transplant* 20[Suppl 2]:ii48–ii53, ii62, 2005.
128. Gruber SA, Katz S, Kaplan B, et al: Initial results of solitary pancreas transplants performed without regard to donor/recipient HLA mismatching. *Transplantation* 70(2):388–391, 2000.
129. Khwaja K, Wijkstrom M, Gruessner A, et al: Pancreas transplantation in cross-match-positive recipients using cyclosporine- or tacrolimus-based immunosuppression. *Transplant Proc* 34(5):1901–1902, 2002.
130. Krishnamurthi V, Philosophe B, Bartlett ST: Pancreas transplantation: contemporary surgical techniques. *Urol Clin North Am* 28(4):833–838, 2001.
131. Gruessner AC, Sutherland DE, Gruessner RW: Pancreas transplantation in the United States: a review. *Curr Opin Organ Transplant* 15(1):93–101, 2010.
132. Stratta RJ, Shokouh-Amiri MH, Egidi MF, et al: A prospective comparison of simultaneous kidney-pancreas transplantation with systemic-enteric versus portal-enteric drainage. *Ann Surg* 233(6):740–751, 2001.
133. Boggi U, Amorese G, Marchetti P: Surgical techniques for pancreas transplantation. *Curr Opin Organ Transplant* 15(1):102–111, 2010.
134. Jimenez-Romero C, Manrigue A, Meneu JC, et al: Compative study of bladder versus enteric drainage in pancreas transplantation. *Transplant Proc* 41(6):2466–2468, 2009.
135. De Roover A, Coimbra C, Detry O, et al: Pancreas graft drainage in recipient duodenum: preliminary experience. *Transplantation* 84(6):795–797, 2007.
136. Quintela J, Aguirrezabalaga J, Alonso A, et al: Portal and systemic venous drainage in pancreas and kidney-pancreas transplantation: early surgical complications and outcomes. *Transplant Proc* 41(6):2460–2462, 2009.
137. Philosophe B, Farney AC, Schweitzer EJ, et al: Superiority of portal venous drainage over systemic venous drainage in pancreas transplantation: a retrospective study. *Ann Surg* 234(5):689–696, 2001.
138. Boggi U, Vistoli F, Signori S, et al: A technique for retroperitoneal pancreas transplantation with portal-enteric drainage. *Transplantation* 79(9):1137–1142, 2005.
139. Sutherland DE, Morel P, Gruessner RW: Transplantation of two diabetic patients with one divided cadaver donor pancreas. *Transplant Proc* 22(2):585, 1990.
140. Saudek F, Malaise J, Boucek P, et al: Efficacy and safety of tacrolimus compared with cyclosporin microemulsion in primary SPK transplantation: 3-year results of the Euro-SPK 001 trial. *Nephrol Dial Transplant* 20[Suppl 2]:ii3–ii10, ii62, 2005.
141. Gruessner RW, Sutherland DE, Parr E, et al: A prospective, randomized, open-label study of steroid withdrawal in pancreas transplantation-a preliminary report with 6-month follow-up. *Transplant Proc* 33(1/2):1663–1664, 2001.
142. Montero N, Webster AC, Royuela A, et al: Steroid avoidance or withdrawal for pancreas and pancreas with kidney transplant recipients. *Cochrane Database Syst Rev* 9:CD007669, 2014.
143. Singh RP, Stratta RJ: Advances in immunosuppression for pancreas transplantation. *Curr Opin Organ Transplant* 13(1):79–84, 2008.
144. Israni AK, Skeans MA, Gustafson SK, et al: OPTN/SRTR 2012 Annual Data Report: pancreas. *Am J Transplant* 14[Suppl 1]:45–68, 2014.
145. Fellmer PT, Pascher A, Kahl A, et al: Influence of donor- and recipient-specific factors on the postoperative course after combined pancreas-kidney transplantation. *Langenbecks Arch Surg* 395(1):19–25, 2010.
146. Humar A, Ramcharan T, Kandaswamy R, et al: The impact of donor obesity on outcomes after cadaver pancreas transplants. *Am J Transplant* 4(4):605–610, 2004.
147. Hill M, Garcia R, Dunn T, et al: What happens to the kidney in an SPK transplant when the pancreas fails due to a technical complication? *Clin Transplant* 22(4):456–461, 2008.

148. Troppmann C: Complications after pancreas transplantation. *Curr Opin Organ Transplant* 15(1):112–118, 2010.
149. Goodman J, Becker YT: Pancreas surgical complications. *Curr Opin Organ Transplant* 14(1):85–89, 2009.
150. Wuthrich RP: Factor V Leiden mutation: potential thrombogenic role in renal vein, dialysis graft and transplant vascular thrombosis. *Curr Opin Nephrol Hypertens* 10(3):409–414, 2001.
151. Friedman GS, Meier-Kriesche HU, Kaplan B, et al: Hypercoagulable states in renal transplant candidates: impact of anticoagulation upon incidence of renal allograft thrombosis. *Transplantation* 72(6):1073–1078, 2001.
152. Zibari GB, Aultman DF, Abreo KD, et al: Roux-en-Y venting jejunostomy in pancreatic transplantation: a novel approach to monitor rejection and prevent anastomotic leak. *Clin Transplant* 14(4 Pt 2):380–385, 2000.
153. Roza AM, Johnson CP, Adams M: Acute torsion of the renal transplant after combined kidney-pancreas transplant. *Transplantation* 67(3):486–488, 1999.
154. West MS, Stevens RB, Metrakos P, et al: Renal pedicle torsion after simultaneous kidney-pancreas transplantation. *J Am Coll Surg* 187(1):80–87, 1998.
155. Troppmann C, Gruessner AC, Dunn DL, et al: Surgical complications requiring early relaparotomy after pancreas transplantation: a multivariate risk factor and economic impact analysis of the cyclosporine era. *Ann Surg* 227(2):255–268, 1998.
156. Gruessner AC, Sutherland DE: Pancreas transplant outcomes for United States (US) cases as reported to the United Network for Organ Sharing (UNOS) and the International Pancreas Transplant Registry (IPTR). *Clin Transpl*:45–56, 2008.
157. Malek SK, Potdar S, Martin JA, et al: Percutaneous ultrasound-guided pancreas allograft biopsy: a single-center experience. *Transplant Proc* 37(10):4436–4437, 2005.
158. Kaplan B, West-Thielke P, Herren H, et al: Reported isolated pancreas rejection is associated with poor kidney outcomes in recipients of a simultaneous pancreas kidney transplant. *Transplantation* 86(9):1229–1233, 2008.
159. Kawecki D, Kwiatkowski A, Michalak G, et al: Etiologic agents of bacteremia in the early period after simultaneous pancreas-kidney transplantation. *Transplant Proc* 41(8):3151–3153, 2009.
160. Gruessner RW, Sutherland DE, Gruessner AC: Mortality assessment for pancreas transplants. *Am J Transplant* 4(12):2018–2026, 2004.
161. Vardanyan M, Parkin E, Gruessner C, et al: Pancreas vs. islet transplantation: a call on the future. *Curr Opin Organ Transplant* 15(1):124–130, 2010.
162. Hering BJ, Wijkstrom M, Graham ML, et al: Prolonged diabetes reversal after intraportal xenotransplantation of wild-type porcine islets in immunosuppressed nonhuman primates. *Nat Med* 12(3):301–303, 2006.

Chapter 62 ■ Critical Care of Intestinal Transplant Recipients

ROBERT M. ESTERL, JR • WILLIAM D. PAYNE • ABHINAV HUMAR • RUY J. CRUZ, JR

INTRODUCTION

The first experimental intestinal transplant was performed by Alexis Carrel in 1901, when he implanted a segment of bowel into the neck of a dog. The first human intestinal transplants occurred in the 1960s, but these transplants were suspended at that time because of dismal graft and patient survival owing to the lack of effective immunosuppressive protocols. The widespread introduction of calcineurin inhibitors (cyclosporine in the 1980s and tacrolimus in the 1990s) renewed interest in intestinal transplantation as a viable surgical option for patients with short bowel syndrome (SBS) who otherwise required chronic total parenteral nutrition (TPN). Newer immunosuppressive regimens, advances in organ preservation, better donor and recipient selection, refinement in surgical techniques, earlier detection and treatment of infections, and improved postoperative critical care management have all played significant roles in the success of intestinal transplantation since the mid-1990s. The advances in this field are presented in Table 62.1. Although intestinal transplantation remains the least frequent of all transplant types, 1-year graft survival rates have significantly improved and now approach those of other nonrenal transplants. As graft losses owing to technical reasons have diminished, immunologic and infectious issues remain primary challenges facing the field today. As the largest lymphoid organ in the human body and a host for potential infectious pathogens, the small bowel continues to be a difficult solid organ to successfully transplant [1–10].

Pretransplant Evaluation

Intestinal failure is defined as the inability of the intestine to maintain nutrition or fluid and electrolyte balance without long-term TPN [2,4,6–8]. The causes of intestinal failure can be divided into two broad groups: (a) SBS (insufficient bowel length) and (b) functional disorders (impaired intestinal motility or absorption with an otherwise sufficient intestinal length and surface area). Currently, an intestinal transplant is indicated for patients suffering from irreversible SBS who present with life-threatening complications secondary to TPN or underlying medical disease [6]. The Centers for Medicare and Medicaid Services have approved coverage for intestinal transplants in patients with SBS who require TPN with these complications: (a) thrombosis of major venous access sites, (b) frequent central line infections and sepsis requiring hospitalization (more than two episodes per year), (c) impending or overt liver failure related to TPN, and (d) severe and frequent episodes of electrolyte imbalance and/or dehydration despite intravenous fluid supplementation and TPN [3,8,11]. Many feel that patients who are stable on TPN without such complications are usually not intestinal transplant candidates, because their estimated annual survival rate could be higher with TPN support than transplantation. Others have suggested that patients with ultrashort bowel remnants, complete portomesenteric thrombosis, slow growing tumors involving the mesenteric root, pseudo-obstruction, and frozen abdomen have indications for intestinal transplantation [4,8].

The most common cause of SBS requiring intestinal transplantation is extensive surgical resection of the small intestine. Uncommon indications for intestinal transplantation for patients with intestinal failure but without SBS are (a) severe gastrointestinal myopathy or neuropathy (hollow visceral myopathy, total intestinal aganglionosis, and pseudo-obstruction syndrome), (b) gut malabsorption syndromes (microvillous inclusion disease, radiation enteritis, and selective autoimmune enteropathy), (c) neoplastic syndromes involving the root of the mesentery (neuroendocrine and desmoid tumors, often associated with familial adenomatous polyposis or Gardener syndrome), and (d) diffuse portomesenteric thrombosis with high risk of gastrointestinal hemorrhage [2,4,7–9].

The causes of intestinal failure and intestinal transplantation differ for adult versus pediatric populations. Gastroschisis, necrotizing enterocolitis, malrotation with mid-gut volvulus, and atresias are the most common causes in pediatric patients; mesenteric arterial thrombosis/embolism, trauma, Crohn disease, and adhesions are the most frequent causes in adult patients [10]. Most patients (53%) who wait for an intestinal transplantation have an underlying diagnosis of SBS [9]. The development of SBS depends not only on the resected length of bowel but also on

TABLE 62.1

Advances in Intestinal Transplantation

Issue	Major advance	References
Indications for intestinal transplantation	Expanded indications for intestinal transplantation over and above CMS approval include ultrashort bowel remnants, complete portomesenteric thrombosis, slow growing tumors involving the mesenteric root, pseudo-obstruction, and frozen abdomen	[4,8]
Surgical options for intestinal transplantation	Standard nomenclature is established to compare unique contributions that surgical procedures play in graft/patient survival	[8,13]
Immunosuppression	Standard immunosuppressive regimens improve graft/patient survival	[9]
Postoperative infections	There exist better methods to diagnose and treat transplant-associated infections, namely, CMV and EBV	[2,8,23,24]
Biomarkers for the diagnosis of acute rejection	There is an increased need to identify biomarkers of intestinal rejection	[8,17–19]
Donor-specific antibodies/ complement activation	There is increased attention to the role of donor-specific antibodies/complement in chronic allograft enteropathy and graft loss and the development of medications/treatments to target various mediators of rejection	[8,16]
Quality of life	Treatment-specific surveys indicate improved global health status/quality of life with intestinal transplants over chronic TPN	[25]
Outcomes	Mortality on the wait list has decreased, and graft/patient survival after intestinal transplantation have increased over last decade	[9]

CMS, Centers for Medicare and Medicaid Services; CMV, cytomegalovirus; EBV, Epstein–Barr virus; TPN, total parenteral nutrition.

the location of the resection and on the retainment (or not) of the ileocecal valve and/or the colon. As a rough guideline, most patients can tolerate up to 50% resection of their intestine with subsequent adaptation, without the need for long-term TPN. Loss of greater than 70% of intestine (considered ultra-short gut syndrome), however, usually necessitates some type of parenteral nutritional support. The development of TPN-induced liver failure is much more fulminant in children than adults. For these reasons, pediatric patients with SBS should be referred early for isolated intestinal transplantation before the development of irreversible TPN-induced liver injury [2,5,7,12].

The pretransplantation evaluation is similar to that of other types of solid organ transplantation. The typical laboratory evaluation includes ABO type, HLA type, panel reactive antibody, complete blood count, comprehensive basic metabolic profile, and coagulation profile. Serology studies should be performed for HIV, hepatitis B and C, cytomegalovirus (CMV), and Epstein–Barr virus (EBV). A clear picture of the anatomy of the patient's gastrointestinal tract is essential [2]. An upper gastrointestinal tract contrast series and abdominal and pelvic computed tomography scan are always necessary in order to plan gastrointestinal tract reconstruction during the transplantation. It is important to estimate actual bowel length and function (transit time with upper gastrointestinal series). Hepatic function should be evaluated carefully, and a transjugular or percutaneous liver biopsy is often required. If there is evidence of significant liver dysfunction, a combined liver-intestinal or multivisceral transplant may be indicated [5,12]. Duplex sonography of the liver and intra-abdominal vascular system can be useful. Patients with thrombotic disorders need specific hematologic tests to define hypercoagulable states (such as protein C and S deficiency, prothrombin G20210 A and factor V Leiden mutation, and hyperhomocysteinemia) [2]. Conventional abdominal visceral angiography and a comprehensive evaluation of the upper and lower central venous system are mandatory in high-risk patients and those with thrombotic disorders. Absolute contraindications, such as advanced malignancy, severe systemic disease, active infection, and marked cardiopulmonary insufficiency, must be ruled out [2,6].

Surgical Procedure

Unfortunately, the nomenclature to describe the technical aspects of intestinal transplantation has not been consistent in the literature, particularly when other organs are transplanted with the intestinal graft [8]. Transplant experts convened at the 2007 International Small Bowel Transplant Symposium and attempted to standardize this nomenclature into two broad categories: with or without simultaneous a liver transplantation. Modifications to these operations then reflect that the transplantation occurs with or without excision of the native foregut. Mazariegos et al. argues that failure to apply standard nomenclature hampers the ability to compare contributions that unique surgical techniques may play in critical data analysis and graft/patient survival [8,13]. The indication for transplantation and the choice of organs to include in the composite graft are defined by the recipient's baseline disease, vascular and gastrointestinal anatomy, associated diseases (such as liver failure, diabetes, exocrine pancreatic insufficiency, or renal failure), and functional quality of the other abdominal organs.

The three most common types of intestinal transplants include (a) isolated intestinal transplants, (b) combined liver–intestine transplants, and (c) multivisceral or modified multivisceral transplants [1–8]. The most common intestinal transplantation is the isolated intestinal graft which includes the entire deceased donor jejunum and ileum, and is used for patients with intestinal failure that is limited to the small bowel. The arterial anastomosis is based on the recipient superior mesenteric artery or using a jump graft from the infrarenal aorta. Venous outflow is usually achieved with the anastomosis of the superior mesenteric vein to the native superior mesenteric vein or splenic vein; however, in some cases, systemic venous drainage to the inferior vena cava is required which can cause metabolic abnormalities. Gastrointestinal continuity occurs with a primary anastomosis between the recipient and donor proximal jejunum and the creation of a distal Bishop-Koop or loop ileostomy with or without anastomosis to the recipient colon. In living donation or in a case of severe donor-to-recipient size mismatch (deceased donor adult to pediatric recipient), a 200-cm length of distal small bowel is used; inflow to the graft is via the ileocolic artery, and outflow is via the ileocolic vein. In patients with combined pancreatic dysfunction (e.g., cystic fibrosis, type I diabetes, or chronic pancreatitis), the inclusion of the pancreas should be considered with intestinal transplantation.

The second most common technique combines the liver and pancreas organs with the intestinal transplantation [1–8]. The liver, pancreas, and intestine (including the duodenum) are procured en bloc from the donor and are transplanted on bloc in the recipient. In the en bloc donor allograft, the arterial inflow is based on an aortic conduit that includes the celiac trunk and the superior mesenteric artery, and the venous outflow that is based on the hepatic veins or the inferior vena cava. The recipient operation includes an arterial anastomosis that occurs between the donor aortic conduit and the recipient suprarenal or infrarenal aorta; a vena caval anastomosis that occurs via standard caval replacement or by the piggyback technique. Gastrointestinal continuity is reestablished with a primary anastomosis between the proximal donor and recipient jejunum or duodenum and distal creation of the Bishop-Koop or loop ileostomy with or without connection to the recipient colon. The clear advantage of the en bloc liver, pancreas, and intestinal transplant is avoidance of hilar dissection and fewer donor-related arterial or biliary complications that can occur especially in pediatric patients. In this configuration, the common bile duct remains intact in the hepatoduodenal ligament along with the second portion of the duodenum and whole pancreas, which obviates biliary reconstruction of the recipient [8].

A technical variation of liver-intestinal transplantation is that the liver and intestine can be transplanted individually without the pancreas [3,6–8]. The advantage of this technique is that one could excise the intestine if severe complications occur (e.g., hyperacute or acute rejection) and leave the liver intact. The disadvantage of this technique is that it requires multiple vascular anastomoses and biliary reconstruction with their potential complications. In the liver-intestinal transplant, the stomach, duodenum, pancreas, and spleen are left intact, and a portocaval shunt is required for venous outflow of these native organs [2,3,6].

The third type of transplantation, including the intestine, is the multivisceral transplant. In the multivisceral transplant, additional gastrointestinal organs can be transplanted in continuity with the intestine, including the donor stomach, duodenum, and colon with or without the liver and/or pancreas. The common indications for multivisceral transplantation include, but are not limited to, hollow visceral myopathy or neuropathy, pseudo-obstruction syndrome, extensive gastrointestinal polyposis, neuroendocrine tumors, and symptomatic total splanchnic vascular thrombosis. The operation involves complete splanchnic evisceration and en bloc transplantation of the stomach, duodenum, pancreas, liver, and small bowel, and, on occasion, the right and transverse colon (full multivisceral transplant). If the stomach is involved in the upper abdominal evisceration, gastrointestinal continuity is achieved by connecting the donor stomach to the recipient distal esophagus or small gastric remnant. In patients with preserved liver function, the native liver is left intact (modified multivisceral transplant). For patients with chronic or impending renal failure, a renal graft (usually right kidney) can also be included in the multivisceral transplant.

As mentioned earlier, the nomenclature for multivisceral transplantation can be somewhat confusing in the literature. Some authors restrict the term "multivisceral" to transplants that contain the stomach, whereas others use the term for any combination of abdominal organs [8]. Other reports use the term "multivisceral" only when native organs are simultaneously excised during the transplantation process. Early series suggested that inclusion of the colon increases the risk of infectious complications, but more recent reports describe that inclusion of the colon is not only safe, but may lead to better absorption of water from stool, resulting in fewer episodes of dehydration from diarrhea and hospital readmission [8]. The inclusion of the stomach is also a controversial topic, in that some centers universally apply this technique and other centers rarely or never do. Evidence regarding the benefits and risks of including the stomach in the multivisceral transplant is limited [8].

The recipient operation can be a challenging procedure because of the presence of abdominal adhesions from multiple previous operations, stomas, gastrojejunostomies, reduced abdominal space, and, in some cases, considerable portal hypertension (if the patient requires a liver transplant). The loss of abdominal domain is a unique problem with intestinal transplants unless the patient has significant ascites from liver failure or hollow visceral myopathy or neuropathy (e.g., pseudo-obstruction syndrome). Loss of domain has been addressed with several innovative techniques, including transplantation of the abdominal wall, placement of tissue expanders, and staged closure of the abdominal wall with musculocutaneous free flaps [8].

Gastrojejunostomy tubes are almost always placed intraoperatively, permitting gastric decompression and enteral nutrition in the early postoperative period [2,6,14]. A Bishop-Koop or loop ileostomy is used to decompress the terminal ileum and to facilitate enteroscopy/biopsy, which is the only reliable method to monitor the allograft for acute rejection. The ileostomy is usually taken down within 1 year after transplantation if there is little need to continue monitoring the graft for rejection. Of note, a prophylactic (donor or native) appendectomy and (donor or native) cholecystectomy are performed in all cases to avoid associated postoperative complications. Finally, for a multivisceral transplantation, a donor pyloroplasty is always performed to enable gastric emptying.

Several factors should be considered in appropriate matching of the donor and the recipient for an intestine transplantation. Usually, ABO-identical grafts are used; ABO nonidentical but compatible grafts are usually avoided because of a higher risk of graft-versus-host disease. Donors are typically young, hemodynamically stable, brain-dead but heartbeating donors. Donors should usually be of similar or smaller size than the recipients, because the latter usually have contracted peritoneal cavities, so that a smaller graft may be more appropriate because of space constraints. Selective bacterial and fungal decontamination of the gut (enteral amphotericin B, polymyxin B, and gentamicin) through a nasogastric tube should be attempted for all donors. CMV enteritis can be a devastating problem in intestinal transplant recipients, so that, if possible, CMV seronegative recipients should receive CMV seronegative intestinal grafts. If possible, similar viral matching should be performed for EBV, when possible, because of the risk for posttransplant lymphoproliferative disorder (PTLD) [2].

Postoperative Care

The early posttransplantation care, in many ways, is similar to that of other solid organ transplantation recipients. Postoperative care for intestinal transplant recipients can be difficult and complicated, especially for those recipients who present with deterioration/malnutrition and organ system failures, when sequelae can persist postoperatively even with improving allograft function. Postoperative management often requires an aggressive, interprofessional approach by medical, nursing, and ancillary health care providers [2]. Initial care is usually in a critical care setting, so that vital signs, urine output, fluid and electrolytes, and blood product replacement can be carefully monitored. Serial hemoglobin measurements are performed to monitor for evidence of hemorrhage. Serum pH and lactate should also be followed for evidence of intestinal ischemia or injury. In patients who received liver-intestinal or multivisceral allografts, pancreatic enzymes and liver function tests should be assessed daily to track organ functional status. Selective bacterial and fungal gut decontamination through a nasogastric tube or gastrojejunostomy tube postoperatively should be performed until enteral nutrition is tolerated. Broad-spectrum antibiotics against bacteria and fungi are routinely administered given the high risk for infectious complications. Routine prophylaxis should also be administered against CMV, EBV, and *Pneumocystis jiroveci* infection [2]. *P. jiroveci* prophylaxis for patients with allergies/intolerance to sulfa medication can be accomplished by monthly inhaled pentamidine.

Continuous intravenous fluids are administered in the postoperative period until the patient is stable from a surgical viewpoint [2]. Postoperative nutritional support initially occurs by resumption of standard TPN solutions. When the gastrointestinal function begins to recover and upper gastrointestinal contrast studies confirm the integrity of gastrointestinal anastomoses, enteral nutrition is initiated via the gastrojejunostomy tube. Most tube feedings are polymeric formulas containing whole complex components instead of a predigested product which can be switched to fiber-containing formulas if significant diarrhea develops [14]. This switch from parenteral to enteral nutrition is gradual and usually occurs in the first 2 weeks after transplantation. Tube feeding is slowly decreased and removed, whereas oral intake is increased proportionately to an unrestricted diet, except in patients with a chylous leak who should receive a low-fat diet. All patients receive antiulcer prophylaxis with proton pump inhibitors, and some patients require antidiarrheal (opiates, loperamide, or soluble fiber supplements) or prokinetic agents (metoclopramide or erythromycin) to modulate stool or stoma output, once rejection or enteritis is ruled out [2].

Most patients can be weaned from TPN and remain TPN free after intestinal transplantation [8]. Matarese reported that enteral nutrition began through a jejunostomy tube at a mean 10.3 days after transplant, that TPN was discontinued at a mean 30.8 days after transplantation and that most patients achieved a regular oral diet at a mean 57 days after transplant [14]. In the early postoperative period, some patients who receive a multivisceral transplantation do not take oral nutrition that is sufficient to meet their nutritional needs. This eating disorder, usually seen in the pediatric population, is caused by many etiologies, including (a) some patients never had the opportunity to eat food before the transplant and never learned the mechanics of food consumption, (b) some patients have associated the act of food consumption with disagreeable and distasteful sentiments with accompanying nausea, vomiting, diarrhea, and abdominal distension and pain, and (c) some patients develop a hyperactive gag reflex evoked by food consumption [2]. Many of these are learned behaviors, and these patients require cognitive redirection of their perceptions around food consumption. They need regular emotional support and nutritional guidance after intestinal transplantation. They often require very slow introduction of new foods. The use of small frequent meals, prokinetic and antidiarrheal agents, and appetite stimulants aid in the transition to regular diets for patients with early satiety, diarrhea, or anorexia [14].

Some intestinal recipients exhibit renal dysfunction in the postoperative period as a result of inadequate intraoperative resuscitation, dehydration from diarrhea/increased stomal output, and high-dose tacrolimus immunotherapy. All patients in the immediate postoperative period have a urinary catheter to monitor the adequacy of resuscitation and appropriate urine output. The increased use of induction immunotherapy for intestinal transplants has led to delayed introduction/decreased target levels for tacrolimus which may translate to more rapid recovery of renal function in the immediate postoperative period and preserved long-term renal function [8].

Immunosuppression should be initiated in the immediate postoperative period [2]. A number of different immunosuppressive protocols have been described. The OPTN/SRTR 2013 Annual Data Report noted that 54% of intestinal recipients received T-cell depleting agents and 11% received interleukin-2 receptor antagonists for induction therapy; yet, 38% received no induction therapy. In this report, the most common initial maintenance immunosuppressive medications were tacrolimus (95%), steroids (73%), mycophenolate (35%), and mTOR inhibitors (15%). Seventy percent of recipients were still maintained on oral steroids 1 year after the intestinal transplantation. Target trough levels for tacrolimus in the whole blood were typically 12 to 15 ng per mL for the first postoperative month, followed by levels of 8 to 12 ng per mL for the next 3 months.

Regardless of the immunosuppressive regimen, intestinal transplants clearly have a high risk of rejection. The ORPN/SRTR 2013 Annual Data Report indicates that the incidence of a first rejection episode increases over time. In adult recipients of isolated intestinal transplants, 45% experience an episode of acute rejection within the first year and 53% within the second year. Although the use of induction agents and tacrolimus-based maintenance therapy have markedly reduced episodes of acute rejection for intestinal transplantation patients, the consequences of steroid resistant rejection carry a 50% mortality in adult intestinal transplant recipients mainly as a result of sepsis [8,15].

Although traditional treatment for acute rejection aims to control the T-cell–mediated response in the intestinal graft with steroid bolus or antilymphocyte therapy, recent attention has been paid to the role of antibody-mediated mechanisms in intestinal graft rejection [8]. Antibody-mediated rejection continues to be a problem in intestinal transplants, because it is relatively resistant to corticosteroid therapy, but donor-specific antibodies in particular are becoming recognized as causes of chronic rejection and late graft loss [16]. This recognition has followed the widespread introduction and implementation of new immunologic technologies, namely, single antigen fluorescent bead assays to detect donor-specific antibodies. The presence of preformed donor-specific antibody and/or increased panel reactive antibody correlates with rejection and graft loss [8,16]. Both preformed and de novo donor-specific antibodies have been associated with antibody-mediated rejection and decreased graft survival; patients with donor-specific antibodies before and after the intestinal transplantation appear to have the lowest long-term graft survival because of not only to episodes of acute rejection but also to chronic allograft enteropathy. Important features of chronic allograft enteropathy are mucosal atrophy and ulceration, mesenteric lymphoid depletion, and mesenteric fibrosis and sclerosis, caused by mesenteric vasculopathy that is highly dependent on donor-specific antibodies [16]. The presence of CD4 and direct evidence of other antibody and complement activity in mesenteric vasculopathy associated with chronic allograft enteropathy may be lacking in the literature, largely because they are best seen on full-thickness intestinal biopsies and not the typical mucosal biopsies. Finally, complement activation appears to play a significant role in the development of late dysfunction and chronic allograft enteropathy [16]. Donor-specific antibodies can bind to the C1q component of complement, activating the full complement cascade. Of note, inclusion of the liver along with the intestine seems to protect the recipient from intestinal rejection, either by inducing a tolerogenic state in the antigen-presenting cells in the liver or providing a reservoir to sequester sensitized T-cells and/or antibodies against the intestine. Larger studies are necessary to define the use of immunosuppressive medications/therapies to target these various mediators of rejection: preformed donor-specific antibodies (plasmapheresis and immunoglobulin), cytokines (infliximab), B cells (rituximab), plasma cells (bortezomab), and early activation of the complement cascade (eclizumab) [8,16].

In a patient with intestinal dysfunction, it is very important to differentiate enteritis (mostly caused by *Clostridium difficile*, adenovirus, CMV, and calicivirus) from rejection, because both conditions may be characterized by low-grade fever, abdominal distension and pain, and diarrhea (or increased stoma output).

The stoma if present should be carefully examined for color, texture, and friability; in the face of rejection, the stoma may appear edematous, erythematous, pale, congested, dusky, or friable. Endoscopy should be performed for inspection of the mucosa and for purposes of biopsy of the most suspicious areas. Endoscopy with biopsy is the primary method to diagnose allograft rejection. Careful evaluation of an intestinal biopsy by an experienced pathologist is always necessary [2].

Because surveillance and diagnostic endoscopy and biopsy are costly and invasive procedures, there is increased interest to identify potential biomarkers of intestinal rejection [8]. Recent studies have shown that several molecules, namely, calprotectin and citrulline, measured in the stool/ileostomy effluent and blood, respectively, are reliable markers of moderate and severe intestinal rejection. Calprotectin is an S100 protein released by infiltrating neutrophils and macrophages into the gut lumen; increased calprotectin levels have been noted prior to the onset of histologic changes of acute rejection, and normal levels are consistently seen with normal intestine graft biopsies [8,17]. Citrulline is an amino acid found almost exclusively in enterocytes, so decreased levels in the blood reflect decreased functional mass of enterocytes [17]. Hibi et al. noted that citrulline levels were inversely proportional to the severity of acute cellular rejection [18]. Negative predictive values for any type of acute cellular rejection (cutoff was 20 μmol per L) and moderate/severe acute cellular rejection (cutoff, 10 μmol per L) were 95% and 99%, respectively. Subgroup analysis showed a strong correlation of citrullene levels (obtained up to 1 week prior to biopsy) with the severity of acute rejection on intestinal biopsy; as the citrulline level decreased, the grade of rejection on biopsy worsened. Other potential markers of intestinal graft dysfunction could include adipsin, C-reactive protein (an inflammatory marker used clinically in Crohn disease), and lathosterol (fecal marker of bile malabsorption when intestinal mucosa is dysfunctional) [17]. Larger studies are needed on all of these potential biomarkers in order to be used widely in clinical practice. Girlanda et al. used liquid chromatography to examine the metabolomic profile of ileostomy effluent of patients who had intestinal graft rejection versus no rejection [19]. These investigators noted the highest-fold change in the proinflammatory mediator leukotriene E4 in patients with rejection, and high-fold changes in taurocholate and water-soluble vitamins B_2, B_5, and B_6 in patients with rejection. Metabolomic analysis could be a promising tool to characterize the pathophysiologic mechanisms of intestinal graft rejection and to identify some potential early noninvasive biomarkers of graft dysfunction.

Short-term results have improved dramatically, mainly because of improvements of surgical techniques and immunosuppression regimens. Nonetheless, intestinal transplants are still associated with fairly high surgical complication rates. Potential complications include enteric leaks with generalized peritonitis or localized intra-abdominal abscesses, biliary leakage and stricture (if a liver transplant occurs), graft vascular thrombosis/stenosis, and life-threatening intraoperative and postoperative hemorrhage [2].

Infectious complications are, unfortunately, very common in intestinal transplantation recipients and are a frequent cause of morbidity/mortality and hospital readmissions [2,8]. There are several factors that contribute to this issue. The intestinal graft itself is a significant source of bacteria, and any process which compromises containment of these bacteria (intraoperative spillage of gastrointestinal contents or postoperative anastomotic leak) can lead to a localized abscess or systemic infection. Because of the higher risk of rejection, intestinal transplantation recipients generally receive higher levels of immunosuppression compared with other organ recipients and they are at greater risk for severe infections, including transplant-associated infections (CMV or EBV) and community-acquired pathogens (respiratory syncytial virus or influenza). The presence of uncorrected surgical/technical/mechanical problems (e.g., biliary leak or stricture for liver transplantation, gastrointestinal anastomotic leak, vesicoureteral reflux for kidney transplant recipients) may predispose intestinal recipients to recurrent infections [20]. If rejection causes disruption of the intestinal mucosal barrier, bacteria and fungi can translocate across the graft directly into the peritoneal cavity, leading to spontaneous bacterial peritonitis. Bacteria can also spread directly into the portal circulation, and subsequently disseminate to distant sites. Patients with indwelling catheters (central catheters for TPN or gastrojejunostomy tubes for enteral nutrition) are at increased risk for infectious complications until the catheter is no longer necessary and is removed [20]. Finally, immunosuppression attenuates the native immune response to vaccines in the postoperative period; when a higher level of immunosuppression is required for an intestinal transplantation recipient (e.g., rejection treatment), it puts pediatric patients at significantly higher risk for vaccine-associated diseases. Live viral vaccines are contraindicated for intestinal recipients in the postoperative period, placing pediatric patients at risk for varicella in addition to measles, mumps, and rubella if they have exposure to these viruses [20].

Bacterial infections are extremely common in the immediate postoperative period after an intestinal transplant. In a study of 40 adult intestinal recipients, Premeggia et al. reported a 30-day postoperative infection rate of 58% with a mean time to first infection of 11 days [21]. In this study, 23 patients developed 36 bacterial infections; of patients with infections, 57% developed one infection, 30% developed two infections, and 13% developed three infections. The most common site of infection was the abdomen, followed by infections in the blood, urine, lung, and surgical site. Of the microbial isolates, 49% were gram-negative bacteria, 39% were gram-positive bacteria, and 11% were fungi. The most common bacterial isolates included *Pseudomonas* (19%), *Enterococcus* (15%), and *Escherichia coli* (13%). Of note, 47% of these infections were caused by multidrug-resistant pathogens. Postoperative bacterial infections remain important complications in intestinal transplantation recipients, and multidrug-resistant pathogens have emerged as a significant clinical challenge.

Fungal infections remain important infectious complications after intestinal transplantation, but data, particularly in pediatric recipients, are lacking in the literature. In a series of 98 pediatric intestinal recipients, Florescu et al. reported that 25 patients developed 59 episodes of *Candida* infections and four episodes of invasive *Aspergillus* infections [22]. Of the *Candida* species, 37% were *Candida albicans*, and 63% were non-*albicans*. Of all fungal infections, 66% were in the blood, 29% were in the intra-abdominal space, 3% were in the urinary tract, and 2% were in the pleural space. Of the *Candida* intra-abdominal infections, 41% developed in the first postoperative month, whereas 80% of fungemia developed after more than 6 months. Median time from intestinal transplant to fungal infection was 9 days for intra-abdominal infections versus 163 days for fungemia. Fungal infections occurred in approximately 25% of pediatric intestinal recipients, and *C. albicans* was the most common species. Intra-abdominal fungal infections occurred much earlier than fungemia after pediatric intestinal transplants.

In addition to bacterial infections, viral infections are also common for intestinal transplant recipients, of which CMV and EBV receive the most attention in the literature [2,8,23]. CMV is the most important viral infection of intestinal recipients. Not only does CMV cause tissue-invasive disease, it is also an independent risk factor for secondary bacterial and fungal infections and PTLD. It can also induce intestinal graft injury and rejection through indirect immunomodulatory causes. The patients who are at highest risk for CMV infection are CMV-negative recipients who receive CMV-positive intestinal organs. CMV-positive recipients are also at risk of CMV infections because of reactivation of latent virus. Antilymphocyte induction therapy further enhances the risk of CMV infections. In patients who receive no prophylaxis, CMV occurs most often within the first 3 months after intestinal transplant, and can present as an asymptomatic infection or as a syndrome, including fever, leukopenia, encephalitis, retinitis, pneumonitis, hepatitis, or enteritis/graft involvement. Antiviral therapy is effective in the prevention and treatment of CMV. For prevention of CMV, patients can receive either universal prophylactic therapy or preemptive therapy. Most experts recommend universal prophylaxis for CMV-negative recipients who receive CMV-positive intestinal organs, and universal prophylaxis or preemptive therapy for CMV-positive recipients for 3 to 6 months postoperatively or during intensified immunosuppressive treatments for rejection. CMV-negative recipients who receive CMV-negative intestinal organs are at the lowest risk of CMV infection, and many experts recommend no CMV-specific antiviral prophylaxis [23]. Historic reports noted CMV to occur in 24% of intestinal recipients, but in a recent study of pediatric intestinal transplants, Florescu et al. reported an 11% incidence of CMV viremia and a 7% incidence of CMV disease; in those patients with CMV disease, there was a high rate of CMV disease relapse and an 11-fold increased risk of postoperative mortality [24].

EBV is also an important viral infection, especially in pediatric patients who have received an intestinal transplantation [2,8,23]. Like CMV, patients with the highest risk for EBV infections are EBV-negative recipients who receive EBV-positive intestinal organs. EBV-positive recipients are at increased risk for reactivation of the latent virus which occurs 2 to 3 months postoperatively. EBV typically causes a syndrome which can include fever, leukopenia, thrombocytopenia, hepatitis, pneumonitis, or PTLD. PTLD can present as a spectrum of diseases ranging from infectious mononucleosis to frank lymphoma that can be nodal or extranodal, localized or disseminated. A positive polymerase chain reaction for EBV in a patient with signs/symptoms of PTLD suggests the diagnosis, but tissue biopsy is mandatory for confirmation. Decreasing the immunosuppression by approximately 50% is the primary treatment which can result in lesion regression. Other treatment options can include surgical resection and radiation therapy for local disease, in addition to rituximab (if CD20 positive) and chemotherapy for disseminated disease. Some centers use antiviral prophylaxis for EBV-negative recipients who received EBV-positive intestinal organs [23].

There is some evidence that intestinal transplantation improves quality of life compared to chronic TPN. In a study of 33 patients on chronic TPN versus 22 patients after intestinal transplantation, Pironi et al. noted that the intestinal recipients had better scores on treatment-specific quality of life questionnaires in the following categories: ability to vacation/travel, fatigue, gastrointestinal symptoms, stoma management/bowel movements, and global health status/quality of life. Subgroup analyses of patients who were employed showed that intestinal transplantation recipients had better scores in the ability to secure and maintain employment and emotional function. These data suggest that a successful intestinal transplant was associated with less uncertainty about employment and, consequently, less anxiety and/or depression [25].

Outcomes

The UNOS Database reported that approximately 2,500 intestinal transplantations have been performed in the United States over the last 25 years [10]. The OPTN/SRTR 2013 Annual Data Report indicated that only 23 centers performed pediatric intestinal transplants, and only 24 centers performed adult intestinal transplants in the United States [9]. According to this report, the most common cause for intestinal failure was short gut syndrome (53%), caused by a host of etiologies. In this report, approximately 170 new candidates were added to the waitlist for an intestinal transplantation in 2013; of these candidates, 49% waited for a liver-intestinal transplant and 51% waited for an intestinal transplant. Since 2008, candidates listed for an intestinal transplantation outnumbered candidates listed for a liver-intestinal transplantation. In the last decade, the age distribution of listed candidates shifted from a pediatric to an adult population, but the race or cause of disease distributions did not changed over that period.

According to the 2013 OPTN/SRTR Annual Report, mortality on the waitlist decreased significantly for all age groups over the last decade [9]. Pretransplant mortality was higher for adult candidates than for pediatric candidates, and was higher for candidates who waited for a liver-intestinal transplant than for an intestinal transplant. This decrease in mortality was likely because of a greater proportion of candidates listed for an intestinal transplantation than a liver-intestinal transplantation (higher mortality risk liver failure patients), improved medical therapies for intestinal failure, and improved organ allocation policies. Regarding 3-year outcomes of intestinal candidates, 69% received intestinal transplantation, 8% were removed from the waitlist, 5% died on the list, and 19% continued to wait on the list. Regarding 3-year outcomes of liver-intestinal candidates, 66% received liver-intestinal transplantation, 11% were removed from the waitlist, 11% died on the list, and 12% continued to wait on the list. Among candidates listed in 2012 to 2013, the median time to adult liver-intestinal transplantation, adult intestinal transplantation, and pediatric liver-intestinal transplantation was 11 months, 4 months, and 7 months, respectively. Among pediatric candidates listed in 2008 to 2009, the median wait time to intestinal transplant was 19 months.

In the 2013 OPTN/SRTR Annual Report, the overall number of liver-intestinal transplantations and intestinal transplantations decreased steadily since 2009 [9]. It was noteworthy that in 2013, the overall number of adult intestinal transplantations was more than double the number of pediatric intestinal recipients. Moreover, liver-intestinal transplantation recipients were younger than intestinal transplantation recipients, were more likely to have a diagnosis of necrotizing enterocolitis or congenital short gut syndrome, and were likely to be hospitalized at the time of the transplant. In 2013, 52% recipients received an intestinal graft with another organ, and 19% of liver-intestinal recipients received a previous intestinal transplantation compared to only 2% of intestinal recipients.

According to the 2013 OPTN/SRTR Annual Report, intestinal graft survival has steadily improved over the last decade [9]. Graft failure within the first 3 months occurred in 14% of intestinal transplants and 11% of liver-intestinal transplants. For all intestinal transplantations in 2008, the 1- and 5-year graft survival rates were 73% and 62%, respectively, for pediatric recipients and 76% and 38% for adult recipients. One- and five-year graft survival rates were 79% and 48%, respectively, for all intestinal recipients and 71% and 49% for all liver-intestinal recipients. The number of recipients who were alive with a functional intestinal graft steadily increased over the last decade. The incidence of acute rejection increased in the postoperative period approaching 53% at 2 years. For transplantations that occurred from 2001 to 2011, 10% of intestinal recipients and 7% liver-intestinal recipients developed PTLD with 5 years postoperatively; and the incidence was highest in EBV-negative intestinal recipients. Regardless of recipient age, patient survival was better for intestinal recipients than for liver-intestinal recipients. Pediatric intestinal recipients had the highest 1- and 5-year patient survival rates at 89% and 81%, respectively, whereas adult liver-intestinal recipients had the lowest 1- and 5-year patient survival rates at 69% and 46%, respectively.

SUMMARY

Intestinal transplantation is a viable option for patients who suffer irreversible, life-threatening intestinal failure. The causes of intestinal failure vary greatly in the pediatric compared to the adult population. Evaluation of a patient who requires an intestinal transplantation is similar to the evaluation of other solid organ recipients, but a very clear picture of the patient's gastrointestinal tract and vascular system is essential. It is important to rule out whether the patient also has hepatic, pancreatic, or renal dysfunction that warrants more detailed investigation. There are several surgical options available to patients, including the isolated intestinal transplantation, the liver-intestinal transplantation, and the multivisceral transplantation. These operations can be complex and challenging with potential for significant medical and surgical postoperative complications. A systematic interprofessional approach is mandatory to manage these patients in the preoperative, intraoperative, and postoperative settings. Despite significant improvements in immunosuppressive therapy, acute rejection of the intestinal graft remains a significant complication. Greater attention has been given to the role of donor-specific antibodies and complement in causes of chronic allograft enteropathy and graft loss, and in potential noninvasive biomarkers to diagnose acute allograft rejection. Because intestinal recipients require increased immunosuppression to prevent rejection, they are at increased risk for bacterial, fungal, and viral infections. Multidrug-resistant bacteria, *Candida*, CMV, and EBV can particularly problematic in the postoperative period. The demographics of the intestinal transplants have changed significantly over the last decade with an increased age of recipient and frequency of isolated intestinal transplantations. With improved graft and patient survival after intestinal transplantation, it does seem counterintuitive that the numbers of intestinal transplantations have decreased over the last few years. With so few US centers performing pediatric or adult intestinal transplants, there could be issues of access to care and financial coverage of medical care/surgical procedures. In conclusion, intestinal transplantation is an attractive alternative option to long-term maintenance therapy with TPN. The future for intestinal transplantation will likely see improvements in surgical techniques and newer medications to treat rejection and infections, which translate into better graft and patient survival. Care of these patients in the critical perioperative period remains a crucial aspect of ensuring a successful outcome.

References

1. Abu-Elmagd KM, Costa G, Bond GJ, et al: Five hundred intestinal and multivisceral transplantations at a Single Center. *Ann Surg* 250(4):567–581, 2009.
2. Scotti-Foglieni C, Marino IR, Cillo U, et al. Human intestinal multivisceral transplantation. In: D'Amico DF, Bassi N, Tedeschi U, Cillo U, editors. *Liver Transplantation: Procedures and Management*. Paris: Masson Publishing Company; pp. 235–254, 1994.
3. Middleton SJ, Jamieson NV: The current status of small bowel transplantation in the UK and internationally. *Gut* 54:1650–1657, 2005.
4. Arruda Pecora RA, David AI, Lee AD, et al: Small bowel transplantation. *ABCD Arq Bras Cir Dig* 26(4):223–229, 2013.
5. Gondolesi GE, Almau HM: Intestinal transplantation outcomes. *Mt Sinai J Med* 79:246–255, 2012.
6. Moon J, Iyer K: Intestinal rehabilitation and transplantation for intestinal failure. *Mt Sinai J Med* 79:256–266, 2012.
7. Fishbein TM: Intestinal transplantation. *N Engl J Med* 361:998–1008, 2009.
8. Sudan D: The current state of intestinal transplantation: indications, techniques, outcomes and challenges. *Am J Transplant* 14:1976–1984, 2014.
9. Smith JM, Skeans MA, Horslen SP, et al: OPTN/SRTR 2013 annual data report: intestine. *Am J Transplant* 15 Suppl 2:1–16, 2015.
10. http://optn.transplant.hrsa.gov. Accessed on May 29, 2015.
11. CMS: Medicare national coverage determinations: intestinal and mutlivisceral transplantation, 2006. Available at www.cms.hhs.gov/transmittals/downloads /R58NCD.pdf. Accessed on May 29, 2015.
12. Diamanti A, Gambarara M, Marcellini M: Prevalence of liver complications in pediatric patients on home nutrition: indications for intestinal or combined liver-intestinal transplantation. *Transplant Proc* 35(8):3047–3049, 2003.
13. Mazariegos GV, Steffick DE, Horslen S, et al: Intestinal transplantation in the United States, 1999–2008. *Amer J Transplant* 10[Pt 2]:1020–1034, 2010.
14. Matarese LE: Nutrition interventions before and after adult intestinal transplantation: the Pittsburgh experience. *Pract Gastroenterol* 35(11):11–26, 2010.
15. Lauro A, Bagni C, Zanfi S, et al: Mortality after steroid-resistant acute cellular rejection and chronic rejection episodes in adult intestinal transplants: report from a single center in induction/preconditioning era. *Transplant Proc* 45:2032–2033, 2013.
16. Berger M, Zeevi A, Farmer DG, et al: Immunologic challenges in small bowel transplantation. *Amer J Transplant* 12:S2–S8, 2012.
17. Christians U, Klawitter J, Klawitter J, et al: Biomarkers of immunosuppressant organ toxicity after transplantation-status, concepts and misconceptions. *Expert Opin Drug Metab Toxicol* 7(2):175–200, 2011.
18. Hibi T, Nishida S, Garcia J, et al: Citrulline level is a potent indicator of acute rejection in long term following pediatric intestinal/multivisceral transplantation. *Amer J Transplant* 12:S27–S32, 2012.
19. Girlanda R, Cheema AK, Kaur P, et al: Metabolics of human intestinal transplant rejection. *Amer J Transplant* 12:S18–S26, 2012.
20. Green M, Michaels MG: Infections in pediatric solid organ transplant recipients. *J Pediatric Infect Dis Soc* 1(2):144–151, 2012.
21. Primeggia J, Matsumoto CS, Fishbein TM, et al: Infection among adult small bowel and multivisceral transplant recipients in the 30-day postoperative period. *Transpl Infect Dis* 15:441–448, 2013.
22. Florescu DF, Islam KM, Grant W, et al: Incidence and outcome of fungal infections in pediatric small bowel recipients. *Transpl Infect Dis* 12:497–504, 2010.
23. Grim SA, Clark NM: Management of infectious complications in solid-organ transplant recipients. *Clin Pharmacol Ther* 90(2):333–342, 2011.
24. Florescu DF, Langnas AN, Sandkowsky U: Opportunistic viral infections in intestinal transplantation. *Expert Rev Ant Infect Ther* 11:367–381, 2014.
25. Pironi L, Baxter JP, Lauro A, et al: Assessment of the quality of life on home parental nutrition and after intestinal transplantation using treatment-specific questionnaires. *Amer J Transplant* 12:S60–S66, 2012.

Chapter 63 ■ Immunosuppression in Solid-Organ Transplantation

MARTIN N. WIJKSTROM • SUNDARAM HARIHARAN • ABHINAV HUMAR

Solid-organ transplantation as routine clinical care required breakthroughs in our understanding of immunology and immunosuppressive therapy. Alexis Carrel, in the early 1900s provided the techniques required (vascular anastomosis); experimental transplants soon followed [1], but the first successful clinical transplant was not done until five decades later. During that interval, it gradually became apparent that early rapid destruction of allografts was due to an immune process, which came to be known as *rejection*.

Organ transplantation is now routine clinical care because results have improved remarkably with the use of more potent, effective, and targeted immunosuppressive agents. Besides the developments in techniques and immunosuppression protocols, progress in tissue typing and cross-matching, progress in organ preservation allowing for transportation of deceased donor organs, effective anti-viral medications, and tests including viral Nucleic acid amplification test (NAAT) testing for screening for viral infection and single-antigen beads for Human Leukocyte Antigen (HLA) antibody detection have played major roles in the development of organ transplantation. This chapter reviews the mechanisms of action, clinical evidence-based use, and the adverse reactions associated with commonly used immunosuppressive agents.

IMMUNOSUPPRESSIVE STRATEGIES

Immunosuppressive strategies must balance the risk of an acute rejection episode with its short- and long-term negative consequences on graft function and survival, the side effects of both long-term immunosuppression on infectious complications and the increased risk of cancers, as well as the individual side effects of the immunosuppressive agents. The relative importance of each factor may vary depending on the organ transplanted. For example, for kidney recipients, an acute rejection episode, possibly antibody-mediated rejection, is a major risk factor for chronic rejection; strategies focus on minimizing the incidence of acute rejection episodes. For liver recipients, an acute rejection episode is usually easily reversed and has little long-term significance; therefore, lower initial doses of immunosuppression can be used and then increased in those patients who suffer a rejection episode. Dialysis can provide backup organ function support if a kidney graft fails, whereas there is no recourse (other than a retransplant) for failure of many other solid-organ grafts. Therefore, particularly for heart and lung recipients, early aggressive immunosuppressive strategies are warranted.

Thus, no single approach applies uniformly across all organs to posttransplant immunosuppressive therapy. Immunosuppressive agents can be categorized according to their use: induction—those used for a limited interval at the time of transplant; maintenance—those used long term for maintenance of immunosuppression; and antirejection—those used for a short time or in high doses to reverse an acute rejection episode. Considerable overlap exists among these categories, however. For example, the monoclonal and polyclonal antibodies can be used for induction or rejection treatment; steroids are used in high doses for induction or antirejection therapy but in lower doses for maintenance therapy.

Finally, many transplant programs individualize immunosuppression depending on the perceived immunologic risk of rejection and graft loss for that recipient. For example, for kidney recipients, immunosuppressive protocols at a single center may vary for a perfectly matched living donor recipients, low-risk cadaver donor recipients, and high risk recipients (e.g., blacks, those with a high panel-reactive antibodies or delayed graft function, or retransplant recipients).

Induction

All recipients (except for identical-twin recipients or those fully chimeric following a bone marrow transplant from the same donor) require immunosuppressive therapy at the time of transplantation. Many transplant centers begin with the same immunosuppression that is used for long-term maintenance. Other centers begin using induction therapy with polyclonal (e.g., thymoglobulin, ATGAM) or monoclonal (e.g., basiliximab, alemtuzumab) antibodies. The purpose of induction immunosuppression is to provide powerful immunosuppression at the time of antigen exposure, with the goal of reduction of the overall incidence of rejection, and if needed, permit a delay in introducing other maintenance agents such as calcineurin inhibitors (CNIs; tacrolimus [TAC] and cyclosporine [CSA]) that may add to graft dysfunction. The frequency of acute rejection episodes is reduced with induction therapy; however, they are expensive, and a long-term benefit has not been well documented for low-risk recipients, although the risk for posttransplant proliferative disorder (PTLD) and viral infections are increased.

Maintenance Therapy

With the introduction of multiple new agents in the 1990s, immunosuppressive protocols have become more varied. At most centers, CNIs form the basis of immunosuppressive protocols. These drugs have been used as monotherapy and/or in combination with PRED or an antimetabolite. Prospective randomized trials have shown a lower incidence of acute rejection when mycophenolate mofetil (MMF) replaces azathioprine (AZA) in these combination protocols [2–4].

Of interest, CNI-free protocols have been devised. The major goal of such protocols is to avoid the nephrotoxicity associated with use of CNIs. The combination of sirolimus (SRL) and MMF has been used to achieve these results. Although nephrotoxicity can be avoided, relatively high doses of both drugs need to be used; as discussed previously, they each have their own side effects and is also associated with high incidence of acute rejection. In other randomized trials of CNI-free protocols, belatacept [5–7] and tofacitinib [8,9] have been used.

PHARMACOLOGIC AGENTS

Calcineurin Inhibitors

Cyclosporine and TAC, although structurally dissimilar, have a similar mechanism of action. Both drugs interfere with the cellular pathway for cytokine production and T-cell proliferation. The protein calcineurin has been validated as part of the calcium-dependent signal transduction pathway of interleukin-2 (IL-2) production in T cells [10]. CSA and TAC bind to two intracellular receptors, CypA and FKBP12, respectively; these receptors are found in virtually all cell types. The resulting receptor complex binds to calcineurin, blocking its phosphatase ability and thereby interrupting the production of IL-2 [10].

Cyclosporine

CSA was isolated from a soil sample in Norway and produced by the fungus *Tolypocladium inflatum*. The first formulation of CSA that was approved by the U.S. Food and Drug Administration (FDA) in 1983 was Sandimmune; this was modified to the microemulsion (ME) formulation called Neoral and was approved by the FDA in 1995.

CSA is a lipophilic decapeptide, consisting of several amino acids in a ring structure. The original oral formulation (Sandimmune) is dependent on the presence of bile in the upper small intestine, which makes it problematic for liver transplant recipients. Neoral self-emulsifies in water, making absorption much more reliable [11]. The side-effect profiles were unchanged. The oral bioavailability of the ME-CSA is approximately 30%. The average half-life of CSA ranges from 6 to 9 hours. It is extensively metabolized by the liver to multiple metabolites via the cytochrome P450 3A4 enzyme system. Significant liver impairment can slow the clearance of CSA by the body. Because very little drug is eliminated by the kidney, renal failure does not change CSA elimination [12].

The extensive side-effect profile of CSA has long been a reason for attempts at minimizing drug exposure. Of most concern is its acute and chronic nephrotoxicity. Acute nephrotoxicity from CSA is initially characterized by vasoconstriction of the intrarenal arterioles, resulting in a reduced glomerular filtration rate [13]. CSA-induced thrombotic microangiopathy (TMA) was first reported in liver allograft recipients and then in kidney and heart recipients [14]. TMA can present as a full-blown syndrome consisting of hemolytic anemia, thrombocytopenia, neurologic abnormalities, fever, and renal failure. Discontinuation of CSA is an important step in management along with plasmapheresis and fresh frozen plasma replacement. TAC or SRL can be substituted as immunosuppressive agents, although TMA can occur with either of these agents. Even in extrarenal transplant recipients, the effect of CSA on long-term kidney function can be significant, leading to proteinuria and end-stage renal disease (ESRD) [15]. Kidney biopsies of their native kidneys reveal wrinkling and thickening of the glomerular basement membrane, with some kidneys exhibiting microthrombotic angiopathy and fibrosis. Most patients receiving CSA develop hypertension, sometimes requiring multiple drug therapy. The mechanism for CSA-induced hypertension is primarily related to small-vessel vasoconstriction, in part by increased endothelin production. Treatment of hypertension has focused on calcium-channel blocker use because calcium-channel activation induces endothelin vasoconstriction and increases blood pressure. CSA has been associated with several neurologic toxicities, including headaches, tremors, seizures, and encephalopathy. Reversible posterior leukoencephalopathy can occur after CSA use and affects the posterior white matter and the frontal lobes and gray matter [16]. It manifests with confusion, coma, cortical blindness, cerebellar syndrome, hemiplegia, and flaccid paralysis or various combinations of these features. Hypertrichosis and gingival hyperplasia can reduce patient compliance to CSA. Electrolyte imbalances may occur with CSA, including hyperkalemia, hyperuricemia, and hypomagnesemia. CSA can increase cholesterol and triglyceride levels, sometimes requiring treatment with lipid-lowering medications [12].

CSA is metabolized by the cytochrome P450 3A4 enzyme system that is found not only in the liver but also in the cells lining the intestine; so CSA levels can be increased or decreased by changes in gut absorption or in liver metabolism [17]. Most centers initiate CSA therapy at 4 to 8 mg/kg/d orally, starting the day after transplant. If the transplanted kidney shows signs of delayed graft function (DGF), the initiation of CSA may be delayed. Monitoring CSA levels is vital because of its narrow therapeutic window.

Tacrolimus

With the success of CSA, researchers studied soil samples from around the world, looking for another compound that might turn out to display immunosuppressive properties. TAC, initially known as FK-506, was isolated from a soil sample in Tsukuba, Japan, in May 1984, from the fungus *Streptomyces tsukubaensis* [18] and was FDA approved in 1994. It has a completely different chemical structure from CSA, yet its effect on the lymphocyte is remarkably similar. A few differences have been found on the cellular level between CSA and TAC. The FKBP12-TAC complex is 10 to 100 times as potent as CSA, possibly because of greater affinity for its binding protein [19].

The pharmacokinetic profile of TAC is similar to that of CSA. TAC has an extremely lipophilic, macrocytic lactone structure. Its oral bioavailability ranges anywhere from 4% to 93% (average 25%). One significant difference between CSA and TAC is that with TAC the presence or absence of bile in the digestive tract does not significantly alter absorption. The metabolism is also similar to CSA, with the cytochrome P450 3A4 system as the primary metabolic pathway. The elimination half-life ranges from 8 to 20 hours, depending on the population studied [20].

The adverse event profile of TAC is similar to CSA in many respects. TAC appears to have the same nephrotoxicity seen with CSA, and the mechanism also appears to be the same. However, in one study, mean or median serum creatinine levels in renal transplant recipients were lower in TAC-treated patients, with 5-year follow-up, than in patients treated with CSA-ME [21]. As with CSA, the nephrotoxicity of TAC is concentration dependent, making drug level monitoring equally important [22]. Hypertension has also been reported with TAC. Immunosuppression with TAC-based regimens is associated with better lipid profiles than is immunosuppression with CSA-based regimens. Neurotoxicity appears to be somewhat worse than with CSA; headache, tremor, neuropathy, seizures, blindness, coma, and various other neurologic complaints have been seen with TAC [23]. Patients usually recover when the drug is stopped. The incidence of hyperkalemia appears to be similar to that with CSA, although hypomagnesemia is more likely to occur with TAC-treated patients [24]. TAC-associated TMA has a reported incidence between 1% and 4.7% [25]. The incidence of posttransplant diabetes mellitus (PTDM) was significantly higher among TAC-treated patients than among CSA-treated patients (9.8% vs. 2.7%) according to a meta-analysis [26]. Many patients with PTDM have reversal of diabetes mellitus, with eventual discontinuation of insulin. In a U.S. trial combining TAC with MMF and corticosteroids, the 10-year incidence was 6.5%, and the 1-year prevalence was 2.2% [27].

TAC is metabolized through the same pathway as CSA and has been subject to the same interactions with the cytochrome P450 3A4 system. As with CSA, careful blood concentration monitoring is required; TAC also has a narrow therapeutic range. The current suggested therapeutic range for TAC is 5 to 20 ng per mL; however, this range is still controversial and under study [19]. TAC is usually initiated at a dose of 0.05 to 0.10 mg/kg/d. Some centers, including ours, use a standard starting dose of 2 mg PO BID and adjust doses on the basis of subsequent trough levels. As with CSA, TAC may be delayed after a kidney transplant in the presence of DGF, especially under the cover of induction therapy.

In studies of TAC and CSA in kidney recipients, results have been similar to those with liver recipients (i.e., same graft and patient survival rates, fewer rejection episodes) [28]. This pattern has also been seen in higher-risk patient populations, such as black recipients [29]. Other transplant categories with historically higher rates of rejection, such as pancreas transplant recipients, have seen benefit with TAC-based immunosuppressive regimens [24]. TAC continues to be the primary maintenance immunosuppressive agent in heart, lung, and bowel recipients and was approved by the FDA for heart transplantation in 2006 [30–33].

Recently, two formulations of tacrolimus with daily administration were approved by the FDA. Astagraf XL, and extended-release capsule, was approved in 2013 for kidney transplant recipients also receiving Mycophenolate Mofetil (MMF) and prednisone (PRED). Envarsus XL was FDA approved in July 2015 for maintenance immunosuppression (IS) after conversion from once-daily tacrolimus. It is possible that extended-release formulations have improved side-effect profile and bioavailability [34]. Phase IV evaluation will further determine their impact on graft and patient survival.

Antiproliferative Agents

Antiproliferative agents have been part of transplant protocols since the first transplant was performed in the 1960s. Early antiproliferative agents included radiation, azaserine, actinomycin D, and cyclophosphamide. AZA, developed in the early 1960s, was part of the first successful transplant series reported in 1963. It continues to be used today in maintenance immunosuppressive regimens and for autoimmune diseases. A major advance in antiproliferative agents has been the development and use of MMF, released for clinical use in 1995. MMF is now a component of most new transplant regimens.

Azathioprine

AZA is a prodrug of 6-mercaptopurine, which interrupts the de novo purine synthesis, leading to inhibition of leukocyte function. It is rapidly absorbed after oral administration, and metabolized by xanthine oxidase and excreted into the kidneys. AZA is relatively well tolerated by most patients. The most common side effect is dose-dependent myelosuppression usually limited to the white blood cells, but occasionally red cell aplasia is observed. Liver function tests must be regularly monitored: AZA has been reported to cause hepatic necrosis and liver failure. Pancreatitis or a skin rash may indicate an allergic reaction, in which case AZA may need to be stopped. Hair loss is bothersome to some patients but is reversible. Gastrointestinal (GI) disturbances, including nausea and vomiting, are mild and usually tolerable. Most recipients are maintained on a daily dose of 1.0 to 2.5 mg per kg. Some centers switched all their recipients when MMF became available, but some are still maintained on AZA because of a significant cost advantage over MMF, or because of improved GI toxicity profile.

Mycophenolate Acid

MMF (CellCept) was approved by the FDA in 1995 to prevent rejection in kidney recipients. Its use has grown to include liver, heart, lung, and pancreas recipients. It has been a major addition to the immunosuppressive arsenal. MMF is also a prodrug, quickly metabolized to the active compound, mycophenolic acid (MPA). In 2004, Myfortic (EC-MPA) an enteric-coated formulation of MPA was FDA approved. MPA acts as a noncompetitive inhibitor of inosine monophosphate dehydrogenase, thereby blocking de novo purine synthesis [35]. The oral bioavailability for MPA approaches 100% and is primarily excreted in the urine.

MMF can cause significant GI problems, including nausea, vomiting, diarrhea, abdominal pain, and gastroesophageal reflux. Persistent diarrhea not accompanied by fever may be associated with an erosive enterocolitis causing malabsorption of nutrients that has been attributed to a toxic action of the acyl mycophenolic acid glucuronide (MPAG) metabolite on absorptive cells [36]. Dividing the total daily dose into four doses instead of two may be effective in reducing GI problems in some recipients. EC-MPA was developed to mitigate the GI toxicities; patients who had GI intolerance on MMF administration required fewer dose changes of EC-MPA [37]. Neutropenia and thrombocytopenia can also occur with MPA, requiring a dosage reduction. At 2 g daily, the occurrence rate in the major trials was comparable to AZA. Coadministration with CSA lowers MPA concentrations [38]. In contrast, coadministration with TAC tends to increase MPA levels because of inhibition of MPA metabolism [39]. Cholestyramine, a bile acid resin, decreases cholesterol by interfering with its enterohepatic cycling and decreases the total area under the curve (AUC) by 40%, and antacids reduce absorption of MMF by 20%.

The success of MPA has allowed it to generally replace AZA in many transplant centers. The results of three major trials were instrumental. The U.S., Tricontinental, and European trials compared MMF, in combination with CSA and steroids, with conventional immunosuppression. The U.S. and Tricontinental trials randomized patients to MMF at a low (2 g per day) or high dose (3 g per day) versus AZA, whereas the European study used a placebo instead of AZA [2–4]. All three trials saw significantly reduced rejection in the MMF arm at 6 months posttransplant. Whether long-term MMF changes survival rates is still controversial. The 3-year data from the U.S. trial periods do not yet show a statistically significant difference in patient or graft survival [2]. A European study using the ME-CSA showed only modest, insignificant reductions in acute rejection episodes with MMF compared with AZA, questioning the value of using the costlier MMF [40]. These findings, which are drawn on low-immunologic-risk patients, ought to be applied cautiously in other situations. A subgroup analysis of the higher immunologic-risk African American patients enrolled in the U.S. pivotal trial showed that the benefit for African American versus White recipients was restricted to the MMF 3 g dose versus the MMF 2 g dose or azathioprine cohorts [41]. Thus, African American recipients should receive 3 g per day unless they are unable to tolerate that dose. In a multicenter trial, using a combination of TAC with MMF, an MMF dose of 2 g per day reduced the incidence of acute rejection episodes compared with MMF 1 g per day or AZA—the low acute rejection rate of 8.6% using a combination with MMF 2 g per day suggest that a combination with TAC produced superior results compared with a combination with CSA [42]. EC-MPA was demonstrated to be therapeutically equivalent to MMF [43]. The combination of TAC and MMF is the most prevalent in the United States; in 2013, almost 95% of patients were maintained on this combination [44]. Based on initial pharmacokinetics studies, MMF doses have not been based on recipient body weight [45]. Determination of MPA levels is not clinical routine.

Sirolimus

Sirolimus (formerly known as rapamycin) belongs to a class of compounds known as the mammalian target of rapamycin (mTOR) inhibitors and was approved in 1999 to prevent rejection in kidney recipients. It is produced by *Streptomyces hygroscopicus*, a fungus isolated from a soil sample found on Easter Island (Rapa Nui). SRL was the first mTOR inhibitor to be approved in the United States. A derivative of rapamycin, everolimus, was approved by the FDA in 2004. SRL binds to FKBP-12, the same binding protein as TAC; however, the target of SRL is not calcineurin, but rather the target protein mTOR [46]. The inhibition of mTOR prevents cell-cycle progression from G1 to S in T lymphocytes; thus, SRL blocks the rejection pathway at a later stage than CSA or TAC [47]. It is rapidly absorbed, but the systemic bioavailability of the current formulation is only approximately 15%. The primary pathway for metabolism is the cytochrome P450 3A4 enzyme system. SRL has a much longer half-life than CSA or TAC, with an average terminal half-life of approximately 60 hours, allowing it to be dosed daily.

SRL has a different profile of adverse events than other immunosuppressive drugs. It is less kidney-toxic and diabetogenic than CSA or TAC. TMA may also occur [48]. Proteinuria is a common manifestation of SRL toxicity in patients converted from CNI for renal impairment. Preexisting renal damage may be necessary before proteinuria manifests, but it is reversible [49]. Hypertriglyceridemia and hypercholesterolemia are dose-related adverse events of SRL that may be exacerbated by the use of steroids or CNI [50]. Fifty-three percent of SRL-treated patients required lipid-lowering agents compared with 24% in the CSA group. SRL causes dose-dependent thrombocytopenia and leukopenia, particularly during initial therapy; their incidence is variable and usually self-limiting; usually only at supertherapeutic serum concentrations ≥16 ng per mL [51]. The incidence of anemia is also increased with the use of mTOR inhibitors and was observed in 16% of recipients taking 2 mg per day and 27% of recipients taking 5 mg per day of SRL [52]. During clinical trials, other adverse events associated with SRL included hypertension, rash, acne, hypokalemia, diarrhea, aphthous ulcers, and arthralgias [53]. Interstitial pneumonitis can occur any time after SRL treatment; mortality up to 12% has been described [54]. Other common adverse effects that occur with de novo SRL use in transplant recipients include wound-healing problems and lymphoceles [55]. Most of the drug interactions that have been reported for SRL are related to P450 enzyme inhibition or induction—the same list of drugs that interact with CSA and TAC. SRL, like TAC, also increases exposure to MPA.

The phase II trials conducted in Europe were among the earliest that used SRL as a principal immunosuppressant. Higher glomerular filtration rates and similar rejection rates were seen in patients receiving SRL as compared with CSA [56,57]. The two large phase III studies of SRL, one conducted in the United States [58] and the second worldwide [52], revealed much about how best to use SRL and its drawbacks: higher incidence of lymphocele formation and wound infections. It was also found that the renal function of patients on a combination of SRL and CSA was worse than patients on CSA alone. Regarding the combination of SRL with TAC, registry data suggest poorer graft survival compared with the combination of TAC with MMF [59]. Phase III studies indicated that the combination of either 1.5 mg per day or 3 mg per day of everolimus was better than MMF in the prevention of acute renal allograft rejection when combined with CSA and steroids after kidney transplantation. The combination of everolimus/CSA was associated with poorer renal function than MMF/CSA combination [60].

Inhibitors of mTOR are known to prevent tumor cell growth. Temsirolimus (and in some cases everolimus), both SRL derivatives, have been used in clinical trials of advanced renal carcinoma, breast cancer, prostate cancer, pancreatic cancer, glioblastoma, and lymphoma. A multivariate analysis of posttransplant malignancies in renal allograft recipients showed a lower incidence of malignancy in patients taking mTOR inhibitors alone or in combination with CNI compared with those taking CNI alone [61]. SRL has also been found to be effective in the treatment of posttransplant lymphoproliferative disorder (PTLD) [62] and Kaposi sarcoma [63]. It is also used to limit scarring on coronary stents. Because of its efficacy/side-effect profile, the clinical use of mTOR inhibitors has decreased from about 20% of kidney recipients in the early 2000s to about 5% of recipients at 1 year posttransplant [44]. Drug level monitoring is important, especially in newer protocols that may not contain CNI or steroids; target trough levels are between 5 and 15 ng per mL.

Corticosteroids

Steroids have been a part of transplantation since its inception. It soon became clear, however, that the toxicities of steroids could overshadow their benefits. The role of steroids in transplantation is changing, as experience is gained in the use of newer immunosuppressive medications that are serving to limit corticosteroid use. Steroids have many different effects on the immune system; they inhibit T-cell proliferation, T-cell–dependent immunity, and the expression of various cytokines, especially IL-2, IL-6, interferon-γ, and tumor necrosis factor-α (TNF-α) [64]. They also suppress antibody formation and the delayed hypersensitivity response found in allograft rejection [65].

For years, steroids have been part of any immunosuppressive regimen to prevent and treat rejection. For use in standard immunosuppression, recipients typically begin on a high initial dose (up to 500 mg IV of methylprednisolone [MP]) on the day of the transplant and then taper over weeks to months to their final maintenance dose. Some centers maintain recipients on 5 to 10 mg daily. Steroids at high doses have successfully reversed rejection episodes [66]. Most centers use 250 to 500 mg of IV MP for three (or more) doses to reverse a suspected or documented rejection episode. Steroid use is associated with a number of problems, acute and long-term, and typically dose-dependent. Acute toxicities of corticosteroids include sodium retention, glucose intolerance, mental status changes, and increase in appetite, acne, and gastritis. The long-term side effects include cataracts, hypertension, osteoporosis, and diabetes. Hypertension, hyperlipidemia, and steroid-induced diabetes may be partly responsible for increasing the risk of cardiovascular death in transplant recipients. Accordingly, many transplant centers are switching to steroid-withdrawal/steroid-free protocols for many of their recipients.

A meta-analysis of trials where steroid withdrawal had been done in the first year after kidney transplantation showed that although the risk of acute rejection was more than twofold when steroids were withdrawn, there was no significant difference in the incidence of graft failure [67]. The European TAC/MMF study group randomly assigned immunologically low-risk patients who had undergone transplantation 3 months earlier to continue triple therapy (TAC, MMF, and steroids), withdraw steroid, or withdraw MMF. Incidence of acute rejection was similar in all three groups at 6 months [68], suggesting TAC enables more effective steroid sparing than does CSA. Graft and patient survival and the incidence of acute rejection were similar between groups at 3 years, and serum creatinine levels remained stable [69]. A 3-year analysis of a large trial was done of 300 patients receiving basiliximab induction, CNI, and MMF or SRL in which patients were assigned to have steroids withdrawn on day 2 or to continue steroids. No difference was noted in graft function, patient and graft survival, biopsy-proven acute rejection, or chronic allograft nephropathy between the two groups [70]. Use of MMF or SRL, with a CNI, may allow safe early withdrawal of steroids.

BIOLOGIC IMMUNOSUPPRESSION

Various antibody preparations, both of polyclonal and monoclonal origin, are currently used in clinical immunosuppression. Polyclonal antibodies directed against lymphocytes were developed first and have been used in transplantation since the 1960s. The production of monoclonal antibodies was later made possible, and, in turn, allowed for the development of targeted therapy. A number of different monoclonal antibodies (mAbs) are currently under development or in various phases of clinical testing; several have been tested and are now in clinical use.

One disadvantage of early murine-based antibody preparations such as OKT3 is the potential for the development of antimouse antibodies by the recipient—antibodies that may then limit further use of the agent. To address this problem, recent efforts have focused on the development of so-called humanized versions of mAbs, either by replacing the murine constant portion (Fc) with a human Fc component, and/or by replacing the hypervariable region of the antibody that determines antigen specificity, thus in both instances creating a chimeric antibody. The remainder of the original murine antibody is replaced by human immunoglobulin G. The advantages of these humanized mAbs are a very long half-life, reduced immunogenicity, and the potential for indefinite and repeated use to confer effects over months rather than days [71]. Owing to their efficacy, biologic induction agents are currently used in about 85% of all kidney transplants in the United States [44].

Polyclonal Antibodies

Polyclonal preparations consist of a wide variety of antibodies and detect specificities including many T-cell molecules involved in antigen recognition. After administration, the transplant recipient's total lymphocyte count will fall, and hence these are known as depleting antibodies. Lymphocytes, especially T cells, are then lysed and cleared from the circulation. Alternatively, their surface antigen may be covered by the antibody. Polyclonal antibodies have been successfully used to prevent rejection and to treat acute rejection episodes. Two main polyclonal antibody agents are available for clinical use in the United States: ATGAM and thymoglobulin.

ATGAM

ATGAM is obtained by immunizing horses with human thymocytes. It is generally administered at a dose of 10 to 15 mg per kg, in a course lasting 7 to 14 days. ATGAM must generally be infused into a central vein because infusion into a peripheral vein is often associated with thrombophlebitis. To avoid the cytokine release syndrome, recipients should be premedicated with MP and diphenhydramine hydrochloride. Side effects include fever, chills, arthralgia, thrombocytopenia, leukopenia, and a serum sickness–like illness. These side effects are more likely related to the release of pyrogenic cytokines such as TNF-α, IL-1, and IL-6, which result from cell lysis due to antibody binding to targeted cellular surface receptors [72]. Increased infection rates are associated with all immunosuppressants, but certain infections, such as cytomegalovirus, are more common after the use of ATGAM and other antibody preparations [73].

Thymoglobulin

Thymoglobulin (ATG) is obtained by immunizing rabbits with human thymocytes. Initial kidney transplant studies show ATG to be statistically superior to ATGAM in preventing acute rejection episodes and in reversing acute rejection episodes [74,75]. Administration before reperfusion is advocated to maximize antiadhesion molecule effects. The side-effect profiles of ATG and ATGAM are similar. With ATG, leukopenia and thrombocytopenia may be quite significant. If a significant drop in platelets or white blood cells is noted, the dosage should be halved or the drug temporarily withheld.

Monoclonal Antibodies

The hybridization of murine antibody–secreting B lymphocytes with a nonsecreting myeloma cell line produces mAbs. A number of mAbs are active against different stages of the immune response.

OKT3

OKT3 was the first monoclonal to be approved by the FDA in 1986. In 2010, the producer, Janssen-Cilag Inc., announced its withdrawal because of lack of sales. The description herein, therefore, will be brief, but it warrants discussion owing to its historical importance. OKT3 binds to CD3 on T cells, and complement-mediated cell lysis and antibody-dependent cell cytotoxicity, leading to rapid clearance of T cells (~95%) from the peripheral circulation [71]. OKT3 was used to treat biopsy-proven acute rejections in patients with steroid-resistant acute rejection associated with vasculitis [76], and also as an induction agent. Human antimouse antibodies developed in at least 30% of patients, which rendered OKT3 ineffective, allowing for the reappearance of CD3+ T cells in the circulation. This scenario is more common with retreatment using OKT3 or with prolonged treatment. A marked cytokine release syndrome was the most common adverse effect. The most serious side effect was a rapidly developing, noncardiogenic pulmonary edema that could be life threatening. It was also associated with a wide spectrum of neurologic complications (headache, aseptic meningitis, and encephalopathy). Nephrotoxicity could also occur, as well as allograft thrombosis, infections (especially with cytomegalovirus), and PTLD.

Anti–Interleukin-2 Monoclonal Antibodies

IL-2 is a cytokine required for the proliferation of cytotoxic T cells. Two mAbs were developed to target the IL-2 receptor α-chain (IL-2Rα; CD25); daclizumab (Zenapax) was FDA approved in 1997, and basiliximab (Simulect) the following year. Daclizumab was withdrawn from clinical use in 2009, leaving basiliximab the only available agent for clinical use. Basiliximab is humanized (75% of the antibody is of human origin), the half-life of which is about 7 days.

Clinical trials in kidney recipients have shown these agents to be effective in preventing acute rejection [77], but it is not indicated for the treatment of acute rejection episodes. For basiliximab, two IV doses of 20 mg (one administered preoperatively and the other on postoperative day 4) are recommended. Comparable outcomes have been seen in studies comparing basiliximab and polyclonal antibodies and maintenance immunosuppression regimens consisting of CSA, MMF, and steroids [78]. Steroid-free maintenance regimens have also been used in kidney transplantation with anti-CD25 induction [79]. In all clinical trials to date, basiliximab has been shown to be remarkably safe, with minimal side effects ascribed directly to its use.

Alemtuzumab (Campath)

The CD52-specific humanized monoclonal antibody alemtuzumab has the advantages of ease of administration, consistency of monoclonal antibodies, and the benefits of humanization. Alemtuzumab rapidly and durably depletes CD52 expressing lymphocytes centrally and peripherally, resulting in near-total T-cell depletion with lesser depletion of B cells and monocytes [80]. It stopped from being commercially available for transplantation in September 2012, but remains available for appropriate patients via the producer (Genzyme). Alemtuzumab is currently being marketed as Lemtrada for the indication of multiple sclerosis.

Although alemtuzumab depletes all T-cell subsets, its action is selective for naive cell types [81]. The T cells that are not depleted exhibit a memory phenotype and are most susceptible to CNI. Maintenance regimens using CNI work best following alemtuzumab induction. Alemtuzumab facilitates reduced-maintenance immunosuppression requirements, without an increase in infections or malignant complications in kidney, pancreas, lung, and liver transplantations as compared with historical controls [82–86].

Rituximab (Humanized Anti-CD20)

This is a chimeric monoclonal antibody specific for CD20, a cell-surface glycoprotein present on B cells (from pre–B cells, but not on terminally differentiated B cells). Rituximab rapidly clears CD20+ cells from the circulation.

Rituximab has been used as an induction agent in lieu of recipient splenectomy in patients undergoing donor desensitization with plasmapheresis and/or intravenous immunoglobulin [87]. Use of rituximab in high-grade rejection remains investigational. Rituximab has a role in the treatment of Banff 2 and 3 rejection and in reducing antibody formations [88]. A recent review indicated the paucity of data supporting its use in transplantation [89].

The most important indication for the area of rituximab in organ transplantation is as treatment of PTLD, as part of R-CHOP chemotherapy.

Fusion Proteins

These are made by the fusion of a single receptor targeting a ligand of interest with a secondary molecule, which is typically the Fc portion of an IgG molecule. Fusion proteins can be composed of humanized components limiting their immune clearance and allowing prolonged administration.

Costimulation-Based Agents

Costimulatory molecules alter the threshold for activation of naive T lymphocytes without having a primary activating or inhibitory function. Fusion proteins have been developed that act by blocking costimulation pathways. The two costimulatory receptors on T cells are CD28 and CD152; these serve reciprocal roles—CD28 facilitates a T-cell response, whereas CD152 reduces it. The fusion proteins that act by inhibiting costimulation-based pathways, and have been studied in renal transplantation, inhibit CD28 and CD152 signaling, and this leads to immunosuppression.

Belatacept (investigative name LEA29Y) is a second-generation (first generation being Abatacept) costimulation-blockade agent that has two amino acid substitutions that give slower dissociation rate for binding to the ligands of CD28. The BENEFIT study reported the primary outcomes from a randomized, phase III study of belatacept versus CSA in kidney transplant recipients [5]. At 12 months, belatacept regimes demonstrated superior renal function and similar patient/graft survival versus CSA, despite an increase in acute rejection in the early posttransplant period. It has also been studies in recipients of extended criteria donor organs [6]. Belatacept is a promising, nonnephrotoxic option in kidney transplant recipients and is being developed with the aim of providing CNI avoidance [90]. It was tested as maintenance together with sirolimus (SIR) (attempted wean at 1 year) immunosuppression in low-risk patients with or without donor bone marrow and Campath induction [7]. The role of bone marrow was not established, but rejection was avoided, in this CNI-free regimen.

It is intended for use as an induction agent as well as for maintenance immunosuppression, but may have increased risk of acute rejection. Belatacept use has been limited owing to cost, monthly IV infusions, and high incidence of acute rejection, especially grade 2 and above.

OTHER IMMUNOSUPPRESSIVE AGENTS

Janus Kinase 3 Inhibitors

Janus kinase 3 (JAK3) is essential for the signal transduction from the cytokine receptors of several cytokines to the nucleus. Being expressed only on immune cell makes it an important target for developing new immunosuppressants. Several JAK3 inhibitors are available, but tofacitinib (CP-690550) is the most potent and selective JAK3 inhibitor. In vivo effects of tofacitinib include reduction in natural killer cell and T-cell numbers, although CD8+ effector memory T cells were unchanged [8]. A randomized, pilot study compared tofacitinib (15 mg BID [CP15] and 30 mg BID [CP30], $n = 20$ each) with TAC ($n = 21$) in de novo kidney transplant recipients [91]. Patients received an IL-2R antagonist, MMF, and steroids. Coadministration of tofacitinib 30 mg BID with MMF was associated with overimmunosuppression. At a dose of 15 mg BID, the efficacy/safety profile was comparable to TAC, although there was a higher rate of viral infection. A recent analysis of previous results demonstrated that patients with lower tofacitinib exposure maintained improved renal function, improved chronic changes on biopsy (IF/TA), and reduced biopsy-proven rejection than did the CSA group [9].

TABLE 63.1

Advances in Immunosuppression of Solid-Organ Transplantation

1. Major emphasis has been in the area of reduction of toxicities of immunosuppressive agents/combinations.
2. With the increasing use of tacrolimus, steroid-free protocols have been used successfully.
3. To circumvent nephrotoxicity of CNIs, several non-nephrotoxic agents like sirolimus, mycophenolate, belatacept, and JAK3 inhibitors have been developed. Use of IL-2 receptor blockers as induction therapy along with combination of nonnephrotoxic agents might one day lead to successful CNI-free immunosuppression.
4. Use of rituximab in the treatment of B-cell (CD20+)–mediated rejection (uncertain efficacy).

CNIs, calcineurin inhibitors; JAK3, janus kinase 3; IL-2, interleukin-2.

CONCLUSIONS

Since 1992, following the introduction of a number of new immunosuppressive agents, short-term graft and patient outcomes improved considerably. However, the side effect of immunosuppressive agents continues to present a major problem. With the increasing use of TAC, steroid-free protocols were used successfully. In kidney transplantation, long-term outcomes have been affected by the nephrotoxicity of CNI. In nonrenal transplant recipients, CNI toxicity has led to renal insufficiency and failure in a significant number of instances. Development of nonnephrotoxic agents like SRL, MMF, belatacept, and JAK3 inhibitors and their use in combination will someday lead to the successful use of CNI-free immunosuppression. A summary of some of the advances in the field of immunosuppression is shown in Table 63.1.

Another major advantage of the availability of several immunosuppressive agents is that immunosuppression can now be tailored for the individual patient. Those having drug-specific toxicity can be switched to another drug with similar efficacy but differing side effects.

ACKNOWLEDGMENT

We are grateful to Melissa Connell for assistance with organizing the manuscript.

References

1. Hamilton D: Kidney transplantation: a history, in Morris PJ, Knechtle S (eds): *Kidney Transplantation, Principles and Practice*. 6th ed. Philadelphia, PA, WB Saunders, 2008, pp 1–8.
2. US Renal Transplant Mycophenolate Mofetil Study Group: Mycophenolate mofetil in cadaveric renal transplantation. *Am J Kidney Dis* 34(2):296–303, 1999.

3. The Tricontinental Mycophenolate Mofetil Renal Transplantation Study Group: A blinded randomized clinical trial of mycophenolate mofetil for the prevention of acute rejection in cadaveric renal transplantation. *Transplantation* 61(7):1029–1037, 1996.
4. European Mycophenolate Mofetil Study Group: Placebo-controlled study of mycophenolate mofetil combined with cyclosporine and corticosteroids for prevention of acute rejection. *Lancet* 345(8961):1321–1325, 1995.
5. Vincenti F, Grinyo JM, Charpentier B, et al: Primary outcomes from a randomized, phase III study of belatacept vs cyclosporine in kidney transplant recipients (BENEFIT Study). *Am J Transplant* 9(S2):191, 2009.
6. Durrbach A, Pestana JM, Pearson T, et al: A phase III study of belatacept versus cyclosporine in kidney transplants from extended criteria donors (BENEFIT-EXT study). *Am J Transplant* 10(3):547–557, 2010.
7. Kirk AD, Guasch A, Xu H, et al: Renal transplantation using belatacept without maintenance steroids or calcineurin inhibitors. *Am J Transplant* 14(5):1142–1151, 2014.
8. Paniagua R, Si MS, Flores MG, et al: Effects of JAK3 inhibition with CP-690550 on immune cell populations and their functions in nonhuman primate recipients of kidney allografts. *Transplantation* 80:1283–1292, 2005.
9. Vicenti F, Silva HT, Busque S, et al: Evaluation of the effect of Tofacitinib exposure on outcomes in kidney transplant patients. *Am J Tranplant* 15(6):1644–1653, 2015.
10. Wiederrecht G, Lam E, Hung S, et al: The mechanism of action of FK-506 and cyclosporine A. *Ann N Y Acad Sci* 696:9–19, 1993.
11. Friman S, Backman L: A new microemulsion of cyclosporin. *Clin Pharmacokinet* 30(3):181–193, 1996.
12. Kahan B: Cyclosporine. *N Engl J Med* 321(25):1725–1737, 1989.
13. Morris ST, McMurray JJ, Roger RS, et al: Endothelial dysfunction in renal transplant recipients maintained on cyclosporine. *Kidney Int* 57:1100–1106, 2000.
14. Pham PTT, Peng A, Williamson AH, et al: Cyclosporine and tacrolimus-associated thrombotic microangiopathy. *Am J Kidney Dis* 36(4):844–850, 2000.
15. Griffith M, Crowe A, Papadaki L, et al: Cyclosporin nephrotoxicity in heart and lung transplant patients. *QJM* 89(10):751–763, 1996.
16. Jarosz JM, Howlett DC, Cox TCS, et al: Cyclosporine-related reversible posterior leukoencephalopathy: MRI. *Neuroradiology* 39:711–715, 1997.
17. Campana C, Regazzi M, Buggia I, et al: Clinically significant drug interactions with cyclosporin. *Clin Pharmacokinet* 30(2):141–179, 1996.
18. Goto T, Kino T, Hatanaka H, et al: FK 506: historical perspectives. *Transplant Proc* 23(6):2713–2717, 1991.
19. Scott LJ, McKeage K, Keown SJ, et al: Tacrolimus: a further update of its use in the management of organ transplantation. *Drugs* 63(12):1247–1297, 2003.
20. Venkataramanan R, Swaminathan A, Prasad T, et al: Clinical pharmacokinetics of tacrolimus. *Clin Pharmacokinet* 29(6):404–430, 1995.
21. Vincenti F, Jensik SC, Filo RS, et al: A long term comparison of tacrolimus (FK506) and cyclosporine in kidney transplantation: evidence for improved allograft survival at 5 years. *Transplantation* 73:775–782, 2002.
22. Shimizu T, Tanabe K, Tokumoto T, et al: Clinical and histological analysis of acute tacrolimus (TAC) nephrotoxicity in renal allografts. *Clin Transplant* 13[Suppl 1]:48–53, 1999.
23. A comparison of tacrolimus (FK 506) and cyclosporine for immunosuppression in liver transplantation. The U.S. Multicenter FK506 Liver Study Group. *N Engl J Med* 331(17):1110–1115, 1994.
24. Webster AC, Woodroffe RC, Taylor RS, et al: Tacrolimus versus ciclosporin as primary immunosuppression for kidney transplant recipients: meta-analysis and meta-regression of randomised trial data. *BMJ* 331:810, 2005.
25. Trimarchi HM, Truong LD, Brennan S, et al: FK 506-associated thrombotic microangiopathy: report of two cases and review of the literature. *Transplantation* 67:539–544, 1999.
26. Heisel O, Heisel R, Batshaw R, et al: New onset diabetes mellitus in patient receiving calcineurin inhibitors: a systematic review and meta-analysis. *Am J Transplant* 4:583–595, 2004.
27. Johnson C, Ahsan N, Gonwa T, et al: Randomized trial of tacrolimus (Prograf) in combination with azathioprine or mycophenolate mofetil versus cyclosporine (Neoral) with mycophenolate mofetil after cadaveric kidney transplantation. *Transplantation* 69:834–841, 2000.
28. Pirsch JD, Miller J, Deierhoi MH, et al: For the FK506 kidney transplant study group: a comparison of tacrolimus (FK506) and cyclosporine for immunosuppression after cadaveric kidney transplantation. *Transplantation* 63:977–983, 1997.
29. Foster CE, Philosophe B, Schweitzer EJ, et al: A decade of experience with renal transplantation in African Americans. *Ann Surg* 236:794–804, 2002.
30. Sutherland DR, Gruessner RWG, Dunn DL, et al: Lessons learned from more than 1000 pancreas transplants at a single institution. *Ann Surg* 233: 463–501, 2001.
31. Meiser BM, Pfeiffer M, Schmidt D, et al: Combination therapy with tacrolimus and mycophenolate mofetil following cardiac transplantation: importance of mycophenolic acid therapeutic drug monitoring. *J Heart Lung Transplant* 18:143–149, 1999.
32. Kur F, Reichenspiner H, Meiser BM, et al: Tacrolimus (FK506) as primary immunosuppressant after lung transplantation. *Thorac Cardiovas Surg* 47:174–178, 1999.
33. Thompson JS: Intestinal transplantation: experience in the United States. *Eur J Pediatric Surg* 9:271–273, 1999.
34. Garnock-Jones KP: Tacrolimus prolonged release (Envarsus®): a review of its use in kidney and liver transplant recipients. *Drugs* 75(3):309–320, 2015.
35. Fulton B, Markham A: Mycophenolate mofetil. *Drugs* 51(2):278–298, 1996.
36. Shipkova M, Armstrong VW, Oellerich M, et al: Acyl glucuronide drug metabolites: toxicological and analytical implications. *Ther Drug Monit* 25:1–16, 2003.
37. Chan L, Mulgaonkar S, Walker R, et al: Patient-reported gastrointestinal symptoms burden and health-related quality of life following conversion from mycophenolate mofetil to enteric-coated mycophenolate sodium. *Transplantation* 81:1290–1297, 2006.
38. Gregoor PJ, de Sevaux RG, Hene RJ, et al: Effect of cyclosporine on mycophenolate acid trough levels in kidney transplant recipients. *Transplantation* 68:1603–1606, 1999.
39. Zucker K, Tsaroucha A, Olson L, et al: Evidence that tacrolimus augments the bioavailability of mycophenolate mofetil through the inhibition of mycophenolic acid glucuronidation. *Ther Drug Monit* 21(1):35–43, 1999.
40. Remuzzi G, Lesti M, Gotti E, et al: Mycophenolate mofetil versus azathioprine for prevention of acute rejection in renal transplantation (MYSS): a randomized trial. *Lancet* 364:503–512, 2004.
41. Neylan J: Immunosuppressive therapy in high-risk transplant patients: dose-dependent efficacy of mycophenolate mofetil in African-American renal allograft recipients. U.S. Renal Transplant Mycophenolate Mofetil Study Group. *Transplantation* 64(9):1277–1282, 1997.
42. Miller J, Mendez R, Pirsch JD, et al: Safety and efficacy of tacrolimus in combination with mycophenolate mofetil (MMF) in cadaveric renal transplant patients. FK506/MMF dose-ranging Kidney Transplant Study Group. *Transplantation* 69:875–880, 2000.
43. Salvadori M, Holzer H, de Mattos, et al; ERL B301 Study Groups: Enteric-coated mycophenolate sodium is therapeutically equivalent to mycophenolate mofetil in de novo renal transplant patients. *Am J Transplant* 4(2):237–243, 2004.
44. Matas AJ, Smith JM, Skeans MA, et al: OPTN/SRTR 2013 Annual Data Report: kidney. *Am J Transplant* 15(S2):1–34, 2015.
45. Pescovitz M, Conti D, Dunn J, et al: Intravenous mycophenolate mofetil: safety, tolerability and pharmacokinetics. *Clin Transplant* 14(3):179–188, 2000.
46. Heitman J, Movva NR, Hall MN: Targets for cell cycle arrest by the immunosuppressant rapamycin in yeast. *Science* 253:905–909, 1991.
47. Sehgal S: Rapamune (RAPA, rapamycin, sirolimus): mechanism of action immunosuppressive effect results from blockade of signal transduction and inhibition of cell cycle progression. *Clin Biochem* 31(5):335–340, 1998.
48. Sartelet H, Toupance O, Lorenzato M, et al: Sirolimus-induced thrombotic microangiopathy is associated with decreased expression of vascular endothelial growth factor in kidneys. *Am J Transplant* 5:2441–2447, 2005.
49. Dittrich E, Schmaldienst S, Soleiman A, et al: Rapamycin-associated post-transplantation glomerulonephritis and its remission after reintroduction of calcineurin-inhibitor therapy. *Transpl Int* 17:215–220, 2004.
50. Kahan B, Napoli K, Kelly P, et al: Therapeutic drug monitoring of sirolimus: correlations with efficacy and toxicity. *Clin Transplant* 14(2):97–109, 2000.
51. Hong J, Kahan B: Sirolimus-induced thrombocytopenia and leukopenia in renal transplant recipients: risk factors, incidence, progression, and management. *Transplantation* 69(10):2085–2090, 2000.
52. MacDonald AS, for the Rapamune Global Study Group (RGS): A worldwide, phase III, randomized, controlled, safety and efficacy study of a sirolimus /cyclosporine regimen for prevention of acute rejection in recipients of primary mismatched renal allografts. *Transplantation* 71(2):271–280, 2001.
53. Anonymous: Rapamune oral solution. Product information. Philadelphia, PA, Wyeth-Ayerst Pharmaceuticals, 1999.
54. Singer S, Tiernan R, Sullivan E: Interstitial pneumonitis associated with sirolimus therapy in renal-transplant recipients. *N Engl J Med* 343(24): 1815–1816, 2000.
55. Tiong HY, Flechner SM, Zhou L, et al: A systemic approach to minimizing wound problems for de novo sirolimus-treated kidney transplant recipients. *Transplantation* 87:296–302, 2009.
56. Morales JM, Wramner L, Kreis H, et al: Sirolimus does not exhibit nephrotoxicity compared to cyclosporine in renal transplant recipients. *Am J Transplant* 2(5):436–442, 2002.
57. Webster AC, Lee VW, Chapman JR, et al: Target of rapamycin inhibitors (sirolimus and everolimus) for primary immunosuppression of kidney transplant recipients: a systematic review and meta-analysis of randomized trials. *Transplantation* 81(9):1234–1248, 2006.
58. Kahan BD: Efficacy of sirolimus compared with azathioprine for reduction of acute renal allograft rejection: a randomized multicenter study. *Lancet* 356:194–202, 2000.
59. Meier-Kriesche HU, Schold JD, Srinivas TR, et al: Sirolimus in combination with tacrolimus is associated with worse renal allograft survival compared to mycophenolate mofetil combined with tacrolimus. *Am J Transplant* 5(9):2273–2280, 2005.
60. Lorber MI, Mulgaonkar S, Butt KMH, et al: Everolimus versus mycophenolate mofetil in the prevention of rejection in de novo renal transplant recipients: a 3-year randomized, multicenter, phase III study. *Transplantation* 80(2):244–252, 2005.
61. Kauffman HM, Cherikh WS, Cheng Y, et al: Maintenance immunosuppression with target-of-rapamycin inhibitors is associated with a reduced incidence of de novo malignancies. *Transplantation* 80(7):883–889, 2005.
62. Cullis B, D'Souza R, McCullagh P, et al: Sirolimus-induced remission of posttransplantation lymphoproliferative disorder. *Am J Kidney Dis* 47(5):e67–e72, 2006.
63. Stallone G, Schena A, Infante B, et al: Sirolimus for Kaposi's sarcoma in renal-transplant recipients. *N Eng J Med* 352:1317–1323, 2005.
64. Suthanthiran M, Strom T: Renal transplantation. *N Engl J Med* 331(6): 365–376, 1994.

65. Popowniak K, Nakamoto S: Immunosuppressive therapy in renal transplantation. *Surg Clin North Am* 51(5):1191–1204, 1971.
66. Alarcon-Zurita A, Ladefoged J: Treatment of acute allograft rejection with high doses of corticosteroids. *Kidney Int* 9(4):351–354, 1976.
67. Pascual J, Quereda C, Zamora J, et al: Steroid withdrawal in renal transplant patients on triple therapy with a calcineurin inhibitor and mycophenolate mofetil: a meta-analysis of randomized, controlled trials. *Transplantation* 78(10):1548–1556, 2004.
68. Vanrenterghem Y, van Hooff JP, Squifflet JP, et al: Minimization of immunosuppressive therapy after renal transplantation: results of a randomized controlled trial. *Am J Transplant* 5(1):87–95, 2005.
69. Pascual J, van Hooff JP, Salmela K, et al: Three-year observational follow-up of a multicenter, randomized trial on tacrolimus-based therapy with withdrawal of steroids or mycophenolate mofetil after renal transplant. *Transplantation* 82(1):55–61, 2006.
70. Kumar MS, Heifets M, Moritz M, et al: Safety and efficacy of steroid withdrawal two days after kidney transplantation: analysis of results at three years. *Transplantation* 81(6):832–839, 2006.
71. Webster A, Pankhurst T, Rinaldi F, et al: Polyclonal and monoclonal antibodies for treating acute rejection episodes in kidney transplant recipients. *Cochrane Database Syst Rev* 19:CD004756, 2006.
72. Vallhonrat H, Williams WW, Cosimi AB, et al: In vivo generation of 4d, Bb, iC3b, and SC5b-9 after OKT3 administration in kidney and lung transplant recipients. *Transplantation* 67(2):253–259, 1999.
73. Jamil B, Nicholls KM, Becker GJ, et al: Influence of anti-rejection therapy on the timing of cytomegalovirus disease and other infections in renal transplant recipients. *Clin Transplant* 14(1):14–18, 2000.
74. Brennan DC, Flavin K, Lowell JA, et al: A randomized, double-blinded comparison of Thymoglobulin versus Atgam for induction immunosuppressive therapy in adult renal transplant recipients. *Transplantation* 67(7):1011–1018, 1999.
75. Gaber AO, First MR, Tesi RJ, et al: Results of the double-blind, randomized, multicenter, phase III clinical trial of Thymoglobulin versus Atgam in the treatment of acute graft rejection episodes after renal transplantation. *Transplantation* 66(1):29–37, 1998.
76. Kamath S, Dean D, Peddi VR, et al: Efficacy of OKT3 as primary therapy for histologically confirmed acute renal allograft rejection. *Transplantation* 64(10):1428–1432, 1997.
77. Thistlethwaite JR Jr, Nashan B, Hall M, et al: Reduced acute rejection and superior 1-year renal allograft survival with basiliximab in patients with diabetes mellitus. The Global Simulect Study Group. *Transplantation* 70(5):784–790, 2000.
78. Sollinger H, Kaplan B, Pescovitz M, et al: Basiliximab versus antithymocyte globulin for prevention of acute renal allograft rejection. *Transplantation* 72(12):1915–1919, 2001.
79. Rostaing L, Cantarovich D, Mourad G, et al: Corticosteroid-free immunosuppression with tacrolimus, mycophenolate mofetil, and daclizumab induction in renal transplantation. *Transplantation* 79(7):807–814, 2005.
80. Kirk AD, Hale DA, Mannon RB, et al: Results from a human renal allograft tolerance trial evaluating the humanized CD52-specific monoclonal antibody alemtuzumab (CAMPATH-1 H). *Transplantation* 76(1):120–129, 2003.
81. Pearl JP, Parris J, Hale DA, et al: Immunocompetent T-cells with a memory-like phenotype are the dominant cell type following antibody-mediated T-cell depletion. *Am J Transplant* 5:465–474, 2005.
82. Bartosh SM, Knechtle SJ, Sollinger HW: Campath 1-H use in pediatric renal transplantation. *Am J Transplant* 5:1569, 2005.
83. Gruessner RW, Kandaswamy R, Humar A, et al: Calcineurin inhibitor-and steroid-free immunosuppression in pancreas-kidney and solitary pancreas transplantation. *Transplantation* 79:1184–1189, 2005.
84. Kaufman DB, Leventhal JR, Gallon LG, et al: Alemtuzumab induction and prednisone-free maintenance immunotherapy in simultaneous pancreas-kidney transplantation comparison with rabbit antithymocyte globulin induction—long-term results. *Am J Transplant* 6:331–339, 2006.
85. McCurry KR, Iacono A, Zeevi A, et al: Early outcomes in human lung transplantation with Thymoglobulin or Campath-1 H for recipient pretreatment followed by posttransplant tacrolimus near-monotherapy. *J Thorac Cardiovasc Surg* 130:528–537, 2005.
86. Tzakis AG, Tryphonopoulos P, Kato T, et al: Preliminary experience with alemtuzumab (Campath-1H) and low-dose tacrolimus immunosuppression in adult liver transplantation. *Transplantation* 77:1209–1214, 2004.
87. Tydén G, Kumlien G, Genberg H, et al: ABO incompatible kidney transplantations without splenectomy, using antigen-specific immunoadsorption and rituximab. *Am J Transplant* 5:145–148, 2005.
88. Becker YT, Samaniego-Picota M, Sollinger HW, et al: The emerging role of rituximab in organ transplantation. *Transpl Int* 19:621–628, 2006.
89. Macklin PS, Morris PJ, Knight SR: A systematic review of the use of rituximab as induction therapy in renal transplantation. *Transplant Rev (Orlando)* 29(2):103–108, 2015. doi:10.1016/j.trre.2014.12.001.
90. Vincenti F, Larsen C, Durrbach A, et al: Costimulation blockade with belatacept in renal transplantation. *N Eng J Med* 353:770–781, 2005.
91. Busque S, Leventhal J, Brennan DC, et al: Calcineurin-inhibitor-free immunosuppression based on the JAK inhibitor CP-690550: a pilot study in de novo kidney allograft recipients. *Am J Transplant* 9:1936–1945, 2009.

Chapter 64 ■ Hematopoietic Cell Transplantation

ANN E. WOOLFREY • MARCO MIELCAREK • PAUL A. CARPENTER

GENERAL PRINCIPLES

Hematopoietic cell transplantation (HCT) is typically performed in patients with life-threatening disorders of the hematopoietic system. The procedure has considerable risks of transplant-related morbidity and mortality with a substantial proportion of patients requiring intensive medical care [1–3]. Thus, knowledge of the basic principles of the transplant procedure and an understanding of potential complications including their differential diagnosis are important for improving the outcomes of critically ill patients after transplantation.

HCT is potentially curative treatment for diseases including leukemia, lymphoma, myelodysplasia, multiple myeloma, aplastic anemia, hemoglobinopathies, and congenital immune deficiencies. In selected cases, HCT may also have a role in the treatment of solid tumors such as germ cell tumors, renal cell cancer, and breast cancer, and as a type of immunosuppression for patients with life-threatening autoimmune diseases (Table 64.1). In preparation for HCT, chemotherapy alone, or combined with irradiation therapy, is used to eradicate the underlying disease and to induce transient immunosuppression in the recipient to prevent graft rejection, a possible complication mediated by immunological host-versus-graft reactions after allogeneic HCT. Chemoradiation is followed by intravenous infusion of the graft, which contains hematopoietic stem cells (HSC) that home to the bone marrow and reconstitute the hematopoietic system of the patient. In contrast to autologous HCT, allogeneic HCT requires prophylactic immunosuppressive therapy after transplant to prevent or mitigate graft-versus-host disease (GVHD), an inflammatory syndrome that primarily affects the skin, gastrointestinal (GI) tract, and liver.

Classification

HCT can be categorized according to the source of stem cells, the type of donor, or the intensity of the preparative regimen. The type of HCT used in an individual patient is a complex decision based on the patient's age, diagnosis, disease stage, prior treatments, donor availability, and presence of comorbidities.

Stem Cell Source

HSCs capable of reconstituting hematopoiesis after HCT can be obtained from bone marrow, peripheral blood, or umbilical cord blood (UCB). The stem cell products obtained from each of these sources are characterized by distinct kinetics of engraftment and

TABLE 64.1

Indications for Allogeneic or Autologous Transplants

Allogeneic	Autologous
High-risk acute leukemia	High-risk lymphoma
Acute myeloid leukemia	Non-Hodgkin lymphoma
Acute lymphoblastic leukemia	Hodgkin lymphoma
Chronic leukemia	Multiple myeloma
Chronic myeloid leukemia	Solid tumors
Chronic lymphocytic leukemia	Neuroblastoma
Juvenile myelomonocytic leukemia	Poor-risk breast cancer
Chronic myelomonocytic leukemia	Poor-risk sarcoma
Myelodysplastic syndromes	Refractory autoimmune disorders
Bone marrow failure syndromes	
Severe aplastic anemia	
Severe immunodeficiency syndromes	
Inborn errors of metabolism	
Hemoglobinopathies	
Thalassemia major	
Symptomatic sickle cell disease	

recovery of immune function after transplantation. These features may affect the risks of developing infectious complications and GVHD during the posttransplant period.

Bone Marrow. Bone marrow was historically the most common source of stem cells for HCT but is now used very infrequently for autologous HCT. Bone marrow is harvested from the iliac crest under general anesthesia, from appropriate volunteer donors. Engraftment after bone marrow transplant is evidenced by rising neutrophil and platelet counts and occurs between 3 and 4 weeks after transplant.

"Mobilized" Peripheral Blood. Growth factor–mobilized peripheral blood stem cells (PBSCs) are the predominant source of HSC for allogeneic HCT in adults and are almost always used as HSC rescue for autologous HCT [4]. Engraftment after PBSC transplantation occurs approximately 1 week earlier compared with bone marrow transplantation. PBSC allografts contain approximately 10 times more T cells than do marrow, which influences the development of GVHD, graft rejection, and rate of relapse for malignancies after HCT. Randomized studies have shown a higher risk for relapse and lower risk for chronic GVHD among recipients of marrow compared with PBSC [5,6].

Umbilical Cord Blood. UCB contains HSC sufficient for reconstitution of hematopoiesis, which can be collected from the placenta and umbilical cord immediately after delivery of a baby. T cells contained in UCB are immunologically naive, which allows for less stringent human leukocyte antigen (HLA) matching between donor and recipient. There generally are smaller numbers of HSC in a typical UCB unit compared with bone marrow or PBSC harvest, which may increase the possibility for delayed engraftment, graft rejection, or infection [7,8]. The infusion of two UCB units appears to mitigate the risk for graft rejection, in part by increasing the total number of HSC delivered to the patient [9].

Donor Type

Autologous. Transplantation of HSC donated by the patient is termed *autologous HCT*. Most commonly, autologous PBSC are cryopreserved and then thawed and reinfused once the high-dose preparative therapy has been completed. High-dose chemoradiation is given to kill tumor cells that may not be susceptible to conventional-dose cytotoxic therapy. The success of the autologous transplant procedures relies exclusively on the tumor-eradicating potential of the preparative regimen [10]. The effect the conditioning regimen has on extrahematopoietic tissues determines the dose-limiting toxicity of the procedure. Relapse after autologous HCT may occur from tumor cells that have survived the conditioning therapy or from those that contaminated the graft, although the former mechanism appears to be more important.

Syngeneic. Transplantation of HSCs donated from identical (monozygotic) twins is termed *syngeneic HCT*. When there is no genetic disparity between donor and recipient, the biology of the transplant is similar to autologous HCT. Compared with allogeneic HCT from HLA-matched related or unrelated donors, relapse rates are higher after syngeneic HCT, which has been attributed to the absence of graft-versus-leukemia reactions.

Allogeneic. Transplantation of HSCs cells donated by another individual is termed *allogeneic HCT*. Allogeneic HCT requires availability of an HLA-compatible related or unrelated donor. Because of the inheritance pattern of HLA haplotypes, the statistical likelihood of two siblings being genotypically HLA identical is 25%. Donor-recipient HLA genotypic identity is associated with the lowest risks for immunologically mediated complications such as graft rejection and GVHD. For patients who do not have an HLA-identical sibling donor, approximately 70% of all patients, a search for a suitable unrelated donor can be considered. HCT from HLA-matched unrelated donors, however, has traditionally been associated with higher risks of transplant-related morbidity and mortality compared with HCT from HLA-identical related donors [11]. Use of unrelated donors who are matched using molecular HLA typing methods can improve outcomes considerably, and, for some diseases, survival of patients with unrelated grafts has approached that with HLA-identical sibling grafts [12,13]. Another alternative source of HSC is a haploidentical relative, such as a parent or child, defined by the inheritance of one identical haplotype and mismatching of one or more HLA loci with the noninherited haplotype. Over the past decade, technological advances have improved the outcome for recipients of HLA-disparate grafts. When more than a single HLA antigen disparity is present, depletion of T cells from the graft is necessary to prevent life-threatening GVHD. Depletion of T cells from the graft may be accomplished *ex vivo* by using immunologic or physical methods to separate HSC from T cells, or *in vivo* by administering cyclophosphamide 3 to 4 days after the transplant [14,15]. Because T cells play an important role in establishment of the graft, early immune reconstitution, and tumor control, T-cell depletion has been associated with higher rates of graft failure, opportunistic infections, and relapse.

Intensity of the Preparative Regimen

Myeloablative. In myeloablative HCT, the preparative regimen ablates the hematopoietic system of the patient and leads to profound myelosuppression with pancytopenia. The transplanted HSC reconstitute the ablated hematopoietic system in the recipient. High-dose chemotherapy regimens, with or without doses of total body irradiation (TBI) that exceed 6 gray (Gy), combine different drug combinations that have nonadditive toxicities with radiation. The aim of high-dose therapy is to overcome the genetic heterogeneity of tumors by employing agents with different mechanisms of action. Although the myeloablative regimens used for autologous HCT typically consist of drugs that provide maximum tumor eradication with tolerable toxicity to the patient, regimens used for allogeneic HCT also must provide sufficient recipient immunosuppression to prevent graft rejection. Myeloablative preparative regimens are associated with substantial risks of transplant-related toxicity and mortality, particularly among older or medically ill patients [16]. Over the past decade, several "reduced-intensity conditioning" (RIC) regimens have been developed that combine lower doses of traditional conditioning agents or substitute less toxic agents, resulting in fewer complications after HCT, although in advanced leukemia the trade-off may be a greater rate of post-HCT relapse [17].

Nonmyeloablative. Nonmyeloablative preparative regimens for allogeneic HCT are mainly immunosuppressive and aimed at preventing graft rejection. The underlying malignancy is eliminated through the ensuing immunologic graft-versus-tumor effects, provided the tumor expresses antigens that make it a target for immune attack. Compared with myeloablative allogeneic HCT, the extrahematopoietic toxicity from nonmyeloablative preparative regimens is considerably milder, an important consideration for older patients or those with comorbidities [18]. Typical post-HCT complications such as GVHD and infections, however, are not prevented by nonmyeloablative conditioning but may have a delayed onset. Not only are RIC regimens highly immunosuppressive, but they also include agents that have marrow-suppressive effects. RIC regimens are generally associated with less morbidity and mortality compared with myeloablative regimens, yet may have greater antitumor effect compared with nonmyeloablative regimens.

Epidemiology

During 2013 more than 21,000 HCT procedures were registered with the Center for International Blood and Marrow Transplant Research (CIBMTR), of which approximately 40% were allogeneic. Allogeneic HCT is most commonly performed in adults using PBSC grafts. In contrast, children now predominantly receive cord blood or marrow grafts (NMDP website: http://www.marrow.org/). PBSC is less used in children because of the difficulties harvesting PBSC from young children and because of the increased risk of chronic GVHD.

Risk Factors for Transplant-Related Morbidity and Mortality

The likelihood of developing transplant-related complications depends on patient age, the intensity of the preparative regimen, the type and stage of the underlying disease, and the presence of comorbidities. Prognosis is most heavily influenced by the underlying disorder. Patients with chronic malignancies and nonmalignant disorders, such as aplastic anemia, have a higher likelihood of survival compared with those with aggressive malignancies, who have a greater tendency to relapse following HCT. Mortality caused by the transplant procedure, and not from disease relapse, termed *transplant-related mortality*, ranges from 15% to 40% for allogeneic HCT recipients compared with 5% to 10% for autologous HCT recipients. HLA disparity between donor and recipient increases the risk of transplant-related mortality owing to the greater likelihood of developing GVHD and graft rejection [13]. The risk for mortality increases significantly with age, although improvements in supportive care and donor selection and the introduction of nonmyeloablative preparative regimens have increased the proportion of patients older than 60 years who benefit from allogeneic HCT. Recent studies have demonstrated that pretransplant assessment of comorbidities using simple but transplant-specific comorbidity scoring systems has improved the ability to predict subsequent transplant-related mortality and survival [16,19].

TRANSPLANT-RELATED COMPLICATIONS

Transplant-related complications include infections, regimen-related toxicity, and alloimmune-mediated graft rejection and GVHD (Fig. 64.1). More intense conditioning regimens and higher degrees of donor-recipient HLA disparity are associated with greater risk for infection. Regimen-related toxicities include profound cytopenias and organ damage that follow myeloablative conditioning. The complications seen after allogeneic HCT that may occur irrespective of the intensity of the conditioning regimen include rejection, GVHD, and hemolysis.

Regimen-Related Pancytopenia

Reconstitution of hematopoiesis after HCT occurs in an orderly pattern; in general, neutrophil recovery occurs first, followed by recovery of platelets and red blood cells (RBCs). The tempo of hematopoietic reconstitution varies according to the type of HSC product, being earlier after PBSC grafts and later after UCB grafts, compared with marrow grafts. Transfusions of platelets and RBCs often are needed until there is marrow recovery. Transfusion of RBCs should be determined by the clinical condition of the patient, including hemodynamic stability and presence of active hemorrhage. RBC transfusions generally are indicated when the hemoglobin falls below 8 g per dL. Platelet transfusions are indicated when the platelet count falls below 10,000 cells per μL to minimize the risk for spontaneous bleeding [20]. Transfusions thresholds should be increased before invasive procedures or in patients with bleeding to a level appropriate for any other intensive care unit patient. Platelet consumption may be increased in patients with fever, disseminated intravascular coagulation (DIC), sinusoidal obstruction syndrome (SOS), or splenomegaly. Patients who have become alloimmunized to platelet antigens demonstrate poor response to platelet transfusions and may achieve higher platelet counts by limiting the number of donor exposures, controlling fever or DIC, or use of nonpooled (single-donor) or HLA-matched platelets [21].

Precautions should be taken in preparation of blood products for transfusion into HCT patients because passenger lymphocytes

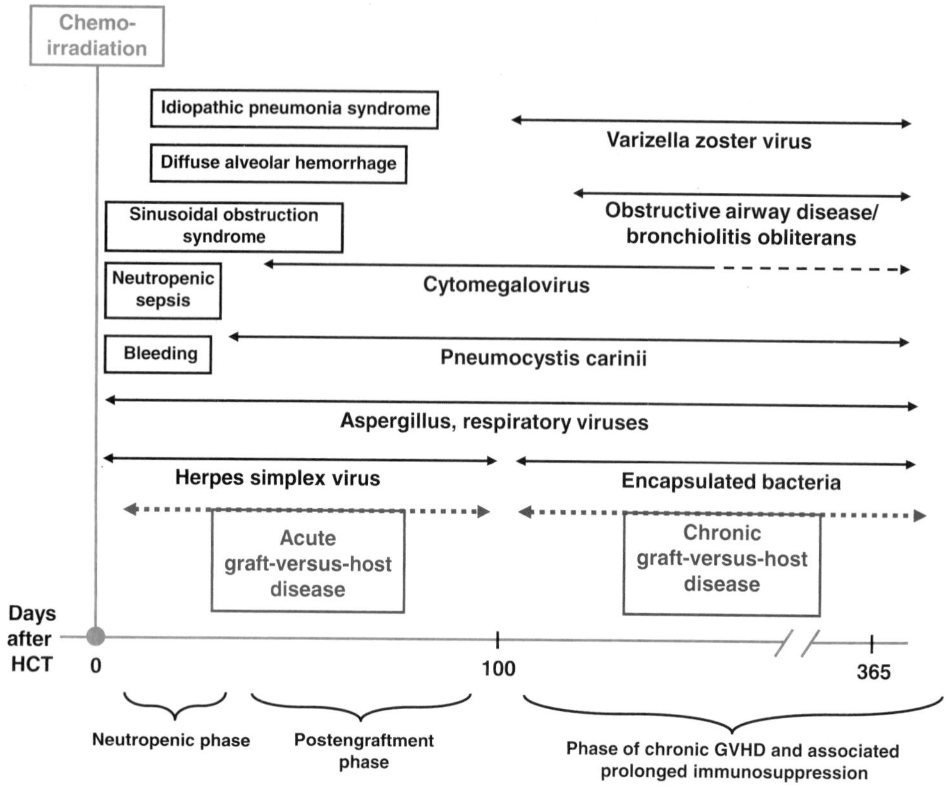

FIGURE 64.1 Complications after myeloablative allogeneic hematopoietic cell transplantation. BOOP, bronchiolitis obliterans with organizing pneumonia (also known as cryptogenic organizing pneumonia); DAH, diffuse alveolar hemorrhage; GVHD, graft-versus-host disease; HHV6, human herpes virus 6; HSV, herpes simplex virus; IPS, idiopathic pneumonia syndrome; SOS, sinusoidal obstruction syndrome.

may cause GVHD and latent viruses may be transferred through leukocytes. Except for the stem cell graft, all other blood product components should be irradiated at a dose of 1,500 to 3,000 cGy to inactivate or eliminate contaminating lymphocytes. Depletion of leukocytes or use of blood components that test seronegative for cytomegalovirus (CMV) are effective for prevention of CMV transmission to CMV-seronegative recipients [22]. Removal of white blood cells from platelet and RBC products also decreases the risk for alloimmunization of the patient.

Regimen-Related Toxicity

High-dose cytotoxic chemotherapy with or without doses of TBI exceeding 6 Gy may severely disrupt mucosal integrity and has the potential to cause regimen-related toxicity (RRT) in the skin, GI tract, liver, bladder, lung, heart, kidney, and nervous system. RRT occurs predominantly within the first 3 to 4 weeks after conditioning and is more common after myeloablative than RIC [23]. RRT increases the risk for opportunistic infection, which is already high because of concomitant profound immunosuppression and regimen-related cytopenias. This section will focus on the noninfectious complications of individual organs specifically attributable to conditioning toxicity. Opportunistic infection or, after allografting, GVHD must strongly be considered as etiologies for organ dysfunction in the differential diagnosis of RRT. These alternative diagnoses are covered elsewhere under the appropriate subsection.

Skin

Generalized skin erythema is common after doses of TBI exceeding 12 Gy, but is self-limiting and rarely associated with skin breakdown. Regimens that contain cytosine arabinoside (Ara-C), thiotepa, busulfan, treosulfan, fludarabine, etoposide, and carmustine may also cause erythema. Hyperpigmentation typically follows the inflammatory dermatitis, with skin folds often being particularly noticeable. Skin biopsies during the first 3 weeks after transplant often show nonspecific inflammatory changes irrespective of cause, making them frequently unhelpful in distinguishing between RRT, drug allergies, or acute GVHD [24].

Gastrointestinal Tract

Mucositis. Most patients who receive high-dose conditioning regimens develop mucositis. Symptoms include inflammation, desquamation, and edema of the oral and pharyngeal epithelial tissue that typically presents within the first several days after HCT and usually resolves by the 3rd week. Anorexia, nausea, or other intestinal symptoms that persist after day 21 are more likely to be caused by GVHD or infection. Severe mucositis places patients at risk for aspiration and, occasionally, airway compromise, indicating the need for endotracheal intubation. Damage to the mucosa of the lower GI tract results in secretory diarrhea, cramping abdominal pain, and anorexia, and it facilitates translocation of intestinal bacteria with sepsis [23,25].

Mucositis is treated supportively with total parenteral nutrition, administration of intravenous fluids, and intravenous narcotics for pain control. It is important to recognize an iatrogenic narcotic bowel syndrome, characterized by abdominal pain and bowel dilatation, which occasionally may be a side effect of efforts to control painful symptoms of mucositis or SOS [26].

Acute Upper Esophageal Bleeding. The combination of mucositis, thrombocytopenia, and severe retching may result in a Mallory–Weiss tear, or esophageal hematoma [27]. The latter condition may have associated symptoms of dysphagia and retrosternal pain, and can be diagnosed by computed tomography

(CT) scan. These conditions are treated supportively with transfusions to maintain platelet counts of greater than 50,000 per μL and optimal management of nausea and vomiting.

Liver

Sinusoidal Obstruction Syndrome. SOS (formerly referred to as veno-occlusive disease) develops in 10% to 60% of patients and is a clinical diagnosis based on the triad of tender hepatomegaly, jaundice, and unexplained weight gain usually within 30 days after HCT and in the absence of other explanations for these symptoms and signs [28–31]. It is more likely to be severe in patients with cirrhosis or fibrosis of the liver, or those with a history of hepatitis or liver irradiation (greater than 12 Gy), or chemotherapy-induced SOS [29,32].

Elevations of total serum bilirubin and serum transaminases are sensitive but nonspecific markers for SOS, and urinary sodium levels are typically low. A hepatobiliary ultrasound may show hepatomegaly, ascites, and dilatation of the hepatic vein or biliary system [33]. Doppler ultrasonography may show attenuation, or diagnostic, reversal of hepatic venous flow, but absence of this pattern does not exclude SOS [34]. If the diagnosis remains unclear, a transvenous liver biopsy may be helpful, and simultaneous measurement of hepatic venous pressure showing a gradient of greater than 10 mm Hg is highly specific for SOS [35].

Other causes of jaundice after HCT seldom lead to renal sodium avidity, rapid weight gain, or hepatomegaly [36]. Cyclosporine, methotrexate, and total parenteral nutrition are iatrogenic causes of hyperbilirubinemia, although rarely cause levels greater than 4 mg per dL [37]. Combinations of illnesses that may mimic SOS are cholangitis lenta (cholestatic effects of endotoxin [38], especially when combined with renal insufficiency), cholestatic liver disease with hemolysis and congestive heart failure, GVHD, and sepsis syndrome.

Once SOS is established, mathematical models can be used to predict prognosis, based on rates of increase in serum bilirubin and weight according to the elapsed time after transplantation [29,39]. The treatment for the 70% to 85% of patients who are predicted to have a mild or moderate course is largely supportive, with attention to management of sodium and water balance to avoid fluid overload [29,40]. Diuretics must be used judiciously to avoid depletion of intravascular volume and renal hypoperfusion. Paracentesis is indicated if the degree of ascites threatens respiratory function. There is no universally effective therapy for severe SOS. Defibrotide is a promising agent that has been shown to reverse SOS in some studies; however, it must be used with caution in patients with low platelet counts or other conditions that predispose to hemorrhage [30,41]. There is no support for insertion of peritoneovenous shunts and limited support for use of portosystemic shunts to reduce ascites [42]. Liver transplantation has been successful in a small number of patients [43].

Lung

Pulmonary complications occur in 40% to 60% of patients after HCT [44,45]. Noninfectious pulmonary problems that may occur within 30 days from the transplant include idiopathic pneumonia syndrome (IPS), diffuse alveolar hemorrhage, pulmonary edema [46] due to excessive sodium and fluid administration or associated with SOS, or acute cardiomyopathy induced by cyclophosphamide, and sepsis with acute respiratory distress syndrome (ARDS) [47]. These complications occur more frequently in older patients, those who receive higher-dose conditioning regimens, and those with allogeneic donors, particularly HLA-disparate donors. Although the incidence of life-threatening pulmonary infections has decreased over the past decade owing to the introduction of routine antimicrobial prophylaxis, pulmonary complications continue to be a leading cause of death.

Idiopathic Pneumonia Syndrome. IPS is defined as a noninfectious inflammatory lung process that may be triggered by TBI and chemotherapies such as carmustine or busulfan. IPS has been reported in 5% to 10% of patients and occurs with a median onset of 2 to 3 weeks after myeloablative HCT [48,49]. Contributing factors to IPS lung injury may be release of inflammatory cytokines due to alloreactivity or sepsis. The clinical symptoms cannot be distinguished from infection and may include fever, nonproductive cough, and tachypnea. Hemoptysis is infrequent and more likely related to invasive fungal disease or diffuse alveolar hemorrhage. Radiographic imaging shows diffuse interstitial or multifocal intra-alveolar infiltrates. Arterial blood gases show hypoxemia and the alveolar–arterial oxygen gradient is increased. In the occasional patient who is not too ill to attempt lung function studies, a new restrictive pattern or a reduced diffusing capacity is characteristic. Measurements of pulmonary artery occlusion pressure or echocardiography may be useful to rule out cardiogenic pulmonary edema. Bronchoalveolar lavage or lung biopsy is necessary to exclude bacterial, fungal, or viral infection because *IPS is a diagnosis of exclusion* [50]. Multifocal bronchiolitis obliterans with organizing pneumonia (BOOP), also known as cryptogenic organizing pneumonia, may mimic late-onset IPS and has been more commonly associated with chronic GVHD [51].

Management of IPS is mainly supportive, including judicious diuresis to decrease pulmonary edema, transfusions of blood components to reverse bleeding diathesis, support of oxygenation, and administration of antibiotics to prevent superinfection with mold and bacteria, particularly in patients receiving high-dose glucocorticoids. Effective therapy for idiopathic pneumonia has not been demonstrated. High-dose glucocorticoids (1 to 2 mg per kg) have been reported to have an adjunctive role in treatment of diffuse alveolar hemorrhage or idiopathic pneumonia [52,53]. Several studies have shown promising results for soluble tumor necrosis factor receptor (etanercept) used with or without glucocorticoids that resulted in an encouraging day-28 survival rate of 73% [53,54]. Historically, IPS has been associated with a mortality rate of 50% to 70% [49,55]. Aggressive management, including initiation of mechanical ventilation to identify and treat reversible causes of respiratory failure, is a reasonable approach for most HCT recipients with diffuse or multifocal pulmonary infiltrates. When hemodynamic instability or sustained hepatic and renal failure develop, survival is extremely unlikely.

Diffuse Alveolar Hemorrhage. DAH may be a manifestation of diffuse alveolar damage. However, the erosion of blood vessels by fungal organisms always needs to be considered [56]. Hemorrhage occurs more frequently in older patients and those with malignancy, severe mucositis, or renal failure [57]. Symptoms and radiographic findings are similar to IPS, and hemoptysis is uncommon. Bronchoalveolar lavage should be performed early to evaluate for concomitant infection, which may be detected in about one-third of patients with DAH [58]. Bloody bronchoalveolar lavage (BAL) fluid with hemosiderin-laden macrophages is characteristic of diffuse alveolar hemorrhage. The treatment is largely supportive, including platelet transfusions and correction of coagulopathies with plasma or cryoprecipitate; however, several studies have also suggested a role for both corticosteroids and soluble tumor necrosis factor receptor [54,59].

Acute Respiratory Distress Syndrome. Sepsis is a common cause of ARDS; however, an ARDS-like syndrome has also been described as a presenting feature of acute GVHD, typically early-onset (hyperacute) GVHD. ARDS has an extremely high mortality rate in the transplant population; recovery depends on aggressive treatment of associated infections and support of respiratory and cardiac function [60]. The diagnosis of ARDS is often complicated by the presence of other illnesses, such as SOS, hemorrhage, or disseminated intravascular hemolysis, which can cause difficulties with fluid management for which pulmonary artery catheterization can be helpful.

Heart

Cardiac complications occur in 5% to 10% of patients after HCT, but death from cardiac failure is uncommon [61,62]. Cardiac injury with hemorrhagic myocardial necrosis is a rare but known adverse effect of high-dose cyclophosphamide, one of the most commonly used chemotherapy agents in conditioning regimens. Risk factors for cyclophosphamide cardiotoxicity include the use of doses equal to or greater than 120 mg per kg, an underlying diagnosis of lymphoma, prior radiation to the mediastinum or left chest wall, older age, and prior abnormally low cardiac ejection fraction [62,63]. Patients who had prior cumulative anthracycline exposures of 550 mg per m^2 doxorubicin equivalents are at an increased risk for developing heart failure. Signs and symptoms of congestive heart failure may occur within a few days of receiving cyclophosphamide, whereas anthracycline-related cardiomyopathy may have a delayed onset. The electrocardiogram (ECG) may show voltage loss or arrhythmia, and echocardiography may reveal systolic dysfunction, pericardial effusion, or tamponade. Management includes attention to fluid and sodium balance, afterload reduction, and inotropes.

Pulmonary hypertension is an uncommon but serious complication of HCT that may lead to right ventricular failure [64]. It may be caused by pulmonary veno-occlusive disease (PVOD), as well as other more typical causes of increased pulmonary artery pressure. The diagnosis is made by cardiac catheterization. Pulmonary biopsy may be helpful in differentiating PVOD from other causes.

Kidney and Bladder

Acute Renal Failure. Acute renal failure (ARF), defined by doubling of baseline serum creatinine, occurs in 30% to 50% of all patients during the first 100 days after HCT, and most often during the first 10 to 30 days [65,66]. Occasionally, ARF develops during conditioning or infusion of HSC, as a consequence of tumor or red-cell lysis. ARF occurs frequently in the setting of SOS and is characterized by low urinary sodium concentration and high blood urea nitrogen–to–creatinine ratio, similar to the hepato-renal syndrome. Renal hypoperfusion, caused by acute hemorrhage, sepsis, or high-volume diarrhea, may result in ARF. Nephrotoxic drugs such as cyclosporine, tacrolimus, all amphotericin products, and aminoglycosides also should be considered as potential causes of ARF.

Thrombotic microangiopathy (TMA), endothelial damage caused by chemoradiotherapy, cyclosporine, tacrolimus, or sirolimus occurs in 5% to 20% of patients, more frequently in allograft recipients [65–68]. The hallmark of TMA is RBC fragmentation (schistocytes) associated with increased RBC turnover (increased reticulocytes; elevations of serum lactate dehydrogenase and indirect bilirubin) without evidence for immune-mediated hemolysis or DIC. The syndrome ranges from subclinical hemolysis to a life-threatening hemolytic syndrome, the latter, being seen more frequently when sirolimus therapy is combined with cyclosporine or tacrolimus (calcineurin inhibitors [CNIs]) and immediately following conditioning with busulfan and cyclophosphamide. High-therapeutic or supratherapeutic serum levels of CNIs or sirolimus are more prone to be associated with TMA [69]. Management involves careful assessment of volume status and discontinuation or adjustment of the drug levels of the offending agent(s). There have been no controlled trials of plasma exchange, and therefore its utility has not been established for correction of TMA in the post-HCT setting [70]. Several other agents, including eculizumab and defibrotide, have been effective in limited numbers of patients [71].

Hypertension. Hypertension develops in approximately 60% of patients after HCT, more often in patients given CNIs for GVHD prophylaxis. Glucocorticoid therapy also contributes to the development of hypertension. Uncontrolled hypertension may lead to fatal intracerebral bleeding in thrombocytopenic patients. Therefore, hypertension should be anticipated and controlled medically. Most patients respond to conventional antihypertensive therapy, such as a calcium-channel blocker, angiotensin-converting enzyme inhibitor, or β-blocker. Correction of hypomagnesemia, which often confounds CNI therapy, may improve control of hypertension [72].

Hemorrhagic Cystitis. High-dose cyclophosphamide is commonly used for conditioning, and one of its toxic metabolites, acrolein, accumulates in the urine and may cause a hemorrhagic chemical cystitis during the conditioning regimen or later after HCT [73]. Measures to prevent hemorrhagic cystitis include aggressive fluid hydration to increase urine volume that dilutes and minimizes contact of acrolein with the mucosa, and administration of the drug mesna, which provides free thiol groups to detoxify acrolein. Viral infections, particularly adenovirus and BK virus, have also been implicated in the development of hemorrhagic cystitis, and the diagnosis is established by viral culture or polymerase chain reaction (PCR) test of a urine sample [74,75]. Unless there is evidence of disseminated infection, viral cystitis is managed with supportive therapy, including hydration and platelet transfusions. Severe hemorrhagic cystitis caused by adenovirus or BK virus that proves refractory to supportive therapy may respond to therapy with cidofovir [76].

Central Nervous System

Noninfectious complications include cerebrovascular events and encephalopathies due to metabolic, toxic, and immune-mediated causes. Focal symptoms are more indicative of infectious or cerebrovascular mechanisms, whereas diffuse symptoms such as delirium or coma may have metabolic causes. Fever is not necessarily associated with central nervous system (CNS) infections. Infection should be considered as the cause of any neurologic symptom and should prompt evaluation, including obtaining CT or magnetic resonance imaging (MRI) scans of the head and a sample of cerebrospinal fluid for appropriate cultures, cytochemistry stains, and PCR tests should be undertaken.

Cerebrovascular Events. Thrombocytopenia poses a risk for intracranial hemorrhage, which usually presents as abrupt onset of focal neurologic deficit or mental status changes [77]. Patients with sickle cell disease have a predisposition to CNS hemorrhage after HCT and should be managed carefully by ensuring sufficient platelet and magnesium levels and strict control of hypertension [78]. Ischemic stroke is an unusual complication after HCT, but has been reported in patients with *Aspergillus* infections, hypercoagulable states, or TMA [79].

Toxic Encephalopathies. Several agents used in conditioning regimens may cause encephalopathy, including high-dose busulfan and high-dose cytarabine. Seizure prophylaxis with Keppra, Ativan, or phenytoin should be considered during conditioning with high-dose busulfan or carmustine, particularly for young children. High-dose cyclophosphamide can be associated with the syndrome of inappropriate antidiuretic hormone (SIADH), rarely causing acute decline in the serum sodium that may prompt seizures. A rare syndrome of encephalopathy and hyperammonemia without other chemical evidence of liver failure has been reported after HCT [80]. Contributing factors may include hypercatabolism induced by conditioning, glucocorticoids, or sepsis, and high nitrogen loads associated with parenteral nutrition or intestinal hemorrhage. The syndrome is difficult to reverse and has a high mortality rate. Treatment involves hemodialysis and administration of ammonia-trapping agents, such as sodium benzoate or sodium phenylacetate. Metabolic encephalopathy may also be associated with gram-negative sepsis, hypoxic encephalopathy with IPS, and hepatic encephalopathy due to SOS or GVHD. Glucocorticoid therapy may be associated with psychosis, mania, or delirium in a dose-dependent fashion. Seizures or altered sensorium may be associated with the use of sedative-hypnotic drugs and have been reported as adverse side effects of many of the commonly used antibiotics and antiviral agents. Treatment of metabolic encephalopathies should be directed at the underlying problem and discontinuation of any offending drugs.

Related to a tendency to accumulate in nervous tissues owing to their lipophilic characteristics, CNIs can cause a range of neurologic toxicities including tremor, neuropathic pain, seizures, headaches, or visual disturbances [81]. Seizures should be managed with anticonvulsant therapy and cessation of the drug. When CNIs are essential for management of GVHD, substitution of one agent for the other, or reinstitution of the offending agent at a lower dose, may be feasible [82]. A unique and usually reversible syndrome of cortical blindness has been reported as a complication of cyclosporine treatment; hypertension and hypomagnesemia are thought to be predisposing factors [83]. Toxicity due to calcineurin inhibitor therapy may occur with "therapeutic" drug levels, and clinical suspicion is often confirmed by MRI scans that show multifocal areas of signal hyperintensity on T2 (time for 63% of transverse relaxation) and fluid-attenuated inversion recovery (FLAIR) sequences, most often in the occipital lobe white matter.

Hemolysis

RBC hemolysis may be encountered after HCT and may include more than one etiology. TMA may present as mild hemolysis or as a more severe form, as described previously [84,85]. Hemolysis mediated by major or minor blood group incompatibilities is only seen in recipients of allografts. *Major* ABO incompatibility occurs in 30% of allograft recipients and is defined by the presence of isohemagglutinins within recipient plasma that are directed against donor A or B antigens [86]. *Minor* ABO incompatibility also occurs in 30% of recipients and is defined by presence of isohemagglutinins within the donor plasma directed against recipient A or B. *Bidirectional* ABO incompatibility may be present as in the case of a type A recipient and type B donor or vice versa. After successful donor engraftment, the conversion of recipient to donor blood type may take weeks to months because of the relatively long half-life of RBCs.

Major ABO incompatibility poses a serious risk of severe hemolytic reactions at the time of infusion of the HSC product if preventative steps are not taken [87]. Immediate hemolytic reactions are more likely in the presence of high-level isoagglutinin titers. Therefore, RBCs are most commonly removed from the graft before infusion to avoid life-threatening hemolysis. Delayed recovery of donor hematopoiesis or hemolysis may occur because recipient plasma cells continue to produce isohemagglutinins for up to several months after HCT [86]. In this case, the diagnosis relies on detection of a positive direct antiglobulin test and the presence of isohemagglutinins directed against donor-type RBCs. Management of major ABO incompatibility includes the transfusion of group O RBCs, donor-type platelets, and donor-type plasma until isohemagglutinins against donor-type RBCs disappear. In the rare cases of ongoing hemolysis due to persistence of donor-directed isohemagglutinins, additional therapy with immunosuppressive agents, erythropoietin, plasma exchange, anti-B-cell antibodies (rituximab), or plasma exchange may be considered [88].

Minor ABO incompatibility poses a risk for mild and self-limited hemolysis at the time of infusion [87]. Delayed hemolysis, seen more commonly after PBSC transplantation, is mediated by clonally expanded donor "passenger lymphocytes" and can present as an abrupt and potentially fatal hemolytic transfusion reaction typically at 1 to 2 weeks after HCT [86,89]. In contrast to major ABO incompatibility, pretransplant donor isohemagglutinin titers do not predict the severity of hemolysis following minor ABO-mismatched HCT. The diagnosis relies again on the detection of a positive direct antiglobulin test and the presence of isohemagglutinins directed against recipient-type RBCs. To prevent hemolysis, plasma should be removed from the donor HSC product if donor hemagglutinin titers are high. Emergence of donor-derived RBC and isohemagglutinin titers should be monitored after allogeneic HCT. Management of minor ABO incompatibility after HCT includes supportive care with judicious fluid management aimed at preventing ARF, and the transfusion of group O RBCs and recipient-type platelets and plasma. There is no convincing evidence to support the use of plasma exchange.

Infection

Conditioning regimens and GVHD severely impair host defense mechanisms, and the process of immune reconstitution necessarily requires many months for completion. Together, these factors place patients at high risk for acquisition of severe infections. Proper medical care of patients after HCT includes measures to monitor and prevent infection, as it is a leading cause of death.

Prevention of infection is of vital importance to the success of HCT procedures. Hospitalized patients should be housed in single rooms that have positive-pressure air flow and ventilation systems with rapid air exchange and high-efficiency particulate air filtration [90]. Strict visitation, hand washing, and isolation policies should be instituted to prevent introduction or spread of communicable disease. A daily program of skin and oral care should include bathing all skin surfaces with mild soap, brushing teeth with a soft brush, frequent rinsing of the oral cavity with saline, and good perineal hygiene. The diet should exclude foods known to contain bacteria or fungi, and patients should avoid exposure to dried or fresh plants or flowers. Caregivers should be trained in the proper handling of central venous catheters.

Immunologic reconstitution after HCT can broadly be categorized into three phases, which are characterized by a spectrum of opportunistic infections. Recommendations for antimicrobial prevention of opportunistic infections after HCT are outlined in Table 64.2.

Before Engraftment Period

The period before engraftment (less than 30 days posttransplant) is characterized by neutropenia and oral and gastrointestinal mucosal damage. The most common infections are bacterial and fungal. The use of indwelling central venous catheters heightens the risk of blood infections with organisms that colonize the skin, such as coagulase-negative *staphylococci* or *Candida* spp., and gastrointestinal mucosal damage increases the risk of infections with enteric organisms, such as *Escherichia coli*. *Clostridium difficile* toxic colitis can be a common infection in transplant patients, particularly those patients in intensive care units. Patients with a history of prolonged neutropenia before HCT are at risk for developing fungal infections involving the skin, lung, and sinuses, which are typically a mold such as *Aspergillus*, or the liver and spleen, typically *Candida* spp. The most likely viral infection in this period is herpes simplex virus. Fever of unknown origin also occurs commonly during the neutropenic period. Prophylactic systemic antibiotics are conventionally administered to reduce the risk of bacteremia during the neutropenic period, although improvement in survival has not been demonstrated [90]. Administration of growth factors, such as granulocyte colony-stimulating factor, shortens the duration of neutropenia, but there is little evidence for improvement in outcome after allogeneic HCT.

Following Engraftment Period

The period following engraftment (30 to 100 days posttransplant) of allogeneic HSC is characterized by skin and mucosal damage and compromised cellular immunity related to GVHD and its treatment. Viral (CMV) and fungal (*Aspergillus*, *Pneumocystis jiroveci*) infections predominate during this period. Gram-negative bacteremias related to GVHD-associated mucosal damage and gram-positive infections due to indwelling catheters remain a risk. Other causes of fever of unknown origin after engraftment include occult sinusitis, hepatosplenic candidiasis, and pulmonary or disseminated *Aspergillus* infection.

Late Phase

The late phase (greater than 100 days posttransplant) after allogeneic HCT is characterized by a persistently impaired cellular immunity in patients with chronic GVHD. Patients with chronic GVHD are highly susceptible to recurrent bacterial infections, especially from encapsulated bacteria, including *Streptococcus pneumonia*, *Hemophilus influenzae*, and *Neisseria meningitides* (functional asplenia). Bronchopulmonary infections, septicemia, and ear, nose, and throat infections occur. Common nonbacterial infections at this time include varicella zoster, CMV, *Pneumocystis jiroveci*, and *Aspergillus*.

Evaluation and Treatment

Signs and symptoms of infection may be diminished in patients who are neutropenic or receiving immunosuppressive drugs. Thus, preemptive antibiotic therapy should be instituted promptly for any fever during the neutropenic period because infections can progress rapidly to a fatal outcome [90]. The febrile patient should be examined thoroughly for source of infection, including the oral cavity, perianal tissue, and skin surrounding the central venous catheter. Cultures should be obtained of blood, urine, and stool if diarrhea is present; and chest radiograph should be performed. Antibiotic therapy should provide empiric coverage for the most common organisms, gram-positive bacteria that colonize the skin and oral cavity, as well as the less common but more virulent gram-negative bacteria that arise from the GI tract. Broad-spectrum antibiotic therapy should be continued through the duration of neutropenia, even if fever resolves. If fever persists, the antibiotic regimen should be broadened after 4 days to provide empiric treatment of fungi. *C. difficile* infection should be considered in patients with diarrhea and can be treated with oral metronidazole or oral vancomycin.

Evaluation of persistent fevers after granulocyte recovery should consider occult sources of bacterial infection, such as sinuses, perirectal tissue, or central venous lines, as well as viral or fungal etiologies. Removal of the central venous catheter is occasionally required. Viral infections must be considered in patients with GI symptoms and may involve the esophagus, upper and lower intestines, or liver [91]. The diagnosis is established by biopsy or brushings taken from the center of the lesions so as to include infected endothelial cells and submucosal tissue. Patients with active chronic GVHD should receive prophylaxis for *P. jiroveci* pneumonia (PJP) with trimethoprim-sulfamethoxazole and for encapsulated organisms with daily trimethoprim-sulfamethoxazole, penicillin, or azithromycin.

Infectious causes of pulmonary infiltrates must be differentiated from noninfectious causes to ensure prompt institution of appropriate therapy [55]. BAL should be performed without delay to establish the etiology of diffuse infiltrates, unless clearly related to pulmonary edema [92,93]. BAL specimens should be assayed for the presence of common nosocomial bacteria as well as *Legionella*, *Mycobacteria*, and *Nocardia*; *P. jiroveci*; fungi other than PJP; respiratory viruses; and herpes group viruses by cultures and immunocytochemical stains. Focal pulmonary infiltrates that occur after HCT are most frequently caused by infection, particularly fungal infection [92,93]. Evaluation of a focal infiltrate should include a CT scan to delineate the number and extent of infiltrates. BAL should be performed as a first step because the procedure is minimally invasive and historically has produced a diagnosis in 50% of patients with fungal lesions using standard diagnostic approaches, although the predictive value of negative results was poor [94]. The increasing use of more sensitive diagnostic approaches like galactomannan antigen testing [95] or molecular methods to detect fungi or viral pathogens continues to improve the yield of BAL [96,97]. Transbronchial biopsy is not recommended because it has not been shown to improve sensitivity in these situations, and often thrombocytopenia precludes the ability to perform the procedure safely. Percutaneous fine-needle aspiration is indicated for diagnosis of peripheral infiltrates that cannot be evaluated by BAL. Fine-needle aspiration has a sensitivity of approximately 67% for diagnosis of fungal infection, but it has a poor negative predictive value. If the diagnosis is not ascertained after BAL or fine-needle aspiration, a biopsy is required [98]. Specimens should be evaluated histologically and undergo testing for bacteria, fungi, and viruses by appropriate cultures and immunocytochemical stains as noted previously. Surgical resection of a solitary fungal lesion may improve the chances for cure [99].

Opportunistic Infections

***Pneumocystis jiroveci* Pneumonia.** Inadequate cell-mediated immunity poses a risk for development of PJP infection after HCT [100]. Recommendations for prevention of PJP are found in Table 64.2 [90].

Fungal Infections

Factors that predispose to invasive yeast infections include neutropenia, mucosal barrier disruption, and broad-spectrum antibiotics that promote colonization of the GI mucosa [101]. Candidal infections generally occur within the first 3 weeks after HCT, coinciding with the period of neutropenia, although a second period of risk occurs during treatment for chronic GVHD. Invasive candidiasis may involve the liver and spleen, with potential for dissemination to kidneys or rarely, the CNS [102]. The diagnosis of invasive candidiasis is difficult because blood cultures are negative in approximately one-half of the cases with organ involvement. Recommendations for prevention of candidiasis are found in Table 64.2 [90,103]. Fluconazole is effective for treatment of the most common *Candida* spp., *C. albicans* and *C. tropicalis* [104,105] (see Table 64.2), but does not prevent or treat infection with *C. glabrata*, *C. krusei*, or *C. parapsilosis*. Lipid-complexed amphotericin products, echinocandins, or other azoles may be useful alternatives [106]. Removal of the central venous catheter should be considered when *Candida* sp. is isolated from blood cultures. Because fungal vegetations on heart valves may occur, echocardiography should be considered to evaluate for this.

Although the era of improved fungal prophylaxis has reduced the incidence of invasive mold infections after HCT to <5% among affected patients, the mortality remains high [107]. The incidence of *Aspergillus* infections is highest within the first month after HCT, and there is a second peak incidence during chronic GVHD. *Aspergillus* infections have been difficult to diagnose by standard methods, and more than 20% of the cases have been diagnosed only at autopsy. Cultures of BAL fluid are negative in 50% of pulmonary disease; therefore, the diagnosis frequently requires a biopsy of affected tissues [108]. The *Aspergillus* Galactomannan Enzyme Immunoassay detects a polysaccharide secreted from *Aspergillus* hyphae and is a useful screening tool, with a sensitivity of 65% and specificity of 95% [109]. High-risk patients, those with severe GVHD treated with high-dose corticosteroids, should be given prophylaxis with agents like voriconazole or

TABLE 64.2

Prevention of Opportunistic Infections after Allogeneic Hematopoietic Cell Transplantation

Infection	Recommendations for prophylaxis (strength of recommendation)[a] All patients	Patients with chronic GVHD
Bacteria	Broad-spectrum antibiotic(s) during period of neutropenia (ANC <500/μL). Choices include a single agent, such as levofloxacin or ceftazidime, or a combination of agents, such as piperacillin. [CIII] Patients with hypogammaglobulinemia: Intravenous immunoglobulin administered at 1- to 4-wk intervals depending on level. [CIII]	Penicillin VK twice daily for encapsulated organisms. [BIIb] Alternatives: TMP/SMX daily, azithromycin three times per week. [CIII] Patients with hypogammaglobulinemia or repeated sinopulmonary infections: Intravenous immunoglobulin administered at monthly intervals depending on level. [CIII]
Fungi	Fluconazole from start of conditioning to day 75 (allogeneic HCT) or day 30 (autologous HCT). [AIa]	Mold-active agents, such as posaconazole when prednisone dose is ≥1 mg/kg. [AI]
PJP	TMP/SMX is the drug of choice and starts 1–2 wk before transplant until 48 h before HCT, then from engraftment until 6 mo after HCT if no chronic GVHD. Alternatives: dapsone, atovoquone, pentamidine. [AIb]	TMP/SMX in a variety schedules. [AIb]
HSV (seropositive patients)	Acyclovir prophylaxis from start of conditioning until day 30. Alternatives: valacyclovir. [AI]	Not indicated
VZV (seropositive)	Acyclovir prophylaxis from start of conditioning until 1 y after HCT for those with a history of natural infection. Alternative: valacyclovir. [AIa]	Acyclovir from start of immune suppression until completion. Alternatives: valacyclovir. [AIa]
CMV (seropositive)	Ganciclovir prophylaxis or preemptive therapy based on plasma CMV DNA detection by PCR between engraftment and day 100. Foscarnet is an equally effective alternative to ganciclovir for preemptive therapy. [AI]	Valganciclovir therapy based on plasma CMV DNA detection by PCR until dose of prednisone is <1 mg/kg. [BIII]
CMV (seronegative)	Preferential use of preemptive therapy with ganciclovir or foscarnet as outlined for seropositive patients. [BII]	Not indicated

Recommendations are: "A," should always be offered; "B," should generally be offered; "C," optional; "D," should generally not be offered. Evidence is "level I" if it is derived from ≥1 properly designed randomized, controlled trial, "level II" if it is derived from ≥1 well-designed clinical trial without randomization, from cohort or case-controlled analytical studies, or from multiple time series or dramatic results from uncontrolled experiments, and "level III" if it is derived from opinions of respected authorities based on clinical experience. Qualifiers, "a," indicates that evidence is directly from study(s) in GVHD, or "b" if the evidence was derived indirectly from study(s) in analogous or other pertinent disease.

[a]Evidence-based grading system adapted from Couriel D, Carpenter PA, Cutler C, et al: Ancillary therapy and supportive care of chronic GVHD: NIH Consensus Development Project on criteria for clinical trials in chronic GVHD: V. Ancillary Therapy and Supportive Care Working Group Report. *Biol Blood Marrow Transplant* 12:375–396, 2006; Aspesberro F, Guthrie KA, Woolfrey AE, et al: Outcome of pediatric hematopoietic stem cell transplant recipients requiring mechanical ventilation. *J Intensive Care Med* 29:31–37, 2012.

ANC, absolute neutrophil count; CMV, cytomegalovirus; DS, double strength; GVHD, graft-versus-host disease; HCT, hematopoietic cell transplantation; HSV, herpes simplex virus; IgG, immunoglobulin G; IV, intravenous; max, maximum dose; MTX, methotrexate; PJP, *Pneumocystis jiroveci* pneumonia; PCR, polymerase chain reaction; SMX, sulfamethoxazole; TMP, trimethoprim; VK, V potassium; VZV, varicella zoster virus.

posaconazole, which is active against aspergillosis and certain other molds. Because invasive aspergillosis is associated with a high mortality rate, documented or suspected infections should be treated aggressively with voriconazole or another mold-active azole, lipid-complexed amphotericin products, or combination therapy [110]. Surgical removal of infected tissue should be restricted to cases of circumscribed disease [111].

Viral Infections

Cytomegalovirus. Protection from exposure by use of seronegative or leukocyte-reduced blood components has reduced the incidence of CMV infection among seronegative patients, whereas ganciclovir has been shown to be an effective agent for prevention of CMV disease in seropositive patients (see Table 64.2). Two approaches have proven successful for reducing the incidence of CMV disease post HCT: (1) ganciclovir prophylaxis initiated after engraftment, with careful monitoring of the patient for marrow suppression, or (2) weekly monitoring for CMV reactivation with serum PCR assays, followed by prompt institution of ganciclovir when the CMV copy number reaches a positive threshold [112]. Generally, surveillance CMV PCR testing is performed weekly from transplant day 0 through day 100; however, monitoring generally is continued for CMV-positive patients on high-dose corticosteroids.

Although prophylaxis greatly reduces the risk for CMV disease, severe pneumonitis, gastroenteritis, hepatitis, or bone marrow failure continue to occur in a small proportion of patients [113]. The diagnosis of CMV pneumonitis can be established in most patients by PCR assay or rapid shell vial culture of BAL fluid [50]. CMV enteritis is often indistinguishable from GVHD clinically, and the diagnosis relies on endoscopic evaluation [114]. CMV enteritis appears as ulcerations of the esophagus, stomach, or intestines. Viral cultures and histologic stains of the affected tissue are used to establish the diagnosis. Treatment of CMV infection includes ganciclovir (foscarnet or cidofovir are acceptable alternatives) in combination with immune globulin [115–117]. Foscarnet can be used in place of ganciclovir if significant marrow toxicity occurs or drug resistance is identified.

Herpes Simplex Virus. Herpes simplex virus (HSV) is the most common cause of infectious mucositis after HCT and may cause life-threatening encephalitis, hepatitis, or pneumonia in immunocompromised patients [118]. HSV pneumonitis or hepatitis is associated with high mortality rates; although less serious, HSV mucositis produces severe local pain and swelling. Acyclovir prophylaxis has been shown to be very effective for prevention of HSV reactivation in seropositive patients and for treatment of established disease [117,119] (see Table 64.2).

Varicella Zoster Virus. Varicella zoster virus (VZV) causes life-threatening disease in immunocompromised patients as a primary infection or reactivation of endogenous virus. Exposed seronegative patients should receive VZV immune globulin within 96 hours if available, and acyclovir should be administered from days 3 to 22 after exposure [120]. Among seropositive patients, VZV reactivation occurs in approximately 40%, with the highest incidence around 5 months after HCT [121]. Prophylaxis with acyclovir is recommended for seropositive patients until 1 year after HCT or until complete discontinuation of immunosuppressive therapy for chronic GVHD immunity [117,122,123] (see Table 64.2). VZV infection typically causes local skin involvement, but it can disseminate in immunocompromised patients, resulting in pneumonitis, esophagitis, pancreatitis, hepatitis, or encephalitis [124–126]. VZV hepatitis may present as a syndrome of fever, severe abdominal pain, and elevated aminotransferase levels, and because it is associated with a high mortality rate, it should be treated presumptively with high-dose acyclovir [36,117]. For localized infection, a short course of intravenous acyclovir for 24 to 48 hours can be followed by oral valacyclovir for the duration of therapy.

Respiratory Viruses. Respiratory viruses may spread quickly within HCT patient populations, causing epidemics of life-threatening infection. Respiratory syncytial virus (RSV), influenza, and parainfluenza are the most frequently encountered respiratory viruses in these situations [127,128]. Symptoms of upper respiratory infection should prompt cultures of nasopharyngeal secretions, careful monitoring for progression of disease, and isolation to prevent spread to other patients. Patients in the period before engraftment are at greatest risk for progression to lower-tract disease with RSV. Once lower-tract disease occurs, however, mortality is high regardless of engraftment status [129]. If lower-tract disease is suspected, BAL should be performed to obtain samples for viral fluorescence antibody and PCR tests and viral cultures [93].

Adenovirus. Adenovirus and polyoma BK virus are common causes of hemorrhagic cystitis after HCT [130,131]. When disseminated, adenovirus can cause hemorrhagic enterocolitis, interstitial pneumonitis, myocarditis, nephritis, meningoencephalitis, or severe hepatitis. Adenoviral infections occur more commonly in children and after allogeneic grafts. Patients with poor T-cell function, such as recipients of T-cell–depleted grafts or those receiving intensive immune-suppressing therapies, are at greatest risk for disseminated infection. Disseminated infections are often difficult to detect by viral cultures, and PCR assays may be more useful [132]. The most promising treatment results have been reported after administration of cidofovir, although renal insufficiency is a potential side effect [133]. Polyoma BK virus should be considered in the differential diagnosis of renal insufficiency in patients on chronic immune suppression and can be diagnosed by renal biopsy.

Epstein–Barr Virus. Epstein–Barr virus (EBV) seropositive immunocompromised patients are at risk for development of life-threatening lymphoproliferative disease (LPD) after HCT [134,135]. The risk for EBV-LPD is highest among patients who receive T-cell–depleted grafts or who are given intensive immune suppression for treatment of GVHD. The diagnosis is made by biopsy of enlarged nodes or affected tissue. A presumptive diagnosis can be made in high-risk patients who have clinical symptoms and elevated plasma or cellular EBV DNA copy number [136]. The mainstay of therapy is reduction or elimination of immunosuppressive therapy to allow reconstitution of EBV-specific T-cell immunity [117]. However, it may not be feasible to eliminate immunosuppression therapy without risking a flare of life-threatening GVHD. Some studies have shown encouraging results with mAb directed against CD20, which targets EBV-infected B cells [137]. EBV-LPD that develops in recipients of T-cell–depleted grafts may be ameliorated by infusion of donor T lymphocytes [138].

Graft Rejection

Graft rejection presents as failure to recover hematopoiesis after transplantation, termed *primary graft failure*, or as the loss of an established donor graft, termed *secondary graft failure*. Persistence of neutropenia (an absolute neutrophil count of more than 100 cells per μL) after day 26 is associated with increased risk of early mortality [139]. Although the molecular and cellular mechanisms are not completely understood, graft rejection appears to be mediated preferentially by recipient T cells [140]. Natural killer cells and host allo-antibodies also have been implicated in graft rejection. Graft rejection is more common after RIC or after transplant of T-cell–depleted grafts, UCB grafts, and grafts containing insufficient numbers of HSC.

Quantitation of donor engraftment (donor chimerism), using PCR-based techniques to detect donor-specific variable nucleotide tandem repeats (VNTR) sequences, may be helpful in determining whether the graft has been rejected, in which case the peripheral blood T cells will be primarily of host origin, or whether the donor graft is not functioning, in which case the cells will be of donor origin. In the latter case, other causes of graft suppression should be considered, including relapse, medications such as ganciclovir or trimethoprim-sulfamethoxazole, mycophenolate mofetil, or viral infections such as CMV, human herpes virus 6, or parvovirus B19. In either case, graft failure after myeloablative conditioning is a life-threatening complication because autologous reconstitution is uncommon and results in death from hemorrhage or infection. A range of cellular therapies have been used to overcome rejection ranging from donor lymphocyte infusions in the case of declining donor T-cell chimerism, possibly combined with immunosuppressive therapy. In fulminant rejection, retransplantation is necessary, using the same or another donor. Preferentially, conditioning should differ from that used at the first transplant to avoid unnecessary toxicity, and a high graft cell dose is recommended.

Graft-Versus-Host Disease

The most significant immunological barrier to successful HCT is the graft-versus-host reaction that can result in life-threatening inflammation and tissue destruction. Donor T cells that recognize disparate recipient alloantigens are the central mediators of GVHD. The most important alloantigens are those encoded by the major histocompatibility complex, or HLA system, although non-HLA antigens may certainly be involved. Despite the significance of GVHD as a complication of HCT, patients who develop GVHD have lower relapse rates than do patients without GVHD, and this can also be explained by an immunologically mediated graft-versus-tumor effect that helps eradicate the underlying malignancy.

Acute GVHD

The incidence and severity of acute GVHD are determined primarily by the degree of HLA disparity and influenced by the nature of GVHD prophylaxis [13]. Severe acute GVHD (grades III to IV) develops in 15% of recipients transplanted from HLA-identical sibling donors and in a greater proportion of those given unrelated or mismatched grafts [141]. Acute GVHD typically begins abruptly at 2 to 4 weeks after myeloablative HCT and generally occurs before day 100, but the onset may be delayed after nonmyeloablative HCT. The clinicopathologic syndrome is consistent with various combinations of inflammatory dermatitis, enteritis, and hepatitis, which reflect the pathophysiology of T-cell activation with generation of cytotoxic lymphocytes and elaboration of inflammatory cytokines that cause tissue damage. The severity of acute GVHD in the three main target organs (skin, liver, and GI tract) is staged 1 through 4 on the basis of accepted criteria that primarily include the extent of rash, magnitude of hyperbilirubinemia, and volume of diarrhea. The various combinations of skin, liver, and GI involvement can then be used to assign an overall grade of GVHD: grade I being mild and grade IV being life threatening (Table 64.3) [142]. When cellular injury is severe, GVHD of the skin may manifest with bulla formation and skin ulceration. In the GI tract, symptoms range from mild anorexia, to nausea and vomiting, or to severe bloody diarrhea with cramping periumbilical pain.

Chronic GVHD

Chronic GVHD (CGVHD) occurs in approximately 30% to 60% of transplant recipients, more often when the donor is not an HLA-identical sibling and when there is a history of acute GVHD [143]. There is a higher risk for developing CGVHD with growth factor–mobilized PBSC grafts compared with marrow grafts [5,6]. CGVHD is also more likely when the recipient or donor is older or CMV seropositive, or in a male patient who receives HSC from a multiparous female donor. Risk factors for mortality at the time of diagnosis of CGVHD include platelet counts less than 100×10^9 per L, greater than 0.5 mg/kg/d prednisone, serum total bilirubin greater than 34 μmol per L, older recipient, prior acute GVHD, older donor, and graft-versus-host HLA mismatching.

CGVHD is defined without reference to time after HCT, but by the presence of hallmark CGVHD features, which resemble autoimmune diseases such as systemic sclerosis, Sjögren syndrome, primary biliary cirrhosis, wasting syndrome, bronchiolitis obliterans, immune cytopenias, and chronic immunodeficiency (Table 64.4) [144]. The overall severity of CGVHD is determined by a 0- to 3-point score (none, mild, moderate, severe) that reflects the clinical effect of CGVHD on the patient's functional status in any number of different organs [145]. CGVHD frequently involves the skin, liver, eyes, mouth, upper respiratory tract, lungs, and esophagus. Less frequently, serosal surfaces, lower GI tract, female genitalia, or

TABLE 64.3

Classification of GVHD

Acute GVHD organ staging			
Organ	**Stage**	**Scores**	**Description**
Skin	1		≤25% body surface area with maculopapular rash
	2		25%–50% body surface area with maculopapular rash
	3		≥50% body surface area with maculopapular rash or erythroderma
	4		Generalized erythroderma with bullae
Liver	1		Bilirubin 2.0–3.0 mg/dL
	2		Bilirubin 3.0–5.9 mg/dL
	3		Bilirubin 6.0–14.9 mg/dL
	4		Bilirubin rise to ≥15 mg/dL
GI tract			Stage is assigned according to a total GI score based on volume of diarrhea, presence of bloody stool, and abdominal pain or cramping
	1		Total GI score of 1
	2		Total GI score of 2
	3		Total GI score of 3–4
	4		Total GI score of 5–7
GI scoring			Diarrhea volume averaged over 3 d Adult (mL/d), child[a] (mL/kg/d)
		+1	>500–999, >10–20
		+2	1,000–1,499, >20–30
		+3	>1,500, >30
		+2	Score additional 2 points for presence of abdominal pain or cramping
		+2	Score additional 2 points for presence of bloody stools

Acute GVHD overall grade	Skin stage	Liver stage	GI stage
I	1–2	0	0
II	3 or	1 or	1
III		2–3	2–3
IV	4 or	4 or	4

[a]Children <17 years of age who are <1.73 m^2.

GI, gastrointestinal; GVHD, graft-versus-host disease.

Adapted from Martin PJ, Nelson BJ, Applebaum FR, et al: Evaluation of a CD5-specific immunotoxin for treatment of acute graft-versus-host disease after allogeneic marrow transplantation. *Blood* 88(3):962–969, 1996, with permission.

TABLE 64.4

Classification of Symptoms and Signs of Chronic GVHD

Organ or site	Diagnostic	Distinctive[a]	Common[b]
Skin	Poikiloderma Lichen-planus–like features Sclerotic features Morphea-like features Lichen-sclerosis–like features	Depigmentation	Erythema Maculopapular rash Pruritis
Nails		Dystrophy Longitudinal ridging, splitting, or brittle features Onycholysis Pterygium unguis Nail loss[c]	
Scalp and body hair		New onset of scalp alopecia Scaling, papulosquamous lesions	
Mouth	Lichentype features Hyperkeratotic plaques Restriction of mouth opening	Xerostomia Mucocele Mucosal atrophy Pseudomembranes[c] Ulcers[c]	Gingivitis Mucositis Erythema Pain
Eyes		New onset dry, gritty, or painful[d] Cicatricial conjunctivitis Keratoconjunctivitis sicca[d] Confluent punctate keratopathy	
Genitalia	Lichen-planus–like features Vaginal scarring or stenosis	Erosions[c] Fissures[c] Ulcers[c]	
GI tract	Esophageal web Esophageal strictures or stenosis in upper to mid-third[c]		Anorexia, nausea vomiting, diarrhea Failure to thrive
Liver			Bilirubin >2 × ULN Alk Phosp >2 × ULN AST/ALT >2 × ULN
Lung	Bronchiolitis obliterans based on lung biopsy	Bronchiolitis obliterans based on PFTs + radiology[d]	COP
Muscles, fascia, joints	Fasciitis Joint stiffness or contractures secondary to sclerosis	Myositis or polymyositis	

Features acknowledged as part of chronic GVHD symptomatology if the diagnosis is already confirmed

Skin	Sweat impairment, ichthyosis, keratosis pilaris, hypopigmentation, hyperpigmentation
Hair	Thinning scalp hair, typically patchy, coarse, dull not explained by endocrine or other causes, premature gray hair
Eyes	Photophobia, periorbital hyperpigmentation, blepharitis
GI tract	Exocrine pancreatic insufficiency
Muscles/joints	Edema, muscle cramps, arthralgia, or arthritis
Hematology	Thrombocytopenia, eosinophilia, lymphopenia
Immune	Lymphopenia, hypo- or hypergammaglobulinemia, autoantibodies (AIHA, ITP)
Other	Pericardial/pleural effusions, ascites, peripheral neuropathy, nephrotic syndrome, myasthenia gravis, cardiac conduction abnormality, or cardiomyopathy

[a]Seen in chronic GVHD, but are insufficient alone to establish the diagnosis.
[b]Seen in both acute and chronic GVHD alone to establish a diagnosis of chronic GVHD.
[c]In all cases must exclude infection, drug effects, malignancy, or other causes.
[d]Diagnosis of chronic GVHD requires biopsy or radiology confirmation (or Schirmer test for eyes).
AIHA, autoimmune hemolytic anemia; ALT, alanine aminotransferase; AST, aspartate aminotransferase; COP, cryptogenic organizing pneumonia; GI, gastrointestinal; ITP, idiopathic (immune) thrombocytopenic purpura; PFTs, pulmonary function tests; ULN, upper limit of normal range for age.
Modified from Filipovich AH, Weisdorf D, Pavletic S, et al: National Institutes of Health consensus development project on criteria for clinical trials in chronic graft-versus-host disease: I. Diagnosis and Staging Working Group report. *Biol Blood Marrow Transplant* 11(12):945–956, 2005, with permission.

TABLE 64.5

Differential Diagnosis of AGVHD

AGVHD manifestation	Differential diagnosis
Rash	Drug reaction Allergic reaction Infection Regimen-related toxicity
Diarrhea	Infection (viral, fungal) Narcotic bowel syndrome (opiate withdrawal)
Abdominal Pain	Acute pancreatitis Acute cholesystitis (biliary sludge, stones, infection) Narcotic bowel syndrome (opiate withdrawal)
Elevated liver enzymes	Sinusoidal obstruction syndrome Medication toxicities (e.g., cyclosporine) Cholangitis lenta (sepsis) Biliary sludge syndrome Viral infections (CMV, EBV, hepatitis B) Hemolysis

AGVHD, acute graft-versus-host disease; CMV, cytomegalovirus; EBV, Epstein–Barr virus.

fascia are involved. Major causes of morbidity include scleroderma, contractures, ulceration, keratoconjunctivitis, strictures, obstructive pulmonary disease, and weight loss. Uncontrolled chronic GVHD interferes with immune reconstitution and is strongly associated with increased risks of opportunistic infections and death.

Confirming the Diagnosis of GVHD

Unlike CGVHD, the clinical signs of acute GVHD are not considered sufficiently pathognomonic to establish the diagnosis, especially when there is isolated organ involvement. However, the combination of rash, nausea, and voluminous diarrhea, occurring at the time of, or early after, neutrophil engraftment makes the diagnosis very likely. The differential diagnosis involves ruling out other causes of rash, diarrhea, or liver toxicity as listed in Table 64.5. Tissue biopsies of the skin, liver, or stomach are recommended to confirm a histologic diagnosis of GVHD and, most importantly, to exclude opportunistic infection; however, the interpretation of biopsies performed within 3 weeks of myeloablative therapy may be problematic because it is difficult to separate cellular injury induced by chemoradiotherapy from GVHD. The gastric antral mucosa provides the most sensitive site for evaluation of intestinal GVHD and is preferred to duodenal biopsy because there is less risk for bleeding complications. The histologic hallmark of GVHD-induced cellular injury is apoptosis, observed in epidermal basal keratinocytes, bile duct, or intestinal crypt epithelial cells, and is often associated with infiltration by lymphocytes [146,147]. Biopsy is unnecessary to confirm the presence of chronic GVHD if at least one diagnostic feature is present, but histologic confirmation or other pertinent testing is necessary when CGVHD features are only distinctive or suggestive (see Table 64.4).

Prevention of GVHD

GVHD prevention strategies are almost always incorporated into the overall treatment plan, and these include optimizing the choice of allogeneic donor and stem cell product based on known risk factors for GVHD, T-cell depletion of the donor HSC graft as discussed earlier, or, most commonly, posttransplant immunosuppression. Ursodeoxycholic acid should be given to all patients irrespective of the approach to GVHD prophylaxis because it improves liver function and reduces the incidence of hepatic GVHD [148].

Postgrafting Immunosuppression. In the absence of T-cell depletion, posttransplant immune suppression must be administered to control donor alloreactive T cells. Most GVHD prophylaxis regimens include a CNI (cyclosporine or tacrolimus) in combination with one or two additional agents, such as methotrexate, mycophenolate mofetil (MMF), or sirolimus [149–152]. In some settings, cyclophosphamide is given on days 3 and 4 after HCT, followed by prophylaxis with a CNI and MMF [15]. Steady-state serum CNI and sirolimus levels require monitoring. Dose reductions should be made when toxicities emerge or when serum trough levels exceed the upper limit of the therapeutic range.

Treatment of GVHD

Despite GVHD prophylaxis regimens, 30% to 80% of allogeneic HCT recipients develop acute GVHD and require additional therapy with glucocorticoids.

Acute GVHD. Glucocorticoids have been the mainstay of primary therapy for acute GVHD. Initial starting doses have been recently calibrated to the severity and extent of organ involvement as demonstrated by one large retrospective study [153]. For the one-third of patients who develop GVHD without liver involvement, and whose GI symptoms are defined as stage 1 (anorexia, nausea, or vomiting with peak stool volume less than 1,000 mL per day), with or without rash involving less than 50% of the body surface, treatment may reasonably begin at 1 mg/kg/d methylprednisolone (or oral equivalent) combined with topical and minimally absorbed glucocorticoids (beclomethasone and/or budesonide). When there is liver involvement, or when intestinal and skin GVHD is greater than defined above, methylprednisolone is typically begun at a dose of 2 mg/kg/d for up to 14 days [154]. Once the symptoms (rash, diarrhea, abdominal pain, and liver dysfunction) are controlled, a glucocorticoid taper should be instituted. For treatment of symptoms that do not respond to the initial treatment, there is no benefit for administration of doses greater than 2 mg/kg/d of methylprednisolone, and alternative approaches to steroid-refractory GVHD must be considered, as discussed below [155].

Chronic GVHD. In practice, systemic therapy is considered when chronic GVHD is present in more than two organs or when there are moderate to severe abnormalities of a single organ with functional impairment (Table 64.6). In contrast,

TABLE 64.6

Indication for Systemic Immunosuppression at Day 80

Global severity of chronic GVHD	High-risk features[a]	Systemic therapy
None	Yes	None[b]
Mild (<3 sites[c], no lung)	No	No
Mild	Yes	Yes
Moderate[d] (or mild lung) or severe[e]	Yes or no	Yes

[a]Less than 100,000 platelets/μL, progressive onset (on prednisone).
[b]Need to balance risks and benefits of graft-versus-tumor against risks of developing more severe chronic GVHD based on the coexistence of risk factors, including unrelated or mismatched-related donor, female donor, and peripheral blood stem cell transplant.
[c]No clinically significant functional impairment (score ≤1 in each site).
[d]At least one site functionally impaired without major disability (Score 2 or 3) or more sites without clinically significant functional impairment (each with score ≤1).
[e]Major disability at any site (score 3, or score ≥2 in lung).
GVHD, graft-versus-host disease.

TABLE 64.7

Therapy Options for Steroid-Refractory Acute Graft-versus-Host Disease

Therapy	Comments
Systemic	
Polyclonal	
Antithymocyte globulin (ATGAM[a], Thymoglobulin[b])	Delayed use appears to be very ineffective. Skin responds best
Monoclonal	
Anti-IL2 (daclizumab[c], basilixumab[e])	Depletes conventional and regulatory T cells
Anti-TNFα (infliximab[e])	Consider early for refractory lower GI tract
Anti-CD52 (alemtuzumab[c])	Depletes T & B cells (lower risk EBV PTLD)
Fusion proteins	
Anti-IL2 (denileukin diftitox)	Anti–T cell but also depletes regulatory T cells
Anti-TNFα (etanercept)	TNF inhibitor
Macrolides and antimetabolites	
Tacrolimus	Inhibits conventional and regulatory T cells
Sirolimus	Inhibits conventional but not regulatory T cells
Mycophenolate mofetil	Enteric-coated formulation may minimize toxicity but liquid formulation not available
Pentostatin	Universal lymphopenia and late infections were dose limiting. Best responses in skin
Extracorporeal photopheresis	Mechanism includes facilitation of regulatory T cells; particularly effective in skin, infrequently associated with opportunistic infections
Mesenchymal stem cells	Mechanism poorly understood but thought to modulate tissue repair
Topical	
Glucocorticoids	
Budesonside	Useful as steroid-sparing agent in lower GI tract
Beclomethasone[d]	Useful as steroid-sparing agent in upper GI tract
PUVA	Useful for skin-only involvement

PUVA, psoralen and ultraviolet A.
[a]Equine
[b]Rabbit
[c]Humanized
[d]Not commercially available]
[e]Chimeric murine-human
Adapted from Carpenter PA, Macmillin ML. Management of acute graft-versus-host disease in children. *Pediatr Clin North Am* 57:273–95, 2010.

systemic therapy is generally not warranted for patients with mild abnormalities of one or two organs that do not cause functional impairment. However, mild chronic GVHD does warrant systemic therapy when either thrombocytopenia or steroid treatment is present at diagnosis.

Standard primary therapy for clinical extensive CGVHD usually begins with glucocorticoids and extended administration of a CNI. After newly diagnosed CGVHD manifestations have been controlled by daily glucocorticoids, the judicious use of glucocorticoids at the lowest effective dose and alternate-day administration can minimize steroid-related side effects. The median duration of systemic immunosuppression for the treatment of CGVHD approximates 2 to 3 years [156,157]. Longer therapy tends to be required for recipients of PBSCs, male patients with female donors, multiple organ involvement at the onset of CGVHD, graft-versus-host HLA mismatch, and hyperbilirubinemia. Infection from a broad array of pathogens is a major cause of mortality among patients with CGVHD; therefore, antibiotic prophylaxis to prevent infection (Table 64.2) and supportive care to minimize morbidity and prevent disability are critically important components of CGVHD management [158,159].

Steroid-Refractory GVHD. Glucocorticoids often fail to control acute GVHD manifestations such that 40% to 60% of patients have steroid-refractory (SR) acute GVHD. SR-GVHD has been defined operationally as the progression of acute GVHD symptoms beyond 3 days after starting methylprednisolone. Persistence of GVHD beyond 7 to 14 days should also be considered failure of response. The prognosis of acute GVHD can be related to its overall severity (grade) and response to glucocorticoids [160]. Grade III and IV SR acute GVHD, especially with visceral involvement, requires urgent initiation of effective secondary therapy [154].

Unfortunately, there is no generally accepted therapy for SR acute GVHD. A full review of the various secondary GVHD therapies is beyond the scope of this review, but various approaches are listed in Table 64.7 [154]. Polyclonal antithymocyte globulins (ATG) or monoclonal antibodies are generally used to treat life-threatening visceral manifestations where urgent control of SR acute GVHD is necessary. Unfortunately, longer term survival has been unusual when visceral manifestations are severe because progressive organ dysfunction is often irreversible and because second-line therapies constitute a "second hit" to an immune system that has already been impaired by cumulative exposure to high-dose prednisone. In this regard, high daily prednisone doses increase the risk for CMV viremia and invasive aspergillosis [161,162].

When CGVHD becomes refractory to steroids, in contrast to SR acute GVHD, secondary therapy generally avoids potent antibody therapies unless the manifestations overlap with the disease features typically associated with severe acute GVHD. The time to complete resolution of classical CGVHD manifestations is in the order of weeks to months, and total duration of therapy spans months to years. Therefore, secondary therapies for SR-CGVHD must try to avoid profound T-cell depletion and must generally be more easily delivered chronically in the outpatient setting. Ideally, second-line agents should promote transplantation tolerance so that the morbidity associated with prolonged use of glucocorticoids and other immunosuppressive agents can be minimized. Agents or strategies that have been used more recently to treat CGVHD, and particularly when fibrotic or sclerotic manifestations are present, include sirolimus, extracorporeal photophoresis, rituximab, low-dose interleukin-2, and imatinib. A number of ancillary measures that are used with topical intent are often used to target specific organ involvement [158].

References

1. Aspesberro F, Guthrie KA, Woolfrey AE, et al: Outcome of pediatric hematopoietic stem cell transplant recipients requiring mechanical ventilation. *J Intensive Care Med* 29:31–37, 2012.
2. Kew AK, Couban S, Patrick W, et al: Outcome of hematopoietic stem cell transplant recipients admitted to the intensive care unit. *Biol Blood Marrow Transplant* 12:301–305, 2006.
3. Duncan CN, Lehmann LE, Cheifetz IM, et al: Clinical outcomes of children receiving intensive cardiopulmonary support during hematopoietic stem cell transplant. *Pediatr Crit Care Med* 14:261–267, 2013.
4. Reddy RL: Mobilization and collection of peripheral blood progenitor cells for transplantation [review]. *Transfus Apher Sci* 32:63–72, 2005.
5. Bensinger WI, Martin PJ, Storer B, et al: Transplantation of bone marrow as compared with peripheral-blood cells from HLA-identical relatives in patients with hematologic cancers. *N Engl J Med* 344:175–181, 2001.
6. Anasetti C, Logan BR, Lee SJ, et al: Peripheral-blood stem cells versus bone marrow from unrelated donors. *N Engl J Med* 367:1487–1496, 2012.
7. Rocha V, Cornish J, Sievers EL, et al: Comparison of outcomes of unrelated bone marrow and umbilical cord blood transplants in children with acute leukemia. *Blood* 97:2962–2971, 2001.
8. Cohen YC, Scaradavou A, Stevens CE, et al: Factors affecting mortality following myeloablative cord blood transplantation in adults: a pooled analysis of three international registries. *Bone Marrow Transplant* 46: 70–76, 2011.
9. Barker JN, Weisdorf DJ, Defor TE, et al: Transplantation of 2 partially HLA-matched umbilical cord blood units to enhance engraftment in adults with hematologic malignancy. *Blood* 105:1343–1347, 2005.
10. Hamadani M: Autologous hematopoietic cell transplantation: an update for clinicians (Review). *Ann Med* 46:619–632, 2014.
11. Arora M, Weisdorf DJ, Spellman SR, et al: HLA-identical sibling versus 8/8 matched and mismatched unrelated donor bone marrow transplant for chronic phase chronic myeloid leukemia. *J Clin Oncol* 27:1644–1652, 2009.
12. Woolfrey A, Lee SJ, Gooley TA, et al: HLA-allele matched unrelated donors compared to HLA-matched sibling donors: role of cell source and disease risk category. *Biol Blood Marrow Transplant* 16:1382–1387, 2010.
13. Lee SJ, Klein J, Haagenson M, et al: High-resolution donor-recipient HLA matching contributes to the success of unrelated donor marrow transplantation. *Blood* 110:4576–4583, 2007.
14. Aversa F, Martelli MF, Velardi A: Haploidentical hematopoietic stem cell transplantation with a megadose T-cell-depleted graft: harnessing natural and adaptive immunity [review]. *Semin Oncol* 39:643–652, 2012.
15. Luznik L, O'Donnell PV, Fuchs EJ: Post-transplantation cyclophosphamide for tolerance induction in HLA-haploidentical bone marrow transplantation. *Semin Oncol* 39:683–693, 2012.
16. Sorror ML, Maris MB, Storer B, et al: Comparing morbidity and mortality of HLA-matched unrelated donor hematopoietic cell transplantation after nonmyeloablative and myeloablative conditioning: influence of pretransplant comorbidities. *Blood* 104:961–968, 2004.
17. Sengsayadeth S, Savani BN, Blaise D, et al: Reduced intensity conditioning allogeneic hematopoietic cell transplantation for adult acute myeloid leukemia in complete remission - a review from the Acute Leukemia Working Party of the EBMT [review]. *Haematologica* 100:859–869, 2015.
18. Storb R, Gyurkocza B, Storer BE, et al: Graft-versus-host disease and graft-versus-tumor effects after allogeneic hematopoietic cell transplantation. *J Clin Oncol* 31:1530–1538, 2013.
19. Sorror ML, Maris MB, Storb R, et al: Hematopoietic cell transplantation (HCT)-specific comorbidity index: a new tool for risk assessment before allogeneic HCT. *Blood* 106:2912–2919, 2005.
20. Stanworth SJ, Hudson CL, Estcourt LJ, et al: Risk of bleeding and use of platelet transfusions in patients with hematologic malignancies: recurrent event analysis. *Haematologica* 100:740–747, 2015.
21. Mishima Y, Tsuno NH, Matsuhashi M, et al: Effects of universal vs bedside leukoreductions on the alloimmunization to platelets and the platelet transfusion refractoriness. *Transfus Apher Sci* 52:112–121, 2015.
22. Ziemann M, Hennig H: Prevention of transfusion-transmitted cytomegalovirus infections: Which is the optimal strategy? [review]. *Transfus Med Hemother* 41:40–44, 2014.
23. McDonald GB, Shulman HM, Sullivan KM, et al: Intestinal and hepatic complications of human bone marrow transplantation. *Gastroenterology* 90:460–477, 770–784, 1986.
24. Sale GE, Shulman HM, Hackman RC: Pathology of hematopoietic cell transplantation, in Blume KG, Forman SJ, Appelbaum FR (eds): *Thomas' Hematopoietic Cell Transplantation.* Oxford, UK: Blackwell, 2004, pp 286–299.
25. Fegan C, Poynton CH, Whittaker JA: The gut mucosal barrier in bone marrow transplantation. *Bone Marrow Transplant* 5:373–377, 1990.
26. Rogers M, Cerda JJ: The narcotic bowel syndrome [review]. *J Clin Gastroenterol* 11:132–135, 1989.
27. Schwartz JM, Strasser SI, Lopez-Cubero SO, et al: Severe gastrointestinal bleeding after marrow transplantation, 1987-1997: incidence, causes and outcome [abstract]. *Gastroenterology* 114:A40, 1998.

28. Bearman SI: The syndrome of hepatic veno-occlusive disease after marrow transplantation. *Blood* 85:3005–3020, 1995.
29. McDonald GB, Hinds MS, Fisher LD, et al: Veno-occlusive disease of the liver and multiorgan failure after bone marrow transplantation: a cohort study of 355 patients. *Ann Intern Med* 118:255–267, 1993.
30. Dignan FL, Wynn RF, Hadzic N, et al: BCSH/BSBMT guideline: diagnosis and management of veno-occlusive disease (sinusoidal obstruction syndrome) following haematopoietic stem cell transplantation. *Br J Haematol* 163:444–457, 2013.
31. Coppell JA, Richardson PG, Soiffer R, et al: Hepatic veno-occlusive disease following stem cell transplantation: incidence, clinical course, and outcome [review]. *Biol Blood Marrow Transplant* 16:157–168, 2010.
32. Slattery JT, Kalhorn TF, McDonald GB, et al: Conditioning regimen-dependent disposition of cyclophosphamide and hydroxycyclophosphamide in human marrow transplantation patients. *J Clin Oncol* 14:1484–1494, 1996.
33. Hommeyer SC, Teefey SA, Jacobson AF, et al: Sonographic evaluation of patients with venoclusive disease of the liver: a prospective study. *Radiology* 184:683–686, 1992.
34. Herbetko J, Grigg AP, Buckley AR, et al: Venoocclusive liver disease after bone marrow transplantation: findings at duplex sonography. *Am J Roentgenol* 158:1001–1005, 1992.
35. Shulman HM, Gooley T, Dudley MD, et al: Utility of transvenous liver biopsies and wedged hepatic venous pressure measurements in sixty marrow transplant recipients. *Transplantation* 59:1015–1022, 1995.
36. Sakai M, Strasser SI, Shulman HM, et al: Severe hepatocellular injury after hematopoietic cell transplant: incidence, etiology and outcome. *Bone Marrow Transplant* 44:441–447, 2009.
37. McDonald GB, Shulman HM, Wolford JL, et al: Liver disease after human marrow transplantation. *Semin Liver Dis* 7:210–220, 1987.
38. Jacobson AF, Teefey SA, Lee SP, et al: Frequent occurrence of new hepatobiliary abnormalities after bone marrow transplantation: results of a prospective study using scintigraphy and sonography. *Am J Gastroenterol* 88:1044–1049, 1993.
39. Bearman SI, Anderson GL, Mori M, et al: Venoocclusive disease of the liver: development of a model for predicting fatal outcome after marrow transplantation. *J Clin Oncol* 11:1729–1736, 1993.
40. Chao N: How I treat sinusoidal obstruction syndrome. *Blood* 123:4023–4026, 2014.
41. Ho VT, Revta C, Richardson PG: Hepatic veno-occlusive disease after hematopoietic stem cell transplantation: update on defibrotide and other current investigational therapies [review]. *Bone Marrow Transplant* 41:229–237, 2008.
42. Fried MW, Connaghan DG, Sharma S, et al: Transjugular intrahepatic portosystemic shunt for the management of severe venoocclusive disease following bone marrow transplantation. *Hepatology* 24:588–591, 1996.
43. Schlitt HJ, Tischler HJ, Ringe B, et al: Allogeneic liver transplantation for hepatic veno-occlusive disease after bone marrow transplantation—clinical and immunological considerations. *Bone Marrow Transplant* 16:473–478, 1995.
44. Soubani AO, Miller KB, Hassoun PM: Pulmonary complications of bone marrow transplantation [review]. *Chest* 109:1066–1077, 1996.
45. Parimon T, Madtes DK, Au DH, et al: Pretransplant lung function, respiratory failure, and mortality after stem cell transplantation. *Am J Respir Crit Care Med* 172:384–390, 2005.
46. Crawford SW: Noninfectious lung disease in the immunocompromised host [review]. *Respiration* 66:385–395, 1999.
47. Clark JG, Crawford SW: Diagnostic approaches to pulmonary complications of marrow transplantation. *Chest* 91:477–479, 1987.
48. Meyers JD, Flournoy N, Thomas ED: Nonbacterial pneumonia after allogeneic marrow transplantation: a review of ten years' experience. *Rev Infect Dis* 4: 1119–1132, 1982.
49. Kantrow SP, Hackman RC, Boeckh M, et al: Idiopathic pneumonia syndrome: changing spectrum of lung injury after marrow transplantation. *Transplantation* 63:1079–1086, 1997.
50. Seo S, Renaud C, Kuypers JM, et al: Idiopathic pneumonia syndrome after hematopoietic cell transplantation: evidence of occult infectious etiologies. *Blood* 125:3789–3797, 2015.
51. Schlemmer F, Chevret S, Lorillon G, et al: Late-onset noninfectious interstitial lung disease after allogeneic hematopoietic stem cell transplantation. *Respir Med* 108:1525–1533, 2014.
52. Metcalf JP, Rennard SI, Reed EC, et al: Corticosteroids as adjunctive therapy for diffuse alveolar hemorrhage associated with bone marrow transplantation. University of Nebraska Medical Center Bone Marrow Transplant Group. *Am J Med* 96:327–334, 1994.
53. Yanik GA, Horowitz MM, Weisdorf DJ, et al: Randomized, double-blind, placebo-controlled trial of soluble tumor necrosis factor receptor: Enbrel (etanercept) for the treatment of idiopathic pneumonia syndrome after allogeneic stem cell transplantation: Blood and Marrow Transplant Clinical Trials Network protocol. *Biol Blood Marrow Transplant* 20:858–864, 2014.
54. Yanik GA, Grupp SA, Pulsipher MA, et al: TNF-receptor inhibitor therapy for the treatment of children with idiopathic pneumonia syndrome. A joint Pediatric Blood and Marrow Transplant Consortium and Children's Oncology Group Study (ASCT0521). *Biol Blood Marrow Transplant* 21:67–73, 2015.
55. Crawford SW, Hackman RC: Clinical course of idiopathic pneumonia after bone marrow transplantation. *Am Rev Respir Dis* 147:1393–1400, 1993.
56. De Lassence A, Fleury-Feith J, Escudier E, et al: Alveolar hemorrhage. Diagnostic criteria and results in 194 immunocompromised hosts. *Am J Respir Crit Care Med* 151:157–163, 1995.
57. Robbins RA, Linder J, Stahl MG, et al: Diffuse alveolar hemorrhage in autologous bone marrow transplant recipients. *Am J Med* 87:511–518, 1989.
58. Gupta S, Jain A, Warneke CL, et al: Outcome of alveolar hemorrhage in hematopoietic stem cell transplant recipients. *Bone Marrow Transplant* 40:71–78, 2007.
59. Rathi NK, Tanner AR, Dinh A, et al: Low-, medium- and high-dose steroids with or without aminocaproic acid in adult hematopoietic SCT patients with diffuse alveolar hemorrhage. *Bone Marrow Transplant* 50:420–426, 2015.
60. Rubenfeld GD, Crawford SW: Withdrawing life support from mechanically ventilated recipients of bone marrow transplants: a case for evidence-based guidelines. *Ann Intern Med* 125:625–633, 1996.
61. Hertenstein B, Stefanic M, Schmeiser T, et al: Cardiac toxicity of bone marrow transplantation: predictive value of cardiologic evaluation before transplant. *J Clin Oncol* 12:998–1004, 1994.
62. Brockstein BE, Smiley C, Al-Sadir J, et al: Cardiac and pulmonary toxicity in patients undergoing high-dose chemotherapy for lymphoma and breast cancer: prognostic factors. *Bone Marrow Transplant* 25:885–894, 2000.
63. Cazin B, Gorin NC, Laporte JP, et al: Cardiac complications after bone marrow transplantation. A report on a series of 63 consecutive transplantations. *Cancer* 57:2061–2069, 1986.
64. Dandoy CE, Hirsch R, Chima R, et al: Pulmonary hypertension after hematopoietic stem cell transplantation [review]. *Biol Blood Marrow Transplant* 19:1546–1556, 2013.
65. Hingorani SR, Guthrie K, Batchelder A, et al: Acute renal failure after myeloablative hematopoietic cell transplant: incidence and risk factors. *Kidney Int* 67:272–277, 2005.
66. Hingorani SR, Seidel K, Pao E, et al: Markers of coagulation activation and acute kidney injury in patients after hematopoietic cell transplantation. *Bone Marrow Transplant* 50:715–720, 2015.
67. Jodele S, Fukuda T, Vinks A, et al: Eculizumab therapy in children with severe hematopoietic stem cell transplantation-associated thrombotic microangiopathy. *Biol Blood Marrow Transplant* 20:518–525, 2014.
68. Jodele S, Laskin BL, Dandoy CE, et al: A new paradigm: diagnosis and management of HSCT-associated thrombotic microangiopathy as multi-system endothelial injury. *Blood Rev* 29:191–204, 2015.
69. Cutler C, Henry NL, Magee C, et al: Sirolimus and thrombotic microangiopathy after allogeneic hematopoietic stem cell transplantation. *Biol Blood Marrow Transplant* 11:551–557, 2005.
70. Ho VT, Cutler C, Carter S, et al: Blood and marrow transplant clinical trials network toxicity committee consensus summary: thrombotic microangiopathy after hematopoietic stem cell transplantation. *Biol Blood Marrow Transplant* 11:571–575, 2005.
71. Kim SS, Patel M, Yum K, et al: Hematopoietic stem cell transplant-associated thrombotic microangiopathy: review of pharmacologic treatment options [review]. *Transfusion* 55:452–458, 2015.
72. June CH, Thompson CB, Kennedy MS, et al: Correlation of hypomagnesemia with the onset of cyclosporine-associated hypertension in marrow transplant patients. *Transplantation* 41:47–51, 1986.
73. Lunde LE, Dasaraju S, Cao Q, et al: Hemorrhagic systitis after allogeneic hematopoietic cell transplantation: risk factors, graft source and survival. *Bone Marrow Transplant* 50(11):1432–1437, 2015.
74. Uhm J, Hamad N, Michelis FV, et al: The risk of polyomavirus BK-associated hemorrhagic cystitis after allogeneic hematopoietic SCT is associated with myeloablative conditioning, CMV viremia and severe acute GVHD. *Bone Marrow Transplant* 49:1528–1534, 2014.
75. Raval M, Gulbis A, Bollard C, et al: Evaluation and management of BK virus-associated nephropathy following allogeneic hematopoietic cell transplantation. *Biol Blood Marrow Transplant* 17:1589–1593, 2011.
76. Cesaro S, Hirsch HH, Faraci M, et al: Cidofovir for BK virus-associated hemorrhagic cystitis: a retrospective study. *Clin Infect Dis* 49:233–240, 2009.
77. Graus F, Saiz A, Sierra J, et al: Neurologic complications of autologous and allogeneic bone marrow transplantation in patients with leukemia: a comparative study. *Neurology* 46:1004–1009, 1996.
78. Walters MC, Sullivan KM, Bernaudin F, et al: Neurologic complications after allogeneic marrow transplantation for sickle cell anemia (Rapid Communication). *Blood* 85:879–884, 1995.
79. Valilis PN, Zeigler ZR, Shadduck RK, et al: A prospective study of bone marrow transplant-associated thrombotic microangiopathy (BMT-TM) in autologous (AUTO) and allogeneic (ALLO) BMT. *Blood* 86:970a, 1995.
80. Davies SM, Szabo E, Wagner JE, et al: Idiopathic hyperammonemia: a frequently lethal complication of bone marrow transplantation. *Bone Marrow Transplant* 17:1119–1125, 1996.
81. Kang JM, Kim YJ, Kim JY, et al: Neurologic complications after allogeneic hematopoietic stem cell transplantation in children: analysis of prognostic factors. *Biol Blood Marrow Transplant* 21:1091–1098, 2015.
82. Furlong T, Storb R, Anasetti C, et al: Clinical outcome after conversion to FK 506 (tacrolimus) therapy for acute graft-versus-host disease resistant to cyclosporine or for cyclosporine-associated toxicities. *Bone Marrow Transplant* 26:985–991, 2000.
83. Drachman BM, DeNofrio D, Acker MA, et al: Cortical blindness secondary to cyclosporine after orthotopic heart transplantation: a case report and review of the literature [review]. *J Heart Lung Transplant* 15:1158–1164, 1996.
84. Pettitt AR, Clark RE: Thrombotic microangiopathy following bone marrow transplantation. *Bone Marrow Transplant* 14:495–504, 1994.
85. Qu L, Kiss JE: Thrombotic microangiopathy in transplantation and malignancy. *Semin Thromb Hemost* 31:691–699, 2005.

86. Rowley SD, Donato ML, Bhattacharyya P: Red blood cell-incompatible allogeneic hematopoietic progenitor cell transplantation [review]. *Bone Marrow Transplant* 46:1167–1185, 2011.
87. Booth GS, Gehrie EA, Bolan CD, et al: Clinical guide to ABO-incompatible allogeneic stem cell transplantation. *Biol Blood Marrow Transplant* 19:1152–1158, 2013.
88. Bolan CD, Leitman SF, Griffith LM, et al: Delayed donor red cell chimerism and pure red cell aplasia following major ABO-incompatible nonmyeloablative hematopoietic stem cell transplantation. *Blood* 98:1687–1694, 2001.
89. Bolan CD, Childs RW, Procter JL, et al: Massive immune haemolysis after allogeneic peripheral blood stem cell transplantation with minor ABO incompatibility. *Br J Haematol* 112:787–795, 2001.
90. Tomblyn M, Chiller T, Einsele H, et al: Guidelines for preventing infectious complications among hematopoietic cell transplant recipients: a global perspective. *Bone Marrow Transplant* 44:453–455, 2009.
91. Wu D, Hockenbery DM, Brentnall TA, et al: Persistent nausea and anorexia after marrow transplantation: a prospective study of 78 patients. *Transplantation* 66:1319–1324, 1998.
92. Brownback KR, Simpson SQ: Association of bronchoalveolar lavage yield with chest computed tomography findings and symptoms in immunocompromised patients. *Ann Thorac Med* 8:153–159, 2013.
93. Brownback KR, Thomas LA, Simpson SQ: Role of bronchoalveolar lavage in the diagnosis of pulmonary infiltrates in immunocompromised patients. *Curr Opin Inf Dis* 27:322–328, 2014.
94. Huaringa AJ, Leyva FJ, Signes-Costa J, et al: Bronchoalveolar lavage in the diagnosis of pulmonary complications of bone marrow transplant patients. *Bone Marrow Transplant* 25:975–979, 2000.
95. Musher B, Fredricks D, Leisenring W, et al: *Aspergillus* galactomannan enzyme immunoassay and quantitative PCR for diagnosis of invasive aspergillosis with bronchoalvolar lavage fluid. *J Clin Microbiol* 42:5517–5522, 2004.
96. Oliveira R, Machado A, Tateno A, et al: Frequency of human metapneumovirus infection in hematopoietic SCT recipients during 3 consecutive years. *Bone Marrow Transplant* 42:265–269, 2008.
97. Englund JA, Boeckh M, Kuypers J, et al: Fatal human metapneumovirus infection in stem cell transplant recipients. *Ann Intern Med* 144:344–349, 2006.
98. Ellis ME, Spence D, Bouchama A, et al: Open lung biopsy provides a higher and more specific diagnostic yield compared to broncho-alveolar lavage in immunocompromised patients. Fungal Study Group. *Scand J Infect Dis* 27:157–162, 1995.
99. Robinson LA, Reed EC, Galbraith TA, et al: Pulmonary resection for invasive Aspergillus infections in immunocompromised patients. *J Thorac Cardiovasc Surg* 109:1182–1196, 1995.
100. Tuan I-Z, Dennison D, Weisdorf DJ: *Pneumocystis carinii* pneumonitis following bone marrow transplantation. *Bone Marrow Transplant* 10:267–272, 1992.
101. Marr KA, Carter RA, Crippa F, et al: Epidemiology and outcome of mould infections in hematopoietic stem cell transplant recipients. *Clin Infect Dis* 34:909–917, 2002.
102. Marr KA, Walsh TJ: Management strategies for infections caused by *candida* species, in Wingard JR, Bowden RA (eds): *Management of Infection in Oncology Patients*. London, UK: Martin Dunitz, 2003, pp 165–177.
103. Girmenia C, Barosi G, Piciocchi A, et al: Primary prophylaxis of invasive fungal diseases in allogeneic stem cell transplantation: revised recommendations from a consensus process by Gruppo Italiano Trapianto Midollo Osseo (GITMO) [review]. *Biol Blood Marrow Transplant* 20:1080–1088, 2014.
104. Goodman JL, Winston DJ, Greenfield RA, et al: A controlled trial of fluconazole to prevent fungal infections in patients undergoing bone marrow transplantation. *N Engl J Med* 326:845–851, 1992.
105. Marr KA, Seidel K, White TC, et al: Candidemia in allogeneic blood and marrow transplant recipients: evolution of risk factors after the adoption of prophylactic fluconazole. *J Infect Dis* 181:309–316, 2000.
106. Marr KA. The changing spectrum of candidemia in oncology patients: therapeutic implications. *Curr Opin Inf Dis* 13:615–620, 2000.
107. Neofytos D, Treadway S, Ostrander D, et al: Epidemiology, outcomes, and mortality predictors of invasive mold infections among transplant recipients: a 10-year, single-center experience. *Transpl Infect Dis* 15:233–242, 2013.
108. Miceli MH, Goggins MI, Chander P, et al: Performance of lateral flow device and galactomannan for the detection of Aspergillus species in bronchoalveolar fluid of patients at risk for invasive pulmonary aspergillosis. *Mycoses* 58:368–374, 2015.
109. Herbrecht R, Letscher-Bru V, Oprea C, et al: Aspergillus galactomannan detection in the diagnosis of invasive aspergillosis in cancer patients. *J Clin Oncol* 20: 1898–1906, 2002.
110. Limper AH, Knox KS, Sarosi GA, et al: An official American Thoracic Society statement: treatment of fungal infections in adult pulmonary and critical care patients. *Am J Respir Crit Care Med* 183:96–128, 2011.
111. Yeghen T, Kibbler CC, Prentice HG, et al: Management of invasive pulmonary aspergillosis in hematology patients: a review of 87 consecutive cases at a single institution. *Clin Infect Dis* 31:859–868, 2000.
112. Green ML, Leisenring W, Stachel D, et al: Efficacy of viral load-based, risk-adapted, preemptive treatment strategy for prevention of cytomegalovirus disease after hematopoietic cell transplantation. *Biol Blood Marrow Transplant* 18:1687–1699, 2012.
113. Boeckh M, Hoy C, Torok-Storb B: Occult cytomegalovirus infection of marrow stroma. *Clin Infect Dis* 26:209–210, 1998.
114. Cox GJ, Matsui SM, Lo RS, et al: Etiology and outcome of diarrhea after marrow transplantation: a prospective study. *Gastroenterology* 107:1398–1407, 1994.
115. Griffiths PD, Boeckh M. Antiviral therapy for human cytomegalovirus, in Arvin A, Campadelli-Flume G, Mocarski E, et al (eds): *Human Herpesviruses: Biology, Therapy, and Immunoprophylaxis*. Cambridge: Cambridge University Press, Chapter 66, 1192-1210, 2007.
116. Ljungman P, Engelhard D, Link H, et al: Treatment of interstitial pneumonitis due to cytomegalovirus with ganciclovir and intravenous immune globulin: experience of European bone marrow transplant group. *Clin Infect Dis* 14:831–835, 1992.
117. Styczynski J, Reusser P, Einsele H, et al: Management of HSV, VZV and EBV infections in patients with hematological malignancies and after SCT: guidelines from the Second European Conference on Infections in Leukemia. *Bone Marrow Transplant* 43:757–770, 2009.
118. Meyers JD, Flournoy N, Thomas ED: Infection with herpes simplex virus and cell-mediated immunity after marrow transplant. *J Infect Dis* 142:338–346, 1980.
119. Wade JC, Newton B, McLaren C, et al: Intravenous acyclovir to treat mucocutaneous herpes simplex virus infection after marrow transplantation: a double-blind trial. *Ann Intern Med* 96:265–269, 1982.
120. Zaia JA, Levin MJ, Preblud SR, et al: Evaluation of varicella-zoster immune globulin: protection of immunosuppressed children after household exposure to varicella. *J Infect Dis* 147:737–743, 1983.
121. Han CS, Miller W, Haake R, et al: Varicella zoster infection after bone marrow transplantation: incidence, risk factors and complications. *Bone Marrow Transplant* 13:277–283, 1994.
122. Boeckh M, Kim HW, Flowers MED, et al: Long-term acyclovir for prevention of varicella zoster virus disease after allogeneic hematopoietic cell transplantation - a randomized double-blind placebo-controlled study. *Blood* 107:1800–1805, 2006.
123. Klein A, Miller KB, Sprague K, et al: A randomized, double-blind, placebo-controlled trial of valacyclovir prophylaxis to prevent zoster recurrence from months 4 to 24 after BMT. *Bone Marrow Transplant* 46:294–299, 2011.
124. Kleinschmidt-DeMasters BK, Amlie-Lefond C, Gilden DH: The patterns of varicella zoster virus encephalitis. *Hum Pathol* 27:927–938, 1996.
125. Morishita K, Kodo H, Asano S, et al: Fulminant varicella hepatitis following bone marrow transplantation. *JAMA* 253:511, 1985.
126. Verdonck LF, Cornelissen JJ, Dekker AW, et al: Acute abdominal pain as a presenting symptom of varicella-zoster virus infection in recipients of bone marrow transplants. *Clin Infect Dis* 16:190–191, 1993.
127. Seo S, Xie H, Karron RA, et al: Parainfluenza virus type 3 Ab in allogeneic hematopoietic cell transplant recipients: factors influencing post-transplant Ab titers and associated outcomes. *Bone Marrow Transplant* 49:1205–1211, 2014.
128. Renaud C, Xie H, Seo S, et al: Mortality rates of human metapneumovirus and respiratory syncytial virus lower respiratory tract infections in hematopoietic cell transplantation recipients. *Biol Blood Marrow Transplant* 19:1220–1226, 2013.
129. Harrington RD, Hooton TM, Hackman R, et al: An outbreak of respiratory syncytial virus in a bone marrow transplant center. *J Infect Dis* 165:987–993, 1992.
130. Yilmaz M, Chemaly RF, Han XY, et al: Adenoviral infections in adult allogeneic hematopoietic SCT recipients: a single center experience. *Bone Marrow Transplant* 48:1218–1223, 2013.
131. Robin M, Marque-Juillet S, Scieux C, et al: Disseminated adenovirus infections after allogeneic hematopoietic stem cell transplantation: incidence, risk factors and outcome. *Haematologica* 92:1254–1257, 2007.
132. Lankester AC, van Tol MJ, Claas EC, et al: Quantification of adenovirus DNA in plasma for management of infection in stem cell graft recipients. *Clin Infect Dis* 34:864–867, 2002.
133. Legrand F, Berrebi D, Houhou N, et al: Early diagnosis of adenovirus infection and treatment with cidofovir after bone marrow transplantation in children. *Bone Marrow Transplant* 27:621–626, 2001.
134. Orazi A, Hromas RA, Neiman RS, et al: Posttransplantation lymphoproliferative disorders in bone marrow transplant recipients are aggressive diseases with a high incidence of adverse histologic and immunobiologic features. *Am J Clin Pathol* 107:419–429, 1997.
135. Rasche L, Kapp M, Einsele H, et al: EBV-induced post transplant lymphoproliferative disorders: a persisting challenge in allogeneic hematopoetic SCT [review]. *Bone Marrow Transplant* 49:163–167, 2014.
136. Hoshino Y, Kimura H, Tanaka N, et al: Prospective monitoring of the Epstein–Barr virus DNA by a real-time quantitative polymerase chain reaction after allogenic stem cell transplantation. *Br J Haematol* 115:105–111, 2001.
137. Kuehnle I, Huls MH, Liu Z, et al: CD20 monoclonal antibody (rituximab) for therapy of Epstein–Barr virus lymphoma after hemopoietic stem-cell transplantation. *Blood* 95:1502–1505, 2000.
138. Papadopoulos EB, Ladanyi M, Emanuel D, et al: Infusions of donor leukocytes to treat Epstein–Barr virus-associated lymphoproliferative disorders after allogeneic bone marrow transplantation. *N Engl J Med* 330:1185–1191, 1994.
139. Offner F, Schoch G, Fisher LD, et al: Mortality hazard functions as related to neutropenia at different times after marrow transplantation. *Blood* 88:4058–4062, 1996.
140. Mattsson J, Ringdén O, Storb R: Graft failure after allogeneic hematopoietic cell transplantation. *Biol Blood Marrow Transplant* 14[Suppl 1]:165–170, 2008.
141. Holtan SG, Pasquini M, Weisdorf DJ: Acute graft-versus-host disease: a bench-to-bedside update [review]. *Blood* 124:363–373, 2014.

142. Przepiorka D, Weisdorf D, Martin P, et al: 1994 Consensus Conference on Acute GVHD Grading. *Bone Marrow Transplant* 15:825–828, 1995.
143. Socié G, Ritz J: Current issues in chronic graft-versus-host disease. *Blood* 124:374–384, 2014.
144. Filipovich AH, Weisdorf D, Pavletic S, et al: National Institutes of Health consensus development project on criteria for clinical trials in chronic graft-versus-host disease: I. Diagnosis and Staging Working Group report. *Biol Blood Marrow Transplant* 11:945–956, 2005.
145. Arai S, Jagasia M, Storer B, et al: Global and organ-specific chronic graft-versus-host disease severity according to the 2005 NIH Consensus Criteria. *Blood* 118:4242–4249, 2011.
146. Sale GE: Pathology and recent pathogenetic studies in human graft-versus-host disease. *Surv Synth Path Res* 3:235–253, 1984.
147. Sale GE, Shulman HM, Gallucci BB, et al: Young rete ridge keratinocytes are preferred targets in cutaneous graft-versus-host disease. *Am J Pathol* 118:278–287, 1985.
148. Ruutu T, Eriksson B, Remes K, et al: Ursodeoxycholic acid for the prevention of hepatic complications in allogeneic stem cell transplantation. *Blood* 100:1977–1983, 2002.
149. Storb R, Deeg HJ, Whitehead J, et al: Methotrexate and cyclosporine compared with cyclosporine alone for prophylaxis of acute graft versus host disease after marrow transplantation for leukemia. *N Engl J Med* 314:729–735, 1986.
150. Yu C, Seidel K, Nash RA, et al: Synergism between mycophenolate mofetil and cyclosporine in preventing graft-versus-host disease among lethally irradiated dogs given DLA-nonidentical unrelated marrow grafts. *Blood* 91:2581–2587, 1998.
151. Alyea EP, Li S, Kim H, et al: Sirolimus, tacrolimus and reduced-dose methotrexate as graft versus host disease (GVHD) prophylaxis after non-myeloablative stem cell transplantation: low incidence of acute GVHD compared with tacrolimus/methotrexate or cyclosporine/prednisone [abstract]. *Blood* 104 [Part 1]:209a, #730, 2004.
152. Antin JH, Kim HT, Cutler C, et al: Sirolimus, tacrolimus, and low-dose methotrexate for graft-versus-host disease prophylaxis in mismatched related donor or unrelated donor transplantation. *Blood* 102:1601–1605, 2003.
153. Mielcarek M, Storer BE, Boeckh M, et al: Initial therapy of acute graft-versus-host disease with low-dose prednisone does not compromise patient outcomes. *Blood* 113:2888–2894, 2009.
154. Martin PJ, Rizzo JD, Wingard JR, et al: First- and second-line systemic treatment of acute graft-versus-host disease: recommendations of the American Society of Blood and Marrow Transplantation. *Biol Blood Marrow Transplant* 18:1150–1163, 2012.
155. van Lint MT, Uderzo C, Locasciulli A, et al: Early treatment of acute graft-versus-host disease with high- or low-dose 6-methylprednisolone: a multicenter randomized trial from the Italian Group for Bone Marrow Transplantation. *Blood* 92:2288–2293, 1998.
156. Stewart BL, Storer B, Storek J, et al: Duration of immunosuppressive treatment for chronic graft-versus-host disease. *Blood* 104:3501–3506, 2004.
157. Carpenter PA, Sanders JE: Steroid-refractory graft-vs.host disease: past, present and future. *Pediatr Transplant* 7[Suppl 3]:19–31, 2003.
158. Carpenter PA, Kitko CL, Elad S, et al: National Institutes of Health Consensus Development Project on Criteria for Clinical Trials in Chronic Graft-versus-Host Disease: V. The 2014 Ancillary Therapy and Supportive Care Working Group Report. *Biol Blood Marrow Transplant* 21:1167–1187, 2015.
159. Couriel D, Carpenter PA, Cutler C, et al: Ancillary therapy and supportive care of chronic graft-versus-host disease: National Institutes of Health consensus development project on criteria for clinical trials in chronic graft-versus-host disease: V. Ancillary Therapy and Supportive Care Working Group report. *Biol Blood Marrow Transplant* 12:375–396, 2006.
160. Martin PJ, Schoch G, Fisher L, et al: A retrospective analysis of therapy for acute graft-versus-host disease: initial treatment. *Blood* 76:1464–1472, 1990.
161. Nichols WG, Corey L, Gooley T, et al: Rising pp65 antigenemia during preemptive anticytomegalovirus therapy after allogeneic hematopoietic stem cell transplantation: risk factors, correlation with DNA load, and outcomes. *Blood* 97:867–874, 2001.
162. Marr KA, Carter RA, Boeckh M, et al: Invasive aspergillosis in allogeneic stem cell transplant recipients: changes in epidemiology and risk factors. *Blood* 100:4358–4366, 2002.

Chapter 65 ■ Management of Graft-versus-Host Disease, Infection, Malignancy, and Rejection in Transplant Recipients

VAUGHN E. WHITTAKER • ABBAS A. RANA • DAVID L. DUNN • RAINER W. G. GRUESSNER

The goal of solid-organ transplantation is maximizing graft survival while minimizing the morbidity and mortality associated with the immunosuppressive regimen necessary to prevent rejection, infection, malignancy, and graft-versus-host disease (GvHD). Allograft rejection in transplant recipients is the feared outcome of the complex and intricate mammalian immune system.

The history of solid-organ transplantation has demonstrated that graft survival depends on successfully manipulating the immune system. However, any modification of the host's defense mechanism can bring unwanted consequences, such as rejection, infection, malignancy, and GvHD. In the early days of solid-organ transplantation during the 1960s, it became clear that suppressing the immune system of the prospective host would be required for sustained graft function. Acute rejection (AR) and graft loss are now largely preventable and effectively treated complications of transplantation in contrast to the earliest experiences just over half a century ago.

Successful antirejection treatment and, more importantly, the ability to markedly reduce the incidence of rejection through preventive strategies with effective immunosuppressive agents has allowed solid-organ transplantation to become routine in clinical practice. Initially, successful allogeneic renal transplantation was achieved using a combination of a high-dose corticosteroid and azathioprine [1]. Contemporaneous observations in the very first transplant recipients demonstrated that nonselective immunosuppressive therapy prolonged graft (and patient) survival but led to an increased susceptibility to infection, often with unusual, opportunistic pathogens [2]. Furthermore, immunosuppressed transplant recipients were noted to have an increased susceptibility to malignancy [3].

In the over 50 years since the report of the initial 12 recipients treated for rejection of allogeneic renal grafts, solid-organ transplantation has become mainstream. Kidney, liver, heart, and lung transplants are now standard-of-care therapies for end-stage renal, hepatic, cardiac, and pulmonary disease, respectively. Pancreas and pancreatic islet-cell transplants restore the β-cell function in patients with diabetes mellitus. The small bowel has also been successfully transplanted as a treatment for patients with short gut syndrome. Such strides have been made possible by the accumulated advances in critical care, organ procurement and preservation, surgical techniques, anesthesia management, tissue typing, immunosuppressive therapy, and the use of antibacterial, antifungal, and antiviral agents for both prophylaxis and treatment of posttransplant infection. Table 65.1 lists some of the major advances in the management of GvHD, infection, malignancy, and rejection in transplant recipients.

Yet even with the expanded immunosuppressive armamentarium of the 21st century, it remains difficult to finely balance the suppression of the host immune system (to allow acceptance and even tolerance of the graft) without oversuppressing immune function (and thereby leaving the host vulnerable to opportunistic infection and malignancy). This chapter reviews the complications (namely, GvHD, infection, malignancy, and graft rejection) of solid-organ transplantation on either side of this delicate balance. Special attention is directed toward opportunistic infections and unusual malignancies that occur in the immunosuppressed patient population.

TABLE 65.1

Major Advances in Management of Rejection, Infection, and Malignancy in Transplant Recipients

Topic	Major advances
Graft-versus-host disease	
Graft rejection	Different types of plasmapheresis [7]
	Desensitization protocols for patients with DSA [72,102,103]
	Flow cytometry, Luminex-based cross-match [73,104]
	Induction therapy and biologics reduce rejections [75,76,105]
Fungal infection	Caspofungin and voriconazole [25,106]
Viral infection	PCR for CMV and EBV detection [31]
	Preemptive CMV therapy [31,107]
	Liver transplants for patients with HBV or HCV [41,43]
	Improved outcomes for recipients with HIV
Malignancy	Chemotherapy and rituximab beneficial for PTLD [56]
	HHV-8 and posttransplant Kaposi sarcoma [108]
	Liver transplant for patients with HCC [69]

DSA, donor-specific antibody; PCR, polymerase chain reaction; CMV, cytomegalovirus; EBV, Epstein–Barr virus; HBV, hepatitis B virus; HCV, hepatitis C virus; HIV, human immunodeficiency virus; PTLD, posttransplant lymphoproliferative disorder; HHV, human herpes virus; HCC, hepatocellular carcinoma.

This chapter focuses on complications in solid-organ transplant recipients. There are also individual chapters devoted to each solid organ. Many of the complications seen in solid-organ transplantation can be seen in hematopoietic transplant recipients, as well. However, these complications are discussed specifically in relation to hematopoietic transplant recipients in Chapter 64.

GRAFT-VERSUS-HOST DISEASE

GvHD is the phenomenon characterized by the immunocompetent donor's cells attacking the tissues of the immunocompromised host. It has an incidence of 0.1% to 2.0% with a mortality rate as high as 75%. It is much more common in patient with bone marrow transplant but still occurs in patients with solid-organ transplants [4,5]. It manifests as fever, rash, diarrhea, or hematocytopenia [4].

The condition typically occurs 2 to 6 weeks after solid-organ transplantation as typified in liver or intestinal transplant recipients, but may occur up to 4 months following the transplant [6]. The mechanism is thought to be related to the engraftment of T cells from the donor graft [6]. There is no standard treatment for GvHD. Treatment options have included almost complete withdrawal of immunosuppressive agents, steroid therapy, antibody therapies, and different types of plasmapherisis. The greatest experience is from bone marrow transplant recipients in whom aside from steroid therapy, extracorporeal photopheresis has also demonstrated therapeutic benefits. This involves subjecting the peripheral blood to phototherapy in an effort to induce apoptosis in mononuclear cells, though this mechanism of action has not been fully validated. The postulated mechanisms involve the following: (1) reduced stimulation of effector T cells; (2) deletion of effector T cells; (3) induction of regulatory T cells; (4) increased anti-inflammatory cytokines; and (5) reduction of proinflammatory cytokines. Photopheresis seems to downregulate the T-cell alloreactivity that plays a significant role in the pathogenesis of GvHD after bone marrow transplant with hemopoetic stem cells [7]. Additional studies and pursuing these therapies with a view to share the results to add to the current cohort of patients who are being treated with this modality are the current recommendations based on a Cochrane review [7].

INFECTIONS

The suppression of the host immune response is required to establish and maintain a functioning solid-organ graft. The development of immunosuppressive therapies has been impressive, leading to the widespread use of solid-organ transplantation as the primary therapy for a number of organ failure syndromes. This success is associated with an increased susceptibility for a number of serious infectious complications. Up to 80% of solid-organ transplant recipients experience an infectious complication during the first year posttransplant, and infections remain a major cause of morbidity and mortality in the transplant population [8].

The range of potential pathogens that can cause disease in the immunosuppressed host is impressive. Not only are the common endogenous and nosocomial flora involved, but "opportunistic" or "atypical" pathogens must also be considered in the differential diagnosis of a solid-organ transplant recipient who has evidence of infection. In considering the epidemiology of infectious complications posttransplant, the clinician must assess numerous factors, including the time posttransplant, the organ transplanted, the type and level of immunosuppression, the need for antirejection therapy, and the potential incidence of surgical complications.

The highest risk of infection corresponds with the period of most intense immunosuppression, which is characteristically during the first 6 to 12 months posttransplant and after antirejection therapy, particularly for recurring episodes of AR. Vidal et al. [8] have characterized periods posttransplant during which certain infection patterns may be seen. Infectious complications in the first month posttransplant are typically caused by endogenous or nosocomial flora that would cause disease in an immunocompetent host [9], including (a) bacterial surgical site infections; (b) postoperative or ventilator-associated pneumonia; (c) urinary tract infections (UTIs) associated with prolonged indwelling urinary catheters; (d) intra-abdominal infections related to surgical complications; and (e) central venous catheter infections.

The infections may be classified as those that affect the graft and those that are systemic in nature. Systemic viral infections such as polyoma virus, BK virus, and cytomegalovirus (CMV) commonly affect the graft as well. CMV may affect other organ systems other than the transplanted graft. These infectious patterns may be categorized into an *early cluster* of viral agents occurring with peak frequency between 2 and 3 months posttransplant and a *late cluster* more commonly occurring between 4 and 9 months posttransplant. The early cluster includes CMV [10], adenoviruses [11], hepatitis B virus (HBV) and hepatitis C virus (HCV), and human herpes virus (HHV)-6. The late cluster includes varicella zoster and polyoma viruses. Epstein–Barr virus (EBV) may cause disease throughout the first year posttransplant [12]. The opportunistic fungi can similarly be observed to cluster with *Candida* and *Aspergillus* species (spp), causing infections in the first 2 to 3 months posttransplant [12], whereas *Cryptococcus*, histoplasmosis, coccidioidomycosis, and *P. jiroveci* most often occur later during the first year [13].

After the first 6 to 12 months, most transplant recipients exhibit patterns of infectious disease morbidity that mirrors the rest of the general population, with frequent respiratory infections secondary to pneumococcal infections and influenza, as well as uncomplicated UTIs. However, opportunistic infections can occur anytime. Increased immunosuppression secondary to AR treatment may slightly increase transplant recipients' susceptibility to, and alter the temporal pattern of, various pathogens. When assessing immunosuppressed transplant recipients for infectious diseases, the clinician must maintain a high index of suspicion at all times. The typical localizing signs of infection and inflammation may be blunted, or even absent, because of the anti-inflammatory action of immunosuppressive regimens.

A key and critical component of the solid-organ transplant process is the preoperative assessment of both the recipient and the donor for any underlying infections, or any disease processes that predispose to infections, that could manifest subsequent to administration of immunosuppressive agents. For the donor, apart from the serologies including HIV, Hepatitis C, and HBV, the most important evaluation is the determination of CMV and EBV status because these two agents are most easily transmitted to a seronegative recipient. For the recipient, a thorough pretransplant history and physical examination are essential to minimize the risk of infectious complications secondary to a latent or indolent infectious process. Routine viral studies should be obtained, vaccinations updated, and prophylaxis administered where indicated (e.g., gut decontamination in liver transplant candidates with end-stage liver disease or prophylactic antibiotics in patients with cystic fibrosis).

Bacterial Infections

The first 30 days posttransplant, bacterial infections are common. Even in the immunocompetent patient population, bacterial infections are common complications of surgery. The risk of a nosocomial bacterial infection is related to the site of surgery as well as to the continued presence of any catheters, lines, endotracheal tubes, or other breaks in the skin. The most common sites of infection are the urinary tract, the surgical site, the lungs, and the bloodstream. The risk of nosocomial bacterial infections is directly related to host factors (including underlying diseases such as diabetes or cirrhosis, obesity, and chronic pulmonary disease) as well as to technical and management factors (including the length and technique of the operation, the development of a hematoma or seroma, and the need for prolonged urinary catheterization, mechanical ventilation, or central venous catheterization).

Renal and bladder-drained pancreas transplant recipients are particularly prone to UTIs. Bacteriuria may be detected in up to 56.7% of renal transplant recipients [14], with an attendant increased risk of systemic sepsis and wound infection. The most common pathogens are gram-negative aerobes, enterococci, and *Candida* spp. The risk factors associated with an increased incidence of UTIs include prolonged catheterization and hemodialysis.

Diagnosis of a UTI in transplant recipients is based on clinical suspicion and on urinalysis and culture results. The typical findings of dysuria, hesitancy, and frequency may be absent; the only clinical manifestations might be minimal fever or an elevated white blood cell count. Treatment is often empiric and, because of the risk of bacteremia, should consist of intravenous administration of a third-generation cephalosporin or a quinolone, particularly during the first month posttransplant. Once the offending organism has been identified and antimicrobial sensitivity data are available, treatment should be targeted.

In recipients of solid-organ grafts besides the kidney and bladder-drained pancreas who do not require a long duration of urinary catheterization, an increased risk of bacterial or fungal UTIs is not seen.

Infections of the surgical site are potentially another source of major morbidity and occasionally graft loss and mortality in solid-organ transplant recipients. Surgical site or wound infections are classified according to the structures involved. Infections above the fascia are superficial, infections below the fascia are deep, and combined infections involve elements of both the superficial and the deep compartments of the wound [15].

In all solid-organ transplant recipients, immediately before their operation begins, a single dose of an antibiotic should be administered within an hour of skin incision, to decrease the risk of surgical site infections. In pancreas, bowel, lung, and liver transplant recipients, significant degrees of wound contamination may occur, and so antibiotics are typically administered for 24 to 72 hours posttransplant, although data to support this practice are lacking [16]. In renal transplant recipients, the surgical site infection rate is very low (1% to 2%) and is comparable to the wound infection rate for other clean-contaminated procedures in immunocompetent patients [15] except in the morbidly obese and diabetic. However, other transplant procedures are associated with higher rates of infection. The wound infection rate after heart transplants is typically below 8%. The rate of wound infections is slightly higher after lung and heart–lung transplants [17]. The rate after liver transplants of superficial wound infections is 6% to 8%; of deep wound infections (most commonly an intra-abdominal abscess secondary to a biliary leak), 15% to 20% [15]. The rate of wound infections after pancreas transplants is high: 10% to 40%, superficial; 15% to 22%, deep; and 8%, combined [18]. Such wound infections confer substantial morbidity, are associated with mortality in some cases, and require a very aggressive approach to diagnosis and therapy.

Pathogenic microorganisms are predictable, according to the type of procedure. In renal transplant recipients, wound infections are caused by the endogenous flora of the skin (gram-positive aerobes) and the bladder (gram-negative aerobes), with occasional *Candida* spp and enterococci.

In heart transplant recipients, wound infections are almost always due to skin flora such as *Staphylococcus aureus* and *Staphylococcus epidermidis*, although some fungal and unusual pathogens are found.

Lung transplants introduce respiratory flora and the potential for grave infections with *Pseudomonas aeruginosa*.

In liver transplant recipients, wound infections are typically associated with either skin or biliary flora, although any preexisting cirrhosis and end-stage liver disease may result in colonization with drug-resistant nosocomial pathogens.

In pancreas transplant recipients, wound infections are invariably polymicrobial, with gram-positive, fungal, and resistant gram-negative pathogens frequently present. Treatment generally requires opening of the wound, reexploration, and/or administration of broad-spectrum antimicrobial therapy (with carbapenem or extended-spectrum penicillin, a β-lactamase inhibitor, and vancomycin) and often antifungal coverage.

Wound infections are often understated, and findings may be limited to fever, elevated white blood cell count, or wound drainage with a deceptively innocuous appearance. Any wound drainage should be examined by Gram stain and culture; any suspicion or evidence of infections should result in opening of the superficial wound. Additionally, imaging should be undertaken to rule out infections in the deep surgical space; if a fluid collection is identified, percutaneous drainage or prompt exploration is needed. Prolonged, broad-spectrum antimicrobial therapy is used, and immunosuppression is significantly reduced in the face of potentially life-threatening infections.

The development of postoperative pneumonia varies with the type of transplant and is associated with a high death rate (20% to 60%). Renal transplants are associated with the lowest incidence of postoperative pneumonia (1% to 2%), and lung transplants the highest (22%). The most common pathogens are gram-negative aerobes, staphylococci, and *Legionella* spp. Frequently, *Candida* spp. or CMV may be identified along with bacterial pathogens, particularly in the first 2 to 3 months posttransplant.

Factors predisposing to the development of pneumonia in solid-organ transplant recipients include prolonged mechanical ventilation, thoracic surgery, pulmonary edema, and intense immunosuppression or treatment for AR. Lung transplant recipients are at increased risk, because of their lungs' preexisting colonization with endogenous flora as well as the loss of mucociliary clearance function associated with denervation [19]. The evaluation of suspected pneumonia in lung transplant recipients should be thorough, including bronchoscopy with biopsies and bronchoalveolar lavage (BAL) to rule out rejection, as will be described. Pleural effusions should be drained and cultured because the progression of an infected effusion to empyema in lung transplant recipients is associated with a very high mortality rate.

Bacteremia in the transplant population, as in the general hospital patients, may occur secondary to seeding along a vascular access device or as a result of hematogenous spread from another source; or, it may be primary (without a source being identified). UTIs, wound infections, and pneumonia are risk factors for the development of bacteremia, as is prolonged vascular catheterization. Other risk factors include receiving a deceased donor graft, leukopenia, and antirejection therapy. Bacteremia in immunosuppressed patients may present as fever, leukocytosis, leukopenia, or hypotension without other significant manifestations. Consequently, routine blood cultures should be part of any workup for fever in this population. Suspicion of bacteremia should prompt removal and culture of intravascular devices and judicious search for a source of other sites of infection. The mortality rate of bacterial sepsis and septic shock in transplant recipients exceeds 50%. Consequently, the use of broad-spectrum antimicrobial therapy, an aggressive approach to source control, and the minimization of immunosuppression are indicated.

There are several atypical bacterial infections that occur in the solid-organ transplant recipients, including mycobacteria such as *Mycobacterium tuberculosis*, *Nocardia* spp, and *Listeria monocytogenes*. Such infections are associated with high rates of morbidity and mortality. Mycobacterial infections are 50 to 100 times more frequent in the transplant population than they are in the general population and are fatal in 30% of cases. Infections are typically due to reactivation of latent disease or transmission from the transplanted graft. Their diagnosis is complicated by the typical lack of reaction to skin testing seen with immunosuppression. Consequently, a high index of clinical suspicion is needed. If mycobacterial pulmonary infection is suspected, bronchoscopic evaluation with biopsy, acid-fast staining, and culture should be performed. Treatment consists of multidrug therapy with isoniazid, ethambutol, pyrazinamide, and rifampin. Preventive strategies should be considered in patient populations in whom infections are common, in patients with a history of significant exposure without subsequent therapy, and in patients with a history of serious or inadequately treated infections.

Nontuberculous mycobacteria (NTM) such as *Mycobacterium avium* complex, *M. ulcerans*, and *M. xenopi* are environmental mycobacteria that rarely caused disease in humans until the AIDS epidemic of the 1980s. NTM infections typically manifest as insidious pulmonary or soft tissue infections in immunosuppressed patients. If NTM infections are suspected, repeat isolations by bronchoscopy or tissue biopsy are required to improve the chance of diagnosis. In addition to acid-fast staining, a special culture for an atypical mycobacterium should be obtained. Besides continuing antimicrobial treatment, wide debridement of the infected site may be required to eradicate such infections [20].

Listeria monocytogenes infection may be associated with pneumonia, bacteremia, or, most worryingly, cerebromeningitis in the transplant population. In renal transplant recipients, *Listeria* spp have been associated with a 26% mortality rate. Consequently, if listeriosis (pulmonary or meningitis) is suspected in any immunosuppressed patient, a thorough evaluation must be performed. Empiric therapy for meningitis should include suitable targeted coverage, such as ampicillin plus an aminoglycoside [21]. The extended-spectrum penicillins also provide adequate coverage.

Nocardial infections most commonly manifest with pulmonary symptoms and signs, but disseminated disease may involve the skin, eyes, and brain, alone or in concert. The clinical manifestations are nonspecific and include fever, chills, malaise, occasional cough, dyspnea, headache, or mental status change. Such infections have a mortality rate of 25% to 50% and must be aggressively diagnosed and treated [21]. The diagnosis is made by microscopic examination of sputum or lung (or occasionally brain) biopsy tissue, or by aspiration of a skin nodule using routine, Kinyoun, and Ziehl-Neelsen staining. Treatment consists of high-dose intravenous TMP-SMX, generally in combination with an aminoglycoside, such as amikacin, with continued treatment with oral TMP-SMX, if possible for life. Concurrently, immunosuppression should be abridged, particularly during treatment of aggressive, disseminated infections.

Fungal Infections

Solid-organ transplants are associated with a significant risk of fungal infections. In the era of broad-spectrum antibacterial prophylaxis and empiric therapy, the incidence of fungi as pathogens is increasing. It is associated with an increased incidence of resistance to azoles as well. Fungal infections are most common after liver and pancreas transplants, with an incidence of 40% [22]. But they are less common after renal transplants (only 5%). Nonetheless, all fungal infections are serious, with an attendant mortality rate, associated with invasive disease, of 30% to 50%. As described previously, most fungal infections occur during the first 3 to 4 months posttransplant, when immunosuppression is greatest. The source of most fungal pathogens is the oral cavity, the gastrointestinal (GI) tract, or the environment.

Candidal overgrowth of the oral and GI tract is common, and prophylaxis consisting of topical nystatin or clotrimazole is often used. Invasive candidal disease is more common in patients with risk factors such as diabetes, neutropenia, intense immunosuppression, and prolonged administration of antibacterial antibiotics, particularly broad-spectrum agents. Long-term TMP-SMX prophylaxis has not been associated with fungal infections. Despite prophylaxis, invasive candidiasis does occur, most often in transplant recipients with a perforation of the GI tract, an anastomotic breakdown, a deep surgical site infection, or a concomitant GI infection, such as CMV gastroenteritis or colitis.

Increasing use of triazoles such as fluconazole has led to more frequent isolation of resistant *Candida* species, such as *C. glabrata* and *C. krusei*. The presence of more resistant strains has necessitated the need for most invasive candidal infections to be treated with amphotericin B or the newer agents like echinocandins (see later). This is a consequence of the attendant morbidity and mortality in the immunosuppressed population [22]. Caspofungin is an echinocandin that acts to block the synthesis of 1,3-β-D-glucan, an essential element of the fungal cell wall. It is well tolerated, with a side-effect profile that compares favorably to amphotericin B. Note that caspofungin and amphotericin B appear to act in an additive manner, and cross-resistance has not been identified [23]. Clinical trials of caspofungin versus amphotericin demonstrated equivalent outcomes in the treatment of candidemia [23]. In solid-organ transplant recipients, caspofungin will be an important drug in treating serious fungal infections, particularly because it lacks the nephrotoxicity of amphotericin. Two of the more recently released triazole drugs, itraconazole and voriconazole, also possess activity in vitro against *Aspergillus* spp; however, the combination of voriconazole and caspofungin has not been shown to enhance clinical efficacy [24].

Disseminated disease is found in over 50% of cases, with a mortality rate in excess of 80% [25]. Most patients with aspergillosis present with what appears to be a bacterial pneumonia. In high-risk lung or liver transplant recipients, or in lower risk patients whose supposed pneumonia fails to respond to appropriate antibiotic therapy, an aggressive diagnostic approach is urgently needed. The diagnosis of aspergillosis is established initially by microscopic examination of samples obtained via bronchoscopy and BAL for the presence of filamentous hyphae. Agents approved by the U.S. Food and Drug Administration (FDA) against invasive aspergillosis include liposomal amphotericin B, itraconazole, voriconazole, posaconazole, and caspofungin. Dissemination to the central nervous system (CNS) may result in brain abscesses, which in the past were nearly uniformly fatal, but more recently have been successfully treated with newer antifungal agents (such as voriconazole) and some require neurosurgical resection [26].

Infections due to a number of other fungi occur in solid-organ transplant recipients, including *Cryptococcus neoformans, Coccidioides immitis, Blastomyces dermatitidis, Histoplasma capsulatum*, and *Zygomycetes*, *Mucor*, and *Rhizopus* spp. Infections caused by those fungi occur in specific settings and present as specific clinical courses that should be considered by the clinician caring for immunosuppressed patients.

Cryptococcus neoformans is the second leading cause of invasive fungal infections in liver transplant recipients. This pathogen may cause pneumonia or meningitis, and patients with pulmonary disease often have CNS involvement as well. A high index of suspicious should be maintained, and it is recommended that immunocompromised patients with cryptococcal infection should undergo lumbar puncture even if asymptomatic neurologically. Skin nodules are occasionally seen. The diagnosis is confirmed by India-ink staining and by testing for cryptococcal antigen in cerebrospinal fluid or sputum. Treatment consists of amphotericin B, followed by oral fluconazole, bearing in mind there is increasing resistance to fluconazole over time [27].

Coccidioides immitis is endemic in the southwestern United States and in Mexico. Between 7% and 9% of solid-organ transplant recipients residing in that area develop coccidioidomycosis, with an associated mortality rate of 25% in pulmonary cases and of up to 70% in disseminated cases. The presentation of disease is variable, as multiple organ systems may be involved. The diagnosis must be made by microscopy, antigen detection, or tissue culture. Lifelong fluconazole prophylaxis for solid-organ transplant recipients who reside in endemic areas is advocated in some centers, though long-term outcome data are lacking. A beneficial adjunct in tackling this disease is a reduction of calcineurin inhibitor dosage. The treatment is prolonged amphotericin B administration or azole therapy [28].

Histoplasmosis and blastomycosis infections occur in endemic areas in the Midwest United States, the Mississippi, and Ohio River valleys. Invasive disease, either reactivation of latent fungi or a new infection, occurs in up to 2% of solid-organ transplant recipients, with the highest incidence in those areas. Invasive disease spreads from the lungs to the skin and bone marrow. Biopsy and samples for culture analysis may be obtained from skin lesions or from a bone marrow aspirate. Amphotericin B or itraconazole are appropriate therapeutic agents [13].

Mucor and *Rhizopus* spp in the Zygomycetes class are soil fungi that, when inhaled, may cause a highly morbid, invasive rhinocerebral infection in profoundly immunosuppressed patients and in diabetic patients with poor glycemic control. The diagnosis is established by biopsy; aggressive surgical debridement is the treatment of choice with adjuvant antifungal therapy (amphotericin B with the occasional addition of 5-flucytosine, itraconazole, or rifampin). The mortality rate associated with those types of infections is in excess of 50% [29].

Pneumocystis jiroveci pneumonia (PJP) is a common cause of pneumonia in immunosuppressed patients. PJP is associated with profound defects in cellular immunity and is normally seen with $CD4^+$ T-cell counts lower than 200 per μL. Those indices are historically seen with OKT3 therapy for AR, which is currently not in use. Prophylaxis with TMP-SMX or atovaquone (if sulfa allergic) makes PJP a rare entity; however, transplant recipients who have a respiratory illness but did not receive prophylaxis (e.g., because of allergy or noncompliance) should be evaluated promptly for PJP. Untreated PJP has a very high mortality rate. The diagnosis is generally established by bronchoscopy and BAL, with methenamine silver staining of washings, or by transbronchial biopsy. Normal findings should not delay further evaluation and therapy, which should be started empirically (the characteristic alveolar and interstitial changes seen on a chest radiograph are late findings). This consists of intravenous TMP-SMX or inhaled pentamidine. Dapsone can be used for patients with sulfa sensitivity.

Viral Infections

Viral infections have frequently been recognized as important causes of morbidity and mortality in solid-organ transplant recipients. Viruses that are endemic and of little clinical concern in the general patient population may produce overwhelming life-threatening infections in the host with suppressed cellular immunity. The recent appreciation of the immunomodulatory effect of several opportunistic viral pathogens gives even more reason for continued development of effective prophylaxis, diagnosis, and treatment modalities for this class of infectious agents. Immunosuppressed transplant recipients may develop serious viral infections by reactivation of latent virus, by transmission of the virus from the donor graft or via blood transfusion, or by exposure to the virus in the environment.

Pathogens known as the HHVs are important in the solid-organ transplant population (Table 65.2). These viruses commonly cause disease during periods of greatest immunosuppression, particularly early posttransplant and after antirejection therapy. They include many of the most important viral pathogens facing immunosuppressed patients, including CMV, EBV, the herpes simplex viruses (HSVs), and the varicella zoster virus (VZV).

CMV infections affect 30% to 75% of solid-organ transplant recipients, primarily within 2 weeks to 3 months posttransplant. The highest hazard for CMV infections is in a CMV-seronegative recipient receiving a graft from a CMV-seropositive donor (the D+/R− graft) [30]. Lung and heart–lung transplant recipients have the highest rate of CMV disease (50% to 80%). The most severe CMV disease is also a primary infection in

TABLE 65.2

Human Herpes Viruses

Virus	Eponym	Clinical syndromes
HHV-1	Herpes simplex virus-1	Mucocutaneous disease Primarily oral–labial symptoms Ocular keratitis Herpes simplex virus encephalitis
HHV-2	Herpes simplex virus-2	Mucocutaneous disease Primarily genital symptoms Ocular keratitis
HHV-3	Varicella zoster virus	Chickenpox, shingles Pneumonitis, encephalitis
HHV-4	Epstein–Barr virus	Infectious mononucleosis Hepatitis, pneumonitis Posttransplant lymphoproliferative disorder Burkitt lymphoma
HHV-5	Cytomegalovirus	Mononucleosis, pneumonitis Hepatitis, gastroenteritis, retinitis
HHV-6	Roseola (6B)	Childhood febrile exanthema Mononucleosis, encephalitis Pneumonitis, disseminated disease
HHV-7		No clear clinical entities
HHV-8	Kaposi agent	Cutaneous lymphomas

HHV, human herpes virus.

the D+/R− population. A superinfection (due to concurrent reactivation of an endogenous strain and transmission of a serotypically distinct strain of CMV) is typically intermediate in severity, whereas reactivation of latent disease is most often comparatively mild [30]. The range of clinical disease is vast: from asymptomatic infections (detected solely by a change in anti-CMV titer or by shedding of virus or viral DNA in blood, urine, or sputum) to tissue-invasive disease (which may affect the lungs, liver, or intestine). Clinically, a mild infection produces a mononucleosis-like syndrome, including fever, malaise, and myalgias, often accompanied by leukopenia. More severe disease clinically manifests with differing signs and symptoms, depending on the site(s) of invasive infection. GI ulceration with occasional hemorrhage is seen in GI disease. CMV pneumonitis may produce respiratory insufficiency and failure. CMV hepatitis may lead to liver failure, severe pancreatitis, and critical deterioration of clinical course. CMV retinitis may produce vision changes, leading to blindness.

Given the high prevalence and significant morbidity of CMV disease, prophylaxis with ganciclovir, valacyclovir, or valganciclovir for 3 to 6 months posttransplant is common, particularly in high-risk patients. Additional prophylaxis is routinely begun with initiation of antirejection therapy. Several randomized clinical trials have shown ganciclovir prophylaxis to be superior to acyclovir prophylaxis in preventing both reactivation and primary CMV disease in solid-organ transplant recipients [31].

A second approach to this problem is the routine close monitoring of at-risk patients with protocol antigenemia or polymerase chain reaction assays followed by empiric (so-called preemptive) therapy with ganciclovir, if levels rise above a predetermined threshold. This approach, though somewhat more cumbersome, has led to reductions in the burden of CMV disease in liver transplant recipients [31]. Prophylaxis, surveillance with empiric therapy, or a combination of both based on calculated risk is currently practiced in most transplant centers. Ganciclovir prophylaxis is used for lung, heart–lung, and heart transplant recipients as well [32], but data on surveillance, preemptive therapy, and efficacy in such recipients are limited. However, there is evidence that there is a tendency toward less CMV disease with the use of mTOR inhibitors [33].

Foscarnet (trisodium phosphonoformate) is used in those rare instances where ganciclovir-resistant strains of CMV are isolated. The data that clearly establish the efficacy of foscarnet in treating CMV disease are limited to CMV retinitis; efficacy equivalent to ganciclovir was observed, but foscarnet was associated with a higher rate of adverse effects (e.g., nephrotoxicity) [30].

The HSVs (HSV-1 and HSV-2) commonly cause mucocutaneous disease of the oropharynx (HSV-1) and the genitalia (HSV-2). In profoundly immunosuppressed patients, they may cause widespread disease, including hepatitis, encephalitis, and pneumonitis. Most such infections are thought to be reactivation of latent virus [34]. The diagnosis is established by identification of the virus by immunofluorescent monoclonal antibody staining or by Tzanck smear. Culture and rising anti-HSV antibody titers provide evidence as well. Treatment consists of acyclovir; most epidermal lesions respond to oral therapy, but any evidence of disseminated disease requires high-dose intravenous acyclovir and minimization of immunosuppression.

Infections associated with EBV are commonly detectable in solid-organ transplant recipients. The most common manifestations include the typical mononucleosis-type syndrome, pneumonitis, and hepatitis. The diagnosis of EBV infections is made by detection of heterophile immunoglobin M antibodies in serum or by following titers of antibodies to viral capsid antigen. Polymerase chain reaction is also used to monitor viral activity and response to therapy. Treatment consists of acyclovir (or ganciclovir, when a CMV infection is also suspected). Immunosuppressive de-escalation is necessary in disseminated disease. In a Cochrane review with the use of Belatacept, there was an increased incidence of posttransplant lymphoproliferative disorder (PTLD) in EBV-naive recipients compared with patients receiving calcinuerin inhibitors [35].

VZV commonly emerges from latency in immunosuppressed transplant recipients and causes an episode of shingles [36]. More rarely, VZV may cause disseminated infections, such as pneumonitis and encephalitis. Pediatric transplant patients are routinely innoculated with the varicella vaccine, which has markedly reduced this type of disease; the vaccine is recommended pretransplant for all pediatric and nonimmunosuppressed transplant candidates. VZV infections are treated with acyclovir; with severe disseminated disease, immunosuppression is reduced in addition [37]. No evidence supports the efficacy of anti-VZV immune globulin for treating severe VZV disease in immunocompromised patients.

Co-infection with HHV-6 and association with severe CMV disease has been reported, but understanding causality in this context is difficult. Treatment of neurologic diseases related to HHV-6 includes ganciclovir and foscarnet, either alone or in combination [38]. HHV-7 is not yet clearly associated with clinical syndromes that pose major problems in solid-organ transplant recipients. HHV-8 is linked to the development of Kaposi sarcoma in transplant recipients (vide infra).

Viral hepatitis is a significant problem, particularly in liver transplant recipients, who may have developed end-stage liver disease as a result of HBV or HCV infections. Primary HBV or HCV infections may occur during the transplant operation itself because of donor graft or blood transfusion transmission.

Would-be donors positive for hepatitis B surface antigen (HBsAg) and/or anti–hepatitis B core antibodies (HBcAbs) are often excluded from donating any organ or tissue [39]. Organs other than the liver have been transplanted from isolated HBcAb-positive donors, without evidence of transmission, and the risk for transmission is very low from a review of the literature [40]. HCV-positive donors are normally allowed to donate their livers and kidneys to recipient who are also HCV-positive. Liver transplant candidates with HBV or HCV disease are transplanted; currently, their graft and patient survival rates, particularly in the short term, are comparable to those for recipients without HBV or HCV disease. HBV disease is no longer a contraindication to a liver transplant; however, the use of lamivudine and HBV-immune globulin (HBIG) has significantly reduced the burden of recurrent HBV disease [41] and has allowed hundreds of patients with end-stage liver disease secondary to HBV to undergo successful transplantation. Continuing HBV prophylaxic therapy appears to be the optimal duration strategy in ensuring low or absent viral levels [41].

Up to 25% of hepatitis C–positive transplant recipients accelerate to cirrhosis within 5 to 10 years posttransplant, likely related to immunosuppressive therapy and rejection [42]. The care of transplant candidates with HCV includes extending the donor pool, tailoring antiviral treatment pre- and posttransplant, and offering a living donor transplant [43]. A very effective interferon-free regimen, which obtains high sustained viral response within 8 to 12 weeks of therapy, has proved effective in managing hepatitis C, although the cost is considered prohibitive, with barriers including insurance denials; however, it is much cheaper than liver transplantation. These drugs are currently available for clinical use with very promising results even in those co-infected with HIV [44].

The transmission of HIV via an organ transplant from an HIV-positive donor was described over two decades ago [45]; HIV-positive status will not be contraindication to either donating or undergoing a transplant after passage of the HOPE Act and the enactment of appropriate policies to support the practice [46]. However, solid-organ transplant recipients infected with HIV have been identified and have enjoyed long-term survival posttransplantation [46], given the success of long-term multidrug therapy for HIV. With the introduction of highly active antiretroviral therapy (HAART), the transplant community has now recognized HIV infections as a chronic condition. In fact, end-organ failure develops in HIV-positive individuals as they age and/or from the side effects of their antiviral treatments. Short-term outcomes for HIV-positive transplant recipients have been good even for those co-infected with hepatitis C [47]: the HIV load remains suppressed, $CD4^+$ T-lymphocyte counts are stable, and the risk of opportunistic infection is acceptable. However, major challenges in the care of HIV-positive transplant recipients include high graft-rejection rates and multiple drug interactions between HAART and maintenance immunosuppression regimes [47].

The polyomavirus, including BK, JC, and SV40, is an omnipresent pathogen that has no clinical significance in immunocompetent hosts. BK virus (BKV) is tropic-specific for human transitional and renal tubular epithelial cells. Primary infection occurs early in life; BKV establishes lifelong latency in the host's renal cells. Reactivation takes place when the host's immune system is compromised, such as during pregnancy or posttransplant immunosuppression. The diagnosis is made by detecting free viral particles in the urine, blood, or intranuclear viral inclusion-bearing cells (decoy cells) in urine cytology specimens. BKV nephropathy (BKN) has been increasingly recognized as an important entity in kidney transplant recipients since the mid-1990s; currently, it is seen in 1% to 9% of them within the first year posttransplant. Depending on the severity of renal tubular injury, clinical presentations of BKN can include fatigue, fever, mild hydronephrosis, or marked graft dysfunction. In bone marrow transplant recipients, hemorrhagic cystitis has been described. The diagnosis of BKV reactivation is made by urinary cytology, quantitative polymerase chain reaction (PCR) analysis to measure the viral load in urine or plasma, and kidney biopsy [48]. The mainstays of caring for patients with BKN are to reduce immunosuppression and to closely monitor disease progression. Given the lack of specific antiviral agents against BKV, low-dose cidofovir or leflunomide or fluoroquinolone has been used, with no appreciable effect, in patients with persistent BKN [49].

Human papilloma viruses may cause disease through the development of tissue-specific growth, leading to benign or malignant processes, including cervical cancer, cancer of the vulva and perineum, condyloma acuminatum, laryngeal polyposis, and nonmelanotic skin cancer (vide infra). Respiratory syncytial virus may produce a fulminant pneumonia in both adult and pediatric transplant recipients. The diagnosis is made by nasopharyngeal washing. More severe cases should be treated with ribavirin.

Parasitic Infections

Numerous common parasitic infections are seen in immunosuppressed solid-organ transplant recipients. *Toxoplasma gondii* presents as a brain abscess with neurologic changes [50]. It is seen late posttransplant, whereas a brain abscess in the early posttransplant period is more likely to be fungal [51]. Heart transplant recipients seem to be at greatest risk, possibly due to the presence of *T. gondii* cysts in donor myocardial tissue. Positive *Toxoplasma* is a not a contraindication for organ donation. However, if the heart donor was seropositive for *T. gondii*, the recipient normally undergoes prophylactic treatment with pyrimethamine and sulfadiazine for 3 to 6 months posttransplantation. Treatment of *T. gondii* infections consists of pyrimethamine and sulfadiazine; the mortality rate is high in transplant recipients who exhibit CNS disease.

MALIGNANCY

Solid-organ transplant recipients have a distinctly increased risk of developing malignancy posttransplantation. The Israel Penn International Transplant Tumor Registry initiated and has maintained an extensive data collection that tracks the epidemiology of tumors in transplant recipients [52]. The increased incidence of malignancy is multifactorial, probably due to a combination of the activation of latent viruses with oncogenic potential, the direct oncogenic effect of immunosuppressive drugs such as cyclosporine, and, perhaps, environmental factors [53]. Strong but indirect evidence points to the loss of immunologic surveillance as a mechanism of increased oncogenesis. The most common neoplasms of solid-organ transplant recipients are skin cancers, PTLD, lung cancer, Kaposi sarcoma, and carcinoma of the cervix. Of those neoplasms, lung cancer appears to occur at the same frequency as in the general population; the other neoplasms occur at increased incidence in solid-organ transplant recipients. PTLD presents the greatest challenge in terms of attendant high morbidity and mortality rates.

Posttransplant Lymphoproliferative Disorder

PTLD encompasses a very broad range of pathologies, from simple lymphoid hyperplasia to very aggressive monoclonal B-cell lymphomas. EBV infections play a central causal role. In particular, primary EBV infections posttransplant (EBV D+/R− match) and immunosuppression markedly increase the risk of PTLD [12]. Other risk factors include active CMV disease [30], CMV D+/R− match, and increasing intensity of immunosuppression.

PTLD is least common in adult kidney transplant recipients and most common in pediatric small-bowel transplant recipients. It is most common early posttransplant, concurrent with the greatest period of immunosuppression and with the use of anti–T-cell therapy for AR, particularly repeated courses. However, a subset of PTLD occurs late (several years) posttransplant. These late occurring neoplasms appear to be related to patient age, duration, and intensity of immunosuppression, and type of graft than to the more typical risk factors seen in early-onset disease.

The clinical presentation of PTLD varies widely, as might be expected from the wide range of pathology encountered with this entity. Many patients experience fever, sweats, and myalgias as the only symptoms. Weight loss, diarrhea, and upper respiratory infection are common symptoms; some, but not all, patients have lymphadenopathy. CNS involvement, which occurs in up to 20% of patients [54], often manifests as mental status changes. GI disease may be silent or may present as abdominal pain, GI bleeding, and perforation with peritonitis, or bowel obstruction. Intrathoracic PTLD has a characteristic radiographic appearance of multiple circumscribed pulmonary nodules, which may or may not be accompanied by mediastinal lymphadenopathy. PTLD in the graft itself can present very similarly to AR; because the therapeutic approach to those two entities is diametrically opposed, a correct diagnosis by biopsy is essential.

The gold standard for establishing the diagnosis of suspected lesions in PTLD is biopsy. These specimens are histologically graded (based on cell morphology and nodal architecture) and assessed for clonality (polyclonal or monoclonal) and for the presence of an EBV genome and copy number. Specific cell marker studies are required to establish the clonality, but most lesions are EBV positive and of B-cell lineage. Experienced pathologists with working knowledge of PTLD as well as with graft rejection and opportunistic infections should review the biopsy. Consensus conference standards for the grading and classification of PTLD have been used [55]. Histologic classification currently uses the Harris standard formulation [56,57]. EBV serology does not typically add to the diagnostic workup of PTLD, with many false-negatives in patients with established primary EBV infections. Similarly, peripheral cytology is not helpful in making the diagnosis and molecular techniques need to be employed [56]. If PTLD is suspected, patients should undergo imaging of the head, thorax, and abdomen. Fluorodeoxyglucose-positron emission tomography (FDG-PET)/CT scanning has high specificity as a diagnostic and/or staging tool and in follow-up studies of PTLD patients [56].

Currently, there is little information to provide direction regarding optimal prophylaxis for PTLD. Clearly, it is important to identify, and closely monitor, high-risk patients (e.g., children; liver and small-bowel transplant recipients; EBV-negative transplant recipients, particularly those with an EBV-positive donor; transplant recipients on intense antilymphocyte therapy for rejection). Both antiviral agents and passive immune transfer with CMV-IVIG immune globulin have been used as prophylaxis against PTLD, with no proven efficacy. Several trials are ongoing to establish the best prophylactic approach. Reduction of the immunosuppressive regimen with evidence of rising EBV titer has shown to be helpful when compared with historical controls [56].

Treatment of established PTLD depends on each patient's clinical situation and histologic diagnosis. With few trials to guide therapy, a gradual, individualized approach is taken. Ordinarily, immunosuppression is reduced to the barest minimum, and specific therapy is directed at the neoplasm. In 25% to 50% of patients, PTLD often regresses after immunosuppression is reduced [56].

Surgical intervention is clearly indicated for patients with GI PTLD that manifests as aggressive disease (e.g., viscus obstruction or perforation). Surgical debulking of the tumor burden has also been used in amenable cases, as has radiotherapy. Isolated CNS disease initially should be treated with external beam irradiation [56].

Medical approaches to treating PTLD include (a) antiviral medications (e.g., acyclovir, ganciclovir); (b) interferon-α2b; (c) immunoglobulins (d) standard, low-dose, and high-dose chemotherapy protocols; and (e) most recently, monoclonal antibodies directed against B-cell surface markers, such as CD19 and CD20 (rituximab). In unusual cases, immunomodulatory therapy with adoptive transfer of cytotoxic T cells sensitized to EBV has been attempted with some success [56].

Late-onset PTLD, occurring more than 1 to 2 years posttransplant, often does not respond to the reduction in immunosuppression and to the medical therapy typically used in patients with early-onset disease. Often EBV-negative, late-onset PTLD is difficult to treat because of side effects, including infectious complications of the aggressive chemotherapy that is often required. Similarly, CNS involvement may be a marker for PTLD that is potentially refractory to therapy, possibly because of the relatively privileged immune site. Therapeutic options include intrathecal administration of interferon-α and anti–B-cell antibody therapy in addition to local radiotherapy, but the prognosis remains guarded [56].

Skin Cancer

Nonmelanotic skin cancers are the most common neoplasms associated with transplantation and immunosuppression. Increased incidence is associated with increasing time posttransplantation and sun exposure. Often-quoted studies show a prevalence of 66% in transplant recipients in Australia after 24 years of surveillance [58] and 40% after 20 years in the Netherlands [59]. Those figures correlate to a 4- to 21-fold increase in prevalence in transplant recipients, as compared with the immunocompetent population, with synergistic increases seen in the areas of highest sunlight exposure in countries such as Australia [53].

Squamous cell carcinoma is the most common skin cancer in transplant recipients. Many recipients develop multiple lesions; the transplant patients are generally younger when compared with members of general population. The incidence of melanoma is also 2.4 times higher than the general population [60]. Even nonmelanotic squamous cell carcinomas behave more aggressively in transplant recipients, with lymph node metastasis and a 6% mortality rate due to disseminated disease [61]. On identification of skin lesions, prompt surgical excision should be undertaken. Solid-organ transplant recipients are instructed to avoid direct exposure to sunlight for any prolonged period of time and to liberally use sunblock. Clearly, close dermatologic counseling, education, and follow-up are warranted in this patient population [62].

Kaposi Sarcoma

Kaposi sarcoma (KS) is a nodular vascular neoplasm commonly seen cutaneously but may be multicentric involving visceral tissues (such as the lungs and GI tract). Endemic in the Mediterranean region and Middle East, it is strongly associated with either endogenous or exogenous immunosuppression, as a result both of AIDS and of immunosuppressive therapy. The incidence of this disease in U.S. transplant recipients is 0.4%, which represents a 20-fold increase over the basal rate in the population at large [63]. Recently, HHV-8 has been implicated as a causal agent in KS.

Cutaneous KS is easily identified by clinical appearance and biopsy. But patients with only visceral KS often present with more advanced disease, usually GI bleeding or viscus perforation, sometimes dyspnea related to pulmonary disease. Immunosuppression should be reduced to the greatest extent possible, after which about 30% to 55% of patients will experience remission. Chemotherapy is reserved for patients with visceral KS and for those who do not experience remission after their immunosuppression is reduced. However, of patients with visceral KS, 45% to 50% die of it [64]. Anecdotal evidence indicates that certain patients may respond to antiviral agents (e.g., ganciclovir).

Cervical Cancer

The incidence of cervical intraepithelial neoplasia is elevated by 10- to 14-fold in solid-organ transplant recipients and may approach 50% [65]. Cervical carcinoma was seen in 10% of all women with posttransplant cancer in the Transplant Tumor Registry [52]. Close surveillance by pelvic examination and Papanicolaou smear is essential in this population, given the increased incidence of disease. In the posttransplant patient with potentially advanced cervical cancer, there is no standardized approach.

Transmitted and Recurrent Malignancy

Thankfully the transmissions of malignancy from grafts are not widespread, but when it does occur it is potentially devastating. Case reports have described patients who received grafts that harbored malignant cells, leading to the development of malignancy. Transmission to transplant recipients of renal cell carcinoma, metastatic cancer of the breast or lung, and melanoma has been reported. Currently, cancer or recent history of cancer is a contraindication to organ donation, with the possible exception of some low-grade skin cancers, noninvasive CNS neoplasms, and small, limited cancers that has been excised and is not likely to recur or spread. Nonetheless, some grafts are found to contain foci of neoplasia, which develop into a clinically significant cancer in recipients. This finding emphasizes the need for a thorough examination of donors during organ procurement, particularly considering the present trend toward the use of older donors.

Patients with a history of malignancy are clearly at risk for recurrent disease posttransplantation, presumably due to the use of immunosuppression. Data from the Transplant Tumor Registry show a 21% recurrence rate, with the highest rates seen in patients with multiple myeloma (67%), nonmelanotic skin cancer (53%), bladder cancer (29%), soft tissue sarcoma (29%), renal cell cancer (27%), and breast cancer (23%) [66], and there is a tendency to using organs with small, incidental renal cell carcinoma may be reasonable [67]. Tumors were least likely to recur if more than 5 years had passed between cancer treatment and the transplantation.

Liver transplantation to treat patients with primary, well-circumscribed liver tumors represent a special case. In this population, liver tumor size and the number of liver tumors are considered indicative of the likelihood of disease recurrence and patient survival posttransplantation. Adjuvant techniques, such as cryoablation and radiofrequency ablation, to reduce the tumor burden pretransplantation have been used, but currently the data are insufficient to clearly define the ability of adjuvant techniques to reduce posttransplant morbidity and mortality secondary to disease recurrence. Risk factors for recurrence include tumor size >6 cm, number of nodules >5, and vascular invasion per the final pathology report [68]. Clearly, tumor biology dictates the risk of disease recurrence [69].

REJECTION

The human immune system is an evolutionarily more advanced, adaptive, efficient, "specific," and versatile host defense mechanism against the invasion of pathogens as compared with the nonspecific innate immune system of invertebrates. However, a side effect of the ability of the host immune system to recognize and attack "nonself" tissues is rejection of grafted tissues posttransplantation. That side effect was observed clinically for centuries before Medawar demonstrated that it was an intrinsic property of the host immune system in response to foreign tissue [70]. The exogenous modulation of the host immune system to allow sustained graft function has proceeded along with—and often preceded—our understanding of the physiologic mechanism of rejection and tolerance.

Understanding the immune system is integral to our understanding of rejection. The immunologic disparity among members of the same species of mammals that leads to lack of recognition of "self" tissue and to rejection of nonself tissue is based on the differences in cell surface molecules that are expressed. In humans, these major histocompatibility antigens were first identified on leukocytes, and hence are termed *human leukocyte antigens* (HLAs). HLAs are subdivided into two classes: class I (HLA-A, -B, and -C), expressed on the surface of all nucleated cells, and class II (HLA-DR, -DQ, and -DP), expressed on the surface of *antigen-presenting cells* (APCs). The recognition of nonself tissue occurs via two distinct immunologic pathways: *direct* and *indirect allorecognition*. Direct allorecognition consists of recipient T-helper cells recognizing donor HLA disparity expressed on the donor cell surface. Indirect allorecognition consists of recipient APCs (e.g., activated macrophages, dendritic cells, B lymphocytes) phagocytosing donor cellular debris, including HLAs, which are then processed and re-presented on the APC surface to be recognized by recipient T-helper cells ($CD4^+$ lymphocytes) (Fig. 65.1).

In either pathway, costimulation signals between $CD4^+$ T-helper lymphocytes and $CD8^+$ cytotoxic T lymphocytes trigger a cascade of immunologic events. Interleukin (IL)-2, an important and early signal in immune activation, is secreted by activated $CD4^+$ T-helper lymphocytes, stimulating increased T-cell responsiveness, clonal expansion of alloreactive T lymphocytes, and acquisition of the cytolytic phenotype by host T lymphocytes. Direct allorecognition leads to a more immediate and vigorous immune response against foreign tissue, but, in both pathways, additional helper T lymphocytes are recruited and secrete a wide array of cytokines (e.g., IL-1, interferon-γ, tumor necrosis factor-α), facilitating the further recruitment of cytotoxic T lymphocytes, natural killer cells, and B lymphocytes. Then, B lymphocytes begin to secrete antibody directed against the allogeneic tissue in ever-increasing quantities. Rejection mechanistically occurs by infiltration of the graft by effector cells, the binding of antibody, and the activation of complement. Unchecked, the phenomenon inexorably leads in graft loss (Table 65.1).

Donor–recipient mismatches between HLAs may produce an immune response by either the direct or indirect pathways;

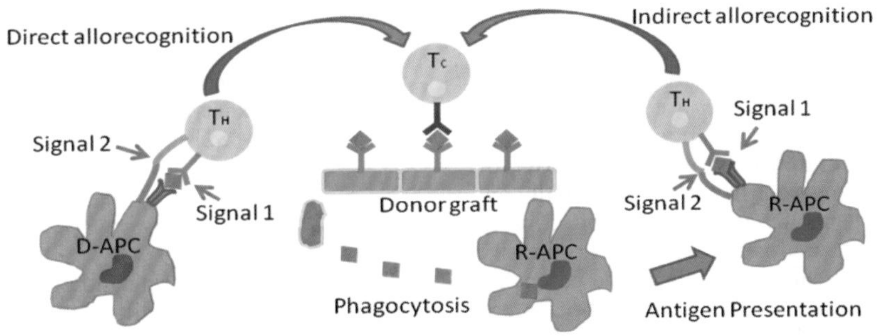

FIGURE 65.1 Direct, indirect pathways of allorecognition. Signal 1 is delivered through the T-cell receptor after engagement by a peptide–HLA complex. Signal 2, also known as costimulatory sign, is delivered by an array of cell surface molecules on the T-helper cell and the antigen-presenting cell (APC). D-APC, donor APC; R-APC, recipient APC; TH, T-helper lymphocyte; Tc, cytotoxic T lymphocytes.

however, minor non-HLA mismatches typically produce an immune response by the indirect pathway only.

Rejection is classified according to the temporal relation between the implantation of the graft and its dysfunction supported by the histologic features seen in allograft. The three main types of rejection are *hyperacute* (HAR), *acute* (AR), and *chronic* (CR). Each type is mediated by a different host immune mechanism. Consequently, each type poses different problems for the patient, clinicians, and pathologists.

Hyperacute Rejection

HAR occurs within a few minutes to a few hours after the reperfusion of the graft. Preformed antibodies directed against antigens presented by the graft mediate activation of complement [71], activation of endothelial cells, and formation of microvascular thrombi, leading to graft thrombosis and loss [71]. The process is irreversible; currently, no treatment is available. Because HAR is mediated by circulating preformed antibodies normally directed against ABO system (comprising the four main blood types, i.e., A, B, AB, and O) antigens or against major HLA antigens, thorough screening of potential transplant recipients and strict adherence to ABO verification policies should prevent nearly all HAR.

The panel-reactive antibody (PRA) assay is a screening test that examines the ability of serum from potential transplant recipients to lyse lymphocytes from a panel of HLA-typed donors. A numerical value, expressed as a percentage, indicates the likelihood of a positive cross-match to the donor population. Therefore, patients lacking preformed antibodies to random donor lymphocytes are defined as having a PRA of 0% and have a very low probability of eliciting a positive lymphocyte cross-match to any donor. The finding of a higher PRA identifies patients at higher immunologic risk for a positive cross-match and thus for HAR and for subsequent graft loss. Most often, such patients were previously sensitized by childbirth, blood transfusions, or prior transplantation.

Pretransplantation, cross-match testing is performed to identify preformed antibodies against class I HLAs (T-lymphocyte cross-match testing) and class II HLAs (B-lymphocyte cross-match testing). In renal and pancreas transplantation, a strong positive class I-HLA cross-match immediately pretransplant is ordinarily an absolute contraindication. At most centers, heart and liver transplantations are performed without a cross-match, unless the recipient is highly sensitized or has previously received a graft possessing major antigens in common with the current donor (i.e., donor-specific antibody [DSA]). A positive B-lymphocyte cross-match indicates preformed antibodies directed against class II HLAs and is a relative, but not absolute, contraindication to a transplant. Recent studies confirmed the efficacy of plasmapheresis followed by administration of immune globulin to reduce PRA levels and to convert strongly positive cross-match results to weakly positive or negative results, thereby allowing organs to be transplanted across what were previously considered as strong immunologic barriers [72].

Cross-match testing helps clinicians to identify the presence of antibodies against potential donor antigens and to assess the risks of posttransplant rejection and subsequent graft loss. However, these cross-matching assays are not standardized. Since the mid-1960s, cross-match testing was based on the complement-dependent cytotoxicity (CDC) assay. The CDC assay was further refined by adding a wash step and an antihuman globulin step, to increase its sensitivity and specificity. Then, with the introduction of technology based on flow cytometry (FC), the presence of recipient antibody on the surface of donor lymphocytes could be detected independent of complement binding.

One of the latest developments in anti-HLA antibody screening was the introduction of Luminex technology, using HLA-coated fluorescent microbeads and FC. This method in theory pinpoints the DSAs in sera of recipients with high PRA levels. Because all transplant donors are currently HLA typed, a negative cross-match for recipients with high PRA levels can be ensured by avoiding the selection of donors carrying unacceptable HLA antigens (virtual cross-match) [73].

The main concerns with these new developments in antibody typing and cross-match testing are between-center test variability and the thresholds of defining false-negative results (results that could deny recipients with high PRA levels a chance for a potential lifesaving transplant). Currently, it is up to an individual transplantation center to implement its own HLA typing and cross-matching policies, depending on the center's experience, clinical outcomes, and risk tolerance.

Although screening has all but eliminated HAR as a clinical problem, active investigation is nonetheless directed at dissecting the underlying pathophysiologic mechanisms of HAR. Another research focus is on the similar rapid rejection of xenoreactive antigens that serve as a barrier to the development of xenotransplantation.

Acute Rejection

AR is the most common form of graft rejection in modern clinical transplantation. It may develop at any time, but is most frequent during the first several months posttransplant. Rarely, it occurs within the first several days posttransplant, a process termed *accelerated acute rejection*, most likely a combination of amnestic immune response driven by sensitized memory B lymphocytes and activation of the direct allorecognition pathway. Under such circumstances, the donor antigen exposure often occurred in the distant past, and so the level of circulating DSAs would have been too low to be detected by conventional cross-matching techniques. Once challenged by the same donor antigens introduced by the organ transplant, dormant memory lymphocytes reactivate, replicate, and differentiate. Within several days, large numbers of antibodies are directed against the donor allograft resulting in graft rejection.

AR may be cell mediated, antibody mediated (AMR), or very occasionally mixed. However, they are not mutually exclusive. Histologically, AR generates an infiltration of activated T lymphocytes into the graft, resulting in gradually progressive endothelial damage, microvascular thrombosis, and parenchymal necrosis. Pathologic grading schemes have been developed regarding the extent to which AR involves vascular damage, cellular infiltration, or a combination of both. Vascular AR is thought to be mediated by the presence of DSAs, albeit not in sufficient numbers to cause HAR. C4d, a complement split product detected immunohistochemically in the capillaries of biopsied graft specimens, is highly correlated with AMR [74]. Without intervention, AR inevitably progresses to graft loss. The clinical presentation of AR varies markedly, depending on the specific organ, on the level of immunosuppression, and on the attendant level of inflammation in the affected tissues.

Unless the host immune system is adequately suppressed pharmacologically, transplantation inevitably leads to AR. A combination of immunosuppressive agents is typically used chronically to prevent AR, including a lymphocyte antagonist (usually a calcineurin inhibitor [CNI] such as cyclosporine or tacrolimus) and an antiproliferative agent (such as azathioprine or mycophenolate mofetil), with or without corticosteroids. Antilymphocyte antibody therapy is often added during induction of immunosuppression or for treatment of "steroid-resistant" AR.

In the last decade, immunosuppression for transplant recipients has been undergoing a paradigm shift. Since the mid-1990s, the use of antibody induction in solid-organ transplant recipients has increased from 25% to more than 90% [75]. Monoclonal antibodies such as basiliximab and daclizumab (both anti-CD25 [IL-2 receptor]) use has declined in the face of increasing use of T-cell depleting agents. Daclizumab is no longer on the market. Furthermore, strategies such as corticosteroid avoidance and CNI-reduced or CNI-free maintenance immunosuppression were shown to be equivalent to traditional triple-drug maintenance [76]. Nonetheless, all immunosuppressive agents carry some risk of toxicity and adverse reactions that may complicate therapy (Table 65.3).

Chronic Rejection

CR is a largely frustrating and poorly understood clinical phenomenon, with slightly different manifestations in each type of graft. Over time, the accumulation of microvascular injury in a graft degrades graft function, with eventual graft loss. This process appears to be mediated by multiple mechanisms, likely including both immune and nonimmune factors. Evidence for the contribution to CR of immune factors includes the observation that AR episodes significantly increase the likelihood of CR as well as the correlation, observed in renal transplant recipients, between a poor response to AR treatment and the subsequent development of CR [77]. A similar association between a poor response to AR treatment and the subsequent development of CR has been observed in liver transplant recipients, although reversible AR has little impact. Nonimmune factors also likely contribute to the development and progression of CR, including the toxic effects of immunosuppressive medication and cumulative injury from infection such as that caused by cytomegalovirus (CMV) [78]. CR nearly always eventuates in graft loss, although the rapidity of the process varies considerably.

Renal Grafts

AR occurs in 10% to 25% of renal transplant recipients. Because most episodes are clinically silent, the diagnosis of AR must be considered in recipients whose serum creatinine, blood urea nitrogen, and urinary output values have normalized and whose graft function has been stable in the outpatient setting, but whose serum creatinine and blood urea nitrogen

TABLE 65.3

Immunosuppressive Medications, Mechanisms of Action, and Common Side Effects

Medications	Mechanisms of action	Side effects
Corticosteroids	Upregulate IκB Decrease IL-1, TNF-α, IFN-γ Exert anti-inflammatory effects	Cushing syndrome, Cataracts Bone demineralization
Azathioprine	Acts as an antimetabolite	Marrow suppression GI, liver toxicity
Mycophenolate mofetil	Acts as an antimetabolite and specifically affects lymphocytes	Marrow suppression GI intolerance
Cyclosporine	Acts as a calcineurin inhibitor Downregulates IL-2	Nephrotoxicity Neurologic symptoms
Tacrolimus (FK506)	Acts as a Calcineurin inhibitor Downregulates IL-2, IFN-γ	Nephrotoxicity Neurotoxicity Diabetogenic
Sirolimus (rapamycin)	Blocks IL-2R, IL-4, IL-6, platelet-derived growth factor signaling	Impaired wound healing Hypertriglyceridemia
Antilymphocyte globulins	Act as a cytolytic antibody Block and deplete T cells	Leukopenia Thrombocytopenia "Serum sickness"
IL-2 receptor blocker (or basiliximab)	Blocks IL-2R Inhibit T-cell activation	Minimal impact

GI, gastrointestinal; IFN, interferon; IL, interleukin; TNF, tumor necrosis factor.

values subsequently rise while their urinary output decreases. The presence of hypovolemia, drug nephrotoxicity (e.g., high calcineurin levels), ureteral obstruction or leak, lymphocele, or vascular anastomotic complications should be excluded, and the diagnosis of AR should be established via histologic examination of a percutaneous graft biopsy specimen. Rarely, tenderness and swelling in the area of the graft occur, and occasionally fever or other signs of systemic inflammation, although such findings used to be common.

A high degree of clinical suspicion should be maintained for recipients who experience delayed graft function, as up to 30% exhibit evidence of AR on biopsy; 20% of recipients who require dialysis posttransplant have AR [79]. Intriguingly, up to 30% of recipients with well-functioning grafts also have AR, per early posttransplant protocol biopsies, but whether such findings are clinically important and whether mild episodes should invariably be treated remain controversial [80]. Recent studies have provided data that may allow prediction of individual risk of AR, with the potential for individualizing immunomodulatory therapy. For example, a donor IL-6 genetic polymorphism is strongly associated with an increased incidence of AR posttransplantation [81].

The diagnostic workup for AR includes studies that may identify alternative causes of recipient graft dysfunction (Table 65.4). It is vital to consider alternative diagnoses, particularly in the early postoperative period, including vascular problems with the arterial or venous anastomoses, ureteral obstruction, or urinary leak. Other common causes of apparent graft dysfunction include the acute tubular necrosis associated with delayed graft function, hypovolemia and attendant prerenal azotemia, and the nephrotoxic effects of cyclosporine and tacrolimus. To rule out the vascular and ureteral problems discussed previously, a duplex ultrasound study of the renal graft is commonly obtained. Several ultrasound findings may suggest the diagnosis of AR: increased size of the graft, increased cortical thickness, enlargement of the renal pyramids, and decreased graft renal artery blood flow [82]. The resistive index has not been shown to be significant in helping with the diagnosis [83]. The diagnosis of AR is clearly established by percutaneous allograft biopsy and histologic examination. Biopsy is generally safe when performed by an experienced practitioner; however, complications include bleeding, hematoma and arteriovenous fistula formation, and ureteral or major vascular injury.

TABLE 65.4

Basic Workup of Recipients with Graft Dysfunction or Acute Rejection

History and physical examination	Establish and order differential diagnosis
Doppler ultrasound	Rule out vascular surgical complication Rule out leak (e.g., biliary, ureteral)
Serum chemistry	Evaluate relative blood urea nitrogen and creatinine, amylase, bilirubin, etc. Detect and treat electrolyte abnormalities
Drug levels	Evaluate for potential drug toxicity Detect inadequate drug levels
Blood cell count, cultures	Evaluate for potential infection
Graft biopsy	Firmly establish and grade graft rejection

Rejection is graded according to the modified Banff Criteria, which may be used to guide therapy that has been expanded to include C4d negative antibody–mediated rejection [84]. Fine-needle aspiration biopsy has been used by some centers to establish the diagnosis of AR; however, some consider the loss of microstructural data, as compared with traditional core biopsy, to be a weakness of the technique. In particular, the diagnoses of acute vascular rejection and CR are difficult to make using fine-needle aspiration biopsy.

The treatment of AR in renal transplant recipients is not standardized and varies between centers. High-dose methylprednisolone (500 to 1,000 mg per day or every other day [2 to 3 doses] is common) is often the initial approach. Corticosteroid-resistant AR, or AR that is histologically graded as severe or vascular, is often treated with potent depleting antilymphocyte antibodies such as polyclonal antithymocyte globulin (antithymocyte gamma globulin, thymoglobulin). Since some AR episodes occurred while the recipients were on stable immunosuppression, their maintenance therapy was switched from cyclosporine to tacrolimus or from azathioprine to mycophenolate mofetil. Most AR episodes are reversible with current therapies; however, as noted previously, the long-term outlook for preservation of graft function is lessened with each episode, especially when the posttreatment serum creatinine level does not return to the pre-AR baseline.

CR in renal transplant recipients is a frustrating clinical problem and appears to be multifactorial, with immunologic and nonimmunologic factors driving the gradual loss of graft function. As described earlier, minimizing the frequency and severity of AR episodes is important in decreasing the likelihood of eventual CR. Nonimmunologic factors thought to contribute to CR include (a) episodes of infection, particularly due to CMV and BK virus (*vide infra*); (b) the nephrotoxicity of CNI therapy; (c) ischemia-reperfusion injury and delayed graft function in the peritransplant period; and (d) innate cell senescence within the graft from donor-derived factors [85]. Attention is being directed toward identifying inflammatory activity within the graft, in response to both immune and nonimmune insults that may contribute to the development of CR. One of the leading causes of kidney retransplants is CR. It remains a formidable problem that is still poorly understood. Chapter 57 is devoted to kidney transplantation.

Hepatic Grafts

The transplanted liver is considered to be immunologically "privileged" in that evidence of some degree of immune tolerance occurs in a substantial number of liver transplant recipients over time. Despite that observation, all forms of rejection can occur posttransplant. At one time, it was thought that HAR did not occur in the hepatic graft; this idea is now known to be incorrect, as anti-HLA antibody–mediated HAR has been described in liver transplant recipients [86]. Unlike the renal graft, the hepatic graft undergoes HAR over a number of days, not minutes to hours, probably secondary to its ability to absorb a large amount of antibody and its functional reserve before the onset of the significant microthrombosis and vascular damage seen in HAR. A more delayed form of antibody-mediated rejection is seen in up to 33% of patients who undergo liver transplants across ABO-incompatible blood groups, but even this barrier appears surmountable with the use of plasmapheresis along with aggressive immunosuppression.

AR remains an important clinical problem in liver transplantation; even with the use of standard multiagent immunosuppression, the incidence of AR ranges from 30% to 80%. In two large, multicenter trials, double therapy with a CNI and steroids resulted in a 60% to 80% incidence of AR [87]. The most common liver transplantation regimen consists of two doses of a monoclonal anti-IL2 receptor (basiliximab) as induction therapy and dual maintenance therapy with the CNI tacrolimus and the antimetabolite mycophenolate mofetil, which lessens the incidence and severity of rejection without increasing infection rates [88].

The diagnosis of AR in liver transplant recipients is normally suggested by elevated levels of transaminases, bilirubin, or alkaline phosphatase. Among patients with T-tube drainage (which is increasingly uncommon), the biliary drainage may be seen to thicken, darken, and decrease in amount. The suspicion of AR mandates graft biopsy and studies to eliminate other possible causes of early hepatic graft failure. Duplex ultrasonography and, in some cases, cholangiography are increasingly being replaced by magnetic resonance imaging. Biopsy findings are classified, according to a standardized set of criteria, as *mild*, *moderate*, and *severe*, with clear implications for prognosis [89]. AR is normally treated with high-dose corticosteroids, but 5% to 10% of cases are steroid resistant; such recipients are then treated with an antilymphocyte antibody or tacrolimus at higher levels.

CR in liver transplant recipients is characterized by vascular obliteration and bile duct loss ("the vanishing duct syndrome"). This is seen in 5% to 10% of recipients, it is more common in those with vasculitic findings during AR episodes; if larger vessels are not seen on biopsy, the diagnosis of CR may be misread as AR. Tacrolimus has been used to salvage grafts in recipients with CR on cyclosporine-based immunosuppression, with a 73% success rate [90]. Chapter 58 is devoted to liver transplantation.

Pancreas Grafts

Diabetic patients undergo pancreas-alone (PTA), pancreas-after-kidney (PAK), or simultaneous pancreas–kidney (SPK) transplants and receive more potent immunosuppression than do renal transplant recipients, supported by initial studies demonstrating a higher rate of AR after pancreas transplantation. Overall success rates continue to improve: the risk of AR has been reduced by standardized induction therapy with antilymphocyte antibody preparations, and it may be further reduced with mammalian target of rapamycin (mTOR) inhibitors and/or with IL-2 receptor monoclonal antibodies [91].

Establishing the diagnosis of AR in pancreas transplant recipients can be difficult. Hyperglycemia is a late finding that only occurs with substantial loss of functional islet-cell mass. By the time hyperglycemia is seen, it may be too late to salvage a functional graft. Clinical findings may include fever and graft tenderness; however, pancreas graft rejection is often clinically silent.

For pancreas grafts transplanted along with a renal graft, a rising creatinine level is often used as a surrogate marker of rejection, with antirejection therapy aimed at both the pancreas and the renal allograft. However, isolated pancreas graft rejection is observed in up to 20% of simultaneous pancreas–kidney transplant recipients who have AR [92,93].

Advantages of a bladder-drained pancreas is the use of a decreasing urinary amylase level as a marker of graft rejection [94]. Other possible markers of rejection (serum anodal trypsinogen, serum amylase, soluble HLA, and analysis of glucose-disappearance kinetics during a brief glucose tolerance test) have been examined but have failed to gain widespread acceptance [93].

The diagnosis of pancreas graft rejection is confirmed by biopsy, which may be performed percutaneously or, in bladder-drained recipients, through a cystoscopic, transduodenal approach. Complications (bleeding, arteriovenous fistula formation, graft pancreatitis) have been described, but most biopsies do not lead to complications. Pancreas transplant recipients with early evidence of graft dysfunction should undergo Doppler ultrasonography to rule out graft thrombosis, which occurs in up to 10% to 20% of grafts [95].

Treatment of AR for pancreas transplantation recipients is similar to that for renal or liver transplantation recipients. High-dose corticosteroids are given initially, with a low threshold maintained for possibly switching to antibody-based therapy, given the relatively common steroid resistance. Most AR episodes are reversed with treatment. Chapter 61 is devoted to pancreas transplantation.

Intestinal Grafts

There is no serum test for intestinal transplantation rejection. As a result, biopsy of the intestinal allograft is the gold standard for diagnosis (via ostomy initially). It has the highest rates of AR and GvHD among all solid-organ transplants. The results have markedly improved over the past two decades: at 1 year, patient survival rates of intestinal transplants alone are >80% and of multivisceral transplants are >70%; the respective graft survival rates are >60% and >50%. Although treatment protocols for AR have significantly improved, chronic rejection remains a major issue because of its poorly understood nature in intestinal transplantation. Chapter 62 is devoted to intestinal transplantation.

Cardiac Grafts

Rejection in heart transplant recipients is a significant cause of morbidity and mortality among these patients and accounts for up to a third of the deaths. All forms of rejection are seen in heart transplant recipients. Albeit rare, HAR due to preformed antigraft antibodies occurs within minutes to days; it manifests with rapid deterioration of cardiac function, with prolonged need for inotropic support. In recipients whose grafts fail to recover rapidly, an attempt to reverse HAR by plasmapheresis may be made, but success is uncommon, and an immediate retransplant is usually required.

AR in heart transplant recipients is common and usually occurs in the first 3 to 4 months posttransplantation. At one time, the diagnosis was made on the basis of the development of congestive heart failure or the elaboration of electrocardiographic abnormalities. However, the present-day routine of protocol endomyocardial biopsies has eliminated such late findings of AR, except in noncompliant recipients. Most centers use frequent percutaneous transjugular right ventricular endomyocardial biopsies as part of a standardized surveillance protocol. Biopsies are evaluated histologically, according to an international grading system [96], and therapy is directed accordingly.

Several investigators have developed noninvasive approaches to establishing the diagnosis of AR, including electrocardiographic frequency analysis, nuclear scintigraphic techniques, and echocardiography; however, no approach has attained sufficient sensitivity to eliminate the need for protocol biopsies. The need for continued endomyocardial biopsies later than 1 year posttransplantation is controversial and center specific, with most choosing to discontinue its performance of biopsies at 1 year unless indicated on clinical grounds.

The treatment of AR is based on histologic findings. High-dose steroid bolus therapy is used in lower-grade rejection without hemodynamic compromise; oral prednisone therapy for mild AR also has been used with success [97]. Salvage therapy with an antilymphocyte antibody agent is most common in recipients with histologic findings of more severe rejection, in recipients with steroid-resistant rejection, and in recipients with signs of hemodynamic compromise.

Other approaches include switching from cyclosporine-based to tacrolimus-based immunosuppression in recipients with refractory AR in an effort to rescue to the graft, a strategy that was proved to be safe and efficacious [97]. Photopheresis has been used in the treatment of recipients with T-cell lymphoma and autoimmune disease. Studies of photopheresis and triple-drug immunosuppression have provided evidence of a decrease in the total number of AR episodes, as compared with triple-drug immunosuppression alone [97].

CR manifests in heart transplantation recipients as cardiac allograft vasculopathy (CAV), an entity that is the major cause of late-term morbidity and mortality. The pathologic findings of CAV include progressive intimal thickening in a concentric manner, which begins distally within the cardiac vasculature. It is associated with the loss of response to endogenous (and pharmacologic) vasodilators [97]. CAV is thought to be immunologically mediated because HLA donor-related matching is clearly associated with reduced rates of CAV but it could be ameliorated with the use of sirolimus [98]. In addition, nonimmunologic mechanisms are thought to be involved; identifiable risk factors for CAV include hyperlipidemia, donor age older than 25 years, recipient weight gain, CMV disease, preexisting donor or recipient coronary artery disease, and increasing time posttransplantation [97]. Another nonimmunologic risk factor for CAV is ischemic time during the peritransplant period. Chapter 60 is devoted to heart transplantation.

Lung Grafts

The lung graft is highly immunologic organ and as a result prone to rejection—nearly all lung transplant recipients experience at least one AR episode. The clinical difficulty posed by rejection is in distinguishing it from other causes of decreased graft function, most commonly infection.

HAR of the lung graft [99] is mediated by recipient-preformed antibodies to the donor graft, in a fashion similar to other organs. The clinical manifestation is similar to the more common ischemia-reperfusion injury, which, unlike HAR, usually resolves. HAR of the lung graft is rare and only described in case reports. HAR is uniformly fatal in lung transplant recipients. It must be prevented via initial cross-match testing and exclusion of immunologically unsuitable donor organs and strict adherence to ABO verification policies.

Most AR episodes occur during the first 3 to 6 months posttransplantation. Some recipients experience symptoms, including fever, cough, and dyspnea. Early diagnosis of AR in lung transplant recipients is essential: untreated AR can lead to respiratory insufficiency or failure, and repeated AR episodes are associated with an increased risk of bronchiolitis obliterans and eventual graft failure [99].

Transbronchial biopsy is the gold standard for establishing the diagnosis of AR, although less invasive techniques continue to be assessed [99]. Bronchoalveolar lavage (BAL) is also performed to rule out infection before increasing immunosuppression; infection and rejection may occur simultaneously in up to 25% of lung transplant recipients with AR [99]. Early diagnosis of AR may be aided by spirometry; decreases in timed forced expiratory volume, in pulmonary capillary blood volume, and in the diffusing capacity of the lungs for carbon monoxide are associated with AR and should prompt investigation. Radiography is not very sensitive. The histologic findings of AR include lymphocytic infiltrates into the perivascular and interstitial spaces; AR is graded according to histologic findings [100].

The initial treatment of AR in lung transplant recipients is similar to other organs with the use of high-dose corticosteroids; if they are not successful, anti–T-cell antibody therapy are the second line for steroid-resistant cases. Many recipients initially respond to the steroid pulse therapy, yet it may not completely clear their AR, and secondary episodes are common, and so additional therapy may be required. For that reason, surveillance bronchoscopy with transbronchial biopsies and BAL are common after initial treatment [99].

CR in lung transplant recipients is extremely common, affecting up to 40% of recipients at 2 years posttransplant and up to 70% of recipients after 5 years [101]. The mean time to diagnosis of graft dysfunction posttransplant is 16 to 20 months. A definitive histologic diagnosis of early bronchiolitis obliterans may be difficult to obtain, and so a high degree of clinical suspicion must be maintained. Radiography, again, is not specific. Typical presenting symptoms are cough, progressive dyspnea, and loss of exercise tolerance. There are myriad of therapeutic modalities that have been attempted for recipients with bronchiolitis obliterans, but with little success. Increases in immunosuppression, antilymphocyte antibody therapy, and inhaled cyclosporine have all been tried. Ultimately, the progress of bronchiolitis obliterans is inexorable, with continued loss of graft function and subsequent death. A lung retransplantation is the only viable option [99]. Chapter 59 is devoted to lung transplantation.

SUMMARY

For more than half a century, substantial advances in the field of solid-organ transplantation have propelled the clinical practice from an experimental to a standardized and routine stage. Dramatic improvements in surgical techniques, immunosuppressive therapy, and medical/critical care have made it possible to increase the pool of potential recipients and now include those who would have been considered too sick or with too many comorbidities even a few years ago. However, despite this progress, until medical science is able to develop immunosuppressive drugs and regimens without side effects, or achieve routine tolerance induction, the predominant challenges in transplantation will remain the prevention, diagnosis, and treatment of GvHD, infection, malignancy, and rejection. These clinical problems have, however, improved in the nearly six decades since the first successful kidney transplant was performed; but they may become more complex throughout the 21st century as we now transplant many more complicated patients.

References

1. Starzl T, Marchioro, TL, Waddell, WR: The Reversal of rejection in human renal homografts with subsequent development of homograft tolerance. *Surg Gynecol Obstet* 117:385–395, 1963.
2. Hill RB, Rowlands DT, Rifkind D: Infectious pulmonary disease in patients receiving immunosuppressive therapy for organ transplantation. *N Engl J Med* 271(20):1021–1027, 1964.
3. Starzl TE, Penn I, Putnam CW, et al: Iatrogenic alterations of immunologic surveillance in man and their influence on malignancy. *Immunol Rev* 7(1):112–145, 1971.
4. Akbulut S, Yilmaz M, Yilmaz S: Graft-versus-host disease after liver transplantation: a comprehensive literature review. *World J Gastroenterol* 18(37):5240–5248, 2012.
5. DePaoli AM, Bitran J: Graft-versus-host disease and liver transplantation. *Ann Intern Med* 117(2):170–171, 1992.
6. Sun B, Zhao C, Xia Y, et al: Late onset of severe graft-versus-host disease following liver transplantation. *Transpl Immunol* 16(3/4):250–253, 2006.
7. Weitz M, Strahm B, Meerpohl JJ, et al: Extracorporeal photopheresis versus alternative treatment for chronic graft-versus-host disease after haematopoietic stem cell transplantation in paediatric patients. *Cochrane Database Syst Rev* (2):CD009898, 2014.
8. Vidal E, Cervera C, Cordero E, et al: Executive summary. Management of urinary tract infection in solid organ transplant recipients: consensus statement of the Group for the Study of Infection in Transplant Recipients (GESITRA) of the Spanish Society of Infectious Diseases and Clinical Microbiology (SEIMC) and the Spanish Network for Research in Infectious Diseases (REIPI). *Enferm Infecc Microbiol Clin* 33:680–687, 2015.
9. Engels EA, Pfeiffer RM, Fraumeni JF Jr, et al: Spectrum of cancer risk among US solid organ transplant recipients. *JAMA* 306(17):1891–1901, 2011.
10. Florescu DF, Qiu F, Schmidt CM, et al: A direct and indirect comparison meta-analysis on the efficacy of cytomegalovirus preventive strategies in solid organ transplant. *Clin Infect Dis* 58(6):785–803, 2014.
11. Park UJ, Hyun SK, Kim HT, et al: Successful treatment of disseminated adenovirus infection with ribavirin and intravenous immunoglobulin in an adult renal transplant recipient: a case report. *Transplant Proc* 47(3):791–793, 2015.
12. Khedmat H, Karbasi-Afshar R, Agah S, et al: A meta-analysis of potential relationship between Epstein-Barr-Encoded-RNA (EBER) and onset time of

post-transplant lymphoproliferative disorders. *Saudi J Kidney Dis Transpl* 26(2):232–237, 2015.

13. Kauffman CA, Miceli MH: Histoplasmosis and blastomycosis in solid organ transplant recipients. *J Fungi* 1(2):94–106, 2015.
14. Parapiboon W, Ingsathit A, Jirasiritham S, et al: High incidence of bacteriuria in early post-kidney transplantation; results from a randomized controlled study. *Transplant Proc* 44(3):734–736, 2012.
15. Gurusamy KS, Nagendran M, Davidson BR: Methods of preventing bacterial sepsis and wound complications after liver transplantation. *Cochrane Database Syst Rev* (3):CD006660, 2014.
16. Orlando G, Manzia TM, Sorge R, et al: One-shot versus multidose perioperative antibiotic prophylaxis after kidney transplantation: a randomized, controlled clinical trial. *Surgery* 157(1):104–110, 2015.
17. de la Torre M, Fernández R, Fieira E, et al: Postoperative surgical complications after lung transplantation. *Rev Port Pneumol* 21(1):36–40, 2015.
18. Tevar A, Humar A, Zureikat A, et al: Pancreas transplantation, in Humar A, Sturdevant ML (eds): *Atlas of Organ Transplantation*: London, Springer, 2015, pp 155–222.
19. Santos C, Brennan DC, Yusen RD, et al: Incidence, risk factors and outcomes of delayed-onset cytomegalovirus disease in a large retrospective cohort of lung transplant recipients. *Transplantation* 99:1658–1666, 2015.
20. Ulubay G, Kupeli E, Duvenci BO, et al: A 10-year experience of tuberculosis in solid-organ transplant recipients. *Exp Clin Transplant* 13:214–218, 2015.
21. Gallagher C, Smith JA: CNS infections in solid organ transplant recipients. *Neurology* 9[Pt 3]:1, 2016.
22. Saliba F, Pascher A, Cointault O, et al: Randomized trial of micafungin for the prevention of invasive fungal infection in high-risk liver transplant recipients. *Clin Infect Dis* 60(7):997–1006, 2015.
23. Lamoth F, Alexander BD: Antifungal Activity of SCY-078 (MK-3118) and Standard Antifungal Agents against Clinical non-Aspergillus Mold Isolates. *Antimicrob Agents Chemother* 59:4308–4311, 2015. doi:10.1128/AAC.00234-15.
24. Raad II, El Zakhem A, El Helou G, et al: Clinical experience of the use of voriconazole, caspofungin or the combination in primary and salvage therapy of invasive aspergillosis in haematological malignancies. *Int J Antimicrob Agents* 45(3):283–288, 2015.
25. Heylen L, Maertens J, Naesens M, et al: Invasive aspergillosis after kidney transplant: case-control study. *Clin Infect Dis* 60:1505–1511, 2015.
26. Cornely OA, Meems L, Herbrecht R, et al: Randomised, multicentre trial of micafungin vs. an institutional standard regimen for salvage treatment of invasive aspergillosis. *Mycoses* 58(1):58–64, 2015.
27. Chen Y-C, Chang T-Y, Liu J-W, et al: Increasing trend of fluconazole-non-susceptible Cryptococcus neoformans in patients with invasive cryptococcosis: a 12-year longitudinal study. *BMC Infect Dis* 15(1):277, 2015.
28. Johnson RH, Heidari A: *Coccidioidomycosis. Diagnosis and Treatment of Fungal Infections*. Switzerland, Springer, 2015, pp 205–216.
29. Miceli MH, Kauffman CA: Treatment options for mucormycosis. *Cur Treat Options Infect Dis* 7(3):142–154, 2015.
30. Tan BH: Cytomegalovirus Treatment. *Cur Treat Options Infect Dis* 6(3):256–270, 2014.
31. Mumtaz K, Faisal N, Husain S, et al: Universal prophylaxis or preemptive strategy for cytomegalovirus disease after liver transplantation: a systematic review and meta-analysis. *Am J Transplant* 15(2):472–481, 2015.
32. Ghassemieh B, Ahya VN, Baz MA, et al: Decreased incidence of cytomegalovirus infection with sirolimus in a post hoc randomized, multicenter study in lung transplantation. *J Heart Lung Transplant* 32(7):701–706, 2013.
33. Potena L, Bianchi G, Chiereghin A, et al: Reconstitution of CMV-specific immunity after heart transplantation may guide customization of immunosuppressive and antiviral strategies: a prospective randomized study. *J Heart Lung Transplant* 33(4):S154–S155, 2014.
34. Ahlenstiel-Grunow T, Koch A, Grosshennig A, et al: A multicenter, randomized, open-labeled study to steer immunosuppressive and antiviral therapy by measurement of virus (CMV, ADV, HSV)-specific T cells in addition to determination of trough levels of immunosuppressants in pediatric kidney allograft recipients (IVIST01-trial): study protocol for a randomized controlled trial. *Trials* 15:324, 2014.
35. Masson P, Henderson L, Chapman JR, et al: Belatacept for kidney transplant recipients. *Cochrane Database Syst Rev* (24):CD010699, 2014.
36. Tan H-H, Goh C-L: Viral infections affecting the skin in organ transplant recipients: epidemiology and current management strategies. *Am J Clin Dermatol* 7(1):13–29, 2006.
37. Yamada N, Sanada Y, Okada N, et al: Successful rescue of disseminated varicella infection with multiple organ failure in a pediatric living donor liver transplant recipient: a case report and literature review. *Virol J* 12(1):91, 2015.
38. Delbue S, Bella R, Ferraresso M: Reactivation of the human herpes virus 6 in kidney transplant recipients: an unsolved question. *J Transplant Technol Res* 5:e134, 2015.
39. Chevaliez S, Pawlotsky J-M: Virology of hepatitis C virus infection. *Best Pract Res Clin Gastroenterol* 26(4):381–389, 2012.
40. Mahboobi N, Tabatabaei SV, Blum HE, et al: Renal grafts from anti-hepatitis B core-positive donors: a quantitative review of the literature. *Transpl Infect Dis* 14(5):445–451, 2012.
41. Buti M, Tabernero D, Mas A, et al: Hepatitis B virus quasispecies evolution after liver transplantation in patients under long-term lamivudine prophylaxis with or without hepatitis B immune globulin. *Transpl Infect Dis* 17(2):208–220, 2015.
42. Duvoux C, Villamil F, Renner EL, et al: Sustained virological response to antiviral therapy in a randomized trial of cyclosporine versus tacrolimus in liver transplant patients with recurrent hepatitis C infection. *Ann Transplant* 20:25–35, 2014.
43. Biggins S, Gralla J, Dodge J, et al: Survival benefit of repeat liver transplantation in the United States: a serial MELD analysis by hepatitis C status and donor risk index. *Am J Transplant* 14(11):2588–2594, 2014.
44. Naggie S, Cooper C, Saag M, et al: Ledipasvir and sofosbuvir for HCV in patients coinfected with HIV-1. *N Engl J Med* 373:705–713, 2015.
45. Simonds RJ: HIV transmission by organ and tissue transplantation. *AIDS* 7:S35–S38, 1993.
46. Miro J, Agüero F, Duclos-Vallée JC, et al: Infections in solid organ transplant HIV-infected patients. *Clin Microbiol Infect* 20[Suppl 7]:119–130, 2014.
47. Sawinski D, Goldberg D, Blumberg E, et al: Beyond the NIH multicenter HIV transplant trial experience: outcomes of HIV+ liver transplant recipients compared to HCV+ or HIV+/HCV+ co-infected recipients in the United States. *Clin Infect Dis* 61:1054–1062, 2015.
48. Gavaldà J, Aguado J, Manuel O, et al: A special issue on infections in solid organ transplant recipients. *Clin Microbiol Infect* 20[Suppl 7]:1–3, 2014.
49. Lee BT, Gabardi S, Grafals M, et al: Efficacy of levofloxacin in the treatment of BK viremia: a multicenter, double-blinded, randomized, placebo-controlled trial. *Clin J Am Soc Nephrol* 9(3):583–589, 2014.
50. Baliu C, Sanclemente G, Cardona M, et al: Toxoplasmic encephalitis associated with meningitis in a heart transplant recipient. *Transpl Infect Dis* 16(4):631–633, 2014.
51. Avila JD, Živković S: The neurology of solid organ transplantation. *Curr Neurol Neurosci Rep* 15(7):1–10, 2015.
52. Penn I. Cancers in renal transplant recipients. *Adv Ren Replace Ther* 7(2):147–156, 2000.
53. Sherston SN, Carroll RP, Harden PN, et al: Predictors of cancer risk in the long-term solid-organ transplant recipient. *Transplantation* 97(6):605–611, 2014.
54. Gifford G, Fay K, Jabbour A, et al: Primary central nervous system posttransplantation lymphoproliferative disorder after heart and lung transplantation. *Intern Med J* 45(5):583–586, 2015.
55. Paya CV, Fung JJ, Nalesnik MA, et al: Epstein–Barr virus-induced posttransplant lymphoproliferative disorders. *Transplantation* 68(10):1517–1525, 1999.
56. Lauro A, Arpinati M, Pinna AD: Managing the challenge of PTLD in liver and bowel transplant recipients. *Br J Haematol* 169(2):157–172, 2015.
57. Harris NL, Ferry JA, Swerdlow SH: Posttransplant lymphoproliferative disorders: summary of society for hematopathology workshop. *Semin Diagn Pathol* 14(1):8–14, 1997.
58. Sheil AG, Disney AP, Mathew TH, et al: De novo malignancy emerges as a major cause of morbidity and late failure in renal transplantation. *Transplant Proc* 25(1, Pt 2):1383–1384, 1993.
59. Bavinck JNB, Vermeer BJ, van der Woude FJ, et al: Relation between skin cancer and HLA antigens in renal-transplant recipients. *N Engl J Med* 325(12):843–848, 1991.
60. Dahlke E, Murray CA, Kitchen J, et al: Systematic review of melanoma incidence and prognosis in solid organ transplant recipients. *Transplant Res* 3:10, 2014.
61. McKnight J, Cen H, Riddler S, et al: EBV gene expression, EBNA antibody responses and EBV+ peripheral blood lymphocytes in post-transplant lymphoproliferative disease. *Leuk Lymphoma* 15(1):9–16, 1994.
62. Robinson JK, Guevara Y, Gaber R, et al: Efficacy of a sun protection workbook for kidney transplant recipients: a randomized controlled trial of a culturally sensitive educational intervention. *Am J Transplant* 14(12):2821–2829, 2014.
63. D'Amico F, Fuxman C, Nachman F, et al: Visceral Kaposi's sarcoma remission after intestinal transplant. First case report and systematic literature review. *Transplantation* 90(5):547–554, 2010.
64. Gutierrez JCL. *Classification of Vascular Tumors. Hemangiomas and Vascular Malformations*. Berlin, Springer, 2015, pp 59–65.
65. Alberu J, Pascoe MD, Campistol JM, et al: Lower malignancy rates in renal allograft recipients converted to sirolimus-based, calcineurin inhibitor-free immunotherapy: 24-months results from the CONVERT trial. *Transplantation* 92(3):303–310, 2011.
66. Penn I: Evaluation of transplant candidates with pre-existing malignancies. *Ann Transplant* 2(4):14–17, 1997.
67. Xiao D, Craig JC, Chapman JR, et al: Donor cancer transmission in kidney transplantation: a systematic review. *Am J Transplant* 13(10):2645–2652, 2013.
68. Onaca N, Klintmalm GB: Liver transplantation for hepatocellular carcinoma: the baylor experience. *J Hepatobiliary Pancreat Surg* 17:559–566, 2010.
69. Halazun KJ, Patzer RE, Rana AA, et al: Standing the test of time: outcomes of a decade of prioritizing patients with hepatocellular carcinoma, results of the UNOS natural geographic experiment. *Hepatology* 60(6):1957–1962, 2014.
70. Medawar PB: Experimental work. *Plast Reconstr Surg* 2(4):387, 1947.
71. Squifflet JP, De Meyer M, Malaise J, et al: Lessons learned from ABO-incompatible living donor kidney transplantation: 20 years later. *Exp Clin Transplant* 2(1):208–213, 2004.
72. Magee CC: Transplantation across previously incompatible immunological barriers. *Transpl Int* 19(2):87–97, 2006.
73. Taylor CJ, Kosmoliaptsis V, Summers DM, et al: Back to the future: application of contemporary technology to long-standing questions about the clinical relevance of human leukocyte antigen-specific alloantibodies in renal transplantation. *Hum Immunol* 70(8):563–568, 2009.
74. Haas M, Rahman MH, Racusen LC, et al: C4d and C3d staining in biopsies of ABO- and HLA-incompatible renal allografts: correlation with histologic findings. *Am J Transplant* 6(8):1829–1840, 2006.

75. Saran R, Robinson B, Ayanian J: United States renal data system, 2014 annual data report: epidemiology of kidney disease in the United States. *Am J Kidney Dis* 66:Svii, S1–S305, 2015.
76. Vincenti F, Schena FP, Paraskevas S, et al: A randomized, multicenter study of steroid avoidance, early steroid withdrawal or standard steroid therapy in kidney transplant recipients. *Am J Transplant* 8(2):307–316, 2008.
77. Matas AJ: Impact of acute rejection on development of chronic rejection in pediatric renal transplant recipients. *Pediatr Transplant* 4(2):92–99, 2000.
78. Sayegh MH: Chronic renal allograft dysfunction (CAD): new frontiers. *Kidney Int* 78:S1, 2010.
79. Jain S, Curwood V, White SA, et al: Weekly protocol renal transplant biopsies allow detection of sub-clinical acute rejection episodes in patients with delayed graft function. *Transplant Proc* 32(1):191, 2000.
80. Dalpiaz T, Nogare ADL, Carpio V, et al: Noninvasive molecular biomarkers of acute antibody mediated rejection in renal transplant patients. *Transplant J* 94:263, 2012.
81. Marshall SE, McLaren AJ, McKinney EF, et al: Donor cytokine genotype influences the development of acute rejection after renal transplantation. *Transplantation* 71(3):469–476, 2001.
82. Kirkpantur A, Yilmaz R, Baydar DE, et al: Utility of the doppler ultrasound parameter, resistive index, in renal transplant histopathology. *Transplant Proc* 40(1):104–106, 2008.
83. Naesens M, Heylen L, Lerut E, et al: Intrarenal resistive index after renal transplantation. *N Engl J Med* 369(19):1797–1806, 2013.
84. Mubarak M: Evolution of the Banff working classification of renal allograft pathology: updates and future directions. *J Transplant Technol Res* 03(02), 2013.
85. Waaga AM, Gasser M, Laskowski I, et al: Mechanisms of chronic rejection. *Curr Opin Immunol* 12(5):517–521, 2000.
86. Demetris AJ, Zeevi A, O'Leary JG: ABO-compatible liver allograft antibody-mediated rejection. *Curr Opin Organ Transplant* 20(3):314–324, 2015.
87. A comparison of tacrolimus (FK 506) and cyclosporine for immunosuppression in liver transplantation. *N Engl J Med* 331(17):1110–1115, 1994.
88. Neuhaus P: Improved treatment response with basiliximab immunoprophylaxis after liver transplantation: results from a double-blind randomized placebo-controlled trial. *Liver Transpl* 8(2):132–142, 2002.
89. Banff Working Group on Liver Allograft Pathology: Importance of liver biopsy findings in immunosuppression management: biopsy monitoring and working criteria for patients with operational tolerance. *Liver Transpl* 18(10):1154–1170, 2012.
90. Wong P, Devlin J, Gane E, et al: FK 506 rescue therapy for intractable liver allograft rejection. *Transpl Int* 7[Suppl 1]:0934–0874, 1994.
91. Gruessner RW, Gruessner AC: The current state of pancreas transplantation. *Nat Rev Endocrinol* 9(9):555–562, 2013.
92. Norman SP, Kommareddi M, Samaniego M, et al: Early pancreas graft loss is associated with increased mortality in simultaneous pancreas and kidney transplant recipients. *Transpl J* 90, 2010.
93. Gruessner RWG, Sutherland DER: Clinical diagnosis in pancreas allograft rejection, in Solez K, Racusen LC, Billingham ME (eds): *Solid Organ Transplant Rejection: Mechanisms, Pathology and Diagnosis*. New York, NY, Marcel Dekker Inc, 1996, pp 455–499.
94. Nghiem DD, Gonwa TA, Corry RJ: Metabolic effects of urinary diversion of exocrine secretions in pancreatic transplantation. *Transplantation* 43(1):70–72, 1987.
95. Gruessner AC: 2011 update on pancreas transplantation: comprehensive trend analysis of 25,000 cases followed up over the course of twenty-four years at the International Pancreas Transplant Registry (IPTR). *Rev Diabet Stud* 8(1):6–16, 2011.
96. Everitt MD, Hammond MEH, Snow GL, et al: Biopsy-diagnosed antibody-mediated rejection based on the proposed International Society for Heart and Lung Transplantation working formulation is associated with adverse cardiovascular outcomes after pediatric heart transplant. *J Heart Lung Transplant* 31(7):686–693, 2012.
97. Hunt SA, Haddad F: The changing face of heart transplantation. *J Am Coll Cardiol* 52(8):587–598, 2008.
98. Matsuo Y, Cassar A, Yoshino S, et al: Attenuation of cardiac allograft vasculopathy by sirolimus: relationship to time interval after heart transplantation. *J Heart Lung Transplant* 32(8):784–791, 2013.
99. Martinu T, Howell DN, Palmer SM: Acute cellular rejection and humoral sensitization in lung transplant recipients. *Semin Respir Crit Care Med* 31(2):179–188, 2010.
100. Berry GJ, Burke MM, Andersen C, et al: The 2013 International Society for Heart and Lung Transplantation Working Formulation for the standardization of nomenclature in the pathologic diagnosis of antibody-mediated rejection in heart transplantation. *J Heart Lung Transplant* 32(12):1147–1162, 2013.
101. Colvin-Adams M, Valapour M, Hertz M, et al: Lung and heart allocation in the United States. *Am J Transplant* 12(12):3213–3234, 2012.
102. Gugenheim J, Samuel D, Bismuth H, et al: Liver transplantation across ABO blood group barriers. *Lancet* 336(8714):519–523, 1990.
103. Mor E, Skerrett D, Manzarbeitia C, et al: Successful use of an enhanced immunosuppressive protocol with plasmapheresis for ABO-incompatible mismatched grafts in liver transplant recipients. *Transplantation* 59(7):986–990, 1995.
104. Pinsky B, Ercole P, Burroughs T, et al: Predicting long-term graft survival in adult kidney transplant recipients. *Saudi J Kidney Dis Transpl* 23(4):693–700, 2012.
105. Ekberg H, Bernasconi C, Tedesco-Silva H, et al: Calcineurin inhibitor minimization in the Symphony study: observational results 3 years after transplantation. *Am J Transplant* 9(8):1876–1885, 2009.
106. Guery BP, Arendrup MC, Auzinger G, et al: Management of invasive candidiasis and candidemia in adult non-neutropenic intensive care unit patients: Part II. Treatment. *Intensive Care Med* 35(2):206–214, 2008.
107. Fernandez-Ruiz M, Arias M, Campistol JM, et al: Cytomegalovirus prevention strategies in seropositive kidney transplant recipients: an insight into current clinical practice. *Transpl Int* 28:1042–1054, 2015.
108. Akerzoul N, Chbicheb S, El Wady W: Kaposi Sarcoma and HHV8. *Oral Surg Oral Med Oral Pathol Oral Radiol* 3(119):e218, 2015.

Section 7
RHEUMATOLOGIC, IMMUNOLOGIC, AND DERMATOLOGIC DISEASES IN THE INTENSIVE CARE UNIT

NANCY Y.N. LIU

Chapter 66 ■ Rheumatologic Diseases in the Intensive Care Unit

NANCY Y.N. LIU • JUDITH A. STEBULIS

Patients with established rheumatologic diseases are rarely admitted to the intensive care unit (ICU) because of their inflammatory joint disease. However, because many of these diseases include systemic involvement, organ system failure and complications of therapy are common reasons for ICU admission. Other musculoskeletal problems frequently encountered in the intensive care setting include (a) patients whose underlying rheumatic diseases may pose certain problems in the planning and execution of some critical care procedures, such as endotracheal intubation, or (b) patients for whom acute rheumatic syndromes develop during their hospitalization.

ACUTE RHEUMATIC DISEASES IN THE INTENSIVE CARE SETTING

Several acute musculoskeletal disorders occur with increasing frequency among selected hospitalized patients, including those in the ICU. The most common is crystal-induced arthritis because of monosodium urate, calcium pyrophosphate dihydrate (CPPD), basic calcium phosphate (BCP)-hydroxyapatite, or calcium oxalate crystals. Two other acute arthritides include septic arthritis from bacteremia and spontaneous hemarthrosis because of complications from anticoagulation therapy or bleeding diathesis.

Gout

Pathogenesis

Gout is characterized by initial and intermittent attacks of mono- or polyarticular arthritis in the setting of prolonged hyperuricemia. Over many years, attacks become more frequent, and chronic arthropathy may develop. Acute gout is triggered by precipitation or shedding of monosodium urate crystals in the joint space or nearby soft tissues, provoking an intense inflammatory reaction. Regardless of a primary or secondary etiology of hyperuricemia, marked fluctuations of serum urate levels increase the risk of acute gout.

Although the specific triggering event that initiates an isolated attack may be difficult to define, many factors cause serum urate fluctuations and result in an increased incidence of secondary gout among ICU patients. A reduction of glomerular filtration rate from either intrinsic renal disease or decreased effective arteriolar blood volume will result in reduced filtered load of urate, hyperuricemia, and an increased risk of gout. In addition, a reduction of effective arteriolar blood volume results in enhanced tubular reabsorption of urate. Because organic acids such as lactic acid, β-hydroxybutyric acid, and acetoacetic acid may competitively inhibit the renal tubular secretion of uric acid, conditions in which these acids accumulate will also lead to hyperuricemia. Mechanisms of hyperlacticacidemia among the critically ill patient are multiple.

Drug-induced hyperuricemia is a common cause of gout in both hospitalized and nonhospitalized patients. Diuretic therapy decreases effective arteriolar blood volume and also may directly inhibit renal tubular secretion of uric acid. Although thiazide diuretics are the most commonly implicated cause of hyperuricemia and gout, other diuretics including furosemide, acetazolamide, ethacrynic acid, and diazoxide are also potential culprits. Furosemide and diazoxide may also induce hyperlacticacidemia.

In addition to diuretics, other drugs associated with hyperuricemia include low-dose salicylates (less than 2.0 g per day), pyrazinamide, levodopa, α-methyldopa, and cyclosporine. Because of the uricosuric effect of radiocontrast media, a contrast study might precipitate an attack of acute gout. Finally, a hyperuricemic patient who undergoes any surgical procedure is at risk for postoperative gout.

Clinical Features

Gout is easily identifiable and treatable. Classically, the patient with acute gout complains of sudden onset of an exquisitely painful joint that involves one or more sites in an asymmetric pattern. The attack is sometimes accompanied by low-grade fever, particularly in a polyarticular presentation. The great toe is involved in more than 50% of the initial acute attacks and in 90% of acute attacks at some time in the course of the disease. Other common sites of involvement in order of observed frequency include insteps, ankles, knees, wrists, fingers, and elbows. Periarticular sites of urate deposition in bursae, tendons, and soft tissues may be similarly inflamed during an acute attack. On examination, the involved area is erythematous, swollen, warm, and exquisitely painful on palpation, sometimes with joint motion. The overlying erythema and edema often extend beyond the joint capsule and can mimic cellulitis or bursitis.

The presence of lymphangitis or lymphadenopathy and the absence of pain on joint motion are more consistent with cellulitis. Bursitis can be distinguished from true arthritis because full joint extension is preserved in bursitis, and the region of erythema is not within the borders of the joint compartment. If clinical suspicion of joint infection is low, then diagnostic arthrocentesis should be avoided until a therapeutic trial of appropriate antibiotics for cellulitis has been completed. Otherwise, there may be a risk of introducing organisms into a sterile joint. However, if motion is restricted or if radiography suggests an effusion, a diagnostic arthrocentesis should be performed before the institution of any therapy.

The diagnosis of gout is confirmed when aspirated synovial fluid or soft tissue site reveals negatively birefringent monosodium urate crystals within polymorphonuclear neutrophils (PMNs) under polarizing light microscopy. Gouty synovial fluid is inflammatory, with more than 2,000 leukocytes per μL, occasionally as high as 100,000 per μL, and PMNs predominate in the cell differential. Because gout and septic arthritis have similar clinical features and can coexist, aspirated synovial fluid should always have a Gram stain for microorganisms and bacterial culture performed. Elevations of the erythrocyte sedimentation rate (ESR), C-reactive protein (CRP), and peripheral leukocytosis cannot distinguish gout from other inflammatory states. Serum urate may be normal during an acute attack, whereas an elevated level does not confirm the diagnosis without crystal identification.

Therapy

Once the diagnosis of acute gout is established, the immediate aim of therapy is to terminate the attack by interruption of the inflammatory response. Long-term management (e.g., prevention of recurrent attacks, sequelae of tophaceous disease, or renal stones) need not be initiated in the ICU setting. In fact, the initiation or discontinuation of any drugs that alter urate levels (i.e., allopurinol, febuxostat, probenecid, or lesinurad) may prolong the acute attack without preventing it. Asymptomatic hyperuricemia should not be treated.

Corticosteroids Systemic and intra-articular steroids are effective for the treatment of gout. Intravenous (IV) methylprednisolone (0.5 to 2 mg per kg IV daily for 3 to 5 days depending on severity and number of joints involved) is the preferred agent in critically ill patients [1]. Oral prednisone may also be effective in doses of 0.5 mg per kg initially and tapered over 7 to 14 days, with decrements of 10 mg every 2 days [1]. Potential complications of steroid treatment include hyperglycemia, fluid retention secondary to mineralocorticoid effects, and hypothalamic–pituitary–adrenal suppression. Intra-articular corticosteroid injection is an excellent choice for acute gouty arthritis if few joints are involved because systemic side effects are avoided. Steroid injection provides rapid resolution of symptoms, usually within 12 to 24 hours, but if infection is suspected, corticosteroid injection should be delayed until culture results are available. Intra-articular corticosteroids are quite effective in small joints if performed by physicians skilled in these injections. Dosing ranges from 10 to 60 mg methylprednisolone or equivalent triamcinolone, depending on the size of the joint involved.

Colchicine Colchicine is one of the established treatments for gout. Its main mechanism of action involves formation of a reversible complex with the tubulin subunit of microtubules, leading to reduced activation and migration of PMNs. Oral colchicine is absorbed in the small intestine and excreted in the bile and urine, reaching a peak serum level in 2 hours. Gastrointestinal side effects, most notably diarrhea, occur among up to 80% of patients, resulting in electrolyte imbalances and fluid losses. In the critically ill patient, oral colchicine may not be feasible and is potentially toxic. Renal and hepatic insufficiencies are risk factors for colchicine-related neuromyopathy and bone marrow suppression. In addition, potential drug–drug interactions, including macrolide antibiotics, HMG-CoA reductase inhibitors, fibric acid derivatives, verapamil and diltiazem, and cyclosporine, may potentiate colchicine toxicities.

Current recommendations for treatment of acute gout with lower dose colchicine (1.2 mg orally followed in 1 hour by another 0.6 mg orally) as opposed to traditional oral loading of colchicine (1.2 mg orally followed by 0.6 mg every hour for 6 hours) are preferred, with fewer toxicities [2]. In addition, the gastrointestinal side effects are significantly reduced with the lower dose regimen. Thus, if an ICU patient with an acute onset of gout has normal renal and hepatic function and is able to take oral colchicine, the low-dose regimen is a reasonable choice. However, if there is renal insufficiency, dose adjustment is necessary and colchicine is probably best avoided if creatinine clearance is less than 10 mL per minute. A more appropriate use of oral colchicine is for the prevention of subsequent attacks once the acute attack is treated. Dosages of 0.6 mg orally once or twice a day have been effective (again dose adjustment is necessary based on GFR) [3]. The most common side effects include nausea, diarrhea, and proximal myopathy with elevated creatinine kinase levels. The risk of myotoxicity correlates with a creatinine clearance of less than 50 mL per minute.

Nonsteroidal Anti-inflammatory Drugs Nonsteroidal anti-inflammatory drugs (NSAIDs) are effective for the treatment of acute gout. However, the mechanism of action involves prostaglandin inhibition, which can interfere with gastric mucosal integrity and worsen renal function by reducing renal perfusion in the setting of volume contraction. NSAIDs may also cause other side effects, including decreased coronary flow and mental status changes. Although the cyclooxygenase-2 inhibitor agents offer the possibility of fewer adverse events, their safety profile is based on outpatient experience. Serious adverse effects with these newer agents have been reported. Given the fact that many patients in the ICU have some degree of renal disease and are at risk for gastrointestinal bleeding, NSAIDs are rarely a first-line agent in the treatment of gout in the ICU.

Other Microcrystalline Arthropathies

Although gout is the best-defined and most common crystalline arthropathy, several other crystalline-induced syndromes may mimic gout and cause potential diagnostic confusion. These include CPPD, BCP-hydroxyapatite, or calcium oxalate crystals.

Pathogenesis

The pathophysiology of these entities appears to be similar to that of gouty arthritis, involving a complex series of biochemical reactions that lead to an inflammatory response within the involved joint or periarticular region.

The acute, self-limited form of CPPD deposition (also known as *pseudogout*) may be precipitated by surgery of any type, and is related to downward fluxes of serum calcium levels that lead to crystal shedding into intra-articular spaces. Attacks commonly occur several days postoperatively and often involve the knee or wrist. Severe medical illnesses, such as ischemic heart disease, cerebral infarction, and thrombophlebitis, may also provoke attacks of CPPD arthritis.

Patients on chronic intermittent peritoneal dialysis have a high incidence of acute arthritis that is secondary to CPPD or BCP-hydroxyapatite deposition in articular cartilage. In contrast, chronic hemodialysis patients are at risk for acute arthritis from calcium oxalate crystals.

Clinical Features

Clinically, each of the above crystalline arthropathies is clinically indistinguishable from acute gout. The presence of radiographic calcification in hyaline or articular cartilage of the involved joint (i.e., chondrocalcinosis) suggests the diagnosis of pseudogout, but the diagnosis is confirmed by visualizing weakly positively birefringent, rhomboid-shaped CPPD crystals within synovial fluid PMNs under polarizing microscopy. Calcium oxalate crystals, likewise, are positively birefringent, but they are pleomorphic, bipyramidal, or rod-like in shape. Smaller BCP-hydroxyapatite crystals, however, are not visible under polarizing microscopy, and a presumptive diagnosis is made given the clinical setting, the exclusion of other diagnoses, and the occasional presence of periarticular, amorphous calcifications on radiographs.

Therapy

Therapeutic options are limited in the ICU patient if NSAIDs are contraindicated. Isolated joints can be aspirated and injected with corticosteroids once infection is excluded. Alternatively, a regimen of tapering corticosteroids similar to acute gout is effective. Pseudogout may also respond dramatically to colchicine in dosing similar to gout. Low-dose colchicine is also used to prevent recurrent attacks for patients who have frequent events.

Septic Arthritis

Joint infection is the most critical diagnosis to establish and treat in any ICU patient who develops acute mono- or oligoarthritis. A delay in the diagnosis and treatment of septic arthritis may lead to destruction of articular cartilage and loss of joint function. Furthermore, a diagnosis of septic arthritis may help identify and initiate early treatment of the source of septicemia, such as endocarditis (see Chapter 78).

Pathogenesis

Risk factors for development of septic arthritis include diabetes mellitus, age over 80, skin infections, rheumatoid arthritis (RA), IV drug abuse, alcoholism, recent joint surgery, low socioeconomic status, and prosthetic joints [4]. In addition, patients in the ICU often have multiple invasive procedures, indwelling lines, or catheters that are potential portals of infection. Acute septic arthritis usually develops from hematogenous seeding from another site of infection. Direct inoculation or local extension from adjacent soft tissue infection or osteomyelitis is less common. Prosthetic joints or damaged joints from rheumatoid or osteoarthritis are particularly susceptible to hematogenous seeding. Once an infection is established within a joint, a complex cascade of physiologic responses occurs that leads to a severe inflammatory reaction, with subsequent cartilage degradation and bone destruction. The rapidity and severity of this process depend on the virulence of the organism and the length of delay before appropriate antibiotics are started.

Clinical Features

Clinically, septic arthritis may be indistinguishable from crystalline arthritis or other inflammatory joint diseases. The presentation is often acute and monoarticular, with physical findings of warmth, swelling, tenderness, erythema within the confines of the joint margins, and markedly limited joint motion. The knee, hip, shoulder, elbow, and ankle are the most frequently involved joints. Atypical joints such as the sternoclavicular or sacroiliac joints, and the symphysis pubis are common sites of infection in younger patients, or those with a history of IV drug use. Polyarticular infections occur in 20% of cases [4], particularly among patients with RA. Fever is a variable finding and may be low grade.

High clinical suspicion remains essential to the diagnosis of septic arthritis. Unless physical examination indicates extra-articular features (e.g., cellulitis), any ICU patient with an acutely swollen, painful joint needs a diagnostic arthrocentesis to exclude infection. In the case of suspected cellulitis, appropriate antibiotics should be administered and arthrocentesis performed only if symptoms or findings do not improve within 48 hours. The diagnosis of septic arthritis is supported by an elevated white blood cell (WBC) count, ESR, and CRP, but these studies cannot reliably differentiate infection from other inflammatory processes. Conversely, the absence of fever or normal ESR or CRP cannot exclude septic arthritis. Synovial fluid analysis can confirm septic arthritis and identify organisms on Gram's stain or in culture. The fluid should be transferred immediately to the laboratory, both anaerobic and aerobic cultures should be ordered routinely, and special requests for fungus or other organisms that require a special growth medium (e.g., *Neisseria gonorrhoeae*) are ordered if clinically indicated. In addition, synovial fluid analysis for WBC with differential and microscopic examination for crystals may support a diagnosis of infection before microbiology results are available. Although leukocyte counts under 20,000 per μL have been associated with septic arthritis, the WBC generally exceeds 50,000 per μL and on occasion may be as high as 200,000 per μL, with a marked PMN predominance. A meta-analysis of various laboratory studies in septic arthritis suggests that the likelihood ratio of septic arthritis increases incrementally with higher synovial leukocyte counts [5]. However, because septic arthritis has been associated with WBC as low as 2,000 to 50,000 per μL, the absolute number cannot differentiate septic arthritis from other inflammatory states such as rheumatoid, psoriatic, or crystalline arthritis.

Although initial radiographs of the infected joint are often normal, baseline x-rays are useful to identify preexisting joint abnormalities and for comparison to identify subsequent damage. Magnetic resonance imaging (MRI) may be helpful to evaluate joints that are difficult to assess clinically (i.e., spine, sacroiliac, or hip) for underlying osteomyelitis and sinus tracts. Classic late radiographic findings include juxta-articular osteopenia, joint-space narrowing, or subchondral bone loss.

Therapy

Treatment of septic arthritis requires adequate drainage in addition to appropriate antibiotics. *N. gonorrhoeae* is the most common cause of septic arthritis in patients under the age of 30, but overall, *Staphylococcus aureus*, including methicillin-resistant *S. aureus* (MRSA), is the most common organism in the immunocompetent patient, followed in frequency by *Streptococcal* species. Gram-negative and anaerobic organisms occur less frequently, but must be suspected in patients at risk (elderly, immunocompromised, recent hospitalization or surgery, prior antibiotics, and possible urogenital or abdominal infections) [4]. For the critically ill patient with multiple risk factors, broad-spectrum antibiotic coverage against *Staphylococcus* and *Streptococcus*, Gram-negative bacteria, and *Pseudomonas* should be initiated until culture results are available. Fungal or mycobacterial septic arthritis is often subacute or chronic, but should be considered in patients failing broad-spectrum antibiotics. *Candida* organisms have caused acute arthritis and the Gram stain or fungal preparation may be positive before cultures are available. The duration of antibiotic therapy varies according to the clinical situation, but antibiotics should be continued intravenously for at least 2 weeks. Further route and duration of therapy depend on the specific type and sensitivity of the identified organism and the patient's clinical response. The length of treatment is usually at least 4 weeks for nongonococcal septic arthritis. Please refer to Chapter 73 for appropriate antibiotic treatment for presumptive or identified infectious organisms.

Drainage of the infected joint with either serial percutaneous needle aspiration or surgical intervention is also crucial. Because there are no prospective studies comparing these options, controversy exists regarding the optimal approach. The physical removal of inflammatory cells, cellular debris, lysosomal enzymes, and bacterial by-products reduces the potential damage to the joint. Prosthetic joints and other native joints such as hip, shoulder, wrist, finger, sacroiliac, or sternoclavicular joints require immediate surgical intervention, whereas native septic knees may respond to serial percutaneous needle aspiration. Arthroscopy or arthrotomy has the advantage of more complete debridement of fibrin, infected synovium, and loculations. However, percutaneous drainage may be the only option for a critically ill patient who is too unstable for surgery. Indications for surgical intervention include initial delay in diagnosis, established joint damage from RA or osteoarthritis, failure to sterilize the joint fluid after 3 to 5 days of antibiotics, difficult percutaneous aspirations because of loculations, or infection with Gram-negative bacterium. Thus, the ideal approach is to consult both an orthopedic surgeon and a rheumatologist at the time of diagnosis to decide on optimal management.

The infected joint should be immobilized in functional position in the first few days. Once antibiotics are given and drainage has been performed, early physical therapy with passive range of motion and graduation to active range of motion will improve outcomes.

Because septic arthritis usually occurs as a consequence of bacteremia from a distant primary source of infection, investigation for these sites must be pursued. Unless an obvious site of local inoculation is present, cultures from blood, urine, sputum, indwelling lines, and catheters should be obtained before the institution of antibiotics. In addition, imaging studies such as echocardiography, computed tomography (CT), or gallium scanning may locate the source of occult infection.

Septic Arthritis of the Prosthetic Joint

Although rates of prosthetic joint infections (PJIs) are generally quite low, 0.8% to 1.9% and 0.3% to 1.7% for knees and hips, respectively [6], RA patients have an increased risk of developing infected prosthetic joints. Risk factors are similar for native joint septic arthritis discussed previously and also include prior infection of a prosthetic joint at the same site or revision arthroplasty. Early infection, usually within 3 months of surgery, is usually due to *S. aureus* or more virulent organisms from direct inoculation at the time of surgery; chronic infections with less aggressive bacterium including coagulase-negative *Staphylococci* occur often months to years after the replacement. Bacteremia with seeding of a prosthetic joint can occur anytime. Causative organisms for PJI are predominantly Gram-positive cocci (65%); aerobic Gram-negative bacilli and anaerobes contribute 10%, whereas 20% are polymicrobial infections [6].

Clinical features of acute PJI include localized pain, fever (occurring in <50%), and elevation of ESR, whereas more chronic infections may present with only pain and loosening of hardware on radiograph. CRP elevation of more than 5 mg per L has a sensitivity of 95% and specificity of 62% in the diagnosis of PJI [7]. Plain radiographs cannot distinguish aseptic periprosthetic loosening from infection. CT and magnetic imaging may be distorted by ferromagnetic prostheses. Synovial fluid studies are as useful for the diagnosis of PJI as they are for native joint infections. A synovial fluid WBC more than 1,700 cells per μL from the prosthetic knee joint or more than 4,200 cells per μL from the prosthetic hip joint with predominantly PMNs is enough to suggest infection [6]. If aspiration is not done before surgery, then intraoperative sampling of multiple periprosthetic tissue sites will increase the yield of an organism. Culture of the removed prosthesis may also provide additional microbial information.

Treatment of suspected PJI should initially cover both Gram-negative and Gram-positive organisms with a regimen such as vancomycin and an aminoglycoside until microbiology results and antibiotic sensitivities are available (see Chapter 73). Infectious disease consultation will help guide therapy.

Antibiotic therapy alone without surgical intervention is rarely successful. If the patient is a surgical candidate, options include: (1) resection arthroplasty, (2) one- or two-stage surgery with prosthesis removal and reimplantation, or (3) surgical debridement with retention of prosthesis with or without long-term oral antibiotic suppression. The first option is rarely performed unless the patient has failed previous surgical attempts at eradicating the infection or is likely to have minimal functional improvement after replacement. Chronic PJI requires resection arthroplasty with one- or two-stage exchanges. The latter usually entails removal of the infected prosthesis, treatment with antibiotics with or without an antibiotic-loaded spacer for a period of 6 to 12 weeks, and then subsequent reimplantation. Debridement with retention of the infected prosthesis is an option only if (i) age of the prosthesis is less than 3 months; (ii) symptoms have been present for less than 3 weeks; (iii) absence of sinus tract communicating with joint space; (iv) no radiographic evidence of prosthetic loosening; (v) infection not involving *S. aureus*, *Pseudomonas aeruginosa*, enterococcus, fungal- or multidrug-resistant organisms; and (vi) absence of comorbidities such as diabetes and RA [8]. Prolonged oral antibiotics (3 months for hips and 6 months for knees) are recommended in patients treated with debridement with implant retention [6].

Hemarthrosis

In the absence of an underlying inherited disorder of coagulation, hemarthrosis in the intensive care setting is most likely a complication of anticoagulation therapy, most frequently described in patients receiving an oral anticoagulant. Because hemarthrosis may occur spontaneously in an anticoagulated patient, a history of trauma is often absent. Clinically, a patient develops a monoarticular, painful, swollen, warm, and tense effusion. Prolongation of coagulation parameters suggests the diagnosis, but diagnostic arthrocentesis is essential to confirm the diagnosis of hemarthrosis and exclude septic arthritis, crystalline disease, or other causes. When performed aseptically and carefully, arthrocentesis is safe and free of significant long-term morbidity. It is unnecessary to reverse the anticoagulant state prior to arthrocentesis.

A precise definition of hemarthrosis has not been established, but the diagnosis is suggested by a synovial fluid hematocrit exceeding 3%. Causes of hemarthrosis other than anticoagulation include trauma (especially with intra-articular fracture), blood dyscrasias, Charcot joint, synovial tumors such as pigmented villonodular synovitis, or other primary or metastatic neoplasms, myeloproliferative disease, CPPD arthropathy, septic arthritis, sickle cell trait or disease, or scurvy.

Despite the fact that hemophiliac patients with repeated hemarthrosis have significant joint abnormalities, an isolated episode of spontaneous hemarthrosis has a benign prognosis. Treatment of hemarthrosis from hemophilia or other bleeding diathesis is discussed elsewhere (see Chapters 88 and 89). Management of spontaneous hemarthrosis from anticoagulation consists of immobilization, analgesia, and, if possible, temporarily reducing or correcting clotting parameters with fresh frozen plasma or reversal agents when the patient is not at high risk of thrombotic complications. If the patient is at high risk (i.e., prosthetic valve), allowing the international normalized ratio (INR) to drift toward the lower therapeutic range is one option. Arthrocentesis may reduce the pressure of joint distension.

ASPECTS OF RHEUMATIC DISEASES COMPLICATING INTENSIVE CARE PROCEDURES

Difficult endotracheal intubations may be encountered among patients with RA, juvenile idiopathic arthritis (JIA), ankylosing spondylitis (AS), or systemic sclerosis (SSc). Involvement of the cervical spine, temporomandibular or cricoarytenoid joints, or oral aperture may limit adequate positioning, visualization, or successful endotracheal intubation with conventional direct laryngoscopy. Advanced airway techniques including fiberoptic intubation, video laryngoscopy, and nasotracheal intubation enable safe airway placement for most patients with difficult airways (see Chapter 8). Laryngeal mask airway is a possible rescue measure for patients who cannot be intubated but can be ventilated and is a good alternative to bag mask ventilation. A surgical airway, cricothyroidotomy or tracheostomy, is required in emergent situations when safe intubation is not possible and the patient cannot be adequately ventilated (see Chapters 8 and 9).

The prevalence of atlantoaxial instability among RA patients is estimated to be 23% to 60% depending on the subpopulation studied and is associated with longer duration and greater severity of disease. This instability also occurs among certain subgroups including patients with JIA and AS. Although the majority of patients with cervical spine involvement are asymptomatic, forced manipulation of the neck (e.g., during intubation, endotracheal suctioning, nasogastric tube placement, bronchoscopy, or endoscopy) may precipitate symptoms and signs of spinal cord compression.

Cervical instability and dislocations most commonly occur at the atlantoaxial (first and second cervical vertebrae) junction because of laxity or erosion of the transverse ligament caused by synovitis. Subsequently, the odontoid (superior peg of the axis) moves more freely and can protrude posteriorly, particularly during neck flexion, and compress the spinal cord, lower medulla, or vertebrobasilar arteries. Fracture or erosive destruction of the odontoid may allow the atlas to slide posteriorly on the axis, a process termed posterior atlantoaxial subluxation. Destruction of the lateral atlantoaxial joints and of the bones of the foramen magnum may allow the axis to sublux cephalad, so-called vertical subluxation. Symptoms suggestive of cervical myelopathy include Lhermitte's sign, neck pain radiating up to the occiput, paresthesias in the hands or feet, loss of arm or leg strength, and urinary incontinence or retention.

Atlantoaxial instability is identified with lateral cervical spine radiographs in flexed and extended views. The normal distance between the odontoid process and the Arch of the Atlantis is less than 4 mm. If this distance is exceeded, care should be taken to avoid sudden or forced neck flexion during any intensive care procedure. A soft cervical collar to maintain the neck in slight extension helps prevent sudden forced flexion and is a reminder to all caregivers that any neck manipulation should proceed with caution. Open-mouth posterior-to-anterior views will exclude odontoid fracture and severe subluxation, but MRI scanning is the best imaging procedure to exclude cord compression.

Among patients with AS with multilevel cervical fusion, large anterior cervical osteophytes can prevent adequate visualization of the larynx or successful endotracheal intubation using standard techniques. Fixed cervical flexion deformities can hinder appropriate neck positioning for intubation. The ankylosed spine is often osteoporotic and brittle. Minor forces in flexing or extending the neck can result in inadvertent fracture. Thus, plain radiographic imaging with lateral views before any procedure can help establish potential barriers to endotracheal intubation and the need for advanced intubation techniques.

Patients with JIA (and less commonly RA) may have micrognathia because of temporomandibular joint disease that restricts lower jaw motion and limits access to the oropharynx. Micrognathia may also cause upper respiratory tract obstruction and sleep apnea, both of which occur more commonly in patients with JIA. In contrast, patients with SSc may have facial tissue fibrosis and atrophy that reduce the oral aperture and make orotracheal intubation difficult or impossible. In these situations, early awareness of the need for nasotracheal intubation or other advanced airway techniques will prevent potential complications in routine or emergency endotracheal intubation.

Nearly 50% to 75% of patients with long-standing RA have involvement of the cricoarytenoid joints on CT scans, but only half have symptoms. These synovial joints allow adduction and abduction of the vocal cords. Symptoms of cricoarytenoid involvement include throat pain, sensation of a foreign object in the throat, odynophagia, dysphagia, hoarseness, shortness of breath, and stridor. As a result of acute or chronic inflammation, the vocal cords may become fixed in adduction, resulting in upper airway obstruction and respiratory failure. The diagnosis may be distinguished from recurrent laryngeal nerve paralysis, tumor, and thyroiditis by visualizing the vocal cords by either direct laryngoscopy or fiberoptic nasopharyngoscopy. For the patient with chronically restricted motion of the cricoarytenoid joints, a superimposed insult, like an upper respiratory tract infection or trauma from intubation, may cause laryngospasm or soft tissue swelling with resultant airway obstruction. Treatment of life-threatening airway obstruction includes establishing an airway by cricothyroidotomy or tracheostomy, administration of high-dose systemic corticosteroids, systemic antirheumatic therapy, or topical aerosolized corticosteroids.

RHEUMATOID ARTHRITIS

RA is a chronic, autoimmune, inflammatory disorder that affects synovial joints and extra-articular organ systems. In the patients with established RA, reasons for admission to the ICU may include airway obstruction because of cricoarytenoid arthritis or atlantoaxial subluxation (discussed previously); septic arthritis; respiratory distress from large pleural effusions or parenchymal lung disease; mononeuritis, or cardiac dysfunction because of pericardial, myocardial, or endocardial involvement; necrotizing vasculitis. The approach to the RA patient in the ICU includes knowledge of the diverse complications of rheumatoid disease and the potential toxicities of RA medications including NSAIDs, corticosteroids, nonbiologic disease-modifying agents, and the newer biologic agents. In addition, RA may be among the differential diagnoses for an acutely ill ICU patient with various organ system involvement, and thus consultation with a rheumatologist is most helpful.

Pathogenesis

RA is characterized by chronic synovial inflammation with subsequent articular cartilage and bone destruction in a genetically susceptible host. The initial triggering antigen, whether exogenous or self, has not been identified, but the initial activation of innate immunity and the subsequent stimulation of T cells initiate the process of recruitment of other cells to the synovium, including macrophages, neutrophils, and B cells. Fibroblast-like and macrophage-like synovial cells perpetuate synovial inflammation through elaboration of cytokines that have paracrine and autocrine activities. In addition to cytokines, the products of several cell types also induce adhesion molecules and stimulate angiogenesis. Activated synovial cells also release metalloproteinases and other enzymes responsible for degradation of articular cartilage and erosion of bone. The disease is characterized by the presence of rheumatoid factor (RF) and anti-citrullinated protein antibodies (ACPA). This latter antibody is more specific for RA and higher titers are associated with more severe disease and some extra-articular organ involvement.

Joint Infections Complicating Rheumatoid Arthritis

One indication for admission of the RA patient to an ICU is sepsis, particularly involving joints. RA patients are more susceptible to developing septic arthritis, often polyarticular and more severe than in patients without RA. A variety of factors, including immunosuppressive drugs, general debility, immobility, and cutaneous ulcers predispose the RA patient to developing bacterial infections in other sites, which hematogenously seed inflamed rheumatoid joints. Normal protective mechanisms, PMN leukocyte bacterial killing, PMN chemotaxis, and complement and serum bactericidal activity of the rheumatoid joint are all decreased. Although joint sepsis after arthrocentesis or intra-articular steroid injection is a rare complication, infection has been reported in this context and may be more resistant to treatment.

A delay in diagnosing joint sepsis for RA patients may also contribute to their increased morbidity and mortality. Other factors include: (1) masking of joint pain and inflammation by NSAIDs, corticosteroids, and immunosuppressive agents; (2) generalized debility and malnutrition; and (3) attributing the joint inflammation to RA rather than infection by the patient or physician. Failure to recognize septic arthritis complicating RA may have disastrous effects. When a single or few joints are more inflamed more than others in a rheumatoid patient, joint sepsis should be excluded by arthrocentesis, Gram's stain, and cultures of synovial fluid, blood, and other appropriate sites guided by the patient's signs and symptoms. Inspection of the skin for a possible portal of bacterial entry and a thorough general examination are of utmost importance.

The microbiology of septic arthritis complicating RA includes a wide range of organisms, but in approximately 80% of cases, the organism is *S. aureus*, with an increasing proportion of MRSA infections. Streptococcal species are also common pathogens. Gram-negative organisms (*P. aeruginosa*, *Escherichia coli*, *Proteus mirabilis*, and others), anaerobes, fungi, mycobacterium, and polymicrobial infection have all been reported as causes of septic arthritis of the rheumatoid joint.

Management of septic arthritis for a rheumatoid patient is identical to that of patients without RA. However, the septic rheumatoid joint more frequently fails percutaneous needle aspiration. Early surgical drainage with synovectomy may be the preferred treatment because there is more proliferative synovitis and an increased tendency for loculations to develop.

Pulmonary Involvement in Rheumatoid Arthritis

The respiratory system of the patient with RA can be involved in numerous ways, including upper airway, bronchi, pleura, parenchyma, vasculature, and diaphragmatic muscles. Pulmonary infections are common, particularly among patients with poor mucociliary clearance, with ineffective cough, on immunosuppressive therapy, or with associated Sjögren syndrome. Table 66.1

TABLE 66.1

Respiratory Involvement in Connective Tissue Diseases

	Common	Rare (<10%)
Upper airway involvement		
Cricoarytenoid arthritis	RA	SLE
Laryngeal nodules	RA	
Bronchial tree		
Obliterative bronchiolitis		RA
Bronchiectasis	SSc	RA, SS, SLE
Follicular or constrictive bronchiolitis		RA, SS
Parenchyma		
Interstitial lung disease	RA, SSc, PM/DM	SLE, SS
Acute pneumonitis		SLE, PM/DM
Cryptogenic organizing pneumonia		RA, SLE, PM/DM, SSc
Rheumatoid nodules ± cavitation	RA	
Aspiration	SSc, PM/DM	RA
Drugs: methotrexate, sulfasalazine, minocycline		All
Infections	All	
Pleura		
Pleuritis	RA, SLE	
Pleural effusions	RA, SLE	
Pleural thickening	RA	SLE
Respiratory muscle disease		
Myositis	PM/DM	RA
Diaphragm dysfunction	PM/DM	SLE
Vascular		
Pulmonary hypertension	SSc	SLE, RA, PM/DM, APS
Vasculitis	SLE	PM/DM, RA
Diffuse alveolar hemorrhage		SLE, RA, PM/DM, APS
Pulmonary embolism	APS, SLE	

RA, rheumatoid arthritis; SLE, systemic lupus erythematosus; SSc, systemic sclerosis; SS, Sjögren syndrome; PM/DM, polymyositis/dermatomyositis; APS, antiphospholipid syndrome.

summarizes respiratory tract involvement in RA and other connective tissue disorders. In addition, certain antirheumatic drugs are associated with pulmonary toxicities. Angioedema and bronchospasm induced or aggravated by aspirin or other NSAIDs are most common, followed by hypersensitivity pneumonitis from methotrexate, sulfasalazine, the newer biologics, or interstitial fibrosis from methotrexate.

Pleural Disease

Pleuritis and interstitial disease are the most common pulmonary manifestations of RA, and the former is most common in a subset of male patients who are seropositive and have nodules. Although involvement may be asymptomatic, acute febrile pleurisy or large pleural effusions impairing respiratory function may occur and result in ICU admission. The differential diagnoses of the pleural effusions include malignancy, pulmonary infarction, viral or bacterial infection, tuberculosis, and empyema. Infectious empyema occurs with increased frequency in patients with preexisting rheumatoid pleural effusions and should be suspected in debilitated, anemic, or hypoproteinemic patients who have been treated with corticosteroids and have persistent fever and pleural effusions. In patients on anti–tumor necrosis factor α (anti-TNFα) therapies, reactivation of (or new infection with) tuberculosis is a major concern and needs to be excluded with pleural biopsy.

Pleural effusions and sterile empyemas associated with RA are exudative and have characteristic features: elevated lactic dehydrogenase (often >700 International Units per L), total protein (>4 g per dL), low glucose (<40 mg per dL), and pH <7.2. Other characteristics include clear yellow to green-yellow appearance, WBC count of 100 to 7,000 cells per μL (predominantly lymphocytes), reduced complement levels, cholesterol crystals, and immune complexes [9]. Chylous effusions may occur if necrotic subpleural nodules rupture into the pleural space.

Once infections including tuberculosis and malignancy are excluded, symptomatic pleural effusions are managed with NSAIDs and thoracentesis. In recurrent pleuritis or sterile empyema, intrapleural corticosteroids, systemic corticosteroids in moderate doses, and additional disease-modifying agents are recommended. Rarely, surgical pleurodesis or decortication is required if chronic adhesive fibrothorax develops. There are no prospective trials to evaluate the efficacy of many of these recommendations [9]. High-dose corticosteroid therapy may not be effective and carries an increased risk of empyema formation.

Lung Disease

RA-associated interstitial lung disease (RA-ILD) occurs among 40% to 60% of patients depending on the subpopulations studied and screening tests used to make the diagnosis. In a review of rheumatoid lung–associated mortality using the US National Center for Health Statistics, clinically significant RA-ILD was 10%; the incidence of mortality was 28.3% for women and 12.5% for men from 1988 to 2004 [10]. In a large UK study, review of RA patients with ILD was estimated to be around 5% to 6%. Males and females were nearly equally affected. Risk factors for poor prognosis included high-titer RF and ACPA, smoking in males, and extent of lung involvement on high-resolution CT (HRCT) scans [11]. Thus, after infection, pulmonary disease is the second most common cause of mortality among RA patients. Pathologically, usual interstitial pneumonia (UIP) is more common (up to 60%), followed by nonspecific interstitial pneumonitis (NSIP). Cryptogenic organizing pneumonia (OP) and acute interstitial pneumonia are less common, whereas lymphocytic interstitial pneumonitis (LIP) and desquamative interstitial pneumonia are rare in RA.

Symptoms include dyspnea on exertion, cough, and chest discomfort. Physical and laboratory findings include dry crackles, diminished diffusion capacity, and restrictive physiology, as well as desaturation with exercise. Chest radiographs may show an interstitial pattern, but HRCT is the most sensitive test in diagnosing UIP and NSIP, with up to 70% correlation with histopathologic findings. Fibrotic changes with honeycombing and traction bronchiectasis are more suggestive of UIP, whereas alveolar infiltrates and ground glass changes are more suggestive of NSIP, acute hemorrhage, or interstitial pneumonia. Bronchoalveolar lavage (BAL) is not particularly helpful except to rule out infection, hemorrhage, or malignancy, whereas thoracoscopy-guided lung biopsy provides the best pathologic material for diagnosis and may be needed when the diagnosis is unclear despite the above evaluations. Treatment of RA-ILD is extremely challenging because there are no randomized trials, and often therapies are extrapolated from idiopathic ILD or treatment for lung disease associated with connective tissue disease. Some patients may respond to corticosteroids alone, but the progressive nature of the disease may require treatment with cytotoxic agents, although it is unclear which immunosuppressants are most effective [12]. In those patients with ground glass opacities on HRCT scanning, IV cyclophosphamide (IVCY) or mycophenolate mofetil (MMF) is frequently used, although no large controlled trial exists to support this approach. Case reports on the use of anti-TNF α medications are conflicting because there are case reports of these drugs being associated with exacerbation of RA-ILD.

Other less common manifestations of rheumatoid lung disease may require treatment in the ICU when patients develop respiratory distress. These include OP, obliterative bronchiolitis (OB), pulmonary vasculitis, spontaneous pneumothorax, and lung toxicities secondary to antirheumatic therapy. It is particularly important to distinguish OP from ILD and OB, and only lung biopsy will provide histologic distinction.

Obliterative alveolitis is often characterized by the abrupt onset of dyspnea and a dry cough with inspiratory crackles, sometimes with a mid-inspiratory squeak, a clear chest radiograph or finding of hyperinflation, irreversible airflow obstruction at low volumes on pulmonary function testing, mild-to-moderate arterial hypoxemia with a respiratory alkalosis, and progressive obliteration of small airways (1 to 6 mm in diameter) with constrictive bronchiolitis [13]. The prognosis is generally poor with a fairly rapid rate of progressive airflow obstruction. Despite the lack of adequate therapeutic trials, when patients present with rapidly progressive deterioration, recommendations based on expert opinion include bronchodilators, inhaled and oral corticosteroids (1 to 1.5 mg/kg/d). Macrolides, pulse IVCY, or etanercept (with methotrexate) may be considered as second-line therapies [13]. Progression to respiratory failure is common.

In contrast, patients with OP present with more systemic symptoms of fevers, malaise, weight loss, and dyspnea but are more responsive to corticosteroid therapy. Rarely, chronic vasculitis may involve pulmonary as well as bronchial arterioles and result in pulmonary hypertension and cor pulmonale. Therapy consists of corticosteroids in combination with cytotoxic agents (see Chapters 67 and 68).

Although pulmonary manifestations of RA are frequent, they are rarely the primary reason for admission to the ICU. Infectious pneumonia is particularly frequent and the major cause of mortality in rheumatoid patients. Since the development and widespread use of anti-TNFα medications, atypical infections and reactivation of tuberculosis have been of great concern. Drug-induced pneumonitis must also be excluded because many of the drugs for treatment of RA have pulmonary toxicities including methotrexate, leflunomide, sulfasalazine, and, less commonly, anti-TNFα, tocilizumab, and rituximab (RTX).

Rheumatoid Cardiac Involvement

RA may involve all structures of the heart as a result of granulomatous proliferation or vasculitis. Pericarditis, myocarditis, endocarditis (valvulitis), coronary arteritis, aortitis, and cardiac conduction abnormalities have all been reported. Cardiac involvement may be the principal reason for intensive care hospitalization, or may complicate the course of the rheumatoid patient hospitalized in the ICU for other medical or surgical problems.

Pericarditis, the most common of the rheumatoid cardiac manifestations (up to 30% by echocardiography but as high as 50% by autopsy studies), rarely causes clinical symptoms. However, constrictive pericarditis or a large pericardial effusion may result in cardiac tamponade. The pericardial fluid has the same characteristics as pleural fluid (see the section "Pulmonary Involvement in Rheumatoid Arthritis"). Pericarditis generally responds to the administration of moderate- to high-dose steroids (0.5 to 1 mg per kg), depending on severity of cardiac impairment. Corticosteroids alone are less likely to be effective in the setting of cardiac tamponade. Pericardiocentesis should be performed early when tamponade is suspected (see Chapter 17) or if there is a question of septic or suppurative pericarditis. Aspiration of pericardial fluid may temporarily improve cardiac function, but often the viscosity of the fluid, loculations, and thickness of the pericardium may necessitate pericardiectomy. In cases of symptomatic constrictive pericarditis, pericardiectomy is the only effective therapy.

The myocardium may be affected by granulomatous inflammation that results in heart failure or conduction system abnormalities. Although myocarditis is clinically rare, newer cardiac MRI with enhancement techniques suggests that myocardial fibrosis and inflammation exist in many asymptomatic RA patients. Arteritis may affect the coronary arteries or the aorta. For patients with active systemic vasculitis, coronary arteritis may be the cause of myocardial infarctions. Involvement of the aorta, either by rheumatoid granulomas or inflammation of the aortic vasa vasorum, may result in dilatation of the aortic root and aortic valvular insufficiency.

RA patients die prematurely from cardiovascular events that include (i) ischemic heart disease, often silent; (ii) congestive failure, often in the setting of preserved ejection fraction; and (iii) sudden death. When compared to non-RA patients, these increased cardiovascular complications and mortality (more than twice that of non-RA populations) are not explained by traditional risk factors alone. Other factors, including chronic inflammation, accelerated atherosclerosis, various drugs used for treatment of RA that affect thrombotic or lipid profiles, and rarely coronary vasculitis, contribute to premature cardiac deaths. Thus, in the ICU setting, silent cardiovascular disease with atypical presentations must be considered for rheumatoid patients.

Rheumatoid Vasculitis

Rheumatoid vasculitis (RV) is a panarteritis involving typically medium size to small arterioles and postcapillary venules with mononuclear cell infiltrates in all layers of the involved blood vessels, fibrinoid necrosis in active lesions, and thrombosis associated with intimal proliferation. Early and more aggressive treatment for RA has improved disease outcome and thus also contributed to decreased prevalence of RV. A retrospective review of RV in a single large center characterized RV patients as having more severe, erosive RA of longer duration that was inactive [14]. Other risk factors included presence of subcutaneous nodules, high-titer RF, active smoking at the time of diagnosis, coexisting cardiovascular disease, and the use of biologic modifiers. The clinical features of RV are variable and include palpable purpura, cutaneous ulcerations, distal arteritis ranging from fingernail-fold infarcts and splinter hemorrhages to digital gangrene, and vasculitic neuropathies. Arteritis of other major organs including the gastrointestinal tract, kidneys, heart, and lungs is clinically similar to polyarteritis nodosa. Patients with RV often present with constitutional symptoms of malaise, weight loss, fevers, and have elevated inflammatory markers, anemia, leukocytosis, hypocomplementia, and elevated RF and/or ACPA. Mortality remains high for RV, and necrotizing forms of RV are associated with a poor prognosis and are treated aggressively with high-dose corticosteroids and cytotoxic agents such as cyclophosphamide similar to treatment for polyarteritis nodosa (see Chapters 67 and 68).

Neurologic Complications of Rheumatoid Arthritis

All components of the nervous system can be affected by RA. The brain and meninges, spinal cord, peripheral nerves, and muscles may be involved with granulomatous inflammation in the form of rheumatoid nodules or vasculitis; the spinal cord and cranial and peripheral nerves may also be compressed by skeletal and soft tissue structures, and the nervous system may be affected by hyperviscosity syndrome and medications.

Spinal cord compression is one of the most common neurologic complications among patients with RA, as discussed in the previous section. Manifestations that require immediate intervention include the sensation of anterior instability of the head during neck flexion, drop attacks, loss of urinary bladder and anal sphincter control, dysphagia, vertigo, hemiplegia, dysarthria, nystagmus, changes in level of consciousness, and peripheral paresthesias without evidence of a peripheral cause. Although RA patients may have radiographic evidence of cervical subluxation without symptoms, once signs of cord compression become apparent, myelopathy may progress rapidly. For patients with manifestations of spinal cord and brain stem compression, surgical stabilization is indicated. For the nonsurgical candidate, a firm collar can be used in an effort to immobilize the neck and prevent further subluxation.

SYSTEMIC LUPUS ERYTHEMATOSUS

Systemic lupus erythematosus (SLE) is an autoimmune disease whose pathogenesis is likely multifactorial, involving genetic predisposition, hormonal factors, environmental triggers, and immune dysregulation. The resultant excessive autoantibody production and immune complex deposition in multiple organ systems manifest in tremendous clinical variations and range from arthralgias, rash, and fatigue to life-threatening renal, central nervous system (CNS), cardiac, pulmonary, or hematologic manifestations. Diagnosis of SLE is based on the clinical criteria set forth by the American College of Rheumatology [15]. Mortality of SLE patients admitted to the ICU is much higher than the general ICU population and is associated with high APACHE scores, older age, multisystem dysfunction, and cytopenias [16]. Among ICU patients with established SLE, it is essential to differentiate problems caused directly by SLE activity from those with secondary causes such as infections, drug-induced lupus (DIL), NSAID-induced renal dysfunction, aseptic meningitis, and corticosteroid-induced psychosis. Diseases associated with SLE include avascular necrosis, hypertensive encephalopathy, pseudotumor cerebri, amyloidosis, myasthenia gravis, and thrombotic thrombocytopenic purpura (TTP). Among ICU patients without a prior history of autoimmune disease, SLE should be considered in the differential diagnosis of patients presenting with acute renal failure, seizures, myocarditis, acute pulmonary deterioration, hemolytic anemia, or thrombocytopenia.

Renal Disease

Renal involvement is the major cause of disease-related mortality in SLE patients. The frequency of renal involvement ranges from 38% to nearly 80% depending on definition, but clinical lupus nephritis (LN) occurs in approximately 50% of the patients. Advances in diagnostic and therapeutic modalities have dramatically improved the survival of lupus patients with renal disease, but 10% to 20% of patients will develop end-stage renal disease. LN constitutes approximately 3% of all end-stage renal failure among patients on dialysis or requiring renal transplantation. Weighted mean of number of renal transplants per study detailed patient survival at 1, 3, 5 years to be 93.3%, 70.1% and 53.3%, respectively, whereas graft survival at 1, 3, 5 years was 85.1%, 60.3%, and 43.9%, respectively [17]. Recurrence of LN has been reported to be around 2.4% in surveillance studies, and risk factors include African American race, young age, and female gender [18].

Classification of LN is based on histopathologic, immunofluorescent, and electron microscopic changes according to the 2003 revised classification by the International Society of Nephrology and the Renal Pathology Society (ISN/RPS) [19]. The classification includes the following: Class I: minimal mesangial LN; Class II: mesangial proliferative LN; Class III: focal proliferative LN; Class IV: diffuse proliferative LN with two subclasses, segmental and global; Class V: membranous LN; and Class VI: advanced sclerosing LN. Classes III and IV are divided into active or chronic, whereas Class IV is further subdivided into segmental or global. Renal lesions are commonly pleomorphic, vary from one glomerulus to another, and temporally transition from one class to another over time. The tubulointerstitium and vasculature are often involved. Semiquantitative scoring to define activity and chronicity may provide information on prognosis and guidelines for therapeutic options. In particular, the presence of proliferative lesions and chronic lesions is associated with greater mortality.

Other SLE renal manifestations aside from immune-mediated glomerular disease include tubulointerstitial disease (usually occurring concurrently with LN but may exist in isolation), vascular disease (vasculitis, thrombotic microangiopathy related to lupus anticoagulant [LA] or antiphospholipid antibodies [aPL], atherosclerotic disease, or thromboembolism). Diagnosis of these processes may require histopathology because treatment may differ from immune complex–mediated LN.

The clinical manifestations of renal involvement vary from rapidly progressive renal failure with attendant fluid overload, to congestive heart failure or accelerated hypertension, and are common events precipitating an ICU admission. A sudden deterioration in an SLE patient's renal function warrants careful consideration of other causes of acute renal insufficiency (see Chapter 200) before attributing the deterioration to active SLE. In particular, hypovolemia, drug-induced interstitial nephritis or renal insufficiency, renal vein thrombosis, and contrast-induced acute tubular necrosis must be excluded. Physical examination may reveal evidence of SLE activity in other organ systems. Laboratory studies should include routine tests to assess renal status and fluid balance, and immunologic studies, including double-stranded DNA (dsDNA) antibody, total hemolytic complement, third (C3) and fourth (C4) complement components and ESR. Active serologies suggest SLE flare, but normal values do not exclude active disease. Renal biopsy is often necessary for diagnosis and informs therapeutic decisions.

Management of LN depends on the patient's renal histopathologic and functional parameters. Thus, a patient with Class I or II LN with normal creatinine clearance requires no specific therapy, whereas a patient with increasing azotemia, active urinary sediment, and impaired clearance requires aggressive therapy. For patients with severe glomerulonephritis (ISN/RPS Class III or IV), induction therapy includes the combination of high-dose corticosteroids with IVCY or oral MMF for 6 months followed by maintenance therapy, which stabilizes renal function and improves survival. The equivalency of MMF up to 3 g per day compared to monthly IVCY as induction therapy for Class III, IV, or V LN has been established by several trials including a large international trial conducted by the ALMS group (Aspreva Lupus Management Study), which confirmed this equivalence of both induction regimens at the end of 24 weeks with a response rate of 56% in each group [20]. However, only 8% from either treatment group reached complete remission. In addition, patients of Hispanic and African descent had a much better response to MMF than IVCY (60% vs. 38%), whereas whites and Asian patients responded equally to either regimen. The risk for gonadal failure was less with MMF, but other toxicities such as infections were similar. Another option for IVCY induction is the low-dose regimen from the Euro-Lupus Nephritis Trial, which demonstrated equal efficacy and less gonadal toxicity between low-dose IVCY (500 mg every 2 weeks for six doses) and high-dose IVCY (500 to 750 mg per m^2 with maximum of 1,500 mg, monthly for 6 months, followed by every 3-month infusion until 1 year) [21]. Both groups then received azathioprine (AZA) at 2 mg/kg/d for maintenance. The long-term outcomes measured by death, end-stage renal disease, and doubling of serum creatinine were similar in both groups after 10 years [22]. This regimen also had less gonadal toxicities.

Although not a pressing decision in SLE patient with acute nephritis, current recommendations for maintenance therapy once induction is completed include either AZA or MMF. A large randomized, double-blind, double-dummy trial for 36 months demonstrated superiority of MMF to AZA in preventing renal relapse and maintaining response [23].

In an acutely ill ICU patient with LN and/or other organ system involvement, IVCY along with pulse IV methylprednisolone at 1,000 mg daily for 3 days may be the regimen of choice because many of the studies have not stratified for disease severity. Patients may not be able to take oral MMF. The protocol for administration of monthly IVCY therapy is outlined in Table 66.7. Dose adjustments for renal insufficiency are outlined and subsequent monthly dosing is based on nadir WBC counts. Alternative regimen would be the low-dose Euro-Lupus regimen [21].

Membranous GN (Class V), which constitutes 20% of LN, is less aggressive than Class IV GN. Although renal survival rate is at 80% at 10 years, it is still associated with significant comorbidities of hyperlipidemia, and cardiovascular and thromboembolic diseases. Angiotensin-converting enzyme (ACE) inhibitors have been used successfully to reduce proteinuria. Treatment with corticosteroids, AZA, and cyclosporine has been studied in small series. More recently, the pooled subset of Class V patients from two prospective randomized studies on treatment of GN demonstrated equivalent efficacy and safety profile of MMF and IVCY [24]. Adjunctive renoprotective therapies that include aspirin, statins, ACE inhibitors, or angiotensin receptor blockers should also be instituted.

Advances of biologic therapies for RA and psoriatic arthritis have also stimulated investigations for SLE. Initial open label studies and case reports suggest promising results with the use of RTX, an anti-CD20 B-cell-depleting monoclonal antibody, for reducing SLE activity. Surprisingly, a randomized trial comparing RTX to placebo with a background of MMF for active proliferative LN revealed no additional benefit, and another study on active nonrenal SLE was also negative [25]. Belimumab, a human immunoglobulin G (IgG)1 λ monoclonal antibody against activity of soluble B-lymphocyte stimulator, whose levels are associated with lupus disease activity, has been approved for use in SLE. Randomized trials have demonstrated decreased lupus activity when compared to placebo among patients receiving standard care. In a post hoc pooled analysis of the trials with belimumab, there appeared to be additional renal benefit for patients receiving MMF and belimumab compared to those receiving placebo [26].

Neuropsychiatric Disease

Neuropsychiatric systemic lupus erythematosus (NPSLE), which encompasses involvement of the central, peripheral, and autonomic nervous systems along with psychiatric syndromes, occurs in 25% to 80% of SLE patients depending on the criteria applied or methods used for diagnosis. Although NPSLE was considered a poor prognostic indicator in the older literature, it does not seem to have significant impact on survival rates. Active CNS disease contributed primarily or secondarily to death in only a small percentage of patients.

Neuropsychiatric manifestations of SLE can be classified into central versus peripheral nervous system involvement. Due to the limitations of the ACR classification criteria of CNS involvement, an ad hoc neuropsychiatric lupus nomenclature committee of the American College of Rheumatology defined 19 manifestations that included 12 in the CNS and 7 in the peripheral nervous system [27] (Table 66.2). The wide range of prevalence for the more diffuse CNS syndromes (cognitive dysfunction, anxiety, acute confusional states, and psychoses) and headache is due to the variable definition, criteria, or diagnostic parameters used among reported studies. This proposed nomenclature attempts to define the spectrum of NPSLE, but is not a substitute for clinical diagnosis. An individual SLE patient may have multiple neuropsychiatric manifestations, and these can develop prior to the formal diagnosis of SLE or during an inactive disease state. Frank psychosis is relatively rare, estimated at 5%. Often, it is difficult to separate active lupus psychosis from other causes such as functional disorders, uremia, illicit drug use, metabolic disturbances, medications, or infections.

Focal CNS disease, including seizures that occur in 15% to 35% of SLE patients, can antedate the diagnosis of SLE or develop any time during the disease course. Grand mal seizures are the most common, but essentially all types have been reported. Secondary causes of seizures must be sought because several prospective studies of SLE patients with neurologic events reported that a majority of seizures were due to associated infections, uremia, hypertension, and metabolic abnormalities.

Cerebrovascular accidents (5% to 18%) include infarctions secondary to intracranial hemorrhage or arteritis, thrombosis from LA or aPL-associated hypercoagulable states (see "Antiphospholipid Syndrome" section), or embolism from Libman–Sacks endocarditis. Movement disorders including chorea, ataxia, and hemiballismus are rare (<1%) [28]. Transverse myelitis is an unusual but devastating complication of SLE characterized by acute or subacute paraplegia or quadriplegia associated with sensory level deficit and loss of sphincter control. Cerebrospinal fluid (CSF) analysis reveals pleocytosis, low CSF glucose, and high CSF protein. T2-weighted MRI usually demonstrates increased signal intensity and cord edema. Meningitis, usually infectious, may develop in SLE patients. However, aseptic meningitis can be idiopathic or secondary to administration of ibuprofen or AZA.

Peripheral nervous system syndromes include cranial neuropathies (4% to 49%) such as facial palsies and ocular muscle dysfunction. Pure sensory or motor abnormalities based on electromyography/nerve conduction studies occur in up to 47%, but plexopathy, Guillain–Barré syndrome, and autonomic neuropathy are rare.

The differentiation of NPSLE from other CNS disorders is difficult and remains a process of elimination. CSF pleocytosis and low glucose require exclusion of infections. Electroencephalography generally reveals diffuse brain wave slowing, but focal activity suggests seizures. The presence of serum antiribosomal P (phosphorylated protein) antibodies are not useful for confirming lupus psychosis, but rather just the diagnosis of SLE. The gold standard for imaging the CNS in SLE is conventional MRI with gadolinium. CT scans are less sensitive and should be reserved for patients in whom MRI is contraindicated or for emergent situations to document bleed, infarct, cerebral edema, or a mass lesion. Focal lesions of the subcortical white matter are the most common MRI findings and correlate with ischemic changes. Changes in the gray matter that brighten on T2-weighted imaging suggest more acute events and may improve with therapy. However, it is often difficult to distinguish acute from chronic MRI lesions, and subcortical lesions are found in up to 50% of patients without any neuropsychiatric symptoms. Angiography is invasive and rarely results in an accurate diagnosis of active CNS lupus. Because the sensitivity of MRI for patients with cognitive or affective symptoms is low, additional imaging techniques have been evaluated. Single-photon emission computerized tomography, which measures functional cerebral blood flow, has low specificity. Magnetic angiography, magnetic resonance spectroscopy, magnetic transfer imaging, and perfusion- and diffusion-weighted imaging are still viewed only as research tools, and their roles in assessment of NPSLE remain to be determined.

Management of SLE patients with neuropsychiatric manifestations should focus on specific neurologic symptoms. Non-SLE causes of CNS disease, including infections, uremia, hypertension, metabolic disturbances, hypoxia, or drug toxicities, must be identified and treated appropriately. If lupus cerebritis is suspected, a brief doubling of the steroid dose for 3 days may exclude the possibility of a diffuse CNS syndrome. If there is no improvement or no evidence of active lupus, the steroid dose should be tapered. Seizures are treated with appropriate

TABLE 66.2

Neuropsychiatric Manifestations of Systemic Lupus Erythematosus

Central nervous system
Diffuse neuropsychiatric syndromes
Cognitive dysfunction (50%–80%)
Anxiety disorders (7%–70%)
Mood disorders (14%–57%)
Psychosis as defined by *DSM-IV* related to medical condition (5%–8%)
Acute confusional state (4%–7%)
Focal neurologic syndromes
Headache (24%–72%): range from migraine, tension, or benign intracranial hypertension
Seizures (15%–35%): grand mal, petit mal, temporal lobe, focal
Cerebrovascular disorders (5%–18%): infarcts, transient ischemic attacks
Movement disorders (<1%): chorea
Transverse myelitis (<1%)
Demyelinating syndrome (<1%)
Aseptic meningitis (<1%)
Peripheral nervous system
Peripheral neuropathy
Polyneuropathy (3%–28%)
Mononeuropathy, single or multiplex
Plexopathy (<1%)
Cranial neuropathies (4%–49%)
Acute inflammatory demyelinating polyradiculoneuropathy (Guillain–Barré syndrome) <1%
Autonomic neuropathy (<1%)
Myasthenia gravis (<1%)

Adapted from The ACR nomenclature and case definitions for neuropsychiatric lupus syndromes. *Arthritis Rheum* 42:599–608, 1999; Hanly JG: Neuropsychiatric lupus. *Rheum Dis Clin N Am* 31:273, 2005.

anticonvulsant medications. Status epilepticus is treated with anticonvulsants and high-dose steroids. Psychotic patients should receive antipsychotic agents. High-dose steroids have been recommended for neuropsychiatric lupus; dosages range from 1.0 to 1.5 mg/kg/d, or its equivalent. In severe cases, pulse IV methylprednisolone in a dose of 1,000 mg per day for 3 days is preferred. As for immunosuppressive agents, few prospective studies of treatment of NPSLE have been performed. A recent Cochrane database review of therapy for neuropsychiatric lupus found only one controlled clinical trial that suggested better outcomes with monthly IVCY than steroids alone [29]. Limited case reports of RTX therapy in NPSLE suggest efficacy, but no randomized studies are available. Transverse myelitis has been treated successfully with pulse methylprednisolone, IVCY, and plasmapheresis.

Pulmonary Disease

The pleuropulmonary manifestations of SLE are common and can involve the pleura, parenchyma, vasculature, diaphragm, or airways (see Table 66.1). Acute pulmonary symptoms can be the initial presentation of SLE that results in an ICU admission, whereas the prevalence of long-term lung damage (11.6% by 10 years of disease duration) can contribute to SLE morbidity and mortality [30].

Pleuritis with or without effusions has been reported in 30% to 50% of patients with SLE, depending on the method of study (i.e., clinical history, radiograph findings, or autopsy findings) [31]. Pleural effusions are usually small and bilateral, but massive collections can occur. Thoracentesis is indicated when the etiology of the fluid is uncertain or if respiratory compromise is present. Pleural fluid is characteristically exudative with high protein, pH is variable but can be low, and glucose slightly decreased in contrast to the uniformly low glucose and pH seen in rheumatoid pleural effusions. WBC counts are elevated and consist predominantly of PMNs or lymphocytes. Mild pleuritis usually responds to NSAIDs or low-dose corticosteroids (0.5 mg/kg/d prednisone or its equivalent). The latter is used only after infection has been excluded.

Acute lupus pneumonitis (ALP), although uncommon (0% to 14%), may be the initial presentation of SLE and can be life threatening [31]. It cannot be differentiated from other forms of bronchopneumonia, and thus infectious etiologies should be excluded by appropriate studies. Clinically, patients present with fever, severe dyspnea, tachypnea, and hypoxemia. Chest radiographs reveal patchy alveolar infiltrates, usually basilar in location. Mortality is as high as 50%. Transbronchial brushings with biopsies and BAL may help exclude infections and malignancies. High frequency of anti-SSA/SSB antibodies has been associated with ALP. Given the poor prognosis, therapy requires high-dose corticosteroids (1 to 2 mg/kg/d) or pulse IV methylprednisolone (1,000 mg IV daily for 3 days) along with broad-spectrum antibiotics until final cultures return. Case reports suggest the use of IVCY, RTX, or IV immunoglobulins in patients who respond poorly to steroids.

Pulmonary hemorrhage is a rare but potentially fatal complication. Patients characteristically present with acute dyspnea, tachycardia, severe hypoxemia, rales, sudden drop in hematocrit, and hemoptysis. Rarely, diagnosis is delayed because of the absence of hemoptysis. BAL provides the most reliable confirmation with the presence of bloody fluid, hemosiderin-laden macrophages, purulent sputum, and absence of pathogenic organisms on culture and Gram stain. Pathologic findings include intra-alveolar hemorrhage sometimes associated with interstitial pneumonitis or capillaritis, but pathology may only be bland hemorrhage. Immunopathologic studies may reveal granular deposition of IgG in alveolar septal walls and pulmonary vessels, thus suggesting a possible immune complex–mediated process. Therapy is generally aggressive with IV methylprednisolone at 1,000 mg daily for 3 days followed by tapering high-dose oral (1 mg/kg/d) corticosteroids. The addition of IVCY should be considered for patients who are critically ill or fail pulse corticosteroids. Plasmapheresis has been added in case reports, but whether it offers any additional benefit is unclear. Mortality remains high at 80% despite such treatment. (See Chapter 175 for an in-depth discussion of intrapulmonary hemorrhage and pulmonary-renal syndromes.)

The prevalence of ILD is less than 3% according to several studies and may occur before or after ALP. Patients usually present with dyspnea on exertion, productive cough, pleuritis, and rales. Pulmonary function tests reveal a restrictive pattern and marked reduction in diffusing capacity. High-resolution thin-section CT may differentiate earlier-stage alveolitis from end-stage fibrosis. The presence of dense alveolar opacities or "ground glass" appearance suggests active inflammation and may guide therapy. The pathology of SLE ILD is similar to those seen in RA and includes NSIP, LIP, and OP. Treatment for ILD is challenging, and there are no prospective randomized trials for specific SLE ILD, but management is similar to rheumatoid lung disease or those with idiopathic interstitial pneumonia. Therapy for symptomatic disease begins with high-dose corticosteroids and again, IVCY, AZA, or MMF has been used in clinically progressive ILD or for steroid sparing.

Pulmonary arterial hypertension (PAH) in SLE is the second most common connective tissue disease–related PAH after SSc, but is a rare complication of SLE, estimated at 4% [32] when other causes of pulmonary hypertension are excluded. Patients usually present with severe dyspnea on exertion, palpitations, and fatigue. Pathologically, changes of intimal thickening and fibrosis, medial hypertrophy, altered elastic laminae, and periadventitial fibrosis have been similar to changes seen in idiopathic pulmonary hypertension, but also findings of inflammatory cell infiltrates and immune deposits have been reported. Other associated factors for PAH include the presence of Raynaud's phenomenon (RP) and aPLs. Often, symptoms develop late in the clinical course, and thus assessment with Doppler echocardiography is useful to monitor for progressive disease requiring therapy.

Therapy for primary pulmonary hypertension is evolving rapidly with the use of prostacyclin agonists, endothelin receptor antagonists, phosphodiesterase inhibitors, soluble guanylate cyclase stimulator, or combination therapies. Most of these drug studies for pulmonary hypertension have included patients with connective disease–associated PAH (see the section "Systemic Sclerosis" and Chapter 174 on pulmonary hypertension). Given the pathologic findings of inflammation and immune deposits, immuosuppression with steroids, cyclophosphamide, and even RTX have been suggested for early-stage PAH along with conventional therapy, but these are based on limited retrospective or case report studies [33]. Pulmonary embolism and peripheral vaso-occlusive disease are well-known risks for SLE patients. One prospective study documented the risk of deep vein thrombosis at approximately 12%, with a 9% risk for pulmonary embolism. The risk of thromboembolic events is increased in patients with LA and aPLs (see "Antiphospholipid Syndrome" section).

Other rare pulmonary syndromes occur in SLE. Dyspnea from shrinking lung syndrome can be either acute or chronic and has a prevalence of 0.5% to 0.9% [30,31]. Postulated mechanisms include myopathy of respiratory skeletal muscles or diaphragm, phrenic neuropathy, or pleural inflammation. Pulmonary function tests reveal reduced total lung volumes with a restrictive pattern, whereas imaging reveals low lung volumes, atelectasis, but no evidence of ILD. Treatment is usually with corticosteroids, but immunosuppressive agents have been used for refractory cases. Acute reversible hypoxemia, possibly secondary to pulmonary leukocyte aggregation, has been described among acutely ill SLE patients. Patients present with severe hypoxemia, hypocapnia, and increased alveolar-arterial PO_2 gradient without obvious parenchymal lung disease. Treatment with high-dose glucocorticoids improves oxygenation. Cricoarytenoid or laryngeal involvement causing upper airway obstruction varies from 0.3% to 30% [31]. Bronchiectasis is common, but usually clinically asymptomatic.

Cardiac Disease

Cardiovascular involvement of SLE ranges from 29% to 66%. This tremendous range reflects whether data are based on clinical parameters or pathologic findings at autopsy. Often, the latter studies document significant findings in the heart without clinical correlation. However, a multisite international SLE cohort study confirmed that circulatory disease (including cardiac, arterial, and cerebral vascular disease) is the major cause of mortality [34].

Pericardial disease is by far the most common cardiac manifestation of SLE but less common than lupus pleuritis, and subclinical pericarditis is often documented only at autopsy. Pericarditis usually presents in association with other organ system activity, rather than as an initial manifestation of SLE. Symptoms, physical exam findings, and diagnostic cardiac testing are similar to idiopathic pericarditis, but some SLE patients may have relatively normal findings.

Life-threatening complications of pericarditis include cardiac tamponade and constriction. Both entities are rare and thus pericardiocentesis fluid data are limited. Typically, pericardial fluid is exudative with high protein and normal-to-low glucose, compared with serum. The total WBC counts from various reports have ranged from 544 to 199,600 cells per μL, with predominantly PMNs [35]. Therefore, suppurative pericarditis becomes a significant and important consideration for SLE patients with pericarditis. Other reported pericardial fluid features of low or absent complement levels, lupus erythematosus cells on Wright stains, and ANA titers are not clinically useful. Constrictive pericarditis may develop after successful treatment of pericarditis with or without corticosteroids.

Once other causes of pericarditis, including uremia, drugs, or viral infections, have been eliminated, hemodynamically stable but symptomatic pericarditis can be successfully treated with NSAIDs or, occasionally, moderate-dose oral corticosteroids (0.5 mg/kg/d). If fever is present and the etiology of the pericardial effusion is not clear, a diagnostic pericardiocentesis may be necessary to rule out bacterial or opportunistic infections. Hemodynamically compromising effusions require pericardiocentesis and high-dose IV corticosteroids (e.g., equivalent of 1 mg/kg/d), and rarely, pericardial window or pericardiectomy may be required.

Another common cardiac manifestation of SLE is valvular heart disease involving the mitral, aortic, or tricuspid valves, often asymptomatic and discovered on echocardiography. Thickened leaflets are common echocardiographic findings but nonbacterial, verrucous lesions (Libman–Sacks endocarditis) may result in embolic events, secondary infectious endocarditis, or valvular insufficiency or stenosis. At autopsy, 15% to 60% of SLE patients have lesions composed of immune complexes, fibrin, platelets, and fibrotic changes on the ventricular surface of the mitral valve (and, less commonly, aortic valve), ventricular endocardium, chordae tendineae, and papillary muscle. Clinically, the presence of these lesions does not correlate with murmurs. Prevalence varies from 11% by transthoracic echocardiogram to 43% by transesophageal approach [36]. In a large meta-analysis to assess the association of aPLs and valvular disease/Libman–Sacks endocarditis in SLE patients, there was a threefold higher risk for any heart valve lesion in SLE patients with aPL than in those without aPL and a 5.3-fold risk for those patients who have both LA and IgG aPL [37]. In patients with aPL and valvular disease, antiplatelet medications are recommended, whereas full anticoagulation is recommended for those with documented embolic events. If significant valvular dysfunction occurs, valve repair or replacement may be required, but complications include rapid calcification of the repaired valve or bioprosthesis.

Myocardial involvement in SLE is the least frequent manifestation of cardiac disease and should be categorized as primary or secondary. Primary myocarditis is rare, clinically occurring in 10% of SLE patients [38]. Myocarditis has been defined as unexplained tachycardia, congestive heart failure, ventricular arrhythmias, conduction defects, ST- or T-wave changes, or cardiomegaly without evidence of valvular or pericardial disease. Congestive heart failure from myocarditis is rare and is estimated to occur among 4% of cases. Echocardiogram may reveal global hypokinesis, whereas cardiac MRI with gadolinium has delayed contrast enhancement. Secondary myocardial dysfunction of SLE includes systemic hypertension, valvular disease, pulmonary disease, coronary artery ischemia (see following discussion), drug toxicity, and amyloidosis. These secondary causes are often more important than true lupus myocarditis. Management of patients with evidence of carditis rests on distinguishing primary from secondary disorders. For the rare patient who has myocarditis from SLE, high-dose corticosteroids are indicated. Data regarding the use of immunosuppressive agents are scarce.

Primary coronary artery involvement in SLE includes embolic events, thromboses, or a true vasculitis of the vessels as opposed to secondary changes of premature atherosclerosis. Coronary arteritis is rare and difficult to distinguish from atherosclerosis on arteriographic studies unless repetitive studies are performed. This can occur in the absence of extracardiac SLE activity. Thrombosis associated with aPL may contribute to myocardial ischemia.

Accelerated atherosclerosis, however, is the most serious cause of morbidity and mortality among SLE patients and especially for the age group between 35 and 44 years. A recent systemic review on the epidemiology of atherosclerotic cardiovascular disease (including coronary artery disease, peripheral vascular disease, congestive heart failure, and cerebral vascular disease) in SLE patients revealed two to threefold risk compared to the general population and even higher risk for young SLE patients (age <45 years) [39]. Traditional risk factors including smoking, diabetes, hypertension, hyperlipidemia, obesity, family history, and sedentary life style are common among the SLE population, but the additional effects of medications such as glucocorticoids, chronic inflammation, and hypercoagulability may also contribute to the significantly higher risk for cardiovascular disease. The management of SLE patients with acute myocardial ischemia initially is similar to any patient with atherosclerotic coronary artery disease. However, the etiology of the ischemia must be determined because management of coronary arteritis differs from management of atherosclerotic disease. Evidence of extracardiac SLE activity may be helpful. Laboratory tests, including ANA, anti-dsDNA, complement levels, complete blood count with differential, and platelet counts may provide some indicators of SLE activity. LA and aPLs should be checked. Coronary arteriogram may be helpful in separating thrombosis and vasculitis from atherosclerosis. However, arteriographic distinction of the latter two may be difficult. If arteriography reveals thrombosis without evident atherosclerosis and the presence of aPLs is documented, therapy should consists of anticoagulation and antiplatelet medications.

Conduction abnormalities and arrhythmias due to SLE are usually clinically insignificant. The incidence of atrioventricular nodal block is estimated to be 5%. Sinus tachycardia without underlying pathology (fever, dehydration, congestive heart failure, thyroid disease, drug abuse) may be a subtle manifestation of lupus activity. If acute conduction disease is suspected clinically to be secondary to myocarditis or arteritis, a short trial of corticosteroids could be initiated in the hemodynamically compromised patient.

Hematologic Disease

Hematologic abnormalities constitute one of the major criteria for SLE. These include hemolytic anemia, thrombocytopenia, leukopenia, and lymphopenia. Anemia is present in the majority of SLE patients, with anemia of chronic disease being the most common etiology. Other causes of anemia include iron deficiency (blood loss from menses or gastrointestinal tract, or poor iron absorption because of increased hepcidin levels), autoimmune hemolytic anemia (AIHA), drug induced (cyclophosphamide or AZA), pure red cell aplasia, and chronic renal insufficiency. Rarely, other syndromes including TTP and macrophage activation syndrome have been reported in SLE patients who have more than two cell lines affected.

Only 8% to 28% of lupus patients develop AIHA sometime during the course of their disease. Although 18% to 65% of SLE patients have a positive direct Coombs assay, significant hemolytic anemia develops in only 10% [40]. The presence of warm IgG autoantibodies and complement on the red cell surface is characteristic of SLE AIHA. Clinically, AIHA is accompanied by an elevated reticulocyte count and indirect bilirubin and decreased haptoglobin levels. Severe hemolytic anemia, defined as hemoglobin <8 g per dL, is often associated with concomitant seizures, nephritis, serositis, and other cytopenias. In addition, 74% of patients with AIHA will have aPLs. Over 75% to 96% of patients with AIHA respond rapidly to high-dose corticosteroids (60 to 100 mg per day prednisone orally or with IV methylprednisolone at 1.5 mg/kg/d) [40]. Prednisone is tapered slowly after 4 weeks, based on laboratory results. If active hemolysis persists after 4 weeks, other therapeutic modalities include danazol, immunosuppressive agents, and splenectomy; however, splenectomy induces permanent remission in fewer than 50% of patients. Combination of high-dose steroids and danazol, 800 to 1,200 mg per day, is an alternative treatment for severe AIHA, with subsequent gradual steroid tapering. One retrospective study of SLE patients treated for AIHA suggests that danazol was the most effective long-term treatment [41]. The short-term efficacy of IVIG is not sustained. Uncontrolled trials or case reports with AZA, RTX, MMF, or cyclophosphamide have shown therapeutic response.

Thrombotic microangiopathy (TMA) pathologically classifies a group of disease that include thrombotic thromboctyopenic purpura (TTP). The latter is characterized by thrombocytopenia, hemolytic anemia and sometimes with renal or neurologic systems and has been described in SLE. Markedly reduced ADAMTS-13 protease (**A** **D**isintegrin **A**nd **M**etalloprotease with a **T**hrombo**S**pondin type 1 motif, member **13**) results in persistence of ultralarge von Willebrand factor multimers on the endothelial surface, which is felt to cause TMA. Among patients with SLE, this deficiency is acquired because of the presence of an inhibitor against the protease. Initial presumptive diagnosis is based on clinical presentation of microangiopathic features, thrombocytopenia, fever, nervous system involvement with mental status changes, and renal insufficiency because ADAMTS-13 results may be delayed. Immediate treatment, similar to idiopathic TTP, with high-dose steroids and plasma exchange is life saving.

Leukopenia, defined as a total WBC count of less than 4,000 per μL, occurs in 50% to 60% of SLE patients, but rarely associated with infectious complications unless CD4 counts are below 200. For febrile, severely neutropenic patient, granulocyte-stimulating factor has been used. *Lymphopenia*, defined as counts lower than 1,500 per μL, is seen among 84% of SLE patients during active disease.

Thrombocytopenia, or platelet counts lower than 100,000 per μL, is observed among 20% to 40% of SLE patients and is severe (less than 50,000 per μL) among 10% of patients. Idiopathic thrombocytopenic purpura (ITP) may be the initial presentation of SLE. When evaluating any patient with thrombocytopenia, underlying causes including drug toxicities, ineffective thrombopoiesis, congestive splenomegaly, dilutional effects, abnormal platelet destruction by disseminated intravascular coagulation (DIC), antiphospholipid syndrome (APS), TTP, hemolytic uremic syndrome (HUS), vasculitis, drug-induced infection, or other hematologic disorders should be excluded. The pathologic mechanism is usually antiplatelet antibodies, with resultant splenic sequestration and decreased platelet life span, although there is association with elevated aPL as well. A bone marrow biopsy is helpful for distinguishing various forms of thrombocytopenia. SLE-associated ITP is characterized by an increased number of megakaryocytes.

Once TTP, HUS, DIC, and drug toxicities are excluded, therapy of severe SLE-associated ITP (less than 30,000 per μL) is similar to that of idiopathic autoimmune thrombocytopenia. Corticosteroid therapy at 1 mg/kg/d is the recommended initial therapy. Subsequent tapering is guided by platelet counts. Administration of IVIG may result in a rapid increase in platelet counts when patients are having acute bleeding or need invasive procedures, but the response is usually not sustained. Recommended dose is 1.0 g per day for 2 to 3 days based on platelet counts. Splenectomy is an option for SLE patients who fail medical therapy, with improved thrombocytopenia in 84% of patients in a median follow-up of 6.6 years after splenectomy [42]. Some of these patients had partial response and required additional medical therapy. For refractory disease, danazol, 800 to 1,200 mg per day alone or in conjunction with corticosteroids, has been effective in several studies. In a meta-analysis, rituximab is effective for idiopathic thrombocytopenia in conjunction with or after failure to respond to glucocorticoids [43]. Given this report and case reports of success in the literature for SLE-associated ITP, it is one of the second-line agents to consider. Other second-line immunosuppressive agents include cyclophosphamide, MMF, and AZA.

LA interferes with the activation of prothrombin activator complex (factors Xa and V, Ca^{2+}, and phospholipid) of the intrinsic and extrinsic pathways. The laboratory findings are markedly prolonged partial thromboplastin time and normal or mildly prolonged prothrombin time that cannot be corrected by mixing with normal plasma. In addition, patients may also have false-positive reactions in the test for syphilis (VDRL). (Please see the section "Antiphospholipid Syndrome" for clinical details.) Although many SLE patients have both LA and aPLs, subsets of patients have only one or the other laboratory abnormality and still develop clinical manifestations of APS.

Gastrointestinal Disease

Gastrointestinal involvement of SLE is not frequently considered because many gastrointestinal symptoms can be attributed to complications of drug therapy, particularly salicylates, NSAIDs, corticosteroids, hydroxychloroquine, and AZA. The prevalence of SLE-related gastrointestinal disease varies from of 8% to 22% and includes serositis, mesenteric vasculitis or thrombosis, pancreatitis, cholecystitis, inflammatory bowel disease, protein-losing enteropathy, intestinal pseudo-obstruction, and pneumatosis intestinalis [44].

The most serious but rare (<1%) gastrointestinal complication of SLE is mesenteric vasculitis or thrombosis with subsequent large or small intestinal ischemia. The severity and extent of involvement vary and symptoms may be chronic or acute in presentation. Intestinal involvement ranges from segmental edema or ulcerations to perforations. Evaluation should include plain films, paracentesis (to rule out perforation or bacterial peritonitis), CT scans, or angiography. Although features of dilated bowel, bowel wall edema or enhancement, or edema of the mesentery or its vessels are nonspecific, multiple vessel involvement, often in the areas of ileum and jejunum, is found in SLE mesenteric vasculitis. However, angiographic results may be normal because of small vessel disease. Direct visualization with endoscopy or colonoscopy may also provide useful information.

Lupus peritonitis is less devastating but often quite dramatic in presentation. Peritoneal fluid may be present, and is usually transudative and sterile with a low cell count. Other causes of ascites must be ruled out, including constrictive pericarditis, nephrotic syndrome, and spontaneous bacterial peritonitis. Pancreatitis attributed to active SLE is rare and more often related to the usual causes of pancreatitis in non-SLE patients (e.g., drugs, hepatobiliary infection, alcohol, etc.) [45]. Protein-losing enteropathy and intestinal pseudo-obstruction were the most common gastrointestinal manifestations among hospitalized SLE patients [44].

Management of the SLE patient with abdominal pain does not differ significantly from that for non-SLE patients. For patients with mild-to-moderate pain with a chronic course, medications and intercurrent disease should be considered first as the cause of pain and surgical consultation obtained. When no etiology is found, peritonitis should be considered and treated with a moderate increase in steroids. For patients who present acutely, supportive care should be started and appropriate laboratory and imaging studies performed. Paracentesis should be done to exclude perforated viscus or infection. A therapeutic trial of high-dose steroids can then be instituted if mesenteric vasculitis is suspected. Rapid (12 to 48 hours) response usually is consistent with vasculitis or peritonitis, although complete response is often delayed; if a patient deteriorates clinically, exploratory laparotomy is necessary. When studies suggest mesenteric vasculitis, IVCY may be necessary along with the corticosteroids.

Drug-Induced Lupus

The syndrome of DIL should be considered for ICU patients when systemic symptoms of fever, arthralgias, arthritis, pleuropericarditis, and, less commonly, rash are present. Because many ICU patients receive medications that potentially induce SLE (see Table 66.3), the diagnosis must be excluded. Although some medications, particularly procainamide, hydralazine, and TNFα inhibitors, produce positive ANA tests, this does not necessarily

TABLE 66.3

Medications Associated with Drug-Related Lupus

Type	Definite	Possible	Rare[a]
Cardiovascular	Methyldopa Hydralazine Procainamide Quinidine Practolol Diltiazem	Captopril β-Blockers Hydrochlorothiazide Amiodarone Ticlopidine	Reserpine Minoxidil Chlorthalidone Clonidine HMG-CoA inhibitors Spironolactone Disopyramide Prazosin
Anticonvulsants or neurologic medications		Phenytoin Mephenytoin Primidone Carbamazepine Trimethadione	Levodopa Ethosuximide Valproate
Psychiatric	Chlorpromazine	Lithium carbonate	Lamotrigine
Antibiotics	Isoniazid Minocycline	Sulfonamides Nitrofurantoin Rifampin Terbinafine	Streptomycin Tetracycline Penicillin Nalidixic acid Griseofulvin
Endocrine		Methimazole Propylthiouracil, methylthiouracil Glyburide	Tolazamide
Rheumatic	Penicillamine TNFα inhibitors	Sulfasalazine	Gold salts Allopurinol *p*-Aminosalicylic acid NSAIDs: tolmetin, ibuprofen, sulindac, diclofenac, tolmetin
Others	Interferon α	Danazol, dapsone Interferon γ Docetaxel	Psoralen Quinine Leuprolide acetate Promethazine Timolol eye drops Olsalazine, mesalamine Zafirlukast Interleukin 2

[a]Rare: usually case reports.

imply that DIL is present. Symptoms typically develop several months after the institution of the offending medication. Although CNS and renal manifestations are rare, case reports of more atypical DIL have been reported. Males and females are equally susceptible. DIL is more common among older patients, except for minocycline-related DIL (younger and more females). Laboratory values reveal an elevated ESR, mild leukopenia or thrombocytopenia, and positive ANA; antihistone antibodies are present in 90% of patients; and specific antibodies to dsDNA and Smith (Sm) antigen are uncommon. However, TNFα inhibitors such as etanercept or infliximab have been associated with anti-dsDNA, anti-Ro, anti-Sm, and antineutrophil cytoplasmic antibodies. Complement levels are normal with DIL.

Subacute cutaneous lupus (SCLE), with characteristic annular or psoriasiform lesions that are photosensitive, is associated with drugs that differ in frequency than those listed in Table 66.3. A review of all patients with SCLE reported that about 38% had exposure to the following drugs that were felt to be causative: terbinafine, TNFα inhibitors, ACE inhibitors, thrombocyte inhibitors, proton pump inhibitors, antiepileptics, and NSAIDs [46]. Discontinuation of the offending medication results in gradual diminution of symptoms that may last as long as a year. NSAIDs or low-dose steroids may control the symptoms, and for patients with severe organ system involvement, treatment is similar to idiopathic lupus. Most rheumatologists believe that patients with idiopathic SLE who require hydralazine, procainamide, isoniazid, phenytoin, β-blockers, or other medications that can potentially induce lupus can take these medications. TNFα inhibitors, however, are relatively contraindicated for SLE. It is advisable to document the clinical and serologic status of the patient before starting the medication.

TABLE 66.4

Modified Sapporo Classification Criteria for Antiphospholipid Syndrome

Clinical criteria
1. Vascular thrombosis involving any size vessel (arterial, venous, or capillary), excluding venous thromboembolism
2. Pregnancy complications
   a. Three or more sequential spontaneous miscarriages before 10 weeks gestation (without obvious causes)
   b. One or more unexplained death of normal fetus beyond 10 weeks gestation
   c. Preterm delivery of normal fetus <34 weeks because of preeclampsia, eclampsia, or placental insufficiency

Laboratory criteria (measured at least on two occasions, 12 weeks apart)
1. Moderate- to high-titer IgM or IgG anticardiolipin antibodies by ELISA
2. Lupus anticoagulant
3. High-titer (>99 percentile) IgM or IgG anti-β_2 glycoprotein I antibody by ELISA

Diagnosis is based on the presence of one clinical and one laboratory criteria. The laboratory finding should not be less than 12 weeks or more than 5 years apart from the clinical event.

Adapted from Miyakis S, Lockshin MD, Atsumi T, et al: International consensus statement on an update of the classification criteria for definite antiphospholipid syndrome. *J Thromb Haemost* 4(2):295–306, 2006.

ANTIPHOSPHOLIPID SYNDROME

APS is defined by vascular thrombosis or pregnancy complications in the presence of LA or moderate- to high-titer aPL, documented at least twice, 12 or more weeks apart (Table 66.4). By definition, aPL includes IgG or IgM anticardiolipin antibodies (aCL) and/or anti-β_2 glycoprotein I antibody (anti-β_2 GPI). The LA, aCL, and anti-β_2 GPI all bind to negatively charged phospholipids. How these antibodies induce thrombosis remains unknown, but interaction with endothelial cells, coagulation factors, and platelets, and complement activation all play a role. Thromboses and emboli occur in all vessel sizes and organ systems. Nonthrombotic associations include valvular lesions similar to Libman–Sacks, hemolytic anemia, thrombocytopenia, livedo reticularis, and false-positive tests for syphilis. Primary APS occurs in the absence of other connective tissue disease. When APS is associated with SLE or other connective tissue disorders, it is referred to as *secondary APS*. Patients with *catastrophic APS* (CAPS) present with acute multiorgan failure from occlusive vasculopathy of small vessels in the kidney, lungs, brain, heart, adrenal glands, and liver. Large vessel occlusions have also been reported.

The APS manifestations that most likely require ICU admission are cerebrovascular disease, pulmonary embolism, major abdominal or extremity arterial or venous thrombosis, myocardial infarctions, severe valvular disease (insufficiency or thrombotic valvular vegetations), and intracardiac thrombosis. Renal manifestations of APS include hypertension, proteinuria, acute or subacute renal insufficiency, and end-stage renal failure [47]. The classical renal lesion is thrombotic microangiopathy, but the entire renal vasculature can be affected; renal artery lesions can cause renal artery stenosis, cortical ischemia, and infarction, whereas thrombosis of the renal vein and inferior vena cava results in nephrotic range proteinuria. Hemodialysis patients with APS are at increased risk of vascular access thrombosis. CAPS, which occurs in less than 1% of APS, is the most serious and devastating subset, with multisystem small vessel thromboses occurring within a short time period [48]. Differentiation from TTP and DIC is imperative but sometimes difficult because microangiopathic hemolytic anemia or elevated fibrin split products are sometimes present in CAPS. Measurement of ADAMTS-13 activity and anti-ADAMTS-13 and anti-heparin antibodies may help clarify the diagnosis. CAPS precipitating factors include infection, surgery, malignancy, subtherapeutic anticoagulation, and SLE flares. Mortality is high, nearly 48%, with death most often associated with renal, pulmonary, splenic, or adrenal involvement, or underlying SLE [49].

APS patients with *venous* thrombosis are treated with heparin anticoagulation followed by conversion to warfarin with an INR target of 2.0 to 3.0. Lifelong anticoagulation is supported by a high incidence of recurrent thrombosis when warfarin is discontinued. Moderate-intensity anticoagulation (INR 2.0 to 3.0) is comparable to high-intensity antocoagulation (INR 3.1 to 4.0) for preventing further venous thromboses and equal in bleeding complications [50]. However, controversy still exists as to whether high-intensity anticoagulation is necessary for patients with arterial clots. Some experts recommend high-intensity warfarin, whereas others recommend moderate-intensity warfarin with or without low-dose aspirin [51]. In APS patients with recurrent thrombosis despite therapeutic anticoagulation, treatment options include standard dose warfarin plus an antiplatelet agent, high-intensity warfarin, unfractionated heparin, or low-molecular-weight heparin. Primary prophylaxis with hydroxychloroquine with or without low-dose aspirin is recommended for patients with SLE and positive LA or persistent moderate- to high-titer aPLs, but there is no evidence to support prophylactic anticoagulation for individuals without SLE who have LA or aPLs in the absence of other thrombotic risk factors [51,52].

Treatment of CAPS requires both anticoagulation and immunosuppressive therapy [51]. Triple therapy with heparin anticoagulation, high-dose corticosteroids, and plasma exchange with or without IVIG has the best survival data [48]. Case reports support the use of RTX (monoclonal antibody to CD20 expressed on B cells) or eculizumab (terminal complement inhibitor) for refractory disease [53,54].

SYSTEMIC SCLEROSIS

SSc, or scleroderma, is an immune-mediated disease characterized by progressive fibrosis of the vasculature and viscera resulting in end-organ damage of the skin, heart, lungs, kidneys, and gastrointestinal tract. There are two subsets of scleroderma: (a) limited cutaneous disease, often associated with the anticentromere antibody, and (b) systemic/diffuse disease, associated with the presence of antitopoisomerase 1 (SCL-70) or anti-RNA polymerase. Both subsets have potential end-organ complications that result in ICU admission, including severe digital ischemia from RP, respiratory failure, cardiac dysfunction, or renal insufficiency. The following discussion is limited to these areas.

Severe Raynaud's Phenomenon

Although primary RP is common in the general population (up to 5%), severe secondary RP associated with connective tissue disease often is more difficult to treat, and digital ulceration or gangrene may occur among 25% of SSc patients. Dihydropyridine-type calcium channel blockers (CCBs), usually nifedipine, reduce the frequency and severity of RP attacks and are considered first-line therapy [55]. For patients with an inadequate response to CCBs, sildenafil and other phosphodiesterase-5 inhibitors reduce the frequency and severity of attacks and promote healing of digital ulcers [56]. Bosentan, a dual endothelin receptor antagonist, is effective for reducing the number of new digital ulcers but, although available in Europe, it has not been approved for use in the United States [57]. Topical nitrates, ACE inhibitors, and α-adrenergic receptor blockade are additional therapies with modest benefits. There is increased interest in the use of botulinum toxin, with several small studies showing pain reduction and improved ulcer healing [58]. IV prostacyclin (epoprostenol) or iloprost (a prostacyclin analog) is effective for patients with critical digital ischemia refractory to other therapies (Table 66.5) [59]. Oral prostanoids are less effective. Use of IV prostaglandins should be avoided for patients with pulmonary hypertension unless closely monitored. Chemical digital sympathectomy with lidocaine provides short-term pain relief, and surgical digital sympathectomy can be a last alternative when medical therapies fail.

Pulmonary Disease

Pulmonary involvement occurs among 25% to 90% of patients with SSc and is now the most frequent cause of death (more than 50%) [60]. ILD and PAH are the two major pulmonary complications of SSc. Patients with diffuse SSc are more likely to develop ILD, whereas isolated PAH is more common in limited scleroderma and patients with anticentromere antibodies, with a prevalence of 12% to 15% [61]. Clinically significant disease from interstitial fibrosis or PAH is estimated to affect 40% of patients (see Table 66.1).

Exertional dyspnea, cough, and basilar crackles are the predominant clinical features of ILD. Radiographs may reveal pulmonary fibrosis among 33% to 40%, with a characteristic basilar reticulonodular or honeycombing pattern [60]. HRCT scans are more sensitive for documenting the reticular and ground glass opacities of ILD when plain radiographs are relatively normal. Pulmonary function tests may reveal restrictive lung disease (decreased total lung capacity and forced vital capacity [FVC]) even before radiographic or clinical findings. A decrease of diffusing capacity (D_LCO) may occur with either ILD or PAH and has been reported in isolation without other pulmonary function test abnormalities. Patients with ILD may develop secondary PAH, but the degree of PAH is disproportionate to the degree of ILD.

Prevention of progressive fibrotic disease is the goal of treatment for SSc-associated ILD. In one study, the extent of disease on CT was predictive of mortality and FVC decline, suggesting that patients with more advanced CT abnormalities should be treated. [62] Patients with less extensive disease should be monitored closely and treated if there is evidence of radiographic progression or decline in pulmonary function. BAL cellularity does not predict disease progression or response to treatment, and currently has a limited role for the evaluation of ILD, but is useful to rule out infection. A randomized, placebo-controlled study of oral cyclophosphamide (1 mg/kg/d titrated to maximum of 2 mg/kg/d) found small but statistically significant improvement in FVC, skin score, and subjective symptoms [63]. Another randomized, placebo-controlled study of IVCY (0.5 to 0.7 g per m^2 monthly) demonstrated improvement of FVC [64]. Although there are no controlled trials to compare efficacy of oral versus IVCY, the IV route is most practical initially for the critically ill ICU patient. Low-dose glucocorticoids (equivalent to prednisone 10 mg per day or less) are usually prescribed with CY. Although debate exists as to the benefit of concomitant high-dose prednisone or prednisolone, high-dose glucocorticoids are usually avoided because of the increased risks of infection and scleroderma renal crisis (SRC) and the lack of clinical trial data.

TABLE 66.5

Drug Therapy for Severe Raynaud's in SSc

Drug	Route of administration	Dose	Side effects
Epoprostenol	Continuous, intravenous	2 ng/kg/min titrated up to 4–8 ng/kg/min over 5 d [59]	Catheter related; flushing, nausea, jaw pain, diarrhea, depression
Iloprost[b]	Intravenous	0.5–2 ng/kg/d for 6 h for over 3–5 d [83]	Infusion site pain, headache, nausea, diarrhea, vomiting, jaw pain
Treprostinil	Continuous infusion, or subcutaneous	2 ng/kg/min titrated up to 40 ng/kg/min (case reports)	Jaw pain, headache, diarrhea, nausea, infusion site pain
Bosentan	Oral	62.5 mg b.i.d. then increased to 125 mg b.i.d. [57]	Hepatotoxicity, anemia, edema, male infertility, teratogenicity
Sildenafil	Oral	50 mg b.i.d. [56]	Headache, diarrhea, dyspepsia, flushing
Botulinum	Injection of digit or palm	Varies, up to 100 units/hand [58]	Pain at the injection site, ecchymosis, or intrinsic muscle weakness

Preliminary results of a large double-blind randomized clinical trial (The Scleroderma Lung Study II) comparing oral CY with MMF suggest that both are effective therapies for SSc ILD, with fewer side effects in the MMF arm [61]. For patients with refractory disease, one small study reported improvement of FVC and D_LCO when RTX was given to patients previously treated with CYC or MMF [65]. Patients with progressive ILD despite medical therapy may be candidates for lung transplantation.

Pulmonary vasospasm and endothelial cell activation with subsequent arterial wall proliferative changes contribute to the development of PAH. Symptoms include exertional dyspnea, fatigue, reduced exercise tolerance, chest pain, syncope, and lower extremity edema, but patients may be asymptomatic until the disease is advanced. The most sensitive tests are decreased diffusing capacity, often with preserved lung volumes, and Doppler echocardiography showing increased pulmonary pressures and right atrial and ventricular hypertrophy. Right heart catheterization is the gold standard for confirmation of suspected PAH and allows vasodilator trials to assess the degree of pulmonary vascular responsiveness to iloprost or epoprostenol, inhaled nitric oxide, or adenosine. General measures include the use of supplemental oxygen for hypoxic patients, diuretics for management of volume overload, and digoxin for atrial arrhythmias. Anticoagulation is recommended when PAH is advanced, but controlled studies have not been reported. Please refer to the section on PAH in Chapter 174 for further discussion of treatment options.

Cardiac Disease

Cardiac involvement of SSc may be a primary process within the heart or secondary to other major organ involvement (i.e., pulmonary, renal, vascular, thyroid). Primary cardiac involvement of SSc includes pericardial disease, myocardial disease, conduction abnormalities, and arrhythmias. Because the most common symptoms are dyspnea, orthopnea, atypical chest pain, palpitations, fatigue, and dizziness, the clinical manifestations of cardiac disease can be confused with those of other organ systemic involvement. Recent studies have also shown an increased burden of atherosclerotic coronary disease with SSc [66].

Pericardial disease is the most common cardiac manifestation, and as in SLE, asymptomatic pericardial disease based on autopsy series or echocardiographic data has a much higher prevalence than symptomatic disease (33% to 71% vs. 7% to 20%). Pericardial effusions are usually small and do not influence prognosis. Larger effusions (>200 mL), however, are associated with a poor prognosis. Pericardial tamponade with hemodynamic compromise is rare. Pericardiocentesis is rarely required unless the patient is hemodynamically compromised or febrile, and an infectious etiology must be excluded. Pericardial fluid tends to be serous with a wide range of leukocyte counts and with normal complement levels. Corticosteroids are rarely required for treatment.

Myocardial involvement is the most common cardiac finding among patients with SSc at autopsy, ranging from 12% to 89%; however, symptomatic disease occurs less frequently than pericarditis. Pathologically, the most common findings are patchy, focal myocardial fibrosis equally distributed in both ventricles and all three layers of the heart [67]. Autonomic cardiac neuropathy may also contribute to the cardiac morbidity of SSc patients.

Clinically, myocardial disease may result in cardiomyopathy, left ventricular diastolic dysfunction, congestive heart failure, angina, conduction abnormalities, or malignant arrhythmias. A high percentage of SSc patients without cardiac symptoms have an abnormal resting ECG, chest radiograph, Holter monitor, or echocardiogram. Electrophysiologic studies reveal a high incidence of reentrant supraventricular tachyarrhythmias and atrioventricular conduction delays. Ventricular tachycardia occurs among 10% to 13% of patients and is a cause of sudden death. Advanced myocardial fibrosis, rather than selective fibrosis of the conduction system, appears to be responsible for conduction abnormalities and arrhythmias.

Evaluation of acutely ill SSc patients for suspected heart disease should include a routine ECG and chest radiograph. Doppler echocardiography provides information regarding the pericardium, valvular function, systolic and diastolic ventricular function, chamber size, wall thickness, and the presence of pulmonary hypertension. Nuclear scanning may reveal subclinical myocardial disease; cardiac catheterization is useful for accurate assessment of pulmonary arterial pressures but is otherwise unremarkable unless the patient has arteriosclerosis. Negative endomyocardial biopsies cannot exclude myocardial fibrosis because the pathologic process tends to be patchy.

Treatment of SSc cardiac disease is tailored to the specific syndrome. Pericarditis is treated similarly to pericarditis because of other causes with NSAIDs or colchicine. Corticosteroids are generally avoided because of the increased risk of renal crisis, but low-dose corticosteroids can be used in refractory cases. Diuresis should be pursued with caution in patients with large pericardial effusions. Renal failure has been reported among patients after vigorous diuresis, presumably secondary to hypovolemia superimposed on low cardiac output, resulting in decreased renal cortical blood flow. Congestive heart failure is treated as outlined in Chapter 33. However, when echocardiography reveals evidence of diastolic dysfunction, ACE inhibitors or CCBs may be more effective than inotropic agents. A high index of suspicion for coronary artery disease and aggressive management of modifiable risk factors are important aspects of therapy for all patients.

Renal Disease

In addition to cardiac and pulmonary involvement of diffuse scleroderma, significant morbidity and mortality result from renal disease. The onset of accelerated hypertension accompanied by signs of microangiopathic hemolytic anemia, hyperreninemia, and rapidly progressive renal failure describes a syndrome referred to as SRC. SRC may develop among up to 10% of patients with diffuse scleroderma [68]. SRC typically occurs early in the course of the disease for patients with diffuse disease, often in the setting of other organ system involvement. Predictors for development of SRC include high skin score, large joint contractures, tendon friction rubs, prednisone use, and anti-RNA polymerase III antibodies [68].

Although the pathophysiology of SRC is unknown, several factors contribute to its evolution. The primary event is endothelial cell injury, leading to intimal proliferation and luminal narrowing. Combined with other contributing factors such as vasospasm, decreased renal blood flow leads to increased renin release and clinical development of malignant hypertension and SRC. Moderate- to high-dose corticosteroid use is associated with the development of SRC, possibly because of the inhibition of prostacyclin production.

The diagnosis of SRC should be strongly considered in the SSc patient with accelerated hypertension, although SRC may occur rarely in normotensive patients. In addition to accelerated hypertension, proposed diagnostic criteria also include increase in serum creatinine >50% over baseline, proteinuria, hematuria, thrombocytopenia, hemolytic anemia, and hypertensive encephalopathy [68].

Since the advent of aggressive management with ACE inhibitors, conservation or improvement of renal function is possible. It is now clear that this class of drugs is the standard of care for SRC. Short-acting ACE inhibitors should be titrated upward every 6 to 12 hours. Blood pressure should be controlled within 48 hours. Additional antihypertensives, including CCBs, can be added. For many patients treated with ACE inhibitors, there may be a transient reduction in glomerular filtration rate and a rise in serum creatinine.

Although ACE inhibitors have markedly improved outcomes in SRC, 1-year mortality is as high as 36%, and 25% remain on dialysis 1 year after SRC onset [69]. Survival data of patients with good outcomes (not requiring dialysis) after SRC are similar to those of SSc patients without renal crisis. For patients with good outcomes after the initial renal crisis, continuing ACE inhibitors indefinitely may provide further benefit to maintain renal function. There is no evidence to support the use of ACE inhibitors for primary prevention of SRC. In fact, exposure to ACE inhibitors prior to onset of SRC is associated with a twofold increased risk of mortality [69].

Gastrointestinal Disease

Gastrointestinal tract involvement is common among SSc, affecting 50% to 80% of patients. The most common physiologic abnormalities, esophageal dysmotility and decreased lower esophageal sphincter pressure, are manifested by symptoms of dysphagia and heartburn, respectively. Impaired microvascular perfusion initially alters myoelectrical function of the smooth muscle layer and results in fibrotic changes in muscularis, submucosa, and lamina propria [70]. Dysphagia and heartburn are treated symptomatically with prokinetic agents (metoclopramide and macrolide antibiotics) and proton pump inhibitors. Serious complications include strictures and Barrett's esophagus.

Gastric involvement is less common but can include gastroparesis and bleeding. Gastroparesis, with symptoms of early satiety, bloating, and vomiting, can lead to malnutrition. Treatment of gastroparesis includes dietary modification, antiemetics, and prokinetic agents. Telangiectasias are a common source of gastrointestinal blood loss. Gastric antral vascular ectasia (GAVE), or "watermelon stomach," may present with acute bleeding and antedate the diagnosis of SSc. Telangiectasias and GAVE are managed with endoscopic coagulation. Partial or total gastrectomy may be required for refractory disease. Supportive measures include iron supplements, blood transfusions, and proton pump inhibitors. Case reports suggest that IVCY is an effective treatment for refractory GAVE [71].

Small and large intestinal involvement usually occurs concomitantly and results in malabsorption, with symptoms of bloating, cramping, and intermittent or severe diarrhea. Hypomotility due to progressive smooth muscle atrophy and fibrosis results in bacterial overgrowth. In addition, adynamic ileus or pseudo-obstruction may occur. Although barium studies reveal wide-mouth sacculations or diverticula on the antimesenteric border, most patients have relatively few symptoms. Fecal incontinence and constipation are common but underreported. Rare complications include obstruction because of fecal impaction, megacolon, and volvulus. Pneumatosis cystoides intestinalis (PCI), or intramural air-filled cysts in the small or large intestines, may be found incidentally or cause abdominal pain, diarrhea, or bloody rectal discharge. Rupture of these cysts results in pneumoperitoneum without peritonitis.

Prokinetic agents have been reported to be useful for treatment of intestinal disease. Intestinal malabsorption has been treated with antibiotics, low-residue diets, medium-chain triglycerides, fat-soluble vitamins, and total parenteral nutrition. Octreotide improves intestinal peristalsis for pseudo-obstruction and, in combination with erythromycin, may have additive benefits [72]. An investigational 5-HT4 receptor agonist, prucalopride, improves symptoms and gut transport in SSc [73]. Prucalopride is approved for use in Europe, but is not yet available in the United States. Cisapride, another 5-HT4 receptor agonist, is severely restricted in the United States because of concerns regarding severe cardiac arrhythmias. PCI is usually managed conservatively without surgery. Malabsorption and PCI are poor prognostic indicators [74].

Primary biliary cirrhosis (PBC) is the most common liver disease associated with SSc. Up to 18% of patients with PBC have SSc, usually the limited cutaneous form, whereas 8% of all SSc patients have antimitochondrial antibodies. PBC most often follows the diagnosis of SSc, but can be the presenting symptom.

IDIOPATHIC INFLAMMATORY MYOPATHIES

Polymyositis (PM), *dermatomyositis* (DM), *inclusion body myositis* (IBM), and *immune-mediated necrotizing myopathy* (IMNM) are the most common acquired inflammatory myopathies, characterized by progressive muscle weakness and elevated muscle enzymes, and some are associated with other organ system involvement. Each subtype also has unique clinical, histologic, and autoantibody features (Table 66.6 provides summary of these features).

In both PM and DM, other organ system involvement is common. Skin involvement is the most visible characteristic finding in DM, with classic findings that may include: heliotrope rash (erythema or violaceous changes on the upper eyelids), Gottron's papules (scaly erythematous patches) overlying the MCP and PIP joints, Gottron's sign (similar to Gottron's papules but located on the extensor surfaces of the knees and elbows), erythema or papules typically in a V shape and mantle distribution on the neck and chest, or scaly lesions in the scalp. "Mechanic's hands" (rough, scaly, cracked lesions in the palm or lateral aspects of the fingers), however, can be found in both DM and PM associated with antisynthetase syndrome. Otherwise, PM and IBM have no skin manifestations, whereas IMNM may have associated skin features if related to SSc or mixed connective tissue disease (MCTD). Both PM and DM may have pulmonary, cardiac, or gastrointestinal involvement (see below).

IBM, however, differs from PM/DM in that age of onset is older and the course is more indolent. Muscle involvement includes distal muscles more than proximal, facial muscles, often in an asymmetric pattern. Atrophy of quadriceps, forearm, or intrinsic hand muscles can be present. Creatine kinase (CK) is often only mildly elevated, and other organ system involvement is rare.

IMNM is characterized by severe proximal muscle weakness, sometimes accompanied by myalgias. IMNM can be idiopathic, associated with statin use, viral infections such as HIV or hepatitis C, scleroderma or MCTD, or malignancies such as adenocarcinoma of colon or lung cancers (both small and non–small cell). Symptom onset is usually subacute but can be acute, and CKs are highly elevated. Other organ systems are rarely involved except the subgroup associated with anti–signal recognition particles (SRPs). Those patients may have ILD, Raynaud's, or dysphagia. If the myositis is associated with connective tissue diseases such as scleroderma, then other organ system involvement can occur [75]. Diagnosis of this subgroup is based on characteristic histopathology and autoantibody profile (see below).

The diagnosis of PM/DM, IBM, and IMNM is based on characteristic clinical, electromyographic, histopathologic, and autoantibody profiles. Other causes of myopathy or myositis need to be excluded. Creatine kinase is elevated anywhere from 10 to 50 times normal, but rhabdomyolysis is rare. Electromyography will identify muscles involved and distinguish myopathic features from neurogenic causes, but it will not be able to differentiate the different types of inflammatory myopathies, or even from toxin-related causes or dystrophies. Muscle biopsy may not be required with classic DM features of skin lesions, proximal muscle weakness, and elevated CPKs. However, for any other presentation that is not classic for DM, a muscle biopsy is important to establish the diagnosis and exclude other causes of muscle weakness (including PM/IBM or IMNM). The biopsy should be taken from a muscle that is affected clinically, usually the quadriceps or deltoid. T2-weighted MRI with fat suppression is useful for identifying an actively inflamed muscle for biopsy. Histopathology of DM is characterized by vascular process with perifascicular atrophy because of inflammation of the perivascular areas, and deposition of aggregates of complement (membrane attack complex) on endothelial cell wall of endomysial. PM and

IBM biopsies, however, reveal inflammation of the perivascular areas and within the endomysium, that is, $CD8^+$ T cell dominant. Inflammatory cells are throughout the normal muscle fibers and fascicles. IBM also has characteristics of inflammatory cells in non-necrotic muscle fibers and presence of rimmed vacuoles, ragged fibers, and inclusion bodies on electron microscopy. In contrast, IMNM histology will reveal the same findings of necrosis as in PM, but only few inflammatory cell infiltrates in the muscle fibers. There may be presence of major histocompatibility complex (MHC) class I expression on noninvolved muscle fibers.

A number of myositis-specific antibodies and myositis-associated antibodies have been identified that correlate with specific clinical presentations and may help with diagnostic and prognostic information [76] Anti-Mi-2, found in up to 10% of patients with myositis, is associated with classic DM, and is a marker for a more favorable prognosis. The presence of anti–histidyl transfer RNA synthetase (anti-Jo-1) or antimelanoma differentiation–associated protein-5 (anti-MDA-5) antibodies is strongly associated with significant ILD (up to 70%) [76]. Antibodies against SRP occur in only 5% of myositis patients, but are associated with acute, severe myositis including IMNM with an overall poor prognosis. Anti–3-hydroxy-3-methylglutaryl-coenzyme A reductase is present among patients who had prior exposure to statins (although some have not), and,

TABLE 66.6

Features of Inflammatory Myopathies

	Polymyositis	Dermatomyositis	Inclusion Body Myositis	Immune-Mediated Necrotizing Myopathy
Mean age at onset	45	Childhood or 40	65	Adults
Sex (M:F)	1:2	1:2	2:1	Unknown
Mode of onset	Subacute over months	Subacute over months	Insidious over years	Acute or subacute
Distribution of muscle involvement	Proximal>>distal, symmetric	Proximal>>distal, symmetric	Variable; distal>proximal asymmetric, finger flexors, facial	Proximal>distal
Dermatologic findings (see text)	No	Yes	No	No[a]
Raynaud's	Yes	Yes	No	No[a]
Pulmonary disease	Yes	Yes	No	No[a] except those with anti-SRP
Cardiac disease	Yes, rare	Yes, rare	No	No[a]
Arthritis	Yes	Yes	No	No[a]
Gastrointestinal tract	Yes	Yes	Cricopharyngeal dysfunction	Dysphagia
Creatine kinase	Highly elevated	Highly elevated—classic DM Normal in amyopathic DM	Normal to mildly elevated (<10× normal)	Highly elevated
EMG/NCS	Myopathic features	Myopathic features	Myopathic features but also neurogenic changes	Myopathic features
Histopathology	Endomysial $CD8^+$ cells invading normal muscle fibers expressing MHC class I, no vascular inflammation or vacuoles	Perivascular, perifascicular, perimysial inflammatory infiltrates; late complements (C_{5-9} membrane attack complex); perifascicular atrophy	Similar to PM but also fiber size variability; ragged-red fibers; rimmed vacuoles and amyloid deposits; EM with tubulofilaments	Widespread myofibril necrosis without many inflammatory cells; MHC class I expression on normal muscle fibers
Antibodies	Anti-synthetase Ab such as Jo-1 (20%), U1-RNP (10%), PM-Scl (10%), SRP (<5%)	Anti-MDA-5[b]; Anti-Jo-1 (5%); Anti-Mi-2[c] (10%), anti-TIF-1[d]; anti-NXP-2[d]; U1-RNP (5%); anti-PM-Scl (0.5%)	Rare	Anti-SRP (15%); anti-HMGCR
Malignancy association	Yes (twofold increase)	Yes (sixfold increase)	No	Yes, associated with colon, lung Ca (small and non–small cell)
Response to therapy	Good	Good	Poor	Sometimes highly resistant

RNP, ribonuclear protein; Scl, scleroderma; SRP, signal recognition peptide; anti-MDA-5, antimelanoma differentiation–associated protein-5; anti-TIF-1γ, antitranscriptional intermediary factor 1γ; anti-NXP-2, anti-nuclear matrix protein 2; anti-HMGCR, anti-3-hydroxy-3-methylglutaryl-coenzyme A reductase.
[a]Unless related connective tissue disease such as systemic sclerosis, mixed connective disease.
[b]Associated with amyopathic DM or rapidly progressive interstitial lung disease.
[c]Associated with typical rash of DM.
[d]Cancer-associated DM.

despite discontinuation, continue to have severe IMNM. Antitranscriptional intermediary factor 1γ (anti-TIF-1γ) is seen with cancer-associated DM. Table 66.6 summarizes the various clinical, laboratory, histopathologic, and serologic features of these idiopathic inflammatory myopathies.

Inflammatory myositis is also associated with inborn errors of metabolism, lipid storage disease, and mitochondrial myopathies, but these will not be discussed here. Numerous drugs can cause myopathy or myositis that is sometimes difficult to distinguish from inflammatory myositis. These drugs include lipid-lowering agents, glucocorticoids, antipsychotics, antimalarials, colchicine, nucleoside reverse transcriptase inhibitors, alcohol, and cocaine. Bacterial infections (*S. aureus*, *Streptococcus pyogenes*, *Clostridium perfringens*, *Borrelia burgdorferi*) and viruses (coxsackievirus A and B, echovirus, influenza A and B, adenovirus 2 and 21, hepatitis B and C, and HIV) can cause a myopathy that may be confused with PM or DM. Parasites including trichinosis, toxoplasmosis, cysticercosis, toxocariasis, and amebiasis may all cause myositis. Muscular dystrophies, neuropathic disease, and metabolic/endocrine diseases also need to be excluded in patients with muscle weakness.

PM and DM are primarily disorders of skeletal muscle, but involvement of the pulmonary, cardiac, articular, gastrointestinal, or vascular systems sometimes leads to catastrophic illness requiring support in an ICU. Moreover, organ dysfunction may occur among patients with overlap syndromes. Respiratory failure, cardiac abnormalities, or comorbidities related to immunosuppression are the most common reasons for ICU admission. A complete discussion of the presentation, diagnosis, management, and differential diagnosis is beyond the scope of this chapter, but excellent reviews exist [76,77].

Pulmonary Involvement

Lung disease in PM/DM patients is common (10% to 40% of patients; see Table 66.1) and includes (a) respiratory insufficiency because of weakness of intercostal or diaphragmatic muscles; (b) aspiration pneumonia; (c) pneumonia from either bacterial, viral, or opportunistic infection; and (d) ILD. Pulmonary vasculitis, pleuritis, pulmonary edema, alveolar hemorrhage, secondary pulmonary hypertension, and OP have also been reported but are uncommon. Dyspnea, cough, and chest pain are the usual symptoms.

Respiratory failure from intercostal muscle weakness or diaphragmatic dysfunction occurs among 7% of PM/DM patients. Thus, pulmonary mechanics (spirometry, inspiratory force) should be evaluated when respiratory symptoms develop. Serial measurements often predict impending respiratory failure that might necessitate intubation and mechanical ventilation. Management of respiratory failure resulting from muscle weakness is supportive (oxygen, mechanical ventilation) and accompanied by therapy directed at the underlying myositis (see Chapter 165).

Bronchopneumonia occurs among up to 24% of PM/DM patients. Contributing factors include pharyngeal incompetence and poor airway protection with subsequent aspiration, iatrogenic immunosuppression, and often a weakened cough. Infectious agents include virulent bacteria and opportunistic organisms. Myositis occurring in the setting of acquired immunodeficiency further expands the possible spectrum of infectious agents. Hence, respiratory symptoms should be evaluated aggressively with chest radiographs and routine and specialized microbiologic techniques (culture for bacteria, mycobacteria, fungi, and smears for *Pneumocystis jiroveci*).

The most common type of parenchymal lung disease in PM/DM is ILD, with a prevalence of 20% to 60%. Patients develop progressive dyspnea with or without a nonproductive cough and bibasilar rales. Pulmonary function tests reveal decreased lung volumes and reduced diffusing capacity. Ground glass opacities, reticulonodular infiltrates, or patchy consolidations may be present on HRCT scans and suggest possible diagnoses. However, histopathology is necessary to diagnose NSIP, UIP, OP, or, less commonly, acute interstitial pneumonia. Patients with Jo-1 and other anti-aminoacyl-tRNA synthetase antibodies have a high incidence of ILD and also described as antisynthetase syndrome that is characterized by prominent arthritis, fever, RP, and mechanic's hands. Fulminant ILD has occurred in amyopathic DM without anti-Jo antibodies but rather with anti-MDA-5.

Myocardial Involvement

Cardiac and pulmonary diseases along with cancer are the main prognostic factors for PM/DM mortality [78]. Up to 70% of patients have cardiac abnormalities on noninvasive testing, but clinically, only less than 10% are symptomatic. However, it is estimated that cardiac disease is the cause of 10% to 20% of deaths in patients with myositis [79]. Myocarditis may manifest as heart failure, arrhythmias, cardiac arrest, or myocardial infarction. It is difficult to diagnose because levels of creatine kinase and muscle brain fractions are elevated as a result of skeletal muscle inflammation. Cardiac troponin I is the most specific marker for myocardial involvement. Cardiac imaging techniques (echocardiogram, gallium citrate- or indium-labeled antimyosin antibody detection, and scintigraphic studies) are insensitive and nonspecific for detecting myocardial involvement. Contrast-enhanced cardiac MRI provides a more sensitive way to differentiate myocarditis from myocardial ischemia.

The extent to which any cardiac abnormality is iatrogenic or arises as a complication of the disease is unclear. For example, steroid therapy accelerates atherosclerosis and may exacerbate hypertension, diabetes mellitus, and electrolyte disturbances. Similarly, hypoxia from pulmonary involvement contributes to arrhythmias, axis shifts, and strain patterns on ECG. However, DM and PM patients have three to fourfold higher risk for myocardial infarction than controls matched for age and other risk factors.

Other Organ System Involvement

The major gastrointestinal manifestation of inflammatory myopathies is weakness of the upper pharyngeal striated muscles, resulting in dysphonia, dysphagia, and regurgitation of fluids. Smooth muscle involvement of the distal esophagus is rare, and intestinal vasculitis, commonly seen in childhood DM, is also uncommon.

Renal failure and its attendant metabolic abnormalities are the result of rhabdomyolysis, myoglobinemia, and subsequent myoglobinuria. Myoglobinuric renal failure is rare, but tends to occur in patients with acute or hyperacute presentations as a result of widespread muscle necrosis and release of sarcoplasmic materials, including myoglobin. Therapy is directed toward the underlying muscle disease while maintaining an adequate urinary output.

Malignancy

The relationship of PM/DM to malignancy has been established by multiple epidemiologic studies from different countries. A meta-analysis recently of all studies up to 2013 confirmed that DM is associated with the highest risk with pooled rate ratio (RR) of 5.5, while PM RR was around 1.6 [80]. The diagnosis of malignancy may precede, be concurrent with, or follow the onset of myositis. The risk decreases with time, but even at 5 years, the risk is still measurable. Identified risk factors include later age at diagnosis, cutaneous necrosis and leukocytoclastic vasculitis, capillary damage on muscle biopsy, and dysphagia. Malignancies commonly associated with DM/PM include breast, ovarian, lung, colon, gastric, pancreatic, nasopharyngeal, and non-Hodgkin's lymphoma. Two myositis-specific antibodies have been associated with malignancy: anti-TIF-1γ and anti-nuclear matrix protein 2 (anti-NXP-2).

Treatment

High-dose corticosteroids are the first-line therapy for PM/DM and IMNM, although there are no published clinical trials to support this approach at this time. Initial treatment is usually with prednisone 1 to 1.5 mg/kg/d for 6 to 8 weeks, then tapered based on clinical response. In more severe cases (dysphagia, alveolitis, myocarditis, or impending respiratory failure from muscle weakness), IV methylprednisolone may be given at a dose of 1,000 mg daily for 3 days followed by the usual high-dose oral corticosteroid regimen. In steroid-responsive patients, a steroid-sparing agent (methotrexate, AZA, MMF, cyclophosphamide, or calcineurin inhibitors) may be added to facilitate steroid tapering, but efficacy is based on small case series or clinical experience as no randomized clinical trials have been done. Therapy for progressive or severe ILD usually requires the use of corticosteroids and cyclophosphamide. Cyclosporine or tacrolimus can be used for refractory cases [81]. Although a placebo-controlled trial of RTX, given either early or late to PM or DM patients unresponsive to steroids or alternative agents, did not show statistically significant differences of disease response, nearly 80% of all patients had improvement and suggested efficacy [81]. IVIG is recommended for patients with severe weakness refractory to steroids based on proven efficacy in a randomized, placebo-controlled trial in patients with DM [82].

Therapy for IBM is more difficult because it responds to steroids poorly and slowly. IVIG and methotrexate have not been effective in double-blind, placebo-controlled trials. Current recommendations include a trial of steroids if muscle biopsies reveal significant inflammation and physical therapy to help maintain strength and function.

Advances in management of rheumatologic diseases, based on randomized controlled trials or meta-analysis of published studies, are summarized in Table 66.7.

TABLE 66.7

Management of Rheumatic Diseases: Available Trials and Strength of Evidence

	Treatment recommendations	Strength of evidence[a]
SLE: LN	MMF is as effective as IVCY in induction of remission of Class III and IV LN without differences in toxicity; MMF more effective than IVCY in patients of Hispanic or African origin [20]	A
	Equivalency of MMF up to 3 g/d compared to monthly IVCY as induction therapy for Class III, IV, or V LN [20]	A
	Superiority of MMF to AZA in preventing renal relapse and maintaining response [23]	A
	Low-dose IVCY is equivalent to high-dose IVCY efficacy for induction, sustained stabilization, toxicity profile over 10 years in LN (Class III, IV, V) [22]	A
	MMF is equivalent to IVCY in induction of remission of Class V LN [24]	A
	Additional renal benefit in patients receiving MMF and belimumab compared to those receiving placebo [26]	B
SLE: NSPLE	IVCY is more effective than pulse methylprednisolone alone for severe NPSLE [29]	A
SLE: thrombocytopenia	Rituximab is effective for idiopathic thrombocytopenia in conjunction with or after failure to respond to glucocorticoid [43]	A
APS	High-intensity warfarin therapy is not superior to moderate-intensity warfarin therapy in patients with APS [50]	B
	Asymptomatic, persistently aPL-positive individuals do not benefit from low-dose aspirin for primary thrombosis prophylaxis [51]	B
SSc: RP	Intravenous prostanoids are effective in healing digital ulcers in patients with SSc RP [59,83]	A
	Bosentan is effective in preventing new digital ulcers in patients with SSc RP [57]	A
	Sildenafil reduces the frequency and severity of attacks and promotes healing of digital ulcers in SSc RP [56]	B
SSc: interstitial lung disease	Both IVCY and oral CY provide modest improvement in SSc lung function, dyspnea, and skin scores compared to placebo [61,64]	A
Inflammatory muscle disease	Rituximab may provide improvement and suggested efficacy in DM/PM patients who failed prednisone and other drugs [81]	A
	Efficacy of IVIG in patients with dermatomyositis [82]	A

Level A recommendation is based on consistent and good-quality patient-oriented evidence; *Level B* recommendation is based on inconsistent or limited-quality patient-oriented evidence.

aPL, antiphospholipid antibody; APS, antiphospholipid syndrome; AZA, azathioprine; IVCY, intravenous cyclophosphamide; LN, lupus nephritis; MMF, mycophenolate mofetil; NSPLE, neuropsychiatric; RP, Raynaud's phenomena; SLE, systemic lupus erythematosus; SSc, systemic sclerosis.

[a]*Strength of Evidence* (based on Ebell MH, Siwek J, Weiss BD, et al: Strength of Recommendation Taxonomy (SORT): A patient-centered approach to grading evidence in the medical literature. *Am Fam Physician* 69:548–556, 2004).

References

1. Khanna D, Khanna PP, Fitzgerald JD, et al: 2012 American college of rheumatology guidelines for management of gout. Part 2: Therapy and antiinflammatory prophylaxis of acute gouty arthritis. *Arthritis Care Res* 64(10):1447–1461, 2012
2. Terkeltaub RA, Furst DE, Bennett K, et al: High versus low dosing of oral colchicine for early acute gout flare: twenty-four-hour outcome of the first multicenter, randomized, double-blind, placebo-controlled, parallel-group, dose-comparison colchicine study. *Arthritis Rheum* 62(4):1060–1068, 2010.
3. Terkeltaub RA: Colchicine update: 2008. *Semin Arthritis Rheum* 38(6):411–419, 2009.
4. Mathews CJ, Weston VC, Jones A, et al: Bacterial septic arthritis in adults. *Lancet* 375(9717):846–855, 2010.
5. Margaretten ME, Kohlwes J, Moore D, et al: Does this adult patient have septic arthritis? *JAMA* 297(13):1478–1488, 2007.
6. Del Pozo JL, Patel R: Clinical practice. infection associated with prosthetic joints. *N Engl J Med* 361(8):787–794, 2009.
7. Muller M, Morawietz L, Hasart O, et al: Diagnosis of periprosthetic infection following total hip arthroplasty—evaluation of the diagnostic values of pre- and intraoperative parameters and the associated strategy to preoperatively select patients with a high probability of joint infection. *J Orthop Surg Res* 3:31-799X-3-31, 2008.
8. Marculescu CE, Berbari EF, Hanssen AD, et al: Outcome of prosthetic joint infections treated with debridement and retention of components. *Clin Infect Dis* 42(4):471–478, 2006.
9. Balbir-Gurman A, Yigla M, Nahir AM, et al: Rheumatoid pleural effusion. *Semin Arthritis Rheum* 35(6):368–378, 2006.
10. Olson AL, Swigris JJ, Sprunger DB, et al: Rheumatoid arthritis-interstitial lung disease-associated mortality. *Am J Respir Crit Care Med* 183(3):372–378, 2011.
11. Kelly CA, Saravanan V, Nisar M, et al: Rheumatoid arthritis-related interstitial lung disease: associations, prognostic factors and physiological and radiological characteristics—a large multicentre UK study. *Rheumatology (Oxford)* 53(9):1676–1682, 2014.
12. Iqbal K, Kelly C: Treatment of rheumatoid arthritis-associated interstitial lung disease: a perspective review. *Ther Adv Musculoskelet Dis* 7(6):247–267, 2015.
13. Devouassoux G, Cottin V, Lioté H, et al: Characterisation of severe obliterative bronchiolitis in rheumatoid arthritis. *Eur Respir J* 33(5):1053–1061, 2009. doi:10.1183/09031936.00091608.
14. Makol A, Crowson CS, Wetter DA, et al: Vasculitis associated with rheumatoid arthritis: a case–control study. *Rheumatology* 53(5):890–899, 2014.
15. Hochberg MC: Updating the American college of rheumatology revised criteria for the classification of systemic lupus erythematosus. *Arthritis Rheum* 40(9):1725, 1997.
16. Quintero OL, Rojas-Villarraga A, Mantilla RD, et al: Autoimmune diseases in the intensive care unit. an update. *Autoimmun Rev* 12(3):380–395, 2013.
17. Hahn BH: Belimumab for systemic lupus erythematosus. *N Engl J Med* 368(16):1528–1535, 2013.
18. Contreras G, Mattiazzi A, Guerra G, et al: Recurrence of lupus nephritis after kidney transplantation. *J Am Soc Nephrol* 21(7):1200–1207, 2010.
19. Weening JJ, D'Agati VD, Schwartz MM, et al: The classification of glomerulonephritis in systemic lupus erythematosus revisited. *Kidney Int* 65(2):521–530, 2004.
20. Appel GB, Contreras G, Dooley MA, et al: Mycophenolate mofetil versus cyclophosphamide for induction treatment of lupus nephritis. *J Am Soc Nephrol* 20(5):1103–1112, 2009.
21. Houssiau FA, Vasconcelos C, D'Cruz D, et al: Immunosuppressive therapy in lupus nephritis: The euro-lupus nephritis trial, a randomized trial of low-dose versus high-dose intravenous cyclophosphamide. *Arthritis Rheum* 46(8):2121–2131, 2002.
22. Houssiau FA, Vasconcelos C, D'Cruz D, et al: The 10-year follow-up data of the euro-lupus nephritis trial comparing low-dose and high-dose intravenous cyclophosphamide. *Ann Rheum Dis* 69(1):61–64, 2010.
23. Dooley MA, Jayne D, Ginzler EM, et al: Mycophenolate versus azathioprine as maintenance therapy for lupus nephritis. *N Engl J Med* 365(20):1886–1895, 2011.
24. Radhakrishnan J, Moutzouris DA, Ginzler EM, et al: Mycophenolate mofetil and intravenous cyclophosphamide are similar as induction therapy for class V lupus nephritis. *Kidney Int* 77(2):152–160, 2010.
25. Merrill JT, Neuwelt CM, Wallace DJ, et al: Efficacy and safety of rituximab in moderately-to-severely active systemic lupus erythematosus: the randomized, double-blind, phase II/III systemic lupus erythematosus evaluation of rituximab trial. *Arthritis Rheum* 62(1):222–233, 2010.
26. Dooley M, Houssiau F, Aranow C, et al: Effect of belimumab treatment on renal outcomes: results from the phase 3 belimumab clinical trials in patients with SLE. *Lupus* 22(1):63–72, 2013.
27. The American college of rheumatology nomenclature and case definitions for neuropsychiatric lupus syndromes. *Arthritis Rheum* 42(4):599–608, 1999.
28. Hanly JG: Neuropsychiatric lupus. *Rheum Dis Clin North Am* 31(2):273–298, vi, 2005.
29. Fernandes Moca Trevisani V, Castro AA, Ferreira Neves Neto J, et al: Cyclophosphamide versus methylprednisolone for treating neuropsychiatric involvement in systemic lupus erythematosus. *Cochrane Database Syst Rev* (2):CD002265, 2013.
30. Bertoli AM, Vila LM, Apte M, et al: Systemic lupus erythematosus in a multiethnic US cohort LUMINA XLVIII: factors predictive of pulmonary damage. *Lupus* 16(6):410–417, 2007.
31. Pego-Reigosa JM, Medeiros DA, Isenberg DA: Respiratory manifestations of systemic lupus erythematosus: old and new concepts. *Best Pract Res Clin Rheumatol* 23(4):469–480, 2009.
32. Prabu A, Patel K, Yee CS, et al: Prevalence and risk factors for pulmonary arterial hypertension in patients with lupus. *Rheumatology (Oxford)* 48(12):1506–1511, 2009.
33. Jais X, Launay D, Yaici A, et al: Immunosuppressive therapy in lupus- and mixed connective tissue disease-associated pulmonary arterial hypertension: a retrospective analysis of twenty-three cases. *Arthritis Rheum* 58(2):521–531, 2008.
34. Bernatsky S, Boivin JF, Joseph L, et al: Mortality in systemic lupus erythematosus. *Arthritis Rheum* 54(8):2550–2557, 2006.
35. Miner JJ, Kim AH: Cardiac manifestations of systemic lupus erythematosus. *Rheum Dis Clin North Am* 40(1):51–60, 2014.
36. Roldan CA, Qualls CR, Sopko KS, et al: Transthoracic versus transesophageal echocardiography for detection of libman-sacks endocarditis: a randomized controlled study. *J Rheumatol* 35(2):224–229, 2008.
37. Zuily S, Regnault V, Selton-Suty C, et al: Increased risk for heart valve disease associated with antiphospholipid antibodies in patients with systemic lupus erythematosus: meta-analysis of echocardiographic studies. *Circulation* 124(2):215–224, 2011.
38. Apte M, McGwin G Jr, Vilá LM, et al: Associated factors and impact of myocarditis in patients with SLE from LUMINA, a multiethnic US cohort. *Rheumatology (Oxford)* 47(3):362–367, 2008.
39. Schoenfeld SR, Kasturi S, Costenbader KH: The epidemiology of atherosclerotic cardiovascular disease among patients with SLE: a systematic review. *Semin Arthritis Rheum* 43(1):77–95, 2013.
40. Newman K, Owlia MB, El-Hemaidi I, et al: Management of immune cytopenias in patients with systemic lupus erythematosus—old and new. *Autoimmun Rev* 12(7):784–791, 2013.
41. Letchumanan P, Thumboo J: Danazol in the treatment of systemic lupus erythematosus: a qualitative systematic review. *Semin Arthritis Rheum* 40(4):298–306, 2011.
42. You YN, Tefferi A, Nagorney DM: Outcome of splenectomy for thrombocytopenia associated with systemic lupus erythematosus. *Ann Surg* 240(2):286–292, 2004.
43. Chugh S, Darvish-Kazem S, Lim W, et al: Rituximab plus standard of care for treatment of primary immune thrombocytopenia: a systematic review and meta-analysis. *Lancet Haematol* 2(2):e75–e81, 2015.
44. Xu D, Yang H, Lai CC, et al: Clinical analysis of systemic lupus erythematosus with gastrointestinal manifestations. *Lupus* 19(7):866–869, 2010.
45. Sultan SM, Ioannou Y, Isenberg DA: A review of gastrointestinal manifestations of systemic lupus erythematosus. *Rheumatology (Oxford)* 38(10):917–932, 1999.
46. Gronhagen CM, Fored CM, Linder M, et al: Subacute cutaneous lupus erythematosus and its association with drugs: a population-based matched case-control study of 234 patients in sweden. *Br J Dermatol* 167(2):296–305, 2012.
47. D'Cruz D: Renal manifestations of the antiphospholipid syndrome. *Curr Rheumatol Rep* 11(1):52–60, 2009.
48. Cervera R, Font J, Gomez-Puerta JA, et al: Validation of the preliminary criteria for the classification of catastrophic antiphospholipid syndrome. *Ann Rheum Dis* 64(8):1205–1209, 2005.
49. Bucciarelli S, Espinosa G, Cervera R, et al: Mortality in the catastrophic antiphospholipid syndrome: causes of death and prognostic factors in a series of 250 patients. *Arthritis Rheum* 54(8):2568–2576, 2006.
50. Crowther MA, Ginsberg JS, Julian J, et al: A comparison of two intensities of warfarin for the prevention of recurrent thrombosis in patients with the antiphospholipid antibody syndrome. *N Engl J Med* 349(12):1133–1138, 2003.
51. Cervera R, Rodriguez-Pinto I, Colafrancesco S, et al: 14th international congress on antiphospholipid antibodies task force report on catastrophic antiphospholipid syndrome. *Autoimmun Rev* 13(7):699–707, 2014.
52. Erkan D, Harrison MJ, Levy R, et al: Aspirin for primary thrombosis prevention in the antiphospholipid syndrome: a randomized, double-blind, placebo-controlled trial in asymptomatic antiphospholipid antibody-positive individuals. *Arthritis Rheum* 56(7):2382–2391, 2007.
53. Berman H, Rodriguez-Pinto I, Cervera R, et al: Rituximab use in the catastrophic antiphospholipid syndrome: descriptive analysis of the CAPS registry patients receiving rituximab. *Autoimmun Rev* 12(11):1085–1090, 2013.
54. Shapira I, Andrade D, Allen SL, et al: Brief report: induction of sustained remission in recurrent catastrophic antiphospholipid syndrome via inhibition of terminal complement with eculizumab. *Arthritis Rheum* 64(8):2719–2723, 2012.
55. Kowal-Bielecka O, Landewe R, Avouac J, et al: EULAR recommendations for the treatment of systemic sclerosis: a report from the EULAR scleroderma trials and research group (EUSTAR). *Ann Rheum Dis* 68(5):620–628, 2009.
56. Roustit M, Blaise S, Allanore Y, et al: Phosphodiesterase-5 inhibitors for the treatment of secondary Raynaud's phenomenon: systematic review and meta-analysis of randomised trials. *Ann Rheum Dis* 72(10):1696–1699, 2013.
57. Matucci-Cerinic M, Denton CP, Furst DE, et al: Bosentan treatment of digital ulcers related to systemic sclerosis: results from the RAPIDS-2 randomised, double-blind, placebo-controlled trial. *Ann Rheum Dis* 70(1):32–38, 2011.
58. Iorio ML, Masden DL, Higgins JP: Botulinum toxin A treatment of Raynaud's phenomenon: a review. *Semin Arthritis Rheum* 41(4):599–603, 2012.
59. Simms R, Farber H, Kissin E, et al: Intravenous epoprostenol for severe digital ischemia in scleroderma. *Arthritis Rheum* 50[Suppl 9]:1702, 2004.
60. White B: Interstitial lung disease in scleroderma. *Rheum Dis Clin North Am* 29(2):371–390, 2003.
61. Clements PJ, Tashkin DP, Roth M, et al: The scleroderma lung study II (SLS II) shows that both oral cyclophosphamide (CYC) and mycophenolate mofetil

(MMF) are efficacious in treating progressive interstitial lung disease (ILD) in patients with systemic sclerosis (SSC) [abstract]. *Arthritis Rheumatol* 67[Suppl 10], 2015.
62. Goh NS, Desai SR, Veeraraghavan S, et al: Interstitial lung disease in systemic sclerosis: a simple staging system. *Am J Respir Crit Care Med* 177(11):1248–1254, 2008.
63. Tashkin DP, Elashoff R, Clements PJ, et al: Cyclophosphamide versus placebo in scleroderma lung disease. *N Engl J Med* 354(25):2655–2666, 2006.
64. Hoyles RK, Ellis RW, Wellsbury J, et al: A multicenter, prospective, randomized, double-blind, placebo-controlled trial of corticosteroids and intravenous cyclophosphamide followed by oral azathioprine for the treatment of pulmonary fibrosis in scleroderma. *Arthritis Rheum* 54(12):3962–3970, 2006.
65. Daoussis D, Liossis SN, Tsamandas AC, et al: Experience with rituximab in scleroderma: results from a 1-year, proof-of-principle study. *Rheumatology (Oxford)* 49(2):271–280, 2010.
66. Nordin A, Jensen-Urstad K, Bjornadal L, et al: Ischemic arterial events and atherosclerosis in patients with systemic sclerosis: a population-based case-control study. *Arthritis Res Ther* 15(4):R87, 2013.
67. Ferri C, Giuggioli D, Sebastiani M, et al: Heart involvement and systemic sclerosis. *Lupus* 14(9):702–707, 2005.
68. Hudson M: Scleroderma renal crisis. *Curr Opin Rheumatol* 2015;27(6):549–554, 2005.
69. Hudson M, Baron M, Tatibouet S, et al: Exposure to ACE inhibitors prior to the onset of scleroderma renal crisis-results from the international scleroderma renal crisis survey. *Semin Arthritis Rheum* 43(5):666–672, 2014.
70. Ebert EC: Gastric and enteric involvement in progressive systemic sclerosis. *J Clin Gastroenterol* 42(1):5–12, 2008.
71. Papachristos DA, Nikpour M, Hair C, et al: Intravenous cyclophosphamide as a therapeutic option for severe refractory gastric antral vascular ectasia in systemic sclerosis. *Intern Med J* 45(10):1077–1081, 2015.
72. Perlemuter G, Cacoub P, Chaussade S, et al: Octreotide treatment of chronic intestinal pseudoobstruction secondary to connective tissue diseases. *Arthritis Rheum* 42(7):1545–1549, 1999.
73. Boeckxstaens GE, Bartelsman JF, Lauwers L, et al: Treatment of GI dysmotility in scleroderma with the new enterokinetic agent prucalopride. *Am J Gastroenterol* 97(1):194–197, 2002.
74. Jaovisidha K, Csuka ME, Almagro UA, et al: Severe gastrointestinal involvement in systemic sclerosis: report of five cases and review of the literature. *Semin Arthritis Rheum* 34(4):689–702, 2005.
75. Basharat P, Christopher-Stine L: Immune-mediated necrotizing myopathy: update on diagnosis and management. *Curr Rheumatol Rep* 17(12):72, 2015.
76. Dalakas MC: Inflammatory muscle diseases. *N Engl J Med* 372(18):1734–1747, 2015.
77. Lazarou IN, Guerne PA: Classification, diagnosis, and management of idiopathic inflammatory myopathies. *J Rheumatol* 40(5):550–564, 2013.
78. Marie I: Morbidity and mortality in adult polymyositis and dermatomyositis. *Curr Rheumatol Rep* 14(3):275–285, 2012.
79. Danieli MG, Gelardi C, Guerra F, et al: Cardiac involvement in polymyositis and dermatomyositis. *Autoimmun Rev* 15(5):462–465, 2016.
80. Yang Z, Lin F, Qin B, et al: Polymyositis/dermatomyositis and malignancy risk: a metaanalysis study. *J Rheumatol* 42(2):282–291, 2015.
81. Oddis CV, Reed AM, Aggarwal R, et al: Rituximab in the treatment of refractory adult and juvenile dermatomyositis and adult polymyositis: a randomized, placebo-phase trial. *Arthritis Rheum* 65(2):314–324, 2013.
82. Dalakas MC, Illa I, Dambrosia JM, et al: A controlled trial of high-dose intravenous immune globulin infusions as treatment for dermatomyositis. *N Engl J Med* 329(27):1993–2000, 1993.
83. Wigley FM, Wise RA, Seibold JR, et al: Intravenous iloprost infusion in patients with Raynaud's phenomenon secondary to systemic sclerosis. A multicenter, placebo-controlled, double-blind study. *Ann Intern Med* 120(3):199–206, 1994.

Chapter 67 ■ Vasculitis in the Intensive Care Unit

PAUL F. DELLARIPA • DONOUGH HOWARD

The vasculitides are a group of disorders characterized by the presence of destructive inflammation in vessel walls [1–4]. The possibility of systemic vasculitis should be considered for a patient with systemic complaints and dysfunction of multiple organ systems, frequently in the context of constitutional symptoms such as fever, malaise, and weight loss (Table 67.1). Patients hospitalized in the intensive care unit (ICU) may present with symptoms related to the clinical features associated with a specific vasculitis but may also present with a known diagnosis of vasculitis and complications of treatment, most notably infection.

Vasculitic syndromes typically are classified by the size of vessel involved. Although there may be an overlap in the vessel size, diseases may affect predominately large vessels (Takayasu's arteritis), medium-size arteries (such as polyarteritis nodosa (PAN) and central nervous system [CNS] vasculitis), and small vessels (granulomatosis with polyangiitis [GPA], formerly known as Wegener's granulomatosis; microscopic polyangiitis; eosinophilic granulomatosis with polyangiitis [EGPA], also known as Churg–Strauss syndrome; cryoglobulinemia; and drug-induced vasculitis). These particular vasculitides are the focus of this chapter. For a more general discussion of vasculitis, other references are noted [1–4].

Disorders not discussed but that may simulate presentation of vasculitis include embolism due to endocarditis; cardiac myxoma; hypercoagulable states including the antiphospholipid antibody syndrome, hyperviscosity syndromes, chronic ergotism, radiation arteriopathy; and, less commonly, Ehlers–Danlos syndrome, neurofibromatosis, Sweet's syndrome, pseudoxanthoma elasticum, and Köhlmeier–Danlos diseases [5,6].

POLYARTERITIS NODOSA

PAN is a systemic necrotizing arteritis involving predominately medium-size vessels, although sometimes affecting smaller vessels. Vasculitic lesions characteristically occur at the bifurcations or branches of vessels and are often segmental. Almost any organ can be involved, but frequently the skin, peripheral nerves, kidneys, gastrointestinal (GI) tract, and joints are the principal organs affected [7].

Clinical manifestations include malaise; weight loss; fevers, abdominal or lower-extremity pain; myalgias; or arthralgias. Clinical parameters include hypertension and azotemia with proteinuria but rarely glomerulonephritis. Peripheral neuropathy occurs in up to 60% of cases, usually involving a mixed sensorimotor and mononeuritis multiplex [8]. Sudden-onset paresthesias associated with motor deficits are common manifestations. CNS involvement, including seizures, focal events, and altered mental status, are less common [9]. Musculoskeletal symptoms including arthralgias (50%), and less frequently, arthritis can occur [7]. Vasculitis of skeletal muscles may cause severe myalgias, and muscle biopsy can be useful diagnostically [10]. Abdominal pain may have a variety of causes, including intestinal angina; mesenteric thrombosis; and localized gallbladder or liver disease. Acute GI bleeding, perforation, and infarction are rare but are associated with a high mortality if the diagnosis is not established promptly [11]. Cardiac involvement, observed in nearly 60% of autopsy series, is often clinically silent and includes congestive heart failure, pericarditis, myocardial infarctions, and conduction abnormalities [12,13]. Cutaneous lesions include nonspecific palpable purpura, livedo reticularis, tender nodular lesions, digital infarcts, and ulcers [14]. Arteritis of the eye, testes, pancreas, ovaries, breasts, and involvement of the temporal arteries may develop rarely.

The pathogenesis of polyarteritis is unknown. Hepatitis B surface antigen has been found in a minority of patients with PAN. The presence of circulating immune complexes of hepatitis B surface antigen and deposition of surface antigen and immunoglobulin in vessel walls has suggested that immune mechanisms may play a role in some forms of polyarteritis [15,16]. Hepatitis C has

TABLE 67.1

Notable Physical Signs, Symptoms, and Laboratory Features of Different Vasculitic Syndromes

Constitutional Symptoms (GPA, MPA, EGPA, BS, TA, PAN, GCA)	Pulmonary infiltrates/nodules (GPA, MPA, EGPA)
Sinusitis/epistaxis (GPA, MPA, EGPA)	Pulmonary hemorrhage (GPA, MPA, rarely EGPA, BS, Cryo)
Cough, hemoptysis (GPA, MPA, EGPA, rarely Cryo)	Subglottic stenosis (GPAG)
Otitis/hearing loss (GPA)	Cardiac involvement (EGPA, PAN, GPA, TA)
Ocular involvement (GPA, BS, GCA, TA)	Mononeuritis (GPA, PAN, MPA, Cryo)
Cutaneous lesions (GPA, PAN, MPA, Cryo, EGPA, BS)	Glomerulonephritis (GPA, MPA, rarely Cryo)
Claudication (TA, GCA)	Hypertension (PAN, TA)
Arthritis/arthralgia (GPA, EGPA, MPA, Cryo, PAN)	ANCA positivity (GPA, MPA, EGPA)
Abdominal pain/GI bleeding (PAN, CSS, BS, MPA)	Angiographic abnormalities (PAN, TA)

ANCA, antineutrophil cytoplasmic antibody; BS, Behcet's syndrome; CSS, Churg–Strauss syndrome; Cryo, cryoglobulinemia; EGPA, eosinophilic granulomatosis with polyangiitis; GCA, giant cell arteritis; MPA, microscopic polyangiitis; PAN, polyarteritis nodosa; TA, Takayasu's arteritis; GPA, granulomatosis with polyangiitis.

rarely been associated with PAN [17]. Pathologically, fibrinoid necrosis and pleomorphic cellular infiltration, predominantly with lymphocytes, macrophages, and varying degrees of polymorphonuclear leukocytes involve the entire wall of small and medium muscular arteries. Thromboses and aneurysms can be found in lesions [18]. Laboratory abnormalities of PAN usually include elevated sedimentation rate, elevated C-reactive protein (CRP), and thrombocytosis. Antineutrophil cytoplasmic antibody (ANCA), antinuclear antibody (ANA), and rheumatoid factor are not typically present in PAN. Mesenteric angiography often shows evidence of aneurysms including the renal, hepatic, and mesenteric arteries, and areas of arterial stenosis alternating with normal or dilated vessels [18]. Sural nerve biopsies are easily accessible sources of nerve tissue when a mononeuritis is present, although the location of biopsy may be guided by electromyography.

Although there is no consensus for treatment of PAN, administration of corticosteroids at 1 mg/kg/d orally is indicated in nearly all cases where there is moderate to severe disease which is defined as the presence of active renal, GI, neurologic, or cardiac disease. In fulminant disease, daily intravenous (IV) methylprednisolone, 1 g/day for 3 days, is reasonable followed by daily oral or intravenous corticosteroids. In the presence of GI involvement, intravenous dosing may need to be continued especially for life-threatening cases. The use of a second drug is guided by the severity of presentation and if there is failure to respond to steroids alone. One prospective trial amongst several retrospective cohorts suggests that those with more severe illness benefit from the use of cyclophosphamide in combination with corticosteroids [19]. Cyclophosphamide may be given orally, usually 2 mg/kg/d, though adjustment should be made for renal failure (Table 67.2), or by intravenous dosing of 500 to 1,000 mg/m^2 monthly (see Table 67.3 on Immunomodulation), or using the IV regimen similar to treatment of GPA (see below). Plasmapheresis in combination with antiviral therapy may be beneficial in hepatitis B-associated PAN [20,21].

TABLE 67.2

Dosage Adjustments of Oral Cyclophosphamide with Renal Impairment

Creatinine clearance (mL/min)	Oral cyclophosphamide dose (mg/kg/d)
>100	2.0
50–99	1.5
25–49	1.2
15–24	1.0
<15 or on dialysis	0.8

From WGET Research Group: Design of the Wegener's Granulomatosis Etanercept Trial (WGET). *Control Clin Trials* 23(4):450–468, 2002, with permission.

A variety of drugs, viral infections, connective tissue diseases such as rheumatoid arthritis, and underlying malignancies may cause a necrotizing angiitis that may be indistinguishable from polyarteritis [22–27].

MICROSCOPIC POLYANGIITIS

Microscopic polyangiitis is a necrotizing vasculitis that involves small vessels, including arterioles, capillaries, and venules. Clinical presentations may involve concomitant capillaritis with or without alveolar hemorrhage and rapidly progressive glomerulonephritis, the so-called pulmonary renal syndrome, although more indolent and slower presentations have been described. Glomerulonephritis occurs in nearly all cases, and pulmonary involvement ranging from cough and dyspnea to frank hemoptysis occurs in up to 30% of cases. Neuropathy and cutaneous vasculitis occur in up to 50% of cases. ANCA is found in about 75% of cases, mostly specific for myeloperoxidase (MPO), though occasionally ANCA proteinase 3 (PR3) has been described [14,26,27].

Diagnosis is typically made with a biopsy of lung, kidney, skin, or nerve in conjunction with a positive ANCA result. Most clinical trials for treatment of ANCA associated vasculitis included both GPA and microscopic PAN. Thus, treatment is identical with corticosteroids at 1 mg/kg/d oral or intravenous methylprednisolone, and intravenous rituximab or cyclophosphamide given orally or intravenously [27–29] (Please refer to following section on treatment of GPA for details). PE may have a role in the treatment of severe renal disease with evidence suggesting a lower frequency of dialysis, but no mortality benefit [30]. There are no prospective data available regarding the efficacy of plasmapheresis in diffuse alveolar hemorrhage (DAH), although retrospective data suggest a benefit [31]. In the face of DAH and severe respiratory failure in the setting of a systemic vasculitis, plasmapheresis in addition to corticosteroids and rituximab or cyclophosphamide is reasonable as long as every effort has been made to exclude infection. In relapsing disease, intravenous immunoglobulin may be of benefit [32].

Eosinophilic Granulomatosis with Polyangiitis (Churg–Strauss Syndrome)

EGPA, formerly Churg–Strauss syndrome (CSS) is characterized by the presence of eosinophilic infiltrates and granulomas in the respiratory tract and necrotizing vasculitis in the setting of asthma and peripheral eosinophilia. Typically, patients have a preceding history of asthma and allergic rhinitis and then develop constitutional symptoms of fatigue and weight loss followed by systemic symptoms such as mononeuritis multiplex, cardiomyopathy, pulmonary infiltrates, or abdominal pain [14]. Pulmonary disease includes fleeting or diffuse infiltrates and nodular lesions [33]. The diagnosis of eosinophilic pneumonia may be suggested in the context of peripheral infiltrates and peripheral eosinophilia. Rarely alveolar hemorrhage may occur. Peripheral neuropathy occurs in up to 75% of patients with EGPA, whereas renal involvement is much less common than in microscopic polyangiitis and GPA. Other sources of morbidity and mortality include GI involvement with bleeding and bowel perforation, cardiac involvement causing arrhythmias, myocarditis, pericarditis, and congestive heart failure [33,34]. The etiology of EGPA is unknown. ANCA is positive in approximately 38% to 60% of cases, mostly myeloperoxidase [35–37]. Distinguishing between EGPA and other types of hypereosinophilic syndromes can be a challenge clinically. Corticosteroids alone in high doses are effective treatment though with severe organ involvement other agents such as cyclophosphamide are utilized [19]. Case reports suggest rituximab may be effective in severe cases of EGPA.

CRYOGLOBULINEMIC VASCULITIS

Cryoglobulins are immunoglobulins that precipitate below 37°C. There are three types: Type I, seen in myeloproliferative disorders; type II, or mixed essential cryoglobulins; and type III, mixed polyclonal. Types II and III are most closely associated with hepatitis C infection. Typical involvement includes cutaneous vasculitis, arthritis, and peripheral neuropathy. Abnormal liver enzymes suggest hepatitis C infection; complement levels, especially C4, are decreased [38,39]. Infrequently, cryoglobulinemic vasculitis may be life threatening with severe renal, GI, and pulmonary involvement including alveolar hemorrhage [40,41]. Therapy in severe cases consists of corticosteroids and rituximab or less frequently cyclophosphamide in conjunction with antiviral therapy for those that are related to hepatitis C, with careful attention to the potential risk of increased hepatitis C replication [42]. For severe cases involving progressive glomerulonephritis, plasmapheresis or cryofiltration may be of additional benefit [43–45].

Granulomatosis with Polyangiitis

GPA, formerly Wegener's granulomatosis, is a disease of unknown etiology characterized by granulomatous vasculitis of the upper and lower respiratory tract, segmental necrotizing glomerulonephritis, and systemic vasculitis of small blood vessels [46]. A subset of patients may have disease isolated to the upper respiratory tract or have less severe organ involvement and are referred to as having "limited" GPA [47,48]. Patients most frequently require intensive care treatment for severe pneumonitis; glomerulonephritis; stroke; myocardial infarction; multiorgan system dysfunction secondary to necrotizing vasculitis; and infection due to immunosuppression and anatomic abnormalities secondary to the granulomatous inflammation.

The etiology of GPA is unknown. Possible infectious etiologic associations with *Staphylococcus aureus* have been proposed but are as yet unproven [49]. ANCA is present in more than 90% of patients with systemic GPA and in 70% to 80% with active limited disease. In GPA, the pattern noted on immunofluorescence is C-ANCA or cytoplasmic staining, and the specific antigen in most cases is the PR3 antigen, although in 10% of cases or more, there may be a P-ANCA or perinuclear staining with MPO (myeloperoxidase) as the specific antigen [50]. Correlation of ANCA titers with clinical remission is controversial, with the most recent data suggesting that relapse is unlikely in treated patients with negative titers, whereas those with rising or recurrently positive titers have a higher risk of relapse, although the timing of relapse is not predictable [51–53]. The pathology of vasculitis includes fibrinoid necrosis with inflammatory mononuclear cell infiltrates of vessel walls, focal destruction of the elastic lamina, and narrowing or obliteration of vessel lumens. Granulomatous lesions are characterized by areas of central necrosis surrounded by epithelial fibroblasts and scattered multinucleated giant cells [54]. Granulomatous vasculitis may involve the lung, skin, CNS, peripheral nerves, heart, and other organs.

Most patients present with symptoms referable to the upper respiratory tract, including sinusitis, nasal obstruction, rhinitis, otitis, hearing loss, ear pain, gingival inflammation, epistaxis, sore throat, laryngitis, and nasal septal deformity. Fever, in addition to being caused by the underlying disease, may be due to suppurative otitis or *S. aureus* sinusitis [55]. Granulomatous vasculitis of the upper respiratory tract may lead to damage of nasal cartilage, resulting in the "saddle-nose" deformity; sore throat; and oral and nasal mucosal ulcers [56]. In addition, chondritis of the nose or ear may develop [57]. Laryngeal involvement may result in severe narrowing of the upper respiratory tract [58–60]. Unusual manifestations of GPA include distinctive punched-out ulcerative skin lesions appearing as pyoderma gangrenosum and painless subcutaneous nodules [61].

Although only one third of patients present with symptomatic lung involvement (including cough, sputum production, dyspnea, chest pain, hemoptysis, and even life-threatening pulmonary hemorrhage), lower respiratory tract disease is found in almost all patients after evaluation. The characteristic chest radiographic findings are multiple, nodular, bilateral cavitary infiltrates, but infiltrates without sharp margins occur more frequently than distinct nodules. Cavitation may occur in distinct nodules and in infiltrates with less-defined borders. Nodules may have thick or thin walls. Infiltrates may involve the lower or upper lobes. In approximately 50% of patients, the infiltrates are bilateral. Infiltrates may be transient [60,62]. Less common chest radiographic abnormalities include paratracheal masses, large cavitary lesions, a miliary pattern, massive pleural effusion, calcified nodule, and masses between the trachea and esophagus [63]. GPA may also be associated with inflammation and subsequent scarring/stenosis of the subglottic region, in about 25% of patients [64]. This complication is distinctly more common in younger adult and pediatric populations and may sometimes be difficult to differentiate from relapsing polychondritis where tracheal and subglottic inflammation is the major presenting feature.

Although renal manifestations are often asymptomatic, urinalysis reveals renal involvement among approximately 80% of patients at presentation. The typical renal lesion is segmental necrotizing glomerulonephritis. Functional renal impairment may progress rapidly if appropriate therapy is not instituted promptly [65,66].

The vasculitis of GPA may cause a variety of other clinical manifestations, including arthralgias and less commonly arthritis, most frequently affecting the knees [67,68]; perinephric hematoma; renal artery aneurysms; ureteral obstruction [69]; a variety of cutaneous lesions, including ulcers, papules, vesicles, and subcutaneous nodules [62]; episcleritis; conjunctivitis; scleritis; uveitis; optic nerve vasculitis [70]; mononeuritis multiplex or polyneuritis; cranial nerve dysfunction; meningitis [71]; cerebral infarction [72]; subarachnoid hemorrhage; abdominal pain; intestinal perforation; and diarrhea [73].

Typically, diagnosis is based on the clinical findings of upper and lower respiratory tract noninfectious inflammation [74] with glomerulonephritis and positive anti-PR3 antibodies and rarely MPO antibodies. For cases with more limited involvement or where ANCA titers are negative or show the less typical MPO specificity, tissue diagnosis may be necessary.

Treatment of GPA have led to the development of a biphasic approach with an initial remission–induction phase using either rituximab or cyclophosphamide in combination with corticosteroids until remission (usually within 3 to 6 months) followed by a remission–maintenance phase using a less toxic immunosuppressive agent, usually methotrexate, azathioprine, or mycophenolate, or continued dosing of rituximab [28,75,76]. At this time, experts in the field are divided on the preferential use of one drug over the other for induction. However, there may be other factors such as fertility concerns, a risk of malignancy, or other issues that favor rituximab as the initial option. In selected patients with early and less severe disease, methotrexate may be used for induction though with a higher risk of relapse [77].

Initial treatment with corticosteroid is generally given as prednisone 1 mg/kg/d orally. For the critically ill patient with severe systemic involvement, pulse corticosteroid with IV methylprednisolone 1 g/day for 3 days is advocated, transitioning to prednisone 1 mg/kg/d orally or its IV equivalent. Prednisone therapy is maintained at 60 mg for 1 month and then weaned to 20 mg over 2 to 3 months and then slowly tapered thereafter.

Two randomized trials explore the efficacy and safety of rituximab versus cyclophosphamide (one study with intravenous dosing and the second with oral dosing) as induction therapy for ANCA-associated vasculitis. The results of both studies suggest equivalency for inducing remission and also similar adverse event profile [29,78]. The precise role of rituximab for rapidly progressive ANCA vasculitis of the critically ill patient (i.e., severe renal failure or pulmonary hemorrhage) is unknown because this was not the focus of the two prospective trials utilizing this agent. Patients should be screened for past exposure to hepatitis B as rituximab can cause fulminant reactivation of latent hepatitis B.

Cyclophosphamide can be administered as intravenous boluses or as a daily oral dose. Both approaches have shown similar rates of remission–induction at 6 months, 78% with daily oral treatment versus 89% with monthly IV boluses [79]. However, relapse rates were much higher among the IV group, 52% compared with 18% in the daily oral group. Follow-up of this group after a mean of 4.3 years revealed that despite the higher relapse rate of the IV group, renal morbidity and overall mortality was equal. The cumulative dose of cyclophosphamide of the IV group was about 50% less than that of the oral group and leukopenia was less frequent. Development of malignancies was not different but the duration of study was likely not long enough to detect changes.

For the clinically ill patient, initial treatment should be with IV cyclophosphamide. One regimen starts with cyclophosphamide 15 mg/kg (maximum dose: 1,200 mg) every 2 weeks for three doses, followed by continued pulses of either 15 mg/kg IV (maximum dose: 1,200 mg) every 3 weeks or 2.5 to 5 mg/kg/d orally on days 1, 2, and 3 every 3 weeks until remission has been achieved and then continued for additional 3 months after remission [79]. Another similar regimen recommends 0.5g/m^2 every 2 weeks for 3 to 6 months until remission. The dose can be increased to 0.75 g/m^2 or lowered based on nadir WBC and absolute neutrophil count. If the oral regimen is chosen, the dose is 2 mg/kg/d in single am dose until remission and then dosing may be decreased to 1.5 mg/kg daily for additional 3 months [79]. Both oral and intravenous doses need to be adjusted for renal impairment. Table 67.2 outlines the renal adjustments in oral cyclophosphamide doses. Although the dosing regimen for IV cyclophosphamide differs for GPA and SLE, Table 68.2, which outlines a standard protocol for the use of monthly IV cyclophosphamide for SLE, provides guidelines on hydration, anti-emetics, dose reduction for renal impairment, and the use of MESNA to prevent bladder toxicities.

Cyclophosphamide therapy is associated with significant morbidity including a 2.4-fold increase of malignancy with 11-fold increase in the risk of leukemia or lymphoma and a significant increased risk of bladder cancer occurring in 1% to 3% of GPA patients treated with cyclophosphamide [80]. Hemorrhage cystitis has been reported in 12% to 43% of patients treated for GPA. In one NIH study, 57% of women of childbearing years became infertile [80]. Opportunistic infection, particularly with *Pneumocystis jiroveci*, was reported among 6% of patients in initial trials with combination cyclophosphamide and corticosteroids and it is now the standard of care for patients to be prophylactically treated with double strength trimethoprim/sulfamethoxazole, three times weekly or atavoquone or dapsone for those intolerant of sulfa.

As in microscopic polyangiitis, plasma exchange may be useful in the context of severe or progressive renal failure or pulmonary hemorrhage, especially in the face of concomitant GBM positivity, and is the focus of an ongoing prospective trial.

In the case of symptomatic subglottic stenosis, optimal treatment of this is best achieved with localized treatment, with bronchoscopic mechanical dilatation, and transbronchial corticosteroid injection of the involved area [81].

DRUG-INDUCED VASCULITIS

Cases of vasculitis associated with the use of certain drugs, vaccines, and toxins have long been recognized. Previously these were described as hypersensitivity reactions causing small vessel vasculitis [82]. Cases ranging from self-limiting cutaneous involvement to severe multiorgan failure have been reported. Diagnosis is based simply on the development of vasculitis where a causal drug/agent can be identified, which in most cases leads to resolution of the vasculitis after drug discontinuation. There is great variation in the length of drug exposure before symptoms develop, with many reports of years of exposure before the apparent sudden onset of vasculitis.

The most commonly reported medications causing drug-induced vasculitis include propylthiouracil, allopurinol, hydralazine, cefaclor, minocycline, D-penicillamine, phenytoin, isotretinoin, and methotrexate with colony-stimulating factors [83]; quinolone antibiotics, and leukotriene inhibitors are more recently added to the list [84]. Other cases have been reported following vaccination, particularly hepatitis B [85] and influenza [86].

The pathophysiology of drug-induced vasculitis appears to be varied. Recently, cases of drug-induced vasculitis have been shown to be associated with temporary production of ANCA antibodies, typically against the MPO antigen and most notable with propylthiouracil and allopurinol [87]. Antibody titers also decrease in these cases following the discontinuation of medication, supporting a causal role [88].

Drug-induced vasculitis can involve medium or small vessels and therefore can present with a variety of clinical features depending on the site and size of vessel involved. Drug-induced vasculitis can present with clinical manifestations similar to any other systemic vasculitis, and there are no clinical findings specific to the syndrome. Skin involvement is common, most commonly in the form of palpable purpura. Although 33% of patients have no symptoms associated with the lesions, 40% complain of burning or pain. Bowel and nervous system involvement is also well recognized along with arthralgias and myalgias. Renal involvement is present in 40% of cases.

Treatment involves the withdrawal of potential causative medications. With mild skin involvement alone, no specific treatment is advocated. Where skin breakdown occurs, skin lesions are very symptomatic, or if internal organ involvement is identified, treatment with corticosteroids is beneficial. For rare cases, particularly those associated with ANCA production, other immunosuppressive agents may be necessary but usually only for short periods of time.

CNS VASCULITIS

CNS vasculitis is a rare condition that can present as a primary form confined to the CNS, known as primary angiitis of the CNS (PACNS) or as a secondary form associated with a systemic vasculitis or other systemic illness. Although many of the systemic vasculitides and rheumatologic diseases can result in CNS involvement and are discussed briefly in other sections, this section focuses on the CNS manifestations of PACNS. Other secondary causes of CNS vasculitis and syndromes mimicking CNS vasculitis include sarcoidosis; antiphospholipid antibody syndrome; lymphoma; atrial myxoma; atheroemboli; reversible vasoconstrictive syndrome; Lyme disease; HIV infection; herpes zoster; tuberculosis; and drugs including cocaine, methamphetamines, ergotamine, pseudoephedrine, and heroin [89].

The clinical presentation associated with PACNS is broad and includes subacute memory loss, acute encephalopathy, and other cognitive and behavioral changes. Seizures, cranial nerve abnormalities, focal deficits involving the cerebrum; cerebellum; and brainstem; spinal cord lesions; meningismus; headache; auditory and vestibular disturbances; intracranial or subarachnoid hemorrhage; and reduced visual acuity or blindness due to retinal and optic nerve vasculitis have been described [90,91]. Frequently, patients have hypertension that aggravates their underlying disease or raises questions about their primary diagnosis. Disease manifestations may develop precipitously but often can present with a long prodrome over months involving subtle mental status changes and cognitive dysfunction [90,91]. The disease has a predilection for the small and medium vessels, especially of the leptomeninges and appears more common in men.

The diagnostic approach to CNS vasculitis includes a careful, frequently repeated neurologic examination; laboratory studies including cultures, viral and bacterial serologies, ANCA, cryoglobulins, antinuclear antibodies, antiphospholipid antibodies, and complement levels, which may help to establish secondary causes of CNS vasculitis related to infections, connective tissue disorders, and systemic vasculitides. CSF abnormalities seen in PACNS, including elevated protein levels and elevated cell counts, mostly lymphocytes, occurs in 80% of patients [91]. Angiographic changes showing alternating areas of stenosis and ectasia are suggestive of the disease but can be seen with other diagnoses including vasospasm and infection. In biopsy proven cases of PACNS, angiography is normal in 40% of cases [91,92]. Magnetic resonance imaging (MRI) can additionally be suggestive of ischemic lesions due to vasculitis if lesions are seen in different vascular distributions, although this finding is not specific for PACNS. A negative MRI and normal CSF make CNS vasculitis less likely, although cases of PACNS have been described with a negative MRI [93,94]. In most cases, unless angiography is highly suggestive in the correct clinical context, pathologic confirmation is necessary. Biopsy of the leptomeninges and other areas guided by previous imaging is necessary to rule out other diagnoses including infection, malignancy, and sarcoidosis, among other diagnoses. In PACNS, the inflammatory infiltrate is predominately mononuclear cells, but neutrophils, plasma cells, and histiocytes may also be noted [95].

Treatment of PACNS involves corticosteroids (CS) as the initial treatment of choice, ranging from doses of 1 mg/kg/d orally to 1 g intravenously daily for 3 days followed by oral CS. Cyclophosphamide is used for most cases or rituximab based on case reports although absolute recommendations are limited by a lack of prospective trials [96].

There are other vasculitic syndromes that can cause similar presentations, as discussed above, although they typically will present with CNS manifestations in the context of other systemic features such as fever, weight loss, peripheral neuropathy, glomerulonephritis, arthritis, or other organ involvement. PAN, GPA, and EGPA can all present with CNS involvement including seizure, cranial nerve deficit, cerebral vascular events, and subarachnoid hemorrhage [97–100].

OTHER VASCULITIDES

Takayasu's arteritis is a large vessel vasculitis that affects the aortic arch and branches, affecting mainly women up to the age of 50. Patients typically present with constitutional symptoms of fatigue, weight loss, elevated erythrocyte sedimentation rate, and evidence of limb claudication and bruits. Patients can present with stroke due to inflammation and subsequent stenosis of the extracranial vessels [101]. Behcet's disease is characterized by aphthous stomatitis, genital ulcers, and can sometimes present with vasculitis that can affect various-sized blood vessels. Meningoencephalitis, seizure, intracranial hemorrhage, and cerebral vascular events have been reported [102]. Connective tissue disease such as systemic lupus erythematosus (SLE), rheumatoid arthritis, and Sjögren syndrome can all be associated with a variety of CNS manifestations including stroke, seizure, encephalopathy, and aseptic meningitis [101–105].

CHOLESTEROL EMBOLISM

Cholesterol crystal embolization can produce a clinical picture very similar to that of a systemic vasculitis [106,107] with the gradual onset of peripheral skin lesions, typically blue toe or livedo reticularis [108], with worsening renal function [109]. Bowel ischemia, acute confusional states [110], and retinal embolization may also be present.

The syndrome occurs due to the release of cholesterol crystals from eroded atherosclerotic plaques. It occurs most frequently following percutaneous endovascular interventions [111,112], but spontaneous episodes or those following anticoagulant [113] or thrombolytic therapy [114] have also been reported.

The chronology of impaired renal function after angiography may help distinguish radiocontrast dye-induced renal failure from renal failure due to atheromatous microemboli. Renal failure caused by radiocontrast dye tends to appear soon after the study, reaches maximal severity within 7 to 10 days, and then improves, with renal function returning to baseline over several weeks. In contrast, renal failure due to atheromatous microemboli to the kidney generally develops over 1 to 4 weeks or even over several months after the angiographic procedure and may not be reversible.

To establish the diagnosis of atheromatous emboli, one must have a high degree of suspicion based on the clinical presentation, history, physical findings, and laboratory results. The diagnosis is confirmed by the demonstration on histologic samples of biopsied skin, muscle, and kidney or amputated tissue of the characteristic biconvex needle-shaped clefts representing the "ghosts" of the cholesterol crystals within arteries and arterioles that are dissolved during routine histologic preparation [115]. With special histologic preparation, the cholesterol crystals display birefringence when viewed with a polarized light microscope.

Treatment of atheromatous emboli consists of controlling pain and blood pressure, and measures to increase local blood flow with topical glyceryl trinitrate (2% Nitrol) ointment, sympathetic blockade, calcium channel blockers to reduce vasospasm, and perhaps pentoxifylline to improve the rheostatic properties of red blood cells. Newer vasodilator agents such as iloprost and phosphodiesterase inhibitors are also being tried [116,117]. There are also case reports of improvements of cholesterol emboli-associated renal disease with statins [118]. Corticosteroid therapy has also been reported to be helpful in several case reports [119]. There are, however, no controlled trials of the use of any of these agents.

A number of modalities are ineffective for the treatment of atheromatous emboli, including the use of antiplatelet drugs and low-molecular-weight dextran. The use of heparin and warfarin is controversial. The general consensus, however, is that these drugs are contraindicated, because by preventing the formation of an organized thrombus over ulcerated atheromatous plaques, anticoagulants may allow continued breakdown and embolization of material [120]. For cases of chronic distal embolization from abdominal aortic aneurysm, surgical repair or endovascular stent-graft repair usually leads to definitive resolution [121].

TREATMENT STRATEGIES IN UNDIFFERENTIATED RHEUMATIC DISEASES PRESENTING WITH CRITICAL ILLNESS AND RELAPSE OR WORSENING KNOWN RHEUMATIC DISEASE

Among certain circumstances, patients present to the hospital or ICU with overwhelming respiratory failure or hemodynamic instability without a previously defined rheumatic disorder. For example, patients with undiagnosed SLE or vasculitis may present with respiratory failure, alveolar hemorrhage, and rapidly progressive renal failure but no specific historical clues or previous serologic data supporting any particular diagnosis, and the results of laboratory and tissue evaluation biopsy may not yet be available. In this situation, one cannot be certain whether the underlying process is an immune complex–mediated disease, such as SLE, Goodpasture's syndrome, or cryoglobulinemia, or a pauci-immune process such as GPA or microscopic polyangiitis. The appropriate laboratory evaluation would include an ANCA, ANA, antiglomerular basement membrane antibody, and cryoglobulins prior to initiating therapy. Initial therapy might include plasmapheresis, which may transiently remove autoantibodies, cytokines, and complement associated with the inflammatory process, in addition to high-dose methylprednisolone, 1 g intravenously per day for 3 days, and then initiation of intravenous or oral cyclophosphamide or rituximab [122,123]. The benefits of intravenous immunoglobulin for relapsing or life-threatening vasculitis are not well understood because of a paucity of controlled trials [124,125].

In the face of known rheumatic disease treatment failure, caution must be exercised to exclude infectious sources that may mimic worsening of the underlying disease process. Especially among patients taking chronic or high-dose corticosteroids and or cyclophosphamide, particular attention must be paid to exclude opportunistic infections such as *P. jiroveci* and fungal infections such as *Aspergillus* while deciding whether disease activity is escalating and becoming unresponsive to therapy. Once infection has been thoroughly excluded, one can consider either higher doses of a standard or novel immunosuppressive agent or addition of other therapies such as immunoglobulin or plasmapheresis.

Owing to the rarity of systemic vasculitis, there have previously been few prospective clinical trials evaluating accepted treatments. In recent years due to establishment of several investigator consortiums, multicenter prospective studies are now beginning to be performed. The more important of these studies are summarized in Table 67.3.

TABLE 67.3

Randomized Trials in the Treatment of Vasculitis

Study	Types of vasculitis	Study design	Results	Comment
Gayraud et al. [19]	PAN, MPA, EGPA	Meta-analysis of randomized trials	Survival benefits of CYC in addition to CS with FFS ≥2	Meta-analysis of four different prospective trials; mixed patient population
Jayne et al. [32]	GPA, MPA	Prospective double-blinded placebo controlled, using IVIG in patients with persistent disease activity	Reduced disease activity in IVIG treated group	Short-term follow-up (3 months)
Gaskin and Jayne [30]	GPA, MPA all with renal failure	Randomized controlled trial using either plasmapheresis or pulse CS in addition to standard CS/CYC	Lower rate of dialysis dependence in plasmapheresis treated group	1 year follow-up data only
de Groot et al. [77]	GPA, MPA	Prospective, randomized, unblinded comparing MTX to CYC in both induction and maintenance of remission in nonrenal AAV	No difference in the number of patients achieving remission, but higher rates of relapse noted in the MTX treated group	MTX may still maintain remission if initial induction is with CYC
Jayne et al. [126]	GPA, MPA	Prospective, randomized, unblinded comparing CYC and AZA in remission maintenance	Relapse rate was not significantly different between the two groups; no difference in AEs	Supports standard of care of changing to AZA once remission induced with CYC
deGroot et al. [79]	ANCA associated vasculitis	Prospective randomized controlled trial using oral or IV CYC for induction of remission	No difference in time to remission or proportion of patients who achieved remission	Total dose of CYC less in IV group. Study not powered to detect differences in relapse rates amongst the two groups.

(*continued*)

TABLE 67.3

Randomized Trials in the Treatment of Vasculitis (*continued*)

Study	Types of vasculitis	Study design	Results	Comment
Jones RB, et al. [29]	GPA, MP: nephritis only	Prospective, open label, multicenter, parallel trial comparing RTX to standard intravenous CYC for induction therapy	Sustained remission rates were similar in both groups and adverse events in both groups were similar	12 months follow-up; small number (44 pts) Patients in RTX group also received IV CYC 15 mg/kg with first and third infusions
Stone et al. [78]	GPA, MP	Randomized, double-blinded, double-dummy multicenter trial comparing RTX to oral CYC for induction therapy	RTX is equivalent to oral CTX in remission induction; no difference in adverse events; RTX may be superior to CYC in relapsing disease	6 months follow-up only and data on maintenance of remission with AZA not available yet 197 patients total
DeVita et al [42]	cryoglobulinemia	Randomized controlled trial with crossover comparing monotherapy RTX to standard therapies for cryoglobulinemic vasculitis	RTX was superior at month 24 in terms of the proportion of patients taking initial therapy and improvement in vasculitic activity score.	Most of the non RTX patients either failed standard therapy or had AEs and crossed over to RTX

AAV, ANCA-associated vasculitis; AEs, adverse events; AZA, azathioprine; CS, corticosteroid; EGPA, eosinophilia with polyangiitis; CYC, cyclophosphamide; IVIG, intravenous immunoglobulin; MPA, microscopic polyangiitis; MTX, methotrexate; PAN, polyarteritis; RTX, rituximab; GPA, granulomatosis with polyangiitis.

References

1. Frankel SK, Sullivan EJ, Brown KK: Vasculitis: Wegener's granulomatosis, Churg-Strauss syndrome, microscopic polyangiitis, polyarteritis nodosa and Takayasu's arteritis. *Crit Care Clin* 18:855–879, 2002.
2. Saleh A, Stone JH: Classification and diagnostic criteria in systemic vasculitis. *Best Pract Res Clin Rheumatol* 19(2):209–221, 2005.
3. Pallan L, Savage CO, Harper L: ANCA associated vasculitis: from bench research to novel treatments. *Nat Rev Nephrol* 5(5):278–286, 2009.
4. Jayne D: The diagnosis of vasculitis. *Best Pract Res Clin Rheumatol* 23(3):445–453, 2009.
5. Lie JT: Vasculitis simulators and vasculitis look-alikes. *Curr Opin Rheumatol* 4:47–55, 1992.
6. O'Keefe ST, Woods BO, Breslin DJ, et al: Blue toe syndrome. Causes and management. *Arch Intern Med* 152:2197–2202, 1992.
7. Guillevin L, Lhote F, Gayraud M, et al: Prognostic factors in polyarteritis nodosa and Churg-Strauss syndrome: a prospective study of 342 patients. *Medicine* 75:17–28, 1996.
8. Griffin J: Vasculitis neuropathies. *Rheum Dis Clin North Am* 27:751–760, 2001.
9. Moore PM, Fauci AS: Neurologic manifestations of systemic vasculitis: a retrospective and prospective study of clinicopathologic features and responses to therapy in 25 patients. *Am J Med* 71:517–524, 1981.
10. Said G, Lacroi-Ciaudo C, Fujimura H, et al: The peripheral neuropathy of necrotizing arteritis: a clinical pathologic study. *Ann Neurol* 23:461–465, 1988.
11. Levine SM, Hellman DB, Stone JH: Gastrointestinal involvement in polyarteritis nodosa (1986–2000); presentation and outcomes in 24 patients. *Am J Med* 112:386–391, 2002.
12. Holsinger DR, Osmundson PJ, Edwards JE: The heart in periarteritis nodosa. *Circulation* 25:610–618, 1962.
13. Schrader ML, Hochman JS, Bulkley BH: The heart in polyarteritis nodosa: a clinicopathologic study. *Am Heart J* 109:1353–1359, 1985.
14. Lhote F, Guilliven L: Polyarteritis nodosa, microscopic polyangiitis, Churg-Strauss syndrome: clinical aspects and treatment. *Rheum Dis Clin North Am* 21:911–947, 1995.
15. Fye KH, Becker MJ, Theofilopoulos AN, et al: Immune complexes in hepatitis B antigen-associated periarteritis nodosa: detection by antibody independent cell–mediated cytotoxicity and the Raji cell assay. *Am J Med* 62:783–791, 1977.
16. Tsukada N, Koh C, Owa M, et al: Chronic neuropathy associated with immune complexes of hepatitis B virus. *J Neurol Sci* 61:193–211, 1983.
17. Carson CW, Conn AJ, Czaja AJ, et al: Frequency and significance of antibodies to hepatitis C virus in polyarteritis nodosa. *J Rheumatol* 20:304–309, 1993.
18. Cid MC, Grau JM, Casademont J, et al: Immunohistochemical characterization of inflammatory cells and immunologic activation markers in muscle and nerve biopsy specimens from patients with polyarteritis nodosa. *Arthritis Rheum* 37:1055–1061, 1994.
19. Guillevin L, Cohen P, Mahr A et al. Treatment of polyarteritis nodosa and microscopic polyangiitis with poor prognosis factors: a prospective trial comparing glucocorticoids and six or twelve cyclophosphamide pulses in sixty five patients. *Arthritis Rheum* 49(1):93-100,2003.
20. Guillevin L, Mahr A, Cohen P, et al: Short-term corticosteroids then lamivudine and plasma exchanges to treat hepatitis B virus related polyarteritis nodosa. *Arthritis Rheum* 51(3):482–487, 2004.
21. Guillevin L, Fain O, Lhote F, et al: Lack of superiority of steroids plus plasma exchange to steroids alone in the treatment of polyarteritis nodosa and Churg-Strauss syndrome. A prospective randomized trial in 78 patients. *Arthritis Rheum* 35:208–215, 1992.
22. Citron BP, Halpern M, McCarron M, et al: Necrotizing angiitis associated with drug abuse. *N Engl J Med* 283(19):1003–1111, 1970.
23. Luqmani R, Watts RA, Scott DGI, et al: Treatment of vasculitis in rheumatoid arthritis. *Ann Intern Med* 145:566–576, 1994.
24. Mertz LE, Conn DL: Vasculitis associated with malignancy. *Curr Opin Rheumatol* 4:39–46, 1992.
25. Somer T, Finegold SM: Vasculitides associated with infections, immunizations, and antimicrobial drugs. *Clin Infect Dis* 20:1010–1036, 1995.
26. Falk RJ, Nachman PH, Hogan SL, et al: ANCA glomerulonephritis and vasculitis: a Chapel Hill perspective. *Semin Nephrol* 20(3):233–243, 2000.
27. Jayne D: Challenges in the management of microscopic polyangiitis: past, present and future. *Curr Opin Rheumatol* 20(1):3–9, 2008.
28. Pagnoux C, Mahr A, Hamidou MA, et al: Azathioprine or methotrexate maintenance for ANCA-associated vasculitis. *N Engl J Med* 359(26):2790–2803, 2008.
29. Jones RB, Tervaert JW, Hauser T, et al: Rituximab versus cyclophosphamide in ANCA-Associated Renal Vasculitis. *N Engl J Med* 363:211–220, 2010.
30. Jayne D, Gaskin G, Rasmussen N. Randomized trial of plasma exchange or high dose methylprednisolone as adjunctive therapy for severe renal vasculitis. *J Am Soc Nephrol* 18(7):2180-2188,2007.
31. Klemmer PJ: Plasmapheresis for diffuse alveolar hemorrhage in patients with systemic vasculitis. *Am J Kidney Dis* 42(6):1149–1153, 2003.
32. Jayne DRW, Chapel H, Adu D, et al: Intravenous immunoglobulin for ANCA-associated systemic vasculitis with persistent disease activity. *Q J Med* 93:433–439, 2000.
33. Guillevin L, Cohen P, Gayraud M, et al: Churg-Strauss syndrome: clinical study and long-term follow-up in 96 patients. *Medicine (Baltimore)* 78:26–37, 1999.
34. Neuman T, Manger B, Schmid M, et al: Cardiac involvement in Churg Strauss syndrome: impact of endomyocarditis. *Medicine (Baltimore)* 88(4):236–243,2009.
35. Guillevin L, Visser H, Noel LH, et al: Antineutrophilic cytoplasm antibodies in systemic polyarteritis nodosa with and without hepatitis B virus infection and Churg-Strauss syndrome—62 patients. *J Rheumatol* 20:1345–1349, 1993.
36. Solans R, Bosch JA, Perez-Bocanegra C, et al: Churg-Strauss syndrome: outcome and long-term follow-up of 32 patients. *Rheumatology* 40:763–771, 2001.
37. Sable-Fourtassou R, Cohen P, Mahr A, et al: Antineutrophil cytoplasmic antibodies and Churg-Strauss syndrome. *Ann Intern Med* 143:632–638, 2005.

38. Agnello V, Ghung RT, Kaplan LM: A role for hepatitis C virus in type II cryoglobulinemia. *N Engl J Med* 327:1490–1495, 1992.
39. Lamprecht P, Moosig F, Gause A, et al: Immunologic and clinical follow-up of hepatitis C virus associated cryoglobulinemic vasculitis. *Ann Rheum Dis* 60:385–390, 2001.
40. Tarantino A, Campise M, Banfi G, et al: Long-term predictors of survival in essential mixed cryoglobulinemic glomerulonephritis. *Kidney Int* 47:618–623, 1995.
41. Bombardieri S, Paoletta P, Ferri C, et al: Lung involvement in essential mixed cryoglobulinemia. *Am J Med* 66:748–756, 1979.
42. DeVita S, Quaartuccio L, Isola M et al. A randomized controlled trial of rituximab for the treatment of severe cryoglobulinemic vasculitis. *Arthritis Rheum* 64(3):843-53,2012
43. Gomez-Tello V, Onoro-Canaveral JJ, de la Casa Monje RM, et al: Diffuse recidivant alveolar hemorrhage in a patient with hepatitis C virus related mixed cryoglobulinemia. *Intensive Care Med* 25(3):319–322, 1999.
44. Rieu V, Cohen P, Andre MH, et al: Characteristics and outcome of 49 patients with symptomatic cryoglobulinemia. *Rheumatology (Oxford)* 41:290–300, 2002.
45. Guillevin L, Pagnoux C: Indications of plasma exchanges for systemic vasculitides. *Ther Apher Dial* 7(2):155–160, 2003.
46. Cupps TR, Fauci AS: *Wegener's Granulomatosis: The Vasculitides*. Philadelphia, WB Saunders, 1981.
47. Fauci AS, Wolff SM: Wegener's granulomatosis: studies in eighteen patients and a review of the literature. *Medicine* 52(6):535–561, 1973.
48. Wolff SM, Fauci AS, Horn RG, et al: Wegener's granulomatosis. *Ann Intern Med* 81(4):513–525, 1974.
49. Popa ER, Tervaert JW: The relationship between *Staphylococcus aureus* and Wegener's granulomatosis: current knowledge and future directions. *Intern Med* 42(9):771–780, 2003.
50. Franssen C, Stegeman CA, Kallenberg CG, et al: Antiproteinase 3 and antimyeloperoxidase-associated vasculitis. *Kidney Int* 57(6):2195–2206, 2000.
51. Finkielman JD, Merkel PA, Schroeder D, et al: Antiproteinase 3 antineutrophil cytoplasmic antibodies and disease activity in Wegener's granulomatosis. *Ann Intern Med* 147(9):611–619, 2007.
52. Sanders JS, Huitma MG, Kallenberg CG, et al: Prediction of relapse in PR3-ANCA-associated vasculitis by assessing responses of ANCA titres to treatment. *Rheumatology (Oxford)* 45(6):724–729, 2006.
53. Birck R, Schmitt WH, Kaelsch IA et al. Serial ANCA determinations for monitoring disease activity in patients with ANCA-associated vasculitis:systemic review. *Am J Kidney Dis* 47(1):15. 2006
54. Godman GC, Churg J: Wegener's granulomatosis: pathology and review of literature. *Arch Pathol* 58:533–553, 1954.
55. Fauci AS, Haynes BF, Katz P, et al: Wegener's granulomatosis: prospective clinical and therapeutic experience with 85 patients for 21 years. *Ann Intern Med* 98(1):76–85, 1983.
56. Schramm VL Jr, Myers EN, Rogerson DR: The masquerade of vasculitis: head and neck diagnosis and management. *Laryngoscope* 88(12):1922–1934, 1978.
57. Goldenberg DL, Goodman ML: Case 26-1985. Case records of the Massachusetts General Hospital: weekly clinicopathological exercises. *N Engl J Med* 312:1695–1697, 1985.
58. Girard C, Charles P, Terrier, B et al. Tracheobronchial stenoses in granulomatosis with polyangiitis (Wegener's): a report of 26 cases. *Medicine* 94(32).1088-1096 2015
59. Harrington JT, McCluskey RT: Case 24-1979. Case records of the Massachusetts General Hospital: weekly clinicopathological exercises. *N Engl J Med* 300:1378–1380, 1979.
60. McDonald TJ, DeRemee RA: Wegener's granulomatosis. *Laryngoscope* 93(2):220–231, 1983.
61. Bernhard JD, Mark EJ: Case 17–1986. Case records of the Massachusetts General Hospital: weekly clinicopathological exercises. *N Engl J Med* 314:1170–1173, 1986.
62. McGregor MG, Sandler G: Wegener's granulomatosis. A clinical and radiological survey. *Br J Radiol* 37:430–439, 1964.
63. Maguire R, Fauci AS, Doppmann JL, et al: Unusual radiographic features of Wegener's granulomatosis. *Am J Roentgenology* 130(2):233–238, 1978.
64. Langford CA, Sneller MC, Hallahan CW, et al: Clinical features and therapeutic management of subglottic stenosis in patients with Wegener's granulomatosis. *Arthritis Rheum* 39(10):1754–1760, 1996.
65. Weiss MA, Crissman JD: Renal biopsy findings in Wegener's granulomatosis: segmental necrotizing glomerulonephritis with glomerular thrombosis. *Hum Pathol* 15(10):943–956, 1984.
66. Horn RG, Fauci AS, Rosenthal AS, et al: Renal biopsy pathology in Wegener's granulomatosis. *Am J Pathol* 74(3):423–440, 1974.
67. Pritchard MH: Wegener's granulomatosis presenting as rheumatoid arthritis (two cases). *Proc R Soc Med* 69(7):501–504, 1976.
68. Noritake DT, Weiner SR, Bassett LW, et al: Rheumatic manifestations of Wegener's granulomatosis. *J Rheumatol* 14(5):949–951, 1987.
69. Baker SB, Robinson DR: Unusual renal manifestations of Wegener's granulomatosis. Report of two cases. *Am J Med* 64(5):883–889, 1978.
70. Haynes BF, Fishman ML, Fauci AS, et al: The ocular manifestations of Wegener's granulomatosis. Fifteen years' experience and review of the literature. *Am J Med* 63(1):131–141, 1977.
71. Parker SW, Sobel RA: Case 12–1988. Case records of the Massachusetts General Hospital: weekly clinicopathological exercises. *N Engl J Med* 318:760, 1988.
72. Satoh J, Miyasaka N, Yamada T, et al: Extensive cerebral infarction due to involvement of both anterior cerebral arteries by Wegener's granulomatosis. *Ann Rheum Dis* 47(7):606–611, 1988.
73. Camilleri M, Pusey CD, Chadwick VS, et al: Gastrointestinal manifestations of systemic vasculitis. *Q J Med* 52(206):141–149, 1983.
74. Lynch JP, Matteson E, McCune WJ: Wegener's granulomatosis: evolving concepts. *Med Rounds* 2:67, 1989.
75. Regan M, Hellmann D, Stone J: Treatment of Wegener's granulomatosis. *Rheum Dis Clin North Am* 27(4):863–886, 2001.
76. Stassen PM, Cohen Tervaert JW, Stegeman CA: Induction of remission in active antineutrophil cytoplasmic antibody-associated vasculitis with mycophenolate mofetil in patients who cannot be treated with cyclophosphamide. *Ann Rheum Dis* 66(6):798–802, 2007.
77. De Groot K, Rasmussen N, Bacon PA, et al: Randomized trial of cyclophosphamide versus methotrexate for induction of remission in early systemic antineutrophil cytoplasmic antibody-associated vasculitis. *Arthritis Rheum* 52(8):2461–2469, 2005.
78. Stone JH, Merkel PA, Spiera R, et al: Rituximab versus cyclophosphamide for ANCA-Associated Vasculitis. *N Engl J Med* 363:221–232, 2010.
79. deGroot K, Harper L, Jayne DR, et al: Pulse versus daily oral cyclophosphamide for induction of remission in antineutrophil cytoplasmic antibody-associated vasculitis. *Ann Int Med* 150(10):670–680, 2009.
80. Hoffman G, Kerr G, Leavitt R: Wegener's granulomatosis: an analysis of 158 patients. *Ann Intern Med* 116:488–498, 1992.
81. Langford CA, Sneller MC, Hallahan CW, et al: Clinical features and therapeutic management of subglottic stenosis in patients with Wegener's granulomatosis. *Arthritis Rheum* 39:1754–1760, 1996.
82. Calabrese LH, Michel BA, Bloch DA, et al: The American College of Rheumatology 1990 criteria for the classification of hypersensitivity vasculitis. *Arthritis Rheum* 33(8):1108–1113, 1990.
83. Bonilla MA, Dale D, Zeidler C, et al: Long-term safety of treatment with recombinant human granulocyte colony-stimulating factor in patients with severe congenital neutropenias. *Br J Haematol* 88(4):723–730, 1994.
84. Merkel P: Drug-induced vasculitis. *Rheum Dis Clin North Am* 27(4):849–862, 2001.
85. Ascherio A, Zhang SM, Hernan MA, et al: Hepatitis B vaccination and the risk of multiple sclerosis. *N Engl J Med* 344(5):327–332, 2001.
86. Blumberg S, Bienfang D, Kantrowitz FG, et al: A possible association between influenza vaccination and small vessel vasculitis. *Arch Intern Med* 140(6):847–848, 1980.
87. Choi HK, Merkel P, Walker AM, et al: Drug-induced ANCA-positive vasculitis: prevalence amongst patients with high titers of anti-myeloper-oxidase antibodies. *Arthritis Rheum* 43(2):405–413, 2000.
88. Dedeoglu F: Drug-induced autoimmunity. *Curr Opin Rheumatol* 21(5): 547–551, 2009.
89. Siva A: Vasculitis of the nervous system. *J Neurol* 248:451–468, 2001.
90. Younger DS, Calabrese LH, Hays AP: Granulomatous angiitis of the nervous system. *Neurol Clin* 15:821–834, 1997.
91. Calabrese LH, Furlan AJ, Gragg LA, et al: Primary angiitis of the central nervous system (PACNS): a reappraisal of diagnostic criteria and revised clinical approach. *Cleve Clin J Med* 59:293–306, 1992.
92. Duna GF, Calabrese LH: Limitations of invasive modalities in the diagnosis of primary angiitis of the central nervous system. *J Rheumatol* 222:662–667, 1995.
93. Harris K, Tram D, Skekels W, et al: Diagnosing intracranial vasculitis: the roles of MRI and angiography. *Am J Neuroradiol* 15:317–330, 1994.
94. Stone JH, Pomper MG, Roubenoff R, et al: Sensitivities of noninvasive tests for central nervous system vasculitis: a comparison of lumbar puncture, computed tomography, and magnetic resonance imaging. *J Rheumatol* 21(7):1277–1282, 1994.
95. Lie JT: Primary (granulomatous) angiitis of the central nervous system: a clinical pathologic analysis of 15 new cases and a review of the literature. *Hum Pathol* 23:164–171, 1992.
96. Rituximab for primary CNS vasculitis:report of 2 patients from the French COVAC cohort and review of the literature. *J Rheumatol* 40(12):2102-3. 2013
97. Moore PM, Cupps T: Neurologic complications of vasculitis. *Ann Neurol* 14:155–157, 1983.
98. Moore PM, Fauci AS: Neurologic manifestations of systemic vasculitis: a retrospective and prospective study of clinicopathologic features and responses to therapy in 25 cases. *Am J Med* 71:517–524, 1981.
99. Sigal LH: The neurologic presentation of vasculitic and rheumatologic syndromes. A review. *Medicine (Baltimore)* 66:157–180, 1987.
100. Nishino H, Rubino F, DeRemee R, et al: Neurological involvement in Wegener's granulomatosis: an analysis of 324 consecutive cases at the Mayo Clinic. *Ann Neurol* 33:4–9, 1993.
101. Takano K, Sadoshima S, Ibayashi S, et al: Altered cerebral hemodynamics and metabolism in Takayasu's arteritis with neurological deficits. *Stroke* 24(10):1501–1506, 1993.
102. Siva A, Altintas A, Saip S: Behcet's syndrome and the nervous system. *Curr Opin Neurol* 17(3):347–357, 2004.Siva A, Altintas A, Saip S: Behcet's syndrome and the nervous system. *Curr Opin Neurol* 17(3):347–357, 2004.
103. Alexander EL: Neurologic disease in Sjögren's syndrome: mononuclear inflammatory vasculopathy affecting the central/peripheral nervous system and muscle. *Rheum Dis Clin North Am* 19:869–908, 1993.
104. Neamtu L, Belmont M, Miller DC, et al: Rheumatoid disease of the central nervous system with meningeal vasculitis presenting with seizure. *Neurology* 56(6):814–815, 2001.

105. Ellis SG, Verity MA: Central nervous system involvement in systemic lupus erythematosus: a review of neuropathologic findings in 57 cases. *Semin Arthritis Rheum* 8:212–221, 1979.
106. Cappiello RA, Espinoza LR, Adelman H, et al: Cholesterol embolism: a pseudovasculitic syndrome. *Semin Arthritis Rheum* 18(4):240–246, 1989.
107. Anderson RW: Necrotizing angiitis associated with embolization of cholesterol. *Am J Clin Pathol* 43:65, 1965.
108. Applebaum RM, Kronzon I: Evaluation and management of cholesterol embolization and the blue toe syndrome. *Curr Opin Cardiol* 11(5):533–542, 1996.
109. Hara S, Asada Y: Atheroembolic renal disease: clinical findings of 11 cases. *J Atheroscler Thromb* 9(6):288–291, 2002.
110. Thadhani RI, Camargo CA, Xavier RJ, et al: Atheroembolic renal failure after invasive procedures. Natural history based on 52 histologically proven cases. *Medicine* 74:350–358, 1995.
111. Paraskevas KI, Koutsias S, Mikhailidis DP, et al: Cholesterol crystal embolization: a possible complication of peripheral endovascular interventions. *J Endovasc Ther* 15(5):614–625, 2008.
112. Fukumoto Y, Tsutsui H, Tsuchihashi M, et al: The incidence and risk factors of cholesterol embolization syndrome, a complication of cardiac catheterization: a prospective study. *J Am Coll Cardiol* 42(2):211–216, 2003.
113. Moll S, Huffman J: Cholesterol emboli associated with warfarin treatment. *Am J Hematol* 77(2):194–195, 2004.
114. Hitti WA, Wali RK, Weinman EJ, et al: Cholesterol embolization syndrome induced by thrombolytic therapy. *Am J Cardiovasc Drugs* 8(1):27–34, 2008.
115. Manganoni AM, Venturini M, Scolari F, et al: The importance of skin biopsy in the diverse clinical manifestations of cholesterol embolism. *Br J Dermatol* 150(6):1230–1231, 2004.
116. Grenader T, Lifschitz M, Shavit L: Iloprost in embolic renal failure. *Mt Sinai J Med* 72(5):339–341, 2005.
117. Elinav E, Chajek-Shaul T, Stern M, et al: Improvement in cholesterol emboli syndrome after iloprost therapy. *BMJ* 324(7332):268–269, 2002.
118. Yonemura K, Ikegaya N: Potential therapeutic effect of simvastatin on progressive renal failure and nephrotic-range proteinuria caused by renal cholesterol embolism. *Am J Med Sci* 322(1):50–52, 2001.
119. Graziani G, Santostasi S, Angelini C, et al: Corticosteroids in cholesterol emboli syndrome. *Nephron* 87(4):371–373, 2001.
120. Belenfant X, d'Auzac C, Bariety J, et al: Cholesterol crystal embolism during treatment with low-molecular-weight heparin. *Presse Med* 26(26):1236–1237, 1997.
121. Carroccio A, Olin JW, Ellozy SH, et al: The role of aortic stent grafting in the treatment of atheromatous embolization syndrome: results after a mean of 15 months follow-up. *J Vasc Surg* 40(3):424–429, 2004.
122. Soding PF, Lockwood CM, Park GR: The intensive care of patients with fulminant vasculitis. *Anaesth Intensive Care* 22:81–89, 1994.
123. Schmitt WH, Gross WL: Vasculitis in the seriously ill patient: diagnostic approaches and therapeutic options in ANCA-associated vasculitis. *Kidney Int* 53(64):S39–S44, 1998.
124. Martinez V, Cohen P, Pagnoux C, et al: Intravenous immunoglobulins for relapses of systemic vasculitides associated with antineutrophil cytoplasmic autoantibodies: results of a multicenter, prospective, open label study of twenty two patients. *Arthritis Rheum* 58(1):308–317, 2008.
125. Fortin PM, Tejani AM, Bassett K, et al: Intravenous immunoglobulins as adjuvant therapy for Wegener's granulomatosis. *Cochrane Database Syst Rev* 8(3):CD007057, 2009.
126. Jayne D, Rasmussen N, Andrassy K, et al: A randomized trial of maintenance therapy for vasculitis associated with antineutrophil cytoplasmic autoantibodies. *N Engl J Med* 349(1):36–44, 2003.

Chapter 68 ▪ Therapeutics for Immune-Mediated Rheumatic Diseases

PEGGY WU

The explosion of immunologic or genetically based therapies has affected all areas of medicine and, most dramatically, the fields of hematology/oncology, rheumatology, and transplantation medicine. Specific areas of dermatology, gastroenterology, neurology, nephrology, and allergy/immunology have also benefited from these therapeutics. Some of the following medications were initially FDA approved for a rheumatologic disease, then shortly thereafter approved for other indications. For example, adalimumab, a TNFα inhibitor initially approved for rheumatoid arthritis (RA), is also used for psoriasis, inflammatory bowel disease, and, most recently, uveitis. The reverse can also occur, and there is much crossover between different fields. Even therapies used for allergic asthma (such as omalizumab) are now also approved for idiopathic urticaria. To review all the immunologic and biologic medications of the various subspecialties is beyond the scope of this chapter. Some medications not discussed in this chapter are addressed in other sections such as hematology/oncology and pulmonary diseases, and in great detail in Chapter 63 on immunosuppression in solid organ transplantation.

NONSTEROIDAL ANTI-INFLAMMATORY DRUGS (NSAIDs)

NSAIDs are very commonly used for rheumatologic diseases for their analgesic, anti-inflammatory, and antipyretic effects. There are numerous NSAIDs with variable dosing regimens available, but in the intensive care setting, comorbidities are common, thus limiting their use. NSAIDs are often contraindicated for critically ill patients because of their potential toxicities (gastrointestinal bleeding, exacerbation of cardiac and renal dysfunction) and also have synergistic toxicities for those on anticoagulation.

CORTICOSTEROID THERAPY

Although NSAIDs are one of the first-line medications given for nonseptic inflammatory joint disease, corticosteroids are commonly given for many rheumatologic and dermatologic diseases for their potent anti-inflammatory effects. However, the physiology and mechanism of action of corticosteroids are beyond the scope of this chapter.

The body typically produces 5.7 mg/m^2/d of cortisol [1]. Exogenous corticosteroids at a dose equivalent of prednisone 5.0 to 7.5 mg per day inhibit the hypothalamic–pituitary–adrenal axis. Guidelines are controversial and suggest that supplementation beyond a patient's baseline dose in times of stress can be deferred for those receiving $<$5 mg of prednisone or its equivalent daily and for those on alternate-day dosing. However, those on corticosteroids chronically (greater than 3 weeks) at $>$10 mg daily or those who have clinical Cushing syndrome require stress doses during situations such as surgery, sepsis, trauma, or serious medical illness. This is especially relevant for patients with systemic rheumatologic disorders with major organ involvement (i.e., newly diagnosed myositis, lupus, vasculitis) because extended courses of medium- to high-dose steroids are the therapeutic mainstay of treatment for these diseases.

Several corticosteroid preparations are available, which differ in potency, half-life, and mineralocorticoid activity. In the ICU, the most commonly used corticosteroids are hydrocortisone, methylprednisolone, and prednisone. Glucocorticoids can be affected by age, severe liver disease, hyperthyroidism, hypoalbuminemia, hemodialysis, and certain medications such as anticonvulsants, erythromycin, or ketoconazole.

The dosage and mode of administration of corticosteroids depend on the clinical situation. As mentioned earlier, rheumatologic diseases with major organ involvement require high doses—typically around 1 to 1.5 mg/kg/d—to achieve disease control. However, for acutely ill patients, high-dose steroids usually with pulse IV methylprednisolone at 1,000 mg daily for 3 consecutive days will often be given prior to initiating a regimen of 1 to 1.5 mg/kg/d. Pulse IV methylprednisolone may produce minor side effects (metallic taste, facial flushing, transient hypertension, and hyperglycemia), but significant (although rare) toxicities such as seizures, psychosis, intractable hiccups, arrhythmias, hemiplegia, and sudden death (more typically from arrhythmias or cardiovascular collapse) can occur. Other toxicities with longer-term use include peptic ulcer disease, fluid retention, dyslipidemia, increased risk for infection, osteonecrosis, and osteoporosis. Tapering regimens vary depending on the disease and dose of steroid.

DISEASE-MODIFYING ANTIRHEUMATIC DRUGS (DMARDs)

DMARDs were initially used for rheumatic diseases as steroid-sparing agents. However, convincing evidence exists that these agents can produce dramatic improvement or induce remission in many different rheumatic diseases. The most commonly used drugs include hydroxychloroquine, sulfasalazine, methotrexate, azathioprine, mycophenolate mofetil, leflunomide, and cyclophosphamide. Cyclosporine and gold are older medications that have fallen out of favor for the treatment of rheumatologic disease as newer agents with less toxicity have emerged. Calcineurin inhibitors have also been used less commonly in rheumatoid arthritis and lupus nephritis as steroid sparing agents. However, these medications are not addressed here. See chapter 63 for more detailed discussion.

DMARDs all typically have immunosuppressive effects except for perhaps hydroxychloroquine, a medication previously used to prevent malaria. In an ICU setting, patients are severely ill perhaps with active infection, sepsis, cytopenias, major organ failure, and/or issues requiring surgery. In all of these cases, cytotoxic therapy is typically held until the acute issues are resolved. If the rheumatologic disease becomes active while the DMARD is held, glucocorticoids can be given in the lowest minimal dose necessary, assuming there is no contraindication. Adjustments to conventional dosing may be necessary depending on renal or hepatic function. Further details for the most common DMARDs will be discussed in the following section.

Mechanism of Action and Metabolism

Hydroxychloroquine works by elevating the pH within intracellular vacuoles, thus altering the environment required for antigenic protein digestion and the molecular assembly of peptide complexes, namely, the formation of peptide–MHC protein complexes. These complexes are required to stimulate CD4$^+$ T cells, so when the complexes are not allowed to form, there is downregulation of the immune response against autoantigenic peptides. The major toxicity is retinal toxicity typically after 7 years, gastrointestinal issues, rash, and myopathy.

The other immunosuppressive agents interfere with the cell cycle, and cytotoxic effects occur through inhibition of cell division.

Sulfasalazine is a combination of sulfapyridine and 5-aminosalicylic acid linked by a diazo bond. Sulfasalazine alters neutrophil function, inhibits the cytotoxicity of the natural killer cells, and decreases levels of IL-1, TNF-α, and IL-6. Sulfasalazine also inhibits matrix metalloproteinase activity and matrix remodeling.

Methotrexate (MTX) inhibits dihydrofolate reductase, thus reducing intracellular tetrahydrofolate levels and interfering with tetrahydrofolate-dependent metabolic pathways, which include purine and pyrimidine metabolism. Potential mechanisms whereby MTX exerts an anti-inflammatory effect include increased extracellular adenosine concentrations, reduction of proinflammatory cytokines (IL-1β and IL-6), inhibition of cyclooxygenase and lipoxygenase activity, and induction of apoptosis. MTX and its metabolites are excreted by the kidney and so should not be used for patients whose estimated glomerular filtration rate is less than 30 mL per minute.

Azathioprine (AZA), a purine analog, prevents the biosynthesis of purine bases. AZA is a prodrug that is metabolized in the liver to 6-mercaptopurine and then, through the enzyme thiopurine S-methyltransferase (TMPT), to its active metabolites. A genetic polymorphism of TMPT results in variable enzyme activity and predicts greater risk of myelosuppression for patients at low or undetectable levels. TMPT genotype testing is recommended before initiating AZA therapy [2]. Because 45% of the prodrug is renally excreted, the dose should be reduced for patients with renal insufficiency, but specific recommendations are not available. AZA should be avoided, or the dose markedly reduced, in patients taking allopurinol, which interferes with its metabolism by inhibiting xanthine oxidase. However there are exceptions to this rule and the combination of AZA and allopurinol is sometimes used in treating inflammatory bowel disease and autoimmune hepatitis to optimize thiopurine therapy.

Mycophenolate mofetil (MMF) is a reversible inhibitor of inosine monophosphate dehydrogenase, resulting in reduced purine synthesis and consequent inhibition of T- and B-cell proliferation. The antiproliferative effects of MMF are relatively specific for lymphocytes. Other potential mechanisms of MMF-induced immunosuppression include the induction of T lymphocyte apoptosis and inhibition of adhesion molecule expression. Most of the MMF dose (90%) is excreted renally and the remainder by enterohepatic elimination. Dose adjustment is necessary in patients with renal insufficiency.

Leflunomide (LEF) selectively inhibits dihydroorotate dehydrogenase, an enzyme critical in the de novo synthesis of pyrimidine ribonucleosides. By reducing the pyrimidine pool and thus inhibiting DNA synthesis, LEF is postulated to modulate pathogenic T-cell proliferation and the subsequent inflammatory cascade. LEF has a very long half-life, is highly protein bound, undergoes enterohepatic recirculation, and is eliminated by the gastrointestinal tract and by excretion in the urine. It should not be used for patients with hepatic impairment.

Cyclophosphamide (CY) is an alkylating agent that can be given by mouth or intravenously. It binds to DNA and prevents cell replication. CY is cytotoxic to both resting and dividing lymphocytes. It globally reduces T-cell function, and reduces B-cell numbers and antibody production. CY is metabolized by the liver to several active and inactive compounds that are also excreted in the urine. Dose adjustment is recommended for patients with renal insufficiency (Table 68.1). Hepatic impairment does not appear to alter CY clearance, although both hepatic and renal function should be monitored.

CY is typically used for organ-threatening manifestations of rheumatologic diseases, primarily for lupus and vasculitis. There are different dosing regimens, depending on the disease and the manifestations. We have provided one of the more typical dosing regimens in Table 68.1. In the rare event that CY has to be given to a critically ill patient, caregivers would need to ensure that there is adequate urinary drainage by catheter to protect the bladder from CY-associated hemorrhage from stasis; an hourly urine flow of 100 mL per hour is recommended. Sometimes, continuous bladder irrigation through a three-way catheter may be needed if patients have a lower urine output.

Certain medications can also affect the hepatic microsomal enzymes, thus altering the metabolism of CY. Those that induce these enzymes (i.e., barbiturates, phenytoin, and rifampin) can potentially increase toxicity, whereas those that inhibit the hepatic microsomal enzymes (allopurinol, antimalarials, corticosteroids, tricyclic antidepressants) can decrease efficacy. Another medication interaction that can have important consequences is succinylcholine. Anesthesiologists need to be aware that both

TABLE 68.1

Intravenous Cyclophosphamide Therapy (IVCY)

1. Initiate IV hydration at 200–500 mL/h
   Normal or ½ NS for 1 L over 1–2 h if CrCl >50 mL/min and depending on cardiac status. (If medical status prevents adequate hydration, MESNA can be substituted—see below.)
2. Antiemetic treatment
   Ondansetron, 8 mg IV 30 min (or PO 60 min), prior to CY and then 8 mg every 8 h for 24 h
3. MESNA (for CrCl <50 mL/min or inadequate prehydration due to cardiopulmonary status)
   Give 100% of total CY dose in divided doses: Infuse each dose over 15 min. Give 20% of CY dose (mixed in 50 mL of D_5 W) 30 min prior to CY, then 40% of CY dose at 4 and 8 h following CY.
4. Cyclophosphamide: Initial dose is 500–750 mg/m^2 in 250 mL NS over 60 min. Subsequent dose is based on WBC nadir obtained 10-14 days after infusion after infusion.
   Dose adjustments
   a. CrCl 10–50 mL/min: 75% of CY dose
   b. CrCl <10 mL/min: 50% of CY dose
   c. Hemodialysis patients: 50% of CY dose after dialysis
   d. Subsequent month dose: increase or decrease by 10%–20% of previous dose based on WBC nadir.
5. Posthydration fluid is identical to prehydration. Monitor adequate urine output and encourage frequent voiding for 24 h after IVCY. In patients without indwelling Foley catheter, avoid CY infusion after 4 PM to reduce prolonged bladder contact with CY metabolites overnight.

CY, cyclophosphamide; D_5W, dextrose 5% in water; IV, intravenous; MESNA, sodium 2-mercaptoethane sulfonate; NS, normal saline; PO, by mouth; WBC, white blood cells.

succinylcholine and CY inhibit plasma pseudocholinesterase activity, thereby leading to the potential for prolonged neuromuscular blockade if given concomitantly.

Toxicities

Toxicities common to all of the foregoing immunosuppressive agents include bone marrow suppression, infections, and gastrointestinal irritation. Bone marrow toxicity may occur at any time. Infections secondary to immunosuppression occur with any drug but do not necessarily correlate with the degree of leukopenia, duration of drug therapy, or concomitant corticosteroid therapy. Prior to starting these medications patients should be screened for hepatitis B and C because these immunosuppressants can reactivate infection in hepatitis B carriers or worsen preexisting disease. In addition, MMF has also been associated with progressive multifocal leukoencephalopathy (PML) which can be fatal.

MTX has similar adverse effects, which include cytopenias, hepatotoxicity, alopecia, and skin photosensitivity, as well as more minor toxicities, which include nausea, vomiting, anorexia, diarrhea, weight loss, and stomatitis. MTX can also be associated with pulmonary toxicities too, most commonly hypersensitivity pneumonitis, which usually improves with discontinuation of methotrexate, supportive care, and glucocorticoids if needed. Other pulmonary toxicities include interstitial fibrosis, pleuritis, noncardiogenic pulmonary edema, and increased pulmonary nodulosis.

Small series have also reported development of lymphoproliferative disorders in MTX-treated patients. However, RA patients are already at greater risk for lymphoma than the general population. A study reviewing a national data bank for rheumatic disease in over 18,000 patients did not identify a significantly higher risk of lymphoma for patients treated with MTX [3]. Risk factors for MTX toxicity include renal insufficiency, viral infections, folic acid deficiency, and concurrent use of trimethoprim-sulfamethoxazole and probenecid. For MTX overdose, folinic acid (leucovorin), in a dose equal to the MTX dose, should be given every 4 to 6 hours until the serum MTX level is no longer detectable.

Toxicities associated with LEF include diarrhea, alopecia, rash, hypertension, weight loss, hepatotoxicity, and anemia. Hepatotoxicity can be significant, and there have been reports of hepatic failure and death. The extended half-life of LEF can be problematic, especially for patients who experience severe side effects or who wish to become pregnant. For these cases, elimination of LEF and its metabolites can be accelerated by the administration of cholestyramine, 8 g three times a day for 11 days.

Specific toxicities of AZA include pancreatitis and hypersensitivity hepatitis with transaminitis and cholestasis that usually resolve after drug discontinuation, although irreversible damage has been reported. Azoospermia, anovulation, and teratogenesis are unusual. TPMT levels do not predict these toxicities, in contrast to the known association of low enzyme levels with risk of myelosuppression. It is uncertain whether neoplasia occurs at a greater incidence among rheumatic patients treated with AZA as compared to transplantation patients. However, relative risk of lymphoproliferative disorders among RA patients receiving AZA is estimated at 2.2% to 8.7%.

The toxicity profile of MMF is similar to AZA and includes hepatoxicity and cytopenias. Hepatic fibrosis is an infrequent but concerning complication. Gastrointestinal intolerance with nausea, vomiting, and diarrhea may improve over time and seldom requires drug discontinuation. Rarely, an enterocolitis has been associated with MMF. A delayed release formulation (mycophenolic acid) is available that may improve gastrointestinal tolerance. As with other immunosuppressive medications, there may be an increased risk of malignancies, including lymphoma.

Similar to the other DMARDS, CY can also cause bone marrow suppression. However, CY can have further major side effects, including infertility, bladder toxicities, and carcinogenicity. Oral and IV regimens can induce gonadal dysfunction in men and women because of injury to germinal epithelium. Azoospermia in males and amenorrhea in premenopausal women is dose related and is usually permanent. The risk may be reduced by the induction of gonadal quiescence during CY treatment, such as using leuprolide to preserve ovarian function in women with lupus nephritis treated with CY [4]. Leuprolide was ineffective for men, but a small study has shown a reduced risk of azoospermia in men treated with testosterone [5]. Sperm banking is also recommended for men undergoing CY therapy. Cryopreservation of ova or embryos can be recommended but is sometimes impractical because it entails hormonal manipulation and significant delay in treatment.

Hemorrhagic cystitis due to acrolein, a metabolite of CY, occurs in 20% to 30% of patients receiving oral CY. Bladder carcinoma occurs in 10% of patients who receive long-term CY therapy, even 20 years after exposure. IV CY may have fewer bladder complications than the oral regimen. Adequate hydration for all patients and concomitant use of sodium 2-mercaptoethane sulfonate (MESNA) during IV CY infusion for patients with renal insufficiency should be used to reduce the risk of hemorrhagic cystitis. The regimen is outlined in Table 68.1. Skin and hematologic malignancies and premalignant and malignant changes of the cervix are also associated with CY. Hepatotoxicity is rare, but nausea or vomiting with IVCY is common. Other toxicities include infections, cardiomyopathy, and pulmonary fibrosis. PJP has also occurred in patients with autoimmune diseases treated with CY and steroids. PJP prophylaxis is recommended for all patients treated with CY.

BIOLOGIC MODIFIERS

In addition to the foregoing traditional immunosuppressive agents, there has been continued growth in the development of biologic modifiers for the treatment of rheumatic diseases. The mechanisms of action vary and include anticytokine therapies, T-cell costimulation blockade, B-cell depletion and inhibition, phosphodiesterase 4 (PDE4) inhibition, and Janus kinase (JAK) enzyme blockade (see Table 68.2.). Biologic agents are increasingly used to treat RA, psoriatic arthritis (PsA), ankylosing spondylitis, inflammatory bowel disease, and even lupus. It is unlikely that the ICU physician will initiate any of these agents for therapeutic indications. However, if a patient is receiving one of these agents chronically, it is important for the ICU team to understand the mechanism of action and the potential complications or toxicities of these therapies [6].

TABLE 68.2

Biologic Agents for the Treatment of Rheumatic Diseases

Drug	Mechanism of action	Half-life	Side effects
Etanercept and etanercept -szzs	Soluble p75 TNF-α receptor fusion protein	72–132 h	Injection site/infusion reaction, TB reactivation, opportunistic infections, fungal and mycobacterial infections, demyelinating syndromes, drug-induced lupus, pancytopenia, aplastic anemia, hepatotoxicity, CHF, possible increased risk of lymphoma and nonmelanoma skin cancer
Infliximab and Infliximab-dyyb	Chimeric anti-TNF-α monoclonal antibody	7–12 d	Same as etanercept
Adalimumab and adalimumab -atto	Human anti-TNF-α monoclonal antibody	7–12 d 10–20 d	Same as etanercept Same as etanercept
Golimumab	Human anti-TNF-α monoclonal antibody	14 d	Same as etanercept
Certolizumab pegol	Human anti-TNF-α antibody Fab' fragment coupled to polyethylene glycol	14 d	Same as etanercept
Abatacept	CTLA4-Ig soluble fusion protein, inhibits T-cell activation by blocking costimulatory signal	8–25 d	Injection site/infusion reactions, infections similar to TNF-α inhibitors, COPD exacerbations, possible increased risk of lung cancer and lymphoma
Tocilizumab and Sarilumab	Humanized IgG1 IL-6 receptor antibody	6–13 d	Injection site/infusion reactions, infections similar to TNF-α inhibitors, hypertension, hypercholesterolemia, hepatotoxicity, gastrointestinal perforation
Anakinra	Human recombinant IL-1 receptor antagonist	4–6 h	Injection site reactions, infections similar to TNF-α inhibitors, neutropenia, hypersensitivity reactions
Canakinumab	Human monoclonal antibody that binds to IL-1	23 to 26 d	Same as anakinra.
Rilonacept	Dimeric fusion protein consisting of IL-1R1 and IL1RAcP linked in-line to the Fc region of IgG1 that binds and neutralizes IL-1	8.6 d	Same as anakinra.
Secukinumab	Human immunoglobulin G1 monoclonal antibody against IL-17A	28.1 d	Injection site/infusion reactions. Increased infections—mostly nasopharyngitis and upper respiratory infections, few increased cardiovascular events
Ustekinumab	IL12/23 p40 neutralizing antibody	15–45 d	Injection site reactions, increased risk for atypical infections, nonmelanoma skin cancers, reversible posterior leukoencephalopathy syndrome (rare), hypersensitivity reactions.
Rituximab	B-cell depleting chimeric monoclonal CD20 antibody	19 d	Infusion reactions, PML, new or reactivated viral infections, including fulminant hepatitis B
Tofacitinib	Pan JAK inhibitor with potent inhibition of JAK3, JAK1, and, to minor degree, JAK2	3 h	Metabolized via CYP3A4, so concern for drug interactions
Apremilast	Small molecule inhibitor of PDE4	6–9 h	Diarrhea, nausea, depression, suicidal ideation, and hypersensitivity.
Belimumab	Human IgG1λ monoclonal antibody that inhibits B-lymphocyte stimulator (BlyS)	19 d	Nausea, vomiting, diarrhea, abdominal pain, insomnia, headaches, myalgias, fever, leukopenia, cough, sore throat.

TNF, tumor necrosis factor; Tb, tuberculosis; Fab, fragment antigen binding; CTLA4, cytotoxic T lymphocyte–associated antigen; IL, interleukin; CHF, congestive heart failure; COPD, chronic obstructive pulmonary disease; PML, progressive multifocal leukoencephalopathy; IL-1R1, human interleukin-1 receptor component; IL-1RAcP, IL-1 receptor accessor protein.

Treatments for RA are diverse and include six TNF-α inhibitors, one IL-6 inhibitor, one JAK inhibitor, and agents that work through T-cell costimulation blockade and B-cell depletion. There are also two IL-1 antagonists, although these are used less commonly.

The TNF-α inhibitors are also used to treat spondyloarthropathies, such as psoriatic arthritis and ankylosing spondylitis. However, newer agents have emerged that work through PDE4 inhibition and the inhibition of cytokines IL-12, IL-23, and IL17A. A brief summary of mechanism of action and toxicity for each of these agents follows.

TNF-α Inhibitors

Eight TNF-α inhibitors (infliximab, infliximab-dyyb (the biosimilar of infliximab), adalimumab, adalimumab-atto (the biosimilar of adalimumab) etanercept, etanercept-szzs (the biosimilar of etanercept) golimumab, and certolizumab pegol) are currently approved for the treatment of moderate to severe RA, psoriatic arthritis, ankylosing spondylitis, and inflammatory bowel disease. Although TNF-α has many diverse cellular effects for RA and other inflammatory arthropathies, it acts as a potent inflammatory cytokine by binding to one of its receptors, p55 or p75, on chondrocytes, fibroblasts, and osteoclasts in the rheumatoid synovium. This binding stimulates the production of metalloproteinases and other effector molecules that damage the joint. In addition, TNF-α–activated endothelial cells express adhesion molecules, which promote the ingress of polymorphonuclear (PMN) cells into the joint. Naturally occurring soluble TNF-α receptors, which theoretically should neutralize TNF-α, exist in high concentrations in rheumatoid synovial fluid but may be inadequate in concentration to neutralize TNF-α in this disease.

Infliximab, a chimeric (human and mouse) monoclonal antibody against TNF-α, is administered intravenously at doses that can be titrated up from 3 to a maximum of 10 mg per kg every 4 weeks to 8 weeks depending on the severity of a patient's disease. On April 5, 2016, the FDA approved a biosimilar to infliximab also given by IV infusion. A biosimilar is a product that is essentially "interchangeable" or "highly similar" to the reference product in terms of mechanism of action, dosage and strength, and route of administration. In addition, the biosimilar product must not have any clinically meaningful differences in efficacy or safety profile compared to the reference drug.

Etanercept, a fusion protein comprising two recombinant p75-soluble TNF-α receptors combined with the Fc portion of human IgG, is administered by SQ injection (25 mg twice a week or 50 mg weekly). Adalimumab and golimumab are recombinant human IgG1 monoclonal antibodies against TNF-α administered as a 40 mg SQ injection every other week, and 50 mg SQ injection every month, respectively. In August of 2016, the FDA approved etanercept-szzs, a biosimilar to etanercept and in September of 2016, adalimumab -atto, a biosimilar to adalimumab, was approved.

Certolizumab is a pegylated human anti-TNF-α antibody Fab' that is given SQ every 2 to 4 weeks. MTX is recommended in combination with infliximab and adalimumab to reduce the frequency of neutralizing human/antichimeric antibodies or human/antihuman antibodies, respectively. However, the role of MTX use with golimumab and certolizumab to prevent these sorts of antibodies is not as clear. Studies have previously shown that the combination of methotrexate with these biologics works better than either one alone, but the self-injections are now often used as monotherapy.

Short-term toxicities of etanercept, adalimumab, golimumab, and certolizumab include injection site reactions with local urticarial lesions that often resolve with subsequent repeated dosing. Mild hypersensitivity reactions with infliximab infusions occur in 20% of patients, but 2% will experience severe infusion reactions. There is an increased risk of serious infections among patients taking all TNF-α inhibitors, including opportunistic, fungal, and mycobacterial infections. All patients should be tested for latent TB before initiating therapy with a TNF-α inhibitor, and patients with known hepatitis B infection should not receive these drugs.

Demyelinating syndromes have been reported in patients treated with TNF-α inhibitors. Immunogenicity, low-titer anti-dsDNA antibody, and drug-induced lupus syndromes have been documented in patients treated with TNF-α inhibitors. Pancytopenia, aplastic anemia, elevated liver function tests, and exacerbation of preexisting or new onset congestive heart failure have all been reported. Long-term toxicities, including an increased risk for malignancy, are ongoing concerns, although the data are inconclusive. Initial surveillance suggested a higher incidence of lymphoma and nonmelanoma skin cancers. However, a Cochrane review looking at the adverse effect of biologics (including not only TNF-α inhibitors but also abatacept, tocilizumab, rituximab, and anakinra) revealed that there was no statistically significant difference in the rate of lymphoma compared to controls [7]. Other studies from large patient data registries from the United States [8] and Europe [9] have also not shown increased malignancy rates associated with TNF-α inhibitors.

IL-1 Inhibitors

IL-1, produced by rheumatoid synovial macrophages, acts synergistically with TNF-α on synovial fibroblasts, chondrocytes, endothelial cells, and osteoclasts. These interactions promote the influx of PMN cells into the joint, release of metalloproteinases and collagenases from chondrocytes, and activation of osteoclastic bone resorption. IL-1 binds to two types of cell-surface receptors, but only type I is capable of intracellular activation. IL-1 inhibition has had modest benefit for RA but has been found to be effective primarily in a group of rare, inherited, autoinflammatory diseases called the cryopyrin-associated periodic syndromes (CAPS).

There are three medications that inhibit IL-1—anakinra, canakinumab, and rilonacept. Anakinra is a recombinant IL-1 receptor antagonist, which blocks the biologic activity of both IL-1α and IL-1β by competitively inhibiting IL-1 binding to the IL-1 type 1 receptor. Anakinra is given once daily and approved for the treatment of moderate to severe RA and CAPS. Canakinumab is a human monoclonal IL-1β antibody, which targets interleukin-1 β (IL-1β), thereby blocking its interaction with IL-1 receptors and neutralizing IL-1β activity. Canakinumab is given once a month and is approved for CAPS and systemic juvenile idiopathic arthritis (SJIA). Rilonacept prevents both IL-1α and IL-1β from binding to the IL-1 receptor complex on the surface of effector cells that mediate the proinflammatory response. It is given once weekly and is only approved to treat CAPS. Toxicities for all of the IL-1 inhibitors include injection site reactions, especially with anakinra, immunosuppression, leading to an increase of serious infections, cytopenias, and hepatotoxicity.

IL-6 Inhibition

IL-6, a proinflammatory cytokine expressed in RA synovial tissues, promotes the activation of B-cells, T cells, and macrophages, and upregulation of endothelial adhesion molecule expression. IL-6 also stimulates osteoclast maturation and promotes bone erosion. There are two FDA approved medications inhibiting IL-6 in rheumatoid arthritis, tocilizumab and sarilumab, the latter just approved May 2017. Tocilizumab, a humanized IgG1 anti-IL-6 receptor antibody, is approved for the treatment of RA, polyarticular JIA, SJIA, and giant cell arteritis. Sarilumab is similar and also a human recombinant monoclonal antibody that binds soluble and membrane-bound IL-6 receptors (sIL-6R and mIL-6R), thus inhibiting IL-6-mediated-signaling. Sarilumab is only approved for adult RA. Typically, both are used for patients who fail to respond to DMARDs and TNF-α inhibitors. Tocilizumab can be administered as a monthly IV infusion or as an injection every

1 to 2 weeks (depending on weight and severity of disease) either alone or in combination with weekly methotrexate. Sarilumab is given as a subcutaneous injection in 2 doses—150mg or 200mg every 2 weeks. The risk of serious infection is similar to that of TNF-α inhibitors. TB has been reported, but there are insufficient data to quantify the risk. To date, there is no evidence of an increased incidence of malignancies among RA patients treated with tocilizumab. In clinical trials, tocilizumab has also been associated with hypertension, hypercholesterolemia, elevated liver transaminases, and intestinal perforation.

IL-12 and IL23 Inhibition

Ustekinumab is a human monoclonal antibody directed against the p40 subunit common to IL-12 and IL-23. Ustekinumab was initially studied for psoriasis because concentrations of IL-12 and IL-23 are higher in psoriatic lesions. In addition, cytokines induced by IL-12 (IFN-γ) and IL-23 (IL-17A, IL-17F, and IL-22) are also elevated in psoriatic plaques [10]. Further studies demonstrated that ustekinumab also benefits PsA and has now been approved to treat both psoriasis and PsA. It is initially given by subcutaneous injection at weeks 0 and 4, and then every 12 weeks. Phase 2 trials of ustekinumab for RA and ankylosing spondylitis are ongoing. Adverse events are similar to the other biologic agents and include injection site reactions; increased risk for atypical infections, including reactivation of tuberculosis; increased risk for nonmelanoma skin cancers; reversible posterior leukoencephalopathy syndrome (rare); and hypersensitivity reactions. There also appears to be a risk for antibody formation to ustekinumab.

IL-17A Inhibition

Secukinumab is a high-affinity human immunoglobulin G1 monoclonal antibody that selectively binds to and neutralizes IL-17A. Cells that produce IL-17A are increased in the circulation, joints, and skin plaques in patients with PsA [11,12]. In addition, levels of IL-17^{+}CD8^{+} T cells have been shown to correlate with disease activity measures and erosions/structural joint damage [11]. Secukinumab was approved for the treatment of moderate to severe plaque psoriasis in January of 2015, and then soon after for the treatment of ankylosing spondylitis and psoriatic arthritis in January of 2016. Adverse reactions include more frequent infections such as nasopharyngitis and upper respiratory tract infections. Four strokes and two myocardial infarctions were also reported in the secukinumab groups versus zero in the placebo group, so more studies need to be done [13].

B-cell Depletion

Rituximab (RTX), a chimeric monoclonal antibody to CD20 that results in the depletion of mature B-cells and disruption of T-cell activation, is now approved for three rheumatologic conditions—moderate to severe RA in a patient who has failed other DMARDS and a TNF inhibitor; granulomatosis with polyangiitis (previously known as Wegener's granulomatosis); and microscopic polyangiitis. Rituximab is usually given with methotrexate when used for RA. For the vasculitides, rituximab is typically given with glucocorticoids as they are being tapered. Toxicities include infusion reactions with hypotension, fever, and nausea. Serious and potentially fatal viral infections include reactivation of hepatitis B with fulminant hepatitis and hepatic failure. In terms of infection risk, respiratory tract infections appear to be the most common with rituximab. In addition, a link has been found between those with preexisting hypogammaglobulinemia and increased risk of further reduction of immunoglobulin G (IgG) levels thus leading to serious infections after rituximab therapy [14]. Rates of opportunistic infections or tuberculosis do not appear to be increased, and no increased risks for malignancies have been reported in the limited follow-up of treated RA patients. Data from the non-Hodgkins lymphoma database as well as a national registry looking primarily at the use of rituximab for autoimmune diseases have been reassuring, in that serious adverse events were infrequent [15]. However, there are case reports of progressive multifocal leukoencephalopathy (PML) in patients with RA and systemic lupus erythematosus (SLE) that has led to death.

B-lymphocyte Stimulator Inhibition

Belimumab is a human IgG1λ monoclonal antibody that effectively targets the soluble form of B-lymphocyte stimulator (BlyS), which in turn inhibits the development and homeostasis of B lymphocytes [16]. This inhibition is thought to block autoantibody production responsible for the clinical features of lupus [16]. Belimumab was approved by the Food and Drug Administration in 2011 for the treatment of active SLE for patients currently receiving standard therapy (e.g., glucocorticoids, antimalarials, immunosuppressants, and NSAIDs). Standard dosing is 10 mg per kg given intravenously on days 0, 14, and 28, and then every 28 days thereafter. Data obtained after 52 weeks from Phase III trials (BLISS-76 and BLISS-52) noted belimumab improved overall SLE disease activity in the most common musculoskeletal and mucocutaneous organ domains [17]. Subjects with severe active lupus nephritis or central nervous system involvement were excluded from these trials, but patients with baseline proteinuria >0.2 g per 24 hours had significantly greater median percent reductions in proteinuria during weeks 12 to 52 than those treated with placebo [18]. Belimumab has been well tolerated with a safety profile that is comparable to placebo in terms of rates of infections and malignancies.

T-cell Costimulation Blockade

Abatacept, a selective modulator of T-cell activation, is approved for the treatment of moderate to severe RA for patients who have an inadequate response to methotrexate, other DMARDs, or TNF-α inhibitors. Abatacept can be given intravenously or by SQ injection once a week. T-cell activation requires two signals. The first is generated by the binding of a T-cell receptor (TCR) to an antigen presented by a major histocompatibility complex (MHC) on an antigen-presenting cell. The second, costimulatory signal is generated through a connection between CD80/86 on APCs and the CD28 receptor on T cells. To balance out T-cell activity, another protein receptor on the surface of T cells, cytotoxic T-lymphocyte-associated protein 4 (CTLA4), downregulates T-cell activation. Abatacept is a soluble fusion protein comprised of the extracellular domain of CTLA4 and the Fc portion of IgG1 (CTLA4-Ig) that interferes with T-cell activation by binding to CD80/86, thereby inhibiting the required costimulatory signal. Toxicities include hypersensitivity infusion reactions, infections, exacerbations of chronic obstructive pulmonary disease (COPD), and potential concerns about malignancies, including lymphoma and lung cancer though as mentioned earlier, data is not clear.

SMALL MOLECULE INHIBITORS

Janus Kinase (JAK) Inhibition

Tofacitinib was approved by the FDA on November 2012 for RA and was the first orally administered Janus kinase (JAK) inhibitor [19]. Tofacitinib works by entering immune cells and binding to the adenosine triphosphate (ATP) binding cleft of JAK1 and JAK3. This binding inhibits the autophosphorylation and phosphorylation of tyrosine residues, thereby preventing the activation of signal transducer and activator of transcription (STAT) molecules. When STAT molecules are not activated, gene transcription and cytokine production are inhibited, leading to decreased synovial inflammation and structural joint damage in

RA patients. Toxicities include cytopenias, dyslipidemia, elevations in creatinine and transaminases, and immunosuppressive effects, including reactivation of latent tuberculosis. Malignancy risk (excluding nonmelanoma skin cancers) was within the expected range for patients with moderate to severe RA [20].

Phosphodiesterase 4 (PDE4) Inhibition

Apremilast is a small molecule inhibitor of PDE4 that was approved for the treatment of moderate to severe plaque psoriasis and psoriatic arthritis. Apremilast is an oral drug that inhibits PDE4, thereby blocking the degradation of cyclic adenosine monophosphate (cAMP). As a result, elevated levels of cAMP downregulate proinflammatory cytokines such as IL-12, IL-23, TNF-α, and IFN-γ, thus decreasing inflammation. Benefit to the skin is more modest, although PDE4 is expressed in cell types present in the joints and skin [21]. The most common adverse events are gastrointestinal (typically diarrhea and nausea), and they usually occur early and are self-limiting. Serious reactions include depression, suicidal ideation, and hypersensitivity. There has been no significant increase in major adverse cardiac events, serious or opportunistic infections, malignancies, or laboratory abnormalities compared to placebo [22]. The favorable infection profile and decreased need for regular lab monitoring make this drug desirable.

INTRAVENOUS IMMUNOGLOBULIN (IVIG)

Immunoglobulin therapy is a blood product made of pooled polyvalent IgG antibodies extracted from the serum of a large number of donors. It is the mainstay therapy for patients with hereditary or acquired immunodeficiency. In addition, IVIG has been used to treat several immune-mediated diseases. There is good supporting evidence for use against Kawasaki disease, immune thrombocytopenia purpura, chronic, demyelinating polyneuropathy (CIDP), and Guillaine Barre syndrome [23]. IVIG is also used as second-line therapy for dermatomyositis and polymyositis, and in some cases of ANCA-associated vasculitides [23]. The mechanism of action is thought to be complex and not completely understood. IVIG has been used in antiphospholipid antibody syndrome and CAPS, but the evidence does not support its use in CAPS unless complicated by significant autoimmune thrombocytopenia [23].

The dosing of IVIG varies depending on the disease being treated. For immunodeficiency states, dosing is usually 300 to 800 mg per kg every 3 to 4 weeks. In contrast, a typical regimen may be 2 g per kg over 5 days for CIDP or polymyositis. IVIG is generally considered safe therapy, but immediate side effects can include malaise, fatigue, headache, arthralgias, myalgias, flushing, chest tightness, fever, chills, gastrointestinal upset, changes in blood pressure, and anaphylactic reactions [24]. Late adverse reactions are quite rare but can include thromboembolic events in up to 2% of patients [24]. Slowing down the infusion rate and giving a lower concentration of IVIG can decrease this risk.

DMARDs, BIOLOGICS, AND PREGNANCY

Most DMARDs are also teratogens and contraindicated in pregnancy, although hydroxychloroquine, sulfasalazine, AZA, and sometimes cyclosporine are tolerated in those with severe disease. MTX and LEF are rated as pregnancy class X (contraindicated, risk outweighs benefits), and should not be used during pregnancy. AZA, although rated as class D (positive evidence of risk), is considered safer than many other immunosuppressive agents during pregnancy, based on the literature in the transplantation population. When the benefit of immunosuppression appears to outweigh the risks (e.g., in renal transplant recipients, active lupus, or inflammatory bowel disease), AZA is preferred over other immunosuppressive medications. We strongly recommend avoidance of CY and MMF (both pregnancy class D) during pregnancy except for life-threatening medical conditions in which no alternative therapy is available.

Data on the safety of biologic agents are limited primarily to case reports largely looking at TNF-α inhibitors. However, collective evidence suggests that exposure to TNF-α inhibitors at conception or during the first trimester does not result in an increased risk of adverse pregnancy and fetal outcomes [25]. There is much less data about other biologic therapies. As of the time of this publication, the TNF-α inhibitors, ustekinumab, and anakinra are rated pregnancy class B (no evidence of risk). Abatacept, rituximab, belimumab, tocilizumab, tofacitinib, and apremilast are all class C (risk cannot be ruled out). Use of these biologic agents should be avoided during pregnancy unless no alternative therapies are available.

SUMMARY

A critically ill patient who has recently received one of the above DMARDs or biologic agents should be approached as an immunocompromised host. Most are immunosuppressive except for perhaps hydroxychloroquine and apremilast. Atypical or opportunistic infections are high on the differential if the patient is febrile. In addition, other toxicities of these drugs can include cytopenias, liver function abnormalities, atypical neurologic symptoms, and congestive heart failure. Given the critical nature of the illness that requires ICU care, it is prudent to postpone patients' scheduled doses of these DMARDs or biologic agents until their medical status is more stable.

References

1. Esteban NV, Loughlin T, Yergey AL, et al: Daily cortisol production rate in man determined by stable isotope dilution/mass spectrometry. *J Clin Endocrinol Metab* 72(1):39–45, 1991.
2. Clunie GP, Lennard L: Relevance of thiopurine methyltransferase status in rheumatology patients receiving azathioprine. *Rheumatology (Oxford)* 43(1):13–18, 2004.
3. Wolfe F, Michaud K: Lymphoma in rheumatoid arthritis: the effect of methotrexate and anti-tumor necrosis factor therapy in 18,572 patients. *Arthritis Rheum* 50(6):1740–1751, 2004.
4. Mersereau J, Dooley MA: Gonadal failure with cyclophosphamide therapy for lupus nephritis: advances in fertility preservation. *Rheum Dis Clin North Am* 36(1):99–108, viii, 2010.
5. Masala A, Faedda R, Alagna S, et al: Use of testosterone to prevent cyclophosphamide-induced azoospermia. *Ann Intern Med* 126(4):292–295, 1997.
6. Furst DE, Keystone EC, So AK, et al: Updated consensus statement on biological agents for the treatment of rheumatic diseases, 2012. *Ann Rheum Dis* 72 Suppl 2:ii2–ii34, 2013.
7. Singh JA, Wells GA, Christensen R, et al: Adverse effects of biologics: a network meta-analysis and cochrane overview. *Cochrane Database Syst Rev* (2):CD008794, 2011. doi:10.1002/14651858.CD008794.pub2.
8. Solomon DH, Kremer JM, Fisher M, et al: Comparative cancer risk associated with methotrexate, other non-biologic and biologic disease-modifying anti-rheumatic drugs. *Semin Arthritis Rheum* 43(4):489–497, 2014.
9. Ramiro S, Gaujoux-Viala C, Nam JL, et al: Safety of synthetic and biological DMARDs: a systematic literature review informing the 2013 update of the EULAR recommendations for management of rheumatoid arthritis. *Ann Rheum Dis* 73(3):529–535, 2014.
10. Quatresooz P, Hermanns-Le T, Pierard GE, et al: Ustekinumab in psoriasis immunopathology with emphasis on the Th17-IL23 axis: a primer. *J Biomed Biotechnol* 2012:147413, 2012.
11. Menon B, Gullick NJ, Walter GJ, et al: Interleukin-17+CD8+ T cells are enriched in the joints of patients with psoriatic arthritis and correlate with disease activity and joint damage progression. *Arthritis Rheumatol* 66(5):1272–1281, 2014.
12. Kagami S, Rizzo HL, Lee JJ, et al: Circulating Th17, Th22, and Th1 cells are increased in psoriasis. *J Invest Dermatol* 130(5):1373–1383, 2010.
13. Mease PJ, McInnes IB, Kirkham B, et al: Secukinumab inhibition of interleukin-17A in patients with psoriatic arthritis. *N Engl J Med* 373(14):1329–1339, 2015.
14. Kado R, Sanders G, McCune WJ: Suppression of normal immune responses after treatment with rituximab. *Curr Opin Rheumatol* 28:251–258, 2016.

15. Tony HP, Burmester G, Schulze-Koops H, et al: Safety and clinical outcomes of rituximab therapy in patients with different autoimmune diseases: experience from a national registry (GRAID). *Arthritis Res Ther* 13(3):R75, 2011.
16. Frieri M, Heuser W, Bliss J: Efficacy of novel monoclonal antibody belimumab in the treatment of lupus nephritis. *J Pharmacol Pharmacother* 6(2):71–76, 2015.
17. Manzi S, Sanchez-Guerrero J, Merrill JT, et al: Effects of belimumab, a B lymphocyte stimulator-specific inhibitor, on disease activity across multiple organ domains in patients with systemic lupus erythematosus: combined results from two phase III trials. *Ann Rheum Dis* 71(11):1833–1838, 2012.
18. Dooley M, Houssiau F, Aranow C, et al: Effect of belimumab treatment on renal outcomes: results from the phase 3 belimumab clinical trials in patients with SLE. *Lupus* 22(1):63–72, 2013.
19. Lundquist LM, Cole SW, Sikes ML: Efficacy and safety of tofacitinib for treatment of rheumatoid arthritis. *World J Orthop* 5(4):504–511, 2014.
20. Curtis JR, Lee EB, Kaplan IV, et al: Tofacitinib, an oral janus kinase inhibitor: analysis of malignancies across the rheumatoid arthritis clinical development programme. *Ann Rheum Dis*, 2015.
21. Genovese MC, Jarosova K, Cieslak D, et al: Apremilast in patients with active rheumatoid arthritis: a phase II, multicenter, randomized, double-blind, placebo-controlled, parallel-group study. *Arthritis Rheumatol* 67(7):1703–1710, 2015.
22. Kavanaugh A, Mease PJ, Gomez-Reino JJ, et al: Longterm (52-week) results of a phase III randomized, controlled trial of apremilast in patients with psoriatic arthritis. *J Rheumatol* 42(3):479–488, 2015.
23. Mulhearn B, Bruce IN: Indications for IVIG in rheumatic diseases. *Rheumatology (Oxford)* 54(3):383–391, 2015.
24. Orbach H, Katz U, Sherer Y, et al: Intravenous immunoglobulin: adverse effects and safe administration. *Clin Rev Allergy Immunol* 29(3):173–184, 2005.
25. Hyrich KL, Verstappen SM: Biologic therapies and pregnancy: the story so far. *Rheumatology (Oxford)* 53(8):1377–1385, 2014.

Chapter 69 ■ Anaphylaxis

FREDERIC F. LITTLE • HELEN M. HOLLINGSWORTH

Anaphylaxis is the most severe and potentially fatal form of the immediate hypersensitivity reactions. The term *anaphylaxis* (antiphylaxis) is derived from Greek and means "against protection" [1]. It describes the shock-like state that is caused by contact with a substance and contrasts with the term *prophylaxis*, which denotes a beneficial or protective state resulting from contact with a substance.

The clinical features of anaphylactic reactions are the physiologic sequelae of release of chemical mediators from tissue-based mast cells and circulating basophils and include a potential for life-threatening vascular collapse and respiratory obstruction [2,3]. A clinically and physiologically indistinguishable hypersensitivity reaction, which is called an anaphylactoid reaction, differs from anaphylactic reactions only because the chemical mediators are released by nonimmunologic mechanisms. Since the clinical features are indistinguishable, both will be referred to collectively as anaphylactic reactions [4].

Estimation of the annual incidence of anaphylactic reactions from administrative sources is hampered by complex coding and incomplete reporting. Anaphylaxis is frequent, with approximately 50 to 103 cases occurring per 100,000 person-years [5]. The case fatality rate from anaphylaxis is estimated at 0.25% to 0.33% of hospitalizations and emergency department visits for anaphylaxis [6]. In a separate study, examination of a United States database identified 2,458 deaths from anaphylaxis from 1999 to 2010 [7].

PATHOPHYSIOLOGY OF ANAPHYLACTIC REACTIONS

Mechanisms of Release of Chemical Mediators

For humans, anaphylaxis involves a series of steps that result in the release of chemical mediators from tissue-based mast cells and circulating basophils. First, contact with an antigen stimulates the generation of antibodies of the immunoglobulin E (IgE) class. Next, the IgE molecules bind by way of their Fc receptor to a glycoprotein receptor on the cell-surface membrane of tissue mast cells and blood-borne basophils, the so-called target cells. As many as 4,000 to 100,000 IgE molecules normally bind to a single target cell, and up to 100,000 to 500,000 among atopic individuals [7,8]. This binding may remain for weeks to months. When two IgE molecules with the same Fab-binding (antigen-recognition) specificity are in close proximity on the surface of mast cells and basophils, the cells are termed *sensitized*.

For subsequent antigenic exposure to stimulate the release of mediators from mast cells and basophils, the specific antigen must bind to the Fab portion of two IgE molecules fixed to the surface of the target cell. This bridging of two IgE molecules initiates a series of biochemical modifications called the activation–secretion response (Fig. 69.1). This sequence causes secretion of preformed primary mediators of anaphylaxis from the cytoplasmic granules of target cells, including histamine, serotonin, eosinophil chemotactic factor of anaphylaxis (ECF-A), heparin, neutrophil chemotactic factor, and proteolytic enzymes that include tryptase [3].

The activation–secretion response also stimulates synthesis of kallikrein and newly generated, secondary lipid mediators, which include platelet-activating factor (PAF); prostaglandin D_2 (PGD_2), a product of the cyclooxygenase pathway of arachidonic acid metabolism; and leukotrienes C_4, D_4, and E_4 (LTC_4, LTD_4, and LTE_4, respectively), products of the lipoxygenase pathway of arachidonic acid metabolism [1,3]. Several cytokines are also released after activation, including interleukins (IL-1, IL-2, IL-3, IL-4, IL-5, and IL-6), tumor necrosis factor, endothelin-1, and granulocyte-macrophage colony–stimulating factor [1].

A variety of substances can induce IgE antibody formation and, on subsequent challenge, provoke anaphylactic reactions [9]. The most common substances are drugs, insect venoms, foods, and allergen extracts used in specific immunotherapy (SIT) [9–11]. These and other less common causes of IgE-mediated anaphylaxis are outlined in Table 69.1.

Non–IgE-mediated anaphylaxis occurs when certain ingested or infused substances cause direct mast cell and basophil activation. Clinically significant examples of non–IgE-mediated anaphylaxis are noted in Table 69.2. The administration of blood, serum, or immunoglobulins to patients who are IgA deficient can result in immune complex formation between donor IgA and recipient IgG anti-IgA antibodies [4,12]. These immune complexes fix complement causing activation of the complement cascade with release of the C3a and C5a complement fragments. C3a and C5a are anaphylatoxins and can directly activate mast cells and basophils.

Physiologic Properties of the Chemical Mediators of Anaphylaxis

The most important chemical mediators of anaphylaxis are histamine, cysteinyl leukotrienes (LTC_4, LTD_4, and LTE_4), PAF,

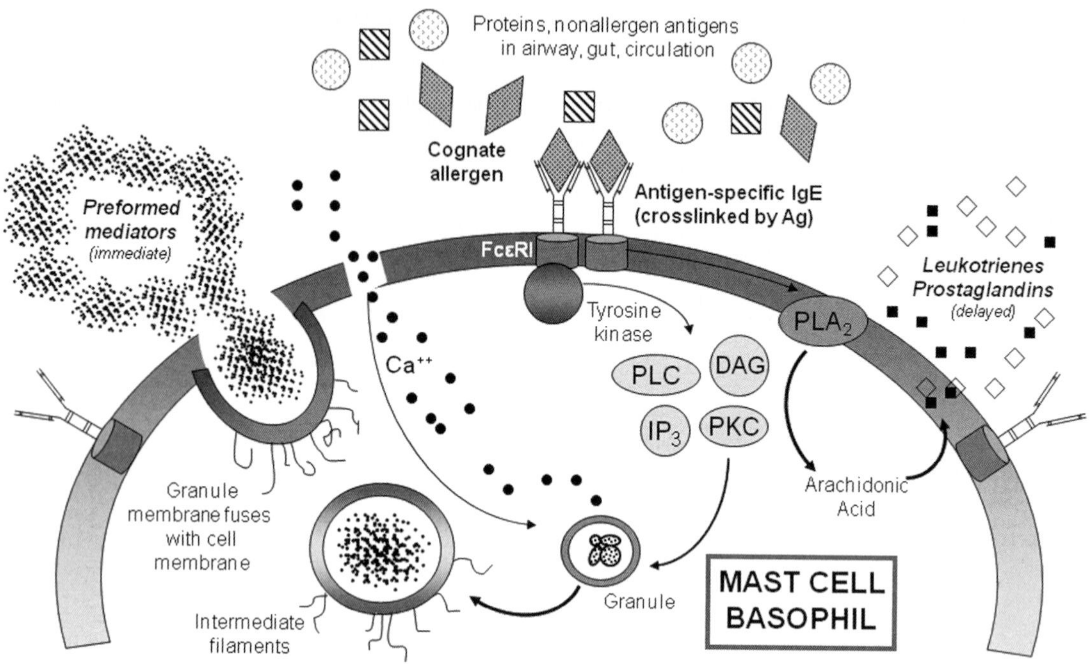

FIGURE 69.1 Chemical mediator release. When two IgE molecules are bridged by an antigen that is specifically recognized by those IgE molecules, a cascade of transmembrane and intracellular events is triggered. The result is the extrusion of granule contents (mediators) into the extracellular space and elaboration of other, newly formed mediators. Tyrosine kinase appears to be an important intramembrane messenger that initiates the intracellular cascades. At least one cascade involves PLC, which mediates calcium influx into the cell and catalyzes hydrolysis of phosphatidylinositol into the secondary messengers 1,4,5-IP_3 and 1,2-DAG. IP_3 plays a role in calcium mobilization; DAG mediates production of arachidonic acid metabolites and activates PKC. PKC, in turn, participates in the fusion of granules within the cell membrane. PLA_2 mediates the conversion of membrane phospholipid into arachidonic acid, resulting in elaboration of prostaglandins and leukotrienes. Ag, antigen; DAG, diacylglycerol; IgE, immunoglobulin E; IP_3, inositol triphosphate; PKC, protein kinase C; PLA_2, phospholipase A_2; PLC, phospholipase C.

TABLE 69.1

Causes of Immunoglobulin E–Mediated Anaphylaxis

Type	Agent	Example
Proteins	Allergen extracts	Pollen, dust mite, mold
	Vaccines	Influenza
	Venoms	Hymenoptera
	Heterologous serum	Tetanus antitoxin [11], antithymocyte globulin, snake antivenom
	Others	Heparin, latex [9], thiobarbiturates, seminal fluid
Hormones		Insulin [118], ACTH, TSH [11], progesterone, salmon calcitonin
Haptens	Antibiotics	β-lactams [11], ethambutol, nitrofurantoin, sulfonamides [11], streptomycin, vancomycin [121]
Disinfectants		Ethylene oxide
Local anesthetics[a]		Benzocaine, tetracaine, lidocaine, mepivacaine [11]
Others		Aminopyrine, sulfobromophthalein

[a]Precise mechanism not established.
ACTH, adrenocorticotropic hormone; TSH, thyroid-stimulating hormone.

and bradykinin. Physiologically, these substances increase arteriolar vasodilatation, enhance capillary permeability, recruit other inflammatory cells, and precipitate bronchoconstriction (reviewed in [13]). The contribution of multiple mediators other than histamine explains the limited benefit of antihistamines *alone* in treating anaphylaxis.

Histamine (reviewed in [14]) acts to (a) increase capillary permeability by stimulating terminal arteriolar dilatation and contraction of endothelial cells in postcapillary venules, which opens intercellular gaps, and, as a result, causes the development of urticaria and angioedema; (b) increase secretion from nasal and bronchial mucous glands; (c) stimulate contraction of smooth muscle; (d) enhance prostaglandin synthesis; (e) chemotactically modulate eosinophil migration; and (f) regulate parasympathetic afferent nerve stimulation (a process blocked by atropine), which increases airway resistance and decreases lung compliance. Studies of histamine infusion into normal human volunteers suggest that vasodilatation is mediated by both H_1 and H_2 receptors, whereas bronchoconstriction and tachycardia are mediated by H_1 receptors alone [15].

During an anaphylactic reaction, LTC_4, LTD_4, and LTE_4 (a) induce a prolonged constrictive effect on bronchial smooth

TABLE 69.2

Causes of Non–immunoglobulin E–Mediated Anaphylaxis

Complement activation
Blood product transfusion in IgA-deficient patient [12]
Hemodialysis with cuprophane membrane [122]
Direct release of chemical mediators of anaphylaxis
Protamine [11][a]
Radiographic contrast media [66]
Dextran [123][a]
Hydroxyethyl starch [124]
Muscle relaxants [125]
Ketamine [126]
Local anesthetics [127][a]
Codeine and other opiate narcotics [11]
Highly charged antibiotics, including amphotericin B [121]
Generation of leukotrienes
Nonsteroidal anti-inflammatory drugs [11]
Indomethacin [111]
Acetylsalicylic acid (aspirin) [128]
Sulindac [112]
Zomepirac sodium [113]
Tolmetin sodium [114]
Other
Antineoplastic agents (e.g., platinum-based [129,130])
Sulfiting agents
Exercise [43]
Idiopathic recurrent anaphylaxis [98,100]

[a]Precise mechanism not established.

muscle, which affects the peripheral more than the central airways, (b) increase vascular permeability, and (c) act as chemotactic agents for other inflammatory cells [16,17]. In fact, leukotrienes are far more potent bronchoconstrictors than is histamine.

Two additional modulators of anaphylaxis are bradykinin, which stimulates a slow, sustained contraction of bronchial and vascular smooth muscles while increasing vascular permeability and secretion from mucous glands, and PAF, which induces platelet aggregation, recruits eosinophils, and can directly increase vascular permeability [3,18].

Thus, the physiologic consequences of chemical mediator release during anaphylaxis are (a) an increased vascular permeability; (b) an increased secretion from nasal and bronchiolar mucous glands; (c) smooth muscle contraction in the blood vessels, the bronchioles, the gastrointestinal tract, and the uterus; (d) migration–attraction of eosinophils and neutrophils; (e) bradykinin generation stimulated by kallikrein substances; and (f) induction of platelet aggregation and degranulation. These events act synergistically to increase the vascular permeability that in turn permits the access of a variety of plasma proteins (antibodies, complement, kinins, and coagulation proteins) to tissue sites, which further contributes to the observed inflammation. Substances such as PAF potentially contribute to local coagulation abnormalities, which may also be seen in anaphylactic reactions [3].

CLINICAL AND LABORATORY FEATURES

Mast cells are concentrated in the skin, in the mucous membranes of the respiratory and gastrointestinal tracts, and in the perivenular tissue, whereas basophils are located in the bloodstream, all of which are potential sites of exposure to offending antigens (e.g., food, drugs, insect venom, diagnostic agents) [1]. These sites are also most commonly involved in the manifestations of an anaphylactic reaction. Urticaria, angioedema, respiratory obstruction (cough, wheezing, stridor, or breathlessness), and vascular collapse are the most important clinical features of anaphylaxis, and these signs and symptoms are due to the direct effects of mast cell and basophil-derived mediators on affected organ systems. Other clinical manifestations may include (a) a sense of fright or impending doom, (b) weakness or dizziness, (c) sweating, (d) sneezing, (e) rhinorrhea, (f) conjunctivitis, (g) generalized pruritus and swelling, (h) flushing, (i) hypoxemia, (j) choking, (k) dysphagia, (l) vomiting or diarrhea, (m) abdominal pain, (n) incontinence, (o) uterine cramps, and (p) loss of consciousness.

Profound hypotension and shock may develop as a result of significant arteriolar vasodilatation, increased vascular permeability, cardiac arrhythmias, or irreversible cardiac failure, even in the absence of respiratory or other symptoms [3,10]. Furthermore, transient or sustained hypotension may result in local tissue ischemia, stroke, myocardial infarction, or death [10]. Intravascular coagulation, evidenced by a fall in the levels of factors V, VIII, fibrinogen, kininogen, and complement components, has also been described [1].

Anaphylaxis-induced fatalities most often result from involvement of the respiratory tract [19,20]. Structures throughout the respiratory tract may be affected, but respiratory failure is generally the result of upper respiratory tract obstruction due to laryngeal edema or obstruction of small airways due to bronchoconstriction, mucosal edema, and hypersecretion of mucus [21,22]. Intra-alveolar hemorrhage and acute respiratory distress syndrome have been reported [22,23].

The physical examination of a patient with anaphylactic shock may reveal one or more of the following: a rapid, weak, irregular, or unobtainable pulse, tachypnea, respiratory distress, cyanosis, hoarseness, stridor, dysphagia, diminished breath sounds, crackles, cough, wheezes, hyperinflated lungs, urticaria, angioedema, or conjunctival edema (Table 69.3) [24]. A given patient may manifest only a subset of these findings, sometimes only cardiovascular collapse or only stridor and breathlessness.

Laboratory findings in anaphylaxis are varied. Biochemical abnormalities in anaphylaxis include elevation of plasma histamine, serum or plasma tryptase, and depression of serum complement components [9,10]. Although these biochemical abnormalities codify our understanding of the pathophysiology of anaphylaxis, they are rarely evaluated in the acute management of clinically established anaphylaxis. Plasma histamine peaks by 15 minutes after the onset of anaphylaxis and returns to baseline by 60 minutes; measurement is generally not feasible unless anaphylaxis develops in the hospital. As discussed in the next section, serum or plasma tryptase may be helpful retrospectively when the diagnosis is uncertain [9,25].

Although there have been no systematic reviews of electrocardiographic findings, reports describe disturbances in rate, rhythm, repolarization, and ectopy [26–28], as well as myocardial infarction [29,30]. Chest radiography may reveal hyperinflation caused by severe bronchoconstriction.

DIAGNOSIS AND DIFFERENTIAL DIAGNOSIS OF ANAPHYLAXIS

Diagnostic Criteria

Development of the characteristic clinical features of anaphylaxis shortly after exposure to an antigen or other inciting agent usually establishes the diagnosis of an anaphylactic reaction [2,9,31]. The setting is often suggestive as well: a patient who has just received an antibiotic or radiographic contrast media

TABLE 69.3

Clinical Manifestations of Anaphylactic Reactions

System	Reaction	Symptoms	Signs
Respiratory tract	Rhinitis	Nasal congestion and itching	Mucosal edema
	Laryngeal edema	Dyspnea	Laryngeal stridor, edema of vocal cords
	Bronchoconstriction	Cough, wheezing, and sensation of chest tightness	Crackles, respiratory distress, tachypnea, and wheezes
Cardiovascular	Hypotension	Syncope, feeling of faintness	Hypotension, tachycardia
	Arrhythmias	Palpitations	ECG changes: nonspecific ST segment and T-wave changes, nodal rhythm, and atrial fibrillation
Skin	Urticaria	Pruritus, hives	Urticarial lesions
	Angioedema	Nonpruritic swelling of extremity or perioral, or periorbital region	Nonpruritic, frequently asymmetric swelling of extremity, perioral, or periorbital region
Gastrointestinal tract	Smooth muscle contraction, mucosal edema	Nausea, vomiting, abdominal pain, and diarrhea	Abdominal tenderness, distention
Eye	Conjunctivitis	Ocular itching, lacrimation	Conjunctival inflammation

ECG, electrocardiogram.
Summarized from McGrath K: Anaphylaxis, in Patterson R, Grammer LC, Greenberger PA (eds): *Patterson's Allergic Diseases - Diagnosis and Management*. Philadelphia, PA, Lippincott-Raven, 2009, pp 439–458; Lieberman P, Nicklas RA, Randolph C, et al: Anaphylaxis—a practice parameter update 2015. *Ann Allergy Asthma Immunol* 115(5):341–384, 2015.

infusion or one who presents to the emergency room after a yellow jacket sting. Clinical criteria have been developed to help clinicians recognize the variable presentations of anaphylaxis [2,31]. A diagnosis of anaphylaxis is likely when any one of the following three criteria is present: (1) the rapid onset (minutes to several hours) of an illness with involvement of skin and/or mucosa (angioedema, flushing, pruritus, urticaria), and either respiratory compromise (dyspnea, wheeze, decreased peak flow, stridor, hypoxemia) or hypotension or end-organ dysfunction (collapse, syncope, incontinence); (2) onset of two or more of the following features after exposure to a likely allergen: skin and/or mucosa (angioedema, flushing, pruritus, urticaria), respiratory compromise (dyspnea, wheeze, decreased peak flow, stridor, hypoxemia), hypotension or end-organ dysfunction (collapse, syncope, incontinence), or persistent gastrointestinal symptoms (vomiting, crampy abdominal pain, diarrhea); or (3) onset of hypotension minutes to several hours after exposure to a known allergen for that patient [31]. Recognition of the early signs and symptoms of anaphylaxis and prompt treatment are imperative to prevent progression to irreversible shock and death [9].

Laboratory Testing

Initial laboratory testing is often not helpful diagnostically, except to exclude other causes of the clinical presentation. However, samples obtained during the acute episode can be assayed subsequently for serum or plasma total tryptase. Total tryptase levels include both α- and β-tryptase; the former is increased in systemic mastocytosis and the latter can be elevated for up to 6 hours after the onset of a suspected anaphylactic reaction [25]. However, the sensitivity of β-tryptase is suboptimal because levels can be normal after documented anaphylaxis, especially when caused by foods [9]. There may be a role for serial measurements for documenting the course of systemic mast cell and basophil degranulation [9]. As noted above, histamine is rarely assessed clinically because it must be obtained within the first hour after a reaction and requires special handling.

Retrospectively, measurement of antigen (allergen)-specific IgE antibodies by an ImmunoCAP (or similar assay, which have replaced radioallergosorbent tests [RAST]) may be helpful. Specific skin tests may also define allergic sensitivity. Skin testing must be done in a carefully controlled setting due to the risk of provoking a severe reaction. Cutaneous assessment for the presence of antigen-specific IgE may be negative for several days after a reaction because mast cell and basophil degranulation at the time of the initial reaction may lead to a refractory period. This can be avoided by delaying testing for 4 to 6 weeks [32].

Differential Diagnosis

Clinical disorders that may be confused with anaphylaxis are sudden, acute bronchoconstriction in an asthmatic, vasovagal syncope, tension pneumothorax, mechanical airway obstruction, pulmonary edema, cardiac arrhythmias, myocardial infarction with cardiogenic shock, aspiration of a food bolus, pulmonary embolism, seizures, acute drug toxicity, septic shock, and toxic shock syndrome [10,31]. Particularly relevant syndromes in the differential diagnosis are the noningestion/medication-triggered urticaria/angioedema disorders—ACEI-induced, idiopathic (spontaneous), hereditary, and acquired. These can present with several of the concerning manifestations of anaphylaxis, including respiratory failure requiring intensive care. While the initial management is similar to that of anaphylaxis, there are several key differentiating clinical and laboratory features to aid in accurate diagnosis. These are discussed in more detail under the "Specific Agents and Precipitants" section later in this chapter.

CLINICAL COURSE OF ANAPHYLACTIC REACTIONS

The constellation of clinical symptoms as well as their severity and duration is variable but will depend to some extent on the mode of antigen exposure. Anaphylaxis may occur within seconds following parenteral introduction of antigen and usually occurs within 30 minutes [1,9,33]. In contrast, the onset of anaphylaxis that follows oral administration of an antigen ranges from minutes to several hours [34]. In a series of 164 fatal episodes of anaphylaxis, the median time between onset of symptoms and cardiac or respiratory arrest was 5 minutes for iatrogenic anaphylaxis, 15 minutes for stinging insect anaphylaxis, and 30 minutes for food-induced anaphylaxis [33].

Generally, the more rapid the onset of symptoms, the more severe will be the reaction [1]. Mild systemic reactions often last for several hours, rarely more than 24 hours. Severe manifestations, such as laryngeal edema, bronchoconstriction, and hypotension, if not fatal, may persist or recur for several days. However, even severe manifestations may resolve within minutes of treatment. Up to 20% of patients will experience biphasic or protracted anaphylaxis, with signs and symptoms recurring up to 24 hours or persisting beyond 24 hours after initial presentation [24]. This highlights the need for close observation after initial response to treatment.

TREATMENT OF ANAPHYLAXIS

The key to successful treatment of anaphylaxis is prompt intervention to support cardiopulmonary function and effective action to prevent further exposure to the inciting stimulus when possible. The prompt administration of epinephrine is critical and should be supplemented, when needed, with aggressive use of vasopressors, fluid replacement, and medications to counteract the effects of released chemical mediators [9]. Injectable epinephrine, intravenous infusion materials and fluids, antihistamines, intubation equipment, a tracheostomy set, and individuals trained to use these materials should be available. Since symptoms of a systemic anaphylactic reaction may be followed by potentially fatal manifestations, patients must be serially examined and continuously monitored [9]. Many therapeutic and diagnostic agents frequently employed in intensive care settings (e.g., antibiotics, radiographic contrast) may induce anaphylactic reactions. Thus, the anticipation and the preparedness to deal with these potential reactions are very important.

Emergency Measures

The evaluation of individuals who are suspected of having anaphylaxis must be performed rapidly. The cause and mechanism of antigen exposure should be ascertained to assess how long the inciting antigen has been present and, when possible, to limit further absorption (e.g., stopping infusion of a medication or contrast media). Epinephrine should be administered intramuscularly, as soon as anaphylaxis is identified. The patient should be placed in a recumbent position with the legs elevated; pregnant patients may be placed in the left lateral decubitus position if inferior vena cava compression is a concern. Intravenous access with one or two large bore catheters should be achieved for fluid resuscitation.

A history of previous allergic reactions and former treatment may help to guide immediate therapy, obviating the need to try previously failed regimens in a life-threatening situation [35].

Supportive Cardiopulmonary Measures

Particular attention to the respiratory and cardiovascular systems is paramount and must include assessment for laryngeal edema and bronchoconstriction, as well as monitoring of oxygenation, blood pressure, and cardiac rhythm [31].

Ensuring adequate ventilation and oxygenation is essential. Supplemental oxygen should be administered and pulse oximetry monitored. Intubation and assisted ventilation may be necessary for cases of severe bronchoconstriction, and ventilator management strategies such as those used for treatment of acute severe asthma exacerbation may be necessary. These techniques are discussed in Chapters 166 and 172.

Oral or nasal endotracheal intubation is usually feasible, but rarely edema of the tongue, larynx, or vocal cords may obstruct the upper airway and preclude oropharyngeal or nasopharyngeal intubation. To ensure a patent airway in such instances, cricothyroidotomy or tracheotomy may be necessary (see Chapters 8 and 9).

Close electrocardiographic monitoring is indicated because the sequelae of anaphylaxis and its therapy are both potentially arrhythmogenic [9]. Hypotension, acidosis, hypoxia, vasopressors, and bronchodilators are well-described predisposing factors for cardiac arrhythmias (see Chapter 189). Adequate intravenous or intraosseous access should be established as soon as possible, preferably with two 18-gauge or larger peripheral catheters or needles.

Pharmacologic Therapy

The mainstay of therapy is parenteral epinephrine (adrenaline), which acts on bronchial and cardiac β-receptors, causing bronchial dilatation and both chronotropic and inotropic cardiac stimulation. An equally important effect of epinephrine is stimulation of α-adrenergic receptors on blood vessels, which causes vasoconstriction. This is important for managing anaphylaxis-induced hypotension [31]. In addition, epinephrine increases intracellular levels of cyclic adenosine monophosphate (AMP) and thereby acts to inhibit the activation of tissue-based mast cells and circulating basophils [3,15]. Inhaled β_2-adrenergic agents, such as albuterol (salbutamol), complement the actions of epinephrine by reversing bronchoconstriction and reducing bronchial mucus secretion [9].

Antihistamines, particularly the H_1-receptor blocker diphenhydramine, are useful for treating cutaneous manifestations of anaphylaxis, but are slower in onset than epinephrine and not helpful for hemodynamic compromise. Thus, they are considered adjunctive therapy to epinephrine. Given their beneficial safety profile, they may be administered empirically unless there is a specific contraindication (e.g., known prior hypersensitivity). Glucocorticoids, although not immediately active in anaphylactic shock, are effective pharmacologic agents that are capable of increasing tissue response to β-adrenergic agonists as well as inhibiting basophil activation and phospholipase-mediated generation of LTC_4, LTD_4, and LTE_4 [1,3].

The guidelines for pharmacologic therapy of anaphylaxis are listed in Table 69.4.

Specific Therapy

Epinephrine. Epinephrine should be administered first to treat all initial manifestations of anaphylaxis [9,10]. When administered alone, it may reverse rhinitis, urticaria, bronchoconstriction, and hypotension. The failure to administer epinephrine or a delay in its administration may be fatal. The intramuscular (IM) route is recommended on the basis of compelling evidence, both from animal and human studies, that epinephrine is more rapidly absorbed when given intramuscularly rather than subcutaneously (SC) [9,31]. The dose is 0.3 to 0.5 mL of a 1:1,000 dilution (0.3 to 0.5 mg) for adults given IM in the anterolateral thigh and should be repeated in 5 to 15 minutes if improvement is equivocal, usually not more than three times [9].

If shock develops, IM epinephrine is unlikely to be well absorbed. In this setting, epinephrine should be given intravenously: 1 mg (1 mL of a 1:1,000 solution or 10 mL of a 1:10,000 solution) diluted in 1,000 mL of D_5W and infused at a rate of 1 μg per minute, titrating up to a maximum of 10 μg per minute, as needed with continuous electrocardiographic monitoring.

TABLE 69.4

Treatment of Anaphylaxis in Adults [9,10,31]

- Mandatory and immediate
  - General measures
    - Aqueous epinephrine (1:1,000), 0.2–0.5 mL IM; up to 3 doses at 1- to 5-min intervals
    - Tourniquet proximal to antigen injection or sting site
    - Aqueous epinephrine (1:1,000), 0.1–0.3 mL infiltrated into antigen injection or sting site (unless anatomic region with terminal circulation, e.g., fingertip)
  - For laryngeal obstruction or respiratory arrest
    - Establish airway: endotracheal intubation, cricothyroidotomy, or tracheotomy
    - Supplemental oxygen
    - Mechanical ventilation
- After clinical appraisal
  - General measures
    - Diphenhydramine, 1.25 mg/kg to maximum of 50 mg, IV or IM
    - Aqueous hydrocortisone, 200 mg, or methylprednisolone, 50 mg, IV every 6 h for 24–48 h
    - Ranitidine, 150 mg, IV over 3–5 min
  - For hypotension
    - Aqueous epinephrine (1:1,000), 1 mL in 500 mL of saline at 0.5–2.0 mL/min, or 1–4 μg/min, preferably by a central venous line
    - Normal saline or lactated Ringer solution for volume expansion
    - Glucagon, if patient is receiving β-blocker therapy and hypotension is refractory, 1–5 mg IV slow bolus, followed by 5–15 mcg/minute IV infusion
  - For bronchoconstriction
    - Supplemental oxygen
    - Albuterol (0.5%), 0.5 mL in 2.5 mL of saline, by nebulizer

D_5W, dextrose in 5% water; IM, intramuscular; IV, intravenous.

Slow continuous infusion is preferred over bolus administration due to an excess risk of toxicity with bolus infusion [36]. If intravenous access is not easily obtained, epinephrine may be given by intraosseous access at the same rate, starting at 1 μg per minute and titrating up to a maximum of 10 μg per minute. Another alternative is to administer epinephrine via endotracheal tube (10 mL of a 1:10,000 solution). If hypotension persists, continuous infusion of a pressor, such as norepinephrine, dopamine, or phenylephrine, is typically initiated (see Chapter 190).

Management of β-Adrenergic Blockade. Preexisting β-adrenergic blockade with noncardioselective or cardioselective agents is another potential cause of refractory anaphylactic shock [37,38]. In the presence of β-blockade, anaphylaxis is characterized by bradycardia with or without atrioventricular nodal delay (in contrast to the usual tachycardia), profound and refractory hypotension, urticaria, and angioedema [37]. Whether β-blockade truly increases the chance of developing anaphylaxis or just the severity is not known. β-Blockade appears to increase anaphylactic mediator synthesis and release, as well as altering end-organ responsiveness. Although α-adrenergic agents may increase in vitro release of mast cell mediators in the presence of β-blockade [39], the drug of first choice for treating anaphylaxis in the presence of β-blockade remains epinephrine [9]. Dopamine, which has combined α, β, and dopaminergic activities, may be useful for shock refractory to epinephrine. The dose of β agonists will likely have to be more than usual to overcome the β-blockade. Several case reports note success in treating refractory shock with glucagon ([off-label] 1–5 mg IV by slow bolus followed by 5–15 microg/minute IV infusion titrated as needed), which is often used in the treatment of β-blocker overdose. Glucagon appears to increase cardiac cyclic AMP independent of β-receptors and to increase heart rate despite β-blockade [37,40].

Bronchodilators. Bronchoconstriction is treated with a nebulized short-acting β-agonist (typically albuterol 2.5 mg in 3 mL [0.083%]), often in addition to parenteral epinephrine, as described above. Nebulizer treatments should be repeated every 15 to 20 minutes until bronchoconstriction abates. Alternatively, albuterol can be administered by continuous nebulization (see chapter on asthma). Methylxanthines are not recommended in hypotensive patients because they may worsen hypotension and cause unpredictable cardiovascular toxicity [1]. Their exact mechanism of action is not well defined, and they are not first-line agents in the treatment of bronchoconstriction.

Volume Resuscitation. Given the distributive nature of shock in anaphylaxis, aggressive volume resuscitation should accompany epinephrine (and other vasoactive medications) when hypotension develops. For adults, normal saline is generally preferred, starting with a rapid infusion of 1 L intravenously, although some patients may require more. If intravenous access cannot be obtained, intraosseous administration of saline is an alternative [31].

If the blood pressure does not improve with pressors and volume resuscitation, the central venous pressure or ultrasonography may provide guidance regarding the adequacy of fluid resuscitation. For refractory hypotension, serial ultrasonography or pulmonary artery catheterization (see Chapter 19) can help guide further fluid, inotropic, and vasopressor therapy, as outlined in Chapter 190.

Antihistamines. Histamine receptor antagonists are considered adjunctive therapies to be administered after epinephrine when needed to relieve itching and hives. Antihistamines are more effective for prevention than in treatment of full-blown anaphylaxis and should never be used as the primary therapy for anaphylactic shock. When administered, parenteral administration is preferred to oral administration. The H_1-receptor-blocker diphenhydramine (1 to 2 mg per kg up to 50 mg for an adult) can be given intravenously as a bolus [1]. The H_2-receptor-blocker ranitidine (150 mg for adults) can be infused over 3 to 5 minutes or given intramuscularly [9]. H_2-receptor-blocking antihistamines prevent the fall in diastolic blood pressure induced by experimental histamine infusion, but the evidence that H_2-receptor-blocking antihistamines are effective in the treatment of anaphylaxis is anecdotal. The H_2-blocker cimetidine has been reported to cause hypotension when given intravenously and should be avoided.

Glucocorticoids. Glucocorticoids are not of immediate clinical benefit and are considered adjunctive therapy to epinephrine and not a substitute. They may help to reduce bronchoconstriction and laryngeal edema and provide blood pressure support when used in high doses and for prolonged attacks (see Table 69.4 for recommended doses). When parenteral glucocorticoids are administered, the initial dose is usually methyl prednisolone 1 to 2 mg per kg up to 125 mg (or the equivalent), intravenously. Subsequent dosing is based on the response to initial therapy; methylprednisolone may be continued every 6 to 12 hours for 72 hours in patients with persistent or recurrent symptoms [1,9,31].

Despite the theoretical basis for glucocorticoids preventing late recurrences of anaphylaxis, biphasic anaphylaxis has been reported to occur in 20% of anaphylactic reactions in spite of glucocorticoid therapy [24,41]. In this report, after an initial response to therapy, life-threatening symptoms recurred up to

8 hours later. Whether glucocorticoid therapy helped prevent recurrences after 8 hours is not known. Because of the possibility of a late recurrence, patients should be monitored in the intensive care setting for 8 to 12 hours after resolution of symptoms. Roughly 30% of anaphylaxis cases may have protracted symptoms for 5 to 32 hours despite vigorous therapy including glucocorticoids [24].

PREVENTION OF ANAPHYLACTIC REACTIONS

In view of the potential morbidity and mortality from anaphylactic reactions, prevention is of primary importance. Prevention includes obtaining a careful history to identify possible precipitants of anaphylaxis. Both physicians and patients should be aware of potential cross-reacting agents. For example, individuals with anaphylaxis secondary to aspirin are frequently sensitive to nonsteroidal anti-inflammatory drugs, such as ibuprofen, naproxen, ketorolac, and sulindac. Preservatives, such as metabisulfite, ethylenediamine, and methylparaben, have been associated with anaphylactic reactions. It is therefore helpful to review the inactive ingredients contained in medications temporally associated with anaphylaxis [42]. In some instances, combined precipitants can trigger anaphylaxis, as in food-exercise– or NSAID-exercise–induced anaphylaxis (discussed later), where each precipitant alone does not trigger anaphylaxis but the combined stress, particularly if temporally close, can cause anaphylaxis. Prevention for these settings involves specific recommendations, usually related to adequate time separation of triggers [43].

Prevention of reactions to specific agents (e.g., antibiotics) is discussed below. In general, patients with a history of anaphylaxis should wear emergency alert jewelry, which details offending precipitants and potential cross-reacting agents. In addition, patients should be provided with and instructed in the use of anaphylaxis kits (e.g., EpiPen) for prompt treatment in future reactions. Finally, consultation with an allergist can clarify the offending trigger (if unknown) and guide appropriate evaluation and treatment plans. These three actions are the most relevant elements of postanaphylaxis care from the intensive care perspective.

MANAGEMENT OF ANAPHYLAXIS TO SPECIFIC AGENTS AND PRECIPITANTS

β-Lactam Antibiotic Anaphylaxis

One of the most common causes of anaphylaxis in the United States is penicillin. Systemic reactions complicate approximately 1% to 2% of penicillin courses. Approximately 10% of the population will have positive skin tests to penicillin. Thus, a substantial portion of the population is at risk for developing anaphylactic reactions to the drug. About 10% of these reactions are life threatening, and 2% to 10% are fatal [11]. Seventy-five percent of the patients who die of penicillin anaphylaxis have experienced previous allergic reactions to the drug. As with other medications, the risk of a severe reaction is greater with parenteral administration than with oral administration [11]. On the other hand, about 85% to 90% of individuals who report penicillin allergy are found to be nonallergic on subsequent evaluation [44].

Skin testing for penicillin hypersensitivity with the major determinant benzylpenicilloyl-poly-L-lysine (BPO, PRE-PEN, and ALK-Abello) and minor determinants benzylpenicillin (Pen-G), benzylpenicilloate, and benzylpenilloate is effective for detecting IgE-mediated sensitivity and thereby identifying individuals at risk for developing acute allergic reactions to penicillin [11]. The minor determinant mixture of the above-noted substances is not commercially available, and it is accepted that Pen-G is adequate to represent the minor determinants. The negative predictive value of skin testing when both major and minor determinants of penicillin are used is excellent for immediate hypersensitivity reactions to penicillin [45]. This testing does not evaluate other types of sensitivity, such as serum sickness reactions, morbilliform rashes, hemolytic anemia, and interstitial nephritis. In addition, it does not evaluate patients who may have specific allergy to a β-lactam side chain of a penicillin derivative, for example, cephalosporins or carbapenems [46]. Cross-reactivity between β-lactams and monobactams, for example, aztreonam, is rare. For critically ill patients, who need a β-lactam drug and who have a convincing history of severe β-lactam antibiotic allergy, the best strategy is to use an alternate, non–cross-reacting antibiotic or to proceed with a rapid desensitization protocol. These have become well established in clinical practice and vary slightly from institution to institution. The essentials, as described [11], are a series of infusions of gradually increasing concentrations (hence drug amount) over several hours with observation between infusions ending in infusion of desired/target dose of medication. A retrospective review of antibiotic desensitization for IgE-mediated allergy found that it was successful in 75% of patients [47]. Patients with a remote or uncertain history of β-lactam allergy can be considered for a graded challenge: 10% of the target dose administered followed by observation for 30 minutes, and the remainder administered with observation. The benefit of this approach, if applicable, is that a successful graded challenge demonstrates *tolerance* to the antibiotic, namely, that allergy has been disproved. In contrast, desensitization success does not disprove allergy.

The incidence of anaphylactic reactions to cephalosporins is infrequent but increasing [53]. Patients with a history of penicillin allergy have been reported to have allergic reactions to cephalosporins at a rate of 5.4% to 16.5%, compared with patients with a negative history, whose reaction rate was 1% to 2% [48,49]. The rate of cross-reactivity is lower with second- and third-generation than with first-generation cephalosporins. However, not all of these reactions reflect true cross-reactivity, as only 15% to 40% of patients with a positive history react to penicillin on subsequent testing [48,50]. In a study of 30 patients with immediate-type hypersensitivity reactions to second- and third-generation cephalosporins, 25 of 36 reactions were anaphylactic shock [51]. Only 13% of individuals had either a positive skin test or in vitro evidence of antigen-specific IgE to penicillin determinants, whereas all but three reactions were correlated with a positive skin test to culprit cephalosporins. Unfortunately, skin testing with cephalosporin derivatives is not reliable; severe allergic reactions have occurred in patients with negative cephalosporin skin tests, and cephalosporin antigenic determinants for skin testing have not been standardized. On the other hand, patients with negative penicillin skin tests have no greater risk of allergic reaction to cephalosporins than the general population [49]. Several protocols for desensitization to cephalosporins have been outlined in a review [52]. Cross-reactivity between cephalosporins appears related to the degree of similarity of the R1 side chains; these similarities do not explicitly predict reactivity, but rather guide the choice of an alternate cephalosporin with a *different* R1 side chain. Ninety percent of patients allergic to second- and third-generation cephalosporins do not react to penicillin derivatives [53].

As noted earlier, monobactams (e.g., aztreonam) do not show cross-reactivity with penicillin, but do show some cross-reactivity with the cephalosporins (i.e., ceftazidime) [53]. Carbapenems (e.g., imipenem, meropenem), in comparison, have historically shown significant in vivo cross-reactivity with penicillin, and desensitization of penicillin-allergic patients was recommended when there was no reasonable alternative [54]. Several highly informative reports from penicillin (PCN) skin test–positive patients have suggested that carbapenems can be given safely to young [55,56] and adult [57] patients, who have negative skin tests to the proposed carbapenem. In urgent settings and/or where skin testing is not feasible, a graded challenge or desensitization protocol should be employed with the same precautions as if giving the patient penicillin [11].

Food Anaphylaxis

Food allergy occurs among approximately 6% of children and 3.7% of adults [34]; however, fatal anaphylactic reactions are much less common. Due to variable patterns of absorption, biphasic and/or prolonged anaphylaxis occurs in about 20% of cases. However, the delayed phase is rarely associated with a mild acute phase, where hypotension and bronchoconstriction are readily apparent [58]. A review of fatal and severe nonfatal anaphylactic reactions to foods revealed several important features of the fatal anaphylactic reactions: all occurred among patients with asthma, all were in a public setting rather than in the home, and all were associated with delayed or nonadministration of epinephrine [2]. The foods that caused these severe reactions were peanuts, cashews, milk, filberts (hazelnuts), walnuts, and eggs. In another review of the causes of anaphylaxis, the five most common foods were pine nuts, peanuts, soy, shellfish, and other nuts [59]. A survey of food-related anaphylactic fatalities reported to an association registry confirmed the association between asthma and severe anaphylaxis; 90% of fatalities among this group were due to peanuts and tree nuts [20]. A methodical approach to the diagnosis and treatment of food hypersensitivity has been outlined by Sicherer and Sampson [34].

Processed foods may contain significant amounts of milk products, despite a lack of mention of this on the label ingredient lists [60]. This is important to remember for patients with milk allergy who appear to experience a cryptogenic anaphylactic episode. Standards for food labeling instituted in 2006 by the U.S. Food and Drug Administration have assisted patients with food allergy and their providers by requiring identification of possible trace allergen contaminants in processed foods. Other food additives, such as preservatives, have been implicated as causes of anaphylaxis [61]. In the critical care setting, evaluation of likely cause, if cryptic, can begin with serum testing for allergen (food)-specific IgE (ImmunoCAP, others) to a broad range of suspected culprits. However, there is no role for skin testing in the acute setting as skin tests can be negative or misleading in the first 4 to 6 weeks following documented anaphylaxis.

Anesthetic Anaphylaxis

Immediate hypersensitivity reactions to local anesthetics are rare, despite their being one of the most commonly used groups of drugs in medicine [62,63]. Cell-mediated reactions that manifest as contact dermatitis are more common. Local anesthetics are divided into two classes: group I (para-aminobenzoic acid ester) consists of benzocaine, tetracaine, and procaine; group II (non–ester-containing) consists of lidocaine, mepivacaine, dibucaine, and cyclomethycaine. Cross-reactivity between the two groups is very rare, and cross-reactivity between the amides is also rare [64,65]. Skin testing, using a progressive challenge protocol, can help determine whether sensitivity exists and which drugs are likely to be safe in the future [63,65].

General anesthetics, such as neuromuscular blocking agents and thiobarbiturates, also cause anaphylaxis [66]. A skin test protocol has been described for evaluating patients with possible allergy to general anesthetics [67]. Other etiologies of perioperative anaphylaxis include allergy to antibiotics, latex, glutaraldehyde, and opioids.

Since neuromuscular blocking agents are used in intensive care units, anaphylaxis to these agents should be considered in the differential diagnosis of unexplained hypotension in the intensive care unit.

Radiocontrast Media Anaphylaxis

Radiocontrast media studies are frequently necessary in critically ill patients, and so it is important to know when a reaction is likely to occur and how to prevent it. Unfortunately, the likelihood of an anaphylactic reaction to radiocontrast media cannot be predicted by pretesting with oral, conjunctival, or intradermal skin tests [68]. Although the overall adverse reaction rate ranges from 1% to 12% [69], patients with a history of a previous anaphylactic reaction to radiocontrast media have a repeat reaction rate of 35% to 60% [70]. Patients with a general history of allergies, whether to inhalant allergens, foods, or medications, also have an increased reaction rate of serious reactions compared with nonallergic individuals [71]. The majority of contrast media reactions are non-IgE mediated, although evidence is accumulating to suggest that an IgE-mediated mechanism may be contributory in some cases [72,73]. Although exceedingly rare, there have been several confirmed reports of anaphylactic reactions to iodinated oral contrast: Gastrografin (sodium and meglumine diatrizoate), Hypaque (sodium diatrizoate), barium sulfate, and gadolinium [74–78].

Nonionic, low-osmolal radiocontrast agents have largely replaced high-ionic contrast media due to a decreased incidence of overall adverse reactions [79,80], although not all studies have found a reduction in life-threatening reactions or death [80,81]. Currently, for patients who have had a prior anaphylactic reaction to contrast media and who require a contrast study, the use of nonionic, low-osmolal contrast is recommended in addition to pretreatment with glucocorticoids and, diphenhydramine with or without ephedrine [10,82], as outlined below. Iso-osmolal and noniodinated contrast are also being explored as alternatives to low-osmolal agents [82,83].

Pretreatment protocols have been developed for patients with a history of a prior anaphylactic reaction who require additional intravascular media studies [68,70,84]. In one study of 192 procedures for patients with previous anaphylactic reactions to contrast media, pretreatment with prednisone, 50 mg orally at 13 hours, 7 hours, and 1 hour before the procedure; diphenhydramine, 50 mg orally or intramuscularly at 1 hour before the procedure; and ephedrine, 25 mg orally at 1 hour before the procedure resulted in a reaction rate of 3.1% [70]. A multicenter study of unselected patients receiving intravenous contrast media reported a reaction rate of 5.4% in 2,513 patients given oral methylprednisolone, 32 mg at 12 hours and again at 2 hours before the procedure [84]. In this same study, a single dose of methylprednisolone, 32 mg 2 hours before the procedure, was no better than placebo, with a reaction rate of 9.4% in 1,759 patients. This finding raises the question of how to manage patients with a prior history of anaphylaxis requiring an urgent radiocontrast study. In a small study, 9 such patients were treated with hydrocortisone, 200 mg intravenously immediately and every 4 hours until the procedure was completed, and diphenhydramine, 50 mg intravenously 1 hour before the procedure [85]. Roughly half of the patients received one dose of hydrocortisone, and the other half received two doses. No reactions occurred among these patients. Given that this study evaluated only nine patients, it remains unknown whether additional therapy with ephedrine or an H_2-receptor blocking agent, or both, would provide better protection.

Latex-Induced Anaphylaxis

Latex allergy, caused by sensitivity to *Hevea brasiliensis* proteins, can take several forms: contact dermatitis, asthma, urticaria, and anaphylaxis. Perioperative anaphylaxis caused by latex exposure has been described in several children with *spina bifida* and in patients with a history of multiple surgical procedures [86]. In addition, latex allergy has become an occupational hazard in the health profession since the institution of universal precautions [87]. Sensitivity seems to be increased among atopic individuals with frequent exposure to latex. Unexplained perioperative or nosocomial urticaria, bronchoconstriction, or hypotension should raise concern for latex anaphylaxis. Mucosal and parenteral exposures have the highest risk of anaphylaxis.

Patients with latex allergy often have cross-sensitivity with certain fruits and vegetables, including banana, kiwi, avocado, chestnut, papaya, potato, and tomato. Latex is found in a wide spectrum of health care products, including elastic thread, rubber bands, condom catheters, Foley catheters, surgical/examination gloves, enema bags, tubing on blood pressure cuffs, rubber stoppers on medication vials and intravenous line tubing, as well as some surgical drapes, drains, and gowns [88–91].

Establishing a diagnosis of latex allergy for a patient who is at high risk on the basis of prior exposures or who may have had latex-induced anaphylaxis is important to guide future prevention efforts. However, skin test extracts are not yet commercially available in the United States and noncommercial latex extracts have been associated with systemic reactions. In addition, the specificity and sensitivity of noncommercial extracts may vary. A preferred alternative is serologic testing by Phadia ImmunoCAP or the Siemens Immulite autoanalyzer; these tests have about 80% sensitivity [90].

The most important steps for the prevention of future anaphylactic reactions to latex are careful patient education and in-hospital latex avoidance through the use of alert bracelets and latex-free kits [66]. Verbal and written information should be provided regarding potential sources of latex exposure and sources of latex-free gloves for patients to take to dentist and doctor visits. In addition, patients should understand the importance of alerting health care professionals who may care for them in the future and the need to carry an EpiPen kit in case of inadvertent exposure.

Stinging Insect Venom Anaphylaxis

Venom extracts for yellow jacket, white-faced hornet, yellow-faced hornet, wasp, honeybee, and fire ant are available for skin testing to confirm specific IgE mediation and for desensitization. Results with venom desensitization suggest more than 95% protection against anaphylaxis on subsequent stings [92]. The duration of desensitization therapy necessary for long-term protection is probably 5 years [92,93]. The geographic distribution of fire ants is expanding, making systemic allergic reactions to these insects a growing concern [94].

Exercise-Induced Anaphylaxis

Exercise-induced anaphylaxis syndrome is distinct from cold and cholinergic urticaria and exercise-induced asthma and usually occurs among individuals who engage in vigorous exercise [43,95]. A subgroup of these patients is allergic to a specific food (wheat is the most common), which acts as a cofactor; manifestations of anaphylaxis only occur if ingestion of the specific food is accompanied by exercise. Other potential cofactors include nonsteroidal anti-inflammatory drugs (NSAIDs), alcoholic beverages, and exposure to high pollen counts [96,97]. Typically, these patients can either ingest the food/NSAID or perform the exercise without adverse effect.

Anaphylaxis can be prevented by delaying exercise by at least 2 and preferably 4 hours after eating (48 hours after ingesting a known food cofactor) and stopping exercise at the onset of pruritus. When NSAIDs are a cofactor, they should not be taken for at least 24 hours before exercise. Exercising with someone who is capable of administering epinephrine is also recommended. Antihistamines and/or leukotriene modifiers (montelukast, zileuton, and others) are occasionally of benefit in prevention.

Idiopathic (Spontaneous) Urticaria/Angioedema/Anaphylaxis

A group of patients has been described who experience recurrent anaphylaxis without an identifiable precipitant, the so-called *idiopathic anaphylaxis* [98]. In these patients, a careful review of all foods, preservatives, and drugs ingested before the episodes, as well as physical factors such as exercise, fails to reveal a cause for recurrent life-threatening anaphylaxis. These patients should be evaluated for possible systemic mastocytosis [99]. Idiopathic anaphylaxis is most likely on the spectrum of diseases of excess mast cell activity with resultant signs and symptoms of excess histamine release and its consequences, whether from autoantibodies to the high-affinity IgE receptor on mast cells or other unknown triggers [100,101]. These patients can have diffuse hives, angioedema including airway involvement, and typically both. Maintenance therapy is directed at reducing histamine responsiveness as well as oral glucocorticoids, and, in refractory cases, anti-IgE therapy (omalizumab) [102,103]. Second-line additional agents (cyclosporine, dapsone, hydroxychloroquine) have been used in individual patients [104].

Bradykinin/Complement-Mediated Angioedema: Angiotensin-Converting Enzyme Inhibitor, Hereditary, and Acquired

Angiotensin converting enzyme (ACE) inhibitors can cause potentially life-threatening facial and oropharyngeal angioedema [105]. Onset of angioedema usually starts within the first several hours or up to a week after beginning therapy, but angioedema can develop after months to years of asymptomatic usage [106]. Subsequent episodes may recur days to weeks after discontinuation. A late onset of symptoms, 12 to 24 hours after the last dose, has been reported with the long-acting ACE inhibitors lisinopril and enalapril [107]. As with ACE-induced cough, cross-reactivity is the rule among different ACE inhibitors. The mechanism is unknown but is suspected to be related to an alteration in bradykinin metabolism, leading to excess bradykinin and resultant vasodilatation or, possibly, an interaction with components of the complement cascade (e.g., complement 1-esterase inhibitor) [106,108].

Diagnostic testing is not available, and so the diagnosis is made clinically on the basis of the characteristic pattern of angioedema in a patient taking an ACE inhibitor. An important distinguishing feature of bradykinin/complement angioedema is that, as a rule, there is no associated urticaria or pruritus. Treatment includes cessation of ACE inhibitor therapy and assessment and maintenance of airway patency. In general, epinephrine, antihistamines, and systemic glucocorticoids are of minimal benefit, although a few studies have suggested an earlier time to extubation among patients treated with antihistamines. For patients with severe or persistent airway swelling, some studies have reported benefit with agents that are approved for use in hereditary angioedema, such as icatibant (off-label, 30 mg given by slow infusion subcutaneously, may be repeated in 6 hours), fresh frozen plasma (2 units), and purified C1 inhibitor concentrate (off-label, dosing per package insert) [106,108].

Hereditary angioedema (HAE) is the result of dysfunction or low levels of C1 esterase inhibitor, causing unchecked complement activation and (1) excess C3a, C4a, and C5a, and (2) excess bradykinin, resulting in angioedema. The disorder is inherited in an autosomal dominant pattern, but up to 15% of cases are new mutations without ancestral history. Onset of disease is typically in early to late adolescence and is marked with three main types of crises: extremity, facial/airway, and abdominal. Although crises can be spontaneous, trauma is a well-recognized precipitant, specifically for extremity and facial/airway crises. Of particular relevance is the development of facial and airway angioedema within 24 hours after invasive dental work or oral surgery because this can be readily misidentified as local anesthetic allergy since these are usually co-administered in these procedures. Abdominal crises are characterized by subacute or acute onset of crampy abdominal pain associated with nausea and vomiting. Due to bowel wall edema, there is often initial constipation from peristaltic dysfunction, which can be followed by diarrhea. Of note, these patients can present with an acute abdomen and radiographic findings suggestive of ischemic bowel. Careful clinical judgment is needed because episodes are typically self-limited and abdominal surgery, as a traumatic trigger, could further exacerbate visceral angioedema.

Acquired angioedema (AAE) occurs in the setting of autoimmune disease (e.g., rheumatoid arthritis) or hematologic malignancy, where there is either excess complement component C1 activation or autoantibodies against C1 esterase inhibitor, leading to angioedema from the same downstream mechanisms as in HAE. These patients typically present after their fourth decade of life, in contrast to patients with HAE.

Diagnostic laboratory evaluation is warranted in patients who present with angioedema *without* urticaria and no clear trigger, especially if there is suggestive underlying autoimmune or lymphoproliferative disorder. In patients with HAE or AAE, complement component C4 is typically decreased at all times, whereas C2 is more typically low during attacks. Tests for quantitative and functional C1 esterase inhibitor should be sent, as well as complement component C1q, as the latter is decreased in AAE but not in HAE. As a rule, C3 levels are of little benefit as they remain normal in HAE/AAE even during attacks, and a low C3 should lead to inquiry of potential comorbid or alternate causes. Of note, a subtype of HAE (HAE-III) has been identified, almost exclusively in women, with a similar clinical presentation as other forms of HAE, but whose laboratory evaluation detailed above is normal. This rare disorder, which is beyond the scope of the current chapter, has been reviewed [105].

Beyond immediate supportive measures, use of epinephrine, antihistamines, and systemic glucocorticoids are of minimal benefit as in ACEI-induced angioedema. Several agents have been approved for use in acute attacks of HAE/AAE focusing on airway crises, including concentrated (plasma-derived) C1 esterase inhibitor (e.g., Berinert, Cinryze), bradykinin B2 receptor antagonists (icatibant [Firazyr]), and kallikrein inhibitor (ecallantide [Kalbitor]) [109]. In the absence of ready availability of these agents, 2 units of fresh frozen plasma [110], with the intent to provide functional exogenous C1 esterase inhibitor, can be used, typically to avert the need to establish an emergency airway for severe laryngeal edema. The approach to treatment of attacks of AAE is similar with respect to clinical assessment and therapeutic measures.

Aspirin and NSAIDs

Acetylsalicylic acid (aspirin) and nonsteroidal anti-inflammatory agents can cause urticaria, flares of urticaria in patients with chronic idiopathic urticaria, anaphylaxis, and aspirin-exacerbated respiratory disease (AERD) [11,111–114]. Most patients have either the urticaria/anaphylaxis pattern or the respiratory disease pattern, but a few patients have both. Some patients with the urticaria/anaphylaxis pattern appear to have sensitivity to a particular NSAID, but most have cross-sensitivity that is related to abnormalities of prostaglandin/leukotriene metabolism [115]. Desensitization protocols for patients with coronary artery disease, who need the antiplatelet effects of aspirin, have been published [116,117].

Miscellaneous Causes of Anaphylaxis

Insulin therapy has been associated with an increased risk of anaphylaxis, particularly when a patient on insulin therapy has a history of local wheal-and-flare reactions at the site of insulin injections and interrupts insulin therapy for more than 48 hours and then resumes it [11,118]. Anaphylaxis has also been described with recombinant DNA insulin [119] and to protamine in neutral protamine Hagedorn insulin [120].

TABLE 69.5

Management of Anaphylaxis—Quality of the Evidence

History of exposures and timing is the most important information to determine whether a set of symptoms was due to anaphylaxis and what tripper precipitated the event. (C)

The appropriate dose of epinephrine should be administered promptly at the onset of anaphylaxis. (A/D)

Intravenous infusion of crystalloid is essential for patients who are unstable or refractory to initial therapy with epinephrine. (B)

Specific situations

The extent of allergic cross-reactivity between penicillin and cephalosporins is low. (C)

Aztreonam cross-reacts with ceftazidime by shared R-group side chain. (B)

The three groups at increased risk for latex anaphylaxis are health care workers, children with *spina bifida* and genitourinary problems, and workers with occupational exposure to latex. (B)

Precautions for latex-allergic patients undergoing anesthesia include avoiding latex gloves, latex blood pressure cuffs, latex tourniquets, latex intravenous tubing ports, and rubber stoppers on vials. (B)

The greatest number of anaphylactic reactions in children has involved peanuts, tree nuts, fish, shellfish, milk, and eggs. (C)

Anaphylactic reactions to foods almost always occur immediately, but may recur hours later. (A)

Strength of recommendation

A. Directly based on meta-analysis of randomized controlled trials or from at least one randomized controlled trial or systematic review of randomized controlled trials/body of evidence.
B. Directly based on at least one controlled trial without randomization or at least one other type of quasi-experimental study or extrapolated recommendation from A.
C. Directly based on at least one other type of quasi-experimental or descriptive/comparative study or extrapolated recommendation from A or B.
D. Directly based on evidence from expert committee report or opinions or clinical experience of respected authorities or both.

Summarized from reference Lieberman P, Nicklas RA, Randolph C, et al: Anaphylaxis—a practice parameter update 2015. *Ann Allergy Asthma Immunol* 115(5):341–384, 2015 and others.

The injection of heterologous serum carries a significant risk of anaphylaxis. Human serum (homologous) should be used whenever available. If heterologous serum must be used (antitoxin for snake bites, passive rabies immunization in developing countries, and antilymphocytic serum for organ transplantation), patients are usually evaluated for cutaneous sensitivity by first performing a scratch test with antitoxin or normal horse serum. If there is no reaction, 0.02 mL of a 1:10 serum dilution can be injected intradermally. As with all skin testing, the physician must be prepared to treat any systemic reactions that arise [1].

Patients with mastocytosis appear to be at greater risk for developing anaphylaxis from Hymenoptera stings (even in the absence of IgE mediation) and from mast cell degranulating agents (see Table 69.2). These patients should carry an epinephrine kit during Hymenoptera season. Administration of diagnostic and therapeutic agents that might cause mast cell activation should be avoided in these patients.

The quality of evidence and recommendations for diagnosis and management of anaphylaxis are summarized in Table 69.5.

References

1. McGrath K: Anaphylaxis, in Patterson R, Grammer LC, Greenberger PA (eds): *Patterson's Allergic Diseases—Diagnosis and Management*. Philadelphia, Lippincott-Raven, 2009, pp 439–458.
2. Sampson HA, Munoz-Furlong A, Campbell RL, et al: Second symposium on the definition and management of anaphylaxis: summary report—Second National Institute of Allergy and Infectious Disease/Food Allergy and Anaphylaxis Network symposium. *J Allergy Clin Immunol* 117(2):391–397, 2006.
3. Kemp SF, Lockey RF: Anaphylaxis: a review of causes and mechanisms. *J Allergy Clin Immunol* 110(3):341–348, 2002.
4. Simons FE: Anaphylaxis. *J Allergy Clin Immunol* 125[2 Suppl 2]:S161–S181, 2010.
5. Tejedor-Alonso MA, Moro-Moro M, Mugica-Garcia MV: Epidemiology of anaphylaxis: contributions from the last 10 years. *J Investig Allergol Clin Immunol* 25(3):163–175, 2015.
6. Ma L, Danoff TM, Borish L: Case fatality and population mortality associated with anaphylaxis in the United States. *J Allergy Clin Immunol* 133(4):1075–1083, 2014.
7. Jerschow E, Lin RY, Scaperotti MM, et al: Fatal anaphylaxis in the United States, 1999-2010: temporal patterns and demographic associations. *J Allergy Clin Immunol* 134(6):1318–1328, 2014.
8. Stone KD, Prussin C, Metcalfe DD: IgE, mast cells, basophils, and eosinophils. *J Allergy Clin Immunol* 125[2 Suppl 2]:S73–S80, 2010.
9. Lieberman P, Nicklas RA, Randolph C, et al: Anaphylaxis—a practice parameter update 2015. *Ann Allergy Asthma Immunol* 115(5):341–384, 2015.
10. Simons FE, Ardusso LR, Bilo MB, et al: World allergy organization guidelines for the assessment and management of anaphylaxis. *World Allergy Organ J* 4(2):13–37, 2011.
11. Joint Task Force on Practice Parameters, American Academy of Allergy, Asthma and Immunology, American College of Allergy, Asthma and Immunology, et al: Drug allergy: an updated practice parameter. *Ann Allergy Asthma Immunol* 105(4):259–273, 2010.
12. Vyas GN, Perkins HA, Fudenberg HH: Anaphylactoid transfusion reactions associated with anti-IgA. *Lancet* 2(7563):312–315, 1968.
13. Busse WW, Lemanske RF Jr: Asthma. *N Engl J Med* 344(5):350–362, 2001.
14. Simons FE: Advances in H1-antihistamines. *N Engl J Med* 351(21):2203–2217, 2004.
15. Kaliner M, Austen KF: Cyclic AMP, ATP, and reversed anaphylactic histamine release from rat mast cells. *J Immunol* 112(2):664–674, 1974.
16. Kanaoka Y, Boyce JA: Cysteinyl leukotrienes and their receptors: cellular distribution and function in immune and inflammatory responses. *J Immunol* 173(3):1503–1510, 2004.
17. Drazen JM: Leukotrienes as mediators of airway obstruction. *Am J Respir Crit Care Med* 158(5 Pt 3):S193–S200, 1998.
18. Gill P, Jindal NL, Jagdis A, et al: Platelets in the immune response: revisiting platelet-activating factor in anaphylaxis. *J Allergy Clin Immunol* 135(6):1424–1432, 2015.
19. Pumphrey R: Anaphylaxis: can we tell who is at risk of a fatal reaction? *Curr Opin Allergy Clin Immunol* 4(4):285–290, 2004.
20. Bock SA, Munoz-Furlong A, Sampson HA: Fatalities due to anaphylactic reactions to foods. *J Allergy Clin Immunol* 107(1):191–193, 2001.
21. Barnard JH: Allergic and pathologic findings in fifty insect-sting fatalities. *J Allergy* 40(2):107–114, 1967.
22. Delage C, Irey NS: Anaphylactic deaths: a clinicopathologic study of 43 cases. *J Forensic Sci* 17(4):525–540, 1972.
23. Edde RR, Burtis BB: Lung injury in anaphylactoid shock. *Chest* 63(4):637–638, 1973.
24. Lieberman P: Biphasic anaphylactic reactions. *Ann Allergy Asthma Immunol* 95(3):217–226, 2005.
25. Sala-Cunill A, Cardona V, Labrador-Horrillo M, et al: Usefulness and limitations of sequential serum tryptase for the diagnosis of anaphylaxis in 102 patients. *Int Arch Allergy Immunol* 160(2):192–199, 2013.
26. Patel SC, Detjen PF: Atrial fibrillation associated with anaphylaxis during venom and pollen immunotherapy. *Ann Allergy Asthma Immunol* 89(2):209–211, 2002.
27. Booth BH, Patterson R: Electrocardiographic changes during human anaphylaxis. *JAMA* 211(4):627–631, 1970.
28. Petsas AA, Kotler MN: Electrocardiographic changes associated with penicillin anaphylaxis. *Chest* 64(1):66–69, 1973.
29. Triggiani M, Patella V, Staiano RI, et al: Allergy and the cardiovascular system. *Clin Exp Immunol* 153[Suppl 1]:7–11, 2008.
30. Yildiz A, Biceroglu S, Yakut N, et al: Acute myocardial infarction in a young man caused by centipede sting. *Emerg Med J* 23(4):e30, 2006.
31. Campbell RL, Li JT, Nicklas RA, et al: Emergency department diagnosis and treatment of anaphylaxis: a practice parameter. *Ann Allergy Asthma Immunol* 113(6):599–608, 2014.
32. Goldberg A, Confino-Cohen R: Timing of venom skin tests and IgE determinations after insect sting anaphylaxis. *J Allergy Clin Immunol* 100(2):182–184, 1997.
33. Pumphrey RS: Lessons for management of anaphylaxis from a study of fatal reactions. *Clin Exp Allergy* 30(8):1144–1150, 2000.
34. Sicherer SH, Sampson HA: 9. Food allergy. *J Allergy Clin Immunol* 117[2 Suppl Mini-Primer]:S470–S475, 2006.
35. Valentine MD: Anaphylaxis and stinging insect hypersensitivity. *JAMA* 268(20):2830–2833, 1992.
36. Campbell RL, Bellolio MF, Knutson BD, et al: Epinephrine in anaphylaxis: higher risk of cardiovascular complications and overdose after administration of intravenous bolus epinephrine compared with intramuscular epinephrine. *J Allergy Clin Immunol Pract* 3(1):76–80, 2015.
37. Toogood JH: Risk of anaphylaxis in patients receiving beta-blocker drugs. *J Allergy Clin Immunol* 81(1):1–5, 1988.
38. Thomas M, Crawford I: Best evidence topic report. Glucagon infusion in refractory anaphylactic shock in patients on beta-blockers. *Emerg Med J* 22(4):272–273, 2005.
39. Jacobs RL, Rake GW Jr, Fournier DC, et al: Potentiated anaphylaxis in patients with drug-induced beta-adrenergic blockade. *J Allergy Clin Immunol* 68(2):125–127, 1981.
40. Zaloga GP, DeLacey W, Holmboe E, et al: Glucagon reversal of hypotension in a case of anaphylactoid shock. *Ann Intern Med* 105(1):65–66, 1986.
41. Ko BS, Kim WY, Ryoo SM, et al: Biphasic reactions in patients with anaphylaxis treated with corticosteroids. *Ann Allergy Asthma Immunol* 115(4):312–316, 2015.
42. Twarog FJ, Leung DY: Anaphylaxis to a component of isoetharine (sodium bisulfite). *JAMA* 248(16):2030–2031, 1982.
43. Feldweg AM: Exercise-induced anaphylaxis. *Immunol Allergy Clin North Am* 35(2):261–275, 2015.
44. Park M, Markus P, Matesic D, et al: Safety and effectiveness of a preoperative allergy clinic in decreasing vancomycin use in patients with a history of penicillin allergy. *Ann Allergy Asthma Immunol* 97(5):681–687, 2006.
45. Sogn DD, Evans R III, Shepherd GM, et al: Results of the National Institute of Allergy and Infectious Diseases Collaborative Clinical Trial to test the predictive value of skin testing with major and minor penicillin derivatives in hospitalized adults. *Arch Intern Med* 152(5):1025–1032, 1992.
46. Torres MJ, Romano A, Mayorga C, et al: Diagnostic evaluation of a large group of patients with immediate allergy to penicillins: the role of skin testing. *Allergy* 56(9):850–856, 2001.
47. Turvey SE, Cronin B, Arnold AD, et al: Antibiotic desensitization for the allergic patient: 5 years of experience and practice. *Ann Allergy Asthma Immunol* 92(4):426–432, 2004.
48. Anderson JA: Cross-sensitivity to cephalosporins in patients allergic to penicillin. *Pediatr Infect Dis* 5(5):557–561, 1986.
49. Saxon A, Beall GN, Rohr AS, et al: Immediate hypersensitivity reactions to beta-lactam antibiotics. *Ann Intern Med* 107(2):204–215, 1987.
50. DeSwarte RD, Patterson R: Drug allergy, in Patterson R, Grammer LC, Greenberger PA (eds): *Allergic Diseases - Diagnosis and Management*. Philadelphia, Lippincott-Raven, 1997, pp 317–401.
51. Romano A, Mayorga C, Torres MJ, et al: Immediate allergic reactions to cephalosporins: cross-reactivity and selective responses. *J Allergy Clin Immunol* 106(6):1177–1183, 2000.
52. Kelkar PS, Li JT: Cephalosporin allergy. *N Engl J Med* 345(11):804–809, 2001.
53. Romano A, Gaeta F, Valluzzi RL, et al: IgE-mediated hypersensitivity to cephalosporins: cross-reactivity and tolerability of penicillins, monobactams, and carbapenems. *J Allergy Clin Immunol* 126(5):994–999, 2010.
54. Saxon A, Adelman DC, Patel A, et al: Imipenem cross-reactivity with penicillin in humans. *J Allergy Clin Immunol* 82(2):213–217, 1988.
55. Atanaskovic-Markovic M, Gaeta F, Medjo B, et al: Tolerability of meropenem in children with IgE-mediated hypersensitivity to penicillins. *Allergy* 63(2):237–240, 2008.
56. Atanaskovic-Markovic M, Gaeta F, Gavrovic-Jankulovic M, et al: Tolerability of imipenem in children with IgE-mediated hypersensitivity to penicillins. *J Allergy Clin Immunol* 124(1):167–169, 2009.

57. Romano A, Viola M, Gueant-Rodriguez RM, et al: Imipenem in patients with immediate hypersensitivity to penicillins. *N Engl J Med* 354(26):2835–2837, 2006.
58. Golden DB: Patterns of anaphylaxis: acute and late phase features of allergic reactions. *Novartis Found Symp* 257:101–110, 2004.
59. Wiggins CA: Characteristics and etiology of 30 patients with anaphylaxis. *Immunol Allergy Practice* 13:313, 1991.
60. Gern JE, Yang E, Evrard HM, et al: Allergic reactions to milk-contaminated "nondairy" products. *N Engl J Med* 324(14):976–979, 1991.
61. Moffitt JE, Golden DB, Reisman RE, et al: Stinging insect hypersensitivity: a practice parameter update. *J Allergy Clin Immunol* 114(4):869–886, 2004.
62. Haugen RN, Brown CW: Case reports: type I hypersensitivity to lidocaine. *J Drugs Dermatol* 6(12):1222–1223, 2007.
63. Gall H, Kaufmann R, Kalveram CM: Adverse reactions to local anesthetics: analysis of 197 cases. *J Allergy Clin Immunol* 97(4):933–937, 1996.
64. Schatz M: Skin testing and incremental challenge in the evaluation of adverse reactions to local anesthetics. *J Allergy Clin Immunol* 74(4 Pt 2):606–616, 1984.
65. Chandler MJ, Grammer LC, Patterson R: Provocative challenge with local anesthetics in patients with a prior history of reaction. *J Allergy Clin Immunol* 79(6):883–886, 1987.
66. Mertes PM, Malinovsky JM, Jouffroy L, et al: Reducing the risk of anaphylaxis during anesthesia: 2011 updated guidelines for clinical practice. *J Investig Allergol Clin Immunol* 21(6):442–453, 2011.
67. Kannan JA, Bernstein JA: Perioperative anaphylaxis: diagnosis, evaluation, and management. *Immunol Allergy Clin North Am* 35(2):321–334, 2015.
68. Shehadi WH: Adverse reactions to intravascularly administered contrast media. A comprehensive study based on a prospective survey. *Am J Roentgenol Radium Ther Nucl Med* 124(1):145–152, 1975.
69. Canter LM: Anaphylactoid reactions to radiocontrast media. *Allergy Asthma Proc* 26(3):199–203, 2005.
70. Greenberger PA: Contrast media reactions. *J Allergy Clin Immunol* 74(4 Pt 2):600–605, 1984.
71. Morcos SK: Review article: acute serious and fatal reactions to contrast media: our current understanding. *Br J Radiol* 78(932):686–693, 2005.
72. Dewachter P, Mouton-Faivre C, Felden F: Allergy and contrast media. *Allergy* 56(3):250–251, 2001.
73. Laroche D, imone-Gastin I, Dubois F, et al: Mechanisms of severe, immediate reactions to iodinated contrast material. *Radiology* 209(1):183–190, 1998.
74. Miller SH: Anaphylactoid reaction after oral administration of diatrizoate meglumine and diatrizoate sodium solution. *AJR Am J Roentgenol* 168(4):959–961, 1997.
75. Marik PE, Patel SY: Anaphylactoid reaction to oral contrast agent. *AJR Am J Roentgenol* 168(6):1623–1624, 1997.
76. Seymour PC, Kesack CD: Anaphylactic shock during a routine upper gastrointestinal series. *AJR Am J Roentgenol* 168(4):957–958, 1997.
77. Skucas J: Anaphylactoid reactions with gastrointestinal contrast media. *AJR Am J Roentgenol* 168(4):962–964, 1997.
78. Li A, Wong CS, Wong MK, et al: Acute adverse reactions to magnetic resonance contrast media—gadolinium chelates. *Br J Radiol* 79(941):368–371, 2006.
79. Barrett BJ, Parfrey PS, McDonald JR, et al: Nonionic low-osmolality versus ionic high-osmolality contrast material for intravenous use in patients perceived to be at high risk: randomized trial. *Radiology* 183(1):105–110, 1992.
80. Cochran ST, Bomyea K, Sayre JW: Trends in adverse events after IV administration of contrast media. *AJR Am J Roentgenol* 176(6):1385–1388, 2001.
81. Wolf GL, Arenson RL, Cross AP: A prospective trial of ionic vs nonionic contrast agents in routine clinical practice: comparison of adverse effects. *AJR Am J Roentgenol* 152(5):939–944, 1989.
82. Greenberger PA, Patterson R: The prevention of immediate generalized reactions to radiocontrast media in high-risk patients. *J Allergy Clin Immunol* 87(4):867–872, 1991.
83. Coche EE, Hammer FD, Goffette PP: Demonstration of pulmonary embolism with gadolinium-enhanced spiral CT. *Eur Radiol* 11(11):2306–2309, 2001.
84. Lasser EC, Berry CC, Talner LB, et al: Pretreatment with corticosteroids to alleviate reactions to intravenous contrast material. *N Engl J Med* 317(14):845–849, 1987.
85. Greenberger PA, Halwig JM, Patterson R, et al: Emergency administration of radiocontrast media in high-risk patients. *J Allergy Clin Immunol* 77(4):630–634, 1986.
86. Landwehr LP, Boguniewicz M: Current perspectives on latex allergy. *J Pediatr* 128(3):305–312, 1996.
87. Liss GM, Sussman GL, Deal K, et al: Latex allergy: epidemiological study of 1351 hospital workers. *Occup Environ Med* 54(5):335–342, 1997.
88. Jaeger D, Kleinhans D, Czuppon AB, et al: Latex-specific proteins causing immediate-type cutaneous, nasal, bronchial, and systemic reactions. *J Allergy Clin Immunol* 89(3):759–768, 1992.
89. Biagini RE, Krieg EF, Pinkerton LE, et al: Receiver operating characteristics analyses of Food and Drug Administration-cleared serological assays for natural rubber latex-specific immunoglobulin E antibody. *Clin Diagn Lab Immunol* 8(6):1145–1149, 2001.
90. Biagini RE, MacKenzie BA, Sammons DL, et al: Latex specific IgE: performance characteristics of the IMMULITE 2000 3gAllergy assay compared with skin testing. *Ann Allergy Asthma Immunol* 97(2):196–202, 2006.
91. Kelly KJ, Sussman G, Fink JN: Rostrum. Stop the sensitization. *J Allergy Clin Immunol* 98(5 Pt 1):857–858, 1996.
92. Golden DB, Kwiterovich KA, Kagey-Sobotka A, et al: Discontinuing venom immunotherapy: outcome after five years. *J Allergy Clin Immunol* 97(2):579–587, 1996.
93. Reisman RE, Lantner R: Further observations of stopping venom immunotherapy: comparison of patients stopped because of a fall in serum venom-specific IgE to insignificant levels with patients stopped prematurely by self-choice. *J Allergy Clin Immunol* 83(6):1049–1054, 1989.
94. Golden DB, Moffitt J, Nicklas RA, et al: Stinging insect hypersensitivity: a practice parameter update 2011. *J Allergy Clin Immunol* 127(4):852–854, 2011.
95. Sheffer AL, Austen KF: Exercise-induced anaphylaxis. *J Allergy Clin Immunol* 66(2):106–111, 1980.
96. van Wijk RG, de GH, Bogaard JM: Drug-dependent exercise-induced anaphylaxis. *Allergy* 50(12):992–994, 1995.
97. Shadick NA, Liang MH, Partridge AJ, et al: The natural history of exercise-induced anaphylaxis: survey results from a 10-year follow-up study. *J Allergy Clin Immunol* 104(1):123–127, 1999.
98. Wong S, Dykewicz MS, Patterson R: Idiopathic anaphylaxis. A clinical summary of 175 patients. *Arch Intern Med* 150(6):1323–1328, 1990.
99. Webb LM, Lieberman P: Anaphylaxis: a review of 601 cases. *Ann Allergy Asthma Immunol* 97(1):39–43, 2006.
100. Wong S, Yarnold PR, Yango C, et al: Outcome of prophylactic therapy for idiopathic anaphylaxis. *Ann Intern Med* 114(2):133–136, 1991.
101. Lenchner KI, Ditto AM: Idiopathic anaphylaxis. *Allergy Asthma Proc* 25[4 Suppl 1]: S54–S56, 2004.
102. Lieberman JA, Chehade M: Use of omalizumab in the treatment of food allergy and anaphylaxis. *Curr Allergy Asthma Rep* 13(1):78–84, 2013.
103. Maurer M, Rosen K, Hsieh HJ, et al: Omalizumab for the treatment of chronic idiopathic or spontaneous urticaria. *N Engl J Med* 368(10):924–935, 2013.
104. Khan DA: Alternative agents in refractory chronic urticaria: evidence and considerations on their selection and use. *J Allergy Clin Immunol Pract* 1(5):433–440, 2013.
105. Riedl MA: Hereditary angioedema with normal C1-INH (HAE type III). *J Allergy Clin Immunol Pract* 1(5):427–432, 2013.
106. Javaud N, Achamlal J, Reuter PG, et al: Angioedema related to angiotensin-converting enzyme inhibitors: attack severity, treatment, and hospital admission in a prospective multicenter study. *Medicine (Baltimore)* 94(45):e1939, 2015.
107. Bielory L, Lee SS, Holland CL, et al: Long-acting ACE inhibitor-induced angioedema. *Allergy Proc* 13(2):85–87, 1992.
108. Bas M, Greve J, Stelter K, et al: A randomized trial of icatibant in ACE-inhibitor-induced angioedema. *N Engl J Med* 372(5):418–425, 2015.
109. Bhardwaj N, Craig TJ: Treatment of hereditary angioedema: a review (CME). *Transfusion* 54(11):2989–2996, 2014.
110. Prematta M, Gibbs JG, Pratt EL, et al: Fresh frozen plasma for the treatment of hereditary angioedema. *Ann Allergy Asthma Immunol* 98(4):383–388, 2007.
111. Vane JR: Inhibition of prostaglandin synthesis as a mechanism of action for aspirin-like drugs. *Nat New Biol* 231(25):232–235, 1971.
112. Burrish GF, Kaatz BL: Sulindac-induced anaphylaxis. *Ann Emerg Med* 10(3):154–155, 1981.
113. Corre KA, Rothstein RJ: Anaphylactic reaction to zomepirac. *Ann Allergy* 48(5):299–301, 1982.
114. Moore ME, Goldsmith DP: Nonsteroidal anti-inflammatory intolerance. An anaphylactic reaction to tolmetin. *Arch Intern Med* 140(8):1105–1106, 1980.
115. Mastalerz L, Setkowicz M, Sanak M, et al: Hypersensitivity to aspirin: common eicosanoid alterations in urticaria and asthma. *J Allergy Clin Immunol* 113(4):771–775, 2004.
116. Gollapudi RR, Teirstein PS, Stevenson DD, et al: Aspirin sensitivity: implications for patients with coronary artery disease. *JAMA* 292(24):3017–3023, 2004.
117. Silberman S, Neukirch-Stoop C, Steg PG: Rapid desensitization procedure for patients with aspirin hypersensitivity undergoing coronary stenting. *Am J Cardiol* 95(4):509–510, 2005.
118. Heinzerling L, Raile K, Rochlitz H, et al: Insulin allergy: clinical manifestations and management strategies. *Allergy* 63(2):148–155, 2008.
119. Grammer LC, Roberts M, Buchanan TA, et al: Specificity of immunoglobulin E and immunoglobulin G against human (recombinant DNA) insulin in human insulin allergy and resistance. *J Lab Clin Med* 109(2):141–146, 1987.
120. Gruchalla RS: 10. Drug allergy. *J Allergy Clin Immunol* 111[2 Suppl]:S548–S559, 2003.
121. Wong JT, Ripple RE, MacLean JA, et al: Vancomycin hypersensitivity: synergism with narcotics and "desensitization" by a rapid continuous intravenous protocol. *J Allergy Clin Immunol* 94(2 Pt 1):189–194, 1994.
122. Craddock PR, Fehr J, Brigham KL, et al: Complement and leukocyte-mediated pulmonary dysfunction in hemodialysis. *N Engl J Med* 296(14):769–774, 1977.
123. Fanous LH, Gray A, Felmingham J: Severe anaphylactoid reactions to dextran 70. *Br Med J* 2(6096):1189–1190, 1977.
124. Ring J, Messmer K: Incidence and severity of anaphylactoid reactions to colloid volume substitutes. *Lancet* 1(8009):466–469, 1977.
125. Fisher MM: Severe histamine mediated reactions to intravenous drugs used in anaesthesia. *Anaesth Intensive Care* 3(3):180–197, 1975.
126. Mathieu A, Goudsouzian N, Snider MT: Reaction to ketamine: anaphylactoid or anaphylactic? *Br J Anaesth* 47(5):624–627, 1975.
127. Thomas AD, Caunt JA: Anaphylactoid reaction following local anaesthesia for epidural block. *Anaesthesia* 48(1):50–52, 1993.
128. Berkes EA: Anaphylactic and anaphylactoid reactions to aspirin and other NSAIDs. *Clin Rev Allergy Immunol* 24(2):137–148, 2003.
129. Basu R, Rajkumar A, Datta NR: Anaphylaxis to cisplatin following nine previous uncomplicated cycles. *Int J Clin Oncol* 7(6):365–367, 2002.
130. Sliesoraitis S, Chikhale PJ: Carboplatin hypersensitivity. *Int J Gynecol Cancer* 15(1):13–18, 2005.

Chapter 70 ■ Dermatology in the Intensive Care Unit

JULIA BALTZ • KRISTEN BERREBI • DORI GOLDBERG • MARY E. MALONEY • HALEY SNADECKI

INTRODUCTION

Patients in the intensive care unit (ICU) often present with cutaneous findings. Their reason for admission to the ICU may be primarily dermatologic, as in the case of toxic epidermal necrolysis (TEN) or pemphigus vulgaris, two diseases in which large areas of the epidermis are shed. Or they may have skin findings that provide diagnostic clues to their internal disease, as when a patient with systemic lupus erythematosus (SLE) presents with a classic malar rash. Patients with life-threatening infections, such as Rocky Mountain spotted fever (RMSF) and meningococcemia, may present with characteristic skin lesions that suggest the correct diagnosis and allow prompt institution of lifesaving treatment.

Skin conditions in ICU patients are often iatrogenic, being caused by drugs (e.g., TEN, drug reaction with eosinophilia and systemic symptoms [DRESS], acute generalized exanthematous pustulosis [AGEP]), procedures (e.g., cholesterol emboli), dressings (e.g., contact dermatitis), or inattentive care (e.g., pressure ulcers). At other times, patients may have skin conditions which, although relatively minor, may complicate their ICU stay, put other patients and health care workers at risk (e.g., scabies), or make patients uncomfortable (e.g., miliaria, Grover's disease).

In this chapter, we give an overview of serious illnesses with prominent cutaneous findings, including drug reactions, exfoliative erythrodermas, infections, blistering disorders, vascular disorders, connective tissue disorders, and graft-versus-host disease (GVHD). In addition, we provide a brief description of more common but less serious dermatoses that may coexist in ICU patients, with suggestions for their management. We emphasize the importance of lesion morphology, that is, the shape, color, size, arrangement, and distribution of skin lesion in making a correct diagnosis. Table 70.1 provides a list of skin

TABLE 70.1

Differential Diagnosis of Skin Eruptions by Morphology

Fever and rash
- Infectious disease (bacterial, fungal, viral)
- Rheumatologic disease (SLE, rheumatoid arthritis, juvenile rheumatoid arthritis, Still's disease, mixed connective tissue disease)
- Pustular psoriasis
- Drug eruption
- Leukemia/lymphoma
- Lofgren's syndrome (acute sarcoidosis with erythema nodosum, hilar adenopathy, fever, and arthritis)
- Sweet's syndrome
- Polyarteritis nodosa

Morbilliform (maculopapular)
- Drug eruption
- Viral exanthem
- Graft-versus-host disease
- Rickettsial infections

Generalized erythema
- Staphylococcal scalded skin syndrome
- Exfoliative erythroderma

Localized erythematous papules and plaques
- Psoriasis
- Seborrheic dermatitis
- Contact dermatitis
- Pityriasis rosea
- Tinea
- Scabies
- Dermatomyositis
- Lupus erythematosus
- Secondary syphilis
- Urticaria
- Still's disease
- Disseminated candidiasis
- Erythema nodosum
- Grover's disease

Annular (ring-shaped) erythematous lesions
- Tinea
- Erythema multiforme
- Urticaria
- Granuloma annulare
- Sarcoid
- Subacute cutaneous lupus
- Sweet's syndrome
- Erythema chronicum migrans (Lyme disease)
- Leprosy

Pustules
- Pustular psoriasis
- Steroid acne
- Folliculitis
- Acute generalized exanthematous pustulosis (AGEP)

Vesicles/Bullae
- Herpes simplex
- Varicella zoster
- Miliaria
- Bullous infections (impetigo, tinea, cellulitis)
- Erythema multiforme/Stevens–Johnson syndrome/TEN
- Pemphigus
- Paraneoplastic pemphigus
- Bullous pemphigoid
- Linear IgA dermatosis
- Epidermolysis bullosa acquisita
- Porphyria cutanea tarda
- Dermatitis herpetiformis

Purpura
- Vasculitis
- Purpura fulminans
- Calciphylaxis
- Heparin or Coumadin necrosis
- Cryoglobulinemia
- Cholesterol emboli
- Myeloproliferative disease
- Antiphospholipid syndrome

Ulcers
- Vasculopathy
- Infectious
- Neoplastic
- Bullous disorders
- Panniculitis
- Neuropathy
- Bites
- Aphthae
- Trauma

diseases arranged by morphology to assist with formulating a differential diagnosis.

Dermatologic consultation is often helpful for diagnosis and management of skin diseases of ICU patients. The dermatologic consultant may be able to help sort out multiple potential differential diagnoses by inspection of morphology, skin biopsy, or use of other diagnostic tests (skin scrapings for scabies, potassium hydroxide preparations for fungus, viral and bacterial cultures, and direct fluorescent antibody [DFA] tests for viral infections). Because morphology evolves with the natural course of disease and with attempted therapeutic measures, it is helpful to request consultation early in the course of cutaneous disease.

DRUG ERUPTIONS

Cutaneous drug reactions are frequently encountered among ICU patients. Certain drug reactions such as TEN, Stevens–Johnson syndrome (SJS), DRESS, and AGEP may be the primary cause for admission to the ICU. These reactions will be discussed in depth following a brief overview of more commonly occurring drug reactions. The exanthematous or morbilliform drug eruption is the most common (Fig. 70.1). It typically appears 7 to 14 days after introduction of the offending agent. Clinically it appears as symmetric macules that may become slightly papular on the trunk and upper extremities, and may become confluent with time. Low-grade fever and pruritus are sometimes present. The differential diagnosis includes viral exanthem, Kawasaki's disease, GVHD, and the more serious drug reactions discussed below (TEN, SJS, DRESS, and AGEP). Facial edema, mucosal lesions, blisters or sloughing of the skin, and laboratory abnormalities such as neutrophilia, eosinophilia, and elevated liver function tests may indicate the presence of a more serious drug reaction. Withdrawal of the causative drug is the most important treatment, although topical corticosteroids and oral antihistamines may be used for symptomatic relief. Exanthematous drug eruptions resolve without sequelae 1 to 2 weeks after the offending drug has been discontinued.

Toxic Epidermal Necrolysis/Stevens–Johnson Syndrome

TEN and SJS are entities on a spectrum of severe cutaneous reactions that are most commonly caused by medications. Patients exhibit severe blistering and sloughing of the skin (Fig. 70.2) with mucosal involvement (Fig. 70.3), and can have

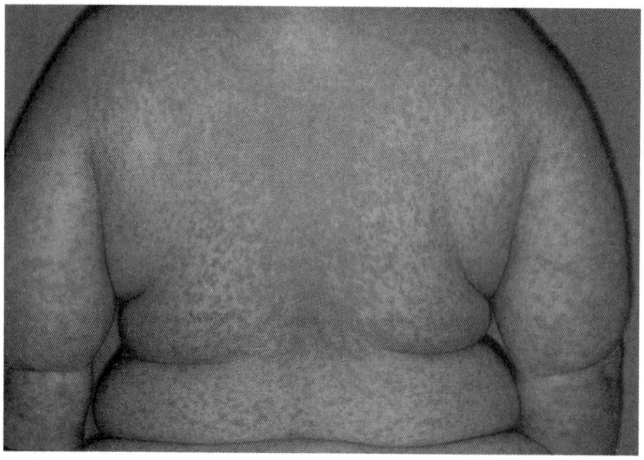

FIGURE 70.1 Morbilliform (maculopapular) drug eruption. Note the pink blanchable papules and plaques with areas of confluence over the trunk and extremities.

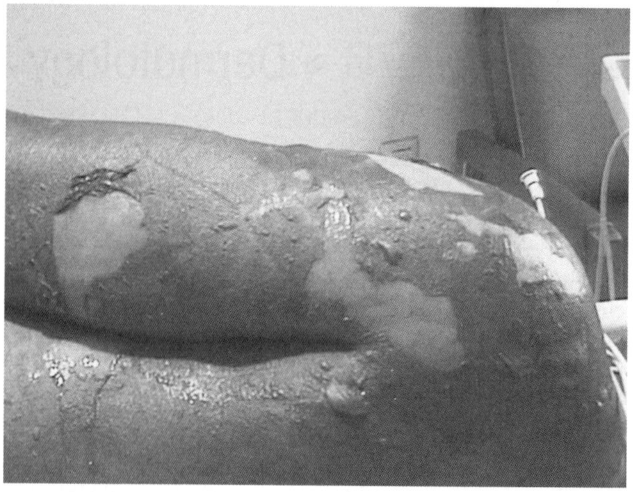

FIGURE 70.2 Toxic epidermal necrolysis. Bullae and sheets of epidermal sloughing leaving behind red denuded areas are seen.

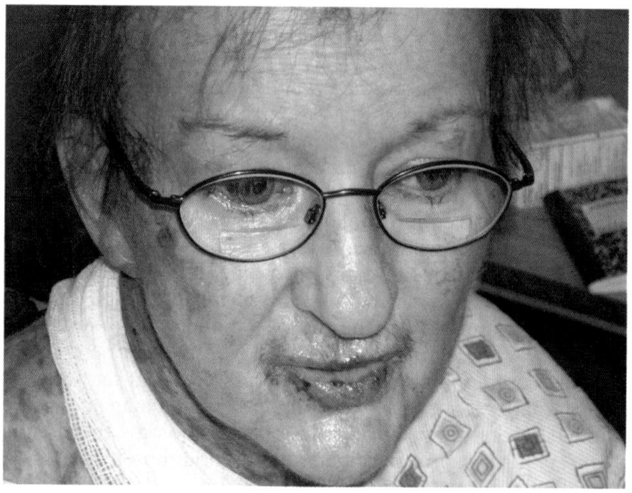

FIGURE 70.3 Stevens–Johnson syndrome. Bullae over the left top eyelid and erythematous and edematous plaques on the neck and shoulders. Note the erosions over the lips.

high morbidity and mortality. The distinction between TEN and SJS is based on the percentage of skin involved with SJS being <10%, TEN being >30%, and SJS/TEN overlap being 10% to 30% of the body surface area affected. The cumulative combined incidence of these entities has been estimated at 2 to 7 per million people annually SJS/TEN occur in all age groups. TEN is more common among women, and incidence increases with age and immunosuppression [1]. HIV infection increases the risk of SJS/TEN with the incidence of TEN in HIV patients receiving trimethoprim–sulfamethoxazole, 8.4 per 100,000 exposures as opposed to 2.6 per 100,000 exposures in non–HIV-infected individuals [2]. Certain human leukocyte antigen (HLA) genotypes render patients more susceptible to SJS/TEN. Currently the FDA recommends HLA-B1502 testing in most East Asian patients prior to prescribing carbamazepine and HLA-B5701 testing on all HIV-positive patients prior to receiving abacavir [3].

Ninety-five percent of patients with TEN have a history of drug exposure and there is a clear relationship to a drug in 80% of cases. The most common causative medications along with relative risks listed in parentheses include: trimethoprim–sulfamethoxazole (172), carbamazepine (90), nonsteroidal antiinflammatory drugs (NSAIDs) (72), corticosteroids (54), phenytoin (53), allopurinol (52), phenobarbital (45), valproic acid (25), cephalosporins (14), quinolones (10), and aminopenicillins (6.7), with more recent reports implicating lamotrigine, rituximab, imatinib, and lenalidomide [4]. The time from drug ingestion to clinical symptoms is generally 1 to 3 weeks, except for the aromatic anticonvulsants that can take up to 2 months to cause disease [5]. Previous classifications included *Mycoplasma pneumoniae* as a cause of SJS; however, it has been recently proposed that the mucocutaneous eruption associated with *mycoplasma* be considered a separate entity: *Mycoplasma*-induced rash and mucositis (MIRM). Patients with a mucocutaneous *mycoplasma*-associated eruption present with oral mucosal erosions (94%), ocular involvement (82%), and urogenital involvement (63%). Cutaneous involvement is absent among 34% of patients, and targetoid lesions not usually seen. Treatment consists of antibiotics and corticosteroids. Intravenous immunoglobulin (IVIG) is not warranted, as prognosis is excellent with few long-term sequelae [6].

The cutaneous eruption of SJS/TEN may be preceded by a 1- to 3-day prodrome of fever and flu-like symptoms. The initial cutaneous finding is irregularly shaped erythematous to purpuric macules distributed on the face and trunk. These may evolve into flaccid blisters that may be easily enlarged with lateral pressure (Nikolsky sign). The skin can become gray, which usually heralds full thickness epidermal sloughing. Mucosal involvement is present in 90% of patients with SJS and TEN, with the most common affected areas being the conjunctiva, oral cavity, and genitalia. Symptoms include severe skin pain and difficulty swallowing and urinating. Respiratory epithelium may also be involved with resultant dyspnea, pulmonary edema, and hypoxia.

The differential diagnosis includes staphylococcal scalded skin syndrome (SSSS), AGEP, severe acute GVHD, drug-induced linear IgA bullous dermatosis, paraneoplastic pemphigus, and MIRM as discussed above. The appropriate clinical setting and skin biopsy easily differentiate SJS/TEN from these entities. Early lesions demonstrate necrotic keratinocytes, whereas advanced lesions reveal full thickness epidermal necrosis, and a 2005 study found that the density of the dermal mononuclear cell infiltrate correlates with the severity of disease and mortality rate [7].

Prompt diagnosis and rapid cessation of the causative medication along with supportive therapy is the cornerstone of treatment. Careful monitoring of fluid volume, electrolytes, renal function, nutritional status, and evaluation for signs of sepsis should be standard. For extensive body surface involvement, care should be provided in an ICU with staff accustomed to caring for patients with fragile and denuded skin, usually a burn unit. Uninvolved skin should not be manipulated, whereas involved skin should be covered with Vaseline-impregnated gauze and a topical antibiotic ointment. Debridement of necrotic skin may be followed by placement of artificial membranes or biologic dressings such as xenografts or allografts. Bacterial cultures should be performed of involved skin and mucosa as well as blood, urine, and any intravenous catheters, as sepsis is the most common cause of mortality among patients with SJS/TEN. Systemic antibiotics should not be started unless signs of sepsis are present because of the risk of selecting for antibiotic-resistant organisms, and prophylactic use of antibiotics has not been shown to improve outcomes. Patients should be followed by an ophthalmologist for management to prevent conjunctival scarring.

Currently, there is no gold standard systemic therapy for TEN/SJS, as much of the available data are based upon case reports, case series, and small retrospective chart reviews. IVIG has been used, based on its ability to bind Fas receptors, thought to be a mediator, along with granulysin, of apoptosis in TEN/SJS. Unfortunately, there are no randomized double-blinded trials to support its use, and while some studies have shown mortality benefit with doses more than 1 g/kg/d, others have shown no benefits or even increased mortality associated with its use [8]. Systemic corticosteroid pulse therapy early in the disease course has been shown to have benefits for preventing ocular complications, and topical high potency corticosteroids appear to prevent corneal epithelial stem cell loss and scarring [9]. Furthermore, evidence suggests that high-dose (1.5 mg/kg/d) pulse corticosteroids decreased TEN-associated mortality [10]. There are emerging data supporting the use of cyclosporine as a possibly superior alternative to IVIG [11]. Despite newer data on alternatives, a recent survey study of 111 US burn centers found that IVIG and systemic corticosteroids are the most commonly used therapeutic interventions, with decision to treat based upon the degree and severity of skin/mucosal involvement as well as the likelihood of ongoing infection [10]. Evidence is further clouded because SJS/TEN is a self-limited disease, with maximal detachment occurring at approximately 8 days after the onset of symptoms [8].

The mortality rate for SJS and TEN is 5% and 30%, respectively, and is directly related to the percentage of skin involved. Risk of mortality can be predicted using the Severity of illness SCOR for TEN (SCORTEN) algorithm. One point each is assigned for the presence of the following seven criteria: age >40 years, presence of malignancy, heart rate >120, initial epidermal detachment >10%, serum urea nitrogen >10 mmol per L, serum glucose >14 mmol per L, and serum bicarbonate <20 mmol per L. The points are added and the predicted mortality based upon this total is 0 to 1 (3.2%), 2 (12.1%), 3 (35.8%), 4 (58.3%), and 5 or more (90%) [12]. Healing of sloughed epidermis usually takes 3 weeks; however, survivors may experience delayed ocular scarring and visual loss, necessitating long-term follow-up with ophthalmology. If the causative medication is reintroduced, the disease may recur in less than 48 hours. Notably, a patient who experiences TEN to one class of medication is not predisposed to TEN in response to other medication classes; however, cross-reactivity may be seen between related drug classes such as penicillins and cephalosporins.

Drug Rash with Eosinophilia and Systemic Symptoms

Drug rash with eosinophilia and systemic symptoms (DRESS), also called drug-induced hypersensitivity syndrome, is a potentially fatal hypersensitivity reaction to medication, most commonly anticonvulsants [13]. The incidence is between 1/1,000 and 1/10,000 exposures and it is thought to occur with higher frequencies in patients of African ancestry [14].

Although the etiology of DRESS is not understood completely, alteration in drug detoxification pathways, reactivation of herpesviruses, association with certain HLA alleles and immunologic mechanisms are all implicated in the pathogenesis [15]. DRESS is most commonly caused by the aromatic anticonvulsants, including phenobarbital, phenytoin, and carbamazepine. Of note, these drugs may cross-react. Other common causes include allopurinol, sulfonamides, minocycline, and dapsone.

In contrast to other drug reactions, DRESS may develop as late as 4 to 6 weeks after the offending medication has been introduced. DRESS has even been reported to occur more than 1 year after initiating allopurinol. The rash is usually morbilliform, though erythroderma, pustules, vesicles, and purpuric areas may also be present. One study suggested that an erythema multiforme-like eruption may be more indicative of severe hepatic involvement [16].

The hallmark features of DRESS are high fever and edema of the face. Initial systemic involvement may include pharyngitis, lymphadenopathy, hepatosplenomegaly, peripheral eosinophilia, abnormal liver function tests, arthralgias, pulmonary infiltrates, and interstitial nephritis. Liver injury is common and the most common pattern of liver injury is cholestatic type. [17] Circulating atypical lymphocytes may also be present [14]. Certain medications are more commonly associated with specific internal organ involvement [15]. Several case series have shown that high eosinophil count is a poor prognostic factor with other indications of poor prognosis including pancytopenia, thrombocytopenia, and multiple medical comorbidities. Septic shock is a significant cause of mortality in patients with DRESS [18,19]. Late sequelae involving the endocrine system, commonly the thyroid and pancreas, may develop weeks to months after drug withdrawal or rebound during corticosteroid taper. Although end-organ involvement is more common among older patients, young patients are more likely to develop autoimmune sequelae [20]. Fulminant myocarditis is underrecognized and can present initially or months later. One study found ampicillin and minocycline to be the most common medications associated with myocarditis [21].

The differential diagnosis includes AGEP, SJS, TEN, Kawasaki's disease, and the hypereosinophilic syndrome. Histopathology of skin biopsies taken from patients with DRESS is variable and therefore not diagnostic [18]. The history of recent initiation of a suspect drug, the presence of atypical lymphocytes, peripheral eosinophilia, increased liver function tests, abnormal serum creatinine or urinalysis, and cutaneous eruption as described above, especially with facial edema, suggest the diagnosis of DRESS.

The most effective treatment is prompt diagnosis and cessation of the offending drug; most patients completely recover after drug withdrawal. A recent study suggests that mild forms of DRESS can be managed without systemic steroids [22] and cutaneous symptoms can be treated with topical steroids. In most cases, other than withdrawing the offending drug, prednisone at 1 mg/kg/d gradually tapered over 3 to 6 months is the current mainstay of treatment. However, there are no controlled clinical trials investigating the risks and benefits of systemic corticosteroids or other systemic treatments [23].

Primary and secondary prevention of DRESS is of utmost importance and one must have knowledge of the most common causative drugs and an understanding of the cross-reactivity among the aromatic hydrocarbons. Mortality rates up to 10% have been reported primarily due to fulminant hepatitis. It is important to monitor for long-term sequelae [23].

Acute Generalized Exanthematous Pustulosis

AGEP, also known as toxic pustuloderma [24] or pustular drug rash [25], is a very rare reaction that presents with fever, leukocytosis, and multiple pustules on a background of generalized erythema. AGEP occurs equally in both males and females, and also occurs at any age. Incidence rates have been estimated at 1 to 5 cases per million per year [26].

Drugs are responsible for at least 90% of AGEP cases. In a report of 97 cases from Europe, aminopenicillins (odds ratio [OR] = 23), macrolides (OR = 11), quinolones (OR = 33), hydroxychloroquine (OR = 39), calcium channel blockers (OR = 15), anticonvulsants (OR = 8), and corticosteroids (OR = 12) were the most common causative agents [27]. Patch testing with the offending agent is frequently positive reflecting the dominant role of T cells in the disorder. Although drug-related in the vast majority of cases, there is some evidence showing the reaction is not always related to medication administration. More recently, spider bites have been reported as triggers in addition to possible viral causes [28–30].

The eruption is frequently of sudden onset and the majority of cases appear within 24 hours to several days of exposure to the offending agent. A fever of more than 38°C is followed by the appearance of tiny nonfollicular pustules on a background of generalized erythema and edema. Petechiae, purpura, vesicles, or target lesions may be present, and oral lesions may be observed among 20% of patients. The face and intertriginous areas are the most common presenting locations. Neutrophilia occurs among 90% and eosinophilia among 30% of patients. Liver function tests are usually normal and there is typically no systemic involvement, but lymphadenopathy is sometimes seen. The differential diagnosis includes pustular psoriasis, subcorneal pustular dermatosis, DRESS, and in severe cases, TEN. An acute onset and clinical history of a new drug favors AGEP over pustular psoriasis, whereas DRESS and TEN exhibit systemic involvement.

Discontinuation of the causative drug is the definitive treatment. Once the diagnosis is made and the causative drug is stopped, the pustules will resolve in less than 15 days with desquamation, and prognosis is excellent. Antipyretics may be used for symptomatic treatment of the fever and topical steroids may be used for symptomatic treatment of the rash, although neither will hasten the resolution of the eruption.

EXFOLIATIVE ERYTHRODERMA

Erythroderma (Fig. 70.4) is a rare, life-threatening skin condition characterized by erythema involving at least 90% of the body surface area with variable degrees of scaling [31–33]. Although age at presentation varies with the underlying cause, patients are typically over 40 or 45 years. Male to female ratio and reported incidence are also variable, and there is no racial predilection [33–35].

The causes of erythroderma may be categorized into preexisting skin conditions (psoriasis, atopic dermatitis, contact dermatitis, and seborrheic dermatitis), drug reactions, malignancy, skin infections and infestations, and idiopathic etiology [31,33]. Over 60 topical and systemic medications have been implicated in erythroderma, including angiotensin-converting enzyme inhibitors, anticonvulsants, penicillin, vancomycin, antifungals, and barbiturates [34,35]. Leukemias and lymphomas constitute up to 40% of malignancy-related erythrodermas. Cutaneous T-cell lymphoma (CTCL) and Sezary syndrome represent most of these cases. Primary blood vessel malignancy and solid organ cancers are also reported in association with erythroderma [35]. Staph scalded skin syndrome (SSSS), HIV seroconversion, superficial dermatophyte and candidal infections, scabies infestation, lupus erythematosus, sarcoidosis, and mastocytosis may rarely cause erythroderma as well. Up to 46% of cases have no identifiable trigger [31,34].

Varying degrees of scaling, which often begin at flexural surfaces, follow intense widespread erythema within 2 to 6 days. Erythroderma associated with psoriasis and atopic dermatitis

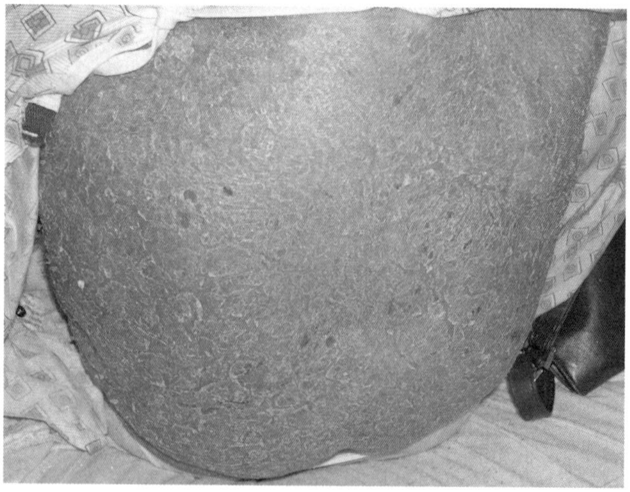

FIGURE 70.4 Exfoliative erythroderma. Widespread red blanchable erythema with scale.

has a more indolent course than the more rapidly progressive form linked to malignancy, drugs, and SSSS [34]. Along with intense erythema, patients may have fever, hyperkeratosis of the palms and soles, nail dystrophy, cheilitis, alopecia, edema of the face and legs, dermatopathic lymphadenopathy, hepatomegaly, and splenomegaly [33,34].

Erythrodermic patients have dramatic disturbances in the body's regulatory mechanisms. Increased cutaneous blood flow results in exaggerated heat and fluid losses with a compensatory increase in the body's basal metabolic rate. This, in conjunction with the shedding of 20 to 30 g per day of proteinaceous scale, can result in a hypoalbuminemia that exacerbates edema and nutritional deficits [34,35]. Complications include electrolyte imbalance, thermoregulation, dehydration, high output cardiac failure, and secondary infections.

Identification of the underlying trigger is important in the evaluation and management of erythrodermic patients. Early examination of the skin with corroborating evidence from skin biopsy may be helpful in establishing the etiology, but in the majority of adult cases, the underlying dermatosis is obscured by widespread erythema and scaling. Skin biopsy has recently been shown to be more useful in detecting some underlying triggers for infantile and neonatal cases of erythroderma [36].

Erythroderma should be managed as a dermatologic emergency in the inpatient setting. Initial treatment, regardless of the underlying cause, consists of temperature regulation (in spite of the skin being warm or hot to the touch, patients become hypothermic), hemodynamic support and monitoring, and skin care. Topical therapies include low-to-mid potency corticosteroids such as triamcinolone 0.025% to 0.1% or mometasone cream under wet dressings. Tap water–soaked gauze dressings may be changed every 2 to 3 hours, and tepid baths may provide additional relief. As the skin condition improves, emollients can be substituted for corticosteroids. Systemic corticosteroids can be helpful, but must be used with caution in atopic dermatitis and are contraindicated in infection and psoriasis. Additional therapy is targeted to the triggering disease and may include systemic retinoids, cyclosporine, or methotrexate in the case of psoriasis, and psoralen with UVA phototherapy in the case of CTCL [34,35]. Regardless of the underlying cause, relapses of erythroderma are common. Mortality rates range from 4.6% to 64% and are influenced by advanced age and comorbidities [33].

INFECTIONS

Toxic Shock Syndrome

Toxic shock syndrome (TSS) is an acute febrile illness caused by toxin-producing strains of *Staphylococcus aureus*, presenting with fever, rash, and hypotension, and often progressing to multiorgan failure [37]. A similar syndrome caused by *Streptococcus pyogenes* has also been described, known as streptococcal toxic shock syndrome (STSS) [38]. TSS was originally seen in young women and was associated with tampon use. Although it is now seen in multiple settings, it is still worthwhile to be sure that in menstruating women, a tampon has not been left in place. Pathophysiology of both entities involves massive release of cytokines due to bacterial toxins acting as superantigens.

Both TSS and STSS present with high fever, headache, nausea and vomiting, and myalgias and arthralgias. Hypotension, metabolic acidosis, acute renal failure, elevated transaminases, thrombocytopenia, leukocytosis, disseminated intravascular coagulation (DIC), cardiomyopathy, and acute respiratory distress syndrome (ARDS) are often seen. Most patients with TSS do not have an obvious localized *S. aureus* infection. In contrast, 80% of patients with STSS have a clinically evident painful streptococcal soft tissue infection, often necrotizing fasciitis (NF), usually of an extremity [37].

Skin findings are especially prominent with TSS, which classically presents with generalized macular erythema, but a scarlatiniform rash with accentuation of the flexures can also be seen. Erythema of the palms and soles, conjunctivae, and mucous membranes is also observed. The patient may develop a bright red "strawberry" tongue. The eruption is followed by desquamation 1 to 2 weeks later, especially of the palms and soles.

The differential diagnosis includes RMSF, meningococcemia, Kawasaki's disease, SSSS, scarlet fever, or a medication hypersensitivity reaction. Blood cultures are positive in 60% of cases of STSS, less often in TSS ($<15\%$) [37]. Diagnosis is on clinical grounds and requires four major criteria (fever $>38.9°C$, erythroderma, desquamation 1 to 2 weeks later, hypotension, and poor peripheral perfusion) and at least three minor criteria (vomiting or diarrhea; severe myalgia or creatine phosphakinase (CPK) twice normal; hyperemic mucous membranes; elevated urea or creatinine; elevated bilirubin, alanine transaminase (ALT), or Aspartate Aminotransferase (AST); platelets $<100 \times 10^9$ per L; and disorientation or altered consciousness). TSS also has a specific T-cell signature with early depletion of the V β-2 subset followed by massive expansion, which can aid in early diagnosis [39]. Skin biopsy shows a neutrophilic and eosinophilic perivascular and interstitial infiltrate with scattered necrotic keratinocytes.

Treatment is with supportive care (intravenous fluids and vasopressors), penicillinase-resistant antibiotics, and IVIG or fresh frozen plasma (FFP). The current recommendation is that all patients with suspected TSS and STSS be treated with empiric clindamycin (900 mg IV every 8 hours) plus vancomycin (15 to 20 mg/kg/dose every 8 to 12 hours) until sensitivities are known. In addition, prompt surgical exploration and drainage of suspected deep tissue infections is critical in cases of STSS in which NF may be present.

TSS has a case fatality rate of less than 5%, whereas mortality in STSS ranges from 30% to 70%, and significant morbidity, including renal failure, amputation, or hysterectomy may also occur [37,38].

Cellulitis and Erysipelas

Cellulitis is an acute bacterial infection of the skin and subcutaneous tissues. Erysipelas is a more superficial skin infection that involves the upper dermis and often superficial lymphatics. It is distinguished from cellulitis and other infections by its very sharply demarcated borders and induration. Cellulitis is common and more frequently affects men than women. The lower extremities are most often involved (73% of cases), followed by the upper extremities (19%), and head and neck (7%) [40]. Cellulitis is usually caused by group A β-hemolytic streptococci or *S. aureus*, including methicillin-resistant *S. aureus* (MRSA) [41], although it may also be caused by Group B streptococci, *Haemophilus influenzae*, *Pseudomonas aeruginosa*, and other bacteria in certain settings. Infection following aquatic injury is often Gram negative and polymicrobial, though nontuberculous mycobacterial infections should also be considered [42]. Erysipelas is almost always caused by Group A streptococci.

Predisposing factors for cellulitis include venous stasis disease, lymphedema, lower extremity ulceration, surgical wounds, tinea pedis, chronic dermatoses, and obesity. Bacteria on the skin surface enter through breaks in the skin and proliferate in the dermis and subcutaneous tissues, causing inflammation.

Patients with cellulitis present with poorly demarcated erythema, swelling, warmth, and tenderness. Cellulitis of the lower extremity commonly occurs in the setting of leg edema or dermatitis. If a line is drawn around the involved area, the area of redness is often seen to spread outward over hours to days. Patients frequently have tender local lymphadenopathy and/or lymphangitis. Fever or myalgias are sometimes present. In erysipelas, the skin is bright red and the borders are elevated and sharply demarcated from the uninvolved skin.

Cellulitis has a broad differential diagnosis, including contact dermatitis, superficial thrombophlebitis, deep venous thrombosis, NF, lipodermatosclerosis, and insect bites or stings [43,44]. One of the most commonly confused entities is simple stasis dermatitis, which is usually bilateral with scaling and hyperpigmentation of the distal lower extremities in addition to erythema and swelling. It is usually not tender unless ulceration is present. Cellulitis (particularly "bilateral cellulitis") is commonly misdiagnosed in the inpatient setting and early involvement of a dermatologist may improve diagnostic accuracy and decrease unnecessary antibiotic use [45].

Diagnosis of cellulitis and erysipelas is generally on clinical grounds. Cultures of blood or cutaneous aspirates and biopsies or swabs are not routinely recommended except in patients with malignancy receiving chemotherapy, neutropenia, cell-mediated immunodeficiency, and history of immersion injury and animal bite [46]. Radiographic studies are usually unnecessary, although plain films or computed tomography (CT) may be of value to evaluate underlying osteomyelitis, and magnetic resonance imaging (MRI) may be used to differentiate cellulitis from NF [43]. If NF is strongly suspected, surgical debridement and intravenous antibiotics should be initiated immediately without waiting for radiologic or microbiologic studies.

Treatment of cellulitis is directed at the most likely bacterial causes, which are streptococci and *S. aureus*. Initial treatment of the hospitalized patient is with β-lactamase-resistant penicillins or cephalosporins such as cefazolin 1 g IV every 6 hours, nafcillin 1 to 1.5 g IV every 4 to 6 hours, or ceftriaxone 1 g IV every 24 hours. Coverage for MRSA should be added if there is evidence of penetrating trauma, MRSA infection elsewhere, nasal colonization with MRSA, injection drug use, signs of sepsis, or if the patient is immunocompromised. Treatment for MRSA can be with IV vancomycin, linezolid, daptomycin, telavancin, or clindamycin and should be started empirically for hospitalized patients with complicated infections [46]. A recent study showed that obese individuals are at risk of clinical failure secondary to inadequate dosing of antimicrobial therapy [47]. As the cellulitis begins to resolve and the patient becomes afebrile, the patient may be converted to oral dicloxacillin or cephalexin 500 mg every 6 hours, for a total course of 7 to 14 days of antibiotics [43]. Otherwise healthy patients without systemic signs of infection can be treated with oral antibiotics as outpatients.

Local treatment of a cellulitic limb with elevation to reduce swelling and saline dressings to any open wounds may be helpful. Prognosis of patients with uncomplicated cellulitis is excellent but recurrences can occur. Patients with a chronic tinea pedis as the probable cause of leg cellulitis should have the tinea treated, and venous stasis or lymphedema should be treated with compression stockings or devices to prevent recurrences [43]. A recent randomized control trial showed that treatment of patients with recurrent cellulitis with low-dose penicillin daily was effective for preventing subsequent infections and this should be considered for patients with 3 to 4 episodes of cellulitis per year [46,48].

Necrotizing Fasciitis

NF is a rapidly progressive infection involving the subcutis and fascia that typically occurs in the elderly, diabetics, alcohol abusers, cirrhotics, those with chronic cardiac disease or peripheral vascular disease and immunosuppression including cancer, organ transplant, HIV, and neutropenia [49,50]. It is increasing in frequency among young, previously healthy individuals. NF may occur de novo, after surgery and injection therapy or injection drug use, or after penetration or even blunt trauma [51]. The extremity is the usual site of involvement. When NF originates in the scrotum, it is known as Fournier's gangrene. Most cases result from a polymicrobial infection. Pathogens may include streptococci, *S. aureus*, enterococci, *Escherichia coli*, *Pseudomonas*, *Bacteroides*, and *Clostridium* spp. Community-acquired MRSA has been reported more recently [52]. Invasive Group A *Streptococcus* is implicated in previously healthy patients and has been reported among patients with a history of outpatient liposuction surgery [53]. Other less frequent pathogens include *P. aeruginosa*, *Aeromonas hydrophila*, and *Vibrio vulnificus*, *Haemophilus influenzae* type b.

The skin is initially shiny, erythematous, hot, tender, swollen, and tense. Pain is out of proportion to physical findings. Within 24 to 36 hours, skin color changes from red to dusky gray-blue, and bullae may develop. Deeper soft tissue may feel firm. With the destruction of cutaneous nerves, skin becomes anesthetic. The area becomes gangrenous by the fourth or fifth day, and patients appear toxic with fever, chills, tachycardia, shock, and leukocytosis.

NF may be difficult to differentiate from cellulitis, especially early in the course of disease. Features that suggest NF include severe pain which may be out of proportion to physical findings, anesthesia of involved skin, rapid spread, edema and bulla formation, associated varicella infection, signs of shock, elevated creatine phosphokinase level, or NSAID use. NSAID use is implicated in disease progression through attenuation of signs and symptoms of inflammation that leads to a delay of diagnosis and treatment. MRI is the preferred diagnostic imaging technique as CT changes may be minimal early on [49]. A newer tool called the laboratory risk indicator for NF uses a scoring system based on C-reactive protein, total white cell count, hemoglobin, sodium, creatinine, and glucose levels to help distinguish between necrotizing soft tissue infections and non-necrotizing infections, and in one retrospective study, was noted to predict mortality and amputation rates [54].

Early fasciotomy and immediate intravenous antimicrobial therapy based on initial Gram stain are crucial. Initial therapy involves vancomycin or linezolid plus either piperacillin–tazobactam, a carbapenem or a both ceftriaxone and metronidazole. Penicillin and clindamycin should be used for the treatment of documented Group A *Streptococcus* infection [46]. Hyperbaric oxygen therapy for anaerobic Gram-negative infection is controversial. Supportive care and attention to nutrition are important in optimizing postoperative wound healing. Even with early treatment, mortality may be between 9% and 25% [55]. Poor prognostic factors include older age, liver cirrhosis, soft tissue air, aeromonas infection, >10% bands, bacteremia, creatinine >2, peripheral vascular disease, hospital-acquired infection, multifocal disease, and severe sepsis or septic shock on admission [56,57].

Staphylococcal Scalded Skin Syndrome

SSSS is a blistering, desquamative skin condition caused by the exfoliative toxins of *S. aureus*. Infants and young children are the most commonly affected, likely because of their immature immune and renal function, resulting in a lack of antitoxin antibodies and accumulation of exfoliative toxin. A few cases have been reported in adults who generally have underlying renal impairment or immunosuppression [58,59].

Two toxins, ETA and ETB, have been detected in human disease, with the majority caused by ETA. These toxins bind to and cleave desmoglein-1, a desmosomal protein in the superficial epidermis critical for binding between keratinocytes. Cleavage of this protein causes separation between keratinocytes in the upper layers of the epidermis and also of the superficial epidermis from deeper layers, with resulting fragile blisters and denuded skin [58,59].

In the localized form of SSSS, bullous impetigo, *S. aureus* enters the skin through a break or tear and introduces exfoliative toxin which results in the development of blisters. Spread of toxin is prevented by antibodies to the toxin. In generalized SSSS, the focus of infection is at a distant site, such as an abscess, pneumonia, osteomyelitis, or endocarditis. Frequently, however, a focus of infection is not found. A lack of protective antibodies allows the toxin to reach the epidermis by hematogenous spread and causes widespread skin disease [58–60].

Whereas bullous impetigo has no associated systemic symptoms, generalized SSSS is associated with a prodrome of fever, malaise, and generalized erythema. This is followed by the formation of large blisters with clear or purulent fluid that easily rupture, leaving extensive areas of denuded skin. The degree of skin involvement may vary from focal blistering to entire body exfoliation. Significant pain and tenderness, hypothermia, fluid losses, secondary infection with *Pseudomonas* and other species, bacteremia, and sepsis may complicate the disease course [58,59].

SSSS should be considered for any presentation of fever and diffuse skin erythema. Although the main differential diagnosis is TEN, other conditions to consider include pemphigus foliaceus, scalding or chemical burns, GVHD, and epidermolysis bullosa. A thorough evaluation should include determination of the degree of denudation, identification of the source of infection, determination of fluid status, and a search for signs of secondary infection. Culture and Gram stain of the skin and focus of infection may identify *S. aureus*, but alone do not confirm the diagnosis of SSSS. Enzyme-linked immunosorbent assay (ELISA) can detect production of exotoxin from isolated *S. aureus* species, but should be used as confirmation of SSSS only, as false negatives can easily result if the pathogenic strain of bacteria is not detected on culture. Blood cultures are frequently positive in adults with SSSS [58,59].

Skin biopsy is the most useful diagnostic test, as it further distinguishes between SSSS and TEN. SSSS shows cleavage in the mid-epidermis with minimal associated inflammation. In TEN, cleavage occurs at the dermoepidermal junction and there is cellular necrosis of the epidermis. TEN can also be distinguished clinically by the presence of mucosal involvement, a finding that is not seen in SSSS. Pemphigus foliaceus, an autoimmune blistering disorder caused by autoantibodies against desmoglein-1, can also be difficult to distinguish both clinically and by routine histology [58,59]. Direct immunofluorescence will demonstrate anti-desmoglein antibodies in the epidermis of pemphigus foliaceus patients [61].

Treatment of generalized SSSS is with intravenous antibiotics targeting penicillin-resistant *S. aureus*. Aminoglycosides may be added if there are signs of secondary infection. Analgesia, fluid resuscitation, and wound care are other key elements of treatment. Use of steroids is contraindicated [58,59].

Exfoliation continues for 24 to 48 hours after institution of appropriate antibiotics. MRSA must be considered for any patient not responding to therapy after this time. Although the disease is rarely fatal in children, mortality in adults, even with treatment, is upward of 50% to 60%, when there are serious underlying medical conditions [58,59].

Meningococcemia

Neisseria meningitidis is a major cause of meningitis and sepsis in the United States, with an annual incidence of approximately 1 in 100,000. Meningococcal disease is often rapidly fatal due to shock and multiorgan failure. The majority of cases occur in winter and early spring. Disease peaks in infants and teenagers. Meningococcal disease often occurs in localized outbreaks such as in schools or military barracks [62]. Most affected patients are previously healthy, but those with HIV, immunoglobulin deficiencies, asplenia, or inherited and acquired deficiencies of terminal complement components C5–C9 are at increased risk [62,63]. *N. meningitidis* is an aerobic Gram-positive diplococcus that only infects humans. Thirteen serotypes have been identified, of which groups A, B, C, Y, and W-135 are the major pathogens. A vaccine against types A, C, Y, and W-135 is available for high-risk individuals. The bacteria inhabit the respiratory mucosa and are spread through respiratory secretions. Virulence factors allow invasion through the respiratory epithelium and into the bloodstream where they damage the endothelium directly and release lipopolysaccharide endotoxin, provoking massive release of tumor necrosis factor α, interleukins-1 and -6, and interferon-γ. These cytokines promote vascular permeability, hypotension, and eventually multiorgan failure and DIC [62,63].

Mild cases may manifest as a viral syndrome with fever, headache, nausea, vomiting, and arthralgias, whereas in fulminant cases, patients are severely ill with high fever, hypotension, and a hemorrhagic rash. Half of the cases will have meningitis with headache, stiff neck, and photophobia. Cutaneous findings are prominent in as many as 60% of patients with meningococcemia, with petechiae or purpura beginning at points of pressure on the trunk and extremities, spreading to involve any body area. Urticarial and maculopapular lesions may also be observed early in the clinical course. As meningococcemia progresses, large areas of irregular gunmetal gray hemorrhage and necrosis may develop (Fig. 70.5) because of DIC. Among 10% to 20% of children with meningococcemia, purpura fulminans (PF) in combination with multiorgan failure and adrenal hemorrhage, Waterhouse–Friderichsen syndrome, may occur [64].

The differential diagnosis of meningococcemia includes RMSF, leukocytoclastic vasculitis, TSS, erythema multiforme, and other forms of bacterial sepsis. Diagnosis is usually based on blood or cerebrospinal fluid (CSF) cultures, and in cases of meningococcal meningitis, Gram staining of CSF is up to 90% sensitive. Newer polymerase chain reaction (PCR) tests for meningococcus are available, including the IS-1106, nspA, and ctrA TaqMan tests [64,65]. Because meningococcal sepsis

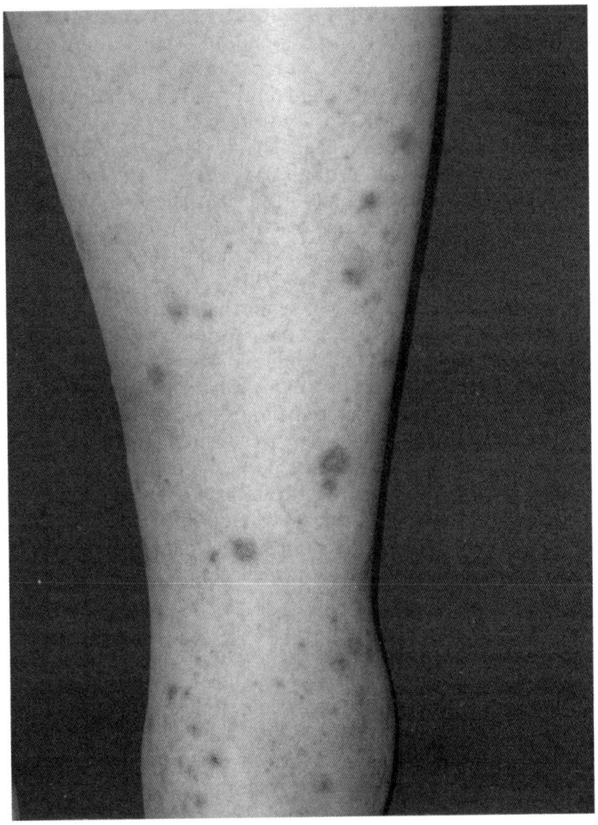

FIGURE 70.5 Meningococcemia. Purpuric papules and plaques, some of which have a dusky or gunmetal gray center.

progresses rapidly and has a case fatality rate of up to 40%, treatment should never be delayed pending diagnosis. Prompt treatment is critical. First-line empiric therapy for adults aged 18 to 50 is a broad-spectrum cephalosporin, such as ceftriaxone (2 g IV q12 hours). In adults over 50 years of age, ampicillin is given concomitantly. Once the diagnosis of meningococcemia is confirmed, patients in the United States may be switched to penicillin G (4 million units IV Q 4 hours), as penicillin-resistant strains are not prevalent [64]. Intensive supportive care with intravenous fluids, pressors, and ventilatory support is usually needed. The prognosis for untreated cases is poor, with 70% dying before antibiotics were available. The overall case fatality of meningococcal disease is now around 10%, though it remains 40% for those with sepsis. Up to 19% of survivors have severe sequelae such as deafness or limb loss [62].

Rocky Mountain Spotted Fever

RMSF is a life-threatening tick-borne febrile illness caused by the intracellular pathogen, *Rickettsia rickettsi*. Despite its name, RMSF is most commonly reported in the Southeast to Midwest states. Cases occur most often in the summer months, when tick exposures are most likely. RMSF is a rare disease, with an annual incidence of seven cases per million, most commonly seen in children. Case fatality rates range from 0.5% to 2.6%, highest on Indian reservations, in the elderly, and the very young. Untreated RMSF has a mortality of 25%, whereas patients receiving appropriate treatment within 5 days of symptom onset have a mortality of 5% [66].

R. rickettsi, a pleomorphic coccobacillary obligate intracellular parasite, is transmitted to humans by the American dog tick (*Dermacentor variabilis*) in the Eastern United States and the wood tick (*Dermacentor andersoni*) in the mountain West. *R. rickettsi* infects vascular endothelium and smooth muscle cells where it can replicate and spread to other cells, causing vascular and tissue injury. Vasculitis may occur in the gastrointestinal tract, lungs, kidneys, liver, heart, brain, and skin, leading to multiorgan failure. In addition, *R. rickettsi* promotes the coagulation cascade, leading to hypercoagulability and thrombocytopenia.

Most patients with RMSF present within 14 days of a tick bite with fever and severe headache. Rash usually occurs 2 to 5 days later. Roughly half of all patients will present with the classic triad of fever, rash, and headache. The rash of RMSF is initially blanching pink to red macules on the wrists and ankles, spreading to the palms and soles and then to the arms, legs, and trunk. The face is usually spared. Over several days, the rash becomes purpuric with areas of hemorrhage and necrosis [67]. In addition to fever and headache, patients frequently present with abdominal pain, nausea and vomiting, myalgias, and shortness of breath. Respiratory failure, myocardial edema, renal failure, liver dysfunction, and altered mental status may occur [68].

The differential diagnosis of RMSF includes other febrile illnesses with rash, such as ehrlichiosis, meningococcemia, TSS, measles, drug fever, idiopathic thrombocytopenic purpura, and various viral syndromes. In cases where no rash occurs, the differential diagnosis would include appendicitis, gastroenteritis, and other causes of acute abdomen. Several diagnostic tests are helpful; however, empiric therapy should be initiated as soon as RMSF is suspected. The indirect fluorescent antibody test for *R. rickettsi* is 94% sensitive and specific but requires 7 to 14 days to become positive. Skin biopsy shows a lymphohistiocytic vasculitis with extravasation of red blood cells and occasional fibrin thrombi. *R. rickettsi* may be identified intracellularly by Giemsa staining. Nonspecific laboratory findings include thrombocytopenia and elevated transaminases.

Treatment of RMSF is with doxycycline 100 mg twice daily (or 3 mg per kg of body weight, whichever is higher) for at least 7 days, given orally for outpatients and intravenously for hospitalized patients. Doxycycline should be used even for children (at a dose of 4.4 mg/kg/d divided into BID doses), as the risk of tooth staining has been shown to be quite low for short-term therapy. This regimen will cover other tick-borne illnesses such as Lyme disease and ehrlichiosis. Chloramphenicol (at a dose of 50 to 75 mg/kg/d divided into four doses) is an alternative choice for pregnant women and patients with documented allergy to doxycycline, but is reportedly less effective. Treatment should be continued until the patient has been afebrile for 2 to 3 days [69].

Disseminated Herpes Simplex Virus Infection

Herpes simplex virus (HSV), a member of the human herpes virus family, is a common cause of dermatologic disease. HSV-1 and HSV-2 have seroprevalence rates as high as 80% and 25% of US adults, respectively [70].

Infection is spread by close physical contact of mucous membranes or open skin with infected fluids or skin that is actively shedding virus. After initial infection, the virus remains latent in the dorsal root ganglion. Reactivation may be triggered by stress, illness, trauma (such as from intubation), intense UV exposure, and pregnancy. Grouped vesicles on an erythematous base, often with associated pain or pruritus, appear with reactivation. Rupture of vesicles leaves characteristic punched-out ulcers with scalloped edges [70,71]. Infection of immunocompetent patients is self-limited [72]. Immunocompromised patients (HIV, malignancy, medications, or pregnancy) have more frequent and more severe reactivations and there is an increased risk of disseminated cutaneous and visceral disease [72]. Reactivation of genital HSV in immunocompromised and pregnant individuals is associated with an increased risk of visceral dissemination and high mortality. Patients with disrupted skin secondary to eczema, TEN, burns and other dermatologic diseases including Grover's disease, Darier disease, and pemphigus vulgaris are at risk of disseminated cutaneous disease known as Kaposi's varicelliform eruption or eczema herpeticum [70,73]. Patients with vesicular eruptions should be examined carefully for clustered lesions or erosions suspicious of HSV. A high index of suspicion is essential. The differential diagnosis includes herpes zoster, varicella, contact dermatitis, bullous impetigo, and other causes of vesiculation of the skin. Confirmatory tests include Tzanck smear, DFA, viral culture, PCR, and ELISA. All studies are most sensitive when performed on vesicles less than 48 hours old. DFA and culture should be performed together to increase sensitivity from approximately 50% for each alone, to almost 80% [74]. PCR is the most sensitive test, but it is not always available.

Although there are no controlled studies for treatment of disseminated disease and no evidence that treatment decreases mortality, intravenous acyclovir at 8 to 10 mg per kg every 8 hours for 7 to 10 days is generally employed [71]. The dose is adjusted for patients with renal insufficiency. Alternatives for acyclovir-resistant cases include foscarnet, vidarabine, and cidofovir [72]. Secondary bacterial infection may complicate the course of HSV infection and should be treated with appropriate antibiotic therapy.

Disseminated Herpes Zoster

Varicella zoster virus (VZV) causes both chicken pox (varicella), representing a primary infection, and shingles (zoster), a manifestation of reactivated latent infection. After initial exposure, the virus remains dormant in the dorsal root ganglion] or in cranial nerve root ganglia [75]. Medications, aging, malignancy, bone marrow transplantation, organ transplantation, HIV, rheumatologic disease, and poor nutrition can affect immune status and thereby increase the risk of reactivation. Since the introduction of the herpes zoster vaccine for patients over the age of 60 who are not immunosuppressed, the incidence of VZV infection in the United States has decreased by up to 90% [76].

Upon reactivation, VZV tracks along sensory nerves to affect a particular dermatome, most commonly the ophthalmic division of the trigeminal nerve (V_1) and the thoracic dermatome. A prodrome of pain, pruritus, and paresthesia in the affected dermatome is noted by up to half of the patients. This is followed by an eruption of erythematous macules and/or papules. Over 24 hours, the lesions begin to vesiculate, and over the next 48 to 72 hours, crust over. Pain is the most common symptom, present in 90% to 95% of patients. Prior to the onset of skin lesions, involvement of the thoracic dermatome may be mistaken for acute coronary syndrome.

Immunocompromised hosts may have atypical presentations with unusual lesion morphology, distribution, greater ulceration, and dissemination. Disseminated zoster occurs among 2% of the general population and has been observed in as many as 35% of hospitalized immunocompromised patients. Disseminated zoster is seven times more frequent among patients with HIV and patients with disseminated zoster should be tested for HIV [75]. Disseminated disease presents 7 to 14 days after classical dermatomal zoster and is defined as more than 20 lesions outside the primary dermatome, in either multiple contiguous or noncontiguous dermatomes. Visceral dissemination can involve the lung, liver, and brain [77]. Cases of VZV reactivation and visceral dissemination without cutaneous lesions have been rarely reported [75,78].

Uveitis, keratitis, corneal ulcers, and blindness may result from reactivation along the ophthalmic division of the trigeminal nerve. Myelitis or encephalitis may result in weakness and altered mental status. Rarely, motor nerves may be involved with resulting weakness [75]. Patients are contagious until lesions become crusted. Transmission is via direct contact or airborne from respiratory secretions or aerosolized skin lesions. Airborne transmission is more likely among patients with disseminated disease and these patients should be under strict isolation precautions [79].

Differential diagnosis includes HSV infections, bullous drug eruption, contact dermatitis, and erythema multiforme. Tzanck smear cannot differentiate VZV from other herpesviruses and has a limited sensitivity; therefore, it should not be used to rule out disease [75]. PCR for viral DNA is the most sensitive and specific diagnostic test and can be performed on vesicular fluid, crusted lesions, blood, plasma, CSF, and bronchoalveolar lavage. PCR results take about 1 day to result. DFA testing is performed on scrapings from non-crusted vesicular lesions, has a high sensitivity (90%) and specificity (95%), and results can return in several hours where available. The sensitivity of viral culture is poor and serologic testing is not helpful in an acute setting [80]. Treatment should not be delayed pending results. Patients should be treated if they present within 1 week of onset of their lesions or if they still have any lesions that have not crusted over [77].

Oral acyclovir or valacyclovir is appropriate for healthy individuals who can take oral treatment and for uncomplicated cases of immunocompromised patients. The dosing regimen is 1 g of valacyclovir or 500 mg of famciclovir every 8 hours, or acyclovir 800 mg 5 times a day, with dose adjustment for renal insufficiency. The duration of treatment is 7 to 10 days. IV acyclovir is the treatment of choice for immunocompromised patients with ophthalmic, disseminated, or HIV-associated disease or those with significant comorbidities [75,77]. Acyclovir resistance is more prevalent among immunocompromised populations and should be suspected if new lesions are forming on acyclovir or a related drug (famciclovir, valacyclovir). Viral sensitivities should be checked in this setting. Resistant strains are treated with foscarnet, 180 mg/kg/d divided into two or three doses and renally adjusted [77]. Central nervous system (CNS), ophthalmologic, or atypical cutaneous presentations should trigger neurology, ophthalmology, and dermatology consultation [75,77]. The mortality for disseminated zoster is between 5% and 15% with most deaths attributable to pneumonia [81].

BLISTERING DISEASES

Pemphigus vulgaris, paraneoplastic pemphigus, and bullous pemphigoid (BP) are autoimmune blistering disorders characterized by autoantibodies directed at cell–cell adhesion molecules or components of the basement membrane zone.

Pemphigus Vulgaris

Pemphigus vulgaris is a rare but potentially fatal bullous disorder that affects the skin and mucous membranes. The worldwide incidence is 0.76 to 5 per million population. However, the incidence is much higher in those of Jewish ancestry [82]. Pemphigus typically affects middle-aged or older individuals. It is caused by autoantibodies against the desmosomal proteins, desmoglein 1 and 3, which are required to maintain cellular adhesion between keratinocytes in the epidermis.

The presenting sign of pemphigus is usually painful oral lesions that occur in virtually all patients. Hoarseness and dysphagia may be a sign of pharyngeal and esophageal involvement, respectively. Mucosal and laryngeal involvement can make intubation and endotracheal tube maintenance more difficult. Cutaneous lesions develop in more than half of the patients, usually after the onset of oral erosions, with fragile vesicles or bullae that rupture easily as blistering is confirmed to the epidermis. Consequently, it is more likely to encounter erosions rather than intact blisters on the skin. Blistering may be induced by rubbing intact, normal appearing skin adjacent to areas of blistering, a phenomenon known as the Nikolsky sign. Extensive loss of epidermal barrier function in pemphigus may be complicated further by secondary systemic bacterial infection and fluid loss.

For patients with only oral disease, the differential diagnosis includes oral HSV, aphthous ulcers, oral lichen planus, and SLE. With cutaneous disease, further consideration should be given to bullous impetigo, bullous drug eruptions, and other autoimmune blistering disorders. Drug-induced pemphigus has been associated with the use of various medications, in particular penicillamine and captopril [82].

Diagnosis of pemphigus is made by routine histology, which demonstrates loss of cell–cell adhesion of keratinocytes (acantholysis) and retained attachment of basal cells to the basement membrane along the dermal–epidermal junction. Immunofluorescence of perilesional tissue shows intercellular deposits of IgG. Serum sent for indirect immunofluorescence or ELISA assays will demonstrate circulating antibodies, and titers in pemphigus usually correlate with disease activity [82].

Standard treatment of pemphigus is oral prednisone at 1 to 1.5 mg/kg/d. Studies of corticosteroid-sparing agents for pemphigus, including azathioprine, mycophenolate mofetil, cyclosporine, cyclophosphamide, and IVIG, are reviewed in Table 70.2 [83–89]. Rituximab has been observed to be beneficial in refractory pemphigus and has been reported to be effective as an adjuvant to topical corticosteroid [90]. A recent randomized controlled trial showed infliximab was not effective in the treatment of pemphigus [91]. Overall, the optimal therapeutic strategy still has not been established [92]. Most patients require maintenance treatment for sustained remission. Prior to treatment with oral corticosteroids, most patients died within 5 years of disease onset. Current mortality rate is about 5% to 15%, mostly due to complications from immunosuppressive therapy such as sepsis [82].

TABLE 70.2

Summary of Recommendations Based upon Randomized Controlled Clinical Trials for Pemphigus Vulgaris

Intervention	Year	Study	No. of patients	Findings	Reference
Oral prednisolone, high-dose (120 mg/d) versus low-dose (60 mg/d) regimens	1990	Prospective, randomized trial over 5 y	22	High-dose regimen had no long-term benefit over low-dose regimen in terms of frequency of relapse or incidence of complications	[83]
Adjuvant oral dexamethasone pulse therapy (300 mg pulses 3 d/mo) versus placebo in conjunction with conventional oral prednisolone (80 mg/d) and azathioprine sodium (3 mg/d)	2006	Multicenter, randomized, placebo-controlled trial	20	No benefit of oral dexamethasone pulse therapy given in addition to conventional treatment	[84]
Comparison of four treatment regimens for pemphigus vulgaris: prednisolone alone, prednisolone plus azathioprine, prednisolone plus mycophenolate mofetil, and prednisolone plus intravenous cyclophosphamide pulse therapy	2007	Randomized, controlled open-label trial over 1 y	120 (30 patients/arm)	Efficacy of prednisolone is enhanced when combined with cytotoxic agent. Azathioprine was found to be the most efficacious cytotoxic drug to reduce steroid, followed by cyclophosphamide and mycophenolate mofetil.	[85]
Comparison of oral methylprednisolone plus azathioprine or mycophenolate mofetil	2006	Prospective, multicenter, randomized, non-blinded trial	33	Azathioprine and mycophenolate mofetil have similar efficacy, corticosteroid-sparing effects, and safety profiles as adjuvant treatments.	[86]
High-dose intravenous immunoglobulin (IVIG) over 5 consecutive days in patients relatively resistant to systemic steroids	2009	Multicenter, randomized, placebo-controlled, double-blind trial	61 (includes pemphigus foliaceus)	IVIG (400 mg/kg/d for 5 d) is safe and effective for relatively steroid-resistant patients.	[87]
Dapsone versus placebo in patients already on conventional systemic steroids	2008	Multicenter, randomized, placebo-controlled, double-blind trial	19	"Trend to efficacy" of dapsone but not statistically significant.	[88]
Cyclosporine as adjuvant to systemic corticosteroids	2000	Concurrently randomized trial	29	Cyclosporine ineffective as adjuvant to corticosteroids.	[89]

Paraneoplastic Pemphigus

Paraneoplastic pemphigus is a variant of pemphigus associated with benign or malignant neoplasms. Most commonly associated conditions include non-Hodgkin's lymphoma, chronic lymphocytic leukemia, Castleman's disease, thymoma, sarcoma, and Waldenstrom's macroglobulinemia. Autoantibodies in paraneoplastic pemphigus are directed against a variety of proteins including desmogleins 1 and 3, bullous pemphigoid antigen 230, as well as the plakin family of proteins [93]. For diagnosis, the detection of autoantibodies against envoplakin and periplakin, or α2-macroglobulin-like-1 protein by immunoprecipitation are 95% sensitive, whereas the combination of rat bladder indirect immunofluorescence and immunoblotting is 100% sensitive and specific [94].

The disease usually presents with a recalcitrant stomatitis involving the mouth and characteristically, the lips. Other mucous membranes, including the eyes, genitalia, nasopharynx, and esophagus, may be involved. Cutaneous lesions are polymorphic and may resemble pemphigus vulgaris, BP, erythema multiforme, or lichen planus. Some patients develop bronchiolitis obliterans, which may be fatal as a result of respiratory failure [93]. Two-thirds of patients diagnosed with paraneoplastic pemphigus have a known underlying neoplasm. In the other third, mucocutaneous disease precedes the diagnosis of an associated neoplasm, and these patients must be carefully followed. Severe, intractable stomatitis is a clue for differentiating paraneoplastic pemphigus from other bullous disorders. Disease associated with benign neoplasms such as thymoma or Castleman's disease may improve or clear completely with treatment of the underlying condition, but the course of disease and prognosis in malignancy-associated paraneoplastic pemphigus is poor. The stomatitis is often refractory to treatment with corticosteroids and immunosuppressants [93]. Patients with extensive skin involvement who present with erythema multiforme–like skin lesions and histologic keratinocyte necrosis often have more severe disease which can rapidly become fatal. These patients must be managed particularly carefully [95].

Bullous Pemphigoid

BP is a chronic subepidermal blistering disorder most prevalent in the elderly, with an incidence of 6 to 7 cases per million. BP often requires long-term use of immunosuppressive agents, which can lead to both morbidity and mortality. BP is characterized as an autoimmune blistering disease. The subepidermal blisters in BP result from autoantibodies directed against the hemidesmosomal proteins BP180 and BP230, located at the epidermal–dermal junction. BP is thought to be induced by an environmental stimulus in genetically predisposed individuals. Viral triggers have been postulated and BP may be induced by medications, the most common of which are penicillamine and furosemide [96].

BP has a variety of clinical manifestations, including a nonbullous prodromal phase characterized by severe pruritus, either alone or associated with excoriated eczematous or urticarial lesions. The bullous phase is characterized by tense vesicles and bullae on normal or erythematous skin. Unlike pemphigus, numerous blisters in BP are found intact. The lesions are frequently symmetrical and are most commonly found in flexural areas on the limbs, the lower trunk, and abdomen. The oral mucosa is involved in 10% to 30% of patients [97].

The differential diagnosis includes pemphigus, bullous lupus erythematosus, dermatitis herpetiformis, bullous erythema multiforme, cicatricial pemphigoid, linear IgA dermatosis, and epidermolysis bullosa acquisita. Diagnosis is made by skin biopsy from the edge of a blister, which shows a subepidermal blister with an eosinophil-rich dermal inflammatory infiltrate. Direct immunofluorescence of perilesional skin shows linear deposits of IgG and/or C3 along the basement membrane zone. Indirect immunofluorescence will detect circulating autoantibodies in 60% to 80% of patients [97].

BP has a tendency toward remission and can be controlled more easily than pemphigus. Treatment with high potency topical corticosteroids has been proven effective with fewer side effects than oral corticosteroids [98]. Other immunosuppressive agents such as azathioprine, mycophenolate mofetil, cyclophosphamide, and methotrexate may be added for recalcitrant cases or for steroid sparing in patients with long-term disease. The combination of nicotinamide and minocycline or tetracycline has been successful in small case series. Dapsone, IVIG, plasmapheresis, and extracorporeal photopheresis have been reported to be effective, and rituximab has shown promise for recalcitrant disease in multiple case series [99].

VASCULAR DISORDERS

Cutaneous Vasculitis

Vasculitis is defined by inflammation of the blood vessel wall and may involve any sized vessel. As medium vessel vasculitides (polyarteritis nodosa, Wegener's granulomatosis, Churg–Strauss syndrome) are covered in more depth in Chapter 196, the present discussion will focus on cutaneous small vessel vasculitis (CSVV) and cutaneous findings in other types of medium and large vasculitis.

CSVV may be limited to the skin, or there may be multiorgan involvement most commonly involving the kidneys, the gastrointestinal tract, and/or the joints. It is important to recognize that skin involvement may be a sign of more serious internal organ involvement. The pathogenesis involves immune complex deposition in the affected vessel walls triggering the activation of complement.

Vasculitis may be secondary to infections (15% to 20%), medications (10% to 15%), malignancy (2% to 5%), or autoimmune connective tissue disease and inflammatory disorders including inflammatory bowel disease, cryoglobulinemia (CG), Anti-neutrophil cytoplasmic antibody (ANCA)-associated vasculitis and Behçet's syndrome (15% to 20%). Henoch–Schönlein purpura (HSP) is a specific subtype of IgA-mediated vasculitis [100,101]. Commonly associated infections include streptococcal and other bacterial acute respiratory infections, bacterial endocarditis, gonococcemia, chronic meningococcemia, hepatitis B and C, HIV, cytomegalovirus (CMV), and mycobacteria. Implicated medications include antibiotics (especially β lactams, sulfonamides, and minocycline), allopurinol, thiazide diuretics, hydantoins, propylthiouracil, NSAIDs, granulocyte macrophage colony stimulating factor (GM-CSF), and anti-tumor necrosis factor (TNF) agents. Malignancies associated with vasculitis include lymphoproliferative, hematologic, and solid organ cancers. Among connective tissue diseases, SLE, rheumatoid arthritis and Sjogren's syndrome are commonly complicated by cutaneous vasculitis [101]. Levamisole-adulterated cocaine is an increasingly common cause of cutaneous vasculitis that commonly presents with purpura of the ears, retiform purpura of the trunk, neutropenia and a positive P-ANCA [102]. More recently, alcohol has been implicated as a potential cause of cutaneous vasculitis presenting with palpable purpura on the lower extremities several hours after consumption [103]. The underlying etiology may remain unidentified in up to 50% of patients [100].

The skin findings of vasculitis correlate with the size of vessels involved. The morphologic hallmark of CSVV is palpable purpura. Red to purple, non-blanching macules and papules are concentrated over dependent areas of the skin such as the ankles and lower legs (Fig. 70.6), or over pressure areas such as the buttocks. There may be significant associated edema. Other morphologies include urticarial lesions, which, unlike hives, last more than 24 hours. Patients may be asymptomatic or have burning, pruritus or pain and associated constitutional symptoms and arthralgias. Cutaneous lesions usually occur within 7 to 10 days of exposure to a drug or infectious trigger and 6 months after the onset of an underlying medical condition, though this is variable. Although most cases of CSVV affect only the skin, further consideration should be given to rule out systemic involvement. HSP is an IgA-mediated CSVV that may have associated abdominal pain, gastrointestinal (GI) bleeding, arthritis, and glomerulonephritis. The initial workup of CSVV without an obvious cause includes complete blood count (CBC), basic metabolic panel (BMP), urinalysis, liver function tests (LTFs), hepatitis studies, HIV test, antistrptolysin O (ASO), anti-nuclear antibody (ANA) and rheumatoid factor (RF) [104] and stool Hemoccult blood testing. Further evaluation, treatment, and specialist referral is guided by laboratory findings.

Histopathologic evaluation is important for diagnosis and early lesions are most revealing on biopsy. Thus, timely consultation of the dermatology service is important. Along with determining the size of vessel disease, microscopic evaluation of tissue vessels distinguishes inflammatory from noninflammatory

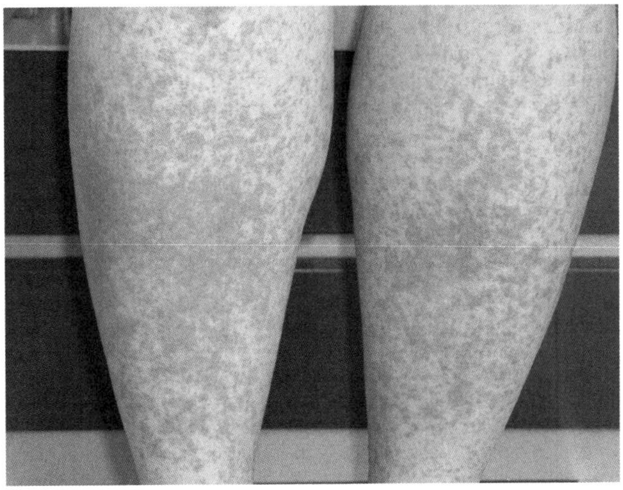

FIGURE 70.6 Vasculitis. Nonblanching, red to purple papules and plaques over the legs associated with edema.

vessel disease. Furthermore, immunofluorescence studies of sampled tissue may help confirm a diagnosis of IgA vasculitis associated with HSP. Patients with HSP need ongoing monitoring of blood pressure and renal function as delayed-onset kidney involvement can occur. It is important to consider coagulopathies and other occlusive vascular diseases in the differential diagnosis of vasculitis as the management of noninflammatory vessel disease differs from that of vasculitis. Purpura, livedo reticularis, ulcers, and necrosis are manifestations of coagulopathies such as immune thrombocytopenic purpura, thrombotic thrombocytopenic purpura, drug-induced thrombocytopenia, inherited platelet dysfunction, warfarin and heparin necrosis, DIC, gammopathies, protein C and S deficiencies, and the antiphospholipid syndrome. In bland occlusive disorders in which vessels may be occluded by fibrin, cryoglobulins, or emboli, the purpura may be palpable as in leukocytoclastic vasculitis, so the clinical distinction is not always apparent.

Treatment is directed at the underlying etiology and preventing the progression of inflammation. It is always important to evaluate and treat any underlying cause, whether it is infection, malignancy, or a drug toxicity. With early intervention, morbidity and mortality from vasculitis may be reduced. For disease limited to the skin, supportive care with rest, leg elevation, topical steroids, and analgesics is usually sufficient. The eruption typically resolves over weeks with hyperpigmentation. It is important to monitor for systemic disease, even after the cutaneous signs have resolved. NSAIDs, colchicine, dapsone, or prednisone can be helpful for patients with recalcitrant or progressive skin disease. Severe intractable skin disease or involvement of organs other than the skin may require immunosuppressive therapy with high-dose prednisone 1 to 2 mg/kg/d, sometimes with steroid-sparing support from methotrexate, cyclosporine, azathioprine, cyclophosphamide, or mycophenolate mofetil [101].

Disorders with large vessel vasculitis are usually diagnosed when bruits, asymmetric pulses, claudication, or neurologic deficits are present. Some patients also have cutaneous findings that serve as clues to underlying pathology. In giant cell arteritis (GCA), the temporal artery is tender, swollen, indurated, or pulseless. The tongue may be tender, atrophic, swollen, or cyanotic. Rarely, patients with GCA may have tender nodules overlying other superficial arteries. In less than 20% of cases of Takayasu's arteritis, erythema nodosum–like nodules or pyoderma gangrenosum–like ulcers may be present. Cutaneous findings, although present in 80% of patients, are nonspecific in Kawasaki's disease, a syndrome associated with coronary artery aneurysms in 12% of affected children. The eruption of Kawasaki's disease is polymorphous, and patients may present with macules, papules, wheals, targetoid plaques, papulovesicles, pustules, or a scarlatiniform eruption most commonly on the abdomen, groin, perineum, and buttocks. There is often desquamation of the fingertips and mucous membrane involvement may include conjunctival injection, dryness of the lips, erythema of the mouth, and prominent tongue papillae (strawberry tongue). Most patients have enlarged cervical lymph nodes and high fever.

Purpura Fulminans

PF is characterized by extensive purpura and necrosis of the skin associated with fever, DIC, sepsis, and hypotension. PF is seen mostly in three clinical settings: acute infections, inherited or acquired coagulopathies, and idiopathic. Meningococcemia, in which 3% of cases develop PF, is the most commonly associated infection. Varicella and pneumococcal sepsis are less frequently associated and rare or isolated reports include *H. influenzae* [105] and other organisms. Asplenism is a risk factor for infection associated with PF. PF in the newborn period is usually due to an inherited coagulopathy and results in high mortality. PF has also been reported in association with acquired coagulopathies seen in inflammatory bowel disease [106,107]. Idiopathic disease is the mildest variant [108–110].

The pathophysiology of PF depends on the underlying trigger. The common end point is that of extensive microvascular thrombosis that affects cutaneous and visceral blood supply. In meningococcemia, endotoxin results in release of cytokines and activation of coagulation pathways, and infection is associated with substantially decreased levels of protein C [108].

Initially in PF, there is pain and erythema of affected areas. Irregular areas of blue–black or dusky discoloration develop within the center of erythematous patches, and lesional skin becomes indurated. There is progression to hemorrhagic vesicles and bullae, and finally to tissue necrosis. Lesions associated with infection tend to involve distal parts first and spread proximally, whereas idiopathic and coagulopathy-associated disease may remain localized to the lower extremities. Idiopathic PF usually affects only the skin; however, other forms may result in widespread necrosis with multiorgan failure. Disease complications include scarring, secondary infections, digital or limb necrosis, and autoamputation [108–110].

The differential diagnosis of PF includes HSP and postinfectious thrombocytopenic purpura, although these are both associated with milder disease than that seen in PF. The presence of DIC helps distinguish PF from other causes of cutaneous necrosis [109].

Early recognition of disease and identification of the underlying trigger is essential in this rapidly progressive condition. Appropriate antimicrobials are instituted for infection. Supportive care includes aggressive fluid resuscitation, electrolyte monitoring, and replacement of blood products. If deficient, protein C and antithrombin III may be replaced. Other treatment options include FFP, heparin, plasmapheresis, topical nitroglycerin (for local vasodilation), and recombinant tissue plasminogen activator [109]. Surgical consultation may be necessary for debridement and grafting.

Antiphospholipid Antibody Syndrome

Antiphospholipid antibody syndrome (APS) is characterized by a hypercoagulable state with venous or arterial thrombosis, recurrent fetal loss, thrombocytopenia, and elevated titers of the antiphospholipid antibodies (anticardiolipin antibodies, lupus anticoagulant, anti-β-2 glycoprotein I antibodies). Up to 2% of the normal population exhibits detectable titers of these antibodies and 0.2% have elevated titers. APS may be primary, or it may be seen in conjunction with SLE, malignancy, drug toxicity, infection, or hematologic disease [111–113].

Cutaneous manifestations in APS, although highly variable, are common and often the presenting sign of disease. Recognition of these findings is therefore essential for early diagnosis and prompt evaluation for more extensive disease. Skin lesions are thought to be a direct result of arterial or venous occlusion and subsequent ischemia. The most common finding is livedo reticularis or livedo racemosa, seen in up to 40% of patients, and up to 70% of patients who have systemic lupus. These present as a netlike pattern of dusky erythema often found on the upper or lower extremities; they are thought to be more common in cases with underlying arterial disease and are less often seen in venoocclusive disease [114]. Other associated findings include cyanotic macules, ecchymosis and purpura, ulcerations of the ears, face, and legs, porcelain-white scars (atrophie blanche) at the ankles, thrombophlebitis, Raynaud's phenomenon, digital ischemia, and gangrene. Any major organ system can be affected by thrombosis [111–113]. A highly morbid variant, catastrophic APS, is characterized by thrombosis of multiple organs developing over a short period of time. Standard therapy is IVIG or plasma exchange, anticoagulation, and corticosteroids (see Chapter 68 for a more detailed discussion) [115].

The differential diagnosis of APS includes other disorders with associated livedo reticularis and cutaneous necrosis including vasculitis, warfarin-induced skin necrosis (WISN), cholesterol emboli, and CG. Similar to other vasoocclusive disorders, APS shows bland thrombosis of small dermal vessels. APS is distinguished from other noninflammatory vasoocclusive disorders by the presence of elevated antiphospholipid antibody titers [111,113]. Although cutaneous findings are common, they are not among the diagnostic criteria for APS, which require positive antibodies on two occasions at least 6 weeks apart in addition to a history of vascular thrombosis or pregnancy complications [116].

Both treatment and prophylaxis consist of anticoagulation. Some advocate the use of aspirin in those without a history of thrombosis or with superficial venous thrombosis only. Otherwise, long-term warfarin anticoagulation with an internal normalized ratio goal of 3 to 4 is recommended. Immunosuppressive agents and immunotherapy (plasmapheresis, IVIG, cyclophosphamide) may help reduce antibody levels, but these are likely to rebound once treatment is discontinued [111,113]. Rituximab has been shown to be effective for decreasing cutaneous ulcerations and thrombocytopenia; however, it has not been shown to decrease thrombotic events [117].

Warfarin-Induced Skin Necrosis

WISN is seen in 0.01% to 0.1% of individuals on warfarin, 3 to 10 days after starting therapy. Women are affected four times more frequently than men, and are most often middle-aged and obese. Three quarters of patients with WISN are being treated for deep venous thrombosis or pulmonary embolism. Atrial fibrillation, valve replacement, and arterial occlusion are disorders in which anticoagulation with warfarin less commonly results in WISN [118].

Although the pathophysiology of WISN is not understood completely, the generally accepted mechanism involves the imbalance between intrinsic procoagulant and anticoagulant factors created early on during warfarin therapy. Because of their short half-lives, anticoagulant protein C and factor VII are depleted before procoagulant factors II, IX, and X, and this results in an initial hypercoagulability that is thought to trigger onset of WISN [118]. Most individuals on warfarin do not experience this complication, and therefore additional risk factors are likely required to induce necrosis. Protein C and S deficiency, activated protein C resistance, factor V Leiden, antithrombin III deficiency, or prothrombin gene mutations, and heparin-induced thrombocytopenia may be contributory. Protein C deficiency, either inherited or acquired, is a significant risk factor [118], and has been implicated in more than 50% of cases of WISN. High loading doses of warfarin and inadequate overlap with heparin therapy are also thought to increase risk of early WISN. There are rare reports of cases occurring up to years after the onset of warfarin therapy, and delayed-onset WISN may be related to poor compliance with warfarin, courses of interacting medications, or changing liver synthetic function [118].

Initially, patients experience pressure or pain in the involved area of skin. Poorly demarcated, indurated erythema develops asymmetrically over fatty areas such as the breast, buttock, thighs, and lower abdomen. Induration progresses over 24 to 72 hours to edema with a *peau d'orange* surface, blue–black discoloration, and hemorrhagic bullae. Localized or widespread full thickness skin necrosis ensues. Histology of involved skin shows noninflammatory thrombosis and fibrin deposition in small dermal vessels with necrosis of the dermis and subcutaneous fat [118]. Differential diagnosis of WISN includes NF, APS, DIC or PF, calciphylaxis, gangrene, embolic disease, cellulitis, and pyoderma gangrenosum. Recent initiation of warfarin should raise suspicion of WISN.

Treatment is discontinuation of warfarin, administration of FFP and vitamin K to reverse its effects, and anticoagulation with heparin. Small lesions may be treated conservatively. Extensive involvement may necessitate debridement, grafting, and in extreme cases, amputation. Deep tissue necrosis, secondary infection, and multiorgan failure are more likely with more widespread disease. Even with treatment, the mortality rate is 15% within 3 months of onset. Prior episodes of WISN are not predictive of future occurrences. In most patients with WISN, future warfarin therapy may be reinstituted with caution, avoiding loading doses and overlapping with heparin initially [118].

Cryoglobulinemia

CG is characterized by precipitation of immunoglobulins from serum in cold temperatures. There are three subtypes. Type I CG constitutes 5% to 25% of cases and presents with monoclonal immunoglobulinemia associated with underlying B-cell lymphoproliferative disorders such as multiple myeloma or Waldenstrom's macroglobulinemia. Types II and III CG are mixed CGs most often associated with connective tissue disorders, lymphoproliferative disorders, and chronic viral infections. Type I disease is notable for more frequent and severe attacks related to hyperviscosity, and may manifest on the skin as livedo reticularis or Raynaud's phenomenon. Vascular occlusion rather than immune complex deposition predominates, as these cryoglobulins have a decreased ability to activate the complement cascade. Further cutaneous consequences include digital ischemia and purpura [119].

The mixed CGs are seen in association with infectious and inflammatory diseases. These underlying conditions are thought to trigger B-cell hyperactivation, which promotes production of cryoglobulins. Meltzer's triad of palpable purpura, arthralgia, and myalgia may be apparent in 25% to 30% of patients. Other findings include fatigue, neuropathy (70% to 80%), and cutaneous vasculitis. Organ systems other than the skin may be involved as well. The kidneys may be affected in any of the three forms. Bone marrow may be involved in Type I disease, whereas the peripheral nervous system may be affected in Types II and III.

Diagnosis is based on clinical signs and symptoms and elevated serum cryoglobulin levels. Blood samples should be collected in prewarmed vials and maintained at 37°C to prevent precipitation of cryoglobulins. Although involved skin characteristically shows noninflammatory occlusion of dermal vessels by immunoglobulin precipitates, leukocytoclastic vasculitis may be apparent in up to 50% of cases.

Treatment of mild disease is supportive and otherwise focused on any underlying disease process. For more severe disease, options include immunosuppressive agents, plasmapheresis, rituximab plus systemic corticosteroids, and radiation or chemotherapy to treat the associated hematologic malignancy.

CG itself does not typically worsen clinical outcomes of associated conditions. Morbidity and mortality are attributed to associated diseases, and death often results from cardiac disease or infection [120].

Embolic Diseases

Embolization of cholesterol or atheromatous material, fat, or tumor may result in striking systemic and cutaneous findings. Cholesterol embolization is typically a result of interventional vascular procedures such as left heart catheterization or angiograms, and can also be associated with cardiac surgery, thrombolysis, and aortic dissection. Less frequently, patients with severe and extensive atherosclerotic disease may experience spontaneous embolization, or emboli triggered by coughing or straining. Showers of cholesterol and atherosclerotic material travel distally and lodge in small arteries of the CNS, lungs, GI tract, kidneys,

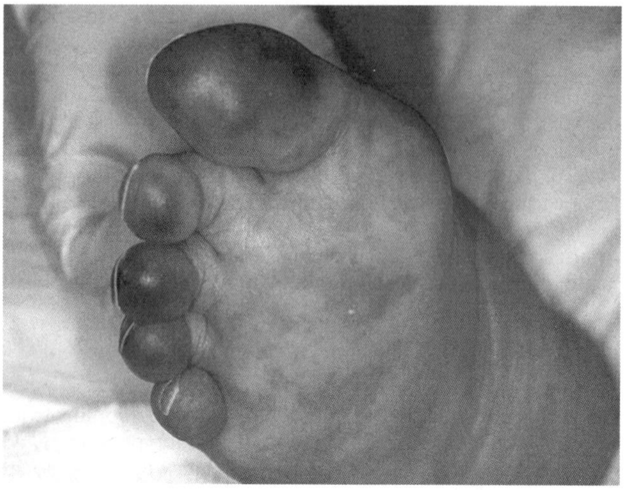

FIGURE 70.7 Cholesterol emboli. Purpuric plaques involving the toes represent areas of necrosis. Note the livedoid (reticulated) pattern on the sole of the foot, an earlier sign of vascular occlusion.

and skin. Presenting signs and symptoms of embolic disease include mental status changes, pulmonary edema, heme-positive stools, and acute renal failure. Cutaneous findings are striking when apparent and include livedo reticularis, a coarse netlike pattern of violaceous erythema evident on the lower extremities and abdomen (Fig. 70.7). The erythema may be more prominent when the patient is standing compared to the supine position. Tender blue discoloration, petechiae, ecchymosis, ulceration, and gangrene of the feet and toes may eventuate. Pedal pulses are generally intact but bruits may be audible over the femoral artery and abdominal aorta. Calf tenderness is variable. Similar findings on the arm and hands may result from aortic embolization to the upper extremities [121–123].

Fat embolization, seen most commonly after fractures of the long bones or following surgical procedures, is a less common source of embolic disease that presents with the classic triad of pulmonary, neurologic, and cutaneous symptoms. It has rarely been reported following liposuction. Petechiae distributed on the upper body (head, neck, chest, and subconjunctiva) are thought to be pathognomonic and are seen about 50% of the time [124]. Emboli from atrial myxoma, a benign cardiac hamartoma, may result in cyanosis, ecchymosis, splinter hemorrhages, and tender violaceous lesions of the digits [125]. There is no specific laboratory test to confirm cholesterol embolization. Biopsy of the area in question is the only means to confirm the diagnosis [126].

The diagnosis of emboli should be highly suspected in any patient with characteristic skin findings, acute onset end-organ failure, and a recent invasive vascular procedure. Biopsy of the affected organ will show occlusion of vessels with needle-shaped clefts representing cholesterol crystals. Skin is the most accessible and easiest tissue to sample. Atrial myxoma is evident on echocardiogram, and sampling of affected skin will demonstrate the embolized myxomatous material. Laboratory parameters such as blood urea nitrogen, creatinine, CBC and erythrocyte sedimentation rate, presence of hematuria, and heme-positive stools will be reflective of the organs involved. Treatments include surgical removal or bypass of emboli, amputation of gangrenous digits, and anticoagulation if disease is not thrombolytic-induced [122,125].

Calciphylaxis

Calciphylaxis, or calcific uremic arteriolopathy, is a rare but serious disorder involving calcification of cutaneous arteries and resultant tissue necrosis, usually in the setting of end-stage renal disease (ESRD) and dialysis. Other risk factors include hyperparathyroidism, obesity, white race, female sex, liver disease, malignancy, hypercoagulability, and use of corticosteroids or vitamin D [127]. An elevated calcium phosphate product is not a prerequisite for calciphylaxis, nor is there a correlation between the degree of elevation of calcium, phosphate, or parathyroid hormone levels and the likelihood of developing calciphylaxis. Among patients with ESRD, 1% to 4% develop this disorder.

Calciphylaxis presents with intensely painful indurated erythematous papules, plaques and subcutaneous nodules that may develop a livedoid pattern. Purpura and skin necrosis may evolve within the background of livedo reticularis. A distal, proximal, or mixed distribution may occur, with distal lesions on the lower legs being most common. Proximal presentations involve the upper thighs, buttocks, and lower abdomen, and are associated with a worse prognosis [128,129]. Lesions may even occur on the digits. The differential diagnosis of calciphylaxis includes vasculitis, warfarin necrosis, atheroemboli, CG, APS, protein C or S deficiency, polyarteritis nodosa, and DIC. A deep incisional skin biopsy is usually diagnostic. Calcification is seen primarily in the medial layer of arterioles in the subcutaneous fat, associated with endovascular fibrosis, thrombosis, and necrosis of the subcutaneous fat and overlying skin. Vasculitis is not seen. Laboratory studies addressing causes of hypercoagulability can be helpful as can plain radiographs or technetium 99 bone scans showing vascular calcification.

Treatment of calciphylaxis is controversial and no controlled studies have been performed. Treatment should be multidisciplinary with involvement of nephrology, dermatology, wound care, pain control, and nutrition. Most sources recommend normalization of calcium and phosphorus levels using diet, binding agents, low-calcium dialysis, and cinacalcet or parathyroidectomy if hyperparathyroidism is present [130]. Good wound care and pain control are important. Precipitating factors such as intravenous infusions, oral calcium supplements, or corticosteroids should be avoided or discontinued. Recent studies show that treatment with IV sodium thiosulfate may improve calciphylaxis outcomes [131]. IV sodium thiosulfate has been effective in cases of both uremic and nonuremic calciphylaxis. Intralesional sodium thiosulfate can aid in the resolution of cutaneous lesions [130,132]. Although the mortality of calciphylaxis is still high at 60% to 80%, it may be changing with more successful therapies [133].

CONNECTIVE TISSUE DISORDERS

Systemic Lupus Erythematosus

Lupus erythematosus may involve the skin in many forms. Patients with the acute form of cutaneous lupus erythematosus are most likely to have systemic disease, which may be encountered in an ICU setting. Approximately 80% of patients with SLE have cutaneous manifestations that, although they appear in a multitude of ways, are helpful for identifying affected patients. In fact, 4 of the 11 American Rheumatism Association criteria for diagnosing SLE are cutaneous findings (malar rash, photosensitivity, discoid rash, and oral ulceration). The most characteristic eruption is transient facial erythema involving the malar area and the bridge of the nose that follows sun exposure (Fig. 70.8). The redness, which may be accompanied by edema, lasts between hours and several weeks before resolving without scarring. This "butterfly" rash may be an indicator of internal disease as it may be associated with anti-dsDNA antibody and lupus nephritis [134]. Classically, there is sparing of the nasolabial folds.

Erythema and poikiloderma (hyperpigmentation, hypopigmentation, telangiectasia, and atrophy) also occur over other sun-exposed surfaces such as the V neck area of the chest and the back. On the hands, erythema characteristically spares the

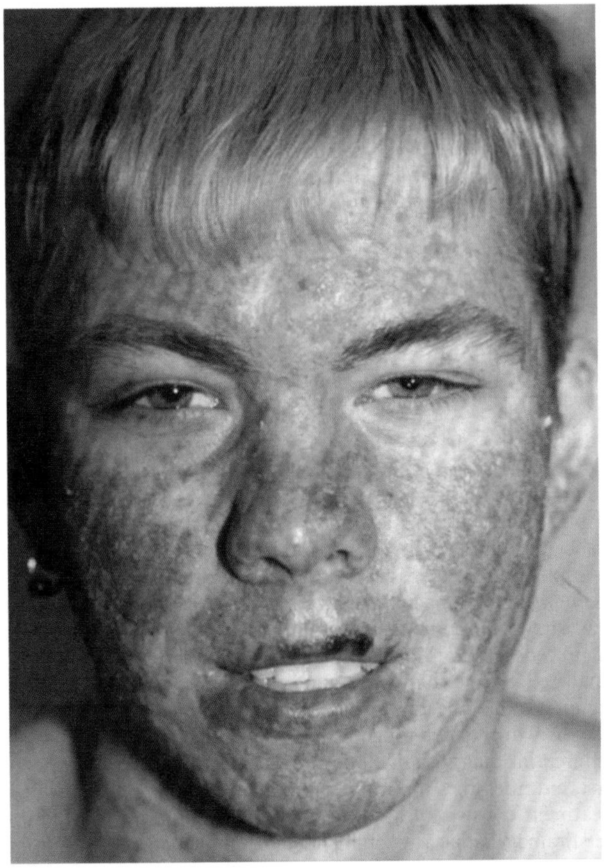

FIGURE 70.8 Cutaneous lupus erythematosus. Marked erythema and telangiectasia involving the malar and other areas of the face.

knuckles. Tense bullae, also triggered or worsened by sun exposure, may appear in a similar distribution. Mucous membrane lesions occur in 20% to 30% of patients with SLE. Petechiae or shallow ulcerations may be noted on the hard palate and may accompany malar erythema. Gingival, nasal, and vaginal ulcerations may also be seen.

Scalp hair shedding occurs diffusely and is not associated with scarring. Fragile hairs on the periphery of the scalp break and appear short. Hair shedding may also result from telogen effluvium associated with chronic illness. Patients with SLE are also more likely to have alopecia areata [134], which typically manifests as oval patches of scalp alopecia.

Vascular lesions, although not specific to SLE, occur in 50% of patients and are highly suggestive of connective tissue disease. The presence of Raynaud's phenomenon, periungual telangiectasias, purplish plaques over the tips of fingers and toes with cold exposure, and persistent erythema over the palms, soles, elbows, knees, or buttocks should prompt a search for systemic disease. Vasculitis involving postcapillary venules in the skin manifests as palpable purpura or hemorrhagic wheals. Nodules that ulcerate along the course of arteries reflect deeper, larger vessel involvement. Vascular thrombosis as a consequence of an associated APS causes punched-out ulcers that typically appear over malleolar and pretibial surfaces. The presence of livedo reticularis, thrombosis, and cutaneous infarction also warrants consideration of a prothrombotic state.

Less common cutaneous findings in SLE include a symmetric eruption of erythematous papules on the extremities, which demonstrate palisaded granulomatous inflammation with or without vasculitis on light microscopy. Calcinosis cutis, rarely present in SLE, presents as reddish or violaceous firm plaques or nodules on the head, trunk, or extremities.

Other connective tissue diseases should be considered in the differential diagnosis of the acute lupus syndrome. Eruptions of lupus localized to the head and neck may be difficult to differentiate from rosacea, dermatomyositis, drug-induced photosensitivity, and sunburn. Drug eruptions or exanthems appear similar when lupus manifests diffusely on the skin.

Strict sun protection along with topical corticosteroids and calcineurin inhibitors are the mainstay of treatment for cutaneous lupus. Antimalarial agents with or without corticosteroids or steroid-sparing immunosuppressants may be required for systemic or severe skin disease [135].

Dermatomyositis

Dermatomyositis is a rare disease characterized by a proximal muscle myositis with skin changes. It has a bimodal age distribution and is more common in female and black patients. Initial cutaneous manifestations include swelling of the face and eyelids with a characteristic violaceous erythema (heliotrope rash). These changes become more widespread with erythema and telangiectasia spreading to the neck, sun-exposed area of the chest and back in a shawl distribution, as well as to the scalp, elbows, and knees. These eruptions are usually photosensitive, and pruritus or burning is a common complaint. Gottron's sign, which consists of scaly reddish papules over the knuckle, is considered pathognomonic of dermatomyositis. Hands may take on the appearance of mechanics' hands with hyperpigmentation, scaling, fissuring of the fingertips, ragged cuticles, and enlarged proximal nail fold capillaries. Intermittent malaise, anorexia, weight loss, and arthralgias are commonly associated symptoms. Cutaneous disease usually precedes myositis by months. Dermatomyositis may be drug-induced, with hydroxyurea being the most common culprit [136].

Aggressive treatment at an early stage allows for better disease control with lower immunosuppression. Early treatment also reduces the development of disfiguring calcium deposition in the skin and muscle. Initial treatment of skin disease includes sunscreens with topical corticosteroids or calcineurin inhibitors, but resistant skin disease may require methotrexate or antimalarials. With evident myositis, therapy requires the use of prednisone (0.5 to 1.5 mg/kg/d tapered slowly over 1 to 2 years) and the addition of a steroid-sparing immunosuppressive such as azathioprine or methotrexate. It is important to also consider the coexistence of other connective tissue diseases such as scleroderma, SLE, and rheumatoid arthritis in a patient with dermatomyositis. With appropriate and timely therapy, patients may become disease-free and off therapy within 2 to 4 years. Of note, patients should be surveyed for an occult visceral malignancy which is associated with dermatomyositis in up to 25% of adult cases. Poor prognostic factors include malignancy, older age, initiating therapy after 24 months of muscle weakness, extensive cutaneous lesions, dysphagia, and cardiac or pulmonary disease [137]. The Cutaneous Dermatomyositis Disease and Severity Index (CDASI) was developed to give an objective basis for disease severity and to judge clinical response to treatment [138]. A discussion of myositis and systemic disease associated with dermatomyositis is detailed in Chapter 66.

DERMATOLOGIC ISSUES RELATED TO BONE MARROW TRANSPLANTATION

Graft-Versus-Host Disease

GVHD continues to be a major cause of morbidity and mortality and the major cause of late non-relapse death in hematopoietic cell transplant recipients [139]. Although it is typically a complication of bone marrow and hematopoietic stem cell transplantations, GVHD may also occur in the setting of unirradiated blood product infusion and solid organ transplantation containing lymphoid tissue [140]. Risk factors for GVHD include unrelated donor, HLA mismatch, older age of recipient, female donor with a male recipient, and suboptimal dosing of immunosuppressive drugs. Patients who develop GVHD appear to be at a reduced risk of recurrence of their malignancy, probably due to graft-versus-leukemia or graft-versus-malignancy reactions. GVHD can occur when immunologically competent donor T cells are transferred to a host that is incapable of rejecting them. The pathogenesis is incompletely understood, but the current model suggests a three-phase process. First, recipient tissue damage from conditioning regimens leads to inflammatory cytokines, this activates donor lymphocytes, and finally, alloreactive T cells expand into cytotoxic T cells [139].

GVHD can be divided into acute and chronic forms, with the acute form developing within the first 100 days after transplantation and the chronic form developing after about day 100. Acute GVHD can further classified into classic acute and persistent, recurrent or late acute where an acute presentation develops after day 100. Similarly, chronic GVHD can be classified as classic or overlap, the latter has features of both acute and chronic GVHD [139]. Hyperacute GVHD occurs within 14 days of transplantation [141].

Acute GVHD

The incidence of acute GVHD varies between 20% and 70%, and this range is lower with HLA-matched siblings. Acute GVHD is classified into four grades based on the extent of skin involvement, serum bilirubin level, and the volume of diarrhea per 24-hour period. Skin findings begin with painful or pruritic erythematous macules which can arise on the palms, soles, and ears, and evolve into a diffuse morbilliform eruption which is often folliculocentric. In severe cases, there may be progression with bullae formation, erythroderma, and skin necrosis. There have been rare reports of acquired ichthyosis as a manifestation of acute GVHD [142]. The differential diagnosis of acute GVHD includes drug eruptions, viral exanthems, and the eruption of lymphocyte recovery. To further complicate the picture, viral reactivation is a common complication of acute GVHD. Common viruses include HHV6, VZV, parvovirus B19, CMV and Epstein–Barr virus, and specific virus may be more likely to reactivate at different times posttransplantation [143]. Mucous membrane lesions may be difficult to distinguish from mucositis caused by chemotherapy. Histopathology of involved skin classically shows an interface dermatitis and apoptotic keratinocytes. However, the utility of a skin biopsy for diagnosing GVHD is controversial. In a small case series, the presence of eosinophils in biopsy specimens was not a reliable marker favoring drug hypersensitivity reaction over GVHD [144]. In three bone marrow transplant recipients with acute skin eruptions, biopsy led to an initial diagnosis of drug eruption, and immunosuppressive therapy was delayed until additional features of GVHD appeared, resulting in considerable morbidity and two deaths. If there is strong clinical suspicion of GVHD, biopsy findings should not delay or preclude treatment.

Chronic GVHD

Chronic GVHD is observed in 33% of HLA-identical sibling transplantations, in 49% of HLA-identical related transplantations, and in 64% of matched unrelated donor transplantations [140]. The model for the pathophysiology of chronic GVHD is autoimmune, and patients with chronic GVHD have a high incidence of antibodies. Lichenoid and sclerodermoid GVHD are the two major forms chronic cutaneous GVHD; however, increasingly variable cutaneous presentations have been reported [139].

The lichenoid variant is characterized by erythematous and violaceous papules and plaques, often distributed on flexural surfaces that resemble lichen planus. The sclerodermoid form presents with sclerotic, indurated white to yellow plaques that involve the dermis. The process may extend to fascia and result in significant tightening of skin and joint contractures. Chronic GVHD most commonly affects the skin but can also affect the oral mucosa, liver, eye, gastrointestinal tract, lungs, esophagus, genitalia, and joints. The oral mucosa is often involved and may demonstrate redness and atrophy of mucosal surfaces, lacy white reticulations of buccal mucosa, and ulcerations. Xerostomia is frequently present as well.

COMMON DERMATOLOGIC CONDITIONS COEXISTING IN ICU PATIENTS

Abscess

A cutaneous abscess is a painful, fluctuant, walled-off collection of pus found within the skin. A furuncle represents an abscess associated with a hair follicle and a carbuncle is a collection of multiple furuncles. Abscesses and furuncles are typically caused by *S. aureus*, though bacteria can vary by anatomic location. Patients may carry *S. aureus* in their nares or have staphylococcal folliculitis as preceding conditions. The clinical presentation consists of a small red papule that evolves into a tender, erythematous deep-seated nodule that may become fluctuant. The surrounding area may be warm to the touch if there is an associated cellulitis. The differential diagnosis includes an inflamed epidermal inclusion cyst, hidradenitis suppurativa, and arthropod bite. Conservative treatment consists of application of warm compresses. Incision and drainage alone is recommended for smaller abscesses (<5 cm), whereas addition of antibiotics with empiric MRSA coverage is recommended for recurrent abscesses or in patients with positive systemic inflammatory response syndrome (SIRS) criteria [46,145]. Performing a culture is recommended to help guide antibiotic choice.

Folliculitis

Folliculitis is a common disorder characterized by inflammation of hair follicles. Infectious folliculitis is usually caused by staphylococci, *Pseudomonas*, or *Malassezia furfur*, whereas noninfectious folliculitis is the result of trauma to or occlusion of the pilosebaceous unit. Herpes virus and dermatophytes are less commonly implicated. Folliculitis presents as papules or pustules on an erythematous base with a centrally extruding hair. The lesions may be pruritic and are most often found on the face, scalp, thighs, axillae, and inguinal area. Pseudomonal folliculitis may be more inflammatory and localized to a distribution that would be covered by a bathing suit. Pityrosporum folliculitis may be localized to the upper back and chest and be extremely pruritic [146]. Diagnostic tools include a potassium hydroxide (KOH) preparation, Gram stain, and bacterial, fungal, and viral cultures. Treatment is directed at the underlying etiology. Most cases will respond to appropriate topical and/or oral antibiotics (most commonly anti-staphylococcal). Pityrosporum folliculitis requires topical or oral antifungals and pseudomonal folliculitis is often self-limited, but may require fluoroquinolones in immunosuppressed patients. The prognosis is generally good, but some patients experience recurrent disease [147].

Peripheral Edema

Peripheral edema, which is commonly seen among elderly and hospitalized patients, occurs when capillary hydrostatic pressure and filtration exceeds the lymphatic drainage rate. Common causes of edema include heart failure, renal failure, nephrotic syndrome, cirrhosis, venous thrombosis, or medications, particularly calcium channel blockers. Acute exacerbations of chronic edema may cause edema blisters which present as asymptomatic, noninflammatory tense vesicles and bullae with clear fluid, usually on the distal lower extremities. Edema blisters can be distinguished from other blistering disorders by clinical history and physical examination. If needed, a biopsy for routine histopathology and immunofluorescence may help exclude other blistering disorders. Acute peripheral edema may also produce local dermal edema, leading to induration of the skin and dimpling, known as peau d'orange.

Stasis Dermatitis

Stasis dermatitis occurs in the setting of venous hypertension due to valvular incompetence. Risk factors include conditions that exacerbate lower extremity edema such as obesity, congestive heart failure, cirrhotic liver disease, and chronic renal insufficiency. Typically, there is reddish mottling and a yellowish or brown discoloration of the medial lower legs, corresponding to the location of major communicating veins. There may be an eczematous component as well that often results from contact sensitization to topical medicaments applied to the legs. There are often other signs of venous hypertension, including edema, varicose veins, and venous leg ulcers. Over years, the legs may develop lipodermatosclerosis, which occurs when adipose tissue becomes indurated and adherent to fascia, and lower legs take on the appearance of an inverted wine bottle. The diagnosis is evident in the right clinical context. However, asteatotic eczema, contact dermatitis, and cellulitis may also be considered in the differential. Of note, bilateral cellulitis of the legs is extremely rare and is often confused with stasis dermatitis. Careful clinical evaluation can lead to the correct diagnosis [148].

Relief of itching is attained through the regular application of emollients and the use of class IV or V topical steroids. Long-term management involves improving venous return through various measures such as leg elevation, elastic compression, and exercises to strengthen calf muscles. Care should be taken to avoid trauma to the leg that would facilitate ulcer formation. In severe cases, ligation of incompetent communicating veins may be necessary. Secondary infection is not uncommon as the barrier function of the skin is lost with chronic stasis dermatitis. The presence of bacteria must be recognized as a secondary event to the stasis, and treatment with antibiotics in conjunction with topical steroids is routine.

Pressure Ulcers

Pressure ulcers are areas of ischemic soft tissue necrosis resulting from prolonged pressure, shearing force, or friction anywhere on the body. Sites that are most frequently involved include skin overlying bony prominences of the sacrum, ischial tuberosities, heels, greater trochanters, and lateral malleoli.

Nonblanching erythema of skin overlying a bony prominence may signify impending ulceration. Other early indicators include warmth, edema, or induration of skin. Initial ulcers appear punched out. Ulceration may occur as partial thickness skin loss, full thickness skin loss involving subcutaneous tissue, or full thickness skin loss extending to muscle, tendon, or bone. Associated pain may be severe and should be managed aggressively. Treatment involves relief of pressure, which may be accomplished through frequent position changes and supportive surfaces such as air, liquid, or foam cushions. Local wound care includes cleansing with normal saline, debridement, and occlusive hydrocolloid dressings or foam dressings to optimize healing [149]. Nutritional supplementation should be considered for malnourished patients. A recent randomized control trial showed improved pressure ulcer healing in malnourished patients given a nutritional formula enriched with arginine, zinc, and antioxidants [150]. The majority of pressure ulcers are superficial and heal by secondary intention, but operative repair is necessary for some cases. Electrical stimulation can be used as an adjunctive therapy [149]. Wounds should be monitored for local infection and treated accordingly. Sepsis and osteomyelitis may further complicate ulceration and lead to mortality.

Psoriasis

In its most common form (chronic plaque psoriasis), psoriasis presents as chronic well-demarcated erythematous plaques with adherent silvery scale, most commonly over the elbows, knees, and scalp. In guttate (raindrop-like) psoriasis, there are smaller psoriatic papules and plaques diffusely over the body, and this is often triggered by streptococcal infections. Sudden onset of sterile pustules that coalesce to form "lakes of pus" at the edges of psoriatic plaques associated with fever typifies the more generalized form of pustular psoriasis (Fig. 70.9).Pustular psoriasis is not infectious in etiology. Hypocalcemia and pregnancy may be triggering factors in pustular psoriasis. In erythrodermic psoriasis, there is bright red erythema involving ≥90% of the skin. These patients are itchy and also complain of chills from the extensive heat loss due to dilatation of cutaneous vessels. In both pustular and erythrodermic forms, patients are generally toxic and may have associated ARDS, congestive heart failure, pneumonia, or viral hepatitis (see "Exfoliative Erythroderma" section). There is a recognized association of psoriasis, particularly severe disease, with increased risk of cardiovascular, cerebrovascular, and peripheral vascular disease [151,152].

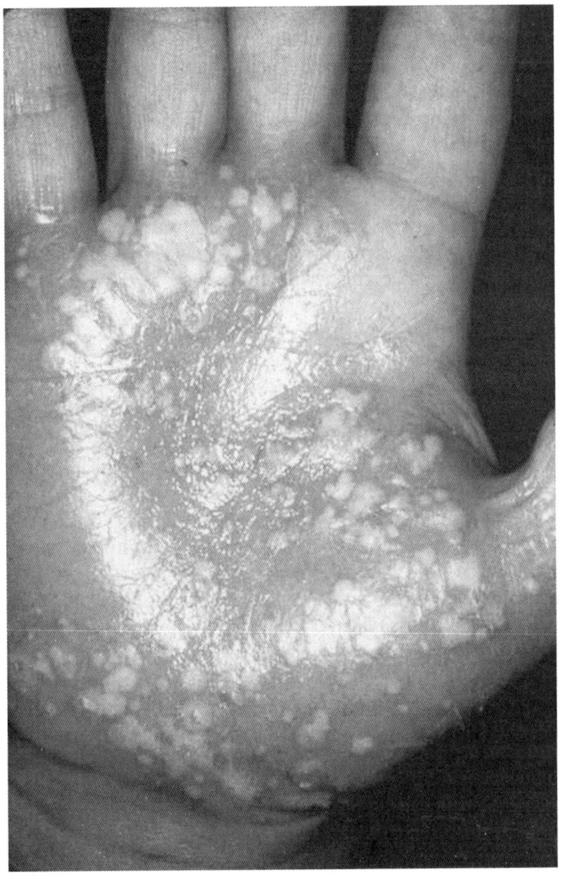

FIGURE 70.9 Pustular psoriasis. Large pustules coalescing to form "lakes of pus" over an area of well-demarcated erythema of the palm.

First-line treatment of mild cases is with topical corticosteroids and the vitamin D derivative, calcipotriene, whereas more severe cases require ultraviolet phototherapy, methotrexate, systemic retinoids, or biologic agents. For erythrodermic psoriasis, cyclosporine and infliximab appear to be the fastest acting agents; however, their use is predicated on severity of presentation and patient comorbidities [153].

Atopic Dermatitis

Atopic dermatitis is characterized by eczematous skin changes and typically involves flexor surfaces in adults, although any body area may be involved. The disease is most common among young children in whom the tendency for atopic dermatitis is to gradually improve with age; however, in a minority of patients, disease persists into or manifests in adulthood. Affected individuals frequently have a personal or family history of seasonal allergies and asthma. In the most severe cases, eczematous dermatitis may evolve into erythroderma (see "Exfoliative Erythroderma" section). Other complications of this disease include secondary bacterial infection (impetigo) or herpetic infection, a condition known as eczema herpeticum. Treatment of atopic dermatitis includes topical corticosteroids, emollients, oral antihistamines, antibiotics as needed, and management of coexisting asthma and allergies.

Contact Dermatitis

Contact dermatitis occurs when direct contact with a substance triggers an inflammatory response in the skin. Irritant contact dermatitis, which accounts for 80% of contact cases, occurs when a chemical directly induces damage to the skin. Common irritants include soap, water, and solvents. Allergic contact dermatitis makes up the remaining 20% of cases, and is an immunologically mediated, delayed (Type IV) hypersensitivity reaction. Causes of allergic contact dermatitis in hospitalized patients include adhesives, topical medications, topical antibiotics, preservatives, fragrances, metals, and rubber components. Older adults have an impaired epidermal barrier and are more susceptible to both irritants and allergens. Patients with stasis dermatitis and lower extremity ulcerations are at increased risk of allergic contact dermatitis [154].

Acute contact dermatitis, whether irritant or allergic in nature, presents with pruritic papules and weepy vesicles on an erythematous base, initially localized to the area of contact. Chronic lesions are erythematous plaques of thickened skin with accentuated skin markings, scale, and occasionally fissuring. The differential diagnosis may vary depending on the location of the eruption, but generally includes atopic dermatitis, seborrheic dermatitis, stasis dermatitis, and tinea. Rarely, systemic contact dermatitis can occur when a sensitized individual is exposed to a cross-reacting substance. This presents with erythema of the buttocks and flexural skin folds. The most common allergens implicated in systemic allergic contact dermatitis are nickel, aminoglycoside antibiotics, corticosteroids, balsam of Peru, and plants [155]. Because contact dermatitis causes a break in the epidermal barrier, secondary infection is common. A common mistake is to attribute the dermatitis to the infection rather than seeing the infection as the result of the dermatitis. History and physical examination are usually sufficient to make the diagnosis. Patch testing may be useful in identifying potentially relevant contact allergens. Treatment involves avoidance of the offending agents. For mild to moderate cases, topical steroids and bland emollients are used. For extensive and severe cases, a 2- to 3-week tapering course of oral prednisone, along with an oral antihistamine to relieve pruritus, is appropriate. For lesions that are oozing and crusting, wet-to-dry or aluminum acetate compresses may be helpful. Treatment of any secondary infection speeds resolution. It is not uncommon to treat patients with both steroids and antibiotics to treat both the cause and the secondary infection.

Seborrheic Dermatitis

Seborrheic dermatitis is a common, usually asymptomatic, scaly eruption of the oil gland–bearing skin of the scalp, face, and trunk. It may present in mild cases as common dandruff and in severe cases as a florid erythematous scaling eruption involving the scalp, eyebrows, eyelids, paranasal folds, chest, and axillae. Seborrheic dermatitis typically occurs in healthy individuals, but is usually most severe among immunocompromised patients and among patients with neuropsychiatric disorders. An acute severe presentation should prompt testing for HIV. Paradoxically, acute severe seborrheic dermatitis is also common following initiation of HAART among patients with baseline low CD4 counts [156]. *Malassezia* yeasts are frequently seen in high levels on the skin of patients with seborrheic dermatitis, but their pathogenic role is unclear. Nonetheless, treatment with antifungals is effective. Diagnosis of seborrheic dermatitis is clinical. The differential diagnosis includes psoriasis, tinea capitis, rosacea, and atopic or contact dermatitis. Treatment is with antidandruff shampoos containing selenium sulfide, zinc pyrithione, ketoconazole, or ciclopirox and topical antifungals (ketoconazole cream, etc.) or mild corticosteroids (hydrocortisone cream) [157]. If the patient is not bothered by this rash, it need not be treated.

Transient Acantholytic Dermatosis (Grover's Disease)

Transient acantholytic dermatosis (TAD) is a common eruption consisting of discrete variably pruritic red to brown nonfollicular scaly keratotic papules of the upper trunk seen typically in middle-aged white men, more often in the wintertime. TAD is often seen in bedbound patients and can be associated with malignancies. Like miliaria, TAD is often associated with heat and excessive sweating; however, its histopathology, clinical appearance, and treatment are different. Lesions of TAD are more keratotic and scaly than those of miliaria, and histopathology reveals epidermal acantholysis rather than spongiosis. TAD may also be confused with folliculitis, which consists of follicular non-scaly papules and pustules. Treatment of TAD consists of mitigation of heat and sweating, application of mid-strength topical corticosteroids (such as triamcinolone cream 0.1% twice daily for up to 2 weeks), topical lotions containing pramoxine or menthol, and oral antihistamines (such as hydroxyzine 10 to 25 mg every 6 hours as needed for itch). In severe cases, oral retinoids such as isotretinoin (0.5 to 1 mg per kg daily) may be used. The condition usually remits slowly over weeks to months but can recur.

Miliaria

Miliaria is a common skin eruption among hospitalized patients. It is caused by blockage of eccrine sweat ducts that occurs in the setting of fever and excessive sweating, often in patients who are largely confined to bed. It occurs in three main forms: miliaria crystallina, which presents as tiny clear asymptomatic superficial vesicles on the trunk, head, and neck; miliaria rubra, which presents as uniform, small pruritic erythematous papules on the trunk, neck, and flexural extremities (Fig. 70.10); and miliaria profunda, which presents as firm, flesh-colored symptomatic nonfollicular papules or pustules on the trunk

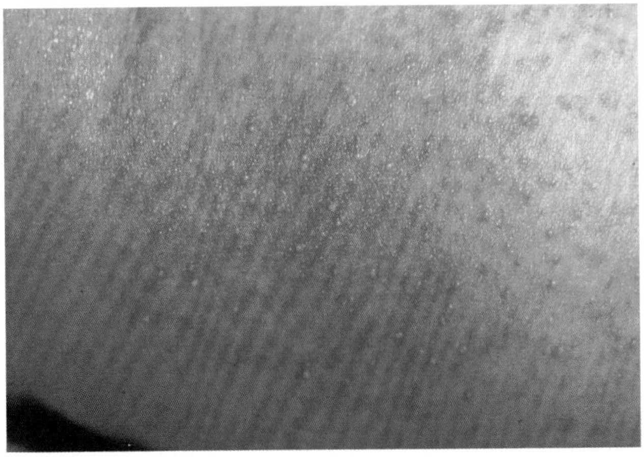

FIGURE 70.10 Miliaria rubra. Tiny nonfollicular inflammatory papules and pustules.

and extremities of patients who have had repeated episodes of miliaria rubra. It is important to be able to recognize miliaria to distinguish it from more medically significant entities such as disseminated herpes simplex, varicella, or candidiasis. The distribution of miliaria in areas where the skin is occluded and where excessive sweating occurs is helpful for the diagnosis.

Miliaria crystalline does not need to be treated, as it is self-limited and asymptomatic. Miliaria rubra may be treated by decreasing the heat and humidity of the patient's environment. Some reports state that oral ascorbic acid and topical lanolin can be helpful, but no controlled trials have been done [158].

Tinea Corporis

Fungal infection is named for the affected body part. Tinea corporis is the common, superficial fungal infection found on any area of the skin excluding the palms, soles, scalp, and groin. *Trichophyton rubrum* is the most common causative organism, although any dermatophyte may be responsible.

Tinea corporis presents as one or multiple annular lesions with erythematous scaly borders that exhibit centrifugal spread and leave a central clearing. Other clinical presentations include tinea profunda, which exhibits a granulomatous or verrucous appearance due to an excessive host inflammatory response, and Majocchi's granuloma, which presents as follicular-based pustules or papules. The differential diagnosis includes nummular eczema, subacute cutaneous lupus erythematosus, and granuloma annulare. The diagnosis is easily confirmed by potassium hydroxide (KOH) examination of scale or fungal culture. Limited disease may be treated with topical agents such as naftifine 1% cream, terbinafine 1% cream, or clotrimazole 1% cream applied twice daily for 2 to 4 weeks in combination with a topical steroid if there is significant local inflammation [159]. More extensive or recalcitrant disease may require systemic treatment such as itraconazole 100 mg daily or terbinafine 250 mg daily for 2 weeks. Prognosis is excellent with 70% to 100% cure after treatment, but recurrence is common [160], especially among the immunosuppressed.

Scabies

Scabies is a common, extremely pruritic dermatosis caused by infestation with the mite, *Sarcoptes scabiei*. It spreads from person to person through direct skin contact, although it can rarely spread through fomites such as bedding or towels. Scabies should be considered in the differential diagnosis of any patient with severe generalized itching, especially if they have had contact with residential institutions such as nursing homes, where it may be endemic.

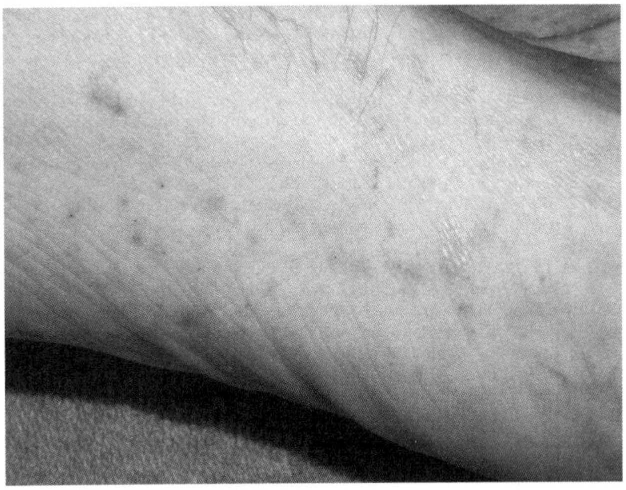

FIGURE 70.11 Scabies. Pink excoriated papules and linear burrows on the foot.

Patients with scabies present with severe generalized pruritus, sparing the head and neck, which is worse at night. The pathognomonic lesions are linear burrows (Fig. 70.11), most often found on the hands and feet, especially in the web spaces. Papules, pustules, vesicles, and nodules may also occur, the last being especially common in children. Scabies has a predilection for the hands, feet, wrists, axillae, abdomen, buttocks, and genitalia. Immunocompromised and neurologically impaired patients may present with the crusted or "Norwegian" variant of scabies, in which the skin is markedly thickened and crusted. These crusts are filled with thousands of mites and the patients are highly infectious.

Definitive diagnosis of scabies is made by observing skin scrapings microscopically for mites, eggs, or mite feces. First-line treatment of scabies is with topical 5% permethrin cream applied from neck down and left on overnight, with special attention to the genitalia, web spaces, and under the fingernails. All household members or suspected contacts over the age of 2 months and nonpregnant individuals should be treated simultaneously. All bedding, clothing, and towels are then laundered. The application is repeated after 1 week. When topical treatment is impractical, oral ivermectin may be given as a single dose of 200 μg per kg of body weight, repeated in 1 week. Itching can persist for up to a month after adequate treatment. Patients can be concurrently treated with topical corticosteroids and oral antihistamines to help alleviate itch [161].

References

1. Scwartz RA, McDonough PH, Lee BW: Toxic epidermal necrolysis. Part I. Introduction, history, classification, clinical features, systemic manifestations, etiology, and aimmunopathogenesis. *J Am Acad Dermatol* 69:173.e1–173.e13, 2013.
2. Lee HY, Dunant A, Sekula P, et al: The role of prior corticosteroid use on the clinical course of Stevens-Johnson syndrome and toxic epidermal necrolysis: a case–control analysis of patients selected from the multinational EuroSCAR and RegiSCAR studies. *Br J Dermatol* 167:555–562, 2012.
3. Scwartz RA, McDonough PH, Lee BW: Toxic epidermal necrolysis. Part II. Prognosis, sequelae, diagnosis, differential diagnosis, prevention, and treatment. *J Am Acad Dermatol* 69:187.e1–187.e16, 2013.
4. Mockenhaupt M, Viboud C, Dunant A, et al: Stevens–Johnson syndrome and toxic epidermal necrolysis: assessment of medication risks with emphasis on recently marketed drugs. The EuroSCAR-Study. *J Invest Derm* 128(1):35–44, 2008.
5. Roujeau JC, Kelly JP, Naldi L, et al: Medication use and the risk of Stevens–Johnson syndrome or toxic epidermal necrolysis. *N Engl J Med* 333(24):1600, 1995.

6. Canavan TN, Mathes EF, Frieden I, et al: Mycoplasma pneumoniae-induced rash and mucositis as a syndrome distinct from Stevens-Johnson syndrome and erythema multiforme: a systematic review. *J Am Acad Dermatol* 72(2):239–245, 2015.
7. Quinn AM, Brown K, Bonish BK, et al: Uncovering histologic criteria with prognostic significance in toxic epidermal necrolysis. *Arch Dermatol* 141:683–687, 2005.
8. Heng YK, Lee HY, Roujeau JC: Epidermal necrolysis: 60 years of errors and advances. *Br J Dermatol* 173(5):1250–1254, 2015.
9. Araki Y, Sotozono C, Inatomi T, et al: Successful treatment of Stevens–Johnson syndrome with steroid pulse therapy at disease onset. *Am J Opthalmol* 147:1004–1011, 2009.
10. Le HG, Saeed H, Mantagos IS, et al: Burn unit care of Stevens Johnson syndrome/toxic epidermal necrolysis: a survey. *Burns* 42(4):830–835, 2016.
11. Kirchhof MG, Miliszewski MA, Sikora S, et al: Retrospective review of Stevens-Johnson syndrome/toxic epidermal necrolysis treatment comparing intravenous immunoglobulin with cyclosporine. *J Am Acad Dermatol* 71:941–947, 2014.
12. Bastuji-Garin S, Fouchard N, Bertocchi M, et al: SCORTEN: a severity-of-illness score for toxic epidermal necrolysis. *J Invest Dermatol* 115(2):149, 2000.
13. Bocquet H, Bagot M, Roujeau JC: Drug-induced pseudolymphoma and drug hypersensitivity syndrome (drug rash with eosinophilia and systemic symptoms: Dress). *Semin Cutan Med Surg* 15(4):250, 1996.
14. Roujeau JC: Clinical heterogeneity of drug hypersensitivity. *Toxicology* 209(2):123, 2005.
15. Husain Z, Reddy BY, Schwarts RA: DRESS syndrome part I: clinical perspectives. *J Am Acad Dermatol* 68(5):693.e1–693.e14, 2013.
16. Walsh S, Diaz-Cano S, Higgins E, et al: Drug reaction with eosinophilia and systemic symptoms: is cutaneous phenotype a prognostic marker for outcome? A review of clinicopathological features of 27 cases. *Br J Dermatol* 168(2):391–401, 2013.
17. Lin IC, Yang HC, Strong C, et al: Liver injury in patients with DRESS: a clinical study of 72 cases. *J Am Acad Dermatol* 72(6):984–991, 2015.
18. Chiou CC, Yang LC, Hung SI, et al: Clinicopathological features and prognosis of DRESS: a study of 30 cases in Taiwan. *J Eur Acad Dermatol Venereol* 22:1044–1049, 2008.
19. Chen YC, Chiu HC, Chu CY: Drug reaction with eosinophilia and systemic symptoms: a retrospective study of 60 cases. *Arch Dermatol* 146(12):1373–1379, 2010.
20. Chen YC, Chang CY, Cho YT, et al: Long-term sequelae of drug reaction with eosinophilia and systemic symptoms: a retrospective cohort study from Taiwan. *J Am Acad Dermatol* 68(3):459–465, 2013.
21. Bourgeosis GP, Cafardi JA, Groysman V, et al: A review of DRESS-associated myocarditis. *J Am Acad Dermatol* 66(6):e229–e236, 2012.
22. Funck-Brentano E, Duong TA, Bouvresse S: Therapeutic management of DRESS: a retrospective study of 38 cases. *J Am Acad Dermatol* 72(2):246–252, 2015.
23. Husain Z, Reddy BY, Schwartz RA: DRESS syndrome: part II management and therapeutics. *J Am Acad Dermatol* 68(5):709e1–709e9, 2013.
24. Staughton RC, Payne CM, Harper JI, et al: Toxic pustuloderma—a new entity? *J R Soc Med* 77[Suppl 4]:6, 1984.
25. Macmillan AL: Generalised pustular drug rash. *Dermatologica* 146(5):285, 1973.
26. Sidoroff A, Halevy S, Bavinck JN, et al: Acute generalized exanthematous pustulosis (AGEP)–a clinical reaction pattern. *J Cutan Pathol* 28(3):113, 2001.
27. Sidoroff A, Dunant A, Viboud C, et al: Risk factors for acute generalized exanthematous pustulosis—results of a multi-national case-control study (EuroSCAR). *Br J Dermatol* 157:989–996, 2007.
28. Davidovici BB, Pavel D, Cagnano E, et al: Acute generalized exanthematous pustulosis following a spider bite: report of 3 cases. *J Am Acad Dermatol* 55(3):525–529, 2006.
29. Lee D, Kang JN, Hwang SH, et al: Acute generalized exanthematous pustulosis induced by parvovirus b19 infection. *Ann Dermatol* 26(3):399–400, 2014.
30. Birnie AJ, Litlewood SM: Acute generalized exanthematous pustulosis does not always have a drug-related cause. *Br J Dermatol* 159(2):492–493, 2008.
31. Sigurdsson V, Toonstra J, Hezemans-Boer M, et al: Erythroderma. A clinical and follow-up study of 102 patients, with special emphasis on survival. *J Am Acad Dermatol* 35(1):53, 1996.
32. Sigurdsson V, Toonstra J, van Vloten WA: Idiopathic erythroderma: a follow-up study of 28 patients. *Dermatology* 194(2):98, 1997.
33. Rym BM, Mourad M, Bechir Z, et al: Erythroderma in adults: a report of 80 cases. *Int J Dermatol* 44(9):731, 2005.
34. Umar SH, Kelly AP: Erythroderma (generalized exfoliative dermatitis). Emedicine, 2014. Available at: http://emedicine.medscape.com/article/1106906-overview. Accessed November 8, 2015.
35. Sehgal VN, Srivastava G, Sardana K: Erythroderma/exfoliative dermatitis: a synopsis. *Int J Dermatol* 43(1):39, 2004.
36. Leclerc-Mercier S, Bodemer C, Bourdon-Lanoy E, et al: Early skin biopsy is helpful for the diagnosis and management of neonatal and infantile erythrodermas. *J Cutan Pathol* 37(2):249–255, 2010.
37. Stevens DL: The toxic shock syndromes. *Infect Dis Clin North Am* 10:727, 1996.
38. Wolf JE, Rabinowitz LG: Streptococcal toxic shock-like syndrome. *Arch Dermatol* 131:73, 1995.
39. Ferry T, Thomas D, Bouchut JC, et al: Early diagnosis of Staphylococcal toxic shock syndrome by detection of the TSST-1 Vbeta signature in peripheral blood of a 12-year-old boy. *Pediatr Infect Dis J* 27(3):274–277, 2008.
40. Baddour LM, Eason JH, Lunde PA, et al: Case report: acute cellulitis and lymphadenitis caused by mucoid streptococcus pyogenes. *Am J Med Sci* 312(1):40, 1996.
41. McKinnon PS, Paladino JA, Grayson ML, et al: Cost-effectiveness of ampicillin/sulbactam versus imipenem/cilastatin in the treatment of limb-threatening foot infections in diabetic patients. *Clin Infect Dis* 24(1):57, 1997.
42. Diaz JH, Lopez FA. Skin, soft tissue and systemic bacterial infections following aquatic injuries and exposures. *Am J Med Sci* 349(3):269–275, 2015.
43. Swartz MN: Clinical practice. Cellulitis. *N Engl J Med* 350(9):904, 2004.
44. Falagas ME, Vergidis PI: Narrative review: diseases that masquerade as infectious cellulitis. *Ann Intern Med* 142(1):47, 2005.
45. Strazzula L, Cotliar J, Fox LP, et al: Inpatient dermatology consultation aids diagnosis of cellulitis among hospitalized patients: a multi-institutional analysis. *J Am Acad Dermatol* 73(1):70–75, 2015.
46. Stevens DL, Bisno AL, Chambers HF, et al: Practice guidelines for the diagnosis and management of skin and soft tissue infections: 2014 update by the infectious diseases society of America. *Clin Infect Dis* 59(2):147–159, 2014.
47. Halilovic J, Heintz BH, Brown J: Risk factors for clinical failure in patients hospitalized with cellulitis and cutaneous abscess. *J Infect* 65(2):128–134, 2012.
48. Thomas KS, Crook AM, Nunn AJ, et al: Penicillin to prevent recurrent leg cellulitis. *N Engl J Med* 368(18):1695–1703, 2013.
49. Edlich R: Necrotizing fasciitis. Emedicine, 2015. Available at: http://emedicine.medscape.com/article/2051157-overview. Accessed December 15, 2015.
50. Hung TH, Tsai CC, Tsai CC, et al: Liver cirrhosis as a real risk factor for necrotising fasciitis: a three-year population-based follow-up study. *Singapore Med J* 55(7):378–382, 2014.
51. Friederichs J, Torka S, Militz M, et al: Necrotizing soft tissue infections after injection therapy: higher mortality and worse outcome compared to other entry mechanisms. *J Infect* 71(3):312–316, 2015.
52. Miller LG, Perdreau-Remington F, Reig G, et al: Necrotizing fasciitis caused by community-acquired methicillin-resistant Staphylococcus aureus in Los Angeles. *N Engl J Med* 352(14):1445, 2005.
53. Beaudoin AL, Torso L, Richards K, et al: Invasive group A Streptococcus infections associated with liposuction surgery at outpatient facilities not subject to state or federal regulation. *JAMA Intern Med* 174(7):1136–1142, 2014.
54. Su Y, Chen H, Hong U, et al: Laboratory risk indicator for necrotizing fasciitis score and the outcomes. *ANZ J Surg* 78(11):968, 2008.
55. Kao LS, Lew DF, Arab SN, et al: Local variations in the epidemiology, microbiology, and outcome of necrotizing soft-tissue infections: a multicenter study. *Am J Surg* 202(2):139–145, 2011.
56. Hua C, Sbidian E, Hemery F, et al: Prognostic factors in necrotizing soft-tissue infections (NSTI): a cohort study. *J Am Acad Dermatol* 73(6):1006–12 e8, 2015.
57. Huang KF, Hung MH, Lin YS, et al: Independent predictors of mortality for necrotizing fasciitis: a retrospective analysis in a single institution. *J Trauma* 71(2):467–473, 2011; discussion 73.
58. Ladhani S: Recent developments in staphylococcal scalded skin syndrome. *Clin Microbiol Infect* 7(6):301, 2001.
59. Ladhani S: Understanding the mechanism of action of the exfoliative toxins of Staphylococcus aureus. *FEMS Immunol Med Microbiol* 39(2):181, 2003.
60. King RW, Victor PDS, Carone HL: Staphylococcal scalded skin syndrome. Emedicine, 2015. Available at: http://emedicine.medscape.com/article/788199-overview. Accessed December 29, 2015.
61. Patel GK, Varma S, Finlay AY: Staphylococcal scalded skin syndrome in healthy adults. *Br J Dermatol* 142(6):1253, 2000.
62. Rosenstein NE, Perkins BA, Stephens DS, et al: Meningococcal disease. *N Engl J Med* 344(18):1378, 2001.
63. Javid, MH: Meningococcemia. Medscape, 2015. Available at: http://emedicine.medscape.com/article/1052846-overview. Accessed December 15, 2015.
64. Hsia RY, Wang E, Thanassi WT: Fever, abdominal pain, and leukopenia in a 13-year-old: a case-based review of meningococcemia. *J Emer Med* 37(1):21–28, 2009.
65. Cummings KC, Louie J, Probert WS, et al: Increased detection of meningococcal infections in California using a polymerase chain reaction assay. *Clin Infect Dis* 46(7):1124–1126, 2008.
66. Openshaw JJ, Swerdlow DL, Krebs JW, et al: Rocky mountain spotted fever in the United States, 2000–2007: interpreting contemporary increases in incidence. *Am J Trop Med Hyg* 83(1):174–182, 2010.
67. McGinley-Smith DE, Tsao SS: Dermatoses from ticks. *J Am Acad Dermatol* 49(3):363, 2003.
68. Singh-Behl D, La Rosa SP, Tomecki KJ: Tick-borne infections. *Dermatol Clin* 21(2):237, 2003.
69. Masters EJ, Olson GS, Weiner SJ, et al: Rocky Mountain spotted fever: a clinician's dilemma. *Arch Intern Med* 163(7):769, 2003.
70. Salvaggio MR: Herpes simplex. Emedicine, 2015. Available at: http://emedicine.medscape.com/article/218580-overview. Accessed December 17, 2015.
71. Corey L: Herpes simplex virus, in Mandell GL, Bennett JE, Dolin R (eds): *Principles and Practice of Infectious Diseases*. 6th ed. New York, Churchill Livingstone, 2005, p 1762.
72. Chilukuri S, Rosen T: Management of acyclovir-resistant herpes simplex virus. *Dermatol Clin* 21(2):311, 2003.
73. Nikkels AF, Delvenne P, Herfs M, et al: Occult herpes simplex virus colonization of bullous dermatitides. *Am J Clin Dermatol* 9(3):163–168, 2008.
74. Lafferty WE, Krofft S, Remington M, et al: Diagnosis of herpes simplex virus by direct immunofluorescence and viral isolation from samples of external genital lesions in a high-prevalence population. *J Clin Microbiol* 25(2):323, 1987.
75. Janniger CK: Herpes zoster. Emedicine 2015. Available at: http://emedicine.medscape.com/article/1132465-overview. Accessed December 17, 2015.
76. Marin M, Meissner HC, Seward JF: Varicella prevention in the United States: a review of successes and challenges. *Pediatrics* 122(3):e744–e751, 2008.

77. Ahmed AM, Brantley JS, Madkan V, et al: Managing herpes zoster in immunocompromised patients. *Herpes* 14(2):32, 2007.
78. Grant RM, Weitzman SS, Sherman CG, et al: Fulminant disseminated varicella zoster virus infection without skin involvement. *J Clin Virol* 24(1–2):7, 2002.
79. O'Connor KM, Paauw DS: Herpes zoster. *Med Clin North Am* 97(4):503–522, ix, 2013.
80. Dworkin RH, Johnson RW, Breuer J, et al: Recommendations for the manage- ment of herpes zoster. *Clin Infect Dis* 44[Suppl 1]:S1–S26, 2007.
81. Sampathkumar P, Drage LA, Martin DP: Herpes zoster (shingles) and posther-petic neuralgia. *Mayo Clin Proc* 84(3):274–280, 2009.
82. Zeina B, Mansour S, Sakka N: Pemphigus vulgaris. Emedicine, 2015. Available at: http://emedicine.medscape.com/article/1064187-overview. Accessed December 29, 2015.
83. Ratnam KV, Phay KL, Tan CK: Pemphigus therapy with oral prednisolone regimens. A 5-year study. *In J Dermatol* 29:363–367, 1990.
84. Mentink LF, Mackenzie MW, Tóth GG, et al: Randomized controlled trial of adjuvant oral dexamethasone pulse therapy in pemphigus vulgaris: PEMPULS trial. *Arch Dermatol* 142:570–576, 2006.
85. Chams-Davatchi C, Esmaili N, Daneshpahooh M, et al: Randomized controlled open-label trial of four treatment regimens for pemphigus vulgaris. *J Am Acad Dermatol* 57:622–628, 2007.
86. Beissert S, Werfel T, Frieling U, et al: A comparison of oral methylprednisolone plus azathioprine or mycophenolate mofetil for the treatment of pemphigus. *Arch Dermatol* 142:1447–1454, 2006.
87. Amagai M, Ikeda S, Shimizu H, et al: A randomized double-blind trial of intravenous immunoglobulin for pemphigus. *J Am Acad Dermatol* 60:595–603, 2009.
88. Werth VP, Fivenson D, Pandya AG, et al: Multicenter randomized, double-blind, placebo-controlled, clinical trial of dapsone as a glucocorticoid-sparing agent in maintenance-phase pemphigus vulgaris. *Arch Dermatol* 144:25–32, 2008.
89. Ioannides D, Chrysomallis F, Bystryn JC: Ineffectiveness of cyclosporine as an adjuvant to corticosteroids in the treatment of pemphigus. *Arch Dermatol* 136:868–872, 2000.
90. Ingen-Housz-Oro S, Valeyrie-Allanore L, Cosnes A, et al: First-line treatment of pemphigus vulgaris with a combination of rituximab and high-potency topical corticosteroids. *JAMA Dermatol* 151(2):200–203, 2015.
91. Hall RP 3rd, Fairley J, Woodley D, et al: A multicentre randomized trial of the treatment of patients with pemphigus vulgaris with infliximab and prednisone compared with prednisone alone. *Br J Dermatol* 172(3):760–768, 2015.
92. Zhao CY, Murrell DF: Pemphigus vulgaris: an evidence-based treatment update. *Drugs* 75(3):271–284, 2015.
93. Goldberg LJ, Nisar N: Paraneoplastic pemphigus. Emedicine, 2015. Available at: http://emedicine.medscape.com/article/1064452-overview. Accessed December 29, 2015.
94. Poot AM, Diercks GF, Kramer D, et al: Laboratory diagnosis of paraneoplastic pemphigus. *Br J Dermatol* 169(5):1016–1024, 2013.
95. Leger S, Picard D, Ingen-Housz-Oro S, et al: Prognostic factors of paraneoplastic pemphigus. *Arch Dermatol* 148(10):1165–1172, 2012.
96. Sagi L, Baum S, Agmon-Levin N, et al: Autoimmune bullous diseases the spectrum of infectious agent antibodies and review of the literature. *Autoimmun Rev* 10(9):527–535, 2011.
97. Chan L: Bullous pemphigoid. Medscape, 2015. Available at: http://emedicine.medscape.com/article/1062391-overview. Accessed December 30, 2015.
98. Joly J, Roujeau JC, Benichou J, et al: A comparison of oral and topical corticosteroids in patients with Bullous Pemphigoid. *N Engl J Med* 346:321–327, 2002.
99. Kasperkiewicz M, Shimanovich I, Ludwig RJ, et al: Rituximab for treatment-refractory pemphigus and pemphigoid: a case series of 17 patients. *J Am Acad Dermatol* 65(3):552, 2011.
100. Eastham BW: Leukocytoclastic vasculitis. Emedicine, 2015. Available at: http://emedicine.medscape.com/article/333891-overview. Accessed December 19, 2015.
101. Goeser MR, Laniosz V, Wetter DA: A practical approach to the diagnosis, evaluation, and management of cutaneous small-vessel vasculitis. *Am J Clin Dermatol* 15(4):299–306, 2014.
102. Chung C, Tumeh PC, Birnbaum R, et al: Characteristic purpura of the ears, vasculitis, and neutropenia—a potential public health epidemic associated with levamisole-adulterated cocaine. *J Am Acad Dermatol* 65(4):722–725, 2011.
103. Abuabara K, Samimi S, Chu EY, et al: Alcohol-induced vasculitis: case report and commentary. *J Am Acad Dermatol* 70(2):e42–e43, 2014.
104. Micheletti RG, Werth VP: Small vessel vasculitis of the skin. *Rheum Dis Clin North Am* 41(1):21–32, vii, 2015.
105. Gast T, Kowal-Vern A, An G, et al: Purpura fulminans in an adult patient with Haemophilus influenzae sepsis: case report and review of the literature. *J Burn Care Res* 27(1):102, 2006.
106. Kennedy KJ, Walker S, Pavli P, et al: What may underlie recurrent purpura fulminans? *Med J Aust* 186(7):373, 2007.
107. Kempton CL, Bagby G, Collins JF: Ulcerative colitis presenting as purpura fulminans. *Inflamm Bowel Dis* 7(4):319, 2001.
108. Smith OP, White B: Infectious purpura fulminans: diagnosis and treatment. *Br J Haematol* 104(2):198, 1999.
109. Nolan J, Sinclair R: Review of management of purpura fulminans and two case reports. *Br J Anaesth* 86(4):581, 2001.
110. Oh DH, Eulau D, Tokugawa DA, et al: Five cases of calciphylaxis and a review of the literature. *J Am Acad Dermatol* 40(6 Pt 1):979, 1999.
111. Gibson GE, Su WP, Pittelkow MR: Antiphospholipid syndrome and the skin. *J Am Acad Dermatol* 36(6):970–982, 1997.
112. Nahass GT: Antiphospholipid antibodies and the antiphospholipid antibody syndrome. *J Am Acad Dermatol* 36(2):149–171, 1997.
113. Sharkey MP, Daryanani II, Gillett MB, et al: Localized cutaneous necrosis associated with the antiphospholipid syndrome. *Australas J Dermatol* 43(3):218–220, 2002.
114. Weinstein S, Piette W: Cutaneous manifestations of antiphospholipid antibody syndrome. *Hematol Oncol Clin North Am* 22(1):67–77, 2008.
115. Berman H, Rodríguez-Pintó I, Cervera R, et al: Catastrophic Antiphospholipid Syndrome (CAPS) Registry Project Group (European Forum on Antiphospholipid Antibodies). Rituximab use in the catastrophic antiphospholipid syndrome: descriptive analysis of the CAPS registry patients receiving rituximab. *Autoimmun Rev* 12(11):1085–1090, 2013.
116. Kriseman YL, Nash JW, Hsu S: Criteria for the diagnosis of antiphospholipid syndrome in patients presenting with dermatologic symptoms. *J Am Acad Dermatol* 57(1):112–115, 2007.
117. Erkan D, Vega J, Ramon G, et al: A pilot open label phase II trial of rituximab for non-criteria manifestations of antiphospholipid syndrome. *Arthritis Rheum* 65(2), 464–471, 2013.
118. Nazarian RM, Van Cott EM, Zembowicz A, et al: Warfarin-induced skin necrosis. *J Am Acad Dermatol* 61(2):325, 2009.
119. Terrier B, Krastinova E, Marie I, et al: Management of noninfectious mixed cryoglobulinemia vasculitis: data from 242 cases included in the CryoVas survey. *Blood* 119(25):5996–6004, 2012.
120. Terrier B, Marie I, Lacraz A, et al: Non HCV-related infectious cryoglobulinemia vasculitis: results from the French nationwide CryoVas survey and systematic review of the literature. *J Autoimmun* 65:74–81, 2015.
121. McGevna LF, Raugi J, Raza SR: Cutaneous manifestations of cholesterol embolism. Emedicine, 2014. Available at: http://emedicine.medscape.com /article/1096593-overview. Accessed December 29, 2015.
122. Donohue KG, Saap L, Falanga V: Cholesterol crystal embolization: an atherosclerotic disease with frequent and varied cutaneous manifestations. *J Eur Acad Dermatol Venereol* 17(5):504, 2003.
123. Hitti WA, Wali RK, Weinman EJ, et al: Cholesterol embolization syndrome induced by thrombolytic therapy. *Am J Cardiovasc Drugs* 8(1):27, 2008.
124. Wang H, Zheng J, Deng C, et al: Fat embolism syndromes following liposuction. *Aesth Plast Surg* 32(5):731, 2008.
125. Garcia FVMJ, Sanz-Sanchez T, Aragues M, et al: Cutaneous embolization of cardiac myxoma. *Br J Dermatol* 147(2):379, 2002.
126. Saric M, Kronzon I: Cholesterol embolization syndrome. *Curr Opin Cardiol* 26(6):472–479, 2011.
127. Kalajian AH, Malhotra PS, Callen JP, et al: Calciphylaxis with normal renal and parathyroid function: not as rare as previously believed. *Arch Dermatol* 145(4):451–458, 2009.
128. Weenig RH, Sewell LD, Davis MD, et al: Calciphylaxis: natural history, risk factor analysis, and outcome. *J Am Acad Dermatol* 56(4):569–579, 2007.
129. Bhambri A, Del Rosso JQ: Calciphylaxis: a review. *J Clin Aesthet Dermatol* 1(2):38–41, 2008.
130. Nigwekar SU, Kroshinsky D, Nazarian RM, et al: Calciphylaxis: risk factors, diagnosis, and treatment. *Am J Kidney Dis* 66(1):133–146, 2015.
131. Nigwekar SU, Brunelli SM, Meade D, et al: Sodium thiosulfate therapy for calcific uremic arteriolopathy. *Clin J Am Soc Nephrol* 8(7):1162–1170, 2013.
132. Strazzula L, Nigwekar SU, Steele D, et al: Intralesional sodium thiosulfate for the treatment of calciphylaxis. *JAMA Dermatol* 149(8):946–949, 2013.
133. Vedvyas C, Winterfield LS, Vleugels RA: Calciphylaxis: a systematic review of existing and emerging therapies. *J Am Acad Dermatol* 67(6):e253–e2560, 2012.
134. Bartels CM, Muller D: Systemic lupus erythematosus. Medscape, 2015. Available at: http://emedicine.medscape.com/article/332244-overview. Accessed December 30, 2015.
135. Kuhn A, Ruland V, Bonsmann G: Cutaneous lupus erythematosus: update of therapeutic options: Part I. *J Amer Acad Derm* 65(6):179–193, 2011.
136. Seidler AM, Gottlieb AB: Dermatomyositis induced by drug therapy: a review of case reports. *J Am Acad Dermatol* 59:872–880, 2008.
137. Jorizzo LJ, Jorizzo JL: The treatment and prognosis of dermatomyositis: an updated review. *J Am Acad Dermatol* 59:99–112, 2008.
138. Anyanwu CO, Fiorentino DF, Chung L, et al: Validation of the cutaneous dermatomyositis disease area and severity index: characterizing disease severity and assessing responsiveness to clinical change. *Br J Dermatol* 173(4):969–974, 2013.
139. Hymes SR, Alousi AM, Cowen EW: Graft-versus-host disease: part I. Pathogenesis and clinical manifestations of graft-versus-host disease. *J Am Acad Dermatol* 66(4):515 e1–515 e18; quiz 33, 34, 2012.
140. Mandanas RA: Graft versus host disease. Emedicine 2015. Available at: http://emedicine.medscape.com/article/429037-overview. Accessed December 19, 2015.
141. Saliba RM, de Lima M, Giralt S, et al: Hyperacute GVHD: risk factors, outcomes, and clinical implications. *Blood* 109(7):2751–2758, 2007.
142. Huang J, Pol-Rodriguez M, Silvers D, et al: Acquired ichthyosis as a manifestation of acute cutaneous graft-versus-host disease. *Pediatr Dermatol* 24(1):49–52, 2007.
143. Tong LX, Worswick SD: Viral infections in acute graft-versus-host disease: a review of diagnostic and therapeutic approaches. *J Am Acad Dermatol* 72(4):696–702, 2015.
144. Marra DE, McKee PH, Nghiem P: Tissue eosinophils and the perils of using skin biopsy specimens to distinguish between drug hypersensitivity and cutaneous graft-versus-host disease. *J Am Acad Dermatol* 51(4):543, 2004.
145. Rajendran PM, Young D, Maurer T, et al: Randomized, double-blind, placebo-controlled trial of cephalexin for treatment of uncomplicated skin abscesses in a population at risk for community-acquired methicillin-resistant Staphylococcus aureus infection. *Antimicrob Agents Chemother* 51(11):4044, 2007.

146. Laureano AC, Schwartz RA, Cohen PJ: *Facial bacterial infections: folliculitis. Clin Dermatol* 32(6):711–714, 2014.
147. Satter EK: Folliculitis. Medscape, 2015. Available at: http://emedicine.medscape.com/article/1070456-overview. Accessed December 23, 2015.
148. Hirschmann JV, Raugi GJ: Lower limb cellulitis and its mimics: part II. Conditions that simulate lower limb cellulitis. *J Am Acad Dermatol* 67(2):177.e1–177.e 9; quiz 185, 186, 2012.
149. Qaseem A, Humphrey LL, Forciea MA, et al: Clinical guidelines committee of the American college of physicians treatment of pressure ulcers: a clinical practice guideline from the American College of Physicians. *Ann Intern Med* 162(5):370–379, 2015.
150. Cereda E, Klersy C, Serioli M, et al: Element Sore Trial Study G. A nutritional formula enriched with arginine, zinc, and antioxidants for the healing of pressure ulcers: a randomized trial. *Ann Intern Med* 162(3):167–174, 2015.
151. Gelfand JM, Neimann AL, Shin DB, et al: Risk of myocardial infarction in patients with psoriasis. *JAMA* 296(14):1735–1741, 2006.
152. Prodanovich S, Kirsner RS, Kravetz JD, et al: Association of psoriasis with coronary artery, cerebrovascular, and peripheral vascular diseases and mortality. *Arch Dermatol* 145(6):700–703, 2009.
153. Rosenbach M, Hsu S, Korman NJ, et al: National Psoriasis Foundation Medical Board. Treatment of erythrodermic psoriasis: from the medical board of the National Psoriasis Foundation. *J Am Acad Dermatol* 62(4):655–662, 2010.
154. Prakash AV, Davis MD: Contact dermatitis in older adults: a review of the literature. *Am J Clin Dermatol* 11(6):373–381,2010.
155. Kulberg A, Schliemann S, Elsner P: Contact dermatitis as a systemic disease. *Clin Dermatol* 32(3):414–419, 2014.
156. Osei-Sekyere B, Karstaedt AS: Immune reconstitution inflammatory syndrome involving the skin. *Clin Exp Dermatol* 35(5):477, 2010.
157. Dessinioti C, Katsambas A: Seborrheic dermatitis: etiology, risk factors, and treatments: facts and controversies. *Clin Dermatol* 31(4):343–351, 2013.
158. Levin NA: Dermatologic manifestations of miliaria. Emedicine 2015. Available at: http://emedicine.medscape.com/article/1070840-overview. Accessed December 19, 2015.
159. Van Zuuren EJ, Fedorowicz Z, El-Gohary M: Evidence-based topical treatments for tinea cruris and tinea corporis: a summary of a Cochrane systematic review. *Br J Dermatol* 172(3):616–641, 2015.
160. Lesher JL, Elston D: Tinea corporis. Medscape 2015. Available at: http://emedicine.medscape.com/article/1091473-overview. Accessed December 22, 2015.
161. Barry M, Wilson BB, Kauffman CL, et al: Scabies: Emedicine, 2015, Available at: http://emedicine.medscape.com/article/1109204-overview. Accessed December 29, 2015.

Section 8
INFECTIOUS DISEASE PROBLEMS IN THE INTENSIVE CARE UNIT

ROBERT W. FINBERG

Chapter 71 ■ Approach to Fever in the ICU Patient

RAUL E. DAVARO • RICHARD H. GLEW

> Humanity has but three great enemies: fever, famine and war; of these by far the greatest, by far the most terrible, is fever [1].
>
> *Sir William Osler*

APPROACH TO THE FEBRILE PATIENT

Fever is a common symptom among hospitalized patients and one-third of all medical patients develop fever [2]. The incidence of fever in the intensive care unit (ICU) ranges from 25% to 70% [3]. In addition to being common, fever has also been shown to be independently associated with mortality for patients admitted to the ICU.

Pathophysiology

As homeothermic organisms, humans must regulate their temperature to maintain fundamental biologic processes [2]. Core temperature typically exhibits diurnal rhythmicity, with a nadir of about 36.2°C in the morning and a peak of approximately 37.7°C in the afternoon [4]. Temperature elevates to >39°C in febrile response to infection or other stress [4].

Fever is the result of an upward adjustment in the thermoregulatory set point involving cytokine-mediated rise in core temperature, generation of acute-phase reactants, and activation of numerous physiologic, endocrinologic, and immunologic systems [5]. In contrast, simple heat illness or malignant hyperthermia is an unregulated rise in body temperature caused by inability to eliminate heat adequately [4]. Physiologically, fever begins with the production of one or more proinflammatory cytokines in response to exogenous pyrogenic substances (such as microorganisms and toxic agents) or immunologic mediators. Interleukin-1 (IL-1) was the first purified protein with demonstrated pyrogenic properties; subsequently, other cytokines such as tumor necrosis factor (TNF), lymphotoxin, interferons (IFNs), and interleukin (IL-6) were also documented to induce fever. Cytokines interact with receptors located at the organum vasculosum of the lamina terminalis, causing synthesis and release of prostaglandins, chiefly prostaglandin E2, which raise body temperature by initiating local cAMP production, which resets the thermoregulatory set point of the hypothalamus, and by coordinating other adaptive responses, such as shivering and peripheral vasoconstriction [5]. Fever induces the production of heat shock proteins (HSPs), a class of proteins critical for cellular survival during stress. HSPs that act as molecular chaperones may have an anti-inflammatory role and indirectly decrease the level of proinflammatory cytokines [4].

Measurement

The Society of Critical Care Medicine and the Infectious Disease Society of America issued a consensus statement recommending that core temperature of higher than 38.3°C (101°F) be considered fever [6].

In the ICU, body temperature can be measured using a number of different methods, including thermistors on intravascular, bladder, esophageal, or rectal probes, in addition to infrared tympanic membrane and temporal artery thermometers. Although the pulmonary artery catheter has been considered the gold standard measurement technique, in most situations, relatively small differences exist between the other commonly used methods [7].

ETIOLOGY OF FEVER IN THE INTENSIVE CARE PATIENT

The prevalence of fever in the ICU depends on the population studied and the definition of fever used. The major causes of abnormally elevated temperatures in critically ill patients can be broadly classified as infectious fevers, noninfectious fevers, and hyperthermia syndromes (Table 71.1) [8].

Noninfectious Causes of Fever

About one-half of all fevers in the ICU are caused by noninfectious etiologies (Table 71.1) [2,8,9]. Noninfectious causes of fever are inflammatory conditions that activate the cytokine system and trigger a systemic inflammatory response syndrome (SIRS) a clinical response to inflammation [10]. Conditions associated with fever as one of the components of SIRS can occur in critically ill patients with large hematomas; acute vasculitis; subarachnoid hemorrhage; dissection of an aortic aneurysm; mesenteric ischemia; heat stroke; pancreatitis; or hyperthyroidism [2,8,9]. Fever may appear in the patient in whom the stress of surgery unmasks adrenal insufficiency or following bilateral adrenal hemorrhage in patients with a history of thromboembolic disease, recent surgery, and/or anticoagulant therapy [11]. Fever is a cardinal manifestation of delirium tremens in patients with acute alcohol withdrawal, although it is necessary to exclude other complications of alcohol abuse such as pneumonia or spontaneous bacterial peritonitis [12]. Likewise, fever associated with seizures must be differentiated from possible underlying causes of seizure, such as meningitis; encephalitis; brain abscess; or stroke.

TABLE 71.1

Noninfectious Sources of Fever in the ICU Patient

A. Inflammatory conditions
   1. Reaction to medications
   2. Reaction to blood products
   3. Collagen vascular diseases
      a. Systemic lupus erythematous
      b. Rheumatoid arthritis
   4. Vasculitis
      a. Hypersensitivity vasculitis
      b. Henoch–Schonlein purpura
      c. Granulomatosis with polyangiitis (formerly Wegener's granulomatosis)
      d. Giant cell arteritis
   5. Microcrystalline arthritis
      a. Gout
      b. Pseudogout
   6. Postpericardiotomy syndrome
   7. Pancreatitis
B. Vascular conditions
   1. Deep venous thrombophlebitis
   2. Pulmonary embolism
   3. Dissecting aortic aneurysm
   4. Mesenteric ischemia/infarction
   5. Hemorrhage into
      a. CNS
      b. Retroperitoneum
      c. Joint
      d. Lung
      e. Adrenals
   6. Myocardial infarction
C. Metabolic conditions
   1. Heat stroke
   2. Malignant hyperthermia secondary to anesthesia or medications
   3. Hyperthyroidism
   4. Adrenal insufficiency/hemorrhage
   5. Alcohol withdrawal
   6. Seizures
   7. Neuroleptic malignant syndrome
D. Neoplasia
   1. Lymphoma
   2. Renal cell carcinoma
   3. Hepatocellular carcinoma
   4. Malignancy metastatic to liver
   5. Colon carcinoma

ICU, intensive care unit; CNS, central nervous system.

Drug fever is a disorder characterized by a febrile response coinciding temporally with the administration of a drug in the absence of underlying conditions that can be responsible for the fever. A key feature that differentiates drug fever from fever of other causes is that it disappears once the offending drug is discontinued. Drug fever tends to be a diagnosis of exclusion, often suspected among patients with otherwise unexplained fevers [13].

Neoplastic fevers are now most commonly encountered in the setting of febrile patients with a known malignancy, and present a diagnostic challenge in differentiating whether fever is attributable to infection, therapy, or disease [14].

Hyperthermia is the unregulated rise in body temperature and a failure of the thermoregulatory homeostasis; malignant hyperthermia, neuroleptic malignant syndrome and serotonin syndrome are conditions that produce a high temperature resulting from hypothermia, not fever [15].

Conspicuously absent from Table 71.1 is atelectasis, a process widely regarded as a cause of fever, especially in the postoperative patient where atelectasis is common, although there is no clear evidence of such a connection [16].

Accurate and timely recognition of noninfectious causes of fever can avoid unnecessary use of antibiotics, reducing the risks of untoward reactions.

Infectious Causes of Fever

On any given day, approximately 1 of every 25 in patients in U.S. acute care hospitals has at least one health care–associated infection. Pneumonia and surgical-site infection are the most common infection types, and *C. difficile* is the most common pathogen. Infections other than those associated with central catheters, urinary catheters, and ventilators account for the majority of the U.S. burden of health care–associated infections and may warrant increased attention (Table 71.2) [17].

Bacteremias

Secondary bacteremia may originate from multiple sources (e.g., lungs, genitourinary tract, abdomen, skin, and soft tissues) or can develop as a consequence of vascular invasion via intravenous and intra-arterial lines and monitors; temporary transvenous pacemakers; and intra-aortic assist devices [17].

Health Care–associated Pneumonia

Respiratory infections continue to be the most common cause of sepsis and septic shock. Mechanical ventilation with an endotracheal tube increases the risk of pneumonia 6- to 20-fold [2]. Ventilator-associated pneumonia (VAP) is the most common infection acquired in the ICU [17].

Intra-abdominal Infections

Abdominal infections represent the third most common cause of sepsis in the intensive care unit and present an important diagnostic and therapeutic challenge.

The spectrum of diseases that can lead to ICU admission or complicate an ICU stay ranges from common, community acquired diseases to severe nosocomial infections. Rarely do intra-abdominal infections present as the only reason for admission to the ICU. Patients may have multiple comorbidities, be at high risk for treatment failure, and may already be septic at the time of admission. Other types of infection classically present during treatment for a different medical problem such as acalculous cholecystitis, or complicated *C difficile* colitis after the extensive use of broad-spectrum antibiotics, an increasing nosocomial problem of the last few years [17–19].

Urinary Tract Infections

Urinary tract infection (UTI) is one of the most common hospital-acquired infections; 70% to 80% of these infections are attributable to an indwelling urethral catheter. Partial or total obstruction or local complications (e.g., intrarenal or perinephric abscesses) must be suspected in patients with bacteremic pyelonephritis if fever and bacteremia persist despite appropriate antibiotic therapy [20].

Nosocomial Sinusitis

Nasogastric and nasotracheal tubes; facial fractures; and nasal packing are common predisposing factors to nosocomial sinusitis, an occasional cause of fever in the ICU [21].

TABLE 71.2

Infectious Sources of Fever in the ICU Patient

A. Urinary tract
  1. Pyelonephritis
  2. Prostatitis, prostatic abscess

B. Vascular devices
  1. Intravenous access site
    a. Phlebitis
    b. Bacteremia or fungemia
    c. Cellulitis
  2. Intra-arterial access site
    a. Bacteremia
    b. Fungemia

C. Respiratory
  1. Tracheobronchitis
  2. Pneumonia
  3. Sinusitis
  4. Empyema
  5. Lung abscess

D. Surgical-related wound
  1. Wound infection (superficial/incisional or deep)
  2. Deep-seated abscess (liver, spleen, kidney, brain, subphrenic, and bowel)

E. Skin/soft tissue
  1. Decubitus ulcer, with cellulitis/fasciitis/myositis
  2. Cellulitis

F. Gastrointestinal
  1. Antibiotic-associated colitis/*Clostridium difficile* colitis
  2. Ischemic colitis (mesenteric ischemia/infarction)
  3. Biliary
    a. Cholecystitis, including acalculous form
    b. Cholangitis
  4. Hepatitis (transfusion related)
    a. Cytomegalovirus
    b. Hepatitis C
    c. Hepatitis B
  5. Intra-abdominal abscess
  6. Diverticulitis

G. Prosthetic device infection
  1. Cardiac valve/pacemaker
  2. Joint replacement prosthesis
  3. Peritoneal dialysis catheter/peritonitis
  4. CNS intraventricular shunt

H. Miscellaneous
  1. Pyarthrosis
  2. Osteomyelitis (including vertebral osteodiscitis in adults)
  3. Meningitis

ICU, intensive care unit; CNS, central nervous system.

DIAGNOSTIC CONSIDERATIONS

In some ICUs, the finding of fever triggers an automatic fever workup, resulting in many tests that are time consuming, costly, and disruptive to the patient and staff. The American College of Critical Care Medicine and the Infectious Disease Society of America convened a task force to provide guidelines for evaluation of new fever in patients older than 18 years in the ICU setting [6].

History and Physical Examination

If able to communicate, the patient should be interviewed to identify localizing complaints. The patient and the patient's electronic medical record should be reviewed thoroughly for a history of relevant antecedent problems (e.g., previous infections, cancer, allergic reactions to drugs). If the patient is unable to communicate, the medical record and medical personnel can provide insightful information concerning duration of intravascular accesses; amount and purulence of sputum or wound drainage; changes in skin condition; apparent abdominal or musculoskeletal pain or tenderness; difficulty in handling respiratory secretions and feedings; and changes in ventilator support parameters. Relatives and friends of the patient can provide epidemiologic information related to the patient's exposures and risk factors for infections.

Physical examination of the febrile ICU patient may be difficult to conduct caused by limitations imposed by wound dressings, catheters, ventilator tubes, and monitors, but nonetheless it should be thorough. Skin examination may demonstrate findings suggestive of drug reaction, vasculitis, endocarditis, or soft tissue necrosis. All intravenous and intra-arterial line sites should be inspected; a tender intravenous access site, with or without purulence, can indicate septic thrombophlebitis. Spreading erythema, warmth, and tenderness that appear to indicate cellulitis of an extremity also can be the hallmarks of deep venous thrombophlebitis; pyarthrosis; or gout. After the first 24 hours postoperatively, wounds should be examined; this may require fenestrating or changing a cast to allow for examination of a fractured extremity if no other source of fever is found.

Head and neck examination can provide important signs of systemic and localized infection. Fundoscopic examination, preferably by an ophthalmologist, can provide clues to systemic fungal or viral infections in the immunocompromised. Hospital-associated sinusitis often develops in patients who required extensive period of intensive care, especially in the setting of nasal intubation and may have a paucity of associated symptoms. Oral lesions of recrudescent herpetic stomatitis are common in the ICU setting and often are obscured by the presence of oral endotracheal tubes or orogastric feeding tubes. These lesions may be extensive; more ulcerated and necrotic; and less vesicular in appearance in a seriously ill patient.

Examination of the lungs can be difficult for the intubated ICU patient and often is unrewardingly nonlocalizing and nonspecific. More sensitive (although nonspecific) indicators of pneumonia include chest imaging studies; occurrence of unexplained deterioration in oxygen exchange; and changes of the character of respiratory secretions. Unfortunately, pulmonary infiltrates and hypoxemia are nonspecific signs, because they can be seen with congestive heart failure; atelectasis; aspiration pneumonitis; pulmonary embolism; acute respiratory distress syndrome; and, less commonly, reactions to medications and pulmonary hemorrhage. Cardiac examination may demonstrate a new or changing murmur possibly due to endocarditis.

Abdominal findings can be misleadingly unremarkable in the elderly, in the patient with obtunded sensorium, and in the patient receiving sedatives. Abdominal examination can be confounding in the patient with recent abdominal or thoracic surgery. Abdominal pain and tenderness may be localized (cholecystitis; intra-abdominal abscess; and diverticulitis) or generalized (diffuse peritonitis, ischemic bowel, and antibiotic-associated colitis). Examination of the genitalia and rectum may demonstrate unsuspected epididymitis; prostatitis; prostatic abscess; or perirectal abscess.

Diagnostic Studies

Because the information provided by positive blood cultures has important prognostic and therapeutic implications, blood cultures should be obtained for patients with new onset of fever when clinical evaluation suggests an infectious cause. The volume of blood that is obtained for each blood culture request is the most important variable in recovering bacteria and fungi from patients with bloodstream infections. For adults, 20 to 30 mL of blood per culture set is recommended and may require more than two bottles depending on the system [6,22].

Rapid identification of microorganisms growing in blood culture bottles using a new proteomic technology, matrix-assisted laser desorption ionization–time of flight mass spectrometry (MALDI-TOF MS) is promising [23]. When urinary tract may be the source of fever, a urine specimen (aspirated from the catheter sampling port) should be obtained and evaluated by microscopy, and quantitative culture [6].

For patients with clinical suspicion of pneumonia, chest imaging with radiograph or CT scan is mandatory, and efforts should be made to obtain secretions for stains and cultures. Microscopic examination of pulmonary secretions may provide timely information about possible causative organisms. Results on Gram's staining and culture of sputum are positive in more than 80% of cases of pneumococcal pneumonia when a good-quality specimen (>10 inflammatory cells per epithelial cell) can be obtained before, or within 6 to 12 hours after, the initiation of antibiotics. The yield diminishes with increasing time after antibiotics have been initiated and with decreasing quality of the sputum sample [24]. Nebulization with hypertonic saline (the so-called induced sputum) may increase the likelihood of obtaining a valid sample. Techniques aimed at obtaining samples of secretions and tissue from the distal respiratory tract include protected and nonprotected bronchoalveolar lavage (BAL); transbronchial biopsy; protected specimen brush and telescoping plugged catheter; video-assisted lung biopsy; and open lung biopsy. Respiratory secretions from these sampling methods may use quantitative culture thresholds to improve the diagnostic accuracy. BAL is the preferred diagnostic approach, with a low rate of complications (2%) and a diagnostic yield between 30% and 90% depending on the type of population studied; prior antibiotic treatment; and the definition of pneumonia used [25].

In general, abnormal fluid collections (pleural effusion, joint effusion, and ascites) should be sampled for microscopic, hematologic, and chemical analysis, as well as microbiologic culture. Microbiologic yield from ascites culture has been shown to be greater when ascitic fluid is placed into blood culture or fungal isolator media [22]. Infection; crystal-induced disease; trauma; and a variety of systemic diseases can create a painful, swollen peripheral joint; arthrocentesis is indicated to establish the nature of the effusion [26]. Nosocomial bacterial meningitis may result from invasive procedures (e.g., craniotomy; placement of internal or external ventricular catheters; lumbar puncture; intrathecal infusions of medications; or spinal anesthesia), complicated head trauma, or in rare cases, metastatic infection in patients with hospital-acquired bacteremia. These cases of meningitis are caused by a different spectrum of microorganisms than cases acquired in the community setting. The diagnostic workup consists of neuroimaging; cerebrospinal fluid analysis (cell counts; Gram's staining; biochemical tests for glucose and protein; and cultures); and cultures of blood [27].

Computed tomography (CT) scan should be considered as one of the most useful imaging techniques in assessing intra-abdominal infections. Image quality and information can be optimized by the application of intravenous, oral, or rectal contrast [28].

Stool samples should be sent for determination of *C. difficile* toxin PCR for patients with diarrhea, fever and leukocytosis who received an antibacterial agent, proton pump inhibitor or *chemotherapy* 60 days before the onset of diarrhea [18].

A novel approach for determining the necessity and optimal duration of antibiotic therapy is the use of biomarkers, such as procalcitonin (PCT) levels, which become upregulated during bacterial infections and appear to mirror the severity of infections. Procalcitonin, the precursor peptide of the hormone calcitonin, is released ubiquitously in response to primarily bacterial toxins and bacteria-specific proinflammatory mediators, particularly interleukin 1b, tumor necrosis factor, and interleukin 6. In previous studies, a strong correlation was observed between the concentration of PCT and the extent and severity of bacterial infections.

PCT levels are routinely used as surrogate marker for bacterial infection to discontinue empiric antibacterial therapy for patients found to have low levels of this marker [29].

Two approaches that have gained particular attention for the diagnosis of invasive fungal infections are detection of 1,3-*β*-D-glucan (BDG) and galactomanan, major constituents of fungal cell walls, and polymerase chain reaction amplification of fungal DNA [30,31].

TREATMENT CONSIDERATIONS

Initial Antibiotic Therapy

Aggressive resuscitation bundles, adequate source control, appropriate antibiotic therapy, and organ support are cornerstones for the successful treatment of patients with severe sepsis [32]. Thus, intravenous antibiotic therapy should be started as early as possible and should cover all likely pathogens. It has not been determined whether combination antimicrobial therapy produces better outcomes than adequate single-agent antibiotic therapy in patients with severe sepsis. Current guidelines recommend combination antimicrobial therapy only for neutropenic sepsis and sepsis caused by *Pseudomonas* species. Empirical antifungal therapy should be used only for patients at high risk for invasive candidiasis. Antimicrobial therapy should be evaluated daily to optimize efficacy, prevent resistance, and avoid toxicity. Positive cultures may permit narrowing of the spectrum of antibiotic coverage or may dictate that additional organisms need to be covered by added antimicrobial therapy. Negative cultures of a patient who is unimproved yet stable on broad therapy indicate that antibiotics should be discontinued and the patient reevaluated. Negative cultures in a febrile patient who is unimproved or worsened may be a clue to disseminated fungal infection, and empiric antifungal therapy should be considered [33].

For an ICU patient, one should assume that in addition to the usual expected pathogens at a given site, infection is likely to involve more opportunistic hospital-associated pathogens, such as *S. aureus* (including methicillin-resistant *S. aureus* or MRSA) and coagulase-negative staphylococci; and multidrug-resistant enteric gram-negative bacilli and lactose nonfermenting gram-negative bacilli (e.g., *Pseudomonas aeruginosa* and *Acinetobacter* species) and yeast (*Candida* species) [34]. In light of possible impairment of mechanical and immunologic defenses and the presence of intravascular lines, the febrile ICU patient should be considered to be bacteremic until proven otherwise. Patients with intravascular lines and bacteremia should have their lines removed, if possible [35].

Once the spectrum of potential infecting organisms has been narrowed to one or a few likely candidates, empiric antibiotic therapy should be changed according to generally accepted principles as outlined later in the chapter (Table 71.3) [36].

Dosage and Route of Administration

A vast array of pathophysiologic changes can occur in critically ill patients that can complicate antibiotic dosing. As a rule, the intravenous route is preferred because of possible unreliable absorption from muscle and the gastrointestinal tract caused by impaired hemodynamics and/or gastrointestinal function [37].

Hydrophilic antibiotics (e.g., aminoglycosides, *β*-lactams, glycopeptides, and colistin) are mostly affected with the pathophysiologic changes observed among critically ill patients with increased volumes of distribution and altered drug clearance (related to changes in creatinine clearance). Lipophilic antibiotics

TABLE 71.3

Presumptive Antibiotic Therapy in the ICU or CCU Patient

Site/diagnosis	Potential causes	Initial therapy	Alternative therapy
Vascular/line-associated bacteremia	*Staphylococcus aureus*, GNR, coagulase-negative *staphylococci*	Vancomycin **plus** a third-generation cephalosporin[a]; suspect MRSA.	Linezolid **plus** a fluoroquinolone
Vascular/acute endocarditis	*S. aureus*, *Enterococcus* spp.	Vancomycin (modify according to susceptibilities MRSA, MSSA, VRE)	Linezolid or daptomycin; consider adding an aminoglycoside in *Enterococcus* spp. is the pathogen
Vascular/bacteremia	GNR	Third-generation cephalosporin[b] or imipenem or piperacillin–tazobactam	Linezolid **plus** fluoroquinolone
Pulmonary/pneumonia	GNR, *Haemophilus influenzae*, *Streptococcus pneumoniae*	Piperacillin–tazobactam or third/fourth-generation cephalosporin[b] **plus** metronidazole if anaerobes suspected	Imipenem or meropenem or ertapenem
Pulmonary/pneumonia	*S. aureus*	Vancomycin or linezolid until MRSA excluded	Cefazolin or oxacillin or nafcillin if MSSA
Pulmonary/pneumonia	*Legionella pneumophila*	Azithromycin or fluoroquinolone	Doxycycline or clarithromycin
Urinary tract/pyelonephritis	GNR, *Enterococcus* spp.	Third-generation cephalosporin[b] or fluoroquinolone	Aztreonam or ampicillin or piperacillin–tazobactam (if *Enterococcus* spp. suspected)
Abdomen/peritonitis, abscess, pelvic infection	GNR, anaerobes, *Enterococcus* spp.	Piperacillin–tazobactam or fluoroquinolone **plus** metronidazole	Vancomycin **plus** metronidazole **plus** aztreonam or imipenem or tigecycline
Abdominal/biliary tract	GNR, enterococcus, anaerobes (less often)	Piperacillin–tazobactam or fluoroquinolone **plus** metronidazole	Vancomycin **plus** metronidazole **plus** aztreonam or imipenem
CNS/meningitis (community acquired)	*Streptococcus pneumoniae*, *Neisseria meningitidis*	Ceftriaxone **plus** vancomycin	Vancomycin **plus** aztreonam
CNS/meningitis (elderly)	*S. pneumoniae*, *Listeria monocytogenes*, GNR	Ampicillin **plus** third-generation cephalosporin[b] possibly **plus** vancomycin	Vancomycin **plus** third-generation cephalosporin[b] or aztreonam **plus** trimethoprim–sulfamethoxazole if *Listeria* suspected
CNS/meningitis (nosocomial)	GNR, *S. aureus*, coagulase-negative *staphylococci*, *S. pneumoniae*	Vancomycin **plus** ceftazidime	Oxacillin[c] or nafcillin[c] **plus** ceftazidime or aztreonam
CNS/abscess	*S. aureus*, GNR, anaerobes, microaerophilic *Streptococcus* spp.	Third-generation cephalosporin[b] **plus** metronidazole **plus** vancomycin if MRSA suspected	Vancomycin **plus** metronidazole **plus** fluoroquinolone[b]
Sepsis syndrome	GNR, *S. aureus*	Piperacillin–tazobactam or ceftazidime **plus** vancomycin	Fluoroquinolone **plus** linezolid

[a]Gentamicin, tobramycin, or amikacin.
[b]Cefotaxime, ceftriaxone, or ceftazidime.
[c]Vancomycin if methicillin-resistant *S. aureus* common.
ICU, intensive care unit; CCU, coronary care unit; GNR, gram-negative rod; MRSA, methicillin-resistant *S. aureus*; MSSA, methicillin-sensitive *S. aureus*; VRE, vancomycin-resistant enterococci.

(e.g., fluoroquinolones, macrolides, tigecycline, and lincosamides) have lesser volume of distribution alterations, but may develop altered drug clearances. Augmented renal clearance (ARC) refers to the enhanced renal elimination of circulating solute (such as waste products and drugs). This is based in part on PK studies demonstrating elevated renal clearances of β-lactams, aminoglycosides, and glycopeptides among subsets of critically ill patients.

Dosing intervals for most antibiotics are selected so that the drugs are administered every three to four serum half-lives ($t_{½}$). Because most of the older parenterally administered β-lactam antibiotics have a $t_{½}$ of about 1 hour, intravenous penicillins and cephalosporins traditionally are given every 4 hours. However, the $t_{½}$ for cefazolin, cefotaxime, and ceftazidime is 1.5 to 2.5 hours, and these agents can be administered less frequently, perhaps ever 6 to 8 hours, even for serious infections; for ceftriaxone, the $t_{½}$ is 8 hours and the administration frequency is every 12 to 24 hours. In the clinical setting, β-lactam optimization strategies often include the use of a prolonged infusion (i.e., same dose administered over 3 to 4 hours) for each dosing interval or as a continuous infusion where the total daily dose is given at a constant rate over 24 hours. Each of these strategies has been reported to enhance the efficacy when compared to conventional regimens. Levofloxacin and the macrolide azithromycin are administered once a day (Table 71.2) [38,39].

Antimicrobial Therapy

Antimicrobial administration within the first hour of documented hypotension is associated with increased survival in adult patients with septic shock, and it should be initiated at maximal recommended doses for all patients with suspected life-threatening infections without delay [32].

Initial Therapy of a Life-Threatening Infection

A variety of studies including infected and septic patients show that inappropriate antimicrobial therapy is a consistent predictor of poor outcomes [6,40]. The choice of empirical therapy depends on the suspected site of infection and local microbial-susceptibility patterns. Inappropriate or delayed antibiotic treatment is associated with increased mortality. Thus, intravenous antibiotic therapy should be started as early as possible and should cover all likely pathogens. For example, suspected acute overwhelming infection of unknown or uncertain source of an ICU patient warrants therapy with vancomycin to cover *S. aureus*, including MRSA, plus a third-generation or fourth-generation cephalosporin or a fluoroquinolone to treat gram-negative bacilli. If hospital-acquired, ventilator-associated, or health care–associated pneumonia is likely, a fluoroquinolone such as levofloxacin or gatifloxacin along with piperacillin–tazobactam and vancomycin provides optimal coverage for gram-negative enteric bacilli; atypical bacterial pathogens, such as *Legionella*, *Chlamydia trachomatis*, and *Mycoplasma*; and MRSA [25,41]. In patients with febrile neutropenia, an antipseudomonal penicillin (piperacillin/tazobactam) or cephalosporin (ceftazidime or cefepime) or carbapenem (meropenem or imipenem) is recommended; vancomycin is added for clinical or bacteriologic evidence of MRSA, such as severe mucositis, catheter-related sepsis, and hypotension [42]. It is important when choosing empiric regimens to consider recent antibiotic therapy that might have resulted in selection of resistant pathogens. Empiric treatment must be streamlined once the cultures confirm a pathogen to avoid selection of resistant flora.

Therapy of Mixed Bacterial Infections

Combination therapy is necessary to provide a broad effective coverage in specific infections expected to involve diverse microorganisms. For example, intra-abdominal and intrapelvic infections frequently involve complex infecting flora, including aerobic and anaerobic pathogens. Definitive treatment of such infections often includes an extended spectrum β-lactam (ESBL) or a fluoroquinolone for members of the *Enterobacteriaceae* family; clindamycin or metronidazole for *Bacteroides fragilis* and other anaerobes; and ampicillin or piperacillin for enterococci. An alternative regimen particularly in the patient with known or suspected (long-term residence in the ICU or recent receipt of broad-spectrum antibiotic therapy) multiresistant gram-negative bacteria is meropenem, imipenem, or piperacillin/tazobactam [28,43].

Fungal Infections

Candida species are among the most common microorganisms isolated from patients with sepsis with 4.6 sepsis cases per 10,000 admissions. *Candida* bloodstream infections are associated with crude hospital mortality in the range of 40%. Trauma; burns; abdominal surgery; parenteral nutrition; broad-spectrum antibiotics; malignancy; cancer chemotherapy; and immunosuppressive therapy following major organ transplantation are factors that increase the risk of invasive fungal infections [43].

For neutropenic and transplant recipients, fungal pathogens like *Aspergillus* sp., *Fusarium* sp., *Trichosporon* sp., *Zygomycetes*, *Pseudallescheria boydii*, and dematiaceous fungi produce severe and often fatal infections [42,44].

Early recognition and aggressive medical therapy are key to the successful treatment of fungal infections.

Multidrug-resistant Organisms

Antimicrobial multidrug resistance (MDR) is now prevalent all over the world with extreme drug resistance (XDR) and pandrug resistance (PDR) being encountered increasingly often, especially among hospital acquired infections occurring in large highly specialized hospitals treating patients. Gram-negative bacilli resistance is a persistent problem in the ICU [34]. ESBLs have been identified for decades in the *Enterobacteriaceae*, particularly *Klebsiella* species, *Escherichia coli*, and *Proteus mirabilis*. CRE, or carbapenem-resistant Enterobacteriaceae, are a family of organisms that are difficult to treat because they have high levels of resistance to antibiotics. *Klebsiella* species and *Escherichia coli (E. coli)* are examples of Enterobacteriaceae, a normal part of the human gut bacteria that can become carbapenem-resistant. Types of CRE are sometimes known as KPC (*Klebsiella pneumoniae* carbapenemase) and NDM (New Delhi metallo-β-lactamase). KPC and NDM are enzymes that break down carbapenems and make them ineffective. Both of these enzymes, as well as the enzyme VIM (Verona integron–encoded Metallo-β-lactamase), have also been reported for Pseudomonas CDC. These organisms also typically carry other resistance genes and are frequently resistant to trimethoprim-sulfamethoxazole, fluoroquinolones, and aminoglycosides [34,45]. *Acinetobacter baumannii* is a major hospital-associated pathogen that causes a spectrum of diseases including respiratory tract, bloodstream, urinary tract, surgical site, and wound infections; *Acinetobacter baumannii* has a propensity to acquire resistance to multiple classes of antimicrobial agents, and treatment of infection by highly resistant strains can be extremely difficult [46].

Vancomycin-resistant *Enterococcus* species have emerged in the recent decades as a major nosocomial pathogen for patients with complications of prolonged hospitalization, intravenous lines, intra-abdominal surgery, on mechanical ventilation; or who received broad-spectrum antibiotics that are devoid of activity against enterococci. Linezolid, daptomycin, ceftaroline, and tigecycline are treatment options for the treatment of serious nosocomial infections caused by vancomycin-resistant enterococci [47].

Treatment of Fever

Several factors must be considered when determining whether to treat fever symptomatically using antipyretics. Although strong arguments exist for and against the treatment of fever, the currently available randomized trial literature does not support an outcome benefit from a particular fever management strategy. However, antipyretic therapy may relieve discomfort and decrease the metabolic rate associated with fever [48].

We recommend that antipyretic therapy be withheld unless the temperature exceeds 41°C.

Physical methods used to reduce temperature such as cooling blankets, ice packs, and intravascular cooling devices may produce shivering with an increase in metabolic demand and cause patient discomfort [9].

References

1. Beam LJ (ed): *Selected Aphorism*. Birmingham, AL, The Classics of Medicine Library, 1985.
2. Rehman T, deBoisblanc BP: Persistent fever in the ICU. *Chest* 145 (1):158–165, 2014.
3. Kiekkas P, Brokakali H, Theodorakopoulou G, et al: Physical antipyresis in critically ill adults. *Am J Nurs* 108(7):40–49, 2008.
4. Hua-Gang Z, Mehta K, Cohen P, et al: Hyperthermia on immune regulation. *Cancer Lett* 271(2):191–204, 2008.
5. Plaisance KL, Mackowiack PA: Antipyretic therapy; physiologic rationale, diagnostic implications and clinical consequences. *Arch Intern Med* 160(4):449–456, 2000.

6. O'Grady NP, Barie PS, Barlett JG, et al: Guidelines for evaluation of new fever in critically ill adult patients: 2008 update from the American College of Critical Care Medicine and the Infectious Disease Society of America. *Crit Care Med* 36(4):1330–1349, 2008.
7. Kushimoto S, Yamanouchi S, Endo T, et al: Body temperature abnormalities in non-neurological critically ill patients: a review of the literature. *J Intensive Care* 2:14, 2014.
8. Niven DJ, Stelfox HT, Shahpori R, et al: Fever in the adult ICUs: an interrupted time series analysis. *Crit Care Med* 41:1863–1869, 2013.
9. Niven DJ, Leger C, Stelfox HT, et al: Fever in the critically ill: a review of epidemiology, immunology, and management. *J Intensive Care Med* 27(5):290–297, 2012.
10. Angus DC, van der Poll T: Severe sepsis and septic shock. *N Engl J Med* 369:840–851, 2013.
11. Cooper MS, Stewart PM: Corticosteroid insufficiency in acutely ill patients. *N Engl J Med* 248(8):727–734, 2003.
12. Kosten TR, O'Connor PG: Management of drug and alcohol withdrawal. *N Engl J Med* 348(18):1786–1795, 2003.
13. Patel RA, Gallagher JC. Drug fever. *Pharmacotherapy* 30(1):57–69, 2010.
14. Foggo, Cavenagh J: Malignant causes of fever of unknown origin. *Clin Med* 15(3):292–294, 2015.
15. Munro N: Fever in acute and critical care: a diagnostic approach. *AACN Adv Crit Care* 25(3):237–248, 2014.
16. Barone JE: Fever: fact and fiction. *J Trauma* 67:406–409, 2009.
17. Magill SS, Edwards JR, Bamberg W, et al: Multistate point prevalence of health care associated infections. *N Engl J Med* 370:1198–1208, 2014.
18. Leffler DA, Lamont JT: Clostridium difficile infection. *N Engl J Med* 372;1539–1548, 2015.
19. Friedrich AK, Cahan M: Intraabdominal infections in the intensive care unit. *J Intensive Care Med* 29(5)247–254, 2013.
20. Lo, E, Nicolle LE, Coffin SE, et al: Strategies to prevent catheter associated urinary tract infections in acute care hospitals: 2014 update. *Infect Control Hosp Epidemiol* 35(5):464–479, 2014.
21. van Zanten ARH, Dixon JM, Nipshagen MD, et al: Hospital acquired sinusitis is a common cause of fever of unknown origin in orotracheally intubated critically ill patients. *Criti Care* 9:R583–R590, 2005.
22. Baron EJ, Miller JM, Weinstein MP, et al: A Guide to utilization of the microbiology laboratory for diagnosis of infectious diseases: 2013. Recommendations by the Infectious Diseases Society of America (IDSA) and the American Society for Microbiology (ASM). *Clin Infect Dis* 57(4):e21–e121, 2013.
23. Patel R: Matrix-assisted laser desorption ionization-time of flight mass spectrometry in clinical microbiology. *Clin Infect Dis* 57(4):564–572, 2013.
24. Musher DM, Thorner AR: Community-acquired pneumonia. *N Engl J Med* 371:1629–1628, 2014.
25. American Thoracic Society; Infectious Diseases Society of America: Guidelines for the management of adults with hospital acquired, ventilator associated, and health care associated pneumonia. *Am J Respir Crit Care Med* 171(4):388–416, 2004.
26. Margaretten ME, Kohlwes J, Moore D, et al: Does this adult patient have septic arthritis? *JAMA* 297(13):1478–1488, 2007.
27. Van de Beek D, Drake JM, Tunkel AR: Nosocomial bacterial meningitis. *N Engl J Med* 362:146–154, 2010.
28. Friedrich AKU, Cahan M: Intraabdominal infections in the intensive care unit. *J Intensive Care Med* 29(5):247–254, 2014.
29. Schuetz P, Chiappa V, Briel M, et al: Procalcitonin algorithms for antibiotic therapy decisions. *Arch Intern Med* 171(5):1322–1331, 2011.
30. Nguyen MH, Wissel MC, Shields RK, et al: Performance of Candida real time polymerase chain reaction, B-D-Glucan assay, and blood cultures in the diagnosis of invasive candidiasis. *Clin Infect Dis* 54(9):1240–1248, 2012.
31. Arvanitis M, Mylonakis E: Diagnosis of invasive aspergillosis: recent developments and ongoing challenges. *Eur J Clin Invest* 45(6):646–652, 2015.
32. Ferrer R, Martin-Loeches I, Phillips G, et al: Empiric antibiotic treatment reduces mortality in severe sepsis and septic shock from the first hour: result from a guideline-based performance improvement program. *Crit Care Med* 42:1749–1755, 2014.
33. Finfer SR, Vincent JL: Severe sepsis and septic shock. *N Engl J Med* 369:840–851, 2013.
34. Bassetti M, De Waele JJ, Eggiman P, et al: Preventive and therapeutic strategies in critically ill patients with highly resistant bacteria. *Intensive Care Med* 41:776–795, 2015.
35. Mermet LA, Allon M, Bouza E, et al: Clinical practice guidelines for the diagnosis and management of intravascular catheter-related infections: 2009 Update by the Infectious Disease Society of America. *Clin Infect Dis* 49(5):491–545, 2009.
36. Bochud PY, Bonten M, Marchetti O, et al: Antimicrobial therapy for patients with severe sepsis and septic shock: an evidence-based review. *Crit Care Med* 32[11, Suppl]:S495–S512, 2004.
37. Udy A, Roberts JA, Lipman J: Clinical implications of antibiotic pharmacokinetic principles in the critically ill. *Intensive Care Med* 39:2070–2082, 2013.
38. Bassetti M, Nicolau DP, Calandra T: What's new in antimicrobial use and resistance in critically ill patients? *Intensive Care Med* 40:422–426, 2014.
39. Roberts JA, Lippman J: Pharmocokinetic issues for antibiotics in the critically ill patient.*Crit Care Med* 37:840–851, 2014.
40. Kumar A, Roberts D, Wood KE, et al: Duration of hypotension before initiation of effective antimicrobial therapy is the critical determinant of survival in human septic shock. *Crit Care Med* 34(6):1589–1596, 2006.
41. File TM: Recommendations for treatment of hospital acquired and ventilator associated pneumonia: review of recent international guidelines. *Clin Infec Dis* 51(S1): S42–S47, 2010.
42. Freifeld AG, Bow EJ, Sepkowitz KA, et al: Clinical practice guideline for the use of antimicrobial agents in neutropenic patients with cancer: 2010 update by the Infectious Disease Society of America. *Clin Infect Dis* 54(4):e53–e96, 2011.
43. Solomkin GS, Mazuski JE, Bradley JS, et al: Diagnosis and management of complicated intraabdominal infections in adults and children: guidelines by the Surgical Infection Society and the Infectious Disease Society of America. *Clin Infec Dis* 50:133–164, 2010.
44. Low CY, Rotstein C: Emerging fungal infection in immunocompromised patients. *F1000 Med Rep* 3:14, 2011. http://f1000.com/reports/m/3/14. Accessed June 1, 2017.
45. Mehrad B, Clark NM, Zhanel GG, et al: Antimicrobial resistance in hospital-acquired gram-negative bacterial infections. *Chest* 147(5):1413–1421, 2015.
46. Qureshi ZA, Hittle LE, O'Hara JA, et al: Colistin-resistant *Acinetobacter baumannii*: beyond carbapenem resistance. *Clin Infec Dis* 60(9):1295–1303, 2015.
47. Arias CA, Murray BE: Emergence and management of drug resistant enterococcal infections. *Expert Rev Anti Infect Ther* 6(5):637–655, 2008.
48. Henker R, Carlson KK: Fever: applying research to bedside practice. *AACN Adv Crit Care* 18(1):76–87, 2007.

Chapter 72 ■ Prevention and Control of Healthcare-Acquired Infections in the Intensive Care Unit

SUMANTH GANDRA • RICHARD T. ELLISON, III

INTRODUCTION

Preventing healthcare-acquired infections in intensive care units (ICUs) is a daily concern of physicians providing care for critically ill patients. Patients in ICUs are at increased risk of infection for multiple reasons including their underlying illness, the use of medical devices for organ system support and hemodynamic monitoring, impaired nutritional status that contributes to immune function compromise, and ongoing exposure to hospital resident antibiotic-resistant bacterial flora. The focus of this chapter is to review the general epidemiology of these infections, the factors contributing to their development, preventive strategies, and important characteristics of key healthcare-acquired pathogens.

EPIDEMIOLOGY OF HEALTHCARE-ACQUIRED ICU INFECTIONS

Studies performed over the last three decades have found that infections in ICU patients are both common and significant. Work by Craven and colleagues in the early 1980s at Boston City Hospital in adult medical and surgical ICUs found that overall, 28% of the patients developed at least one nosocomial infection, and that infected patients had threefold increases in mortality compared to those not infected [1]. In another single medical ICU study performed in the United States over 20 months in 2000 to 2001, 42% of patients requiring at least 48 hours of ICU care had a microbiologically confirmed infection, and patients with infection had a 1.9-fold increased risk of in-hospital mortality ($p < 0.001$) [2]. Similarly, in 2007, European investigators assessed the prevalence of infections among adults ICUs in a multinational survey involving 14,414 patients in 1,265 ICUs from 75 countries on one single day (the EPIC II Study), and found that 51% of patients were infected [3]. In the same study, the mortality was twice among patients infected than those not infected (25% vs. 11%; $p < 0.001$). More recently, in 2011, a multistate point prevalence survey of healthcare-associated infections by the Centers for Disease Control and Prevention (CDC) from 183 hospitals in the United States involving 11,282 patients found that 34.5% of healthcare-associated infections occurred in ICUs [4].

The types of infection seen in ICU patients have varied slightly over time and between types of ICU units, but several types of infections have predominated. In the Boston City Hospital study, pneumonia, surgical wound infections, urinary tract infections (UTIs), and bloodstream infections (BSIs) were the most frequent infections [1]. Klevens and colleagues, using a multi-step approach, estimated 394,288 hospital-associated infections among adults and children in ICU in 2002 from US hospitals. The infection rate per 1,000 patient-days was 13.0, among all, UTI was the highest (3.38) followed by pneumonia (3.33) and BSI (2.71) [5]. In the EPIC II study, among 7, 087 patients with infection in adult ICUs, the principal site of infections were respiratory tract (63.5%), abdomen (19.6%), bloodstream (15.1%) and urinary tract (14.3%) [3]. The use of medical devices is a predominant cause of infection in the ICU setting, and major concerns are pneumonia associated with mechanical ventilation, UTIs associated with urinary catheterization, and primary BSIs linked to central venous catheters.

The National Healthcare Safety Network (NHSN) of the CDC assesses device-associated infections in various types of ICUs in the US yearly using standardized surveillance definitions. According to NHSN data, in 2013 the pooled mean of central line–associated bloodstream infections (CLABSIs) in various ICUs was 0.99 per 1,000 central line days [6]. Similarly, for catheter-associated urinary tract infections (CAUTI) in 2013, the pooled mean was 2.3 per 1,000 urinary catheter days but with a higher mean of 5.3 per 1,000 central line days in neurosurgical units [6]. For ventilator-associated pneumonia (VAP), in 2012, the pooled mean was 1.32 per ventilator days with the highest rate in in burn units and lowest in pediatric cardiothoracic units [7]. The variation of rates for device-associated infections between different types of critical care units is likely related to the size of the unit (small vs. large), the type of more predominant device use (urinary catheters, endotracheal tubes, and vascular catheters), the age group of the patients (pediatric vs. adults), and the most predominant illness of the patients (coronary, surgical, burn, medical, pediatric). Pediatric ICUs differ from adult ICUs in many ways. First, they are typically combined units (medical and surgical). Second, their beds are not commonly physically separated as in adult ICU beds. Third, pediatric patients usually have less comorbid conditions than adults.

Infections rates in ICUs among developing countries are high when compared to developed countries. A systematic review of studies on healthcare-associated infections in developing countries from 1995 through 2008 reported a healthcare-associated infection density in adult ICUs as 47.9 per 1,000 patient-days, which is three times that of US ICUs [8]. More recently, the International Nosocomial Infection Control Consortium (INICC) surveillance study from January 2007 through December 2012 reported on device-associated healthcare-associated infections in 503 ICUs in 43 countries from Latin America, Asia, Africa, and Europe [9]. In this study, the device utilization rates in ICUs in developing countries were similar to those of the United States; however, infection rates were significantly higher. In corresponding ICUs, the pooled rate of VAP was nearly 16 times (16.8 vs. 1.1 per 1,000 ventilator days), CLABSI was five times (4.9 vs. 0.9 per 1,000 central line days) and CAUTI was nearly four times (5.5 vs. 1.3 per 1,000 catheter days) the US rates in 2012 [9].

MICROBIOLOGY OF ICU INFECTIONS

The predominant causes of ICU infections are a limited number of bacterial and fungal pathogens. In general, the pathogens that are seen can be characterized as those that survive well in a moist environment (e.g., gram-negative bacteria including *Enterobacter* strains, *Pseudomonas aeruginosa*, and *Acinetobacter* species), those that colonize the skin and produce biofilm to allow adherence to catheters and other devices (e.g., *Staphylococcus aureus* and coagulase-negative staphylococci), and those which are resistant to commonly used antibiotics (e.g., methicillin-resistant *S. aureus* [MRSA], vancomycin-resistant enterococci [VRE], multidrug-resistant [MDR] gram-negative bacteria, and Candida species). In the EPIC II study, gram-negative organisms were predominantly isolated (62%), followed by gram-positive (47%) and fungal organisms (19%). Among gram-positives, *S. aureus* was most common (20%), and among gram-negative organisms *Pseudomonas* species were most commonly isolated

(20%) followed by *Escherichia coli* (16%). Overall, *S. aureus* was the single most common organism isolated (20%) and 50% of these strains were MRSA [3]. The NHSN 2009 to 2010 data on healthcare-associated infections occurring in both ICU and non-ICU settings show that *S. aureus* was the most common (15.6%) organism isolated, followed by *E. coli* (11.5%) and coagulase-negative *Staphylococci* (11.4%) [10]. When reviewed by type of infection, in CLABSIs, the coagulase-negative *Staphylococci* were the most common organisms followed by *S. aureus*. In CAUTIs, *E. coli* was the most common pathogen followed by *P. aeruginosa*, and in VAP, *S. aureus* was the most common organism followed by *P. aeruginosa*. In contrast to US NHSN data, the INICC surveillance study of developing countries showed that all device-associated infections were predominantly caused by gram-negative organisms. In CLABSIs, *Klebsiella pneumoniae* was the most common organism followed by *Acinetobacter baumannii*; for CAUTIs, *E. coli* was the most common organism followed by *K. pneumoniae*; and for VAP, *A. baumannii* was the most common organism followed by *P. aeruginosa* [9].

Antimicrobial resistance patterns among the pathogens seen with device-associated infections for both the United States and developing countries show a high frequency of MDR organisms [9,10]. Although there is variation among institutions and sites of infections, common pathogens reported in the NHSN and INICC data include MRSA, VRE, third-generation cephalosporin-resistant Enterobacteriaceae, and MDR *P. aeruginosa* and *A. baumannii*. In addition, carbapenem-resistant Enterobacteriaceae are being seen more frequently.

RISK FACTORS

The length of ICU stay is the predominant risk factor for nosocomial infection followed by the use of medical devices. In the EPIC II study, the infection rate increased from 32% for patients with ICU stay of 0 or 1 day prior to the study day to more than 70% in patients with ICU stay of more than 7 days prior to the study day [3]. The NHSN nosocomial infection rates for pneumonia, BSIs, and UTIs have correlated strongly with device usage [5,11]. Other risk factors identified in the EPIC II study include the severity of patient's underlying illness, increasing age, renal replacement therapy, and presence of comorbid conditions (like chronic obstructive pulmonary disease (COPD), cancer, HIV, and immunosuppression). Teaching hospitals with higher rates of device utilization have had higher device-associated infection rates [5,11]. Similar to adults, risk factors for nosocomial infection for pediatric ICU patients include length of stay in ICU, rate of device utilization, severity of underlying illness, and parenteral nutrition [12].

Hyperglycemia has also been considered a risk factor for infections in the ICU. Hyperglycemia is common in the ICU setting because of underlying disease, physiologic stress, and parenteral nutritional support. In vitro investigations suggest that hyperglycemia can impair polymorphonuclear leukocyte and monocyte phagocytic and bactericidal activities [13]. However, this assumption has not been confirmed as both systematic reviews and meta-analyses have found no effect of intensive glucose control on the infection rates of ICUs [14,15].

PREVENTIVE AND CONTROL MEASURES

A number of approaches have been found to help prevent ICU-associated infections. The comprehensive use of standard infection control practices as well as enhanced infection control precautions for selected pathogens, limiting the use of medical devices, and careful attention to architectural design are key components of strategies to prevent ICU infections. Additionally, the implementation of targeted quality improvement programs for central vascular catheter infections and VAP has been shown to be an highly effective approach for decreasing infection rates.

Infection Control Precautions

Isolation Precautions

The CDC and the Hospital Infection Control Practices Advisory Committee have prepared guidelines on isolation precautions to prevent the transmission of microorganisms from colonized or infected patients to other patients, visitors, and health care workers (HCWs) [16]. The current guidelines were last updated in 2007, and recommend a two-tiered approach to patient care. Standard precautions are used for the care for all patients. Additional more stringent transmission-based precautions are used for the care of patients who are suspected or known to be colonized or infected with specific pathogens that are readily transmitted either through direct contact, through large respiratory droplets, or through smaller airborne particles. The current guidelines are summarized in Table 72.1. Contact precautions are commonly

TABLE 72.1

Isolation Precautions

		Transmission-based		
	Standard	**Airborne**	**Droplet**	**Contact**
Definition	Reduce risk of transmission of bloodborne pathogens and pathogens from moist body substances, and apply to all patients	Prevent transmission of disease by airborne droplet nuclei ($\leq 5\ \mu m$ size)	Reduce risk of transmission of microorganisms by droplets ($\geq 5\ \mu m$ size) generated by the patient sneezing, coughing, talking, or performance of procedure	Reduce transmission of epidemiologic important organisms from an infected or colonized patient through direct or indirect contact
Room		Private-negative pressure room with air exhausted to outdoors or through high-efficient filtration; door kept closed	Private room; door may remain open	Private room or cohorted with a patient with similar organism. Patient care items should be dedicated to a single patient

(continued)

TABLE 72.1 (*continued*)

Isolation Precautions

	Standard	Transmission-based: Airborne	Transmission-based: Droplet	Transmission-based: Contact
Mask	Mask, goggles, and face shields provide barrier protection to reduce the transmission of pathogens when splashes or spray of blood, body fluids, secretions, or excretions are likely	N95 mask or comparable respirator. Surgical mask should be worn by the patient during transportation outside the negative pressure room	Mask if entering the room	
Gowns	Provide barrier protection, prevent contamination of clothing, and protect the skin of personnel from blood and body fluid exposures			
Gloves	Anticipated blood, body fluid, secretions/excretions, nonintact skin, contaminated items, and mucous membranes			
Hand hygiene	Before and after patient contact; immediately after glove removal; after contact with blood, body fluids, secretions/excretions, or mucous membranes			
Suspected or Confirmed Pathogens	Used for all patients independent of the presence of known pathogens	Tuberculosis Varicella SARS Measles Disseminated Zoster Viral hemorrhagic fevers (including Ebola) Smallpox Monkeypox Avian influenza	Meningitis due to *Neisseria meningitides* or *Haemophilus influenzae* Diphtheria (pharyngeal) Pertussis Mumps *Mycoplasma pneumoniae* Pneumonic plague Streptococcal (Group A) pharyngitis, pneumonia Influenza Rubella Parvovirus B19	MDR bacterial (MRSA, VRE, GISA, VRSA, gram-negative bacilli) *C. difficile* Viral hemorrhagic fevers (including Ebola) Scabies Lice HSV (neonatal; disseminated) Disseminated Zoster

SARS, severe acute respiratory syndrome; MDR, multidrug-resistant; MRSA, methicillin-resistant *Staphylococcus aureus*; VRE, vancomycin-resistant enterococci; GISA, glycopeptide-intermediate *Staphylococcus aureus*; VRSA, vancomycin-resistant *Staphylococcus aureus*; HSV, herpes simplex virus.

used in ICUs to decrease the transmission of MDR bacteria such as MRSA, VRE, extended-spectrum beta-lactamase (ESBL)-producing bacteria, and carbapenem-resistant gram-negative bacteria. However, routine use of contact precautions for all patients in ICUs is debatable. A recent large cluster randomized study found that the universal use of contact precautions for all ICU patients did not reduce the primary combined end point of MRSA or VRE acquisition compared to baseline rates, although this study did not assess acquisition of other antibiotic-resistant organisms [17].

Hand Hygiene

A key component of these infection control guidelines is the need for healthcare workers to practice good hand hygiene [16,18]. Approaches that have been shown to improve compliance with this practice have included the provision of water-free alcohol-based hand rubs throughout institutions, an intensified educational programs on hand hygiene, and electronic monitoring programs [19,20] Alcohols have excellent in vitro germicidal activity against gram-positive and gram-negative pathogens, fungi, and many viruses including HIV, influenza virus, and respiratory syncytial virus (RSV). Alcohol-based hand rubbing is recommended in all clinical situations except when the hands are visibly soiled. Alcohol is inactive against *Clostridium difficile* spores. However, there has been no association between the use of alcohol-based hand hygiene and the incidence of *C. difficile* disease [21]. Consequently, other than in outbreak settings, routine alcohol-based hand hygiene is still recommended when caring for *C. difficile* patients [22]. An ongoing issue remains the relatively low rate of hand hygiene activity by healthcare workers and ongoing effort is necessary to promote this practice.

Antimicrobial Bathing

Patients in the ICU are major reservoirs of MDR organisms and decreasing this reservoir would lead to a decrease in the risk of nosocomial transmission. Accordingly, recent work has assessed the performance of daily bathing of patients with chlorhexidine gluconate using either impregnated clothes or dilute bathing solutions. Both a meta-analysis and several multicenter trials have found that this approach can decrease the incidence of BSIs and contribute to reducing transmission of MDR organisms [23–26]. However, a recent pragmatic trial in a single center that already had a low incidence of healthcare-acquired infections did not find additional benefit to this practice [27].

Environmental Cleaning

Although not associated with alterations in infection rates, the institution of programs to monitor the actual performance of housekeeping staff has been found to improve disinfection in the hospital environment in ICUs, including disinfection of computer stations [28]. "No touch" automated room disinfection methods using hydrogen peroxide vapor or ultraviolet (UV) light have been shown to reduce the rate of pathogen transmission between patients compared to conventional cleaning methods [29–32]. Whether this reduced rate of pathogen transmission among ICU patients using automated room disinfection methods would result in a significant reduction in the occurrence of healthcare-associated infections is yet to be shown. Still, several single-center retrospective studies using automated room disinfection methods have reported a significant decrease in hospital acquisition of MDR organisms and *C. difficile*, and there is a need for prospective multicenter cluster randomized studies to confirm these findings [33–36].

In addition to these automated disinfection methods, there has been interest in self-disinfecting antimicrobial surfaces because of the potential ability to prevent recolonization by microorganisms. Recently, a randomized control study in the United States in three ICUs in three hospitals showed a significant reduction in the incidence of hospital-acquired infections and or MRSA or VRE colonization (0.071 vs. 0.128; p = .020) among patients admitted to patient rooms with copper alloy on high touch surfaces [37]. However, additional randomized control studies are needed to confirm the efficacy of this expensive approach.

Randomized control trials involving various infection prevention measures and their findings are summarized in Table 72.2.

Architectural Design and Hospital Construction

Modern ICU design includes the use of single patient rooms, adequate physical space for equipment and personnel, individual patient sinks, adequate hand hygiene stations, and adequate room ventilation with filtered air and at least six air changes per hour [38]. Additionally, there are defined guidelines for the design of airborne isolation infection rooms for patients requiring management of tuberculosis or other infections readily transmitted by the airborne route.

Ongoing construction and renovation activities in healthcare facilities have also been recognized as significant risk factors for infections with environmental pathogens. There can be concerns with environmental gram-negative organisms, particularly *Legionella* species. More frequent is a concern with disease caused by environmental molds, in particular *Aspergillus* species [38,39]. US healthcare institutions are now required to have procedures in place to ascertain that construction and renovation activities are performed in a manner that protects patients from being exposed to environmental pathogens [38].

Infection Control Surveillance Programs

In 1970, the CDC initiated the National Nosocomial Infection Surveillance system (NNIS) as an approach to identifying secular trends in these infections. The program initially included 10 to 20 hospitals, but expanded to nearly 300 hospitals. Subsequent studies that analyzed healthcare-acquired infection rates at differing institutions before and after the distribution of infection rate data found that institutional infection rates diminished after institutions were made aware of their infection rates [40,41]. In the last 5 years, all US hospitals have been required to report hospital-acquired infection rates to the second-generation

TABLE 72.2

Summary of Randomized Control Trials of Various Infection Prevention Measures in Preventing ICU Acquired Infections

Chlorhexidine Gluconate (CHG) bathing and risk of ICU acquired infections

Intervention	Year	Study	Patients	Findings	References
CHG bathing +nasal mupirocin + SDD with polymixin E & tobramycin	1996–1998	multicenter placebo-controlled randomized double-blind study	416	Lower incidence of all ICU acquired infections in the intervention group	[89]
Daily CHG bathing	2007–2009	multicenter cluster-randomized crossover	7727	Nosocomial bacteremia decreased in CHG group	[24]
Daily CHG bathing in pediatric patients	2008–2010	multicenter cluster-randomized crossover	4947	Lower incidence of bacteremia in CHG group	[25]
Daily CHG bathing + nasal mupirocin for 5 days	2010–2011	multicenter cluster-randomized	74,256	Lower incidence of bacteremia due to any pathogen in CHG+ nasal mupirocin group	[26]
Daily CHG bathing	2012–2013	single center cluster-randomized crossover	9340	No benefit	[27]

Contact Precautions for all ICU patients and acquisition of MRSA and VRE

Intervention	Year	Study	Patients	Findings	References
Contact isolation precautions for all ICU patients	2012	matched pair cluster randomized trial	26,180	No benefit	[17]

Copper surfaces in ICU and risk of ICU acquired infections

Intervention	Year	Study	Patients	Findings	References
Copper alloy surfaces for six high touched areas	2010–2011	multicenter randomized trial	614	Lower incidence of ICU acquired infections including MRSA and VRE colonization	[37]

ICU = Intensive care unit; SDD = Selective digestive decontamination surveillance program, the NHSN, and with this requirement there has been an ongoing reduction in the rate of CLABSIs nationally [11,42]. Disseminating data in a simple and routine manner, to those who need to know, enables clinicians to make decisions on the basis of scientific data and to alter practice.

Quality Improvement Initiatives

A major advance in medical care in the last decade has been the adoption of quality improvement strategies used in other industries such as air transportation. The development of standardized approaches to the provision of care has been particularly effective in the prevention of device-related infections in the ICU stetting. Several institutions have documented a significant reduction in BSIs linked to central venous catheters after the implementation of quality improvement programs targeted against these infections [43,44]. Principal components of these programs have included providing education on appropriate infection control practices to staff involved in central catheter placement and care, standardizing the location of catheter placement to preferentially use the subclavian location and avoid femoral lines when possible, centralizing the location of all equipment required for catheter placement, the use of maximal sterile-barrier precautions (i.e., use of cap, surgical masks, sterile gowns, sterile gloves, and large sterile drapes) during catheter insertion, and trying to remove these catheters as quickly as possible [44–47].

A similar approach has been taken to prevent VAP in the ICU with the use of targeted education programs [48–50]. These quality improvement education programs have in general followed CDC guidelines on measures to prevent healthcare-acquired pneumonia and have been directed at medical staff, ICU nursing staff, and respiratory therapists. Key elements of the program include a focus on hand hygiene, maintaining the patient in a semi-recumbent position with the head of the bed elevated 30 degrees, standardizing the approach to changing ventilator circuitry, avoiding nasal intubations, avoiding gastric distension, removing nasogastric tubes, and weaning patients as rapidly as possible [48].

SELECTED HEALTHCARE-ACQUIRED PATHOGENS

Clostridium difficile-Associated Colitis

C. difficile is the most frequent etiology for healthcare-acquired diarrhea. In 2011, an estimated 453,000 cases and 29,300 deaths occurred in the United States with more than two-thirds of cases being healthcare associated [51]. The organism may asymptomatically colonize the gut or cause illness extending from watery diarrhea through pseudomembranous colitis, toxic megacolon, perforation, and even death [52,53]. Transmission in the healthcare setting appears to occur through transient hand carriage of HCW, close contact with other colonized or infected patients, or exposure to spores present on contaminated environmental surfaces [53,54]. Exposure to antibiotics increases the risk of developing disease. Practically all antibiotics have been implicated in the development of clostridium difficile associated diarrhea (CDAD), but disease is especially common with clindamycin, penicillins, and cephalosporins.

At least part of the increasing incidence can be linked to the spread of a specific *C. difficile* strain, BI/NAP1/027, which is associated with severe disease, excess mortality, and epidemic outbreaks [55,56]. In 2011, among 453,000 *C. difficile* cases, NAP1/027 accounted for an estimated 30.7% and 18.8% of the healthcare and community-associated infections, respectively [51]. It is unclear why this strain has spread so widely; however, there is evidence that it has increased virulence because of increased production of the *C. difficile* A and B toxins, and has also acquired resistance to fluoroquinolone antibiotics which are used widely for treatment of UTI and community-acquired pneumonia [57].

Approaches to the prevention of CDAD are directed toward preventing horizontal transmission of the pathogen, as well as reducing the individual patient's risks of disease if they acquire the organism through the judicious use of antibiotic therapy. Barrier methods remain fundamental to prevention of spread, as well as the use of private rooms or cohorting CDAD patients. Alcohol hand hygiene preparations are not active against bacterial spores, including those of *C. difficile*, but clinical studies have shown no association between the use of alcohol-based hand hygiene and the incidence of *C. difficile* [21]. Therefore, the use of soap and water for enhanced mechanical clearance during hand hygiene should be considered in the setting of increased transmission of *C. difficile* [22]. Healthcare workers should wear gloves when caring for patients with CDAD, and the use of gowns is also recommended when soiling of the patient's cloth is likely [18,58]. In addition to the above infection control measures, implementing antimicrobial stewardship programs which limit inappropriate antibiotic use has been associated with decreases in the incidence of CDAD [59,60].

Thorough environmental cleaning is critical, as *C. difficile* spores can live for several months on hospital dry surfaces. Commonly used hospital cleaning agents such as quaternary ammonium–based detergents are ineffective in killing *C. difficile* spores [61]. Use of 10% sodium hypochlorite solution is effective in reducing environmental contamination with *C. difficile* spores and is associated with decreased clostridium difficile infection (CDI) rates [62,63]. Other novel strategies reported for environmental decontamination include hydrogen peroxide vapor, UV light decontamination, and copper-coated surfaces [36,64,65]. Whether these approaches will decrease nosocomial CDI rates remains to be studied in clinical trials.

Methicillin-Resistant *Staphylococcus aureus*

The prevalence of MRSA in ICUs in the United States has risen, from an incidence of 30% to 40% in the middle of the 1990s to over 60% in 2004 [66]. However, compared to 2005, the estimated national incidence of hospital-onset MRSA infections in the United States in 2011 decreased by 54% (9.91 vs. 4.54 cases per 100,000 persons) [67]. Similarly, all-cause mortality rates due to hospital-onset invasive MRSA infections decreased from 2.7 per 100, 000 persons in 2005 to 1 per 100, 000 persons in 2011 [67]. The decrease in incidence is likely due to increased implementation of infection prevention measures, especially targeting intravascular catheter-related infections [68]. There has been also a change in the frequency of infections caused by different MRSA strains. Infections due to community-associated MRSA strains are increasing in hospital settings (including ICUs), are becoming endemic, and are replacing the traditional hospital strains of MRSA [69,70]. Risk factors associated with acquisition of healthcare-acquired strains of MRSA include recent hospitalization, hemodialysis, and residence in a long-term facility or injection drug use.

Current CDC guidelines recommend the use of "contact precautions" for patients known or suspected to be colonized with epidemiologically important organisms [16]. However, the use of contact precautions for endemic MRSA remains controversial [71,72]. Contact precautions have been used as a part of multiple control measures and unfortunately, there are no randomized control trials comparing contact precautions versus standard precautions alone in the acquisition of MDR organisms. Few quasi-experimental before and after studies report no change in MRSA or VRE transmission and no change in rates of MRSA or VRE device-associated infections with removal of contact precautions for MRSA and VRE-colonized or infected patients [73,74]. In addition, a recent cluster randomized study on measures to prevent MRSA infections found that "vertical" measures targeting a specific organism were inferior to "horizontal" measures active against multiple organisms such as universal decolonization and daily chlorhexidine bathing [26]. However, in the setting of outbreaks of MRSA, institutions may also consider instituting patient/staff cohorting, decolonization of patients with topical nasal mupirocin and total body chlorhexidine baths/showers, and screening healthcare workers for MRSA colonization [75]. Enhanced infection control policy with stringent contact precautions has been recommended for patients with vancomycin-resistant *S. aureus* (VRSA) [76].

Vancomycin-Resistant Enterococci

VRE was first recognized in Europe in 1988 and in the United States soon thereafter. By 1993, there was a 20-fold increase in VRE prevalence in ICUs in the United States [77]. A recent meta-analysis of 37 published studies estimated that the prevalence of VRE on admission to adult ICUs was 8.8% [78]. In 2009 to 2010 NHSN data, 84% and 82% of *Enterococcus faecium* isolates obtained from CLABSI and CAUTI, respectively, were vancomycin resistant. Whereas, 9% and 6% of *Enterococcus faecalis* isolates obtained from CLABSI and CAUTI, respectively, were vancomycin resistant [10]. Although not as virulent a pathogen as MRSA, VRE can cause infections in the debilitated ICU patient. Also, as the gene inducing vancomycin resistance in VRE, *vanA*, can be transferred to *S. aureus*, the presence of VRE in ICU patients increases the potential for the emergence of VRSA strains [79]. Risk factors for VRE colonization are previous hospitalization, glycopeptide administration, colonization pressure, and patients with comorbid conditions [80]. Similar to MRSA, the use of contact precautions for endemic VRE remains controversial and there are no randomized control trials comparing contact precautions versus standard precautions alone in the acquisition of VRE. Quasi-experimental studies involving removal of contact precautions for patients colonized or infected with VRE did not have effects on VRE transmission or device-associated infection rates [73,74]. Horizontal measures probably play a more significant role than contact precautions in limiting the transmission of VRE.

Multidrug-Resistant Gram-Negative Bacilli

According to NHSN, gram-negative bacteria belonging to Enterobacteriaceae family and organisms like *P. aeruginosa* and *A. baumannii* are frequent cause of healthcare-associated infections in 2009 to 2010 in the United States [10]. There is a growing concern of increasing multidrug resistance among gram-negative bacteria, particularly the rapid global spread of carbapenem-resistance caused by carbapenemases in Enterobacteriaceae (CRE) [81]. This has been facilitated by mobile genetic elements harboring genes encoding for carbapenemases such as *Klebsiella pneumoniae* carbapenemase (KPC) and metallo-β-lactamases (like New Delhi Metallo-β-lactamase-1—NDM1). The proportion of CRE isolation in healthcare-associated infections increased from 1.2% in 2001 to 4.2% in 2011 in NNIS/NHSN [82]. This is concerning because of the frequency of infections caused by the Enterobacteriaceae family, limited number of options for treating CRE infections, and high mortality associated with these infections. The risk factors for acquisition of CRE include ICU stay, residence in long-term acute care (LTAC) facilities, presence of indwelling devices, antimicrobial exposure (carbapenems, extended-spectrum cephalosporins, fluoroquinolones), CRE colonization pressure, severity of illness, and immunosuppression/organ transplantation [83–86]. Current CDC interim surveillance definition (which could be subjected to change soon) for CRE includes any Enterobacteriaceae that is non-susceptible to one of the three carbapenems (doripenem, meropenem, imipenem) and resistant to all three third-generation cephalosporins (ceftriaxone, cefotaxime, and ceftazidime) [87]. Currently, active surveillance for asymptomatic rectal CRE colonization is not recommended routinely. However, it can be considered in the setting of an outbreak and for high-risk patients (admission to LTAC facilities, ICUs). Infection control measures for patients colonized or infected with CRE should include strict contact precautions, minimizing use of invasive devices, antimicrobial stewardship, and other general measures like hand hygiene and chlorhexidine bathing [87].

P. aeruginosa is the fifth most common pathogen isolated from device-associated healthcare-associated infections in 2009 to 2010 NHSN data. MDR *P. aeruginosa* isolates ranged from a minimum of 5% in surgical site infections to a maximum of 18% in VAP [10]. Similarly, *A. baumannii* is one of the most common pathogens isolated from device-associated healthcare-associated infections. Overall, it is the fourteenth most common organism isolated from device-associated infections and it is the fifth most common gram-negative pathogen isolated from VAP in 2009 to 2010 NHSN data. MDR *A. baumannii* isolates ranged from a minimum of 44% for surgical site infections to a maximum of 78% for CAUTI [10]. Unfortunately, this organism survives well in the environment, and has been associated with significant ICU outbreaks. Infections due to this organism are associated with poor outcomes, including higher rates of morbidity and mortality, and higher medical expenses. Control measures involve the use of "contact precautions" and enhanced environmental cleaning efforts [16,88].

Given this rapidly increasing incidence of resistant gram-negative strains, it is important for institutions to track rates of antibiotic resistance in their ICUs independent of overall institutional antibiotic resistance rates. Empiric antibiotic coverage for gram-negative pathogens in given ICUs should be targeted at the known gram-negative pathogens present in the environment. Enhanced infection control contact precautions should be used for patients who are colonized or infected with ESBL- or KPC- or NDM-positive gram-negative pathogens or MDR *P. aeruginosa* or *A. baumannii*.

References

1. Craven DE, Kunches LM, Lichtenberg DA, et al: Nosocomial infection and fatality in medical and surgical intensive care unit patients. *Arch Internal Med* 148(5):1161–1168, 1988.
2. Osmon S, Warren D, Seiler SM, et al: The influence of infection on hospital mortality for patients requiring > 48 h of intensive care. *Chest* 124(3):1021–1029, 2003.
3. Vincent JL, Rello J, Marshall J, et al: International study of the prevalence and outcomes of infection in intensive care units. *JAMA* 302(21):2323–2329, 2009.
4. Magill SS, Edwards JR, Bamberg W, et al: Multistate point-prevalence survey of health care–associated infections. *N Eng J Med* 370(13):1198–1208, 2014.
5. Klevens RM, Edwards JR, Richards CL Jr, et al: Estimating health care-associated infections and deaths in U.S. hospitals, 2002. *Public Health Rep* 122(2):160–166, 2007.
6. Dudeck MA, Edwards JR, Allen-Bridson K, et al: National Healthcare Safety Network report, data summary for 2013, Device-associated Module. *Am J Infect Control* 43(3):206–221, 2015.
7. Dudeck MA, Weiner LM, Allen-Bridson K, et al: National Healthcare Safety Network (NHSN) report, data summary for 2012, Device-associated module. *Am J Infect Control* 41(12):1148–1166, 2013.
8. Allegranzi B, Bagheri Nejad S, Combescure C, et al: Burden of endemic health-care-associated infection in developing countries: systematic review and meta-analysis. *Lancet* 377(9761):228–241, 2011.
9. Rosenthal VD, Maki DG, Mehta Y, et al: International Nosocomial Infection Control Consortium (INICC) report, data summary of 43 countries for 2007-2012. Device-associated module. *Am J Infect Control* 42(9):942–956, 2014.
10. Sievert DM, Ricks P, Edwards JR, et al: Antimicrobial-resistant pathogens associated with healthcare-associated infections: summary of data reported to the National Healthcare Safety Network at the Centers for Disease Control and Prevention, 2009–2010. *Infect Control Hosp Epidemiol* 34(1):1–14, 2013.

11. Edwards JR, Peterson KD, Mu Y, et al: National Healthcare Safety Network (NHSN) report: data summary for 2006 through 2008, issued December 2009. *Am J Infect Control* 37(10):783–805, 2009.
12. Mello MJ, Albuquerque Mde F, Lacerda HR, et al: Risk factors for healthcare-associated infection in pediatric intensive care units: a systematic review. *Cad Saude Publica* 25(3):S373–S391, 2009.
13. Van den Berghe G: How does blood glucose control with insulin save lives in intensive care? *J Clin Invest* 114(9):1187–1195, 2004.
14. Kansagara D, Fu R, Freeman M, et al: Intensive insulin therapy in hospitalized patients: a systematic review. *Ann Intern Med* 154(4):268–282, 2011.
15. Ling Y, Li X, Gao X: Intensive versus conventional glucose control in critically ill patients: a meta-analysis of randomized controlled trials. *Eur J Intern Med* 23(6):564–574, 2012.
16. Siegel JD, Rhinehart E, Jackson M, et al: 2007 guideline for isolation precautions: preventing transmission of infectious agents in health care settings. *Am J Infect Control* 35[10 Suppl 2]:S65–S164, 2007.
17. Harris AD, Pineles L, Belton B, et al: Universal glove and gown use and acquisition of antibiotic-resistant bacteria in the ICU: a randomized trial. *JAMA* 310(15):1571–1580, 2013.
18. Boyce JM, Pittet D, Healthcare Infection Control Practices Advisory Committee, et al: Guideline for hand hygiene in health-care settings: recommendations of the Healthcare Infection Control Practices Advisory Committee and the HICPAC/SHEA/APIC/IDSA Hand Hygiene Task Force. *Infect Control Hosp Epidemiol* 23[12 Suppl]:S3–S40, 2002.
19. Armellino D, Hussain E, Schilling ME, et al: Using high-technology to enforce low-technology safety measures: the use of third-party remote video auditing and real-time feedback in healthcare. *Clin Infect Dis* 54(1):1–7, 2012.
20. Marra AR, Sampaio Camargo TZ, Magnus TP, et al: The use of real-time feedback via wireless technology to improve hand hygiene compliance. *Am J Infect Control* 42(6):608–611, 2014.
21. Boyce JM, Ligi C, Kohan C, et al: Lack of association between the increased incidence of Clostridium difficile-associated disease and the increasing use of alcohol-based hand rubs. *Infect Control Hosp Epidemiol* 27(5):479–483, 2006.
22. Dubberke ER, Carling P, Carrico R, et al: Strategies to prevent Clostridium difficile infections in acute care hospitals: 2014 update. *Infect Control Hosp Epidemiol* 35[Suppl 2]:S48–S65, 2014.
23. O'Horo JC, Silva GL, Munoz-Price LS, et al: The efficacy of daily bathing with chlorhexidine for reducing healthcare-associated bloodstream infections: a meta-analysis. *Infect Control Hosp Epidemiol* 33(3):257–267, 2012.
24. Climo MW, Yokoe DS, Warren DK, et al: Effect of daily chlorhexidine bathing on hospital-acquired infection. *N Eng J Med* 368(6):533–542, 2013.
25. Milstone AM, Elward A, Song X, et al: Daily chlorhexidine bathing to reduce bacteraemia in critically ill children: a multicentre, cluster-randomised, crossover trial. *Lancet* 381(9872):1099–1106, 2013.
26. Huang SS, Septimus E, Kleinman K, et al: Targeted versus universal decolonization to prevent ICU infection. *N Eng J Med* 368(24):2255–2265, 2013.
27. Noto MJ, Domenico HJ, Byrne DW, et al: Chlorhexidine bathing and health care-associated infections: a randomized clinical trial. *JAMA* 313(4):369–378, 2015.
28. Carling PC, Parry MF, Bruno-Murtha LA, et al: Improving environmental hygiene in 27 intensive care units to decrease multidrug-resistant bacterial transmission. *Crit Care Med* 38(4):1054–1059, 2010.
29. Blazejewski C, Wallet F, Rouze A, et al: Efficiency of hydrogen peroxide in improving disinfection of ICU rooms. *Crit Care* 19:30, 2015.
30. Chan HT, White P, Sheorey H, et al: Evaluation of the biological efficacy of hydrogen peroxide vapour decontamination in wards of an Australian hospital. *J Hosp Infect* 79(2):125–128, 2011.
31. Rutala WA, Gergen MF, Tande BM, et al: Rapid hospital room decontamination using ultraviolet (UV) light with a nanostructured UV-reflective wall coating. *Infect Control Hosp Epidemiol* 34(5):527–529, 2013.
32. Boyce JM, Havill NL, Moore BA: Terminal decontamination of patient rooms using an automated mobile UV light unit. *Infect Control Hosp Epidemiol* 32(8):737–742, 2011; discussion 743–737.
33. Haas JP, Menz J, Dusza S, et al: Implementation and impact of ultraviolet environmental disinfection in an acute care setting. *Am J Infect Control* 42(6):586–590, 2014.
34. Mitchell BG, Digney W, Locket P, et al: Controlling methicillin-resistant Staphylococcus aureus (MRSA) in a hospital and the role of hydrogen peroxide decontamination: an interrupted time series analysis. *BMJ Open* 4(4):e004522, 2014.
35. Manian FA, Griesnauer S, Bryant A: Implementation of hospital-wide enhanced terminal cleaning of targeted patient rooms and its impact on endemic Clostridium difficile infection rates. *Am J Infect Control* 41(6):537–541, 2013.
36. Levin J, Riley LS, Parrish C, et al: The effect of portable pulsed xenon ultraviolet light after terminal cleaning on hospital-associated Clostridium difficile infection in a community hospital. *Am J Infect Control* 41(8):746–748, 2013.
37. Salgado CD, Sepkowitz KA, John JF, et al: Copper surfaces reduce the rate of healthcare-acquired infections in the intensive care unit. *Infect Control Hosp Epidemiol* 34(5):479–486, 2013.
38. Sehulster L, Chinn RY: Guidelines for environmental infection control in health-care facilities. Recommendations of CDC and the Healthcare Infection Control Practices Advisory Committee (HICPAC). *MMWR Recomm Rep* 52(RR-10):1–42, 2003.
39. Panackal AA, Dahlman A, Keil KT, et al: Outbreak of invasive aspergillosis among renal transplant recipients. *Transplantation* 75(7):1050–1053, 2003.
40. Gaynes RP. Surveillance of nosocomial infections: a fundamental ingredient for quality. *Infect Control Hosp Epidemiol* 18(7):475–478, 1997.
41. Centers for Disease Control and Prevention: Monitoring hospital-acquired infections to promote patient safety—United States, 1990-1999. *MMWR Morb Mortal Wkly Rep* 49(8):149–153, 2000.
42. Fagan RP, Edwards JR, Park BJ, et al: Incidence trends in pathogen-specific central line-associated bloodstream infections in US intensive care units, 1990-2010. *Infect Control Hosp Epidemiol* 34(9):893–899, 2013.
43. Pronovost P, Needham D, Berenholtz S, et al: An intervention to decrease catheter-related bloodstream infections in the ICU. *N Engl J Med* 355(26):2725–2732, 2006.
44. Berenholtz SM, Pronovost PJ, Lipsett PA, et al: Eliminating catheter-related bloodstream infections in the intensive care unit. *Crit Care Med* 32(10):2014–2020, 2004.
45. Warren DK, Yokoe DS, Climo MW, et al: Preventing catheter-associated bloodstream infections: a survey of policies for insertion and care of central venous catheters from hospitals in the prevention epicenter program. *Infect Control Hosp Epidemiol* 27(1):8–13, 2006.
46. Sherertz RJ, Ely EW, Westbrook DM, et al: Education of physicians-in-training can decrease the risk for vascular catheter infection. *Ann Intern Med* 132(8):641–648, 2000.
47. Warren DK, Zack JE, Mayfield JL, et al: The effect of an education program on the incidence of central venous catheter-associated bloodstream infection in a medical ICU. *Chest* 126(5):1612–1618, 2004.
48. Babcock HM, Zack JE, Garrison T, et al: An educational intervention to reduce ventilator-associated pneumonia in an integrated health system: a comparison of effects. *Chest* 125(6):2224–2231, 2004.
49. Baxter AD, Allan J, Bedard J, et al: Adherence to simple and effective measures reduces the incidence of ventilator-associated pneumonia. *Can J Anaesth* 52(5):535–541, 2005.
50. Salahuddin N, Zafar A, Sukhyani L, et al: Reducing ventilator-associated pneumonia rates through a staff education programme. *J Hosp Infect* 57(3):223–227, 2004.
51. Lessa FC, Winston LG, McDonald LC: Burden of Clostridium difficile infection in the United States. *N Eng J Med* 372(24):2369–2370, 2015.
52. Dallal RM, Harbrecht BG, Boujoukas AJ, et al: Fulminant Clostridium difficile: an underappreciated and increasing cause of death and complications. *Ann Surg* 235(3):363–372, 2002.
53. Gerding DN, Johnson S, Peterson LR, et al: Clostridium difficile-associated diarrhea and colitis. *Infect Control Hosp Epidemiol* 16(8):459–477, 1995.
54. Brooks SE, Veal RO, Kramer M, et al: Reduction in the incidence of Clostridium difficile-associated diarrhea in an acute care hospital and a skilled nursing facility following replacement of electronic thermometers with single-use disposables. *Infect Control Hosp Epidemiol* 13(2):98–103, 1992.
55. O'Connor JR, Johnson S, Gerding DN: Clostridium difficile infection caused by the epidemic BI/NAP1/027 strain. *Gastroenterology* 136(6):1913–1924, 2009.
56. See I, Mu Y, Cohen J, et al: NAP1 strain type predicts outcomes from Clostridium difficile infection. *Clin Infect Dis* 58(10):1394–1400, 2014.
57. Drudy D, Kyne L, O'Mahony R, et al: gyrA mutations in fluoroquinolone-resistant Clostridium difficile PCR-027. *Emerg Infect Dis* 13(3):504–505, 2007.
58. Johnson S, Gerding DN, Olson MM, et al: Prospective, controlled study of vinyl glove use to interrupt Clostridium difficile nosocomial transmission. *Am J Med* 88(2):137–140, 1990.
59. Carling P, Fung T, Killion A, et al: Favorable impact of a multidisciplinary antibiotic management program conducted during 7 years. *Infect Control Hosp Epidemiol* 24(9):699–706, 2003.
60. Valiquette L, Cossette B, Garant MP, et al: Impact of a reduction in the use of high-risk antibiotics on the course of an epidemic of Clostridium difficile-associated disease caused by the hypervirulent NAP1/027 strain. *Clin Infect Dis* 45[Suppl 2]:S112–S121, 2007.
61. Wilcox MH, Fawley WN: Hospital disinfectants and spore formation by Clostridium difficile. *Lancet* 356(9238):1324, 2000.
62. Mayfield JL, Leet T, Miller J, et al: Environmental control to reduce transmission of Clostridium difficile. *Clin Infect Dis* 31(4):995–1000, 2000.
63. Wilcox MH, Fawley WN, Wigglesworth N, et al: Comparison of the effect of detergent versus hypochlorite cleaning on environmental contamination and incidence of Clostridium difficile infection. *J Hosp Infect* 54(2):109–114, 2003.
64. Best EL, Parnell P, Thirkell G, et al: Effectiveness of deep cleaning followed by hydrogen peroxide decontamination during high Clostridium difficile infection incidence. *J Hosp Infect* 87(1):25–33, 2014.
65. Wheeldon LJ, Worthington T, Lambert PA, et al: Antimicrobial efficacy of copper surfaces against spores and vegetative cells of Clostridium difficile: the germination theory. *J Antimicrob Chemother* 62(3):522–525, 2008.
66. National Nosocomial Infections Surveillance System: National Nosocomial Infections Surveillance (NNIS) System Report, data summary from January 1992 through June 2004, issued October 2004. *Am J Infect Control* 32(8):470–485, 2004.
67. Dantes R, Mu Y, Belflower R, et al: National burden of invasive methicillin-resistant Staphylococcus aureus infections, United States, 2011. *JAMA Intern Med* 173(21):1970–1978, 2013.
68. Wise ME, Scott RD 2nd, Baggs JM, et al: National estimates of central line-associated bloodstream infections in critical care patients. *Infect Control Hospital Epidemiol* 34(6):547–554, 2013.
69. Popovich KJ, Weinstein RA, Hota B: Are community-associated methicillin-resistant Staphylococcus aureus (MRSA) strains replacing traditional nosocomial MRSA strains? *Clin Infect Dis* 46(6):787–794, 2008.

70. Milstone AM, Carroll KC, Ross T, et al: Community-associated methicillin-resistant Staphylococcus aureus strains in pediatric intensive care unit. *Emerg Infect Dis* 16(4):647–655, 2010.
71. Morgan DJ, Murthy R, Munoz-Price LS, et al: Reconsidering contact precautions for endemic methicillin-resistant staphylococcus aureus and vancomycin-resistant enterococcus. *Infect Control Hosp Epidemiol* 36(10):1163–1172, 2015.
72. Edmond MB, Wenzel RP: Screening inpatients for MRSA—case closed. *N Eng J Med* 368(24):2314–2315, 2013.
73. Gandra S, Barysauskas CM, Mack DA, et al: Impact of contact precautions on falls, pressure ulcers and transmission of MRSA and VRE in hospitalized patients. *J Hosp Infect* 88(3):170–176, 2014.
74. Edmond MB, Masroor N, Stevens MP, et al: The impact of discontinuing contact precautions for VRE and MRSA on device-associated infections. *Infect Control Hosp Epidemiol* 36(8):978–980, 2015.
75. Calfee DP, Salgado CD, Milstone AM, et al: Strategies to prevent methicillin-resistant Staphylococcus aureus transmission and infection in acute care hospitals: 2014 update. *Infect Control Hosp Epidemiol* 35[Suppl 2]:S108–S132, 2014.
76. Edmond MB, Wenzel RP, Pasculle AW: Vancomycin-resistant Staphylococcus aureus: perspectives on measures needed for control. *Ann Intern Med* 124(3):329–334, 1996.
77. Centers for Disease Control and Prevention: Nosocomial enterococci resistant to vancomycin—United States, 1989-1993. *MMWR Morb Mortal Wkly Rep* 42(30):597–599, 1993.
78. Ziakas PD, Thapa R, Rice LB, et al: Trends and significance of VRE colonization in the ICU: a meta-analysis of published studies. *PloS One* 8(9):e75658, 2013.
79. de Niederhausern S, Bondi M, Messi P, et al: Vancomycin-resistance transferability from VanA enterococci to Staphylococcus aureus. *Curr Microbiol* 62(5):1363–1367, 2011.
80. Papadimitriou-Olivgeris M, Drougka E, Fligou F, et al: Risk factors for enterococcal infection and colonization by vancomycin-resistant enterococci in critically ill patients. *Infection* 42(6):1013–1022, 2014.
81. Nordmann P, Naas T, Poirel L: Global spread of Carbapenemase-producing Enterobacteriaceae. *Emerg Infect Dis* 17(10):1791–1798, 2011.
82. Centers for Disease Control and Prevention: Vital signs: carbapenem-resistant Enterobacteriaceae. *MMWR Morb Mortal Wkly Rep* 62(9):165–170, 2013.
83. Swaminathan M, Sharma S, Poliansky Blash S, et al: Prevalence and risk factors for acquisition of carbapenem-resistant Enterobacteriaceae in the setting of endemicity. *Infect Control Hosp Epidemiol* 34(8):809–817, 2013.
84. Bhargava A, Hayakawa K, Silverman E, et al: Risk factors for colonization due to carbapenem-resistant Enterobacteriaceae among patients exposed to long-term acute care and acute care facilities. *Infect Control Hosp Epidemiol* 35(4):398–405, 2014.
85. Routsi C, Pratikaki M, Platsouka E, et al: Risk factors for carbapenem-resistant Gram-negative bacteremia in intensive care unit patients. *Intensive Care Med* 39(7):1253–1261, 2013.
86. Nordmann P, Cuzon G, Naas T: The real threat of Klebsiella pneumoniae carbapenemase-producing bacteria. *Lancet Infect Dis* 9(4):228–236, 2009.
87. Centers for Disease Control and Prevention. *Facility Guidance for Control of Carbapenem-resistant Enterobacteriaceae (CRE), 2015 Update CRE Toolkit.* https://www.cdc.gov/hai/pdfs/cre/CRE-guidance-508.pdf. Accessed on September 28, 2017.
88. Karageorgopoulos DE, Falagas ME: Current control and treatment of multidrug-resistant Acinetobacter baumannii infections. *Lancet Infect Dis* 8(12):751–762, 2008.
89. Camus C, Bellissant E, Sebille V, et al: Prevention of acquired infections in intubated patients with the combination of two decontamination regimens. *Crit Care Med* 33(2):307–314, 2005.

Chapter 73 ■ Use of Antimicrobials in the Treatment of Infection in the Critically Ill Patient

IVA ZIVNA • RICHARD H. GLEW • JENNIFER S. DALY

This chapter reviews antimicrobial agents used in the treatment of bacterial, viral, fungal, and protozoan infections in the intensive care unit (ICU).

PENICILLINS

The classes of penicillins include penicillin G, ampicillin, the antistaphylococcal (semisynthetic) penicillins, and the expanded spectrum (antipseudomonal) penicillins alone and in combination with a β-lactamase inhibitor [1]. The serum half-life ($t_{1/2}$) of most penicillins is short, and rapid clearance occurs via the kidneys. Some semisynthetic penicillins, particularly nafcillin and oxacillin, are metabolized to a large extent by the liver; therefore, adjustment in dosage is not required in patients with renal insufficiency; for piperacillin, dosing adjustment is necessary only in severe renal insufficiency. For most other penicillins, moderate adjustments should be made in dosage for patients with severe renal insufficiency (Table 73.1). Penicillins are relatively nontoxic at usual doses, and side effects most commonly involve hypersensitivity reactions. Bone marrow and hepatic toxicity caused by semisynthetic penicillins have been described, with neutropenia more commonly seen with nafcillin and hepatitis more likely to occur with oxacillin.

Penicillin G

In the ICU, aqueous penicillin G is appropriate in the therapy of severe, overwhelming infections caused by susceptible organisms, including pneumococcal pneumonia and bacteremia caused by penicillin-susceptible strains [1], such as necrotizing fasciitis due to group A *Streptococcus* (in combination with clindamycin), and for streptococcal bacteremia. Because of the prevalence of penicillin-resistant pneumococci, life-threatening infections (especially meningitis) due to these organisms should be treated initially with ceftriaxone, cefotaxime, or vancomycin [2]. Although aspiration pneumonia commonly involves mouth anaerobes that are susceptible to penicillin G, penicillin-resistant anaerobes can be found in putrid, cavitary pneumonia and empyema, and clindamycin with or without a third-generation cephalosporin (or an extended-spectrum β-lactam plus metronidazole) is the preferred regimen [3,4]. Therapy for penicillin-susceptible *Enterococcus* spp causing endocarditis is penicillin G or ampicillin plus an aminoglycoside, generally gentamicin [5]. The activity of penicillin G and ampicillin against most Gram-negative bacilli is poor. *Staphylococcus aureus* should be presumed to be resistant to penicillin, ampicillin, and piperacillin, as most strains produce a penicillinase.

Penicillinase-resistant Semisynthetic Penicillins

Because most strains of *S. aureus* are resistant to penicillin G by virtue of β-lactamase production, treatment of severe infections caused by these organisms involves one of the β-lactamase–resistant penicillins (see Table 73.1). Nafcillin and oxacillin are interchangeable. Both exhibit excellent in vitro activity against most susceptible isolates of *S. aureus*, but are less active (although generally effective) than penicillin G against streptococci. Both are sufficiently metabolized by the hepatic route such that no adjustment in dose is necessary for patients with renal insufficiency. Because of the high prevalence of community-acquired methicillin-resistant *S. aureus* (MRSA), vancomycin should be used for empiric therapy of suspected staphylococcal infections

TABLE 73.1

Examples of Parenteral Penicillins

		Dose based on creatinine clearance			
Penicillin	Indication	>80 mL/min (normal)	50–80 mL/min	10–50 mL/min	<10 mL/min
Penicillin G	Meningitis	2 million U q2h	4 million U q4h	4 million U q4h	2 million U q6h
	Endocarditis	3–4 million U q4h	3–4 million U q4h	3 million U q4h	2 million U q6h
Ampicillin	Meningitis	2–3 g q4h	2–3 g q6h	2–3 g q8h	2–3 g q12h
	Endocarditis	2 g q4h	2 g q6h	2 g q8h	2 g q12h
Nafcillin or oxacillin	*Staphylococcus aureus* bacteremia, meningitis	2 g q4h	2 g q4h	2 g q4h	2 g q4h
	Skin, soft tissue infections	1–2 g q4–6h	1–2 g q4–6h	1–2 g q4–6h	1–2 g q4–6h

[6]. In patients with overwhelming or disseminated infection caused by β-lactam–susceptible *S. aureus*, therapy should be instituted with 9 to 12 g per day of intravenous (IV) oxacillin or nafcillin, in divided doses every 4 hours (see Table 73.1).

Anti–gram-negative Penicillins

The expanded-spectrum penicillin (piperacillin) and the combination agent piperacillin/tazobactam exhibit activity against many *Enterobacteriaceae* that are resistant to ampicillin [7].

In the ICU patient with suspected bacteremia or overwhelming infection due to Gram-negative bacilli, therapy should be chosen with knowledge of local ICU resistance patterns and include agents that the patient has not received recently. Pharyngeal colonization with Gram-negative bacilli develops rapidly among patients in the ICU, and initial therapy of nosocomial aspiration pneumonia requires the addition of an antipseudomonal penicillin, carbapenem, or cephalosporin, usually in combination with an aminoglycoside or fluoroquinolone [8,9]. For patients with *Pseudomonas aeruginosa* infections, the intensivist should consider using higher dosages or continuous infusions of piperacillin/tazobactam or piperacillin, with or without an aminoglycoside. The addition of the aminoglycoside to extended-spectrum penicillins is controversial [10] but has been shown to provide broader Gram-negative coverage and synergistic killing against *P. aeruginosa*.

β-Lactamase–inhibitor Combinations

Clavulanic acid, sulbactam, and tazobactam are β-lactamase inhibitors that bind irreversibly to β-lactamases derived from *S. aureus* and anaerobes, as well as some β-lactamases from Gram-negative bacilli. Thus, the combination of one of these β-lactamase inhibitors with ampicillin or piperacillin results in a drug combination that is active against β-lactamase–producing strains of *S. aureus*, *Bacteroides* sp, *Haemophilus influenzae*, *Neisseria gonorrhoeae*, and enteric Gram-negative bacilli such as *Escherichia coli*, *Klebsiella* spp. and *Proteus* spp. However, chromosomally mediated β-lactamases of other Gram-negative bacilli are unaffected by these β-lactamase inhibitors, and therefore these combinations are ineffective against many isolates of *P. aeruginosa*, *Enterobacter cloacae*, *Citrobacter freundii*, and *Serratia marcescens*.

Formulations of β-lactamase combinations available parenterally include ampicillin/sulbactam and piperacillin/tazobactam. Piperacillin/tazobactam can be effective in the treatment of mixed infections, such as nosocomial pneumonia, intra-abdominal infections, and synergistic skin soft tissue infections. However, depending on local resistance patterns, the lack of efficacy against multiple-resistant Gram-negative bacilli commonly found in the ICU warrants monitoring of local resistance patterns and use of a carbapenem, or adding an aminoglycoside as part of a combination regimen to ensure broad efficacy against nosocomial Gram-negative bacilli [8,9].

The usual suggested dosages of the available combinations are presented in Table 73.1. For treatment of *P. aeruginosa* infections, the dosage of piperacillin/tazobactam should be increased to 3.375 g IV every 4 hours or 4.5 g IV every 6 hours for pneumonia. The pharmacology of the β-lactamase inhibitors is similar to that for other β-lactams: Clearance is by renal mechanisms, and dosage adjustments must be made with these combinations in the setting of renal impairment. Continuous infusion of piperacillin/tazobactam after a bolus has a pharmacodynamic advantage for organisms with relatively high minimum inhibitory concentrations (MICs) to piperacillin and for patients on continuous venovenous hemofiltration (CVVH).

CEPHALOSPORINS

Cephalosporin antibiotics exhibit relative safety and an antibacterial spectrum that includes activity against Gram-positive and Gram-negative bacteria. Examples of parenteral cephalosporins that are currently available are listed in Table 73.2. Cephalosporins are not active against MRSA, *Enterococcus* spp, or *Stenotrophomonas maltophilia*. Many strains of *Enterobacter* possess an inducible chromosomal β-lactamase and may become resistant during therapy.

First-generation Cephalosporins

First-generation cephalosporins exhibit a virtually identical spectrum of antibacterial activity, and they differ only in their pharmacokinetic properties. These agents are active against staphylococci (β-lactam–susceptible staphylococci) but are not effective against enterococci, *Listeria monocytogenes*, MRSA, or the majority of coagulase-negative staphylococci. Community-acquired strains of *E. coli*, *Proteus mirabilis*, and *Klebsiella pneumoniae* often are susceptible to the first-generation cephalosporins, but in general, third-generation agents are far more potent against Gram-negative bacilli and are preferred in the treatment of such infections in ICU patients. Nosocomial isolates of *Enterobacteriaceae* usually are resistant to first-generation cephalosporins, as are *Pseudomonas* and *Acinetobacter* spp.

Second-generation Cephalosporins

Second-generation cephalosporins (e.g., cefuroxime) have only limited activity against hospital-acquired Gram-negative bacilli

TABLE 73.2

Examples of Parenteral Cephalosporins and Related β-Lactams

Antibiotic	Dosage based on creatinine clearance		
	>50 mL/min	10–50 mL/min	<10 mL/min
Ampicillin-sulbactam	3 g q6h	3 g q12h	3 g q24h
Piperacillin-tazobactam	3.375 g or 4.5 g q6h	2.25 g q6h	2.25 g q8h
First-generation cephalosporins			
Cefazolin	1–2 g q8h	0.5–1 g q12h	0.5–1 g q24h
Second-generation cephalosporins			
Cefuroxime	0.75–1.5 g q6–8h	0.75–1.50 g q8–12h	0.75 g q24h
Third-generation cephalosporins			
Cefotaxime	1–2 g q6h	1–2 g q8–12h	1–2 g q12–24h
Ceftriaxone	1–2 g q12–24h	1–2 g q24h	1–2 g q24h
Ceftizoxime	1–2 g q6–8h	0.25–1 g q8–12h	0.25–1 g q24h
Ceftazidime	1–2 g q8h	1–2 g q12–24h	0.5–1 g q24–48h
Newest-generation cephalosporins			
Cefepime	1–2 g q8–12h	0.5–2 g q12–24h	0.25–1 g q24h
Ceftaroline	0.6 g q12h	0.3–0.4 g q12h	0.2–0.4 g q12h
Ceftolozane-tazobactam	1.5 g q8h	GFR 30–50; 0.75 g q8h GFR 15–29; 0.375 g q8h	No data for use
Ceftazidime-avibactam	2.5 g q8h	GFR 31–50; 1.25 g q8h GFR 16–30; 0.94 g q12h	GFR 6–15; 0.94 g q24h GFR <5; 0.94 g q48h
Monobactams/Carbapenems			
Aztreonam	1–2 g q8h	1 g q8h	0.5 g q8h
Imipenem/cilastatin	0.5–1.0 g q6h	0.5 g q8–12h	0.25–0.5 g q12h
Ertapenem	1 g q24h	0.5–1 g q24h	0.5 g q24h
Meropenem	1–2 g q8h	0.5–1 g q12h	0.5–1 g q24h
Doripenem	0.5 g q8h	0.25 g q8–12h	No data for use

and therefore are not recommended for treatment of Gram negatives in the ICU setting.

Third-generation Cephalosporins

Third-generation cephalosporins exhibit an expanded spectrum and increased potency against Gram-negative organisms, especially *Enterobacteriaceae*. A number of these agents, particularly ceftazidime, are less active than first-generation cephalosporins against Gram-positive cocci. However, ceftriaxone has significant activity against *Streptococcus pneumoniae* and other oral streptococci, and has been recommended for use in severely ill patients with community-acquired pneumonia (CAP), bacterial meningitis, and bacterial endocarditis [5,11,12].

The activity of most third-generation cephalosporins against *P. aeruginosa* is variable and unpredictable; only ceftazidime and cefepime, a fourth-generation cephalosporin, are considered active against this organism and should be used in combination with an aminoglycoside when infection with *P. aeruginosa* is likely [13]. If a third-generation cephalosporin is used as a single agent, gaps in coverage may occur, including: (a) enterococcal superinfection; (b) *P. aeruginosa* infections in neutropenic patients; (c) emergence of broad-spectrum resistance by means of chromosomally mediated inducible β-lactamases during cephalosporin monotherapy of deep-seated infections by species of *Enterobacter*, *Providencia*, *Serratia*, *Pseudomonas*, and *Acinetobacter*; (d) intra-abdominal or intrapelvic infections likely to involve *Bacteroides fragilis*; and (e) *S. aureus* bacteremia, endocarditis, or meningitis. Thus, in ICU patients, third-generation cephalosporins generally should be used empirically as part of combination therapy or as specific single-agent treatment of Gram-negative bacillary infections involving organisms documented to be susceptible to the agent in vitro.

Newer Cephalosporins

Cefepime, a fourth-generation cephalosporin [14], has activity against Gram-positive organisms similar to that of cefotaxime and ceftriaxone and activity against *Pseudomonas* similar to that of ceftazidime. Compared with third-generation cephalosporins, cefepime has a lower affinity for β-lactamases and is not an inducer of chromosomal β-lactamases. The pharmacokinetics of cefepime are similar to those of ceftazidime: $t_{1/2}$ is 2.1 hours, and 80% to 90% of the dose is recovered in the urine. For treatment of infections due to *P. aeruginosa*, cefepime (often in conjunction with an aminoglycoside) should be dosed every 8 hours, but for moderate infections due to more susceptible species, it can be dosed every 12 hours (see Table 73.2).

Ceftaroline is indicated for treatment of acute bacterial skin and skin structure infections caused by susceptible isolates of the following Gram-positive and Gram-negative microorganisms: *S. aureus* (including methicillin-resistant isolates), *S. pyogenes*, *S. agalactiae*, *E. coli*, *K. pneumoniae*, and *K. oxytoca* [15]. It is also approved for the treatment of community-acquired bacterial pneumonia caused by susceptible isolates of *S. pneumoniae* (including cases with concurrent bacteremia), *S. aureus* (methicillin-susceptible isolates only), *H. influenzae*, *K. pneumoniae*, *K. oxytoca*, and *E. coli*. Ceftaroline is infused over 1 hour at dose 600 mg IV every 12 hours. Ceftaroline is primarily excreted by urine (88%). In patients with renal impairment dose adjustment is needed (Table 73.2).

Adverse Reactions

Cephalosporins are relatively nontoxic agents. The most commonly noted adverse effects are hypersensitivity reactions, including rashes, fever, interstitial nephritis, and anaphylaxis. In patients with documented penicillin allergy, the risk of cross-reactive allergic reactions to the cephalosporins is cited as 5% to 10%, and generally it is felt that cephalosporins should be avoided for patients with a history of documented anaphylaxis or immediate hypersensitivity (urticaria) reaction to the penicillins, but can be given to patients with a history of other types of reactions to penicillins, including morbilliform rash and fever. Enterococcal superinfections occur with any of the extended-spectrum cephalosporins because none of these agents has significant activity against enterococci [16].

Dosage

When used in the treatment of severe infections in ICU patients, all cephalosporins should be used, at least initially, at maximal doses and short dosing intervals (Table 73.2). In patients with severe impairment of renal function, dosages of all cephalosporins except ceftriaxone must be adjusted to avoid accumulation.

Cephalosporins with β-Lactamase Inhibitor Activity

Ceftazidime/avibactam is a combination of a third generation cephalosporin with a novel non-β-lactam β-lactamase inhibitor (avibactam) [17]. Ceftazidime has bactericidal activity against most Gram negative organism including *P. aeruginosa* as it arrests bacterial growth by binding to one or more penicillin-binding proteins, thereby inhibiting final transpeptidation steps of peptidoglycan synthesis in bacterial cell-wall. The addition of avibactam protects ceftazidime from degradation by β-lactamase enzymes and effectively extends the antibiotic spectrum of ceftazidime against isolates which are carbapenem resistant due to KPC (Ambler classes A, C, D) or that express ESBL's or AmpC. Currently, ceftazidime/avibactam is approved by US Food and Drug Administration (FDA) for treatment of complicated intraabdominal infections and complicated urinary tract infection. In a phase 2 clinical trial in patients with complicated intraabdominal infections, ceftazidime/avibactam at a dose 2.5 g (2 g ceftazidime and 0.5 g avibactam) IV every 8 hours in combination with metronidazole (500 mg IV every 8 hours) provided similar efficacy to meropenem. In patients with complex urinary tract infection, ceftazidime/avibactam (500 mg ceftazidime and 125 mg of avibactam) IV every 8 hours and imipenem-cilastatin provided similar efficacy and safety profile. In patients with ceftazidime-resistant pathogens, 85.7 (6/7) and 81.8% (9/11) had favorable microbiological response at test of cure for the ceftazidime-avibactam and imipenem/cilastatin groups, respectively. Since ceftazidime/avibactam is excreted primarily by the kidney, renal dose adjustment is required in patients with renal impairment (Table 73.2).

Ceftolozane/tazobactam is a novel antipseudomonal cephalosporin combined with a well-established β-lactamase inhibitor. The chemical structure of ceftolozane is similar to that of ceftazidime, with the exception of a modified side-chain at the 3-position of the cephem nucleus, which confers potent antipseudomonal activity. Ceftolozane is distinguished from other cephalosporins by its potent activity versus *P. aeruginosa*, as well as *A. baumanii* and carbapenem-, piperacillin/tazobactam-, and ceftazidime-resistant isolates. The addition of tazobactam extends the activity of ceftolozane to include most ESBL producers as well as some anaerobic species. Ceftolozane/tazobactam is approved for treatment of complicated intraabdominal infections at a dose of 1.5 g (1 g ceftolozane and 0.5 g tazobactam) IV every 8 hours in combination with metronidazole (500 mg IV every 8 hours) and for treatment of patients with complicated urinary tract infections [18]. In a phase 3 clinical trial for treatment of complicated intraabdominal infection ceftolozane/tazobactam 1.5 g IV every 8 hours with metronidazole was noninferior to meropenem by clinical cure rates [19]. Overall, incidence of adverse events were similar for both groups. Ceftolozane/tazobactam is excreted primarily by the kidney, with ceftozolane being eliminated unchanged and tazobactam being hydrolyzed to inactive metabolite. Renal dose adjustment is required (Table 73.2).

CARBAPENEMS

Four carbapenem antibiotics—imipenem, meropenem, ertapenem, and doripenem—are approved for clinical use [20,21]. Imipenem is administered in combination with cilastatin, an enzymatic inhibitor of a renal dehydropeptidase, which inhibits metabolism of imipenem by the kidney, increasing the $t_{1/2}$ and decreasing the nephrotoxicity of imipenem. Imipenem exhibits activity against Gram-negative bacilli at least equal to that of the third-generation cephalosporins (including anti-*Pseudomonas* potency equal to that of ceftazidime); against Gram-positive cocci similar to that of oxacillin, nafcillin, and cefazolin; and against anaerobic bacteria equal to metronidazole and clindamycin. MRSA are resistant to imipenem. *Enterococcus faecalis* appears susceptible in vitro, but *Enterococcus faecium* usually is resistant, and imipenem should not be regarded as effective therapy for serious infections caused by enterococci. Among nonfermentative Gram-negative bacilli associated with nosocomial infections, *S. maltophilia*, *Burkholderia cepacia*, and *Flavobacterium* spp usually are resistant to imipenem. Resistance to imipenem arises infrequently (most commonly with *P. aeruginosa*) during therapy, usually via alteration in porin channels in the bacterial cell outer membrane, resulting in diminished intracellular concentrations of the drug. The usual dosage of imipenem/cilastatin is 2 g per day in four divided doses, with up to 4 g per day in life-threatening infections by less susceptible organisms (e.g., *P. aeruginosa*). Dosage adjustment (see Table 73.2) is necessary for patients with renal dysfunction because serum concentration-related myoclonus and seizures can occur. Treatment of highly resistant Gram-negative bacilli (e.g., *P. aeruginosa*, *E. cloacae*, and *Acinetobacter* spp) with imipenem may involve initial coadministration of a second agent, such as an aminoglycoside.

Adverse reactions to imipenem include rash and fever. The frequency of cross-reactivity with other classes of β-lactams is estimated to be approximately that observed with penicillins and cephalosporins. Risk of seizures can be minimized by adjustment of dosing in the elderly and in patients with reduced renal function; usage should be avoided when possible in patients with a history of seizures or central nervous system (CNS) lesions.

Meropenem and ertapenem are broad-spectrum carbapenem antibiotics similar to imipenem. Meropenem is more active against Gram-negative rods, including *Pseudomonas* spp, and slightly less active against Gram-positive cocci, including *S. aureus*. Ertapenem is not active against *Pseudomonas* spp or *Enterococcus* spp but has activity against extended-spectrum β-lactamase (ESBL) producing *Klebsiella*. The standard dosing for ertapenem is 1 g IV every 24 hours and for meropenem 1 g IV every 8 hours (see Table 73.2). Meropenem and ertapenem are excreted via the kidney but, in contrast to imipenem, their renal metabolism is negligible and cilastatin is not coadministered. Meropenem and ertapenem are less likely than imipenem to cause seizures.

Doripenem is a novel carbapenem with a broad spectrum of activity against Gram-positive pathogens, anaerobes, and Gram-negative bacteria, including *P. aeruginosa*. Doripenem exhibits rapid bactericidal activity with two- to fourfold lower MIC values for Gram-negative bacteria, compared with other carbapenems. It has significant in vitro activity against

Enterobacteriaceae (including ESBL+ strains), *P. aeruginosa*, *Acinetobacter* spp, and *B. fragilis*. Doripenem is dosed at 500 mg IV every 8 hours; dose and/or interval adjustment is required based on creatinine clearance (see Table 73.2). Low risk of seizures has been demonstrated in clinical studies [21].

AZTREONAM

Aztreonam is a monobactam, differing from penicillins and cephalosporins in that it has a monocyclic rather than a bicyclic nucleus, granting aztreonam little cross-allergenicity with other β-lactams. Although skin rashes occur occasionally with this drug, aztreonam has been given safely to patients with immediate hypersensitivity-type reactions (anaphylaxis, urticaria) to penicillins or cephalosporins. Aztreonam has no activity against Gram-positive or anaerobic bacteria. Against most facultative aerobic Gram-negative bacilli, aztreonam exhibits a spectrum and potency much like that of third-generation cephalosporins, including activity against some strains of *Pseudomonas* spp. The usual dosage of aztreonam is 1 to 2 g IV every 6 to 8 hours. Aztreonam is cleared by the kidneys, and dosage must be reduced in patients with renal insufficiency.

AMINOGLYCOSIDES

Aminoglycoside antibiotics are anti-bactericidal agents of value in the treatment of Gram-negative infections in ICU patients [22]. Aminoglycosides in common clinical use for the critically ill patient include gentamicin, tobramycin, and amikacin. Streptomycin occasionally is used for treatment of enterococcal or mycobacterial infections.

Pharmacology

All available aminoglycosides exhibit similar pharmacologic properties: (a) absorption from the gastrointestinal (GI) tract is negligible, and adequate serum levels are obtained only by the IV or intramuscular routes; (b) volume of distribution is similar to that of total volume of extracellular fluid and therefore can be unpredictable under conditions of abnormal extracellular fluid, such as dehydration, third-space losses, congestive heart failure, or ascites; (c) protein binding is minimal; (d) penetration into the cerebrospinal fluid (CSF) is poor even in the presence of meningeal inflammation; (e) drug levels in bronchial secretions are only two thirds of those in serum and are poor in vitreous fluid, prostate, and bile; (f) excretion is predominantly by glomerular filtration, and $t_{½}$ of the aminoglycosides in the presence of normal renal function is approximately 2 to 3 hours (longest for amikacin) and is prolonged in patients with renal impairment, approaching 24 hours in those with end-stage renal failure; (g) all aminoglycosides are dialyzable, and greater efficacy of removal occurs with hemodialysis (approximately 60% to 75% cleared in 6 hours) than with peritoneal dialysis; and (h) aminoglycoside activity is reduced under conditions of reduced pH and oxygen tension, such as in purulent, particularly anaerobic, fluids, and tissues [22].

Spectrum of Action and Indications for Therapy

The primary clinical indication for aminoglycoside therapy is serious infection caused by Gram-negative bacilli. Aminoglycosides also are used in combination with a cell wall agent for therapy of enterococcal endocarditis. Another indication is treatment of mycobacterial disease. Although more toxic than penicillins and cephalosporins, aminoglycosides provide the broadest range of potent, bactericidal antibiotic activity against Gram-negative bacilli, particularly when multiply-resistant enteric Gram-negative bacilli (e.g., *Enterobacter* spp) or nonfermentative Gram-negative organisms such as *Pseudomonas* and *Acinetobacter* spp are considered possible pathogens. Resistance to aminoglycosides generally emerges slowly and infrequently. However, resistance to aminoglycosides has increased dramatically among *Enterococcus* spp, and currently in many hospitals, up to one fourth of isolates are gentamicin-resistant [23]. Some high-level gentamicin-resistant isolates remain susceptible to high levels of streptomycin.

Gentamicin and Tobramycin

In many ICUs, gentamicin (and tobramycin) resistance is prevalent among local isolates of Gram-negative bacilli, and amikacin may be preferred in the initial management of Gram-negative bacillary infections, pending results of susceptibility testing. In addition, gentamicin in combination with ampicillin, penicillin, or vancomycin is indicated for treatment of endocarditis due to enterococci or viridans group streptococci and can be used with vancomycin and rifampin for treatment of prosthetic valve endocarditis caused by coagulase-negative staphylococci. Tobramycin is more potent than gentamicin against *P. aeruginosa* in vitro and, along with amikacin, may be effective against gentamicin-resistant strains of this organism. However, the frequency of cross-resistance is unpredictable and may be alarmingly common. In addition, tobramycin is less active than gentamicin against some organisms, such as *Serratia* spp and *Acinetobacter* spp.

Amikacin

Amikacin is the semisynthetic aminoglycoside most resistant to aminoglycoside-inactivating enzymes. For most gentamicin-resistant Gram-negative bacilli such as multiresistant ESBL-producing *Klebsiella*, amikacin is the most active aminoglycoside and should be the empiric aminoglycoside of choice in hospitals or ICUs in which gentamicin and tobramycin resistance is prevalent.

Adverse Reactions

Unlike β-lactam antibiotics, aminoglycosides are characterized by a narrow therapeutic–toxic ratio, and therapy with these agents can be associated with considerable toxicity. Hypersensitivity reactions such as fever and rash are uncommon and anaphylaxis has been observed rarely. Neuromuscular blockade has been described uncommonly and appears to be of concern only in patients with myasthenia gravis or severe hypocalcemia or those who are receiving neuromuscular blocking agents. Ototoxicity appears to occur with equal frequency (up to 10% of patients) among the modern aminoglycosides. Vestibular damage has been described more commonly with gentamicin and tobramycin, whereas impairment of auditory acuity seems more common with amikacin [22]. Ototoxicity occurs unpredictably (either early or late in therapy), is related only partially to elevated serum levels, most closely correlates with duration of therapy and total dosage administered, and often is irreversible. Patients expected to receive aminoglycoside therapy for extended duration and who are conscious and communicative should be questioned periodically about symptoms of eighth cranial nerve dysfunction, such as tinnitus, diminished auditory acuity, lightheadedness, and dizziness.

Nephrotoxicity has been reported to occur in 2% to 10% of all patients receiving aminoglycoside therapy and in up to 10% to 25% of critically ill patients. However, renal damage usually is mild and reversible promptly with cessation of therapy. Aminoglycoside-induced nephrotoxicity is related to dose and duration of therapy as well as to serum concentrations,

TABLE 73.3

Recommended Dosage Regimens and Serum Concentrations of Aminoglycosides in Intensive Care Unit Patients Based on Calculated Creatinine Clearance

				Target serum concentration (μg/mL)[a]		
Drug/renal function	**Route**	**Loading dose (mg/kg)**	**Regimen (mg/kg)**	**Peak**[b]	**Trough**[b]	**8 h after dose**
Traditional regimen						
Gentamicin, tobramycin						
>80 mL/min	IV, IM	2.0–2.5	1.3–1.7 q8h	4–8	1.0–1.5	
60–79 mL/min		2.0–2.5	1.3–1.7 q12h	4–8	1.0–1.5	
40–59 mL/min		2.0–2.5	3 q24h	4–8	1.0–1.5	
30–39 mL/min		2.0–2.5	2 q24h	4–8	1.0–1.5	
10–29 mL/min		2.0–2.5	2–3 q48h	4–8	1.0–1.5	
<10 mL/min		2.0–2.5	1–2 q48h	4–8	1.0–1.5	
Amikacin	IV, IM					
>80 mL/min		7.5–10.0	7.5 q12h	20–25	5–10	
60–79 mL/min		7.5–10.0	5.0 q12h	20–25	5–10	
40–59 mL/min		7.5–10.0	7.5 q24h	20–25	5–10	
30–39 mL/min		7.5–10.0	5.0 q24h	20–25	5–10	
10–29 mL/min		7.5–10.0	7.5 q48h	20–25	5–10	
<10 mL/min		7.5–10.0	5.0 q48h	20–25	5–10	
Once-daily dosing[c]						
Gentamicin, tobramycin						
80 mL/min	IV	Not needed	5–7 q24h	NA[d]	Undetectable (<0.3)	2–6
60–79 mL/min	IV	Not needed	5–7 q36–48h (based on serum concentration at 6–14 h after dose)	NA[d] [29]	Undetectable (<0.3)	6–11
Amikacin	IV	Not needed	15–20 q24h	NA[d]	Undetectable (<0.3)	6–18

Creatinine clearance; for women, multiply the result by 0.85.
[a]Lower concentrations are desired when using aminoglycosides for treatment of gram-positive infections
[b]Serum for peak levels should be drawn 30 min after a 30-min infusion, and trough levels should be obtained within the 30 min before the next dose.
[c]Patient exclusions—age <12 y, pregnancy, burns >20% body surface area, ascites, dialysis, endocarditis, creatinine clearance <60 mL/min.
[d]NA—with once-daily dosing, peak concentrations are high transiently and measurement of peaks is not applicable.

especially elevated trough levels. It occurs more commonly among elderly patients, those with preexisting renal disease, those with diminished tissue perfusion caused by cardiogenic or peripheral vascular factors, and patients receiving other nephrotoxic agents. The most useful laboratory tests available to reduce and detect aminoglycoside nephrotoxicity are the serum creatinine levels and determinations of trough serum aminoglycoside concentrations.

Therapy and Determination of Serum Levels

Recommended dosage schedules and desired serum concentrations for the aminoglycosides are shown in Table 73.3. The use of the once-daily dosing method for aminoglycosides (see Table 73.3) may reduce nephrotoxicity and enhance efficacy against Gram-negative bacilli [24]. These agents induce a postantibiotic effect, and hence are suited for less frequent dosing. Postantibiotic effect is uncertain for Gram-positive bacteria, and the desired peak and trough levels are lower when aminoglycosides are employed for synergistic activity against Gram-positive pathogens. For patients with impaired renal function, serum concentrations (and serum creatinine and blood urea nitrogen values) should be monitored to ensure safe and effective concentrations. Trough concentrations should be monitored frequently (and dosage/frequency adjusted accordingly) in patients with fluctuating cardiovascular function/fluid volumes or renal function and in those who are anticipated to receive prolonged therapy. Trough serum concentrations should be less than 1 μg per mL (or undetectable) when large doses are given at intervals of 24 hours or greater. In patients undergoing hemodialysis, it can be estimated that approximately two thirds to three fourths of a dose (i.e., 1 mg per kg gentamicin or tobramycin or 5 mg per kg amikacin) is required at the end of each hemodialysis session, and serum concentrations (trough before dialysis, peak after supplemental dose given) should be monitored. In patients undergoing peritoneal dialysis, instillation of the aminoglycoside into the dialysate at a therapeutic concentration (i.e., 4 μg per mL = 4 mg per L for gentamicin and tobramycin and 20 μg per mL = 20 mg per L for amikacin) eliminates a serum-dialysis concentration gradient and minimizes loss of drug through dialysis.

FLUOROQUINOLONES

Fluoroquinolones are broad-spectrum agents that exert their antimicrobial activity by inhibiting deoxyribonucleic acid (DNA) synthesis via binding to two enzymes, bacterial DNA gyrase and topoisomerase IV, enzymes that induce superhelical twists into double-stranded bacterial DNA. Fluoroquinolones broadly in use include ciprofloxacin, levofloxacin, and moxifloxacin. These agents are active and generally bactericidal against susceptible enteric Gram-negative bacilli (including enteric pathogens such as *Salmonella* spp and *Shigella* spp), *H. influenzae*. Resistance to these agents is increasing among Gram-negative bacteria such as *P. aeruginosa*, *Acinetobacter* spp, and *Aeromonas hydrophila;* non–lactose-fermenting Gram-negative bacilli, such as *B. cepacia*, *Pseudomonas fluorescens*, and *S. maltophilia*, often are resistant to the quinolones. Of the quinolones, ciprofloxacin has greatest potency against *P. aeruginosa*. Activity of quinolones against aerobic Gram-positive cocci is variable, and activity against methicillin-susceptible *S. aureus* and coagulase-negative staphylococci has diminished; MRSA commonly are resistant [25]. Although, in general, streptococci (particularly *S. pneumoniae*, *Streptococcus pyogenes*) and enterococci exhibit poor susceptibility to older quinolones (i.e., ciprofloxacin), moxifloxacin and levofloxacin are considered efficacious in treatment of pneumococcal pneumonia. Moxifloxacin has in vitro activity against *B. fragilis*, but there is little clinical experience with its use against this pathogen. Quinolones have activity against mycobacteria, including *Mycobacterium tuberculosis*, *Mycobacterium kansasii*, and *Mycobacterium fortuitum*, but susceptibility results should be used to guide therapy. Levofloxacin and moxifloxacin are more active than ciprofloxacin against *Mycoplasma* spp, *Chlamydophilia trachomatis*, and *Ureaplasma urealyticum*. All demonstrate activity against *Legionella pneumophila*. The $t_{1/2}$ of the fluoroquinolones is relatively long (3 to 4 hours for ciprofloxacin and levofloxacin, and 9 to 10 hours for moxifloxacin). Levofloxacin is cleared primarily by the kidneys and requires dosage adjustment for patients with renal insufficiency. Moxifloxacin is cleared by the liver, and dosage adjustments in renal failure are unnecessary. Some hepatic excretion occurs with ciprofloxacin, and major dosage adjustment (50% of dose, 12-hour interval) is required only at creatinine clearance rates of less than 20 mL per minute. The fluoroquinolones are not eliminated by hemodialysis or peritoneal dialysis. Although available oral fluoroquinolone formulations can achieve adequate serum and tissue concentrations to treat infections outside the urinary tract, parenteral therapy is preferred in the acute management of serious infections in the ICU, as oral absorption may be unreliable due to problems with intestinal motility or perfusion. Ciprofloxacin, moxifloxacin, and levofloxacin are available in IV preparations. GI tract absorption of fluoroquinolones can be impaired by concomitant administration of antacids, sucralfate, and multivitamins containing zinc or iron.

Adverse Reactions

In general, fluoroquinolones are safe and well tolerated. The most common adverse reactions include GI tract symptoms (nausea, vomiting, dyspepsia, abdominal pain, and diarrhea), CNS symptoms (insomnia, restlessness, headache, dizziness, confusion, and, rarely, seizures), tendon rupture, and occasional hypersensitivity reactions (rash, pruritus, and drug fever). Ciprofloxacin increases serum concentrations and potentiates the effects of theophylline, warfarin, and cyclosporine.

Indications

The fluoroquinolones are indicated for the treatment of (a) complicated urinary tract infections involving susceptible Gram-negative bacilli; (b) prostatitis; (c) bacterial pneumonia, especially due to Gram-negative bacilli, *H. influenzae*, *Legionella* sp, or high-level penicillin-resistant *S. pneumoniae*; (d) bacterial diarrhea of diverse etiologies, including traveler's diarrhea and enteritis due to *Shigella*, *Salmonella*, and *Campylobacter* spp; (e) invasive (malignant) external otitis; (f) intra-abdominal and intrapelvic infections (in combination with anaerobic coverage); (g) outpatient treatment of CAP; and (h) septic shock due to urinary tract infections, in combination with a β-lactam agent. For treating nosocomial pneumonia, it must be remembered that the older fluoroquinolones (e.g., ciprofloxacin) have limited activity against streptococci and no activity against anaerobes, and addition of an agent active against these organisms should be considered. In addition, resistance to fluoroquinolones is becoming increasingly common in *S. aureus* and among Gram-negative bacilli, especially *P. aeruginosa*.

VANCOMYCIN

Vancomycin is bactericidal at low concentrations against most Gram-positive cocci and bacilli, including *S. aureus* (including MRSA), coagulase-negative staphylococci, *S. pneumoniae* (including drug-resistant strains), viridans group *Streptococcus* spp, *Streptococcus bovis*, *Clostridium* sp, and *Diphtheroid* spp. Although most enterococci are inhibited by low concentrations of vancomycin, bactericidal killing of these organisms requires the addition of an aminoglycoside such as gentamicin or streptomycin. Resistance to vancomycin is an emerging problem, particularly in strains of *E. faecium*. Because of poor absorption from the GI tract and severe pain with intramuscular injection, vancomycin is given IV for the treatment of systemic infections. Oral vancomycin is used only for patients with antibiotic-associated colitis caused by *Clostridium difficile*. In severely ill patients with *C. difficile* infection, oral vancomycin or a combination of oral vancomycin and IV metronidazole is recommended. Vancomycin is excreted primarily by the kidneys. In patients with normal renal function, serum $t_{1/2}$ of IV-administered vancomycin varies from 2.7 to 13.3 hours, and peak and trough serum concentrations are unpredictable. The usual recommended dose for adults with normal renal function is 2 to 3 g per day in divided doses every 8 to 12 hours. The dose should be administered IV over 60 minutes. For complicated infections in seriously ill patients, a loading dose of 25 to 30 mg per kg (based on actual body weight) may be used to achieve target concentration rapidly, followed with 15 to 20 mg/kg/dose every 8 to 12 hours. Nomograms are available to guide vancomycin dosing in patients with varying degrees of renal insufficiency. Serum trough concentrations should be monitored for patients with reduced renal function or unstable hemodynamics; monitoring of peak concentrations usually is not helpful. For pneumonia due to MRSA and meningitis, dosing to achieve higher troughs of 15 to 20 μg per mL should be used. For endocarditis dosing to achieve troughs of 10 to 15 μg per mL are recommended [26].

Adverse Reactions

Because there is no cross-reaction with β-lactam allergy, vancomycin is the drug of choice in the therapy of serious Gram-positive infections in patients who are allergic to penicillins and cephalosporins. Vancomycin is associated with hypersensitivity reactions such as rash and fever in approximately 3% to 5% of patients. Rapid IV administration of vancomycin can produce a histamine-associated reaction characterized by flushing, tingling, pruritus, tachycardia, hypotension, and an erythematous rash over the upper trunk and face. This Red-Person Syndrome is a histamine-release phenomenon, not a manifestation of hypersensitivity, and can be avoided by slow IV administration of the drug (i.e., at a rate no faster than 15 mg per minute or 0.5 g over 60 minutes and 1 g over 60 to 90 minutes) or by pretreatment with an antihistamine. Neutropenia occurs occasionally [27]. Ototoxicity occurs uncommonly in patients who receive vancomycin, usually in association with elevated serum levels (at least 50 μg per mL), and generally is reversible with discontinuation of therapy. Nephrotoxicity occurs rarely in patients who receive vancomycin alone, is usually associated with elevated serum vancomycin levels, and is more common in patients with recent concomitant aminoglycoside administration.

LIPOGLYCOPEPTIDE

First-generation Lipoglycopeptide

Telavancin, a glycopeptide analog of vancomycin, telavancin, shows promise as alternative treatment for patients with serious infections caused by Gram-positive pathogens [28]. Telavancin exhibits low potential for resistance development and is active against resistant pathogens, including MRSA. Telavancin currently is approved only for treatment of complicated skin and skin structure infections (cSSSIs). Similar to vancomycin, it demonstrates activity in vitro against a variety of Gram-positive pathogens, including but not limited to MRSA and penicillin-resistant *S. pneumoniae*. Modifications to vancomycin's structure expanded telavancin's spectrum of activity in vitro to include organisms such as glycopeptide-intermediate *S. aureus* (GISA), vancomycin-resistant *S. aureus* (VRSA), and vancomycin-resistant enterococci (VRE). Dosing at 10 mg/kg/d is recommended for patients with normal renal function. Since telavancin is cleared extensively by the kidneys, dosage adjustments will be required in patients with moderate-to-severe renal impairment. Renal toxicity was reported more frequently with telavancin than with vancomycin in two phase III clinical trials (3% vs. 1%). Potential teratogenicity of this agent must be considered in women who are pregnant or may become pregnant.

Second-generation Lipoglycopeptide

Oritavancin and dalbavancin are indicated for treatment of acute bacterial skin and skin structure infections caused by susceptible Gram-positive organism including MRSA [29,30]. Oritavancin and dalbavancin, like other lipoglycopeptides, exert concentration-dependent bactericidal activity by disruption of bacterial membrane integrity, leading to cell death. Oritavancin is used in a single 1,200 mg dose administered IV over 3 hours. Oritavancin is not metabolized and it is extensively distributed into tissues. In patients with mild-to-moderate renal impairment no dosage adjustment is required. Oritavancin as well as dalbavancin has not been studied in patients with severe hepatic impairment. Dalbavancin is infused over 30 minutes as a 2-dose regimen of 1,000 mg IV followed 1 week later by 500 mg. Excretion of dalbavancin is by urine (55%) and by feces (20%).

THERAPY OF ANAEROBIC INFECTIONS

As reviewed previously, excellent efficacy against anaerobes is provided by carbapenems as well as *β*-lactam/*β*-lactamase combination agents. Additional agents with anaerobic activity include metronidazole and clindamycin.

Metronidazole

Metronidazole is highly active against obligate anaerobes. Although orally administered metronidazole is absorbed nearly completely, critically ill patients with infections other than *C. difficile*–associated diarrhea should receive therapy by the IV route. Metronidazole is administered at 500 mg (7.5 mg per kg) IV every 8 hours [31]. Metronidazole is metabolized by the liver; no dose adjustment is required in patients with renal insufficiency, but dosages must be reduced in individuals with severe hepatic insufficiency. Penetration into CSF and brain is excellent. Reported serious adverse events include neutropenia, pancreatitis, peripheral neuropathy, and hepatitis. Metallic taste (dysgeusia) occurs commonly, and up to 12% of patients have minor GI tract side effects. A disulfiram-like reaction can occur with concomitant alcohol intake.

Metronidazole is active in vitro against anaerobic Gram-negative bacilli and is probably the most potent agent for treatment of infections caused by *B. fragilis*. Metronidazole must be used in conjunction with an agent active against aerobic organisms in the treatment of intra-abdominal, intrapelvic, and pulmonary infections where aerobic organisms can be expected to be concurrent pathogens. It has become the drug of first choice for treatment of *C. difficile*–associated diarrhea because of limitations on the use of oral vancomycin in an attempt to decrease selective pressure for the emergence of VRE, although oral vancomycin, often with IV metronidazole, is preferred for critically ill patients [31].

Clindamycin

Clindamycin is active in vitro against a wide variety of anaerobic bacteria. It has been used with great success in the treatment of anaerobic infections of the head, neck, and lungs/pleural space. The use of clindamycin in addition to penicillin is recommended in the treatment of necrotizing fasciitis due to *β*-hemolytic *Streptococcus* spp because of its apparent activity against organisms that are present in very high inoculum [32]. Clindamycin-resistant strains of *B. fragilis* group are becoming more prevalent, with 29% of isolates resistant in 2001 versus 10% in 1988. Usual parenteral therapy with clindamycin for severe infections consists of 600 to 900 mg IV every 8 hours (25 to 40 mg/kg/d). Because clindamycin is metabolized by the liver and excreted in inactive form in bile, no adjustment in dosage is required in patients with renal insufficiency. The most important side effects of clindamycin are gastrointestinal. The incidence of diarrhea during therapy with clindamycin has been reported to range from 3% to 30%. Pseudomembranous colitis due to *C. difficile* has been reported to occur in up to 10% of patients who receive clindamycin [33].

MACROLIDES

The macrolides are bacteriostatic antibiotics that act on the 50 S ribosome subunit. The most common use of macrolides is to treat primary atypical pneumonia due to *Mycoplasma pneumoniae*, *Chlamydophilia pneumoniae*, or *Legionella* spp; pharyngitis due to *S. pyogenes*; *Bordetella pertussis* infections; enteritis due to *Campylobacter* spp; and eradication of the diphtheria carrier state. Erythromycin is the oldest agent in current use in this class, and now is used rarely, with azithromycin or Clarithromycin the preferred agents. Erythromycin is used occasionally in the ICU setting to enhance gut motility.

Azithromycin is available in oral and IV preparations and Clarithromycin only in oral form. In addition to sharing the microbiologic spectrum of activity of erythromycin, azithromycin is more active against *C. trachomatis* but is less active than erythromycin or clarithromycin against staphylococci and streptococci. Clarithromycin shares the antimicrobial spectrum of erythromycin but is more active against Gram-positive cocci. Both agents have activity against *Mycobacterium avium-intracellulare* and *Mycobacterium chelonae* and are used prophylactically and therapeutically for disseminated *M. avium* complex infection in patients with advanced human immunodeficiency virus (HIV) disease. These agents are bacteriostatic and not usually used as first-line agents for treatment of Gram-positive infections in the ICU.

OXAZOLIDINONES

First-generation Oxazolidinones

Linezolid, the first available oxazolidinone antimicrobial, exerts its action by inhibiting the initiation of protein synthesis by stopping assembly of bacterial ribosomes [34]. Linezolid has bacteriostatic activity against MRSA, VRSA, and VRE and is bactericidal against penicillin-resistant *S. pneumoniae*. It is approved for treatment of nosocomial pneumonia and cSSSIs caused by *S. aureus* (including MRSA). It is available for IV or oral use at a dosage of 600 mg every 12 hours and has excellent oral bioavailability. Dosage adjustments are not necessary for patients with renal insufficiency. The oxazolidinones have the potential for interaction with monoamine oxidase inhibitors, selective serotonin receptor uptake inhibitors (SSRIs), adrenergic agents used to support blood pressure in the ICU, and foods that contain a high tyramine content, with potential to trigger the serotonin syndrome, which can involve cognitive, autonomic, and somatic manifestations, presenting variously as confusion, agitation, coma, autonomic instability, flushing, low-grade fever, nausea, diarrhea, diaphoresis, myoclonus, rigidity, and rarely myoclonus and death [35]. Reversible thrombocytopenia may occur if treatment is given longer than 14 days. Resistance may develop in enterococci with long-term use and has been reported in *S. aureus* [36,37].

Second-generation Oxazolidinones

Tedizolid is approved for treatment of bacterial skin and skin structure infection with susceptible isolates of Gram-positive microorganisms including methicillin-sensitive and methicillin-resistant *S.aureus* and *E. fecalis* [38]. Tedizlolide is either infused over 1 hour or given orally in a dose of 200 mg every day. Tedizolide is excreted 82% in feces; 18% in urine. No dosage adjustment required for patients with renal or hepatic impairment.

Quinupristin/Dalfopristin

Quinupristin/dalfopristin is a combination of two streptogramin antibiotics used to treat infections due to vancomycin-resistant *E. faecium* and other Gram-positive bacteria, including *S. aureus*. This agent is given by the IV route and, due to a high incidence of phlebitis, has to be administered through a central vascular catheter. It has bacteriostatic activity against *E. faecium*. The dose is 7.5 mg per kg every 8 hours for serious infections and 7.5 mg per kg every 12 hours for skin and skin structure infections. This drug is reserved for patients with difficult-to-treat infections. Quinupristin/dalfopristin has been used for a few patients with meningitis, and CSF concentrations appear to be higher than the MIC for susceptible organisms. Myalgias and arthralgias occur in up to 10% of patients and may limit its use [39].

Daptomycin

Daptomycin, a cyclic lipopeptide antimicrobial agent with rapid, concentration-dependent bactericidal activity against aerobic and facultative Gram-positive microorganisms, is active against a range of Gram-positive bacteria, including many multidrug-resistant isolates. Daptomycin is approved for treatment of cSSSIs caused by susceptible strains of *S. aureus* (including MRSA), *S. pyogenes*, and other *Streptococcus* and *Enterococcus species*. The dosage of daptomycin for soft tissue infections is 4 mg per kg every 24 hours by IV infusion given over 30 minutes for patients with a creatinine clearance greater than 30 mL per minute. A dose of 6-8 mg per kg every 24 hours is recommended for bacteremia and right-sided endocarditis caused by susceptible strains of *S. aureus* (including MRSA). In the lung, daptomycin is bound to surfactant, and thus it is not clinically effective for treatment of pneumonia [40]. The drug is excreted primarily via the kidney, with low potential for interference with hepatically metabolized drugs. If the creatinine clearance is less than 30 mL per minute, the dosage interval should be extended to 48 hours. Reported adverse effects include diarrhea, vomiting, sickle-cell crisis, hypersensitivity reactions, dermatitis, myalgias, and creatinine kinase elevations [41,42].

Tigecycline

Tigecycline, a minocycline derivative, is the first antibiotic in the glycylcycline class [43]. Tigecycline is one of the few new antimicrobials with activity against Gram-negative bacteria, including multiresistant *Acinetobacter* spp and organisms that produce ESBL. In addition, it is active against Gram positives such as MRSA and enterococci including VRE. Tigecycline is approved treatment of cSSSIs and complicated intra-abdominal infections. Tigecycline is available only for IV administration, given as a 100-mg initial dose, then 50 mg every 12 hours. The most common treatment adverse effects are nausea and vomiting which occur generally during the first 2 days of therapy.

THERAPY OF FUNGAL INFECTIONS

Invasive and disseminated fungal infections are increasingly common in ICU patients, especially those who receive immunosuppressive therapy or broad-spectrum antibiotics; in patients with lymphoreticular malignancies or transplants; and in individuals with advanced HIV disease. Newer antifungals of the triazole class (fluconazole, itraconazole, voriconazole, and posaconazole) and echinocandin class (caspofungin, micafungin, and anidulafungin) have become available for the treatment of systemic mycoses. However, amphotericin B remains important for empiric initial therapy for life-threatening fungal infections when the infecting organism is not yet identified or is resistant to triazoles.

Amphotericin B

Amphotericin B is a polyene antibiotic, insoluble in water, and solubilized by the addition of sodium deoxycholate, forming a colloidal dispersion. Its mechanism of action is due to its binding to ergosterol, a sterol present in the cell membrane of susceptible fungi, resulting in altered membrane permeability and causing leakage of cell components and resultant cell death. Amphotericin B is effective against most species of fungi that are pathogenic in humans [44]. Either amphotericin B deoxycholate or one of the liposomal preparations is the initial drug of choice for empiric therapy of life-threatening, invasive, or systemic fungal infections including mucormycosis, cryptococcosis, histoplasmosis, and coccidioidomycosis and is effective for blastomycosis and extracutaneous sporotrichosis. Although *Candida albicans* generally is susceptible to amphotericin B, non-*albicans* species of *Candida* often are less susceptible, and fluconazole or an echinocandin is the drug of choice once the infecting species is identified and susceptibility is known. Amphotericin B preparations have variable activity against *Aspergillus* spp, *Zygomycetes* spp, *Scedosporium boydii*, *Fusarium* spp, and dematiaceous fungi. The combination of amphotericin B plus flucytosine is synergistic against *Candida* spp and *Cryptococcus neoformans* and is used to treat meningitis due to these fungi.

Amphotericin B for IV administration should be prepared in 5% dextrose because saline solutions result in drug precipitation. The drug is highly protein bound and is distributed into many tissues (liver, spleen, lung, muscle, kidney, skin, and adrenals); because penetration into CSF is poor, intrathecal/intracisternal administration or the use of triazoles may be necessary for some CNS mycoses. The metabolism of amphotericin B is obscure, but renal and hepatic insufficiency has little effect on serum levels of the drug and hemodialysis does not affect serum levels.

Amphotericin B usually is given by IV infusion once a day over 2 to 6 hours, at a concentration of 0.1 mg per mL. Daily and total doses are adjusted according to the fungal species, sites, and extent of infection and the individual tolerance of the patient. A test dose of 1 mg (in 25 to 100 mL 5% dextrose) is infused over 30 minutes. For patients who are critically ill with apparently rapidly progressive fungal disease, the full daily dose of 0.5 to 1.0 mg per kg can be given immediately following the test dose. For patients who exhibit poor tolerance with the test dose or subsequent increased doses, amphotericin B dosing can be increased in a gradual fashion, with increase in the dosage by 5 to 10 mg per day until the final daily dose is reached. The usual duration of amphotericin B therapy for systemic mycoses is 4 to 12 weeks, to a total dose of 1 to 2 g. For infections caused by less susceptible fungi (e.g., *Aspergillus* spp, *Zygomycetes* spp [*Mucor*], and *Coccidioides immitis*), treatment warrants daily doses of up to 1.0 to 1.5 mg per kg and a total dose of 2 g. Cryptococcosis can be treated successfully with reduced (0.3 mg/kg/d) dosages of amphotericin B plus flucytosine (150 mg/kg/d orally) for 6 weeks.

Adverse Reactions

Adverse effects of amphotericin B most frequently include infusion-associated constitutional symptoms such as fever, chills, hypotension, and tachypnea, most common and most severe with the first few doses of the drug and during escalation of dosage and can be minimized by increasing daily dosage slowly (if the clinical situation permits) or by pretreatment with acetaminophen, hydrocortisone (25 to 50 mg IV), or meperidine (25 mg IV). Dantrolene (10 mg IV) has been used successfully as an alternative or adjunctive agent in patients with severe rigors [45]. Nephrotoxicity occurs frequently with amphotericin B deoxycholate therapy, and thus patients with renal insufficiency or administration of other nephrotoxic agents should be given one of the liposomal preparations. Potassium levels should be monitored closely and supplementation with potassium begun as soon as serum potassium decreases toward the low end of normal range. Mild anemia occurs commonly during amphotericin B therapy, but thrombocytopenia, leukopenia, and severe hepatitis are rare. Alternative lipid preparations of amphotericin B have become available in an attempt to decrease renal toxicity [46]. The lipid formulations are more expensive than amphotericin B deoxycholate but are advantageous in patients with, or at risk of, renal insufficiency, those on other nephrotoxic medications, or those whose renal function worsens during treatment with amphotericin B. The ability to deliver a higher dose with the lipid complex than with amphotericin B alone has resulted in reports of patients responding to the lipid formulation at high dose (5 to 10 mg per kg) when traditional therapy with amphotericin B had been ineffective.

Flucytosine

Flucytosine is an orally administered pyrimidine analog with a narrow spectrum of action, generally used in combination with an amphotericin preparation for therapy of *C. neoformans* and *Candida* meningitis. Most strains of *C. neoformans* and *Candida* spp are susceptible initially, whereas most other fungi that are pathogenic for humans are resistant. The use of combination therapy with flucytosine allows a reduction in dosage and duration (0.3 mg/kg/d for 6 weeks) of amphotericin B in treatment of cryptococcal meningitis and improves efficacy in the treatment of *Candida* meningitis because of its excellent penetration into this site. The drug is cleared by the kidneys, with a serum $t_{1/2}$ of 3 hours in patients with normal renal function and 85 hours in anuric patients. The usual recommended dosage in patients with normal renal function is 150 mg per kg daily in four divided doses; the interval between doses should be doubled (every 12 hours) when the creatinine clearance rate is 20 to 40 mL per minute and quadrupled (every 24 hours) when the creatinine clearance rate is 10 to 20 mL per minute. The serum level of flucytosine should be monitored, particularly in patients with renal impairment, and the dose should be adjusted to maintain a level of 50 to 100 μg per mL. Leukopenia is the most serious complication of flucytosine therapy and occurs most commonly in patients with renal insufficiency and when serum levels exceed 100 μg per mL. GI tract intolerance (nausea, vomiting, anorexia, or diarrhea), hepatitis, and rash occur occasionally.

TRIAZOLES

Fluconazole

Fluconazole is a water-soluble triazole available for IV and oral use and exhibits good activity in vitro against *Candida* spp and *C. neoformans* [47]. As with all the triazoles, its mode of action is mediated through inhibition of ergosterol synthesis. Oral absorption is excellent, resulting in serum levels nearly as high as with IV administration, and is independent of gastric acidity. Fluconazole penetrates well into bodily fluids, including CSF (50% to 90% of serum concentrations) and the eye. Fluconazole has a long (30 hours) $t_{1/2}$; because of its renal clearance, adjustments must be made in dosing in patients with renal impairment. For patients with oropharyngeal or esophageal candidiasis, the usual dosage of fluconazole is 200 mg (oral or IV) on the first day of therapy, followed by 100 mg once a day; therapy is continued until clinical findings resolve and for a total of 2 to 3 weeks. Fluconazole (800 mg loading dose, then 400 mg once daily) is effective in the treatment of systemic or hepatic candidiasis due to susceptible strains of *C. albicans* [48]. Non-albicans species of *Candida* may be less susceptible. For severe systemic mycoses (i.e., coccidioidomycosis, cryptococcosis) or candidemia, the usual daily dosage is 800 mg then 400 mg IV daily. Side effects of fluconazole are relatively minor and uncommon, with GI tract symptoms (nausea) most frequent. Mild, transient elevation of serum transaminase levels occurs occasionally. Fluconazole inhibits the metabolism and potentiates the effects of warfarin, phenytoin, cyclosporine, tacrolimus, and oral hypoglycemic agents.

Itraconazole

Itraconazole, a broad-spectrum triazole antifungal with notable activity against *Aspergillus* spp, *H. capsulatum*, *C. immitis*, and *Sporothrix schenckii*, is available for IV or oral use. Itraconazole is widely distributed in most tissues but with poor penetration into CSF. Itraconazole has a role in the treatment of sporotrichosis, blastomycosis, histoplasmosis, paracoccidioidomycosis, and chromomycosis and may be of use in treating patients with coccidioidomycosis, cryptococcosis, or aspergillosis who have failed prior therapy with amphotericin B or other azoles. Daily dosage is 200 to 800 mg orally, with the higher doses indicated in patients with CNS infection. Clearance is by hepatic metabolism, and no adjustment of dosage is required in patients with renal failure. Like voriconazole, the IV form of itraconazole includes cyclodextrin to improve solubility; since cyclodextrin is cleared by the kidney, the IV formulation should not be used if creatinine clearance is less than 30 mL per minute. Itraconazole is well tolerated, with occasional GI tract symptoms (abdominal discomfort, nausea, and diarrhea) or minor elevation of liver chemistry values noted. Itraconazole requires an acidic environment for optimal GI tract absorption. Absorption of the elixir form of the drug is greater than with the capsules, and absorption is better with multiple daily dosing. Itraconazole has only a minimal effect on the synthesis of androgens or cortisol but can produce a picture of mineralocorticoid excess with hypokalemia, edema, and hypertension.

Voriconazole

Voriconazole is a second-generation, broad-spectrum triazole that is a synthetic derivative of fluconazole. Voriconazole is active against strains of *C. krusei* and *C. glabrata* that are inherently fluconazole resistant and against strains of *C. albicans* that have acquired resistance to fluconazole. Voriconazole has a broad activity against many species of *Aspergillus* spp, including *Aspergillus terreus*, which often is resistant to amphotericin B [49]. It is a drug of choice for invasive aspergillosis and refractory infections with *Pseudoallescheria/Scedosporium* and *Fusarium* spp.

Voriconazole is available in oral and IV formulations. The standard loading dose is 6 mg per kg repeated in 12 hours. Patients who weigh more than 40 kg should receive 200 mg every 12 hours for maintenance therapy, and the dosage should be adjusted in patients with mild-to-moderate liver disease. Because the azoles are metabolized by the hepatic cytochrome P450 systems, a variety of drug interactions can occur; however, voriconazole generally is well tolerated. Reported toxicities include elevations in liver enzymes, rash, and, in a third of patients, transient ocular toxicity [50]. The IV form contains cyclodextrin and should be used for short periods (<2 weeks) in patients with renal insufficiency due to accumulation of the metabolites.

Posaconazole

Posaconazole is a second-generation triazole approved for the treatment of oropharyngeal candidiasis, including infections refractory to itraconazole and/or fluconazole [51]. It is approved also as prophylaxis for invasive *Aspergillus* and *Candida* infections in patients older than 13 years who are at high risk of developing fungal infections, such as hematopoietic stem cell transplant recipients with graft-versus-host disease and neutropenic patients with hematologic malignancies [52,53]. Limited clinical experience suggests efficacy for the treatment of infections due to Zygomycetes and as salvage therapy for patients with invasive aspergillosis and coccidioidomycosis. Posaconazole currently is available only as an oral tablet or suspension and requires administration with food or a nutritional supplement to assure adequate bioavailability. Dose adjustment is not required in the presence of renal or hepatic insufficiency. Although not a substrate of hepatic CYP450 3A4, posaconazole inhibits this enzyme and thus has the potential for significant pharmacokinetic interactions with drugs metabolized by this isoform. Its use in combination with CYP450 substrates that prolong the QTc interval is contraindicated, as is its use with ergot alkaloids. The recommended dosage for posaconazole antifungal prophylaxis is 200 mg (5 mL) three times daily. Recommended therapy of oropharyngeal candidiasis is a loading dose of 200 mg (100 mg twice daily), followed by 100 mg daily for 13 days. Refractory oropharyngeal candidiasis may be treated with 400 mg twice daily, with the duration based on clinical response and the patient's underlying disease. Experimental treatment of invasive fungal infections with posaconazole at 200 mg orally four times daily and maintenance therapy at 400 mg orally twice daily is based on pharmacokinetic data; however, package labeling does not include this indication. The most common adverse effects associated with the use of posaconazole include headache, fever, nausea, vomiting, and diarrhea.

Isavuconazole

Isavuconazole is indicated for treatment of invasive aspergillosis and mucormycosis. Isavuconazole has activity against most strains of the *A. flavus*, *A. fumigatus*, and *A. niger* as well as invasive mucormycosis caused by Mucorales and fungi such as *Rhizopus oryzae* and *Mucormycetes* spp. In a phase 3 clinical trial, isavuconazole demonstrated non-inferiority to voriconazole on the primary endpoint of all-cause mortality at day 42 for the treatment of adult patients with invasive aspergillosis or other filamentous fungi [54]. The overall safety profile for isavuconazole demonstrated similar rates of mortality and non-fatal adverse events as the comparator, voriconazole. Isavuconazole is given at initial dose of 372 mg PO or IV every 8 hours for 6 doses over 48 hours and continues at maintenance dose of 372 mg PO or IV every day. Excretion of isavuconazole is 46.1% by feces; 45.5% by urine. Similar to posaconazole, dose adjustment is not required in the presence of renal and/or hepatic insufficiency. Use of isavuconazole is contraindicated in combination with CYP450 substrates and in patients with familial short QT syndrome.

ECHINOCANDINS

Caspofungin/Micafungin/Anidulafungin

Caspofungin, micafungin, and anidulafungin are echinocandins, a class of antifungal agents that act on the fungal cell wall by inhibiting glucan synthesis. Echinocandins are available only for IV administration and are active against most species of Candida. Caspofungin can be used for refractory cases of invasive aspergillosis in patients intolerant of voriconazole and amphotericin B. All these agents may be used to treat candidemia with similar success but with fewer side effects than amphotericin B [55]. These agents are highly protein bound and distribute into all major organ sites including the brain; however, concentration in uninfected CSF is low. For caspofungin, the recommended dosage for adults is 70 mg as a loading dose, then 50 mg per day. Dose alteration is recommended in the presence of moderate hepatic insufficiency. Caspofungin is metabolized by the liver, and dose adjustment is required when it is given with other drugs that alter cytochrome P450 activity. In general, caspofungin is well tolerated, with the most frequently reported adverse effects being increased serum transaminases, GI upset, and headaches. Caspofungin is classified as pregnancy category C and should be used during pregnancy only if the potential benefit outweighs the potential fetal risk. These three agents exhibit a fungicidal effect against most *Candida* spp and have become the drugs of choice for empiric therapy of candidemia in the ICU. However, they are not active against *C. neoformans*. They have a fungistatic effect against *Aspergillus* spp. Micafungin appears comparable to fluconazole as antifungal prophylaxis in patients undergoing hematopoietic stem-cell transplantation [56] and anidulafungin has been used in neutropenic children. Absence of antagonism in combination with other antifungal agents suggests that combination antifungal therapy warrants further study, particularly for severe aspergillosis and candidiasis [57].

Trimethoprim–Sulfamethoxazole

Trimethoprim–sulfamethoxazole (cotrimoxazole) works through sequential, two-stage inhibition of folate synthesis. It has activity against Gram-positive and Gram-negative bacteria, *Nocardia* spp, and *Pneumocystis jiroveci* (previously known as *P. carinii*). Trimethoprim–sulfamethoxazole can be used in the therapy of Gram-negative infections in the ICU patient, including those caused by *Enterobacter* spp. The dose for serious bacterial infections is 8 to 10 mg/kg/d (of the trimethoprim component), divided every 6 to 12 hours.

Trimethoprim–sulfamethoxazole is the drug of choice for *Pneumocystis jiroveci* pneumonia [58]. In moderately to severely ill patients, it is administered IV or orally at a dosage of 15 to 20 mg/kg/d of the trimethoprim component in three to four divided doses for a total course of 14 days in non-AIDS patients and at a dosage of 15 mg per kg of the trimethoprim component daily (or 75 mg per kg of the sulfa component daily) for 21 days in patients with AIDS. Failure to obtain satisfactory response in 5 days (7 days in individuals with HIV infection) warrants change to an alternative regimen (see HIV Chapter 76 for *Pneumocystis* pneumonia therapy). Adverse reactions to trimethoprim–sulfamethoxazole occur in approximately 10% to 15% of patients who are uninfected with HIV-1 and in up to two thirds of patients with AIDS. The most common problems are neutropenia, thrombocytopenia, or both (particularly in patients with advanced HIV-1–induced immunodeficiency or receiving zidovudine); rash or fever; nausea or vomiting; and abnormalities of hepatic enzymes.

Pyrimethamine–Sulfadiazine

For the treatment of systemic and invasive (including encephalitis) toxoplasmosis in the compromised host, the alternate double-antifolate combination of pyrimethamine–sulfadiazine usually is used. Pyrimethamine is administered orally with a loading dose of 200 mg, then at 75 mg daily (with folinic acid 5 mg daily) together with sulfadiazine orally at 6 g daily in four divided doses. Adverse reactions occur in similar frequency and type as with cotrimoxazole. Alternative therapy for CNS toxoplasmosis is clindamycin (900 mg IV every 6 hours) plus pyrimethamine [59].

THERAPY OF VIRAL INFECTIONS

As viral infections have become more common and more severe in an era of expanding populations of immunocompromised hosts, several antiviral agents have become available (Table 73.4). Nevertheless, antiviral therapy remains problematic and limited in scope as compared with antibacterial treatments. Antiretroviral therapy is discussed in Chapter 76.

Acyclovir and Related Compounds

Acyclovir is a nucleoside analog of guanosine with antiviral activity against herpes viruses, particularly herpes simplex virus (HSV) types 1 and 2 and varicella-zoster virus (VZV) [60]. Administered as a prodrug, acyclovir requires phosphorylation to a monophosphate form by a virus-generated thymidine kinase and then to a triphosphate form by host cellular enzymes. Because cytomegalovirus (CMV) lacks a thymidine kinase, acyclovir has poor activity against this virus. Acyclovir is available in topical, oral, and IV preparations, with the last route preferred for serious infections in critically ill patients and for milder illnesses in those unable to take medications by mouth. After oral administration, absorption is slow and incomplete, with oral bioavailability of only 15% to 30%. Serum $t_{1/2}$ is 2 to 3 hours in patients with normal

TABLE 73.4

Antiviral Therapy

Antiviral agent	Indication	Dose	Route	Duration of treatment	Adjust for renal failure
Acyclovir	Herpes simplex virus				
	Encephalitis	10–12 mg/kg q8h	IV	10–14 d	Yes
	Neonatal infection	10 mg/kg q8h	IV	10–14 d	Yes
	Mucocutaneous disease	5 mg/kg q8h	IV	7–10 d	Yes
	Herpes varicella-zoster	10 mg/kg q8h	IV	7–10 d	Yes
Ganciclovir	Cytomegalovirus				
	Induction	5 mg/kg q12h	IV	14–21 d	Yes
	Maintenance	5 mg/kg qd or	IV	Indefinite	
		6 mg/kg 5 d/wk	IV	Indefinite	
		3,000 mg qd	PO	Indefinite	
Foscarnet	Cytomegalovirus				
	Induction	60 mg/kg q8h or	IV	14–21 d	Yes
		90 mg/kg q12h	IV		
	Maintenance	90 mg/kg qd	IV	Indefinite	
Cidofovir (+probenecid premedication)	Cytomegalovirus Induction	5 mg/kg q wk 5 mg/kg q 2 wk	IV	14 d Indefinite	Contraindicated in patients with baseline creatinine >1.5 mg/dL or increase to >2.0 mg/dL

renal function. Because 85% of clearance is renal, dosage must be reduced in patients with impaired renal function. Acyclovir is well tolerated. Reversible renal impairment, due to crystalluria, occurs occasionally, usually in patients who are receiving high doses by rapid IV infusion or those who are elderly, dehydrated, or have antecedent renal insufficiency. At high doses, especially IV, neurologic reactions (confusion, delirium, hallucinations, seizures, and tremors) have occurred in approximately 1% of patients. Occasionally, patients experience nausea, vomiting, or rash. Dosage varies according to the condition under treatment. Intravenous acyclovir at 10 to 12 mg per kg every 8 hours is the drug of choice for HSV encephalitis (for a course of 14 to 21 days), for congenital HSV infection (10 to 14 days), and for VZV infections (chickenpox or shingles) in immunocompromised patients (7 to 10 days). Acyclovir at 5 mg per kg IV every 8 hours is effective against mucocutaneous HSV in immunocompromised patients.

Valacyclovir, a prodrug for acyclovir, is more completely absorbed via the oral route than acyclovir and is hydrolyzed rapidly to acyclovir in the intestinal wall and the liver [61]. In general, it is well tolerated, but thrombocytopenia and hemolytic-uremic syndrome have been reported in immunocompromised patients. Other side effects are similar to those of acyclovir and include encephalopathy, fevers, seizures, and rash. Acyclovir, or valacyclovir, is used prophylactically in patients who are undergoing bone marrow or solid organ transplantation.

Famciclovir, a prodrug for penciclovir, is active against VZV and HSV. Side effects are similar to those of acyclovir. Both of the newer oral agents, famciclovir and valacyclovir, are dosed three times a day orally rather than the five times a day that is needed with acyclovir for VZV infections.

Ganciclovir

Ganciclovir is highly active against CMV, in part because of the high concentration of the triphosphorylated form of the drug in infected cells. The most problematic adverse effect is myelosuppression, particularly neutropenia. Other side effects include nausea and vomiting and CNS abnormalities. Ganciclovir is effective in the treatment of disseminated CMV and CMV retinitis, GI tract infection (colitis, esophagitis, and gastritis), and pneumonitis. In bone marrow transplant patients, the drug sometimes is used in combination with CMV hyperimmune globulin IV for the treatment of CMV pneumonitis [62]. Valganciclovir is a prodrug for ganciclovir [63]. It is more completely absorbed from the GI tract, achieving higher serum levels than possible with oral therapy with the parent drug.

Treatment with ganciclovir for AIDS patients with CMV retinitis usually involves induction therapy with 5 mg per kg IV twice a day for 14 to 21 days, followed by maintenance therapy with oral valganciclovir. It is given for 3 weeks or until serum CMV molecular assays are negative for immunocompromised patient with disseminated CMV infection. Ganciclovir and valganciclovir are cleared by the kidney and dosage adjustments must be made in patients with renal impairment, especially in light of the relationship between drug serum levels and myelosuppression. Valganciclovir is used as prophylaxis or preemptive therapy for CMV in transplant patients.

Cidofovir

Cidofovir is a nucleotide analog that is active against herpes viruses, including CMV, HSV, and VZV. It is a prodrug that is converted to cidofovir diphosphate by host cellular enzymes. In contrast to ganciclovir and acyclovir, activation by viral-encoded enzymes is not required, so it may be used to treat CMV infections when the virus is resistant to ganciclovir because of its UL97 mutation.

Foscarnet

Foscarnet (trisodium phosphonoformate) is an inorganic pyrophosphate analog that acts by inhibiting viral DNA polymerases of most human herpes viruses (particularly CMV) and reverse transcriptases of human retroviruses (particularly HIV-1) [62]. Foscarnet is effective for the therapy of CMV retinitis for patients with AIDS and has been used alone and in combination with ganciclovir to treat ganciclovir-resistant CMV of immunocompromised patients (especially transplant recipients). Foscarnet is associated with a significant (25%) incidence of nephrotoxicity. Therapy involves IV administration at a dosage of 60 mg per kg three times a day for induction and at 90 to 120 mg per kg once a day for maintenance therapy. Clearance is by renal excretion, and dosage adjustment is required in patients with renal impairment. Nonrenal adverse effects include nausea, vomiting, anemia, seizures, and metabolic abnormalities (hyperphosphatemia and hypophosphatemia, hypercalcemia and hypocalcemia, hypokalemia, and hypomagnesemia).

Anti-influenza Agents

Amantadine and rimantadine are oral antiviral compounds that inhibit influenza A, and zanamivir, oseltamivir, and peramivir are neuraminidase inhibitors that inhibit both influenza A and B viruses. If initiated within 48 hours of the onset of symptoms, all four agents may reduce the intensity of influenza infection in patients infected with susceptible viruses [45,64]. For patients who are immunocompromised or who have ongoing viral replication and progressive symptoms, therapy after 48 hours may also be beneficial, although supporting data are not available. Zanamivir is given by the inhaled route and oseltamivir by the oral route. The dose of oseltamivir is 100 mg per day and for zanamivir 20 mg by inhalation daily. Peramivir is given intravenously as a single dose of 600 mg. Resistance to the antiviral agents has occurred in influenza viruses, and clinicians need to be aware of the susceptibility of prevailing influenza strains in their communities to appropriately choose an agent for use in their ICUs.

References

1. Tleyjeh IM, Tlaygeh HM, Hejal R, et al: The impact of penicillin resistance on short-term mortality in hospitalized adults with pneumococcal pneumonia: a systematic review and meta-analysis. *Clin Infect Dis* 42(6):788–797, 2006.
2. van de Beek D, de Gans J, Tunkel AR, et al: Community-acquired bacterial meningitis in adults. *N Engl J Med* 354(1):44–53, 2006.
3. Erwin ME, Fix AM, Jones RN: Three independent yearly analyses of the spectrum and potency of metronidazole: a multicenter study of 1,108 contemporary anaerobic clinical isolates. *Diagn Microbiol Infect Dis* 39(2):129–132, 2001.
4. Allewelt M, Schuler P, Bolcskei PL, et al: Ampicillin + sulbactam vs clindamycin +/- cephalosporin for the treatment of aspiration pneumonia and primary lung abscess. *Clin Microbiol Infect* 10(2):163–170, 2004.
5. Baddour LM, Wilson WR, Bayer AS, et al: Infective endocarditis: diagnosis, antimicrobial therapy, and management of complications: a statement for healthcare professionals from the Committee on Rheumatic Fever, Endocarditis, and Kawasaki Disease, Council on Cardiovascular Disease in the Young, and the Councils on Clinical Cardiology, Stroke, and Cardiovascular Surgery and Anesthesia, American Heart Association: endorsed by the Infectious Diseases Society of America.[Erratum appears in *Circulation* 115(15):e408, 2007], [Erratum appears in *Circulation* 116(21):e547, 2007], [Erratum appears in *Circulation* 112(15):2373, 2005], [Erratum appears in *Circulation* 118(12):e497, 2008]. *Circulation* 111(23):e394–e434, 2005.
6. Francis JS, Doherty MC, Lopatin U, et al: Severe community-onset pneumonia in healthy adults caused by methicillin-resistant Staphylococcus aureus carrying the Panton-Valentine leukocidin genes. *Clin Infect Dis* 40(1):100–107, 2005.
7. Perry CM, Markham A: Piperacillin/tazobactam: an updated review of its use in the treatment of bacterial infections. *Drugs* 57(5):805–843, 1999.
8. American Thoracic S; Infectious Diseases Society of America: Guidelines for the management of adults with hospital-acquired, ventilator-associated, and health-care-associated pneumonia. *Am J Respir Crit Care Med* 171(4):388–416, 2005.

9. Jacoby GA, Munoz-Price LS: The new beta-lactamases. *N Engl J Med* 352(4):380–391, 2005.
10. Paul M, Lador A, Grozinsky-Glasberg S, et al: Beta lactam antibiotic monotherapy versus beta lactam-aminoglycoside antibiotic combination therapy for sepsis. *Cochrane Database Syst Rev* 1:CD003344, 2014.
11. Tunkel AR, Hartman BJ, Kaplan SL, et al: Practice guidelines for the management of bacterial meningitis. *Clin Infect Dis* 39(9):1267–1284, 2004.
12. Wunderink RG, Waterer GW: Clinical practice. Community-acquired pneumonia. *N Engl J Med* 370(6):543–551, 2014.
13. Safdar N, Handelsman J, Maki DG: Does combination antimicrobial therapy reduce mortality in Gram-negative bacteraemia? A meta-analysis. *Lancet Infect Dis* 4(8):519–527, 2004.
14. Siedner MJ, Galar A, Guzman-Suarez BB, et al: Cefepime vs other antibacterial agents for the treatment of Enterobacter species bacteremia. *Clin Infect Dis* 58(11):1554–1563, 2014.
15. File TM Jr, Wilcox MH, Stein GE: Summary of ceftaroline fosamil clinical trial studies and clinical safety. *Clin Infect Dis* 55 Suppl 3:S173–S180, 2012.
16. Marshall WF, Blair JE: The cephalosporins. *Mayo Clin Proc* 74(2):187–195, 1999.
17. Lucasti C, Popescu I, Ramesh MK, et al: Comparative study of the efficacy and safety of ceftazidime/avibactam plus metronidazole versus meropenem in the treatment of complicated intra-abdominal infections in hospitalized adults: results of a randomized, double-blind, Phase II trial. *J Antimicrob Chemother* 68(5):1183–1192, 2013.
18. Wagenlehner FM, Umeh O, Steenbergen J, et al: Ceftolozane-tazobactam compared with levofloxacin in the treatment of complicated urinary-tract infections, including pyelonephritis: a randomised, double-blind, phase 3 trial (ASPECT-cUTI). *Lancet* 385(9981):1949–1956, 2015.
19. Maseda E, Aguilar L, Gimenez MJ, et al: Ceftolozane/tazobactam (CXA 201) for the treatment of intra-abdominal infections. *Expert Rev Anti Infect Ther* 12(11):1311–1324, 2014.
20. Keating GM, Perry CM: Ertapenem: a review of its use in the treatment of bacterial infections. *Drugs* 65(15):2151–2178, 2005.
21. Lucasti C, Jasovich A, Umeh O, et al: Efficacy and tolerability of IV doripenem versus meropenem in adults with complicated intra-abdominal infection: a phase III, prospective, multicenter, randomized, double-blind, noninferiority study. *Clin Ther* 30(5):868–883, 2008.
22. Edson RS, Terrell CL: The aminoglycosides. *Mayo Clin Proc* 74(5):519–528, 1999.
23. Chow JW: Aminoglycoside resistance in enterococci. *Clin Infect Dis* 31(2):586–589, 2000.
24. Barclay ML, Kirkpatrick CM, Begg EJ: Once daily aminoglycoside therapy. Is it less toxic than multiple daily doses and how should it be monitored? *Clin Pharmacokinet* 36(2):89–98, 1999.
25. Van Bambeke F, Michot JM, Van Eldere J, et al: Quinolones in 2005: an update. *Clin Microbiol Infect* 11(4):256–280, 2005.
26. Rybak M, Lomaestro B, Rotschafer JC, et al: Therapeutic monitoring of vancomycin in adult patients: a consensus review of the American Society of Health-System Pharmacists, the Infectious Diseases Society of America, and the Society of Infectious Diseases Pharmacists. *Am J Health Syst Pharm* 66(1):82–98, 2009.
27. Segarra-Newnham M, Tagoff SS: Probable vancomycin-induced neutropenia. *Ann Pharmacother* 38(11):1855–1859, 2004.
28. Corey GR, Rubinstein E, Stryjewski ME, et al: Potential role for telavancin in bacteremic infections due to gram-positive pathogens: focus on Staphylococcus aureus. *Clin Infect Dis* 60(5):787–796, 2015.
29. Corey GR, Good S, Jiang H, et al: Single-dose oritavancin versus 7–10 days of vancomycin in the treatment of gram-positive acute bacterial skin and skin structure infections: the SOLO II noninferiority study. *Clin Infect Dis* 60(2):254–262, 2015.
30. Boucher HW, Wilcox M, Talbot GH, et al: Once-weekly dalbavancin versus daily conventional therapy for skin infection. *N Engl J Med* 370(23):2169–2179, 2014.
31. Zar FA, Bakkanagari SR, Moorthi KM, et al: A comparison of vancomycin and metronidazole for the treatment of Clostridium difficile-associated diarrhea, stratified by disease severity. *Clin Infect Dis* 45(3):302–307, 2007.
32. Bisno AL, Stevens DL: Streptococcal infections of skin and soft tissues. *N Engl J Med* 334(4):240–245, 1996.
33. Riddle DJ, Dubberke ER: Clostridium difficile infection in the intensive care unit. *Infect Dis Clin North Am* 23(3):727–743, 2009.
34. Perry CM, Jarvis B: Linezolid: a review of its use in the management of serious gram-positive infections. *Drugs* 61(4):525–551, 2001.
35. Lawrence KR, Adra M, Gillman PK: Serotonin toxicity associated with the use of linezolid: a review of postmarketing data. *Clin Infect Dis* 42(11):1578–1583, 2006.
36. Schulte B, Heininger A, Autenrieth IB, et al: Emergence of increasing linezolid-resistance in enterococci in a post-outbreak situation with vancomycin-resistant Enterococcus faecium. *Epidemiol Infect* 136(8):1131–1133, 2008.
37. Miller K, O'Neill AJ, Wilcox MH, et al: Delayed development of linezolid resistance in Staphylococcus aureus following exposure to low levels of antimicrobial agents. *Antimicrob Agents Chemother* 52(6):1940–1944, 2008.
38. Moellering RC Jr: Tedizolid: a novel oxazolidinone for Gram-positive infections. *Clin Infect Dis* 58 Suppl 1:S1–S3, 2014.
39. Olsen KM, Rebuck JA, Rupp ME: Arthralgias and myalgias related to quinupristin-dalfopristin administration. *Clin Infect Dis* 32(4):e83–e86, 2001.
40. Silverman JA, Mortin LI, Vanpraagh AD, et al: Inhibition of daptomycin by pulmonary surfactant: in vitro modeling and clinical impact. *J Infect Dis* 191(12):2149–2152, 2005.
41. Levine DP: Clinical experience with daptomycin: bacteraemia and endocarditis. *J Antimicrob Chemother* 62 Suppl 3:iii35–iii39, 2008.
42. Arbeit RD, Maki D, Tally FP, et al: The safety and efficacy of daptomycin for the treatment of complicated skin and skin-structure infections. *Clin Infect Dis* 38(12):1673–1681, 2004.
43. Montravers P, Dupont H, Bedos JP, et al: Tigecycline use in critically ill patients: a multicentre prospective observational study in the intensive care setting. *Intensive Care Med* 40(7):988–997, 2014.
44. Barrett JP, Vardulaki KA, Conlon C, et al: A systematic review of the antifungal effectiveness and tolerability of amphotericin B formulations. *Clin Ther* 25(5):1295–1320, 2003.
45. Libraty D: *Serious viral epidemic pneumonias. Irwin and Rippe Intensive Care Medicine.* Chapter 83, 2016.
46. Sun HY, Alexander BD, Lortholary O, et al: Lipid formulations of amphotericin B significantly improve outcome in solid organ transplant recipients with central nervous system cryptococcosis. *Clin Infect Dis* 49(11):1721–1728, 2009.
47. Charlier C, Hart E, Lefort A, et al: Fluconazole for the management of invasive candidiasis: where do we stand after 15 years? *J Antimicrob Chemother* 57(3):384–410, 2006.
48. Eggimann P, Garbino J, Pittet D: Management of Candida species infections in critically ill patients. *Lancet Infect Dis* 3(12):772–785, 2003.
49. Denning DW, Ribaud P, Milpied N, et al: Efficacy and safety of voriconazole in the treatment of acute invasive aspergillosis. *Clin Infect Dis* 34(5):563–571, 2002.
50. Lazarus HM, Blumer JL, Yanovich S, et al: Safety and pharmacokinetics of oral voriconazole in patients at risk of fungal infection: a dose escalation study. *J Clin Pharmacol* 42(4):395–402, 2002.
51. Nagappan V, Deresinski S: Reviews of anti-infective agents: posaconazole: a broad-spectrum triazole antifungal agent. *Clin Infect Dis* 45(12):1610–1617, 2007.
52. Cornely OA, Maertens J, Winston DJ, et al: Posaconazole vs. fluconazole or itraconazole prophylaxis in patients with neutropenia. *N Engl J Med* 356(4):348–359, 2007.
53. Ullmann AJ, Lipton JH, Vesole DH, et al: Posaconazole or fluconazole for prophylaxis in severe graft-versus-host disease.[Erratum appears in *N Engl J Med* 357(4):428, 2007]. *N Engl J Med* 356(4):335–347, 2007.
54. Pettit NN, Carver PL: Isavuconazole: a new option for the management of invasive fungal infections. *Ann Pharmacother* 49(7):825–842, 2015.
55. Morrison VA: Caspofungin: an overview. *Expert Rev Anti Infect Ther.* 3(5):697–705, 2005.
56. Hiramatsu Y, Maeda Y, Fujii N, et al: Use of micafungin versus fluconazole for antifungal prophylaxis in neutropenic patients receiving hematopoietic stem cell transplantation. *Int J Hematol* 88(5):588–595, 2008.
57. Chandrasekar PH, Sobel JD: Micafungin: a new echinocandin. *Clin Infect Dis* 42(8):1171–1178, 2006.
58. Masters PA, O'Bryan TA, Zurlo J, et al: Trimethoprim-sulfamethoxazole revisited. *Arch Intern Med* 163(4):402–410, 2003.
59. Katlama C, De Wit S, O'Doherty E, et al: Pyrimethamine-clindamycin vs. pyrimethamine-sulfadiazine as acute and long-term therapy for toxoplasmic encephalitis in patients with AIDS. *Clin Infect Dis* 22(2):268–275, 1996.
60. Whitley RJ, Gnann JW Jr: Acyclovir: a decade later. *N Engl J Med* 327(11):782–789, 1992.
61. Acosta EP, Fletcher CV: Valacyclovir. *Ann Pharmacother* 31(2):185–191, 1997.
62. Balfour HH Jr: Management of cytomegalovirus disease with antiviral drugs. *Rev Infect Dis* 12 Suppl 7:S849–S860, 1990.
63. Pescovitz MD, Rabkin J, Merion RM, et al: Valganciclovir results in improved oral absorption of ganciclovir in liver transplant recipients. *Antimicrob Agents Chemother* 44(10):2811–2815, 2000.
64. Anonymous: Antiviral drugs prophylaxis and treatment of influenza. *Med Lett Drugs Ther* 48(1246):87–88, 2006.

Chapter 74 ■ Life-Threatening Community-Acquired Infections: Toxic Shock Syndrome, Meningococcemia, Overwhelming Postsplenectomy Infection, Malaria, Rocky Mountain Spotted Fever, and Others

MISHA HUANG • MARY T. BESSESEN

This chapter covers several infections of low incidence and high mortality, a combination of factors that challenges the physician to recognize a life-threatening disease he or she may never have seen before and institute appropriate therapy promptly. To assist in this challenge, as these diseases are discussed, key historical points and clinical clues will be emphasized.

The critically ill febrile patient should undergo a thorough history and physical examination. Family members may need to be interviewed if the patient is too ill to participate fully in the history. Key points of the exposure history include travel, employment, hobbies, and exposure to pets, wildlife, and livestock. This portion of the interview will yield better results if it is carried out in a slow-paced conversational manner, allowing the patient or family member to chat a bit. It is less focused than a standard social history and review of symptoms, owing to the heterogeneous nature of the exposures being sought. A complete physical examination should be performed. In assessing vital signs, one must evaluate hypothermia (temperature less than 36°C) in the same light as fever (temperature higher than 38°C). Laboratory studies should include a complete blood count with platelet and differential counts; prothrombin and partial thromboplastin times; electrolytes, including calcium and magnesium; blood glucose; renal and liver functions; two sets of blood cultures, urine for culture and urinalysis; and a chest radiograph. If a serious infection is under diagnostic consideration, the hematology laboratory should supplement the automated differential leukocyte count with a manual differential count by microscopic examination of the peripheral blood film. This may require a specific request from the physician, especially if the total leukocyte count falls within the normal range.

TOXIC SHOCK SYNDROMES

There are two toxic shock syndromes (TSSs) commonly recognized, one caused by *Staphylococcus aureus* and the other caused by *Streptococcus pyogenes* (group A streptococcus). To further complicate this picture, it has recently been reported that group C and group G streptococci may occasionally cause TSS [1]. In addition, *Clostridium sordellii* has been reported to cause a similar, but clinically distinct, TSS in obstetric patients, injection drug users, and recipients of musculoskeletal tissue allografts. Each of these three syndromes are discussed in the subsequent sections.

Staphylococcal Toxic Shock Syndrome

Staphylococcal TSS was first described in 1978 [2], and gained notoriety in the early 1980s when menstrual-associated cases struck large numbers of young women [3]. It is a multisystem disease characterized by acute onset of high fever, hypotension, diffuse macular rash, severe myalgia, vomiting, diarrhea, headache, and nonfocal neurologic abnormalities. The primary focus of staphylococcal infection may be mucosal, typically vaginal, associated with tampon or diaphragm use, or a wound. Currently, there are four well-recognized forms of staphylococcal TSS: menstrual [3], postsurgical [4], influenza associated [5], and recalcitrant erythematous desquamating syndrome in acquired immunodeficiency syndrome [6].

Etiology

Staphylococcal TSS is a toxin-mediated illness caused by *S. aureus* strains that produce superantigens (SAgs). Menstrual-associated TSS is almost always caused by a strain that carries the SAg TSS toxin 1 (TSST-1), which is able to cross intact mucous membranes. Nonmenstrual TSS may be caused by any of 15 described SAgs, but is most commonly associated with TSST-1, staphylococcal enterotoxin B, or staphylococcal enterotoxin C [7]. Staphylococcal enterotoxins B and C are not absorbed across mucous membranes, but can cause TSS in cases of staphylococcal infection of wounds. There are rare case reports of staphylococcal TSS associated with nosocomial strains of methicillin-resistant *Staphylococcus aureus* (MRSA) [8]. MRSA strains producing TSST-1 have been implicated in the development of a related disease, neonatal TSS-like exanthematous disease (NTED), first described as part of an epidemic in Japanese neonatal intensive care units in the early 2000s, with only isolated case reports in Europe since that time [9–11]. TSS has not been a feature of the epidemic of the community-associated MRSA strain, USA300, nor was TSST-1 identified in a large collection of USA300 isolates [12].

Pathogenesis

In TSS, bacterial toxins function as SAgs. Conventional antigens presented in the context of major histocompatibility molecules on antigen-presenting cells (APCs) must be processed by the APC and recognized by multiple elements of the T-cell receptor (TCR). In contrast, SAgs do not require processing by an APC but instead bind directly to the TCR to activate T cells. Expansion of T-cell populations expressing particular TCR Vβ chains results in massive release of proinflammatory cytokines, such as γ-interferon, tumor necrosis factor α (TNF-α), interleukin 1-β (IL-1β), and interleukin-2 (IL-2), leading to a capillary leak syndrome [7]. The absence of preexisting antibody to the pertinent bacterial toxin is a critical host factor of TSS. Among cases of menstruation-associated TSS, 90% do not have preexisting antibody to TSST-1. In contrast, more than 90% of healthy persons older than 25 years of age have antibody to TSST-1. It is also hypothesized that a lack of antibody to TSST-1 in pregnant women may contribute to the development of NTED [10]. Recently, it has been postulated that an altered vaginal microbiome may contribute to the hyperproduction of TSST-1 by commensal *S. aureus* organisms and present a risk factor for the TSS [13].

Diagnosis

Clinical Features. The classic case profile is a young (15 to 25 years old), menstruating female. However, any staphylococcal infection can predispose to TSS, including surgical wound infections, furuncles, and abscesses. Postpartum cases can occur after vaginal or cesarean delivery. Nasal reconstructive surgery carries an especially high risk of TSS. Cases may also occur after nasal packing for epistaxis.

The typical presentation is one of high fever, rash, and confusion. There may be a prodromal period of 2 to 3 days, consisting of malaise, myalgia, and chills. Patients are listless, but focal neurologic findings are not seen. Examination of patients with menstruation-associated TSS reveals vaginal hyperemia and exudate that yields *S. aureus* on culture. In nonmenstrual cases, a careful examination usually reveals a focus of staphylococcal infection. It is important to note that this focus may be subtle, with only serous drainage [4]. This is a toxin-mediated disease, and the local appearance is not one of intense purulence. Drainage of local infections is essential to a favorable outcome.

Laboratory Findings. Leukocytosis with marked left shift, thrombocytopenia, azotemia, sterile pyuria, and elevated transaminases are common, although nonspecific findings. Cultures of blood and cerebrospinal fluid (CSF) are usually sterile. Cultures of the local site of infection are usually, but not invariably, positive for *S. aureus*.

Differential Diagnosis. Streptococcal scarlet fever, measles, leptospirosis, Rocky Mountain spotted fever (RMSF), Stevens–Johnson syndrome, and Kawasaki disease can mimic TSS. Multiorgan involvement is usually absent in streptococcal scarlet fever, and the primary focus yields *S. pyogenes*. Exclusion of measles, leptospirosis, ehrlichiosis, and RMSF requires a careful history for potential exposures and serologic testing. Stevens–Johnson syndrome is characterized by target lesions and is commonly associated with exposure to medications. Kawasaki disease is characterized by fever and rash without multisystem involvement, is most commonly seen in children younger than 6 years of age, and is associated with thrombocytosis rather than thrombocytopenia.

The US Centers for Disease Control and Prevention (CDC) case definition of nonstreptococcal TSS consists of both clinical and laboratory criteria, as outlined in Table 74.1 [14].

TABLE 74.1

CDC Case Definition for Nonstreptococcal Toxic Shock Syndrome

Clinical criteria:

- Fever ≥102°F or ≥38.9°C
- Diffuse macular erythroderma
- Desquamation (unless death occurs before the onset of desquamation)
- Hypotension (systolic blood pressure ≤ 90 mm Hg for adults or less than fifth percentile by age for children aged less than 16 y)
- Involvement of three or more organ systems

Laboratory criteria (if obtained):

- Negative blood and cerebrospinal fluid cultures for another pathogen (blood cultures may be positive for *Staphylococcus aureus*)
- Negative serologies for Rocky Mountain Spotted Fever, leptospirosis, and measles

A confirmed case meets the laboratory criteria and all five clinical criteria; a probable case meets the laboratory criteria and four of the five clinical criteria.

CDC, Centers for Disease Control and Prevention.

A confirmed case meets the laboratory criteria and all five clinical criteria; a probable case meets the laboratory criteria and four of the five clinical criteria. The CDC case definition is useful for surveillance purposes, but it identifies the most severe cases and may underestimate the true burden of disease. TSS should be empirically treated when there is a clinical suspicion, even if not all of the clinical criteria are met.

Treatment

The primary intervention consists of fluid resuscitation and supportive care. Any focus of staphylococcal infection must be drained. For women, a vaginal examination must be performed as soon as the patient is stabilized, and any foreign bodies (such as tampon or diaphragm) should be removed. After cultures of the local site and the blood are obtained, antistaphylococcal therapy should be administered intravenously.

Empiric antibacterial therapy for the critically ill patient should include an agent that is active against 100% of suspected pathogens, if feasible. At this time, the antibiotic that is most likely to cover all *S. aureus* isolates is vancomycin. There is in vitro evidence that clindamycin [15] and linezolid [16] inhibit staphylococcal toxin production, whereas β-lactam agents increase TSST-1 in culture supernatants, probably because of cell lysis–releasing toxin [17]. One retrospective study showed improved outcomes for children with TSS who received therapy with clindamycin or erythromycin in the first 48 hours [18]. Initial empiric treatment for TSS when the pathogen has not yet been identified should consist of vancomycin combined with clindamycin. If methicillin-susceptible *S. aureus* is isolated, the vancomycin should be switched to nafcillin or oxacillin, and after 48 hours the clindamycin can be discontinued. First-generation cephalosporins (cefazolin) may be substituted for an antistaphylococcal penicillin in patients with a history of non–life-threatening allergy to penicillins.

Intravenous immunoglobulin (IVIG) may be a useful adjunctive therapy. Higher doses of IVIG may be required for staphylococcal TSS than for streptococcal TSS [19].

Outcomes

The mortality of menstrual staphylococcal TSS is 3%, and two to three times higher in nonmenstrual-associated cases. Poor outcomes are associated with prolonged and refractory hypovolemic shock, acute respiratory distress syndrome, acute renal failure, electrolyte and acid–base imbalances, cardiac dysrhythmia, and disseminated intravascular coagulation (DIC) with thrombocytopenia.

Staphylococcal TSS may recur among patients with menstrual or nonmenstrual disease [20,21]. Recurrence is associated with continued use of tampons and absence of antistaphylococcal therapy for the initial episode.

Streptococcal Toxic Shock Syndrome

The clinical presentation and pathophysiology of streptococcal TSS are similar to staphylococcal TSS with a few notable differences: bacteremia is commonly seen, rash is less common, and mortality is markedly higher (30% to 70%) [7].

Like staphylococcal TSS, streptococcal TSS is a toxin-mediated disease. Streptococcal toxins that function as SAgs are streptococcal pyrogenic exotoxin A (SPE A) and streptococcal pyrogenic exotoxin B (SPE B). In addition, M-protein, a classic streptococcal virulence factor, may be released from the cell surface, bind to fibrinogen, and form large aggregates that activate intravascular polymorphonuclear leukocytes, leading to a vascular leak syndrome [22]. Blood cultures are usually positive for patients with streptococcal TSS. Underlying infections are varied and include cellulitis, necrotizing fasciitis, postpartum myometritis, surgical wound infection, and, occasionally, pharyngitis [23]. Diagnosis is made by gram stain and culture of blood and other bodily fluids.

Treatment is similar to that for staphylococcal TSS in that supportive care, including fluids, vasopressors, and ventilatory assistance, should be administered as needed, and surgical drainage of pyogenic sites is imperative. For confirmed streptococcal TSS, the antibiotic of choice is intravenous penicillin. For those who are intolerant to penicillin, other suitable agents are cephalosporins and vancomycin. Until the bacteriologic diagnosis is confirmed by culture, staphylococcal coverage should be included in the antibiotic regimen. Clindamycin is also very active against *S. pyogenes*. In an animal model of streptococcal myositis, clindamycin was more effective than penicillin [24]. This may be owing to greater activity against high burdens of organisms (inoculum effect). An alternative explanation is that inhibition of protein synthesis blocks toxin production by the pathogen and reduces TNF production by the host [25]. A case–control study has shown improved outcomes among children with invasive *S. pyogenes* infections whose therapy included clindamycin or erythromycin in the first 24 hours [18]. Another observational study of patients with invasive *S. pyogenes* infection showed lower mortality associated with clindamycin use, despite higher severity of illness. Clindamycin is, therefore, often recommended to be used in combination with a β-lactam or other cell-wall active agent. The usual adult dose of clindamycin in this setting is 900 mg every 8 hours. Adjunctive therapy of streptococcal TSS with IVIG is recommended by many experts, based on retrospective and observational studies employing doses ranging from 400 to 2 g per kg for variable durations [26–29]. A randomized controlled trial was attempted but halted prior to completion, and it showed a trend toward improved survival in the treatment group [30]. In that trial, the dose of IVIG was 1 g per kg on day 1 and 0.5 g per kg on days 2 and 3.

Outbreaks of infections caused by *S. pyogenes* have previously been reported, and a recent surveillance study noted an increased incidence of invasive *S. pyogenes* infection in household contacts of index cases [28]. However, cases of invasive *S. pyogenes* infections among contacts of index cases remain rare overall. The use of antibiotic prophylaxis for household contacts has not been studied. Although one may consider offering chemoprophylaxis to household contacts with underlying conditions who are at increased risk of sporadic *S. pyogenes* infection or are at increased risk of mortality as a result of this infection (age $\geq$ 65 or other immunosuppression), its routine use is currently not recommended [31]. Infection control measures in the hospital should include droplet precautions for the first 24 hours after the initiation of appropriate antimicrobial therapy if pharyngitis and/or pneumonia are possible etiologies; otherwise, standard precautions are sufficient [32].

C. sordellii Toxic Shock Syndrome

C. sordellii is an anaerobic, gram-positive spore-forming bacillus that has been an occasional cause of obstetric infections for many years [33]. Recently, there have been reports of a TSS caused by this pathogen in association with surgical and medical abortion [33–35], subcutaneous injection of black-tar heroin [36], and musculoskeletal tissue allografts [37]. The distinctive features of this syndrome are hypothermia, and profound hemoconcentration and leukemoid reaction. In one review of *C. sordellii* cases, a marked leukocytosis was highly predictive of death [38]. Management consists of supportive care, including aggressive volume resuscitation, drainage of purulent foci, and broad-spectrum antibacterial therapy, to include anaerobic organisms. Antitoxin therapy is of theoretic interest, but clinically unproven.

MENINGOCOCCEMIA

The CDC estimated that between 800 and 1,200 cases of invasive meningococcal disease occurred each year during the years 2005 to 2011 in the United States, which represents a decline in incidence since a peak during the late 1990s [39,40]. This section covers *Neisseria meningitidis* bacteremia. Meningitis is covered in Chapter 81. Although infants are at highest risk for meningococcal disease, case rates also rise in the early teenage years, and 32% of cases occur among persons aged 30 years or older [40]. There are five serogroups, A, B, C, Y, and W-135. In the United States, serogroups B, C, and Y cause 93% of cases, with each representing about one-third of cases. Serogroup B disease is more common among infants. Disease rates vary seasonally, with the lowest rates in the summer and early autumn months [40]. Despite overall decrease in incidence in the United States, recent outbreaks have been reported among men who have sex with men in New York City, Los Angeles, and Chicago [41–44].

Pathophysiology

N. meningitidis colonizes the nasopharynx in normal individuals by adherence to epithelial cells via pili and other adhesion factors. For the majority of individuals, it never causes disease. Invasive disease has been associated with a variety of factors, including antecedent viral infection, exposure to passive smoking, and inhalation of dry, dusty air [45]. Specific antibody and the complement system are key protective components of the host immune system. Deficiency of components of the complement system because of genetic defects or underlying disease predisposes to invasive meningococcal disease [46]. When bacteria invade the bloodstream, endotoxin activates the host immune system and proinflammatory cytokines cause a vascular leak syndrome. The endothelial thrombomodulin–endothelial protein C receptor pathway is downregulated, leading to thrombosis and purpura fulminans [47]. Profound vasoconstriction leads to peripheral ischemia and gangrene [45], and depression of myocardial contractility by cytokines contributes to shock.

Diagnosis

Clinical Manifestations

Few disease states are as impressive as full-blown meningococcal sepsis. The challenge is early recognition, and intervention before irreversible damage occurs. Early in the course of meningococcal sepsis, nonspecific symptoms and signs are the only manifestations. Fever, malaise, myalgias, vomiting, tachypnea, and tachycardia are typical. The rash begins as an erythema, progressing to the characteristic petechiae and purpura only later in the course of disease. As the disease progresses, it evolves to septic shock, with hypotension, poor peripheral perfusion, impaired mentation, and anuria or oliguria. Other manifestations include hemorrhage, cardiac failure, acute renal failure, and thrombocytopenia with or without DIC [48]. Other, less common complications of meningococcal sepsis include adrenal hemorrhage and failure (Waterhouse–Friderichsen syndrome), chronic renal failure necessitating hemodialysis, cutaneous necrosis with sloughing requiring skin grafting, extremity gangrene requiring subsequent amputation, and often several surgical revisions, septic arthritis, endophthalmitis, and pericarditis. Mortality remains high, despite antibiotics and intensive care; 20% to 50% of children who develop shock from meningococcal sepsis die. Transfer to a specialist unit is associated with a marked reduction of mortality [49].

Laboratory Findings

Leukocytosis or leukopenia, with a shift to immature forms, and thrombocytopenia are typical. There may be laboratory evidence of DIC. Chemistries may demonstrate acidemia, hypoglycemia, decreased cortisol levels, and elevated blood urea nitrogen and creatinine. Diagnosis is confirmed by isolation of *N. meningitidis* from cultures of blood or other normally sterile body fluids. If the diagnosis of meningococcal sepsis is clinically apparent, some experts caution against performing a lumbar puncture for CSF culture because of concerns for brain herniation or clinical deterioration related to positioning the patient for the procedure. Latex agglutination and polymerase chain reaction (PCR) assays provide increased sensitivity [50].

Differential Diagnosis

Purpura fulminans is characteristic of meningococcemia, but may also be caused by *Streptococcus pneumoniae* or *Haemophilus influenzae* type B. Other infections that may mimic meningococcemia are fulminant *S. aureus* sepsis, *S. pyogenes* bacteremia, gram-negative sepsis, RMSF, vasculitis, thrombotic thrombocytopenic purpura, Henoch–Schonlein purpura, and any febrile illness of a patient with thrombocytopenia.

Therapy

Third-generation cephalosporins are the treatment of choice for meningococcemia owing to reports of penicillin resistance [51]. Ceftriaxone, 4 g intravenously daily in one or two divided doses or cefotaxime 8 to 12 g intravenously daily in four to six divided doses, should be administered to adults with suspected meningococcal disease. There is limited clinical experience with alternative antibacterial agents for patients with a history of cephalosporin allergy. Based on in vitro susceptibility data, options include meropenem and chloramphenicol [51,52]. Fluoroquinolones may be useful for postpubertal persons, but rare cases of fluoroquinolone resistance have been reported [53].

Patients should be admitted to an intensive care unit and placed in respiratory isolation until 24 hours of appropriate antibiotic therapy has been administered. Supportive care is critical to a favorable outcome. Surgical intervention may be indicated for necrotic skin lesions and gangrenous limbs. Early fasciotomy appears to limit the extent of amputation that is ultimately required [54]. Adrenal insufficiency may occur; in hypotensive patients, corticosteroids should be administered pending return of results of cosyntropin stimulation test. Use of plasmapheresis has been reported in uncontrolled series [55,56].

Prophylaxis

The CDC recommends chemoprophylaxis after exposure to people with *N. meningitidis* infection for household, day care, and other close contacts; for people in close contact with infected respiratory secretions, such as those performing mouth-to-mouth resuscitation or endotracheal intubation, and for travelers in contact with respiratory secretions of, or seated next to, an index case for 8 hours or more [39]. The agents recommended for chemoprophylaxis are rifampin (600 mg orally for adults, 10 mg per kg orally for children) given every 12 hours for four doses; ciprofloxacin 500 mg orally once, for adults; or ceftriaxone, 125 mg intramuscularly in children younger than 15 years of age or 250 mg intramuscularly in people aged 15 years or older [39]. Resistance to ciprofloxacin, which has been widely used for prophylaxis, was reported among several cases of meningococcal infection in North Dakota and Minnesota between 2007 and 2008, leading to a recommendation to use alternative agents for prophylaxis in those areas, either rifampin, ceftriaxone, or azithromycin 500 mg orally once [39,57]. Since that time, two additional isolates of ciprofloxacin-resistant *N. meningitidis* have been identified in the United States through susceptibility testing of isolates previously collected by an active population-based surveillance system operating in 10 states or metropolitan areas, although detection of these strains may be limited because susceptibility testing is not routinely done in the United States [58]. Nevertheless, this same analysis of 466 *N. meningitidis* isolates collected in the years 2004, 2008, 2010, and 2011 revealed no instances of ceftriaxone or azithromycin resistance, and rare isolates with rifampin resistance [58]. Routine chemoprophylaxis is recommended for medical staff only if they had managed an airway or were exposed to respiratory secretions before the institution of antibiotic therapy. When indicated, postexposure prophylaxis should be given as soon as possible, although it is likely not useful if given greater than 14 days after exposure [39].

Immunization with the tetravalent vaccine MenACWY is indicated for the following populations: children at their 11- to 12-year-old preadolescent health care visit, college freshmen living in dormitories, travelers to areas where *N. meningitidis* is epidemic or hyperendemic, microbiologists with frequent exposure to *N. meningitidis*, military recruits, those at risk during an outbreak (such as school or dormitory mates), and those with increased susceptibility (e.g., persons with complement deficiencies or asplenia) [39]. Meningococcal serogroup B (MenB) vaccines have recently been made available and are now recommended for a subset of populations who are also eligible to receive MenACWY (persons with complement deficiencies or asplenia, microbiologists routinely exposed to *N. meningitidis*, and persons at risk because of an outbreak of serogroup B meningococcal disease; MenB vaccines are not licensed for use in children younger than 10 years of age [59].

OVERWHELMING POSTSPLENECTOMY INFECTION

Overwhelming postsplenectomy sepsis is a catastrophic illness with high morbidity and mortality among patients who have undergone splenectomy or who have severe splenic dysfunction. The spleen provides three major functions for protection from infection. It acts as a mechanical filter for infected or senescent erythrocytes; it participates in the production of soluble immune factors, including immunoglobulins and tuftsin, and it provides a site for components of the cellular immune system to act in proximity to one another [60].

Splenic function may be lost owing to surgical removal, irradiation, several disease processes, and therapies [61], including sickle cell anemia, systemic lupus erythematosus, celiac disease, liver disease, acute alcoholism, high-dose corticosteroid therapy, splenic irradiation [62], and bone marrow transplantation. Normal aging has also been associated with a decrease in splenic function [63].

Splenectomy was the accepted procedure for splenic trauma for centuries, owing to the belief that it served no important physiologic function, repair of trauma was difficult because of the friable nature of the organ, and expected high mortality of attempted conservative management. This prevailing wisdom was challenged in the 1970s, and, currently, splenic salvage is reported in 90% of cases of splenic rupture [64]. Splenic salvage in the trauma setting is associated with marked reductions in the risk of infection during the acute hospitalization, including surgical site infections and pneumonia [65]. Implantation of splenic fragments into the peritoneum has been performed in an attempt to maintain splenic function. Immune protection by these splenic fragments is incomplete at best, because of the loss of the normal splenic circulation. The presence of

Howell–Jolly bodies on the peripheral blood smear indicates decreased splenic function, placing the patient at risk for overwhelming postsplenectomy infection (OPSI) [66]. Although Howell–Jolly bodies may be detected by autoanalysers, a manual blood film should be reviewed if there is a clinical question of hyposplenism.

Epidemiology

The incidence of OPSI is impacted by many factors, including underlying disease, patient age, age at time of splenectomy, time elapsed since splenectomy, pneumococcal vaccination, and antibiotic prophylaxis. Reported incidence rates are highest among patients with underlying thalassemia, intermediate in patients with sickle cell anemia, malignancy, or hematologic disorders, and lowest among patients who undergo splenectomy for trauma.

Encapsulated bacteria are the most common organisms causing OPSI. *S. pneumoniae, N. meningitidis,* and *H. influenzae* are the organisms of greatest concern. *S. pneumoniae* is the most frequently isolated pathogen, representing over 50% of cases of OPSI. Other bacterial pathogens include *Salmonella* spp. [60], *Capnocytophaga canimorsus* [67,68], which is associated with dog bites, and *Campylobacter* spp [69]. There has been one reported case each of OPSI as a result of *Mycobacterium tuberculosis* [70] and *Mycoplasma pneumonia* [71].

Asplenic individuals are also at risk for severe infection with the intraerythrocytic pathogens *Babesia microti* and *Babesia bovi*. Both organisms are transmitted by tick bites; *B. microti* is endemic on islands off the northeastern coast of the United States (Long Island, Nantucket Island, Martha's Vineyard), whereas *B. bovi* is found in Europe. The acute phase of malaria may be more severe in splenectomized individuals, but splenectomy may be protective in the chronic phase. Atypically, severe cases of *Plasmodium vivax* and *Plasmodium ovale* have been reported in splenectomized individuals, and relapse of malaria following splenectomy has occurred [60].

Diagnosis

Clinical Presentation

OPSI should be considered in any febrile patient with a history or abdominal scar consistent with splenectomy or disease process associated with hyposplenism. The initial symptoms of OPSI are fever, headache abdominal pain, vomiting, and diarrhea. There may be a nonspecific prodrome characterized by low grade fever and myalgias. If untreated, the disease evolves into fulminant septic shock and death over 2 to 5 days [72]. In advanced cases, acute tubular necrosis, adrenal cortical necrosis, and DIC may occur. A petechial or purpuric rash may be seen. Meningitis or pneumonia occurs in approximately one-half of cases; in the remaining cases, septicemia occurs, which is presumed to arise from colonization of the pharynx.

Laboratory Features

Blood cultures yield the causative organism for most cases of OPSI. Infections of lesser severity also occur and may not be associated with detectable bacteremia. Hematologic findings of DIC (thrombocytopenia, elevated prothrombin time, D-dimer, and fibrin split products), elevated serum creatinine, and blood urea nitrogen are frequently seen. Howell–Jolly bodies are found on a peripheral blood film. During the immediate postsplenectomy period, mild elevation in the platelet and leukocyte counts are physiologic, but a leukocyte count higher than 15,000 cells per μL after the fourth postoperative day suggests that infection is likely the cause [73].

Differential Diagnosis

OPSI may be mistaken for uncomplicated sepsis if the history asplenia or hyposplenism are not appreciated. Thrombotic thrombocytopenic purpura may also have a similar presentation, with fever, thrombocytopenia, and acute renal failure.

Management

In addition to supportive care, antimicrobial therapy should be initiated promptly. Third-generation cephalosporins are active against *S. pneumoniae*, *N. meningitidis*, and *H. influenzae* in most locales. Cefotaxime 2 g intravenously every 8 hours or ceftriaxone 1 to 2 g intravenously once daily may be used for uncomplicated cases [74]. If meningitis is suspected, the dose of cefotaxime should be increased to 2 g every 4 to 6 hours, and ceftriaxone should be given in a dose of 2 g twice daily. If pneumococci with high-grade resistance to penicillin and cephalosporins are prevalent in the region, vancomycin should be added until culture and susceptibility data become available. Patients with a severe allergy to penicillins and cephalosporins may be treated with vancomycin given with chloramphenicol or a fluoroquinolone [61]. Expert consultation should be sought in such cases.

Prevention

Prevention of OPSI entails ensuring adequate vaccination, prompt evaluation and empiric antimicrobial treatment for febrile episodes, and, possibly, prophylactic antibiotics. Current recommendations include vaccination with the 13-valent pneumococcal conjugate vaccine (PCV13) followed by the 23-valent pneumococcal polysaccharide vaccine (PPSV23) at least 8 weeks later [75]. If possible, the series should be completed 2 weeks or longer prior to splenectomy. If that is impractical, it is recommended that patients be immunized as soon as possible postoperatively. Recent observations that antibody levels are improved if vaccination is delayed until 14 days postoperatively [76] must be weighed against the risk that vaccination may be overlooked if it is not carried out prior to hospital discharge. A reasonable compromise may be to immunize the patient at hospital discharge. A second dose of PPSV23 should be administered 5 years later [75]. Meningococcal conjugate vaccine (MenACWY) should be administered to patients who are asplenic or who have splenic dysfunction [39]. In addition, serogroup B meningococcal vaccines have recently been made available and are now recommended for use in patients aged 10 years or older with anatomic or functional aspenia [59]. Owing to the ongoing risk for meningococcal disease in asplenic persons, MenACWY vaccination should be repeated at 3- to 5-year intervals [39,77]. The conjugate *H. influenzae* vaccine should be administered to asplenic patients according to the standard schedule for all children [78]; unvaccinated persons aged 5 or older should receive one dose [75]. Influenza vaccine should be administered annually owing to the risk of secondary bacterial infection [79].

Lifelong antibiotic prophylaxis is recommended by some authors [78], whereas others question this approach [60]. The data supporting prophylaxis are stronger for the pediatric population than for adults [61]. In the first 2 years following splenectomy of a child, or of a patient with thalassemia or immune deficiency, antibiotic prophylaxis is recommended by most experts. Penicillin remains the drug of choice, despite emergence of resistance among some isolates. Ideally, it should be dosed twice daily, but if adherence is an issue, it may be given once daily. Erythromycin may be substituted for patients who are allergic to penicillin. "Stand-by" antibiotics, to be taken early in the course of a febrile illness, is a strategy favored by all [60,78]. Amoxicillin-clavulanate is a good choice for this indication. Patients must be counseled to seek medical care when they have a suspected infection, and not rely on stand-by antibiotics alone.

MALARIA

In developed countries, malaria is primarily seen among travelers, immigrants, and military personnel, but, in the developing world, it is a major cause of morbidity and mortality. There are between 300 and 660 million cases that occur annually worldwide, resulting in 700,000 to 2.7 million deaths each year [80]. Imported cases have increased throughout the world; in the United States, over 1,600 cases were reported to the National Malaria Surveillance System, a passive reporting system administered by the CDC in 2012 [81]. This represents an overall increasing trend of malaria cases in the United States since the 1970s [81]. In 2003, *Plasmodium falciparum* was identified as the causative species for 53% of cases; 70% of the cases were acquired in Africa. Virtually, all of the fatal cases of malaria in the United States are caused by *P. falciparum*. Although the great majority of cases occurred among persons who did not follow a CDC–recommended prophylaxis regimen, it must be noted that approximately 20% of patients with malaria reported taking appropriate chemoprophylaxis. Failure to take a recommended regimen resulted in fatal malaria in seven reported cases since 1992 [82]. There have been small clusters of mosquito-borne malaria transmission within the United States as well as occasional congenital cases and transmission via blood transfusion [83]. This discussion will focus on severe malaria, and its management in critical care settings.

Etiology

Plasmodium is an intracellular parasite that sequentially infects hepatocytes and then erythrocytes, resulting in clinical malaria. Four species cause disease in humans: *P. falciparum*, *P. malariae*, *P. ovale*, and *P. vivax*. *Plasmodium* is transmitted to human hosts by its vector, the female *Anopheles* mosquito.

Pathophysiology

Severe malaria is almost always caused by *P. falciparum*, which, because of its ability to infect erythrocytes of all ages, can produce very high levels of parasitemia. Cerebral malaria is the most common clinical presentation of severe malaria. Many factors can contribute to diminished brain function in severe malaria, including obstruction of microvascular flow, elevated intracranial pressure, cerebral edema, disruption of the blood–brain barrier, hypoglycemia, hypovolemia, and seizure activity.

Obstruction of microvascular flow is caused by sequestration of erythrocytes in brain capillaries, autoagglutination, and decreased erythrocyte deformability caused by intracellular parasites. Cytoadherence, a process in which *P. falciparum* derived proteins on infected erythrocytes attach to the CD36 receptor on vascular endothelial cells, appears to mediate sequestration [84].

In endemic areas, malaria is largely a disease of children. By the time they reach adulthood, residents of endemic areas develop partial immunity to *Plasmodium* infections, limiting the severity of disease. Travelers, conversely, are generally not immune; nonimmune adults who become infected are almost always symptomatic, and severe disease may develop.

Diagnosis

Clinical Features

Although imported malaria may occur at any time after leaving an endemic area, there are epidemiologic clues to help guide the evaluation. Among returning travelers presenting with fever, the most common specific diagnosis is malaria, occurring among 9% of cases [85]. Among cases diagnosed in New York, 80% of patients had symptom onset within 1 month of leaving the endemic area. Most of the cases presenting later than 1 month postdeparture had *P. vivax*, which rarely causes life-threatening disease.

Patients with malaria present with a history of fever and chills, but fever may not be present at the time of the initial examination. The classic descriptions of tertian and quartan fever are rarely seen; their absence is not evidence against the diagnosis of malaria. Chills, headache, fatigue, and myalgias are common complaints. Signs include hypotension, jaundice, and hepatosplenomegaly, but these are seen in a minority of patients [86]. If hypotension is present, gram-negative bacteremia must be excluded and treated empirically until cultures return. Cough, dyspnea, and tachypnea may dominate the clinical picture in children, causing confusion with pneumonia in areas of the developing world where chest radiography is not readily available [87].

Malaria during pregnancy presents with similar, although more severe, manifestations. Hypoglycemia and lactic acidosis are more frequently seen in maternal malaria, and the mortality of cerebral malaria is increased [88]. The partial immunity of residents of endemic areas is blunted during pregnancy [89]. Other complications include preterm delivery, intrauterine growth retardation, anemia, postpartum hemorrhage, and eclampsia [88]. Human immunodeficiency virus (HIV)–infected gravida are both at increased risk of infection with *Plasmodium* species, and have a more severe course of malaria. Additionally, malaria is associated with an increased maternal HIV viral load, and may increase HIV transmission to the fetus [90]. Placental malaria may be present even if peripheral blood films are negative for parasites [91].

Complications

The most common complications of malaria are cerebral malaria, severe anemia, metabolic acidosis, and noncardiogenic pulmonary edema. Gram-negative sepsis is a less common, but potentially grave complication of severe malaria.

Variability of host susceptibility and of the definition of cerebral malaria may account for the wide range of reported incidence. The World Health Organization (WHO) defines cerebral malaria as coma that cannot be explained by hypoglycemia, postictal state, or other nonmalarial causes, such as sedative drugs, for a patient with parasitemia. Common findings are decerebrate or decorticate posturing, flaccid tone, seizures, and retinal hemorrhages. A recent study of imported severe *falciparum* malaria reported cerebral malaria in 37% of cases [92]. Overall, mortality of severe malaria in that series of cases treated in a highly experienced intensive care unit setting was 11%. Cerebral malaria was present among 90% of nonsurvivors.

Laboratory Features

Common laboratory findings are anemia, thrombocytopenia, and hyperbilirubinemia. Hypoglycemia, elevated creatinine, and hypothrombinemia may also be present [92].

Microscopic examination for parasites on thick and thin films of peripheral blood remains the standard for diagnosis of malaria. Sensitivity is increased when blood for malaria smears are obtained from a capillary-rich area, such as the fingertip or earlobe, rather than by venipuncture. A thick smear examined by an experienced microscopist can detect 50 parasites per μL of blood, which is equivalent to 0.001% of erythrocytes infected [91]. Sensitivity is approximately 10-fold lower for routine clinical laboratories. In addition, patients with *falciparum* malaria may have parasites sequestered in deep capillaries of the spleen, liver, bone marrow, or placenta, with a false-negative peripheral smear. Because the sensitivity of the smear is imperfect, empiric therapy for malaria should be administered when clinical suspicion is high. The thin blood film is used to identify the species and to quantitatively follow the parasitemia on serial samples. Real-time PCR is more sensitive than microscopy, especially at low levels of parasitemia, and although it is not Food and Drug Administration (FDA) approved, the assay is readily available from reference laboratories. The CDC currently encourages specimens from confirmed cases of malaria diagnosed in the United States to be submitted to their laboratories for PCR testing for species confirmation and antimalarial resistance, for surveillance purposes [93]. Many rapid diagnostic tests (RDTs) have been developed which detect *Plasmodium* antigens and may provide a rapid diagnosis of malaria when access to high-quality microscopy is not readily available, although these tests do not provide information regarding species or degree of parasitemia; currently, only one RDT is approved for use in the United States [94].

Differential Diagnosis

Cerebral malaria may mimic meningoencephalitis owing to viral, bacterial, fungal, or other parasitic causes. Dengue, typhoid, *Rickettsial* infection, or mononucleosis may present with an undifferentiated fever in a returned traveler. The differential diagnosis of jaundice in this population includes leptospirosis, yellow fever, viral hepatitis, sepsis, and relapsing fevers [87]. Bacterial sepsis must also be considered as a separate or a complicating diagnosis.

Treatment

Management in an intensive care unit is indicated for patients with severe malaria. Careful management of fluids and electrolytes is critical, as well as monitoring for hypoglycemia. Renal, cardiac, and neurologic function should also be carefully monitored.

Intravenous quinidine has been used in the United States for the treatment of severe malaria since 1991, when the CDC stopped providing intravenous quinine [95]. At that time, quinidine was readily available on most hospital formularies, and therapy could be initiated rapidly. The declining use of intravenous quinidine for cardiac dysrhythmias has reduced the ready availability of quinidine, but a replacement strategy has not yet been developed for malaria [96], and it remains the drug of choice. It should be initiated for severe malaria, defined as a positive blood smear with any one of the following criteria: impaired consciousness/coma, severe normocytic anemia, renal failure, pulmonary edema, acute respiratory distress syndrome, circulatory shock, DIC, spontaneous bleeding, acidosis, hemoglobinuria, jaundice, repeated generalized convulsions, or parasitemia greater than 5%.

Hypoglycemia, QT interval prolongation, cardiac dysrhythmias, and hypotension may complicate quinidine infusion. Intensive care unit monitoring and consultation with an infectious disease specialist and a cardiologist are recommended. Cardiac complications may require slowing or stopping the infusion. When dosage is calculated, it is important to distinguish the salt from the base to ensure accuracy. The usual dose is 6.25 mg base per kg (10 mg salt per kg) loading dose intravenously over 1 to 2 hours, then 0.0125 mg base/kg/min (0.02 mg salt/kg/min) continuous infusion for at least 24 hours. If the patient has received mefloquine or more than 40 mg per kg of quinine in the 12 hours prior to beginning quinidine infusion, the loading dose should be omitted. Dosage adjustment for renal failure is not necessary during the first 48 hours of therapy [97]. Thin smears to assess the degree of parasitemia should be performed every 12 to 24 hours. Oral quinine 542 mg base (650 mg salt) three times daily for 3 to 7 days should be substituted when the patient is able to swallow, parasitemia is less than 1%, and mental status is normal. For infections acquired in Southeast Asia CDC recommends that therapy continue for 7 days; for disease acquired in Africa, therapy should be stopped after 3 days.

Patients with malaria normally show improvement in 1 to 3 days [98]. If the course is more prolonged, drug resistance or inadequate serum drug levels should be suspected. In addition to quinine, the patient should be treated with one of the following: doxycycline 100 mg orally twice daily for 7 days, tetracycline 250 mg four times daily for 7 days, or clindamycin 20 mg base/kg/d orally in three divided doses for 7 days.

Artesunate, a new agent that was developed in China, has been shown in a randomized controlled trial to be superior to quinine for therapy of severe malaria [99]. Although it is not FDA approved for use in the United States, it is available on a treatment investigational new drug protocol from the CDC for cases of severe malaria. Physicians who encounter a case of *falciparum* malaria should contact the CDC malaria hotline (770-488-7788) to report the case and to obtain artesunate; parenteral quinidine (in combination with doxycycline, tetracycline, or clindamycin) should be initiated while awaiting artesunate. If quinidine is not on the hospital formulary, the hospital pharmacy should attempt to obtain it from a nearby facility.

Treatment of a pregnant woman with malaria requires additional considerations [88]. High doses of quinine are reported to be abortifacient. Nevertheless, treatment with quinine has not been associated with an increased risk of congenital abnormalities, low birth weight, or stillbirth, and it is considered to be safe in the first trimester [100]. As discussed earlier, quinidine is substituted for quinine in the United States. Quinidine is listed as category C and is considered safe for breastfeeding women. Clindamycin should be given in conjunction with quinidine or oral quinine treatment [94]. Chloroquine is safe for use in pregnant women for the treatment of non-*falciparum* or chloroquine-sensitive *falciparum* malaria. Artesunate-atovaquone-proguanil has been shown to be superior to quinine during the second and third trimesters, with no differences in birth weight, duration of gestation, or congenital abnormality rates in newborns [101]. If fetal distress is observed on monitoring, emergency cesarean delivery may be necessary [87,102].

Exchange transfusion is controversial owing to the lack of randomized trial data. Although its use was previously recommended by the WHO and CDC for patients with severe disease [87], a recent retrospective propensity score-matched study of patients with severe malaria reported to the National Malaria Surveillance System revealed no survival benefit of exchange transfusion [103]. Although some still advocate for its use in cases of severe malaria [104], the CDC has since revised its guidelines and currently does not recommend using exchange transfusion as an adjunct therapy; the WHO also does not make any recommendations regarding its use [94,105].

A randomized controlled trial has shown that corticosteroids were of no benefit and potentially harmful in the treatment of cerebral malaria [106]. Other adjunctive therapies that should not be used include heparin, sodium bicarbonate, mannitol, immunoglobulins, and iron chelators [87,106].

Advances in cerebral malaria, based on randomized controlled trials or meta-analyses of such trials, are summarized in Table 74.2.

ROCKY MOUNTAIN SPOTTED FEVER

RMSF is a potentially fatal zoonosis caused by the bacterium *Rickettsia rickettsii*, which is transmitted by ticks. Although the classic constellation of findings is fever, rash, and tick bite occurring in the summer months, it is important to consider the disease even when some of these features are lacking. A history of tick bite is reported in only 60% of documented cases [107], and rash may be absent in 20%. Recognition of RMSF is critical, because outcome is much improved with timely, appropriate therapy [108].

RMSF is transmitted by the hard ticks *Dermacentor andersoni, Dermacentor variabilis, Amblyomma cajennense,* and *Rhipicephalus*

TABLE 74.2

Summary Recommendations for Management of Cerebral Malaria Based on Randomized Controlled Clinical Trials

- Corticosteroids are harmful and should not be used.[a]
- Artesunate is the antimalarial of choice for cerebral malaria. When it becomes available in the United States, it should replace quinidine for this indication. Physicians who encounter a case of cerebral malaria should contact the CDC for an update on availability of aretsunate.[b]

[a]Warrell DA, Looareesuwan S, Warrell MJ, et al: Dexamethasone proves deleterious in cerebral malaria. A double-blind trial in 100 comatose patients. *N Engl J Med* 306(6):313–319, 1982.
[b]Dondorp A, Nosten F, Stepniewska K, et al: Artesunate versus quinine for treatment of severe *falciparum* malaria: a randomised trial. *Lancet* 366(9487):717–725, 2005.
CDC, Centers for Disease Control and Prevention.

sanguineus. The latter tick, previously a recognized vector for RMSF in Mexico, was implicated in a recent outbreak of RMSF in Arizona, an area that had previously been spared this disease. A review of cases of RMSF that were reported to the CDC's National Notifiable Diseases Surveillance system from 2000 to 2007 revealed a greater than fourfold increase in incidence over this time period, although the majority of reported cases were probable, rather than confirmed cases, and a change in case definition in 2004 to allow the use of enzyme-linked immunosorbent assay tests in the reporting of probable cases is postulated to have contributed to this increased incidence [109]. Yet, another change in case definition and reporting standards occurred in 2010, such that RMSF is reported along with other clinically similar *Rickettsial* infections as "Spotted Fever Rickettsiosis," which may influence future surveillance reports [110]. Although the peak incidence is in the summer months, cases occur throughout the year. Classically, it has been considered that children and males are at highest risk, but recent CDC data show that females and adults have only a slightly lower incidence. Native Americans have a higher incidence than other ethnic groups. RMSF was first described in Montana, thus its name, but is more frequently seen in the Southeastern United States, especially the Carolinas, Oklahoma, Arkansas, and Missouri.

Pathophysiology

R. rickettsii parasitize endothelial cells of many organs and vascular smooth muscle. The organisms cause a direct cytopathic effect, leading to vascular injury, clotting activation, and a vascular leak syndrome. In severe cases, this manifests as multiorgan failure. Renal failure, respiratory failure, and coma may ensue.

Diagnosis

Clinical Features

The presentation of RMSF is protean, owing to the multisystem nature of the disease. Symptoms include fever, malaise, headache, rash, myalgia, nausea, vomiting, abdominal pain, and diarrhea. Two-thirds of cases have a temperature above 102°F at presentation; 90% have temperature above 102°F within 48 hours of presentation. Rash generally appears by the second or third day of illness and classically starts at the wrists and ankles, but is frequently generalized. It may involve the palms and soles; the face is spared. Rash may be missed in persons with dark skin. Gastrointestinal symptoms may be prominent, despite the systemic nature of the disease. Headache is typically present and is often severe. The key to the diagnosis is to consider it in any febrile patient who has been spent time outdoors in an endemic area. Investigations into the Arizona outbreak which reviewed 205 cases that occurred in multiple tribal Native American communities between 2002 and 2011 revealed that cases occurring in this region were more often atypical in presentation, and case fatality was higher, than cases reported from other regions in the United States [111,112]. Thus, clinicians practicing in this region should remain vigilant about the possibility of RMSF in febrile or otherwise ill-appearing patients and institute empiric treatment promptly.

Laboratory Features

Laboratory findings include a white blood cell count that is typically in the normal range, although a manual differential count reveals a shift to immature neutrophils. Platelets are usually decreased. Other nonspecific findings reflect the multisystem nature of the process and include hyponatremia, elevated creatine phosphokinase, hepatic transaminases, and creatinine and clotting indices (prothrombin time, partial thromboplastin time, and fibrin degradation products). CSF examination commonly demonstrates a mononuclear pleocytosis and, occasionally, an elevated CSF protein and low CSF glucose levels [108].

Differential Diagnosis

R. rickettsii cannot be cultured in most clinical laboratories; therefore, the diagnosis is most often based on clinical grounds. Diagnosis may be confirmed by biopsy of skin involved with rash and processed with immunofluorescence or immunoperoxidase staining or by PCR. Confirmation can also be made by serologic testing of acute and convalescent serum, 2 to 4 weeks apart. These methods usually provide retrospective confirmation of the diagnosis, and although this is important for accurate epidemiologic surveillance, these tests do not help in clinical decision-making at the point of care. A single elevated immunoglobin M (IgM) antibody titer is likely not helpful, either, because false positives can occur [113].

Differential Diagnosis

RMSF is frequently misdiagnosed as pharyngitis or scarlet fever, despite the low incidence of sore throat [114]. Gastroenteritis is also a common initial diagnosis, owing to prominent gastrointestinal symptoms. RMSF must also be distinguished from rheumatic fever, encephalitis, meningitis, pneumonia, measles, meningococcemia, leptospirosis, acute abdominal illness, idiopathic thrombocytopenic purpura, thrombotic thrombocytopenic purpura, drug reaction, ehrlichiosis, and vasculitis [108,114,115].

Therapy

Specific therapy should not be delayed while awaiting confirmation of the diagnosis. Most broad-spectrum antibacterial agents such as cephalosporins, penicillins, and sulfa drugs are inactive against *R. rickettsii*. The treatment of choice for nonpregnant adults and children weighing more than 45 kg is doxycycline [116], 100 mg twice daily for 7 to 10 days. Children who weigh less than 45 kg should be given 2.2 mg per kg twice daily [107,117]. The risk of dental staining by tetracyclines in children is small for short courses of therapy; this consideration should not delay treatment [118]. A recent retrospective cohort study of children on a Native American reservation in Arizona who were treated with doxycycline for RMSF when they were less than 8 years of age demonstrated that these children had no differences in dental staining or enamel hypoplasia, compared to other children in the same community who did not have doxycycline exposure [119]. Therapy of pregnant women is problematic because tetracyclines are associated with maternal hepatotoxicity and fluorescent yellow discoloration of fetal deciduous teeth. Calcification of permanent teeth does not begin until after birth; discoloration of permanent teeth would not be expected. The US FDA and the Australian Drug Evaluation Committee have assigned pregnancy category D to doxycycline. Chloramphenicol is considered pregnancy category A by the Australian Drug Evaluation Committee [120]. Although teratogenicity has not been proven with chloramphenicol, maternal aplastic anemia or reversible bone marrow suppression may occur. Gray baby syndrome has occurred in neonates treated with chloramphenicol, and may occur in infants born to women treated with chloramphenicol near term. Doxycycline may be used for women presenting with RMSF near term [121]. Most authorities recommend therapy of pregnant women in the first or second trimester with chloramphenicol, 50 to 75 mg/kg/d in divided doses. Corticosteroid therapy has not been studied in a controlled manner, although older literature has recommended it for patients with widespread vasculitis and encephalitis [122].

Prognosis

Outcomes are directly related to timely, appropriate therapy. Mortality rates are as high as 20% for untreated cases, and 5% with proper therapy [123,124]. Risk factors for mortality include central nervous system involvement, renal dysfunction at presentation, a delay in the institution of therapy, therapy with an agent other than a tetracycline [116], and increased age.

MISCELLANEOUS INFECTIOUS DISEASES

There are many unusual infectious diseases that occasionally lead to intensive care unit admission. Several of these diseases are discussed briefly below and others are discussed in other chapters, such as serious epidemic viral pneumonias (Chapter 83) and biologic agents of mass destruction (Chapter 130).

Ehrlichiosis and *anaplasmosis* are tick-borne *Rickettsial* diseases that present as a fever with few localizing symptoms or signs. Headache, myalgias, malaise, and rigors are seen in nearly all cases; gastrointestinal or respiratory symptoms may occur in a minority of cases [125]. Human monocytic ehrlichiosis (HME), caused by *Ehrlichia chaffeensis* and transmitted by the Lone Star tick (*Amblyomma americanum*), is most commonly seen in the Southeastern United States. HME may present with meningoencephalitis, acute respiratory distress syndrome, and a toxic shock–like illness [126]. Human granulocytic anaplasmosis (HGA), caused by *Anaplasma phagocytophilum* is most commonly seen in the upper Midwestern states and the Northeastern United States [115]. HGA is typically a less severe disease than HME. It is found in the same geographic areas as babesiosis and Lyme disease and transmitted by *Ixodes scapularis* and by *Ixodes pacificus,* the same ticks that transmit *Borrelia burgdorferi* and *Babesia* species. Coinfection with *A. phagocytophilum*, *Babesia* spp, and *B. burgdorferi* has been reported [115,127]. *Ehrlichia ewingii* infection has been reported to cause a granulocytic ehrlichiosis in the Southeastern United States, primarily in immunocompromised hosts [115]. In contrast to most tick-borne illnesses, ehrlichiosis and anaplasmosis are more frequently seen in middle-aged and older individuals [126,127]. Cases most often present in spring and summer, but have been reported in every month of the year [126]. HME may follow a fulminant course in HIV-infected individuals [128]. Leukocyte counts are generally low or normal with a shift to immature forms; elevated transaminases and thrombocytopenia are typically found if patients are followed carefully [125,127]. The diagnosis may be confirmed by the observation of clumps of organisms within leukocytes, termed morulae, but the sensitivity of microscopy in the first week of illness is only 60%, even in very experienced hands [127]. Sensitivity is even lower later in the course. The diagnosis may be confirmed serologically or by a PCR assay at a reference laboratory [115], but therapy may need to be initiated while awaiting results if suspicion is high. The treatment of choice for both HME and HGA is doxycycline; rifampin has been used if doxycycline is contraindicated [127]. Owing to the overlap in clinical syndromes and the uncertainty of diagnosis early in the course, it is important to be certain that RMSF has been ruled out if an alternative agent to doxycycline is selected.

Capnocytophaga spp. are fastidious gram-negative rods that cause soft tissue infections (including gangrene), fever of unknown origin, bacteremia, endovascular infections including endocarditis, and meningitis [129–131]. *C. canimorsus* is normal oral flora in dogs, and infection is often associated with a dog bite. Cases have been reported in association with cat bites and with nontraumatic exposure to the oral secretions of dogs. Several other species of the *Capnocytophaga* genus are normal oral flora of humans, and may cause bacteremia in the setting of cancer chemotherapy [132,133]. Compromised hosts, particularly those with anatomic or functional asplenia or alcoholism, may follow a severe course of illness, especially if bacteremia is complicated by DIC [129]. *Capnocytophaga* spp. are resistant to many antibacterial agents that are commonly used to treat skin and soft tissue infections, including oxacillin and cefazolin. Ampicillin-sulbactam is a good empiric choice for serious soft tissue infection when there is a history of a dog bite. Clindamycin can be used for culture-proven cases of monomicrobial infection with *Capnocytophaga* in the case of penicillin allergy [132], but it is not active against *Pasteurella multocida*, which is a common pathogen in cases of dog or cat bites. Imipenem-cilastin is another alternative active against *Capnocytophaga* and *P. multocida* as well as other common pathogens of skin and soft tissue except MRSA.

References

1. Hashikawa S, Iinuma Y, Furushita M, et al: Characterization of group C and G streptococcal strains that cause streptococcal toxic shock syndrome. *J Clin Microbiol* 42(1):186–192, 2004.
2. Todd J, Fishaut M, Kapral F, et al: Toxic-shock syndrome associated with phage-group-I Staphylococci. *Lancet* 2(8100):1116–1118, 1978.
3. Chesney PJ, Davis JP, Purdy WK, et al: Clinical manifestations of toxic shock syndrome. *JAMA* 246(7):741–748, 1981.
4. Bartlett P, Reingold AL, Graham DR, et al: Toxic shock syndrome associated with surgical wound infections. *JAMA* 247(10):1448–1450, 1982.
5. Todd JK: Toxic shock syndrome, *Staphylococcus aureus*, and influenza. *JAMA* 257(22):3070–3071, 1987.
6. Cone LA, Woodard DR, Byrd RG, et al: A recalcitrant, erythematous, desquamating disorder associated with toxin-producing staphylococci in patients with AIDS. *J Infect Dis* 165(4):638–643, 1992.
7. McCormick JK, Yarwood JM, Schlievert PM: Toxic shock syndrome and bacterial superantigens: an update. *Annu Rev Microbiol* 55:77–104, 2001.
8. Jamart S, Denis O, Deplano A, et al: Methicillin-resistant *Staphylococcus aureus* toxic shock syndrome. *Emerg Infect Dis* 11(4):636–637, 2005.
9. van der Mee-Marquet N, Lina G, Quentin R, et al: Staphylococcal exanthematous disease in a newborn due to a virulent methicillin-resistant *Staphylococcus aureus* strain containing the TSST-1 gene in Europe: an alert for neonatologists. *J Clin Microbiol* 41(10):4883–4884, 2003.
10. Takahashi N, Imanishi K, Uchiyama T: Overall picture of an emerging neonatal infectious disease induced by a superantigenic exotoxin mainly produced by methicillin-resistant *Staphylococcus aureus*. *Microbiol Immunol* 57(11):737–745, 2013.
11. Durand G, Bes M, Meugnier H, et al: Detection of new methicillin-resistant *Staphylococcus aureus* clones containing the toxic shock syndrome toxin 1 gene responsible for hospital- and community-acquired infections in France. *J Clin Microbiol* 44(3):847–853, 2006.
12. Limbago B, Fosheim GE, Schoonover V, et al: Characterization of methicillin-resistant *Staphylococcus aureus* isolates collected in 2005 and 2006 from patients with invasive disease: a population-based analysis. *J Clin Microbiol* 47(5):1344–1351, 2009.
13. MacPhee RA, Miller WL, Gloor GB, et al: Influence of the vaginal microbiota on toxic shock syndrome toxin 1 production by *Staphylococcus aureus*. *Appl Environ Microbiol* 79(6):1835–1842, 2013.
14. Centers for Disease Control and Prevention: Toxic Shock Syndrome (other than Streptococcal) (TSS) 2011 Case Definition. http://wwwn.cdc.gov/nndss/

conditions/toxic-shock-syndrome-other-than-streptococcal/case-definition/2011/. Accessed September 8, 2015.
15. Dickgiesser N, Wallach U: Toxic shock syndrome toxin-1 (TSST-1): influence of its production by subinhibitory antibiotic concentrations. *Infection* 15(5):351–353, 1987.
16. Stevens DL, Wallace RJ, Hamilton SM, et al: Successful treatment of staphylococcal toxic shock syndrome with linezolid: a case report and in vitro evaluation of the production of toxic shock syndrome toxin type 1 in the presence of antibiotics. *Clin Infect Dis* 42(5):729–730, 2006.
17. Stevens DL: The toxic shock syndromes. *Infect Dis Clin North Am* 10(4):727–746, 1996.
18. Zimbelman J, Palmer A, Todd J: Improved outcome of clindamycin compared with beta-lactam antibiotic treatment for invasive *Streptococcus pyogenes* infection. *Pediatr Infect Dis J* 18(12):1096–1100, 1999.
19. Darenberg J, Soderquist B, Normark BH, et al: Differences in potency of intravenous polyspecific immunoglobulin G against streptococcal and staphylococcal superantigens: implications for therapy of toxic shock syndrome. *Clin Infect Dis* 38(6):836–842, 2004.
20. Andrews MM, Parent EM, Barry M, et al: Recurrent nonmenstrual toxic shock syndrome: clinical manifestations, diagnosis, and treatment. *Clin Infect Dis* 32(10):1470–1479, 2001.
21. Kass EH: Toxic shock syndrome: a reprise. *Ann Intern Med* 97(4):608–611, 1982.
22. Brown EJ: The molecular basis of streptococcal toxic shock syndrome. *N Engl J Med* 350(20):2093–2094, 2004.
23. Chiang MC, Jaing TH, Wu CT, et al: Streptococcal toxic shock syndrome in children without skin and soft tissue infection: report of four cases. *Acta Paediatr* 94(6):763–765, 2005.
24. Stevens DL, Gibbons AE, Bergstrom R, et al: The Eagle effect revisited: efficacy of clindamycin, erythromycin, and penicillin in the treatment of streptococcal myositis. *J Infect Dis* 158(1):23–28, 1988.
25. Stevens DL, Bryant AE, Hackett SP Antibiotic effects on bacterial viability, toxin production, and host response. *Clin Infect Dis* 20 Suppl 2:S154–S157, 1995.
26. Kaul R, McGeer A, Norrby-Teglund A, et al: Intravenous immunoglobulin therapy for streptococcal toxic shock syndrome—a comparative observational study. The Canadian Streptococcal Study Group. *Clin Infect Dis* 28(4):800–807, 1999.
27. Cawley MJ, Briggs M, Haith LR Jr, et al: Intravenous immunoglobulin as adjunctive treatment for streptococcal toxic shock syndrome associated with necrotizing fasciitis: case report and review. *Pharmacotherapy* 19(9):1094–1098, 1999.
28. Carapetis JR, Jacoby P, Carville K, et al: Effectiveness of clindamycin and intravenous immunoglobulin, and risk of disease in contacts, in invasive group a streptococcal infections. *Clin Infect Dis* 59(3):358–365, 2014.
29. Linner A, Darenberg J, Sjolin J, et al: Clinical efficacy of polyspecific intravenous immunoglobulin therapy in patients with streptococcal toxic shock syndrome: a comparative observational study. *Clin Infect Dis* 59(6):851–857, 2014.
30. Darenberg J, Ihendyane N, Sjolin J, et al: Intravenous immunoglobulin G therapy in streptococcal toxic shock syndrome: a European randomized, double-blind, placebo-controlled trial. *Clin Infect Dis* 37(3):333–340, 2003.
31. Prevention of Invasive Group A Streptococcal Infections Workshop Participants: Prevention of invasive group A streptococcal disease among household contacts of case patients and among postpartum and postsurgical patients: recommendations from the Centers for Disease Control and Prevention. *Clin Infect Dis* 35(8):950–959, 2002.
32. Siegel JD, Rhinehart E, Jackson M, et al; Health Care Infection Control Practices Advisory Committee: 2007 guideline for isolation precautions: preventing transmission of infectious agents in health care settings. *Am J Infect Control* 35[10 Suppl 2]:S65–S164, 2007.
33. Sinave C, Le Templier G, Blouin D, et al: Toxic shock syndrome due to *Clostridium sordellii*: a dramatic postpartum and postabortion disease. *Clin Infect Dis* 35(11):1441–1443, 2002.
34. Fischer M, Bhatnagar J, Guarner J, et al: Fatal toxic shock syndrome associated with *Clostridium sordellii* after medical abortion. *N Engl J Med* 353(22):2352–2360, 2005.
35. Meites E, Zane S, Gould C; *Clostridium sordellii* Investigators. Fatal *Clostridium sordellii* infections after medical abortions. *N Engl J Med* 363(14):1382–1383, 2010.
36. Kimura AC, Higa JI, Levin RM, et al: Outbreak of necrotizing fasciitis due to *Clostridium sordellii* among black-tar heroin users. *Clin Infect Dis* 38(9):e87–e91, 2004.
37. Kainer MA, Linden JV, Whaley DN, et al: Clostridium infections associated with musculoskeletal-tissue allografts. *N Engl J Med* 350(25):2564–2571, 2004.
38. Aldape MJ, Bryant AE, Stevens DL: *Clostridium sordellii* infection: epidemiology, clinical findings, and current perspectives on diagnosis and treatment. *Clin Infect Dis* 43(11):1436–1446, 2006.
39. Cohn AC, MacNeil JR, Clark TA, et al: Prevention and control of meningococcal disease: recommendations of the Advisory Committee on Immunization Practices (ACIP). *MMWR Recomm Rep* 62(RR-2):1–28, 2013.
40. Rosenstein NE, Perkins BA, Stephens DS, et al: The changing epidemiology of meningococcal disease in the United States, 1992–1996. *J Infect Dis* 180(6):1894–1901, 1999.
41. Chicago Department of Public Health: Meningococcal Vaccine Recommendations for HIV-positive individuals. 2015. https://www.chicagohan.org/mening;jsessionid=26A202153B93BCF32DCEBE782223277B. Accessed September 16, 2015.
42. LAC DPH Health Alert: Invasive Meningococcal disease update: new vaccine recommendations for Men who Have Sex with Men (MSM) [press release]. April 2, 2014.
43. Kratz MM, Weiss D, Ridpath A, et al: Community-based outbreak of *Neisseria meningitidis* serogroup C infection in men who have sex with men, New York City, New York, USA, 2010–2013. *Emerg Infect Dis* 21(8):1379–1386, 2015.
44. Simon MS, Weiss D, Gulick RM: Invasive meningococcal disease in men who have sex with men. *Ann Intern Med* 159(4):300–301, 2013.
45. Pathan N, Faust SN, Levin M: Pathophysiology of meningococcal meningitis and septicaemia. *Arch Dis Child* 88(7):601–607, 2003.
46. Ellison RT 3rd, Kohler PF, Curd JG, et al: Prevalence of congenital or acquired complement deficiency in patients with sporadic meningocococcal disease. *N Engl J Med* 308(16):913–916, 1983.
47. Faust SN, Levin M, Harrison OB, et al: Dysfunction of endothelial protein C activation in severe meningococcal sepsis. *N Engl J Med* 345(6):408–416, 2001.
48. Havens PL, Garland JS, Brook MM, et al: Trends in mortality in children hospitalized with meningococcal infections, 1957 to 1987. *Pediatr Infect Dis J* 8(1):8–11, 1989.
49. Booy R, Habibi P, Nadel S, et al: Reduction in case fatality rate from meningococcal disease associated with improved healthcare delivery. *Arch Dis Child* 85(5):386–390, 2001.
50. Hazelzet JA: Diagnosing meningococcemia as a cause of sepsis. *Pediatr Crit Care Med* 6[3 Suppl]:S50–S54, 2005.
51. Jorgensen JH, Crawford SA, Fiebelkorn KR: Susceptibility of *Neisseria meningitidis* to 16 antimicrobial agents and characterization of resistance mechanisms affecting some agents. *J Clin Microbiol* 43(7):3162–3171, 2005.
52. Brigham KS, Sandora TJ: *Neisseria meningitidis*: epidemiology, treatment and prevention in adolescents. *Curr Opin Pediatr* 21(4):437–443, 2009.
53. Centers for Disease Control and Prevention (CDC): Emergence of fluoroquinolone-resistant *Neisseria meningitidis*—Minnesota and North Dakota, 2007–2008. *MMWR Morb Mortal Wkly Rep* 57(7):173–175, 2008.
54. Warner PM, Kagan RJ, Yakuboff KP, et al: Current management of purpura fulminans: a multicenter study. *J Burn Care Rehabil* 24(3):119–126, 2003.
55. Churchwell KB, McManus ML, Kent P, et al: Intensive blood and plasma exchange for treatment of coagulopathy in meningococcemia. *J Clin Apher* 10(4):171–177, 1995.
56. Valbonesi M, Pallavicini FB, Cannella G, et al: MOF induced by meningococcal sepsis: successful outcome after intensive multidisciplinary approaches. *Transfus Apher Sci* 33(1):75–77, 2005.
57. Wu HM, Harcourt BH, Hatcher CP, et al: Emergence of ciprofloxacin-resistant *Neisseria meningitidis* in North America. *N Engl J Med* 360(9):886–892, 2009.
58. Harcourt BH, Anderson RD, Wu HM, et al: Population-based surveillance of *Neisseria meningitidis* antimicrobial resistance in the United States. *Open Forum Infect Dis* 2(3):ofv117, 2015.
59. Folaranmi T, Rubin L, Martin SW, et al: Use of serogroup B meningococcal vaccines in persons aged ≥10 years at increased risk for serogroup B meningococcal disease: recommendations of the Advisory Committee on Immunization Practices, 2015. *MMWR Morb Mortal Wkly Rep* 64(22):608–612, 2015.
60. Styrt B: Infection associated with asplenia: risks, mechanisms, and prevention. *Am J Med* 88(5N):33N–42N, 1990.
61. Brigden ML, Pattullo AL: Prevention and management of overwhelming postsplenectomy infection—an update. *Crit Care Med* 27(4):836–842, 1999.
62. Coleman CN, McDougall IR, Dailey MO, et al: Functional hyposplenia after splenic irradiation for Hodgkin's disease. *Ann Intern Med* 96(1):44–47, 1982.
63. Markus HS, Toghill PJ: Impaired splenic function in elderly people. *Age Ageing* 20(4):287–290, 1991.
64. Upadhyaya P: Conservative management of splenic trauma: history and current trends. *Pediatr Surg Int* 19(9–10):617–627, 2003.
65. Gauer JM, Gerber-Paulet S, Seiler C, et al: Twenty years of splenic preservation in trauma: lower early infection rate than in splenectomy. *World J Surg* 32(12):2730–2735, 2008.
66. Corazza GR, Ginaldi L, Zoli G, et al: Howell-Jolly body counting as a measure of splenic function. A reassessment. *Clin Lab Haematol* 12(3):269–275, 1990.
67. Chiappa V, Chang CY, Sellas MI, et al: Case records of the Massachusetts General Hospital. Case 10-2014. A 45-year-old man with a rash. *N Engl J Med* 370(13):1238–1248, 2014.
68. Sawmiller CJ, Dudrick SJ, Hamzi M: Postsplenectomy *Capnocytophaga canimorsus* sepsis presenting as an acute abdomen. *Arch Surg* 133(12):1362–1365, 1998.
69. Sakran W, Raz R, Levi Y, et al: Campylobacter bacteremia and pneumonia in two splenectomized patients. *Eur J Clin Microbiol Infect Dis* 18(7):496–498, 1999.
70. Sheng CF, Liu BY, Zhang HM, et al: Overwhelming postsplenectomy infection. *Genet Mol Res* 14(1):2702–2706, 2015.
71. Xu F, Dai CL, Wu XM, et al: Overwhelming postsplenectomy infection due to *Mycoplasma pneumoniae* in an asplenic cirrhotic patient: case report. *BMC Infect Dis* 11:162, 2011.
72. Hansen K, Singer DB: Asplenic-hyposplenic overwhelming sepsis: postsplenectomy sepsis revisited. *Pediatr Dev Pathol* 4(2):105–121, 2001.
73. Toutouzas KG, Velmahos GC, Kaminski A, et al: Leukocytosis after posttraumatic splenectomy: a physiologic event or sign of sepsis? *Arch Surg* 137(8):924–928, 2002; discussion 928-929.
74. Working Party of the British Committee for Standards in Haematology Clinical Haematology Task Force: Guidelines for the prevention and treatment of infection in patients with an absent or dysfunctional spleen. *BMJ* 312(7028):430–434, 1996.

75. Rubin LG, Levin MJ, Ljungman P, et al: 2013 IDSA clinical practice guideline for vaccination of the immunocompromised host. *Clin Infect Dis* 58(3):e44–e100, 2014.
76. Shatz DV, Schinsky MF, Pais LB, et al: Immune responses of splenectomized trauma patients to the 23-valent pneumococcal polysaccharide vaccine at 1 versus 7 versus 14 days after splenectomy. *J Trauma* 44(5):760–765, 1998; discussion 765–766.
77. Centers for Disease Control and Prevention (CDC): Updated recommendation from the Advisory Committee on Immunization Practices (ACIP) for revaccination of persons at prolonged increased risk for meningococcal disease. *MMWR Morb Mortal Wkly Rep* 58(37):1042–1043, 2009.
78. Davies JM, Lewis MP, Wimperis J, et al: Review of guidelines for the prevention and treatment of infection in patients with an absent or dysfunctional spleen: prepared on behalf of the British Committee for Standards in Haematology by a working party of the Haemato-Oncology task force. *Br J Haematol* 155(3):308–317, 2011.
79. Rubin LG, Schaffner W: Clinical practice. Care of the asplenic patient. *N Engl J Med* 371(4):349–356, 2014.
80. Snow RW, Guerra CA, Noor AM, et al: The global distribution of clinical episodes of *Plasmodium falciparum* malaria. *Nature* 434(7030):214–217, 2005.
81. Cullen KA, Arguin PM: Malaria surveillance—United States, 2012. *MMWR Surveill Summ* 63(12):1–22, 2014.
82. Centers for Disease Control and Prevention (CDC): Malaria deaths following inappropriate malaria chemoprophylaxis—United States, 2001. *MMWR Morb Mortal Wkly Rep* 50(28):597–599, 2001.
83. Zucker JR: Changing patterns of autochthonous malaria transmission in the United States: a review of recent outbreaks. *Emerg Infect Dis* 2(1):37–43, 1996.
84. Ho M, White NJ: Molecular mechanisms of cytoadherence in malaria. *Am J Physiol* 276[6 Pt 1]:C1231–C1242, 1999.
85. Freedman DO, Weld LH, Kozarsky PE, et al: Spectrum of disease and relation to place of exposure among ill returned travelers. *N Engl J Med* 354(2):119–130, 2006.
86. Winters RA, Murray HW: Malaria—the mime revisited: fifteen more years of experience at a New York City teaching hospital. *Am J Med* 93(3):243–246, 1992.
87. Severe falciparum malaria. World Health Organization, Communicable Diseases Cluster. *Trans R Soc Trop Med Hyg* 94 Suppl 1:S1–S90, 2000.
88. Alvarez JR, Al-Khan A, Apuzzio JJ: Malaria in pregnancy. *Infect Dis Obstet Gynecol* 13(4):229–236, 2005.
89. Whitty CJ, Edmonds S, Mutabingwa TK: Malaria in pregnancy. *BJOG* 112(9):1189–1195, 2005.
90. Brentlinger PE, Behrens CB, Micek MA: Challenges in the concurrent management of malaria and HIV in pregnancy in sub-Saharan Africa. *Lancet Infect Dis* 6(2):100–111, 2006.
91. Rogerson SJ, Mkundika P, Kanjala MK: Diagnosis of *Plasmodium falciparum* malaria at delivery: comparison of blood film preparation methods and of blood films with histology. *J Clin Microbiol* 41(4):1370–1374, 2003.
92. Bruneel F, Hocqueloux L, Alberti C, et al: The clinical spectrum of severe imported falciparum malaria in the intensive care unit: report of 188 cases in adults. *Am J Respir Crit Care Med* 167(5):684–689, 2003.
93. Centers for Disease Control and Prevention: CDC Now Provides Malaria Drug Resistance Testing Services. http://www.cdc.gov/malaria/features/ars.html. Accessed September 20, 2015.
94. Centers for Disease Control and Prevention: Treatment of Malaria (Guidelines For Clinicians). 2013.
95. Centers for Disease Control and Prevention (CDC): Availability and use of parenteral quinidine gluconate for severe or complicated malaria. *MMWR Morb Mortal Wkly Rep* 49(50):1138–1140, 2000.
96. Magill A, Panosian C: Making antimalarial agents available in the United States. *N Engl J Med* 353(4):335–337, 2005.
97. Griffith KS, Lewis LS, Mali S, et al: Treatment of malaria in the United States: a systematic review. *JAMA* 297(20):2264–2277, 2007.
98. Miller KD, Greenberg AE, Campbell CC: Treatment of severe malaria in the United States with a continuous infusion of quinidine gluconate and exchange transfusion. *N Engl J Med* 321(2):65–70, 1989.
99. Dondorp A, Nosten F, Stepniewska K, et al; South East Asian Quinine Artesunate Malaria Trial group: Artesunate versus quinine for treatment of severe falciparum malaria: a randomised trial. *Lancet* 366(9487):717–725, 2005.
100. McGready R, Thwai KL, Cho T, et al: The effects of quinine and chloroquine antimalarial treatments in the first trimester of pregnancy. *Trans R Soc Trop Med Hyg* 96(2):180–184, 2002.
101. McGready R, Ashley EA, Moo E, et al: A randomized comparison of artesunate-atovaquone-proguanil versus quinine in treatment for uncomplicated falciparum malaria during pregnancy. *J Infect Dis* 192(5):846–853, 2005.
102. Wong RD, Murthy AR, Mathisen GE, et al: Treatment of severe falciparum malaria during pregnancy with quinidine and exchange transfusion. *Am J Med* 92(5):561–562, 1992.
103. Tan KR, Wiegand RE, Arguin PM: Exchange transfusion for severe malaria: evidence base and literature review. *Clin Infect Dis* 57(7):923–928, 2013.
104. Shaz BH, Schwartz J, Winters JL, et al: American society for apheresis guidelines support use of red cell exchange transfusion for severe malaria with high parasitemia. *Clin Infect Dis* 58(2):302–303, 2014.
105. WHO Guidelines Approved by the Guidelines Review Committee: *Guidelines for the Treatment of Malaria*. Geneva, World Health Organization Copyright (c) World Health Organization, 2015.
106. Warrell DA, Looareesuwan S, Warrell MJ, et al: Dexamethasone proves deleterious in cerebral malaria. A double-blind trial in 100 comatose patients. *N Engl J Med* 306(6):313–319, 1982.
107. Masters EJ, Olson GS, Weiner SJ, et al: Rocky Mountain spotted fever: a clinician's dilemma. *Arch Intern Med* 163(7):769–774, 2003.
108. Kirk JL, Fine DP, Sexton DJ, et al: Rocky Mountain spotted fever. A clinical review based on 48 confirmed cases, 1943–1986. *Medicine (Baltimore)* 69(1):35–45, 1990.
109. Openshaw JJ, Swerdlow DL, Krebs JW, et al: Rocky mountain spotted fever in the United States, 2000–2007: interpreting contemporary increases in incidence. *Am J Trop Med Hyg* 83(1):174–182, 2010.
110. Centers for Disease Control and Prevention: Spotted Fever Rickettsiosis (*Rickettsia* spp.) 2010 Case Definition. http://wwwn.cdc.gov/nndss/conditions/spotted-fever-rickettsiosis/case-definition/2010/. Accessed September 20, 2015.
111. Traeger MS, Regan JJ, Humpherys D, et al: Rocky mountain spotted fever characterization and comparison to similar illnesses in a highly endemic area-Arizona, 2002–2011. *Clin Infect Dis* 60(11):1650–1658, 2015.
112. Regan JJ, Traeger MS, Humpherys D, et al: Risk factors for fatal outcome from rocky mountain spotted Fever in a highly endemic area-Arizona, 2002–2011. *Clin Infect Dis* 60(11):1659–1666, 2015.
113. McQuiston JH, Wiedeman C, Singleton J, et al: Inadequacy of IgM antibody tests for diagnosis of Rocky Mountain Spotted Fever. *Am J Trop Med Hyg* 91(4):767–770, 2014.
114. Helmick CG, Bernard KW, D'Angelo LJ: Rocky Mountain spotted fever: clinical, laboratory, and epidemiological features of 262 cases. *J Infect Dis* 150(4):480–488, 1984.
115. Chapman AS, Bakken JS, Folk SM, et al: Diagnosis and management of tickborne rickettsial diseases: Rocky Mountain spotted fever, ehrlichioses, and anaplasmosis—United States: a practical guide for physicians and other health-care and public health professionals. *MMWR Recomm Rep* 55(RR-4):1–27, 2006.
116. Holman RC, Paddock CD, Curns AT, et al: Analysis of risk factors for fatal Rocky Mountain Spotted Fever: evidence for superiority of tetracyclines for therapy. *J Infect Dis* 184(11):1437–1444, 2001.
117. Centers for Disease Control and Prevention (CDC): Fatal cases of Rocky Mountain spotted fever in family clusters—three states, 2003. *MMWR Morb Mortal Wkly Rep* 53(19):407–410, 2004.
118. Lochary ME, Lockhart PB, Williams WT Jr: Doxycycline and staining of permanent teeth. *Pediatr Infect Dis J* 17(5):429–431, 1998.
119. Todd SR, Dahlgren FS, Traeger MS, et al: No visible dental staining in children treated with doxycycline for suspected Rocky Mountain Spotted Fever. *J Pediatr* 166(5):1246–1251, 2015.
120. Chloramphenicol Sodium Succinate. In *Micromedex®* 2.0, (electronic version). Truven Health Analytics, Greenwood Village, Colorado, USA. Available at: http://www.micromedexsolutions.com.proxy.hsl.ucdenver.edu/ (cited: *09/25/2017*).
121. Stallings SP: Rocky Mountain spotted fever and pregnancy: a case report and review of the literature. *Obstet Gynecol Surv* 56(1):37–42, 2001.
122. Woodward TE: Rocky Mountain spotted fever: epidemiological and early clinical signs are keys to treatment and reduced mortality. *J Infect Dis* 150(4):465–468, 1984.
123. Kirkland KB, Wilkinson WE, Sexton DJ: Therapeutic delay and mortality in cases of Rocky Mountain spotted fever. *Clin Infect Dis* 20(5):1118–1121, 1995.
124. Dalton MJ, Clarke MJ, Holman RC, et al: National surveillance for Rocky Mountain spotted fever, 1981–1992: epidemiologic summary and evaluation of risk factors for fatal outcome. *Am J Trop Med Hyg* 52(5):405–413, 1995.
125. Bakken JS, Krueth J, Wilson-Nordskog C, et al: Clinical and laboratory characteristics of human granulocytic ehrlichiosis. *JAMA* 275(3):199–205, 1996.
126. Demma LJ, Holman RC, McQuiston JH, et al: Epidemiology of human ehrlichiosis and anaplasmosis in the United States, 2001–2002. *Am J Trop Med Hyg* 73(2):400–409, 2005.
127. Bakken JS, Dumler JS: Human granulocytic ehrlichiosis. *Clin Infect Dis* 31(2):554–560, 2000.
128. Paddock CD, Suchard DP, Grumbach KL, et al: Brief report: fatal seronegative ehrlichiosis in a patient with HIV infection. *N Engl J Med* 329(16):1164–1167, 1993.
129. Butler T: *Capnocytophaga canimorsus*: an emerging cause of sepsis, meningitis, and post-splenectomy infection after dog bites. *Eur J Clin Microbiol Infect Dis* 34(7):1271–1280, 2015.
130. Brenner DJ, Hollis DG, Fanning GR, et al: *Capnocytophaga canimorsus* sp. nov. (formerly CDC group DF-2), a cause of septicemia following dog bite, and C. cynodegmi sp. nov., a cause of localized wound infection following dog bite. *J Clin Microbiol* 27(2):231–235, 1989.
131. Janda JM, Graves MH, Lindquist D, et al: Diagnosing *Capnocytophaga canimorsus* infections. *Emerg Infect Dis* 12(2):340–342, 2006.
132. Bonatti H, Rossboth DW, Nachbaur D, et al: A series of infections due to Capnocytophaga spp in immunosuppressed and immunocompetent patients. *Clin Microbiol Infect* 9(5):380–387, 2003.
133. Martino R, Ramila E, Capdevila JA, et al: Bacteremia caused by Capnocytophaga species in patients with neutropenia and cancer: results of a multicenter study. *Clin Infect Dis* 33(4):E20–E22, 2001.

Chapter 75 ■ Acute Infection in the Immunocompromised Host

JENNIFER S. DALY • ROBERT W. FINBERG

Advances in the management of neoplastic diseases, transplant immunology, and the therapy of autoimmune diseases have resulted in marked improvements in life expectancy and the quality of patients' lives. However, patients with autoimmune diseases, neoplasia, or transplantation become highly susceptible to infection by virtue of their associated therapies or by the nature of their underlying illness. Infection has been and remains a leading cause of death among patients with leukemia and lymphoma and a major cause of morbidity and mortality in patients with solid tumors or transplants [1–4]. Rapid progression of fungal, bacterial, and mycobacterial infections occurs in patients given monoclonal antibodies to treat Crohn's disease and autoimmune diseases such as rheumatoid arthritis [5–7]. The epidemic of human immunodeficiency virus (HIV)-1 infection has added to the numbers of immunocompromised hosts by virtue of the central event of the virus's pathogenesis: a progressive, irreversible weakening of cell-mediated immunity unless the patient responds to antiretroviral agents (see Chapter 76).

Traditionally, infection has accounted for up to 75% of deaths in patients with acute leukemia or Hodgkin's disease [1,8] or in transplant recipients [3,9], but with advances in prophylaxis and management, deaths because of infections have decreased to about 50%, whereas death owing to graft versus host disease, relapse of malignancy, and multiorgan failure have increased [10–13]. Once patients require intensive care unit (ICU) care, the mortality increases, and the 1-year survival of cancer patients that require mechanical ventilation in the ICU is below 11% for some centers [14], with acute mortality between 44% and 74% [15–17]. Although intensive efforts are clearly beneficial for stem cell transplantation patients requiring ICU care for the pre-engraftment period, patients with graft versus host disease following engraftment have the worst prognosis [14]. Early ICU admission has been advocated based on one small study demonstrating that among patients initially thought to be too sick to benefit from ICU care, many were subsequently admitted to the ICU, and did well [18].

Although a great variety of microorganisms have been noted to cause severe, life-threatening infections in immunocompromised hosts, the clinician can formulate a diagnostic plan and decide on empiric therapy by giving careful consideration to the nature, duration, and severity of the immunosuppression that is causing the patient's predisposition to infection. Infection can arise as a consequence of derangements in host defenses that result from the primary disease, the medical and surgical treatment of the condition, or a combination of these factors. Additionally, immunocompromised patients are likely to manifest their infections in ways that are characteristically different from those of patients with intact immune responses.

IMMUNE DEFECTS AND ASSOCIATED ORGANISMS AND INFECTIONS

Underlying disease or treatments affect different aspects of the immune system and, depending on the type of defect, are associated with predisposition to infection with specific classes of organisms or disease syndromes. A level of suspicion of infection with certain organisms depends on the specific immune defect, the duration of immunosuppression, surgical and medical interventions, colonization with nosocomial pathogens, and previous latent or asymptomatic infections that may reactivate after immunosuppression. In general, the most common sites of serious, definable infection in the immunocompromised host are the bloodstream (including infection related to intravenous [IV] access devices), lung, and mucocutaneous surfaces (including oral, gastrointestinal, skin, and perirectal areas). The diverse organisms frequently or uniquely associated with infections in the compromised host are listed in Table 75.1. As a general rule, patients whose underlying disease or treatment leads to a lack of T cells or any abnormality in T cell–macrophage activation will be subject to infections with organisms that live intracellularly such as viruses, fungi, and intracellular bacteria (e.g., *Listeria*, *Legionella*, mycobacteria). Patients with profound neutropenia will be subject to infection with aerobic Gram-positive and Gram-negative bacteria that live on the skin and within the gut. Patients lacking antibodies or a spleen will be unusually susceptible to infection with encapsulated bacteria (*Streptococcus pneumoniae*, *Haemophilus influenzae*, and *Neisseria meningitidis*). As for any patient in the ICU, the immunocompromised patient is susceptible to infection with bacteria that are found in ventilators or spread in the ICU. The most common organisms found in patients with bloodstream infections vary by center and whether or not patients are on prophylactic antimicrobials [19]. *Escherichia coli* and *Staphylococcus aureus*, including methicillin-resistant *S. aureus* (MRSA), continue to be common, followed by coagulase-negative staphylococci, enterococci including vancomycin-resistant enterococci, *Pseudomonas aeruginosa*, *Klebsiella* species, *Enterobacter* species, and various streptococci [20–23]. In patients with neutropenia and documented bacteremia, Gram-positive organisms predominate over Gram-negative bacilli in most centers, and the presence of an intravascular device is associated with having a positive blood culture [24], although some centers have noted an increase in patients with bacteremia because of multiply resistant Gram-negative bacilli [25]. Fungal infections increase in frequency with increasing duration of the immunocompromised state and therapy with broad-spectrum antibiotics and choice of antifungal prophylaxis.

Anatomic Barriers

The skin and mucosal surfaces serve a primary role in the defense of the host against invasion by endogenous and exogenous microorganisms. Mucous membrane ulceration in the mouth and gastrointestinal tract can occur spontaneously in patients with acute leukemia, although this complication more commonly arises after chemotherapy. In patients with solid tumors, disruption of mucocutaneous barriers can result from invasion, obstruction, or perforation by the malignancy. Iatrogenic disruption of the normal skin and mucosal barriers results from medical and surgical support interventions common to the ICU, including intravascular and urinary catheters [26] (see Chapter 79 on catheter infections). Organisms that most frequently cause infection of intravascular catheters include coagulase-negative staphylococci, *S. aureus*, enterococci, *Corynebacterium* species (including *C. jeikeium*), and *Candida* species [1,26,27]. Percutaneously inserted central catheters are associated with an

TABLE 75.1

Organisms Commonly or Uniquely Associated with Acute Infection in the Immunocompromised Host

Organism	Type of immune deficiency most likely to predispose to this organism
Bacteria	
Enteric Gram-negative bacilli (*Escherichia coli*, *Klebsiella*, *Enterobacter*, or *Proteus* species)	All immunocompromised patients, especially those with neutropenia and those on mechanical ventilation or medications that suppress gastric acid
Staphylococcus aureus	All immunocompromised patients, especially those with skin infections or intravascular catheters
Pseudomonas aeruginosa	Especially common in neutropenic patients and those on mechanical ventilation
Listeria monocytogenes	Patients with T-cell or macrophage deficiencies, HIV/AIDS patients
Legionella pneumophila and related organisms	Patients with T-cell or macrophage deficiencies and anyone exposed to water sources contaminated with Legionella
Skin/mucous membrane saprophytes	All immunocompromised patients
Corynebacterium jeikeium	Neutropenic patients, especially those with indwelling catheters, splenectomized patients
Capnocytophaga species	Splenectomized patients
Coagulase-negative staphylococci	Patients with indwelling vascular catheters or prosthetic material
Nocardia species	Patients with T-cell or macrophage abnormalities
Streptococcus pneumoniae	Patients with immunoglobulin deficiencies or hyposplenism
Haemophilus influenzae	Patients with immunoglobulin deficiencies or hyposplenism
Neisseria meningitidis	Patients with immunoglobulin deficiencies or hyposplenism
Mycobacteria	Patients with a history of high-risk exposure for tuberculosis (lived in an endemic area or history of a positive tuberculin skin test) or long-standing immune defects and/or chronic lung disease
Fungi	
Candida albicans and other *Candida* species	Patients with vascular catheters, after abdominal surgery including liver transplantation, patients with prolonged neutropenia, and those receiving intravenous hyperalimentation
Candida glabrata	Same as candidiasis, increased in patients with diabetes and urinary tract colonization
Aspergillus species	Patients with prolonged neutropenia, after transplantation, or on medications such as steroids and cytotoxic agents
Zygomycetes species	Patients with neutropenia, after transplantation, with diabetes, or on medications such as steroids and cytotoxic agents
Trichosporon species	Patients with neutropenia, after transplantation, or on medications such as steroids and cytotoxic agents, with vascular catheters and those receiving intravenous hyperalimentation
Fusarium species	Patients with neutropenia, after transplantation, or on medications such as steroids and cytotoxic agents, with vascular catheters and those receiving intravenous hyperalimentation
Pneumocystis jiroveci	Patients with T-cell or macrophage deficiencies, especially those receiving steroids, antirejection agents, or with lymphocytic leukemia or HIV/AIDS
Endemic fungi and yeasts	
Cryptococcus neoformans	Patients with HIV/AIDS, after transplantation, or receiving steroids
Histoplasma capsulatum	Patients from an endemic area
Coccidioides immitis	Patients from an endemic area
Protozoa	
Toxoplasma gondii	Patients with HIV/AIDS, after transplantation, or on medications such as steroids and cytotoxic agents
Parasites	
Strongyloides stercoralis	Patients from an endemic area and after transplantation, or on medications such as steroids and cytotoxic agents
Viruses	
Cytomegalovirus	Patients after bone marrow or solid organ transplantation
Varicella-zoster virus	Patients with T-cell or macrophage abnormalities, especially those not receiving antiviral prophylaxis with cancer, or after bone marrow or solid organ transplantation
Herpes simplex virus	Patients with T-cell or macrophage abnormalities and ICU patients, especially those not receiving antiviral prophylaxis with cancer, or after bone marrow or solid organ transplantation

increased risk of both infection and thrombosis [28]. The risk of these infections can be reduced, although not eliminated, through the use of permanent, subcutaneously tunneled catheters (e.g., Hickman, Broviac, Groshung, or Portacath systems) [29]. Genitourinary tract infections are associated with disruption of the urinary tract integrity, as occurs with urinary catheter drainage, pelvic tumors, or radiation with resultant ureteral obstruction, or after renal transplant.

The gastrointestinal tract is a source of occult bacteremia or fungemia, because chemotherapy and neutropenia cause breakdown in normal mucosal defenses of the gut, facilitating entry of bacteria or yeast into the bloodstream. Clinically apparent intestinal problems seen in neutropenic patients include typhlitis, anorectal cellulitis/fasciitis/abscess, necrotizing colitis, and *Clostridium difficile*–associated colitis caused by chemotherapy or antibiotics [30]. Typhlitis, an inflammatory disease of the cecum, may lead to toxic megacolon and perforation and requires a high index of suspicion, and prompt diagnosis. Unusually severe and prolonged viral gastroenteritis caused by cytomegalovirus, adenovirus, rotavirus, and Coxsackie virus has been observed in marrow transplant recipients [31–33]. Herpes simplex virus (HSV) should be suspected as a possible cause for any lesion of mucous membranes of an immunocompromised host, and may also cause fatal hepatitis [34]. Adenovirus may cause hepatitis, pneumonitis, or hemorrhagic cystitis [33], and BK and JC viruses may cause persistent fever and renal insufficiency [35,36]. Necrotizing gingivostomatitis caused by oral anaerobes as well as severe periodontal infection may also complicate neutropenia.

Defective Phagocytosis

Neutrophils and macrophages provide defense against infection by bacteria and many fungi. Patients with leukemia, particularly an acute type of leukemia, commonly have a reduction in their absolute number of circulating neutrophils; qualitative defects of neutrophil function have also been described in these patients. Aplastic anemia, as well as extensive bone marrow involvement caused by lymphoma or metastatic solid tumors, may result in neutropenia. By far the most common cause of neutropenia, however, is cytotoxic chemotherapy. Patients whose neutrophils are reduced in number by malignancy or chemotherapy are at risk for the development of spontaneous bacteremia. The risk becomes significant at absolute neutrophil counts that are persistently below 500 per μL (or below 1,000 per μL and falling) and increases dramatically at counts below 100 per μL [33,37].

Invasive and disseminated fungal infections also may be a consequence of neutropenia and become more common after the neutropenic patient has received broad-spectrum antibiotic therapy [33,38]. *Candida* and *Aspergillus* species are the most common fungal pathogens observed in neutropenic hosts, but unusual genera such as *Fusarium*, *Trichosporon*, *Scedosporium* (*Pseudallescheria*), mucormycoses, and *Cunninghamella* have been described with increasing frequency [39–41].

Altered Humoral Immunity

B-cell lymphocytic function and antibody production may be impaired in untreated patients with chronic lymphocytic leukemia, multiple myeloma, and lymphoma. Acquired deficits in antibody production may also be encountered in otherwise healthy patients (e.g., immunoglobulin A deficiency, common variable immunodeficiency). Hypogammaglobulinemia or impaired antibody response predisposes patients to infections attributable to encapsulated bacteria such as *S. pneumoniae*, *H. influenzae*, and *N. meningitidis*; moreover, these infections are likely to be sudden, severe, and associated with fulminant bacteremia [33]. Infections caused by enteric Gram-negative bacilli and *P. aeruginosa* also may be seen in previously untreated patients with defective humoral immunity secondary to B-cell malignancies.

Impaired Cell-Mediated Immunity

T cell–mediated immunity includes cytotoxic (killer) T cells, activated macrophages, and antibody-dependent cellular cytotoxicity. These critical components of immunity are impaired in patients with Hodgkin's disease [42] and other lymphomas and in those taking antirejection drugs (e.g., cyclosporine, mycophenolate mofetil, tacrolimus, sirolimus, and antilymphocyte antibodies), antibodies against tumor necrosis factor (TNF)-α, or corticosteroids [3,6,7,43]. Patients infected with HIV-1 experience a progressive and devastating loss of T cell–mediated immunity. This virus selectively infects and lyses $CD4^+$ lymphocytes that play a central role in governing humeral and cellular immune responses. Defects in cell-mediated immunity are commonly associated with primary or reactivation of infection by herpes viruses (varicella-zoster virus, cytomegalovirus, HSV), protozoa (*Toxoplasma gondii* and *Cryptosporidium* species), fungi (*Pneumocystis jiroveci*, *Cryptococcus neoformans*, *Histoplasma capsulatum*, *Coccidioides immitis*, and *Candida* species), helminths (*Strongyloides stercoralis*), mycobacteria (*M. tuberculosis*, *M. avium-intracellulare*, *M. kansasii*, *M. chelonae*), and other intracellular bacteria (*Listeria monocytogenes*, *Salmonella*, and *Legionella* species) [3,42,44].

Immunosuppressive Medications

Cytotoxic chemotherapy, corticosteroids, anticytokine antibodies, and other immunosuppressive therapeutic regimens can alter host defenses in several ways. Immunosuppressive effects depend on the class of drug, dose and duration of therapy, and timing relative to other therapeutic modalities (e.g., radiation, which may contribute to neutropenia). Several new inhibitors of cytokines and cytokine activation (including anti-TNF and anti-IL-1 antibodies) used to treat autoimmune disorders have resulted in the reactivation of latent tuberculosis and histoplasmosis as well as invasive aspergillosis [6,45,46]. Physicians need to be aware of the fact that patients on such agents have a risk of reactivation of intracellular organisms [47].

Antimicrobial Therapy

Antibiotic therapy is highly effective in the management of documented infections and febrile episodes in the compromised host. These agents are double-edged swords, however, and promote a shift toward increasing frequency of infections caused by progressively more resistant organisms, including *P. aeruginosa*, *Enterobacter* species, extended spectrum β-lactamase–producing *Klebsiella* species, multiply resistant enterococci, MRSA, and fluconazole-resistant *Candida* species. Unusual, intrinsically resistant bacteria (e.g., *Capnocytophaga* and *Corynebacterium* species) and fungi (e.g., *Scedosporium* and *Fusarium* species) are being seen with increasing frequency in oncology centers.

Splenectomy

Splenectomy, which results in the loss of the reticuloendothelial capacity to clear organisms from the bloodstream, predisposes patients to fulminant, overwhelming bacteremia caused by encapsulated bacteria (*S. pneumoniae*, *H. influenzae*, and

N. meningitidis) as well as *S. aureus*. Although the syndrome of overwhelming postsplenectomy infection is most common among patients whose splenectomy was for malignancy or reticuloendothelial disease, overwhelming postsplenectomy infection can occur in any splenectomized patient regardless of underlying disease or interval since surgery (see Chapter 74). Accordingly, fever higher than 38°C in the splenectomized patient warrants immediate investigation and empiric therapy for possible bacteremia or focal bacterial infection. Consideration of ICU admission and presumptive antibiotic therapy is appropriate if the patient appears systemically toxic. A third-generation cephalosporin (e.g., ceftriaxone or cefotaxime) is reasonable empiric therapy, although if skin or skin structure infection is present, vancomycin should be added because of the increasing likelihood of community-acquired MRSA.

DIAGNOSTIC APPROACH TO FEVER

In the evaluation of acutely ill, immunocompromised patients with fever in the ICU, a meticulous and thorough history and physical examination must be performed initially and repeated daily. Particular attention should be directed to sites of high risk, such as the oropharynx, anorectal region, lungs, skin, optic fundi, and vascular catheter sites. Patients with focal abnormalities such as solid tumors, organ transplantation, or recent surgery need to have these specific sites investigated with special care. Patients with neutropenia and infection exhibit fewer and less striking physical findings of infection (e.g., local warmth, swelling, adenopathy, exudate, or fluctuance) than are ordinarily encountered in immunocompetent individuals (see Chapter 71).

Initial laboratory studies that should be performed in the evaluation of the acutely ill, febrile, compromised host include (a) cultures of blood, (b) cultures of urine if symptoms or abnormal urinalysis, (c) routine sputum culture, if the patient has symptoms or signs of pulmonary disease, (d) swab, aspiration, or biopsy of suspect skin, mucous membrane, or other lesions for smears, cultures, and pathologic examination, (e) semiquantitative culture of IV catheters in place when fever develops; if possible (if the cannula is a critical lifeline or a subcutaneously tunneled device that shows no local signs of infection, removal can be deferred pending results of routine blood cultures), (f) chest radiography, and (g) serum chemistries (i.e., electrolytes, liver chemistries, creatinine), in part to detect possible visceral involvement or multiorgan failure caused by disseminated infection and also to serve as baselines for monitoring possible adverse reactions to subsequent antimicrobial therapy.

Patients with defects of cell-mediated immunity (e.g., HIV-1 infection, lymphoma, transplant recipients) often harbor organisms that are best diagnosed by histologic examination (e.g., *Pneumocystis jiroveci*, *T. gondii*) or special culture techniques (e.g., mycobacteria, viruses). In instances in which such organisms are high in the differential diagnosis, initial evaluation often entails immediate biopsy of the pathologic process. Localizing symptoms and signs may indicate the need for other studies, such as computed tomography (CT), magnetic resonance imaging (MRI), or nuclear medicine scans (e.g., gallium-67 scan to detect *P. jiroveci* pneumonia [PCP]). Tachypnea warrants arterial blood gas studies because progressive hypoxemia in the absence of radiographic findings can be an early indicator of pulmonary infection, especially PCP, and may indicate a need for bronchoscopy. Depending on the nature of the abnormality and the state of immunosuppression, consider lung biopsy and/or quantitative culture of washings or protected brushings obtained through the bronchoscope if patient presents with pulmonary symptoms and a new finding on chest X-ray [48,49].

APPROACH TO SPECIFIC INFECTIOUS DISEASE PRESENTATIONS

Acute Fever without Obvious Source: Neutropenia

In patients with fever and neutropenia, shock may be an early complication of bacteremia. Although now that antibiotic prophylaxis during episodes of neutropenia is widely used, only 20% to 30% of febrile neutropenic patients have documented infection [50,51]; multiple randomized trials and consensus guidelines support the initiation of empiric broad-spectrum antibiotic therapy for all patients with fever greater than 38°C and absolute neutrophil counts less than 500 per μL (or less than 1,000 per μL and falling) [37,38,52,53]. The immediate institution of such therapy in these patients (even in the absence of documentation of bacterial infection) dramatically reduces morbidity and mortality. The most rapidly fatal infectious agents that are documented to cause acute fever in the critically ill neutropenic cancer patient are enteric Gram-negative bacilli (e.g., *E. coli*, *Klebsiella* species, *Proteus* species), *P. aeruginosa*, and *S. aureus* [37,38]. In the patient without an obvious site of infection, initial empiric antibiotic therapy should be directed against these pathogens (Table 75.2). Such therapy should take into consideration idiosyncrasies of the antimicrobial susceptibility

TABLE 75.2

Empiric Regimens for Initial Therapy of Critically Ill, Febrile, Adult ICU Patients with Neutropenia and Cancer (Dosages Provided for Patients with Normal Renal Function)

Choice of β-lactam or monobactam[a]	Plus or minus additional antimicrobial to treat skin/soft tissue infections if present (must use for patients given aztreonam) or patients suspected of having staphylococcal infection[a]
Piperacillin/tazobactam 3.375 g IV q4h or 4.5 g IV q6h OR Ceftazidime 2 g IV q8h OR Imipenem/cilastatin 500–750 mg IV q6h OR Meropenem 1 g IV q8h For penicillin and cephalosporin allergic patients: Aztreonam, 2 g IV q6–8h, plus vancomycin, 2 g/d (divided q6–12h)	Vancomycin 1 g–1.5 g IV q 12 (weight based—15 mg/kg q12h) (alternatives for allergic patients include linezolid, daptomycin, quinupristin/dalfopristin, or clindamycin)

[a]The choice of regimen should be based on local resistance patterns and the individual patient's most recent prior antimicrobial therapy.

patterns of organisms in the institutions where the patient has resided in the months before infection and recent antibiotic use in a particular patient.

Despite the testing of hundreds of antibacterial regimens for use in patients with fever and neutropenia, there is no consensus on one best regimen. For patients who have not received prior antibiotic prophylaxis or therapy, a single antipseudomonal third-generation cephalosporin (e.g., ceftazidime), piperacillin/tazobactam, or a carbapenem (imipenem, or meropenem) constitutes an appropriate regimen [54–56]. Although the use of piperacillin/tazobactam alone or cefepime is somewhat controversial, none of the β-lactam agents above are clearly preferred except as dictated by local resistance patterns or cost [52,54,56]. Another review provides the evidence from meta-analyses that empiric use of aminoglycosides with broad-spectrum β-lactam agents is not needed [55] (Table 75.4).

For a patient in septic shock who is admitted to the ICU or in institutions with endemic resistant Gram-negative bacteria, a multidrug regimen may be indicated. For patients with immediate hypersensitivity reactions to cephalosporins and penicillins, aztreonam has activity against Gram-negative bacilli and can be used with an antimicrobial agent with activity against a broad spectrum of Gram-positive organisms (e.g., vancomycin typically is added to this regimen because aztreonam has no Gram-positive activity). Because of the increased prevalence of methicillin-resistant staphylococci, recent guidelines have recommended routine initial inclusion of vancomycin in empiric regimens for patients in shock, particularly in patients on antimicrobial prophylaxis and those with evidence of skin or skin structure infections or with inflammation at the site of or dysfunction of indwelling plastic venous access catheters [52]. Randomized controlled trials have demonstrated no benefit to continuing vancomycin after 72 hours unless patients demonstrated a Gram-positive infection [52,57].

Most standard regimens are designed for patients who have not previously received antibiotics. The development of fever with systemic symptoms such as shock or respiratory distress in a patient on antibiotic therapy requires a change in therapy to include organisms that are known to be resistant to classes of antibacterials the patient has received. For example, in a patient who recently has received cephalosporins, the choice of piperacillin/tazobactam or imipenem may be preferable to ceftazidime especially if expanded spectrum β-lactamase–producing organisms are established flora in the local ICU.

After initial evaluation of the patient and initiation of empiric antibiotic therapy, subsequent management is based on (a) identification of a focus of infection, (b) isolation of an etiologic agent, (c) defervescence versus continued fever, and (d) duration of neutropenia. In the patient for whom an infection has been documented clinically or by culture, antibiotics should be continued as appropriate for the site of infection, susceptibility profile of pathogens, and the patient's clinical response. Even when a specific pathogen is identified by culture, in patients who are neutropenic, a broad-spectrum regimen usually is maintained for the duration of neutropenia [38,52,58]. For patients likely to have permanent or extremely prolonged granulocytopenia, attempts to stop therapy are reasonable but should be made with continuing close clinical observation [52,59].

If fever has not been eliminated or the patient continues to have evidence of ongoing sepsis, the search should continue for potential sites of focal infection (skin, optic fundi, oropharynx, chest, abdomen, and perirectal area). The serial, empiric addition of one antibiotic after another without culture data is not efficacious in most settings and may lead to confusion in the event that an adverse reaction occurs [52]. Cephalosporins and vancomycin can cause bone marrow suppression and lead to colonization with resistant organisms. The addition or sequential substitution of multiple cephalosporins may induce β-lactamase production by some organisms.

Persistent or Recurrent Fever without Obvious Source: Neutropenia

Should fevers persist for 4 to 7 days of neutropenia, randomized controlled trials have found that empiric antifungal therapy with an amphotericin B preparation, voriconazole, or an echinocandin [60–62] is appropriate. The rationale for such therapy is that it is difficult to culture fungi before they cause disseminated disease and that the mortality from disseminated fungal disease among neutropenic hosts is high. *Candida* and *Aspergillus* species are common pathogens, and *Fusarium*, *Trichosporon*, and *Bipolaris* species are seen occasionally but are becoming more common [63–66]. The use of the serum assay for galactomannan as a marker for aspergillus infection is controversial because sensitivity is low and there may be false-positive results in patients receiving piperacillin [67,68]. Another serum assay that tests for 1,3 β-D-glucan antigenemia shows promise, but serial monitoring is needed and predictive value for invasive fungal infections varies in different centers [69,70]. More research is needed on both of these assays.

Patients at particularly high risk of disseminated fungal disease include those with (a) prolonged granulocytopenia, (b) parenteral nutrition, (c) *Candida* colonization in oropharynx or urine, (d) corticosteroid therapy, and (e) advancing multiple organ dysfunction (renal, hepatic, pulmonary). Moreover, multiorgan failure often is a reflection of disseminated candidiasis [71]. The use of antifungal prophylaxis with the imidazoles (fluconazole) has caused a shift in the species of *Candida*-causing infection from *C. albicans* and *C. tropicalis* to the more imidazole-resistant *C. krusei* and *C. glabrata* [72], and with the use of posaconazole or voriconazole, a shift has started to occur to more infections because of Zygomycetes [73,74]. Hepatosplenic (also called *chronic disseminated*) candidiasis presents with fevers and elevation of serum alkaline phosphatase that continue through the return of neutrophils to greater than 1,000 cells per mm^3 [75]. Multiple embolic lesions are present in liver and spleen, and prolonged therapy with amphotericin B, itraconazole, fluconazole, or an echinocandin depending on the susceptibility of the organism, is beneficial [76]. Use of biomarkers and direct testing are controversial and not uniformly available [77,78].

Based on the findings from a randomized clinical trial of primary therapy and randomized studies of salvage therapy, voriconazole is the drug of choice for infections caused by *Aspergillus* [79,80]. However, an amphotericin preparation continues to be the drug of choice when a fungal infection is suspected in patients already receiving an azole antifungal [74]. Amphotericin has activity against *Aspergillus*, the zygomycetes, and many other filamentous fungi. According to data from randomized clinical trials, the newer preparations of amphotericin B appear to decrease renal toxicity while maintaining efficacy: therefore, amphotericin B complexed with cholesteryl sulfate, with liposomal vesicles, or with a bilayered lipid membrane has become standard for use in patients on other nephrotoxic drugs or those with impaired renal function, despite their higher cost [81] (see Chapter 73). Prognosis remains poor, however, for patients treated for documented invasive fungal infection in the setting of persistent neutropenia [63,82]. Most ICU patients who remain febrile and neutropenic after 4 to 7 days of broad-spectrum antibacterials should be treated with voriconazole, an amphotericin B preparation or an echinocandin, although in selected low-risk patients (where the risk of Aspergillus or Zygomyces is low), itraconazole or fluconazole is equally efficacious as shown in open randomized clinical trials and endorsed in expert reviews of these studies [62,83–86].

Pneumonia in the Compromised Host

The lung is one of the most common identifiable sites of infection in immunocompromised patients [2,48,87]. Pulmonary disease can be caused by a wide variety of agents, including bacteria, protozoa, helminths, viruses, fungi, and mycobacteria (Table 75.3) (see Chapter 181). The differential diagnosis is made even more difficult by the various noninfectious pulmonary complications that can present abruptly with acute respiratory symptoms and fever. These include underlying malignancy or vasculitis, drug toxicity, interstitial fibrosis, diffuse alveolar hemorrhage, radiation pneumonitis, cardiogenic pulmonary edema, bronchiolitis obliterans organizing pneumonia, pulmonary alveolar proteinosis, and pulmonary embolism [48,87].

Pneumonia in the immunocompromised patient often presents without the symptoms and signs seen in normal hosts. Regardless of cause, fever and progressive shortness of breath (and concomitant tachypnea and arterial hypoxemia) tend to be common symptoms; in the neutropenic patient, cough, sputum production, and physical examination (as well as radiographic) findings are likely to be unimpressive or absent. Chest radiographs should be obtained promptly in the compromised patient with fever or dyspnea. High-resolution CT or MRIs will often reveal infiltrates or masses that cannot be appreciated on conventional X-rays and thus are recommended in cases in which there is question about the diagnosis [88].

TABLE 75.3

Common Causes of Acute Pulmonary Disease in Immunocompromised Patients

Infectious causes
Bacteria
• *Streptococcus pneumoniae*
• *Haemophilus influenzae*
• *Pseudomonas aeruginosa*
• Enteric Gram-negative bacilli
• *Staphylococcus aureus*
• *Legionella* species
• *Nocardia* species
• Mycobacteria
Fungi
• *Aspergillus* species
• *Pneumocystis jiroveci*
• *Candida* species
• *Zygomycetes* species
• *Cryptococcus neoformans*
Viruses
• Cytomegalovirus
• Herpes simplex virus
Protozoa
• *Toxoplasma gondii*
Parasite
• *Strongyloides stercoralis*
Noninfectious causes
Primary disease
Malignancy
Primary
Metastatic
Vasculitis
Drug toxicity
• Bleomycin
• Busulfan
• Cyclophosphamide
Hemorrhage
Congestive heart failure
Radiation

Differential Diagnosis

Developing an appropriate differential diagnosis for the causative agents of pneumonia in the immunocompromised host rests first on an appreciation of the nature, severity, and duration of the immune suppression. In addition to being susceptible to conventional respiratory tract pathogens (*S. pneumoniae*, *H. influenzae*) hospitalized immunocompromised hosts are prone to Gram-negative bacillary pneumonia; those with prolonged (greater than 7 days) or profound (less than 100 neutrophils per μL) neutropenia may become infected with *Aspergillus* or *Zygomycetes* spp [2]. T-cell–deficient hosts (e.g., patients with HIV infection, transplant, or lymphoma) are more likely to acquire PCP [89] or infection with CMV, HSV [90–92], endemic fungi (*Cryptococcus, Histoplasma*) [46,93,94], *Nocardia* spp, or intracellular bacteria (mycobacteria, *Legionella* spp) [95–97]. Patients who have resided in tropical countries may reactivate latent infection by *Strongyloides stercoralis* in the setting of altered cell-mediated immunity. Pulmonary infiltrates, polymicrobial bacteremia, and bacterial meningitis are the hallmarks of this syndrome [98]. Patients with deficient neutrophil and T-cell function (e.g., bone marrow transplant recipients) may be at risk for all of these pathogens.

Chest radiographs may provide useful clues; focal or multifocal infiltrates tend to suggest infections by bacteria or fungi, but are unlikely to provide a definitive diagnosis. CT scanning often provides more information, including the detection of lesions not seen on routine chest radiograph [48]. Diffuse disease is more characteristic of viral causes (HSV, CMV), PCP, or noninfectious processes (drug toxicity, lymphangitic carcinomatosis, and radiation pneumonitis). Cavitary disease can be seen with some of the necrotizing Gram-negative bacilli such as *P. aeruginosa* as well as *S. aureus* and anaerobes (e.g., postaspiration or postobstructive). Cavities also can be a late finding with pneumonia because of *Aspergillus*, *Zygomycetes*, and *Nocardia* spp. It is impossible, however, to make firm rules with regard to radiographic patterns. Gram-negative bacilli or *Legionella* may progress to diffuse disease or incite the acute respiratory distress syndrome. Patients with severe defects in cell-mediated immunity may manifest a miliary pattern caused by disseminated tuberculosis or histoplasmosis. Conversely, radiation pneumonitis may present as focal, sharply demarcated infiltrates confined to the irradiated portion of the lung.

Diagnostic Approach and Empiric Therapy

The diagnostic approach to pulmonary disease in the immunocompromised host also depends on the nature of the immune deficit. As a general rule, all accessible sites (blood, urine, and sputum) should be cultured, although sputum of high quality is obtained rarely in these circumstances. In neutropenic hosts, empiric antibacterial therapy is begun at the outset regardless of radiographic pattern, using one of the regimens discussed previously for fever and neutropenia [37,38]. In the case of ventilated inpatients, treatment of pneumonia must include antibiotic(s) that are effective against organisms that are likely to be present in the ICU (some of these organisms are resistant to antibiotics typically used in treating febrile, neutropenic patients). These regimens typically contain more than one antibiotic and they should be adjusted based on the cumulative susceptibility report of the hospital or unit. Although logical, the use of "protected specimen brushes" has not been shown to be of clear clinical value and should not be a reason to perform an invasive procedure in an immunocompromised patient [99].

TABLE 75.4

Advances in Management Based upon Randomized Controlled Clinical Trials and Meta-Analyses of These Trials

Acute fever without obvious source: Neutropenia
- Broad-spectrum antibiotic therapy should be started for all immunocompromised patients with fever greater than 38°C and absolute neutrophil counts less than 500 per mm^3 (or less than 1,000 per mm^3 and falling) [37,38,52,53]
- There is no benefit to continuing vancomycin after 72 h unless a Gram-positive infection is documented [60–62,76,114–116]
- There is no benefit to adding an aminoglycoside to a β-lactam agent in patients with fever and neutropenia [55]

Persistent fever or recurrent fever with obvious source: Neutropenia
- Empiric antifungal with an amphotericin B preparation, voriconazole, or caspofungin should be started for the immunocompromised patient with neutropenia and fever of 4–7 d duration [60–62,114,115,117]

Treatment of aspergillosis
- Voriconazole is the drug of choice for documented infections because of Aspergillus [79]

Prophylaxis of fungal infections
- In patients undergoing chemotherapy for acute myelogenous leukemia or myelodysplastic syndrome, posaconazole prevented invasive fungal infections more effectively than did either fluconazole or itraconazole and improved overall survival. There were more serious adverse events possibly or probably related to treatment in the posaconazole group [110,118]
- Both fluconazole and itraconazole have shown benefit for prophylaxis in patients after allogeneic stem cell transplant [119]

If a clinical response occurs in a neutropenic patient, therapy is continued until neutropenia resolves. In the setting of persistent neutropenia, a clinical picture of progressive pulmonary disease despite antibiotic therapy suggests invasive disease caused by fungi found in the environment (a variety of "saprophytic" fungi are a major concern: especially *Aspergillus*, but also *Rhizopus*, *Fusarium*, and *Trichosporon* spp) [39,65,66]. Expectorated sputum, bronchial brush specimen cultures, or bronchial lavage fluid may provide presumptive evidence of these pathogens, but prompt definitive diagnosis often requires open or thoracoscopically guided lung biopsy. Transbronchial biopsy is often nondiagnostic. Typically, pneumonia caused by *Aspergillus* or *Zygomycetes* spp causes areas of lung infarction that may be missed by transbronchial biopsy [100,101]. CT scans may show the classic "crescent" sign in patients with aspergillosis, but this is a sign of late disease, and although it may be helpful diagnostically in patients who are recovering, early diagnosis is important to prevent mortality in persistently neutropenic patients. Unlike bacteria, which are usually easy to culture, fungi are often not isolated from cases where histopathology eventually demonstrates their presence. Although PCR-based techniques have yet to be of demonstrated clinical usefulness in these clinical situations, measurements of polysaccharide antigen in serum or other body fluids have been of demonstrated utility for the diagnosis of both *Cryptococcus*- and *Histoplasma*-associated pneumonia.

The standard approach to therapy of confirmed pulmonary disease caused by *Aspergillus* is to treat with voriconazole because this agent has been shown to be superior to treatment with amphotericin B preparations [80,102]. Although the use of combinations of antifungal agents (including echinocandins and azoles as well as echinocandins and amphotericin) has rationale, support from animal data, and anecdotal human experience, large trials have yet to be performed, making it difficult to recommend this approach at this time unless single agents have failed. There is no established therapy for some emerging fungal pathogens such as *Trichosporon* or *Fusarium* spp, although encouraging results have been reported in a few cases using posaconazole, voriconazole, or isavuconazole [102,103].

For patients with compromised T-cell immunity, the list of diagnostic possibilities is longer and more diverse, making a single formula for empiric therapy a virtual impossibility. Clinicians caring for these patients should be guided by both the type of the underlying immunodeficiency and the patient's previous experiences with both pathogens and antimicrobial agents. Expectorated or induced sputum may demonstrate the organism by special stains in a minority of cases (*P. jiroveci*, *M. tuberculosis*, *Nocardia asteroides*), but flexible bronchoscopy with lavage or transbronchial biopsy and open or thoracoscopically assisted lung biopsy may be required in order to make a diagnosis for these patients [48,104,105] (see Chapter 10). Bronchoscopy is particularly helpful for diffuse or interstitial disease, in which it provides not only lavage fluid with reasonable diagnostic accuracy for infectious agents such as *P. jiroveci* and bacteria but pathologic specimens that may allow diagnosis of CMV infection, drug pneumonitis, hemorrhage, or lymphangitic carcinomatosis. In patients with focal or nodular disease, thoracoscopically assisted biopsy is likely to yield the best results.

For the immunocompromised host (non–HIV infected), the diagnosis of PCP often requires bronchoscopy with bronchoalveolar lavage with or without biopsy. A variety of other infections also require biopsy for diagnosis. It is reasonable to treat (empirically) with trimethoprim–sulfamethoxazole (15 per kg of the trimethoprim component IV daily divided every 6 or 8 hours) while arrangements are made for diagnostic procedures, because the organisms persist for the first few days of treatment. It is usually an error to postpone performing bronchoscopy (with biopsy) or thoracoscopically guided lung biopsy for severely ill immunocompromised patients with pulmonary infiltrates in the hope that they will improve, because clinical deterioration may make the procedure (and the diagnosis) impossible. If PCP is confirmed and the patient has severe renal insufficiency, serum drug concentration monitoring, if available, should be used to adjust therapy to obtain a peak serum sulfamethoxazole level of 100 μg per mL or trimethoprim levels of 5 to 8 mg per μL [106]. An alternative diagnosis, established by histologic or microbiologic techniques, allows institution of specific therapy, such as acyclovir for HSV pneumonia; ganciclovir for CMV pneumonia; trimethoprim–sulfamethoxazole for nocardiosis; or corticosteroids for radiation pneumonitis, bronchiolitis obliterans with organizing pneumonia, acute fibrinous and organizing pneumonia, or drug-induced disease [48,104,107,108].

PREVENTION OF INFECTION

Increasing emphasis is being placed on the prevention of opportunistic infections in immunocompromised hosts. These strategies have taken many different forms. Early efforts were directed at modifications of the environment of neutropenic patients through laminar airflow, nonabsorbable antibiotics, and elaborate efforts at disinfecting the inanimate environment. These approaches have proven expensive and laborious, and because they did not affect either disease remission or mortality, they have been abandoned by most centers.

Oral fluoroquinolone (and trimethoprim–sulfamethoxazole) administration has been studied in patients with prolonged neutropenia. These agents reduce levels of aerobic Gram-negative bacilli in the gut lumen, the major reservoir for dissemination of infection in the neutropenic host, and studies document the efficacy of levofloxacin for preventing infections and hospitalizations in patients with chemotherapy-induced neutropenia [109].

Antifungal prophylaxis with oral fluconazole (400 mg orally daily or 200 mg IV every 12 hours) has proved effective in reducing infection by *Candida* spp in bone marrow transplant recipients [81] (see Chapter 64). Recent studies suggest that posaconazole, which has a much broader spectrum than fluconazole (including aspergillus), is efficacious in preventing fungal infections in severely neutropenic patients, hematopoietic stem cell transplant patients, and those with graft versus host disease [110].

Antiviral prophylaxis with acyclovir has been shown to reduce mucositis and mucocutaneous infections by HSV in transplant recipients and in patients with leukemia [111,112]. Although prophylactic administration of ganciclovir has been demonstrated to decrease CMV disease in solid organ transplant recipients, the administration of this agent to bone marrow transplant patients resulted in neutropenia. Consequently, most centers are now using "preemptive" treatment with ganciclovir (beginning treatment only when DNA levels are increased in the serum of patients at risk) (see Chapters 63 and 64).

Administration of granulocyte–colony stimulating factors hastens bone marrow recovery and shortens the duration of neutropenia in some patients receiving chemotherapy. Consensus guidelines suggest that they should be used to support dose-intense chemotherapy and have little impact on mortality in patients with existing neutropenia and fever and should not be used as a routine adjunct to antimicrobials [113].

References

1. Bodey GP, Bolivar R, Fainstein V: Infectious complications in leukemic patients. *Semin Hematol* 19:193, 1982.
2. Winston DJ, Emmanouilides C, Busuttil RW: Infections in liver transplant recipients. *Clin Infect Dis* 21:1077, 1995.
3. Fishman JA: Infection in solid-organ transplant recipients. *N Engl J Med* 357:2601, 2007.
4. Tolsma V, Schwebel C, Azoulay E, et al: Sepsis severe or septic shock: outcome according to immune status and immunodeficiency profile. *Chest* 146:1205, 2014.
5. Warris A, Bjorneklett A, Gaustad P: Invasive pulmonary aspergillosis associated with infliximab therapy. *N Engl J Med* 344:1099, 2001.
6. Keane J, Gershon S, Wise RP, et al: Tuberculosis associated with infliximab, a tumor necrosis factor alpha-neutralizing agent. *N Engl J Med* 345:1098, 2001.
7. Crum NF, Lederman ER, Wallace MR: Infections associated with tumor necrosis factor-alpha antagonists. *Medicine (Baltimore)* 84:291, 2005.
8. Notter DT, Grossman PL, Rosenberg SA, et al: Infections in patients with Hodgkin's disease: a clinical study of 300 consecutive adult patients. *Rev Infect Dis* 2:761, 1980.
9. Zander DS, Baz MA, Visner GA, et al: Analysis of early deaths after isolated lung transplantation. *Chest* 120:225, 2001.
10. Jurado M, Deeg HJ, Storer B, et al: Hematopoietic stem cell transplantation for advanced myelodysplastic syndrome after conditioning with busulfan and fractionated total body irradiation is associated with low relapse rate but considerable nonrelapse mortality. *Biol Blood Marrow Transplant* 8:161, 2002.
11. Kobayashi K, Kami M, Murashige N, et al: Outcomes of patients with acute leukaemia who relapsed after reduced-intensity stem cell transplantation from HLA-identical or one antigen-mismatched related donors. *Br J Haematol* 129:795, 2005.
12. Yoo JH, Choi SM, Lee DG, et al: Prognostic factors influencing infection-related mortality in patients with acute leukemia in Korea. *J Korean Med Sci* 20:31, 2005.
13. Gratwohl A, Brand R, Frassoni F, et al: Cause of death after allogeneic haematopoietic stem cell transplantation (HSCT) in early leukaemias: an EBMT analysis of lethal infectious complications and changes over calendar time. *Bone Marrow Transplant* 36:757, 2005.
14. Pene F, Aubron C, Azoulay E, et al: Outcome of critically Ill allogeneic hematopoietic stem-cell transplantation recipients: a reappraisal of indications for organ failure supports. *J Clin Oncol* 24:643, 2006.
15. Azoulay E, Thiery G, Chevret S, et al: The prognosis of acute respiratory failure in critically ill cancer patients. *Medicine (Baltimore)* 83:360, 2004.
16. Huynh TN, Weigt SS, Belperio JA, et al: Outcome and prognostic indicators of patients with hematopoietic stem cell transplants admitted to the intensive care unit. *J Transplant* 2009:917294, 2009.
17. Nishida K, Palalay MP: Prognostic factors and utility of scoring systems in patients with hematological malignancies admitted to the intensive care unit and required a mechanical ventilator. *Hawaii Med J* 67:264, 2008.
18. Thiery G, Azoulay E, Darmon M, et al: Outcome of cancer patients considered for intensive care unit admission: a hospital-wide prospective study. *J Clin Oncol* 23:4406, 2005.
19. Reuter S, Kern WV, Sigge A, et al: Impact of fluoroquinolone prophylaxis on reduced infection-related mortality among patients with neutropenia and hematologic malignancies. *Clin Infect Dis* 40:1087, 2005.
20. Paul M, Gafter-Gvili A, Leibovici L, et al: The epidemiology of bacteremia with febrile neutropenia: experience from a single center, 1988-2004. *Isr Med Assoc J* 9:424, 2007.
21. Ramphal R. Changes in the etiology of bacteremia in febrile neutropenic patients and the susceptibilities of the currently isolated pathogens. *Clin Infect Dis* 39[Suppl 1]:S25, 2004.
22. Wisplinghoff H, Seifert H, Wenzel RP, et al: Current trends in the epidemiology of nosocomial bloodstream infections in patients with hematological malignancies and solid neoplasms in hospitals in the United States. *Clin Infect Dis* 36:1103, 2003.
23. Avery R, Kalaycio M, Pohlman B, et al: Early vancomycin-resistant enterococcus (VRE) bacteremia after allogeneic bone marrow transplantation is associated with a rapidly deteriorating clinical course. *Bone Marrow Transplant* 35:497, 2005.
24. Zinner SH: Fluoroquinolone prophylaxis in patients with neutropenia. *Clin Infect Dis* 40:1094, 2005.
25. Gudiol C, Bodro M, Simonetti A, et al: Changing aetiology, clinical features, antimicrobial resistance, and outcomes of bloodstream infection in neutropenic cancer patients. *Clin Microbiol Infect* 19:474, 2013.
26. Fatkenheuer G, Buchheidt D, Cornely OA, et al: Central venous catheter (CVC)-related infections in neutropenic patients--guidelines of the Infectious Diseases Working Party (AGIHO) of the German Society of Hematology and Oncology (DGHO). *Ann Hematol* 82[Suppl 2]:S149, 2003.
27. Sepkowitz KA: Treatment of patients with hematologic neoplasm, fever, and neutropenia. *Clin Infect Dis* 40[Suppl 4]:S253, 2005.
28. Cheong K, Perry D, Karapetis C, et al: High rate of complications associated with peripherally inserted central venous catheters in patients with solid tumours. *Intern Med J* 34:234, 2004.
29. Mermel LA, Allon M, Bouza E, et al: Clinical practice guidelines for the diagnosis and management of intravascular catheter-related infection: 2009 Update by the Infectious Diseases Society of America. *Clin Infect Dis* 49:1, 2009.
30. Maschmeyer G, Haas A: The epidemiology and treatment of infections in cancer patients. *Int J Antimicrob Agents* 31:193, 2008.
31. Sandherr M, Einsele H, Hebart H, et al: Antiviral prophylaxis in patients with haematological malignancies and solid tumours: guidelines of the Infectious Diseases Working Party (AGIHO) of the German Society for Hematology and Oncology (DGHO). *Ann Oncol* 17(7):1051–1059, 2006.
32. Yolken RH, Bishop CA, Townsend TR, et al: Infectious gastroenteritis in bone-marrow-transplant recipients. *N Engl J Med* 306:1010, 1982.
33. Pizzo PA: Fever in immunocompromised patients. *N Engl J Med* 341:893, 1999.
34. Herget GW, Riede UN, Schmitt-Graff A, et al: Generalized herpes simplex virus infection in an immunocompromised patient--report of a case and review of the literature. *Pathol Res Pract* 201:123, 2005.
35. Hirsch HH, Randhawa P: BK virus in solid organ transplant recipients. *Am J Transplant* 9[Suppl 4]:S136, 2009.
36. Drachenberg CB, Hirsch HH, Papadimitriou JC, et al: Polyomavirus BK versus JC replication and nephropathy in renal transplant recipients: a prospective evaluation. *Transplantation* 84:323, 2007.
37. Pizzo PA: Management of fever in patients with cancer and treatment-induced neutropenia. *N Engl J Med* 328:1323, 1993.
38. Hughes WT, Armstrong D, Bodey GP, et al: 2002 guidelines for the use of antimicrobial agents in neutropenic patients with cancer. *Clin Infect Dis* 34:730, 2002.
39. Husain S, Munoz P, Forrest G, et al: Infections due to Scedosporium apiospermum and Scedosporium prolificans in transplant recipients: clinical characteristics and impact of antifungal agent therapy on outcome. *Clin Infect Dis* 40:89, 2005.
40. Park BJ, Pappas PG, Wannemuehler KA, et al: Invasive non-aspergillus mold infections in transplant recipients, United States, 2001-2006. *Emerg Infect Dis* 17:1855, 2011.
41. Walsh TJ, Groll A, Hiemenz J, et al: Infections due to emerging and uncommon medically important fungal pathogens. *Clin Microbiol Infect* 10[Suppl 1]:48, 2004.
42. Fisher RI, DeVita VT Jr, Bostick F, et al: Persistent immunologic abnormalities in long-term survivors of advanced Hodgkin's disease. *Ann Intern Med* 92:595, 1980.
43. Hellmann DB, Petri M, Whiting-O'Keefe Q: Fatal infections in systemic lupus erythematosus: the role of opportunistic organisms. *Medicine (Baltimore)* 66:341, 1987.

44. Patel R, Roberts GD, Keating MR, et al: Infections due to nontuberculous mycobacteria in kidney, heart, and liver transplant recipients. *Clin Infect Dis* 19:263, 1994.
45. Giles JT, Bathon JM: Serious infections associated with anticytokine therapies in the rheumatic diseases. *J Intensive Care Med* 19:320, 2004.
46. Wood KL, Hage CA, Knox KS, et al: Histoplasmosis after treatment with anti-tumor necrosis factor-alpha therapy. *Am J Respir Crit Care Med* 167:1279, 2003.
47. Murdaca G, Spano F, Contatore M, et al: Infection risk associated with anti-TNF-alpha agents: a review. *Expert Opin Drug Saf* 14:571, 2015.
48. Shorr AF, Susla GM, O'Grady NP: Pulmonary infiltrates in the non-HIV-infected immunocompromised patient: etiologies, diagnostic strategies, and outcomes. *Chest* 125:260, 2004.
49. Fagon JY, Chastre J, Wolff M, et al: Invasive and noninvasive strategies for management of suspected ventilator-associated pneumonia. A randomized trial. *Ann Intern Med* 132:621, 2000.
50. Klastersky J, Ameye L, Maertens J, et al: Bacteraemia in febrile neutropenic cancer patients. *Int J Antimicrob Agents* 30[Suppl 1]:S51, 2007.
51. Zinner SH: New pathogens in neutropenic patients with cancer: an update for the new millennium. *Int J Antimicrob Agents* 16:97, 2000.
52. Baden LR, Bensinger W, Angarone M, et al: Prevention and treatment of cancer-related infections Version 2.2015, NCCN Clinical Practice Guidelines in Oncology. *Natl Compr Canc Netw*, 2015.
53. Pizzo PA, Hathorn JW, Hiemenz J, et al: A randomized trial comparing ceftazidime alone with combination antibiotic therapy in cancer patients with fever and neutropenia. *N Engl J Med* 315:552, 1986.
54. Paul M, Yahav D, Fraser A, et al: Empirical antibiotic monotherapy for febrile neutropenia: systematic review and meta-analysis of randomized controlled trials. *J Antimicrob Chemother* 57:176, 2006.
55. Paul M, Grozinsky-Glasberg S, Soares-Weiser K, et al: Beta-lactam versus beta-lactam-aminoglycoside combination therapy in cancer patients with neutropenia. *Cochrane Database Syst Rev*, 2010.
56. Pereira CA, Petrilli AS, Carlesse FA, et al: Cefepime monotherapy is as effective as ceftriaxone plus amikacin in pediatric patients with cancer and high-risk febrile neutropenia in a randomized comparison. *J Microbiol Immunol Infect* 42:141, 2009.
57. Wade JC, Glasmacher A: Vancomycin does not benefit persistently febrile neutropenic people with cancer. *Cancer Treat Rev* 30:119, 2004.
58. Pizzo PA, Robichaud KJ, Gill FA, et al: Duration of empiric antibiotic therapy in granulocytopenic patients with cancer. *Am J Med* 67:194, 1979.
59. DiNubile MJ: Stopping antibiotic therapy in neutropenic patients. *Ann Intern Med* 108:289, 1988.
60. Pizzo PA, Robichaud KJ, Gill FA, et al: Empiric antibiotic and antifungal therapy for cancer patients with prolonged fever and granulocytopenia. *Am J Med* 72:101, 1982.
61. Walsh TJ, Pappas P, Winston DJ, et al: Voriconazole compared with liposomal amphotericin B for empirical antifungal therapy in patients with neutropenia and persistent fever. *N Engl J Med* 346:225, 2002.
62. Martino R, Viscoli C: Empirical antifungal therapy in patients with neutropenia and persistent or recurrent fever of unknown origin. *Br J Haematol* 132:138, 2006.
63. Shaukat A, Bakri F, Young P, et al: Invasive filamentous fungal infections in allogeneic hematopoietic stem cell transplant recipients after recovery from neutropenia: clinical, radiologic, and pathologic characteristics. *Mycopathologia* 159:181, 2005.
64. Pagano L, Offidani M, Fianchi L, et al: Mucormycosis in hematologic patients. *Haematologica* 89:207, 2004.
65. Husain S, Alexander BD, Munoz P, et al: Opportunistic mycelial fungal infections in organ transplant recipients: emerging importance of non-Aspergillus mycelial fungi. *Clin Infect Dis* 37:221, 2003.
66. Singh N: Trends in the epidemiology of opportunistic fungal infections: predisposing factors and the impact of antimicrobial use practices. *Clin Infect Dis* 33:1692, 2001.
67. Weisser M, Rausch C, Droll A, et al: Galactomannan does not precede major signs on a pulmonary computerized tomographic scan suggestive of invasive aspergillosis in patients with hematological malignancies. *Clin Infect Dis* 41:1143, 2005.
68. Marr KA, Laverdiere M, Gugel A, et al: Antifungal therapy decreases sensitivity of the Aspergillus galactomannan enzyme immunoassay. *Clin Infect Dis* 40:1762, 2005.
69. Ellis M, Al-Ramadi B, Finkelman M, et al: Assessment of the clinical utility of serial beta-D-glucan concentrations in patients with persistent neutropenic fever. *J Med Microbiol* 57:287, 2008.
70. Senn L, Robinson JO, Schmidt S, et al: 1,3-Beta-D-glucan antigenemia for early diagnosis of invasive fungal infections in neutropenic patients with acute leukemia. *Clin Infect Dis* 46:878, 2008.
71. Maksymiuk AW, Thongprasert S, Hopfer R, et al: Systemic candidiasis in cancer patients. *Am J Med* 77:20, 1984.
72. Rex JH, Pappas PG, Karchmer AW, et al: A randomized and blinded multicenter trial of high-dose fluconazole plus placebo versus fluconazole plus amphotericin B as therapy for candidemia and its consequences in nonneutropenic subjects. *Clin Infect Dis* 36:1221, 2003.
73. Smith WJ, Drew RH, Perfect JR: Posaconazole's impact on prophylaxis and treatment of invasive fungal infections: an update. *Expert Rev Anti Infect Ther* 7:165, 2009.
74. Chamilos G, Marom EM, Lewis RE, et al: Predictors of pulmonary zygomycosis versus invasive pulmonary aspergillosis in patients with cancer. *Clin Infect Dis* 41:60, 2005.
75. Thaler M, Pastakia B, Shawker TH, et al: Hepatic candidiasis in cancer patients: the evolving picture of the syndrome. *Ann Intern Med* 108:88, 1988.
76. Pappas PG, Kauffman CA, Andes D, et al: Clinical practice guidelines for the management of candidiasis: 2009 update by the Infectious Diseases Society of America. *Clin Infect Dis* 48:503, 2009.
77. Martin-Mazuelos E, Loza A, Castro C, et al: Beta-D-Glucan and Candida albicans germ tube antibody in ICU patients with invasive candidiasis. *Intensive Care Med* 41:1424, 2015.
78. Idelevich EA, Grunewald CM, Wullenweber J, et al: Rapid identification and susceptibility testing of Candida spp. from positive blood cultures by combination of direct MALDI-TOF mass spectrometry and direct inoculation of Vitek 2. *PLoS One* 9:e114834, 2014.
79. Herbrecht R, Denning DW, Patterson TF, et al: Voriconazole versus amphotericin B for primary therapy of invasive aspergillosis. *N Engl J Med* 347:408, 2002.
80. Walsh TJ, Anaissie EJ, Denning DW, et al: Treatment of aspergillosis: clinical practice guidelines of the Infectious Diseases Society of America. *Clin Infect Dis* 46:327, 2008.
81. Herbrecht R, Natarajan-Ame S, Nivoix Y, et al: The lipid formulations of amphotericin B. *Expert Opin Pharmacother* 4:1277, 2003.
82. Cordonnier C, Ribaud P, Herbrecht R, et al: Prognostic factors for death due to invasive aspergillosis after hematopoietic stem cell transplantation: a 1-year retrospective study of consecutive patients at French transplantation centers. *Clin Infect Dis* 42:955, 2006.
83. Winston DJ, Hathorn JW, Schuster MG, et al: A multicenter, randomized trial of fluconazole versus amphotericin B for empiric antifungal therapy of febrile neutropenic patients with cancer. *Am J Med* 108:282, 2000.
84. Boogaerts M, Winston DJ, Bow EJ, et al: Intravenous and oral itraconazole versus intravenous amphotericin B deoxycholate as empirical antifungal therapy for persistent fever in neutropenic patients with cancer who are receiving broad-spectrum antibacterial therapy. A randomized, controlled trial. *Ann Intern Med* 135:412, 2001.
85. Bennett JE, Powers J, Walsh T, et al: Forum report: issues in clinical trials of empirical antifungal therapy in treating febrile neutropenic patients. *Clin Infect Dis* 36:S117, 2003.
86. Perfect JR: Management of invasive mycoses in hematology patients: current approaches. *Oncology (Williston Park)* 18:5, 2004.
87. Sharma S, Nadrous HF, Peters SG, et al: Pulmonary complications in adult blood and marrow transplant recipients: autopsy findings. *Chest* 128:1385, 2005.
88. Franquet T: High-resolution computed tomography (HRCT) of lung infections in non-AIDS immunocompromised patients. *Eur Radiol* 16:707, 2006.
89. Sepkowitz KA, Brown AE, Telzak EE, et al: Pneumocystis carinii pneumonia among patients without AIDS at a cancer hospital. *JAMA* 267:832, 1992.
90. Sia IG, Patel R: New strategies for prevention and therapy of cytomegalovirus infection and disease in solid-organ transplant recipients. *Clin Microbiol Rev* 13:83, 2000.
91. Graham BS, Snell JD Jr: Herpes simplex virus infection of the adult lower respiratory tract. *Medicine (Baltimore)* 62:384, 1983.
92. Ramsey PG, Rubin RH, Tolkoff-Rubin NE, et al: The renal transplant patient with fever and pulmonary infiltrates: etiology, clinical manifestations, and management. *Medicine (Baltimore)* 59:206, 1980.
93. Wheat LJ: Diagnosis and management of histoplasmosis. *Eur J Clin Microbiol Infect Dis* 8:480, 1989.
94. Chang WC, Tzao C, Hsu HH, et al: Pulmonary cryptococcosis: comparison of clinical and radiographic characteristics in immunocompetent and immunocompromised patients. *Chest* 129:333, 2006.
95. Wiesmayr S, Stelzmueller I, Tabarelli W, et al: Nocardiosis following solid organ transplantation: a single-centre experience. *Transpl Int* 18:1048, 2005.
96. Alp E, Yildiz O, Aygen B, et al: Disseminated nocardiosis due to unusual species: Two case reports. *Scand J Infect Dis* 38:545, 2006.
97. O'Reilly KM, Urban MA, Barriero T, et al: Persistent culture-positive Legionella infection in an immunocompromised host. *Clin Infect Dis* 40:e87, 2005.
98. Nucci M, Portugal R, Pulcheri W, et al: Strongyloidiasis in patients with hematologic malignancies. *Clin Infect Dis* 21:675, 1995.
99. Fujitani S, Yu VL: Diagnosis of ventilator-associated pneumonia: focus on nonbronchoscopic techniques (nonbronchoscopic bronchoalveolar lavage, including mini-BAL, blinded protected specimen brush, and blinded bronchial sampling) and endotracheal aspirates. *J Intensive Care Med* 21:17, 2006.
100. Shelhamer JH, Toews GB, Masur H, et al: NIH conference. Respiratory disease in the immunosuppressed patient. *Ann Intern Med* 117:415, 1992.
101. Rosenow EC 3rd, Wilson WR, Cockerill FR 3rd: Pulmonary disease in the immunocompromised host. 1. *Mayo Clin Proc* 60:473, 1985.
102. Pfaller MA, Messer SA, Hollis RJ, et al: Antifungal activities of posaconazole, ravuconazole, and voriconazole compared to those of itraconazole and amphotericin B against 239 clinical isolates of Aspergillus spp. and other filamentous fungi: report from SENTRY Antimicrobial Surveillance Program, 2000. *Antimicrob Agents Chemother* 46:1032, 2002.
103. Maertens JA, Raad II, Marr KA, et al: Isavuconazole versus voriconazole for primary treatment of invasive mould disease caused by Aspergillus and other filamentous fungi (SECURE): a phase 3, randomised-controlled, non-inferiority trial. *Lancet* 387(10020):760–769, 2015.
104. Maschmeyer G, Beinert T, Buchheidt D, et al: Diagnosis and antimicrobial therapy of pulmonary infiltrates in febrile neutropenic patients--guidelines of the Infectious Diseases Working Party (AGIHO) of the German Society of Hematology and Oncology (DGHO). *Ann Hematol* 82[Suppl 2]:S118, 2003.

105. Patel NR, Lee P-S, Kim JH, et al: The influence of diagnostic bronchoscopy on clinical outcomes comparing adult autologous and allogeneic bone marrow transplant patients. *Chest* 127:1388, 2005.
106. Sattler FR, Cowan R, Nielsen DM, et al: Trimethoprim-sulfamethoxazole compared with pentamidine for treatment of Pneumocystis carinii pneumonia in the acquired immunodeficiency syndrome: a prospective, noncrossover study. *Ann Intern Med* 109:280, 1988.
107. Bhatti S, Hakeem A, Torrealba J, et al: Severe acute fibrinous and organizing pneumonia (AFOP) causing ventilatory failure: successful treatment with mycophenolate mofetil and corticosteroids. *Respir Med* 103:1764, 2009.
108. Peikert T, Rana S, Edell ES: Safety, diagnostic yield, and therapeutic implications of flexible bronchoscopy in patients with febrile neutropenia and pulmonary infiltrates. *Mayo Clin Proc* 80:1414, 2005.
109. Bucaneve G, Micozzi A, Menichetti F, et al: Levofloxacin to prevent bacterial infection in patients with cancer and neutropenia. *N Engl J Med* 353:977, 2005.
110. Cornely OA, Maertens J, Winston DJ, et al: Posaconazole vs. fluconazole or itraconazole prophylaxis in patients with neutropenia. *N Engl J Med* 356:348, 2007.
111. Seale L, Jones CJ, Kathpalia S, et al: Prevention of herpesvirus infections in renal allograft recipients by low-dose oral acyclovir. *JAMA* 254:3435, 1985.
112. Wade JC, Newton B, Flournoy N, et al: Oral acyclovir for prevention of herpes simplex virus reactivation after marrow transplantation. *Ann Intern Med* 100:823, 1984.
113. Aapro MS, Cameron DA, Pettengell R, et al: EORTC guidelines for the use of granulocyte-colony stimulating factor to reduce the incidence of chemotherapy-induced febrile neutropenia in adult patients with lymphomas and solid tumours. *Eur J Cancer* 42:2433, 2006.
114. Walsh TJ, Finberg RW, Arndt C, et al: Liposomal amphotericin B for empirical therapy in patients with persistent fever and neutropenia. National Institute of Allergy and Infectious Diseases Mycoses Study Group. *N Engl J Med* 340:764, 1999.
115. Wingard JR: Empirical antifungal therapy in treating febrile neutropenic patients. *Clin Infect Dis* 39[Suppl 1]:S38, 2004.
116. Paul M, Borok S, Fraser A, et al: Empirical antibiotics against Gram-positive infections for febrile neutropenia: systematic review and meta-analysis of randomized controlled trials. *J Antimicrob Chemother* 55:436, 2005.
117. Walsh TJ, Teppler H, Donowitz GR, et al: Caspofungin versus liposomal amphotericin B for empirical antifungal therapy in patients with persistent fever and neutropenia. *N Engl J Med* 351:1391, 2004.
118. Winston DJ, Cornely OA, Maertens J, et al: A multicenter, randomized trial of posaconazole versus fluconazole or intraconazole for prophylaxis of invasive fungal infections in neutropenic patients with acute myelogenous leukemia or myelodysplastic syndrome receiving intensive chemotherapy. *Biol Blood Marrow Transplant* 12[Suppl]:141, 2006.
119. Glasmacher A, Prentice AG: Evidence-based review of antifungal prophylaxis in neutropenic patients with haematological malignancies. *J Antimicrob Chemother* 56[Suppl 1]:i23, 2005.

Chapter 76 ■ Intensive Care of Patients with HIV Infection

THOMAS C. GREENOUGH • SARAH H. CHEESEMAN • MARK J. ROSEN

At the start of the pandemic in the 1980s, AIDS was considered to be rapidly fatal in almost all cases, and the benefits of aggressive interventions, including treatment in the intensive care unit (ICU), were questioned for patients with advanced disease. Respiratory failure because of *Pneumocystis jirovecii* pneumonia (PCP) was by far the most common disorder that prompted ICU admission, outcomes were uniformly dismal, and ICU admission was often discouraged by clinicians and declined by patients. HIV-infected persons who now have access to effective combination antiretroviral therapy (ART) enjoy much better outcomes. The use of these drugs became the standard of care in 1996, and as a result U.S. mortality rates declined dramatically. For people with HIV infection, mortality reached a peak of around 50,000 per year in 1995, and declined rapidly in the era of effective ART. More recently, death rates have shown a more gradual decline, and were estimated at around 14,000 in 2012 [1]. The improved prognosis in the United States and the developed nations is hampered by limitations to diagnosis and care. In 2011, it was estimated that roughly 25% of HIV-infected individuals in the United States were on treatment with ART and have an undetectable viral load. In this analysis, upward of 20% of people with HIV infection in the United States were undiagnosed [2]. Moreover, improvements of care and survival observed among developed nations still stand in sharp contrast to the global epidemic. In 2014 an estimated 2.0 million people acquired HIV infection, and 1.2 million died [3]. Despite these grim statistics, dramatically scaled-up access to combination ART is now reducing HIV-related mortality and HIV transmission worldwide. Worldwide, an estimated 15 million of the 36.9 million people living with HIV had access to ART as of March 2015 [3].

With the use of effective ART, the spectrum of critical illness related to HIV infection is changing, along with the short- and long-term prognosis for these illnesses. Increasingly, infected individuals who are receiving effective ART have critical illnesses more related to their age than their HIV infection. For some illness such as cardiovascular disease, the risk may be elevated by HIV or its treatment [4]. The use of antiretrovirals entails risk of drug interactions and toxicity, requiring vigilance in the multidrug complexity of ICU care.

REASONS FOR INTENSIVE CARE UNIT ADMISSION

The literature on the frequency and reasons for ICU admission in patients with HIV infection must be interpreted with the understanding that with rare exception, each study reviews the experience of a single center and reflects local ICU admission criteria and practice patterns. Care of patients with HIV infection and with critical illness in general may vary widely, so the conclusions from these reports cannot be generalized [5]. The decision on whether to admit HIV-infected patients to the ICU or withhold such treatment varies by hospital characteristics (county/state, Veterans Affairs Medical Centers, church affiliated, voluntary, and for profit) and geographic location, and these differences are maintained after controlling for severity of illness and patient demographic and socioeconomic characteristics. Thus, data on diseases and outcomes from one center cannot be applied reliably to others. Endemic fungi and other pathogens influence ICU admission rates for different diseases; this is important in the United States, where regional differences in HIV/AIDS incidence and prevalence are notable, and may shift over time [1].

Nevertheless, there is evidence that the reasons for ICU admission have changed over the last three decades of the AIDS epidemic, largely because of reduced incidence of opportunistic infections owing to ART. In the era before ART, an estimated 5% to 10% of hospitalizations of patients with HIV infection involved an ICU admission; most patients were admitted for respiratory failure, and PCP was the most common diagnosis

[6–8]. Although PCP has always been the most common cause of respiratory failure in patients with HIV infection, it appears that ICU admissions for PCP, and for respiratory failure in general, continue to decline [9,10]. The few studies of intensive care in the era of ART suggest that overall ICU utilization by HIV-infected persons has not declined; respiratory failure is still the most common reason for admission, but its relative frequency is declining as other organ failures are increasing [10]. Patients are also less likely to be admitted for PCP and other HIV-associated opportunistic infections, and are now more likely to have life-threatening bacterial pneumonia, sepsis, neurologic disorders, and complications of end-stage liver disease [9–14]. Patients may also become critically ill from the toxic effects of antiretroviral medications, or drug interactions, or from an accelerated inflammatory response related to immune reconstitution resulting from the use of ART [15–17].

PULMONARY DISORDERS

Pneumocystis Pneumonia

Pneumonia caused by *Pneumocystis jirovecii* (formerly classified as *Pneumocystis carinii* f. sp. *hominis*) has always been a major cause of illness and death in patients with HIV infection. Once thought to be a parasite, genomic analysis revealed that *P. jirovecii* is in fact a fungus that is species specific and infects only humans [18]. Although the taxonomy of this pathogen has changed, the term PCP is still acceptable shorthand for *Pneumocystis* pneumonia.

Despite immune restoration from ART and effective specific chemoprophylaxis for PCP, this infection still occurs for several reasons: many patients do not know that they have HIV infection until disease advances to a stage where they develop an opportunistic infection; others know that they have HIV but are not receiving medical care; and still others are in care but are either not prescribed or choose not to take prophylaxis or ART [2,19]. Although newer combinations of ART are coformulated and less likely to cause adverse effects, suboptimal adherence leads to selection of HIV mutations that confer drug resistance, and adherence to complex "salvage" regimens with difficult-to-tolerate side effects is often problematic. Some patients take prophylaxis for PCP, but are still so profoundly immunocompromised that it is ineffective [20]. Nevertheless, the incidence of PCP has declined in the era of ART [21].

PCP should be suspected for a patient with known or suspected HIV infection, fever, and progressive cough and dyspnea. Radiographically, the diagnosis is strongly suggested by perihilar or diffuse ground glass opacities, but this pattern is not specific for PCP. Other radiographic findings include pneumatoceles, pneumothorax, nodules, lobar consolidation, and normal images [22]. The diagnosis can be confirmed only by identifying the organism in specimens obtained from the respiratory tract, either in sputum induced by inhalation of hypertonic saline or by bronchoscopy. Although establishing a diagnosis is not difficult, many clinicians treat patients with suspected PCP empirically, reserving bronchoscopy for patients who do not respond to treatment. A decision-analysis model and a retrospective study comparing these two strategies suggest that the outcomes are similar, but no clinical trial has ever evaluated whether initial empiric therapy or a more aggressive diagnostic strategy that includes bronchoscopy is preferable [23,24]. Among intubated patients, the diagnosis may be established easily with bronchoalveolar lavage. A test that has gained acceptance as an indicator of PCP is the plasma β-D-glucan (BDG) assay. When high values are observed in the context of typical radiographic findings, fever, cough, and respiratory failure in a patient with AIDS, the positive predictive value for PCP is high (negative predictive values are high when BDG levels are low in this context) [25]. It is important to emphasize that this is not a specific test, and other fungal pathogens may present similarly with high BDG and respiratory failure.

The treatment of moderate to severe PCP is outlined in Table 76.1 [26]. Trimethoprim–sulfamethoxazole (TMP-SMX) is the preferred treatment for PCP in patients who have not had an adverse reaction to this drug [26]. Many physicians are willing to use TMP-SMX despite a history of a prior adverse reaction in patients receiving adjunctive corticosteroid therapy and ICU support, because it is not clear whether any of the alternatives is as effective for moderate-to-severe disease. Patients with severe PCP who do not respond, or who are intolerant of this medication

TABLE 76.1

Treatment of Moderate-to-Severe *Pneumocystis* Pneumonia ($PaO_2 < 70$ mm Hg at room air, or A-a O_2 gradient ≥ 35 mm Hg)

Drug	Dose	Comments
Preferred:		
Trimethoprim–sulfamethoxazole	15–20 mg/kg/d TMP plus 75–100 mg/kg/d SMX IV or PO in 3 or 4 divided doses	Drug of choice, but toxicity (rash, fever, nausea, leukopenia) is frequent
Alternate:		
Pentamidine isethionate	4 mg/kg IV daily, infused over at least 60 min; may reduce to 3 mg/kg IV daily for toxicities	Toxicity: dysglycemia, renal failure, QT interval prolongation, arrhythmias, pancreatitis, hypotension; 50% dextrose must be available
Clindamycin plus primaquine	Clindamycin 600–900 mg q6–8 h IV or PO plus 30 mg primaquine base *qd* (15 mg primaquine base = 26.3 mg primaquine phosphate)	Screen for glucose-6-phosphate dehydrogenase deficiency
Adjunctive Therapy:		
Prednisone	40 mg PO *bid* days 1–5, 20 mg PO *bid* or 40 mg PO daily, days 6–10 20 mg PO daily, days 11–21 (IV methylprednisolone can be given as 75% of prednisone dose)	Recommended as early as possible and within 72 h of initiation of PCP therapy, for moderate to severe disease

IV, intravenous; PO, by mouth; SMX, sulfamethoxazole; TMP, trimethoprim.

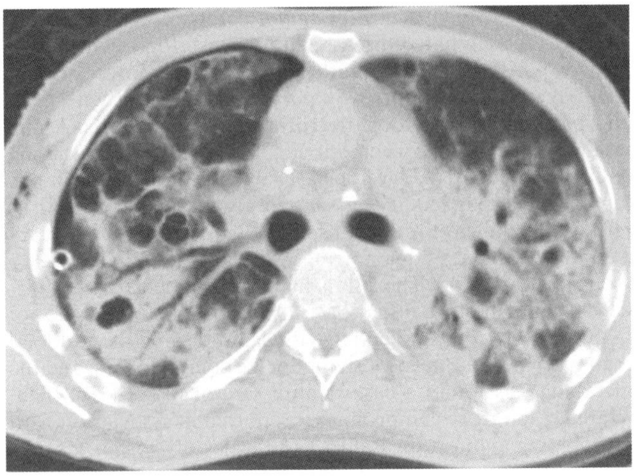

FIGURE 76.1 Selected computerized tomographic image of a patient with severe *Pneumocystis* pneumonia. This patient has significant cystic changes, as well as areas of dense pulmonary consolidation. Note the pneumothorax and chest tube in the right lung.

are usually given pentamidine, but this drug is associated with adverse reactions that are more serious than those associated with TMP-SMX. Clindamycin with primaquine is effective for moderate-to-severe PCP, but primaquine cannot be administered parenterally, potentially limiting its use.

When treatment of PCP is delayed or ineffective, patients may develop hypoxemic respiratory failure. The clinical and radiographic features of severe PCP resemble the acute respiratory distress syndrome (ARDS), with hypoxemia, intrapulmonary shunting, reduced pulmonary compliance, and diffuse radiographic opacities [27]. As the disease progresses and pulmonary compliance diminishes, pneumothorax is common and is associated with a particularly poor prognosis [28,29] (Fig. 76.1). Just as severe PCP resembles ARDS clinically, the supportive treatment is similar, including intubation, mechanical ventilation, application of positive end-expiratory pressure, and lung-protective ventilation strategies [30].

Animal models of PCP indicate that the clinical severity of infection correlates more closely with markers of inflammation than with the organism burden, suggesting that the immune response and its attendant inflammation account for the clinical manifestations of pneumonia [31]. Respiratory compromise is believed to be mediated by activated $CD8^+$ cells and neutrophils in the lung in response to killed organisms, and patients with PCP typically have deterioration of gas exchange during the first few days of treatment with anti-*Pneumocystis* agents alone [32]. When corticosteroids (administered as a taper described in Table 76.1) are administered to patients with moderate-to-severe PCP (defined as a PaO_2 less than 70 mm Hg while breathing room air or an arterial-alveolar oxygen difference greater than or equal to 35 mm Hg) at the start of anti-*Pneumocystis* treatment, there is a reduced likelihood of respiratory failure, deterioration of oxygenation, and death [33,34]. Corticosteroids may attenuate lung injury caused by the inflammatory response to killed organisms, allowing the patient to survive to receive more antimicrobial therapy. Corticosteroids offer no benefit for patients with less severe abnormalities in gas exchange at the start of therapy, or in whom they are administered more than 72 hours after anti-*Pneumocystis* treatment has begun.

Other Pulmonary Disorders

A wide variety of infectious and noninfectious HIV-associated pulmonary disorders may lead to respiratory failure. Bacterial pneumonias, most commonly caused by *Streptococcus pneumoniae*, have probably surpassed PCP as the cause of respiratory failure in the era of ART [35–37]. In patients with severe immune compromise, pulmonary infection or disseminated disease with *Pseudomonas aeruginosa*, *Mycobacterium tuberculosis*, cytomegalovirus, endemic fungi, and *Aspergillus* spp may also lead to respiratory failure [38]. Similarly, influenza-related morbidity and mortality are increased in severely immunocompromised patients. During active seasonal influenza cycles, empiric treatment with appropriate antivirals (e.g., oseltamivir) should be considered as diagnostic samples are acquired (e.g., nasopharyngeal swabs to detect respiratory viruses by PCR) [39].

CENTRAL NERVOUS SYSTEM DISORDERS

Because a substantial percentage of individuals with HIV present with advanced disease for reasons described earlier, other severe opportunistic diseases may require intensive care. Prominent among these are diseases of the central nervous system (CNS).

Meningitis caused by *Cryptococcus neoformans* often presents in a subacute manner, sometimes with headache and typical meningeal symptoms and signs, and occasionally with altered mental status thought to relate to elevated intracranial pressure (ICP) [40,41]. Infection is usually disseminated at the time of presentation with CNS disease, and there may be pulmonary and cutaneous manifestations as well. Given the tendency for elevated ICP to develop, imaging prior to lumbar puncture is generally recommended if cryptococcal meningitis (CM) is suspected. A lumbar puncture should include measurement of the opening pressure. Diagnosis is usually made by CSF analysis that includes cryptococcal antigen detection. Most often, the CSF will have a relatively low white blood (mononuclear) cell count, mildly elevated protein, and low glucose. A substantial minority will have a normal CSF profile. Features that are associated with severe disease and higher mortality are presentation with altered mental status, low CSF white blood cell count (<20 per μL), and high cryptococcal antigen titer ($>$1:1024) [42]. Treatment for severe disease is complicated by the tendency for elevated intracerebral pressure to develop. Repeated therapeutic lumbar punctures (LP) are sometimes required to improve clinical outcomes [43]. Treatment occurs in stages; the first stage is induction (duration $\geq$ 2 weeks), which involves infusion of an amphotericin B formulation together with oral flucytosine [44,45]. Close monitoring of renal function and CBC is necessary, given the toxicities of these agents. Therapeutic drug monitoring of flucytosine should be included, if available. With CM, the timing of initiation of ART is delayed because early treatment is associated with worse outcome [46,47]. Most clinicians wait until well after the induction stage of treatment of CM before starting ART (delaying ART initiation by 4 to 10 weeks). Later stages of CM treatment include consolidation with high-dose fluconazole for 8 weeks, and maintenance with lower dose fluconazole for 2 or more years following initiation of ART [48].

Focal encephalitis caused by *Toxoplasma gondii* most often presents with headache, altered mental status, seizures, and focal neurologic signs [49], occasionally requiring intensive care management. A diagnosis is made using a combination of imaging modalities and CSF sampling. MRI is the most useful, but findings usually cannot distinguish between toxoplasmosis, CNS lymphoma, or abscess; all may present with one or more ring-enhancing lesions. A brain biopsy can establish the diagnosis, but lesions are often relatively inaccessible. If imaging suggests that lumbar puncture can be performed safely, CSF should be sent for *Toxoplasma* PCR, and studies to rule out other opportunistic diseases of the CNS (cytology, Epstein–Barr virus [EBV] PCR, *M. tuberculosis* PCR, cryptococcal antigen, JC virus PCR, etc.). Empiric treatment is often prescribed for patients with advanced immunocompromise, positive *Toxoplasma* serology, and characteristic CNS lesions. The treatment of choice is pyrimethamine and sulfadiazine, with leukovorin [50]. Individuals with sulfa allergies may be managed with clindamycin substituted for sulfadiazine. Adjunctive corticosteroids and/or anticonvulsants (see Chapters 81 and 151) may be needed in individuals with significant mass effect and/or presentation with seizures. With empiric treatment, a response should be expected within 2 weeks.

Other opportunistic diseases of the CNS observed with AIDS are lymphoma (usually EBV related) and progressive multifocal leukoencephalopathy (PML) caused by JC virus. These may present as severe disease, and treatment is largely supportive. In the case of PML, the optimal treatment is rapid initiation of ART. As immune reconstitution occurs in response to ART, CNS inflammation may worsen leading to clinical deterioration. Close monitoring and administration of corticosteroids may be required if there is paradoxical worsening of neurologic function.

HEPATIC DISORDERS

Coinfection with HIV and Hepatitis Viruses

With improved treatment of HIV with antiretroviral agents, complications of hepatitis B (HBV) and C viruses (HCV) have emerged as a major cause of mortality for HIV-infected persons [51–53]. An estimated 15% to 30% of patients with HIV in the United States are coinfected with HCV, an eightfold increase in HCV infection compared with the general population [54]. Patients coinfected with HCV and HIV are more likely to develop cirrhosis than those with HCV alone [55]. Thus, many patients with HIV infection are admitted to ICUs with end-stage liver disease and associated encephalopathy and gastrointestinal hemorrhage.

A number of antiretroviral agents are also active against HBV, permitting construction of regimens effective against both pathogens for HIV–HBV coinfected patients. The management of coinfection with HIV and HCV entails separate combination drug regimens with interactions and overlapping toxicities. Recent advances in HCV treatment have improved the outlook for infected individuals, with cure rates well in excess of 90% in many studies. Direct acting antivirals (DAAs) now include inhibitors of the HCV protease, NS5a and NS5b (polymerase). Evolving recommendations require frequent updates to guidelines ([56] http://www.hcvguidelines.org). The treatment approach for HIV and HCV coinfected individuals is the same as for those with HCV infection alone; however, drug interactions with ART agents often limit options. Drug interactions with HCV-specific DAAs extend beyond ART agents, and careful review of medications is necessary for individuals receiving these agents during hospitalizations. Despite the high HCV cure rates, and relatively short and simplified treatment regimens, therapy continues to require close supervision by experienced specialists. Treatment with these agents may be associated with exacerbation of liver dysfunction and decompensation, particularly in individuals with advanced stages of cirrhosis (http://www.hcvguidelines.org).

IMMUNE RECONSTITUTION DISORDERS

Initiation of ART may be followed by paradoxical worsening of known opportunistic infections after an initial response to therapy, characterized by a robust inflammatory reaction. Alternatively, patients with an unrecognized infection, not yet manifested clinically, may develop an inflammatory reaction at the infected site (so-called unmasking). These reactions are not typical of the usual clinical presentation of the infectious agent, and are now termed "immune reconstitution inflammatory syndrome" (IRIS) or "immune restoration disease" [57,58]. For instance, *Mycobacterium avium* complex, which usually produces disseminated disease with no histologic evidence of host response in persons with advanced HIV infection and $CD4^+$ lymphocyte counts <50 per μL, may present with fever and pain because of focal necrotizing lymphadenitis. A meta-analysis of 64 reports comprising 13,103 persons initiating ART found that 13% developed IRIS; some series report much higher rates, particularly in patients with cytomegalovirus retinitis [16]. The time to onset of IRIS is reported to vary from 3 to 658 days after starting ART, with a median of 29 to 49 days [15–17,58]. The risk is higher for patients with lower $CD4^+$ counts before initiation of ART, but the occurrence of IRIS seems to correlate better with rapid decline in viral load than with increase in $CD4^+$ lymphocyte count [15,17], and the meta-analysis found a case-fatality rate of 6.7% [16]. IRIS-related respiratory compromise is reported in association with mycobacterial infection and PCP [59,60]. Corticosteroids may be used to suppress the aberrant inflammatory reaction, but there are no guidelines as to when to use them or the optimal dose and duration. Corticosteroids are usually reserved for patients with severe inflammatory disease.

OTHER CRITICAL ILLNESSES

HIV-infected persons are not spared any of the diseases that can bring non–HIV-infected persons with otherwise similar characteristics to the ICU, including gastrointestinal hemorrhage, trauma, drug overdose, violence, and cardiovascular diseases. Injection drug users are obviously at increased risk of developing infective endocarditis. With advances made in ART, HIV-infected individuals can have a life expectancy that approaches that of uninfected individuals [61]. The usual diseases associated with aging are seen with increasing frequency as the HIV-infected population on effective ART grows older [62]. Some diseases of aging are seen with higher frequency among HIV-infected populations.

Patients with HIV infection have accelerated atherosclerosis and increased risk of coronary artery disease; this was previously attributed to therapy, particularly protease inhibitors which are known to increase plasma lipid levels [63,64]. However, the risk of major cardiovascular disease outcomes increased among patients randomized to interrupt ART when $CD4^+$ lymphocyte count rose above 400 compared to those who continued therapy and who had more drug exposure [65]. Subsequent analyses have correlated cardiovascular disease risk to higher levels of viremia [66] and abnormalities of endothelial function that improve with ART [67].

Laboratory abnormalities, including pancytopenia, eosinophilia, and transaminase elevations, may either represent the patient's baseline or indicate significant disease or drug toxicity. Among laboratory abnormalities that may safely be followed are macrocytosis as a normal accompaniment of zidovudine, stavudine, or tenofovir therapy (provided there are no hypersegmented polymorphonuclear leukocytes), mild indirect hyperbilirubinemia of patients on atazanavir or indinavir, and hyperuricemia of patients taking didanosine. Note that the use of stavudine, indinavir, and didanosine is increasingly rare, with the availability of less toxic alternative ART. Elevations of creatine phosphokinase in patients taking zidovudine or tenofovir may also be asymptomatic and benign, but some reflect clinical myositis caused by these drugs. Hyponatremia seems to be relatively common and well tolerated in advanced HIV infection, but frank adrenal insufficiency or isolated hypoaldosteronism may require specific diagnosis and management.

TOXIC EFFECTS OF ANTIRETROVIRAL THERAPY

The drugs used for ART are associated with several life-threatening toxicities that may prompt admission to the ICU. Older nucleoside analog reverse transcriptase inhibitors (NRTIs), especially didanosine and stavudine (and zalcitabine, which is no longer available in the United States), can cause pancreatitis, which may be severe. In a retrospective study of 73 HIV-infected patients with pancreatitis, 46% of cases were attributed to drug toxicity, with didanosine and pentamidine (used to treat PCP) the most common offending agents [68]. Didanosine may cause portal hypertension without cirrhosis [69]. Patients who received this drug even many years before may present with life-threatening hemorrhage from esophageal varices.

NRTIs can cause lactic acidosis by inhibiting DNA polymerase-γ, disrupting mitochondrial DNA. This may also cause hepatic steatosis or mitochondrial myopathy [70]. Lactic acidosis is the consequence of increased anaerobic glycolysis by damaged mitochondria, coupled with decreased lactate clearance by the fatty liver. Mild hyperlactatemia occurs commonly among patients receiving NRTIs and is not clinically important, but severe lactic acidosis occurs at a rate of 1.3 to 3.2 cases per 1,000 person-years of nucleoside exposure and may be life threatening [71,72]. The appearance of nausea, vomiting, abdominal pain, dyspnea, or weakness in persons on long-term therapy with these agents may herald the onset of this life-threatening illness and should prompt measurement of serum lactate. This entity should be considered in the differential diagnosis of apparent sepsis, hepatic failure, and pancreatitis requiring ICU admission of patients on ART. Because patients may also develop severe lactic acidosis as a result of sepsis, empiric antibiotics should be administered, pending the results of microbiologic evaluations. If severe hyperlactatemia or lactic acidosis is found, all ART must be stopped immediately because continuation of a partial regimen may lead to viral resistance. In addition to standard care, case reports suggest that this disorder may improve with use of riboflavin, thiamine, L-carnitine, and coenzyme Q [73–75]. The same drugs and mechanism underlie a syndrome of severe neuromuscular weakness and respiratory failure that may mimic Guillain–Barré syndrome or botulism, and the same therapies have been proposed [76]. The newer NRTIs (tenofovir, emtricitabine, lamivudine, and abacavir) produce less inhibition of DNA polymerase-γ and have largely replaced the agents most commonly implicated (stavudine, didanosine, and zidovudine); this seems to have reduced the incidence of syndromes related to mitochondrial toxicity.

Abacavir hypersensitivity is a protean syndrome that may include fever, chills, nausea, diarrhea, rash, myalgia, aseptic meningitis, hepatitis, cough, or influenza-like illness within a few weeks of starting treatment. Discontinuation of the drug leads to resolution of symptoms, but rechallenge can produce an anaphylactic reaction with cardiovascular collapse and high fever [77,78]. This syndrome should be virtually eliminated by the introduction of screening for the HLA-B*5701 allele and avoidance of abacavir in persons who carry it [79,80].

Tenofovir nephrotoxicity rarely presents as Fanconi syndrome; with increases in serum creatinine, glycosuria, hypophosphatemia, and acute tubular necrosis. Electrolyte imbalance because of tubular dysfunction may be severe and require intensive repletion [81].

Severe rash, including Stevens–Johnson syndrome, is most notably associated with nevirapine, but can occur with other nonnucleoside reverse transcriptase inhibitors (NNRTIs) and rarely with protease inhibitors and NRTIs.

MANAGEMENT OF PROPHYLACTIC AND ANTIRETROVIRAL AGENTS

Even when critically ill, patients with advanced HIV disease who received prophylaxis against opportunistic infections like PCP before ICU admission should continue to receive it unless contraindicated. Initiation of appropriate prophylactic measures should be considered in those who have not. Judging whether prophylaxis is indicated may be difficult in acutely ill patients because of effects that stress, infections, and medications may have on $CD4^+$ T-cell counts. Even a single dose of glucocorticoids can reduce the $CD4^+$ T-cell count dramatically. In general, decisions regarding prophylaxis should be based on $CD4^+$ T-cell values recently obtained, but prior to acute illness or receiving corticosteroids if they are available. In patients who stopped taking ART for more than a month, it is usually best to assume that the risk of a patient developing opportunistic infections corresponds to that before starting ART.

The use of ART for critically ill patients requires expertise in selection of drugs and consideration of their doses, toxicity, and interactions with other treatments. The critical care clinician is well-advised to manage these patients in close collaboration with an expert in antiretroviral treatment. Patients receiving ART should continue to receive these drugs whenever possible, because discontinuing therapy is associated with viral replication, emergence of resistance, and clinical progression of HIV infection. In patients coinfected with HBV, discontinuation of lamivudine (and presumably emtricitabine and tenofovir, the other antivirals active against HBV) may result in exacerbations of hepatitis B that may be fatal [82,83].

The feasibility of continuing ART depends on that of enteral administration. When the gastrointestinal tract is significantly dysfunctional, all of the drugs in a patient's regimen will inevitably be stopped at the same time, and no harm is likely if they can be resumed in a few days. Still, the NNRTIs (efavirenz, nevirapine, and etravirine) are eliminated very slowly, and stopping all agents at the same time may lead to a prolonged period of inadvertent NNRTI monotherapy and selection for virus with drug resistance mutations. When ART therapy must be interrupted for more than a few days, consultation with an HIV specialist is recommended.

Continuing ART entails potentially complex interactions with other drugs prescribed, including effects on absorption and metabolism that result in either suboptimal or toxic levels of both the antiretrovirals and other drugs. For example, administration of proton-pump inhibitors causes significant reductions in the protease inhibitor atazanavir; an H_2 blocker can be given safely 12 hours before or after atazanavir. Protease inhibitors significantly reduce the metabolism and increase the activity of midazolam. Lorazepam and temazepam may be safer alternatives for sedation, but dose titration with close monitoring of effect in the ICU setting may suffice to overcome the potential risks of midazolam administration. Given the frequency of cardiovascular disease as a cause of ICU admission among HIV-infected persons, HMG-CoA reductase inhibitors may be prescribed, but protease inhibitors have significant and varying interactions with most of these drugs; simvastatin and lovastatin are contraindicated with all of the protease inhibitors because of massive increases in their plasma levels.

The presence of acute kidney injury necessitates dose adjustments of all the nucleoside analogs except abacavir, and the components of fixed-dose combinations require individual adjustments. If renal function varies or is impaired for several days, the best way to assure consistently adequate and nontoxic levels of antiretrovirals is to change the regimen to drugs that do not require adjustment for renal insufficiency, when possible.

When considering whether to start ART for a critically ill patient who did not receive it before, a few questions may guide the decision. First, is the enteral route expected to remain available to permit consistent and continuous drug administration? If not, ART must wait. Second, does the patient have an infection for which there is no effective therapy other than the potential offered by improved immunologic status (e.g., cryptosporidiosis or PML)? In this situation, all other care is futile unless ART is begun, and it should be. Third, did the patient not receive ART because the diagnosis of HIV infection was never established, by choosing not to take ART because of personal reasons, or because of repeatedly opting to stop ART? The latter two do not lend themselves to easy answers, and it may be well to wait at least until the patient has decisional capacity and able to share in decision making. Patients with advanced neurocognitive disease may have marked improvement on ART and may regain functional independence; for them, treatment is as imperative as for those with otherwise untreatable infections. When therapy is started for patients who are deemed to be at high risk of abandoning it, the chosen regimen should have minimal adverse consequences if discontinued abruptly (e.g., NNRTIs should be avoided).

The risk of IRIS has been a deterrent to starting ART early for patients with opportunistic infection, but more recent studies have clarified this issue considerably. A randomized trial of early versus deferred ART in patients with acute opportunistic infections excluding tuberculosis found that fewer patients who received early therapy had progression of AIDS or death, with no difference in the rate of IRIS [84]. Other studies support a survival advantage for patients who started on ART in the ICU [85,86]. For patients with tuberculosis, IRIS occurred among 12.4% of patients randomized to early ART (started at a mean of 70 days after the initiation of antituberculous therapy) and only 3.8% of those whose ART was delayed until completion of treatment for tuberculosis (mean of 260 days), but mortality was significantly higher among the delayed ART group (12.1% vs. 5.4%), and no deaths were attributed to IRIS [87]. However, among patients with CM treated with a suboptimal fluconazole regimen that is the only one commonly available in Africa, early initiation of ART (within 72 hours of diagnosis) resulted in nearly threefold increased mortality compared to initiation after 10 weeks, with median survivals of 28 and 637 days, respectively [47]. Although firm conclusions are not yet available about the timing of ART in patients with serious opportunistic infections, it seems that the opportunistic infection should be under good control before initiating ART and that the clinician must anticipate the potential emergence of serious effects from IRIS [88].

PREDICTORS OF OUTCOME

Overall, it seems that critically ill patients with HIV infection have similar short-term outcomes as other patients with a comparable severity of illness, and survival rates seem to be improving [9–11,89,90]. Most studies in patients with HIV infection are limited by selection bias, because they are usually retrospective analyses where the admitting physician's knowledge of the patient's serostatus may have affected the decision to admit to ICU or the vigor or goals of care. In a study conducted in a South African surgical ICU, HIV testing was performed but results not divulged and there were no differences in ICU or hospital mortality or duration of stay when outcome was adjusted for age, despite a higher incidence of sepsis and organ failure in the HIV-infected patients [91]. Thus, evidence from a variety of settings supports the concept that HIV-infected and uninfected persons have similar outcomes of intensive care, and that decisions regarding the appropriateness of ICU interventions should not use HIV status alone as a criterion.

Studies examining the value of laboratory testing and scoring systems for predicting ICU outcomes of HIV-infected patients, including lactate dehydrogenase, serum albumin, $CD4^+$ lymphocyte count, APACHE II score, and multisystem organ failure scores, yield conflicting data on their reliability. It now seems clear that patients with HIV/AIDS have similar short-term outcomes to those of other patients with a similar severity of illness. Long-term survival is related to the severity of the HIV disease, other comorbid illness, and whether the patient has been treated with ART. In addition to the patient's illness, the experience of the hospital and healthcare providers with treating HIV-associated infections and managing complications also influences mortality. In one large study, adjusted mortality for patients with AIDS was 30% lower among hospitals with the most experience treating these patients [92].

Because the outcomes for intensive care do not depend directly on the patient's HIV status, determination of whether or not a patient has HIV infection or determination of $CD4^+$ lymphocyte counts should not be overriding considerations in deciding whether to offer or withhold intensive care. Rather, these decisions should be made using the same criteria as for all patients, namely, the likelihood of benefit and the patient's values.

RISK TO HEALTHCARE WORKERS AND POSTEXPOSURE PROPHYLAXIS

Intensive care of patients carries an increased risk of exposure to bloodborne pathogens, including HIV. The risk of acquiring HIV-1 infection by mucous membrane exposure is approximately 0.09% (just under 1 in 10,000) and by percutaneous (e.g., needlestick) exposure, approximately 0.3%, or 1 in 300 instances [93,94]. Virtually all documented infections have involved accidents with hollow-bore needles. The risk is higher when inflicted by a device that came directly from the HIV-infected patient's artery or vein, had visible blood on it, produced deep injury, or came from a source patient with terminal illness (defined as death because of AIDS within 60 days of the healthcare worker's exposure). Each of these features increases the risk of infection independently. In a case–control study where healthcare workers infected by needlestick exposures were compared with healthcare workers who sustained exposures from HIV-infected patients but did not become infected, the only factor that was shown to reduce the risk of infection was postexposure use of zidovudine by the healthcare worker [95]. Zidovudine prophylaxis appeared to reduce the risk of infection by 81%. This study led to much stronger recommendations for ART for healthcare workers with percutaneous or mucous membrane exposure to HIV-1.

Current recommendations reflect the failure rate of single-agent postexposure prophylaxis, the prevalence of ART-resistant virus, the proven antiviral efficacy of three-drug regimens in infected individuals, and the importance of tolerability of the regimen to ensure completion of a full 4-week course [96]. The US Public Health Service now recommends three or more drugs for high-risk exposures from a known HIV-positive source. Examples of high-risk exposures include percutaneous injury involving a contaminated needle, or exposure to blood, tissue, or potentially infectious bodily fluid on mucous membranes or nonintact skin from patients with symptomatic HIV infection, AIDS, acute seroconversion, or known high viral load. The National Institutes of Health AIDS Information Web site (https://aidsinfo.nih.gov/) provides the most current drug recommendations and links to current PHS recommendations [96]. Expert consultation is advised, especially for cases involving drug-resistant virus, and pregnant or breastfeeding personnel. Recommendations for postexposure prophylaxis emphasize initiating treatment within an hour or two of exposure, and data from infants of HIV-positive mothers not treated during pregnancy and delivery suggest little benefit to therapy delayed beyond 48 to 72 hours [97]. However, the time after which therapy will not be successful has not been defined.

The list of potential side effects of antiretroviral drugs is daunting, but newer regimens are better tolerated. Many healthcare workers receiving PEP will experience adverse effects, along with justifiable anxiety. They should be reassured that most HIV-infected people tolerate these regimens with the help of adequate psychosocial support and proper medical follow-up.

SUMMARY

In summary, the evolution of the AIDS epidemic and the continuing improvements of effective ART have changed the spectrum of critical illnesses for patients with HIV infection. The use of ART

TABLE 76.2

Summary of Recommendations for Management of Complications of Human Immunodeficiency Virus Infection Based on Randomized Clinical Trials

- Early adjunctive treatment with corticosteroids reduces the risks of respiratory failure and death in patients with acquired immunodeficiency syndrome (AIDS) and moderate-to-severe *Pneumocystis* pneumonia [26,33,34].
- Combination treatment with amphotericin B and flucytosine versus fluconazole improves outcome in individuals with cryptococcal meningitis [44].
- Early versus delayed ART in patients with cryptococcal meningitis increases risk of death in patients receiving suboptimal treatment with amphotericin B and/or fluconazole [46,47].
- Early versus deferred ART in patients with acute opportunistic infections excluding tuberculosis decreases progression to AIDS or death, with no difference in the rate of IRIS [84].
- Early versus deferred ART in patients with tuberculosis decreases mortality, but increases risk of IRIS [87].

ART, antiretroviral therapy; IRIS, immune reconstitution inflammatory syndrome.

has led to reduced risk of AIDS-associated illness and improved survival, but raises new and complex questions about how best to use these treatments in patients with critical illness. Clearly, large-scale multidisciplinary studies of critical care of patients with HIV infection would yield valuable insights, but until the important clinical questions are answered, critical care clinicians must work closely not only with the ICU multidisciplinary team, but also with colleagues with backgrounds in infectious diseases, pharmacology, and palliative care. Advances in the management of opportunistic disease associated with HIV infection, based on randomized controlled trials or meta-analyses of such trials, are summarized in treatment guidelines that are maintained as living documents available to the public (https://aidsinfo.nih.gov) [26] and Table 76.2.

References

1. Centers for Disease Control and Prevention: HIV Surveillance Report, 2013. http://www.cdc.gov/hiv/library/reports/surveillance/. Published February, 2015. Accessed February 9, 2017.
2. Gardner EM, McLees MP, Steiner JF, et al: The spectrum of engagement in HIV care and its relevance to test-and-treat strategies for prevention of HIV infection. *Clin Infect Dis* 52(6):793–800, 2011.
3. UNAIDS: Fact Sheet 2015. http://www.unaids.org/en/resources/documents/2015/20150714_factsheet. 2015. Accessed February 9, 2017.
4. Martin-Iguacel R, Llibre JM, Friis-Moller N: Risk of cardiovascular disease in an aging HIV population: where are we now? *Curr HIV/AIDS Rep* 12(4):375–387, 2015.
5. Curtis JR, Bennett CL, Horner RD, et al: Variations in intensive care unit utilization for patients with human immunodeficiency virus-related Pneumocystis carinii pneumonia: importance of hospital characteristics and geographic location. *Crit Care Med* 26(4):668–675, 1998.
6. Afessa B, Green B: Clinical course, prognostic factors, and outcome prediction for HIV patients in the ICU. The PIP (Pulmonary complications, ICU support, and prognostic factors in hospitalized patients with HIV) study. *Chest* 118(1):138–145, 2000.
7. Rosen MJ, Clayton K, Schneider RF, et al: Intensive care of patients with HIV infection: utilization, critical illnesses, and outcomes. Pulmonary Complications of HIV Infection Study Group. *Am J Respir Crit Care Med* 155(1):67–71, 1997.
8. Rosen MJ, De Palo VA: Outcome of intensive care for patients with AIDS. *Crit Care Clin* 9(1):107–114, 1993.
9. Narasimhan M, Posner AJ, DePalo VA, et al: Intensive care in patients with HIV infection in the era of highly active antiretroviral therapy. *Chest* 125(5):1800–1804, 2004.
10. Powell K, Davis JL, Morris AM, et al: Survival for patients with HIV admitted to the ICU continues to improve in the current era of combination antiretroviral therapy. *Chest* 135(1):11–17, 2009.
11. Huang L, Quartin A, Jones D, et al: Intensive care of patients with HIV infection. *N Engl J Med* 355(2):173–181, 2006.
12. Rosenberg AL, Seneff MG, Atiyeh L, et al: The importance of bacterial sepsis in intensive care unit patients with acquired immunodeficiency syndrome: implications for future care in the age of increasing antiretroviral resistance. *Crit Care Med* 29(3):548–556, 2001.
13. Valdez H, Chowdhry TK, Asaad R, et al: Changing spectrum of mortality due to human immunodeficiency virus: analysis of 260 deaths during 1995–1999. *Clin Infect Dis* 32(10):1487–1493, 2001.
14. Akgun KM, Pisani M, Crothers K: The changing epidemiology of HIV-infected patients in the intensive care unit. *J Intensive Care Med* 26(3):151–164, 2011.
15. Manabe YC, Campbell JD, Sydnor E, et al: Immune reconstitution inflammatory syndrome: risk factors and treatment implications. *J Acquir Immune Defic Syndr* 46(4):456–462, 2007.
16. Muller M, Wandel S, Colebunders R, et al: Immune reconstitution inflammatory syndrome in patients starting antiretroviral therapy for HIV infection: a systematic review and meta-analysis. *Lancet Infect Dis* 10(4):251–261, 2010.
17. Murdoch DM, Venter WD, Feldman C, et al: Incidence and risk factors for the immune reconstitution inflammatory syndrome in HIV patients in South Africa: a prospective study. *AIDS* 22(5):601–610, 2008.
18. Stringer JR, Beard CB, Miller RF, et al: A new name (Pneumocystis jirovecii) for Pneumocystis from humans. *Emerg Infect Dis* 8(9):891–896, 2002.
19. Kaplan JE, Hanson D, Dworkin MS, et al: Epidemiology of human immunodeficiency virus-associated opportunistic infections in the United States in the era of highly active antiretroviral therapy. *Clin Infect Dis* 30[Suppl 1]:S5–S14, 2000.
20. Saah AJ, Hoover DR, Peng Y, et al: Predictors for failure of Pneumocystis carinii pneumonia prophylaxis. Multicenter AIDS Cohort Study. *JAMA* 273(15):1197–1202, 1995.
21. Morris A, Lundgren JD, Masur H, et al: Current epidemiology of Pneumocystis pneumonia. *Emerg Infect Dis* 10(10):1713–1720, 2004.
22. Thomas CF Jr, Limper AH: Pneumocystis pneumonia. *N Engl J Med* 350(24):2487–2498, 2004.
23. Parada JP, Deloria-Knoll M, Chmiel JS, et al: Relationship between health insurance and medical care for patients hospitalized with human immunodeficiency virus-related Pneumocystis carinii pneumonia, 1995–1997: medicaid, bronchoscopy, and survival. *Clin Infect Dis* 37(11):1549–1555, 2003.
24. Tu JV, Biem HJ, Detsky AS: Bronchoscopy versus empirical therapy in HIV-infected patients with presumptive Pneumocystis carinii pneumonia. A decision analysis. *Am Rev Respir Dis* 148(2):370–377, 1993.
25. Sax PE, Komarow L, Finkelman MA, et al: Blood (1->3)-beta-D-glucan as a diagnostic test for HIV-related Pneumocystis jirovecii pneumonia. *Clin Infect Dis* 53(2):197–202, 2011.
26. Panel on Opportunistic Infections in HIV-Infected Adults and Adolescents: Guidelines for the prevention and treatment of opportunistic infections in HIV-infected adults and adolescents: recommendations from the Centers for Disease Control and Prevention, the National Institutes of Health, and the HIV Medicine Association of the Infectious Diseases Society of America. http://aidsinfo.nih.gov/contentfiles/lvguidelines/adult_oi.pdf (at http://aidsinfo.nih.gov). 2015. Accessed February 9, 2017.
27. Maxfield RA, Sorkin IB, Fazzini EP, et al: Respiratory failure in patients with acquired immunodeficiency syndrome and Pneumocystis carinii pneumonia. *Crit Care Med* 14(5):443–449, 1986.
28. Afessa B: Pleural effusion and pneumothorax in hospitalized patients with HIV infection: the pulmonary complications, ICU support, and prognostic factors of hospitalized patients with HIV (PIP) study. *Chest* 117(4):1031–1037, 2000.
29. Wachter RM, Luce JM, Safrin S, et al: Cost and outcome of intensive care for patients with AIDS, Pneumocystis carinii pneumonia, and severe respiratory failure. *JAMA* 273(3):230–235, 1995.
30. Davis JL, Morris A, Kallet RH, et al: Low tidal volume ventilation is associated with reduced mortality in HIV-infected patients with acute lung injury. *Thorax* 63(11):988–993, 2008.
31. Beck JM, Rosen MJ, Peavy HH: Pulmonary complications of HIV infection. Report of the Fourth NHLBI Workshop. *Am J Respir Crit Care Med* 164(11):2120–2126, 2001.
32. Montaner JS, Russell JA, Lawson L, et al: Acute respiratory failure secondary to Pneumocystis carinii pneumonia in the acquired immunodeficiency syndrome. A potential role for systemic corticosteroids. *Chest* 95(4):881–884, 1989.
33. Bozzette SA, Sattler FR, Chiu J, et al: A controlled trial of early adjunctive treatment with corticosteroids for Pneumocystis carinii pneumonia in the acquired immunodeficiency syndrome. California Collaborative Treatment Group. *N Engl J Med* 323(21):1451–1457, 1990.
34. Gagnon S, Boota AM, Fischl MA, et al: Corticosteroids as adjunctive therapy for severe Pneumocystis carinii pneumonia in the acquired immunodeficiency syndrome. A double-blind, placebo-controlled trial. *N Engl J Med* 323(21):1444–1450, 1990.
35. Baddour LM, Yu VL, Klugman KP, et al: Combination antibiotic therapy lowers mortality among severely ill patients with pneumococcal bacteremia. *Am J Respir Crit Care Med* 170(4):440–444, 2004.
36. Barbier F, Coquet I, Legriel S, et al: Etiologies and outcome of acute respiratory failure in HIV-infected patients. *Intensive Care Med* 35(10):1678–1686, 2009.
37. Heffernan RT, Barrett NL, Gallagher KM, et al: Declining incidence of invasive Streptococcus pneumoniae infections among persons with AIDS in an era of highly active antiretroviral therapy, 1995–2000. *J Infect Dis* 191(12):2038–2045, 2005.
38. Masur H: Management of patients with HIV in the intensive care unit. *Proc Am Thorac Soc* 3(1):96–102, 2006.
39. Sheth AN, Althoff KN, Brooks JT: Influenza susceptibility, severity, and shedding in HIV-infected adults: a review of the literature. *Clin Infect Dis* 52(2):219–227, 2011.

40. Bicanic T, Brouwer AE, Meintjes G, et al: Relationship of cerebrospinal fluid pressure, fungal burden and outcome in patients with cryptococcal meningitis undergoing serial lumbar punctures. *AIDS* 23(6):701–706, 2009.
41. Graybill JR, Sobel J, Saag M, et al: Diagnosis and management of increased intracranial pressure in patients with AIDS and cryptococcal meningitis. The NIAID Mycoses Study Group and AIDS Cooperative Treatment Groups. *Clin Infect Dis* 30(1):47–54, 2000.
42. Saag MS, Powderly WG, Cloud GA, et al: Comparison of amphotericin B with fluconazole in the treatment of acute AIDS-associated cryptococcal meningitis. The NIAID Mycoses Study Group and the AIDS Clinical Trials Group. *N Engl J Med* 326(2):83–89, 1992.
43. Rolfes MA, Hullsiek KH, Rhein J, et al: The effect of therapeutic lumbar punctures on acute mortality from cryptococcal meningitis. *Clin Infect Dis* 59(11):1607–1614, 2014.
44. Day JN, Chau TT, Wolbers M, et al: Combination antifungal therapy for cryptococcal meningitis. *N Engl J Med* 368(14):1291–1302, 2013.
45. van der Horst CM, Saag MS, Cloud GA, et al: Treatment of cryptococcal meningitis associated with the acquired immunodeficiency syndrome. National Institute of Allergy and Infectious Diseases Mycoses Study Group and AIDS Clinical Trials Group. *N Engl J Med* 337(1):15–21, 1997.
46. Boulware DR, Meya DB, Muzoora C, et al: Timing of antiretroviral therapy after diagnosis of cryptococcal meningitis. *N Engl J Med* 370(26):2487–2498, 2014.
47. Makadzange AT, Ndhlovu CE, Takarinda K, et al: Early versus delayed initiation of antiretroviral therapy for concurrent HIV infection and cryptococcal meningitis in sub-saharan Africa. *Clin Infect Dis* 50(11):1532–1538, 2010.
48. Perfect JR, Dismukes WE, Dromer F, et al: Clinical practice guidelines for the management of cryptococcal disease: 2010 update by the infectious diseases society of america. *Clin Infect Dis* 50(3):291–322, 2010.
49. Navia BA, Petito CK, Gold JW, et al: Cerebral toxoplasmosis complicating the acquired immune deficiency syndrome: clinical and neuropathological findings in 27 patients. *Ann Neurol* 19(3):224–238, 1986.
50. Katlama C, De Wit S, O'Doherty E, et al: Pyrimethamine-clindamycin vs. pyrimethamine-sulfadiazine as acute and long-term therapy for toxoplasmic encephalitis in patients with AIDS. *Clin Infect Dis* 22(2):268–275, 1996.
51. Bica I, McGovern B, Dhar R, et al: Increasing mortality due to end-stage liver disease in patients with human immunodeficiency virus infection. *Clin Infect Dis* 32(3):492–497, 2001.
52. Monga HK, Rodriguez-Barradas MC, Breaux K, et al: Hepatitis C virus infection-related morbidity and mortality among patients with human immunodeficiency virus infection. *Clin Infect Dis* 33(2):240–247, 2001.
53. Sulkowski MS, Thomas DL: Hepatitis C in the HIV-infected patient. *Clin Liver Dis* 7(1):179–194, 2003.
54. Sherman KE, Rouster SD, Chung RT, et al: Hepatitis C virus prevalence among patients infected with human immunodeficiency virus: a cross-sectional analysis of the US adult AIDS Clinical Trials Group. *Clin Infect Dis* 34(6):831–837, 2002.
55. Lo Re V 3rd, Kallan MJ, Tate JP, et al: Hepatic decompensation in antiretroviral-treated patients co-infected with HIV and hepatitis C virus compared with hepatitis C virus-monoinfected patients: a cohort study. *Ann Intern Med* 160(6):369–379, 2014.
56. AASLD/IDSA HCV Guidance Panel: Hepatitis C guidance: AASLD-IDSA recommendations for testing, managing, and treating adults infected with hepatitis C virus. *Hepatology* 62(3):932–954, 2015. www.hcvguidelines.org. Accessed February 9, 2017.
57. Shelburne SA 3rd, Hamill RJ, Rodriguez-Barradas MC, et al: Immune reconstitution inflammatory syndrome: emergence of a unique syndrome during highly active antiretroviral therapy. *Medicine (Baltimore)* 81(3):213–227, 2002.
58. Shelburne SA, Visnegarwala F, Darcourt J, et al: Incidence and risk factors for immune reconstitution inflammatory syndrome during highly active antiretroviral therapy. *AIDS* 19(4):399–406, 2005.
59. Narita M, Ashkin D, Hollender ES, et al: Paradoxical worsening of tuberculosis following antiretroviral therapy in patients with AIDS. *Am J Respir Crit Care Med* 158(1):157–161, 1998.
60. Wislez M, Bergot E, Antoine M, et al: Acute respiratory failure following HAART introduction in patients treated for Pneumocystis carinii pneumonia. *Am J Respir Crit Care Med* 164(5):847–851, 2001.
61. May MT, Gompels M, Delpech V, et al: Impact on life expectancy of HIV-1 positive individuals of $CD4^+$ cell count and viral load response to antiretroviral therapy. *AIDS* 28(8):1193–1202, 2014.
62. Brooks JT, Buchacz K, Gebo KA, et al: HIV infection and older Americans: the public health perspective. *Am J Public Health* 102(8):1516–1526, 2012.
63. Barbaro G, Di Lorenzo G, Cirelli A, et al: An open-label, prospective, observational study of the incidence of coronary artery disease in patients with HIV infection receiving highly active antiretroviral therapy. *Clin Ther* 25(9):2405–2418, 2003.
64. Friis-Moller N, Sabin CA, Weber R, et al: Combination antiretroviral therapy and the risk of myocardial infarction. *N Engl J Med* 349(21):1993–2003, 2003.
65. Strategies for Management of Antiretroviral Therapy Study Group; El-Sadr WM, Lundgren J, Neaton JD, et al: $CD4^+$ count-guided interruption of antiretroviral treatment. *N Engl J Med* 355(22):2283–2296, 2006.
66. Marin B, Thiebaut R, Bucher HC, et al: Non-AIDS-defining deaths and immunodeficiency in the era of combination antiretroviral therapy. *AIDS* 23(13):1743–1753, 2009.
67. Torriani FJ, Komarow L, Parker RA, et al: Endothelial function in human immunodeficiency virus-infected antiretroviral-naive subjects before and after starting potent antiretroviral therapy: The ACTG (AIDS Clinical Trials Group) Study 5152s. *J Am Coll Cardiol* 52(7):569–576, 2008.
68. Gan I, May G, Raboud J, et al: Pancreatitis in HIV infection: predictors of severity. *Am J Gastroenterol* 98(6):1278–1283, 2003.
69. Kovari H, Ledergerber B, Peter U, et al: Association of noncirrhotic portal hypertension in HIV-infected persons and antiretroviral therapy with didanosine: a nested case-control study. *Clin Infect Dis* 49(4):626–635, 2009.
70. Miller KD, Cameron M, Wood LV, et al: Lactic acidosis and hepatic steatosis associated with use of stavudine: report of four cases. *Ann Intern Med* 133(3):192–196, 2000.
71. Moyle GJ, Datta D, Mandalia S, et al: Hyperlactataemia and lactic acidosis during antiretroviral therapy: relevance, reproducibility and possible risk factors. *AIDS* 16(10):1341–1349, 2002.
72. Sundar K, Suarez M, Banogon PE, et al: Zidovudine-induced fatal lactic acidosis and hepatic failure in patients with acquired immunodeficiency syndrome: report of two patients and review of the literature. *Crit Care Med* 25(8):1425–1430, 1997.
73. Brinkman K, ter Hofstede HJ, Burger DM, et al: Adverse effects of reverse transcriptase inhibitors: mitochondrial toxicity as common pathway. *AIDS* 12(14):1735–1744, 1998.
74. Fouty B, Frerman F, Reves R: Riboflavin to treat nucleoside analogue-induced lactic acidosis. *Lancet* 352(9124):291–292, 1998.
75. Schramm C, Wanitschke R, Galle PR: Thiamine for the treatment of nucleoside analogue-induced severe lactic acidosis. *Eur J Anaesthesiol* 16(10):733–735, 1999.
76. H. I. V. Neuromuscular Syndrome Study Group: HIV-associated neuromuscular weakness syndrome. *AIDS* 18(10):1403–1412, 2004.
77. Escaut L, Liotier JY, Albengres E, et al: Abacavir rechallenge has to be avoided in case of hypersensitivity reaction. *AIDS* 13(11):1419–1420, 1999.
78. Walensky RP, Goldberg JH, Daily JP: Anaphylaxis after rechallenge with abacavir. *AIDS* 13(8):999–1000, 1999.
79. Mallal S, Phillips E, Carosi G, et al: HLA-B*5701 screening for hypersensitivity to abacavir. *N Engl J Med* 358(6):568–579, 2008.
80. Saag M, Balu R, Phillips E, et al: High sensitivity of human leukocyte antigen-b*5701 as a marker for immunologically confirmed abacavir hypersensitivity in white and black patients. *Clin Infect Dis* 46(7):1111–1118, 2008.
81. Karras A, Lafaurie M, Furco A, et al: Tenofovir-related nephrotoxicity in human immunodeficiency virus-infected patients: three cases of renal failure, Fanconi syndrome, and nephrogenic diabetes insipidus. *Clin Infect Dis* 36(8):1070–1073, 2003.
82. Bessesen M, Ives D, Condreay L, et al: Chronic active hepatitis B exacerbations in human immunodeficiency virus-infected patients following development of resistance to or withdrawal of lamivudine. *Clin Infect Dis* 28(5):1032–1035, 1999.
83. Sellier P, Clevenbergh P, Mazeron MC, et al: Fatal interruption of a 3TC-containing regimen in a HIV-infected patient due to re-activation of chronic hepatitis B virus infection. *Scand J Infect Dis* 36(6–7):533–535, 2004.
84. Zolopa A, Andersen J, Powderly W, et al: Early antiretroviral therapy reduces AIDS progression/death in individuals with acute opportunistic infections: a multicenter randomized strategy trial. *PLoS One* 4(5):e5575, 2009.
85. Croda J, Croda MG, Neves A, et al: Benefit of antiretroviral therapy on survival of human immunodeficiency virus-infected patients admitted to an intensive care unit. *Crit Care Med* 37(5):1605–1611, 2009.
86. Morris A, Wachter RM, Luce J, et al: Improved survival with highly active antiretroviral therapy in HIV-infected patients with severe Pneumocystis carinii pneumonia. *AIDS* 17(1):73–80, 2003.
87. Abdool Karim SS, Naidoo K, et al: Timing of initiation of antiretroviral drugs during tuberculosis therapy. *N Engl J Med* 362(8):697–706, 2010.
88. Bicanic T, Meintjes G, Rebe K, et al: Immune reconstitution inflammatory syndrome in HIV-associated cryptococcal meningitis: a prospective study. *J Acquir Immune Defic Syndr* 51(2):130–134, 2009.
89. Casalino E, Mendoza-Sassi G, Wolff M, et al: Predictors of short- and long-term survival in HIV-infected patients admitted to the ICU. *Chest* 113(2):421–429, 1998.
90. Dickson SJ, Batson S, Copas AJ, et al: Survival of HIV-infected patients in the intensive care unit in the era of highly active antiretroviral therapy. *Thorax* 62(11):964–968, 2007.
91. Bhagwanjee S, Muckart DJ, Jeena PM, et al: Does HIV status influence the outcome of patients admitted to a surgical intensive care unit? A prospective double blind study. *BMJ* 314(7087):1077–1081, 1997; discussion 1081-1074.
92. Cunningham WE, Tisnado DM, Lui HH, et al: The effect of hospital experience on mortality among patients hospitalized with acquired immunodeficiency syndrome in California. *Am J Med* 107(2):137–143, 1999.
93. Bell DM: Occupational risk of human immunodeficiency virus infection in healthcare workers: an overview. *Am J Med* 102(5B):9–15, 1997.
94. Ippolito G, Puro V, De Carli G: The risk of occupational human immunodeficiency virus infection in health care workers. Italian Multicenter Study. The Italian Study Group on Occupational Risk of HIV infection. *Arch Intern Med* 153(12):1451–1458, 1993.
95. Cardo DM, Culver DH, Ciesielski CA, et al: A case-control study of HIV seroconversion in health care workers after percutaneous exposure. Centers for Disease Control and Prevention Needlestick Surveillance Group. *N Engl J Med* 337(21):1485–1490, 1997.
96. Kuhar DT, Henderson DK, Struble KA, et al: Updated US Public Health Service guidelines for the management of occupational exposures to human immunodeficiency virus and recommendations for postexposure prophylaxis. *Infect Control Hosp Epidemiol* 34(9):875–892, 2013.
97. Wade NA, Birkhead GS, Warren BL, et al: Abbreviated regimens of zidovudine prophylaxis and perinatal transmission of the human immunodeficiency virus. *N Engl J Med* 339(20):1409–1414, 1998.

Chapter 77 ■ Infectious Complications of Drug Abuse

AFROZA LITON • WILLIAM L. MARSHALL

Drug abuse, the deliberate taking of an unprescribed drug dose or illicit substance, is a pervasive problem in our society [1]. A variety of drugs are abused, including opiates, depressants, stimulants, and hallucinogens. This chapter will focus on infections that occur as a consequence of drugs that are either explicitly illegal or those which are legal but are used by the patient for purposes other than for which they were prescribed. Abused drugs can be administered by a variety of means, including "snorting" through the nasal mucosa, via inhalation through smoking, orally, and by parenteral routes, including injection into the soft tissues, called "skin popping," or directly into the vascular system.

Drug abuse is attended by an increased risk in a number of infections, some of which may lead patients to be admitted to the intensive care unit [2]. Infections associated with parenteral drug abuse include skin and soft tissue infection, endocarditis, bone and joint infections, pneumonia, ophthalmologic infections, and hepatitis [2–4]. Illicit drugs are often "cut" or mixed with adulterants, which may be contaminated with bacteria or may suppress the immune response—as is the case with agranulocytosis caused by levamisole-containing cocaine leading to bacterial or fungal infection [5]. Illicit drug injection occurs under unsanitary conditions using drugs that are not sterile and injection equipment that has often been used more than once. Such practices provide a mechanism for the passage of a variety of infectious agents. Although in some instances, particularly for the hepatitis viruses and human immunodeficiency virus (HIV), the infectious agent is passed directly from blood-contaminated drug paraphernalia to the patient, the mode of spread is less clear for other agents. Prevention of infectious complications of drug use is directed at treating addiction, or failing that, mitigating infectious complications via needle exchange programs [6]. Finally, many patients with substance abuse problems are homeless, have poor nutrition, and live under crowded conditions, placing them at increased risk of tuberculosis (TB).

FEVER

Fever is one of the most common complaints of parenteral drug users presenting to the hospital. Self-limited illnesses are the most common causes of fever in this population. More significant etiologies include pneumonia, cellulitis, and soft tissue abscesses. Endocarditis accounts for fewer than 15% of all cases of fever [7].

All febrile parenteral drug users should undergo a thorough history, physical examination, and have routine blood laboratories and chest radiographs taken. Particular attention should be paid to abnormalities of the skin and soft tissues, cardiac valvular abnormalities, bony tenderness, and pulmonary abnormalities. However, clinical evaluation alone often does not differentiate major disease from trivial illness in these patients. Parenteral drug users who are febrile should be admitted to the hospital for further observation.

Weisse et al. [7] have developed an algorithm for febrile parenteral drug abusers with no apparent source of infection. In this approach, blood cultures are obtained from all patients and empiric antibiotic therapy is started. If blood cultures are positive or if the patient has clinical stigmata indicative of endocarditis, an echocardiogram is performed. If valvular vegetations are seen, the diagnosis of endocarditis is considered established. On the other hand, if blood cultures are negative and the patient is clinically well, antibiotic therapy may be discontinued. However, parenteral drug users commonly self-administer antibiotics and this practice may substantially reduce the likelihood of positive blood cultures, as can prophylactic antibiotics in HIV+ patients [8]. Hence, careful clinical evaluation is advised when making antibiotic decisions for these patients.

BACTEREMIA

Bacteremia is a frequent occurrence among febrile parenteral drug users [9]. Approximately 60% of bacteremias in parenteral drug abusers are due to causes other than endocarditis [10]. Of these, the majority are caused by either skin or soft tissue infections or to mycotic aneurysms of peripheral arteries. A smaller number of bacteremias result from miscellaneous causes, such as septic arthritis, septic thrombophlebitis, or pneumonia. In about 3% of cases, the source of the bacteremia is undiscovered.

Although the organisms associated with bacteremias among parenteral drug users may vary based on geographic location and the type of drug abused, some generalizations can be made [10]. Drug users have an increased incidence of staphylococcal carriage of the skin, nose, or throat. Bacterial infection derives principally from the user's own flora, so that *Staphylococcus aureus* constitutes the majority of bacteremias among these patients. In this regard, methicillin-resistant *S. aureus* (MRSA) infections are now being encountered with increasing frequency in parenteral drug users and in the community [11,12].

Streptococci and Gram-negative aerobic bacilli are the next most frequently isolated organisms. Polymicrobial bacteremias occur in about 10% of cases, and in about two-thirds of these cases at least one of the organisms isolated is a *Staphylococcus* spp. Bacteremia and other infections caused by the facultative anaerobe *Eikenella corrodens* are particularly associated with injecting drug users (IDUs) who contaminate the injection needle or the injection site with saliva [10,13].

The approach toward the bacteremic parenteral drug user should be to search for an underlying etiology and to begin empiric antibiotic treatment. The isolation of a group A β-hemolytic streptococci from the blood should prompt a search for a cutaneous or soft tissue focus of infection [14]. Empiric antibiotic therapy may be based on local antimicrobial sensitivities but should generally include agents directed against staphylococci and streptococci as well as aerobic Gram-negative bacilli. If MRSA infections have previously occurred among parenteral drug users in the community, vancomycin should be considered.

SOFT TISSUE INFECTIONS

Skin and soft tissue infections occur commonly in the parenteral drug user and are increasing in frequency [15,16]. Such infections are often polymicrobial and appear to derive from either the skin or oral cavity. The most common pathogens are *S. aureus*, streptococci, oral anaerobes, and aerobic Gram-negative bacilli [13–17]. Cutaneous infection in the intravenous drug user generally occurs in the antecubital fossa, forearm, and hand as these are the sites of the most accessible veins. However, intravenous drug users may also avail themselves of other, less available sites with infection occurring in the feet, legs, anterior neck, groin, and axilla [18,19].

The most common skin infections among IDUs are simple cellulitis and localized skin abscess. These occur more frequently among those who "skin pop" compared to those who inject intravenously [20]. Simple cellulitis usually requires only antibiotic therapy directed against staphylococci and streptococci. IDUs are particularly at risk of MRSA infections of the skin and soft tissues [11]; patients requiring intravenous therapy should receive vancomycin. Localized soft tissue abscesses that do not penetrate into the deep subcutaneous tissue should be drained. Given the risk of occult bacteremia for this population, antibiotic therapy should be given as directed by Gram stain of the drained material. In all patients with a history of injection drug use, blood cultures should be obtained as part of the workup of skin and soft tissue infections.

The presence of vesicles or bullae, an area of central necrosis within a larger area of erythema, and the presence of subcutaneous crepitation in a patient with systemic toxicity is suggestive of necrotizing fasciitis [21]. Gas seen in the soft tissues on radiographs is also indicative of deep infection [22]. However, extensive necrosis may be present even in the absence of these signs, and surgical exploration should be considered in any case that manifests local erythema, fluctuance, and induration [21]. Suspicion for needles or other foreign bodies should similarly prompt surgical exploration. Any abnormal material from this exploration should be immediately examined using Gram stain to provide the basis for empiric antimicrobial therapy. Examination of a sample of tissue using frozen-section biopsy may also be useful [23]. Magnetic resonance imaging (MRI) typically reveals increased T2 signal along fascial planes and gadolinium enhancement, whereas contrast-enhanced computed tomography (CT) scanning is a less sensitive diagnostic tool for necrotizing fasciitis [22].

Necrotizing fasciitis, pyomyositis, or gangrene requires immediate, aggressive debridement in the operating room in association with parenteral antibiotics [21]. Gram stain and culture are imperative to guide antimicrobial therapy. Empiric therapy should be directed against staphylococci, streptococci, anaerobes, and aerobic Gram-negative bacilli. Surgical debridement may be required on multiple occasions before the infection is controlled. There have been multiple outbreaks of soft tissue infection with or without systemic symptoms associated with *Clostridium* spp. discussed later in this chapter.

PERIPHERAL VASCULAR INFECTIONS

Because parenteral drug use often involves vascular injection of material under nonsterile conditions, it is not surprising that a wide range of vascular complications may result from these practices [24]. The most frequent manifestations of such infections are fever associated with pain, redness, and swelling over the involved area. When the injecting site is into the deep tissues of the groin or neck, it may be difficult to distinguish involvement of vascular structures from simple cellulitis, soft tissue abscess, or fasciitis. If there is any question, angiography should be performed to determine if vascular tissue is involved. Septic thrombophlebitis usually presents as fever, bacteremia, and swelling over the involved vein. This can often be treated with antibiotics alone, although incision, drainage, and removal of the vein are sometimes necessary. Anticoagulation is generally not required [10].

Mycotic aneurysms result when the user injects directly into the artery [10,24]. Aneurysms most frequently occur in the femoral arteries. Carotid aneurysms and brachial artery aneurysms occasionally occur [24]. The classic presentation of this syndrome is a febrile patient with a tender, pulsatile mass, usually in the groin or the neck. Sometimes, there is a small amount of bleeding at the site. If there is any question of an aneurysm, a vascular surgical consultation should be obtained prior to any exploration of the lesion. Angiography will confirm the site and extent of the aneurysm. The most frequent microbiologic agents isolated are *S. aureus* and streptococci, with aerobic Gram-negative bacilli occasionally being identified [10]. Empiric antibiotic therapy should be directed against these organisms. Ligation and excision of the involved arterial segment is usually successful [25].

ENDOCARDITIS

Endocarditis in the parenteral drug abuser differs in several respects from endocarditis in the nonaddict. It is more likely to occur in persons without underlying valvular heart disease, to involve the tricuspid valve, to be caused by *S. aureus*, and to have a more benign outcome [3,26]. Certain types of intravenous drug abuse may predispose to the development of endocarditis. Heroin use has long been associated with this complication.

Tricuspid valve endocarditis is the prototypical presentation of endocarditis in the parenteral drug user [27]. The patient complains of fever, usually for less than 1 week. There may be a history of chills and pleuritic chest pain and occasionally hemoptysis. On physical examination, fever is a nearly universal finding. A systolic murmur may or may not be present on admission, but often develops during the course of therapy. Signs of peripheral embolization, such as petechiae, splinter hemorrhages, Janeway lesions, or Roth spots, are uncommon. Osler's nodes are frequently absent. On chest radiograph, multiple patchy infiltrates indicative of pulmonary emboli are strongly suggestive of the diagnosis of tricuspid endocarditis. Blood cultures are usually positive and in the majority of instances, *S. aureus* is isolated. When blood cultures are negative in the face of the appropriate clinical syndrome, one should suspect that the patient has recently taken antibiotics.

Endocarditis involving the valves of the left side of the heart may also occur in the parenteral drug user. Compared to patients with tricuspid valve endocarditis alone, there is more likely to be a history of underlying heart disease [10]. On examination, a heart murmur is usually evident on presentation, and peripheral emboli are frequent. Streptococci are more likely to be isolated from the blood, but *S. aureus* is still frequently isolated [3,10,27].

In addition to staphylococci and streptococci, a variety of other organisms have been associated with endocarditis in the parenteral drug user, including aerobic Gram-negative bacilli, particularly *Pseudomonas aeruginosa*, and fungi, notably *Candida* spp. [3]. Moreover, polymicrobial bacteremia is a well-recognized complication of endocarditis in this population and is usually indistinguishable on clinical grounds from that caused by a single organism [28].

Bacteremia and pulmonary emboli on chest radiograph are highly predictive of tricuspid valve endocarditis among parenteral drug users [3,10]. However, all individuals with clinically suspected endocarditis should have echocardiography performed. Transesophageal echocardiography is more sensitive than transthoracic echocardiography in identifying valvular vegetations [29]. When echocardiographic findings are combined with clinical manifestations, the diagnosis of endocarditis can usually be established with high sensitivity and specificity using the Duke criteria or modifications of the Duke criteria, even among IDUs with HIV infection [30].

Empiric therapy for endocarditis of the parenteral drug user should be directed against staphylococci, streptococci, and, rarely, aerobic Gram-negative bacilli. Nafcillin, oxacillin, and cefazolin are reasonable choices only if methicillin resistance among staphylococci has not been encountered. Vancomycin is the current alternative for the treatment of MRSA infections and for the β-lactam–allergic patient.

The prognosis for tricuspid valve staphylococcal endocarditis of the parenteral drug user is good, with a mortality of less than

10% employing a choice of several therapies [3,10,30]. There was no difference of outcome between treatments with a β-lactam antibiotic alone and in combination with an aminoglycoside for 4 weeks [31]. Although a combination of a penicillinase-resistant penicillin with an aminoglycoside has been advocated for 2-week therapy for right-sided endocarditis [32], one study found that results for combination therapy were no different from those when a penicillinase-resistant penicillin was used alone [33] (see Table 77.1).

Nonstaphylococcal endocarditis, particularly that involving the aortic and mitral valves, has a significantly worse prognosis. Left-sided endocarditis secondary to *P. aeruginosa* has a particularly poor outcome, with a mortality rate of nearly 70% [10]. To achieve cure, a 6-week course of intravenous therapy with an antipseudomonal β-lactam antibiotic plus an aminoglycoside, both at high doses, combined with early surgical removal of the involved valve is usually required [34]. *Candida* endocarditis also has an extremely high mortality rate even with prompt valve replacement and systemic antifungal therapy [35].

The role of surgery for endocarditis of the parenteral drug user is no different from endocarditis in the general population. Hemodynamic decompensation, persistently positive blood cultures in the face of appropriate antimicrobial therapy, multiple embolic episodes after therapy is initiated, fungal endocarditis, and evidence of extravalvular extension of infection constitute major criteria for valve replacement [36]. Tricuspid valvulotomy is successful in the majority of patients with isolated tricuspid valve involvement and intractable infection. Only about 10% of patients require a subsequent prosthetic valve to control congestive right-sided heart failure [37].

SKELETAL INFECTIONS

Infections of the bones and joints represent a distinct clinical syndrome in the drug abuser. Most cases have been reported among intravenous heroin users, and many cases occur in association with endocarditis [38]. Bacterial osteomyelitis of the vertebral column is the most frequent skeletal infection reported. The lumbar, cervical, and thoracic spine are involved, in that order. Patients generally present with weeks to months of pain in the involved area. High fevers are unusual, and many patients are

TABLE 77.1

Summary of Recommendations Based on Randomized Controlled Trials of Interventions to Control Infectious Diseases in Drug Users

Intervention	Year	Study	No. of patients	Findings	Reference
Accelerated HBV vaccine schedule: (0, 1, 6 mo) or accelerated (0, 1, 2 mo) vaccination schedule	2015	Randomized controlled trial (RCT)	707	Accelerated vaccine schedule improves hepatitis B vaccination adherence among IDU.	[64]
Daily oral antiretroviral preexposure prophylaxis (PrEP) for preventing human immunodeficiency virus (HIV) infection	2013	RCT	2,413	49% decrease in HIV infection (note that CDC recommends TDF/FTC for this type of PrEP)	[54]
INH treatment of latent TB in IDUs	2003	Observational	2,212	Treatment with isoniazid was beneficial in HIV-infected, tuberculin-positive IDUs	[68]
Patients were randomized to 2 wks of therapy for MSSA endocarditis with gentamicin (1.5 mg/kg every 8 h) AND either cloxacillin (11 patients, 2 g every 4 h) OR vancomycin (11 patients, 500 mg every 6 h) OR with teicoplanin (12 patients, 24 mg/kg for 1 d, then 12 mg/kg every 24 h).	2001	RCT	34	RR of failure of cloxacillin plus gentamicin versus a glycopeptide plus gentamicin IV for 2 wks was 0.12	[77]
For right-sided endocarditis: cloxacillin (2 g every 4 h for 2 wks) and gentamicin (1 mg/kg every 8 h for 1 wk) were compared with cloxacillin (2 g every 4 h for 2 wks)	1996	RCT	90	RR of failure for cloxacillin and gentamicin compared with cloxacillin alone was 1.27 (95% CI 0.65–2.49).	[33]
All patients with MRSA triscupid valve endocarditis were randomized to either 3 wks of trimethoprim/sulfamethoxazole (320/1,600 mg every 12 h) OR 3 wks of vancomycin (1 g every 12 h).	1992	RCT	15	4/7 receiving trimethoprim/sulfamethoxazole versus 1/8 receiving vancomycin demonstrated microbiologic failure (RR 4.57, 95% CI 0.66–31.89).	[76]

afebrile. There is usually tenderness over the involved vertebral bodies and radiographic evidence of osteomyelitis. Laboratory values are generally normal, although the peripheral white blood cell count may be modestly elevated. The erythrocyte sedimentation rate and/or C-reactive protein are almost always elevated and may serve as useful markers of a response to therapy [39]. Because of the chronicity of symptoms and the general lack of toxicity of these patients, it is not unusual for the diagnosis to be missed for weeks or even months. The complaint of low back or neck pain in an intravenous drug user should always suggest the diagnosis of vertebral osteomyelitis. Septic arthritis often involves the sacroiliac and sternoarticular joints and the symphysis pubis. There is usually weeks to months of pain at the site and tenderness to palpation at the site of involvement. Radiographs are usually normal at presentation. MRI is preferable to contrast-enhanced CT of the spine to make the diagnosis of vertebral osteomyelitis [40].

The bacteriology of skeletal infections among drug users is quite different from that seen in other patients. Gram-positive cocci, such as staphylococci and streptococci, are frequently isolated, as well as aerobic Gram-negative bacilli, particularly *P. aeruginosa* [38]. Skeletal infections caused by *Candida* spp. may also occur, either alone or as part of a dissemination syndrome [41]. Because of this, it is imperative that a bacteriologic diagnosis be established in such patients. In most cases, this can be achieved by needle aspirate of the involved bone or joint. For sternoarticular infections, open surgical exploration is often required. Therapy involves long-term antibiotic therapy and in some cases surgical debridement [42].

SYSTEMIC SYNDROMES WITH SPORE-FORMING BACTERIA

Anaerobic spore-forming bacilli of the genus *Clostridium* are ubiquitous in the environment; exospores can remain viable indefinitely. If illicit substances become contaminated with these spores, subsequent injection of the substances may result in severe illness or death. The first reports of infections in people addicted to morphine injection were of tetanus in 1876. By the 1950s in New York, drug addiction accounted for the majority of cases of tetanus. Wound botulism caused by *Clostridium botulinum* was first observed in IDUs in the United States in 1982. Cases increased during the 1990s with the use of black-tar heroin, and a similar outbreak was seen in Germany in 2005. These patients presented with abscesses associated with symmetrical descending paralysis, some requiring mechanical ventilation. Treatment included antitoxin, antimicrobials, and surgical drainage of abscesses [43]. In the last decade, there have been outbreaks of serious illness and death among IDUs in the United Kingdom due to *Clostridium novyi* and *Clostridium histolyticum* [44]. Skin poppers using subcutaneous and intramuscular injection appear to be particularly at risk [45].

Similar to infections with *Clostridium* spp., since 2009, there have been cases of anthrax confirmed in heroin users in Scotland [46]. All injection routes have been implicated, but smoking or snorting may also pose a significant risk. Most had severe soft tissue infections with significant soft tissue edema but differed from classic necrotizing fasciitis or classic cutaneous anthrax. Patients had vague prodromal symptoms, appeared very ill, but their symptoms had nonspecific systemic features. Some developed septic shock leading to multiorgan failure.

HUMAN IMMUNODEFICIENCY VIRUS INFECTION

Injecting drug use represents the third most common risk behavior for infection with HIV in the United States and is associated with 75% of HIV cases among heterosexual men. Black and Hispanic ethnic groups are disproportionately represented among IDUs with HIV infection [47]. In some metropolitan regions, notably Atlanta, Detroit, and San Francisco, the rate of HIV infection among IDUs is approximately 10%. There is great geographic variability in the prevalence of HIV infection among IDUs. The highest rates are in the northeastern United States and Puerto Rico.

Certain practices increase the risk for a drug user to acquire HIV infection. These include frequent intravenous drug injections, injection in "shooting galleries," places where users rent the injecting paraphernalia and return it after use, injection with used needles, or sharing needles. Additional factors associated with an increased risk include use of cocaine or other drugs that prompts HIV risk behaviors and having sex partners who use intravenous drugs. The latter is significantly associated with HIV infection in women [48]. Finally, the use of methamphetamine, "crystal meth," has been linked to an increase in the sexual transmission of HIV, including highly antiretroviral-resistant strains [49]. In vitro studies show that opiates, methamphetamine, and cocaine can potentiate HIV replication and can enhance neurotoxicity [50].

HIV-positive IDUs are more likely to develop infections that are not AIDS-defining illnesses. Disease patterns in this group may differ from the other HIV-infected groups [51]. In particular, they have a high risk of developing bacterial pneumonia and bacterial sepsis, especially because of encapsulated organisms such as *Streptococcus pneumoniae* or *Haemophilus influenzae*. This observation highlights the importance of pneumococcal and *H. influenzae* type B vaccines in this group. Progressive decline of CD4 lymphocyte counts to less than 200 per μL, and smoking illicit drugs significantly increase the risk of bacterial pneumonia [52]. In one study, *Pneumocystis* pneumonia, community-acquired bacterial pneumonia, and TB were the three most frequent pulmonary diseases seen among a group of illicit drug users in Washington, DC [53].

Any intravenous drug user should be considered at risk of HIV infection, and such patients should be offered testing for infection [47]. In addition, one study demonstrated the effectiveness of preexposure prophylaxis with daily administration of tenofovir in IDUs, although public health authorities suggest that emtricitabine be coadministered with tenofovir for HIV prophylaxis in IDUs ([54], see Table 77.1). In areas of high prevalence, the clinician should be aware that HIV-related immunodeficiency might be complicating the clinical course in an IDU. In the United States, IDUs are also the highest risk group for human T-cell lymphotropic virus type I or II (HTLV-I or HTLV-II) infection [4]. The impact of this on HIV-related mortality is unclear, but coinfection with HIV and HTLV-I has been associated with myelopathy [55].

VIRAL HEPATITIS

Acute and chronic hepatitis have long been recognized as common reasons for hospital admission among drug users [4]. Of the infectious causes, hepatitis B virus (HBV) remains a principal pathogen. It is estimated that from 60% to 80% of parenteral drug users in the United States are infected with hepatitis B, and that nearly 10% are chronic carriers [56]. Moreover, coinfection with the hepatitis delta virus, a hepatotropic agent that requires hepatitis B for replication, has been reported in 8% to 40% of IDUs infected with hepatitis B and is associated with a more fulminant course [57]. Hepatitis A has also been documented as a cause of acute hepatitis among intravenous drug users [58].

After HIV infection, infection with hepatitis C virus (HCV) is the next emerging infectious disease epidemic in the United States. The vast majority of cases of HCV infection are associated with injecting drug use. Acute infection, which occurs relatively soon after injection drug practices begin, is rarely symptomatic, but chronic infection occurs in about 85% of all infections. A subset of patients may develop chronic liver disease, cirrhosis, and hepatocellular carcinoma. Recent studies report a decrease in HCV seroprevalence among IDUs from 65% to 35% [59]. Parenteral drug abusers may suffer multiple attacks of acute hepatitis and are also likely to have significant structural and functional abnormalities of their liver, even if they are asymptomatic. Noninfectious factors, particularly the use of alcohol and other drugs, may act synergistically with the hepatitis viruses to lead to a poorer outcome [56].

Concomitant HCV and either HBV or hepatitis A virus (HAV) can lead to severe hepatitis or death, underlining the importance of vaccinating eligible parenteral drug users for HAV and HBV [60]. Special attention is required to choose therapies in patients with HIV and HBV coinfection. Antiretroviral medications like lamivudine or tenofovir are only partially active as monotherapy against both viruses, requiring thoughtful combination therapy to be effective against both viruses. There is an increase in the incidence of hepatocellular carcinoma and hepatotoxic effects associated with antiretroviral drugs in patients with HIV and HCV/HBV coinfection [61]. Newer, interferon-free oral HCV therapies are becoming available to cure HCV infection in 12 to 24 weeks in IDUs and potentially halt the HCV epidemic [62].

Prevention services recommended for injection-drug users include annual testing for HIV infection, hepatitis A vaccination, accelerated hepatitis B vaccination, and testing for HCV infection [63,64].

Sexually Transmitted Diseases

Sexually transmitted infections such as Chlamydia and gonorrhea are closely associated with substance abuse, both because of frequent exchange of sex for money or drugs and because of the sexual disinhibition that result from the use of psychoactive substances, especially alcohol and cocaine. Freebase ("crack") cocaine use has also been linked to an increased risk of syphilis and other ulcerative genital infections [65]. The high false-positive rate of nontreponemal tests for syphilis (rapid plasma reagin test and the Venereal Disease Research Laboratory test) in IDUs requires use of specific treponemal tests (e.g., the fluorescent treponemal antibody absorption test). Standard therapy for syphilis appears to be effective in both HIV-seropositive and HIV-seronegative IDUs. HIV-infected women have higher risk of cervical dysplasia and cancer associated with concurrent human papillomavirus infection that warrants at least yearly Papanicolaou smears in this group [51].

PULMONARY DISEASE AND TUBERCULOSIS

As noted earlier, community-acquired pneumonia, TB, HIV-associated *Pneumocystis* pneumonia, and septic pulmonary emboli caused by right-sided endocarditis are the major pulmonary complications of illicit drug use [10,53]. In addition, pulmonary edema may acutely attend drug injection. This is not associated with infection and usually clears in 1 to 2 days.

A unilateral infiltrate on chest radiograph in a drug abuser should suggest a bacterial pneumonia. Antibiotic therapy should be directed against community-acquired pathogens, such as *S. pneumoniae*, *S. aureus*, and nonpseudomonal Gram-negative bacilli, such as *H. influenzae* and *Klebsiella pneumoniae*. If there is a recent history of unconsciousness suggesting aspiration of oropharyngeal contents, antimicrobial therapy directed against anaerobes should be considered.

Nearly one out of three U.S.-born persons older than 15 years of age who has TB is a substance abuser. In addition to poor socioeconomic condition, substance abuse often takes place in enclosed spaces with poor ventilation and high volumes of human traffic, and increases the likelihood of TB transmission [66]. The risk of developing active TB among IDUs is significant, particularly if they are coinfected with HIV. Many drug users with HIV infection and TB may not demonstrate cutaneous tuberculin reactivity probably because of anergy. These patients have a high risk of developing active TB that is more likely to be extrapulmonary [67]. Data indicate the effectiveness of preventive isoniazid therapy for all drug users who are HIV infected and live in areas of high prevalence of TB [68]. Some experts advocate treatment of latent TB regardless of tuberculin skin test reaction, but the spread of multidrug-resistant TB in HIV+, drug-using populations suggests that this approach may not always be successful [69].

The clinician should maintain a high index of suspicion of TB in any drug user with pulmonary disease, particularly if the patient is infected with HIV. If there is any possibility of pulmonary TB, patients should be placed in respiratory isolation. Acid-fast smears should be performed on at least three respiratory specimens before active pulmonary TB is ruled out. If smears are positive, antituberculous therapy should be initiated [70] (see Chapter 82). Clinicians must address barrier to treatment adherence to reduce the risk of treatment failure that will lead to developing drug resistance [51].

DISSEMINATED CANDIDIASIS

A distinctive form of disseminated candidiasis has been described in injecting drug abusers who use brown heroin. *Candida albicans* has been specifically implicated in these cases. The source of infection is unclear but appears to be derived from the drug user's own flora. The syndrome is characterized by fever within hours after injection, followed days to weeks later by skin, eye, and osteoarticular lesions. The skin lesions consist of deep subcutaneous nodules confined to the scalp or other hairy areas, and painful pustules on an erythematous base found in all areas of the body. Direct examination of expressed material from these pustules will demonstrate budding yeast. Costochondral tumors are a unique part of the syndrome, presenting as pain and swelling over the involved ribs. Biopsy of such lesions is often diagnostic, demonstrating both pseudohyphae and yeast. Optimal therapy is not established. Azole antifungals have been used successfully in many cases of skin involvement alone, but amphotericin B or surgery has been required with ocular or osteoarticular involvement [71].

OCULAR INFECTIONS

IDUs have an increased risk of eye infections, usually secondary to hematogenous spread from another site. Most cases are secondary to *Candida* spp., either as part of the disseminated candidiasis syndrome described earlier or with eye involvement alone. *Aspergillus* and *Fusarium* spp. have also been associated with endophthalmitis in the parenteral drug user. Usually only one eye is involved, and there are no other sites of infection. Treatment generally requires vitrectomy combined with systemic antifungal therapy such as voriconazole or amphotericin B.

Endophthalmitis due to bacteria is far less common than that due to fungi. Unlike fungal endophthalmitis, which often presents indolently, the onset of bacterial endophthalmitis is usually explosive with acute pain, redness, and decreased visual acuity. It may be mistaken initially for conjunctivitis. Progressive destruction of the eye may occur rapidly and immediate ophthalmologic consultation is requisite. Unusual organisms have been frequently isolated in this disease, such as *Bacillus* spp. and *Staphylococcus epidermidis* [72].

CENTRAL NERVOUS SYSTEM INFECTIONS

Epidural abscess is the most frequent central nervous system infection in IDUs. A common presentation is indolent radicular pain associated with an underlying vertebral osteomyelitis. Imaging studies, such as myelography, CT scan, or MRI, are useful in defining the extent of the infectious process. Needle aspiration under radiographic visualization can establish the microbiologic etiology. Staphylococci are the most frequent cause, although other pathogens, including *P. aeruginosa* and *Mycobacterium tuberculosis*, have also been recognized. Neurosurgical consultation should be obtained at the time the diagnosis is first suspected [2,73].

Brain abscesses may occur, usually as a result of embolization from either endocarditis or a mycotic aneurysm. They are usually multiple and generally caused by *S. aureus*. Antibiotic therapy alone has led to cure in some cases [74]. Cerebral mucormycosis is another complication of intravenous drug use and is suggested by the finding of lesions in the basal ganglia [75].

References

1. Schulden JD, Thomas YF, Compton WM: Substance abuse in the United States: findings from recent epidemiologic studies. *Curr Psychiatry Rep* 11(5):353–359, 2009.
2. Calder KK, Severyn FA: Surgical emergencies in the intravenous drug user. *Emerg Med Clin North Am* 21(4):1089–1116, 2003.
3. Brown PD, Levine DP: Infective endocarditis in the injection drug user. *Infect Dis Clin North Am* 16(3):645–665, viii–ix, 2002.
4. Contoreggi C, Rexroad VE, Lange WR: Current management of infectious complications in the injecting drug user. *J Subst Abuse Treat* 15(2):95–106, 1998.
5. Knowles L, Buxton JA, Skuridina N, et al: Levamisole tainted cocaine causing severe neutropenia in Alberta and British Columbia. *Harm Reduct J* 6:30, 2009.
6. Des Jarlais DC, Perlis T, Arasteh K, et al: Reductions in hepatitis C virus and HIV infections among injecting drug users in New York City, 1990–2001. *AIDS* 19[Suppl 3]:S20–S25, 2005.
7. Weisse AB, Heller DR, Schimenti RJ, et al: The febrile parenteral drug user: a prospective study in 121 patients. *Am J Med* 94(3):274–280, 1993.
8. Styrt BA, Chaisson RE, Moore RD: Prior antimicrobials and staphylococcal bacteremia in HIV-infected patients. *AIDS* 11(10):1243–1248, 1997.
9. Manfredi R, Costigliola P, Ricchi E, et al: Sepsis-bacteraemia and other infections due to non-opportunistic bacterial pathogens in a consecutive series of 788 patients hospitalized for HIV infection. *Clin Ter* 143(4):279–290, 1993.
10. Levine DP, Crane LR, Zervos MJ: Bacteremia in narcotic addicts at the Detroit Medical Center. II. Infectious endocarditis: a prospective comparative study. *Rev Infect Dis* 8(3):374–396, 1986.
11. El-Sharif A, Ashour HM: Community-acquired methicillin-resistant Staphylococcus aureus (CA-MRSA) colonization and infection in intravenous and inhalational opiate drug abusers. *Exp Biol Med (Maywood)* 233(7):874–880, 2008.
12. Frazee BW, Lynn J, Charlebois ED, et al: High prevalence of methicillin-resistant Staphylococcus aureus in emergency department skin and soft tissue infections. *Ann Emerg Med* 45(3):311–320, 2005.
13. Armstrong O, Fisher M: The treatment of Eikenella corrodens soft tissue infection in an injection drug user. *W V Med J* 92(3):138–139,1996.
14. Bernaldo de Quiros JC, Moreno S, Cercenado E, et al: Group A streptococcal bacteremia. A 10-year prospective study. *Medicine (Baltimore)* 76(4):238–248, 1997.
15. Irish C, Maxwell R, Dancox M, et al: Skin and soft tissue infections and vascular disease among drug users, England. *Emerg Infect Dis* 13(10):1510–1511, 2007.
16. Centers for Disease Control and Prevention (CDC): Soft tissue infections among injection drug users—San Francisco, California, 1996–2000. *MMWR Morb Mortal Wkly Rep* 50(19):381–384, 2001.
17. Ebright JR, Pieper B: Skin and soft tissue infections in injection drug users. *Infect Dis Clin North Am* 16(3):697–712, 2002.
18. Espiritu MB, Medina JE: Complications of heroin injections of the neck. *Laryngoscope* 90(7, Pt 1):1111–1119, 1980.
19. Somers WJ, Lowe FC: Localized gangrene of the scrotum and penis: a complication of heroin injection into the femoral vessels. *J Urol* 136(1):111–113, 1986.
20. Thomas WO III, Almand JD, Stark GB, et al: Hand injuries secondary to subcutaneous illicit drug injections. *Ann Plast Surg* 34(1):27–31, 1995.
21. Smolyakov R, Riesenberg K, Schlaeffer F, et al: Streptococcal septic arthritis and necrotizing fasciitis in an intravenous drug user couple sharing needles. *Isr Med Assoc J* 4(4):302–303, 2002.
22. Johnston C, Keogan MT: Imaging features of soft-tissue infections and other complications in drug users after direct subcutaneous injection ("skin popping"). *AJR Am J Roentgenol* 182(5):1195–1202, 2004.
23. Majeski J, Majeski E: Necrotizing fasciitis: improved survival with early recognition by tissue biopsy and aggressive surgical treatment. *South Med J* 90(11):1065–1068, 1997.
24. al Zahrani HA: Vascular complications following intravascular self-injection of addictive drugs. *J R Coll Surg Edinb* 42(1):50–53, 1997.
25. Tsao JW, Marder SR, Goldstone J, et al: Presentation, diagnosis, and management of arterial mycotic pseudoaneurysms in injection drug users. *Ann Vasc Surg* 16(5):652–662, 2002.
26. Martin-Davila P, Navas E, Fortun J, et al: Analysis of mortality and risk factors associated with native valve endocarditis in drug users: the importance of vegetation size. *Am Heart J* 150(5):1099–1106, 2005.
27. Jain V, Yang MH, Kovacicova-Lezcano G, et al: Infective endocarditis in an urban medical center: association of individual drugs with valvular involvement. *J Infect* 57(2):132–138, 2008.
28. Baddour LM, Meyer J, Henry B: Polymicrobial infective endocarditis in the 1980s. *Rev Infect Dis* 13(5):963–970, 1991.
29. Habib G, Badano L: Recommendations for the practice of echocardiography in infective endocarditis. *Eur J Echocardiogr* 11(2):202–219, 2010.
30. Cecchi E, Imazio M, Tidu M, et al: Infective endocarditis in drug addicts: role of HIV infection and the diagnostic accuracy of Duke criteria. *J Cardiovasc Med (Hagerstown)* 8(3):169–175, 2007.
31. Abrams B, Sklaver A, Hoffman T, et al: Single or combination therapy of staphylococcal endocarditis in intravenous drug abusers. *Ann Intern Med* 90(5):789–791, 1979.
32. DiNubile MJ: Short-course antibiotic therapy for right-sided endocarditis caused by Staphylococcus aureus in injection drug users. *Ann Intern Med* 121(11):873–876, 1994.
33. Ribera E, Gomez-Jimenez J, Cortes E, et al: Effectiveness of cloxacillin with and without gentamicin in short-term therapy for right-sided Staphylococcus aureus endocarditis. A randomized, controlled trial. *Ann Intern Med* 125(12):969–974, 1996.
34. Levitsky S, Mammana RB, Silverman NA, et al: Acute endocarditis in drug addicts: surgical treatment for gram-negative sepsis. *Circulation* 66(2, Pt 2):I135–I138, 1982.
35. Popescu GA, Prazuck T, Poisson D, et al: A "true" polymicrobial endocarditis: Candida tropicalis and Staphylococcus aureus–to a drug user. Case presentation and literature review. *Rom J Intern Med* 43(1–2):157–161, 2005.
36. Baddour LM, Wilson WR, Bayer AS, et al: Infective endocarditis: diagnosis, antimicrobial therapy, and management of complications: a statement for healthcare professionals from the Committee on Rheumatic Fever, Endocarditis, and Kawasaki Disease, Council on Cardiovascular Disease in the Young, and the Councils on Clinical Cardiology, Stroke, and Cardiovascular Surgery and Anesthesia, American Heart Association: endorsed by the Infectious Diseases Society of America. *Circulation* 111(23):e394–e434, 2005.
37. Arbulu A, Holmes RJ, Asfaw I: Surgical treatment of intractable right-sided infective endocarditis in drug addicts: 25 years experience. *J Heart Valve Dis* 2(2):129–137, 1993; discussion 138–139.
38. Sapico FL, Liquete JA, Sarma RJ: Bone and joint infections in patients with infective endocarditis: review of a 4-year experience. *Clin Infect Dis* 22(5):783–787, 1996.
39. Beronius M, Bergman B, Andersson R: Vertebral osteomyelitis in Goteborg, Sweden: a retrospective study of patients during 1990–95. *Scand J Infect Dis* 33(7):527–532, 2001.
40. Gotway MB, Marder SR, Hanks DK, et al: Thoracic complications of illicit drug use: an organ system approach. *Radiographics* 22 Spec No:S119–S135, 2002.
41. Lafont A, Olive A, Gelman M, et al: Candida albicans spondylodiscitis and vertebral osteomyelitis in patients with intravenous heroin drug addiction. Report of 3 new cases. *J Rheumatol* 21(5):953–956, 1994.
42. Brancos MA, Peris P, Miro JM, et al: Septic arthritis in heroin addicts. *Semin Arthritis Rheum* 21(2):81–87, 1991.
43. Cooper JG, Spilke CE, Denton M, et al: Clostridium botulinum: an increasing complication of heroin misuse. *Eur J Emerg Med* 12(5):251–252, 2005.
44. Brazier JS, Gal M, Hall V, et al: Outbreak of clostridium histolyticum infections in injecting drug users in England and Scotland. *Euro Surveill* 9(9):15–16, 2004.
45. Brazier JS, Duerden BI, Hall V, et al: Isolation and identification of Clostridium spp. from infections associated with the injection of drugs: experiences of a microbiological investigation team. *J Med Microbiol* 51(11):985–989, 2002.
46. Booth MG, Hood J, Brooks TJ, et al: Anthrax infection in drug users. *Lancet* 375(9723):1345–1346, 2010.
47. Centers for Disease Control and Prevention (CDC): Trends in HIV/AIDS diagnoses—33 states, 2001–2004. *MMWR Morb Mortal Wkly Rep* 54(45):1149–1153, 2005.
48. Schoenbaum EE, Hartel D, Selwyn PA, et al: Risk factors for human immunodeficiency virus infection in intravenous drug users. *N Engl J Med* 321(13):874–879, 1989.
49. Nakamura N, Mausbach BT, Ulibarri MD, et al: Methamphetamine use, attitudes about condoms, and sexual risk behavior among HIV-positive men who have sex with men. *Arch Sex Behav* 40(2):267–272, 2009.
50. Nath A: Human immunodeficiency virus-associated neurocognitive disorder: pathophysiology in relation to drug addiction. *Ann N Y Acad Sci* 1187:122–128, 2010.
51. O'Connor PG, Selwyn PA, Schottenfeld RS: Medical care for injection-drug users with human immunodeficiency virus infection. *N Engl J Med* 331(7):450–459, 1994.
52. Caiaffa WT, Vlahov D, Graham NM, et al: Drug smoking, Pneumocystis carinii pneumonia, and immunosuppression increase risk of bacterial pneumonia in human immunodeficiency virus-seropositive injection drug users. *Am J Respir Crit Care Med* 150(6, Pt 1):1493–1498, 1994.

53. O'Donnell AE, Selig J, Aravamuthan M, et al: Pulmonary complications associated with illicit drug use. An update. *Chest* 108(2):460–463, 1995.
54. Choopanya K, Martin M, Suntharasamai P, et al: Antiretroviral prophylaxis for HIV infection in injecting drug users in Bangkok, Thailand (the Bangkok Tenofovir Study): a randomised, double-blind, placebo-controlled phase 3 trial. *Lancet* 381:2083–2090, 2013.
55. Beilke MA, Theall KP, O'Brien M, et al: Clinical outcomes and disease progression among patients coinfected with HIV and human T lymphotropic virus types 1 and 2. *Clin Infect Dis* 39(2):256–263, 2004.
56. Haverkos HW, Lange WR: From the alcohol, drug abuse, and mental health administration. Serious infections other than human immunodeficiency virus among intravenous drug abusers. *J Infect Dis* 161(5):894–902, 1990.
57. Kreek MJ, Des Jarlais DC, Trepo CL, et al: Contrasting prevalence of delta hepatitis markers in parenteral drug abusers with and without AIDS. *J Infect Dis* 162(2):538–541, 1990.
58. Centers for Disease Control (CDC): Hepatitis A among drug abusers. *MMWR Morb Mortal Wkly Rep* 37(19):297–300, 305, 1988.
59. Amon JJ, Garfein RS, Ahdieh-Grant L, et al: Prevalence of hepatitis C virus infection among injection drug users in the United States, 1994–2004. *Clin Infect Dis* 46(12):1852–1858, 2008.
60. Soriano V, Vispo E, Labarga P, et al: Viral hepatitis and HIV co-infection. *Antiviral Res* 85(1):303–315, 2010.
61. Koziel MJ, Peters MG: Viral hepatitis in HIV infection. *N Engl J Med* 356(14):1445–1454, 2007.
62. Aspinall EJ, Corson S, Doyle JS et al: Treatment of hepatitis C virus infection among people who are actively injecting drugs: a systematic review and meta-analysis. *Clin Infect Dis* 57[Suppl 2]:S80–S89, 2013.
63. Mast EE, Weinbaum CM, Fiore AE, et al; Advisory Committee on Immunization Practices (ACIP) Centers for Disease Control and Prevention (CDC): A comprehensive immunization strategy to eliminate transmission of hepatitis B virus infection in the United States. *MMWR Recomm Rep* 55(RR-16):1–33, 2006.
64. Shah DP, Grimes CZ, Nguyen AT, et al: Long-term effectiveness of accelerated hepatitis B vaccination schedule in drug users. *Am J Public Health* 105(6):e36–e43, 2015.
65. Siegal HA, Falck RS, Wang J, et al: History of sexually transmitted diseases infection, drug-sex behaviors, and the use of condoms among midwestern users of injection drugs and crack cocaine. *Sex Transm Dis* 23(4):277–282, 1996.
66. Pevzner ES, Robison S, Donovan J, et al: Tuberculosis transmission and use of methamphetamines and other drugs in Snohomish County, WA, 1991–2006. *Am J Public Health* 100(12):2481–2486, 2010.
67. Selwyn PA, Sckell BM, Alcabes P, et al: High risk of active tuberculosis in HIV-infected drug users with cutaneous anergy. *JAMA* 268(4):504–509, 1992.
68. Scholten JN, Driver CR, Munsiff SS, et al: Effectiveness of isoniazid treatment for latent tuberculosis infection among human immunodeficiency virus (HIV)-infected and HIV-uninfected injection drug users in methadone programs. *Clin Infect Dis* 37(12):1686–1692, 2003.
69. Hannan MM, Peres H, Maltez F, et al: Investigation and control of a large outbreak of multi-drug resistant tuberculosis at a central Lisbon hospital. *J Hosp Infect* 47(2):91–97, 2001.
70. Aaron L, Saadoun D, Calatroni I, et al: Tuberculosis in HIV-infected patients: a comprehensive review. *Clin Microbiol Infect* 10(5):388–398, 2004.
71. Bisbe J, Miro JM, Latorre X, et al: Disseminated candidiasis in addicts who use brown heroin: report of 83 cases and review. *Clin Infect Dis* 15(6):910–923, 1992.
72. Kim RW, Juzych MS, Eliott D: Ocular manifestations of injection drug use. *Infect Dis Clin North Am* 16(3):607–622, 2002.
73. Chuo CY, Fu YC, Lu YM, et al: Spinal infection in intravenous drug abusers. *J Spinal Disord Tech* 20(4):324–328, 2007.
74. Tunkel AR, Pradhan SK: Central nervous system infections in injection drug users. *Infect Dis Clin North Am* 16(3):589–605, 2002.
75. Hopkins RJ, Rothman M, Fiore A, et al: Cerebral mucormycosis associated with intravenous drug use: three case reports and review. *Clin Infect Dis* 19(6):1133–1137, 1994.
76. Markowitz N, Quinn EL, Saravolatz LD: Trimethoprimsulfamethoxazole compared with vancomycin for the treatment of Staphylococcus aureus infection. *Ann Intern Med* 117:390–398, 1992.
77. Fortun J, Navas E, Martínez-Beltrán J, et al: Short-course therapy for right-side endocarditis due to Staphylococcus aureus in drug abuser: Cloxacillin versus glycopeptides in combination with Gentamicin. *Clin Infect Dis* 33:120–125, 2001.

Chapter 78 ▪ Infective Endocarditis and Infections of Intracardiac Prosthetic Devices

SARAH H. CHEESEMAN • KAREN C. CARROLL • SARA E. COSGROVE

Infective endocarditis (IE) is an infection of the endothelial lining of the heart, characterized on pathologic study by vegetations. The infected site is usually a valve, but endocarditis may be situated on mural thrombi (rare) or the endothelial surface on which the jet stream from a stenotic lesion (patent ductus, ventricular septal defect, or stenotic valve) impinges. The term encompasses infection of the endothelial surface of any blood vessel, which most frequently occurs on hemodynamically or structurally abnormal ones such as abdominal aortic aneurysms, arteriovenous fistulas, and prosthetic grafts. The peculiarities of these infections are beyond the scope of this chapter, but the general principles of diagnosis and treatment are the same.

Significant changes in the epidemiology and character of IE have been noted since 1990 [1–10]. Shifting demographics, an expanding pool of elderly, chronically ill and immunocompromised patients, and rising rates of nosocomial bacteremia have been observed [1–10]. Unanticipated increases in societal behaviors that predispose to bacteremia, such as injection drug use, body art (including piercing and tattooing) [11], and acupuncture [12], have also contributed to the steady incidence of IE. All of the above have contributed to changes in the microbiology of IE [1–10]. Simultaneously, advances in diagnostic criteria and methods and improvements in cardiothoracic surgery have occurred. Taken together, there has not been a noticeable decline in either the incidence of or the mortality from IE [1–10].

Among published series of more than 100 patients between 1994 and 2008, reported mortality ranged from 10% to 37% [1–4,9,10], with the lowest mortality rates attributed to earlier and higher rates of surgery, short delay before treatment, or high doses of bactericidal drugs. Decline in mortality has occurred predominantly among young patients. Mortality remains high for the elderly [2,3,10,13], diabetics [14], patients with other predisposing diseases such as chronic renal failure requiring hemodialysis and immunosuppression [1,2,9,10,15–18], patients with discernible valvular vegetations [16], patients with healthcare-associated infections [10,17], and those infected with staphylococci, particularly methicillin-resistant *Staphylococcus aureus* (MRSA) [2,8,10,16,19].

Traditionally two clinical forms of endocarditis have been delineated: acute and subacute. Subacute disease denotes insidious onset, with slow development of the characteristic lesions and absence of marked toxicity for a long period. A high proportion of these cases occur on previously damaged valves and many are caused by organisms of relatively low virulence, such as α-hemolytic streptococci (viridans streptococci). In contrast, acute bacterial endocarditis presents as a fulminant infection, with abrupt onset, high fever, more frequent leukocytosis, and rapid downhill course with respect to both valve destruction and systemic toxicity. This is most frequently secondary to *S. aureus* and may occur on previously normal valves. Among patients who require intensive care, the acute form of infection will be the more frequent problem.

"Surgery during initial hospitalization independently of the completion of a full therapeutic course of antibiotics is indicated in patients with left-sided IE caused by *S. aureus*, fungal, or other highly resistant microorganisms" (http://www.jtcvsonline.org/article/S0022-5223(17)30116-2/pdf).

A classification that more accurately characterizes current trends in IE has been proposed [6]. Dividing IE into four major categories as follows may provide better delineation of clinical conditions and microbial pathogens [6]. These categories are (a) native valve endocarditis (NVE); (b) prosthetic valve endocarditis (PVE)—early (<12 months following surgery) and late (>12 months following surgery); (c) IE in the injection drug user; and (d) nosocomial IE.

All observers of IE have noted a decrease in the frequency of rheumatic heart disease as a predisposing lesion and an increase in degenerative diseases [3,6,7,9] and other previously unrecognized conditions such as mitral valve prolapse and idiopathic hypertrophic subaortic stenosis [15,16]. Taking these trends together, the universal observation of an increasing proportion of cases among older age groups is not surprising. The incidence of IE is higher among men compared with women among patients younger than 65 years and has remained relatively stable over the last several decades. In contrast, the incidence among women has significantly increased since 2000, especially among the elderly (>65 years) [8,9,13].

Populations particularly at risk of endocarditis are injection drug users and patients with prosthetic valves. Since the 1990s, other populations at risk have increased: transplant recipients [20,21], burn patients [22], patients with medical devices that put them at risk of bacteremia [9,17,23,24], and, most notably, persons on chronic hemodialysis [17,18,25,26].

Problems of endocarditis particularly relevant to patients in cardiac or intensive care units (ICUs) include the following:

1. Acute bacterial endocarditis,
2. Prosthetic valve endocarditis,
3. Endocarditis in patients with intravascular foreign bodies, such as pacemakers and indwelling vascular catheters,
4. Indications for surgery for endocarditis.

TABLE 78.1

Etiology of Endocarditis from Reported Large Series 1985 to 2005

Etiologic agents	Attributable range[a,b] (%)
Staphylococcus aureus	18–57
Viridans streptococci	11–53
Coagulase-negative staphylococci	1–15
Enterococci	4–10
Streptococcus gallolyticus (bovis)	1–13
β-Hemolytic streptococci	3–9
Streptococcus pneumoniae	1–3
Other streptococci	3–7
HACEK[c]	1–6
Enterobacteriaceae	1–4
Yeast	1–2
Molds	<1
Polymicrobial	1–6
Other bacteria[d]	2–11
Culture negative	2–39

[a]All figures are the percentage ranges of episodes reported.
[b]Rounded to nearest whole percentage.
[c]HACEK = *Haemophilus* sp., *Aggregatibacter actinomycetemcomitans, Cardiobacterium hominis, Eikenella corrodens, Kingella kingae.*
[d]Includes a variety of single isolates of species not represented by above genera, including *Neisseria* sp., *Pseudomonas, Legionella, Lactobacilli.*
Compiled from references [1–4,8,9,15,27–31].

ETIOLOGY

The term *infective endocarditis* properly includes the whole world of microorganisms that can cause the disease. Fungi, rickettsiae (*Coxiella burnetii*, which causes Q fever), *Chlamydia* sp., and perhaps even viruses have been implicated in endocarditis, although bacteria are still the predominant cause. Substantial advances in the isolation of microorganisms and improvements in serologic testing and molecular detection have widened the spectrum of causative organisms. Uncommon species of streptococci, emerging pathogens such as *Bartonella* sp. and *Tropheryma whipplei*, the increase in fungal pathogens among nosocomial cases and immunocompromised patients, and increasing resistance among "typical" endocarditis pathogens such as enterococci present unique diagnostic or therapeutic challenges [5,6,17,20–23,26].

Table 78.1 summarizes the most common pathogens from a large series of endocarditis cases that occurred between 1985 and 2005 [1–4,6–9,15,27–30]. Series with a large number of injection drug users [1,6,15,19,28], patients on chronic hemodialysis [1,2,10,18,23], transplant recipients [20,21], and those reporting healthcare-associated IE [1,6,7,10,17,23,24,26] tend to report more cases caused by *S. aureus*. Viridans streptococci occur more frequently but no longer predominate among non-injection drug user populations and the elderly [9]. Identification to species level among the viridans streptococci may have important therapeutic and prognostic implications. The *Streptococcus anginosus* (*milleri*) groups (*S. anginosus*, *S. constellatus*, and *S. intermedius*) are frequently associated with abscess formation and tend to cause severe disease but cause endocarditis less often than other viridans streptococci [31,32]. *S. anginosus* is the least likely among the three species to cause abscesses and the most likely to be associated with endocarditis [32,33]. The nutritionally deficient streptococci include the following genera and species: *Abiotrophia defectiva*, *Granulicatella adiacens*, *Granulicatella para-adiacens*, *Granulicatella balaenopterae*, and *Granulicatella elegans* [34,35]. Together these organisms constitute 3% to 5% of cases of endocarditis caused by viridans streptococci [35]. These organisms require pyridoxal, the active form of vitamin B_6, for growth. Unlike other species of viridans streptococci, these organisms are tolerant to penicillin, and at least one series [34] has found decreased susceptibility to penicillin, extended-spectrum cephalosporins, and macrolide antibiotics. High relapse rates are described especially when patients are treated with penicillin alone [35]. Most cases of viridans streptococcal endocarditis (80%) are caused by *Streptococcus sanguis*, *Streptococcus mitis*, or *Streptococcus mutans* [15,19,30,31]. There do not appear to be any statistically significant differences in the symptoms, demographics, or complications among patients with infections caused by this group of organisms. Newer species of viridans streptococci continue to be described.

Enterococci rank third in frequency of isolation for most series, including healthcare-associated cases and those among patients on hemodialysis. Among the non–viridans streptococci, pneumococci are still relatively uncommon causes of endocarditis (1% to 3% of all cases) [36]. The proportion of cases caused by β-hemolytic streptococci has not increased since 1980; infections with group B and group G are seen most frequently [33,37,38]. Patients with these infections usually have underlying valvular disease (including prosthetic valves) [39], numerous predisposing factors, most notably diabetes mellitus, and acute onset of their infection [33,37,38]. The organism formerly called *Streptococcus bovis,* a non-enterococcal group D streptococcus, belongs to a larger group including *Streptococcus gallolyticus*, based upon DNA–DNA reassociation studies [39]. Some of the newly described species and subspecies (e.g., *S. gallolyticus* subsp. *pasteurianus*) are more frequently associated with meningitis, while *S. gallolyticus*, subsp. *gallolyticus* is associated with endocarditis and with benign and malignant disorders of the gastrointestinal tract. In some series, this organism group has been increasing in frequency in Europe and South America [9], particularly among the elderly and among patients with chronic liver disease [4,40–42]. When this organism is isolated, the patient should be carefully evaluated for gastrointestinal tract malignancy, although it may occur months to years after the bacteremic episode [41]. In fact, colonoscopy during the admission for endocarditis found premalignant or malignant lesions in 49% of patients with this organism [43], which we will hereafter refer to as *Streptococcus gallolyticus (bovis)*, consistent with the usage in the American Heart Association (AHA) guidelines on IE [44]. *S. aureus* has increased in frequency and accounts for more than 50% of cases in more recent series [1,2,6,9,17,18,20,26,28]. In several recent prospective studies, including data from the International Collaboration on Endocarditis-Prospective Cohort Study (ICE-PCS), patients with *S. aureus* endocarditis were more likely than patients with IE due to other pathogens to have a shorter duration of symptoms before diagnosis, to be hemodialysis dependent, and to have other serious comorbidities such as diabetes mellitus or other chronic illnesses [9,10,45–48]. Patients with *S. aureus* IE were also more likely to have severe sepsis with persistent bacteremia, major neurologic events, systemic embolization, and death than patients with IE caused by other bacteria [46–48]. In these studies, patients with *S. aureus* IE frequently had healthcare-associated or nosocomial acquisition and were more likely to have MRSA infection than patients with community-acquired *S. aureus*. In the ICE-PCS series [41], a multivariate model identified the following patient characteristics associated with MRSA IE: persistent bacteremia, chronic immunosuppressive therapy, intravascular devices as sources, and diabetes mellitus. Overall, MRSA now accounts for 25% to 50% of the cases attributable to *S. aureus* [2,26,45–48]. Persistent bacteremia correlated with infection caused by MRSA, and risk of embolic phenomena was negatively associated with oxacillin resistance [45–48].

Coagulase-negative staphylococci (CoNS) are recognized pathogens on prosthetic valves and close to 8% of cases on native valves are now caused by these organisms [49]. The majority of the CoNS species recovered are *Staphylococcus epidermidis* [49]. *Staphylococcus lugdunensis* has emerged as a particularly aggressive pathogen that causes a destructive NVE, frequently following vasectomy or other procedures involving breaks in the skin in the perineal area [50]. In spite of universal susceptibility to *β*-lactams and other agents, mortality attributable to this pathogen is high, possibly related to the large vegetations frequently seen with this organism, leading to valvular dehiscence, abscess formation, and systemic embolization [50].

Before 1980, endocarditis caused by Gram-negative organisms comprised less than 3% of cases. Recent series report that Gram-negative organisms now account for 4% to 10% of all NVE [3,6,16,51], but these rates vary by geographic location, whether the infection is community or healthcare associated and the type of Gram-negative pathogen involved. Within this subset is the HACEK group (*Haemophilus* sp., *Aggregatibacter* [previously *Actinobacillus*] *actinomycetemcomitans*, *Cardiobacterium hominis*, *Eikenella corrodens*, *Kingella kingae*), which accounts for 2% to 5% of cases [8,9,27,51]. *A. actinomycetemcomitans* is the HACEK species most frequently involved in IE [51]. HACEK organisms are fastidious, nonmotile, slow-growing coccobacilli that require a mean of 3.3 days of incubation in automated blood culture systems for growth [51]. The HACEK organisms rarely cause endocarditis among patients without preexisting valvular disease or in the absence of predisposing factors [51].

Non-HACEK Gram-negative endocarditis (*Enterobacteriaceae* and others) remains relatively rare and is seen primarily among debilitated patients with healthcare-associated infections related to medical devices or surgery [22,52,53], including PVE. The same epidemiologic features are associated with polymicrobial endocarditis, but at least in one series of polymicrobial endocarditis, Gram-negative bacilli were isolated less often than CoNS and enterococci [54]. However, 12 cases of endocarditis due to non-HACEK Gram-negative bacilli (eight on prosthetic valves and two in injection drug users) and only seven due to HACEK organisms were seen at one hospital in Paris during the years 2009 to 2014 [55].

Bartonella quintana [56,57], the agent of trench fever, *Rochilimaea* subsp. nov. *elizabethae* [58], and *Bartonella henselae* [58], the agent of cat scratch disease, were first reported as causes of endocarditis in 1993. In 1995, *Bartonella quintana*, the agent of trench fever, was identified in middle-aged, homeless male alcoholics without known underlying valvular disease [59]. Since then, multiple additional species of *Bartonella* have been discovered [60–62]. Seven species and subspecies, namely *B. quintana*, *B. henselae* (the agent of cat scratch disease), *B. elizabethae*, *B. vinsonii* spp. *berkhoffii*, *B. vinsonii* spp. *arupensis*, *B. koehlerae*, and *B. alsatica* have been implicated in cases of endocarditis [60,61]. Contact with animals is a frequent association, and ectoparasites such as scabies, lice, and fleas are proposed as possible vectors of disease [60–62]. The majority of patients with *B. henselae* endocarditis have a previous history of underlying valvular disease and report contact with cats [60–62]. Characteristically, patients with *Bartonella* endocarditis present with a subacute course and large vegetations [60–62]. Diagnosis based on serology and molecular methods has established *Bartonella* spp. as the cause of 1.1% of cases of IE in the United Kingdom, 3% in France, Germany, and Brazil [63,64], and 4.5% in Egypt [65]. The laboratory that has diagnosed the largest number of cases reports that the frequency of this organism appears to be stable over time [63]. Because of the fastidious nature of the organism and serologic cross-reactivity between antibodies to *B. quintana* and *Chlamydia* sp., it is likely that cases of *Bartonella* endocarditis constitute a proportion of cases previously diagnosed as culture negative or due to *Chlamydia* sp. [60–62].

In spite of improvements in blood culture and serologic techniques, negative blood cultures can occur in up to 31% of cases [1–3,7,66]. There are several reasons cited for negative blood cultures in IE: (a) prior antibiotic administration; (b) infection with fastidious, slow-growing organisms (e.g., *Bartonella* sp., fungi, *Chlamydia* and *Coxiella* spp.); (c) infection with nonbacterial organisms such as fungi; or (d) endocarditis of patients with an indwelling cardiac device such as a pacemaker [66,67]. Two surveys [66,67] of culture-negative cases in France over two decades used serologic studies and molecular methods to augment blood cultures in determining the etiology for more than 348 [66] and 740 [67] patients, respectively. In the initial study of definite cases of IE, among the 79% of patients with blood culture–negative disease in whom an etiologic agent was identified, *C. burnetii* and *Bartonella* sp. predominated, accounting for 76% of the total [66]. Other rare bacteria included *T. whipplei*, *Mycoplasma hominis*, various streptococci, and *Legionella pneumophila* [66]. Twenty-one percent did not have an etiology determined, of whom 79% had received prior administration of antibiotics [66]. In the more recent prospective series, both definite and possible cases were included and an etiologic diagnosis was determined for 64.6%. The same group of organisms predominated [67].

IE among injection drug users has increased in the new millennium and *S. aureus* is by far the most common cause [68,69]. Enterococci, enteric Gram-negative bacilli, *Pseudomonas*, *Candida*, and other yeasts are also important [6,9,68]. Polymicrobial endocarditis is more common among injection drug users than in non-injection drug users in most series [6,9,19], but in a series from Spain, only one out of 60 cases of polymicrobial endocarditis was in an injection drug user [54].

The common causes of early-onset PVE are CoNS (mostly *S. epidermidis*), *S. aureus*, enterococci, diphtheroids, Gram-negative bacilli, and fungi. In 11 (44%) of 25 cases, enterococci caused endocarditis with onset <12 months after transcatheter aortic valve implantation (TAVI) in a review of the literature [70] and 21% of all cases of endocarditis in a multicenter registry of 7944 patients who underwent this procedure [71]. The incidence of endocarditis in the first year after TAVI appears similar to that after surgical valve replacement, 0.50% [71]. Among the fungi, *Candida* sp. are the most common cause of PVE and have emerged as causes of both early- and late-onset disease, especially among patients with healthcare-associated infection [72]. However, late-onset disease is still caused mainly by organisms such as CoNS and streptococci, although *S. aureus* accounts for about 11% of cases [9,19,73,74]. This difference is thought to be explained by intraoperative or early postoperative contamination of the prosthesis with resistant hospital flora in early PVE. Late cases represent either smoldering infections with relatively avirulent organisms seeded at the original surgery or subsequent transient bacteremias, such as those that induce endocarditis on native valves [74].

PATHOPHYSIOLOGY

The laboratory model of endocarditis is a rabbit in which a catheter passed through a valve produces mild trauma with the elaboration of a fibrin–platelet thrombus. Subsequent injection of bacteria either through the catheter or at a distant vascular site leads to infection of the traumatized valve [75]. It appears that the fibrin–platelet thrombus allows for avid binding of the bacteria [6]. Adherent bacteria induce blood monocytes to produce cytokines that contribute to further enlargement of the vegetation [76]. As the vegetation matures, the bacteria become fully enveloped, which allows for persistence by avoiding host defenses.

This model conforms to the propensity of damaged human valves toward endocarditis. Transient bacteremia with mouth flora, predominantly viridans streptococci, during chewing, toothbrushing, and the like, explains the pattern observed with subacute bacterial endocarditis [6]. More virulent organisms such as *S. aureus* seem to be able to invade even normal hearts. There are several factors expressed by this pathogen that make it more virulent. In addition to surface fibronectin-binding proteins that facilitate adherence, *S. aureus* produces exoenzymes and exotoxins that are controlled by global regulators, such as accessory gene regulator (*agr*) and staphylococcal accessory regulator (*sar*), the expression of which permits tissue invasion and destruction [6]. Intravenous drug users combine the injection of contaminated materials with particulate and often irritant matter, probably accounting for the frequency of endocarditis in this setting and the propensity for right heart involvement [68,77,78]. The use of intravascular central lines reaching near the tricuspid valve or even crossing tricuspid and pulmonic valves reproduces the rabbit model of endocarditis in humans. The introduction of bacteria through these lines causes the specter of iatrogenic endocarditis.

Once the fibrin–platelet thrombus has become infected, the pathologic process is the enlargement of this mass into a vegetation and invasion of tissue by the infection with eventual disruption. In addition to the mass of the vegetation, there are perforations or total erosions of valve cusps, rupture of chordae tendineae, fistulas from the sinus of Valsalva to atrium or pericardium, and burrowing myocardial abscesses.

Depending on the valve involved, the physiologic consequences may be predicted. Rarely, a vegetation will be so large as to function as an occlusive or stenotic lesion [78]. More often, the tissue destruction process predominates and valvular incompetence results. New regurgitant murmurs of mitral, tricuspid, or aortic origin may acutely stress the heart with resultant congestive failure. Aortic valve disease carries the worst prognosis [78] for several reasons: (a) the heart tolerates acute aortic insufficiency least well; (b) pericardial tamponade or massive left-to-right shunt may develop if a sinus of Valsalva aneurysm erodes into the pericardium or right atrium, respectively; (c) heart block may occur if a myocardial abscess invades the conducting system; and (d) aortic valve ring vegetations are most likely to be flipped into the coronary arteries, infarcting already overworked muscle. These catastrophes are all even more likely in the presence of a prosthetic aortic valve, in which case the infection has its seat at the annulus. Tricuspid valve endocarditis is the most benign. Even total tricuspid insufficiency can be tolerated for a time, and acute right-sided heart failure is not as life threatening as is the pulmonary edema of left-sided failure.

The vegetations themselves may break off in whole or part as emboli to the brain, viscera (spleen and kidney are particularly common targets), coronary arteries, and notably in fungal endocarditis, large arteries of the extremities. Septic emboli to the lungs can result in pulmonary infiltrates, often nodular and sometimes cavitating. Emboli to other organs produce infarction, which is usually bland, although splenic abscess, brain abscess, and even purulent meningitis may occur in staphylococcal endocarditis. The most common cerebral lesion, however, is embolic infarct with the clinical appearance of a stroke [78,79]. The smaller vascular lesions of endocarditis may be of an immunologic, vasculitic nature or truly embolic and suppurative in character. Emboli to the vasa vasorum or vasculitis of the arteries lead to mycotic aneurysms of both cerebral and peripheral vessels. The cerebral aneurysms are generally asymptomatic until they rupture and present as subarachnoid or intracerebral hemorrhage. Peripheral mycotic aneurysms may come to attention because of their obvious enlargement, pulsation, and frequent overlying inflammation. Other phenomena that fall into this category are the cutaneous stigmata of endocarditis—Osler's nodes, Janeway lesions, splinter hemorrhages, and petechiae—as well as the frequent renal involvement. Kidney pathology may take several forms: localized renal infarcts, vasculitic glomerulonephritis, acute diffuse glomerulonephritis thought to represent immune complex disease, renal cortical necrosis, and interstitial nephritis likely related to antibiotic administration [78].

DIAGNOSIS

Endocarditis is diagnosed on the basis of signs and symptoms that reflect the pathology: fever, embolic phenomena, and evidence of valvular dysfunction. A continuous bacteremia is characteristic and, indeed, highly suggestive of endovascular infection, although the entity of culture-negative endocarditis also exists. The frequency of various findings in IE is shown in Table 78.2 [1,3,4,9,15,19,28].

Criteria

Proof of the diagnosis, in terms of histopathologic confirmation of vegetation with infecting organisms on the affected valve, may be obtained only in cases requiring cardiac surgery or, in the event of death, with autopsy. Clinical criteria for the diagnosis sufficiently stringent to allow for analysis of case characteristics, epidemiology, and the outcome of therapy have been devised and revised over the years with the latest version known as the Duke criteria [27]. The Duke criteria incorporate echocardiographic findings in addition to giving heavy weight to clinical circumstances such as the type of organisms recovered from blood and injection drug use as a predisposing factor. Major and minor criteria analogous to the Jones criteria for diagnosis of rheumatic fever are summarized in Table 78.3. A definite diagnosis requires the presence of two major criteria, one major and three minor criteria, or five minor criteria. The diagnosis is rejected if a firm alternate diagnosis adequately explains the clinical findings, they resolve with less than 4 days of antibiotic therapy, or histopathologic evidence is lacking at autopsy or surgery performed after no more than 4 days of antibiotic

TABLE 78.2

Clinical Features of Endocarditis

Feature	Frequency range (%)
History	
Fever	81–98
Malaise/weakness	49–96
Weight loss	6–30
Musculoskeletal complaints	9–25
Mental status change/neurologic event	11–32
Previous heart disease	25–55
Physical examination	
Fever	54–95
Murmur	76–95
Change in murmur	10–67
Splenomegaly	1–29
Petechiae	12–16
Osler's nodes	3–16
Janeway lesions	3–5
Splinters	3–35
Fundoscopic abnormalities	0–3
Clubbing	6–20
Lab tests	
Hematuria	26–53
↑ESR	22–89
Rheumatoid factor	5–51
Anemia	66–68
Echocardiographic vegetations[a]	60–86

[a]Combined transthoracic and transesophageal results.
↑ESR, elevated erythrocyte sedimentation rate.
Data compiled from references [1,3,4,15,19,28].

therapy. All other clinically suspect cases meriting more than 4 days of antibiotic treatment are classified as possible [27].

Several studies have demonstrated very good sensitivity and excellent specificity (92% to 99%) for the Duke criteria [80–82]. Moreover, these criteria have been evaluated for the diagnosis of IE in children [83] and the elderly [84], as well as in patients with PVE [85]. Several criticisms and proposed modifications have followed these rigorous studies. The inability of the Duke criteria to reject cases that receive more than 4 days of antibiotic therapy may lead to occasional overdiagnosis of endocarditis [86]. Modifications to the major and minor criteria, including serologic evidence of *Coxiella burnetii* (the agent of Q fever) infection and the category of "possible" endocarditis, requiring one major and one minor criterion or three minor criteria, as proposed by Li [87], are now recognized, as listed in Table 78.3.

History

The most frequent symptoms reported by patients with endocarditis are fever and malaise, but some present with acute musculoskeletal symptoms, most frequently lower back pain or polyarthralgia [88], and others, because of an embolus, without complaining of or even noticing fever [89]. A common feature of endocarditis is loss of appetite, and its return may be the first clinical sign of response to treatment. Any febrile illness of a patient with known valvular heart disease must bring to mind the question of endocarditis, as should fever in an injection drug user, especially with pleuritic pain. Other clinical scenarios in which endocarditis should be strongly considered include fever and back pain, stroke (particularly with fever or in a young person), acute unexplained renal failure, persistent bacteremia, and bacteremia with a suspect organism (especially *S. aureus* or enterococcus) and no source. Similarly, a history of recent

TABLE 78.3

Duke Criteria and Proposed Modified Duke Criteria for Definitive Clinical Diagnosis of Endocarditis

Major criteria

1. Positive blood culture for infective endocarditis
   - Typical microorganisms for infective endocarditis from two separate blood cultures
   - Viridans streptococci, *Streptococcus bovis*, HACEK group, or *Staphylococcus aureus* or community-acquired enterococci in the absence of a primary focus, or
   - Persistently positive blood culture, defined as recovery of a microorganism consistent with infective endocarditis from
     - A. Blood cultures drawn more than 12 h apart, or
     - B. All of three or a majority of four or more separate blood cultures, with first and last drawn at least 1 h apart
     - C. Single positive blood culture for *Coxiella burnetii* or anti-phase 1 IgG antibody titer ≥ 1:800
2. Evidence of endocardial involvement
   - Positive echocardiogram for IE (TEE recommended in patients with prosthetic valves, rated at least "possible IE" by clinical criteria, or complicated IE [paravalvular abscess]; TTE as first test in other patients), defined as:
     - A. Oscillating intracardiac mass on valve or supporting structures, or in the path of regurgitant jets, or on implanted material, in the absence of an alternative anatomic explanation, or
     - B. Abscess, or
     - C. New partial dehiscence of prosthetic valve, or new valvular regurgitation (increase or change in preexisting murmur not sufficient)

Minor criteria

1. Predisposition: predisposing heart condition or injection drug use
2. Fever: >38.0°C (100.4°F)
3. Vascular phenomena: major arterial emboli, septic pulmonary infarcts, mycotic aneurysm, intracranial hemorrhage, conjunctival hemorrhages, Janeway lesions
4. Immunologic phenomena: glomerulonephritis, Osler's nodes, Roth spots, rheumatoid factor
5. Microbiologic evidence: positive blood culture but not meeting major criterion as noted previously or serologic evidence of active infection with organism[a] consistent with infective endocarditis

A definite diagnosis requires the presence of two major criteria, one major and three minor criteria, or five minor criteria. A possible diagnosis requires one major and one minor criterion, or thee minor criteria.
[a]Excluding single positive blood cultures for coagulase-negative staphylococci and organisms that do not cause endocarditis.
HACEK, *Haemophilus sp., Aggregatibacter actinomycetemcomitans, Cardiobacterium hominis, Eikenella corrodens, Kingella kingae*; IE, infective endocarditis; TEE, transesophageal echocardiography.
Modified from Durack DT, Lukes AS, Bright DK: New criteria for diagnosis of infective endocarditis: utilization of specific echocardiographic findings. Duke Endocarditis Service. *Am J Med* 96:200–209, 1994 and Li JS, Sexton DJ, Mick N, et al: Proposed modifications to the Duke criteria for the diagnosis of infective endocarditis. *Clin Infect Dis* 30:633–638, 2000.

dental cleaning or extraction or genitourinary manipulation may indicate an opportunity for bacteremia and seeding of the valve and should be sought, as should suggestions of injection drug abuse. The history of appropriate antibiotic prophylaxis for these procedures is not sufficient to exclude the possibility of endocarditis, because failures occasionally occur with currently recommended regimens.

It is important to establish the duration and tempo of the illness by history. Abrupt onset of symptoms, shaking chills, and body temperature greater than 38.9°C (102°F) strongly suggest acute endocarditis. Subacute bacterial endocarditis, in contrast, is characterized by a vague illness occurring over a period of several weeks or months.

Physical Examination

In contrast to the vagueness of the symptoms of endocarditis, many findings on physical examination are characteristic. Most pertinent to the diagnosis are cardiac murmurs and mucocutaneous embolic phenomena. Any heart murmur is compatible with a diagnosis of endocarditis because it is evidence of the turbulent flow that provides the proper nidus for infection. The fact that a murmur has been documented for a long time in no way excludes the possibility of active endocarditis. Changing murmurs, particularly new regurgitant murmurs, are much less commonly observed but are highly significant with respect to both certainty of the diagnosis and functional consequences. Thus, patients must be examined both supine and sitting up leaning forward so that an aortic regurgitant murmur is not missed. Careful listening on both sides of the sternum during inspiration is important to detect tricuspid insufficiency. Signs of congestive heart failure are not early findings in endocarditis, but must be watched for, because the onset of failure signals a need to consider cardiac surgical intervention.

The most commonly observed mucocutaneous lesions of endocarditis are petechiae. They most often appear on the plantar surface of the toes and fingertips, as well as the conjunctival and buccal mucosa (see Fig. 78.1B). They may be larger and more irregular in outline than conventional petechiae and sometimes have a white or even pustular center. Conjunctival petechiae commonly occur in patients on cardiopulmonary bypass [90], so it is necessary to record their presence or absence on first encounter with a patient after cardiac surgery and to interpret only those that develop under observation. The same necessity applies to subungual splinter hemorrhages, which are so commonly a result of trauma that many patients will have one or two on admission; only those which appear subsequently, while the patient is at rest in the hospital, have diagnostic usefulness [91].

Osler's nodes and Janeway lesions favor the plantar and palmar surfaces but are uncommon in recent series of endocarditis. Osler's node is a painful, tender, bluish-purple nodular lesion located on the pads of the fingers or toes. The Janeway lesion is a painless, pink, nontender macular lesion that is located commonly on the palms or soles [91,92].

Fundoscopic examination may also show evidence of endocarditis. Showering of emboli often occurs, as in the patient whose findings are illustrated in Figure 78.1. The fingertip, subungual, conjunctival, and retinal lesions all developed the day after admission for acute renal failure, subsequently found

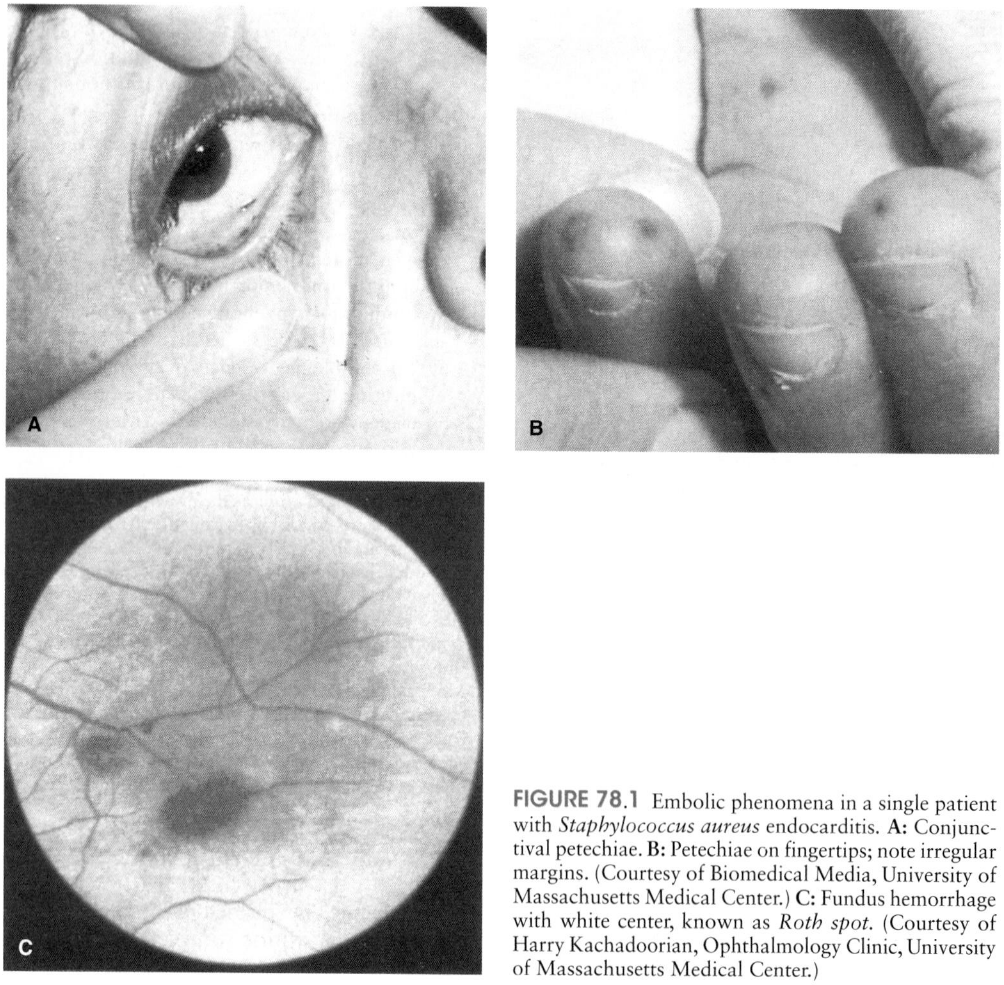

FIGURE 78.1 Embolic phenomena in a single patient with *Staphylococcus aureus* endocarditis. **A:** Conjunctival petechiae. **B:** Petechiae on fingertips; note irregular margins. (Courtesy of Biomedical Media, University of Massachusetts Medical Center.) **C:** Fundus hemorrhage with white center, known as *Roth spot.* (Courtesy of Harry Kachadoorian, Ophthalmology Clinic, University of Massachusetts Medical Center.)

to be due to *S. aureus* endocarditis. Splenomegaly is found in nearly half of the patients with subacute bacterial endocarditis and in very few of those with acute disease.

Laboratory Tests

The key to the diagnosis of endocarditis is blood cultures. The current practice of early initiation of antimicrobial therapy for acutely ill patients has led to the recommendation that at least three separate blood cultures be drawn from separate sites with a minimum of 1 hour between the first and the last [44]. Strict aseptic technique and optimal skin preparation should be used when collecting blood cultures and the blood cultures should be obtained prior to administration of antibiotics [44]. In adults, 20 to 30 mL of blood per culture is optimal [44]. In cases that appear to be culture negative [66,67,93], the advice of a clinical microbiologist should be sought regarding the need for special media, such as those adequate for the propagation of *Brucella* sp., *Bartonella* organisms, or other nonculture-based tests such as serology and molecular methods (see later). Prolonging the incubation of standard blood culture bottles beyond 7 days has not been demonstrated to be necessary for successful recovery of HACEK organisms, nor does it significantly improve diagnostic yield of other fastidious pathogens [93–95].

Diphtheroids and CoNS should not be disregarded as skin contaminants if isolated repeatedly; they are well established causes of endocarditis. A particularly troublesome problem is the recovery of CoNS of different colony types or susceptibility patterns from different blood cultures. This is not necessarily evidence for multiple contaminated cultures because the pattern can be observed in true coagulase-negative staphylococcal endocarditis.

Fungal endocarditis has become more frequent. Fungi most commonly isolated include *Candida albicans*, followed by *Candida parapsilosis*, then other non-albicans species of *Candida* [96], *Aspergillus* sp., and *Histoplasma* sp. [72,97]. In one review, emerging fungi accounted for 25% of cases [97]. Among patients with fungal endocarditis, the overall frequency of positive blood cultures is 54% [97]. Among cases of endocarditis caused by *Candida* sp., the percentage of positive blood cultures may be as high as 83% to 95% if appropriate methods are used [93].

Current commercially available routine manual and automated blood culture systems are usually able to recover yeasts within 5 to 7 days of incubation. The best chances for recovery of filamentous fungi such as *Aspergillus* or *Histoplasma* require the use of the lysis centrifugation method (Isolator, Wampole Laboratories, Cranbury, NJ) [93]. Premortem microbiologic diagnosis may often be made by culture and special histologic stains of large arterial emboli or cardiac vegetations [66,97].

Noncultivatable or difficult to cultivate organisms may be detected by serologic or molecular studies. Such organisms include *C. burnetii*, the agent of Q fever endocarditis, *Chlamydia* sp., *Bartonella* sp., and some fungi [60–62,66,67,97,98]. Timely inclusion of serologic studies, particularly in environments where Q fever, *Brucella*, and *Bartonella* sp. are prevalent, can enhance the definitive diagnosis of cases of endocarditis as demonstrated in the studies by Raoult et al. [67,99].

Molecular techniques such as polymerase chain reaction and sequence analysis of the amplified DNA have been applied to blood cultures, whole (EDTA) blood, and to valvular tissue removed at the time of surgery [63,67,100,101]. Several studies have demonstrated the utility of these methods in assessing patients with high pretest probability of endocarditis but who have negative blood cultures by standard methods. Many of these studies are well summarized in the review by Syed et al. [100]. Advantages include high sensitivity, rapid results, and accurate identification. Limitations include potential for contamination and lack of an organism to test for antimicrobial susceptibility [67,100,101].

Other Diagnostic Tests

The electrocardiogram (ECG) is the simplest test for evaluation of perivalvular extension of infection in endocarditis [102]. Persistent (2 to 3 days) prolongation of the PR interval in the absence of digitalis toxicity, new persistent bundle-branch block, or complete heart block is quite specific for predicting extension into myocardial or aortic root tissue and the subsequent need for surgery [102]. However, the absence of PR prolongation does not rule out perivalvular extension.

Echocardiography plays an essential role in the diagnosis and management of IE and should be performed in all cases of suspected endocarditis [44,103,104]. Current roles for echocardiography include (a) diagnosis of IE by demonstration of vegetations, (b) characterization of underlying valvular disease, (c) clarification of the destructive nature of endocarditis, (d) assessment of the persistently febrile patient for evidence of perivalvular extension of infection, and (e) assessment of valvular function for PVE.

Studies performed in the period between 1988 and 1998 demonstrated that transthoracic two-dimensional (2D) echocardiography (TTE) has an overall sensitivity of vegetation detection of 50%, with a range of 14% to 78% in published series [105–107]. Sensitivity is affected by vegetation size, with 25% of vegetations less than 5 mm and 70% between 6 and 10 mm detected [108]. Obesity, chronic lung disease, and thoracic deformity may preclude obtaining the high-quality images needed to detect vegetations in as many as 30% of patients [108,109]. Equivocal results due to thickening or myxomatous degeneration of native valves and artifact from prosthetic valves are problems with TTE [106,109]. Diagnostic yield is also influenced by experience and skill of the person performing the procedure and the pretest probability of endocarditis. TTE has very limited ability to detect valve perforations and abscess extension, especially on prosthetic heart valves. Technologic advances such as harmonic imaging and digital processing and storage have improved TTE image quality [100,110]. At least one report describes improved sensitivity to more than 80% using contemporary TTE [110]. Transesophageal echocardiography (TEE) is a significant advance for the evaluation of the patient with IE [100,106,111]. Unlike TTE, TEE has a high negative predictive value for patients with suspect NVE (86% to 97%) [100,106,111]. Despite the somewhat invasive nature of TEE, the procedure is quite safe when performed by a skilled physician, with interruption of the procedure or complications occurring less than 1% of the time [112]. Relative contraindications include esophageal diseases, severe atlantoaxial joint disease, prior irradiation to the chest, and perforated viscus [113].

Image quality of the TEE benefits from the high-resolution transducer and unobstructed view of cardiac structures [102,106–109]. The TEE is much more sensitive than TTE for the detection of valvular vegetations; sensitivity with current biplane TEE is 90%, with vegetations as small as 1 mm being seen [112,114–116]. Early studies on 3D TEE demonstrate the potential of this technology to enhance localization of vegetations [117]. Like the situation with 3D TTE, however, large series demonstrating superiority are lacking.

TEE is also superior to TTE for detection of perivalvular abscess, with approximately 87% sensitivity [105,114]. TEE appears to be the optimal tool to detect vegetations on prosthetic valves and to assess valve dysfunction. Likewise, TEE is superior to TTE for detecting infections of pacemaker leads [109,116–119]. TEE also appears superior to TTE in the intraoperative assessment of cardiac structure and hemodynamics [116,118].

The AHA guidelines [44] prefer TEE for all patients with suspected endocarditis, but do accept that it may be omitted when TTE is diagnostic for endocarditis and the likelihood of complications is felt to be low. TEE is definitely indicated for the diagnosis of endocarditis in the presence of a prosthetic valve and when clinical suspicion of endocarditis is high but TTE is negative [44,103,104]. Whenever TEE is positive, TTE views of the areas with abnormal findings should be obtained for comparison during follow-up [44]. The European Society of Cardiology (ESC) practice guidelines [103] similarly recommend TEE for all cases except those for whom good quality TTE images and unequivocal findings demonstrate isolated right-sided endocarditis. All of the guidelines agree that echocardiography should be repeated when the initial imaging is negative and clinical suspicion remains high: TTE or TEE in 3 to 5 days [103], TEE in 5 to 7 days [44], TTE or TEE in 7 to 10 days [104]. TEE should also be obtained when the TTE is positive but the patient's clinical course suggests the development of cardiac complications [44,103,104].

Investigators have attempted to determine cost-effective uses of echocardiography for patients with suspected endocarditis [120,121]. Some advocate that if the pretest probability is high (ranging from 4% to 60%), it is more cost-effective to proceed directly to TEE as the first and only study [120]. For determination of duration of therapy for catheter-associated *S. aureus* bacteremia (SAB), TEE is probably most cost-effective when used to stratify patients to short (2 weeks) or long (4 weeks) course therapy, when long-course therapy would have otherwise been chosen for an at-risk, native valve population without immunocompromise [121].

The prognostic implications of vegetations identified by echocardiographic studies remain controversial. Some recent studies have indicated an increased risk of embolization in patients with vegetations greater than or equal to 10 mm in size, particularly in patients with mitral valve disease [122,123]. Still others have found that the predictive value of size for embolization depended on the organism and the mobility of the vegetation [122–124]. Most investigators agree that the presence of a vegetation alone is not an independent indication for valve replacement [122,123].

Although emboli may occur in as many as 16% of patients with Duke definite endocarditis who do not have vegetations on echocardiography [125], vegetations greater than or equal to 10 mm in size are associated with an increased risk of embolization [122,123,125]. Mitral location, causative organism, and the mobility of the vegetation also contribute to embolic risk, and echocardiography may be useful for stratifying patients to high-risk subgroups where early surgery should be considered [122–125].

TEE is inconclusive in 10% to 20% of patients with suspected IE [126]. Adjunctive imaging modalities such as multislice computed tomography (CT) are complementary to TEE and may improve diagnosis rates in difficult-to-detect cases. Further, CT may have advantages in detecting perivalvular diseases associated with IE such as root abscess, pseudoaneurysm, or fistula, as well as in the evaluation of patients with extensive valvular calcifications. CT is inferior to TEE in detecting small vegetations and valve perforations, and its use is limited among patients with poor renal function or who cannot tolerate iodinated contrast [127]. Molecular imaging modalities such as ^{18}F-fluorodesoxyglucose (^{18}F-FDG) positron emission tomography or single photon emission computed tomography have also shown promise in confirming the diagnosis in patients with suspected IE by Duke criteria, nearly doubling the diagnostic sensitivity for IE compared to using the Duke criteria alone [127]. However, these molecular modalities are time-consuming, expensive, and may not be able to differentiate IE from inflammatory changes due to surgery or other conditions such as vasculitis [126]. Neither U.S. nor European guidelines currently recommend the routine use of alternative imaging modalities such as CT or nuclear imaging in the diagnosis of IE [44,103], but their adjunctive use alongside traditional cardiac imaging modalities may prove useful in the evaluation of patients with perivalvular extension of disease or with inconclusive echocardiographic findings.

DIFFERENTIAL DIAGNOSIS

By far, the most common difficulty confronting the present-day practitioner is deciding which episodes of bacteremia represent endocarditis. The question becomes particularly acute for patients with intravascular foreign bodies, such as pacemakers, valves, and patches, and when the organism is *S. aureus*. The approach to this problem must take into account the propensity for the foreign body to become infected, the propensity of the organism to cause endocarditis, and the duration of bacteremia. Because sustained bacteremia characterizes infection of endovascular sites, the longer the bacteremia lasts, the greater the concern for an endothelial origin. In addition, even if the origin is distant and known, the longer the organisms circulate, the greater is the risk that they have settled out and seeded the intravascular foreign body secondarily.

Prosthetic valves, both mechanical and of biologic origin, have a very high risk of becoming infected, whereas permanent pacemakers (PPMs), once endothelialized, appear to carry a relatively low risk. Infection usually occurs at the skin–catheter junction and thus is most likely to invade the circulation when the vessel is in close proximity to the skin wound. However, for patients with a PPM, sustained bacteremia without an obvious focus implies infection of the pacemaker electrode, the tricuspid valve, or fibrotic endocardial regions in contact with the electrode tip [128].

Enteric Gram-negative bacilli are among the most common blood culture isolates at most hospitals but are less common as a cause of endocarditis (see Table 78.1). Notable exceptions to this characterization of enteric Gram-negative bacilli are salmonellae, particularly *S. typhimurium* and *S. choleraesuis*, which seem to have an affinity for damaged vascular endothelium and have infected aortic aneurysms as well as cardiac devices [129]. AIDS patients older than 50 years who develop salmonella bacteremia in the setting of predisposing valvular disease appear to be at particular risk of endocarditis [53,130].

Nosocomial bacteremia with Gram-negative bacilli has been shown to constitute a risk for development of PVE. Fang et al. [131] found that 26% of new cases of PVE occurred among patients who developed nosocomial Gram-negative bacteremia, in most cases from an identifiable portal of entry. Thus, patients with Gram-negative bacteremia in the setting of a prosthetic valve should receive antibiotic therapy adequate for possible endocarditis.

SAB always raises the question of whether treatment as endocarditis is warranted. A classical study reported that 64% of all bacteremias with *S. aureus* from 1940 to 1954 represented endocarditis, proved by autopsy in 38% of cases [132]. A subsequent report from the same center defined 16% of 134 patients with SAB from 1975 to 1977 as having definite or probable endocarditis [133]. These and other studies have amply demonstrated the ability of *S. aureus* to produce endocarditis on a valve previously presumed normal and have shown that established endocarditis may be found at postmortem examination in patients in whom no murmur was ever heard during their lifetime [48,132]. The changing demographics of staphylococcal endocarditis have been discussed in detail in the "Etiology" section of this chapter.

The absence of a primary focus appears to be a powerful predictor of endocarditis from community-acquired staphylococcal bacteremia [48,134]. Injection drug users are also at high risk of endocarditis and metastatic abscesses, and SAB should be treated in a fashion appropriate to endocarditis whenever it occurs in this group.

IE has been shown to be clinically occult in a high proportion of patients with staphylococcal bacteremia [135]. TEE has been valuable for identifying which patients have endocarditis in the setting of staphylococcal bacteremia [45,121,135]. One study examined the use of a scrupulous definition of negative TTE plus clinical criteria (absence of any of the following high-risk features: community-acquired *S. aureus* bacteremia [SAB], prosthetic valves or valve repair materials, intracardiac devices, history of prior endocarditis, or injection drug use) among patients with SAB [136]. A TTE was called negative only if it was not suboptimal or indeterminate in any way and had no abnormality, even if that abnormality did not fulfill any criteria for endocarditis, strictures that excluded 22% of the TTEs performed. In their validation cohort of 268 patients with SAB and a 14.2% prevalence of endocarditis, these rules would have missed only one case of IE, a negative predictive value of 99% [136].

Several studies support the use of a 2-week course of antibiotic therapy for catheter-associated SAB in patients at low risk of endocarditis. This would include patients without valvular heart disease (or prosthetic valves) and in whom the catheter has been removed promptly, subsequent blood cultures are negative, defervescence occurred within 72 hours, and TEE is normal [121,137,138]. Failures may still occur in up to 16% of cases assessed as low risk using these criteria [138]; recurrences are reported in 5% to 24% of patients with catheter-associated SAB, usually within 10 weeks of discontinuing therapy [139,140]. Clearly, patients who have prolonged fever or bacteremia after catheter removal should receive the longer course of antibiotic therapy because of the high mortality from catheter-associated *S. aureus* endocarditis [46,139,140]. All patients with SAB, whether treated with short or longer courses of therapy, should be followed closely for at least 3 months following treatment, preferably by an infectious diseases specialist [141].

The overall mortality rate for staphylococcal endocarditis in one multicenter study ranged from 16.7% to 23.7% [46]. Overall mortality rates of 36% to 48% have been reported during the last decade [142]. In contrast, human immunodeficiency virus (HIV)–seronegative parenteral drug users with this disease have a 2% to 4% mortality rate, although considerable morbidity, including congestive heart failure, occurs in 23% [142]. The more favorable outcome of injecting drug users is generally attributed to their younger age and absence of underlying systemic illness, as well as the location of their valve involvement (right-sided valvular disease). In the HIV-seropositive injection drug user, mortality is related to the degree of immunosuppression [143]. In one study, for patients with CD4 counts of 200 or more, there was no difference in mortality between HIV-positive and HIV-negative individuals and mortality was directly related to the valve involved [142].

The epidemiology of enterococcal bacteremia has also changed [144]. Enterococci have emerged as major causes of healthcare-associated infections and in so doing have become increasingly resistant to antimicrobial agents, most importantly the penicillins, aminoglycosides, and glycopeptides [17,144–146]. Frequently, the enterococcus occurs in polymicrobial bacteremic infections along with enteric Gram-negative bacilli [146], but it may also accompany other Gram-positive organisms, particularly CoNS [54]. Mortality attributed to enterococcal bacteremia is high, ranging from 13% to 42%, and seems to correlate directly with the severity of underlying illness as well as with antimicrobial resistance [146,147]. Higher mortality rates are seen among patients infected with strains that have high-level aminoglycoside resistance and resistance to vancomycin [146–148].

Two case series of patients with enterococcal bacteremia examined the risk factors for development of endocarditis [144,145]. These studies refute previous reports that nosocomial bacteremia and polymicrobial infections with enterococci are rarely associated with endocarditis. In both studies, *E. faecalis* was the predominant enterococcal species. Approximately 60% of the patients had nosocomial infections and polymicrobial bacteremia varied from 17% to 37%. Factors that were significantly associated with endocarditis included three or more positive blood cultures, the presence of a prosthetic valve, underlying valvular disease, and infection with *E. faecalis* [144,145].

INFECTIONS OF CARDIOVASCULAR IMPLANTABLE ELECTRONIC DEVICES: PACEMAKERS, AUTOMATIC IMPLANTABLE CARDIOVERTER DEFIBRILLATORS, AND VENTRICULAR ASSIST DEVICES

Cardiovascular implantable electronic devices (CIEDs) are essential for the management of cardiac disease, and their use has increased significantly in the United States [149,150]. A recent population-based survey on the use of CIEDs reported that 70% of device recipients are elderly and many of these patients have multiple coexisting illnesses placing them at risk of CIED infections [151]. Despite improvements in the technology and greater ease of implantation, CIED infections appear to be increasing with the probability of infection being higher among patients with implantable cardioverter defibrillators (ICDs) than with PPMs [149,152,153]. Nearly 50% of patients in one series had undergone invasive procedures or hospitalization within the 6 months preceding their CIED infections [153].

Several recent studies have identified risk factors for PPM infection including long-term corticosteroid use, the presence of more than two pacing leads versus two leads, fever within 24 hours of implantation, early reinterventions, and the use of temporary pacing before the implantation [154,155]. Other patients at risk include those individuals with diabetes mellitus, renal dysfunction, heart failure, and oral anticoagulant use [149,153]. Studies that examined this outcome showed a lower risk of infection among patients given perioperative antimicrobial prophylaxis for the implantation procedure [149,154,155].

Infections of pacemakers can be divided into the following distinct syndromes:

- Generator pocket infections, which tend to occur within 2 months of surgery and are usually caused by *S. aureus*.
- Infections associated with the lead wire and electrode, which generally present months later and are more typically caused by CoNS.
- Endocarditis, which usually follows contiguous spread of infection along the pacer system.

Inflammation at the generator pocket may be absent or detectable only at surgery in patients with the latter two syndromes [150].

Local erythema, erosion over the generator site, or drainage characterizes pocket infections, whereas electrode infections and endocarditis present more typically with sepsis and sustained bacteremia. Among cases of pacemaker endocarditis, TEE is a useful diagnostic tool for defining the pacemaker as the source of bacteremia by visualizing vegetations on the leads or the tricuspid valve, as well as the possibility of left-sided valvular involvement, myocardial abscess, and other cardiac complications [103,119,149,150,156].

Infections that involve pacemaker wires and electrodes are almost never cured with antibiotics alone, and the entire system should be removed [103,149,156]. This usually can be accomplished in a one-stage procedure in which the old system is removed and the new system placed at a site remote from the infection (usually the contralateral side), followed by a course of antibiotics [149]. However, temporary pacing is not recommended and new device placement should be delayed until blood cultures have been negative for at least 72 hours in cases of bacteremia, and only if reevaluation of the indications determines that it is still required [103,149]. The optimal duration of antimicrobial therapy depends upon the extent of infection and whether bacteremia is present. Short-course therapy following extraction may be possible for infections confined to the pacer pocket in the absence of bacteremia, whereas much longer duration of treatment is essential in patients with bacteremia. Patients with *S. aureus* bacteremia and no obvious source should have all hardware removed. Guidelines for management are discussed in detail elsewhere [103,149].

Removal of the old system may not always be easy to accomplish. Sometimes defective or infected electrodes become firmly enclosed by fibrous tissue and are adherent to the vessel endothelium, precluding easy extraction through the venous system. Removal of a retained wire using traction devices has been successful in some instances, but serious complications such as avulsion of the tricuspid valve and creation of atrioventricular fistulae have been reported [156].

Specialized tools have been developed to remove leads from fibrotic tissue. The newest technologies are laser sheath devices. A multicenter study reviewed the experience with laser sheath extraction in the United States where 1,684 patients (2,561 leads) were treated with a laser sheath [157]. Complete success, defined as removal of all lead material from the vasculature, was seen in 90% of the patients. The most predictive factor for failure to remove a lead by this procedure was lead implant duration of more than 10 years. Cardiopulmonary bypass surgery with dissection of the electrode may be required for patients who can tolerate surgery when percutaneous approaches are not successful or intracardiac complications, including valvular involvement, are present [103,149,156].

Infection is one of the most serious complications of automatic implantable cardioverter defibrillators (AICDs). Infection rates of older AICDs, in which one of the electrodes is a surgically implanted epicardial patch, range from 1% to 7% [158]. Early infections typically involve the generator pocket and are caused by *S. aureus* [158]. Late infections tend to involve the patch with resultant purulent pericarditis, usually caused by CoNS and corynebacteria [159]. There is now agreement that these infections, whether early or late, require removal of the entire system [149,159]. Radical debridement of the pericardium is necessary if infection extends beyond the electrode patch capsule [159]. Prolonged antibiotic therapy (i.e., 6 weeks) follows these procedures. Reimplantation of the generator following disinfection and appropriate gas sterilization using new electrodes and wires after the patient has been on antibiotic therapy for 2 weeks has been successful [158] but is not recommended [149]. More recent AICDs use intracardiac defibrillating electrodes placed transvenously; management of infections involving these systems is similar to that of PPMs [149].

Ventricular assist devices have revolutionized the management of patients with end-stage cardiac pump failure. They may be used temporarily in patients who are expected to have recovery of natural heart function, as a "bridge" in the group who are awaiting cardiac transplantation, or as destination therapy in patients ineligible for transplantation. A ventricular assist device consists of an encased pumping chamber usually placed in a preperitoneal or intraabdominal position, a driveline tunneled to an exit point in the lower quadrant, and inflow and outflow conduits with unidirectional valves attached with a Dacron graft to the left ventricular apex and the ascending aorta, respectively, each of which locations has its own peculiarities and propensity to infection [160]. Incidence of infection following left ventricular assist device (LVAD) implantation ranges from 18% to 59% [160]. Infections range in severity from local driveline exit site infections to pocket (meaning the body cavity, either preperitoneal or intra-abdominal, in which the device is placed) infection and bacteremia, for which determining whether the device is, in fact, seeded is the key question [161]. A series published in 2006 reported that most infections occurred between 2 weeks and 2 months of implantation [160], but a more recent report of infections in LVADs placed from 2005 to 2011 found endovascular infections occurred early (0.3 to 7.3 months, median 1.6 months) postimplantation, whereas "local" infections, predominantly involving the driveline exit site, tended to occur later (3 to 19.8, median 7.1, months) [161].

The most serious of these infections is LVAD endocarditis, defined as infection of the LVAD surface or valves associated with persistent bacteremia or fungemia [160]. Clinical features include persistent fever, cachexia, septic cerebral embolization, and device failure [160–162]. Pathogens are typical nosocomial organisms: Gram-positive cocci, particularly staphylococci, are the most frequent etiologies, followed by Gram-negative bacilli including *Pseudomonas aeruginosa* and *Candida* sp. [160,161]. Mortality with LVAD endocarditis is high, approaching 50% in one series [162]. All-cause mortality was 43% at 2 years from the time of implantation in a series that included all LVAD-related infections; 47% of the 30 patients whose LVADs were intended as bridge to transplant actually received heart transplants [161]. A recent paper proposes an algorithm to guide workup and therapy of these infections; the authors stress that chronic suppressive antimicrobial therapy is indicated when the LVAD is believed to be seeded and recommend continuation of that therapy even if the device is explanted and replaced [161].

TREATMENT

Treatment of IE encompasses antimicrobial therapy, close clinical monitoring, and the decision as to whether and when surgical intervention should be undertaken. In a consecutive series of patients admitted to medical ICUs at a single hospital in France between 1993 and 2000, the in-hospital mortality rate was 45% (102 of 228) [163]. In an international collaborative study of NVE managed between 2000 and 2005 at 61 centers in 28 countries, the in-hospital mortality was 143 of 1,065 (13%) in patients with community-associated disease and 138 of 557 (25%) in patients with healthcare-associated infection [17]. Mortality for PVE is higher and ranges from 13% to 45% [164]. In the years since 2000, antimicrobial resistance has increased among the usual causative organisms, particularly staphylococci and enterococci, increasing the challenge of treating these infections.

Antimicrobial Therapy

Antimicrobials used to treat IE must provide bactericidal activity in the bloodstream, bathing the infected vegetation and heart valve, since neither possesses an intrinsic vascular supply, and bacteria within the vegetation may be shielded by the surrounding fibrin–platelet thrombus. Certain organisms also produce a slime around indwelling devices that provides a further barrier to antimicrobial penetration and alters killing conditions. In vitro and animal model systems can suggest potential approaches to therapy, but clinical outcomes are the final arbiter of whether a particular drug or combination of drugs has worked for the patient with endocarditis. There have been very few controlled clinical trials [165–168]. Rather, regimens have been evaluated by comparing cure rates to those expected. In the clearest case, "Bacteriologic cure rates ≥ 98% may be anticipated in patients who complete 4 weeks of therapy with parenteral penicillin or ceftriaxone for endocarditis caused by highly penicillin-susceptible viridans group streptococci or *S. gallolyticus (bovis)*" [44]. For other etiologies of IE, the expectation of successful therapy is less uniform. Extensive reviews of published data and the clinical wisdom of experts in the field provide the basis for the therapeutic recommendations of various guidelines ([44], United

States; [103], Europe; [104], United Kingdom [see individual references for Web site addresses]).

In the following discussion, we review the major U.S. recommendations [44] but urge the reader to consult the most up-to-date version of them at the time of need and take care to note the specifics of the organism, valve type, and dosing recommendations.

Streptococci

For the highly penicillin-susceptible viridans group streptococci and *S. gallolyticus (bovis)* with penicillin MIC ≤0.12 μg per mL, the dose of aqueous crystalline penicillin G is 12 to 18 million units IV given either continuously or divided into four to six daily doses, or ceftriaxone 2 g IV or IM given as a single daily dose. Duration of treatment is 4 weeks for NVE. A randomized controlled trial has shown that the addition of gentamicin, 3 mg per kg IV once daily, given in close temporal proximity to the dose of the cell-wall active agent (penicillin or ceftriaxone), can reduce the duration of treatment to 2 weeks for patients without cardiac complications or extracardiac sites of infection [165]. For prosthetic valve infections, 6-week therapy with the β-lactam is recommended, and gentamicin is optional [44]. Endocarditis due to group A β-hemolytic streptococcus (*S. pyogenes* or GAS) is treated similarly, with penicillin, ceftriaxone, or vancomycin (when the patient cannot tolerate β-lactams) for 4 to 6 weeks [44].

Note that the 2015 version of the U.S. guidelines [44] includes continuous infusion of penicillin among the recommended dosing schedules, and that one study has demonstrated significantly better outcomes (odds ratio for successful therapy 2.79, CI 1.43 to 5.62) for patients who received penicillin on a q4h schedule compared to those dosed at 6-hour intervals [169]. Ampicillin, 2 g IV every 4 hours, may be used in place of penicillin. Vancomycin is recommended for patients with endocarditis due to streptococci only if they are unable to tolerate penicillin or ceftriaxone. The vancomycin dose is 15 mg per kg IV every 12 hours, adjusted to yield trough levels of 10 to 15 μg per mL [44]. Desensitization to a β-lactam antibiotic, rather than use of vancomycin, should be strongly considered for patients with anaphylactic β-lactam allergies. These comments apply to all regimens using these drugs.

For strains of viridans group streptococci and *S. gallolyticus (bovis)* with penicillin MIC greater than 0.12 but less than or equal to 0.5 μg per mL, the penicillin dose is higher (24 million units per day), 2-week therapy is not an option, and a single daily dose of gentamicin is recommended for the first 2 weeks of a 4-week course in NVE and for the entire 6-week course for prosthetic valve disease. Ceftriaxone may be used if the organism is susceptible, in which case gentamicin may be omitted from the treatment of native valve disease but should be given for the full course in PVE. If vancomycin must be used because the patient is intolerant to β-lactams, gentamicin is not recommended [44]. Highly penicillin-resistant viridans group streptococci (penicillin MIC ≥ 0.5 μg per mL) may be treated with combination penicillin or ampicillin plus gentamicin (see regimen for enterococci, below), or if susceptible to ceftriaxone, with that drug plus gentamicin. If vancomycin is required, gentamicin is not given [44]. Patients with pneumococcal endocarditis may have concomitant meningitis (present in 40.8% of cases in a recent series [36]), in which case the β-lactam or vancomycin dose must be appropriate for the latter indication [44]. The European guidelines recommend use of ceftriaxone rather than penicillin or ampicillin in this circumstance (unless the susceptibility of the organism requires addition of vancomycin) [103]. Even in the absence of meningitis, high-dose penicillin or ceftriaxone should be used, and the addition of vancomycin and rifampin may be considered if the *S. pneumoniae* MIC is greater than 2 μg per mL [44]. Treatment duration is 4 weeks for native valve disease and 6 weeks for PVE [44]. For groups B, C, and G β-hemolytic streptococcal endocarditis, including the *S. anginosus (milleri)* group, recommended treatment is penicillin or ceftriaxone with the addition of gentamicin for at least the first 2 weeks of a 4- to 6-week course [44].

Staphylococci

Most centers must now use vancomycin as the initial therapy for suspected *S. aureus* infection, despite slower killing and inferior clinical response, due to the frequency of oxacillin resistance in both healthcare-associated and community-acquired strains. Empiric vancomycin should be changed to nafcillin or oxacillin, 2 g IV every 4 hours (or cefazolin, 2 g IV every 8 hours, for patients with non-anaphylactoid β-lactam hypersensitivity) when *S. aureus* is determined to be susceptible to oxacillin; desensitization to oxacillin or nafcillin should be strongly considered for patients with anaphylactic β-lactam allergies. Controlled trials have shown that the addition of gentamicin does not improve outcome in native valve *S. aureus* endocarditis [166–168]. Recent data also suggest that even short courses of low doses of gentamicin are associated with nephrotoxicity in patients with SAB and endocarditis, particularly in patients with any degree of baseline renal dysfunction, advanced age, or diabetes [170]. Gentamicin is no longer recommended for treatment of NVE due to *S. aureus* in any of the major guidelines [44,103,104]. However, gentamicin is recommended for the first 2 weeks of therapy of PVE caused by gentamicin-susceptible staphylococci. U.S. guidelines favor q8–12h gentamicin dosing [44], whereas the European recommendation is a single daily dose [103]; both recommend 3 mg/kg/d. If the organism is gentamicin resistant but susceptible to a fluoroquinolone, then addition of a fluoroquinolone to the β-lactam or vancomycin can be considered for PVE. Rifampin has a special role in PVE because of its ability to sterilize devices (probably due to activity within the slime); the dose is 300 mg by mouth (preferred) or IV every 8 hours. Rifampin should be given for the entirety of the course, if the organism isolated is susceptible. The European guidelines [103] recommend waiting 3 to 5 days before starting rifampin; this provides time to be sure the organism is susceptible, and may decrease the likelihood of selecting for rifampin resistance while the organism is still replicating rapidly. The usual duration of therapy for *S. aureus* endocarditis is 4 weeks for uncomplicated cases, 6 weeks for complicated cases, and 6 or more weeks for PVE, although a 2-week course of nafcillin or oxacillin can be used for selected cases of native valve *S. aureus* endocarditis limited to the right side of the heart [44].

For MRSA endocarditis, vancomycin is still the current first-line recommendation, but there is growing dissatisfaction with its efficacy. A review of multiple case series established that mortality and treatment failure are significantly more frequent among bloodstream infections caused by MRSA with vancomycin MICs ≥ 1.5 μg per mL which are considered vancomycin-susceptible using the current standard susceptibility cutoff [169]. The European guidelines have responded to this by urging higher doses of vancomycin (aiming at trough levels >20 μg per mL) and recommending alternative agents, including daptomycin at a dose of ≥10 mg/kg/d along with a β-lactam or fosfomycin, or cotrimoxazole (trimethoprim-sulfamethoxazole) plus clindamycin for MRSA endocarditis [103]. The U.S. guidelines discuss some of these options, as well as noting that none of the treatment failures in an early study of trimethoprim-sulfamethoxazole occurred in patients infected with MRSA ([44], referring to [171]). The difficulty with treating these strains may not be entirely due to their resistance to vancomycin: higher in-hospital mortality was also found among patients with endocarditis due to methicillin-susceptible *S. aureus* with vancomycin MICs ≥ 1.5 μg per mL, even though they were treated with a β-lactam [172].

Staphylococci with vancomycin MICs < 2 μg per mL are still generally treated with that agent. The addition of synergistic gentamicin is not thought to be more useful in this situation than for oxacillin-susceptible disease, and coadministration with vancomycin may increase toxicity. Addition of rifampin to vancomycin therapy is not recommended due to a lack of benefit on either survival or duration of bacteremia [173].

CoNS, best known for causing prosthetic valve and other device infections, should be assumed to be oxacillin resistant until proven otherwise by rigorous testing (not available in all laboratories). The same antimicrobial regimens are recommended as for MRSA, although there are occasional reports of successful therapy with linezolid [174,175].

Enterococci

For many years, enterococcal endocarditis has been the one instance where the combination of penicillin, ampicillin, or vancomycin with an aminoglycoside (streptomycin or gentamicin) was required for clinical efficacy [176]. These recommendations have recently changed. The demonstration that ceftriaxone could be used for synergy in cases of endocarditis caused by high-level aminoglycoside-resistant (HLAR) *Enterococcus faecalis* was extended to include patients with non-HLAR enterococcal endocarditis with renal failure or a risk for nephrotoxicity [177]. An observational study comparing outcomes for patients who received ampicillin plus ceftriaxone or ampicillin plus gentamicin, as chosen by their treating physicians, found equivalent efficacy and much less toxicity for the double β-lactam combination [177,178]. Ceftriaxone provides synergy by binding to additional penicillin-binding proteins. This regimen is now recommended at the same level as the traditional combination of ampicillin plus an aminoglycoside in both U.S. [44] and European guidelines [103] and is the recommended therapy for HLAR strains of *E. faecalis*. However, it is not active against *E. faecium*. If the enterococcus is ampicillin-resistant due to β-lactamase production, one of the drugs that combine ampicillin or amoxicillin with a β-lactamase inhibitor (e.g., ampicillin–sulbactam) can be substituted, but if ampicillin resistance is not due to β-lactamase production, vancomycin must be used along with an aminoglycoside. Although the aminoglycoside has conventionally been recommended for the full duration of therapy, a retrospective study in Sweden found good results for patients who received only 15 days of aminoglycoside [179]. A subsequent study in Denmark, looking at outcomes before and after limiting the duration of aminoglycoside therapy to 2 weeks while continuing the β-lactam for a total of 4 to 6 weeks, found that patients receiving 2 and 6 weeks of aminoglycoside therapy had equivalent outcomes [180]. Recommended duration of combination therapy using penicillin or ampicillin with gentamicin for enterococcal NVE of less than 3 months' duration is 4 weeks [44,103]. For disease of longer duration, prosthetic valve involvement, or vancomycin-based therapy, treatment is prolonged to 6 weeks with both drugs [44,103]. A 6-week course is also recommended for double β-lactam therapy for both native and prosthetic valve disease, as well as intracardiac device infection. The ceftriaxone dose is 2 g IV q12h, and that of ampicillin is 2 g IV q4h [44,103].

Endocarditis due to vancomycin-resistant enterococci (VRE) warrants infectious disease consultation and may require specialized laboratory investigation [44,181,182]. Daptomycin has in vitro activity against VRE, and time–kill curves demonstrated synergy with gentamicin and rifampin in a case where that combination was used [183]. Quinupristin–dalfopristin is active only against *E. faecium*, and in this series was never the sole component of successful therapy [183]. The quinupristin–dalfopristin compassionate-plea program reported clinical and bacteriologic response in only 2 out of 10 (0 of 1 evaluable) patients [184]. Linezolid 600 mg IV or orally every 12 hours proved successful in 10 (77%) of 13 evaluable cases of VRE endocarditis (nine courses of therapy were not evaluable) [185].

HACEK organisms

First-choice therapy for HACEK endocarditis is ceftriaxone 2 g IV every 24 hours (or other third- or fourth-generation cephalosporin) for 4 weeks in native valve disease and 6 weeks with prosthetic valves [44]. Ampicillin–sulbactam may be used, but the combination of ampicillin and gentamicin is no longer recommended. Therapeutic failures with this combination in *A. actinomycetemcomitans* endocarditis include a nearly 30% mortality in one series [186,187]. Ciprofloxacin at 500 mg orally every 12 hours or 400 mg IV every 8 hours is the suggested alternative for patients who cannot tolerate ceftriaxone or ampicillin–sulbactam [44].

Candida

Candida endocarditis has generally been regarded as an indication for valve replacement surgery, but often the patients who get this infection have been too ill for surgery. Factors associated with survival of some of these high-risk patients in the absence of cardiac surgery include receiving initial combination antifungal therapy (most often amphotericin B plus 5-flucytosine) followed by long-term suppressive therapy with fluconazole [188,189]. Case reports of good outcomes for patients treated with caspofungin, including four who did not have valve replacement [190–192], are now supported by a larger experience indicating that echinocandins are equally effective [96]. Unfortunately, the mortality rate remains high (36% in hospital and 59% at 1 year), with no impact by choice of drug or performance of surgery in this series of 70 cases from 2000 to 2010 [96].

Empiric therapy

Patients with endocarditis who require intensive care at admission will most likely have the acute form of the disease due to virulent pathogens such as *S. aureus* or, more rarely, *Streptococcus pneumoniae* or pyogenic streptococci, unless they have undiagnosed subacute endocarditis and require intensive care due to cardiac or neurologic complications. Large emboli are a particular feature of HACEK, non-group A β-hemolytic streptococcal and candidal endocarditis. The British guideline is the only one that specifically addresses empiric therapy for the critically ill patient; it recommends vancomycin plus meropenem [104]. The AHA guideline suggests vancomycin and cefepime as the initial regimen for acute IE on native valves, to insure activity against aerobic Gram-negative bacilli [44], but given the small proportion of endocarditis cases (1% to 4%, Table 78.1) due to these organisms, providing treatment for enterococci may be a more important priority. Among patients with endocarditis admitted to ICUs in France from 2002 to 2012, enterococci were the etiology in 10.2% and Enterobacteriaceae in 4.7%. [39]. Enterococcus is the third most common etiology among injection drug users [9] and the cause of more than 10% (13% in North America [9]) of all cases of endocarditis in recent series [9,96]. The European guideline [103] suggests ampicillin, oxacillin, and gentamicin for community-acquired NVE while awaiting documentation of the etiology from blood cultures, but this would not be adequate in settings where oxacillin-resistant *S. aureus* (MRSA) is a major concern. Where that is the case, initial empiric therapy for community-acquired NVE for patients requiring intensive care, including injection drug users, might well consist of vancomycin, ceftriaxone (at the 2 g q12h dose), and ampicillin. This regimen should provide activity against staphylococci, viridans group (oral) and other streptococci, *Enterococcus faecalis*, and HACEK organisms.

Those who develop endocarditis after prolonged hospitalization have high rates of MRSA, enterococcal, and fungal endocarditis and may be the group at highest risk of non-HACEK Gram-negative bacillary endocarditis. Empiric anticandidal therapy may also be considered for ICU patients who are on or have recently received prolonged courses of antimicrobial therapy. The lesser toxicity of echinocandin would favor use of one of these agents over amphotericin in this setting; they appeared to be equally efficacious in a study by the ICE investigators [96]. The same patients are among those with risk factors for extended-spectrum β-lactamase-producing Enterobacteriaceae or *P. aeruginosa*, for whom the British guideline recommendation may well have been intended.

All of the guidelines [44,103,104] agree on empiric therapy for PVE: vancomycin, gentamicin, plus rifampin (with the suggestion that rifampin be deferred for the first several days in the European guideline) [103]. The U.S. guideline recommends the addition of cefepime for patients within the first year after prosthetic valve placement [44].

Supportive Care and Monitoring

Careful clinical monitoring of the patient on therapy for endocarditis includes surveillance for fever, evidence of congestive heart failure or other cardiac complication, metastatic infection, adverse effects of antimicrobial drugs (and levels, when appropriate), changes in renal function, and superinfection. Follow-up blood cultures should be obtained every 48 hours until they are repeatedly sterile. The duration of antimicrobial therapy is counted from the first day of blood culture negativity [44]. For aortic and mitral valve endocarditis, serial ECGs should be obtained to look for prolongation of the PR interval or other conduction abnormality that would signal invasion of the interventricular septum by the infection. Echocardiographic imaging should be repeated as described above to better define disease in patients whose initial echocardiography was unrevealing. It should also be repeated at any time when clinical changes, such as new murmur, embolism, persisting fever, heart failure, or atrioventricular block suggest poor control of disease or complications [44,103]; it may also be wise to repeat this study to detect new silent complications and follow vegetation size, especially for endocarditis caused by virulent organisms [103]. Echocardiography should also be repeated at the end of therapy as to define the patient's new baseline [44,103].

Recrudescence of fever after initial resolution most often indicates a new problem outside the heart, such as catheter-associated sepsis, drug fever, or antibiotic-associated *Clostridium difficile* colitis, but superinfection of the endocarditic valve may occur. Unless there is another immediately obvious cause, persistent or recurrent fever should prompt repeat echocardiography.

The possible need for cardiac surgery mandates discontinuation of warfarin and substitution of heparin when the diagnosis of endocarditis is made for patients on anticoagulant therapy for prosthetic valves or other indications [44]. Anticoagulation in endocarditis carries the risk of converting bland emboli (infarcts) to hemorrhagic ones, and thus should be carefully monitored and continued with caution. When emboli with hemorrhage occur, anticoagulant therapy should be withheld for a period of time. The risk of central nervous system (CNS) hemorrhage in *S. aureus* PVE is so high that some recommend discontinuation of all anticoagulation during the acute phase of this illness [193].

Role of Cardiac Surgery

At times, failure of antibiotics to sterilize the blood necessitates surgical debridement and removal of the infected focus—the valve. Even if bacteriologic cure is achieved, some patients have sufficient valvular damage that they will die of hemodynamic compromise unless a valve is replaced. The surprisingly favorable outcomes of a number of patients operated on in these desperate circumstances have led to consideration of cardiac surgery much earlier in the course of endocarditis [194–197]. The two indications for surgery already mentioned—microbiologic failure and congestive heart failure—are now well accepted. The challenge is to identify patients who would eventually meet these criteria before their clinical condition deteriorates.

Harbingers of microbiologic failure include difficult-to-treat and aggressive organisms, such as *S. lugdunensis*, *S. aureus*, *P. aeruginosa* or other Gram-negative bacilli involving the aortic or mitral valve, and fungi, particularly molds. *C. burnetii*, *Bartonella*, *Brucella*, and other unusual organisms associated with true culture-negative endocarditis are also difficult to eradicate with antimicrobial therapy alone. The risk of microbiologic failure or relapse is elevated in the presence of prosthetic material, resulting in the recommendation for valve replacement in most cases of early PVE and the necessity of removing infected intracardiac devices such as pacemakers and other CIEDs. Conventional blood cultures should become sterile within 7 days after the institution of appropriate antibiotic therapy [44,93,192,197]. The median time for clearance of *S. aureus* varies among studies but may be as long as 9 days [167] but the surgical indication would be the duration of positive cultures, not simply the identification of this organism. Patients should defervesce within 9 to 10 days. Persistent fever may indicate continued active infection, myocardial abscess, or an embolic complication.

Many patients with endocarditis have preexisting congestive failure as a result of their underlying valvular disease, but new-onset or worsening heart failure carries an ominous prognosis—a mortality of 56% in one series [196]. Urgent surgery is indicated for these patients, and a number of authors have noted that medical stabilization may be impossible once severe progressive failure begins [196]. Acute aortic and mitral regurgitation, due to perforation, valve rupture, or paravalvular leak (in the case of PVE), are frequent mechanisms of congestive failure [197]. Valvular obstruction is less common but does occur on prosthetic valves and is an equally urgent indication for surgery. Rupture of sinus of Valsalva aneurysm into the right heart or pericardium also mandates surgery [198]. It cannot be overemphasized that once surgery is clearly indicated, it should not be delayed, because of the unpredictability of the clinical course and the increasing risk of the operation as failure progresses [196,197,199].

Echocardiography can be very helpful for defining the presence of complications that do require surgery, including destruction of the valve or extension of infection beyond the valve ring as a myocardial abscess. Myocardial abscess may be the reason for prolonged fever [197,200], lead to conduction defects [102,197], or cavitate into the pericardium with resultant purulent pericarditis [197]. Myocardial abscess is generally an indication for surgery to extirpate all infected tissue as well as correct the accompanying hemodynamic abnormalities [44,103,197,198]. Occasionally, abscesses that are less than 1 cm, that do not progress on therapy, and that are not complicated by disruption of other structures, may be followed with serial TEE and do not require surgery [44,197].

The risk of embolization is the most debatable indication for surgery. Although often viewed as an indication for surgery, this risk diminishes greatly over the first 2 weeks of antimicrobial therapy [44,103,197,198]. In one large study, 56% of embolic events in 629 patients with IE occurred before hospital admission or on the day antibiotic treatment started [201], and in another, only 7.3% of 384 patients had new embolic events after the initiation of therapy [202]. The difficulty lies in for defining when there is sufficient risk of clinically significant systemic or cerebral embolization to justify cardiac surgery not required for any other reason but before serious target organ damage has already occurred. There have been many attempts to establish echocardiographic predictors of embolization; vegetation length more than 10 mm by TEE was associated with a ninefold increase in risk of systemic or cerebral embolization on therapy and "severe mobility," defined as "prolapsing vegetation that crosses the coaptation plane of the leaflets during the cardiac cycle," with a 2.4-fold increase [202]. The U.S. guidelines deem one or more embolic events during the first 2 weeks of therapy a class I indication for surgery (condition for which there is evidence, general agreement, or both that a given procedure or treatment is useful and effective) [44]. Anterior mitral valve leaflet vegetations, especially those greater than 10 mm, and the presence of persistent vegetations after systemic embolization are class IIa indications (the weight of evidence/opinion is in favor of usefulness/efficacy), but increase in size of vegetation despite therapy is less well established as an indication for surgery [44]. European guidelines advise consideration of surgery for recurrent emboli despite adequate antibiotic therapy or mobile vegetations greater than 10 mm before or during the first week of antibiotic therapy [181]. U.S. experts recommend delaying valve surgery for a minimum of 2 weeks after a CNS embolic event [44,197] and at least a month after CNS hemorrhage [197], but European guidelines suggest that surgery can be performed within the first 72 hours of CNS embolism if a computed tomographic scan of the brain performed immediately preoperatively shows no hemorrhage [103].

Right-sided endocarditis requires surgical intervention much less frequently than left-sided disease. In patients with isolated right-sided lesions, most often injection drug users, tricuspid vegetectomy, valve repair, or valvulectomy may permit cure of endocarditis due to resistant organisms without the risk of subsequent PVE. In the absence of pulmonary hypertension, tricuspid regurgitation may be tolerated without valve replacement [181,197].

The surgical approach for endocarditis is changing, with increasing interest in vegetectomy and valve repair rather than replacement. Repair is most often performed on the mitral valve and offers improved outcome over replacement [203,204]. Complete debridement of all infected tissue is mandatory. The reconstructive techniques developed for valve repair may also facilitate the surgical approach for cases with extensive perivalvular infection, where homografts and pericardial patches may be used to construct an annulus to which to attach a prosthetic valve when large amounts of normal tissue have been lost. The current view is that the risk of recurrent endocarditis on bioprosthetic and mechanical valve replacements is comparable, about 2% to 3% [44,181]. If valve cultures from surgery are negative, the duration of the antibiotic course originally planned should be completed, as long as it extends at least 7 to 15 days postoperatively. If intraoperative cultures are positive, the full recommended duration of antibiotics for the infecting organism should be administered counting from the day of surgery [44].

There is little difference in the clinical indications for surgery in native and PVE, but the proportion of patients requiring surgery is higher among those with prosthetic valves, approximately 50% [164,197,203,205–209]. Staphylococcal etiology and CNS embolization are uniformly identified as poor prognostic features. Early surgical intervention reduces the overall mortality of PVE [197,207,209]. Some studies have identified patients with PVE in whom medical therapy has equivalent outcomes to surgery as those with late-onset streptococcal disease who have no significant heart failure, no new valvular regurgitation or other intracardiac complication, and no CNS or systemic embolization [165,205,206]. Most important is that cardiac surgical treatment reduces the mortality rate among patients with poor prognostic factors to the level experienced by the patients with more favorable disease characteristics [164].

Comparison of outcomes of IE treated surgically versus medically have become more sophisticated, with matching for many variables, such as age and comorbidities, propensity scores grading the likelihood of surgical therapy, and correction for survival bias, which is the negative impact of patients who die early in their hospital course(s) and are categorized as having received medical therapy alone, thus prejudicing the outcome of the nonsurgically treated group. Studies of the impacts of surgery using these methods do not present a uniform picture of its benefits. Apparent improvement in mortality became nonsignificant after these adjustments for some studies [210–212], but persisted in others [213–215], at least for some indications. For instance, patients with heart failure seemed to benefit from surgery (performed at a median of day 7) in one study [213], but not in another (also with surgery at a median of day 7 after admission), for which patients with valve perforation also did not benefit, although those with paravalvular complications, systemic embolization, *S. aureus* NVE, and stroke did [214]. Even at sites involved in major multicenter studies of endocarditis, substantially fewer patients had surgery than had conditions listed as surgical indications, but there is no way to determine how many of those had simultaneous contraindications or refused a recommendation for surgery [215,216].

A single randomized study of early surgery, performed within 48 hours of randomization (the discussion says "within 48 hours of diagnosis," but the protocol excluded patients referred from another hospital more than 7 days after diagnosis, suggesting that patients would have been eligible as late as 7 days after diagnosis) enrolled patients with left-sided NVE, severe mitral or aortic valve disease, and a vegetation greater than 10 mm (thus, thought to be at high risk of emboli) [217]. The primary end point was in-hospital death or symptomatic embolic events confirmed by imaging within 6 weeks after randomization. Secondary end points at 6 months included death from any cause, embolic events, recurrence of IE, and need for readmission to the hospital for congestive heart failure. Of those randomized to conventional treatment, 77% underwent surgery during the initial hospitalization or follow-up (eight required surgery on an urgent basis, at a median of 6.5 days after randomization; 22 had elective procedures more than 2 weeks after randomization). One patient in each group died in the hospital, and eight patients in the conventional treatment group had emboli (all before valve surgery), a result favoring early surgery with $p = 0.03$ (hazard ratio 0.10, confidence interval [CI] 0.01 to 0.82). There was no significant difference in all-cause mortality at 6 months (3% vs. 5%); rate of the secondary end point at 6 months was 3% in the early surgery group and 28% in the conventional treatment group, $p = 0.02$ (hazard ratio 0.08, CI 0.02 to 0.65) [217]. The author of this study argues strongly in favor of surgery within 48 hours of diagnosis for endocarditis of those with "moderate to severe heart failure, uncontrolled infection, and large vegetations associated with severe valvular disease," except for cases with intracerebral hemorrhage or large cerebral infarction [218].

It is noteworthy that the mean (interquartile range) interval from admission to surgery was 18 [10–44,211] and 21 [9–37,212] days in two of the studies that showed no benefit for surgery after adjustment for survival bias (information on time to surgery not provided in [210]). In a direct comparison of surgery within the first week of antimicrobial therapy with procedures after that time, there was a decrease in 6-month mortality only for the quintile with the highest propensity for surgery (odds ratio 0.18, 95% CI 0.04 to 0.83, $p = 0.03$). The patients in this group were younger, more likely to have *S. aureus* endocarditis, congestive heart failure, and larger vegetations; they were at higher risk of relapse and prosthetic valve dysfunction, as well [219]. By contrast, 59 patients with left-sided NVE and vegetations $\geq$ 10 mm as the only indication for surgery who underwent early surgery at a mean of 5 $\pm$ 6 days following initiation of antimicrobial therapy had higher in-hospital (42% vs. 8%, $p = 0.03$) as well as long-term mortality (59% vs 17, $p = 0.007$, at 6.0 $\pm$ 2.9 years) [220]. It should be noted that these patients appear to have had delayed diagnoses, with first symptoms of IE nearly 4 weeks before the start of antimicrobial therapy, so their surgery may not really have been early in the course; more than half had already had systemic emboli by the time of surgery and 16 (27%) had impaired mental status on admission. *S. aureus* was the etiology of endocarditis in 18 (32%) of the patients treated surgically, but only one (8%) of those treated medically. The decision for surgery was made on clinical grounds, presumably because of the severity of illness.

The variability of definition of "early surgery" is also a factor, as stressed by the only randomized clinical trial, in which patients with IE and severe aortic or mitral regurgitation were randomized to surgery within 48 hours or later, with improved 6-month survival for those who had valve replacement within the first 48 hours [217]. A retrospective review of patients who met criteria for valve replacement but did not undergo early surgery found endocarditis due to *S. aureus* less often treated surgically, largely because of the ongoing septic picture due to that organism [215]. High-risk surgical scores were another reason patients who had indications did not have cardiac surgery, but those at high risk who had surgery had marked improvement in survival compared to similar patients who did not, while patients with less than median surgical risk who underwent surgery fared at least as well as patients who had no indication for surgery and thus were treated only medically [215,216].

A meta-analysis of 21 reports from 1996 to 2015 [221] found that early surgery at ≤20 days was associated with decreased all-cause mortality compared to the group that did not receive surgery within the first 3 weeks, at a high level of statistical significance ($p < 0.001$), and also statistically significantly better than with medical therapy alone ($p < 0.001$). When the early surgery group was separated into those with surgery at ≤7 days and those with surgery at 8 to 20 days, both surgical groups had statistically significantly lower all-cause mortality than patients treated with medical therapy alone. Those who had surgery at ≥21 days had lower all-cause mortality than those who never had surgery, but the difference was not statistically significant. Analysis restricted to studies that used propensity weighting yielded the same findings, except that surgery at ≤20 days was statistically significantly better than later surgery ($p = 0.008$). In-hospital mortality was not different for groups receiving early (at <21 days) surgical intervention versus conventional therapy (meaning medical treatment with or without surgery at ≥21 days) in the 11 studies for which this outcome was available.

PVE has been thought to warrant surgery most of the time, but that may not always be true. A study of 1,025 patients, approximately half of whom had "early" surgery (during the initial hospitalization for endocarditis) found no difference in in-hospital or 1-year mortality when corrected for survival bias [222]. However, in-hospital mortality was lower with early surgery in the highest propensity quintile, and 1-year mortality was lower for both the fourth and fifth quintiles of surgical propensity (24.8% vs. 42.9% and 27.9% vs. 50.0%, respectively; $p = 0.007$ for both comparisons); however, these values were not corrected for survival bias [222]. More patients in the surgical group had congestive heart failure (36% vs. 29%), NYHA class III or IV heart failure (28% vs. 22%), and CoNS etiology (20% vs. 11%), but more patients in the medical therapy group had Enterococcus (17% vs. 9%). In a study limited to patients with *S. aureus* left-sided PVE, those who had surgery appeared to have significantly reduced 1-year mortality, but the significance did not persist in multivariate, propensity-based models (risk ratio 0.67, CI 0.39 to 1.15, $p = 0.15$) [223]. The fact is that for many cases, surgery for PVE is not elective but mandated by congestive failure, uncontrolled infection, and persistent sepsis. In this situation, current 30-day mortality rates are 12% to 14% and 5-year survival around 75% [224]. A prolonged period of symptoms without diagnosis and treatment increased risk, but duration of antibiotic therapy prior to surgery did not [224].

Neurologic complications of endocarditis do affect the decision on timing of surgery, but not necessarily whether it should be done. Given that valve surgery requires cardiopulmonary bypass with anticoagulation and may result in placement of a prosthetic valve requiring lifelong anticoagulation, there is justifiable concern that the cerebral lesions of endocarditis could be worsened by bleeding during or after surgery. Consideration of valve surgery for endocarditis is one of the reasons to perform cerebral imaging, even in the absence of neurologic symptoms. Neuroimaging may also provide additional diagnostic information that mandates therapy, as in the case of discovery of unruptured mycotic aneurysms (also called infective intracranial aneurysms). Mycotic aneurysms were found in 32% of patients in a series from Egypt in which the mean duration of symptoms was 52.6 days (± standard deviation of 56.4 days) prior to presentation; 36% of patients with cerebral mycotic aneurysms were asymptomatic [225]. By comparison, a study in France using magnetic resonance imaging (MRI) found mycotic aneurysms in 8% (10 of 130 patients), confirmed by CT angiography in only four of the six in whom that was performed, for a corrected prevalence of 6% [226]. A study from Sweden using MRI with contrast (and CT with and without contrast in patients for whom MRI was contraindicated) identified mycotic aneurysm in only one patient (1.6% of a series of 60), who had subarachnoid bleeding due to its rupture at presentation after a 3-month delay of treatment [79]. These rates certainly suggest an association of mycotic cerebral aneurysm with prolonged duration of endocarditis prior to therapy. Obviously, unruptured aneurysms should be addressed before they bleed.

Studies using systematic neuroimaging have demonstrated cerebrovascular complications in 65% to 82% of patients with left-sided IE, of which 41% to 85% were silent [223,225–227]. In one series, four (16%) out of 25 patients with preoperative embolic stroke who had surgery during the active phase of endocarditis (while still on antimicrobial therapy) died in hospital, but the remaining 21 were long-term survivors (84%, compared to 95% of 166 patients without stroke) [228]. A larger series, comparing outcomes of valve surgery in 375 patients with IE and symptomatic or silent cerebral embolism over the period 1995 to 2012, found that 21.6% died within 30 days of surgery or while still in hospital, no different from the 19.7% of 1,196 patients undergoing valve surgery for endocarditis who had normal preoperative cranial CT scans [229]. The major cause of postoperative mortality was septic shock with multiple organ failure, followed by low cardiac output syndrome. Only 12 of the 375 patients died from cerebral complications, seven (less than 2% of the 375) of whom had severe intracerebral bleeding, the complication that is feared as a result of the surgery itself. In this study, there was no difference in either early (in-hospital) or late mortality between patients with silent and those with symptomatic cerebral emboli [229]. In a consecutive series of 64 patients with acute cerebral infarct due to endocarditis who underwent cardiac surgery, one patient who had cardiac surgery 2 days after multiple small cerebral infarcts had thalamic bleeding resulting in hemiplegia, one with surgery at day 15 had small hemorrhagic transformation without neurologic deterioration, and one with surgery at 20 days suffered a new cerebral hemorrhage that proved fatal [227]. Three patients had ectopic hemorrhage detected only on postoperative neuroimaging: a small subarachnoid hemorrhage in a patient who had surgery on day 5 after infarct, and small subdural hemorrhages in two, following surgery at days 24 and 81 [227].

A large international study of 4,794 cases of IE from 2000 to 2006 [230] identified 857 patients with clinically overt stroke (defined as neurologic deficit of vascular origin lasting more than 24 hours), 556 of which were found to be ischemic on neuroimaging. 198 of these patients had cardiac surgery, 58 at 1 to 7 days after the stroke and the remainder later. Surgery within the first 7 days was not associated with higher in-hospital or 1-year mortality than later surgery after adjusting for other risk factors. The authors did not comment on hemorrhagic complications of surgery, but did state that their findings support performing cardiac surgery without delay when there is an indication for it [230]. A nationwide database study from Japan came to the same conclusion, based on a review of 253 patients with ischemic stroke due to endocarditis, using the same definitions of early and late surgery and both propensity-adjusted and inverse probability-weighted models [231].

The question of bleeding as a result of surgery is even more pressing for patients who have already had intracranial hemorrhage due to their endocarditis. A study from Japan included 30 such patients among 246 who underwent valve surgery for IE 2004 to 2012 [232]. Among the 30, 18 had cerebral hemorrhage, 8 subarachnoid hemorrhage, and 4 hemorrhagic infarction; 21 were symptomatic; all patients had preoperative brain CT on which the diagnoses were based. Eight had mycotic aneurysms, which were treated prior to valve surgery by either clipping or resection. Timing of valve surgery was decided by the individual patients' surgeons, and was within 7 days of onset of the intracranial hemorrhage in five, 8 to 14 days in six, 15 to 28 days for nine, and more than 29 days for 10. There were no deaths from cerebrovascular complications and none of the patients had neurologic deterioration; however, four patients who underwent surgery 4, 25, 31, and 47 days after onset of intracranial hemorrhage died after surgery of cardiac failure or multiple organ dysfunction. Postoperative imaging showed no enlargement of any of the preexisting hemorrhagic areas, although some patients had new small areas of hemorrhage [232]. This study also includes a literature review, indicating that neurologic deterioration occurred in 1/9 previously reported patients who had valve surgery within 0 to 14 days of intracranial hemorrhage, in 0/15 with surgery at 15 to 28 days, and in 1/29 with surgery at 29 days or later.

Both the AHA and the European Heart Society (EHS) published revised treatment guidelines for IE, including the role of surgery and its timing after neurologic events, in the fall of 2015. The AHA [44] and EHS [103] guidelines are in complete agreement about the indications for surgery in right-sided endocarditis. These are:

1. Right-sided heart failure due to severe tricuspid regurgitation with poor response to medical (diuretic) therapy.
2. Organisms that are difficult to eradicate: EHS would base this on the organism isolated (e.g., persistent fungi), whereas the AHA specifies sustained infection (presumably, prolonged duration of positive blood cultures) caused by difficult-to-treat organisms (i.e., fungi, multidrug-resistant bacteria).
3. Clinical failure: EHS specifies bacteremia for at least 7 days despite adequate antimicrobial therapy, which would meet the AHA criterion of lack of response to appropriate antimicrobial therapy.
4. Large tricuspid vegetation (>20 mm) with recurrent pulmonary embolism. EHS specifies that the vegetation persists after pulmonary emboli, whereas AHA defines this as recurrent pulmonary embolism despite antimicrobial therapy.

They both recommend repair over valve replacement whenever possible, because of the risk of reinfection from continued injection drug use.

Their conclusions regarding the indications for surgery in left-sided IE are also very similar, although their views of the strength of the evidence differ slightly, and only the EHS guidelines specify timing of surgery. Table 78.4 presents the indications for surgery as well as the class of recommendation for each and the timing for intervention recommended by the EHS. The AHA guidelines use the term "early surgery" to mean valve surgery during the initial hospitalization and before completion of a full course of antibiotics for endocarditis, whereas the EHS is more specific: "emergent" means within 24 hours, "urgent" means "within a few days, <7 days," and elective means after at least 1 to 2 weeks of antibiotic therapy. They both classify the level of recommendation based on the robustness of the studies; the EHS also considers the degree of agreement among experts in their system. Both provide suggested wording to describe the strength of each recommendation:

- Class I means the procedure "is recommended/is indicated" in the EHS document and "should be performed/administered" in the AHA one.
- Class IIa means "should be considered" (EHS) or "is reasonable," "can be useful/effective/beneficial," "is probably recommended or indicated" (AHA).
- Class IIb means "may be considered" in both.

Thus, both consider heart failure due to severe regurgitation, obstruction, or fistula a class I indication; if this is causing refractory pulmonary edema or cardiogenic shock, it requires immediate surgery, whereas if the regurgitation or obstruction is causing symptoms of heart failure or echocardiographic signs of poor hemodynamic tolerance, surgery should be performed within a few days, no more than a week.

The category of uncontrolled infection includes anatomic evidence of progression, such as the development of annular or aortic abscess (which may be evidenced by heart block), destructive penetrating lesions (fistulae), aneurysms and false aneurysms, which both guidelines consider a class I indication for surgery. The EHS also includes enlarging vegetations in this group and considers these findings to require urgent, but not emergent, surgery. Organisms known to be difficult to control, including fungi, VRE, and multidrug-resistant Gram-negative bacilli, are class I indications for surgery for both AHA and EHS, with timing that may be urgent or elective. Clinical evidence of uncontrolled infection, such as persistent positive blood cultures despite appropriate antimicrobial therapy and drainage or extirpation of sites of metastatic infection (e.g., splenic abscess) are class I indications in the U.S. guidelines, along with persistence of fever beyond 5 to 7 days, but IIa in the European ones, with timing of surgery urgent (EHS). The EHS considers PVE caused by staphylococci or non-HACEK Gram-negative bacilli to be a class IIa indication for surgery which may be either urgent or elective, but the AHA does not, although PVE caused by staphylococci or non-HACEK Gram-negative bacilli is a class IIa indication for urgent or elective surgery in both guidelines. The U.S. guidelines also consider relapsing PVE a class IIa indication, but this criterion is not mentioned in the European ones.

Both sources also see prevention of embolism as an indication for surgery. The specific criteria differ a little, as do the interpretations of the strength of the evidence. Persistent vegetations > 10 mm after one or more embolic episodes occurring despite appropriate antibiotic therapy are a class I indication for urgent surgery according to EHS and class IIa for the AHA. NVE with vegetations >10 mm associated with severe valvular stenosis or regurgitation is a class IIa indication in patients with low operative risk (EHS; timing urgent) or when the vegetation is mobile (AHA). Isolated vegetations > 15 mm with no other indication for surgery is a class IIb indication for the EHS (urgent), while a mobile vegetation > 10 mm, especially on the anterior leaflet of the mitral valve, along with other relative indications for surgery, is a class IIb indication for the AHA.

Individual patient situations may modify the readiness to resort to surgery. For instance, for a patient with another condition that makes the risk of general anesthesia prohibitive, such as severe restrictive lung disease, one might elect to operate only in the event of congestive heart failure. The guidelines for surgical intervention are not absolute predictors of failure of medical management but overall can predict low rates of success.

In summary, therapy for endocarditis requires skillful manipulation of antibiotics and careful day-to-day judgments of

TABLE 78.4

Indications and Timing of Surgery in Patients with Left-sided Infective Endocarditis

Indications for Surgery	AHA Class	EHS Class	EHS Timing[a]
1. Heart failure			
Severe acute regurgitation, obstruction, or fistula causing refractory pulmonary edema or cardiogenic shock	I	I	Emergency
Severe regurgitation or obstruction causing symptoms of heart failure or echocardiographic signs of poor hemodynamic tolerance	I	I	Urgent
2. Uncontrolled infection			
Locally uncontrolled abscess, false aneurysm, fistula, enlarging vegetation (AHA: PVE complicated by heart block)	I	I	Urgent
Infection caused by fungi or multiresistant organisms (AHA: e.g., VRE, multidrug-resistant Gram-negative bacilli, etc.)	I	I	Urgent/Elective
Persisting positive blood cultures (AHA: or fever, >5–7 d) despite appropriate antibiotic therapy and control of septic metastatic foci	I	IIa	Urgent
PVE caused by staphylococci or non-HACEK Gram-negative bacilli	NA	IIa	Urgent/Elective
Relapsing PVE	IIa	NA	
3. Prevention of embolism			
Persistent vegetations > 10 mm after ≥ 1 embolic episode despite appropriate antibiotic therapy	IIa	I	Urgent
NVE with vegetations >10 mm associated with severe valve stenosis or regurgitation and low operative risk (EHS), mobile vegetation (AHA)	IIa	IIa	Urgent
Isolated very large vegetations (>30 mm)	NA	IIa	Urgent
Isolated large vegetations (>15 mm) and no other indication for surgery (EHS) Mobile vegetation > 10 mm in PVE or NVE esp. on anterior leaflet mitral valve, with other relative indications for surgery (AHA)	IIb	IIb	Urgent

[a]Both guidelines recommend that cardiac surgery be postponed for at least 4 weeks (AHA)/1 month (EHS) following intracranial hemorrhage or presence of coma following (AHA "major") ischemic stroke (class IIa), but may proceed without delay after ischemic stroke if presence of cerebral hemorrhage has been excluded by cranial CT or MRI and coma is absent (EHS, class IIa; AHA wording "if neurologic damage is not severe [i.e., coma]" class IIb).

NA = not addressed.

AHA, American Heart Association; EHS, European Heart Society, PVE, prosthetic valve endocarditis

Modified from Baddour LM, Wilson WR, Bayer AS, et al: Infective endocarditis in adults: diagnosis, antimicrobial therapy, and management of complications: a scientific statement for healthcare professionals from the American Heart Association. *Circulation* 132:1466, 2015 and Habib G, Lancellotti P, Antunes MJ, et al: 2015 ESC Guidelines for the management of infective endocarditis: The Task Force for the Management of Infective Endocarditis of the European Society of Cardiology (ESC). Endorsed by: European Association for Cardio-Thoracic Surgery (EACTS), the European Association of Nuclear Medicine (EANM). *Eur Heart J* 36:3099, 2015.

the relative risks of expectant versus surgical management. It should be stressed that among cases with any adverse prognostic features, including all patients with staphylococcal or PVE, it is wise to make provisions for possible urgent surgery early in the course. This includes discussions of surgery with the patient and family and consultation with the cardiac surgical team. Table 78.5 provides a summary of recommendations for management of endocarditis supported by randomized controlled clinical trials.

TABLE 78.5

Summary Recommendations for Management of Endocarditis Based on Randomized Clinical Trials

- NVE caused by highly penicillin-susceptible viridans streptococci or *Streptococcus bovis* is effectively treated with a 2-wk regimen of ceftriaxone 2 g every 24 h IV with gentamicin 3 mg/kg/24 h IV given in a single dose [165]
- Addition of 2 wk of gentamicin to 4 wk of oxacillin or nafcillin therapy for methicillin-susceptible *Staphylococcus aureus* endocarditis does not improve outcome [166,167]
- Uncomplicated tricuspid valve endocarditis caused by methicillin-susceptible *Staphylococcus aureus* is effectively treated with a 2-wk regimen of either nafcillin or oxacillin 12 g/24 h IV in four to six equally divided doses [44], based on a trial comparing cloxacillin 2 g IV q4h with and without gentamicin 1 mg/kg IV q8h in injection drug users [168]

References

1. Bouza E, Menasalvas A, Munoz P, et al: Infective endocarditis–a prospective study at the end of the twentieth century: new predisposing conditions, new etiologic agents, and still a high mortality. *Medicine (Baltimore)* 80:298–307, 2001.
2. Cabell CH, Jollis JG, Peterson GE, et al: Changing patient characteristics and the effect on mortality in endocarditis. *Arch Intern Med* 162:90–94, 2002.
3. Fefer P, Raveh D, Rudensky B, et al: Changing epidemiology of infective endocarditis: a retrospective survey of 108 cases, 1990–1999. *Eur J Clin Microbiol Infect Dis* 21:432–437, 2002.
4. Hoen B, Alla F, Selton-Suty C, et al: Changing profile of infective endocarditis: results of a 1-year survey in France. *JAMA* 288:75–81, 2002.
5. Millar BC, Moore JE: Emerging issues in infective endocarditis. *Emerg Infect Dis* 10:1110–1116, 2004.
6. Moreillon P, Que YA: Infective endocarditis. *Lancet* 363:139–149, 2004.
7. Mouly S, Ruimy R, Launay O, et al: The changing clinical aspects of infective endocarditis: descriptive review of 90 episodes in a French teaching hospital and risk factors for death. *J Infect* 45:246–256, 2002.
8. Correa de Sa DD, Tleyjeh IM, Anavekar NS, et al: Epidemiological trends of infective endocarditis: a population-based study in Olmsted County, Minnesota. *Mayo Clin Proc* 85:422–426, 2010.
9. Murdoch DR, Corey GR, Hoen B, et al: Clinical presentation, etiology, and outcome of infective endocarditis in the 21st century: the International

Collaboration on Endocarditis-Prospective Cohort Study. *Arch Intern Med* 169:463–473, 2009.
10. Selton-Suty C, Celard M, Le Moing V, et al: Preeminence of Staphylococcus aureus in infective endocarditis: a 1-year population-based survey. *Clin Infect Dis* 54:1230–1239, 2012.
11. Armstrong ML, DeBoer S, Cetta F: Infective endocarditis after body art: a review of the literature and concerns. *J Adolesc Health* 43:217–225, 2008.
12. Cheng TO: Infective endocarditis, cardiac tamponade, and AIDS as serious complications of acupuncture. *Arch Intern Med* 164:1464, 2004.
13. Durante-Mangoni E, Bradley S, Selton-Suty C, et al: Current features of infective endocarditis in elderly patients: results of the International Collaboration on Endocarditis Prospective Cohort Study. *Arch Intern Med* 168:2095–2103, 2008.
14. Kourany WM, Miro JM, Moreno A, et al: Influence of diabetes mellitus on the clinical manifestations and prognosis of infective endocarditis: a report from the International Collaboration on Endocarditis-Merged Database. *Scand J Infect Dis* 38:613–619, 2006.
15. Hogevik H, Olaison L, Andersson R, et al: Epidemiologic aspects of infective endocarditis in an urban population. A 5-year prospective study. *Medicine (Baltimore)* 74:324–339, 1995.
16. Weng MC, Chang FY, Young TG, et al: Analysis of 109 cases of infective endocarditis in a tertiary care hospital. *Zhonghua Yi Xue Za Zhi (Taipei)* 58:18–23, 1996.
17. Benito N, Miro JM, de Lazzari E, et al: Health care-associated native valve endocarditis: importance of non-nosocomial acquisition. *Ann Intern Med* 150:586–594, 2009.
18. Kamalakannan D, Pai RM, Johnson LB, et al: Epidemiology and clinical outcomes of infective endocarditis in hemodialysis patients. *Ann Thorac Surg* 83:2081–2086, 2007.
19. Sandre RM, Shafran SD: Infective endocarditis: review of 135 cases over 9 years. *Clin Infect Dis* 22:276–286, 1996.
20. Ruttmann E, Bonatti H, Legit C, et al: Severe endocarditis in transplant recipients–an epidemiologic study. *Transpl Int* 18:690–696, 2005.
21. Sherman-Weber S, Axelrod P, Suh B, et al: Infective endocarditis following orthotopic heart transplantation: 10 cases and a review of the literature. *Transpl Infect Dis* 6:165–170, 2004.
22. Regules JA, Glasser JS, Wolf SE, et al: Endocarditis in burn patients: clinical and diagnostic considerations. *Burns* 34:610–616, 2008.
23. Ben-Ami R, Giladi M, Carmeli Y, et al: Hospital-acquired infective endocarditis: should the definition be broadened? *Clin Infect Dis* 38:843–850, 2004.
24. Martin-Davila P, Fortun J, Navas E, et al: Nosocomial endocarditis in a tertiary hospital: an increasing trend in native valve cases. *Chest* 128:772–779, 2005.
25. Chang CF, Kuo BI, Chen TL, et al: Infective endocarditis in maintenance hemodialysis patients: fifteen years experience in one medical center. *J Nephrol* 17:228–235, 2004.
26. Nucifora G, Badano LP, Viale P, et al: Infective endocarditis in chronic haemodialysis patients: an increasing clinical challenge. *Eur Heart J* 28:2307–2312, 2007.
27. Durack DT, Lukes AS, Bright DK: New criteria for diagnosis of infective endocarditis: utilization of specific echocardiographic findings. Duke Endocarditis Service. *Am J Med* 96:200–209, 1994.
28. Siddiq S, Missri J, Silverman DI: Endocarditis in an urban hospital in the 1990s. *Arch Intern Med* 156:2454–2458, 1996.
29. Olaison L, Hogevik H: Comparison of the von Reyn and Duke criteria for the diagnosis of infective endocarditis: a critical analysis of 161 episodes. *Scand J Infect Dis* 28:399–406, 1996.
30. Kjerulf A, Tvede M, Aldershvile J, et al: Bacterial endocarditis at a tertiary hospital–how do we improve diagnosis and delay of treatment? A retrospective study of 140 patients. *Cardiology* 89:79–86, 1998.
31. Kurland S, Enghoff E, Landelius J, et al: A 10-year retrospective study of infective endocarditis at a university hospital with special regard to the timing of surgical evaluation in S. viridans endocarditis. *Scand J Infect Dis* 31:87–91, 1999.
32. Woo PC, Tse H, Chan KM, et al: "Streptococcus milleri" endocarditis caused by Streptococcus anginosus. *Diagn Microbiol Infect Dis* 48:81–88, 2004.
33. Lefort A, Lortholary O, Casassus P, et al: Comparison between adult endocarditis due to beta-hemolytic streptococci (serogroups A, B, C, and G) and Streptococcus milleri: a multicenter study in France. *Arch Intern Med* 162:2450–2456, 2002.
34. Liao CH, Teng LJ, Hsueh PR, et al: Nutritionally variant streptococcal infections at a University Hospital in Taiwan: disease emergence and high prevalence of beta-lactam and macrolide resistance. *Clin Infect Dis* 38:452–455, 2004.
35. Lin CH, Hsu RB: Infective endocarditis caused by nutritionally variant streptococci. *Am J Med Sci* 334:235–239, 2007.
36. de Egea V, Munoz P, Valerio M, et al: Characteristics and outcome of Streptococcus pneumoniae Endocarditis in the XXI century: a systematic review of 111 cases (2000–2013). *Medicine (Baltimore)* 94:e1562, 2015.
37. Gallagher PG, Watanakunakorn C: Group B streptococcal endocarditis: report of seven cases and review of the literature, 1962–1985. *Rev Infect Dis* 8:175–188, 1986.
38. Baddour LM: Infective endocarditis caused by beta-hemolytic streptococci. The Infectious Diseases Society of America's Emerging Infections Network. *Clin Infect Dis* 26:66–71, 1998.
39. Leroy O, Georges H, Devos P, et al: Infective endocarditis requiring ICU admission: epidemiology and prognosis. *Ann Intensive Care* 5:45, 2015.
40. Beck M, Frodl R, Funke G: Comprehensive study of strains previously designated Streptococcus bovis consecutively isolated from human blood cultures and emended description of Streptococcus gallolyticus and Streptococcus infantarius subsp. coli. *J Clin Microbiol* 46:2966–2972, 2008.
41. Hoen B, Chirouze C, Cabell CH, et al: Emergence of endocarditis due to group D streptococci: findings derived from the merged database of the International Collaboration on Endocarditis. *Eur J Clin Microbiol Infect Dis* 24:12–16, 2005.
42. Tripodi MF, Adinolfi LE, Ragone E, et al: Streptococcus bovis endocarditis and its association with chronic liver disease: an underestimated risk factor. *Clin Infect Dis* 38:1394–1400, 2004.
43. Corredoira-Sanchez J, Garcia-Garrote F, Rabunal R, et al: Association between bacteremia due to Streptococcus gallolyticus subsp. gallolyticus (Streptococcus bovis I) and colorectal neoplasia: a case-control study. *Clin Infect Dis* 55:491–496, 2012.
44. Baddour LM, Wilson WR, Bayer AS, et al: Infective endocarditis in adults: diagnosis, antimicrobial therapy, and management of complications: a scientific statement for healthcare professionals from the American Heart Association. *Circulation* 132:1435–1486, 2015.
45. Fowler VG Jr, Sanders LL, Kong LK, et al: Infective endocarditis due to Staphylococcus aureus: 59 prospectively identified cases with follow-up. *Clin Infect Dis* 28:106–114, 1999.
46. Fowler VG Jr, Miro JM, Hoen B, et al: Staphylococcus aureus endocarditis: a consequence of medical progress. *JAMA* 293:3012–3021, 2005.
47. Nadji G, Remadi JP, Coviaux F, et al: Comparison of clinical and morphological characteristics of Staphylococcus aureus endocarditis with endocarditis caused by other pathogens. *Heart* 91:932–937, 2005.
48. Chang FY, MacDonald BB, Peacock JE Jr, et al: A prospective multicenter study of Staphylococcus aureus bacteremia: incidence of endocarditis, risk factors for mortality, and clinical impact of methicillin resistance. *Medicine (Baltimore)* 82:322–332, 2003.
49. Chu VH, Woods CW, Miro JM, et al: Emergence of coagulase-negative staphylococci as a cause of native valve endocarditis. *Clin Infect Dis* 46:232–242, 2008.
50. Frank KL, Del Pozo JL, Patel R: From clinical microbiology to infection pathogenesis: how daring to be different works for Staphylococcus lugdunensis. *Clin Microbiol Rev* 21:111–133, 2008.
51. Paturel L, Casalta JP, Habib G, et al: Actinobacillus actinomycetemcomitans endocarditis. *Clin Microbiol Infect* 10:98–118, 2004.
52. Morpeth S, Murdoch D, Cabell CH, et al: Non-HACEK gram-negative bacillus endocarditis. *Ann Intern Med* 147:829–835, 2007.
53. Aubron C, Charpentier J, Trouillet JL, et al: Native-valve infective endocarditis caused by Enterobacteriaceae: report on 9 cases and literature review. *Scand J Infect Dis* 38:873–881, 2006.
54. Garcia-Granja PE, Lopez J, Vilacosta I, et al: Polymicrobial infective endocarditis: clinical features and prognosis. *Medicine (Baltimore)* 94:e2000, 2015.
55. Loubet P, Lescure FX, Lepage L, et al: Endocarditis due to gram-negative bacilli at a French teaching hospital over a 6-year period: clinical characteristics and outcome. *Infect Dis (Lond)* 47:889–895, 2015.
56. Spach DH, Callis KP, Paauw DS, et al: Endocarditis caused by Rochalimaea quintana in a patient infected with human immunodeficiency virus. *J Clin Microbiol* 31:692–694, 1993.
57. Daly JS, Worthington MG, Brenner DJ, et al: Rochalimaea elizabethae sp. nov. isolated from a patient with endocarditis. *J Clin Microbiol* 31:872–881, 1993.
58. Hadfield TL, Warren R, Kass M, et al: Endocarditis caused by Rochalimaea henselae. *Hum Pathol* 24:1140–1141, 1993.
59. Drancourt M, Mainardi JL, Brouqui P, et al: Bartonella (Rochalimaea) quintana endocarditis in three homeless men. *N Engl J Med* 332:419–423, 1995.
60. Avidor B, Graidy M, Efrat G, et al: Bartonella koehlerae, a new cat-associated agent of culture-negative human endocarditis. *J Clin Microbiol* 42:3462–3468, 2004.
61. Dreier J, Vollmer T, Freytag CC, et al: Culture-negative infectious endocarditis caused by Bartonella spp.: 2 case reports and a review of the literature. *Diagn Microbiol Infect Dis* 61:476–483, 2008.
62. Raoult D, Fournier PE, Drancourt M, et al: Diagnosis of 22 new cases of Bartonella endocarditis. *Ann Intern Med* 125:646–652, 1996.
63. Edouard S, Nabet C, Lepidi H, et al: Bartonella, a common cause of endocarditis: a report on 106 cases and review. *J Clin Microbiol* 53:824–829, 2015.
64. Siciliano RF, Castelli JB, Mansur AJ, et al: Bartonella spp. and Coxiella burnetii associated with community-acquired, culture-negative endocarditis, Brazil. *Emerg Infect Dis* 21:1429–1432, 2015.
65. El-Kholy AA, El-Rachidi NG, El-Enany MG, et al: Impact of serology and molecular methods on improving the microbiologic diagnosis of infective endocarditis in Egypt. *Infection* 43:523–529, 2015.
66. Houpikian P, Raoult D: Blood culture-negative endocarditis in a reference center: etiologic diagnosis of 348 cases. *Medicine (Baltimore)* 84:162–173, 2005.
67. Fournier PE, Thuny F, Richet H, et al: Comprehensive diagnostic strategy for blood culture-negative endocarditis: a prospective study of 819 new cases. *Clin Infect Dis* 51:131–140, 2010.
68. Wilson LE, Thomas DL, Astemborski J, et al: Prospective study of infective endocarditis among injection drug users. *J Infect Dis* 185:1761–1766, 2002.
69. Cooper HL, Brady JE, Ciccarone D, et al: Nationwide increase in the number of hospitalizations for illicit injection drug use-related infective endocarditis. *Clin Infect Dis* 45:1200–1203, 2007.
70. Amat-Santos IJ, Ribeiro HB, Urena M, et al: Prosthetic valve endocarditis after transcatheter valve replacement: a systematic review. *JACC Cardiovasc Interv* 8:334–346, 2015.
71. Amat-Santos IJ, Messika-Zeitoun D, Eltchaninoff H, et al: Infective endocarditis after transcatheter aortic valve implantation: results from a large multicenter registry. *Circulation* 131:1566–1574, 2015.

72. Baddley JW, Benjamin DK Jr, Patel M, et al: Candida infective endocarditis. *Eur J Clin Microbiol Infect Dis* 27:519–529, 2008.
73. Castillo JC, Anguita MP, Torres F, et al: Long-term prognosis of early and late prosthetic valve endocarditis. *Am J Cardiol* 93:1185–1187, 2004.
74. Alonso-Valle H, Farinas-Alvarez C, Garcia-Palomo JD, et al: Clinical course and predictors of death in prosthetic valve endocarditis over a 20-year period. *J Thorac Cardiovasc Surg* 139:887–893, 2010.
75. Wright AJ, Wilson WR: Experimental animal endocarditis. *Mayo Clin Proc* 57:10–14, 1982.
76. Veltrop MH, Bancsi MJ, Bertina RM, et al: Role of monocytes in experimental Staphylococcus aureus endocarditis. *Infect Immun* 68:4818–4821, 2000.
77. Frontera JA, Gradon JD: Right-side endocarditis in injection drug users: review of proposed mechanisms of pathogenesis. *Clin Infect Dis* 30:374–379, 2000.
78. Bashore TM, Cabell C, Fowler V Jr: Update on infective endocarditis. *Curr Probl Cardiol* 31:274–352, 2006.
79. Snygg-Martin U, Gustafsson L, Rosengren L, et al: Cerebrovascular complications in patients with left-sided infective endocarditis are common: a prospective study using magnetic resonance imaging and neurochemical brain damage markers. *Clin Infect Dis* 47:23–30, 2008.
80. Bayer AS, Ward JI, Ginzton LE, et al: Evaluation of new clinical criteria for the diagnosis of infective endocarditis. *Am J Med* 96:211–219, 1994.
81. Hoen B, Beguinot I, Rabaud C, et al: The Duke criteria for diagnosing infective endocarditis are specific: analysis of 100 patients with acute fever or fever of unknown origin. *Clin Infect Dis* 23:298–302, 1996.
82. Dodds GA, Sexton DJ, Durack DT, et al: Negative predictive value of the Duke criteria for infective endocarditis. *Am J Cardiol* 77:403–407, 1996.
83. Stockheim JA, Chadwick EG, Kessler S, et al: Are the Duke criteria superior to the Beth Israel criteria for the diagnosis of infective endocarditis in children? *Clin Infect Dis* 27:1451–1456, 1998.
84. Gagliardi JP, Nettles RE, McCarty DE, et al: Native valve infective endocarditis in elderly and younger adult patients: comparison of clinical features and outcomes with use of the Duke criteria and the Duke Endocarditis Database. *Clin Infect Dis* 26:1165–1168, 1998.
85. Perez-Vazquez A, Farinas MC, Garcia-Palomo JD, et al: Evaluation of the Duke criteria in 93 episodes of prosthetic valve endocarditis: could sensitivity be improved? *Arch Intern Med* 160:1185–1191, 2000.
86. Sekeres MA, Abrutyn E, Berlin JA, et al: An assessment of the usefulness of the Duke criteria for diagnosing active infective endocarditis. *Clin Infect Dis* 24:1185–1190, 1997.
87. Li JS, Sexton DJ, Mick N, et al: Proposed modifications to the Duke criteria for the diagnosis of infective endocarditis. *Clin Infect Dis* 30:633–638, 2000.
88. Llinas L, Harrington T: Musculoskeletal manifestations as the initial presentation of infective endocarditis. *South Med J* 98:127–128, 2005.
89. Habib G, Derumeaux G, Avierinos JF, et al: Value and limitations of the Duke criteria for the diagnosis of infective endocarditis. *J Am Coll Cardiol* 33:2023–2029, 1999.
90. Willerson JT, Moellering RC Jr, Buckley MJ, et al: Conjunctival petechiae after open-heart surgery. *N Engl J Med* 284:539–540, 1971.
91. Silverman ME, Upshaw CB Jr: Extracardiac manifestations of infective endocarditis and their historical descriptions. *Am J Cardiol* 100:1802–1807, 2007.
92. Marrie TJ: Osler's nodes and Janeway lesions. *Am J Med* 121:105–106, 2008.
93. Anonymous: *CLSI: Principles and Procedures for Blood Cultures; Approved Guideline, CLSI document M47-A*. Wayne, PA, Clinical and Laboratory Standards Institute, 2007.
94. Petti CA, Bhally HS, Weinstein MP, et al: Utility of extended blood culture incubation for isolation of Haemophilus, Actinobacillus, Cardiobacterium, Eikenella, and Kingella organisms: a retrospective multicenter evaluation. *J Clin Microbiol* 44:257–259, 2006.
95. Baron EJ, Scott JD, Tompkins LS: Prolonged incubation and extensive subculturing do not increase recovery of clinically significant microorganisms from standard automated blood cultures. *Clin Infect Dis* 41:1677–1680, 2005.
96. Arnold CJ, Johnson M, Bayer AS, et al: Candida infective endocarditis: an observational cohort study with a focus on therapy. *Antimicrob Agents Chemother* 59:2365–2373, 2015.
97. Ellis ME, Al-Abdely H, Sandridge A, et al: Fungal endocarditis: evidence in the world literature, 1965–1995. *Clin Infect Dis* 32:50–62, 2001.
98. Houpikian P, Raoult D: Diagnostic methods current best practices and guidelines for identification of difficult-to-culture pathogens in infective endocarditis. *Infect Dis Clin North Am* 16:377–392, x, 2002.
99. Raoult D, Casalta JP, Richet H, et al: Contribution of systematic serological testing in diagnosis of infective endocarditis. *J Clin Microbiol* 43:5238–5242, 2005.
100. Syed FF, Millar BC, Prendergast BD: Molecular technology in context: a current review of diagnosis and management of infective endocarditis. *Prog Cardiovasc Dis* 50:181–197, 2007.
101. Millar BC, Moore JE: Current trends in the molecular diagnosis of infective endocarditis. *Eur J Clin Microbiol Infect Dis* 23:353–365, 2004.
102. Carpenter JL: Perivalvular extension of infection in patients with infectious endocarditis. *Rev Infect Dis* 13:127–138, 1991.
103. Habib G, Lancellotti P, Antunes MJ, et al: 2015 ESC Guidelines for the management of infective endocarditis: The Task Force for the Management of Infective Endocarditis of the European Society of Cardiology (ESC). Endorsed by: European Association for Cardio-Thoracic Surgery (EACTS), the European Association of Nuclear Medicine (EANM). *Eur Heart J* 36:3075–3128, 2015.
104. Gould FK, Denning DW, Elliott TS, et al; Working Party of the British Society for Antimicrobial Chemotherapy: Guidelines for the diagnosis and antibiotic treatment of endocarditis in adults: a report of the Working Party of the British Society for Antimicrobial Chemotherapy. *J Antimicrob Chemother* 67:269–289, 2012.
105. Daniel WG, Mugge A, Martin RP, et al: Improvement in the diagnosis of abscesses associated with endocarditis by transesophageal echocardiography. *N Engl J Med* 324:795–800, 1991.
106. Kemp WE Jr, Citrin B, Byrd BF 3rd: Echocardiography in infective endocarditis. *South Med J* 92:744–754, 1999.
107. Bayer AS, Bolger AF, Taubert KA, et al: Diagnosis and management of infective endocarditis and its complications. *Circulation* 98:2936–2948, 1998.
108. Erbel R, Rohmann S, Drexler M, et al: Improved diagnostic value of echocardiography in patients with infective endocarditis by transoesophageal approach. A prospective study. *Eur Heart J* 9:43–53, 1988.
109. Birmingham GD, Rahko PS, Ballantyne F 3rd: Improved detection of infective endocarditis with transesophageal echocardiography. *Am Heart J* 123:774–781, 1992.
110. Casella F, Rana B, Casazza G, et al: The potential impact of contemporary transthoracic echocardiography on the management of patients with native valve endocarditis: a comparison with transesophageal echocardiography. *Echocardiography* 26:900–906, 2009.
111. Daniel WG, Mugge A, Grote J, et al: Evaluation of endocarditis and its complications by biplane and multiplane transesophageal echocardiography. *Am J Card Imaging* 9:100–105, 1995.
112. Daniel WG, Erbel R, Kasper W, et al: Safety of transesophageal echocardiography. A multicenter survey of 10,419 examinations. *Circulation* 83:817–821, 1991.
113. Spier BJ, Larue SJ, Teelin TC, et al: Review of complications in a series of patients with known gastro-esophageal varices undergoing transesophageal echocardiography. *J Am Soc Echocardiogr* 22:396–400, 2009.
114. Shapiro SM, Young E, De Guzman S, et al: Transesophageal echocardiography in diagnosis of infective endocarditis. *Chest* 105:377–382, 1994.
115. Pedersen WR, Walker M, Olson JD, et al: Value of transesophageal echocardiography as an adjunct to transthoracic echocardiography in evaluation of native and prosthetic valve endocarditis. *Chest* 100:351–356, 1991.
116. Shively BK, Gurule FT, Roldan CA, et al: Diagnostic value of transesophageal compared with transthoracic echocardiography in infective endocarditis. *J Am Coll Cardiol* 18:391–397, 1991.
117. Hansalia S, Biswas M, Dutta R, et al: The value of live/real time three-dimensional transesophageal echocardiography in the assessment of valvular vegetations. *Echocardiography* 26:1264–1273, 2009.
118. Daniel WG, Mugge A, Grote J, et al: Comparison of transthoracic and transesophageal echocardiography for detection of abnormalities of prosthetic and bioprosthetic valves in the mitral and aortic positions. *Am J Cardiol* 71:210–215, 1993.
119. Evangelista A, Gonzalez-Alujas MT: Echocardiography in infective endocarditis. *Heart* 90:614–617, 2004.
120. Heidenreich PA, Masoudi FA, Maini B, et al: Echocardiography in patients with suspected endocarditis: a cost-effectiveness analysis. *Am J Med* 107:198–208, 1999.
121. Rosen AB, Fowler VG Jr, Corey GR, et al: Cost-effectiveness of transesophageal echocardiography to determine the duration of therapy for intravascular catheter-associated Staphylococcus aureus bacteremia. *Ann Intern Med* 130:810–820, 1999.
122. Sachdev M, Peterson GE, Jollis JG: Imaging techniques for diagnosis of infective endocarditis. *Cardiol Clin* 21:185–195, 2003.
123. Jacob S, Tong AT: Role of echocardiography in the diagnosis and management of infective endocarditis. *Curr Opin Cardiol* 17:478–485, 2002.
124. Hill EE, Herijgers P, Claus P, et al: Clinical and echocardiographic risk factors for embolism and mortality in infective endocarditis. *Eur J Clin Microbiol Infect Dis* 27:1159–1164, 2008.
125. Hubert S, Thuny F, Resseguier N, et al: Prediction of symptomatic embolism in infective endocarditis: construction and validation of a risk calculator in a multicenter cohort. *J Am Coll Cardiol* 62:1384–1392, 2013.
126. Bruun NE, Habib G, Thuny F, et al: Cardiac imaging in infectious endocarditis. *Eur Heart J* 35:624–632, 2014.
127. Cahill TJ, Prendergast BD: Current controversies in infective endocarditis. *F1000Res* 4, 2015.
128. Arber N, Pras E, Copperman Y, et al: Pacemaker endocarditis. Report of 44 cases and review of the literature. *Medicine (Baltimore)* 73:299–305, 1994.
129. Fernandez Guerrero ML, Aguado JM, Arribas A, et al: The spectrum of cardiovascular infections due to Salmonella enterica: a review of clinical features and factors determining outcome. *Medicine (Baltimore)* 83:123–138, 2004.
130. Fernandez Guerrero ML, Torres Perea R, Gomez Rodrigo J, et al: Infectious endocarditis due to non-typhi Salmonella in patients infected with human immunodeficiency virus: report of two cases and review. *Clin Infect Dis* 22:853–855, 1996.
131. Fang G, Keys TF, Gentry LO, et al: Prosthetic valve endocarditis resulting from nosocomial bacteremia. A prospective, multicenter study. *Ann Intern Med* 119:560–567, 1993.
132. Wilson R, Hamburger M: Fifteen years' experience with staphylococcus septicemia in a large city hospital; analysis of fifty-five cases in the Cincinnati General Hospital 1940 to 1954. *Am J Med* 22:437–457, 1957.
133. Shah M, Watanakunakorn C: Changing patterns of Staphylococcus aureus bacteremia. *Am J Med Sci* 278:115–121, 1979.

134. del Rio A, Cervera C, Moreno A, et al: Patients at risk of complications of Staphylococcus aureus bloodstream infection. *Clin Infect Dis* 48[Suppl 4]:S246–S253, 2009.
135. Abraham J, Mansour C, Veledar E, et al: Staphylococcus aureus bacteremia and endocarditis: the Grady Memorial Hospital experience with methicillin-sensitive S aureus and methicillin-resistant S aureus bacteremia. *Am Heart J* 147:536–539, 2004.
136. Showler A, Burry L, Bai AD, et al: Use of transthoracic echocardiography in the management of low-risk Staphylococcus aureus bacteremia: results from a Retrospective Multicenter Cohort Study. *JACC Cardiovasc Imaging* 8:924–931, 2015.
137. Fowler VG Jr, Li J, Corey GR, et al: Role of echocardiography in evaluation of patients with Staphylococcus aureus bacteremia: experience in 103 patients. *J Am Coll Cardiol* 30:1072–1078, 1997.
138. Fowler VG Jr, Olsen MK, Corey GR, et al: Clinical identifiers of complicated Staphylococcus aureus bacteremia. *Arch Intern Med* 163:2066–2072, 2003.
139. Jernigan JA, Farr BM: Short-course therapy of catheter-related Staphylococcus aureus bacteremia: a meta-analysis. *Ann Intern Med* 119:304–311, 1993.
140. Raad II, Sabbagh MF: Optimal duration of therapy for catheter-related Staphylococcus aureus bacteremia: a study of 55 cases and review. *Clin Infect Dis* 14:75–82, 1992.
141. Mitchell DH, Howden BP: Diagnosis and management of Staphylococcus aureus bacteraemia. *Intern Med J* 35[Suppl 2]:S17–S24, 2005.
142. Fernandez Guerrero ML, Gonzalez Lopez JJ, Goyenechea A, et al: Endocarditis caused by Staphylococcus aureus: a reappraisal of the epidemiologic, clinical, and pathologic manifestations with analysis of factors determining outcome. *Medicine (Baltimore)* 88:1–22, 2009.
143. Gebo KA, Burkey MD, Lucas GM, et al: Incidence of, risk factors for, clinical presentation, and 1-year outcomes of infective endocarditis in an urban HIV cohort. *J Acquir Immune Defic Syndr* 43:426–432, 2006.
144. Fernandez-Guerrero ML, Herrero L, Bellver M, et al: Nosocomial enterococcal endocarditis: a serious hazard for hospitalized patients with enterococcal bacteraemia. *J Intern Med* 252:510–515, 2002.
145. Anderson DJ, Murdoch DR, Sexton DJ, et al: Risk factors for infective endocarditis in patients with enterococcal bacteremia: a case-control study. *Infection* 32:72–77, 2004.
146. McBride SJ, Upton A, Roberts SA: Clinical characteristics and outcomes of patients with vancomycin-susceptible Enterococcus faecalis and Enterococcus faecium bacteraemia–a five-year retrospective review. *Eur J Clin Microbiol Infect Dis* 29:107–114, 2010.
147. Shaked H, Carmeli Y, Schwartz D, et al: Enterococcal bacteraemia: epidemiological, microbiological, clinical and prognostic characteristics, and the impact of high level gentamicin resistance. *Scand J Infect Dis* 38:995–1000, 2006.
148. Chou YY, Lin TY, Lin JC, et al: Vancomycin-resistant enterococcal bacteremia: comparison of clinical features and outcome between Enterococcus faecium and Enterococcus faecalis. *J Microbiol Immunol Infect* 41:124–129, 2008.
149. Baddour LM, Epstein AE, Erickson CC, et al: Update on cardiovascular implantable electronic device infections and their management: a scientific statement from the American Heart Association. *Circulation* 121:458–477, 2010.
150. Baddour LM, Cha YM, Wilson WR: Clinical practice. Infections of cardiovascular implantable electronic devices. *N Engl J Med* 367:842–849, 2012.
151. Zhan C, Baine WB, Sedrakyan A, et al: Cardiac device implantation in the United States from 1997 through 2004: a population-based analysis. *J Gen Intern Med* 23[Suppl 1]:13–19, 2008.
152. Uslan DZ, Sohail MR, St Sauver JL, et al: Permanent pacemaker and implantable cardioverter defibrillator infection: a population-based study. *Arch Intern Med* 167:669–675, 2007.
153. Carrasco F, Anguita M, Ruiz M, et al: Clinical features and changes in epidemiology of infective endocarditis on pacemaker devices over a 27-year period (1987–2013). *Europace* 18:836–841, 2015. doi:10.1093/europace/euv377.
154. Sohail MR, Uslan DZ, Khan AH, et al: Risk factor analysis of permanent pacemaker infection. *Clin Infect Dis* 45:166–173, 2007.
155. Klug D, Balde M, Pavin D, et al: Risk factors related to infections of implanted pacemakers and cardioverter-defibrillators: results of a large prospective study. *Circulation* 116:1349–1355, 2007.
156. del Rio A, Anguera I, Miro JM, et al: Surgical treatment of pacemaker and defibrillator lead endocarditis: the impact of electrode lead extraction on outcome. *Chest* 124:1451–1459, 2003.
157. Byrd CL, Wilkoff BL, Love CJ, et al: Clinical study of the laser sheath for lead extraction: the total experience in the United States. *Pacing Clin Electrophysiol* 25:804–808, 2002.
158. Wunderly D, Maloney J, Edel T, et al: Infections in implantable cardioverter defibrillator patients. *Pacing Clin Electrophysiol* 13:1360–1364, 1990.
159. Almassi GH, Olinger GN, Troup PJ, et al: Delayed infection of the automatic implantable cardioverter-defibrillator. Current recognition and management. *J Thorac Cardiovasc Surg* 95:908–911, 1988.
160. Gordon RJ, Quagliarello B, Lowy FD: Ventricular assist device-related infections. *Lancet Infect Dis* 6:426–437, 2006.
161. Nienaber JJ, Kusne S, Riaz T, et al: Clinical manifestations and management of left ventricular assist device-associated infections. *Clin Infect Dis* 57:1438–1448, 2013.
162. Oz MC, Argenziano M, Catanese KA, et al: Bridge experience with long-term implantable left ventricular assist devices. Are they an alternative to transplantation? *Circulation* 95:1844–1852, 1997.
163. Mourvillier B, Trouillet JL, Timsit JF, et al: Infective endocarditis in the intensive care unit: clinical spectrum and prognostic factors in 228 consecutive patients. *Intensive Care Med* 30:2046–2052, 2004.
164. Wang A, Pappas P, Anstrom KJ, et al: The use and effect of surgical therapy for prosthetic valve infective endocarditis: a propensity analysis of a multicenter, international cohort. *Am Heart J* 150:1086–1091, 2005.
165. Sexton DJ, Tenenbaum MJ, Wilson WR, et al: Ceftriaxone once daily for four weeks compared with ceftriaxone plus gentamicin once daily for two weeks for treatment of endocarditis due to penicillin-susceptible streptococci. Endocarditis Treatment Consortium Group. *Clin Infect Dis* 27:1470–1474, 1998.
166. Korzeniowski O, Sande MA: Combination antimicrobial therapy for Staphylococcus aureus endocarditis in patients addicted to parenteral drugs and in nonaddicts: a prospective study. *Ann Intern Med* 97:496–503, 1982.
167. Abrams B, Sklaver A, Hoffman T, et al: Single or combination therapy of staphylococcal endocarditis in intravenous drug abusers. *Ann Intern Med* 90:789–791, 1979.
168. Ribera E, Gomez-Jimenez J, Cortes E, et al: Effectiveness of cloxacillin with and without gentamicin in short-term therapy for right-sided Staphylococcus aureus endocarditis. A randomized, controlled trial. *Ann Intern Med* 125:969–974, 1996.
169. van Hal SJ, Lodise TP, Paterson DL: The clinical significance of vancomycin minimum inhibitory concentration in Staphylococcus aureus infections: a systematic review and meta-analysis. *Clin Infect Dis* 54:755–771, 2012.
170. Cosgrove SE, Vigliani GA, Fowler VG Jr, et al: Initial low-dose gentamicin for Staphylococcus aureus bacteremia and endocarditis is nephrotoxic. *Clin Infect Dis* 48:713–721, 2009.
171. Markowitz N, Quinn EL, Saravolatz LD: Trimethoprim-sulfamethoxazole compared with vancomycin for the treatment of Staphylococcus aureus infection. *Ann Intern Med* 117:390–398, 1992.
172. Cervera C, Castaneda X, de la Maria CG, et al: Effect of vancomycin minimal inhibitory concentration on the outcome of methicillin-susceptible Staphylococcus aureus endocarditis. *Clin Infect Dis* 58:1668–1675, 2014.
173. Levine DP, Fromm BS, Reddy BR: Slow response to vancomycin or vancomycin plus rifampin in methicillin-resistant Staphylococcus aureus endocarditis. *Ann Intern Med* 115:674–680, 1991.
174. de Feiter PW, Jacobs JA, Jacobs MJ, et al: Successful treatment of Staphylococcus epidermidis prosthetic valve endocarditis with linezolid after failure of treatment with oxacillin, gentamicin, rifampicin, vancomycin, and fusidic acid regimens. *Scand J Infect Dis* 37:173–176, 2005.
175. Wareham DW, Abbas H, Karcher AM, et al: Treatment of prosthetic valve infective endocarditis due to multi-resistant Gram-positive bacteria with linezolid. *J Infect* 52:300–304, 2006.
176. Sande MA, Scheld WM: Combination antibiotic therapy of bacterial endocarditis. *Ann Intern Med* 92:390–395, 1980.
177. Gavalda J, Len O, Miro JM, et al: Brief communication: treatment of Enterococcus faecalis endocarditis with ampicillin plus ceftriaxone. *Ann Intern Med* 146:574–579, 2007.
178. Fernandez-Hidalgo N, Almirante B, Gavalda J, et al: Ampicillin plus ceftriaxone is as effective as ampicillin plus gentamicin for treating enterococcus faecalis infective endocarditis. *Clin Infect Dis* 56:1261–1268, 2013.
179. Olaison L, Schadewitz K: Enterococcal endocarditis in Sweden, 1995–1999: can shorter therapy with aminoglycosides be used? *Clin Infect Dis* 34:159–166, 2002.
180. Dahl A, Rasmussen RV, Bundgaard H, et al: Enterococcus faecalis infective endocarditis: a pilot study of the relationship between duration of gentamicin treatment and outcome. *Circulation* 127:1810–1817, 2013.
181. Habib G, Hoen B, Tornos P, et al: Guidelines on the prevention, diagnosis, and treatment of infective endocarditis (new version 2009): the Task Force on the Prevention, Diagnosis, and Treatment of Infective Endocarditis of the European Society of Cardiology (ESC). Endorsed by the European Society of Clinical Microbiology and Infectious Diseases (ESCMID) and the International Society of Chemotherapy (ISC) for Infection and Cancer. *Eur Heart J* 30:2369–2413, 2009.
182. Elliott TS, Foweraker J, Gould FK, et al: Guidelines for the antibiotic treatment of endocarditis in adults: report of the Working Party of the British Society for Antimicrobial Chemotherapy. *J Antimicrob Chemother* 54:971–981, 2004.
183. Stevens MP, Edmond MB: Endocarditis due to vancomycin-resistant enterococci: case report and review of the literature. *Clin Infect Dis* 41:1134–1142, 2005.
184. Linden PK, Moellering RC Jr, Wood CA, et al: Treatment of vancomycin-resistant Enterococcus faecium infections with quinupristin/dalfopristin. *Clin Infect Dis* 33:1816–1823, 2001.
185. Birmingham MC, Rayner CR, Meagher AK, et al: Linezolid for the treatment of multidrug-resistant, gram-positive infections: experience from a compassionate-use program. *Clin Infect Dis* 36:159–168, 2003.
186. Kaplan AH, Weber DJ, Oddone EZ, et al: Infection due to Actinobacillus actinomycetemcomitans: 15 cases and review. *Rev Infect Dis* 11:46–63, 1989.
187. Schack SH, Smith PW, Penn RG, et al: Endocarditis caused by Actinobacillus actinomycetemcomitans. *J Clin Microbiol* 20:579–581, 1984.
188. Steinbach WJ, Perfect JR, Cabell CH, et al: A meta-analysis of medical versus surgical therapy for Candida endocarditis. *J Infect* 51:230–247, 2005.
189. Pappas PG, Kauffman CA, Andes D, et al: Clinical practice guidelines for the management of candidiasis: 2009 update by the Infectious Diseases Society of America. *Clin Infect Dis* 48:503–535, 2009.

190. Rajendram R, Alp NJ, Mitchell AR, et al: Candida prosthetic valve endocarditis cured by caspofungin therapy without valve replacement. *Clin Infect Dis* 40:e72–e74, 2005.
191. Lye DC, Hughes A, O'Brien D, et al: Candida glabrata prosthetic valve endocarditis treated successfully with fluconazole plus caspofungin without surgery: a case report and literature review. *Eur J Clin Microbiol Infect Dis* 24:753–755, 2005.
192. Bacak V, Biocina B, Starcevic B, et al: Candida albicans endocarditis treatment with caspofungin in an HIV-infected patient–case report and review of literature. *J Infect* 53:e11–e14, 2006.
193. Tornos P, Almirante B, Mirabet S, et al: Infective endocarditis due to Staphylococcus aureus: deleterious effect of anticoagulant therapy. *Arch Intern Med* 159:473–475, 1999.
194. Olaison L, Hogevik H, Myken P, et al: Early surgery in infective endocarditis. *QJM* 89:267–278, 1996.
195. Mullany CJ, Chua YL, Schaff HV, et al: Early and late survival after surgical treatment of culture-positive active endocarditis. *Mayo Clin Proc* 70:517–525, 1995.
196. Middlemost S, Wisenbaugh T, Meyerowitz C, et al: A case for early surgery in native left-sided endocarditis complicated by heart failure: results in 203 patients. *J Am Coll Cardiol* 18:663–667, 1991.
197. Prendergast BD, Tornos P: Surgery for infective endocarditis: who and when? *Circulation* 121:1141–1152, 2010.
198. Olaison L, Pettersson G: Current best practices and guidelines indications for surgical intervention in infective endocarditis. *Infect Dis Clin North Am* 16:453–475, xi, 2002.
199. Larbalestier RI, Kinchla NM, Aranki SF, et al: Acute bacterial endocarditis. Optimizing surgical results. *Circulation* 86:II68–II74, 1992.
200. Blumberg EA, Robbins N, Adimora A, et al: Persistent fever in association with infective endocarditis. *Clin Infect Dis* 15:983–990, 1992.
201. Fabri J Jr, Issa VS, Pomerantzeff PM, et al: Time-related distribution, risk factors and prognostic influence of embolism in patients with left-sided infective endocarditis. *Int J Cardiol* 110:334–339, 2006.
202. Thuny F, Di Salvo G, Belliard O, et al: Risk of embolism and death in infective endocarditis: prognostic value of echocardiography: a prospective multicenter study. *Circulation* 112:69–75, 2005.
203. Gammie JS, O'Brien SM, Griffith BP, et al: Surgical treatment of mitral valve endocarditis in North America. *Ann Thorac Surg* 80:2199–2204, 2005.
204. Ruttmann E, Legit C, Poelzl G, et al: Mitral valve repair provides improved outcome over replacement in active infective endocarditis. *J Thorac Cardiovasc Surg* 130:765–771, 2005.
205. Truninger K, Attenhofer Jost CH, Seifert B, et al: Long term follow up of prosthetic valve endocarditis: what characteristics identify patients who were treated successfully with antibiotics alone? *Heart* 82:714–720, 1999.
206. Habib G, Tribouilloy C, Thuny F, et al: Prosthetic valve endocarditis: who needs surgery? A multicentre study of 104 cases. *Heart* 91:954–959, 2005.
207. Wolff M, Witchitz S, Chastang C, et al: Prosthetic valve endocarditis in the ICU. Prognostic factors of overall survival in a series of 122 cases and consequences for treatment decision. *Chest* 108:688–694, 1995.
208. John MD, Hibberd PL, Karchmer AW, et al: Staphylococcus aureus prosthetic valve endocarditis: optimal management and risk factors for death. *Clin Infect Dis* 26:1302–1309, 1998.
209. Bonow RO, Carabello BA, Kanu C, et al: ACC/AHA 2006 guidelines for the management of patients with valvular heart disease: a report of the American College of Cardiology/American Heart Association Task Force on Practice Guidelines (writing committee to revise the 1998 Guidelines for the Management of Patients With Valvular Heart Disease): developed in collaboration with the Society of Cardiovascular Anesthesiologists: endorsed by the Society for Cardiovascular Angiography and Interventions and the Society of Thoracic Surgeons. *Circulation* 114:e84–e231, 1998.
210. Tleyjeh IM, Ghomrawi HM, Steckelberg JM, et al: The impact of valve surgery on 6-month mortality in left-sided infective endocarditis. *Circulation* 115:1721–1728, 2007.
211. Sy RW, Bannon PG, Bayfield MS, et al: Survivor treatment selection bias and outcomes research: a case study of surgery in infective endocarditis. *Circ Cardiovasc Qual Outcomes* 2:469–474, 2009.
212. Bannay A, Hoen B, Duval X, et al: The impact of valve surgery on short- and long-term mortality in left-sided infective endocarditis: do differences in methodological approaches explain previous conflicting results? *Eur Heart J* 32:2003–2015, 2011.
213. Kiefer T, Park L, Tribouilloy C, et al: Association between valvular surgery and mortality among patients with infective endocarditis complicated by heart failure. *JAMA* 306:2239–2247, 2011.
214. Lalani T, Cabell CH, Benjamin DK, et al: Analysis of the impact of early surgery on in-hospital mortality of native valve endocarditis: use of propensity score and instrumental variable methods to adjust for treatment-selection bias. *Circulation* 121:1005–1013, 2010.
215. Chu VH, Park LP, Athan E, et al: Association between surgical indications, operative risk, and clinical outcome in infective endocarditis: a prospective study from the International Collaboration on Endocarditis. *Circulation* 131:131–140, 2015.
216. Iung B, Doco-Lecompte T, Chocron S, et al: Cardiac surgery during the acute phase of infective endocarditis: discrepancies between European Society of Cardiology guidelines and practices. *Eur Heart J* 37:840–848, 2016.
217. Kang DH, Kim YJ, Kim SH, et al: Early surgery versus conventional treatment for infective endocarditis. *N Engl J Med* 366:2466–2473, 2012.
218. Kang DH: Timing of surgery in infective endocarditis. *Heart* 101:1786–1791, 2015.
219. Thuny F, Beurtheret S, Mancini J, et al: The timing of surgery influences mortality and morbidity in adults with severe complicated infective endocarditis: a propensity analysis. *Eur Heart J* 32:2027–2033, 2011.
220. Desch S, Freund A, de Waha S, et al: Outcome in patients with left-sided native-valve infective endocarditis and isolated large vegetations. *Clin Cardiol* 37:626–633, 2014.
221. Anantha Narayanan M, Mahfood Haddad T, Kalil AC, et al: Early versus late surgical intervention or medical management for infective endocarditis: a systematic review and meta-analysis. *Heart* 102:950–957, 2016. doi:10.1136/heartjnl-2015-308589.
222. Lalani T, Chu VH, Park LP, et al: In-hospital and 1-year mortality in patients undergoing early surgery for prosthetic valve endocarditis. *JAMA Intern Med* 173:1495–1504, 2013.
223. Chirouze C, Alla F, Fowler VG Jr, et al: Impact of early valve surgery on outcome of Staphylococcus aureus prosthetic valve infective endocarditis: analysis in the International Collaboration of Endocarditis-Prospective Cohort Study. *Clin Infect Dis* 60:741–749, 2015.
224. Grubitzsch H, Schaefer A, Melzer C, et al: Outcome after surgery for prosthetic valve endocarditis and the impact of preoperative treatment. *J Thorac Cardiovasc Surg* 148:2052–2059, 2014.
225. Meshaal MS, Kassem HH, Samir A, et al: Impact of routine cerebral CT angiography on treatment decisions in infective endocarditis. *PLoS One* 10:e0118616, 2015.
226. Duval X, Iung B, Klein I, et al: Effect of early cerebral magnetic resonance imaging on clinical decisions in infective endocarditis: a prospective study. *Ann Intern Med* 152:497–504, W175, 2010.
227. Yoshioka D, Sakaguchi T, Yamauchi T, et al: Impact of early surgical treatment on postoperative neurologic outcome for active infective endocarditis complicated by cerebral infarction. *Ann Thorac Surg* 94:489–495, 2012; discussion 496.
228. Pang PY, Sin YK, Lim CH, et al: Surgical management of infective endocarditis: an analysis of early and late outcomes. *Eur J Cardiothorac Surg* 47:826–832, 2015.
229. Misfeld M, Girrbach F, Etz CD, et al: Surgery for infective endocarditis complicated by cerebral embolism: a consecutive series of 375 patients. *J Thorac Cardiovasc Surg* 147:1837–1844, 2014.
230. Barsic B, Dickerman S, Krajinovic V, et al: Influence of the timing of cardiac surgery on the outcome of patients with infective endocarditis and stroke. *Clin Infect Dis* 56:209–217, 2013.
231. Morita K, Sasabuchi Y, Matsui H, et al: Outcomes after early or late timing of surgery for infective endocarditis with ischaemic stroke: a retrospective cohort study. *Interact Cardiovasc Thorac Surg* 21:604–609, 2015.
232. Yoshioka D, Toda K, Sakaguchi T, et al: Valve surgery in active endocarditis patients complicated by intracranial haemorrhage: the influence of the timing of surgery on neurological outcomes. *Eur J Cardiothorac Surg* 45:1082–1088, 2014.

Chapter 79 ■ Infections Associated with Vascular Catheters

PAYAL K. PATEL • SUZANNE F. BRADLEY • CAROL A. KAUFFMAN

INTRODUCTION

As US health care payment structures are shifting toward quality rather than quantity of care, health care-associated infections have come to the forefront as targets for infection prevention. Significant efforts to reduce the burden of health care-associated infections have included multistep prevention bundles and encouraging line removal wherever possible, but despite these efforts, 1 in 25 inpatients has a health care-associated infection [1]. Intensive care unit (ICU) patients account for 80,000 central line-associated bloodstream infections (CLABSI) per year. Each infection can cost up to $56,000 and have an attributable mortality of up to 40% [2]. Groups such as the National Healthcare Safety Network (NHSN) compare hospital CLABSI rates, and hospitals in the lowest-performing quartile can have funds withheld because of these performance measures.

Guidelines for the prevention and treatment of catheter-associated infections have been updated in the past few years [3–5]. Recommendations in this chapter are based on these published guidelines. The reader is referred to these publications for a more in-depth review of the topics of prevention, diagnosis, and treatment of catheter-associated infections.

PATHOGENESIS OF CATHETER-RELATED INFECTION

Foreign bodies that penetrate the cutaneous barriers of the host induce a chronic inflammatory response and are coated with host proteins, including fibronectin, fibrin, and laminin [6]. The coated catheter provides a niche for microorganisms that adhere by fimbriae and adhesins that bind to surface receptors present on some of the coating proteins, or by electromagnetic interactions leading to the formation of biofilms within days of insertion [6].

Microorganisms gain entry to the catheter primarily at the insertion site. Particularly in catheters used short term, there is a correlation between organisms isolated from the catheter and those obtained from the insertion site [3]. Contamination of the catheter hub and ultimately the internal lumen of the catheter plays a larger role in the development of infections of catheters remaining in place for more than a month [3,6]. Less commonly, catheter-associated infections occur as a result of hematogenous seeding from a distant focus of infection or from a contaminated infusate.

DIAGNOSIS OF CATHETER-RELATED INFECTION

The diagnosis of catheter-associated infection still relies primarily on the recognition of clinical signs and symptoms of a patient who has an intravascular device in place, absence of an alternative cause for those clinical findings, and microbiological evidence for infection [5]. The clinical signs noted for some, but not all, patients with a catheter-associated infection are development of warmth, erythema, and pain at the site of current or recent catheter placement. Patients with catheter-associated bloodstream infection generally have fever, with or without hypotension and other signs of sepsis. Finding microorganisms when a catheter tip is submitted for culture from an asymptomatic patient is not indicative of infection; conversely, impressive local findings may reflect only phlebitis or reaction to the infusate. Thus, differentiating catheter-associated infection from colonization of the catheter can be difficult, and no perfect diagnostic method has been established.

Blood Culture with Catheter Retention

Positive blood cultures from a patient who has an indwelling vascular catheter and no other obvious source of infection raises the possibility of a catheter-associated infection. A variety of approaches have been devised to help differentiate whether a positive blood culture represents catheter-associated infection or has arisen from another source. Quantitative cultures of blood taken simultaneously from the catheter and from peripheral blood that demonstrate a difference of at least threefold more microorganisms from the catheter is probably the most accurate method to determine if catheter-associated infection is present without removing the catheter [7,8]. However, few clinical laboratories routinely perform quantitative blood cultures.

Differential time to positivity of blood cultures taken from a central line compared with those taken from a peripheral vein is another diagnostic method. Blood cultures obtained from an infected central catheter may turn positive at least 2 hours sooner than blood drawn simultaneously from a peripheral vein [8]. Another method that does not require the removal of the catheter involves culture of peripheral blood as well as the insertion site and hub. Growth of more than 15 colonies of the same organism from all three sites suggests catheter-related infection [5,9].

It is important to minimize the possibility of contamination when obtaining blood for culture by having specifically trained personnel obtain the samples. Disinfection of the skin and hub using an alcoholic chlorhexidine antiseptic, not povidone–iodine, is recommended [3,4]. Blood samples taken from a peripheral vein are less likely to be contaminated than blood samples obtained from the catheter [10]. All of the techniques listed above require sampling from the catheter as well as from a peripheral vein. Additionally, all catheter lumens should be sampled to increase the sensitivity of diagnosis of catheter-related infection [11].

Catheter Culture Following Catheter Removal

Although culture of the catheter is very helpful for the diagnosis of catheter-associated infection, it necessitates removal of the catheter before the diagnosis can be made. For optimum culture, the catheter tip should be cultured. Quantitative cultures obtained by sonication of the catheter tip have been advocated as a more accurate method to determine the numbers of microorganisms present on both the internal and external surfaces of the catheter [5]. However, others have shown no benefit of the more complicated sonication method over the roll-plate method [12].

Rolling the distal segment of the catheter on an agar plate yields semiquantitative results that compare favorably with quantitative methods and has gained the greatest acceptance [5,7]. The presence of ≥15 bacterial colonies on an agar plate correlates significantly with the presence of local inflammation and signs and symptoms of bloodstream infection. No similar cutoff has been established when yeasts are grown from the catheter tip.

A drawback of this technique is that only the external portion of the catheter is cultured, not the lumen, which may be the primary site of infection for long-term catheters. For short-term catheters, the roll-plate technique is the recommended microbiologic method for diagnosis of catheter-related infection [5,7].

Types of Catheters

Nontunneled Central Venous Catheters

These catheters are inserted into the subclavian vein, the internal jugular vein, and rarely the femoral vein. They can be single or multilumen depending on the specific needs of each patient. Some studies, but not all, have shown that multilumen catheters are associated with a higher rate of colonization and infection than single-lumen catheters, particularly when used for an extended period of time [13–15]. Increased risk for infection, especially with multilumen catheters, occurs with the frequent manipulations that are required in the care of critically ill patients. It is recommended that a central venous catheter be chosen with the minimum number of ports or lumens required for the care of the patient [4]. Care of these multilumen lines should be limited to a few well-trained personnel [4]. Multiple indwelling central venous catheters also increase the risk of infection, and removal of unnecessary lines should be considered on a daily basis [4,16–18]. Nontunneled central venous catheters should be used predominantly for patients in the ICU.

Antimicrobial Impregnated or Coated Central Venous Catheters

Numerous antimicrobial agents (tetracyclines, rifamycins, glycopeptides, β-lactams, and echinocandins), antiseptics (benzalkonium chloride, chlorhexidine, tridodecylmethylammonium chloride, iodine, gentian violet, and silver molecules), and antithrombotic agents (heparin and ethylenediaminetetraacetate [EDTA]) alone or in various combinations have been bound to polymer material or used to coat the surfaces of catheters in the hope of reducing colonization, thrombosis, and subsequent infection [3,4,7,19–21]. Heparin-coated catheters should not be used because of concerns for developing heparin-induced thrombocytopenia [21].

Minocycline–rifampin-coated catheters (Cook Medical, Bloomington, IN), chlorhexidine–silver sulfadiazine-coated catheters (Arrow International, Reading, PA), and a silver–platinum–carbon impregnated catheter (Vantex, Edwards Life Sciences, Irvine, CA) are currently available. All of these catheters have been shown to reduce catheter-associated colonization [4,7,19]. In some controlled trials, the rates of catheter-associated bacteremia were sufficient to demonstrate significant reductions of infection rates when antimicrobial catheters were compared with standard catheters [4,7,22,23]. The recommendations are to strongly consider the use of antimicrobial-coated catheters for adult patients who will likely require a central catheter for 5 to 14 days, if the local rate of catheter-associated bloodstream infections is unacceptably high in spite of adherence to other measures, such as maximal sterile barriers and use of chlorhexidine antisepsis [3,7,19]. Use of these catheters also could be considered for patients who have limited venous access and a history of recurrent catheter-related infections and for those with increased risk for severe sequelae if they develop systemic infections, such as patients with recently implanted devices [3]. Each hospital must decide, based on their rates of catheter-associated bloodstream infection, whether the higher costs of purchasing antimicrobial-coated catheters are justified.

Peripherally Inserted Central Venous Catheters

Peripherally inserted central venous catheters (PICC) have become increasingly common for venous access. PICCs were initially thought to have lower rates of infectious complications when compared to other central venous catheters. PICCs may have a lower risk of infection in outpatients, but the infection risk in hospitalized patients is comparable to that with central venous catheters [4,11,24,25]. Initial insertion costs are lower than those for tunneled central venous catheters, but rates of mechanical complications and phlebitis can be higher. These catheters must be inserted by specially trained health care workers or interventional radiologists. A PICC can be left in place for weeks to months as long as there is no malfunction; evidence of phlebitis; or infection.

Semipermanent Tunneled Catheters (Long-Term Central Venous Catheters)

Cuffed double-lumen subclavian catheters tunneled subcutaneously are used primarily for infusing parenteral nutrition solutions and cancer chemotherapy. The risk of infection with semipermanent tunneled catheters appears to be low [5,7]. Routine use in the ICU is not practical.

Pulmonary Artery Catheters

Use of pulmonary artery catheters has decreased markedly in the last decade because of the introduction of new hemodynamic monitoring technologies. The approach to placement and maintenance of these catheters in patients who have an appropriate indication should generally follow established guidelines for central line placement [3].

Peripheral Arterial Catheters

Although peripheral arterial catheters were initially believed to have lower risk of catheter-related infection, indwelling arterial catheters appear to have rates of complications similar to those for venous catheters [3,26]. Signs and symptoms of infection for arterial catheters are similar to those for venous catheters; however, the absence of local signs of inflammation does not preclude infection. Distal embolic lesions and hemorrhage are highly predictive of arterial catheter-associated bloodstream infection. Late complications such as pseudoaneurysm formation and rupture of the artery may occur [27]. The longer the catheter remains in place, the higher the rate of bloodstream infection.

Midline Catheters

Midline catheters are 3 to 8 inches in length, are inserted into the antecubital fossa or upper arm veins, and extend no further than the distal portion of the subclavian vein. These catheters are ideal if infusions are required for 6 to 14 days for non–critically ill patients [25]. They can remain in place for 4 weeks, are convenient to insert, are associated with fewer infections than central venous catheters, and cause less phlebitis than peripheral catheters [3]. However, infusions that irritate the vascular endothelium, such as vancomycin, nafcillin, and amphotericin B, cannot be given through this type of catheter.

Catheter Insertion

Choice of Insertion Site

Regardless of the type of catheter inserted, the major risk factor for the development of catheter-associated infection is the breach of a major host defense against infection—the skin. Catheter-associated infections are usually because of organisms colonizing the skin, particularly gram-positive cocci, such as coagulase-negative staphylococci and *Staphylococcus aureus*. However, the distribution of microorganisms on the skin varies. For example, gram-negative bacilli, *Candida* spp., and anaerobes are increased in the groin area and on the lower extremities.

The human microbiome is altered by illness, hospitalization, and the presence of foreign bodies.

The use of antimicrobial agents contributes to the emergence of resistant gram-positive and gram-negative organisms and yeasts. Daily disinfection of patient skin with chlorhexidine wipes or baths has been effective for reducing colonization and ultimately bloodstream infections in ICU patients [28,29]. Patients who have a productive cough or a tracheostomy can easily contaminate their skin with organisms from their respiratory tract [30].

The site of catheter insertion influences the risk of infection. Central venous catheters inserted in the internal jugular and femoral veins are associated with bloodstream infection significantly more often than those inserted into the subclavian vein [31]. Increased risk of thrombosis, contamination, and difficulties in dressing the site may play a role [4,31]. Insertion site colonization risk is particularly increased among obese patients with femoral catheters and for patients with tracheostomies with jugular catheters [3,30,32]. Risk of pneumothorax is more common among patients who have subclavian catheters; insertion using ultrasound guidance may help limit this complication [4,33]. Decisions regarding insertion site must be based on the risks of mechanical complications versus infectious and thrombotic risks. For long-term catheters, for which the risks of infection and thrombosis increase with duration of catheterization, use of the subclavian site is preferred [4,31]. All catheters should be removed as promptly as possible especially if they are inserted emergently under less than sterile conditions or if the catheter is no longer needed [3,4].

Insertion Techniques

It is essential that health care personnel perform hand hygiene with an alcohol-based waterless product or washing with antiseptic soap and water prior to insertion of a catheter [3,4,34]. Use of gloves is not a substitute for hand hygiene. Catheter-associated phlebitis and infection are more likely to occur when catheters are inserted by inexperienced personnel rather than personnel who are trained in these techniques.

Prospective, randomized trials have shown that strict adherence to sterile technique (i.e., mask, cap, and large sterile drape, gloves, and gown) is beneficial for preventing central venous catheter infections, and also highly cost-effective [3,4]. The importance of sterile techniques using maximal barrier precautions for short-term central catheters cannot be overemphasized and should become a part of house staff training [3,4]. Use of a standardized catheter cart or kit that contains all of the equipment necessary to insert a central venous catheter and use of a hospital-specific bundle or catheter insertion checklist filled out by a trained observer to ensure and document adherence to infection prevention practices at the time of insertion are recommended [3,4,16]. Health care personnel should be empowered to stop the catheter insertion if any breach in aseptic technique is observed.

Ultrasound guidance for the insertion of central vascular catheters, especially internal jugular catheters, has been shown to reduce the risk of infection [3,4,33].

Cutaneous Antisepsis

Chlorhexidine and iodine-based solutions, alone or in combination with alcohol, have been used to reduce microbial contamination at the insertion site of the catheter [3,4]. Current recommendations include the application of alcoholic chlorhexidine antiseptic (0.5% chlorhexidine gluconate) to the insertion site; the site should be allowed to dry before catheter insertion [3,4,35]. Chlorhexidine products should be used with care in children less than 2 months of age [3].

Antimicrobial ointments have been shown to increase the risk of infection with *Candida* and antibiotic-resistant bacteria and may affect the integrity of some catheters. With the exception of povidone–iodine ointment for some hemodialysis catheters, routine use of ointments at the catheter insertion site is discouraged [3,4].

A chlorhexidine-impregnated patch (BIOPATCH, Ethicon, Somerville, NJ) has been shown by a randomized controlled trial to reduce colonization at the catheter site and to reduce catheter-related bloodstream infections [36]. However, several guidelines do not recommend routine use of this patch, but rather suggest that it can be considered for use when the rates of catheter-associated infection remain high despite consistent use of evidence-based prevention bundles [3,4]. Use of these patches could be considered for patients who have limited access and a history of recurrent catheter-associated infections and for those who have a heightened risk of severe sequelae if infection should occur [3]. The use of systemic antibiotics as prophylaxis before the placement of central venous devices is strongly discouraged because selection for antibiotic-resistant microorganisms is highly likely [3,4].

Care of the Catheter and Insertion Site

Insertion Site Dressings

Either gauze and tape bandages or transparent semi-permeable dressings can be used for peripheral and central catheters. Transparent dressings are changed every 5 to 7 days and gauze dressings every 2 days or more frequently if the dressing is soiled, loose, or damp [3]. Site care should be performed with a chlorhexidine-based antiseptic with each dressing change [3]. At some centers, chlorhexidine patches are placed over catheters during routine dressing changes.

Catheter Hub Disinfection

Local disinfection of the hubs of central venous catheters must be performed using either a chlorhexidine-based preparation or 70% alcohol before attempting access [3,4]. With either preparation, it is very important to allow the antiseptic to dry to ensure antimicrobial activity before accessing the catheter. Maintenance of the catheter hub should be performed with strict standards, similar to those for insertion of catheters, to decrease the risk of contamination and infection [4]. A randomized controlled trial found that reducing the frequency of changing unsoiled adherent dressings from 3 to 7 days, and thus decreasing manipulation of the site, did not increase the risk of infection [36].

Catheter Replacement

Peripheral Catheters

Phlebitis of a peripheral vein is a well-recognized harbinger of infection and may be quite uncomfortable for the patient. A catheter causing phlebitis should be removed promptly and the tip cultured. Complications of peripheral venous catheter insertion, including phlebitis and catheter-associated infection, increase after 72 hours of insertion. Recommendations to remove and change these catheters to another site every 72 hours are aimed at decreasing the risk for infection and the discomfort associated with phlebitis [4]. Midline catheters and PICC lines should not be removed and changed routinely unless phlebitis or signs of infection develop [4].

Central Catheters

The risk of infection increases during the time that a central catheter is in place, but several studies have shown that routine replacement of these catheters does not reduce rates of catheter-associated bloodstream infections [3,4]. Routine rotation of a central catheter to a different site is associated with increased risk for pneumothorax, laceration of a vessel with hemothorax, and arrhythmias and thus, is not recommended [5].

The use of routine catheter change over a guidewire has also been tried as a means to decrease catheter-related infections. However, a meta-analysis of studies employing this technique failed to show an effect on decreasing infections, and routine catheter changes over a guidewire are not recommended [4,37].

Thrombosis requires removal of an indwelling catheter [38]. An exception is made for the patient who has poor access and is dependent on a surgically implanted semipermanent central catheter. Under these circumstances, an attempt to salvage the catheter is reasonable [5].

Infusion-Related Issues

Local Effects

Intravenous solutions and drugs that are acidic, hypertonic, or directly irritating to vascular endothelium (KCl, certain antibiotics, and chemotherapeutic agents) may lead to a local inflammatory response, thrombosis, and phlebitis, with an increased risk of infection. When such infusions are necessary, a central catheter should be used.

In-Line Devices and Filters

In-line devices can be a significant source of catheter-associated infections. Pressure transducers have been implicated during outbreaks of catheter-associated bloodstream infection, particularly those due to water-associated gram-negative bacilli, including *Pseudomonas*, *Serratia*, *Enterobacter*, *Citrobacter*, and *Acinetobacter* spp. [39]. Stopcocks are easily contaminated through manipulation by personnel or by injection with contaminated syringes and may be an important source of infection; use of a closed system rather than stopcocks has been shown to lead to less contamination of the line. Some studies suggest that needleless mechanical valve devices may pose a greater risk of infection than split septum devices [40,41]. Disposable transducer domes, stopcocks, needleless components, and other in-line devices should be changed with the rest of the infusion set. In-line filters do not decrease the rate of infection, and their use is not recommended [4]. All catheter hubs, needleless connectors, and injection ports should be disinfected with a chlorhexidine preparation before accessing the device [3].

Contamination of Infusates

Breaks in sterile technique by hospital personnel can cause bloodstream infection. Gram-negative bacilli, such as *Enterobacter*, *Klebsiella*, *Serratia*, and *Citrobacter*, can proliferate in the acidic environment of intravenous fluids containing minimal nutrients, and other organisms, including fungi, can grow in parenteral nutrition infusates containing lipids [42,43].

Multifaceted Approach to Prevention of Catheter Infection

An optimal approach to prevent catheter-associated infection involves the use of multiple infection control strategies, often termed a bundle. In Michigan, 108 ICUs assessed the impact of five-evidence based procedures recommended by the Centers for Disease Control and Prevention to prevent catheter-associated bloodstream infection [44]. This bundle consisted of full-barrier precautions for catheter insertion; hand washing; insertion site cleansing with chlorhexidine; avoidance of femoral insertion site; and removal of unnecessary catheters. This was implemented

TABLE 79.1

Summary of Recommendations for Prevention of Central Venous Catheter-Associated Infections Based on SHEA/IDSA Guidelines [3]

- Bathe intensive care unit patients with chlorhexidine daily (grade of evidence: I)
- Document adherence to infection prevention practices at the time of catheter insertion by a checklist filled out by a trained observer (II)
- Perform hand hygiene prior to insertion or manipulation of the catheter (grade of evidence: II)
- Use maximal sterile barriers (sterile full-sized drape, sterile gown, sterile gloves, face mask, and head cap) during insertion (II)
- Perform insertion site antisepsis with chlorhexidine (grade of evidence: I)
- Consider the use of a chlorhexidine-impregnated patch at the insertion site (grade of evidence: I)
- Change transparent dressings and perform site care with chlorhexidine-based antiseptic every 5–7 days or immediately if dressing is soiled, loose, or damp (grade of evidence: II)
- Do not routinely replace central intravascular catheters (grade of evidence: I)
- Consider use of central intravascular catheters coated with antimicrobial agents (minocycline–rifampin) or chlorhexidine–silver sulfadiazine when infection rates are high (grade of evidence: I)

I, high quality; II, moderate quality.
Grade of quality of evidence is from SHEA/IDSA Practice Recommendation [3].

in conjunction with clinician education, use of a designated central-line cart, a checklist to ensure adherence, and empowerment of the assistant to stop the procedure if the practices in the bundle were not being followed. This intervention led to a sustained 66% reduction in catheter-associated bloodstream infections over 18 months. Subsequent reports verified the efficacy of this approach [45–47]. The "bundle" approach has become standard of care and has been incorporated into practice guidelines [3,4,16]. Advances of prevention of infections associated with vascular catheters are summarized in Table 79.1.

CATHETER-ASSOCIATED INFECTIONS

Microbiology

Coagulase-negative staphylococci (*S. epidermidis* and other species) are the most common organisms implicated in catheter-associated infections, followed by *S. aureus*; a variety of gram-negative bacilli; other gram-positive cocci and bacilli; and *Candida* and other yeasts [5]. Coagulase-negative staphylococci are associated with less severe disease than most other organisms. *S. aureus* bloodstream infection is most likely to cause complications, including endocarditis, and *Candida* spp. have a propensity to seed to other structures, such as the eye [48,49].

Complications

Major complications of catheter-associated infections include septic shock, suppurative phlebitis, metastatic infection, endocarditis, and arteritis. These complications often require aggressive management that combines appropriate antimicrobial therapy and surgical intervention. Complications of bloodstream infection should be suspected, especially if the catheter has been removed, when a patient has persistence or relapse of the same organism by blood cultures after 72 hours of appropriate medical therapy and no alternative explanation can be found.

Suppurative Phlebitis

Suppurative phlebitis associated with vascular catheters is manifested by fever and positive blood cultures; signs of phlebitis may not be obvious. For peripheral catheters, old healed insertion sites may require exploration by needle aspiration or incision. Suppurative phlebitis of central veins, particularly of the subclavian veins and superior vena cava, should be confirmed by detection of a thrombus by computerized tomography, magnetic resonance imaging, venography, or ultrasound. Surgical or interventional radiological procedures to remove the thrombus are technically difficult, but should be considered when bloodstream infection persists despite conservative management. Most patients will respond to 3 to 4 weeks of treatment with systemic antimicrobial therapy.

Endocarditis

Endocarditis is a dreaded complication of catheter-associated infections, and is most likely to occur with infection with *S. aureus*. The aortic and mitral valves are involved most often; normal valves, as well as previously damaged valves, can be infected. Right atrial catheters that cross the tricuspid valve can cause endothelial damage and turbulence, predisposing the patient to the development of right-sided endocarditis if bacteremia or fungemia occurs. Persistent or intermittent bacteremia or fungemia despite catheter removal; and evidence of pulmonary, cutaneous, central nervous system, or other embolic phenomena suggest a diagnosis of endocarditis.

Initial Treatment

In the febrile patient in whom catheter-associated bloodstream infection is suspected, empiric treatment should include antimicrobial agents that cover both gram-positive cocci and gram-negative bacilli [5]. Vancomycin is chosen most frequently because of its activity against methicillin-resistant *Staphylococcus aureus* (MRSA) and coagulase-negative staphylococci. An alternative agent, such as daptomycin, should be considered in settings in which MRSA isolates commonly have vancomycin minimum inhibitory concentrations (MICs) $\geq 2\ \mu g$ per mL. For gram-negative bacilli, the choice of a β-lactam–β-lactamase inhibitor combination, an anti-pseudomonal cephalosporin, or a carbapenem should be based on local antimicrobial susceptibility data.

Use of an antifungal agent, preferably an echinocandin, should be considered for patients who have risk factors for candidemia, including a hematologic malignancy or solid organ transplant, presence of a femoral catheter; who are receiving parenteral nutrition and/or broad-spectrum antibiotic therapy; who have had recent abdominal surgery; and who are known to be colonized with *Candida* spp. [49]. Once the organism has been identified, the appropriate antimicrobial therapy should be chosen based on antimicrobial susceptibilities (Table 79.2).

Staphylococcus aureus Infections

It is difficult to distinguish uncomplicated from complicated catheter-associated *S. aureus* bloodstream infections and to predict which patients have endocarditis [50,51]. It is recommended that transthoracic echocardiography (TTE) be performed in all cases of catheter-associated *S. aureus* bacteremia [52]. For many patients, the TTE is equivocal, and transesophageal echocardiography (TEE) should be performed to better define the presence of vegetations and other cardiac abnormalities. Because TEE is invasive, several experts have suggested that a TEE might best be done only for those patients at highest risk for having endocarditis, which in one study was defined as those who have persistent bacteremia ≥4 days duration or in whom there is a permanent intracardiac device [51,53]. If the catheter is promptly removed and TEE is negative for vegetations, *S. aureus* bacteremia can be treated with a minimum of 2 weeks of a penicillinase-resistant β-lactam antibiotic or a first-generation cephalosporin; vancomycin or daptomycin should be used for

TABLE 79.2

Systemic Treatment of Intravascular Catheter-Associated Bloodstream Infection

Pathogen	First-line agent	Alternative agents
Coagulase (−) staphylococci		
Methicillin-susceptible	Nafcillin, oxacillin	Cefazolin, vancomycin
Methicillin-resistant	Vancomycin	Daptomycin, ceftaroline
Staphylococcus aureus		
Methicillin-susceptible	Nafcillin, oxacillin	Cefazolin, vancomycin
Methicillin-resistant	Vancomycin[a]	Daptomycin, ceftaroline
Gram-negative bacilli		
Enterobacteriaceae[b]		
ESBL (−)	Ceftriaxone, ceftazidime Ampicillin + sulbactam Piperacillin + tazobactam	Ciprofloxacin, aztreonam, cefepime
ESBL (+)	Carbapenem	Ciprofloxacin
Pseudomonas[b]	Cefepime, carbapenem Piperacillin + tazobactam	Ciprofloxacin, aztreonam
Candida spp.	Echinocandin	Fluconazole (if susceptible) Lipid amphotericin formulation without prior exposure

[a]Use an alternative agent if the vancomycin minimum inhibitory concentrations $\geq 2\ \mu g$ per mL.
[b]See local hospital antibiogram.
ESBL, extended spectrum β-lactamase.

MRSA. However, even those patients who appear to be appropriate candidates for short-course therapy may later present with metastatic foci, so it is essential to reassess "uncomplicated" cases if fever or embolic phenomena occur and certainly when follow-up blood cultures also yield *S. aureus* [5].

Candida spp. Infections

Current recommendations are to treat all patients with catheter-associated fungemia with an antifungal agent [49]. The possibility that the organism has seeded to distant sites, especially the eye, is high, leading to the recommendation that all candidemic patients should have a dilated retinal examination, preferably by an ophthalmologist [49]. Most studies have found that outcomes are improved when the catheter is promptly removed, but the argument has been made that for most many patients with neutropenia, the gut is the source of candidemia, and the catheter does not have to be removed. Many of these patients are thrombocytopenic, and the tunneled catheter or indwelling port cannot be removed easily. However, in the non-neutropenic patient, the recommendation is to remove all central catheters as soon as possible when feasible [49]. Treatment with an echinocandin (anidulafungin, caspofungin, and micafungin) is recommended; fluconazole can be used when the organism has been shown to be susceptible. The treatment should continue for 2 weeks after the first negative blood culture is obtained; however, if a metastatic focus of infection is noted, a prolonged therapy will be required.

Should the Catheter Be Removed?

Catheters in which the insertion site is painful, erythematous, indurated, or with exudate; and tunneled catheters that manifest a tunnel infection should be removed as soon as possible [5]. For exit site infections not accompanied by gross purulence, systemic signs of infection, or positive blood cultures, treatment with local topical antimicrobial agents, as well as systemic antibiotics can be tried based on culture data from a sample taken at the exit site. If treatment fails, then the catheter should be removed.

In the febrile patient who is clinically stable and without localizing signs of infection along the catheter insertion site, central catheters should not be removed until a microbiological assessment that includes samples of blood, with or without culture of insertion sites and hubs, is performed. Cultures that are positive from a single blood sample for organisms that are part of the normal skin flora, such as coagulase-negative staphylococci, diphtheroids, *Micrococcus*, or *Propionobacterium* spp., should be repeated to establish whether a true bloodstream infection is present [5,7]. If true bacteremia has been established, and there is no alternative source, catheters should be removed. Catheter-related infections due to coagulase staphylococci are a special case in that antibiotics alone without catheter removal are usually adequate to treat the acute infection [5]. However, recurrent infection is highly likely if the catheter is retained; unless there are cogent reasons for keeping the catheter in place, it should be removed [54]. If a catheter has been changed over a guide wire, and there is growth of $\geq$15 organisms from the tip of the removed catheter, the newly placed catheter is almost certainly infected and should be removed [3–5].

Catheter Salvage

In the case of long-term, tunneled, semipermanent catheters or ports that cannot be easily removed or for patients who have limited vascular access, treatment of catheter-associated infection with antibiotics without catheter removal can be tried. Catheter salvage is not recommended for patients with complications of catheter infection, such as suppurative phlebitis, endocarditis, tunnel infection, or for patients who have severe sepsis or have an implanted intravascular device, such as a prosthetic cardiac valve [5].

If salvage is considered, most success has occurred with coagulase-negative staphylococcal infections [5,7,54]. For bloodstream infections due to *S. aureus* and *Candida* spp., catheter salvage should be reserved for extenuating circumstances, i.e., when there is no alternative access. These infections and those due to gram-negative bacilli almost always require catheter removal [5]. Thrombolytics are not recommended as an adjunct to the treatment of catheter-associated bloodstream infection [38].

Antibiotic lock therapy, as an adjunct to systemic antimicrobial therapy, has been used for salvage of long-term catheters. In general, lock therapy involves the instillation of 2 to 5 mL of an antibiotic, often with an anticoagulant, into the catheter, allowing it to dwell until the catheter is reaccessed [7]. Ethanol and EDTA have also been used for lock therapy [55–57]. Compatibility issues are important as some solutions may influence the integrity of the catheter structure. Short-term catheters are less likely to have an intraluminal source of infection and are less likely to benefit from antibiotic lock therapy. The lock therapy antimicrobial agents and systemic antibiotics should be used concomitantly. In general, the duration of lock and systemic therapy ranges from 7 to 14 days. If antibiotic lock therapy cannot be given, then systemic treatment should be administered directly through the infected catheter. If patients with no alternative access do not respond to the antibiotic treatment, exchange over a guidewire can be attempted [5].

For treatment of infections due to gram-positive cocci, an antibiotic lock solution containing a combination of vancomycin plus heparin or saline is used most often; the vancomycin instilled should be 1,000-fold higher than the MICs for the bacteria involved [7]. A small randomized placebo-controlled trial of antibiotic lock therapy using vancomycin or ceftazidime for gram-positive or gram-negative organisms, respectively, found a trend to successful outcome associated with lock therapy, and anecdotal reports of successful cure of infection with gentamicin, amikacin, ciprofloxacin, ampicillin, cefazolin, ceftazidime, and minocycline–EDTA, have been reported [5,58].

References

1. Magill SS, Edwards JR, Bamberg W, et al: Multistate point-prevalence of health care-associated infections. *N Engl J Med* 370:1198–1208, 2014.
2. Herzer KR, Niessen L, O Constenla, et al: Cost-effectiveness of a quality improvement programme to reduce central line-associated bloodstream infections in intensive care units in the USA. *BMJ Open* 4:e006065, 2014.
3. Marschall J, Mermel LA, Fakih M, et al: Strategies to prevent central line-associated bloodstream infections in acute care hospitals: 2014 update. *Infect Control Hosp Epidemiol* 35:753–771, 2014.
4. O'Grady NP, Alexander M, Burns LA, et al: Summary of recommendations: guidelines for the prevention of intravascular catheter-related infections. *Clin Infect Dis* 52:1087–1099, 2011.
5. Mermel LA, Allon M, Bouza E, et al: Clinical practice guidelines for the diagnosis and management of intravascular catheter-related infection: 2009 Update by the Infectious Diseases Society of America. *Clin Infect Dis* 49:1–45, 2009.
6. Donlan RM: Biofilm elimination on intravascular catheters: important considerations for the Infectious Diseases practitioner. *Clin Infect Dis* 52:1038–1045, 2011.
7. Raad I, Hanna H, Maki D: Intravascular catheter-related infections: advances in diagnosis, prevention, and management. *Lancet Infect Dis* 7:645–657, 2007.
8. Al Wohoush I, Cairo J, Rangaraj G, et al: Comparing quantitative culture of a blood sample obtained through the catheter with differential time to positivity in establishing a diagnosis of catheter-related bloodstream infection. *Infect Control Hosp Epidemiol* 31:1089–1091, 2010.
9. Bouza E, Alvarado N, Alcala L, et al: A randomized and prospective study of 3 procedures for the diagnosis of catheter-related bloodstream infection without catheter withdrawal. *Clin Infect Dis* 44:820–826, 2007.
10. Boyce JM, Nadeau J, Dumigan D, et al: Obtaining blood cultures by venipuncture versus from central lines: impact on blood culture contamination rates and potential effect on central line-associated bloodstream infection reporting. *Infect Control Hosp Epidemiol* 34:1042–1047, 2013.
11. Guembe M, Rodriquez-Creixems M, Sanchez-Carrillo C, et al: How many lumens should be cultured in the conservative diagnosis of catheter-related bloodstream infections? *Clin Infect Dis* 50:1575–1579, 2010.
12. Erb S, Frei R, Schregenberger K, et al: Sonication for diagnosis of catheter-related infection is not better than traditional roll-plate culture: a prospective cohort study with 975 central venous catheters. *Clin Infect Dis* 59:541–544, 2014.

13. Bouza E, Guembe M, Munoz P: Selection of the vascular catheter: can it minimize the risk of infection? *Int J Antimicrob Agents* 36:S22–S25, 2010.
14. Templeton A, Schlegel M, Fleisch F, et al: Multilumen central venous catheters increase risk or catheter-related bloodstream infection: prospective surveillance study. *Infection* 36:322–327, 2008.
15. Dezfulian C, Lavelle J, Nallamothu B, et al: Rates of infection for single-lumen versus multilumen central venous catheters: a meta-analysis. *Crit Care Med* 31:2385–2390, 2003.
16. Latif A, Halim M, Pronovost P: Eliminating infections in the ICU: CLABSI. *Curr Infect Dis Rep* 17:1–9, 2015.
17. Concannon C, van Wijngaarden E, Stevens V, et al: The effect of multiple concurrent central venous catheters on central line-associated bloodstream infections. *Infect Control Hosp Epidemiol* 35:1140–1146, 2014.
18. Fong K, Banks M, Benish R, et al: Intensity of vascular catheter use in critical care: impact on catheter associated bloodstream infection rates and association with severity of illness. *Infect Control Hosp Epidemiol* 33:1268–1270, 2012.
19. Casey AL, Mermel LA, Nightingale P, et al: Antimicrobial central venous catheters in adults: a systematic review and meta-analysis. *Lancet Infect Dis* 8:763–776, 2007.
20. Hanna H, Bahna P, Reitzel R, et al: Comparative in vitro efficacies and antimicrobial durabilities of novel antimicrobial central venous catheters. *Antimicrob Agents Chemother* 50:3283–3288, 2006.
21. Mitchell M, Anderson B, Williams K, et al: Heparin flushing and other interventions to maintain patency of central venous catheters: a systematic review. *J Adv Nurs* 65:2007–2021, 2009.
22. Bonne S, Mazuski J, Sona C, et al: Effectiveness of minocycline and rifampin versus chlorhexidine and silver sulfadiazine-impregnated central venous catheters in preventing central line-associated bloodstream infection in a high-volume academic intensive care unit: a before and after trial. *J Am Coll Surg* 221:739–747, 2015.
23. Lai NM, Chaiyakunapruk N, Lai NA, et al: Catheter impregnation, coating or bonding for reducing central venous catheter-related infections in adults. *Cochrane Database Syst Rev* 6:CD007878, 2013.
24. Chopra V, O'Horo J, Rogers M, et al: The risk of bloodstream infection associated with peripherally inserted central catheters compared with central venous catheters in adults: a systematic review and meta-analysis. *Infect Control Hosp Epidemiol* 34:908–918, 2013.
25. Chopra V, Flanders S, Saint S, et al: The Michigan Appropriateness Guide for Intravenous Catheters (MAGIC): results from a multispecialty panel using the RAND/UCLA appropriateness method. *Ann Intern Med* 15:S1–S40, 2015.
26. Lucet J, Bouadma L, Zahar J, et al: Infectious risk associated with arterial catheters compared with central venous catheters. *Crit Care Med* 38:1030–1035, 2010.
27. Ganchi P, Wilhelmi B, Fujita K, et al: Ruptured pseudoaneurysm complicating an infected radial artery catheter: case report and review of the literature. *Ann Plast Surg* 46:647–649, 2001.
28. Huang SS, Septimus E, Kleinman K, et al: Targeted versus universal decolonization to prevent ICU infection. *N Engl J Med* 368:2255–2265, 2013.
29. Bleasdale SC, Trick WE, Gonzalez IM, et al: Effectiveness of chlorhexidine bathing to reduce catheter-associated bloodstream infections in medical intensive care unit patients. *Arch Intern Med* 167:2073–2079, 2007.
30. Lorente L, Jimenez A, Roca I, et al: Influence of tracheostomy on the incidence of catheter-related bloodstream infection in the catheterization of jugular vein by posterior access. *Eur J Clin Microbiol Infect Dis* 30:1049–1051, 2011.
31. Parienti J-J, Mongardon N, Megarbane B, et al: Intravascular complications of central venous catheterization by insertion site. *N Engl J Med* 373:1220–119, 2015.
32. Parienti JJ, du Cheyron D, Timsit JF, et al: Meta-analysis of subclavian insertion and nontunneled central venous catheter–associated infection risk reduction in critically ill adults. *Crit Care Med* 40:1627–1634, 2012.
33. Frankel HL, Kirkpatrick AW, Elbarbary M, et al: Guidelines for the appropriate use of bedside general and cardiac ultrasonography in the evaluation of critically ill patients—Part I: General ultrasonography. *Crit Care Med* 43:2479–2502, 2015.
34. Ellingson K, Haas JP, Allison AE, et al: Strategies to prevent healthcare-associated infections through hand hygiene. *Infect Control Hosp Epidemiol* 35:937–960, 2014.
35. Maiwald M, Chan ESY: The forgotten role of alcohol: a systematic review and meta-analysis of the clinical efficacy and perceived role of chlorhexidine in skin antisepsis. *PLoS One* 9:e44277, 2012.
36. Timsit J-F, Schwebel C, Bouadma L, et al: Clorhexidine-impregnated sponges and less frequent dressing changes for prevention of catheter-related infections in critically ill adults: a randomized controlled trial. *JAMA* 301:1231–1241, 2009.
37. Cook D, Randolph A, Kernerman P, et al: Central venous catheter replacement strategies: a systematic review of the literature. *Crit Care Med* 25:1417–1424, 1997.
38. Baskin JL, Pui C-H, Reiss U, et al: Management of occlusion and thrombosis associated with long-term indwelling central venous catheters. *Lancet* 374:159–169, 2009.
39. Archibald L, Jarvis WR: Health care-associated infection outbreak investigations by the Centers for Disease Control and Prevention, 1946–2005. *Am J Epidemiol* 174:S47–S64, 2011.
40. Field K, McFarlane C, Cheng AC, et al: Incidence of catheter-related bloodstream infection among patients with a needleless, mechanical valve-based intravenous connector in an Australian hematology-oncology unit. *Infect Control Hosp Epidemiol* 28:610–613, 2007.
41. Salgado CD, Chinnes L, Paczesny TH, et al: Increased rate of catheter-related bloodstream infection associated with use of a needleless mechanical valve device at a long-term acute care hospital. *Infect Control Hosp Epidemiol* 28:684–688, 2007.
42. Macias A, Huertas M, Ponce de Leon S, et al: Contamination of intravenous fluids: a continuing cause of hospital bacteremia. *Am J Infect Control* 38:217–221, 2010.
43. Kuwahara T, Shimono K, Kaneda S, et al: Growth of Microorganisms in total parenteral nutrition solutions containing lipid. *Int J Med Sci* 7:101–109, 2010.
44. Pronovost P, Needham D, Berenholtz S, et al: An intervention to decrease catheter-related bloodstream infections in the ICU. *N Engl J Med* 355:2725, 2006.
45. Shuman EK, Washer LL, Arndt JL, et al: Analysis of central line-associated bloodstream infections in the intensive care unit after implementation of central line bundles. *Infect Control Hosp Epidemiol* 31:551–553, 2010.
46. Weber DJ, Brown VM, Sickbert-Bennett EE, et al: Sustained and prolonged reduction in central line-associated bloodstream infections as a result of multiple interventions. *Infect Control Hosp Epidemiol* 31:875–877, 2010.
47. Blot K, Bergs J, Vogelaers D, et al: Prevention of central line-associated bloodstream infections through quality improvement interventions: a systematic review and meta-analysis. *Clin Infect Dis* 59:96–105, 2014.
48. Fowler VG, Justice A, Moore C, et al: Risk factors for hematogenous complications of intravenous catheter-associated *Staphylococcus aureus*. *Clin Infect Dis* 40:695–703, 2005.
49. Pappas PG, Kauffman CA, Andes D, et al: Clinical practice guideline for the management of candidiasis: 2015 Update by the Infectious Diseases Society of America. *Clin Infect Dis* 62:e1–e50, 2016.
50. Fowler VG, Olsen MK, Corey GR, et al: Clinical identifiers of complicated *Staphylococcus aureus* bacteremia. *Arch Intern Med* 163:2066–2072, 2003.
51. Kaasch AJ, Fowler VG, Rieg S, et al: Use of a simple criteria set for guiding echocardiography in nosocomial *Staphylococcus aureus* bacteremia. *Clin Infect Dis* 53:1–9, 2011.
52. Baddour LM, Wilson WR, Bayer AS, et al: Infective endocarditis in adults: diagnosis, antimicrobial therapy, and management of complications. *Circulation* 132:1435–1486, 2015.
53. Khatib R, Sharma M: Echocardiography is dispensable in uncomplicated *Staphylococcus aureus* bacteremia. *Medicine* 92:182–188, 2013.
54. Raad I, Kassar R, Ghannam D, et al: Management of catheter in documented catheter-related coagulase-negative staphylococcal bacteremia: remove or retain? *Clin Infect Dis* 49:1187–1194, 2009.
55. Raad I, Hanna H, Dvorak T, et al: Optimal antimicrobial lock solution, using different combinations of minocycline, EDTA, and 25-percent ethanol, rapidly eradicates organisms embedded in biofilm. *Antimicrob Agents Chemother* 51:78–83, 2007.
56. Raad I, Rosenblatt J, Reitzel R, et al: Chelator-based catheter lock solutions in eradicating organisms in biofilm. *Antimicrob Agents Chemother* 57:586–588, 2013.
57. Maiefski M, Rupp ME, Hermsen ED: Ethanol lock technique: review of the literature. *Infect Control Hosp Epidemiol* 30:1096–1108, 2009.
58. Rijinders BJ, Van Wijngaerden E, Vandecasteele SJ, et al: Treatment of long-term intravascular catheter-related bacteraemia with antibiotic lock: randomized, placebo-controlled trial. *J Antimicrob Chemother* 55:90–94, 2005.

Chapter 80 ■ Urinary Tract Infections

STEVEN M. OPAL

Urinary tract infection (UTI) remains a common nosocomially acquired infection, accounting for approximately 25% to 40% of all infectious complications in hospitalized patients [1–4]. In a nation-wide surveillance study in the USA of nearly one half million intensive care unit (ICU) patients, UTI accounted for 23% of all infections and was associated with urinary catheters in 97% of patients [1]. Similar findings have recently been reported from surveys from Spain [2], Germany [3], and Brazil [4] with an overall incidence of urinary catheter-associated UTI of about 1 to 10 episodes per 1000 catheter days. Furthermore, the urinary tract is the most frequently recognized source of gram-negative bacteremia, which constitutes a major cause of infectious morbidity and mortality for the critically ill patient [5,6]. Approximately 100,000 annual admissions to acute care hospitals in the USA have been attributed to severe infections of the urinary tract [7]. Complicated UTI, progressive antimicrobial resistance, and the prevention of UTIs with the widespread use of indwelling urinary catheters remain major challenges for critical care practice.

THE PATHOPHYSIOLOGY OF UTIs

UTIs are primarily caused by gram-negative bacilli (71%) with gram-positive pathogens and fungi accounting for the remainder of microorganisms [5]. *Escherichia coli* is by far the most common cause of community-acquired and nosocomially acquired UTI. Most UTIs arise from ascending infection by enteric organisms that colonize the perineum and distal urethra. Specific clones of *E. coli* have evolved that readily colonize the uroepithelium and cause UTIs. These clones possess the requisite set of virulence genes needed to successfully attach, survive, and invade the urinary tract in nonimmunocompromised patients with anatomically normal genitourinary (GU) tracts [8].

An essential characteristic of uropathogenic *E. coli* is its ability to adhere to uroepithelial membranes. Urinary isolates of *E. coli* possess an array of adhesins including: type I (common pili), S pili, FIC pili, and P pili. These pili (also known as fimbria) are bacterial surface structures that facilitate attachment to epithelial surfaces. Type I pili bind to mannose-containing polysaccharides on the cell surface of epithelial membranes. This allows the organism to attach and persist within the urinary tract and avoid elimination during micturition [9].

Another important characteristic of uropathogenic *E. coli* is the expression of P pili on the bacteria's outer membrane [10]. P pili bind to α-D-galactose 1 $\rightarrow$ 4 β-D-galactose (Gal–Gal) containing disaccharides of the globoseries of glycolipids found in blood group P antigens. These glycolipids are also found on the epithelial surfaces of the upper urinary tract and enterocytes. The ability of *E. coli* to express P pili is particularly important in the establishment of upper UTIs where Gal–Gal disaccharide-containing glycolipids are found in large concentration. Recent genetic analysis reveals that bacterial pathogens cluster their virulence factors in discreet loci along the chromosome known as pathogenicity associated islands (PAIs). These genetic elements contain a large number of genes associated with virulence and distinguish uropathogenic strains from nonpathogenic colonizing strains [8].

Other genera of the Enterobacteriaceae, including *Citrobacter*, *Klebsiella*, *Enterobacter*, *Serratia*, *Proteus*, *Morganella*, and *Providencia* spp., become more common causes of UTI when patients receive antibiotics or have anatomic or functional abnormalities in urine flow [11–13]. The microbiology of UTIs after short-term urinary catheterization is similar to that observed in the noncatheterized patient. However, long-term (>30 days) catheterization generates an environment that supports a complex and often polymicrobial microflora. An extensive extracellular array of microbial-derived polysaccharides surrounds bacterial microcolonies within the lumen of the long-term urinary catheter. This biofilm structure protects bacterial populations from immune, phagocytic, or antibacterial clearance [12]. Bacteria found in the urine of chronically catheterized patients differ from noncatheterized patients. *Proteus*, *Providencia*, *Morganella*, and *Pseudomonas* species become more common, whereas *E. coli* and *Klebsiella* species become less common (Fig. 80.1). *Proteus* species, some other gram-negative enteric organisms, and *Staphylococcus saprophyticus* synthesize the enzyme urease, a known bacterial virulence factor for the urinary tract. The generation of ammonia from the breakdown of urea increases regional pH, favoring the generation of the "triple-phosphate crystals" struvite and apatite in urine. Struvite crystals can block urinary catheter flow and promote the formation of urinary calculi [13].

Gram-positive bacteria occasionally cause UTIs in critically ill patients. The isolation of *Staphylococcus aureus* in the urine is significant as it often accompanies staphylococcal bacteremia. *S. aureus* isolation from urine cultures, particularly of noncatheterized patients, should prompt a search for extrarenal sources of staphylococcal infection. *S. aureus* may also colonize chronically catheterized patients. This is particularly true for methicillin-resistant *S. aureus* strains, which may thrive in hospital settings with many elderly, catheterized patients [1,2].

Enterococci are prevalent in the GU tract of elderly populations and among patients with long-term urinary catheters [11,12,14]. The remarkable ability of this organism to rapidly evolve resistance to antimicrobial agents, including β-lactam antibiotics, aminoglycosides, quinolones, and recently vancomycin, contributes to making this organism a frequent cause of health care associated infection [1,7]. It should be noted, however,

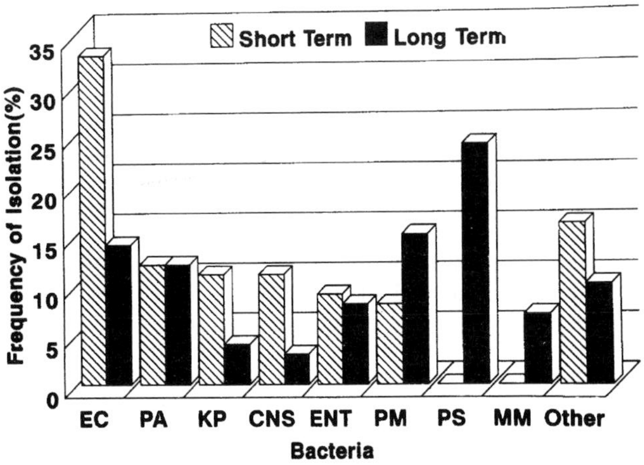

FIGURE 80.1 Distribution of bacterial isolation associated with catheter-related UTI. CNS, coagulase-negative staphylococci; EC, *Escherichia coli*; ENT, Enterococci; KP, *Klebsiella pneumoniae*; MM, *Morganella morganii*; PA, *Pseudomonas aeruginosa*; PM, *Proteus mirabilis*; PS, *Providencia stuartii*.

that at least in premenopausal women with symptomatic UTI, poor correlations were found between voided and catheterized urine cultures when either enterococci or group B streptococci were detected [15]. In a recent study comparing urinary culture derived from midstream voiding urine with immediate straight catheterization of the bladder urine, the positive predictive value (likelihood that catheterized bladder urine would have enterococci present when it was found in voided midstream urine) of a positive culture for enterococci in voided urine was only 10% to 33% [15]. How relevant this discrepancy is to determining the frequency of enterococcal UTI in critical care units remains unclear at present.

Candida species and other fungal organisms may colonize or infect the GU tract. Candiduria may be associated with hematogenous dissemination ("descending UTI") or ascending UTIs from perineal surfaces. The unique problems associated with the isolation of *Candida* species of the urinary tract are considered in the final section of this chapter.

HOST DEFENSE MECHANISMS AGAINST UTI

The human GU tract is remarkably resistant to UTI by mechanical, mucosal, and immunologic mechanisms. The flushing action of urinary flow itself is an important defense against UTI. The frequent occurrence of UTIs after obstruction or incomplete bladder emptying attests to the importance of micturition in clearing potential pathogens. Patients with neurogenic bladder or vesicoureteral reflux are highly susceptible to UTI and renal scarring. While urinary pathogens must possess a full complement of virulence factors to cause infection in the anatomically normal urinary tract, UTI in the obstructed urinary tract occurs with bacterial species devoid of special urinary virulence factors [8].

Urinary osmolarity, urea concentration, pH, and oxygen concentration limit the growth potential of many bacterial pathogens in the urinary tract. Continuous sloughing of uroepithelial cells, urinary mucosal glycocalyx (slime), and secretion of the Tamm-Horsfall protein assist in the mechanical removal of adherent bacteria that have entered the urinary tract [14].

The mucosal surfaces of uroepithelial cells of patients vary in their ability to attach bacteria depending upon the nature of mucopolysaccharide content and its chemical composition. Patients with high concentrations of Gal–Gal disaccharides on the cell surfaces of the urinary tract are predisposed to UTI from P-piliated *E. coli* [8]. Patients who are nonsecretors of blood group antigens have an increased risk of UTI [9,10,16]. Blood group antigens coat uroepithelial cells when secreted onto the mucosal surface. These antigens prevent attachment of bacteria to adhesin-receptor oligosaccharides on the surface of epithelial cells. Individuals who fail to secrete blood group antigens are rendered infection prone to UTI.

Although secretory immunoglobulin, neutrophils, and cell-mediated immunity contribute to the host defense against UTI, their roles are secondary to mechanical and physical barriers to infection. Uroepithelial cells produce the chemokine interleukin-8 (IL-8) in response to *E. coli* infection. IL-8 promotes neutrophil migration to the urinary tract which reduces the risk of disseminated infection. Patients differ in their level of expression of the IL-8 receptor CXCR1. Decreased CXCR1 expression in the urinary tract might contribute to increased susceptibility to pyelonephritis in some patients [16].

Adult women are much more likely to develop UTI than men. Women are more likely to develop pyelonephritis if they are sexually active, use spermicidal agents, experience urinary incontinence, have diabetes mellitus, or a family history of UTI [17]. The increased anatomic distance from the urethral orifice to the urinary bladder, the infrequent presence of gram-negative bacteria around the male urethra, and the production of inhibitory prostatic secretions protect men from UTI until they become elderly [18]. Bladder neck obstruction from age-related benign prostatic hypertrophy causes urinary obstruction and UTI in elderly men.

Asymptomatic bacteriuria is a commonplace occurrence for adult women, particularly elderly women, despite the absence of any recognized anatomic defect or immune deficiency. Our understanding of the role of asymptomatic bacteriuria in disease causation or recurrent symptomatic UTI has evolved significantly over the past few decades [19–21]. Epidemiologic studies now demonstrate that with exception of pregnancy, severe neutropenia, or diabetes mellitus in women or preceding urologic procedures in men, treatment of asymptomatic bacteriuria is not only ineffective, it may well do more harm than good [22]. Treatment alters the urinary and intestinal microbiome thereby increasing the risk of subsequent symptomatic UTI and promotes acquisition and infection by antibiotic-resistant uropathogens. Asymptomatic bacteriuria microorganisms might actually prevent infection of more pathogenic organisms, although this has yet to be definitively established. Unless specific indications exist, treatment of asymptomatic bacteriuria is discouraged in existing guidelines [20,23]. This recommendation holds true in the presence or absence of an indwelling urinary catheter.

SEVERE UTI

Acute Pyelonephritis

Acute pyelonephritis can precipitate severe sepsis/septic shock when complicated by urinary obstruction, papillary necrosis, or other local suppurative complications. Failure of the patient to respond clinically within 72 hours to seemingly appropriate antimicrobial therapy should prompt a search for complications of UTI. Functional or mechanical obstruction to urinary flow is the principal underlying cause of treatment failure in UTI. Obstruction may arise from extrarenal causes such as retroperitoneal or pelvic masses or abnormalities intrinsic to the GU tract such as renal calculi or ureteral obstruction. Alleviation of obstruction facilitates antimicrobial treatment and is often essential to successfully eradicate infections in the upper urinary tract system [24].

Suppurative Complications of UTI

Abscess formation within the GU tract may take several forms and pose a diagnostic and therapeutic challenge. It is important to distinguish between these entities because the clinical implications and medical–surgical management of each process differs substantially (see Table 80.1). Radiographic findings in a typical case of emphysematous pyelonephritis (usually caused by enteric bacteria, not *Clostridium* spp. or other anaerobes) are seen in Figure 80.2 A,B. Suppurative complications of UTI necessitate urgent intervention with percutaneous or surgical drainage [24].

Diagnostic Methods for UTI

The clinical diagnosis of acute UTI of the upper urinary tract in the noncatheterized patient is usually straightforward, with a history of urinary frequency and dysuria accompanied with costovertebral angle (CVA) tenderness and signs of systemic toxicity. The urinalysis often shows positive "dipstick" results for leukocyte esterase and nitrite, markers for leukocytes and enteric bacteria. The presence of excess numbers of urinary leukocytes and bacteria in the urinary sediment, in the absence of contamination by epithelial cells, is indicative of a UTI in symptomatic patients.

The Gram stain of unspun urine is helpful for determining the most likely agent causing the UTI. Gram-negative rods in the urine are readily identifiable and this confirms the presence of significant bacteriuria. The finding of more than one organism

TABLE 80.1

Suppurative Complications of UTI

Disease process	Pathogenesis	Predisposing factors	Common pathogens	Radiographic features	Standard treatment
Papillary necrosis	Ischemia, necrosis, infection	Analgesics, diabetes, obstruction	Gram-negative enterics	Sloughed papilla in calyx	Antibiotics alone
Pyonephritis	Infection with hydronephrosis	Ureteral obstruction, calculi	Gram-negative enterics	Hydronephrosis with gas, debris in collecting system	Nephrostomy tube, antibiotics
Focal bacterial nephritis	Ascending UTI with focal renal inflammation	UTI with upper tract involvement	Gram-negative enterics	Focal defect on contrast-enhanced CT scan	Antibiotics alone
Corticomedullary abscess	Ascending UTI with focal renal liquefaction	UTI with obstruction, diabetes	Gram-negative enterics	Focal fluid-filled defect on CT or ultrasound	Antibiotics alone or percutaneous drainage
Xanthogranulomatous pyelonephritis	Enlarging granulomatous process with cholesterol laden macrophages	Chronic obstruction with infection	*Proteus* spp., *Klebsiella* spp.	Large heterogenous mass	Partial or complete nephrectomy
Emphysematous pyelonephritis	Ischemic necrosis with infection from gas-forming organisms	Elderly diabetic	Gram-negative enterics, rarely anaerobes	Gas on plain film, CT	Closed or open drainage or nephrectomy, antibiotics
Cortical abscess (renal carbuncle)	Hematogenous seeding of kidney	Extrarenal infection with *Staphylococcus aureus*	*S. aureus*	Semisolid intrarenal mass with caliceal distortion	Antibiotics alone or with percutaneous drainage
Perinephritic abscess	Rupture of intrarenal abscess	Obstruction, diabetes, renal transplants	*Escherichia coli*, *Proteus* spp., *S. aureus*, others	Displaced renal tissue, perinepheric mass	Closed or open surgical drainage, antibiotics

CT, computed tomography; UTI, urinary tract infection.

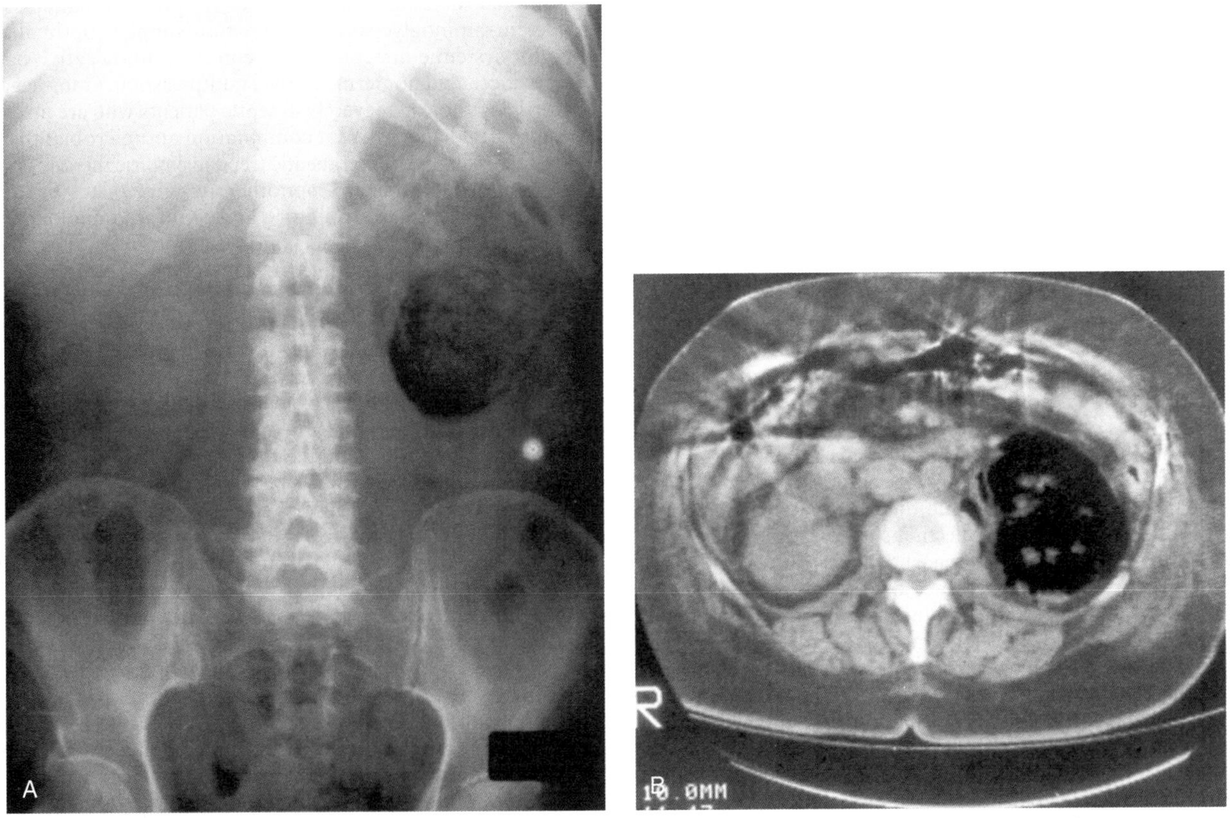

FIGURE 80.2 Radiographic findings in a diabetic woman with emphysematous pyelonephritis caused by *Escherichia coli*. **A:** Plain abdominal radiograph with evidence for gas in the left renal fossa. **B:** Computed tomography scan confirming gas in the left kidney. This patient recovered following emergency nephrectomy and antimicrobial therapy.

per high-powered field in unspun urine equates with $>10^5$ colony-forming units (CFU) per mL [24]. Urinary Gram stain can also detect gram-positive microorganisms such as enterococci and staphylococci, and fungal elements. Polymicrobial bacteriuria is often apparent by urinary Gram stain and may be seen in UTI from long-standing urinary catheterization, enterovesical fistula, or complicated UTI associated with obstruction or foreign bodies.

Patients with severe UTIs requiring critical care management should have quantitative urinary culture performed, preferably before the initiation of antimicrobial therapy. The urine culture confirms the diagnosis and defines the most appropriate antimicrobial agent for treatment. The progressive increase of antimicrobial resistance makes it imperative to carefully select antimicrobial agents based on susceptibility patterns of the infecting microorganism. Greater than 10^5 CFU per mL in clean catch, mid-stream urine is generally diagnostic. The quantitative level of bacteriuria diagnostic for acute UTI varies depending on the clinical situation [24–27].

In clinical surveys of symptomatic women with UTI repeated isolation of as few as $>10^2$ pathogenic microorganisms per mL is diagnostic [15,25]. Catheterized patients may also have UTI with $<10^5$ CFU per mL. The presence of an indwelling urinary catheter may not allow ongoing replication of microorganisms in the urinary tract to achieve levels greater than 10^5 CFU per mL. Moreover, urinary cultures from non-instrumented men are significant with as little as 10^3 CFU per mL [28].

The absence of pyuria and significant bacteriuria does not exclude the possibility of a potentially serious UTI. Patients with severe neutropenia may not have significant levels of pyuria. Urine cultures may be negative in more than 40% of patients with perinephric abscess, and most patients with renal cortical abscesses have urinalyses without significant bacteriuria [29]. Complete unilateral urinary obstruction associated with pyonephrosis can fail to show the primary pathogen within voided urine. Urinary stent placement increases the risk of UTI. In a recent survey voided urine specimens taken at the time of stent removal were negative in the presence of microbial colonization in 40% of the patients [30].

Blood cultures should be obtained for all patients who are septic in the setting of a UTI. Urine cultures should also be performed from nephrostomy tube drainage in patients with prior urinary diversion procedures. It is generally unnecessary to change a urinary catheter before the acquisition of urine cultures in patients with acute symptomatic UTI.

IMAGING PROCEDURES FOR THE DIAGNOSIS OF UTI

Complicated UTIs often require radiologic methods to establish the correct diagnosis. Routine abdominal radiographs may assist in the diagnosis of complicated forms of UTI. The presence of radiopaque renal calculi can be readily detected on abdominal radiography. Emphysematous pyelonephritis appears as an abnormal collection of gas within the renal parenchyma. Gas is detectable in the urinary collecting system in many patients with pyonephrosis. Abnormal renal shadows and loss of psoas margins may suggest the presence of a perinephric abscess. Renal ultrasonography and computed tomography (CT) have replaced the intravenous pyelogram (or excretory urogram) as the principal radiographic technique in the detection of complicated UTI. The anatomic definition of the kidney and perirenal tissues is superior with a contrast-enhanced abdominal CT scan and is generally the preferred imaging method for complicated UTI (see Table 80.1). Renal ultrasound provides another rapid method of detecting hydronephrosis and anatomic detail of the renal parenchyma. Ultrasonography can also determine the solid or cystic nature of a renal mass detected on abdominal CT. Ultrasound can image the kidney on any plane and may be performed urgently in the absence of intravenous contrast media. The CT scan or renal ultrasound is indispensable for the localization of inflammatory processes during diagnostic aspiration or percutaneous drainage procedures. Magnetic resonance imaging (MRI) provides detailed information about the renal structures and retroperitoneal space, but the CT has sufficient resolving power for most forms of renal inflammatory disease.

The gallium-67–scan or indium-111–labeled leukocyte studies can occasionally be useful in the diagnosis of complicated UTI. These nuclear medicine studies assist in the differentiation between a renal neoplasm and a focal inflammatory process of the kidney. These studies are useful for the evaluation of patients with fever of unknown origin secondary to perinephric abscess or renal cortical abscess [31].

MEDICAL MANAGEMENT OF UTI

Patients admitted to the intensive care unit for management of UTI usually suffer from severe infections complicated by a systemic inflammatory response (sepsis) or suppurative complications of the GU tract. Medical management initially consists of stabilization of the patient's hemodynamic parameters and supportive measures in the management of septic shock. After the completion of appropriate diagnostic studies, empiric antimicrobial therapy should be directed toward the most likely infecting urinary pathogen(s). A urinary Gram stain usually provides evidence of either a gram-negative or gram-positive bacterial pathogen. If this is unavailable or nondiagnostic, then broad-spectrum, empiric antimicrobial therapy is indicated.

For the septic patient presenting with septic shock from a UTI, the initial use of a β-lactam antibiotic (assuming there is no history of allergic reactions to β-lactams) in combination with an aminoglycoside or a fluoroquinolone have been the traditional therapeutic regimens for hospitalized patients. The β-lactam–aminoglycoside combination supplies optimal therapy for systemic infections with enteric gram-negative bacilli, enterococci, and nonfermentative, multiresistant, gram-negative bacterial pathogens. Severely ill septic patients who are immunocompromised also warrant combination antimicrobial therapy [32]. Increasingly, the therapeutic trend in empiric therapy is away from aminoglycosides to monotherapy with β-lactams alone, β-lactam–β-lactamase inhibitors, and/or fluoroquinolones [33].

Community-acquired UTIs of nonimmunocompromised patients who have not received antimicrobial agents infrequently harbor multiresistant gram-negative bacilli or *Pseudomonas* sp. Should the urinary Gram stain exclude enterococci as a potential pathogen, then single therapy with a third-generation cephalosporin, extended-spectrum penicillin, carbapenem (e.g., imipenem or meropenem), β-lactam–β-lactamase inhibitor (e.g., piperacillin–tazobactam) trimethoprim–sulfamethoxazole, or a fluoroquinolone is acceptable therapy while awaiting culture results. Local susceptibility patterns of urinary pathogens should guide the selection of antimicrobial therapy until specific susceptibility data are available. There is no evidence that combination antimicrobial therapy is necessary for UTIs caused by gram-negative bacilli unless *Pseudomonas aeruginosa* infection with neutropenia is present. A single antimicrobial agent known to be active against the infecting uropathogen should be employed once the causative organism is known. Parenteral therapy is generally administered until the patient has been rendered nontoxic and afebrile for 24 to 48 hours. Therapy may then be administered orally and should be given for a total of approximately 2 weeks [32,33]. Patients with obstructive lesions and complicated UTIs not amenable to corrective surgery may require prolonged courses of antimicrobial therapy as indicated by their underlying urologic disorder.

Treatment options to treat UTIs have become much more complicated recently as a result of increasing prevalence of antimicrobial resistance among both hospital-acquired and community-acquired uropathogens. Fortunately, at least some new antimicrobial agents have entered the market recently to treat severe UTI from multidrug resistant (MDR) pathogens. Both of these new agents are β-lactam–β-lactamase inhibitor combinations: ceftolozone–tazobactam [34] and ceftazidime–avibactam [35]. Both these combination drugs are now available and are specifically indicated to treat UTIs in patients requiring intravenous antibiotic therapy caused by MDR gram-negative bacteria. Common antimicrobial agents useful for the treatment of severe UTIs and their relative merits are listed in Table 80.2.

Standard therapy for severe enterococcal UTIs has been ampicillin and an aminoglycoside. Although this regimen remains active against most enterococcal isolates, progressive antimicrobial resistance to aminoglycosides, ampicillin, and other β lactams and vancomycin has complicated the antimicrobial therapy for enterococcal infections [36]. Rare strains of β-lactamase–producing enterococci are susceptible to β-lactam inhibitors such as ampicillin/sulbactam or piperacillin/tazobactam. High-level aminoglycoside-resistant strains of enterococci are problematic, as the addition of an aminoglycoside no longer contributes to synergistic clearance of these infections. Aminoglycosides should not be used in this situation.

Glycopeptide-resistant strains of enterococci pose a serious threat to the antimicrobial management of enterococcal infections. Some of these isolates remain susceptible to β-lactam agents. Newer fluoroquinolones occasionally have activity against enterococci and may be useful in the treatment of glycopeptide- and β-lactam–resistant strains of enterococci. Tetracyclines and nitrofurantoin are useful alternatives for uncomplicated, enterococcal UTI if susceptibility testing indicates activity. Linezolid, an oxazolidinone that inhibits the initiation of translation at the 30S ribosome of bacteria, has activity against vancomycin-resistant enterococci [37]. Multidrug resistant enterococci are an infection control hazard in the ICU and contact precautions are recommended.

Antistaphylococcal penicillins such as nafcillin or oxacillin are indicated for the empiric therapy of renal cortical abscesses (renal carbuncle). Vancomycin should be instituted if there is a

TABLE 80.2

Common Antimicrobial Agents for Severe UTI

Agent	Dose and frequency[a]	Principal indications	Comments
Ampicillin–sulbactam	3.0 g IV q6–8h	Gram-negative enterics	Other β-lactam–inhibitor combinations also effective
Aztreonam	1 g IV q8h[c]	Gram-negative enterics *Pseudomonas* spp.	Useful in penicillin-allergic patients
Cefazolin	1.0 g IV q8h		
Cefotaxime	1–2 g IV q8h	Gram-negative enterics	Other second- and third-generation cephalosporins also effective
Ciprofloxacin	400 mg IV q12h	Gram-negative enterics *Pseudomonas* spp.	Other fluoroquinolones may not be as effective, moxifloxacin does not achieve high levels in urine
Fluconazole	200 mg loading 100 mg q24h	*Candida* spp. UTI	If non-*albicans Candida* spp., check susceptibility or use Amphotericin B
Gentamicin[b]	1.5 mg/kg IV q12h or 5 mg/kg/d	Gram-negative enterics *Pseudomonas* spp. enterococci	Dosing interval dependent on renal function
Piperacillin/tazobactam	3.375 g IV q8h[d]	Gram-negative enterics *Pseudomonas* spp.	Other extended-spectrum penicillins also effective
Trimethoprim/sulfamethoxazole	160/800 mg IV q12h	Gram-negative enterics	Watch for sulfa allergies
Vancomycin	500 mg IV q12h	MRSA, vancomycin-sensitive enterococci	Watch renal function carefully
Linezolid	600 mg IV or PO q12h	MRSA, VRE	Monitor complete blood counts
Ceftolozane/tazobactam	1.5 g every 8 h	MDR-enterics and *Pseudomonas* spp.	Useful against ESBL-producing gram-negative bacilli but not KPC or NDM
Ceftazidime/avibactam	2.5 g (2.0 g. ceftazidime +0.5 g avibactam) q8h	MDR-enterics and *Pseudomonas* spp.	The β-lactamase inhibitor avibactam is active against many ESBLs, and KPCs but not NDM
Meropenem	1.0 g every 8 h	MDR-enterics, bowel anaerobes and *Pseudomonas* spp.	Broad-spectrum agent but not active in gram-negative bacilli expressing carbapenemase or porin mutants

[a] Adult dosing in patients with normal renal function; follow susceptibility test results and treat parenterally until systemic toxicity resolves.
[b] Gentamicin or other aminoglycosides often given with a β-lactam agent in gram-negative septic shock or severe enterococcal infections.
[c] Aztreonam dose can be increased to 2 g q8h for *P. aeruginosa* infection.
[d] Piperacillin/tazobactam dose can be increased to 4.5 g q8h for *P. aeruginosa* infection.
MRSA, Methicillin-resistant *S. aureus*; UTI, Urinary tract infections; VRE, vancomycin-resistant enterococci; MDR, Multidrug resistant; ESBL, extended spectrum β-lactamase; KPC, *Klebsiella pneumoniae* carbapenemase; NDM, New Delhi metallo-β-lactamase.

suspicion of the presence of methicillin-resistant staphylococcal isolates in a patient with a cortical abscess or perinephric abscess.

Urgent percutaneous nephrotomy tube placement for urinary drainage and abscess management is indicated foe severely septic patients with obstructed urinary collecting systems. Percutaneous catheter drainage of perinephric abscesses, renal carbuncles, and infected urinary cysts are often necessary in combination with antimicrobial therapy to manage these complicated UTIs. Open surgical drainage is reserved for patients who fail to respond to attempted percutaneous drainage.

PREVENTIVE MEASURES AGAINST UTI IN THE ICU SETTING

The most efficacious method of preventing UTIs among critically ill patients is not using urinary catheters at all or limiting their duration of use as much as possible [27,38]. Asymptomatic bacteriuria should generally not be treated whether an indwelling urinary catheter is present or not. Asymptomatic bacteriuria among pregnant women and severely immunocompromised patients should be treated with specific antimicrobial agents as the risk of ascending UTI in such patients is considerable and can be avoided by early medical intervention [39,40].

The Management of Catheter-Related UTI

The ubiquitous presence of the indwelling urinary catheter among hospitalized patients provides microbial pathogens ready access to the urinary tract with subsequent development of UTI. It is estimated that 10% of all hospitalized patients in the USA will have a urinary catheter inserted during their hospitalization, resulting in over 1 million UTIs and 40% of all hospital-acquired infection per year [27]. The overall incidence of catheter-acquired UTI among patients within critical care units varies from 0.5 to 10 UTI per 1,000 catheter days [27,40]. The risk factors for acquisition of catheter-related UTI include duration of catheter placement, increasing patient age, female gender, severity of underlying illness, and perhaps obesity [40,41]. The estimated risk of bacteriuria after urinary tract catheterization is approximately 5% for each day of catheterization. Chronically catheterized (more than 30 days) patients almost invariably have bacteriuria, and their admission to the ICU poses a threat of cross-contamination of urinary pathogens to other ICU patients. Despite continued infection control efforts to decrease the frequency of contamination, UTI remains the major complication of urinary catheters. The average, calculated, incremental cost associated with the hospital care of a patient with a catheter related UTI is $589.00 [38,42].

Pathogenesis

The catheter itself interferes with physiological host defense mechanisms against UTI. Trauma produced by an indwelling catheter may damage the bladder mucosa and the mucous layer that coats uroepithelial cells [27]. This exposes the cell surface of epithelial cells to bacterial adhesions and increases the risk of UTI. Indwelling catheters prevent complete bladder emptying. Residual urine serves as a culture medium for bacteria in an inadequately drained urinary bladder. Additionally, temporary obstruction of urine flow caused by kinking or clamping of the urinary catheter can lead to bladder distension, vesicoureteral reflux, and infection.

Bacteria gain access to the urinary tract of catheterized patients by one of three mechanisms: (1) during insertion, (2) along the external surface after insertion, or (3) via the inner lumen of the urinary catheter. Implantation of bacteria into the bladder during catheter placement occurs at a frequency of approximately 0.5% to 8% [27]. This risk varies with the experience of the health care worker placing the catheter and with the level of periurethral colonization by potential uropathogens. Ascending infection from within the lumen accounts for approximately 20% of catheter-related UTIs [24]. The use of sterile, closed urinary collecting devices with a sterile vent to avoid a standing column of urine from the bladder to the collecting bag has decreased the frequency of UTIs. Optimal catheter design includes a sterile sampling port that obviates the need to open the system to collect urine samples. The collecting bag should have a large reservoir with a device to measure urine output with minimal manipulation of the catheter system.

Most catheter-related UTIs are derived from microorganisms that enter the urinary bladder along the external surface of the catheter [27,43]. The periurethral space becomes colonized with enteric organisms, which then migrate along the periurethral mucous sheath that surrounds the surface of the catheter. Continued movement of the catheter in and out of the urinary bladder occurs upon repositioning of the patient or catheter manipulations. This process provides ample opportunity for organisms coating the catheter surface to gain access to the urinary bladder and cause infection.

Numerous enteric organisms avidly adhere to the mucosal surface of the urinary bladder. Some organisms, such as *Providencia stuartii* and *P. aeruginosa,* also possess surface adhesins that bind directly to the urinary catheter itself. The urinary catheter becomes an ecologic niche for these organisms, resulting in prolonged infections that may persist for months in the catheterized patient [44]. Over 90% of *P. stuartii* bacteremias occur as the result of urinary catheter-induced UTIs [45]. The urease produced by *Proteus* species affects the local pH surrounding the catheter, which facilitates the deposition of struvite microcrystals on the surface of the catheter. These encrustations serve as a nidus for persistent colonization with urinary pathogens. Adherent bacteria establish microcolonies coated with extracellular polysaccharides. The continued buildup of this biofilm within the lumen of the urinary catheter eventually leads to obstruction of urinary flow [12,46]. The presence of a foreign body within the urinary bladder interferes with the penetration and antimicrobial action of antibiotics. Bactericidal agents inhibit, but often fail to kill, microorganisms that adhere to catheter materials. Furthermore, the catheter serves as a foreign body inducing early degranulation and loss of bactericidal activity of neutrophils. These factors contribute to the difficulties eradicating urinary pathogens in the catheterized patient.

Diagnosis

The presence of bacteriuria in the catheterized patient documents colonization of the urinary tract but does not necessarily confirm the presence of an actual UTI. A UTI develops when a host response occurs to the presence of microbial pathogens in the urine. As many as 70% of patients who develop catheter-related bacteriuria remain symptom free and resolve spontaneously with the catheter removal [47]. It is generally acknowledged that the treatment of asymptomatic bacteriuria in the catheterized patient is not warranted, except in some specific circumstances [20,27]. The severely neutropenic patient with asymptomatic bacteriuria should be treated because of the risk of systemic infection in this patient population.

It is often difficult to recognize that a symptomatic UTI is present in the catheterized patient. Altered levels of consciousness may interfere with the patient's awareness of the UTI. Furthermore, the presence of a urinary catheter removes the symptoms of urinary frequency and the perception of dysuria. Hematuria and pyuria may be found in the catheterized patient in the absence of urinary colonization with bacteria. Isolated pyuria in patients with asymptomatic bacteriuria is not an indication for antimicrobial treatment [20]. This is presumably related to sterile inflammation and trauma induced by the catheter itself. High-grade pyuria with fever supports the diagnosis of a UTI in the catheterized patient [48].

The presence of lower numbers of bacteria than the traditional $>10^5$ CFU per mL can indicate infection in catheterized patients [49]. Quantitative counts as low as 10^2 CFU per mL may be significant in the catheterized patient. Low colony counts in catheterized urine can progress to high-grade bacteriuria in catheterized patients. Clinical laboratories should isolate and characterize urinary isolates from catheterized patients with low grade bacteriuria. A recent consensus review recommended the cutoff of $>10^3$ CFU per mL for significant bacteriuria in catheterized patients [48]. The high flow rate of catheterized urine, presence of inhibitors to bacterial growth, and significance of slow-growing organisms such as enterococci and *Candida* make it incumbent on the laboratory to characterize even low numbers of uropathogens in these patients. Moreover, polymicrobial bacteriuria occurs in more than 15% of patients with catheter-related UTI [49]. Multiple organisms obtained from a recently inserted urinary catheter (<72 hours) should be isolated, characterized, and subjected to susceptibility testing to ensure adequate treatment of catheter-related UTIs.

Most patients with catheter-associated UTIs have lower urinary tract involvement. Upper tract involvement occurs in up to one third of catheter-related UTIs and may have serious consequences [50]. The clinical and laboratory recognition of upper urinary tract involvement in persons with UTI (with or without a catheter) remains imprecise and unsatisfactory. ICU patients with UTIs may have altered levels of consciousness and may not be able to relate the symptoms of upper tract involvement. Radiographic indicators of upper tract involvement by ultrasound and CT include enlarged kidneys and focal nephritis these are reliable diagnostic techniques in ICU patients. Evidence of systemic toxicity from a UTI is highly indicative of upper tract disease and should be treated accordingly. Bacteria confined to the urinary bladder, in contrast, readily clear with removal of the catheter and a short course of antimicrobial therapy, if necessary.

Treatment

The most important therapeutic modality in catheter-related UTIs is the removal of the urinary catheter itself. Up to two-thirds of patients with asymptomatic bacteriuria associated with urinary catheterization spontaneously resolve within 1 week after catheter removal [20]. Persistent bacteriuria longer than 48 hours after catheter removal should be treated with a short course (3 days) of an appropriate antimicrobial agent. If patients have persistent bacteriuria after short-course therapy, upper tract infection is assumed to be present and a 14-day course of an active antimicrobial agent is indicated [27,48].

If a patient becomes systemically ill from a UTI, treatment is warranted even if the catheter must remain in place. It is possible to successfully treat UTIs in patients with indwelling catheters, although treatment failures and reinfection occur at a greater frequency than in noncatheterized patients [24]. Antimicrobial agents useful in the treatment of catheter-related UTI are described in Table 80.2.

Routine replacement of indwelling urinary catheters complicated by UTI is generally unnecessary. Nonetheless, some organisms such as *Proteus*, *Providencia*, *Morganella*, and *Pseudomonas* species and enterococci may colonize the urinary catheter in greater quantities than the bladder itself. Despite the fact that the microbiology of urine samples from indwelling catheters and replacement catheters does not differ markedly in the presence of a UTI [51], indwelling catheters should be replaced and urine cultures obtained if they malfunction, leak, or have been in place for prolonged periods (longer than 2 weeks) as a guide to antibiotic therapy for catheter-related infections. Leaking urinary catheters generally indicate luminal obstruction and require replacement.

Long-term urinary catheterization may be associated with other local suppurative complications, particularly in adult men. These include prostatitis, prostatic abscess, epididymitis, scrotal abscess, and other urethral complications [52]. These local complications require urologic management and necessitate the removal of the urethral catheter.

Prevention

Alternatives to Urethral Catheterization

The high frequency of catheter-related UTIs has led to concerted efforts to find alternative methods to manage the incontinent patient and patients with urinary outflow obstruction. Bladder training, meticulous nursing care, special linens, and adult diapers may assist some incontinent patients and avoid long-term catheterization.

Condom catheterization has been used for men with urinary incontinence and consists of the application of an external collector about the penis with a collection tube and drainage bag. Condom catheterization may be a reasonable alternative in highly motivated, cooperative, selected patients. However, leakage of the catheter, kinking and disruption of the collecting system, and maceration and ulceration of the epithelium of the penis are frequent complications of condom drainage. Regrettably, the overall incidence of UTIs with condom drainage does not differ significantly from indwelling catheter drainage [27,53].

Catheter Design, Maintenance, and Care

Because most catheter-related infections are derived from endogenous perineal organisms adherent to the exterior surface of the catheter itself, daily application of antimicrobial materials at the urethral orifice would seem to be a logical preventive measure. However, randomized, controlled, clinical trials with meatal care and application of povidone-iodine solution or topical polyantimicrobial applications have failed to convincingly demonstrate a reduction in catheter-related infections [43]. This procedure cannot be recommended as a means of prevention of catheter-associated UTI.

Considerable effort is under way to develop a urinary catheter that prevents binding with bacteria, inhibits biofilm formation, or possesses antibacterial properties. Existing studies and a recent evidence-based systematic review of the existing literature indicates that antibiotic-coated catheters reduce the incidence of asymptomatic bacteriuria following short-term catheterization; however, there is no clear evidence of reduced symptomatic UTI or major complications such as bacteremia [54–56]. Such catheters may be considered for selected patients at great risk of complications for UTI such as a patient with severe neutropenia, but such patients are uncommon in most critical care units.

Exogenous contamination of urine within the collection bag remains a potential problem associated with indwelling urethral catheters. The instillation of antiseptic agents within the drainage bag as a means of prevention of catheter-related UTIs has met with conflicting results [55,56] and this infection control strategy for UTI is not recommended based upon current clinical evidence [27,57,58]. The urinary collection bag should not be allowed to be elevated above the urinary bladder. This results in reflux of voided urine back into the bladder with its attendant risk of inducing UTI. Collecting bags with antireflux valves should be used to avoid this complication of urinary catheterization.

TABLE 80.3

Evidence-Based Recommendations for UTI

Summary of recommendations for the prevention and management of bacteriuria and UTIs in catheterized patients

- Screening for asymptomatic bacteriuria in a patient with an indwelling urinary catheter is not recommended [20].
- Treatment of asymptomatic bacteriuria is not recommended in the chronically catheterized patient [20,27].
- Pyuria is a frequent occurrence in patients with urinary catheters with or without asymptomatic bacteriuria; this finding is *not* sufficient evidence of catheter associated UTI to warrant the use of antibiotic therapy.
- The clinical value and cost-effectiveness from the use of antimicrobial-coated urinary catheters to prevent catheter-associated urinary tract or other complications (e.g., bacteremia, sepsis, or suppurative lesions) remains unclear [54–56].
- There are insufficient data to support the use of chemical disinfection, cranberry product antiseptics, or locally applied antibiotics within the urinary drainage system as a means of preventing catheter-associated UTIs [57,58].
- Daily meatal care to prevent contamination of the external surface of the urinary catheter is *not* recommended as a means of preventing catheter-associated UTIs [43].
- Persistent bacteriuria >48 hours after removal of a urinary catheter should be treated with antimicrobial agents [27].

Summary of recommendations in the management of candiduria in the ICU patient

- Quantitative cultures with $>10^3$ CFU/mL of *Candida* spp in a catheterized patient or $>10^4$ CFU/mL of *Candida* spp in a noncatheterized patient is considered clinically significant [48,67].
- The finding of a fungus ball within the urinary collecting system, papillary necrosis, fungal casts in the urine, or renal abscess in the presence of candiduria is considered clinically significant [48,68,70].
- In medically stable patients without major immunocompromised states, simple removal of an indwelling urinary catheter without specific antifungal therapy may be an acceptable treatment option [48,60,61].
- Because of high levels of urinary excretion, fluconazole is generally preferred over caspofungin, other *β*-glucan inhibitors, and other triazoles (such as voriconzole, itraconazole, or posaconzole) in the treatment of genitourinary candidiasis [48,70].
- Bladder irrigation with a short course of amphotericin B (2 days) remains a viable treatment option in catheterized patients with candiduria in the absence of evidence of disseminated candidiasis [72].
- A short course of fluconazole (5–7 days) is usually sufficient to treat UTIs due to *Candida* spp. [75,76].

UTI, urinary tract infections; CFU, colony-forming units.

Short-term systemic antimicrobial prophylaxis against catheter-related UTI might be useful in special circumstances such as renal transplantation or foreign body implant surgery. A summary of evidence to support prevention and treatment recommendations for urinary catheter-associated UTI is listed in Table 80.3.

THE PROBLEM OF CANDIDURIA

The clinical interpretation of the isolation of *Candida* species from the urine is problematic in that candiduria may occur in a spectrum of illnesses ranging from simple urinary contamination to life-threatening systemic candidiasis. *Candida* species are normal inhabitants of the vaginal tract of women and may contaminate inadequately collected urine specimens. This is particularly true for older women, diabetics, and patients receiving antibacterial therapy. Additionally, *Candida* species frequently colonize the urinary tract of catheterized patients. These organisms are of marginal clinical significance and frequently disappear on removal of the urinary catheter without any specific antifungal therapy [59]. In a detailed survey of 861 patients with funguria by the national mycoses study group, no treatment was given in 155 patients and funguria resolved spontaneously in 76% of these patients [60]. Even for ICU patients, simply changing an indwelling catheter with a new one will spontaneously clear candiduria in 20 to 40% of cases [61].

However, tissue invasive infection of the urinary bladder has been documented cystoscopically for patients with GU candidiasis. *Candida* cystitis may produce a friable white pseudomembrane on the bladder mucosa similar to the findings of oral thrush. Furthermore, ascending urinary infection of the kidney and renal pelvis may follow GU candidiasis. Papillary necrosis, fungus ball formation, urinary obstruction, bladder rupture, and perinephric abscess have all been described from ascending infection with *Candida* species [62,63]. *Candida* infection of the upper urinary tract may arise from hematogenous dissemination of *Candida* organisms from extrarenal sites. Microabscesses of the renal parenchyma with subsequent candiduria are frequently present among those with disseminated candidiasis. A positive urine culture for *Candida* species may be the first indication of disseminated candidiasis for the critically ill patient. Therefore, the clinical significance of *Candida* in the urine remains a diagnostic dilemma.

Quantitative culture of the urine has been used in an attempt to determine the clinical ramifications of candiduria. Unfortunately, the quantitative colony counts of *Candida* species in the urine do not have the same diagnostic and prognostic implications as quantitative bacteriology of the urine [48,63]. Large studies and review of this topic [48,64,65] indicate that quantitative values for candiduria of clinical significance are seen at more than 10^3 CFU per mL (catheterized patients) or more than 10^4 CFU per mL (noncatheterized patients). The finding of urinary casts made up of *Candida* elements is of diagnostic significance and indicates invasive upper tract candidiasis. Candiduria associated with a fungus ball in the urinary collecting system dictates the need for antifungal therapy, as does papillary necrosis or abscess formation within the renal parenchyma. Recurrent isolation of *Candida* species from urine cultures of immunocompromised patients, or patients with unexplained fever and pyuria, suggests UTI with *Candida* species. Evidence of concomitant infection with *Candida* organisms in other organ systems increases the likelihood of the significance of *Candida* isolates in the urine. Disseminated candidiasis should be considered for patients with repeated and unexplained *Candida* isolates in the urinary tract [66–68]. Biomarker plasma sample evidence of disseminated candidemia such as an elevated *β*-D-glucan level can assist in early detection of systemic candidiasis in septic patients [32].

THE TREATMENT OF GU CANDIDIASIS

There are several management options available for candiduria, depending on the clinical circumstances of each patient. The discontinuation of antibacterial agents, removal of immunosuppression, or removal of urinary catheters may be sufficient to spontaneously clear candiduria in medically stable patients [69].

Published treatment guidelines for GU candidiasis recommend fluconazole in place of amphotericin B as the preferred treatment in the ICU setting [61,70]. This triazole compound is water soluble, available as oral or intravenous formulations, and is excreted as the active compound in the urine. Posaconazole, itraconazole, caspofungin, and voriconazole might be useful despite the fact that they are excreted by the kidney and do not uniformly achieve fungicidal levels in the urine. Tissue levels in the upper urinary tract might still be sufficient to treat genitourinary candidiasis for selected patients, but clinical experience is limited [61]. Fluconazole also provides systemic antifungal activity when unrecognized disseminated candidiasis is present.

It is now recommended that antifungal susceptibility testing be performed for serious *Candida* infections for fluconazole, itraconazole, and flucytosine [71]. Resistance among *Candida albicans* isolates is increasingly recognized and these findings emphasize the necessity of antifungal susceptibility testing [72]. *Candida krusei* is intrinsically resistant to fluconazole; *Candida lusitaniae* is resistant to amphotericin B; and *Candida glabrata* is variably sensitive to azole antifungal agents. *C. parapsilosis* appears to be less susceptible to the echinocandins although the clinical significance of this finding is debatable [70]. Amphotericin B in vitro susceptibility testing is technically difficult and the methodology has not yet been standardized for routine clinical laboratory testing [71]. High doses of amphotericin B instilled into the bladder is potentially toxic to uroepithelial cells; however, a 2-day infusion of 50 mg of amphotericin B in 1,000 cc of sterile water per day is effective [72]; a single systemic dose of amphotericin B can also clear candiduria [73]. Systemic fluconazole or amphotericin B is indicated in candiduria patients with suspected systemic candidiasis, renal abscess formation, and fungus balls within the urinary collecting system [74]. *Candida* UTI may be readily treated with oral or intravenous fluconazole. A short course of fluconazole at 200 mg orally followed by 100 mg daily for 5 to 7 days is generally sufficient for the treatment of *Candida* [75] cystitis while upper urinary tract disease is generally treated with 200 to 400 mg fluconazole for 2 weeks [76]. Clinical evidence in support of the current management strategies for GU candidiasis is provided in Table 80.3.

Utility of Ultrasonography for Diagnosis of UTI

Ultrasonography is an important imaging modality for diagnosis of UTI, particularly if there may be a complication such as obstructive uropathy, perinephric abscess, kidney stone, or emphysematous pyelonephritis. As it can be performed rapidly at point of care, ultrasonography is the first line imaging technique where there is clinical suspicion of complicated UTI. Equipment and scanning technique for ultrasonography of the kidney and bladder are reviewed elsewhere in this textbook (Chapter 200, Acute Kidney Injury).

Characteristic Ultrasonography Findings

Uncomplicated pyelonephritis results in enlargement of the kidney but otherwise has no specific findings. Normal kidney length is 9 to 12 cm. Hydronephrosis is readily detected with ultrasonography (Video 80.1). When associated with clinical evidence of UTI, its presence mandates consideration of decompression of the infected space. Perinephric abscess results in a heterogeneous crescent-shaped collection that surrounds the kidney, while renal abscess appears as a complex hypoechoic mass with irregular thick walls. Kidney stones may complicate a kidney infection; they are identified as strongly hyperechoic structures within the kidney with associated acoustic shadowing. Emphysematous pyelonephritis results in hyperechoic foci within the parenchymal/pelvocalyceal area with associated comet tail artifact or mild acoustic shadowing. Bladder infection has no characteristic features on ultrasonography examination.

References

1. Richards MJ, Edwards JR, Culver DH, et al: Nosocomial infections in combined medical-surgical intensive care units in the United States. *Infect Control Hosp Epidemiol* 21:510–515, 2000.
2. Lizan-Garcia M, Peyro R, Cortina M, et al: Nosocomial surveillance in a surgical intensive care unit in Spain, 1996–2000: a time-trend analysis. *Infect Control Hosp Epidemiol* 27(1):54–59, 2006.
3. Wagenlehner FM, Loibl E, Vogel H, et al: Incidence of nosocomial urinary tract infections on a surgical intensive care unit and implications for management. *Int J Antimicrob Agents* 28(Suppl 1):S86–S90, 2006.
4. Salomao R, Rosenthal VD, Grimberg G, et al: Device-associated infection rates in intensive care units of Brazilian hospitals: findings of the International Nosocomial Infection Control Consortium. *Rev Panam Salud Publica* 24(3):195–202, 2008.
5. Gaynes R, Edwards JR: Overview of nosocomial infections caused by gram-negative bacilli. *Clin Infect Dis* 41(6):848–854, 2005.
6. Rosenthal VD: Device-associated nosocomial infections in limited-resources countries: findings of the International Nosocomial Infection Control Consortium (INICC). *Am J Infect Control* 36(10):7–12, 2008.
7. Richards MJ, Edwards JR, Culver DH, et al: Nosocomial infections in medical intensive care units in the United States: national nosocomial infections surveillance system. *Crit Care Med* 27:887–892, 1999.
8. Johnson JR, Kuskowski MA, Gajewske A, et al: Virulence characteristics and phylogenetic background of multidrug-resistant and antimicrobial-susceptible clinical isolates of *Escherichia coli* from across the United States, 2000–2001. *J Infect Dis* 190:1739–1744, 2004.
9. De Man P, Jodal U, Lincoln K, et al: Bacterial attachment and inflammation in the urinary tract. *J Infect Dis* 158:29–35, 1988.
10. Dominque GJ, Roberts JA, Laucirica R, et al: Pathogenic significance of P fimbriated *Escherichia coli* in urinary tract infections. *J Urol* 133:983–989, 1985.
11. Warren JW, Tenney JH, Woopes JM, et al: A prospective microbiologic study of bacteriuria in patients with chronic indwelling urethral catheters. *J Infect Dis* 146:719–723, 1982.
12. Casterton JW, Stewart PS, Greenberg ED: Bacterial biofilms: a common cause of persistent infections. *Science* 284:1318–1322, 1999.
13. McLean R, Nickel JC, Noakes VC, et al: An in vitro ultrastructural study of infectious kidney stone genesis. *Infect Immun* 49:805–811, 1985.
14. Sobel JD, Kaye D: Reduced uromucoid excretion in the elderly. *J Infect Dis* 152:653, 1985.
15. Hooton TM, Roberts PL, Cox ME, et al: Voided midstream urine culture and acute cystitis in premenopausal women. *N Engl J Med* 369(20):1883–1891, 2013.
16. Svanborg C, Frendeus B, Godaly L, et al: Toll-like receptor signaling and chemokine receptor expression influence the severity of urinary tract infection. *J Infect Dis* 183(1):S61, 2001.
17. Scholes D, Hooton TM, Roberts PL, et al: Risk factors associated with acute pyelonephritis in healthy women. *Ann Intern Med* 142:20–27, 2005.
18. Stamey TA, Fair WR, Timothy MM: Antibacterial nature of prostatic fluid. *Nature* 218:444–447, 1968.
19. Cai T, Mazzoli S, Mondaini N, et al: The role of asymptomatic bacteriuria in young sexually active with recurrent urinary tract infection: to treat or not to treat? *Clin Infect Dis* 55:771–777, 2012.
20. Nicolle LE, Bradley S, Colgan R, et al: Infectious Diseases Society of America guidelines for the diagnosis and treatment of asymptomatic bacteriuria in adults. *Clin Infect Dis* 40:643–654, 2005.
21. Raz R: Asymptomatic bacteriuria: clinical significance and management. *Int J Antimicrob Agents* 22(Suppl 2):45–47, 2003.
22. Cai T, Nesi G, Mazzoli S, et al: Asymptomatic bacteriuria treatment is associated with a higher prevalence of antibiotic resistant strains in women with urinary tract infections. *Clin Infect Dis* 61(11):1655–1661, 2015.
23. Wagenlehner FM, Naber KG: Treatment of asymptomatic bacteriuria might be harmful. *Clin Infect Dis* 66(11):1662–1663, 2015.
24. Stamm WE, Hooten TM: Management of urinary tract infections in adults. *N Engl J Med* 329:1328–1334, 1993.
25. Stamm WE, Counts GW, Running KR, et al: Diagnosis of coliform infection in acutely dysuric women. *N Engl J Med* 307:463–468, 1982.
26. Gupta K, Hooton TM, Naber KG, et al: International clinical practice guidelines for the treatment of acute uncomplicated cystitis and pyelonephritis in women: 2010 update by the Infectious Diseases Society of America and the European Society of Microbiology and Infectious Diseases. *Clin Infect Dis* 52(5):e103–e120, 2011.

27. Hooton TM, Bradley SF, Cardenas DD, et al: Diagnosis, prevention, and treatment of catheter-associated urinary tract infections in adults: 2009 International clinical practice guidelines from the Infectious Diseases Society of America. *Clin Infect Dis* 50:625–663, 2010.
28. Lipsky BA: Urinary tract infection in men: epidemiology, pathophysiology, diagnosis and treatment. *Ann Intern Med* 110:138–150, 1989.
29. Meng MV, Mario LA, McAninch JW: Current treatment and outcomes of perinephric abscesses. *J Urol* 168(4 Pt 1):1337–1340, 2002.
30. Kehinda EO, Rotimi VO, Al Hunayan A, et al: Bacteriology of urinary tract infection associated with indwelling J ureteral stents. *J Endourol* 18(9):891, 2004.
31. Piccirillo M, Rigsby C, Rosenfield AT: Contemporary imaging of renal inflammatory disease. *Infect Dis Clin North Am* 1:927–964, 1987.
32. Dellinger P, Levy MM, Rhodes A, et al: The surviving sepsis guidelines: 2012. *Crit Care Med* 41(2):580–637, 2013.
33. Czaja CA, Scholes D, Hooton TM, et al: Population-based epidemiologic analysis of acute pyelonephritis. *Clin Infect Dis* 45:273–280, 2007.
34. Sorbera M, Chung E, Ho CW, et al: Ceftolozane/tazobactam: a new option in the treatment of complicated gram-negative infections. *Pharm Ther* 39(12):828–832, 2014.
35. Lagace-Wiens P, Walkty A, Karlowsky JA: Ceftazidime/avibactam: an evidence-based review of its pharmacology and potential use in the treatment of gram-negative infections. *Core Evid* 9:13–25, 2014.
36. Linden PK: Clinical implications of nosocomial gram-positive bacteremia and superimposed antimicrobial resistance. *Am J Med* 104:24S–33S, 1998.
37. Noskin G, Siddique F, Stosor V, et al: Successful treatment of persistent vancomycin-resistant *Enterococcus faecium* bacteremia with linezolid and gentamicin. *Clin Infect Dis* 28:689–690, 1999.
38. Wald HL, Kramer AM: Nonpayment for harms resulting from medical care. *JAMA* 298 (23):2782–2784, 2007.
39. Millar LK, Cox SM: Urinary tract infections complicating pregnancy. *Infect Dis Clin North Am* 11:13–26, 1997.
40. Laupland KB, Zygun DA, Davies HD, et al: Incidence and risk factors for acquiring nosocomial urinary tract infection in the critically ill. *J Crit Care* 17(1):50–57, 2002.
41. Bochicchio GV, Joshi M, Bochicchio SD, et al: Reclassification of urinary tract infections in critically ill trauma patients: a time-dependent analysis. *Surg Infect* 4(4):379–385, 2003.
42. Tambyah PA, Knasinski V, Maki DG: The direct costs of nosocomial catheter-associated urinary tract infection in the era of managed care. *Infect Control Hosp Epidemiol* 23(1):27–31, 2002.
43. Garibaldi RA, Burke JP, Britt MR, et al: Meatal colonization and catheter-associated bacteriuria. *N Engl J Med* 303:316–318, 1980.
44. Mobley HL, Chippendale GR, Tenney JH, et al: MR/K hemagglutination of *Providencia stuartii* correlates with adherence to catheters and with persistence in catheter-associated bacteriuria. *J Infect Dis* 157:264–271, 1988.
45. Woods TD, Watanakunakorn C: Bacteremia due to *Providencia stuartii*: a review of 49 episodes. *South Med J* 89:221–224, 1996.
46. Mobley HL, Warren JW: Urease-positive bacteriuria and obstruction of long-term urinary catheters. *J Clin Micro* 25(11):2216–2217, 1987.
47. Harding GKM, Nicolle LE, Ronald AR, et al: How long should catheter-acquired urinary tract infection in women be treated. *Ann Intern Med* 114:713–719, 1991.
48. Calandra T, Cohen J: The international sepsis forum definition of infection in the ICU consensus conference. *Crit Care Med* 33(7):1538–1548, 2005.
49. Stark RP, Maki D: Bacteriuria in the catheterized patient: what quantitative level of bacteriuria is relevant? *N Engl J Med* 311:560–564, 1984.
50. Warren JW, Damron D, Tenney JH, et al: Fever, bacteremia, and death as complications of bacteriuria in women with long-term urethral catheters. *J Infect Dis* 155:1151–1158, 1987.
51. Grahn D, Norman DC, White ML, et al: Validity of urinary catheter specimens for the diagnosis of urinary tract infection in the elderly. *Arch Intern Med* 145:1858–1860, 1985.
52. Weinberger M, Cytron S, Servadio C, et al: Prostatic abscess in the antibiotic era. *Rev Infect Dis* 10:239–249, 1988.
53. Warren JW: Urethral catheters, condom catheters, and nosocomial urinary tract infections. *Infect Control Hosp Epidemiol* 17:212–214, 1996.
54. López-López G, Pascual A, Martínez-Martínez L, et al: Effect of a siliconized latex urinary catheter on bacterial adherence in human neutrophil activity. *Diagn Microbiol Infect Dis* 14:1–6, 1991.
55. Johnson JR, Roberts PL, Olsen RJ, et al: Prevention of catheter-associated urinary tract infection with a silver oxide-coated urinary catheter: clinical and microbiologic correlates. *J Infect Dis* 162:1145–1150, 1990.
56. Johnson JR, Kushowski MA, Wilt TJ: Systemic review: antimicrobial urinary catheters to prevent catheter-associated urinary tract infection in hospitalized patients. *Ann Intern Med* 144:116–126, 2006.
57. Thompson RL, Haley CE, Searcey MA, et al: Catheter-associated bacteriuria: failure to reduce attack rates using periodic instillations of a disinfectant into urinary drainage systems. *JAMA* 251:747–751, 1984.
58. Holliman RC, Seal DV, Archer H, et al: Controlled trial of chemical disinfection of urinary drainage bags: reduction in hospital-acquired, catheter-associated infection. *Br J Urol* 60(5):419–422, 1987.
59. Jacobs LG: Fungal urinary tract infections in the elderly: treatment guidelines. *Drugs Aging* 8(2):89–96, 1996.
60. Kauffman CA, Vazquez JA, Sobel JD, et al: Prospective multicenter surveillance study of funguria in hospitalized patients. The National Institute of Allergy (NIAID) mycoses study group. *Clin Infect Dis* 30:14–18, 2000.
61. Fisher JE, Sobel JD, Kauffman CA, et al: Candida urinary tract infections-treatment. *Clin Infect Dis* 52(Suppl 6):S457–S466, 2011.
62. Paul N, Mathai E, Abraham OC, et al: Factors associated with candiduria and related mortality. *J Infect* 55(5):450–455, 2007.
63. Carvalho J, Guimarães CM, Mayer JR, et al: Hospital-associated funguria: analysis of risk factors, clinical presentation and outcome. *Braz J Infect Dis* 5(6):313–318, 2001.
64. Kauffman CA: Candiduria. *Clin Infect Dis* 41(Suppl 6):S371–S376.
65. Tambyah PA, Maki DG: The relationship between pyuria and infection in patients with indwelling urinary catheters: a prospective study of 761 patients. *Arch Intern Med* 160:673–677, 2000.
66. Magill SS, Swoboda SM, Johnson EA, et al: The association between anatomic site of Candida colonization, invasive candidiasis, and mortality in critically ill surgical patients. *Diagn Microbiol Infect Dis* 55(4):293–301, 2006.
67. Lundstrom T, Sobel J: Nosocomial candiduria: a review. *Clin Infect Dis* 32:1602–1607, 2001.
68. Martino P, Girmenia C, Venditti M, et al: *Candida* colonization and systemic infection in neutropenic patients. *Cancer* 64:2030–2034, 1989.
69. Apisarnthanarak A, Rutjanawech S, Wichansawakun S, et al: Initial inappropriate urinary catheters use in a tertiary-care center: incidence, risk factors, and outcomes. *Am J Infect Control* 35(9):594–599, 2007.
70. Pappas PG, Kauffman CA, Andes D, et al: Clinical Practice guidelines for the management of candidiasis: 2009 update by the Infectious Disease Society of America. *Clin Infect Dis* 48:503–535, 2009.
71. Rex JH, Pfaller MA, Gulgiani JN, et al: Development of interpretive breakpoints for antifungal susceptibility testing: conceptual framework and analysis of in vitro–in vivo correlation data for fluconazole, itraconazole, and *Candida* infections. *Clin Infect Dis* 24:235–247, 1997.
72. Hsu CCS, Chang R: Two-day continuous bladder irrigation with amphotericin B. *Clin Infect Dis* 20:1570–1571, 1995.
73. Fisher JF, Woeltje K, Espinel-Ingroff A, et al: Efficacy of a single intravenous dose of amphotericin B for Candida urinary tract infections: further favorable experience. *Clin Microbiol Infect* 9(10):1024–1027, 2003.
74. Rex JH, Bennett JE, Sugar AM, et al: A randomized trial comparing fluconazole with amphotericin B for the treatment of candidemia in patients without neutropenia. *N Engl J Med* 331:1325–1330, 1994.
75. Boodeker KS, Kilzoi WJ: Fluconazole dose recommendation in urinary tract infection. *Ann Pharmacother* 35(3):369–372, 2001.
76. Sobel JD: When and how to treat candiduria. *Infect Dis Clin Pract* 14:125–126, 2006.

Chapter 81 ■ Central Nervous System Infections

HEIDI L. SMITH

The central nervous system (CNS) infections of major interest in the intensive care unit (ICU) are bacterial meningitis, encephalitis, brain abscess, and other parameningeal foci of infection. The clinical presentations of these diseases may overlap. *Meningitis* means inflammation of the leptomeninges; its hallmark is stiff neck. *Encephalitis* is a syndrome consisting of disturbance of cerebral function and inflammation of the brain parenchyma, usually associated with cerebrospinal fluid (CSF) pleocytosis. Many cases of bacterial meningitis also fit this definition of encephalitis due to the occurrence of mental status changes, seizures, or coma. Focal infections, such as brain abscesses, may present more as space-occupying lesions than with classical infectious signs or symptoms.

CSF examination is the major tool used for the diagnosis of CNS infections. The terms *purulent* and *aseptic* describe contrasting CSF formulas, though overlap exists. The typical purulent CSF has a white blood cell count of more than 1,000 cells per μL (most of which are neutrophils), a depressed glucose concentration (<40 mg per dL), and an elevated protein level (>100 mg per dL); it is most commonly seen in bacterial meningitis. In contrast, an "aseptic" formula has a lower total leukocyte count with a predominance of mononuclear cells, a glucose concentration greater than 40% to 50% of the blood level, and less marked elevation of protein; this picture characterizes most other CNS infections. An intermediate CSF formula, in which a moderate lymphocytic pleocytosis is accompanied by depressed glucose and elevated protein, suggests granulomatous disease.

GENERAL CLINICAL APPROACH

Initial evaluation of the patient with suspected CNS infection should focus on defining the nature of the symptoms (meningitic vs. encephalitic) and the presence and pattern of neurologic involvement (focal vs. diffuse).

If bacterial meningitis is suspected, expeditious analysis of CSF is critical. This must be balanced with the need to administer antibiotics promptly; delays as short as 3 hours have been shown to lead to unfavorable outcomes [1,2]. If lumbar puncture (LP) is delayed, antibiotics (and dexamethasone; see later) should be started as soon as blood cultures have been obtained while efforts to obtain CSF proceed [3].

LP is not without risk. In patients with bleeding disorders, it should be delayed until the defect(s) can be corrected [4]. LP may be hazardous in the settings of intracranial mass lesion. Concern for cerebral herniation as a consequence of the procedure has led to the common practice of routinely performing computed tomography (CT) scanning prior to LP. This practice is not well founded, however [5]. A prospective study confirmed that CT scans rarely discover abnormalities that would represent a contraindication to LP except among patients who have a prior history of CNS disease, immunosuppressive disorders, seizures, moderate-to-severe impairment of consciousness, papilledema, or focal neurological findings [6].

BACTERIAL MENINGITIS

Bacterial meningitis is perhaps the most clear-cut emergency in the field of infectious diseases. Delayed or inadequate treatment increases the risk of death or significant neurological impairment [1].

Etiology

The predominant organisms vary based on the age and underlying condition of the host. Historically, bacterial meningitis in the United States has been primarily caused by five organisms: *Streptococcus pneumoniae*, *Neisseria meningitidis*, *Listeria monocytogenes*, *Haemophilus influenzae*, and group B streptococcus. However, immunization of young children against *H. influenzae* and *S. pneumoniae* has had a marked impact, raising the average age of meningitis from 15 months old to 42 years old [7].

S. pneumoniae accounts for more than half of all community-acquired bacterial meningitis cases in the United States after the neonatal period [7,8]. The case fatality rate is 20% to 30% in adults and survivors have approximately a 30% risk of sequelae [9,10]. Pneumococcal meningitis is more common in the setting of a CSF leak, hypogammaglobulinemia, asplenia, alcoholism, head trauma, or cochlear implant [11]. Routine infant immunization has also reduced the incidence of pneumococcal meningitis in older children and adults due to a reduction in *S. pneumoniae* carriage in the younger population [12,13], though there has been an increase in pneumococal meningitis caused by nonvaccine strains [14].

N. meningitidis incidence has declined substantially in recent years, but still causes more than 10% of bacterial meningitis in the United States [7,15]. Incidence peaks in three age groups: infants and children under 5 years, adolsescents/young adults (16 to 21 years), and adults over 65 years [16]. It is the one form of bacterial meningitis associated with epidemic spread, though the majority of cases in the United States are sporadic [9,16]. Routine immunization with a meningococcal conjugate vaccine directed against serogroups A, C, W, and Y is currently recommended for preadolescents, freshman entering college, and military recruits as well as special populations at increased risk of meningococcal disease [16]. Vaccines providing protection from serogroup B have recently been licensed and are currently recommended for individuals over 10 years of age at increased risk [17]. To date, there does not appear to have been replacement with nonvaccine meningococcal serotypes in the United States [18].

L. monocytogenes is a common cause of meningitis in the neonatal period or in the setting of malignancy, immunosuppression, or alcoholism. Approximately 30% of patients have no apparent immunocompromising condition; most of these individuals are older than 50 years [7,19]. Listeria may be associated with lower CSF WBC counts and higher CSF glucose than other bacterial meningitides [9,20].

H. influenzae type B was formerly the most common cause of bacterial meningitis among young children. Childhood vaccination has reduced the incidence of invasive *H. influenzae* type B disease by more than 90% [7,9,21]. Sporadic cases have been reported in unimmunized and partially immunized children and *H. influenzae* strains not covered by the vaccine can also cause meningitis [22]. *H. influenzae* in adults is uncommon and is usually associated with predisposing factors, particularly defects in humoral immunity [21].

Gram-negative bacillary meningitis occurs in the neonatal period or after neurosurgery or trauma [7,23]. Craniotomy is associated with a 1% to 2% rate of bacterial meningitis [24]. Increased infection rates are associated with perioperative steroids, CSF leak, and ventricular drainage [25]. Spontaneous gram-negative bacillary meningitis is associated with advanced age, cancer, and bacteremic urinary tract infection; *Escherichia coli* and *Pseudomonas* sp. are the most frequent pathogens [23].

Staphylococcus aureus meningitis is associated with neurosurgery or trauma. Community-acquired cases occur in the presence of a focus of infection outside the CNS, such as endocarditis or soft tissue infections, and have a worse prognosis [26]. Meningitis in patients with CSF shunts or other hardware such as Omaya reservoirs and deep brain stimulators is most commonly caused by skin flora (*S. aureus*, *Staphylococcus epidermidis*, and *Propionibacterium acnes*) and Gram-negative bacilli [27–30]. These infections can have an indolent presentation and milder CSF abnormalities [3,24,28]. Use of shunt catheters impregnated with antimicrobials reduces the rates of infection [31].

Several additional species of streptococci can cause meningitis. Group B streptococcus, *Streptococcus agalactiae*, is the most common cause of neonatal meningitis, though rates of early-onset disease have decreased with use of intrapartum penicillin prophylaxis [7,9]. Rates of group B streptococcal invasive disease in adults are increasing, particularly in diabetic patients, but only a small proportion present as meningitis [32]. *Streptococcus suis* is an increasingly common cause of meningitis in Asia and should be considered in travelers who may have ingested raw pork or had contact with pigs [33]. The use of catheters for anesthesia and imaging procedures has been associated with the introduction of α-hemolytic streptococci [24,34]. Anaerobic bacteria and other streptococci are otherwise uncommon causes of meningitis that are usually related to spread from brain abscess or parameningeal foci [35].

Pathogenesis

Bacterial seeding of the meninges can arise from hematogenous spread or spread from contiguous foci of infection. Direct invasion can be facilitated by anatomic defects secondary to trauma, such as when basilar skull fractures create a communication between the sinuses and the subarachnoid space [9,24]. Bacteremia can arise from simple colonization of the nasopharynx, though colonization alone is obviously not sufficient, since up to 40% of the population can be colonized with *N. meningitidis* and surveys in daycare centers show up to 60% *S. pneumoniae* carriage [36,37]. The bacterial species most commonly associated with meningitis bind receptors on microvascular endothelial cells, facilitating entry to the CNS [38]. Most meningitis pathogens also secrete immunoglobulin A proteases, facilitating immune evasion at mucosal sites [39]. Inadequate levels of antibody specific for the invading organism (such as occurs at the extremes of age or in acquired immunodeficiencies) and opsonophagocytic deficiencies (such as in asplenia, diabetes, or alcoholism) are the most commonly recognized risk factors for meningitis [36]. Individuals with terminal complement component deficiencies may experience recurrent episodes of meningococcal meningitis [16,37,40].

Once bacteria reach the CSF, both bacterial and host factors contribute to disease. Recognition of bacterial components leads to elaboration of inflammatory mediators such as tumor necrosis factor-α (TNF-α), interleukin-1, and interleukin-6; intrathecal TNF-α levels correlate with severity in the disruption of the blood-brain barrier [36]. Additional inflammation, triggers release of tissue factor (which aids thrombus formation and disrupts cerebral perfusion), nitric oxide (which disrupts autoregulation of blood flow and can have direct toxic effects on neurons), and matrix metalloproteinases (which can also disrupt endothelial junctions and impair neuronal function) [36,41]. Neuronal damage is further worsened by increases in intracranial pressure [41].

Antibiotics that rapidly lyse bacteria transiently increase in inflammation as a response to the release of bacterial cell wall components [36]. Adjunctive steroid therapy acts to decrease inflammation associated with bacterial lysis [36,42]. The body also deploys endogenous immunomodulators such as interleukin-10 and TNF-related apoptosis-inducing ligand (TRAIL), which has been shown to reduce neuronal damage in animal models [36,43].

The clinical consequence of these pathologic processes is a generalized disturbance of cerebral function. Early agitation, delirium, or mania may be noted. Lethargy progresses to obtundation and sometimes coma. Seizures and increased intracranial pressure can further depress levels of consciousness. Hyponatremia, which can be caused by the syndrome of inappropriate antidiuretic hormone (SIADH) secretion, cerebral salt wasting, or aggressive fluid resuscitation, may contribute to obtundation and seizures. Focal neurologic deficits may be observed; sensorineural deafness is particularly common [36,44].

Diagnosis

History

Patients with meningitis may be unable to give a coherent history. Patients found unresponsive should be evaluated with a high level of suspicion for meningitis. Patients with fever and derangement of cerebral function, even if there is another cause for the latter, must have meningitis excluded. Persons with coexistent alcoholism, general debility, head trauma, or neurosurgery are at higher risk for meningitis.

Classic meningeal symptoms are headache (often with photophobia), neck pain, fever, and mental status changes; in a case series, 95% of patients with bacterial meningitis had at least two of these four symptoms [45]. Symptoms of other foci of infection, such as pneumonia, otitis, or sinusitis, may also be present [46]. Any history of head trauma (including remote events) or recent clear nasal or ear discharges should be obtained. Recent antibiotics, which could interfere with culture results, should be noted. A history of exposure to a patient with known meningococcal disease is usually forthcoming if present. Travel history may aid the identification of regionally endemic pathogens.

Physical Examination

Nuchal rigidity suggests meningitis when present. Kernig's and Brudzinski's signs have low sensitivity but high specificity [46]. The initial neurologic examination should evaluate the mental status and the presence of focal deficits. Papilledema is rarely observed at presentation but alters the approach to LP when present. Serial examinations document any functional progression or improvement.

The systemic examination may give clues to the cause of meningitis. A thorough ear, nose, and throat examination can reveal possible foci leading to contiguous extension to the meninges. Petechiae or purpuric lesions strongly suggest meningococcal disease, though they may also be seen in other bacterial infections or in aseptic meningitis caused by enteroviruses or rickettsiae. Needle aspiration or punch biopsy of skin lesions should be used to obtain material for Gram stain and culture. *N. meningitidis* can be detected on either culture or stain of skin specimens [9].

Laboratory Tests

Evaluation of the CSF is essential for the diagnosis of meningitis. The typical features of purulent CSF have been noted earlier. Neutrophil counts greater than 1,000 cells per μL are strongly associated with bacterial meningitis [9]. In rare cases, the CSF shows many organisms on Gram stain but few cells, implying rapidly progressive disease [9,45]. Elevated protein is also almost always present [9]. Severe depression of the CSF glucose

(<20 mg per dL) is strong evidence for a pyogenic process, but CSF glucose is normal in over 50% of patients with bacterial meningitis [9]. Treatment with antibiotics prior to LP may alter CSF chemistries, resulting in higher glucose levels and lower protein levels, though cell counts are usually unaffected [47].

Cultures remain the mainstays of diagnosis. Blood cultures can be useful in identifying the causative agent of meningitis in cases where CSF cultures are unrevealing [48]. Ultimately, 60% to 90% of patients with community-acquired meningitis and purulent CSF have an organism isolated in culture [46]. CSF cryptococcal antigen assay should be considered; bacterial antigen detection tests offer little additional information [3,49]. Polymerase chain reaction (PCR) detection of bacterial DNA may provide more rapid and sensitive diagnosis, particularly in the setting of antibiotic pretreatment; however, these assays are not yet available in all settings [46,50].

Imaging studies are of secondary importance in the diagnosis of meningitis. Imaging of the chest and paranasal sinuses may identify other foci of infection. CT and magnetic resonance imaging (MRI) of the brain are most useful for evaluating complications of meningitis. Rapid deterioration should lead to consideration of subdural empyema, a collection between the dura and the arachnoid membrane [44,51]. A new focal neurologic abnormality, decreased level of consciousness, or cerebrovascular accident with a nonarterial distribution should prompt imaging for venous thrombophlebitis [44,51]. In post-neurosurgical meningitis, imaging should evaluate for ventricular size, CSF leaks, and shunt malfunction [24].

Differential Diagnosis

Several pathogens other than pyogenic bacteria can cause clinical presentations and/or spinal fluid formulas that overlap with bacterial meningitis.

Viral meningitis can have initial clinical presentations similar to bacterial meningitis, with an early neutrophil predominance and a shift to lymphocytes over time [3]. Viral meningitis can be caused by a wide range of pathogens including enteroviruses, arboviruses such as West Nile virus (WNV) [52], herpes viruses such as herpes simplex virus (HSV) [53], and acute HIV infection [54].

Tuberculous meningitis most commonly presents with a mononuclear predominance in the CSF along with low glucose and high protein. However, some cases have a total leukocyte count in the range of purulent meningitis with a polymorphonuclear predominance [55]. A history of tuberculosis, risk factors for exposure, or the presence of an immunocompromising condition should raise suspicion, particularly in the setting of a subacute meningitis presentation [56]. If an initial diagnosis of bacterial meningitis is not confirmed by culture and the patient's condition does not improve, repeat LP with studies for acid-fast bacilli should be performed. A switch to lymphocytic predominance, additional decrease in CSF glucose and increase in protein, positive chest radiograph, or well-founded clinical suspicion mandates institution of antituberculous therapy [55]. Acid-fast stains of CSF are positive in, at most, 60% of cases [56]. Nucleic acid amplification tests may facilitate earlier diagnosis, but there is a wide variability in their availability and sensitivity [57]. MRI is more likely than CT to visualize tuberculomas [58].

Parasitic infections can cause purulent meningitis. Primary amebic meningitis with *Naegleria fowleri* is acquired through freshwater exposure and presents similarly to acute bacterial meningitis. Diagnosis can be made on wet mount of CSF, though trophozoites are often mistaken for leukocytes; Centers for Disease Control and Prevention (CDC) can provide additional diagnostic modalities for suspected cases [59]. The nematode *Strongyloides stercoralis* is capable of establishing a cycle of autoinfection in immunosuppressed hosts, including those on oral corticosteroids. Migration of larvae from the gut can result in the deposition of enteric bacteria in the CNS, causing Gram-negative or polymicrobial meningitis [60].

Fungal meningitis may present with hypoglycorrhachia. An indolent course and lymphocytic CSF pleocytosis usually distinguish these from pyogenic infections, but *Coccidioides immitis*, an endemic fungus of the southwest United States, can have neutrophil predominance [61]. *Cryptococcus neoformans* is a major cause of meningitis in patients with immunosuppressive conditions, though it can occur in normal hosts; *Cryptococcus gatti* is an emerging cause of cryptococcal meningitis in immunocompetent hosts [62]. Cryptococcal antigen assay of the CSF provides a sensitive means of diagnosis [63].

Parameningeal foci of infection, including epidural abscess, can present a purulent picture, usually with elevated protein and a normal glucose concentration [64]. Brain abscess that has ruptured into the ventricles may duplicate the clinical picture of bacterial meningitis. Localizing neurologic findings or isolation of an anaerobe or multiple organisms from the CSF should suggest one of these diagnoses [35].

Noninfectious conditions can cause meningeal signs and CSF findings that overlap with those of bacterial meningitis. Drug-induced meningitis may have a CSF formula indistinguishable from pyogenic infection; the most commonly implicated agents are nonsteroidal anti-inflammatories, antibiotics, immunomodulatory agents, and antiepileptics [65]. Postneurosurgical chemical meningitis, believed to be an inflammatory reaction to surgical manipulation, blood, or bone dust, can present with a CSF profile similar to bacterial meningitis. Although symptoms, CSF leukocytosis, and hypoglycorrhachia are usually less severe, no single parameter has been proven to distinguish between the two conditions. Given the risk of bacterial meningitis in the postneurosurgical population, antibiotics are often administered until CSF culture results are finalized [24,25,66].

Therapy

Bacterial meningitis requires prompt initiation of antimicrobial and anti-inflammatory therapy, aggressive control of the potential complications, and prevention of disease spread [3]. Overall mortality from bacterial meningitis is in the range of 20% to 30% [45,67]. However, mortality rates are significantly influenced by both the pathogen, with *S. pneumoniae* among the most deadly, and the host, with elderly patients among the most susceptible [9,45]. Consequently, most patients should be treated in an intensive care setting.

Antimicrobial Therapy

The principal consideration for choosing an antibiotic regimen for bacterial meningitis is that the agent(s) reach the CSF in concentrations that are bactericidal for the likely pathogens. Table 81.1 lists recommendations for therapy of bacterial meningitis in a variety of clinical settings. Initial therapy is usually selected empirically based on the age and underlying condition of the patient. Once the CSF Gram stain result is available, antimicrobial therapy can be targeted appropriately.

The third-generation cephalosporins (ceftriaxone or cefotaxime) are the mainstays of therapy for community-acquired meningitis. These agents are active against most strains of *S. pneumoniae* and provide excellent coverage against *N. meningitidis* and Gram-negative bacilli (except *Pseudomonas aeruginosa*). *S. pneumoniae* with reduced susceptibility to the cephalosporins has been reported; this organism remains universally susceptible to vancomycin [68]. If the CSF Gram stain suggests pneumococci or is unrevealing, vancomycin should be given in addition to the cephalosporin until culture and sensitivity results are available [3]. Meropenem also demonstrates activity against many, but not all, cephalosporin-resistant strains of *S. pneumoniae*

TABLE 81.1

Antimicrobial Agents Recommended for Therapy of Bacterial Meningitis

Clinical situation	Recommended therapy[a]
Initial cerebrospinal fluid (CSF) Gram stain negative or delayed	
Age < 3 mo	Ampicillin plus ceftriaxone[b]
Age 3 mo to 50 y	Ceftriaxone[b] plus vancomycin[c]
Age > 50 y	Ampicillin plus ceftriaxone[b] plus vancomycin[c]
After neurosurgery or penetrating cranial trauma	Vancomycin[c] plus ceftazidime[d]
Immunosuppression, alcoholism, debilitation	Ampicillin plus ceftriaxone[b] plus vancomycin[c]
Initial CSF Gram stain positive (community-acquired bacterial meningitis)	
Gram-positive cocci	Vancomycin[c] plus ceftriaxone[b]
Gram-negative cocci	Ceftriaxone[b]
Gram-positive bacilli	Ampicillin ± gentamicin[e]
Gram-negative bacilli	Ceftazidime[d] ± aminoglycoside[f]
Organism known, susceptibility not yet known	
Streptococcus pneumoniae	Vancomycin[c] plus ceftriaxone[b]
Streptococcus, group A or B	Penicillin G ± gentamicin[e]
Enterococcus	Penicillin G ± gentamicin[e]
Staphylococcus aureus	Vancomycin[c] (and/or nafcillin[g])
Listeria monocytogenes	Ampicillin ± gentamicin[e]
Neisseria meningitidis	Penicillin G
Haemophilus influenzae	Ceftriaxone[b]
Pseudomonas aeruginosa	Ceftazidime[d] plus tobramycin[f]
Other Gram-negative bacilli (e.g., *Escherichia coli, Klebsiella, Proteus*)	Ceftriaxone[b] plus gentamicin[f]

[a]Usual daily doses (schedules) for adults are as follows: ampicillin, 12 g/d (q4h); ceftriaxone, 4 g/d (q12h); ceftazidime, 6 g/d (q8h); nafcillin, 12 g/d (q4h); penicillin G, 24 million U/d (q2–4h).
[b]Cefotaxime, 8–12 g/d, given q4–6h, is equally effective.
[c]Usual daily dose of vancomycin for adults is 2–3 g/d, given q8–12h, with body weight guiding dose and creatinine clearance guiding frequency of dosing. Troughs should be monitored with a goal of 15–20 mg/dL.
[d]Cefepime, 6 g/d given q8h, may be used as an alternative.
[e]Although CSF penetration of aminoglycosides is poor, some specialists recommend their use in these settings.
[f]Consideration should be given to initial intrathecal administration in addition to intravenous administration.
[g]In most areas, where methicillin resistance is common among isolates of *S. aureus*, vancomycin should be used and addition of nafcillin can be considered. In areas where methicillin resistance among *S. aureus* is still rare, nafcillin is the preferred agent.

and has demonstrated clinical effectiveness for treatment of meningitis [68,69].

Ampicillin (or penicillin) should be included in the regimen for empiric therapy in neonates (<1 month old), individuals older than 50 years, patients with alcoholism, or those who are debilitated or immunosuppressed, for coverage of *L. monocytogenes* [19,70]. Initial therapy for postneurosurgical bacterial meningitis should include vancomycin plus either ceftazidime or cefepime to provide adequate coverage for methicillin-resistant staphylococci and *P. aeruginosa.* Resistance to antimicrobials, either at the outset or developing during treatment, can complicate therapy for Gram-negative organisms [71]. An increasing number of cases due to multidrug-resistant hospital-acquired organisms such as *Acinetobacter* sp. have been reported [72].

Few good treatment regimens exist for the cephalosporin-intolerant patient. Consequently, a trial of the third-generation cephalosporins (or meropenem) should be strongly considered unless there is a documented, serious intolerance. Vancomycin is the preferred alternative for treatment of pneumococcal meningitis. Moxifloxacin has activity against pneumococci, meningococci, and *H. influenzae* and has shown promise in animal models, but clinical experience is limited [3]. Trimethoprim–sulfamethoxazole is effective for the treatment of meningitis caused by *L. monocytogenes* and many Gram-negative bacilli other than *P. aeruginosa* [73].

If *S. pneumoniae* is isolated, therapy should be adjusted based on the results of drug susceptibility testing. Fully susceptible organisms can be treated with third-generation cephalosporin alone. For resistant organisms, vancomycin and cephalosporin should be continued and the addition of rifampin considered [3]. Continued clinical instability after 48 hours of appropriate antibiotic therapy is an indication for repeat LP [3]. Repeat CSF samples should have a negative Gram stain and culture after at least 24 hours of effective antibiotic therapy [44].

The recommended duration of antimicrobial therapy for meningitis depends on the etiology and the clinical response. For infection with *H. influenzae* or meningococci, 7 to 10 days of therapy is adequate. *S. pneumoniae* is usually treated for 10 to 14 days, but longer durations may be needed for drug-resistant organisms. Gram-negative bacillary meningitis is typically treated for 3 weeks and staphylococcal disease, when accompanied by bacteremia, for 4 to 6 weeks [3].

Anti-Inflammatory Therapy

The role of endogenous mediators of inflammation in the pathogenesis of meningitis has provided a rationale for the use of anti-inflammatory agents. Dexamethasone, 0.15 mg per kg every 6 hours for 4 days, has been shown to reduce both mortality and neurologic sequelae [42,67]. However, the benefit appears to be primarily for pneumococcal meningitis [74,75]. Dexamethasone therapy should be initiated before or simultaneously with the first antimicrobial dose in patients with suspected or confirmed pneumococcal meningitis [3,67].

The recommended duration of steroid therapy is 4 days, but some studies in children suggest that 2 days may be adequate [42,76]. Current guidelines recommend discontinuing steroids when bacteria other than *S. pneumoniae* are isolated [3].

The benefits of steroid therapy seen in studies performed in industrialized countries have not been consistently observed in the developing world [77,78]; therefore, adjunctive dexamethasone is not routinely recommended in these settings.

Supportive Therapy

Treatment of meningitis also requires management of seizures and increased intracranial pressure. Seizures should be controlled by anticonvulsants as necessary (see Chapter 151), and aspiration and hypoxia must be prevented. Severe cerebral edema with evidence of uncal or cerebellar herniation can be managed with CSF drainage, osmotherapy, and steroids [5]. Fluid management should be directed at maintenance of euvolemia [44].

Bacterial meningitis in the setting of CSF shunts presents additional considerations. The highest rates of cure (>80%) are obtained with initiation of antibiotics, removal of the entire shunt, temporary external drainage, and replacement of the shunt when follow-up CSF cultures are negative. One stage removal with immediate replacement of the device followed by antibiotics is associated with a 65% rate of cure. Antibiotics alone, usually only considered for less virulent organisms such as *P. acnes* and non-aureus staphylococci, are successful 35% of the time [3,24].

Infection Control

Patients with *N. meningitidis* or *H. influenzae* type B meningitis should be managed with droplet precautions until 24 hours after initiation of antibiotics. Chemoprophylaxis is recommended for the situations described below. Dosing and duration are detailed in Table 81.2.

For *N. meningitidis*, household and day care contacts as well as hospital personnel who have performed unprotected cardiopulmonary resuscitation, intubation, or suctioning should receive chemoprophylaxis. Rifampin, ciprofloxacin, or ceftriaxone are the recommended agents [16]. A small number of ciprofloxacin-resistant *N. meningitidis* isolates have been reported in North Dakota and Minnesota [79]. Primary rifampin resistance is similarly rare but may develop secondarily in individuals who receive rifampin for prophylaxis [80]. Meningococcal vaccines (quadrivalent or serogroup B, depending on the setting) can be used as an adjunct to chemoprophylaxis to prevent late secondary cases in contacts or to control outbreaks of disease [16,17].

For *H. influenzae* type B disease, chemoprophylaxis is recommended for household contacts only if there is at least one child younger than 4 years who is not fully vaccinated or if there is an immunocompromised child in the household. In addition, if two or more cases have occurred in the same day-care group within 60 days, chemoprophylaxis is recommended. Rifampin is the recommended agent [21].

ENCEPHALITIS

Encephalitis is a more rare infection than meningitis and a far less uniform one. Although a specific diagnosis provides important prognostic and epidemiologic information, there are only a handful of treatable causes of encephalitis. Efforts should focus on identifying and addressing these causes. Infections of the brain that do not present as acute encephalitis but rather as subacute to chronic processes are not discussed further in this chapter.

Etiology

For almost half of all encephalitis cases in the United States, the etiology is not identified. Among the cases with a defined diagnosis, 50% are caused by viruses, with HSV and varicella zoster virus (VZV) being the most common [81–86]. Part of the diagnostic challenge stems from the sheer number and diversity of causative organisms. With improved diagnostic techniques, there is increased recognition of viruses such as Jamestown Canyon virus [87] and Powassan virus [88] as well as newly identified causative agents [89]. Many nonviral pathogens, including Mycobacterium tuberculosis, rickettsiae, *Mycoplasma pneumoniae*, *Bartonella* sp., *Treponema pallidum*, *Borrelia burgdorferi*, amoebae, *L. monocytogenes*, and *Toxoplasma gondii*, have all been associated with the syndrome [81–86]. In addition, immune-mediated encephalitis may have a similar presentation to infectious encephalitis. Autoimmune processes, such as anti-*N*-methyl-D-aspartate (NMDA) receptor and voltage gated potassium channel (VGKC) antibodies, are increasingly recognized causes of encephalitis, particularly in young women [84,90]. Table 81.3 lists the causes of infectious encephalitis that are indigenous to the United States in general prognostic categories. Despite the favorable prognosis, encephalitis caused by organisms listed in group 1 may be extremely severe, with prolonged unresponsiveness followed by gradual clearing.

Pathogenesis

Although HSV is the most common organism identified in encephalitis cases, the pathogenesis of herpes simplex encephalitis (HSE) is not entirely clear. The characteristic feature of HSE is its focal nature, an acute hemorrhagic necrotizing process with a predilection for the temporal lobe [91]. HSV persists in the

TABLE 81.2

Chemoprophylaxis for *Neisseria meningitidis* and *Haemophilus influenzae*

Pathogen	Antibiotic	Dose and duration
N. meningitidis	Ceftriaxone[a]	125 mg for children or 250 mg for adults as a single intramuscular injection
	Ciprofloxacin[b]	500 mg as a single dose in adults
	Rifampin	10 mg/kg (maximum dose, 600 mg) by mouth twice a day for 2 d
H. influenzae	Rifampin	20 mg/kg (maximum dose, 600 mg) by mouth once a day for 4 d

[a]Preferred agent in pregnant women.
[b]In geographic areas where ciprofloxacin-resistant *N. meningitidis* has been reported, azithromycin 10 mg/kg for children or 500 mg for adults as a single dose can be used as an alternative.

TABLE 81.3

Prognostic Categorization of Encephalitides Indigenous to the United States

Agent	Comments
Group 1: Causes of encephalitis that tend to resolve spontaneously and rarely leave neurologic residua	
Epstein-Barr virus	
Human herpes virus type 6	
Enteroviruses	
Lymphocytic choriomeningitis virus	
Mumps	
California encephalitis	Arbovirus
St. Louis encephalitis	Arbovirus
Colorado tick fever	Arbovirus
Herpes zoster	
Bartonellosis (cat scratch disease)	Especially acute cerebellar ataxia
Mycoplasma pneumonia	Especially acute cerebellar ataxia
Rocky Mountain spotted fever	Contingent on recovery from the systemic illness
Leptospirosis	Contingent on recovery from the systemic illness
Group 2: Causes of encephalitis that carry a small but definite risk of death and a sizable risk of sequelae	
Measles	
Powassan virus	Arbovirus
Western equine encephalitis	Arbovirus
West Nile virus	Arbovirus
Venezuelan equine encephalitis	Arbovirus
Group 3: Causes of encephalitis with a large risk of death; most survivors have significant residua	
Herpes simplex	
Cytomegalovirus	Immunosuppressed hosts
Eastern equine encephalitis	Arbovirus
Rabies	Six reported survivors

trigeminal ganglia and is thought to travel up to the trigeminal or olfactory nerves at the time of reactivation [91]. Studies of children with HSE have revealed defects in innate immunity [92,93].

Arboviruses are transmitted by the bite of their insect vector [94]. The insect vector inoculates the arboviruses, producing viremia. The organisms replicate in reticuloendothelial tissues, where a secondary viremia arises and infects the CNS. By the time encephalitic symptoms develop, the virus has usually been cleared from the circulation and specific antibody is present, facilitating diagnosis [94]. Blood transfusions and organ transplantation have also been a mechanism for transmission of WNV [52]. The mosquito-borne infections have seasonal prevalence in late summer and early fall. Prevalence in a given year can depend on weather trends affecting vectors. All arboviruses affect young children and the elderly more severely. Eastern equine encephalitis is the most virulent, causing death or severe neurologic sequelae in more than 60% of cases [95].

Rabies virus reaches the brain by spreading up neural pathways from its site of inoculation, a process that may take weeks to years. Saliva contains the virus, which is usually introduced by a bite or salivary contamination of an open wound [96]. In the past 30 years, the majority of cases in North America have been caused by bat rabies [97]. Human-to-human transmission has occurred through organ transplantation from donors with undiagnosed rabies [98]. Although it has never been documented, human-to-human transmission through saliva is theoretically possible; therefore, patients should be placed in strict isolation. Prophylaxis for rabies exposure consists of a combination of passive immunization with rabies immunoglobulin plus active immunization with rabies vaccine [99].

There are numerous noninfectious processes that can produce a clinical picture overlapping with infection-related encephalitis. Encephalitis associated with antineuronal antibodies fall into two main subtypes based on whether they bind intracellular targets or cell surface antigens [100,101]. The clinical presentation of the two forms overlap, frequently presenting with psychiatric symptoms, sleep disruption, movement disorders, and seizures. Antibodies associated with intracellular targets such as anti-Hu and anti-Ma2 are responsible for classic paraneoplastic syndromes and are strongly associated with underlying malignancy. The antibodies themselves are usually not pathogenic, but rather markers of a destructive cell-mediated response [101]. Antibodies to cell surface antigens, such as anti-NMDA and anti-VGKC, are directly pathogenic [101]. While they may occur in the setting of some malignancies (such as ovarian teratoma), the association with cancer is weaker [100,101]. Postinfectious encephalitis can present with encephalopathy and demyelination days to weeks following a minor infection [102]. CNS vasculitis or sarcoidosis may manifest as acute or subacute encephalitis. Although the underlying etiologies are diverse, they share the common feature of vessel wall inflammation leading to ischemia and infarction [103].

Diagnosis

The diagnostic process is directed principally at identifying treatable causes of encephalitis, especially HSE or nonviral pathogens [84,86,104].

History

The epidemiologic features reviewed earlier (see Pathogenesis) are major contributors to diagnosis. A history of foreign travel may widen the differential diagnosis beyond the considerations reviewed here. Establishing the host's immune status, and potential for occult HIV infection, will also help guide the diagnostic workup [104,105]. A history of recent infection or a prominent component of psychiatric disturbance or movement disorder raises the likelihood of immune-mediated processes [100,102].

Fever and headache are common. A neurologic presentation may occur, with seizures, mania, personality change, or another neuropsychiatric disorder as the principal signs [104,105]. Focal neurologic findings, including aphasia, suggest a diagnosis of HSE [106]. Aversion to water, refusal to swallow, and delirious behavior are classic features of "furious" rabies but are absent in 20% to 40% of cases presenting with flaccid paralysis [96,107]. Flaccid paralysis mimicking poliomyelitis has also been observed in WNV encephalitis and with certain enteroviruses [52,108].

Physical Examination

The critical component of the physical examination is to determine whether an anatomic focus of abnormality is present, increasing the likelihood of HSE. Typical skin findings may suggest diagnoses such as Rocky Mountain spotted fever, measles, or herpes zoster.

Laboratory Tests

Analysis of CSF is the most important diagnostic procedure; 20 mL should be obtained if possible with 5 to 10 mL frozen for possible future studies [104]. Opening pressure should be measured [104]. The CSF in encephalitis usually fits the aseptic picture described earlier. It may be normal early in the course of infection or in immunocompromised patients [104]. The presence of red blood cells suggests a hemorrhagic type of encephalitis, such as HSE, but is not diagnostic [91]. Eosinophils suggest infection with helminths, treponemes, rickettsiae, coccidiomycosis, toxoplasmosis, or *M. pneumoniae* [86].

Given its prevalence and the availability of specific therapy, PCR for HSV should be performed on CSF in all cases [86]. False-negative results can occur early in the disease. A repeat HSV PCR in 3 to 7 days is recommended if the clinical scenario remains consistent with HSV and no alternative diagnosis has emerged; testing for HSV intrathecal antibody production can be considered in cases with negative PCR despite high clinical suspicion [104,109].

Enteroviral PCR and VZV PCR should be sent from CSF for most adult cases, given their frequency as causative agents of encephalitis. VZV CSF IgG and IgM may also be necessary as the sensitivity of PCR may be low [104]. Treponemal testing (VDRL) and cryptococcal antigen testing of CSF should also be considered in initial evaluation [104]. When evidence of involvement outside the CNS is present, evaluation of other tissues may be helpful. Respiratory viral testing or cultures should be pursued in patient with respiratory symptoms, culture and enteroviral testing of stool in patients with diarrhea, and skin biopsy in patients with lesions [104]. PCR of serum can aid the diagnosis of ehrlichiosis, whereas PCR of lymph node tissue can detect *B. henselae* [86].

Diagnosis of most other causes of encephalitis relies on serologic testing. In arboviral infection, antibody is usually present at the onset of neurologic signs and is sufficiently rare in the general population to permit presumptive diagnosis [86]. The presence of antibody to *T. pallidum*, *B. burgdorferi*, rickettsia, or ehrlichia may reflect prior infection but is sufficient evidence to warrant treatment [86,105]. Detection of pathogen-specific antibody in the CSF can provide more convincing evidence of the etiology of encephalitis, with a serum to CSF antibody ratio of less than 20 suggesting intrathecal production of antibody. For most causes of encephalitis listed in Table 81.3, the demonstration of a significant increase in antibody titer is required for diagnosis. The preferred approach is the comparison of a stored sample from the acute phase of infection to a sample obtained 2 to 4 weeks later [86].

For rabies, the reference standard is detection of viral nucleocapsid by fluorescent antibody staining of brain tissue, but this is often only obtained postmortem. Premortem diagnostic techniques exploit the fact that rabies virus nucleocapsids are concentrated in the nerve endings surrounding the base of hair follicles; nuchal skin biopsy followed by fluorescent staining or RT-PCR for virus has the highest sensitivity [110].

Diagnosis of amebic encephalitis due to *N. fowleri*, *Balamuthia mandrillaris*, and *Acanthamoeba* spp. remains challenging. *N. fowleri* can be observed on CSF wet mount [104]. *B. mandrillaris* may be accompanied by nodular skin lesions with evidence of the organism on biopsy [111]. The CDC can support diagnostic testing which can include immunohistochemistry and PCR testing [59,104].

Although they share no distinct profile, patients with encephalitis due to noninfectious causes generally have lower CSF white blood cell counts and protein levels [82]. Recurrent encephalitis, patients with cerebellar dysfunction, and presentations with psychotic features are somewhat more likely to be secondary to noninfectious etiologies [82]. Oligoclonal bands and abnormal IgG index are often present in the CSF in immune-mediated encephalitis, prompting the recommendation to include these tests in initial encephalitis evaluations in recent guidelines [104]. CSF assay for known antineuronal antibodies should be performed [100,101].

Neuroimaging, preferably MRI, is recommended for the evaluation of all patients with suspected encephalitis [86,104]. The findings in viral encephalitis are most often nonspecific, but the identification of mass lesions or infarcts will redirect the diagnostic workup toward brain abscess, vasculitis, or endocarditis. The finding of focal encephalitis, particularly involving the temporal lobes, is suggestive of HSE [86,104], though VZV encephalitis can have similar neuroimaging features [112]. Characteristic abnormalities may not be seen initially; if the clinical suspicion is high, imaging studies should also be repeated after several days.

Electroencephalography (EEG) may provide early clues to a diagnosis before imaging changes are apparent, but the abnormalities usually are less specific. In patients with HSE, 80% have a temporal focus, although serial studies are often required to detect these changes [104,105]. EEG may also identify epileptiform discharges as a cause of obtundation in patients without overt seizure activity [104]. Normal EEG is associated with better prognosis [113].

With the advent of new molecular approaches and improved serologic diagnostics, brain biopsy is less commonly performed. However, it should be considered in selected situations, such as when a patient continues to deteriorate on acyclovir [109]. In the largest brain biopsy series reported, 9% of all patients with suspected HSE had another treatable disorder [114]. Neuroimaging should be used to guide sampling of abnormal tissue. Yield is likely to be higher earlier in disease. Specimens should be sent directly for culture, PCR, and immunofluorescence as well as fixed for routine histology with staining for pathogen detection [86].

Therapy

Empiric therapy with acyclovir (10 mg per kg every 8 hours in adults) should be initiated in all patients with encephalitis pending results of the diagnostic workup for HSE [86]. Subsequent management depends on the clinical response and HSV PCR results. Total duration of therapy in confirmed HSE is at least 14 to 21 days [86]. Repeat HSV PCR is recommended prior to stopping therapy in HSE patients who continue to exhibit encephalitic features, with continuation of acyclovir if the repeat PCR is positive [86]. HSV resistance to acyclovir in immunocompetent adults is extremely rare [115]. There is no benefit to continuing extended oral therapy with valacyclovir after completion of intravenous acyclovir therapy [116].

Empiric doxycycline therapy (100 mg twice a day) should be considered for patients presenting with clinical suspicion of rickettsial or ehrlichial diseases in the summer months [86]. Early institution of tetracyclines reduces mortality in Rocky Mountain spotted fever. Therapy should be given in confirmed cases until the patient has been afebrile for 2 to 3 days [117].

Specific therapy is available for most nonviral microbial causes of encephalitis. Neurosyphilis should be treated with 10 to 14 days of high-dose penicillin G [118]. Meningoencephalitis caused by the Lyme disease spirochete is treated with ceftriaxone (2 g IV once daily) for 14 days [119]. Treatment for toxoplasmic encephalitis consists of pyrimethamine plus either sulfadiazine or clindamycin [120]. Neurologic disease in the setting of *Bartonella* sp. is treated with doxycycline and rifampin in adults [121].

Antiviral therapy may be efficacious for some non-HSE forms of viral encephalitis. Although efficacy has not been established in large clinical trials, acyclovir therapy is recommended for VZV encephalitis based on limited evidence of improved outcomes in small case series [86]. Ribavirin can be considered for cases of encephalitis secondary to rabies or measles viruses, but there is little published experience. In influenza-related encephalitis with a susceptible strain, oseltamivir is recommended [86].

For immune-mediated encephalitis, treatment of paraneoplastic syndromes relies upon treatment of the underlying malignancy triggering the cross-reactive response in combination with immune modulating therapies [101]. For syndromes caused by antibodies binding cell surface antigens, antibody removal and/or suppression of the immune response can yield clinical improvement. Current treatments rely on high dose steroids, intravenous immunoglobulin, and/or plasma exchange, with rituximab and cyclosphosphamide deployed as second-line treatment [101].

Treatment for most cases of encephalitis is supportive, with particular attention to the management of cerebral edema and seizures [122]. Status epilepticus (see Chapter 151) may produce additional neurologic damage. Intubation may frequently be necessary to prevent aspiration and to provide ventilatory assistance. The risks of nosocomial infection, particularly pneumonia, are very high for patients with prolonged periods of unconsciousness.

BRAIN ABSCESS

Etiology and Pathogenesis

Brain abscesses most commonly arise in the setting of a predisposing factor such as immunosuppression, contiguous focus of infection, disruption of the natural protective barriers of the brain, or bacteremia. The abscess etiology is strongly influenced by these predisposing factors. In the setting of immunosuppression, brain abscesses are more likely to be caused by atypical bacteria such as *M. tuberculosis* and Nocardia or nonbacterial causes such as fungi (*Aspergillus*, sp.) or parasites (*Toxoplasma gondii*, *Ancathamoeba* sp.). Infections following neurosurgical procedures or head trauma are commonly caused by skin flora or gram-negative bacilli. Abscesses caused by spread from contiguous foci are often streptocci, though *S. aureus* and polymicrobial infections including anaerobes are also seen. Hematogenously seeded abscesses are commonly staphylococcal and streptococcal species, though anaerobes (such as *Fusobacterium necroforum* in Lemierre's syndrome), Nocardia, and other pathogens can also hematogenously seed the CNS [35]. Sequencing of 16S ribosomal RNA from brain abscess aspirates has revealed a more diverse array of organisms than had previously been isolated in culture [123].

For the development of brain abscesses, initial infection of brain tissue leads to a focus of inflammation known as early cerebritis. This area appears hypodense on CT scan and will enhance with contrast administration. The area of cerebritis expands and develops a central area of necrosis in the late cerebritis stage. A ring-enhancing wall of well-vascularized tissue then separates the necrotic, infected area from healthy surrounding tissue as the abscess matures into the capsule stage [35,51].

Diagnosis

Brain abscess usually presents more as a focal mass lesion—with headache, seizures, or neurological deficit—than as an infectious disease; fever is often not present [35]. Cranial CT or MRI aids localization of abscesses, staging the disease, and evaluation of the underlying cause [51]. Blood cultures and CSF cultures are positive in 25% of brain abscesses, but LP is contraindicated for most cases due to potential mass effects. Drainage of contiguous foci with material sent for culture is crucial for both treatment and diagnosis. If the causative agent has not been identified from other sources, aspiration of the brain abscess itself is indicated. Aspirate should be sent for gram stain, aerobic, and anaerobic cultures in all cases. If risk factors for tuberculosis are present, mycobacterial stain and culture should be performed. If the patient is immunosuppressed, cultures for Nocardia and fungus should be performed along with PCR for *T. gondii* [35].

Therapy

Initial antimicrobial therapy should be based on the pathogens predicted by the probable underlying source. Unless a diagnostic aspiration is imminent and the patient is stable, empiric therapy should not be delayed pending culture as rapid decompensation can occur. Standard empiric therapy consists of ceftriaxone plus metronidazole to provide coverage for aerobic Gram-positive cocci, anaerobes, and aerobic Gram-negative bacilli. Antistaphylococcal therapy may also be required if *S. aureus* is in the differential diagnosis. Postneurosurgical abscesses should be treated with vancomycin, cefepime, and metronidazole as initial therapy. Patients with HIV should have therapy for toxoplasmosis added if they have a history of a positive serology and empiric therapy for Nocardia and fungi should be considered in initial management of transplant patients. Duration of therapy is not well defined. Most bacterial brain abscesses require a prolonged 6- to 8-week course of intravenous antibiotics with serial cranial imaging to assess response to therapy [35,124].

Prolonged antimicrobial therapy alone is curative for some patients, especially when the lesions are small (<2.5 cm) and do not have a well-defined capsule by CT criteria. However, in the absence of a contraindication, prompt aspiration of the abscess contents using CT-guided stereotactic techniques is usually recommended. This provides confirmation of the diagnosis, material for culture, and possible adequate drainage of the focus of infection. In patients with multiple abscesses, the largest lesions are usually aspirated [35].

PARAMENINGEAL FOCI

Subdural Empyema

Subdural empyema usually arises from the same foci as brain abscess or as a complication of meningitis [44,125]. The infection spreads through venous drainage into intracranial vessels, which course through the subdural space. The clinical features of subdural empyema are caused by local inflammation and cerebral edema, leading to increased intracranial pressure and herniation. Patients demonstrate depression of consciousness, hemiplegia, focal seizures, papilledema, and meningitic signs [125]. MRI is the most sensitive diagnostic modality [51]. Surgical decompression and drainage are urgent adjuncts to antibiotic therapy [125].

Dural Sinus Thrombophlebitis

Major dural sinus thrombophlebitis may occur in pyogenic meningitis but more often arises from contiguous spread of sinusitis, mastoiditis, otitis, or cranial skin and soft tissue infection. The microbiology reflects that of acute infection at these sites: *S. aureus*, *S. pneumoniae* or other streptococci, and anaerobes. Clinical signs and symptoms vary with the thrombus location. For instance, sagittal sinus thrombophlebitis may cause seizures and hemiplegia, whereas cavernous sinus thrombophlebitis presents with proptosis, marked chemosis, and ophthalmoplegia. Sigmoid sinus thrombophlebitis may give no neurologic signs but produce persistent fever in a case of chronic otitis media and mastoiditis. CT and MRI often can demonstrate thrombosis in the dural sinuses. Antibiotics and drainage or excision of the focus from which the problem originates are the mainstays of therapy. The merits of anticoagulation are controversial due to the propensity of venous infarcts to become hemorrhagic [126].

Spinal Epidural Abscess

Spinal epidural abscess is an infection that may be seeded during bacteremia or occur as a complication of vertebral osteomyelitis or surgery. More than half of cases are caused by *S. aureus* [64,127].

The classic triad of symptoms is back pain, fever, and neurologic deficit, though many patients do not demonstrate all three [127]. Percussion tenderness is not always present [127]. Most patients have elevated C-reactive protein or erythrocyte sedimentation rate and approximately 60% have positive blood cultures [127]. Early recognition of epidural abscess is critical because neurologic progression may be rapid and irreversible. MRI should be performed quickly to distinguish the extent of spinal involvement and to evaluate adjacent structures [64].

Immediate neurosurgical consultation is mandatory. The goals of prompt surgical intervention are to prevent or relieve paraplegia and to obtain material for microbiological diagnosis. A nonoperative approach has been used with increasing frequency, particularly in patients with poor medical condition or if the neurologic condition is stable and a microbial etiology is identified quickly from cultures of blood or aspirated material [128]. However, the neurological condition may deteriorate rapidly even after several weeks of antimicrobial therapy. MRI scanning and neurosurgical consultation should be available on an urgent basis for patients who are managed nonoperatively.

Blood cultures and image-guided abscess aspirate cultures should be obtained prior to initiation of antibiotic therapy in neurologically stable patients unless signs of impending sepsis are present [64]. Antistaphylococcal antibiotics should be started after cultures are obtained; Gram-negative coverage should be considered in intravenous drug abusers or patients with a documented Gram-negative focus elsewhere, such as the urinary tract. Therapy is adjusted based on the results of Gram stains and cultures. There are no controlled studies to support a specific duration of antibiotic therapy. Six weeks of therapy with close clinical monitoring and serial measurement of inflammatory markers is recommended. Repeat imaging should be obtained only if clinical improvement is not observed [64].

Advances in CNS infections, based on randomized controlled trials or meta-analyses, are summarized in Table 81.4.

TABLE 81.4

Summary Recommendations for Management of Central Nervous System Infections Based on Randomized Controlled Clinical Trials

- Dexamethasone treatment begun just prior to the institution of antibiotic therapy reduces the incidence of hearing loss in children with acute bacterial meningitis [129].
- Outcome of 2 versus 4 days of therapy with dexamethasone was equivalent in childhood bacterial meningitis [76].
- Dexamethasone treatment begun just prior to the institution of antibiotic therapy reduces mortality and the incidence of neurologic sequelae in adults with acute bacterial meningitis [67].
- Silver impregnated external ventricular catheters reduce the incidence of central nervous system infection compared with plain catheters [31].
- Acyclovir treatment reduces the mortality and the incidence of neurologic sequelae in herpes simplex virus encephalitis [130].
- Following completion of a standard course of intravenous acyclovir for herpes simplex encephalitis, an extended course of oral valacyclovir did not improve neurologic outcomes [116].

References

1. Auburtin M, Wolff M, Charpentier J, et al: Detrimental role of delayed antibiotic administration and penicillin-nonsusceptible strains in adult intensive care unit patients with pneumococcal meningitis: the PNEUMOREA prospective multicenter study. *Crit Care Med* 34:2758–2765, 2006.
2. Lepur D, Barsic B: Community-acquired bacterial meningitis in adults: antibiotic timing in disease course and outcome. *Infection* 35:225–231, 2007.
3. Tunkel AR, Hartman BJ, Kaplan SL, et al: Practice guidelines for the management of bacterial meningitis. *Clin Infect Dis* 39:1267–1284, 2004.
4. Straus SE, Thorpe KE, Holroyd-Leduc J: How do I perform a lumbar puncture and analyze the results to diagnose bacterial meningitis? *JAMA* 296:2012–2022, 2006.
5. Glimåker M, Johansson B, Halldorsdottir H, et al: Neuro-intensive treatment targeting intracranial hypertension improves outcome in severe bacterial meningitis: an intervention-control study. *PLoS One* 9:e91976, 2014.
6. Hasbun R, Abrahams J, Jekel J, et al: Computed tomography of the head before lumbar puncture in adults with suspected meningitis. *N Engl J Med* 345:1727–1733, 2001.
7. Thigpen MC, Whitney CG, Messonnier NE, et al: Bacterial meningitis in the United States, 1998–2007. *N Engl J Med* 364:2016–2025, 2011.
8. Castelblanco RL, Lee M, Hasbun R: Epidemiology of bacterial meningitis in the USA from 1997 to 2010: a population-based observational study. *Lancet Infect Dis* 14:813–819, 2014.
9. Brouwer MC, Tunkel AR, van de Beek D: Epidemiology, diagnosis, and antimicrobial treatment of acute bacterial meningitis. *Clin Microbiol Rev* 23:467–492, 2010.
10. Jit M: The risk of sequelae due to pneumococcal meningitis in high-income countries: a systematic review and meta-analysis. *J Infect* 61:114–124, 2010.
11. Wei BP, Robins-Browne RM, Shepherd RK, et al: Can we prevent cochlear implant recipients from developing pneumococcal meningitis? *Clin Infect Dis* 46:e1–e7, 2008.
12. Hsu HE, Shutt KA, Moore MR, et al: Effect of pneumococcal conjugate vaccine on pneumococcal meningitis. *N Engl J Med* 360:244–256, 2009.
13. Tsai CJ, Griffin MR, Nuorti JP, et al: Changing epidemiology of pneumococcal meningitis after the introduction of pneumococcal conjugate vaccine in the United States. *Clin Infect Dis* 46:1664–1672, 2008.
14. Olarte L, Barson WJ, Barson RM, et al: Impact of the 13-valent pneumococcal conjugate vaccine on pneumococcal meningitis in US children. *Clin Infect Dis* 61:767–775, 2015.
15. Cohn AC, MacNeil JR, Harrison LH, et al: Changes in Neisseria meningitidis disease epidemiology in the United States, 1998-2007: implications for prevention of meningococcal disease. *Clin Infect Dis* 50:184–191, 2010.
16. Cohn AC, MacNeil JR, Clark TA, et al: Prevention and control of meningococcal disease: recommendations of the Advisory Committee on Immunization Practices (ACIP). *MMWR Recomm Rep* 62:1–28, 2013.
17. Folaranmi T, Rubin L, Martin SW, et al; Centers for Disease Control (CDC): Use of serogroup B meningococcal vaccines in persons aged ≥10 years at increased risk for serogroup B meningococcal disease: recommendations of

the Advisory Committee on Immunization Practices, 2015. *MMWR Morb Mortal Wkly Rep* 64:608–612, 2015.
18. Wang X, Shutt KA, Vuong JT, et al: Changes in the population structure of invasive Neisseria meningitidis in the United States after quadrivalent meningococcal conjugate vaccine licensure. *J Infect Dis* 211:1887–1894, 2015.
19. Brouwer MC, van de Beek D, Heckenberg SG, et al: Community-acquired Listeria monocytogenes meningitis in adults. *Clin Infect Dis* 43:1233–1238, 2006.
20. Pagliano P, Attanasio V, Rossi M, et al: Listeria monocytogenes meningitis in the elderly: distinctive characteristics of the clinical and laboratory presentation. *J Infect* 71:134–136, 2015.
21. Briere EC, Rubin L, Moro PL, et al: Prevention and control of haemophilus influenzae type b disease: recommendations of the advisory committee on immunization practices (ACIP). *MMWR Recomm Rep* 63:1–14, 2014.
22. Center for Disease Control and Prevention: Invasive Haemophilus influenzae Type B disease in five young children–Minnesota, 2008. *MMWR Morb Mortal Wkly Rep* 58:58–60, 2009.
23. Pomar V, Benito N, López-Contreras J, et al: Spontaneous gram-negative bacillary meningitis in adult patients: characteristics and outcome. *BMC Infect Dis* 13:451, 2013.
24. van de Beek D, Drake JM, Tunkel AR: Nosocomial bacterial meningitis. *N Engl J Med* 362:146–154, 2010.
25. Kourbeti IS, Vakis AF, Ziakas P, et al: Infections in patients undergoing craniotomy: risk factors associated with post-craniotomy meningitis. *J Neurosurg* 122:1113–1119, 2015.
26. Aguilar J, Urday-Cornejo V, Donabedian S, et al: Staphylococcus aureus meningitis: case series and literature review. *Medicine (Baltimore)* 89:117–125, 2010.
27. Brouwer MC, McIntyre P, de Gans J, et al: Corticosteroids for acute bacterial meningitis. *Cochrane Database Syst Rev*:CD004405, 2010.
28. Conen A, Walti LN, Merlo A, et al: Characteristics and treatment outcome of cerebrospinal fluid shunt-associated infections in adults: a retrospective analysis over an 11-year period. *Clin Infect Dis* 47:73–82, 2008.
29. Fily F, Haegelen C, Tattevin P, et al: Deep brain stimulation hardware-related infections: a report of 12 cases and review of the literature. *Clin Infect Dis* 52:1020–1023, 2011.
30. Mead PA, Safdieh JE, Nizza P, et al: Ommaya reservoir infections: a 16-year retrospective analysis. *J Infect* 68:225–230, 2014.
31. Keong NCH, Bulters DO, Richards HK, et al: The SILVER (Silver Impregnated Line Versus EVD Randomized trial): a double-blind, prospective, randomized, controlled trial of an intervention to reduce the rate of external ventricular drain infection. *Neurosurgery* 71:394–403, 2012; discussion 403–404.
32. Skoff TH, Farley MM, Petit S, et al: Increasing burden of invasive group B streptococcal disease in nonpregnant adults, 1990–2007. *Clin Infect Dis* 49:85–92, 2009.
33. Huong VTL, Ha N, Huy NT, et al: Epidemiology, clinical manifestations, and outcomes of Streptococcus suis infection in humans. *Emerg Infect Dis* 20:1105–1114, 2014.
34. Centers for Disease Control and Prevention (CDC): Bacterial meningitis after intrapartum spinal anesthesia—New York and Ohio, 2008–2009. *MMWR Morb Mortal Wkly Rep* 59:65–69, 2010.
35. Brouwer MC, Tunkel AR, McKhann GM, et al: Brain abscess. *N Engl J Med* 371:447–456, 2014.
36. Mook-Kanamori BB, Geldhoff M, van der Poll T, et al: Pathogenesis and pathophysiology of pneumococcal meningitis. *Clin Microbiol Rev* 24:557–591, 2011.
37. Tan LKK, Carlone GM, Borrow R: Advances in the development of vaccines against Neisseria meningitidis. *N Engl J Med* 362:1511–1520, 2010.
38. Coureuil M, Lécuyer H, Scott MGH, et al: Meningococcus Hijacks a β2-adrenoceptor/β-Arrestin pathway to cross brain microvasculature endothelium. *Cell* 143:1149–1160, 2010.
39. Virji M: Pathogenic neisseriae: surface modulation, pathogenesis and infection control. *Nat Rev Microbiol* 7:274–286, 2009.
40. Tebruegge M, Curtis N: Epidemiology, etiology, pathogenesis, and diagnosis of recurrent bacterial meningitis. *Clin Microbiol Rev* 21:519–537, 2008.
41. Gerber J, Nau R: Mechanisms of injury in bacterial meningitis. *Curr Opin Neurol* 23:312–318, 2010.
42. van de Beek D, de Gans J, McIntyre P, et al: Corticosteroids for acute bacterial meningitis. *Cochrane Database Syst Rev*:CD004405, 2007.
43. Hoffmann O, Priller J, Prozorovski T, et al: TRAIL limits excessive host immune responses in bacterial meningitis. *J Clin Invest* 117:2004–2013, 2007.
44. van de Beek D, de Gans J, Tunkel AR, et al: Community-acquired bacterial meningitis in adults. *N Engl J Med* 354:44–53, 2006.
45. van de Beek D, de Gans J, Spanjaard L, et al: Clinical features and prognostic factors in adults with bacterial meningitis. *N Engl J Med* 351:1849–1859, 2004.
46. Brouwer MC, Thwaites GE, Tunkel AR, et al: Dilemmas in the diagnosis of acute community-acquired bacterial meningitis. *Lancet Lond Engl* 380:1684–1692, 2012.
47. Nigrovic LE, Malley R, Macias CG, et al: Effect of antibiotic pretreatment on cerebrospinal fluid profiles of children with bacterial meningitis. *Pediatrics* 122:726–730, 2008.
48. Fuglsang-Damgaard D, Pedersen G, Schonheyder HC: Positive blood cultures and diagnosis of bacterial meningitis in cases with negative culture of cerebrospinal fluid. *Scand J Infect Dis* 40:229–233, 2008.
49. Karre T, Vetter EA, Mandrekar JN, et al: Comparison of bacterial antigen test and gram stain for detecting classic meningitis bacteria in cerebrospinal fluid. *J Clin Microbiol* 48:1504–1505, 2010.
50. Wang X, Theodore MJ, Mair R, et al: Clinical validation of multiplex real-time PCR assays for detection of bacterial meningitis pathogens. *J Clin Microbiol* 50:702–708, 2012.
51. Foerster BR, Thurnher MM, Malani PN, et al: Intracranial infections: clinical and imaging characteristics. *Acta Radiol* 48:875–893, 2007.
52. Lindsey NP, Lehman JA, Staples JE, et al; Division of Vector-Borne Diseases, National Center for Emerging and Zoonotic Infectious Diseases, CDC: West nile virus and other arboviral diseases—United States, 2013. *MMWR Morb Mortal Wkly Rep* 63:521–526, 2014.
53. Shalabi M, Whitley RJ: Recurrent benign lymphocytic meningitis. *Clin Infect Dis* 43:1194–1197, 2006.
54. Hanson KE, Reckleff J, Hicks L, et al: Unsuspected HIV infection in patients presenting with acute meningitis. *Clin Infect Dis* 47:433–434, 2008.
55. Christie LJ, Loeffler AM, Honarmand S, et al: Diagnostic challenges of central nervous system tuberculosis. *Emerg Infect Dis* 14:1473–1475, 2008.
56. Thwaites GE, van Toorn R, Schoeman J: Tuberculous meningitis: more questions, still too few answers. *Lancet Neurol* 12:999–1010, 2013.
57. Nhu NTQ, Heemskerk D, Thu DDA, et al: Evaluation of GeneXpert MTB/RIF for diagnosis of tuberculous meningitis. *J Clin Microbiol* 52:226–233, 2014.
58. Abdelmalek R, Kanoun F, Kilani B, et al: Tuberculous meningitis in adults: MRI contribution to the diagnosis in 29 patients. *Int J Infect Dis* 10:372–377, 2006.
59. Lopez C, Budge P, Chen J, et al: Primary amebic meningoencephalitis: a case report and literature review. *Pediatr Emerg Care* 28:272–276, 2012.
60. Shimasaki T, Chung H, Shiiki S: Five cases of recurrent meningitis associated with chronic strongyloidiasis. *Am J Trop Med Hyg* 92:601–604, 2015.
61. Johnson RH, Einstein HE: Coccidioidal meningitis. *Clin Infect Dis* 42:103–107, 2006.
62. Franco-Paredes C, Womack T, Bohlmeyer T, et al: Management of Cryptococcus gattii meningoencephalitis. *Lancet Infect Dis* 15:348–355, 2015.
63. Sloan DJ, Parris V: Cryptococcal meningitis: epidemiology and therapeutic options. *Clin Epidemiol* 6:169–182, 2014.
64. Berbari EF, Kanj SS, Kowalski TJ, et al: 2015 Infectious Diseases Society of America (IDSA) clinical practice guidelines for the diagnosis and treatment of native vertebral osteomyelitis in adultsa. *Clin Infect Dis* 61:e26–e46, 2015.
65. Morís G, Garcia-Monco JC: The challenge of drug-induced aseptic meningitis revisited. *JAMA Intern Med* 174:1511–1512, 2014.
66. Brown EM, de Louvois J, Bayston R, et al: Distinguishing between chemical and bacterial meningitis in patients who have undergone neurosurgery. *Clin Infect Dis* 34:556–558, 2002.
67. de Gans J, van de Beek D: Dexamethasone in adults with bacterial meningitis. *N Engl J Med* 347:1549–1556, 2002.
68. Jones ME, Draghi DC, Karlowsky JA, et al: Prevalence of antimicrobial resistance in bacteria isolated from central nervous system specimens as reported by U.S. hospital laboratories from 2000 to 2002. *Ann Clin Microbiol Antimicrob* 3:3, 2004.
69. Odio CM, Puig JR, Feris JM, et al: Prospective, randomized, investigator-blinded study of the efficacy and safety of meropenem vs. cefotaxime therapy in bacterial meningitis in children. Meropenem Meningitis Study Group. *Pediatr Infect J* 18:581–590, 1999.
70. Safdar A, Armstrong D: Antimicrobial activities against 84 Listeria monocytogenes isolates from patients with systemic listeriosis at a comprehensive cancer center (1955–1997). *J Clin Microbiol* 41:483–485, 2003.
71. O'Neill E, Humphreys H, Phillips J, et al: Third-generation cephalosporin resistance among Gram-negative bacilli causing meningitis in neurosurgical patients: significant challenges in ensuring effective antibiotic therapy. *J Antimicrob Chemother* 57:356–359, 2006.
72. Kim BN, Peleg AY, Lodise TP, et al: Management of meningitis due to antibiotic-resistant Acinetobacter species. *Lancet Infect Dis* 9:245–255, 2009.
73. Levitz RE, Quintiliani R: Trimethoprim-sulfamethoxazole for bacterial meningitis. *Ann Intern Med* 100:881–890, 1984.
74. Brouwer MC, Heckenberg SGB, de Gans J, et al: Nationwide implementation of adjunctive dexamethasone therapy for pneumococcal meningitis. *Neurology* 75:1533–1539, 2010.
75. Heckenberg SGB, Brouwer MC, van der Ende A, et al: Adjunctive dexamethasone in adults with meningococcal meningitis. *Neurology* 79:1563–1569, 2012.
76. Syrogiannopoulos GA, Lourida AN, Theodoridou MC, et al: Dexamethasone therapy for bacterial meningitis in children: 2- versus 4-day regimen. *J Infect Dis* 169:853–858, 1994.
77. Nguyen TH, Tran TH, Thwaites G, et al: Dexamethasone in Vietnamese adolescents and adults with bacterial meningitis. *N Engl J Med* 357:2431–2440, 2007.
78. Scarborough M, Gordon SB, Whitty CJ, et al: Corticosteroids for bacterial meningitis in adults in sub-Saharan Africa. *N Engl J Med* 357:2441–2450, 2007.
79. Wu HM, Harcourt BH, Hatcher CP, et al: Emergence of ciprofloxacin-resistant Neisseria meningitidis in North America. *N Engl J Med* 360:886–892, 2009.
80. Delaune D, Andriamanantena D, Mérens A, et al: Management of a rifampicin-resistant meningococcal infection in a teenager. *Infection* 41:705–708, 2013.
81. George BP, Schneider EB, Venkatesan A: Encephalitis hospitalization rates and inpatient mortality in the United States, 2000–2010. *PLoS One* 9:e104169, 2014.
82. Glaser CA, Honarmand S, Anderson LJ, et al: Beyond viruses: clinical profiles and etiologies associated with encephalitis. *Clin Infect Dis* 43:1565–1577, 2006.
83. Glaser C, Bloch KC: Encephalitis: why we need to keep pushing the envelope. *Clin Infect Dis* 49:1848–1850, 2009.
84. Granerod J, Cunningham R, Zuckerman M, et al: Causality in acute encephalitis: defining aetiologies. *Epidemiol Infect* 138:783–800, 2010.

85. Mailles A, Stahl J-P; Steering Committee and Investigators Group: Infectious encephalitis in France in 2007: a national prospective study. *Clin Infect Dis* 49:1838–1847, 2009.
86. Tunkel AR, Glaser CA, Bloch KC, et al: The management of encephalitis: clinical practice guidelines by the Infectious Diseases Society of America. *Clin Infect Dis* 47:303–327, 2008.
87. Pastula DM, Hoang Johnson DK, White JL, et al: Jamestown canyon virus disease in the United States-2000–2013. *Am J Trop Med Hyg* 93:384–389, 2015.
88. Raval M, Singhal M, Guerrero D, et al: Powassan virus infection: case series and literature review from a single institution. *BMC Res Notes* 5:594, 2012.
89. Hoffmann B, Tappe D, Höper D, et al: A variegated squirrel bornavirus associated with fatal human encephalitis. *N Engl J Med* 373:154–162, 2015.
90. Gable MS, Sheriff H, Dalmau J, et al: The frequency of autoimmune N-methyl-D-aspartate receptor encephalitis surpasses that of individual viral etiologies in young individuals enrolled in the California Encephalitis Project. *Clin Infect Dis* 54:899–904, 2012.
91. Whitley RJ: Herpes simplex encephalitis: adolescents and adults. *Antiviral Res* 71:141–148, 2006.
92. Casrouge A, Zhang SY, Eidenschenk C, et al: Herpes simplex virus encephalitis in human UNC-93B deficiency. *Science* 314:308–312, 2006.
93. Zhang SY, Jouanguy E, Ugolini S, et al: TLR3 deficiency in patients with herpes simplex encephalitis. *Science* 317:1522–1527, 2007.
94. Davis LE, Beckham JD, Tyler KL: North American encephalitic arboviruses. *Neurol Clin* 26:727–757, ix, 2008.
95. Deresiewicz RL, Thaler SJ, Hsu L, et al: Clinical and neuroradiographic manifestations of eastern equine encephalitis. *N Engl J Med* 336:1867–1874, 1997.
96. Jackson AC: Rabies. *Neurol Clin* 26:717–726, ix, 2008.
97. De Serres G, Dallaire F, Cote M, et al: Bat rabies in the United States and Canada from 1950 through 2007: human cases with and without bat contact. *Clin Infect Dis* 46:1329–1337, 2008.
98. Vora NM, Basavaraju SV, Feldman KA, et al: Raccoon rabies virus variant transmission through solid organ transplantation. *JAMA* 310:398–407, 2013.
99. Rupprecht CE, Briggs D, Brown CM, et al: Use of a reduced (4-dose) vaccine schedule for postexposure prophylaxis to prevent human rabies: recommendations of the advisory committee on immunization practices. *MMWR Recomm Rep* 59:1–9, 2010.
100. Armangue T, Leypoldt F, Dalmau J: Autoimmune encephalitis as differential diagnosis of infectious encephalitis. *Curr Opin Neurol* 27:361–368, 2014.
101. O'Toole O, Clardy S, Lin Quek AM: Paraneoplastic and autoimmune encephalopathies. *Semin Neurol* 33:357–364, 2013.
102. Sonneville R, Klein I, de Broucker T, et al: Post-infectious encephalitis in adults: diagnosis and management. *J Infect* 58:321–328, 2009.
103. Scolding NJ: Central nervous system vasculitis. *Semin Immunopathol* 31:527–536, 2009.
104. Venkatesan A, Tunkel AR, Bloch KC, et al: Case definitions, diagnostic algorithms, and priorities in encephalitis: consensus statement of the international encephalitis consortium. *Clin Infect Dis* 57:1114–1128, 2013.
105. Steiner I, Budka H, Chaudhuri A, et al: Viral encephalitis: a review of diagnostic methods and guidelines for management. *Eur J Neurol* 12:331–343, 2005.
106. Whitley RJ, Soong SJ, Linneman C Jr, et al: Herpes simplex encephalitis. Clinical assessment. *JAMA* 247:317–320, 1982.
107. Gadre G, Satishchandra P, Mahadevan A, et al: Rabies viral encephalitis: clinical determinants in diagnosis with special reference to paralytic form. *J Neurol Neurosurg Psychiatry* 81:812–820, 2010.
108. Greninger AL, Naccache SN, Messacar K, et al: A novel outbreak enterovirus D68 strain associated with acute flaccid myelitis cases in the USA (2012-14): a retrospective cohort study. *Lancet Infect Dis* 15:671–682, 2015.
109. Rice CM, Yadav S, Boyanton B, et al: Clinical problem-solving. A creeping suspicion. *N Engl J Med* 371:68–73, 2014.
110. Dacheux L, Reynes JM, Buchy P, et al: A reliable diagnosis of human rabies based on analysis of skin biopsy specimens. *Clin Infect Dis* 47:1410–1417, 2008.
111. Schuster FL, Yagi S, Gavali S, et al: Under the radar: balamuthia amebic encephalitis. *Clin Infect Dis* 48:879–887, 2009.
112. Pahud BA, Glaser CA, Dekker CL, et al: Varicella zoster disease of the central nervous system: epidemiological, clinical, and laboratory features 10 years after the introduction of the varicella vaccine. *J Infect Dis* 203: 316–323, 2011.
113. Sutter R, Kaplan PW, Cervenka MC, et al: Electroencephalography for diagnosis and prognosis of acute encephalitis. *Clin Neurophysiol* 126: 1524–1531, 2015.
114. Whitley RJ, Cobbs CG, Alford CA Jr, et al: Diseases that mimic herpes simplex encephalitis. Diagnosis, presentation, and outcome. NIAD Collaborative Antiviral Study Group. *JAMA* 262:234–239, 1989.
115. Schulte EC, Sauerbrei A, Hoffmann D, et al: Acyclovir resistance in herpes simplex encephalitis. *Ann Neurol* 67:830–833, 2010.
116. Gnann JW, Sköldenberg B, Hart J, et al: Herpes simplex encephalitis: lack of clinical benefit of long-term valacyclovir therapy. *Clin Infect Dis* 61:683–691, 2015.
117. Dantas-Torres F: Rocky Mountain spotted fever. *Lancet Infect Dis* 7:724–732, 2007.
118. Workowski KA, Bolan GA; Centers for Disease Control and Prevention: Sexually transmitted diseases treatment guidelines, 2015. *MMWR Recomm Rep* 64:1–137, 2015.
119. Shapiro ED: Lyme disease. *N Engl J Med* 370:1724–1731, 2014.
120. Kaplan JE, Benson C, Holmes KH, et al; Centers for Disease Control and Prevention (CDC); National Institutes of Health; HIV Medicine Association of the Infectious Diseases Society of America: Guidelines for prevention and treatment of opportunistic infections in HIV-infected adults and adolescents: recommendations from CDC, the National Institutes of Health, and the HIV Medicine Association of the Infectious Diseases Society of America. *MMWR Recomm Rep* 58:1–207, 2009.
121. Rolain JM, Brouqui P, Koehler JE, et al: Recommendations for treatment of human infections caused by Bartonella species. *Antimicrob Agents Chemother* 48:1921–1933, 2004.
122. Thakur KT, Motta M, Asemota AO, et al: Predictors of outcome in acute encephalitis. *Neurology* 81:793–800, 2013.
123. Al Masalma M, Armougom F, Scheld WM, et al: The expansion of the microbiological spectrum of brain abscesses with use of multiple 16S ribosomal DNA sequencing. *Clin Infect Dis* 48:1169–1178, 2009.
124. Arlotti M, Grossi P, Pea F, et al: Consensus document on controversial issues for the treatment of infections of the central nervous system: bacterial brain abscesses. *Int J Infect Dis* 14[Suppl 4]:S79–S92, 2010.
125. Greenlee JE: Subdural empyema. *Curr Treat Options Neurol* 5:13–22, 2003.
126. Stam J: Thrombosis of the cerebral veins and sinuses. *N Engl J Med* 352:1791–1798, 2005.
127. Zimmerli W: Clinical practice. Vertebral osteomyelitis. *N Engl J Med* 362:1022–1029, 2010.
128. Siddiq F, Chowfin A, Tight R, et al: Medical vs surgical management of spinal epidural abscess. *Arch Intern Med* 164:2409–2412, 2004.
129. Schaad UB, Lips U, Gnehm HE, et al: Dexamethasone therapy for bacterial meningitis in children. *Lancet* 342:457–461, 1993.
130. Whitley RJ, Alford CA, Hirsch MS, et al: Vidarabine versus acyclovir therapy in herpes simplex encephalitis. *N Engl J Med* 314:144–149, 1986.

Chapter 82 ■ Tuberculosis

MICHELLE K. HAAS • ROBERT W. BELKNAP

EPIDEMIOLOGY

Tuberculosis (TB) continues to cause significant morbidity and mortality worldwide. In 2013, there were an estimated 9.0 million new cases and 1.5 million deaths due to tuberculosis [1]. Globally, the total number of tuberculosis cases is declining, with an estimated 37 million lives saved since 2000 due to intensified diagnosis and treatment. Between 1990 and 2013, the TB prevalence rate fell by 41% globally. In the United States, incident tuberculosis cases have been declining since 1992 and reached a historic low in 2014 at 9,412 [2]. However, the rate of decline in incidence is the lowest in a decade. Foreign-born individuals continue to shoulder a disproportionate burden of TB, with a rate 13.4 times higher than U.S.-born persons. Racial and ethnic disparities persist, signaling a need to increase access to TB care services for our vulnerable populations.

A threat to TB control efforts worldwide has been the rise of multidrug-resistant (MDR) and extensively drug-resistant (XDR) forms of tuberculosis. Since the outbreak of XDR tuberculosis in rural South Africa associated with a high and rapid mortality, MDR and XDR TB epidemics are increasingly recognized globally [1,3]. In 2013, there were an estimated 480,000 cases of MDR-TB globally, 9% of which were estimated to be XDR. Even more worrisome is the gap between identification of cases and treatment: only 45% of cases who could have been detected were identified, with only 20% estimated to have initiated treatment [1]. If all TB patients were able to be tested for MDR-TB, more than half of the detected MDR-TB cases would have been identified from India, China, and the Russian Federation. While the accuracy of these estimates is limited by the availability of diagnostic testing, they have implications for choosing empiric TB regimens for individuals who hail from areas with larger burdens of drug-resistant TB.

The proportion of newly diagnosed tuberculosis patients who require hospitalization each year is poorly characterized. One large urban hospital reported that tuberculosis accounted for 1% of medical intensive care unit (ICU) admissions over a 15-year period [4]. Epidemiologic studies show that between 3% and 24% of hospitalized tuberculosis patients require treatment in an ICU and that between 2% and 13% require mechanical ventilation [4,5]. Although overall mortality from tuberculosis in the United States has been around 5% for the past decade [6], mortality remains particularly high (50% to 60%) among patients with tuberculosis-associated respiratory failure requiring mechanical ventilation [5,7,8]. Factors associated with mortality include multiorgan failure, malnutrition, renal failure, immunosuppression, and delayed diagnosis [5,7–10].

PATHOGENESIS

The pathogenesis of tuberculosis is a two-stage process, which can be divided into tuberculosis infection and progression to disease [11,12]. These stages are reflective of the risk factors that should be considered when determining the likelihood a patient has tuberculosis (Table 82.1). Tuberculosis infection, with rare exceptions, results from the airborne transmission of tubercle bacilli. Upon reaching the alveoli of a susceptible host, the tubercle bacilli multiply to produce a localized pneumonia, spread to involve the hilar lymph nodes, then enter the bloodstream through the thoracic duct, and disseminate throughout the body. This primary infection is usually clinically unapparent. Most patients develop cell-mediated immunity to *M. tuberculosis,* which brings the infection under control over a period of weeks. Despite initial immunologic control of tuberculosis infection, viable tubercle bacilli remain in scattered foci as latent tuberculosis infection that is left untreated may persist for life [13].

The second stage is the development of active tuberculosis, which occurs at a variable rate dependent upon the person's age at infection and other medical conditions [12]. Progression from latent to active tuberculosis, termed *reactivation*, is much more frequent in people with certain conditions, particularly HIV infection (Table 82.1) [12,14]. Patients with advanced HIV have a 10 times greater risk, whereas those on effective antiretroviral therapy (ART) still have twice the risk of an uninfected person [12]. In most cases, reactivation of tuberculosis causes pulmonary disease, but reactivation can occur at any site where a latent focus was established during the initial infection [11]. Disseminated disease may also occur and is believed to result from the erosion of a tuberculous focus directly into a blood vessel [15]. In a critically ill patient, the presence of any risk factor for infection or progression should prompt consideration of tuberculosis in the differential diagnosis.

TABLE 82.1

Factors That Should Prompt Consideration of Tuberculosis in the Differential Diagnosis

Risks for tuberculosis infection

1. History of active tuberculosis, particularly if never or inadequately treated
2. History of a positive tuberculin skin test or positive interferon-γ release assay (IGRA) test
3. Other risk factors for infection (tuberculin status unknown)
   - Prior residence in a country with ongoing TB transmission as reflected by a TB incidence of >= 20/100,000
   - Contact with known or suspected tuberculosis
   - Presence of fibrotic lung lesions compatible with inactive tuberculosis
   - Advanced age (living at a time in the United States in which TB incidence was higher)
   - Homeless shelters or living in another congregate setting
   - Correctional facilities

Risks for progression to active tuberculosis (tuberculin/IGRA status positive or unknown)

1. Known or suspected HIV infection
2. Other immunosuppressive conditions
   - Tumor necrosis factor-α inhibitors, high-dose corticosteroids, and other immunosuppressive therapy
3. Recent tuberculosis infection
4. Presence of upper-lobe scars compatible with inactive tuberculosis
5. Certain medical conditions
   - Diabetes mellitus
   - Silicosis
   - Chronic renal failure
   - Gastrectomy or other conditions associated with weight loss

CLINICAL MANIFESTATIONS AND DIAGNOSIS

Physicians in intensive care settings face the challenge of maintaining an appropriate index of suspicion for tuberculosis when it is a relatively rare cause of critical illness. Prompt recognition of tuberculosis and early institution of effective multiple-drug therapy are required to achieve the dual goals of successfully treating patients and preventing nosocomial tuberculosis transmission. Delays in diagnosis are unfortunately common and have been noted in more than half of patients admitted to community hospitals [16]. Concomitant nontuberculous infections occur in up to a third of patients and can lead to delays in diagnosis [8]. Fluoroquinolones are a well-established therapy for *M. tuberculosis* [17] and should be avoided in patients in whom tuberculosis is suspected. Use of fluoroquinolones can be associated with clinical improvement, delaying the diagnosis of tuberculosis, which is associated with worsened outcomes, including excess mortality [18,19–25]. Linezolid also has activity against *M. tuberculosis* and is one of the agents utilized to treat drug-resistant tuberculosis [26,27]. Linezolid is used to treat resistant gram-positive bacteria including methicillin-resistant *Staphylococcus aureus* (MRSA). MRSA pneumonia can present with cavitary pneumonia similar to TB, and so linezolid should be avoided in patients in whom tuberculosis is suspected.

Tuberculosis may present as the primary cause of a life-threatening illness, but it may also be a coincidental illness in patients being treated for another condition [8] (Fig. 82.1). The symptoms and signs of tuberculosis are variable and depend upon the site and extent of the disease [5,7,8]. The history of a chronic, progressive illness with fever, night sweats, and weight loss, with or without a chronic cough, is most suggestive of tuberculosis. However, obtaining an accurate history can be difficult and tuberculosis patients often report the acute onset of symptoms [7,28,29]. Cough duration is a poor predictor of tuberculosis, particularly in the context of underlying HIV disease, and should not be used to differentiate a respiratory syndrome due to pulmonary tuberculosis from other etiologies [30]. A variety of laboratory abnormalities have been associated with tuberculosis, including anemia, hypoalbuminemia, elevated alkaline phosphatase, and hyponatremia, but are nonspecific [11,31].

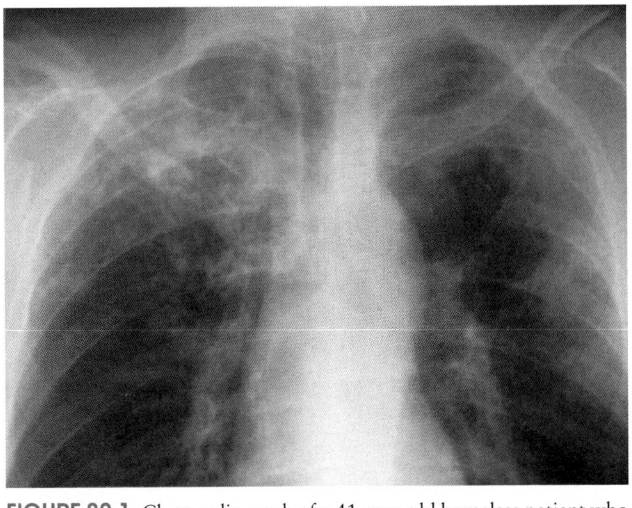

FIGURE 82.1 Chest radiograph of a 41-year-old homeless patient who was hospitalized with multiple fractures, including the right clavicle, after being hit by a car. The patient denied all respiratory symptoms despite having extensive bilateral upper-lobe fibronodular and cavitary disease. Sputum samples were smear positive and grew *M. tuberculosis*.

Pulmonary Tuberculosis

Pulmonary tuberculosis is the most common form of the disease, accounting for 79% of cases in the United States in 2013, with 9% of those with both pulmonary and extrapulmonary disease [6]. Extrapulmonary tuberculosis is more common among patients who are female, born outside the United States, and who have HIV disease [32]. Acute respiratory failure, which occurs in 2% to 13% of hospitalized tuberculosis cases, is the most common reason for admission to an ICU [4,5,10,29]. Although chronic cough and fevers are usually present, other symptoms suggestive of pulmonary tuberculosis include weight loss, dyspnea, and hemoptysis [11]. Of note, dyspnea may be minimal despite fairly extensive lung destruction. Hemoptysis occurs in about 20% of patients and occasionally can be massive [33]. Pulmonary tuberculosis may also be asymptomatic, occurring in patients with primarily extrapulmonary disease, or may be a coincidental finding (Fig. 82.1).

Definitively diagnosing pulmonary tuberculosis relies upon the collection of respiratory samples for smear and culture. More recently, there has been an increasing role for the use of nucleic acid amplification tests for diagnosing pulmonary tuberculosis at the point of care [34]. Sputum samples should be considered for symptomatic patients at risk for tuberculosis even when the chest radiograph appears normal. Positive sputum cultures for M.tuberculosis in the absence of radiographic abnormalities appear more commonly among individuals with underlying HIV disease [35–37]. The proportion of hospitalized tuberculosis patients who have a positive sputum smear ranges between 35% and 65% [7,9]. A minimum of three sputa or other lower respiratory tract specimens should be collected when pulmonary, pleural, or disseminated tuberculosis is suspected. The samples should be collected 8 hours apart, preferably with at least one early morning specimen [38].

Patients who are unable to spontaneously produce sputum should have samples induced using nebulized hypertonic saline [11]. Bronchoscopic specimens are not more sensitive and should not be considered a replacement for three expectorated or induced sputa [39]. Bronchoscopy is generally helpful if alternative diagnoses are being sought or if a tissue biopsy is needed. For selected patients, including young children, who either can't tolerate the nebulizer or still don't produce an adequate sputum sample, gastric aspirates should be obtained. When acid-fast bacilli (AFB) smears of respiratory secretions are negative, other specimens that may yield a diagnosis include pleural fluid, pleural biopsy, or transbronchial biopsy [11,40]. More invasive procedures such as transthoracic needle biopsy of the lung or mediastinal lymph nodes or open lung biopsy may be necessary under certain circumstances.

Pleural Tuberculosis

Pleural tuberculosis presents in two forms, commonly as tuberculous pleuritis and rarely as tuberculous empyema [11,41]. Tuberculous pleuritis occurs in 6% of HIV-negative and 11% of HIV-positive patients [42], and the incidence increases with declining CD4 cell counts [43]. It results from the rupture of a granuloma into the pleural space and may occur alone or in conjunction with pulmonary disease [41]. Often patients are asymptomatic but some present with acute symptoms of fever and chest pain, suggesting a viral or bacterial cause. The pathogenesis is primarily an immunologic reaction with very few tubercle bacilli actually present in the pleural space. Radiographically, a unilateral effusion covering less than half the hemithorax is typical. Untreated, tuberculous pleuritis often resolves but these patients are at high risk for recurrent pulmonary disease. Tuberculous empyema is much less common and results from the entry of large numbers of bacilli into the pleural space due the rupture of an adjacent cavity or development of a bronchopleural fistula [44].

Pleural fluid and tissue biopsy are typically needed to definitively diagnose tuberculous pleuritis. Sputum specimens should also be collected to evaluate for concurrent pulmonary disease. The pleural fluid most often shows a serous exudate with elevated protein and lactate dehydrogenase levels, low to normal glucose levels, and a pH range between 7.05 and 7.45 [42,45]. Early in the process, the fluid has a predominance of polymorphonuclear leukocytes that are replaced by lymphocytes within days. Adenosine deaminase (ADA) and other biochemical markers have been studied extensively, alone and in combination, as markers for diagnosing tuberculous pleuritis. Studies have supported measuring ADA levels, especially isoenzyme 2, showing additive diagnostic sensitivity and specificity when combined with other tests [46]. ADA levels may be useful in settings that lack the capacity to do cultures, but should not replace a pleural biopsy, which provides tissue for culture and pathology review.

AFB smears of pleural fluid and pleural biopsies are rarely positive (10% to 20%). The earliest presumptive diagnosis is provided by pathologic findings of granulomas with or without caseation, which are seen histologically in 60% of specimens [41]. Pleural fluid cultures are positive in only 20% to 30%. The yield increases slightly with multiple samples but waiting for positive cultures will delay the initiation of tuberculosis treatment [47]. Pleural biopsies are culture positive in 55% to 85% of specimens and should be sought whenever tuberculosis is considered a likely diagnosis.

Disseminated Tuberculosis

Disseminated tuberculosis refers to multiorgan involvement and may occur during progressive primary infection or as a complication of chronic tuberculosis [40,48]. The term *miliary tuberculosis*, which refers to the histologic appearance of diffuse nodular lesions resembling millet seeds, has historically been used interchangeably with disseminated disease. Now the term miliary is generally reserved to describe a diffuse micronodular infiltrate on the chest radiograph (Fig. 82.2). Young children and immunocompromised patients are at greatest risk for disseminated tuberculosis. However, a chronic, cryptic form of disease, termed *late generalized tuberculosis*, can occur in the elderly or those with other underlying illnesses [15]. In this cryptic form of disseminated tuberculosis, miliary infiltrates are rare and a diagnosis is often made postmortem.

Clinical evidence of dissemination is common among HIV-positive individuals living in hyperendemic tuberculosis settings [49–51] and thus vigilance for this presentation is critical when managing patients who are from these areas. Dissemination is also seen in up to 33% of solid-organ transplantation associated tuberculosis cases [52,53]. The presentations range from generalized lymphadenopathy to sepsis [49,50] and fulminant respiratory failure [54]. The duration of symptoms before diagnosis may vary from 1 week to over a year. Fever and other constitutional symptoms are seen in over 90%, respiratory symptoms in 75%, abdominal symptoms in 25%, and central nervous system symptoms in 20%. In some reports, the presentation of disseminated tuberculosis has been similar to that of gram-negative sepsis [55]. Acute respiratory failure is uncommon but a well-characterized complication of disseminated or miliary tuberculosis [29,56]. Laboratory abnormalities in disseminated disease are nonspecific. Anemia is common, but leukocyte and platelet counts range from markedly elevated to severely depressed [48]. Alkaline phosphatase levels are frequently elevated, likely related to granulomatous hepatitis. Chest radiographic findings are variable and may demonstrate miliary nodules of 1 to 3 mm in diameter or larger nodules of 5 to 7 mm. In about 10% of disseminated cases, radiographs will be normal, particularly early in the illness.

Virtually any body fluid, tissue, or organ may yield a diagnosis, particularly with clinical or laboratory abnormalities that suggest an extrapulmonary site of disease. Because extrapulmonary tuberculosis usually involves a lower burden of organisms compared with pulmonary disease, histological examination and culture of biopsy specimens often provides the greatest diagnostic yield. Sputum smears should be examined for AFB, but are positive in less than a third of patients with miliary tuberculosis. Histology and cultures of transbronchial, thoracoscopic, or traditional open lung biopsy will usually confirm the diagnosis. However, a careful search for chronic skin lesions, scrotal involvement,

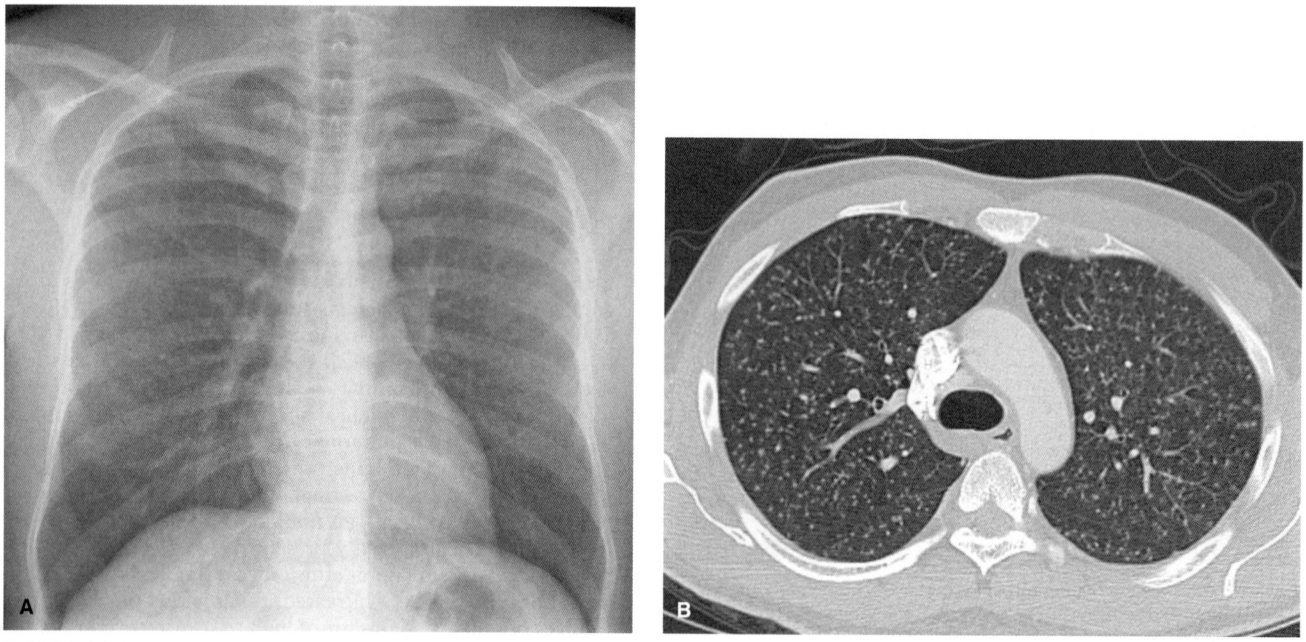

FIGURE 82.2 Chest radiograph (**A**) and CT scan (**B**) showing miliary disease in a 36-year-old patient who presented with several months of fever, weight loss, and abdominal pain.

or lymphadenopathy may disclose other more accessible sites for a diagnostic biopsy [57]. Urine and stool cultures are easily obtainable and also may provide the diagnosis. Lumbar puncture should be considered for patients with headache or other central nervous system symptoms because meningitis is found in nearly 20% of patients with disseminated tuberculosis. Mycobacterial blood cultures are positive for 26% to 42% of HIV-positive individuals and is the only culture-positive specimen in some [49,50,58]. Other potentially useful diagnostic tests include culture of gastric aspirates and biopsy specimens of liver or bone marrow. Among those with disseminated tuberculosis, granulomas are seen in about 90% of liver biopsies; the yield is lower from bone marrow biopsy unless pancytopenia is present [59].

Central Nervous System Tuberculosis

Tuberculosis involving the central nervous system may present as meningitis, as one or more parenchymal tuberculomas, or as a combination of both [60,61]. The clinical presentation varies from an indolent illness with headache and subtle changes in mental status to more acute presentations. Focal neurologic symptoms and signs may result from a tuberculoma causing a localized mass effect or from basilar meningitis affecting the cranial nerves directly or causing infarction of intracranial arteries [60]. Evidence of active or inactive tuberculosis at another site is noted in about three-fourths of cases, most often miliary infiltrates on chest radiographs. Tuberculomas of the central nervous system are readily detected by computed tomography (Fig. 82.3), but magnetic resonance imaging is often needed to detect basilar meningitis [61]. Tuberculous meningitis and tuberculomas are more common among HIV-positive individuals and present with signs, symptoms, and laboratory findings that are similar to those found in individuals who are HIV-negative [62].

Rapid diagnosis and treatment is critical to patient survival and favorable neurologic outcomes after tuberculous meningitis. A definitive diagnosis can be difficult though, and antituberculous treatment should be initiated immediately in individuals suspected of neurologic disease because delays in therapy are correlated with outcomes. Evaluation of cerebral spinal fluid (CSF), although often nonspecific, is important for diagnosing central nervous system (CNS) tuberculosis. The CSF findings classically described are a lymphocytic pleocytosis, low glucose, and an elevated protein. However, the absence of these findings does not exclude the diagnosis because the white cell count may range widely, a polymorphonuclear predominance occurs in up to 30%, and the protein and glucose may be normal [60,61]. AFB smears of CSF are positive in only 10% to 20% of cases, and cultures are positive in <50%. Because disseminated disease is common with tuberculous meningitis, AFB cultures sent from other sources, including sputum, urine, and stool, may provide a diagnostic smear or culture. CNS tuberculomas may be diagnosed by a typical radiographic appearance and response to treatment, but definitive diagnosis usually requires biopsy or surgical excision.

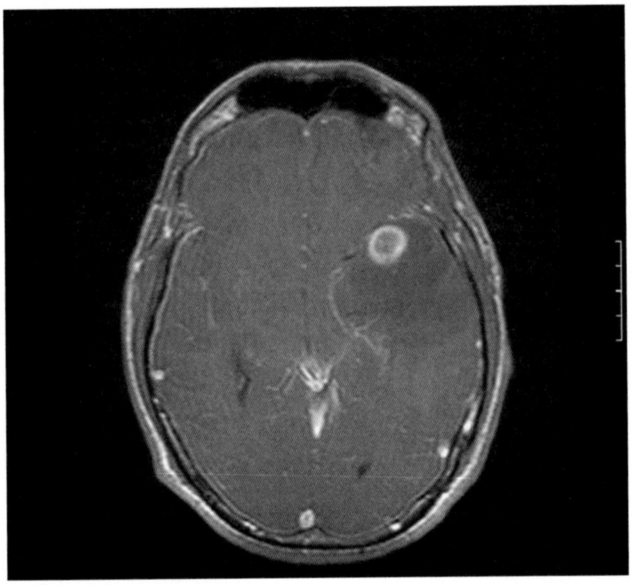

FIGURE 82.3 Computed tomographic scan of a 45-year-old patient with AIDS, known to be TST (+) but never completed latent treatment, who presented with a headache, expressive aphasia, and neologisms. The scan shows a tuberculoma with marked surrounding edema. Cerebral spinal fluid showed a white blood cell count of 675 (100% lymphocytes), glucose 42 mg/dL, and protein 246 mg/dL. CSF cultures were negative, but the diagnosis of isoniazid-resistant tuberculosis was confirmed by excisional biopsy.

Other Forms of Extrapulmonary Tuberculosis

Other forms of tuberculosis, such as lymphatic, pericardial, gastrointestinal, cutaneous, skeletal, and genitourinary, may be either coincidental findings or may provide clues to the diagnosis of disseminated disease in critically ill patients [11].

Tuberculosis patients on therapy may also present to the ICU after developing an immune reconstitution syndrome or paradoxical reaction. This syndrome is characterized by a worsening of symptoms and/or radiographic studies despite effective chemotherapy with microbiologic improvement [63]. Typical manifestations are the recurrence or development of fever and other systemic manifestations, enlargement and suppuration of lymphatic tissue, worsening of pulmonary infiltrates, and life-threatening complications such as respiratory failure or enlargement of intracranial lesions. These reactions can occur in any tuberculosis patient but are most common in patients with tuberculosis and HIV coinfection who are started on ART within the first few months of tuberculosis treatment [64].

Chest Radiography

Routine chest radiography is an invaluable screening and diagnostic tool for patients at risk for tuberculosis. Radiographs are able to detect most active pulmonary tuberculosis cases, particularly the most infectious cases with extensive parenchymal disease and cavitation. Radiographs can demonstrate fibrosis from previously active tuberculosis that identifies patients at higher risk for reactivation and can provide clues to the diagnosis in patients with extrapulmonary disease. The classic radiographic appearance of active tuberculosis is a fibrotic, cavitary upper-lobe opacity (Fig. 82.1), but pulmonary tuberculosis can present with a variety of findings on chest radiograph, including a normal film. The radiographic appearance of tuberculosis depends primarily upon the duration of illness and the host's immune function. For example, primary tuberculosis typically presents as a lower lobe infiltrate often with ipsilateral hilar adenopathy. Primary tuberculosis occurs most often in young children but can be seen at any age including the elderly, as described among recently infected nursing home residents [65]. Other radiographic appearances, which can be seen alone or in combination, are alveolar opacities, mixed alveolar-interstitial infiltrates, miliary disease, and intrathoracic adenopathy (Figs. 82.2 and 82.4) [8]. These "atypical" presentations of pulmonary tuberculosis have been reported in up to 34% to 45% of HIV-negative individuals in some series [66,67]. In the presence of advanced immunodeficiency, there is greater variation in the radiographic patterns of tuberculosis with more frequently lower lobe involvement, diffuse infiltrates, hilar or mediastinal adenopathy, and pleural effusions [52,68].

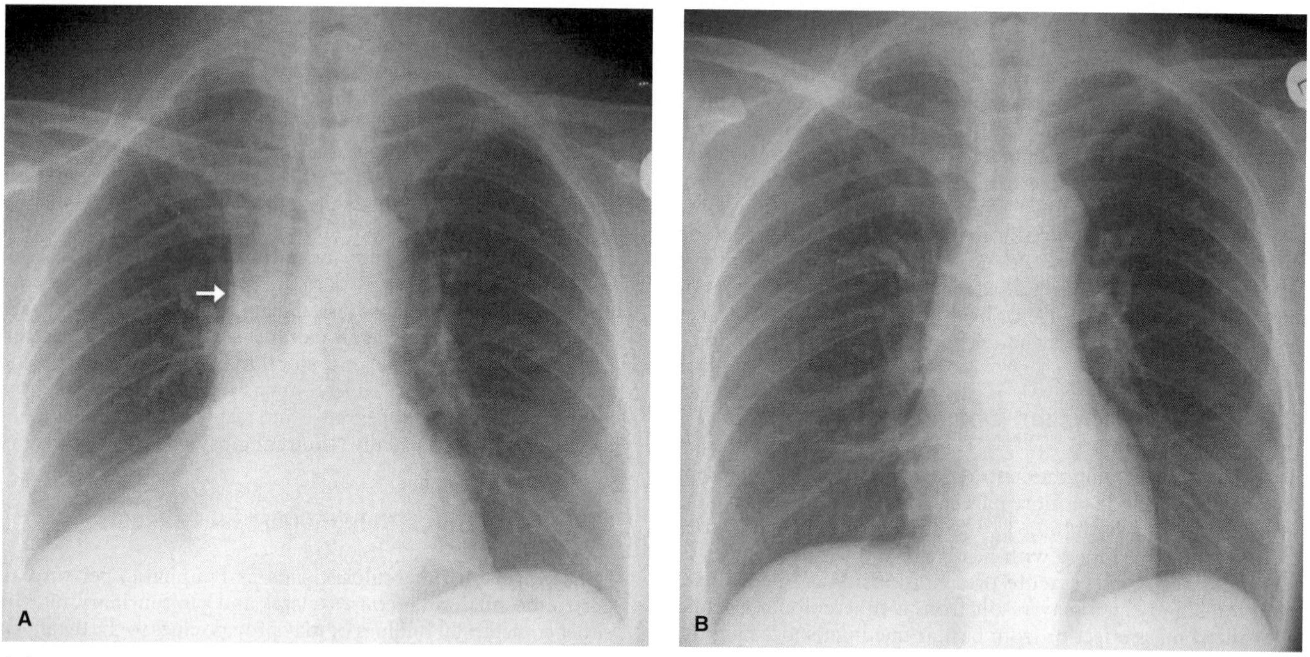

FIGURE 82.4 Chest radiographs of a 49-year-old patient who had undergone a liver transplant 6 months prior for hepatitis B–associated liver disease. The initial radiograph (**A**) showed right paratracheal adenopathy (*arrow*) with partial right lower lobe collapse that resolved by the end of treatment (**B**). The patient received standard tuberculosis therapy with the substitution of rifabutin for rifampin to minimize the drug interaction with tacrolimus.

Tuberculin Skin Testing and Interferon-γ Release Assays

The tuberculin skin test (TST) had been the only licensed test for detecting tuberculosis infection, but newer blood tests, interferon-γ release assays (IGRAs), are now commercially available [11,69]. IGRAs measure the interferon-γ produced by peripheral blood lymphocytes after stimulation with mycobacterial antigens. Both the TST and IGRAs are useful adjunctive tests but must be interpreted with caution. A positive result indicates the patient has been infected and may increase your clinical suspicion for active disease but is nondiagnostic. Similarly, a negative test does not rule out active tuberculosis since between 10% and 25% of patients with culture-confirmed disease will have a negative TST or IGRA [70,71].

Nucleic Acid Amplification Tests

Culture remains the gold standard for diagnosing all forms of tuberculosis, although it is limited by the duration of growth needed to identify *M. tuberculosis*. One approach to overcome these limitations has been the development of nucleic acid amplification (NAA) tests [72]. These tests offer several advantages including a rapid result, high specificity, and broad application to tissue samples, in some cases even formalin-fixed tissue [73]. The "first generation" of these tests were limited by a sensitivity of approximately 50% for smear-negative pulmonary, pleural, and meningeal tuberculosis [61,74]. Later-generation NAA tests such as Gene Xpert MTB/RIF and Line Probe assays can identify tuberculosis in <24 hours on either smear-negative or smear-positive sputum specimens. Current guidelines for the use of nucleic acid tests published by the Centers for Disease Control and Prevention (CDC) are to perform NAA testing on at least one specimen from individuals in whom TB remains high on the differential and where the result would alter management [75]. The sensitivity of these more recently developed NAA tests is greater than 95% in smear-positive specimens but only 50% to 80% in smear-negative, culture-positive specimens [76–79]. Importantly, these NAA tests not only determine if a specimen contains *M. tuberculosis*, but also give information about drug resistance. In individuals who have previously been treated for tuberculosis or who are from countries with a substantial amount of drug resistance, this information is critical to designing tuberculosis treatment regimens. Rapid susceptibility testing is most important for identifying *M. tuberculosis* isolates with resistance to at least isoniazid and rifampin. These isolates are referred to as multidrug resistant because tuberculosis due to these strains can be expected to fail standard therapy [80].

Rifampin susceptibility or resistance is determined by the *rpoB* gene, making it the most accurate target for molecular testing. Line probe assays utilize DNA probes to amplify genetic mutations that then undergo reverse hybridization with probes that can detect both rifampin and isoniazid resistance [81]. The MTBDR*plus* (Hain Lifescience) detects resistance to isoniazid and rifampin, whereas MTBDR*sl* can detect resistance to fluoroquinolones, aminoglycosides/cyclic peptides, and ethambutol, with good correlation to culture-based drug susceptibility testing [82]. Probes using molecular beacons such as GeneXpert MTB/RIF TB assay (Cepheid) will emit light when tuberculosis is present and can detect rifampin resistance [34]. Similar to sputum smears, a negative NAA test does not exclude tuberculosis. Therefore, empiric treatment should be considered when an alternative diagnosis has not been made, there is no clinical improvement, and the patient is at risk for tuberculosis.

Culture and Drug Susceptibility Testing

The importance of using rapid diagnostic techniques in clinical mycobacteriology has been tragically illustrated in outbreaks of drug-resistant tuberculosis among immunocompromised hosts whose median survival with standard, ineffective therapy was 16 days [3]. Liquid culture systems containing radiometric or colorimetric material permit detection of mycobacterial growth in 2 to 6 days with an average of 2 weeks [83]. The traditional use of biochemical testing for identification of isolates as

M. tuberculosis has been largely replaced by the more accurate and rapid methods using commercial nucleic acid probes. Drug susceptibility testing can also be done more rapidly with the commercial liquid cultures systems. Many hospital laboratories now lack the expertise and the number of specimens to conduct the full range of testing on a daily basis [11]. More timely results may be achieved by sending specimens, particularly those that are AFB smear positive to a full-service mycobacteriology laboratory. It is critical to pair molecular testing for resistance with standard phenotypic culture-based drug susceptibility testing, to ensure that resistance mediated through mutations not detected through NAA testing are also identified.

TREATMENT

Principles of Therapy for Tuberculosis

Two characteristics of *M. tuberculosis* dictate the requirements for successful therapy: a high frequency of spontaneous mutations and a slow, intermittent growth cycle. Overcoming these characteristics requires multiple drugs to prevent the selection of drug-resistant mutants and an extended duration of therapy to kill the dormant mycobacteria [80]. Culture confirmation should always be pursued aggressively, but empiric therapy for tuberculosis based on clinical suspicion should be considered and may be important for the survival of critically ill patients.

Recommendations for Initial Therapy

The choice of initial tuberculosis therapy in the ICU should be made after considering the risk for multidrug-resistant disease. The potential for drug-resistant tuberculosis can be estimated by knowing the patient's country of birth and whether he or she has a history of prior tuberculosis treatment. In 2013, the percentage of patients with multidrug-resistant tuberculosis among U.S.-born and foreign-born persons with no prior tuberculosis treatment was low at 0.3% and 1.7%, respectively. Among those with a history of prior treatment, these rates increased to 2.2% in U.S.-born and 5.1% in foreign-born persons [84]. Drug resistance should also be suspected for patients who fail while on treatment or who relapse after treatment has ended, particularly patients who did not get directly observed therapy [85,86].

For most patients, the four-drug, oral regimen of isoniazid, rifampin, pyrazinamide, and ethambutol will be appropriate [80]. The choice of therapy, when drug resistance is suspected, should be made in consultation with a physician experienced in treating multidrug-resistant tuberculosis and generally should include two or more agents likely to have activity. The agents usually chosen include an aminoglycoside (amikacin, kanamycin, or capreomycin), a fluoroquinolone (typically levofloxacin or moxifloxacin), and one or two of the "second-line" agents such as ethionamide, cycloserine, or *p*-aminosalicylic acid (PAS) [80,87]. Of note, ethambutolpyrazinamide, ethionamide, cycloserine, and PAS can only be given orally, and of these all except PAS can be given enterally via a feeding tube because PAS can clog enteral feeding tubes [80,87]. Due to the relatively poor antituberculosis activity of second-line drugs, some experts have recommended measuring serum drug levels to allow dose increases in order to achieve concentrations above the in vitro minimum inhibitory concentration [88]. Although not examined in a comparative trial, surgical resection may be a useful adjunct in the therapy of multidrug-resistant tuberculosis after weeks or months of medical therapy [87].

More detailed information regarding tuberculosis treatment is available on the CDC website (http://www.cdc.gov/tb/publications/guidelines/Treatment.htm). Other complicating factors that may need consideration when starting tuberculosis therapy in a critically ill patient are shown in Table 82.2.

TABLE 82.2

Select Therapeutic Challenges in Treating Critically Ill Tuberculosis Patients (When Drug-Susceptible Disease Is Known or Expected)

1. Documented or anticipated malabsorption—medications that can be given parenterally
   a. Rifampin
   b. Fluoroquinolone—levofloxacin or moxifloxacin
   c. Aminoglycoside—amikacin (streptomycin can be used if drug susceptibility is known); second-line agents are kanamycin and capreomycin
   d. Isoniazid—when available but it may be difficult to obtain as a parenteral medication
   e. Linezolid
2. Hepatic failure—acute or severe
   a. Empiric therapy: aminoglycoside, fluoroquinolone (levofloxacin may be preferred since moxifloxacin is hepatically cleared), ethambutol, (consider including rifampin if not fulminant hepatic failure)
   b. Avoid: isoniazid and pyrazinamide
3. Renal failure
   a. Dose adjust: ethambutol, pyrazinamide, aminoglycosides, and levofloxacin
   b. No change in dosing: isoniazid, rifampin, linezolid, and moxifloxacin
4. Pregnancy
   a. Empiric therapy: isoniazid, rifampin, ethambutol. Pyrazinamide is generally avoided in the United States; however, use in pregnancy is recommended by WHO [103], particularly in severely ill individuals with underlying HIV disease. Therefore, its use should be considered in pregnant women with severe disease or who are immunocompromised.
   b. Avoid: aminoglycosides and if possible, limit the use of fluoroquinolones given limited data for their use in pregnancy

Adjunctive Corticosteroids

In certain circumstances, corticosteroids may be useful for adjunctive tuberculosis treatment by reducing the intensity of the inflammatory response [80]. In a randomized, placebo-controlled trial, corticosteroids were shown to lower the mortality and morbidity of patients with tuberculous meningitis [89]. Corticosteroids also reduce the need for pericardiocentesis in patients being treated for tuberculous pericarditis [90], but there does not appear to be a long-term benefit in reducing the late complication of constrictive pericarditis. Corticosteroids also appear beneficial for treating severe pulmonary tuberculosis with more rapid defervescence, weight gain, and radiographic improvement [91]. The initial corticosteroid dose in most studies has been the equivalent of 40 to 80 mg of daily prednisone, tapering off over 1 to 3 months.

Management of Adverse Drug Effects

During the treatment of tuberculosis, serious mistakes can result from the failure to appropriately recognize and manage adverse drug effects [92]. Most mistakes fall into three categories: (1) failing to discontinue therapy in the face of a serious adverse effect; (2) abandoning important first-line drugs because of minor adverse effects; and (3) failing to recognize serious drug–drug interactions. Drug-induced hepatitis is probably the greatest concern for clinicians treating tuberculosis, particularly when patients have underlying liver disease. Fortunately, the risk of fulminant hepatitis is low and generally occurs when tuberculosis medications are continued despite evidence of toxicity.

While clinically significant or fulminant hepatitis is rare, increased transaminase levels are common with the combination of isoniazid, rifampin, and pyrazinamide. Clinicians should also remember that patients with severe or disseminated tuberculosis might have elevated liver function tests, particularly alkaline phosphatase, as a result of their disease. Patients with abnormal liver function tests and no known cause should have tuberculosis treatment held if transaminases are three times the upper limit of normal and the patient has symptoms of toxicity (i.e., nausea, vomiting, loss of appetite, or jaundice) or if transaminases are five times the upper limit in asymptomatic patients [93]. Patients with underlying liver disease and/or baseline liver function abnormalities should generally start standard tuberculosis treatment with close monitoring of symptoms and liver function tests.

The decision to stop or change therapy due to liver dysfunction must be made on a case-by-case basis. When therapy is held due to hepatotoxicity, the drugs are usually restarted cautiously, resuming one drug at a time. Pyrazinamide is the most frequent cause of liver injury in patients receiving the standard four-drug regimen and may best be avoided if rifampin and isoniazid are reintroduced without difficulty. Among critically ill patients for whom holding therapy may pose a significant risk, reasonable short-term therapy can be achieved with an aminoglycoside, fluoroquinolone, and ethambutol (Table 82.2). Patients who develop a rapid rise in transaminases to levels of 10 to 20 times normal should probably not be rechallenged with pyrazinamine or isoniazid. Other serious side effects that should result in the permanent discontinuation of the offending medication are severe rifampin-associated hypersensitivity reactions like acute renal failure, hemolysis, or thrombocytopenia.

When minor side effects occur, all attempts should be made to treat the symptoms and to determine if an alternative cause exists before discontinuing standard first-line tuberculosis medications. Minor side effects such as gastrointestinal upset can often be managed by adjusting the dosing schedule or by prescribing an antiemetic. Isolated bilirubin elevation caused by rifampin-associated cholestasis may occur but resolves despite continued therapy. Transient minor rashes or pruritus are often associated with pyrazinamide and may be managed using antihistamines without interrupting therapy.

Finally, recognizing potentially serious drug–drug interactions and adjusting therapy accordingly can avoid many drug-associated adverse events. Rifampin and to a lesser extent rifabutin are inducers of the hepatic cytochrome P-450 enzyme system. Therefore, particular caution should be used when HIV-infected tuberculosis patients are taking or may be starting ART [94]. The optimal timing for antiretrovirals has been controversial, but three recent trials have greatly improved our understanding of when to start ART in individuals with tuberculosis [95–98]. When initiating ART for individuals with CD4 counts <50 cells per μL, there was a mortality benefit to initiating after 2 weeks of tuberculosis treatment despite the higher risk of immune reconstitution syndrome in this group. Otherwise, there was no mortality benefit to delaying the initiation of ART to near the end of the initial 8-week phase of tuberculosis treatment. However, the optimal timing of ART in highly immunosuppressed individuals with CNS disease is uncertain, but early therapy in one trial did not show a benefit [99].

Updated recommendations for the combined use of tuberculosis and HIV drugs can be found on the CDC website at (http://www.cdc.gov/tb/publications/guidelines/TB_HIV_Drugs/default.htm). Other notable interactions with rifamycins include warfarin, most antiseizure medications, and many antirejection medications given for bone marrow and solid-organ transplants. The safest practice is to review all medications when treating someone with a rifamycin.

INFECTION CONTROL AND RESPIRATORY ISOLATION

Preventing Nosocomial Transmission

Early suspicion for tuberculosis is the most important step in preventing transmission because it allows the appropriate use of effective respiratory isolation, prompt diagnostic evaluation, and initiation of effective treatment. Screening for active tuberculosis is generally achieved through the collection of three sputa for AFB smear. In 2015, the Food and Drug Administration (FDA) approved use of Xpert MTB/RIF to evaluate for tuberculosis within hospitalized patients because a recent study demonstrated that the negative predictive value of 1 to 2 Xpert tests is high [100]. However, pulmonary tuberculosis with smear-negative disease is transmittable, and although data are limited, the potential exists for transmission to occur in tuberculosis patients who are Xpert negative and culture positive [101]. Therefore, hospitalized patients with negative sputum smears or negative Xpert testing but are at high risk for tuberculosis should be kept in respiratory isolation until an alternative diagnosis is made or empiric TB treatment has been initiated for several days. The infectiousness of tuberculosis begins to decrease within days after initiating effective therapy, probably by decreasing the cough as well as by reducing the number of tubercle bacilli. Decisions about discontinuing isolation once treatment is instituted should be carefully individualized considering the initial burden of disease and the clinical and microbiologic response to treatment, avoiding a decision based only on the number of days on therapy. Other measures that may be of benefit in intubated patient include the use of a closed suctioning system to avoid generating infectious aerosols and the use of submicron filters for air exhausted from ventilators [38].

All health care workers who will be exposed to potentially infectious tuberculosis patients should use personal protective devices. Properly fitted masks capable of filtering at least 95% of particles 1 μm in size are recommended with fit-testing to ensure a face-seal leakage of less than 10%. Powered air-purifying respirators with a helmet or hood are a more effective and more expensive option. These could be considered for certain high-risk situations such as an unavoidable bronchoscopy of an infectious case of tuberculosis. Periodic tuberculin testing or IGRA testing [102] of hospital personnel should be continued as a means of monitoring the effectiveness of other measures and of evaluating tuberculin converters and providing treatment when appropriate [38].

Public Health Aspects

Presumptive and confirmed cases of tuberculosis should be promptly reported to the local public health department as required by law in every state. The function of this reporting is to provide the opportunity to conduct timely contact investigations, which may be critical to preventing life-threatening complications of tuberculosis among small children or immunocompromised household members. In addition, many health departments can assist in ensuring completion of outpatient therapy and thus prevent a hospital readmission for treatment failure or relapse with drug-resistant tuberculosis.

Treatment recommendations for tuberculosis, based on randomized controlled trials, are summarized in Table 82.3.

TABLE 82.3

Summary of Recommendations for Tuberculosis Treatment That Are Supported by Randomized Controlled Trials

Treatment for known or suspected drug-susceptible tuberculosis, initial phase

1. Isoniazid, rifampin, pyrazinamide and ethambutol 7 d/wk for 56 doses (8 wk) [80]

Adjunctive corticosteroids are recommended for:

1. Tuberculous meningitis—improved survival and fewer serious adverse events [89]
2. Tuberculosis pericarditis--there is no improved survival with the routine addition of corticosteroids for pericardial TB", however corticosteriods may be considered in individuals who have large effusions or who are unable to undergo a pericardial window [90]

References

1. World Health Organization: *Global Tuberculosis Report 2014*. Geneva, Switzerland, World Health Organization, 2014.
2. Scott C, Kirking HL, Jeffries C, et al: Tuberculosis trends—United States, 2014. *MMWR Morb Mortal Wkly Rep* 64(10):265–269, 2015.
3. Gandhi NR, Moll A, Sturm AW, et al: Extensively drug-resistant tuberculosis as a cause of death in patients co-infected with tuberculosis and HIV in a rural area of South Africa. *Lancet* 368(9547):1575–1580, 2006.
4. Frame RN, Johnson MC, Eichenhorn MS, et al: Active tuberculosis in the medical intensive care unit: a 15-year retrospective analysis. *Crit Care Med* 15(11):1012–1014, 1987.
5. Rao VK, Iademarco EP, Fraser VJ, et al: The impact of comorbidity on mortality following in-hospital diagnosis of tuberculosis. *Chest* 114(5):1244–1252, 1998.
6. Centers for Disease Control and Prevention: *Reported Tuberculosis in the United States, 2013*. Atlanta, GA: US Department of Health and Human Services, CDC, 2014, pp 1–204.
7. Lee PL, Jerng JS, Chang YL, et al: Patient mortality of active pulmonary tuberculosis requiring mechanical ventilation. *Eur Respir J* 22(1):141–147, 2003.
8. Zahar JR, Azoulay E, Klement E, et al: Delayed treatment contributes to mortality in ICU patients with severe active pulmonary tuberculosis and acute respiratory failure. *Intensive Care Med* 27(3):513–520, 2001.
9. Sacks LV, Pendle S: Factors related to in-hospital deaths in patients with tuberculosis. *Arch Intern Med* 158(17):1916–1922, 1998.
10. Erbes R, Oettel K, Raffenberg M, et al: Characteristics and outcome of patients with active pulmonary tuberculosis requiring intensive care. *Eur Respir J* 27(6):1223–1228, 2006.
11. American Thoracic Society/Centers for Disease Control and Prevention: Diagnostic standards and classification of tuberculosis in adults and children. *Am J Respir Crit Care Med* 161(4 Pt 1):1376–1395, 2000.
12. Horsburgh CR Jr: Priorities for the treatment of latent tuberculosis infection in the United States. *N Eng J Med* 350(20):2060–2067, 2004.
13. Lillebaek T, Dirksen A, Baess I, et al: Molecular evidence of endogenous reactivation of Mycobacterium tuberculosis after 33 years of latent infection. *J Infect Dis* 185(3):401–404, 2002.
14. Centers for Disease Control and Prevention: Targeted tuberculin testing and treatment of latent tuberculosis infection. *MMWR Recomm Rep* 49(RR-6):1–51, 2000.
15. Slavin RE, Walsh TJ, Pollack AD: Late generalized tuberculosis: a clinical pathologic analysis and comparison of 100 cases in the preantibiotic and antibiotic eras. *Medicine* 59:352–366, 1980.
16. Greenaway C, Menzies D, Fanning A, et al: Delay in diagnosis among hospitalized patients with active tuberculosis—predictors and outcomes. *Am J Respir Crit Care Med* 165(7):927–933, 2002.
17. Jindani A, Harrison TS, Nunn AJ, et al: High-dose rifapentine with moxifloxacin for pulmonary tuberculosis. *N Eng J Med* 371(17):1599–1608, 2014.
18. Dooley KE, Golub J, Goes FS, et al: Empiric treatment of community-acquired pneumonia with fluoroquinolones, and delays in the treatment of tuberculosis. *Clin Infect Dis* 34(12):1607–1612, 2002.
19. Yoon YS, Yoon HI, Yoo CG, et al: Impact of fluoroquinolones on the diagnosis of pulmonary tuberculosis initially treated as bacterial pneumonia. *Int J Tuberc Lung Dis* 9(11):1215–1219, 2005.
20. Wang JY, Hsueh PR, Jan IS, et al: Empirical treatment with a fluoroquinolone delays the treatment for tuberculosis and is associated with a poor prognosis in endemic areas. *Thorax* 61(10):903–908, 2006.
21. Long R, Chong H, Hoeppner V, et al: Empirical treatment of community-acquired pneumonia and the development of fluoroquinolone-resistant tuberculosis. *Clin Infect Dis* 48(10):1354–1360, 2009.
22. Chang KC, Leung C, Yew WW, et al: Newer fluoroquinolones for treating respiratory infection: do they mask tuberculosis? *Eur Respir J* 35(3):606–613, 2010.
23. Jeon CY, Calver AD, Victor TC, et al: Use of fluoroquinolone antibiotics leads to tuberculosis treatment delay in a South African gold mining community. *Int J Tuberc Lung Dis* 15(1):77–83, 2011.
24. Wang M, Fitzgerald JM, Richardson K, et al: Is the delay in diagnosis of pulmonary tuberculosis related to exposure to fluoroquinolones or any antibiotic? *Int J Tuberc Lung Dis* 15(8):1062–1068, 2011.
25. van der Heijden YF, Maruri F, Blackman A, et al: Fluoroquinolone exposure prior to tuberculosis diagnosis is associated with an increased risk of death. *Int J Tuberc Lung Dis* 16(9):1162–1167, 2012.
26. Blumberg HM, Burman WJ, Chaisson RE, et al: American Thoracic Society/Centers for Disease Control and Prevention/Infectious Disease Society of America: treatment of tuberculosis. *Am J Respir Crit Care Med* 167(4):603–662, 2003.
27. Lee M, Lee J, Carroll MW, et al: Linezolid for treatment of chronic extensively drug-resistant tuberculosis. *N Eng J Med* 367(16):1508–1518, 2012.
28. Penner C, Roberts D, Kunimoto D, et al: Tuberculosis as a primary cause of respiratory failure requiring mechanical ventilation. *Am J Respir Crit Care Med* 151(3 Pt 1):867–872, 1995.
29. Levy H, Kallenbach JM, Feldman C, et al: Acute respiratory failure in active tuberculosis. *Crit Care Med* 15(3):221–225, 1987.
30. Cain KP, McCarthy KD, Heilig CM, et al: An algorithm for tuberculosis screening and diagnosis in people with HIV. *N Eng J Med* 362(8):707–716, 2010.
31. Braidy J, Pothel C, Amra S: Miliary tuberculosis presenting as adrenal failure. *Can Med Assoc J* 124(6):748–749, 1981.
32. Peto HM, Pratt RH, Harrington TA, et al: Epidemiology of extrapulmonary tuberculosis in the United States, 1993-2006. *Clin Infect Dis* 49(9):1350–1357, 2009.
33. Sanyika C, Corr P, Royston D, et al: Pulmonary angiography and embolization for severe hemoptysis due to cavitary pulmonary tuberculosis. *Cardiovasc Intervent Radiol* 22(6):457–460, 1999.
34. Boehme CC, Nabeta P, Hillemann D, et al: Rapid molecular detection of tuberculosis and rifampin resistance. *N Engl J Med* 363(11):1005–1015, 2010.
35. Pedro-Botet J, Gutierrez J, Miralles R, et al: Pulmonary tuberculosis in HIV-infected patients with normal chest radiographs. *AIDS (London, England)* 6(1):91–93, 1992.
36. Wood R, Middelkoop K, Myer L, et al: Undiagnosed tuberculosis in a community with high HIV prevalence: implications for tuberculosis control. *Am J Respir Crit Care Med* 175(1):87–93, 2007.
37. Lawn SD, Kerkhoff AD, Wood R: Progression of subclinical culture-positive tuberculosis to symptomatic disease in HIV-infected individuals. *AIDS (London, England)* 25(17):2190–2191, 2011.
38. Jensen PA, Lambert LA, Iademarco MF, et al: Guidelines for preventing the transmission of *Mycobacterium tuberculosis* in Health-Care Settings, 2005. *MMWR Recomm Rep* 54(RR-17):1–141, 2005.
39. Brown M, Varia H, Bassett P, et al: Prospective study of sputum induction, gastric washing, and bronchoalveolar lavage for the diagnosis of pulmonary tuberculosis in patients who are unable to expectorate. *Clin Infect Dis* 44(11):1415–1420, 2007.
40. Sharma SK, Mohan A, Sharma A, et al: Miliary tuberculosis: new insights into an old disease. *Lancet Infect Dis* 5(7):415–430, 2005.
41. Ferrer J: Tuberculous pleural effusion and tuberculous empyema. *Semin Respir Crit Care Med* 22(6):637–646, 2001.
42. Frye MD, Pozsik CJ, Sahn SA: Tuberculous pleurisy is more common in AIDS than in non-AIDS patients with tuberculosis. *Chest* 112(2):393–397, 1997.
43. Keiper MD, Beumont M, Elshami A, et al: CD4 T lymphocyte count and the radiographic presentation of pulmonary tuberculosis. A study of the relationship between these factors in patients with human immunodeficiency virus infection. *Chest* 107(1):74–80, 1995.
44. Johnson TM, McCann W, Davey WN: Tuberculous bronchopleural fistula. *Am Rev Respir Dis* 107(1):30–41, 1973.
45. Epstein DM, Kline LR, Albelda SM, et al: Tuberculous pleural effusions. *Chest* 91(1):106–109, 1987.
46. Zemlin AE, Burgess LJ, Carstens ME: The diagnostic utility of adenosine deaminase isoenzymes in tuberculous pleural effusions. *Int J Tuberc Lung Dis* 13(2):214–220, 2009.
47. Kirsch CM, Kroe DM, Azzi RL, et al: The optimal number of pleural biopsy specimens for a diagnosis of tuberculous pleurisy. *Chest* 112(3):702–706, 1997.
48. Maartens G, Willcox PA, Benatar SR: Miliary tuberculosis: rapid diagnosis, hematologic abnormalities, and outcome in 109 treated adults. *Am J Med* 89(3):291–296, 1990.
49. Crump JA, Ramadhani HO, Morrissey AB, et al: Bacteremic disseminated tuberculosis in sub-saharan Africa: a prospective cohort study. *Clin Infect Dis* 55(2):242–250, 2012.
50. Jacob ST, Pavlinac PB, Nakiyingi L, et al: Mycobacterium tuberculosis bacteremia in a cohort of HIV-infected patients hospitalized with severe sepsis in Uganda-high frequency, low clinical suspicion and derivation of a clinical prediction score. *PloS One* 8(8):e70305, 2013.
51. McDonald LC, Archibald LK, Rheanpumikankit S, et al: Unrecognised mycobacterium tuberculosis bacteraemia among hospital inpatients in less developed countries. *Lancet* 354(9185):1159–1163, 1999.

52. Singh N, Paterson DL: *Mycobacterium tuberculosis* infection in solid-organ transplant recipients: impact and implications for management. *Clin Infect Dis* 27(5):1266–1277, 1998.
53. Hill AR, Premkumar S, Brustein S, et al: Disseminated tuberculosis in the acquired immunodeficiency syndrome era. *Am Rev Respir Dis* 144(5):1164–1170, 1991.
54. Gachot B, Wolff M, Clair B, et al: Severe tuberculosis in patients with human immunodeficiency virus infection. *Intensive Care Med* 16(8):491–493, 1990.
55. Ahuja SS, Ahuja SK, Phelps KR, et al: Hemodynamic confirmation of septic shock in disseminated tuberculosis. *Crit Care Med* 20(6):901–903, 1992.
56. Kim JY, Park YB, Kim YS, et al: Miliary tuberculosis and acute respiratory distress syndrome. *Int J Tuberc Lung Dis* 7(4):359–364, 2003.
57. Kennedy C, Knowles GK: Miliary tuberculosis presenting with skin lesions. *Br Med J* 3:356, 1975.
58. Bouza E, Diaz-Lopez MD, Moreno S, et al: *Mycobacterium tuberculosis* bacteremia in patients with and without human immunodeficiency virus infection. *Arch Intern Med* 153(4):496–500, 1993.
59. Cucin RL, Coleman M, Eckardt JJ, et al: The diagnosis of miliary tuberculosis: utility of peripheral blood abnormalities, bone marrow and liver needle biopsy. *J Chronic Dis* 26(6):355–361, 1973.
60. Rock RB, Olin M, Baker CA, et al: Central nervous system tuberculosis: pathogenesis and clinical aspects. *Clin Microbiol Rev* 21(2):243–261, 2008, table of contents.
61. Thwaites G, Fisher M, Hemingway C, et al: British Infection Society guidelines for the diagnosis and treatment of tuberculosis of the central nervous system in adults and children. *J Infect* 59(3):167–187, 2009.
62. Dube MP, Holtom PD, Larsen RA: Tuberculous meningitis in patients with and without human immunodeficiency virus infection. *Am J Med* 93(5):520–524, 1992.
63. Breen RA, Smith CJ, Bettinson H, et al: Paradoxical reactions during tuberculosis treatment in patients with and without HIV co-infection. *Thorax* 59(8):704–707, 2004.
64. Lawn SD, Bekker LG, Miller RF: Immune reconstitution disease associated with mycobacterial infections in HIV-infected individuals receiving antiretrovirals. *Lancet Infect Dis* 5(6):361–373, 2005.
65. Stead WW: Tuberculosis among elderly persons: an outbreak in a nursing home. *Ann Intern Med* 94(5):606–610, 1981.
66. Khan MA, Kovnat DM, Bachus B, et al: Clinical and roentgenographic spectrum of pulmonary tuberculosis in the adult. *Am J Med* 62(1):31–38, 1977.
67. Miller WT, MacGregor RR: Tuberculosis: frequency of unusual radiographic findings. *Am J Roentgenol* 130(5):867–875, 1978.
68. Burman WJ, Jones BE: Clinical and radiographic features of HIV-related tuberculosis. *Semin Respir Infect* 18(4):263–271, 2003.
69. Centers for Disease Control and Prevention: Guidelines for using the quantiFERON-TB Gold test for detecting *Mycobacterium tuberculosis* infection, United States. *MMWR Recomm Rep* 54(RR-15):49–55, 2005.
70. Holden M, Dubin MR, Diamond PH: Frequency of negative intermediate-strength tuberculin sensitivity in patients with active tuberculosis. *N Eng J Med* 285(27):1506–1509, 1971.
71. Pai M, Zwerling A, Menzies D: Systematic review: T-cell-based assays for the diagnosis of latent tuberculosis infection: an update. *Ann Intern Med* 149(3):177–184, 2008.
72. Piersimoni C, Scarparo C: Relevance of commercial amplification methods for direct detection of *Mycobacterium tuberculosis* complex in clinical samples. *J Clin Microbiol* 41(12):5355–5365, 2003.
73. Ruiz-Manzano J, Manterola JM, Gamboa F, et al: Detection of mycobacterium tuberculosis in paraffin-embedded pleural biopsy specimens by commercial ribosomal RNA and DNA amplification kits. *Chest* 118(3): 648–655, 2000.
74. Pai M, Flores LL, Pai N, et al: Diagnostic accuracy of nucleic acid amplification tests for tuberculous meningitis: a systematic review and meta-analysis. *Lancet Infect Dis* 3(10):633–643, 2003.
75. Centers for Disease Control and Prevention: Updated guidelines for the use of nucleic acid amplification tests in the diagnosis of tuberculosis. *MMWR Morb Mortal Wkly Rep* 58(1):7–10, 2009.
76. Moore DF, Guzman JA, Mikhail LT: Reduction in turnaround time for laboratory diagnosis of pulmonary tuberculosis by routine use of nucleic acid amplification test. *Diagn Microbiol Infect Dis* 53(3):247–254, 2005.
77. Guerra RL, Hooper NM, Baker JF, et al: Use of the amplified mycobacterium tuberculosis direct test in a publich health laboratory: test performance and impact on clinical care. *Chest* 132(3):946–951, 2007.
78. Dinnes J, Deeks J, Kunst H, et al: A systematic review of rapid diagnostic tests for the detection of tuberculosis infection. *Health Technol Assess* 11(1):1–196, 2007.
79. Flores LL, Pai M, Colford JM Jr, et al: In house nucleic acid amplifcation tests for the detection of Mycobacterium tuberculosis in sputum specimens: meta-analysis and meta-regression. *BMC Microbiol* 5:55, 2005.
80. Nahid P, et al. Official American Thoracic Society/Centers for Disease Control and Prevention/Infectious Diseases Society of America Clinical Practice Guidelines: Treatment of Drug-Susceptible Tuberculosis. Clinical Infectious Diseases, August 10, 2016..
81. Kalokhe AS, Shafiq M, Lee JC, et al: Multidrug-resistant tuberculosis drug susceptibility and molecular diagnostic testing. *Am J Med Sci* 345(2):143–148, 2013.
82. Barnard M, Warren R, Van Pittius NG, et al: Genotype MTBDRsl line probe assay shortens time to diagnosis of extensively drug-resistant tuberculosis in a high-throughput diagnostic laboratory. *Am J Respir Crit Care Med* 186(12):1298–1305, 2012.
83. Shinnick TM, Iademarco MF, Ridderhof JC: National Plan for reliable tuberculosis laboratory services using a systems approach: recommendations from CDC and the Association of Public Health Laboratories Task Force on Tuberculosis Laboratory Services. *MMWR Recomm Rep* 54(RR-6):1–12, 2005.
84. Centers for Disease Control and Prevention: Trends in tuberculosis—United States, 2008. *MMWR Morb Mortal Wkly Rep* 58(10):249–253, 2009.
85. Centers for Disease Control and Prevention: *Reported Tuberculosis in the United States, 2004*. Atlanta, GA: U.S. Department of Health and Human Services, CDC, 2005.
86. Weis SE, Slocum PC, Blais FX, et al: The effect of directly observed therapy on the rates of drug resistance and relapse in tuberculosis. *N Eng J Med* 330:1179–1184, 1994.
87. Iseman MD: Treatment of multidrug-resistant tuberculosis. *N Eng J Med* 329:784–791, 1993.
88. Peloquin CA: Using therapeutic drug monitoring to dose the antimycobacterial drugs. *Clin Chest Med* 18:79–87, 1997.
89. Thwaites GE, Nguyen DB, Nguyen HD, et al: Dexamethasone for the treatment of tuberculous meningitis in adolescents and adults. *N Engl J Med* 351(17):1741–1751, 2004.
90. Mayosi B et al. N Engl J Med. 371(12):1121-1130, 2014..
91. Smego RA, Ahmed N: A systematic review of the adjunctive use of systemic corticosteroids for pulmonary tuberculosis. *Int J Tuberc Lung Dis* 7(3):208–213, 2003.
92. Davidson PT, Le HQ: Drug treatment of tuberculosis—1992. *Drugs* 43(5):651–673, 1992.
93. Saukkonen JJ, Cohn DL, Jasmer RM, et al: An official ATS statement: hepatotoxicity of antituberculosis therapy. *Am J Respir Crit Care Med* 174(8):935–952, 2006.
94. Burman WJ, Jones BE: Treatment of HIV-related tuberculosis in the era of effective antiretroviral therapy. *Am J Respir Crit Care Med* 164(1):7–12, 2001.
95. Blanc FX, Sok T, Laureillard D, et al: Earlier versus later start of antiretroviral therapy in HIV-infected adults with tuberculosis. *N Eng J Med* 365(16):1471–1481, 2011.
96. Abdool Karim SS, Naidoo K, Grobler A, et al: Timing of initiation of antiretroviral drugs during tuberculosis therapy. *N Eng J Med* 362(8):697–706, 2010.
97. Abdool Karim SS, Naidoo K, Grobler A, et al: Integration of antiretroviral therapy with tuberculosis treatment. *N Eng J Med* 365(16):1492–1501, 2011.
98. Havlir DV, Kendall MA, Ive P, et al: Timing of antiretroviral therapy for HIV-1 infection and tuberculosis. *N Eng J Med* 365(16):1482–1491, 2011.
99. Torok ME, Yen NT, Chau TT, et al: Timing of initiation of antiretroviral therapy in human immunodeficiency virus (HIV)—associated tuberculous meningitis. *Clin Infect Dis* 52(11):1374–1383, 2011.
100. Division of Microbiology Devices, Office of In Vitro Diagnostics and Radiological Health, Center for Devices and Radiological Health, Food and Drug Administration, Centers for Disease Control and Prevention (CDC): Revised device labeling for the Cepheid Xpert MTB/RIF assay for detecting Mycobacterium tuberculosis. *MMWR Morb Mortal Wkly Rep* 64(7):193, 2015.
101. Behr MA, Warren SA, Salamon H, et al: Transmission of Mycobacterium tuberculosis from patients smear-negative for acid-fast bacilli. *Lancet* 353(9151):444–449, 1999.
102. Dorman SE, Belknap R, Graviss EA, et al: Interferon-γ release assays and tuberculin skin testing for diagnosis of latent tuberculosis infection in healthcare workers in the United States. *Am J Respir Crit Care Med* 189(1):77–87, 2013.
103. World Health Organization: *Treatment of Tuberculosis: Guidelines*. 4th ed. Geneva, Switzerland, World Health Organization, 2010.

Chapter 83 ■ Serious Epidemic Viral Pneumonias

DANIEL H. LIBRATY

There are a number of established, emerging, and reemerging viruses that can lead to severe respiratory illness in immunocompetent individuals. The etiologic agents of serious viral pneumonias can generally be divided into three groups:

1. *Human-adapted respiratory viruses.* The primary site of entry, replication, and disease for these viruses is the human respiratory tract. They are spread efficiently by person-to-person transmission. The most significant members of this group are the human influenza A and B viruses; others are respiratory syncytial virus (RSV) and adenovirus.
2. *Human-adapted viruses—respiratory disease after a viremic phase.* Viral entry and person-to-person spread of these viruses are via the respiratory tract. However, these viruses cause respiratory illness after a phase of systemic viral replication and dissemination. Members of this group include varicella zoster virus (chickenpox) and rubeola virus (measles).
3. *Zoonotic viruses.* Viruses in this group include the New World hantaviruses producing the hantavirus cardiopulmonary syndrome (HCPS), H5N1, and other avian influenza A viruses, and the severe acute respiratory syndrome (SARS) coronavirus.

PATHOGENESIS

A virus must first gain access to the lower respiratory tract in order to produce severe pneumonia. The most common mode of entry is via droplet transmission. Airborne virus-containing droplets 5 to 10 μm in diameter are filtered and deposited in the upper respiratory tract. Virus reaches the lower respiratory tract after efficient replication and spread within squamous epithelial cells, often in the setting of impaired mucociliary clearance (due to extremes of age, antecedent or concurrent infections, and drugs). This is the usual mode of entry for many human-adapted respiratory viruses, such as influenza, RSV, adenovirus, and coronavirus. Person-to-person spread via droplets is limited to a distance of approximately 1 m. Other viruses such as varicella and rubeola are transmitted via aerosols (particles 1 to 5 μm in diameter) that can deposit directly in the lower respiratory tract. As such, they are highly infectious and can be transmitted over greater distances and time than agents transmitted by droplets. Although deposited directly in alveoli, viral dissemination to the lung typically occurs hematogenously after a viremic phase [1,2].

Once in the lower respiratory tract, there are a limited number of ways that the lung can respond to a viral infection and produce respiratory illness. Viral invasion and replication can directly produce a necrotizing bronchopneumonia with highly inflammatory, purulent, and exudative reactions. This is not common, but can be seen with influenza and adenovirus infections. Respiratory viral infections can impair host lung defenses in a way that leads to secondary bacterial pneumonias, particularly with *Streptococcus pneumoniae* or *Staphylococcus aureus*. The classic examples are postinfluenza or measles pneumonias. Finally, viral infection of the lower respiratory tract may produce severe disease by triggering a common tissue response to acute lung injuries termed *diffuse alveolar damage* or *acute respiratory distress syndrome*. The acute lung injury may progress from an early exudative phase, often with profound noncardiogenic pulmonary edema (especially in HCPS); to a proliferative or organizing phase that produces interstitial inflammation, and a late resolving phase [3].

CLINICAL MANIFESTATIONS

The limited host-response patterns to virus-induced lung injury mean that there is significant overlap of the clinical manifestations of viral pneumonias. The clues to a specific viral etiology are often found in assessing host risk factors and epidemiology on presentation. A summary of the common clinical manifestations for specific viral pneumonias is presented in Table 83.1. Many of the viral infections discussed in this chapter are characterized by a "flu-like illness" prodrome. Symptoms begin with the acute onset of headache, chills, and myalgias. Within a few days, a cough and sore throat develop along with upper respiratory tract infection. The presence or absence of upper respiratory symptoms at this stage may provide one clue to the specific viral etiology. The human-adapted respiratory viruses (human influenza, RSV, adenovirus, and non-SARS coronavirus) generally all produce upper respiratory symptoms. Measles is characterized by coryza and conjunctivitis in the prodrome. The absence of upper respiratory symptoms has been reported to be characteristic of infections with several of the zoonotic viruses: SARS coronavirus, hantaviruses, and H5N1 and other avian influenza viruses [4–6]. The lower respiratory tract signs and symptoms in viral pneumonias are generally nonspecific and progress to dyspnea, tachypnea, and inspiratory crackles (rales). Sputum production is variable. If the clinical course is biphasic (dyspnea and productive cough after improvement of a flu-like illness), then a secondary bacterial pneumonia should be suspected.

Routine laboratory tests are generally of little help in distinguishing among the viruses that can produce severe respiratory illness. Total leukocyte counts are typically within the normal range or slightly elevated. One exception is measles virus infection, which can produce a marked leukopenia [7]. The most common hematologic finding in the viral pneumonias is a relative lymphopenia. The complete blood count may be useful for diagnosing HCPS. In HCPS caused by Sin Nombre virus (a New World hantavirus), the triad of thrombocytopenia (platelet count less than 150 K per mm^3), absolute neutrophilia, and the presence of immunoblasts was a sensitive and specific predictor of HCPS in one study [5]. Electrolyte abnormalities and hepatic transaminase elevation can occur among any of the severe viral pneumonias.

The radiographic findings of the viral pneumonias are also broad and nonspecific. Radiographic infiltrates can have interstitial, alveolar, or combined patterns. The presence of only a diffuse alveolar pattern might suggest primary influenza pneumonia with hemorrhagic alveolitis [8] or the capillary leak syndrome of acute respiratory distress syndrome, especially due to HCPS. Peribronchial nodular infiltrates is a pattern often reported with varicella pneumonia [9]. Computed tomography (CT) scans are better at detecting the presence, extent, and complications of respiratory infections than chest radiographs. However, they are no better at defining particular radiographic patterns of specific viral or bacterial causes [9].

TABLE 83.1

Presentation and Manifestations of Specific Viral Pneumonias

Virus	Transmission	Epidemiology/settings	Pulmonary manifestations	Extrapulmonary manifestations	Laboratory findings	Radiographic findings
Human influenza A and B viruses	Airborne droplet transmission (≥10 μm) Small aerosol (rare) Fomite contact	Yearly and seasonal (peak season November–April in temperate climates) Attack rates highest at extremes of age Predisposing risk factors for pulmonary complications: chronic heart, lung, renal disease; pregnancy Nosocomial transmission in hospitals and institutional settings	Flu-like illness prodrome (see text) with upper respiratory signs/symptoms Bronchitis Croup Unilateral and bilateral primary viral pneumonia Secondary bacterial pneumonias (*Streptococcus pneumoniae* and *Staphylococcus aureus*)	Secondary bacterial otitis media Myositis (early convalescence) Myocarditis/pericarditis Reye's syndrome (children)	(Nonspecific) Relative lymphopenia in adults Leukocytosis in children	(Nonspecific) Segmental and bilateral alveolar and/or interstitial infiltrates Consolidation suggests superimposed bacterial process Diffuse hemorrhagic alveolitis seen in primary influenza pneumonia
Respiratory syncytial virus	Airborne droplet transmission (≥10 μm)	Yearly and seasonal (overlaps with human influenza) Severe illness at extremes of age: <2 and >65 y old High-risk individuals: children with underlying cardiopulmonary disorders; adults with congestive heart failure or chronic pulmonary disease Outbreaks in long-term care facilities	Prodrome with upper respiratory signs/symptoms as with human influenza Bronchiolitis (common in infants) Pneumonia, unilateral and bilateral	Otitis media	(Nonspecific) Same as influenza	(Nonspecific) Segmental and multiple areas of interstitial and/or alveolar infiltrates In children, hyperaeration is reported as common finding
Adenovirus	Airborne droplet transmission (≥10 μm)	Endemic: mild respiratory disease year round Epidemic: outbreaks in military barracks, hospitals, and institutional settings	Flu-like illness prodrome with upper respiratory signs/symptoms Progression to severe pneumonia, can be necrotizing	The adenovirus serotypes that produce severe pneumonia are generally not the ones that produce extrapulmonary disease such as diarrhea, epidemic keratoconjunctivitis, or hemorrhagic cystitis	(Nonspecific) Relative lymphopenia	(Nonspecific) Segmental and multiple areas of interstitial and/or alveolar infiltrates Focal infiltrates reported as a common presentation
Varicella virus	Airborne: aerosol transmission	Year-round transmission with peaks in late winter and early spring in temperate climates Intimate contact with index case of primary varicella infection (chickenpox) Incubation period is 10–20 d after infection	Pneumonia presents 1–6 d after onset of typical rash (chickenpox) Fever, dyspnea, tachypnea in absence of upper respiratory symptoms	Cutaneous lesions (chickenpox) CNS involvement (uncommon): acute cerebellar ataxia, encephalitis, CNS vasculitis	(Nonspecific)	Nodular or interstitial pneumonitis common

		Risk factors for developing pneumonia: nonimmune adults; smoking; chronic obstructive pulmonary disease; >100 skin lesions; pregnancy, third trimester				
Rubeola virus	Fomite and direct contact with respiratory droplets Airborne: aerosol transmission	Epidemic transmission, localized outbreaks in household and community settings Outbreaks in doctor's offices and emergency departments Infectivity greatest in the 3 d before onset of rash in index case (incubation period 10–14 d) Risk factors for severe illness: nonimmune adults and children <5 y old; crowding; pregnancy; HIV infection; malnourished children, developing countries; vitamin A deficiency	Prodrome: cough, coryza, conjunctivitis Unilateral and bilateral primary viral pneumonia Secondary bacterial pneumonias (*S. pneumoniae*, *S. aureus*, and others)	Typical morbilliform rash (see text) CNS involvement: acute or chronic encephalitis (typically after respiratory disease)	Leukopenia	(Nonspecific)
SARS coronavirus	Airborne droplet transmission (≥10 μm) Fomites	Epidemic/outbreak settings Originated in Asia Person-to-person transmission after contact with symptomatic, SARS CoV-infected person No transmission seen since 2003	Fever, myalgias, cough Upper respiratory signs/symptoms are uncommon Dyspnea, tachypnea, respiratory decompensation develop around second week of illness	Watery diarrhea in 25% of patients around second week of illness	Absolute lymphopenia common	Ground-glass opacifications Unilateral and bilateral focal infiltrates Pneumomediastinum without preceding intubation or positive pressure ventilation reported as characteristic sign
New World hantaviruses	Small-particle aerosols generated from rodent excreta	Sporadic, clustered cases in Americas Exposure to rodents, their droppings and urine, especially in closed spaces In general, no person-to-person transmission (except possibly with Andes virus)	Febrile/flu-like prodrome usually without any upper respiratory signs/symptoms Rapid progression to noncardiogenic pulmonary edema/ARDS with hypotension	Renal dysfunction with proteinuria and microscopic hematuria	Thrombocytopenia (early and nearly all cases) Absolute neutrophilia Relative lymphopenia with immunoblasts on peripheral smear Elevated hepatic transaminases (nearly all cases)	Bilateral noncardiogenic pulmonary edema/ ARDS
Avian influenza A viruses (e.g., H5N1)	Presumed droplet transmission and/or direct contact from bird to human	Sporadic cases in countries with animal influenza A H5N1 Close contact/exposure to live or dead domestic fowl or wild birds or domestic ducks Few reports of limited person-to-person transmission by intimate contact only	Flu-like prodrome often without upper respiratory signs/symptoms Early development of primary viral pneumonia	Watery diarrhea Multiorgan failure	(Nonspecific) Lymphopenia Mild-to-moderate thrombocytopenia Elevated hepatic transaminases	(Nonspecific) Unilateral and bilateral infiltrates Multifocal consolidations ARDS

ARDS, acute respiratory distress syndrome; CNS, central nervous system; HIV, human immunodeficiency virus; SARS CoV, severe acute respiratory syndrome coronavirus.

DIAGNOSIS

The diagnostic modalities available for viral pneumonias rely on the detection of a viral component (nucleic acid or protein), growth of the virus in vitro, or development of a virus-specific antibody response. Definitive serologic evidence of a viral infection requires a rise in virus-specific antibody titers between paired acute illness and convalescent sera. With a few exceptions, serologic assays are therefore not generally helpful for the clinician in the acute setting of a severe viral pneumonia. This section will focus on diagnostic tests that may assist the clinician faced with a critically ill patient and suspected viral pneumonia.

Human Influenza A and B

Rapid, direct, antigen-detection assays are commercially available for diagnosing human influenza A and B virus infections. These assays rely on detection of the influenza virus nucleoprotein in respiratory secretions, and results can be obtained within 1 hour. Because they are based on the viral nucleoprotein, none of the rapid antigen tests provide information about influenza A hemagglutinin subtypes (e.g., H1, H3). Details regarding the available rapid antigen tests for influenza are provided by the Centers for Disease Control and Prevention (CDC) (http://www.cdc.gov/flu/professionals/diagnosis/rapidclin.htm). The test specificities for diagnosing an influenza virus infection are generally high (more than 90%), but reported sensitivities are lower (33% to 80%) and may vary for different human influenza A virus subtypes [10–12]. In clinical practice, the timing and method of sample collection can greatly affect test sensitivity. Influenza A virus shedding from the upper respiratory tract typically peaks 2 to 3 days after symptom onset [13,14]. The window available to reliably detect viral antigen from upper respiratory tract secretions may extend only 5 to 6 days after symptom onset. Influenza virus nucleoprotein is most abundant in the columnar respiratory epithelium. Posterior nasopharyngeal swabs or aspirates that collect columnar epithelial cells are usually the preferred samples for rapid antigen detection assays [10,15,16], even for mechanically ventilated patients in the intensive care unit (ICU).

Reverse transcriptase polymerase chain reaction (RT-PCR) assays and viral cultures are the next most commonly used diagnostic tests for human influenza virus infections. Posterior nasopharyngeal swabs or washes, and samples of lower respiratory tract secretions such as endotracheal aspirates or bronchoalveolar lavages, are acceptable samples. Virus typing and influenza A subtyping can be accomplished with either method. Due to its high sensitivity, specificity, and throughput, RT-PCR assays have generally supplanted virus culture in most clinical microbiology laboratories. Unlike viral culture, the detection of influenza viral RNA by RT-PCR cannot assess the presence of live virus in respiratory secretions.

Respiratory Syncytial Virus (RSV)

Rapid antigen-detection assays and direct immunofluorescent staining for RSV from respiratory secretions have been the primary diagnostic tests used in children. These tests have >80% sensitivity and >90% specificity [17]. RT-PCR assays and respiratory viral culture are the other common diagnostic approaches in pediatric populations. Among adults, the RSV rapid antigen assays and viral cultures are generally insensitive due to low virus shedding and preexisting anti-RSV antibody in respiratory secretions [18,19]. Direct fluorescent antibody staining in nasopharyngeal specimens was reported to be the only rapid assay at least equivalent to viral culture in adults [17]. A RT-PCR assay on respiratory secretions is the preferred acute illness diagnostic method for RSV infection in adults [20,21].

Adenovirus

PCR of adenovirus DNA or respiratory viral culture from a nasopharyngeal swab or aspirate, sputum, or lower respiratory tract secretions is the diagnostic test of choice for adenoviral pneumonia. Direct adenovirus antigen assays that cover most serotypes, such as immunofluorescent antibody staining, are not as sensitive as PCR assays or viral culture.

Varicella

Varicella pneumonia typically develops within 1 to 6 days after the characteristic rash of chickenpox has appeared [22]. If desired, a specific microbiological diagnosis can be obtained by PCR assay or viral culture from a swab or scraping at the base of an unroofed vesicle. Viral detection in respiratory secretions is generally not required.

Rubeola (Measles)

Pulmonary involvement with measles is generally diagnosed on the basis of history and physical findings. In outbreak settings, pneumonia should be suspected for patients who develop respiratory distress and persistent or recurrent fevers during the course of typical measles. Measles is characterized by malaise and fever, followed rapidly by coryza, conjunctivitis, and cough [23]. Early in illness, the presence of Koplik spots on the buccal mucosa is pathognomonic of measles. The classic morbilliform rash begins 3 to 4 days after onset of illness and starts to fade after another 3 days. Worsening respiratory symptoms as the rash is fading is suspicious for rubeola pneumonia. Laboratory confirmation may be useful, particularly for suspected sporadic cases within a highly immunized population. Viral isolation or rapid detection of measles antigen in nasopharyngeal secretions is difficult and not readily available. A presumptive serologic diagnosis can be made by detection of serum anti-measles virus immunoglobulin M (IgM) or immunoglobulin G (IgG) in unimmunized individuals. Serum antibodies appear 1 to 3 days after onset of the rash [24]. Definitive serologic diagnosis requires paired acute and convalescent sera. In immunocompromised patients with overwhelming pneumonia, the antibody response may be minimal. Viral antigen staining of cells or RT-PCR assays on nasal exudates or urinary sediment may be useful in this setting [23].

Severe Acute Respiratory Syndrome (SARS) Coronavirus

The most practical diagnostic approach for SARS coronavirus is a RT-PCR assay on nasopharyngeal specimens within 2 weeks after symptom onset [25]. The other primary site where SARS coronavirus RNA can be detected is stool (week 2 onward). Lower respiratory tract secretions harbor a greater viral load than upper respiratory tract secretions early in illness. However, lower respiratory tract aspiration, lavage, or intubation pose serious nosocomial transmission risks and should not be pursued solely for diagnostic purposes. IgM seroconversion does not occur until after the first week of illness and therefore is also of limited diagnostic utility [4]. With resolution of SARS viral transmission in 2003, and the apparent subsequent mutation of the virus [26], any initial positive test for SARS coronavirus must be viewed as a potential false-positive finding. Middle Eastern Respiratory Syndrome (MERS) is another coronavirus associated with transmission by camels. This virus and its manifestations are discussed in Chapter 84.

Hantaviruses

There are nearly a dozen New World hantaviruses that have been associated with HCPS. Sin Nombre virus (in the southwestern United States) and Andes virus (in South America) are the two best known HCPS-associated hantaviruses. The diagnosis of HCPS can be made by detection of anti-hantavirus IgM antibodies in acute illness serum. Nearly all patients with HCPS have detectable IgM in their sera at the onset of pulmonary edema. The currently available IgM capture enzyme-linked immunosorbent assay using a recombinant Sin Nombre virus antigen can be used to diagnose all New World hantavirus infections [27]. RT-PCR assay on blood or lung tissue is a research assay of limited utility and not widely available. Because of low yield and biosafety issues, attempted culture of hantaviruses in clinical microbiology laboratories is not recommended.

Avian Influenza Viruses (e.g., H5N1)

If H5N1 influenza A virus infection is suspected on epidemiologic grounds, then all avenues for making a definitive diagnosis should be pursued. The diagnostic approach to H5N1 influenza is to collect nasopharyngeal and lower respiratory tract specimens for rapid antigen detection, RT-PCR assay, and viral culture. Aerosol-generating procedures for specimen collection should be performed with appropriate infection control precautions. Detection of viral RNA in respiratory specimens by RT-PCR is the most sensitive and rapid method for detecting influenza A/H5N1. A hallmark of H5N1 influenza has been a higher frequency of virus detection and viral loads in pharyngeal and lower respiratory tract samples than in nasal samples between 2 and 16 days after the onset of illness [6,28]. Viral RNA has also been detected in fecal samples. The CDC has provided guidance for the laboratory testing of suspected H5N1 and other avian influenza cases (http://www.cdc.gov/flu/avianflu/). The clinical microbiology laboratory should be notified, if H5N1 or another avian influenza A virus infection is suspected and specimens are collected for viral culture. This is to ensure that the specimens will be handled and processed with the appropriate biosafety containment level.

TREATMENT AND MANAGEMENT

Caring for a patient with a severe viral pneumonia can be complex; however, the approach to such a patient is often identical to that of other acute severe pneumonias. First, a clinical assessment of disease severity is made so that an appropriate level of care can be established. This process can be assisted by standardized scoring algorithms established for critically ill patients or community-acquired pneumonias [29,30]. Supportive care with maintenance of ventilation, oxygenation, and hemodynamic parameters is based on general principles previously outlined in Chapter 181. Next, diagnostic procedures to try to establish the cause of the severe pneumonia can be pursued. Finally, one needs to evaluate the role of specific antiviral and/or immunomodulatory therapies in the care of the patient. As with most infectious pneumonias, the decision to treat with these therapies is often made empirically or with limited diagnostic information. A summary of potential therapeutic options, dosages, and adverse effects is presented in Table 83.2.

Human Influenza A and B

There are two classes of antiviral drugs currently available for the treatment of human influenza virus infections: adamantanes (amantadine and rimantadine) and neuraminidase inhibitors (oseltamivir, zanamivir, and peramivir). The adamantanes are older, established compounds, but they are not active against influenza B. In placebo-controlled trials, when amantadine or rimantadine therapy was initiated within 48 hours of symptom onset in influenza A virus infections, there was a 1-to-2-day reduction in duration of fever and overall illness symptom scores [31]. However, there are no controlled data on the utility of adamantanes in the treatment of severe influenza A lower respiratory tract infections, and several factors make them less than ideal for patients in the ICU. In several studies, rimantadine treatment produced small initial decreases in viral titers, but later in therapy, similar or higher frequencies of viral shedding compared with placebo [32]. The incidence of adamantane resistance among influenza A viruses worldwide has increased in recent years [33]. Resistance emerges at a high frequency during treatment with adamantanes, and resistant virus can be transmitted to the close contacts of patients in community and nosocomial settings [32,34].

The neuraminidase inhibitors have activity against influenza A and B. As with the adamantanes, oseltamivir and zanamivir decrease the duration and severity of generalized symptoms by approximately 1 day when started within 48 hours after onset of illness [35]. Some lines of evidence make the neuraminidase inhibitors attractive for treatment of patients with severe influenza virus pneumonias. They markedly reduce viral load during the first 48 hours of treatment, can decrease viral shedding, and may lower the incidence of influenza-related lower respiratory tract complications [36–38]. However, the latter benefit has been questioned by a meta-analysis [39]. Development of resistance to oseltamivir or zanamivir has been uncommon in immunocompetent adults, but appears to be higher in children and immunocompromised individuals [40,41]. Importantly, person-to-person transmission of resistant virus has not been documented. Zanamivir may be active against some oseltamivir-resistant strains.

Despite the lack of randomized controlled trials in the ICU setting, most practitioners would initiate treatment with a neuraminidase inhibitor in patients with suspected or confirmed severe influenza pneumonia. Recent trials have not identified a clinical benefit of higher (double) dose oseltamivir [42,43]. Zanamivir should not be nebulized for patients on mechanical ventilation due to possible obstruction of the ventilation circuit (http://www.fda.gov/safety/medwatch/safetyinformation/safetyalertsforhumanmedicalproducts/ucm186081.htm). Peramivir is an intravenous neuraminidase inhibitor.

Pregnant women, infants, and children younger than 2 years, individuals with chronic cardiopulmonary or renal disease, and those immunosuppressed were at higher risk of developing severe illness during the 2009 H1N1 influenza pandemic (same as in all human influenza outbreaks). The 2009 H1N1 virus has become the dominant circulating influenza A H1N1 strain worldwide. There are no data to support the use of corticosteroids in the treatment of influenza pneumonia, and inhaled ribavirin is not beneficial [44]. An important addition to the treatment of influenza pneumonia is antibacterial therapy. There is a high incidence of secondary bacterial infections complicating influenza pneumonia, particularly with *S. pneumoniae* or *S. aureus* [45]. In this setting, antibiotic therapy directed against *S. aureus* should be added to the antibiotic regimen used for community-acquired pneumonia bacterial pathogens. In areas where there is a high prevalence of community-acquired methicillin-resistant *S. aureus*, vancomycin should be used as the initial antistaphylococcal antibiotic.

Respiratory Syncytial Virus

Because respiratory syncytial virus (RSV) is a frequent cause of serious lower respiratory tract infections among infants and young children, data on potential therapies come from pediatric studies. There have been no trials of anti-RSV therapies in adults. The current

TABLE 83.2

Summary of Antiviral Agents and Therapeutic Options for Specific Viral Pneumonias

Virus	Drug	Adult dosage (duration)	Dosage adjustments[a]	Potential adverse effects	Comments
Human influenza viruses	Oseltamivir	75 mg PO b.i.d (5 d)	Decrease to 75 mg PO qd in patients with CrCl between 10 and 30 mL/min	Nausea, vomiting, headache	Neuraminidase inhibitors effective against human influenza A and B viruses
	Zanamivir	2 × 5 mg oral inhalations bid (5 d)	None	Cough, nasal and throat discomfort, bronchospasm, decreased lung function	Use with caution in patients with asthma or COPD
	Amantadine	100 mg PO b.i.d or 200 mg PO qd (3–5 d)	Decrease to 100 mg/d for patients >65 y old or CrCl <50 mL/min	Anticholinergic effects: CNS effects can include insomnia, delirium, hallucinations, and seizures	Adamantanes not effective against human influenza B viruses
	Rimantadine	100 mg PO b.i.d or 200 mg PO qd (3–5 d)	Decrease to 100 mg/d for patients >65 y old, CrCl <10 mL/min, or with severe hepatic dysfunction	Same as amantadine, except CNS adverse effects less common	
Adenovirus	Cidofovir	5 mg/kg IV × 1	Contraindicated in patients with CrCl ≤55 mL/min	Renal toxicity: acute renal failure, proteinuria Neutropenia Metabolic acidosis Uveitis	Cidofovir given with probenecid (2 g PO 3 h before cidofovir infusion, and 1 g PO 2 and 8 h after the infusion) Also, prehydrate with 1 L IV NS IV hydration to avoid renal toxicity
Varicella	Acyclovir	10 mg/kg IV q8 h × 7–10 d	Decrease to 10 mg/kg IV q12 h for CrCl 10–50 mL/min 10 mg/kg IV q24 h for CrCl <10 mL/min	Occasional mild nausea, vomiting, diarrhea Crystal formation and renal tubular obstruction Dizziness, delirium, obtundation (rare)	CNS toxicity seen with high drug levels
Rubeola (measles)	Vitamin A	200,000 IU PO qd × 1–2 d (100,000 IU PO qd if ≤1 y old)	None		
	Ribavirin?	20–35 mg/kg/d IV × 7 d	None	Dose-related hemolytic anemia (common) Cough, dyspnea, nausea, headache, fatigue Hypocalcemia with IV ribavirin	Data from small case series; no randomized trial
New World hantaviruses	Ribavirin?	33 mg/kg IV load, then 16 mg/kg IV q6 h × 4 d, 8 mg/kg IV q8 h × 3 d	None	Same as previously noted	No suggestion of benefit if ribavirin started in cardiopulmonary phase of HCPS; unknown if there would be benefit if initiated earlier during prodromal phase
Avian influenza A viruses (e.g. H5N1)	Oseltamivir	75 mg PO b.i.d × 5 d or consider increase to 150 mg PO b.i.d × 7–10 d	Same as previously noted	Same as previously noted	Most experience to date in treating H5N1 infections has been with oseltamivir, but no randomized trials
	Zanamivir	2 × 5 mg oral inhalations b.i.d (5 d)	None	Same as previously noted	Same cautions as previously noted

Zanamavir may be useful for oseltamivir-resistant H5N1 strains, but no experience as either single agent or in combination with other antivirals.
[a]Consult appropriate references for potential drug–drug interactions.
b.i.d, twice daily; CrCl, creatinine clearance; COPD, chronic obstructive pulmonary disease; CNS, central nervous system; HCPS, hantavirus cardiopulmonary syndrome; IV, intravenous; PO, orally; NS, normal saline.

treatment strategies for RSV lower respiratory tract infections are essentially supportive. Aerosolized ribavirin therapy of infants with RSV lower respiratory tract infections had no significant effects on clinical outcome in two randomized trials [46,47]. Palivizumab, a humanized anti-RSV neutralizing monoclonal antibody, has been successful in reducing hospitalizations of high risk children for RSV lower respiratory tract infections when given prophylactically [48]. However, the utility of palivizumab or anti-RSV immune globulin as a potential treatment of serious RSV infections is unknown. Clinical observations and a mouse model of RSV infection have demonstrated airway hyperresponsiveness and other asthmatic changes in RSV-infected lungs [49], and prompted trials of anti-inflammatory therapies. Unfortunately, two randomized trials failed to demonstrate any overall beneficial effect of intravenous dexamethasone in RSV lower respiratory tract infections [50,51]. On subgroup analysis in one study, dexamethasone treatment was beneficial in mechanically ventilated patients with bronchiolitis and mild gas exchange abnormalities (PaO_2/FIO_2 more than 200 mm Hg or mean airway pressure ≤10 cm H_2O) [50]. These findings have yet to be confirmed in a prospective fashion.

Adenovirus

Adenoviral pneumonia occurs in isolated outbreaks among immunocompetent adults or sporadically in immunocompromised individuals. As such, there are no prospective randomized trials of antiviral medications. Cidofovir is an antiviral drug with potent in vitro activity against adenovirus. Cidofovir has been reported to be successful for treating adenoviral pneumonia in small case series [52–54], and is currently considered the antiviral agent of choice. Because severe adenovirus disease is associated with defects in cellular or humoral immunity, donor lymphocyte infusions, and intravenous immunoglobulin have been used as adjunctive therapy [52]. Their efficacy for the treatment of adenoviral pneumonia is unknown.

Varicella

Intravenous acyclovir is considered standard therapy for the treatment of varicella pneumonia. There have been no randomized controlled trials of acyclovir for varicella pneumonia. Its efficacy for reducing the severity of pox lesions [55,56] and apparent benefit in numerous case series of varicella pneumonia support its use. A compilation of 46 case reports and 227 patients with varicella pneumonia suggested that mortality was 3.6-fold higher in untreated compared with acyclovir-treated patients [22]. In a small uncontrolled retrospective study, patients who received adjunctive corticosteroids had shorter ICU and hospital stays than those who did not receive corticosteroids [57]. There are no prospective controlled studies supporting the use of adjunctive corticosteroid therapy in varicella pneumonia.

Rubeola (Measles)

Pneumonia is the most common severe complication of measles and accounts for most measles-associated deaths [58]. There is no specific antiviral therapy for measles. In developing countries, treatment with vitamin A has been associated with a 50% reduction in the mortality of severe measles. Hospitalized children with measles in the United States often have a measurable deficiency in vitamin A, and they are more likely to have pneumonia or diarrhea. The World Health Organization recommends vitamin A therapy for all children with measles, and the American Academy of Pediatrics recommends vitamin A therapy for hospitalized children older than 2 years with measles in the United States [58]. Data for older children and adults are lacking, but vitamin A treatment should probably be provided for all individuals with severe measles [59,60]. Intravenous ribavirin was reported to have beneficial effects in a small case series of measles pneumonia in adults [61], but there are no data from prospective randomized studies. Another important point in the treatment of measles pneumonia is antibacterial therapy. Secondary bacterial pneumonia and laryngotracheobronchitis are frequent complications of measles. As with influenza, *S. aureus* and *S. pneumoniae* are the most commonly isolated bacterial pathogens. Less frequent bacterial causes of pneumonia following measles include *Neisseria meningitidis, Klebsiella pneumoniae, Escherichia coli, Haemophilus influenzae*, and *Pseudomonas* species [58]. Broad-spectrum antibiotic therapy, including coverage for *S. aureus* and *S. pneumoniae*, should be instituted.

Severe Acute Respiratory Syndrome (SARS) Coronavirus

The SARS epidemic of 2003 was marked by the empiric use of several antiviral and immunomodulatory strategies because controlled trials were not possible. Ribavirin was the most commonly used antiviral agent, but its poor in vitro activity against the SARS coronavirus and its apparent limited ability to reduce early viral shedding in patients makes its usefulness questionable [62]. Corticosteroids were used extensively during the SARS outbreak of 2003 at varying doses and durations. Retrospective analyses on the effects of corticosteroids in SARS suggest that they did not provide any significant benefits and may have been associated with some adverse outcomes [62,63].

Hantaviruses

There has been only one placebo-controlled, double-blind trial of intravenous ribavirin for the treatment of HCPS due to Sin Nombre virus [64]. The accrual of study subjects was low and inadequate to clearly assess the efficacy of ribavirin. There were no trends to support the use of ribavirin in patients presenting in the cardiopulmonary phase of HCPS. Whether ribavirin may have a beneficial effect if initiated during the prodromal phase is unknown. Intravenous ribavirin was beneficial when given early to patients with another hantavirus disease, hemorrhagic fever with renal syndrome caused by Hantaan virus [65]. There is no evidence that pharmacologic doses of corticosteroids provide any benefit in HCPS.

At the present time, clinical management of HCPS involves supportive care with several caveats. Excessive fluid resuscitation will exacerbate the pulmonary edema of HCPS without commensurate improvement in cardiac output. Recommendations are to fluid resuscitate with 1 to 2 L of isotonic crystalloid and then maintain as low a wedge pressure (8 to 12 mm Hg) as is compatible with satisfactory cardiac output (cardiac index more than 2.2 L/min/m^2). The use of loop diuretics is discouraged. Inotropic agents (e.g., dobutamine, dopamine, and norepinephrine) should be initiated earlier in resuscitation than in other conditions, instead of continued fluid boluses [5].

Avian Influenza Viruses (e.g., H5N1)

The H5N1 influenza A viruses are susceptible in vitro to the neuraminidase inhibitors, and neuraminidase inhibitors have been protective in animal models of influenza A H5N1 infection [66–68]. Although prospective clinical trials have not been performed, the current recommendation is that patients with suspected influenza A H5N1 infection promptly receive a neuraminidase inhibitor, preferably within 48 hours of infection [6,69]. Emergence of resistance to oseltamivir has been documented in a few patients with H5N1 infections treated with oseltamivir [70]. These strains remain susceptible to zanamivir. Whether combination therapy with zanamivir or other antivirals is beneficial and would reduce the emergence of oseltamivir resistance is unknown. The influenza A H5N1 isolates from Asia are highly resistant to the adamantanes, and therefore these drugs do not play a therapeutic role [6]. Corticosteroids have been used in the treatment of sporadic influenza A H5N1 infections, but their routine use cannot be recommended. In a randomized trial in Vietnam, all four patients given dexamethasone died [71].

INFECTION CONTROL ISSUES FOR THE INTENSIVE CARE UNIT

Most of the viruses presented in this chapter can be transmitted in the nosocomial setting via direct contact with an infected patient and through inhalation of droplets or aerosols. Efforts to reduce transmission to healthcare workers and other patients are often guided by the transmission efficiency of the specific viral agents. Human influenza, RSV, adenovirus, varicella, and measles are efficiently transmitted person to person. SARS coronavirus and avian influenza A H5N1 virus are transmitted less efficiently, but nosocomial transmission may be promoted by aerosol-generating procedures. The New World hantaviruses are generally not transmitted person to person, except possibly the Andes virus.

Strategies to prevent nosocomial transmission include isolation precautions for patients, chemoprophylaxis and immunization of healthcare workers if possible, and surveillance and rapid identification of healthcare workers' exposures. In general, patients with suspected epidemic viral pneumonias should be housed with a combination of standard, contact, droplet, and airborne isolation precautions. When feasible, limit the number of healthcare workers with direct access to the patient and limit their contact with other patients. Restrict visitors to a minimum and provide them appropriate personal protective equipment. High-efficiency N-95 masks or powered air-purifying respirators are preferred for healthcare workers. If high-efficiency masks are limited or unavailable, surgical masks may be considered if the primary mode of agent transmission is via droplets and no aerosol-generating procedures are performed. Detailed guidelines can be found on the CDC Web site (http://www.cdc.gov/ncidod/dhqp/guidelines.html).

Advances of antiviral or immunomodulatory therapy of viral pneumonias based on randomized controlled trials or meta-analyses of such trials is summarized in Table 83.3.

TABLE 83.3

Summary of Recommendations for Antiviral or Immunomodulatory Therapies of Viral Pneumonias Based on Randomized Controlled Clinical Trials

Human influenza

- Neuraminidase inhibitors given within 48 h of flu symptom onset decrease the duration of symptoms, viral load, and viral shedding; controversy as to whether they lower the incidence of influenza-related lower respiratory tract complications [35,39]; no randomized controlled trials for treatment of severe pneumonia.
- Aerosolized ribavirin does not provide any clinical benefit [44].

Respiratory syncytial virus (RSV)

- Aerosolized ribavirin has no significant effect on outcome in infants with RSV lower respiratory tract infections [46,47].
- Intravenous dexamethasone does not provide any overall beneficial effect in RSV lower respiratory tract infections [50,51].
- On post-hoc analysis, dexamethasone (0.6 mg/kg IV q6 h × 48 h) may be beneficial in mechanically ventilated patients with bronchiolitis and mild gas exchange abnormalities (PaO_2/FIO_2 >200 mm Hg or mean airway pressure ≤10 cm H_2O) [50].

Adenovirus

- No randomized controlled trials of cidofovir for adenovirus pneumonia.

Varicella

- No randomized controlled trials of IV acyclovir for varicella pneumonia. A meta-analysis of published case series suggests that IV acyclovir decreases mortality [22].

Rubeola (measles)

- Oral vitamin A therapy decreases mortality and improves recovery from pneumonia in children [58,59].

SARS coronavirus

- No randomized controlled trials for antivirals or corticosteroids.

Hantavirus cardiopulmonary syndrome (HCPS)

- No trends to support the use of ribavirin in patients presenting in the cardiopulmonary phase of HCPS [64].

Avian influenza A viruses (e.g., H5N1)

- Neuraminidase inhibitors have been protective in animal models of influenza A H5N1 infection. There are no patient-based randomized controlled trials.
- No trends to support the use of dexamethasone from a small, unpublished, randomized trial [71].

IV, intravenous; SARS, severe acute respiratory syndrome.

References

1. Bryant RE: Viral pneumonia, in Braude AI, Davis CE, Fierer J (eds): *Infectious Diseases and Medical Microbiology*. Philadelphia, WB Saunders, 1986, p 815.
2. Dermody TS, Tyler KL: Introduction to viruses and viral diseases, in Mandell GL, Bennett JE, Dolin R (eds): *Principles and Practice of Infectious Diseases*. Philadelphia, Churchill Livingstone, 2000, p 1536.
3. Barrios R: Diffuse alveolar damage, in Cagle PT (ed): *Color Atlas and Text of Pulmonary Pathology*. Philadelphia, Lippincott Williams & Wilkins, 2005, p 361.
4. Peiris JS, Yuen KY, Osterhaus AD, et al: The severe acute respiratory syndrome. *N Engl J Med* 349:2431, 2003.
5. Hantavirus in the Americas [in English, French]. *Wkly Epidemiol Rec* 74(22):173, 1999.
6. Beigel JH, Farrar J, Han AM, et al: Avian influenza A (H5N1) infection in humans. *N Engl J Med* 353:1374, 2005.
7. Bernstein DL, Reuman PD, Schiff GM: Rubeola (measles) and subacute sclerosing panencephalitis virus, in Gorbach SL, Bartlett JG, Blacklow NR (eds): *Infectious Diseases*. Philadelphia, WB Saunders, 1992, p 1754.
8. Lindsay MI Jr, Morrow GW Jr: Primary influenzal pneumonia. *Postgrad Med* 49:173, 1971.
9. Donowitz GR, Mandell GL: Acute pneumonia, in Mandell GL, Bennett JE, Dolin R (eds): *Principles and Practice of Infectious Diseases*. Philadelphia, Churchill Livingstone, 2000, p 717.
10. Fiore AE, Shay DK, Broder K, et al: Prevention and control of seasonal influenza with vaccines: recommendations of the Advisory Committee on Immunization Practices (ACIP), 2009. *MMWR Recomm Rep* 58(RR-8):1–52, 2009.
11. Kok J, Blyth CC, Foo H, et al: Comparison of a rapid antigen test with nucleic acid testing during cocirculation of pandemic influenza A/H1N1 2009 and seasonal influenza A/H3N2. *J Clin Microbiol* 48(1):290–291, 2010.
12. Faix DJ, Sherman SS, Waterman SH: Rapid-test sensitivity for novel swine-origin influenza A (H1N1) virus in humans. *N Engl J Med* 361(7):728–729, 2009.
13. Dolin R: Influenza: current concepts. *Am Fam Physician* 14:72, 1976.
14. Douglas RGJ: Influenza in man, in Kilbourne ED (ed): *The Influenza Viruses and Influenza*. New York, Academic Press, 1975, p 395.
15. Hers JF: Disturbances of the ciliated epithelium due to influenza virus. *Am Rev Respir Dis* 93[Suppl]:162, 1996.

16. Schmid ML, Kudesia G, Wake S, et al: Prospective comparative study of culture specimens and methods in diagnosing influenza in adults. *BMJ* 316:275, 1998.
17. Ohm-Smith MJ, Nassos PS, Haller BL: Evaluation of the Binax NOW, BD Directigen, and BD Directigen EZ assays for detection of respiratory syncytial virus. *J Clin Microbiol* 42:2996, 2004.
18. Casiano-Colon AE, Hulbert BB, Mayer TK, et al: Lack of sensitivity of rapid antigen tests for the diagnosis of respiratory syncytial virus infection in adults. *J Clin Virol* 28:169, 2003.
19. Falsey AR, Formica MA, Treanor JJ, et al: Comparison of quantitative reverse transcription-PCR to viral culture for assessment of respiratory syncytial virus shedding. *J Clin Microbiol* 41:4160, 2003.
20. Falsey AR, Formica MA, Walsh EE: Diagnosis of respiratory syncytial virus infection: comparison of reverse transcription-PCR to viral culture and serology in adults with respiratory illness. *J Clin Microbiol* 40:817, 2002.
21. Falsey AR, Hennessey PA, Formica MA, et al: Respiratory syncytial virus infection in elderly and high-risk adults. *N Engl J Med* 352:1749, 2005.
22. Mohsen AH, McKendrick M: Varicella pneumonia in adults. *Eur Respir J* 21:886, 2003.
23. Gershon AA: Measles virus (rubeola), in Mandell GL, Bennett JE, Dolin R (eds): *Principles and Practice of Infectious Diseases*. Philadelphia, Churchill Livingstone, 2000, p 1801.
24. Bernstein DI, Schiff GM: Measles, in Gorbach SL, Bartlett JG, Blacklow NR (eds): *Infectious Diseases*. Philadelphia, WB Saunders, 1992, p 1088.
25. Lau SK, Che XY, Woo PC, et al: SARS coronavirus detection methods. *Emerg Infect Dis* 11:1108, 2005.
26. Li F, Li W, Farzan M, et al: Structure of SARS coronavirus spike receptor-binding domain complexed with receptor. *Science* 309:1864, 2005.
27. Organization PAHO: *Hantavirus in the Americas: Guidelines for Diagnosis, Treatment, Prevention, and Control*. Washington, DC, PAHO, 1999.
28. Peiris JS, Yu WC, Leung CW, et al: Re-emergence of fatal human influenza A subtype H5N1 disease. *Lancet* 363:617, 2004.
29. Knaus WA, Draper EA, Wagner DP, et al: APACHE II: a severity of disease classification system. *Crit Care Med* 13:818, 1985.
30. Buising KL, Thursky KA, Black JF, et al: A prospective comparison of severity scores for identifying patients with severe community acquired pneumonia: reconsidering what is meant by severe pneumonia. *Thorax* 61:419, 2006.
31. Jefferson T, Deeks JJ, Demicheli V, et al: Amantadine and rimantadine for preventing and treating influenza A in adults. *Cochrane Database Syst Rev* 3:CD001169, 2004.
32. Hayden FG, Sperber SJ, Belshe RB, et al: Recovery of drug-resistant influenza A virus during therapeutic use of rimantadine. *Antimicrob Agents Chemother* 35:1741, 1991.
33. Bright RA, Medina MJ, Xu X, et al: Incidence of adamantane resistance among influenza A (H3N2) viruses isolated worldwide from 1994 to 2005: a cause for concern. *Lancet* 366:1175, 2005.
34. Shiraishi K, Mitamura K, Sakai-Tagawa Y, et al: High frequency of resistant viruses harboring different mutations in amantadine-treated children with influenza. *J Infect Dis* 188:57, 2003.
35. Cooper NJ, Sutton AJ, Abrams KR, et al: Effectiveness of neuraminidase inhibitors in treatment and prevention of influenza A and B: systematic review and meta-analyses of randomised controlled trials. *BMJ* 326(7401):1235, 2003.
36. Puhakka T, Lehti H, Vainionpaa R, et al: Zanamivir: a significant reduction in viral load during treatment in military conscripts with influenza. *Scand J Infect Dis* 35:52, 2003.
37. Nicholson KG, Aoki FY, Osterhaus AD, et al: Efficacy and safety of oseltamivir in treatment of acute influenza: a randomised controlled trial. Neuraminidase Inhibitor Flu Treatment Investigator Group. *Lancet* 355:1845, 2000.
38. Kaiser L, Wat C, Mills T, et al: Impact of oseltamivir treatment on influenza-related lower respiratory tract complications and hospitalizations. *Arch Intern Med* 163:1667, 2003.
39. Jefferson T, Jones M, Doshi P, et al: Neuraminidase inhibitors for preventing and treating influenza in healthy adults: systematic review and meta-analysis. *BMJ* 339:b5106, 2009.
40. Kiso M, Mitamura K, Sakai-Tagawa Y, et al: Resistant influenza A viruses in children treated with oseltamivir: descriptive study. *Lancet* 364:759, 2004.
41. Ison MG, Gubareva LV, Atmar RL, et al: Recovery of drug-resistant influenza virus from immunocompromised patients: a case series. *J Infect Dis* 193:760, 2006.
42. Lee N, Hui DS, Zuo Z, et al: A prospective intervention study on higher-dose oseltamivir treatment in adults hospitalized with influenza A and B infections. *Clin Infect Dis*. 2013;57(11):1511–1519.
43. South East Asia Infectious Disease Clinical Research Network: Effect of double dose oseltamivir on clinical and virological outcomes in children and adults admitted to hospital with severe influenza: double blind randomised controlled trial. *BMJ* 346:f3039, 2013.
44. Rodriguez WJ, Hall CB, Welliver R, et al: Efficacy and safety of aerosolized ribavirin in young children hospitalized with influenza: a double-blind, multicenter, placebo-controlled trial. *J Pediatr* 125:129, 1994.
45. Oliveira EC, Lee B, Colice GL: Influenza in the intensive care unit. *J Intensive Care Med* 18:80, 2003.
46. Guerguerian AM, Gauthier M, Lebel MH, et al: Ribavirin in ventilated respiratory syncytial virus bronchiolitis. A randomized, placebo-controlled trial. *Am J Respir Crit Care Med* 160:829, 1999.
47. Rodriguez WJ, Kim HW, Brandt CD, et al: Aerosolized ribavirin in the treatment of patients with respiratory syncytial virus disease. *Pediatr Infect Dis J* 6:159, 1987.
48. Feltes TF, Cabalka AK, Meissner HC, et al: Palivizumab prophylaxis reduces hospitalization due to respiratory syncytial virus in young children with hemodynamically significant congenital heart disease. *J Pediatr* 143:532, 2003.
49. Mejias A, Chavez-Bueno S, Jafri HS, et al: Respiratory syncytial virus infections: old challenges and new opportunities. *Pediatr Infect Dis J* 24[Suppl 11]:S189, 2005.
50. van Woensel JB, van Aalderen WM, de Weerd W, et al: Dexamethasone for treatment of patients mechanically ventilated for lower respiratory tract infection caused by respiratory syncytial virus. *Thorax* 58:383, 2003.
51. Buckingham SC, Jafri HS, Bush AJ, et al: A randomized, double-blind, placebo-controlled trial of dexamethasone in severe respiratory syncytial virus (RSV) infection: effects on RSV quantity and clinical outcome. *J Infect Dis* 185:1222, 2002.
52. Bordigoni P, Carret AS, Venard V, et al: Treatment of adenovirus infections in patients undergoing allogeneic hematopoietic stem cell transplantation. *Clin Infect Dis* 32:1290, 2001.
53. Ribaud P, Scieux C, Freymuth F, et al: Successful treatment of adenovirus disease with intravenous cidofovir in an unrelated stem-cell transplant recipient. *Clin Infect Dis* 28:690, 1999.
54. Barker JH, Luby JP, Sean Dalley A, et al: Fatal type 3 adenoviral pneumonia in immunocompetent adult identical twins. *Clin Infect Dis* 37:e142, 2003.
55. Dunkle LM, Arvin AM, Whitley RJ, et al: A controlled trial of acyclovir for chickenpox in normal children. *N Engl J Med* 325:1539, 1991.
56. Wallace MR, Bowler WA, Murray NB, et al: Treatment of adult varicella with oral acyclovir. A randomized, placebo-controlled trial. *Ann Intern Med* 117:358, 1992.
57. Mer M, Richards GA: Corticosteroids in life-threatening varicella pneumonia. *Chest* 114:426, 1998.
58. Perry RT, Halsey NA: The clinical significance of measles: a review. *J Infect Dis* 189[Suppl 1]:S4, 2004.
59. Rupp ME, Schwartz ML, Bechard DE: Measles pneumonia. Treatment of a near-fatal case with corticosteroids and vitamin A. *Chest* 103:1625, 1993.
60. Tatsukawa M, Sawayama Y, Nabeshima S, et al: A case of severe adult measles pneumonia—efficacy of combination of steroid pulse therapy, high-dose vitamin A and gamma globulins. *Kansenshogaku Zasshi* 75:989, 2001.
61. Forni AL, Schluger NW, Roberts RB: Severe measles pneumonitis in adults: evaluation of clinical characteristics and therapy with intravenous ribavirin. *Clin Infect Dis* 19:454, 1994.
62. Yu WC, Hui DS, Chan-Yeung M: Antiviral agents and corticosteroids in the treatment of severe acute respiratory syndrome (SARS). *Thorax* 59:643, 2004.
63. Auyeung TW, Lee JS, Lai WK, et al: The use of corticosteroid as treatment in SARS was associated with adverse outcomes: a retrospective cohort study. *J Infect* 51:98, 2005.
64. Mertz GJ, Miedzinski L, Goade D, et al: Placebo-controlled, double-blind trial of intravenous ribavirin for the treatment of hantavirus cardiopulmonary syndrome in North America. *Clin Infect Dis* 39:1307, 2004.
65. Huggins JW, Hsiang CM, Cosgriff TM, et al: Prospective, double-blind, concurrent, placebo-controlled clinical trial of intravenous ribavirin therapy of hemorrhagic fever with renal syndrome. *J Infect Dis* 164:1119, 1991.
66. Govorkova EA, Leneva IA, Goloubeva OG, et al: Comparison of efficacies of RWJ-270201, zanamivir, and oseltamivir against H5N1, H9N2, and other avian influenza viruses. *Antimicrob Agents Chemother* 45:2723, 2001.
67. Gubareva LV, McCullers JA, Bethell RC, et al: Characterization of influenza A/HongKong/156/97 (H5N1) virus in a mouse model and protective effect of zanamivir on H5N1 infection in mice. *J Infect Dis* 178:1592, 1998.
68. Leneva IA, Goloubeva O, Fenton RJ, et al: Efficacy of zanamivir against avian influenza A viruses that possess genes encoding H5N1 internal proteins and are pathogenic in mammals. *Antimicrob Agents Chemother* 45:1216, 2001.
69. Chotpitayasunondh T, Ungchusak K, Hanshaoworakul W, et al: Human disease from influenza A (H5N1), Thailand, 2004. *Emerg Infect Dis* 11:201, 2005.
70. de Jong MD, Tran TT, Truong HK, et al: Oseltamivir resistance during treatment of influenza A (H5N1) infection. *N Engl J Med* 353:2667, 2005.
71. Tran TH, Nguyen TL, Nguyen TD, et al: Avian influenza A (H5N1) in 10 patients in Vietnam. *N Engl J Med* 350:1179, 2004.

Chapter 84 ■ Middle East Respiratory Syndrome (MERS) Coronavirus

CHRISTOPHER M. COLEMAN • MATTHEW B. FRIEMAN

CORONAVIRUSES ARE IMPORTANT EMERGING PATHOGENS

The *Coronaviridae* are a family of viruses that infect a wide-range of animal species, including humans. Coronaviruses (CoV) are large positive-sense RNA viruses. The virion is enveloped with cellular membrane and is formed of the virus-encoded structural proteins, of which spike (S) protein is the main attachment factor responsible for entry of the virion into the host cell [1]. Of the known human coronaviruses (hCoV), all cause respiratory tract infections of varying severity. There are a number of less pathogenic coronaviruses, namely hCoV-229E, hCoV-HKU1, hCoV-OC43, and hCoV-NL63, that cause common-cold–like symptoms in healthy adults, though all of these coronaviruses have been associated with more severe diseases in particularly susceptible populations, such as those with immune deficiencies, the young or the elderly [2,3]. However, since 2003 there have been two incidences of highly pathogenic coronaviruses in humans, emerging from zoonotic reservoirs: severe acute respiratory syndrome (SARS)-CoV and Middle East respiratory syndrome (MERS)-CoV, which cause severe respiratory infections that can lead to lethal disease in previously healthy adults [4,5].

SARS-CoV was the first identified coronavirus that developed into highly lethal severe respiratory tract infection. The first confirmed case was in November 2002, after which it spread around the world to 26 countries, causing 8,096 confirmed cases and 774 deaths (a case fatality rate of 9.6%) [4,6]. The last reported community-acquired infection was in July 2003 because SARS-CoV was eventually controlled by effective quarantine of infected persons and elimination of the direct animal reservoir. During the SARS-CoV epidemic, therapy for severe cases was restricted to standard respiratory support and there were, and still are not, any approved treatments or vaccines for specific use against SARS-CoV [7].

All known human coronaviruses, except for hCoV-229E, have strong evidence of a zoonotic origin. SARS-CoV emerged in 2003 in the Guangdong province of China from Chinese horseshoe bats of the *Rhinolophidae* family [8] and passed into humans via raccoon dogs and civet cats [9] in the wet markets of China, where all of these species interact with each other.

EMERGENCE OF MERS-CoV

In November 2012, the first report of MERS-CoV infection in humans was of a case that presented with severe respiratory infection in July 2012 [5]. As of March 2016, MERS-CoV has spread to 27 countries, causing 1,625 confirmed cases and 585 deaths (a case fatality rate of 36%; www.who.org). It was suggested that the high case fatality rate was due to underreporting of asymptomatic or mild MERS-CoV infection; however, large-scale screens of populations of the Middle East have so far failed to show large numbers of people exposed to MERS-CoV [10].

The vast majority of MERS-CoV cases are in the Middle East, in particular the Kingdom of Saudi Arabia, and most cases reported outside of the Middle East are in people who travelled to the Middle East, became infected with MERS-CoV and then returned home prior to developing symptoms, resulting in small numbers of case reports in countries such as the United States [11]. There is evidence of human-to-human transmission of MERS-CoV, though community-acquired MERS-CoV infections do not appear to be a significant aspect of MERS-CoV transmission. However, once in a hospital setting with many comorbid patients, MERS-CoV spreads efficiently, causing lethal disease as well as asymptomatic cases, including healthy adults.

A prime example of the transmissibility of MERS-CoV was a recent outbreak in the Republic of Korea (ROK) in 2015 [12]. In ROK, a patient travelled to the Middle East became infected with MERS-CoV and then returned home to Seoul. After returning home, he fell ill and became patient 0 in the outbreak that occurred there. Once symptoms developed, the patient travelled through the ROK medical system, and it has been possible to track the spread of MERS-CoV through other patients and medical staff in that system [13,14]. The ROK outbreak eventually caused a total of 186 confirmed cases and 33 deaths, none of whom, other than patient 0, had any other recent travel to the Middle East. This suggests that human-to-human transmission can and does occur when there is close and sustained contact with a MERS-CoV–infected individual [15].

There is evidence that MERS-CoV exists in bat populations in the Middle East, particularly the Egyptian tomb bat (*Taphozous perforates*) [16], and, therefore, this is the ultimate reservoir of MERS-CoV. There is also evidence that dromedary camels (*Camelus dromedaries*) act as an intermediate between bats and humans [17,18]. Camels are an extremely important species in the Middle East, where they are a source of meat, fabric, and milk, and camel racing is an important part of the cultural and economic development in the region.

MERS-CoV RECEPTOR USAGE AND TROPISM

The cell surface receptor for MERS-CoV has been identified as dipeptidyl peptidase-4 (DPP4) [19]. DPP4 is a promiscuous enzyme with a wide-range of substrates, including cytokines [20], growth factors [21], and incretins such as glucagon-like protein 1 (GLP1) [22]. DPP4 is widely expressed in many organs, but levels of expression vary, even within an organ. DPP4 is expressed in the human respiratory tract [23], in particular in alveolar epithelial cells (both type I and type II), alveolar macrophages and less so in the upper respiratory tract [23]. This suggests that MERS-CoV has a particular affinity for the lower respiratory tract, the site usually associated with more severe respiratory infections. Interestingly, DPP4 in the lower respiratory tract was shown to be unregulated in patients with chronic lung diseases [23], suggesting that there are conditions that can predispose a patient to a higher burden of pulmonary MERS-CoV infection.

DPP4 is also highly expressed in the kidney [24], kidney cells are susceptible to MERS-CoV infection *in vitro* [25] and individual case reports have reported kidney problems as a results of MERS-CoV infection, including in the first reported MERS-CoV infection [5]. There is also *in vitro* evidence that MERS-CoV can infect circulating T cells [26], which suggest that MERS-CoV can be found in the blood. However, there is currently no evidence of direct infection by MERS-CoV of any cell outside the lung during human infections.

TABLE 84.1

Presenting Symptoms of MERS-CoV Patients

Symptoms of MERS-CoV infection at presentation	
Common symptoms (>30% of cases)	**Less common symptoms (<30% of cases)**
Arthralgia	Diarrhea
Chills	Headache
Cough (dry or productive)	Hemoptysis
Fever	Nausea
Malaise	Rhinorrhea
Myalgia	Sore throat
Shortness of breath	Vomiting

Information in this table is derived from a review of MERS-CoV–associated symptoms [31].

The interaction between the MERS-CoV S protein and DPP4 is highly dependent on the posttranslational modification of DPP4. Mice cannot be infected with MERS-CoV [27] and it has been shown that mouse DPP4 is not a functional receptor for MERS-CoV [28], because mouse DPP4 contains a glycosylated residue that conflicts with MERS-CoV S binding [29].

MERS-CoV CLINICAL SYMPTOMS AND RISK FACTORS

After a predicted incubation period of 5 to 14 days [30], severe MERS-CoV–induced disease typically begins with fever, cough, chills, sore throat, myalgia, and arthralgia that progresses to pneumonia that often requires mechanical ventilation of other support within the first week (Table 84.1) [31]. Though respiratory symptoms are the major feature of MERS-CoV infection, some patients also develop gastrointestinal symptoms, such as vomiting or diarrhea [31] and there is evidence that MERS-CoV RNA can be isolated from blood, urine and stool of infected patients [32]. Furthermore, there are suggestions that kidney failure was a result of MERS-CoV infection, including in the first reported case [5] and epidemiological analysis has shown a correlation between MERS-CoV and kidney failure [33,34], however, it remains unclear if this is a direct result of MERS-CoV replication in any organ outside the lung, or is a result of the multi-organ failure caused by a severe pneumonia.

There has only been a single autopsy report of a fatal human MERS-CoV infection [35]. The lungs displayed extensive damage, with diffuse alveolar damage, denuding of the bronchiolar epithelium and type II pneumocyte hyperplasia [35]. There is also evidence of edema and the alveolar septa were thickened with lymphocytes (but not plasma cells), neutrophils, and macrophages [35]. The authors also observed damage to other organs, such as the kidney and spleen, but did not observe any MERS-CoV antigen or RNA in these areas [35], suggesting that these features were not a direct result of MERS-CoV infection and may also be due to an extended time from death to autopsy.

Direct exposure to dromedary camels is a risk factor for developing MERS-CoV infection [36], which further suggests that camels, or animals closely linked to them, are the intermediate reservoir of MERS-CoV. Epidemiological studies of risk factors for developing severe symptoms of MERS-CoV infection have suggested that comorbidities have a strong correlation with severe MERS-CoV infection (Table 84.2) [34,36,37]. In particular, preexisting diabetes is strongly associated with a more severe outcome from MERS-CoV infection [34]. Some have suggested that age is a factor in severe MERS-CoV infection [37]; however, others have not shown a strong correlation [34] and age may be a factor only in the sense that other comorbidities increase with age. Later analyses have suggested that there is no significant association between severe MERS-CoV and gender [34,37], despite data occasionally showing a significant correlation between severe MERS-CoV disease and being male [38,39] that were most likely a result of external factors, such as males usually being responsible for handling camels and therefore more exposed to MERS-CoV [36,39].

TABLE 84.2

Risk Factors and Comorbidities for Severe MERS-CoV–Associated Disease

Age
Diabetes
Direct exposure to dromedary camels
End-stage renal disease
Heart disease
Obesity
Pneumonia
Pulmonary infiltrate on chest X-ray
Smoking
Travel to the Middle East

Information is this table is derived from epidemiological analyses of MERS-CoV risk factors and comorbidities [34,36,37]. Each factor in the table has been associated with MERS-CoV in at least one of these studies. Gender, specifically being male, is excluded from the table, as this factor has been specifically identified with access to dromedary camels [36,39].

ISOLATION OF INFECTED PATIENTS AND CONTAINMENT OF SECRETIONS

Because human-to-human transmission does occur, isolation of infected patients in isolation rooms with negative pressure is recommended. All medical staff attending to suspected MERS-CoV–infected patients should wear personal protective equipment to protect against transmission, including gowns, gloves, and face shield or goggles that are either disposable or able to be cleaned with disinfectants [40]. Additionally, all equipment used on MERS-CoV–infected patients should be thoroughly sterilized, or disposed of in a fully contained waste receptacle after use and patients who need to leave isolation should wear the same protective equipment as the medical staff [40]. It is also important to establish a clear infection control plan for use in the hospital setting, including rapid diagnostic and safety protocols [41].

TREATMENTS FOR MERS-CoV

There are currently no approved treatments or vaccines for MERS-CoV and use of antivirals to treat MERS-CoV is limited to advisory opinions for the most severe cases (Table 84.3) [42]. There have been no specific guidelines issued on the use of specific supportive therapies, such as steroids, colloid, or electrolytes for MERS-CoV–associated pneumonia; however, any therapy with immunosuppressive activity should be used with care in MERS-CoV–infected patients, as this may exacerbate the disease.

In vitro screens of FDA-approved compounds have identified a number of inhibitors of MERS-CoV [43,44], but none has been tested in human clinical trials as a treatment for MERS-CoV infection. A number of small-scale trials, however, have been

TABLE 84.3

Summary of Clinical Trials for MERS-CoV Therapeutics

Intervention	Year	Study	Number of patients	Findings	Reference
Ribavirin + IFN-α2b	2014	Observational	5	No improvement in outcome	[48]
Ribavirin + IFN-α2a	2014	Retrospective	20	Improvement at 14 d posttreatment but higher mortality at 28 d posttreatment	[47]
Ribavirin + IFN-α2b	2014	Observational	2 (first RT-PCR positive for MERS-CoV, second was close contact, never MERS-CoV positive, but had clinical symptoms)	First patient improved with treatment, second patient started prophylactically and never developed MERS-CoV	[49]

attempted in severe cases of MERS-CoV using treatments that show efficacy against other viruses. Ribavirin and type I interferons (IFN) have been shown to be effective against viruses such as hepatitis C virus [45] and in an animal model of MERS-CoV infection [46]. Therefore, these have been used for a small number of cases to attempt to treat MERS-CoV. A retrospective study suggested that treatment with ribavirin and IFN-α2a correlated with enhanced survival at 14 days posttreatment, though not at 28 days posttreatment [47], however, as acknowledged by the authors themselves, the sample size was low and there have been no placebo controlled trials of this combination in the treatment of MERS-CoV. Additionally, in at least one study, use of ribavirin and IFN-α2b was shown to have no effect on outcome of MERS-CoV infection [48]. In a third study, two patients were also treated with ribavirin and IFN-α2b. The first patient developed respiratory symptoms and was treated with ribavirin and IFN-α2b at first symptom development, 72 hours before being shown to be MERS-CoV positive by RT-PCR. This patient recovered and was discharged. The second patient, the wife of the first, was given ribavirin and IFN-α2b prophylactically and developed respiratory symptoms, but was never MERS-CoV RT-PCR positive. This patient also recovered and was discharged. In total, these studies suggest no effect of ribavirin and IFN-α2b and potentially a worse outcome from this treatment. Interestingly, ribavirin and IFN-α2b treatment is still being used in KSA and further analysis of larger cohorts of patients is forthcoming. No other treatments are currently approved for use in MERS patients.

Novel treatments designed to specifically inhibit MERS-CoV are still in the very early stages of development, but several have shown promise *in vitro* and in animal models. However, none of these have yet entered clinical trials and, therefore, are some time away from being used in clinics to treat MERS-CoV infection.

References

1. Perlman S, Dandekar AA: Immunopathogenesis of coronavirus infections: implications for SARS. *Nat Rev Immunol* 5(12):917–927, 2005.
2. Talbot HK, Crowe JE Jr, Edwards KM, et al: Coronavirus infection and hospitalizations for acute respiratory illness in young children. *J Med Virol* 81(5):853–856, 2009.
3. Gorse GJ, O'Connor TZ, Hall SL, et al: Human coronavirus and acute respiratory illness in older adults with chronic obstructive pulmonary disease. *J Infect Dis* 199(6):847–857, 2009.
4. Peiris JS, Lai ST, Poon LL, et al: Coronavirus as a possible cause of severe acute respiratory syndrome. *Lancet* 361(9366):1319–1325, 2003.
5. Zaki AM, van Boheemen S, Bestebroer TM, et al: Isolation of a novel coronavirus from a man with pneumonia in Saudi Arabia. *N Engl J Med* 367(19):1814–1820, 2012.
6. Marra MA, Jones SJ, Astell CR, et al: The genome sequence of the SARS-associated coronavirus. *Science* 300(5624):1399–1404, 2003.
7. Coleman CM, Frieman MB: Coronaviruses: important emerging human pathogens. *J Virol* 88(10):5209–5212, 2014.
8. Ge XY, Li JL, Yang XL, et al: Isolation and characterization of a bat SARS-like coronavirus that uses the ACE2 receptor. *Nature* 503(7477):535–538, 2013.
9. Guan Y, Zheng BJ, He YQ, et al: Isolation and characterization of viruses related to the SARS coronavirus from animals in southern China. *Science* 302(5643):276–278, 2003.
10. Muller MA, Meyer B, Corman VM, et al: Presence of Middle East respiratory syndrome coronavirus antibodies in Saudi Arabia: a nationwide, cross-sectional, serological study. *Lancet Infect Dis* 15(5):559–564, 2015.
11. Bialek SR, Allen D, Alvarado-Ramy F, et al: First confirmed cases of Middle East respiratory syndrome coronavirus (MERS-CoV) infection in the United States, updated information on the epidemiology of MERS-CoV infection, and guidance for the public, clinicians, and public health authorities - May 2014. *MMWR Morb Mortal Wkly Rep* 63(19):431–436, 2014.
12. Lee SS, Wong NS: Probable transmission chains of Middle East respiratory syndrome coronavirus and the multiple generations of secondary infection in South Korea. *Int J Infect Dis* 38:65–67, 2015.
13. Ki M: 2015 MERS outbreak in Korea: hospital-to-hospital transmission. *Epidemiol Health* 37:e2015033, 2015.
14. Kim KM, Ki M, Cho SI, et al: Epidemiologic features of the first MERS outbreak in Korea: focus on Pyeongtaek St. Mary's Hospital. *Epidemiol Health* 37:e2015041, 2015.
15. Korea Centers for Disease Control and Prevention: Middle East Respiratory Syndrome Coronavirus Outbreak in the Republic of Korea, 2015. *Osong Public Health Res Perspect* 6(4):269–278, 2015.
16. Memish ZA, Mishra N, Olival KJ, et al: Middle East respiratory syndrome coronavirus in bats, Saudi Arabia. *Emerg Infect Dis* 19(11):1819–1823, 2013.
17. Haagmans BL, Al Dhahiry SH, Reusken CB, et al: Middle East respiratory syndrome coronavirus in dromedary camels: an outbreak investigation. *Lancet Infect Dis* 14(2):140–145, 2014.
18. Alagaili AN, Briese T, Mishra N, et al: Middle East respiratory syndrome coronavirus infection in dromedary camels in Saudi Arabia. *MBio* 5(2):e00884–14.
19. Raj VS, Mou H, Smits SL, et al: Dipeptidyl peptidase 4 is a functional receptor for the emerging human coronavirus-EMC. *Nature* 495(7440):251–254, 2013.
20. O'Leary H, Ou X, Broxmeyer HE, et al: The role of dipeptidyl peptidase 4 in hematopoiesis and transplantation. *Curr Opin Hematol* 20(4):314–319, 2013.
21. Ou X, O'Leary HA, Broxmeyer HE: Implications of DPP4 modification of proteins that regulate stem/progenitor and more mature cell types. *Blood* 122(2):161–169, 2013.
22. Barnett A: DPP-4 inhibitors and their potential role in the management of type 2 diabetes. *Int J Clin Pract* 60(11):1454–1470, 2006.
23. Meyerholz DK, Lambertz AM, McCray PB Jr: Dipeptidyl peptidase 4 distribution in the human respiratory tract: implications for the Middle East respiratory syndrome. *Am J Pathol* 186(1):78–86, 2016.
24. von Websky K, Reichetzeder C, Hocher B: Physiology and pathophysiology of incretins in the kidney. *Curr Opin Nephrol Hypertens* 23(1):54–60, 2014.
25. Eckerle I, Müller MA, Kallies S, et al: In-vitro renal epithelial cell infection reveals a viral kidney tropism as a potential mechanism for acute renal failure during Middle East Respiratory Syndrome (MERS) coronavirus infection. *Virol J* 10:359, 2013.
26. Chu H, Zhou J, Wong BH, et al: Middle east respiratory syndrome coronavirus efficiently infects human primary T lymphocytes and activates the extrinsic and intrinsic apoptosis pathways. *J Infect Dis* 213(6):904–914, 2016.
27. Coleman CM, Matthews KL, Goicochea L, et al: Wild type and innate immune deficient mice are not susceptible to the Middle East Respiratory Syndrome coronavirus. *J Gen Virol* 95:408–412, 2013.
28. Cockrell AS, Peck KM, Yount BL, et al: Mouse dipeptidyl peptidase 4 is not a functional receptor for Middle East respiratory syndrome coronavirus infection. *J Virol* 88(9):5195–5199, 2014.

29. Peck KM, Cockrell AS, Yount BL, et al: Glycosylation of mouse DPP4 plays a role in inhibiting Middle East Respiratory Syndrome Coronavirus Infection. *J Virol* 89(8):4696–4699, 2015.
30. Assiri A, Al-Tawfiq JA, Al-Rabeeah AA, et al: Epidemiological, demographic, and clinical characteristics of 47 cases of Middle East respiratory syndrome coronavirus disease from Saudi Arabia: a descriptive study. *Lancet Infect Dis* 13(9):752–761, 2013.
31. Zumla A, Hui DS, Perlman S: Middle East respiratory syndrome. *Lancet* 386(9997):995–1007, 2015.
32. Poissy J, Goffard A, Parmentier-Decrucq E, et al: Kinetics and pattern of viral excretion in biological specimens of two MERS-CoV cases. *J Clin Virol* 61(2):275–278, 2014.
33. Cha RH, Joh JS, Jeong I, et al: Renal complications and their prognosis in Korean patients with Middle East respiratory syndrome-coronavirus from the Central MERS-CoV Designated Hospital. *J Korean Med Sci* 30(12):1807–1814, 2015.
34. Al-Tawfiq JA, Hinedi K, Ghandour J, et al: Middle East respiratory syndrome coronavirus: a case-control study of hospitalized patients. *Clin Infect Dis* 59(2):160–165, 2014.
35. Ng DL, Al Hosani F, Keating MK, et al: Clinicopathologic, immunohistochemical, and ultrastructural findings of a fatal case of Middle East respiratory syndrome coronavirus infection in United Arab Emirates, April 2014. *Am J Pathol* 186(3):652–658, 2016.
36. Alraddadi BM, Watson JT, Almarashi A, et al: Risk factors for primary Middle East respiratory syndrome coronavirus illness in humans, Saudi Arabia, 2014. *Emerg Infectious Dis* 22(1):49–55, 2016.
37. Alsahafi AJ, Cheng AC: The epidemiology of Middle East Respiratory Syndrome (MERS) coronavirus in the Kingdom of Saudi Arabia, 2012-2015. *Int J Infect Dis* 45:1–4, 2016.
38. Alghamdi IG, Hussain II, Almalki SS, et al: The pattern of Middle East respiratory syndrome coronavirus in Saudi Arabia: a descriptive epidemiological analysis of data from the Saudi Ministry of Health. *Int J Gen Med* 7:417–423, 2014.
39. Banik GR, Alqahtani AS, Booy R, et al: Risk factors for severity and mortality in patients with MERS-CoV: analysis of publicly available data from Saudi Arabia. *Virol Sin* 31(1):81–84, 2016.
40. Kim JY, Song JY, Yoon YK, et al: Middle East respiratory syndrome infection control and prevention guideline for healthcare facilities. *Infect Chemother* 47(4):278–302, 2015.
41. Butt TS, Koutlakis-Barron I, AlJumaah S, et al: Infection control and prevention practices implemented to reduce transmission risk of Middle East respiratory syndrome-coronavirus in a tertiary care institution in Saudi Arabia. *Am J Infect Control* 44(5):605–611, 2016.
42. Chong YP, Song JY, Seo YB, et al: Antiviral treatment guidelines for Middle East respiratory syndrome. *Infect Chemother* 47(3):212–222, 2015.
43. Dyall J, Coleman CM, Hart BJ, et al: Repurposing of clinically developed drugs for treatment of middle East respiratory syndrome coronavirus infection. *Antimicrob Agents Chemother* 58(8):4885–4893, 2014.
44. de Wilde AH, Coleman CM, Hart BJ, et al: Screening of an FDA-approved compound library identifies four small-molecule inhibitors of Middle East respiratory syndrome coronavirus replication in cell culture. *Antimicrob Agents Chemother* 58(8):4875–4884, 2014.
45. Hauser G, Awad T, Brok J, et al: Peginterferon plus ribavirin versus interferon plus ribavirin for chronic hepatitis C. *Cochrane Database Syst Rev* 2:CD005441, 2014.
46. Falzarano D, de Wit E, Feldmann F, et al: Infection with MERS-CoV causes lethal pneumonia in the common marmoset. *PLoS Pathog* 10(8):e1004250, 2014.
47. Omrani AS, Saad MM, Baig K, et al: Ribavirin and interferon alfa-2a for severe Middle East respiratory syndrome coronavirus infection: a retrospective cohort study. *Lancet Infect Dis* 14(11):1090–1095, 2014.
48. Al-Tawfiq JA , Momattin H, Dib J, et al: Ribavirin and interferon therapy in patients infected with the Middle East respiratory syndrome coronavirus: an observational study. *Int J Infect Dis* 20:42–46, 2014.
49. Khalid M, Al Rabiah F, Khan B, et al: Ribavirin and interferon (IFN)-alpha-2b as primary and preventive treatment for Middle East respiratory syndrome coronavirus (MERS-CoV): a preliminary report of two cases. *Antivir Ther* 20(1):87–91, 2015.

Chapter 85 ■ Critical Care of Patients Infected with Ebola Virus

STEVEN HATCH

Ebola virus disease (EVD), a severe illness caused by various strains of the filovirus Ebola, represents a major concern for critical care units in resource-rich settings not only because of the lethality of the infection but also because of issues pertaining to infection control, resource allocation, and treatment ethics. EVD had previously been confined to small outbreaks in Central Africa; however, the West African Outbreak that began in 2014 ultimately spread to ten countries on three different continents and affected more than 10 times the number of people from all previous Ebola outbreaks combined [1]. The size and worldwide nature of this outbreak demonstrates that health care facilities require protocols for the care of patients who might be or are definitively harboring Biosafety Level 4 agents such as Ebola.

The following chapter will review special considerations for the diagnosis and care of patients with Ebola virus infection. Given its similar taxonomy and clinical features, the principles discussed here almost certainly apply in like manner to patients suffering from Marburg virus disease, which since its original episode in Germany has not been observed outside of sub-Saharan Africa, but is equally likely to present off the African continent given the ease and increase of international travel.

EPIDEMIOLOGY AND PATHOGENESIS

There are four principal strains of the virus that are known to cause virus in humans: Zaire (ZEBOV), Sudan (SEBOV), Bundibugyo (BDBV), and Taï Forest (TAFV), the last of which has only had one known human case [2]. ZEBOV and SEBOV outbreaks are associated with a significantly higher mortality rate (approximately 50% to 90%) than BDBV (approximately 25%) [3,4]. A fifth strain, the Reston Ebolavirus (RESTV), has thus far not been associated with human disease, although antibody responses of humans exposed to the virus have been observed [5].

The transmission of Ebola primarily takes place by direct contact with body fluids, where virions enter into the host via mucous membranes or skin breaks [6]. Ebola virus has been detected in virtually every body fluid [7]. The virus has now been shown to persist for months in semen, effectively making EVD a sexually transmitted disease well past the time when outbreaks have traditionally been considered to have run their course [8]. Parenteral introduction of the virus, such as seen with needlestick exposures, often cause severe disease and represent a major hazard for medical personnel caring for patients with EVD in high-resource settings [9].

Incubation of the virus typically lasts between 2 and 21 days; most cases present in the second week following exposure [10]. The relatively long incubation times coupled with highly efficient transcontinental travel underscores the importance of heightened surveillance and the need for health care facilities everywhere to have response plans in place. Of the four cases of Ebola diagnosed in the United States, two had acquired the virus in Africa [11]. Therefore, patients from Ebola-endemic countries presenting with circulatory collapse in the setting of a febrile illness may require rapid isolation and testing for Ebola and Marburg.

The bulk of pathophysiologic studies have been performed on nonhuman primates (NHPs) in Biosafety Level 4 facilities; the presentation of EVD in NHPs is similar to that of humans and the fatality rate is likewise similar [12]. NHP studies have demonstrated that significant disruption of the endothelial and epithelial barriers of the colon takes place, leading to diffuse mucosal injury and inflammation [13]. This, in turn, may lead to gut translocation of gram-negative organisms, potentially leading to bacterial sepsis as a major cause of mortality [14]. Moreover, the cytokine cascade induced by EVD (which includes a complex interplay of TNF-α, IL-1-β, IL-6, IL-10, and various interferons) probably produces intravascular coagulation and may account for the hemorrhage of EVD cases when hemorrhage occurs [15].

CLINICAL PRESENTATION

EVD typically presents initially as a viral prodrome with nonspecific symptoms, making clinical diagnosis essentially impossible except in large outbreaks. The overwhelming majority of patients present with fever [16]. Some previous studies have noted that body temperatures in EVD can fluctuate [17]. Other common early symptoms include fatigue, arthralgias and myalgias, anorexia, headache, and abdominal pain. A diffuse, erythematous nonpruritic maculopapular rash was only rarely reported in the West African Outbreak, although it appeared to have been more prevalent among the whites who became infected and thus may have been underdiagnosed in Africans with darker skin [18].

Confirmation of EVD is done via reverse transcription polymerase chain reaction (RT-PCR). Because the test may not be positive in the early stages of the illness, a patient with suspected EVD and a negative RT-PCR test less than 72 hours after onset of symptoms does not necessarily rule out infection. If the patient is no longer symptomatic after 72 hours, repeat testing is not required; however, patients with ongoing symptoms must be retested. Similarly, if a patient with symptoms greater than 72 hours in duration tests negative, EVD is ruled out.

Laboratory values in the setting of EVD resemble those of other acute viral illnesses, with common findings including leukopenia (with or without atypical lymphocytosis), thrombocytopenia, transaminitis (AST > ALT), hyponatremia, hypocalcemia, elevated creatinine, elevated lactate, hypoalbuminemia, and prolonged prothrombin time (PT) and partial thromboplastin time (PTT) values. Potassium regulation can be difficult, as one study indicated that equal numbers of patients developed hypo- or hyperkalemia [19]. As with symptoms of EVD, pathognomonic clinical signs do not exist, although a pulse-temperature dissociation similar to that seen in typhoid fever has been observed, and a saddleback fever curve has also been reported for some patients. Hiccups may also be seen and should prompt suspicion in the setting of other appropriate epidemiologic clues [20].

EVD is primarily a gastrointestinal syndrome that can cause massive fluid losses. For instance, during the West African Outbreak an epidemiologist working for the WHO became infected and was flown to Germany on the 10th day after onset of symptoms; the patient was recorded to have total fluid losses of nearly 10 L per day, mainly in the form of diarrhea and, to a smaller extent, vomiting [21]. Coupled with insensible losses from fevers, the significant fluid depletion often leads to circulatory collapse and likely accounts at least in part for the high mortality of the disease.

Despite its reputation as a disease with a massive bleeding diathesis, EVD does not typically present with frank hemorrhage. The prevalence of bleeding of any kind before the West African Outbreak was reported to be in the range of approximately 50%; during the West African Outbreak, at least one study reported a prevalence of less than 20% [22]. Studies in previous outbreaks indicated that, although less common, hemorrhage was typically associated with a worse prognosis [23]. Similarly, mental status changes such as encephalopathy probably reflects end-organ damage and carries a high mortality. The clinical presentation, laboratory symptoms, and prognostic factors associated with EVD are summarized in Table 85.1.

Survival and convalescence are prolonged. While many patients experience rapid improvement, they remain viremic for as long as 21 days or more [24]. Therefore, provisions need to be made for convalescing patients who must remain in isolation during this time, and psychosocial needs may outweigh physiologic considerations, as survivors commonly cope with fear, grief, and anxiety about the social stigma that may await them following discharge [25]. Current WHO guidelines for discharge is that the patient meet the criteria of having no signs and symptoms of EVD, as well as two negative Ebola PCR tests on whole blood separated by at least 48 hours [26].

Following discharge, patients experience a range of complications that can be debilitating and last for months or even years. These complications are summarized in Table 85.2. The persistence of Ebola virus in immunologically privileged "sanctuary" sites, such as semen [27] and ocular fluid [28], indicates that special precautions must be taken when evaluating survivors

TABLE 85.1

Common Symptoms, Laboratory Abnormalities, and Mortality Risk Factors Associated with Ebola Virus Disease [19,51–54]

Symptoms	Laboratory test abnormalities	Factors associated with increased mortality
Fever	Leukopenia	Age >40
Vomiting	Thrombocytopenia	Viral load >10^6 copies/mL
Diarrhea	Elevated AST	Confusion
Malaise or fatigue	Hyponatremia	RIFLE-3 acute kidney injury
Anorexia	Hypokalemia	Hyperkalemia
Abdominal pain	Hypocalcemia	AST >525 U/L
Myalgia or arthralgia	Elevated creatinine	Elevated hematocrit
Conjunctivitis	Elevated creatinine kinase	
Confusion	Elevated C-reactive protein	
Hiccups	Lactic acidosis	
Sore throat	Prolonged PT and PTT	

PT, prothrombin time; PTT, partial thromboplastin time

TABLE 85.2

Common Symptomatic Complications and Objective Clinical Sequelae of Ebola Virus Infection [55,56]

Complications	Clinical sequelae
Anorexia (80%–100%)	Auditory symptoms (25%)
Arthralgia (75%)	Uveitis (20%)
Fatigue (75%)	Persistence of virus in semen and ocular fluid
Ocular symptoms (60%)	
Difficulty concentrating (40%)	
Headaches (25%)	
Insomnia (20%)	

in routine follow-up care, with Biosafety Level 4 protocols being used in the event that providers might be exposed to fluids from these viral reservoirs.

INFECTION CONTROL AND OTHER SAFETY CONSIDERATIONS

The management of patients with EVD must be carried out with maximum adherence to infection control procedures and health care worker safety considerations. In critical care settings, the need for safety protocols is even greater due to the larger number of opportunities for occupational exposure.

If faced with the care of a patient with suspected or confirmed EVD, health care facilities should have a specialized, fully trained team of health care workers assigned to such patients. The team would include all personnel whose work is necessary in intensive care settings. Periodic training and "dry run" simulations should be considered, especially due to the physically demanding nature of Ebola care brought on by the sensory deprivations of personal protective equipment (PPE).

The Centers for Disease Control and Prevention (CDC) recommends standard, contact, and droplet precautions for isolation of and care for patients with suspected or known EVD [29]. PPE should ensure the health care worker has no skin exposed. Donning and doffing should always take place in a single decontamination area that is clearly demarcated. Only staff involved in entering or leaving the high-risk area, or those who are supervising such workers, should be allowed in such areas. The entry and exit process should proceed according to a strict step-by-step protocol provided by either the CDC or WHO. Owing to the multistep nature of the donning and doffing procedures, the protocol should be simulated multiple times by the staff. Before entering a high-risk area, the health care worker should have their PPE examined for any exposed areas. Special care should be given to evaluation of the face if goggles are being worn on top of a hood instead of a single headpiece, as the corners of the mask may not overlap.

Perfect adherence to protocol during doffing in particular is critical because this is when the outer surface of PPE may be coated in virus, and protocol deviations place health care workers at possibly the highest risk of exposure. Multiple disinfection steps with bleach solution are essential. Doffing should be supervised by a trained observer who calls out each step of the protocol. If the worker "gets lost" in the multistep process, the supervisor/observer should always spray the worker down with a bleach solution before proceeding to the next step.

Once inside a high-risk area, the care of patients with EVD proceeds as it would with any other patient. Because standard PPE in EVD care typically involves two layers of gloves, special care should be taken to any tasks requiring fine motor skill, such as IV line placement (either peripherally or centrally), hooking and unhooking IV lines, withdrawing blood for laboratory analysis, and so on.

Currently, there is controversy as to whether EVD can be transmitted through aerosols, and whether negative pressure rooms are completely necessary is a topic of debate at the time of this writing. A statement by the WHO notes that there have been no documented cases of aerosolized transmission of Ebola [30], but other specialists counter that this may be possible given findings in animal models of EVD [31]. Consequently, PPE should include either N95 respirators or powered air purifying respirators. The latter, while more expensive, have the advantages of not requiring fit testing and may provide better protection in the event of splashes.

Laboratory testing presents a special challenge in Ebola care. Because commonly tested body fluids used in clinical specimens should be regarded as highly infectious and require at least as much care with respect to decontamination as health care workers, testing should be minimized to the greatest extent possible. Point-of-care testing, when possible, should be utilized, particularly as clinical Ebola management involves monitoring and adjusting standard laboratory parameters, especially sodium and potassium, for which point-of-care products are generally found with ease.

Health care workers identified for work in a high-risk area with suspect or confirmed EVD cases should be considered candidates for Ebola vaccines if they are available. At present, multiple candidate vaccines have been studied, although no definitive results with respect to vaccine efficacy have been established at the time of this writing [32]. Consultation with CDC or WHO health officials should take place immediately in confirmed EVD cases to assess the availability of vaccines for health care staff planning on caring for such patients [33].

CRITICAL CARE MANAGEMENT

Supportive care, while not having any direct action against the Ebola virus, almost certainly has a significant impact on mortality. Of the many thousands of cases of EVD in the West African Outbreak, 24 were treated in Western countries, with five deaths, which represented a much lower case fatality rate than those infected in Africa. Moreover, of the 7 EVD cases whose symptoms began in the West, only one patient died, and this patient's diagnosis was delayed [34]. Although nearly all of these patients underwent experimental therapies, the fact that they were all provided supportive care as a single common denominator, coupled with the much lower mortality rates both in the current outbreak and in the past, indicates that such care is critically important.

Empiric antibiotics may be beneficial. As noted previously, NHP models indicate that EVD causes a massive inflammatory response in the gut mucosa, potentially leading to translocation of gut organisms and ultimately bacterial sepsis late in the course of EVD infection. Therefore, institution of broad-spectrum antibiotics may have a mortality impact. Although no definitive clinical data exist to support this, one observational study of 581 patients with EVD in Sierra Leone in 2014 showed a lower case fatality rate compared with the overall rate; all such patients were given intravenous ceftriaxone along with oral metronidazole for the first 72 hours following admission to the Ebola Treatment Unit. Coupled with the pathophysiologic studies of NHPs, the Sierra Leone data suggest that empiric broad-spectrum antibiotics should be instituted at the time of diagnosis and continued for a minimum of 72 hours [35].

No randomized trials have been performed on the value of intravenous access in EVD. However, the evidence available strongly supports the idea that parenteral access is likely to have at least a moderate, and possibly profound, favorable impact on patient care. One review concluded that the ability to infuse large volumes of fluid in order to counteract the intravascular collapse brought on by EVD is likely to yield significant benefits with respect to morbidity and mortality. If routine intravenous access cannot be obtained, intraosseous or even subcutaneous routes could be considered viable alternatives [36]. Once fluid repletion is instituted, care should be given to frequent monitoring of electrolyte levels, particularly sodium and potassium, whose values can fluctuate dramatically. There is no evidence for which crystalloid solution is superior (e.g., normal saline vs. Lactated Ringer's).

Less is known about other tools in the arsenal of critical care medicine, such as intubation and hemodialysis, as effectively the entire literature on these interventions is limited to case reports [37,38]. Still, the evidence would suggest that patients should be treated for sepsis syndrome with such technologies provided the risk to health care providers is sufficiently minimized. Noninvasive mechanical ventilation is not a recommended strategy due to the possibility of aerosolized transmission.

Other supportive care measures include antipyretics, antiemetics, and analgesics. Antipyretics should favor acetaminophen over nonsteroidal anti-inflammatory drugs (NSAIDs) due to nephrotoxicity of the latter as well as antiplatelet effects, although dosage adjustments must be considered on the basis of hepatic function. Antimotility agents are controversial because the benefits of fluid retention are balanced by the risks of translocation of gut organisms that could result in gram-negative septicemia, which has been documented in at least one case report. If the patient became infected in a malaria-endemic region, then evaluation for and treatment of malaria is indicated [39].

SPECIFIC THERAPY

In the absence of approved treatments for EVD, during the West African Outbreak, multiple drugs were provided under compassionate-use doctrines with the goal of decreasing the mortality of the disease.

Favipiravir, an oral medication used for influenza and that has been shown to have anti-Ebola activity both with in vitro and in vivo models [40], was administered in a Phase II study in Guinea, but the study was fraught with numerous experimental design flaws, preventing a comprehensive assessment of its value [41].

Unlike the "repurposed" drug favipiravir, TKM-Ebola was designed specifically with EVD treatment in mind. TKM-Ebola is a cocktail of three small interfering (si)RNA molecules intended to disrupt viral replication, transcription, assembly, and evasion of the host immune response. The drug was found to be effective in a nonhuman primate model, preventing death in 100% of animals following a lethal challenge [42]. A Phase I trial was launched during the West African Outbreak, but was put on partial hold following the discovery of high cytokine release in the study subjects [43]. It was administered under compassionate-use protocols for two other patients, both of whom survived, but their reactions during infusions (including fevers, rigors, and a general health decline) make it difficult to assess its clinical value [44].

The monoclonal antibody mixture ZMapp is designed to neutralize the virus by binding to discrete regions of the surface glycoprotein. As with TKM-Ebola, ZMapp was shown to be effective in a nonhuman primate model. However, large-scale production of ZMapp proved challenging, and its use was mainly limited to compassionate-use instances in the West. Generally, patients fared well, but other intensive care measures may have been primarily responsible for the low mortality [45]. However, a clinical trial of ZMapp in West Africa has just been completed as this book is going to press, and results should be available by its publication [46].

Two novel therapeutic approaches were not studied in humans during the West African Outbreak, but are being investigated in animal models. First, antisense oligonucleotides, referred to as "PMOs" (phosphorodiamidate morpholino oligomers) have been evaluated in Phase I trials and appear to be safe [47]. Second, the nucleoside analog BCX4430 is designed to act as a viral RNA chain terminator, and studies are ongoing as to its feasibility in humans [48].

In situations where the above drugs have not been scaled up for mass production, as well as in resource-limited settings, the use of convalescent whole blood or convalescent plasma may be considered if EVD survivors are available for donation. This strategy has been used in previous EVD outbreaks, although concerns about alloimmunization, febrile transfusion reactions, graft-versus-host disease, and other side effects would suggest this approach be considered as second-line at best [49]. Furthermore, infection control procedures surrounding the donation, manipulation, and infusion of survivor blood products, but done while minimizing the amount of equipment required in a BL-4 setting, make fast implementation a major challenge and thus may create more problems than they solve.

ETHICAL CONSIDERATIONS

The challenges of intensive care of patients with EVD not only is limited to the technical matters described above, but also impact the relationship between patient and provider, for the occupational exposure risks involved in end-of-life situations (such as cardiopulmonary resuscitation) raise the question of just how much should providers be obligated to do in such circumstances. Although no clear consensus exists at this time as to whether or not certain heroic measures can be jettisoned for EVD care, current guidelines of critically ill patients already account for the need to individualize goals of care [50], and in this respect EVD is simply one factor in the decision-making process. When possible, medical staff responsible for the care of patients with EVD should discuss with one another potential scenarios that could reasonably be postulated and how team members will react in such instances. Mobilization of a hospital ethical committee for the express purpose of considering these matters also has the potential to prevent misunderstandings so that all providers have uniform expectations of their roles and the roles of their colleagues.

Author Disclosure

The author has served as a paid consultant by Medivector, Inc., which produces the drug favipiravir and is discussed in this review.

References

1. World Health Organization: *Ebola Situation Report, 20 January 2016*.
2. Le Guenno B, Formenty P, Wyers M, et al: Isolation and partial characterisation of a new strain of Ebola virus. *Lancet* 345(8960):1271–1274, 1995.
3. Feldmann H, Geisbert TW: Ebola haemorrhagic fever. *Lancet* 377:849–862, 2011.
4. Wamala JF, Lukwago L, Malimbo M, et al: Ebola hemorrhagic fever associated with novel virus strain, Uganda, 2007–2008. *Emerg Infect Dis* 16(7):1087–1092, 2010.
5. Miranda M, Miranda J: Reston Ebolavirus in humans and animals in the Phillipines: a review. *J Infect Dis* 204[Suppl 3]:S757–S760, 2011.
6. Dowell S, Mukunu R, Ksiazek TG, et al: Transmission of Ebola hemorrhagic fever: a study of risk factors in family members, Kikwit, Democratic Republic of the Congo, 1995. *J Infect Dis* 179[Suppl 1]:S87–S91, 1999.
7. Bausch D, Towner J, Dowell S, et al: Assessment of the risk of Ebola virus transmission from bodily fluids and fomites. *J Infect Dis* 196:S142–S147, 2007.
8. Thorson A, Fomenty P, Lofthouse C, et al: Systematic review of the literature on viral persistence and sexual transmission from recovered Ebola survivors: evidence and recommendations. *BMJ Open* 6:1 e008859, 2016.
9. Gunther S, Feldmann H, Geisbert T, et al: Management of accidental exposure to Ebola virus in the biosafety level 4 laboratory, Hamburg, Germany. *J Infect Dis* 204[Suppl 3]:S785–S790, 2011.

10. Schieffelin JS, Shaffer JG, Goba A, et al: Clinical illness and outcomes in patients with Ebola in Sierra Leone. *N Engl J Med* 371(22):2092–2100, 2014.
11. Centers for Disease Control: Cases of Ebola diagnosed in the United States. Available at: http://www.cdc.gov/vhf/ebola/outbreaks/2014-west-africa/united-states-imported-case.html. Retrieved January, 2016.
12. Ebihara H, Rockx B, Marzi A, et al: Host response dynamics following lethal infection of rhesus macaques with Zaire ebolavirus. *J Infect Dis* 204[Suppl 3]:S991–S999, 2011.
13. Geisbert T, Hensley L, Larsen T, et al: Pathogenesis of Ebola hemorrhagic fever in cynomolgus macaques: evidence that dendritic cells are early and sustained targets of infection. *Am J Pathol* 163(6):2347–2370, 2003.
14. Lynn L: Combined endothelial and epithelial barrier disruption of the colon may be a contributing factor to the Ebola sepsis-like syndrome. *Patient Saf Surg* 9:1, 2015.
15. Fletcher T, Fowler R, Beeching N: Understanding organ dysfunction in Ebola virus disease. *Int Care Med* 40:1936–1939, 2014.
16. Bausch D, Sprecher A, Jeffs B: Treatment of Marburg and Ebola hemorrhagic fevers: a strategy for nesting new drugs and vaccines under outbreak conditions. *Antiviral Res* 78:150–161, 2008.
17. Kortepeter M, Bausch D, Bray M: Basic clinical and laboratory features of filoviral hemorrhagic fever. *J Infect Dis* 204:S810–S816, 2011.
18. Parra JM, Salmerón OJ, Velasco M: The first case of Ebola virus disease acquired outside Africa. *N Engl J Med* 371(25):2439–2440, 2014.
19. Hunt L, Gupta-Wright A, Simms V, et al: Clinical presentation, biochemical, and haematological parameters and their association with outcome in patients with Ebola virus disease: an observational cohort study. *Lancet Infect Dis* 15(11):1292–1299, 2015.
20. Bwaka MA, Bonnet MJ, Calain P, et al: Ebola hemorrhagic fever in Kikwit, Democratic Republic of the Congo: clinical observations in 103 patients. *J Infect Dis* 179[Suppl 1]:S1–S7, 1999.
21. Kreuels M, Wichmann D, Emmerich P, et al: A case of severe Ebola virus infection complicated by gram-negative septicemia. *N Engl J Med* 371:2394–2401, 2014.
22. WHO Ebola Response Team: Ebola virus disease in West Africa: the first 9 months of the epidemic and forward projections. *N Engl J Med* 371:1481–1495, 2014.
23. Roddy P, Howard N, Van Kerkhove M, et al: Clinical manifestations and case management of Ebola haemorrhagic fever caused by a newly identified virus strain, Bundibugyo, Uganda, 2007–2008. *PLoS One* 7(12):e52986, 2012.
24. Towner J, Rollin P, Bausch D, et al: Rapid diagnosis of Ebola hemorrhagic fever by reverse transcription-PCR in an outbreak setting and assessment of patient viral load as a predictor of outcome. *J Virol* 78(8):4330–4341, 2004.
25. Yadav S, Rawal G: The current mental health status of Ebola survivors in Western Africa. *J Clin Diagn Res* 9(10):LA01–LA02, 2015.
26. World Health Organization: Laboratory diagnosis of Ebola virus disease. Available at: http://apps.who.int/iris/bitstream/10665/134009/1/WHO_EVD_GUIDANCE_LAB_14.1_eng.pdf?ua=1. Accessed January, 2016.
27. Deen G, Knust B, Broutet N, et al: Ebola RNA persistence in semen of Ebola virus disease survivors - preliminary report. *N Engl J Med*, 2015, doi:10.1056/NEJMoa1511410,
28. Varkey JB, Shantha JG, Crozier I, et al: Persistence of Ebola virus in ocular fluid during convalescence. *N Engl J Med* 372(25):2423–2427, 2015.
29. Centers for Disease Control: Infection prevention and control recommendations for hospitalized patients under investigation (PUIs) for Ebola virus disease (EVD) in US Hospitals. Available at: http://www.cdc.gov/vhf/ebola/healthcare-us/hospitals/infection-control.html. Retrieved January, 2016.
30. World Health Organization: What we know about transmission of the Ebola virus among humans. Available at: http://www.who.int/mediacentre/news/ebola/06-october-2014/en/. Accessed January, 2016.
31. Kobinger G, Leung A, Neufeld J, et al: Replication, pathogenicity, shedding, and transmission of *Zaire ebolavirus* in pigs. *J Infect Dis* 204(2):200–208, 2011.
32. Sridhar S: Clinical development of Ebola vaccines. *Ther Adv Vaccines* 3(5–6):125–138, 2015.
33. Levine MM, Tapia M, Hill AV, et al: How the current West African Ebola virus disease epidemic is altering views on the need for vaccines and is galvanizing a global effort to field-test leading candidate vaccines. *J Infect Dis* 211(4):504, 2015.
34. New York Times staff: How many patients have been treated outside of Africa? New York Times online interactive feature. Available at: http://www.nytimes.com/interactive/2014/07/31/world/africa/ebola-virus-outbreak-qa.html?_r=0. Accessed January, 2016 (last updated January 26, 2015).
35. Ansumana R, Jacobsen K, Idris M, et al: Ebola in Freetown area, Sierra Leone—a case study of 581 patients. *N Engl J Med* 372:587–588, 2015.
36. Ker K, Tansley G, Beecher D, et al: Comparison of routes for achieving parenteral access with a focus on the management of patients with Ebola virus disease. *Cochrane Database Syst Rev* (2):CD011386, 2015, doi:10.1002/14651858.CD011386.pub2.
37. Wolf T, Kann G, Becker S, et al: Severe Ebola virus disease with vascular leakage and multiorgan failure: treatment of a patient in intensive care. *Lancet* 385(9976):1428–1435, 2015.
38. West TE, von Saint André-von Arnim A: Clinical presentation and management of severe Ebola virus disease. *Ann Am Thorac Soc* 11(9):1341–1350, 2014.
39. Fowler RA, Fletcher T, Fischer WA, et al: Caring for critically ill patients with ebola virus disease. Perspectives from West Africa. *Am J Respir Crit Care Med* 190(7):733–737, 2014.
40. Smither S, Estaugh L, Steward J, et al: Post-exposure efficacy of oral T-705 (Favipiravir) against inhalational Ebola virus infection in a mouse model. *Antiviral Res* 104:153–155, 2014.
41. Bouazza N, Treluyer J, Foissac F: Favipiravir for children with Ebola. *Lancet* 385(9968):603–604, 2015.
42. Thi EP, Mire CE, Lee AC, et al: Lipid nanoparticle siRNA treatment of Ebola-virus-Makona-infected nonhuman primates. *Nature* 521(7552):362–365, 2015.
43. Gao J, Yin L: Drug development for controlling Ebola epidemic—a race against time. *Drug Discov Ther* 8(5):229–231, 2014.
44. Kraft CS, Hewlett AL, Koepsell S: The use of TKM-100802 and convalescent plasma in 2 patients with Ebola virus disease in the United States. *Clin Infect Dis* 61(4):496–502, 2015.
45. Madelain V, Nguyen TH, Olivo A, et al: Ebola virus infection: review of the pharmacokinetic and pharmacodynamic properties of drugs considered for testing in human efficacy trials. *Clin Pharmacokinet* 55(8):907–923, 2016.
46. National Institute of Allergy and Infectious Diseases: Putative investigational therapeutics in the treatment of patients with known Ebola infection. Available at: https://clinicaltrials.gov/ct2/show/study/NCT02363322?term=zmapp+ebola&rank=1. Accessed January, 2016.
47. Heald A, Iversen P, Saoud J, et al: Safety and pharmacokinetic profiles of phosphorodiamidate morpholino oligomers with activity against ebola virus and marburg virus: results of two single-ascending-dose studies. *Antimicrob Agents Chemother* 58(11):6639, 2014.
48. Warren T, Wells J, Panchal R, et al: Protection against filovirus diseases by a novel broad-spectrum nucleoside analogue BCX4430. *Nature* 508(7496):402–405, 2014.
49. Mendoza E, Qiu X, Kobinger G: Progression of Ebola therapeutics during the 2014-2015 outbreak. *Trends Mol Med* 22(2):164–173, 2016.
50. Halpern S, Becker D, Curtis J, et al: An official American Thoracic Society/American Association of Critical-Care Nurses/American College of Chest Physicians/Society of Critical Care Medicine policy statement: the Choosing Wisely® top 5 list in critical care medicine. *Am J Resp Crit Care Med* 190(7):818–826, 2014.
51. Mattia J, Vandy M, Chang J, et al: Early clinical sequelae of Ebola virus disease in Sierra Leone: a cross-sectional study. *Lancet Infect Dis*, 2015, doi:10.1016/S1473-3099(15)00489-2.
52. Zhang X, Rong Y, Sun L, et al: Prognostic analysis of patients with Ebola virus disease. *PLoS Negl Trop Dis* 9(9):e0004113, 2015.
53. Lado M, Walker NF, Baker P: Clinical features of patients isolated for suspected Ebola virus disease at Connaught Hospital, Freetown, Sierra Leone: a retrospective cohort study. *Lancet Infect Dis* 15(9):1024–1033, 2015.
54. Fischer W, Uyeki T, Tauxe R: Ebola virus disease: what clinicians in the United States need to know. *Am J Infect Control* 43(8):788–793, 2015.
55. Qureshi A, Chughtai M, Loua T, et al: Study of Ebola virus disease survivors in Guinea. *Clin Infect Dis* 61(7):1035–1042, 2015.
56. Clark D, Kibuuka H, Millard M, et al: Long-term sequelae after Ebola virus disease in Bundibugyo, Uganda: a retrospective cohort study. *Lancet Infect Dis* 15(8):905–912, 2015.

Chapter 86 ■ Botulism

DAVID M. BEBINGER • RICHARD T. ELLISON, III

Botulism remains a rare disease but a potential threat to many people across the world. Recognition of the disease is important as it is life-threatening and treatable. Early recognition and prompt treatment improves outcomes and are essential to initiate surveillance for other potential cases in an outbreak or bioterrorism event.

The name botulism is derived from the Latin term *botulus* for sausage. Justinus Kerner (1786 to 1862) first recognized the association between the mysterious "sausage poison" and paralytic illnesses in 1820. *Clostridium botulinum*, the etiologic agent of botulism, is an anaerobic, spore-forming organism that elaborates a neurotoxin that prevents the release of acetylcholine. Genetic studies have revealed heterogeneity of the organisms containing the botulism toxin genes indicating that traditional forms of nomenclature defining the organism by the presence of the toxin gene or gene product are too simplistic. Currently, the organisms that carry the gene and produce the toxin are divided into four subspecies and two related species. This helps to explain why the toxin is seen in environments beyond the traditional loamy soils where potatoes and other vegetables implicated in outbreaks are grown [1].

Illness develops after toxin exposure, and patients present with a symmetric descending paralysis that characteristically begins with dysarthria, diplopia, dysphonia, or dysphagia. The most common botulism syndromes include food-borne, wound, and infant botulism. Botulism toxin is also now used therapeutically in neuromuscular and ophthalmologic disorders as well as a cosmetic enhancement tool, and cases of iatrogenic botulism have occurred. Although the majority of cases are due to infant botulism, food-borne botulism is considered a public health emergency, as there is always a potential that a large number of individuals may have been exposed. Additionally, botulinum is a category A biological agent, and any case must initially be considered as potentially linked to a bioterrorist event (see Chapter 130).

PATHOGENESIS

C. botulinum is an anaerobic Gram-positive bacillus that produces heat resistant spores that can survive boiling. Under conditions of an anaerobic environment, low acidity (pH greater than 4.6), and low temperature the organism can germinate, grow, and produce a neurotoxin that itself is readily inactivated by heat (greater than 85°C for 5 minutes) [2].

Seven distinct antigenic neurotoxins (A through G) may be produced by *C. botulinum* but only four types—A, B, E, and F—are associated with human disease. Food-borne botulism occurs after the ingestion of preformed toxin in foods contaminated by spores. Wound botulism occurs when spores infect traumatized or contaminated skin. Infant botulism occurs in infants 3 to 26 weeks old after intestinal colonization by *C. botulinum* [3]. Botulism of undetermined etiology occurs among adults whose intestinal flora has been altered or whose gastric barrier has been compromised because of intestinal surgery, gastric achlorhydria, or antibiotic therapy [3,4].

All botulinum toxins have the same mechanism of action [3]. The toxin is carried via the bloodstream to the neuromuscular junction where it binds irreversibly and thereby produces paralysis. However, it does not affect the central nervous system or the adrenergic nervous system [2]. The toxin is a zinc-containing endopeptidase that cleaves to specific sites on three proteins (VAMP, SNAP25, and syntaxin), interfering with the release of acetylcholine [5]. Paralysis correlates with the amount of toxin ingested and the length of the affected nerve with short cranial nerves affected first and long lower extremity nerves last.

EPIDEMIOLOGY

There have been approximately 20 cases of food-borne botulism annually in the United States, with the majority of cases caused by toxin type A (50%), followed by toxin type E (37%), and then toxin type B (10%) [2]. Food-borne botulism has traditionally been associated with home-processed foods. However, a number of cases have been associated with commercially prepared foods that have inadvertently been processed in a manner that allowed the production of the toxin. Recently, small outbreaks have been reported in prisons associated with the production of Pruno, an alcoholic beverage made from foodstuffs that in the reported outbreaks included potatoes [6].

Wound botulism has primarily been seen in intravenous drug users who present with cranial nerve palsies in the setting of abscesses from heroin use [7]. California has accounted for over 75% of US cases, with an epidemic noted in individuals injecting black tar heroin [8].

Iatrogenic botulism has rarely developed after botulinum toxin (Botox) has been injected for cosmetic or neurologic purposes [9,10]. Although, the normal concentration of botulinum toxin A in the therapeutic preparation allows for a large margin of safety with minimal treatment side effects, therapeutic doses have been reported to cause generalized muscle weakness with widespread electromyogram (EMG) abnormalities typical of botulism [11]. In addition, four individuals have contracted botulism after receiving unlicensed preparations of botulinum toxin for cosmetic purposes [12].

Botulism toxin is the most poisonous substance known to man with 1 g of toxin able to potentially kill one million people [10]. Given its ease of production and transport, it is a major bioterrorism threat and is classified as a category A biological agent. Botulism toxin was used as a bioweapon in the 1930s by the Japanese military who fed cultures of *C. botulinum* to prisoners during that country's occupation of Manchuria [13]. Aerosols derived from botulism toxin were also dispersed in Japan on at least three different occasions by a Japanese cult, although for unclear reasons these terrorist attempts failed [13] (see Chapter 130).

CLINICAL MANIFESTATIONS

Clinical manifestations of all forms of botulism are similar. Cardinal features include (a) cranial nerve palsies, (b) descending paralysis, (c) symmetry in symptoms, (d) absence of fever, (e) clear sensorium, and (f) lack of sensory findings [2]. Food-borne botulism may be preceded by gastrointestinal symptoms such as cramps, nausea, vomiting, and diarrhea [3,14]. Infant botulism is usually characterized by a history of constipation and feeding difficulties [3,14].

Patients may complain of dry mouth secondary to parasympathetic blockade as well as neurologic symptoms such as dysphagia, dysphonia, diplopia, and dysarthria related to palsies of the bulbar musculature. Symptoms then progress to involve lower extremity weakness and loss of the protective gag reflex requiring respiratory support. Physical examination is significant for a lack of fever except in cases of wound botulism with secondarily infected wounds. Sensory findings are absent except for periorbital paresthesias secondary to hyperventilation. Deep tendon reflexes, although present initially, usually disappear. Ocular findings are common and include dilated, poorly reactive, or fixed pupils, ptosis, nystagmus, and sixth cranial nerve dysfunction. A clear sensorium is usually present because the toxin does not usually penetrate the central nervous system [3,14].

The incubation period of food-borne botulism is usually 12 to 36 hours after toxin ingestion but may be as short as 2 hours [3,14]. Severity of disease depends on the amount of toxin that is absorbed into the system. Mortality has improved with the advances in critical care, and eventual recovery is seen in 95% of cases in the United States [9]. The recovery period may be protracted and is dependent on the reinnervation of paralyzed muscle fibers [13,15].

DIAGNOSIS

Successful diagnosis of botulism requires a high index of suspicion for the disease given that the symptoms and laboratory values are often nonspecific. If there is a suspected case of botulism, the local state health department should be notified [16]. The Centers for Disease Control and Prevention (CDC) can also be contacted through its 24-hour botulism consultation service for additional information at 770-488-7100. Prior to the administration of antitoxin, a serum sample (10 to 15 mL) should be collected and refrigerated. Anaerobic cultures and toxin assays of stool, serum, and gastric aspirates, suspected foodstuff, or wounds should be collected. Early cases are more likely to be diagnosed by toxin detection, while later cases are confirmed by culture [17]. The only acceptable method for the detection of the botulism neurotoxin is the mouse bioassay in which a patient's serum or supernatant from a culture of the patient specimens suspected to contain toxin is administered to pairs of mice with and without toxin, serving to confirm the diagnosis and define the circulating toxin. However, a study of clinical wound botulism revealed the sensitivity of the assay to be only 68% [18].

DIFFERENTIAL DIAGNOSIS

Diseases mistaken for botulism include brainstem infarction, polyradiculopathies such as the Guillain-Barre syndrome or its Miller Fisher variant, myasthenia gravis (MG), brainstem infarction, tick paralysis, polio, meningitis, or encephalitis and poisonings such as carbon monoxide, shellfish, or organophosphate poisoning [2,9]. An improvement of strength after the edrophonium test is suggestive of MG but has also been reported in botulism [19]. The Guillain-Barre syndrome is characterized by an ascending paralysis and usually, but not always, an elevated cerebrospinal fluid protein level initially. Electrophysiologic studies may be helpful in distinguishing between causes of flaccid paralysis such as myasthenia gravis, the Guillain-Barre syndrome, and the Lambert Eaton syndrome. Normal nerve conduction velocity, absence of sensory deficits, and a small increment of motor response seen on repetitive nerve stimulation at 20 Hz (as compared with the 4 Hz in MG) are characteristic of botulism. Tick paralysis is diagnosed by the presence of an embedded *Dermacentor* tick. Altered mental status is usually seen in encephalitis, organophosphate, and carbon monoxide poisonings rather than botulism. Shellfish poisoning presents with tremors and paresthesias that are usually absent in botulism [2].

TREATMENT

The mortality rate from botulism has decreased dramatically since the first decades of the 20th century to its current rate of 3% to 5% with the advent of intensive care units [20], and all patients suspected of botulism should initially be monitored in an intensive care setting.

Therapy consists of toxin removal, supportive care, including nutritional support, and passive immunization with equine antitoxin [3]. Patients should be assessed and monitored for the adequacy of cough, the control of oropharyngeal secretions, and ventilation. Please refer to the chapter on extrapulmonary causes of respiratory failure for guidelines on how to monitor for the adequacy of ventilation and when to consider endotracheal intubation (Chapter 165); and to the chapter on invasive mechanical ventilation for guidelines on how to ventilate patients with respiratory failure due to neuromuscular diseases.

For adults and older children, passive immunization with equine antitoxin should be administered as soon as botulism is diagnosed. Antitoxin will only neutralize toxin molecules that have not bound to nerve endings. Timely administration minimizes subsequent nerve damage and severity of disease but will not reverse existing paralytic damage [21]. The preferred antitoxin is the heptavalent equine antitoxin available through the CDC [22]. Clinicians should contact their local state health departments or the CDC (770-488-7100). Additional assistance can be obtained through the US Army, USAMRIID (888-872-7443). Patients should be skin tested prior to antitoxin administration and desensitized using the protocol enclosed with the antitoxin if there is any evidence of a wheal and flare reaction. A single case of intestinal botulism is documented as being refractory to toxin administration. This is explained by the shorter half-life of the heptavalent preparation and ongoing toxin production from the intestinal bacterium [23]. This is not an issue with the more common food-borne cases in which continued toxin production does not occur.

Equine antitoxin is not recommended for treatment of infants suspected of botulism because of the potential serious side effects of serum sickness and anaphylaxis. However, a 2006 study found that the administration of human botulism immune globulin intravenous within 72 hours of hospitalization for suspected infant botulism decreased illness severity, shortened hospital stays, and reduced costs [24]. This preparation, human botulism immune globulin (Baby-BIG), is now FDA agent approved and available through the California Department of Public Health.

Patients with wound botulism also require aggressive wound debridement regardless of how well the wound appears as toxin is produced until the infection is eliminated. Antitoxin should be administered prior to surgery to neutralize toxin released by the procedure. Penicillin therapy, 10 to 20 million units per day, is appropriate [5,8]. Aminoglycosides and clindamycin should be avoided because of the potential for neuromuscular blockade [25,26].

Because botulinum toxin is not absorbed through intact skin, standard precautions should be undertaken when caring for patients suspected of botulism. There have been no cases of human-to-human transmission described [9].

A number of potential vaccine candidates remain investigational with no phase 3 studies reported to date.

Advances in botulism, based on randomized controlled trials, are summarized in Table 86.1.

TABLE 86.1

Recommendations for the Treatment of Botulism Based on Randomized Clinical Trials

Treatment with the drug Human Botulism Immune Globulin Intravenous (BIG-IV) given within 3 d of hospital admission for infant botulism shortens length and cost of the hospital stay and the length of illness.

Arnon SS, Schechter R, Maslanka SE, et al: Human botulism immune globulin for the treatment of infant botulism. *N Engl J Med* 354(5):-462–471, 2006.

References

1. Lindstrom M, Korkeala H: Laboratory diagnostics of botulism. *Clin Mic Rev* 19(2): 298–314, 2006.
2. Sobel J, Tucker N, Sulka A, et al: Foodborne botulism in the United States, 1990–2000. *Emerg Infect Dis* 10:1606–1611, 2004.
3. Center for Disease Control: *Botulism in the United States 1899–1996: Handbook for Epidemiologists, Clinicians and Laboratory Workers*. Atlanta, CDC, 1998.
4. Bartlett JC: Infant botulism in adults. *N Engl J Med* 1315:254–255, 1986.
5. Arnon SS, Schechter R, Inglesby TV, et al: Botulinum toxin as a biological weapon: medical and public health management. *JAMA* 285:1059–1070, 2001.
6. Vugia DJ, Mase SR, Inami G, et al: Botulism from drinking pruno. *Emerg Infect Dis* 15:69–71, 2009.
7. MacDonald KL, Rutherford GW, Friedman SM, et al: Botulism and botulism-like illness in chronic drug abusers. *Ann Intern Med* 102:616–618, 1985.
8. Werner SB, Passaro D, McGee J, et al: Wound botulism in California 1951–1998: recent epidemic in heroin injectors. *Clin Infect Dis* 31:1018–1024, 2000.
9. Sobel J: Botulism. *Clin Infect Dis* 41:1167–1173, 2005.
10. Ting PT, Freiman A: The story of Clostridium botulinum: from food poisoning to Botox. *Clin Med* 4:258–261, 2004.
11. Bakheit AM, Ward CD, McLellan DL: Generalised botulism-like syndrome after intramuscular injections of botulinum toxin type A: a report of two cases. *J Neurol Neurosurg Psychiatry* 62:198, 1997.
12. Chertow DS, Tan ET, Maslanka, SE, et al: Botulism in 4 adults following cosmetic injections with an unlicensed, highly concentrated botulinum preparation. *JAMA* 296:2476–2479, 2006.
13. Duchen LW: Motor nerve growth induced by botulinum toxin as a regenerative phenomenon. *Proc R Soc Med* 65:196–197, 1972.
14. Dembek ZF, Smith LA, Rusnak JM: Botulism: cause, effects, diagnosis, clinical and laboratory identification, and treatment modalities. *Disaster Med Public Health Prep* 1:122–134, 2007.
15. Mann JM, Martin S, Hoffman R, et al: Patient recovery from type A botulism: morbidity assessment following a large outbreak. *Am J Public Health* 71:266–269, 1981.
16. Shapiro RL, Hatheway C, Becher J, et al: Botulism surveillance and emergency response. A public health strategy for a global challenge. *JAMA* 278:433–435, 1997.
17. Woodruff BA, Griffin PM, McCroskey LM, et al: Clinical and laboratory comparison of botulism from toxin types A, B, and E in the United States, 1975–1988. *J Infect Dis* 166:1281–1286, 1992.
18. Wheeler C, Inami G, Mohle-Boetani J, et al: Sensitivity of mouse bioassay in clinical wound botulism. *Clin Infect Dis* 48:1669–1673, 2009.
19. Cherington M: Electrophysiologic methods as an aid in diagnosis of botulism: a review. *Muscle Nerve* 5:S28–S29, 1982.
20. Gangarosa EJ, Donadio JA, Armstrong RW, et al: Botulism in the United States, 1899–1969. *Am J Epidemiol* 93:93–101, 1971.
21. Tacket CO, Shandera WX, Mann JM, et al: Equine antitoxin use and other factors that predict outcome in type A foodborne botulism. *Am J Med* 76: 794–798, 1984.
22. Centers for Disease Control and Prevention (CDC): Investigational heptavalent botulinum antitoxin (HBAT) to replace licensed botulinum antitoxin AB and investigational botulinum antitoxin E. *MMWR Morb Mortal Wkly Rep* 59: 299, 2010.
23. Fagan RP, Neil FP, Khalil W, et al: Initial recovery and reboud of type F intestinal colonization botulism after administration of investigational heptavalent botulinum antitoxin. *Clin Infect Dis* 53:e125–e128, 2011.
24. Arnon SS, Schechter R, Maslanka SE, et al: Human botulism immune globulin for the treatment of infant botulism. *N Engl J Med* 354:462–471, 2006.
25. Santos JI, Swensen P, Glasgow LA: Potentiation of Clostridium botulinum toxin aminoglycoside antibiotics: clinical and laboratory observations. *Pediatrics* 68:50–54, 1981.
26. Schulze J, Toepfer M, Schroff KC, et al: Clindamycin and nicotinic neuromuscular transmission. *Lancet* 354:1792–1793, 1999.

Chapter 87 ■ Tetanus

MARY DAWN T. CO • RICHARD T. ELLISON, III

Tetanus, caused by the neurotoxin tetanospasmin, is produced by the anaerobic spore-forming gram-positive bacterium *Clostridium tetani*. Clinically, tetanus presents with skeletal muscle rigidity and spasms that classically involve the muscles of the face (lockjaw). It is a relatively rare clinical entity in developed countries because of the broad use of tetanus toxoid (TT) immunization. However, tetanus still occurs frequently in the third world, and in individuals who have never been or have been inadequately vaccinated in the setting of a wound infection or another portal of entry. Diagnosis is based on clinical suspicion and the exclusion of other entities because of a lack of timely confirmatory testing. Treatment relies mainly on respiratory support and symptomatic management of the muscular rigidity and spasms and the autonomic manifestations of the disease.

PATHOGENESIS

Clostridium tetani is an obligate anaerobic spore-forming bacillus which is ubiquitous in the environment. Mature organisms develop spores that are widely distributed in soil and dust as well as in the intestines and feces of animals. The vegetative form of *C. tetani* produces two types of zinc metalloproteinase toxins, tetanospasmin and tetanolysin, with tetanospasmin playing a more prominent role in pathogenesis. The *C. tetani* neurotoxin is of a single antigenic type and specifically targets the central nervous system (CNS), including the peripheral motor end plates, spinal cord, brain, and the sympathetic nervous system [1,2]. Although this toxin can exert an excitatory effect, it acts primarily by blocking the release of neurotransmitters such as glycine and gamma-amino butyric acid, which normally act to inhibit the transmission of motor nerve impulses. Specifically, the toxin degrades synaptobrevin, a protein required for contact of inhibitory neurotransmitter vesicles with their release site on the presynaptic membrane [3].

Antitoxin is of therapeutic value only for protecting neurons that have not already bound the toxin. As the effect of the toxin on a synapse does not appear reversible, recovery from tetanus depends on the generation of new nerve terminals and new synapse formation.

EPIDEMIOLOGY

Tetanus is endemic in the developing world with neonatal tetanus accounting for the majority (>50%) of deaths due to tetanus [4]. Tetanus is a rare disease in the developed world with morbidity and mortality in the United States declining steadily, due to the availability of tetanus vaccines, improved wound management and the use of tetanus immunoglobulin for postexposure prophylaxis [4]. According to 2001 to 2008 surveillance data, a history of incomplete TT immunization and inadequate wound prophylaxis remain the most important factors associated with tetanus [5]. Age ≥ 65 years old remained the highest risk factor for fatal tetanus with a case fatality rate of 31.3%. [5]. Sporadic cases of tetanus have been reported in those with a tetanus antibody level adequate for protective immunity [6].

CLINICAL MANIFESTATIONS

Tetanus usually occurs in the setting of either a penetrating wound, foreign body or necrotic or infected tissue in which anaerobic bacterial growth is facilitated [7]. However, in up to 30% of cases, no acute injury is reported [8]. The incubation period for tetanus varies from 3 to 21 days, with the length of the incubation period dependent on how far the injury site is from the CNS [9]. The first nerves affected are the shortest, accounting for the early symptoms of facial distortion and neck stiffness. The shorter the incubation period, the worse the prognosis [10].

Clinical tetanus can present in three forms—local, cephalic, and generalized—with 80% of cases being generalized. Local tetanus presents as a focal region of muscle contraction at a site of spore inoculation [1]. Symptoms may persist but usually resolve spontaneously. Cephalic tetanus develops after a traumatic head injury, but has been reported after otitis media when *C. tetanus* was present in the middle ear [11]. Typically, there is involvement of the cranial nerves, especially cranial nerve VII in the facial area.

Generalized tetanus typically presents with involvement of facial musculature, starting with masseter rigidity (lockjaw or trismus) and risus sardonicus (orbicularis oris), and then progresses in a descending fashion with difficulty swallowing and abdominal rigidity [1]. Spasms, which are often triggered by sensory stimuli, are common and may resemble seizures with flexion of the arms and the extension of legs (opisthotonus). Loss of consciousness is uncommon and severe pain usually accompanies the spasms. Laryngospasm and respiratory compromise may result from vocal cord or diaphragmatic spasms and upper airway obstruction. Fractures of the spine or the long bones, dislocations, and rhabdomyolysis may occur as a result of spasms. The course of this illness occurs over 2 weeks, reflecting the time it takes for intraaxonal toxin to travel to the CNS. Spasms occur within the first 2 weeks of illness followed by autonomic disturbances such as extremes in blood pressure and cardiac arrhythmias including sinus tachycardia and cardiac arrest [12,13]. Individuals with tetanus are at high risk of nosocomial pneumonia with an incidence of approximately 35%. Autonomic dysfunction is an independent risk factor for pneumonia in patients with tetanus [14].

Neonatal tetanus, more often seen in developing countries, is a form of generalized tetanus that commonly arises when an unhealed umbilical stump becomes infected after an incision with an unsterile instrument and if the mother had not been adequately immunized [1,9].

DIAGNOSIS

No laboratory test is available that provides a definitive diagnosis of tetanus. Diagnosis is clinical and primarily based on the presence of trismus, dysphagia, muscular rigidity, and spasm. Unusual presentations such as meningitis should be considered in the setting of risk factors such as a history of a contaminated wound [15].

Few other conditions present with muscular rigidity and sympathetic hyperreactivity except for strychnine poisoning. Strychnine blocks the inhibitory glycine receptor in the spinal cord and the brain. Unlike tetanus, however, the sudden contraction of all striated muscles is usually followed by complete relaxation of these muscles. Additional conditions that can mimic the spasms seen in tetanus include hypocalcemia and reactions to certain medications including neuroleptic drugs and central dopamine antagonists. Odontogenic infections can produce trismus but not the other manifestations of tetanus [1].

TREATMENT

The mortality rate in tetanus varies from 6% in mild to moderate tetanus up to 60% in the severest of cases [1,16]. Autonomic nervous system dysfunction has been shown to predict a poor outcome in mild to moderate cases of tetanus [17]. Illness is less severe among patients who have received a complete immunization series of TT compared with those who were never or inadequately vaccinated [18].

Individuals suspected of generalized tetanus should be observed in an intensive care setting with minimal stimuli. Initial management consists of airway stabilization and general intensive care support including mechanical ventilation, nutritional support, and deep venous thrombosis prophylaxis. Benzodiazepines such as midazolam, lorazepam, and diazepam have been the mainstay of treatment [1]. This class of agents acts as γ-aminobutyric acid (GABA) agonists, thus indirectly opposing the effects of the toxin by competing for receptor sites [2]. Doses are initially titrated to produce sedation and limit reflex spasms. Propofol (alone or in combination with benzodiazepines) and intrathecal baclofen are alternative options that have been used [19,20]. Intravenous diazepam and lorazepam contain propylene glycol, which may increase the risk of lactic acidosis at the recommended doses of treatment [21]. If the muscle spasms cannot be controlled with these agents, a neuromuscular paralytic agent such as vecuronium can be added [1]. Once the symptoms have resolved, benzodiazepines should be tapered to prevent withdrawal.

Botulinum toxin acts mainly on lower motor neurons by inhibiting acetylcholine release and muscle activity. Direct injection of botulinum toxin into the muscle has been successfully used in a small number of patients to reduce tetanus induced rigidity and spasm [22].

If a portal of entry can be identified, the wound should be debrided and an antibiotic active against anaerobic organisms should be administered with metronidazole for 7 to 10 days now considered to be the first line of therapy. Treatment courses of 7 to 10 days using regimens of penicillin, either as a single-dose intramuscular benzathine dose or intravenous benzyl penicillin are alternative regimens [1,23]. Alternative regimens such as doxycycline, clindamycin, vancomycin, and chloramphenicol are likely to be effective given susceptibility data against *C. tetani* [24]. Passive immunization with human tetanus immunoglobulin (at a dose of 500 units) may shorten the course and severity of tetanus by neutralizing toxin that has not reached the CNS [25]. In a randomized clinical trial, patients treated with intrathecal rather than intramuscular administration of human antitetanus immunoglobulin showed better clinical progression including fewer respiratory complications and significantly shorter duration of spasms [26], though methodical issues with the study have been raised [7].

Autonomic dysfunction is usually related to excessive catecholamine release and can be treated by a combined α- and β-blocker such as labetalol. Beta-blockade alone may result in severe hypertension due to an unopposed α effect [27]. Magnesium sulfate has been studied in a randomized controlled trial and found to reduce the requirements of other drugs to control spasms and cardiac instability [28].

As the amount of toxin causing disease may be too small to induce a consistent immunological response, active immunization with three doses of TT should be given at diagnosis, at 4 to 6 weeks and 1 year later to prevent future attacks [1,9]. TT should be given at a site different than tetanus immunoglobulin [7].

Over the past 30 years, there have only been nine randomized clinical trials that have addressed therapeutic interventions [29]. Advances in tetanus, based on randomized controlled trials are summarized in Table 87.1.

TABLE 87.1

Recommendations for the Treatment of *Clostridium tetanus* Based on Randomized Clinical Trials

- Treatment with metronidazole, benzyl penicillin, or intramuscular benzathine penicillin has a comparable impact on the need for tracheostomy, the use of neuromuscular blockade, the need for mechanical ventilation, and the incidence of dysautonomia, nosocomial pneumonia, and in-hospital death) [23].
- Treatment with intrathecal rather than intramuscular administration of antitetanus immunoglobulin showed better clinical progression including fewer respiratory complications and a significantly shorter duration of spasms [26]
- Magnesium infusion for 7 d did not reduce the need for mechanical ventilation in adults with severe tetanus but did reduce the requirement for other drugs to control muscle spasms and cardiovascular instability [28]

References

1. Bleck T: Clostridium tetani, in Bennett JE, Mandell GL, Dolin R, (eds): *Principles and Practice of Infectious Diseases*. 6th ed. Philadelphia, Elsevier-Churchill Livingstone, 2005, pp 2817–2822.
2. Akbulut D, Grant KA, McLauchlin J: Improvement in laboratory diagnosis of wound botulism and tetanus among injecting illicit-drug users by use of real-time PCR assays for neurotoxin gene fragments. *J Clin Microbiol* 43(9):4342–4348, 2005.
3. Cornille F, Martin L, Lenoir C, et al: Cooperative exosite-dependent cleavage of synaptobrevin by tetanus toxin light chain. *J Biol Chem* 272(6):3459–3464, 1997.
4. Kretsinger K, Srivastava P: Tetanus, in Roush SW, McIntyre LM, Baldy LM, (eds): *Manual for the Surveillance of Vaccine-Preventable Diseases, Chapter 16-1*. 4th ed. Atlanta, GA, Center for Disease Control and Prevention, 2008.
5. Center for Disease Control and Prevention: Tetanus surveillance—United States, 2001–2008. *MMWR Morb Mortal Wkly Rep* 60(12):365–369, 2011.
6. Vollman KE, Acquisto NM, Bodkin RP: A case of tetanus infection in an adult with a protective tetanus antibody level. *Am J Emerg Med* 32(4):392 e3–4, 2014.
7. Sexton DJ: Tetanus, in UpToDate, Post TW (ed): *UpToDate*, Waltham, MA (Accessed on July 13, 2015).
8. Pascual FB, McGinley EL, Zanardi LR, et al: Tetanus surveillance–United States, 1998–2000. *MMWR Surveill Summ* 52(3):1–8, 2003.
9. Centers for Disease Control and Prevention: Tetanus, in Atkinson W, Wolfe S, Hamborsky J, et al, (eds): *Epidemiology and Prevention of Vaccine-Preventable Diseases*. 11th ed. Washington DC, Public Health Foundation, 2009, pp 273–282.
10. Veronesi R, Focaccia R: The clinical picture, in Veronesi R, (ed): *Tetanus: Important New Concepts*. Amsterdam, Excerpta Medica, 1981, pp 183–206.
11. Raghuram J, Ong YY, Wong SY: Tetanus in Singapore: report of three cases. *Ann Acad Med Singapore* 24(6):869–873, 1995.
12. Mitra RC, Gupta RD, Sack RB: Electrocardiographic changes in tetanus: a serial study. *J Indian Med Assoc* 89(6):164–167, 1991.
13. Kanarek DJ, Kaufman B, Zwi S: Severe sympathetic hyperactivity associated with tetanus. *Arch Intern Med* 132(4):602–604, 1973.
14. Cavalcante NJ, Sandeville ML, Medeiros EA: Incidence of and risk factors for nosocomial pneumonia in patients with tetanus. *Clin Infect Dis* 33(11):1842–1846, 2001.
15. Moniuszko A, Zajkowska A, Tumiel E, et al: Meningitis, clinical presentation of tetanus. *Case Rep Infect Dis* 372–375, 2015.
16. Nolla-Salas M, Garces-Bruses J: Severity of tetanus in patients older than 80 years: comparative study with younger patients. *Clin Infect Dis* 16(4):591–592, 1993.
17. Wasay M, Khealani BA, Talati N, et al: Autonomic nervous system dysfunction predicts poor prognosis in patients with mild to moderate tetanus. *BMC Neurol* 5(1):2, 2005.
18. Wassilak S, Orenstein W, Sutter R: Tetanus toxoid, in Plotkin S, Orenstein W, (eds): *Vaccines*. 3rd ed. Philadelphia, WB Saunders, 1999, pp 441–474.
19. Borgeat A, Popovic V, Schwander D: Efficiency of a continuous infusion of propofol in a patient with tetanus. *Crit Care Med* 19(2):295–297, 1991.
20. Santos ML, Mota-Miranda A, Alves-Pereira A, et al: Intrathecal baclofen for the treatment of tetanus. *Clin Infect Dis* 38(3):321–328, 2004.
21. Kapoor W, Carey P, Karpf M: Induction of lactic acidosis with intravenous diazepam in a patient with tetanus. *Arch Intern Med* 141(7):944–945, 1981.
22. Hassel B: Tetanus: pathophysiology, treatment, and the possibility of using botulinum toxin against tetanus-induced rigidity and spasms. *Toxins (Basel)* 5(1):73–83, 2013.
23. Ganesh Kumar AV, Kothari VM, Krishnan A, et al: Benzathine penicillin, metronidazole and benzyl penicillin in the treatment of tetanus: a randomized, controlled trial. *Ann Trop Med Parasitol* 98(1):59–63, 2004.
24. Afshar M, Raju M, Ansell D, et al: Narrative review: tetanus-a health threat after-natural disasters in developing countries. *Ann Intern Med* 154(5):329–335, 2011.
25. Blake PA, Feldman RA, Buchanan TM, et al: Serologic therapy of tetanus in the United States, 1965–1971. *JAMA* 235(1):42–44,1976.
26. Miranda-Filho Dde B, Ximenes RA, Barone AA, et al: Randomised controlled trial of tetanus treatment with antitetanus immunoglobulin by the intrathecal or intramuscular route. *BMJ* 328(7440):615, 2004.
27. Domenighetti GM, Savary G, Stricker H: Hyperadrenergic syndrome in severe tetanus: extreme rise in catecholamines responsive to labetalol. *Br Med J (Clin Res Ed)* 288(6429):1483–1484,1984.
28. Thwaites CL, Yen LM, Loan HT, et al: Magnesium sulphate for treatment of severe tetanus: a randomised controlled trial. *Lancet* 368(9545):1436–1443, 2006.
29. Thwaites CL, Farrar JJ: Preventing and treating tetanus. *BMJ* 326(7381): 117–118, 2003.

Section 9

HEMATOLOGIC AND ONCOLOGIC PROBLEMS IN THE INTENSIVE CARE UNIT

PATRICK F. FOGARTY

Chapter 88 ■ Disorders of Hemostasis in Critically Ill Patients

ALICE D. MA

Disorders of hemostasis are common in critically ill patients. This chapter will review hemostasis, pathophysiology of commonly encountered congenital and acquired bleeding disorders along with their associated symptoms, laboratory findings, and management.

REVIEW OF NORMAL HEMOSTASIS

Hemostasis can be broken into a series of steps occurring in overlapping sequence. Primary hemostasis refers to the interactions between the platelet and the injured vessel wall, culminating in the formation of a platelet plug. The humoral phase of clotting, or secondary hemostasis, encompasses a series of enzymatic reactions, resulting in a hemostatic fibrin plug. Finally, fibrinolysis and wound repair occur. Each of these steps is carefully regulated, and perturbations can predispose to either hemorrhage or thrombosis. Depending on the nature of the defect, the hemorrhagic or thrombotic tendency can be either profound or subtle.

Primary hemostasis begins at the site of vascular injury, with platelets adhering to the subendothelium, utilizing interactions between molecules such as collagen and von Willebrand factor (vWF) in the vessel wall with glycoprotein (GP) receptors on the platelet surface. Upon exposure to agonists present at a wounded vessel, signal transduction leads to platelet activation. Via a process known as inside-out signaling, the platelet membrane integrin $\alpha_{2b}\beta_3$ (also known as GP IIbIIIa) undergoes a conformational change to be able to bind fibrinogen, which cross-links adjacent platelets, leading to platelet aggregation. Secretion of granular contents is also triggered by outside signals, potentiating further platelet activation (Fig. 88.1). Lastly, the surface of the platelet changes to serve as an adequate scaffold for the series of biochemical reactions resulting in thrombin generation.

Following platelet activation, a series of enzymatic reactions take place on phospholipid surfaces, culminating in the formation of a stable fibrin clot. Several models have attempted to make sense of these reactions. The cascade model was developed by two groups nearly simultaneously in 1964 and explained the extrinsic, intrinsic, and common pathways leading to fibrin formation (Fig. 88.2). Although the cascade model accounts for the physiologic reactions underlying the prothrombin time (PT) and the activated partial thromboplastin time (aPTT), it fails to explain completely the bleeding diathesis seen in individuals deficient in factors XI, IX, and VIII, as well as the lack of bleeding in those deficient only in contact factors. A cell-based model of hemostasis has been developed to address these deficiencies [1]. In this model, upon vascular injury, the membrane of a tissue factor (TF)-bearing cell such as an activated monocyte or fibroblast serves as a platform for generation of a small amount of thrombin and FIXa, which then serves to activate platelets and cleave FVIII from vWF. Newly formed FVIIIa participates in the tenase complex on the surface of activated platelets to form FXa that interacts with the FVa generated on the platelet surface to form the prothrombinase complex. This complex generates a large burst of thrombin which is sufficient to cleave fibrinogen, activate FXIII, and activate the thrombin-activatable fibrinolysis inhibitor, thus allowing for formation of a stable fibrin clot (Fig. 88.2).

Fibrinolysis leads to clot dissolution once wound healing has occurred, in order to restore normal blood flow. Plasminogen is activated to plasmin by the action of either tissue plasminogen activator (t-PA) or urokinase plasminogen activator. Plasmin degrades fibrin and fibrinogen and can thus dissolve both formed clot as well as its soluble precursor. Plasmin is inhibited by a number of inhibitors, of which α_2-plasmin inhibitor is the most significant. Plasminogen activation is also inhibited by a number of molecules; chief among them is plasminogen activator inhibitor-1. Lastly, cellular receptors act to localize and potentiate or clear plasmin and plasminogen activators (see Chapter 93 for further discussion).

APPROACH TO THE BLEEDING PATIENT

Physicians in the intensive care unit (ICU) often encounter bleeding patients and it can be difficult to identify which of these patients require further evaluation. Patients who experience bleeding that is excessive, spontaneous, or delayed following surgery or tissue injury require further investigation, which must begin with a thorough clinical history. A bleeding history should assess a patient's exposure and response to all hemostatic challenges in the past such as trauma, surgery, and childbirth. Characterization of menses in females also may be revealing. Several bleeding assessment tools have been developed and are useful in the evaluation for an underlying coagulopathy, particularly von Willebrand disease (vWD) [2]. This history should also identify coexisting medical conditions such as liver, kidney, or thyroid disorders. A careful medication history is also important, including use of all over-the-counter medications which may contain aspirin, as well as any herbal preparations. Also of importance is an evaluation for a family history of abnormal bleeding. An inherited or congenital bleeding disorder is suggested by abnormal bleeding with onset shortly after birth and persistence throughout life. It is further supported by a family history with a consistent genetic pattern. However, it is important to note that a negative family history does not exclude a congenital bleeding disorder. For instance, approximately one-third of all cases of hemophilia A arise from spontaneous mutations. Many of the rare coagulation disorders, including deficiency of factors II, V, VII, X, as well as vWD type 2 N, among others, are inherited in an autosomal recessive fashion, and the parents of the patient may be entirely asymptomatic.

A bleeding history should also ascertain past sites/mechanisms of bleeding. Surgical bleeding in patients with an underlying hemorrhagic condition is typically described as "diffuse oozing," without the readily identifiable bleeding source seen with a surgical mishap such as a severed vessel. Patients with platelet disorders typically manifest mucocutaneous bleeding such as gingival bleeding and epistaxis as well as menorrhagia, petechiae, and ecchymoses. Platelet defects impact primary hemostasis and therefore the bleeding in these disorders is often immediate

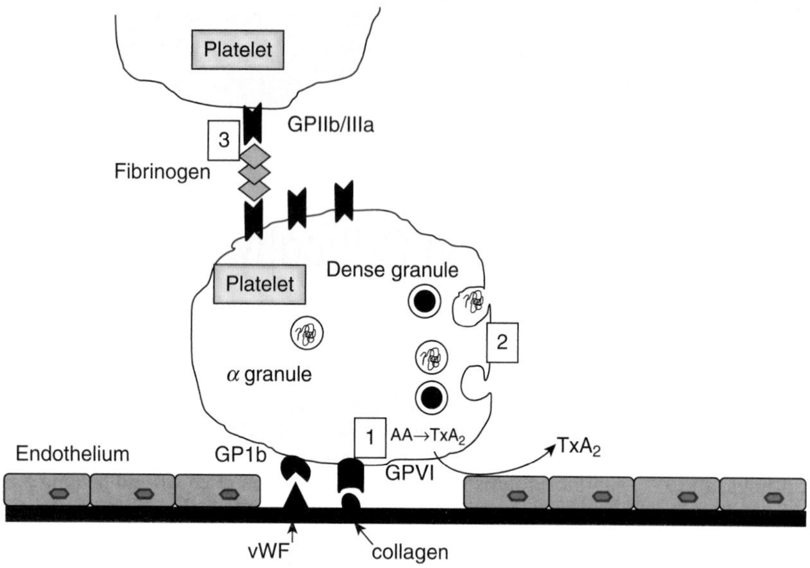

FIGURE 88.1 Primary hemostasis. (*1*) Exposure of subendothelium at sites of vascular disruption results in platelet adhesion via GPIb and GP VI with exposed von Willebrand factor (vWF) and collagen, respectively. Following platelet adhesion, TxA_2 is produced and released, which promotes vasoconstriction and platelet aggregation. (*2*) Platelet adhesion also results in fusion of cytoplasmic granules to the plasma membrane. Release of alpha and dense granules activates nearby platelets. (*3*) Platelet activation results in exposure of GPIIb/IIIa on the platelet surface allowing fibrinogen to cross bridge platelets resulting in a platelet plug.

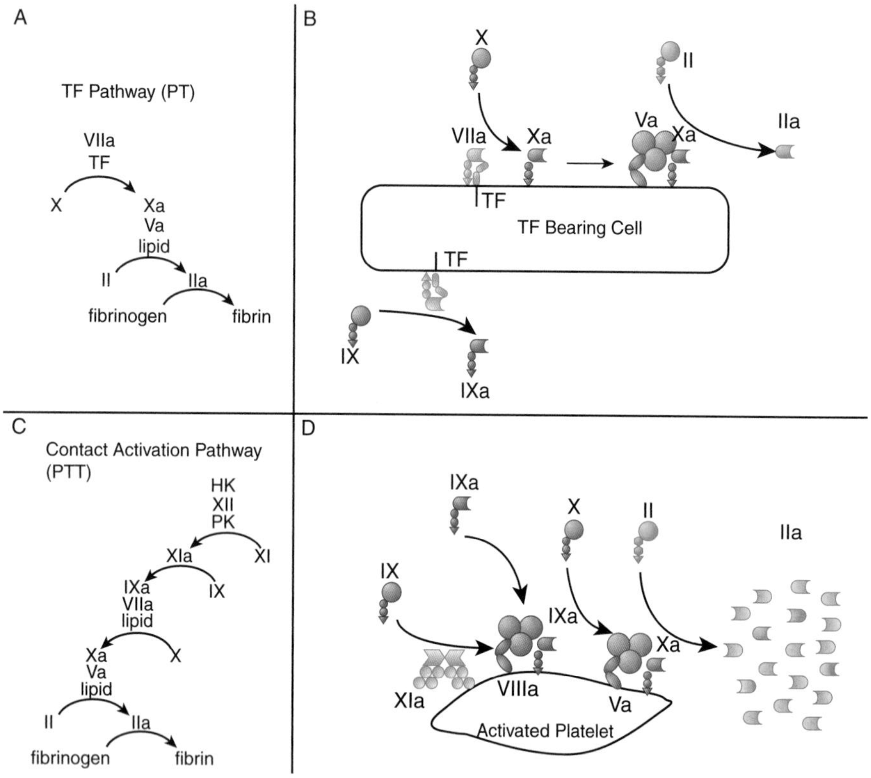

FIGURE 88.2 Secondary hemostasis. **A:** Tissue factor (TF) pathway cascade model of coagulation—basis for prothrombin time (PT) laboratory assay. **B:** Circulating FVIIa binds TF on a TF-bearing cell. TF/FVIIa along with calcium (Ca) and phospholipid (lipid) form the "extrinsic tenase" complex and converts FX to FXa. FXa combines with FVa, calcium, and phospholipid, "prothrombinase" complex, to activate FII to FIIa which in turn converts fibrinogen into fibrin. **C:** Contact activation pathway model of coagulation—basis for partial thromboplastin time (PTT) laboratory assay. **D:** On an activated platelet surface, FXIa activates FIXa. FIXa is also formed on the surface of a TF-bearing cell (**B**). FIXa, along with FVIIIa, Ca, and lipid, constitute the "intrinsic tenase" complex. This complex converts FX to FXa with subsequent FIIIa generation through the prothrombinase complex. (Courtesy of Dougald Monroe.)

following surgery or trauma, whereas delayed bleeding is more classically associated with coagulation disorders. Patients with coagulation defects typically present with hemorrhages into soft tissues such as muscles and joints.

LABORATORY ASSAYS OF PRIMARY AND SECONDARY HEMOSTASIS

Although the history and physical examination can increase suspicion for the presence of a bleeding disorder, laboratory confirmation is required for precise diagnosis and treatment. Laboratory evaluation is particularly crucial in individuals who are suspected of having a bleeding disorder but in whom prior bleeding is absent, such as those with mild congenital bleeding disorders who never previously underwent a sufficient hemostatic challenge, or those with acquired hemorrhagic disorders.

Initial Evaluation of Primary Hemostasis—Platelet Function

An assessment of a patient's platelet count is fundamental in evaluating primary hemostasis. This is typically part of a complete blood count. Reduced platelet counts, or thrombocytopenia, may be seen in a large number of acquired and congenital conditions. Evaluation and management of thrombocytopenia is further discussed in Chapter 91.

An evaluation of the peripheral smear is also cardinal in any evaluation of a bleeding patient. It allows one to assess platelet size and morphology, presence of platelet clumping (pseudothrombocytopenia), leukocyte inclusions, and red cell fragments, among other aberrancies, which may further direct workup and treatment.

Traditionally, platelet function was evaluated by bleeding time (BT). However, many institutions have discontinued using this test given the difficulty in standardization. Furthermore, the BT has been shown to be an inadequate predictor of bleeding, particularly in preoperative risk assessment [3]. More recently, automated tests have been developed to assess platelet function. The most widely used is the platelet function analyzer (PFA-100). This assay measures the time required (closure time) for flowing whole, citrated blood to occlude an aperture in a membrane impregnated with a combination of either collagen and epinephrine or collagen and adenosine diphosphate (ADP). Closure time is affected by platelet count, hematocrit, platelet function, and vWF [4]. The PFA-100 appears to assess platelet function with greater sensitivity and reproducibility than the BT; however, it may not have sufficient sensitivity or specificity to be used as a screening tool for platelet disorders [5].

Evaluation of Secondary Hemostasis—Coagulation

The PT and the aPTT are assays performed on citrated plasma, which require enzymatic generation of thrombin on a phospholipid surface. Prolongation of the PT and the aPTT can be seen in individuals with either deficiencies of, or inhibitors to, humoral clotting factors, though not all patients with prolongations of these assays will have bleeding diatheses (Table 88.1).

The PT measures the time needed for formation of an insoluble fibrin clot once citrated plasma has been recalcified and thromboplastin has been added, indicating activity of factors VII, V, X, and II, and fibrinogen. It is commonly used to monitor anticoagulation with vitamin K antagonists such as warfarin. As thromboplastin from various sources and different lots can affect the rates of clotting reactions, the International Normalized Ratio (INR) measurement was developed to avoid some of this variability in PT measurement. Each batch of thromboplastin reagent has assigned to it a numerical International Sensitivity Index (ISI) value, which is used in the formula:

$$\text{INR} = (\text{PT}_{\text{patient}}/\text{PT}_{\text{normal}})^{\text{ISI}}$$

The INR is less predictive of bleeding in patients with liver disease, and can be inaccurate in patients with lupus anticoagulants that are strong enough to affect the PT.

The aPTT tests the activity of factors XII, XI, IX, VIII, X, V, and II, and fibrinogen, high-molecular-weight (HMW) kininogen, and plasma prekallikrein [6]. Citrated plasma is recalcified, and phospholipids (to provide a scaffold for the clotting reactions) and an activator of the intrinsic system such as kaolin, celite, or silica are added. The reagents used show variable sensitivities to inhibitors such as lupus anticoagulants and heparin, and to deficiencies (if any) in involved clotting factors, and normal ranges will vary from laboratory to laboratory. aPTT values that are vastly different from one laboratory to another should prompt suspicion of a lupus anticoagulant.

The Thrombin Clotting Time and Reptilase Time

The thrombin clotting time or thrombin time (TT) measures the time needed for clot formation once thrombin is added to citrated plasma. Thrombin enzymatically cleaves fibrinopeptides A and B from the α and β-chains of fibrinogen, allowing for polymerization into fibrin. The TT is prolonged in the presence of any thrombin inhibitor such as heparin, lepirudin, or argatroban; by low levels of fibrinogen or structurally abnormal fibrinogen (dysfibrinogens); and by elevated levels of fibrinogen or fibrin degradation products, which can serve as nonspecific inhibitors of the reaction. Patients with paraproteins can have a prolonged TT because of the inhibitory effect of the paraprotein on fibrin polymerization.

TABLE 88.1

Laboratory Test Abnormalities in Common Acquired and Congenital Bleeding Disorders

	Acquired bleeding disorders	Congenital bleeding disorders
PT elevated, aPTT wnl	Liver disease DIC Vitamin K deficiency Vitamin K antagonists (e.g., warfarin)	FVII deficiency
PT wnl, aPTT elevated	Heparin Lupus inhibitor Acquired FVIII inhibitor	Hemophilia A and B FXI deficiency Severe vWD
Both PT and aPTT elevated	Heparin overdose Warfarin overdose FVI inhibitors FX inhibitors Severe DIC Severe vitamin K deficiency Severe liver disease Direct thrombin inhibitors	Afibrinogenemia Hypo- or dysfibrinogenemia Prothrombin deficiency FV deficiency Combined deficiency of FV and FVIII
Both PT and aPTT wnl	LMWH therapy Fondaparinux therapy Antiplatelet agents Acquired vWD Scurvy Acquired thrombocytopenia	vWD FXIII deficiency Congenital platelet dysfunction Congenital thrombocytopenia Collagen disorders (e.g., Ehlers–Danlos syndrome)

wnl, within normal limits; DIC, disseminated intravascular coagulation; LMWH, low-molecular-weight heparin; PT, prothrombin time; PTT; partial thromboplastin time; vWD, von Willebrand disease.

Reptilase is snake venom from *Bothrops atrox* which also enzymatically cleaves fibrinogen. Reptilase cleaves only fibrinopeptide A from the α-chain of fibrinogen, but fibrin polymerization still occurs. Reptilase time (RT) is not affected by heparin but may be more sensitive than the TT to the presence of a dysfibrinogenemia.

Mixing Studies

Mixing studies are used to evaluate prolongations of the aPTT (less commonly the PT or the TT) and are useful in making the distinction between an inhibitor and a clotting factor deficiency. The patient's plasma is mixed 1:1 with normal control plasma, and the assay is repeated (with or without prolonged incubation at 37°C). Correction of the clotting test signifies factor deficiency, as the normal plasma will supply the deficient factor. Incomplete correction of the clotting test after mixing suggests the presence of an inhibitor, as an inhibitor will prolong clotting in normal plasma. Incomplete correction can sometimes be seen with nonspecific inhibitors such as lupus anticoagulants, elevated fibrin split products, or a paraprotein. Less commonly, deficiencies of multiple clotting factors can lead to incomplete correction of the mixing study, as the mixing study was designed to correct deficiency of a single factor.

Tests of specific factor activity levels as well as evaluation for vWD will be discussed in the following sections.

CONGENITAL DISORDERS OF HEMOSTASIS

Due to a requirement for specialized management, all cases of suspected or proven congenital hemostatic defects require consultation with a hematologist upon admission to the critical care setting.

von Willebrand Disease

It has been estimated that lower-than-reference levels of vWF occur in 1% of the population worldwide and therefore vWD is the most common congenital bleeding disorder. However, only a fraction of the aforementioned individuals are symptomatic (approximately 5% of those with low levels) [7]. vWD is inherited in an autosomal manner with the more common type I disease being autosomal dominant.

vWD constitutes a quantitative or qualitative deficiency in vWF, and is divided into three subtypes according to the pathophysiology. Types 1 and 3 are the result of a partial (type 1) or virtually a complete (type 3) quantitative deficiency of vWF, whereas type 2 is a qualitative defect in vWF. Type 1 vWD represents the most common subtype accounting for approximately 70% of patients, whereas type 2 accounts for 15% to 20% and type 3 for only 2% to 5% of vWD patients [6].

Because bleeding symptoms in persons with vWD may be absent or overlooked until a major hemorrhage due to surgery or trauma has occurred, the diagnosis should be considered in an ICU patient with otherwise unexplained excessive bleeding, particularly if there is a significant family history including an autosomal pattern of inheritance. The most common historical bleeding symptoms include epistaxis, increased bleeding after dental extractions, and menorrhagia. A validated bleeding assessment tool has been developed to screen outpatients who may benefit from formal vWD laboratory testing, but its usefulness in the critical care setting has not been established.

A formal diagnosis of vWD should be based on three components: (a) a history of excessive bleeding, either spontaneous, mucocutaneous and/or postsurgical, (b) a positive family history for excessive bleeding, and (c) confirmatory laboratory testing. Diagnostic tests for vWD, reviewed elsewhere [6], should be performed in a specialized laboratory and are summarized in Table 88.2.

TABLE 88.2

Expected Laboratory Values in vWD from the NHLBI

	Normal	Type 1	Type 2A	Type 2B	Type 2M	Type 2N	Type 3	PLT-vWD[a]
vWF:Ag	N	L, ↓ or ↓↓	↓ or L	↓ or L	↓ or L	N or L	Absent	↓ or L
vWF:RCo	N	L, ↓ or ↓↓	↓↓ or ↓↓↓	↓↓	↓↓	N or L	Absent	↓↓
FVIII	N	N or ↓	N or ↓	N or ↓	N or ↓	↓↓	1–9 IU/dL	N or L
RIPA	N	Often N	↓	Often N	↓	N	Absent	Often N
LD RIPA	Absent	Absent	Absent	↑↑↑	Absent	Absent	Absent	↑↑↑
PFA-100 CT	N	N or ↑	↑	↑	↑	N	↑↑↑	↑
BT	N	N or ↑	↑	↑	↑	N	↑↑↑↑	↑
Platelet count	N	N	N	↓ or N	N	N	N	↓
vWF Multimer Pattern	N	N	Abnormal	Abnormal	N	N	Absent	Abnormal

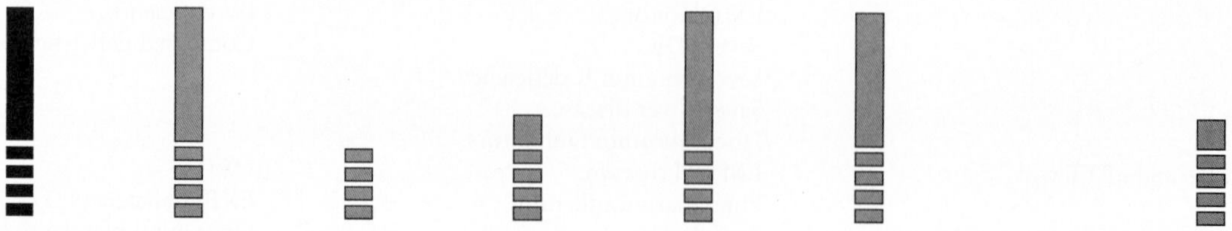

L, 30–50 IU/dL; ↓, ↓↓, ↓↓↓, relative decrease; ↑, ↑↑, ↑↑↑, relative increase; BT, bleeding time; FVIII, factor VIII activity; LD RIPA, low-dose ristocetin-induced platelet aggregation (concentration of ristocetin ≤ 0.6 mg/mL); N, normal; PFA-100 CT, platelet function analyzer closure time; RIPA, ristocetin-induced platelet aggregation; vWF, von Willebrand factor; vWF:Ag, vWF antigen; vWF:RCo, vWF ristocetin cofactor activity.

[a]The symbols and values represent prototypical cases. In practice, laboratory studies in certain patients may deviate slightly from these expectations.

Reprinted from The National Heart, Lung, and Blood Institute: *The Diagnosis, Evaluation, and Management of von Willebrand Disease*. Bethesda, MD, National Institutes of Health Publication 08-5832, 2008.

The goals of treatment in vWD are to correct the quantitative or qualitative deficiencies in vWF, platelets, and FVIII. Treatment options include desmopressin (DDAVP), vWF-containing concentrates, and/or antifibrinolytics. See Tables 88.3 and 88.4 for general treatment guidelines.

In normal volunteers, DDAVP increases plasma levels of FVIII, vWF, and t-PA [8]. It may be given by the intravenous, subcutaneous, or intranasal route [9]. When given intravenously, the FVIII and vWF levels are usually increased three- to fivefold above basal levels within 30 minutes. vWD patients should undergo a DDAVP trial to gauge their individual response as there is considerable interindividual variability. Dosing of DDAVP for vWD is generally recommended at 0.3 μg per kg (IV or SQ), or 300 μg intranasally, which can be repeated at intervals of 12 to 24 hours. Tachyphylaxis (due to depletion of FVIII/vWF from repeated endothelial exocytosis into plasma) following repeated dosing is expected; DDAVP given as a second dose is 30% less effective than the first dose [10]. For this reason, and because of the risk of hyponatremia (which can lead to seizures), serial dosing should be limited to two to three doses

TABLE 88.3

Dosing Guidelines for von Willebrand Disease (vWD) Treatment

Medication	Dose	Comments
DDAVP	Nasal spray: 300 μg (1 spray in each nostril) If weight <50 kg 150 μg (1 spray in 1 nostril) IV: 0.3 μg/kg (not to exceed 20–25 μg)	Most useful in type 1 vWD, ineffective in type 3. Requires challenge to document efficacy. Relatively contraindicated in type 2B as may exacerbate thrombocytopenia May repeat dose in 12 h and/or 24 h. Tachyphylaxis occurs with repeat dosing. Due to risk of hyponatremia, if dosing serially, limit doses to no more than 2–3 in a 72-h period, restrict fluid, and follow serum sodium levels. Avoid in patients with coronary disease.
Antifibrinolytic agents: epsilon aminocaproic acid (EACA) Tranexamic acid	50 mg/kg PO up to q6h (lower doses may be effective) or 1 g/h IV continuous infusion Do not exceed 24 g/24 h 25 mg/kg q8h (not yet available in the United States)	Especially useful for mucocutaneous bleeding, especially for dental procedures May be used as adjunctive treatment (DDAVP, factor concentrates) Avoid in upper urinary tract bleeding
vWF-containing FVIII concentrates (e.g., Humate-P, Alphanate)	60–80 RCoF U/kg as an initial dose, then 40–60 U/kg IV every 12 h (see Table 88.4)	FVIII activity levels are often used in the monitoring of response to vWF-containing products as real-time vWF activity measures are not always available Dosed in RCoF units. Individual product is labeled with ratio of RCoF units:FVIII

DDAVP, desmopressin; vWD, von Willebrand disease; vWF, von Willebrand factor; RCoF, ristocetin cofactor.

TABLE 88.4

Suggested Initial Dosing of vWF Concentrates for Prevention or Management of Bleeding

Major surgery/bleeding	
Loading dose[a]	60–80 RCoF U/kg
Maintenance dose	40–60 RCoF U/kg, typically every 12 h initially
Monitoring	vWF:RCo and FVIII trough and peak, at least daily
Therapeutic goal	Trough vWF:RCo and FVIII >50 IU/dL for 7–14 d
Safety parameter	Do not exceed vWF:RCo 200 IU/dL or FVIII 250–300 IU/dL
May alternate with DDAVP for latter part of treatment	
Minor surgery/bleeding	
Loading dose[a]	30–60 U/kg
Maintenance dose	20–40 U/kg every 12–48 h
Monitoring	vWF:RCo and FVIII trough and peak, at least once
Therapeutic goal	Trough vWF:RCo and FVIII >50 IU/dL for 3–5 d
Safety parameter	Do not exceed vWF:RCo 200 IU/dL or FVIII 250–300 IU/dL
May alternate with DDAVP for latter part of treatment	

[a]Loading dose is in vWF:RCo IU/dL.
Adapted from The National Heart, Lung, and Blood Institute: *The Diagnosis, Evaluation, and Management of von Willebrand Disease*. Bethesda, MD, National Institutes of Health Publication 08-5832, 2008.

in a 72-hour period with concurrent free water restriction and monitoring of serum sodium levels. DDAVP is most effective in type 1 vWD. It is relatively contraindicated in type 2B vWD because of the transient induction of thrombocytopenia. Patients with type 3 vWD are usually unresponsive to DDAVP. Certain hemophilia treatment centers caution against the use of DDAVP in patients with coronary artery disease, as this agent may also activate platelets.

Antifibrinolytic agents (epsilon aminocaproic acid and tranexamic acid) can be used alone or as adjunctive treatment in vWD patients with mucosal bleeding. These drugs inhibit fibrinolysis by inhibiting plasminogen activation, thereby promoting clot stability. They are contraindicated in the setting of gross hematuria as resultant ureteral obstruction by insoluble clot has been described. Given a concern for thrombosis, antifibrinolytics should be avoided in patients with prothrombotic conditions, disseminated intravascular coagulation (DIC), or when receiving prothrombin complex concentrates (PCCs).

vWF factor-containing FVIII concentrates are appropriate for patients with severe vWD or in situations when other therapies (including DDAVP) are ineffective and are preferred to cryoprecipitate, which contains vWF, but has not undergone viral inactivation. When used in the treatment of vWD, they are dosed in ristocetin cofactor (RCoF) units, as opposed to FVIII units (Table 88.4). Limited data suggest a role for rFVIIa in patients with type 3 vWD who have developed alloantibodies to vWF.

The National Heart Lung and Blood Institute has published guidelines for the diagnosis, evaluation, and management of vWD [6].

Hemophilia

The hemophilias are congenital bleeding disorders characterized by X-linked inheritance and result in a deficiency of FVIII (hemophilia A) or FIX (hemophilia B). In the United States, they have a combined incidence of 1 in 5,000 male births. Hemophilia A is more common than hemophilia B and accounts for approximately 80% of cases. Because hemophilia is an X-linked disorder, all daughters of affected males are obligate carriers and all sons are healthy. Females may rarely manifest bleeding symptoms if they (a) are the homozygous offspring from a carrier mother and affected father, (b) have a high degree of lyonization, or (c) are a carrier with concomitant Turner's syndrome (XO).

The clinical phenotype of hemophilia patients depends on the residual level of circulating procoagulant protein (FVIII or FIX). It is possible to differentiate three degrees of clinical severity: (a) mild hemophilia (5% to 50% factor activity) in which bleeding is prolonged but typically only occurs following trauma or surgery, (b) moderate hemophilia (1% to 5% factor activity) in which prolonged bleeding follows minor trauma, and (c) severe hemophilia (<1% factor activity) where patients experience spontaneous hemorrhage into joints (hemarthrosis) and muscles.

In severe and moderate hemophilia, the PT is normal and the aPTT is prolonged. However, the PTT may be normal in patients with mild hemophilia whose residual factor activity is >20%. If the aPTT is prolonged, it should correct with a mixing study, as hemophilia is a factor deficiency syndrome. Specific factor assays should be performed to confirm a diagnosis of hemophilia A or B.

The management of most cases of hemophilia, thanks to the availability of replacement clotting factor concentrates, occurs in the outpatient setting, but individuals who previously have escaped diagnosis (mild or moderate hemophilia) or who have sustained major trauma or complications from a bleeding episode (compartment syndrome) may present to critical care. If not previously diagnosed, hemophilia should be suspected in male patients who have a personal history of bleeding into joints or muscles, a history of excessive bleeding upon surgical challenge, and/or a positive sex-linked family history of bleeding.

Hemarthrosis, a hallmark of hemophilia, accounts for approximately 85% of all bleeding events in severe hemophilia and most commonly involves the ankles, knees, and elbows. Intramuscular hematomas in persons with hemophilia may expand to the point where blood flow is compromised to surrounding neurovascular structures resulting in tissue gangrene and compartment syndrome; the condition requires surgery and aggressive clotting factor replacement therapy [11] (Table 88.5). Gastrointestinal bleeding is uncommon in hemophilia. However, patients with an underlying structural lesion may present with hematemesis, hematochezia, or melena. Hemophilia patients who present with evidence for gastrointestinal bleeding should have a complete endoscopic evaluation to assess for and treat any underlying lesion. Approximately 90% of persons with severe hemophilia will develop hematuria during their life, although the condition is typically painless, benign, and unassociated with a structural lesion. As discussed earlier, antifibrinolytic agents are contraindicated in patients with genitourinary bleeding.

Hemorrhage into head and neck structures is a medical emergency in persons with hemophilia. Retropharyngeal hematoma, which may occur spontaneously or following dental or surgical procedures, may present with inability to control saliva, neck swelling, and pain. If untreated, it may result in airway compromise and in some cases may require tracheostomy. Hemorrhage into the central nervous system is a severe and potentially fatal (albeit rare) complication of hemophilia. Intracranial hemorrhage (ICH) may occur spontaneously in severe hemophilia or as the result of trauma. Prompt recognition of ICH is paramount and factor replacement therapy should be given immediately while the diagnostic workup is underway (Table 88.5).

The approach to treating major bleeding episodes in hemophilia A and B is similar. The clinical scenario dictates the target factor activity level (Table 88.5). For example, an ICH requires a target activity level of 100% initially, whereas levels of 30% to 40% may be sufficient for minor bleeds such as uncomplicated hemarthrosis. Prior to completion of the diagnostic (radiologic or otherwise) workup, clotting factor concentrate should be administered immediately to a person with hemophilia and a suspected life- or limb-threatening bleed. Plasma-derived and recombinant factor concentrates contain much higher concentrations of the desired factor compared to fresh frozen plasma (FFP) or cryoprecipitate. If possible, avoidance of FFP or cryoprecipitate is advised to avoid volume overload, transfusion-related lung injury (TRALI), and potential transmission of infectious agents (see Chapter 89).

DDAVP may be used instead of factor concentrate in selected patients with mild hemophilia A who have minor bleeding or a requirement for an enhanced FVIII activity level prior to a short-lived bleeding challenge. Any mild hemophilia A patient

TABLE 88.5

Recommended Hemostatic Levels in Hemophilia[a]

Clinical situation	Hemophilia target factor activity (%)[a]
Mild hemorrhage (joint, muscle)	30–40
Mucosal hemorrhage (oral, dental)	30–40 with EACA
Major hemorrhage	>50
Life-threatening hemorrhage or perioperative management (major and orthopedic procedures)	100

[a]Minimum recommended goal factor activity levels.
EACA, epsilon aminocaproic acid.

should undergo a DDAVP trial to gauge his individual response in lieu of assuming efficacy of the agent. FVIII levels in plasma increase two- to sixfold following administration. For mild hemophilia A, the recommended dose is 0.3 μg per kg (IV or SQ) or 300 μg intranasally; as previously discussed, tachyphylaxis and hyponatremia may develop after serial dosing.

Antifibrinolytic agents are a useful adjunctive treatment in hemophilia patients with mucosal bleeding. However, hemophilic patients with hematuria, DIC, receiving a PCC, or other prothrombotic conditions should not be treated with antifibrinolytics.

One of the most significant complications of hemophilia treatment is the development of an inhibitor. Inhibitors are alloantibodies against exogenously administered clotting factor that neutralize the factor. The development of a new inhibitor is more common in hemophilia A than in hemophilia B, in severe hemophilia, and among previously untreated patients (as opposed to adults who typically have been extensively exposed to clotting factor concentrate) [12].

Inhibitors, if present at high titer, neutralize exogenous factor rendering factor concentrates ineffective. Therefore, an inhibitor should be suspected when administration of factor concentrate at a dose previously sufficient to achieve hemostasis, or improve bleeding, fails to do so. Once suspected, a Bethesda assay should be performed to document the titer of the inhibitor (reported in Bethesda units, BU). Of the two goals of treatment in patients with inhibitors, namely, to achieve adequate hemostasis and to eradicate the inhibitor, only the former is typically relevant to the critical care setting. Bleeding should be treated with bypassing agents, typically an activated prothrombin complex concentrate (aPCC) or rFVIIa [13]. If the titer is <5 BU, high doses of FVIII or FIX may be given as initial treatment in cases of life- or limb-threatening bleeding episodes. In patients with a long-standing inhibitor, however, the anamnestic response negates factor activity after 5 to 7 days, at which point bypassing agents become necessary.

RARE CONGENITAL COAGULATION DISORDERS

Less Common Coagulation Factor Deficiencies

The hemophilias and vWD represent approximately 85% of congenital bleeding disorders. The remaining disorders will be briefly discussed next.

Disorders of Fibrinogen

Congenital fibrinogen disorders result from a quantitative (afibrinogenemia) or qualitative (dysfibrinogenemia) defect in fibrinogen synthesis. Congenital afibrinogenemia has a variable bleeding phenotype with the majority of patients experiencing moderate bleeding [9]. Afflicted individuals present typically in the neonatal period with umbilical stump bleeding or bleeding following circumcision. Patients may also experience hemarthrosis, intramuscular hemorrhage, spontaneous abortion, mucosal surface bleeds, ICH, or spontaneous splenic rupture [14]. Heterozygotes are typically asymptomatic. The clinical phenotype in patients with congenital dysfibrinogenemia is variable and includes (a) asymptomatic (55%), (b) hemorrhagic (25%), (c) thrombotic (10% to 20%), or (d) a combination of both hemorrhagic and thrombotic complications (1% to 2%) [15]. Treatment of congenital fibrinogen disorders should be individualized given the clinical variability. In general, replacement therapy in the form of fibrinogen concentrates, cryoprecipitate, or (not recommended) FFP should be given to patients with a hemorrhagic presentation to achieve a goal fibrinogen level of 50 to 100 mg per dL [16].

Prothrombin (FII) Deficiency

Congenital prothrombin deficiency is characterized by a concordant decrease in prothrombin antigen and activity. Aprothrombinemia has not been reported. Patients with hypoprothrombinemia present with severe hemorrhage including ICH, mucocutaneous bleeding, hemarthrosis, spontaneous abortions, and significant postoperative bleeding. Heterozygotes are usually asymptomatic; however, they may experience increased postoperative bleeding [17]. Prothrombin deficiency is treated with factor replacement in the form of FFP or PCC to a goal prothrombin level of 30% [18].

Factor V Deficiency

FV deficiency is associated with mucocutaneous bleeding and rarely with ICH [19]. There are mild, moderate, and severe deficiency states. Patients with severe deficiency usually present with umbilical stump and mucocutaneous bleeding. Older individuals may present with postoperative bleeding or menorrhagia. FV deficiency is treated with FFP to a goal activity level of 20% to 30% [20]. Alpha granules in platelets contain FV, and platelet transfusions have been used in the treatment of FV deficiency when patients have developed neutralizing inhibitors to FV with varying success [21]. Combined deficiency of FV and FVIII should always be considered in the differential diagnosis of patients who present with FV deficiency. This is discussed next.

Combined Factor V and VIII Deficiency

Combined FV and FVIII deficiency (F5F8D) is a rare disorder where patients have detectable, but low antigen and activity levels of both factors, typically in the 5% to 15% range. Patients present with increased bleeding following trauma or surgery. Patients are treated with a combination of FFP and FVIII concentrates [22].

Factor VII Deficiency

Patients with less than 1% FVII activity manifest a severe bleeding disorder, predominantly involving the mucous membranes, muscles, joints, and following surgery or trauma, whereas those with more than 5% have relatively mild symptoms. Factor VII activity correlates poorly with bleeding severity, but in general, only modest amounts of circulating FVII are required for adequate hemostasis, and bleeding is uncommon, even with surgery, in individuals with FVII activity levels >15% to 20% [23]. In the United States, rFVIIa is used to treat FVII deficiency. Plasma-derived FVII concentrates are available in Europe to treat this disorder [24,25]. When rFVIIa and/or FVII concentrates are unavailable, 4-factor PCC or FFP may be used.

Factor X Deficiency

In congenital FX deficiency, severity of bleeding appears to correlate with residual FX activity and may be quite severe. The most common symptoms appear to be epistaxis, menorrhagia, and hemarthrosis [26]. FX deficiency is treated with PCCs.

Factor XI Deficiency

FXI deficiency, previously known as hemophilia C, is common among Ashkenazi Jews where the gene frequency is 8% to 9% [27]. The inheritance is autosomal rather than X linked as with hemophilia A and B. Severe FXI deficiency (<15% to 20% FXI activity) occurs in homozygotes or compound heterozygotes. Heterozygous individuals have a partial FXI deficiency (20% to 70% FXI activity) [27]. Bleeding is unpredictable as some severe FXI-deficient patients are asymptomatic, whereas an analysis of 50 kindreds demonstrated that 30% to 50% of heterozygotes experienced significant bleeding [28].

Treatment for FXI deficiency includes FFP, antifibrinolytic agents [29], FXI concentrates (not available in the United States), and rFVIIa (not FDA approved for this purpose) [30]. There is concern of a prothrombotic potential associated with FXI concentrates as DIC and arterial thrombosis have been described in up to 10% of patients. Heparin has been added to these concentrates to reduce this thrombotic potential, but there is a general recommendation to maintain FXI levels at no greater than 70 IU per dL [30].

Factor XIII Deficiency

The most common presentation for FXIII-deficient patients is umbilical stump bleeding, but FXIII-deficient patients may also experience ICH, hemarthrosis, menorrhagia, and increased bleeding following surgery or trauma [31]. FXIII has a half-life of 8 to 12 days, and levels required to maintain hemostasis are only in the range of 2% to 5%. Treatment includes FXIII concentrates, FFP, or cryoprecipitate. Given FXIII's long half-life, factor concentrates may be given once every several weeks as prophylactic therapy [17].

Vitamin K-Dependent Factor Deficiencies

Patients with combined deficiency of the vitamin K-dependent factors (FII, FVII, FIX, FX, proteins C and S) may present with umbilical stump bleeding or ICH [32]. Factor activity levels are variable and generally range from 1% to 30%. High doses of supplemental vitamin K may significantly improve or completely correct deficient factor activities. In acute bleeding episodes, patients may be treated with FFP or PCCs.

Congenital Qualitative Platelet Disorders

Defects in Platelet Adhesion

Bernard–Soulier syndrome (BSS) is a rare, autosomal recessive, severe bleeding disorder characterized by thrombocytopenia, giant platelets, and severe mucocutaneous bleeding [19]. Deficient platelet binding to subendothelial vWF is caused by abnormalities (either qualitative or quantitative) in the GP Ib/IX/V complex. The mainstay of treatment in BSS is platelet transfusion during clinically significant hemorrhagic episodes. However, alloimmunization to transfused platelets is often encountered when patients develop neutralizing antibodies to GP Ib/IX/V on transfused platelets which renders those platelets useless. rFVIIa has been used to treat patients with these inhibitors and has proven successful in many cases [33].

Defects in Platelet Aggregation

Glanzmann thrombasthenia is a rare, autosomal recessive disorder characterized by absent platelet aggregation secondary to defective GP IIb/IIIa on the platelet surface. Affected patients present with severe to life-threatening mucocutaneous bleeding. Treatment includes platelet transfusion. However, many patients may become refractory as alloantibodies to transfused platelet forms. rFVIIa has been used to treat bleeding in this disorder [34].

Disorders of Platelet Secretion: The Storage Pool Diseases

Platelets contain two types of intracellular granules, alpha and delta (or dense), which are required for an optimal secondary wave of platelet aggregation. The gray platelet syndrome is the most common alpha granule storage pool disease (SPD) and may predispose to early onset myelofibrosis, a probable consequence of the impaired storage of growth factors such as platelet-derived growth factor [35]. Hermansky–Pudlak syndrome and Chédiak–Higashi syndrome are SPDs affecting dense granules [36]. The Hermansky–Pudlak syndrome is associated with oculocutaneous albinism and increased accumulation of an abnormal fat-protein compound, ceroid, in the reticuloendothelial system. The Chédiak–Higashi syndrome is characterized by oculocutaneous albinism, neurologic abnormalities, immune deficiency with a tendency to infections, and giant inclusions in the cytoplasm of platelets and leukocytes. The primary treatment for clinically significant bleeding in patients with SPDs is platelet transfusion.

ACQUIRED COAGULATION DISORDERS

Anticoagulant Drugs

Use of anticoagulants in the critical care setting is ubiquitous. The pharmacology, monitoring, and appropriate reversal of anticoagulant drugs are reviewed in detail in Chapter 110.

Generally, patients on anticoagulants who develop clinically insignificant bleeding may be closely monitored while the drug is continued; appropriate therapeutic monitoring (e.g., INR, aPTT, TT, anti-Xa) should also be obtained and followed closely. Major bleeding, except in rare instances, typically should prompt discontinuation of anticoagulant drugs. Consideration should also be given to holding subsequent doses or reducing doses based on laboratory or clinical evolution.

Heparins, Low-Molecular-Weight Heparins, and Fondaparinux

These agents, and management of associated bleeding complications, are discussed in Chapter 93.

Warfarin (Coumadin)

Given its widespread use, warfarin is a common cause of iatrogenic, serious bleeding that frequently requires critical care. Warfarin is an oral vitamin K antagonist that exerts its anticoagulant effects through inhibition of vitamin K-dependent γ carboxylation of the vitamin K-dependent factors (FII, FVII, FIX, and FX). γ carboxylation is required for these coagulation factors to become biologically active. Warfarin also inhibits γ carboxylation of the vitamin K-dependent regulatory proteins C and S. Treatment with warfarin reduces the biologically active levels of all these vitamin K-dependent factors, both procoagulant and anticoagulant. However, the net effect at steady state is anticoagulation. Given the half-life of the independent factors affected by warfarin, patients may become relatively prothrombotic in the first several days after warfarin initiation as proteins C and S are the first to become significantly reduced. This is the rationale for "bridging" with unfractionated heparin (UFH) or low-molecular-weight heparin (LMWH) for the first several days of warfarin administration to abrogate extension of existing thrombosis or development of new ones.

Warfarin is monitored via the PT and INR with a typical therapeutic range of 2.0 to 3.0 but this is patient and indication

TABLE 88.6

Reversal of Warfarin-induced Anticoagulation Management of Supratherapeutic INR

Clinical situation	INR	Actions
No significant bleeding	<5.0	• Lower dose, or • Hold dose and restart at a lower dose once INR in desired range, or • Check INR in 24 h if INR only mildly prolonged
	5.0–9.0	• Hold warfarin, repeat INR in 24 h • Give vitamin K_1 1–2.5 mg PO × 1 if at increased risk of bleeding • Check INR in 24 h—when INR in desired range, restart warfarin at adjusted dose
	≥9.0	• Hold warfarin and give vitamin K_1 2.5–5 mg PO × 1 (may repeat in 24 h if INR not improved) • When INR in desired range, restart warfarin at adjusted dose
Serious or life-threatening bleeding	Any prolongation in INR due to warfarin administration	• Hold warfarin • Give vitamin K_1 10 mg slow IV push (over 30 min); may repeat in 12–24 h • Give FFP, prothrombin complex concentrate (PCC), or rFVIIa for acute reversal • Monitor INR and repeat intervention as necessary

Adapted from Ansell J, Hirsh J, Hylek E, et al: Pharmacology and management of the vitamin K antagonists: American College of Chest Physicians Evidence-Based Clinical Practice Guidelines (8th Edition). *Chest* [6, Suppl]:175s, 2008.

specific [24]. At supratherapeutic doses, the aPTT may also become prolonged.

When asymptomatic, supratherapeutic anticoagulation with warfarin does not generally require treatment beyond reducing the dose or holding warfarin for a period of time to allow for correction in the INR. Consideration may also be given to administering a small dose of vitamin K (1 to 5 mg) which will significantly lower the INR within 24 hours, depending on the INR and clinical scenario. If the patient is experiencing significant or life-threatening bleeding, reversal of anticoagulation is indicated and accomplished by replenishing the vitamin K-dependent factors. This can be best achieved using the 4-factor PCC (Table 88.6).

PCCs are plasma-derived products enriched in vitamin K-dependent factors. The typical dose is 25 to 50 U per kg depending on the degree of anticoagulation. There are two types of PCCs available, activated PCC (aPCC) and nonactivated (simply referred to as PCC). The activated form contains activated coagulation proteases that are used in the treatment of hemophilia with inhibitors. The nonactivated formulations were originally licensed for the treatment of hemophilia B, given their high FIX content. Furthermore, there are two types of nonactivated PCCs: a 4-factor (FII, FVII, FIX, FX)–containing product and 3-factor (FII, FIX, FX) products. Although the 3-factor products do contain some FVII, it is at a low concentration (less than one-third that of FIX) and therefore is considered a 3-factor concentrate. Recently, a 4-factor PCC was approved for reversal of oral vitamin K antagonist–induced bleeding. Both activated and nonactivated PCCs contain heparin and are therefore contraindicated in patients with heparin-induced thrombocytopenia [24]. As the effects of FFP, PCC, and rFVIIa are transient, 10 mg of parenteral vitamin K (IV over 30 minutes) should also be given to reverse the INR more durably. When available, PCCs are preferred over FFP because they are concentrated into much smaller volumes, can be virally inactivated, and have a lower risk of TRALI (see Chapter 89). The pharmacodynamics of warfarin is discussed further in Chapter 93.

Superwarfarins

The superwarfarins are a group of pharmacologic compounds that are long-acting rat poisons. They have considerably longer half-lives than warfarin (weeks to months vs. 1 to 2 days) and are considerably more potent. Superwarfarin poisoning has been associated with homicide and suicide attempts, accidental ingestion, and occupational exposure. Patients typically present with bleeding symptoms and laboratory findings similar to those of warfarin overdose; however, the PT/INR does not appropriately normalize with standard doses of vitamin K. An assay for each of the superwarfarins is necessary to confirm the diagnosis. Patients require high doses of vitamin K for prolonged periods to control bleeding risk. FFP or PCCs may be required in episodes of life-threatening bleeding [25].

Direct Thrombin Inhibitors (Argatroban, Bivalirudin, and Dabigatran)

Reversal of anticoagulation due to direct thrombin inhibitors (DTIs) in cases of clinically significant bleeding is typically achieved through cessation of drug given a short half-life (<1 hour). A specific reversal agent for dabigatran has been approved for use in bleeding patients or those who need urgent surgery. This agent, Idarucizumab, is a F(ab)2 against dabigatran, which binds and clears active drug from the circulation. The pharmacodynamics of DTIs is discussed in greater detail in Chapter 93.

Vitamin K Deficiency

Vitamin K deficiency is a frequently encountered problem in hospitalized medical patients. It is particularly common in those with chronic malabsorption syndromes (e.g., cystic fibrosis), malnutrition, and those on broad-spectrum antibiotics [37]. Patients on warfarin and with vitamin K deficiency present with similar laboratory and physical findings, namely prolongation primarily of the PT as well as easy bruising or soft tissue bleeding. Vitamin K deficiency is managed by supplementation of vitamin K. If a patient has a malabsorptive syndrome, parenteral vitamin K is typically recommended.

As vitamin K-dependent coagulation factors are synthesized in the liver, it can be difficult to distinguish between vitamin K deficiency and a coagulopathy of liver disease (decreased hepatic synthesis of coagulation factors). In clinical scenarios where underlying liver disease is present, it may be beneficial to evaluate coagulation factor levels, both vitamin K dependent and independent (e.g., FII and FV, respectively). In this example, if both FII and FV levels are decreased, then the patient likely has hepatic synthetic dysfunction. If FV is normal and FII is decreased, then the patient likely has vitamin K deficiency.

Coagulopathy of Liver Disease

An unfortunate hallmark of liver disease is coagulopathy. It stands to reason that as all of the coagulation factors (except FVIII, which is also synthesized in extrahepatic endothelial cells) are made in the liver, end-stage liver disease (ESLD) is marked by multiple coagulation factor deficiencies [38]. However, increased extravascular redistribution and increased factor consumption also contribute. The degree of coagulation factor reduction as well as the number of factors reduced typically parallel the severity of liver disease. Factors V and VII appear to be sensitive markers of hepatic synthetic dysfunction with FVII levels typically the most notably affected secondary to its short half-life [39]. A prolongation in the PT is therefore an early marker of liver disease. As hepatic dysfunction progresses and other coagulation factors in the common and contact activation pathway are decreased, the aPTT prolongs. In contrast, FVIII levels are typically elevated in compensated cirrhosis. This may be secondary to an increase in vWF that is seen in cirrhotics. In addition, proteins required for FVIII clearance such as low-density lipoprotein receptor-related protein are present in decreased amounts, thus raising FVIII levels. Patients with liver disease may have normal fibrinogen levels, given its long half-life, but they may develop an acquired dysfibrinogenemia associated with abnormal fibrinogen glycosylation that disrupts fibrin polymerization. This may be reflected by a normal fibrinogen quantitative assay but an abnormal functional assay such as the TT or RT.

In addition to coagulation factor deficiency, a number of other variables associated with advanced liver disease may contribute to coagulopathy in this population. These include (a) vitamin K deficiency secondary to malnutrition, malabsorption/maldigestion from bile salt insufficiency, and altered intestinal motility; (b) portal hypertension with resultant hypersplenism and secondary thrombocytopenia; (c) decreased thrombopoietin (the principal regulator of platelet production) synthesis by hepatocytes with resultant thrombocytopenia; (d) impaired platelet function as demonstrated by abnormal platelet function, as assessed by PFA-100; and (e) hyperfibrinolysis secondary to impaired synthesis of plasminogen activator inhibitors and decreased clearance of plasminogen activators. Chronic, low-grade DIC may also contribute to coagulopathy (discussed later).

Despite evidence for a significant coagulopathy based on laboratory tests as well as evident petechiae, ecchymosis, purpura, and bleeding after invasive procedures, patients with ESLD rarely bleed spontaneously. It is much more common for them to present with hemorrhage as a result of an underlying anatomic lesion such as from an esophageal varix. There remains active debate as to the actual net degree of coagulopathy in these patients. For instance, Mannucci has argued that defects in platelet number and function may be balanced by increased levels of vWF. Furthermore, decreased levels of coagulation factors and inhibitors of fibrinolysis are balanced by decreased levels of inhibitors of coagulation and profibrinolytic factors [40]. The end result is a potential rebalancing of hemostasis. The fact that the degree of PT and aPTT prolongation correlates poorly with bleeding after liver biopsy and other potentially hemorrhagic procedures supports this rebalancing notion [41,42]. Ultimately, a more comprehensive assessment of hemostasis is needed as PT and aPTT only assess thrombin generation in a closed system devoid of anticoagulant factors and do not address fibrinolysis at all.

Given that we lack a comprehensive hemostatic assessment tool, many physicians prefer to prophylactically give FFP or other hemostatic agents to patients with ESLD who are to undergo procedures or who have significantly abnormal coagulation laboratory values. Unfortunately, we have little data to support these measures. The current guidelines recommend FFP transfusions only when hemostasis is needed for bleeding or invasive procedures and the PT or aPTT is >1.5 times normal (reviewed in reference [43]). FFP is generally given at a dose of 10 to 15 mL per kg repeated every 8 hours. Notably, despite repeated infusions of FFP, the PT may not completely correct and therefore clinical response should be monitored rather than relying on the PT as a measure of efficacy. As discussed earlier, patients with ESLD may also develop hypofibrinogenemia or a dysfibrinogenemia. This should be suspected in a patient with a prolonged TT or RT or in a patient who continues to bleed despite FFP infusion. Cryoprecipitate may be required to treat hypo/dysfibrinogenemia as FFP typically does not sufficiently replace fibrinogen. Cryoprecipitate is typically given in doses of 10 pooled units. Patients should be transfused to a goal fibrinogen level of >100 mg per dL. There are a number of human fibrinogen concentrates available in Europe, and in 2009 the Food and Drug Administration approved the first human fibrinogen concentrate in the United States. It is currently indicated for the treatment of patients with congenital afibrinogenemia and hypofibrinogenemia. Some authors have reported beneficial outcomes in patients given rFVIIa and PCCs in ESLD. However, there are currently no guidelines or randomized trials that address dosing or efficacy. However, given the hypervolemia typical of patients with ESLD, multiple infusions of FFP may not be possible and treatment with PCCs may be considered to reduce volume overload as well as decrease the risk of TRALI. Many have argued for controlled trials to evaluate the role of prophylactic hemostatic agents in this patient population as current practice typically involves using expert opinion and case series data.

Disseminated Intravascular Coagulation

DIC is a well-recognized syndrome characterized by both thrombotic and hemorrhagic complications in the setting of a number of defined disorders that are typically associated with systemic inflammation (Table 88.7). The pathogenesis of DIC is complex and is characterized by widespread activation of the TF coagulation pathway with a marked imbalance between procoagulant and anticoagulant processes resulting in unopposed thrombin generation and diffuse fibrin clot formation with subsequent microvascular occlusion and tissue hypoxia [44]. When severe, these changes may culminate in multiple organ dysfunction syndrome.

The clinical presentation of DIC is variable and the majority of patients do not demonstrate a significant hemorrhagic phenotype. A clinical suspicion for DIC is paramount in establishing its diagnosis. In addition to a compatible underlying condition (e.g., sepsis), abnormal laboratory studies consistent with increased thrombin generation and fibrinolysis (consumptive coagulopathy) are also required. A DIC screening panel is typically composed of PT, aPTT, platelet count, fibrinogen, and D-dimer. DIC is suggested when the laboratories demonstrate increased activation of coagulation (elevated PT/aPTT, decreased fibrinogen) as well as evidence of fibrinolysis (elevated D-dimer or fibrin

TABLE 88.7

Disorders Associated with Disseminated Intravascular Coagulation

Infection
- Gram-negative or gram-positive septicemia
- Rickettsiae—especially Rocky Mountain spotted fever
- Spirochetes
- Fungi
- Viruses—especially herpes
- Protozoa—especially malaria

Tissue damage
- Trauma
- Crush injury
- Burn
- Heat stroke
- Hemolytic transfusion reaction

Neoplasia
- Metastatic carcinoma
- Leukemia—especially acute promyelocytic leukemia
- Chemotherapy

Obstetric disasters
- *Abruptio placentae*
- Retained dead fetus
- Preeclampsia/eclampsia
- Amniotic fluid embolism
- Placenta previa, accreta, and percreta

Miscellaneous
- Fat embolism
- Shock
- Cardiac arrest
- Giant hemangioma (Kasabach–Merritt syndrome)
- Vasculitis
- Toxins (snake venom, brown recluse spider bite)
- Near drowning—especially fresh water

degradation products). An elevation in PT is a very sensitive measure of DIC but has lower specificity as it may be normal, especially in chronic DIC [44]. As fibrinogen is an acute phase reactant, it may be normal or even elevated in chronic DIC, thereby limiting its specificity in low-grade DIC. Elevation of D-dimer is a sensitive marker for DIC, in the range of 90% to 100% in one report; however, its specificity limits its utility as a single screening test [45].

The International Society on Thrombosis and Hemostasis established a subcommittee on DIC to develop and validate a scoring system to aid in the diagnosis of DIC. This system is based on platelet count, fibrin degradation products, PT, and fibrinogen level [46]. A prospective validation study demonstrated this scoring system to be 91% sensitive and 97% specific for the diagnosis of DIC, with higher scores correlated with higher 28-day mortality (Table 88.8) [47].

Identification and treatment of the underlying disorder remains the hallmark of treatment for DIC. Treatment of DIC should be based on both the clinical presentation as well as the laboratory results. Recommendations for the management of DIC are based on expert opinion given a lack of published, randomized data. In general, patients who experience significant bleeding or who require invasive procedures should be treated with FFP to replace coagulation factors. PCCs may also be considered when hypervolemia complicates FFP administration, but they may lack certain depleted factors such as FV [48]. Cryoprecipitate should be used to replace fibrinogen if the plasma level is <100 g per dL. Although there is no established threshold at which to transfuse platelets in DIC, in the setting of active bleeding or in anticipation of invasive procedures, platelet transfusions may be indicated.

TABLE 88.8

Diagnostic Score for Disseminated Intravascular Coagulation

1. Underlying disorder associated with DIC—if yes → proceed, if no → do not proceed, search for alternative process
2. Obtain global coagulation tests: platelet count, PT, fibrinogen, D-dimer
3. Assign score based on laboratory tests
   a. Platelet count
      i. >100 = 0, <100 = 1, <50 = 2
   b. D-dimer or fibrin degradation products
      i. No increase = 0, moderate increase = 2, strong increase = 3
   c. Prolonged PT
      i. <3 s = 0, >3 s but <6 s = 1, >6 s = 2
   d. Fibrinogen level
      i. >1.0 g/L = 0, <1.0 g/L = 1
4. Calculate score
   a. If ≥5, compatible for DIC
   b. If <5, suggestive, but not confirmed DIC, repeat in 1–2 d

Adapted from Bakhtiara K, Meijers JC, de Jonge E, et al: Prospective validation of the International Society of Thrombosis and Haemostasis scoring system for disseminated intravascular coagulation. *Crit Care Med* 32(12):2416–2421, 2004.

In contrast to replacing coagulation factors, fibrinogen, and platelets, some investigators have evaluated the role of anticoagulants, namely UFH, in the treatment of DIC. This putative measure is based on the pathologic activation of coagulation associated with DIC as well as the depletion of endogenous anticoagulants. Initial animal studies evaluating anticoagulants in DIC suggested a benefit [49]; however, subsequent human trials have yielded conflicting results [50,51]. To date there are no data from randomized, controlled trials to support the use of UFH in the management of DIC.

DIC is discussed in further detail in Chapters 91 and 94.

Trauma-Induced Coagulopathy

Trauma-induced coagulopathy includes the coagulopathy associated with the stresses of trauma as well as unintended consequences of its treatment. Historically it was felt that the coagulopathy associated with trauma was largely secondary to dilution of the coagulation system with volume and blood replacement. However, it is becoming increasingly apparent that this process is much more dynamic and complicated. Traumatic events requiring massive transfusion of blood lead to significant coagulopathy through a number of mechanisms that include (a) dilution of coagulation proteins and platelets from volume resuscitation, (b) consumptive coagulopathy and thrombocytopenia (through DIC associated with trauma), (c) acidemia which impairs function of the coagulation cascade, (d) hypothermia which impairs function of platelets and coagulation factors, and (e) electrolyte perturbations, particularly hypocalcemia which impairs the calcium-dependent coagulation processes [52]. Prompt attention is required to mitigate the coagulopathy associated with trauma and to rapidly correct it. Clinically, patients have a compatible history of massive trauma requiring aggressive resuscitation and typically have a prolongation of PT and aPTT that corrects on mixing study, as well as thrombocytopenia and often hypofibrinogenemia. Treatment is targeted at correcting or preventing the occurrence of the aforementioned mechanisms that have been associated with the development of trauma-induced coagulopathy. Most guidelines recommend transfusion of red blood cells to a target hemoglobin of 7 to 10 g per dL to maintain rheology, FFP administration to a goal PT/aPTT of $<1.5 \times$ upper limit of normal, platelet transfusion to keep platelets $>50 \times 10^9$ per L (or $>100 \times 10^9$ in patients with brain injury), and fibrinogen >100 mg per dL [53]. More recently, ratio-driven transfusion protocols utilizing equal volumes of FFP, packed red cells, and platelets have been utilized to treat hemorrhagic shock in both trauma and non-trauma patients [54]. The use of factor concentrates (fibrinogen, PCCs) to target specific phases of coagulation may offer benefit over blood product ratio-driven transfusion. The outcome benefit of factor concentrates, however, has not yet been demonstrated in well-powered prospective trials [55].

Acquired Hemophilia A

The most common antibodies that affect clotting factor activity with a resultant hemorrhagic phenotype are directed against FVIII. Acquired hemophilia A, or acquired FVIII deficiency, is a rare disorder with an estimated incidence of 1.0 per million that is caused by autoantibodies directed against a patient's endogenous FVIII, resulting in low FVIII activity levels [56]. Acquired hemophilia A is most commonly an idiopathic condition that occurs in the elderly but can also be associated with malignancy, drugs, autoimmune disorders, and the postpartum state.

Acquired hemophilia should be suspected in patients without a prior bleeding history who present later in life with significant, large ecchymoses, hematomas, mucosal, gastrointestinal bleeding, or who experience significant bleeding following surgery or trauma. Hemarthroses that are a hallmark of congenital hemophilia are not typical of acquired hemophilia.

Patients with acquired hemophilia present with bleeding symptoms and a prolonged aPTT in contrast to patients with a lupus anticoagulant who typically present with a prolonged aPTT and thrombotic complications [57,58]. Once acquired hemophilia is suspected based on clinical presentation and a prolonged aPTT, an incubated aPTT mixing study should be performed. As FVIII inhibitors are commonly time and temperature dependent, the mixing study should be performed at 37°C for 1 to 2 hours. In the case of an acquired FVIII inhibitor, the incubated aPTT will not completely correct into the normal range which indicates the presence of an inhibitor. A FVIII activity level may also be helpful to identify the inhibitor as FVIII specific. The strength of the inhibitor may be quantified in a Bethesda assay. The strength of the inhibitor has treatment implications.

Treatment goals of these patients are twofold: (a) control of bleeding and (b) eradication of the inhibitor. Bleeding in patients with low-titer inhibitors (<5 BU) can often be treated with high doses of FVIII concentrates. Bleeding in patients with high-titer inhibitors is treated with a FVIII inhibitor bypassing agent, such as an aPCC or rFVIIa [59,60]. Recombinant porcine FVIII has been recently approved for treatment of acquired hemophilia [61]. Inhibitor eradication typically involves immunosuppression, though spontaneous resolution of the inhibitor can occur [62,63].

ACQUIRED PLATELET DISORDERS/DYSFUNCTION

Medications

The antiplatelet effect of medications is the most common cause for acquired platelet dysfunction. Aspirin and nonsteroidal antiinflammatory drugs (NSAIDs) are the most commonly used medications that affect platelet function (Table 88.9) [64]. Their predominant antiplatelet effect is achieved through the inhibition of platelet cyclooxygenase (COX-1) which in turn ultimately inhibits vasoconstriction and platelet aggregation. Inhibition of COX-1 by aspirin is irreversible for the life of the platelet and is dose dependent. There is an increased risk of bleeding in patients taking aspirin, and two meta-analyses described an approximate 1% increase in absolute risk of bleeding in patients taking aspirin compared to placebo [65,66]. Notably, this bleeding risk does not appear to be dose dependent when the total daily dose is ≤325 mg per day but does increase with concomitant administration of other anticoagulants or antiplatelet agents [67,68]. The primary site of bleeding associated with aspirin is gastrointestinal. NSAIDs, on the other hand, reversibly inhibit COX-1 for the length of time that the medication remains metabolically active. Platelet function is not substantially affected by the COX-2 specific inhibitor, celecoxib, or acetaminophen.

TABLE 88.9

Drugs that Commonly Affect Platelet Function

- Analgesics
  - Aspirin
  - NSAIDs
- Cardiovascular medications
  - Dipyridamole
- $P2Y_{12}$ receptor blockers—thienopyridines
  - Ticlid (ticlopidine)
  - Plavix (clopidogrel)
  - Effient (prasugrel)
- GP IIb/IIIa inhibitors
  - ReoPro (abciximab)
  - Aggrastat (tirofiban)
  - Integrilin (eptifibatide)
- Antibiotics
  - β-Lactam antibiotics—e.g., PCN, cephalosporins
- Psychotropic
  - Antidepressants (fluoxetine)
  - Phenothiazines
- Herbal supplements
  - Fish oil
  - Cumin
  - Garlic
  - *Ginkgo biloba*
  - Turmeric

Dipyridamole is a less frequently used antiplatelet drug with an unclear mechanism of action. It has historically been used for stroke prophylaxis. There does not appear to be a significant increase in bleeding risk for patients taking dipyridamole versus placebo in several randomized trials evaluating the efficacy of dipyridamole in stroke prevention [69].

Clopidogrel (Plavix), ticlopidine (Ticlid) and prasugrel (Effient) belong to a class of antiplatelet agents known as the thienopyridines and are in the treatment of cardio- and cerebrovascular disease. Thienopyridines are irreversible antagonists to the platelet $P2Y_{12}$ receptor which inhibits ADP-mediated platelet aggregation. The thienopyridines, particularly ticlopidine (Ticlid), have been implicated in the development of thrombotic thrombocytopenic purpura [40]. Ticagrelor (Brilinta) is often listed with thienopyridine inhibitors and has similar indications for use but is not a thienopyridine. It is a cyclo-pentyltriazolo-pyrimidine that reversibly inhibits the $P2Y_{12}$ receptor.

The GP IIb/IIIa antagonists are a group of antiplatelet agents that are primarily used during coronary procedures. These drugs impair aggregation by inhibiting the cross bridging of platelets by fibrinogen. This class is associated with an increased risk of bleeding, particularly at the puncture site for percutaneous coronary intervention. There does not appear to be an increased risk for intracerebral hemorrhage for patients receiving GP IIb/IIIa inhibitors versus heparin [70]. These agents are also associated with thrombocytopenia, often profound, that may result in significant bleeding complications [71].

Many other medications including large doses of penicillins, psychotropic drugs such as fluoxetine, dietary supplements such as fish oil, gingko, garlic, and cumin may impair platelet function, although not typically to a significant degree [72].

Laboratory testing to confirm an acquired platelet defect secondary to medication is rarely necessary as clinical history and medication record usually suffice. However, if needed for confirmation, platelet function testing may be useful. Treatment for drug-induced platelet dysfunction depends on the severity of bleeding as well as the medication involved. In most cases, minor bleeding may be addressed by withholding the medication. In more severe cases, platelet transfusion may be indicated depending on timing of the last dose as well as its specific platelet effect. In general, platelets have an average life span of 7 to 10 days. As a result, the bone marrow replaces approximately 10% of the body's platelets each day. Therefore, if a medication irreversibly inhibits platelet function, platelet transfusion may be needed to reverse the antiplatelet effect until the bone marrow has sufficiently replenished the affected platelets. For most situations, a single platelet transfusion is sufficient to correct bleeding association with disordered platelets.

Acquired platelet dysfunction due to antiplatelet agents is discussed in further detail in Chapter 91.

Uremia

The multisystem organ dysfunction encountered in critically ill patients often includes acute kidney injury and subsequent uremia. Bleeding associated with uremia has long been recognized and has historically been associated with a prolonged BT. However, the degree of BT prolongation neither correlates with the degree of azotemia nor the severity of bleeding symptoms. The clinical manifestations of uremic bleeding are predominantly mucocutaneous, though patients may present with epistaxis, gastrointestinal bleeding, hematuria, or increased bleeding following surgery or procedures.

Despite this long-recognized association between uremia and a bleeding diathesis, the exact pathophysiology remains poorly defined, though impairment in platelet function appears integral [73]. There are data to suggest that this is a multifactorial process and includes an acquired platelet defect as well as impairment in platelet–endothelium interaction. Additional factors include vWF abnormalities, anemia which affects rheology, thrombocytopenia, uremic toxins, and increased nitrous oxide (NO) production [74]. The presence of a uremic toxin is supported by the improvement in platelet function in patients following dialysis. Notably, urea is unlikely to be the primary toxin as there is no positive correlation between blood urea nitrogen and bleeding risk [75].

Treatment for uremic bleeding often includes aggressive dialysis which may correct the bleeding and has been suggested to prevent uremic bleeding [76]. DDAVP has been recommended as the first-line therapy for uremic bleeding (2 to 4 μg per kg intranasally or 0.3 μg per kg by slow intravenous infusion); it improves platelet function in uremia, most likely due to release of FVIII and vWF [77]. If no improvement is noted after the first dose, further doses should not be given. If DDAVP is ineffective or contraindicated, cryoprecipitate may be given (10 units every 12 to 14 hours). Improvement in bleeding in response to cryoprecipitate is likely related to FVIII and vWF [78]. Correction of anemia to a goal hematocrit of 30% corrects the BT in many patients through improved rheology. This may be accomplished via red cell transfusions in the acute period or erythropoietin over prolonged periods. Erythropoietin may also have beneficial effects on platelet function [79]. Conjugated estrogens may improve uremic bleeding and appears to do so in a dose-dependent manner presumably by reducing NO production (reviewed in reference [76]).

Hematologic Disorders

Abnormal platelet function is frequently noted in patients with a number of primary hematologic disorders, including myelodysplastic syndromes and myeloproliferative disorders. The bleeding diathesis occurs out of proportion to that expected in patients with similar quantitative platelet defects. In general, the mechanisms underlying the platelet dysfunction seen in these disorders are poorly understood but probably reflect the genetic and developmental abnormalities in stem cells that underlie these disorders. The severity of the predisposition to bleeding cannot be reliably predicted from the results of the BT, platelet count, or in vitro platelet function tests.

The bleeding complications of the myeloproliferative disorders have been estimated in the literature to range from 1.7% to 37%, depending on the disorder and population screened [80]. The bleeding manifestations in both polycythemia vera and essential thrombocythemia involve the skin and mucous membranes and include menorrhagia, epistaxis, ecchymosis, and gastrointestinal bleeding. This pattern of bleeding suggests an underlying platelet or vWD defect. It has long been assumed that dysfunctional platelets derived from abnormal stem cells were responsible for increased bleeding with these disorders. Extreme thrombocytosis has been recognized to paradoxically result in an acquired type 2 vWD which contributes to the bleeding diathesis [81]. Other conditions associated with acquired vWD include Heyde's syndrome, which is the association of tight aortic stenosis with gastrointestinal arteriovenous malformations. In this condition, the shear stress associated with the stenotic aortic valve consumes the HMW multimers of vWF [82]. The pathophysiology is the same in bleeding patients with left ventricular assist devices [47].

Treatment of the underlying disorder remains the mainstay, though platelet transfusions may be needed for clinically significant bleeding. If acquired vWD is suspected, it should be confirmed through appropriate testing (to be discussed later) prior to initiating directed treatment. Treatment depends largely on the degree of defect and could include intravenous immune globulin, DDAVP, or vWF replacement [83].

OTHER ACQUIRED BLEEDING DISORDERS

Acquired vWD

Acquired vWD is a heterogenous disorder that is associated with a number of different disease states. Several distinct pathophysiologic mechanisms are involved which include increased vWF clearance or proteolysis, vWF adsorption to cells with subsequent increased clearance, decreased synthesis, and antibody formation against vWF [83]. Lymphoproliferative and autoimmune disorders are most commonly associated with acquired vWD.

In general, mechanisms underlying acquired vWD are divided into immune- and nonimmune-mediated categories. Immune-mediated acquired vWD is suggested by mixing studies which show an inhibition of vWF in a functional assay. Proposed nonimmune mechanisms include (a) vWF being adsorbed onto cells (e.g., Wilm's tumor, platelets in myeloproliferative disorders, plasma cells in multiple myeloma, and Waldenström's macroglobulinemia); (b) increased proteolysis of HMW multimers at sites of high blood shear flow rates in patients with aortic stenosis, angiodysplasia, and congenital heart disease;

(c) decreased synthesis in hypothyroidism; and (d) proteolysis by plasmin during increased periods of fibrinolysis such as with thrombolytic therapy and DIC. A diagnosis should be expected if a patient has a bleeding phenotype similar to a patient with vWD, a compatible underlying disorder, an absence of lifelong bleeding symptoms, and a negative family history [84]. Treatment for acquired vWD is aimed at correcting the underlying disorder if possible and promoting hemostasis as one would in patients with congenital vWD (e.g., DDAVP, factor concentrates, antifibrinolytics).

Acquired FII (Prothrombin) Inhibitors

Clinically, patients with antiphospholipid antibodies most commonly have a thrombotic phenotype; however, rarely these patients may also have an antibody directed against prothrombin. This antibody binds to prothrombin and increases its clearance, which results in low FII activity levels and clinically significant bleeding. This disorder should be considered in a bleeding patient with evidence for prolongation in PT and PTT. The PT should correct with mixing, the PTT will not. Tests for the lupus inhibitor will be positive, and measurements of FII activity as well as FII antigen will be low. Treatment for acute hemorrhage involves FFP, typically at a dose of 15 to 20 mL per kg with a goal FII activity of >30%. PCCs may also be used [85].

Acquired FV Inhibitors

Acquired FV inhibitors in the past were noted to occur most frequently following exposure to topical bovine thrombin or fibrin-glue preparations. These preparations were contaminated with bovine FV and antibodies cross-reacted with human FV. These preparations are no longer used. A systematic review showed that acquired FV inhibitors now occur more commonly in conjunction with autoimmune disorders, cancer, and drugs [86]. Patients typically present with a significant prolongation in both the PT and PTT. This prolongation fails to correct in a mixing study. Inhibitor specificity to FV is demonstrated with a low FV activity. FFP is not recommended as a treatment as FV is present in such a low concentration that it is quickly neutralized by the inhibitor. PCCs are likewise felt to be unhelpful given their low FV content. Plasma exchange and platelet transfusions have been used successfully to control bleeding. It is thought that FV contained in the alpha granules of circulating platelets is protected from inhibition until the platelet becomes activated at the site of vessel damage. rFVIIa has been reported to successfully promote hemostasis.

Acquired FX Deficiency

Acquired FX deficiency is associated with amyloidosis. It is thought that amyloid fibrils bind to FX and thereby remove it from circulation. Treatment of the underlying amyloidosis and/or splenectomy has been shown to improve the circulating FX level [87]. PCCs are the preferred treatment for acute bleeding episodes, and pharmacokinetic studies should be done on each individual to provide guidance as to optimal dose and interval [88].

References

1. Roberts HR, Hoffman M, Monroe DM: A cell-based model of thrombin generation. *Semin Thromb Hemost* 32[Suppl 1]:32–38, 2006.
2. Rodeghiero F, Tosetto A, Abshire T, et al; ISTH/SSC joint VWF and Perinatal/Pediatric Hemostasis Subcommittees Working Group: ISTH/SSC bleeding assessment tool: a standardized questionnaire and a proposal for a new bleeding score for inherited bleeding disorders. *J Thromb Haemost* 8(9):2063–2065, 2010.
3. De Caterina R, Lanza M, Manca G, et al: Bleeding time and bleeding: an analysis of the relationship of the bleeding time test with parameters of surgical bleeding. *Blood* 84:3363–3370, 1994.
4. Franchini M, Gandini G, Di Paolantonio T, et al: Acquired hemophilia A: a concise review. *Am J Hematol* 80:55–63, 2005.
5. Hayward CP, Harrison P, Cattaneo M, et al; Platelet Physiology Subcommittee of the Scientific and Standardization Committee of the International Society on Thrombosis and Haemostasis: Platelet function analyzer (PFA)-100 closure time in the evaluation of platelet disorders and platelet function. *J Thromb Haemost* 4:312–319, 2006.
6. Nichols WL, Hultin MB, James AH, et al: von Willebrand disease (VWD): evidence-based diagnosis and management guidelines, the National Heart, Lung, and Blood Institute (NHLBI) Expert Panel report (USA). *Haemophilia* 14:171–232, 2008.
7. Sadler JE, Budde U, Eikenboom JC, et al: Update on the pathophysiology and classification of von Willebrand disease: a report of the Subcommittee on von Willebrand Factor. *J Thromb Haemost* 4:2103–2114, 2006.
8. Mannucci PM, Ruggeri ZM, Pareti FI, et al: 1-Deamino-8-d-arginine vasopressin: a new pharmacological approach to the management of haemophilia and von Willebrands' diseases. *Lancet* 1:869–872, , 1977.
9. al-Mondhiry H, Ehmann WC: Congenital afibrinogenemia. *Am J Hematol* 46:343–347, 1994.
10. Mannucci PM, Bettega D, Cattaneo M: Patterns of development of tachyphylaxis in patients with haemophilia and von Willebrand disease after repeated doses of desmopressin (DDAVP). *Br J Haematol* 82:87–93, 1992.
11. Rodriguez-Merchan EC: Acute compartment syndrome in haemophilia. *Blood Coagul Fibrinolysis* 24(7):677–682, 2013.
12. Astermark J: FVIII inhibitors: pathogenesis and avoidance. *Blood* 125: 2045–2051, 2015.
13. Kempton CL, Meeks SL: Toward optimal therapy for inhibitors in hemophilia. *Blood* 124:3365–3372, 2014.
14. Shima M, Tanaka I, Sawamoto Y, et al: Successful treatment of two brothers with congenital afibrinogenemia for splenic rupture using heat- and solvent detergent-treated fibrinogen concentrates. *J Pediatr Hematol Oncol* 19:462–465, 1997.
15. Roberts HR, Stinchcombe T, Gabriel DA: The dysfibrinogenaemias. *Br J Haematol* 114:249–257, 2001.
16. Bornikova L, Peyvandi F, Allen G, et al: Fibrinogen replacement therapy for congenital fibrinogen deficiency. *J Thromb Haemost* 9:1687–1704, 2011.
17. Nugent DJ, Ashley C, García-Talavera J, et al: Pharmacokinetics and safety of plasma-derived factor XIII concentrate (human) in patients with congenital factor XIII deficiency. *Haemophilia* 21(1):95–101, 2015.
18. Lancellotti S, Basso M, De Cristofaro R: Congenital prothrombin deficiency: an update. *Semin Thromb Hemost* 39:596–606, 2013.
19. Andrews RK, Berndt MC: Bernard-Soulier syndrome: an update. *Semin Thromb Hemost* 39:656–662, 2013.
20. Thalji N, Camire RM: Parahemophilia: new insights into factor v deficiency. *Semin Thromb Hemost* 39:607–612, 2013.
21. Franchini M, Lippi G: Acquired factor V inhibitors: a systematic review. *J Thromb Thrombolysis* 31:449–457, 2011.
22. Zheng C, Zhang B: Combined deficiency of coagulation factors V and VIII: an update. *Semin Thromb Hemost* 39:613–620, 2013.
23. Mariani G, Bernardi F: Factor VII deficiency. *Semin Thromb Hemost* 35:400–406, 2009.
24. Ageno W, Gallus A, Wittkowsky A, et al: Oral anticoagulant therapy. *Chest* 141:e44S–e88S, 2012.
25. King N, Tran MH: Long-acting anticoagulant rodenticide (Superwarfarin) poisoning: a review of its historical development, epidemiology, and clinical management. *Transfus Med Rev* 6:S0887–S7963, 2015.
26. Menegatti M, Peyvandi F: Factor X deficiency. *Semin Thromb Hemost* 35:407–415, 2009.
27. Seligsohn U: Factor XI deficiency. *Thromb Haemost* 70:68–71, 1993.
28. Bolton-Maggs PH, Patterson DA, Wensley RT, et al: Definition of the bleeding tendency in factor XI-deficient kindreds—a clinical and laboratory study. *Thromb Haemost* 73:192–202, 1995.
29. Berliner S, Horowitz I, Martinowitz U, et al: Dental surgery in patients with severe factor XI deficiency without plasma replacement. *Blood Coagul Fibrinolysis* 3:465–468, 1992.
30. Duga S, Salomon O: Congenital factor XI deficiency: an update. *Semin Thromb Hemost* 39:621–631, 2013.
31. de Jager T, Pericleous L, Kokot-Kierepa M, et al: The burden and management of FXIII deficiency. *Haemophilia* 20:733–740, 2014.
32. Weston BW, Monahan PE: Familial deficiency of vitamin K-dependent clotting factors. *Haemophilia* 14:1209–1213, 2008.
33. Tefre KL, Ingerslev J, Sorensen B: Clinical benefit of recombinant factor VIIa in management of bleeds and surgery in two brothers suffering from the Bernard–Soulier syndrome. *Haemophilia* 15:281–284, 2009.
34. Solh T, Botsford A, Solh M: Glanzmann's thrombasthenia: pathogenesis, diagnosis, and current and emerging treatment options. *J Blood Med* 6:219–227, 2015.
35. Di Paola J, Johnson J: Thrombocytopenias due to gray platelet syndrome or THC2 mutations. *Semin Thromb Hemost* 37:690–697, 2011.
36. Nurden AT, Nurden P: Inherited disorders of platelet function: selected updates. *J Thromb Haemost* 13[Suppl 1]:S2–S9, 2015.
37. Vermeer C, Hamulyák K: Pathophysiology of vitamin K-deficiency and oral anticoagulants. *Thromb Haemost* 66:153–159, 1991.

38. Tripodi A, Mannucci PM: The coagulopathy of chronic liver disease. *N Engl J Med* 365:147–156, 2011.
39. Green G, Poller L, Thomson JM, et al: Factor VII as a marker of hepatocellular synthetic function in liver disease. *J Clin Pathol* 29:981–975, 1976.
40. Bennett CL, Kim B, Zakarija A, et al: Two mechanistic pathways for thienopyridine-associated thrombotic thrombocytopenic purpura: a report from the SERF-TTP Research Group and the RADAR Project. *J Am Coll Cardiol* 50:1138–1143, 2007.
41. Boks AL, Brommer EJ, Schalm SW, et al: Hemostasis and fibrinolysis in severe liver failure and their relation to hemorrhage. *Hepatology* 6:79–86, 1986.
42. Ewe K: Bleeding after liver biopsy does not correlate with indices of peripheral coagulation. *Dig Dis Sci* 26:388–393, 1981.
43. Caldwell SH: Management of coagulopathy in liver disease. *Gastroenterol Hepatol (N Y)* 10:330–332, 2014.
44. Levi M: Diagnosis and treatment of disseminated intravascular coagulation. *Int J Lab Hematol* 36:228–236, 2014.
45. Wada H, Matsumoto T, Aota T, et al: Progress in diagnosis and treatment for disseminated intravascular coagulation [in Japanese]. *Rinsho Ketsueki* 56:169–176, 2015.
46. Taylor FB Jr, Toh CH, Hoots WK, et al: Towards definition, clinical and laboratory criteria, and a scoring system for disseminated intravascular coagulation. *Thromb Haemost* 86:1327–1330, 2001.
47. Czul F, Barkin JS: Continuous-flow left ventricular assist device, valvular disease, and acquired von Willebrand Syndrome. *Clin Gastroenterol Hepatol* 13:1376–1377, 2015.
48. Franchini M, Crestani S, Frattini F, et al: Hemostatic agents for bleeding: recombinant-activated factor VII and beyond. *Semin Thromb Hemost* 41:342–347, 2015.
49. Slofstra SH, van't Veer C, Buurman WA, et al: Low molecular weight heparin attenuates multiple organ failure in a murine model of disseminated intravascular coagulation. *Crit Care Med* 33:1365–1370, 2005.
50. Levi M: Disseminated intravascular coagulation: what's new? *Crit Care Clin* 21:449–467, 2005.
51. Feinstein DI: Diagnosis and management of disseminated intravascular coagulation: the role of heparin therapy. *Blood* 60:284–287, 1982.
52. Gando S: Hemostasis and thrombosis in trauma patients. *Semin Thromb Hemost* 41:26–34, 2015.
53. Armand R, Hess JR: Treating coagulopathy in trauma patients. *Transfus Med Rev* 17:223–231, 2003.
54. McDaniel LM, Etchill EW, Raval JS, et al: State of the art: massive transfusion. *Transfus Med Rev* 24:138–144, 2014.
55. Tobin JM, Tanaka K, Smith CE: Factor concentrates in trauma. *Curr Opin Anaesthesiol* 28:217–226, 2015.
56. Franchini M, Mannucci P: Acquired haemophilia A: a 2013 update. *Thromb Haemost* 110:1114–1120, 2013.
57. Kershaw G, Favaloro EJ: Laboratory identification of factor inhibitors: an update. *Pathology* 44:293–302, 2012.
58. Tiede A, Werwitzke S, Scharf RE: Laboratory diagnosis of acquired hemophilia A: limitations, consequences, and challenges. *Semin Thromb Hemost* 40:803–811, 2014.
59. Tiede A, Amano K, Ma A, et al: The use of recombinant activated factor VII in patients with acquired haemophilia. *Blood Rev* 29[Suppl 1]:S19–S25, 2015.
60. Borg JY, Négrier C, Durieu I, et al; FEIBHAC Study Group: FEIBA in the treatment of acquired haemophilia A: results from the prospective multicentre French 'FEIBA dans l'hémophilie A acquise' (FEIBHAC) registry. *Haemophilia* 21:330–337, 2015.
61. Janbain M, Leissinger C, Kruse-Jarres R: Acquired hemophilia A: emerging treatment options. *J Blood Med* 8:143–150, 2015.
62. Collins P, Baudo F, Knoebl P, et al; EACH2 Registry Collaborators: Immunosuppression for acquired hemophilia A: results from the European Acquired Haemophilia Registry (EACH2). *Blood* 120:47–55, 2012.
63. Boles JC, Key NS, Kasthuri R, et al: Single-center experience with rituximab as first-line immunosuppression for acquired hemophilia. *J Thromb Haemost* 9:1429–1431, 2011.
64. Konkle BA: Acquired disorders of platelet function. *Hematology Am Soc Hematol Educ Program* 2011:391–396, 2011.
65. Derry S, Loke YK: Risk of gastrointestinal haemorrhage with long term use of aspirin: meta-analysis. *BMJ* 321:1183–1187, 2000.
66. Weisman SM, Graham DY: Evaluation of the benefits and risks of low-dose aspirin in the secondary prevention of cardiovascular and cerebrovascular events. *Arch Intern Med* 162:2197–2202, 2002.
67. Delaney JA, Opatrny L, Brophy JM: Drug drug interactions between antithrombotic medications and the risk of gastrointestinal bleeding. *CMAJ* 177:347–351, 2007.
68. McQuaid KR, Laine L: Systematic review and meta-analysis of adverse events of low-dose aspirin and clopidogrel in randomized controlled trials. *Am J Med* 119:624–638, 2006.
69. Guthrie R: Review and management of side effects associated with antiplatelet therapy for prevention of recurrent cerebrovascular events. *Adv Ther* 28:473–482, 2011.
70. Memon MA, Blankenship JC, Wood GC, et al: Incidence of intracranial hemorrhage complicating treatment with glycoprotein IIb/IIIa receptor inhibitors: a pooled analysis of major clinical trials. *Am J Med* 109:213–217, 2000.
71. Merlini PA, Rossi M, Menozzi A, et al: Thrombocytopenia caused by abciximab or tirofiban and its association with clinical outcome in patients undergoing coronary stenting. *Circulation* 109:2203–2206, 2004.
72. Shen YM, Frenkel EP: Acquired platelet dysfunction. *Hematol Oncol Clin North Am* 21:647–661, 2007.
73. Ho SJ, Gemmell R, Brighton TA: Platelet function testing in uraemic patients. *Hematology* 13(1):49–58, 2008.
74. Sohal AS, Gangji AS, Crowther MA, et al: Uremic bleeding: pathophysiology and clinical risk factors. *Thromb Res* 118:417–422, 2006.
75. Steiner RW, Coggins C, Carvalho AC: Bleeding time in uremia: a useful test to assess clinical bleeding. *Am J Hematol* 7:107–117, 1979.
76. Hedges SJ, Dehoney SB, Hooper JS, et al: Evidence-based treatment recommendations for uremic bleeding. *Nat Clin Pract Nephrol* 3:138–153, 2007.
77. Lee HK, Kim YJ, Jeong JU, et al: Desmopressin improves platelet dysfunction measured by in vitro closure time in uremic patients. *Nephron Clin Pract* 114:c248–c52, 2010.
78. Davenport R: Cryoprecipitate for uremic bleeding. *Clin Pharm* 10:429, 1991.
79. Zhou XJ, Vaziri ND: Defective calcium signalling in uraemic platelets and its amelioration with long-term erythropoietin therapy. *Nephrol Dial Transplant* 17:992–997, 2002.
80. Elliott MA, Tefferi A: Thrombosis and haemorrhage in polycythaemia vera and essential thrombocythaemia. *Br J Haematol* 128:275–290, 2005.
81. Tefferi A, Barbui T: Polycythemia vera and essential thrombocythemia: 2015 update on diagnosis, risk-stratification and management. *Am J Hematol* 90:162–173, 2015.
82. Vincentelli A, Susen S, Le Tourneau T, et al: Acquired von Willebrand syndrome in aortic stenosis. *N Engl J Med* 349:343–349, 2003.
83. Federici AB, Budde U, Castaman G, et al: Current diagnostic and therapeutic approaches to patients with acquired von Willebrand syndrome: a 2013 update. *Semin Thromb Hemost* 39:191–202, 2013.
84. Saif MA, Thachil J, Brown R, et al: Is it congenital or acquired von Willebrands disease? *Haemophilia* 21:338–342, 2015.
85. Mulliez SM, De Keyser F, Verbist C, et al: Lupus anticoagulant-hypoprothrombinemia syndrome: report of two cases and review of the literature. *Lupus* 24:736–745, 2015.
86. Franchini M, Lippi G: Acquired factor V inhibitors: a systematic review. *J Thromb Thrombolysis* 2011:449–457, 2011.
87. Furie B, Voo L, McAdam KP, et al: Mechanism of factor X deficiency in systemic amyloidosis. *N Engl J Med* 304:827–830, 1981.
88. Lim MY, McCarthy T, Chen SL, et al: Importance of pharmacokinetic studies in the management of acquired factor X deficiency. *Eur J Haematol* 96:60–64, 2015.

Chapter 89 ■ Transfusion Therapy: Blood Components and Transfusion Complications

TERRY GERNSHEIMER

Transfusion support can be a key element in decreasing morbidity and mortality of the critically ill patient by the support of oxygen delivery and correction of hemostatic abnormalities. An understanding of the benefits, limitations, and risks of blood component therapy is of fundamental importance in the intensive care setting. This chapter outlines blood components available for transfusion, their appropriate dosages, and therapeutic effects. Complications of transfusion therapy, including infectious risks, transfusion reactions, effects of storage, and immunomodulatory effects, as well as methods to minimize these complications, are also discussed.

BLOOD COMPONENT THERAPY

Cellular Blood Components

Red Blood Cells

A thoughtful transfusion policy depends on the time the anemia developed over and can be expected to continue; additional medical problems that may make a patient more susceptible to anemia, such as tissue ischemia and pulmonary disease; and whether there is rapid, ongoing blood loss.

One unit of "packed" red blood cells (pRBCs) is processed by the removal of platelet-rich plasma from a donated unit of whole blood and contains approximately 200 mL RBCs, usually less than 50 mL plasma, and an additive that brings the component to 300 to 350 mL in total volume. Depending upon the additive, the storage life at 4°C will be from 35 to 42 days. RBC storage has multiple theoretic and measurable effects. Any platelets still present in the component are rendered inactive by the cold storage. As RBCs are stored, intracellular potassium leaks into the plasma space. 2,3-Diphosphoglyceric acid (2,3-DPG) may also be depleted from the RBCs, which theoretically could cause increased oxygen affinity and decreased release of oxygen at the tissues [1]. This effect reverses after several hours in vivo, but may be clinically significant in the patient undergoing massive transfusion. Stored pRBC also have elevated plasma ammonia levels, elevated pCO_2, lowered pH, and increased amounts of microaggregates, and the RBCs undergo changes in shape and deformability, thereby making transit through small vessels more difficult. These all have theoretic effects on oxygen delivery when given rapidly in large amounts. Massive transfusion can also theoretically result in hypocalcemia and hyperkalemia.

In 1993, Marik and Sibald [2] reported the incidental finding of increased gastric pH in 23 patients with septic shock transfused with 3 units of pRBC, but Walsh failed to find a similar effect in a small randomized control trial in 22 patients with septic shock transfused with pRBC stored for <5 or >20 days [3]. Since that time, small prospective trials and retrospective studies examining the effects of RBC age at transfusion have yielded conflicting results [4–6]. A prospective, blinded randomized trial of 2,400 critically ill patients comparing RBCs stored for less than 8 days or standard issue (mean 22.0 ± 8.4 days) showed no difference in 90-day mortality nor adverse outcomes between the groups [7]. A prospective trial in nearly 1,100 patients undergoing complex cardiac surgery randomized patients aged 12 years or older to receive red cells stored for 10 days or less or 21 days or more [8]. No difference between the groups was found in Multiple Organ Dysfunction Score, 7- and 28-day mortality or adverse events, although hyperbilirubinemia was more common in the longer term storage group. The effect of storage age remains controversial, particularly in neonates and pediatric patients [9] and will require additional prospective randomized clinical trials before the true clinical significance of storage age and the nature of the effect becomes clear [10].

Other than factors V and VIII, the activity of most coagulation factors are quite stable during storage, even after 2 weeks, and, therefore, whole blood (without the plasma removed), when available, may be used in selected patients with coagulopathy and bleeding, and can reduce donor exposure by limiting administration of multiple products (e.g., red cells and plasma) during massive transfusion [11]. Factor V levels in stored whole blood are well above 50% and, therefore, adequate for hemostasis. Factor VIII is produced by endothelial cells as well as by the liver, and the levels increase in the setting of inflammation, so a decrease with storage may be less clinically relevant. Whole blood may also be the preferred form of red cell transfusion in patients who require intravascular volume expansion as well as increased oxygen-carrying capacity.

The primary function of hemoglobin in RBCs is to transport oxygen efficiently from the lungs to the various tissues of the body. Oxygen transport is a complex process regulated by several control mechanisms, involving the heart and vascular system. The most important functional feature of the hemoglobin molecule is its ability to combine loosely and reversibly with oxygen. Decreased hemoglobin oxygen affinity and increased tissue oxygen delivery occurs with increased temperature and decreased pH, when there are increased tissue requirements. Oxygen is also less tightly bound when 2,3-DPG levels are increased, which are increased in chronically ill patients [12]. In the seriously ill patient with severe acidosis and septic shock, however, 2,3-DPG levels may decrease, resulting in decreased tissue oxygen delivery.

Transfusion Threshold. In a normovolemic, otherwise healthy individual, the effect of a decreased hematocrit is decreased blood viscosity and a compensatory augmentation of cardiac output and blood flow to most organs [13]. Human and animal studies reveal remarkable tolerance for hematocrit levels as low as 15% [14,15], but an optimum value has not been well defined and is very dependent on the patient's physiologic state. Advocates of restrictive transfusion strategies point out that transfusing to normal hemoglobin concentrations does not improve organ failure and mortality in the critically ill patient [16] and, to data, suggesting transfusion may actually be associated with increased infection rates, morbidity, and mortality [17]. The proponents of more liberal transfusion strategies point out the possible detrimental effects that may be associated with oxygen debt [18].

A decrease in the hematocrit also involves a redistribution of blood flow away from the endocardium and may have adverse effects on ischemic cardiac tissue. Postoperative patients with known vascular disease and hematocrits <28% have been shown to have a significant increase in myocardial ischemia and morbid cardiac events [19], and in one study that retrospectively evaluated patients refusing transfusion on religious grounds, low preoperative hemoglobin was associated with increased morbidity and mortality in patients with cardiovascular disease undergoing surgery [20]. However, in a large multicenter, randomized trial, there were no differences in adverse outcomes when patients with cardiac disease were transfused at a hemoglobin threshold of 7.0 versus 10 g [21]. In this study of more than 800 patients, less acutely ill, younger patients (<55 years of age) without cardiac disease who were randomized to the more liberal (higher) transfusion trigger had a higher overall mortality rate. A restrictive RBC transfusion strategy also did not adversely affect outcomes related to mechanical ventilation [22]. In postoperative patients without cardiovascular disease, few studies support interference with wound healing or increased anesthesia risk at hemoglobin levels of <10 g per dL [23], and hemoglobin values as low as 7 g per dL, appear to be safe in otherwise healthy individuals [24].

A systematic review of 11 observational studies of RBC transfusion involving more than 290,000 patients with acute coronary syndromes suggested that transfusion thresholds less than 8 g per dL of hemoglobin appeared to be beneficial or, at worst, neutral, whereas there was a suggestion of harm when transfusion was undertaken at hemoglobin levels above 11.0 g per dL. Elderly patients with known cardiovascular risk factors undergoing hip surgery do not experience improvements in mortality, in-hospital morbidity, or mobility when transfused at a hemoglobin threshold of 10 versus 8 g per dL [25]. A prospective randomized trial of 2,000 patients in the United Kingdom compared a hemoglobin transfusion threshold of <9 g per dL to a threshold <7.5 g per dL [26]. Although there were more deaths in the restrictive-threshold group (4.2% vs. 2.6%; hazard ratio, 1.64; 95% confidence interval, 1.00 to 2.67; $p = 0.045$), the primary outcomes of serious infection or an ischemic event did not differ between the groups. Further study in this patient population is needed to determine optimum transfusion thresholds, particularly in the setting of cardiac surgery and intracardiac devices and major vascular surgery where perioperative transfusion may be independently associated with increased morbidity and mortality [27].

Other patient populations have specifically been evaluated in prospective randomized trials for optimum hemoglobin threshold for red cell transfusion. Restrictive transfusion thresholds of <7.0 g per dL were not associated with increased mortality or adverse outcomes in patients with septic shock [28] and significantly improved outcomes in patients with acute upper gastrointestinal bleeding [29]. Studies in animal models [30] and in humans [31,32] reveal that platelet function and interaction with subendothelium decline at lower hematocrits; however, whether higher hematocrits protect against bleeding in the thrombocytopenic or thrombocytopathic (e.g., uremic) patient is not known and that further studies are needed [33].

Blunted erythropoietin responses have been noted in critically ill pediatric [34] and adult patients [35]. Long-term intensive care patients may not only fail to increase their erythropoietin level in response to anemia, but may have correctable nutritional deficiencies and iron profiles consistent with anemia of chronic disease. Although erythropoietin therapy increases RBC production and appears to decrease transfusion needs [36–38], the effect can take weeks and may reduce blood cell transfusion only minimally. It is an expensive alternative to more restrictive transfusion strategies to reduce transfusion exposure in appropriately chosen patients.

Therapeutic Effects. The response to red cell transfusion will depend on intravascular volume, but it can be estimated that 1 unit of pRBC will increase the hematocrit by approximately 3%. It may take up to 24 hours while intravascular volume equilibrates for full effect. A stable patient should be transfused only 1 unit of red cells before rechecking. Rapid ongoing red cell destruction or splenic sequestration may also affect hematocrit increment and red cell survival.

Emergency Blood Usage. Uncrossmatched type O RBCs can be used for a bleeding patient when it is judged to be life- or organ saving. Type O, Rh-negative RBCs can be transfused to people of any blood type with only a slight risk of hemolysis. This risk increases in patients who have previously been transfused or pregnant and may have formed antibodies [39]. Type O, Rh-positive RBCs are sometimes used for women who are beyond childbearing age and in adult males. When Rh-positive RBCs are used in an Rh-negative patient, there is a chance of a D immunization, and if the patient requires emergency transfusion in the future, they may have preformed antibodies. Anti-D antibodies do not generally cause immediately intravascular hemolysis, but rather a slow extravascular hemolysis with relatively low risk. Anti-RhD (Rhogam) may be given within 48 hours of giving transfusion of Rh-positive blood to an Rh-negative woman of childbearing age, but the amounts required limit its use in prevention of alloimmunization. A strategy of equal numbers of red cells units to plasma and platelets (see "Platelets" section) appears to be beneficial in the resuscitation of the trauma patient requiring massive transfusion [40].

Platelets

Platelets are essential for the initial phase of hemostasis. Following exposure of subendothelial substances, platelets adhere to the subendothelial tissues by von Willebrand Factor and other adhesive proteins. This initial adhesion activates platelets, causing release of platelet α and dense granules. Some of these granule contents, including Factor V, fibrinogen, von Willebrand Factor, and calcium, move to the extracellular space via the open canalicular system, increasing their concentrations in the immediate "neighborhood" of the platelet. With platelet activation, anionic phospholipids move to the outer membrane surface, forming binding sites collectively known as Platelet Factor 3, upon which coagulation factors can interact with calcium to form factors IXa, Xa, and thrombin. Glycoprotein IIb-IIIa is exposed and binds fibrinogen, forming links between platelets. Thrombin generation causes further platelet activation and converts fibrinogen to fibrin, resulting in a platelet-fibrin mass that can effectively cease bleeding from a break in the endothelium. Fifteen percent of the platelet's protein is actin and myosin, coupling in the presence of increased concentrations of adenosine triphosphate and calcium, leading to cytoskeletal movement and clot retraction.

The threshold of thrombocytopenia at which bleeding may occur will vary depending on the patient's clinical condition. In general, spontaneous bleeding does not occur until the platelet count falls below 5,000 to 10,000 per μL [41–44]. In a prospective clinical trial of 600 patients with hematologic malignancy, waiting to transfuse platelets therapeutically upon observation of bleeding is associated with increased bleeding [45]. The recommended "trigger" by the AABB for prophylactic platelet transfusions in patients undergoing chemotherapy or hematopoietic stem cell transplantation without bleeding or other comorbid conditions is <10,000 per μL [46]. Lower doses seem to be as effective in preventing bleeding as higher doses, but patients who receive smaller doses require more frequent transfusions, making this strategy less appropriate for outpatient transfusion [47]. For the majority of invasive procedures, including lumbar puncture, a platelet count of 30 to 50,000 per μL will be adequate. For high-risk procedures, such as neurologic or ophthalmologic surgeries, a platelet count of 100,000 per μL is recommended by the American Society of Anesthesiology [48]. Technique and experience appear to be as least important predictors of bleeding following placement of catheters as clotting abnormalities, even in patients with isolated platelet counts <20,000 per μL [49]. The risk of bleeding with thrombocytopenia increases when complicated by other hemostatic abnormalities.

Platelet counts less than 50,000 per μL are associated with increased risk of microvascular bleeding in the massively transfused patient [50]. For this reason, platelet transfusion has been advocated with replacement of every blood volume to avoid the effect of dilutional thrombocytopenia [51]. In the pragmatic, randomized optimal platelet and plasma ratios (PROPPR) trial, platelet concentrates were transfused in equal numbers to units of red cells and plasma [40]. However, it is important to note that up to six platelet concentrates or their equivalent are generally present in a platelet component prepared by the transfusion service. Therefore, one platelet transfusion should accompany every 5 or 6 units of red cells and plasma.

Higher transfusion triggers may be indicated with abnormal platelet function [52]. Platelet function abnormalities may be congenital or acquired. Medications, sepsis, malignancy, tissue trauma, obstetric complications, and extracorporeal circulation may all adversely affect platelet function. Liver and kidney disease may be associated with severe thrombocytopathy. Hypothermia prolongs bleeding time in trauma patients [53] and arterial hemorrhage in animals [54]. Glycoprotein IIb-IIIa inhibitors may affect platelet number and function. If platelet dysfunction is present, the patient with a disrupted vascular system (e.g., trauma or surgery) will require a higher platelet count to achieve hemostasis. Higher counts may be necessary to prevent spontaneous bleeding as well. The transfused platelets may quickly become dysfunctional in the patient, and other therapy may be necessary, such as dialysis, desmopressin acetate (DDAVP) and estrogen for bleeding in renal failure [55], rewarming of the hypothermic patient, or correction of acidosis.

In several situations, platelet transfusions may not be indicated unless there is significant bleeding. In autoimmune thrombocytopenias (e.g., immune thrombocytopenic purpura and post-transfusion purpura), transfusion increments are usually poor, and platelet survival is short. Administration of intravenous immune globulin in high doses may improve transfusion response and survival, as well as treat the underlying disease [56]. Because of reports of rapid exacerbation of the thrombotic process in the cerebrovascular circulation in patients with thrombotic thrombocytopenic purpura (TTP) following platelet transfusion [57] and the association of arterial thrombosis and in-hospital mortality with platelet transfusion in a large retrospective study of patients with TTP or heparin-induced thrombocytopenia [58] make platelet transfusions relatively contraindicated in TTP unless there is clinically significant bleeding.

Pooled random donor platelet concentrates are prepared from platelets that have been harvested by centrifuging units of donated whole blood. Up to 8 units of platelets, each from a separate donor, can be pooled into a single bag for transfusion. All units are from the same ABO type. If ABO compatible platelets are unavailable, in most cases, pooled ABO incompatible platelets can be substituted with very little risk. The usual adult dose is 1 unit per 15 kg of body weight for a bleeding patient.

In a 70-kg patient with a normal sized spleen, each unit is expected to increase the platelet count by approximately 7,000 per μL (Table 89.1) when checked 10 minutes to 1 hour after transfusion [59]. The survival of transfused platelets averages 3 to 5 days, but will decrease if a consumptive process is present. Platelet concentrates also contain about 60 mL of plasma per unit and small numbers of RBCs and leukocytes. Platelet units must be maintained at room temperature because platelets lose shape and release their granular contents when refrigerated. Apheresis platelets, collected from a single donor, are prepared in components equivalent to 4 to 6 pooled units. An apheresis platelet concentrate contains 200 to 400 mL of plasma and, if the plasma is of an incompatible type, may be reduced in volume by centrifugation, although this results in an approximate 10% to 15% loss of platelets and, probably, some loss of function. Apheresis platelets may be collected for a specific recipient from a family member or other human leukocyte antigen (HLA)-compatible donor for patients that have become refractory to random donor platelet transfusions owing to alloimmunization. Leukocyte reduction of transfused cellular blood components has been clearly shown to reduce the rate of alloimmunization in patients undergoing chemotherapy for acute myelocytic leukemia [60].

Granulocytes

The degree of granulocytopenia is directly related to the risk of infection [61]. Although antibiotics have improved morbidity and mortality in patients affected by prolonged periods of neutropenia, most antimicrobials are less effective in the presence of granulocytopenia. Bacterial and, more particularly, fungal infections remain a major cause of death in hematopoietic stem cell transplantation patients despite shortening of the period of neutropenia with hematopoietic growth factors [62]. Granulocytes collected by continuous flow centrifugation and filtration leukapheresis function normally in vitro in the quantitative nitroblue tetrazollium, oxygen consumption, and chemotaxis assays [63]. Bacterial killing by filtration leukopheresis granulocytes, which circulate for several hours post-transfusion, is only slightly decreased compared to granulocytes collected by continuous flow centrifugation. Transfused granulocytes rapidly migrate to sites of infection [64].

Early studies showed promise for the use of granulocyte transfusion for treatment of documented infections in neutropenic patients [65–67]. However, their usefulness in the prevention of infection has been more controversial [68] owing to limitations in the inability to collect cells in sufficient amounts to provide an effective transfusion dose, poor response to granulocytes in heavily transfused, alloimmunized patients [69], and the early development of alloimmunization in patients transfused with granulocytes [70]. To this end, HLA-compatible donors

TABLE 89.1

Expected Platelet Increment with Transfusion[a]

	1 unit[b]	4 units	6 units
	0.8×10^{11}	3.2×10^{11}	4.8×10^{11}
50 lb/23 kg	17,600/μL	70,400/μL	105,600/μL
100 lb/45 kg	8,800	35,200	52,800
150 lb/68 kg	5,900	23,500	35,200
200 lb/91 kg	4,400	17,600	26,400

[a]In a patient with a normal sized spleen and without platelet antibodies.
[b]Whole blood platelets. An apheresis platelet component contains the equivalent of 4–8 units of whole blood platelets.

have been administered corticosteroids prior to granulocyte collection with some limited success. The administration of granulocyte colony-stimulating factor (G-CSF) has been shown to be safe when given to normal donors [71] and has been administered to donors prior to collection to increase collection and post-transfusion increments [72]. A study of granulocyte transfusion from G-CSF–stimulated donors failed to show improvement in mortality when compared to no transfusion; however, when data from centers that collected higher doses of granulocytes were evaluated, there appeared to be a benefit [73].

Plasma Components

Plasma

One unit of plasma is the plasma taken from a unit of whole blood. It may be frozen within 8 hours of collection and contain all coagulation factors in normal concentrations. It is free of RBCs, leukocytes, and platelets. Plasma may also be provided as "frozen plasma" or "thawed plasma". These components are prepared by methods similar to plasma, and their factor concentrations differ only slightly. All will be considered here collectively as "Plasma." One unit contains approximately 200 to 250 mL and must be ABO compatible (type AB is the universal donor type). Rh factor need not be considered. Because there are no viable leukocytes, plasma carries minimal risk of cytomegalovirus (CMV) transmission or graft-versus-host disease (GVHD).

Plasma transfusion is indicated in patients with documented coagulation factor deficiencies and active bleeding. Plasma should not be used to correct isolated deficiencies in clotting factors when a concentrated replacement source, such as factor VIII or IX, is available, because these concentrates are either recombinant or have undergone processing to inactivate viruses and can correct the deficiency using a much smaller infused volume. Factor deficiencies may be congenital or acquired, secondary to liver disease, warfarin anticoagulation, disseminated intravascular coagulation (DIC), or massive replacement with RBCs and crystalloid/colloid solutions. Usually, there is an increase of at least 1.6 times the normal prothrombin time (PT) or activated partial thromboplastin time (aPTT) before clinically important factor deficiency exists. This corresponds to levels of most factors <20% of normal. Above these levels, most routine nonmajor invasive procedures such as line placement, liver biopsy [74], and thoracentesis [75] are not associated with an increased risk of bleeding complications; however, the acceptable upper limits of PT and PTT prior to invasive procedures have not been evaluated in a large prospective randomized study to date [76–78].

In the massively transfused patient, consumption and dilution of coagulation factors may cause rapid development of coagulopathy. Patients with a PT or aPTT ratio (reference midrange normal value divided by actual) ≥1.8 had an 80% to 85% chance of exhibiting microvascular bleeding, and either of these tests should be closely monitored during resuscitation of the bleeding patient [48]. Plasma transfusion is indicated when the ratio exceeds 1.5 times the midrange normal value in these patients. Usually, an increase in factor levels of at least 10% will be needed for any significant change in coagulation status, so the usual dose is 3 to 4 units (approximately 10 to 15 mL per kg), but the amount will vary depending on the patient's size and clotting factor levels (Table 89.2). Reversal of warfarin anticoagulation is indicated only if significant bleeding or risk of bleeding is present. Plasma may be used for this purpose, but, often, recurrent transfusion is required to maintain normal factor levels. Many patients receiving warfarin will not tolerate the volume of plasma required or require more rapid replacement for life-threatening bleeding in which case a prothrombin complex concentrate may be more appropriate.

TABLE 89.2

Plasma—Dosage for Transfusion

Volume of 1 Unit PLASMA: 200–250 mL

1 mL plasma contains 1 unit coagulation factors

1 Unit PLASMA contains 220 units coagulation factors

Factor recovery with transfusion = 40%

1 Unit PLASMA provides ~80 units coagulation factors

70 kg × 0.05 = plasma volume of 35 dL (3.5 L)

$\frac{80 \text{ units}}{35 \text{ dL}}$ = 2.3 unit/dL = 2.3% (of normal 100 unit/dL)

In a 70-kg patient:

1 Unit PLASMA increases most factors ~2.5%

4 Units PLASMA increase most factors ~10%

Plasma is indicated in the treatment of TTP, most commonly in conjunction with plasmapheresis. Many other disorders are treated by plasmapheresis, but, usually, plasma replacement is not used. Plasma should not be used for volume expansion unless the patient also has a significant coagulopathy and is bleeding.

Cryoprecipitate

Cryoprecipitate is prepared from plasma and contains fibrinogen, von Willebrand factor, factor VIII, factor XIII, and fibronectin. Cryoprecipitate is supplied in bags (each made from 1 whole blood unit) from multiple donors that have been resuspended in saline or plasma and pooled prior to transfusion. It must be kept at room temperature. The concentration of fibrinogen in cryoprecipitate units is up to 10 times that in plasma, and, therefore, blood levels can be increased rapidly with much smaller volumes.

Fibrinogen levels can drop rapidly in DIC, and is usually associated with other coagulation abnormalities that may in combination be treated with plasma. Isolated hypofibrinogenemia is infrequently associated with bleeding in adults, and correction should be reserved for patients with clinical bleeding or patients who are a risk of bleeding as a result of imminent invasive procedures or trauma [26] with significant hypofibrinogenemia (<100 mg per dL).

Cryoprecipitate should not be used for patients with von Willebrand disease or hemophilia A (factor VIII deficiency) unless they do not (or are not known to) respond to DDAVP, and recombinant and/or virally inactivated preparations are not available. It is usually given for factor XIII deficiency, when virus-inactivated concentrates of this protein are not available. Cryoprecipitate is sometimes useful if platelet dysfunction associated with renal failure does not respond to dialysis or DDAVP and in other platelet function defects [79].

The amount of fibrinogen per bag of cryoprecipitate can vary widely between blood centers and depending on the donor's fibrinogen concentration. The approximate fibrinogen increment with each bag of cryoprecipitate transfused can be calculated by the formula: 25 mg per plasma volume (in liters). Six bags will increase the fibrinogen level of a 70-kg patient approximately 45 mg per dL. To replace factor VIII or von Willebrand factor when specific factor concentrates are unavailable, the usual dose is 1 bag per 10 kg of body weight. Approximately 150 units of factor VIII and von Willebrand factor are provided per bag. Although single units of cryoprecipitate can be used in the preparation of locally applied fibrin glue for surgery, commercially available, virally inactivated concentrates have a higher fibrinogen concentration and are preferred for this purpose. A patient may donate autologous plasma for processing into cryoprecipitate prior to a planned surgical procedure.

Human fibrinogen concentrate (RiaSTAP) is a heat-treated, lyophilized fibrinogen (coagulation factor I) powder made from pooled human plasma. It is indicated for bleeding or procedure prophylaxis in patients with congenital hypofibrinogenemia or dysfibrinogenemia.

COMPLICATIONS OF TRANSFUSION

Transfusion-related Risks

Infectious Complications

Because the recognition that human immunodeficiency virus (HIV) could be transmitted by blood transfusion in the mid-1980s, exclusion of donors with high risk has done more to decrease transfusion transmitted infection than any testing that has been implemented since that time [80]. Enzyme-linked immunosorbent assay testing for anti-HIV antibody was instituted in 1985 dropping the risk of HIV transmitted infection to 1 in 667,000 units [81]. The addition of P24 antigen decreased the window period between infection and detection to approximately 16 days [82], and polymerase chain reaction screening for HIV has decreased the current estimated risks/unit to as low as 1 in 2,000,000 [83].

As of early 2014, testing for infectious disease screening is performed for the following agents: HIV-1, HIV-2, human T-lymphotropic virus (HTLV)-I, HTLV-II, hepatitis C virus, hepatitis B virus, West Nile virus, *Treponema pallidum* (syphilis), and *Treponema cruzi*. In addition to these tests, platelet units are tested for bacterial contamination. Current risk estimates per unit for hepatitis B virus, hepatitis C virus, and HTLV are 1:1 million, 1:1.2 million, and 1:2.7 million, respectively [84].

CMV is a DNA virus acquired as a primary infection with body secretions, blood products, or organ allografts. Infection in a normal host usually is asymptomatic, but remains latent for life and can cause recurrent infection when it reactivates. CMV infection and seropositivity is extremely common, being 40% in highly industrialized areas, and is close to 100% in warmer climates, densely populated areas, and developing countries [85]. Transfusion-associated CMV infection in the immunocompetent patient with a normal immune system is usually asymptomatic, occurring 4 to 12 weeks after blood component exposure in 0.9% to 17% of patients [86]. In CMV negative, immunosuppressed neonates, transplant, and HIV-positive patients, the risk of CMV infection and severe end-organ disease and organ allograft rejection is high [87]. Leukocyte depletion of blood is similar to CMV seronegative blood in preventing CMV infection through transfusion [88].

Bacterial contamination of RBC and platelet units may occur during collection. RBC units may be contaminated with cold-loving organisms, such as Yersinia. Platelets are stored at room temperature, and multiple organisms can grow in those conditions. Although *Staphylococcus* and *Streptococcus* are the most frequently implicated, gram-negative organisms have also been identified [89]. The incidence of bacterial contamination of platelets has been estimated to be as high as 0.1% [90]. The institution of bacterial testing of platelets in 2004 in the United States is expected to decrease this risk [91], and septic transfusion reactions are estimated to occur in less than 1:50,000 transfusions, but these are likely underreported. Symptoms of hypotension, fever, and chills almost always occur within 3 hours of the transfusion and may be complicated by severe shock and DIC [92]. Both the patient and the blood component bag should be cultured if bacterial contamination is suspected.

Other organisms that can be transmitted by blood transfusion include other hepatitis viruses, malaria and, rarely, syphilis. *T. cruzi*, the parasite responsible for Chagas disease is becoming a commonly transfusion transmitted disease in Central and South America, and has been reported in some Southern US states. Fear of transfusion transmission of new variant Creutzfeldt–Jakob disease has led to stringent criteria on blood donor eligibility and institution of universal leukoreduction in some European countries, but the risk of infection by transfusion is low [93] and testing is not universal.

In 2014, pathogen inactivation of platelets and plasma has been approved in the United States and has been used in some European countries since 2003. Units are photochemically treated using a psoralen compound and exposure to long-wavelength ultraviolet light to inactivate viruses, bacteria, protozoa, and leukocytes. Another inactivation process is sometimes used in Europe utilizing riboflavin and ultraviolet light.

Transfusion Reactions

A transfusion should be stopped immediately whenever a transfusion reaction is suspected.

An **acute hemolytic transfusion reaction** (AHTR) occurs following transfusion of an incompatible blood component. Most are caused by naturally occurring antibodies in the ABO antigen system, but AHTR may occur with incompatibility of Rh, Kell, Kidd, Lewis, and other RBC antigen systems. The vast majority of cases are caused by failure of appropriate systems to identify the correct transfusion recipient [94]. Signs and symptoms include fever, hypotension, tachycardia, dyspnea, chest or back pain, flushing, and severe anxiety. Release of cytokines, such as tumor necrosis factor, interleukin 8, and monocyte chemoattractant protein-1 [95], is followed by fever, capillary leak, and activation of the hemostatic mechanism. If the reaction is severe, it may go on to cause a consumptive coagulopathy (DIC) and renal failure as a result of shock and deposition of thrombi in arterioles. Hemoglobinuria may be the first sign of hemolysis in the sedated patient. Centrifuging a tube of blood and examining the plasma for a reddish discoloration can quickly make the diagnosis. Treatment should first of all be immediate discontinuation of the transfusion as soon as AHTR is suspected and then maintenance of venous access and fluid resuscitation if necessary. Pressor support may be necessary along with central venous pressure monitoring. AHTR is rare, estimated at 1:77,000 units [96].

Delayed hemolytic transfusion reactions (DHTRs) usually occur in patients who have been previously sensitized to an antigen through transfusion or pregnancy. A fall in titer over time may make incompatibility undetectable. A subsequent transfusion causes recall of the antibody, followed by a falling hematocrit 5 to 10 days later. The hematocrit will continue to fall until all of the incompatible transfused cells have been destroyed. DHTR can result in symptomatic or asymptomatic hemolysis, but has only rarely been reported to cause severe morbidity or mortality [97]. Once recognized, the patient is usually easily supported by transfusion of compatible RBCs.

Febrile nonhemolytic transfusion reaction (FNHTR) is a 1°C rise in temperature or greater that cannot be explained by the patient's clinical condition. FNHTR usually occurs within 1 hour of completion of the transfusion. Reactions are more common with platelet transfusions and for patients who have been heavily transfused, and can be quite severe. FNHTR is often caused by sensitization to antigens on donor leukocytes [98]. Cytokines, released from the white cells during storage of cellular blood components, also appear to play a role [99]. Prestorage leukocyte depletion of RBCs and platelets by filtration may be helpful in patients for whom this is a problem. Leukocyte-reduced single-donor apheresis platelets are a possible alternative to leukocyte depletion by filtration of pooled random donor platelets. Occasionally, patients with persistent febrile reactions will require removal of most of the plasma (volume reduction) from platelet preparations. Apheresis platelets prepared with platelet additive solutions (PASs) may also decrease their occurrence. FNHTR should be differentiated from bacterial contamination, which is usually associated with higher fevers and other symptoms of sepsis. Antipyretics can be used to prevent or treat FNHTR. Some clinicians feel meperidine may be useful in the treatment of rigors, although this has not been shown to be beneficial in clinical trials.

Transfusion-related acute lung injury (TRALI) can be indistinguishable from adult respiratory distress syndrome [100,101], involving severe bilateral pulmonary edema and hypoxemia. Symptoms of dyspnea, hypotension, and fever typically begin 30 minutes to 6 hours after transfusion, and the chest X-ray shows diffuse nonspecific infiltrates. Ventilatory support may be required for several days before resolution, but approximately 80% of patients improve within 48 to 96 hours. TRALI occurs when donor plasma contains an antibody, usually against the patient's HLA or leukocyte-specific antigens. Lipids generated during prior storage of the transfused product and preexisting lung damage also appear to play parts in the pathogenesis of TRALI. Less often, the patient may have antibodies against donor leukocytes in the component. The blood center should be notified promptly so that components from the donor can be quarantined and the donor tested for antibodies against the patient.

Transfusion-associated cardiovascular overload may occur in patients sensitive to increased amounts of intravascular volume with transfusion and may initially present a clinical picture similar to TRALI. Unlike TRALI, diuresis is usually effective treatment.

Allergic and anaphylactic reactions are common and usually because of preformed immunoglobin E antibodies to specific proteins in the donor's plasma. Mild urticaria complicates up to 3% of plasma infusions [102] and can be avoided with future transfusions by pretreatment with antihistamines and, in severe cases, with corticosteroids. Only in cases of severe reactions (anaphylaxis), washing of RBCs and platelets to remove all plasma is indicated. Slowing of the rate of transfusion and centrifugation to remove some of the plasma in a platelet component or the use of PAS will sometimes be effective in preventing future reactions among patients for whom this is a recurrent problem.

Transfusion-related GVHD (TRGVHD) is caused by infusion of donor lymphocytes that engraft and then proliferate in response to stimulation by foreign (host) antigens. TRGVHD typically begins 2 to 50 days after transfusion with rash, diarrhea, signs of hepatic inflammation, and pancytopenia [103]. TRGVHD occurs in patients with severe defects of cellular immunity, most notably hematopoietic stem cell transplantation patients, neonates, and patients with lymphoproliferative disorders. Transfusion from relatives and HLA-compatible donors is at risk of causing GVHD. It can be prevented by γ irradiation of cellular blood components.

Immune Modulation

Transfusions have been known to induce immune tolerance following the observation made more than 20 years ago that multiply transfused kidney transplant recipients had an increased graft survival rate [104]. Transfusion-induced immunosuppression has been implicated in postoperative infection, increased cancer recurrence rates, and development of non-Hodgkin lymphoma [105,106]. There is also evidence from animal studies that transfusion increases the risk of metastatic disease, although data in humans are inconclusive. Removal of donor leukocytes has been shown to decrease the immunomodulatory effects of blood transfusions. The clinical usefulness is clear only for prevention of alloimmunization in patients undergoing chemotherapy for acute myelocytic leukemia [50]. A prospective randomized study in patients undergoing cardiac surgery showed a decrease in infection rates when leukocyte reduced blood components were used [107]. This has led some centers to adopt policies of universal leukoreduction, but this remains controversial.

Table 89.3 summarizes some of the most important recent advances in transfusion medicine based on randomized controlled trials or meta-analyses of such trials.

TABLE 89.3

Randomized Clinical Trials in Transfusion Medicine That Have Resulted in Changes in Clinical Practice

Appropriate hemoglobin threshold for RBC transfusion	Hebert et al., [21] Hebert et al., [22] Holst et al., [28] Villanueva et al., [29]	A hemoglobin threshold of 7.0 g/dL vs. 9.0 g/dL is not associated with increased morbidity, mortality, or prolonged ventilatory support in intensive care patients, in septic shock, or in acute gastrointestinal bleeding.
Appropriate platelet count threshold for prophylactic platelet transfusion	Gmur et al., [42] Wandt et al., [43] Rebulla et al., [44]	Platelet transfusion "triggers" of <10,000/μL are safe for the prevention of bleeding in chemotherapy-induced thrombocytopenia in patients without comorbid conditions.
Prevention of transfusion transmitted CMV infection	Bowden et al., [88]	Leukocyte reduction of cellular blood components is as effective in reducing the risk of CMV transmission as the use of CMV seronegative blood components.
Prevention of platelet alloimmunization	TRAP Study Group, [60]	Leukoreduction of cellular blood components prevents HLA alloimmunization in patients with acute leukemia undergoing induction chemotherapy.
Use of leukoreduction to decrease postoperative infection	van de Watering et al., [107]	Leukoreduction of cellular blood components decreases postoperative infection in patients undergoing cardiac surgery.
Appropriate platelet transfusion dose for prophylactic transfusion of thrombocytopenia	Slichter et al., [47]	Low-dose platelet transfusion results in an overall decrease in the number of total platelets transfused and no increase in bleeding. Platelet transfusion frequency is increased.

CMV, cytomegalovirus; HLA, human leukocyte antigen.

References

1. Valeri CR, Hirsch NM: Restoration in vivo of erythrocyte adenosine triphosphate, 2,3-diphosphoglycerate, potassium ion, and sodium ion concentrations following the transfusion of acid-citrate-dextrose stored human blood cells. *J Lab Clin Med* 73:722–733, 1969.
2. Marik PE, Sibbald WJ: Effect of stored-blood transfusion on oxygen delivery in patients with sepsis. *JAMA* 269:3024–3029, 1993.
3. Walsh TS, McArdle F, McLellan SA, et al: Does the storage time of transfused red blood cells influence regional or global indexes of tissue oxygenation in anemic critically ill patients? *Crit Care Med* 32:364–371, 2004.
4. Hébert PC, Chin-Yee I, Fergusson D, et al: A pilot trial evaluating the clinical effects of prolonged storage of red cells. *Anesth Analg* 100:1433–1438, 2005.
5. van de Watering L, Lorinser J, Versteegh M, et al: Effects of storage time of red blood cell transfusions on the prognosis of coronary artery bypass graft patients.*Transfusion* 46:1712–1718, 2006.
6. Koch CG, Li L, Sessler, DI: Duration of red-cell storage and complications after cardiac Surgery. *N Engl J Med* 358:1229–1239, 2008.
7. Lacroix J, Hébert PC, Fergusson DA, et al: Age of transfused blood in critically ill adults. *N Engl J Med* 372:1410–1418, 2015.
8. Steiner ME, Ness PM, Assmann SF, et al: Effects of red-cell storage duration on patients undergoing cardiac surgery. *N Engl J Med* 372:1419–1429, 2015.
9. Gauvin F, Spinella PC, Lacroix J, et al: Association between length of storage of transfused red blood cells and multiple organ dysfunction syndrome in pediatric intensive care patients. *Transfusion* 50:1902–1913, 2010.
10. Lee J S, Gladwin MT: The risks of red cell storage. *Nat Med* 16:381–382, 2010.
11. Counts RB, Haisch C, Simon TL et al: Hemostasis in massively transfused trauma patients. *Ann Surg* 190:91–99, 1979.
12. Allen JB, Allen FB: The minimum acceptable level of hemoglobin. *Int Anesthesiol Clin* 20:1–22, 1982.
13. Messmer KFW: Acceptable hematocrit levels in surgical patients. *World J Surg* 11:41–46, 1987.
14. Jan KM, Chien S: Effect of hematocrit variations on coronary hemodynamics and oxygen utilization. *Am J Physiol* 233:H106–H113, 1977.
15. Brazier J, Cooper N, Maloney JV Jr, et al: The adequacy of myocardial oxygen delivery in acute normovolemic anemia. *Surgery* 75:508–516, 1974.
16. Alvarez G, Hebert PC: Debate: transfusing to normal hemoglobin levels will not improve outcome. *Crit Care* 5:56–63, 2001.
17. Vincent JL, Baron JF, Reinhart K, et al: Anemia and blood transfusion in critically ill patients. *JAMA* 288:1499–1507, 2002.
18. Haupt MT: Debate: transfusing to normal hemoglobin levels improves outcome. *Crit Care* 5:64–66, 2001.
19. Nelson AH, Fleisher LA, Rosenbaum SH: Relationship between postoperative anemia and cardiac morbidity in high-risk vascular patients in the intensive care unit. *Crit Care Med* 21:860–866, 1993.
20. Carson JL, Duff A, Poses RM, et al: Effect of anaemia and cardiovascular disease on surgical mortality and morbidity. *Lancet* 348:1055–1060, 1996.
21. Hebert PC, Wells G, Blajchman MA, et al: A multicenter, randomized, controlled clinical trial of transfusion requirements in critical care. *N Engl J Med* 340:409–417, 1999.
22. Hebert PC, Blajchman MA, Cook DJ, et al: Do blood transfusions improve outcomes related to mechanical ventilation? *Chest* 119:1850–1857, 2001.
23. Perioperative Red Cell Transfusion: National Institute of Health Consensus Development Conference Statement June 27–29, 1988. https://consensus.nih.gov/1988/1988redcelltransfusion070html.htm.
24. Carson JL, Hill S, Carless P, et al: Transfusion triggers: a systematic review of the literature. *Transfus Med Rev* 16:187–199, 2002.
25. Carson JL, Terrin ML, Noveck H, et al: Liberal or restrictive transfusion in high-risk patients after hip surgery. *N Engl J Med* 365:2453–2462, 2011.
26. Murphy GJ, Pike K, Rogers CA, et al: Liberal or restrictive transfusion after cardiac surgery. *N Engl J Med* 372:997–1008, 2015.
27. Obi AT, Park YJ, Bove P, et al: The association of perioperative transfusion with 30-day morbidity and mortality in patients undergoing major vascular surgery. *J Vasc Surg* 61:1000–1009, 2015.
28. Holst LB, Haase N, Wetterslev J, et al: Lower versus higher hemoglobin threshold for transfusion in septic shock. *N Engl J Med* 371:1381–1391, 2014.
29. Villanueva C, Colomo A, Bosch A, et al: Transfusion strategies for acute upper gastrointestinal bleeding. *N Engl J Med* 368:11–21, 2013.
30. Blajchman MA, Bordin JO, Bardossy L, et al: The contribution of the haematocrit to thrombocytopenic bleeding in experimental animals. *Br J Haematol* 86:347–350, 1994.
31. Anand A, Feffer SE: Hematocrit and bleeding time: an update. *South Med J* 87:299–301, 1994.
32. Valeri CR, Cassidy G, Pivicek LE, et al: Anemia-induced increase in the bleeding time: implications for treatment of nonsurgical blood loss. *Transfusion* 41:977–983, 2001.
33. Webert KE, Cook RJ, Couban S, et al: A multicenter pilot-randomized controlled trial of the feasibility of an augmented red blood cell transfusion strategy for patients treated with induction chemotherapy for acute leukemia or stem cell transplantation. *Transfusion* 48:81–91, 2008.
34. Krafte-Jacobs B, Levetown ML, Bray GL, et al: Erythropoietin response to critical illness. *Crit Care Med* 22:821–826, 1994.
35. Rogiers P, Zhang H, Leeman M, et al: Erythropoietin response is blunted in critically ill patients. *Intensive Care Med* 23:159–162, 1997.
36. Gabriel A, Chiari K, Grabner FR, et al: High dose recombinant human erythropoietin stimulates reticulocyte production in patients with multiple organ dysfunction syndrome. *J Trauma* 44:361–367, 1998.
37. van Iperen CE, Gaillard CA, Kraaijenhagen RJ, et al: Response of erythropoiesis and iron metabolism to recombinant human erythropoietin in intensive care unit patients. *Crit Care Med* 28:2773–2778, 2000.
38. Corwin HL, Gettinger A, Rodriguez RM, et al: Efficacy of recombinant human erythropoietin in the critically ill patient: a randomized, double blind, placebo-controlled trial. *Crit Care Med* 27:2346–2350, 1999.
39. Oberman HA, Barnes BA, Friedman BA: The risk of abbreviating the major crossmatch in urgent or massive transfusion. *Transfusion* 18:137–141, 1978.
40. Holcomb JB, Tilley BC, Baraniuk S: Transfusion of plasma, platelets and red blood cells in a 1:1:1 vs a 1:1:2 ratio and mortality in patients with severe trauma. The PROPPR randomized clinical trial. *JAMA* 313:471–482, 2015.
41. Slichter SJ, Harker LA: Thrombocytopenia: mechanisms and management of defects in platelet function. *Clin Haematol* 7:523–529, 1978.
42. Gmur J, Burger J, Schanz U, et al: Safety of stringent prophylactic platelet transfusion policy for patients with acute leukaemia. *Lancet* 338:1223–1236, 1991.
43. Wandt H, Frank M, Ehninger G, et al: Safety and cost effectiveness of a 10 X 10^9/L trigger for prophylactic platelet transfusions compared to the traditional 20 X 10^9/L: a prospective comparative trial in 105 patients with acute myeloid leukemia. *Blood* 91:3601–3606, 1998.
44. Rebulla P, Finazzi G, Marangoni F, et al: The threshold for prophylactic platelet transfusions in adults with acute myeloid leukemia. *N Engl J Med* 337:1870–1875, 1997.
45. Stanworth SJ, Estcourt LJ, Powter G, et al: A no-prophylaxis platelet-transfusion strategy for hematologic cancers. *N Engl J Med* 368:1771–1780, 2013.
46. Kaufman RM, Djulbegovic B, Gernsheimer T, et al: Platelet transfusion: a clinical practice guideline from the AABB. *Ann Intern Med* 162:205–213, 2015.
47. Slichter SJ, Kaufman RL, Assmann SF, et al: Dose of prophylactic platelet transfusion and prevention of hemorrhage. *N Engl J Med* 362:600–613, 2010.
48. ASA Task Force on Blood Transfusion and Adjuvant Therapies: Practice guidelines for perioperative blood transfusion and adjuvant therapies. *Anesthesiology* 105:198–208, 2006.
49. DeLoughery TG, Liebler JM, Simonds V, et al: Invasive line placement in critically ill patients: do hemostatic defects matter? *Transfusion* 36:827–831, 1996.
50. Ciavarella D, Reed RL, Counts RB, et al: Clotting factor levels and the risk of diffuse microvascular bleeding in the massively transfused patient. *Br J Haematol* 67:365–368, 1987.
51. Leslie SD, Toy PT: Laboratory hemostatic abnormalities in massively transfused patients given red blood cells and crystalloid. *Am J Clin Pathol* 96:770–773, 1991.
52. Contreras M: The appropriate use of platelets: an update from the Edinburgh consensus conference. *Br J Haematol* 101[Suppl 1]:10–12, 1998.
53. Leben J, Tryba M, Bading B, et al: Clinical consequences of hypothermia in trauma patients. *Acta Anaesthesiol Scand Suppl* 109:39–41, 1996.
54. Oung CM, Li MS, Shum-Tim D, et al: In vivo study of bleeding time and arterial hemorrhage in hypothermic versus normothermic animals. *J Trauma* 32:251–254, 1993.
55. Hedges SJ, Dehoney SB, Hooper JS, et al: Evidence-based treatment recommendations for uremic bleeding. *Nature Clin Pract* 3:138–153, 2007.
56. Spahr JE, Rodgers GM: Treatment of immune-mediated thrombocytopenia purpura with concurrent intravenous immunoglobulin and platelet transfusion: a retrospective review of 40 patients. *Am J Hematol* 83(2):122–125, 2008.
57. Gordon LI, Kwaan HC, Rossi EC: Deleterious effects of platelet transfusions and recovery thrombocytosis in patients with thrombotic microangiopathy. *Semin Hematol* 24:194–201, 1987.
58. Goel R, Ness PM, Takemoto CM, et al: Platelet transfusions in platelet consumptive disorders are associated with arterial thrombosis and in-hospital mortality. *Blood* 125:1470–1476, 2015.
59. Slichter SJ: Principles of platelet transfusion therapy, in Hoffman R, Benz EJ, Shattil SJ, et al (eds): *Hematology Basic Principles and Practice*. New York, NY, Churchill-Livingstone, 1991, pp 1610–1622.
60. The Trial to Reduce Alloimmunization to Platelets Study Group: Leukocyte reduction and ultraviolet B Irradiation of Platelets to Prevent Alloimmunization and Refractoriness to Platelet Transfusions. *N Eng J Med* 337:1861–1869, 1997.
61. Pizzo PA: Management of fever in patients with cancer and treatment-induced neutropenia. *N Engl J Med* 328:1323–1332, 1993.
62. Engels EA, Ellis CA, Supran SE, et al: Early infection in bone marrow transplantation: quantitative study of clinical factors that affect risk. *Clin Infect Dis* 28:256–266, 1999.
63. McCullough J, Weiblen B, Deinard AR, et al: In vitro function and post-transfusion survival of granulocytes collected by continuous-flow centrifugation and by filtration leukapheresis. *Blood* 2:315–326, 1976.
64. Dutcher J, Schiffer C, Johnston G: Rapid migration of 111indium-labeled granulocytes to sites of infection. *N Eng J Med* 304:586–589, 1981.
65. Lowenthal RM, Grossman L, Goldman JM, et al: Granulocyte transfusions in treatment of infections in patients with acute leukemia and aplastic anemia. *Lancet* i:353–358, 1975.
66. Alavi J, Root R, Djerassi I, et al: A randomized clinical trial of granulocyte transfusions for infection in acute leukemia. *N Engl J Med* 13:706–711, 1977.
67. Vogler W, Winton E: A controlled study of the efficacy of granulocyte transfusions in patients with neutropenia. *Am J Med* 4:548–555, 1977.
68. Clift RA, Sanders JE, Thomas ED, et al: Granulocyte transfusions for the prevention of infection in patients receiving bone marrow transplants. *N Engl J Med* 298:1052–1057, 1978.

69. Adkins D, Goodnough L, Shenoy S, et al: Effect of leukocyte compatibility on neutrophil increment after transfusion of Granulocyte Colony-Stimulating Factor-mobilized prophylactic granulocyte transfusions and on clinical outcomes after stem cell transplantation. *Blood* 11:3605–3612, 2000.
70. Schiffer C, Aisner J, et al: Alloimmunization following prophylactic granulocyte transfusion. *Blood* 54:766–774, 1979.
71. Bensinger WI, Price TH, Dale DC: The effects of daily recombinant human granulocyte colony-stimulating factor administration on normal granulocyte donors undergoing leukapheresis. *Blood* 81:1883–1888, 1993.
72. Price TH, Bowden RA, Boeckh M, et al: Phase I/II trial of neutrophil transfusions from donors stimulated with G-CSF and Dexamethasone for treatment of patients with infections in hematopoietic stem cell transplantation. *Blood* 95:3302–3309, 2000.
73. Price TH, Boeckh M, Harrison RW, et al: Efficacy of transfusion with granulocytes from G-CSF/dexamethasone-treated donors in neutropenic patients with infection. *Blood* 126:2153–2161, 2015.
74. McVay PA, Toy PT: Lack of increased bleeding after liver biopsy in patients with mild hemostatic abnormalities. *Am J Clin Pathol* 94:747–753, 1990.
75. McVay PA, Toy PT: Lack of increased bleeding after Paracentesis and Thoracentesis in patients with mild coagulation abnormalities. *Transfusion* 31:164–171, 1991.
76. Wallis J, Dzik W: Is FFP over-transfused in the USA? *Transfusion* 44: 1674–1675, 2004.
77. Müller MC, Straat M, Meijers JC, et al: Fresh frozen plasma transfusion fails to influence the hemostatic balance in critically ill patients with a coagulopathy. *J Thromb Haemost* 13:989–97, 2015.
78. Contreras M, Ala FA, Greaves M, et al: Guidelines for the use of fresh frozen plasma. British Committee for Standards in Haematology, Working Party of the Blood Transfusion Task Force. *Transfus Med* 2:57–63, 1992.
79. Weigert AL, Schafer AL: Uremic bleeding: pathogenesis and therapy. *Am J Med Sci* 316:94–104, 1998.
80. Busch MP, Young MJ, Samson SM, et al: Risk of human immunodeficiency virus (HIV) transmission by blood transfusions before the implementation of HIV-1 antibody screening. The Transfusion Safety Study Group. *Transfusion* 31(1):4–11, 1991.
81. Schreiber GB, Busch MP, Kleinman, SH, et al: The risk of transfusion-transmitted viral infections. *N Eng J Med* 337(26):1685–1690, 1996.
82. Benjamin RJ: Nucleic acid testing: update and applications. *Sem Hematol* 38:11–16, 2001.
83. Busch MP, Glynn SA, Stramer SL, et al; NHLBI-REDS NAT Study Group: A new strategy for estimating risks of transfusion-transmitted viral infections based on rates of detection of recently infected donors. *Transfusion* 45:254–264, 2005.
84. Zou S, Stramer SL, Dodd RY: Donor testing and risk: current prevalence, incidence, and residual risk of transfusion-transmissible agents in US allogeneic donations. *Transfus Med Rev* 26:119, 2012.
85. Clair P, Embil J, Fahey J: A seroepidemiologic study of cytomegalovirus infection in a Canadian recruit population. *Mil Med* 155(10):489–492, 1990.
86. Tegtmeier GE: Post transfusion cytomegalovirus infections. *Arch Pathol Lab Med* 113:236–245, 1989.
87. Bowden RA: Transfusion-transmitted cytomegalovirus infection. *Hematol Onc Clin N A* 9:155–166, 1995.
88. Bowden RA, Slichter SJ, Sayers MH, et al: A comparison of filtered leukocyte-reduced and cytomegalovirus (CMV) seronegative blood products for the prevention of transfusion-associated CMV infection after marrow transplant. *Blood* 86:3598–3603, 1995.
89. Perez P, Salmi LR, Follea G, et al: BACTHEM Group; French Haemovigilance Network: Determinants of transfusion-associated bacterial contamination: results of the French BACTHEM Case-Control Study. *Transfusion* 41:862–872, 2001.
90. Blajchman MA: Bacterial contamination of blood products and the value of pre-transfusion testing. *Immunol Invest* 24:163–170, 1995.
91. Centers for Disease Control and Prevention: Fatal bacterial infections associated with platelet transfusions—United States, 2004. *MMWR Morb Mortal Wkly Rep* 54:168–170, 2005.
92. Goldman M, Sher G, Blajchman M: Bacterial contamination of cellular blood products: the Canadian perspective. *Transfus Sci* 23:17–19, 2000.
93. Krailadsiri P, Seghatchian J, MacGregor I, et al: The effects of leukodepletion on the generation and removal of microvesicles and prion protein in blood components. *Transfusion* 46:407–417, 2006.
94. Lumadue JA, Manabe YC, Moore RD, et al: Adherence to a strict specimen-labeling policy decreases the incidence of erroneous blood grouping of blood bank specimens. *Transfusion* 37:1169–1172, 1997.
95. Capon SM, Goldfinger D: Acute hemolytic transfusion reaction, a paradigm of the systemic inflammatory response: new insights into pathophysiology and treatment. *Transfusion* 35:513–520, 1995.
96. Linden JV, Wagner K, Voytovich AE, et al: Transfusion errors in New York State: an analysis of 10 years' experience. *Transfusion* 40:1207–1213, 2000.
97. Sazama K: Reports of 355 transfusion-associated deaths: 1976 through 1985. *Transfusion* 30:583–590, 1990.
98. Brubaker DB: Clinical significance of white cell antibodies in febrile nonhemolytic transfusion reactions. *Transfusion* 30:733–737, 1990.
99. Heddle NM, Kelton JG: Febrile Nonhemolytic transfusion reactions, in Popovsky MA (ed): *Transfusion Reactions*. 2nd ed. Bethesda, MD, AABB Press, 2001, pp 55–62.
100. Kleinman S, Caulfield T, Chan P, et al: Toward an understanding of transfusion-related acute lung injury: statement of a consensus panel. *Transfusion* 44:1774–1789, 2004.
101. Moore SB: Transfusion-related acute lung injury (TRALI): clinical presentation, treatment, and prognosis. *Crit Care Med* 34[5 Suppl]:S114–S117, 2006.
102. Stephen CR, Martin RC, Bourgeois-Cavardin M: Antihistaminic drugs in the treatment of nonhemolytic transfusion reactions. *JAMA* 158:525–529, 1955.
103. Gorlin JB, Mintz PD in Mintz PD (ed): *Transfusion Therapy: Clinical Principles and Practice*. Bethesda, MD, AABB Press, 1999, 341–357.
104. Opelz G, Sengar DP, Michkey MR, et al: Effect of blood transfusions on subsequent kidney transplants. *Transplant Proc* 5:253–259, 1973.
105. Vamvakas EC, Blajchman MA: Deleterious clinical effects of transfusion-associated Immunomodulation: fact or fiction? *Blood* 97:1180–1195, 2001.
106. Vamvakas EC: Allogeneic blood transfusion as a risk factor for the subsequent development of non-Hodgkin's lymphoma. *Transfu Med Rev* 14:258–268, 2000.
107. van de Watering LM, Hermans J, Houbiers JG, et al: Beneficial effects of leukocyte depletion of transfused blood on postoperative complications in patients undergoing cardiac surgery: a randomized clinical trial. *Circulation* 97:562–568, 1998.

Chapter 90 ■ Anemia in the Critical Care Setting

MARC S. ZUMBERG • MARC J. KAHN • ALICE D. MA

GENERAL PRINCIPLES

Anemia is common in the critical care setting. Up to 60% of patients are anemic upon admission to an intensive care unit (ICU) with a first hemoglobin concentration <9 g per dL [1,2]. Anemia will develop in nearly all patients at some point during the course of a prolonged ICU stay, and as a result, the majority of patients admitted more than 7 days receive a red blood cell (RBC) transfusion [1,3]. Anemia in the critically ill patient has been shown to be associated with poor outcomes; however, many interventions including red cell transfusion, erythropoietin (EPO), and iron supplementation have not been shown to consistently improve these same outcomes [2–4].

Certain anemias may be encountered more frequently in patients who are admitted to critical care units than in other settings, including anemias arising from iatrogenic sources (e.g., mechanical hemolysis caused by ventricular assist devices or intraaortic balloon pumps); those producing hemodynamic or systemic compromise that leads to a requirement for critical care (e.g., massive blood loss due to trauma, gastrointestinal lesions, or surgical invasion; thrombotic microangiopathies); and those arising in the context of prolonged critical illness (e.g., anemia of chronic disease/inflammation [ACD]). Losses from an enhanced frequency of phlebotomy for diagnostic testing in the critical care unit may contribute to the development or maintenance of anemia and has been estimated to account for 1 to 2 units lost during a typical hospital stay [4–6]. It has been reported that there is an additional 18% risk for development of moderate to severe hospital-acquired anemia for every 50 mL of phlebotomized blood [7].

This chapter provides an overview of the evaluation and laboratory testing for anemia, with a focus on diagnoses that are the most clinically concerning, are important to recognize quickly, and are the most likely to be encountered in the critical care setting. Accordingly, the hemolytic anemias, including the microangiopathic hemolytic anemias, autoimmune hemolytic anemia (AIHA), and sickle cell syndromes, will be covered in more detail (Table 90.1). The ACD often develops in patients in the ICU and will also be a focus of this chapter. Anemia due to massive blood loss including trauma and gastrointestinal bleeding is essential to recognize, obtain proper consultation for, and treat appropriately, but the diagnosis is usually self-evident and will be covered in other areas of this textbook (Chapters 37 and 203) .

Initial Evaluation

The etiologies of anemia in the critical care setting are diverse, but the evaluation of anemia in a critically ill patient initially should be approached in a manner similar to the noncritical care setting.

The patient's volume status should be considered first, as an increase in the plasma volume may lead to a decrease in the measured hemoglobin or hematocrit that does not represent a true decrease in the red cell mass or oxygen carrying capacity. This situation is known as dilutional or spurious anemia and is particularly common in ICU patients who have been in positive fluid balance. Dilutional anemia does not require treatment, other than correcting the underlying deficit.

To more accurately develop a differential diagnosis, it should be determined whether the anemia predated the patient's critical illness, developed in conjunction with the critical illness, or developed during the ICU stay (Table 90.2).

TABLE 90.1

Classification of the Hemolytic Anemias: Congenital versus Acquired

Congenital hemolytic anemias
Defects in the erythrocyte membrane
• e.g., hereditary spherocytosis
Deficiencies in erythrocyte metabolic enzymes
• e.g., pyruvate kinase deficiency
• e.g., glucose-6-phosphate dehydrogenase deficiency
Defects in globin structure and synthesis
• e.g., sickle cell disease
• e.g., thalassemia
Acquired hemolytic anemias
Autoimmune hemolytic anemias
• e.g., warm autoimmune hemolytic anemia
• e.g., cold agglutinin disease
• e.g., paroxysmal cold hemoglobinuria
• e.g., drug-induced hemolytic anemia
Microangiopathic hemolytic anemia
• e.g., thrombotic thrombocytopenic purpura
• e.g., hemolytic uremic syndrome
• e.g., disseminated intravascular coagulation
Hemolytic transfusion reaction
Paroxysmal nocturnal hemoglobinuria
Infectious agents
• e.g., malaria
Chemicals, drugs, and physical agents
• e.g., arsenic
Advanced liver disease

TABLE 90.2

Sample Differential Diagnosis of Anemia Based on the Time Course of Anemia in Relation to the Critical Illness

Anemia predating the critical illness
- Primary bone marrow disorders
- Vitamin deficiencies
- Hemoglobinopathies
- Congenital anemias

Anemia developing in conjunction or part of the critical illness
- Anemia of chronic disease/inflammation
- Hemolytic anemias
- TTP
- DIC

Anemia developing during the course of the intensive care unit stay
- Gastrointestinal bleeding
- Frequent phlebotomies
- Drug-induced hemolytic anemia
- Anemia of chronic disease/inflammation
- DIC

DIC, disseminated intravascular coagulation; TTP, thrombotic thrombocytopenic purpura.

TABLE 90.3

Differential Diagnosis of Selected Anemias Based on Red Cell MCV

Microcytic (MCV <80 fL)
- Fe deficiency
- α-Thalassemia
- β-Thalassemia
- Anemia of chronic disease/inflammation
- Lead poisoning
- Sideroblastic anemia

Normocytic (MCV 80–100 fL)
- Acute blood loss
- Primary bone marrow disorders
- Anemia of chronic disease/inflammation
- Splenomegaly
- Hemolytic anemia with low or normal reticulocyte count
- Endocrine disorders

Macrocytic (MCV >100 fL)
- Megaloblastic anemia
  - B_{12} deficiency
  - Folic acid deficiency
  - Drug induced
- Hypothyroidism
- Liver disease
- Hemolytic anemia with reticulocytosis
- Myelodysplastic syndrome or other primary bone marrow disorders

MCV, mean corpuscular volume.

Laboratory Studies

Anemias can be classified by the size of the RBCs as reflected by the mean corpuscular volume (MCV): microcytic (MCV, <80 fL), normocytic (80 to 100 fL), and macrocytic (>100 fL). A finite number of diagnoses constitute each of these categories, allowing the practitioner to narrow the differential diagnosis (Table 90.3). One should take caution to review the MCV prior to

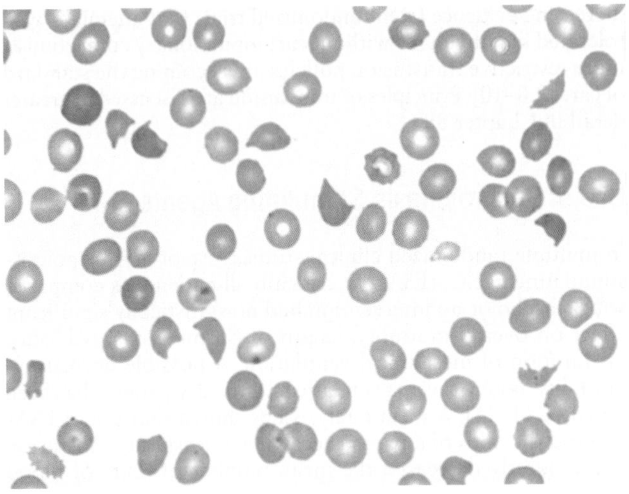

FIGURE 90.1 Peripheral smear from a patient with disseminated intravascular coagulation shows characteristic "helmet" cells. (Reused with permission from Maslak P. ASH Image Bank 2008;2008:8-00102.)

the transfusion of RBCs, as transfused donor RBCs may increase or decrease the MCV depending on the pretransfusion value.

Several additional tests may be helpful for the evaluation of anemia. The reticulocyte count, which is a measure of the bone marrow's ability to produce new RBCs, should be the initial test performed. The reticulocyte count is typically elevated in hemolytic anemias, acute gastrointestinal bleeding, or after supplementation of a missing nutrient such as iron or vitamin B_{12}. The reticulocyte count is typically low in primary bone marrow disorders, nutritional deficiencies, the ACD, and any condition leading to the underproduction of or resistance to EPO (e.g., renal disease). If a hemolytic anemia is suspected (i.e., due to consistently hemolyzed blood specimens, characteristic findings on physical examination [see later], or refractoriness to erythrocyte transfusion), measurement of total and unfractionated bilirubin (elevated), lactate dehydrogenase (LDH) (elevated), and haptoglobin (decreased) may be useful, although the results

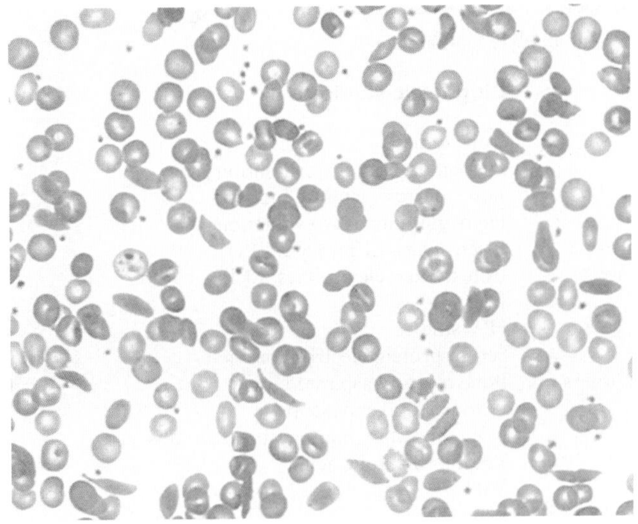

FIGURE 90.2 Peripheral smear from a patient with sickle cell disease illustrates the spectrum of RBC findings in this disorder including sickle cells, polychromatophilic RBCs, target cells, and Howell–Jolly bodies. (Reused with permission from Lazarchick J. ASH Image Bank 2009;2009:9-00044.)
RBC, red blood cell.

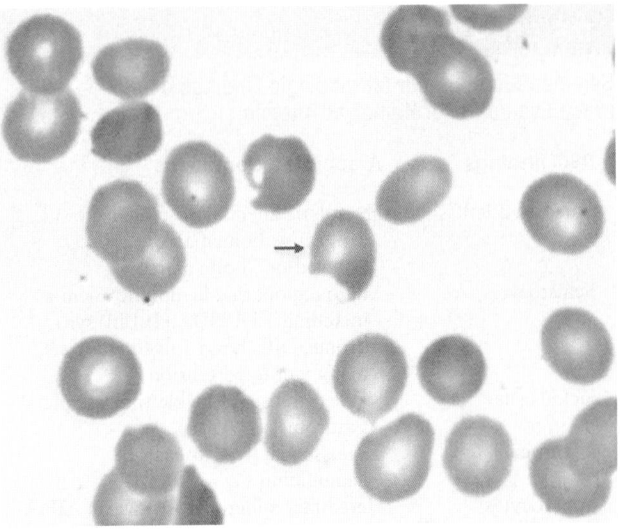

FIGURE 90.3 The RBC deformity (*arrow*) shown in this image is referred to as a "bite" cell. (Reused with permission from Lazarchick J. ASH Image Bank 2008;2008:8-00151.)
RBC, red blood cells.

are not specific to hemolysis and may show a similar pattern in patients with advanced liver disease.

A review of the blood smear will often help to narrow the differential diagnosis and quickly identify anemias due to causes that require expeditious, specialized management (e.g., thrombotic microangiopathies). Examples of erythrocyte abnormalities with classic blood smear findings include schistocytes (Fig. 90.1), sickle cells (Fig. 90.2), bite cells (Fig. 90.3), or spherocytes (Fig. 90.4), and identification of these aberrant forms is critical in making the correct diagnosis (Table 90.4).

Further laboratory testing should be guided by the results of the MCV, reticulocyte count, review of the blood smear, and clinical suspicion of any possible underlying diagnoses (Table 90.5).

Therapeutic Red Cell Transfusion

Clinicians caring for patients in critical care settings are often confronted with the decision to transfuse RBCs even before

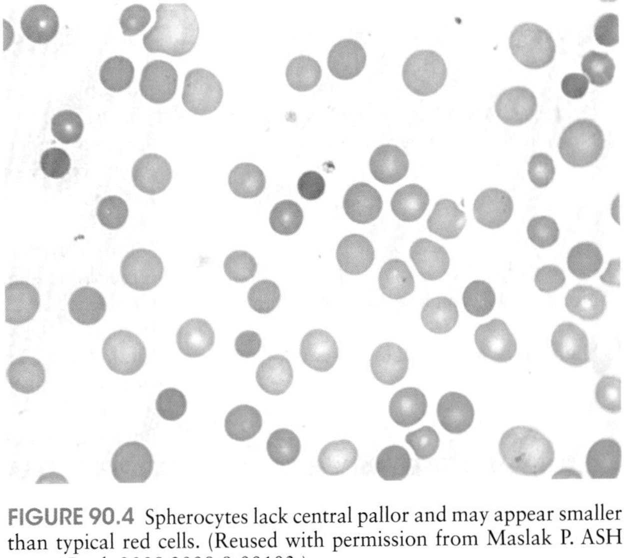

FIGURE 90.4 Spherocytes lack central pallor and may appear smaller than typical red cells. (Reused with permission from Maslak P. ASH Image Bank 2008;2008:8-00103.)

TABLE 90.4

Selected Blood Smear Morphologic Findings Useful in the Evaluation of Hemolytic Anemia

RBC findings	Associated conditions
Nucleated RBCs	Hemolytic anemia, postsplenectomy, infiltrative bone marrow process, "revved-up" bone marrow
Schistocytes	Microangiopathic hemolytic anemia including TTP, HUS, HELLP syndrome, DIC, heart valve hemolysis, malignant hypertension
Sickle cells	Sickle cell disease, sickle-thalassemic syndromes
Target cells	Thalassemia, liver disease, hemoglobin C
Spherocytes	Hereditary spherocytosis, warm AIHA
Bite cells	G6PD deficiency
Tear drop cells	Myelofibrosis, infiltrative bone marrow process
RBC agglutination	CAD
Rouleaux formation	Multiple myeloma, Waldenstrom's macroglobulinemia

CAD, cold agglutinin disese; DIC, disseminated intravascular coagulation; G6PD, glucose 6 phosphate AIHA, autoimmune hemolytic anemia dehydrogenase; HELLP syndrome, hemolysis, elevated liver enzymes, low platelets; HUS, hemolytic uremic syndrome; RBC, red blood cell; TTP, thrombotic thrombocytopenic purpura.

results of laboratory testing or other evaluation have elucidated the cause of the anemia. Erythrocyte transfusion in this setting should be guided by hemodynamic considerations, rather than a finite transfusion trigger [8]. Because of the (albeit low) risk of transmission of infectious pathogens and the potential for transfusion reactions and immunomodulation, and in light of increasing evidence from randomized trials that anemia is well tolerated in individuals without cardiopulmonary compromise, more restrictive transfusion policies are becoming the standard of care [2,8–10]. Principles of transfusion are discussed in greater detail in Chapter 89.

Use of Erythropoiesis-Stimulating Agents

In multiple randomized clinical studies, use of erythropoiesis-stimulating agents (ESAs) in critically ill patients as compared with placebo or no intervention had no statistically significant effect on overall mortality, length of hospital stay, ICU stay, or duration of mechanical ventilation. A possible decrease in mortality among severe traumatic brain injury patients has been noted [2,11–15]. A meta-analysis has shown that use of ESAs reduced the odds of a patient receiving at least one transfusion and modestly decreased the mean number of units of blood transfused by 0.41 units [13]. The optimal dosing and schedule of EPO remain to be determined [13,16], and the benefits of concomitant supplemental intravenous iron, which may be considered when the serum ferritin drops below 100 to 200 ng per mL or iron saturation drops below 20% [2], still is debated. A meta-analysis of off-label use of ESAs in critically ill patients showed an increase in thrombotic vascular events, but not other adverse events or death [17]. Thus, at the present time, there remains insufficient evidence to recommend the routine use of ESAs in critically ill anemic patients [1,13].

Hematology Consultation

If the etiology of the anemia is not apparent despite the above evaluation or if treatment options remain uncertain, hematology consultation should be initiated. A bone marrow aspirate and biopsy may be useful if the diagnosis remains in question or if a primary bone marrow disorder is suspected because of unexplained abnormalities (morphologic or quantitative) in other blood cell lineages.

TABLE 90.5

Suggested Initial Sample Laboratory Evaluation Based on the MCV and Reticulocyte Count

Laboratory finding	Suspected diagnoses	Diagnostic studies[a]
Decreased MCV/low reticulocyte count	Iron deficiency	Iron studies
	Thalassemia minor	Hemoglobinopathy evaluation
	Sideroblastic anemia	Bone marrow aspirate/biopsy
Decreased MCV/high reticulocyte count	Thalassemia	Hemoglobinopathy evaluation
Normal MCV/low reticulocyte count	Organ dysfunction	Electrolytes, LFTs, TSH, EPO
	Anemia of chronic disease	Iron studies, electrolytes, LFTs
	Early iron deficiency	Iron studies
	HIV	HIV studies
	Multiple myeloma	Serum protein electrophoresis
	Other bone marrow disorders	Bone marrow aspirate/biopsy
Normal MCV/high reticulocyte count	GI bleed	Guaiac stool, endoscopy
	Hemolytic anemia	LDH, bilirubin, haptoglobin, Coombs test
High MCV/low reticulocyte count	Vitamin deficiencies	Vitamin B_{12}, folic acid
	Hypothyroidism	TSH
	Advanced liver disease	LFTs
	Bone marrow disorders	Bone marrow aspirate/biopsy
High MCV/high reticulocyte count	Hemolytic anemia	LDH, bilirubin, haptoglobin, Coombs test

[a]Diagnostic studies may be ordered in succession until diagnostic result is reached.
EPO, erythropoietin; GI, gastrointestinal; HIV, human immunodeficiency virus; LDH, lactate dehydrogenase; LFTs, liver function tests; MCV, mean corpuscular volume; TSH, thyroid stimulating hormone.

HEMOLYTIC ANEMIAS

The hemolytic anemias are characterized by a decreased red cell life span. The physiologic sequelae of these disorders, in addition to the ability of the hemolytic process to cause a decrease in hemoglobin and oxygen carrying capacity in a short period of time, may lead to a requirement for critical care. The patient with hemolysis may be very or only minimally symptomatic, depending on the rate of red cell destruction and the degree of compensation by the bone marrow, which produces young red cells (reticulocytes) in response to the decreased hemoglobin.

Overview of Laboratory Features

Pathologic features of hemolysis differ greatly depending on whether the red cell destruction is primarily intravascular or extravascular. Biochemical evidence for intravascular hemolysis includes elevated levels of LDH and unconjugated bilirubin and decreased levels of haptoglobin, which is cleared from the circulation after binding free hemoglobin. Hemoglobinuria results when free hemoglobin is filtered through the glomerulus and is released into the urine, imparting a reddish color. Some hemoglobin in the urine is taken up by tubular cells and is converted to hemosiderin. This can be detected by checking for intracellular iron in the urine by staining the urine with Prussian blue stain. Extravascular hemolysis may be evidenced by only a declining hemoglobin level, although cases of brisk destruction of red cells may show elevations in LDH and unconjugated bilirubin.

Increased red cell production is evidenced by an increase in the number of circulating reticulocytes, which are young red cells whose large size typically results in an elevated red cell MCV and red cell distribution width. Circulating nucleated red blood cells (NRBCs) may be seen in cases of brisk hemolysis. Morphologic evidence of red cell destruction may be evident on the blood smear (see following sections and Figs. 90.1 to 90.4).

Immune-Mediated Hemolysis

The pathophysiology of immune-mediated hemolysis involves antibodies binding to red cells, with or without the activation of complement, leading to red cell destruction. If the antibody on the red cell surface is immunoglobulin G (IgG), then red cell destruction is mediated via Fc receptors on macrophages within the reticuloendothelial (RE) system. Complete or partial phagocytosis occurs causing the red cells to take a spherocytic shape as opposed to the normal, more pliable, biconcave disc shape.

Antibodies which lead to hemolysis can be divided into two categories: Warm and cold, referring to the temperature at which the antibody optimally reacts with the red cell. Warm antibodies react optimally with red cells at temperatures 37°C and typically do not agglutinate red cells [18]. Cold antibodies typically react best at temperatures less than 32°C, with maximal reactivity at 4°C and lead to red cell agglutination [19]. The hallmark of AIHA is a positive direct Coombs test, which will detect the presence of either IgG or C3 bound to red cells (Table 90.6).

Warm Autoimmune Hemolytic Anemia

In warm autoimmune hemolytic anemia (WAIHA), IgG antibodies are directed against red cell surface membrane antigens [18]. Most commonly, these antibodies are directed against members of the Rh blood group, but the specificity of the pathogenic IgG antibodies is not always identified. The IgG antibodies coat the red cells and may or may not fix complement (C3). IgG-coated red cell membrane fragments are engulfed by macrophages in the RE system (usually the spleen) [18,20]. As the red cell loses surface area, it loses the ability to retain its biconcave disc shape. As the shape with the smallest surface area-to-volume ratio is a sphere, the red cell becomes progressively more spherocytic with each pass through the splenic circulation [18].

WAIHA can manifest as a primary disorder, or alternatively, it can be secondary to an underlying disorder, such as collagen vascular disease (e.g., lupus) or a lymphoproliferative disorder (e.g., lymphoma). Approximately 30% of patients with chronic lymphocytic leukemia have a positive Coombs test, although a much lower proportion develops hemolysis [21]. AIHA may be associated with immune thrombocytopenia, a condition called Evans syndrome. AIHA can also be provoked by infection or can be induced by various drugs. Causes of WAIHA are listed in Table 90.7.

Clinical Features. Almost all patients present with worsening and often debilitating fatigue. Older patients, and those with rapid hemolysis and ensuing severe anemia, may present with evidence of organ compromise such as dyspnea, angina, or syncope and can suffer myocardial ischemia, hypotension, and/or renal failure. Physical findings can include pallor, jaundice, and splenomegaly. Laboratory findings include an increased reticulocyte count, increased bilirubin (total and indirect), and increased LDH. The direct Coombs test should be positive (Table 90.6), and typically spherocytes, microspherocytes, NRBCs, and/or anisocytosis are seen on the blood smear.

TABLE 90.6

Interpretation of the Coombs Test and Differential Diagnosis

	IgG positive	IgG negative
C3 positive	WAIHA	Drug-induced hemolysis
	Drug-induced hemolysis	CAD
		PCH
C3 negative	WAIHA	WAIHA (rare)

In performing this test, red cells from the patient are washed to remove nonspecific proteins and antibodies. Next, antibodies to human IgG, human C3, or both are added to the cells. If the patient's red cells have either IgG or C3 attached to them, the red cells will agglutinate, indicating a positive test. The specificity of the antibody can be tested by testing the patient's serum against panels of red cells that express different subsets of red cell antigens. CAD, cold agglutinin disease; IgG, immunoglobulin G; PCH, paroxysmal cold hemoglobinuria; WAIHA, warm autoimmune hemolytic anemia.

TABLE 90.7

Causes of Immune Hemolytic Anemias

WAIHA
- Idiopathic
- Lymphoproliferative disease
- Autoimmune disease
- Drugs
- Infections
- Solid tumors

CAD
- Idiopathic
- Lymphoproliferative disease
- Infections

CAD, cold agglutinin disease; WAIHA, warm autoimmune hemolytic anemia.

Transfusion in Patients with Warm Autoimmune Hemolytic Anemia. If the patient has heart failure, angina, shock, or evidence of hypoperfusion to vital organs, or if compensatory erythrocytosis is absent or inadequate because of an underlying illness that suppresses the bone marrow, such as leukemia, prior chemotherapy, or renal failure, then red cell transfusion should be performed [18]. The anti-erythrocyte autoantibody itself can also be occasionally directed against red cell precursors in the marrow, leading to an inappropriately low reticulocyte count [18,22]. Any transfusion in patients with WAIHA needs to be coordinated closely with the blood bank or transfusion service. The offending antibody will frequently interfere with performing a crossmatch to identify compatible blood for transfusion. It is critical to obtain a thorough transfusion and pregnancy history to determine the likelihood of an underlying alloantibody which may be masked by the autoantibody; testing a red cell eluate may be helpful in this regard. Crossmatching can be done using low ionic strength solution which will minimize nonspecific interactions, allowing the stronger alloantibody interactions to appear. If time allows, phenotyping can be performed; such a maneuver may help to minimize the risk of a delayed hemolytic transfusion reaction (DHTR). If crossmatched units are not available, phenotypically matched red cells are preferred. If not available, due to time constraints or the patient's condition, then ABO and Rh type-specific, noncrossmatched, or "least incompatible" units should be used. Each unit should be transfused slowly, while the patient's clinical status is closely assessed for evidence of worsening hemolysis. The blood bank may require that samples of the patient's blood be drawn soon after the transfusion begins to record any evidence of hemolysis. This is termed an in vivo crossmatch.

Treatment. After hemostatic instability has been addressed through transfusion of RBCs, the initial treatment of WAIHA consists of immunosuppression which, if successful, may attenuate antibody production and allow the patient's RBCs to survive normally in the circulation. First-line therapy consists of glucocorticosteroids, either intravenously such as methylprednisolone or oral prednisone, typically at 1 to 2 mg per kg daily [19]. Intravenous immunoglobulin (IVIG) has also been used but is less effective than in immune thrombocytopenic purpura [18,23]. If steroids are ineffective, or if relapse occurs, then alternative immunosuppression should be considered. Agents which have been reported to be useful in WAIHA include rituximab, cyclophosphamide, mycophenolate mofetil, and azathioprine [18,24–26]. Splenectomy should also be considered as a reasonable second-line treatment option in eligible patients [18]. As with all hemolytic anemias, the administration of folic acid 1 to 5 mg per day, at least as long as hemolysis is ongoing, is recommended. The reticulocyte count and complete blood cell count (CBC) should be followed closely to monitor the effectiveness of therapy. The amount of blood drawn may be minimized by using pediatric tubes or "bullet" tubes, if available.

Cold Agglutinin Disease

In cold agglutinin disease (CAD), immunoglobulin M (IgM) antibodies target red cell surface antigens, typically with specificity to either "I" or "i." These IgM antibodies optimally bind to red cells at "cold" temperatures (typically <32°C and most strongly at 4°C) [20], and, given their ability to bind more than one RBC simultaneously, lead to the agglutination and clumping of RBCs in the distal microvasculature. IgM anti-erythrocyte antibodies fix complement to the red cell, leading to either intravascular or extravascular hemolysis. CAD may be primary or secondary due to lymphoproliferative disorders or infection [27,28].

Clinical Features. In most patients, CAD is a chronic condition characterized by mild to moderate hemolysis and episodic cyanosis and ischemia of the ears, tip of the nose, and digits [28]. When episodic, cold-induced hemolytic episodes occur, intravascular hemolysis may be associated with shock, rigors, back pain, and renal failure.

Laboratory Evaluation. Cold agglutinin titers can be measured. On Coombs testing, complement (C3) is typically positive whereas IgG is negative, reflecting the underlying IgM autoantibody which more efficiently fixes complement (Table 90.6). The thermal amplitude of the autoantibody, not the antibody titer, however, best determines the severity of clinical symptoms. If binding occurs only at 4°C to 30°C, it is less clinically important than if significant binding occurs at temperatures more than 34°C, approximating more physiologic conditions. In fact, many normal individuals will have cold agglutinins detected at 4°C but have no clinical symptoms.

Treatment. In patients with chronic, mild CAD, the mainstay of treatment is avoidance of cold temperatures. Corticosteroids and splenectomy are typically less effective in CAD as compared with WAIHA. Other agents, such as chlorambucil, cyclophosphamide, and rituximab, have been used successfully [19,29]. In patients who present with impending or actual end-organ damage such as myocardial ischemia or stroke, plasmapheresis may be effective because IgM remains primarily intravascular and can be efficiently removed. Plasmapheresis may need to be performed preoperatively in surgeries requiring cardiopulmonary bypass or cardioplegia [19,30]. In all patients, care must be taken to keep the extracorporeal tubing warm and to warm intravenous fluids and blood products, or hemolysis may worsen. Folic acid repletion is recommended in all patients.

Paroxysmal Cold Hemoglobinuria

IgG is the pathogenic antibody in this rare condition. Similar to IgM antibodies in CAD, the IgG antibody in paroxysmal cold hemoglobinuria (PCH) binds to red cells only at cold temperatures where it fixes complement. Unlike the antibody in CAD, however, it is activated at warmer temperatures and does not agglutinate red cells. This antibody is called the Donath–Landsteiner antibody and is directed against the "P" red cell antigen [19]. Red cell destruction occurs primarily via activation of the complement cascade and leads to subsequent intravascular hemolysis. In the past, PCH was primarily a disease associated with tertiary syphilis and, therefore, has become much less common in the penicillin era. Currently, PCH is primarily a pediatric disorder (often following a viral infection), only rarely affecting adults. Patients suffer episodic, cold-induced hemolysis. There is no cold-induced digital ischemia.

The diagnosis is made by detection of the Donath–Landsteiner antibody. The Coombs test is typically negative for IgG and positive for C3 (Table 90.6). The blood bank should be alerted to the possibility of this diagnosis, as special considerations are required for detection. Serum is collected from the patient and kept at 37°C. Patient serum and normal red cells are next chilled to 4°C, then warmed to 37°C. The presence of lysis is revealed by the detection of free hemoglobin in the sample. Controls must be performed where red cells and serum are incubated at 37°C and in a separate test tube at 4°C. In both of these scenarios, there should be no lysis detected [31], as a positive test requires the extremes of temperature.

Drug-Induced Hemolytic Anemias

More than 130 drugs have been reported to cause immune-mediated hemolytic anemia [32]. Drugs can induce hemolytic anemia by three general mechanisms: the innocent bystander mechanism,

TABLE 90.8

Mechanisms of Drug-Induced Hemolysis

Mechanism	Pathophysiology	Examples
Innocent bystander mechanism	Antibodies develop against the drug. The drug and antibody bind together to form immune complexes, which deposit on the surface of the red cell, where they are recognized by the RE system. The drug must be present in order for hemolysis to occur	Quinine Quinidine Isoniazid
Hapten mechanism	Drug binds to the red cell surface, and antibodies form which are directed against the complex of RBC/drug	Penicillins Cephalosporins, especially Cefotetan
True autoimmune mechanism	Certain drugs appear to induce formation of antibodies directed against red cell surface components, independent of any binding to the RBC surface. Once the process has been initiated, antibody production can continue, even in the absence of drug	Alpha methyldopa Levodopa Procainamide Fludarabine

RBC, red blood cell; RE, reticuloendothelial.

hapten mechanism, and a true autoimmune mechanism [33,34]. These are described in Table 90.8. It should be noted that many drugs may lead to a positive direct Coombs test in the absence of overt hemolysis. Thus, a positive direct Coombs test should not be inferred to represent hemolysis unless there is worsening anemia in conjunction with consistent laboratory evaluation. Currently, piperacillin is the most common drug to cause immune hemolytic anemia [35].

Other drugs may cause hemolysis by alternative mechanisms. Oxidant agents such as dapsone and other sulfa drugs may cause hemolysis in a dose-dependent fashion, especially in individuals with glucose 6-phosphate dehydrogenase (G6PD) deficiency who are impaired in their ability to detoxify the oxidant damage to hemoglobin (see "Glucose 6-Phosphate Dehydrogenase Deficiency" section later in the chapter). Ribavirin, used to treat hepatitis C, causes hemolysis in a dose-dependent fashion. Its mechanism of red cell damage is unclear, but it may relate to nucleotide depletion. Other agents such as cyclosporine and tacrolimus may cause a microangiopathic hemolytic anemia due to endothelial damage (see "Microangiopathic Hemolytic Anemia" section).

MICROANGIOPATHIC HEMOLYTIC ANEMIA

The microangiopathic hemolytic anemias are a heterogeneous group of disorders defined by vascular damage leading to thrombosis of small arterioles and capillaries resulting in distortion and fragmentation of erythrocytes, hemolysis, subsequent anemia, and thrombocytopenia [36,37]. The hallmark finding on the blood smear is the schistocyte, a fragmented RBC (Fig. 90.1). It is essential that the intensivist recognize the differential diagnosis of microangiopathic hemolytic anemia as many of the diagnoses require prompt recognition and treatment (Table 90.9) [36]. If the underlying etiology of a microangiopathic hemolytic anemia is in question, immediate hematology consultation is strongly recommended to evaluate for life-threatening diagnosis such as thrombotic thrombocytopenic purpura (TTP).

TTP, once almost uniformly fatal, can now be treated effectively in the majority of patients with prompt recognition and initiation of therapeutic plasma exchange (TPE) [36]. The diagnosis should be suspected in any patient who presents with unexplained microangiopathic hemolytic anemia and thrombocytopenia [36,38–40]. The "classic pentad" of microangiopathic hemolytic anemia, thrombocytopenia, mental status changes, renal failure, and fever is present in fewer than 25% of patients at presentation. Only unexplained microangiopathic hemolytic anemia and thrombocytopenia are required to begin TPE; the aforementioned clinical sequela are likely late manifestations of the disease [36,39–41].

TABLE 90.9

Differential Diagnosis of Microangiopathic Hemolytic Anemia

- TTP
- Hemolytic uremic syndrome
- Disseminated intravascular coagulation
- HELLP syndrome
- Preeclampsia
- Malignant hypertension
- Malfunctioning prosthetic heart valve with turbulent flow
- Severe vasculitis
- Scleroderma renal crisis
- Catastrophic antiphospholipid antibody syndrome
- Malignancy
- Intravascular foreign bodies
  - Left ventricular assist device
  - Intraaortic balloon pump
- Drugs
  - Cyclosporine
  - Tacrolimus
  - Ticlopidine
  - Clopidogrel
  - Chemotherapeutic agents such as mitomycin C, gemcitabine, and VEGF inhibitors

HELLP, hemolysis, elevated liver enzymes, low platelets; TTP, thrombotic thrombocytopenic purpura; VEGF, vascular endothelial growth factor.

Moake and others first noted unusually large von Willebrand factor (vWF) multimers in the plasma of affected patients and proposed them to be central in the pathophysiology of the disorder [42]. In the late 1990s, two groups reported that a vWF-cleaving protease (later termed ADAMTS-13, as a member of a disintegrin and metalloproteinase with thrombospondin components family of proteins) was found to be absent in familial TTP and inhibited by an antibody in the majority of cases of acquired TTP [43,44]. The absence of ADAMTS-13 was subsequently shown to prevent the breakdown and lead to the accumulation of ultra large molecular weight vWF multimers [42,45,46]. These ultra large vWF multimers efficiently bind to glycoprotein receptors on platelet surfaces leading to adhesion of platelets to the blood vessel endothelium and subsequently to small vessel occlusion affecting a variety of organs [36,42]. Hemolytic anemia occurs because of the mechanical shearing of RBCs as they transverse the turbulent and occluded microvasculature, thus leading to the classic findings of schistocytes seen on the peripheral blood smear (Fig. 90.1).

Clinical Manifestations

As discussed earlier, the clinical manifestations of TTP can be quite varied. Neurologic symptoms may range from subtle confusion to frank seizures or coma. Renal dysfunction may range from mild proteinuria or azotemia to acute renal failure. Occlusion in blood vessels of the cardiac conduction system may lead to arrhythmias and sudden cardiac death. Pancreatitis has been described and should be considered in patients with abdominal pain. Fever is often noted. Essentially any organ system may be affected leading to a wide range of symptoms.

Laboratory Features

Laboratory evaluation usually reveals a hemolytic anemia with at least (and often much more than) two schistocytes or greater than 1% of RBCs per 100 × field on microscopic examination (Table 90.4 and Fig. 90.1). Coagulation studies such as the activated partial thromboplastin time and the prothrombin time are typically normal, whereas they are usually prolonged in disseminated intravascular coagulation (DIC). The Coombs test is typically negative. Most cases of classic acquired TTP are associated with a severe deficiency of ADAMTS-13 (<5%), and an inhibitory antibody can be demonstrated [36,39–41]. ADAMTS-13 results are often not available in real time, are not required to make the diagnosis, and therefore not routinely used to make initial therapeutic decisions regarding the initiation of plasma exchange. ADAMTS-13 levels have prognostic value regarding the risk of relapse but are less useful in determining the likelihood of initial response to plasma exchange. Mild to moderate decreases in ADAMTS-13 are not specific and may be seen in a variety of disorders including sepsis [34,37,39,41].

Schistocytes may be seen in conditions other than TTP (Table 90.9). These conditions usually have in common damage to the blood vessel endothelium, leading to the release of ultra large vWF multimers. The presentation of these syndromes may mimic TTP. The hemolytic uremic syndrome (HUS) often presents with a primary component of renal failure [47]. Conditions other than TTP are not associated with severe (<5%) deficiency of ADAMTS-13 and TPE is typically much less or ineffective. When atypical HUS is suspected, TPE is often initiated until the ADAMTS-13 results become available [36,40,41].

The distinction between TTP and HUS may be difficult, although it has been reported that a serum creatinine >150 to 200 μmol per L or a platelet count >30 × 10^9 per L is rarely associated with severe ADAMTS-13 deficiency as seen in TTP [41,47]. Classic childhood HUS is usually preceded by hemorrhagic diarrhea caused by *Escherichia coli* O157:H7. In atypical HUS, renal failure is more severe and extrarenal manifestations are less common or absent as compared to TTP [41,47]. ADAMTS-13 is not usually severely depressed in HUS, suggesting a different pathophysiology between these two related conditions [36]. Atypical HUS has been linked to uncontrolled activation of the complement system due to either congenital or acquired mutations or antibodies against various factors in the complement pathway [36,48]. As the ability to differentiate between TTP and atypical HUS is often unclear, prompt TPE is often initiated in atypical HUS, even though efficacy is less as compared to TTP [36,41]. Eculizumab, a terminal complement inhibitor, was approved and has become the standard of care for the treatment of atypical HUS since 2011 [36,47,49]. As soon as the diagnosis is confirmed/deemed highly likely or if there is high suspicion and TPE is ineffective, eculizumab should be promptly initiated. Meningococcal vaccination is recommended prior to the first dose. Both nephrology and hematology consultation should be sought when the diagnosis of atypical HUS is suspected.

Treatment

TPE with fresh frozen plasma (FFP) at a 1.0 to 1.5 × plasma volume should be initiated as soon as idiopathic TTP is suspected [36–41]. A dual-lumen, large-bore, dialysis-type catheter is often needed for the procedure, despite the coexisting thrombocytopenia. With prompt TPE, 80% to 90% of patients with classic TTP survive this once uniformly fatal disease [36]. The effectiveness of TPE is thought to be due to both the removal of an anti-ADAMTS-13 antibody and the replacement of ADAMTS-13 in donor FFP. If TPE is not readily available, FFP should be infused at a rate of 30 mL/kg/d while arrangements for TPE are made [41]. Randomized trials have supported the efficacy of TPE over simple plasma infusion which is often problematic given the large volume of FFP required [36,39–41].

TPE should be continued until the platelet count and LDH have normalized for 2 days [36,39,41]. Plasma exchange is often tapered down to every other day upon remission, but this practice has not been critically studied and its efficacy in preventing relapse is uncertain [41]. In refractory or relapsing patients, cryosupernatant plasma, devoid of vWF, should be considered [38]. Catheter-related infections should also be investigated and have been documented to lead to relapse. Immunosuppressants such as glucocorticoids and cyclosporine as adjuncts to plasma exchange have been used, but efficacy remains uncertain [36,38–41]. Platelet transfusion is generally avoided, as it is thought to possibly exacerbate thrombosis, although evidence is conflicting [50,51].

Rituximab has been increasingly used as adjuvant therapy to TPE in both the initial and refractory settings [52]. Recent guidelines have stated that rituximab should be considered along with TPE and steroids during an acute event and recommended in patients who have a refractory episode of TPE despite plasma exchange [52]. Recombinant ADAMTS-13 is under development and may prove to be effective in the future.

Disseminated Intravascular Coagulation

Although microangiopathic hemolytic anemia may be present in patients with DIC, typically the thrombotic or bleeding manifestations of DIC are more clinically significant. DIC, which is often due to an underlying serious or catastrophic event such as septicemia or an obstetric emergency, will be covered in greater detail in Chapter 94.

Other Causes of Microangiopathic Hemolytic Anemia

The differential diagnosis of microangiopathic hemolytic anemia includes other diagnoses listed in Table 90.9. Appropriate consultation and treatment should be pursued dependent on the most likely diagnosis.

HEMOGLOBINOPATHIES

Sickle Cell Anemia

Sickle cell anemia results from the presence of a point mutation leading to an amino acid substitution (valine for glutamic acid) in the sixth position of the beta chain of hemoglobin. An unstable form of hemoglobin (hemoglobin S) is produced which polymerizes in the setting of dehydration or hypoxia, leading to irreversible sickling of erythrocytes. Erythrocyte sickling is responsible for a variety of clinical conditions including extremely painful episodes in the back and extremities. Patients may be symptomatic if they are homozygous for hemoglobin S; if they are compound heterozygotes for hemoglobin S, hemoglobin C, hemoglobin D, and hemoglobin E; or if they also have concomitant β-thalassemia. The most common complications of sickling disorders leading to ICU admission are listed in Table 90.10.

Transfusion

Although patients with sickling disorders are nearly always anemic, routine transfusions are not indicated for hemodynamically stable anemia, routine vasoocclusive crisis, routine pregnancies, or simple surgical procedures that do not require general anesthesia. In general, hematology consultation is indicated if transfusion is considered, as the need for transfusion usually suggests a more complicated clinical scenario. Transfusion therapy can be simple, chronic, or performed via RBC exchange. Simple transfusion involves infusion of a sufficient volume of red cells to improve tissue oxygenation. Chronic simple transfusions are primarily used to prevent stroke recurrence. RBC exchange, performed (where available) via erythrocytapheresis using a non-collapsible, large-bore, dialysis-type catheter, involves the removal of the patient's hemoglobin S red cells, followed by replacement of RBCs from a non–hemoglobin S donor targeting a final hemoglobin no higher than 8 to 10 g per dL with hemoglobin S less than 30%. RBC exchange is often used in the management of acute stroke, severe acute chest syndrome (ACS), or multiorgan failure as a more rapid and efficient way to remove hemoglobin S and improve oxygen delivery. As opposed to simple transfusion, which can further increase iron load, exchange transfusion is also helpful in iron-overloaded patients because iron is removed with removal of hemoglobin S red cells. As an alternative to pheresis, manual exchange transfusion involves removing 500 mL of blood, followed by infusion of 300 mL normal saline, followed by another 500 mL removal of blood, and subsequent transfusion of 4 to 5 units of packed red cells. However if possible, automated exchange by pheresis is more effective at achieving targeted hemoglobin concentrations [53]. With both exchange modalities, care should be taken to keep the end hemoglobin value no higher than 10 g per dL to minimize the risk of hyperviscosity.

Alloimmunization, typically to the Rh (E, C), Kell (K), Duffy (Fya, Fyb), and Kidd (Jk) antigens, occurs in up to 30% of patients [54]. Alloimmunization can be minimized by transfusing red cells that have been phenotypically matched for these red cell antigens. If phenotypically matched units are not available, crossmatched red cell units that are negative for C, E, and Kell are recommended.

TABLE 90.10

Critical Care Complications of Sickle Cell Disease

ACS
Acute stroke
Acute cholecystitis
Congestive heart failure
Hyperhemolysis
Pulmonary hypertension
Sepsis
Severe aplastic crisis
Delayed transfusion reaction

ACS, acute chest syndrome.

Acute Chest Syndrome

Pulmonary complications frequently cause significant morbidity and mortality in patients with sickling disorders and are a common reason for ICU admission. Among the pulmonary complications, the ACS is among the most frequently observed in the ICU setting.

Clinical Features. ACS can be defined by a constellation of fever, hypoxemia, chest pain, leukocytosis, and new pulmonary infiltrate in a patient with a sickling disorder [55]. Although most common in patients homozygous for hemoglobin S, ACS can also be seen in decreasing frequency in patients with hemoglobin SC disease and S/β+ thalassemia. Importantly, the clinical definition of ACS does not indicate a specific etiology. ACS can be caused by infection, thrombosis, fat embolism, or any combination of these conditions. A large multicenter study showed that a specific cause of ACS could be identified in more than 50% of patients studied [56]. The most common etiologies observed were fat embolism and infection. Specific etiologies of ACS from this study of 671 episodes are listed in Table 90.11.

Physiologic Markers. Secretory phospholipase A_2, a potent inflammatory mediator, has been implicated as a cause of lung damage in patients with ACS [57], and serum levels may be predictive of impending ACS [58]. In addition, circulating activated endothelial progenitor cells have been proposed as a potential etiology of ACS [59], as have levels of pentraxin 3, an acute phase reactant and key component of innate immunity [60].

Treatment. Treatment of ACS depends in part on the clinical presentation. If the sputum Gram stain suggests infection with a particular organism, targeted antibiotic therapy should be initiated without delay. Interestingly, although pneumococcus is a frequent cause of infection in children with ACS, it is much less common in adults, in whom mycoplasma is more frequently implicated [55]. However, when an infectious etiology of ACS is suspected, empiric coverage for pneumococcus remains appropriate. In addition, because of the high mortality associated with ACS, empiric antibiotic coverage for mycoplasma and chlamydia should also be strongly considered. A recently published NIH expert panel report strongly recommends treatment of ACS with cephalosporins, a macrolide, and oxygen to maintain a saturation of greater than 95% [61]. Similarly, the use of incentive spirometry was strongly encouraged by this same expert panel. Maintaining hydration and oxygenation during episodes of ACS

TABLE 90.11

Causes of the ACS in a 30-Center Study

Cause	Percentage
Fat embolism, with or without infection	8.8
Chlamydia	7.2
Mycoplasma	6.6
Virus	6.4
Bacteria	4.5
Mixed infections	3.7
Legionella	0.6
Miscellaneous infections	0.4
Infarction	16.1
Unknown	45.7

ACS, acute chest syndrome.
Adapted from Vichinsky EP, Neumayr LD, Earles AN, et al: Causes and outcomes of the acute chest syndrome in sickle cell disease. *N Engl J Med* 342:1855–1865, 2000.

are imperative to prevent further sickling. However, fluids must be administered carefully to avoid fluid overload. There are no data to support the routine use of anticoagulants in ACS, and in the absence of data, this practice should be avoided.

Patients with ACS and hypoxia (PO_2 <75 mm Hg) should be transfused red cells by either simple or exchange transfusion [61]. One small single-institution study found no difference between the two transfusion modalities [62]. The NIH expert panel recommends simple transfusion to a hemoglobin of 10 g per dL unless there is rapid progression of ACS as demonstrated by oxygen saturation below 90% despite supplemental oxygen, increasing respiratory distress, worsening chest X-ray, or decline in hemoglobin despite supplemental oxygen [61]. Because patients with hemoglobin SC disease typically have baseline hemoglobin levels in the 10 to 11 g per dL range, exchange transfusion is the preferred means of red cell administration. In addition to providing a source of oxygen delivery, exchange transfusion also decreases levels of inflammatory mediators such as soluble vascular cell adhesion molecule-1 [63].

Acute Stroke

Stroke is one of the most morbid complications of sickle cell disease, with a prevalence of more than 20% in some series [64]. In addition to overt stroke, more than 60% of patients with sickle cell disease have evidence of brain damage from occult infarction that is incidentally found on magnetic resonance imaging [65]. The pathophysiology of stroke in sickle cell patients is complicated. Stroke is related to nitric oxide depletion, hypercoagulability, and abnormalities of the major cerebral arteries. Unfortunately, stroke recurrence is common with more than 50% of cases occurring within 36 months following the initial event [66]. The presence of constricted cerebral arteries with collateralization (moyamoya syndrome) is associated with recurrent stroke and may be alleviated by surgical vascular bypass [67]. Although transcranial Doppler measurement of blood velocity has predictive value for stroke in pediatric patients with sickle cell disease, the measurement of cranial blood flow velocity is less able to stratify the risk of stroke for adults [68].

Treatment. Although there have been no specific trials addressing the issue, antiplatelet agents can be used in the treatment of acute stroke in adults with sickle cell disease, similar to patients without sickle cell disease [69]. Even in the absence of large randomized studies, an NIH expert panel recommends exchange transfusion for sickle cell patients with confirmed acute stroke on neuroimaging studies [61]. In the setting of acute stroke, emergent red cell exchange transfusion to reduce hemoglobin S to less than 30% is recommended. Similarly, consensus opinion suggests that conventional angiography can be used in sickle cell patients suspected of having an aneurysmal subarachnoid hemorrhage [70]. Because of the osmotic dye load which might increase intracerebral sickling, experts also suggest exchange transfusion prior to angiography [71]. Acute retinal artery occlusion can be considered as an ophthalmic stroke. The exact pathophysiology of retinal artery occlusion in sickle cell disease and risk factors for the condition are not known [72]. Similarly, there are scant data on the treatment of retinal artery occlusion in sickle cell anemia. At this time, it is reasonable for sickle cell patients presenting with acute thrombotic stroke or acute retinal artery occlusion to undergo red cell exchange transfusion. In addition, antiplatelet agent administration appears reasonable.

Acute Cholecystitis

Patients with hemolytic disorders, including sickle cell disease, form gallstones composed of the insoluble salt, calcium bilirubinate. It is estimated that up to 75% of adults with sickle cell disease have ultrasound-identified gallstones [73]. An NIH expert panel recommends treating acute cholecystitis with antibiotics and surgical consultation (consensus opinion) [61]. This group also recommends a laparoscopic approach if surgery is indicated and recommends simple transfusion to a hemoglobin of 10 g per dL prior to surgery. This recommendation is based on a randomized trial that suggested that simple preoperative transfusion to a hemoglobin level of 10 g per dL is not associated with more complications than preoperative red cell exchange transfusion to a target hemoglobin S less than 30% [74]. In addition, simple transfusion is associated with a lower rate of alloantibody formation, as fewer units of RBCs are transfused. The use of postoperative incentive spirometry is strongly encouraged because of a decreased incidence of ACS [75].

Pulmonary Hypertension

Pulmonary hypertension is a recently recognized cause of morbidity and mortality in sickle cell disease occurring in more than 30% of patients and conferring an increased death rate ratio of 10.1 [76]. Pulmonary hypertension may be secondary to nitric oxide scavenging by free hemoglobin released during hemolysis. Such scavenging can lead to the synthesis of vasoconstrictors such as vascular cell adhesion molecule 1 and E-selectin. Hemolysis also leads to the release of arginase from hemolyzed red cells, reducing nitric oxide synthesis. The formation of reactive oxygen and nitrogen species catalyzed by free hemoglobin may also lead to pulmonary vasoconstriction. Pulmonary hypertension, in conjunction with high cardiac output, is a major cause of congestive heart failure in patients with sickle cell disease.

The management of patients with sickle cell disease and pulmonary hypertension remains controversial. Some authors have noted a decreased incidence of pulmonary hypertension in retrospective studies of patients treated with hydroxyurea [77], but this finding is not universal. A small study found that therapy with sildenafil improved exercise capacity in patients with sickle cell disease and pulmonary hypertension [78]. However, a recent trial using sildenafil in children with sickle cell disease and pulmonary hypertension was prematurely suspended because of an increased incidence of adverse events including painful crisis. Speculation exists that endothelin antagonists, such as bosentan, may also be effective in reducing pulmonary pressures, although prospective trials are lacking. Similar is also the case for epoprostenol and oral arginine [79].

Currently, there is insufficient evidence in the medical literature to suggest specific treatment strategies for patients with sickle cell disease and pulmonary hypertension. At a minimum, conservative management including oxygen therapy to treat hypoxia and echocardiographic documentation and aggressive treatment of right heart failure are recommended [61].

Hyperhemolysis

Patients with hyperhemolysis, characterized by a lower posttransfusion hemoglobin compared with the pretransfusion value, present with profound anemia and hemolysis despite red cell transfusion support [80]. The pathophysiology of hyperhemolysis in sickle cell disease remains unclear but may be related to a combination of bystander hemolysis, suppression of erythropoiesis, and destruction of RBCs due to contact lysis via activated macrophages [81]. There are case reports supporting the use of IVIG or corticosteroids in addition to plasma to red cell exchange transfusion to maintain enough RBCs to support the circulation [82]. EPO administration may also be of benefit in cases where the reticulocyte count is inadequate. Rituximab has been reported as an effective treatment for this condition [83]. Although hyperhemolysis can recur, typically it occurs as an isolated event. Prompt recognition is important to avoid life-threatening anemia in the setting of continued erythrocyte transfusion.

Aplastic Crisis

Aplastic crisis in sickle cell disease is usually secondary to either folic acid deficiency or infection with parvovirus B19. Aplasia secondary to folic acid deficiency is more common in late pregnancy when folic acid requirements are increased. Infection with parvovirus can be accompanied by marked marrow necrosis [84]. Treatment of parvovirus infection–induced aplasia in immunocompetent individuals is supportive using red cell transfusion to restore the hemoglobin to a safe level and resolves upon clearance of the virus.

Sepsis

Because patients with sickling disorders are functionally asplenic, infection remains a common reason for hospitalization. Pneumonia is the most common infection and may be caused by pneumococcal species, especially if the patient did not receive appropriate immunizations. Treatment of the patient with sickle cell disease and sepsis parallels the treatment of similar patients without a coexistent hemoglobinopathy. Broad-spectrum antibiotics which can later be tailored to the most likely organism should be administered immediately. Adequate hydration must be maintained during an infectious episode to prevent further sickling of erythrocytes. Organisms responsible for sepsis in the sickle cell population can be found in Table 90.12. Consideration of immunization status is important when considering the most likely organism.

Iron Overload

Because patients with sickle cell disease are transfused throughout their lifetime, these patients run the risk of iron overload. The liver, heart, and pancreas are particularly vulnerable to the effects of excess iron. Iron chelation is particularly important in iron-overloaded patients (serum ferritin > 1,000 ng per mL or liver iron concentrations of greater than 2.2 mg iron per g dry weight of liver tissue). Oral iron chelators including deferasirox or deferiprone have increased tolerability as compared with parenteral deferoxamine and appear as effective at removing iron [85].

Thalassemia

Patients with thalassemia can develop high output heart failure that can lead to ICU admissions. Treatment of heart failure in thalassemic patients is similar to the management of heart failure in other patient populations including the use of diuretics, angiotensin-converting enzyme inhibitors, and β-blockers. Chelation therapy with deferasirox is recommended in patients with thalassemia major and iron overload, especially if iron overload has caused cardiac toxicity. Transfusion support is required in symptomatic anemia. Unless a coexistent hemoglobinopathy is present, stroke, ACS, and other common complications of sickle cell disease are not typically seen.

TABLE 90.12

Organisms Responsible for Blood-Borne Infections in Patients with Sickling Disorders

Gram-positive cocci
Staphylococcus aureus
Coagulase-negative staphylococci
Streptococcus pneumoniae
Viridans streptococci
Enterococci
Streptococcus bovis
Gram-negative bacilli
Acinetobacter baumannii
Escherichia coli
Klebsiella spp.
Anaerobes
Bacteroides spp.
Fusobacterium sp.
Fungi

Adapted from Chulamokha L, Scholand SJ, Riggio JM, et al: Bloodstream infections in hospitalized adults with sickle cell disease: a retrospective analysis. *Am J Hematol* 81:723–728, 2006.

Hemolytic Transfusion Reactions

Patients may experience hemolytic transfusion reactions that are either immediate (acute) or delayed. Acute hemolytic transfusion reactions (AHTRs) typically manifest with a feeling of impending doom. Subsequently, back pain, hypotension, red urine, and shock develop. Renal failure due to the massive hemoglobin load may occur, and DIC often ensues. Between 1990 and 1992, the majority of the 150 preventable transfusion-related fatalities reported to the Food and Drug Administration (FDA) were due to ABO-incompatible RBC transfusions leading to an AHTR [86–88]. Indeed, AHTR is typically the result of human error, in specimen collection, labeling, or transfusion [87]. Errors within the laboratory are much less common. Although this dramatic presentation is classic, it is important to note that a rise in temperature of 1°C above baseline may be the sole initial presentation of a hemolytic transfusion reaction and necessitates the cessation of transfusion of that unit of red cells and initiation of workup for transfusion reaction. In the case of an immediate hemolytic transfusion reaction, hemoglobinuria and hemoglobinemia may be seen, and reaction between the remnant of the transfused unit and the patient's pretransfusion serum can be identified. Treatment consists of stopping the transfusion as soon as the reaction is suspected and maintenance of blood pressure with fluids and pressors as needed.

DHTRs typically present 1 to 4 weeks after transfusion of a unit of red cells. The patient may present with fatigue, jaundice, pallor, or red- or tea-colored urine. Patients with sickling disorders may come to medical attention because of a new or worsening pain crisis. The hemoglobin will be lower than that seen posttransfusion. The LDH and bilirubin will be increased, the reticulocyte count will likely be elevated, and the antibody screen will be positive, and a new alloantibody often identified. The DHTR is typically due to mismatches of non-ABO red cell antigens. Patients should be issued a card stating the antigen to which they have made a new alloantibody and told to present this card prior to all future transfusions. This is especially important in cases of antibodies to the Kidd antigen, as these alloantibodies are typically transient and may not be detectable on future antibody screens.

Glucose 6-Phosphate Dehydrogenase Deficiency

G6PD deficiency, a sex-linked trait primarily affecting men most commonly of African American or Mediterranean descent, is the most common erythrocyte enzyme defect in the world [89]. G6PD is necessary to maintain glutathione in its reduced state in the erythrocyte. Patients deficient in this enzyme are subject to oxidative hemolysis when exposed to certain drugs and toxins, or during episodes of infection. A sample list of drugs to be avoided in G6PD-deficient patients is provided in Table 90.13. Because acute infection makes oxidative hemolysis more likely, there has been confusion about the safety of certain drugs in G6PD-deficient patients. A list of drugs that can be safely administered to G6PD-deficient patients is shown in Table 90.14. A more exhaustive drug list can be found at many Web sites dedicated to G6PD deficiency (e.g., www.g6pd.org). G6PD deficiency is seldom a major issue in critically ill patients because the anemia

TABLE 90.13

Drugs to be Avoided in G6PD-Deficient Patients

Dapsone
Methylene blue
Nalidixic acid
Nitrofurantoin
Phenazopyridine
Primaquine
Sulfacetamide
Sulfanilamide
Sulfapyridine
Toluidine blue
Urate oxidase

List is not intended to be all inclusive.
G6PD, glucose 6-phosphate dehydrogenase.
Adapted from Lichtman MA, Beutler E, Kipps TJ, et al: *Williams Hematology.* 7th ed. New York, McGraw-Hill Medical, 2006.

TABLE 90.14

Drugs That Are Safe in G6PD-Deficient Patients

Acetaminophen
Acetylsalicylic acid
Ascorbic acid
Chloramphenicol
Chloroquine
Colchicine
Diphenhydramine
Isoniazid
Phenytoin
Procainamide
Pyrimethamine
Quinine
Streptomycin
Sulfadiazine
Sulfamethoxazole
Trimethoprim
Vitamin K

List is not intended to be all inclusive.
G6PD, glucose 6-phosphate dehydrogenase.
Adapted from Lichtman MA, Beutler E, Kipps TJ, et al: *Williams Hematology.* 7th ed. New York, McGraw-Hill Medical, 2006.

is typically not severe, and the patients are closely monitored. However, in solid organ transplant recipients who are exposed to oxidant drugs such as trimethoprim–sulfamethoxazole or dapsone, the diagnosis should be strongly considered in the setting of a new hemolytic or unexplained acute anemia [90].

In the more common African American variant of G6PD, enzyme levels are elevated in young reticulocytes, and therefore measurement of this enzyme should not be attempted in the setting of an acute hemolytic episode, where the majority of circulating red cells are young.

Paroxysmal Nocturnal Hemoglobinuria

Paroxysmal nocturnal hemoglobinuria (PNH) is an acquired disease in which an abnormal stem cell clone gives rise to red cells, white cells, and platelets that lack proteins which are normally attached to the cell surface by a glycosylphosphatidylinositol (GPI) anchor. Among these proteins are CD55 and CD59, which are responsible for inactivating complement on the surface of red cells. PNH cells are therefore more susceptible to complement-mediated lysis [91]. Patients with PNH may come to the attention of the intensivist with complications such as hemolysis, pancytopenia, arterial, or venous thrombosis (including the Budd–Chiari syndrome/hepatic vein thrombosis). Patients may also develop pancytopenia due to marrow hypoplasia, as there is an association with primary bone marrow disorders such as aplastic anemia, myelodysplastic syndrome (MDS), and acute myelogenous leukemia [92,93].

Flow cytometry showing the absence of GPI-linked surface molecules CD55 and CD59 on erythrocytes and granulocytes has supplanted older testing (such as the Ham's test) for the diagnosis of PNH [93]. Eculizumab has been FDA approved for the treatment of hemolysis due to PNH. Patients treated with eculizumab show markedly lower rates of hemolysis and also thrombosis [94–98] but are at increased risk of infection with meningococcus, requiring immunization prior to use [93].

Hereditary Spherocytosis

Hereditary spherocytosis (HS) is an autosomal dominant disorder of red cell membrane skeletal proteins leading to a lack of anchoring of the red cell lipid bilayer to its skeletal backbone [99–101], leading to a characteristic spherocytic shape. Patients have lifelong hemolysis which is often well compensated. However, with even mild infections, the hemolysis can accelerate, and the patient can become more anemic. Splenomegaly is present in many patients and splenic rupture may occur after trauma. Patients with HS may present with an aplastic crisis manifested by severe reticulocytopenia and anemia often due to parvovirus B-19 infection which transiently suppresses the bone marrow's ability to produce red cells and compensate for the accelerated hemolysis [101,102]. The Coombs test will be negative and should be used to differentiate HS from WAIHA, which can present similarly. Diagnosis is made by showing an increase in osmotic fragility and a decrease in eosin-5'-maleimide binding to band 3 [103]. RBC transfusion may be administered to patients with aplastic crisis.

Hemolysis from Infectious Agents

Certain infectious pathogens cause hemolysis that can be severe or life threatening. Malaria is prototypic; infection with falciparum malaria is known as blackwater fever, due to the massive hemolysis caused by this agent. *Babesia microti* is another intracellular parasite that can lead to hemolysis. It is carried by the same tick as Lyme disease and can look like malarial forms on peripheral smear. *Bartonella bacilliformis*, the agent responsible for Oroya fever, and *Verruca peruviana*, an extracellular parasite, can lyse red cells leading to dramatic hemolysis. In endemic regions of the world, these organisms are leading causes of hemolysis in critically ill patients. The toxin of *Clostridium welchii*, an agent of gas gangrene, may cause severe hemolysis. The bacterium produces a lysolecithinase, which attacks the red cell membrane bilayer. *Clostridium perfringens*, another agent causing gas gangrene, also leads to hemolysis via the action of phospholipases produced in its exotoxin [104]. In certain cases, the hemolysis can be severe enough to produce a disparity between the hemoglobin and the hematocrit. This infectious complication typically follows bowel or gynecologic surgery.

Hemolysis Associated with Chemical and Physical Agents

Arsenic, especially arsine gas, can lead to hemolysis, as it can elevate levels of copper in the blood. Wilson's disease, which is a disorder of copper metabolism, may present with hemolysis as part of its clinical picture [105]. Some dialysis centers have had difficulty with copper contamination of their water supply, leading to severe hemolysis [106]. Insect and spider bites, especially the bite of the brown recluse spider (*Loxosceles reclusa*), can lead to hemolysis, as can certain snakebites [107]. Severe burns can lead to hemolysis, as the red cell membrane is sensitive to temperatures more than 55°C.

Other Causes of Anemia in the Critical Care Setting

Iron deficiency leads to a hypoproliferative anemia due to the inability to synthesize hemoglobin. Iron deficiency may be caused by chronic blood loss, decreased iron intake (either from dietary reasons or from iron malabsorption as occurs in celiac sprue or following gastrointestinal bypass), or both. In the ICU, red cell transfusion is the most immediate way to correct the anemia, but in patients with low hemoglobin but without hemodynamic compromise, oral or intravenous iron is preferred. Parenteral iron may be preferred in iron-deficient patients who have undergone gastrointestinal bypass, those with inflammatory bowel disease, cancer patients, those who suffer from functional iron deficiency, patients undergoing treatment with EPO, or patients with chronic kidney disease [108–111]. Iron dextran, iron sucrose, iron gluconate, ferumoxytol, and iron carboxymaltose are all available for intravenous use. The newer formulations of iron dextran have a lower rate of severe allergic reactions compared with older dextran preparations, but the incidence continues to remain higher than with the newer non-dextran iron preparations [112–119]. Ferumoxytol is not approved for inpatient use and has recently been given a black box warning to avoid use in anyone with a history of prior allergic reaction to ANY other iron preparation. The iron deficit can be calculated by the following formula: (desired hemoglobin − actual hemoglobin) × (weight in pounds) + storage iron. Storage iron is estimated at 1,000 g for men and 600 mg for women.

Megaloblastic Anemia

Megaloblastic anemia is a rare cause of anemia in the ICU but should be suspected in individuals presenting with a macrocytic, hypoproliferative anemia (high MCV, low reticulocyte count) (Table 90.5). Vitamin B_{12} and folic acid levels should be measured, but accuracy may be affected in the acute setting. The measurement of homocysteine and methylmalonic acid (MMA) is a more sensitive way to assess for these nutritional deficiencies but can also be altered in the critically ill patient [120]. Typically, both homocysteine and MMA are elevated in B_{12} deficiency, although homocysteine alone is elevated in folic acid deficiency. Elevation of homocysteine and MMA may be the first laboratory signs of subclinical B_{12} deficiency. The peripheral smear may show oval macrocytes and hypersegmented neutrophils. Other anemias which are hypoproliferative and macrocytic include the MDSs, aplastic anemia, the anemia of hypothyroidism, and liver disease (Table 90.5). Additionally, medications such as hydroxyurea, methotrexate, and zidovudine may lead to macrocytosis.

Anemia of Chronic Disease (ACD)/Inflammation

The ACD/inflammation is common in the ICU and its etiology is multifactorial (Table 90.15) [121]. Once thought to occur over weeks to months, the ACD has been shown to occur in less than a week and is thus thought to be a major contributor to anemia in critically ill patients [121,122]. Several studies have shown elevated levels of pro-inflammatory mediators such as tumor necrosis factor-alpha; interleukin-6; C-reactive protein; and interferons-α, -β, and -γ in ACD [121,123,124].

TABLE 90.15

Mechanisms of the Anemia of Chronic Disease/Critical Illness

Blood loss
Phlebotomy
Active bleeding
Decreased red cell production
Decreased production of EPO
Blunted response to EPO
Sequestration of iron through upregulation of hepcidin
Renal dysfunction
Increased red cell destruction
Reduced red blood cell deformability

EPO,erythropoietin.

This acute-phase reactant response has been shown to inhibit EPO production, blunt the erythropoietic response, and play a central role in iron metabolism, leading to the sequestration of iron. Iron metabolism is primarily mediated by the antimicrobial peptide hepcidin, which impairs the ability to export iron from gut epithelial cells and hepatocytes into the bloodstream [125]. Hepcidin is upregulated in the ACD, leading to the sequestration of iron. In the ACD, the serum iron (Fe), total iron-binding capacity (TIBC), and percentage iron saturation (iron/TIBC) are typically low. Ferritin, an acute-phase reactant, is often normal or elevated, as opposed to iron deficiency where it is low. Renal failure is common in the ICU and also may contribute to the ACD, especially when progressive [121,126]. Increased red cell destruction has also been noted in the ACD because of decreased RBC deformability [121].

CONCLUSIONS

As demonstrated in this chapter, anemia is exceedingly common in the critical care setting, but its etiology remains diverse. A rational approach to the evaluation of anemia includes review of the white blood count, platelet count, MCV, reticulocyte count, peripheral blood smear, and any prior CBCs that may be available. If hemolysis is suspected, LDH, bilirubin, and haptoglobin will provide additional information to support or refute this diagnosis. A Coombs test is often sent if the etiology of hemolysis remains in question. As highlighted in the chapter, certain causes of anemia such as blood loss, microangiopathic hemolytic anemia, complications of sickle cell disease, hemolysis from drugs as well as foreign devices, and ACD are frequently present in critically ill patients and should be considered in the ICU patient population. Specific treatment recommendations are based on the underlying diagnosis. Minimizing the volume and frequency of blood draws is essential. Conservative transfusion thresholds are increasingly being used in the absence of hemodynamic compromise or acute blood loss. The role of ESAs has been investigated but remains uncertain. If the etiology of the anemia remains obscure, or the management of an underlying diagnosis remains uncertain, hematology consultation is recommended.

References

1. Corwin HL, Gettinger A, Pearl RG, et al: The CRIT study: anemia and blood transfusion in the critically ill-current clinical practice in the United States*. *Crit Care Med* 32(1):39–52, 2004.
2. Retter A, Wyncoll D, Pearse R, et al: Guidelines on the management of anaemia and red cell transfusion in adult critically ill patients. *Br J Haematol* 160(4):445–464, 2013.

3. Corwin HL, Napolitano LM: Anemia in the critically ill: do we need to live with it? *Crit Care Med* 42(9):2140–2141, 2014.
4. Koch CG, Li L, Sun Z, et al: Hospital-acquired anemia: prevalence, outcomes, and healthcare implications. *J Hosp Med* 8(9):506–512, 2013.
5. Koch CG, Reineks EZ, Tang AS, et al: Contemporary bloodletting in cardiac surgical care. *Ann Thorac Surg* 99(3):779–784, 2015.
6. Levi ML: Twenty-five million liters of blood into the sewer. *J Thromb Haemost* 12(10):1592–1592, 2014.
7. Salisbury AC, Reid KJ, Alexander KP, et al: Diagnostic blood loss from phlebotomy and hospital-acquired anemia during acute myocardial infarction. *Arch Intern Med* 171(18):1646–1653, 2011.
8. Carson JL, Grossman BJ, Kleinman S, et al: Red blood cell transfusion: a clinical practice guideline from the AABB*. *Ann Int Med* 157(1):49–58, 2012.
9. Salpeter SR, Buckley JS, Chatterjee S: Impact of more restrictive blood transfusion strategies on clinical outcomes: a meta-analysis and systematic review. *Am J Med* 127(2):124–131.e3, 2014.
10. Holst LB, Haase N, Wettersley J, et al: Lower versus higher hemoglobin threshold for transfusion in septic shock. *N Eng J Med* 371(15):1381–1391, 2014.
11. Talving P, Lustenberger T, Inaba K, et al: Erythropoiesis-stimulating agent administration and survival after severe traumatic brain injury: a prospective study. *Arch Surg* 147(3):251–255, 2012.
12. Luchette FA, Pasquale MD, Fabian TC, et al: A randomized, double-blind, placebo-controlled study to assess the effect of recombinant human erythropoietin on functional outcomes in anemic, critically ill, trauma subjects: the Long Term Trauma Outcomes Study. *Am J Surg* 203(4):508–516, 2012.
13. Zarychanski R, Turgeon AF, McIntyre L, et al: Erythropoietin-receptor agonists in critically ill patients: a meta-analysis of randomized controlled trials. *CMAJ* 177(7):725–734, 2007.
14. Corwin HL, Gettinger A, Fabian TC, et al: Efficacy and safety of epoetin alfa in critically ill patients. *N Eng J Med* 357(10):965–976, 2007.
15. Jelkmann I, Jelkmann W: Impact of erythropoietin on intensive care unit patients. *Transfus Med Hemother* 40(5):310–318, 2013.
16. Cook D, Crowther M: Targeting anemia with erythropoietin during critical illness. *N Eng J Med* 357(10):1037–1039, 2007.
17. Mesgarpour B, Heidinger BH, Schwameis M, et al: Safety of off-label erythropoiesis stimulating agents in critically ill patients: a meta-analysis. *Intensive Care Med* 39(11):1896–1908, 2013.
18. Packman CH: Hemolytic anemia due to warm autoantibodies. *Blood Rev* 22(1):17–31, 2008.
19. Petz LD: Cold antibody autoimmune hemolytic anemias. *Blood Rev* 22(1):1–15, 2008.
20. Mollison PL: Measurement of survival and destruction of red cells in haemolytic syndromes. *Br Med Bull* 15(1):59–66, 1959.
21. Gribben JG: How I treat CLL up front. *Blood* 115:187–197, 2010.
22. Conley C, Lippman SM, Ness P: Autoimmune hemolytic anemia with reticulocytopenia: a medical emergency. *JAMA* 244(15):1688–1690, 1980.
23. Flores G, Cunningham-Rundles C, Newland AC, et al: Efficacy of intravenous immunoglobulin in the treatment of autoimmune hemolytic anemia: results in 73 patients. *Am J Hematol* 44(4):237–242, 1993.
24. Valent P, Lechner K: Diagnosis and treatment of autoimmune haemolytic anaemias in adults: a clinical review. *Wien Klin Wochenschr* 120(5–6): 136–151, 2008.
25. Hoffman PC: Immune hemolytic anemia—selected topics. *Hematology Am Soc Hematol Educ Program* 2009(1):80–86, 2009.
26. Bussone G, Ribeiro E, Dechartres A, et al: Efficacy and safety of rituximab in adults' warm antibody autoimmune haemolytic anemia: retrospective analysis of 27 cases. *Am J Hematol* 84(3):153–157, 2009.
27. Berentsen S, Bø K, Shammas FV, et al: Chronic cold agglutinin disease of the "idiopathic" type is a premalignant or low-grade malignant lymphoproliferative disease. *APMIS* 105(1–6):354–362, 1997.
28. Berentsen S, Beiske K, Tjønnfjord GE: Primary chronic cold agglutinin disease: an update on pathogenesis, clinical features and therapy. *Hematology* 12(5):361–370, 2007.
29. Berentsen S, Ulvestad E, Gjertsen BT, et al: Rituximab for primary chronic cold agglutinin disease: a prospective study of 37 courses of therapy in 27 patients. *Blood* 103:2925–2928, 2004.
30. Gertz MA: Management of cold haemolytic syndrome. *Br J Haematol* 138(4):422–429, 2007.
31. Eder AF: Review: acute Donath-Landsteiner hemolytic anemia. *Immunohematology* 21(3):132, 2005.
32. Salama A: Drug-induced immune hemolytic anemia. *Expert Opin Drug Saf* 8(1):73–79, 2009.
33. Johnson ST, Fueger JT, Gottschall JL: One center's experience: the serology and drugs associated with drug-induced immune hemolytic anemia—a new paradigm. *Transfusion* 47(4):697–702, 2007.
34. Garratty G: Drug-induced immune hemolytic anemia. *ASH Educ Program Book* 2009(1):73–79, 2009.
35. Garratty G, Arndt PA: Drugs that have been shown to cause drug-induced immune hemolytic anemia or positive direct antiglobulin tests: some interesting findings since 2007. *Immunohematology* 30(2):66–79, 2014.
36. George JN, Nester CM: Syndromes of thrombotic microangiopathy. *N Eng J Med* 371(7):654–666, 2014.
37. Knöbl PN: Treatment of thrombotic microangiopathy with a focus on new treatment options. *Hamostaseologie* 33(2):149–159, 2013.
38. Sayani FA, Abrams CS: How I treat refractory thrombotic thrombocytopenic purpura. *Blood* 125(25):3860–3867, 2015.
39. Scully M, Hunt BJ, Benjamin S, et al: Guidelines on the diagnosis and management of thrombotic thrombocytopenic purpura and other thrombotic microangiopathies. *Br J Haematol* 158(3):323–335, 2012.
40. Sarode R, Bandarenko N, Brecher ME, et al: Thrombotic thrombocytopenic purpura: 2012 American Society for Apheresis (ASFA) consensus conference on classification, diagnosis, management, and future research. *J Clin Apher* 29(3):148–167, 2014.
41. Scully M, Goodship T: How I treat thrombotic thrombocytopenic purpura and atypical haemolytic uraemic syndrome. *Br J Haematol* 164(6):759–766, 2014.
42. Moake JL, Rudy CK, Troll JH, et al: Unusually large plasma factor VIII: von Willebrand factor multimers in chronic relapsing thrombotic thrombocytopenic purpura. *N Eng J Med* 307(23):1432–1435, 1982.
43. Furlan M: von Willebrand factor–cleaving protease in thrombotic thrombocytopenic purpura and the hemolytic–uremic syndrome. *N Eng J Med* 339(22):1578–1584, 1998.
44. Tsai HM, Lian EC: Antibodies to von Willebrand factor–cleaving protease in acute thrombotic thrombocytopenic purpura. *N Eng J Med* 339(22):1585–1594, 1998.
45. Lämmle B, Kremer Hovinga JA, George JN: Acquired thrombotic thrombocytopenic purpura: ADAMTS13 activity, anti-ADAMTS13 autoantibodies and risk of recurrent disease. *Haematologica* 93:172–177, 2008.
46. Sadler JE: Von Willebrand factor, ADAMTS13, and thrombotic thrombocytopenic purpura. *Blood* 90:11–18, 2008.
47. Zuber J, Fakhouri F, Roumenina LT, et al: Use of eculizumab for atypical haemolytic uraemic syndrome and C3 glomerulopathies. *Nat Rev Nephrol* 8(11):643–657, 2012.
48. Noris M, Remuzzi G: Atypical hemolytic–uremic syndrome. *N Eng J Med* 361(17):1676–1687, 2009.
49. Legendre CM, Licht C, Muus P, et al: Terminal complement inhibitor eculizumab in atypical hemolytic–uremic syndrome. *N Eng J Med* 368(23):2169–2181, 2013.
50. Zhou A, Mehta R, Smith R: Outcomes of platelet transfusion in patients with thrombotic thrombocytopenic purpura: a retrospective case series study. *Ann Hematol* 94(3):467–472, 2015.
51. Goel R, Ness PM, Takemoto CM, et al: Platelet transfusions in platelet consumptive disorders are associated with arterial thrombosis and in-hospital mortality. *Blood* 125:1470–1476, 2015.
52. Lim W, Vesely SK,George JN: The role of rituximab in the management of patients with acquired thrombotic thrombocytopenic purpura. *Blood* 125:1526–1531, 2015.
53. Kuo KHM, Ward R, Kaya B, et al: A comparison of chronic manual and automated red blood cell exchange transfusion in sickle cell disease patients. *Br J Haematol* 170(3):425–428, 2015.
54. Campbell-Lee SA, Kittles RA: Red blood cell alloimmunization in sickle cell disease: listen to your ancestors. *Transfus Med Hemother* 41(6):431–435, 2014.
55. Charache S, Scott JC, Charache P: "Acute chest syndrome" in adults with sickle cell anemia: Microbiology, treatment, and prevention. *Arch Intern Med* 139(1):67–69, 1979.
56. Vichinsky EP, Neumayr LD, Earles AN, et al: Causes and outcomes of the acute chest syndrome in sickle cell disease. *N Eng J Med* 342(25):1855–1865, 2000.
57. Ball JB, Khan SY, McLaughlin NJ, et al: A two-event in vitro model of acute chest syndrome: the role of secretory phospholipase A2 and neutrophils. *Pediatr Blood Cancer* 58(3):399–405, 2012.
58. Styles L, Wager CG, Labotka RJ, et al: Refining the value of secretory phospholipase A(2) as a predictor of acute chest syndrome in sickle cell disease: results of a feasibility study (PROACTIVE). *Br J Haematol* 157(5):627–636, 2012.
59. van Beem RT, Nur E, Zwaginga JJ, et al: Elevated endothelial progenitor cells during painful sickle cell crisis. *Exp Hematol* 37(9):1054–1059, 2009.
60. Elshazly SA, Heiba NM, Abdelmageed WM: Plasma PTX3 levels in sickle cell disease patients, during vaso occlusion and acute chest syndrome (data from Saudi population). *Hematology* 19(1):52–59, 2014.
61. US Department of Health & Human Services: *Evidence-Based Management of Sickle Cell Disease: Expert Panel Report, 2014*. Washington, DC, National Institute of Health, 2014, pp 46–48.
62. Turner JM, Kaplan JB, Cohen HW, et al: Exchange versus simple transfusion for acute chest syndrome in sickle cell anemia adults. *Transfusion* 49(5):863–868, 2009.
63. Liem RI, O'Gorman MR, Brown DL: Effect of red cell exchange transfusion on plasma levels of inflammatory mediators in sickle cell patients with acute chest syndrome. *Am J Hematol* 76(1):19–25, 2004.
64. Verduzco LA, Nathan DG: Sickle cell disease and stroke. *Blood* 114:5117–5125, 2009.
65. van der Land V, Zwanenburg JJ, Fijnvandraat K, et al: Cerebral lesions on 7 tesla MRI in patients with sickle cell anemia. *Cerebrovasc Dis* 39(3–4): 181–189, 2015.
66. Kirkham FJ: Therapy insight: stroke risk and its management in patients with sickle cell disease. *Nat Clin Pract Neurol* 3(5):264–278, 2007.
67. Fryer RH, Anderson RC, Chiriboga CA, et al: Sickle cell anemia with moyamoya disease: outcomes after EDAS procedure. *Pediatr Neurol* 29(2):124–130, 2003.
68. Valadi N, Silva GS, Bowman LS, et al: Transcranial doppler ultrasonography in adults with sickle cell disease. *Neurology* 67(4):572–574, 2006.
69. Sacco RL, Adams R, Albers G, et al: Guidelines for prevention of stroke in patients with ischemic stroke or transient ischemic attack: a statement for healthcare professionals from the American Heart Association/American Stroke Association Council on Stroke: co-Sponsored by the Council on Cardiovascular Radiology and Intervention: the American Academy of Neurology affirms the value of this guideline. *Stroke* 37(2):577–617, 2006.

70. Nabavizadeh SA, Vossough A, Ichord RN, et al: Intracranial aneurysms in sickle cell anemia: clinical and imaging findings. *J NeuroInterv Surg* 8(4):434–440, 2015.
71. Danielson CF: The role of red blood cell exchange transfusion in the treatment and prevention of complications of sickle cell disease. *Ther Apher* 6(1):24–31, 2002.
72. Liem RI, Calamaras DM, Chhabra MS, et al: Sudden onset blindness in sickle cell disease due to retinal artery occlusion. *Pediatr Blood Cancer* 50(3):624–627, 2008.
73. Ahn H, Li CS, Wang W: Sickle cell hepatopathy: clinical presentation, treatment, and outcome in pediatric and adult patients. *Pediatr Blood Cancer* 45(2):184–190, 2005.
74. Haberkern CM, Neumayr LD, Orringer EP, et al: Cholecystectomy in sickle cell anemia patients: perioperative outcome of 364 cases from the National Preoperative Transfusion Study. *Blood* 89:1533–1542, 1997.
75. Bellet PS, Kalinyak KA, Shukla R, et al: Incentive spirometry to prevent acute pulmonary complications in sickle cell diseases. *N Eng J Med* 333(11):699–703, 1995.
76. Gladwin MT, Sachdev V, Jison ML, et al: Pulmonary hypertension as a risk factor for death in patients with sickle cell disease. *N Eng J Med* 350(9):886–895, 2004.
77. Ataga KI, Moore CG, Jones S, et al: Pulmonary hypertension in patients with sickle cell disease: a longitudinal study. *Br J Haematol* 134(1):109–115, 2006.
78. Machado RF, Martyr S, Kato GJ, et al: Sildenafil therapy in patients with sickle cell disease and pulmonary hypertension. *Br J Haematol* 130(3):445–453, 2005.
79. Benza R: Pulmonary hypertension associated with sickle cell disease: pathophysiology and rationale for treatment. *Lung* 186(4):247–254, 2008.
80. Santos B, Portugal R, Nogueira C, et al: Hyperhemolysis syndrome in patients with sickle cell anemia: report of three cases. *Transfusion* 55(6 Pt 2):1394–1398, 2015.
81. Win N, New H, Lee E, et al: Hyperhemolysis syndrome in sickle cell disease: case report (recurrent episode) and literature review. *Transfusion* 48(6):1231–1238, 2008.
82. Uhlmann EJ, Shenoy S, Goodnough LT: Successful treatment of recurrent hyperhemolysis syndrome with immunosuppression and plasma-to-red blood cell exchange transfusion. *Transfusion* 54(2):384–388, 2014.
83. Bachmeyer C, Maury J, Parrot A, et al: Rituximab as an effective treatment of hyperhemolysis syndrome in sickle cell anemia. *Am J Hematol* 85(1):91–92, 2010.
84. Godeau B, Galacteros F, Schaeffer A, et al: Aplastic crisis due to extensive bone marrow necrosis and human parvovirus infection in sickle cell disease. *Am J Med* 91(5):557–558, 1991.
85. Vichinsky E, Onyekwere O, Porter J, et al: A randomised comparison of deferasirox versus deferoxamine for the treatment of transfusional iron overload in sickle cell disease. *Br J Haematol* 136(3):501–508, 2007.
86. Goodnough LT, Brecher ME, Kanter MH, et al: Transfusion medicine—blood transfusion. *N Eng J Med* 340(6):438–447, 1999.
87. Linden JV: Errors in transfusion medicine: scope of the problem. *Arch Pathol Lab Med* 123(7):563–565, 1999.
88. Mummert TB, Tourault MA: Transfusion-related fatality reports—a summary. *Nurs Manage* 25(10):80I, 80L, 80O, 1994.
89. Nkhoma ET, Poole C, Vannappagari V, et al: The global prevalence of glucose-6-phosphate dehydrogenase deficiency: a systematic review and meta-analysis. *Blood Cells Mol Dis* 42(3):267–278, 2009.
90. Cappellini MD, Fiorelli G: Glucose-6-phosphate dehydrogenase deficiency. *Lancet* 371(9606):64–74, 2008.
91. Brodsky RA: Advances in the diagnosis and therapy of paroxysmal nocturnal hemoglobinuria. *Blood Rev* 22(2):65–74, 2008.
92. Hillmen P, Lewis SM, Bessler M, et al: Natural history of paroxysmal nocturnal hemoglobinuria. *N Eng J Med* 333(19):1253–1259, 1995.
93. Hill A: Eculizumab in the treatment of paroxysmal nocturnal hemoglobinuria. *Clin Med Insights Ther* 1:1467, 2009.
94. Brodsky RA, Young NS, Antonioli E, et al: Multicenter phase 3 study of the complement inhibitor eculizumab for the treatment of patients with paroxysmal nocturnal hemoglobinuria. *Blood* 111:1840–1847, 2008.
95. Hill A, Hillmen P, Richards SJ, et al: Sustained response and long-term safety of eculizumab in paroxysmal nocturnal hemoglobinuria. *Blood* 106:2559–2565, 2005.
96. Hillmen P, Hall C, Marsh JC, et al: Effect of eculizumab on hemolysis and transfusion requirements in patients with paroxysmal nocturnal hemoglobinuria. *N Eng J Med* 350(6):552–559, 2004.
97. Hillmen P, Young NS, Schubert J, et al: The complement inhibitor eculizumab in paroxysmal nocturnal hemoglobinuria. *N Eng J Med* 355(12):1233–1243, 2006.
98. Young NS, Antonioli E, Rotoli B, et al: Safety and efficacy of the terminal complement inhibitor eculizumab in patients with paroxysmal nocturnal hemoglobinuria: interim shepherd phase III clinical study. *Blood* 108(11):971.
99. Gallagher PG, Ferriera JD: Molecular basis of erythrocyte membrane disorders. *Curr Opin Hematol* 4(2):128–135, 1997.
100. Mohandas N, Gallagher PG: Red cell membrane: past, present, and future. *Blood* 112(10):3939–3948, 2008.
101. Perrotta S, Gallagher PG, Mohandas N: Hereditary spherocytosis. *Lancet* 372(9647):1411–1426.
102. Summerfield GP, Wyatt GP: Human parvovirus infection revealing hereditary spherocytosis. *Lancet* 326(8463):1070, 1985.
103. King MJ, Zanella A: Hereditary red cell membrane disorders and laboratory diagnostic testing. *Int J Lab Hematol* 35(3):237–243, 2013.
104. Boyd SD, Mobley BC, Regula DP, et al: Features of hemolysis due to Clostridium perfringens infection. *Int J Lab Hematol* 31(3):364–367, 2009.
105. Balkema S, Hamaker ME, Visser HP, et al: Haemolytic anaemia as a first sign of Wilson's disease. *Neth J Med* 66(8):344–347, 2008.
106. Ivanovich P, Manzler A, Drake R: Acute hemolysis following hemodialysis. *ASAIO J* 15(1):316–318, 1969.
107. McDade J, Aygun B, Ware RE: Brown recluse spider (loxosceles reclusa) envenomation leading to acute hemolytic anemia in six adolescents. *J Pediatr* 156(1):155–157, 2010.
108. Aggarwal HK, Nand N, Singh S, et al: Comparison of oral versus intravenous iron therapy in predialysis patients of chronic renal failure receiving recombinant human erythropoietin. *J Assoc Physicians India* 51:170–174, 2003.
109. Auerbach M, Ballard H, Trout JR, et al: Intravenous iron optimizes the response to recombinant human erythropoietin in cancer patients with chemotherapy-related anemia: a multicenter, open-label, randomized trial. *J Clin Oncol* 22(7):1301–1307, 2004.
110. Henry DH, Dahl NV, Auerbach M, et al: Intravenous ferric gluconate significantly improves response to epoetin alfa versus oral iron or no iron in anemic patients with cancer receiving chemotherapy. *Oncologist* 12(2):231–242, 2007.
111. Van Wyck DB, Roppolo M, Martinez CO, et al: A randomized, controlled trial comparing IV iron sucrose to oral iron in anemic patients with nondialysis-dependent CKD. *Kidney Int* 68(6):2846–2856, 2005.
112. Chertow GM, Mason PD, Vaage-Nilsen O, et al: Update on adverse drug events associated with parenteral iron. *Nephrol Dial Transplant* 21(2):378–382, 2006.
113. Faich G, Strobos J: Sodium ferric gluconate complex in sucrose: safer intravenous iron therapy than iron dextrans. *Am J Kidney Dis* 33(3):464–470, 1999.
114. Kosch M, Bahner U, Bettger H, et al: A randomized, controlled parallel-group trial on efficacy and safety of iron sucrose (Venofer) vs iron gluconate (Ferrlecit) in haemodialysis patients treated with rHuEpo. *Nephrol Dial Transplant* 16(6):1239–1244, 2001.
115. Laman CA, Silverstein SB, Rodgers GM: Parenteral iron therapy: a single institution's experience over a 5-year period. *J Natl Compr Canc Netw* 3(6):791–795, 2005.
116. Michael B, Coyne DW, Fishbane S, et al: Sodium ferric gluconate complex in hemodialysis patients: adverse reactions compared to placebo and iron dextran. *Kidney Int* 61(5):1830–1839, 2002.
117. Michael B, Coyne DW, Folkert VW, et al: Sodium ferric gluconate complex in haemodialysis patients: a prospective evaluation of long-term safety. *Nephrol Dial Transplant* 19(6):1576–1580, 2004.
118. Silverstein SB, Rodgers GM: Parenteral iron therapy options. *Am J Hematol* 76(1):74–78, 2004.
119. Zumberg MS, Kahn MJ: Acquired anemias: iron deficiency, cobalamin deficiency, and autoimmune hemolytic anemia, in *Evidence-Based Hematology*. Eds. Crowther MA, Ginsberg J, Schunemann HJ, Meyer RM, and Lottenberg R. Wiley-Blackwell, 2009, pp 197–205.
120. Wickramasinghe SN: Diagnosis of megaloblastic anaemias. *Blood Rev* 20(6):299–318, 2006.
121. Asare K: Anemia of critical illness. *Pharmacotherapy* 28(10):1267–1282, 2008.
122. Patteril MV, Davey-Quinn AP, Gedney JA, et al: Functional iron deficiency, infection and systemic inflammatory response syndrome in critical illness. *Anaesth Intensive Care* 29(5): 473–478, 2001.
123. Jelkmann W: Proinflammatory cytokines lowering erythropoietin production. *J Interferon Cytokine Res* 18(8):555–559, 1998.
124. von Ahsen N, Müller C, Serke S, et al: Important role of nondiagnostic blood loss and blunted erythropoietic response in the anemia of medical intensive care patients. *Crit Care Med* 27(12):2630–2639, 1999.
125. Ganz T: Molecular pathogenesis of anemia of chronic disease. *Pediatr Blood Cancer* 46(5):554–557, 2006.
126. Radtke HW, Claussner A, Erbes PM, et al: Serum erythropoietin concentration in chronic renal failure: relationship to degree of anemia and excretory renal function. *Blood* 54(4):877–884, 1979.

Chapter 91 ■ Thrombocytopenia

THOMAS G. DELOUGHERY

Thrombocytopenia is common in the intensive care unit (ICU) with platelet counts below 50×10^9 per L occurring in 12% to 13% of ICU patients and below 10×10^9 per L in 2% to 3% [1–3]. A variety of disease processes can lead to thrombocytopenia, ranging from an epiphenomenon of the illness that led to the ICU admission to a devastating complication of therapy. The differential diagnosis of thrombocytopenia is very broad. Table 91.1 lists some causes of special interest to the intensivist.

The immediate priorities in thrombocytopenic patients are to establish the validity and severity of the thrombocytopenia, evaluate for life-threatening processes such as heparin-induced thrombocytopenia (HIT) or thrombotic thrombocytopenic purpura (TTP), and initiate therapy. In the critical care setting, therapeutic decisions often have to be made before a definitive cause of the thrombocytopenia is established.

TABLE 91.2

Typical Platelet Counts in Various Disease States

Moderate thrombocytopenia (50–100 × 10⁹/L)
Disseminated intravascular coagulation
Hemophagocytic syndrome
Heparin-induced thrombocytopenia
Thrombotic thrombocytopenic purpura
Severe thrombocytopenia (<20 × 10⁹/L)
Drug-induced thrombocytopenia
Immune thrombocytopenia
Posttransfusion purpura

INITIAL EVALUATION

The initial assessment should be rapid, focusing on whether the patient is bleeding or experiencing thrombosis; the underlying disorder(s) leading to the ICU admission; current medications; and (if available) past medical history.

In the assessment of bleeding, one should distinguish whether the patient is suffering from "structural" aberrancies (e.g., bleeding from a gastric ulcer) or generalized bleeding, which may suggest a hemostatic defect such as may occur due to thrombocytopenia. One should inspect sites of instrumentation such as intravenous (IV) sites or chest tube drainage, and the mucosa for bleeding. The fingertips and toes should be examined for evidence of emboli or ischemia.

Exposure to medication is a common cause of thrombocytopenia. One should carefully review the record of current and recently administered medications and ask the patient (if possible) and family about medications (prescribed, over the counter, and "natural" [4]) that the patient has recently taken.

Laboratory Testing

In thrombocytopenic patients, examination of the blood smear can quickly reveal whether pseudothrombocytopenia (artifactual platelet clumping) is present and verify the degree of thrombocytopenia. Although exceptions do exist, the magnitude of thrombocytopenia can be an aid in the differential diagnosis of low platelet counts (Table 91.2). HIT and thrombotic microangiopathy (including TTP) often present with modest thrombocytopenia (50 to 100×10^9 per L). The smear should be carefully reviewed for the presence of fragmented red cells (schistocytes). Laboratory assessment of liver function and renal function also should be assessed. A markedly elevated level of lactate dehydrogenase (LDH) level out of proportion to other liver function abnormalities characteristically occurs in TTP and Hantavirus infection. If there is any suspicion of HIT, all heparin should be stopped and alternative antithrombotic agents should be started. Assessment of platelet function can be difficult and must be based largely on clinical judgment. The bleeding time or the platelet function assay are rarely useful in the evaluation of a thrombocytopenic patient, because the low platelet count lead to prolongations in the test end point.

TABLE 91.1

Causes of Thrombocytopenia of Special Interest to the Intensivist

Disseminated intravascular coagulation
Drug-induced thrombocytopenia
HELLP syndrome
Hemophagocytic syndrome
Heparin-induced thrombocytopenia
Liver disease
Posttransfusion purpura
Pseudothrombocytopenia
Thrombotic thrombocytopenia purpura

HELLP, Hemolysis, Elevated Liver tests, and Low Platelets.

Diagnostic clues

The reason for the ICU admission is an important step in evaluation of thrombocytopenia [5] (Table 91.3). For example, thrombocytopenia in patients who present with sudden-onset multiorgan system failure may indicate TTP or sepsis. In long-term critical care patients, new-onset thrombocytopenia may be a manifestation of HIT, drug-induced thrombocytopenia, occult or established sepsis, or bacteremia [6].

IMMEDIATE THERAPY—PLATELET TRANSFUSION

Although platelet thresholds below which critically ill patients are at risk of severe bleeding are likely to vary among patients, clinical practice generally dictates that a platelet count above 10×10^9 per L does not require platelet transfusion; as long as the patient is stable without signs of bleeding, is not receiving platelet inhibitors, has preserved renal function, does not require an invasive procedure, and does not have aggressive disseminated intravascular coagulation (DIC) [7].

TABLE 91.3

Diagnostic Clues to Thrombocytopenia

Private clinical setting	Differential diagnosis
Cardiac surgery	Cardiopulmonary bypass, HIT, dilutional thrombocytopenia, TTP
Interventional cardiac procedure	Abciximab or other IIb/IIIa blockers, HIT
Sepsis syndrome	DIC, ehrlichiosis, sepsis hemophagocytosis syndrome, drug-induced, misdiagnosed TTP, mechanical ventilation, pulmonary artery catheters
Pulmonary failure	DIC, H1N1, HUS, mechanical ventilation, pulmonary artery catheters
Mental status changes/seizures	TTP, ehrlichiosis
Renal failure	TTP, dengue, HIT, DIC
Cardiac failure	HIT, drug-induced, pulmonary artery catheter
Post-surgery	Dilutional, drug-induced, HIT, TTP
Pregnancy	HELLP syndrome, fatty liver of pregnancy, TTP/HUS
Acute liver failure	Splenic sequestration, HIT, drug-induced, DIC

HIT, heparin-induced thrombocytopenia; DIC, disseminated intravascular coagulation; TTP, thrombotic thrombocytopenic purpura; HUS, hemolytic uremic syndrome; HELLP, Hemolysis, Elevated Liver tests, and Low Platelets.

If any of these are present, especially major or life-threatening hemorrhage (such as intracranial), then a threshold of greater than 50×10^9 per L is reasonable. An exception is thrombocytopenia caused by thrombotic microangiopathy (TTP), wherein platelet transfusion is contraindicated [8]. Platelet transfusions should comprise six platelet concentrates or one single-donor plateletpheresis unit. Additional discussion regarding transfusion of blood products in critically ill patients is found in Chapter 89.

CAUSES OF THROMBOCYTOPENIA

Heparin-Induced Thrombocytopenia

HIT occurs because of the formation of antibodies directed against the complex of heparin and platelet factor 4 [9]. This complex in a minority of cases binds to the FcγRIIA receptor, activating platelets and macrophages leading to a procoagulant state. The frequency of HIT is 1% to 5% when unfractionated heparin is used but less than 1% with low molecular-weight heparin [10]. HIT is more common in women and in postsurgical patients [11].

HIT should be suspected when there is a sudden onset of thrombocytopenia with either at least a 50% drop in the platelet count from baseline or the platelet count falling to less than 100×10^9 per L in a patient receiving heparin in *any* form. HIT usually occurs at least 4 days after starting heparin but may occur suddenly in patients with recent (less than 3 months) exposure [12]. An often overlooked feature of HIT is recurrent thrombosis in a patient receiving heparin despite a normal platelet count [13]. Another clinical clue is a biphasic pattern of thrombocytopenia following cardiac surgery; recovery from the postsurgical thrombocytopenia followed by recurrent thrombocytopenia is strongly predictive of HIT [14]. A scoring system (the four Ts) has been validated in several studies as a means of assessing the pretest probability of HIT [15] (Table 91.4). Patients with scores of 0 to 3 are very unlikely to have HIT and can forego PF4-heparin antibody testing and empiric therapy.

The diagnosis of HIT can be challenging in the critical care patient who has multiple reasons for being thrombocytopenic. In this situation, the laboratory assay for HIT is helpful. Two levels of HIT testing exist. A widely available ELISA assay that detects the presumed pathogenic anti-heparin-platelet factor 4 antibodies is evaluated initially [16]. This test is very sensitive but in some populations not specific. For example, 10% to 50%

TABLE 91.4

Prediction Rule for Heparin-Induced Thrombocytopenia

Points	2	1	0
Thrombocytopenia	>50% fall from baseline and nadir 20–100,000/μL	30–50% fall or nadir 10–19,000/μL	Fall < 30% or nadir < 10,000/μL
Timing of platelet fall	Onset day 5–10 of heparin or <1 d if patient recently exposed to heparin	Consistent but not clear records or count falls after day 10	Platelets falls < 5 d and no recent (100 d) heparin
Thrombosis	New thrombosis or skin necrosis or systemic reaction with heparin	Progressive or recurrent thrombosis or suspected but not proven thrombosis	None
Other cause for thrombocytopenia	No	Possible	Definite

Patients with a low probability score are very unlikely to have HIT and can forgo PF4-heparin antibody testing and empiric therapy. Patients with intermediate and high scores should receive empiric therapy until definitive testing can be obtained.
Score 6–8 high, 4–5 intermediate, 0–3 low.
Adapted from [103,104].

of cardiac surgery, dialysis, or ICU patients will show positive results. The value of testing is that a negative test rules out HIT in all but the highest risk patients.

A second type of test is a functional platelet aggregation assay that consists of patient plasma, donor platelets, and heparin. If added heparin induces platelet aggregation, the test is considered to be positive. The test is technically demanding; but, if performed carefully, can be sensitive and specific [16]. Because of substantial frequency of false positivity of PF4-heparin ELISA, a positive test should be confirmed by a functional assay, even if treatment for HIT already has been initiated.

The first step in therapy of HIT consists of stopping *all* heparin. Low-molecular-weight heparins cross-react with the HIT antibodies, and therefore these agents are also contraindicated. Institution of warfarin therapy alone following a diagnosis of HIT has been associated with an increased risk of thromboses and is also contraindicated. Because of the high risk of thrombosis (53% in one study) [10] among HIT patients, antithrombotic therapy should be administered to all patients [17]. For immediate therapy of HIT patients, several antithrombotic agents are available [18] (Table 91.5).

Argatroban is a direct thrombin inhibitor with a short half-life of 40 to 50 minutes. Dosing is 2 μg/kg/min with the infusion adjusted to keep the activated partial thromboplastin time (aPTT) 1.5 to 3 times normal. One advantage of argatroban is that it is not renally excreted, so no dose adjustment is necessary in renal disease [19]. These characteristics make it the most useful agent for patients in the critical care unit. However, argatroban must be used with caution in patients with severe liver disease by using an initial dose of 0.5 μg/kg/min [20]. Also, metabolism appears to be decreased in patients with multiorgan system failure and these patients should receive a dose of μg/kg/min [21]. Argatroban (like all thrombin inhibitors) prolongs the prothrombin time/international normalized ratio (PT/INR) making initiation of warfarin therapy difficult. Options for converting a patient from argatroban to warfarin include:

1. Use the chromogenic Xa assay to adjust warfarin therapy aiming for a factor X level of 15% to 25%.
2. If the dose of argatroban is 2 μg/kg/min or less, one can simply aim for a PT/INR of more than 4.0 as therapeutic.
3. When platelets recover, change the patient to fondaparinux and initiate warfarin.
4. When platelets recover, change the patient to a direct oral anticoagulant.

Bivalirudin is a semisynthetic direct thrombin inhibitor that has been tested mostly in the setting of cardiac disease. This agent is an option for patients with HIT who need cardiac procedures and is especially an option for cardiac bypass with the most common dose being a 1 mg per kg bolus and infusion at 1.75 to 2.5 mg/kg/h to keep the activated clotting time > 300 seconds [22].

The indirect anti-Xa inhibitor fondaparinux does not cross-react with HIT antibodies suggesting a potential role in therapy of HIT [23]. However, it has not been studied as extensively in HIT as there are rare reports of a syndrome similar to delayed-onset HIT [24]. In addition, its long half-life of 19 hours and renal clearance do not make it practical to use in most ICU patients.

Theoretically, direct oral anticoagulants may be an option, but there are no substantial data on their use in acute HIT [25]. They are best used in patients with a history of HIT or for long-term anticoagulation when the platelet count has returned to normal.

The issue of platelet transfusion remains controversial [26]. Patients with HIT rarely bleed, which reduces clinical concern over the potential for platelet transfusions; but a prudent approach is to reserve transfusion of platelets for the rare patient with severe thrombocytopenia who also has life-threatening bleeding.

As mentioned above, initiation of warfarin as the sole antithrombotic agent in the initial treatment of HIT has been associated with limb gangrene. In patients to be started on warfarin, it should be started in small doses (2 to 5 mg daily) once the platelet count has recovered. These often malnourished patients tend to have a dramatic response to warfarin therapy, and excessive anticoagulation can easily occur. One should overlap warfarin and parental therapy by 2 to 3 days, as there is evidence that patients may do worse if therapy with a direct thrombin inhibtor is truncated [20].

Patients with HIT should be carefully screened for any thrombosis, at least by performing lower extremity Doppler ultrasound. If thrombosis is present, a minimum of 3 months of therapeutic anticoagulation is required, whereas HIT without thrombosis usually is treated with 30 days of therapeutic anticoagulation.

TABLE 91.5

Treatment of Heparin-Induced Thrombocytopenia

Argatroban
Therapy: initial dose of 2 μg/kg/min adjusted to an aPTT of 1.5–3.0 times normal.
Reversal: no antidote but $T_{1/2} \sim 40$ min
In severe liver disease (jaundice), dose at 0.5 μg/kg/min adjusted to an aPTT 1.5–3.0 times normal.
For patients with multiorgan system failure, 1 μg/kg/min adjusted to aPTT 1.5–3.0 times normal
Post-CABG, 0.5–1 μg/kg/min adjusted to aPTT 1.5–3.0 times normal
Indication: Prevention and treatment of thrombosis in HIT
Bivalirudin
Bolus: 1 mg/kg
Infusion: 2.5 mg/kg/h for 4 h and then 0.2 mg/kg/h for 14–20 h.
Renal adjustment:
For creatinine clearance of 30–59 mL/min, decrease dose by 20%
For creatinine clearance of 10–29 mL/min, decrease dose by 60%
For creatinine clearances less than 10 mg/min, decrease dose by 90%
Indication: Percutaneous coronary intervention in patients with or without HIT
Fondaparinux[a]
Therapy: 7.5 mg every 24 h (consider 5.0 mg in patients under 50 kg and 10 mg in patients over 100 kg)
Reversal: Protamine ineffective; see Chapter 93.

aPTT, activated partial thromboplastin time; CABG, coronary artery bypass grafting; HIT, heparin-induced thrombocytopenia.

[a]Fondaparinux is not approved for treatment of HIT. Its use, however, may be considered after initial anticoagulation with a direct thrombin inhibitor has been administered and the platelet count has recovered, while awaiting a therapeutic INR from therapy with warfarin [18].

Thrombotic Thrombocytopenic Purpura

TTP should be suspected when any patient presents with thrombocytopenia and microangiopathic hemolytic anemia, as evidenced by schistocytes on the blood smear and biochemical evidence of hemolysis); end-organ damage, manifesting as renal insufficiency or neurologic phenomena; and fever. Patients with TTP may not present with all of the aforementioned features. Critical care patients with TTP often present with intractable seizures, strokes, or sequela of renal insufficiency. Postsurgical TTP may occur 1 to 2 weeks after major surgery, and is heralded by decreasing platelet counts and renal insufficiency [27]. Many patients who present to the critical care unit with TTP have been misdiagnosed as having sepsis, "lupus flare," or vasculitis.

The majority of patients with the classic form of TTP have an inhibitor against an enzyme that is responsible for cleaving newly synthesized von Willebrand factor (VWF) [28]. VWF is synthesized as an ultra large multimer that can spontaneously aggregate platelets. The enzyme, ADAMTS13, cleaves VWF into a smaller form that can circulate without spontaneously binding platelets [29]. Presumably in TTP, when ADAMTS13 is inhibited, the ultra large multimers spontaneously aggregate platelets leading to the clinical syndrome of TTP. However, some patients with classic TTP have normal activity of ADAMTS13, implying other factors are important in pathogenesis of the disease.

There is currently no single diagnostic test for TTP; rather, the diagnosis is based on the clinical presentation [30]. Patients uniformly will have a microangiopathic hemolytic anemia with the presence of schistocytes on the peripheral smear. Renal insufficiency without severe renal failure is the most common renal manifestation. Thrombocytopenia may range from a mild decrease in platelet number to platelets being undetectable. The finding of thrombocytopenia with a relative normal PT helps eliminate DIC from the differential [31]. The LDH is often very elevated and is a prognostic factor in TTP. Finding very low levels of ADAMTS13 (<10%) is specific to TTP; but, as testing can take time and the test is not sensitive, initiation of therapy should not depend on assay results.

Untreated TTP is rapidly fatal. Mortality in the pre-plasma exchange era ranged from 95% to 100%. Plasma exchange therapy is presently the cornerstone of TTP treatment and has reduced mortality to less than 20% [32].

Glucocorticoid therapy, either 1 to 2 mg per kg of methylprednisolone until remission or 1 gm of methylprednisolone initially, may be given to patients who have TTP [33,34]. Glucocorticoids may be continued until the patient has fully recovered or longer, given the presumed autoimmune nature of the disease and the high relapse rates. Plasma infusion is beneficial, but plasma exchange has been shown to be superior to simple plasma infusion in therapy of TTP [35]. This may be due to the ability of plasma exchange to give large volumes of fresh frozen plasma and removal of inhibitory antibodies. In patients in whom plasma exchange is not readily available, plasma infusions should be started at a dose of 1 unit every 4 hours. Patients with all but the mildest cases of TTP should receive 1 to 1.5 plasma volume exchange each day for at least 5 days (see Chapter 96). Daily plasma exchange should be continued daily until the LDH has normalized, at which point the frequency of exchange may be tapered, starting with every other day exchange. If the platelet count falls or LDH level rises, daily exchange should be reinstated. Although the platelet count can be affected by a variety of external influences, the LDH level tends to be the most reliable marker of disease activity. There is evidence that the use of anti-CD20 therapy may reduce the incidence of relapses and shorten the duration of therapy in refractory disease [36]. In patients with refractory TTP, aggressive measures such as twice a day exchanges, splenectomy, or immunosuppression need to be considered [37].

Hemolytic Uremic Syndrome

Classically, hemolytic uremic syndrome (HUS) comprises the triad of renal failure, microangiopathic anemia, and thrombocytopenia. Two major forms are recognized: a "typical" form, which occurs in young children with an antecedent diarrheal illness, and an "atypical" form, which is increasingly being recognized as a disease of complement activation [33].

Typical HUS

Typical HUS occurs when HUS occurs after a prodrome of bloody diarrhea [38]. Most often, etiology is infection with *Escherichia coli* O157:H7 but increasingly other serotypes such as O26 and O104:H4 are being reported. Patients come to medical attention either because of the diarrhea or because of symptoms of renal failure. In HUS, thrombocytopenia can be mild in the 50×10^9 per L range. Extrarenal involvement is common in typical HUS. Neurologic involvement can be seen in 40% of patients with seizure being the predominant feature. Elevated liver function tests are seen in 40% of patients and 10% of patients have pancreatitis. Patients with classic HUS respond to conservative therapy and renal replacement therapy. Treatment of severe cases or those with prominent extrarenal manifestations is controversial, as studies suggest no benefit with plasma exchange [39]. Although benefit in atypical HUS, data currently suggest no role for eculizumab in typical HUS. Most patients recover some renal function, though some patients have long-term renal damage.

Atypical HUS

Atypical HUS is associated with excess complement activation that leads to renal damage with resultant renal failure [40]. Some patients may transiently respond to plasma exchange, but then relapse with relentless decline in renal function. Atypical HUS may recur following renal transplant. Proof of the role of complement activation is the dramatic response seen in patients with complement inhibitor treatment. Atypical HUS is a clinical diagnosis and should be considered in the patient with HUS that has no preceding diarrheal syndrome or in the patient with suspected TTP who has normal ADAMTS13 levels and prominent renal disease. Patients with atypical HUS should receive therapy with the C5a inhibitor eculizumab, as this has consistent and long-term clinical benefits in atypical HUS [41]. Patients receiving this agent should be vaccinated for meningococcal infections as the risk of these infections is increased with blockade of the terminal part of complement.

Therapy-Related Thrombotic Microangiopathies

Thrombotic microangiopathies (TM) syndromes can complicate a variety of therapies [42]. TMs can be associated with medications such as cyclosporine, tacrolimus, gemcitabine, and thienopyridines. Cyclosporine/tacrolimus-associated TM occurs within days after the agent is started manifesting as a falling platelet count, falling hematocrit, and rising serum LDH level. Some cases have been fatal, but often the TM resolves with decreasing the dose of the calcineurin inhibitor or changing to another agent.

In the past TM, was most commonly seen with the antineoplastic agent mitomycin C, with a frequency of 10% when a dose of more than 60 mg was used [43]. Presently, the most common antineoplastic drug causing TM is gemcitabine with an incidence of 0.1% to 1% [44]. The appearance of the TM syndrome associated with gemcitabine can be delayed, and the condition can be fatal. Severe hypertension often precedes the clinical appearance of TM [45]. The use of plasma exchange is controversial [46], and there are reports of the use of the complement inhibitor eculizumab halting TM [47]. The increasing use of vascular endothelial growth factor inhibitors such as bevacizumab and sunitinib has been associated with TM syndromes as well [48].

TM has been reported with other drugs including the thienopyridines: ticlopidine, clopidogrel, and prasugrel. The frequency of ticlopidine-associated TM may be as high as 1:1600; and, as this drug is often prescribed for the patient with vascular disease, the patient may be initially misdiagnosed as having recurrent strokes or angina [49]. The frequency of TTP using clopidogrel and prasugrel is low at 0.0001%; but, as they are widely prescribed, it is the second most common cause of drug-induced TM [50]. Almost all cases of clopidogrel-induced TTP occur within 2 weeks of starting the drug. All patients with thienopyridine-associated TM should receive plasma exchange.

TMs can complicate both autologous and allogeneic stem cell transplants [51]. The incidence ranges from 15% for allogeneic to 5% for autologous stem cell transplants. Several types of TMs are recognized in stem cell transplantations [51,52]. One is "multiorgan fulminant" which occurs early (20 to 60 days posttransplant), has multiorgan system involvement, and is often fatal. Another type of TM is similar to calcineurin inhibitor TM. A "conditioning" TM, which occurs 6 months or more after total body irradiation, is associated with primary renal involvement. Finally, patients with systemic cytomegalovirus (CMV) infections can present with a TM syndrome related to vascular infection with CMV. The etiology of bone marrow transplant–related TM appears to be different from that of "classic" TTP, as autoantibodies to ADAMTS13 have not been found in stem cell transplant TM–related vascular damage [53]. The therapy of stem cell transplant TM is uncertain. Patients should have their calcineurin inhibitors doses decreased. The response to plasma exchange is poor with fulminant or conditioning-related TM.

Pregnancy-Related Thrombocytopenic Syndromes

One should consider three syndromes in the critically ill pregnant woman who presents with thrombocytopenia. These are the HELLP syndrome, fatty liver of pregnancy, and TTP (Table 91.6) [54,55].

The acronym HELLP syndrome (**H**emolysis, **E**levated **L**iver tests, **L**ow **P**latelets) describes a variant of preeclampsia [56]. Classically, HELLP syndrome occurs after 28 weeks of gestation in the patient with preeclampsia but can occur as early as 22 weeks in patients with the antiphospholipid antibody syndrome [57]. The preeclampsia need not be severe. The first sign of HELLP is a decrease in the platelet count followed by abnormal liver function tests. Signs of hemolysis are present with abundant schistocytes on the smear and a high LDH. HELLP can progress to liver failure, and deaths are also reported due to hepatic rupture. Unlike TTP, fetal involvement is present in the HELLP syndrome with fetal thrombocytopenia reported in 30% of cases. In severe cases, elevated D-dimers consistent with DIC are also found. Delivery of the child will often result in cessation of the HELLP syndrome, but refractory cases require dexamethasone (most commonly dosed as 10 mg every 12 hours) and, rarely, plasma exchange [58]. About a quarter of women who suffer from HELLP will have a recurrence with a later pregnancy.

Fatty liver of pregnancy also occurs late in pregnancy and is only associated with preeclampsia in 50% of cases [55,59]. Patients present with nonspecific symptoms of nausea and vomiting, but can progress to fulminant liver failure. Patients develop thrombocytopenia early in the course; but, in later stage, can develop DIC and very low fibrinogen levels. Mortality rates without therapy can be as high as 90%. Hypoglycemia, low antithrombin, and high ammonia levels can help distinguish fatty liver from other pregnancy complications [59]. Treatment consists of prompt delivery of the child and aggressive blood product support.

TTP can occur anytime during pregnancy often leading to diagnostic confusion because of the overlap of symptoms between TTP and HELLP syndrome [60]. A unique presentation of TTP occurs in the second trimester at 20 to 22 weeks [61]. The fetus is uninvolved with no evidence of infarction or thrombocytopenia, if the mother survives. The pregnancy appears to promote TTP, as TTP will resolve with termination of the pregnancy and can recur with the next pregnancy [62]. Therapy includes termination of pregnancy or supporting the patient with plasma exchange until the fetus is viable. Pregnancy-related TTP is a common presentation of congenital TTP; and, if ADAMTS13 inhibitors are not found, the patients should undergo genetic testing. An unusual complication of pregnancy is a HUS-type syndrome seen up to 28 weeks postpartum. This form of HUS is severe, and permanent renal failure often results despite aggressive therapy. Many of these patients have defects in regulatory proteins of complement such as factor H deficiency. This may explain the severity of their renal failure [63].

Disseminated Intravascular Coagulation

At the most basic level, DIC is the clinical manifestation of inappropriate thrombin activation [64]. Inappropriate thrombin activation can be caused by sepsis or obstetric disasters. The activation of thrombin leads to (1) conversion of fibrinogen to fibrin, (2) activation of platelets (and their consumption), (3) activation of factors V and VIII, (4) activation of protein C (and degradation of factors Va and VIIIa), (5) activation of endothelial cells, and (6) activation of fibrinolysis.

The clinical manifestations of DIC depend on the balance of thrombin activations and secondary fibrinolysis balanced by the ability of the patient to compensate for the DIC. Patients with DIC can present in one of four patterns:

TABLE 91.6

Pregnancy-Related Diseases—TTP/HUS, HELLP Syndrome, and AFLP

Private	HELLP	TTP/HUS	AFLP
Hypertension	Always present	Sometimes present	Sometimes present
Proteinuria	Always present	Sometimes present	Sometimes present
Thrombocytopenia	Always	Always	Always
LDH elevation	Present	Marked	Present
Fibrinogen	Normal to low	Normal	Normal to very low
Schistocytes	Present	Present	Absent
Liver tests	Elevated	Normal	Elevated
Ammonia	Normal	Normal	Elevated
Glucose	Normal	Normal	Low

HELLP, Hemolysis, Elevated Liver tests, and Low Platelets; TTP/HUS, thrombotic thrombocytopenic purpura/hemolytic uremia syndrome; AFLP, acute fatty liver of pregnancy; LDH, lactate dehydrogenase.

1. Asymptomatic. Patients can present with laboratory evidence of DIC but no bleeding or thrombosis. This is often seen in patients with sepsis or cancer. With further progression of the underlying disease, these patients can rapidly become symptomatic.
2. Bleeding. The bleeding is caused by a combination of factor depletion, platelet dysfunction, thrombocytopenia, and excessive fibrinolysis. These patients may present with diffuse bleeding from multiple sites such as IV sites, areas of instrumentation, and surgical wounds.
3. Thrombosis. Despite the general activation of the coagulation process, thrombosis is unusual with acute DIC. Exceptions include cancer patients, trauma patients, and certain obstetric patients. Most often the thrombosis is venous, but arterial thrombosis and nonbacterial thrombotic endocarditis have been reported [65].
4. Purpura fulminans. This severe form of DIC is described in more detail later.

The most effective way to treat DIC is to treat the underlying cause that is driving thrombin generation [66]. In the past, there was concern about replacement of depleted blood cells and coagulation proteins in DIC because of fears of "feeding the fire." This has not been well validated, and replacement is mandatory, if depletion occurs and bleeding ensues. Measurement of laboratory tests that will reflect the basic parameters essential for both blood volume and hemostasis is helpful. Replacement therapy is based on the results of these laboratories and the clinical situation of the patient (Table 91.7). Additional discussion regarding transfusion of blood products in critically ill patients is found in Chapter 116.

Heparin therapy is reserved for the patient who has thrombosis as a component of their DIC. Given the coagulopathy that is often present, specific heparin levels instead of the aPTT are monitored to guide anticoagulation therapy.

TABLE 91.7

Management of DIC: Transfusion

The five basic tests of hemostasis[a]

Hematocrit
Platelet count
Prothrombin time (PT)
Activated partial thromboplastin time (aPTT)
Fibrinogen level

Guidelines for transfusion in patients at high risk of bleeding[b]

A. Platelets $<50 \times 10^9$/L: give platelet concentrates or 1 unit of single-donor platelets.
B. Fibrinogen < 150/dL: give 10 units of cryoprecipitate[c]
C. Hematocrit below 30%: give red cells
D. Protime > twofold the upper limit of normal *and* aPTT abnormal: give 2–4 units of FFP[d]

[a]These laboratory tests should be repeated after administering blood products serially. A record of the test and the blood products administered should be maintained.
[b]Patients with DIC who are not actively bleeding generally do not require replacement of platelets or coagulation factors, unless an invasive procedure is planned or other circumstances are present; see text.
[c]For a fibrinogen level less than 150 mg/dL, transfusion of 10 units of cryoprecipitate is expected to increase the plasma fibrinogen level by 100 mg/dL.
[d]In patients with DIC and a markedly prolonged PT and aPTT, one can give 2-4 units of fresh frozen plasma (FFP) initially.

Purpura Fulminans

DIC in association with necrosis of the skin may occur in two situations [67]. Primary purpura fulminans is most often seen following a viral infection [68]. In this case, the purpura fulminans starts with a painful red area on the lower extremities that rapidly progresses to a black ischemic lesion. Acquired deficiency of protein S may be present [69].

Secondary purpura fulminans is most often associated with meningococcemia infections, but it can occur in any patient with overwhelming infection [70]. Post-splenectomy sepsis syndrome patients and those with functional hyposplenism due to chronic liver diseases are also at risk [71]. Patients present with signs of sepsis, and the skin lesions often involve the extremities and may lead to amputation. As opposed to primary purpura fulminans, those with secondary purpura fulminans will have symmetrical ischemic lesions at the distal parts of the body (toes and fingers) that ascend as the process progresses. Adrenal infarction (Waterhouse–Friderichsen syndrome) can occur which leads to severe hypotension [72].

Therapy for purpura fulminans is controversial. Primary purpura fulminans, especially cases with post-varicella autoimmune protein S deficiency, may respond to plasma infusion titrated to keep the protein S level more than 25% [67]. Intravenous immune globulin has also been reported to help decrease the anti-protein S antibodies. Heparin has been reported to control the DIC and the extent of necrosis. The starting dose in these patients is 5 to 8 units/kg/h [73].

Critically ill patients with secondary purpura fulminans have been treated with plasma drips, plasmapheresis, and continuous plasma ultrafiltration. Heparin therapy alone has not been shown to improve survival [74]. Much attention has been given to replacement of natural anticoagulants such as antithrombin as therapy for purpura fulminans, but randomized trials using antithrombin have shown mostly negative results [75]. Many patients need debridement and amputation; in one review, approximately 66% of patient required amputation [76].

Drug-Induced Hemolytic-DIC Syndromes

A severe variant of drug-induced immune complex hemolysis, which may be associated with DIC, has been recognized. The syndrome has occurred in association with the use of advanced-generation cephalosporins (notably cefotetan and ceftriaxone), and it has been reported with carboplatin and oxaliplatin [77]. The clinical syndrome associated with cephalosporin starts 7 to 10 days after receiving the drug and may occur following a single dose given as surgical prophylaxis. The patient develops severe Coombs-positive hemolysis with hypotension and DIC. The patient may be misdiagnosed as having sepsis and be reexposed to the cephalosporin, resulting in worsening of the clinical picture. The outcome may be fatal because of massive hemolysis and thrombosis.

Quinine is associated with a unique syndrome of drug-induced DIC [78]. Approximately 24 to 96 hours after quinine exposure, the patient becomes acutely ill with nausea and vomiting. The patient then develops a microangiopathic hemolytic anemia, DIC, and renal failure. Some patients, besides having antiplatelet antibodies, also have antibodies that bind to red cells and neutrophils that may lead to the more severe syndrome. Despite therapy, patients will frequently progress to chronic renal failure.

Treatment of the drug-induced hemolytic-DIC syndrome is based on anecdotal reports. Patients have responded to aggressive therapy including plasma exchange, dialysis, and prednisone. Early recognition of the hemolytic anemia (and the suspicion that it is drug-related) is important for early diagnosis so that the culprit drug can be discontinued.

Drug-Induced Thrombocytopenia

Patients with drug-induced thrombocytopenia typically present with very low platelet counts 1 to 3 weeks after starting a new medication [79]. One of the agents most commonly associated with drug-induced thrombocytopenia in the critical care setting is vancomycin. The thrombocytopenia is acute and severe (below $<10 \times 10^9$ per L), is durably refractory to platelet transfusions, and resolves within days of stopping the drug [80]. In patients with a possible drug-induced thrombocytopenia, the primary therapy is to stop the suspect drug. Patients with severe thrombocytopenia should receive platelet transfusions because of the risk of fatal bleeding [81]. However, with vancomycin-induced thrombocytopenia, the patient may be refractory to platelet transfusion [80]. If there are multiple risk medications, the best approach is to stop any drug that is strongly associated with thrombocytopenia (Table 91.8). Immune globulin or corticosteroids have been suggested as useful in drug-related thrombocytopenia. As most patients recover when the agent is cleared from the body, this therapy may not be necessary.

Sepsis

Thrombocytopenia associated with sepsis syndromes classically has been attributed to DIC or destruction by autoimmune mechanisms. Increasing evidence points to cytokine-driven hemophagocytosis of platelets [82]. Patients with hemophagocytosis appear to have higher rates of multiple organ system failure and higher mortality rates. Inflammatory cytokines, especially monocyte-colony stimulating factor, are thought responsible for inducing the hemophagocytosis. Some patients, because of infection, tumors, or autoimmune disease, may develop an overwhelming hemophagocytic syndrome (HPS) [83]. The patient will have pancytopenia, fevers, high ferritins and triglycerides, and low fibrinogens. Mortality is high with HPS, unless there is aggressive treatment.

Thrombocytopenia may be a diagnostic clue to infection with unusual organisms [84]. Three members of the Ehrlichia/anaplasma family have been reported to cause infections in humans [85]. They are transmitted by ticks, and the diseases that they produce are similar. Most patients have a febrile illness with high fevers, headaches, and myalgias [86]. Patients may have central nervous system signs and marked elevation of the serum levels of liver enzymes. Rarely, patients may present with a toxic shock-like syndrome [87]. Although many cases are mild, severe disease is common in immunosuppressed patients. The case fatality rate is 2% to 5% [88]. The typical hematologic picture is leukopenia (1.3 to 4×10^9 per L) and mild thrombocytopenia (30 to 60×10^9 per L). In many patients, the buffy coat reveals the organisms bundled in a 2 to 5 μm morula in the cytoplasm of the granulocytes or monocytes. Consideration of ehrlichiosis is important because highly specific therapy is doxycycline, which is a drug not routinely used for therapy of sepsis syndrome.

The classical hematologic presentation of Hantavirus pulmonary syndrome (HPS) can be helpful in the diagnosis of this severe illness (see Chapter 83). Patients suffer a flu-like prodrome and then rapidly develop a noncardiac pulmonary edema resulting in profound respiratory failure [89]. Ventilatory support is required in 75% of cases and the mortality is approximately 50%. A powerful indicator of the presence of Hantavirus is found on the peripheral smear. The triad of thrombocytopenia, increased and left-shifted white cell count, and more than 10% circulating immunoblasts can identify all cases of HPS and was seen in only 2.6% non-HPS controls. Marked hemoconcentration is also present because of capillary leak syndrome with the hematocrit reaching in some patients as high as 68%.

TABLE 91.8

Critical Care Drugs Commonly Implicated in Thrombocytopenia

- Antiarrhythmics
  - Procainamide
  - Quinidine
- Anti-GP IIb/IIIa agents
  - Abciximab
  - Eptifibatide
  - Tirofiban
- Antimicrobial
  - Amphotericin B
  - Piperacillin
  - Rifampin
  - Trimethoprim–sulfamethoxazole
  - Vancomycin
- H_2-blockers
  - Cimetidine
  - Ranitidine
- Acetaminophen
- Amiodarone
- Carbamazepine
- Haloperidol
- Gold
- Heparin
- Hydrochlorothiazide
- Nonsteroidal antiinflammatory agents
- Oxaliplatin
- Phenytoin
- Quinine
- Valproic acid

From [81,105,106].

Viral Hemorrhagic Fevers

Viral hemorrhagic fevers (VHF) are a diverse group of viral infections that can result in massive bleeding [90–92]. VHF are an important problem in certain parts of the world, but travelers may carry the disease anywhere. In the southern United States, dengue is becoming an increasing problem, and fatal cases of arenavirus have been reported in California [93]. As described in Table 91.9, there are four groups of viruses which can lead to VHF [94]. The typical pattern is a febrile illness that proceeds over a few days to shock and diffuse bleeding with the patient developing signs of thrombocytopenia and in some cases DIC. Patients at first presentation often have pharyngitis, conjunctivitis, and a skin rash. A key sign is that patients will experience profuse bleeding from the gastrointestinal tract and mucosal bleeding often out of proportion to the observed coagulation defects. This finding should serve as a diagnostic clue. Most VHF are also associated with leukopenia and hemoconcentration. Therapy is aggressive supportive care of the patients and replacement of coagulation factors. As noted in Table 91.9, ribavirin can treat certain VHF. Given the propensity of many of these infections to spread to health care workers, precautions should be taken to prevent nosocomial spread [95].

Bleeding in the Platelet-Refractory Patient

Bleeding in patients who are refractory to platelet transfusion presents a difficult clinical problem (Table 91.10) [96]. If patients are demonstrated to have human leukocyte antigen antibodies, one can transfuse HLA-matched platelets. Although matched

TABLE 91.9

Viral Hemorrhagic Fever–Associated Thrombocytopenia

Arenaviridae

Diseases: Lassa fever, New World arenaviruses
Distribution: West Africa (Lassa), South America (rare California) (New world)
Vector: Rodents
Incubation: 5–16 d
Therapy: Ribavirin
Unique clinical features: pharyngitis, late deafness (Lassa); neurologic involvement—seizures (New World)

Bunyaviridae

Diseases: Crimean-Congo hemorrhagic virus (CCHF), Rift Valley fever, hemorrhagic fever with renal syndrome (HFRS)
Distribution: Africa, Central Asia, Eastern Europe, Middle East (CCHF), Africa, Middle East (Rift), Asia, Balkans, Europe (HFRS)
Vector: ticks (CCHF), mosquitoes (Rift Valley), rodents (HFRS)
Incubation: 1–6 d (CHHF), 2 wk to 2 mo (HFRS)
Therapy: Ribavirin
Unique clinical features: retinitis, hepatitis (Rift Valley), prominent bleeding with DIC, jaundice (CCHF); renal disease (CCHF)

Filoviridae

Diseases: Ebola, Marburg viruses
Distribution: Africa
Vector: Bats and other wild animals
Incubation: 2–21 d
Unique clinical feature: maculopapular rash, high mortality

Flaviviridae

Diseases: dengue, yellow fever
Distribution: widespread (dengue), Africa, Tropical Americans (yellow)
Vector: mosquitoes
Incubation: 3–15 d
Unique clinic feature: liver involvement (yellow)

From [94,107,108]

TABLE 91.10

Evaluation and Management of Platelet Alloimmunization

1. Check platelet count 15 min after platelet transfusion.
2. If rise in platelet count is less than 5×10^9/L, check for HLA antibodies.
3. Administer HLA-matched platelets and evaluate for response.
4. If three sequential HLA-matched platelet transfusions are ineffective, discontinue HLA-matched platelets.
5. In completely refractory patients:
   A. Evaluate for other causes of thrombocytopenia (HIT, drugs).
   B. Consider institution of antifibrinolytic therapy
      1. Epsilon aminocaproic acid 1 gm/h IV, or
      2. Tranexamic acid 10 mg/kg IV every 8 h.
   C. Platelet "drip"—continuous infusion of platelets at the rate 1 unit over 6 h
   D. Recombinant activated VII for life-threatening bleeding

HLA, human leukocyte antigen; HIT, heparin-induced thrombocytopenia; IV, intravenous.

TABLE 91.11

Key Recent Articles for ICU Thrombocytopenia

Platelet transfusions
- AABB practice guidelines [7]

Heparin-induced thrombocytopenia
- Four T scoring system in ICU patients [15]
- Use of fondaparinux [23]
- Use of direct oral anticoagulants [25]

Thrombotic microangiopathies
- Treatment of refractory TTP [37]
- Lack of value for aggressive therapy in typical HUS [39]
- Use of eculizumab in atypical HUS [41]

Hemophagocytic syndrome
- Treatment of acquired cases [83]

AABB, American Association of Blood Banks; ICU, intensive care unit; TTP, thrombotic thrombocytopenic purpura; HUS, hemolytic uremic syndrome.

platelet transfusions do not work in 20% to 70% of these patients. Some loci are difficult to match, so effective products may not be available. As many as 25% of patients have antiplatelet antibodies in which HLA-matched products will be ineffective. Platelet cross-matching to find compatible units may not always be successful. In the patient who is totally refractory to platelet transfusion, it is important to consider whether a drug has resulted in antiplatelet antibodies (especially vancomycin) [97]. Use of antifibrinolytic agents such as epsilon aminocaproic acid or tranexamic acid may decrease the incidence of minor bleeding but are ineffective for major bleeding [98]. "Platelet drips" consisting of infusing either a platelet concentrate per hour or one plateletpheresis unit every 6 hours may be given as a continuous infusion [99].

Catastrophic Antiphospholipid Antibody Syndrome

The patient with catastrophic antiphospholipid antibody syndrome (CAPS) can present with fulminant multiorgan system failure [100]. CAPS is caused by widespread microthrombi in multiple vascular fields. These patients develop renal failure, encephalopathy, adult respiratory distress syndrome (often with pulmonary hemorrhage), cardiac failure, dramatic livedo reticularis, and worsening thrombocytopenia. Many of these patients have preexisting autoimmune disorders and high titer anticardiolipin antibodies. Therapy for these patients includes aggressive immunosuppression, plasmapheresis, and anticoagulation, with consideration of monthly IV cyclophosphamide [100]. Early recognition of this syndrome can lead to quick therapy and resolution of the multiorgan system failure.

Posttransfusion Purpura

Patients with this rare disorder develop severe thrombocytopenia ($<10 \times 10^9$ per L), and often severe bleeding, 1 to 2 weeks after receiving blood products [101]. Affected patients usually lack the platelet antigen PLA1. For unknown reasons, exposure to the antigens from the transfusion leads to rapid destruction of the patient's own platelets. The diagnostic clue is thrombocytopenia in a patient, typically female, who has received a red cell or platelet blood product in the past 7 to 10 days. Treatment consists of intravenous immunoglobulin [102] and plasmapheresis to remove the offending antibody (see Chapter 96). If patients with a history of posttransfusion purpura require further transfusions, only PLA1-negative platelets should be given.

References

1. Williamson DR, Lesur O, Tetrault JP, et al: Thrombocytopenia in the critically ill: prevalence, incidence, risk factors, and clinical outcomes. *Can J Anaesth* 60(7):641–651, 2013.
2. Stanworth SJ, Walsh TS, Prescott RJ, et al: Thrombocytopenia and platelet transfusion in UK critical care: a multicenter observational study. *Transfusion* 53(5):1050–1058, 2013.
3. Williamson DR, Albert M, Heels-Ansdell D et al: Thrombocytopenia in critically ill patients receiving thromboprophylaxis: frequency, risk factors, and outcomes. *Chest* 144(4):1207–1215, 2013.
4. Royer DJ, George JN, Terrell DR: Thrombocytopenia as an adverse effect of complementary and alternative medicines, herbal remedies, nutritional supplements, foods, and beverages. *Eur J Haematol* 84:421–429, 2010.
5. Alving BM, Spivak JL, DeLoughery TG: Consultive hematology: hemostasis and transfusion issues in surgery and critical care medicine. *Hematology* 1998:320–341, 1998.
6. Oguzulgen IK, Ozis T, Gursel G: Is the fall in platelet count associated with intensive care unit acquired pneumonia? *Swiss Med Wkly* 134(29/30):430–434, 2004.
7. Kaufman RM, Djulbegovic B, Gernsheimer T, et al: Platelet transfusion: a clinical practice guideline from the AABB. *Ann Intern Med* 162(3):205–213, 2015.
8. Kumar A, Mhaskar R, Grossman BJ, et al: Platelet transfusion: a systematic review of the clinical evidence. *Transfusion* 55(5):1116–1127, 2015.
9. Linkins LA: Heparin induced thrombocytopenia. *Brit Med J* 350:g7566, 2015.
10. Warkentin TE, Levine MN, Hirsh J et al: Heparin-induced thrombocytopenia in patients treated with low-molecular-weight heparin or unfractionated heparin. *N Engl J Med* 332:1330–1335, 1995.
11. Warkentin TE, Sheppard JA, Sigouin CS, et al: Gender imbalance and risk factor interactions in heparin-induced thrombocytopenia. *Blood* 108(9):2937–2941, 2006.
12. Warkentin TE, Kelton JG: Temporal aspects of heparin-induced thrombocytopenia. *N Engl J Med* 344(17):1286–1292, 2001.
13. Hach-Wunderle V, Kainer K, Krug B, et al: Heparin-associated thrombosis despite normal platelet counts. *Lancet* 344:469–470, 1994.
14. Pouplard C, May MA, Regina S, et al: Changes in platelet count after cardiac surgery can effectively predict the development of pathogenic heparin-dependent antibodies. *Br J Haematol* 128(6):837–841, 2005.
15. Cuker A, Gimotty PA, Crowther MA, et al: Predictive value of the 4Ts scoring system for heparin-induced thrombocytopenia: a systematic review and meta-analysis. *Blood* 120(20):4160–4167, 2012.
16. Arepally GM, Ortel TL: Heparin-induced thrombocytopenia. *Annu Rev Med* 61:77–90, 2010.
17. Cuker A, Cines DB: How I treat heparin-induced thrombocytopenia. *Blood* 119(10):2209–2218, 2012.
18. Kelton JG, Arnold DM, Bates SM: Nonheparin anticoagulants for heparin-induced thrombocytopenia. *N Engl J Med* 368(8):737–744, 2013.
19. Swan SK, Hursting MJ: The pharmacokinetics and pharmacodynamics of argatroban: effects of age, gender, and hepatic or renal dysfunction. *Pharmacotherapy* 20(3):318–329, 2000.
20. Kondo LM, Wittkowsky AK, Wiggins BS: Argatroban for prevention and treatment of thromboembolism in heparin-induced thrombocytopenia. *Ann Pharmacother* 35(4):440–451, 2001.
21. Baghdasarin SB, Singh I, Militello MA, et al: Argatroban dosage in crtically ill patients with HIT. *Blood* 104(11):1779, 2004.
22. Czosnowski QA, Finks SW, Rogers KC: Bivalirudin for patients with heparin-induced thrombocytopenia undergoing cardiovascular surgery. *Ann Pharmacother* 42(9):1304–1309, 2008.
23. Kang M, Alahmadi M, Sawh S, et al: Fondaparinux for the treatment of suspected heparin-induced thrombocytopenia: a propensity score-matched study. *Blood* 125(6):924–929, 2015.
24. Warkentin TE, Maurer BT, Aster RH: Heparin-induced thrombocytopenia associated with fondaparinux. *N Engl J Med* 356(25):2653–2655, 2007.
25. Miyares MA, Davis KA: Direct-acting oral anticoagulants as emerging treatment options for heparin-induced thrombocytopenia. *Ann Pharmacother* 49(6):735–739, 2015.
26. Hopkins CK, Goldfinger D: Platelet transfusions in heparin-induced thrombocytopenia: a report of four cases and review of the literature. *Transfusion* 48(10):2128–2132, 2008.
27. Saltzman DJ, Chang JC, Jimenez JC, et al: Postoperative thrombotic thrombocytopenic purpura after open heart operations. *Ann Thorac Surg* 89(1):119–123, 2010.
28. Chapman K, Seldon M, Richards R: Thrombotic microangiopathies, thrombotic thrombocytopenic purpura, and ADAMTS-13. *Semin Thromb Hemost* 38(1):47–54, 2012.
29. Sadler JE: Von Willebrand factor, ADAMTS13, and thrombotic thrombocytopenic purpura. *Blood* 112(1):11–18, 2008.
30. George JN, Nester CM: Syndromes of thrombotic microangiopathy. *N Engl J Med* 371(7):654–666, 2014.
31. Park YA, Waldrum MR, Marques MB: Platelet count and prothrombin time help distinguish thrombotic thrombocytopenic purpura-hemolytic uremic syndrome from disseminated intravascular coagulation in adults. *Am J Clin Pathol* 133(3):460–465, 2010.
32. Bittencourt CE, Ha JP, Maitta RW: Re-examination of 30-day survival and relapse rates in patients with thrombotic thrombocytopenic purpura-hemolytic uremic syndrome. *PLoS One* 10(5):e0127744, 2015.
33. Donegani E, Hillebrandt D, Windsor J, et al: Pre-existing cardiovascular conditions and high altitude travel. Consensus statement of the Medical Commission of the Union Internationale des Associations d'Alpinisme (UIAA MedCom) Travel Medicine and Infectious Disease. *Travel Med Infect Dis* 12(3):237–252, 2014.
34. Balduini CL, Gugliotta L, Luppi M, et al: High versus standard dose methylprednisolone in the acute phase of idiopathic thrombotic thrombocytopenic purpura: a randomized study. *Ann Hematol* 89(6):591–596, 2010.
35. Rock GA, Shumak KH, Buskard NA, et al: Comparison of plasma exchange with plasma infusion in the treatment of thrombotic thrombocytopenic purpura. *N Engl J Med* 325:393–397, 1991.
36. Lim W, Vesely SK, George JN: The role of rituximab in the management of patients with acquired thrombotic thrombocytopenic purpura. *Blood* 125(10):1526–1531, 2015.
37. Sayani FA, Abrams CS: How I treat refractory thrombotic thrombocytopenic purpura. *Blood* 125(25):3860–3867, 2015.
38. Karch H, Friedrich AW, Gerber A, et al: New aspects in the pathogenesis of enteropathic hemolytic uremic syndrome. *Semin Thromb Hemost* 32(2):105–112, 2006.
39. Menne J, Nitschke M, Stingele R, et al: Validation of treatment strategies for enterohaemorrhagic Escherichia coli O104:H4 induced haemolytic uraemic syndrome: case-control study. *Brit Med J* 345:e4565, 2012.
40. Joseph C, Gattineni J: Complement disorders and hemolytic uremic syndrome. *Curr Opin Pediatr* 25(2):209–215, 2013.
41. Licht C, Greenbaum LA, Muus P, et al: Efficacy and safety of eculizumab in atypical hemolytic uremic syndrome from 2-year extensions of phase 2 studies. *Kidney Int* 87(5):1061–1073, 2015.
42. Kreuter J, Winters JL: Drug-associated thrombotic microangiopathies. *Semin Thromb Hemost* 38(8):839–844, 2012.
43. Wu DC, Liu JM, Chen YM, et al: Mitomycin-C induced hemolytic uremic syndrome: a case report and literature review. *Jpn J Clin Oncol* 27(2):115–118, 1997.
44. Izzedine H, Isnard-Bagnis C, Launay-Vacher V, et al: Gemcitabine-induced thrombotic microangiopathy: a systematic review. *Nephrol Dial Transplant* 21(11):3038–3045, 2006.
45. Walter RB, Joerger M, Pestalozzi BC: Gemcitabine-associated hemolytic-uremic syndrome. *Am J Kidney Dis* 40(4):E16, 2002.
46. Gore EM, Jones BS, Marques MB: Is therapeutic plasma exchange indicated for patients with gemcitabine-induced hemolytic uremic syndrome? *J Clin Apher* 24(5):209–214, 2009.
47. Al Ustwani O, Lohr J, Dy G, et al: Eculizumab therapy for gemicitabine induced hemolytic uremic syndrome: case seriers and concise review. *J Gastrointest Oncol* 5(1):E30–E33, 2014.
48. Eremina V, Jefferson JA, Kowalewska J, et al: VEGF inhibition and renal thrombotic microangiopathy. *N Engl J Med* 358(11):1129–1136, 2008.
49. Jacob S, Dunn BL, Qureshi ZP, et al: Ticlopidine-, clopidogrel-, and prasugrel-associated thrombotic thrombocytopenic purpura: a 20-year review from the Southern Network on Adverse Reactions (SONAR). *Semin Thromb Hemost* 38(8):845–853, 2012.
50. Zakarija A, Kwaan HC, Moake JL, et al: Ticlopidine- and clopidogrel-associated thrombotic thrombocytopenic purpura (TTP): review of clinical, laboratory, epidemiological, and pharmacovigilance findings (1989–2008). *Kidney Int Suppl* (112):S20–S24, 2009.
51. Clark RE: Thrombotic microangiopathy following bone marrow transplantation. *Bone Marrow Transplant* 14(4):495–504, 1994.
52. Fuge R, Bird JM, Fraser A, et al: The clinical features, risk factors and outcome of thrombotic thrombocytopenic purpura occurring after bone marrow transplantation. *Br J Haematol* 113(1):58–64, 2001.
53. Van der Plas RM, Schiphorst ME, Huizinga EG, et al: von Willebrand factor proteolysis is deficient in classic, but not in bone marrow transplantation-associated, thrombotic thrombocytopenic purpura. *Blood* 93(11):3798–3802, 1999.
54. Joshi D, James A, Quaglia A, et al: Liver disease in pregnancy. *Lancet* 375(9714):594–605, 2010.
55. Goel A, Jamwal KD, Ramachandran A, et al: Pregnancy-related liver disorders. *J Clin Exp Hepatol* 4(2):151–162, 2014.
56. Aloizos S, Seretis C, Liakos N, et al: HELLP syndrome: understanding and management of a pregnancy-specific disease. *J Obstet Gynaecol* 33(4):331–337, 2013.
57. Le Thi TD, Tieulie N, Costedoat N, et al: The HELLP syndrome in the antiphospholipid syndrome: retrospective study of 16 cases in 15 women. *Ann Rheum Dis* 64(2):273–278, 2005.
58. Martin JN Jr, Perry KG Jr, Blake PG, et al: Better maternal outcomes are achieved with dexamethasone therapy for postpartum HELLP (hemolysis, elevated liver enzymes, and thrombocytopenia) syndrome. *Am J Obstet Gynecol* 177(5):1011–1017, 1997.

59. Minakami H, Morikawa M, Yamada T, et al: Differentiation of acute fatty liver of pregnancy from syndrome of hemolysis, elevated liver enzymes and low platelet counts. *J Obstet Gynaecol Res* 40(3):641–649, 2014.
60. Scully M, Thomas M, Underwood M, et al: Thrombotic thrombocytopenic purpura and pregnancy: presentation, management, and subsequent pregnancy outcomes. *Blood* 124(2):211–219, 2014.
61. Esplin MS, Branch DW: Diagnosis and management of thrombotic microangiopathies during pregnancy. *Clin Obstet Gynecol* 42(2):360–367, 1999.
62. Dashe JS, Ramin SM, Cunningham FG: The long-term consequences of thrombotic microangiopathy (thrombotic thrombocytopenic purpura and hemolytic uremic syndrome) in pregnancy. *Obstet Gynecol* 91(5, Pt 1):662–668, 1998.
63. Fakhouri F, Roumenina L, Provot F, et al: Pregnancy-associated hemolytic uremic syndrome revisited in the era of complement gene mutations. *J Am Soc Nephrol* 21(5):859–867, 2010.
64. Levi M, ten Cate H: Disseminated intravascular coagulation. *N Engl J Med* 341(8):586–592, 1999.
65. Sharma S, Mayberry JC, DeLoughery TG, et al: Fatal cerebroembolism from nonbacterial thrombotic endocarditis in a trauma patient: case report and review. *Mil Med* 165(1):83–85, 2000.
66. Wada H, Asakura H, Okamoto K, et al: Expert consensus for the treatment of disseminated intravascular coagulation in Japan. *Thromb Res* 125(1):6–11, 2009.
67. Darmstadt GL: Acute infectious purpura fulminans: pathogenesis and medical management. *Pediatr Dermatol* 15(3):169–183, 1998.
68. Spicer TE, Rau JM: Purpura fulminans. *Am J Med* 61(4):566–571, 1976.
69. Josephson C, Nuss R, Jacobson L, et al: The varicella-autoantibody syndrome. *Pediatr Res* 50(3):345–352, 2001.
70. Gamper G, Oschatz E, Herkner H, et al: Sepsis-associated purpura fulminans in adults. *Wien Klin Wochenschr* 113(3/4):107–112, 2001.
71. Carpenter CT, Kaiser AB: Purpura fulminans in pneumococcal sepsis: case report and review. *Scand J Infect Dis* 29(5):479–483, 1997.
72. Zeerleder S, Hack CE, Wuillemin WA: Disseminated intravascular coagulation in sepsis. *Chest* 128(4):2864–2875, 2005.
73. De Jonge E, Levi M, Stoutenbeek CP, et al: Current drug treatment strategies for disseminated intravascular coagulation. *Drugs* 55:767–777, 1998.
74. Manios SG, Kanakoudi F, Maniati E: Fulminant meningococcemia. Heparin therapy and survival rate. *Scand J Infect Dis* 3(2):127–133, 1971.
75. Afshari A, Wetterslev J, Brok J, et al: Antithrombin III in critically ill patients: systematic review with meta-analysis and trial sequential analysis. *Brit Med J* 335(7632):1248–1251, 2007.
76. Davis MD, Dy KM, Nelson S: Presentation and outcome of purpura fulminans associated with peripheral gangrene in 12 patients at Mayo Clinic. *J Am Acad Dermatol* 57(6):944–956, 2007.
77. Haley KM, Russell TB, Boshkov L, et al: Fatal carboplatin-induced immune hemolytic anemia in a child with a brain tumor. *J Blood Med* 5:55–58, 2014.
78. Reese JA, Bougie DW, Curtis BR, et al: Drug-induced thrombotic microangiopathy: experience of the Oklahoma registry and the BloodCenter of Wisconsin. *Am J Hematol* 90(5):406–410, 2015.
79. Arnold DM, Nazi I, Warkentin TE, et al: Approach to the diagnosis and management of drug-induced immune thrombocytopenia. *Transfus Med Rev* 27(3):137–145, 2013.
80. Von DA, Curtis BR, Bougie DW, et al: Vancomycin-induced immune thrombocytopenia. *N Engl J Med* 356(9):904–910, 2007.
81. Aster RH, Bougie DW: Drug-induced immune thrombocytopenia. *N Engl J Med* 357(6):580–587, 2007.
82. Francois B, Trimoreau F, Vignon P, et al: Thrombocytopenia in the sepsis syndrome: role of hemophagocytosis and macrophage colony-stimulating factor. *Am J Med* 103(2):114–120, 1997.
83. Schram AM, Berliner N: How I treat hemophagocytic lymphohistiocytosis in the adult patient. *Blood* 125(19):2908–2914, 2015.
84. Amsden JR, Warmack S, Gubbins PO: Tick-borne bacterial, rickettsial, spirochetal, and protozoal infectious diseases in the United States: a comprehensive review. *Pharmacotherapy* 25(2):191–210, 2005.
85. Ismail N, Bloch KC, McBride JW: Human ehrlichiosis and anaplasmosis. *Clin Lab Med* 30(1):261–292, 2010.
86. Dumler JS, Bakken JS: Human ehrlichiosis: newly recognized infections transmitted by ticks. *Annu Rev Med* 49:201–213, 1998.
87. Fichtenbaum CJ, Peterson LR, Weil GJ: Ehrlichiosis presenting as a life-threatening illness with features of the toxic shock syndrome. *Am J Med* 95(4):351–357, 1993.
88. Sachdev SH, Joshi V, Cox ER, et al: Severe life-threatening Ehrlichia chaffeensis infections transmitted through solid organ transplantation. *Transpl Infect Dis* 16(1):119–124, 2014.
89. Hartline J, Mierek C, Knutson T, et al: Hantavirus infection in North America: a clinical review. *Am J Emerg Med* 31(6):978–982, 2013.
90. Schnittler HJ, Feldmann H: Viral hemorrhagic fever—a vascular disease? *Thromb Haemost* 89(6):967–972, 2003.
91. Geisbert TW: Emerging viruses: advances and challenges. *Curr Mol Med* 5(8):733–734, 2005.
92. Paessler S, Walker DH: Pathogenesis of the viral hemorrhagic fevers. *Annu Rev Pathol* 8:411–440, 2013.
93. Centers for Disease Control and Prevention (CDC): Fatal illnesses associated with a new world arenavirus–California, 1999–2000. *MMWR Morb Mortal Wkly Rep* 49(31):709–711, 2000.
94. DeLoughery TG: Critical care clotting catastrophies. *Crit Care Clin* 21(3):531-562, 2005.
95. Beeching NJ, Fenech M, Houlihan CF: Ebola virus disease. *Brit Med J* 349:g7348, 2014.
96. Dan ME, Schiffer CA: Strategies for managing refractoriness to platelet transfusions. *Curr Hematol Rep* 2(2):158–164, 2003.
97. Christie DJ, van Buren N, Lennon SS, et al: Vancomycin-dependent antibodies associated with thrombocytopenia and refractoriness to platelet transfusion in patients with leukemia. *Blood* 75(2):518–523, 1990.
98. Fricke W, Alling D, Kimball J, et al: Lack of efficacy of tranexamic acid in thrombocytopenic bleeding. *Transfusion* 31:345–348, 1991.
99. Hod E, Schwartz J: Platelet transfusion refractoriness. *Br J Haematol* 142(3):348–360, 2008.
100. Merrill JT, Asherson RA: Catastrophic antiphospholipid syndrome. *Nat Clin Pract Rhuem* 2:81–89, 2006.
101. Gonzalez CE, Pengetze YM: Post-transfusion purpura. *Curr Hematol Rep* 4:154–159, 2005.
102. Mueller-Eckhardt C, Kiefel V: High-dose IgG for post-transfusion purpura-revisited. *Blut* 57(4):163–167, 1988.
103. Crowther MA, Cook DJ, Albert M, et al: The 4Ts scoring system for heparin-induced thrombocytopenia in medical-surgical intensive care unit patients. *J Crit Care* 25:287–293, 2010.
104. Lo GK, Juhl D, Warkentin TE, et al: Evaluation of pretest clinical score (4 T's) for the diagnosis of heparin-induced thrombocytopenia in two clinical settings. *J Thromb Haemost* 4(4):759–765, 2006.
105. George JN, Raskob GE, Shah SR, et al: Drug-induced thrombocytopenia: a systematic review of published case reports. *Ann Intern Med* 129:886–890, 1998.
106. Green D, Hougie C, Kazmier FJ, et al: Report of the working party on acquired inhibitors of coagulation: studies of the "lupus" anticoagulant. *Thromb Haemost* 49:144–146, 1983.
107. Cook GC, Zumla A, (eds): *Manson's Tropical Diseases*. W.B. Saunders, 2004.
108. Hunter GW, Strickland TG, Magill AJ, et al, (eds): *Hunter's Tropical Medicine and Emerging Infectious Diseases*. 8th ed. W.B. Saunders, 2004.

Chapter 92 ■ Venous Thromboembolism and Associated Prothrombotic Disorders in the Intensive Care Unit

ERIC S. CHRISTENSON • SHEETAL KARNE • ASHKAN EMADI • MICHAEL B. STREIFF

INCIDENCE

Venous thromboembolism (VTE), which includes deep vein thrombosis (DVT) and pulmonary embolism (PE), is a common cause of morbidity and mortality affecting over 600,000 Americans each year and causing up to 50,000 deaths [1]. The risk of VTE is particularly high among critical care patients. In the PROTECT trial, a prospective multicenter study of thromboprophylaxis in the intensive care unit (ICU) patients, 7.7% of patients developed VTE despite thromboprophylaxis [2]. Therefore, knowledge of risk factors, as well as evidence-based approaches to prevention and treatment of VTE, is essential for critical care physicians.

RISK FACTORS

Recognizing the conditions that predispose patients to VTE is essential because more than 60% of PE-related deaths occur in patients who go untreated, because the diagnosis was unsuspected and, therefore, undetected [3]. Virtually, all the identified risk factors for VTE can be classified into one of the three classic components of Virchow triad of stasis, venous injury, and hypercoagulability described nearly 150 years ago (Table 92.1) [4,5]. Inherited or acquired thrombophilia states are present in more than 20% of patients with VTE and occur at higher frequency among patients with idiopathic or recurrent VTE (see Table 92.3) [4–6].

TABLE 92.1

Risk Factors for First Episode of Venous Thromboembolism

Genetic Risk Factors
Antithrombin deficiency
Protein C deficiency
Protein S deficiency[a]
Factor V Leiden
Prothrombin gene mutation
Non-O ABO blood group
Dysfibrinogenemia[a]
Elevated factor VIII
Elevated factor IX
Elevated factor XI
Hyperhomocysteinemia (including homocystinuria)[a]
Acquired Risk Factors
Increasing age[a]
Cancer[a]
Antiphospholipid syndrome[a]
Infections (HIV, sepsis, etc.)[a]
Inflammatory disorders (e.g., SLE, IBD, vasculitis, etc.)[a]
Nephrotic syndrome
Obesity
Smoking
Environmental
Surgery (major inpatient, ambulatory)[a]
Trauma[a]
Immobilization
Central venous catheter
Pregnancy/postpartum
Hormonal therapy (e.g., oral, transcutaneous, vaginal ring contraceptive, Depot progestin injections, hormone replacement, etc.)
Chemotherapy
Vena cava filter
Travel

[a]Associated with arterial thromboembolism in the absence of patent foramen ovale.
SLE, systemic lupus erythematosus; IBD, inflammatory bowel disease.

Inherited Hypercoagulable Disorders

Factor V Leiden

Factor V Leiden (FVL) is the most common inherited thrombophilic state affecting 5% of European Americans, 2% of Hispanic Americans, 1% of African Americans and Native Americans, and 0.5% of Asian Americans [7]. FVL refers to a point mutation (G1691A), which results in a single amino acid change (Arg506Gln) at the site in the factor V protein where it is cleaved by activated protein C (PC). The mutation markedly slows the rate of inactivation of factor Va by activated PC, leading to more thrombin generation. FVL heterozygosity is associated with a fivefold increased risk of first-ever VTE, whereas homozygosity imparts 80-fold increased risk. FVL does not increase the risk of arterial thromboembolism [8]. FVL heterozygosity and homozygosity increase the risk of *recurrent* VTE by 1.6-fold and 2.7-fold, respectively [9]. The activated PC resistance assay is used to screen for the presence of FVL. Commercially available polymerase chain reaction (PCR)–based assays are used to confirm the diagnosis [10].

Prothrombin G20210A Mutation

The prothrombin G20210A mutation (PGM) is present in approximately 1% of non-Hispanic whites and Mexican Americans and in 0.3% of African Americans [11]. It is associated with a 30% increase in prothrombin levels in heterozygotes, resulting in a 2.8-fold increased risk of VTE [12]. Although homozygosity is rare, it is associated with a 70% increase in prothrombin levels and imparts a 3.8-fold increased risk of first-ever VTE among carriers [8]. Similar to FVL, the PGM does not increase the risk of arterial thromboembolism [13]. Diagnosis of both FVL and PGM are diagnosed via PCR-based testing of peripheral blood with excellent analytical validity [10].

Compound Heterozygotes for the Factor V Leiden and Prothrombin G20210A Mutations

Given the relatively high frequency of the FVL mutation and PGM in the population, compound heterozygosity occasionally is identified. In a systematic review, Segal et al. estimated that the pooled odds ratio (OR) for recurrent VTE in compound heterozygotes was 4.8% [9].

Protein C deficiency

PC is an important endogenous anticoagulant protein that inactivates activated factors V and VIII. Heterozygous PC deficiency affects 0.2% of the general population and 3.2% of unselected patients with their first episode of VTE [14]. It is associated with a sevenfold increased risk of VTE [15]. Homozygous PC deficiency is a rare serious thrombophilic syndrome that causes life-threatening thrombotic complications shortly after birth, a condition called *neonatal purpura fulminans*. Deficiency of PC may by quantitative (type I deficiency) or qualitative (type II). Therefore, accurate diagnostic testing should include both PC activity and antigen levels. Acquired causes of PC deficiency include disseminated intravascular coagulation (DIC), acute thrombosis, vitamin K deficiency, vitamin K antagonist (VKA) therapy (e.g., warfarin), and liver disease. Therefore, diagnostic testing should be performed in the absence of these conditions to ensure accurate interpretation [16].

Protein S deficiency

Protein S (PS) is the nonenzymatic cofactor for activated PC. PS circulates in two forms: approximately 60% is bound to C4b protein whereas the remaining 40% is free. Only free PS has cofactor activity. The incidence of PS deficiency in the general population has been estimated to be 0.03% to 0.13%. PS deficiency affects 7.3% of unselected patients with venous thrombosis [14]. PS deficiency is associated with an eightfold increased risk of VTE [15], and may be a risk factor for arterial thromboembolism [17,18].

Deficiency of PS may by quantitative (type I deficiency) or qualitative (type II). An additional type of PS deficiency (type III) can be acquired during pregnancy, inflammatory states, and estrogen therapy, which increase C4b protein levels, leading to reduced free PS. Other acquired causes of PS deficiency include vitamin K deficiency, VKA therapy, acute thrombosis, and liver disease. For accurate diagnosis of PS deficiency, tests, including PS activity, total PS antigen, and free PS antigen, should be measured in the absence of conditions associated with acquired PS deficiency [19].

Antithrombin deficiency

Antithrombin (AT) inhibits serine protease coagulation factors by binding to the active site of the target serine protease (e.g., thrombin, activated factors X and IX, etc.) and forming an inactive complex. Heterozygous type I AT deficiency is rare, affecting 1 in 2,000 individuals in the population. It is associated with an 8- to 10-fold increased risk of thrombosis and is present in 1% to 2% of patients with thrombosis [20]. AT deficiency does not increase the risk of arterial thromboembolism [17,18]. Deficiency of AT may be quantitative (type I) or qualitative (type II). Complete AT deficiency is incompatible with life. The diagnosis of AT deficiency is made by measuring AT activity and antigen levels. Acquired AT deficiency may occur in acute thrombosis, DIC, and during heparin therapy. Spurious increases in AT can be seen during therapy with VKA [20].

The use of AT complex (ATC) concentrates as replacement therapy should be limited to conditions with low levels of functional AT and with associated thrombotic imbalance. For example, administration of ATC is recommended for individuals with congenital AT deficiency and for prophylaxis of VTE or treatment of ongoing thrombosis. ATC may also be considered in situations of increased consumption, such as DIC; however, evidence for its use in DIC associated with trauma, burns, or pregnancy, as well as individuals on extracorporeal circulation, is limited [21].

Dysfibrinogenemia

Dysfibrinogenemia is a rare inherited thrombophilic state caused by mutations in the Aα, Bβ, or γ fibrinogen genes. It affects fewer than 1% of individuals with VTE. Acquired dysfibrinogenemia is associated with chronic liver disease and cirrhosis as well as hepatocellular and renal cell carcinoma. Approximately one-third of cases of dysfibrinogenemia are complicated by thrombosis (venous more commonly than arterial), possibly because of reduced binding to thrombin or inhibition of fibrinolysis. Diagnosis of dysfibrinogenemia is made by measuring fibrinogen function (e.g., Clauss fibrinogen assay) and fibrinogen antigen levels. In dysfibrinogenemia, typically the fibrinogen activity is much lower than the fibrinogen level [22].

Hyperhomocysteinemia

Homocysteine is a thiol-containing amino acid that is converted to methionine by methionine synthase with vitamin B_{12} and 5-methyltetrahydrofolate as cofactors. Homocysteine is also converted to cysteine by cystathionine β-synthase (CBS) which requires pyridoxine (vitamin B_6) as a cofactor. Congenital causes of hyperhomocysteinemia include homocystinuria (deficiency of CBS) and inheritance of the thermolabile mutation in the methylene tetrahydrofolate reductase (MTHFR) gene [23]. Acquired causes of hyperhomocysteinemia include deficiency of vitamin B_{12}, folate, and pyridoxine, as well as renal insufficiency [24].

Hyperhomocysteinemia has been associated with a 20% increase in cardiovascular disease for each 5 μmol per L increase in fasting homocysteine levels [25]. Homozygosity for the MTHFR mutation is associated with an approximately 1.2-fold increased risk of coronary artery disease [23]. This risk appears to be significantly modified by folate status. Hyperhomocystenemia is also associated with a twofold to threefold higher risk of initial and recurrent VTE [26,27]. However, randomized studies of vitamin supplementation in patients with venous and arterial thrombotic disease did not demonstrate improved clinical outcomes [28]. The diagnosis of hyperhomocysteinemia is based upon demonstrating elevated levels of homocysteine in a fasting blood sample. Methionine loading prior to sampling can increase the sensitivity of testing.

Elevated Coagulation Factor Levels

Elevated factor VIII (>95 percentile) has been associated with an increased risk of initial and recurrent VTE [29,30]. Elevated factor VIII levels appear to be inherited, but the responsible genetic alterations have yet to be completely characterized. Inflammatory conditions, which are common among patients in the critical care setting, may also transiently raise factor VIII. Elevated factor IX and XI antigen levels have been associated with a 2.5- and 2.2-fold increased risk of initial VTE, respectively [31,32].

Acquired Hypercoagulable Disorders

Surgery

In the first 6 weeks after an operation, the risk of VTE is 70-fold that of the general population. The risk of VTE gradually declines over time to 20-fold that of the general population in postoperative weeks 7 to 12, 9.4-fold at 4 to 6 months postoperation, and 3.7-fold at 10 to 12 months postoperation. In the Million Women study, hip and knee replacement surgery (7.7 per 1,000 persons-months), cancer surgery (4.4 per 1,000 person-months), hip fracture surgery (3.8 per 1,000 person-months), and vascular surgery (3.1 per 1,000 person-months) were associated with a high risk of VTE [33].

Ethnicity and Medical Illness

Ethnicity is an important risk factor for VTE, with Caucasians and African Americans having a higher incidence of VTE than Hispanics and Asians [34]. Immobility is associated with a 9-fold increased risk of VTE [4]. Increased risk is also associated with infectious illnesses such as HIV and autoimmune disorders such as inflammatory bowel disease and systemic lupus erythematosus (SLE) [5]. Chronic hemolytic anemia such as sickle cell anemia and paroxysmal nocturnal hemoglobinuria (PNH) are associated with an increased risk of VTE [35,36].

Central Venous Catheters

Indwelling central venous catheters (CVCs), particularly common in critically ill patients, increase the propensity for venous thrombosis through a variety of mechanisms, including endothelial damage, blood flow impedance, and serving as a nidus for clot formation. Symptomatic CVC-associated deep venous thrombosis occurs in 2% to 6% of patients [37]. The risk is even higher with peripherally inserted central catheters (PICCs) which are associated with thrombosis in 14% of critical care patients [38]. Risk factors for CVC-associated DVT include femoral and subclavian insertion sites, number of catheter lumens and catheter size, PICC versus other CVC, location of catheter tip, history of previous VTE, and presence of active cancer [37]. Among hospitalized patients, the critically ill are at especially high risk for VTE as a result of severe underlying disease, immobility, and CVCs with the incidence of VTE corresponding to the number of risk factors present.

Cancer

Cancer is associated with a fourfold to sevenfold increased risk of VTE that varies with the type and extent of cancer and the use of chemotherapy, radiation therapy and growth factors, such as erythropoietic stimulatory agents. Neoplasms of the pancreas, brain, and stomach place patients at high risk for development of thromboembolism, whereas lung and colon cancers are associated with intermediate risk and breast and prostate cancer are associated with a lower risk. Compared to squamous cell carcinoma, adenocarcinoma is associated with a higher risk of thromboembolism. Metastatic disease is associated with a higher risk of thromboembolism than localized cancer [39–41].

Unlike most of the inherited hypercoagulable conditions, cancer is associated with both arterial thromboembolism and VTE. Thromboembolism can be the first sign of an occult malignancy. Unprovoked thromboembolic events are 4.8-fold more commonly associated with the presence of occult malignancy than provoked episodes of thromboembolism [42]. Although routine imaging to detect occult cancer is not associated with a survival benefit in patients with unprovoked VTE [43], we recommend age-appropriate cancer screening (e.g., colonoscopy). Cancer patients are twofold to threefold more likely to suffer recurrent VTE [44]. Low molecular weight heparin (LMWH) has been shown to reduce the incidence of recurrent VTE by 50% in patients with cancer [45]. Therefore, LMWH rather than oral VKAs is considered the agent of choice for long-term management of VTE in cancer patients.

Myeloproliferative Neoplasms

Myeloproliferative neoplasms, in particular polycythemia vera (PV), are associated with an increased risk of arterial thromboembolism and VTE that is mediated, at least in part, by erythrocytosis and the associated increased whole blood viscosity, as well as functional abnormalities in leukocytes and platelets. Risk factors for thromboembolism include age older than 60 years, a previous history of thromboembolism, poorly controlled erythrocytosis, leukocytosis, thrombocytosis, the presence of additional thrombophilic conditions, the JAK2-V617F mutation, and the presence of cardiovascular risk factors, including diabetes, hypertension, hyperlipidemia, and smoking. It is essential to control erythrocytosis in patients with PV, particularly if they are scheduled for surgery. In patients with PV and essential thrombocythemia, aspirin decreases the probability of arterial thromboembolism. In patients older than 60 years of age or those who have prior thromboembolic events, cytoreductive therapy with hydroxyurea, anagrelide, or α-interferon should be strongly considered. Anticoagulation is appropriate for patients who suffer VTE [46,47].

Paroxysmal Nocturnal Hemogobinuria

PNH is a rare clonal hematopoietic stem cell disorder associated with decreased expression of complement regulatory proteins (CD55 and CD59) on blood cell membranes. This acquired genetic alteration results in chronic intravascular hemolysis, pancytopenia, and a strong predisposition to venous (more common) and arterial (less common) thromboses [48,49]. Unusual locations for thrombosis (e.g., mesenteric vein thrombosis) are not uncommon in PNH patients. The diagnosis of PNH can be confirmed with flow cytometry to detect the presence/absence of CD55 and CD59 (using antibodies) or glycosylphosphatidlyinositol-anchored proteins on the surface of blood cell membranes. Symptomatic patients with significant hemolysis, fatigue, or end-organ damage or thromboembolism should be treated with eculizumab (monoclonal antibody against complement protein C5a). For patients with thromboembolism, conventional anticoagulation is appropriate although it is not always effective in preventing recurrent events. Eculizumab therapy reduces the risk of recurrent thromboembolism by more than 90% [49].

Pregnancy and Postpartum

VTE is a leading cause of death in pregnant women. The age-adjusted risk of VTE is at least fivefold higher compared with nonpregnant women [50]. Pregnancy is accompanied by hormonal changes that increase the prothrombotic potential of the blood that include increases in factor VIII, fibrinogen, von Willebrand factor, and plasminogen activator inhibitor 1 and decreases in free PS. In addition, decreased mobility, increased venous distensibility, and compression of the inferior vena cava (IVC) and iliac veins by the uterus lead to venous stasis. Left leg DVT is more common owing to disproportionate compression of the left venous system by the gravid uterus [51,52].

The antepartum risk of VTE is highest in the third trimester. The immediate postpartum period is associated with the highest risk which declines to baseline by 12 weeks postpartum [53,54]. Risk factors for VTE during pregnancy include a previous history of VTE, thrombophilia, surgical delivery, age greater than 35 years, obesity, and comorbid medical illness, such as sickle cell anemia [55].

Heparin-Induced Thrombocytopenia

Thrombocytopenia affects approximately 20% of patients in the ICU [56]. Although heparin-induced thrombocytopenia (HIT) is uncommon in the ICU [57], prompt recognition and treatment are essential because of the adverse consequences associated with this condition. Surgical patients (particularly, orthopedic and cardiothoracic) are at high risk for HIT, whereas medical patients are at intermediate risk and obstetric and pediatric patients are at low risk [58]. The pretest probability of HIT can be assessed using the "4T score," a validated clinical prediction rule (see Chapter 91 for the elements of the 4T score and newer proposed clinical tools) [59]. Without treatment, the mortality of HIT is as high as 20% to 25% with a similar percentage of patients surviving with major complications (e.g., stroke or limb loss). Early diagnosis and treatment has improved mortality and morbidity to 5% to 10% [60]. Additional information regarding the pathophysiology and management of HIT is discussed in Chapter 91, "Thrombocytopenia."

Major Trauma

Major trauma is an important cause of VTE in the ICU. Fifty-eight percent of trauma patients develop venographic VTE in the absence of thromboprophylaxis [61]. Trauma is a potent stimulus for clot formation because it impacts all three elements of Virchow' triad. Patients are immobilized (stasis) for a prolonged period of time and have extensive vascular and tissue damage (vascular wall injury), leading to tissue factor and collagen exposure resulting in activated coagulation (hypercoagulability) [62]. Thromboprophylaxis with enoxaparin (30 mg subcutaneously twice daily), which appears to be more effective than unfractionated heparin (UFH) (5,000 units twice daily), can reduce the incidence of VTE by 50% in major trauma patients [63]. Mechanical prophylaxis with intermittent pneumatic compression devices are a useful adjunctive measure, if feasible, based on the patient's injuries.

Given the high incidence of VTE, critical care physicians should maintain a high index of suspicion and confirm any clinical findings indicative of thrombosis with objective radiologic testing. Although some have advocated routine radiologic surveillance and prophylactic vena cava filter placement as strategies to reduce VTE in trauma patients, the value of these strategies remains unproven [64,65]. Acute VTE should be managed by conventional anticoagulation. If contraindications present, an optional vena cava filter can be placed until the patient can tolerate anticoagulation.

Drug-induced hypercoagulable conditions

Hormonal therapies, including combined estrogen–progestin oral contraceptives and estrogen replacement therapy, are associated with a threefold to fourfold and twofold increased risk of VTE, respectively [66]. The estrogen vaginal ring and oral, as well as depot medroxyprogesterone, also appears to be associated with increased risk. The low-dose progestin intrauterine device thus far has not been associated with increased risk [67]. Selective estrogen receptor modulators tamoxifen and raloxifene; immunomodulatory imide drugs, including thalidomide, lenalidomide, and pomalidomide; erythropoietic stimulatory agents; and atypical antipsychotics, including clozapine, quetiapine, olanzapine, and risperidone; have been associated with an increased risk of thromboembolism [42,68].

Detection of acute thrombosis in a patient receiving one of these medications typically is a sufficient criterion for discontinuation, and the use of such agents in patients with a prior history of thromboembolism must be considered very carefully, weighing the potential benefit against the potential for recurrent thrombosis. In patients whose condition warrants continued treatment with the medication, concomitant anticoagulation should be considered to prevent recurrent thromboembolism. In the MEGA study, resumption of oral contraceptives was associated with more than a twofold increase in recurrence rates compared with patients who did not resume hormonal therapy after an initial hormone-associated VTE [69].

Antiphospholipid Antibody Syndrome

The antiphospholipid antibody syndrome (APS) is an acquired, autoimmune thrombophilic disorder that is associated with an increased risk of venous and/or arterial thromboembolism, recurrent pregnancy losses, thrombocytopenia, renal insufficiency, vasculitis, and cardiac valvular abnormalities. APS may be primary (not as a result of any immediately apparent underlying autoimmune disorder) or secondary, most commonly in association with rheumatologic diseases such as SLE. The diagnostic criteria for APS require the occurrence of one or more objectively documented episodes of thromboembolism or recurrent pregnancy losses in association with positive laboratory testing for lupus anticoagulants (LA) or immunoglobin G (IgG)/IgM anticardiolipin antibodies or β-2 glycoprotein I antibody performed on at least two occasions 12 or more weeks apart, and at least 23 weeks after the thrombotic event [70].

The prevalence of elevated anticardiolipin antibodies or LAs in the general population varies from 1% to 5%. Approximately 15% to 30% of patients with SLE have an elevated LA and 20% to 40% have an elevated anticardiolipin antibody. The mean age of onset of APS is 31 years. Onset after age 50 is uncommon [71]. In a mixed population of patients with and without SLE, the incidence of thromboembolism in patients with APS was 2.8% per year [72]. In a cohort of SLE patients, 50% suffered a thromboembolic event over 20 years (2.5% per year) [73]. Patients with a positive LA or β-2 glycoprotein I antibodies appear to be at higher risk for thromboembolism than patients with anticardiolipin antibodies [70]. In addition, IgG β-2 glycoprotein I antibodies appear to confer a greater risk of thrombosis than IgM antibodies [72,74]. Triple-positive patients (i.e., patients positive for LAs, β-2 glycoprotein I antibodies, and anticardiolipin antibodies) appear to be at particularly high risk for thromboembolism with 44% suffering thromboembolism over 10 years [75].

The most common manifestation of APS that would bring patients to the ICU is VTE or arterial thromboembolism. A retrospective review of APS patients noted that 59% had VTE, 28% arterial thromboembolism, and 13% both VTE and arterial thromboembolism [76]. In the ICU, the diagnosis of APS is made by objectively confirming clinical manifestations (thromboembolism and pregnancy morbidity) and documenting laboratory evidence of antiphospholipid antibodies.

Treatment of VTE in patients with APS is similar to that for patients with other thrombophilic disorders with several important caveats. APS patients who have an abnormal LA often have baseline prolongation of their activated thromboplastin time (aPTT). If the standard therapeutic range is used in these patients', UFH may be underdosed. Therefore, patients with a prolonged aPTT at baseline should be treated with an LMWH or have their UFH therapy monitored with an anti-Xa heparin activity assay.

Similar precautions should be taken when considering chronic anticoagulation with a VKA in an LA-positive APS patient. These patients' LA can prolong the PT/international normalized ratio (INR), giving health care providers the false impression of therapeutic anticoagulation. Therefore, LA-positive patients starting VKA therapy should have their INR correlated with a chromogenic factor X activity assay (therapeutic range, 20% to 40%) [71,77,78]. This test may also be useful if an APS patient experiences a recurrent thromboembolic event despite conventional intensity anticoagulation. A higher INR target range or alternative anticoagulants (e.g., LMWH, fondaparinux) may be necessary [71,79].

For patients with APS and arterial thromboembolism, we also prefer therapeutic anticoagulation rather than antiplatelet agents. Although one study suggested that aspirin and warfarin were equally effective for arterial thromboembolism, participants did not fulfill criteria for APS [80].

Catastrophic Antiphospholipid Syndrome

Catastrophic antiphospholipid syndrome (CAPS) is a rare (<1% of APS patients) and potentially life-threatening manifestation of APS characterized by multiorgan (kidneys, brain, skin, liver, etc.) dysfunction as a result of diffuse microvascular thrombosis. CAPS is often triggered by infections, major surgery, or discontinuation of immunosuppression or anticoagulation.

TABLE 92.2

Clinical Manifestations of Catastrophic Antiphospholipid Syndrome

Organ system	Manifestations
Blood	Coombs positive hemolytic anemia, autoimmune thrombocytopenia, DIC, bone marrow infarct
Brain	Infarcts, encephalopathy, seizure, transient ischemic attack
Heart	Valvular lesions (Libman–Sacks endocarditis), myocardial infarction, heart failure
Kidney	A 50% increase in serum creatinine, severe systemic hypertension (>180/100 mm Hg), and/or proteinuria (>500 mg/24 h)
Lung	Acute respiratory distress syndrome (most common) [68], pulmonary hypertension with normal cardiac output and pulmonary capillary wedge pressure, pulmonary hemorrhage
Skin	Livedo reticularis, skin ulcers, digital ischemia, purpura, skin necrosis
Vasculature	Venous and/or arterial thromboembolism, including deep venous thrombosis, pulmonary embolism, extremity artery thromboembolism, portal vein and inferior vena cava thrombosis, retinal artery and vein thrombosis

DIC, disseminated intravascular coagulation.

Almost all patients with CAPS require an ICU level of care. Common manifestations of CAPS-associated organ involvement are displayed in Table 92.2 [81].

CAPS is thought to be the result of widespread activation of the endothelium, monocytes, and platelets with tissue factor expression and diffuse activation of the coagulation cascade, resulting in widespread microvascular thrombosis and tissue infarction. The differential diagnosis in patients suspected to have CAPS usually includes severe sepsis, thrombotic thrombocytopenic purpura, hemolytic uremic syndrome, DIC, infectious purpura fulminans, and HIT.

Multimodality therapy is necessary for effective treatment of CAPS. The mainstay of therapy includes anticoagulation (e.g., weight-based UFH titrated to a therapeutic aPTT or anti-Xa heparin level) and immunosuppression with corticosteroids (e.g., intravenous [IV] pulse methylprednisolone 1,000 mg per day for 3 to 5 days followed 1 to 2 mg/kg/d for 2 to 3 weeks). Second-line therapies that are frequently employed in addition to anticoagulation and corticosteroids include IV immunoglobulins (total dose 2,000 mg per kg [400 mg/kg/d for 5 days or 1,000 mg/kg/d for 2 days]), plasmapheresis, and rituximab (375 mg per m^2 weekly for 4 weeks). Fibrinolytic agents are often used to treat life- or limb-threatening venous or arterial thrombosis. Third-line therapies include cyclophosphamide, prostacyclin (5 ng/kg/min for 7 days [per case reports]), and defibrotide (100 to 275 mg/kg/d for a minimum of 3 weeks). Emerging data suggest that eculizumab may be an effective treatment for CAPS [82].

Treatment of potential precipitating factors of CAPS is also extremely important. Such measures include broad-spectrum antibiotics for infections, aggressive hemodynamic resuscitation in case of shock, debridement or amputation for necrotic tissues, mechanical ventilation, renal replacement therapy, tight glycemic control, stomach acid suppression, and control of malignant hypertension in case of renal artery/vein thromboses. Intravascular instrumentation, especially arterial, should be minimized because of the potential for new clot formation [83].

CAPS mortality rate remains as high as 48% despite all therapies. The clinical manifestations related to poor prognosis and mortality include involvement of the kidney, spleen, lung, and adrenal, as well as history of SLE. Approximately 25% of the survivors will develop further APS-related events, but it is rare to develop recurrent CAPS [83].

Diagnostic Approach to Hypercoagulable Conditions

Because testing for inherited hypercoagulable conditions is expensive and has yet to be demonstrated to significantly influence patient outcomes, there should a strong clinical rationale for considering thrombophilia testing focusing on individuals likely to benefit from the results.

Testing in the setting of an acute thrombosis (including in the critical care setting) is rarely appropriate, with the exception of HIT and APS in patients with suspected CAPS, because acute thrombosis and its treatment can influence test results. The summary of appropriate laboratory tests for hypercoagulable conditions is demonstrated in Table 92.3.

PATHOPHYSIOLOGY

The precise sequence of events that leads to venous thrombosis is not fully understood and likely varies based on dynamic interactions between genetic and acquired risk factors. In one proposed scheme, blood stasis–induced hypoxia or direct vein wall injury results in endothelial disruption or activation with the exposure of tissue factor on the luminal surface of the vessel triggering initiation of the coagulation cascade, leading to thrombin generation and fibrin deposition [84,85]. Therefore, it is not surprising that many venous thrombi arise in valve pockets where blood flow tends to stagnate, or at a specific area of vascular disruption such as at a CVC insertion site.

Proximal lower extremity DVT is the most frequent source of PE. In untreated patients with proximal DVT, approximately half will go on to develop PE. Other sources of PE include pelvic, renal, or upper extremity veins, as well as the right heart. Embolism to the lungs typically occurs 3 to 7 days after the development of a DVT. After traveling to the lungs, a large thrombus may occlude a major pulmonary artery and cause significant cardiovascular symptoms, or it may break up into smaller clots traveling distally, where it is more likely to produce pleuritic chest pain. Thrombi are most frequently carried to the lower lobes because of preferential blood flow to this location [86].

Hypoxemia results from occlusion of pulmonary vessels and intrapulmonary shunting of blood which leads to an increase in ventilation/perfusion ($\dot{V}/\dot{Q}$) mismatch frequently producing an elevated alveolar-to-arteriolar oxygen gradient. For patients with a patent foramen ovale, progressive pulmonary hypertension may lead to a right-to-left intra-atrial shunt precipitating worsening hypoxemia and, rarely, paradoxic embolization [87,88]. The hemodynamic response to PE varies, depending on the degree of vascular occlusion and the presence of underlying cardiopulmonary disease. The decrease in the cross-sectional area of the pulmonary arterial bed that results from PE leads to increased pulmonary vascular resistance. Pulmonary hypertension suppresses right ventricular (RV) outflow precipitating a reduction in left ventricular (LV) preload and, ultimately, diminished cardiac output and systemic hypotension. Progressive vascular obstruction and hypoxemia promote a vicious cycle of increasing vasoconstriction and further rises

TABLE 92.3

Laboratory Testing for Prothrombotic Conditions

Condition	Test	Timing	Potential causes of erroneous results
Factor V Leiden	Activated protein C resistance	Anytime	anti-Xa level >1.0 units/mL
	Factor V Leiden PCR based	Anytime	DNA contamination
Prothrombin gene mutation	Factor II PCR-based testing	Anytime	DNA contamination
Protein C deficiency	PC activity (if abnormal, then protein C antigen)	Prior to anticoagulation or after discontinuation	Acute thrombosis, DIC, warfarin, vitamin K deficiency, anti-Xa level >1.0 units/mL, lupus anticoagulant, elevated factor VIII concentrations, liver disease
Protein S deficiency	Protein S activity (if abnormal, then total and free protein S antigen)	Prior to anticoagulation or after discontinuation	Acute thrombosis, DIC, warfarin, vitamin K deficiency, estrogen therapy, pregnancy/postpartum, anti-Xa level >1.0 units/mL, lupus anticoagulant, elevated factor VIII concentrations, liver disease
Antithrombin deficiency	Antithrombin activity (if abnormal, then antithrombin antigen)	Prior to anticoagulation or after discontinuation	Acute thrombosis, DIC, warfarin, vitamin K deficiency, anti-Xa level >1.0 units/mL, lupus anticoagulant, elevated factor VIII concentrations, liver disease, nephrotic syndrome
Dysfibrinogenemia	Fibrinogen activity (i.e., standard Clauss fibrinogen assay), thrombin time, fibrinogen antigen, Reptilase time	Prior to anticoagulation with heparin or direct thrombin inhibitors	Heparin (thrombin time is very sensitive to heparin, fibrinogen less sensitive, Reptilase time and fibrinogen antigen insensitive), direct thrombin inhibitors affect thrombin time and fibrinogen activity, myeloma proteins, liver disease
Hyperhomocysteinemia	Homocysteine level	Fasting, with or without methionine loading at anytime	Renal insufficiency, vitamin B12 deficiency, folate deficiency
Elevated factor VIII levels	Factor VIII activity	At least 6 mo after thrombotic event in the absence of inflammation	Acute phase response (e.g., infection, inflammation, postsurgery), heparin, direct thrombin inhibitors, DIC
Elevated factor IX levels	Factor IX antigen	At least 6 mo after thrombotic event after discontinuation of warfarin	Acute thrombosis, DIC, warfarin, vitamin K deficiency, liver disease
Elevated factor XI levels	Factor XI antigen	At least 6 mo after thrombotic event	Acute thrombosis, DIC, severe liver disease
Heparin-induced thrombocytopenia	ELISA assay	Anytime	Elevated immunoglobulin level
	Serotonin release assay	Anytime	
Antiphospholipid syndrome	Activated partial thromboplastin time (low phospholipid reagent) + mixing studies with normal plasma	At diagnosis of thrombotic event and at least 12 wk later	Heparin, direct thrombin inhibitors
	Dilute Russell viper venom time with confirm procedure	At diagnosis of thrombotic event and at least 12 wk later	anti-Xa level >1.0 units/mL, direct thrombin inhibitor, fondaparinux, warfarin, factors X, V, and II inhibitors
	Platelet neutralization procedure	At diagnosis of thrombotic event and at least 12 wk later	Heparin, factor V deficiency/inhibitors
	Anticardiolipin antibody ELISA	At diagnosis of thrombotic event and at least 12 wk later	Rheumatoid factor, Syphilis and HIV can result in positive test and must be ruled out
	β-2 Glycoprotein I antibody ELISA	At diagnosis of thrombotic event and at least 12 wk later	Rheumatoid factor can produce false-positive results

ELISA, enzyme-linked immunosorbent assay; PCR, polymerase chain reaction.

in pulmonary artery pressure. The normal right ventricle fails acutely when it cannot generate sufficient systolic pressure to maintain pulmonary perfusion. RV failure typically occurs when mean pulmonary artery pressures rise to greater than 40 mm Hg. Because the pulmonary circulation has a large reserve capacity, more than 50% obstruction is generally required to precipitate a significant increase in the mean pulmonary artery pressure. Patients with preexisting cardiopulmonary disease have less physiologic reserve than healthy individuals, so they may develop right heart failure with a less significant degrees of pulmonary vascular occlusion [89,90].

PREVENTION

Meta-analyses have demonstrated that pharmacologic VTE prophylaxis reduces the risk of symptomatic DVT, PE, and fatal PE by approximately 50% at the expense of a modest increase in major bleeding [91]. UFH, LMWH, and fondaparinux have all been demonstrated to be effective in medically ill patients [92–95]. Three times-daily UFH may be associated with a greater risk of bleeding than twice-daily UFH [96]. In critically ill patients, dalteparin was associated with a lower risk of DVT than twice-daily UFH [97].

Large prospective multicenter surveys have demonstrated that VTE prophylaxis is underprescribed [98]. Strategies that have been demonstrated to improve prescription of VTE prophylaxis and reduce VTE include computer alerts and mandatory clinical decision support smart order sets [99–101]. Prescription of VTE prophylaxis does not ensure its administration. Retrospective studies have demonstrated that 12% of prescribed doses of VTE prophylaxis are not administrated primarily owing to refusal. In 5% of patients, 75% or more of prescribed doses of VTE prophyaxis are not administered [102]. A retrospective study of general surgery and trauma patients found that omission of two or more doses of prophylaxis was associated with a significantly increased risk of VTE [103]. Therefore, identification of strategies to increase VTE prophylaxis administration is an important patient safety priority.

It is important to note that VTE prophylaxis may not have a favorable risk to benefit ratio for all hospitalized patients. Several risk assessment tools have been developed for hospitalized medical (Padua score-expert opinion based and Improve score-evidence based) and surgical patients (Caprini model and Rogers score) [104–107]. The Padua, Improve, and Caprini models have been validated in independent patient populations [108–110]. Given their severity of illness, all ICU patients are likely to benefit from VTE prophylaxis. However, implementation of a VTE prophylaxis order sets that include one of these risk stratification models is likely to improve the risk–benefit balance of VTE prophylaxis and should be considered at all health care facilities (Tables 92.4 to 92.6). Table 92.7 outlines available pharmacologic VTE prophylaxis options.

Pharmacologic VTE prophylaxis is associated with an increased risk of bleeding which may outweigh its benefits in patients at high risk for bleeding. The IMPROVE survey identified a number of variable associated with an increased risk of bleeding associated with anticoagulants [111]. A validation study of the IMPROVE bleeding risk score is underway. For patients at increased risk for bleeding, intermittent pneumatic compression devices have been shown to reduce the risk of DVT [112]. In contrast, graduated compression stockings do not appear to reduce VTE but do increase the risk of skin breakdown complications [113].

DIAGNOSIS

Recognizing the presence of VTE can be challenging because the signs and symptoms are neither sensitive nor specific for the diagnosis. Consequently, the most important step in diagnosis is maintaining adequate clinical suspicion [86,114]. This goal is best achieved by careful attention to each patient's constellation of risk factors, symptoms, and signs. Although clinical assessment alone is inadequate to confirm the diagnosis of VTE, both clinical gestalt and clinical prediction rules are useful in establishing the pretest probability of disease in outpatients [45–49]. Clinical pretest probability models such as the Wells criteria and pulmonary embolism rule-out criteria (PERC) serve as the foundation for diagnostic algorithms for DVT and PE (Tables 92.8 to 92.10) [115–117].

Diagnosis of VTE in the critically ill patient can be particularly challenging because underlying chronic systemic illnesses, as well as superimposed acute illnesses may mimic or mask the typical signs and symptoms of VTE. In addition, common clinical

TABLE 92.4

Padua VTE Risk Assessment Model

Clinical characteristic	Score
Active cancer (patient with local or distant metastases and/or in whom chemotherapy or radiotherapy has been performed within 6 mo)	3
Previous VTE (with the exclusion of superficial vein thrombosis)	3
Reduced mobility (bedrest with bathroom privileges for 3 d or more)	3
Known thrombophilia	3
Recent (within 1 mo) surgery or trauma	2
Age ≥70 y	1
Heart and/or respiratory failure	1
Acute myocardial infarction or ischemic stroke	1
Acute infection and/or rheumatologic disorder	1
Obesity (BMI ≥ 30)	1
Ongoing hormonal therapy	1

Low risk 3 points or less; high risk ≥4 points.
BMI, body mass index; VTE, venous thromboembolism.
Adapted from Barbar S, Noventa F, Rossetto V, et al: A risk assessment model for the identification of hospitalized medical patients at risk for venous thromboembolism: The padua prediction score. *J Thromb Haemost* 8:2450–2457, 2010.

TABLE 92.5

IMPROVE VTE Risk Assessment Score

Clinical characteristic	Score
Previous VTE	3
Known thrombophilia	2
Lower limb paralysis	2
Active cancer	2
Immobility ≥7 d (including days prior to and during hospital admission)	1
ICU/CCU stay	1
Age >60 y	1

Low risk = 0 to 1 points; moderate risk 2 to 3 points, and high risk 4 or more points.
CCU, coronary care unit; ICU, intensive care unit; VTE, venous thromboembolism.
Adapted from Mahan CE, Liu Y, Turpie AG, et al: External validation of a risk assessment model for venous thromboembolism in the hospitalised acutely-ill medical patient (VTE-VALOURR). *Thromb Haemost* 112:692–699, 2014.

TABLE 92.6

Caprini VTE Risk Assessment Model

Clinical characteristic	Score
Stroke (<1 mo)	5
Elective major lower extremity arthroplasty	5
Hip, pelvis, or leg fracture (<1 mo)	5
Acute spinal cord injury (paralysis) (<1 mo)	5
Multiple trauma (<1 mo)	5
Age 75 y or older	3
History of DVT/PE	3
Positive factor V Leiden	3
Positive prothrombin gene G20210A mutation	3
Elevated serum homocysteine	3
Positive lupus anticoagulant	3
Elevated anticardiolipin antibodies	3
HIT (do not use heparin or low molecular weight heparin)	3
Other congenital or acquired thrombophilia	3
Family history of thrombosis	3
Age 61–74 y	2
Arthroscopic surgery	2
Malignancy (present or previous)	2
Laparoscopic surgery (>45 min)	2
Patient confined to bed (>72 h)	2
Immobilizing plaster cast (<1 mo)	2
Central venous access	2
Major surgery (>45 min)	2
Age 41–60 y	1
Swollen legs (current)	1
Varicose veins	1
Overweight/obesity (BMI >25)	1
Minor surgery planned	1
Sepsis (<1 mo)	1
Acute myocardial infarction	1
Congestive heart failure (<1 mo)	1
Medical patient at bedrest	1
History of inflammatory bowel disease	1
History of prior major surgery (<1 mo)	1
Chronic obstructive pulmonary disease	1
Serious lung disease including pneumonia (<1 mo)	1
Oral contraceptive or hormone replacement therapy	1
Pregnancy or postpartum (<1 mo)	1
History of unexplained fetal death or recurrent spontaneous abortion (≥3), premature birth with toxemia or growth-restricted infant	1

Low risk 0–1 point early ambulation; moderate risk 2 points heparin 5 000 units sc q12h or pneumatic compression device; high risk 3 to 4 points heparin 5,000 units sc q8h or enoxaparin 40 mg q24h (weight <150 kg) (30 mg sc q24h with creatinine clearance <30 mL/min and weight <150 kg) or enoxaparin 30 mg sc q12h (weight >150 kg) with option to add pneumatic compression device; very high risk 5 or more points high-risk pharmacologic options PLUS pneumatic compression device.

BMI, body mass index; DVT, deep vein thrombosis; HIT, heparin-induced thrombocytopenia PE, pulmonary embolism; VTE, venous thromboembolism.

Adapted from Caprini JA, Arcelus JI, Hasty JH, et al: Clinical assessment of venous thromboembolic risk in surgical patients. *Semin Thromb Hemost* 17[Suppl 3]:304–312, 1991.

TABLE 92.7

VTE Prophylaxis Options

Unfractionated heparin: 5,000 units sc q8–12h
7,500 units sc q8 h (obesity dosing BMI ≥40)
Low Molecular Weight Heparin
Dalteparin 5,000 units sc q24h
7,500 units q24h (obesity dosing BMI ≥40) (limited data)
Enoxaparin 40 mg sc q24h (general medical and surgical prophylaxis)
Enoxaparin 30 mg sc q24h (renal dosing; creatinine clearance 20–30 mL/min)
Enoxaparin 40 mg sc q12h (obesity dosing BMI ≥40)
Enoxaparin 30 mg sc q12h (orthopedic surgery prophylaxis)
Pentasaccharide
Fondaparinux 2.5 mg sc q24h
Renal dosing: avoid in patients with CrCl <30 mL/min; caution in patients with CrCl 30–50 mL/min
Direct Thrombin Inhibitors
Dabigatran (oral direct thrombin inhibitor)
110 mg orally 1–4 h after hip replacement surgery when hemostasis has been secured, then 220 mg orally once daily for 28–35 d
(Avoid in patients with CrCl <30 mL/min or epidural/neuraxial analgesia)
Direct Factor Xa Inhibitors
Apixaban (oral direct factor Xa inhibitor)
2.5 mg orally BID ×35 d starting 12–24 h after hip replacement surgery once hemostasis is secured
2.5 mg orally BID ×12 d starting 12–24 h after knee replacement surgery once hemostasis is secured.
Would avoid in patients with CrCl <25 mL/min or in presence of neuraxial analgesia)
Rivaroxaban (oral direct factor Xa inhibitor)
10 mg orally once daily ×35 d starting 6–10 h after hip replacement surgery once hemostasis is achieved
10 mg orally once daily ×12 d starting 6–10 h after knee replacement surgery once hemostasis is achieved
Avoid in patients with CrCl <30 mL/min and those with neuraxial analgesia

BID, twice a day; BMI, body mass index; CrCl, creatinine clearance; q, every; sc, subcutaneously; VTE, venous thromboembolism.

prediction models for VTE may not be valid in the ICU setting [118]. Furthermore, objective testing for VTE may be precluded by relative contraindications, such as mechanical ventilation, shock, and renal failure.

Symptoms and Signs

Although most DVT begin in the calf, the presenting symptoms and signs are often not noted until more proximal veins are involved [86]. The initial clinical manifestations of DVT may include warmth, erythema, swelling, and pain or tenderness and may be acute, progressive, or resolve spontaneously. Cellulitis, trauma, Baker cyst, or musculoskeletal pain can all cause signs and symptoms similar to acute DVT.

Most patients with acute PE present with at least one of the following: dyspnea, pleuritic chest pain, or tachypnea. Other findings may include tachycardia, a loud pulmonic component of the second heart sound, fever, crackles, pleural rub, and/or wheezing. Pleuritic chest pain and hemoptysis occur more commonly with pulmonary infarction as a result of smaller, peripheral emboli. PE must always be considered in cases of unexplained

TABLE 92.8

Wells Clinical DVT Model

Clinical characteristic	Score
Active cancer (patient receiving treatment for cancer within 6 m or currently receiving palliative treatment)	1
Paralysis, paresis, or recent plaster cast immobilization of the lower extremities	1
Recently bedridden for 3 d or more, or major surgery within the previous 12 wk requiring general or regional anesthesia	1
Localized tenderness along the distribution of the deep venous system	1
Entire leg swollen	1
Calf swelling at least 3 cm larger than the asymptomatic side (measured 10 cm below the tibial tuberosity)	1
Pitting edema confined to the symptomatic leg	1
Collateral superficial veins (nonvaricose)	1
Previously documented deep vein thrombosis	1
Alternative diagnosis at least as likely as deep vein thrombosis	−2

A score of ≤ 0 indicates that a low pretest probability of deep vein thrombosis. A score of 1 or 2 points indicates a moderate risk of DVT and a score of 3 or higher indicates a high risk of deep vein thrombosis.
DVT, deep vein thrombosis.
Wells PS, Anderson DR, Rodger M, et al: Evaluation of D-dimer in the diagnosis of suspected deep-vein thrombosis. *N Engl J Med* 349:1227–1235, 2003.

TABLE 92.9

Wells Clinical Pulmonary Embolism Model

Clinical characteristic	Score
Active cancer (patient receiving treatment for cancer within 6 m or currently receiving palliative treatment)	1
Surgery or bedridden for 3 d or more during the past 4 wk	1.5
History of deep venous thrombosis or pulmonary embolism	1.5
Hemoptysis	1
Heart rate >100 beats/min	1.5
Pulmonary embolism judged to be the most likely diagnosis	3
Clinical signs and symptoms compatible with deep venous thrombosis	3

A score of <2 indicates a low probability of pulmonary embolism. A score of 2 to 6 indicates an intermediate probability of PE. A score of more than 6 indicates a high probability of pulmonary embolism.
Kearon C, Ginsberg JS, Douketis J, et al: An evaluation of D-dimer in the diagnosis of pulmonary embolism: a randomized trial. *Ann Intern Med* 144(11):812–821, 2006.

TABLE 92.10

Revised Geneva Score Pulmonary Embolism Model (Simplified Version)

Clinical characteristic	Score
Previous PE or DVT	1
Heart rate	
75–94 beats/min	1
≥95 beats/min	2
Surgery or fracture within last month	1
Hemoptysis	1
Active cancer	1
Unilateral lower limb pain	1
Pain on lower limb deep venous palpation and unilateral edema	1
Age >65y	1

A score of <2 indicates a low probability of pulmonary embolism. A score of 2 to 4 indicates an intermediate probability of PE. A score of 5 or more indicates a high probability of pulmonary embolism.
DVT, deep vein thrombosis; PE, pulmonary embolism.
Klok FA, Mos IC, Nijkeuter M, et al: Simplification of the revised Geneva score for assessing clinical probability of pulmonary embolism. *Arch Intern Med* 168(19):2131–2136, 2008.

dyspnea, syncope, or sudden hypotension. Symptoms and signs of PE are nonspecific and can be frequently seen in patients with other cardiopulmonary diseases, including pneumonia, chronic obstructive lung disease exacerbation, pneumothorax, myocardial infarction, heart failure, pericarditis, musculoskeletal pain or trauma, pleuritis, malignancy, and, occasionally, intra-abdominal processes such as acute cholecystitis or nephrolithiasis.

Given the potential for rapid clinical decompensation and the significant associated morbidity and mortality, clinicians must maintain a high index of suspicion for PE in the ICU. Subtle signs such as worsening hypoxemia, a reduction in arterial carbon dioxide with spontaneous respirations (especially in a patient with chronic lung disease), increased central venous or pulmonary artery pressure, or unexplained fever should all be considered potential heralds of PE. Even in the presence of alternative diagnoses, evaluation for possible VTE may still be appropriate when suggestive signs, symptoms, and risk factors are present [119,120].

Clinical Prediction Models

Clinical pretest probability models are useful for assessing a patient's risk for VTE and determining the appropriate course for further evaluation. The most widely studied and validated models are the Wells score and the Geneva Rule (Tables 92.8 to 92.10) [115,116,121]. The major distinction between these two preclinical probability models is that the Geneva Rule consists of completely objective criteria whereas the Wells score incorporates clinical judgment as to whether PE is the most likely etiology of the patient's symptoms. When these models were compared head-to-head, there were no major differences in diagnostic accuracy or negative predictive value for the exclusion of VTE [122]. All scoring systems performed well in combination with D-dimer measurement to identify a low-risk population that did not require radiologic testing to exclude VTE [123]. The PERC is a clinical decision support tool developed by Kline and coworkers to identify outpatients presenting with chest pain who are thought to be at low risk for PE in whom further diagnostic testing can be avoided (Table 92.11) [117]. A recent meta-analysis of 12 studies encompassing over 14,000 patients confirmed the accuracy of the PERC [124]. Consequently, the PERC was included in the American College of Physician's Practice Guideline on the diagnosis of PE [125].

TABLE 92.11

Pulmonary Embolism Rule-Out Criteria

Clinical characteristic	Meets criterion	Does not meet criterion
Age <50 y	0	1
Initial heart rate <100 beats/min	0	1
Initial oxygen saturation >94% on room air	0	1
No unilateral leg swelling	0	1
No hemoptysis	0	1
No surgery or trauma within 4 wk	0	1
No history of venous thromboembolism	0	1
No estrogen use	0	1

Pretest probability with a score of 0 is less than 1%.
Derived from Kline JA, Courtney DM, Kabrhel C, et al: Prospective multicenter evaluation of the pulmonary embolism rule-out criteria. *J Thromb Haemost* 6(5):772–780, 2008.

D-Dimer

Quantitative plasma measurements of D-dimer (a fragment of cross-linked fibrin) have been extensively studied in patients with acute DVT and PE. Although multiple inexpensive D-dimer tests are available, rapid quantitative enzyme-linked immunosorbent assays are preferred because of their high sensitivity [126]. In conjunction with pretest probability models, sensitive enzyme-linked immunosorbent assay D-dimer tests measurements have been demonstrated to safely exclude the presence of DVT and PE in outpatients judged to be at low risk for VTE [115,116,121]. Unfortunately, D-dimer levels are elevated by a large number of clinical conditions (including cancer, inflammation, infection, pregnancy, and recent surgery) which makes the test less useful in unselected and hospitalized patients [127]. For these cases, objective radiologic testing is necessary to confirm/exclude the diagnosis [128]. Because D-dimer levels increase with age, age-specific D-dimer cutoffs have been proposed to increase the utility of D-dimer testing in older adults. This approach has been noted in a meta-analysis by Schouten et al. to lead to increased specificity for individuals older than 50 years of age while maintaining excellent sensitivity [129].

Diagnosis of Acute Deep Venous Thrombosis

Compression venous ultrasonography is the preferred noninvasive test for the diagnosis of symptomatic proximal DVT, where it has a weighted sensitivity and specificity of 95% and 98%, respectively [130]. Although it is generally appropriate to initiate or withhold treatment based on the result of the examination, an exception would be when the result is discordant with the clinical assessment. For instance, a negative compression ultrasound in the context of a high clinical suspicion for DVT would warrant further investigation, such as venography, magnetic resonance imaging (MRI), or computed tomographic venography (CTV). Duplex ultrasonography is also useful for detecting upper extremity DVT. Limitations of venous ultrasonography include insensitivity for asymptomatic DVT and pelvic vein clots, dependence on operator skill, and difficulty distinguishing acute from chronic DVT in symptomatic patients [131].

MRI and CTV are being increasingly employed to diagnose DVT. MRI is highly accurate and has multiple advantages, including excellent resolution of the IVC and pelvic veins, accuracy in diagnosing upper extremity DVT, concurrent thoracic as well as bilateral examination, differentiating acute from chronic disease, and lack of exposure to ionizing radiation [132]. However, MRI is expensive, time-consuming, not portable, and is restricted in patients with metallic devices or claustrophobia. As with MRI, computed tomographic angiography (CTA)/CTV has the advantage of evaluating both PE and DVT in a single study. CTV is accurate in the detection of DVT and may be particularly useful in imaging the pelvis and upper thighs [132]. In the PIOPED II, concurrent leg evaluation with CTV increased the sensitivity of CTA from 83% to 90%, although the small improvement in overall diagnostic yield may not warrant the additional irradiation associated with CTV [133]. Contrast venography is rarely done anymore.

Diagnosis of Acute Pulmonary Embolism

Contrast-enhanced chest CTA is the imaging procedure of choice for PE because it has the capacity to reveal emboli in the main, lobar, segmental, and subsegmental pulmonary arteries, as well as other diseases of the thorax that can mimic PE. In patients with an intermediate or high probability of PE, an abnormal CTA has a positive predictive value of 92% and 96%, respectively. In patients with a low clinical likelihood of PE, normal findings on CTA had a 96% negative predictive value supporting the use of multidetector CTA as stand-alone imaging for suspected PE in the majority of patients. This modality can be used in combination with D-dimer to screen low- to intermediate-risk patients with excellent negative predictive value [134].

Unfortunately, 5% to 8% of CTAs are technically inadequate owing to motion artifact or inappropriate contrast timing [128]. Therefore, in such an instance, PE should not be prematurely dismissed as a diagnostic possibility in the context of a high clinical probability. When compared head-to-head with ($\dot{V}/\dot{Q}$) scanning, CTA was shown to identify more patients with PE although the clinical significance of these additional identified PE has not been elucidated [135]. CTA also has the advantage of rapid performance. The disadvantages of CTA include the risk of adverse reactions to contrast (such as anaphylaxis or nephrotoxicity) and lack of portability. ICU patients frequently have a prohibitive creatinine clearance.

Although chest CTA is a superior imaging test for PE, $\dot{V}/\dot{Q}$ scanning is still utilized in select cases of suspected PE. $\dot{V}/\dot{Q}$ scans are typically interpreted as being normal or low, intermediate, or high probability of PE. A normal scan essentially excludes the diagnosis of PE. In the PIOPED study, when the clinical suspicion of PE was high, PE was present in 96% of patients with high-probability lung scans. However, in patients with a high clinical pretest probability for PE, 66% of patients with intermediate-probability scans and 40% of patients with low-probability scans were subsequently diagnosed with PE by pulmonary angiography [136]. This emphasizes that low- and intermediate-probability $\dot{V}/\dot{Q}$ scans are frequently nondiagnostic when there is a high clinical suspicion for PE. However, in the setting of a low clinical pretest probability for PE, a normal or low-probability $\dot{V}/\dot{Q}$ scan correctly excluded PE in more than 95% of cases. $\dot{V}/\dot{Q}$ scans are typically used for PE imaging in patients with contrast allergies or those at risk for contrast nephrotoxicity and in pregnant patients to reduce radiation exposure [128].

MRI has excellent sensitivity and specificity and may allow the simultaneous detection of DVT and PE. However, MR angiography and MR venography are technically difficult, leading to inadequate results in 52% of patients in the PIOPED III study [137]. This modality should, therefore, only be considered in centers that routinely perform this study in patients with contraindications to standard testing.

Pulmonary artery angiography is sensitive and specific test for confirming or excluding acute PE and remains the "gold standard" diagnostic technique. In 1,111 cases from the PIOPED study, 3% of studies were nondiagnostic and 1% were incomplete, usually owing to a complication. Although complications are more common in the ICU, angiography is generally deemed quite safe, with major morbidity and mortality rates of 1% and 0.5%, respectively. Serious complications include respiratory failure (0.4%), renal failure (0.3%), and hemorrhage requiring blood transfusion [138]. Pulmonary angiography is generally reserved for patients in whom less invasive testing has been nondiagnostic. To avoid the potential complications associated with angiography, lower extremity duplex ultrasound is often performed in lieu of angiography in the diagnosis of patients with suspected but unconfirmed PE.

An Integrated Approach to Venous Thromboembolism Diagnosis

To minimize patient exposure to ionizing radiation and overall health care costs, an efficient and cost-effective approach to VTE diagnosis integrates pretest probability models such as the Wells criteria and PERC, D-dimer testing, and imaging. In conjunction with D-dimer testing, the Wells criteria have been demonstrated to safely exclude VTE in outpatients with suspected thromboembolism. The PERC facilitate identification of low-risk patients in whom PE can be ruled out without imaging. A schematic depiction of the use of the Wells criteria and the Geneva Score in conjunction with the PERC and D-dimer testing in the diagnosis of DVT and PE is displayed in Figures 92.1 and 92.2.

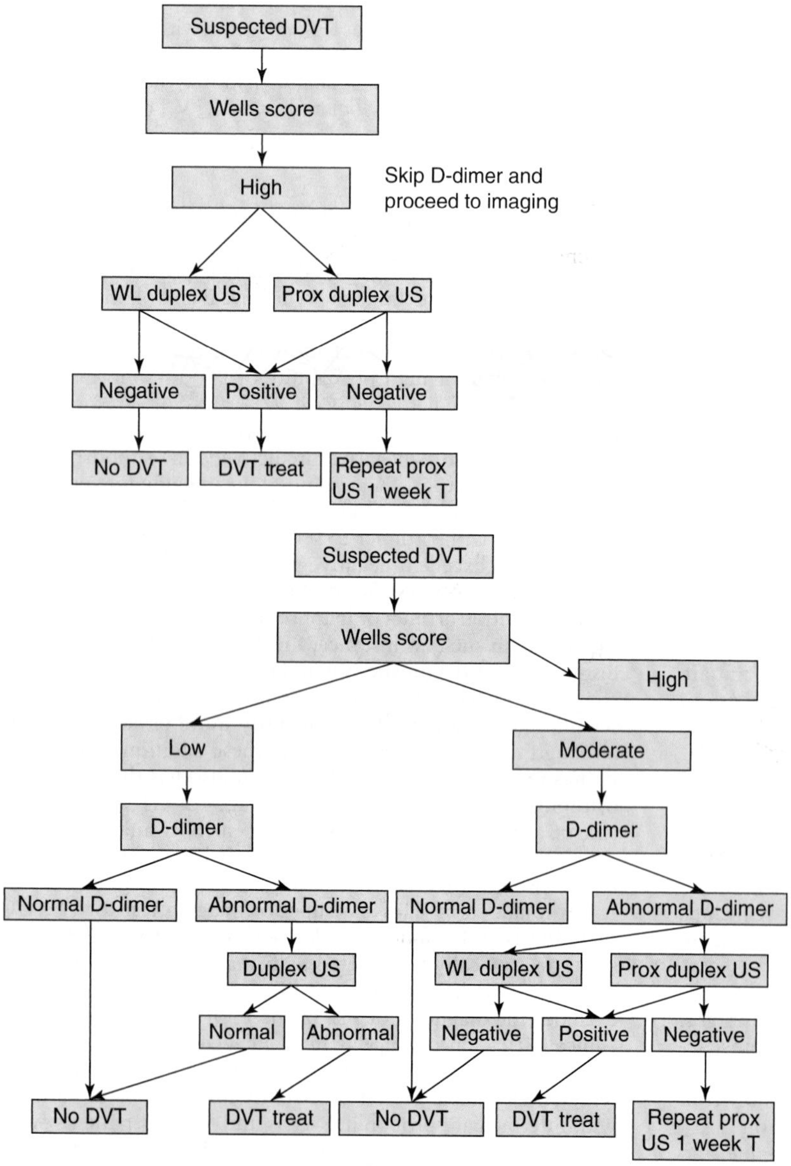

FIGURE 92.1 Diagnostic algorithm for DVT. DVT, deep vein thrombosis.

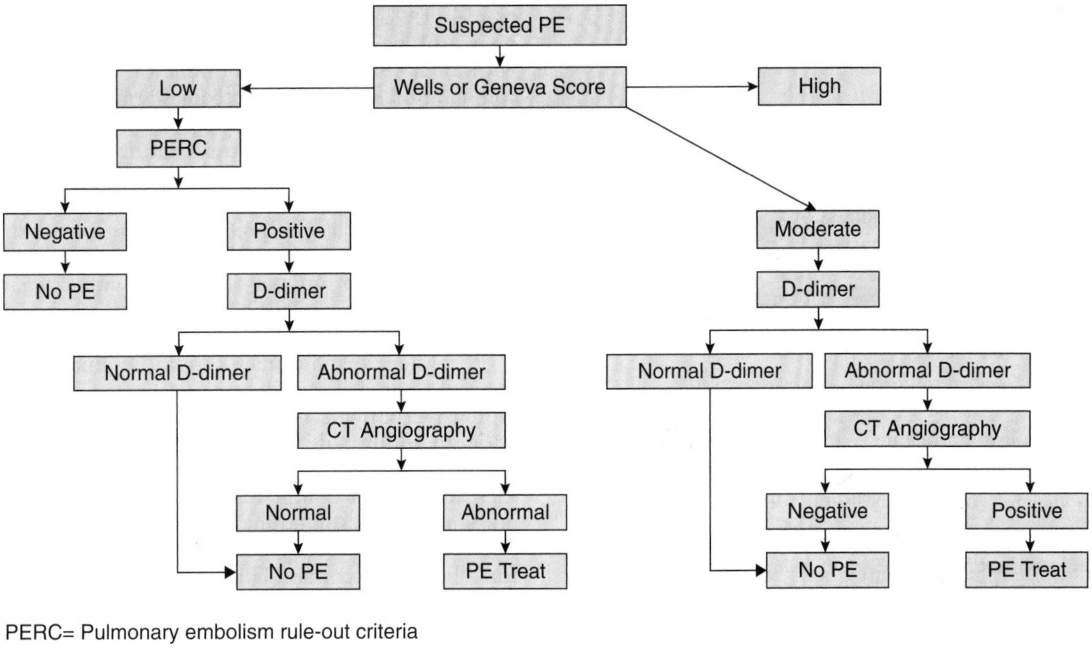

FIGURE 92.2 Diagnostic algorithm for PE. PE, pulmonary embolism.

Risk Stratification

Risk stratification is essential to selection of the appropriate treatment strategy. PE has traditionally been classified into massive, submassive, and normal risk on the basis of hemodynamic compromise along with the presence/absence of ventricular strain. Massive PE is defined by the presence of hypotension with a systolic blood pressure of 90 mm Hg or less or the need for vasopressors to maintain adequate end-organ perfusion. Massive PE necessitates prompt intervention and constitutes a medical emergency [128].

Submassive PE is characterized by evidence of RV dysfunction as documented by echocardiography, CT scan, elevated right heart pressure on cardiac catheterization, or elevated natriuretic peptide or troponin measurements. These patients are at increased risk for the development of hemodynamic compromise and are often monitored as inpatients initially. Patients without these features are considered normal risk and can be discharged for outpatient management [128].

Several evidence-based risk stratification tools have been developed to identify PE patients at low risk for complications who can be managed as outpatients, including the Pulmonary Embolism Severity Index (PESI) (Table 92.12) and the HESTIA criteria (Table 92.13) [139,140]. Of these, the PESI score and a simplified version, sPESI, have been the most extensively validated. In a multicenter, prospective, open randomized clinical management study, Aujesky et al. found that the PESI score was able to identify low-risk PE patients who did equally well whether managed as inpatients or outpatients [141]. The HESTIA criteria have also been demonstrated to be useful in identifying patients for outpatient management [142].

Because right ventricular enlargement (RVE) is an important marker of thrombus burden and hemodynamic compromise resulting from PE, imaging studies such as echocardiography and CT have also been used for risk stratification of PE patients. In a retrospective study of 431 patients with PE, RVE on CT was an independent predictor of 30-day mortality (hazard ratio: 5.17; 95% CI 1.63 to 16.35) [143]. A meta-analysis of 10 studies of normotensive PE patients determined that CT RVE was associated with an overall increased risk of death (OR 1.8; 95% CI 1.3 to 2.6), death as a result of PE (OR 7.4; 95% CI 1.4 to 39.5), and PE-related complications (OR 2.4; 95% CI 1.2 to 4.7) [144]. However, CT only demonstrated modest utility in identifying patients at risk for complications and, therefore, should not be used in isolation for determining management.

Echocardiography has also been used to determine RV overload for the purposes of PE prognostication. However,

TABLE 92.12

PESI Score

Predictors	Points assigned
Age in years	Age, in years
Altered mental status[b]	+60
Systolic blood pressure <100 mm Hg	+30
History of cancer	+30
Arterial oxygen saturation <90%[a]	+20
Temp <36°C	+20
Respiratory rate ≥30/min	+20
Pulse ≥110/min	+20
Male sex	+10
History of heart failure	+10
History of chronic lung disease	+10

A total point score for a given patient is obtained by summing the patient's age in years and the points for each applicable predictor. Points assignments correspond with the following risk classes: Class 1 (very low risk): ≤65; Class II (low risk): 65–85; Class III (intermediate risk): 86–105; Class IV (high risk): 106–125; Class V (very high risk): >125.

[a]Chronic obstructive pulmonary disease with and without supplemental oxygen administration.

[b]Altered mental status was defined as confusion, disorientation, somnolence, lethargy, stupor, or coma.

PESI, Pulmonary Embolism Severity Index.

Adapted from Aujesky D, Obrosky DS, Stone RA, et al: Derivation and validation of a prognostic model for pulmonary embolism. *Am J Respir Crit Care Med* 172:1041–1046, 2005.

TABLE 92.13

HESTIA Criteria

Criteria
Hemodynamically instable (e.g., HR >100 beats/min, systolic BP <100 mm Hg, needs ICU admission)
Thrombolysis or embolectomy necessary
High risk of bleeding (e.g., GI bleed within 14 d, recent stroke within 4 wk, recent surgery within 2 wk, platelets <75,000/μL, uncontrolled HTN: systolic BP >180 mm Hg, diastolic BP >110 mm Hg)
Supplemental O_2 needed to keep O_2 saturation >90% for >24 h
Pulmonary embolism during anticoagulation treatment
Intravenous pain medication >24 h
Medical or social reason for in-hospital treatment >24 h
Creatinine clearance <30 mL/min
Severe liver impairment
Pregnant
Documented history of HIT

The presence of any criterion precludes outpatient treatment.
BP, blood pressure; ICU, intensive care unit; GI, gastrointestinal; HIT, heparin-induced thrombocytopenia; HR, hazard rate; HTN, hypertension.
Adapted from Zondag W, den Exter PL, Crobach MJ, et al: Comparison of two methods for selection of out of hospital treatment in patients with acute pulmonary embolism. *Thromb Haemost* 109:47–52, 2013.

a meta-analysis noted that echocardiography had an unsatisfactory negative likelihood ratio for early all-cause mortality (0.62; 95% CI 0.41 to 0.92) and PE-related mortality (0.36; 95% CI 0.20 to 0.80). This outcome may reflect the lack of standardized echocardiographic criteria for RV dysfunction and the difficulty in differentiating between acute and chronic RV overload [145]. Therefore, it is currently premature to rely upon echocardiography to identify low-risk patients with PE.

Cardiac biomarkers such as troponin I and T and NT-pro-BNP that are released from myocytes during RV strain have also proven useful for prognostication of PE patients. In a multicenter prospective study, Vuilleumier and colleagues found that an NT-pro-BNP level <300 pg per mL had a negative predictive value of 100% (95% CI 91 to 100) for adverse outcomes from PE at 3 months [146]. In a prospective validation study 7 of 526 normotensive PE patients, Lankeit et al. noted that only 4 of 214 (1.9%) patients with a high sensitive troponin T <14 pg per mL had adverse outcomes at 30 days. When combined with an sPESI score of zero, none of 127 patients with this combination had adverse outcomes [147].

A combination of clinical and laboratory biomarkers may represent the ideal strategy for identification of normotensive patients at low risk for adverse outcomes. Jimenez et al. conducted a multicenter cohort study of normotensive PE patients to identify a multimarker prognostic score for risk stratification. The combination of an sPESI and a brain natriuretic peptide level <100 pg per mL was associated with a negative predictive value of 99% and 100% in the derivation and validation cohorts, respectively [148].

PE patient management should be guided by an assessment of their risk for adverse outcomes (Table 92.14). Normotensive patients in PESI class ≥ II or sPESI ≥1 should undergo additional imaging and laboratory risk assessment and warrant initial inpatient management until the results of these studies are complete. Patients in this group who have no sign of RV dysfunction on echocardiography or abnormal cardiac biomarkers are considered at low intermediate risk for adverse outcomes. This group of patients can be considered for early discharge from the hospital. Patients with abnormal echocardiography or cardiac biomarkers are consider intermediate–low-risk patients and are often managed in the hospital. Patients with abnormal echocardiography and cardiac biomarkers are considered at intermediate high risk of adverse outcomes and are generally managed as inpatients. Intermediate–high-risk PE patients are considered for thrombolytic therapy on a case-by-case basis. PE patients with hypotension are at high risk for adverse outcomes. They routinely undergo echocardiography and are strongly considered for thrombolytic therapy (Table 92.12) [128].

TREATMENT

Treatment for VTE centers on the use of anticoagulation to prevent clot propagation and promote the body's natural thrombolytic processes to resorb the clot and allow for vessel recanalization (Table 92.15) Other treatment options include thrombolytic therapy, IVC filter placement, and surgical embolectomy. Each approach has specific indications as well as advantages and disadvantages. Initiation of therapy should usually be delayed for confirmatory testing in most clinical scenarios. Exceptions to this principle includes patients with high clinical pretest probability, moderate pretest probability where the results of diagnostic testing will be delayed for hours, or clinical scenarios where delaying therapy would lead to high likelihood of an adverse outcome [149].

TABLE 92.14

Mortality Risk Categories for Patients with Acute Pulmonary Embolism

	Risk Factors			
30-D Mortality Risk	**Hypotension**	**PESI Class III through V**	**RV Dysfunction**	**Abnormal Cardiac Biomarkers**
High	Present	Optional assessment	Present	Optional test
Intermediate-high	Absent	Present	Present	Present
Intermediate-low	Absent	Present	Either one or neither present	Either one or neither present
Low	Absent	Absent	Absent but test not necessary	Absent but test not necessary

PESI, Pulmonary Embolism Severity Index; RV, right ventricular.
Adapted from: Konstantinides SV, Torbicki A, Agnelli G, et al: 2014 ESC guidelines on the diagnosis and management of acute pulmonary embolism. *Eur Heart J* 14;35(43):3033,69, 3069a–3069k, 2014.

TABLE 92.15

Treatment Options for VTE

Unfractionated heparin: 80 unit/kg IV bolus followed by 18 units/kg/h infusion adjusted to aPTT ratio

Low Molecular Weight Heparin (LMWH)

Dalteparin 100 units/kg sc q12h or 200 units/kg sc q24h

Renal dosing: no official recommendation-use with caution, consider LMWH anti-Xa levels monitoring and dose adjustment

Enoxaparin 1 mg/kg sc q12h or 1.5 mg/kg sc q24h

FDA approved renal dosing- 1mg/kg sc q24h (CrCl <30 mL/min)

Tinzaparin 175 units/kg sc q24h

Renal dose: same (no evidence of bioaccumulation in the IRIS study)

Pentasaccharide

Fondaparinux 5–10 mg sc q24h (5 mg for weight <50 kg, 7.5 mg for weight 50–100 kg, and 10 mg for weight >100 kg)

Renal dosing: avoid in patients with CrCl <30 mL/min; caution in patients with CrCl 30–50 mL/min

Direct Thrombin Inhibitors

Argatroban[a]

2 g/kg/min continuous IV infusion adjusted to an aPTT ratio of 1.5–3.0 (check first aPTT after 2 h initiation and after each dose change (normal hepatic function)

0.5 μg/kg/min continuous IV infusion (Child–Pugh Classes B and C patients)

Bivalirudin[b]

CrCl >60 mL/min 0.15 mg/kg/h IV infusion

CrCl 45–60 mL/min 0.075 mg/kg/h IV

CrCl 30–44 mL/min 0.05 mg/kg/h IV

CrCl <30 mL/min or renal replacement therapy 0.025 mg/kg/h IV

Dabigatran (oral direct thrombin inhibitor)

150 mg orally BID after 5–10 d of initial parenteral anticoagulation

(Avoid in patients with CrCl <30 mL/min and liver impairment with transaminase >2× ULN))

Direct Factor Xa Inhibitors

Apixaban (oral direct factor Xa inhibitor)

10 mg orally BID ×7 d then 5 mg orally BID

In patients with at least two of the following characteristics: age ≥80 y, body weight ≤60 kg, or serum creatinine ≥1.5 mg/dL, the recommended dose is 2.5 mg orally BID.

Would avoid in patients with CrCl <25 mL/min or sCr >2.5 mg/dL or hepatic dysfunction (AST/ALT >2X ULN or bilirubin >1.5× ULN)

Edoxaban (oral direct factor Xa inhibitor)

60 mg orally once daily

30 mg once daily if CrCl 15–50 mL/min or body weight ≤60 kg or avoid in patients with CrCl <15 mL/min or Child–Pugh class B/C hepatic impairment

Rivaroxaban (oral direct factor Xa inhibitor)

15 mg orally BID ×3 wk followed by 20 mg once daily

Avoid in patients with CrCl <30 mL/min and Child–Pugh class B/C

Vena cava filter

[a]Argatroban dosing per package insert at: https://www.gsksource.com/pharma/content/dam/GlaxoSmithKline/US/en/Prescribing_Information/Argatroban/pdf/ARGATROBAN.PDF. Accessed December 29, 2015.

[b]Adapted from Kiser TH, Mann AM, Trujillo TC, et al: Evaluation of empiric versus nomogram-based direct thrombin inhibitor management in patients with suspected heparin-induced thrombocytopenia. *Am J Hematol* 86:267–272, 2011.

ALT, alanine transaminase; aPTT, activated partial thromboplastin time; AST, aspartate transaminase; BID, twice a day; CrCl, creatinine clearance; FDA, Food and Drug Administration; IV, intravenous; sc, subcutaneously; q, every; ULN, upper limit of normal; VTE, venous thromboembolism.

Anticoagulation

Anticoagulants do not directly dissolve preexisting clot; instead, they prevent thrombus extension and indirectly decrease clot burden through the body's endogenous fibrinolytic system. Information regarding pharmacokinetics and dosing of traditional anticoagulants such as UFH, the LMWH, fondaparinux, and warfarin can be found in Chapter 93. For critically ill ICU patients, UFH is the parenteral anticoagulant of choice given its short half-life and complete reversibility with protamine. Multiple clinical trials have demonstrated that LMWH is a safe and effective alternative to UFH for the treatment of acute VTE that does not require laboratory monitoring [150]. Similarly, fondaparinux, a synthetic pentasaccharide, is as effective as LMWH and UFH in the initial treatment and prevention of VTE [151]. Although fondaparinux is an attractive agent for outpatient anticoagulation because of its extremely rare association with HIT, it is often an impractical anticoagulant in ICU patients owing to its long half-life, renal elimination, and the absence of an available reversal agent.

Except for those with active cancer, most VTE patients will be transitioned from parenteral therapy to warfarin or a direct oral anticoagulant for short- or long-term treatment. Because warfarin requires at least 5 days to achieve therapeutic anticoagulation, initial coadministration with a rapid-onset parenteral anticoagulant such as UFH or LMWH is necessary when initiating therapy. Failure to employ a parenteral agent during initial warfarin therapy is occasionally complicated by warfarin skin necrosis, a procoagulant state characterized by thrombosis of dermal vessels and skin ulceration with a predilection for adipose-laden areas of the body. Therefore, it is recommended that parenteral anticoagulants continue until an INR of 2 or more has been achieved for at least 24 hours [152,153].

Dabigatran is an oral direct thrombin inhibitor that is the Food and Drug Administration (FDA) approved for treatment of VTE and thromboprophylaxis in nonvalvular atrial fibrillation and orthopedic VTE prophylaxis (see Chapter 93 for information regarding pharmacokinetics and approved dosing). In the RECOVER trials, dabigatran was demonstrated to be as effective and safe as warfarin for prevention of recurrent thromboembolism in patients with acute VTE following at least 5 days of therapy with a parenteral anticoagulant [154,155]. In the past 4 years, three oral direct factor Xa inhibitors have been approved by the FDA for treatment of VTE, apixaban, edoxaban, and rivaroxaban (see Chapter 93). In the AMPLIFY study, apixaban was as effective as LMWH/warfarin for the first 6 months of therapy of acute VTE [156]. In the AMPLIFY-EXT study, Agnelli and colleagues demonstrated that apixaban 2.5 mg twice daily was superior to placebo in prevention of recurrent VTE and associated with a similar risk of clinically relevant nonmajor bleeding for long-term therapy (>6 months) of VTE [157]. In the EINSTEIN studies, rivaroxaban was demonstrated to be as effective as LMWH/VKA in the treatment of initial and long-term therapy of VTE [158,159]. Edoxaban is an oral factor Xa inhibitor that was compared with warfarin for treatment of VTE in the HOKUSAI study. Similar to dabigatran, edoxaban was preceded by a 5- to 10-day course of parenteral therapy [160]. Therefore, initial parenteral therapy should be employed for at least 5 days when using edoxaban or dabigatran for treatment of VTE.

Although each of the direct oral anticoagulants have been demonstrated to be as safe and effective as conventional anticoagulation for treatment of VTE, the long half-lives of these medications, their dependence on renal and/or hepatic function for clearance, and the absence of readily available laboratory tests for monitoring and a reversal agent for bleeding complications makes them less attractive agents for critically ill patients.

Thrombolytic Therapy

In patients with PE, systemic thrombolytic therapy is reserved for patients with massive PE characterized by the presence of hypotension (systolic blood pressure <90 mm Hg) and hypoxemia (room air O_2 saturation <90%) in whom mortality rates can be as high as 58% [161]. Thrombolytic therapy is not generally used in patients with submassive PE. In two randomized controlled trials in patients with submassive PE, thrombolytic therapy prevented clinical deterioration but was not associated with a mortality benefit and increased bleeding complications so it should be reserved for patients with massive PE [162,163]. The standard thrombolytic regimen for PE is alteplase 100 mg over 2 hours with 10 mg administered as a bolus at the initiation of therapy. (Table 92.14) Lower dose alteplase regimens should be considered for older patients (age >65 years) who are at higher risk for bleeding complications [128]. The decision for thrombolysis should be made on a case-by-case basis. Even in the setting of a relative contraindication, thrombolytic therapy may be reasonable when a patient is extremely unstable from life-threatening PE.

Catheter-directed thrombolysis (CDT) using the EKOS ultrasound catheter may be a useful option for patients with massive or submassive PE deemed at high risk for bleeding who are also at high risk for clinical deterioration as a result of their PE. The EKOS catheter uses ultrasound to disrupt the structure of the thrombus while spraying the thrombolytic agent locally into the substance of the clot via side holes in the catheter. Preliminary studies of the "EKOS" catheter indicate that it may accelerate clot resolution with a low risk of major bleeding [164,165]. Further investigation of the EKOS catheter is warranted to confirm its impact on clinical outcomes.

In an arrest or a periarrest situation, the use of thrombolytics is often considered in an attempt to improve hemodynamics and reverse/prevent hemodynamic collapse. There is some evidence for improved outcomes with this approach in patients with a confirmed or strongly suspected PE [128,166]. However, empiric use in a trial evaluating administration in undifferentiated out-of-hospital arrests showed no significant improvement in mortality [167].

Each of the FDA–approved thrombolytic agents is administered at a fixed dose, making measurements of coagulation unnecessary during infusion (Table 92.16). Tissue-type plasminogen activator (2-hour infusion) is most commonly used. Shorter regimens and even bolus dosing may be favored in cases of unstable patients with massive PE. Following infusion of thrombolytics, the aPTT should be measured and repeated at 4-hour intervals until the aPTT is less than twice the upper limit of normal, after which continuous IV UFH should be administered without a loading bolus dose.

Thrombolytic therapy is contraindicated in patients at high risk for bleeding (Table 92.17). Intracranial hemorrhage is the most devastating (and often fatal) complication of thrombolytic therapy and occurs in 1% to 3% of patients [161,168,169].

TABLE 92.16

Thrombolytic Treatment Regimens for PE

Streptokinase 250,000 units IV (loading dose during 30 min); then 100,000 units/h for 24 h
Urokinase[a] 2,000 units/lb (or 4,400 units/kg) IV (loading dose during 10 min); then 2,000 units/lb/h (or 4,400 units/kg/h) for 12–24 h
Alteplase tPA 100 mg IV during 2 h

[a]Limited availability.
IV, intravenous; PE, pulmonary embolism; tPA, tissue plasminogen activator.

TABLE 92.17

Contraindications to Thrombolysis

Absolute
History of hemorrhagic stroke or stroke of unknown origin
Intracranial tumor
Ischemic stroke in previous 3 mo
History of major surgery, trauma, head injury within previous 3 wk
Platelet count below 100,000/μL
Active bleeding
Bleeding diathesis
Relative
Age >75 y
Pregnancy or first postpartum week
Noncompressible puncture sites
Traumatic resuscitation
Refractory hypertension (systolic blood pressure >180 mm Hg; diastolic blood pressure >100 mm Hg)
Advanced liver disease
Infective endocarditis
Recent gastrointestinal bleed (within 3 mo)
Life expectancy ≤1 y

Invasive procedures should be minimized around the time of therapy to decrease the risk of bleeding.

In patients with deep venous thrombosis, CDT is generally reserved for patients with massive or limb-threatening iliofemoral deep venous thrombosis. In the CAVENT study, an open randomized controlled trial of CDT versus conventional anticoagulation in iliofemoral DVT, CDT was associated with more rapid resolution of thrombus burden and a reduced incidence of post-thrombotic syndrome [170]. In patients with May–Thurner syndrome (iliac vein compression syndrome), CDT in conjunction with angioplasty and venous stenting has been advocated as the preferred approach to therapy although supportive data are limited to retrospective case series [171]. Randomized studies should be performed before this is considered standard therapy. The benefits of CDT include more rapid and complete reduction of thrombus burden and associated clinical symptoms, as well as the potential to reduce venous valvular damage and the incidence of post-thrombotic syndrome. The primary risk associated with thrombolytic therapy is an increase in bleeding complications. The ongoing ATTRACT trial should help to answer some of the outstanding questions surrounding thrombolytic therapy for DVT [172]. Until these data are available, CDT should be reserved for patients with extensive proximal clots with low bleeding risk.

Inferior Vena Cava Interruption

IVC filters are metallic wire devices often constructed of flexible nonferromagnetic alloys that designed to catch large clots that could cause life-threatening pulmonary emboli. Although originally designed for permanent placement, most current IVC filters are designed to be retrieved. Because permanent and retrievable filters appear to have similar efficacy and safety and most patients have transient contraindications to anticoagulation, it is preferable to use retrievable filters that afford the option of later retrieval [173].

The only widely accepted indication for IVC filter placement is a contraindication to anticoagulation in a patient with acute (within 1 month) proximal deep venous thrombosis with or without PE. Because the risk of recurrent VTE is substantially lower in patients with less acute DVT (10% during months 2 to 3), the use of IVC filters in this patient population is likely to be associated with less attractive risk to benefit balance particularly if the contraindication to anticoagulation is temporary. It remains unclear if IVC filters are beneficial in patients with isolated PE without evidence of proximal DVT or IVC thrombosis [173].

Although the data are not conclusive, several studies suggest that the Trapease (permanent filter) and Optease (retrievable filter) are associated with a greater risk for filter-related IVC thrombosis perhaps owing to its opposing dual cone filter design [174]. Therefore, we would suggest that health care providers avoid use of these filters. If a retrievable filter is placed, it is incumbent upon the responsible physicians to ensure that the filter is removed as soon as it is no longer needed because many filters are left in place unnecessarily. It is particularly important to retrieve filters with a short retrieval window such as the Optease filter (within 3 weeks).

IVC filters are likely to reduce the incidence of PE in patients who cannot be anticoagulated [175]. In patients who can be treated with anticoagulation, filters do not reduce the incidence of PE or improve mortality [176]. They are associated with a 1.5-fold increased risk of deep venous thrombosis and a cumulative incidence of IVC thrombosis of 14% at 8 years of follow-up [177]. Anticoagulation likely reduces the risk of deep venous thrombosis associated with IVC filters, therefore anticoagulation should be considered in appropriate candidates. There is limited literature on the risks and benefits of SVC filters. Because the PE is less common in patients with upper extremity thrombosis, the use of filters in this position is discouraged [173].

Pulmonary Embolectomy

Given its high morbidity and mortality, surgical embolectomy has traditionally been a treatment of last resort, often reserved for patients with documented central PE and refractory cardiogenic shock despite maximal therapy. Contemporary studies show improved outcomes with in-hospital mortality as low as 5% to 6% and suggest that emergency surgical pulmonary embolectomy may be feasible in carefully selected patients and with an experienced surgical team [178]. Catheter-directed embolectomy and/or the localized administration of thromblytics is an emerging treatment modality shown to improve hemodynamics by reducing the burden of central pulmonary artery thromboembolism. Ultrasound has been used as an adjunct to this approach with the idea of destabilizing the clot and increasing the efficacy of thrombolytic therapy [164,165,179].

Adjunctive Care for Massive Pulmonary Embolism

The mere suspicion of massive PE warrants immediate supportive therapy. A cautious fluid challenge of IV saline may augment preload and improve impaired RV function. Dopamine and norepinephrine are favored if hypotension remains, and combination therapy with dobutamine may boost RV output, although it may exacerbate hypotension. Additionally, clinicians must be cautious that augmenting cardiac output above physiologic levels may exacerbate ($\dot{V}/\dot{Q}$) mismatch by shunting blood from areas with partially obstructed vessels. Supplemental oxygen and mechanical ventilation may be instituted as needed to support respiratory failure. Inhaled nitric oxide may improve the hemodynamic status of patients while avoiding the potentially deleterious effects of IV agents on systemic blood pressure [128]. Thrombolytic therapy or pulmonary embolectomy should be considered followed by anticoagulation as previously described.

SPECIAL THERAPEUTIC CONSIDERATIONS

Central Venous Catheter–Associated Thrombosis

Symptomatic catheter-related thrombosis are felt to occur in up to 6% of adults with conventional CVC and 14% with PICC [37,38], and upper extremity thrombosis is common complication in critically ill patients primarily because of the wide spread use of CVCs. CVC-associated DVT is generally treated with anticoagulation for at least 3 months or until the CVC is removed whichever is longer. If the CVC is still needed for patient care, there is no need to remove the catheter unless symptoms fail to improve with anticoagulation. Thrombolytic therapy is reserved for limb-threatening or extremely symptomatic CVC-associated DVT that has not responded to standard therapy in candidates without contraindications. CVC removal is consider as primary therapy for patients who are not candidates for anticoagulation although it should be noted that this approach is probably associated with a higher risk of embolization in the absence of at least a week of anticoagulation. Complications of CVC-associated thrombosis include catheter infections, PE, post-thrombotic syndrome, catheter dysfunction, and persistent vascular compromise [180]. Symptomatic PE occurs in 3% to 12% of adult patients with an upper extremity DVT. The risk of clot embolization that accompanies CVC extraction is outweighed by the risk for chronic thrombotic complications and potential infection. Upper extremity DVTs have a substantially lower rate of recurrence than those in the lower extremities [37].

Pregnancy-Associated VTE

The diagnosis of VTE during pregnancy is complicated by physiologic changes in the mother and the presence of the fetus which limit the use of radiographic imaging. D-Dimer levels tend to be elevated during pregnancy which limits the diagnostic utility of the test. Chan and colleagues developed a pretest probability score for DVT diagnosis called the LEFT model [181] that may reduce the need for diagnostic testing; if testing is required, however, noninvasive methods such as lower extremity duplex ultrasonography should be used initially. If the duplex ultrasound is nondiagnostic, to assess for PE, a chest radiograph should be ordered to look for active pulmonary disease. In the setting of a normal chest X-ray, a ($\dot{V}/\dot{Q}$) scan may be performed. Conversely, a CTA with abdominal shielding should be ordered if the chest radiograph is abnormal [182]. Interestingly, data suggest that a chest CT may deliver less radiation to a fetus than a ($\dot{V}/\dot{Q}$) scan when performed during the first or second trimester [128].

Weight-adjusted LMWH is the principal therapy for VTE during pregnancy because warfarin and direct oral anticoagulants are contraindicated. UFH is preferred by some health care providers after 36 weeks of gestation because of its complete reversibility with protamine. Warfarin can be used in the postpartum period because it does not appear to be secreted in clinically relevant concentrations in breast milk. Thrombolytic therapy is relatively contraindicated because of the potential risk of maternal hemorrhage and fetal demise. However, thrombolytic therapy should not be withheld in cases of massive PE when its use may be lifesaving. IVC filters are limited to pregnant patients with acute proximal DVT and contraindications to anticoagulation. Prophylactic anticoagulation is used in patients who are at high risk for recurrent VTE during pregnancy, such as those on anticoagulation prior to pregnancy, patients with a history of estrogen- or pregnancy-associated VTE, and patients with high-risk thrombophilia [183].

SEQUELAE OF VENOUS THROMBOEMBOLISM

VTE is associated with several sequelae, including nonfatal recurrent VTE, post-thrombotic syndrome, chronic thromboembolic pulmonary hypertension, and fatal PE. Death occurs in approximately 6% of DVT cases and 12% of PE cases within 1 month of diagnosis [184]. In the ICOPER study, the all-cause 3-month mortality rate was 17.4% [161]. In the PIOPED study, all-cause mortality at 3 months was 15%, but only 10% of deaths during the first year of follow-up were attributable to PE [185]. The risk of death is as high as 58% in patients with massive PE [161].

During the initial 3 months of therapeutic anticoagulation, 4% of patients with proximal DVT will suffer a recurrent episode of VTE, and about 1 in 250 will develop fatal PE [186]. In addition, about 3% to 4% of PE patients will develop chronic thromboembolic pulmonary hypertension. Chronic thromboembolic pulmonary hypertension (CTEPH) is increased in patients with larger perfusion defects, younger patients, and patients with recurrent PE. In patients with suspected CTEPH or at high risk for CTEPH should undergo echocardiography and ($\dot{V}/\dot{Q}$) scanning. Right heart catheterization is recommended for accurate determination of pulmonary artery pressures. CTEPH can be managed medically with vasodilators such as IV epoprostenol and oral bosentan and sildenafil. For patients with severe pulmonary hypertension not responsive to medical therapy, pulmonary thromboendarterectomy is recommended. The University of California at San Diego has the world's largest experience with this surgery and has published very good outcomes with this procedure [187].

Duration of Anticoagulation

Although decision-making regarding the appropriate duration of therapy for VTE is not often an immediate concern for critical care physicians, an understanding of the current treatment approach can be valuable when caring for critically ill patients who suffer complications of anticoagulant therapy. Currently, the duration of therapy for VTE is largely dictated by the clinical circumstances of the thrombotic event. Unprovoked VTE is associated with a high risk of recurrence (~7% per year) after completion of a standard course of anticoagulation, whereas VTE associated with a major surgical procedure are associated with a low risk of recurrence (0.7% per patient-year). VTE that occurs during a medical illness has an intermediate risk of recurrence (4.5% per patient-year) [188]. Therefore, indefinite therapy is often considered for patients with unprovoked VTE whereas patients with surgically provoked events discontinue anticoagulation after 3 to 6 months of therapy once they have recovered from their surgery and any attendant complications. Patients who develop VTE in conjunction with a medical illness continue anticoagulation for an intermediate duration that generally is continued until the inciting medical illness has been treated into remission or at least 3 months whichever is longer [189].

The presence of thrombophilia does not automatically indicate the need for long-term therapy although indefinite therapy is often considered for patients with known high-risk thrombophilia (e.g., deficiency of AT, PC, or PS, antiphospholipid syndrome, homozygous FVL or prothrombin gene mutation or compound heterozygosity of FVL, and the prothrombin gene mutation). Cancer patients who develop VTE are treated with anticoagulation as long as their cancer remains active or under therapy [189].

Complications of Anticoagulation

The principal complication of anticoagulation is major bleeding. A pooled analysis of 11 clinical trials involving approximately 15,000 patients treated with either UFH or LMWH reported the frequency of major bleeding at 1.9% and 1.1% and a fatal hemorrhage rate of 0.2% and 0.1%, respectively [190]. Given the wide use of anticoagulants for the prevention of thromboembolism in ambulatory and hospitalized patients, bleeding complications related to anticoagulants are likely to be treated by clinicians working in critical care environments.

Reversal of antithrombotic agents is addressed in Chapter 93. A few reversal agents in development, however, deserve special mention. Idarucizumab, a humanized mouse monoclonal antibody directed against dabigatran, has been evaluated clinically for reversal of dabigatran in patients with life-threatening bleeding or in need of an emergent invasive procedure. When administered as a 5-g IV bolus, idarucizumab rapidly reversed dabigatran's anticoagulant activity, and its effects lasted 12 to 24 hours after administration [191].

Andexanet alfa is a genetically engineered form of factor Xa that binds and inactivates direct and indirect factor Xa inhibitors. Following a bolus and IV infusion, it reduced rivaroxaban and apixaban levels by 90% [192]. FDA approval is expected in 2016. PER977, a small molecule cationic inhibitor that binds to direct oral anticoagulants as well as UFH and LMWH has been shown to reverse the anticoagulant effects of edoxaban in normal volunteers [193]. Once approved, these reversal agents are likely to be invaluable in the treatment of patients with bleeding complications associated with direct oral anticoagulants as well as conventional anticoagulant.

Utility of Ultrasonography for Evaluation of Venous Thromboembolism

Utility of Ultrasonography for Diagnosis of Deep Vein Thrombosis

Ultrasonography is the primary imaging modality used for the diagnosis of DVT. With appropriate training, intensivists and emergency medicine physicians can perform compression studies with results that are as accurate as those performed by consultative radiology or vascular services; where there is often delay in performance of the examination [194–196]. The frontline intensivist who performs the DVT study accrues major advantage: the examination is done immediately at point of care, it can be repeated as often as required, and it provides important clinical information that is promptly integrated into management plan [194]. The intensivist who is competent in the two-dimensional (2-D) compression examination can perform the examination in a few minutes. The addition of Doppler to the examination (duplex and triplex) affords no improvement in accuracy over the simpler 2-D compression ultrasound test [197]. Proficiency in the 2-D compression examination for DVT is, therefore, a key part of competence in critical care ultrasonography.

Equipment Requirements

The 2-D compression examination is performed with a linear vascular probe (7.5 MHz) of the type that is used to guide vascular access. Lower frequency probes used for cardiac, thoracic, and abdominal scanning do not usually have adequate resolution to examine for venous thrombosis. The width of the scanning field of a linear vascular probe varies according to probe design. The choice of a narrow or wide width is determined by operator preference.

Scanning Technique

Scanning technique is standard regardless of the vessel under examination. The target vein is scanned in its transverse axis. The examiner positions the transducer over the target vessel perpendicular to the skin surface, and the vessel is centered beneath the transducer by adjusting the position of the transducer. Depth and gain are set for optimal image quality. By standard convention, the orientation marker is set on the right side of the screen, and the probe marker is always directed to the right side of the patient. The vessel is examined for visible thrombus. If no thrombus is visible, an isoechoic thrombus may be present. To examine for this possibility, the transducer is pressed into the skin with the force vector perpendicular to the vein. The amount of applied force is sufficient to deform the adjacent artery. Normal veins are fully compressible with moderate pressure applied with the transducer; such that, with compression, the visible lumen disappears as the opposing venous walls come into full contact (Video 92.1). Thrombus will prevent full compression of the vein. Frequently, the thrombus will only become visible with the compression maneuver. Although the compression maneuver is best performed with transverse view of the vein, the longitudinal view may be used to supplement to examination.

Examination for Deep Vein Thrombosis of the Lower Extremity

The patient is in supine position with the leg externally rotated. The examination proceeds in a proximal to distal direction using an imaging sequence that requires identification and compression at defined anatomic levels of the venous system (Video 92.2) (Fig. 92.3) The mandatory image sequence is as follows:

1. Identification and compression of the proximal common femoral vein (CFV) and its paired artery). In slender individuals, it may be possible to image the distal iliac vein. The CFV is medial to the common femoral artery (CFA).

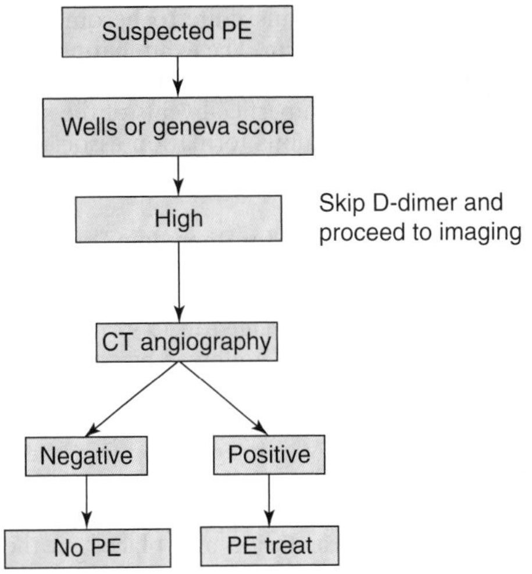

FIGURE 92.3 Anatomic points for venous compression study of the leg.

2. Identification and compression of the junction of the saphenous vein and the CFV. This is common site for thrombus formation.
3. Identification and compression of the CFV at the level of the bifurcation of the CFA into the femoral artery (FA) and profunda femoris artery. There is often a lateral perforating vein that runs between the FA and profunda femoris artery.
4. Identification and compression at the level of the junction of the CFV and the profunda femoris vein. Below this point, the CFV becomes the femoral vein (FV). (The FV may be referred to as the superficial FV. This is confusing; it is actually a deep vein).
5. Identification and compression of the FV. The FV is posterior to the FA. It is very uncommon to find a DVT in the FV in the absence of thrombus at the inguinal level, so there is debate as to how far down the thigh to continue the examination and compression of the SV. However, it does take much time to examine the FV at several points.
6. Identification and compression of the popliteal vein (PV). The knee is flexed with the leg externally rotated, and the probe is placed in the popliteal fossa in order to image and compress the PV. Several points along the PV may be examined. The PV is superficial to the popliteal artery.

Ultrasonography Findings

An intraluminal mass within the vein is diagnostic of thrombus because of the absence of compressibility of the vessel (Video 92.3). Isoechoic thrombus (i.e., noncompressible vessel) suggests that the clot is new. Older clots are echoic. Freely moving thrombus implies instability with risk of dislodgement and resulting PE. As the thrombus ages, it becomes incorporated into the vessel wall, progressively more echoic, and may eventually calcify. An intraluminal mass within the IVC may be thrombus, but intravascular spread of malignancy is a consideration. Renal cell carcinoma is frequently the culprit tumor in this situation.

Examination for Deep Vein Thrombosis of the Upper Extremity

The patient is in supine position with the arm abducted and externally rotated. Starting at the antecubital fossa, the brachial artery is identified in its transverse axis at the cubital fossa. This allows identification of the accompanying brachial veins that are usually paired. The transducer is moved proximally along the brachial veins with examination for visible thrombus followed by compression at multiple points along the medial arm. The paired brachial veins unite to become the axillary vein in the proximal upper arm. The examination continues as far into axilla as possible. Using similar technique, ultrasonography visualization of the superficial veins of the arm is useful in order to assess for thrombus formation associated with IV access (Video 92.4).

Ultrasonography Examination for Deep Vein Thrombosis of the Great Vessels

The internal jugular vein is imaged in its transverse axis and examined for visible thrombus, followed by compression study along its length (Video 92.5). This is a standard part of assessment in preparation for central venous access.

The subclavian vein (SCV) is imaged in its transverse axis and examined for visible thrombus, followed by compression study along its length (Video 92.6). To locate the vessel, the transducer is held in longitudinal orientation and placed on the clavicle using a sagittal scanning plane directed through the medial third of the clavicle. The transducer is then moved laterally on the clavicle until the SCV appears from underneath the clavicle. With further lateral movement of the probe, the target vessel and its paired artery are visualized in the subpectoral area away from the clavicle. The subclavian becomes the axillary vein when it crosses the lateral part of the first rib. Although visible thrombus is diagnostic, the SCV may be difficult to compress so that absence of compression does not indicate that there is thrombus in the vessel. Difficulty with compressing the vein occurs in obese or muscular patients. If the SCV is fully compressible along its course, no thrombus is present. The absence of compression may be because of patient-specific factors or owing to the presence of an isoechoic thrombus.

The IVC is imaged in its transverse axis and examined for visible thrombus (Video 92.7). A transhepatic approach is used to image the proximal IVC. The longitudinal axis view may also be used. Bowel gas may degrade image quality when attempting to scan the distal IVC, and patient-specific factors such as obesity, anasarca, or heavy musculature limit visualization as well. If the IVC is visible in its extrahepatic course, a compression maneuver is performed. This is may only be possible in slender individuals. In its intrahepatic course, the IVC is not compressible. The proximal superior vena cava (SVC) may be imaged using transesophageal echocardiography. The midesophageal bicaval view can detect an SVC thrombus. This may be associated with CVC.

Limitations

1. Training is required for the intensivist to be competent in the examination for DVT. The anatomic basis for the examination is a key component of the examination because it is mastery of machine control and image acquisition. An overgained image may give the false impression of a thrombus, whereas an undergained image may cause the operator to miss a thrombus. Misorientation of the image may cause confusion between the artery and the vein.
2. Off-axis force application during the compression maneuver may give the false impression that the vein is not compressible. The compression is performed in a direction straight down onto the vessel.
3. There is concern that a compression of a vein with thrombus carries the risk of dislodgement with resultant PE. This has been reported as a very rare complication of the examination. The definitive identification of a thrombus on the 2-D examination does not require compression for verification of a venous thrombosis.
4. If the operator exerts too much pressure on the probe while trying to locate a vessel, the vein may not be visible because it is inadvertently compressed. This is common error at the junction of the CFV and the saphenous vein, as well when examining the PV.
5. When compressing the PV, the probe often slips to one side so the correct image is lost. An alternative method of performing compression of the PV is to center the target vessel on the screen and then apply counterpressure to the overlying patella instead of direct pressure with the probe.
6. The results of the intensivist examination may be not diagnostic. This occurs when patient-specific factors degrade image quality. Expert-level radiology or vascular service consultation is then necessary.
7. Lymph nodes, particularly in the inguinal area, may be mistaken for intraluminal thrombus (Video 92.8). The distinction is made visualizing the structure in both transverse and sagittal planes. The lymph node will not elongate as will the vein in sagittal scanning plane.
8. Internal echoes ("smoke") are frequently encountered in patent veins in the presence of low-flow states. This should not be confused with true thrombi. Venous valves may be mistaken for thrombi. Valves are thin linear echogenic structures that have respirophasic movement and are within a compressible vessel (Video 92.8).
9. Minor anatomic variants are common, particularly with leg veins. For example, the FV may be lateral or medial to the FA instead of posterior to the artery. The profunda femoris vein may be difficult to identify because its junction with the CFV is not at a constant level in the upper thigh.
10. The results of the examination require documentation. One simple method is to obtain an adequate view at the appropriate anatomic level. The operator then activates the video clip function of the machine with a preset of 4-second duration. The compression maneuver is performed during this period. Each anatomic point is documented in similar manner.
11. The standard DVT examination does not include the lower leg or lower arm. Although the venous system of these areas can be examined, it requires specific training and adds considerable time to the examination, particularly for the calf veins. In addition, the finding of DVT in calf or forearm veins has uncertain value for management of the acutely ill patient. Radiology or vascular consultative services have the expertise required for this type of examination.

Echocardiography for Evaluation of Pulmonary Embolism

The main utility of ultrasonography for evaluation of PE derives from its use for diagnosis of DVT. The finding of a DVT is strong evidence that the patient has a PE, given the appropriate clinical circumstance. For this reason, the initial imaging study for patients with suspicion of PE is an immediate DVT study. If this is negative, further imaging such as CT pulmonary angiogram (CTPA) or ($\dot{V}/\dot{Q}$) scan may then be considered. The intensivist who is competent in critical care ultrasonography has, by definition, the ability to perform the DVT study immediately at point of care.

Critical care echocardiography has several applications for the diagnosis and management of PE.

1. Although uncommon, transthoracic echocardiography (TTE) may detect a thrombus in transit through the heart or in the main pulmonary artery [198]. Direct observation of the thrombus is diagnostic and allows the team to take immediate life-saving action, because a visible intracardiac thrombus is often associated with severe hemodynamic failure (Video 92.9). The right apical four-chamber view, subcostal long-axis view, and RV inflow view are useful for identification of a thrombus in transit. Rarely, a PE may be visualized in the main pulmonary artery with TTE from the parasternal short-axis view of the pulmonary artery or from

the subcostal short-axis view. A PE may be visualized using transesophageal echocardiography in the main and right pulmonary arteries but not often in the left pulmonary artery on account of tracheal air shadowing [199] (Video 92.9).

2. PE is always a consideration for the patient with hemodynamic failure. Goal-directed echocardiography (GDE) is useful in identification of cardiac dysfunction that is consistent with modynamically significant PE. The occurrence of hemodynamic failure from the RV afterload effect of PE is strongly associated with RV dilatation [200]. The patient who is in shock from PE has characteristic features on GDE that are consistent with acute cor pulmonale (APE) (Video 92.10).
   a. Parasternal long-axis view: The findings include a rounded and dilated RV outflow tract and paradoxic septal movement (typically, an end-systolic posterior movement of the interventricular septum).
   b. Parasternal short-axis view: The findings include flattening of interventricular septum, dilation of the RV, and paradoxic septal movement (typically, an end-systolic movement of the interventricular septum toward the LV cavity).
   c. Apical four-chamber view: The RV to LV size ratio is greater than 1. A ratio that is greater than 1 is consistent with APE. Submassive PE may be associated with moderate RV dilation (RV to LV size ratio >0.6).
   d. Subcostal long-axis view: The RV to LV size ratio is greater than 1.
   e. IVC long-axis view: The IVC is dilated.

The intensivist who is competent in advanced critical care echocardiography utilizes Doppler based measurements of RV function that are relevant to assessment of the PE, such as pulmonary artery pressures, tissue Doppler tricuspid annular velocity, tricuspid annular planar systolic excursion, respirophasic variation of pulmonary artery stroke volume, reduced main pulmonary artery acceleration time, and biphasic systolic velocity time interval of the pulmonary outflow in the proximal pulmonary artery. All of the TEE views described above have equivalent views that may be obtained with TEE.

Except for the unusual circumstance where the PE is directly visualized by echocardiography, the echocardiography examination is mainly useful to support the diagnosis of PE and to aid in categorizing the severity. In the acute situation where the patient presents with an undifferentiated shock state, GDE is useful because it may identify a dilated RV or APE, which, absent other explanation, immediately suggests the possibility of a hemodynamically consequential PE. This directs the care team to obtain further confirmatory studies. GDE is helpful for categorization of submassive PE, and, through serial examinations, it can is used to follow response to therapy. The GDE examination is considered within the context of the entire clinical picture, and is combined with other aspect of critical care ultrasonography such as DVT study and lung ultrasonography. There are other causes of RV dysfunction other than PE, and the patient may have alternative or coexisting diagnosis that will complicate the management of PE. Echocardiography cannot be used to exclude PE because the echocardiography results may be normal if the clot burden is low.

The combination of echocardiography, thoracic ultrasonography, and DVT study may be useful to reduce the need for unnecessary CTPA, when there is clinical suspicion for PE. Koenig et al. have reported that the finding of negative DVT study, absence of RV dilation, and the finding of an alternative diagnosis with ultrasonography for the clinical presentation (e.g., lung or cardiac abnormality) predicted that the patient would have a negative CTPA [201]. Nazerian et al. reported similar results with the addition of comprehensive lung ultrasonography [202]. Multisystem ultrasonography in combination with clinical scoring systems and D-dimer results may be useful in reducing the rate of negative CTPA, although it is clear that some patients will still require CTPA when ultrasonography results are equivacol. Mathis et al. reported that pulmonary emboli commonly result in small areas of consolidation immediately deep to the pleural interface with preferential distribution to the lower lobes of the lung [203]. This is a difficult area to image in the critically ill patient who is generally in supine position, so their results have uncertain application for the intensivist.

References

1. Heit JA: Epidemiology of venous thromboembolism. *Nat Rev Cardiol* 12:464–474, 2015.
2. Lim W, Meade M, Lauzier F, et al: Failure of anticoagulant thromboprophylaxis: Risk factors in medical-surgical critically ill patients. *Crit Care Med* 43(2):401–410, 2015.
3. Sandler DA, Martin JF: Autopsy proven pulmonary embolism in hospital patients: Are we detecting enough deep vein thrombosis? *J R Soc Med.* 82:203–205, 1989.
4. Rosendaal FR: Risk factors for venous thrombotic disease. *Thromb Haemost* 82:610–619, 1999
5. Lijfering WM, Rosendaal FR, Cannegieter SC: Risk factors for venous thrombosis—current understanding from an epidemiological point of view. *Br J Haematol* 149:824–833, 2010.
6. Seligsohn U, Lubetsky A: Genetic susceptibility to venous thrombosis. *N Engl J Med* 344:1222–1231, 2001.
7. Ridker PM, Miletich JP, Hennekens CH, et al: Ethnic distribution of factor V leiden in 4047 men and women. implications for venous thromboembolism screening. *JAMA* 277:1305–1307, 1997.
8. Emmerich J, Rosendaal FR, Cattaneo M, et al: Combined effect of factor V leiden and prothrombin 20210A on the risk of venous thromboembolism—pooled analysis of 8 case-control studies including 2310 cases and 3204 controls. study group for pooled-analysis in venous thromboembolism. *Thromb Haemost* 86:809–816, 2001.
9. Segal JB, Brotman DJ, Necochea AJ, et al: Predictive value of factor V leiden and prothrombin G20210A in adults with venous thromboembolism and in family members of those with a mutation: a systematic review. *JAMA* 301:2472–2485, 2009.
10. Emadi A, Crim MT, Brotman DJ, et al: Analytic validity of genetic tests to identify factor V leiden and prothrombin G20210A. *Am J Hematol* 85:264–270, 2010.
11. Chang MH, Lindegren ML, Butler MA, et al: Prevalence in the united states of selected candidate gene variants: Third national health and nutrition examination survey, 1991–1994. *Am J Epidemiol* 169:54–66, 2009.
12. Poort SR, Rosendaal FR, Reitsma PH, et al: A common genetic variation in the 3'-untranslated region of the prothrombin gene is associated with elevated plasma prothrombin levels and an increase in venous thrombosis. *Blood* 88:3698–3703, 1996.
13. Ridker PM, Hennekens CH, Miletich JP: G20210A mutation in prothrombin gene and risk of myocardial infarction, stroke, and venous thrombosis in a large cohort of US men. *Circulation* 99:999-1004, 1999.
14. Mateo J, Oliver A, Borrell M, et al: Laboratory evaluation and clinical characteristics of 2,132 consecutive unselected patients with venous thromboembolism—results of the Spanish multicentric study on thrombophilia (EMET-study). *Thromb Haemost* 77:444–451, 1997.
15. Martinelli I, Mannucci PM, De Stefano V, et al: Different risks of thrombosis in four coagulation defects associated with inherited thrombophilia: a study of 150 families. *Blood* 92:2353–2358, 1998.
16. Khor B, Van Cott EM: Laboratory tests for protein C deficiency. *Am J Hematol* 85:440–442, 2010.
17. Douay X, Lucas C, Caron C, et al: Antithrombin, protein C and protein S levels in 127 consecutive young adults with ischemic stroke. *Acta Neurol Scand* 98:124–127, 1998.
18. Mahmoodi BK, Brouwer JL, Veeger NJ, et al: Hereditary deficiency of protein C or protein S confers increased risk of arterial thromboembolic events at a young age: results from a large family cohort study. *Circulation* 118:1659–1667, 2008.
19. Castoldi E, Hackeng TM: Regulation of coagulation by protein S. *Curr Opin Hematol* 15:529–536, 2008.
20. Patnaik MM, Moll S: Inherited antithrombin deficiency: a review. *Haemophilia* 14:1229–1239, 2008.
21. Liumbruno G, Bennardello F, Lattanzio A, et al: Recommendations for the use of antithrombin concentrates and prothrombin complex concentrates. *Blood Transfus* 7:325–334, 2009.
22. Cunningham MT, Brandt JT, Laposata M, et al: Laboratory diagnosis of dysfibrinogenemia. *Arch Pathol Lab Med* 126:499–505, 2002.
23. Klerk M, Verhoef P, Clarke R, et al: MTHFR 677C-->T polymorphism and risk of coronary heart disease: a meta-analysis. *JAMA* 288:2023–2031, 2002.
24. Ray JG: Hyperhomocysteinemia: no longer a consideration in the management of venous thromboembolism. *Curr Opin Pulm Med* 14:369–373, 2008.
25. Humphrey LL, Fu R, Rogers K, et al: Homocysteine level and coronary heart disease incidence: A systematic review and meta-analysis. *Mayo Clin Proc* 83:1203–1212, 2008.

26. Eichinger S, Stumpflen A, Hirschl M, et al: Hyperhomocysteinemia is a risk factor of recurrent venous thromboembolism. *Thromb Haemost* 80:566–569, 1998.
27. Ray JG: Meta-analysis of hyperhomocysteinemia as a risk factor for venous thromboembolic disease. *Arch Intern Med* 158:2101–2106, 1998.
28. Ray JG, Kearon C, Yi Q, et al: Homocysteine-lowering therapy and risk for venous thromboembolism: a randomized trial. *Ann Intern Med* 146:761–767, 2007.
29. Koster T, Blann AD, Briet E, et al: Role of clotting factor VIII in effect of von willebrand factor on occurrence of deep-vein thrombosis. *Lancet* 345:152–155, 1995.
30. Kyrle PA, Minar E, Hirschl M, et al: High plasma levels of factor VIII and the risk of recurrent venous thromboembolism. *N Engl J Med* 343:457–462, 2000.
31. Meijers JC, Tekelenburg WL, Bouma BN, et al: High levels of coagulation factor XI as a risk factor for venous thrombosis. *N Engl J Med* 342:696–701, 2000.
32. van Hylckama Vlieg A, van der Linden IK, Bertina RM, et al: High levels of factor IX increase the risk of venous thrombosis. *Blood* 95:3678–3682, 2000.
33. Sweetland S, Green J, Liu B, et al: Duration and magnitude of the postoperative risk of venous thromboembolism in middle aged women: prospective cohort study. *BMJ* 339:b4583, 2009.
34. White RH, Zhou H, Murin S, et al: Effect of ethnicity and gender on the incidence of venous thromboembolism in a diverse population in California in 1996. *Thromb Haemost* 93:298–305, 2005.
35. Naik RP, Streiff MB, Haywood C Jr, et al: Venous thromboembolism in adults with sickle cell disease: A serious and under-recognized complication. *Am J Med* 126:443–449, 2013.
36. Brodsky RA: Paroxysmal nocturnal hemoglobinuria. *Blood* 124:2804–2811, 2014.
37. Grant JD, Stevens SM, Woller SC, et al: Diagnosis and management of upper extremity deep-vein thrombosis in adults. *Thromb Haemost* 108:1097–1108, 2012.
38. Chopra V, Anand S, Hickner A, et al: Risk of venous thromboembolism associated with peripherally inserted central catheters: a systematic review and meta-analysis. *Lancet* 382:311–325, 2013
39. Heit JA, Silverstein MD, Mohr DN, et al: Risk factors for deep vein thrombosis and pulmonary embolism: A population-based case-control study. *Arch Intern Med* 160:809–815, 2000
40. Blom JW, Doggen CJ, Osanto S, et al: Malignancies, prothrombotic mutations, and the risk of venous thrombosis. *JAMA* 293:715–722, 2005.
41. Wun T, White RH: Venous thromboembolism (VTE) in patients with cancer: Epidemiology and risk factors. *Cancer Invest* 27 Suppl 1:63–74, 2009.
42. Khorana AA, Connolly GC: Assessing risk of venous thromboembolism in the patient with cancer. *J Clin Oncol* 27:4839–4847, 2009.
43. Carrier M, Lazo-Langner A, Shivakumar S, et al: Screening for occult cancer in unprovoked venous thromboembolism. *N Engl J Med* 373:697–704, 2015.
44. Prandoni P, Lensing AW, Piccioli A, et al: Recurrent venous thromboembolism and bleeding complications during anticoagulant treatment in patients with cancer and venous thrombosis. *Blood* 100:3484–3488, 2002.
45. Lee AY, Levine MN, Baker RI, et al: Low-molecular-weight heparin versus a coumarin for the prevention of recurrent venous thromboembolism in patients with cancer. *N Engl J Med* 349:146–153, 2003.
46. Tefferi A, Elliott M: Thrombosis in myeloproliferative disorders: Prevalence, prognostic factors, and the role of leukocytes and JAK2V617F. *Semin Thromb Hemost* 33:313–320, 2007.
47. Spivak JL: Polycythemia vera: Myths, mechanisms, and management. *Blood* 100:4272–4290, 2002.
48. Hillmen P, Muus P, Duhrsen U, et al: Effect of the complement inhibitor eculizumab on thromboembolism in patients with paroxysmal nocturnal hemoglobinuria. *Blood* 110:4123–4128, 2007.
49. Brodsky RA: How I treat paroxysmal nocturnal hemoglobinuria. *Blood* 113:6522–6527, 2009.
50. Heit JA, Kobbervig CE, James AH, et al: Trends in the incidence of venous thromboembolism during pregnancy or postpartum: a 30-year population-based study. *Ann Intern Med* 143:697–706, 2005.
51. James AH: Venous thromboembolism in pregnancy. *Arterioscler Thromb Vasc Biol* 29:326–331, 2009.
52. Marik PE, Plante LA: Venous thromboembolic disease and pregnancy. *N Engl J Med* 359:2025–2033, 2008.
53. Pomp ER, Lenselink AM, Rosendaal FR, et al: Pregnancy, the postpartum period and prothrombotic defects: risk of venous thrombosis in the MEGA study. *J Thromb Haemost* 6:632–637, 2008.
54. Kamel H, Navi BB, Sriram N, et al: Risk of a thrombotic event after the 6-week postpartum period. *N Engl J Med* 370:1307–1315, 2014.
55. James AH, Jamison MG, Brancazio LR, et al: Venous thromboembolism during pregnancy and the postpartum period: incidence, risk factors, and mortality. *Am J Obstet Gynecol* 194:1311–1315, 2006.
56. Crowther MA, Cook DJ, Meade MO, et al: Thrombocytopenia in medical-surgical critically ill patients: Prevalence, incidence, and risk factors. *J Crit Care* 20:348–353, 2005.
57. Crowther MA, Cook DJ, Albert M, et al: The 4Ts scoring system for heparin-induced thrombocytopenia in medical-surgical intensive care unit patients. *J Crit Care* 25:287–293, 2010.
58. Warkentin TE, Greinacher A, Koster A, et al: Treatment and prevention of heparin-induced thrombocytopenia: American college of chest physicians evidence-based clinical practice guidelines (8th edition). *Chest* 133:340S–380S, 2008.
59. Lo GK, Juhl D, Warkentin TE, et al: Evaluation of pretest clinical score (4 T's) for the diagnosis of heparin-induced thrombocytopenia in two clinical settings. *J Thromb Haemost* 4:759–765, 2006.
60. Warkentin TE: Heparin-induced thrombocytopenia. *Hematol Oncol Clin North Am* 21:589–607, 2007.
61. Geerts WH, Code KI, Jay RM, et al: A prospective study of venous thromboembolism after major trauma. *N Engl J Med* 331:1601–1606, 1994.
62. Knudson MM, Ikossi DG, Khaw L, et al: Thromboembolism after trauma: an analysis of 1602 episodes from the American college of surgeons national trauma data bank. *Ann Surg* 240:490–496; discussion 496–498, 2004.
63. Geerts WH, Jay RM, Code KI, et al: A comparison of low-dose heparin with low-molecular-weight heparin as prophylaxis against venous thromboembolism after major trauma. *N Engl J Med* 335:701–707, 1996.
64. Adams RC, Hamrick M, Berenguer C, et al: Four years of an aggressive prophylaxis and screening protocol for venous thromboembolism in a large trauma population. *J Trauma* 65:300–306; discussion 306–308, 2008.
65. Greenfield LJ, Proctor MC, Rodriguez JL, et al: Posttrauma thromboembolism prophylaxis. *J Trauma* 42:100–103, 1997.
66. Jacobsen AF, Sandset PM: Venous thromboembolism associated with pregnancy and hormonal therapy. *Best Pract Res Clin Haematol* 25:319–332, 2012.
67. Lidegaard O, Nielsen LH, Skovlund CW, et al: Venous thrombosis in users of non-oral hormonal contraception: follow-up study, Denmark 2001–2010. *BMJ* 344:e2990, 2012.
68. Liperoti R, Pedone C, Lapane KL, et al: Venous thromboembolism among elderly patients treated with atypical and conventional antipsychotic agents. *Arch Intern Med* 165:2677–2682, 2005.
69. Christiansen SC, Cannegieter SC, Koster T, et al: Thrombophilia, clinical factors, and recurrent venous thrombotic events. *JAMA* 293:2352–2361, 2005.
70. Giannakopoulos B, Passam F, Ioannou Y, et al: How we diagnose the antiphospholipid syndrome. *Blood* 113:985–994, 2009.
71. Giannakopoulos B, Krilis SA: How I treat the antiphospholipid syndrome. *Blood* 114:2020–2030, 2009.
72. Forastiero R, Martinuzzo M, Pombo G, et al: A prospective study of antibodies to beta2-glycoprotein I and prothrombin, and risk of thrombosis. *J Thromb Haemost* 3:1231–1238, 2005.
73. Somers E, Magder LS, Petri M: Antiphospholipid antibodies and incidence of venous thrombosis in a cohort of patients with systemic lupus erythematosus. *J Rheumatol* 29:2531–2536, 2002.
74. Galli M, Luciani D, Bertolini G, et al: Anti-beta 2-glycoprotein I, antiprothrombin antibodies, and the risk of thrombosis in the antiphospholipid syndrome. *Blood* 102:2717–2723, 2003.
75. Pengo V, Ruffatti A, Legnani C, et al: Clinical course of high-risk patients diagnosed with antiphospholipid syndrome. *J Thromb Haemost* 8:237–242, 2010.
76. Provenzale JM, Ortel TL, Allen NB: Systemic thrombosis in patients with antiphospholipid antibodies: Lesion distribution and imaging findings. *Am J Roentgenol* 170:285–290, 1998.
77. Crowther MA, Ginsberg JS, Julian J, et al: A comparison of two intensities of warfarin for the prevention of recurrent thrombosis in patients with the antiphospholipid antibody syndrome. *N Engl J Med* 349:1133–1138, 2003.
78. Finazzi G, Marchioli R, Brancaccio V, et al: A randomized clinical trial of high-intensity warfarin vs. conventional antithrombotic therapy for the prevention of recurrent thrombosis in patients with the antiphospholipid syndrome (WAPS). *J Thromb Haemost* 3:848–853, 2005.
79. Lim W, Crowther MA, Eikelboom JW: Management of antiphospholipid antibody syndrome: A systematic review. *JAMA* 295:1050–1057, 2006.
80. Levine SR, Brey RL, Tilley BC, et al: Antiphospholipid antibodies and subsequent thrombo-occlusive events in patients with ischemic stroke. *JAMA* 291:576–584, 2004.
81. Bucciarelli S, Espinosa G, Cervera R: The CAPS registry: Morbidity and mortality of the catastrophic antiphospholipid syndrome. *Lupus* 18:905–912, 2009.
82. Strakhan M, Hurtado-Sbordoni M, Galeas N, et al: 36-year-old female with catastrophic antiphospholipid syndrome treated with eculizumab: a case report and review of literature. *Case Rep Hematol* 2014:704371, 2014.
83. Cervera R: Update on the diagnosis, treatment, and prognosis of the catastrophic antiphospholipid syndrome. *Curr Rheumatol Rep* 12:70–76, 2010.
84. Furie B, Furie BC: Mechanisms of thrombus formation. *N Engl J Med* 359:938–949, 2008.
85. Versteeg HH, Heemskerk JW, Levi M, et al: New fundamentals in hemostasis. *Physiol Rev* 93:327–358, 2013.
86. Kearon C: Natural history of venous thromboembolism. *Circulation* 107:I22–I30, 2003.
87. D'Alonzo GE, Bower JS, DeHart P, et al: The mechanisms of abnormal gas exchange in acute massive pulmonary embolism. *Am Rev Respir Dis* 128:170–172, 1983.
88. D'Alonzo GE, Dantzker DR: Gas exchange alterations following pulmonary thromboembolism. *Clin Chest Med* 5:411–419, 1984.
89. McIntyre KM, Sasahara AA: The hemodynamic response to pulmonary embolism in patients without prior cardiopulmonary disease. *Am J Cardiol* 28:288–294, 1971.
90. McIntyre KM, Sasahara AA: Hemodynamic and ventricular responses to pulmonary embolism. *Prog Cardiovasc Dis* 17:175–190, 1974.
91. Streiff MB, Lau BD: Thromboprophylaxis in nonsurgical patients. *Hematol Am Soc Hematol Educ Prog* 2012:631–637, 2012.
92. Kleber FX, Witt C, Vogel G, et al: Randomized comparison of enoxaparin with unfractionated heparin for the prevention of venous thromboembolism in medical patients with heart failure or severe respiratory disease. *Am Heart J* 145:614–621, 2003.
93. Samama MM, Cohen AT, Darmon JY, et al: A comparison of enoxaparin with placebo for the prevention of venous thromboembolism in acutely ill medical patients. prophylaxis in medical patients with enoxaparin study group. *N Engl J Med* 341:793–800, 1999.

94. Leizorovicz A, Cohen AT, Turpie AG, et al: Randomized, placebo-controlled trial of dalteparin for the prevention of venous thromboembolism in acutely ill medical patients. *Circulation* 110:874–879, 2004.
95. Cohen AT, Davidson BL, Gallus AS, et al: Efficacy and safety of fondaparinux for the prevention of venous thromboembolism in older acute medical patients: randomised placebo controlled trial. *BMJ* 332:325–329, 2006.
96. King CS, Holley AB, Jackson JL, et al: Twice vs three times daily heparin dosing for thromboembolism prophylaxis in the general medical population: a metaanalysis. *Chest* 131:507–516, 2007.
97. PROTECT Investigators for the Canadian Critical Care Trials Group and the Australian and New Zealand Intensive Care Society Clinical Trials Group, Cook D, Meade M, et al: Dalteparin versus unfractionated heparin in critically ill patients. *N Engl J Med* 364:1305–1314, 2011.
98. Cohen AT, Tapson VF, Bergmann JF, et al: Venous thromboembolism risk and prophylaxis in the acute hospital care setting (ENDORSE study): a multinational cross-sectional study. *Lancet* 371:387–394, 2008.
99. Kucher N, Koo S, Quiroz R, et al: Electronic alerts to prevent venous thromboembolism among hospitalized patients. *N Engl J Med* 352:969–977, 2005.
100. Zeidan AM, Streiff MB, Lau BD, et al: Impact of a venous thromboembolism prophylaxis "smart order set": improved compliance, fewer events. *Am J Hematol.* 88(7):545–549, 2013.
101. Haut ER, Lau BD, Kraenzlin FS, et al: Improved prophylaxis and decreased rates of preventable harm with the use of a mandatory computerized clinical decision support tool for prophylaxis for venous thromboembolism in trauma. *Arch Surg* 147:901–907, 2012.
102. Shermock KM, Lau BD, Haut ER, et al: Patterns of non-administration of ordered doses of venous thromboembolism prophylaxis: implications for novel intervention strategies. *PLoS One* 8:e66311, 2013.
103. Louis SG, Sato M, Geraci T, et al: Correlation of missed doses of enoxaparin with increased incidence of deep vein thrombosis in trauma and general surgery patients. *JAMA Surg* 149:365–370, 2014.
104. Barbar S, Noventa F, Rossetto V, et al: A risk assessment model for the identification of hospitalized medical patients at risk for venous thromboembolism: the padua prediction score. *J Thromb Haemost* 8:2450–2457, 2010.
105. Spyropoulos AC, Anderson FA Jr, Fitzgerald G, et al: Predictive and associative models to identify hospitalized medical patients at risk for VTE. *Chest* 140:706–714, 2011.
106. Caprini JA, Arcelus JI, Hasty JH, et al: Clinical assessment of venous thromboembolic risk in surgical patients. *Semin Thromb Hemost* 17[Suppl 3]:304–312, 1991.
107. Rogers SO Jr, Kilaru RK, Hosokawa P, et al: Multivariable predictors of postoperative venous thromboembolic events after general and vascular surgery: results from the patient safety in surgery study. *J Am Coll Surg* 204:1211–1221, 2007.
108. Obi AT, Pannucci CJ, Nackashi A, et al: Validation of the caprini venous thromboembolism risk assessment model in critically ill surgical patients. *JAMA Surg* 150:941–948, 2015.
109. Nendaz M, Spirk D, Kucher N, et al: Multicentre validation of the geneva risk score for hospitalised medical patients at risk of venous thromboembolism. Explicit assessment of thromboembolic risk and prophylaxis for medical patients in Switzerland (ESTIMATE). *Thromb Haemost* 111:531–538, 2014.
110. Mahan CE, Liu Y, Turpie AG, et al: External validation of a risk assessment model for venous thromboembolism in the hospitalised acutely-ill medical patient (VTE-VALOURR). *Thromb Haemost* 112:692–699, 2014.
111. Decousus H, Tapson VF, Bergmann JF, et al: Factors at admission associated with bleeding risk in medical patients: Findings from the IMPROVE investigators. *Chest* 139:69–79, 2011.
112. CLOTS (Clots in Legs Or sTockings after Stroke) Trials Collaboration, Dennis M, Sandercock P, et al: Effectiveness of intermittent pneumatic compression in reduction of risk of deep vein thrombosis in patients who have had a stroke (CLOTS 3): a multicentre randomised controlled trial. *Lancet* 382:516–524, 2013.
113. CLOTS Trials Collaboration, Dennis M, Sandercock PA, et al: Effectiveness of thigh-length graduated compression stockings to reduce the risk of deep vein thrombosis after stroke (CLOTS trial 1): a multicentre, randomised controlled trial. *Lancet* 373:1958–1965, 2009.
114. Agnelli G, Becattini C: Acute pulmonary embolism. *N Engl J Med* 363:266–274, 2010.
115. Wells PS, Anderson DR, Rodger M, et al: Evaluation of D-dimer in the diagnosis of suspected deep-vein thrombosis. *N Engl J Med* 349:1227–1235, 2003.
116. Kearon C, Ginsberg JS, Douketis J, et al: An evaluation of D-dimer in the diagnosis of pulmonary embolism: a randomized trial. *Ann Intern Med* 144:812–821, 2006.
117. Kline JA, Courtney DM, Kabrhel C, et al: Prospective multicenter evaluation of the pulmonary embolism rule-out criteria. *J Thromb Haemost* 6:772–780, 2008.
118. Ollenberger GP, Worsley DF: Effect of patient location on the performance of clinical models to predict pulmonary embolism. *Thromb Res* 118:685–690, 2006.
119. Lapner ST, Kearon C: Diagnosis and management of pulmonary embolism. *BMJ* 346:f757, 2013.
120. Huisman MV, Klok FA: How I diagnose acute pulmonary embolism. *Blood* 121:4443–4448, 2013.
121. Klok FA, Mos IC, Nijkeuter M, et al: Simplification of the revised geneva score for assessing clinical probability of pulmonary embolism. *Arch Intern Med* 168:2131–2136, 2008.
122. Lucassen W, Geersing GJ, Erkens PM, et al: Clinical decision rules for excluding pulmonary embolism: a meta-analysis. *Ann Intern Med* 155:448–460, 2011.
123. Douma RA, Mos IC, Erkens PM, et al: Performance of 4 clinical decision rules in the diagnostic management of acute pulmonary embolism: a prospective cohort study. *Ann Intern Med* 154:709–718, 2011.
124. Singh B, Mommer SK, Erwin PJ, et al: Pulmonary embolism rule-out criteria (PERC) in pulmonary embolism—revisited: a systematic review and meta-analysis. *Emerg Med J* 30:701–706, 2013.
125. Raja AS, Greenberg JO, Qaseem A, et al: Evaluation of patients with suspected acute pulmonary embolism: best practice advice from the clinical guidelines committee of the American college of physicians. *Ann Intern Med* 163(9):701–711, 2015.
126. Stein PD, Hull RD, Patel KC, et al: D-dimer for the exclusion of acute venous thrombosis and pulmonary embolism: a systematic review. *Ann Intern Med* 140:589–602, 2004.
127. Brotman DJ, Segal JB, Jani JT, et al: Limitations of D-dimer testing in unselected inpatients with suspected venous thromboembolism. *Am J Med* 114:276–282, 2003.
128. Konstantinides SV, Torbicki A, Agnelli G, et al: 2014 ESC guidelines on the diagnosis and management of acute pulmonary embolism. *Eur Heart J* 35:3033–3069, 3069a–3069k, 2014.
129. Schouten HJ, Geersing GJ, Koek HL, et al: Diagnostic accuracy of conventional or age adjusted D-dimer cut-off values in older patients with suspected venous thromboembolism: Systematic review and meta-analysis. *BMJ* 346:f2492, 2013.
130. Kearon C, Julian JA, Newman TE, et al: Noninvasive diagnosis of deep venous thrombosis. McMaster diagnostic imaging practice guidelines initiative. *Ann Intern Med* 128:663–677, 1998.
131. Bates SM, Jaeschke R, Stevens SM, et al: Diagnosis of DVT: antithrombotic therapy and prevention of thrombosis, 9th ed: American college of chest physicians evidence-based clinical practice guidelines. *Chest* 141:e351S–418S, 2012.
132. Huisman MV, Klok FA: Diagnostic management of acute deep vein thrombosis and pulmonary embolism. *J Thromb Haemost* 11:412–422, 2013.
133. Stein PD, Woodard PK, Weg JG, et al: Diagnostic pathways in acute pulmonary embolism: Recommendations of the PIOPED II investigators. *Radiology.* 242:15–21, 2007.
134. Righini M, Le Gal G, Aujesky D, et al: Diagnosis of pulmonary embolism by multidetector CT alone or combined with venous ultrasonography of the leg: a randomised non-inferiority trial. *Lancet.* 371:1343–1352, 2008.
135. Anderson DR, Kahn SR, Rodger MA, et al: Computed tomographic pulmonary angiography vs ventilation-perfusion lung scanning in patients with suspected pulmonary embolism: A randomized controlled trial. *JAMA* 298:2743–2753, 2007.
136. PIOPED Investigators: Value of the ventilation/perfusion scan in acute pulmonary embolism. results of the prospective investigation of pulmonary embolism diagnosis (PIOPED). *JAMA* 263:2753–2759, 1990.
137. Stein PD, Chenevert TL, Fowler SE, et al: Gadolinium-enhanced magnetic resonance angiography for pulmonary embolism: a multicenter prospective study (PIOPED III). *Ann Intern Med* 152:434–443, W142–W143, 2010.
138. Stein PD, Athanasoulis C, Alavi A, et al: Complications and validity of pulmonary angiography in acute pulmonary embolism. *Circulation* 85:462–468, 1992.
139. Aujesky D, Obrosky DS, Stone RA, et al: Derivation and validation of a prognostic model for pulmonary embolism. *Am J Respir Crit Care Med* 172:1041–1046, 2005.
140. Zondag W, Mos IC, Creemers-Schild D, et al: Outpatient treatment in patients with acute pulmonary embolism: The HESTIA study. *J Thromb Haemost* 9:1500–1507, 2011.
141. Aujesky D, Roy PM, Verschuren F, et al: Outpatient versus inpatient treatment for patients with acute pulmonary embolism: An international, open-label, randomised, non-inferiority trial. *Lancet* 378:41–48, 2011.
142. Zondag W, den Exter PL, Crobach MJ, et al: Comparison of two methods for selection of out of hospital treatment in patients with acute pulmonary embolism. *Thromb Haemost* 109:47–52, 2013.
143. Schoepf UJ, Kucher N, Kipfmueller F, et al: Right ventricular enlargement on chest computed tomography: a predictor of early death in acute pulmonary embolism. *Circulation* 110:3276–3280, 2004.
144. Trujillo-Santos J, den Exter PL, Gomez V, et al: Computed tomography-assessed right ventricular dysfunction and risk stratification of patients with acute non-massive pulmonary embolism: systematic review and meta-analysis. *J Thromb Haemost* 11:1823–1832, 2013.
145. Coutance G, Cauderlier E, Ehtisham J, et al: The prognostic value of markers of right ventricular dysfunction in pulmonary embolism: a meta-analysis. *Crit Care* 15:R103, 2011.
146. Vuilleumier N, Le Gal L, Verschuren F, et al: Cardiac biomarkers for risk stratification in non-massive pulmonary embolism: a multicenter prospective study. *J Thromb Haemost* 7:391–398, 2009.
147. Lankeit M, Jimenez D, Kostrubiec M, et al: Predictive value of the high-sensitivity troponin T assay and the simplified pulmonary embolism severity index in hemodynamically stable patients with acute pulmonary embolism: a prospective validation study. *Circulation* 124:2716–2724, 2011.
148. Jimenez D, Kopecna D, Tapson V, et al: Derivation and validation of multimarker prognostication for normotensive patients with acute symptomatic pulmonary embolism. *Am J Respir Crit Care Med* 189:718–726, 2014.

149. Kearon C, Akl EA, Comerota AJ, et al: Antithrombotic therapy for VTE disease: Antithrombotic therapy and prevention of thrombosis, 9th ed: American college of chest physicians evidence-based clinical practice guidelines. *Chest* 141:e419S–e494S, 2012.
150. Dolovich LR, Ginsberg JS, Douketis JD, et al: A meta-analysis comparing low-molecular-weight heparins with unfractionated heparin in the treatment of venous thromboembolism: Examining some unanswered questions regarding location of treatment, product type, and dosing frequency. *Arch Intern Med* 160:181–188, 2000.
151. Garcia DA, Baglin TP, Weitz JI, et al: Parenteral anticoagulants: Antithrombotic therapy and prevention of thrombosis, 9th ed: American college of chest physicians evidence-based clinical practice guidelines. *Chest* 141:e24S–e43S, 2012.
152. Ageno W, Gallus AS, Wittkowsky A, et al: Oral anticoagulant therapy: Antithrombotic therapy and prevention of thrombosis, 9th ed: American college of chest physicians evidence-based clinical practice guidelines. *Chest* 141:e44S–e88S, 2012.
153. Holbrook A, Schulman S, Witt DM, et al: Evidence-based management of anticoagulant therapy: Antithrombotic therapy and prevention of thrombosis, 9th ed: American college of chest physicians evidence-based clinical practice guidelines. *Chest* 141:e152S–e184S, 2012
154. Schulman S, Kearon C, Kakkar AK, et al: Dabigatran versus warfarin in the treatment of acute venous thromboembolism. *N Engl J Med* 361:2342–2352, 2009.
155. Schulman S, Kearon C, Kakkar AK, et al: Extended use of dabigatran, warfarin, or placebo in venous thromboembolism. *N Engl J Med* 368:709–718, 2013.
156. Agnelli G, Buller HR, Cohen A, et al: Oral apixaban for the treatment of acute venous thromboembolism. *N Engl J Med* 369:799–808, 2013.
157. Agnelli G, Buller HR, Cohen A, et al: Apixaban for extended treatment of venous thromboembolism. *N Engl J Med* 368(8):699–708; 2012.
158. EINSTEIN Investigators, Bauersachs R, Berkowitz SD, et al: Oral rivaroxaban for symptomatic venous thromboembolism. *N Engl J Med* 363:2499–2510, 2010.
159. EINSTEIN-PE Investigators, Buller HR, Prins MH, et al: Oral rivaroxaban for the treatment of symptomatic pulmonary embolism. *N Engl J Med* 366:1287–1297, 2012.
160. Hokusai-VTE Investigators, Buller HR, Decousus H, et al: Edoxaban versus warfarin for the treatment of symptomatic venous thromboembolism. *N Engl J Med* 369:1406–1415, 2013.
161. Goldhaber SZ, Visani L, De Rosa M: Acute pulmonary embolism: clinical outcomes in the international cooperative pulmonary embolism registry (ICOPER). *Lancet.* 353:1386–1389, 1999.
162. Konstantinides S, Geibel A, Heusel G, et al: Heparin plus alteplase compared with heparin alone in patients with submassive pulmonary embolism. *N Engl J Med* 347:1143–1150, 2002.
163. Meyer G, Vicaut E, Danays T, et al: Fibrinolysis for patients with intermediate-risk pulmonary embolism. *N Engl J Med* 370:1402–1411, 2014.
164. Kucher N, Boekstegers P, Muller OJ, et al: Randomized, controlled trial of ultrasound-assisted catheter-directed thrombolysis for acute intermediate-risk pulmonary embolism. *Circulation* 129:479–486, 2014.
165. Kuo WT, Banerjee A, Kim PS, et al: Pulmonary embolism response to fragmentation, embolectomy, and catheter thrombolysis (PERFECT): Initial results from a prospective multicenter registry. *Chest* 148:667–673, 2015.
166. Er F, Nia AM, Gassanov N, et al: Impact of rescue-thrombolysis during cardiopulmonary resuscitation in patients with pulmonary embolism. *PLoS One* 4:e8323, 2009.
167. Bottiger BW, Arntz HR, Chamberlain DA, et al: Thrombolysis during resuscitation for out-of-hospital cardiac arrest. *N Engl J Med* 359:2651–2662, 2008.
168. Stein PD, Matta F, Steinberger DS, et al: Intracerebral hemorrhage with thrombolytic therapy for acute pulmonary embolism. *Am J Med* 125:50–56, 2012.
169. Chatterjee S, Chakraborty A, Weinberg I, et al: Thrombolysis for pulmonary embolism and risk of all-cause mortality, major bleeding, and intracranial hemorrhage: a meta-analysis. *JAMA* 311:2414–2421, 2014.
170. Enden T, Klow NE, Sandvik L, et al: Catheter-directed thrombolysis vs. anticoagulant therapy alone in deep vein thrombosis: Results of an open randomized, controlled trial reporting on short-term patency. *J Thromb Haemost* 7:1268–1275, 2009.
171. Birn J, Vedantham S: May-thurner syndrome and other obstructive iliac vein lesions: Meaning, myth, and mystery. *Vasc Med* 20:74–83, 2015.
172. Vedantham S: Interventional therapy for venous thromboembolism. *J Thromb Haemost* 13[Suppl 1]:S245–S251, 2015.
173. Rajasekhar A, Streiff MB: Vena cava filters for management of venous thromboembolism: a clinical review. *Blood Rev* 27:225–241, 2013.
174. Usoh F, Hingorani A, Ascher E, et al: Prospective randomized study comparing the clinical outcomes between inferior vena cava greenfield and TrapEase filters. *J Vasc Surg* 52:394–399, 2010.
175. Decousus H, Leizorovicz A, Parent F, et al: A clinical trial of vena caval filters in the prevention of pulmonary embolism in patients with proximal deep-vein thrombosis. prevention du risque d'embolie pulmonaire par interruption cave study group. *N Engl J Med* 338:409–415, 1998.
176. Mismetti P: PREPIC 2: Interruption of inferior vena cava by a retrievable filter for the prevention of recurrent pulmonary embolism: a randomised, open label study.
177. PREPIC Study Group: Eight-year follow-up of patients with permanent vena cava filters in the prevention of pulmonary embolism: The PREPIC (prevention du risque d'embolie pulmonaire par interruption cave) randomized study. *Circulation* 112:416–422, 2005.
178. He C, Von Segesser LK, Kappetein PA, et al: Acute pulmonary embolectomy. *Eur J Cardiothorac Surg* 43:1087–1095, 2013.
179. Kuo WT, Gould MK, Louie JD, et al: Catheter-directed therapy for the treatment of massive pulmonary embolism: Systematic review and meta-analysis of modern techniques. *J Vasc Interv Radiol* 20:1431–1440, 2009.
180. Jasti N, Streiff MB: Prevention and treatment of thrombosis associated with central venous catheters in cancer patients. *Expert Rev Hematol* 7:599–616, 2014.
181. Chan WS, Lee A, Spencer FA, et al: Predicting deep venous thrombosis in pregnancy: Out in "LEFt" field? *Ann Intern Med* 151:85–92, 2009.
182. Leung AN, Bull TM, Jaeschke R, et al: An official American thoracic Society/Society of thoracic radiology clinical practice guideline: evaluation of suspected pulmonary embolism in pregnancy. *Am J Respir Crit Care Med* 184:1200–1208, 2011.
183. Bates SM, Greer IA, Middeldorp S, et al: VTE, thrombophilia, antithrombotic therapy, and pregnancy: Antithrombotic therapy and prevention of thrombosis, 9th ed: American college of chest physicians evidence-based clinical practice guidelines. *Chest* 141:e691S–e736S, 2012.
184. White RH: The epidemiology of venous thromboembolism. *Circulation* 107:I4–I8, 2003.
185. Carson JL, Kelley MA, Duff A, et al: The clinical course of pulmonary embolism. *N Engl J Med* 326:1240–1245, 1992.
186. Douketis JD, Kearon C, Bates S, et al: Risk of fatal pulmonary embolism in patients with treated venous thromboembolism. *JAMA* 279:458–462, 1998.
187. Piazza G, Goldhaber SZ: Chronic thromboembolic pulmonary hypertension. *N Engl J Med* 364:351–360, 2011.
188. Iorio A, Kearon C, Filippucci E, et al: Risk of recurrence after a first episode of symptomatic venous thromboembolism provoked by a transient risk factor: a systematic review. *Arch Intern Med* 170:1710–1716, 2010.
189. Streiff MB: Predicting the risk of recurrent venous thromboembolism (VTE). *J Thromb Thrombolysis* 39:353–366, 2015.
190. Gould MK, Dembitzer AD, Doyle RL, et al: Low-molecular-weight heparins compared with unfractionated heparin for treatment of acute deep venous thrombosis: a meta-analysis of randomized, controlled trials. *Ann Intern Med* 130:800–809, 1999.
191. Pollack CV Jr, Reilly PA, Eikelboom J, et al: Idarucizumab for dabigatran reversal. *N Engl J Med* 373:511–520, 2015.
192. Siegal DM, Curnutte JT, Connolly SJ, et al: Andexanet alfa for the reversal of factor xa inhibitor activity. *N Engl J Med* 373:2413–2424, 2015.
193. Ansell JE, Bakhru SH, Laulicht BE, et al: Use of PER977 to reverse the anticoagulant effect of edoxaban. *N Engl J Med* 371:2141–2142, 2014.
194. Kory PD, Pellecchia CM, Shiloh AL, et al: Accuracy of ultrasonography performed by critical care physicians for the diagnosis of DVT. *Chest* 139:538–542, 2011.
195. Theodoro D, Blaivas M, Duggal S, et al: Real-time B-mode ultrasound in the ED saves time in the diagnosis of deep vein thrombosis (DVT). *Am J Emerg Med* 22:197–200, 2004.
196. Jang T, Docherty M, Aubin C, et al: Resident-performed compression ultrasonography for the detection of proximal deep vein thrombosis: fast and accurate. *Acad Emerg Med* 11:319–322, 2004.
197. Lensing AW, Doris CI, McGrath FP, et al: A comparison of compression ultrasound with color Doppler ultrasound for the diagnosis of symptomless postoperative deep vein thrombosis. *Arch Intern Med* 157:765–776, 1997.
198. Agarwal V, Nalluri N, Shariff MA, et al: Large embolus in transit - an unresolved therapeutic dilemma (case report and review of literature). *Heart Lung*. 2014;43:152–154.
199. Vieillard-Baron A, Page B, Augarde R, et al: Acute cor pulmonale in massive pulmonary embolism: incidence, echocardiographic pattern, clinical implications and recovery rate. *Intensive Care Med* 2001;27:1481–1486.
200. Vieillard-Baron A, Qanadli SD, Antakly Y, et al: Transesophageal echocardiography for the diagnosis of pulmonary embolism with acute cor pulmonale: a comparison with radiological procedures. *Intensive Care Med* 24:429–433, 1998.
201. Koenig S, Chandra S, Alaverdian A, et al: Ultrasound assessment of pulmonary embolism in patients receiving CT pulmonary angiography. *Chest* 145(4):818–823, 2014.
202. Nazerian P, Vanni S, Volpicelli G, et al: Accuracy of point-of-care multi-organ ultrasonography for the diagnosis of pulmonary embolism. *Chest* 145:950–957, 2014.
203. Mathis G, Blank W, Reissig A, et al: Thoracic ultrasound for diagnosing pulmonary embolism: a prospective multicenter study of 352 patients. *Chest* 2005;128:1531–1538.

Chapter 93 ■ Antithrombotic Pharmacotherapy

KEVIN E. ANGER • CHRISTOPHER D. ADAMS • BONNIE C. GREENWOOD • JEREMY R. DEGRADO • JOHN FANIKOS

INTRODUCTION

Thromboembolic disease is commonly encountered among critically ill patients [1]. While these patients are at high risk for developing arterial and venous thrombosis due to underlying comorbidities, central venous catheter placement, and immobility, they are also at high risk for hemorrhagic complications resulting from gastrointestinal stress ulcerations, invasive procedures, liver dysfunction, uremia, or coagulopathy [2]. These divergent features often complicate antithrombotic treatments for the prevention or management of thrombosis. Limitations in administration routes, hemodynamic instability, alterations in renal and hepatic function, and drug interactions further complicate the administration of these high-risk medications [3].

This chapter focuses on the mechanisms of action, pharmacokinetics, pharmacodynamics, clinical indications, complications of therapy, and reversal options for antithrombotic pharmacotherapy in critically ill patients.

ANTIPLATELET PHARMACOTHERAPY

Overview of Antiplatelet Pharmacotherapy

Antiplatelet agents target mechanisms in platelet activation, adhesion, and aggregation. Pharmacological inhibitors of platelet function fall into five general categories: thromboxane (TXA) inhibitors, antagonists of adenosine diphosphate (ADP)-mediated platelet activation, glycoprotein (GP) IIb/IIIa complex inhibitors, thrombin receptor antagonists, and phosphodiesterase inhibitors (Fig. 93.1).

Antiplatelet 'resistance' and 'nonresponse' are terms applied to clinical outcomes characterized by failure to prevent a thrombotic event due to inadequate platelet inhibition [4]. Resistance is conferred by underlying clinical, cellular, and genetic mechanisms. It is best confirmed by platelet function testing [4]. While several methods are available for measuring the overall and drug-specific platelet aggregation, standard testing protocols have yet to be established [5].

Aspirin and Aspirin Derivatives

Pharmacology, Pharmacodynamics, and Monitoring

Aspirin, or acetylsalicylic acid, is a prodrug of salicylic acid that blocks platelet activation. Aspirin irreversibly inhibits cyclooxygenase enzymes (COX-1, COX-2), reducing prostaglandin and TXA by-products generated from arachidonic acid. Thromboxane A_2 stimulates platelet activation, aggregation, and recruitment [6]. COX-1 enzymes are present in most tissues, but larger amounts are found in the stomach, kidneys, and platelets. The prostaglandin products of COX enzyme activity provide protection from gastrointestinal mucosal injury. COX-2 is found in both nucleated and nonnucleated cells and is responsive to inflammatory stimuli. Inhibition of COX-1 appears to be the primary mechanism by which aspirin inhibits hemostasis. Aspirin's acetylation of platelet COX-1 enzymes causes inhibition of platelet TXA_2 production. The irreversible antiplatelet effect lasts for the lifespan of the platelet (7 to 10 days). Saturation of aspirin's antithrombotic mechanisms occurs at doses as low as 30 mg with larger doses (>3,000 mg daily) required to inhibit COX-2 and produce systemic anti-inflammatory effects. Consequently, there is a 50- to 100-fold variation between the daily doses required to suppress inflammation and inhibit platelet function [7].

Enteric-coated and delayed release formulations have diminished bioavailability, take 3 to 4 hours to reach peak plasma levels, and have delayed onset. Rectally administered aspirin has variable absorption with a bioavailability of 20% to 60% over a 2- to 5-hour retention time [8]. For acute thrombosis, immediate-release enteral aspirin is preferred [9].

The optimal aspirin dose that maximizes efficacy and minimizes toxicity is controversial. Evidence-based recommendations vary from 75 to 325 mg daily. There are currently no data suggesting inferiority of lower (75 to 100 mg) to higher (>100 mg) maintenance dosing in preventing thromboembolic events [9,10].

Recurrent vascular thrombotic episodes despite aspirin therapy occur at rates between 2% and 6% of patients per year [11] Aspirin resistance occurs in 5.5% to 45% of aspirin-treated patients. Possible mechanisms of aspirin resistance include extrinsic factors (adherence, absorption, dosage formulation, and smoking) and intrinsic factors (pharmacodynamic alterations, receptor polymorphisms, up regulation of nontargeted platelet activation pathways). In clinical trials, aspirin resistance has been associated with an increased risk of death, acute coronary syndromes (ACS), and stroke [12].

Clinical Indications

Aspirin is indicated for the primary and secondary prevention of arterial and venous thrombosis (Table 93.1). Aspirin is effective in reducing atherothrombotic disease morbidity and mortality in ACS, stable angina, coronary bypass surgery, peripheral arterial disease (PAD), transient ischemic attack, acute ischemic stroke, and polycythemia vera. Aspirin provides effective thromboprophylaxis in patients on warfarin with prosthetic heart valves and in patients with nonvalvular atrial fibrillation [13].

Complications and Reversal of Effect

Aspirin increases the incidence of major, gastrointestinal, and intracranial bleeding [6]. The recommended interval for discontinuation of aspirin prior to elective surgery or procedures is 7 to 10 days. Therapy can be resumed approximately 24 hours or the next morning after surgery when there is adequate hemostasis [14]. For patients exhibiting clinically significant bleeding or requiring emergent surgery, platelet transfusion may be warranted (Table 93.2). Intravenous desmopressin antagonizes aspirin's effect, suggesting a role in emergent situations as well [15].

Aspirin produces gastrointestinal ulcerations and hemorrhage through direct irritation of the gastric mucosa and via inhibition of prostaglandin synthesis. Aspirin, in recommended doses, increases the risk of gastrointestinal bleeding 1.5- to 3-fold [16]. Enteric-coated and buffered aspirin doses ≤325 mg do not reduce the incidence of gastrointestinal bleeding [17]. Aspirin-induced gastric toxicity can be prevented with concurrent use of acid-suppressive therapy [16].

Underlying aspirin allergy can exacerbate respiratory tract disease, angioedema, urticaria, or anaphylaxis and is estimated to occur in 10% of the general population. These patients

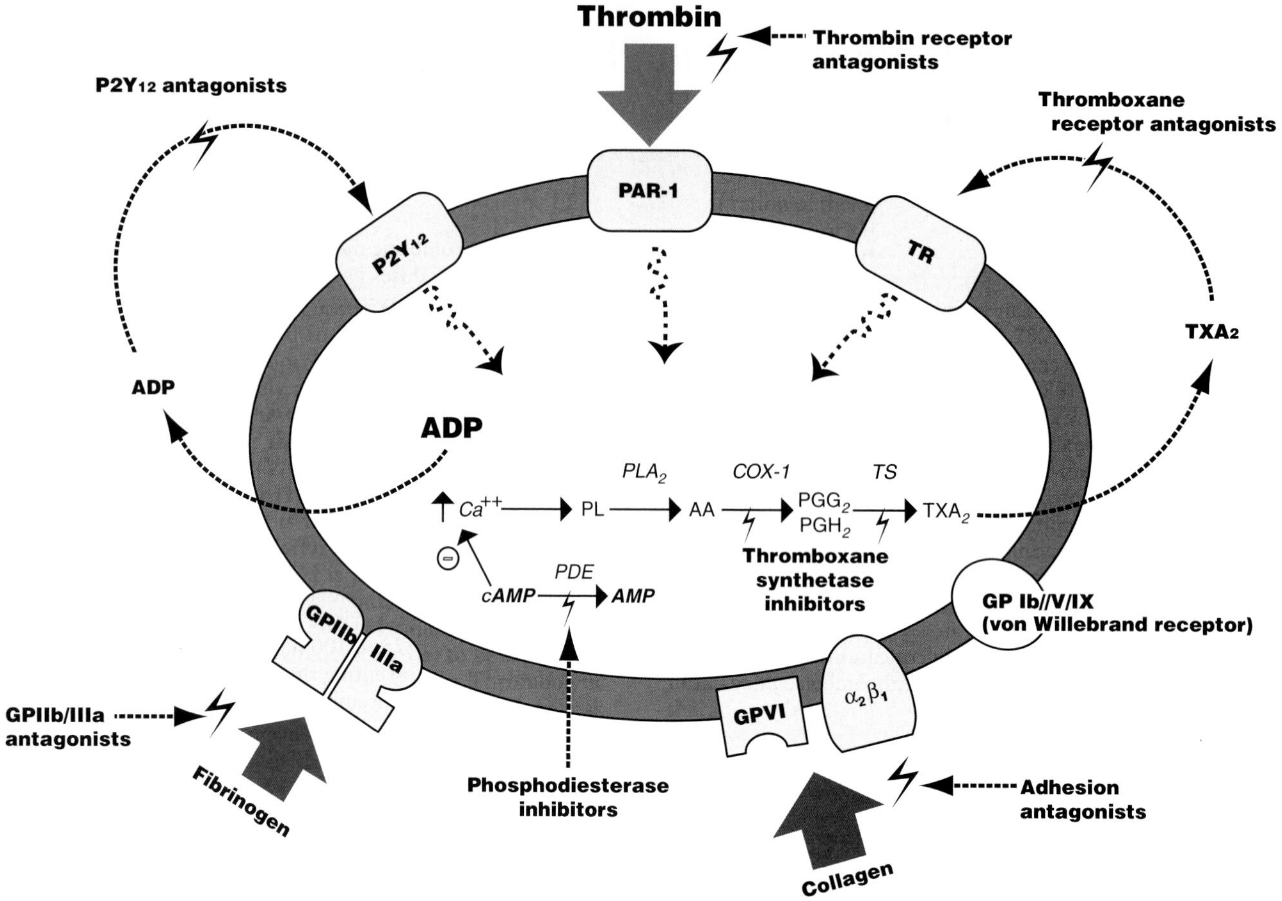

FIGURE 93.1 Platelet activation and pharmacological inhibitors of platelet function. Platelet activation involves four mechanisms: adhesion to sites of vascular injury, release of stimulatory compounds, aggregation, and priming of coagulation. Pharmacological inhibitors of platelet function target adhesion, release, and aggregation mechanisms. Platelet adhesion is a four-step process involving tethering of von Willebrand factor (VWF) to glycoprotein (GP) IIb platelet receptors, a potential target of investigational agents. The rolling phase of adhesion involves interaction between vascular collagen with GP VI and GP Ia/IIa receptors, another potential target of investigational agents. The activation phase of adhesion involves release of thromboxane A_2 (TXA_2) and adenosine diphosphate (ADP) which can be blocked with use of aspirin, $P2Y_{12}$ inhibitors, and thromboxane (TR) receptor antagonists. The stable adhesion phase involves the interaction of GP IIb/IIIa receptors with fibrinogen and VWF, which can be blocked with the use of GP IIb/IIIa inhibitors. Thrombin receptor antagonists block platelet aggregation by selectively blocking PAR-1 thrombin receptors.

may be converted to alternative antiplatelet therapies. Leukotriene-modifying agents may reduce aspirin-provoked respiratory reactions but do not eliminate the risk. For patients with a compelling indication for therapy, aspirin desensitization may be considered [18].

$P2Y_{12}$ Inhibitors

Pharmacology, Pharmacodynamics, and Monitoring

$P2Y_{12}$ inhibitors prevent platelet activation by blocking adenosine diphosphate (ADP) binding to $P2Y_{12}$ receptors. This action prevents activation of the GP IIb/IIIa receptor complex on the platelet surface [9]. Thienopyridine derivatives, clopidogrel, prasugrel, and ticlopidine, are prodrugs requiring hepatic activation via the cytochrome P450 (CYP450) isoenzyme system (Table 93.3). Metabolism by CYP450 plays a key role in the onset of action, potency, and drug interaction profile of these agents [19,20]. A loading dose provides a rapid increase in plasma concentration and a faster onset of action. Both clopidogrel and ticlopidine require a two-step activation process via CYP450. Prasugrel undergoes one-step oxidation by multiple CYP450 isoenzyme pathways which are believed to be responsible for its more predictable action.

While thienopyridine metabolites have a short plasma elimination half-life (1 to 8 hours), their irreversible activity at $P2Y_{12}$ receptors spans the life of the platelet (7 to 10 days). The onset of action, duration of antiplatelet effect, and unpredictable levels of platelet inhibition led to the development of newer agents [21]. Ticagrelor is a nonthienopyridine $P2Y_{12}$ inhibitor that does not require hepatic activation resulting in immediate, short-acting, dose-dependent inhibition of platelet activation aggregation [22]. Ticagrelor binds reversibly at $P2Y_{12}$ receptors resulting in a shorter duration of antiplatelet activity compared to thienopyridines [22]. Cangrelor in an intravenous (IV) agent with a very short half-life and rapid onset that lends itself useful in the procedural setting [23].

Resistance to clopidogrel occurs in 4% to 34% of patients and depends on the agent, type, and timing of platelet function test, as well as underlying comorbidities such as diabetes and obesity [20]. Possible mechanisms of $P2Y_{12}$ inhibitor resistance include extrinsic factors and intrinsic factors. Recent literature highlighted the importance of genetic and drug-induced alterations of CYP3A4 enzymes, the pathway responsible for thienopyridine activation [21]. Clopidogrel resistance has been associated with an increased risk of death, myocardial infarction (MI), and stroke. Monitoring the antiplatelet effect of $P2Y_{12}$ inhibitors using platelet function testing is an evolving area of research [5].

TABLE 93.1

Aspirin Containing Product Clinical Pharmacology

Drug	Indications	Dosing, timing, duration	Monitoring, precautions, and contraindications
Acetylsalicylic Acid (Aspirin)	Treatment of ACS ± PCI	Loading dose: 325 mg orally 81 mg if on prior antiplatelet therapy Maintenance: 81–325 mg/day orally	**Monitoring** • CBC • Signs of bleeding • Blood pressure • LFTs • Renal function **Precautions** • Thrombocytopenia • Bleeding disorders • Alcohol use (3 or more drinks/day) • Pregnancy (third trimester) • Gastrointestinal disorders • Renal failure • Severe hepatic insufficiency • Concomitant antithrombotic medication use • Alcohol consumption **Contraindications** • Hypersensitivity to salicylates • Children and teenagers with chickenpox or flu symptoms (risk of Reye's syndrome)
	Primary and secondary prevention of MI in patients with chronic stable angina, previous MI, or UA	81–325 mg/day orally	
	Secondary prevention in stroke and TIA patients	75–325 mg/day orally	
	Acute thrombotic stroke	160–325 mg/day, initiated within 48 h (in patients who are not candidates for thrombolytics and are not receiving systemic anticoagulation)	
	Secondary prevention in CABG, Carotid endarterectomy patients	75–325 mg/day starting 6 h following procedure; if bleeding prevents administration at 6 h after CABG, initiate as soon as possible	

ACS, acute coronary syndromes; CABG, coronary artery bypass graft; LFT, liver function tests; MI, myocardial infarction; PCI, percutaneous coronary intervention; TIA, transient ischemic attack; UA, unstable angina

While the high incidence of varied responses to thienopyridines due to CYP450 polymorphisms and potential drug interactions has suggested a strategy for improving response, the routine use of point-of-care platelet function testing has not been established [24]. Recent literature does not show significant improvements in clinical outcomes with platelet-function monitoring and treatment adjustment for coronary stenting, as compared with standard antiplatelet therapy without monitoring [24]. For patients with threatened in-stent thrombosis and presumed or confirmed clopidogrel resistance, maintenance dosing up to 150 mg daily could be attempted with platelet function testing. Higher maintenance dosing has not shown to improve antiplatelet activity in all patients with established CYP450 polymorphisms [5,10]. In patients with an acute coronary syndrome who were referred for an invasive strategy, there was no significant difference between a 7-day, double-dose clopidogrel regimen and the standard-dose regimen, or between higher-dose aspirin and lower-dose aspirin, with respect to the primary outcome of cardiovascular death, MI, or stroke [10]. Availability of newer agents and unavailability of platelet function testing capacity make switching to agents such as prasugrel and ticagrelor with less pharmacokinetic variability more practical.

Clinical Indications

$P2Y_{12}$ inhibitors are indicated for primary and secondary thrombosis prevention in a variety of disease states (Table 93.4). Ticlopidine reduces thrombotic events in patients with stroke, but is associated with neutropenia, thrombocytopenia, and thrombotic thrombocytopenic purpura [21]. Clopidogrel is indicated alone or in combination with aspirin for primary and secondary prevention of ischemic events in ACS, PAD, stroke, and coronary artery disease. Prasugrel is indicated alone or in combination with aspirin for the prevention of thrombotic cardiovascular events, including in-stent thrombosis, in ACS patients who are managed with percutaneous coronary intervention (PCI) [20]. Ticagrelor is indicated in combination with aspirin for primary and secondary prevention of ischemic events in patients experiencing ACS. Ticagrelor may be used in preference to clopidogrel in NSTEMI patients (or ACS) patients undergoing early invasive reperfusion procedures [25]. Cangrelor is indicated for the reduction of cardiovascular (CV) events in select patients undergoing PCI [26].

Complications and Reversal of Effect

The incidence of major bleeding with $P2Y_{12}$ inhibitors varies between agents, dosing, patient populations, and concomitant antithrombotic therapies. Gastrointestinal hemorrhage is a common complication of $P2Y_{12}$ inhibitor therapy [16]. For patients exhibiting clinically significant bleeding, platelet transfusion may be warranted in combination with IV desmopressin (Table 93.2) [15]. $P2Y_{12}$ inhibitors should be avoided in patients undergoing neuraxial analgesia due to the risk of subdural hematoma [27]. Therapy should be discontinued 7 to 10 days prior to elective surgery or invasive procedure and resumed approximately 24 hours or the next morning after surgery.

Due to the unique structure of ticagrelor, it has been associated with adverse effects not seen with thienopyridine derivatives. An increased rate of dyspnea, ventricular pauses, and hyperuricemia has been reported with ticagrelor in clinical trials likely due to its capacity to delay adenosine metabolism [22].

Glycoprotein IIb/IIIa Inhibitors

Pharmacology, Pharmacodynamics, and Monitoring

GP IIb/IIIa receptors are expressed on the platelet surface, with approximately 50,000 to 80,000 copies per platelet. Blocking

TABLE 93.2

Reversal Strategies for Select Antithrombotic Agents

Agents	Reversal strategies	Additional considerations
Aspirin	Desmopressin 0.3–0.4 mcg/kg IV bolus and/or platelet transfusion	• Interruption of therapy may warrant consultation of specialist in select patient care scenarios (i.e., recent placement of drug eluting stent)
$P2Y_{12}$ Inhibitors	Platelet transfusion and/or desmopressin 0.3–0.4 mcg/kg IV bolus	
Warfarin	INR 4–10 (no signs of bleeding) • Vitamin K; 1–2.5 mg by mouth INR >10 (no signs of bleeding) • Vitamin K; 2.5–5 mg by mouth Surgery within 24 h: • Interrupt warfarin • Vitamin K 2.5–5 mg IV Surgery within 48 h: • Interrupt warfarin • Vitamin K 2.5 mg orally Urgent surgery or invasive procedure: • Four-factor PCC (Kcentra) • Vitamin K 10 mg IV	• Close monitoring of INR is needed for patients demonstrating elevations in INR on warfarin therapy and to assess need for supplemental vitamin K • Repeat testing of the INR at 24 h and pre-operation may be needed to assess need for supplemental vitamin K or FFP • IV and oral therapy are preferred over subcutaneous administration due to erratic absorption

	Severe or life-threatening bleed:
	• Interrupt warfarin therapy
	• Vitamin K 10 mg IV + FFP 15–30 mL/kg
	• Four-factor PCC (Kcentra)
	  • INR <4 = 25 units/kg
	  • INR 4–6 = 35 units/kg
	  • INR >6 = 50 units/kg
	  • Maximum dosing weight = 100 kg
	• Consider administering three-factor PCC 25–50 units/kg (product specific dosing) if four factor unavailable or rVIIa 10-90 mcg/kg IV (if no PCC available) as alterative or adjunct therapy
		• PCCs and rVIIa have been associated with thromboembolic events

Indirect Factor Xa Inhibitors[a] (Fondaparinux)	• Interrupt fondaparinux
	• rVIIa 90 mcg/kg IV[b,c]
	• Prothrombin complex concentrates
	  • FEIBA 20–50 units/kg IV[b,c]
	  • Kcentra 25–50 units/kg IV[b,c]
		• Duration of effect is dependent upon renal function/clearance and can range from 13 to 21 h in healthy persons, and be prolonged in renal dysfunction
		• PCCs and rVIIa have been associated with thromboembolic events
		• FEIBA is derived from human plasma, thus risk of immune-mediated reaction and infection transmission

Direct Factor Xa inhibitors[a] (Apixaban, Betrixaban, Edoxaban, and Rivaroxaban)	• Interrupt therapy
	• rVIIa 90 mcg/kg IV[b,c]
	• Prothrombin complex concentrates
	  • FEIBA 50—100 units/kg IV[b,c]
	  • Kcentra 50 units/kg[b,c]
		• Duration of effect is dependent upon renal function/clearance and hepatic function, and can be prolonged in organ dysfunction
		• PCCs and rVIIa have been associated with thromboembolic events
		• FEIBA is derived from human plasma, thus risk of immune-mediated reaction and infection transmission

Direct thrombin inhibitors[a]	• Interrupt therapy • Idarucizumab (PraxBind) 5g IV bolus (Dabigatran reversal only) • Hemofiltration and hemodialysis may be effective in the removal of bivalirudin and dabigatran • Desmopressin 0.3–0.4 mcg/kg IV bolus[c] • Prothrombin complex concentrates • FEIBA 50–100 units/kg IV[b,c]	

[a]No specific antidote exists; beneficial effects described in the literature limited to animal models, human laboratory studies, and case reports
[b]Reversal data based on laboratory endpoints, no experience in actively bleeding patients
[c]Data based upon animal models, laboratory studies, or case reports
APCC, prothrombin complex concentrates; FEIBA, Factor VIII inhibitor bypassing activity; FFP, fresh frozen plasma; PCC, prothrombin complex concentrates; rVIIa, recombinant human factor 7a.

TABLE 93.3

P2Y$_{12}$ Inhibitor Pharmacokinetics and Pharmacodynamics

	Ticlopidine	Clopidogrel	Prasugrel	Ticagrelor	Cangrelor
Route	Oral	Oral	Oral	Oral	IV
Receptor binding	Irreversible	Irreversible	Irreversible	Reversible	Reversible
Prodrug	Yes	Yes	Yes	No	No
Metabolism	CYP3A4	CYP3A4, 2B6	CYP3A4, 2B6, 2C9, 2C19	CYP3A4	Plasma esterase
Clearance	Renal 60% Fecal 23%	Renal 50% Fecal 46%	Renal 68% Fecal 27%	Renal 1%	–
Time to peak platelet inhibition	2–5 d	300 mg LD: 6 h 600 mg LD: 2 h	1–2 h	2 h	30 min
Duration of antiplatelet effect	7–10 d	7–10 d	7–10 d	1 d	20–60 min
Genetic polymorphisms	Yes	Yes	No	No	Not reported

IV, intravenous; CYP, cytochrome P; LD, loading dose.

TABLE 93.4

P2Y$_{12}$ Inhibitor Clinical Pharmacology

Drug	Indications	Dosing, timing, duration	Monitoring, precautions, and contraindications
Cangrelor (Kengreal)	Reduction in cardiovascular events in patients undergoing PCI	30 mcg/kg bolus followed by 4 mcg/kg/min during PCI for 2 h or duration of PCI	**Monitoring** • Signs of bleeding • CBC with differential • Bleeding time • LFTs • Lipid panel (ticlopidine) • Platelet function testing may be warranted in select patients (Platelet aggregometry and/or Vasodilator-stimulated phosphoprotein [VASP] phosphorylation) • CYP2C19 genotyping if suspicion of poor metabolizer (clopidogrel) **Precautions** • Interruption of clopidogrel may cause in-stent thrombosis with subsequent fatal and nonfatal myocardial infarction • Indwelling epidural catheter • Combination of aspirin and clopidogrel in patients with recent TIA or stroke • Liver disease • Thrombotic thrombocytopenic purpura may occur (rare) • Recent trauma, surgery/biopsy, or other pathological condition • Concomitant use with potent CYP3A inducers and inhibitors (ticagrelor) • Use of daily maintenance doses of aspirin above 100 mg not recommended (ticagrelor) • Underlying hematologic disorders • Discontinue if ANC less than 1,200/mm^3 or platelet count less than 80000/mm^3 (ticlopidine) • Elevated Triglycerides (ticlopidine) • Clopidogrel concentrations may be reduced in poor metabolizers of CYP2C19 **Contraindications** • Hypersensitivity to agent or any component of their product • Recent stroke or TIA (prasugrel) • Severe active bleeding (such as peptic ulcer or intracranial hemorrhage) • Neutropenia/thrombocytopenia • Severe liver impairment
Clopidogrel (Plavix)	Treatment of ACS ± PCI	ACS LD: 300 mg × 1 PCI LD: 300–600 mg × 1 Maintenance: 75 mg orally once daily	
	Primary and secondary prevention of MI in patients with chronic stable angina, previous MI, or UA Cerebrovascular accident	75 mg orally once daily	
	Peripheral arterial occlusive disease		
Prasugrel (Effient)	Treatment of ACS ± PCI	LD 60 mg X1 Maintenance: 10 mg/day orally, consider 5 mg orally once daily in patients weighing less than 60 kg	
Ticagrelor (Brilinta)	Treatment of ACS ± PCI	LD 180 mg X1 Maintenance: 90 mg twice daily	
Ticlopidine (Ticlid)	Placement of stent in coronary artery Secondary prevention in thromboembolic stroke	250 mg orally twice daily; LD of 500 mg if initiated prior to PCI	

ACS, acute coronary syndromes; ANC, absolute neutrophil count; CABG, coronary artery bypass graft; CBC, complete blood count; LD, loading dose; LFT, liver function tests; MI, myocardial infarction; PCI, percutaneous coronary intervention; TIA, transient ischemic attack; UA, unstable angina.

TABLE 93.5

Glycoprotein IIB/IIIA Inhibitor Clinical Pharmacology

	Abciximab	Eptifibatide	Tirofiban
Agent type	Fab fragment of human–mouse chimeric monoclonal antibody	Cyclic heptapeptide	Nonpeptide, small molecule
Antigenicity	Yes	No	No
Receptor binding effect	Reversible	Reversible	Reversible
Receptor affinity	High	Moderate	Moderate
Excretion	Renal and reticuloendothelial system	50% renal	39%–69% renal
Dosage reduction in renal failure	No	Yes, decrease infusion dose by 50% if CrCl <50 mL/min	Yes, decrease infusion dose by 50% if CrCl <60 mL/min
Removable by dialysis	No	Yes	Yes
Duration of antiplatelet effect	24–48 h	4–8 h	4–8 h

CrCl; creatinine clearance using Cockcroft–Gault equation.

GP IIb/IIIa receptors prevents platelet activation, aggregation, and fibrinogen-mediated platelet-to-platelet bridging. Intravenous GP IIb/IIIa inhibitors (abciximab, eptifibatide, and tirofiban) vary in their structure and pharmacokinetic properties (Table 93.5) [9,28].

Although the exact threshold required for efficacy with these agents has not been established, >80% platelet inhibition is thought to be a target associated with adequate antiplatelet activity in patients with ACS and in those undergoing PCI [29]. Abciximab is a human–murine chimeric monoclonal antibody that demonstrates a dose-dependent inhibition of GP IIb/IIIa receptors. After an initial intravenous bolus and infusion, the onset of platelet inhibition is rapid (5 minutes) and 80% to 90% of ADP-induced platelet aggregation is suppressed [28,29]. Abciximab has a strong affinity for the receptor, resulting in occupancy that persists for weeks. Once discontinued, platelet function recovers gradually, with bleeding time normalizing at 12 hours and ADP-induced aggregation returning at 24 to 48 hours [28,29].

Both eptifibatide, a synthetic peptide, and tirofiban, a synthetic small molecule, demonstrate high selectivity, but reduced affinity for the GP IIb/IIIa receptor when compared to abciximab; both exhibit platelet inhibition that is linear and dose dependent. An intravenous eptifibatide or tirofiban bolus dose followed by an infusion provides >80% inhibition of ADP-induced platelet aggregation. For patients undergoing PCI, a second eptifibatide bolus 10 minutes after the initial dose further enhances platelet inhibition at 1 hour. Since both agents dissociate from the GP IIb/IIIa receptor rapidly, normal platelet aggregation is restored within 4 to 8 hours after drug discontinuation [28,29]. Platelet counts should be monitored within the first 24 hours while taking GP IIb/IIIa inhibitors. For abciximab, platelet counts should be evaluated within 2 to 4 hours of initiation due to a higher risk of thrombocytopenia.

Clinical Indication

GP IIb/IIIa inhibitors are included in evidence-based guidelines as adjunctive therapy for patients with ACS and those undergoing PCI (Table 93.6). Optimal use of GP IIb/IIIa inhibitors involves appropriate patient risk stratification, use with other antithrombotic agents, appropriate dose, and duration of therapy [25,29].

Complications and Reversal of Effect

The frequency of major bleeding with GP IIb/IIIa therapy ranges from 1% to 14% of patients and depends on the agent, concomitant therapies, and settings of ACS or PCI [28,29]. Failure to adjust dosing in renal dysfunction further increases the risk of bleeding [30]. Factors associated with bleeding risk include age, female gender, body weight, diabetes, congestive heart failure, renal function, concomitant fibrinolytic use, prolonged femoral sheath placement, and heparin dosing [29,31,32].

The duration of the antiplatelet effect is agent specific and is influenced by platelet binding (abciximab binds to platelets for up to 10 days) and renal function (tirofiban and eptifibatide have half-lives of 1.5 to 3 hours with normal renal function). An intravenous desmopressin bolus of 0.3 μg per kg may be beneficial in reducing bleeding time (Table 93.2) [33].

Nonhemorrhagic side effects of GP IIb/IIIa inhibitors include severe thrombocytopenia. The incidence of thrombocytopenia with eptifibatide and tirofiban is similar to placebo, with rates ranging from 0.2% to 0.3% of treated patients. With abciximab, the incidence is reported as 5%; however, up to 4% of cases can be due to pseudothrombocytopenia as a result of platelet clumping. The onset of thrombocytopenia usually occurs within the first 24 hours of infusion, but delayed onset has been reported [34].

Platelet or red blood cell transfusions may be warranted for patients with persistent thrombocytopenia or clinically significant bleeding and must take into account drug concentrations in the plasma or drug bound to platelets [28]. Abciximab has been associated with antibody formation in 6% of patients. The risk of thrombocytopenia and immune-mediated reactions may limit repeat use [9,34]. GP IIb/IIIa inhibitor administration should be avoided in patients requiring neuraxial analgesia due to risk of subdural hematoma [27].

Other Antiplatelet Targets

Pharmacology, Pharmacodynamics, and Monitoring

While aspirin, P2Y12 receptor antagonists, and GP IIb/IIIa inhibitors are the predominant targets of antiplatelet pharmacotherapy, several other targets with varying degrees of potency are available. Vorapaxar is a thrombin receptor (protease-activated receptor-1) antagonist that inhibits thrombin-mediated and thrombin receptor agonist peptide (TRAP)-mediated platelet aggregation [35]. Other available oral drugs that effect platelet function include cilostazol and dipyridamole. Cilostazol blocks platelet activation via phosphodiesterase 3 (PDE3) inhibition. PDE3 inhibition increases cAMP concentrations resulting in inhibition of platelet aggregation and an increase

TABLE 93.6

Glycoprotein IIB/IIIA Inhibitor Indications and Dosing

Drug	Indications	Dosing, timing, duration	Monitoring, precautions, and contraindications
Abciximab (Reopro)	Treatment of ACS ± PCI	LD: 0.25 mg/kg IV bolus (over 5 min), followed by 0.125 mcg/kg/min (maximum 10 mcg/min) IV infusion for 12 h in combination with fibrinolytic treatment or after PCI, unless complications	*Monitoring* • Signs of bleeding • CBC • aPTT while on heparin • Activated clotting time (ACT) during PCI and prior to sheath removal Serum creatinine *Precautions*
Eptifibatide (Integrilin)	Treatment of ACS ± PCI	LD: 180 mcg/kg IV bolus based on actual body weight (ABW) (maximum 22.6 mg) as soon as possible, followed by 2 mcg/kg ABW/min (maximum 15 mg/h) infusion until discharge or CABG surgery, up to 72 h If undergoing PCI, administer a second 180 mcg/kg IV bolus 10 minutes after the first and continue the infusion up to discharge, or for up to 18–24 h after procedure, whichever comes first, allowing for up to 96 h of therapy Renal impairment: CrCl <50 mL/min, 180 mcg/kg actual body weight (maximum 22.6 mg) IV bolus as soon as possible, followed by 1 mcg/kg/min (maximum 7.5 mg/h) infusion	• Indwelling epidural catheter • Do not remove arterial sheath unless activated partial thromboplastin time (aPTT) is less than 45 s or ACT less than 150 s and heparin discontinued for 3–4 h • Platelet count below 150,000/mm^3 • Renal insufficiency (eptifibatide and tirofiban) • Re-administration of abciximab may result in hypersensitivity, thrombocytopenia, or diminished benefit due to formation of human anti-chimeric antibodies • Hemorrhagic retinopathy *Contraindications* • Active internal bleeding • Abnormal bleeding within the previous 30 d or a history of bleeding diathesis • Concomitant or planned administration of other parenteral glycoprotein IIb/IIIa inhibitors
Tirofiban (Aggrastat)	Treatment of ACS ± PCI	LD: 25 mcg/kg IV within 5 minutes and then 0.15 mcg/kg/min for up to 18 h. Renal impairment: CrCl ≤60 mL/min, give LD 25 mcg/kg within 5 minutes and then 0.075 mcg/kg/min for up to 18 h.	• Hypersensitivity to active ingredient or any other product component • Hypersensitivity to murine proteins (abciximab) • Major surgery (within the previous 6 wk) • Stroke (within previous 30 d) • Severe hypertension (systolic pressure over 180–200 mm Hg or diastolic pressure above 110 mm Hg) • History or clinical suspicion of intracranial bleeding, tumor, arteriovenous malformation, or aneurysm • Pericarditis • Aortic dissection • Thrombocytopenia following prior tirofiban administration

ACS, acute coronary syndromes; CABG, coronary artery bypass graft; CrCl, creatinine clearance; LD, loading dose; MI, myocardial infarction; PCI, percutaneous coronary intervention; UA, unstable angina.

in vasodilation [36]. Cilostazol is extensively metabolized by the CYP 450-3A4 subclass. Avoidance of therapy or reduced dosing may be required for patients taking potent CYP3A4 inhibitors [37]. Dipyridamole inhibits adenosine binding to platelets and endothelial cells. The increase in adenosine leads to a rise in cyclic adenosine monophosphate (cAMP), which in turn decreases platelet responsiveness to various stimuli. Dipyridamole is metabolized hepatically and has a half-life of approximately 10 hours [9].

Clinical Indications

Vorapaxar is indicated for the reduction of CV events in patients with a MI or PAD [35]. Cilostazol is indicated for treatment of intermittent claudication symptoms and has shown benefit in reducing symptoms and improving walking distance [37]. Dipyridamole is indicated as adjunctive therapy for the prevention of thromboembolism in patients with cardiac valve replacement. Combined with aspirin, dipyridamole is indicated for secondary prevention of cerebrovascular accidents and TIA. The combination of aspirin and extended-release dipyridamole was associated with reductions in major vascular events in patients with stroke or TIA (Table 93.7) [9,38].

Complications and Reversal of Effect

Vorapaxar has a long half-life (165 to 311 hours) with 50% inhibition of platelet aggregation recorded for as long as 4 weeks after discontinuation of therapy [21,35]. Nonhemorrhagic complications of cilostazol therapy include headache, peripheral edema, and tachycardia [37]. While headache is the most common adverse effect associated with dipyridamole therapy,

TABLE 93.7

Other Antiplatelet Agent Clinical Pharmacology

Drug	Indications	Dosing, timing, duration	Monitoring, precautions, and contraindications
Cilostazol (Pletal)	Intermittent claudication	100 mg orally twice daily	**Monitoring** • Signs of bleeding • CBC • Coagulation panel • Blood pressure • Heart rate • LFTs Signs of congestive heart failure (Cilostazol) **Precautions** • Hypotension • Severe coronary artery disease, abnormal cardiac rhythm • Avoid in patients with severe hepatic insufficiency (Aggrenox) • Avoid in patients with severe renal failure (Aggrenox and cilostazol) • Coagulation abnormalities • Low body weight, older age (Vorapaxar) • Concomitant use with other anticoagulants, strong CYP3A inducers/inhibitors (vorapaxar) **Contraindications** • Hypersensitivity to agent or any components of the product • CHF of any severity (cilostazol) • Hemostatic disorders or active pathological bleeding (bleeding peptic ulcer or intracranial bleeding) • History of stroke, TIA, ICH. Discontinue with occurrence (vorapaxar)
Dipyridamole (Persantine)	Thromboembolic prophylaxis after heart valve replacement	With concomitant warfarin therapy: 75–100 mg orally four times daily	
Dipyridamole extended-release/Aspirin (Aggrenox)	Secondary prevention in stroke and TIA patients	200 mg dipyridamole, 25 mg aspirin (1 capsule) orally twice daily Patients with intolerable headache 200 mg dipyridamole, 25 mg aspirin orally daily at bedtime, with 81 mg of aspirin in the morning. Return to usual dose as soon as tolerance to headache develops (usually within a week)	
Vorapaxar (**Zontivity**)	Treatment/prophylaxis of thrombosis in patients with history of MI/PAD	2.08 mg orally once daily	

CHF, congestive heart failure; LFT, liver function tests; TIA, transient ischemic attack.

hemorrhage may also occur. For patients exhibiting clinically significant bleeding, platelet transfusion may be warranted.

Overview of Anticoagulant Pharmacotherapy

Blood coagulation has been summarized previously in Chapter 88. Anticoagulant agents inhibit thrombosis and propagation by inhibiting thrombin directly or indirectly by attenuating thrombin generation (Fig. 93.2). Anticoagulants work with traditional agents including warfarin and heparin derivatives. Newer agents such dabigatran, rivaroxaban, apixaban, and edoxaban have a more fined mechanism of action and often referred to as target-specific oral anticoagulants (TSOACs) and direct acting oral anticoagulants (DOACs) [39].

Unfractionated heparin (UFH) and low-molecular-weight heparin (LMWH) are effective in acute thrombosis due to their rapid onset. Since they are dependent on the presence of antithrombin (AT) for clotting factor inhibition, they are considered indirect anticoagulants. Heparins contain a pentasaccharide sequence that binds to AT, producing a conformational change that accelerates AT inactivation of coagulation factors XIIa, IXa, XIa, Xa, and IIa (thrombin). Of these, thrombin and Xa play the most critical role in the coagulation cascade. The active pentasaccharide sequence responsible for catalyzing AT is found on one-third and one-fifth of the chains of UFH and LMWH, respectively. Fondaparinux is a synthetic analog of this naturally occurring pentasaccharide [40].

Unfractionated Heparin

Pharmacology, Pharmacodynamics, and Monitoring

UFH is composed of a heterogeneous mixture of highly sulfated polysaccharide chains that vary in molecular weight, anticoagulant activity, and pharmacokinetic properties. A minimum of 18 saccharide units are required for UFH to form a ternary complex with AT and inhibit thrombin. Once bound to AT molecules, UFH can readily dissociate and bind to other AT molecules. Alternatively, the only requirement for factor Xa inhibition is for the heparin-AT complex to be formed. UFH has equal inhibitory activity against factor Xa and thrombin, binding in a 1:1 ratio. The heparin-AT complex also catalyzes the inhibition of factors such as IXa, XIa and XIIa.

Since UFH is poorly absorbed orally, intravenous or subcutaneous injections are the preferred administration routes [41]. When given as subcutaneous injection with therapeutic intent, UFH doses need to be large enough (>30,000 units per day) to overcome erratic bioavailability. UFH readily binds to plasma

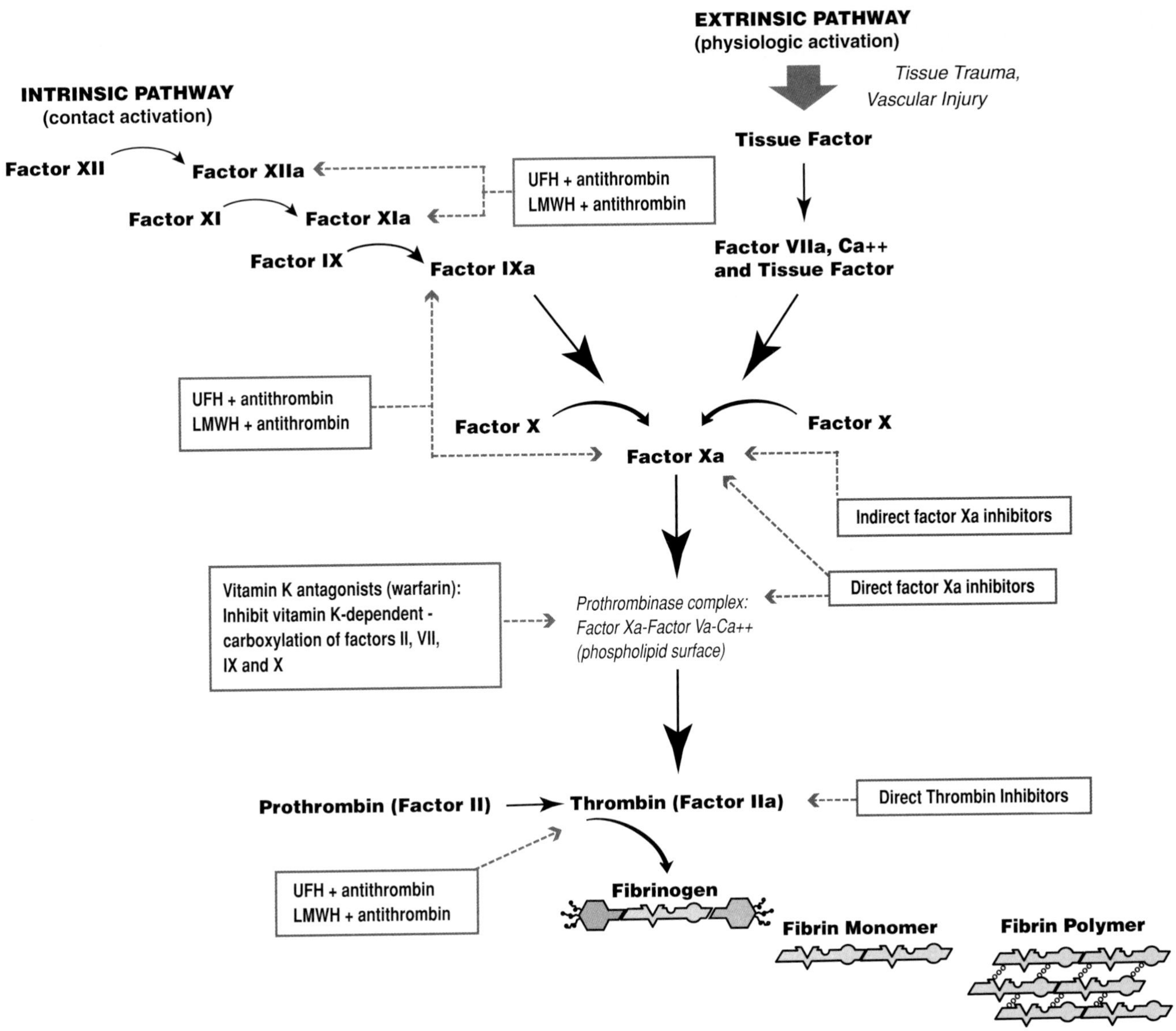

FIGURE 93.2 The coagulation cascade comprises the intrinsic (contact activation) pathway and the extrinsic (tissue factor) pathway. Each pathway generates a series of reactions in which inactive circulating enzymes and their cofactors are activated. These activated factors then catalyze the next reaction in the cascade. Thrombin plays a pivotal role by triggering the conversion of soluble fibrinogen in insoluble fibrin monomers, which serve as the foundation for thrombus formation. Thrombin also activates factors VIII, V, and XIII. Factor XIII generates the covalent bonds that link fibrin strands, ensuring structural integrity. Anticoagulants, either through their interaction with antithrombin, or through a direct inhibition of thrombin, interrupt these enzymatic reactions.

proteins after parenteral administration which contributes to variable anticoagulant response. Despite these limitations, intravenous administration rapidly achieves therapeutic plasma concentrations that can be monitored and adjusted based on infusion rates [42].

UFH clearance from systemic circulation is dose related and occurs through two independent mechanisms [42]. The initial phase is rapid and saturable binding to endothelial cells, macrophages, and local proteins where UFH is depolymerized. The second phase is a slower, nonsaturable, renal-mediated clearance. At therapeutic doses, UFH is cleared primarily in the initial phase with higher-molecular-weight chains being cleared more rapidly than lower-weight counterparts. As elimination becomes dependent on renal clearance, increased or prolonged UFH dosing provides a disproportionate increase in both the intensity and duration of anticoagulant effect. With therapeutic intravenous doses, the half-life of UFH is approximately 60 minutes [41,42].

The anticoagulant response to UFH is monitored using activated partial thromboplastin time (aPTT), a measurement sensitive to the inhibitory effects of thrombin. The aPTT should be measured every 6 hours, and doses adjusted accordingly, until the patient sustains therapeutic levels. Once steady state is reached, the frequency of monitoring can be extended.

Weight-based dosing nomograms are recommended for treatment of thromboembolic disease. Such nomograms have been associated with a shorter time to reach a therapeutic level without an increase in bleeding events. UFH dosing nomograms differ between hospitals due to differences in thromboplastin agents and inter-laboratory standards in aPTT measurements [43].

Clinical Indications

Clinical indications for UFH include treatment of ACS, treatment or prevention of venous thromboembolism (VTE), bridge

TABLE 93.8

Unfractionated Heparin Clinical Pharmacology

Drug	Indications	Dosing, timing, duration	Monitoring, precautions, and contraindications
Unfractionated heparin	VTE treatment	LD: 80 units/kg bolus 18 units/kg/h infusion adjusted per local heparin nomogram	**Monitoring** • Signs of bleeding • CBC • aPTT: at least 4 h after initiation, then at least once daily • Anti-Xa levels (alternative if available, consider in patients with heparin resistance or antiphospholipid antibody syndromes) HIT antibody testing (not warranted in the absence of thrombocytopenia, thrombosis, heparin-induced skin lesions, or other signs pointing to a potential diagnosis of immune-mediated HIT) **Precautions** • Allergic or hypersensitivity-type reactions • Congenital or acquired bleeding disorders • Indwelling epidural catheter • Gastrointestinal ulceration and ongoing tube drainage of the small intestine or stomach • Hepatic disease with impaired hemostasis • Hereditary antithrombin III deficiency and concurrent use of antithrombin • Neonates and infants weighing <10 kg • Premature infants weighing less than 1 kg • Risk of delayed onset of HIT and HITT **Contraindications** • Uncontrollable active bleeding, except when due to disseminated intravascular coagulation • Instances in which blood coagulation tests cannot be performed at necessary intervals • Severe thrombocytopenia • Positive test for immune-mediated HIT • Patients within a remote history of HIT (>100 d) could be considered for a rechallenge with heparin provided a negative antibody test
	ACS treatment	LD: 60 units/kg (max 4,000 units) 12 units/kg/h (max initial dosing 1,000 units/h) ± fibrin specific adjusted to maintain aPTT 1.5–2 times control or per local heparin nomogram	
	Bridge therapy for atrial fibrillation, cardioversion	IV infusion: 60–80 units/kg bolus Target aPTT, 60s (range 50–70 s)	
	Prophylaxis of VTE in the medically ill or surgical population	5,000 units SC Q8h	
	Prophylaxis of VTE in pregnancy (with prior VTE)	7,500–15,000 units SC every 12 h	

ACS, acute coronary syndromes; HIT, heparin-induced thrombocytopenia; HITT, heparin-induced thrombocytopenia with thrombosis; LD, loading dose; VTE, venous thromboembolism.

therapy for atrial fibrillation, and cardioversion (Table 93.8) [41,44]. Due to UFH's short half-life and reversibility, it remains the best option in patients with bleeding risk or organ dysfunction. Patients with fluctuating renal function or a calculated creatinine clearance less than 30 mL per minute are generally not good candidates for LMWH or fondaparinux due to the risk of accumulation and increased bleeding risk, and should be given UFH [45]. When used for thromboprophylaxis in medical patients, three times daily heparin dosing provides better efficacy in reducing VTE events compared to twice daily dosing, but generates more major, but not minor, bleeding episodes [46].

Complications and Reversal of Effect

The major complications of UFH therapy include bleeding (major bleeding, 0% to 7%; fatal bleeding, 0% to 3%), heparin-induced thrombocytopenia (1% to 5%), and osteoporosis (2% to 3% risk of vertebral fracture with less than 1 month of treatment) [47]. Hemorrhagic episodes are associated with anticoagulation intensity, route of administration (continuous infusions are associated with lower rates), and concomitant use of GP IIb/IIIa inhibitors, aspirin or fibrinolytic agents [47].

Patient-specific risk factors for bleeding include age, gender, renal failure, low body weight, and excessive alcohol consumption [47]. Perioperative anticoagulation must be individualized based on the surgery or procedure and the patient's risks for thrombosis and bleeding. Discontinuing therapeutic doses of heparin 4 hours before surgery and measuring an aPTT is usually sufficient since normal hemostasis is restored in this time frame [14]. Therapeutic-dose UFH therapy can be restarted 12 hours after major surgery, but should be delayed if evidence of bleeding is present. There is no contraindication to neuraxial techniques in patients receiving twice daily, low-dose UFH subcutaneously, as the risk for developing spinal hematoma appears to be minimal [14,27].

Treatment of UFH-related bleeding includes protamine sulfate, transfusion, and supportive care. Protamine sulfate binds to UFH to form a stable salt, which renders UFH inactive. Protamine dosing is dependent on timing of the last UFH dose (Table 93.9) [41,48]. If the dose of UFH is unknown, the maximal tolerated protamine dose of 50 mg can be slowly administered followed by serial measurements of aPTT. Adverse reactions, such as hypotension and bradycardia, are common. However, reaction severity can be reduced by slowly administering protamine over 1 to 3 minutes. Allergic responses to protamine are more common in patients who have been previously exposed to the drug, but patients can be pre-treated with corticosteroids and antihistamines [41,49].

TABLE 93.9

Protamine Dose Calculation for Heparin and Low Molecular Weight Heparin Reversal

UFH delivery time (h)	Heparin dose	Patient weight (kg)	Intravenous UFH dose administered (units)	UFH accumulation at 1 hour[a,b] (units)	UFH remaining at 2 h[a,b] (units)	UFH remaining at 3 h[a,b] (units)	Protamine dose (mg) required to reverse UFH[c]
0	80 units/kg Bolus	80	6,400	3,200	1,600	800	8
0	18 units/kg/h Infusion	80	1,440	1,440	720	360	3.6
1	18 units/kg/h Infusion	80	1,440	(0)	1,440	720	7.2
2	18 units/kg/h Infusion	80	1,440	(0)	(0)	1,440	14.4
Approximate amount of unfractionated heparin remaining in circulation→						3,320	33.2

LMWH delivery time (h)	LMWH dose	Patient weight (kg)	LMWH dose administered (mg)	LMWH remaining within 8 h[a] (mg)	LMWH remaining at 8–12 h[a] (mg)	LMWH remaining after 12 h (mg)	Protamine Dose (mg) required to reverse LMWH[c]
0	1 mg/kg every 12 h	80	80	80	–	–	80
8	(0)	80	–	–	40	–	40
12	(0)	80	–	–	–	≤20	0–20

Illustration assumes an 80-kg patient given a bolus and infusion for 3 hours that developed clinically significant bleeding
[a]Assumes half-life of heparin to be 1 hour
[b]Calculated amounts of heparin remaining at 1 hour following the initiation of continuous infusion may be overestimated in this model
[c]Administer no more than 20 mg of protamine per minute, with a max of 50 mg over any 10 minute period
Adapted from Irwin RS, Rippe JM: *Manual of Intensive Care Medicine*. 5th ed. Philadelphia, PA: Lippincott Williams and Wilkins; 2009.

Low-Molecular-Weight Heparins

Pharmacology, Pharmacodynamics, and Monitoring

LMWHs are derived from UFH by chemical or enzymatic depolymerization, yielding fragments approximately one-third the molecular weight of UFH. All LMWH molecules contain the active pentasaccharides that catalyze AT inhibition of factor Xa. Because of their smaller size, LMWHs have decreased affinity for plasma proteins and cellular binding sites, resulting in a superior pharmacokinetic profile compared to UFH. LMWHs also have increased bioavailability after subcutaneous injection, renal clearance that is dose-independent, and a longer half-life (17 to 21 hours). LMWHs are administered in fixed doses for thromboprophylaxis or in total body weight-adjusted doses for therapeutic anticoagulation (Table 93.10) [41,42].

With their predictable dose response (peak anti-Xa activity occurs 3 to 5 hours after injection), laboratory monitoring is usually not necessary. Anti-Xa monitoring is optional in high-risk patient populations, specifically renal insufficiency, obesity, and pregnancy. In these cases, peak anti-Xa plasma levels are drawn 4 hours after administration, and subsequent doses are adjusted to a target range of 0.5 to 1.1 IU per mL [50]. Trough levels can be assessed to determine clearance in surgical, procedural, and patient bleeding scenarios.

Clinical Indications

LMWHs require fewer injections and produce fewer adverse events compared to subcutaneous UFH. In hospitalized medical patients receiving thromboprophylaxis, LMWH was associated with a lower risk of deep vein thrombosis (DVT), fewer injection-site hematomas, and no difference in bleeding when compared with UFH [51]. LMWHs have largely replaced intravenous UFH in patients with acute VTE who are able to receive unmonitored anticoagulation in the ambulatory setting. UFH remains the preferred option for ACS patients, those who may require an urgent surgical intervention, those with compromised renal function, or those requiring intensive monitoring for other reasons [41]. Recent data suggest reduction in pulmonary embolism (PE) rates with LMWH vs heparin prophylaxis for VTE prophylaxis in the ICU [52].

Complications and Reversal of Effect

Hemorrhage is the major complication of LMWH therapy, with data suggesting lower rates when compared to UFH. Major bleeding is reported to occur in 0% to 3% of patients [41,47]. Periprocedural thromboembolic risk assessment, bleeding risk assessment, and physician preference will play a role in determining whether LMWH prophylaxis is continued or withheld in the surgical setting. For patients receiving therapeutic LMWH, therapy should be discontinued 12 to 24 hours prior to the procedure, or earlier in patients with renal dysfunction. Therapeutic doses of LMWH should not be restarted for 24 hours after a major procedure or with neuraxial anesthesia [14].

In the setting of overdose or hemorrhage, protamine completely reverses the antithrombin activity of LMWH, but only reverses 60% of the antifactor Xa activity (Table 93.9). If immediate reversal is warranted within 8 hours of LMWH administration, a protamine dose of 1 mg neutralizes 100 anti-Xa units or 1 mg of LMWH (Table 93.9). Initial dosing should max at 50 mg. Should bleeding continue, a second dose of 0.5 mg of protamine per 100 anti-Xa units or 1 mg of LMWH may be administered. Smaller protamine doses are required if the LMWH administration interval is beyond 8 hours [41]. Andexanet alfa is a modified recombinant form of factor Xa currently under investigation for reversal of LMWH [53,54]. This agent acts as

TABLE 93.10

Low Molecular Weight Heparin Clinical Pharmacology

Drug	Indications	Dosing, timing, duration	Monitoring, precautions, and contraindications
Dalteparin (Fragmin)	Treatment of VTE	<56 kg: 10,000 IU SC daily 57–68 kg: 12,500 IU SC daily 83–98 kg: 18,000 IU SC daily >99 kg: 18,000 IU SC daily	**Monitoring** • Signs of bleeding • Anti-Xa levels in patients with mechanical prosthetic heart valves, significant renal impairment, those experiencing bleeding or abnormal coagulation parameters, pregnant patients, obese or low-weight patients, and children • CBC • Serum creatinine HIT antibody testing (not warranted in the absence of thrombocytopenia, thrombosis, heparin-induced skin lesions, or other signs pointing to a potential diagnosis of HIT) **Precautions** • Indwelling epidural catheter • Recent spinal or ophthalmologic surgery • History of recent major bleed (GI, intracranial, etc.) • Congenital or acquired bleeding disorders • Bacterial endocarditis • History of heparin-induced thrombocytopenia • Liver disease • Renal impairment (CrCl <30 mL/min), consider UFH • Concomitant use of antithrombotic drugs • Diabetic retinopathy • Uncontrolled hypertension **Contraindications** • Severe active bleeding • Hypersensitivity to enoxaparin, dalteparin, tinzaparin, heparin, or pork products, sulfites (tinzaparin), or formulation excipients • Positive test for immune-mediated HIT • Patients within a remote history of HIT (>100 d) could be considered for a re challenge with heparin provided a negative antibody test
	Treatment of ACS	120 IU/kg SC Q12h (MAX 10,000 IU/dose)	
	Prophylaxis of VTE after hip or other major surgery (first month)	Maintenance: 5,000 IU SC Q24h	
	Prophylaxis of VTE in the medically ill or surgical population	5,000 IU SC Q24h	
Enoxaparin (Lovenox)	Treatment of VTE	1 mg/kg SC Q12h OR 1.5 mg/kg SC Q24h CrCl <30 mL/min: 1 mg/kg SC Q24h	
	Treatment of ACS	STEMI: 30 mg bolus IV followed by 1 mg/kg SC Q12h + fibrinolytic NSTEMI/UA: 1 mg/kg SC Q12h CrCl <30 mL/min: not recommended	
	Prophylaxis/bridge therapy for atrial fibrillation/cardioversion	1 mg/kg SC Q12h OR 1.5 mg/kg SC Q24h CrCl <30 mL/min: 1 mg/kg SC Q24	
	Prophylaxis of VTE in the medically ill or surgical population	40 mg SC Q24h CrCl <30 mL/min: 1 mg/kg SC daily	
	Prophylaxis of VTE in the trauma patients	30 mg SC Q12h *Or* 40 mg SC Q24h	
Tinzaparin (**Innohep**)	Treatment of DVT	175 IU anti-Xa/kg SC daily	
	VTE prophylaxis	75 IU anti-Xa/kg SC daily (initial dose given post-op) for 7–10 d 50 IU anti-Xa/kg SC daily (initial dose given 2 h pre-op) for 7–10 d	

ACS, acute coronary syndromes; CrCl, creatinine clearance; DVT, deep vein thrombosis; HIT, heparin-induced thrombocytopenia; HITT, heparin-induced thrombocytopenia with thrombosis; MI, myocardial infarction; VTE, venous thromboembolism

a hemostatically inactive factor Xa decoy that binds free oral direct Xa inhibitors [54].

Heparin-induced thrombocytopenia (HIT) is an immune-mediated, hypercoagulable disorder that results from antibodies formed against the heparin-platelet factor 4 complex. The incidence in critically ill patients ranges from 0.3% to 0.5% and is associated with thrombocytopenia and life-threatening thrombosis in antibody-positive patients [55]. HIT typically occurs in patients who have been exposed to UFH or LMWH for 5 to 7 days, or even sooner in patients with prior exposure. A 30% to 50% decrease in platelet count occurring 5 to 14 days after the initiation of UFH or LMWH therapy or formation of a new thrombus during therapy may be indicative of HIT [55,56]. Platelet counts should be measured prior to the initiation of UFH or LMWH and monitored every other day for the first 4 to 10 days of therapy. Since heparin alternatives must be used in patients with HIT, direct thrombin inhibitors are the treatment of choice [56].

Patients receiving heparin for a period of greater than 1 month are at risk for developing osteoporosis and vertebral fractures.

Osteoporosis reportedly occurs less frequently in patients treated with LMWHs as compared to UFH [41].

Fondaparinux

Pharmacology, Pharmacodynamics, and Monitoring

Fondaparinux is a synthetic analog of the naturally occurring pentasaccharide found in heparins. Fondaparinux selectively and irreversibly binds to AT. This results in neutralization of factor Xa, which ultimately inhibits thrombin formation and thrombus development [41]. After subcutaneous administration, fondaparinux has a half-life of 17 to 21 hours in patients with normal renal function. Fondaparinux is excreted in the urine; clearance is reduced in patients with renal impairment. Laboratory monitoring of fondaparinux-specific anti-Xa assays is not recommended on a routine basis, although high-risk patients may warrant monitoring (Table 93.12) [41].

Clinical Indications

Fondaparinux is as safe and effective as heparins for treatment of DVT and PE and for thromboprophylaxis in surgical and medically ill patients [40]. Fondaparinux may be an option for thromboprophylaxis in the setting of HIT but conclusive data are not available [56].

Complications and Reversal of Effect

Fondaparinux is contraindicated in patients with severe renal impairment (calculated creatinine clearance <30 mL per minute) and should not be used for VTE prophylaxis in patients weighing less than 50 kg. No antidote exists for fondaparinux-related hemorrhage and reversal is further complicated by its prolonged half-life (Table 93.2) [15]. Recombinant factor VIIa (rVIIa) reverses the coagulation parameter alterations induced by fondaparinux, but the clinical utility is unknown [15]. With a short half-life (2 to 3 hours), rVIIa may require repeat dosing. The use of fondaparinux and neuraxial anesthesia or analgesia should follow the conditions used in clinical trials as closely as possible [27].

Direct acting FXa-inhibitors

Pharmacology, Pharmacodynamics, and Monitoring

Direct oral direct Xa inhibitors are the newest class of anticoagulants to clinical practice. They selectively bind to the active site of factor Xa and prevent the interaction with prothrombin [40]. Compared to indirect Xa inhibitors such as fondaparinux, these agents do not require antithrombin as a cofactor and inactivate both free and clot-bound factor Xa [40].

The oral direct Xa inhibitors differ in their pharmacokinetic parameters (Table 93.11). These agents have varying degrees of renal and hepatic elimination, elimination half-life, and susceptibility to drug interactions [40,57]. Oral direct Xa inhibitors were developed to provide more stable pharmacokinetic and dynamic profiles that eliminate the need for routine monitoring. Nevertheless, for patients undergoing invasive procedures or for critically ill patients with altered organ function, drug monitoring may be necessary [39]. Oral direct Xa inhibitors alter aPTT and INR values; however, these tests cannot be used to monitor therapy. Calibrated chromogenic anti-Xa assays provide a means to potentially monitor activity; however, exact therapeutic targets have yet to be described in practice [39].

Clinical Indications

Available agents include apixaban, edoxaban, and rivaroxaban, which are approved for the prophylaxis and treatment of thromboembolism in a variety of clinical settings (Table 93.12) [21,39,58]. Betrixaban is another oral agent under clinical investigation.

Complications and Reversal of Effect

Bleeding is the major complication of oral direct Xa inhibitors. These agents have demonstrated a lower rate of intracranial bleeding compared to warfarin; however, the rates of gastrointestinal bleeding were higher compared to warfarin [21,39]. Currently there are no available agents for the reversal of oral direct Xa inhibitors. Administration of activated and inactivated prothrombin complex concentrates (PCC) and recombinant factor VIIa may lower PT/INR values; however, impact on reversing bleeding and prothrombotic complications with these

TABLE 93.11

Factor Xa Inhibitor Pharmacokinetics and Pharmacodynamics

	Apixaban	Betrixaban	Edoxaban	Fondaparinux	Rivaroxaban
Molecular weight (Da)	460	567	548	1,728	436
Bioavailability	50%	34%	>60%	100%	60%–100% (increased w/food)
Protein binding	87%	60%	54%	94%–97%	>90%
Half-life (h)	8–15	37	9–11	17–21	5–9
Cmax (h)	1–4	3–4	1–3	2–3	2–4
Metabolism	>50% unchanged; <32% CYP w/no active metabolites	Minimal	Minimal	Minimal	43% unchanged; ~30% metabolites in urine
P-glycoprotein	Yes	Yes	Yes	No	Yes
CYP	15% (CYP3A4)	<1%	<4% (CYP3A4)	None	30% (CYP3A4, CYP2J2)
Clearance	Renal 25%—27% Fecal >50% (unchanged)	Renal 6%–13% Fecal 82%–89%	Renal 35%–50% Fecal 50%–65%	Renal 77%	Renal 66% (33–36% unchanged) Fecal/biliary 28% (7% unchanged)

Da, daltons; CYP, cytochrome P; Cmax, time to maximum concentration.

TABLE 93.12

Factor Xa Inhibitor Clinical Pharmacology

Drug	Indications	Dosing, timing, duration	Monitoring, precautions, and contraindications
Apixaban (Eliquis)	Reduce the risk of stroke and systemic embolism in patients with nonvalvular atrial fibrillation	5 mg orally twice daily. Reduce dose to 2.5 mg orally twice daily in patients with at least 2 of the following characteristics: age ≥80 years, body weight ≤60 kg, or serum creatinine ≥1.5 mg/dL	**Monitoring** • Signs of bleeding • CBC • Serum creatinine • Anti-Xa levels in patients with significant renal/hepatic impairment, those experiencing bleeding or abnormal coagulation parameters, pregnant patients, obese or low-weight patients, and children (agent specific assay calibration required) • LFTs (apixaban and rivaroxaban) Signs of neurological impairment, especially in patients receiving epidural/spinal anesthesia or puncture **Precautions** • Indwelling epidural catheter • Neuraxial anesthesia or spinal puncture • Recent spinal or ophthalmologic surgery • History of recent major bleed • Congenital or acquired bleeding disorders • Hepatic dysfunction (apixaban and rivaroxaban) • Concomitant use with strong CYP3A4 and P-glycoprotein inhibitors and inducers (apixaban, betrixaban, rivaroxaban, and edoxaban) • Mechanical heart valves or moderate-severe mitral stenosis (apixaban and edoxaban). **Contraindications** • Severe active bleeding • Bacterial endocarditis • Body weight less than 50 kg for prophylactic therapy of hip fracture, hip replacement or knee replacement surgery, or abdominal surgery; increased risk for major bleeding episodes • Fondaparinux-related thrombocytopenia • Hypersensitivity to agent or formulation excipients • CrCl <30 mL/min (fondaparinux) • Severe liver failure (apixaban) • Hepatic dysfunction with coagulopathy (rivaroxaban & edoxaban)
	Treatment of DVT and PE, and for the reduction in the risk of recurrent DVT and PE following initial therapy	10 mg orally twice daily ×7 days, then 5 mg orally twice daily. After at least 6 months of treatment for DVT or PE then 2.5 mg orally twice daily	
	DVT prophylaxis in patients undergoing knee or hip replacement surgery	2.5 mg orally twice daily Initial dose 12–24 h after surgery ×12 days (knee) ×35 days (hip)	
Betrixaban (Bevyxxa)	Venous thromboembolism, In patients with restricted mobility from acute illness and other risk factors	Initial, 160 mg orally as a single dose, followed by 80 mg once daily with food P-glycoprotein inhibitors and renal dose adjustment for CrCl 15–30 mL/min: Initial, 80 mg orally as a single dose, followed by 40 mg once daily with food	
Edoxaban (Savaysa)	Reduce the risk of stroke and systemic embolism in patients with nonvalvular atrial fibrillation	60 mg once daily in patients with CrCL >50 to ≤95 mL/min Do not use in patients with CrCL >95 mL/min 30 mg once daily in patients with CrCL 15–50 mL/min	
	Treatment of DVT and PE	>60 kg: 60 mg orally daily after 5–10 days of parenteral anticoagulant ≤60kg: 30 mg orally daily 5–10 days of parenteral anticoagulant P-glycoprotein inhibitors: 30 mg orally daily Renal dose adjustment: CrCl >95 mL/min: not recommended CrCl 95–51 mL/min: no adjustment CrCl 15–50 mL/min: 30 mg daily CrCl <15 mL/min: not recommended	
Fondaparinux (Arixtra)	Treatment of VTE	<50 kg: 5 mg SC daily 50–100 kg: 7.5 mg SC daily >100 kg: 10 mg SC daily Renal impairment: consider empiric dosage reduction CrCl 50–80 mL/min: 25% reduction in total clearance CrCl 30–50 mL/min: 40% reduction in total clearance CrCL<30 mL/min: contraindicated	
	Prophylaxis of VTE in major surgery and acute medically ill[a]	2.5 mg SC QD	

TABLE 93.12

Factor Xa Inhibitor Clinical Pharmacology (*continued*)

Drug	Indications	Dosing, timing, duration	Monitoring, precautions, and contraindications
Rivaroxaban (Xarelto)	Reduce the risk of stroke and systemic embolism in patients with nonvalvular atrial fibrillation	20 mg orally daily with meal Renal impairment: CrCl 15–49 mL/min: 15 mg orally daily with meal CrCl <15 mL/min: avoid use	
	Treatment of DVT and PE, and for the reduction in the risk of recurrent DVT and PE following initial therapy.	15 mg orally twice daily for 3 wk, then 20 mg orally daily Renal impairment: CrCl <30 mL/min: avoid use	
	DVT prophylaxis in patients undergoing knee or hip replacement surgery	10 mg orally daily for 5 wk (hip) 2 wk (knee) [a]1st dose within 6–10 h postsurgery	

[a]Indicates off-label use of medication.
ACS, acute coronary syndromes; CrCl, creatinine clearance; DVT, deep vein thrombosis; LFT, liver function tests; VTE, venous thromboembolism.

agents has not been evaluated (Table 93.2) [54]. Andexanet alfa is a modified recombinant form of factor Xa currently under investigation for reversal of oral direct acting Xa inhibitors [53,54]. This agent acts as a hemostatically inactive factor Xa decoy that binds free oral direct Xa inhibitors [54].

Direct Thrombin Inhibitors

Pharmacology, Pharmacodynamics, and Monitoring

Direct thrombin inhibitors (DTIs) include the older IV agents such as argatroban and bivalirudin, and the newest agent to the class, dabigatran, which is orally administered. They exert their antithrombotic effect by binding to the active site of thrombin and inhibiting thrombin-catalyzed reactions. This prevents fibrin formation, activation of coagulant factors V, VIII, XIII, protein C, and platelet aggregation [41].

Dabigatran etexilate is a small molecule oral prodrug with low bioavailability. After oral administration, it is converted to its active form dabigatran. The DTIs differ considerably in their pharmacokinetic parameters (Table 93.13) [59,60]. Bivalirudin has the shortest half-life, making it a particularly useful agent in the procedural or periprocedural period. DTI selection is predicated on patient-specific characteristics such as hemodynamic stability, hepatic function, and renal function. Critically ill patients typically require lower doses than those recommended by the manufacturer [41,59,60]. Intravenous DTIs are monitored using aPTT measured every 6 hours until the patient has sustainable therapeutic levels, and then the monitoring frequency can be extended [56]. Similar to the IV DTI's, dabigatran prolongs the aPTT and the International Normalized Ration (INR); however, no recommendations are available on using this parameter to guide therapy. While ecarin clotting time (ECT) or thrombin time (TT) may be useful laboratory tests for monitoring coagulation during DTI therapy, these tests are often not widely available in the clinical setting [39].

TABLE 93.13

Direct Thrombin Inhibitor Pharmacokinetic and Pharmacodynamics

Feature	Dabigatran	Argatroban	Bivalirudin
Molecular weight (Da)	628	526	2,180
FDA-approved indication	Stroke prevention in nonvalvular AF; VTE treatment after 5–10 d of parenteral therapy	Management of HIT, or use in patients with HIT who are undergoing PCI	Use in patients with or at risk for HIT or HITTS who are undergoing PCI
Bioavailability	3%–7%	N/A	N/A
Primary elimination route	Renal	Hepatic	Enzymatic
Elimination half-life	12–17 h	39–51 min	10–24 min
Fraction eliminated unchanged by kidney (%)	~80	16	20
P-glycoprotein	Yes	No	No
Laboratory test to monitor	aPTT, ECT	aPTT, ECT	aPTT, ACT, ECT
Target range	N/A	aPTT: 1.5–3 × control	aPTT: 1.5–2.5 × control
Effects on INR	Minimal to moderate	Moderate to clinically significant	Minimal to moderate

ACT, activated clotting time; AF, atrial fibrillation, aPTT, activated partial thromboplastin time; Da, dalton; ECT, ecarin clotting time; FDA, Food and Drug Administration; HIT, heparin-induced thrombocytopenia; HITTS, HIT with thrombosis syndrome; INR, international normalized ratio; PCI, percutaneous coronary intervention; VTE, venous thromboembolism

Clinical Indications

Argatroban and bivalirudin are indicated for prophylaxis of thrombosis in patients with, or at risk for, HIT undergoing PCI. Bivalirudin is also indicated in the treatment of patients undergoing PCI as well as those with unstable angina/non-ST segment elevation MI undergoing PCI (Table 93.14) [60]. Dabigatran is indicated for the prevention of stroke and systemic embolism in patients with atrial fibrillation, for the treatment of VTE and to reduce the risk of recurrence [39].

Complications and Reversal of Effect

Bleeding is one the most serious adverse effects of DTI therapy. A humanized monoclonal antibody fragment (Fab) that selectively binds to and inhibits the activity of dabigatran (idarucizumab) only is currently commercially available [53,61]. No specific reversal agents are available for other agents (Table 93.2). Recombinant factor VIIa has been reported to be a potential option in the reversal of DTI bleeding [54]. Removal of dabigatran with hemodialysis or hemoperfusion has been reported to reverse its effects [54].

DTIs can produce elevation in the INR, an effect that is most pronounced with argatroban, and magnified when coadministered with warfarin. This laboratory interaction has misled clinicians to discontinue argatroban therapy prematurely, predisposing patients to venous limb gangrene [60]. With concurrent administration, the argatroban infusion should be stopped and the INR measured 4 to 6 hours. If the INR is within therapeutic range on warfarin alone, warfarin monotherapy can be continued, otherwise argatroban therapy should be resumed [60].

Oral Anticoagulants—Vitamin K Antagonists

Pharmacology, Pharmacodynamics, and Monitoring

Warfarin, a vitamin K antagonist (VKA), inhibits the enzyme vitamin K epoxide reductase complex (VKORC), which converts

TABLE 93.14

Direct Thrombin Inhibitor Clinical Pharmacology

Drug	Indications	Dosing, timing, duration	Monitoring, precautions, and contraindications
Argatroban	Treatment and prophylaxis of HITT	0.5–1.2 mcg/kg/min continuous IV infusion to start titration to goal aPTT between 50 and 85 seconds Begin VKA therapy, measure INR daily. Stop argatroban when INR >4. Repeat INR in 4–6 h, if INR is below desired range then resume argatroban infusion	**Monitoring** • Signs of bleeding • CBC • aPTT (argatroban and bivalirudin) (not reliable marker with dabigatran) • ACT • PT/INR (false elevation) • Modified thrombin clotting time (dabigatran) • Ecarin clotting time (ECT) (dabigatran) • Renal function (Bivalirudin and argatroban, desirudin and dabigatran) LFTs (argatroban) **Precautions** • Indwelling epidural catheter • Recent major, spinal or ophthalmologic surgery • History of recent major bleed (GI, intracranial, etc.) • Congenital or acquired bleeding disorders • Recent cerebrovascular accident • Hepatic impairment (argatroban) • Renal dysfunction (all agents) **Contraindications** • Hypersensitivity to agent or formulation excipients • Severe active bleeding • Mechanical prosthetic valve or valvular heart disease (dabigatran).
	Treatment of ACS	LD: 100 mcg/kg IV bolus Initial infusion: 1–3 mcg/kg/min for 6–72 h; maintain aPTT between 50 and 85 seconds	
Bivalirudin (Angiomax)	PCI	LD: 0.75 mg/kg IV bolus dose, followed by an infusion of 1.75 mg/kg/h for the duration of the procedure Renal impairment: CrCL <30 mL/min, 0.75 mg/kg IV bolus dose, then 1 mg/kg/h should be considered Hemodialysis: 0.75 mg/kg IV bolus dose, then 0.25 mg/kg/h should be considered	
	Treatment of ACS[a]	LD: 0.1 mg/kg IV bolus, followed by 0.25 mg/kg/h. Titration to aPTT 1.5–2 times control	
	Treatment and prophylaxis of HITT[a]	0.1–0.2 mg/kg/h, titration to aPTT 1.5–2 times control	
Dabigatran (Pradaxa)	Reduce the risk of stroke and systemic embolism in patients with nonvalvular atrial fibrillation.	150 mg orally twice daily for patients with CrCl >30 mL/min 75 mg orally twice daily for patients with CrCl 15–30 mL/min	
	Treatment of DVT and PE in patients who have been treated with a parenteral anticoagulant for 5–10 days	150 mg orally twice daily after 5–10 days of parenteral anticoagulation for patients with CrCl >30 mL/min	
	To reduce the risk of recurrence of DVT and PE in patients who have been previously treated		
	To reduce the risk of recurrence of DVT and PE following hip replacement	110 mg orally 1–4 h after surgery and after hemostasis is achieved, then 220 mg orally once daily for 28–35 days for patients with a CrCl >30 mL/min	

[a]Indicates off-label use of medication.
ACS, acute coronary syndromes; CrCl, creatinine clearance; HIT, heparin-induced thrombocytopenia; HITT, heparin-induced thrombocytopenia with thrombosis; LD, loading dose; LFT, liver function tests; MI, myocardial infarction; VTE, venous thromboembolism

vitamin K to an active form. The absence of vitamin K reduces the hepatic production of functional coagulation thrombin, VII, IX, and X and the regulatory anticoagulant proteins C, S, and Z. Since thrombin has a longer half-life (60 to 72 hours) compared to the other factors (6 to 24 hours), at least 6 days of warfarin treatment is required for an antithrombotic effect [62].

Warfarin is extensively metabolized by the CYP450 isoenzyme system including CYP2C9, CYP1A1, CYP1A2, and CYP3A4. Several genetic polymorphisms have been identified with CYP2C9 and VKORC that may influence warfarin clearance and dose sensitivity [62].

In critically ill patients, alterations in coagulation factors, caused by reduced dietary vitamin K intake, hypoalbuminemia, antibiotic administration, acute hepatic injury, or hypermetabolic states, will impact the effects of warfarin. Furthermore, drug interactions alter warfarin absorption, clearance, and plasma protein binding. The interactions could have either synergistic or antagonistic effects [62].

Warfarin's anticoagulant effect is measured using the INR [62]. The INR uses the international sensitivity index of the local thromboplastin reagent to standardize the laboratory result. The INR target range will vary based on indication and the patient's risk for thromboembolic and bleeding complications (Table 93.15). Nomogram-based warfarin dosing is considered safer and more effective for reaching target INR goals. To prevent excessive anticoagulation, loading doses are avoided

TABLE 93.15

Vitamin K Antagonist: Warfarin Clinical Pharmacology

Drug	Indications	Dosing, timing, duration	Monitoring, precautions, and contraindications
Warfarin (coumadin)	Treatment of VTE	Initial dosing: 2.5–10 mg Q24h (see precautions) titrated to range INR: 2.0–3.0; target of 2.5	**Monitoring** • Signs of bleeding • CBC • PT/INR • Genetic testing may be warranted **Precautions** • Lower initial dosing (less than 5 mg) may be warranted in patients who are debilitated, are malnourished, have congestive heart failure (CHF), have liver disease, have had recent major surgery, or are taking medications known to increase sensitivity to warfarin • Cerebrovascular disease • Coronary disease • CYP2C9 and VKORC1 genetic variation • Moderate to severe hypertension • Malignancy • Renal impairment • Recent trauma • Malignancy • Collagen vascular disease • Conditions that increase risk of hemorrhage, necrosis, and/or gangrene, preexisting • Congestive heart failure • Severe diabetes • Excessive dietary vitamin K • Elderly or debilitated patients (lower dosing may be required) • Hepatic impairment • Thyroid disorders • Epidural catheters • Infectious diseases or disturbances of intestinal flora, such as sprue or antibiotic therapy • Poor nutritional state • Protein C deficiency • HITT • Vitamin K deficiency **Contraindications** • Hypersensitivity to warfarin or any component of the product • Pregnancy, known or suspected • Spinal puncture and other procedures with potential for uncontrollable bleeding • Pericarditis and pericardial effusion • Bleeding tendencies of the gastrointestinal, genitourinary, or respiratory tract • Gastrointestinal, genitourinary or respiratory tract ulcerations or overt bleeding • Cerebrovascular hemorrhage
	Atrial fibrillation	Initial dosing: 2.5–10 mg Q24h (see precautions) titrated to range INR: 2.0–3.0; target of 2.5	
	s/p MI	Initial dosing: 2.5–10 mg Q24h (see precautions) titrated to range INR: 2.0–3.0; target of 2.5	
	Mechanical valve in the atrial position	Initial dosing: 2.5–5 mg Q24h (see precautions) titrated to range INR 2.0–3.0; target of 2.5	
	Mechanical valve in the mitral position	Initial dosing: 2.5–5 mg Q24h (see precautions) titrated to range INR 2.5–3.5; target of 3.0	
	Mechanical valve in *both* the atrial and mitral position	Initial dosing: 2.5–5 mg Q24h (see precautions) titrated to target INR 2.5–3.5; target of 3.0	
	Bioprosthetic valve in the mitral position	Initial dosing: 2.5–5 mg Q24h (see precautions) titrated to target INR 2.0–3.0; target of 2.5 × 3 months	

HITT, heparin-induced thrombocytopenia with thrombosis; MI, myocardial infarction; VTE, venous thromboembolism and low doses are employed for the elderly [44]. Frequent INR monitoring is necessary during initiation of therapy until steady state is reached.

Clinical Indications

Warfarin is effective for primary and secondary prevention of venous thromboembolism, for prevention of systemic embolism in patients with prosthetic heart valves or atrial fibrillation, and for prevention of stroke, recurrent infarction, or death in patients with acute MI [62,63].

Complications and Reversal of Effect

Treatment with warfarin increases the risk of major bleeding by 0.3% to 0.5% per year and the risk of intracerebral hemorrhage by approximately 0.2% per year compared to controls [54]. Important risk factors for hemorrhage include anticoagulant intensity, time within therapeutic range, and patient age. Higher goal INR (INR >3) has been directly associated with increased hemorrhage rates. Based upon the clinical scenario, an elevated INR can be managed by withholding therapy, decreasing dosing, or administration of reversal therapy (Table 93.2). For patients requiring reversal, available therapies include vitamin K, fresh frozen plasma (FFP), PCC, and rVIIa [54]. Vitamin K is given orally or parenterally. Oral vitamin K normalizes supratherapeutic INRs more rapidly than subcutaneous vitamin K, and the correction of INR is faster with IV route compared to oral administration and is both faster and more complete than subcutaneous administration [15,44,54,64]. For patients with an INR >4.5 but <10.0 and no significant bleeding, the next two doses of warfarin should be held, and low-dose (1 to 2.5 mg) oral vitamin K administered [44]. For patients with an INR >10, the vitamin K dose can be increased to 2.5 to 5 mg [62]. While 2.5 mg of vitamin K can reverse the effects of warfarin, in the setting of serious or life-threatening hemorrhage, warfarin should be held and vitamin K dosing up to 10 mg should administered by slow IV infusion [54].

The supplementation of coagulation factors with FFP or PCC's may be more effective in cases of severe bleeding or where immediate reversal of the INR is necessary [54,65]. PCCs are available in several products globally with varying degrees of factor type and quantities. PCCs offer faster reversal than vitamin K and reduced intravenous fluid volume compared to FFP. PCCs with activated factors (i.e., FEIBA) may have an increased risk of thrombosis compared to nonactivated PCC's [66]. Recombinant factor VIIa may be an option in patients with refractory bleeding; however, risk of prothrombotic events such as stroke and MI limits its use to life-threatening bleeds [54,67]. Nonhemorrhagic adverse events of warfarin include acute skin necrosis and limb gangrene. These complications are typically observed on the third to eighth day of therapy [62].

In patients scheduled for surgery, warfarin may be continued, interrupted for approximately 5 days, or replaced with short-term parenteral or subcutaneous heparinoid bridge therapy depending on the patient's risk for venous or arterial thromboembolism [14]. Warfarin can be re-initiated with or without bridge therapy after surgery. Recent findings suggest that the thromboembolism risk during warfarin treatment interruption may be overstated and bridging anticoagulation unnecessary in selected patient populations [68,69].

For warfarin-treated patients receiving neuraxial anesthesia with an indwelling catheter, the catheter should be removed when the INR is less than 1.5. Patients with a low risk of bleeding may undergo surgery with an INR of 1.3 to 1.5 [27,70].

FIBRINOLYTIC THERAPY

Pharmacology, Pharmacodynamics, and Monitoring

Fibrinolytic agents have been used clinically since the 1950s when streptokinase was shown to be effective in dissolving occlusive thrombi. Fibrinolytic agents promote the conversion of plasminogen to plasmin, which subsequently causes the degradation of fibrin clots [71]. Streptokinase and urokinase are naturally occurring first-generation fibrinolytic agents [72]. Recombinant tissue plasminogen activator (rt-PA) is a second-generation fibrinolytic that causes less overall systemic depletion of fibrinogen and plasminogen compared with streptokinase and urokinase. The half-life of rt-PA is less than 5 minutes when administered as a bolus followed by rapid continuous infusion (Table 93.16). Third-generation fibrinolytic agents are synthetic agents with increased fibrin specificity compared to first-generation fibrinolytics and extended half-lives compared to rt-PA [72].

Clinical Indications

Fibrinolytic therapy is administered to patients with acute ischemic stroke, VTE, acute MI, peripheral arterial occlusion, and in those patients requiring venous catheter maintenance (Table 93.17). A clear role for fibrinolytic therapy, compared with surgical revascularization, for acute limb ischemia has yet to be defined. There is wide variation in fibrinolytic agents employed, doses studied, patient populations, and endpoints of therapy. The greatest benefit has been shown for patients presenting with acute ischemia <14 days who are at low risk

TABLE 93.16

Fibrinolytic Pharmacokinetics and Pharmacodynamics

	Streptokinase	Urokinase	Alteplase	Reteplase	Tenecteplase
	First-generation		Second-generation	Third-generation	
Source	Group C β-hemolytic strep	Synthesized from urine or kidney cell tissue	Recombinant DNA technology	Recombinant DNA technology	Recombinant DNA technology
Molecular weight (Da)	47,000	Variable	70,000	39,000	70,000
Administration	Continuous infusion	Continuous infusion	Rapid continuous infusion	Sequential bolus	Single bolus
Half-life	20–80 min	15–20 min	5 min	15–18 min	20 min

Da, dalton; DNA, deoxyribonucleic acid.

TABLE 93.17

Fibrinolytic Clinical Pharmacology

Drug	Indications	Dosing, timing, duration	Monitoring, precautions, and contraindications
Alteplase (Activase and Cathflo Activase)	Acute ST elevation MI	>67 kg LD: 15 mg IV bolus, followed by 50 mg infusion over 30 min, then 35 mg infusion over 60 min (total = 100 mg) ≤67 kg LD: 15 mg IV bolus, followed by 0.75 mg/kg infusion over 30min (max 50 mg), then 0.5 mg/kg over 60 min (max 35 mg)	**Monitoring** • Signs of bleeding • CBC • Blood pressure • ECG • Cranial CT scan, improved neurological recovery (Acute ischemic stroke) • Cardiac enzymes, ECG, resolution of chest pain (acute myocardial infarction) Fibrinogen, thrombin time (TT), activated partial thromboplastin time (APTT), prothrombin time (PT); at baseline, 4 h after therapy initiation, and TT only within 3–4 h after therapy **Precautions** • Recent major or minor surgery (within 10 days) • Cerebrovascular diseases • Recent gastrointestinal or genitourinary bleeding • Recent trauma • Hypertension: systolic BP greater than or equal to 175–180 mm Hg and/or diastolic BP greater than or equal to 110 mm Hg • High likelihood of left heart thrombus • Acute pericarditis • Subacute bacterial endocarditis • Hemostatic defects • Severe hepatic or renal dysfunction • Pregnancy • Diabetic hemorrhagic retinopathy or other hemorrhagic ophthalmic conditions • Septic thrombophlebitis or occluded AV cannula at a seriously infected site • Advanced age • Patients currently receiving oral anticoagulants • Known or suspected infection in the catheter during use for catheter clearance • Severe neurological deficit (NIHSS greater than 22) (ischemic stroke) • Patients with major early infarct signs on computerized cranial tomography (ischemic stroke) **Contraindications** • Hypersensitivity to agent or formulation excipients • Active internal bleeding • Severe uncontrolled hypertension • Recent intracranial or intraspinal surgery or trauma (within 3 months) • Intracranial neoplasm, arteriovenous malformation, or aneurysm • Known bleeding diathesis • History of cerebrovascular accident • Evidence, suspicion, or history of intracranial hemorrhage • Seizure at the onset of stroke (ischemic stroke) • Platelet count less than 100,000/μL (ischemic stroke) • Administration of heparin with 48 h preceding the onset of stroke and have an elevated activated partial thromboplastin time at presentation (ischemic stroke)
	Lysis of massive and submassive PE	Routine administration for PE (*non-cardiac arrest*): 100 mg IV administered over 2 h During cardiopulmonary resuscitation: 50 mg IV single dose administered over 5 minutes	
	Acute ischemic stroke (within 3 h of symptom onset) Acute ischemic stroke (within 3–4.5 h of symptom onset) Exclusions: Age >80 years: evidence of taking oral anticoagulant therapy, baseline NIHSS score >25; history of stroke and diabetes	0.9 mg/kg IV (not to exceed 90 mg total dose) infused over 60 minutes with 10% of the total dose administered as an initial intravenous bolus over 1 minute	
	Peripheral Arterial or venous thrombosis	Catheter-directed administration: 1.5 mg/h by transcatheter intra-arterial infusion until lysis of thrombus	
	Venous catheter occlusion	Weight >30 kg 2 mg/2 mL Patient weight >10 kg but <30 kg—110% of the internal lumen volume, not to exceed 2 mg/2 mL	
Reteplase (Retavase)	Acute ST elevation MI	10 units IV bolus, two doses give 30 minutes apart	
	Venous catheter occlusion[a]	0.4 units/2 mL	
Tenecteplase (TNKase)	Acute ST elevation MI	<60 kg: 30 mg dose ≥60 to <70 kg: 35 mg ≥70 to <80 kg: 40 mg ≥80 to <90 kg: 45 mg ≥90 kg: 50 mg	
	Lysis of high and intermediate risk PE due to right ventricular dysfunction and myocardial injury[a]	30–50 mg (based on patient weight) single IV bolus given over 5–10 s in conjunction with heparin adjusted to therapeutic levels	

[a]Indicates off-label use of medication.
LD, loading dose; MI, myocardial infarction; NIHSS, National Institutes of Health Stroke Scale; PE, pulmonary embolism.

for irreversible ischemia [73]. A common use for fibrinolytic agents is to clear thrombotic occlusions within central venous and dialysis catheters. This therapy is both effective and safe since little to no active drug reaches the systemic circulation [74].

Complications and Reversal of Effect

Bleeding is the most common and severe complication of fibrinolytic therapy. The most common areas of bleeding are the gastrointestinal and genitourinary tracts as well as sites of interrupted vascular integrity, including catheter access sites, gingiva, and skin [75–77]. Various risk factors for hemorrhage have been identified, but application to clinical practice is limited [78].

Patients receiving fibrinolytic therapy should be closely monitored for intracerebral hemorrhage. Intracerebral hemorrhage should be suspected in patients with sudden focal neurological deterioration (over minutes to hours), decreased level of consciousness, new-onset headache, nausea, vomiting, or acute increases in blood pressure during and within 24 hours of fibrinolytic treatment. Prompt treatment should ensue with replacement of coagulation factors, platelets, FFP, red blood cells, and aminocaproic acid. Due to its derivation from *Streptococcus*, patients may have performed antibodies to streptokinase from prior streptococcal infections. Adverse drug events include allergic reactions, anaphylaxis, fever, and hypotension.

References

1. Boonyawat K, Crowther MA: Venous thromboembolism prophylaxis in critically ill patients. *Semin Thromb Hemost* 41:68–74, 2015.
2. Hunt BJ: Bleeding and coagulopathies in critical care. *N Engl J Med* 370:847–859, 2014.
3. Smith BS, Yogaratnam D, Levasseur-Franklin KE, et al: Introduction to drug pharmacokinetics in the critically ill patient. *Chest* 141:1327–1336, 2012.
4. Airee A, Draper HM, Finks SW: Aspirin resistance: disparities and clinical implications. *Pharmacotherapy* 28:999–1018, 2008.
5. Gurbel PA, Tantry US: Do platelet function testing and genotyping improve outcome in patients treated with antithrombotic agents? Platelet function testing and genotyping improve outcome in patients treated with antithrombotic agents. *Circulation* 125:1276–1287; discussion 87, 2012.
6. Fuster V, Sweeny JM: Aspirin: a historical and contemporary therapeutic overview. *Circulation* 123:768–778, 2011.
7. Patrono C, Rocca B: Aspirin, 110 years later. *J Thromb Haemost* 7[Suppl 1]:258–261, 2009.
8. Nowak MM, Brundhofer B, Gibaldi M: Rectal absorption from aspirin suppositories in children and adults. *Pediatrics* 54:23–26, 1974.
9. Eikelboom JW, Hirsh J, Spencer FA, et al: Antiplatelet drugs: Antithrombotic Therapy and Prevention of Thrombosis, 9th ed: American College of Chest Physicians Evidence-Based Clinical Practice Guidelines. *Chest* 141:e89S–119S, 2012.
10. Mehta SR, Bassand JP, Chrolavicius S, et al: Dose comparisons of clopidogrel and aspirin in acute coronary syndromes. *N Engl J Med* 363:930–942, 2010.
11. Sanderson S, Emery J, Baglin T, et al: Narrative review: aspirin resistance and its clinical implications. *Ann Intern Med* 142:370–380, 2005.
12. Krasopoulos G, Brister SJ, Beattie WS, et al: Aspirin "resistance" and risk of cardiovascular morbidity: systematic review and meta-analysis. *BMJ* 336:195–198, 2008.
13. Loualidi A, Bredie SH, Janssen MC: Indications of combined vitamin K antagonists and aspirin therapy. *J Thromb Thrombolysis* 27:421–429, 2009.
14. Douketis JD, Spyropoulos AC, Spencer FA, et al: Perioperative management of antithrombotic therapy: Antithrombotic Therapy and Prevention of Thrombosis, 9th ed: American College of Chest Physicians Evidence-Based Clinical Practice Guidelines. *Chest* 141:e326S–e350S, 2012.
15. Levi M, Eerenberg E, Kamphuisen PW: Bleeding risk and reversal strategies for old and new anticoagulants and antiplatelet agents. *J Thromb Haemost* 9:1705–1712, 2011.
16. Cryer B: Management of patients with high gastrointestinal risk on antiplatelet therapy. *Gastroenterol Clin North Am* 38:289–303, 2009.
17. Kelly JP, Kaufman DW, Jurgelon JM, et al: Risk of aspirin-associated major upper-gastrointestinal bleeding with enteric-coated or buffered product. *Lancet* 348:1413–1416, 1996.
18. Gollapudi RR, Teirstein PS, Stevenson DD, et al: Aspirin sensitivity: implications for patients with coronary artery disease. *JAMA*. 292:3017–3023, 2004.
19. Cattaneo M: New P2Y(12) inhibitors. *Circulation* 121:171–179, 2010.
20. Reinhart KM, White CM, Baker WL: Prasugrel: a critical comparison with clopidogrel. *Pharmacotherapy* 29:1441–1451, 2009.
21. Mega JL, Simon T: Pharmacology of antithrombotic drugs: an assessment of oral antiplatelet and anticoagulant treatments. *Lancet* 386:281–291, 2015.
22. Dobesh PP, Oestreich JH: Ticagrelor: pharmacokinetics, pharmacodynamics, clinical efficacy, and safety. *Pharmacotherapy* 34:1077–1090; 2014.
23. Waite LH, Phan YL, Spinler SA: Cangrelor: a novel intravenous antiplatelet agent with a questionable future. *Pharmacotherapy* 34:1061–1076, 2014.
24. Collet JP, Cuisset T, Range G, et al: Bedside monitoring to adjust antiplatelet therapy for coronary stenting. *N Engl J Med* 367:2100–2109, 2012.
25. Amsterdam EA, Wenger NK, Brindis RG, et al: 2014 AHA/ACC guideline for the management of patients with non-ST-elevation acute coronary syndromes: executive summary: a report of the American College of Cardiology/American Heart Association Task Force on Practice Guidelines. *Circulation* 130:2354–2394, 2014.
26. Company TM: Kengreal™ (Cangrelor), 2015.
27. Horlocker TT, Wedel DJ, Rowlingson JC, et al: Regional anesthesia in the patient receiving antithrombotic or thrombolytic therapy: American Society of Regional Anesthesia and Pain Medicine Evidence-Based Guidelines (Third Edition). *Reg Anesth Pain Med* 35:64–101, 2010.
28. Crouch MA, Nappi JM, Cheang KI: Glycoprotein IIb/IIIa receptor inhibitors in percutaneous coronary intervention and acute coronary syndrome. *Ann Pharmacotherapy* 37:860–875, 2003.
29. Atwater BD, Roe MT, Mahaffey KW: Platelet glycoprotein IIb/IIIa receptor antagonists in non-ST segment elevation acute coronary syndromes: a review and guide to patient selection. *Drugs* 65:313–324, 2005.
30. Alexander KP, Chen AY, Roe MT, et al: Excess dosing of antiplatelet and antithrombin agents in the treatment of non-ST-segment elevation acute coronary syndromes. *JAMA* 294:3108–3116, 2005.
31. Kirtane AJ, Piazza G, Murphy SA, et al: Correlates of bleeding events among moderate- to high-risk patients undergoing percutaneous coronary intervention and treated with eptifibatide: observations from the PROTECT-TIMI-30 trial. *J Am Coll Cardiol* 47:2374–2379, 2006.
32. Hernandez AV, Westerhout CM, Steyerberg EW, et al: Effects of platelet glycoprotein IIb/IIIa receptor blockers in non-ST segment elevation acute coronary syndromes: benefit and harm in different age subgroups. *Heart* 93:450–455, 2007.
33. Reiter RA, Mayr F, Blazicek H, et al: Desmopressin antagonizes the in vitro platelet dysfunction induced by GPIIb/IIIa inhibitors and aspirin. *Blood* 102:4594–4599, 2003.
34. Aster RH: Immune thrombocytopenia caused by glycoprotein IIb/IIIa inhibitors. *Chest* 127:53S–59S, 2005.
35. Frampton JE: Vorapaxar: a review of its use in the long-term secondary prevention of atherothrombotic events. *Drugs* 75:797–808, 2015.
36. Ansara AJ, Shiltz DL, Slavens JB: Use of cilostazol for secondary stroke prevention: an old dog with new tricks? *Ann Pharmacother* 46:394–402, 2012.
37. Jacoby D, Mohler ER, 3rd: Drug treatment of intermittent claudication. *Drugs* 64:1657–1670, 2004.
38. Sacco RL, Diener HC, Yusuf S, et al: Aspirin and extended-release dipyridamole versus clopidogrel for recurrent stroke. *N Engl J Med* 359:1238–1251, 2008.
39. Nutescu EA: Oral anticoagulant therapies: balancing the risks. *Am J Health Syst Pharm* 70:S3–S11, 2013.
40. Rupprecht HJ, Blank R: Clinical pharmacology of direct and indirect factor Xa inhibitors. *Drugs* 70:2153–2170, 2010.
41. Garcia DA, Baglin TP, Weitz JI, et al: Parenteral anticoagulants: Antithrombotic Therapy and Prevention of Thrombosis, 9th ed: American College of Chest Physicians Evidence-Based Clinical Practice Guidelines. *Chest* 141:e24S–e43S, 2012.
42. Weitz DS, Weitz JI: Update on heparin: what do we need to know? *J Thromb Thrombolysis* 29:199–207, 2010.
43. Raschke RA, Reilly BM, Guidry JR, et al: The weight-based heparin dosing nomogram compared with a "standard care" nomogram. A randomized controlled trial. *Ann Intern Med* 119:874–881, 1993.
44. Holbrook A, Schulman S, Witt DM, et al: Evidence-based management of anticoagulant therapy: Antithrombotic Therapy and Prevention of Thrombosis, 9th ed: American College of Chest Physicians Evidence-Based Clinical Practice Guidelines. *Chest* 141:e152S–e84S, 2012.
45. Lim W, Dentali F, Eikelboom JW, et al: Meta-analysis: low-molecular-weight heparin and bleeding in patients with severe renal insufficiency. *Ann Intern Med* 144:673–684, 2006.
46. King CS, Holley AB, Jackson JL, et al: Twice vs three times daily heparin dosing for thromboembolism prophylaxis in the general medical population: a metaanalysis. *Chest* 131:507–516, 2007.
47. Schulman S, Beyth RJ, Kearon C, et al: Hemorrhagic complications of anticoagulant and thrombolytic treatment: American College of Chest Physicians Evidence-Based Clinical Practice Guidelines (8th Edition). *Chest* 133:257S–298S, 2008.
48. Cuker A SS, Lilly C: Hematologic problems in the intensive care unit, in Irwin RS, Rippe JM (eds): *Manual of Intensive Care Medicine*. Philadelphia, PA, Lippincott Williams & Wilkins, 2010, p 563.
49. Carr JA, Silverman N: The heparin-protamine interaction. A review. *J Cardiovasc Surg* 1999;40:659–666.
50. Nutescu EA, Spinler SA, Wittkowsky A, et al: Low-molecular-weight heparins in renal impairment and obesity: available evidence and clinical practice recommendations across medical and surgical settings. *Ann Pharmacother* 43:1064–1083, 2009.
51. Wein L, Wein S, Haas SJ, et al: Pharmacological venous thromboembolism prophylaxis in hospitalized medical patients: a meta-analysis of randomized controlled trials. *Arch Intern Med* 167:1476–1486, 2007.

52. PROTECT Investigators for the Canadian Critical Care Trials Group and the Australian and New Zealand Intensive Care Society Clinical Trials Group, Cook D, Meade M, et al: Dalteparin versus unfractionated heparin in critically ill patients. *N Engl J Med* 364:1305–1314, 2011.
53. Mo Y, Yam FK: Recent advances in the development of specific antidotes for target-specific oral anticoagulants. *Pharmacotherapy* 35:198–207, 2015.
54. Suryanarayan D, Schulman S: Potential antidotes for reversal of old and new oral anticoagulants. *Thromb Res* 133[Suppl 2]:S158–S166, 2014.
55. Warkentin TE: Heparin-induced thrombocytopenia in critically ill patients. *Crit Care Clin* 27:805–823, 2011.
56. Linkins LA, Dans AL, Moores LK, et al: Treatment and prevention of heparin-induced thrombocytopenia: Antithrombotic Therapy and Prevention of Thrombosis, 9th ed: American College of Chest Physicians Evidence-Based Clinical Practice Guidelines. *Chest* 141:e495S–e530S, 2012.
57. Chan NC, Bhagirath V, Eikelboom JW: Profile of betrixaban and its potential in the prevention and treatment of venous thromboembolism. *Vasc Health Risk Manag* 11:343–351, 2015.
58. Dobesh PP, Fanikos J: New oral anticoagulants for the treatment of venous thromboembolism: understanding differences and similarities. *Drugs* 74:2015–2032, 2014.
59. Hursting MJ, Soffer J: Reducing harm associated with anticoagulation: practical considerations of argatroban therapy in heparin-induced thrombocytopenia. *Drug Saf* 32:203–218, 2009.
60. Schaden E, Kozek-Langenecker SA: Direct thrombin inhibitors: pharmacology and application in intensive care medicine. *Intensive Care Med* 36:1127–1137, 2010.
61. Pollack CV Jr, Reilly PA, Eikelboom J, et al: Idarucizumab for dabigatran reversal. *N Engl J Med* 373(6):511–520, 2015.
62. Ageno W, Gallus AS, Wittkowsky A, et al: Oral anticoagulant therapy: Antithrombotic Therapy and Prevention of Thrombosis, 9th ed: American College of Chest Physicians Evidence-Based Clinical Practice Guidelines. *Chest* 141:e44S–e88S, 2012.
63. Guyatt GH, Akl EA, Crowther M, et al: Executive summary: Antithrombotic Therapy and Prevention of Thrombosis, 9th ed: American College of Chest Physicians Evidence-Based Clinical Practice Guidelines. *Chest* 141:7S–47S, 2012.
64. Thigpen JL, Limdi NA: Reversal of oral anticoagulation. *Pharmacotherapy* 33:1199–1213, 2013.
65. Sarode R, Milling TJ Jr, Refaai MA, et al: Efficacy and safety of a 4-factor prothrombin complex concentrate in patients on vitamin K antagonists presenting with major bleeding: a randomized, plasma-controlled, phase IIIb study. *Circulation* 128:1234–1243, 2013.
66. Garcia DA, Crowther MA: Reversal of warfarin: case-based practice recommendations. *Circulation* 125:2944–2947, 2012.
67. Makris M, van Veen JJ, Maclean R: Warfarin anticoagulation reversal: management of the asymptomatic and bleeding patient. *J Thromb Thrombolysis* 2010;29:171–181.
68. Douketis JD, Spyropoulos AC, Kaatz S, et al: Perioperative bridging anticoagulation in patients with atrial fibrillation. *N Engl J Med* 373:823–833, 2015.
69. Siegal D, Yudin J, Kaatz S, et al: Periprocedural heparin bridging in patients receiving vitamin K antagonists: systematic review and meta-analysis of bleeding and thromboembolic rates. *Circulation* 126:1630–1639, 2012.
70. O'Donnell M, Kearon C: Perioperative management of oral anticoagulation. *Cardiol Clin* 26:299–309, viii, 2008.
71. Haire WD: Pharmacology of fibrinolysis. *Chest* 101:91S–7S, 1992.
72. Verstraete M: Third-generation thrombolytic drugs. *Am J Med* 109:52–58, 2000.
73. Ouriel K, Kandarpa K: Safety of thrombolytic therapy with urokinase or recombinant tissue plasminogen activator for peripheral arterial occlusion: a comprehensive compilation of published work. *J Endovasc Ther* 11:436–446, 2004.
74. Baskin JL, Pui CH, Reiss U, et al: Management of occlusion and thrombosis associated with long-term indwelling central venous catheters. *Lancet* 374:159–169, 2009.
75. Donovan BC: How to give thrombolytic therapy safely. *Chest* 95:290S–292S, 1989.
76. Broderick J, Connolly S, Feldmann E, et al: Guidelines for the management of spontaneous intracerebral hemorrhage in adults: 2007 update: a guideline from the American Heart Association/American Stroke Association Stroke Council, High Blood Pressure Research Council, and the Quality of Care and Outcomes in Research Interdisciplinary Working Group. *Circulation* 116:e391–413, 2007.
77. Emberson J, Lees KR, Lyden P, et al: Effect of treatment delay, age, and stroke severity on the effects of intravenous thrombolysis with alteplase for acute ischaemic stroke: a meta-analysis of individual patient data from randomised trials. *Lancet* 384:1929–1935, 2014.
78. Fiumara K, Kucher N, Fanikos J, et al: Predictors of major hemorrhage following fibrinolysis for acute pulmonary embolism. *Am J Cardiol* 97:127–129, 2006.

Chapter 94 ■ Critical Care of Patients with Hematologic Malignancies

MATTHEW J. WIEDUWILT • LLOYD E. DAMON

INTRODUCTION

Although the incidence of aggressive hematologic malignancies like acute myeloid leukemia (AML), acute lymphoblastic leukemia (ALL), and intermediate- and high-grade non-Hodgkin lymphomas is low, these potentially curable diseases frequently require intensive care unit (ICU) management at presentation to prevent early mortality and achieve disease remission. Patients with hematologic malignancies account for approximately 2% of all ICU admissions [1,2]. Approximately 7% of patients with hematologic malignancies admitted to the hospital will become critically ill [3]. The most frequently reported indications for ICU admission in patients with hematologic malignancies are respiratory failure (26% to 91%), severe sepsis (8% to 64%), neurologic impairment (14% to 23%), and acute renal failure (14% to 23%). For all critically ill patients with hematologic malignancies, ICU mortality, in-hospital mortality and 6-month mortality rates are 23% to 62%, 54% to 82%, and 66% to 83%, respectively [1–12]. Risk factors for death in the ICU include high disease severity score (APACHE II, SAPS II, SOFA), poor performance status, vasopressor use, leukopenia, increasing number of organ failures, and acute renal failure (see Table 94.1). In a large prospective study of 1,100 critically ill patients with hematologic malignancies, earlier admission to the ICU and cancer in remission were associated with improved hospital survival [12]. Notably, mechanical ventilation has not been consistently associated with increased risk of death in this patient population, and some studies suggest improved outcomes with early endotracheal intubation [2,13]. In addition, survival in patients with hematologic malignancies admitted to the ICU after chemotherapy alone versus hematopoietic cell transplant (HCT) are not different, suggesting that critically ill HCT patients should be treated aggressively on ICU admission [14,15]. In fact, when matched for severity of acute illness upon ICU admission, survival of patients with hematologic malignancies and nononcologic patients appears to be similar [1].

OVERVIEW OF HEMATOLOGIC MALIGNANCIES

Acute Myeloid Leukemia

AML accounts for 22% to 54% of hematologic malignancy admissions to the ICU [1,2,4,6–11]. Patients with AML may require ICU admission for disease- or treatment-related complications including sepsis (frequently complicated by neutropenia), bleeding caused by thrombocytopenia and occasionally acute disseminated intravascular coagulation (DIC) and multiple organ failure.

The incidence of AML in the United States is 3.5 cases per 100,000 persons per year with approximately 12,000 new cases diagnosed annually. More than half of newly diagnosed AML patients are over 65 years of age and a third are older than 75

TABLE 94.1

Outcomes of Patients with Hematologic Malignancies Admitted to the ICU

Number of patients	ICU mortality (%)	In-hospital mortality (%)	Risk factors for death	Reference
7,689	43	59	HCT, Hodgkin lymphoma, severe sepsis, age, length of hospital stay prior to ICU admission, respiratory failure, neurologic failure, renal failure, anemia	[2]
22	55	82	APACHE II score, number of failing organs, mechanical ventilation	[4]
60	—	78	APACHE II score >30, number of failing organs, resistant disease, leukopenia	[5]
92	—	77	Progression of underlying malignancy	[6]
78	26	—	Number of failing organs, liver failure	[7]
104	44	—	SAPS II score, mechanical ventilation	[8]
124	42	54	Leukopenia, vasopressors, renal failure	[9]
58	62	—	SAPS II score, SOFA score	[10]
24	—	75	SAPS II score >66, liver failure, neurologic failure, number of failing organs	[3]
92	50	55	SAPS II, SOFA, ODIN, and LODS scores, allogeneic HCT, neutropenia, severe sepsis, vasopressor use, invasive mechanical ventilation	[11]
101	23	—	SAPS II score, SOFA score, mechanical ventilation, renal replacement therapy	[1]
1,011		49	Multivariate: cancer not in remission, time to ICU admission >24 h	[12]

HCT, hematopoietic stem cell transplant; SAPS II, Simplified Acute Physiology Score II; APACHE II, Acute Physiology and Chronic Health Evaluation II; SOFA, Sequential Organ Failure Assessment; ODIN, Organ Dysfunction and/or Infection Score; LODS, Logistic Organ Dysfunction Score.

years. Five-year survival rates are approximately 50% in adults under the age of 45 years but drop to less than 10% in patients over the age of 65 [16].

AML arises from the acquisition of genetic mutations in myeloid precursors or stem cells leading to various degrees of maturation arrest, unregulated proliferation, and resistance to apoptosis. By the World Health Organization 2008 classification system, the diagnosis of AML requires myeloid blasts to comprise 20% or more of nucleated cells in the peripheral blood or bone marrow except in cases of AML with the recurrent cytogenetic abnormalities t(15;17), t(8;21), inv(16)/t(16;16), myeloid sarcoma (a tumor of myeloblasts), and some cases of erythroleukemia. The recurrent cytogenetic abnormalities t(15;17), t(8;21), inv(16)/t(16;16) and normal cytogenetics accompanied by gene mutations in NPM1 or both alleles of CEBP-α confer a better prognosis in terms of risk of relapse, and the majority of patients obtain durable complete remissions with chemotherapy alone [17]. Conversely, patients with poor risk cytogenetics and those with normal cytogenetics accompanied by mutations in the FLT3 protooncogene have a low likelihood of durable remission with chemotherapy alone and typically undergo allogeneic HCT in first complete remission [17].

Standard induction chemotherapy for AML using 3 days of intravenous (IV) anthracycline (daunorubicin, idarubicin) or anthracenedione (mitoxantrone) and 7 days of cytarabine by continuous IV infusion, ideally initiated within 5 days of diagnosis for de novo AML, leads to complete remission rates of 60% to 80% in young adults under 60 years of age and 50% in patients over 60 years of age. Postremission therapy is tailored to pretreatment risk status, performance status, comorbidities, and age, and may consist of chemotherapy alone or myeloablative or reduced-intensity conditioning allogeneic HCT [18].

Acute Promyelocytic Leukemia

Acute promyelocytic leukemia (APL) accounts for 5% to 6% of all AML with approximately 600 to 800 new diagnoses made each year in the United States. APL frequently presents with acute DIC that can be rapidly fatal due to intracerebral, pulmonary, or gastrointestinal (GI) hemorrhage, in all accounting for 50% to 60% of early deaths. Early suspicion and treatment of APL, even prior to definitive genetic diagnosis, is important to reduce the risk of life-threatening hemorrhage [19]. Paradoxically, patients are also at risk of thrombotic events that complicate about 10% to 12% of cases, frequently in those with expression of CD2, CD15, and FLT3-ITD mutation APL occurs due to arrest of myeloid differentiation at the promyelocyte stage leading to accumulation of leukemic promyelocytes in the bone marrow, blood, and tissues. Morphologically, leukemic promyelocytes typically have variable nuclear morphology with bilobed or reniform nuclei, prominent cytoplasmic granules, and numerous large Auer rods, frequently in bundles. Approximately 5% of APL presents as a microgranular variant characterized by few or absent granules. Patients with this microgranular variant tend to have higher presenting white blood cell counts, placing them at higher risk of complications and relapse. Except in rare instances, APL is characterized by the presence of the recurrent cytogenetic abnormality t(15;17)(q22;q12) leading to a PML-RAR-α fusion gene that can be demonstrated by cytogenetic analysis, fluorescence in situ hybridization (FISH) and quantitative reverse transcription polymerase chain reaction (RT-PCR). The chimeric PML-RAR-α protein is the target of therapy with all-*trans*-retinoic acid (ATRA) and arsenic trioxide (ATO), agents that cause degradation of the PML-RAR-α oncoprotein thereby promoting terminal differentiation of leukemic promyelocytes [20,21].

The diagnosis of APL should be considered in any patient with a new diagnosis of leukemia, especially if accompanied by clinical and laboratory evidence of acute DIC. Early institution of treatment with the differentiating agent ATRA is indicated upon suspicion of APL to reduce the risk of fatal bleeding [19]. Careful review of the peripheral blood smear from new leukemia patients in consultation with hematologists and hematopathologists should be performed to look for characteristic hypergranular leukemic promyelocytes. Expedited performance of flow cytometry, specifically evaluating for coexpression of CD34, CD15, and CD13 on the surface of leukemic cells can aid in diagnosing the microgranular variant of APL.

Greater than 70% of APL patients attain prolonged remissions with current treatment strategies. Induction chemotherapy regimens generally combine ATRA with ATO or ATRA with an anthracycline, typically idarubicin or daunorubicin [19,22]. ATO is highly active against APL and in combination with ATRA produces complete response rates over 90% [22]. ATRA or ATO, however, may cause a fatal differentiation syndrome (DS) characterized by fever, dyspnea, pulmonary infiltrates, pleuropericardial effusions, weight gain, peripheral edema, renal failure, and hypotension.

Acute Lymphoblastic Leukemia

ALL results from the acquisition of genetic mutations in lymphoid progenitor or stem cells resulting in the arrest of cells at an early stage of differentiation. In 2009, about 5,760 people were diagnosed with ALL in the United States with a median age of 13 years. ALL patients comprise 9% to 27% of ICU admissions for hematologic malignancies [1,2,4,6–11]. The 10-year survival among all adults with ALL is less than 30%. Favorable disease characteristics in ALL include ages 1 to 15 years, presenting WBC <30,000 per μL for B-cell ALL or <50-100,000 per μL for T-cell ALL, rapid achievement of complete remission, and minimal residual disease negativity whereas age >35 years is unfavorable. Cases with t(9;22)/BCR-ABL (Philadelphia chromosome, Ph), representing 15% to 20% of adult cases of ALL, or t(4;11)/MLL-AF4 translocations typically fare poorly, with historical survival rates of less than 10% with chemotherapy alone and long-term survival after allogeneic HCT ranging 20% to 45%. The addition of tyrosine kinase inhibitors targeting BCR-ABL1 (e.g., imatinib, dasatinib, nilotinib) to chemotherapy for Ph+ ALL has dramatically improved survival in patients not undergoing allogeneic HCT.

Clinical trial regimens in the last decade have improved complete remission rates to 74% to 93% with 5-year survival rates as high as 48%. Therapy for ALL typically spans 2 to 3 years and includes induction therapy, postremission therapy, central nervous system (CNS) prophylaxis and maintenance chemotherapy in patients who do not undergo HCT. Induction therapy for ALL typically combines vincristine, an anthracycline (e.g., daunorubicin), and a corticosteroid (prednisone or dexamethasone) typically with L-asparginase and/or cyclophosphamide. Prophylaxis against CNS relapse includes intrathecal chemotherapy with methotrexate with or without cytarabine and frequently high-dose IV methotrexate. Postremission therapy typically includes the same agents used in induction as well as methotrexate, cytarabine, and 6-mercaptopurine, among other agents. Maintenance therapy consists of oral methotrexate and 6-mercaptopurine often with pulses of vincristine and corticosteroids. Imatinib, dasatinib, and nilotinib inhibit the chimeric BCR-ABL1 tyrosine kinase produced by the Ph chromosome and improve complete remission and survival rates in Ph+ ALL. Allogeneic HCT is often performed in adult patients with ALL, although recent data suggests that patients who are negative for minimal residual disease at the completion of induction chemotherapy may not require allogeneic HCT to maximize likelihood of survival [23].

Aggressive Non-Hodgkin Lymphomas

Diffuse large B-cell lymphoma (DLBCL) is an aggressive non-Hodgkin lymphoma of intermediate histologic grade that typically presents with rapidly enlarging lymph nodes or extranodal masses frequently with symptoms of organ compromise from lymphomatous involvement of extranodal sites. Diagnosis is typically made by excisional biopsy of a lymph node or mass showing large lymphoid cells that completely efface lymph node architecture. Malignant B cells express CD19, CD20, and CD22 with variable expression of surface immunoglobulin, CD5, and CD10. Common genetic abnormalities in DLBCL include constitutive expression of the transcriptional repressor Bcl-6, the antiapoptotic protein Bcl-2, and/or the transcription factor c-myc. The International Prognostic Index for aggressive lymphomas uses five unfavorable variables to establish risk status: age greater than 60 years, poor performance status, advanced stage (Ann Arbor Stage III or IV disease), extranodal involvement at more than one site, and elevated serum lactate dehydrogenase. First-line combination chemotherapy with cyclophosphamide, doxorubicin, vincristine, and prednisone (CHOP) in combination with the humanized monoclonal anti-CD20 antibody rituximab results in 2-year overall survival rates of 70% to 90%.

Burkitt lymphoma (BL), which has the fastest growth rate of any human malignancy, is an aggressive non-Hodgkin lymphoma with endemic, sporadic, and immunodeficiency-associated clinical variants. BL typically presents with rapidly progressive nodal and extranodal disease, commonly in the abdomen and GI tract leading to nausea, vomiting, anorexia, bowel obstruction, and GI bleeding. Advanced stage is common at diagnosis with bone marrow involvement in 30% to 38% and CNS involvement in 13% to 17% of adults. Morphologically, lymphoma cells are medium-sized with deeply basophilic cytoplasm containing cytoplasmic lipid vacuoles and a high proliferative index of greater than 90%. A leukemic variant exists and can be distinguished from ALL by surface expression of immunoglobulin, CD20, and CD10, without coexpression of TdT or CD34. BL is genetically characterized by chromosomal translocations that lead to constitutive expression of c-myc, typically t(8;14) and rarely t(2;8) or t(8;22). High-intensity, brief-duration chemotherapy, typically with cyclophosphamide, doxorubicin, vincristine, and antimetabolite-containing regimens, with intensive CNS prophylaxis, have led to 1-year remission rates as high as 86%. The bulky disease and high cell proliferation rates seen in both DLBCL and BL place patients at high risk of tumor lysis syndrome, and prophylactic treatment with allopurinol to prevent hyperuricemia is typically given prior to chemotherapy.

Other Malignancies

Other notable hematologic malignancies frequently requiring ICU level care are multiple myeloma, Waldenstrom macroglobulinemia and myeloproliferative neoplasms such as chronic myeloid leukemia, essential thrombocythemia, polycythemia vera, and chronic idiopathic myelofibrosis. In multiple myeloma, spinal cord compression may occur due to encroachment of the spinal canal by epidural plasmacytomas and/or from pathologic fracture of spinal vertebrae. Emergent imaging of the entire spine with magnetic resonance imaging is required for diagnosis (see Chapter 95). In Waldenstrom macroglobulinemia, high concentrations of monoclonal immunoglobulin M (IgM) paraprotein in the serum can lead to the hyperviscosity syndrome manifest as mucosal bleeding, confusion, seizures, coma, visual disturbance, and/or headache as well as cryoglobulinemia, cold agglutinin hemolytic anemia, and plasma volume expansion leading to congestive heart failure. Myeloproliferative neoplasms may lead to life-threatening hemorrhage or thrombosis, requiring critical care (see Chapter 95).

DISEASE AND TREATMENT-RELATED COMPLICATIONS

Hyperleukocytosis and Leukostasis

In AML, hyperleukocytosis, generally defined as a circulating blast count greater than 100,000 per μL, occurs in 5% to 18% of patients at initial presentation. Early mortality during initial treatment of patients with hyperleukocytic AML ranges from 5% to 30% with advanced age, poor performance status, coagulopathy, respiratory compromise, and organ failure associated with early death [24]. Hyperleukocytosis in AML is frequently associated with leukostasis manifesting as respiratory failure, visual disturbances, intracranial hemorrhage, and renal failure.

Leukostasis, although typically associated with hyperleukocytosis, can occur at white blood cell counts less than 50,000 per μL (likely caused by interpatient variability in leukemia cell biology and individual susceptibility). Myeloid leukemic blasts are less deformable than mature white blood cells possibly predisposing to formation of aggregates of cells in the small blood vessels, tissue ischemia, endothelial damage, and tissue infiltration. In addition, expression of specific cell surface adhesion molecules on leukemia cells and endothelial cell activation by cytokines secreted by leukemic blasts may play important roles in promoting leukostasis. For instance, the expression of CD56/NCAM on the surface of leukemia cells in myelomonocytic AML correlates with the development of leukostasis [25]. In vitro, myeloid blasts promote their own adhesion to the vascular endothelium by upregulating expression of ICAM-1, VCAM-1, and E-selectin on endothelial cells [26]. Expression of the cell surface integrin CD11c on the surface of AML blasts is associated with increased early death risk in the setting of hyperleukocytosis [27]. In ALL, hyperleukocytosis is rarely associated with symptomatic leukostasis except with extreme hyperleukocytosis (WBC >400,000 per μL) possibly due to the smaller size, easier deformability, and decreased vascular endothelium adherence of lymphoblasts. In AML with hyperleukocytosis, most studies have not shown a demonstrable difference in complete response rates, disease-free survival or overall survival after treatment. However, the presence of pulmonary leukostasis, hepatomegaly, hyperbilirubinemia, and hypofibrinogenemia are predictors of poor outcome in patients with hyperleukocytosis [24].

Hydroxyurea at doses of 20 to 30 mg/kg/d or more can reduce peripheral leukocyte counts, and generally requires 1 to 2 days to take effect. Red blood cell transfusions should be avoided until the leukocyte count is less than 50,000 per μL to avoid ischemic events such as stroke or acute coronary syndrome. Although invasive, leukapheresis is a relatively safe procedure and is frequently used in combination with hydroxyurea to rapidly lower circulating blast counts and theoretically decrease the risk of tumor lysis syndrome and progressive leukostasis (see Chapters 89 and 96). Two blood volumes (140 mL per kg) are processed in the typical leukapheresis procedure. Studies have failed to show a consistent clinical benefit with the use of leukapheresis in hyperleukocytic leukemia [28,29], although some uncontrolled retrospective single institution studies show reduction in early mortality in patients undergoing leukapheresis without an overall survival benefit [28]. A recent meta-analysis of 21 studies of hyperleukocytic AML failed to show an early mortality benefit with leukapheresis or early institution of chemotherapy including hydroxyurea [29]. In APL patients presenting with hyperleukocytosis and organ failure, leukapheresis is contraindicated due to the risk of exacerbating acute DIC, initiating vasomotor instability, and increasing induction death [19].

Hyperviscosity Syndrome

The hyperviscosity syndrome occurs in 30% of patients with Waldenstrom macroglobulinemia (also called lymphoplasmacytic lymphoma with IgM monoclonal gammopathy) at presentation and is defined by the presence of increased serum viscosity with neurologic symptoms related to impaired blood flow including headache, vertigo, dizziness, visual impairment, hearing impairment, tinnitus, nystagmus, stupor, stroke, dementia, and coma [30]. In addition, mucosal bleeding, including GI hemorrhage, renal failure, and congestive heart failure because of plasma volume expansion and concomitant anemia may occur. Elevated serum IgM, with its large pentameric structure, is most commonly associated with hyperviscosity, although the syndrome has been reported with immunoglobulin A, immunoglobulin G, and κ light chain multiple myeloma. Normal serum viscosity measures 1.4 to 1.8 centipoises and symptomatic hyperviscosity typically occurs at greater than 4 centipoises.

Emergent plasmapheresis is indicated for symptomatic hyperviscosity. One to two plasma volumes are typically exchanged and replaced with 5% albumin in patients with low bleeding risk or fresh frozen plasma (FFP) in patients at high risk of bleeding. Symptoms typically resolve quickly but neurologic deficits can remain. Red blood cell transfusions should be avoided if possible until serum viscosity is lowered (see Chapter 89). Definitive treatment for the underlying malignancy should be instituted quickly to control paraprotein production. Procedural risks include depletion of clotting factors when 5% albumin is used as the exchange fluid, hypocalcemia from citrate anticoagulant use, dialysis catheter-related infection, pneumothorax or thrombosis, and complications from FFP administration including anaphylaxis, blood-borne infections, and transfusion-related acute lung injury.

Bleeding

Bleeding in hematologic malignancies is a common cause of morbidity and mortality. DIC and thrombocytopenia are common etiologies, but acquired clotting factor deficiencies can also predispose to life-threatening hemorrhage.

Disseminated Intravascular Coagulation

Acute DIC is a common cause of morbidity and mortality during the treatment of many hematologic malignancies and is especially characteristic of APL and to a lesser degree other forms of acute leukemia. Sepsis, especially gram-negative sepsis occurring in the setting of disease or treatment-related neutropenia, is a common cause of DIC as well. Complicating the diagnosis of DIC is the frequent presence of hepatic failure due to malignant infiltration of the liver or treatment-related hepatotoxicity. Clinically, patients are at high risk of death from bleeding and can develop oozing from IV lines and surgical sites, purpura, pulmonary hemorrhage, intracranial hemorrhage, GI bleeding, and multiple organ failure.

Acute DIC results from pathologic coagulation within small blood vessels, typically from the release of tissue factor or endotoxin exposure, leading to unmitigated activation of coagulation and consumption of coagulation factors and platelets. Depletion of clotting factors and platelets, activation of plasmin, and the production of anticoagulant fibrin split products can lead to severe bleeding. Laboratory hallmarks of acute DIC include thrombocytopenia, prolongation of clotting times, hypofibrinogenemia, elevated fibrin split products, and sometimes schistocytes on the peripheral blood smear.

The coagulopathy observed in APL resembles acute DIC but with some subtle differences. In APL, leukemic cells produce tissue factor and high levels of a cysteine protease called cancer procoagulant, both of which are downregulated by ATRA treatment in primary and cultured leukemic APL blasts [31–34]. Tissue factor in conjunction with activated Factor VII activates Factor X, whereas cancer procoagulant can directly activate Factor X leading to pathologic coagulation. In addition, rapid death of malignant cells leads to increased thrombin generation [35]. Unlike acute DIC, antithrombin and protein C levels are maintained in the coagulopathy of APL [36]. Increased fibrinolysis also complicates APL and can lead to bleeding. APL cells express both cell surface u-PA (urokinase-plasminogen activator) and t-PA (tissue-plasminogen activator). u-PA is transiently upregulated upon differentiation of leukemic cells with ATRA [37,38]. Dexamethasone administered with ATRA suppresses the upregulation of u-PA. Annexin II is highly expressed on leukemic promyelocytes and interacts with plasminogen and t-PA to increase plasmin production [39]. In addition, annexin II is highly expressed on cerebral endothelial cells potentially explaining the high rates of intracerebral hemorrhage in APL [40]. Notably, treatment with ATRA downregulates the expression of annexin II on leukemic promyelocytes [39].

Reversal of acute DIC requires effective treatment of the underlying cause. Supportive care includes early management of sepsis including the administration of broad-spectrum antibiotic coverage with antipseudomonal activity in neutropenic patients and reversal of organ dysfunction when possible. In the setting of APL, early institution of ATRA combined with cytotoxic chemotherapy in high-risk patients with WBC >10,000 per μL is indicated to reduce the burden of leukemic promyelocytes. DIC typically resolves within 48 hours of initiation of ATRA in this setting.

With acute DIC, frequent monitoring of complete blood count, prothrombin time (PT), partial thromboplastin time (PTT), and fibrinogen three to four times a day is prudent to monitor the consumptive process and guide replacement of platelets and coagulation factors. In patients with APL-associated DIC who are bleeding or who are at high risk of bleeding, maintenance of platelet count above 30,000 to 50,000 per μL and fibrinogen above 100 to 150 mg per dL with platelet and cryoprecipitate transfusions has been recommended [19]. FFP also may be given to reduce the prolonged PT and PTT. By inhibiting thrombin and Factor Xa, low-dose heparin (4 to 5 U/kg/h) could theoretically improve severe bleeding in acute DIC by limiting fibrinogen and platelet consumption, plasminogen activation, and fibrin split product production. Results of clinical studies, however, have been equivocal, and routine use of heparin to prevent or treat acute DIC-related bleeding is not universally standard. Conversely, thrombosis may occur in acute DIC, and in this setting, the administration of low-dose heparin may be beneficial. The role of activated protein C, soluble thrombomodulin, tranexamic acid, and aminocaproic acid in the management of DIC in hematologic malignancy patients is unclear. A meta-analysis of four randomized controlled trials in patients with acute or chronic leukemias was unable to show any benefit to the use of activated protein C, soluble thrombomodulin, and tranexamic acid in treating leukemia patients with DIC [41]. Rare patients with intractable bleeding despite standard measures may benefit from tranexamic acid or aminocaproic acid but with a risk of microvascular thrombosis and organ failure.

Thrombocytopenia

Thrombocytopenia in patients with hematologic malignancies can be caused by bone marrow infiltration by malignant cells, myelosuppression from chemotherapy and other medications, bacterial sepsis, acute DIC, immune thrombocytopenia, and/or hypersplenism from splenomegaly. The risk of major hemorrhage dramatically increases at platelet counts less than 5,000 per μL and the use of prophylactic platelet transfusions, starting in the 1970s, typically with a transfusion threshold of 20,000 per μL, reduced the frequency of fatal bleeding in this population to less than 1%. However, this strategy led to an increased demand for platelet concentrates.

The issue of the optimal platelet count to trigger a prophylactic platelet transfusion has been addressed. A 2004 Cochrane Database systematic review included three prospective randomized studies comparing prophylactic platelet transfusions at platelet counts of 10,000 per μL versus 20,000 per μL. None of these studies showed significant differences in severe bleeding events or mortality but the studies were small and possibly underpowered to show noninferiority of the lower transfusion threshold [42]. The risk of spontaneous hemorrhage in patients without concomitant coagulopathy or acute DIC, platelet dysfunction, fever, mucositis, or uncontrolled hypertension appears acceptable until platelets are below 10,000 per μL. Safely minimizing the platelet dose per prophylactic transfusion has been studied as well. A 2010 study randomized 1,272 patients undergoing chemotherapy or HCT for hematologic and nonhematologic malignancies to receive 1.1×10^{11}, 2.2×10^{11}, or 4.4×10^{11} platelets per m^2 of body surface area to be given prophylactically for platelet counts less than 10,000 per μL. The lowest dose group required fewer platelets overall but required more transfusions (five vs. three per patient per treatment course). Bleeding rates of all grades were similar between the groups with no deaths from hemorrhage in the low- and medium-dose groups supporting the use of low-dose platelet transfusions [43]. Avoiding drugs that cause platelet dysfunction (especially aspirin, nonsteroidal antiinflammatory drugs [NSAIDs], Cox-2 inhibitors, and clopidogrel), treating underlying coagulopathy, and reversing renal dysfunction are important adjuncts to preventing bleeding in thrombocytopenic patients as well.

Acquired von Willebrand Syndrome

The acquired von Willebrand syndrome (aVWS) results from a reduction in the level of von Willebrand factor (VWF) and may rarely occur in monoclonal gammopathy of undetermined significance, Waldenstrom macroglobulinemia, multiple myeloma, non-Hodgkin lymphomas, and myeloproliferative neoplasms, especially essential thrombocythemia. Treatment of the underlying malignancy to decrease tumor burden or reduce elevated platelet counts is generally effective in resolving acquired von Willebrand disease. Management may include platelet apheresis in the setting of extreme thrombocytosis and active bleeding. High-dose intravenous immunoglobulin (dose, 1 g/kg/d for 2 days) may be considered in patients with lymphoid neoplasms who have inhibitory antibodies to VWF. For treatment of acute bleeding, desmopressin (dose, 0.03 μg per kg IV) or purified plasma-derived vWF/FVIII concentrates may be considered. Aspirin and NSAIDs should be avoided until aVWS has resolved.

Pulmonary Complications

Mechanical ventilation is associated with poor outcomes in patients with hematologic malignancies. Mortality ranges from 39% to 82%, although most studies of respiratory failure in patients with hematologic malignancies are retrospective and have failed to match mechanically ventilated and nonventilated patients for degree of respiratory compromise. Hampshire et al. retrospectively studied 7,689 cases of hematologic malignancies requiring ICU admission in England, Wales, and Northern Ireland. When matched for PaO_2:FiO_2 ratios, mechanically ventilated hematologic malignancy patients had reduced mortality compared with nonventilated hematologic malignancy patients (mortality 67% vs. 85% for PaO_2:FiO_2 <100 mm Hg, 50% vs. 69% for PaO_2:FiO_2 100 to 199 mm Hg) [2]. In a smaller study, invasive mechanical ventilation within 24 hours after ICU admission was associated with lower mortality rates compared with patients receiving noninvasive positive pressure ventilation [13]. After

HCT, however, patients who require mechanical ventilation appear to fare less well. Short-term mortality is 82% to 96% and worsens to 98% to 100% in the setting of combined renal and hepatic failure. Only 9% to 14% of mechanically ventilated HCT patients are alive 6 months after ICU admission.

Diagnostic approaches to identify the etiology of respiratory failure include blood, urine, and sputum cultures, blood and urine infectious serologies, diagnostic imaging, bronchoscopy, and surgical lung biopsy. Flexible bronchoscopy with bronchoalveolar lavage (BAL) detects pulmonary infections in approximately 50% of patients with hematologic malignancies presenting with respiratory deterioration leading to a change in antimicrobial therapy in 38% of patients [44,45]. In one study, there was no survival advantage to BAL, and respiratory deterioration requiring mechanical ventilation occurred in 36% of patients as a short-term consequence of BAL highlighting the need for careful patient selection and the broad use of noninvasive diagnostic tests prior to pursuing BAL [45]. In two retrospective studies of surgical lung biopsy among hematologic malignancy patients with unexplained pulmonary infiltrates, a specific diagnosis was made in 62% to 67% of patients and led to change in therapy 40% to 57% of the time. A specific diagnosis was significantly associated with decreased mortality in both studies (absolute reduction in mortality, 29% to 33%) [46,47].

Infection is the most common identifiable cause of respiratory distress in hematologic malignancies. Pulmonary hemorrhage, diffuse alveolar damage, pulmonary embolism, and congestive heart failure are the most common identifiable noninfectious causes. Pulmonary infections are typically caused by *Pseudomonas aeruginosa*, *Staphylococcus aureus*, and streptococcal species with *Legionella pneumophila* and mycobacterial infections being less common pathogens. Prolonged neutropenia from underlying disease or myelotoxic chemotherapy places patients at risk of mycelial fungal pneumonia with *Aspergillus* spp. being the most common offenders. Patients with lymphoid malignancies and those treated with allogeneic HCT are also at risk of *Pneumocystis jirovecii* pneumonia and viral pneumonias including cytomegalovirus (CMV) infection. Effective antimicrobial treatment can be difficult in this group of patients as mixed infections and antimicrobial resistance are common. Ganciclovir and related antiviral agents in combination with IV immunoglobulin have reduced the mortality of CMV pneumonia in HCT patients [48].

Noninfectious etiologies of respiratory failure in patients with hematologic malignancies, including those undergoing HCT, include cardiogenic pulmonary edema, diffuse alveolar hemorrhage (DAH), engraftment syndrome, idiopathic pneumonia syndrome (IPS), bronchiolitis obliterans syndrome (BOS), cryptogenic organizing pneumonia (COP), granulomatous inflammation and malignant infiltration of the lungs. Chemotherapeutic agents such as carmustine (BCNU), busulfan, and bleomycin are known to cause lung injury. ICU patients with hematologic malignancies are also at high risk of pulmonary embolism given immobility, active malignancy, and frequently DIC.

DAH accounts for 20% to 30% of pulmonary complications after allogeneic HCT and is a cause of early death in 1.5% of patients with APL. DAH occurs with hematopoietic engraftment in allogeneic HCT patients and presents with cough, hemoptysis, declining hemoglobin, and hypoxemia with diffuse alveolar filling on lung imaging. Serial lavage during BAL classically shows increasingly bloody fluid return. Treatment for DAH includes replacement of platelets and coagulation factors to maintain hemostasis, supportive mechanical ventilation as needed, and corticosteroids. Small retrospective studies support the use of high-dose corticosteroids (methylprednisolone 30 to 1,500 mg per day) for treatment of DAH after allogeneic HCT. However, a recent retrospective single-center study of 119 patients found that the use of medium to high doses of corticosteroids was associated with higher ICU mortality [49]. Administration of parenteral recombinant activated Factor VII has been associated with resolution of DAH occurring after HCT in case reports and series [50,51].

In addition to DAH, early-onset noninfectious pulmonary complications after allogeneic HCT include pulmonary engraftment syndrome and IPS. Pulmonary engraftment syndrome mimics DAH and is characterized by fever, pulmonary infiltrates, hypoxia, and a skin rash developing early after HCT, coinciding with recovery of circulating neutrophils (ANC >500 per μL). It is typically a self-limited process lasting 1 to 2 weeks that is treated with supportive care and a short course of standard-dose corticosteroids (approximately 1 mg per kg prednisone or equivalent) [52]. IPS, which occurs in about 10% of HCT patients, presents with fever, cough, shortness of breath, hypoxemia, and diffuse bilateral pulmonary infiltrates without an identifiable infection by BAL. IPS occurs after hematopoietic engraftment with a median onset of 21 to 52 days after HCT and carries a 60% to 90% mortality. Pathologically, the syndrome is characterized by an interstitial infiltrate comprised primarily of lymphocytes. In a study of 15 patients with IPS, the combination of etanercept, a tissue necrosis factor-α antagonist, and corticosteroids given at 2 mg per kg daily (methylprednisolone equivalent) resulted in 10 complete responses and a 28-day survival of 73% [53].

Late-onset noninfectious pulmonary complications after HCT typically occur more than 3 months after stem cell infusion and include BOS and COP (formerly referred to as bronchiolitis obliterans with organizing pneumonia). BOS occurs in 14% of allogeneic HCT patients with chronic graft-versus-host disease (cGVHD). BOS is a manifestation of cGVHD whereby alloreactive donor T cells generate fibromuscular proliferation of the walls of small airways. This produces an obstructive physiology with air trapping and occasionally the need for supplemental oxygen. There is no standard treatment for BOS beyond immunosuppression for cGVHD, although aerosolized corticosteroids, oral azithromycin, have been used and montelukast (a leukotriene receptor antagonist). COP tends to occur late after allogeneic HCT and demonstrates restrictive pulmonary physiology. COP is associated with GVHD and may be a manifestation of the disease itself. Some insult triggers inflammation of the small airways causing a proliferative bronchiolitis and deposition of cellular matrix materials into alveoli leading to hypoxemia. Unlike BOS, COP is reversible and corticosteroid responsive.

Common pulmonary processes complicating hematologic malignancies are summarized in Table 94.2.

Infection

Chemotherapy for high-grade hematologic malignancies commonly causes neutropenia and cellular and/or humoral immunosuppression. Unless receiving immunosuppressive chemotherapy agents (e.g., fludarabine, cladribine), AML patients typically retain adequate cellular and humoral immunity even during periods of severe bone marrow suppression. Neutropenic patients are susceptible to infections by endogenous skin, genitourinary and GI tract flora as well as hospital-acquired infections including nosocomial and ventilator-associated pneumonias, central venous line infections, *Clostridium difficile* colitis, and infections with *Pseudomonas* spp., *Stenotrophomonas* spp., *Burkholderia* spp., vancomycin-resistant enterococcus, methicillin-resistant *S. aureus* (MRSA), and extended-spectrum β-lactamase-producing gram-negative organisms. Prolonged neutropenia, especially with concomitant corticosteroid administration or diabetes mellitus, places patients at risk of invasive fungal infections, especially *Aspergillus* spp. Immunosuppressed patients, particularly those with lymphoid malignancies and those undergoing allogeneic HCT, are at additional risk of

TABLE 94.2

Frequently Encountered Pulmonary Complications in Hematologic Malignancies

Complication	Context	Timing	Diagnosis	Management
Infection	Neutropenia	Variable: ≤7 d of neutropenia: bacterial, *Candida* spp. >7 d of neutropenia: bacterial, fungal including *Aspergillus* spp.	Blood cultures, fungal serologies, BAL, lung biopsy (transbronchial, VATS, open) CXR/CT/HRCT	Empiric antimicrobials may include coverage of MRSA, GNRs, *Pseudomonas* spp., typical and atypical bacterial pathogens, *Candida* spp., *Aspergillus* spp.
	HCT	After engraftment: viral including CMV, RSV, Herpesviridae, fungal, bacterial, mycobacterial, *Pneumocystis jirovecii*	Blood cultures, fungal serologies, respiratory virus DFA and PCR, CMV PCR (blood), BAL, lung biopsy (transbronchial, VATS, open) CMV shell culture, viral PCR, fungal, bacterial, and mycobacterial cultures with BAL and lung biopsy CXR/CT/HRCT	Prophylaxis: Herpesviridae: Acyclovir/valacyclovir. PCP: TMP/SMX, dapsone, atovaquone or inhaled pentamidine Treatment: Empiric coverage of MRSA, GNRs, *Pseudomonas* spp., typical and atypical bacterial pathogens, *Candida* spp., *Aspergillus* spp. pending diagnosis Targeted therapy for diagnosed infection
Diffuse alveolar hemorrhage	DIC, APL, HCT	Anytime until DIC resolves First 3–4 wk after transplant, around engraftment	Cough, hemoptysis, hemoglobin drop CXR/CT/HRCT: diffuse ground glass opacities, consolidations BAL: increasingly bloody return on serial lavage	DIC: treat underlying cause Platelet goal >50,000/μL Fibrinogen goal >100–150 mg/dL HCT: high-dose corticosteroids, platelet goal >50,000/μL, correct coagulopathy, consider recombinant activated Factor VII
Drug toxicity	HCT (carmustine, busulfan) Busulfan	3 mo–2 y after exposure	CXR/CT/HRCT: ground glass opacities, interstitial pneumonitis PFTs: decreased DLCO	Corticosteroids, supportive care
Pulmonary engraftment syndrome	HCT	At count recovery (ANC >500/μL)	Associated findings: fever, rash	Self-limited lasting 1–2 wk Corticosteroids
Idiopathic pneumonia syndrome	HCT	3 wk–4 mo after HCT	CXR/CT/HRCT: interstitial pulmonary infiltrate	Corticosteroids Consider etanercept
Cryptogenic organizing pneumonia	HCT	Late (>100 d after HCT)	CXR/CT/HRCT: bilateral patchy alveolar filling, areas of ground glass opacities and consolidation PFTs: restrictive physiology	Corticosteroid responsive Reversible
Bronchiolitis obliterans syndrome	HCT, chronic GVHD	Late (>100 d after HCT)	CT/HRCT: air trapping, bronchiolitis PFTs: obstructive physiology Irreversible, corticosteroids may slow progression	Treat underlying GVHD Azithromycin, inhaled corticosteroids, and montelukast

BAL, bronchoalveolar lavage; VATS, video-assisted thoracoscopic surgery, CXR, chest X-ray; CT, computed tomography; HRCT, high-resolution computed tomography; MRSA, methicillin-resistant *Staphylococcus aureus*; GNR, gram-negative rod; HCT, hematopoietic cell transplant; CMV, cytomegalovirus; RSV, respiratory syncytial virus; DFA, direct fluorescence assay; PCR, polymerase chain reaction; PCP, *Pneumocystis jirovecii* pneumonia; TMP/SMX, trimethoprim/sulfamethoxazole; DIC, disseminated intravascular coagulation; APL, acute promyelocytic leukemia; PFTs, pulmonary function tests; DLCO, diffusing capacity; ANC, absolute neutrophil count; GVHD, graft-versus-host disease.

opportunistic infections such as *P. jirovecii*, herpes simplex virus, varicella zoster virus, and CMV. Treatment of febrile patients with neutropenia or immunosuppression involves rapid evaluation for infectious causes and initiation of empiric broad-spectrum antibiotic therapy with adequate coverage of *P. aeruginosa* and MRSA. For patients with persistent fever and prolonged neutropenia (>7 days), the addition of antifungal therapy targeting *Aspergillus* spp. is indicated. Afebrile neutropenic patients with an absolute neutrophil count less than 500 per μL should receive daily prophylactic treatment with a fluoroquinolone antibiotic. A meta-analysis of 95 trials including 52 trials using fluoroquinolone prophylaxis showed that neutropenic patients receiving fluoroquinolone prophylaxis had significant decreases in all-cause mortality, infection-related mortality, fever and documented infection with a nonsignificant trend toward increasing antimicrobial resistance [54]. The use of granulocyte-stimulating growth factors (e.g., G-CSF) in patients receiving myelotoxic chemotherapy reduces total days of neutropenia and hospital length of stay without promoting tumor cell growth or affecting overall survival.

Differentiation Syndrome

DS, formerly referred to as retinoic acid syndrome, is a potentially fatal process of unclear mechanism (likely, detrimental cytokine storm) that occurs in 2% to 27% of APL patients treated with ATRA or ATO [55]. Symptoms include fever, peripheral edema, weight gain more than 5 kg, pleuropericardial effusions, shortness of breath, interstitial pulmonary infiltrates, acute renal failure, and hypotension after initiating APL treatment with the differentiating agents ATRA or ATO. The diagnosis requires at least two of the above findings. Moderate DS is defined as having two to three of the above findings, whereas severe DS has four or more findings. Elevation of liver transaminases may also occur. Symptoms can develop at any time within the first 4 weeks of treatment with the highest incidence in the first and third weeks of treatment. Risk factors for the development of severe DS include WBC >5,000 per μL and elevated serum creatinine [55].

The diagnosis of DS is difficult at times as frequent complications of APL and its treatment, such as pneumonia, pulmonary hemorrhage, heart failure, acute renal failure, and sepsis, can mimic the syndrome. Early consideration of DS is important, however, so that prompt treatment with dexamethasone can be initiated. In both moderate and severe cases, dexamethasone is given at 10 mg per os (PO) or IV twice a day. Although no controlled studies of dexamethasone treatment have been published, since the inception of this practice the mortality rate from DS has dropped to less than 1% in recent studies. In moderate cases, ATRA and/or ATO can be continued safely with close monitoring for worsening symptoms. In severe cases, ATRA and/or ATO are held until symptoms resolve at which point it is generally safe to resume treatment. Administration of chemotherapy early in ATRA treatment has been shown to reduce the incidence of DS [56]. Patients with high suspicion of APL and a WBC >10,000 per μL should be treated immediately with cytotoxic chemotherapy in addition to ATRA prior to molecular diagnosis as these patients are at especially high risk of severe DS and death during induction therapy. Even with improved recognition and treatment, 26% of patients in the LPA96 and LPA99 trials developing severe DS died during induction therapy, 11% from DS alone [55].

Cytokine Release Syndrome

In recent years, therapies attempting to engage T cells with target cancer cells have shown impressive activity in hematologic malignancies. The bifunctional T-cell engaging antibody blinatumomab joins anti-CD3 and anti-CD19 variable regions of monoclonal antibodies with a peptide linker to create an molecule that is able to engage T cells (through CD3) directly with CD19-expressing target cells such as B-cell lymphoblasts and B-cell lymphoma cells. Autologous T cells taken from patients and engineered to express chimeric antigen receptors composed of an extracellular short chain variable fragment of a monoclonal antibody against CD19 combined the CD3 intracellular signaling domain and a costimulatory domain are highly active against CD19-expressing malignancies such as B-cell ALL and chronic lymphocytic leukemia where response rates are approximately 90% and 45%, respectively [57].

Both of these therapies can cause a potentially fatal cytokine release syndrome (CRS) of variable severity ranging from fevers and flu-like symptoms to cardiovascular collapse requiring vasopressor support and even intubation for respiratory failure. CRS occurs with the release of cytokines such as IL-6, IFN-γ, IL-10, and others seen with robust activation and proliferation of T cells. Neurotoxicity is also frequently seen with both therapies and can manifest as encephalopathy, seizures, and neuropathies. Optimal treatment for CRS is still being defined and although corticosteroids have been used with success, the anti-IL-6 antibody tocilizumab appears particularly effective at reversing CRS [58].

Therapeutic Agents

Treatment of aggressive hematologic malignancies typically requires toxic, myelosuppressive chemotherapy regimens. Patients are prone to life-threatening bacterial and fungal infections as a result of prolonged neutropenia, bleeding from thrombocytopenia, and organ failure from the toxic effects of chemotherapy. Selected toxicities of agents commonly used in the treatment of hematologic malignancies and their management are given in Table 94.3.

Additional complications of malignant hematologic diseases or their treatment, including tumor lysis syndrome and malignant epidural cord compression, are discussed in detail in Chapter 95.

Selected evidenced-based approaches for managing patients with hematologic malignancies are presented in Table 94.4.

TABLE 94.3

Overview of Therapeutic Agents for Hematologic Malignancies

Drug	Indication	Mechanism	Major toxicities	Management
Anthracyclines, anthracenediones	AML, APL, ALL, lymphomas, myeloma	Topoisomerase II inhibition, reactive oxygen species generation	1. Vesicant 2. Cardiac toxicity 3. Myelosuppression 4. t-AML, t-MDS at 1–5 y after treatment	1. CVC preferred 2. Dexrazoxane for prophylaxis 3. G-CSF support
Cytosine arabinoside (cytarabine, AraC)	AML, ALL, high-grade lymphomas	Inhibits DNA polymerase, incorporation into DNA	1. Myelosuppression 2. Acute cytarabine syndrome: fever, rash, conjunctivitis, myalgias and bone pain 6–12 h after infusion. 3. High dose ($\geq$1 g/m^2): mucositis, conjunctivitis, enterocolitis, rash, neurotoxicity, cerebellar toxicity (2%–3%, >40% with CrCl <60 mL/min)	1. G-CSF support 2. Corticosteroids 3. Ophthalmic corticosteroids, systemic corticosteroids
All-*trans*-retinoic acid (ATRA)	APL	Promotes degradation of PML-RARα oncoprotein	1. Differentiation syndrome: fever, peripheral edema, weight gain more than 5 kg, pleuropericardial effusions, shortness of breath, interstitial pulmonary infiltrates, acute renal failure, and hypotension 2. Bone pain, arthralgias, headache, dry skin, rash, nausea, edema, mouth sores, flu-like symptoms, pseudotumor cerebri, Sweet's syndrome	1. Dexamethasone 10 mg PO or IV twice daily, hold ATRA for severe symptoms
Arsenic trioxide (ATO)	APL	Promotes degradation of PML-RAR α oncoprotein	1. Differentiation syndrome identical to ATRA 2. QTc prolongation 3. Hypokalemia, hypomagnesemia 4. Myelosuppression, fatigue, fever, headache, nausea, vomiting, diarrhea, abdominal pain, chest pain, myalgias, bone pain, hyperglycemia, atrial arrhythmias	1. Dexamethasone 10 mg PO or IV twice daily, hold ATO for severe symptoms 2. Frequent EKGs, correct electrolyte abnormalities, hold ATO
Ifosfamide, cyclophosphamide	High-grade lymphomas, myeloma, hematopoietic cell transplant conditioning	DNA alkylation causing inter- and intrastrand DNA cross-linking	1. Hemorrhagic cystitis due to acrolein metabolite 2. Myelosuppression 3. Ifosfamide: CNS toxicity 4. Cyclophosphamide: SIADH, cardiotoxicity (>200 mg/kg) 5. t-MDS and t-AML 3–5 y after treatment	1. MESNA prophylaxis 2. G-CSF support 3. Drug cessation, methylene blue
Vincristine	Lymphomas, ALL		1. Vesicant 2. Sensory motor and autonomic neuropathy, severe constipation, ileus, small bowel obstruction, hyponatremia	1. CVC preferred 2. Aggressive bowel regimen
Methotrexate (MTX)	ALL, lymphomas	Inhibits dihydrofolate reductase	1. Myelosuppression, hepatitis, acute renal failure, mucositis, seizure	1. Urine alkalinization, hydration, leucovorin rescue, carboxypeptidase G-2 (cleaves MTX)

(continued)

TABLE 94.3 (*continued*)

Overview of Therapeutic Agents for Hematologic Malignancies

Drug	Indication	Mechanism	Major toxicities	Management
6-Mercaptopurine	ALL, APL maintenance therapy	Inhibits de novo purine synthesis, DNA and RNA synthesis	1. Myelosuppression, immunosuppression, GI irritation, biliary stasis, transaminitis	1. Dose reduction
Escherichia coli L-asparaginase	ALL	Deamination of plasma asparagine and glutamine	1. Venous thrombosis from decreased antithrombotic factors, cerebral venous sinus thrombosis 2. Hypersensitivity reactions 3. Hepatotoxicity, pancreatitis, hypoinsulinemia/hyperglycemia, hypertriglyceridemia	1. 3–6 mo of anticoagulation 2. *Erwinia* asparaginase
Rituximab	$CD20^+$ B-cell lymphomas, CLL	Binds to CD20 on the surface of malignant and benign B cells	1. Hypersensitivity reactions 2. Tumor lysis syndrome (high risk with circulating lymphoma/leukemia cells >10,000/μL)	1. Acetaminophen, antihistamine, corticosteroids, slow infusion 2. Allopurinol, hydration, rasburicase
Blinatumomab	B-cell ALL	Bifunctional T-cell engaging chimeric antibody binding CD3 and CD19	1. Cytokine release syndrome 2. Neurotoxicity	1. Corticosteroids, tocilizumab
CAR19 T cells	B-cell ALL, B-cell non-Hodgkin lymphomas	T cells genetically modified to express a chimeric antigen receptor against CD19	1. Cytokine release syndrome 2. Neurotoxicity 3. Prolonged B-cell aplasia	1. Corticosteroids, tocilizumab 2. IVIG

AML, acute myeloid leukemia; APL, acute promyelocytic leukemia; ALL, acute lymphoblastic leukemia; t-AML, treatment-related AML; t-MDS, treatment-related myelodysplastic syndrome; CVC, central venous catheter; G-CSF, granulocyte colony-stimulating factor; SIADH, syndrome of inappropriate ADH; CLL, chronic lymphocytic leukemia; IVIG, intravenous immunoglobulin; CAR, chimeric antigen receptor.

TABLE 94.4

Selected Evidence-Based Approaches for Hematologic Malignancies

Clinical relevance	Comparison	Results	Reference
ICU outcomes			
Patients with hematologic malignancies have similar mortality to nononcologic patients when matched for disease severity.	Retrospective study of 101 consecutive ICU admissions of patients with hematologic malignancies vs. 3,808 nononcologic admissions.	Mortality of hematologic malignancy and nononcologic patients similar when matched for SAPS II score (OR = 0.59, 95% CI = 0.32–1.08, $p = 0.09$).	[1]
Hyperleukocytosis			
Improved short-term but not long-term survival with leukapheresis in hyperleukocytic AML.	Retrospective analysis of leukapheresis in 53 vs. no leukapheresis in 28 AML patients with hyperleukocytosis (WBC >100,000/μL).	Reduced 21-d mortality in leukapheresis group vs. no leukapheresis (16% vs. 32%, $p = 0.015$). No difference in overall survival (median 6.5 vs. 7.5 mo).	[28]
Prophylactic platelet transfusion			
Equivalent bleeding rates with platelet transfusion threshold 10,000/μL vs. 20,000/μL.	Meta-analysis of three prospective randomized trials.	No difference in mortality, remission rates, severe bleeding events, or RBC transfusion requirements between two threshold levels. Studies potentially underpowered.	[42]

TABLE 94.4 (continued)

Selected Evidence-Based Approaches for Hematologic Malignancies

Clinical relevance	Comparison	Results	Reference
Noninvasive positive pressure ventilation			
Improved survival with addition of noninvasive positive pressure ventilation to standard care alone in patients with early hypoxemia.	Prospective, randomized trial of 52 immunosuppressed patients with fever, pulmonary infiltrates, and early hypoxemic respiratory failure treated with NIPPV vs. supplemental oxygen-based therapy alone.	NIPPV superior to supplemental oxygen-based therapy alone for incidence of endotracheal intubation (2 vs. 20 patients, $p = 0.03$), serious complications (13 vs. 21, $p = 0.02$), death in the ICU (10 vs. 18, $p = 0.03$), and death in the hospital (13 vs. 21, $p = 0.02$).	[59]
Invasive ventilation			
Improved survival with early intubation of hypoxemic patients.	Retrospective analysis of 166 consecutive admits requiring mechanical ventilation with NIPPV vs. IMV.	Intubation within 24 h of ICU admission associated with improved survival (OR = 0.29, 95% CI = 0.11–0.78). Survival equivalent between NIPPV and IMV when matched for SAPS II score.	[13]
Prophylactic antibiotics during neutropenia			
Use of prophylactic antibiotics in afebrile neutropenic patients improves survival and supports use of fluoroquinolone prophylaxis.	Meta-analysis of 100 trials (10,275 patients).	Compared to placebo, antibiotic prophylaxis associated with reduced risk of death (RR = 0.66, 95% CI = 0.54–0.81), infection-related death (RR = 0.58, 95% CI = 0.45–0.74), and fever (RR = 0.52, 95% CI = 0.37–0.84). Fluoroquinolone prophylaxis with reduced all-cause mortality (RR = 0.52, 95% CI = 0.37–0.84).	[54]
Growth factors for neutropenia			
G-CSF shortens duration of neutropenia without improving overall survival.	Prospective, randomized trial of G-CSF vs. placebo following AML induction chemotherapy.	Neutrophil recovery 15% earlier in G-CSF–treated patients ($p = 0.014$). No difference in complete remission rates or 6-mo survival.	[60]
Differentiation syndrome			
Early institution of chemotherapy after starting ATRA for APL reduces the incidence of differentiation syndrome.	Randomized, prospective analysis of rates of differentiation syndrome in APL patients with WBC <5,000/μL treated with ATRA until complete remission followed by chemotherapy vs. ATRA with chemotherapy starting day 3.	Incidence of differentiation syndrome 18% in ATRA with delayed chemotherapy vs. 9.2% in ATRA with early chemotherapy ($p = 0.035$).	[56]

SAPS II, Simplified Acute Physiology Score II; AUC, area under the curve; CI, confidence interval; NIPPV, noninvasive positive pressure ventilation; IMV, invasive mechanical ventilation; OR, odds ratio; RR, relative risk; G-CSF, granulocyte colony-stimulating factor; ATRA, all-*trans*-retinoic acid; APL, acute promyelocytic leukemia.

References

1. Merz TM, Schär P, Bühlmann M, et al: Resource use and outcome in critically ill patients with hematological malignancy: a retrospective cohort study. *Crit Care* 12:R75, 2008.
2. Hampshire PA, Welch CA, McCrossan LA, et al: Admission factors associated with hospital mortality in patients with haematological malignancy admitted to UK adult, general critical care units: a secondary analysis of the ICNARC Case Mix Programme Database. *Crit Care* 13:R137, 2009.
3. Gordon AC, Oakervee HE, Kaya B, et al: Incidence and outcome of critical illness amongst hospitalised patients with haematological malignancy: a prospective observational study of ward and intensive care unit based care. *Anaesthesia* 60:340–347, 2005.
4. Lloyd-Thomas A, Dhaliwal H, Lister T, et al: Intensive therapy for life-threatening medical complications of haematological malignancy. *Intensive Care Med* 12:317–324, 1986.
5. Lloyd-Thomas AR, Wright I, Lister TA, et al: Prognosis of patients receiving intensive care for life-threatening medical complications of haematological malignancy. *BMJ* 296:1025–1029, 1988.
6. Yau E, Rohatiner AZ, Lister TA, et al: Long term prognosis and quality of life following intensive care for life-threatening complications of haematological malignancy. *Br J Cancer* 64:938–942, 1991.
7. Evison J, Rickenbacher P, Ritz R, et al: Intensive care unit admission in patients with haematological disease: incidence, outcome and prognostic factors. *Swiss Med Wkly* 131:681–686, 2001.
8. Kroschinsky F, Weise M, Illmer T, et al: Outcome and prognostic features of intensive care unit treatment in patients with hematological malignancies. *Intensive Care Med* 28:1294–1300, 2002.
9. Benoit D, Vandewoude K, Decruyenaere J, et al: Outcome and early prognostic indicators in patients with a hematologic malignancy admitted to the ICU for a life-threatening complication. *Crit Care Med* 31:104–112, 2003.
10. Cornet AD, Issa AI, Loosdrecht AA, et al: Sequential organ failure predicts mortality of patients with a haematological malignancy needing intensive care. *Eur J Haematol* 74:511–516, 2005.
11. Lamia B, Hellot M, Girault C, et al: Changes in severity and organ failure scores as prognostic factors in onco-hematological malignancy patients admitted to the ICU. *Intensive Care Med* 32:1560–1568, 2006.
12. Azoulay E, Mokart D, Pene F, et al: Outcomes of critically ill patients with hematologic malignancies: prospective multicenter data from France and

Belgium—A Groupe de Recherche Respiratoire en Réanimation Onco-Hematologique Study. *J Clin Oncol* 31:2810–2818, 2013.
13. Depuydt PO, Benoit DD, Vandewoude KH, et al: Outcome in noninvasively and invasively ventilated hematologic patients with acute respiratory failure. *Chest* 126:1299–1306, 2004.
14. Lim Z, Pagliuca A, Simpson S, et al: Outcomes of patients with haematological malignancies admitted to intensive care unit. A comparative review of allogeneic haematopoietic stem cell transplantation data. *Br J Haematol* 136:448–450, 2007.
15. Bruennler T, Mandraka F, Zierhut S, et al: Outcome of hemato-oncologic patients with and without stem cell transplantation in a medical ICU. *Eur J Med Res* 12(8):323–330, 2007.
16. Pulte D, Gondos A, Brenner H: Expected long-term survival of patients diagnosed with acute myeloblastic leukemia during 2006–2010. *Ann Oncol* 21(2):335–341, 2010.
17. Schlenk RF, Dohner K, Krauter J, et al: Mutations and treatment outcome in cytogenetically normal acute myeloid leukemia. *N Engl J Med* 358:1909–1918, 2008.
18. Dohner H, Estey EH, Amadori S, et al: Diagnosis and management of acute myeloid leukemia in adults: recommendations from an international expert panel, on behalf of the European LeukemiaNet. *Blood* 115(3):453–474, 2010.
19. Sanz MA, Grimwade D, Tallman MS, et al: Management of acute promyelocytic leukemia: recommendations from an expert panel on behalf of the European LeukemiaNet. *Blood* 113(9):1875–1890, 2009.
20. Raelson JV, Nervi C, Rosenauer A, et al: The PML/RAR alpha oncoprotein is a direct molecular target of retinoic acid in acute promyelocytic leukemia cells. *Blood* 88:2826–2832, 1996.
21. Lallemand-Breitenbach V, Jeanne M, Benhenda S, et al: Arsenic degrades PML or PML-RARalpha through a SUMO-triggered RNF4/ubiquitin-mediated pathway. *Nat Cell Biol* 10:547–555, 2008.
22. Lo-Coco F, Avvisati G, Vignetti, M, et al: Retinoic acid and arsenic trioxide for acute promyelocytic leukemia. *N Engl J Med* 369:111–121, 2013
23. Dhedin N, Huynh A, Maury S, et al: Role of allogeneic stem cell transplantation in adult patients with Ph-negative acute lymphoblastic leukemia. *Blood* 125:2486–2496, 2015.
24. Lester TJ, Johnson JW, Cuttner J: Pulmonary leukostasis as the single worst prognostic factor in patients with acute myelocytic leukemia and hyperleukocytosis. *Am J Med* 79(1):43–48, 1985.
25. Novotny JR, Nuckel H, Duhrsen U: Correlation between expression of CD56/NCAM and severe leukostasis in hyperleukocytic acute myelomonocytic leukaemia. *Eur J Haematol* 76:299–308, 2006.
26. Stucki A, Rivier AS, Gikic M, et al: Endothelial cell activation by myeloblasts: molecular mechanisms of leukostasis and leukemic cell dissemination. *Blood* 97:2121–2129, 2001.
27. Bug G, Anargyrou K, Tonn T, et al: Impact of leukapheresis on early death rate in adult acute myeloid leukemia presenting with hyperleukocytosis. *Transfusion* 47(10):1843–1850, 2007.
28. Giles FJ, Shen Y, Kantarjian HM, et al: Leukapheresis reduces early mortality in patients with acute myeloid leukaemia with high white cell counts but does not improve long-term survival. *Leuk Lymphoma* 42:67–73, 2001.
29. Oberoi S, Lehrnbecher T, Phillips B, et al. Leukapheresis and low-dose chemotherapy do not reduce early mortality in acute myeloid leukemia hyperleukocytosis: a systematic review and metaanalysis. *Leuk Res* 38(4):460–468, 2014.
30. Garcia-Sanz R, Montoto S, Torrequebrada A, et al: Waldenstrom macroglobulinaemia: presenting features and outcome in a series with 217 cases. *Br J Haematol* 115(3):575–582, 2001.
31. Falanga A, Consonni R, Marchetti M, et al: Cancer procoagulant in the human promyelocytic cell line NB4 and its modulation by retinoic acid. *Leukemia* 8:156–159, 1994.
32. Koyama T, Hirosawa S, Kawamata N, et al: All-trans retinoic acid upregulates thrombomodulin and downregulates tissue factor expression in acute promyelocytic leukemia cells: distinct expression of thrombomodulin and tissue factor in human leukemic cells. *Blood* 84:3001–3009, 1994.
33. Falanga A, Iacoviello L, Evangelista V, et al: Loss of blast cell procoagulant activity and improvement of hemostatic variables in patients with acute promyelocytic leukemia administered all-trans retinoic acid. *Blood* 86:1072–1081, 1995.
34. De Stefano V, Teofili L, Sica S, et al: Effect of all-trans retinoic acid on procoagulant and fibrinolytic activities of cultured blast cell from patients with acute promyelocytic leukemia. *Blood* 86:3535–3541, 1995.
35. Wang J, Weiss I, Svoboda K, et al: Thrombogenic role of cells undergoing apoptosis. *Br J Haematol* 115:382–391, 2001.
36. Rodeghiero F, Mannucci PM, Vigano S, et al: Liver dysfunction rather than intravascular coagulation as the main cause of low protein C and antithrombin III in acute leukemia. *Blood* 63:965–969, 1984.
37. Tapiovaara H, Alitalo R, Stephens R, et al: Abundant urokinase activity on the surface of mononuclear cells from blood and bone marrow of acute leukemia patients. *Blood* 82:914–919, 1993.
38. Tapiovaara H, Matikainen S, Hurme M, et al: Induction of differentiation of promyelocytic NB4 cells by retinoic acid is associated with rapid increase in urokinase activity subsequently downregulated by production of inhibitors. *Blood* 83:1883–1891, 1994.
39. Menell JS, Cesarman GM, Jacovina AT, et al: Annexin II and bleeding in acute promyelocytic leukemia. *N Engl J Med* 340:994–1004, 1999.
40. Kwaan HC, Wang J, Weiss I: Expression of receptors for plasminogen activators on endothelial cell surface depends on their origin. *J Thromb Haemost* 2:306–312, 2004.
41. Martí-Carvajal AJ, Anand V, Solà I: Treatment for disseminated intravascular coagulation in patients with acute and chronic leukemia. *Cochrane Database Syst Rev* 6:CD008562, 2015. doi:10.1002/14651858.CD008562.pub3.
42. Stanworth SJ, Hyde C, Heddle N, et al: Prophylactic platelet transfusion for haemorrhage after chemotherapy and stem cell transplantation. *Cochrane Database Syst Rev* (4):CD004269, 2004. doi:10.1002/14651858.CD004269.pub2.
43. Slichter SJ, Kaufman RM, Assmann SF, et al: Dose of prophylactic platelet transfusions and prevention of hemorrhage. *N Engl J Med* 362(7):600–613, 2010.
44. Hummel M, Rudert S, Hof H, et al: Diagnostic yield of bronchoscopy with bronchoalveolar lavage in febrile patients with hematologic malignancies and pulmonary infiltrates. *Ann Hematol* 87:291–297, 2008.
45. Azoulay E, Mokart D, Rabbat A, et al: Diagnostic bronchoscopy in hematology and oncology patients with acute respiratory failure: prospective multicenter data. *Crit Care Med* 36:100–107, 2008.
46. Zihlif M, Khanchandani G, Ahmed HP, et al: Surgical lung biopsy in patients with hematological malignancy or hematopoietic stem cell transplantation and unexplained pulmonary infiltrates: improved outcome with specific diagnosis. *Am J Hematol* 78:94–99, 2005.
47. White DA, Wong PW, Downey R: The utility of open lung biopsy in patients with hematologic malignancies. *Am J Respir Crit Care Med* 161:723–729, 2000.
48. Enright H, Haake R, Weisdorf D, et al: Cytomegalovirus pneumonia after bone marrow transplantation. Risk factors and response to therapy. *Transplantation* 55(6):1339–1346, 1993.
49. Rathi NK, Tanner AR, Dinh A, et al: Low-, medium- and high-dose steroids with or without aminocaproic acid in adult hematopoietic SCT patients with diffuse alveolar hemorrhage. *Bone Marrow Transplant* 50:420–426, 2015.
50. Shenoy A, Savani BN, Barrett AJ: Recombinant factor VIIa to treat diffuse alveolar hemorrhage following allogeneic stem cell transplantation. *Biol Blood Marrow Transplant* 13(5):622–623, 2007.
51. Pathak V, Kuhn J, Gabriel D, et al: Use of activated factor VII in patients with diffuse alveolar hemorrhage: a 10 years institutional experience. *Lung* 193(3):375–379, 2015.
52. Lee CK, Gingrich RD, Hohl RJ, et al: Engraftment syndrome in autologous bone marrow and peripheral stem cell treransplantation. *Bone Marrow Transplant* 16(1):175–182, 1995.
53. Yanik GA, Ho VT, Levine JE, et al: The impact of soluble tumor necrosis factor receptor etanercept on the treatment of idiopathic pneumonia syndrome after allogeneic hematopoietic stem cell transplantation. *Blood* 112(8):3073–3081, 2008.
54. Gafter-Gvili A, Fraser A, Paul M, et al: Meta-analysis: antibiotic prophylaxis reduces mortality in neutropenic patients. *Ann Intern Med* 142(12 Pt 1):979–995, 2005.
55. Montesinos P, Bergua JM, Vellenga E, et al: Differentiation syndrome in patients with acute promyelocytic leukemia treated with all-trans retinoic acid and anthracycline chemotherapy: characteristics, outcome, and prognostic factors. *Blood* 113(4):775–783, 2009.
56. de Botton S, Chevret S, Coiteux V, et al: Early onset of chemotherapy can reduce the incidence of ATRA syndrome in newly diagnosed acute promyelocytic leukemia (APL) with low white blood cell counts: results from APL 93 trial. *Leukemia* 17(2):339–342, 2003.
57. Maude SL, Teachey DT, Porter DL, et al: CD19-targeted chimeric antigen receptor T cell therapy for acute lymphoblastic leukemia. *Blood* 125(26):4017–4023, 2015.
58. Teachey DT, Rheingold SR, Maude SL, et al: Cytokine release syndrome after blinatumomab treatment related to abnormal macrophage activation and ameliorated with cytokine-directed therapy. *Blood* 121(26):5154–5157, 2013.
59. Hilbert G, Gruson D, Vargas F, et al: Noninvasive ventilation in immunosuppressed patients with pulmonary infiltrates, fever, and acute respiratory failure. *N Engl J Med* 344:481–487, 2001.
60. Godwin JE, Kopecky KJ, Head DR, et al: A double-blind placebo-controlled trial of granulocyte-colony stimulating factor in elderly patients with previously untreated acute myeloid leukemia: a Southwest oncology group study (9031). *Blood* 91:3607–3613, 1998.

Chapter 95 ■ Oncologic Emergencies

EUNPI CHO • BRUCE MONTGOMERY • COLLEEN TIMLIN • JOHN A. THOMPSON • DAMIAN J. GREEN

The clinical presentation of oncologic emergencies has not changed dramatically over the past 50 years; however, the efficacy and variety of therapeutic interventions have improved considerably. Because a patient's prognosis has a significant impact on the choice of treatments, it is of paramount importance for the intensivist and the care team to determine the following:

a. Is the clinical scenario truly emergent?
b. Is the syndrome related to malignancy, a side effect of treatment, or a benign process?
c. What is the specific tumor type that is responsible for the syndrome?
d. What is the stage of disease?
e. What studies are necessary to establish the diagnosis?
f. What are the wishes of the patient and family?

The prognostic implications and the expected impact of treatment are then weighed and appropriate therapy instituted or modified.

SUPERIOR VENA CAVA SYNDROME

Physiology

The superior vena cava (SVC) syndrome develops as a result of impaired blood return through the SVC to the right atrium caused by extrinsic compression or internal thrombus. Obstruction results in venous hypertension, with the severity of ensuing signs and symptoms dependent on the site of obstruction and the rapidity with which the block occurs. The SVC is formed by the union of the left and right brachiocephalic veins in the middle third of the mediastinum and extends inferiorly for 5 to 8 cm, terminating in the right atrium (Fig. 95.1). The SVC serves as the principal venous drainage for the head, neck, and upper extremities. The major collateral, the azygous vein, joins posteriorly just over the right mainstem bronchus and drains the posterior thorax. The SVC is thin walled and is bounded by the mediastinal parietal pleura and the right paratracheal, azygous, hilar, and subcarinal lymph nodes. As a result, it is extremely susceptible to extrinsic compression by adjacent lymph nodes or the aorta, with subsequent stasis, occlusion, or thrombosis. If obstruction occurs distal to the azygous vein, collateral flow through the azygous can adequately compensate for diminished return. However, if the obstruction is proximal to the azygous, flow must completely bypass the SVC and return via internal mammary, superficial thoracoabdominal, and vertebral venous systems to the inferior vena cava. This more circuitous route results in significantly higher venous pressures, which can result in interstitial edema of the head and neck as well as extrinsic compression of the larynx or trachea.

Etiology

The vast majority of patients with the SVC syndrome have bronchogenic carcinoma, most commonly of the small cell histology (Table 95.1). Non-Hodgkin lymphoma, breast cancer, and other neoplasms make up the remainder of the malignant causes. Despite a high frequency of mediastinal involvement, Hodgkin lymphoma patients rarely present with SVC compression. Benign causes of SVC syndrome exist in up to 40% of all cases and include thrombosis due to indwelling intravenous catheters or fibrosing mediastinitis from infectious causes [1].

Clinical Manifestations

The presentation of SVC syndrome depends largely on the acuity of the obstruction to flow. In patients with benign causes, extensive collateral flow often develops that minimizes symptoms for months to years. Acute compression by tumor or thrombosis does not allow time for collateralization, and venous hypertension inevitably results in symptoms, which include dyspnea, cough, dysphagia, and edema of the face, neck, upper torso, and extremities. Physical signs include jugular venous distention, edema of the face or upper extremities, dilated venous collaterals, plethora, stridor, and tachypnea. Rarely, SVC syndrome can lead to the serious sequela of cerebral edema resulting in headaches, confusion, and possibly coma.

Diagnosis

Initial evaluation should include a chest radiograph and contrast-enhanced computed tomography (CT) to confirm the clinical diagnosis, identify a potential etiology, and localize the obstruction. Venography or magnetic resonance imaging (MRI) may be appropriate in subsequent evaluation to better define the extent of obstruction, particularly if stenting of the obstruction is considered (Fig. 95.2). Of note, focal hepatic contrast enhancement on CT has been noted in patients with SVC syndrome due to collateralization through patent remnants of the umbilical vein or of the musculophrenic venous system [2]. These abnormalities could be mistaken for metastatic disease and should be further evaluated in patients in whom therapy would be changed in the presence of isolated metastases. If a malignant cause of SVC obstruction is considered, all reasonable efforts should be made to obtain diagnostic material, as treatment depends on the underlying histology. The approach may include sputum cytology, bronchoscopy using endobronchial ultrasound-guided needle aspiration, transthoracic needle aspiration, biopsy of palpable lymph nodes, mediastinoscopy, thoracotomy, or video-assisted thoracoscopy. Despite concerns regarding surgical complications, morbidity associated with surgical procedures necessary to procure a diagnosis is not substantially different from that in patients without the SVC syndrome [3]. With rare exceptions, it is safe to wait to institute treatment until the underlying cause of the syndrome has been established. Clinicians at Yale University have proposed a grading scheme for severity of SVC syndrome spanning from asymptomatic to life threatening based on the presence of significant cerebral edema, laryngeal edema, or hemodynamic compromise. They estimated that life-threatening symptoms requiring immediate intervention prior to diagnostic evaluation occur in only 5% of cases of SVC syndrome [4].

Treatment

Once the diagnosis is established, initiation of therapy depends on the etiology, the severity of symptoms, the acuity of presentation, and the goals of treatment. If patients are minimally

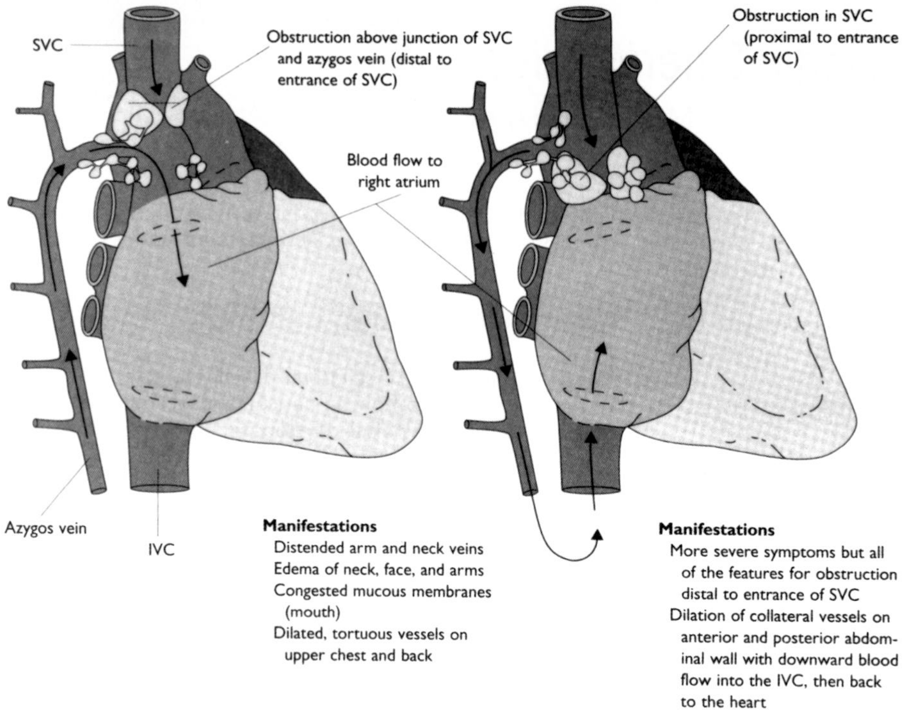

FIGURE 95.1 Anatomic locations of superior vena cava (SVC) obstruction leading to the SVC syndrome. IVC, inferior vena cava. (Reprinted from Skarin AT (ed): *Atlas of Diagnostic Oncology*. 2nd ed. St. Louis, Mosby, 1996, with permission.)

symptomatic, the azygous is patent, and treatment is focused on palliation, observation is a reasonable option. Chemotherapy is the treatment of choice for SVC syndrome due to small cell lung carcinoma, non-Hodgkin lymphoma, and germ cell tumors. Although radiation is often considered in addition to chemotherapy even in the palliative setting, 80% of these patients have a complete or partial response of their symptoms to chemotherapy alone [5]. Other histologies should be treated with endovascular stent placement, radiation therapy, or both. Radiation therapy prior to biopsy has been associated with a significant reduction in rates of histologic diagnosis and should be avoided [6]. Although external beam radiation effectively palliates symptoms in more than 70% of patients within 2 weeks [7], relapse after radiotherapy occurs in 15% to 30% of cases.

TABLE 95.1

Primary Diagnosis in 125 Cases of SVC Syndrome

Histology	% of Cases	Total (%)
Lung carcinoma		79
Small cell	34	
Squamous cell	21	
Adenocarcinoma	14	
Large cell/other	11	
Lymphoma		14
Non-Hodgkin's lymphoma		
Hodgkin's lymphoma		
Other malignancy		6
Adenocarcinoma		
Kaposi's sarcoma		
Seminoma		
Acute myelomonocytic leukemia		
Leiomyosarcoma		

From Armstrong BA, Perez CA, Simpson JR, et al: Role of irradiation in the management of superior vena cava syndrome. *Int J Radiat Oncol Biol Phys* 13:531–539, 1987.

Endovascular stent placement, as a primary intervention, is a particularly attractive option for patients who lack a tissue diagnosis and whose symptoms on presentation require a rapid palliative intervention; this includes all patients, regardless of histology, who present with airway compromise or cerebral edema. SVC stent placement can provide rapid relief of symptoms (within 48 hours of placement) in up to 95% of patients with a primary patency rate of 80% at 6 months [8]. Some authors have suggested a role for stent placement for first-line management of all SVC syndrome patients as outcomes are encouraging with low rates of complications, but no randomized controlled trials have been published [9]. Anticoagulation after stent placement is controversial with recent publications advocating the use of antiplatelet agents such as aspirin for 3 to 6 months following insertion [8,9].

In patients with an established diagnosis, radiation therapy remains an appropriate intervention. Many fractionation protocols have been used, with the majority of patients receiving 30 Gy in 10 fractions, whereas patients treated with curative intent often receive 50 Gy in 25 fractions. Although high doses of radiation have often been given early in the treatment course to achieve rapid tumor response, there is little evidence to suggest that this

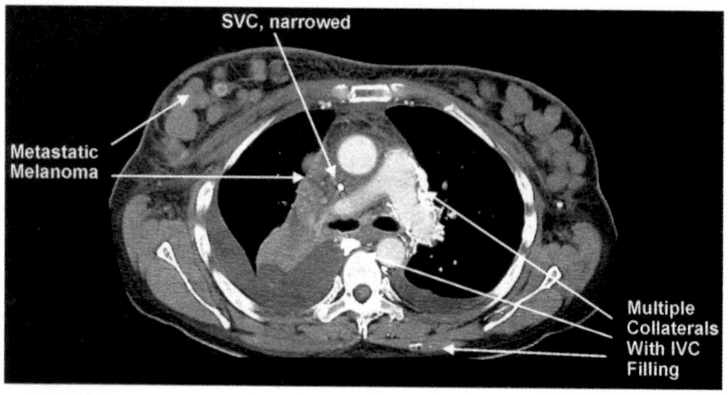

FIGURE 95.2 Upper extremity contrast injection demonstrating severe narrowing of the superior vena cava (SVC) with the development of multiple collaterals and inferior vena cava (IVC) filling.

is necessary [10]. In cases of SVC thrombosis with an indwelling catheter or pacemaker, thrombolytic agents may be useful as primary therapy or as an adjunct to stent placement [11]. The additional benefit of thrombolytics or anticoagulation in patients treated for malignant SVC syndrome is not well established.

Surgical resection and reconstruction of the SVC is reserved for patients with benign disease or the rare patient with tracheal obstruction in the setting of chemotherapy or radiotherapy-resistant disease.

SVC syndrome has been thought to predict poor outcomes. However, the presence of SVC syndrome is not a negative prognostic factor in small cell carcinoma and lymphoma independent of the stage and bulk of disease, and patients should be treated with curative intent if otherwise appropriate [12].

CARDIAC TAMPONADE

Physiology

Cardiac tamponade results from accumulation of fluid within the pericardium that impairs left ventricular expansion and diastolic filling. As stroke volume drops, compensatory tachycardia occurs to offset progressive hypotension. Ultimately, pressures equalize in the left atrium, pulmonary vasculature, right atrium, and SVC, and circulatory collapse ensues. As with SVC syndrome, the severity of symptoms is dependent on the speed of progression. Tamponade occurs when the pericardium cannot expand with resultant impedance to venous inflow.

Etiology

Malignancy is identified as the cause in up to 40% of unselected patients presenting with cardiac tamponade; the frequency with which tamponade develops as the initial manifestation of the patient's disease has led to standard cytologic examination of all significant effusions [13,14]. Tumors may involve the pericardium by direct extension from intrathoracic organs or hematogenous spread. Malignancies most often associated with pericardial effusions are lung, breast, lymphoma, and leukemia. Pericardial effusions in patients with cancer are due to pericardial or cardiac involvement in 60% of cases, with idiopathic pericarditis and radiation-induced pericarditis causing 32% and 10% of cases, respectively [15].

Clinical Manifestations

Common symptoms of pericardial effusion include dyspnea (85%), cough (30%), orthopnea (25%), and chest pain (20%). The common signs of pericardial effusion are jugular venous distention (100%), tachycardia (100%), pulsus paradoxus (89%), systolic blood pressure of less than 90 (52%), and pericardial friction rub (22%) [16]. Plain films may demonstrate cardiac enlargement in at least half of all cases, and electrocardiography may reveal abnormalities suggestive of pericarditis (low-voltage, ST-segment elevation) or electrical alternans.

Diagnosis

Echocardiography is the most useful means of rapidly detecting a hemodynamically significant effusion. The echocardiographic findings of pericardial tamponade are reviewed in Chapter 17 (Pericardiocentesis). Echocardiography also allows estimation of the volume, fluidity, and contents of the effusion, although it is difficult to distinguish tumor, thrombus, or fibrinous material from one another. Emergent treatment of tamponade invariably involves drainage of the effusion, and cytologic evaluation of the fluid provides a very specific means of establishing a malignant etiology. The detection rate for malignancy by pericardial fluid cytology ranges from 66% to 90%, and certain histologies, such as lymphoma and mesothelioma, are more difficult to demonstrate in pericardial fluid [17,18]. Hemorrhagic effusions are more likely to be related to malignancy [17]. Pericardial biopsy is occasionally required to establish a diagnosis in difficult cases and can be performed under local anesthesia using a subxiphoid approach.

Treatment

Cardiac tamponade requires immediate treatment to relieve the increased end-diastolic pressure and inadequate ventricular filling. Oxygen, pressor agents, and intravenous fluids to improve cardiac output should be provided as appropriate. Inotropic agents are frequently ineffective, however, because a state of intense adrenergic stimulation is already present [19]. When airway management is required, significant caution should be exercised because the positive intrathoracic pressure that results from initiation of mechanical ventilation places tamponade patients at particularly high risk of profound post-intubation hypotension [19]. Emergent pericardiocentesis is indicated for significant hypotension, and it has been suggested that a pulse pressure of less than 20 mm Hg, a paradoxic pulse greater than 50% of the pulse pressure, or a peripheral venous pressure above 13 mm are other absolute indications for emergent intervention [20]. Because of the high rate of recurrent effusions after a simple pericardiocentesis in patients with tamponade from malignancy, additional therapy is generally indicated. One option is to perform a pericardiostomy (pericardial window) via a surgical approach or a balloon catheter to drain the pericardial fluid. In one retrospective study that compared outcomes of 118 patients undergoing simple pericardiocentesis alone to 18 patients undergoing pericardiocentesis followed by pericardial surgery, the patients in the former group had a recurrence rate of 36% whereas none of the patients in the latter group had recurrence [21]. A recent retrospective multicenter study also suggested that patients had superior outcomes when systemic chemotherapy was combined with a pericardiostomy rather than simple pericardiocentesis or pericardial drainage [22].

Radiation therapy is noninvasive and allows treatment of the majority of the pericardium but carries a theoretical risk of radiation-induced pericarditis. As a single modality, radiation controls pericardial effusion in 67% of cases, with a particularly high success in hematopoietic tumors (93%) [23]. Systemic therapy is generally used only for diseases that are considered to be chemosensitive, such as breast cancer or lymphoma; in these individuals, it prevented recurrence in 73% of treated patients[23].

Instillation of sclerosing agents, radionuclides, and chemotherapy through indwelling catheters has been widely used with the intent to induce nonspecific inflammation with obliteration of the pericardial space or to achieve specific antineoplastic effects. Typically, a catheter is placed into the pericardial sac and drainage continued until output is less than 100 mL per day. Sclerosing agent or chemotherapy is injected into the catheter every 24 to 48 hours until fluid output is less than 25 to 50 mL per day, and the catheter is removed. A review of 20 different studies reported an overall control rate of 82% with common toxicities, including fever, pain, arrhythmias, and occasional cytopenias [23]. A wide variety of agents have been used including tetracycline, doxycycline, minocycline, bleomycin, and talc. However, use of sclerosing agents has not shown a definitive benefit over drainage alone and this technique is used infrequently [24].

Prognosis

The development of malignant pericardial effusion and tamponade usually reflects uncontrolled metastatic disease and portends a dire prognosis. Median survivals for patients treated for tamponade range from 2 to 4 months [25]. Nonrandomized studies suggest that patients with hematologic malignancies and breast cancer have substantially better survival rates if systemic therapy can be instituted [26,27]. The decision to intervene in a patient with malignant cardiac tamponade depends on the patient's histology and sensitivity to treatment as well as the patient's condition. Patients for whom treatment of tamponade provides meaningful palliative benefit should be considered for the treatment that is likely to provide durable relief of symptoms with the minimum of morbidity and requirement for hospitalization.

MALIGNANT EPIDURAL CORD COMPRESSION

Few complications of malignancy are more dreaded than epidural cord compression. The associated pain, neurologic deficits, and dramatically impaired quality of life are serious problems for the patients who develop this condition and by extension, for their families. Early recognition of the signs and symptoms of cord compression may prevent serious compromise in survival and functional capacity. Epidural cord compression is defined by compression of the dural sac and its contents by an extradural tumor mass. Minimum radiologic evidence for compression is indentation of the theca at the level of clinical features, which include pain, weakness, sensory disturbance, or evidence of sphincter dysfunction [28]. Approximately 20% of cases are the initial manifestation of malignancy [29].

Physiology

Epidural cord compression by malignancy occurs as a result of metastasis or primary tumor involvement of the vertebral column, paravertebral space, or epidural space. Damage to the cord occurs when the tumor compromises the vertebral venous plexus or compresses neural tissue directly or when compromised bone impinges on the cord. The resulting vasogenic edema and hemorrhage induce further ischemic damage. The vertebral body is the most common source of compressive lesions, predominantly in the thoracic (60%), followed by the lumbar (25%) and cervical (15%) regions [30]. Tumor invasion through the intervertebral foramen and cord compression without bone involvement is most often seen with lymphoma, leading to normal plain films and radionuclide scans despite clinical compression. Multiple noncontiguous levels are involved in 10% to 40% of cases [31].

Etiology

The most common causes of malignant cord compression are tumors with a propensity for bony metastases, including breast and lung, followed by hematopoietic, gastrointestinal, and genitourinary malignancies [32] (Table 95.2). Nonmalignant causes of cord compression include stenosis, epidural abscess, or hematoma.

TABLE 95.2

Primary Diagnosis Causing Epidural Cord Compression ($N = 896$)

Histology	% of Cases
Lung	25
Breast	7
Unknown primary	7
Lymphoma	9
Myeloma	11
Sarcoma	2
Prostate	16
Gastrointestinal tract	4
Renal	4
Other	15

Data from Mak KS, Lee LK, Mak RH, et al: Incidence and treatment patterns in hospitalizations for malignant spinal cord compression in the United Sates 1998–2006. *Int J of Radiat Oncol Biol Phys* 80:824–831, 2011.

Clinical Manifestations

The cardinal sign of malignant cord compression is pain, present in 95% of patients at diagnosis. The median time from pain onset to a diagnosis of cord compression is approximately 2 months. Pain is typically worse with recumbency, coughing, straining, or exercise. Radicular pain develops later and is an important localizing sign. Weakness, autonomic dysfunction, and sensory changes are present in more than 50% of cases [30]. Isolated bowel or bladder dysfunction is rarely the presenting symptom of cord compression; however, 50% to 60% of patients can have bowel or bladder symptoms at the time of diagnosis ranging from urgency to incontinence or retention, which can indicate more severe cord involvement [30].

Diagnosis

The diagnosis of cord compression relies primarily on MRI, given its sensitivity, speed, and the ability to detect compression at multiple levels. MRI allows evaluation of the entire spine including vertebral bones and soft tissues in the paravertebral space. It has a sensitivity and specificity of 93% and 97% respectively in detection of cord compression [33]. Other imaging techniques including plain films and radionuclide bone scans can be used but cannot match the accuracy of MRI. A prospective study analyzed the expected outcome with treatment planning on the basis of plain films and clinical examination versus use of MRI, and found that MRI changed the radiotherapy plan in 53% of patients [34]. These changes included 21% of patients in whom all paraspinal disease would not have been treated and 5% of those in whom additional levels of true cord compression would not have been treated. In 30% of patients, the demonstrated level of compression on MRI was more than two vertebral levels away from the level indicated by neurologic examination. If patients are unable to undergo MRI because of claustrophobia, the presence of metal implants, or access, myelography can be performed instead. CT scanning is superior to MRI for definition of vertebral body anatomy and may be useful before consideration of surgical intervention.

Treatment

Therapeutic options include corticosteroids, surgery, and radiation. In emergent situations, corticosteroids are generally given while awaiting MRI to decrease peritumoral edema and to prevent edema formation during radiation. On the basis of laboratory studies and a single randomized controlled trial that compared high-dose dexamethasone with radiation to radiation alone, some authors support the use of high-dose dexamethasone, defined as a 96-mg intravenous bolus followed by 96 mg per day tapered over a 2-week period [35]. A reasonable alternative is a moderate dose approach with a 10-mg intravenous loading dose followed by 4 mg every 6 hours tapered over 2 weeks [36], especially in patients who are clinically stable. Ambulatory patients without progressive deficit may forgo steroids altogether during radiotherapy without undue risk [37].

Historically, radiation therapy and direct decompressive surgery were felt to be equally effective as initial interventions in patients with metastatic spinal cord compression. However, a randomized trial published in 2005 compared direct decompressive surgery plus postoperative radiotherapy to radiotherapy alone, demonstrating a statistically significant outcome benefit to the combined approach for patients who had less radiosensitive tumors and only one area of spinal cord compression [38]. Compared with patients who received radiotherapy alone, more patients who underwent surgery were able to walk after treatment (84% vs. 57%) and were ambulatory for a significantly longer duration (median: 122 vs. 13 days). First-line radiation therapy remains an important option for patients with radiosensitive tumors, nonsurgical candidates, patients with multiple areas of spinal cord compression, and those who experienced symptoms of total paraplegia for longer than 48 hours at presentation. Because surgical complication rates approach 20%, radiation therapy should generally be used as the first-line intervention in patients over age 65 [39]. Specific radiation treatment plans for cord compression vary between centers. In patients with metastatic spinal canal compression, a single fraction of 8 Gy can effectively improve neurologic function and treat pain [40].

Prognosis

Early intervention is vital to preserving function. For patients who are ambulatory at the time of treatment, at least 80% remain ambulatory. The development of paraparesis decreases the ambulation rate to 50%, and patients who are paraplegic at the time of therapy recover ambulation only 10% to 19% of the time after radiation therapy alone [38,41]. In paraplegic patients, outcomes appeared to be better for individuals who were candidates for upfront surgical decompression (62% of patients randomized to combined surgery plus radiation regained the ability to walk compared with 19% of those who received radiation alone), the difference was statistically significant, but the sample size was small (n = 32) [38].

TABLE 95.3

Algorithm for Clinical Management of Hypercalcemia of Malignancy

Calcium Level (mg/dL)	Symptoms	Therapy
<12	None	Observation, or hydration followed by observation
<12	Present	Hydration, bisphosphonate
12–14	Present	Hydration, bisphosphonate
>14	Present	Hydration, bisphosphonate
>14	Severe	Hydration, loop diuretics, calcitonin, bisphosphonate Alternatives: prednisone, denosumab, dialysis

HYPERCALCEMIA

Hypercalcemia of malignancy (HCM) is the most common emergent metabolic disorder associated with cancer, affecting 20% to 30% of patients with malignancy at some time during their clinical course [42]. Although hypercalcemia has been associated with nearly all malignancies, it is most frequently associated with multiple myeloma, breast, lung, and kidney cancers.

Physiology

In healthy persons, vitamin D and parathyroid hormone (PTH) control absorption and mobilization of calcium. Calcitriol, the active form of vitamin D, enhances gastrointestinal absorption and mobilizes calcium from bone. PTH increases renal calcium resorption in the distal tubule and also mobilizes calcium from bone. In patients with HCM, increased calcium mobilization combines with renal insufficiency to cause symptomatic hypercalcemia. At least two mechanisms are proposed: direct osteolysis by tumor or increased osteoclastic resorption as a result of humoral mediators such as PTH-related protein (PTHrP), calcitriol, and PTH. Both mechanisms may be active in many patients.

PTHrP is postulated to play a role in the majority of patients with HCM, as levels are elevated in at least 80% of cases [43]. PTHrP is a normal gene product expressed in a variety of tissues and it appears to have important roles in calcium transport and developmental biology. The N-terminal 13 amino acids of PTHrP share amino acid sequence and homology with intact PTH and it can bind to PTH-1 receptor leading to hypercalcemia when pathologically secreted in excess by cancer cells. PTHrP stimulates osteoblasts to produce receptor activator of nuclear factor-κB ligand (RANKL) which in turn activates osteoclast precursors and leads to both osteolysis and the release of bone-derived growth factors. These growth factors, including transforming growth factor-β and insulin like growth factor-1, are known to both promote tumor cell proliferation and further increase production of PTHrP [44]. Circulating vitamin D metabolites may be increased in some lymphomas, enhancing intestinal calcium absorption and causing or exacerbating hypercalcemia [45].

Normal kidneys are capable of filtering and excreting four to five times the normal calcium concentration in the serum to maintain serum calcium homeostasis. PTHrP increases renal tubular resorption and osteolytic calcium release, causing rapid and persistent elevation of extracellular calcium. The subsequent calciuria and osmotic diuresis result in volume depletion. Decreased glomerular filtration limits the kidney's ability to filter and excrete calcium, and proximal tubular calcium and sodium reabsorption increase, leading to further increases in serum calcium concentrations. Symptoms of nausea and vomiting worsen the dehydration. If the concentration of calcium in the glomerular filtrate exceeds its solubility, calcium may precipitate in the renal tubules, further compromising renal function.

The direct osteolytic effect of tumors leads to hypercalcemia in about 20% of cases; and this phenomenon is seen most frequently in breast cancer, multiple myeloma, and lymphomas. In rare cases, tumors can secrete calcitriol or PTH leading to hypercalcemia.

Etiology

HCM occurs most frequently in patients with breast cancer, multiple myeloma, and squamous cell malignancies of the lung, head and neck, and esophagus. Some malignancies are rarely associated with hypercalcemia despite a propensity for widespread metastases, including prostate cancer and small cell lung cancer. A recent case series of 138 cases of PTHrP-mediated hypercalcemia identified squamous cell lung cancer as the single most common etiology (10.9%) followed by urothelial carcinoma (8.7%), other non-small cell lung cancers (8.7%), adenocarcinomas of unknown primary (8.0%) and breast cancer (7.2%) [46].

Clinical Manifestations

As with other oncologic emergencies, the rapidity with which hypercalcemia develops often determines the severity of symptoms. Some patients may have significant symptoms with minimally elevated calcium and require therapy, whereas other patients are minimally symptomatic despite long-standing hypercalcemia. Many of the symptoms of hypercalcemia are relatively nonspecific, and the possibility of hypercalcemia must be kept in mind when considering patients with nausea, fatigue, lethargy, and mental status changes. Decreased intravascular volume and hypercalcemia cause malaise, fatigue, anorexia, and polyuria. Hypercalcemia decreases neuromuscular excitability and decreased muscle tone. Neuromuscular symptoms include weakness and diminished deep tendon reflexes. Neuropsychiatric manifestations may include confusion, lethargy, psychosis, or even coma. Hypercalcemia heightens cardiac contractility and irritability, and this is reflected by electrocardiographic changes, such as prolonged PR interval, widened QRS complex, and a shortened QT. With progressive hypercalcemia, bradyarrhythmias and bundle-branch block may develop, which can evolve to complete heart block and asystole.

Diagnosis

The diagnosis of hypercalcemia is documented by the presence of elevated corrected serum calcium, defined by the following formula:

$$[4.0 - \text{patient (Alb)}] \times 0.8 + [\text{Ca}],$$

where Alb signifies albumin. Alternatively, an elevation of serum ionized calcium documents hypercalcemia and does not require the concomitant measurement of serum albumin. Other laboratory studies that should be considered include PTH, PTHrP, blood urea nitrogen and creatinine, phosphate, and magnesium. The assessment of a patient presenting with hypercalcemia should include several important aspects of disease history. Although hypercalcemia is a common complication of malignancy, other nonmalignant causes (including hyperparathyroidism, intravenous fluids, total parenteral nutrition, milk-alkali syndrome, thiazide diuretics, vitamins A and D, and lithium) are present in 10% to 15% of cancer patients who present with hypercalcemia and should be considered in the differential diagnosis.

Treatment

The decision to treat hypercalcemia should be dictated by the patient's history, current disease status, quality of life, and the wishes of the patient and family. The prognosis for most patients with HCM is poor with the median overall survival reported at 52 days from one case series [46]. Severe pain, obstruction, or irreversible structural symptoms may be an indication not to pursue therapy. However, relief of the symptoms of hypercalcemia may improve quality of life and functional status for many patients during the remainder of their lifetimes. Patients who are symptomatic and who have no other potential etiology of hypercalcemia should be treated. If calcium is elevated but the patient is asymptomatic, specific hypocalcemic therapy can be held, with close observation, particularly if effective systemic therapy is to be initiated. Because most symptoms and the underlying physiology of hypercalcemia are due in part to volume depletion, intravenous hydration is the initial therapy of choice (Table 95.3). Although no randomized controlled clinical trials have been conducted to inform the approach to hydration, in general patients require repletion with 3 to 7 L intravenous saline over 24 to 36 hours to achieve euvolemia. If congestive heart failure is a concern or if the patient has severe hypercalcemia, loop diuretics can be used, but only after it is clear that adequate volume expansion has been achieved. If diuretics are used before the glomerular filtration rate has been restored, renal clearance of calcium is impaired further, and hypercalcemia may worsen despite the best intentions. Loop diuretics suppress proximal absorption of sodium and calcium, augmenting calciuresis.

Bisphosphonates are the most useful hypocalcemic agents available for controlling HCM. They inhibit prenylation of small guanosine triphosphatases, which are necessary for osteoclast function and are cytotoxic to osteoclasts through a number of different mechanisms [47]. Zoledronic acid and pamidronate are the bisphosphonates currently in clinical use. Two randomized trials comparing pamidronate and zoledronic acid demonstrated improved response rates for zoledronic acid, 4- and 8-mg infusions; complete response rates by day 10 were 88.4%, 86.7%, and 69.7% for zoledronic acid, 4 and 8 mg, and pamidronate, 90 mg, respectively [48]. Normalization of calcium occurred by day 4 in 50% of patients treated with zoledronic acid and 33% of those given pamidronate. Median duration of complete response favored zoledronic acid, 4 and 8 mg, over pamidronate, with response durations of 32, 43, and 18 days, respectively. Optimal zoledronic acid dosage and administration schedules have not been established; the standard dose is 4 mg, with 8 mg reserved for patients with recurrent or refractory hypercalcemia. The onset of zoledronic acid's effect is apparent within 3 to 4 days, with maximal effect within 7 to 10 days, and lasts for 14 days to 2 months. Adverse effects include transient low-grade temperature elevations that typically occur within 24 to 36 hours after administration and persist for up to 2 days (≤20% of patients). New-onset hypophosphatemia and hypomagnesemia may occur; preexisting abnormalities in the same electrolytes may be exacerbated by treatment. Serum calcium may fall below the normal range, although symptoms are rare. Acute kidney injury has been reported with zoledronic acid, and renal function should be monitored routinely during administration [49]. A relatively uncommon but potentially serious side effect of bisphosphate treatment is osteonecrosis of the jaw, a form of avascular necrosis. The overall risk of this complication is <2%, and the risk is

TABLE 95.4

Algorithm for Treatment of Symptomatic Hyponatremia

Acute	Mildly symptomatic	Na <125 mg/dL	Free water restriction 500–1,000 mL/d demeclocycline
Acute	Severe symptoms	Na <115 mg/dL	3% saline Furosemide diuresis Vasopressin analogs (conivaptan; tolvaptan)

significantly increased in individuals with underlying dental conditions or those undergoing dental procedures during treatment.

Other treatments for HCM include corticosteroids, calcitonin, and denosumab. Calcitonin rapidly inhibits bone resorption and decreases renal calcium reabsorption. Salmon calcitonin is administered at 4 IU per kg subcutaneously or intramuscularly every 12 hours, and tachyphylaxis occurs rapidly, necessitating dosing increases to 8 IU every 6 to 12 hours. Efficacy is limited to the first 24 to 48 hours after initiation of therapy, and additional treatment with bisphosphonate should be considered concurrent with calcitonin. Corticosteroids are effective in lymphoma and multiple myeloma, tumors in which steroids are often cytotoxic. The onset of action is slow, over several weeks, and the mechanism of effect is through treatment of the underlying malignancy and suppression of gastrointestinal calcium absorption. Therapies designed to interfere with RANKL binding, including the monoclonal antibody denosumab and a decoy RANKL receptor, osteoprotegerin, appear to decrease serum calcium levels in preclinical and clinical settings; however, no randomized clinical trials have been performed to evaluate these agents in patients with hypercalcemia. Denosumab may have a role in the treatment of HCM that is refractory to bisphosphonates or in patients with renal dysfunction as unlike bisphosphonates, it is not cleared by the kidneys [50,51]. Dialysis should be considered for patients with severe renal insufficiency and associated electrolyte abnormalities, particularly in patients for whom effective therapy is available.

Hypercalcemia reflects biologically aggressive, advanced disease. For patients with solid tumors, particularly those with chemotherapy-resistant disease, the prognosis is extremely grim, with median survivals of 30 to 60 days in most studies [52]. By contrast, hypercalcemia in patients with multiple myeloma and breast cancer is associated with relatively longer survival. The argument has been made that treatment of HCM prolongs survival in patients in whom other morbid complications of their disease will develop. In fact, it is clear that hypocalcemic agents do not prolong survival but can have impressive palliative benefit in relieving symptoms from hypercalcemia, such as nausea, emesis, and constipation, and improving pain control for some patients who achieve normocalcemia.

LEUKOSTASIS

Physiology

Leukostasis is a potentially devastating complication of leukemia in patients who present with hyperleukocytosis, defined as a leukocyte count greater than 100,000 per μL. The syndrome of leukostasis is related to obstruction of flow in capillary beds of the central nervous system, lungs, and heart by immature, rigid blasts. Although viscosity might be expected to play a role, it is rarely elevated because the principal determinant of viscosity, red blood cells, is often low due to marrow replacement by leukemic blasts. The obstruction of capillary beds by blasts and restricted flow results in tissue hypoxia, cytokine release, and coagulation. Tissue invasion also occurs and is not affected by leukapheresis. The risk of leukostasis was evaluated by Lichtman and Rowe [53], who demonstrated that the leukocrit, which is proportional to the number and volume of circulating leukocytes and blasts, was the parameter most closely associated with the development of leukostasis.

Etiology

Hyperleukocytosis occurs in 10% to 20% of patients with acute myelogenous leukemia (AML) at presentation and is much less common in patients with chronic myelogenous leukemia, acute lymphoblastic leukemia, or chronic lymphocytic leukemia. For equivalent degrees of leukocytosis, the risk of leukostasis is much higher with AML than with other diagnoses because of the larger size and adhesion characteristics of AML blasts. The risk of developing leukostasis depends on total white blood cell count, the percentage of blasts, and the rate at which counts are rising. The clinical presentation, diagnosis, and management of hyperleukocytosis are discussed in further detail in Chapter 94 and apheresis treatment in Chapter 96.

HYPONATREMIA

Physiology

Clinically symptomatic hyponatremia is a relatively rare complication of malignancy affecting only 1% to 2% of cancer patients. In the majority of these individuals, the syndrome of inappropriate antidiuretic hormone (SIADH) develops. Secretion of ectopic ADH occurs almost solely in patients with small cell bronchogenic carcinoma, and the majority of other patients have coincident central nervous system or pulmonary disease. As a result of excess ADH, excessive water resorption occurs in the collecting ducts, and extracellular fluid osmolality decreases inappropriately. Water is able to move freely, and the decrease in extracellular osmolality results in a shift to the intracellular compartment with associated cellular edema. When hyponatremia occurs acutely, this edema causes dramatic neuronal edema and subsequent neurologic symptoms. Plasma volume expands, and urinary sodium excretion parallels the rate of oral sodium intake. Typically, the patient with SIADH is euvolemic to slightly hypervolemic, urine sodium is greater than 20 mEq per L, and plasma urea, uric acid, creatinine, and rennin activity are normal or low.

Etiology

Hyponatremia occurs most frequently in small cell lung cancer with approximately 25% of patients noted to have a serum sodium of <136 mEq per L [54]. SIADH has also been reported in a broad variety of other malignancies but is most commonly found in the setting of central nervous system or pulmonary metastases. SIADH may also develop in patients with malignancy because of other conditions, including the use of opiates, vinca alkaloids, β agonists, chlorpropamide, and cyclophosphamide. Hypoadrenalism caused by rapid tapering of therapeutic corticosteroids is another common etiology for mild hyponatremia. Other etiologies include volume contraction resulting from emesis or diarrhea, renal wasting resulting from diuretics or intrinsic renal disease, and pseudohyponatremia resulting from excess serum lipids or paraproteins. Hypothyroidism and pulmonary or central nervous system disease are also potential causes of SIADH.

Diagnosis

Hyponatremia is often manifested as fatigue, nausea, myalgia, headaches, and subtle neurologic symptoms. Rapid drops in serum sodium or levels less than 115 mg per dL cause altered mental status, seizures, coma, pathologic reflexes, and papilledema. The diagnostic evaluation includes a review of medications and assessment of volume status as well as serum and urine electrolytes, osmolality, and creatinine. Patients with SIADH have inappropriately elevated urine sodium, and urine osmolality is greater than plasma osmolality but never reaches maximal dilution (<100 μOsm per L). Thyroid and adrenal dysfunction cause similar electrolyte imbalances and must be ruled out if laboratory studies suggest SIADH. CT or radiographs of the chest and brain may be necessary to eliminate pulmonary or central nervous system disease as causes of excessive ADH secretion.

Treatment

Treatment of the hyponatremia is tailored to the time course of its development and the extent of symptoms that the patient is experiencing. Asymptomatic hyponatremia can be managed with fluid restriction alone. Treatment of the underlying malignancy may alleviate SIADH due to small cell carcinoma. Local therapy to brain or pulmonary metastases may improve serum sodium, and discontinuing offending medications should be effective. Acute symptomatic hyponatremia can be treated as indicated in Table 95.4.

Free water restriction is expected to improve hyponatremia within 7 to 10 days. Demeclocycline induces a dose-dependent, reversible nephrogenic diabetes insipidus and is expected to correct sodium within 3 to 4 days. The primary side effect of demeclocycline is renal toxicity, and the risk of toxicity is increased by renal or hepatic dysfunction. The initial dose of demeclocycline is 600 mg daily to a maximum of 1,200 mg per day in two- to three-times-a-day dosing. Unfortunately, this approach is only effective in approximately 60% of patients [55]. Tolvaptan is an oral vasopressin receptor antagonist approved for the treatment of euvolemic or hypervolemic hyponatremia, and does not require severe fluid restriction. It increases urine water excretion by blocking the effects of endogenous vasopressin in the renal collecting duct. The starting dose is 15 mg per day and close monitoring in a hospital setting is required to ensure that serum sodium is corrected in a controlled manner. Patients should be provided access to sufficient amounts of water to ensure that they do not become overly dehydrated [56]. A small case series has demonstrated efficacy in patients with SIADH from small cell lung cancer [57]. Conivaptan is an intravenous vasopressin receptor antagonist, which also has demonstrated efficacy in SIADH.

Patients who are seizing, comatose, or rapidly decompensating should be treated with hypertonic saline and furosemide to induce an isotonic diuresis as originally proposed by Gross et al. [58] and Hantman et al. [59]. Once the sodium level is above 120 mg per dL, more conservative measures are appropriate. The primary risk of rapid correction of hyponatremia is central pontine myelinolysis, which typically occurs 3 to 5 days after repletion with corticobulbar spinal dysfunction, dysphasia, quadriparesis, and delirium. Although controversial, most data support the idea that the risk of pontine myelinolysis is greatest for patients with chronic, severe hyponatremia who are treated too rapidly. Generally, the sodium level should not be corrected at a rate faster than 6 mEq per L within 6 hours even in acute circumstances.

ONCOLOGIC THERAPEUTICS

Chemotherapeutic and supportive care agents may themselves lead to toxic effects that require critical care. Potentially offending agents, and the physiologic impact, are summarized in Table 95.5.

TUMOR LYSIS SYNDROME

Physiology

Tumor lysis syndrome (TLS) is a metabolic emergency that remains a significant risk for patients with hematopoietic malignancy and is being recognized with greater frequency in patients with solid tumors. TLS results from the release of intracellular purines, phosphate, and potassium from rapidly proliferating tumor cells, which may occur spontaneously or with the initiation of therapy. The massive tumor necrosis that initiates the syndrome may occur as a result of tumor hypoxia or with the use of chemotherapy, radiation, or embolization of tumor. Tumor lysis is followed by hyperuricemia, hyperkalemia, hyperphosphatemia, hypocalcemia, and renal insufficiency. Hyperuricemia, combined with metabolic acidosis, results in crystallization of uric acid in the collecting ducts of the kidneys and ureters, leading to obstructive uropathy. Hyperphosphatemia may also cause metastatic calcification in the renal tubules. The resultant renal insufficiency worsens hyperkalemia and hypocalcemia.

Etiology

Patients at highest risk include those with Burkitt lymphoma, bulky, aggressive non-Burkitt non-Hodgkin lymphoma, and acute leukemia presenting with an initial leukocytosis greater than 100×10^9 per L [60]. The frequency of TLS depends on the criteria used, which are not well established or accepted. New agents in CLL have also been associated with high rates of tumor lysis syndrome including ibrutinib and venetoclax. In Burkitt lymphoma, the incidence may be as high as 30%, and in patients with acute leukemia with hyperleukocytosis, electrolyte disturbances develop consistent with TLS in 50% of cases [61,62]. A variety of solid tumors have been reported to cause the syndrome, but the most common appear to be small cell lung carcinoma, germ cell tumors, and neuroblastoma [60]. Generally, these malignancies are clinically aggressive and sensitive to chemotherapy or radiation. The International Tumor Lysis Syndrome consensus panel also recommends incorporating renal function into risk assessment by classifying low-risk patients as intermediate risk and intermediate-risk patients as high risk if there is evidence of renal dysfunction, renal involvement, or elevated uric acid, phosphate, or potassium at presentation [60].

Diagnosis

The diagnosis of TLS is a clinical one, as there is no specific pathognomonic finding or laboratory value that is specific to the syndrome. The diagnosis of TLS is made on the basis of the presence of azotemia, hyperuricemia, hyperphosphatemia, and hypocalcemia in a patient with extensive, rapidly proliferating tumor. Profound metabolic acidosis out of proportion to the degree of renal insufficiency is common. Many of the metabolic abnormalities of TLS may occur as a result of acute renal failure alone, and a urinary uric acid to creatinine ratio greater than 1 helps to distinguish acute uric acid nephropathy from other catabolic forms of acute renal failure.

Treatment

Management can be grouped into prevention/conservative therapy and hemodialysis. Allopurinol in doses of 200 to 600 mg/m^2/d should be initiated before therapy to decrease uric acid production [63]. Intravenous allopurinol can be used for patients who are unable to take oral allopurinol. Allopurinol is associated with a significant number of side effects and should be discontinued within 3 days of completion of treatment if there is no evidence of tumor lysis. Intravenous hydration of 2 to 3L/m^2/d should be given with close monitoring of urine output with a target of 2 mL/kg/h [63]. Urinary alkalinization is controversial and it is recommended only in patients with metabolic acidosis [63]. Hyperkalemia should be aggressively managed with potassium restriction and sodium polystyrene sulfonate as appropriate. Hemodialysis is often necessary and

TABLE 95.5

Agents Associated with a Probability of Severe, Life-Threatening Reactions

Drug Class/Name	Type of Reaction	Comments
Platinum agents: Carboplatin Cisplatin Oxaliplatin	Anaphylaxis Type I reaction Type II reaction	• IgE-mediated hypersensitivity • Commonly presents with classic hypersensitivity symptoms such as pruritus, urticaria, diffuse erythroderma, chest tightness, bronchospasm, facial swelling, and hypotension • Incidence increases with repeated exposure (i.e., after six to seven cycles of chemotherapy; with disease recurrence, break in therapy, then retreatment) • Typically occurs when drug is rechallenged • Desensitization can potentially be performed
Taxanes: Docetaxel Paclitaxel Cabazitaxel (semi-synthetic taxane derivative)	Anaphylaxis Hypersensitivity	• Direct release of mast cells such as histamine and tryptase, complement activation, IgE-mediated anaphylaxis • Thought to be caused by both the medication and the medication diluents (Paclitaxel—polyoxyethylated castor oil (Cremophor); Docetaxel—tween 80) • Most reactions present within minutes of the start of the first or second infusion. • Common reactions reported include dyspnea, bronchospasm, urticaria, rash, hypotension, fluid retention, and angioedema. • Premedication regimens consisting of glucocorticoids, H1 and H2 receptor blockers may be used to reduce the severity and incidence of reactions (both hypersensitivity and fluid retention)
Epothilones: Ixabepilone	Anaphylaxis Hypersensitivity	• Formulated in Cremophor (similar to paclitaxel) • May premedicate with glucocorticoids, H1 receptor antagonist, and H2 receptor antagonist
Topoisomerase II inhibitors Teniposide Etoposide	Anaphylaxis	• Thought to be due to the drug vehicle (polysorbate 80, same as docetaxel) • Presents with angioedema, dyspnea, wheezing, hypotension/hypertension, urticaria, angioedema, facial flushing, chest pain • May premedicate with glucocorticoid and antihistamine • May switch to etoposide phosphate if hypersensitivity develops
Monoclonal antibodies: Alemtuzumab Bevacizumab Cetuximab Ofatumumab Panitumumab Rituximab Trastuzumab	Anaphylaxis Hypersensitivity	• IgE-mediated allergic responses or cytokine-release syndrome • Murine >> chimeric > humanized • Presents with fever, chills, rash, urticaria, nausea, chest pain, hypoxia, bronchospasm, angioedema, hypotension, ventricular fibrillation, cardiogenic shock, anaphylaxis • Premedication suggested to decrease incidence • Consider withholding antihypertensives 12 hours prior to therapy to reduce the severity of hypotension • Incidence highest during initial therapy and/or high disease burden • Severe reactions seen more commonly in females, elderly, patients with pulmonary infiltrates, and in the treatment of chronic lymphocytic leukemia or mantle-cell lymphoma
Immune globulin (IVIG)	Hypersensitivity Infusion-related reaction	• Increased risk in IgA deficiency with anti-IgA antibodies • Increased risk with corn allergy • Premedicate with antipyretic and H1-blocker to minimize chance of reaction • May change products if hypersensitivity to one product occurs
Melphalan	Hypersensitivity	• Type I hypersensitivity • Intravenous > oral • Typically does not manifest until at least two doses
Blinatumomab Clofarabine Dinutuximab Gemcitabine Filgrastim Filgrastim-sndz Tbo-filgrastim Sargramostim	Capillary leak syndrome	• Leakage of plasma and proteins into the interstitial compartment • Patients may present with tachypnea, tachycardia, hypotension, pulmonary edema, rapid-onset respiratory distress, pleural/pericardial effusion, multiorgan failure • Consider premedication with corticosteroid

(continued)

TABLE 95.5

Agents Associated with a Probability of Severe, Life-Threatening Reactions(*continued*)

Drug Class/Name	Type of Reaction	Comments
Acitretin	Capillary leak syndrome	• Possibly an indication of retinoic acid syndrome
Aldesleukin (IL-2)	Capillary leak syndrome	• Consider premedication with antipyretic, H2 antagonist, antiemetic, antidiarrheal, and continue for 12 hours after the last dose • High-dose therapy recommended to be administered in a hospital setting with access to an intensive care unit
Alemtuzumab Anti-CD3 (OKT3) Antithymocyte Globulin Rabbit Blinatumomab Lymphocyte Immune Globulin Rituximab TGN1412	Cytokine-release syndrome Anaphylaxis	• Non–antigen-specific toxicity • Characterized by release of inflammatory markers (i.e., IFN-γ, IL-1β, IL-2, IL-6, IL-8 and/or TNF-α) • May present with fever, rigors, tachypnea, tachycardia, headache, mental status change, tremor, seizure, myalgias, arthralgias, nausea, vomiting, diarrhea, rash, hypotension, transaminitis, hyperbilirubinemia • Symptoms typically occur within minutes to hours after the infusion begins • Treatment may consist of corticosteroids and/or cytokine antagonists
Ifosamide	Neurotoxicity	• Encephalopathy characterized by confusion, blurred vision, mutism, hallucinations, seizures • Accumulation of drug metabolite (chloroacetaldehyde) causing direct central nervous system effects • Potentially reversible (spontaneously with cessation of drug within 48–72 hours; scant data with reversal drug therapy) • Increased incidence with presence of low serum albumin concentrations, high serum creatinine concentrations and the presence of pelvic carcinomatosis
Nelarabine	Neurotoxicity	• Higher correlation with higher doses • Mechanism of toxicity suspected to be due to high intracellular accumulation of Ara-G/AraGTP in nerve tissue • Often reversible with drug discontinuation or dose reduction • Patients may present with somnolence, malaise, fatigue, hypoesthesias, paresthesias, peripheral neuropathies, seizures, myoclonic jerking, paralysis, coma
Bleomycin	Hyperpyrexia syndrome	• Resembles the systemic inflammatory response, involving pyrogenic cytokine release • Do not appear to be allergic in nature • Hyperpyrexia syndrome rare but serious ($<$1% of patients)—characterized by excessive sweating, high fever, mental status change, hypotension • Reaction can be immediate to delayed by hours to days • Highest at the early doses (first and second doses) • Successful rechallenge can be performed with premedications
Arsenic trioxide Tretinoin	Differentiation syndrome	• Presents with unexplained fever, weight gain, peripheral edema, dyspnea with pulmonary infiltrates, pleuropericardial effusion, hypotension, acute renal failure • Prophylaxis/preemptive approach may include use of prednisone, methylprednisolone, or dexamethasone • Occurs more frequently with higher disease burden

Ig, immunoglobulin; IVIG, intravenous immunoglobulin; IFN, interferon; IL, interleukin; TNF, tumor necrosis factor.

is indicated to control volume, reduce phosphorus and uric acid levels, and manage uremia. Some proposed criteria for initiation of hemodialysis are persistent hyperkalemia despite conventional treatment, rapidly rising phosphate, symptomatic hypocalcemia, fluid overload, severe metabolic acidosis, and hyperuricemia. Typically, daily dialysis is necessary because the catabolic rate is sharply increased in patients with TLS. Daily weights, close monitoring of fluid intake and output, and serum electrolytes, including potassium, calcium, phosphorus, and uric acid, should be performed at least twice a day in a patient at high risk and more frequently if dialysis is instituted. Rasburicase is a recombinant urate oxidase that converts uric acid to more soluble allantoin. A randomized study of rasburicase and allopurinol in pediatric patients at high risk of tumor lysis demonstrated that uric acid levels were substantially lower in patients receiving prophylactic rasburicase. The size of the trial was too small to demonstrate a significant difference in renal failure, and the incidence of tumor lysis was not reported [64]. A phase III study compared rasburicase alone to rasburicase plus allopurinol to allopurinol alone in 280 adults with hematologic malignancies at risk of TLS. Both rasburicase groups were superior to allopurinol alone in normalization of serum uric acid, but there were no differences in the incidence of clinical TLS or acute kidney injury [65]. The most common rasburicase-associated toxicities included rash and hypersensitivity. When rasburicase is used, it is important to recognize that the enzyme can continue to degrade uric acid in blood samples at room temperature. Samples must be collected in prechilled heparinized tubes, transported on ice, and analyzed within 4 hours of collection. Rasburicase is contraindicated in patients with glucose-6-phosphate dehydrogenase deficiency.

Outcomes with development of full-blown TLS are variable. In the reported cases of solid tumor TLS, the fatality rate was very high (36%) [66]. Institution of prophylaxis in patients identified as high risk (even those with solid tumors), which includes both rasburicase and consideration for early use of hemodialysis, is highly recommended [60]. Advances in oncologic emergencies, based on randomized, controlled trials or meta-analyses of such trials, are summarized in Table 95.6.

TABLE 95.6

Advances in Management Based on Randomized Controlled Clinical Trials in Oncologic Emergencies

Clinical description	Comparison	Results	Significance	Reference
Spinal cord compression	Radiation +/− high-dose dexamethasone	High-dose dexamethasone improved functional outcome initially and at 6 months.	Little morbidity was associated with dexamethasone with major benefit when used with radiation.	[35]
Spinal cord compression	Operable candidates: decompressive surgery followed by radiation vs. radiation alone	Surgery followed by radiation therapy gave a superior functional outcome compared to radiation therapy alone.	For operable candidates whose life expectancy is more than weeks or a few months, surgery followed by radiation should be an initial consideration.	[38]
Spinal cord compression	Age stratification: decompressive surgery followed by radiation vs. radiation alone	Secondary data analysis demonstrates a strong relationship between age and treatment benefit.	Age is an important variable in predicting which patients will benefit from surgical decompression in patients with epidural cord compression; no surgery benefit is seen in individuals >age 65.	[39]
Hypercalcemia	Zoledronic acid (4 vs. 8 mg) vs. pamidronate (three-arm randomized study)	Zoledronic acid at 4 mg produced more rapid and sustained response compared to pamidronate with excellent side effect profile compared to pamidronate; 8 mg did not add to response effect.	Zoledronic acid is the bisphosphonate of choice in the treatment of hypercalcemia of malignancy.	[48]
Tumor lysis syndrome	Rasburicase vs. allopurinol for prophylaxis of tumor lysis in lymphoma patients (children)	Four hours after the first dose, patients randomized to rasburicase compared to allopurinol achieved an 86% vs. 12% reduction ($p < 0.0001$) of initial plasma uric acid levels; sample size was small; adult trial results not available.	In patients who have evidence of pretreatment tumor lysis syndrome or patients who are allergic to allopurinol, rasburicase may be a suitable alternative to allopurinol.	[64]
Tumor lysis syndrome	Rasburicase vs. rasburicase + allopurinol vs. allopurinol monotherapy	Trial demonstrated a significant improvement in uric acid response rates (the proportion of patients with plasma uric acid levels less than 7.5 mg/dL from day 3 through day 7 following initiation of antihyperuricemic treatment) among rasburicase-treated patients compared to *allopurinol*-treated patients.	Rasburicase was approved by the FDA for the initial management of patients with malignancy at high risk of developing tumor lysis syndrome.	[65]

References

1. Rice TW, Rodriguez RM, Light RW: The superior vena cava syndrome: clinical characteristics and evolving etiology. *Medicine (Baltimore)* 85(1):37–42, 2006.
2. Baba Y, Ohkubo K, Nakai H, et al: Focal enhanced areas of the liver on computed tomography in a patient with superior vena cava obstruction. *Cardiovasc Intervent Radiol* 22(1):69–70, 1999.
3. Ahmann FR: A reassessment of the clinical implications of the superior vena caval syndrome. *J Clin Oncol* 2(8):961–969, 1984.
4. Yu JB, Wilson LD, Detterbeck FC: Superior vena cava syndrome—a proposed classification system and algorithm for management. *J Thorac Oncol* 3(8):811–814, 2008.
5. Urban T, Lebeau B, Chastang C, et al: Superior vena cava syndrome in small-cell lung cancer. *Arch Intern Med* 153(3):384–387, 1993.
6. Loeffler JS, Leopold KA, Recht A, et al: Emergency prebiopsy radiation for mediastinal masses: impact on subsequent pathologic diagnosis and outcome. *J Clin Oncol* 4(5):716–721, 1986.
7. Armstrong BA, Perez CA, Simpson JR, et al: Role of irradiation in the management of superior vena cava syndrome. *Int J Radiat Oncol Biol Phys*13(4):531–539, 1987.
8. Fagedet D, Thony F, Timsit JF, et al: Endovascular treatment of malignant superior vena cava syndrome: results and predictive factors of clinical efficacy. *Cardiovasc Intervent Radiol* 36(1):140–149, 2013.
9. Lanciego C, Pangua C, Chacon JI, et al: Endovascular stenting as the first step in the overall management of malignant superior vena cava syndrome. *Am J Roentgenol* 193(2):549–558, 2009.
10. Chan RH, Dar AR, Yu E, et al: Superior vena cava obstruction in small-cell lung cancer. *Int J Radiat Oncol Biol Phys* 38(3):513–520, 1997.
11. Gray BH, Olin JW, Graor RA, et al: Safety and efficacy of thrombolytic therapy for superior vena cava syndrome. *Chest* 99(1):54–59, 1991.
12. Wurschmidt F, Bunemann H, Heilmann HP: Small cell lung cancer with and without superior vena cava syndrome: a multivariate analysis of prognostic factors in 408 cases. *Int J Radiat Oncol Biol Phys* 33(1):77–82, 1995.
13. Ben-Horin S, Bank I, Guetta V, et al: Large symptomatic pericardial effusion as the presentation of unrecognized cancer: a study in 173 consecutive patients undergoing pericardiocentesis. *Medicine (Baltimore)* 85(1):49–53, 2006.
14. Dragoescu EA, Liu L: Pericardial fluid cytology: an analysis of 128 specimens over a 6-year period. *Cancer cytopathology* 121(5):242–251, 2013.
15. Posner MR, Cohen GI, Skarin AT: Pericardial disease in patients with cancer. The differentiation of malignant from idiopathic and radiation-induced pericarditis. *Am J Med* 71(3):407–413, 1981.
16. Markiewicz W, Borovik R, Ecker S: Cardiac tamponade in medical patients: treatment and prognosis in the echocardiographic era. *Am Heart J* 111(6):1138–1142, 1986.
17. Atar S, Chiu J, Forrester JS, et al: Bloody pericardial effusion in patients with cardiac tamponade: is the cause cancerous, tuberculous, or iatrogenic in the 1990s? *Chest* 116(6):1564–1569, 1999.
18. Wiener HG, Kristensen IB, Haubek A, et al: The diagnostic value of pericardial cytology. An analysis of 95 cases. *Acta Cytol* 35(2):149–153, 1991.
19. Little WC, Freeman GL: Pericardial disease. *Circulation* 113(12):1622–1632, 2006.
20. Spodick DH: Acute cardiac tamponade. *N Engl J Med* 349(7):684–690, 2003.
21. Tsang TS, Seward JB, Barnes ME, et al: Outcomes of primary and secondary treatment of pericardial effusion in patients with malignancy. *Mayo Clin Proc* 75(3):248–253, 2000.
22. Celik S, Lestuzzi C, Cervesato E, et al: Systemic chemotherapy in combination with pericardial window has better outcomes in malignant pericardial effusions. *J Thorac Cardiovasc Surg* 148(5):2288–2293, 2014.
23. Vaitkus PT, Herrmann HC, LeWinter MM: Treatment of malignant pericardial effusion. *JAMA* 272(1):59–64, 1994.
24. McDonald JM, Meyers BF, Guthrie TJ, et al: Comparison of open subxiphoid pericardial drainage with percutaneous catheter drainage for symptomatic pericardial effusion. *Ann Thorac Surg* 76(3):811–815; discussion 816, 2003.
25. Dequanter D, Lothaire P, Berghmans T, et al: Severe pericardial effusion in patients with concurrent malignancy: a retrospective analysis of prognostic factors influencing survival. *Ann Surg Oncol* 15(11):3268–3271, 2008.
26. Dosios T, Theakos N, Angouras D, et al: Risk factors affecting the survival of patients with pericardial effusion submitted to subxiphoid pericardiostomy. *Chest* 124(1):242–246, 2003.
27. Girardi LN, Ginsberg RJ, Burt ME: Pericardiocentesis and intrapericardial sclerosis: effective therapy for malignant pericardial effusions. *Ann Thorac Surg* 64(5):1422–1427; discussion 1427–1428, 1997.
28. Loblaw DA, Laperriere NJ: Emergency treatment of malignant extradural spinal cord compression: an evidence-based guideline. *J Clin Oncol* 16(4):1613–1624, 1998.
29. Schiff D, O'Neill BP, Suman VJ: Spinal epidural metastasis as the initial manifestation of malignancy: clinical features and diagnostic approach. *Neurology* 49(2):452–456, 1997.
30. Cole JS, Patchell RA: Metastatic epidural spinal cord compression. *Lancet Neurol* 7(5):459–466, 2008.
31. Schiff D, O'Neill BP, Wang CH, et al: Neuroimaging and treatment implications of patients with multiple epidural spinal metastases. *Cancer* 83(8):1593–1601, 1998.
32. Mak KS, Lee LK, Mak RH, et al: Incidence and treatment patterns in hospitalizations for malignant spinal cord compression in the United States, 1998-2006. *Int J Radiat Oncol Biol Phys* 80(3):824–831, 2011.
33. Li KC, Poon PY: Sensitivity and specificity of MRI in detecting malignant spinal cord compression and in distinguishing malignant from benign compression fractures of vertebrae. *Magn Reson Imaging* 6(5):547–556, 1988.
34. Husband DJ, Grant KA, Romaniuk CS: MRI in the diagnosis and treatment of suspected malignant spinal cord compression. *Br J Radiol* 74(877):15–23, 2001.
35. Sorensen S, Helweg-Larsen S, Mouridsen H, et al: Effect of high-dose dexamethasone in carcinomatous metastatic spinal cord compression treated with radiotherapy: a randomised trial. *Eur J Cancer* 30A(1):22–27, 1994.
36. Vecht CJ, Haaxma-Reiche H, van Putten WL, et al: Initial bolus of conventional versus high-dose dexamethasone in metastatic spinal cord compression. *Neurology* 39(9):1255–1257, 1989.
37. Maranzano E, Latini P, Beneventi S, et al: Radiotherapy without steroids in selected metastatic spinal cord compression patients. A phase II trial. *Am J Clin Oncol* 19(2):179–183, 1996.
38. Patchell RA, Tibbs PA, Regine WF, et al: Direct decompressive surgical resection in the treatment of spinal cord compression caused by metastatic cancer: a randomised trial. *Lancet* 366(9486):643–648, 2005.
39. Chi JH, Gokaslan Z, McCormick P, et al: Selecting treatment for patients with malignant epidural spinal cord compression-does age matter?: results from a randomized clinical trial. *Spine (Phila Pa 1976)* 34(5):431–435, 2009.
40. Loblaw DA, Mitera G, Ford M, et al: A 2011 updated systematic review and clinical practice guideline for the management of malignant extradural spinal cord compression. *Int J Radiat Oncol Biol Phys* 84(2):312–317, 2012.
41. Maranzano E, Latini P: Effectiveness of radiation therapy without surgery in metastatic spinal cord compression: final results from a prospective trial. *Int J Radiat Oncol Biol Phys* 32(4):959–967, 1995.
42. Stewart AF: Clinical practice. Hypercalcemia associated with cancer. *N Engl J Med* 352(4):373–379, 2005.
43. Ratcliffe WA, Hutchesson AC, Bundred NJ, et al: Role of assays for parathyroid-hormone-related protein in investigation of hypercalcaemia. *Lancet* 339(8786):164–167, 1992.
44. Horwitz MJ, Tedesco MB, Sereika SM, et al: Direct comparison of sustained infusion of human parathyroid hormone-related protein-(1-36) [hPTHrP-(1-36)] versus hPTH-(1-34) on serum calcium, plasma 1,25-dihydroxyvitamin D concentrations, and fractional calcium excretion in healthy human volunteers. *J Clin Endocrinol Metab* 88(4):1603–1609, 2003.
45. Roodman GD: Mechanisms of bone lesions in multiple myeloma and lymphoma. *Cancer* 80[8, Suppl]:1557–1563, 1997.
46. Donovan PJ, Achong N, Griffin K, et al: PTHrP-mediated hypercalcemia: causes and survival in 138 patients. *J Clin Endocrinol Metab* 100(5):2024–2029, 2015.
47. Rogers MJ, Gordon S, Benford HL, et al: Cellular and molecular mechanisms of action of bisphosphonates. *Cancer* 88[12, Suppl]:2961–2978, 2000.
48. Major P, Lortholary A, Hon J, et al: Zoledronic acid is superior to pamidronate in the treatment of hypercalcemia of malignancy: a pooled analysis of two randomized, controlled clinical trials. *J Clin Oncol* 19(2):558–567, 2001.
49. Chang JT, Green L, Beitz J: Renal failure with the use of zoledronic acid. *N Engl J Med* 349(17):1676–1679; discussion 1676–1679, 2003.
50. Hu MI, Glezerman IG, Leboulleux S, et al: Denosumab for treatment of hypercalcemia of malignancy. *J Clin Endocrinol Metab* 99(9):3144–3152, 2014.
51. Bech A, de Boer H: Denosumab for tumor-induced hypercalcemia complicated by renal failure. *Ann Intern Med* 156(12):906–907, 2012.
52. Ralston SH, Gallacher SJ, Patel U, et al: Cancer-associated hypercalcemia: morbidity and mortality. Clinical experience in 126 treated patients. *Ann Intern Med* 112(7):499–504, 1990.
53. Rowe JM, Lichtman MA: Hyperleukocytosis and leukostasis: common features of childhood chronic myelogenous leukemia. *Blood* 63(5):1230–1234, 1984.
54. Lassen U, Osterlind K, Hansen M, et al: Long-term survival in small-cell lung cancer: posttreatment characteristics in patients surviving 5 to 18+ years--an analysis of 1,714 consecutive patients. *J Clin Oncol* 13(5):1215–1220, 1995.
55. Sherlock M, Thompson CJ: The syndrome of inappropriate antidiuretic hormone: current and future management options. *Eur J Endocrinol* 162[Suppl 1]:S13–S18, 2010.
56. Castillo JJ, Vincent M, Justice E: Diagnosis and management of hyponatremia in cancer patients. *Oncologist* 17(6):756–765, 2012.
57. Petereit C, Zaba O, Teber I, et al: A rapid and efficient way to manage hyponatremia in patients with SIADH and small cell lung cancer: treatment with tolvaptan. *BMC Pulm Med* 13:55, 2013.
58. Gross P, Reimann D, Neidel J, et al: The treatment of severe hyponatremia. *Kidney Int Suppl* 64:S6–S11, 1998.
59. Sterns RH, Hix JK, Silver S: Treatment of hyponatremia. *Curr Opin Nephrol Hypertens* 19(5):493–498, 2010.
60. Cairo MS, Coiffier B, Reiter A, et al: Recommendations for the evaluation of risk and prophylaxis of tumour lysis syndrome (TLS) in adults and children with malignant diseases: an expert TLS panel consensus. *Br J Haematol* 149(4):578–586, 2010.
61. Thiebaut A, Thomas X, Belhabri A, et al: Impact of pre-induction therapy leukapheresis on treatment outcome in adult acute myelogenous leukemia presenting with hyperleukocytosis. *Ann Hematol* 79(9):501–506, 2000.
62. Kemeny MM, Magrath IT, Brennan MF: The role of surgery in the management of American Burkitt's lymphoma and its treatment. *Ann Surg* 196(1):82–86, 1982.
63. Coiffier B, Altman A, Pui CH, et al: Guidelines for the management of pediatric and adult tumor lysis syndrome: an evidence-based review. *J Clin Oncol* 26(16):2767–2778, 2008.
64. Goldman SC, Holcenberg JS, Finklestein JZ, et al: A randomized comparison between rasburicase and allopurinol in children with lymphoma or leukemia at high risk for tumor lysis. *Blood* 97(10):2998–3003, 2001.
65. Cortes J, Moore JO, Maziarz RT, et al: Control of plasma uric acid in adults at risk for tumor Lysis syndrome: efficacy and safety of rasburicase alone and rasburicase followed by allopurinol compared with allopurinol alone—results of a multicenter phase III study. *J Clin Oncol* 28(27):4207–4213, 2010.
66. Kalemkerian GP, Darwish B, Varterasian ML: Tumor lysis syndrome in small cell carcinoma and other solid tumors. *Am J Med* 103(5):363–367, 1997.

Chapter 96 ■ Therapeutic Apheresis: Technical Considerations and Indications in Critical Care

LAURA S. CONNELLY-SMITH • THERESA A. NESTER

TECHNICAL RATIONALE AND INSTRUMENTS

Apheresis means *to remove*. Apheresis instruments are designed to separate whole blood into its component parts to selectively remove one component and return the remaining components to the patient. By processing one or more blood volumes, a significant amount of pathologic solutes or cells may be removed while the intravascular compartment remains relatively euvolemic. In an exchange procedure, replacement fluid or blood is given back to the patient to allow plasma or red cells to be removed. With any apheresis procedure, some type of anticoagulant is added to the circuit to ensure that blood flows freely.

Centrifugation apheresis instruments use either a continuous or a discontinuous flow method to deliver blood to the separation device where blood cells and plasma are differentially sedimented according to their specific gravity. Continuous flow methods draw blood into the extracorporeal circuit, separate blood into components in the centrifugation chamber, divert the unwanted component into a collection bag, and return nonpathologic components to the patient without interruption (Fig. 96.1). Dual venous/catheter access is required for these procedures. Discontinuous, or intermittent, flow methods accomplish the same steps but draw and process a discrete amount of blood into the extracorporeal circuit and then return the processed effluent before another discrete volume of blood is removed. Discontinuous procedures take a longer time than continuous procedures but require only single vein/catheter access [1].

Some apheresis instruments, predominantly used in Asia and Europe, use a membrane filtration technique to isolate plasma. The extracorporeal membrane consists of either a flat plate or a hollow fiber with a pore size that excludes cellular components from the filtrate. The plasma that is separated in the instrument is diverted for disposal or treatment, whereas the other blood components are returned to the patient [2].

Specialized columns and instruments have been developed over the years to treat separated plasma, with the goal of selectively removing pathogenic proteins or other solutes [2,3]. One example is hypercholesterolemia therapy. Two different columns are approved for patients with familial hypercholesterolemia who have failed combination drug therapy. The heparin-induced extracorporeal low-density lipoprotein (LDL) precipitation (HELP) system and Liposorber LA-15 system target the removal

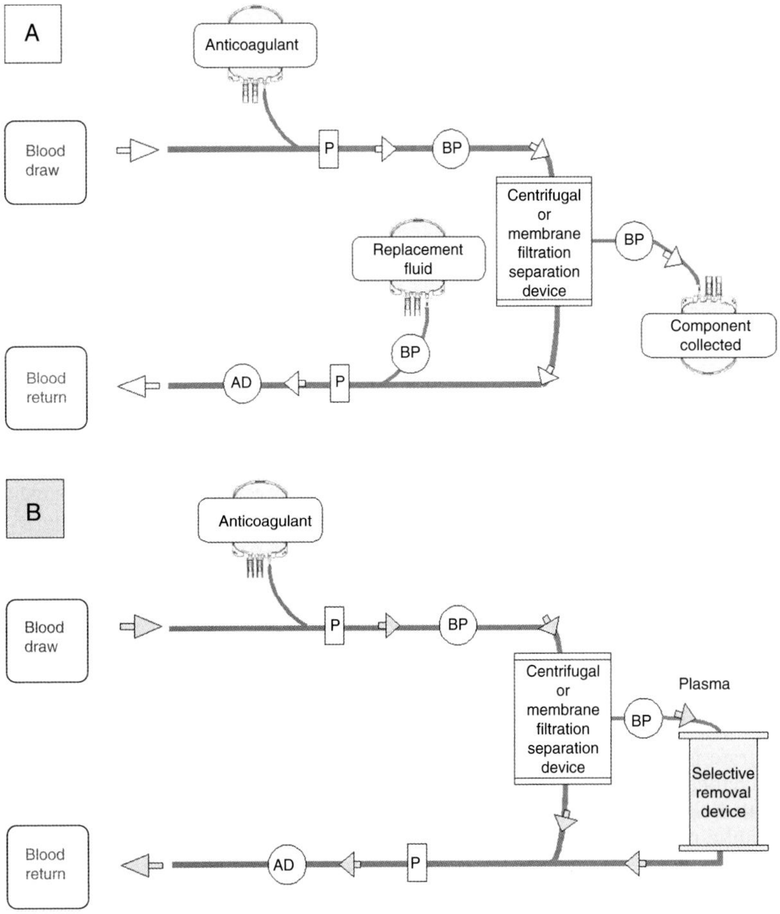

FIGURE 96.1 **A:** Basic circuitry and instrumentation of component removal in a therapeutic apheresis procedure. Anticoagulant is added to the patient's blood as it is drawn and pumped to the separation device. The component to be collected is pumped from the device to a collection bag, and the remainder of the blood is returned, along with appropriate replacement fluid, to the patient. **B:** Circuitry and instrumentation for selective removal of pathogenic substance from the patient's plasma. The patient's anticoagulated blood is pumped to the separation device, and separated plasma is then delivered to the selective removal device. The purified plasma is then combined with the cellular portion of the patient's blood and returned to the patient. AD, air detector; BP, blood pump; P, pressure monitor. (From Linenberger ML, Price TH: Use of cellular and plasma apheresis in the critically ill patient. Part 1: technical and physiological considerations. *J Intensive Care Med* 20:18–27, 2005, with permission.)

of LDLs from separated plasma [3]. Additional columns and systems have been tested and used outside the United States. These include a dextran sulfate column to remove anti-DNA and anticardiolipin antibodies and immobilized polymyxin B or other adsorbers to remove inflammatory cytokines and mediators of sepsis [3]. One specialized methodology, called extracorporeal photopheresis (ECP), involves isolating peripheral white blood cells by leukapheresis, treating the cells with a psoralen drug, and exposing them to ultraviolet A light before returning the photoactivated cells to the patient [4]. A dedicated instrument approved by the Food and Drug Administration is used to perform ECP, which is beneficial for some patients with cutaneous T-cell lymphoma, graft-versus-host disease after hematopoietic stem cell transplantation, systemic sclerosis, and solid organ transplant allorejection [5]. Although ECP is usually an elective procedure, a critically ill patient may undergo treatment as part of a multimodality therapeutic approach.

PHYSIOLOGIC PRINCIPLES

The effectiveness of an apheresis procedure in reducing a plasma molecule or cellular component depends on two factors: (a) the distribution of that component between the intravascular and extravascular space and (b) the rate of regeneration of the component [6]. For solutes that move freely between intravascular and extravascular compartments, complete reequilibration between the compartments occurs at approximately 48 hours after a plasma exchange. Circulating blood cells also traffic between sites of vascular margination and/or splenic sequestration and this, in turn, can affect the efficiency of a therapeutic cytapheresis procedure.

The rate of intravascular regeneration of a pathologic solute or blood cell population after apheresis also depends on the rates of synthesis or production and decay or cell death. Plasma exchange typically removes large molecules at a rate that greatly exceeds their natural synthetic rate; thus, a simple one-compartment mathematical model is used to predict the depletion of soluble plasma substances. Assumptions of the model are that the plasma removed is replaced with a fluid devoid of the target substance, and that complete mixing of the replacement fluid with the remaining intravascular plasma volume occurs [6]. Figure 96.2 depicts the kinetics of removal and regeneration of plasma immunoglobulin G (IgG) and IgM after therapeutic plasma exchange (TPE). The reliability of the one-compartment model to predict removal of soluble substances may be limited by conditions that cause an expanded plasma volume, such as paraproteinemia, molecules with rapid synthetic rates, and situations where rebound IgG production occurs, such as in the setting of humoral solid organ rejection due to a preformed antibody [7].

The efficiency of cell depletion by cytapheresis is less predictable than soluble substance removal by plasma exchange. Factors that may hinder the prediction include a rapid rate of cell production, such as occurs with untreated acute leukemia; the propensity of the spleen to sequester abnormal circulating cells or platelets; and miscalculation of the plasma volume of the patient. In general, a cytapheresis procedure in which 1.5 to 2.0 blood volumes are processed can be expected to remove approximately 35% to 85% of the target cells [8].

ANTICOAGULATION AND FLUID REPLACEMENT

Citrate is the most commonly used anticoagulant for plasma exchange and cytapheresis procedures. Heparin is often used with ECP, specialized column extraction systems, and plasma membrane filtration. Current apheresis instruments limit both the anticoagulant (citrate or heparin) dose and rate of blood return based on the patient's total blood volume. The operator can also adjust the ratio of anticoagulant to whole blood being processed [9].

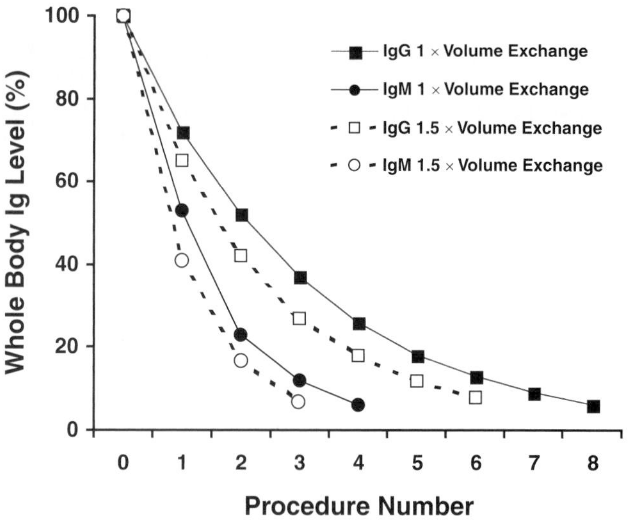

FIGURE 96.2 Hypothetical depletion of whole body immunoglobulin (Ig) levels by therapeutic plasma exchange. The one-compartment model predicts that approximately 60% of the soluble substance will be removed from the plasma with a 1× plasma volume therapeutic exchange, and approximately 80% will be removed with a 1.5× volume exchange. Because roughly 50% of IgG distributes to the extravascular space, reequilibration between the intravascular and extravascular compartments occurs between sequential procedures, and 6 or 7 1× volume exchanges are needed to deplete whole body IgG to less than 10% of the pretreatment level. By comparison, IgM is predominantly intravascular, and, therefore, only 3 or 4 1× volume exchanges are needed to deplete whole body IgM to less than 10%. By increasing the processing to 1.5× plasma volumes, the same therapeutic goal would require three procedures to deplete IgM and five procedures to deplete IgG. (From Linenberger ML, Price TH: Use of cellular and plasma apheresis in the critically ill patient. Part 1: technical and physiological considerations. *J Intensive Care Med* 20:18–27, 2005, with permission.)

The acid-citrate-dextrose (ACD) solution effectively chelates free or ionized plasma calcium, thereby preventing coagulation of blood and plasma in the apheresis circuit. The precise decrease in ionized calcium in vivo during an apheresis procedure is difficult to predict, as this depends on dilution, metabolism, redistribution, and excretion of infused citrate [9]. Fluid replacement with plasma or albumin may decrease the ionized calcium further because of citrate in the plasma or calcium binding by albumin. Ionized calcium may typically decrease by 25% to 35%, as measured during donor apheresis procedures [9].

Citrate does not produce an anticoagulant effect in vivo. The half-life in patients with normal renal and hepatic function is approximately 30 minutes. In a patient with severe liver disease, where citrate will not be as quickly metabolized, the operator should reduce the amount and/or rate of ACD used during an exchange. In critically ill patients needing plasma exchange, it is advised that ionized calcium be monitored and intravenous calcium replacement be provided as needed. Some apheresis services use protocols for the infusion of intravenous calcium gluconate or calcium chloride during all TPEs [10].

Continuous reinfusion of extracorporeal heparin during an apheresis procedure will affect the patient's hemostatic parameters. The effect is measurable until the drug is metabolized, usually within 60 to 120 minutes of finishing the procedure. For patients already therapeutically anticoagulated with heparin, the anticoagulation normally used with apheresis may be reduced or eliminated. The primary providers of critically ill patients must communicate with the apheresis team all information regarding systemic anticoagulation, coagulopathy, and contraindications to anticoagulation, especially when heparin is planned for a therapeutic procedure. It is particularly important to document if the patient has known or suspected heparin-induced thrombocytopenia.

Replacement fluid used in plasma exchange may consist of plasma, albumin, or saline. The type of fluid depends on (a) the patient's baseline hemostatic parameters, particularly fibrinogen; (b) the anticipated number and frequency of procedures; and (c) the condition being treated. For a patient with a neurologic illness, such as acute Guillain–Barré syndrome, 1 to 1.5 plasma volume exchanges are typically performed every other day with 5% albumin as replacement fluid. This regimen and schedule allows the fibrinogen level to recover between procedures. Alternatively, if a condition requires that plasma exchange be performed daily, some plasma replacement will likely be needed to maintain the patient's fibrinogen at a hemostatic level. For conditions where a plasma component is felt to be an important part of the therapy, such as with thrombotic thrombocytopenic purpura, plasma should comprise at least half of the replacement fluid [11]. In such cases, fibrinogen and other coagulation factors will not be depleted.

An apheresis instrument that uses a centrifugation technique must deliver a specific volume of packed red cells to the separation chamber to maintain the cell/plasma density gradient necessary for efficient selective extraction. The extracorporeal blood volume (ECV) necessary for this purpose varies according to the specifications of the instrument and disposable tubing kit and the hematocrit of the patient. The AABB (formerly American Association of Blood Banks) recommends that the ECV for a general procedure should not exceed 15% of a patient's total blood volume [12]. The implications for a therapeutic apheresis procedure can be illustrated by the following example. A 60-kg adult with a hematocrit of 40% has a total blood volume of: 60 kg × 70 mL per kg (the standard conversion factor for an adult male) = 4,200 mL; and a red cell volume of 4,200 mL × 40/100 = 1,680 mL. If the instrument requires 200 mL of extracorporeal red cell volume, then the ECV required to deliver that 200 mL will be 200/1,680 = 0.12, or 12% of the total blood volume. If, however, the same patient has a hematocrit of 20%, the red cell volume will be 4,200 mL × 20/100 = 840 mL; and the required ECV will be 200/840 = 0.24 or 24% of the total blood volume, which exceeds the AABB safety limit. Allogeneic red cells are required when the ECV exceeds 15%. These are either given to the patient as a transfusion prior to the procedure (to increase their pretreatment red cell volume), or used to "prime" the apheresis circuit at the beginning of the procedure (and returned to the patient as part of the return fluid).

VASCULAR ACCESS

The type of vascular access required for therapeutic apheresis depends on the status of the patient's peripheral veins, the condition being treated, and the anticipated frequency and duration of treatment. The vein or catheter must be able to withstand negative pressures associated with inlet rates ranging from 50 to 150 mL per minute for the draw line and up to 150 mL per minute for blood being returned to the patient. For a patient needing only one exchange, it may be possible to use antecubital or forearm veins. A 16- to 18-gauge Teflon or silicone-coated steel, back-eye apheresis, or dialysis-type needle is required for the draw line [13]. The patient ideally will be able to help by squeezing a ball during the exchange.

A large bore central venous catheter is often required for critically ill patients, especially those requiring daily procedures [14]. Temporary or long-term tunneled catheters for adults weighing more than 40 kg should be at least 10-Fr size (Table 96.1). Smaller diameter short-term catheters are acceptable for smaller adults and pediatric patients. Plastic central venous catheters such as those used for cardiac pressure monitoring are not adequate for the draw line because they collapse under the negative pressure generated from the high inlet flow rate. These catheters or a peripheral vein may be useful as return access under certain circumstances.

Peripherally inserted central venous catheter lines and standard port-a-catheters are also not suitable options to accommodate the negative pressures and blood flow rates required. Subcutaneous ports with a reservoir-type chamber can accommodate flow rates required for some apheresis procedures, typically, chronic red blood cell exchanges rather than plasma exchanges [15]. Arteriovenous fistulas created for dialysis access can be used for therapeutic apheresis [13]. The critical care team should consult with the apheresis team prior to placing venous access for the procedure.

LIMITATIONS AND POTENTIAL ADVERSE EVENTS

When considering therapeutic apheresis, certain limitations should be remembered. First, apheresis is not the same as dialysis. It is not usually possible to end a procedure with a large net negative fluid balance (i.e., >200 to 400 mL) because the deficit is colloid rather than crystalloid, and hypotension is likely to occur. A safe end fluid balance is plus or minus 10% to 15% of the total blood volume. In addition, it is not recommended that red cells be transfused during the apheresis procedure (other than at the start as a blood "prime") because the cell separation gradient and cell/plasma interface in the separation chamber may be disturbed. Second, the procedure is almost always an adjunctive, rather than definitive therapy for the condition being treated. Thus, although apheresis can be performed in very ill patients, one must carefully consider the risks that are associated with hemodynamic instability, hematologic abnormalities, the need for vascular access, and the priorities for more urgent primary treatments.

Possible adverse complications related to therapeutic apheresis are shown in Table 96.2. Central line complications include procedure-related events, infection, and bleeding (Chapter 6). Citrate toxicity occurs in 1.5% to 9.0% of therapeutic procedures [16]. Higher risk is associated with larger process volumes, longer procedure duration, nonphysiologic bleeding, severe anemia, unstable vital signs, liver failure, alkalosis due to hyperventilation, and use of replacement fluid consisting of blood components that contain citrate as the anticoagulant [16,17]. Signs and symptoms of hypocalcemia can include a metallic taste in the mouth, muscle or gastrointestinal cramps, perioral numbness, distal paresthesias, and chest tightness. In sedated or unconscious patients, severe citrate toxicity may manifest as tetany, muscle spasm including laryngospasm, a prolonged QTc interval, and decreased myocardial contractility [16]. Hypomagnesemia and hypokalemia may also occur, as the kidneys increase cation excretion into the urine to facilitate excretion of the citrate load. Although rare, fatal arrhythmias have occurred during therapeutic apheresis. To avoid these complications, ionized calcium should be monitored and intravenous calcium infused, as indicated, either through the return line or as an additive with the albumin replacement fluid. Some apheresis practitioners will add small amounts of potassium to albumin to minimize the risk of hypokalemia; otherwise, one should consider monitoring of serum potassium for intensive regimens that use albumin as the replacement fluid [17].

Hypotension or vasovagal reactions have a reported incidence of 1.7% [17]. Patients with preexisting hemodynamic instability or diminished vascular tone, as seen in certain neurologic disorders, may be at particular risk. In such patients, a net negative end fluid balance must be avoided. Transfusion reactions may occur if blood components are part of the replacement fluid. Allergic reactions have also been reported in some patients receiving albumin as the replacement fluid.

Hemostatic alterations and bleeding may occur in severely ill patients with baseline coagulopathy and/or severe thrombocytopenia. A typical 1.3-volume plasma exchange using albumin depletes most coagulation factors to approximately 25% to 45% of their preprocedure values [18]. Repletion time of these coagulation

TABLE 96.1

Catheter Recommendations Based on Patient Weight

Patient weight (kg)	Catheter name	Manufacturer	Size/Gauge (Fr)
Short-term non-tunneled catheters			
35–70	Mahurkar	Covidien	8, 10, and 11.5 12 (triple lumen)
	Duo-Flow XTP	MedComp	9, 11.5
>70	Mahurkar	Covidien	10, 11.5 12 (triple lumen)
	Hemo-Cath ST	MedComp	8, 11.5
Tunneled catheters for long-term apheresis			
35–70	Hemo-Cath LT	MedComp	8, 12.5
	Permcath	Covidien	10
>70	Hickman TriFusion	BARD	12 (triple lumen)
	HemoStar (VasCath)	BARD	14.5
	Split Cath	MedComp	14, 16
	Mahurkar Cuffed	Covidien	13.5
	Tal Palindrome	Covidien	14.5

TABLE 96.2

Possible Adverse Effects of Therapeutic Apheresis

- Central venous catheter-associated complications
- Signs and symptoms of hypocalcemia and/or hypomagnesemia
- Hypotension related to vasovagal reactions or fluid shifts
- Transfusion reactions
- Altered hemostatic parameters
- Bradykinin reaction in patients on ACE inhibitors undergoing plasma exchange or plasma treatment
- Removal of highly protein-bound drugs or immunoglobulins (with frequent plasma exchanges)

ACE, angiotensin-converting enzyme.

factors depends on their respective rates of synthesis, with most factors returning to baseline values by 24 hours. The exception is fibrinogen, which takes about 3 days to return to baseline values. Because fibrinogen levels are the most severely affected during the course of a series of plasma exchanges, preprocedure fibrinogen levels should be monitored, especially if the replacement fluid does not include at least 50% plasma. Therapeutic leukapheresis removes a portion of circulating platelets, and this decrement could be clinically significant in a patient with preprocedure severe thrombocytopenia. The postprocedure platelet count and coagulation status should be monitored in a critically ill patient, particularly if an invasive procedure is needed shortly after apheresis.

In some patients undergoing plasma exchange with albumin as the replacement fluid, a severe reaction consisting of flushing, hypotension, bradycardia, and dyspnea has been linked to concomitant use of angiotensin-converting enzyme (ACE) inhibitors [19]. This reaction is mediated by bradykinin, which is thought to be generated by prekallikrein-activating factor in the albumin preparation. These reports have led to the recommendation that ACE inhibitors be withheld for 24 to 48 hours (depending on the half-life of the specific drug) before plasma exchange using albumin [19]. If an emergency exchange is required in a patient on an ACE inhibitor, fresh frozen plasma (FFP) should be used as the replacement fluid to avoid this reaction. Similar reactions involving ACE inhibitors have been seen in patients undergoing plasma treatment with specialized columns; thus, similar precautions must be followed [20].

An additional potential adverse effect of repeated plasma exchange is the removal of highly protein-bound therapeutic drugs and plasma immunoglobulins. The exact effects of exchange on individual drug levels have not been delineated. To avoid this complication, medications should be administered following a plasma exchange procedure whenever possible. Immunoglobulin levels should also be measured periodically in immunosuppressed patients undergoing a series of plasma exchanges, as these proteins will be nonselectively depleted from the circulation, and severe hypogammaglobulinemia could further predispose the patient to infections [17].

INDICATIONS IN CRITICAL CARE

Evidence-based guidelines for clinical applications are published by the American Society for Apheresis (ASFA) every few years [21]. Medical conditions are placed into categories from I to IV, with I indicating that therapeutic apheresis is known to be an effective primary or adjunct therapy based on randomized controlled clinical trials or broad noncontroversial experience, and category IV indicating no demonstrated efficacy, and possibly even a negative impact of therapeutic apheresis for the condition [5]. Examples of evidence-based indications for therapeutic apheresis are shown in Table 96.3.

Therapeutic Plasma Exchange

In the intensive care unit, TPE is likely to be the most frequent apheresis procedure used. Antibody-mediated conditions known to respond to plasma exchange include thrombotic thrombocytopenic purpura [11,22,23]; demyelinating diseases including acute inflammatory demyelinating polyneuropathy/Guillain–Barré syndrome [24–27]; severe, acute idiopathic inflammatory demyelinating diseases [24,28]; myasthenic crisis [24,29–32]; demyelinating polyneuropathy with IgG and IgA [24]; anti-glomerular basement membrane (anti-GBM) (Goodpasture's) disease; and pulmonary hemorrhage associated with other forms of rapidly progressive glomerulonephritis (RPGN) [33,34,35].

Randomized trials and systematic reviews have directed decision-making in the use of therapeutic apheresis as a treatment

TABLE 96.3

Evidence-Based Indication Categories for Therapeutic Apheresis for Disorders Potentially Affecting Critically Ill Patients

Disease	Apheresis procedure	Indication Category	Recommendation Grade
Renal			
Antiglomerular basement membrane antibody disease			
Diffuse Alveolar Haemorrhage (DAH)	Plasma exchange	I	1C
Dialysis independence	Plasma exchange	I	IB
Dialysis dependence and no DAH	Plasma exchange	III	2B
ANCA-associated rapidly progressive glomerulonephritis			
Dialysis dependence	Plasma exchange	I	1A
DAH	Plasma exchange	I	1C
Dialysis independence	Plasma exchange	III	2C
Focal segmental glomerulosclerosis	Plasma exchange	I	1B
Myeloma cast nephropathy	Plasma exchange	II	2B
Thrombotic microangiopathy, Shiga toxin mediated			
Severe neurological symptoms	Plasma exchange	III	2C
Absence of severe neurological symptoms	Plasma exchange	IV	1C
Streptococcus pneumonia	Plasma exchange	III	2C
Thrombotic microangiopathy, coagulation mediated			
Factor H autoantibodies	Plasma exchange	I	2C
Complement factor gene mutations	Plasma exchange	III	2C
MCP mutations	Plasma exchange	III	2C
Allograft rejection (antibody mediated)			
ABO Compatible	Plasma exchange	I	IB
ABO Incompatible	Plasma exchange	II	1B
Immunoglobulin A nephropathy	Plasma exchange	III	2B
Nephrogenic systemic fibrosis	Plasma exchange	III	2C
Autoimmune and rheumatologic			
Cryoglobulinemia (severe/symptomatic)	Plasma exchange	II	2A
Idiopathic thrombocytopenic purpura	Plasma exchange	III	2C
Systemic lupus erythematosus (severe)	Plasma exchange	II	2C
Systemic lupus erythematosus nephritis	Plasma exchange	IV	1B
Catastrophic antiphospholipid syndrome	Plasma exchange	II	2C
Dermatomyositis or polymyositis	Plasma exchange	IV	2B
Hematologic			
Thrombotic thrombocytopenic purpura	Plasma exchange	I	1A
Hyperleukocytosis with leukostasis	Leukapheresis	II	1B
Sickle cell disease with acute stroke	Red cell exchange	I	1C
Sickle cell disease with acute chest syndrome	Red cell exchange	II	1C
Thrombocytosis (symptomatic, myeloproliferative origin)	Plateletpheresis	II	2C
Posttransfusion purpura	Plasma exchange	III	2C
Polycythemia vera	Erythrocytapheresis	I	IB
Secondary erythrocytosis	Erythrocytapheresis	III	1C
Hyperviscosity (monoclonal IgM, IgA, IgG)	Plasma exchange	I	1B
Coagulation factor inhibitors (alloantibody)	Plasma exchange	IV	2C
Coagulation factor inhibitors (autoantibody)	Plasma exchange	III	2C
Babesiosis (severe)	Red cell exchange	II	2C
Malaria (severe)	Red cell exchange	III	2B
Heparin Induced thrombocytopenia	Plasma exchange	III	2C
Neurologic			
Acute inflammatory demyelinating polyradiculopathy/ Guillain–Barre syndrome (primary treatment)	Plasma exchange	I	1A
Acute disseminated encephalomyelitis	Plasma exchange	II	2C
Chronic inflammatory demyelinating polyradiculopathy	Plasma exchange	I	1B
Myasthenia crisis	Plasma exchange	I	1B
Demyelinating polyneuropathy with IgG and IgA	Plasma exchange	I	1B
Demyelinating polyneuropathy with IgM	Plasma exchange	I	1C
Lambert-Eaton myasthenia syndrome	Plasma exchange	II	2C

(continued)

TABLE 96.3

Evidence-Based Indication Categories for Therapeutic Apheresis for Disorders Potentially Affecting Critically Ill Patients (*continued*)

Disease	Apheresis procedure	Indication Category	Recommendation Grade
Multiple sclerosis (acute, fulminant)	Plasma exchange	II	1B
Neuromyelitis optica (acute)	Plasma exchange	II	1B
PANDAS (exacerbation)	Plasma exchange	II	1B
Sydenenhams chorea (severe)	Plasma exchange	III	2B
Other disorders			
Drug overdose, poisoning and envenomation	Plasma exchange	III	2C
Mushroom poisoning	Plasma exchange	II	2C
Dilated cardiomyopathy, idiopathic	Plasma exchange	III	2C
Acute liver failure	Plasma exchange	III	2B
Toxic epidermal necrolysis (refractory)	Plasma exchange	III	2B
Sepsis and multiple-organ failure	Plasma exchange	III	2B
Wilson disease (fulminant)	Plasma exchange	I	IC
Hashimoto's encephalopathy	Plasma exchange	II	2C
Burn shock resuscitation	Plasma exchange	III	2B

Category I: Disorders for which apheresis is accepted as first-line therapy, either as a primary standalone treatment or in conjunction with other modes of treatment. *Category II*: Disorders for which apheresis is accepted as second-line therapy, either as a standalone treatment or in conjunction with other modes of treatment. *Category III*: Disorders for which the optimum role of apheresis therapy is not established. Decision-making should be individualized. *Category IV*: Disorders in which published evidence demonstrates or suggests apheresis to be ineffective or harmful. Institutional review board approval is desirable if apheresis treatment is undertaken in these circumstances.

Note: The grade system has also been assigned in an effort to parallel an approach more commonly used to evaluate therapeutic recommendations.

ANCA, antineutrophil cytoplasmic antibody; IgA, immunoglobulin A; IgG, immunoglobulin G; IgM, immunoglobulin M.

Adapted from Guyatt G, Gutterman D, Baumann MH, et al: Grading strength of recommendations and quality of evidence in clinical guidelines: report from an American college of chest physicians task force. *Chest* 129:174–181, 2006; also adapted from evidence-based indications categorizations generated by the American Society for Apheresis (ASFA) Apheresis Applications Committee. Shaz B (ed): *Clinical Applications of Therapeutic Apheresis: An Evidence Based Approach*. 6th ed. *J Clin Apher* 28(3), 2013.

modality (Table 96.4); however, in certain conditions, there limited data are available with its effectiveness and optimal role yet to be determined.

With the muscle-specific receptor tyrosine kinase antibody (MuSK-Ab) form of myasthenia gravis, TPE appears to be a more effective therapy than intravenous immunoglobulin (IVIg) infusion [29,36]. By comparison, with the acetyl cholinesterase receptor (AChR-Ab) form of myasthenia gravis, and with Guillain–Barré syndrome, plasma exchange is effective but not superior to or as tolerable as IVIg infusion [26,27,31] (see Table 96.4). For patients with acute attacks of demyelination, plasma exchange may be useful. Although there is only one randomized controlled trial [28], observations from this study and retrospective data indicate that at least 50% of patients with neuromyelitis optica (NMO), characterized by spinal and visual involvement, achieve increased function with plasma exchange, and that patients with steroid-refractory optic neuritis may also achieve some benefit [37]. A potential mechanism of action of TPE with NMO is modulation of the serum autoantibody NMO-IgG, which has been implicated in disease pathophysiology [38].

The optimum role of TPE in the setting of severe sepsis and multiorgan dysfunction is not established. Two randomized controlled trials in adults using either continuous plasma filtration versus supportive care [39] or plasma exchange versus standard care [40] have been published. No differences were observed in the 14-day mortality rates of 14 patients with sepsis syndrome receiving 34 hours of continuous plasma filtration and 16 untreated control patients (57% vs. 50%) [39] (see Table 96.4). By comparison, the 28-day mortality rate was 33.3% among 54 patients with sepsis and septic shock treated with one or two TPE treatments compared with 53.8% among 52 nontreated control patients ($p = 0.05$) [40] (see Table 96.4). When differences between the control and experimental groups were considered using multiple logistic regression, the significance of the treatment variable on mortality was $p = 0.07$. A recent meta-analysis of these two trials demonstrated insufficient evidence to recommend plasma exchange as an adjunctive therapy for patients with sepsis or septic shock [41].

A nonrandomized observational cohort study evaluated hemodynamic and mortality outcomes in critically ill surgical patients with sepsis treated with TPE and continuous venovenous hemofiltration [42]. No overall difference in mortality was observed between treated patients and an untreated historical control group (42% vs. 46%); however, patients with organ failure limited to one or two systems appeared to benefit, with mortality rates of 10% among 10 treated patients versus 38% among 16 untreated control patients [42]. Although encouraging, these data must be supported by results from additional well-designed randomized controlled trials before plasma exchange can be recommended as a noninvestigational therapy for this indication [41,43].

A meta-analysis of the available limited data on plasma exchange for patients with renal vasculitis and RPGN suggests that TPE may reduce the composite end point for end-stage renal failure or death [44]. The evidence supporting a potential benefit of plasma exchange derives from retrospective and case–control studies among more severely affected patients [45,46], whereas randomized controlled trials have yielded supportive results in some studies [47] but not others [48,49] (see Table 96.4). For patients with renal vasculitis due to causes other than anti-GBM disease, a review of randomized controlled clinical trials demonstrated a significant reduction in end-stage renal disease with use of TPE [50].

Red Blood Cell Exchange

Use of red blood cell exchange may be warranted for selected patients with sickle cell disease who are experiencing stroke, acute chest syndrome (ACS), priapism, splenic/hepatic sequestration,

TABLE 96.4

Randomized Controlled Trials and Systematic Reviews of Randomized Controlled Trials That Utilized Therapeutic Apheresis for Disorders in Critical Care Patients

Disease category [Ref.]	*n*	Intervention	Outcome
Severe sepsis and septic shock [40]	106	Plasma exchange (PE) vs. standard therapy	**28-d mortality** 18/54 (33%) PE 28/52 (54%) Control ($p = 0.05$)
Sepsis syndrome [39]	30	Plasma filtration (PF) vs. standard therapy	**14-d mortality** 8/14 (57%) PF 8/16 (50%) Control ($p = 0.73$)
Acute inflammatory demyelinating polyradiculopathy/Guillain–Barré syndrome (systematic review of 6 trials) [26]	649	PE vs. supportive care	**Mechanical ventilation at 4 wk** 85/315 (27%) Control 44/308 (14%) PE (RR 0.53; 95% CI 0.39–0.74, $p = 0.0001$) **Severe sequelae at 1 y** 55/328 (17%) Control 35/321 (11%) PE (RR 0.65; 95% CI 0.44–0.96, $p = 0.03$) **1-y mortality** 18/328 (5.5%) Control 15/321 (4.7%) PE (RR 0.85; 95% CI 0.42–1.45, $p = 0.70$)
Acute inflammatory demyelinating polyradiculopathy/Guillain–Barré syndrome (systematic review of five trials) [27]	582	PE vs. intravenous immunoglobulin (IVIg)	**Median time to discontinuation of mechanical ventilation (2 studies)** 34 d ($n = 34$) PE vs. 27 d ($n = 29$) IVIg (p = NS) 29 d ($n = 40$) PE vs. 26 d ($n = 44$) IVIg (p = NS) **Mortality during follow-up** 9/286 (3.1%) PE 7/296 (2.4%) IVIg (RR 0.78; 95% CI 0.31–1.95, p = NS)
Severe, acute idiopathic inflammatory demyelinating diseases of the central nervous system, including multiple sclerosis [28]	22	Active PE vs. sham PE (crossover allowed)	**≥Moderate acute improvement** 8/19 (42%) Active PE therapy 1/17 (6%) Sham PE therapy
Rapidly progressive glomerulonephritis (RPGN), including antiglomerular basement membrane (anti-GBM) disease and antineutrophil cytoplasmic antibody (ANCA)-associated disease [47]	44	PE vs. immunoadsorption (IA)	**6-mo median creatinine clearance** 49 mL/min PE 49 mL/min IA **6-mo mortality** 1/23 (4.3%) PE 2/21 (9.5%) IA (p = NS)
RPGN, including anti-GBM disease and ANCA-associated disease [48]	33	PE vs. standard therapy with immunosuppression	Dialysis-free survival among patients with type III RPGN 42% PE ($n = 18$) 49% Control ($n = 15$; p = NS)
RPGN, including anti-GBM disease and ANCA-associated disease [49]	32	PE vs. standard therapy with immunosuppression	**Patients on dialysis at study end** 3/16 (19%) PE 5/16 (31%) Control (p = NS)
Renal vasculitis (adult) other than anti-GBM (systematic review of six trials) [50]		Use of PE	**3-mo response rate** Significant reduction in risk of end-stage renal disease ($p = 0.01$) **12-mo response rate** Significant reduction in risk of end-stage renal disease ($p = 0.002$)
Thrombotic thrombocytopenic purpura [11]	102	PE vs. plasma infusion (PI)	**6-mo response rate** 40/51 (78%) PE 25/51 (49%) PI ($p = 0.002$) **6-mo mortality** 11/51 (22%) PE 19/51 (37%) PI ($p = 0.036$)
Myasthenia gravis [31]	87	PE vs. intravenous immunoglobulin (IVIg)	**Day 15 variation of myasthenic muscular score** +18 PE ($n = 41$) +15.5 IVIg ($n = 46$; $p = 0.65$)
Myasthenia gravis [32]	84	PE vs. intravenous immunoglobulin (IVIg)	**Day 14 variation of quantitative myasthenia gravis score** −3.2 IVIg ($n = 41$) −4.7 PE ($n = 43$; $p = 0.13$)

CI, confidence interval; *n*, number; NS, not significant; RR, relative risk.

or multiple organ failure as a complication of their disease [51]. Because automated red cell exchange (also called erythrocytapheresis) can more rapidly reduce the level of hemoglobin S-positive cells (to the goal of <30%) [5]. Although maintaining euvolemia and minimizing hyperviscosity complications, this modality has been utilized in preference to simple transfusion by many centers. Although this makes intuitive sense, the data needed to show a clear advantage of automated red cell exchange over simple transfusion are lacking. An observational, retrospective cohort analysis found no differences in postprocedure and total lengths of stay for patients with ACS treated with automated red cell exchange ($n = 20$) compared with those who received simple transfusion support ($n = 20$) [52]. Moreover, the apheresis group required, on average, four times as many units of donor red cells.

Manual exchange transfusion, in which phlebotomized blood is replaced by simple transfusions of allogeneic red cells and FFP, has the added theoretical advantage of reducing the levels of plasma inflammatory mediators, which might augment vasoocclusive tissue injury in patients with ACS [53]. One nonrandomized trial used a combination of TPE and automated red cell exchange for seven patients with severe ACS and multiorgan failure, and observed an 86% 1-year survival [54]. Despite these observations, the optimal approach for critically ill patients with ACS and other severe complications remains undefined, in part because crossmatch-compatible blood may be very difficult to locate for heavily transfused sickle cell patients with multiple alloantibodies. Adequately powered randomized clinical trials are sorely needed to clarify the indications for automated or manual red cell exchange versus simple transfusion support and the potential role of TPE [51].

Red cell exchange may also be useful in patients with severe clinical manifestations of falciparum malaria or babesiosis [55]. Although a meta-analysis performed in 2002 showed no survival benefit of red cell exchange compared with antimalarials and aggressive supportive care alone [56], many case reports and series suggest a benefit in clinical status with rapid reduction of hyperparasitemia using adjunctive manual or automated red cell exchange [57–59]. In 2013, however, the Centers for Disease Control and Prevention (CDC) revised their previous recommendation on the use of red cell exchange as adjunctive therapy for the treatment of severe malaria [60].They now no longer recommend its use based on a review of the published literature that found no evidence of overall survival benefit for exchange transfusion as adjunctive therapy [61]. ASFA currently continues to support certain indications for the use of exchange transfusion in severe malaria [62] but recognizes that quinidine (or artesunate) administration should not be delayed and may be given concurrently with the exchange. As in fulminant malaria, several case reports demonstrate that patients with overwhelming parasitemia from Babesia also quickly respond to red cell exchange [63].

Automated red cell exchange may be considered as an alternative to large volume phlebotomy in selected patients with uncontrolled erythrocytosis and polycythemia vera with acute thromboembolism, severe microvascular complications, or bleeding [64]. This method can quickly and more safely normalize the hematocrit in patients who are hemodynamically unstable.

Leukapheresis

Leukapheresis (i.e., selective removal of white blood cells) is commonly used in patients with acute myeloid leukemia (AML) and hyperleukocytosis experiencing symptoms of leukostasis. Signs and symptoms typically manifest as neurologic alterations (confusion, mental status changes, altered level of consciousness) or pulmonary compromise (hypoxemia, diffuse lung infiltrates). Leukapheresis is indicated in patients with AML and a circulating blast count greater than 50,000 per μL who are clearly demonstrating signs of intravascular leukostasis (i.e., symptoms not attributable to infection, bleeding, or metabolic derangements) [65,66]. Leukapheresis may be warranted sooner in monocytic subtypes of AML, as signs of intravascular leukostasis may be seen at blast counts less than 50,000 per μL [66] after the start of chemotherapy. Because of the high mortality rate associated with leukostasis, leukapheresis is often considered an urgent, lifesaving procedure and is recognized as a Category II indication according to ASFA [5]. Metaanalysis on the use of leukapheresis in hyperleukocytosis (retrospective data) has however found no impact on the early death rate in AML [67]. The potential benefits of urgent leukapheresis should be discussed with the apheresis physician; however, definitive treatment with chemotherapy should not be delayed by the leukapheresis procedure and is required to prevent the rapid reaccumulation of blasts. Prophylactic leukapheresis could be considered in AML patients with circulating blast counts greater than 100,000 per μL, particularly if the count is rapidly rising but definitive therapy with induction chemotherapy should not be delayed [5]. In comparison with AML, leukostasis complications are rare in patients with acute lymphoblastic leukemia (ALL) and circulating blast counts less than 400,000 per μL. Studies have shown that prophylactic leukapheresis for asymptomatic patients with ALL and hyperleukocytosis does not offer additional benefit above aggressive supportive care and chemotherapy [68].

Plateletpheresis

Plateletpheresis should be considered as an urgent intervention in patients experiencing thrombosis or hemorrhage in the setting of uncontrolled thrombocytosis associated with a stem cell disorder [69]. Such stem cell disorders include essential thrombocythemia, polycythemia vera, idiopathic myelofibrosis, chronic myeloid leukemia, or unclassified myeloproliferative neoplasm. The goal of plateletpheresis is to decrease the platelet count (ideally below 600,000 per μL) and to maintain the count until pharmacologic cytoreductive therapy takes effect [5]. Plateletpheresis may also be electively considered for the prevention of perioperative thrombohemorrhagic complications in patients with myeloproliferative neoplasms undergoing splenectomy [70].

APHERESIS CONSULTATION

For any apheresis procedure, consultation with the apheresis team can be useful in assessing experience and available data for a given condition. The apheresis physician and team should be viewed as partners in determining the treatment plan. Initial discussion with the apheresis physician will include whether the indication is urgent or routine, the impact of apheresis on other treatment modalities, volume management, fluid replacement, and vascular access. Ongoing discussions should continue through the patient's course so that appropriate adjustments can be made to optimize the therapy.

References

1. Burgstaler EA: Current instrumentation for apheresis, in McLeod BC, Szczepiorkowski ZM, Price TH, Weinstein R, Winters JL (eds): *Apheresis: Principles and Practice*. 3rd ed. Bethesda, MD, AABB, 2010, pp 71–108.
2. Ward DM: Conventional apheresis therapies: a review. *J Clin Apher* 26:230–238, 2011
3. Sanchez AP, Cunard R, Ward DM: The selective therapeutic apheresis procedures. *J Clin Apher* 28:20–29, 2013.
4. Ward DM: Extracorporeal photopheresis: how, when, and why. *J Clin Apher* 26:276–285, 2011.
5. Schwartz J, Padmanabhan A, Aqui N, et al: Guidelines on the use of therapeutic apheresis in clinical practice-evidence-based approach from the Writing Committee of the American Society for Apheresis: the seventh special issue. *J Clin Apher* 31:149–341, 2016.
6. Okafor C, Ward DM, Mokrzycki MH, et al: Introduction and overview of therapeutic apheresis. *J Clin Apher* 25:240–249, 2010.

7. Tobian AA, Shirey RS, Montogomery RA, et al: The critical role of plasmapheresis in ABO-incompatible renal transplantation. *Transfusion* 48: 2453–2460, 2008.
8. Hester J: Therapeutic cell depletion, in McLeod BC, Price TH, Weinstein R (eds): *Apheresis: Principles and Practice*. 2nd ed. Bethesda, MD, AABB, 2003, pp 283–294.
9. Lee G, Arepally GM. Anticoagulation techniques in apheresis: from heparin to citrate and beyond. *J Clin Apher* 27:117–125, 2012.
10. Weinstein R: Prevention of citrate reactions during therapeutic plasma exchange by constant infusion of calcium gluconate with the return fluid. *J Clin Apher* 11:204–210, 1996.
11. Rock GA, Shumak KH, Buskard NA, et al: Comparison of plasma exchange with plasma infusion in the treatment of thrombotic thrombocytopenic purpura. The Canadian Apheresis Study Group. *N Engl J Med* 325:393–397, 1991.
12. Chhibber V, King KE: Management of the therapeutic apheresis patient, in McLeod BC, Szczepiorkowski ZM, Price TH, Weinstein R, et al (eds): *Apheresis: Principles and Practice*. 3rd ed. Bethesda, MD, AABB, 2010, pp 229–249
13. Golestaneh L, Mokrzycki MH: Vascular access in therapeutic apheresis: update 2013. *J Clin Apher* 28:64–72, 2013.
14. Linenberger ML, Price TH. Use of cellular and plasma apheresis in the critically ill patient: part 1: technical and physiological considerations. *J Intensive Care Med* 20:18–27, 2005.
15. Shrestha A, Jawa Z, Koch KL et al. Use of a dual lumen port for automated red cell exchange in adults with sickle cell disease. *J Clin Apher* 30(6):353–358.
16. Mokrzycki MH, Balogun RA: Therapeutic apheresis: A review of complications and recommendations for prevention and management. *J Clin Apher* 26:243–248, 2011.
17. Kaplan A: Complications of apheresis. *Semin Dial* 25:152–158, 2012.
18. Chirnside A, Urbaniak SJ, Prowse CV, et al: Coagulation abnormalities following intensive plasma exchange on the cell separator, II: effects on factors I, II, V, VII, VIII, IX, X, and antithrombin III. *Br J Haematol* 48:627–634, 1981.
19. Owen HG, Brecher ME: Atypical reactions associated with use of angiotensin-converting enzyme inhibitors and apheresis. *Transfusion* 34:891–894, 1994.
20. Olbricht CJ, Schaumann D, Fischer D: Anaphylactoid reactions, LDL apheresis with dextran sulfate, and ACE inhibitors [letter]. *Lancet* 340:908–909, 1992.
21. Shaz BH, Schwartz J, Winters JL. How we developed and use the American Society for Apheresis guidelines for therapeutic apheresis procedures. *Transfusion*.54:17–25, 2014.
22. Sarode R, Bandarenko N, Brecher ME et al: Thrombotic thrombocytopenic purpura: 2012 American Society for Apheresis (ASFA) consensus conference on classification, diagnosis, management, and future research. *J Clin Apher* 29:148–167, 2014.
23. Michael M, Elilott EJ, Ridley GF, et al: Interventions for haemolytic uremic syndrome and thrombotic thrombocytopenic purpura. *Cochrane Database Syst Rev* (1):CD003595, 2009.
24. Gwathmey K, Balogun RA, Burns T: Neurologic indications for therapeutic plasma exchange: 2013 update. *J Clin Apher* 29:211–219, 2014.
25. Cortese I, Chaudhry V, So YT, et al. Evidence-based guideline update: plasmapheresis in neurologic disorders: report of the Therapeutics and Technology Assessment Subcommittee of the American Academy of Neurology. *Neurology* 76:294–300, 2011.
26. Raphael JC, Chevret S, Hughes RAC, et al: Plasma exchange for Guillain–Barré syndrome. *Cochrane Database Syst Rev* (2):CD001798, 2012.
27. Hughes RA, Raphael JC, Swan AV, et al: Intravenous immunoglobulin for Guillain–Barré syndrome. *Cochrane Database Syst Rev* (1):CD002063, 2006.
28. Weinshenker BG, O'Brien PC, Petterson TM, et al: A randomized trial of plasma exchange in acute central nervous system inflammatory demyelinating disease. *Ann Neurol* 46:878–886, 1999.
29. El-Salem K, Yassin A, Al-Hayk K, et al. Treatment of MuSK-associated myasthenia gravis. *Curr Treat Options Neurol* 16:283, 2014.
30. Köhler W1, Bucka C, Klingel R. A randomized and controlled study comparing immunoadsorption and plasma exchange in myasthenic crisis. *J Clin Apher* 26:347–355, 2011.
31. Gajdos P, Chevret S, Clair B, et al: Clinical trial of plasma exchange and high-dose intravenous immunoglobulin in myasthenia gravis. Myasthenia Gravis Clinical Study Group. *Ann Neurol* 41:789–796, 1997.
32. Dhawan PS, Goodman BP, Harper CM, et al. IVIG Versus PLEX in the treatment of worsening myasthenia gravis: what is the evidence? A critically appraised topic. *Neurologist* 19:145–148, 2015
33. Nguyen TC, Kiss JE, Goldman JR, et al: The role of plasmapheresis in critical illness. *Crit Care Clin* 28:453–468, 2012.
34. Walters GD, Willis NS, Craig JC: Interventions for renal vasculitis in adults. A systematic review. *BMC Nephrol* 11:12, 2010.
35. Walsh M, Catapano F, Szpirt W, et al: Plasma exchange for renal vasculitis and idiopathic rapidly progressive glomerulonephritis: a meta-analysis. *Am J Kidney Dis* 57:566–574, 2011.
36. Oh SJ: Muscle-specific receptor tyrosine kinase antibody positive myasthenia gravis current status. *J Clin Neurol* 5:53–64, 2009.
37. Ruprecht K, Klinker E, Dintelmann T, et al: Plasma exchange for severe optic neuritis. *Neurology* 63:1081–1083, 2004.
38. Watanabe S, Nakashima I, Misu T, et al: Therapeutic efficacy of plasma exchange in NMO-IgG-positive patients with neuromyelitis optica. *Mult Scler* 13:128–132, 2007.
39. Reeves JH, Butt WW, Sham F, et al: Continuous plasmafiltration in sepsis syndrome. Plasmafiltration in Sepsis Study Group. *Crit Care Med* 27: 2096–2104, 1999.
40. Busund R, Koukline V, Utrobin U, et al: Plasmapheresis in severe sepsis and septic shock: a prospective, randomized, controlled trial. *Intensive Care Med* 28:1434–1439, 2002.
41. Zarychanski R, Abou-Setta AM, Kanji S, et al: The efficacy and safety of heparin in patients with sepsis: a systematic review and metaanalysis. *Crit Care Med* 43:511–518, 2015.
42. Schmidt J, Mann S, Mohr VD, et al: Plasmapheresis combined with continuous venovenous hemofiltration in surgical patients with sepsis. *Intensive Care Med* 26:532–537, 2000.
43. Stegmayer B: Apheresis in patients with severe sepsis and multi organ dysfunction syndrome. *Transfus Apher Sci* 38:203–208, 2008.
44. Walsh M, Catapano F, Szpirt W, et al: Plasma exchange for renal vasculitis and idiopathic rapidly progressive glomerulonephritis: a meta-analysis. *Am J Kidney Dis* 57:566–574, 2011.
45. Frasca GM, Soverini ML, Falaschini A, et al: Plasma exchange treatment improves prognosis oantineutrophil cytoplasmic antibody-associated crescentic glomerulonephritis: a case-control study in 26 patients from a single center. *Ther Apher Dial* 7:540–546, 2003.
46. Klemmer PJ, Chalermskulrat W, Reif MS, et al: Plasmapheresis therapy for diffuse alveolar hemorrhage in patients with small-vessel vasculitis. *Am J Kidney Dis* 42:1149–1153, 2003.
47. Stegmayr BG, Almroth G, Berlin G, et al: Plasma exchange or immunoadsorption in patients with rapidly progressive crescentic glomerulonephritis. A Swedish multicenter study. *Int J Artif Organs* 22:81–87, 1999.
48. Zauner I, Bach D, Braun N, et al: Predictive value of initial histology and effect of plasmapheresis on long-term prognosis of rapidly progressive glomerulonephritis. *Am J Kidney Dis* 39:28–35, 2002.
49. Cole E, Cattran D, Magil A, et al: A prospective randomized trial of plasma exchange as additive therapy in idiopathic crescentic glomerulonephritis. The Canadian Apheresis Study Group. *Am J Kidney Dis* 20:261–269, 1992.
50. Walters G, Willis NS, Graig JC: Interventions for renal vasculitis in adults. *Cochrane Database System Rev* (3):CD003232, 2008.
51. Kim HC. Red cell exchange: special focus on sickle cell disease. *Hematology* 2014:450–456.
52. Turner JM, Kaplan JB, Cohen HW, et al: Exchange versus simple transfusion for acute chest syndrome in sickle cell anemia adults. *Transfusion* 49:863–868, 2009.
53. Liem RI, O'Gorman MR, Brown DL: Effect of red cell exchange transfusion on plasma levels of inflammatory mediators in sickle cell patients with acute chest syndrome. *Am J Hematol* 76:19–25, 2004.
54. Boga C, Kozanoglu I, Ozdogu H, et al: Plasma exchange in critically ill patients with sickle cell disease. *Transfus Apher Sci* 37:17–22, 2007.
55. Marques MB, Singh N, Reddy VV. Out with the bad and in with the good; red cell exchange, white cell reduction, and platelet reduction. *J Clin Apher* 29:220–227, 2014.
56. Riddle MS, Jackson JL, Sanders JW, et al: Exchange transfusion as an adjunct therapy in severe Plasmodium falciparum malaria: a meta-analysis. *Clin Infect Dis* 34:1192–1198, 2002.
57. Shelat SG, Lott JP, Braga MS, et al: Considerations on the use of adjunct red blood cell exchange transfusion in the treatment of severe plasmodium falciparum malaria. *Transfusion* 50(4):875–880, 2009.
58. Nieuwenhuis JA, Meertens JHJM, Zijlstra JG, et al: Automated erythrocytapheresis in severe falciparum malaria: a critical appraisal. *Acta Trop* 98:201–206, 2006.
59. van Genderen PJJ, Hesselink DA, Bezemer JM, et al: Efficacy and safety of exchange transfusion as an adjunct therapy for severe Plasmodium falciparum malaria in non immune travelers: a 10-year single-center experience with a standardized treatment protocol. *Transfusion* 50(4):787–794, 2009.
60. Centers for Disease Control and Prevention: Available at http://www.cdc.gov/malaria/facts.htm.
61. Tan KR, Wiegand RE, Arguin PM: Exchange transfusion for severe malaria: evidence base and literature review. *Clin Infect Dis* 57:923–928, 2013.
62. Shaz BH, Schwartz J, Winters JL, et al. American society for apheresis guidelines support use of red cell exchange transfusion for severe malaria with high parasitemia. *Clin Infect Dis* 58:302–303, 2014.
63. Spaete J, Patrozou E, Rich JD, et al: Red cell exchange transfusion for babesiosis in Rhode Island. *J Clin Apher* 24:97–105, 2009.
64. Connelly-Smith LS, Linenberger ML. Therapeutic apheresis for patients with cancer. *Cancer Control* 1:60–78, 2015.
65. Blum W, Porcu P: Therapeutic apheresis in hyperleukocytosis and hyperviscosity syndrome. *Semin Thromb Hemost* 33:350–354, 2007.
66. Bug G, Anargyrou K, Tonn T, et al: Impact of leukapheresis on early death rate in adult acute myeloid leukemia presenting with hyperleukocytosis. *Transfusion* 47:1843–1850, 2007.
67. Oberoi S, Lehrnbecher T, Phillips B, et al. Leukapheresis and low-dose chemotherapy do not reduce early mortality in acute myeloid leukemia hyperleukocytosis: a systematic review and meta-analysis. *Leuk Res* 38:460–468, 2014.
68. Lowe EJ, Pui CH, Hancock ML, et al: Early complications in children with acute lymphoblastic leukemia presenting with hyperleukocytosis. *Pediatr Blood Cancer* 45:10–15, 2005.
69. Zarkovic M, Kwaan HC: Correction of hyperviscosity by apheresis. *Semin Thromb Hemost* 29:535–542, 2003.
70. Mesa R, Nagorney DS, Schwager S, et al: Palliative goals, patient selection, and perioperative platelet management. Outcomes and lessons from 3 decades of splenectomy for myelofibrosis with myeloid metaplasia at the Mayo Clinic. *Cancer* 107:361–370, 2006.

Section 10 PHARMACOLOGY, OVERDOSES, AND POISONINGS

STEVEN B. BIRD • LUKE YIP • KENNON HEARD

Chapter 97 ■ General Considerations in the Evaluation and Treatment of Poisoning

IAN M. BALL

The objective of this chapter is to provide the general intensivist with both an overview and an approach to the management of the critically ill poisoned patient. General concepts germane to the intensive care unit (ICU) will be introduced and explored. Every attempt has been made to be as evidence based as possible, within the intrinsic limitations of the medical toxicology literature.

Because overdose studies cannot ethically be performed in humans and animal data may not be available or applicable to humans, predicting the severity of poisoning must be based on toxicodynamic data from previously published reports of human poisonings. However, such data are often incomplete or altogether unavailable and are always limited by the accuracy of the overdose history.

Poisoning or *intoxication* is defined as the occurrence of harmful effects resulting from exposure to a foreign chemical or xenobiotic. Such effects may be local (i.e., limited to exposed body surfaces), subjective (i.e., symptoms only) or systemic and objective (e.g., behavioral, biochemical, cognitive, or physiological). In the absence of signs or symptoms, external or internal body contact with a potentially harmful amount of a chemical is merely an exposure. An *overdose* is an excessive exposure to a chemical that in specified (e.g., therapeutic) amounts is normally intended for human use. Whether an exposure or overdose results in poisoning depends more on the conditions of exposure (primarily the dose) than the identity of the agent involved. Ordinarily safe chemicals, even those essential for life such as oxygen and water, in excessive amounts or by an inappropriate route can result in harmful effects. Conversely, by limiting the dose, chemicals usually thought of as poisons can be rendered harmless. Poisoning is distinguished from adverse allergic, intolerance, and idiosyncratic pharmacogenetic reactions in that effects are concentration or dose related and, hence, predictable. As such, it includes adverse drug reactions due to unwanted secondary effects and pharmacokinetic and pharmacodynamic interactions.

Poisonings, exposures, and overdoses may be characterized by the route, duration, and intent of exposure. Ingestion, dermal or ophthalmic contact, inhalation, and parenteral injection (including bites and stings) are the most common routes, but rectal, urethral, vaginal, bladder, peritoneal, intraocular, and intrathecal exposures can also occur. Events that occur once or during a short period of time are considered acute, whereas those that occur repeatedly or over a prolonged time interval are said to be chronic.

EPIDEMIOLOGY

Although the true incidence of poisoning is difficult to accurately quantify, it is clearly a significant medical problem. Just over 2 million human exposures were reported to the National Poison Data System in 2013 [1]. Of these, 20% to 25% are treated at a health care facility, and approximately 6% are admitted to a hospital. Half of those admitted are treated in an ICU. In other countries, the ICU admission rate for those evaluated at a health care facility varies from 5% to 22% [2].

Exposures and poisonings are responsible for 1% to 5% of emergency department visits, 5% to 10% of all ambulance transports, 5% to 14% of adult ICU admissions, and 2% to 5% of pediatric hospital admissions [2–4]. In addition, 25% of routine medical admissions involve some form of drug-related adverse patient event (an adverse drug reaction or noncompliance), and up to 30% of acute psychiatric admissions are prompted by attempted self-harm via chemical exposure. Although the incidence of poisoning in children has decreased since the introduction of the Poison Prevention Packaging Act in 1970 [5], the overall incidence of poisoning increased over the past decade, particularly that due to suicide attempts in teens, middle-aged adults, and the elderly. The volume of calls handled by United States Poison Centers has flattened out over the past year [2]. Poisonings with less serious outcomes have decreased by 3.7% per year since 2008, while the incidence of more serious outcomes and death has increased by 4.7% per year since 2000 [2]. Poisoning is second only to firearms as the leading cause of suicide [2]. Poisoning is the second leading cause of injury death [1]. The yearly medical cost for the treatment of poisoning in the United States is estimated to be 26 billion [6]. Poisoning accounts for 6% of the economic costs of all injuries in the United States [6].

Most exposures reported to US poison centers are acute (90.9%), unintentional (83.2%), occur at home (92.9%), cause minor or no harmful effects (95%), result from ingestion (78.4%), and involve children 6 years of age or younger (51.2%) [1].

Poisoning accounts for 2% to 14% of all ICU admissions, with an average length of stay of about 3 days [2,4]. The mortality rate for such patients varies from 0.6% to 6.1% [3,4]. Although only 1,218 poisoning fatalities were reported by US poison centers in 2013 [1], death certificate data indicate that the true number of poisoning deaths is 20 to 50 times higher [7]. Poison center statistics vastly underestimate mortality from poisoning because they rarely capture cases in which the victim is found dead and goes directly to the medical examiner.

PHARMACOLOGICAL CONCEPTS

Toxic exposures all undergo the same pharmacological steps, as outlined in Table 97.1. Clinician familiarity with toxicokinetics is essential for predicting the effect of a particular exposure and guiding appropriate treatment and disposition. Only a brief overview of these concepts is presented here. The reader is referred to other sources for additional information [8–10]. Details regarding the disposition and toxic effects of specific agents can be found in subsequent chapters and other references [9–16].

TABLE 97.1

Toxicokinetic Stages

1. Absorption
2. Distribution
3. Metabolism
4. Excretion

Mechanism of Action

Most chemicals are absorbed and cause systemic poisoning by selectively binding to and disrupting the function of specific targets (e.g., enzymes, proteins, membrane lipids, or neurohumoral receptors). Effects may be systemic or limited to a specific organ or tissue, depending on the distribution and location of target site.

Poisoning is usually functional and reversible. Hence, if end-organ function can be supported, complete patient recovery is possible upon toxin elimination. However, if normal activity of the target site is essential for cell viability, a toxic exposure may result in necrosis. Agents that can cause fatal cellular damage include acetaminophen, carbon monoxide, corrosives, toxic alcohols, heavy metals, and neurotoxic hydrocarbons.

Absorption

Absorption involves the translocation of chemicals across the membranes of cells that make up mucosal surfaces, pulmonary epithelium, and skin, all of which function as biological barriers. Translocation occurs by filtration or passive diffusion through gaps or membrane pores by dissolving in and diffusing through the membrane itself (e.g., lipid-soluble chemicals), or by attaching to carrier molecules in the membrane, which actively or passively facilitate diffusion (e.g., water-soluble chemicals). The rate and extent of absorption depends on physical properties of the chemical and the route of exposure. In general, only chemicals that are small (i.e., <4 nm in diameter), have low molecular weight (i.e., <50 Da), and are soluble in both water and lipids at the pH of body fluids can readily cross membranes.

Absorption after intravenous injection is complete and almost instantaneous. Peak arterial and venous blood concentrations occur within 30 to 90 seconds. Most toxins cross biological membranes by simple passive diffusion. The rate at which this occurs is governed by Fick's law of diffusion.

$$\text{Rate of Diffusion} = dQ/dt = [DAK(C1 - C2)]/d$$

where D is the diffusion constant (constant for each toxin), A is the membrane surface area, K is the partition coefficient (represents the lipid: water partitioning of the toxin), d is the membrane thickness, and C is the toxin concentration. Pulmonary absorption is rapid but incomplete. Blood concentrations peak within seconds to minutes. The absorption of chemicals after intramuscular or subcutaneous injection is slower but relatively complete. Peak blood levels generally occur within an hour of administration. Poor water solubility (low K) is responsible for the slow absorption and long duration of action of intramuscular depot formulations (e.g., neuroleptics).

The rate and extent of absorption after ingestion are variable. Peak blood levels are typically noted within 0.5 to 2.0 hours of a therapeutic dose. The absorbed dose is proportional to, but not necessarily equal to, the administered dose. The rate and extent of absorption after contact with other mucosal surfaces (e.g., oral, nasal, ophthalmic, and rectal) is similar to ingestion. Skin absorption, if it occurs at all, is usually considerably slower. Regardless of route, absorption tends to follow first-order kinetics (i.e., the amount of chemical absorbed per unit of time is directly proportional to its concentration). *Hence, threshold tissue concentrations are usually reached more quickly and effects begin sooner after an overdose than after a therapeutic dose.*

Zero-Order Kinetics: rate of reaction is not proportional to toxin concentration

First-Order Kinetics: rate of reaction is proportional to toxin concentration

The dissolution and solvation of particulate material is often a rate-limiting step in gastrointestinal (GI) drug absorption. Hence, pill, solid, and suppository formulations tend to be absorbed more slowly than liquids, powders, or suspensions. Slow dissolution and solvation also account for the delayed and prolonged absorption of enteric-coated tablets (e.g., aspirin, potassium), sustained-release preparations (e.g., cardiovascular drugs, lithium, phenytoin, and theophylline), drugs that tend to form concretions (e.g., ethchlorvynol, glutethimide, heavy metals, iron, lithium, and meprobamate), and those with poor water solubility (e.g., carbamazepine and digoxin). The rate of dissolution is also inversely related to the tablet concentration. *Hence, absorption generally takes longer and peak effects occur later after an overdose than after a therapeutic one.*

Ingested chemicals are predominantly absorbed from the small intestine rather than the stomach, because the small intestine has a larger surface area. Hence, decreased gastric emptying or bowel activity caused by the presence of food, disease, or the effects of ingested agents (e.g., anticholinergics, opioids, sedative–hypnotics, and salicylates) can also delay or prolong absorption. Food and coingestants may decrease absorption by binding to the chemical within the gut lumen or by competitively inhibiting its dissolution and translocation. Absorption may also be decreased if intestinal motility is excessive.

Distribution

During distribution, chemicals may become bound to and inactivated by endogenous nontarget molecules such as serum proteins. The final distribution of chemical is uneven and reflects its affinity for active and inactive binding sites and the locations of such sites. It is also influenced by biological variables such as age, sex, weight, and disease states as they relate to body composition (e.g., water, fat, and muscle content) and serum protein concentrations. The extent of distribution of a chemical is reflected by its apparent volume of distribution, measured in liters per kilogram of body weight, and calculated most simply by dividing the amount of chemical in the body (i.e., the absorbed or bioavailable dose) by its plasma concentration.

Volume of Distribution = Bioavailable Dose/Plasma Concentration

Because distribution is also a translocation process, it is influenced by the same chemical characteristics as absorption and follows first-order kinetics. Distribution generally occurs much faster than absorption, as evidenced by the occurrence of peak effects within minutes of an IV drug injection. Slow distribution is partly responsible for the delayed onset of action of some agents (e.g., digitalis, heavy metals, lithium, and salicylates).

Tissue Concentration

The severity of poisoning reflects the concentration of a chemical at its site(s) of action and is proportional to the dose. Because the blood concentration of a chemical is also proportional to the dose, blood levels are sometimes used as a surrogate to assess the severity of poisoning. However, blood and target site concentrations are not always in steady-state equilibrium. When distribution occurs more slowly than absorption (e.g., after IV administration, inhalational exposure, and the ingestion of agents with inherently slow distribution), blood levels may be higher than those in tissue. Conversely, when redistribution of a chemical from tissue to blood occurs more slowly than elimination (e.g., after extracorporeal removal), blood levels may be lower than those in tissue. In both instances, blood levels do not accurately reflect those in tissue and do not correlate with the severity of poisoning.

Age, genetic influences, tolerance, underlying disease, and the presence or absence of other chemicals may have synergistic or antagonistic effects and may also influence the response to a given level of toxin exposure. The effect of metabolites must also be considered. Many chemicals have metabolites that remain pharmacologically active. Some (e.g., acetaminophen, toxic alcohols, chlorinated hydrocarbons, meperidine, paraquat, and certain organophosphate insecticides) undergo metabolic activation, resulting in the production of compounds that are more toxic than the parent one.

Metabolism/Elimination

Elimination of chemicals from the body (detoxification) is accomplished by urinary, pulmonary, GI, and glandular (e.g., bile, milk, tears, saliva, and sweat) excretion or metabolic inactivation. Hepatic metabolism and renal excretion are the major routes of elimination for most agents. Pulmonary excretion also plays a major role in the elimination of gases and volatile chemicals. Elimination generally follows first-order kinetics. For some toxins, hepatic metabolism has a finite capacity (i.e., becomes "saturated") and proceeds at a constant rate (zero-order kinetics). When the primary route of elimination is a zero-order metabolism, a small increase in dose can result in a large increase in blood and tissue concentrations and potential poisoning. Chemicals exhibiting such metabolism include alcohols, phenytoin, salicylate, and theophylline.

Renal excretion is accomplished by translocation processes (e.g., glomerular filtration, tubular secretion, and reabsorption) and is therefore influenced by the same factors as absorption and distribution. Any condition that impairs hepatic or renal blood flow or function can decrease toxin elimination. Metabolic enzymes are also subject to genetic influences and to induction or inhibition resulting from past or current chemical exposures. Regardless of the kinetics and route of elimination, the time required for elimination increases as the tissue concentration of chemical increases. *Hence, the duration of the effect tends to be longer after an overdose than after a therapeutic dose.*

CLINICAL CONSIDERATIONS

The principal objectives in the diagnosis and evaluation of the poisoning are recognition of an exposure or poisoning, identification of the offending agent(s), prediction of potential toxicity, and assessment of the severity of clinical effects. Treatment objectives include resuscitation, prevention of further absorption, enhancement of elimination, and the administration of antidotal or novel therapy (Table 97.2).

TABLE 97.2

Treatment Objectives—General Principles

1. Resuscitation
2. Prevention of further exposure
3. Enhanced elimination
4. Novel/antidotal therapy

Early accurate diagnosis is a prerequisite for optimal management.

The priority of assessment and treatment objectives depends on the phase of poisoning [17]. During the preclinical phase (the time between exposure and the onset of clinical or laboratory evidence of toxicity), management priorities include chemical identification, prediction of toxicity, and prevention of absorption (decontamination). The sooner decontamination is accomplished, the greater its efficacy. Hence, the physical examination and gathering of ancillary data should initially be brief. Assessment should focus on the exposure history, whether or not poisoning is likely to ensue, and whether or not decontamination is indicated.

During the toxic phase (the time between the onset of toxicity and its peak), assessment of the severity of poisoning, resuscitation, prevention of further absorption, enhancement of elimination, and antidotal/novel therapy are the primary objectives. If the patient is critically ill, the history, physical examination, and diagnostic testing must be conducted concurrently with resuscitation.

During the resolution phase (the time between peak toxicity and full recovery), continued supportive care, enhancement of elimination, antidotal therapy, and reassessment of severity (evaluation of the response to treatment) are the most important management considerations. Measures to prevent subsequent reexposure should also be initiated before discharge.

Recognition of Poisoning

Although poisoning can cause a wide variety of nonspecific signs and symptoms, the diagnosis can usually be established by the history, physical examination, routine and toxicologic laboratory evaluation, and the clinical course. Ideally, criteria similar to Koch's postulates for infectious disease should be met: A chemical is identified in or on the body in an amount known to cause the observed signs and symptoms within the reported time frame. In reality, the diagnosis is often made on the basis of a history of exposure, a clinical course consistent with poisoning, and exclusion of other etiologies.

Making the diagnosis can be easy when an accurate history of exposure is available. However, patients may be unaware of an exposure, unwilling to admit to one, or unable to give a history at all. Patients may give a history that is vague, confusing, or intentionally disguised.

Circumstances that should arouse suspicion of occult poisoning include sudden or unexplained illness in a previously healthy individual; similar unexplained symptoms in a group of individuals; a psychiatric history, alcoholism, or drug abuse; a recent change in health, economic status, or social relationships; and the onset of illness shortly after ingesting food, drink, or medication. Poisoning should always be considered in patients with metabolic abnormalities (especially acid–base disturbances), gastroenteritis, or changes in behavior or mental status of unclear etiology. Leakage of illicit drug packets that have been ingested or concealed in body cavities should be suspected in patients with altered mental status or unusual behavior who have just arrived from abroad (especially Asia and South America) or who have recently been arrested or incarcerated for criminal activity [18,19]. Drug intoxication is a risk factor for trauma and suicide and should also be considered in all injured patients.

To avoid missing the diagnosis of poisoning, the physician must specifically inquire about toxin exposure. In suspicious cases, the physician should assume the role of detective to elicit historical support for the diagnosis. Paramedics, police, and family, friends, employer, pharmacist, or personal physician can be questioned regarding the circumstances and events surrounding the illness, particularly the availability of chemicals and the likelihood of exposure. The patient's clothes and place of discovery should be searched for a suicide note, xenobiotics, and open or empty medication containers. Third parties should be instructed to search the house for such evidence and to bring it in for inspection.

In the absence of a history of exposure, the characteristic clinical course of poisoning may also suggest the diagnosis. Signs and symptoms of poisoning typically develop within minutes to an hour of an acute exposure, progress to a maximum within several hours, and gradually resolve over a period of hours to a few days. In such situations, toxicology screening may allow for a positive diagnosis if signs and symptoms are consistent with the known toxicity of the toxin(s) detected and other etiologies have been excluded.

Identification of the Offending Agent

History

The etiology of poisoning may or may not be disclosed by the patient history. Even when a history is available, its accuracy and reliability must be carefully assessed. The identity and amount of the toxin involved is frequently incorrectly reported by patients with intentional ingestions. Layperson misidentification of acetaminophen as aspirin and vice versa is relatively common. To avoid misdiagnosis, the presence or absence of both drugs should be confirmed by laboratory analysis when an overdose of any kind is suspected.

Pill, Product, Plant, and Animal Identification

Drugs in pill form can often be identified by the imprint code; the alphabetical and numeric markings on tablets and capsules. A listing of imprint codes with the corresponding trade name and ingredient(s) can be found in the Identidex portion of *Poisindex* [16], which is available at virtually all poison centers in the United States. It also provides the identities of street drugs based on their slang names. Prescription drugs may be identified by contacting the dispensing pharmacy. Drug samples can sometimes be identified by direct chemical analysis (see "Toxicology Screening" section). Police and government toxicology laboratories may be of assistance when illicit drug use is involved.

By US law [20], the ingredients of potentially hazardous commercial products used in and around the home must be stated on their labels. This information, however, is not always present or accurate, and labels may be missing or unreadable. In such cases, the ingredients may be identified by consulting *Poisindex* [16] or a regional poison center. Alternatively, the manufacturer or distributor may be called to obtain information. This may be particularly helpful when the product is an outdated formulation or a recently reformulated or released one. Most large companies maintain 24-hour emergency telephone numbers for such purposes, and many employ medical consultants to provide management advice. Although industrial products do not have the same labelling requirements as household ones, right-to-know legislation requires that companies make information regarding the ingredients and potential toxicity of products they make, distribute, or use available to workers and health care providers. Such information can be obtained by requesting a Material Safety Data Sheet (MSDS).

Information on drugs and chemical products manufactured or obtained outside the United States can be found in *Poisindex* [16] and *Martindale: The Complete Drug Reference* [12], or obtained from a domestic or foreign poison center. Information on drugs undergoing clinical trials in the United States may also be found in *Martindale*, since such drugs are often already available in other countries. Most foreign poison centers have English-speaking staff or translators available.

Plants (including fungi or mushrooms), along with their active parts and chemical constituents, can be identified by consulting *Poisindex* [16] if either their common or botanical name is known. If the name is not known but a sample is available, a representative from a local nursery, horticultural or mycologic society, or university botany department may be of assistance in identifying it. Similarly, pet stores, zoos, veterinarians, amateur or academic entomologists, herpetologists, zoologists, and field guides can be helpful in identifying potentially venomous insects, reptiles, snakes, and other animals. Poison centers usually maintain lists of local experts who are willing to help with such identifications.

Toxidrome Recognition

A toxidrome is a clinical syndrome that involves multiple physiologic systems and facilitates bedside identification of the culprit toxin's drug class. The physiological state of the patient can usually be characterized as excited (central nervous system [CNS] excitation with increased blood pressure, pulse, respirations, and temperature), depressed (decreased level of consciousness and decreased vital signs), discordant (inconsistent, mixed, or opposing CNS and vital sign abnormalities), or normal. The differential diagnosis can then be narrowed to the common or characteristic causes of these physiologic states (Table 97.3).

The *excited state* is primarily caused by sympathomimetics (agents that directly or indirectly stimulate α- and β-adrenergic receptors), anticholinergics (agents that block parasympathetic muscarinic receptors), hallucinogens, and withdrawal syndromes. The *depressed state* is primarily caused by sympatholytics (agents that block adrenergic receptors or depress cardiovascular activity), cholinergics (agents that directly or indirectly stimulate muscarinic receptors), opioids, or sedative hypnotics (which enhance the effect of the inhibitory CNS neurotransmitter γ-aminobutyric acid [GABA] or depress neuronal membrane excitability). The *discordant state* is primarily due to asphyxiants (agents that decrease the availability, absorption, transport, or use of oxygen), membrane active agents (those that block sodium channels or otherwise alter the activity of excitable cell membranes), and agents that cause a variety of CNS syndromes due to interference with dopamine, GABA, glycine, or the synthesis, metabolism, or function of serotonin. A *normal physiological state* may be due to a nontoxic exposure (Table 97.4), psychogenic illness, or presentation during the preclinical phase of poisoning. Agents that have a long preclinical phase (delayed onset of toxicity) are known as toxic "time bombs." Delayed onset of toxicity may result from slow absorption or distribution, metabolic activation, or a mechanism of action that involves the disruption of metabolic or synthetic pathways. Psychogenic illness should be considered when symptoms are inconsistent with the reported exposure and cannot be substantiated by objective physical findings, laboratory abnormalities, and toxicologic testing and other etiologies have been excluded [21].

An excited or depressed state may be mischaracterized as a discordant one when the activity of a stimulant or depressant is selective for a receptor subtype or results in a compensatory or opposing autonomic response. For example, hypotension caused by an α-blocker, β_2-agonist, or vasodilator may be accompanied by tachycardia, and hypertension due to a selective α-agonist (phenylpropanolamine) may be accompanied by bradycardia. Severe stimulant or depressant poisoning can also cause what appears to be a discordant state (Table 97.5). For example, prolonged seizures and extreme hyperthermia caused by sympathomimetics can culminate in cardiovascular collapse as a consequence of anaerobic metabolism, acidosis, or depletion of neurotransmitters. Similarly, marked hypotension and hypoventilation caused by physiologic depressants can precipitate seizures and tachyarrhythmias as a result of ischemia, anoxia, and acidosis. In addition, paradoxic excitation can result from the preferential inhibition of cortical function that normally controls social activity by low doses of CNS depressants, most

TABLE 97.3

Differential Diagnosis of Poisoning Based on Physiological Assessment and Underlying Mechanisms

Excited (CNS stimulation with increased vital signs)	Depressed (CNS depression with decreased vital signs)	Discordant (mixed CNS and vital sign abnormalities)	Normal
Sympathomimetics	**Sympatholytics**	**Asphyxiants**	**Nontoxic exposure**
Amphetamines	α-Adrenergic antagonists	Carbon monoxide	**Psychogenic illness**
Bronchodilators (β-agonists)	Angiotensin-converting enzyme inhibitors	Cyanide	**Toxic time bombs**
Catecholamine analogues	β-Adrenergic blockers	Hydrogen sulfide	Acetaminophen
Cocaine	Calcium channel blockers	Inert (simple) gases	Agents that form concretions
Decongestants	Clonidine gestants	Irritant gases	Amanita phalloides and related mushrooms
Ergot alkaloids	Cyclic antidepressants	Methemoglobinemia	Anticholinergics
Methylxanthines	Decongestants (imidazolines)	Oxidative phosphorylation inhibitors	Cancer therapeutics
Monoamine oxidase inhibitors	Digitalis	Herbicides (nitrophenols)	Carbamazepine
Thyroid hormones	Neuroleptics	**AGMA inducers**	Chloramphenicol
Anticholinergics	**Cholinergics**	Alcoholic ketoacidosis	Chlorinated hydrocarbons
Antihistamines	Bethanechol	Ethylene glycol	Colchicine
Antispasmodics (GI-GU)	Carbamate insecticides	Iron	Digitalis preparations
Atropine and other belladonna alkaloids	Echothiophate	Methanol (formaldehyde)	Dilantin kapseals
Cyclic antidepressants	Myasthenia gravis therapeutics	Paraldehyde	Disulfiram
Cyclobenzaprine	Nicotine	Metformin/phenformin (chronic)	Enteric-coated pills
Mydriatics (topical)	Organophosphate insecticides	Salicylate	Ethylene glycol
Nonprescription sleep aids	Physostigmine	Toluene	Heavy metals
Orphenadrine	Pilocarpine	Valproic acid	Fluoride
Parkinsonian therapeutics	Urecholine	**CNS syndromes**	Immunosuppressive agents
Phenothiazines	**Opioids**	Disulfiram	Lithium
Plants/mushrooms	Analgesics	Extrapyramidal reactions	Lomotil (atropine and diphenoxylate)
Hallucinogens	Antidiarrheal drugs	Isoniazid (GABA lytic)	Methanol
LSD and tryptamine derivatives	Fentanyl and derivatives	Neuroleptic malignant syndrome	Methemoglobin inducers(some)
Marijuana	Heroin	Serotonin syndrome	Monoamine oxidase inhibitors
Mescaline and amphetamine derivatives	Opium	Solvents (hydrocarbons)	Paraquat
Psilocybin mushrooms	**Sedative-hypnotics**	Strychnine (glycinergic)	Opioids
Phencyclidine	Alcohols	**Membrane active agents**	Organophosphate insecticides (some)
Withdrawal syndromes	Anticonvulsants	Amantadine	Podophyllin
Baclofen	Barbiturates	Antiarrhythmics	Salicylates
β-Adrenergic blockers	Benzodiazepines	β-Blockers	Sustained-release formulations
Clonidine	Bromide	Cyclic antidepressants	Thyroid hormone synthesis inhibitors
Cyclic antidepressants	Ethchlorvynol	Fluoride	Thyroxine valproic acid
Ethanol	GHB	Heavy metals	Viral antimicrobials
Opioids	Glutethimide	Lithium	
Sedative hypnotics	Methyprylon	Local anesthetics	
	Muscle relaxants	Meperidine/propoxyphene	
		Neuroleptics	
		Quinine (antimalarials)	

AGMA, anion gap metabolic acidosis; CNS, central nervous system; GABA, γ-aminobutyric acid; GHB, γ-hydroxybutyrate; GI–GU, gastrointestinal–genitourinary; LSD, lysergic acid diethylamide.

TABLE 97.4

Criteria for a Nontoxic Exposure

Patient is asymptomatic by both history and physical examination
Amount and identity of all chemicals and time of exposure are known with high degree of certainty
Exposure dose is less than the smallest dose known or predicted to cause toxicity

notably alcohol and other sedative hypnotics. In such cases, the physiologic state and its cause can often be correctly identified by the overall clinical picture and course of events.

The severity of mental status changes and the nature of associated autonomic findings can be used to narrow the differential diagnosis of physiological stimulation and depression to one of four subcategories (see Table 97.3). For the excited patient, marked vital sign abnormalities (severe hypertension with end-organ ischemia, tachyarrhythmias, hyperthermia, and cardiovascular collapse) with minor mental status changes suggest an agent with peripheral sympathomimetic activity as

TABLE 97.5

Physiological Grading of the Severity of Poisoning

Severity	Signs and symptoms: Stimulant poisoning	Signs and symptoms: Depressant poisoning
Grade 1	Agitation, anxiety, diaphoresis, hyperreflexia, mydriasis, tremors	Ataxia, confusion, lethargy, weakness, verbal, able to follow commands
Grade 2	Confusion, fever, hyperactivity, hypertension, tachycardia, tachypnea	Mild coma (nonverbal but responsive to pain); brainstem and deep tendon reflexes intact
Grade 3	Delirium, hallucinations, hyperpyrexia, tachyarrhythmias	Moderate coma (respiratory depression, unresponsive to pain); some but not all reflexes absent
Grade 4	Coma, cardiovascular collapse, seizures	Deep coma (apnea, cardiovascular depression); all reflexes absent

the cause. Conversely, marked mental status abnormalities with nearly normal vital signs suggest a centrally acting hallucinogen. Anticholinergic poisoning (Table 97.6) can be differentiated from sympathomimetic (Table 97.7), hallucinogen, and withdrawal syndromes by the presence of dry, flushed, and hot skin; decreased or absent bowel sounds; and urinary retention. Other causes of excitation are usually accompanied by pallor, diaphoresis, and increased bowel or bladder activity.

In the patient with physiological depression, marked cardiovascular abnormalities (hypotension and bradycardia) with relatively clear sensorium suggest a peripherally acting sympatholytic, whereas marked CNS and respiratory depression with minimal pulse and blood pressure abnormalities suggest a centrally acting agent (opioid or sedative hypnotic). Cholinergic poisoning (Table 97.8) can be distinguished from other causes of physiologic depression by the presence of characteristic autonomic findings: *S*alivation, *l*acrimation, *u*rination, *d*efecation, *G*I cramps, and *e*mesis (SLUDGE syndrome). In addition, cholinergic poisoning causes pallor and diaphoresis, whereas the skin is usually warm and dry with opioid and sedative–hypnotic poisoning.

TABLE 97.6

Anticholinergic Toxidrome

Tachycardia
Hyperthermia
Hallucination/confusion
Dry mouth/garbled speech
Mydriasis
Ileus
Urinary retention
Dry, flushed skin

TABLE 97.7

Sympathomimetic Toxidrome

Mydriasis
Agitation
Diaphoresis
Hypertension
Hyperthermia
Tachycardia

TABLE 97.8

Cholinergic Toxidrome

Salivation
Lacrimation
Urination
Defecation
GI cramps
Emesis

Other findings can sometimes help narrow the differential diagnosis further. Only the most common and diagnostically useful ones are noted here. Because of limited specificity and sensitivity, the presence or absence of a particular sign or symptom cannot be used to confirm or exclude a given etiology.

Ocular findings can sometimes help narrow the diagnostic possibilities. Although mydriasis can be caused by any agent or condition that results in physiologic excitation (see Table 97.3), it is most pronounced in anticholinergic poisoning, in which it is associated with minimal pupil response to light and accommodation. Similarly, although miosis is a nonspecific manifestation of physiological depression, it is usually most pronounced in opioid poisoning. Notable miosis can, however, also be caused by cholinergic agents and sympatholytics with α-blocking effects (e.g., phenothiazines). Visual disturbances suggest anticholinergic, cholinergic, digitalis, hallucinogen, methanol, and quinine poisoning. Horizontal nystagmus and disconjugate gaze are nonspecific manifestations of sedative–hypnotic poisoning. Although vertical and rotary nystagmus can be seen in patients with lithium and phenytoin poisoning, they are classical findings of phencyclidine intoxication. These etiologies should be readily distinguishable by assessing the physiological state. Rapidly alternating lateral "ping-pong" gaze has been described in monoamine oxidase inhibitor poisoning. Except for abnormalities due to topical chemical exposure, both eyes are equally affected. Although failure to respond to topical miotics has been said to be diagnostic of drug-induced pupillary dilatation, this is only true for topical exposures. Hence, unilateral pupillary abnormalities should generally prompt evaluation for a central, structural lesion.

Dermatological abnormalities may also be helpful. Flushed skin can be caused by anticholinergics, boric acid, a disulfiram-ethanol reaction, monosodium glutamate, niacin, scombroid (fish poisoning), and rapid infusion of vancomycin (red man syndrome). The skin is hot and dry in anticholinergic poisoning but normal or moist with other etiologies. Flushing should not be confused with the orange skin discoloration caused by rifampin. Pallor and diaphoresis may be due to cholinergics, hallucinogens, hypoglycemics, sympathomimetics, and drug withdrawal (see Table 97.3). As noted previously, manifestations of the SLUDGE syndrome distinguish cholinergic poisoning from other etiologies. Cyanosis may be due to agents that cause cardiovascular or respiratory depression, methemoglobinemia, pneumonitis, or simple asphyxia. For methemoglobinemia, skin may have a slate-gray hue that is unaffected by oxygen administration. Cyanosis should not be confused with the blue discoloration of the skin caused by amiodarone or by topical exposure to blue dyes. The latter condition can be diagnosed by wiping the skin with acetone or alcohol. Hair loss, mucosal pigmentation, and nail abnormalities are suggestive of heavy metal poisoning (arsenic, lead, mercury, and thallium).

Finally, the presence of neuromuscular abnormalities may suggest certain etiologies. Seizures and tremors can be caused by cholinergics, hypoglycemic agents, lithium, membrane-active agents, some narcotics (meperidine, propoxyphene), and stimulants (see Table 97.3). They can also occur in patients poisoned by agents that cause asphyxia, low lactate increased anion gap metabolic acidosis (AGMA; see later), and cerebral hypoperfusion or hypoventilation (physiologic depressants; see Table 97.3). The most common causes of seizures due to poisoning are tricyclic antidepressants, sympathomimetics, antihistamines (primarily diphenhydramine), theophylline, and isoniazid. Although carbon monoxide, hypoglycemics, lithium, and theophylline can cause focal seizures, seizures due to poisoning are usually generalized. Because hypertensive and traumatic CNS hemorrhages are known complications of poisoning, the possibility structural lesions should always be considered. Myoclonus suggests anticholinergic, sympathomimetic poisoning, or Serotonin syndrome. Fasciculations are typical of cholinergic insecticide poisoning but can also be caused by sympathomimetics. Rigidity may be seen in phencyclidine and sympathomimetic poisoning and in those with CNS syndromes (see Table 97.3). Dystonic posturing is most often caused by antipsychotic agents. It is also a characteristic feature of strychnine poisoning.

Laboratory Findings

Acid–base status, anion gap, serum osmolality, ketone, electrolyte, glucose, and organ function abnormalities identified by routine laboratory tests can be extremely helpful in the differential diagnosis of poisoning. As with clinical manifestations, the diagnostic sensitivity and specificity of a single finding is not sufficiently high for its presence or absence to confirm or exclude a specific etiology. The use of anion and osmolar gaps and serum ketone and lactate levels in the diagnosis of poisoning of unknown etiology is summarized in Figure 97.1.

Assessing acid–base status and calculating the anion gap is particularly important because an increased AGMA may be due to advanced ethylene glycol, methanol, and salicylate poisoning. In such cases, prompt initiation of specific therapies is essential to prevent progressive, irreversible, or fatal poisoning [22]. The normal anion gap is 13 ± 4 mEq per L in unselected acutely hospitalized patients. In ethylene glycol and methanol poisoning, AGMA is primarily due to the accumulation of acid metabolites. In salicylate poisoning, it is caused by the accumulation of a variety of endogenous organic acids resulting from salicylate's interference with intermediary metabolism. Agents that cause hypoxemia, cellular asphyxia, seizures, shock, or extensive tissue necrosis can also cause an AGMA, but in these instances, the accumulation of lactic acid generated by anaerobic metabolism is responsible for the AGMA. When the underlying cause is unclear, measuring the serum lactate level may be helpful. The lactate concentration is usually low (<5 mEq per L) or significantly less than the anion gap in ethylene glycol, methanol, and salicylate poisoning, but higher in conditions associated with anaerobic metabolism.

Other common toxicologic causes of a low-lactate AGMA include ethanol, which can cause ketoacidosis by disrupting intermediary metabolism in susceptible alcoholics, and toluene,

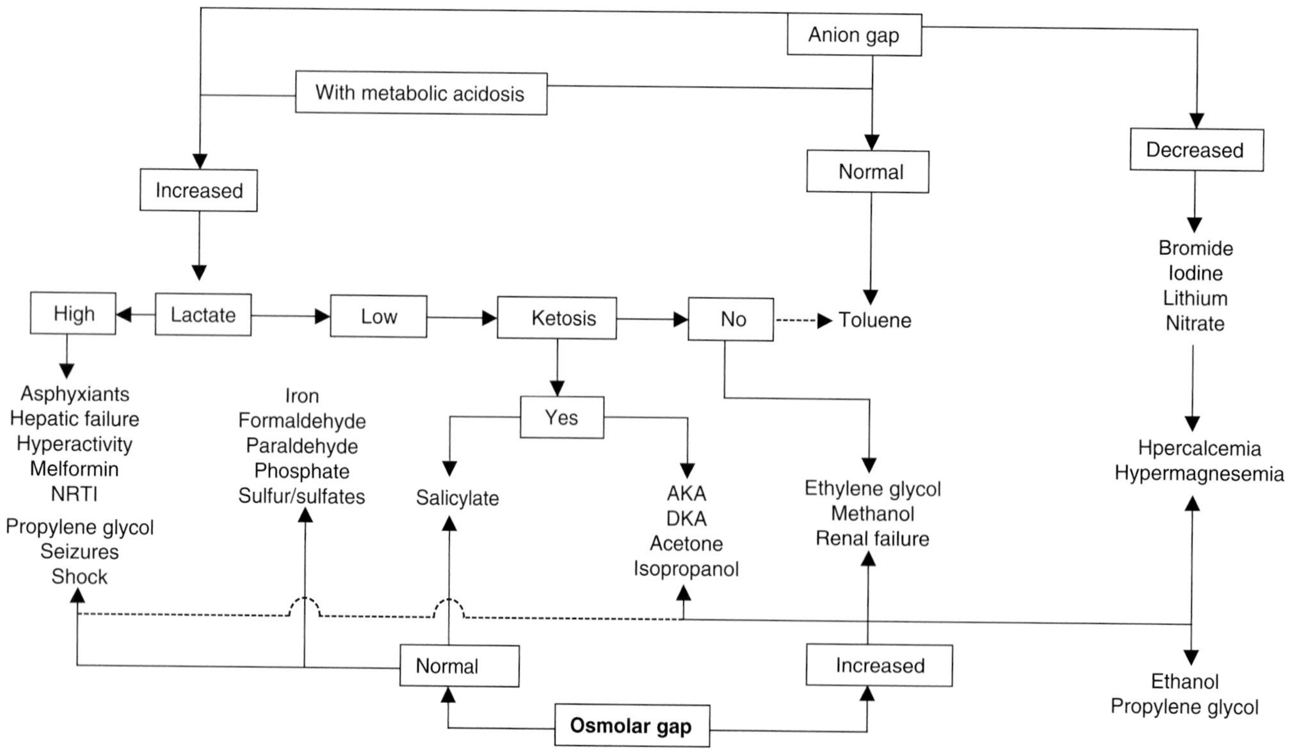

FIGURE 97.1 Use of routine laboratory findings and calculated gaps in the differential diagnosis of poisonings. AKA, alcoholic ketoacidosis; DKA, diabetic ketoacidosis; NRTI, nucleoside/nucleotide reverse transcriptase inhibitors.

which can cause renal tubular acidosis with bicarbonate wasting. Rarely, this metabolic picture occurs in poisoning by formaldehyde (which is metabolized to formic acid), paraldehyde (presumably as a result of its metabolism to acetic acid), phosphate, and sulfur (and possibly sulfates). It can also be seen with large overdoses of ibuprofen (and probably all nonsteroidal anti-inflammatory agents) and valproic acid (due to high levels of these acidic drugs and their metabolites). Metformin and nucleoside reverse transcriptase inhibitor antiretroviral agents (e.g., zidovudine or azidothymidine) can interfere with normal-lactate metabolism and cause a high-lactate AGMA at therapeutic as well as excessive doses. A high-lactate AGMA can occur soon after massive acetaminophen ingestion [23].

An abnormally low anion gap may be seen in severe bromide, calcium, iodine, lithium, magnesium, and nitrate intoxication [24]. In bromide, iodine, and lithium intoxication, the low anion gap results from spuriously elevated chloride levels, and with nitrate poisoning, it is due to falsely elevated bicarbonate levels.

Serum osmolality can help differentiate the toxic causes of a low-lactate AGMA. An increased osmole gap may be seen early in the course of ethylene glycol and methanol (when high serum levels of the parent compounds are present) but not salicylate poisoning. Although not strictly accurate from a physical chemistry perspective [25], the osmole gap is typically defined as the difference between the measured serum osmolality and the calculated serum osmolality.

$$\text{Serum Osmolality } (\mu\text{mol/L}) = 2\ (\text{serum Na}) + \text{serum glucose} + \text{serum BUN}$$

where normal serum osmolality is 290 ± 10 mOsm per kg of H_2O normal osmole gap is 5 ± 7 mOsm per kg (in unselected acutely hospitalized patients [22]).

$$\text{Osmole gap} = [\text{calculated serum osmolality} - \text{measured serum osmolality}]$$

Normal osmole gap is 5 ± 7 mOsm per kg (in unselected hospitalized patients [22]).

This formula assumes that all concentrations are measured in millimoles per liter. If the glucose and BUN concentrations are measured in milligrams per deciliter, dividing them by 18 and 3, respectively, gives their approximate concentrations in millimoles.

Additional causes of an increased osmolar gap include other low-molecular-weight solutes, such as acetone, ethanol, isopropyl alcohol, magnesium, mannitol, and propylene glycol [26]. The approximate concentration of these substances that will increase the serum osmolality by 1 mOsm per kg of H_2O, calculated on the basis of their molecular weights, is shown in Table 97.9. When direct measurements are not readily available, the serum concentration of these agents can be estimated by multiplying this amount by the osmolar gap. Serum osmolality must be measured by freezing point depression (rather than the headspace or vapor pressure method) to detect the presence of volatile agents such as acetone and toxic alcohols. An increased osmolar gap can be seen in alcoholic ketoacidosis and other conditions causing lactic acidosis.

Serum ketones can also help to differentiate the toxic causes of a low-lactate AGMA. Ketosis, as defined by a positive nitroprusside reaction, is relatively common in salicylate poisoning but unusual in ethylene glycol and methanol poisoning. Ketosis is also seen in alcoholic ketoacidosis and in acetone or isopropyl alcohol poisoning.

The urinalysis, serum calcium concentration, and the overall clinical picture can also be helpful in differentiating the toxic causes of a low-lactate AGMA. Crystalluria, hypocalcemia, and back pain or flank tenderness suggest ethylene glycol; visual symptoms implicate methanol; and tinnitus or impaired hearing point to salicylates. Crystalluria can also be caused by acyclovir [27], felbamate [28], indinavir [29], oxalate [18], primidone [19], and sulfa drugs [30]. Hypocalcemia is also seen in fluoride and oxalate [18] intoxication.

TABLE 97.9

Effects of Some Solutes on Serum Osmolality

Solute	Approximate concentration required to increase serum osmolality by 1 mOsm/kg
Alcohols, glycols, and ketones	
Acetone	5.8 mg/dL
Ethanol	4.6 mg/dL
Ethylene glycol	5.2 mg/dL
Isopropanol	6.0 mg/dL
Methanol	2.6 mg/dL
Propylene glycol	7.6 mg/dL
Electrolytes	
Calcium	4.0 mg/dL (1 mEq/L)
Magnesium	2.4 mg/dL (1 mEq/L)
Sugars	
Mannitol	18 mg/dL
Sorbitol	18 mg/dL

Serum potassium and glucose abnormalities may also provide clues to the etiology of the poisoning [11]. Toxicologic causes of hypokalemia include barium, β_2-adrenergic agonists, calcium channel blockers, chloroquine, diuretics, insulin, licorice, methylxanthines, and toluene. Hyperkalemia can be caused by α-adrenergic agonists, angiotensin-converting enzyme inhibitors, β-blockers, digitalis, fluoride, potassium-sparing diuretics, and trimethoprim. Common toxicologic causes of hypoglycemia are ethanol, β-blockers, hypoglycemics, quinine, and salicylate. Common causes of hyperglycemia include acetone, β-agonists, calcium channel blockers, iron, and methylxanthines.

Common toxicologic causes of acute liver dysfunction are acetaminophen, ethanol, halogenated hydrocarbons (carbon tetrachloride), heavy metals, and mushrooms (*Amanita phalloides* and related species). Acute renal toxicity is most often due to ethylene glycol, halogenated hydrocarbons, heavy metals, nonsteroidal anti-inflammatory drugs, toluene, envenomations, and agents that cause hemolysis or rhabdomyolysis. An elevated creatinine with a normal BUN can be seen in acetone and isopropyl alcohol poisoning because acetone interferes with colorimetric assays for creatinine, resulting in falsely high results. Acute hemolysis (in the absence of glucose-6-phosphate dehydrogenase deficiency) can result from poisoning by arsine gas, naphthalene, and inducers of methemoglobinemia. Rhabdomyolysis is associated with toluene abuse, CNS syndromes (see Table 97.3), and severe physiological dysfunction (extreme agitation, deep or prolonged coma, hyperthermia, and seizures) of any etiology. The most common agents involved are sympathomimetics, ethanol, and MDMA.

Electrocardiographic Findings

The ECG may provide clues to the cause of poisoning [11]. Ventricular tachyarrhythmias that occur in patients with normal QRS and QT intervals suggest myocardial irritation (increased automaticity) as the underlying mechanism. Sympathomimetics, digitalis, and cardiac-sensitizing agents such as chloral hydrate and aliphatic or halogenated hydrocarbons, which potentiate the action of endogenous catecholamines, are potential causes. In contrast, ventricular tachyarrhythmias that occur in the setting of depolarization and repolarization abnormalities, reflected by QRS and QT interval prolongation, respectively, suggest a reentrant mechanism. Causes include electrolyte abnormalities, organophosphate insecticides, and other membrane active agents (see Table 97.1). Torsades de pointes (polymorphous) ventricular tachycardia strongly implicates a QTc prolonging agent.

Atrioventricular conduction abnormalities and bradyarrhythmias can be caused by β-blockers, calcium channel blockers, digitalis, membrane-active psychotherapeutic agents, organophosphate insecticides, and α-agonists such as phenylpropanolamine.

Radiographic Findings

Ingested chemicals can sometimes be visualized within the GI tract by abdominal radiographic imaging, and such imaging can occasionally be helpful in suggesting the etiology or amount of an unknown ingestion. Agents most likely to be visible on plain films are indicated by the mnemonic CHIPES (Table 97.10) [11].

Ingested drug packets may appear as uniform, marble-sized densities scattered along the GI tract [31,32]. Ingested hydrocarbons may sometimes appear as a double gastric fluid level or "double bubble" because of the air–fluid and fluid–fluid interface lines created when less dense hydrocarbons layer on top of gastric fluids. Computed tomography may be superior to plain films in detecting ingested drug packets but the optimal test in this setting remains unclear [33]. Whether or not contrast should be used remains controversial. Abdominal ultrasound can detect ingested pills, particularly enteric-coated and sustained-released formulations. Such imaging may be useful in confirming or refuting some recent specific (CHIPES) ingestions. Because the volume of pills can be determined, plain radiography may be used to guide GI decontamination.

Abnormal findings on chest radiography can be caused by a wide variety of chemicals [11]. Diffuse or patchy infiltrates (pneumonitis or acute lung injury) can be due to the inhalation of irritant gases (ammonia, chlorine, hydrogen sulfide, nitrogen oxides, phosgene, smoke, and sulfur dioxide), fumes (beryllium, metal oxides, and polymers), and vapors (acids, aldehydes, hydrocarbons, isocyanates, and mercury). They can also be seen among patients who have ingested or injected cholinergic agents (carbamate and organophosphate insecticides), metabolic poisons (cyanide, carbon monoxide, heavy metals, and hydrogen sulfide), paraquat, phencyclidine, salicylates, thiazide diuretics, and tocolytics, and in patients with envenomations. Aspiration pneumonitis is quite common and can occur in patients with coma or seizures. Acute lung injury can also develop among patients with prolonged or pronounced anoxia, hyperthermia, or hypotension. Chronic chemical exposure can cause pulmonary fibrosis, granulomas, or pleural plaques.

Response to Antidotes

The use of antidotes for diagnostic purposes has largely fallen from favor. The availability of point of care blood glucose measurement negates the need for empiric intravenous dextrose in altered patients. Many antidotes may be harmful if used inappropriately, including flumazenil physostigmine, glucagon, nitrites, chelators, and lipid emulsions. Naloxone remains a reasonably safe therapy for a patient with clinical signs of opiate intoxication. Clinicians should be prepared to manage acute withdrawal and its sequelae.

Toxicology Screening

Analyses of a sample of the toxin itself, or patient urine, blood, or gastric contents can sometimes be helpful for identifying the cause of poisoning. Urine is generally the best specimen to analyze, because large quantities can be obtained for extraction procedures and many chemicals are concentrated in urine. However, toxicology testing can detect only a small fraction of all chemicals (primarily drugs) and is not always reliable. Immunoassay screens are inexpensive and provide results within minutes, but they are only capable of detecting a few agents. They suffer from many false positives and false negatives. Patients may be misdiagnosed and potentially harmed by clinicians acting solely on the results of immunoassay screens [34]. Comprehensive screens are expensive and require 2 to 6 hours for completion (excluding transportation times). Although results may increase diagnostic certainty or specificity, they rarely change disposition or treatment in patients who are asymptomatic or who have signs and symptoms consistent with the reported exposure [34–37]. Noteworthy exceptions are acetaminophen and salicylate, which are widely available, commonly ingested, sometimes misidentified, require specific treatment, and cause few or nonspecific early signs and symptoms. Hence, in most overdose patients, quantitative acetaminophen and salicylate levels are the only *screening* toxicology tests likely to be clinically useful.

Critically ill poisoned patients suffering seizures, cardiovascular instability, acid–base abnormalities, multiple-organ dysfunction, nonsinus cardiac rhythms, or cardiac conduction disturbance without a toxicologic diagnosis should generally have comprehensive toxicology screening.

Knowledge of the methods used for chemical detection (colorimetric spot tests, thin-layer chromatography, gas or high-pressure liquid chromatography, absorbance, atomic absorption, flame ionization, or fluorometric assays, enzyme-multiplied and radionuclide immunoassays, and gas chromatography with mass spectrometry) is required for optimum interpretation of screening tests results [21,34,38]. A positive result on one assay should always be confirmed by repeat analysis using a different technique. The physician should communicate directly with the laboratory technician to determine which chemicals can be detected by the screening methods used and the sensitivity and specificity of each assay. In addition, directed analysis (coma, hallucinogen, or stimulant screen), with more rapidly available results, can be performed when the technician and clinician communicate.

A negative result from a screen should never be used to exclude the diagnosis of poisoning when clinical findings suggest otherwise. It may simply mean a chemical is not detectable by the assay(s) used, its concentration is below the limit of detection of the assay(s), or its concentration is too low to be confirmed. It may also mean the timing of sampling or the specimen submitted is inappropriate for testing (the chemical may be undergoing absorption and is not yet present in urine or it may already have been metabolized or eliminated). In such cases, repeating the test on a sample obtained at an earlier or later time may be revealing.

TABLE 97.10

Xenobiotics Visible on Plain Stomach Radiographs

Chlorinated hydrocarbons
Heavy metals
Iodinated compounds
Packets of drugs
Enteric-coated drugs
Salicylates

Prediction of Potential Toxicity

The prediction of toxicity requires knowledge of the dose, time, and identity of an exposure and helps optimize treatment. For commercial products, the amount and concentration of every ingredient should be identified. Household products deemed hazardous by the US Consumer Product Safety Committee are required by law to bear a label describing the nature of their toxicity and first aid measures as well as a "keep out of reach of children" warning and a signal word that indicates the degree or severity of potential toxicity [20]. The signal words "caution," "warning," and "danger" identify a product or its constituent(s) as a weak irritant (may damage mucosal surfaces), strong irritant (can damage skin and mucosa), or corrosive (can cause permanent tissue damage or death) after topical exposure or moderately toxic, highly toxic, or extremely toxic (oral median lethal dose: 50 to 500 mg per kg, 1 to 50 mg per kg, or <1 mg per kg, respectively) after ingestion. Label information is frequently inaccurate or incomplete [20] and should generally be confirmed by consulting an independent information source.

The dose of drug in a pill or tablet can be determined using the resources cited in "Identification of the Offending Agent" section of this chapter. For liquids and powders, the dose can be estimated or measured using the container or the weights and volumes listed on the label. An exposure may also be reported in tablespoons or swallows. Standard flatware volumes can vary from 3 to 7 mL for a teaspoon and from 7 to 14 mL for a tablespoon. The volume of a swallow varies with age, height, weight, sex, the orifice size of the container, and the viscosity of the ingested liquid and ranges from 1 to 5 mL in infants to 4 to 40 mL in adults [39].

The accuracy and reliability of the history must be evaluated when assessing potential toxicity. The amount and time of ingestion are frequently erroneous when reported by patients with intentional self-poisoning. It is always best to assume a worst-case scenario: that the maximum possible dose (the entire amount available or not clearly accounted for) was ingested. The potential toxicity can then be estimated from previously reported toxicodynamic data. For drugs with CNS and cardiovascular activity, the ingestion of 5 to 10 therapeutic doses by an adult and one adult dose by a young child can result in significant toxicity. β-Blockers, calcium channel blockers, and oral hypoglycemics can cause toxicity after only one or two therapeutic doses, particularly in those physiologically naive to their effects. The ingestion of only one to two tablets, capsules, or teaspoonfuls of an antimalarial (chloroquine, hydroxychloroquine), antipsychotic, camphor, calcium channel blocker, methyl salicylate, opioid, oral hypoglycemic, theophylline, or tricyclic antidepressant can be fatal to a toddler [40].

The time of exposure is important because it helps to predict the times of toxicity onset and of peak toxicity. Only when the time elapsed since exposure clearly exceeds the longest reported or predicted interval between exposure and peak toxicity should the possibility of subsequent poisoning be excluded (see Table 97.5). Peak toxicity usually occurs within 4 to 6 hours of an oral overdose. Important exceptions to this generalization are the toxic time bombs described earlier. For some of these agents (acetaminophen, ethylene glycol, methanol, and paraquat), the serum concentration measured during the preclinical phase can be used to predict subsequent toxicity. Peak toxicity may also be delayed (up to 12 to 24 hours) after exposure to irritants and corrosives. The possibility of pregnancy and potential toxicity to the fetus should also be considered.

Assessment of Severity

The severity of poisoning is primarily determined by the clinical picture. Because poisoning is far more dynamic than most diseases and illnesses, frequent reevaluations are required. Poisoned patients can rapidly deteriorate, with few or no warning signs.

A complete physical examination should be performed in all patients. The examination should initially be directed toward assessment of cardiovascular stability, respiratory function, and neurologic status. Accurate and timely measurement of all vital signs is essential. The respiratory rate should be measured accurately. A core temperature should be obtained to detect severe or occult abnormalities. The most severe patients are most likely to have significant temperature abnormalities. Preoccupation with their cardiovascular and respiratory therapy may lead to delayed temperature measurement. An abbreviated mental status examination is usually sufficient.

The number and type of ancillary tests required to assess metabolic or organ function is determined primarily by clinical severity and secondarily by the history. Asymptomatic but potentially poisoned patients with reliable histories and unintentional exposures should have blood and urine samples obtained on presentation. Samples can be saved and subsequently sent for (baseline) analysis in the event of deterioration. Pregnancy testing is recommended in all susceptible women of childbearing age. Patients who are symptomatic or suicidal should have serum electrolytes, BUN, creatinine, glucose, urinalysis, and 12-lead ECG. Arterial blood gas, serum osmolality, and ketone and methemoglobin analyses may be indicated. Anion, osmolal, and oxygen saturation gaps should be calculated whenever their determinants are measured. Assessment of patients with respiratory complaints or grade 2 or greater stimulant or depressant poisoning (see Table 97.5) should include a chest radiograph. A complete blood cell count, coagulation studies, serum amylase, calcium, magnesium, creatine phosphokinase, and hepatic enzyme levels should also be determined in any patient with grade 2 or greater physiological dysfunction. Additional testing should be individualized and based on the history, physical examination findings, and the results of routine ancillary studies.

The measurement of chemical concentrations in serum or urine can sometimes help in assessing the severity of poisoning. Agents for which quantitative measurements are necessary or desirable for optimal patient management include acetaminophen, acetone, alcohols, antiarrhythmics, antiepileptics, barbiturates, carbon monoxide, digoxin, electrolytes (including calcium and magnesium), toxic alcohols, heavy metals, lithium, salicylate, and theophylline [21,34]. Quantitative or qualitative assays for other toxins are not generally helpful because they serve only to confirm the clinical impression and do not affect treatment (which is either supportive or must be initiated long before laboratory results are available in order to be effective).

Provision of Supportive Care

Meticulous supportive care is necessary to maintain physiological and biochemical homeostasis and to prevent secondary complications (anoxia, aspiration, and secondary organ injury) until detoxification is complete. Despite advances in preventing absorption, enhancing elimination, and antidotal treatment, supportive care remains the mainstay of therapy for most poisoned patients. Details of supportive therapy by organ system can be found in the delineated chapters. Only considerations of special relevance to the poisoned patient are discussed here.

Monitoring

Unless toxicity is minimal and predicted with a high degree of certainty to remain so, venous access should be established and continuous cardiac monitoring initiated. Pulse oximetry should be performed on presentation and monitored frequently if abnormal or significant (grade 2 or greater) physiologic dysfunction (see Table 97.5) is present. Until the ultimate severity of poisoning is known, frequent or continuous visual observation is also necessary. Patients with intentional self-poisoning also need close behavioral observation until the possibility of a repeat suicide attempt has been evaluated in detail and assessed to be unlikely.

Respiratory Care

Aspiration of gastric contents is a relatively common complication of poisoning and its treatment (during GI decontamination procedures). Patients with CNS depression or seizures are at particularly high risk. For patients deemed high risk for aspiration, or whose clinical conditions are likely to progress to requiring airway protection, endotracheal intubation should be performed early. Prophylactic or therapeutic intubation may also be required for patients with extreme behavioral agitation or physiological over activity who require aggressive pharmacologic therapy with a sedative, antipsychotic, anticonvulsant, or the combination of a neuromuscular blocking agent with a sedative.

Cardiovascular Therapy

Because of adverse drug interactions, therapy intended to maintain or restore normal blood pressure, pulse, and sinus rhythm may paradoxically worsen cardiovascular toxicity. Hence, the severity and trend of cardiovascular abnormalities and the potential complications of treatment should be considered before instituting pharmacological therapy. In addition, because the causes of cardiovascular toxicity are varied and multiple mechanisms may be concurrently operative, invasive hemodynamic monitoring may be necessary for accurate diagnosis and optimal treatment. Aggressive supportive measures, such as transvenous cardiac pacing and intra-aortic balloon pump or extracorporeal membrane oxygenation should be considered in patients with reversible poisoning who are unresponsive to less aggressive therapeutic measures [41]. Intoxicated patients tend to deteriorate more quickly than standard ICU patients, so the necessary consults to initiate ECMO should be made as early as possible. The required duration of ECMO will be much shorter for intoxicated patients than for other ICU patients.

In the absence of extremes of heart rate, hypotension due to poisoning is most often caused by loss of peripheral vascular tone rather than pump failure. Bedside echocardiography can also be useful to assess cardiac output. Norepinephrine is generally considered the first line vasopressor for patients who do not respond to fluid administration.

When hypertension causes end-organ dysfunction, therapy is indicated. For patients with sympathomimetic poisoning, β-blockade may result in unopposed α-receptor stimulation. This leads to increased peripheral vascular resistance, increasing the demand on a β-blocked heart. Hence, treatment with a nonselective sympatholytic or with an arteriodilator followed by a β-blocker is preferred.

Sinus tachycardia can usually be managed with sympatholytics. In patients with sympathomimetic poisoning and signs or symptoms of myocardial ischemia, a β-blocker (with or without an arteriodilator, depending on the presence or absence of coexisting hypertension) or a calcium channel blocker can be used.

Amiodarone is generally first line therapy for ventricular tachyarrhythmias. Underlying electrolyte and metabolic abnormalities should be corrected. Sodium bicarbonate or hypertonic saline may be effective in treating wide-complex tachycardias due to toxins with sodium channel blocking properties.

Normalizing electrolytes and continuous electrocardiographic monitoring is the mainstay of treatment for toxins that prolong the QT interval. The clinician must be prepared to manage Torsades des Pointes. Antibodies are available to treat serious dysrhythmias caused by cardiac glycosides. Magnesium may also be effective in digitalis poisoning. Procainamide, other class 1 A agents (including Phenytoin), β-blockers, and physostigmine should not be used for arrhythmias caused by membrane-active agents or those associated with prolonged QRS or QT intervals because of the potential for worsening rhythm disturbances and conduction abnormalities.

Bradycardia requires treatment only if it is associated with hemodynamic instability. In most cases, atropine, dopamine, and epinephrine are the agents of choice. Glucagon, Calcium, high dose insulin, and lipid therapy can be effective in β-blocker poisoning. Calcium, high dose insulin, and lipid therapy can be effective in calcium channel blocker poisoning.

Treatment of Neuromuscular Hyperactivity

Profound metabolic acidosis and sudden cardiac arrest can occur in patients with severe agitation who continue to struggle while being physically restrained. Prompt pharmacologic treatment of behavioral and muscular hyperactivity in such patients is critical. In general, benzodiazepines are preferred to antipsychotic agents because the latter lower the seizure threshold and prolong QTc. We have decades of experience and safety data supporting the use of benzodiazepines in this setting. For agitation and hallucinations due to anticholinergic poisoning, physostigmine may be considered.

Seizures can usually be effectively treated with GABA agonists such as benzodiazepines or propofol. Pyridoxine is usually necessary in isoniazid poisoning. Phenytoin, a Vaughn–Williams class 1 anticonvulsant, should be avoided in all cases where a toxin with sodium channel blocking properties may have been ingested. Seizures due to cyanide, hydrogen sulfide, and organophosphate insecticides usually require specific antidotes. Please see Chapter 151 for detailed discussion of the treatment of seizures.

Severe agitation or prolonged convulsions can also cause rhabdomyolysis and hyperthermia. Because these complications can result in additional organ dysfunction, neuromuscular blocking agents should be given to patients after they do not respond to sedatives alone. During such therapy, vigilant monitoring for seizures is important (electroencephalography is recommended) because urgent effective treatment can prevent permanent neurologic damage.

Prevention of Absorption

Early and effective decontamination can limit the surface exposure and systemic absorption of chemicals and reduce toxicity. Decontamination should be considered in all patients unless the exposure is clearly nontoxic (see Table 97.4), the time of predicted peak toxicity has passed, or the benefit of decontamination is minimal.

Body Cavity Exposure

The removal of chemicals from body cavities (bladder, external auditory canal, nose, rectum, and vagina) can be accomplished by aspiration and irrigation using normal saline. Particulate matter (pills, suppositories, and drug packages) should be manually removed, preferably under direct visualization. The removal of ingested drug packages from the GI tract is discussed in "Ingestion" section of this chapter.

Eye and Skin Exposure

Decontamination after topical exposure includes manual removal of particulate material, irrigation of exposed surfaces, and a scrub for skin exposed to noncorrosive chemicals. Because "time is damage," particularly with corrosives, tap water or any other readily available liquid that is clear and drinkable can be used in the prehospital setting. If exposure involves an unknown chemical, its pH should be measured. Searching for pH paper (pHydrion), usually available in the emergency department or the labor and delivery area, should not delay treatment. Irrigation should initially be performed for about 20 minutes. Prolonged irrigation (up to 24 hours) may be beneficial for corrosive exposures, especially those involving strong alkali.

With ocular exposures, blepharospasm secondary to pain can prevent effective irrigation unless treatment is preceded by the instillation of a topical anesthetic. Particulate material should be removed with a moist cotton-tipped swab or eye spud. Normal saline and lactated Ringer's solution are traditionally used irrigation fluids. Irrigating solutions can be administered via an IV infusion setup, directly through the tubing, or via an irrigating (Morgan) lens attachment. A low-pressure squeeze bottle also may be used. One or two liters is usually sufficient. For acid or alkali exposures, the tear pH (normally 7.3 to 7.7) should be determined before and after irrigation. Irrigation should continue until the pH is between 5 and 8.

For skin exposures, treatment should begin with the removal of contaminated clothing. Gloves should be worn to prevent contamination of caretakers. Particulate matter should be removed from the skin using a soft brush, forceps, or hand-held vacuum cleaner before irrigation. Washing the skin with soap and water or isopropyl alcohol more effectively prevents pesticide absorption than using water alone. For some toxins, a triple wash (irrigation and washing with soap before and after an alcohol scrub) may provide better decontamination than irrigation alone.

Ingestion

GI decontamination can be accomplished with activated charcoal, gastric lavage, whole-bowel irrigation, and endoscopic or surgical removal of the ingested chemical. There is little to no role for Ipecac [42,43]. Cathartics, although previously used in conjunction with other treatments, are not an effective method of decontamination [44]. Except for cases of corrosive ingestion, the same is true for diluents.

Despite extensive experimental data documenting the efficacy of GI decontamination measures for preventing chemical absorption in animals and in human volunteers, there is no conclusive evidence that these interventions improve the outcome in actual overdose patients [42,44–48]. Clinical efficacy is difficult to prove because the overdose history is frequently unreliable, and most overdoses do not cause severe or life-threatening toxicity. In addition, the efficacy of GI decontamination decreases as the time between ingestion and treatment increases. Experimental data showing that GI decontamination is effective in preventing chemical absorption when initiated more than 1 hour after ingestion is limited. Since the mean time between ingestion and arrival at a hospital is more than 1 hour in children and more than 3 hours in adults [49–52], most patients present for treatment at a time when the efficacy of GI decontamination remains unproven.

With the sophisticated monitoring and supportive techniques available today, it is more likely that most poisoned patients will recover fully without any decontamination therapy [51]. However, since experimental studies show that decontamination can limit toxin absorption and shorten the duration of toxicity, and since absorption is prolonged after overdose, decontamination may be effective longer after ingestion than experimentally proven. It is therefore recommended that it be performed unless the exposure is nontoxic (see Table 97.4), or the risk of decontamination outweighs the potential benefit.

The choice of decontamination method should be based on the relative efficacy, and contraindications of the available options. Activated charcoal has equal or greater efficacy, fewer contraindications, less frequent and less serious complications than other methods of decontamination, and is the preferred treatment for most overdoses [48–53]. Emptying the stomach via lavage has rare, specific indications.

Gastric lavage is indicated for recent life-threatening ingestions, when the toxin is small in size or easily dissolved in the stomach, not well adsorbed by activated charcoal and not responsive to other therapies. Whole-bowel irrigation should be considered for patients who have ingested toxic amounts of agents that are slowly absorbed or not amenable to decontamination by other techniques. Endoscopy and surgery should be reserved for patients with potentially severe poisoning in whom alternative methods of decontamination are unsuccessful or contraindicated.

Activated Charcoal. Activated charcoal can prevent absorption of ingested chemicals by binding them within the gut lumen. Its clinical efficacy remains controversial [48] because it is neither absorbed nor metabolized, the toxin bound to it is normally eliminated with stool [47,54]. Activated charcoal is a fine black powder produced by the activation (pyrolysis, oxidation, and purification) of carbon-containing materials such as bone, coal, peat, petroleum, and wood. It is odorless, tasteless, and insoluble in liquids. The activation process yields particles that have an extensive internal network of minute, branching, irregular, interconnecting channels that range in size from approximately 10 to 100 nm in diameter and account for the extremely large surface area of activated charcoal. The surface area of activated charcoal in clinical use ranges from 600 to 2,000 m^2 per g.

The absorption or adherence of chemical molecules to the external and internal surfaces of activated charcoal is rapid (within minutes of contact). It is due to relatively weak van der Waals forces and can be described by the following reversible equilibrium: activated charcoal + toxin ↔ activated charcoal – toxin complex. Hence, as the amount of activated charcoal is increased, the fraction of unbound or free chemical decreases (the equilibrium shifts to the right according to the law of mass action). At an activated charcoal to chemical ratio of 10 to 1 or greater, 90% or more of most chemicals is adsorbed into charcoal in vitro. The absorptive capacity (the amount of chemical that can be absorbed by 1 g of charcoal in vitro) ranges from a few milligrams to more than 1 g depending on the molecular size, structure, and solubility of the chemical, the pore size and surface area of activated charcoal, the negative logarithm of acid ionization constant of the chemical and the pH of the solution, and the presence or absence of competing solutes. Small, highly ionized molecules of inorganic compounds, such as acids, alkali, electrolytes, and the readily dissociable salts of arsenic, bromide, cyanide, fluoride, iron, and lithium, are not well adsorbed by activated charcoal [54].

In animal studies and in simulated overdoses using therapeutic or slightly greater doses in human volunteers, activated charcoal prevents the GI absorption of nearly all chemicals [55]. In agreement with in vitro studies, as the ratio of activated charcoal to chemical increases, its efficacy increases; with simultaneous dosing of activated charcoal and chemical at a ratio of 10 to 1 or greater, charcoal prevents the absorption of most chemicals by more than 90%. At a constant charcoal to chemical ratio, the efficacy of activated charcoal in preventing chemical absorption increases as the amount and concentration of either agent increases [54,55], suggesting that the efficacy of activated charcoal may be relatively greater after actual overdose than it is after a simulated one. Diluting a dose of activated charcoal and administering it in aliquots by gastric lavage is less effective than administering the same dose as a single concentrated bolus [54]. Administering a dose before and after gastric lavage is more effective than giving one only after lavage.

The interval between administration of toxin and activated charcoal also has a significant effect on the in vivo efficacy of charcoal. As this interval increases, the ability of activated charcoal to prevent chemical absorption decreases. In controlled studies using doses of activated charcoal many times greater than those of toxin, charcoal decreased chemical absorption an average of 71% (range 10% to 100%) when it was given within 5 minutes, 52% (range 17% to 75%) when given at 30 minutes, and 38%, 34%, 21%, 29%, and 14% when given at 1, 2, 3, 4, and 6 hours, respectively [47].

The ability of activated charcoal to prevent the absorption of a toxin in vivo generally correlates with its ability to absorb that chemical in vitro [55]. However, the absorption of some toxins that are poorly adherent to activated charcoal (e.g., cyanide, malathion, and tolbutamide) is significantly reduced. Conversely, the absorption of some toxins that are relatively adherent to activated charcoal in vitro (ethanol, ipecac, and *N*-acetylcysteine) is not significantly inhibited in vivo. The presence of food in the stomach appears to enhance the efficacy of activated charcoal in preventing the absorption of ingested agents, possibly by slowing gastric emptying. Coingested antacids, cathartics, chocolate, ethanol, and excipients have variable but relatively minor or no effect on its efficacy.

Activated charcoal is administered as an aqueous suspension; a minimum of 8 mL of water should be added to each gram of powdered charcoal if a premixed formulation is not available. Premixed product containers should be thoroughly agitated to resuspend sedimented charcoal before use.

Activated charcoal can be given orally to awake patients or by gastric tube to comatose or uncooperative patients. A nipple bottle can be used for infants. The recommended dose is at least 10 times the weight of the ingested toxin. Because of volume constraints, the maximum single dose is generally limited to 1 to 2 g per kg of body weight.

Compared with other methods of GI decontamination, the advantages of activated charcoal are ease of administration, rapidity of action, extensively documented safety and efficacy, lack of absolute contraindications, and its ability to enhance toxin elimination (see "Multiple-Dose Activated Charcoal" section of this chapter). The main disadvantages are its dark color (significantly impairs bronchoscopy if aspirated), and low or reversible binding of some chemicals. It can also prevent the enteral absorption and enhance elimination of drugs administered for therapeutic purposes. Aspiration of activated charcoal along with gastric contents can result in large and small airway obstruction, pneumonitis, and death [56,57].

Although there are no absolute contraindications, activated charcoal is not recommended for ingestions of acids, alkali, and hydrocarbons that are poorly absorbed and have low systemic toxicity (low-viscosity petroleum distillates and turpentine) [47,48,54]. It does not adsorb these corrosives and obscures endoscopic assessment of the extent of injury. With hydrocarbons, it may promote vomiting and increase the risk of pulmonary aspiration.

Gastric Lavage. Gastric lavage can directly remove ingested chemicals from the stomach and thereby prevent their absorption [45]. As with activated charcoal, the efficacy of gastric lavage decreases as the time between ingestion and treatment increases. In animal studies and in simulated overdoses in human volunteers, gastric lavage decreased chemical absorption an average of 42% (range 29% to 90%) when performed within 20 minutes of chemical administration, 26% (13% to 38%) when performed at 30 minutes, and 17% (8% to 32%) when performed at 60 minutes [45]. Efficacy is enhanced if activated charcoal is given before and after lavage, but not if it is only given afterward [43].

Gastric lavage is performed by first aspirating stomach contents and then repetitively instilling and withdrawing fluid through a large orogastric tube. It appears to be most effective if the patient is placed in a left lateral decubitus Trendelenburg position. The left lateral decubitus position has also been shown to delay spontaneous drug absorption [58].

The simplest, quickest, and least expensive method to use is a funnel connected to the lavage tube, raising it 2 to 3 feet above the level of the stomach when administering fluid and lowering it 2 to 3 feet below the stomach to allow drainage [59]. Tap water is the lavage fluid of choice for patients older than 2 years. The optimal volume of fluid for each lavage cycle is unclear. Recommended amounts range from 60 to 800 mL for adults and up to 10 mL per kg of body weight for children [45]. Larger aliquots (5 to 10 mL per kg body weight) are superior to smaller ones. It is recommended that lavage be continued until the return is relatively clear.

Although endotracheal intubation does not completely prevent aspiration during gastric lavage, it is recommended to reduce the risk of aspiration, facilitate other investigations and for the patient's predicted clinical course [45].

As in experimental studies, the clinical efficacy of gastric lavage decreases as the time between overdose and initiation of treatment increases. The efficacy of gastric lavage increases in cases of toxin induced gastroparesis or decreased intestinal motility.

Although there are no absolute contraindications to gastric lavage, its use for corrosive and hydrocarbon ingestions is not recommended [45,57]. With corrosives, insertion of a tube may increase the risk of esophageal perforation. Gastric lavage should be reserved for large ingestions of liquid acid or alkali and for agents that can cause systemic toxicity (heavy metals, hydrazine), and only if it can be performed within 1 to 2 hours of exposure. Because lavage may increase the risk of pulmonary aspiration after hydrocarbon ingestion, it should only be considered for large ingestions of agents that have systemic toxicity (camphor, halogenated and aromatic derivatives, and those that contain heavy metals or pesticides) and in conjunction with the advice of a poison center.

Syrup of Ipecac. Although syrup of ipecac is simple to use, and was once widely available for home administration, it is less effective than activated charcoal in preventing chemical absorption in experimental studies and has more contraindications [42]. Vomiting exposes patients to aspiration risks and may preclude the administration of activated charcoal or other oral antidotes. There is virtually no role for Ipecac in the critically ill poisoned patient.

Whole-Bowel Irrigation. *Whole-bowel irrigation* refers to the enteral administration of large volumes of an electrolyte solution. It is commonly used to cleanse the GI tract before colonoscopy, barium enema radiography, and bowel surgery and can prevent the absorption of ingested chemicals by increasing gut motility [46,60].

In experimental studies, whole-bowel irrigation decreased chemical absorption by about 70% (range, 67% to 73%) when initiated 1 hour after simulated overdose of ampicillin, paraquat, and sustained-release formulations of aspirin and lithium and 4 hours after a supratherapeutic dose of enteric-coated aspirin [60–62]. Whole-bowel irrigation solutions have been found both to enhance [63,64] and to interfere [60,62] with the in vitro adsorptive capacity of activated charcoal.

Whole-bowel irrigation is performed by administering a solution of electrolytes and polyethylene glycol by nasogastric tube at a rate of 0.5 L per hour in children 9 months to 6 years of age, 1 L per hour for 6- to 12-year-olds, and 2 L per hour for those older than 12 years, until the rectal effluent is clear, which typically takes 2 to 4 hours.

In human volunteer studies, whole-bowel irrigation was more effective than gastric lavage [60,65]. The combination of charcoal followed by whole-bowel irrigation was more effective than whole-bowel irrigation alone [61,62]. Although no controlled studies addressing efficacy in overdose patients have been performed, it may be useful for ingestions of enteric-coated or sustained-release pharmaceuticals, foreign bodies (bezoars, button batteries, drug packets, and lead paint chips), and agents that are poorly adsorbed by activated charcoal (iron and other metals), and for patients with extremely large ingestions or delayed presentations [47,64–70]. Potential complications of whole-bowel irrigation include regurgitation and aspiration of gastric contents and abdominal distension with cramping [47,61]. Whole-bowel irrigation does not cause fluid and/or electrolyte abnormalities. Disadvantages of whole-bowel irrigation are that it is unpleasant, labor intensive, and time-consuming. Contraindications include bowel obstruction, perforation or ileus, and hemodynamic instability. It can be safely performed in intubated obtunded patients.

Endoscopy and Surgery. Gastric endoscopy, using baskets or snares to grasp or break up particulate chemicals, can be used to remove foreign bodies (button batteries that break apart or fail to pass beyond the pylorus) and gastric pill bezoars (see "Absorption" section). It should be reserved for patients with severe or potentially lethal poisoning, such as those with large amounts of heavy metal visible in the stomach on radiograph and those who continue to deteriorate and have rising drug levels despite attempts at GI decontamination by other methods. Endoscopy should never be used for the removal of drug packets, because it may cause rupture and lethal toxicity.

Immediate retrieval by laparotomy is indicated for patients who develop toxicity after the ingestion of packets containing cocaine. Surgery should also be considered when endoscopic removal is unsuccessful or impossible because of the location of the toxin or foreign body [71].

Cathartics. Cathartics are osmotically active saccharides (mannitol, sorbitol) or salts (magnesium citrate, magnesium sulfate, and disodium phosphate) that cause retention of fluids within the gut, thereby stimulating GI motility and the evacuation of intestinal contents [44,72]. In animal and human volunteer studies, cathartics have variable but clinically insignificant effects on chemical absorption [44]. Their effect on the efficacy of activated charcoal is also minimal and clinically insignificant [73,74]. There is currently no role for cathartics in the critically ill poisoned patient.

Dilution. The administration of water, milk, or other drinkable liquids is now recommended as a primary treatment only for corrosive ingestions. In this setting, dilution may lower the concentration of chemical and limit its toxicity. To be effective, dilution should be accomplished as soon as possible. The volume of fluid should not exceed 5 mL per kg, because larger amounts may induce vomiting and cause further esophageal exposure. Dilution is no longer recommended to prevent toxin absorption. It may facilitate the dissolution of solid chemicals, increase the amount of chemical in solution, and stimulate gastric emptying, thereby enhancing chemical absorption.

Antidotal Therapy

Antidotes directly or indirectly counteract the effects of toxins [10,11]. They can be classified as *selective* or *nonselective*. Selective antidotes act by competing with chemicals for target sites or metabolic pathways, by binding and neutralizing them, by promoting their metabolic detoxification, and by antagonizing their autonomic effects via activation or inhibition of opposing neuronal pathways (see Table 97.11). Nonselective antidotes act by correcting metabolic derangements or enhancing nonmetabolic toxin elimination.

Although antidotes can reduce morbidity and mortality, few are available and most are potentially harmful. Reasonable diagnostic certainty is necessary for their safe and effective use. Specific indications, contraindications, dosing, and potential complications are discussed in the following chapters. A summary Table of antidotes can be found in the Appendix.

Enhancement of Elimination

The nonmetabolic elimination of most toxins can be accelerated by therapeutic interventions such as diuresis, urine alkalization, GI dialysis (i.e., multiple-dose activated charcoal or whole-bowel irrigation), and extracorporeal techniques.

All enhanced elimination procedures are associated with potential complications, and some require specialized equipment and expertise. Reasonable diagnostic certainty is generally a prerequisite to their use. In general, invasive elimination procedures should be reserved for patients with severe poisoning and/or those who deteriorate or fail to improve despite aggressive supportive care, antidotal therapy, and noninvasive methods of toxin removal.

TABLE 97.11

Chemicals and Toxic Syndromes with Specific Antidotes

Agent/condition	Antidotes
Acetaminophen	*N*-acetylcysteine
Anticholinergic poisoning	Physostigmine
Anticoagulants	Phytonadione (vitamin K), protamine
Benzodiazepines	Flumazenil
β-adrenergic antagonists	Glucagon, calcium salts
Calcium channel blockers	Calcium salts, glucagons
Carbon monoxide	Oxygen, hyperbaric oxygen
Cholinergic syndrome	Atropine, pralidoxime
Cyanide	Nitrites, thiosulfate, hydroxycobal
Digoxin (digitalis)	Fab antibody fragments, magnesium
Dystonic reactions	Benztropine, diphenhydramine
Ethylene glycol	Ethanol, 4-methylpyrazole, pyridoxine, thiamine
Envenomations (arthropod, snake)	Antivenins
Fluoride	Calcium and magnesium salts
Heavy metals (arsenic, mercury, lead)	British antilewisite (dimercaprol), dimercaptosuccinic acid, D-penicillamine, calcium disodium, ethylenediaminetetraacetic acid
Hydrogen sulfide	Oxygen, nitrites
Iron	Deferoxamine
Isoniazid (hydrazines)	*γ*-Aminobutyric acid agonists, pyridoxine
Methanol	Ethanol, 4-methylpyrazole, folate
Methemoglobinemia	Methylene blue
Opioids	Naloxone, nalmefene, naltrexone
Sympathomimetics	Adrenergic blockers
Vacor (*N*-3-pyridylmethyl-*N*′–P-nitrophenylurea)	Nicotinamide (niacinamide)

Diuresis and Manipulation of Urinary pH

Maintenance of a dilute urine flow enhances toxin excretion by decreasing the passive distal tubular reabsorption of toxins that have undergone glomerular filtration and proximal tubular secretion [9–11]. Increasing urinary pH (considered neutral at a pH of 6) can enhance the renal excretion of acidic toxins by a mechanism known as ion trapping. Like all membranes, those of the nephron, particularly the distal tubule, are generally more permeable to nonionized and nonpolar molecules than to ionized and polar ones. After filtration and secretion, nonionized forms of weak acids become ionized and trapped in an alkaline urine. Diuresis and urinary alkalinization act synergistically [75].

Diuresis alone can enhance the renal excretion of alcohols, bromide, calcium, fluoride, lithium, meprobamate, potassium, and isoniazid. Except for calcium and potassium, however, clinical efficacy remains unproven.

Alkalinization of the urine can enhance the excretion of the chlorophenoxy acetic acid herbicide 2,4-D (and probably 2,4,5-T), chlorpropamide, diflunisal, fluoride, methotrexate, phenobarbital (and probably other long-acting barbiturates), sulfonamides, and salicylates. Only for phenobarbital and salicylate poisoning is urinary alkalization accepted as clinically effective [76].

The goal of urinary alkalinization is a urine pH of 7.5 or greater. An alkaline diuresis solution can be prepared by adding three ampules (132 mEq) of sodium bicarbonate to dextrose 5% in water such that the final solution is nearly isotonic. Fluids are administered at roughly the same rate as the desired urine output. Acetazolamide should not be used to produce an alkaline urine because it may worsen toxicity by causing a concomitant systemic acidosis, resulting in an increase in the amount of unionized drug in the blood and enhanced tissue distribution. It may also compete with acidic drugs for tubular secretion and thereby inhibit their elimination. Systemic hypokalemia will prevent effective urine alkalinization by retention of potassium and excretion of hydrogen ions into the urine at the level of the hydrogen potassium ATPase.

Acid–base status, fluid balance, electrolyte parameters, and clinical response must be carefully monitored during therapy. Urine pH should be measured hourly.

Multiple-Dose Activated Charcoal

Repetitive activated charcoal administration can enhance the elimination of previously absorbed chemicals by binding them within the GI tract as they are excreted in the bile, secreted by cells of the stomach or intestine, or passively diffuse into the lumen of the gut [55,77–79]. The charcoal–chemical complex is then excreted with stool. Multidose activated charcoal works by reverse absorption, using the entire surface of the gut acting as a dialysis membrane. Activated charcoal keeps the concentration of free toxin in gut fluids near zero, and chemicals diffuse from blood perfusing the gut into luminal fluids as a result of concentration gradients. Interruption of enterohepatic or enteroenteric recirculation appears to be the underlying mechanism of action for a minority of toxins. Theoretically, multiple-dose charcoal can enhance the elimination of any chemical whose absorption is decreased by a single dose. Efficacy is predicted to be greatest for chemicals with a high charcoal binding capacity, physical, and pharmacokinetic characteristics that make them amenable to removal by extracorporeal methods (see later), and a long intrinsic elimination half-life (amiodarone, isotretinoin, organochlorine pesticides, and organometallic compounds) [80].

Multiple-dose activated charcoal enhances the elimination of most chemicals regardless of whether the chemical is administered orally or parenterally [79]. As with most forms of decontamination, the clinical efficacy of this therapy is difficult to prove. Although clinically significant reductions in half-life have been noted in patients with carbamazepine, dapsone, phenobarbital, quinine, and theophylline overdose, there are no prospective studies showing that this therapy reduces morbidity or mortality [79].

The efficacy of multiple-dose activated charcoal increases as the cumulative amount of charcoal administered increases. When the cumulative amount of charcoal remains constant, there is no difference in the efficacy of different dosing regimens (25 g every 2 hours vs. 50 g every 4 hours) [81]. With normal bowel activity, doses of activated charcoal of 0.5 to 1.0 g per kg every 4 hours are generally well tolerated. In those with decreased GI motility, smaller doses or less frequent intervals should be used. Alternatively, charcoal can be given by a slow, continuous nasogastric infusion. This method of administration may also be better for patients who cannot retain charcoal because of vomiting. Metoclopramide and ondansetron (or other serotonergic antiemetics) can also be given to control or prevent vomiting. Gastric aspiration should be performed before repeating the dose of charcoal.

Complications of multiple-dose activated charcoal are similar to those for charcoal used for GI decontamination. In addition, intestinal obstruction, pseudo-obstruction, and nonocclusive intestinal infarction have been reported in patients with decreased bowel motility treated with multiple doses of activated charcoal [82,83].

Extracorporeal Methods

Peritoneal dialysis, hemodialysis, hemoperfusion, hemofiltration, plasmapheresis, and exchange transfusion are theoretically capable of removing any chemical from the blood [81]. Most toxins undergo significant tissue distribution, and few remain in the blood in amounts high enough to warrant extracorporeal removal. Hemodialysis is therefore most effective for toxins with volumes of distribution less than 1 L per kg. In addition, with dialysis techniques, only toxins that are small (molecular weight less than 500 to 1,500 Da), water soluble, and not highly bound to serum proteins (90% to 95% or less) readily diffuse across dialysis membranes. (Table 97.12) There remains very little evidence regarding the efficacy of continuous renal replacement therapy (CRRT) in the management of human poisonings. Even at high flow rates, CRRT's ability to clear toxins is a fraction of that of traditional intermittent hemodialysis (IHD).

The clearance of a toxin by extracorporeal removal must be significantly greater than its intrinsic total body clearance (the sum of metabolic, renal, and other routes of clearance) to be considered effective from a pharmacokinetic perspective. As with other treatments, renal replacement therapy's efficacy (ability to decrease morbidity and mortality) is based on observation, experience, and retrospective comparisons rather than on controlled prospective studies.

Hemodialysis is considered effective for the treatment of barbiturate, bromide, chloral hydrate, ethanol, ethylene glycol, isopropyl alcohol, lithium, methanol, procainamide, acetaminophen, theophylline, and salicylate poisoning. Because hemodialysis can remove toxins from the blood faster than they can redistribute from tissue to blood, a rebound increase in blood concentration and clinical relapse may occur within 1 or 2 hours of treatment.

TABLE 97.12

Properties of a Dialyzable Toxin

1. Small volume of distribution
2. Low molecular weight
3. Water soluble
4. Uncharged
5. Low protein binding

Other techniques are less effective than hemodialysis. Peritoneal dialysis may be useful when these methods are not available or technically difficult (in neonates) or when anticoagulation may be hazardous. Complications include infection, injury to intra-abdominal organs, and hypothermia. Plasma exchange may also be a useful alternative in neonates. It is effective for treating hemolysis (arsine poisoning) and methemoglobinemia. Two blood-volume exchanges are usually performed using central or peripheral arteriovenous or venovenous access. Complications include transfusion reactions and hypothermia.

Safe Disposition

ICU admission is recommended for patients with coma, refractory hemodynamic instability, respiratory depression, seizures, and/or dysrhythmias. Patients with extremes of temperature, severe agitation, or life-threatening metabolic abnormalities also benefit from intensive care. Patients who are less ill, stable, or even asymptomatic are frequently unnecessarily admitted to the ICU because of physician uncertainty, fear of late deterioration and potential litigation, and lack of an alternative monitored setting. Some patients may require close observation and cardiac monitoring; but unless active interventions are likely to be necessary, admission to an intermediate care unit, telemetry unit, or emergency department observation unit is appropriate. Length of hospital stay for patients with self-poisoning can be reduced by use of a multidisciplinary team that involves a toxicologist and psychiatrist as well as medical personnel [84].

Prevention of Recurrence

Suicidal patients require psychiatric assessment. If they are given prescriptions, the amount of drug (1 to 2 week supply) and number of refills should be limited. Substance abusers should be counseled regarding attendant medical risks and given the opportunity for rehabilitation through referral for behavior modification, supervised withdrawal, and abstinence or maintenance therapy.

Adults with accidental poisoning should be educated regarding the safe use of drugs and other chemicals. Assistance with the administration of medications may be required for visually impaired, elderly, developmentally delayed, or confused patients. Preventive education may be indicated for health care providers who have committed dosing errors or who are unaware of adverse drug interactions. When poisoning results from environmental or workplace exposure, the appropriate governmental agency (Environmental Protection Agency, Occupational Safety and Health Administration, National Institute of Occupational Safety and Health, or local state, or federal health departments) should be notified. Unsafe working conditions should be brought to the attention of employers. Industrial hygiene and occupational health services should be offered if available. Finally, physicians have a duty to warn the general public (via press releases) of acute environmental hazards.

References

1. Bronstein AC, Spyker DA, Cantilena LR, et al: 2013 Annual Report of the American Association of Poison Control Centers' National Poison Data System: 31st Annual Report. *Clin Toxicol* 52:1032–1283, 2014.
2. Henderson A, Wright M, Pond SM: Experience with 732 acute overdose patients admitted to an intensive care unit over six years. *Med J Aust* 158:28, 1993.
3. McCaig LF, Burt CW: Poisoning-related visits to emergency departments in the United States, 1993–1996. *Clin Toxicol* 37:817, 1999.
4. Bosch TM, van der Werf TS, Uges DRA, et al: Antidepressants self-poisoning and ICU admissions in a university hospital in the Netherlands. *Pharm World Sci* 22:92–95, 2000.
5. Walton WW: An evaluation of the Poison Packaging Act. *Pediatrics* 69:363, 1982.
6. Centers for Disease Control and Prevention: Unintentional poisoning deaths—United States, 1999–2004. *MMWR Morb Mortal Wkly Rep* 56:93–96, 2007.
7. Hoppe-Roberts JM, Lloyd LM, Chyka PA: Poisoning mortality in the United States: comparison of national mortality statistics and poison control center reports. *Ann Emerg Med* 35:440, 2000.
8. Kearns GL, Abdel-Rahman SM, Alander SW, et al: Developmental pharmacology—drug disposition, action, and therapy in infants and children. *N Engl J Med* 349:1157, 2003.
9. Hardman JG, Limbird LE, Goodman AG (eds): *Goodman and Gilman's The Pharmacological Basis of Therapeutics*. 10th ed. New York, McGraw-Hill, 2001.
10. Klassen CD (ed): Casarett and Doull's Toxicology: The Basic Science of Poisons. 6th ed. New York, McGraw-Hill, 2001.
11. Hoffman R, Howland MA, Lewin N, et al (eds): *Goldfrank's Toxicologic Emergencies*. 10th ed. New York, McGraw-Hill, 2014.
12. Brayfield (ed): *Martindale: The Complete Drug Reference*. 38th ed. London, Pharmaceutical Press, 2014.
13. Dart RC (ed): *Medical Toxicology*. 3rd ed. Philadelphia, Lippincott Williams & Wilkins, 2004.
14. McEvoy GK (ed): *AHFS Drug Information*. Bethesda, MD, American Society of Health-System Pharmacists, 2015.
15. Brent J, Wallace KL, Burkhart KK, et al (eds): Critical Care Toxicology: Diagnosis and Management of the Critically Poisoned Patient. Philadelphia, Elsevier Mosby, 2005.
16. *Poisindex System*. Greenwood Village, CO, Thomson Micromedex, updated quarterly.
17. Kulig K: Initial management of ingestions of toxic substances. *N Engl J Med* 326:1677, 1992.
18. Sanz P, Reig R: Clinical and pathological findings in fatal plant oxalosis. A review. *Am J Forensic Med Pathol* 13:342, 1992.
19. Van Heijst ANP, deJong W, Seldenrijk R, et al: Coma and crystalluria: a massive primidone intoxication treated with hemoperfusion. *Clin Toxicol* 20:307, 1983.
20. Consumer Product Safety Commission. *Federal Hazardous Substances Act*. 2011.
21. Hepler BR, Sutheimer CA, Sunshine I: Role of the toxicology laboratory in the treatment of acute poisoning. *Med Toxicol* 1:61, 1986.
22. Aabakken L, Johansen KS, Rydningen EB, et al: Osmolal and anion gaps in patients admitted to an emergency medical department. *Hum Exp Toxicol* 13:131, 1994.
23. Roth B, Woo O, Blanc P: Early metabolic acidosis and coma after acetaminophen ingestion. *Ann Emerg Med* 33:452, 1999.
24. Senecal PE, Dyer JE, Osterloh JD: Nitrate as a cause of decreased anion gap. *Vet Hum Toxicol* 33:375, 1991.
25. Koga Y, Purssell RA, Lynd LD: The irrationality of the present use of the osmole gap: applicable physical chemistry principle and recommendations to improve validity of current practices. *Toxicol Rev* 23:203, 2004.
26. Purssell RA, Lynd LD, Koga Y: The use of the osmole gap as a screening test for the presence of exogenous substances. *Toxicol Rev* 23:189, 2004.
27. Blossom AP, Cleary JD, Daley WP: Acyclovir-induced crystalluria. *Ann Pharmacother* 36:526, 2002.
28. Rengstorff DS, Milstone AP, Seger DL, et al: Felbamate overdose complicated by massive crystalluria and acute renal failure. *Clin Toxicol* 38:667, 2000.
29. Tsao JW, Kogan SC: Indinavir crystalluria. *N Engl J Med* 340:1329, 1999.
30. Simon DI, Brosius FC, Rothstein DM: Sulfadiazine crystalluria revisited. *Arch Intern Med* 150:2379, 1990.
31. June R, Aks SE, Keys N, et al: Medical outcome of cocaine bodystuffers. *J Emerg Med* 18:221, 2000.
32. Traub SJ, Hoffman RS, Nelson LS: Body packing—the internal concealment of illicit drugs. *N Engl J Med* 349:2519, 2003.
33. Hergan K, Kofler K, Oser W: Drug smuggling by body packing: what radiologists should know about it. *Eur Radiol* 14(4):736–742, 2004.
34. Kozer E, Vergee Z, Koren G: Misdiagnosis of a mexiletine overdose because of a nonspecific result of urinary toxicologic screening. *N Engl J Med* 343:1971, 2000.
35. Fabbri A, Ruggeri S, Marchesni G, et al: A combined HPLC-immunoenzymatic comprehensive screening for suspected drug poisoning in the emergency department. *Emerg Med J* 21:317, 2004.
36. Eisen JS: Screening urine for drugs of abuse in the emergency department: do test results affect physician's patient care decisions? *Can J Emerg Med* 6:104, 2004.
37. Tomaszewski C, Runge J, Gibbs M, et al: Evaluation of a rapid bedside toxicology screen in patients suspected of drug toxicity. *J Emerg* 28:389, 2005.
38. Nice A, Leikin JB, Maturen A: Toxidrome recognition to improve efficiency of emergency urine drug screens. *Ann Emerg Med* 17:676, 1988.
39. Saylor JH: Volume of a swallow: role of orifice size and viscosity. *Vet Hum Toxicol* 29:79, 1987.
40. Bar-Oz B, Levichek Z, Koren G: Medications that can be fatal for a toddler with one tablet or teaspoonful: a 2004 update. *Paediatr Drugs* 6:123, 2004.
41. Purkayastha S, Bhangoo P, Athanasiou T, et al: Treatment of poisoning induced cardiac impairment using cardiopulmonary bypass: a review. *Emerg Med J* 23:246, 2006.
42. American Academy of Clinical Toxicology and European Association of Poisons Centre and Clinical Toxicologists: Position paper: ipecac syrup. *Clin Toxicol* 42:133, 2004.
43. Manoguerra AS, Cobaugh DJ, and Members of the Guidelines for the Management of Poisonings Consensus Panel of the American Association of Poison

Control Centers: Guideline on the use of ipecac syrup in the out-of-hospital management of ingested poisons. *Clin Toxicol* 1:1, 2005.
44. American Academy of Clinical Toxicology and European Association of Poisons Centre and Clinical Toxicologists: Position paper: cathartics. *Clin Toxicol* 42:243, 2004.
45. American Academy of Clinical Toxicology and European Association of Poisons Centre and Clinical Toxicologists: Position paper: gastric lavage. *Clin Toxicol* 42:933, 2004.
46. American Academy of Clinical Toxicology and European Association of Poisons Centre and Clinical Toxicologists: Position paper: whole bowel irrigation. *Clin Toxicol* 42:843, 2004.
47. American Academy of Clinical Toxicology and European Association of Poisons Centre and Clinical Toxicologists: Position paper: single-dose activated charcoal. *Clin Toxicol* 43:61, 2005.
48. Eddleston M, Juszczak E, Buckley N, et al: Multiple-dose activated charcoal in acute self-poisoning: a randomized controlled trial. *Lancet* 371:597–607, 2008.
49. Bosse GM, Barefoot JA, Pfeifer MP, et al: Comparison of three methods of gut decontamination in tricyclic antidepressant overdose. *J Emerg Med* 13:203, 1995.
50. Pond SM, Lewos-Driver DJ, Williams GM, et al: Gastric emptying in acute overdose: a prospective randomised controlled trial. *Med J Aust* 163:345, 1995.
51. Cooper GM, Le Couteur DG, Richardson D, et al: A randomized clinical trial of activated charcoal for the routine management of oral drug overdose. *Clin Toxicol* 40:313, 2002.
52. Merigian KS, Blaho K: Single dose activated charcoal in the treatment of the self-poisoned patient: a prospective controlled trial. *Am J Ther* 9:301, 2002.
53. Bond GR: The role of activated charcoal and gastric lavage in gastrointestinal decontamination: a state-of-the-art review. *Ann Emerg Med* 39:273, 2002.
54. Graudins A, Linden CH: The effect of charcoal and drug concentrations on the adsorption of acetaminophen to activated charcoal. *Clin Toxicol* 34:594, 1996.
55. Palatnick W, Tenenbein M: Activated charcoal in the treatment of drug overdose: an update. *Drug Saf* 7:3, 1992.
56. Seger D: Single-dose activated charcoal—backup and re-assess. *Clin Toxicol* 42:101, 2004.
57. Arnold TC, Willis BH, Xiao F, et al: Aspiration of activated charcoal elicits an increase in lung microvascular permeability. *Clin Toxicol* 37:9, 1999.
58. Vance MV, Selden BS, Clark RF: Optimal patient position for transport and initial management of toxic ingestions. *Ann Emerg Med* 21:243, 1992.
59. Shrestha M, George J, Chiu MJ, et al: A comparison of three gastric lavage methods using the radionuclide gastric emptying study. *J Emerg Med* 14:413, 1996.
60. Tenenbein M, Cohen S, Sitar DS: Whole bowel irrigation as a decontamination procedure after acute drug overdose. *Arch Intern Med* 147:905, 1987.
61. Mizutani T, Yamashita M, Okubo N, et al: Efficacy of whole bowel irrigation using solutions with or without adsorbent in the removal of paraquat in dogs. *Hum Exp Toxicol* 11:495, 1992.
62. Kirshenbaum LA, Sitar DS, Tenenbein M: Interaction between whole-bowel irrigation solution and activated charcoal: implications for the treatment of toxic ingestions. *Ann Emerg Med* 19:1129, 1990.
63. Arimori K, Furukawa E, Nakano M: Adsorption of imipramine onto activated charcoal and a cation exchange resin in macrogel-electrolyte solution. *Chem Pharm Bull* 40:3105, 1992.
64. Arimori K, Deshimaru M, Furukawa E, et al: Adsorption of mexiletine onto activated charcoal in macrogel-electrolyte solution. *Chem Pharm Bull* 41:766, 1993.
65. Rosenberg PJ, Livingstone DJ, McLellan BA: Effect of whole bowel irrigation on the antidotal efficacy of oral activated charcoal. *Ann Emerg Med* 17:681, 1988.
66. Hoffman RS, Chiang WK, Howland MA, et al: Theophylline desorption from activated charcoal caused by whole bowel irrigation solution. *Clin Toxicol* 29:191, 1991.
67. Makosiej FJ, Hoffman RS, Howland MA, et al: An in vitro evaluation of cocaine hydrochloride adsorption by activated charcoal and desorption upon addition of polyethylene glycol electrolyte lavage solution. *Clin Toxicol* 31:381, 1993.
68. Burkhart KK, Wuerz RC, Donovan JW: Whole bowel irrigation as an adjunctive treatment for sustained-released theophylline overdose. *Ann Emerg Med* 21:1316, 1992.
69. Buckley N, Dawson AH, Howarth D, et al: Slow-release verapamil poisoning. Use of polyethylene glycol whole-bowel irrigation lavage and high-dose calcium. *Med J Aust* 158:202, 1993.
70. Melandri R, Re G, Morigi A, et al: Whole bowel irrigation after delayed release fenfluramine overdose. *Clin Toxicol* 33:161, 1995.
71. Tenenbein M, Wiseman N, Yatscoff RW: Gastrotomy and whole bowel irrigation in iron poisoning. *Pediatr Emerg Care* 7:286, 1991.
72. Tenenbein M: Cathartics for drug overdose. *Ann Emerg Med* 16:832, 1987.
73. Al-Shareef AH, Buss DC, Allen EM, et al: The effects of charcoal and sorbitol (alone and in combination) on plasma theophylline concentrations after a sustained-release formulation. *Hum Exp Toxicol* 9:179, 1990.
74. Keller RE, Schwab RA, Krenzelok EP: Contribution of sorbitol combined with activated charcoal in prevention of salicylate absorption. *Ann Emerg Med* 19:654, 1990.
75. Garrettson LK, Geller RJ: Acid and alkaline diuresis: when are they of value in the treatment of poisoning? *Drug Saf* 5:220, 1990.
76. Proudfoot AT, Krenzelok EP, Vale JA: Position paper on urine alkalinization. *Clin Toxicol* 42:1, 2004.
77. Chyka PA: Multiple-dose activated charcoal and enhancement of systemic drug clearance: summary of studies in animal and human volunteers. *Clin Toxicol* 33:399, 1995.
78. Bradberry SM, Vale JA: Multiple-dose activated charcoal: a review of relevant clinical studies. *Clin Toxicol* 33:407, 1995.
79. American Academy of Clinical Toxicology and European Association of Poisons Centre and Clinical Toxicologists: Position statement and practice guidelines on the use of multi-dose activated charcoal in the treatment of acute poisoning. *Clin Toxicol* 37:731, 1999.
80. Campbell JW, Chyka PA: Physiochemical characteristics of drugs and response to repeat-dose activated charcoal. *Am J Emerg Med* 10:208, 1992.
81. Ilkhanipourk K, Yealy DM, Kronzelok EP: The comparative efficacy of various multiple-dose activated charcoal regimens. *Am J Emerg Med* 10:298, 1992.
82. Longdon P, Henderson A: Intestinal pseudo-obstruction following the use of enteral charcoal and sorbitol and mechanical ventilation with papaveretum sedation for theophylline poisoning. *Drug Saf* 7:74, 1992.
83. Goulbourne KB, Cisek JE: Small-bowel obstruction secondary to activated charcoal and adhesions. *Ann Emerg Med* 24:108, 1994.
84. Whyte IM, Dawson AH, Buckley NA, et al: Model for the management of self-poisoning. *Med J Aust* 167:142, 1997.

Chapter 98 ▪ Acetaminophen Poisoning

STEVEN B. BIRD

PHARMACOLOGY

Acetaminophen (*N*-acetyl-para-aminophenol [APAP]) is a nonopiate analgesic with excellent antipyretic activity but few anti-inflammatory effects. It belongs to the same drug family as phenacetin and acetanilid, the coal tar or aminobenzene analgesics [1,2]. Although APAP is the active metabolite of phenacetin, unlike phenacetin, it rarely, causes nephrotoxicity and does not cause methemoglobinemia or hemolytic anemia. Unlike aspirin, APAP has no barrier-breaker effect on the gastrointestinal tract and no effect on platelet function, has a high therapeutic index, and has not been implicated as a factor in Reye's syndrome. As a result, APAP is the preferred agent for the treatment of fever and mild to moderate pain when anti-inflammatory and antiplatelet action is not important.

Acetaminophen is an active ingredient in several hundred products, including pure APAP formulations, combinations with opioid analgesics, and numerous combination cough and cold preparations. It is also available in an extended-release (ER) formulation (which contains 325 mg of immediate-release and 325 mg of delayed-release acetaminophen per tablet) as a suppository, and a recently available intravenous formulation.

Acetaminophen has a pK_a of 9.5 and is quickly and almost completely absorbed after ingestion of therapeutic doses of immediate-release formulations (10 to 15 mg per kg every 4 hours), yielding peak plasma concentrations between 5 and 20 μg per mL within 30 to 120 minutes. Clinical effects are noted within 30 minutes. Liquid preparations are absorbed slightly faster than solid formulations. Rectal absorption is similar to that of oral ingestion. The volume of distribution of APAP is 0.9 to 1.0 L per kg, and protein binding is negligible. Therapeutic plasma concentrations range from 10 to 20 μg per L, and elimination after therapeutic dosing follows first-order kinetics, with an average half-life of 2 to 4 hours [1]. Elimination is slower in neonates and young infants [3], the elderly[2], and in patients with hepatic dysfunction [4]. Clinical effects persist for 3 to 4 hours after therapeutic doses.

After overdose, peak acetaminophen levels are usually noted within 4 hours. The ingestion of very large doses and the concomitant ingestion of agents that delay gastric emptying (e.g., anticholinergics and opioids) may result in peak levels occurring later. Prolonged absorption with a late rise in the acetaminophen level has also been reported after an ER overdose [5].

TOXICOLOGY

The short- or long-term therapeutic use of APAP is rarely associated with adverse effects. Hypersensitivity reactions, such as urticaria, fixed drug eruption, angioedema, laryngeal edema, and anaphylaxis, are extremely rare [6]. Although high-dose APAP has been associated with chronic renal impairment [7], a cause–effect relationship has not been established.

Despite remarkable safety in appropriate doses, APAP can cause fatal hepatic necrosis after overdosage. This was first recognized in Europe more than 50 years ago, and the first cases of hepatotoxicity in the United States were reported in 1975. Since that time, the incidence of APAP poisoning has increased dramatically in parallel with its increased availability and use; APAP is now the most common drug involved in exposures reported to US poison control centers, accounting for more than 141,000 calls in 2015 [8]. The incidence of occult poisoning is unknown, but based on retrospective data approximately 1 of every 70 overdose patients may have a detectable acetaminophen concentration and approximately 1 in 300 a potentially toxic APAP ingestion [9].

The metabolism of APAP explains its toxicity and the rationale for the current treatment of overdose (Fig. 98.1) [2]. After therapeutic doses, approximately 90% of APAP metabolism occurs by hepatic conjugation with sulfate or glucuronide to form inactive, nontoxic, renally eliminated metabolites. In adults, glucuronidation is the predominant route; in infants and young children, sulfation is the major pathway. Less than 5% of APAP is eliminated unchanged in the urine. The small remaining fraction (approximately 5%) undergoes oxidation by the P450 mixed-function oxidase enzyme system (CYP2E1) to yield the highly reactive, potentially toxic, electrophilic intermediate *N*-acetyl-para-benzoquinoneimine (NAPQI) [10]. NAPQI is quickly detoxified by reduced glutathione (GSH) to form nontoxic cysteine and mercapturic acid conjugates that are excreted in the urine.

After overdose, the amount of drug metabolized by the P450 route increases, because of a greater total drug burden and saturation of alternative enzymatic pathways [11]. As a result, GSH utilization increases. If GSH regeneration is inadequate to meet demand and becomes significantly depleted, NAPQI can persist and react with hepatocyte macromolecules, resulting in the death of hepatocytes. In animal studies, such injury occurs when GSH stores reach less than 30% of normal [12]. Hepatocyte necrosis is most pronounced in areas of highest CYP2E1 activity: the centrilobular (central venule) zones of the liver. The degree of injury can range from asymptomatic elevations in aminotransferase levels to fulminant liver failure. Although far less common, the same process can occur in the kidney [13]. Very rarely, renal toxicity can occur in the absence of serious hepatotoxicity [14].

Pancreatitis can occur, and diffuse myocardial necrosis has been noted in fatal cases. Very rarely, with massive ingestions, early coma and metabolic acidosis may be seen [15]. Although uncommon, thrombocytopenia after acute overdose has also been described [16]. The mechanisms causing these atypical toxicities are unknown, and it is unclear to what extent these effects are directly due to APAP.

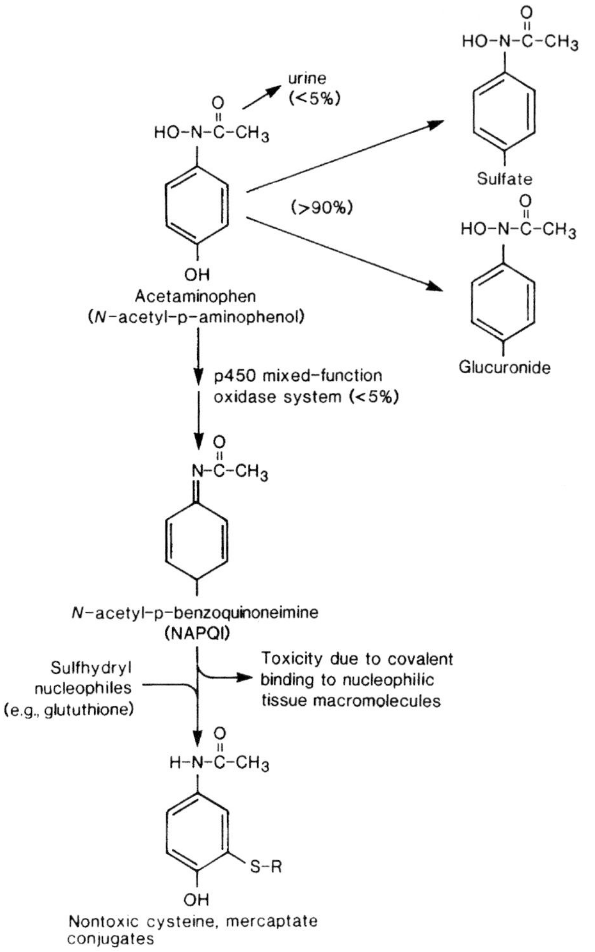

FIGURE 98.1 Postulated metabolism of acetaminophen. Toxicity occurs when the supply of sulfhydryl nucleophiles (e.g., glutathione) is inadequate to prevent the persistence of *N*-acetyl-para-benzoquinoneimine (NAPQI) and subsequent binding to hepatocyte macromolecules.

The precise dosage required to produce hepatotoxicity is unknown and almost certainly varies to some degree with individual differences in CYP2E1 activity, GSH stores, and capacity for GSH regeneration. Retrospective data suggest that significant toxicity is likely only after acute overdoses of greater than 250 mg per kg in adults [13], and prospective studies have suggested that toxicity is unlikely in unintentional pediatric ingestions of up to 200 mg per kg [17]. The possibility of toxicity at lower doses and skepticism regarding the accuracy of overdose histories have led to acceptance of a more conservative definition of risk, particularly in the United States. On the basis of APAP's volume of distribution and the well-established accuracy of APAP blood levels in predicting toxicity (see later), it is currently recommended that single ingestions of greater than 140 to 150 mg per kg be considered potentially toxic.

Elevated aminotransferase concentrations have also been reported after repeated ingestions of therapeutic or slightly greater doses of APAP [18]. Individuals who have conditions associated with increased CYP2E1 activity (e.g., chronic alcoholics) or glutathione depletion such as children younger than 10 years of age [19], those with chronic malnutrition, recent fasting (due to intercurrent illness), or recent ethanol use [20] may be at increased risk for such toxicity, but the accuracy of these reports has been challenged, and their therapeutic implications remain controversial. Such individuals are likely to have low hepatic carbohydrate and sulfate stores and, hence, decreased capacity for APAP metabolism via the glucuronidation and sulfation.

TABLE 98.1

Treatment of Acetaminophen Poisoning or Associated Hepatotoxicity

1. Administer activated charcoal if ingestion within 1–2 h
2. Administer NAC either IV (preferred) or orally
3. Early consultation with hepatology and or transplant services for critically ill patients
4. Psychiatric evaluation for all intentional overdoses

There is currently no valid estimation of the amount, frequency, or duration of the dosing that defines risk. It appears that after repeated doses, accumulation of APAP to concentrations associated with toxicity after acute overdose is not required and that sustained moderate elevations are sufficient to cause GSH depletion and toxicity [21]. Such observations suggest that the APAP level at which NAPQI production exceeds GSH regeneration is near, or possibly within, the therapeutic range and that GSH stores and the capacity for its regeneration are the most important factors in the development of hepatotoxicity. They also support the concept that hepatotoxicity is more dependent on the area under the curve (time vs. concentration) of APAP than the peak drug level.

Intentional acute overdose is the most common cause of toxicity and fatalities, but accidental therapeutic overdosing and the abuse of opioids with unintentional coingestion of APAP (e.g., with codeine or propoxyphene) have also been reported. Therapeutic overdoses may result from dosing calculation errors, excessive self-treatment, the use of adult formulations or extrastrength formulations when lower dosage formulations were intended, and errors involving substitution of higher dose rectal suppositories for similar-appearing lower dosage forms.

The importance of accurately diagnosing APAP toxicity soon after overdose extends beyond the high frequency with which it is encountered and its potential for causing morbidity and mortality. Acetaminophen is unique among common toxic exposures because effective treatment requires recognition of potential poisoning and initiation of therapy when no reliable clinical signs of overdose are present. Physicians must therefore consider occult APAP ingestion and liberally obtain APAP levels on all overdose patients to avoid missing the diagnosis.

CLINICAL MANIFESTATIONS

Acetaminophen hepatotoxicity can be divided into four clinical stages based on the time interval after ingestion: stage I (0 to 24 hours), the latent period; stage II (24 to 48 hours), the onset of hepatotoxicity; stage III (72 to 96 hours), maximal hepatic injury; and stage IV (4 days to 2 weeks), recovery [2,13].

During stage I, patients may be completely asymptomatic but often experience nausea, vomiting, and malaise, which may be accompanied by pallor and mild diaphoresis. There is no known correlation between presence or absence of early symptoms and the risk of hepatotoxicity. Although late in stage I very sensitive indicators of hepatic injury, such as γ-glutamyltransferase level, may be elevated, more widely used laboratory studies (e.g., aspartate aminotransferase [AST], alanine aminotransferase, prothrombin time, bilirubin) are completely normal. Early coma and metabolic acidosis have been reported in patients with massive ingestions [15], but these findings are so atypical that other causes should be suspected. They should be attributed to APAP only if the APAP concentration is extremely high and other etiologies have been excluded.

Symptoms during stage II are typical of hepatitis and include right upper-quadrant abdominal pain, nausea, fatigue, and malaise. Physical examination often reveals right upper-quadrant tenderness and hepatomegaly. The first elevation of aminotransferase levels usually occurs between 24 and 36 hours after APAP ingestion, but in the most severe cases, it can occur by 16 hours or earlier. Early in stage II, tests reflecting liver function, such as bilirubin and prothrombin time, are most often normal or only slightly elevated. Marked elevations of aminotransferase levels (greater than 1,000 IU per L) within 24 hours or of bilirubin and prothrombin time within 36 hours should suggest that the time of ingestion was earlier than reported. Although unusual, in severe cases, marked liver function abnormalities may be evident by 36 to 48 hours. Complications during stage II are directly related to the degree of liver injury and may include coagulopathy, encephalopathy, acidosis, and hypoglycemia. With few exceptions, life-threatening problems are not seen earlier than 48 hours, and death in this period is distinctly rare. Renal dysfunction, manifested by rising creatinine and an active urinary sediment, may become evident during this stage but usually lags somewhat behind the hepatic injury. The blood urea nitrogen may also be elevated, but it can be normal in the presence of hepatic failure and resultant decreased urea formation.

Biochemical evidence of liver injury becomes most pronounced during stage III. With successful treatment, however, peak aminotransferase levels may sometimes occur earlier (Fig. 98.2). Most patients, even those with markedly elevated aminotransferase levels, go on to recover fully. Most deaths occur 3 to 7 days after ingestion and result from intractable metabolic disturbances, secondary complications such as cerebral edema or dysrhythmias, or exsanguination due to coagulopathy. Renal failure may result from acute tubular necrosis. Some degree of renal dysfunction occurs in approximately 25% of patients with significant hepatotoxicity [15]. Even when severe, renal failure is almost always reversible.

During stage IV, if sufficient hepatocytes remain viable and the patient survives, the liver regenerates. Recovery is often complete by day 5 or 6 in patients with minimal toxicity, but those with more serious poisoning may not be clinically normal for 2 weeks or more. It is interesting that even patients with severe toxicity who survive regain normal liver function. There are no known cases of chronic or persistent liver abnormalities from APAP poisoning. In those who ultimately die, a slow decline in aminotransferase levels without clinical improvement may be seen. Declining enzyme levels merely represent a washout of those released at the time of the initial insult, not a recovery of normal liver function. These patients can be identified by persistent or increasing marked elevations of bilirubin and

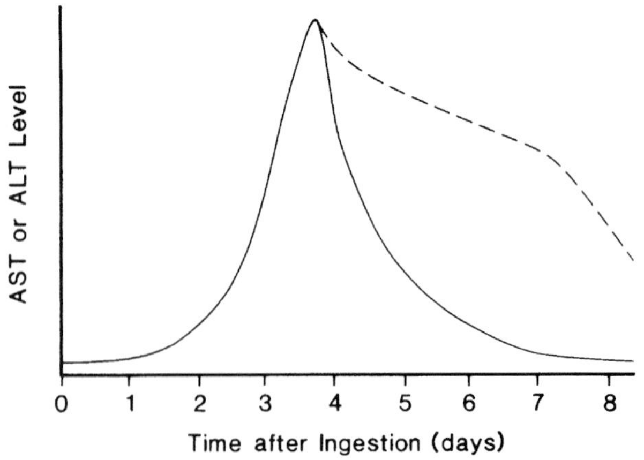

FIGURE 98.2 Expected time course of aminotransferase elevation due to acetaminophen-induced hepatotoxicity. The solid line represents typical course; the dashed line represents course of severe toxicity. ALT, alanine aminotransferase; AST, aspartate aminotransferase (Adapted from Jaeschke H, Mitchell JR: Neutrophil accumulation exacerbates acetaminophen-induced liver injury [abstract]. *FASEB J* 3:A920, 1989, with permission.)

prothrombin time. Although this pattern is occasionally seen in patients who recover, most survivors do not have significant or persistent bilirubin or prothrombin time elevation after aminotransferase levels fall.

Because of variations in dosing patterns and patient characteristics, the time course of toxicity in patients with repeated ingestions is not well defined. With chronic toxicity, dose–response patterns differ from those of acute overdose, but the clinical manifestations are the same.

DIAGNOSTIC EVALUATION

The diagnostic evaluation consists of determining the risk of toxicity and assessing for it. The serum APAP concentration is used to predict toxicity after acute overdose. If the APAP concentration between 4 and 24 hours after ingestion falls on or above the acetaminophen treatment nomogram line (Fig. 98.3), the patient should be considered at risk for hepatotoxicity, and hence in need of antidotal therapy (see later). Conversely, if the APAP concentration is even slightly below the nomogram line, the risk of hepatotoxicity is negligible and antidotal therapy is not necessary. The original Rumack–Matthew nomogram line, which defined the risk of toxicity based on the natural course of untreated patients [22], was actually 25% higher than the line now used in the United States. Hence, the nomogram has a 25% safety margin that allows one to be rigid when using the nomogram to make treatment decisions.

There are, however, some important caveats regarding use of the nomogram. First and foremost, it applies only to single acute ingestions. Second, when there is uncertainty about the exact time of ingestion, the worst-case scenario should be assumed. For example, if the ingestion was between 4 and 6 hours earlier, the 6-hour value on the nomogram should be used. And finally, when levels are obtained 20 to 24 hours after overdose, the limit

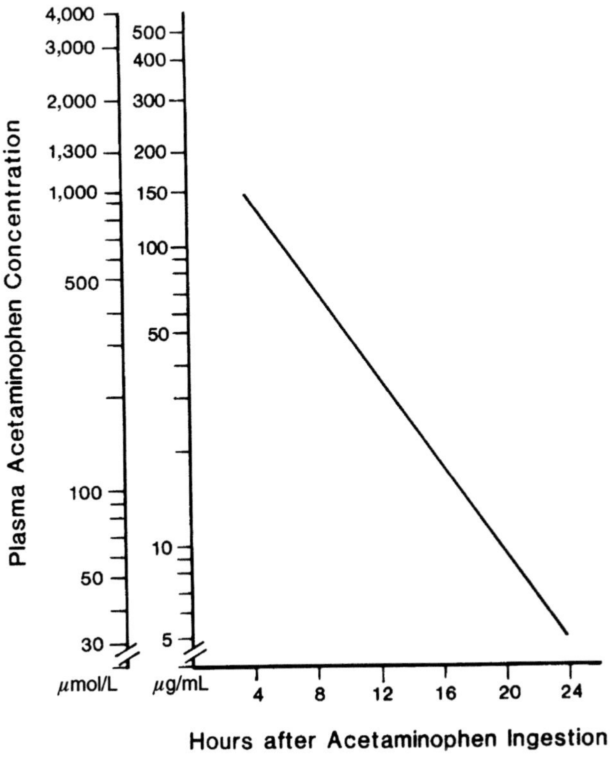

FIGURE 98.3 Acetaminophen treatment nomogram. Patients with acetaminophen concentrations on or above the line require treatment with *N*-acetylcysteine. (Adapted from Jaeschke H, Mitchell JR: Neutrophil accumulation exacerbates acetaminophen-induced liver injury [abstract]. *FASEB J* 3:A920, 1989, with permission.)

of detection of the APAP assay must also be considered. Because most hospitals use immunoassays with a detection limit of 10 μg per mL, potentially toxic APAP levels during this period will be below this limit and reported as nondetectable, which does not necessarily mean nontoxic. Again, a worst-case scenario should be assumed, and antidotal treatment should be given until the level is confirmed to be nontoxic by a more sensitive assay, or until it has been determined that the patient is asymptomatic and has no laboratory evidence of hepatotoxicity.

With rare exceptions (see later), a single APAP concentration within the time specified by the nomogram is sufficient to plan appropriate therapy. Although it is true that the elimination half-life of APAP is related to the likelihood of toxicity, half-lives should not be relied on in making therapeutic decisions. The observations that half-lives greater than 4 hours were associated with toxicity and that toxicity was negligible if APAP half-life was less than 4 hours [23] were based on multiple APAP determinations in untreated patients over a 36-hour period. Because treatment must be started as early as possible [24] and treatment may alter APAP elimination [11], half-life determinations are not relevant to current standards of care.

There are three situations in which repeat measurements may be of value. The first is in the patient with a time of ingestion that is unknown, but that was within 4 hours. In this situation, an increasing APAP level indicates ongoing absorption from a recent ingestion. To detect a rising level and define the peak value, repeat determinations must be frequent (every hour) until the level declines. This prevents underestimation of the peak value due to incomplete absorption at the time of the first level. It also may rule out toxicity by detecting a peak value less than 150 μg per mL.

The second situation in which repeating the APAP may be useful is after an overdose of an ER formula. Because of prolonged absorption, patients with nontoxic APAP levels soon after ingestion may have subsequent concentrations that are toxic by the nomogram [25]. The optimal time to repeat drug levels to detect such nomogram line-crossers is unknown. In one patient, a potentially toxic APAP level did not occur until 14 hours after ingestion [5]. The manufacturer recommends obtaining a second APAP level 4 to 6 hours after the initial one [26]. Others have recommended that to avoid missing a potentially toxic level, drug levels should be measured every 2 hours from 4 to 16 hours after overdose [27].

Finally, repeat APAP levels may be of value in the patient with very high levels and slow elimination in whom it is possible that APAP may still be present at the completion of therapy. Antidotal treatment should not be discontinued while APAP is still present. This is particularly relevant as shorter courses of antidotal therapy have become the routine.

In assessing the patient who is found to be at risk for toxicity and hence requires hospitalization and antidotal treatment, a complete blood count, electrolytes, blood urea nitrogen, creatinine, glucose, prothrombin time, aminotransferase levels, and bilirubin should be obtained at admission and repeated every 24 hours until resolution of toxicity is noted. If liver failure develops, laboratory values, particularly prothrombin time and glucose, must be obtained more frequently. Renal function, acid–base status, amylase, and electrocardiogram may also need to be evaluated or repeated. Assessment of renal, pancreatic, and myocardial toxicity should follow the same guidelines as those for other etiologies.

MANAGEMENT

Treatment includes gastrointestinal decontamination, antidotal treatment (if indicated), and support of organ function. Unless clinically significant hepatic or renal failure develops, management consists only of antidote administration and monitoring of signs, symptoms, and laboratory parameters. Although this can be accomplished outside the intensive care unit, patients often require monitoring or treatment for toxicity owing to coingestions or constant observation because of suicide risk. If significant hepatic failure ensues, intensive care unit admission is required for close monitoring and treatment of complications. Invasive monitoring is infrequently required, but may be useful if multisystem failure occurs.

Gastrointestinal Decontamination

Gastrointestinal decontamination is recommended for patients who can be treated within 1 to 2 hours of APAP overdose. Although once considered controversial and even contraindicated, activated charcoal is now considered the method of choice for gastrointestinal decontamination. As routine treatment of APAP poisoning has moved from oral *N*-acetylcysteine (NAC) to intravenous administration, this formerly contentious point has been rendered moot.

Antidotal Treatment

The observation that hepatotoxicity occurs only when GSH is depleted led to a search for agents that might increase available sulfhydryl groups either by increasing GSH or by providing alternative sulfhydryl sources. Exogenous GSH does not readily enter cells, so various precursors and substitutes, including cysteamine, methionine, and NAC [24,28], have been tried. Although all regimens are effective when started within 8 to 10 hours of ingestion, cysteamine was abandoned because of its toxicity, and methionine has been replaced by NAC, which is more effective and probably carries less risk of worsening hepatic encephalopathy when liver failure is present.

There are several suggested mechanisms of action of NAC. In cells, NAC is converted to cysteine, a GSH precursor, and thus increases GSH stores. Second, NAC or cysteine can substitute directly for GSH because it has available sulfhydryl groups. Third, NAC augments the sulfation of APAP to nontoxic metabolite by providing sulfur substrate [11]. Fourth, NAC may promote the back conversion of NAPQI to its precursors, although this has not been demonstrated in humans. Finally, there is accumulating evidence that NAC may be beneficial, even after liver injury has occurred, through mechanisms other than its effects on APAP metabolism [29]. Suggested mechanisms for these late effects of NAC include direct antioxidant action to modify postinflammatory radical-mediated destruction, restoration of enzyme function in injured tissue, and correction of microvascular function by restoring endothelial-derived relaxing factor [29]. It is likely that the relative importance of each of the previously described effects of NAC in any given patient varies with the severity of the overdose and the delay to NAC initiation. These variations may explain apparent differences in efficacy between different NAC protocols.

Two treatment regimens are currently approved for use in the United States. The first consists of a 72-hour course of oral NAC given as a 140-mg-per-kg loading dose, followed by 17 doses of 70 mg per kg every 4 hours beginning 4 hours after the loading dose, for a total NAC dose of 1,330 mg per kg [30]. The second regimen consists of an intravenous loading dose of acetylcysteine of 150 mg per kg in 200 mL dextrose 5% in water (D_5W) over 15 minutes, followed by 50 mg per kg in 500 mL D_5W over 4 hours, then 100 mg per kg in 1 L D_5W over the next 16 hours [31]. This is identical to the standard treatment regimens in Europe and Canada [28]. Because the FDA-approved dosing requires three separate intravenous formulations, some poison control centers, hospitals, and medical toxicologists have simplified NAC protocols that differ from the FDA-approved dosing [32].

For oral therapy, NAC is usually supplied as a 20% solution (20 g per 100 mL), which should be diluted 3 to 1 to yield a 5% mixture with juice or a soft drink to increase its palatability and decrease gastrointestinal side effects. Antiemetics are frequently required to treat antecedent vomiting or vomiting due to NAC. If antiemetics fail, NAC can be given by gastric or duodenal tube. Various other methods may prove helpful in decreasing emesis after dosing: chilling the solution with ice chips, using a straw and covering the container, diluting to a 10% solution, or administering the solution over 15 to 60 minutes instead of as a bolus. If vomiting occurs within 1 hour of any dose, that dose should be repeated.

The use of oral or IV NAC is dependent on the experience of the clinician, the local hospital formulary, severity of the patient, and physician preference. Most patients can be adequately treated with oral NAC if it is begun within 8 to 10 hours of ingestion. Other patients, particularly those who present after 8 to 10 hours or those with encephalopathy, should receive IV NAC therapy.

There are no well-documented serious side effects of oral NAC, although nausea and vomiting are extremely common [33]. Side effects from intravenous NAC are far less common but potentially more serious. There are several reports of serious or fatal anaphylactoid reactions (e.g., hypotension, bronchospasm, rash, death) to intravenous NAC during the 20-hour protocol, and minor dermatologic reactions are common [34,35]. It is important to recognize that adverse effects of intravenous NAC are not truly anaphylactic; they are dose and concentration dependent [34]. As a result, more dilute and slowly administered doses are better tolerated [36]. Except for an anaphylactoid reaction in one patient after an NAC overdose, there were no serious adverse reactions reported during the 48-hour intravenous protocol [36]. Transient skin rash occurred in approximately 15% of patients during the loading dose but did not necessitate discontinuing treatment. Even with more serious reactions, NAC therapy can often be continued or resumed after treatment with diphenhydramine [35].

All dosing protocols appear to be equivalent when NAC is started within 8 hours of ingestion. Efficacy decreases with longer delays in therapy, with apparent differences between the dosing regimens when NAC is started after 16 hours. With late treatment, 82% of high-risk patients treated with the 20-hour regimen developed aminotransferase values above 1,000 IU per L, an incidence not significantly different from the 89% incidence reported in untreated historical control subjects [28]. After treatment with 48 hours of intravenous NAC, only 58% of late-treated patients developed hepatotoxicity, a result that was significantly better than that with the 20-hour course or no treatment [36]. After 72 hours of oral NAC, only 41% of late-treated patients developed hepatotoxicity [24], although this was not statistically different from the 48-hour protocol [36]. These studies included only patients receiving NAC within 24 hours of ingestion.

In the first controlled study of NAC started more than 24 hours after overdose, intravenous NAC started after onset of liver failure (median 53 hours after APAP) reduced cerebral edema, need for vaso pressors, and mortality [37]. It is interesting that this study used the same NAC dosing that had earlier been found ineffective more than 15 hours after overdose [28], but instead of discontinuing NAC after 20 hours, therapy was continued until either recovery or death occurred.

The numerous actions of NAC may explain why various NAC protocols are equivalent when started early but not when started late. When started within 8 hours of overdose, NAC probably exclusively affects APAP metabolism and GSH turnover, and its role is preventative before GSH depletion and NAPQI covalent binding. In this setting, NAC may be needed only until APAP metabolism is complete; thus, shorter courses of NAC are effective. With further treatment delay, the role of NAC may increasingly be to ameliorate the effects of NAPQI covalent binding, and by 16 hours after ingestion, this may be its sole action and would explain why longer courses of NAC, continued during the period of maximal liver injury, appear to be superior. These considerations have led to selective management, such as short-course NAC for those treated early who do not develop aminotransferase elevations or late treatment with NAC for any patient who develops liver injury (see later).

Cimetidine has been suggested as a possible antidote for APAP because of its inhibitory effect on P450 activity. Animal studies showed efficacy of high-dose cimetidine given before or soon after APAP, but there is no evidence of efficacy in humans [38]. Even if the massive dose suggested by animal studies proved to be safe and effective in humans, its theoretical effect would require early administration. In problematic cases, such as late presentation, there is no theoretical or experimental support for cimetidine use. Hence, although cimetidine is not contraindicated, it has no proven role and should never be considered an alternative to NAC.

Supportive Care

The management of hepatic failure, renal failure, or other end-organ manifestations of APAP toxicity should be treated according to usual guidelines. In view of the increased availability and success of liver transplantation, the most severely ill patients deserve this consideration. Several successful transplants have been done after APAP overdose. The greatest challenge is early identification of patients destined for irreversible hepatic failure (see the section Prognosis and Outcome).

SPECIAL CONSIDERATIONS

Acute Overdose in Alcoholics and Other High-Risk Patients

Certain subgroups of patients appear to be at greater or lesser risk for APAP toxicity, but this fact is of more theoretic than practical value in the management of acute overdose. Higher risk is expected in patients with increased CYP2E1 enzyme activity from chronic use of agents that induce this enzyme (e.g., ethanol, barbiturates, phenytoin, sedative–hypnotics, griseofulvin, haloperidol, tolbutamide)[39] or decreased GSH stores or low GSH turnover rates (e.g., malnourished patients or those with liver disease). Lower toxicity might be expected when CYP2E1 activity is inhibited by chronic use of agents such as cimetidine or when a patient has coingested an agent that is metabolized by this enzyme, thus competing with APAP and decreasing NAPQI formation [2].

Acute overdose studies in animals demonstrated increased toxicity after chronic ethanol use and decreased toxicity when ethanol and APAP were coingested [40]. The protective effect of ethanol coingestion appears to be due to competitive inhibition of NAPQI formation by P450 ethanol metabolism. Chronic ethanol use, particularly in an alcoholic that is currently abstinent [41] could worsen toxicity by causing P450 induction, GSH depletion, or some other unknown mechanism. For example, an alcoholic might be protected by the acute coingestion of ethanol or be nutritionally deprived and have lower P450 activity. Despite suggestions that some of these factors may be important [42], the amount of chronic ethanol or drug use that is clinically significant is unknown and certain to be variable.

Because the treatment nomogram line is conservative, treatment decisions after acute overdose should be made in the same manner as described previously, regardless of chronic coingestants.

Acute Overdose in Pediatric Patients

Of 417 children with acute APAP overdose, 49 of whom had plasma APAP levels over the nomogram line, indicating potential toxicity, only three (6.1%) developed an AST or ALT greater than 1,000 IU per L [43]. This incidence is less than that reported in adults, leading to speculation that children are relatively protected from APAP toxicity.

Several pharmacokinetic differences between children and adults have been noted. The most consistent finding is that the ratio of APAP-sulfate to APAP-glucuronide is higher in children than in adults [44], but this difference in nontoxic routes of metabolism has not been shown to be associated with a decrease in production of NAPQI. Thus, increased sulfation has not been proven favorably to alter NAPQI formation. Decreased P450 activity, and thus decreased NAPQI formation, has also been postulated in children, but decreased P450 activity is noted only in fetal and neonatal subjects [45]. Most APAP poisonings occur outside the newborn period, when P450 activity may be even greater than in adults. Hence, this theory cannot explain a hepatoprotective effect in older children. If children are actually less susceptible to APAP toxicity, it may be because of an increased ability to regenerate GSH, but this, too, is unproven.

Perhaps the most likely explanation is that pediatric overdoses are quantitatively less severe. In adults, particularly those treated late, the outcome is worse in patients with very high APAP levels [24]. Substantial toxicity has also developed in children with very high concentrations, but there are too few cases to allow for any conclusions. Until larger numbers of children with very high APAP levels are studied, patients of all ages with a significant overdose must still be considered at substantial risk and managed accordingly. As with adults, the longer the time between ingestion and presentation or treatment in children with potentially toxic drug levels, the greater the incidence of hepatotoxicity and the worse the prognosis [21].

Acute Overdose in Pregnancy

Although experience with overdose in pregnancy is limited [46], certain conclusions seem valid. First, there is clear evidence that APAP overdose can result in morbidity and mortality to women and the fetus at all stages of pregnancy. Second, there currently is no evidence that NAC is harmful to a pregnant woman or her fetus. Third, NAC is hepatoprotective to the women. Fourth, NAC crosses the human placenta [47], and this is likely to be beneficial to the fetus. On the basis of these observations, it is recommended that pregnant women be treated according to standard guidelines regardless of gestational age of the fetus and that newborns delivered during a course of maternal NAC treatment should also complete a course of NAC after delivery.

Acute Overdose of Extended-Release Acetaminophen

Because experience with ER APAP overdose is limited, the applicability of the nomogram, which was derived from clinical outcome data in patients with immediate-release APAP overdose, to those with ER APAP overdose remains to be determined [25–27]. Although it is agreed that patients who have a potentially toxic APAP level after acute acetaminophen ER overdose require NAC, the management of those with levels that are elevated but nontoxic is controversial. Some have suggested that such patients do not require NAC [48]. Given that peak drug levels after supratherapeutic but nontoxic doses of ER acetaminophen are only two-thirds of those seen after equivalent doses of an immediate-release formulation, despite nearly identical areas under the curve [49], others recommend treatment if any APAP level is two-thirds or more of the one that is indicated toxic by the nomogram [27].

Chronic Overdose

There are occasional reports of serious toxicity from chronic overdose in infants with acute febrile illness [19,21]. Chronic toxicity has also been reported after doses only slightly higher than recommended and even with therapeutic ones in adults with fasting and alcohol use [50]. Although alcoholics do appear to be at greater risk for toxicity from therapeutic doses, the validity of data on fasting has been questioned [51]. There is no evidence that this occurs in otherwise healthy individuals. Similarly, in the absence of continued ethanol abuse, there is no evidence that therapeutic dosing carries an increased risk in patients with cirrhosis or other forms of chronic liver disease [52]. On the basis of current knowledge, there is no reason to avoid APAP in any of these groups, although patients must be clearly instructed to avoid overdosing.

Evaluation of patients with chronic overdose should include a detailed history of the timing of doses, particularly the last dose; the amount ingested at each dose; possible increased risk factors (e.g., chronic alcoholism, use of other P450 inducers); symptomatology; an APAP level at least 4 hours after the last dose; and aminotransferase levels. In such cases, the nomogram has never been studied and has little or no validity. Because there are currently no reliable guidelines to assess risk, it is best then to consult with a toxicologist or regional poison center to determine the best course of action. One approach is to treat according to the guidelines discussed in the next section.

Late Treatment

Treatment decisions in patients who present more than 24 hours after an overdose are problematic. Initial studies of the 20-hour intravenous NAC protocol suggested that NAC was of no value if started more than 12 to 15 hours after ingestion [28], and initial results of the 72-hour oral protocol indicated that treatment more than 16 hours after ingestion was ineffective [30]. As a result, studies of treatment initiated after 24 hours were not performed initially. More extensive data and analyses of patients treated with 72 hours of oral NAC revealed that patients first treated between 16 and 24 hours after overdose experienced less hepatotoxicity than untreated historical control subjects or historical control subjects treated late with a 20-hour course of intravenous NAC [24].

Subsequently, a series of studies showed theoretical and clinical benefit to late NAC administration [29,53,54]. In the most remarkable of these, NAC started a median of 53 hours after ingestion and after evidence of severe liver injury reduced morbidity and mortality [29]. Although the issue of which cases warrant late treatment is not well defined, the following approach to the treatment of patients who present late is offered: If the APAP level is undetectable and aminotransferase levels are normal, NAC is not indicated, because the possibility of hepatotoxicity is extremely low. If hepatotoxicity is evident, a full course of NAC is indicated. For patients who have detectable APAP levels and no hepatotoxicity, NAC therapy should be started. It can be discontinued before completing a full course of therapy when the APAP concentration falls to zero, if aminotransferase levels remain normal.

Short-Course ORAL Treatment

Treatment of acute APAP overdose with an abbreviated course of oral NAC is based on the observation that treatment for 20 hours with intravenous NAC [28] and for 48 hours with oral NAC [36] is just as effective as treatment with oral NAC for 72 hours [24] when treatment is started within 8 to 16 hours of ingestion (see previous section), and that patients who develop hepatotoxicity exhibit laboratory evidence of such toxicity within 24 to 36 hours of ingestion [9,55]. In short-course protocols, oral NAC is initiated in patients with toxic or potentially toxic APAP levels (by the nomogram) in the same dose as used in the standard 72-hour regimen, and APAP levels and aminotransferases are obtained at 24 and 36 hours postingestion. As with late treatment, if the APAP level becomes undetectable and aminotransferase levels are normal at either point in time, NAC is stopped, whereas if hepatotoxicity becomes evident, a full course of NAC is indicated. For patients who have detectable APAP levels and no hepatotoxicity, NAC therapy should be continued. It can be discontinued before completing a full course of therapy if the APAP concentration subsequently becomes undetectable and if aminotransferase levels remain normal. Although toxicologists have been successfully using short-course NAC therapy for years, published data are limited [56], and poison centers have been slow to adopt this approach. Hence, consultation with a toxicologist is advised when contemplating such treatment.

PROGNOSIS AND OUTCOME

Severe hepatotoxicity after APAP overdose has traditionally been defined by an ALT or AST greater than 1,000 IU per L, although most patients with such elevations have no significant short- or long-term sequelae. Using this definition, the risk of hepatotoxicity can be estimated on the basis of the initial APAP concentration. Without NAC therapy, hepatotoxicity develops in less than 8% of all overdose patients, in 60% of probable risk cases (APAP concentration above a nomogram line intersecting 200 μg per mL at 4 hours and 50 μg per mL at 12 hours), and in 89% of high-risk cases (APAP concentration above a nomogram line intersecting 300 µg per mL at 4 hours and 75 μg per mL at 12 hours) [13].

Far less toxicity occurs in patients treated with NAC, although outcome depends on APAP concentration and the time NAC was started. Even in high-risk late-treated cases, only 41% of patients treated with oral NAC for 72 hours developed toxicity. Most important is that regardless of APAP level, NAC is extremely effective when started within 8 hours [24]. Hepatotoxicity occurred in less than 5% of patients in this subset.

Death is unusual after APAP overdose. When patients at probable risk for hepatotoxicity are considered, the reported mortality rate in untreated cases varies from 5.3% [28] to 24% [57]. A mortality rate of 1.1% has been noted in similar patients treated with the 20-hour intravenous NAC protocol [29], and it was found to be 0.68% in patients treated with the 72-hour oral NAC protocol [24]. In fact, even among high-risk cases first treated between 16 and 24 hours after overdose, the mortality rate was only 3.1% after oral NAC therapy [24].

It is not uncommon to see aminotransferase elevations greater than 10,000 IU per L during stage III, with eventual complete recovery [2]. As a result, aminotransferase levels alone are inadequate to judge prognosis. Evidence of hepatic dysfunction, such as marked elevations in prothrombin time and bilirubin, or evidence of persistent hypoglycemia, lactic acidosis, or hepatic encephalopathy, indicates true hepatic failure and a poor prognosis. Previous reports suggested that a bilirubin greater than 4 mg per dL or a prothrombin time greater than twice control indicates a poor prognosis [58]. More recently, a pH less than 7.30, prothrombin time greater than 100 seconds, serum creatinine greater than 3.4 mg per dL, and grade III or higher encephalopathy have been used to define poor prognosis [59], as has the single criterion of an increasing prothrombin time on day 4 after overdose (60) or a lactate of greater than 3.5 mmol per L shorter after admission [61]. More recently, Schmidt and Dalhoff [62] demonstrated that an increasing alpha-fetoprotein serum concentration (particularly a concentration of more than 3.9 μg per L on the day after peak ALT) is associated with survival. As noted previously, patients meeting these criteria may benefit from NAC treatment [29,53]. Standard measures for the treatment of liver failure, including arrangements for possible liver transplantation, should also be provided.

The presence or absence of aminotransferase elevation at the time of treatment initiation appears to be the most sensitive early prognostic indicator. To date, all reported patients who died from APAP toxicity already had some degree of AST or ALT elevation at the time a 72-hour course of oral NAC was started [24]. Hence, all patients with liver enzyme values that are normal when oral NAC is started would be expected to survive.

ACKNOWLEDGMENT

Christopher H. Linden, M.D., contributed to this chapter in a previous edition.

References

1. Burke A, Smyth E, Fitzgerald GA. Analgesic-antipyretic and antiinflammatory agents; pharmacotherapy of gout. In: Brunton LL, Lazo JS, Parker KL, eds. *Goodman and Gilman's The Pharmacological Basis of Therapeutics*. 11th ed. New York, NY: McGraw Hill; 2006.
2. Linden CH, Rumack BH. Acetaminophen overdose. *Emerg Med Clin North Am* 2(1):103–119, 1984.
3. Peterson RG, Rumack BH. Pharmacokinetics of acetaminophen in children. *Pediatrics* 62[5 Pt 2 Suppl]:877–879, 1978.
4. Andreasen PB, Hutters L. Paracetamol (acetaminophen) clearance in patients with cirrhosis of the liver. *Acta Med Scand Suppl* 624:99–105, 1979.
5. Bizovi KE, Aks SE, Paloucek F, et al. Late increase in acetaminophen concentration after overdose of tylenol extended relief. *Ann Emerg Med* 28(5):549–551, 1996.
6. Stricker BH, Meyboom RH, Lindquist M. Acute hypersensitivity reactions to paracetamol. *Br Med J (Clin Res Ed)* 291(6500):938–939, 1985.
7. Fored CM, Ejerblad E, Lindblad P, et al. Acetaminophen, aspirin, and chronic renal failure. *N Engl J Med* 345(25):1801–1808, 2001.
8. Mowry JB, Spyker DA, Brooks DE, et al. 2015 Annual report of the American Association of Poison Control Centers' National Poison Data System (NPDS). *Clin Toxicol* 54(10):924–1109, 2016.
9. Ashbourne JF, Olson KR, Khayam-Bashi H. Value of rapid screening for acetaminophen in all patients with intentional drug overdose. *Ann Emerg Med* 18(10):1035–1038, 1989.
10. Corcoran GB, Mitchell JR, Vaishnav YN, et al. Evidence that acetaminophen and N-hydroxyacetaminophen form a common arylating intermediate, N-acetyl-p-benzoquinoneimine. *Mol Pharmacol* 18(3):536–542, 1980.
11. Slattery JT, Wilson JM, Kalhorn TF, et al. Dose-dependent pharmacokinetics of acetaminophen: evidence of glutathione depletion in humans. *Clin Pharmacol Ther* 41(4):413–418, 1987.
12. Mitchell JR, Thorgeirsson SS, Potter WZ, et al. Acetaminophen-induced hepatic injury: protective role of glutathione in man and rationale for therapy. *Clin Pharmacol Ther* 16(4):676–684, 1974.
13. Prescott LF. Paracetamol overdosage. Pharmacological considerations and clinical management. *Drugs* 25(3):290–314, 1983.
14. Davenport A, Finn R. Paracetamol (acetaminophen) poisoning resulting in acute renal failure without hepatic coma. *Nephron* 50(1):55–56, 1988.
15. Roth B, Woo O, Blanc P. Early metabolic acidosis and coma after acetaminophen ingestion. *Ann Emerg Med* 33(4):452–456, 1999.
16. Fischereder M, Jaffe JP. Thrombocytopenia following acute acetaminophen overdose. *Am J Hematol* 45(3):258–259, 1994.
17. Mohler CR, Nordt SP, Williams SR, et al. Prospective evaluation of mild to moderate pediatric acetaminophen exposures. *Ann Emerg Med* 35(3):239–244, 2000.
18. Watkins PB, Kaplowitz N, Slattery JT, et al. Aminotransferase elevations in healthy adults receiving 4 grams of acetaminophen daily: a randomized controlled trial. *JAMA* 296(1):87–93, 2006.
19. Heubi JE, Barbacci MB, Zimmerman HJ. Therapeutic misadventures with acetaminophen: hepatoxicity after multiple doses in children. *J Pediatr* 132(1):22–27, 1998.
20. Whitcomb DC, Block GD. Association of acetaminophen hepatotoxicity with fasting and ethanol use. *JAMA* 272(23):1845–1850, 1994.
21. Rivera-Penera T, Gugig R, Davis J, et al. Outcome of acetaminophen overdose in pediatric patients and factors contributing to hepatotoxicity. *J Pediatr* 130(2):300–304, 1997.
22. Rumack BH, Matthew H. Acetaminophen poisoning and toxicity. *Pediatrics* 55(6):871–876, 1975.
23. Prescott LF, Roscoe P, Wright N, et al. Plasma-paracetamol half-life and hepatic necrosis in patients with paracetamol overdosage. *Lancet* 13;1(7698):519–522, 1971.
24. Smilkstein MJ, Knapp GL, Kulig KW, et al. Efficacy of oral N-acetylcysteine in the treatment of acetaminophen overdose. Analysis of the national multicenter study (1976 to 1985). *N Engl J Med* 319(24):1557–1562, 1988.
25. Cetaruk EW, Dart RC, Horowitz RS, et al. Extended-release acetaminophen overdose. *JAMA* 275(9):686, 1996.
26. Temple AR, Mrazik TJ. More on extended-release acetaminophen. *N Engl J Med* 333(22):1508–1509, 1995.
27. Graudins A, Aaron CK, Linden CH. Overdose of extended-release acetaminophen. *N Engl J Med* 333(3):196, 1995`.
28. Prescott LF, Illingworth RN, Critchley JA, et al. Intravenous N-acetylcystine: the treatment of choice for paracetamol poisoning. *Br Med J* 2(6198):1097–1100, 1979.
29. Harrison PM, Wendon JA, Gimson AE, et al. Improvement by acetylcysteine of hemodynamics and oxygen transport in fulminant hepatic failure. *N Engl J Med* 324(26):1852–1857, 1991.
30. Rumack BH, Peterson RC, Koch GG, et al. Acetaminophen overdose. 662 cases with evaluation of oral acetylcysteine treatment. *Arch Intern Med* 141(3 Spec No):380–385, 1981.
31. Acetadote [package insert]. Nashville, TN: Cumberland Pharmaceuticals Inc. Available at www.acetadote.com/acetadote-prescribing-information-11-2016.pdf
32. Kao LW, Kirk MA, Furbee RB, et al. What is the rate of adverse events after oral N-acetylcysteine administered by the intravenous route to patients with suspected acetaminophen poisoning? *Ann Emerg Med* 42(6):741–750, 2003.
33. Miller LF, Rumack BH. Clinical safety of high oral doses of acetylcysteine. *Semin Oncol* 10[1 Suppl 1]:76–85, 1983.
34. Dawson AH, Henry DA, McEwen J. Adverse reactions to N-acetylcysteine during treatment for paracetamol poisoning. *Med J Aust* 150(6):329–331, 1989.
35. Bailey B, McGuigan MA. Management of anaphylactoid reactions to intravenous N-acetylcysteine. *Ann Emerg Med* 31(6):710–715, 1998.
36. Smilkstein MJ, Bronstein AC, Linden C, et al. Acetaminophen overdose: a 48-hour intravenous N-acetylcysteine treatment protocol. *Ann Emerg Med* 20(10):1058–1063, 1991.
37. Keays R, Harrison PM, Wendon JA, et al. Intravenous acetylcysteine in paracetamol induced fulminant hepatic failure: a prospective controlled trial. *BMJ* 303(6809):1026–1029, 1991.
38. Burkhart KK, Janco N, Kulig KW, et al. Cimetidine as adjunctive treatment for acetaminophen overdose. *Hum Exp Toxicol* 14(3):299–304, 1995.
39. Coon MJ, Koop DR, Reeve LE, et al. Alcohol metabolism and toxicity: role of cytochrome P-450. *Fundam Appl Toxicol* 4[2 Pt 1]:134–143, 1984.
40. Tredger JM, Smith HM, Read RB, et al. Effects of ethanol ingestion on the metabolism of a hepatotoxic dose of paracetamol in mice. *Xenobiotica* 16(7):661–670, 1986.
41. Ali FM, Boyer EW, Bird SB. Estimated risk of hepatotoxicity after an acute acetaminophen overdose in alcoholics. *Alcohol* 42(3):213–218, 2008.
42. Bray GP, Harrison PM, O'Grady JG, et al. Long-term anticonvulsant therapy worsens outcome in paracetamol-induced fulminant hepatic failure. *Hum Exp Toxicol* 11(4):265–270, 1992.
43. Rumack BH. Acetaminophen overdose in young children. Treatment and effects of alcohol and other additional ingestants in 417 cases. *Am J Dis Child* 138(5):428–433, 1984.
44. Miller RP, Roberts RJ, Fischer LJ. Acetaminophen elimination kinetics in neonates, children, and adults. *Clin Pharmacol Ther* 19(3):284–294, 1976.
45. Roberts I, Robinson MJ, Mughal MZ, et al. Paracetamol metabolites in the neonate following maternal overdose. *Br J Clin Pharmacol* 18(2):201–206, 1984.
46. Riggs BS, Bronstein AC, Kulig K, et al. Acute acetaminophen overdose during pregnancy. *Obstet Gynecol* 74(2):247–253, 1989.
47. Horowitz RS, Dart RC, Jarvie DR, et al. Placental transfer of N-acetylcysteine following human maternal acetaminophen toxicity. *J Toxicol Clin Toxicol* 35(5):447–451, 1997.
48. Douglas D, Smilkstein M, Sholar JB. Overdose with extended-relief acetaminophen: is a new approach necessary? *Acad Emerg Med* 2:397, 1995.
49. Stork DG, Rees S, Howland MA, et al. Pharmacokinetics of extended relief vs. regular release Tylenol in simulated human overdsoe. *J Toxicol* 34:157, 1996.
50. Seeff LB, Cuccherini BA, Zimmerman HJ, et al. Acetaminophen hepatotoxicity in alcoholics. A therapeutic misadventure. *Ann Intern Med* 104(3):399–404, 1986.
51. Hall AH, Kulig KW, Rumack BH. Acetaminophen hepatotoxicity. *JAMA* 256(14):1893–1894, 1986.
52. Benson GD. Acetaminophen in chronic liver disease. *Clin Pharmacol Ther* 33(1):95–101, 1983.
53. Harrison PM, Keays R, Bray GP, et al. Improved outcome of paracetamol-induced fulminant hepatic failure by late administration of acetylcysteine. *Lancet* 335(8705):1572–1573, 1990.
54. Bruno MK, Cohen SD, Khairallah EA. Antidotal effectiveness of N-acetylcysteine in reversing acetaminophen-induced hepatotoxicity. Enhancement of the proteolysis of arylated proteins. *Biochem Pharmacol* 37(22):4319–25, 1988.
55. Singer AJ, Carracio TR, Mofenson HC. The temporal profile of increased transaminase levels in patients with acetaminophen-induced liver dysfunction. *Ann Emerg Med* 26(1):49–53, 1995.
56. Yip L, Dart RC. A 20-hour treatment for acute acetaminophen overdose. *N Engl J Med* 348(24):2471–2472, 2003.
57. Hamlyn AN, Douglas AP, James O. The spectrum of paracetamol (acetaminophen) overdose: clinical and epidemiological studies. *Postgrad Med J* 54(632):400–404, 1978.
58. Clark R, Borirakchanyavat V, Davidson AR, et al. Hepatic damage and death from overdose of paracetamol. *Lancet* 1(7794):66–70, 1973.
59. O'Grady JG, Wendon J, Tan KC, et al. Liver transplantation after paracetamol overdose. *BMJ* 303(6796):221–223, 1991.
60. James O, Lesna M, Roberts SH, et al. Liver damage after paracetamol overdose. Comparison of liver-function tests, fasting serum bile acids, and liver histology. *Lancet* 2(7935):579–581, 1975.
61. Bernal W, Donaldson N, Wyncoll D, et al. Blood lactate as an early predictor of outcome in paracetamol-induced acute liver failure: a cohort study. *Lancet* 359(9306):558–563, 2002.
62. Schmidt LE, Dalhoff K. Alpha-fetoprotein is a predictor of outcome in acetaminophen-induced liver injury. *Hepatology* 41(1):26–31, 2005.

Chapter 99 ■ Alcohols and Glycol Poisoning

JENNIFER L. ENGLUND • MARCO L. A. SIVILOTTI • MARSHA D. FORD

The accidental or deliberate consumption of alcohols and glycols is a major cause of health problems. Although light consumption of ethanol may be associated with health benefits for some populations, heavy consumption increases overall mortality, especially mortality due to trauma, suicide, cirrhosis, and malignancies [1]. Ethanol is estimated to contribute to nearly 90,000 deaths each year in the United States, with economic costs in excess of $200 billion per annum [2]. The so-called toxic alcohols, namely, methanol and ethylene glycol, are usually involved in sporadic poisonings, often involving the accidental exposure of a young child to automotive or household products or the intentional suicidal ingestion of adults. Furthermore, multiple-victim poisonings can occur after recreational substitution for ethanol, during illicit manufacture of ethanol, or after the addition of other glycol products (see further discussion later).

ETHANOL

Ethanol is consumed by most adults and is the most serious drug of abuse among Western societies. Approximately one-third of the US population can be categorized as moderate-to-heavy drinkers, consuming four or more alcoholic drinks per week and of these, about one in five can be considered problem drinkers or alcoholics. Ethanol use is a factor in about 8% of emergency department visits [3] and 10% to 50% of hospital admissions, and its projected economic costs due to job absenteeism and poor job performance are substantial. Chronic ethanol consumption can cause multiorgan system disease, nutritional disorders, and teratogenic effects. In addition to beverages (typically 4% to 50% ethanol by volume), ethanol can be found in a myriad of other things such as colognes, perfumes, mouthwashes, aftershaves, and over-the-counter medicinals. Many of these products contain ethanol and can be sources of intoxication, especially among children.

The chemical properties and kinetics of ethanol are summarized in Table 99.1. Ethanol is a small, slightly polar aliphatic alcohol with a weak electric charge and is miscible in water and lipids. It diffuses easily into all body tissues. It is postulated that ethanol influences multiple ion channels, possibly by causing subtle alterations in their tertiary structure or their dynamic interaction with cell membranes. The behavioral effects of ethanol may result from its ability to antagonize the excitatory *N*-methyl-D-aspartate–glutamate receptor and to potentiate the inhibitory γ-aminobutyric acid A receptor [4–7]. Ethanol is also known to interact

TABLE 99.1

Comparative Data on the Toxic Alcohols and Glycols

Substance	Formula	Molecular weight	Specific gravity	V_d (L/kg)	Elimination half-life	Boiling point (°C)	Onset of toxicity	Important metabolites
Ethanol	CH_3CH_2OH	46	0.79	0.6	Zero order at 15–30 mg/dL/h	78.5	30–60 min	Acetaldehyde Acetic acid
Methanol	CH_3OH	32	0.79	0.7	Zero order at 8.5 mg/dL/h without ethanol; first order: $t½$ = 46.5 h with ethanol or fomepizole and 2.5 h with hemodialysis	64.7	12–24 h[a]	Formaldehyde Formic acid
Ethylene glycol		62	1.11	0.68	First order: $t½$ = 2.5–4.5 h without ethanol and with normal kidneys, 17 h with ethanol or fomepizole and <3 h with hemodialysis	197.6	4–12 h[a]	Glycoaldehyde Glyoxylic acid Glycolic acid Oxalic acid

(*continued*)

TABLE 99.1

Comparative Data on the Toxic Alcohols and Glycols (*continued*)

Substance	Formula	Molecular weight	Specific gravity	V_d (L/kg)	Elimination half-life	Boiling point (°C)	Onset of toxicity	Important metabolites
Isopropanol		60	0.79	0.6–0.7	First order: $t½$ = 2.5–3.5 h	82.5	30–60 min	Acetone
Propylene glycol		76	1.04	0.55	First order: $t½$ = 2–5 h in adults, 19.3 h in infants	188.2	Seconds with intravenous, ? with dermal	Pyruvate Lactate Acetate
Benzyl alcohol		108	1.04	?	?	204.7	?	Benzoic acid Hippuric acid
Diethylene glycol		106	1.12	?	?	245	?	2-Hydroxyethoxyacetic acid

V_d, volume of distribution.
[a]For metabolite effects; may be longer if ethanol coingested.
Data from references [75,80,81,86,91,92,94,103,104,107,110,127–129,145].

with glycine, nicotinic acetylcholine, 5-HT_3, and P_{2X} purinergic receptors, as well as the L-type calcium- and potassium-channel proteins [8,9]. The major metabolite, acetate, has been shown to mimic adenosine's effects via the P_1 receptor [10]. The precise role of these and other effects in producing intoxication, dependence, and withdrawal (see Chapter 126) is uncertain.

Ethanol is readily absorbed from the gastrointestinal tract, with 70% occurring in the stomach and 25% within the duodenum [11]. Peak ethanol levels typically occur 30 to 60 minutes after ingestion. Women have higher peak ethanol concentrations after a given dose because of smaller body mass and smaller relative body water, rather than gender differences of gastric mucosal alcohol dehydrogenase (ADH) activity [12].

Metabolism of ethanol occurs predominantly in the liver by three enzymatic systems: the cytosolic ADH enzyme family (especially class I), the cytochrome P450 enzymes (microsomal ethanol oxidizing system, largely CYP2E1 but also 3A4 and 1A2), and peroxisomal catalase [13,14]. Metabolism is Michaelis–Menten with zero-order kinetics prevailing at levels over 100 mg per dL [15]. Only a small fraction of ethanol is exhaled or secreted in urine and sweat [16].

ADH is responsible for greater than 57% of ethanol metabolism at low doses. In the ADH metabolic pathway (Fig. 99.1), ethanol is oxidized to acetaldehyde and then to acetate in a process that reduces oxidized nicotinamide adenine dinucleotide (NAD^+) to nicotinamide adenine dinucleotide (NADH). The increased ratio of NADH to NAD^+ can inhibit NAD^+-dependent reactions, such as gluconeogenesis, as well as slowing subsequent ethanol oxidation and clearance [17]. Acetate is linked to coenzyme A (acetyl-CoA), which can then participate in the citric acid cycle, fatty acid synthesis, or ketone formation [16]. Genetic variations of ADH and aldehyde dehydrogenase have been extensively characterized and may play a role in determining susceptibility to alcoholism [18,19]. Normally, the cytochrome P450 and catalase systems play minor roles in ethanol metabolism. Chronic ethanol use can induce CYP2E1 activity 4- to 10-fold, allowing habitual users to metabolize ethanol twice as quickly as occasional drinkers [20].

Ethanol is a central nervous system (CNS) depressant. After acute ingestion, there is often an initial stage of paradoxical excitation because of release of inhibitions. For nontolerant individuals,

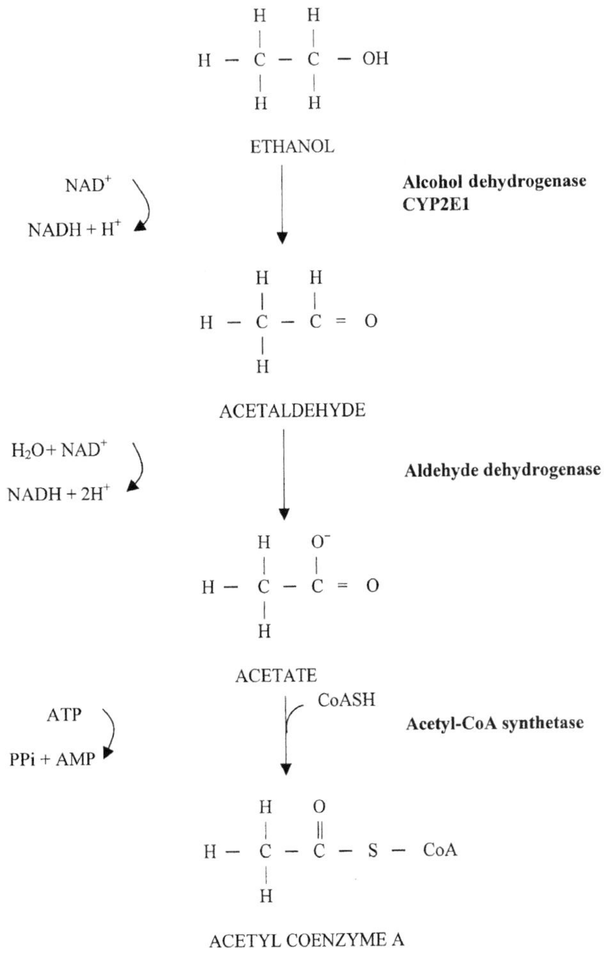

FIGURE 99.1 Ethanol metabolism. AMP, adenosine monophosphate; ATP, adenosine triphosphate; Co, coenzyme; NAD^+, oxidized form of nicotinamide adenine dinucleotide; NADH, nicotinamide adenine dinucleotide; PPi, inorganic pyrophosphate.

a blood ethanol concentration as low as 20 mg per dL impairs driving-related skills involving perception and attention [21]. At concentrations of 50 mg per dL, gross motor control and orientation may be affected, and intoxication may become apparent [22]. Lethargy, ataxia, and muscular incoordination may be seen at serum levels of 150 mg per dL or greater, coma at approximately 250 mg per dL, and death with levels greater than 450 mg per dL [23,24]. Tolerant drinkers can achieve higher levels before developing similar symptoms, and survival has been reported despite a serum level of 1,500 mg per dL [11,25]. At high doses, ethanol functions as an anesthetic, causing CNS depression, autonomic dysfunction (e.g., hypotension, hypothermia), coma, and death from respiratory depression and cardiovascular collapse. The estimated LD_{50} in adults is 5 to 8 g per kg and 3 g per kg for children [23].

Tolerance to ethanol's effects develops both acutely and after chronic consumption. With acute consumption, the physiologic effects at a given serum level of ethanol have been noted to be less when ethanol concentrations are declining rather than when levels are rising (Mellanby effect). Compared with inexperienced drinkers, chronic drinkers experience diminished effects to a given amount of ethanol. Tolerance is accompanied by changes in membrane-associated receptors.

Clinical Manifestations

Patients may present with varying degrees of altered consciousness, including agitation, stupor, and coma. The odor of ethanol or its congeners on their breath is usually present. Slurred speech, ataxia, and nystagmus are noted in patients with mild to moderate intoxication. Disconjugate gaze is frequently seen in comatose patients. Acute intoxication may be accompanied by vomiting, particularly in novice drinkers.

Diagnostic Evaluation

The physical examination should be directed toward evaluation of the airway and a search for complicating or contributing factors such as trauma, infection, and hemorrhage. For patients with moderate-to-severe poisoning, laboratory studies including complete blood cell count; serum electrolytes, blood urea nitrogen, creatinine, glucose, ethanol, magnesium, calcium, and phosphorus level; liver function tests; prothrombin time; electrocardiogram; chest radiograph; arterial or venous blood gas; and urinalysis should be obtained as clinically indicated. Blood alcohol levels may be helpful to support the diagnosis, but it does not predict clinical severity or overall outcomes [11]. If the level of consciousness is inconsistent with the serum ethanol level or does not improve over a few hours, the physician should reconsider the diagnosis of ethanol intoxication (Table 99.2).

Management

Patients with stupor or coma who cannot be aroused to a verbal (but not necessarily coherent) state or who have a poor respiratory effort should be intubated to ensure airway patency and to protect against pulmonary aspiration. Intravenous (IV) naloxone (0.1 to 2 mg), dextrose (25 to 50 g), and thiamine hydrochloride (100 mg) should be administered when opioid toxicity, hypoglycemia, or Wernicke's encephalopathy are considerations.

Activated charcoal should be withheld unless potentially toxic coingestants are suspected. Hypothermia, when present, is usually mild in the absence of environmental exposure and can be managed with warm blankets. Nutritional, electrolyte, and fluid deficiencies should be corrected. A variety of interventions trying to increase ethanol clearance or decrease its effects are neither clinically useful nor recommended.

TABLE 99.2

Differential Diagnoses for Acute Ethanol Intoxication

- Metabolic
  - Hypoglycemia
  - Hyperglycemia
  - Hyponatremia
  - Hypothermia
  - Hepatic encephalopathy
- Disulfiram reaction
  - Hypercalcemia
  - Hypoxia
  - Drug intoxication
  - Phencyclidine
  - Opioids
  - Cyclic antidepressants
  - Other alcohols (methanol, isopropanol, ethylene glycol)
  - Other sedative-hypnotics (meprobamate, methaqualone, glutethimide, benzodiazepines, barbiturates, chloral hydrate, ethchlorvynol, methyprylon)
  - Anticholinergics
  - Carbon monoxide
- Trauma
  - Intracranial hemorrhage (subdural, epidural, intracerebral bleed)
- Infections
  - Central nervous system infections
  - Acquired immunodeficiency syndrome
  - Sepsis
- Neurologic
  - Postictal
  - Delirium tremens
  - Wernicke's encephalopathy

Adapted from Adinoff B, Bone GHA, Linnoila M: Acute ethanol poisoning and the ethanol withdrawal syndrome. *Med Toxicol* 3:172, 1988.

ALCOHOLIC KETOACIDOSIS

Alcoholic ketoacidosis (AKA) develops as a result of hormonal, nutritional, and metabolic changes caused by ethanol (Fig. 99.2). Because ethanol retards ketogenesis, AKA usually occurs when ethanol levels are low to absent [16]. Ethanol metabolism indirectly impairs gluconeogenesis and increases fatty acid and ketone formation. Inadequate nutritional intake of alcoholics depletes glycogen, mineral, and vitamin stores. Vomiting results in decreased intravascular volume and increased catecholamine levels that blunt insulin release [26] activate lipase and accelerate free fatty acid oxidation. Glucagon activates the carnitine acyltransferase system, producing excess acetyl-CoA.

Acetyl-CoA cannot be used by mammals to form pyruvate or higher carbohydrates. Instead, it can undergo only three metabolic fates: fatty acid synthesis, oxidation to CO_2 in the citric acid cycle, and cholesterol or ketone body formation via 3-hydroxy-3-methylglutaryl-CoA. The ketogenic pathway has the largest capacity and requires the least adenosine triphosphate for handling acetyl-CoA overload [26]. Nutritional deficiencies impair acetyl-CoA conversion to triglycerides and its entrance into the citric acid cycle [16]. Finally, the increased NADH-to-NAD^+ redox ratio caused by ethanol oxidation favors the conversion of acetoacetate to β-hydroxybutyrate, which is largely responsible for the ketoacidosis.

Other acid–base abnormalities may occur among alcoholics. Respiratory acidosis may be caused by hypoglycemia or

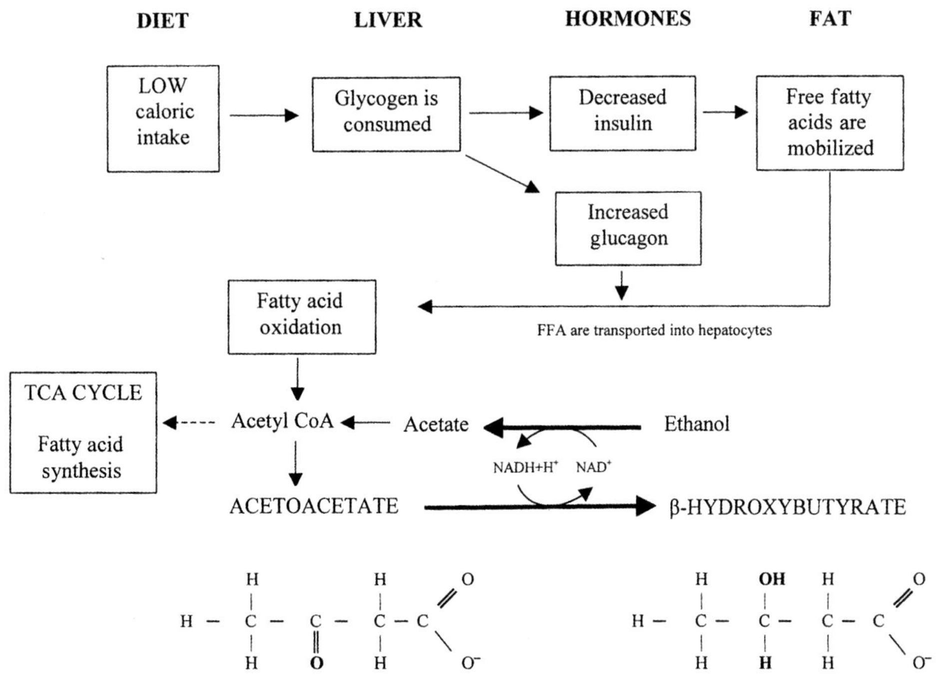

FIGURE 99.2 Mechanism of alcoholic ketoacidosis. Co, coenzyme; FFA, free fatty acids; NAD^+, oxidized form of nicotinamide adenine dinucleotide; NADH, nicotinamide adenine dinucleotide; TCA, tricarboxylic acid cycle (also known as *citric acid cycle*). (Adapted from Eckardt MJ, Harford TC, Kaelber CT, et al: Health hazards associated with alcohol consumption. *JAMA* 246:648, 1981, with permission.)

ethanol-induced respiratory depression. Lactic acidosis can occur secondary to seizure activity, an increase in the NADH-to-NAD^+ ratio that favors lactate formation from pyruvate, decreased gluconeogenesis, thiamine deficiency impairing pyruvate's entry into the citric acid cycle, and liver dysfunction [14,27]. Vomiting may cause volume contraction, hypokalemia, and metabolic alkalosis [14,26]. A mild acetic acidosis may be seen when peripheral tissues incompletely oxidize acetate. A hyperchloremic metabolic acidosis has been observed among acutely intoxicated patients who have excreted β-hydroxybutyrate in their urine [27].

Clinical Manifestations

Patients with AKA usually present with a recent history of binge alcohol drinking in the setting of chronic alcohol use and poor nutritional intake followed by vomiting and abdominal pain. The fruity odor of ketones may be detected along with Kussmaul's breathing, dry mucous membranes, tachycardia, orthostatic hypotension, and poor skin turgor [16]. Abdominal pain is typical, with nonspecific tenderness on examination [14].

Diagnostic Evaluation

The diagnosis of AKA is a diagnosis of exclusion. Signs and symptoms of concomitant gastritis, pancreatitis, hepatitis, gastrointestinal hemorrhage, and vitamin and mineral deficiencies are often present. Laboratory studies should include those listed for acute ethanol intoxication plus serum ketones, lactate, and osmolality. Ethanol levels are often low to undetectable, and hypoglycemia may be present [28]. A respiratory or metabolic alkalosis may be present in addition to the anion gap metabolic acidosis. At presentation, the predominant serum ketone is usually β-hydroxybutyrate because of the altered redox state, which results in falsely low serum ketones by the semiquantitative nitroprusside test for acetoacetate [16]. Many laboratories now measure β-hydroxybutyrate directly to mitigate this concern. Hypokalemia is uncommon, in part because acidosis shifts potassium out of the cell. The osmol gap may be elevated from glycerol, acetone, and its metabolites [29], even after correcting for the serum ethanol concentration [30,31].

The differential diagnosis of an anion gap metabolic acidosis includes lactic acidosis, salicylate poisoning, uremia, diabetic ketoacidosis, and intoxication from iron, ibuprofen, toluene, methanol, ethylene glycol, and diethylene glycol. AKA can usually be differentiated from diabetic ketoacidosis by the lack of significant hyperglycemia, minimal alteration of consciousness, a relatively mild acidosis, and rapid improvement with supportive therapy [32]. The presence of more than mild tenderness on abdominal examination should prompt investigation for other pathology such as pancreatitis, hepatitis, sepsis, or pneumonia [14].

Management

Supportive therapy is the same as that noted for acute intoxication. IV fluid resuscitation, glucose (25 to 50 g), and thiamine (100 mg) reverse the ketogenic process and are the mainstays of therapy. Maintenance fluids should consist of dextrose (5%) in normal saline [14,30]. Thiamine facilitates the entry of pyruvate into the citric acid cycle and protects against Wernicke's encephalopathy [33]. Once urine output is established, supplemental potassium and magnesium should be administered. Hypophosphatemia may develop with increased glycolysis and carbohydrate refeeding and should be corrected with potassium phosphate [32,34]. Hospitalization and refeeding of malnourished patients may be required.

ETHYLENE GLYCOL AND METHANOL

Ethylene Glycol

Ethylene glycol (1,2-ethanediol) is a colorless, sweet liquid [35] that imparts a warm sensation to the tongue and esophagus when swallowed. It is found primarily in automotive antifreeze and de-icing solutions. Ingestions usually result from suicide attempts, intentional substitution of ethylene glycol for ethanol, or accidental exposure. According to the Annual Report of the American Association of Poison Control Centers' National Poison Data System (NPDS) during 2014 poison centers received 6,078 calls about ethylene glycol [36], including 2,134 cases treated in a health care facility and 16 deaths. Ethylene glycol itself causes little toxicity other than ethanol-like inebriation until it is metabolized in the liver into its toxic acid metabolites (Fig. 99.3). Ethylene glycol is first metabolized in the liver by ADH to glycoaldehyde, which is rapidly transformed via aldehyde dehydrogenase to glycolic acid. Glycolic acid is slowly converted to glyoxylic acid, which in turn is converted to multiple metabolites, including oxalic acid [37,38]. It is uncertain which of these metabolites is most directly responsible for renal tubular toxicity, though recent studies suggest that internalization of calcium oxalate crystals by proximal tubule cells may be directly related to renal damage [39].

The anion gap metabolic acidosis seen in ethylene glycol poisoning is due predominantly to elevated glycolic acid levels [37,40], although oxalic acid, glyoxylic acid, and glycoaldehyde may be more toxic [39]. Elevated lactic acid levels contribute to the acidosis [40,41] and have been attributed to the increased NADH-to-NAD$^+$ ratio caused by metabolism of ethylene glycol [42,43] and to the toxicity of glyoxylic acid on mitochondrial respiration [37]. Some lactate assays may misinterpret glycolate as lactate and report falsely elevated lactate levels [44–46].

Pathologic changes are noted in the CNS, kidneys, lungs, heart, liver, muscles, and retina [23,47]. Renal findings include dilation of the proximal tubules with swelling and vacuolization of the epithelial cells, distal tubular dilation, intratubular deposition of calcium oxalate crystals, and interstitial edema [42]. Pulmonary edema, interstitial pneumonitis, and hemorrhagic bronchopneumonia may occur. In some cases, interstitial myocarditis, skeletal muscle inflammation, and centrilobular hepatic fatty infiltration may develop. CNS findings include cerebral edema, meningoencephalitis, and cerebellar changes, including focal loss of Purkinje cells [47].

The chemical properties and kinetics of ethylene glycol are summarized in Table 99.1. Oral absorption of ethylene glycol occurs rapidly. Percutaneous absorption through intact skin is negligible. Ethylene glycol has a high boiling point and toxicity from vapor inhalation does not occur. Hepatic metabolism predominates, yet renal elimination of the parent compound is initially substantial. The ensuing renal failure markedly prolongs the elimination of ethylene glycol and its metabolites [42,48,49].

The estimated minimum lethal dose is 1.4 mL per kg body weight for humans [35]. With early and intensive treatment, survival has been reported in patients with serum ethylene glycol concentrations as high as 1,889 mg per dL [50].

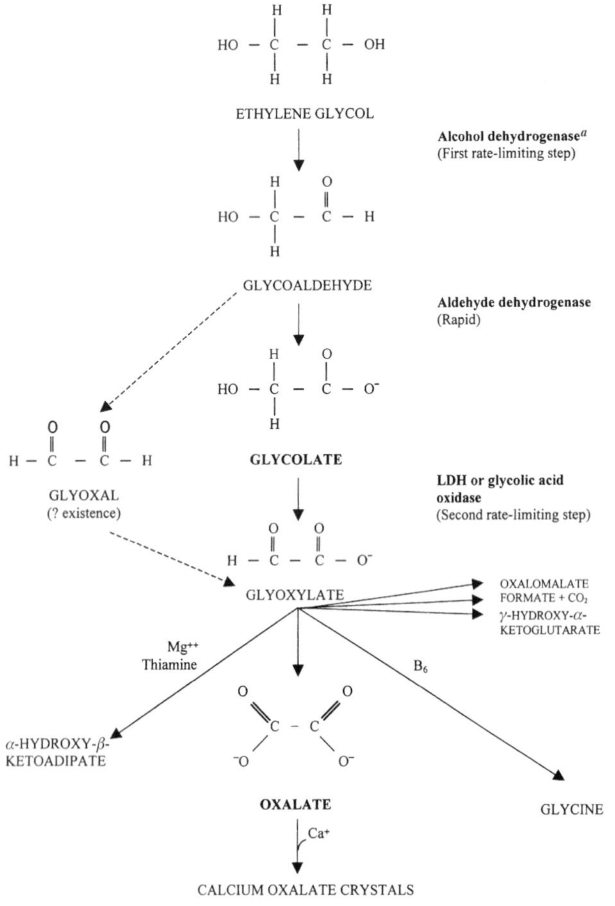

FIGURE 99.3 Ethylene glycol metabolism. [a]Blocked by ethanol and fomepizole. LDH, lactate dehydrogenase.

Methanol

Methanol is a colorless liquid and has an odor distinct from that of ethanol. Dietary sources and endogenous metabolism can produce serum methanol levels of 0.15 mg per dL [51]. Exogenous sources of methanol include windshield washing fluid, de-icing fluids, carburetor cleaners, paint removers, and paint thinners. The NPDS reports that during 2014 there were 1,825 calls to poison centers regarding methanol and 9 associated deaths [36].

Methanol is oxidized in the liver by ADH to formaldehyde, which is quickly converted to formic acid (formate) by hepatic aldehyde dehydrogenase (Fig. 99.4). In primates, formate accumulates because of saturation of one-carbon metabolism. High levels of formate, an inhibitor of mitochondrial cytochrome oxidase, cause histotoxic hypoxia and are responsible for the characteristic metabolic acidosis and ocular toxicity seen with methanol toxicity [52]. Formaldehyde is also very toxic, but it has a very short half-life [53].

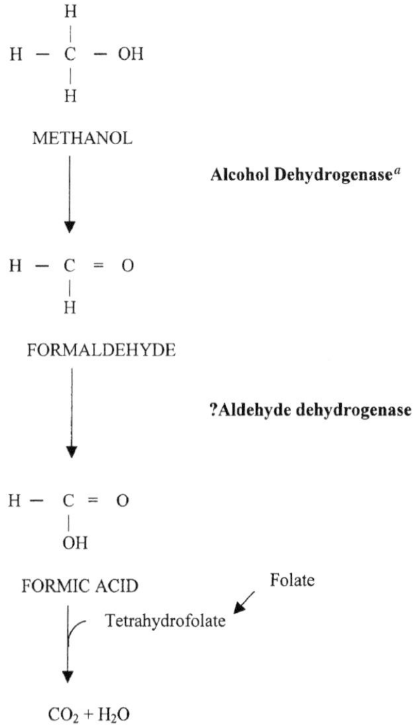

FIGURE 99.4 Methanol metabolism. [a]Blocked by ethanol and fomepizole.

Formate plays a pivotal role in methanol toxicity. Blood formate concentrations account for nearly the entire observed anion gap and base deficit [54]. Symptoms and prognosis also correlate better with formate than with methanol levels [55,56]. Primates infused with formic acid develop ocular toxicity, even when the acidosis is controlled with sodium bicarbonate [57]. Ocular toxicity results from the inhibition of cytochrome oxidase by formic acid in the optic nerve, leading to disruption of mitochondrial electron transport and decreased axoplasmic flow and electrical conduction [58]. Direct retinal toxicity can also occur [59].

The chemical properties and kinetics of methanol are summarized in Table 99.1. Methanol is absorbed orally, dermally, and via inhalation [60]. Exposure can occur intentionally or accidentally, including mass outbreaks, as occurred in Estonia in 2001 when 68 patients died after consuming illegal spirits contaminated with methanol [61]. Adults who abuse carburetor cleaning fluid by inhalation can achieve serum methanol levels greater than 50 mg per dL [62]. Methanol's metabolism is slower than that of ethylene glycol or ethanol [42,53]. Hepatic oxidation predominates, with only trivial amounts eliminated via the lungs and kidneys [53]. Elimination follows first-order kinetics at low doses and during hemodialysis [63–65]. At higher doses, zero-order (Michaelis–Menten) kinetics may prevail. In one untreated patient, methanol elimination occurred at a rate of 8.5 mg/dL/h [66]. The elimination half-life of formate in one untreated patient was 3.7 hours [67] and averaged 3.4 ± 1.5 hours in eight patients treated with fomepizole (4-methylpyrazole) and leucovorin [54]. With hemodialysis, the formate elimination half-life was estimated to be between 1.8 and 3.1 hours [54,67].

Reported lethal doses for patients with inadequate, delayed, or no therapy vary considerably and are not well established. In one epidemic, the minimal lethal dose was 15 mL of a 40%-by-weight methanol solution. Yet, in a case report a 27-year-old man with a blood methanol concentration of 1,290 mg per dL (12.9 g per L), possibly ingesting up to 1,000 mL of a 60%-by-weight methanol solution, survived with moderate visual sequelae and esophageal stenosis [68].

Clinical Manifestations

Ethylene Glycol

Ethanol-like intoxication usually begins within an hour of ingestion. Symptoms due to toxic metabolites usually occur 4 to 12 hours after ingestion, but are delayed further if ethanol was coingested by delaying the metabolism of ethylene glycol. Patients may present alert, intoxicated, or in a coma, depending on the time since ingestion, the dose of ethylene glycol, coingestion of ethanol, and cross-tolerance [42,47]. Vital signs can be normal. Ocular exposure can produce a chemical conjunctivitis and chemosis [47], but systemic toxicity does not occur.

The classic division of ethylene glycol poisoning into three stages is primarily of historical interest. In reality, patients rarely exhibit sequential toxicity that can be readily divided into distinct stages. Shortly after ingestion and before significant metabolism of ethylene glycol has occurred, CNS effects such as ethanol-like intoxication, stupor, nausea, and vomiting predominate. As toxic metabolites begin to accumulate, a metabolic acidosis ensues with associated cardiovascular and pulmonary signs, including Kussmaul's respirations, tachycardia, cyanosis, and cardiogenic or noncardiogenic pulmonary edema. As renal injury progresses, flank pain and tenderness, proteinuria, and anuria may occur. Acute renal failure occurs in nearly all untreated patients who manifest metabolic acidosis (serum bicarbonate <10 mmol per L). Renal dysfunction can develop within 9 hours of ingestion [69]. Patients may also develop myositis with muscle tenderness and elevated creatine kinase [42]. Death may result from severe metabolic derangements, cardiovascular or respiratory failure, or progressive CNS depression. Prolonged seizures, coma, and a cerebral herniation syndrome have also been reported [70]. Preterminal dysrhythmias and hypotension are rare. The presence of hyperkalemia, severe acidemia, seizures, and coma at presentation demonstrate severe toxicity.

Seizures are usually generalized but do not occur in all cases. Jacksonian seizures have been reported, as have myoclonic jerks and tetanic contractions due to hypocalcemia [47]. Progressive CNS depression and prolonged seizures usually result from cerebral edema [42]. Transient nystagmus and cranial nerve (II, V, VI, VII, VIII, IX, and X) palsies have been reported to occur 4 to 18 days postingestion [35,50,70–73].

Methanol

Onset of toxicity usually occurs within 30 hours of methanol ingestion. In one epidemic, a range of 40 minutes to 72 hours was reported. Factors influencing time to symptoms include the dose, ethanol coingestion, and folate stores.

Neurologic, ophthalmologic, and gastrointestinal symptoms predominate. Methanol is a less potent CNS depressant than ethanol. Patients may be alert on admission and complain only of headache and dizziness. Amnesia, restlessness, acute mania, lethargy, confusion, coma, and convulsions may follow. Cases mimicking subarachnoid hemorrhage with severe headache, vomiting, hypertension, and bradycardia followed by loss of consciousness have been described. Dyspnea is reported by only 8% to 25% of patients [61].

Early on, many patients offer no visual complaints. Visual symptoms accompany the metabolic acidosis and usually develop when the blood pH falls below 7.2. Blurred vision, photophobia, scotomata, eye pain, partial or complete loss of vision, and visual hallucinations (e.g., bright lights, "skin over eyes," "snowstorm," dancing spots, flashes) have been reported. These disturbances can persist after formate has been completely eliminated and the acidosis has resolved.

Methanol can produce severe hemorrhagic gastritis and pancreatitis, causing upper abdominal pain, nausea, vomiting, and diarrhea. Liver function abnormalities have been documented in moderately to severely ill patients.

Vital signs may reveal tachycardia and Kussmaul's respirations, but the blood pressure is usually maintained. Untreated, patients can die from sudden respiratory arrest [74]. The skin may be cool and diaphoretic, and abdominal muscles rigid without rebound tenderness.

The most notable physical findings are those discovered on ophthalmologic examination, but these are late findings. Pupils may react sluggishly or may be fixed and dilated. Funduscopic examination may show hyperemia of the optic discs followed by retinal edema, which develops initially along the retinal vessels and then spreads to the central areas of the fundus. Retinal vessel engorgement accompanies the retinal edema [52]. Papilledema may develop [7]. Ophthalmologic findings do not necessarily correlate with visual complaints.

Diagnostic Evaluation

Poisoning by ethylene glycol and methanol should be suspected for all patients with a history of ingesting ethanol substitutes or who have an unexplained anion gap metabolic acidosis.

Ethylene Glycol

Laboratory studies should include complete blood cell count; serum electrolytes; glucose; blood urea nitrogen; creatinine; arterial or venous blood gas; calcium; serum osmolality; ethanol, methanol, and ethylene glycol levels; and urinalysis. Additional laboratory studies may include electrocardiogram, chest radiograph, and head computed tomography as clinically indicated. Early after ingestion, before significant metabolism of ethylene glycol, an osmol gap may be present with neither metabolic acidosis nor an anion gap (see later discussion on osmol gap). As ethylene glycol is metabolized, the osmol gap decreases and an anion gap metabolic acidosis develops. Patients who present very late may have renal failure with normal osmol and anion gaps, normal pH, and unmeasurable ethylene glycol levels.

Perhaps the greatest diagnostic challenge of managing a patient suspected to have ingested a toxic alcohol or glycol is the limited availability of methanol and ethylene glycol testing. Gas chromatography can reliably quantify the presence of ethylene glycol or methanol, but most hospitals are unable to obtain these tests in a timely fashion. Moreover, some hospitals offer a "toxic alcohol screen" that detects methanol, ethanol, and isopropanol but not ethylene glycol, which is a diol. This nomenclature can mislead a clinician into interpreting a negative "toxic alcohol screen" as excluding the presence of ethylene glycol. Interference due to propionic acid, propylene glycol, glycerol, 2,3-butanediol, and β-hydroxybutyrate has been described [75–78]. Testing for glycolic acid or formic acid is even less available. A rapid bedside qualitative test for ethylene glycol is available but not yet approved for diagnostic use in humans [79]. Breath alcohol analysis can mistake methanol for ethanol, providing indirect evidence of exposure. Therefore, diagnostic and therapeutic decisions are often based on circumstantial evidence derived from the history and available laboratory testing, pending confirmatory testing. It is essential for the physician to understand the strengths and the limitations of these indirect markers of toxicity.

Arterial pH measurements in ethylene glycol–exposed patients can range from 6.7 to 7.5 [69]. Ethylene glycol poisoning often results in higher anion gaps than other causes of this abnormality [56,43,80,81]. The differential diagnosis of an increased anion gap metabolic acidosis is discussed above (see "Alcoholic Ketoacidosis" section). In young children, child abuse and inborn errors of organic acid metabolism should be considered in the differential diagnosis [78,82]. Hyperkalemia may be seen in association with acidosis and with renal failure [47,83,84]. The creatinine and blood urea nitrogen are normal unless renal failure has supervened. Calcium levels are initially normal but may drop significantly as calcium complexes with oxalic acid to form calcium oxalate. The electrocardiogram may show ST-T wave and QTc changes consistent with hypocalcemia, hyperkalemia, or both.

The osmol gap (refer to Chapters 97, 137, and 198) is frequently used as a diagnostic test in the evaluation of these patients. Extreme caution must be used when interpreting the osmol gap, however. First, the serum osmolality should be measured by the freezing point depression, as vapor pressure osmometry will not detect methanol, ethanol, and isopropanol.

Although an osmol gap greater than 10 mOsm is often sought as indirect evidence of the presence of an exogenous alcohol or glycol, *failure to find an elevated osmol gap does not rule out significant alcohol or glycol ingestion* [80]. Cumulative measurement error in the formula parameters, variations of the formula itself, and the natural variability in the osmol gap at baseline contribute to imprecision in the calculated osmol gap [30,85,86]. This variability can hide a significant amount of an alcohol or glycol. Furthermore, as the parent alcohol or glycol is oxidized to the toxic-charged metabolite, the osmol gap disappears. Conversely, an elevated osmol gap is not specific for alcohols or glycols, as lactic acidosis, ketoacidosis, and sepsis can also increase the osmol gap [80].

In studies of various control populations not exposed to methanol, isopropanol, or ethylene glycol, osmol gaps averaged approximately −1 to −2 mOsm per kg [31,87,88]. The variability was substantial, however, with standard deviations of between 5 and 8 mOsm per kg. Thus, although an arbitrary upper limit of 10 mOsm per kg has historically been used for the normal osmol gap, an osmol gap of 10 mOsm per kg in a patient whose usual baseline gap is 0 could represent substantial serum concentrations of ethylene glycol (62 mg per dL) or methanol (32 mg per dL) [81]. One patient with an osmol gap of only 11 mOsm per kg had an ethylene glycol level of 38 mg per dL and subsequently developed renal failure [43], whereas another patient with an osmol gap of 7.2 mOsm per kg required hemodialysis for ethylene glycol toxicity [89]. Thus, an elevated osmol gap may suggest the presence of an alcohol or glycol, but a normal gap does not rule out a small ingestion or a late presentation.

Microscopic examination of the urine for crystals is another indirect diagnostic test frequently recommended. Less than 50% of patients have crystalluria at presentation, however. Calcium oxalate monohydrate (needle-shaped) and calcium oxalate dihydrate (envelope-shaped) crystals can both be seen, but the monohydrate may be confused with uric or hippuric acid crystals [43,90]. The dihydrate crystals tend to occur at higher concentrations and convert to the monohydrate form within 24 hours [91], but are also nonspecific and can be found in the urine after ingestion of oxalate-containing foods such as rhubarb. Other nonspecific urinary findings can include low specific gravity, proteinuria, hematuria, and pyuria. Some antifreeze manufacturers add fluorescein to their products to facilitate the detection of radiator leaks. Wood's lamp examination of the urine or gastric aspirate to detect fluorescence is unreliable and should not be used to make or exclude the diagnosis. Other drugs, food products, toxins, and even endogenous compounds cause urine to fluoresce, as do the containers used to collect urine [92,93].

Methanol

The laboratory studies listed for ethylene glycol evaluation should be obtained. Methanol can also cause an anion gap metabolic acidosis and an osmol gap [35]. The caveats noted under ethylene glycol for the evaluation and interpretation of these parameters apply equally to methanol. Elevated lactate levels, mild hypokalemia, and leukocytosis may occur. Lactic acidosis may be seen late in the course of methanol poisoning and may result from inhibition of the mitochondrial electron transport system or from poor tissue perfusion [42]. Serum lactate concentrations of 11.5 and 23 mmol per L have been reported 24 hours or more after ingestion. Amylase elevations and pancreatitis can occur in up to one-half of severely poisoned patients [66,94]. Computed tomography scanning can demonstrate cerebral edema, as well as frontal lobe and basal ganglia hemorrhages and infarcts associated with poor clinical outcomes.

Management

The focus of treatment for ethylene glycol and methanol poisoning is to prevent the formation of toxic metabolites by inhibiting liver ADH and enhancing the removal of the parent compound and metabolites. Antidotal therapy, cofactor therapy, and hemodialysis may be necessary in addition to supportive care to achieve these goals.

Initial treatment includes airway management in the comatose patient, IV fluids, cardiac monitoring, and appropriate laboratory studies. Gastric aspiration via a nasogastric tube may be beneficial when performed within an hour of an intentional ingestion. Oral activated charcoal is ineffective, but may be considered when coingestants are suspected [95,96].

IV sodium bicarbonate should be administered to correct serum pH to at least 7.3 [66,96]. Large doses of sodium bicarbonate may be required. Sodium bicarbonate is useful in ethylene glycol and methanol poisonings for three reasons. First, unlike the metabolites in lactic acidosis and ketoacidosis, the metabolites of ethylene glycol and methanol cannot be transformed to regenerate bicarbonate [43], and the acidosis must be corrected with exogenous alkali. Second, increasing the serum pH enhances the ionization of acid metabolites, making them less diffusible, trapping them in the blood and extracellular fluid, and limiting their tissue penetration [42]. Third, urinary alkalinization may increase excretion of acid metabolites through ion trapping, provided renal function remains normal [35,90]. In ethylene glycol poisoning, however, the hypocalcemia that occurs as calcium complexes with oxalate may be worsened by alkali administration. Calcium chloride/gluconate should be administered to correct symptomatic hypocalcemia including seizures, but the indiscriminate use of calcium salts to correct a laboratory value should be avoided because it may increase the precipitation of calcium oxalate crystals [97]. In methanol poisoning, increasing the serum pH may increase the concentration of ionized formate, thus diminishing formic acid access to the CNS and possibly ameliorating retinal toxicity [42].

Seizures should initially be treated with standard anticonvulsants, such as benzodiazepines and barbiturates. Hypocalcemia and hypoglycemia should be excluded. Recurrent or persistent coma or seizures should prompt evaluation for underlying cerebral edema. Cerebral edema should be managed acutely with hyperventilation, mannitol (provided renal function is intact), and potentially intracranial pressure monitoring and decompression. Cardiopulmonary complications may require inotropes and vasopressors.

Ethanol and fomepizole are antidotes for ethylene glycol and methanol poisoning. These agents inhibit liver ADH, and block the initial oxidation of ethylene glycol and methanol to their more toxic metabolites. After ADH is inhibited, ethylene glycol and methanol can be eliminated via endogenous or extracorporeal routes [49,98,99]. Antidotal therapy has no effect on the elimination of the acid metabolites. Indications for antidotal therapy in cases of known or possible methanol or ethylene glycol intoxication are outlined in Table 99.3 [69,84,96,100].

Recognition that ethanol is the preferred substrate for ADH (10 to 20 times greater affinity for ADH than other alcohols) [35] suggested its clinical use as a competitive inhibitor of this enzyme. Although most sources recommend administering sufficient ethanol to maintain serum ethanol concentrations between 100 and 150 mg per dL [63], limited data support this target concentration. Because ethanol is a competitive inhibitor of ADH, extremely high levels of ethylene glycol or methanol must by necessity be met with higher doses of ethanol. Targeting a 1:4 molar ratio [42,101] a serum ethanol concentration of 100 mg per dL should suffice for methanol concentrations as high as 257 mg per dL or ethylene glycol as high as 540 mg per dL. Dosage guidelines to achieve an ethanol concentration of 100 mg per dL are outlined in Table 99.4.

There are disadvantages to using ethanol therapeutically. Perhaps the most important limitation is the toxicity of ethanol itself, including coma, airway compromise, respiratory depression, and agitation [16,102,103]. At recommended doses, ethanol induces inebriation in the nontolerant individual. Subsequent behavioral effects and severe mental status depression may require interventions, such as sedation and endotracheal intubation shortly after initiation of therapy. The need for these interventions as well as the continuous infusion of ethanol itself can complicate and delay interfacility transfer. Although IV ethanol administration is generally preferred to oral ethanol, this requires extemporaneous compounding from dehydrated ethanol and an infusion of a hypertonic solution (10% ethanol by volume is 1,700 mOsm per kg), usually via a central venous catheter. Maintaining an adequate ethanol level can be difficult and interindividual variation in metabolism and removal during hemodialysis necessitate frequent monitoring of serum concentrations and dosage adjustments [102]. This allows for more opportunity for ethanol-related medication errors, such as excessive ethanol dose, inadequate monitoring, and inappropriate antidote duration, as compared with fomepizole therapy [104]. Finally, ethanol therapy is relatively contraindicated in patients on disulfiram or similar medications, patients with hepatic disease, and patients with alcohol addiction. Admission to an intensive care setting is considered mandatory for an individual receiving ethanol therapy.

Given these limitations to ethanol therapy, fomepizole has emerged as the preferred antidote. It is a more potent competitive inhibitor of ADH, with 500 to 1,000 times greater affinity for ADH than is ethanol [35,90,97,105,106]. Fomepizole

TABLE 99.3

Indications for Alcohol Dehydrogenase Inhibitor Therapy

A serum methanol or ethylene glycol concentration >20 mg/dL[a]
When serum methanol or ethylene glycol levels are not readily available:
- Documented ingestion of a consequential amount of methanol or ethylene glycol, especially when it is associated with a falling serum bicarbonate level or serum osmol gap >10 mOsm/kg by freezing point depression
- History or strong clinical suspicion of methanol or ethylene glycol ingestion and one of the following:
  - A falling serum bicarbonate level or a serum bicarbonate <20 mmol
  - Arterial pH <7.3
  - Renal dysfunction or ocular toxicity

[a]Attempts should be made to obtain confirmatory methanol or ethylene glycol concentrations as soon as possible when contemplating alcohol dehydrogenase inhibitor therapy. In all cases, consultation with a medical toxicologist is strongly recommended.

TABLE 99.4

Ethanol Dosing for Ethylene Glycol or Methanol Poisoning

Loading dose of ethanol:
- 0.8 g/kg (1 mL/kg) of 100% ethanol
- Oral or via nasogastric tube: Use 20%–30% concentration (e.g., 5 mL/kg of 20% ethanol; recall "80 proof" = 40% by volume)
- Intravenous: use 5%–10% concentration, load over 1 h (e.g., 10 mL/kg of 10% ethanol in D_5 W over 1 h)

If ethanol is already present, the amount of ethanol required to achieve a serum ethanol level of 100–150 mg/dL may be calculated as follows:
- Amount ethanol (mg) = [desired concentration (mg/dL) – known concentration (mg/dL)] V_d of ethanol (0.6 L/kg) × body weight (kg) × 10 dL/L

Maintenance doses of ethanol:
- Begin during administration of the loading dose.
- Give 80 mg/kg/h of ethanol orally or intravenously (as above). For a patient on hemodialysis, the maintenance dose should be higher: 250–350 mg/kg/h. Chronic alcoholics also require higher doses (average 150 mg/kg/h). Because of potential hypoglycemia, glucose should be given along with ethanol. Serum ethanol and glucose levels must be monitored frequently.

D_5 W, dextrose 5% in water; V_d, volume of distribution.
Adapted from Ekins BR, Rollins DE, Duffy DP, et al: Standardized treatment of severe methanol poisoning with ethanol and hemodialysis. *West J Med* 142:337, 1985.

has many advantages over ethanol: wide therapeutic margin, ease of administration, fixed dosing schedule, lack of CNS or behavioral toxicity, lack of metabolic or fluid balance effects, patient and provider safety, and no need for drug concentration monitoring [95,103,105, 107,108]. Despite these advantages, ethanol should not be overlooked as a viable treatment option during mass outbreaks or times of limited resources or drug availability [109]. Currently, fomepizole is only available in a parenteral formulation, although oral administration of this same formulation has similar pharmacokinetics and efficacy [110]. Highly selected patients treated with fomepizole may also avoid hemodialysis (discussed later), intensive care unit admission, or even interfacility transfer [48,49,90,95,106,107,110–115]. These advantages are even more important in the setting of mass epidemics and in pediatric exposures [116].

A minimum serum fomepizole concentration of 10 μM (0.8 mg per dL) [117] effectively halts ethylene glycol and methanol oxidation [49,118] and is much higher than the in vitro K_i of fomepizole for human ADH of 1 μM [119]. Recommended dosing (Table 99.5) achieves and maintains serum fomepizole concentrations greater than 100 μM, eliminating the need for drug concentration monitoring [120]. Adverse drug events associated with fomepizole therapy are infrequent, but include rash, eosinophilia, minimal hepatic transaminase elevations, nausea, vomiting, and abdominal pain [121]. Hypersensitivity to pyrazoles, such as celecoxib and zaleplon, is the only contraindication to its use. Fomepizole does not appear to affect retinol dehydrogenases involved in vision [122]. Its dosing protocol is based on zero-order elimination kinetics, increased clearance during hemodialysis, and potential autoinduction of metabolism via cytochrome P450–2E1 [123,124] (Table 99.5).

The main disadvantage to fomepizole therapy is the higher acquisition cost of the drug compared with ethanol [125,126], although this acquisition cost must be balanced against improved patient safety and reduced intensity of monitoring and therapy [107,113,127]. Although there are no prospective clinical studies directly comparing the safety of ethanol with fomepizole, there are retrospective evaluations that have reported fewer adverse drug events with fomepizole [102,128]. Fomepizole is the antidote of choice, when available [126], especially for a patient who has coingested other CNS depressants, for the critically ill patient with a profound anion gap metabolic acidosis of uncertain etiology, and for the patient in whom hemodialysis may be technically challenging (e.g., infants) or unnecessary [95,108,129].

Fomepizole has also been successfully used to treat combined methanol/isopropanol [130] and diethylene glycol/triethylene glycol [112] overdose in humans. Treatment with fomepizole or ethanol should be continued until the metabolic acidosis has resolved and serum methanol or ethylene glycol levels fall below 20 mg per dL (200 mg per L).

Cofactor therapy for patients poisoned by ethylene glycol includes IV pyridoxine (100 mg) and thiamine (100 mg) once a day until ethylene glycol levels are unmeasurable and acidemia has cleared. Pyridoxine is required for the conversion of glyoxylic acid to glycine, whereas thiamine and magnesium are required for the conversion of glycolic acid to γ-hydroxy-α-ketoadipate. Administering these cofactors may shunt metabolism away from the formation of oxalic acid [83,131], although benefit has not been documented in human poisonings. Magnesium should be administered to patients with hypomagnesemia.

Patients poisoned with methanol should receive IV folinic acid (leucovorin), 1 to 2 mg per kg every 4 to 6 hours until methanol and metabolic acidosis have been cleared [67,97]. Folic acid (folate) can be substituted if leucovorin is unavailable. Hepatic formate metabolism occurs through a folate-dependent mechanism (see Fig. 99.4). The susceptibility of primates to methanol toxicity correlates with reduced hepatic 5,6,7,8-tetrahydrofolate (THF, or reduced folate) stores compared with lower mammals [97], and exogenous folinic acid (5-formyl-THF) or folate may increase their capacity to remove formate. Although human data are limited, monkeys pretreated with folic or folinic acid resulted in marked attenuation of serum formate levels and metabolic acidosis after methanol administration [132]. Folinic acid given after the onset of methanol toxicity was also beneficial.

Hemodialysis effectively removes ethylene glycol, methanol, glycolic acid, formic acid, and probably the other toxic metabolites and should be used in nearly all cases with acidosis or end-organ toxicity [35,48,53,54,56,63,133]. Early hemodialysis can prevent subsequent toxicity [8,91]. Addition of extra sodium bicarbonate to the dialysate can assist in correcting acidosis, and hemodialysis may assist in controlling volume status. The frequency of fomepizole dosing must be increased during hemodialysis to compensate for its removal. When using ethanol, its infusion rate should be empirically doubled at the start of hemodialysis, and serum ethanol levels should be monitored hourly.

Recommendations for hemodialysis are outlined in Table 99.6 [35,48,50,53,97,98,107,108]. Traditional criteria for hemodialysis have included a serum ethylene glycol or methanol concentration >50 mg per dL (500 mg per L), independent of symptoms,

TABLE 99.5

Fomepizole Intravenous Dosing Protocol

Loading dose: 15 mg/kg
Maintenance dose (beginning 12 h after loading dose):
- 10 mg/kg every 12 h; increase dose to 15 mg/kg every 12 h if more than 48 h after loading dose

Dosing during hemodialysis:
- At initiation of dialysis:
  - If <6 h since last dose, no additional dose
  - If >6 h since last dose, next scheduled dose
- During hemodialysis: next scheduled dose every 4 h
- At completion of hemodialysis:
  - If <1 h since last dose, no additional dose
  - If 1–3 h since last dose, half of next scheduled dose
  - If >3 h since last dose, next scheduled dose

Each dose diluted in 100 mL normal saline and infused over 30 min

TABLE 99.6

Indications for Hemodialysis in Methanol or Ethylene Glycol Poisoning

Renal dysfunction as evidenced by increased serum creatinine concentration[a]

Severe metabolic acidosis (pH <7.25) with evidence of end-organ toxicity (abnormal renal function for ethylene glycol, visual toxicity for methanol) independent of parent compound concentration

Serum methanol or ethylene glycol concentration >50 mg/dL

[a]Selected patients with ethylene glycol concentrations above 50 mg/dL *and* normal creatinine and arterial pH at initiation of fomepizole treatment may be eligible for conservative treatment without hemodialysis. In all cases, consultation with a medical toxicologist is strongly recommended.

Adapted from Barceloux DG, Krenzelok EP, Olson K, et al: American Academy of Clinical Toxicology practice guidelines on the treatment of ethylene glycol poisoning. *J Toxicol Clin Toxicol* 37:537, 1999.

acid–base status, or other markers of end-organ toxicity [97], but selected patients have been successfully managed with fomepizole, cofactors, and IV fluid hydration *alone* despite serum ethylene glycol concentrations >400 mg per dL, although consultation with a toxicologist is strongly recommended [49]. Such patients must be hemodynamically stabile and have near normal acid–base status and renal function. If minimal ethylene glycol metabolism has occurred before initiation of fomepizole therapy, the endogenous ethylene glycol elimination half-life is expected to be less than 18 hours [48,49]. Thus, patients with a normal serum creatinine and arterial pH at the start of fomepizole therapy may forgo hemodialysis despite high serum ethylene glycol concentrations [48,95,114]. Although a similar strategy has been reported for a patient with combined methanol/isopropanol ingestion [130], the prolonged methanol elimination half-life (approximately 50 hours) after ADH inhibition [53,134] would favor hemodialysis when readily available and technically feasible [53]. Intermittent hemodialysis is preferred when available, especially for acidemic patients, because of the much higher elimination of the toxic acid metabolites [53]. During mass outbreaks, however, both continuous and intermittent hemodialysis have been utilized, with no reported significant differences of mortality rates between these two dialytic modalities [135]. Therefore, although intermittent hemodialysis is suggested as the most effective method to decrease serum alcohol levels and for removing organic acid anions [35], in the setting of limited resources, continuous hemodialysis should also be considered. Acid–base status, renal function, and serum ethylene glycol or methanol levels must be closely monitored for patients in whom hemodialysis is withheld [107].

Ethylene glycol clearance rates of 156 to 226 mL per minute (fractional excretion 43% to 92%; half-life 2.3 to 3.5 hours) can be expected during hemodialysis, as compared with renal clearance rates of 27.5 ± 4.1 mL per minute (fractional excretion 26% ± 9%) in patients with normal renal function, and clearance rates of 1 to 6 mL per minute in patients with renal dysfunction [48,136]. Glycolic acid is removed by hemodialysis, with a clearance of 105 to 170 mL per minute (half-life 2.5 hours) [37,40,43]. The hemodialysis elimination rate for methanol is 142 to 286 mL per minute; for formate, it is 148 to 203 mL per minute [7,54,63,84,137].

Hemodialysis should be continued until serum ethylene glycol or methanol levels are below 20 mg per dL (200 mg per liter) and acid–base derangements has been corrected [35,53,42,95]. The required duration of hemodialysis in hours can be estimated using the formula $[-V \ln (20/A)/0.06\,k]$, where V is total body water in liters, A is the initial alcohol concentration in mg per dL, and k is 57% of the dialyzer urea clearance in milliliters per minute at the observed blood flow rate [138–140]. More than one round of hemodialysis may be necessary for those with massive overdoses and for ethylene glycol–poisoned patients with renal failure.

Peritoneal dialysis is markedly inferior to hemodialysis because of its low clearance of alcohols and organic acid anions [35]. Continuous arteriovenous hemofiltration with dialysis has been used in a hemodynamically unstable patient, but is less efficient at toxin removal [141]. Sorbent-based hemodialysis systems were inadvertently shown to be ineffective for methanol removal because of rapid saturation of the sorbent cartridge [142] and charcoal cartridges saturate within a few hours [132].

Patients with ethylene glycol poisoning who have acute renal failure may require hemodialysis for several months. Recovery of renal function is the expected course, although renal dysfunction may be permanent [37,42,83,90,128,143]. Full neurological recovery is possible even after prolonged coma and seizures. Transient cranial nerve palsies developing 4 to 18 days after ingestion have been reported in under- or untreated patients [71–73,136]. Bilateral basal ganglia and brainstem infarction can occur in severely ethylene glycol–poisoned patients [144].

Seizures, coma, and severe acidosis among patients with methanol poisoning portend a poor prognosis [56,145]. Cerebral edema is a common postmortem methanol toxicity finding [114]. The development of dilated, unresponsive pupils may indicate either severe optic nerve damage or cerebral edema [52]. Other neurologic sequelae include a parkinsonian-like syndrome, spasticity, transient resting tremor, cognitive defects, and paraplegia. Computed tomography, magnetic resonance imaging, and autopsy studies have documented frontal lobe and basal ganglia hemorrhages and infarcts, especially in the putamen [146,147]. Bilateral putaminal hemorrhage and/or insular subcortex white matter necrosis correlate with a poor clinical outcome following methanol toxicity. The etiology of these lesions remains uncertain, but they are likely due to the direct toxicity of methanol and/or its metabolites. These abnormalities usually occur among severely acidemic patients with delayed presentation or diagnosis.

Harvesting of organs for transplant is not precluded for patients who die from ethylene glycol or methanol poisoning. Several centers have reported successful experience with kidney, heart, lung, pancreatic β cell, and liver procurement from methanol-poisoned patients [127,148].

ISOPROPANOL

Isopropanol (isopropyl alcohol) is a clear, colorless, volatile liquid with a disagreeable taste and characteristic odor [149]. It is commonly available over the counter in 70% solutions of "rubbing alcohol," but it is also used in cleaners, disinfectants, hand sanitizers, cosmetics, solvents, inks, and pharmaceuticals [150]. Because of its ready availability at an inexpensive price, abusers of alcohol often ingest isopropanol as an ethanol substitute. Cases of toxicity have been reported among children who were sponge bathed with the compound [151]. The NPDS reports that during 2014 the poison centers received 12,479 calls related to isopropanol exposures [36].

Isopropanol produces CNS depression, coma, and death from respiratory depression. In this respect, it has twice the potency of ethanol [152], a phenomenon attributed to its higher molecular weight [149] and possibly the CNS depressant effects of its metabolite, acetone. Depending on individual tolerance, serum concentrations of 150 mg per dL or greater may induce coma, and levels of 200 mg per dL or greater can be fatal in untreated patients, although lower concentrations may produce severe adverse effects [35,153].

The chemical properties and kinetics of isopropanol are summarized in Table 99.1. Oral absorption occurs quickly, and peak plasma concentrations can occur within 30 minutes [150]. Eighty percent of an absorbed dose is oxidized to acetone via ADH (Fig. 99.5) [149]. Acetone cannot undergo further oxidation to a carboxylic acid, however. Therefore, metabolic acidosis is not a feature of isopropanol toxicity unless respiratory depression with hypoxia or hypotension results in lactate production. Excretion of acetone and unchanged isopropanol (20% of an absorbed dose) is predominantly renal, with some excretion by respiratory, gastric, and salivary routes. Acetone can be detected in the urine within 3 hours of ingestion [154]. The elimination half-life of isopropanol can be as long as 5.8 hours for infants [155]. Serum acetone levels frequently remain elevated after isopropanol levels are undetectable because acetone is eliminated slowly, with a half-life of 10.8 to 31.0 hours. The contribution of acetone to the prolonged duration of CNS depression remains speculative [149].

Clinical Presentation

An "intoxicated" patient without acidemia, yet with positive serum or urinary ketones and a fruity breath odor, should be suspected of isopropanol intoxication. Initial signs and symptoms usually

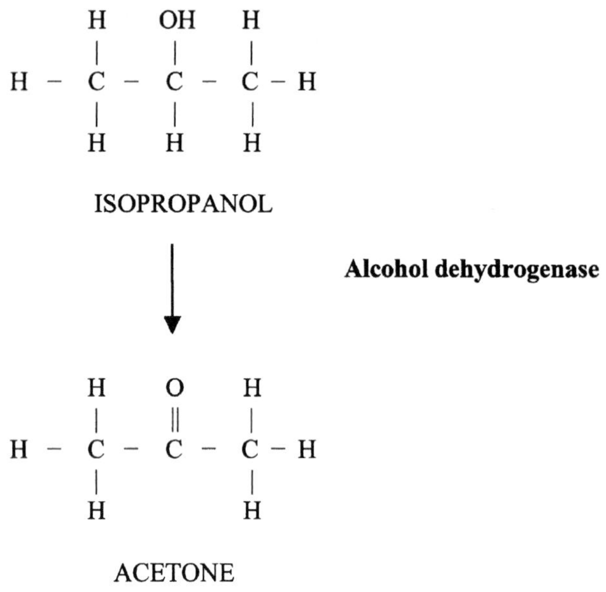

FIGURE 99.5 Isopropanol metabolism.

consist of mild intoxication followed by gastritis, abdominal pain, nausea, vomiting, and possibly hematemesis [149]. Hemorrhagic tracheobronchitis may occur. As CNS depression progresses, patients become ataxic, dysarthric, confused, stuporous, and comatose. Pupils are typically miotic, but mydriasis has been reported [149,156]. Respiratory depression and hypotension may occur with severe intoxication [157]. Because of the profound and prolonged cerebral depressive effects of isopropanol, comatose patients may develop compartment syndromes and rhabdomyolysis with myoglobinuria.

Many patients who ingest isopropanol are ethanol abusers who have a multitude of associated diseases, including chronic liver disease, pancreatitis, traumatic injuries, and chronic obstructive pulmonary disease, which may complicate the clinical picture.

Diagnostic Evaluation

Patients with known or suspected isopropanol poisoning should have quantitative isopropanol and acetone serum levels along with the laboratory studies noted for acute ethanol intoxication. The presence of high levels of acetone can interfere with older creatinine assays based on a colorimetric method, producing a falsely high creatinine value in the presence of a normal BUN [158]. In patients who may have also ingested other toxic alcohols, serum osmolality, ethanol, ethylene glycol, and methanol levels should also be obtained.

The differential diagnosis of isopropanol poisoning includes toxic and metabolic states in which ketonemia may develop, such as alcoholic, diabetic, and starvation ketoacidosis. Patients with these conditions have elevated acetoacetate, β-hydroxybutyrate, and acetone levels compared with the isolated acetonemia seen with isopropanol intoxication. Traces of isopropanol may be detected among patients with diabetic or AKA because of the back reduction of acetone to isopropanol [159]. Poisoning by salicylate, cyanide, and acetone itself (which is found in nail polish and super glue remover) and inborn errors of metabolism should also be considered in the differential diagnosis of unexplained ketosis. Some degree of metabolic acidosis is expected in most of these conditions, whereas it is absent in uncomplicated isopropanol or acetone poisoning cases.

Management

Treatment is similar to that described for acute ethanol intoxication. Airway management and evaluation for hemorrhagic gastritis are particularly important. IV fluids should contain glucose, and serum glucose levels should be periodically checked. Isopropanol and acetone are removed by hemodialysis, but such therapy is rarely indicated. Occasionally, patients with serum isopropanol concentration >200 mg per dL accompanied by hemodynamic instability despite IV fluids may benefit from hemodialysis [35,149]. Since acetone is less toxic than isopropanol, there is no indication for either fomepizole or ethanol therapy [130,150,160].

Most patients recover with appropriate airway management and treatment of complicating factors. CNS depression and volume depletion secondary to vomiting can cause hypotension [149]. Pulmonary edema and hemorrhage are common findings on autopsy and should be anticipated in severely ill patients.

PROPYLENE GLYCOL

Propylene glycol (1,2-propanediol) is commonly used as a solvent (e.g., in laundry stain removers), as an antifreeze, in hydraulic fluids, and as a diluent for a number of pharmaceuticals, including IV formulations of chlordiazepoxide, lorazepam, diazepam, etomidate, phenobarbital, pentobarbital, phenytoin, procainamide, nitroglycerin, and theophylline and topical silver sulfadiazine cream. Oral and dermal absorption is usually poor, but toxic amounts may be absorbed through abraded or burned skin [161]. Approximately one-half of a dose undergoes hepatic oxidation via ADH to lactate, and then to pyruvate and acetate. The rest is excreted unchanged in the urine [162].

Although oral doses of as much as 1 g per kg are essentially nontoxic, toxicity can occur following rapid or prolonged infusion of higher doses. Rapid IV infusion, as might occur during phenytoin loading, can cause prolonged PR and QRS duration, idioventricular rhythms, and cardiorespiratory depression and arrest [163]. Infusion of smaller doses has also precipitated cardiac standstill [164]. Propylene glycol, rather than phenytoin, is responsible for such toxicity [163]. Elderly patients, especially those with severe underlying cardiac disease, are at increased risk and should be infused with medications containing propylene glycol at rates slower than those usually recommended.

More commonly in the intensive care setting, frequent repeat IV dosing of medications containing propylene glycol can lead to accumulation of propylene glycol and its metabolites, resulting in seizures and decreased level of consciousness. Propylene glycol toxicity has been described following extremely high doses of diazepam for ethanol withdrawal, massive ingestion of products containing propylene glycol, or the chronic dermal absorption of silver sulfadiazine through damaged skin [165–167]. On laboratory testing, an osmolar gap and high serum lactate concentrations are expected. Propylene glycol can be mistaken for ethylene glycol on gas chromatography [168].

Management of this iatrogenic condition consists of immediately stopping IV infusion or dermal application and supportive therapy. Although theoretically fomepizole may be beneficial to block the metabolism of propylene glycol, this therapy cannot be universally recommended at this time without more information, including information on the relative toxicity of the parent compound to its metabolites [35,169]. Hemodialysis and continuous venovenous hemofiltration have reportedly been used to treat patients with propylene glycol toxicity, especially in the setting of renal failure, high blood concentrations, or severe metabolic acidosis [35,170,171].

DIETHYLENE GLYCOL

Diethylene glycol (2,2′-dihydroxydiethyl ether, ethylene diglycol, 2,2′-oxydiethanol, 3-oxapentane-1,5-diol; DEG) is a viscous and sweet-tasting liquid found in resins, antifreeze, brake fluids, cosmetics, wallpaper strippers, inks, lubricants, liquid heating/cooking fuels, plasticizers, adhesives, paper, and packaging materials [172,173]. Over the years, diethylene glycol has resulted in tragic outbreaks of renal failure and death following its substitution for propylene glycol in medications [174,175]. Unlike propylene glycol, diethylene glycol can cause acute renal failure, elevated liver enzymes, encephalopathy, and delayed neurologic toxicity. Since the first reported outbreak that occurred in the United States in 1937, there have been other outbreaks worldwide, including South Africa (1969), Spain (1985), India (1986 and 1998), Nigeria (1990 and 2008), Bangladesh (1990 to 1992), Argentina (1992), Haiti (1996), Panama (2006), and China (2006). These outbreaks often involved medications, such as acetaminophen, cough syrup, or teething syrup, ingested by children. The number of identified deaths during each outbreak ranged from 5 to 236. The median toxic dose is estimated to be approximately 0.14 mg per kg [35,176].

Following diethylene glycol ingestion, patients may present with gastrointestinal symptoms, inebriation, CNS depression, acidosis, and acute renal failure. Interestingly, additional neurologic symptoms may develop up to several weeks after the ingestion and include cranial nerve palsy, peripheral neuropathy, dysphonia, lethargy, mental status changes, quadriparesis, and seizures [174,177]. Metabolism of diethylene glycol via hepatic ADH leads to 2-hydroxyethoxyacetic acid (HEAA) [173]. Although HEAA is believed to be the primary toxic metabolite, the parent glycol itself may also be directly toxic. Although the name suggests the potential to be metabolized to two ethylene glycol molecules, this does not occur in vivo [173]. Survivors with renal failure tend to remain dialysis dependent, and the degree of renal injury may be a predictor of delayed neurologic sequelae. Treatment is similar to ethylene glycol, including ADH inhibition using fomepazole or ethanol, extracorporeal elimination, and supportive care [35]. Fomepizole alone without hemodialysis, however, is not recommended given the uncertain toxicity of the diethylene glycol itself, the frequency of associated renal failure, and the theoretical dialyzability of diethylene glycol and HEAA [35,113,173,174]. Case reports exist of successful treatment of pediatric patients with fomepizole for diethylene glycol toxicity using the same dosing regimen as adults [35,116].

References

1. Thun MJ, Peto R, Lopez AD, et al: Alcohol consumption and mortality among middle-aged and elderly U.S. adults. *N Engl J Med* 337:1705, 1997.
2. Stahre M, Roeber J, Kanny D, et al: Contribution of excessive alcohol consumption to deaths and years of potential life lost in the United States. *Prev Chronic Dis* 11:130293, 2014.
3. McDonald AJ III: US emergency department visits for alcohol-related diseases and injuries between 1992 and 2000. *Arch Intern Med* 164:531, 2004.
4. Ueno S, Harris RA, Messing RO, et al: Alcohol actions on GABA(A) receptors: from protein structure to mouse behavior. *Alcohol Clin Exp Res* 25[Suppl 5]:81S, 2001.
5. Chester JA, Cunningham CL: GABA(A) receptor modulation of the rewarding and aversive effects of ethanol. *Alcohol* 26(3):131, 2002.
6. Aguayo LG, Peoples RW, Yeh HH, et al: GABA(A) receptors as molecular sites of ethanol action. Direct or indirect actions? *Curr Top Med Chem* 2(8):869, 2002.
7. Allgaier C: Ethanol sensitivity of NMDA receptors. *Neurochem Int* 41(6):377, 2002.
8. Nutt DJ, Peters TJ: Alcohol: the drug. *Br Med Bull* 50:5, 1994.
9. Crews FT, Morrow AL, Criswell H, et al: Effects of ethanol on ion channels. *Int Rev Neurobiol* 39:283, 1996.
10. Israel Y, Orrego H, Carmichael FJ: Acetate-mediated effects of ethanol. *Alcohol Clin Exp Res* 18:144, 1994.
11. Vonghia L, Leggio L, Ferrulli A, et al: Review article acute alcohol intoxication. *Eur J Intern Med* 19:561, 2008.
12. Levitt MD, Levitt DG: Appropriate use and misuse of blood concentration measurements to quantitate first-pass metabolism. *J Lab Clin Med* 136(4):275, 2000.
13. Ramchandani VA, Bosron WF, Li TK: Research advances in ethanol metabolism. *Pathol Biol (Paris)* 49(9):676, 2001.
14. McGuire LC, Cruickshank AM, Munro PT: Alcoholic ketoacidosis. *Emerg Med J* 23:417, 2006.
15. Brennan DR, Betzelos S, Reed R, et al: Ethanol elimination in an ED population. *Am J Emerg Med* 13:276, 1995.
16. Hoffman RS, Goldfrank LR: Ethanol-associated metabolic disorders. *Emerg Med Clin North Am* 7:943, 1989.
17. Lands WE: A review of alcohol clearance in humans. *Alcohol* 15:147, 1998.
18. Crabb DW: Ethanol oxidizing enzymes: roles in alcohol metabolism and alcoholic liver disease. *Prog Liver Dis* 13:151, 1995.
19. Agarwal DP: Genetic polymorphisms of alcohol metabolizing enzymes. *Pathol Biol (Paris)* 49(9):703, 2001.
20. Norberg A, Jones AW, Hahn RG, et al: Role of variability in explaining ethanol pharmacokinetics: research and forensic applications. *Clin Pharmacokinet* 42(1):1, 2003.
21. Ogden EJ, Moskowitz H: Effects of alcohol and other drugs on driver performance. *Traffic Inj Prev* 5(3):185–198, 2004.
22. Crabb DW, Bosrom WF, Li TK: Ethanol metabolism. *Pharmacol Ther* 34:59, 1987.
23. Scherger DL, Wruk KM, Kulig KW, et al: Ethyl alcohol (ethanol)-containing cologne, perfume, and after-shave ingestions in children. *Am J Dis Child* 142:630, 1988.
24. Charness ME, Simon RP, Greenberg DA: Ethanol and the nervous system. *N Engl J Med* 321:442, 1989.
25. Johnson RA, Noll EC, Rodney WM: Survival after a serum ethanol concentration of 1 1/2%. *Lancet* 2(8312):1394, 1982.
26. Halperin ML, Hammeke M, Josse RG, et al: Metabolic acidosis in the alcoholic: a pathophysiologic approach. *Metabolism* 32:308, 1983.
27. Fulop M, Bock J, Ben-Ezra J, et al: Plasma lactate and 3-hydroxybutyrate levels in patients with acute ethanol intoxication. *Am J Med* 57:191, 1986.
28. Marinella MA: Alcoholic ketoacidosis presenting with extreme hypoglycemia. *Am J Emerg Med* 15:257, 1997.
29. Braden GL, Strayhorn CH, Germain MJ, et al: Increased osmolal gap in alcoholic acidosis. *Arch Intern Med* 153:2377, 1993.
30. Purssell RA, Pudek M, Brubacher J, et al: Derivation of a formula to calculate the contribution of ethanol to the osmolar gap. *Ann Emerg Med* 38:653, 2001.
31. Sivilotti MLA, Collier CP, Choi SB: Ethanol and the osmolal gap. *Ann Emerg Med* 39:656, 2002.
32. Wrenn KD, Slovis CM, Minion GE, et al: The syndrome of alcoholic ketoacidosis. *Am J Med* 2:119, 1991.
33. Watson AJS, Walker JF, Tomkin GH, et al: Acute Wernicke's encephalopathy precipitated by glucose loading. *Ir J Med Sci* 150:301, 1981.
34. Bluntzer ME, Blachley JD: Acid-base and electrolyte disturbances induced by alcohol. *J Crit Illn* 1:19, 1986.
35. Kraut JA, Kurtz I: Toxic alcohol ingestions: clinical features, diagnosis, and management. *Clin J Am Soc Nephrol* 3:208, 2008.
36. Mowry JB, Spyker DA, Brooks DE, et al: 2014 Annual Report of the American Association of Poison Control Centers' National Poison Data System (NPDS): 32nd Annual Report. *Clin Toxicol (Phila)* 53(10):962, 2015.
37. Jacobsen D, Ovrebo S, Ostborg J, et al: Glycolate causes the acidosis in ethylene glycol poisoning and is effectively removed by hemodialysis. *Acta Med Scand* 216:409, 1984.
38. Ekka M, Aggarwal P: Review Article toxic alcohols. *J Mahatma Gandhi Inst of Med Sci* 20(1):38, 2015.
39. Hovda KE, Guo C, Austin R, et al: Renal toxicity of ethylene glycol results from internalization of calcium oxalate crystals by proximal tubule cells. *Toxicol Lett* 192:365, 2010.
40. Moreau CL, Kerns W, Tomaszewski CA, et al: Glycolate kinetics and hemodialysis clearance. *J Toxicol Clin Toxicol* 36:659, 1998.
41. Jacobsen D: Organic acids in ethylene glycol intoxication [letter]. *Ann Intern Med* 105:799, 1986.
42. Jacobsen D, McMartin KE: Methanol and ethylene glycol poisonings: mechanism of toxicity, clinical course, diagnosis and treatment. *Med Toxicol* 1:309, 1986.
43. Gabow PA, Clay K, Sullivan JB, et al: Organic acids in ethylene glycol intoxication. *Ann Intern Med* 105:16, 1986.
44. Morgan TJ, Clark C, Clague A: Artifactual elevation of measured plasma L-lactate concentration in the presence of glycolate. *Crit Care Med* 27:2177, 1999.
45. Shirey T, Sivilotti M: Reaction of lactate electrodes to glycolate. *Crit Care Med* 27:2305, 1999.
46. Manini AF, Hoffman RS, McMartin KE, et al: Relationship between serum glycolate and falsely elevated lactate in severe ethylene glycol poisoning. *J Anal Toxicol* 33(3):174–176, 2009.
47. Friedman EA, Greenberg JB, Merrill JP, et al: Consequences of ethylene glycol poisoning. *Am J Med* 32:891, 1962.
48. Sivilotti MLA, Burns MJ, McMartin KE, et al: Toxicokinetics of ethylene glycol during fomepizole therapy: implications for management. *Ann Emerg Med* 36:114, 2000.
49. Levine M, Curry SC, Ruha AM, et al: Ethylene glycol elimination kinetics and outcomes in patients managed without hemodialysis. *Ann Emerg Med* 59(6):527, 2012.
50. Johnson B, Meggs WJ, Bentzel CJ: Emergency department hemodialysis in a case of severe ethylene glycol poisoning. *Ann Emerg Med* 33:108, 1999.

51. Eriksen SP, Kulkarni AB: Methanol in normal human breath. *Science* 141:639, 1963.
52. Ingemansson SO: Clinical observations on ten cases of methanol poisoning with particular reference to ocular manifestations. *Acta Ophthalmol* 62:15, 1984.
53. Roberts DM, Yates C, Megarbane B, et al: Recommendations for the role of extracorporeal treatments in the management of acute methanol poisoning: a systematic review and consensus statement. *Crit Care Med* 43(2):461, 2015.
54. Kerns W II, Tomaszewski C, McMartin K, et al: Formate kinetics in methanol poisoning. *J Toxicol Clin Toxicol* 40:137, 2002.
55. Kostic MA, Dart RC: Rethinking the toxic methanol level. *J Toxicol Clin Toxicol* 41:793, 2003.
56. Coulter CV, Farquhar SE, McSherry CM, et al: Methanol and ethylene glycol acute poisonings - predictors of mortality. *Clin Toxicol (Phila)* 49:900, 2011.
57. Martin-Amat G, McMartin KE, Hayreh SS, et al: Methanol poisoning: ocular toxicity produced by formate. *Toxicol Appl Pharmacol* 45:201, 1978.
58. Hayreh MS, Hayreh SS, Baumbach GL, et al: Methyl alcohol poisoning. III. Ocular toxicity. *Arch Ophthalmol* 95:1851, 1977.
59. Eells JT: Methanol-induced visual toxicity in the rat. *J Pharmacol Exp Ther* 257:56, 1991.
60. Kahn A, Blum D: Methyl alcohol poisoning in an 8-month-old boy: an unusual route of intoxication. *J Pediatr* 94:841, 1979.
61. Paasma R, Hovda KE, Tikkerberi A, et al. Methanol mass poisoning in Estonia: outbreak in 154 patients. *Clin Toxicol (Phila)* 45(2):152–157, 2007.
62. Wallace EA, Green AS: Methanol toxicity secondary to inhalant abuse in adult men. *Clin Toxicol (Phila)* 47(3):239–242, 2009.
63. Jacobsen D, Ovrebo S, Sejersted OM: Toxicokinetics of formate during hemodialysis. *Acta Med Scand* 214:409, 1983.
64. McCoy HG, Cipolle RJ, Ehlers SM, et al: Severe methanol poisoning: application of a pharmacokinetic model for ethanol therapy and hemodialysis. *Am J Med* 67:574, 1979.
65. Jones AW: Elimination half-life of methanol during hangover. *Pharmacol Toxicol* 60:217, 1987.
66. Jacobsen D, Webb R, Collins TD, et al: Methanol and formate kinetics in late diagnosed methanol intoxication. *Med Toxicol Adverse Drug Exp* 3:418, 1988.
67. Osterloh JD, Pond SM, Grady S, et al: Serum formate concentrations in methanol intoxication as a criterion for hemodialysis. *Ann Intern Med* 104:200, 1986.
68. Hantson P, Haufroid V, Mahieu P: Survival with extremely high blood methanol concentration. *Eur J Emerg Med* 7:237, 2000.
69. Brent J, McMartin K, Phillips S, et al: Fomepizole for the treatment of ethylene glycol poisoning. *N Engl J Med* 340:832, 1999.
70. Morgan B, Ford MD, Fullmer R: Ethylene glycol ingestion resulting in brainstem and midbrain dysfunction. *J Toxicol Clin Toxicol* 38:445, 2000.
71. Berger JR, Syyar DR: Neurological complications of ethylene glycol intoxication: report of a case. *Arch Neurol* 38:724, 1981.
72. Anderson B: Facial-auditory nerve oxalosis. *Am J Med* 88:87, 1990.
73. Spillane L, Roberts JR, Meyer AE: Multiple cranial nerve deficits after ethylene glycol poisoning. *Ann Emerg Med* 20:208, 1991.
74. Becker CE: Methanol poisoning. *J Emerg Med* 1:51, 1983.
75. Blandford DE, Desjardins PR: A rapid method for measurement of ethylene glycol. *Clin Biochem* 27:25, 1994.
76. Jones AW, Nilsson L, Gladh SA, et al: 2,3-butanediol in plasma from an alcoholic mistakenly identified as ethylene glycol by gas chromatographic analysis. *Clin Chem* 37:1453, 1991.
77. Malandain H, Cano Y: Interference of glycerol, propylene glycol and other diols in enzymatic assays of ethylene glycol [abstract]. *Clin Chem* 41:S120, 1995.
78. Shoemaker JD, Lynch RE, Hoffman JW, et al: Misidentification of propionic acid as ethylene glycol in a patient with methylmalonic acidemia. *J Pediatr* 120:417, 1992.
79. Long H, Nelson LS, Hoffman RS: A rapid qualitative test for suspected ethylene glycol poisoning. *Acad Emerg Med* 15(7):688–690, 2008.
80. Lynd LD, Richardson KJ, Purssell RA, et al: An evaluation of the osmole gap as a screening test for toxic alcohol poisoning. *BMC Emerg Med* 8:5, 2008.
81. Purssell RA, Lynd LD, Koga Y: The use of the osmole gap as a screening test for the presence of exogenous substances. *Toxicol Rev* 23:189, 2004.
82. Woolf AD, Wynshaw-Boris A, Rinalso P, et al: Intentional infantile ethylene glycol poisoning presenting as an inherited metabolic disorder. *J Pediatr* 120:421, 1992.
83. Beasley VR, Buck WB: Acute ethylene glycol toxicosis: a review. *Vet Hum Toxicol* 22:255, 1957.
84. Catchings TT, Beamer WC, Lundy L, et al: Adult respiratory distress syndrome secondary to ethylene glycol ingestion. *Ann Emerg Med* 14:594, 1985.
85. Koga Y, Purssell RA, Lynd LD: The irrationality of the present use of the osmole gap. *Toxicol Rev* 23:203, 2004.
86. Krahn J, Khajuria A: Osmolality gaps: diagnostic accuracy and long-term variability. *Clin Chem* 52(4):737–739, 2006.
87. Schelling JR, Howard RL, Winter SD, et al: Increased osmolal gap in alcoholic ketoacidosis and lactic acidosis. *Ann Intern Med* 113:557, 1990.
88. Hoffman RS, Smilkstein MJ, Howland MA, et al: Osmol gaps revisited: normal values and limitations. *J Toxicol Clin Toxicol* 31:81, 1993.
89. Jobard E, Harry P, Turcant A, et al: 4-methylpyrazole and hemodialysis in ethylene glycol poisoning. *J Toxicol Clin Toxicol* 34:379, 1996.
90. Jacobsen D, Hewlett TR, Webb R, et al: Ethylene glycol intoxication: evaluation of kinetics and crystalluria. *Am J Med* 84:145, 1988.
91. Burns JR, Finlayson B: Changes in calcium oxalate crystal morphology as a function of concentration. *Invest Urol* 18:174, 1980.
92. McStay CM, Gordon PE: Images in clinical medicine. Urine fluorescence in ethylene glycol poisoning. *N Engl J Med* 356(6):611, 2007.
93. Winter ML, Snodgrass WR, Theelen T, et al: Urine fluorescence in ethylene glycol poisoning. *N Engl J Med* 356(19):2006, 2007.
94. Naraqi S, Dethlefs RF, Slobodniuk RA, et al: An outbreak of acute methyl alcohol intoxication. *Aust N Z J Med* 9:65, 1979.
95. Barceloux DG, Krenzelok EP, Olson K, et al: American Academy of Clinical Toxicology practice guidelines on the treatment of ethylene glycol poisoning. *J Toxicol Clin Toxicol* 37:537, 1999.
96. Barceloux DG, Bond GR, Krenzelok EP, et al: American Academy of Clinical Toxicology practice guidelines on the treatment of methanol poisoning. *J Toxicol Clin Toxicol* 40:415, 2002.
97. Jacobsen D, McMartin KE: Antidotes for methanol and ethylene glycol poisoning. *J Toxicol Clin Toxicol* 35:127, 1997.
98. Frederick LJ, Schulte PA, Apol A: Investigation and control of occupational hazards associated with the use of spirit duplicators. *Am Ind Hyg Assoc J* 45:51, 1984.
99. Palatnick W, Redman LW, Sitar DS, et al: Methanol half-life during ethanol administration: implications for management of methanol poisoning. *Ann Emerg Med* 26:202, 1995.
100. Brent J, McMartin K, Phillips S, et al: Fomepizole for the treatment of methanol poisoning. *N Engl J Med* 344:424, 2001.
101. Tephly TR, McMartin KE: Methanol metabolism and toxicity, in Stegink L, File LJ (eds): *Aspartame: Physiology and Biochemistry.* New York, Marcel Dekker Inc, 1984, p 111.
102. Lepik KJ, Levy AR, Sobolev BG, et al: Adverse drug events associated with the antidotes for methanol and ethylene glycol poisoning: a comparison of ethanol and fomepizole. *Ann Emerg Med* 53(4):439–450 e10, 2009.
103. Sivilotti ML: Ethanol: tastes great! Fomepizole: less filling! *Ann Emerg Med* 53(4):451–453, 2009.
104. Lepik KJ, Sobolev BG, Levy AR, et al: Medication errors associated with the use of ethanol and fomepizole for methanol and ethylene glycol poisoning. *Clin Toxicol (Phila)* 49:391, 2011.
105. Bestic M, Blackford M, Reed M: Fomepizole: a critical assessment of current dosing recommendations. *J Clin Pharmacol* 49(2):130–137, 2009.
106. Baud FJ, Bismuth C, Garnier R, et al: 4-methylpyrazole may be an alternative to ethanol therapy for ethylene glycol intoxication in man. *J Toxicol Clin Toxicol* 24:463, 1986.
107. Jacobsen D: New treatment for ethylene glycol poisoning. *N Engl J Med* 340:879, 1999.
108. Tenenbein M: Recent advancements in pediatric toxicology. *Pediatr Clin North Am* 46:1179, 1999.
109. Zakharov S, Pelclova D, Navratil T, et al: Fomepizole vs ethanol in the treatment of acute methanol poisoning: comparison of clinical effectiveness in a mass poisoning outbreak. *Clin Toxicol (Phila)* 53:797, 2015.
110. Megarbane B, Houze P, Baud FJ: Oral fomepizole administration to treat ethylene glycol and methanol poisonings: advantages and limitations. *Clin Toxicol (Phila)* 46(10):1097, 2008.
111. Harry P, Turcant A, Bouachour G, et al: Efficacy of 4-methylpyrazole in ethylene glycol poisoning: clinical and toxicokinetic aspects. *Hum Exp Toxicol* 13:61, 1994.
112. Borron SW, Baud FJ, Garnier R: Intravenous 4-methylpyrazole as an antidote for diethylene glycol and triethylene glycol poisoning: a case report. *Vet Human Toxicol* 39:26, 1997.
113. Boyer EW, Mejia M, Woolf A, et al: Severe ethylene glycol ingestion treated without hemodialysis. *Pediatrics* 107:172, 2001.
114. Cheng JT, Beysolow TD, Kaul B, et al: Clearance of ethylene glycol by kidneys and hemodialysis. *J Toxicol Clin Toxicol* 25:95, 1987.
115. Ghannoum M, Hoffman RS, Mowry JB, et al: Trends in toxic alcohol exposures in the United States from 2000 to 2013: a focus on the use of antidotes and extracorporeal treatments. *Semin Dial* 27(4):395–401, 2014.
116. Brendt J: Fomepizole for the treatment of pediatric ethylene and diethylene glycol, butoxyethanol, and methanol poisonings. *Clin Toxicol (Phila)* 48:401, 2010.
117. McMartin KE, Hedstrom KG, Tolf BR, et al: Studies on the metabolic interaction between 4-methylpyrazole and methanol using the monkey as an animal model. *Arch Biochem Biophys* 199:606, 1980.
118. Sivilotti ML, Burns MJ, McMartin KE, et al: Toxicokinetics of ethylene glycol during fomepizole therapy: implications for management. For the methylpyrazole for Toxic Alcohols Study Group. *Ann Emerg Med* 36(2):114–125, 2000.
119. Li TK, Theorell H: Human liver alcohol dehydrogenase: inhibition by pyrazole and pyrazole analogues. *Acta Chem Scand* 23:892, 1969.
120. McMartin KE, Brent J, META Study Group: Pharmacokinetics of fomepizole (4MP) in patients. *J Toxicol Clin Toxicol* 36:450, 1998.
121. Lepik KJ, Brubacher JR, DeWitt CR, et al: Bradycardia and hypotension associated with fomepizole infusion during hemodialysis. *Clin Toxicol (Phila)* 46(6):570–573, 2008.
122. Sivilotti MLA, Burns MJ, Aaron CK, et al: Reversal of severe methanol-induced visual impairment: no evidence of retinal toxicity due to fomepizole. *J Toxicol Clin Toxicol* 39:627, 2001.
123. Jacobsen D, Barron SK, Sebastian CS, et al: Non-linear kinetics of 4-methylpyrazole in healthy human subjects. *Eur J Clin Pharmacol* 37:599, 1989.
124. Jacobsen D, Ostensen J, Bredesen L, et al: 4-Methylpyrazole (4-MP) is effectively removed by hemodialysis in the pig model. *Hum Exp Toxicol* 15:494, 1996.
125. Sivilotti MLA, Eisen JS, Less JS, et al: Can emergency departments not afford to carry essential antidotes? *CJEM* 4:23, 2002.

126. Dart RC, Borron SW, Caravati EM, et al: Expert consensus guidelines for stocking of antidotes in hospitals that provide emergency care. *Ann Emerg Med* 54(3):386–394.e1, 2009.
127. Caballero F, Cabrer C, Gonzalez-Segura C, et al: Short- and long-term success of organs transplanted from donors dying of acute methanol intoxication. *Transplant Proc* 31:2591, 1999.
128. Rasic S, Cengic M, Golemac S, et al: Acute renal insufficiency after poisoning with ethylene glycol. *Nephron* 81:119, 1999.
129. Baum CR, Langman CB, Oker EE, et al: Fomepizole treatment of ethylene glycol poisoning in an infant. *Pediatrics* 106:1489, 2000.
130. Bekka R, Borron SW, Astier A, et al: Treatment of methanol and isopropanol poisoning with intravenous fomepizole. *J Toxicol Clin Toxicol* 39:59, 2001.
131. Haupt MC, Zull DN, Adams SL: Massive ethylene glycol poisoning without evidence of crystalluria: a case for early intervention. *J Emerg Med* 6:295, 1988.
132. Noker PE, Eells JT, Tephly TR: Methanol toxicity: treatment with folic acid and 5-formyl tetrahydrofolic acid. *Alcohol Clin Exp Res* 4:378, 1980.
133. Clay KL, Murphy RC: On the metabolic acidosis of ethylene glycol intoxication. *Toxicol Appl Pharmacol* 39:39, 1977.
134. Burns MJ, Graudins A, Aaron CK, et al: Treatment of methanol poisoning with intravenous 4-methylpyrazole. *Ann Emerg Med* 30:829, 1997.
135. Zakharov S, Pelclova D, Urban P, et al: Czech mass methanol outbreak 2012: epidemiology, challenges and clinical features. *Clin Toxicol (Phila)* 52:1013, 2014.
136. Peterson CD, Collins AJ, Himes JM, et al: Ethylene glycol poisoning: pharmacokinetics during therapy with ethanol and hemodialysis. *N Engl J Med* 304:21, 1981.
137. Ekins BR, Rollins DE, Duffy DP, et al: Standardized treatment of severe methanol poisoning with ethanol and hemodialysis. *West J Med* 142:337, 1985.
138. Youssef GM, Hirsch DJ: Validation of a method to predict required dialysis time for cases of methanol and ethylene glycol poisoning. *Am J Kidney Dis* 46:509, 2005.
139. McMurray M, Carty D, Toffelmire EB: Predicting methanol clearance during hemodialysis when direct measurement is not available [in English, French]. *CAANT J* 12:29, 2002.
140. Burns AB, Bailie GR, Eisele G, et al: Use of pharmacokinetics to determine the duration of dialysis in management of methanol poisoning. *Am J Emerg Med* 16:538, 1998.
141. Christiansson LK, Kaspersson KE, Kulling PE, et al: Treatment of severe ethylene glycol intoxication with continuous arteriovenous hemofiltration dialysis. *J Toxicol Clin Toxicol* 33:267, 1995.
142. Whalen JE, Richards CJ, Ambre J: Inadequate removal of methanol and formate using the sorbent based regeneration hemodialysis delivery system. *Clin Nephrol* 11:318, 1979.
143. Stokes JB, Aueron F: Prevention of organ damage in massive ethylene glycol ingestion. *JAMA* 243:2065, 1980.
144. Dribben W, Furbee B, Kirk M: Brainstem infarction and quadriplegia associated with ethylene glycol ingestion. *J Toxicol Clin Toxicol* 37:657, 1999.
145. Jacobsen D, Bredesen JE, Eide I, et al: Anion and osmolal gaps in the diagnosis of methanol and ethylene glycol poisoning. *Acta Med Scand* 212:17, 1982.
146. Phang PT, Passerini L, Mielke B, et al: Brain hemorrhage associated with methanol poisoning. *Crit Care Med* 16:137, 1988.
147. Hantson P, Duprez T, Mahieu P: Neurotoxicity to the basal ganglia shown by magnetic resonance imaging (MRI) following poisoning by methanol and other substances. *J Toxicol Clin Toxicol* 35:151, 1997.
148. Bentley MJ, Mullen JC, Lopushinsky SR, et al: Successful cardiac transplantation with methanol or carbon monoxide-poisoned donors. *Ann Thorac Surg* 71:1194, 2001.
149. LaCouture PG, Wason S, Abrams A, et al: Acute isopropyl alcohol intoxication: diagnosis and management. *Am J Med* 75:657, 1983.
150. Slaughter RJ, Mason RW, Beasley DMG, et al: Isopropanol poisoning. *Clin Toxicol (Phila)* 52:470, 2014.
151. Vivier PM, Lewander WJ, Martin HF, et al: Isopropyl alcohol intoxication in a neonate through chronic dermal exposure: a complication of culturally based umbilical care practice. *Pediatr Emerg Care* 10:91, 1994.
152. Martinez TT, Jaeger RW, deCastro FJ, et al: A comparison of the absorption and metabolism of isopropyl alcohol by oral, dermal and inhalation routes. *Vet Hum Toxicol* 28:233, 1986.
153. Alexander CB, McBay AJ, Hudson RP: Isopropanol and isopropanol deaths: ten years' experience. *J Forensic Sci* 27:541, 1982.
154. LaCouture PG, Heldreth DD, Shannon M, et al: The generation of acetonemia/acetonuria following ingestion of a subtoxic dose of isopropyl alcohol. *Am J Emerg Med* 7:38, 1989.
155. Parker KM, Lera TA: Acute isopropanol ingestion: pharmacokinetic parameters in the infant. *Am J Emerg Med* 10:542, 1992.
156. Kelner M, Bailey DN: Isopropanol ingestion: interpretation of blood concentrations and clinical findings. *J Toxicol Clin Toxicol* 20:497, 1983.
157. Pappas AA, Ackerman BH, Olsen KM, et al: Isopropanol ingestion: a report of six episodes with isopropanol and acetone serum concentration time data. *J Toxicol Clin Toxicol* 29:11, 1991.
158. Linden CH: Unknown alcohol. *Ann Emerg Med* 28:371, 1996.
159. Bailey DN: Detection of isopropanol in acetonemic patients not exposed to isopropanol. *J Toxicol Clin Toxicol* 28:459, 1990.
160. Su M, Hoffman RS, Nelson LS: Error in an emergency medicine textbook: isopropyl alcohol toxicity. *Acad Emerg Med* 9:175, 2002.
161. Fligner CL, Jack R, Twiggs GA, et al: Hyperosmolality induced by propylene glycol: a complication of silver sulfadiazine therapy. *JAMA* 253:1606, 1985.
162. Ruddick JA: Toxicology, metabolism, and biochemistry of 1,2-propanediol. *Toxicol Appl Pharmacol* 21:102, 1972.
163. Unger AH, Sklaroff HJ: Fatalities following intravenous use of sodium diphenylhydantoin for cardiac arrhythmias. *JAMA* 200:335, 1967.
164. York RC, Coleridge ST: Cardiopulmonary arrest following intravenous phenytoin loading. *Am J Emerg Med* 6:255, 1988.
165. Wilson KC, Reardon C, Farber HW: Propylene glycol toxicity in a patient receiving intravenous diazepam. *N Engl J Med* 343:815, 2000.
166. Arulanantham K, Genel M: Central nervous system toxicity associated with ingestion of propylene glycol. *J Pediatr* 93:515, 1978.
167. Cate JC, Hedrick R: Propylene glycol intoxication and lactic acidosis. *N Engl J Med* 303:1237, 1980.
168. Robinson CA Jr, Scott JW, Ketchum C: Propylene glycol interference with ethylene glycol procedures. *Clin Chem* 29:727, 1983.
169. Mullins ME, Barnes BJ: Hyperosmolar metabolic acidosis and intravenous lorazepam. *N Engl J Med* 347:857–858, 2002.
170. Parker MG, Fraser GL, Watson DM, et al: Removal of propylene glycol and correction of increased osmolar gap by hemodialysis in a patient on high dose lorazepam infusion therapy. *Intensive Care Med* 28:81, 2002.
171. Al Khafaji AH, Dewhirst WE, Manning HL: Propylene glycol toxicity associated with lorazepam infusion in a patient receiving continuous veno-venous hemofiltration with dialysis. *Anesth Analg* 94:1583, 2002.
172. Rentz ED, Lewis L, Mujica OJ, et al: Outbreak of acute renal failure in Panama in 2006: a case-control study. *Bull World Health Organ* 86(10):749–756, 2008.
173. Schep LJ, Slaughter RJ, Temple WA, et al: Diethylene glycol poisoning. *Clin Toxicol (Phila)* 47(6):525–535, 2009.
174. Alfred S, Coleman P, Harris D, et al: Delayed neurologic sequelae resulting from epidemic diethylene glycol poisoning. *Clin Toxicol (Phila)* 43(3):155–159, 2005.
175. Hari P, Jain Y, Kabra SK: Fatal encephalopathy and renal failure caused by diethylene glycol poisoning. *J Trop Pediatr* 52(6):442–444, 2006.
176. O'Brien KL, Selanikio JD, Hecdivert C, et al: Epidemic of pediatric deaths from acute renal failure caused by diethylene glycol poisoning. Acute Renal Failure Investigation Team. *JAMA* 279(15):1175–1180, 1998.
177. Rollins YD, Filley CM, McNutt JT, et al: Fulminant ascending paralysis as a delayed sequela of diethylene glycol (Sterno) ingestion. *Neurology* 59(9):1460–1463, 2002.

Chapter 100 ■ Amphetamines

MICHAEL C. BEUHLER

INTRODUCTION

The term "amphetamine" includes a wide range of amine compounds with sympathetic-like effects. The simplest member of this group is amphetamine, but hundreds of related molecules have similar clinical effects. This chapter will focus on the more important and commonly used licit and illicit members of this group.

Amphetamine and methamphetamine are the most well-known members of this class. Amphetamine or **a**lpha-**m**ethyl **phe**nylethyl**amine** was first synthesized over 125 years ago, and it was widely used by many (including the United States military) as the stimulant Benzedrine, beginning in the 1930s. Restricting use to prescription only has decreased the prevalence slightly, but amphetamines continue to be used for both licit (attention deficit hyperactivity disorder [ADHD], narcolepsy, and weight loss) and illicit reasons. Currently, Adderall (a mixture of *l* and *d* amphetamine) and Vyvanse (lisdexamfetamine; hydrolyzed to *d*-amphetamine) are two commonly used medicinal amphetamine preparations.

Methamphetamine (or *N*-methyl amphetamine) is available for prescription use in generic form and under the trade name Desoxyn(R) for ADHD and obesity. The illicit abuse of methamphetamine is undergoing a surge in the US and worldwide popularity. One reason for its popularity over amphetamine is its longer duration of action. Another reason is that the Drug Enforcement Agency has taken actions to limit the availability of precursor compounds for the synthesis of amphetamine, including the unrelated removal of phenylpropanolamine from the market. Finally, synthesis can be conducted by individuals without training using materials that are easily obtainable, potentially resulting in a relatively pure product.

Several other medicinal compounds have clinical effects similar to amphetamines; a select few are discussed here. Methylphenidate (Ritalin(R)) is commonly used in children for ADHD and is occasionally abused. Phenylpropanolamine (Dexatrim(R)) was used more extensively in the past as a decongestant and weight loss agent; in 2005, the Federal Drug Administration (FDA) deemed phenylpropanolamine unsafe owing to concerns for increased stroke risk, removing it from the human market. Ephedrine has been used extensively in the past in herbal weight loss/energy preparations as well as a decongestant in cough/cold preparations; but in 2004, the FDA prohibited the sale of dietary supplements containing ephedra (ephedrine and pseudoephedrine) over safety concerns. In addition, in 2006, requirements regulating the sale of ephedrine were enacted in an attempt to limit its diversion for methamphetamine synthesis. Phentermine is an amphetamine derivative that is used for appetite suppression. Selegiline is an amphetamine derivative with selective monoamine oxidase inhibitor (MAOI)-B effects that is metabolized to l-methamphetamine. Propylhexedrine (Benzedrex(R) nasal inhaler), although not a true amphetamine, has sympathomimetic and vasoconstrictor properties and is occasionally abused.

Some amphetamine analogs with aromatic ring substitutions have direct affinity for serotonin receptors as well as increased inhibition of serotonin uptake, thereby exerting both sympathomimetic and serotonergic effects manifested by hallucinatory properties. One of the more popular compounds in this group is 3,4-methylenedioxymethamphetamine (MDMA or Ecstasy). Other similar ring-substituted amphetamine compounds include 3,4-methylenedioxyamphetamine (MDA), 3,4-methylenedioxy-*N*-ethylamphetamine (MDEA or Eve), 2,5-dimethoxy-4-bromo-phenethylamine (2-CB; not strictly an amphetamine), para-methoxy-amphetamine (PMA), 2,5-dimethoxy-4-methyl-amphetamine (DOM), and 2,5-dimethoxy-4-bromo-amphetamine (DOB; also the chlorine and iodine derivatives DOC and DOI exist). The 2,5-dimethoxy halogenated amphetamine derivatives (DOB, DOC, DOI) are common substitutions for lysergine acid diethylamide (LSD) found on blotter paper in the United States [1].

There has been a recent surge in the availability and abuse of synthetic cathinones; these compounds all have a β-keto phenylalkylamine group. Bupropion is a cathinone derivative used therapeutically for depression and smoking cessation that has sympathomimetic properties; most notably for causing seizures and ventricular dysrhythmias in supratherapeutic doses. The illicit cathinones are also referred to as "bath salts" and represent a large number of compounds such as methylone, α-pyrrolidinopentiophenone (PVP), and 3,4-methylenedioxypyrovalerone (MDPV) [2]. Although many of these are Schedule I Controlled Substances (i.e., high abuse potential with no recognized therapeutic indications), there is a constant flux of new derivatives. Because of the constant change in which compounds are observed, limited clinical experience with specific compounds and chapter space restrictions, the synthetic cathinones will not be specifically discussed, although notable class cathinone effects will be covered. However, the principles in this chapter can be applied to treating exposures to these compounds because they share many of the clinical effects of amphetamines [3].

Recent increases in clandestine methamphetamine production facilities ("meth labs") have resulted in concern for environmental contamination and bystander toxicity from laboratory chemicals. The vast majority of illicit amphetamine laboratories currently produce methamphetamine by reductive dehydroxylation of ephedrine or pseudoephedrine. Methamphetamine laboratories are often discovered after a chemical mishap or explosion, and health risks from these chemicals include respiratory irritation and caustic injury.

Alternatively, methcathinone is a potent, occasionally used cathinone produced from the *oxidation* of ephedrine in amateur labs, instead of the usual *reduction* to methamphetamine; toxicity from it is similar to the amphetamines except that cases of Parkinson-like neurotoxicity from intravenous (IV) exposure to the manganese in the impure product have been reported.

Methamphetamine is synthesized most commonly by two methods. The probably more dangerous one is the Birch or "Nazi" method, which utilizes lithium metal as the reducing agent dissolved in either anhydrous ammonia or a modified method using ammonium nitrate and solvent in a bottle ("shake and bake"). The other method is the hydriodic acid method, which usually utilizes red phosphorus and iodine.

Depending upon the illicit amphetamine purchased, there is a chance that it will contain one or more contaminants, or possibly be substituted by another drug. Street purchased methamphetamine tends to be of better purity than cocaine, whereas MDMA is very commonly substituted or combined with other psychoactive substances. "Crystal Meth" is a nearly pure crystalline form of methamphetamine. The exact "contaminants" or other chemicals present in street purchased amphetamines are highly variable, based on drug, year, and location. Previously reported substitutions include acetaminophen, anesthetics (benzocaine, lidocaine, and procaine), cocaine, caffeine, ephedrine, ketamine, lead (rare), talc, phencyclidine, piperazine compounds (benzylpiperazine and others), phenylpropanolamine, pseudoephedrine, strychnine, and quinine [4]. Depending on the quantity of the adulterant, it may contribute to the effect or toxicity of the sympathomimetic drugs.

Occasionally, an individual will ingest an amphetamine while it is wrapped in plastic or other nonpermeable material. Body *packers*, or "mules," are people who transport large quantities of specially prepared drug packets in their gastrointestinal (GI) tract. Each packet usually contains drugs in sufficient quantity and purity to cause life-threatening toxicity if rupture occurs. Body *stuffers* are people who quickly swallow ("stuff") drug-containing packets in an attempt to get rid of evidence and avoid arrest by the police. These packets are usually poorly prepared and are at increased risk of leakage and rupture, but often contain far less drug than a packet from a body packer. Body *pushers* are people that hide drug packets in their vagina or rectum; serious illness has been observed in some cases. Rarely, individuals will ingest a plastic bag containing a drug with holes or a corner of the bag cut off in an attempt to produce a sustained release effect ("parachuting") [5].

PHARMACOLOGY

Amphetamine and methamphetamine are similar in their pharmacokinetic properties and have similar physiologic effects in humans [6]. They do not have significant direct effects at adrenergic or dopamine receptors; rather, their effects are mediated by an increase in the concentration of synaptic dopamine and, to a lesser extent, serotonin, and norepinephrine. This increase in biogenic amines occurs by several mechanisms. Amphetamine and methamphetamine enter the presynaptic cytoplasm through both passive diffusion and active uptake by biogenic amine uptake transporters. Amphetamine moves into the synaptic vesicles by diffusion and by the vesicular monoamine transporters (VMAT), subsequently causing release of stored dopamine and norepinephrine, most likely by raising the pH and effecting VMAT. This increases the cytosolic levels of these biogenic amines, resulting in increased synaptic levels due to reverse transport activity by the amine transporters, especially the dopamine transporter. Part of the mechanism of action of amphetamines' raising synaptic levels is also caused by competitive inhibition of biogenic amine reuptake from the synapse into the presynaptic terminal. Finally, some amphetamines have MAOI activity, which inhibits the breakdown of dopamine, serotonin, and norepinephrine, with a few (PMA for example) having significant MAOI activity [7,8].

The mechanism of action of MDMA toxicity includes a direct effect at some serotonin receptors, as well as some of the indirect effects from serotonin release, as described above. Additionally, human and animal studies have shown that MDMA produces a dose-related depletion of serotonin and serotonin transporter activity, as well as serotonergic neuronal degeneration [9]. Methamphetamine causes dopamine and serotonergic neuronal toxicity as well as a decrease in dopamine, VMAT, and serotonin transporter activity in the brain, at least in part by free radical injury [10,11].

Peak plasma concentrations of methamphetamine are reported within 4 hours for an intranasal (insufflated, snorted) dose, within 2 to 3 hours for a smoked (inhaled) dose, and nearly immediately for an IV dose [12]; however, levels do not correlate with the degree of clinical toxicity [13]. Methamphetamine and amphetamine have a *l*- and *d*-isomer; the *d* form is more potent in causing pleasurable central nervous system (CNS) stimulation and persistent cardiovascular activation than the *l* form [14]. Most abused methamphetamine is the *d* isomer, having been synthesized from ephedrine or pseudoephedrine. However, the *d* form of methamphetamine has a shorter half-life (10 to 11 hours) than the *l* form (13 to 15 hours) [14].

The majority of methamphetamine is either eliminated unchanged, *N*-demethylated to amphetamine (active) or hydroxylated to *p*-hydroxymethamphetamine (active) with contribution from CYP2D6 [15]. The a-carbon on the ethyl side chain protects it against MAO degradation. Amphetamine undergoes a similar metabolism, except that it is deaminated to an inactive metabolite as well as hydroxylated to *p*-hydroxyamphetamine (active). Excretion of both is increased in acidic urine, but this fact has limited clinical utility as the risks of urinary acidification outweigh potential benefits. The urine drug screen usually remains positive for at least 24 hours in high-dose, chronic abusers. The serotonergic amphetamine and amphetamine-like compounds (MDMA, PMA, 2-CB) are not metabolized to amphetamine or methamphetamine and have a variable, unpredictable effect on the typical amphetamine urine drug screen..

CLINICAL PRESENTATION

Methamphetamine toxicity has been reported following ingestion, inhalation, insufflation, rectal, subcutaneous, intramuscular, or intravenous exposure [16]. The onset and duration of methamphetamine toxicity depends on factors such as dose, route of exposure, individual tolerance, pattern of use, ambient temperature, and crowding/stimulation level. Most people develop signs and symptoms within a few minutes of parenteral drug use, whereas signs and symptoms may be delayed for hours or days after ingestion with body packers and body stuffers. In most patients, the majority of sympathomimetic effects are expected to resolve within 24 to 36 hours postexposure [16]. Life-threatening toxicity is more common in drug abusers and in people who overdose with suicidal intent, and it can also occur in body packers and body stuffers.

Methamphetamine toxicity usually results in a group of signs and symptoms known as the "sympathomimetic toxidrome," including hypertension, tachycardia, tachypnea, hyperthermia, diaphoresis, mydriasis, hyperactive bowel sounds, agitation, anxiety, and toxic psychosis. This pattern of symptoms is seen in other members of the amphetamine group, as well as the cathinones and other sympathomimetics such as cocaine and to some extent caffeine; but this pattern of symptoms can be variable depending on the sympathomimetic agent involved. For example, phenylpropanolamine has peripheral alpha vasoconstrictive effects that can result in a reflex bradycardia.

Airway and breathing abnormalities are uncommon with ingestion. Transient cough, pleuritic chest pain, and shortness of breath are common after insufflation or smoking. People presenting from illicit drug laboratory fires may have thermal injury to their oropharynx or upper airway, specific toxic issues from drug laboratory fires are extremely uncommon. Insufflation or smoking methamphetamine may result in bronchospasm, pneumothorax, pneumomediastinum, pneumonitis, and noncardiogenic pulmonary edema. Noncardiogenic pulmonary edema and acute respiratory distress syndrome may be associated with multisystem organ failure. Tachypnea is common secondary to agitation or metabolic acidosis. Hypoventilation is rare but may occur secondary to intracranial pathology or the end stage of multisystem organ failure.

Many of the adverse cardiovascular effects result from increases in peripheral catecholamines, which result in a mismatch of oxygen consumption and delivery; there may be a direct cardiotoxic effect of methamphetamine as well. Palpitations and chest pain are common complaints. Acute myocardial infarction due to vasospasm, plaque rupture, and/or thrombosis can occur [17]. Life-threatening atrial or ventricular dysrhythmias, sudden death, and aortic dissection have been reported, with potential synergy if cocaine is also present [17]. Coronary artery disease and cardiomyopathy have been reported with chronic amphetamine abuse [14,18–20]. Peripheral vascular ischemia can result from oral sympathomimetic abuse but is uncommon; however, inadvertent intra-arterial injections can result in significant injury. Hypotension is unusual but may be secondary to dehydration, myocardial depression, intestinal ischemia, or sepsis.

Several important findings may be apparent on the head-eyes-ears-nose-throat exam. Mydriasis is common, and various forms of nystagmus have been reported. Patients who abuse and binge on sympathomimetic agents are often dehydrated and have dry mucous membranes; this can complicate the diagnosis by incorrectly suggesting anticholinergic toxicity. Nasal mucosal abnormalities, including nasal septal perforations, are well reported in patients who chronically insufflate cocaine and are possible with insufflation of other sympathomimetics. An increase in dental pathology has been noted in users of methamphetamines, manifested by a distinctive pattern of caries on the buccal smooth surfaces of the posterior teeth and the interproximal surfaces of the anterior teeth. The teeth may be loose, rotting, or crumbling, and are usually beyond salvage. The pathology of these changes is uncertain, but is believed to result from a combination of decrease in salivation (xerostomia) along with increased ingestion of sugar- and acid-containing sodas, poor hygiene, poor nutrition, localized vasospasm, and bruxism, a side effect especially seen with MDMA [21].

Central nervous system effects are the reason for abuse as well as often the reason for medical care. Methamphetamine produces a euphoric and anorexic effect, with smoked and injected administration producing a greater "rush." The most common presenting symptoms include agitation and altered mental status; other symptoms include headache, hyperactivity, toxic psychosis, loss of consciousness, focal neurologic deficits, or seizures [16,22]. Hyperthermia may be more common and worse in patients with uncontrolled psychomotor agitation, especially when patients are physically but not chemically restrained. The cathinones or "bath salts" are notorious for causing extreme agitation, hyperthermia, and rapid demise. Deaths due to excited delirium from amphetamines and cathinones have been reported. Altered mental status may be secondary to hypoglycemia or an acute intracranial process. Headache may be secondary to intracranial or subarachnoid hemorrhage [23]. Focal neurologic deficit may be secondary to cerebral ischemia or infarction, vasospasm, or direct injection trauma. On arteriography, multiple occlusions or "beading" of the arteries has been observed; this is thought to represent some combination of local vasospasm or vasculitis [23,24]. Seizures may occur in association with and independent of intracranial hemorrhage or cerebral infarction. Prolonged methamphetamine (and probably MDMA) use may lead to cognitive decline represented by attention and memory changes [11].

Some abusers develop stereotyped, compulsive behavior such as cleaning or buttoning shirts; in some cases, it has been observed that addicts compulsively disassemble appliances, usually without reassembly. Psychosis from amphetamines can present as paranoid delusions and perceptual disturbances; these may persist long after the drug has been stopped and can result in homicidal or self-destructive behavior [16,25,26]. Severe and prolonged psychosis following cathinones or "bath salts" abuse may be more common than from amphetamines. After binge use of amphetamines, patients may develop a withdrawal pattern of symptoms consisting of generalized fatigue, dysphoria, decreased level of consciousness, and profound lethargy.

One occasionally sees choreiform, ballistic, bruxism, torticollis, or athetoid involuntary movements with amphetamine, methamphetamine, and cathinone abuse [27]. These movements can be fast or slow, and they can involve the facial, extremity, or trunk muscles. Ataxia may result if the trunk or limb movements are severe enough. These movements usually begin after prolonged abuse of amphetamine or methamphetamine and may worsen or reoccur with additional drug abuse. Usually, the symptoms resolve over several hours to a week following abstinence. However, they may only diminish in magnitude and persist for months or, rarely, even years. The movements may be diminished with voluntary motor activity or during sleep. The mechanism for these movements is not well understood, and may involve a disruption of the normal dopamine neurotransmitter system [28].

Abdominal findings may include increased bowel sounds, bowel obstruction from body packing, and abdominal pain due to intestinal ischemia or bowel perforation [29]. Rhabdomyolysis can result from psychomotor agitation and seizures. Hyperthermia and multisystem organ failure may result in coagulopathy and disseminated intravascular coagulation (DIC). Dehydration, increased anion gap metabolic acidosis associated with increased lactate, and hypokalemia are common in patients with significant sympathomimetic toxicity. Urinary retention has been reported from amphetamine toxicity. Acute tubular necrosis may occur secondary to hyperthermia, hypovolemia, hypotension, and rhabdomyolysis.

Diaphoresis with either warm or cool skin is common. Scarring and hyperpigmentation ("track marks") in areas above veins suggest chronic intravenous drug use. Subcutaneous injection of the drug ("skin popping") can result in scabs, circular scars, and lesions in a variety of areas. Additional excoriations and rashes can result from skin picking and scratching. Abscesses and infection are common.

Medical complications from drug abuse include endocarditis, infectious hepatitis, human immunodeficiency virus infection (HIV), cellulitis, septic emboli, abscesses, tetanus, or wound botulism. Methamphetamine abuse is associated with an increased risk of HIV infection because of both increase in risk-taking behavior (IVDA, unprotected intercourse, untreated STDs) and probable enhancement of HIV infectivity [30].

In general, the toxicity observed in patients using methamphetamine is attributable to the drug and not to any adulterants. Adulterants are not usually present in large enough quantities, and methamphetamine is relatively pure and sufficiently toxic in its own right. However, some important exceptions should be noted. The addition of benzocaine has caused methemoglobinemia [31]. Intra-arterial injection of a drug may cause injury, possibly potentiated by any talc present. Talc pulmonary emboli have been reported as well, which probably contribute to pulmonary hypertension. Lastly, substitution is more of a problem with the ring-modified amphetamines (MDMA); the real substance present in the street purchased product is likely to be contaminated with or entirely comprised of something else such as a piperazine (e.g., benzylpiperazine), caffeine, methamphetamine, cathinone (e.g., methylone), or some other substituted amphetamine such as the very dangerous PMA.

In addition to having some sympathomimetic qualities, nearly all of the ring-substituted amphetamines (e.g., MDMA and DOM) also have hallucinogenic properties likely owing to their direct and indirect effect at serotonin receptors. The route of abuse for MDMA is usually ingestion. MDA, an analog of MDMA, has similar effects to those of MDMA. Serious autonomic reactions include many of the sympathomimetic symptoms discussed earlier as well as seizures, rigidity, dysrhythmias, and profound hyperthermia with grave consequences (rhabdomyolysis, renal failure, DIC) [32]. Given the increased serotonin levels produced, at least part of this toxicity should be characterized as serotonin syndrome.

Some of the ring-substituted amphetamines have specific toxicities. There are several reports of hepatotoxicity resulting in hepatomegaly, jaundice, and death caused by MDMA that did not stem from hyperthermia or shock liver; this probably resulted from an immunologic component [32,33]. Hyperthermia is more common with the ring-substituted amphetamines, likely from contribution from serotonin toxicity and possibly from mitochondrial uncoupling [34]. Hyponatremia resulting in altered mental status, coma, seizures, cerebral edema, and death is also sometimes seen following MDMA use. This probably results from some combination of inappropriate antidiuretic hormone secretion (SIADH) and from excessive water drinking. This SIADH may be more commonly observed in young women using MDMA as an inappropriately large number of cases are reported in this age/gender group. The observed clinical toxicity from PMA (street name "death") includes hyperthermia, hypoglycemia, hyperkalemia, and EKG changes. PMA effects are similar to MDMA but may be more severe because of the steep dose–response curve for elevating brain serotonin levels and significant MAOI activity [7,35]. PMA exposures are often unintentional, with accidental or purposeful substitution for MDMA causing most exposure, and the long onset time sometimes results in users taking multiple doses. DOB is highly potent, enough so that a dose (2 to 5 mg) can be found on a small piece of paper possibly being sold as LSD. Large doses of DOB have been reported to result in significant vasospasm, resulting in seizures, gangrenous amputations, and deaths [36].

DIAGNOSTIC EVALUATION

Patients with amphetamine toxicity (sympathomimetic toxicity) should have frequent vital sign determinations including core or rectal temperature measurement, intravenous access, and continuous cardiac monitoring. Patients with abnormal vital signs or mental status should have an electrocardiogram, complete blood cell count, electrolyte, blood urea nitrogen, creatinine, glucose, and arterial blood gas determinations. Patients with chest pain, dysrhythmias, or persistent pulse or blood pressure abnormalities should be evaluated for acute coronary or vascular syndromes. Patients with prolonged immobilization, uncontrolled psychomotor agitation, or hyperthermia should have serial CPKs to evaluate for rhabdomyolysis and consider the possibility of compartment syndrome. Those that either have or have had significant hyperthermia or shock should also have liver injury and function tests (lactate dehydrogenase, aspartate aminotransferase, alanine aminotransferase, and coagulation profile) to screen for multisystem organ failure and DIC.

Several imaging studies may be warranted for an amphetamine toxic patient, depending on his or her clinical presentation. Those with respiratory symptoms or chest pain should have a chest radiograph and potentially a chest computed tomography (CT) when there is concern for aortic dissection. Patients with headache or seizures should be evaluated for intracranial hemorrhage with CT of the brain. Those with continued suspicion for subarachnoid hemorrhage with a negative CT scan should also have a lumbar puncture [23]. Plain and oral contrast abdominal radiographs may be helpful in detecting drug-containing packets in the GI tract of body packers, but their sensitivity is quite low for stuffers. Experience with abdominal CT and abdominal ultrasound for detection of stuffer packets is limited. A negative imaging study cannot definitively rule out drug packets in the GI tract.

The results of toxicology screening for most drugs of abuse rarely contribute to or alter patient management. However, in the case of sympathomimetic toxicity, the urine drug screen is reasonably sensitive to the recent use of methamphetamine/amphetamine as well as cocaine and can assist in differentiating these syndromes, which can be important in management. If toxicology drug screening is essential, health care providers should contact their clinical laboratory to determine included substances as well as causes of false-positive and false-negative results. For example, the ability of immunologically based amphetamine drug screens to detect MDMA (or similar ring-substituted amphetamines) is highly variable, but specific immunologically based MDMA drug screens are available. Detection of the cathinones requires special specimen handling and testing.

A positive drug screen can confirm the presence of amphetamine or a similar structured drug, whereas a negative drug screen is nondiagnostic. For amphetamines, the screen is typically reasonably sensitive for use within the last few days, but has limited specificity. A sampling of some common substances that may cause a positive amphetamine screen are bupropion, chloroquine, clobenzorex, ephedrine, methylphenidate, phenelzine, phentermine, phenylpropanolamine, pseudoephedrine, selegiline, tranylcypromine, trazodone, and Vicks(R) inhaler [37]. One should remember that if the result of a toxicology screen is to be used for forensic purposes, the chain of custody should be maintained, and results will need to be confirmed using a more rigorous analytical method such as gas chromatography/mass spectrometry.

Toxicologic and nontoxicologic conditions that may have a similar presentation or that present concomitantly (Table 100.1) should be evaluated for and excluded. A serum lactate level may be helpful for patients with increased anion gap metabolic acidosis of unclear origin. An elevated lactate level would be expected for patients with compromised tissue perfusion (e.g., occurring with shock and intestinal or limb ischemia), for those with hypermetabolic states in which metabolic demands exceed available substrates, or for those with cellular dysfunction in whom normal substrates cannot be used. Other causes of increased anion gap metabolic acidosis (e.g., ethylene glycol, methanol, iron, and salicylate) should be investigated when the lactate level is normal or near normal. The possibility of concomitant poisoning with by-products or impurities related to the illicit synthesis of methamphetamine (e.g., phenethylamine derivatives, caffeine, ephedrine, mercury, strychnine, or lead) would be rare, but should also be considered.

TABLE 100.1

Differential Diagnosis of Amphetamine Toxicity

Toxicologic
- β-Agonists toxicity (clenbuterol and others)
- Black widow envenomation
- Cathinones or "bath salts"
- Cocaine
- Dextromethorphan
- Methylxanthine toxicity (caffeine, theophylline)
- Monamine oxidase inhibitor toxicity
- Neuroleptic malignant syndrome
- Piperazine compounds (benzylpiperazine and others)
- Phencyclidine toxicity (PCP)
- Bark scorpion envenomation (found mostly in Arizona/Sonoran Desert)
- Salicylates
- Serotonin toxicity
- Strychnine
- Withdrawal from sedative–hypnotics, including baclofen, barbiturates, benzodiazepines, clonidine, chloral hydrate, ethanol, γ-hydroxybutyrate, γ-butyrolactone, meprobamate, as well as from β-antagonists such as propofol

Nontoxicologic
- Endocarditis
- Encephalitis and meningitis
- Heat stroke
- Intracranial bleed or mass lesion
- Pheochromocytoma
- Sepsis
- Thyrotoxicosis

MANAGEMENT

Patients who present with life-threatening effects from amphetamine toxicity or those that are at increased risk for developing them (such as

TABLE 100.2

Indications for Admitting Patients to an Intensive Care Unit

Acute coronary syndromes	Multisystem organ failure
Aortic dissection	Peripheral ischemia
Body packer or body stuffer	Persistent psychomotor agitation
Cerebral ischemia or infarction	Pneumothorax
Dysrhythmias	Rhabdomyolysis
Hyperthermia	Seizure
Intracranial bleed	
Myocardial infarction	

a packer) should be managed in an intensive care unit (Table 100.2). The overall approach to these patients is aggressive supportive care with supplemental oxygen, sedation, fluid administration, prevention and treatment of hyperthermia, and close monitoring while addressing the specific myriad complications that can occur.

The hemodynamic effects of amphetamines are primarily caused by release of catecholamines and not by a direct effect at receptors. Mild sinus tachycardia and hypertension not associated with psychomotor agitation or evidence of end-organ damage usually do not require pharmacologic treatment. Treatment of psychomotor agitation utilizing occasionally large benzodiazepine doses (e.g., 100 mg of diazepam or its equivalent over 30 minutes with appropriate airway monitoring) will often result in improvement or resolution of tachycardia and hypertension. If sufficient benzodiazepines do not provide adequate improvement, rate-related cardiac ischemia may be treated with a β-blocker, preferably a short-acting and easily titratable agent such as esmolol, or a calcium channel blocker, being cautious to exclude cocaine toxicity if a β-blocker is being used. Patients with life-threatening dysrhythmias who are hemodynamically unstable should be cardioverted or defibrillated. However in the author's experience interventions specifically directed at reducing the heart rate have occasionally precipitated cardiovascular collapse. Persistent hypertension, especially if there is evidence of end-organ damage or hyperthermia, should be treated with benzodiazepines as well as phentolamine, nitroprusside, or nitroglycerin with careful dose titration.

Patients presenting with chest pain should be evaluated for acute coronary syndromes and managed accordingly [20]. Thrombolytic therapy or procedural coronary intervention may be indicated as per current guidelines. In these circumstances, cardiology consultation is recommended, especially since coronary vasospasm is a possibility. Other important potential causes of chest pain such as pneumothorax, pneumomediastinum, infection, septic emboli, and aortic dissection should be ruled out.

Hypotension should be treated with fluids and assessed for comorbid potential life-threatening conditions such as dysrhythmias, acute coronary syndromes, pneumothorax, aortic dissection, hyperkalemia, GI hemorrhage, and sepsis. Persistent symptomatic hypotension that is refractory to fluids necessitates treatment with a direct acting vasopressor such as norepinephrine, epinephrine, or phenylephrine. At times, the choice and dose of vasopressor should be guided by their different pharmacological properties as well as potentially pulmonary artery catheter hemodynamic monitoring or bedside ultrasound.

Management of bronchospasm should include nebulized β_2 agonists (such as albuterol) and anticholinergic agents (such as ipratropium bromide). Noncardiogenic pulmonary edema and acute respiratory distress syndrome should be managed according to current guidelines. The benefit of corticosteroids in patients with sympathomimetic-induced bronchospasm, pneumonitis, and noncardiogenic pulmonary edema has not been well studied, but may be considered in patients with severe or persistent symptoms. Occasionally, pneumomediastinum and pneumothorax following smoking methamphetamine is observed. Patients with pneumothorax may require tube thoracostomy depending on the size of the pneumothorax. Evaluation for a pneumomediastinum usually involves a nonbarium oral contrast imaging study to rule out esophageal perforation, but, surprisingly, these commonly have a completely benign course.

The initial management of a patient with an altered mental status includes assessing and treating all readily reversible causes such as hypoxia, hypoglycemia, electrolyte abnormalities (especially hyponatremia), opioid toxicity, and thiamine deficiency. Imaging studies of the head should be performed on patients with persistent altered mental status, potentially followed by lumbar puncture if indicated. Mild agitation or anxiety may be treated with oral benzodiazepines. Psychomotor agitation that poses a danger to the patient or others requires more aggressive sedation. Incremental doses of intravenous benzodiazepine should be used to achieve the desired effect. The use of antipsychotics for controlling agitation should be as an adjunctive therapy and not as the primary means of control, but does appear to be safe and efficacious in adult and pediatric populations [16,38,39]. One should recognize the other clinical precautions that accompany the use of the antipsychotic drug class (e.g., EKG changes and neuroleptic malignant syndrome). If agitation is severe, more aggressive measures such as sedation, intubation, and paralysis may be required to protect the patient and the staff. Restraints should be used only during the relatively short time of gaining control of the agitation using pharmaceutical methods, as the restrained agitated patient is at risk for several adverse outcomes, including sudden death. Deaths from excited delirium occur quickly, and close cardiac and core temperature monitoring are essential.

Patients presenting with seizures should be treated with incremental doses of intravenous benzodiazepines. If seizures are not rapidly controlled, intravenous propofol (being watchful for hypotension) or phenobarbital is indicated usually along with intubation to secure the airway. The role of phenytoin is limited in the patient with toxin induced seizures and probablyshould be avoided. Seizures refractory to sedative–hypnotic drugs should be managed in consultation with an experienced neurologist with continuous electroencephalogram monitoring. The workup of seizures should include a CT scan and potentially lumbar puncture to evaluate for potential physical causes. Patients with intracranial hemorrhage or cerebral infarction should have neurosurgery consultation. As the etiology of the "beading" seen on angiography is uncertain, the role of calcium channel blockers (e.g., nimodipine) and/or steroids for such patients is equally uncertain.

Patients with peripheral vascular ischemia should be managed in conjunction with a vascular service. Intra-arterial administration of α-adrenergic receptor antagonists such as phentolamine may relieve localized arterial vasospasm. If multiple areas of vasospasm are observed, there may be a role for intravenous nitroprusside with caution not to lower systemic blood pressure significantly. This adverse effect may be observed more typically with some of the substituted hallucinogenic amphetamines such as DOB [36]. Accidental intra-arterial injection during intravenous abuse may lead to significant tissue destruction through emboli (e.g., talc and the other cutting agents), thrombosis, and vasoconstriction. There is no consensus regarding managing these patients, although adequate fluid resuscitation, acetylsalicylate, and heparin appear to be reasonable; other interventions that have been used for intra-arterial injection accidents with heroin include intra-arterial phentolamine, thrombolytics, and systemic steroids (dexamethasone).

Core temperature approaching or more than 104°F (40°C) should be aggressively managed, as the risk for multisystem organ failure rises exponentially with the temperature. One should undress the patient, initiate active cooling measures, and continuously monitor the patient's core temperature. Active cooling techniques include spraying the patient with cool water, draping with cold water–soaked sheets along with the use of large fans for evaporation, ice packs in the axilla and groin, or a cooling blanket placed *under* the patient while utilizing evaporative cooling from above. Active cooling should be terminated when the patient's core temperature approaches 101°F (38.3°C). Benzodiazepines are useful for decreasing motor agitation or seizure activity contributing to the hyperthermia. Paralysis and intubation would be a last resort in the treatment of persistent rigidity associated with hyperthermia. Antipyretics (e.g., acetaminophen, aspirin, nonsteroidal anti-inflammatory drugs) are not useful, and there is limited evidence that dantrolene, bromocriptine, or amantadine enhances the cooling process in these patients with life-threatening hyperthermia.

Fluid management should address any electrolyte and acid–base abnormalities and dehydration. Management of rhabdomyolysis should include generous intravenous crystalloid fluids to maintain urine output of at least 2 to 3 mL/kg/h to minimize the risk of acute tubular necrosis. The role of alkalinizing the urine to provide renal protection from rhabdomyolysis is controversial, but may be performed as desired. Because serum myoglobin levels are not usually rapidly available, serum CPK may be monitored instead. Although no longer recommended for amphetamine toxicity, urinary acidification would increase the urinary excretion of amphetamine, but the risks outweigh the potential benefits.

The serotonergic amphetamines MDMA and related compounds can cause significant serotonergic toxicity when combined with other pharmaceuticals that have serotonin effects such as selective serotonin reuptake inhibitors, MAOIs, and cocaine. Differentiating the degree of concomitant serotonin toxicity can be difficult, but the physical examination findings of myoclonus and hyperreflexia with the lower extremity reflexes more pronounced than the upper extremity reflexes would be suggestive of serotonin toxicity. Treatment involves benzodiazepines and supportive care, although cyproheptadine may be of some benefit. An adult dose of cyproheptadine for serotonin toxicity is 8 mg orally every 6 to 8 hours to a maximum of 32 mg per day. The hyponatremia arising from SIADH should be treated with water restriction and may require hypertonic 3% normal saline. These fluid requirements should be balanced with other fluid issues such as the possible presence of rhabdomyolysis.

The involuntary abnormal choreiform and athetoid movements following abuse may be the reason for presentation and can be a source of great anxiety for the patient. When the symptom onset is rapid and not present for a long period of time, antipsychotics such as haloperidol may be effective [27]. When the involuntary movements have lasted for a long time (e.g., days to weeks), antipsychotics may be less effective. Sedatives have been observed to increase the movements in some patients. There has been some success in alleviating symptoms using centrally acting antimuscarinic drugs (e.g., benztropine) [28].

No treatment consensus is available for the management of asymptomatic body stuffers. Sometimes, individuals claim to have ingested drug packets in an attempt to avoid going to jail, a technique that often works in the short term. The packet count or the amount of drugs in the packet is usually unreliable. Even when bags or packets are ingested, they are rarely seen on imaging studies. An abdominal CT scan is more reliable than plain abdominal imaging, but false-negatives do occur. GI decontamination using activated charcoal (AC) at a dose of 1 to 2 g per kg should be considered for these patients. Multiple doses of AC have no proven benefit and may be harmful in potentially causing obstruction. The risks of forced AC administration usually outweigh any potential benefit when a patient will not voluntarily drink the AC. However, this risk/benefit ratio should be reassessed should a patient clinically deteriorate to the point of requiring intubation. Occasionally, whole bowel irrigation (WBI) is also employed for these patients (see below). Given the lack of end point (i.e., passed packets) in most of these patients, they will require a period of sufficient observation. The safest approach to these patients would be admission for a minimum of 24 hours of close hemodynamic observation, with additional observation time should any unexplained increase in pulse or blood pressure occur. Note this observation period may not be sufficient for all patients; cases of toxicity have resulted from more than 36 hours from ingestion of a sealed baggie [5].

Asymptomatic body packers should also be conservatively managed. One proposed guideline involves the oral administration of a water-soluble contrast solution followed by serial abdominal radiographs (see Chapter 97). Whole bowel irrigation with isotonic polyethylene glycol electrolyte solution has also been advocated for GI decontamination based on case reports. Some clinicians advocate administering polyethylene glycol solution, 1 L per hour, to adults until there is no longer significant concern for retained packets in the GI tract. This is usually signalled by a clear rectal effluent, no radiographic evidence of drug packets in the GI tract, a negative rectal examination for packets, and an accurate accounting of the number of ingested packets. It does appear that the packet count for body packers is sometimes more reliable than for body stuffers, but still may not be correct. Administration of multiple doses of cathartics is not considered whole bowel irrigation and may result in severe fluid and electrolyte abnormalities [40,41].

Body packers and body stuffers who develop sympathomimetic toxicity should be suspected of having leakage or rupture of the drug packets in their GI tract [42]. In the case of a body packer, this is an absolute indication for emergent surgical intervention owing to the massive amount of drug present and profound subsequent local (e.g., bowel ischemia) and systemic effects. Surgical intervention is also indicated for patients with intestinal obstruction, ischemia, or perforation and may be indicated when packets fail to progress through the GI tract after conservative management. Endoscopic retrieval of packets retained in the stomach is rarely performed owing to risk of rupture, but if attempted, it should be by an experienced endoscopist.

The proper management of patients exposed to methamphetamine laboratories varies depending on the exposure scenario and the type of laboratory. Most of the times, the only treatment required is adequate burn care because many of these patients present with thermal burns from a laboratory fire. The most dangerous components to a methamphetamine laboratory not on fire (besides the occasional armed psychotic inhabitant) are the potential gases: anhydrous ammonia, hydrochloric acid (HCl), and phosphine. Of note, the type of possible gases present depends on the type of lab as well as the activity state of lab because generally the HCl and phosphine levels are present only in high enough levels to cause injury during the process of the "cook" [43,44]. All three gases can cause significant acute lung injury, with the injury from phosphine potentially being delayed by several hours and anhydrous ammonia potentially causing significant ocular and dermal injury as well. Methamphetamine laboratories also use caustics and solvents that on contact with skin or eyes can cause significant injury. Variations in the synthesis methods, exposure duration, and preexisting conditions as well as chapter space make it difficult to give further exacting treatment recommendations. It should be noted that despite the subjective complaints, a minor transient exposure to a methamphetamine laboratory is unlikely to cause significant injury, and that unless gross contamination is present, a gentle cleaning with soap and water is adequate for nearly all exposures [45].

ACKNOWLEDGMENT

Edwin K. Kuffner, MD, contributed to previous versions of this chapter.

References

1. U.S. Department of Justice, Drug Enforcement Administration, Office of Forensic Sciences: *Microgram Bulletin*, Issues 4/09, 3/09, 6/08, 3/08, 12/07, 12/06, 11/06, and 5/06.
2. U.S. Drug Enforcement Administration, Office of Diversion Control, National Forensic Laboratory Information System Special Report: *Synthetic Cannabinoids and Synthetic Cathinones Reported in NFLIS, 2010–2013*. Springfield, VA, U.S. Drug Enforcement Administration, 2014.
3. Murphy CM, Dulaney AR, Beuhler MC, et al: "Bath salts" and "plant food" products: the experience of one regional US poison center. *J Med Toxicol* 9(1):42–48, 2013.
4. Klatt EC, Montgomery S, Nemiki T, et al: Misrepresentation of stimulant street drugs: a decade of experience in analysis program. *J Toxicol Clin Toxicol* 24:441, 1986.
5. Hendrickson RG, Horowitz Z, Norton RL: "Parachuting" meth: a novel delivery method for methamphetamine and delayed-onset toxicity from "body stuffing." *Clin Toxicol* 44:379–382, 2006.
6. Lamb RJ, Henningfield JE: Human D-amphetamine drug discrimination: methamphetamine and hydromorphone. *J Exp Anal Behav* 61:169–180, 1994.
7. Green AL, El Hait MAS: p-Methoxyamphetamine, a potent reversible inhibitor of type A-monoamine oxidase in vitro and in vivo. *J Pharm Pharmacol* 32:262–266, 1980.
8. Sulzer D, Sonders MS, Poulsen NW, et al: Mechanisms of Neurotransmitter release by amphetamines: a review. *Prog Neurobiol* 75:406–433, 2005.
9. Ricaurte GA, Forno LS, Wilson MA, et al: (+/-) 3,4-Methylenedioxymethamphetamine selectively damages central serotonergic neurons in nonhuman primates. *JAMA* 260:51, 1988.
10. Krasnova IN, Cadet JL: Methamphetamine toxicity and messengers of death. *Brain Res Rev* 60(2):379–407, 2009.
11. McCann UD, Kuwabara H, Kumar A, et al: Persistent cognitive and dopamine transporter deficits in abstinent methamphetamine users. *Synapse* 62:91–100, 2008.
12. Hart CL, Gunderson EW, Perez A, et al: Acute physiological and behavioral effects on intranasal methamphetamine in humans. *Neuropsychopharmacology* 33(8):1847–1855, 2008.
13. Karch SB, Stephens BG, Ho CH: Methamphetamine-related deaths in San Francisco: demographic, pathologic and toxicologic profiles. *J Forensic Sci* 44(2):359–367, 1999.
14. Mendelson J, Uemura N, Harris D, et al: Human pharmacology of the methamphetamine stereoisomers. *Clin Pharmacol Ther* 80:403–420, 2006.
15. Lin LY, Di Stefano EW, Schmitz DA, et al: Oxidation of methamphetamine and methylenedioxymethamphetamine by CYP 2D6. *Drug Metab Dispos* 25(9):1059–1064, 1997.
16. Derlet RW, Rice P, Horowitz BZ, et al: Amphetamine toxicity: experience with 127 cases. *J Emerg Med* 7:157, 1989.
17. Kaye S, McKetin R, Duflou J, et al: Methamphetamine and cardiovascular pathology: a review of the evidence. *Addiction* 102:1204–1211, 2007.
18. Hong R, Matsuyama E, Nur K: Cardiomyopathy associated with the smoking of crystal methamphetamine. *JAMA* 265(9):1162–1154, 1991.
19. Shao-hua Y, Ren L, Yang T, et al: Myocardial lesions after long term administration of methamphetamine in rats. *Chin Med Sci J* 23(4):239–243, 2008.
20. Turnipseed SD, Richards JR, Kirk JD, et al: Frequency of acute coronary syndrome in patients presenting to the emergency department with chest pain after methamphetamine use. *J Emerg Med* 24(4):369–373, 2003.
21. Hamamoto DT, Rhodus NL: Methamphetamine abuse and dentistry. *Oral Dis* 15:27–35, 2009.
22. Kolecki P: Inadvertent methamphetamine poisoning in pediatric patients. *Pediatr Emerg Care* 14(6):385–387, 1998.
23. Buxton N, McConachie NS: Amphetamine abuse and intracranial haemorrhage. *J R Soc Med* 93:472–477, 2000.
24. Rothrock JF, Rubenstein R, Lyden PD: Ischemic stroke associated with methamphetamine inhalation. *Neurology* 38:589, 1988.
25. Mahoney JJ III, Kalechstein AD, De La Garza R II, et al: Presence and persistence of psychotic symptoms in cocaine versus methamphetamine-dependent participants. *Am J Addict* 17:83–98, 2008.
26. Kratofil PH, Baberg HT, Dimsdale JE: Self-mutilation and severe self-injurious behavior associated with amphetamine psychosis. *Gen Hosp Psychiatry* 18:117–120, 1996.
27. Rhee KJ, Albertson TE, Douglas JC: Choreoathetoid disorder associated with amphetamine-like drugs. *Am J Emerg Med* 6:131, 1988.
28. Lundh H, Tunving K: An extrapyramidal choreiform syndrome caused by amphetamine addiction. *J Neurol Neurosurg Psychiatry* 44:728–730, 1981.
29. Brannan TA, Soundararajan S, Houghton BL: Methamphetamine-associated shock with intestinal infarction. *MedGenMed* 6:6, 2004.
30. Liang, H, Wang X, Chen H, et al: Methamphetamine enhances HIV infection of macrophages. *Am J Pathol* 172(6):1467–1470, 2008.
31. McKinney CK, Postiglione KF, Herold DA: Benzocaine-adulterated cocaine in association with methemoglobinemia. *Clin Chem* 38(4):596–597, 1992.
32. Henry JA, Jeffreys KJ, Dawling S: Toxicity and deaths from 3,4-methylenedioxymethamphetamine ("ecstasy"). *Lancet* 340:384, 1992.
33. Brauer RB, Heidecke CD, Nathrath W, et al: Liver transplantation for the treatment of fulminant hepatic failure induced by the ingestion of ecstasy. *Transpl Int* 10:229–233, 1997.
34. Rusyniak DE, Tandy SL, Hekmatyar SK, et al: The role of mitochondrial uncoupling in 3,4-methylenedioxymethamphetamine-mediated skeletal muscle hyperthermia and rhabdomyolysis. *J Pharmacol Exp Ther* 313: 629–639, 2005.
35. Ling LH, Marchant C, Buckley NA, et al: Poisoning with the recreational drug paramethoxyamphetamine ("death"). *Med J Aust* 174(7):453–455, 2001.
36. Bowen JS, Davis GB, Kearney TE, et al: Diffuse vascular spasm associated with 4-bromo-2,5-dimethoxyamphetamine ingestion. *JAMA* 249:1477, 1983.
37. Weintraub D, Linder MW: Amphetamine positive toxicology screen secondary to bupropion. *Depress Anxiety* 12:53–54, 2000.
38. Ruha AM, Yarema MC: Pharmacologic treatment of acute pediatric methamphetamine toxicity. *Pediatr Emerg Care* 22(12):782–785, 2006.
39. Richards JR, Derlet RW, Duncan DR: Methamphetamine toxicity: treatment with a benzodiazepine versus a butyrophenone. *Eur J Emerg Med* 4:130–135, 1997.
40. Farmer JW, Chan SB: Whole bowel irrigation for contraband body packers. *J Clin Gastroenterol* 37(2):147–150. 2003.
41. Traub SJ, Hoffman RS, Nelson LS: Body packing–the internal concealment of illicit drugs. *N Engl J Med* 349:2519–2526, 2003.
42. Watson CJE, Thompson HJ, Johnston PS: Body-packing with amphetamines—an indication for surgery. *J R Soc Med* 84:311, 1991.
43. Van Dyke M, Erb N, Arbuckle S, et al: A 24 hour study to investigate persistent chemical exposures associated with clandestine methamphetamine laboratories. *J Occup Environ Hyg* 6:82–89, 2009.
44. Willers-Russo LJ: Three fatalities involving phosphine gas, produced as a result of methamphetamine manufacturing. *J Forensic Sci* 44(3):647–652, 1999.
45. Burgess JL, Barnhart S, Checkoway H: Investigating clandestine drug laboratories: adverse medical effects in law enforcement personnel. *Am J Ind Med* 30:488–494, 1996.

Chapter 101 ▪ Antiarrhythmic Agents

STEVEN B. BIRD

The therapeutic use, misuse, and intentional overdose of antiarrhythmic drugs are associated with severe morbidity and mortality [1]. The recognition, management, and prevention of antiarrhythmic toxicity require an understanding of the pharmacology of these drugs as they relate to cardiac electrophysiology. A general review of the mechanisms involved as well as the principles of management of poisoning is followed by a discussion of individual agents.

PHARMACOLOGY

Antiarrhythmic drugs are most commonly classified on the basis of their predominant physiologic effects and mechanism of action as originally proposed by Vaughan Williams [2] and Campbell [3] (Tables 101.1 and 101.2; Fig. 101.1).

The major effect of class I agents is blockade of the fast inward sodium current responsible for the rapid upstroke and conduction of the action potential [4] (see Fig. 101.1). This effect is also known as *local anesthetic* or *membrane stabilizing action*. Class I drugs depress automaticity, particularly in Purkinje fibers. Class I drugs comprise a large group of antiarrhythmic agents, many of which have diverse electrophysiologic properties; consequently, this class has been subdivided into classes IA, IB, and IC (see Table 101.2) [3].

The class II antiarrhythmic drugs are β-adrenergic antagonists; they inhibit the proarrhythmic effects of catecholamines, which shorten refractory periods and facilitate reentrant circuits. The slowly conducting, calcium channel–dependent action potentials of the normal sinoatrial (SA) and atrioventricular (AV) nodes (see Fig. 101.1) rely partially on sympathetic tone. Class II drugs depress conduction and automaticity through these specialized tissues, leading to bradycardia and AV block. Toxicity due to β-blockers is covered further in Chapter 106.

TABLE 101.1

Vaughan Williams Classification of Antiarrhythmic Actions

Class	Drugs	Actions
I	Quinidine Procainamide Disopyramide Moricizine Lidocaine Tocainide Mexiletine Flecainide Propafenone	Block fast sodium current (hence slow conduction)
II	β-blockers	Block effects of catecholamines
III	Amiodarone Sotalol Ibutilide Bretylium	Prolong action potential and, hence, refractoriness by blocking K^+ current
IV	Verapamil Diltiazem	Block cardiac calcium channel

Class III agents prolong the refractory period by increasing the cardiac action potential duration (APD), especially in phases 2 and 3 (see Fig. 101.1). This effect is produced by blockade of the major outward potassium-rectifying (repolarizing) current, of which amiodarone is the prototypic class III agent.

Class IV drugs (calcium antagonists or calcium channel blockers) antagonize the slow inward calcium current responsible for the slow upstroke and conduction of the action potentials of SA and AV nodal cells [4] (see Fig. 101.1). Verapamil, diltiazem, and nifedipine represent the three subclasses of calcium channel antagonists. Both verapamil and diltiazem have negative inotropic and chronotropic properties and are useful for slowing the ventricular response rate for patients with atrial fibrillation. During therapeutic dosing, calcium channel antagonists such as nifedipine have little effect on cardiac conduction or inotropic state and are, therefore, not used for their antiarrhythmic properties. Calcium channel blocker toxicity is discussed in Chapter 107.

Adenosine and digoxin are two drugs with antiarrhythmic effects that do not fall within the Vaughan Williams classification. Adenosine is an endogenous nucleoside that produces AV nodal conduction block and vasodilation via specific adenosine-sensitive receptors. The antiarrhythmic properties and toxicity of digoxin are discussed in Chapter 108.

The cellular electropharmacology of antiarrhythmic agents involves suppression of automaticity, decreased cardiac conduction, and refractory period prolongation. Automaticity, the spontaneous depolarization of pacemaker myocytes, occurs in the SA and AV nodes as well as in Purkinje fibers. In SA and AV nodal cells, the rate of firing depends on several different inward and outward currents; the combination of currents renders these cells relatively insensitive to depression by antiarrhythmic drugs [1,4]. In Purkinje fibers, however, automaticity occurs as an escape phenomenon that arises in the presence of AV block. Escape beats probably result from the action of a single inward sodium channel (the "pacemaker current") and are suppressed by therapeutic concentrations of most class I antiarrhythmic agents. Therefore, Purkinje fiber automaticity is more susceptible to depression by antiarrhythmic agents than is sinus node automaticity. Nonetheless, clinical suppression of the sinus node leading to asystole, particularly in the presence of the high vagal tone commonly seen in the early phases of acute myocardial infarction, is an uncommon but well-recognized complication of therapy with antiarrhythmic agents such as lidocaine.

Reentrant circuit arrhythmias depend on conduction rates around the circuit and the refractory periods of pathway components. If the conduction time falls below the refractory period of part of the circuit, the "excitable gap" disappears, the advancing wavefront meets only refractory tissue, and the arrhythmia terminates. An ideal antiarrhythmic agent would, therefore, accelerate conduction and prolong refractoriness within the substrate for reentry. Many antiarrhythmic agents prolong refractory periods in myocardium, but none accelerates conduction at therapeutic concentrations. Almost invariably, conduction tends to slow. This combination of decreasing conduction and refractory period prolongation can be either proarrhythmic or antiarrhythmic. However, clinicians cannot predict which outcome will occur for a given drug in a given patient. Some antiarrhythmic agents (in particular, class IB drugs and amiodarone [3]) show selectivity for depressing conduction of ischemic or otherwise abnormal myocardium by binding preferentially to the inactivated state of the sodium channel. A complete conduction block through an

TABLE 101.2

Subgroups of Class I Drugs

Class	Drugs	Effects on Action Potential	Summary of Clinical Effects
IA	Quinidine Procainamide Disopyramide Moricizine	Reduce rate of depolarization; prolong duration of action potential	Moderate slowing of cardiac conduction; prolongation of refractory periods
IB	Lidocaine Mexiletine Tocainide	Reduce rate of depolarization selectively in ischemic cells; shorten action potential duration	Selective depression of ischemic tissue; may shorten refractory periods
IC	Flecainide Propafenone	Marked depression of depolarization rate	Marked slowing of cardiac conduction; small increase in refractory periods

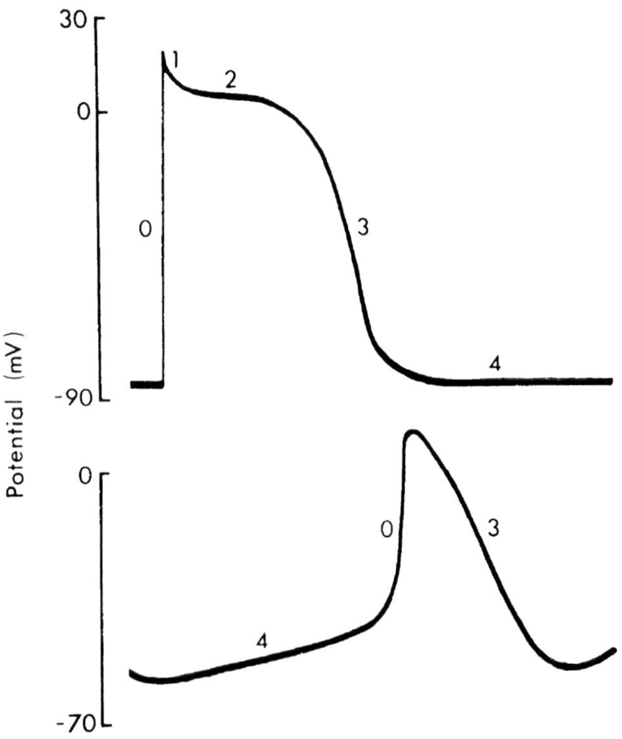

FIGURE 101.1 Typical cellular action potentials recorded from working myocardium (*upper trace*) and the atrioventricular node (*lower trace*). The nodal cell has an action potential of smaller amplitude, with a much slower rate of depolarization in phase 0. The nodal cell exhibits spontaneous diastolic (phase 4) depolarization ("pacemaker" activity). Rapid depolarization in phase 0 (atrial and ventricular cells and Purkinje fibers) is produced by a fast inward sodium current (depressed by class I drugs). A slower inward calcium current is also present but is the only inward current found in sinoatrial and atrioventricular nodal cells. This explains their slower rate of depolarization in phase 0 and their sensitivity to calcium channel blockers. Repolarization (phase 3) is produced by a number of outward potassium currents; the rapid component of the delayed rectifier potassium current is the most important. Blockade of this current by antiarrhythmic or other drugs prolongs repolarization and action potential duration (class III action).

ischemic segment of a reentrant circuit may be the mechanism of arrhythmia termination; this could occur without slowing conduction in healthy myocardium. Other drugs tend to show less selectivity and depress conduction in normal myocardium at therapeutic concentrations, probably explaining the greater propensity of class IC drugs to be proarrhythmic during both therapeutic use and overdose [3].

Although most antiarrhythmic agents prolong refractoriness, lidocaine, mexiletine, and tocainide tend to shorten it, particularly at low concentrations; this may explain some cases of drug-associated arrhythmogenesis of patients with reentrant tachycardias. Lengthening of refractoriness should be proarrhythmic, but if conduction is slowed simultaneously, the net effect on the reentrant circuit determines the outcome.

Antiarrhythmic drugs suppress most forms of automaticity known to cause tachyarrhythmias. The major exception to this rule is the form of triggered automaticity due to *early after-depolarizations* (EADs). EADs can be defined as a marked slowing of repolarization, visible on the action potential recording and due to reduction of the normal repolarizing outward potassium current. If voltage conditions are appropriate, prolonged depolarization may trigger a series of automatic action potentials. The upstrokes of these action potentials are due to inward current flow through the normal calcium channels that had been inactivated, had recovered from inactivation, and had found the membrane potential still within their activation range. The channels then reactivate and produce a secondary upstroke. Increased intracellular calcium concentrations activate calcium-sensitive potassium channels and accelerate repolarization. This process can occur as a single event or as an oscillatory series of action potentials, depending on the prevailing conditions of voltage and calcium levels [5].

The induction of EADs may be the basis of arrhythmias, including torsade de pointes associated with long QT syndromes [6]. According to this theory, the slowing of repolarization leads directly to the QT wave prolongation, often with associated prominent, bizarre TU waves. Any triggered activity, should it occur, results in ventricular tachyarrhythmias.

The class IA antiarrhythmic agents quinidine, disopyramide, and procainamide are all capable of producing EADs and torsade de pointes. This is also true of the class III drugs, such as amiodarone, sotalol, ibutilide, and dofetilide. The class IB agents, lidocaine, mexiletine, and tocainide, do not produce EADs and do not cause torsade de pointes. Class IC compounds infrequently cause significant slowing of repolarization and have not been shown to cause torsade de pointes. Of the class IV agents, only mibefradil has an effect on repolarization, which usually manifests as TU-wave changes. Experimental models suggest that this effect is not proarrhythmic; however, there has been a report of torsade due to QT prolongation from therapeutic dosing of mibefradil [7].

CLINICAL PRESENTATION

Toxicity common to therapeutic doses and overdoses of antiarrhythmic agents include depression of automaticity and cardiac conduction, which may be caused by a combination of direct electrophysiologic and secondary metabolic effects. Symptoms following acute overdose usually begin within 4 hours and can occur at any time during chronic therapy. Drug absorption may continue for many hours following the ingestion of large doses, sustained-release preparations, or agents with anticholinergic effects, resulting in delayed or progressive toxicity. Respiratory depression and hypotension produce acidosis and myocardial ischemia that further aggravate depressed conduction. Cardiac manifestations include QRS prolongation, QTc prolongation, sinus node dysfunction, bradycardia, AV block, ventricular arrhythmias, and poor ventricular function. These derangements can culminate in intractable arrhythmias, cardiogenic shock, or death. Manifestations of acute toxicity may also include dizziness, visual disturbances, psychosis, anticholinergic symptoms, hypoglycemia, hyperglycemia, and hypokalemia. Seizures may result from class I (particularly IB) toxicity. Procainamide and quinidine can cause hypotension if infused too rapidly.

Warning signs that indicate an increased risk of torsade include a QTc interval greater than 560 ms, previous history of torsade, bradycardia, increased frequency and complexity of ventricular premature beats, or a ventricular premature beat falling on the T wave [8].

The electrocardiogram (ECG) may provide a clue to the agent or class involved for cases where the drug ingested is not known. Class IB drugs usually have no effects on the QT interval; whereas class IA, IC, and III agents prolong it. With class IA agents, QT prolongation is due to slowing of both depolarization and repolarization. Hence, both the QRS duration and JT interval are increased. In contrast, QT prolongation primarily results from slowed depolarization with class IC agents, resulting in an increased QRS (but not JT) duration and from prolonged repolarization with class III agents, resulting in an increased JT (but not QRS) interval.

The differential diagnosis of bradyarrhythmias includes β-blocker, calcium channel blocker, cholinergic agent (carbamate and organophosphate insecticides), clonidine, cyclic antidepressant, and digitalis poisoning. Other agents that cause QRS and QT interval prolongation include antihistamines, antipsychotic agents, cyclic antidepressants, magnesium, and potassium. Ventricular tachyarrhythmias may occur with poisoning from sympathomimetics. Hypoglycemia, hypoxia, and metabolic disturbances should be considered in the differential diagnosis of patients with neurologic symptoms.

TABLE 101.3

Management of Life-Threatening Antiarrhythmic Drug Overdose

- Supportive care
  - Activated charcoal for acute (<1 h) oral ingestions
  - Correct acidosis, hypoxia
  - Benzodiazepines for seizure control
- Enhance drug elimination
  - Activated charcoal
  - Consider extracorporeal elimination if appropriate
- Hypotension
  - Fluid administration
  - Alkalinization (hypertonic $NaHCO_3$) for class I drugs
  - Inotropes, vasopressors
  - Consider pulmonary artery catheter for monitoring
  - Circulatory assist devices
- Impaired conduction
  - Temporary pacing for atrioventricular block or bradycardia
  - Alkalinization (hypertonic $NaHCO_3$) for class I drugs
- Ventricular arrhythmias
  - Torsade de pointes
    - Temporary pacing
    - $MgSO_4$
    - Isoproterenol
- Monomorphic ventricular tachycardia
  - Cardioversion, if causing hypotension
  - Hypertonic $NaHCO_3$ for class I drugs
  - Lidocaine, except for class IB drugs
  - Overdrive pacing
- PEA cardiac arrest
  - Intravenous lipid emulsion for bupivicaine (may consider for other lipophilic agents or in refractory cases). Loading dose of 1.5 mL/kg administered over 1 min, repeated 1–2 times every 3–5 min as needed. If hemodynamic improvement is noted, the loading dose should be followed by a continuous infusion at a rate of 0.25–0.5 mL/kg/min.

DIAGNOSTIC EVALUATION

Physical examination should focus on vital signs and respiratory, cardiovascular, and central nervous system (CNS) function. Frequent vital signs and continuous cardiac monitoring should be performed. Essential tests include an ECG and serum electrolytes, blood urea nitrogen, creatinine, and magnesium measurement; liver function tests and serum drug levels, if available, may also be helpful. A chest radiograph should be obtained as clinically indicated. Patients with hypotension and hypoxemia should have arterial blood gas and serum lactate measurements.

MANAGEMENT

The general features of antiarrhythmic drug overdose and their management are discussed below (Table 101.3). Care of the antiarrhythmic poisoned patient centers on general supportive and critical care principles. Unique aspects pertinent to individual drugs are discussed in later sections. All patients suspected of ingesting an overdose of an antiarrhythmic agent should receive oral activated charcoal. Patients with complications of therapeutic dosing may also benefit from oral activated charcoal to reduce absorption of a recently administered drug dose. The greatest amount of absorption to charcoal will occur when it is given within 1 to 2 hours of the ingestion. CNS and respiratory depression commonly require airway support by endotracheal intubation. Seizures are managed by benzodiazepine therapy. Phenytoin should never be used to treat seizures secondary to drug toxicity because of the risk of increased mortality.

Initial therapy for hypotension involves administration of intravenous fluids. Because poisoned patients are infrequently hypovolemic, fluid administration should be monitored closely. In general, if a response in blood pressure is not seen with 2 L of intravenous fluids, pressors such as norepinephrine should be administered. Early consideration should be given to providing a circulatory assist device for patients with cardiogenic shock. Intra-aortic balloon pump counterpulsation has been used successfully to treat patients with severe quinidine or disopyramide toxicity, and partial cardiac bypass has been used to maintain circulation during massive lidocaine or flecainide toxicity [9].

Decreased ventricular conduction, as measured by QRS prolongation during quinidine, procainamide, flecainide, and encainide toxicity, are often treated with sodium bicarbonate infusion [10,11]. In animal studies, hypertonic sodium bicarbonate reverses ventricular arrhythmias caused by flecainide toxicity [12] and reverses hypotension due to tricyclic antidepressants with class IA antiarrhythmic effects. Hypertonic sodium bicarbonate should be considered for the treatment of QRS widening greater than 100 ms or ventricular tachyarrhythmias in the setting of class IA or IC drug toxicity. Common practice is to administer intravenous boluses of sodium bicarbonate (50 mEq of 1 mEq per mL solution) as needed to increase and maintain blood pH between 7.45 and 7.55. As an alternative, a continuous infusion of 1,000 mL of 5% dextrose in water containing 2 to 3 ampoules of sodium bicarbonate and potassium chloride is an option. Bicarbonate should be administered for 12 to 24 hours and then gradually withdrawn while watching for QRS lengthening to recur. At present, there is no evidence that prophylactic alkalinization before QRS widening changes outcome. For the most severely poisoned patients, however, alkalinization may be ineffective, especially if there is persistent metabolic acidosis. In a series of patients with class I antiarrhythmic drug overdose requiring cardiopulmonary resuscitation, only 2 of 29 survived despite the use of hypertonic sodium bicarbonate [13].

Sodium bicarbonate appears to act by increasing the extracellular sodium concentration and reducing the drug-induced sodium channel blockade [14]. Hypertonic sodium chloride has proven effective for animals and, anecdotally, in humans, but sodium bicarbonate is generally preferable because increasing pH is equally or more important in some models [14] (see Chapter 97 for more detail).

The treatment of recalcitrant ventricular tachycardia typically consists of repeated cardioversions, cardiopulmonary resuscitation, vasopressor support, and mechanical ventilation. Treatment with other class IA and IC antiarrhythmic drugs is contraindicated, given the potential for further arrhythmia aggravation [15]. Lidocaine may be considered because it does not depress conduction, but it is often ineffective. Suppression of ventricular tachycardia and hemodynamic improvement has been anecdotally described with sodium bicarbonate [10,11]. Overdrive pacing may also be effective.

The treatment of torsade de pointes should include 1 to 2 g of a 25% solution of intravenous magnesium sulfate. Direct-current cardioversion is often effective in terminating torsade de pointes, but it frequently recurs. Increasing the ventricular rate to greater than 90 to 110 beats per minute by an infusion of isoproterenol or ventricular pacing may also be effective [16]. In one study, infusion of potassium chloride at 0.5 mEq per kg for 60 to 90 minutes normalized excessive quinidine-induced QT prolongation, but simply correcting hypokalemia did not suppress torsade de pointes [17]. Lidocaine is inconsistently effective [18]. Treatment with class IA or III antiarrhythmic drugs is contraindicated because further prolongation of repolarization and the QT interval may exacerbate torsade de pointes. Magnesium therapy should also be considered for patients at increased risk for this arrhythmia (see above); it has been found to prevent occurrence of torsade in a dog model (dose of 30 to 60 mg per kg) [19].

Although most antiarrhythmic drugs are weak bases, urine acidification is contraindicated because systemic acidosis may aggravate cardiotoxicity; treatment with hypertonic alkaline solution to reduce cardiotoxicity is likely to be of greater benefit. Hemodialysis is of limited benefit for antiarrhythmic toxicity because drug clearance is limited by protein binding and high lipid solubility [20]. Hemoperfusion using charcoal resin is more effective for removing drugs with high protein binding and high lipid solubility; however, this modality is rarely available. Hemoperfusion is of greatest value for disopyramide [21] or *N*-acetylprocainamide (NAPA) toxicity [22].

INDIVIDUAL AGENTS

Class IA Agents

Quinidine

Quinidine is administered orally as sulfate or gluconate. The usual dose of immediate-release quinidine sulfate is 200 to 400 mg, 4 times per day, with gluconate doses being approximately 30% higher. Bioavailability is approximately 70% for both forms; peak plasma levels are reached earlier for the sulfate (60 to 90 minutes) than for the gluconate. Quinidine is metabolized by CYP3A4 to 3-OH quinidine and quinidine-*N*-oxide; these metabolites have less electrophysiologic activity than do quinidine [23]. Details of pharmacokinetics are listed in Table 101.4.

Torsade de pointes is an adverse effect of therapeutic doses of quinidine (also known as *quinidine syncope*). Risk factors for this arrhythmia are recent initiation of quinidine therapy, concurrent digoxin therapy, female gender, structural heart disease, hypokalemia, and hypomagnesemia. Possible mechanisms include prolongation of the QTc interval and potentiation of EADs [23].

At therapeutic doses, sustained-release quinidine formulations produce therapeutic plasma concentrations for up to 8 hours for most patients. In overdose, however, saturation of enzymes that metabolize the drug may dramatically prolong serum concentrations. Consequently, serial serum drug monitoring is warranted (see Table 101.4), especially when potentially interactive agents, are coadministered. Agents that are CYP3A4 inhibitors, such as cimetidine, can increase quinidine serum concentration. Mild quinidine overdose presents as cinchonism (headache, tinnitus, deafness, diplopia, confusion), vertigo, visual disturbances (blurred vision, photophobia, scotomata, contracted visual fields, yellow vision), or delirium. Severe toxicity is characterized by CNS toxicity (lethargy, coma, respiratory depression, seizures), gastrointestinal tract toxicity (nausea, vomiting, diarrhea), and cardiovascular collapse [24]. Noncardiac side effects include nausea, cinchonism, thrombocytopenia, and drug-induced fever.

Initial therapy for acute quinidine overdose should include gastric decontamination with activated charcoal. Treatment of CNS toxicity is supportive, with intubation and ventilation for CNS depression and benzodiazepines for seizures. Deaths from quinidine overdose are usually secondary to arrhythmias or hypotension. When pacing is indicated for bradycardia, failure to capture is common in the face of drug-induced myocardial depression. QRS prolongation should be treated with bicarbonate infusion. Hypotension may result from vasodilation from β-adrenergic blockade, impaired contractility from sodium channel blockade, or arrhythmias. Vasodilation may be treated with fluid administration and β-acting vasopressors such as norepinephrine; large doses may be required. Refractory hypotension has been successfully treated with an intra-aortic balloon pump and partial circulatory bypass.

Procainamide

Procainamide is eliminated by hepatic metabolism and renal excretion [25]. The major metabolite is NAPA, which has potent class III and some class I antiarrhythmic activity [26]. In fast acetylators or in renal failure, as much as 40% of a dose of procainamide may be excreted as NAPA. Because the prevalence of the fast and slow acetylator phenotypes varies between ethnic groups, widely variable procainamide and NAPA concentrations may occur in specific populations. Blood concentrations of NAPA may exceed those of the parent drug, given its dependence on renal elimination.

The cardiovascular side effects of procainamide are very similar to those of quinidine except that the drug has no α-adrenergic antagonist activity. Acute procainamide toxicity is manifested primarily by hypotension, but QRS widening and ventricular arrhythmias may also occur [27]. Inappropriate drug dosing in renal insufficiency or before achieving steady-state concentrations is the most common cause of procainamide toxicity. Toxic levels of NAPA (>25 μg per mL) may begin to accumulate as a result of acute or chronic renal insufficiency, potentially leading to torsade. Approximately 40% of patients receiving long-term oral therapy with procainamide develop a syndrome resembling

TABLE 101.4

Dose and Pharmacokinetics of Class I and III Antiarrhythmic Agents

Drug	Usual daily dose	Therapeutic or usual plasma concentration (μg/mL)	Volume of distribution (L/kg)	Elimination half-life	% excreted unchanged in urine	% bound in plasma	Active metabolites	Methods of enhancing elimination
Class IA								
Quinidine	Depends on formulation (see text)	2–7	2.0–3.5	7 h	17–50[a]	80–90	3-OH quinidine	—
Procainamide	3–6 g	4–8 (NAPA, 7–15)	2 (NAPA, 1.4)	2.5–4.5 h (NAPA, 5–9 h)	40–60 (NAPA, 80)	10–20 (NAPA, 10)	NAPA	HD, HP
Disopyramide	300–600 mg	2–6	1.0–1.5	4–10 h	40–60	50–65	—	HD, HP
Moricizine	600–900 mg	0.1–3.0[b]	8–11	1.5–13.0 h	1	95	—	—
Class IB								
Lidocaine	1–3 μg/min	1.5–6.0	1.0–1.7	1.5–2.5 h[c]	<10	60–80	Monoethyl-glycinex-ylidide, glycine xylidide	?HP
Tocainide	1.2–2.4 g	3–10	1.5–3.2	11–20 h	40	10	—	HD, HP
Mexiletine	600–1,200 mg	0.5–2.0	5–7	6–17 h	8–15	50–70	—	—
Class IC								
Flecainide	100–300 mg	0.07–0.50	9	12–18 h[a,d]	70	50	—	—
Propafenone	400–800 mg	0.2–1.8	1.9–3.0	3.6 h (17 h)[e]	—	—	5-hydroxy-propafenone	—
Class III								
Amiodarone	100–400 mg	1.0–2.5[b]	70	40–49 d	<1	99	Desethyl-amiodarone	—
Sotalol	160–320 mg	0.6–3.2	2	12–15 h	>75	0	—	HD, HP

[a]Shorter with lower urine pH.
[b]Correlates poorly with therapeutic effect.
[c]Longer in patients with congestive heart failure.
[d]Dose dependent.
[e]Slow metabolizers at CYP2D6 locus.
HD, hemodialysis; HP, hemoperfusion; NAPA, *N*-acetylprocainamide.

systemic lupus erythematosus that usually resolves after drug withdrawal [28].

Signs and symptoms of acute procainamide overdose are similar to those of quinidine overdose. Patients with non–life-threatening procainamide toxicity (e.g., hypotension) and adequate renal function can be managed with supportive care. Seizure has been reported after a pediatric ingestion. Hypertonic sodium bicarbonate may be useful for QRS prolongation, monomorphic ventricular tachycardia, or hypotension. This therapy has minimal benefit in NAPA toxicity because this metabolite has primarily class III effects. Torsade de pointes should be treated as discussed above. Anecdotal reports have showed increased procainamide and NAPA clearance with hemodialysis or hemoperfusion; however, clinical significance is unclear [22,27].

Disopyramide

Disopyramide, unlike most other antiarrhythmic drugs, has protein binding that shows nonlinear, saturable characteristics [29]. This is clinically important because small increases in total plasma level within the therapeutic range (see Table 101.3) may mask larger rises in free (active) drug concentration. When administered intravenously, disopyramide produces hypotension less frequently than does quinidine or procainamide. Widening of the QRS complex, prolongation of the QT interval, and drug-induced ventricular tachyarrhythmias have all been reported as side effects [30]. There are numerous reports of either QTc prolongation, torsade, or monomorphic ventricular tachycardia from the interaction of disopyramide and macrolide antibiotics. Erythromycin, clarithromycin, and azithromycin have all been implicated; a possible mechanism is inhibition of hepatic CYP3A4.

Acute disopyramide overdose is similar to that of quinidine or procainamide, with QRS prolongation, severe refractory hypotension, and arrhythmias [31,32]. Hypoglycemia is a recognized adverse effect. Data regarding management are limited, but an approach similar to that for quinidine toxicity is appropriate. Hypotension refractory to intravenous fluids and vasopressors has been treated with an intra-aortic balloon pump. Because of its relatively small volume of distribution, disopyramide clearance is substantially increased by hemoperfusion [21].

Class IB Agents

Lidocaine (and Other Local Anesthetics)

Amide-type local anesthetics (e.g., articaine, bupivacaine, etidocaine, lidocaine, mepivacaine, prilocaine, ropivacaine) are extensively metabolized by hepatic dealkylation, hydrolysis, ring hydroxylation, and conjugation. Ester-type agents are metabolized by hepatic and plasma esterases. Derivatives of para-aminobenzoic acid (e.g., benzocaine, procaine, tetracaine) are predominantly hydrolyzed by plasma pseudocholinesterase, whereas other esters (e.g., cocaine, dyclonine, proparacaine) are predominantly metabolized in the liver [33]. Allergic cross-reactivity occurs within the amide and ester groups but not between them.

Extensive first-pass metabolism prevents effective oral therapy with lidocaine and local anesthetics, but toxicity can occur after ingestion [33]. The maintenance infusion rate of lidocaine must be reduced for patients with cardiac failure or hepatic dysfunction and among the elderly. Plasma concentrations should be monitored for infusions lasting longer than 24 hours. Lidocaine has two active metabolites, monoethylglycinexylidide (MEGX) and glycine xylidide (GX). Although these metabolites have short elimination half-lives of 2 hours and 1 hour, respectively, they may contribute significantly to toxicity, which can occur several hours after an infusion is started [33]. Most lidocaine toxicity is caused by errors of dosing and administration [34]. Life-threatening toxicity and death have occurred after inadvertent overdose, surgical procedures such as liposuction, and parenteral, mucosal, and topical anesthesia [35]. The safety of tumescent liposuction, in which large volumes of lidocaine solutions are infused subcutaneously, has been called into question following several reported deaths [36].

All local anesthetics have toxicity similar to lidocaine, with neurologic signs and symptoms usually preceding cardiac manifestations, except in massive acute overdose [37]. Neurologic symptoms, the most significant of which is seizures, include auditory disturbances, visual disturbances, paresthesias, and ataxia. Lidocaine has a bimodal concentration-dependent effect on seizures; lidocaine suppresses seizures at concentrations between 0.5 to 5 μg per mL but increases the risk at levels above 8 to 9 μg per mL. The relative contribution to epileptogenicity of the parent compound compared with the metabolites MEGX and GX is still unclear [38]. Adverse cardiac effects from lidocaine administration are unusual in the absence of severe underlying conduction-system disease, acute myocardial ischemia, or massive overdose. Persons with third-degree heart block requiring ventricular arrhythmia suppression should have a prophylactic pacemaker inserted before lidocaine administration. However, lidocaine administration to asymptomatic patients with bundle-branch block or intraventricular conduction disease carries a low risk [39].

Acute massive overdose of lidocaine is characterized by seizures, coma, respiratory arrest, and cardiovascular collapse [37,40]. Hypotension is due to myocardial depression [41]. Lidocaine has little or no effect on the QT interval; however, QRS prolongation, AV block, and depressed automaticity with bradycardia or asystole can occur. Data regarding management are anecdotal. Seizures should be managed using intravenous diazepam; phenytoin should be avoided. Bradyarrhythmias may respond to isoproterenol infusion or cardiac pacing. Hypotension and shock respond to fluid administration and vasopressors such as dopamine. If QRS prolongation is present, hypertonic sodium bicarbonate may be useful. Intra-aortic balloon pump and cardiopulmonary bypass have been used successfully in patients with circulatory collapse.

Amide-type local anesthetics can also induce methemoglobinemia [33,42]. This effect has been described after percutaneous absorption of benzocaine-containing formulations, during use of prilocaine as an epidural anesthetic agent, and due to prilocaine found in eutectic mixture of local anesthetics (EMLA) cream. Amide agents are hydrolyzed to an amino group that exerts an oxidizing stress in susceptible individuals—such as those with G-6-PD deficiency—to produce methemoglobinemia. In some cases, patients may also exhibit red blood cell hemolysis. Methemoglobinemia is treated with methylene blue (see Chapter 125).

Bupivicaine intoxication can lead to PEA cardiac arrest that is not responsive to standard ACLS protocols. This is a dreaded complication of regional anesthesia after inadvertent intravenous injection of bupivicaine. Intravenous lipid emulsion (Intralipid) is rapidly becoming accepted as standard treatment for bupivicaine-induced cardiac arrest. Even though no human trials exist, there is excellent animal evidence and several human case reports [43]. The mechanism is still unclear, but effects are likely from partitioning of bupivicaine away from cardiac receptors and into an intravenous lipid phase. Therefore, intralipid may be an effective therapy for other lipophilic anesthetic agents. The initial loading dose is 1.5 mL per kg (typically 100 mL in an average adult) administered over 1 minute, which can be repeated 1 to 2 times every 3 to 5 minutes. If hemodynamic improvement is noted, the loading dose should be followed by a continuous infusion at a rate of 0.25 to 0.5 mL/kg/min [44].

Tocainide

Adverse effects are common during tocainide therapy, with up to 50% of patients requiring dosage adjustments or discontinuation [45]. The most common side effects are nausea, vomiting, and anorexia, and neurologic effects such as dizziness, paresthesias, tremor, ataxia, and confusion. Tremor suggests that the maximum tolerable dose of tocainide has been reached. Serious toxicity resulting from pulmonary fibrosis in up to 0.1% and agranulocytosis and leukopenia in 0.2% of patients has been reported [46]. Monitoring for clinical or laboratory signs of agranulocytosis has been recommended, particularly during the first 12 weeks of therapy.

Massive tocainide overdose causes effects similar to those of lidocaine overdose: loss of consciousness, seizures, high-degree AV block, asystole, and ventricular fibrillation [45,47]. Treatment considerations are also similar. Because 40% of tocainide elimination is renal, urine acidification theoretically increases tocainide excretion, but is not recommended because of enhanced systemic toxicity.

Mexiletine

Mexiletine is structurally similar to lidocaine and undergoes extensive metabolism in the liver to largely inactive compounds [48,49]. Hepatic impairment can significantly prolong the elimination half-life to 25 hours or longer. Patients with chronic liver disease, such as hepatic cirrhosis, undergo a marked reduction in the hepatic metabolism of mexiletine [50].

Mexiletine is generally well tolerated, with little effect on hemodynamics, even in patients with congestive heart failure [51]. Mexiletine shares much of the side-effect profile of lidocaine, including cross-reactivity in allergic individuals. Dizziness, ataxia, and tremor are relatively common. Overdose effects resemble those of lidocaine. Heart block or asystole accompanied by hypotension occur with massive overdose. Seizures have been reported to occur in the absence of cardiovascular abnormalities, and the prolonged duration of seizures compared with lidocaine overdose may be due to mexiletine's longer elimination half-life of 5.5 to 12 hours. A urine drug immunoassay was reported as positive for amphetamines in the setting of a mexiletine overdose, likely from cross-reactivity due to structural similarity of these compounds [52].

Class IC Agents

Flecainide

Flecainide is very well absorbed orally, with negligible hepatic first-pass effect. Flecainide displays polymorphic drug metabolism because it is metabolized via CYP2D6 to active metabolites. This phenomenon effectively results in two distinct populations of patients having very different clearance rates. The average half-life is between 8 and 10 hours, with substantial individual variability. Inhibitors of the CYP2D6 pathway, such as INH, quinidine, selective serotonin-uptake inhibitors, and other agents metabolized by this pathway, may decrease or increase the clearance of flecainide when added to or deleted from therapy. Amiodarone can double the serum concentration of flecainide when the two drugs are concomitantly administered; the flecainide dose should be reduced by 50% when these drugs are coadministered. Serum concentrations can be followed but are rarely used. The proposed therapeutic range is 200 to 1,000 ng per mL.

Flecainide is approved for the management of paroxysmal atrial fibrillation or flutter associated with disabling symptoms, but there are many restrictions owing to its adverse effects. Flecainide has a very narrow therapeutic index and can be toxic even at therapeutic concentrations [53]. In the Cardiac Arrhythmia Suppression Trial (CAST) [54], postinfarction patients being treated for ventricular arrhythmias demonstrated an increased mortality relative to patients treated with placebo. Furthermore, flecainide possesses considerable negative inotropic effects that limit its usefulness in the setting of congestive heart failure. Other dose-related side effects occur, including CNS toxicity such as blurred vision, dizziness, headache, nausea, and paresthesias. Flecainide also increases the ventricular pacing threshold.

Flecainide is highly toxic in overdose; in one series, the mortality rate was 10% [13]. Overdose is characterized by QRS prolongation with a normal JT interval, hypotension, coma, or seizures [13]. Serious cardiac effects that can occur include severe bradycardia, high-grade conduction blocks, and ventricular arrhythmias. Cardiac arrest is not uncommon after overdose; survival after full arrest is rare [53]. Data regarding management are mostly anecdotal. In studies of rats, hypertonic sodium bicarbonate, 3 to 6 mEq per kg, reduced flecainide-induced QRS prolongation [55], and for dogs this treatment largely abolished ventricular tachycardia [12]. For overdose patients, both hypertonic sodium bicarbonate and sodium lactate have been reported to be effective [56]. Hypertonic sodium bicarbonate or sodium lactate should be considered for patients with evidence of disturbed ventricular conduction. Cardiopulmonary bypass and extracorporeal membrane oxygenation (ECMO) have been used to support perfusion until spontaneous perfusion has returned [9,57]. In one report, a patient who developed refractory ventricular fibrillation because of a flecainide overdose was successfully resuscitated after a 300-mg amiodarone bolus was given [53].

Propafenone

Propafenone is used for selected patients with atrial fibrillation and for refractory ventricular tachycardia and fibrillation. Like flecainide, propafenone undergoes significant first-pass hepatic metabolism via the CYP2D6 isoenzyme pathway. Bioavailability ranges from 5% to 50%, depending on the patient's phenotype; agents that inhibit CYP2D6 lower its clearance rate. Administering propafenone with food may significantly increase bioavailability among extensive metabolizers by diminishing first-pass drug extraction [58].

Propafenone has other drug interactions as well. Propafenone administration may increase digoxin concentrations between 35% and 85% because of impairment of nonrenal digoxin clearance. Quinidine is a specific and potent inhibitor of CYP2D6 and can significantly increase propafenone concentration [59]. Coadministration of propafenone with warfarin may result in a 25% increase in prothrombin time from unknown mechanisms. Similar to flecainide, propafenone has a narrow therapeutic index.

Propafenone overdose is similar to that of flecainide; toxicity includes QRS prolongation, hypotension, bradycardia, coma, and seizures [13,60]. Seizures appear to be more common with propafenone overdose than with flecainide overdose. PR interval prolongation is a characteristic finding of propafenone toxicity [61]. Hypertonic sodium bicarbonate has been beneficial for QRS prolongations and aberrant ventricular conduction [62]. Benzodiazepines should be used for seizures; phenytoin should be avoided [63]. Management of cardiovascular toxicity is similar to that of flecainide overdose. Transvenous cardiac pacing was successful in a case with severe bradycardia due to a high-grade conduction block [61].

Class III Agents

Amiodarone

Amiodarone was first used as a vascular smooth-muscle relaxant. In addition to its class III activity (prolonging the cardiac APD), amiodarone possesses properties common to all Vaughan Williams classifications. These include calcium channel–smooth-muscle relaxant (class IV), noncompetitive antiadrenergic (class II), and some sodium channel–blocking (class I) activity.

Amiodarone is generally considered the most effective antiarrhythmic agent for treatment and prophylaxis of most types of arrhythmia [64]. Its clinical use, however, is complicated by unusual pharmacokinetics (see Table 101.4) and prevalent side effects [65]. After oral administration, amiodarone widely distributes into body tissues where drug concentration generally exceeds that of the plasma. It is highly lipophilic, highly bound to plasma proteins, and has an extremely long (average, 53 days) elimination half-life [66]. Metabolism occurs in the liver and possibly in the gastrointestinal tract. The major metabolite, desethylamiodarone, accumulates in plasma and tissues and has electrophysiologic properties that are similar to the parent compound [67].

Many side effects are dose dependent, but therapeutic drug monitoring is of little benefit, except to determine compliance. Evidence suggests a limited correlation between drug level and antiarrhythmic effects [68], and serious noncardiac toxicity seems to be more likely at levels above 2.5 μg per mL [69].

Pulmonary fibrosis is an important and potentially life-threatening side effect of long-term therapy [70]. Pulmonary toxicity is somewhat dose dependant; its prevalence ranges from 5% to 15% in patients who take at least 500 mg per day, but is 0.1% to 0.5% when the dose is less than 200 mg per day [71]. Common presenting features include dyspnea, nonproductive cough, fever, and general malaise. A diffuse interstitial pattern on the chest film, similar to congestive heart failure, is the most typical radiographic finding. Symptoms usually resolve with withdrawal of amiodarone therapy. Corticosteroids may improve prognosis and prevent relapse [71].

Amiodarone generally does not produce congestive heart failure, even in patients with poor ventricular function, because its vasodilator properties may offset negative inotropic effects. Sinus bradycardia is common during therapy, and symptomatic sinus pauses or sinus arrest can occur in 2% to 4% of patients. AV block may occur in patients with underlying conduction-system disease. Torsade de pointes has been reported, but is much less likely than with other class III agents.

Amiodarone is iodinated and interferes with conversion of thyroxine to triiodothyronine, causing significant elevations of thyroxine and slight reductions in triiodothyronine concentrations [72]. Most patients are typically euthyroid, with normal thyroid-stimulating hormone levels. Peripheral neuropathy, tremor, and nervousness develop initially in up to 30% of patients, but these symptoms often improve over time. Asymptomatic corneal microdeposits are present among almost all patients on long-term therapy. Dermatologic effects include increased photosensitivity and blue-gray skin discoloration.

Asymptomatic elevation of hepatic transaminases are relatively common with long-term amiodarone therapy; the reported incidence is 24% to 26%. Transaminases can reach up to 3 times the normal level and resolve with or without discontinuation of therapy [73]. Acute hepatitis following intravenous loading of amiodarone is much less common but not infrequently described in the literature [73]. Transaminitis can be severe and rarely lead to fatality. Postulated mechanisms include a polysorbate 80 additive used in the intravenous preparation, immunologically mediated injury, or a direct hepatotoxic effect [74].

Acute amiodarone overdoses generally tend to follow a benign course. There are several reports of ingestions developing self-limited episodes of ventricular tachycardia, QT prolongation, or mild bradycardia [75]. No CNS depression or seizures have been reported. Cholestyramine modestly reduces the elimination half-life of amiodarone from 44 to 28 days, perhaps by interrupting enterohepatic recirculation [76]. There is likely a role for multidose activated charcoal, even up to 12 hours after the ingestion, because amiodarone has delayed an erratic enteral absorption [77].

Sotalol

Sotalol is a β-adrenergic antagonist with class III activity. It is used for the prophylaxis and treatment of AV reentrant and ventricular tachycardias. It has excellent oral bioavailability and is mostly renally excreted unchanged. Overdoses manifest the pharmacologic properties of sotalol; β-adrenergic antagonism causes bradycardia, hypotension, low cardiac output, and CNS depression, whereas the class III activity causes QT prolongation, ventricular ectopy, and arrhythmias, especially torsade de pointes. Reported cases of ventricular arrhythmias due to sotalol overdose are typically associated with bradycardia [77]. Management should include treatment of the β-blocker toxicity (see Chapter 106 for discussion) and control of QT prolongation and torsade de pointes with agents such as magnesium or isoproterenol (see earlier discussion). There are reports of lidocaine suppressing torsade from sotalol overdose [77,78].

Ibutilide and Dofetilide

Ibutilide and dofetilide, the first "pure" action potential–prolonging agents, are approved for termination of atrial fibrillation and flutter [79]. Both drugs are structurally similar to sotalol but have no β-blockade effect. They prolong APD by a dual mode of action, initially blocking the rapid component of the delayed rectifier potassium current and enhancing the noninactivating component of the inward sodium current that flows during the plateau (phase 2) of the action potential. The net effect is to increase atrial and ventricular refractory period of APD. Although very little information is available about overdose toxicity, development of torsade de pointes is the major concern. With therapeutic doses, the incidence of this arrhythmia ranged from 3.6% to 12.5% in clinical trials. Most episodes were self-limited, but some were sustained and required cardioversion. Nonsustained monomorphic ventricular tachycardia may also be provoked by ibutilide [80].

Adenosine

Adenosine is an endogenous purine nucleoside normally present in all cells of the human body. Intravenous adenosine, administered as a rapid infusion, is used for termination of supraventricular arrhythmias. An increased heart rate as compensation for peripheral vasodilation has been reported among patients with atrial fibrillation and flutter or if an atrial impulse is conducted via an accessory pathway [81]. Adenosine may also induce atrial fibrillation as a result of the decrease of atrial APD. It should be used with caution among patients with asthma because it can provoke bronchospasm. Short periods (longer than 6 seconds) of asystole are commonly seen after termination of supraventricular arrhythmias.

Therapeutic and toxic doses of adenosine induce intense vasodilation, flushing, and a feeling of pressure or pain in the chest that patients often describe as extremely unpleasant. The duration of these effects is extremely short (measured in seconds) with bolus therapy, but can be prolonged among patients receiving continuous infusions during radionuclide studies or those patients taking dipyridamole [82].

ACKNOWLEDGMENT

The contributions of Dr. Michael Ganetsky on a previous edition of this chapter are appreciated and acknowledged.

References

1. Roden DM, George AL: The cardiac ion channels: relevance to management of arrhythmias. *Annu Rev Med* 47:135–148, 1996.
2. Vaughn Williams E: A classification of antiarrhythmic actions reassessed after a decade of new drugs. *J Clin Pharmacol* 24:129–147, 1984.
3. Campbell TJ: Subclassification of class I antiarrhythmic drugs: enhanced relevance after CAST. *Cardiovasc Drugs Ther* 6(5):519–528, 1992.
4. Katz AM: Cardiac ion channels. *N Engl J Med* 328(17):1244–1251, 1993.
5. January CT, Riddle JM: Early after depolarizations: mechanism of induction and block. A role for L-type Ca2+ current. *Circ Res* 64(5):977–990, 1989.
6. Roden DM, Hoffman BF: Action potential prolongation and induction of abnormal automaticity by low quinidine concentrations in canine Purkinje fibers. Relationship to potassium and cycle length. *Circ Res* 56(6):857–867, 1985.
7. Glaser S, Steinbach M, Opitz C, et al: Torsades de pointes caused by Mibefradil. *Eur J Heart Fail* 3(5):627–630, 2001.
8. Keren A, Tzivoni D: Torsades de pointes: prevention and therapy. *Cardiovasc Drugs Ther* 5(2):509–513, 1991.
9. Yasui RK, Culclasure TF, Kaufman D, et al: Flecainide overdose: is cardiopulmonary support the treatment? *Ann Emerg Med* 29(5):680–682, 1997.
10. Winkelmann BR, Leinberger H: Life-threatening flecainide toxicity. A pharmacodynamic approach. *Ann Intern Med* 106(6):807–814, 1987.
11. Gardner ML, Brett-Smith H, Batsford WP: Treatment of encainide proarrhythmia with hypertonic saline. *Pacing Clin Electrophysiol* 13(10):1232–1235, 1990.
12. Salerno DM, Murakami MM, Johnston RB, et al: Reversal of flecainide-induced ventricular arrhythmia by hypertonic sodium bicarbonate in dogs. *Am J Emerg Med* 13(3):285–293, 1995.
13. Koppel C, Oberdisse U, Heinemeyer G: Clinical course and outcome in class IC antiarrhythmic overdose. *J Toxicol Clin Toxicol* 28(4):433–444, 1990.
14. Sasyniuk BI, Jhamandas V: Mechanism of reversal of toxic effects of amitriptyline on cardiac Purkinje fibers by sodium bicarbonate. *J Pharmacol Exp Ther* 231(2):387–394, 1984.
15. Yang T, Roden DM: Extracellular potassium modulation of drug block of IKr. Implications for torsade de pointes and reverse use-dependence. *Circulation* 93(3):407–411, 1996.
16. Kay GN, Plumb VJ, Arciniegas JG, et al: Torsade de pointes: the long-short initiating sequence and other clinical features: observations in 32 patients. *J Am Coll Cardiol* 2(5):806–817, 1983.
17. Choy AM, Lang CC, Chomsky DM, et al: Normalization of acquired QT prolongation in humans by intravenous potassium. *Circulation* 96(7):2149–2154, 1997.
18. Stratmann HG, Kennedy HL: Torsades de pointes associated with drugs and toxins: recognition and management. *Am Heart J* 113(6):1470–1482, 1987.
19. Yamamoto H, Bando S, Nishikado A, et al: Efficacy of isoproterenol, magnesium sulfate and verapamil for torsade de pointes [in Japanese]. *Kokyu To Junkan* 39(3):261–265, 1991.
20. Singh SN, Lazin A, Cohen A, et al: Sotalol-induced torsades de pointes successfully treated with hemodialysis after failure of conventional therapy. *Am Heart J* 121(2 Pt 1):601–602, 1991.
21. Gosselin B, Mathieu D, Chopin C, et al: Acute intoxication with diisopyramide: clinical and experimental study by hemoperfusion an Amberlite XAD 4 resin. *Clin Toxicol* 17(3):439–449, 1980.
22. Braden GL, Fitzgibbons JP, Germain MJ, et al: Hemoperfusion for treatment of N-acetylprocainamide intoxication. *Ann Intern Med* 105(1):64–65, 1986.
23. Grace AA, Camm AJ: Quinidine. *N Engl J Med* 338(1):35–45, 1998.
24. Kerr F, Kenoyer G, Bilitch M: Quinidine overdose. Neurological and cardiovascular toxicity in a normal person. *Br Heart J* 33(4):629–631, 1971.
25. Giardina EG, Fenster PE, Bigger JT Jr, et al: Efficacy, plasma concentrations and adverse effects of a new sustained release procainamide preparation. *Am J Cardiol* 46(5):855–862, 1980.
26. Roden DM, Reele SB, Higgins SB, et al: Antiarrhythmic efficacy, pharmacokinetics and safety of N-acetylprocainamide in human subjects: comparison with procainamide. *Am J Cardiol* 46(3):463–468, 1980.
27. Raja R, Kramer M, Alvis R, et al: Resin hemoperfusion for severe N-acetylprocainamide toxicity in patients with renal failure. *Trans Am Soc Artif Intern Organs* 30:18–20, 1984.
28. Hoffman BF, Rosen MR, Wit AL: Electrophysiology and pharmacology of cardiac arrhythmias. VII. Cardiac effects of quinidine and procaine amide. A. *Am Heart J* 89(6):804–808, 1975.
29. Meffin PJ, Robert EW, Winkle RA, et al: Role of concentration-dependent plasma protein binding in disopyramide disposition. *J Pharmacokinet Biopharm* 7(1):29–46, 1979.
30. Fechter P, Ha HR, Follath F, et al: The antiarrhythmic effects of controlled release disopyramide phosphate and long acting propranolol in patients with ventricular arrhythmias. *Eur J Clin Pharmacol* 25(6):729–734, 1983.
31. Podrid PJ, Schoeneberger A, Lown B: Congestive heart failure caused by oral disopyramide. *N Engl J Med* 302(11):614–617, 1980.

32. Kotter V, Linderer T, Schroder R: Effects of disopyramide on systemic and coronary hemodynamics and myocardial metabolism in patients with coronary artery disease: comparison with lidocaine. *Am J Cardiol* 46(3):469–475, 1980.
33. Blumer J, Strong JM, Atkinson AJ Jr: The convulsant potency of lidocaine and its N-dealkylated metabolites. *J Pharmacol Exp Ther* 186(1):31–36, 1973.
34. Davison R, Parker M, Atkinson AJ: Excessive serum lidocaine levels during maintenance infusions: mechanisms and prevention. *Am Heart J* 104(2 Pt 1):203–208, 1982.
35. Brosh-Nissimov T, Ingbir M, Weintal I, et al: Central nervous system toxicity following topical skin application of lidocaine. *Eur J Clin Pharmacol* 60(9):683–684, 2004.
36. Rao RB, Ely SF, Hoffman RS: Deaths related to liposuction. *N Engl J Med* 340(19):1471–1475, 1999.
37. Denaro CP, Benowitz NL: Poisoning due to class 1B antiarrhythmic drugs. Lignocaine, mexiletine and tocainide. *Med Toxicol Adverse Drug Exp* 4(6):412–428, 1989.
38. DeToledo JC: Lidocaine and seizures. *Ther Drug Monit* 22(3):320–322, 2000.
39. Gupta PK, Lichstein E, Chadda KD: Lidocaine-induced heart block in patients with bundle branch block. *Am J Cardiol* 33(4):487–492, 1974.
40. Hess GP, Walson PD: Seizures secondary to oral viscous lidocaine. *Ann Emerg Med* 17(7):725–727, 1988.
41. Groban L, Deal DD, Vernon JC, et al: Cardiac resuscitation after incremental overdosage with lidocaine, bupivacaine, levobupivacaine, and ropivacaine in anesthetized dogs. *Anesth Analg* 92(1):37–43, 2001.
42. Haselbarth V, Doevendans JE, Wolf M: Kinetics and bioavailability of mexiletine in healthy subjects. *Clin Pharmacol Ther* 29(6):729–736, 1981.
43. Ludot H, Tharin JY, Belouadah M, et al: Successful resuscitation after ropivacaine and lidocaine-induced ventricular arrhythmia following posterior lumbar plexus block in a child. *Anesth Analg* 106(5):1572–1574, 2008, table of contents.
44. Weinberg G: Lipid rescue resuscitation from local anesthetic cardiac toxicity. *Toxicol Rev* 25(3):139–145, 2006.
45. Roden DM, Woosley RL: Drug therapy. Flecainide. *N Engl J Med* 315(1):36–41, 1986.
46. Volosin KJ, Greenspon AJ: Tocainide: a new drug for ventricular arrhythmias. *Am Fam Physician* 33(1):233–235, 1986.
47. Cohen A: Accidental overdose of tocainide successfully treated. *Angiology* 38(8):614, 1987.
48. Pringle T, Fox J, McNeill JA, et al: Dose independent pharmacokinetics of mexiletine in healthy volunteers. *Br J Clin Pharmacol* 21(3):319–321, 1986.
49. Upward JW, Holt DW, Jackson G: A study to compare the efficacy, plasma concentration profile and tolerability of conventional mexiletine and slow-release mexiletine. *Eur Heart J* 5(3):247–252, 1984.
50. Wang T, Wuellner D, Woosley RL, et al: Pharmacokinetics and nondialyzability of mexiletine in renal failure. *Clin Pharmacol Ther* 37(6):649–653, 1985.
51. Shanks RG: Hemodynamic effects of mexiletine. *Am Heart J* 107(5 Pt 2):1065–1071, 1984.
52. Kozer E, Verjee Z, Koren G: Misdiagnosis of a mexiletine overdose because of a nonspecific result of urinary toxicologic screening. *N Engl J Med* 343(26):1971, 1972, 2000.
53. Siegers A, Board PN: Amiodarone used in successful resuscitation after near-fatal flecainide overdose. *Resuscitation* 53(1):105–108, 2002.
54. Echt DS, Liebson PR, Mitchell LB, et al: Mortality and morbidity in patients receiving encainide, flecainide, or placebo. The Cardiac Arrhythmia Suppression Trial. *N Engl J Med* 324(12):781–788, 1991.
55. Keyler DE, Pentel PR: Hypertonic sodium bicarbonate partially reverses QRS prolongation due to flecainide in rats. *Life Sci* 45(17):1575–1580, 1989.
56. Hudson CJ, Whitner TE, Rinaldi MJ, et al: Brugada electrocardiographic pattern elicited by inadvertent flecainide overdose. *Pacing Clin Electrophysiol* 27(9):1311–1313, 2004.
57. Auzinger GM, Scheinkestel CD: Successful extracorporeal life support in a case of severe flecainide intoxication. *Crit Care Med* 29(4):887–890, 2001.
58. Straka RJ, Hansen SR, Walker PF: Comparison of the prevalence of the poor metabolizer phenotype for CYP2D6 between 203 Hmong subjects and 280 white subjects residing in Minnesota. *Clin Pharmacol Ther* 58(1):29–34, 1995.
59. Funck-Brentano C, Kroemer HK, Pavlou H, et al: Genetically-determined interaction between propafenone and low dose quinidine: role of active metabolites in modulating net drug effect. *Br J Clin Pharmacol* 27(4):435–444, 1989.
60. Buss J, Neuss H, Bilgin Y, et al: Malignant ventricular tachyarrhythmias in association with propafenone treatment. *Eur Heart J* 6(5):424–428, 1985.
61. Eray O, Fowler J: Severe propafenone poisoning responded to temporary internal pacemaker. *Vet Hum Toxicol* 42(5):289, 2000.
62. Molia AC, Tholon J-P, Lamiable DL, et al: Unintentional pediatric overdose of propafenone. *Ann Pharmacother* 37(7–8):1147, 1148, 2003.
63. Ellison DW, Pentel PR: Clinical features and consequences of seizures due to cyclic antidepressant overdose. *Am J Emerg Med* 7(1):5–10, 1989.
64. Salerno DM, Gillingham KJ, Berry DA, et al: A comparison of antiarrhythmic drugs for the suppression of ventricular ectopic depolarizations: a meta-analysis. *Am Heart J* 120(2):340–353, 1990.
65. Bauman JL, Berk SI, Hariman RJ, et al: Amiodarone for sustained ventricular tachycardia: efficacy, safety, and factors influencing long-term outcome. *Am Heart J* 114(6):1436–1444, 1987.
66. Holt DW, Tucker GT, Jackson PR, et al: Amiodarone pharmacokinetics. *Am Heart J* 106(4 Pt 2):840–847, 1983.
67. Barbieri E, Conti F, Zampieri P, et al: Amiodarone and desethylamiodarone distribution in the atrium and adipose tissue of patients undergoing short- and long-term treatment with amiodarone. *J Am Coll Cardiol* 8(1):210–213, 1986.
68. Mitchell LB, Wyse DG, Gillis AM, et al: Electropharmacology of amiodarone therapy initiation. Time courses of onset of electrophysiologic and antiarrhythmic effects. *Circulation* 80(1):34–42, 1989.
69. Rotmensch HH, Belhassen B, Swanson BN, et al: Steady-state serum amiodarone concentrations: relationships with antiarrhythmic efficacy and toxicity. *Ann Intern Med* 101(4):462–469, 1984.
70. Magro SA, Lawrence EC, Wheeler SH, et al: Amiodarone pulmonary toxicity: prospective evaluation of serial pulmonary function tests. *J Am Coll Cardiol* 12(3):781–788, 1988.
71. Camus P, Bonniaud P, Fanton A, et al: Drug-induced and iatrogenic infiltrative lung disease. *Clin Chest Med* 25(3):479–519, 2004.
72. Nademanee K, Singh BN, Callahan B, et al: Amiodarone, thyroid hormone indexes, and altered thyroid function: long-term serial effects in patients with cardiac arrhythmias. *Am J Cardiol* 58(10):981–986, 1986.
73. Ratz Bravo AE, Drewe J, Schlienger RG, et al: Hepatotoxicity during rapid intravenous loading with amiodarone: description of three cases and review of the literature. *Crit Care Med* 33(1):128–134, 2005; discussion 245–246.
74. Gregory SA, Webster JB, Chapman GD: Acute hepatitis induced by parenteral amiodarone. *Am J Med* 113(3):254–255, 2002.
75. Goddard CJ, Whorwell PJ: Amiodarone overdose and its management. *Br J Clin Pract* 43(5):184–186, 1989.
76. Nitsch J, Luderitz B: Acceleration of amiodarone elimination by cholestyramine [in German]. *Dtsch Med Wochenschr* 111(33):1241–1244, 1986.
77. Leatham EW, Holt DW, McKenna WJ: Class III antiarrhythmics in overdose. Presenting features and management principles. *Drug Saf* 9(6):450–462, 1993.
78. Assimes TL, Malcolm I: Torsade de pointes with sotalol overdose treated successfully with lidocaine. *Can J Cardiol* 14(5):753–756, 1998.
79. Cropp JS, Antal EG, Talbert RL: Ibutilide: a new class III antiarrhythmic agent. *Pharmacotherapy* 17(1):1–9, 1997.
80. Stambler BS, Wood MA, Ellenbogen KA, et al: Efficacy and safety of repeated intravenous doses of ibutilide for rapid conversion of atrial flutter or fibrillation. Ibutilide Repeat Dose Study Investigators. *Circulation* 94(7):1613–1621, 1996.
81. Slade AK, Garratt CJ: Proarrhythmic effect of adenosine in a patient with atrial flutter. *Br Heart J* 70(1):91–92, 1993.
82. Klabunde RE: Dipyridamole inhibition of adenosine metabolism in human blood. *Eur J Pharmacol* 93(1–2):21–26, 1983.

Chapter 102 ■ Anticholinergic Poisoning*

KEITH K. BURKHART

The classic anticholinergic syndrome manifests an easily recognizable toxidrome, but patients may present with some, not all, of the classic symptoms. Decreased secretions, tachycardia, mydriasis, and delirium are those most commonly seen. The presence of coingestants and the multiple pharmacologic actions of many anticholinergic drugs may mask anticholinergic manifestations, although anticholinergic effects often persist longer than other pharmacologic actions [1]. The anticholinergic syndrome is more accurately an antimuscarinic syndrome. However, it is conventionally called anticholinergic, and will be referred to as such herein.

Anticholinergic poisoning may result in seizures, delirium, and coma, along with their associated complications. Anticholinergic-induced coma and respiratory failure may require mechanical ventilation. As with any toxicologic emergency, supportive care is of paramount importance. Physostigmine is an effective antidote with proven benefits, but also has a risk for serious adverse events.

EPIDEMIOLOGY AND SOURCES

A variety of pharmaceuticals and naturally occurring products can produce an anticholinergic syndrome (Table 102.1). Many drugs have off-target anticholinergic effects (e.g., histamine-1

TABLE 102.1

Some Agents That Cause Anticholinergic Syndrome[a]

Pharmaceuticals	Plants
Antihistamines (H_1-blockers)	*Atropa belladonna* (deadly nightshade)
Brompheniramine	*Brugmansia arborea* (angel's trumpet)
Chlorpheniramine	*Brugmansia suaveolens* (angel's trumpet)
Clemastine	*Cestrum diurnum* (day-blooming jessamine)
Cyclizine	*Cestrum nocturnum* (night-blooming jessamine)
Cyproheptadine	*Cestrum parqui* (willow-leaved jessamine)
Dimenhydrinate	*Datura metel* (downy thorn apple)
Diphenhydramine	*Datura stramonium* (jimson weed)
Doxylamine	
Hydroxyzine	*Hyoscyamus niger* (black henbane)
Meclizine	*Lantana camara* (wild sage)
Promethazine	*Lycium halimifolium* (matrimony vine)
Pyrilamine	*Myristica fragrans* (nutmeg)
Tripelennamine	Myristicaceae
Triprolidine	
Antiparkinsonian drugs	Mushrooms
Benztropine	*Amanita muscaria* (fly agaric)
Biperiden	*Amanita pantherina* (panther mushroom)
	Physalis heterophylla (ground cherry)
	Solanaceae
Trihexyphenidyl	*Solanum carolinense* (wild tomato)
Antipsychotics	*Solanum dulcamara* (bitter-sweet)
Acetophenazine	*Solanum nigrum* (black nightshade)
Chlorpromazine	*Solanum pseudocapsicum* (Jerusalem cherry)
Clozapine	
Fluphenazine	*Solanum tuberosum* (potato)
Haloperidol	Verbenaceae
Loxapine	
Molindone	
Olanzapine	
Perphenazine	
Prochlorperazine	
Quetiapine	
Thioridazine	
Thiothixene	
Trifluoperazine	
Antispasmodics	
Anisotropine	
Clidinium	
Dicyclomine	
Isometheptene	
Methantheline	
Propantheline	
Stramonium	
Tridihexethyl	
Belladonna alkaloids and related synthetic congeners	
Atropine (racemic hyoscyamine)	
Glycopyrrolate	
Ipratropium	
Methscopolamine	
Scopolamine	
Cyclic antidepressants	
Amitriptyline	
Amoxapine	
Clomipramine	
Desipramine	
Doxepin	
Imipramine	
Maprotiline	
Nortriptyline	
Protriptyline	
Trimipramine	
Muscle relaxants	
Cyclobenzaprine	
Orphenadrine	
Mydriatics	
Cyclopentolate	
Homatropine	
Tropicamide	

[a]Many of these agents have other significant toxic manifestations in addition to their anticholinergic effects.

*The views expressed in this chapter do not necessarily represent the views of the Food and Drug Administration or the United States.

$[H_1]$–blockers, gastrointestinal and genitourinary tract antispasmodics, cough and cold preparations, over-the-counter sleep aids, some opioids, and anticholinergic plants).

Pharmaceuticals and plants with anticholinergic action may be intentionally abused for mind-altering effects; especially common is the use of *Datura stramonium* (jimsonweed). Anticholinergic toxicity has occurred by a number of routes other than ingestion, including inhalation of nebulized medication, inhalation of pyrolysis products (e.g., the smoking of plant parts), transdermal use, and ocular instillation.

PHARMACOLOGY

Anticholinergic agents antagonize the effects of the endogenous neurotransmitter acetylcholine (ACh). Receptors for ACh are widely distributed in the body, including the central nervous system and the sympathetic and parasympathetic ganglia, postganglionic parasympathetic terminals, and motor end plates of the peripheral nervous system.

ACh receptors are divided into two types, muscarinic and nicotinic, based on their ability to bind muscarine or nicotine. This division has a functional significance as well, best described in the peripheral nervous system, where muscarinic receptors predominate in the parasympathetic terminals and nicotinic receptors in autonomic ganglia and motor end plates. Most drugs have predominant effects on one of the two main ACh receptors, but at high doses, there may be some crossover effect. For example, nicotine primarily stimulates nicotinic receptors. Stimulation produces tachycardia, hypertension, muscle fasciculations, and receptor fatigue, with consequent paralysis at high doses. Nicotinic antagonists, such as the nondepolarizing muscle relaxants (e.g., pancuronium), block the action of ACh at the motor end plate and produce skeletal muscle paralysis. Excessive muscarinic receptor stimulation (e.g., organophosphate poisoning) leads to the cholinergic toxidrome (see Chapter 109). Agents that block muscarinic receptors may cause anticholinergic toxicity, the focus of this chapter.

Many drugs with anticholinergic properties undergo extensive hepatic metabolism into active and inactive metabolites. A number of these drugs may have half-lives greater than 12 to 24 hours (e.g., tricyclic antidepressants). More important may be the persistence of muscarinic receptor binding. In the intensive care unit (ICU), many patients emerge from coma into a delirious state. Reversal by physostigmine suggests persistent anticholinergic delirium rather than ICU psychosis [1].

CLINICAL PRESENTATION

Anticholinergic effects have been classically described by the mnemonic "Blind as a bat, Hot as Hades, Dry as a bone, Red as a beet, and Mad as a hatter" in reference to the consequences of ciliary muscle paralysis, hyperthermia, anhidrosis, vasodilation, and delirium, respectively. The toxidrome has been subdivided into the peripheral anticholinergic syndrome and the central anticholinergic syndrome (Table 102.2). The former is caused by quaternary amines (e.g., glycopyrrolate), which are charged molecules that poorly penetrate the blood–brain barrier, whereas the latter is caused by tertiary amines (e.g., atropine), which are uncharged and reach the central nervous system. The most serious anticholinergic manifestations include agitated delirium, hyperthermia, and seizures. Patients may present with primarily peripheral signs and symptoms, primarily central ones, or both. In addition, central symptoms may persist longer than the peripheral manifestations.

The clinical presentation may be complicated by other pharmacologic actions of the intoxicant (e.g., tricyclic antidepressants and reuptake inhibition of norepinephrine and serotonin or sodium/potassium channel blockade) or the actions of other potentially toxic substances (e.g., salicylates, sympathomimetics).

TABLE 102.2

Manifestations of the Anticholinergic Syndrome

- Peripheral anticholinergic signs and symptoms
  - Cardiovascular: hypertension and tachycardia
  - Skin: dry and flushed with dry mucous membranes
  - Eyes: mydriasis (variable)
  - Genitourinary: urinary retention and decreased bowel sounds (ileus)
- Central anticholinergic signs and symptoms
  - Loss of short-term memory and confusion, disorientation, psychomotor agitation, muffled or garbled speech
  - Visual/auditory hallucinations or frank psychosis
  - Incoordination and ataxia
  - Picking or grasping movements and extrapyramidal reactions
  - Seizures
  - Coma with respiratory failure

MANAGEMENT

Traditionally, anticholinergic-poisoned patients have been managed with conservative supportive care. Obtaining and assessing historical and physical data confirms or provides the diagnoses that guide management decisions. Historical data may be simple in terms of a single agent, such as jimsonweed, or complex, as in a polydrug overdose. An analysis of the pharmacologic properties of the known intoxicants guides management decisions.

Delirium and coma are typically the most serious anticholinergic consequences that would require ICU admission. Shortly after exposure, most patients demonstrate sinus tachycardia and hypertension. These abnormalities are usually mild, but occasionally require medical intervention. Patients' respiratory status should be continuously monitored because of potential for respiratory failure. Hyperthermia, although not often present, is occasionally severe and may require rapid cooling measures. Hyperthermia has also resolved after physostigmine administration. Foley catheter insertion may be needed for urinary retention.

Laboratory studies that should be considered for patients with moderate to severe anticholinergic toxicity include serum electrolytes; blood urea nitrogen; creatinine; and creatine phosphokinase, urinalysis, and electrocardiogram. Rhabdomyolysis and dehydration may be diagnosed. A urine toxicology screen does not detect most anticholinergic agents and typically contributes little to the diagnostic workup or patient management. Many anticholinergic agents are not detected even on comprehensive toxicology screens that take hours to return. Resolution of mental status changes after physostigmine administration may be the most rapid and cost-effective way to arrive at the diagnosis and simultaneously treat the poisoning.

Gastrointestinal decontamination (see Chapters 97 and 125) should be considered, especially for plant ingestions where symptoms persist for days. Administration of activated charcoal is recommended. Its administration, however, may be problematic for the agitated or delirious patient. Physostigmine administration has also been recommended to facilitate activated charcoal administration [2].

Hallucinations, agitation, and delirium have been traditionally treated with benzodiazepines (e.g., diazepam, lorazepam) and butyrophenones (e.g., haloperidol). Heavily sedating doses may often be required such that endotracheal intubation becomes necessary [1]. Furthermore, haloperidol use often worsens the anticholinergic delirium and should not be used. Physostigmine, as an antidote, reversibly binds to acetylcholinesterase and prevents this enzyme from degrading ACh, thereby allowing the neurotransmitter to persist, accumulate, and competitively reverse muscarinic receptor inhibition at its postsynaptic sites of action. Physostigmine, as opposed to similar drugs such as neostigmine and pyridostigmine, is a tertiary rather than a quaternary amine and effectively crosses the blood–brain barrier. As a result, it is effective in reversing central as well as peripheral anticholinergic effects. A more liberal use of physostigmine has the potential to help many patients and save resources. Use as a diagnostic tool may avoid an expensive workup. It may also avoid alternative treatment with other drugs and the costs of potentially having to intubate the heavily sedated patient [1].

Physostigmine administration allegedly has contributed to poor outcomes, asystole, seizures, and death, mostly reported after cyclic antidepressant poisoning. When administered in excessive amounts or to a patient not in an anticholinergic state, signs and symptoms of cholinergic excess may appear. A retrospective series of 39 patients treated with physostigmine included cyclic antidepressant poisoned patients [3]. None of these patients developed dysrhythmias or needed atropine, while one patient had a self-limited seizure. Reports have also described the benefits of physostigmine administration following atypical neuroleptics, including clozapine, olanzapine, and quetiapine poisoning [3,4]. Close observation is mandatory following reversal of anticholinergic-induced respiratory or CNS depression, especially early in the course of intoxication. The awakening and cholinergic effects theoretically could enhance gut activity and further absorption of ingested drugs such that when physostigmine is cleared, the patient might have greater toxicity than at the time of first administration.

Physostigmine can be both diagnostic and therapeutic. Administration to the confused, febrile patient may return mental status to normal and reduce fever. A head computerized axial tomogram and lumbar puncture may be avoided if the patient awakens and provides a history that is consistent with the anticholinergic toxicity. On theoretical grounds, it has been suggested that physostigmine may be useful for seizures unresponsive to conventional treatment; severe hypertension resulting in acute symptoms or end-organ dysfunction; and supraventricular tachycardia resulting in hemodynamic instability, cardiac ischemia, or other organ dysfunction. In clinical practice, these indications rarely arise and physostigmine is almost exclusively used as a diagnostic aid and for the treatment of central nervous system excitation (psychomotor agitation) and coma. In a case series of patients treated by medical toxicologists, physostigmine use was associated with lower rates of intubation [5].

Contraindications to the use of physostigmine include bronchospasm and mechanical obstruction of the intestine or urogenital tract. It should be used with caution among patients with asthma, gangrene, diabetes, cardiovascular disease, or any vagotonic state, and with choline esters or depolarizing neuromuscular-blocking agents (e.g., succinylcholine). Physostigmine should also be used cautiously after cyclic antidepressant overdose and is contraindicated for patients with evidence of cardiac conduction delay (e.g., atrioventricular block and prolonged QRS interval) on electrocardiogram.

Patients receiving physostigmine should be placed on continuous cardiac monitoring and be under continuous careful observation (see Table 102.3). Recommendations for the safe use of physostigmine center on its slow intravenous infusion at a rate not to exceed 0.5 mg per minute to avoid adverse drug events such as bradydysrhythmia and seizures. Slower rates of administration may further reduce the risk for adverse events [6]. The average dose needed for adults is 1 to 2 mg [1,6]. Mental status improvement is usually seen within 5 to 20 minutes of administration. If no reversal of anticholinergic effect has occurred after 10 to 20 minutes, an additional 1 to 2 mg may be administered. Administration by continuous infusion has been used [4]. The recommended dose for pediatric patients is 0.01 to 0.02 mg per kg not to exceed 0.5 mg per minute [5]. The half-life of physostigmine is short, and its duration of action after the 2-mg dose typically is only 1 to 6 hours. The action of many anticholinergic agents persists longer and, therefore, additional doses may be needed [7]. If cholinergic toxicity emerges, atropine is not needed unless severe toxicity develops. Seizures are rare and usually self-limited [3]; an intravenous benzodiazepine is recommended (see Chapter 109). Anecdotally, some physicians have administered lorazepam, 1 mg, before physostigmine as an additional safety measure [8].

TABLE 102.3

Summary Treatment Recommendations for Anticholinergic Toxicity and Use of Physostigmine

Place patient on cardiac and pulmonary monitor
Obtain electrocardiogram—If QRS prolonged more than 100–110 ms, physostigmine should not be used
Consider a urinary catheter
Consider pretreatment with 1 mg lorazepam IV before physostigmine
If no QRS prolongation, administer 2 mg physostigmine IV over 4 min
If no resolution of delirium and no bradycardia or seizures, consider repeat dosing of 1–2 mg physostigmine IV
If appropriate response, repeat 1–2 mg physostigmine as necessary, continuous infusion may be useful in rare circumstances

References

1. Burns MJ, Linden CH, Graudins A, et al: A comparison of physostigmine and benzodiazepines for the treatment of anticholinergic poisoning. *Ann Emerg Med* 35(4):374–381, 2000.
2. Burkhart KK, Magalski AE, Donovan JW: A retrospective review of the use of activated charcoal and physostigmine in the treatment of jimson weed poisoning [abstract]. *J Toxicol Clin Toxicol* 37:389, 1999.
3. Schneir AB, Offerman SR, Ly BT, et al: Complications of diagnostic physostigmine administration to emergency department patients. *Ann Emerg Med* 42(1):14–19, 2003.
4. Eyer F, Pfab R, Felgenhauer N, et al: Clinical and analytical features of severe suicidal quetiapine overdoses—a retrospective cohort study. *Clin Toxicol* 49:846–853, 2011.
5. Watkins JW, Schwarz ES, Arroyo-Plasencia AM, et al: The use of physostigmine by toxicologists in anticholinergic toxicity. *J Med Toxicol* 2014. doi:10.1007/s13181-014-0452-x.
6. Dawson A, Buckley N: Pharmacological management of anticholinergic delirium—theory, evidence and practice. *Br J Clin Pharmacol* 2015. doi:10.1111/bcp.12839.
7. Rosenbaum CD, Bird SB: Frequency and timing of physostigmine redosing in anticholinergic toxidrome. *Clin Toxicol* 46(7):634, 2008.
8. Rasimas JJ, Sachdeva KK, Donovan JW: Revival of an antidote: bedside experience with physostigmine. *J Association for Emergency Psychiatry* 12(2):5–24, 2014.

Chapter 103 ■ Anticonvulsant Poisoning

STEVEN B. BIRD

Anticonvulsants can be divided into four groups based on their primary mechanism of action: those that primarily act on neuronal membranes (membrane-active agents), those that act on neurotransmitters or their receptor sites (synaptic agents), those with multiple sites of action, and those that are not yet understood. Membrane-active agents alter ion fluxes and include carbamazepine (CBZ), oxcarbazepine, ethosuximide, zonisamide, phenytoin, and lamotrigine (LTG). Synaptic agents primarily affect the activity of gamma-aminobutyric acid (GABA) and include barbiturates, benzodiazepines, gabapentin (GBP), tiagabine, and vigabatrin. Agents that have multiple sites of action include valproate, GBP, felbamate, and topiramate, and those for which mechanisms of action still are not understood are levetiracetam, stiripentol, and remacemide [1,2]. (Barbiturates and benzodiazepines are discussed in Chapter 123.) The precise action mechanisms of many of the newer anticonvulsants also remain unknown. Even within groups, the site or mechanism of action may differ. Pharmacologic differences are important from a therapeutic standpoint. For the treatment of seizures, combining agents from different groups may be effective whenever a single agent is ineffective or requires a toxic dose for efficacy. Therapeutic synergism may also occur when different agents of the same group are combined (e.g., benzodiazepines and barbiturates).

PHENYTOIN

Phenytoin (diphenylhydantoin) is the most commonly used anticonvulsant medication. It is also used in the treatment of trigeminal neuralgia. Iatrogenic intoxications can occur with drug interactions because distribution, protein binding, and clearance of phenytoin are affected by other medications and disease states. Toxicity may occur when the daily administered dose exceeds endogenous metabolism and elimination [3]. Toxicity may also result when switching dosage forms or between generic and proprietary forms of the drug because of different release and absorption characteristics. Idiosyncratic and hypersensitivity reactions associated with therapeutic use are unrelated to dose, and are most commonly seen among patients with underlying neurologic disorders [4].

Pharmacology

Phenytoin is the prototypical membrane-active anticonvulsant. It acts on sodium pumps and channels in excitable cell membranes and is classified as a type 1B antidysrhythmic agent. By blocking the accumulation of intracellular sodium during tetanic stimulation, it limits the posttetanic potentiation of synaptic transmission and prevents seizure foci from detonating adjacent areas.

Phenytoin is a weak acid, with a pK_a of 8.5. The intravenous (IV) form has a pH of 10 to 12, contains 50 mg per mL, and is dissolved in a 40% propylene glycol and 10% ethanol vehicle. The phenytoin prodrug fosphenytoin (Cerebyx) has a pH between 8.6 and 9.0 and greater solubility. It is compatible with common IV preparations, lacks the cardiotoxic diluent propylene glycol, and may be administered intramuscularly as well as intravenously. It has a conversion half-life of 8.4 to 32.7 minutes to active phenytoin and is dosed in phenytoin equivalent (PE) units (75 mg per mL of fosphenytoin equals 50 mg per mL of phenytoin) [5]. In many institutions, fosphenytoin has replaced phenytoin.

Absorption occurs in the duodenum but depends on dosage form, gastric emptying, and bowel motility. Peak levels occur between 2.6 and 8.9 hours after oral dosing of an extended-release capsule. During overdosage, absorption may continue for up to 7 days, possibly due to decreased gastric motility and pharmacobezoar formation. The volume of distribution (V_d) of phenytoin is 0.6 L per kg, and it distributes preferentially into the brainstem and cerebellum, which explains the effects seen in overdose. Phenytoin is highly protein bound; decreased protein binding increases the free, pharmacologically active form of the drug and the V_d. Because usually only total phenytoin levels are measured, toxicity from increased free phenytoin may occur at lower total phenytoin levels [3].

Hepatic metabolism of phenytoin follows first-order elimination kinetics, with an average half-life of 22 hours (range: 7 to 55 hours). When plasma levels exceed 10 μg per mL, metabolism follows zero-order elimination kinetics, yielding a much longer half-life. The enzyme system may be induced or inhibited by other drugs, inherited genetic disturbances, or liver disease [6,7].

The anticonvulsant effects of phenytoin occur with plasma levels between 10 and 20 μg per mL. This can be achieved within 45 to 60 minutes by an IV-loading dose of 15 to 20 mg per kg of phenytoin or PE units of fosphenytoin. The rate of IV phenytoin administration should not exceed 50 mg per minute because of propylene glycol toxicity [8]. To avoid hypotension, fosphenytoin administration should not exceed 150 PE units per minute. Phenytoin has been successfully administered by the interosseous route in children with poor venous access. Maintenance dosing is usually 4 to 6 mg/kg/d in single or divided doses, although neonates may require higher doses (5 to 8 mg/kg/d) [9]. Death from isolated phenytoin ingestions is unusual but has been reported in young children with ingestions of 100 to 220 mg per kg. Death results from central nervous system (CNS) depression with respiratory insufficiency and hypoxia-related complications.

Clinical Manifestations

Toxicity resulting from acute and chronic intoxication has a similar presentation. Patients with serum phenytoin concentrations between 20 and 40 μg per mL typically have nausea, vomiting, normal to dilated pupils, nystagmus in all directions, blurred vision, diplopia, slurred speech, dizziness, ataxia, tremor, and lethargy [10]. They may also be excited and agitated. As phenytoin serum concentration increases, confusion, hallucinations, and apparent psychosis may develop. Progressive CNS depression occurs, and nystagmus may improve. Pupillary response becomes sluggish, and deep tendon reflexes diminish. Severe toxicity with coma and respiratory depression occurs with serum concentration exceeding 90 μg per mL [11]. Slowing of alpha wave activity is seen on electroencephalograms. As toxicity increases, brainstem-evoked potentials are suppressed and may be absent. Paradoxical hyperactivity has been reported among patients with underlying neurologic deficits, with findings of dystonia, dyskinesia, choreoathetoid movements, decerebrate rigidity, and increased seizure activity [12]. Patients with baseline focal neurologic deficits may show contralateral abnormalities, including hemianopia, hemianesthesia, and hemiparesis. Patients recover completely if no anoxic or hypoxic complications develop during acute toxicity. Cerebellar atrophy after acute intoxication with phenytoin that was not known to be attributed to hypoxia has been reported, however. Recovery may take 1 week or longer.

In rare instances, chronic toxicity has been associated with a syndrome of inappropriate antidiuretic hormone, encephalopathy, and cerebellar degeneration [13]. Chronic use of phenytoin causes hyperglycemia, vitamin D deficiency and osteomalacia, folate depletion, megaloblastic anemia, and peripheral neuropathy. Other adverse drug events include altered collagen metabolism that causes hirsutism, gingival hyperplasia, keratoconus, and hypertrichosis [14].

Non–dose-dependent phenytoin adverse drug events include hypersensitivity reactions such as fever, rash eosinophilia, hepatitis, lymphadenopathy, myositis, a lupus-like syndrome, rhabdomyolysis, nephritis, vasculitis, and hemolytic anemia [4]. Phenytoin administration during pregnancy has resulted in fetal hydantoin syndrome.

Phenytoin-induced dysrhythmias, hypotension, congestive failure, respiratory arrest, and asystole result predominately from propylene glycol toxicity during rapid IV phenytoin administration (e.g., >50 mg per minute). If the rate of infusion is slowed or temporarily halted, these effects usually resolve spontaneously but may persist for 1 to 2 hours [15]. Cardiovascular toxicity from phenytoin intoxication itself is rare, represents significant toxicity, and primarily occurs in patients with underlying cardiac disorders [16].

Diagnostic Evaluation

Essential laboratory studies should include sequential serum phenytoin levels (free and total, if available) and levels of other anticonvulsant medications, particularly when enteric-coated dosage form is involved. The interval between drug levels should be based on factors such as severity of intoxication, rate of rise of levels, and time since exposure. Intervals should be more frequent during the initial evaluation phase, while absorption is still occurring, than later, during the postabsorptive phase. In stable patients whose drug levels have peaked or started to decline, it may be appropriate to obtain levels every 12 to 24 hours until they return to the therapeutic range. Recommended laboratory studies include serum complete blood cell count, electrolytes, blood urea nitrogen, creatinine, glucose, albumin, and liver function tests. In hypoalbuminemic patients, the corrected phenytoin concentration is equal to the measured phenytoin concentration multiplied by 4.4 and divided by the serum albumin level. In all deliberate overdoses, an electrocardiogram (ECG) and acetaminophen and salicylate levels should be obtained. Arterial blood gas, chest radiograph, head computed tomography, and lumbar puncture should be obtained as clinically indicated.

The differential diagnosis of phenytoin intoxication includes sedative–hypnotic agents, other anticonvulsants, phencyclidine, neuroleptic agents, and other CNS depressant drugs. Other conditions such as diabetic ketoacidosis; hyperosmolar nonketotic coma; sepsis; CNS infection, tumor, and trauma; seizure disorders; extrapyramidal syndromes; postictal states; and cerebellar abnormalities may also mimic phenytoin intoxication.

Management

Patients should have a rapid evaluation of respiratory status followed by intubation if hypoxia or risk of aspiration is present. Vascular access should be established and the patient placed on continuous cardiac monitoring. If the mental status is abnormal, a fingerstick blood sugar should be obtained. Patients who are hyperglycemic from phenytoin intoxication can be treated with discontinuation of the drug; insulin therapy is rarely required. Flumazenil, the benzodiazepine antagonist, has no role in managing phenytoin intoxication, even if benzodiazepines are part of the polypharmacy overdose, as its use may increase the risk of status epilepticus, particularly in patients with a preexisting seizure disorder.

Hypotension occurring during phenytoin infusion is treated with discontinuation of the infusion and administration of crystalloid. Pressors are rarely necessary. Treatment of cardiac dysrhythmias is supportive, with use of the appropriate antidysrhythmics when indicated. Type IB antidysrhythmic agents should be avoided [17].

Patients with a seizure disorder should be placed on seizure precautions because of the possibility of paradoxical seizures during the acute intoxication phase or breakthrough seizures during the recovery phase when phenytoin levels may be in the subtherapeutic range. Seizures should be treated with benzodiazepines or a different anticonvulsant.

Because phenytoin has a long elimination half-life, measures to increase the rate of elimination should be considered. Gastrointestinal (GI) tract decontamination uses oral-activated charcoal administration. Phenytoin undergoes enterohepatic recirculation with active gut secretion; multiple-dose oral-activated charcoal (MDAC) can increase the rate of elimination and may decrease hospital stay [18] (see Chapter 97). MDAC is indicated for patients with a phenytoin concentration greater than 40 μg per mL, moderate neurologic toxicity, or rising levels after GI tract decontamination. As drug levels may continue to decline for many hours after stopping MDAC, such therapy should be discontinued before drug levels reach the therapeutic range for patients who require phenytoin for therapeutic purposes. Serum levels of concurrent anticonvulsant medications may also decline when MDAC is administered, increasing the risk of breakthrough seizures. An observation period is necessary to ensure establishment of a therapeutic anticonvulsant regimen and documentation of stable therapeutic serum levels even after passage of charcoal stools. Because phenytoin has a high degree of protein binding and hepatic elimination, forced diuresis, hemodialysis, and hemoperfusion are not useful and it is likely that hemofiltration would not be useful for similar reasons.

Disposition

Because the majority of patients with phenytoin poisoning do well with supportive therapy alone, determining the degree of toxicity is important. After adequate GI decontamination, the patient should be assessed for progression of toxicity. Patients who are not suicidal or ataxic, have no underlying cardiac dysrhythmias, can feed themselves, and are not at risk of hurting themselves can be discharged, providing serum phenytoin levels are not rising and a reliable caretaker is available. Patients who do not meet these criteria should be admitted. Severely toxic patients, those with an underlying cardiac or CNS disorder, intubated patients, or patients with rapidly progressive signs of toxicity require intensive care monitoring.

VALPROIC ACID

Valproic acid (VA; 2-propylpentanoic or 2-propyl valeric acid) is structurally unique among the anticonvulsants. VA is a branched-chain carboxylic acid with a pK_a of 4.8. In addition to being an anticonvulsant medication, VA is commonly used for the treatment of acute manic episodes, mood stabilization, and prophylaxis of migraine and affective disorders.

VA is marketed as a sodium salt (Depakene); in a syrup solution; in a prodrug form, divalproex sodium (Depakote); and as a sustained-release form of divalproex sodium (Depakote ER). The latter is a molecular complex that dissociates in the GI tract into two molecules of VA. There is also a parenteral form for VA.

Pharmacology

VA is thought to mediate its anticonvulsant effect by increasing cerebral and cerebellar levels of GABA [19] by blocking its metabolism through inhibition of GABA transferase and succinic aldehyde dehydrogenase. It may also prolong the recovery of inactivated sodium channels and have effects on potassium channels in neuronal cell membranes.

The pharmacokinetic profile of VA is significantly altered in an overdose setting. Within its therapeutic range (50 to 100 mg per mL), VA is 80% to 95% serum protein bound [20]. The degree of protein binding decreases and the V_d (0.13 to 0.22 L per kg) increases as VA levels exceed 90 μg per mL [20]. The resultant increase in free VA levels is evident by enhanced distribution into target organ systems and better than predicted extracorporeal drug removal. This has been demonstrated by a higher cerebrospinal fluid-to-serum level and hemodialysis extraction ratio in the VA-poisoned patient [21]. Protein binding of VA may also be decreased in uremic patients or in the presence of other highly protein-bound agents (e.g., acetylsalicylic acid), which displace VA from its binding sites.

VA is highly bioavailable, with the time to peak serum levels after ingestion dependent on the dosage form and VA species. In capsule form, VA itself achieves peak serum levels after 1 to 4 hours with therapeutic dosing, whereas peak serum levels may be delayed 4 to 5 hours after ingestion of the enteric-coated divalproex sodium tablets. Peak serum levels may be delayed out to 17 hours with overdose [22]. This may be explained by the enteric-coating dissolution time and the sequential process of intestinal conversion of divalproex to the sodium salt. This is followed by the final conversion to the free acid, the only form absorbed from the GI tract. There is no evidence suggesting formation of pharmacobezoars from large numbers of VA tablets.

VA is metabolized predominantly by the liver, with 1% to 4% excreted unchanged in the urine [20]. It undergoes beta and omega oxidation to several metabolites: hydroxylvalproate, 2-propylglutarate, 2-propylpent-4-enoate, 5-hydroxyvalproate, and 4-hydroxyvalproate. At high doses of VA, the omega oxidation pathway may become saturated, leading to a decrease in total VA body clearance [21]. The metabolites undergo glucuronidation and biliary excretion, with a possible enterohepatic recirculation [21]. At therapeutic levels, VA elimination half-life averages 10.6 hours (range: 5 to 20 hours), but during an overdose it may extend to 30 hours.

VA disrupts amino acid and fatty acid metabolism, sequesters acetyl coenzyme A by forming valproyl coenzyme A, and interrupts the ornithine–citrulline shuttle and carnitine transport [23,24]. This may result in encephalopathy associated with hyperammonemia at therapeutic levels of VA [25], acutely contribute indirectly to the CNS depressant effects, and chronically contribute to other target organ toxicity. VA metabolites have been implicated in the metabolic perturbations associated with VA poisoning [25,26], interfere with urine ketone determinations, and may be the hepatotoxic mediators of VA. There may be a link between VA- and opiate-induced CNS toxicity because of their similar influence on the GABAnergic systems [11,27]. Because VA and its metabolites are low molecular weight, branched-chain carboxylic acids, they may be used as substrates for several enzymatic processes. This leads to inhibition of critical biochemical pathways, such as the urea cycle, and subsequent fatalities in some sensitive patient populations. Death has occurred after therapeutic doses of VA among patients with a congenital deficiency of ornithine carbamoyltransferase. In addition, a frequently fatal Reye-like hepatitis has been observed in patients receiving therapeutic doses. Those at greatest risk appear to be very young patients (younger than 2 years of age), those being treated with multiple anticonvulsants, and those with other long-term neurologic complications. The fatality rate is 1 per 500 in this patient population [28]. This hepatotoxic reaction occurs with chronic exposure and may be mediated by metabolites formed via the cytochrome P450 pathway. These metabolites in turn depress fatty acid oxidation in the hepatocyte mitochondria. This effect may parallel that seen after ingestion of ackee fruit containing hypoglycin, causing Jamaican vomiting sickness. VA can produce a hyperammonemia and encephalopathy exclusive of the hepatotoxic reaction. This may be associated with VA-induced carnitine deficiency [25].

Valproate as the sodium salt provides a significant sodium load (13.8 mg sodium per 100 mg VA) in overdose. VA and its metabolites are low molecular weight, osmotically active, free acid, or anionic species. They may produce a slightly elevated osmolar gap and an elevated anion gap metabolic acidosis with a reduction in circulating endogenous cations, particularly calcium [21,23,29]. Valproate may have a dose-related toxic effect on bone marrow and platelet function, with resultant hematologic consequences such as thrombocytopenia, anemia, and leukopenia [30].

The morbidity and mortality from dose-related acute or acute-on-chronic VA poisoning appear to be related to hypoxic sequelae from respiratory failure, aspiration, or terminal cardiorespiratory arrest [21,29,31]. Although it has been speculated that VA has a direct, irreversible, neurotoxic effect, this has not been substantiated and it is indistinguishable from hypoxic injury.

Patients ingesting greater than 200 mg per kg are at high risk of significant CNS depression, but poor correlation exists between peak serum level and dose of VA ingested [31]. Patients who die from acute VA poisoning have had peak serum VA levels ranging from 106 to 2,728 μg per mL, whereas survival has been reported in a patient with a peak serum level of 2,120 μg per mL [23]. Although serum VA levels may not correlate with clinical effects, in general, serum levels of 180 μg per mL are usually associated with serious CNS toxicity (e.g., coma and apnea) and significant metabolic derangements (e.g., acidosis and hypocalcemia) [23,32]. The duration of toxicity is proportional to the peak serum VA level.

On the basis of endogenous VA clearance, it will take 3 days for the serum level to drop within the therapeutic range for a patient with a serum level greater than 1,000 μg per mL.

Clinical Manifestations

During acute intoxication, hypotension, mild tachycardia, decreased respiratory rate, and elevated or depressed temperature may be seen. Miosis may be present. The hallmarks of VA toxicity are global CNS-related depression in conjunction with unique metabolic changes. The mental status varies on a continuum from confusion and disorientation to obtundation and deep coma with respiratory failure. Tremor, hallucinations, and hyperactivity have been reported, but there is a notable lack of cerebellar–vestibular effects. Patients with an underlying seizure disorder may have breakthrough seizures. Most patients with serious acute VA poisoning manifest CNS toxicity for at least 24 hours and this may extend to several days. Laboratory abnormalities observed among patients with high serum VA levels include an anion gap metabolic acidosis, hypocalcemia, hyperosmolality, and hypernatremia. Transient rises in serum transaminase levels have been observed without evidence of functional liver toxicity. Hyperammonemia associated with vomiting, lethargy, and encephalopathy may occur at therapeutic serum levels. Although rare, complications or delayed sequelae associated with severe VA intoxication include optic nerve atrophy, cerebral edema, acute respiratory distress syndrome, and hemorrhagic pancreatitis.

Non–dose-related toxicities include hepatic failure, pancreatitis, red blood cell aplasia, neutropenia, and alopecia. Pancreatitis is usually considered a non–dose-related effect but has been observed. Alopecia, thrombocytopenia, leukopenia, and anemia have been associated with acute and chronic VA intoxication.

The differential diagnosis should include opioid toxicity and a list of substances causing an increased anion gap metabolic acidosis. VA intoxication can be indistinguishable from opioid poisoning by signs and symptoms, and VA-poisoned patients may occasionally respond to naloxone. VA may cause a false-positive urine ketone determination, thereby misdirecting the clinician to causes of ketosis [23].

Diagnostic Evaluation

Essential laboratory studies should include sequential serum VA levels and levels of other anticonvulsant medications, particularly when the enteric-coated dosage form is involved. It should be recognized that VA metabolites are highly cross-reactive on enzyme-multiplied immunoassay technique assay for VA [21], and there may be an overestimation of serum VA levels as high as 50%. Recommended laboratory studies include complete blood cell count, reticulocyte count, serum electrolytes, blood urea nitrogen, creatinine, glucose, calcium, ammonia, and liver function tests. In addition, serum amylase and lipase levels should be obtained to rule out pancreatitis.

In all deliberate overdoses, an ECG and acetaminophen and salicylate levels should be obtained. Arterial blood gas, chest radiograph, head computed tomography, and lumbar puncture should be obtained when clinically indicated.

Management

As with any consequential CNS depressant ingestion, the patient's airway and respiratory status should be frequently assessed; early intubation and ventilation help prevent hypoxic sequelae. Vascular access and continuous cardiac monitoring should be established. Patients with altered mental status should have a fingerstick blood sugar determination or receive IV dextrose, followed by naloxone and thiamine as clinically indicated.

Naloxone (0.8 to 2.0 mg) has been reported to be effective in increasing the level of consciousness of patients with signs and symptoms of opioid toxicity and serum VA levels between 185 and 190 μg per mL [32]. Patients with higher VA serum levels have not responded to larger doses of naloxone [33]. Naloxone has been shown experimentally to antagonize GABA, the inhibitory neurotransmitter increased by VA [11,27]. It is therefore worth trying naloxone (up to 10 mg) for all comatose patients with suspected VA poisoning. Flumazenil, the benzodiazepine antagonist, should be avoided for patients with a preexisting seizure disorder.

Carnitine has been used for the treatment of hyperammonemia because VA interferes with the citrulline–ornithine cycle and carnitine's availability to shuttle fatty acids across the mitochondrial membrane. There are some pediatric data suggesting that carnitine may improve mental status [24,34]. The oral and parenteral carnitine doses range from 1.5 to 2.0 g, divided into three to four doses per day.

GI decontamination should be performed for patients with suspected VA, even if several hours have elapsed since ingestion [35]. Activated charcoal is preferred; gastric lavage and whole-bowel irrigation for enteric-coated preparations are additional options. Methods to enhance elimination may be effective as an increase in the free serum drug fraction, decreased protein binding, and marked prolongation in elimination half-life occur after overdose. MDAC may enhance the clearance and reduce the VA half-life by interrupting enterohepatic recirculation and GI tract dialysis [36]. Extracorporeal removal by hemodialysis or hemoperfusion is also effective. Indications for extracorporeal removal are not clearly defined, requiring a risk–benefit analysis on a case-by-case basis. It should be considered when the VA level exceeds 1,000 μg per mL and is recommended for patients with levels exceeding 2,000 μg per mL. In a patient with a level exceeding 2,000 μg per mL, prompt institution of hemodialysis led to complete resolution of toxicity within 3 days, whereas a similar patient managed with only supportive care died [23]. Patients not responding to conventional therapy or who have severe acid–base derangement may also benefit from hemodialysis. VA clearance during hemodialysis has been as high as 270 mL per minute, with a four- to fivefold decrease in elimination half-life. Hemodialysis has the added benefit of correcting acid–base derangements secondary to VA and removal of its metabolites. Because of VA's extensive protein binding and predominate hepatic elimination, it is anticipated that forced diuresis, manipulation of urine pH, and hemofiltration would not be useful in the management of VA intoxication. Charcoal hemoperfusion used for VA intoxication has demonstrated clearance similar to that of hemodialysis [28]. Use of hemodialysis and hemoperfusion in series may be more advantageous because of a more consistent extraction of VA as its degree of protein binding increases coincident with declining levels and desaturation of binding sites [37].

Disposition

The disposition of the VA-poisoned patient is based on the severity of CNS toxicity, quantitative serum levels, evidence of hypoxic insult, risk of secondary complications, and the amount of VA ingested. Patients with serum VA levels exceeding 150 μg per mL are at risk of CNS and respiratory depression and should be observed until levels return to the therapeutic range. Patients with VA serum levels exceeding 1,000 μg per mL are at high risk of serious prolonged toxicity and should be admitted to an intensive care unit.

CARBAMAZEPINE

CBZ is an iminostilbene compound with a chemical structural backbone resembling that of the tricyclic antidepressants. It is stereochemically similar to phenytoin. CBZ has long been recognized as a well-tolerated and effective agent for the management of various types of seizure disorders. It is also used for the treatment of trigeminal and glossopharyngeal neuralgias, tabetic pain, and affective disorders [38]. A sustained-release formulation is available.

Pharmacology

Because CBZ is unionized and highly lipophilic, there is no parenteral dosage form, and the rate-limiting step for systemic absorption is tablet dissolution time. Consequently, the pharmacokinetics and toxicokinetics of CBZ are not well defined and are subject to significant inter- and intrapatient variability. CBZ is 80% protein bound and may have twice the V_d of other anticonvulsants, such as phenytoin and phenobarbital.

In overdose, systemic absorption of CBZ may be inconsistent over time. This leads to intermittent surges of drug released into the circulation and may cause unexpected clinical deterioration of patients. This may explain the "cyclic coma" associated with CBZ poisoning [39]. Patients have been reported to relapse into deep coma as late as 2 days after admission to the hospital coincident with a marked increase in plasma levels of CBZ, even after the patient's condition has appeared to stabilize or improve clinically. CBZ's V_d ranges from 1.4 to 3.0 L per kg at toxic levels [40].

CBZ is predominantly metabolized in the liver, with 1% to 3% excreted unchanged in the urine. Endogenous clearance is 0.6 to 1.3 mL/kg/min [38]. The variability in clearance may be attributed to alteration in the metabolic capabilities of hepatic enzymes, particularly the cytochrome P450 system [38]. This system is sensitive to autoinduction during chronic administration or, conversely, inhibition with concurrent administration of enzyme inhibitors such as erythromycin [41]. The elimination half-life of CBZ in naive users may exceed 24 hours, whereas in chronic users it may be less than 15 hours [38,42]. Half-life determinations of CBZ, especially during an overdose, often are misleading because of erratic absorption and inability to determine the contribution of sustained absorption from the GI tract [42]. Most evidence suggests that CBZ undergoes first-order kinetics, although it is postulated that some of its metabolic pathways, such as epoxidation, may follow Michaelis–Menten kinetics and saturate at high levels [42].

Forty percent of CBZ is converted to the active metabolite CBZ-10,11-epoxide (CBZ-epoxide), further complicating the kinetic and toxicity profile of CBZ [38]. An inactive metabolite is also formed. CBZ-epoxide elimination half-life is 5.0 to 9.8 hours and is in turn converted to 10,11-dihydroxide [40,42]. CBZ-epoxide is much less protein bound than CBZ (50% vs. 80%) [38]. The therapeutic CBZ concentration is 3 to 14 μg per mL. Within this range, adverse drug events including nystagmus, ataxia, dizziness, and anorexia have been noted [43].

CBZ may be best described as a CNS depressant with mild anticholinergic activity and a proclivity for alteration in the cerebellar–vestibular brainstem function. CBZ mediates its pharmacologic effects by mechanisms that include stabilizing the inactive sodium channel, alteration in neurotransmitter activity (norepinephrine, acetylcholine), enhancement of adenosine, stimulation of benzodiazepine receptors, and depression of evoked repetitive firings in neurons and the brainstem reticular formation [38].

CBZ has been described as similar to tricyclic antidepressants in its toxicity profile [39,44,45]. Although these agents share sedative, anticholinergic, and sodium channel blocking activity, CBZ has a higher therapeutic index, and malignant cardiac dysrhythmias and seizures do not usually occur among patients with normal cardiac and neurologic function. During overdose with extremely high CBZ levels, however, fatal dysrhythmias may develop [43,46].

CBZ toxicity can be defined as dose dependent or non–dose dependent. Non–dose-dependent toxicity includes idiosyncratic and immunologic-mediated reactions such as bone marrow suppression, hepatitis, tubulointerstitial renal disease, cardiomyopathy, hyponatremia, and exfoliative dermatitis. Dose-related effects for sensitive populations include those with existing neurologic deficits and myocardial disease. Dose-related toxicity has been reported for acute overdoses, with survival of adults after 80-g ingestions. Death has been reported after acute ingestion of 60 g and after a 6-g ingestion by a patient receiving long-term maintenance therapy [45,47].

Respiratory depression and significant neurologic toxicity and death have been reported, with peak serum CBZ levels ranging from 20 to 65 μg per mL [39,40,43,45,47–51]. Patients with serum levels in the range of 10 to 20 μg per mL usually respond to verbal stimuli unless other coexisting medical complications or additional sedative–hypnotic substances are present [43].

There is poor correlation of serum CBZ levels with clinical outcomes. Prognosis appears to depend on the occurrence of respiratory depression and aspiration of gastric contents [43,45,47–52]. All reported deaths occurred among patients with a history of seizure disorders. Surviving patients may have a protracted course (days to weeks) because of secondary complications arising from hypoxic-related sequelae from respiratory and CNS depression, prolonged GI tract absorption, and a prolonged elimination half-life.

The kinetics of CBZ toxicity are affected by the active metabolite CBZ-epoxide, which may partially account for the lack of correlation between peak CBZ levels and the severity of symptoms. The concentration of CBZ-epoxide is only 40% that of CBZ; however, CBZ-epoxide concentration in the free, unbound form may be equal to or greater than that of CBZ [53].

Toxicity may occur by gradual accumulation of CBZ among patients receiving therapeutic dosing because of improper dosing protocols or as a result of a drug interaction with enzyme inhibitors such as erythromycin or verapamil [41] or from generic substitution [54].

Clinical Manifestations

Patients with acute and chronic exposures have similar findings. Key findings suggestive of CBZ poisoning include the triad of coma, anticholinergic syndrome, and adventitious movements. Physical findings include CNS depression with pronounced effects on the cerebellar–vestibular system (e.g., nystagmus, ataxia, ophthalmoplegia, diplopia, absent doll's eye reflex, and absent caloric reflexes), central and peripheral anticholinergic toxicity (e.g., hyperthermia, sinus tachycardia, hypertension, urinary retention, mydriasis, and ileus), and neuroleptic-type movement disorders (e.g., oculogyric crisis, dystonia, opisthotonus, choreoathetosis, and ballismus), which can occur in patients without preexisting neurologic disorders.

Other effects, which are not clearly reproducible and may be indirectly related to hypoxia or occur in patients with preexisting disease, include cardiac conduction disturbances, hypotension, hypothermia, respiratory depression, deep coma, diminished or exaggerated deep tendon reflexes, and dysarthria. Some patients may be agitated and restless, combative, or irritable, experience hallucinations, or have seizures. Because CBZ has prolonged absorption from the GI tract and prolonged elimination half-life, the clinical course may be extremely protracted and deceptive, and sudden deterioration may occur days after admission [39].

Seizures associated with high levels of CBZ appear to occur predominantly in patients with preexisting neurologic disorders. In many reports, it is unclear whether witnessed motor activity was a true seizure or another movement disorder and whether the seizure occurred primarily or was secondary to hypoxic insult [39,43,44,53].

Cardiac conduction disturbances such as prolongation of the PR, QRS, and QTC intervals and complete heart block have been reported [55]. Patients with an underlying abnormal cardiac conduction system may be at particular risk for the development of complete heart block [56]. For most patients, conduction defects are not seen or there is marginal prolongation of intervals without progression to malignant dysrhythmia despite extremely high CBZ levels [44,45,57].

Diagnostic Evaluation

Essential laboratory studies should include sequential serum CBZ levels and levels of other anticonvulsant medications, serum electrolytes, blood urea nitrogen, creatinine, and ECG. Recommended laboratory studies include complete blood cell count and liver function tests. For all deliberate overdoses, acetaminophen and salicylate levels should be obtained. Arterial blood gas, chest radiograph, head computed tomography, and lumbar puncture should be obtained as clinically indicated.

CBZ and CBZ-epoxide are highly cross-reactive on enzyme-multiplied immunoassay technique assays for CBZ and can result in a falsely elevated CBZ level. The clinical consequence of this is debatable, however. High-pressure liquid chromatography assay has the ability to distinguish between CBZ and

CBZ-epoxide. Using the ratio of CBZ to CBZ-epoxide, an index can be generated that may reflect the rapidity of absorption of CBZ from the GI tract. A ratio greater than 2.5 is evidence of rapid or continued CBZ absorption from the GI tract. Cases in which patients appear to relapse or deteriorate may be due to an abrupt increase in absorption occurring as late as 48 hours after the initial ingestion [45,51]. For cases in which serial CBZ and CBZ-epoxide levels were monitored, the ratio greatly increased just before and coincident with the clinical deterioration [39].

Patients whose serum CBZ level continues to significantly rise, manifesting delayed symptoms, or who appear to relapse or deteriorate after appropriate GI decontamination should be suspect for harboring pharmacobezoars in their GI tract. Radiographic contrast study should be considered to confirm this diagnosis; CBZ is not radiopaque [57]. The differential diagnosis of CBZ toxicity includes tricyclic antidepressants, neuroleptics, sedative–hypnotics, anticholinergic agents, and other anticonvulsant poisonings.

Management

Management begins with treatment of respiratory, neurologic, and cardiovascular derangements. Early intubation and ventilation should be considered, as poor outcomes with CBZ-poisoned patients are primarily associated with pulmonary complications. Vascular access and continuous cardiac monitoring [38,39,43] should be established. Hypotension should be initially managed with crystalloid fluid challenges followed by pressor agents [39,45]. There is no specific antidysrhythmic regimen for CBZ-induced cardiac toxicity. IV sodium bicarbonate therapy should be considered for patients whose QRS is greater than 100 ms. Patients with altered mental status should have a fingerstick blood sugar determination or receive IV dextrose, followed by naloxone and thiamine as clinically indicated. Seizures are usually self-limited but respond to IV diazepam or phenytoin [40].

GI decontamination should be initiated as soon as possible with activated charcoal. MDAC may double the elimination of systematically absorbed CBZ [58] (see Chapter 97) and should also be considered for patients with serum CBZ concentration greater than 20 μg per mL. MDAC should be discontinued before CBZ levels decline to the therapeutic range for those with an underlying seizure disorder. Although MDAC therapy significantly reduces serum CBZ levels, it has not been shown to improve patient outcomes [59]. For patients with rising drug levels despite initial GI tract decontamination, whole-bowel irrigation may also be useful (see Chapter 125).

Hemoperfusion has been used to enhance CBZ clearance in overdose cases but with modest results, usually no more than the increase achieved by MDAC, which is less invasive [45,48]. In one case, it was equivalent to an increase in CBZ excretion of 200 mg per hour [45]. If used at all, extracorporeal removal should be reserved for those with greatly elevated serum levels and concomitant deep coma. Neither urinary manipulation nor hemodialysis is useful.

Although there is one case report of a CBZ-poisoned patient (serum level: 27.8 μg per mL) who responded to a dose of flumazenil [50], this agent may precipitate seizures and is contraindicated for CBZ overdose. Physostigmine has been reported to be effective in the treatment of dystonia associated with CBZ poisoning [44]. Given that CBZ-associated dystonias are self-limited, the risks of physostigmine therapy likely outweigh its potential benefits.

Disposition

Because CBZ displays erratic absorption, the decision should be in favor of admission and a prolonged observation period in an intensive care setting for patients with a history suggestive of a large ingestion. CBZ-poisoned patients at greatest risk of significant sequelae should also be admitted to the intensive care unit. This would include patients whose CBZ levels exceed 20 μg per mL or are rapidly rising, who are obtunded or comatose, those with cardiovascular symptoms, whose ECG shows a QRS greater than 100 ms, and those with seizures. The majority of patients at risk of significant sequelae require observation for a minimum of 48 hours.

NEWER ANTICONVULSANTS

Felbamate (Felbatol)

Felbamate is a phenyl dicarbamate with a structure similar to that of the sedative–hypnotic agent meprobamate. Its mechanism of action is believed to have some indirect effect on the $GABA_A$-receptor supramolecular complex [60], block repetitive neuronal firing, and affect the sodium channel of the neuronal membrane. Felbamate is rapidly absorbed, with a bioavailability of 90% and peak plasma concentrations occurring 1 to 4 hours after oral dosing. Its V_d is 0.75 L per kg. The drug circulates as the free drug and is only 20% to 30% protein bound. Absorption and elimination are linear and plateau at high levels. The drug undergoes partial hepatic metabolism with an inactive metabolite and renal excretion. Approximately 40% of a dose is eliminated unchanged in the urine. The elimination half-life is 20 to 23 hours. Felbamate does not induce its own metabolism [61].

Felbamate has significant drug interactions. It can inhibit and induce the cytochrome P450 system. This affects the metabolism of coadministered medications. Felbamate induces the metabolism of CBZ and inhibits the metabolism of phenytoin and VA. The effect of felbamate on metabolism takes 2 to 3 weeks to clear after discontinuation of the drug [61].

Although uncommon, serious adverse drug events include aplastic anemia and hepatic failure, which is associated with a 20% mortality rate. Other adverse drug events include nausea, vomiting, abdominal pains, headache, insomnia, palpitations, tachycardia, blurred vision, diplopia, tremors, and ataxia. Children are likely to demonstrate anorexia and somnolence [61].

There is limited information regarding deliberate felbamate overdose. A 20-year-old woman developed altered mental status, massive crystalluria, and acute renal failure after an overdose of felbamate and VA. Macroscopic urinary crystals were identified by gas chromatography as containing felbamate. Crystalluria and acute renal failure resolved with hydration. A 44-year-old man who ingested an unknown amount of felbamate, haloperidol, and benztropine recovered with supportive care. Symptoms were predominately neurologic, with ataxia, nystagmus, weakness, abnormal movements, and agitation [62]. The management of felbamate overdose is supportive care. Gut decontamination with activated charcoal would appear to be reasonable. There are no data on hemodialysis, hemoperfusion, or urinary manipulation [62].

Lamotrigine (Lamictal)

LTG, or 3–5-diamino-6 (2,3-dichlorophenyl)-1,2,4-triazine, is not structurally related to other anticonvulsants. The mechanism of action of LTG is believed to involve voltage-sensitive sodium channels and stabilizes neuronal membranes. Lamotrigine has no effect on the release of GABA, acetylcholine, norepinephrine, or dopamine. In oral dosing, LTG is rapidly absorbed, with a bioavailability of 98%. Peak plasma levels are reached 1 to 4 hours after dosing. Protein binding is 55%, and the V_d ranges from 0.9 to 1.4 L per kg. LTG is metabolized in the liver and excreted as the glucuronide metabolite. LTG does not induce its own metabolism. The elimination half-life of the parent compound is 12 to 50 hours (mean: 30 hours) [61].

Adverse drug events include Stevens–Johnson syndrome, toxic epidermal necrolysis, drowsiness, dizziness, headache, unsteady gait, tremor, ataxia, somnolence, diplopia, blurred vision, and nausea [61].

There is increasing information regarding deliberate LTG overdose [63,64]. One patient presented with nystagmus and ataxia 1 hour after ingestion. The initial ECG showed a normal sinus rhythm with a QRS of 112 ms, which gradually resolved over 48 hours. In another case, ataxia, rotary nystagmus, and a normal ECG were noted. A 2-year-old boy developed tremor, muscle weakness, ataxia, hypertonia, and generalized tonic–clonic seizure after ingesting 800 mg of LTG.

The management of acute LTG overdose should include GI decontamination, continuous cardiac monitoring, and supportive care. It would be prudent to closely monitor a patient with serial ECGs for 24 to 48 hours if the initial ECG shows a prolonged QRS duration (greater than 100 ms). IV sodium bicarbonate therapy has not been studied but should be considered. Benzodiazepines are appropriate for the treatment of seizures. There are no data on hemodialysis or hemoperfusion.

Gabapentin (Neurontin)

GBP is an engineered molecule based on GABA and altered to increase membrane permeability and entrance through the blood–brain barrier. Chemically, GBP is GABA with a cyclohexane ring (1-[aminomethyl]-cyclohexane) [61].

Gabapentin appears to bind to a specific site in the CNS but does not affect ligand binding to $GABA_A$, $GABA_B$, benzodiazepine, glutamate, glycine, and *N*-methyl-D-aspartate sites on the neuronal membrane [61].

GBP is 50% to 60% absorbed from the GI tract, with peak serum levels occurring 1 to 3 hours after oral administration. Its V_d is 0.8 to 1.0 L per kg. GBP is not protein bound and does not appear to be metabolized; all of a dose is excreted unchanged in the urine. The terminal elimination half-life is 5 to 7 hours. Renal elimination and half-life are proportional to renal function. The elimination rate can neither be induced, nor can the elimination half-life be altered with repetitive dosing [61].

Adverse drug events include CNS depression, nystagmus, blurred vision, diplopia, mood changes, headache, weight gain, seizures, fatigue, nausea, dizziness, slurred speech, and unsteady gait. Lethargy, somnolence, dizziness, drowsiness, dysarthria, diplopia, sedation, ataxia, slurred speech, and GI distress have been observed after overdose [65,66]. Signs and symptoms resolved within 48 hours without specific therapy. Treatment is supportive. There are no data on binding to activated charcoal, urinary manipulation, hemodialysis, or hemoperfusion.

Oxcarbazepine (Trileptal)

Oxcarbazepine is the dihydro derivative of CBZ and can be thought of as being a prodrug, which is almost 100% biotransformed during hepatic first-pass metabolism to the active metabolite 10,11-dihydro-10-hydroxycarbamazepine. It has the same anticonvulsant effect as CBZ. The parent and the metabolite are lipophilic and pass into the CNS. Its advantages are that it has better tolerability and does not form the CBZ-epoxide. Peak serum drug levels occur 4.5 hours after an oral dose. The V_d is 49 L per kg. The elimination half-lives of oxcarbazepine and its metabolite are 1.0 to 2.5 hours and 8 to 11 hours, respectively. Adverse drug events include hyponatremia (in up to 30% of patients), headache, ataxia, dizziness, nausea, memory impairment, concentration difficulties, anorexia, and weight gain [67]. Evaluation and treatment considerations are the same as for CBZ. CBZ assays cannot be used to measure oxcarbazepine levels. Oxcarbazepine concentrations are not routinely available and are generally not useful for patient management.

Tiagabine (Gabitril)

Tiagabine is a GABA reuptake inhibitor derived from nipecotic acid to which a lipophilic moiety has been added to improve passage into the CNS. By selectively inhibiting neuronal GABA reuptake, it prolongs the action of GABA in the synapse. It is rapidly absorbed orally, with a peak level by 0.5 to 1.0 hours after ingestion. The drug is 96% protein bound and is metabolized by the CYP3A4 isoform to inactive metabolites. There is some degree of enterohepatic circulation. The elimination half-life ranges from 4 to 7 hours in patients receiving enzyme-inducing drugs.

Adverse drug events include CNS depression, nausea, hypertension, tachycardia, asthenia, sedation, dizziness, mild memory impairment, abdominal pain, and nausea. Some patients develop status epilepticus after overdose. Symptoms typically resolve within 12 to 24 hours [68]. Treatment is supportive.

Topiramate (Topamax)

Topiramate is a sulfamate-substituted monosaccharide compound different from other anticonvulsants. Its mechanism of action may be in part due to sodium channel blockade, enhancing the action of GABA, and diminishing kainate-induced excitatory receptor stimulation. Oral absorption is rapid, with a peak serum level at 1.8 to 4.3 hours. The plasma protein binding of topiramate is 9% to 17%, and its V_d is 0.7 L per kg. It is 70% to 97% eliminated unchanged in the urine. The elimination half-life is 18 to 24 hours.

Development of a nonanion-gap metabolic acidosis is a relative common occurrence with topiramate use, both in therapeutic dosing and in overdose [69]. This occurs by impairing both the normal reabsorption of filtered bicarbonate by the proximal renal tubule and the excretion of hydrogen ions by the distal renal tubule. This combination of defects is termed mixed renal tubular acidosis [70]. Treatment of the metabolic acidosis includes cessation of the topiramate and fluid resuscitation as needed. The use of parenteral sodium bicarbonate is rarely needed. Other adverse drug events include sedation, cognitive dysfunction, paresthesias, dizziness, fatigue, weight loss, diarrhea, and urolithiasis. Treatment is supportive.

Levetiracetam (Keppra)

Levetiracetam (Keppra) is a newer anticonvulsant that is now used nearly as often as phenytoin. Although its precise mechanism of action is unknown, levetiracetam does not appear to directly interact with the GABA system. The most common adverse effects in overdose are sedation, vertigo, and ataxia, although respiratory depression may also occur [71]. Therapeutic concentrations of levetiracetam are generally considered to be 10 to 40 μg per mL, but because its therapeutic window is so large, monitoring of blood concentrations is generally not performed. There is no specific antidotal therapy for levetiracetam overdose. Treatment is supportive care.

Vigabatrin (Sabril)

Vigabatrin is an engineered GABA-related anticonvulsant with limited availability in the United States. Chemically, it is gamma-vinyl-GABA. It is a stereospecific GABA transaminase inhibitor, the S(+) enantiomer being biologically active. Its peak serum level occurs 0.5 to 3.0 hours after ingestion, and its V_d is 0.8 L per kg. There is virtually no plasma protein binding of the drug, and more than 80% of the drug is eliminated unchanged. The plasma half-life ranges from 4 to 8 hours. The cerebrospinal fluid level is 0% to 15% of the serum level [65]. Adverse drug events include visual field defects, diplopia, drowsiness, irritability, agitation, anxiety, psychomotor effects, depression, sedation, confusion, and ataxia. A patient who ingested 8 to 12 g in an overdose developed a psychotic episode lasting 36 hours. Supportive care is the mainstay of management.

References

1. Kwan P, Sills GJ, Brodie MJ: The mechanisms of action of commonly used antiepileptic drugs. *Pharmacol Ther* 90:21–34, 2001.
2. Wallace SJ: Newer antiepileptic drugs: advantages and disadvantages. *Brain Dev* 23(5):277–283, 2001.
3. Reidenberg MM, Affrime M: Influence of disease on binding of drugs to plasma proteins. *Ann N Y Acad Sci* 226:115–126, 1973.
4. Powers NG, Carson SH: Idiosyncratic reactions to phenytoin. *Clin Pediatr (Phila)* 26(3):120–124, 1987.
5. Boucher BA, Feler CA, Dean JC, et al: The safety, tolerability, and pharmacokinetics of fosphenytoin after intramuscular and intravenous administration in neurosurgery patients. *Pharmacotherapy* 16(4):638–645, 1996.
6. Reynolds EH: Chronic antiepileptic toxicity: a review. *Epilepsia* 16(2):319–352, 1975.
7. Kutt H: Interactions of antiepileptic drugs. *Epilepsia* 16(2):393–402, 1975.
8. Louis S, Kutt H, McDowell F: The cardiocirculatory changes caused by intravenous Dilantin and its solvent. *Am Heart J* 74(4):523–529, 1967.
9. Borofsky LG, Louis S, Kutt H, et al: Diphenylhydantoin: efficacy, toxicity, and dose-serum level relationships in children. *J Pediatr* 81(5):995–1002, 1972.
10. Kutt H, Winters W, Kikenge R: Metabolism of diphenylhydantoin, blood levels and toxicity. *Arch Neurol* 11:642–648, 1964.
11. Dingledine R, Iversen LL, Breuker E: Naloxone as a GABA antagonist: evidence from iontophoretic, receptor binding and convulsant studies. *Eur J Pharmacol* 47(1):19–27, 1978.
12. Stilman N, Masdeu JC: Incidence of seizures with phenytoin toxicity. *Neurology* 35:1769–1772, 1985.
13. Luscher TF, Siegenthaler-Zuber G, Kuhlmann U: Severe hypernatremic coma due to diphenylhydantoin intoxication. *Clin Nephrol* 20(5):268–269, 1983.
14. Wagner KJ, Zell M, Leikin JB: Metabolic effects of phenytoin toxicity. *Ann Emerg Med* 15(4):509–510, 1986.
15. Garrettson LK, Jusko WJ: Diphenylhydantoin elimination kinetics in overdosed children. *Clin Pharmacol Ther* 17(4):481–491, 1975.
16. Wyte CD, Berk WA: Severe oral phenytoin overdose does not cause cardiovascular morbidity. *Ann Emerg Med* 20(5):508–512, 1991.
17. Rizzon P, Di Biase M, Favale S, et al: Class 1B agents lidocaine, mexiletine, tocainide, phenytoin. *Eur Heart J* 8[Suppl A]:21–25, 1987.
18. Howard CE, Roberts RS, Ely DS, et al: Use of multiple-dose activated charcoal in phenytoin toxicity. *Ann Pharmacother* 28(2):201–203, 1994.
19. Faingold CL, Browning RA: Mechanisms of anticonvulsant drug action. *Eur J Pediatr* 146:8–14, 1987.
20. Chadwick DW: Concentration-effect relationships of valproic acid. *Clin Pharmacokinet* 10(2):155–163, 1985.
21. Dupuis RE, Lichtman SN, Pollack GM: Acute valproic acid overdose. Clinical course and pharmacokinetic disposition of valproic acid and metabolites. *Drug Saf* 5(1):65–71, 1990.
22. Graudins A, Aaron CK: Delayed peak serum valproic acid in massive divalproex overdose—treatment with charcoal hemoperfusion. *J Toxicol Clin Toxicol* 34(3):335–341, 1996.
23. Mortensen PB, Hansen HE, Pedersen B, et al: Acute valproate intoxication: biochemical investigations and hemodialysis treatment. *Int J Clin Pharmacol Ther Toxicol* 21(2):64–68, 1983.
24. Cotariu D, Zaidman JL: Valproic acid and the liver. *Clin Chem* 34(5):890–897, 1988.
25. Riva R, Albani F, Gobbi G, et al: Carnitine disposition before and during valproate therapy in patients with epilepsy. *Epilepsia* 34(1):184–187, 1993.
26. Coulter DL, Allen RJ: Hyperammonemia with valproic acid therapy. *J Pediatr* 99(2):317–319, 1981.
27. Hyden H, Cupello A, Palm A: Naloxone reverses the inhibition by sodium valproate of GABA transport across the Deiters' neuronal plasma membrane. *Ann Neurol* 21(4):416–417, 1987.
28. Dreifuss FE, Santilli N, Langer DH, et al: Valproic acid hepatic fatalities: a retrospective review. *Neurology* 37(3):379–385, 1987.
29. Schnabel R, Rambeck B, Janssen F: Fatal intoxication with sodium valproate. *Lancet* 1(8370):221–222, 1984.
30. Gidal B, Spencer N, Maly M, et al: Valproate-mediated disturbances of hemostasis: relationship to dose and plasma concentration. *Neurology* 44(8):1418–1422, 1994.
31. Garnier R, Boudignat O, Fournier PE: Valproate poisoning. *Lancet* 2(8289):97, 1982.
32. Alberto G, Erickson T, Popiel R, et al: Central nervous system manifestations of a valproic acid overdose responsive to naloxone. *Ann Emerg Med* 18(8):889–891, 1989.
33. Palatrick, W, Honcharik N, Roberts D, et al: Coma, anion gap and metabolic derangements associated with a massive valproic acid poisoning. *J Anal Toxicol* 12:35, 1988.
34. Raskind JY, El-Chaar GM: The role of carnitine supplementation during valproic acid therapy. *Ann Pharmacother* 34(5):630–638, 2000.
35. Lokan RJ, Dinan AC: An apparent fatal valproic acid poisoning. *J Anal Toxicol* 12(1):35–37, 1988.
36. Farrar HC, Herold DA, Reed MD: Acute valproic acid intoxication: enhanced drug clearance with oral-activated charcoal. *Crit Care Med* 21(2):299–301, 1993.
37. Tank JE, Palmer BF: Simultaneous "in series" hemodialysis and hemoperfusion in the management of valproic acid overdose. *Am J Kidney Dis* 22(2):341–344, 1993.
38. Durelli L, Massazza U, Cavallo R: Carbamazepine toxicity and poisoning. Incidence, clinical features and management. *Med Toxicol Adverse Drug Exp* 4(2):95–107, 1989.
39. Sethna M, Solomon G, Cedarbaum J, et al: Successful treatment of massive carbamazepine overdose. *Epilepsia* 30(1):71–73, 1989.
40. Deng JF, Shipe JR Jr, Rogol AD, et al: Carbamazepine toxicity: comparison of measurement of drug levels by HPLC and EMIT and model of carbamazepine kinetics. *J Toxicol Clin Toxicol* 24(4):281–294, 1986.
41. Goulden KJ, Camfield P, Dooley JM, et al: Severe carbamazepine intoxication after coadministration of erythromycin. *J Pediatr* 109(1):135–138, 1986.
42. Vree TB, Janssen TJ, Hekster YA, et al: Clinical pharmacokinetics of carbamazepine and its epoxy and hydroxy metabolites in humans after an overdose. *Ther Drug Monit* 8(3):297–304, 1986.
43. May DC: Acute carbamazepine intoxication: clinical spectrum and management. *South Med J* 77(1):24–26, 1984.
44. O'Neal W Jr, Whitten KM, Baumann RJ, et al: Lack of serious toxicity following carbamazepine overdosage. *Clin Pharm* 3(5):545–547, 1984.
45. Nilsson C, Sterner G, Idvall J: Charcoal hemoperfusion for treatment of serious carbamazepine poisoning. *Acta Med Scand* 216(1):137–140, 1984.
46. Kenneback G, Bergfeldt L, Vallin H, et al: Electrophysiologic effects and clinical hazards of carbamazepine treatment for neurologic disorders in patients with abnormalities of the cardiac conduction system. *Am Heart J* 121(5):1421–1429, 1991.
47. Denning DW, Matheson L, Bryson SM, et al: Death due to carbamazepine self-poisoning: remedies reviewed. *Hum Toxicol* 4(3):255–260, 1985.
48. Chan KM, Aguanno JJ, Jansen R, et al: Charcoal hemoperfusion for treatment of carbamazepine poisoning. *Clin Chem* 27(7):1300–1302, 1981.
49. Leslie PJ, Heyworth R, Prescott LF: Cardiac complications of carbamazepine intoxication: treatment by haemoperfusion. *BMJ (Clin Res Ed)* 286(6370):1018, 1983.
50. Watson WA, Cremer KF, Chapman JA: Gastrointestinal obstruction associated with multiple-dose activated charcoal. *J Emerg Med* 4(5):401–407, 1986.
51. Zuber M, Elsasser S, Ritz R, et al: Flumazenil (Anexate) in severe intoxication with carbamazepine (Tegretol). *Eur Neurol* 28(3):161–163, 1988.
52. Kossoy AF, Weir MR: Therapeutic indications in carbamazepine overdose. *South Med J* 78(8):999–1000, 1985.
53. Patsalos PN, Krishna S, Elyas AA, et al: Carbamazepine and carbamazepine-10,11-epoxide pharmacokinetics in an overdose patient. *Hum Toxicol* 6(3):241–244, 1987.
54. Gilman JT, Alvarez LA, Duchowny M: Carbamazepine toxicity resulting from generic substitution. *Neurology* 43(12):2696–2697, 1993.
55. Beermann B, Edhag O, Vallin H: Advanced heart block aggravated by carbamazepine. *Br Heart J* 37(6):668–671, 1975.
56. Durelli L, Mutani R, Sechi GP, et al: Cardiac side effects of phenytoin and carbamazepine. A dose-related phenomenon? *Arch Neurol* 42(11):1067–1068, 1985.
57. Coutselinis A, Poulos L: An unusual case of carbamazepine poisoning with a near-fatal relapse after two days. *Clin Toxicol* 16(3):385–387, 1980.
58. Neuvonen PJ, Elonen E: Effect of activated charcoal on absorption and elimination of phenobarbitone, carbamazepine and phenylbutazone in man. *Eur J Clin Pharmacol* 17(1):51–57, 1980.
59. Wason S, Baker RC, Carolan P, et al: Carbamazepine overdose—the effects of multiple dose activated charcoal. *J Toxicol Clin Toxicol* 30(1):39–48, 1992.
60. White HS, Wolf HH, Swinyard EA, et al: A neuropharmacological evaluation of felbamate as a novel anticonvulsant. *Epilepsia* 33(3):564–572, 1992.
61. Ramsay RE: Advances in the pharmacotherapy of epilepsy. *Epilepsia* 34[Suppl 5]:S9, 1993.
62. Hwang TL, Still CN, Jones JE: Reversible downbeat nystagmus and ataxia in felbamate intoxication. *Neurology* 45(4):846, 1995.
63. O'Donnell J, Bateman DN: Lamotrigine overdose in an adult. *J Toxicol Clin Toxicol* 38:659–660, 2000.
64. Briassoulis G, Kalabalikis T, Tamiolaki M, et al: Lamotrigine childhood overdose. *Pediatr Neurol* 19:239–242, 1998.
65. Fischer JH, Barr AN, Rogers SL, et al: Lack of serious toxicity following gabapentin overdose. *Neurology* 44(5):982–983, 1994.
66. Verma A, St Clair EW, Radtke RA: A case of sustained massive gabapentin overdose without serious side effects. *Therap Drug Monit* 21:615–617, 1999.
67. Dong X, Leppik IE, White J, et al: Hyponatremia from oxcarbazepine and carbamazepine. *Neurology* 65:1976–1978, 2005.
68. Spiller HA, Winter ML, Ryan M, et al: Retrospective evaluation of tiagabine overdoses. *J Toxicol Clin Toxicol* 43:855–859, 2005.
69. Garris SS, Oles KS: Impact of topiramate on serum bicarbonate concentrations in adults. *Ann Pharmacother* 39:424–426, 2005.
70. Mirza N, Marson AG, Pirmohamed M: Effect of topiramate on acid-base balance: extent, mechanism and effects. *Br J Clin Pharmacol* 68:655–661, 2009.
71. Barrueto F Jr, Williams K, Howland MA, et al: A case of levetiracetam (Keppra) poisoning with clinical and toxicokinetic data. *J Toxicol Clin Toxicol* 40:881–884, 2002.

Chapter 104 ■ Antidepressant Poisoning

ANDREW M. KING • LUKE BISOSKI • CYNTHIA K. AARON

Antidepressants comprise a group of substances primarily indicated in the treatment of major depression. However, since their development in the 20th century, FDA-approved indications for the use of antidepressants for psychiatric and nonpsychiatric illnesses have greatly expanded and so has their consumption. Some indications for the use of cyclic antidepressants (CAs) include treatment of depression, therapy of enuresis in children, treatment of migraine headaches, chronic pain control, smoking cessation, panic disorders, premenstrual dysphoric syndrome, and cocaine detoxification [1,2]. The Center for Disease Control, based on data collected via the National Health and Nutrition Examination Surveys, estimates that approximately 1 in 10 Americans over the age of 12 take antidepressant medications [3]. Given the numerous prescriptions for antidepressants, these medications are freely available to patients who are at high risk for suicide or overdose. The consequences of overdose are severe and predominantly affect the central nervous system (CNS) and cardiovascular system. In 2014, there were over 110,000 antidepressant exposures reported to US poison control centers that resulted in more than 8,600 moderate or major outcomes and 32 deaths [4].

HISTORY

Although the first antidepressants were synthesized in the late 19th century as iminodibenzyl, the pharmacology of CAs was not detailed until the 1940s. These compounds were initially designed to have antihistaminic, sedative, analgesic, and antiparkinsonian properties. Imipramine (Tofranil), the first of the dibenzazepines, was synthesized as a phenothiazine derivative in the late 1950s, but was found to be ineffective as a neuroleptic agent. Patients taking imipramine reported having mood-elevating effects; hence, imipramine and later congeners became the mainstay in the treatment of endogenous depression. As their use increased, the toxicity of CA became more relevant in overdose. In the 1980s, newer generations of CAs were developed in hopes to eliminate some of the adverse effects. These include the tetracylcic antidepressants (e.g., mirtazepine) and the atypical antidepressants (e.g., buproprion). More recently, a newer class of antidepressants called selective serotonin reuptake inhibitors (SSRIs) have been developed followed by the serotonin–norepinephrine reuptake inhibitors (SNRIs) agents.

Monoamine oxidase inhibitors (MAOIs) were first used clinically in the mid 1950s but became popular as first-line therapy for depression as late as the 1970s. Iproniazid was first developed as an antituberculosis medication but after its antidepressant effects were noted, it became the first antidepressant used clinically in the 1950s. Although they remain potent and effective medications, their many food and drug interactions have limited their use so that reports of toxic exposures are becoming much less common.

TYPES OF ANTIDEPRESSANTS

Antidepressants are generally grouped by their mechanism of action or chemical structure. The most common categories include CAs, SSRIs, SNRIs, norepinephrine reuptake inhibitors (NRIs), MAOIs, and lithium salts. Classic tricyclic antidepressants have a seven-membered central ring with a terminal nitrogen containing either three constituents (tertiary amines) or two constituents (secondary amines) [5]. Tertiary amines include amitriptyline, imipramine, doxepin, trimipramine, and chlorimipramine (clomipramine). Secondary amines include desipramine, protriptyline, and nortriptyline. Included with CAs are two dibenzoxazepine compounds that contain the central seven-membered ring with a heterocyclic constituent: loxapine and its demethylated metabolite amoxapine.

Maprotiline, a dibenzobicyclooctadiene, mianserin, and mirtazapine (Remeron) are tetracyclic antidepressants [6,7]. Mirtazapine, a derivative of mianserin, has additional α_2-antagonist activity. Bicyclic compounds include viloxazine, venlafaxine, and zimeldine.

CAs that are not available in the USA because of side effects include mianserin (agranulocytosis), nomifensine (hepatotoxicity and hemolytic anemia), lofepramine (hepatotoxicity and hyponatremia), and zimeldine (Guillain-Barré syndrome) [13–15].

Selective serotonin reuptake inhibitors include fluoxetine, paroxetine, sertraline; fluvoxamine; citalopram; and scitalopram and have various chemical structures. Trazodone, nefazodone, and vilazodone are serotonin antagonist and reuptake inhibitors that are riazolopyridine derivatives. They are structurally and pharmacologically different from the other antidepressants. Similarly, vortioxetine is a new serotonergic agent that acts via inhibiting serotonin reuptake as well as showing mixed antagonist and agonist effects at various serotonin receptors [12]. Bupropion is a unicyclic phenylethylaminoketone classified as a norepinephrine and dopamine reuptake inhibitor (NDRI) [8,9].

Venlafaxine and duloxetine are considered SNRIs since they have norepinephrine-reuptake inhibition effects. Desvenlafaxine is the major active metabolite of venlafaxine [10]. Levomilnacipran is the more active enantiomer of milnacipran, which is approved in Europe and Japan, and has relatively greater norepinephrine uptake compared to serotonin [11]. Although not classically considered SSRIs, some antidepressant agents that have serotonergic activity include mirtazapine, trazodone, nefazodone, and clomipramine. Vortioxetine is a new serotonergic agent that acts via inhibiting serotonin reuptake as well as showing mixed antagonist and agonist effects at various serotonin receptors [12].

The MAOIs are a third class of antidepressants and include moclobemide, pargyline, phenelzine, tranylcypromine, selegiline, and isocarboxazid. They are used to treat depression, panic disorders, phobias, and obsessive-compulsive behavior. A group of MAOIs that selectively inhibit the monoamine oxidase (MAO) isoenzyme type B (MAO-B) are being used as agents to treat Parkinson's disease [16].

PHARMACOLOGY

TCAs

The CAs act as neurotransmitter postsynaptic receptor blockers for histamine, dopamine, acetylcholine, serotonin, and norepinephrine (NE). They inhibit the reuptake of neurotransmitter biogenic amines and have quinidine-like membrane-stabilizing effects [2,6,7,13,17,18] (Tables 104.1–104.3). These agents may induce atrioventricular blocks [19,20] and have direct negative cardiac inotropic effect, demonstrated by decrease in the rate of change in left ventricular pressure and an increase in left ventricular end-diastolic pressure [21,22]. CNS effects may be related to both neurotransmitter and direct membrane effects [23–26]. All tricyclic antidepressants increase the density of β adrenoreceptors.

TABLE 104.1

Cyclic Antidepressant Effects on Neurotransmitters

Antidepressant	Effect
Receptor blockade	
Acetylcholine (antimuscarinic)	Sinus tachycardia, gastrointestinal hypomotility, warm dry skin, urinary retention, mydriasis, lethargy, hallucinations, seizures, coma
Norepinephrine	Hypotension, reflex tachycardia, orthostasis, seizures
Histamine	Antihistamine effects, sedation, hypotension
Serotonin	Hypotension, ejaculation disturbances
Dopamine	Endocrine disturbances (galactorrhea, impotence), dystonias
Biogenic amine reuptake blockade	
Dopamine	Hypotension, psychomotor retardation, antiparkinsonian effects
Norepinephrine	Transient hyperadrenergic state (tremor, tachycardia), adrenergic depletion (hypotension, antidepressant effects), ejaculation disturbances
Serotonin	Seizures, ejaculation disturbances, antidepressant effects

TABLE 104.2

Relative Potencies of Cyclic Antidepressants: Receptor Blockade

Compound	ACh	H_1	α	5-HT	DA
Tertiary amines					
Amitriptyline	4+	3+	4+	2+	1+
Imipramine	3+	2+	4+	1+	1+
Secondary amines					
Nortriptyline	3+	3+	3+	1+	1+
Desipramine	1+	2+	2+	0	0
Dibenzoxazepines					
Amoxapine	±	2+	3+	0	2+
Tetracyclics					
Maprotiline	±	3+	3+	2+	2+
Triazolopyridines					
Trazodone	0	±	3+	0	0
SSRIs					
Fluoxetine	0	0	0	1+	0
Paroxetine	0	0	0	0	1+
Sertraline	0	0	0	0	0
Atypical					
Bupropion	0	1+	0	0	0
Venlafaxine	0	0	0	0	0

ACh, acetylcholine; DA, dopamine; H_1, histamine; 5-HT, serotonin; SSRIs, selective serotonin reuptake inhibitors.

SSRIs and SSNRIs alter serotonergic neurotransmission. The International Union of Pharmacological Societies Commission on Serotonin Nomenclature has classified at least 14 5-hydroxytryptamine (5-HT) receptors based on operational criteria (Table 104.4). SSRIs block some serotonin receptors and inhibit the reuptake of serotonin at other receptor subtypes. Buspirone, a nonbenzodiazepine sedative-hypnotic, is a 5-HT_{1A} partial agonist and is inhibitory on serotonin neuronal firing [27]. It has anxiolytic and antidepressant activity. Excessive stimulation can lead to hypotension. Antagonists at 5-HT_{1C}, such as ritanserin, may be anxiolytic. The 5-HT_{1D} receptor subtype stimulation leads to inhibition of neurotransmitter release, and the representative agonist is sumatriptan, an antimigraine medication. Stimulation at 5-HT_2 can cause vasoconstriction, and 5-HT_3 antagonists have antiemetic and antipsychotic activity (ondansetron) [27–29]. Classic tricyclic antidepressants affect serotonin neurotransmission by enhancing the sensitivity of 5-HT_{1A} postsynaptic receptors. The SSRIs alter the release of serotonin presynaptically, leading to an increase in the amount of serotonin that is available for neurotransmission without changing the sensitivity of the 5-HT_{1A} postsynaptic receptors [30]. In general, the SSRIs normalize the number and function of 5-HT_{1A} and 5-HT_2 receptors [28,29]. As a group, the predominant difference between SSRIs is in their effect on the hepatic cytochrome P450 system and drug–drug interactions.

Venlafaxine and duloxetine are considered selective serotonergic and NE reuptake inhibitors. Blockade of NE-α_2 receptors leads to decrease in 5-HT release. Selective serotonergic and NE reuptake inhibitors induce desensitization and downregulation of 5-HT and NE receptors, leading to disinhibition of

TABLE 104.3

Relative Potencies of Cyclic Antidepressant Reuptake Blockade

Compound	NE	5-HT	DA	ACh
Tertiary amines				
Amitriptyline	2+	1+	1+	3+
Imipramine	2+	2+	1+	3+
Secondary amines				
Nortriptyline	3+	1+	3+	3+
Desipramine	4+	±	1+	2+
Dibenzoxazepines				
Amoxapine	3+	±	3+	2+
Tetracyclics				
Maprotiline	3+	0	1+	±
Triazolopyridines				
Trazodone	0	1+	±	0
SSRIs				
Fluoxetine	±	3+	3+	0
Paroxetine	0	4+	1+	1+
Sertraline	±	3+	0	1+
Atypical				
Bupropion	0	0	2+	1+
Venlafaxine	±	3+	0	0

ACh, acetylcholine; DA, dopamine; 5-HT, serotonin; NE, norepinephrine; SSRIs, selective serotonin reuptake inhibitors.

TABLE 104.4

International Union of Pharmacological Societies Commission on Serotonin Nomenclature

Receptor[a]	Second messenger	Location	Agonist	Effect	Antagonist	Effect
5-HT_{1A}	cAMP	CNS	Buspirone	Anxiolytic	—	—
5-HT_{1B} (rodent only)	cAMP	CNS, PNS	mCPP	—	—	—
5-HT_{1C}	cAMP	CNS	—	—	Ritanserin	Anxiolytic
5-HT_{1D}	cAMP	CNS and extracerebral vascular smooth muscle	Sumatriptan, methylsergide	Antimigraine	—	—
5-HT_{1E}	cAMP	CNS	Ergotamine	—	Methylsergide	—
5-HT_{1F}	cAMP	CNS	Ergotamine	—	Methylsergide, yohimbine	—
5-HT_{2A}	IP_3DG	Vascular smooth muscle	—	Hypertension	Ketanserin, ritanserin	Hypotension
5-HT_{2B}	IP_3DG	Stomach	Tryptamine	—	—	—
5-HT_{2C}	IP_3DG	CNS, choroid plexus	mCPP (trazodone metabolite)	—	—	—
5-HT_3	Ionic channel	CNS, PNS	—	—	Ondansetron, granisetron	Antiemetic
5-HT_4	cAMP	Cardiac (nonventricular), gastrointestinal tract, bladder	Renazapride, cisapride	Gastric motility	—	—
5-HT_5–5-HT_7	cAMP	—	—	—	—	—

[a] All 5-HT receptors are G-proteins except for 5-HT_3 receptors, which are ionic channel receptors. 5-HT_1 receptors are negatively coupled to adenylyl cyclase; 5-HT_2 receptors are coupled to protein kinase C via phosphoinositide breakdown; 5-HT_3 receptors are ionic channels; 5-HT_4, 5-HT_6, and 5-HT_7 receptors are positively coupled to adenylyl cyclase.

cAMP, 3′,5′-cyclic adenosine monophosphate; CNS, central nervous system; 5-HT, serotonin; IP_3DG, inositol triphosphodiglyceride; mCPP, *m*-chlorophenyl piperazine; PNS, peripheral nervous system.

serotonergic neurons, interruption of feedback inhibition, and increased release of synaptic 5-HT.

MAOIs inhibit the activity of MAO, a flavin-containing enzyme located in the mitochondrial membranes of most tissues [31]. MAO enzymes are divided into two families: MAO-A, which uses 5-HT as its predominant substrate, and MAO-B, whose primary substrates include 2-phenylethylamine and O-tyramine. Monoaminergic neurons contain predominantly MAO-A; serotonergic neurons have both. MAO-A metabolizes epinephrine, NE, metanephrine, and 5-HT. MAO-A and MAO-B both metabolize tyramine, octopamine, and tryptamine [32]. MAO regulates intraneuronal catecholamine metabolism and mediates the oxidative deamination of epinephrine, NE, dopamine, and 5-HT. MAO also regulates ingested monoamine (tyramine, ethanolamine) in the gut that would normally be absorbed into the portal circulation [33,34]. The effect of MAOs is to increase the catecholamine storage pool by preventing intraneuronal degradation of catecholamines and 5-HT. These catecholamines can be released by indirectly acting sympathomimetic agents (e.g., amphetamine, tyramine, and dopamine). MAO-A is predominantly found in the intestinal mucosa, placenta, biogenic nerve terminals, liver, and brain; whereas MAO-B is found in the brain, platelets, and liver [35]. Exogenously administered catecholamines are metabolized through catechol-O-methyl transferase (COMT).

MAOIs can be divided into reversible agents (moclobemide) or irreversible (selegiline, phenelzine, isocarboxazid, and tranylcypromine). They may also be selective to MAO-A (moclobemide) or MAO-B (pargyline, selegiline) [36–38]. The original MAOIs (e.g., phenelzine, isocarboxazid, and tranylcypromine) are nonselective irreversible MAO-A and MAO-B inhibitors [39]. Selegiline and tranylcypromine are metabolized to desmethylselegiline, levoamphetamine, and levomethamphetamine and will give a positive amphetamine on drugs of abuse urine screening [40]. The selective MAO-B and the reversible inhibitors of MAO-A (RIMA) are unlikely to cause hypertensive crisis. They are not currently available in the USA.

PHARMACOKINETICS

CAs are well absorbed orally in therapeutic dosing; peak serum levels occur 2 to 6 hours after ingestion. In overdose, gastrointestinal (GI) absorption may be delayed secondary to anticholinergic and antihistaminic properties of these drugs [41]. Metabolism is predominately hepatic with a small enterohepatic circulation [42,43]. Some CAs have active metabolites. The volume of distribution is large, with distribution occurring within the first several hours after ingestion [44–46]. Elimination half-life averages 8 to 30 hours but may be prolonged in overdose [41,42]. Elimination is hepatic, with minimal renal involvement. Since some tertiary CAs are metabolized into their secondary amines toxicity may be prolonged after overdose because of synergistic effect and active metabolites (imipramine is metabolized to desipramine and amitriptyline is metabolized to nortriptyline). CAs are extensively bound to serum proteins, particularly α_1-acid glycoprotein (AAG), and binding appears to be pH dependent [47–49]. MAO inhibitors are well absorbed orally. They have relatively short elimination half-lives [36–38,40] but since the irreversible agents permanently inhibit the activity of MAO, their effects can last for 4 to 6 weeks [36].

In therapeutic doses, CA agents and SSRIs may interact with other medications, increasing the effect of one or both agents. This effect may be magnified after an overdose. Drug interactions may alter metabolism, elimination, or the free fraction of the drug. Most antidepressants are metabolized through the CYP2D6 microsomal agents and are subject to induction and interference. Agents that stimulate the hepatic P450 microsomal system (phenobarbital, carbamazepine, phenytoin, and rifampin; and cigarette smoking) increase the clearance of CAs. Cimetidine is an inhibitor of 2D6 and can lead to elevated TCA levels. Paroxetine, fluoxetine, and norfluoxetine inhibit CYP2D6. The coadministration of CAs and antipsychotic agents may lead to competitive inhibition of the metabolism of both drugs. Other medications that increase the steady-state levels of CAs include chloramphenicol and disulfiram, whereas erythromycin decreases the level. Acute ethanol intoxication may decrease CA metabolism, resulting in markedly prolonged serum drug half-life [50].

MAOIs are both oxidized by CYP2D6 and 2C19 and acetylated by N-acetyltransferase. A large portion of the population are defined as "slow acetylators" which can lead to exaggerated and/or prolonged clinical effects. Irreversible MAOIs can have very long durations of action since new enzymes need to be synthesized to overcome their effects. Phenelzine and isocarboxazid are hydrazides and metabolized to hydrazines. These hydrazine compounds inactivate pyridoxal 5′ phosphate, create a functional low pyridoxine state, and prevent formation of GABA from glutamate.

CLINICAL TOXICITY

General

Antidepressant toxicity predominately involves the CNS and/or the cardiovascular system. The pattern and severity of clinical effects, the clinical course, and treatment may vary significantly. Dependent on the ingested agent, progression of toxicity may be precipitous and lead to coma, hypotension, seizures, dysrhythmia, and death [51]. The newer agents (e.g., nefazodone, trazodone, and the SSRIs) are more likely to be sedating and less likely to exhibit cardiovascular toxicity [9,52–54]. Maprotiline, venlafaxine, amoxapine, and loxapine tend to cause CNS toxicity before cardiovascular toxicity [8,55–60]. Bupropion may cause seizures in therapeutic dosing and exhibits a dose-dependent increase in toxicity (greater than 450 mg per 24 hours) [55,61–63]. With the CAs, if marked myoclonus or seizures develop, severe hyperthermia may result [20,51,64–66].

TCA toxicity

Overview

Toxicity from CAs results in CNS depression, seizures, hypotension, dysrhythmias, and cardiac conduction abnormalities because of its interactions with a number of different receptors and ion channels [6,47–49,67]. Hyperthermia may occur as a result of increased muscle activity, seizures, and autonomic dysfunction [64,66]. The onset of symptoms from CA overdose is rapid. Historically, most patients who die from overdose do so before arriving at the hospital and after having ingested large (greater than 1 g) amounts of a drug [51]. Signs and symptoms usually occur within the first 6 hours after ingestion. Patients who survive the first 24 hours without hypoxic insult generally do well [51]. The progression of toxicity is rapid and unpredictable with patients capable of deteriorating from an awake, alert state to seizures, hypotension, and dysrhythmias within 30 to 60 minutes and with minimal warning signs [13,51,53,54]. Cardiac arrest due to CA poisoning may sometimes respond to prolonged resuscitative efforts. One case reports a patient who survived after a resuscitation of approximately 70 minutes [68].

CNS Manifestations

The CNS effects in CA overdose can be quite profound. Although some of the newer CAs are less toxic in overdose, they can cause seizures and alteration in mental status. The etiology of coma, seizures, and myoclonus is multifactorial and involves $GABA_A$- and $GABA_B$-chloride ion channel, muscarinic receptor blockade, serotonin agonism, and direct sodium channel effects [2,5,6, 17,23,24,26,31,42,45,69,70]. Seizures typically occur early in poisoning and are generalized. Status epilepticus is uncommon. Doxepin is particularly sedating, likely because of its strong histamine antagonism. Antimuscarinic delirium—characterized by mumbling and incoherent speech; inattention; hallucinations; akisthesia; and a characteristic picking behavior—may predominate in some individuals. Other antimuscarinic effects may cause mydriasis, urinary retention, ileus, and cutaneous vasodilation (see Table 104.2). Absence of these signs does not rule out CA ingestion; however, it is unusual for patients to have significant cardiovascular disturbances without an altered mental status. Although rare, tardive dyskinesia, neuroleptic malignant syndrome, and the syndrome of inappropriate antidiuretic hormone secretion have all been reported in association with CA overdose [9,71–73].

Cardiovascular Manifestations

Signs of cardiovascular toxicity may exist even with therapeutic dosing of classic CAs. A prolonged QTc interval and sinus tachycardia may be observed on the electrocardiogram (ECG) in nonoverdose states [74]. Even in therapeutic dosing, the frontal plane axis may shift rightward; the terminal 40 ms of the frontal plane QRS complex may shift to a rightward vector of 130 to 270 degrees. If computerized vector analysis is not available, a widened slurred S wave in leads I and aVL and an R wave in aVR represent this vector. As cardiovascular toxicity progresses, the ECG changes also progress. This would include a gradual progression to repolarization abnormalities, intraventricular conduction delays, ventricular dysrhythmia, high-grade atrioventricular blocks, profound bradycardias, and asystole [54,75–79]. Looking for these changes in overdosed or comatose patients may help in establishing a diagnosis. However, a small portion of the population normally has this unusual vector at baseline and some patients with extreme leftward axis deviation as a baseline may not show the rightward change with CA toxicity [22,54,79]. The absence of this finding does not rule out a classic CA poisoning; its presence with coma, seizures, dysrhythmias, or hypotension is very suggestive of CA toxicity [54].

Dysrhythmias and conduction abnormalities often provide a clue to the recognition of CA overdose. These drugs significantly affect action potential propagation (particularly in ventricular myocardial cells) and the conduction system in general [80]. CAs blunt phase 0 of the action potential depolarization by blocking the fast inward flux of sodium through the sodium channel [43]. This in turn, slows the rate of rise of phase 0 ($\dot{V}\_max$) and slows depolarization. As ventricular conduction slows, the QRS complex widens and there the QTc prolongs because of contributions from the prolonged QRS. This also contributes to unidirectional blocks and reentrant dysrhythmias [81]. Because inward sodium flux is coupled to the calcium excitation in myocardial cells, the myocardial cells are unable to contract fully and lose inotropy [82]. Because CAs have their tightest myocardial binding during diastole, toxicity appears to be directly related to heart rate. This was elegantly demonstrated in amitriptyline-poisoned dogs where increasing heart rate caused a decrease in $\dot{V}\_max$ and widened the QRS complex [43,83,84]. Interventions that slowed the heart rate, such as β-blockers, improved conduction but led to irreversible hypotension [85,86]. Brugada Type I patterns are possible but rare [87].

A secondary effect is seen on phase 4 of the action potential (spontaneous diastolic depolarization), leading to decreased automaticity [82,88]. Delayed repolarization occurs and may contribute to QTc interval prolongation, which has been associated with torsade de pointes [89]. Trazodone, citalopram, and escitalopram may cause marked QTc interval prolongation without QRS effect and may permit torsade de pointes (polymorphous) ventricular tachycardia in the absence of other ECG abnormalities [52,90,91].

Patients who ingest large amounts of CAs frequently present with hypotension. Several mechanisms have been suggested, including direct negative inotropic effects and dysrhythmias [92,93], with subsequent decreases in filling time and cardiac output [64,75,94,95]. α-adrenergic receptor blockade produces vasodilation and autonomic dysfunction. In addition, blockade of the biogenic amine pump prevents adequate uptake and release of these neurotransmitters as active substances, thereby contributing to hypotension [13,20,67,75,95,96]. Tachycardia is common and is because of muscarinic antagonism and reflex tachycardia from vasodilation and antihistaminic effects.

SSRI Toxicity

In contrast to cyclic and atypical antidepressants, SSRIs have little other receptor classes and thus toxicity occurs mainly through serotonergic effects. The pathophysiology of serotonin toxicity or serotonin syndrome is not fully understood but is believed to result from excessive $5\text{-}HT_{1A}$ stimulation, although dopamine and other neurotransmitters may be involved [97]. The Serotonin syndrome is associated with SSRI use, either alone, or in combination with other agents (e.g., serotonin precursor or agonists, lithium, tricyclic antidepressants, 5-HT analogs, other SSRIs, meperidine, pentazocine, tramadol, cocaine, 3,4-methylenedioxy-*N*-methylamphetamine [Ecstasy], MAOIs, and herbal remedies such as Saint John's wort) or with change in dose (increasing or decreasing), and in overdose.

Serotonin toxicity classically manifests as a clinical triad of altered mental status, autonomic dysfunction, and neuromuscular abnormalities. Toxicity exists on a spectrum from mild to life-threatening and mild toxicity may be misidentified as "side effects." Diagnostic criteria have been proposed to aid clinicians considering the diagnosis and severe toxicity is much easier to recognize than mild or moderate toxicity. Additionally, most criteria proposed from presumed serotonin syndrome require that other disease processes first be excluded. Mental status changes range from mood abnormalities to coma. Autonomic signs and symptoms include tachycardia, hypertension, hypotension, diaphoresis, diarrhea, hyperthermia, and tachypnea. Neurologic signs include shivering, tremor, akisthesia, mydriasis, myoclonus, hyperreflexia, and greater rigidity in lower extremity compared to upper extremity. Lactic acidosis, rhabdomyolysis, myoglobinuria, and multiorgan failure may develop in severe cases [97–99]. No gold standard laboratory measurement is currently available.

SSRIs, except for citalopram and escitalopram [91,99], are expected to have minimal cardiac effects. Citalopram, escitalopram, and ritanserin may significantly affect the QTc. QT prolongation via Ikr inhibition may not be seen for up to 24 hours post-ingestion. However polymorphic ventricular dysrhythmias are uncommon but cases of arrhythmia are reported from citalopram [100,101]. Overdoses with extremely large amounts of fluoxetine and citalopram have caused atrial fibrillation and bradycardias. Evidence of Na^+ and Ca^{2+} channel blockade has been shown at extremely high serum levels [102]. Animal experiments with paroxetine required much larger doses, compared to amitriptyline, to induce dysrhythmias [103–105].

Other adverse effects of SSRIs include sexual dysfunction, platelet dysfunction, movement disorders, SIADH, and decreased bone density.

SNRI and Bupropion Toxicity

Seizures and cardiovascular effects are extremely common with bupropion and venlafaxine. These patients almost always have abnormalities of vital signs, reflecting a hyperadrenergic state [55]. Large ingestions of bupropion can prolong the QRS. Sodium channel blockade likely occurs via a different mechanism than CAs, and a recent review concluded that sodium bicarbonate is unlikely to be effective in treating QRS widening from bupropion [106]. Status epilepticus and refractory shock have been reported [61–63,107–109]. Delirium can resemble severe antimuscarinic delirium with severe agitation, akisthesia, incoordination, and hallucinations. Bupropion most commonly exists as extended-release formulations and symptoms can be prolonged. In addition to causing seizures and cardiovascular toxicity, venlafaxine may cause direct muscle toxicity leading to severe rhabdomyolysis [110].

MAOI Toxicity

There are two forms of toxicity caused by MAOI: acute overdose and drug and food interactions. Toxicity from acute MAOI overdose results from the exaggerated pharmacologic effects of MAOI and may be associated with secondary complications [111]. Classic severe MAOI toxicity is biphasic with an initial excitatory and hyperadrenergic syndrome followed by profound CNS depression as monoamine neurotransmitters become depleted. Patients with acute MAOI overdoses may be asymptomatic upon presentation. Signs and symptoms typically develop within 6 to 12 hours of ingestion if the person is on the medication chronically but may be delayed for 24 hours if this is a new medication for the patient. The hallmark of MAOI overdose is rapidly fluctuating autonomic dysfunction.

The primary drug–drug interaction occurs when MAOI is taken with an indirectly acting sympathomimetic agent (e.g., ephedrine, phenylephrine, phenylpropanolamine, or amphetamine), which causes an NE surge in the peripheral sympathetic nerve terminals. MAOI and food interaction primarily involve the small amounts of tyramine or tryptophan that are normally present in certain foods (e.g., aged cheeses; smoked or pickled meats; yeast and meat extracts; red wines; Italian broad beans; pasteurized light and pale beers; and ripe avocados) and are often termed the *cheese reaction*. These indirectly acting agents are usually metabolized by MAO-A in the gut. When MAO-A is inhibited, tyramine absorption is unregulated, enters into the portal circulation, and causes release of stored catecholamines with resultant hypertensive response [33,34]. The onset of MAOI and food or drug interaction usually occurs within 30 to 60 minutes of ingesting the offending substance. Signs and symptoms of both food and drug interaction-induced reaction include hypertension; tachycardia or reflex bradycardia; severe (occipital) headache; nausea and vomiting; hyperthermia; altered mental status; seizures; intracranial hemorrhage; and death.

CNS Manifestations

Early CNS manifestations are generally excitatory and are a result of increased synaptic biogenic amines possibly with increased glutamatergic transmission and decreased GABA effect. Effects include seizures, headache, stroke, agitation, akathisia, shivering, tremor, ocular clonus, hallucincations, nystagmus (ping-pong nystagmus) [112], myoclonus, posturing, hypertonia, hyperreflexia, and muscular rigidity. Coma is a late finding.

Cardiovascular Manifestations

Early cardiovascular manifestations include hypertension, tachycardia, dysrthythmias, myonecrosis, and myocarditis. Cardiovascular collapse can ensure with hypotension, bradycardia, and sudden death. ECG changes may be evident and reflect ischemic changes due to supply and demand mismatch.

If the patient survives this progression, there may be secondary complications from rhabdomyolysis, electrolyte abnormalities, lactic acidosis, and multiple organ system failure. Toxicity may last for up to 72 hours [113]. MAOI poisoning can be very challenging to manage as the patient's vital signs can swing from a hyperadrenergic state to cardiovascular collapse resulting from rapidly and unexpectedly depleted catecholamines [114]. Hyperthermia is multifactorial and can lead to further autonomic dysregulation including acidosis and disseminated intravascular coagulation. Other effects include nausea, vomiting, diarrhea, diaphoresis, and flushing. In cases of MAOI overdose or in conjunction with serotonergic agents, marked muscle rigidity can be seen with opistothonus and secondary hyperthermia, lactic acidemia and rhabdomyolysis.

DIAGNOSTIC EVALUATION

Patients with suspected antidepressant overdose should have routine blood analyses. Stress leukocytosis may occur with any antidepressant overdoses, especially if seizures have occurred. Electrolyte, blood urea nitrogen, creatinine, and glucose levels should be determined, with special attention to the anion gap. Because rhabdomyolysis may occur, most frequently with seizures, creatinine kinase should be followed. Urinalysis is also useful in the diagnosis of rhabdomyolysis and possible myoglobinuric renal failure. Frequent ECGs are a necessity and should be done any time the patient has a change in clinical status. Arterial blood gas and chest radiograph should be obtained as clinically indicated. Since serial measurement of serum pH may be required to gauge toxicity and arterial sampling may be extremely painful and is sometimes associated to complications such as infection, injury, and thrombosis, venous or capillary blood can be used and trended. Venous pH has been shown to strongly correlate that of an arterial sample in CA overdose [115].

Quantitative tricyclic antidepressant levels rarely, if ever, contribute to the clinical patient management. Although total tricyclic levels of more than 1,000 ng per mL have been associated with significant toxicity [41,46,53,54,76,77], there is poor correlation between toxicity and serum level. Repeated levels during resolution of toxicity may be misleading; physical signs of toxicity abate before a significant drop in serum levels because of the prolonged elimination half-life and extensive protein binding [46]. A qualitative screen using a tricyclic antidepressant immunoassay is usually sufficient. However, other drugs that have structural similarity can produce a false positive result (Table 104.5) [116], and if clinical findings are inconsistent with immunoassay results, it may be necessary to perform a more specific test such as gas chromatography with mass spectrometry. Although toxicology testing is discretionary, acetaminophen and salicylate levels and a pregnancy test in a woman of childbearing age should always be checked.

Although the differential diagnosis includes many substances that share some of the effects of CAs, duplicating the entire constellation of signs and symptoms is relatively unusual. Like CAs, anticholinergic and antihistaminic medications can cause dilated pupils, GI hypomotility, confusion, and seizures. Phenothiazines also cause these effects and may increase the QTc. Thioridazine and mesoridazine, two phenothiazines, prolong the QRS and QTc. The atypical neuroleptics (risperidone and olanzapine) have similar sedative, cardiac, and movement effects. Other drugs that affect QRS width include type IA antiarrhythmics (quinidine, procainamide, and disopyramide) and type IC antiarrhythmics (flecainide, encainide, and propafenone). Hyperkalemia and hypocalcemia also widen the QRS complex, and the latter can cause muscle twitching and myoclonus. β-blockers, particularly propranolol, cause seizures and conduction abnormalities in overdose. Tramadol, an opiate analgesic that also causes biogenic amine reuptake inhibition, may cause opioid and serotonergic toxicity, especially when given in conjunction with an SSRI or MAOI as well as seizures. Cyclobenzaprine, a muscle relaxant,

TABLE 104.5

Drugs that May Interfere with the Tricyclic Antidepressant Qualitative Drug Screen

Drugs	Min serum concentration for positive TCA screen
Carbamazepine	Therapeutic range
Chlorpromazine	Therapeutic range
Cyclobenzaprine	10–20 μg/L
Cyproheptadine	390–400 μg/L
Diphenhydramine	>120 μg/L
Quetiapine	Therapeutic range
Thioridazine	Therapeutic range

and carbamazepine share the CA structure, and can cause a similar picture with sedation, hypotension, and prolonged QTc interval.

MANAGEMENT

Patients who ingest antidepressants require immediate evaluation and stabilization. Those who are awake and alert should receive an oral dose of activated charcoal if conditions are appropriate. Patients who have ingested a classic TCA (amitriptyline, nortriptyline, imipramine, desipramine, clomipramine, doxepin, dothiepin, protriptyline, and maprotiline) can be safely observed in the emergency department if they are asymptomatic. An asymptomatic patient implies one with a normal ECG throughout the observation period, a mild sinus tachycardia that resolves within the first 1 to 2 hours, clear mental status, and a nontoxic acetaminophen level. This observation period is defined as a 6-hour interval during which the patient is on continuous ECG monitoring and has intravenous access in place [51,67,77,117,118]. In addition, these patients should have adequate GI decontamination and, preferably, have passed a charcoal stool. Patients should always be referred for psychiatric evaluation, and pregnant women should be directed to prenatal counseling.

No consensus has been reached on emergency department observation for patients with ingestions of immediate-release trazodone, nefazodone, venlafaxine, and the SSRIs because of the paucity of overdose data for these medications, but guidelines exist [68,119]. Observation of asymptomatic patients for 6 to 8 hours or until the ECG returns to normal or baseline is reasonable. Any patient with signs or symptoms of toxicity should be admitted to the intensive care unit (ICU). Admission (or prolonged observation) is also prudent for patients with sustained-release bupropion overdose, as seizures have been reported as far as 12 to 16 hours after ingestion. Intentional MAOI ingestions should be admitted to an ICU or monitored setting since onset of toxicity may be significantly delayed.

All symptomatic patients should have a rapid evaluation of the airway and, if obtunded or hypoventilating, be immediately intubated. Because CA toxicity increases with acidemia, an ABG demonstrating a pH less than 7.4 or hypercarbia should prompt intubation and hyperventilation even in the patient who is able to protect his or her airway. Once an airway is established, the patient should be appropriately ventilated to prevent respiratory acidosis and subsequent deterioration of his or her condition.

GI decontamination for severely ill patients presenting within an hour of ingestion, should consist of oral activated charcoal. Because some CAs have a small enterohepatic circulation, an additional one to two doses of aqueous charcoal (25 g) may be considered [120–122] if clinical conditions are appropriate. This dose should not be administered in the presence of an ileus, gastric distention, or altered mental status with an unsecured airway. Because the majority of these agents are extensively protein bound, hemodialysis and hemoperfusion are not effective in reducing the toxic effects of CAs.

Single or brief flurries of seizures should be treated with a benzodiazepine [23,25]. Seizures are frequently isolated, and the additional use of an anticonvulsant is not indicated in this situation. Status epilepticus should be aggressively managed to prevent the development of acidosis, hyperthermia, and rhabdomyolysis [62,63,66,123–126]. As cardiotoxicity worsens dramatically in the presence of acidemia, rapid control of seizures is mandatory. Status epilepticus should be managed with large doses of benzodiazepines. In the setting of hydrazine-derived MAOI overdose and refractory seizures, empiric pyridoxine should be administered (1 to 5 gm IV). If seizures persist despite appropriate benzodiazepine dosing, propofol may be useful since it has both GABA and *N*-methyl-D-aspartate activity, but there are no data on its use in this setting. Barbiturates should also be considered since they directly open chloride channels. Failing this, management becomes controversial. Administering a nondepolarizing short-acting neuromuscular blocking agent such as vecuronium along with a barbiturate anticonvulsant (e.g., phenobarbital, 15 to 20 mg per kg, or thiopental, 3 to 5 mg per kg) is one option but continuous electroencephalographic monitoring should be used. Chemical paralysis helps treat or prevent hyperthermia, rhabdomyolysis, acidosis, and further deterioration. If the patient continues to have seizure activity once the paralytic has worn off, an additional dose of vecuronium should be given and more aggressive anticonvulsant or general anesthesia should be administered [25,42,127–130]. Serum alkalinization does not affect seizure activity. There is no data to suggest that other anticonvulsants such as phenytoin, levetiracetam, and valproate are effective in terminating seizures; animal data is suggestive of worsening outcomes with phenytoin.

Hypotension often responds to fluid resuscitation. Because concomitant acidosis or abnormal cardiac conduction is often present, a sodium bicarbonate solution can be used for both fluid resuscitation and serum alkalinization. A solution of 1,000 mL dextrose 5% in water with 150 mEq $NaHCO_3$ (roughly equivalent to 0.9% NaCl) is suggested. The rate of fluid administration should be adjusted to maintain a serum pH of 7.45 to 7.55 without causing hypernatremia. In an adult, an initial rate of approximately 200 to 300 mL per hour (1.5 to 2.0 times maintenance fluids) is usually adequate. Many clinicians give boluses of sodium bicarbonate (44 to 50 mEq per bolus) to achieve the same effect. It is difficult to adequately alkalinize the serum in the face of hypokalemia. Since IV bicarbonate will force potassium into the cells, larger potassium doses than anticipated, will be needed to keep the patient normokalemic.

In the event of refractory hypotension, cardiovascular monitoring (arterial line, central venous pressure, systemic vascular resistance, and cardiac index by invasive or noninvasive modalities) may be necessary. Pressor therapy with direct-acting sympathomimetics, such as NE, phenylephrine, or epinephrine, has been shown to be more effective than indirect-acting agents, such as dopamine [131–133]. In experimental rat models, the combination of epinephrine and sodium bicarbonate increased survival and decreased the frequency of arrhythmias. Moreover, this duo drug regimen was found to be more efficacious than the combination of sodium bicarbonate and norepinephrine [132]. If hypotension remains refractory, an inotropic agent such as dobutamine may be required and can be directed by the cardiovascular parameters. Failing optimum medical therapy, mechanical options including intra-aortic balloon pumps and extracorporeal circulatory support is recommended.

Abnormal conduction (QRS complex greater than 120 ms in the limb leads) and ventricular dysrhythmias are treated with alkalinization. A combination of sodium bicarbonate infusion and hyperventilation may be more useful than either alone, although hyperventilation is effective if the patient cannot tolerate the sodium load [83,84,86,134–137]. By combining the two modalities, the arterial partial pressure of carbon dioxide can be maintained at approximately 30 to 35 mm Hg, which prevents cerebral vasoconstriction, while serum sodium is kept within reasonable limits. Optimal arterial pH is between 7.45 and 7.55. Ventricular dysrhythmias that are not responsive to alkalinization may respond to lidocaine. Other than β-adrenergic blockers, no antidysrhythmics have been studied; although phenytoin has been used anecdotally in the 1970s and 1980s. In animal studies, propranolol was effective in improving conduction but led to intractable hypotension [5,83,85,86,134]. Other type IA and IC antidysrhythmics are contraindicated because they worsen cardiotoxicity. Amiodarone, a class III antidysrhythmic, was found to be of no benefit in tricyclic antidepressant-poisoned animal models. In addition, it was felt that the use of amiodarone might have been detrimental because it can further prolong the QTc interval and cause negative inotropy [138]. The successful use of magnesium sulfate was reported in a 23-month-old child who presented with ventricular tachycardia after ingesting unknown amounts of amitriptyline. The child had received normal saline, lidocaine, bicarbonate infusion, and cardioversion without effect. Subsequent magnesium sulfate resulted in normalization of the cardiac rhythm and clinical improvement [68]. Overdrive pacing is another option, but controlled studies are lacking [89].

More recently, the use of lipid emulsion therapy in the clinical scenario of lipid-soluble drug toxicity such as local anesthetics and calcium channel blockers has been gaining wide acceptance in the practice of critical care and emergency medicine [139–142]. Numerous studies have demonstrated significant cardiovascular improvement with severe lipid-soluble drug toxicity when infused with lipid emulsions. Most CAs are lipid soluble and produce significant cardiovascular instability with collapse that may be refractory to standard measures and sodium bicarbonate therapy. In animal models, infusion with lipid emulsion therapy proved to be more potent in reversing cardiac arrest and hypotension and also preventing further cardiovascular collapse [139]. Currently, there are two theories that explain why lipid emulsions may be effective. The first theory is based on the fact that the lipid emulsions create a lipid basin that sequesters lipid soluble drugs away from their site of action. The second theory is that lipid emulsions provide relief to a stressed myocardium by providing high energy to the heart [139,141]. This concept is similar to the use of high-dose insulin regimen for calcium channel blockers toxicity. In conclusion, lipid emulsion infusion should be strongly considered when conventional treatments such as oxygen therapy, fluids, inopressors, and sodium bicarbonate have failed to provide significant results.

Treatment of serotonin syndrome is primarily supportive. Sedation, paralysis, intubation and ventilation, anticonvulsants, antihypertensives, and aggressive rapid cooling may all be necessary. Some success has been achieved with the nonspecific serotonin antagonist cyproheptadine (4 to 12 mg every 8 hours orally or 4 mg per hour to a maximum of 24 mg in 24 hours) [98], but cyproheptadine has significant antimuscarinic effects. Dopamine-2-receptor antagonists, such as haloperidol, have occasionally been effective, but safety and efficacy data are lacking. Bromocriptine increases brain serotonin levels and is contraindicated, and dantrolene may enhance brain 5-HT metabolism and should not be used.

Any patient with an acute MAOI overdose or persistent signs and symptoms from food or drug interactions should be admitted to an intensive care setting for at least 24 hours. Therapy for food or drug interactions is aimed at lowering the blood pressure. A rapidly direct-acting agent that is easy to titrate is recommended (e.g., nitroprusside or nitroglycerine) [143].

Treatment of MAOI overdose is entirely supportive. Muscular hyperactivity and seizures are treated with high-dose benzodiazepines. Hyperthermia that does not respond to benzodiazepine therapy and cooling requires rapid-sequence intubation and paralysis with a nondepolarizing agent to completely shut down muscle activity. Bromocriptine should not be used, as it has drug interactions and is an uncontrolled D_2 agonist and stimulant. Dantrolene is ineffective as it works peripherally and does not affect the central causes of hyperthermia [111,144]. Symptomatic or severe cardiovascular (sympathetic) hyperactivity should be treated with agents that have readily reversible effects and can be titrated to response. Agents such as nitroprusside, nitroglycerine, and esmolol are recommended. Nicardipine can also be used. For cardiovascular depression, direct-acting agents, such as epinephrine, NE, and isoproterenol, are preferred. Although MAO inhibition may prolong their effects, these agents are predominantly metabolized by catechol-O-methyltransferase.

With the exception of MAOI overdose, patients who survive the first 24 hours without major complications (hypoxia, prolonged seizures, profound acidosis, and hyperthermia) generally do well. Most patients show some improvement within 24 hours. Once cardiac conduction improves (narrowing of QRS complex to 110 ms) alkalinization can be discontinued (usually within 12 hours) and the pH allowed to normalize. If the QRS complex again widens, alkalinization should be resumed and the weaning process repeated. Once the ECG has normalized without alkalinization, the patient should be monitored for an additional 12 to 24 hours in the ICU. The patient should be awake and alert, and have passed a charcoal stool before transfer out of the unit. All overdose patients should be referred for psychiatric evaluation before discharge.

Other Management Considerations

Controversial or investigational therapies for CA poisoning include phenytoin, physostigmine, prophylactic alkalinization, mechanical cardiovascular support, antibody therapy, and adenosine antagonists [145–147]. Although phenytoin binds to voltage-dependent Na^+ channels and prevents propagation of seizures, it has no GABA effect and does not prevent toxic seizures [148]. Some animal studies suggested that phenytoin was effective but others did not [129,148]. Studies using phenytoin to improve cardiac conduction were poorly controlled and not reproducible [117,129,149]. Canine data showed that phenytoin transiently facilitates conduction but then increases the incidence and duration of ventricular tachycardia and does not improve survival, suggesting that phenytoin is potentially detrimental [150].

Physostigmine (see Chapter 102) has been used to antagonize the antimuscarinic effects of CAs such as agitated delirium [151,152]. However, bradycardia and asystole have been reported with physostigmine in the presence of aberrant conduction, and as a carbamate pesticide, it may precipitate seizures [152]. Thus, physostigmine is not advocated to treat acute CA overdose and is contraindicated in those with cardiac conduction disturbances.

No studies have been done regarding prophylactic alkalinization in patients with normal cardiac condition. Because altering the pH alters the reliability of the QRS width as a predictor of cardiotoxicity, such therapy is not recommended. Alkalinization is also not without risks, including hyperosmolality, cerebral vasoconstriction, hypokalemia, and alterations in ionized calcium concentrations. There is no evidence that it affects the seizure threshold.

In moribund patients in whom conventional therapy has failed, the use of mechanical circulatory support, such as intra-aortic balloon pump assist or partial cardiac bypass, may be life-saving. In this situation, the use of extracorporeal measures supports myocardial, hepatic, and cerebral perfusion while allowing the liver endogenously to detoxify the CA [107,153–155].

ACKNOWLEDGMENTS

Thank you to Dr. Khatiyar his contributions to the previous version of this chapter.

References

1. Kosten TR, Schumann B, Wright D, et al: A preliminary study of desipramine in the treatment of cocaine abuse in methadone maintenance patients. *J Clin Psychiatry* 48(11):442–444, 1987.
2. Richardson JW 3rd, Richelson E: Antidepressants: a clinical update for medical practitioners. *Mayo Clin Proc* 59(5):330–337, 1984.
3. Pratt LA, Brody D, Gu Q: Antidepressant use in persons aged 12 and over: United States, 2005–2008. *NCHS Data Brief* (76):1–8, 2011.
4. Mowry JB, Spyker DA, Brooks DE, et al: 2014 Annual report of the American Association of poison control centers' national poison data system (NPDS): 32nd annual report. *Clin Toxicol (Phila)* 53(10):962–1147, 2015.
5. Hollister LE: Tricyclic antidepressants (first of two parts). *N Engl J Med* 299(20):1106–1109, 1978.
6. Richelson E: Antimuscarinic and other receptor-blocking properties of antidepressants. *Mayo Clin Proc* 58(1):40–46, 1983.
7. Richelson E: Tricyclic antidepressants and histamine H1 receptors. *Mayo Clin Proc* 54(10):669–674, 1979.
8. Bryant SG, Guernsey BG, Ingrim NB: Review of bupropion. *Clin Pharm* 2(6):525–537, 1983.
9. Hayes PE, Kristoff CA: Adverse reactions to five new antidepressants. *Clin Pharm* 5(6):471–480, 1986.
10. Perry R, Cassagnol M: Desvenlafaxine: a new serotonin-norepinephrine reuptake inhibitor for the treatment of adults with major depressive disorder. *Clin Ther* 31 Pt 1:1374–1404, 2009.
11. Bruno A, Morabito P, Spina E, et al: The role of levomilnacipran in the management of major depressive disorder: a comprehensive review. *Curr Neuropharmacol* 14(2):191–199, 2016.
12. Sanchez C, Asin KE, Artigas F: Vortioxetine, a novel antidepressant with multimodal activity: review of preclinical and clinical data. *Pharmacol Ther* 145:43–57, 2015.
13. Richelson E: Pharmacology of antidepressants. *Mayo Clin Proc* 76(5):511–527, 2001.
14. Richelson E: The newer antidepressants: structures, pharmacokinetics, pharmacodynamics, and proposed mechanisms of action. *Psychopharmacol Bull* 20(2):213–223, 1984.
15. Richelson E: Alcohol and the elderly. Psychotropics and the elderly: interactions to watch for. *Geriatrics* 39(12):30–36, 39–42, 1984.
16. Tetrud JW, Langston JW: The effect of deprenyl (selegiline) on the natural history of Parkinson's disease. *Science* 245(4917):519–522, 1989.
17. Wander TJ, Nelson O, Okazaki H, et al: Antagonism by antidepressants of serotonin S1 and S2 receptors of normal human brain in vitro. *Eur J Pharmacol* 132(2/3):115–121, 1986.
18. Snyder SH, Yamamura HI: Antidepressants and the muscarinic acetylcholine receptor. *Arch Gen Psychiatry* 34(2):236–239, 1977.
19. Freeman JW, Mundy GR, Beattie RR, et al: Cardiac abnormalities in poisoning with tricyclic antidepressants. *Br Med J* 2(5657):610–611, 1969.
20. Shannon M, Merola J, Lovejoy FH Jr: Hypotension in severe tricyclic antidepressant overdose. *Am J Emerg Med* 6(5):439–442, 1988.
21. Jandhyala BS, Steenberg ML, Perel JM, et al: Effects of several tricyclic antidepressants on the hemodynamics and myocardial contractility of the anesthetized dogs. *Eur J Pharmacol* 42(4):403–410, 1977.
22. Thanacoody HK, Thomas SH: Tricyclic antidepressant poisoning: cardiovascular toxicity. *Toxicol Rev* 24(3):205–214, 2005.
23. Malatynska E, Knapp RJ, Ikeda M, et al: Antidepressants and seizure-interactions at the GABA-receptor chloride-ionophore complex. *Life Sci* 43(4):303–307, 1988.
24. Freeman JM, Lietman PS: A basic approach to the understanding of seizures and the mechanism of action and metabolism of anticonvulsants. *Adv Pediatr* 20(0):291–321, 1973.
25. Roszkowski AP, Schuler ME, Schultz R: Augmentation of pentylenetetrazol induced seizures by tricyclic antidepressants. *Mater Med Pol* 8(2):141–145, 1976.
26. Weinberger J, Nicklas WJ, Berl S: Mechanism of action of anticonvulsants. Role of the differential effects on the active uptake of putative neurotransmitters. *Neurology* 26(2):162–166, 1976.
27. Rickels K, Schweizer E: Clinical overview of serotonin reuptake inhibitors. *J Clin Psychiatry* 51 Suppl B:9–12, 1990.
28. Dechant KL, Clissold SP: Sumatriptan. A review of its pharmacodynamic and pharmacokinetic properties, and therapeutic efficacy in the acute treatment of migraine and cluster headache. *Drugs* 43(5):776–798, 1992.
29. Leonard BE: Pharmacological differences of serotonin reuptake inhibitors and possible clinical relevance. *Drugs* 43 Suppl 2:3–9; discussion 9-10, 1992.
30. Dechant KL, Clissold SP: Paroxetine. A review of its pharmacodynamic and pharmacokinetic properties, and therapeutic potential in depressive illness. *Drugs* 41(2):225–253, 1991.
31. Baldessarini R: Drugs and treatment of psychiatric disorders, in Hardman J, Limbird LE, Molinoff PB (eds): *Goodman and Gilman's The Pharmacological Basis of Therapeutics*. New York, NY, McGraw Hill, 1996, p 1.
32. Wells DG, Bjorksten AR: Monoamine oxidase inhibitors revisited. *Can J Anaesth* 36(1):64–74, 1989.
33. Blackwell B: Adverse effects of antidepressant drugs. Part 1: monoamine oxidase inhibitors and tricyclics. *Drugs* 21(3):201–219, 1981.
34. Blackwell B, Marley E: Interactions of cheese and of its constituents with monoamine oxidase inhibitors. *Br J Pharmacol Chemother* 26(1):120–141, 1966.
35. Smith CB: The role of monoamine oxidase in the intraneuronal metabolism of norepinephrine released by indirectly-acting sympathomimetic amines or by adrenergic nerve stimulation. *J Pharmacol Exp Ther* 151(2):207–220, 1966.
36. Tollefson GD: Monoamine oxidase inhibitors: a review. *J Clin Psychiatry* 44(8):280–288, 1983.
37. Crome P: Antidepressant overdosage. *Drugs* 23(6):431–461, 1982.
38. Crome P: Antidepressant poisoning. *Acta Psychiatr Scand Suppl* 302:95–101, 1983.
39. Hill S, Yau K, Whitwam J: MAOIs to RIMAs in anaesthesia—a literature review. *Psychopharmacology (Berl)* 106 Suppl:S43–S45, 1992.
40. Mahmood I: Clinical pharmacokinetics and pharmacodynamics of selegiline. An update. *Clin Pharmacokinet* 33(2):91–102, 1997.
41. Perry PJ, Pfohl BM, Holstad SG: The relationship between antidepressant response and tricyclic antidepressant plasma concentrations. A retrospective analysis of the literature using logistic regression analysis. *Clin Pharmacokinet* 13(6):381–392, 1987.
42. Pentel P, Keyler DE, Haddad LM: Tricyclic, tetracyclic, and atypical antidepressants, in Haddad L, Shannon MW, Winchester JF (eds): *Clinical Management of Poisoning and Drug Overdose*. Philadelphia, PA, WB Saunders, 1977, p 1.
43. Marshall JB, Forker AD: Cardiovascular effects of tricyclic antidepressant drugs: therapeutic usage, overdose, and management of complications. *Am Heart J* 103(3):401–414, 1982.
44. Trimble M, Anlezark G, Meldrum B: Seizure activity in photosensitive baboons following antidepressant drugs and the role of serotoninergic mechanisms. *Psychopharmacology (Berl)* 51(2):159–164, 1977.
45. Malatynska E, Giroux ML, Dilsaver SC, et al: Chronic treatment with amitriptyline alters the GABA-mediated uptake of 36Cl- in the rat brain. *Pharmacol Biochem Behav* 39(2):553–556, 1991.
46. Gard H, Knapp D, Walle T, et al: Qualitative and quantitative studies on the disposition of amitriptyline and other tricyclic antidepressant drugs in man as it relates to the management of the overdosed patient. *Clin Toxicol* 6(4):571–584, 1973.
47. Freilich DI, Giardina EG: Imipramine binding to alpha-1-acid glycoprotein in normal subjects and cardiac patients. *Clin Pharmacol Ther* 35(5):670–674, 1984.
48. Javaid JI, Hendricks K, Davis JM: Alpha 1-acid glycoprotein involvement in high affinity binding of tricyclic antidepressants to human plasma. *Biochem Pharmacol* 32(7):1149–1153, 1983.
49. Levitt MA, Sullivan JB Jr, Owens SM, et al: Amitriptyline plasma protein binding: effect of plasma pH and relevance to clinical overdose. *Am J Emerg Med* 4(2):121–125, 1986.
50. Ereshefsky L, Tran-Johnson T, Davis CM, et al: Pharmacokinetic factors affecting antidepressant drug clearance and clinical effect: evaluation of doxepin and imipramine—new data and review. *Clin Chem* 34(5):863–880, 1988.
51. Callaham M, Kassel D: Epidemiology of fatal tricyclic antidepressant ingestion: implications for management. *Ann Emerg Med* 14(1):1–9, 1985.
52. Chung KJ, Wang YC, Liu BM, et al: Management of ventricular dysrhythmia secondary to trazodone overdose. *J Emerg Med* 35(2):171–174, 2008.
53. Foulke GE, Albertson TE: QRS interval in tricyclic antidepressant overdosage: inaccuracy as a toxicity indicator in emergency settings. *Ann Emerg Med* 16(2):160–163, 1987.
54. Groleau G, Jotte R, Barish R: The electrocardiographic manifestations of cyclic antidepressant therapy and overdose: a review. *J Emerg Med* 8(5):597–605, 1990.
55. Davidson J: Seizures and bupropion: a review. *J Clin Psychiatry* 50(7):256–261, 1989.
56. Bateman DN, Chaplin S, Ferner RE: Safety of mianserin. *Lancet* 2(8607):401–402, 1988.
57. Kulig K, Rumack BH, Sullivan JB Jr, et al: Amoxapine overdose. Coma and seizures without cardiotoxic effects. *JAMA* 248(9):1092–1094, 1982.
58. Holliday W, Brasfield KH Jr, Powers B: Grand mal seizures induced by maprotiline. *Am J Psychiatry* 139(5):673–674, 1982.
59. Peterson CD: Seizures induced by acute loxapine overdose. *Am J Psychiatry* 138(8):1089–1091, 1981.

60. White CM, Gailey RA, Levin GM, et al: Seizure resulting from a venlafaxine overdose. *Ann Pharmacother* 31(2):178–180, 1997.
61. Sheehan DV, Welch JB, Fishman SM: A case of bupropion-induced seizure. *J Nerv Ment Dis* 174(8):496–498, 1986.
62. Morazin F, Lumbroso A, Harry P, et al: Cardiogenic shock and status epilepticus after massive bupropion overdose. *Clin Toxicol (Phila)* 45(7):794–797, 2007.
63. Jepsen F, Matthews J, Andrews FJ: Sustained release bupropion overdose: an important cause of prolonged symptoms after an overdose. *Emerg Med J* 20(6):560–561, 2003.
64. Rosenberg J, Pentel P, Pond S, et al: Hyperthermia associated with drug intoxication. *Crit Care Med* 14(11):964–969, 1986.
65. Goldberg RJ, Capone RJ, Hunt JD: Cardiac complications following tricyclic antidepressant overdose. Issues for monitoring policy. *JAMA* 254(13):1772–1775, 1985.
66. Hantson P, Benaissa M, Clemessy JL, et al: Hyperthermia complicating tricyclic antidepressant overdose. *Intensive Care Med* 22(5):453–455, 1996.
67. Kerr GW, McGuffie AC, Wilkie S: Tricyclic antidepressant overdose: a review. *Emerg Med J* 18(4):236–241, 2001.
68. Citak A, Soysal DD, Uçsel R, et al: Efficacy of long duration resuscitation and magnesium sulphate treatment in amitriptyline poisoning. *Eur J Emerg Med* 9(1):63–66, 2002.
69. Pratt GD, Bowery NG: Repeated administration of desipramine and a GABAB receptor antagonist, CGP 36742, discretely up-regulates GABAB receptor binding sites in rat frontal cortex. *Br J Pharmacol* 110(2):724–735, 1993.
70. Suzdak PD, Gianutsos G: Effect of chronic imipramine or baclofen on GABA-B binding and cyclic AMP production in cerebral cortex. *Eur J Pharmacol* 131(1):129–133, 1986.
71. Abbott R: Hyponatremia due to antidepressant medications. *Ann Emerg Med* 12(11):708–710, 1983.
72. Tao GK, Harada DT, Kootsikas ME, et al: Amoxapine-induced tardive dyskinesia. *Drug Intell Clin Pharm* 19(7/8):548–549, 1985.
73. Baca L, Martinelli L: Neuroleptic malignant syndrome: a unique association with a tricyclic antidepressant. *Neurology* 40(11):1797–1798, 1990.
74. Borganelli M, Forman MB: Simulation of acute myocardial infarction by desipramine hydrochloride. *Am Heart J* 119(6):1413–1414, 1990.
75. Langou RA, Van Dyke C, Tahan SR, et al: Cardiovascular manifestations of tricyclic antidepressant overdose. *Am Heart J* 100(4):458–464, 1980.
76. Salzman C: Clinical use of antidepressant blood levels and the electrocardiogram. *N Engl J Med* 313(8):512–513, 1985.
77. Boehnert MT, Lovejoy FH Jr: Value of the QRS duration versus the serum drug level in predicting seizures and ventricular arrhythmias after an acute overdose of tricyclic antidepressants. *N Engl J Med* 313(8):474–479, 1985.
78. Niemann JT, Bessen HA, Rothstein RJ, et al: Electrocardiographic criteria for tricyclic antidepressant cardiotoxicity. *Am J Cardiol* 57(13):1154–1159, 1986.
79. Wolfe TR, Caravati EM, Rollins DE: Terminal 40-ms frontal plane QRS axis as a marker for tricyclic antidepressant overdose. *Ann Emerg Med* 18(4):348–351, 1989.
80. Pentel PR, Benowitz NL: Tricyclic antidepressant poisoning. Management of arrhythmias. *Med Toxicol* 1(2):101–121, 1986.
81. Pentel P, Benowitz N: Efficacy and mechanism of action of sodium bicarbonate in the treatment of desipramine toxicity in rats. *J Pharmacol Exp Ther* 230(1):12–19, 1984.
82. Tamargo J, Rodriguez S, Garcia de Jalon P: Electrophysiological effects of desipramine on guinea pig papillary muscles. *Eur J Pharmacol* 55(2):171–179, 1979.
83. Nattel S, Keable H, Sasyniuk BI: Experimental amitriptyline intoxication: electrophysiologic manifestations and management. *J Cardiovasc Pharmacol* 6(1):83–89, 1984.
84. Nattel S, Mittleman M: Treatment of ventricular tachyarrhythmias resulting from amitriptyline toxicity in dogs. *J Pharmacol Exp Ther* 231(2):430–435, 1984.
85. Freeman JW, Loughhead MG: Beta blockade in the treatment of tricyclic antidepressant overdosage. *Med J Aust* 1(25):1233–1235, 1973.
86. Sasyniuk BI, Jhamandas V: Mechanism of reversal of toxic effects of amitriptyline on cardiac Purkinje fibers by sodium bicarbonate. *J Pharmacol Exp Ther* 231(2):387–394, 1984.
87. Akhtar M, Goldschlager NF: Brugada electrocardiographic pattern due to tricyclic antidepressant overdose. *J Electrocardiol* 39(3):336–339, 2006.
88. Pentel PR, Keyler DE: Effects of high dose alpha-1-acid glycoprotein on desipramine toxicity in rats. *J Pharmacol Exp Ther* 246(3):1061–1066, 1988.
89. Davison ET: Amitriptyline-induced Torsade de Pointes. Successful therapy with atrial pacing. *J Electrocardiol* 18(3):299–301, 1985.
90. Alderton HR: Tricyclic medication in children and the QT interval: case report and discussion. *Can J Psychiatry* 40(6):325–329, 1995.
91. Catalano G, Catalano MC, Epstein MA, et al: QTc interval prolongation associated with citalopram overdose: a case report and literature review. *Clin Neuropharmacol* 24(3):158–162, 2001.
92. Nicotra MB, Rivera M, Pool JL, et al: Tricyclic antidepressant overdose: clinical and pharmacologic observations. *Clin Toxicol* 18(5):599–613, 1981.
93. Rudorfer MV: Cardiovascular changes and plasma drug levels after amitriptyline overdose. *J Toxicol Clin Toxicol* 19(1):67–78, 1982.
94. Janowsky D, Curtis G, Zisook S, et al: Trazodone-aggravated ventricular arrhythmias. *J Clin Psychopharmacol* 3(6):372–376, 1983.
95. Harvengt C, Desager JP, Vanderbist M, et al: Sympathetic nervous system response in acute cardiovascular toxicity induced by amitriptyline in conscious rabbits. *Toxicol Appl Pharmacol* 44(1):115–126, 1978.
96. Collis MG, Shepherd JT: Antidepressant drug action and presynaptic alpha-receptors. *Mayo Clin Proc* 55(9):567–572, 1980.
97. Buckley NA, Dawson AH, Isbister GK: Serotonin syndrome. *BMJ* 348:g1626, 2014.
98. Graudins A, Stearman A, Chan B: Treatment of the serotonin syndrome with cyproheptadine. *J Emerg Med* 16(4):615–619, 1998.
99. Kelly CA, Dhaun N, Laing WJ, et al: Comparative toxicity of citalopram and the newer antidepressants after overdose. *J Toxicol Clin Toxicol* 42(1):67–71, 2004.
100. Maddry JK, Breyer K, Cook KM, et al: Monomorphic ventricular tachycardia after intentional citalopram overdose. *Am J Emerg Med* 31(2):447e5–447e8, 2013.
101. Kraai EP, Seifert SA: Citalopram overdose: a fatal case. *J Med Toxicol* 11(2):232–236, 2015.
102. Pacher P, Ungvari Z, Nanasi PP, et al: Speculations on difference between tricyclic and selective serotonin reuptake inhibitor antidepressants on their cardiac effects. Is there any? *Curr Med Chem* 6(6):469–480, 1999.
103. Schatzberg AF, Dessain E, O'Neil P, et al: Recent studies on selective serotonergic antidepressants: trazodone, fluoxetine, and fluvoxamine. *J Clin Psychopharmacol* 7(6 Suppl):44S–49S, 1987.
104. Steinberg MI, Smallwood JK, Holland DR, et al: Hemodynamic and electrocardiographic effects of fluoxetine and its major metabolite, norfluoxetine, in anesthetized dogs. *Toxicol Appl Pharmacol* 82(1):70–79, 1986.
105. Fisch C: Effect of fluoxetine on the electrocardiogram. *J Clin Psychiatry* 46(3 Pt 2):42–44, 1985.
106. Bruccoleri RE, Burns MM: A literature review of the use of sodium bicarbonate for the treatment of QRS widening. *J Med Toxicol* 12(1):121–129, 2016.
107. Heise CW, Skolnik AB, Raschke RA, et al: Two cases of refractory cardiogenic shock secondary to bupropion successfully treated with veno-arterial extracorporeal membrane oxygenation. *J Med Toxicol* 12:301–304, 2016.
108. Rivas-Coppola MS, Patterson AL, Morgan R, et al: Bupropion overdose presenting as status epilepticus in an infant. *Pediatr Neurol* 53(3):257–261, 2015.
109. Shenoi AN, Gertz SJ, Mikkilineni S, et al: Refractory hypotension from massive bupropion overdose successfully treated with extracorporeal membrane oxygenation. *Pediatr Emerg Care* 27(1):43–45, 2011.
110. Pascale P, Oddo M, Pacher P, et al: Severe rhabdomyolysis following venlafaxine overdose. *Ther Drug Monit* 27(5):562–564, 2005.
111. Thorp M, Toombs D, Harmon B: Monoamine oxidase inhibitor overdose. *West J Med* 166(4):275–277, 1997.
112. Attaway A, Sroujieh L, Mersfelder TL, et al: "Ping-pong gaze" secondary to monoamine oxidase inhibitor overdose. *J Pharmacol Pharmacother* 7(1):34–37, 2016.
113. Izumi T, Iwamoto N, Kitachi Y, et al: Effects of co-administration of a selective serotonin reuptake inhibitor and monoamine oxidase inhibitors on 5-HT-related behavior in rats. *Eur J Pharmacol* 532(3):258–264, 2006.
114. Giroud C, Horisberger B, Eap C, et al: Death following acute poisoning by moclobemide. *Forensic Sci Int* 140(1):101–107, 2004.
115. Eizadi-Mood N, Moein N, Saghaei M: Evaluation of relationship between arterial and venous blood gas values in the patients with tricyclic antidepressant poisoning. *Clin Toxicol (Phila)* 43(5):357–360, 2005.
116. Nelson ZJ, Stellpflug SJ, Engebretsen KM: What can a urine drug screening immunoassay really tell us? *J Pharm Pract* 29(5):516–526, 2016.
117. Callaham M: Admission criteria for tricyclic antidepressant ingestion. *West J Med* 137(5):425–429, 1982.
118. Pentel P, Olson KR, Becker CE, et al: Late complications of tricyclic antidepressant overdose. *West J Med* 138(3):423–424, 1983.
119. Nelson LS, Erdman AR, Booze LL, et al: Selective serotonin reuptake inhibitor poisoning: An evidence-based consensus guideline for out-of-hospital management. *Clin Toxicol (Phila)* 45(4):315–332, 2007.
120. Crome P, Adams R, Ali C, et al: Activated charcoal in tricyclic antidepressant poisoning: pilot controlled clinical trial. *Hum Toxicol* 2(2):205–209, 1983.
121. Goldberg MJ, Park GD, Spector R, et al: Lack of effect of oral activated charcoal on imipramine clearance. *Clin Pharmacol Ther* 38(3):350–353, 1985.
122. Rinder HM, Murphy JW, Higgins GL: Impact of unusual gastrointestinal problems on the treatment of tricyclic antidepressant overdose. *Ann Emerg Med* 17(10):1079–1081, 1988.
123. Taboulet P, Michard F, Muszynski J, et al: Cardiovascular repercussions of seizures during cyclic antidepressant poisoning. *J Toxicol Clin Toxicol* 33(3):205–211, 1995.
124. Borek HA, Holstege CP: Hyperthermia and multiorgan failure after abuse of "bath salts" containing 3,4-methylenedioxypyrovalerone. *Ann Emerg Med* 60(1):103–105, 2012.
125. Degner D, Porzig J, Rüther E, et al: Serotonin syndrome with severe hyperthermia after ingestion of tranylcypromine combined with serotonin reuptake inhibitors and tyramine-rich food in a case of suicide. *Pharmacopsychiatry* 43(7):284–285, 2010.
126. Richards JR, Colby DK: Stimulant-induced hyperthermia and ice-water submersion: practical considerations. *Clin Toxicol (Phila)* 54(1):69–70, 2016.
127. Bender AS, Hertz L: Evidence for involvement of the astrocytic benzodiazepine receptor in the mechanism of action of convulsant and anticonvulsant drugs. *Life Sci* 43(6):477–484, 1988.
128. Bartholini G: GABA receptor agonists: pharmacological spectrum and therapeutic actions. *Med Res Rev* 5(1):55–75, 1985.
129. Blake KV, Massey KL, Hendeles L, et al: Relative efficacy of phenytoin and phenobarbital for the prevention of theophylline-induced seizures in mice. *Ann Emerg Med* 17(10):1024–1028, 1988.
130. Young JA, Galloway WH: Treatment of severe imipramine poisoning. *Arch Dis Child* 46(247):353–355, 1971.

131. Knudsen K, Abrahamsson J: Effects of epinephrine and norepinephrine on hemodynamic parameters and arrhythmias during a continuous infusion of amitriptyline in rats. *J Toxicol Clin Toxicol* 31(3):461–471, 1993.
132. Knudsen K, Abrahamsson J: Epinephrine and sodium bicarbonate independently and additively increase survival in experimental amitriptyline poisoning. *Crit Care Med* 25(4):669–674, 1997.
133. Buchman AL, Dauer J, Geiderman J: The use of vasoactive agents in the treatment of refractory hypotension seen in tricyclic antidepressant overdose. *J Clin Psychopharmacol* 10(6):409–413, 1990.
134. Bajaj AK, Woosley RL, Roden DM: Acute electrophysiologic effects of sodium administration in dogs treated with O-desmethyl encainide. *Circulation* 80(4):994–1002, 1989.
135. Brown TC: Sodium bicarbonate treatment for tricyclic antidepressant arrhythmias in children. *Med J Aust* 2(10):380–382, 1976.
136. Hoffman JR, McElroy CR: Bicarbonate therapy for dysrhythmia and hypotension in tricyclic antidepressant overdose. *West J Med* 134(1):60–64, 1981.
137. Kingston ME: Hyperventilation in tricyclic antidepressant poisoning. *Crit Care Med* 7(12):550–551, 1979.
138. Barrueto F Jr, Chuang A, Cotter BW, et al: Amiodarone fails to improve survival in amitriptyline-poisoned mice. *Clin Toxicol (Phila)* 43(3):147–149, 2005.
139. Harvey M, Cave G: Intralipid outperforms sodium bicarbonate in a rabbit model of clomipramine toxicity. *Ann Emerg Med* 49(2):178–185, 185e1–185e4, 2007.
140. Tebbutt S, Harvey M, Nicholson T, et al: Intralipid prolongs survival in a rat model of verapamil toxicity. *Acad Emerg Med* 13(2):134–139, 2006.
141. Weinberg GL: Current concepts in resuscitation of patients with local anesthetic cardiac toxicity. *Reg Anesth Pain Med* 27(6):568–575, 2002.
142. Yoav G, Odelia G, Shaltiel C: A lipid emulsion reduces mortality from clomipramine overdose in rats. *Vet Hum Toxicol* 44(1):30, 2002.
143. Cramer C: Emergency! Hypertensive crisis from drug-food interaction. *Am J Nurs* 97(5):32, 1997.
144. Vassallo SU, Delaney KA: Pharmacologic effects on thermoregulation: mechanisms of drug-related heatstroke. *J Toxicol Clin Toxicol* 27(4/5):199–224, 1989.
145. Hannon JP, Pfannkuche HJ, Fozard JR: A role for mast cells in adenosine A3 receptor-mediated hypotension in the rat. *Br J Pharmacol* 115(6):945–952, 1995.
146. Kalkan S, Aygoren O, Akgun A, et al: Do adenosine receptors play a role in amitriptyline-induced cardiovascular toxicity in rats? *J Toxicol Clin Toxicol* 42(7):945–954, 2004.
147. Webb RL, Barclay BW, Graybill SC: Cardiovascular effects of adenosine A2 agonists in the conscious spontaneously hypertensive rat: a comparative study of three structurally distinct ligands. *J Pharmacol Exp Ther* 259(3):1203–1212, 1991.
148. Callaham M, Schumaker H, Pentel P: Phenytoin prophylaxis of cardiotoxicity in experimental amitriptyline poisoning. *J Pharmacol Exp Ther* 245(1):216–220, 1988.
149. Foianini A, Joseph Wiegand T, Benowitz N: What is the role of lidocaine or phenytoin in tricyclic antidepressant-induced cardiotoxicity? *Clin Toxicol (Phila)* 48(4):325–330, 2010.
150. Kulig K, Baror D, Marx J, et al: Phenytoin as treatment for tricyclic antidepressant cardiotoxicity in a canine model. *Vet Hum Toxicol (Abstract)* 26:399, 1984.
151. Bigger JT Jr, Kantor SJ, Glassman AH, et al: Is physostigmine effective for cardiac toxicity of tricyclic antidepressant drugs. *JAMA* 237(13):1311, 1977.
152. Pentel P, Peterson CD: Asystole complicating physostigmine treatment of tricyclic antidepressant overdose. *Ann Emerg Med* 9(11):588–590, 1980.
153. Freedberg RS, Friedman GR, Palu RN, et al: *Cardiogenic shock due to antihistamine overdose. Reversal with intra-aortic balloon counterpulsation. JAMA* 257(5):660–661, 1987.
154. Southall DP, Kilpatrick SM: Imipramine poisoning: survival of a child after prolonged cardiac massage. *Br Med J* 4(5943):508, 1974.
155. Wang GS, Levitan R, Wiegand TJ, et al: Extracorporeal Membrane Oxygenation (ECMO) for severe toxicological exposures: review of the Toxicology Investigators Consortium (ToxIC). *J Med Toxicol* 12(1):95–99, 2016.

Chapter 105 ■ Antipsychotic Poisoning

STEVEN B. BIRD

Antipsychotic agents, sometimes termed *neuroleptics* and *major tranquilizers*, are primarily used to treat schizophrenia, the manic phase of bipolar disorder, and agitated behaviors. They are also used as preanesthetics and to treat drug-associated delirium and hallucinations, nausea, vomiting, headaches, hiccups, pruritus, Tourette syndrome, and a variety of extrapyramidal movement disorders (e.g., chorea, dystonias, hemiballismus, spasms, tics, and torticollis). Antipsychotics are a structurally diverse group of heterocyclic compounds; more than 50 different drugs are available for clinical use worldwide with numerous others are in various stages of development. Classes include benzamide, benzepine, butyrophenone (phenylbutylpiperidine), dibenzo-oxepino pyrrole, diphenylbutylpiperidine, indole, phenothiazine, quinolinone, rauwolfia alkaloid, and thioxanthene derivatives (Table 105.1). The phenothiazine and thioxanthene classes are further subdivided into three groups (aliphatic, piperazine, and piperidine) based on central ring side-chain substitution.

Although traditionally classified by structure, antipsychotics are more ideally classified by pharmacologic profile. Each agent has a unique receptor-binding profile (Table 105.2), and this profile can be used to predict adverse effects in both therapeutic and overdose situations [1,2]. Clinical toxicity is the result of exaggerated pharmacologic activity. Antipsychotics are also classified as *typical* or *atypical* (Tables 105.1 and 105.2). Traditional or conventional antipsychotics, which readily produce extrapyramidal signs and symptoms (EPS) at antipsychotic doses, are considered typical. Newer agents that have minimal extrapyramidal side effects at clinically effective antipsychotic doses are effective for treating the negative symptoms (e.g., alogia, avolition, social withdrawal, and flattened affect) of schizophrenia and have a low propensity to cause tardive dyskinesia with long-term treatment are considered atypical [1,2]. The characterization of antipsychotics as typical or atypical is ultimately determined by receptor binding. One or more of several different receptor-binding characteristics are associated with drug atypia, and each agent is atypical for different reasons [3]. Understanding how specific receptor-binding characteristics produce clinical effects has facilitated the development of antipsychotics that separate antipsychotic activity from other activities; thus, minimizing adverse effects and maximizing patients' compliance.

Antipsychotic toxicity may occur as an idiosyncratic reaction during therapeutic use or following accidental or intentional overdose. Central nervous system (CNS) and cardiovascular disturbances are the most common dose-related toxic manifestations, but other effects include the anticholinergic syndrome (see Chapter 102 and various extrapyramidal syndromes). Therapeutic use has been associated with agranulocytosis, aplastic anemia, diabetes mellitus, hepatotoxicity, hypertriglyceridemia, fatal myocardial infarction, myocarditis, neuroleptic malignant syndrome (NMS) (see Chapter 185), pancreatitis, seizures, sleep apnea, sudden infant death syndrome, sudden adult death, venous thromboembolism, and vasculitis [5–8]. Most deaths are the consequence of suicidal overdose by psychotic or depressed adults and frequently involve mixed ingestions or ingestion of the agents chlorpromazine, loxapine, mesoridazine, quetiapine, or thioridazine [10,11]. Because of a large toxic to therapeutic ratio

TABLE 105.1

Classification and Dosing of Neuroleptic Agents

Structural class	Generic name (trade name)	Affinity of neuroleptic agent for dopamine (D_2) receptor (potency)[a]	Daily dose range (mg)
Typical agents			
Butyrophenone (phenyl-butylpiperidine)	Droperidol (Inapsine)	3+	1.25–30
	Haloperidol (Haldol)		
	Other: benperidol, bromperidol, melperone, pipamperone, trifluperidol[c]	2+	1–30
Diphenylbutylpiperidine	Pimozide (Orap)	2+	1–20
	Other: fluspirilene, penfluridol[c]		
Indole	Molindone (Moban)	1+	15–225
	Other: oxypertine[c]		
Phenothiazine			
Aliphatic	Chlorpromazine (Thorazine)	2+	25–2,000
	Promazine (Sparine)[b]	—	50–1,000
	Promethazine (Phenergan)	2+	25–150
	Triflupromazine (Vesprin)	—	5–90
Piperazine	Acetophenazine (Tindal)	—	40–400
	Fluphenazine (Prolixin)	3+	0.5–30
	Perphenazine (Trilafon)	3+	4–64
	Prochlorperazine (Compazine)	2+	10–150
	Trifluoperazine (Stelazine)	3+	2–40
	Thiethylperazine (Torecan)	—	10–30
Piperidine	Mesoridazine (Serentil)	2+	30–400
	Thioridazine (Mellaril, Millazine)	2+	20–800
	Other: diethazine, ethopropazine, levomepromazine, perazine, pipotiazine thiopropazate, thioproperazine, and pericyazinec		
Thioxanthene	Chlorprothixene (Taractan)	2+	30–600
	Clopenthixol[c]	—	—
	Flupenthixol[c]	3+	4
	Thiothixene (Navane)	3+	6–60
	Zuclopenthixol (Cisordinol, Clopixol)[c]	3+	10–50
Atypical agents			
Benzamides	Amisulpride[c]	2+	100–1,200
	Raclopride[c]	3+	5–8
	Remoxipride[c]	1+	150–600
	Sulpiride[c]	2+	100–1,600
	Sultopride[c]	2+	100–1,200
	Trimethobenzamide (Tigan)[b]	—	100–600
	Other: epidepride, eticlopride levosulpiride, nemonapride, and tiapridec		
Benzepine			
Dibenzodiazepine	Clozapine (Clozaril, Leponex)	1+	150–900
Dibenzo-oxazepine	Loxapine (Loxitane)	1+	20–250
Thienobenzodiazepine	Olanzapine (Zyprexa)	2+	5–20
Dibenzothiazepine	Quetiapine (Seroquel)	1+	300–600
Dibenzothiazepine	Zotepine[c]	2+	100–300
	Other: butaclamol, fluperlapine, clothiapine, metiapine, and savoxepinec		
Indole			
Benzisoxazole	Risperidone (Risperdal)	3+	2–16
	Paliperidone (Invega)	3+	3–12
Imidazolidinone	Sertindole (Serlect)[c]	3+	12–24
Benzisothiazole	Ziprasidone (Zeldox)	3+	40–160
	Other: iloperidonec		
Pyrrole	Asenapine (Saphris)	3+	10–20
Quinolinone	Aripiprazole (Abilify, Abitat)		
	Bifeprunox[c]	3+	10–30

0, minimal to none; 1+, low; 2+, moderate; 3+, high to very high.

[a]A higher numerical value indicates greater binding affinity (greater antagonism) at D_2 receptor. Binding affinity (potency) at D_2 receptor correlates with daily dose range.

[b]Antiemetic only.

[c]Not available for clinical use in the United States.

TABLE 105.2

Relative Neuroreceptor Affinities for Neuroleptics

Neuroleptic agent	Receptor: H_1 histaminergic	α_1-Adrenergic	α_2-Adrenergic	M_1 muscarinic	5-HT_{2A} serotonergic	EPS risk[a]
Typical agents						
Chlorpromazine	2+	3+	0	1+	3+	1+
Fluphenazine	0	0	0	0	0	3+
Haloperidol	0	1+	0	0	1+	3+
Loxapine	3+	3+	0	2+	3+	1+
Mesoridazine	3+	3+	—	1+	—	1+
Molindone	0	0	1+	0	0	3+
Perphenazine	1+	1+	0	0	—	3+
Pimozide	0	1+	—	0	1+	3+
Prochlorperazine	1+	1+	0	0	0	3+
Thioridazine	2+	3+	0	3+	2+	1+
Thiothixene	0	0	0	0	0	3+
Trifluoperazine	0	1+	0	0	1+	3+
Atypical agents						
(Ami)sulpiride	0	0	0	0	0	1+
Asenapine	3+	2+	2+	0	3+	1+
Aripiprazole	2+	2+	0	0	3+	0
Clozapine	3+	3+	3+	3+	3+	0
Olanzapine	2+	2+	0	3+	3+	0
Paliperidone	1+	2+	1+	0	3+	1+[b]
Quetiapine	3+	3+	0	3+	1+	0
Remoxipride	0	0	0	0	0	1+
Risperidone	1+	2+	1+	0	3+	1+[b]
Sertindole	0	1+	0	0	3+	0
Ziprasidone	0	3+	0	0	3+	1+
Zotepine	2+	0	2+	0	3+	1+

Relative neuroreceptor affinity (neuroreceptor affinity at receptor X/dopamine [D_2]-receptor affinity) indicates relative receptor antagonism at therapeutic (D_2-blocking) antipsychotic doses.
0, minimal to none; 1+, low; 2+, moderate; 3+, high; 4+, very high; EPS, extrapyramidal side effects.
[a]A higher M_1 and 5-HT_2 relative neuroreceptor affinity confers a lower EPS risk.
[b]Dose-dependent incidence of extra EPS.
Adapted from references [1–20].

for most antipsychotics, fatalities rarely occur. From one study, the most toxic antipsychotics result in death from poisoning for every 100 patient-years of use [10]. Dose-related effects are most pronounced in nonhabituated patients at the extremes of age.

Data have demonstrated that users of antipsychotic drugs have higher rates of sudden cardiac death than do nonusers and former users of antipsychotic drugs. For both classes of drugs, the risk of sudden cardiac death increases significantly with an increasing dose. Users of clozapine and thioridazine are associated with the greatest risk of sudden cardiac death.

PHARMACOLOGY

Antipsychotics bind to and antagonize presynaptic (autoreceptors) and postsynaptic type 2 dopamine (D_2) receptors in the CNS and peripheral nervous system. Initially, dopaminergic neurons increase the synthesis and release of dopamine in response to autoreceptor antagonism. With repeated dosing, however, depolarization inactivation of the neuron occurs, and decreased synthesis and release of dopamine occur despite ongoing postsynaptic receptor blockade.

All antipsychotics produce their therapeutic antipsychotic effect from mesolimbic D_2-receptor antagonism. D_2-receptor affinity (potency) in this region strongly correlates with the daily therapeutic dose (see Table 105.1) [1]. Simultaneous antagonism of other D_2 receptors produces additional clinical effects, the majority of which are undesirable. Mesocortical receptor blockade appears to create cognitive impairment and further worsens the negative symptoms of schizophrenia. Excessive D_2-receptor blockade in mesocortical and mesolimbic areas, as occurs after neuroleptic overdose, may partly mediate CNS depression from these agents. Antagonism of nigrostriatal D_2 receptors produces EPS (e.g., acute dystonia, akathisia, and parkinsonism). D_2-receptor potency in nigrostriatal relative to mesolimbic areas correlates with the likelihood of developing EPS [1]. Typical antipsychotics antagonize basal ganglia D_2 receptors in the same dose range necessary for limbic D_2-receptor blockade, thus creating high EPS liability. The high-potency or typical agents (i.e., fluphenazine, haloperidol, perphenazine, thiothixene, and trifluoperazine) are most commonly associated with EPS [1]. Atypical agents have low D_2-receptor potency and occupancy (i.e., clozapine, olanzapine, and quetiapine) at therapeutic doses, are partial D_2-receptor agonists (e.g., aripiprazole), or are more site selective (i.e., sulpiride and raclopride) and preferentially antagonize limbic D_2 receptors [2]. Thus, they are less likely to cause EPS or worsen negative symptoms of schizophrenia at therapeutic doses.

D_2-receptor blockade in the anterior hypothalamus (preoptic area) may alter core temperature set point and block thermosensitive neuronal inputs and thermoregulatory responses. Hypothermia or hyperthermia may result. D_2-receptor blockade in the pituitary (tuberoinfundibular pathway) results in sustained elevated prolactin secretion, which may cause galactorrhea, gynecomastia, menstrual changes, and sexual dysfunction (impotence in men) [1]. The antiemetic activity of antipsychotics results from similar inhibition of dopaminergic receptors in the chemoreceptor trigger zone (area postrema) of the medulla oblongata. Antagonism of dopamine receptors presents on peripheral sympathetic nerve terminals and vascular smooth muscle cells may produce autonomic dysfunction (i.e., tachycardia, hypertension, diaphoresis, and pallor) [12]. Simultaneous blockade of D_2 receptors in the hypothalamus, striatum, mesocortical and mesolimbic areas, peripheral sympathetic nerve terminals, and vasculature mediates the NMS in susceptible individuals.

In addition to D_2 receptors, antipsychotics are competitive antagonists at a wide range of neuroreceptors; varied binding affinities exist at α-adrenergic ($\alpha_{1,2}$), dopaminergic (D_{1-5}), histaminergic (H_{1-3}), muscarinic (M_{1-5}), and serotonergic ($5\text{-}HT_{1-7}$) receptors (see Table 105.2) [1]. The neuroreceptor-binding profile for each agent predicts clinical effects. The ratio of other neuroreceptor-binding affinities to D_2-receptor–binding affinity (relative binding affinity) predicts the likelihood of producing those receptor-mediated effects at clinically effective antipsychotic (D_2-blocking) doses and with overdose [1]. A ratio similar to or greater than 1 makes other receptor-mediated effects likely. High relative α_1-adrenergic antagonism (i.e., aliphatic and piperidine phenothiazines, asenapine, clozapine, olanzapine, risperidone, and ziprasidone) correlates with the incidence and severity of orthostatic hypotension, reflex tachycardia, nasal congestion, and miosis. Significant relative α_2-adrenergic blockade, as occurs with asenapine, clozapine, paliperidone, and risperidone, may result in sympathomimetic effects (e.g., tachycardia). High relative H_1-receptor blockade (e.g., aliphatic and piperidine phenothiazines, asenapine, clozapine, olanzapine, and quetiapine) produces sedation, appetite stimulation, and hypotension [1]. Relative potency at M_1 receptors correlates directly with anticholinergic effects (i.e., tachycardia, hypertension, mydriasis, blurred vision, ileus, urinary retention, dry skin and mucous membranes, cutaneous flushing, sedation, memory dysfunction, hallucinations, agitation, delirium, and hyperthermia) and inversely with the incidence of extrapyramidal reactions [1]. Olanzapine, clozapine, and aliphatic and piperidine phenothiazines are associated with clinically significant anticholinergic effects. The ability of clozapine to produce sialorrhea is likely mediated by its partial agonism at M_1 and M_4 receptors [1]. High relative antagonism at $5\text{-}HT_{1A}$ and $5\text{-}HT_{2A}$ receptors appears to predict a low EPS risk [1,13]. The clinical effects that occur with other neuroreceptor subtype binding are not well understood.

The advent of atypical agents, which provide an improved motor side-effect profile, marks significant progress in the neuroleptic development. Atypical agents may be subdivided into four functional groups: (a) the D_2- and D_3-receptor antagonists (i.e., amisulpride, raclopride, remoxipride, and sulpiride); (b) the D_2-, $5HT_{2A}$-, and α_1-receptor antagonists (i.e., paliperidone, risperidone, and ziprasidone); (c) the broad-spectrum, multireceptor antagonists (i.e., asenapine, clozapine, olanzapine, and quetiapine); and (d) the D_2- and $5\text{-}HT_{1A}$-receptor partial agonists (i.e., aripiprazole and bifeprunox), also known as dopamine and serotonin system stabilizers [2] (see Table 105.2). One or more of several different pharmacologic mechanisms define drug atypia. Low D_2-receptor potency (high-milligram dosing), low (less than 70%) D_2-receptor occupancy in mesolimbic and nigrostriatal areas at therapeutic drug doses, partial agonist activity at D_2 receptors, selective mesolimbic D_2-receptor antagonism, and high D_1-, D_4-, M_1-, $5HT_{1A}$-, and $5HT_{2A}$-receptor potencies relative to D_2-receptor–binding are pharmacologic characteristics that alone or in the combination may be responsible for the atypical nature of these agents [1,2,13]. Conversely, typical antipsychotics are characterized by high D_2-receptor potency (low-milligram dosing) and a narrow receptor profile in the brain [1]. Unlike typical agents, atypical agents also appear to have a minimal propensity to elevate serum prolactin concentrations.

Serotonin antagonism enhances antipsychotic efficacy and reduces the incidence of EPS [13]. $5HT_{2A}$-receptor antagonism in the striatum and prefrontal cortex offsets neuroleptic-induced D_2-receptor blockade and reduces EPS and negative symptoms of schizophrenia, respectively [13,14]. $5HT_{2A}$-receptor antagonism also increases serotonin levels in the limbic system, which may have direct antipsychotic effects. Drugs with high relative $5HT_{2A}$-receptor antagonism as compared to D_2-receptor antagonism (i.e., amperozide, asenapine, clozapine, olanzapine, paliperidone, risperidone, and ziprasidone) can be given in smaller clinically effective antipsychotic doses, and thus, have a smaller risk of inducing EPS [1,14]. In addition, antipsychotics that stimulate $5HT_{1A}$ autoreceptors in the striatum (i.e., aripiprazole, clozapine, and ziprasidone) reduce striatal D_2-receptor blockade, thereby decreasing the likelihood of EPS [13].

Aliphatic and piperidine phenothiazines (e.g., chlorpromazine, thioridazine, and mesoridazine) have local anesthetic, quinidine-like (type IA) antiarrhythmic, and myocardial depressant effects. These agents block both fast-sodium channels responsible for myocardial membrane depolarization [15]. Sodium-channel blockade is voltage and frequency dependent; blockade is augmented at less negative membrane potentials and faster heart rates [15]. Thus, the anticholinergic properties (e.g., tachycardia) and tissue acidemia-producing effects (e.g., seizures and hypotension) of these drugs potentiate their sodium-channel blocking effects. Although specifically demonstrated for sertindole and thioridazine only, all neuroleptics appear to variably antagonize delayed-rectifier, voltage-gated, potassium channels responsible for myocardial membrane repolarization; antagonism occurs specifically at the potassium channel encoded by the human ether-a-go-go (*hERG*) gene [16]. Potassium-channel blockade is concentration-, voltage-, and reverse-frequency dependent; blockade is increased at higher tissue concentrations, less negative membrane potentials, and slower heart rates [16]. Potassium-channel blockade may result in early after depolarizations and subsequent torsade de pointes (TdP)–type ventricular tachycardia. Haloperidol, mesoridazine, thioridazine, and pimozide share an added property of calcium-channel blockade [17].

Electrophysiologic effects variably include a depressed rate of phase 0 depolarization, depressed amplitude and duration of phase 2, and prolongation of phase 3 repolarization. Ventricular repolarization abnormalities, such as T-wave changes (blunting, notching, and inversion), increased U-wave amplitude, and prolongation of the QT interval, are the earliest and most consistent electrocardiographic changes produced by neuroleptics [17,18]. Dose-related prolongation of the QT interval has been described with droperidol, haloperidol, loxapine, phenothiazines, pimozide, quetiapine, risperidone, sertindole, and ziprasidone [11,16,18–23]. Conduction disturbances (i.e., bundle-branch, fascicular, intraventricular, and atrioventricular [AV] blocks) and supraventricular and ventricular tachyarrhythmias (i.e., monomorphic and polymorphic TdP ventricular tachycardia, ventricular fibrillation) have been reported [11,20,24]. Cardiac effects are dose and concentration dependent but can occur with therapeutic as well as toxic doses. Ventricular tachyarrhythmias and asphyxia (caused by seizures, aspiration, or respiratory depression) have been postulated as etiologies of sudden death for patients taking therapeutic doses of antipsychotics, particularly phenothiazines [9,25].

Antipsychotics produce dose-related electroencephalographic changes, and some agents have been shown to lower the seizure threshold [26,27]. The risk of seizures is dose related, and thus, greatest after overdose [27]. Chlorpromazine, clozapine, and loxapine are the most likely agents to produce seizures [26,27]. Most other agents, however, are uncommonly associated with seizures, even after overdose. The mechanism by which antipsychotics produce seizures is not well understood but likely involves dose-related blockade of norepinephrine reuptake, antagonism of γ-aminobutyric acid type A receptors, and altered neuronal transmembrane ionic currents.

Antipsychotics have a relatively flat dose–response curve. Effective therapeutic doses vary over a wide range (see Table 105.1). The optimal dose is determined by the clinical response, but not by serum drug levels. Pharmacologic effects generally last 24 hours or more, allowing for once-daily dosing. Tablet, capsule, and liquid oral preparations, suppository, and injectable immediate-release and sustained-release (depot) solutions are available. Oral preparations include both rapidly disintegrating (sublingual absorption) and sustained-release formulations. Paliperidone, the active metabolite of risperidone, is commercially available in an extended-release oral preparation (Invega). Following a single dose, plasma concentrations gradually rise and do not peak until approximately 24 hours after dosing [28]. Slow-release, highly lipophilic depot formulations (i.e., fluphenazine enanthate and decanoate, haloperidol decanoate, and paliperidone palmitate) for intramuscular (IM) injection are created by esterifying the hydroxyl group of an antipsychotic with a long-chain fatty acid and dissolving it in a sesame oil vehicle.

Antipsychotic pharmacokinetics are complex and incompletely understood. When administered orally, they are well absorbed, but bioavailability is unpredictable (range 10% to 70%) owing to large interindividual variability and presystemic (hepatic and intestinal) metabolism [29,30]. After parenteral administration, drug bioavailability is 4 to 10 times greater than with oral dosing because of the absence of first-pass metabolism [29,30]. Hence, therapeutic intravenous (IV) or IM doses are substantially less than oral ones. Plasma concentrations peak for 1 to 6 hours after therapeutic oral and sublingual dosing, 30 minutes to 1 hour after immediate-release IM injection, and within 24 hours after oral dosing of extended-release preparations. After a single IM dose of a depot preparation, plasma concentrations peak variably from a few days to over 2 weeks after initial injection [28–30]. After oral overdose, absorption should occur more rapidly (first-order kinetics), but peak plasma concentrations are delayed, because more time is required for complete absorption. As a result, clinical effects are expected to occur sooner and last longer. Erratic absorption may occur after ingestion of agents with significant anticholinergic effects.

After absorption, antipsychotics are highly bound to plasma proteins (75% to 99%) [29,30]. However, because they are also highly lipophilic, volumes of distribution are large (10 to 40 L per kg), and serum drug levels after therapeutic doses are quite low (one to several hundred ng per mL). These pharmacokinetic characteristics make extracorporeal removal by hemodialysis or hemoperfusion impractical. Antipsychotics tend to accumulate in the brain, easily cross the placenta, and are found in breast milk. Elimination occurs slowly and extensively by hepatic metabolism, with serum concentration half-lives averaging 20 to 40 hours. Depot antipsychotics have an apparent elimination half-life of 1 to 3 weeks due to slow tissue absorption [29]. Small amounts (1% to 3%) are excreted unchanged by the kidney. As a rule, hepatic metabolism yields multiple metabolites, some of which are pharmacologically active and likely to extend parent drug effects after therapeutic or toxic dosing [31,32]. Metabolites are eliminated by urinary and biliary excretion and can be detected in the urine for several days after a single ingestion and for a month or more after cessation of long-term therapy [30]. Large interindividual variations in the metabolism of neuroleptics result in significant differences of steady-state plasma concentrations with fixed, therapeutic dosing [29,30,33]. There is often little correlation among neuroleptic dose, serum concentrations, and clinical effects.

Renal insufficiency may rarely result from drug accumulation and toxicity [34]. Renal excretion accounts for a significant proportion of total drug elimination for the benzamide (e.g., remoxipride and sulpiride) and benzisoxazole derivatives (e.g., paliperidone and risperidone) [28–30]. Thus, dose alteration is recommended for patients with renal insufficiency who regularly take these agents. Other neuroleptics, however, do not routinely require dose alteration for patients with renal impairment. Dose adjustment is also recommended for those patients who have a diminished ability to clear neuroleptics, such as the elderly and those with significant hepatic disease or specific cytochrome P450 enzyme deficiencies (i.e., CYP2D6 and CYP1A2) [30]. Most antipsychotics are pregnancy category C and should be used in pregnancy only if the potential benefit justifies the potential risk to the fetus. Breast feeding is not recommended for women taking neuroleptics because most neuroleptics are secreted into breast milk, and their safety for infants is not established.

The majority of the patients who take an accidental or intentional overdose of an antipsychotic agent remain asymptomatic or develop only mild toxicity [3]. Toxic effects result from exaggerated pharmacologic activity and include CNS and consequent respiratory depression, miosis or mydriasis, cardiovascular abnormalities, agitation, confusion, delirium, anticholinergic stigmata, seizures, EPS, and myoclonic jerking. Hypothermia and, less commonly, hyperthermia have occurred. Hypothermia may result from α_1-adrenergic–mediated peripheral vasodilation at low ambient temperature, hypotension, coma, loss of shivering capabilities, and disrupted hypothalamic thermoregulation. Peripheral vasodilation at high ambient temperature, seizures, neuromuscular agitation, loss of sweating capabilities, and hypothalamic dysfunction may contribute to hyperthermia. Seizures are uncommon and occur mainly among the patients with underlying epilepsy and those with clozapine and loxapine overdoses. In one study of 299 patients with neuroleptic overdose, the incidence of seizure was only 1% [11]. Rhabdomyolysis, myoglobinuria, and acute renal failure may occur after prolonged convulsions [35]. CNS depression is the most frequent clinical finding after neuroleptic overdose [11,36,37]. Sinus tachycardia and orthostatic hypotension are the most frequent cardiovascular findings [36–38]. Other cardiovascular effects include hypertension, cardiac conduction disturbances, tachyarrhythmias, bradyarrhythmias, and, rarely, pulmonary edema [39,40]. Anticholinergic stigmata (see Chapter 102) may occur after overdose with aliphatic and piperidine phenothiazines, clozapine, and olanzapine [3,38,41–43].

Of the thousands of antipsychotic overdoses reported each year, less than 1% result in fatal toxicity [10]. Fatality is most often due to respiratory arrest before medical intervention, arrhythmias, or aspiration-induced respiratory failure [3,9]. Toxic and lethal doses are highly variable and are influenced by the agent ingested, the presence of coingestants and comorbid illness, the age and habituation of the patients, and the time to treatment. Nonhabituated patients at the extremes of age are more sensitive to the toxic effects of these drugs than those who have taken this drug chronically before an acute overdose. The ingestion of a single tablet of chlorpromazine, clozapine, loxapine, mesoridazine, olanzapine, quetiapine, or thioridazine may cause CNS and respiratory depression of young children [3,34,35,41]. Death of an infant was reported after the ingestion of only 350 mg of chlorpromazine. In general, acute ingestion of greater than twice a maximal therapeutic dose is potentially serious.

Unintended adverse effects that occur during therapeutic use may be idiosyncratic or dose related, occur early or late during the course of therapy, or result from interactions with other drugs, and are often due to receptor antagonism. The major adverse side effect, in terms of both prevalence and distress that it causes, is the tendency to induce extrapyramidal dysfunction.

Extrapyramidal syndromes are a group of movement disorders that result from the interference with neurotransmitter (primarily D_2-receptor blockade) function in the basal ganglia. EPS occur in up to 75% of the patients treated with low-milligram, high-potency traditional agents (e.g., fluphenazine, haloperidol, and thiothixene), but an incidence not significantly different from placebo (<5%) has been described with newer atypical agents (e.g., aripiprazole, olanzapine, and quetiapine) [44]. EPS may occur early (i.e., within a few hours to days), at an intermediate stage (i.e., a few days to months), or late (i.e., after >3 months) in the course of therapy. Early EPS include acute dyskinesia (acute dystonic reactions [ADRs]), intermediate syndromes include akathisia and parkinsonism, and late disorders include tardive dyskinesia, tardive dystonia, and focal perioral tremor (rabbit syndrome). EPS are more commonly associated with therapeutic doses of neuroleptics but may follow acute overdose (e.g., ADRs), particularly among children [3,36,45]. Only ADRs, the acute syndrome most likely to develop in the intensive care unit, are discussed.

ADRs are reversible motor disturbances consisting of sustained, uncoordinated, and involuntary spasmodic movements of various muscle groups. Although ADRs most often occur after administration of therapeutic doses of antipsychotics [46], they have also been described after administration of antihistamines (both H_1- and H_2-blockers), anticholinergics (e.g., benztropine and diphenhydramine), anticonvulsants (e.g., carbamazepine and phenytoin), calcium-channel blockers (e.g., nifedipine and verapamil), metoclopramide, cyclic antidepressants (e.g., amitriptyline, amoxapine, doxepin, and imipramine), selective serotonin reuptake inhibitors (e.g., fluoxetine and sertraline), monoamine oxidase inhibitors (e.g., phenelzine and tranylcypromine), anesthetic induction agents (e.g., ketamine, etomidate, and thiopental), cholinergics (e.g., bethanechol and insecticides), and cocaine. ADRs can also occur as a primary (non-drug–related) disorder [47].

The pathophysiology of ADRs is not fully elucidated but involves a disruption of cholinergic (interstriatal) and dopaminergic (nigrostriatal) pathways in the basal ganglia. Normally, dopamine is an excitatory neurotransmitter and acetylcholine is an inhibitory neurotransmitter [48]. Normal balance between these closely linked pathways is necessary for coordinated muscular activity. Dopaminergic D_1-, γ-aminobutyric acid-(striatonigral), glutaminergic-(corticostriatal), noradrenergic-, $5HT_{1A}$- and $5HT_{2A}$-(raphe-striatal and raphe-nigral), and sigma (σ)- (red nucleus, substantia nigra, and cranial nerve motor nuclei) receptor inputs modulate this balance [13,49]. Blockade of striatal D_2 receptors by high-potency neuroleptics disrupts the dopaminergic–cholinergic balance in favor of cholinergic excess and dystonia results [50,51]. Agents that balance D_2-receptor antagonism with D_1-, M_1-, or $5HT_{2A}$-receptor antagonism or $5HT_{1A}$-receptor agonism prevents striatal cholinergic excess and are less likely to precipitate acute dystonia [1,13,52]. γ-aminobutyric acid–receptor affinity correlates inversely, whereas σ- and N-methyl-D-aspartate-glutamate receptor–binding affinities correlate directly with the clinical incidence of acute dystonia [49].

Paradoxically, ADRs may also result from hyperdopaminergic function induced by D_2-receptor blockade in the basal ganglia [53,54]. Acute D_2-receptor blockade may stimulate increased dopamine synthesis and release from nigrostriatal neurons and postsynaptic receptor upregulation (supersensitivity). Because brain concentration of drug declines hours to days after a dose, a state of dopamine excess develops, and dystonia results [53,54].

ADRs usually occur soon after initiation of therapy or after an increase in dose. Fifty percent of ADRs occur within 48 hours of initiating therapy, and 90% within 5 days [55]. Peak incidence occurs when drug levels are declining in the serum. Although the absolute incidence of ADRs is unknown, they are estimated to occur in 25% of the patients treated with IM depot preparations, 16% of the patients who have been given haloperidol, 8% of the patients treated with thiothixene, 2% to 12% of all patients who take phenothiazines, 3.5% of the patients treated with chlorpromazine, and 1% or less in patients taking atypical agents [50,55]. Phenothiazines that contain a piperazine side chain (i.e., prochlorperazine, trifluoperazine, perphenazine, fluphenazine, and acetophenazine) are associated with a higher incidence of dystonic reactions than are other phenothiazines [55]. Atypical agents (particularly clozapine) are unequivocally associated with a reduced incidence of ADRs. The likelihood of an ADR is more dependent on individual susceptibility than on neuroleptic structure, potency, dose, and duration of therapy [56]. ADRs most commonly occur among men, patients 5 to 45 years of age (particularly those younger than 15 years old), and those with a personal or family history of dystonia or a recent history of drug (i.e., cocaine) or alcohol abuse [55,57].

Seizures are an uncommon side effect of certain antipsychotics (e.g., clozapine, chlorpromazine, and loxapine). They typically occur at higher therapeutic doses and after overdose of susceptible patients. Seizures are usually generalized and of the major motor type. Clozapine, the most epileptogenic agent at therapeutic dosing, is associated with a seizure rate of approximately 1% at doses lower than 300 mg per day, a rate of 2.7% at doses between 300 and 600 mg per day, and a rate of 4.4% with doses larger than 600 mg per day. A cumulative seizure risk of 10% after 3.8 years of treatment has been demonstrated with clozapine [38,39]. Newer, atypical agents show no increase of seizure risk when compared with haloperidol or placebo. Other risk factors for seizures include a history of organic brain disease, epilepsy, electroconvulsive therapy, abnormal baseline electroencephalogram, polypharmacy, and initiation and rapid dose titration of neuroleptics [27]. After overdose, the incidence of seizures is as high as 60% and 10% for loxapine and clozapine, respectively, whereas the incidence for most other neuroleptics is approximately 1% [3,11].

Agranulocytosis (absolute neutrophil count < 500 cells per μL) is a serious idiosyncratic side effect of clozapine and phenothiazine therapy. It is rare (0.1 to 1.0 per 1,000 persons) with phenothiazines and usually occurs in the first 12 weeks of therapy [58,59]. A cumulative risk of 0.91% (9 per 1,000 persons) at 18 months is reported with clozapine; more than 80% of the cases occur in the first 3 months [5,60]. Initial mortality rates associated with agranulocytosis ranged from 30% to 85%, but with regular white blood cell count monitoring and treatment with granulocyte colony stimulating factor (G-CSF), mortality rates have dropped to 3% to 4% [5,60,61]. The mechanism underlying clozapine-induced agranulocytosis may be both immune-mediated and the result of direct myelotoxicity from the drug. G-CSF has been useful for treatment, halving recovery time from 16 to 8 days [62]. Agranulocytosis has not been reported after acute overdose. Neutropenia has also been associated with the therapeutic use of olanzapine, quetiapine, and risperidone [63].

Hepatic transaminitis is an adverse side effect of most antipsychotics [7]. Hepatotoxicity is idiosyncratic, often occurs within the first 3 months of treatment, and is usually mild and self-limiting (most patients remain asymptomatic). The patterns of hepatoxicity are both hepatitic (including nonalcoholic steatohepatitis) and cholestatic [63,64].

Most atypical neuroleptics result in an increased appetite and weight gain. More importantly, and perhaps causally related, the therapeutic use of atypical agents has been associated with an increased risk of developing type II diabetes mellitus [57–67]. Several cases of fatal diabetic ketoacidosis and hyperglycemic hyperosmolar nonketotic coma have been reported among the patients taking clozapine and olanzapine [68,69]. Pancreatitis has been associated with the use of clozapine, and hypertriglyceridemia has been reported among patients treated with clozapine, olanzapine, and quetiapine [56,70–72].

Allergic dermatitis, cholestatic jaundice, irreversible pigmentary retinopathy, photosensitivity reactions, and priapism are uncommon idiosyncratic reactions associated with phenothiazine therapy [7]. Myocarditis and cardiomyopathy have been rarely associated with the use of clozapine; these conditions are idiosyncratic, frequently fatal, often occur within the first 2 weeks of treatment, and are likely the result of acute hypersensitivity [8,73].

Drug interactions and adverse effects may be pharmacodynamic (i.e., receptor or channel mediated) or pharmacokinetic (i.e., altered absorption, metabolism, or protein binding) [74]. Combining antipsychotics with other CNS depressants (i.e., antihistamines, cyclic antidepressants, ethanol, opiates, and sedative–hypnotics) may produce enhanced CNS and respiratory depression. Respiratory depression and arrest have been reported with the coadministration of clozapine and lorazepam or diazepam [75,76]. Exaggerated anticholinergic effects may occur with concurrent use of tricyclic antidepressants, certain skeletal muscle relaxants, antihistamines, and antiparkinson agents. The combination of antipsychotics with significant α_1-adrenergic blockade and certain antihypertensive agents (e.g., hydralazine and prazosin) may precipitate hypotension. Enhanced cardiotoxicity may occur when mesoridazine or thioridazine is combined with type IA antiarrhythmic agents or tricyclic antidepressants. High-dose droperidol, haloperidol, sertindole, thioridazine, and ziprasidone may potentiate QT prolongation produced by other cardioactive agents.

Most antipsychotic agents are extensively metabolized by the hepatic cytochrome P450 (CYP) enzyme system, particularly the CYP2D6 and CYP1A2 isoenzymes. Other drugs that are substrates (i.e., cyclic antidepressants), inhibitors (i.e., cimetidine, erythromycin, and selective serotonin reuptake inhibitors), or inducers (i.e., anticonvulsants) of similar CYP isoenzymes may alter antipsychotic metabolism and precipitate adverse effects. These interactions often go unnoticed, but they may be clinically significant. Cimetidine, erythromycin, and fluvoxamine have precipitated clinical clozapine toxicity from hepatic CYP1A2 isoenzyme inhibition [77,78]. Paroxetine may precipitate risperidone toxicity from CYP2D6 isoenzyme inhibition. Knowledge of antipsychotic-associated drug interactions facilitates recognition and treatment of these increasingly common iatrogenic events.

CLINICAL TOXICITY

Acute overdose may result in nausea and vomiting soon after ingestion. CNS and cardiovascular effects, however, usually dominate the clinical picture [3,11,23,36,37]. For mild intoxication, findings include ataxia, confusion, lethargy, slurred speech, tachycardia, and hypertension or orthostatic hypotension. Anticholinergic signs (e.g., dry skin and mucosa, decreased bowel sounds, and urinary retention) and hyperreflexia may also be present. Although usually considered an idiosyncratic reaction, EPS (e.g., ADRs) have been described after acute neuroleptic overdose, particularly among children [3,36,45]. Electrocardiographic changes such as prolonged PR and QT intervals, ST-segment depression, T-wave abnormalities (biphasic, blunting, inversion, notching, and widening), and increased U waves can occur [11,18,19]. Other than sinus tachycardia, repolarization abnormalities are the earliest and most common electrocardiographic findings associated with neuroleptic poisoning [11,18,19,79].

Signs and symptoms of moderate poisoning include low-grade coma (see Chapters 145 and 146, respiratory depression, and hypotension). Miosis or mydriasis may occur. Miosis is more likely to occur following overdose of both atypical and typical agents; it has been described in 75% of the adults and 72% of the children after phenothiazine overdose [3,37,38,41,80]. Internuclear ophthalmoplegia has been reported. Paradoxical agitation, delirium, hallucinations, psychosis, myoclonic jerking, and tachypnea may occur [3,38,41–43,81]. Central and peripheral anticholinergic stigmata frequently occur after overdose with chlorpromazine, clozapine, mesoridazine, olanzapine, and thioridazine [3,38,41–43].

With severe poisoning, high-grade coma with loss of most or all reflexes, apnea, hypotension, seizures, and a variety of cardiac conduction disturbances and arrhythmias may develop. Conduction disturbances include all degrees of AV block, bundle-branch and fascicular block, and nonspecific intraventricular conduction delay [11,19,20,24,79]. Bradyarrhythmias occur uncommonly and, when present, may signify impending respiratory arrest. Tachyarrhythmias include sinus and supraventricular tachycardias, supraventricular and ventricular premature beats, ventricular tachycardia and fibrillation, and TdP [3,11,18–20,24,82]. The latter arrhythmia typically occurs in the setting of QT-interval prolongation and has been described with amisulpride, droperidol, haloperidol, mesoridazine, pimozide, and thioridazine [83]. TdP has also been described when critically ill patients are given haloperidol for sedation. In one study, TdP occurred in 3.6% of such patients; the incidence was 64% in those given greater than 35 mg of haloperidol in less than 6 hours and 84% when given to those with a corrected QT (QTc) interval greater than 500 milliseconds [84]. TdP has been rarely associated with therapeutic (usually large) doses of droperidol [20,85]. Discovery of this association prompted the Federal Drug Administration to issue a "black box" warning to US health care personnel for droperidol in 2001 [86]. Serious cardiovascular toxicity occurs more commonly when piperidine phenothiazines have been ingested [11]. In one study of 299 patients with neuroleptic overdose, thioridazine was associated with a significantly greater incidence of prolonged QRS, prolonged QTc, and arrhythmia as compared to other neuroleptics [11]. Electrocardiographic abnormalities or obvious cardiotoxicity should be evident within several hours of overdose. Newer agents alter cardiac conduction less frequently but are not entirely void of cardiotoxicity. Prolonged QRS and QT intervals and hypotension have been described after risperidone overdose, and ventricular tachycardia has occurred after remoxipride overdose. The new drug approval application for sertindole was withdrawn in the United States due to dose-related prolongation of the QT interval that occurred during premarketing trials with the drug [22].

Although the overall seizure incidence is about 1% for patients that overdose on neuroleptics, the incidence is much greater following ingestion of chlorpromazine, clozapine, loxapine, mesoridazine, and thioridazine [3,10,11]. Occasionally, hypothermia or hyperthermia may be seen [87]. Pulmonary edema has been reported rarely as a complication of overdose with chlorpromazine, clozapine, haloperidol, and perphenazine [3,39,40]. NMS is an idiosyncratic reaction that rarely occurs after acute overdose. Acute overdose, however, may infrequently produce a clinical picture (i.e., the presence of hyperthermia, autonomic instability, neuromuscular hyperreactivity, and hypertonia) that could be misinterpreted as NMS. Agents that produce anticholinergic effects (e.g., clozapine, mesoridazine, olanzapine, and thioridazine) would be more likely to do this.

Loxapine poisoning results in an atypical clinical picture. Cardiovascular effects are mild or absent, but convulsions are common and often lead to rhabdomyolysis and subsequent renal failure [88].

Following overdose, toxic effects (e.g., CNS depression) begin within 1 to 2 hours, maximal severity is usually evident by 2 to 6 hours, and resolution usually occurs by 24 to 48 hours after ingestion. The presentation is the same regardless of age and whether the overdose is acute or chronic. Early deaths are due to respiratory arrest, arrhythmias, shock, or aspiration-associated respiratory failure. Later complications include cerebral and pulmonary edema, disseminated intravascular coagulation, rhabdomyolysis, myoglobinuric renal failure, and infection.

ADRs are characterized by abrupt onset, intermittent and repetitive nature, normal physical examination except for muscular findings, a history of recent neuroleptic use, and rapid response to anticholinergic drug therapy [50,55]. Muscle contractions may sometimes be sustained but usually last from seconds to minutes. They may be focal at the onset and then spread to contiguous muscles; occasionally, they are generalized [89]. The patients remain alert and oriented during these reactions.

Although dystonia may occur in any striated muscle, one of the five areas is typically affected [50,55,90]. ADRs involving the muscles of the eye (oculogyric crisis) cause upward gazing, rotation of the eyes, and spasm of the lids. Those involving muscles of the tongue and jaw (buccolingual crisis) produce trismus, protrusion of the tongue, dysphagia, dysarthria, and facial grimacing. Contractions of muscles of the neck or back result in abnormal head positioning (torticollic reactions) or arching and twisting of the torso (opisthotonic posturing), respectively. When muscles of the abdominal wall are involved, the patients present with abdominal wall pain and spasm, bizarre gait patterns, kyphosis, and lordosis (tortipelvic and gait crises). Buccolingual and torticollic ADRs are the most common [55].

Although ADRs are rarely life threatening, those involving the tongue, jaw, neck, and chest can result in upper airway compromise and impaired respiratory mechanics. Stridor can occur in those with buccolingual and torticollic reactions. Death from respiratory failure has been reported [91].

DIAGNOSTIC EVALUATION

The diagnosis of antipsychotic poisoning is made from a history of exposure, physical findings, and supporting evidence from electrocardiographic, laboratory, and other ancillary studies. A complete history should be obtained from the patient as well as the person(s) who found or brought the patient (to corroborate the patient's history). As with all drug ingestions, the name, quantity, and time of ingestion of the drug(s) should be determined. For patients who become toxic during chronic therapy, a recent medication or dose change or an illness may be responsible. The patients and family members should be specifically questioned about the possibility of antipsychotic exposure when signs of an EPS are present.

Physical examination should focus on the vital signs, respiratory function, and neurologic status. Physical findings that suggest neuroleptic poisoning include CNS and respiratory depression, sinus tachycardia, miosis, anticholinergic stigmata, orthostatic hypotension, and the presence of EPS. The patients should be examined for evidence of coexisting trauma. An initial rhythm strip and subsequent 12-lead electrocardiogram (ECG) should be evaluated. Arterial blood gas determinations and a chest radiograph should be ordered for patients with significant CNS depression. An abdominal radiograph showing radiopaque densities in the gastrointestinal (GI) tract may suggest butyrophenone or phenothiazine poisoning if the etiology of symptoms is unknown. The absence of this finding, however, does not rule out poisoning by these agents. Routine laboratory evaluation should include a complete blood cell count and electrolyte count and blood urea nitrogen, creatinine, and glucose tests. Measurements of serum acetaminophen and salicylate should be performed on all patients with intentional overdose. Among the patients with seizures, hyperthermia, and severe poisoning, laboratory evaluation should include urinalysis (routine and for myoglobin); creatinine phosphokinase, calcium, magnesium, and phosphate tests; and a coagulation profile. Women of childbearing age should have a pregnancy test performed.

Toxicologic analyses of the urine and serum by immunoassay and chromatography–mass spectrometry may be performed to confirm the identity of the offending agent and to rule out other ingestants [92]. Quantitative drug levels are not helpful for predicting clinical toxicity or guiding treatment [29,30,33]. Although neither sensitive nor specific, or readily available, the Forrest, Mason, and Phenistix colorimetric tests are rapid urine screens that may be positive with phenothiazine ingestions [93]. These tests, however, do not detect nonphenothiazine neuroleptic agents. Certain neuroleptics (e.g., chlorpromazine, mesoridazine, quetiapine, and thioridazine) will commonly produce false positive results for tricyclic antidepressants on most commercially available immunoassay screens used by hospitals to test for drugs of abuse [94].

The patients with ADRs should be questioned regarding current medications, previous ADRs, recreational drug use, and change in the dose of a neuroleptic or other medication associated with this syndrome. The diagnosis is made on the basis of history of drug exposure and the physical examination.

A complete blood cell count should be performed for patients who develop a fever or infection while taking clozapine or phenothiazines.

Agents that cause CNS and cardiovascular effects similar to those resulting from antipsychotic poisoning include antiarrhythmic, anticholinergic, anticonvulsant, antidepressant, antihistamine, opioid, other psychotropic agents (e.g., lithium, bupropion) and sedative–hypnotics, and skeletal muscle relaxants. It may be impossible to distinguish cyclic antidepressant or type IA antiarrhythmic agent poisoning from poisoning due to chlorpromazine, thioridazine, or mesoridazine without toxicologic analysis. CNS infection, cerebrovascular accident, occult head trauma, and metabolic abnormalities should also be considered in the differential diagnosis.

The differential diagnosis of an ADR includes primary dystonias, seizures, cerebrovascular accident, encephalitis, tetanus, hypocalcemia, drug intoxication (especially anticholinergic, anticonvulsant, and strychnine), hysterical conversion reactions, joint dislocations, meningitis, hypomagnesemia, torticollis, and alkalosis.

MANAGEMENT

All patients who are symptomatic after acute overdose should be observed until they are alert. Those with mild toxicity can often be managed in the emergency department or a similarly equipped observation unit. Those with protracted hypotension, significant CNS depression or agitation, seizures, acid–base disturbances, nonsinus arrhythmias, and cardiac conduction disturbances should be admitted to an intensive care unit. The patients with ECG abnormalities (e.g., prolonged QRS or QTc intervals) who are otherwise asymptomatic should be admitted to a cardiac monitored bed; such findings have been implicated in sudden death.

Treatment is primarily supportive. The tempo and sequence of interventions depend on the clinical severity. Advanced life support measures should be instituted as necessary, and underlying metabolic abnormalities corrected. All patients require cardiac and respiratory monitoring. Vital signs should be obtained frequently. Endotracheal intubation for airway protection or ventilatory support may be required. The patients with seizures or hyperthermia should have continuous (rectal probe) temperature monitoring. Those with altered mental status should receive supplemental oxygen and be given a diagnostic trial of naloxone (2 mg IV), dextrose (25 g IV), and thiamine (100 mg IV). Although reversal of CNS depression after naloxone administration has been reported [95], such a response is inconsistent with the pharmacology of neuroleptics and should not be expected.

Hypotension should be initially treated with Trendelenburg position and several liters (10 to 40 mL per kg IV) of normal saline. α_1-Adrenergic agonists (i.e., norepinephrine and phenylephrine) are first-line agents for treating refractory hypotension, particularly in the patients who have been poisoned by antipsychotics with significant α_1-adrenergic blockade. Central venous, intra-arterial, and echocardiographic monitoring may be necessary for optimal management of the patients who are hemodynamically unstable.

Sinus and supraventricular tachycardias rarely require specific treatment. If they are associated with hypotension, correction of this abnormality is often all that is necessary. Sodium bicarbonate (1 to 2 mEq per kg IV) may be effective and is strongly recommended for patients who have wide QRS complexes or ventricular tachyarrhythmias. Amiodarone and electrical cardioversion are alternative treatments for patients with ventricular tachyarrhythmias, depending on hemodynamic stability. Type IA (i.e., disopyramide, quinidine, and procainamide), type IC (i.e., propafenone), and type III (i.e., amiodarone) antiarrhythmic drugs are not recommended and are potentially dangerous; they may worsen cardiac conduction abnormalities [96]. TdP ventricular tachycardia should be treated with magnesium (50 to 100 mg per kg IV over 1 hour); or an increase in heart rate (overdrive pacing) should be treated using isoproterenol or a pacemaker [97]. Increasing the heart rate may shorten a prolonged QT interval and thus facilitate conversion of this arrhythmia. The blood pressure should be carefully monitored during isoproterenol administration, as it may cause or worsen hypotension. A search for and correction of hypokalemia, hypomagnesemia, and other electrolyte disturbances is requisite to the management of TdP. Bradyarrhythmias associated with hemodynamic compromise should be treated with atropine, epinephrine, dopamine, or isoproterenol according to current advanced cardiac life support protocols. Complete heart block may require temporary cardiac pacing.

Recent literature supports the antidotal use of intravenous fat emulsions (IFE) for severe CNS or cardiovascular toxicity from highly lipophilic drugs [98]. IFE infusions may create a "lipid sink" whereby lipophilic drugs are sequestered in a newly created intravascular lipid compartment, thereby reducing tissue binding. Alternatively, IFE infusions may restore myocardial function by providing exogenous fatty acid substrate or by increasing intracellular calcium for myocyte function [98]. In clinical case reports, IFE administration has been temporally associated with attenuation of QTc prolongation and CNS depression from quetiapine overdose [99]. The overwhelming majority of the antipsychotic-overdose patients do well with good supportive care and would not necessitate IFE infusion therapy. IFE treatment, however, should be strongly considered and is recommended for patients with severe and refractory cardiovascular or CNS toxicity from antipsychotic drugs. IFE is commonly administered an IV bolus followed by a 3 to 24 hour continuous infusion. A reasonable dosing algorithm for both adults and children is a 1 to 2 mL per kg IV bolus of 20% IFE over 1 minute followed by 0.25 to 0.5 mL/kg/min continuous IV infusion (total dose 2 g/kg/d IFE) [98].

Seizures are often self-limited and may not require specific treatment. If prolonged or recurrent, seizures should be treated with incremental doses of diazepam or lorazepam (initial dose, 0.05 to 0.10 mg per kg IV). A short-acting barbiturate (e.g., amobarbital, 10 to 15 mg per kg IV at a maximal rate of 100 mg per minute) or a long-acting one (e.g., phenobarbital, 20 mg per kg IV at a maximal rate of 30 mg per minute) may sometimes be necessary. The effectiveness of phenytoin is not established for neuroleptic-associated seizures. Refractory convulsions may require the use of a paralyzing agent to prevent complications such as hyperthermia and rhabdomyolysis. A nondepolarizing neuromuscular blocker, such as pancuronium (0.06 to 0.10 mg per kg IV) or rocuronium(0.6 to 1.2 mg per kg IV) is recommended over succinylcholine. Continued treatment of seizures, as indicated by electroencephalogram monitoring, is necessary during therapeutic paralysis. Diuresis and alkalinization of urine may be useful in preventing myoglobinuric renal failure for patients with rhabdomyolysis (see Chapter 200).

Physostigmine may be used safely and effectively in poisoned patients who have significant peripheral or central anticholinergic stigmata (i.e., agitated delirium) and normal PR and QRS intervals on ECG [43]. Physostigmine should be given slowly intravenously (0.02 mg per kg in children or 2 mg in adults) over 3 minutes. Alternatively, agitated delirium from the anticholinergic syndrome may be treated with benzodiazepines.

After stabilization, GI decontamination should be performed for patients with acute ingestions. Oral activated charcoal (1 g per kg) with or without a cathartic is the preferred method for the majority of the patients. Although gastric lavage may possibly benefit comatose patients who present within 1 hour of drug ingestion, it is not routinely recommended for neuroleptic overdose for which the mortality rate is very low [100]. If performed, gastric lavage should always be followed with activated charcoal administration. Because of decreased GI tract motility resulting from poisoning, decontamination (activated charcoal administration) may be of benefit many hours after overdose.

Although clinical improvement was reported during combined hemodialysis and charcoal hemoperfusion [101], the effect was transient, and measures to enhance the elimination of neuroleptic agents, such as diuresis, dialysis, and hemoperfusion, have not been shown to be pharmacokinetically effective [102,103]. Repeated oral doses of activated charcoal are of potential but unproved benefit. Use of multidose charcoal is not recommended and potentially harmful for patients who have developed an ileus.

The vast majority of the patients with neuroleptic poisoning recover completely within several hours to several days, depending on severity. Patients with intentional overdosage require psychiatric evaluation before discharge.

Patients with respiratory distress secondary to ADRs should be given supplemental oxygen. Those with buccolingual and torticollic crises should be given nothing by mouth, because doing so could precipitate choking. Because ADRs rarely result from an overdose, GI tract decontamination is usually not indicated and may, in fact, be hazardous because of the potential for airway complications.

Administration of an anticholinergic agent readily reverses ADRs, presumably by restoring the balance between cholinergic and dopaminergic pathways in the basal ganglia [50]. Benztropine mesylate, 1 to 2 mg, or diphenhydramine, 50 to 100 mg, given intravenously over 1 to 2 minutes, can be used. Reversal of signs and symptoms usually occurs within a few minutes. In some cases, a second dose is needed for complete resolution. Benztropine appears to be more effective and is less likely to cause sedation and hypotension than diphenhydramine and is the preferred agent in adults [104]. Although benztropine is contraindicated in children younger than 3 years of age because of its anticholinergic effects [105], this is precisely the desired effect, and its administration in small doses (e.g., 0.25 to 0.50 mg) is appropriate in this situation. As an alternative, diphenhydramine (1 mg per kg IV) can be used. Benztropine and diphenhydramine can also be given intramuscularly, but it may take 30 to 90 minutes for the ADR to resolve when this route is used. Cases resistant to anticholinergic agents may respond to diazepam (0.1 mg per kg IV) or lorazepam (0.05 to 0.10 mg per kg IV).

Subsequent therapy with an oral anticholinergic agent should be continued for 48 to 72 hours. Without such therapy, the ADR may recur because it may take several days to eliminate completely the agent that caused it and the duration of action of drugs used to treat it is much shorter. In addition to benztropine and diphenhydramine, biperiden (2 mg one to three times a day), trihexyphenidyl (2 mg twice per day), or amantadine (100 to 200 mg twice per day) can be used for oral therapy. For reasons already noted, benztropine (1 to 2 mg twice per day) is the preferred agent for adults. Children younger than 3 years can be given diphenhydramine (1 mg per kg orally three or four times per day). Although patients who have had an ADR are at increased risk for future ADRs, those requiring continued antipsychotic therapy can usually continue or resume taking the offending agent provided they are also maintained on anticholinergic therapy. As an alternative, they can be switched to atypical antipsychotic with less dopaminergic-blocking activity.

References

1. Richelson E: Receptor pharmacology of neuroleptics: relation to clinical effects. *J Clin Psychiatry* 60[Suppl 10]:5–14, 1999.
2. Blin O: A comparative review of new antipsychotics. *Can J Psychiatry* 44:235–244, 1999.
3. Burns MJ: The pharmacology and toxicology of atypical antipsychotic agents. *J Tox Clin Toxicol* 39(1):1–14, 2001.
4. Ray WA, Chung CP, Murray KT, et al: Atypical antipsychotic drugs and the risk of sudden cardiac death. *NEJM* 360:225–235, 2009.
5. Alvir J, Lieberman J, Safferman A, et al: Clozapine-induced agranulocytosis: incidence and risk factors in the United States. *N Engl J Med* 329:162–167, 1993.
6. Laidlaw ST, Snowden JA, Brown MJ: Aplastic anemia and remoxipride. *Lancet* 342:1245, 1993.
7. Selim K, Kaplowitz N: Hepatotoxicity of psychotropic drugs. *Hepatology* 29:1347–1351, 1999.
8. Grenade LL, Graham D, Trontell A: Myocarditis and cardiomyopathy associated with clozapine use in the United States [letter]. *N Engl J Med* 345(3):224, 2001.
9. Mehtonen OP, Aranko K, Malkonen L, et al: A survey of sudden death associated with the use of antipsychotic or antidepressant drugs: 49 cases in Finland. *Acta Psychiatr Scand* 84:58–64, 1991.
10. Buckley N, McManus P: Fatal toxicity of drugs used in the treatment of psychotic illnesses. *Br J Psychiatry* 172:461–464, 1998.
11. Buckley NA, Whyte IM, Dawson AH: Thioridazine has greater cardiotoxicity in overdose than other neuroleptics. *J Toxicol Clin Toxicol* 33:199–204, 1995.
12. Stoof JC, Kebabian JW: Two dopamine receptors: biochemistry, physiology and pharmacology. *Life Sci* 34:2281–2286, 1984.
13. Lieberman JA, Mailman RB, Duncan G, et al: Serotonergic basis of antipsychotic drug effects in schizophrenia. *Biol Psychiatry* 44:1099–1117, 1998.
14. Leysen JE, Janssen PMF, Schotte A, et al: Interaction of antipsychotic drugs with neurotransmitter receptor sites in vitro and in vivo in relation to pharmacologic and clinical effects: role of 5-HT_2 receptors. *Psychopharmacol (Berl)* 112[Suppl 1]:S40–S54, 1993.
15. Ogata N, Narahashi T: Block of sodium channels by psychotropic drugs in single guinea-pig cardiac myocytes. *Br J Pharmacol* 97:905–913, 1989.
16. Rampe D, Murawsky K, Grau J, et al: The antipsychotic agent sertindole is a high affinity antagonist of the human cardiac potassium channel hERG. *J Pharm Exp Ther* 286:788–793, 1998.
17. Gould RJ, Murphy KMM, Reynolds IJ, et al: Calcium channel blockade: possible explanation for thioridazine's peripheral side effects. *Am J Psychiatry* 141:352–357, 1984.
18. Flugelman MY, Tal A, Pollack S, et al: Psychotropic drugs and long QT syndromes: case reports. *J Clin Psychiatry* 46:290–291, 1985.
19. Elkayam U, Frishman W: Cardiovascular effects of phenothiazines. *Am Heart J* 100:397–401, 1980.
20. Lawrence KR, Nasraway SA: Conduction disturbances associated with administration of butyrophenone antipsychotics in the critically ill: a review of the literature. *Pharmacotherapy* 17:531–537, 1997.
21. Riker RR, Fraser GL, Cox PM: Continuous infusion of haloperidol controls agitation in critically ill patients. *Crit Care Med* 22:433–440, 1994.
22. Lee AM, Knoll JL, Suppes R: The atypical antipsychotic sertindole: a case series. *J Clin Psychiatry* 58:410–416, 1997.
23. Hustey FM: Acute quetiapine poisoning. *J Emerg Med* 17:995–997, 1999.
24. Wilt JL, Minnema AM, Johnson RF, et al: Torsades de pointes associated with the use of intravenous haloperidol. *Ann Intern Med* 119:391–394, 1993.
25. Hollister LE, Kosek JV: Sudden death during treatment with phenothiazine derivatives. *JAMA* 192:1035–1038, 1965.
26. Marks RC, Luchins DJ: Antipsychotic medications and seizures. *Psychiatr Med* 9:37–52, 1991.
27. Alldredge BK: Seizure risk associated with psychotropic drugs: clinical and pharmacokinetic considerations. *Neurology* 53[Suppl 2]:S68–S75, 1999.
28. Invega Sustenna. Janssen, Division of Ortho-McNeil-Janssen Pharmaceuticals, Inc. Titusville, NJ, [cited May 25, 2016]. Available at: www.invega.com/prescribing-information.
29. Javaid JI: Clinical pharmacokinetics of antipsychotics. *J Pharmacol* 34:286–295, 1994.
30. Ereshefsky L: Pharmacokinetics and drug interactions: update for new antipsychotics. *J Clin Psychiatry* 57[Suppl 11]:12–25, 1996.
31. Heath A, Svensson C, Martensson E: Thioridazine toxicity: an experimental cardiovascular study of thioridazine and its major metabolites in overdose. *Vet Hum Toxicol* 27:100–105, 1985.
32. Axelsson R, Martensson E: Side effects of thioridazine and their relationship with the serum concentrations of the drug and its main metabolites. *Curr Ther Res* 28:463, 1980.
33. Fang J, Gorrod JW: Metabolism, pharmacogenetics, and metabolic drug-drug interactions of antipsychotic drugs. *Cell Mol Neurobiol* 19:491–510, 1999.
34. Bond GR, Thompson JD: Olanzapine pediatric overdose [letter]. *Ann Emerg Med* 34:292–293, 1999.
35. Parsons M, Buckley NA: Antipsychotic drugs in overdose: practical management guidelines. *CNS Drugs* 6:427–441, 1997.
36. O'Malley GF, Seifert S, Heard K, et al: Olanzapine overdose mimicking opioid intoxication. *Ann Emerg Med* 34:279–281, 1999.
37. Barry D, Meyskens FL, Becker CE: Phenothiazine poisoning: a review of 48 cases. *Calif Med* 118:1–5, 1973.
38. Acri AA, Henretig FM: Effects of risperidone in overdose. *Am J Emerg Med* 16:498–501, 1998.
39. Mahutte CK, Nakassuto SK, Light RW: Haloperidol and sudden death due to pulmonary edema. *Arch Intern Med* 142:1951–1952, 1982.
40. Li C, Gefter WB: Acute pulmonary edema induced by overdosage of phenothiazines. *Chest* 101:102–104, 1992.
41. Yip L, Dart RC, Graham K: Olanzapine toxicity in a toddler [letter]. *Pediatrics* 102:1494, 1998.
42. Burns MJ, Linden CH, Graudins A, et al: A comparison of physostigmine and benzodiazepines for the treatment of anticholinergic poisoning. *Ann Emerg Med* 35:374–381, 2000.
43. Rosenbaum C, Bird SB: Timing and frequency of physostigmine redosing for antimuscarinic toxicity. *J Med Toxicol* 6(4):386–392, 2010.
44. Balestrieri M, Vampini C, Bellantuono C: Efficacy and safety of novel antipsychotics: a critical review. *Hum Psychopharmacol Clin Exp* 15:499–512, 2000.
45. Bonin MM, Burkhart KK: Olanzapine overdose in a 1-year-old male. *Ped Emerg Care* 15:266–267, 1999.
46. McGeer PL, Boulding JE, Gibson WC, et al: Drug-induced extrapyramidal reactions. *JAMA* 177:665–670, 1961.
47. Stahl SM, Berger PA: Bromocriptine, physostigmine, and neurotransmitter mechanisms in the dystonias. *Neurology* 32:889–892, 1982.
48. Young AB, Albion RL, Penney JB: Neuropharmacology of basal ganglia function: relationship to pathophysiology of movement disorders, in Grossman AR, Sambrook MA (eds): *Neural Mechanisms in Disorders of Movement*, London, Libbey, 1989, p 17.
49. Carlsson A, Walters N, Carlsson ML: Neurotransmitter interactions in schizophrenia—therapeutic implications. *Biol Psychiatry* 46:1388–1395, 1999.
50. Rupniak NMJ, Jenner P, Marsden CD: Acute dystonia induced by neuroleptic drugs. *Psychopharmacol* 88:403–419, 1986.
51. Baldessarini RJ, Tarsy D: Dopamine and the pathophysiology of dyskinesia induced by antipsychotic drugs. *Annu Rev Neurosci* 3:23–41, 1980.
52. Stockmeier CA, DiCarlo JJ, Zhang Y, et al: Characterization of typical and atypical antipsychotic drugs based on in vivo occupancy of $serotonin_2$ and $dopamine_2$ receptors. *J Pharmacol Exp Ther* 266:1374–1384, 1993.
53. Kolbe H, Clow A, Jenner P, et al: Neuroleptic-induced acute dystonic reactions may be due to enhanced dopamine release or to supersensitive postsynaptic receptors. *Neurology* 31:434–439, 1981.
54. Marsden CD, Jenner P: The pathophysiology of extrapyramidal side-effects of neuroleptic drugs. *Psychol Med* 10:55–72, 1980.
55. Swett C: Drug-induced dystonia. *Am J Psychiatry* 132:532–534, 1982.
56. Kingsbury SJ, Fayek M, Trufasiu D: The apparent effects of ziprasidone on plasma lipids and glucose. *J Clin Psychiatry* 62:347–349, 2001.
57. Lebovitz HE: Metabolic consequences of atypical antipsychotic drugs. *Psychiatr Q* 74:277–290, 2003.
58. Litvak R, Kaelbling R: Agranulocytosis, leukopenia and psychotropic drugs. *Arch Gen Psychiatry* 24:265–267, 1971.
59. Trayle WH: Phenothiazine-induced agranulocytosis [letter]. *JAMA* 256:1957, 1986.
60. Safferman A, Lieberman JA, Kane JM, et al: Update on the clinical efficacy and side effects of clozapine. *Schizophr Bull* 17:247–261, 1991.
61. Iqbal MM, Rahman A, Husain K, et al: Clozapine: a clinical review of adverse effects and management. *Ann Clin Psychiatry* 15:33–48, 2003.
62. Gerson SL: G-CSF and the management of clozapine-induced agranulocytosis. *J Clin Psychiatry* 55[Suppl B]:139–142, 1994.
63. Ruhe HG, Becker HE, Jessurun P: Agranulocytosis and granulocytopenia associated with quetiapine. *Acta Psychiatr Scand* 104:311–313, 2001.
64. Haberfellner EM, Honsig T: Nonalcoholic steatohepatitis: a possible side effect of atypical antipsychotics. *J Clin Psychiatry* 64:851, 2003.
65. Liebzeit KA: New onset diabetes and atypical antipsychotics. *Eur Neuropsychopharmacol* 11:25–32, 2001.
66. Gianfrancesco F, White R, Ruey-hua W, et al: Antipsychotic-induced type 2 diabetes: evidence from a large health plan database. *J Clin Psychopharmacol* 23:328–335, 2003.
67. Torrey EF, Swalwell CI: Fatal olanzapine-induced ketoacidosis. *Am J Psychiatry*160:2241, 2003.
68. Meatherall R, Younes J: Fatality from olanzapine-induced hyperglycemia. *J Forensic Sci* 47:893–896, 2002.
69. Wehring HJ, Kelly DL, Love RC, et al: Deaths from diabetic ketoacidosis after long-term clozapine treatment. *Am J Psychiatry* 160:2241–2242, 2003.
70. Haupt DW, Newcomer JW: Hyperglycemia and antipsychotic medications. *J Clin Psychiatry* 62[Suppl 27]:15–26, 2001.
71. Meyer JM: Novel antipsychotics and severe hyperlipidemia. *J Clin Psychopharmacol* 21:369–374, 2001.
72. Domon SE, Webber JC: Hyperglycemia and hypertriglyceridemia secondary to olanzapine. *J Clin Adolesc Psychopharmacol* 11:285–288, 2001.
73. Merrill DB, Dec GW, Goff DC: Adverse cardiac effects associated with clozapine. *J Clin Psychopharmacol* 25:32–41, 2005.
74. DeVane CL: Drug interactions and antipsychotic therapy. *Pharmacotherapy* 16[Suppl]:15–20, 1996.
75. Cobb CD, Anderson CB, Seidel DR: Possible interaction between clozapine and lorazepam [letter]. *Am J Psychiatry* 148:1606–1607, 1991.
76. Edge SC, Markowitz JS, DeVane CL: Clozapine drug interactions: a review of the literature. *Hum Psychopharmacol* 12:5–20, 1997.

77. Cohen LG, Chesley S, Eugenio L, et al: Erythromycin-induced clozapine toxic reaction. *Arch Intern Med* 156:675–677, 1996.
78. Funderberg LG, Vertrees JE, True JE, et al: Seizure following addition of erythromycin to clozapine treatment. *Am J Psychiatry* 151:1840–1841, 1994.
79. Axelsson R, Aspenstrom G: Electrocardiographic changes and serum concentrations in thioridazine-treated patients. *J Clin Psychiatry* 43:332–335, 1982.
80. Mitchell AA, Lovejoy FH, Goldman P: Drug ingestions associated with miosis in comatose children. *J Pediatr* 89:303–305, 1976.
81. Knight ME, Roberts RJ: Phenothiazine and butyrophenone intoxication in children. *Pediatr Clin North Am* 33:299–309, 1986.
82. Zee-cheng CS, Mueller CE, Seifert CF, et al: Haloperidol and torsades de pointes [letter]. *Ann Intern Med* 102:418, 1985.
83. Isbister GK, Murray L, John S, et al: Amisulpride deliberate self-poisoning causing severe cardiac toxicity including QT prolongation and torsades de pointes. *Med J Aust* 184(7):354–356, 2006.
84. Sharma ND, Rosman HS, Padhi D, et al: Torsades de pointes associated with intravenous haloperidol in critically ill patients. *Am J Cardiol* 81:238–240, 1998.
85. Lischke V, Behne M, Doelken P, et al: Droperidol causes a dose-dependent prolongation of the QT interval. *Anesth Analg* 79:983–986, 1994.
86. Jackson CW, Sheehan AH, Reddan JG: Evidence-based review of the black-box warning for droperidol. *Am J Health Syst Pharm* 64:1174–1186, 2007.
87. Baker PB, Merigian KS, Roberts JR, et al: Hyperthermia, hypotension, hypertonia, and coma in a massive thioridazine overdose. *Am J Emerg Med* 6:346–349, 1988.
88. Tam CW, Olin BR, Ruiz AE: Loxapine-associated rhabdomyolysis and acute renal failure. *Arch Intern Med* 140:975–976, 1980.
89. Hoffman AS, Schwartz HI, Novick RM: Catatonic reaction to accidental haloperidol overdose: an unrecognized drug abuse risk. *J Nerv Ment Dis* 174:428–430, 1986.
90. Fahn S: The varied clinical expressions of dystonia. *Neurol Clin* 2:541–554, 1984.
91. Koek RJ, Edmond HP: Acute laryngeal dystonic reactions to neuroleptics. *Psychosomatics* 30:359–364, 1989.
92. Baselt RC (ed): *Disposition of Toxic Drugs and Chemicals in Man.* 7th ed. Foster City, CA, Biomedical Publications, 2004.
93. Forrest FM, Forrest IS, Mason AS: Review of rapid urine tests for phenothiazine and related drugs. *Am J Psychiatry* 118:300–307, 1961.
94. Sloan KL, Haver VM, Saxon AJ: Quetiapine and false-positive urine drug testing for tricyclic antidepressants [letter]. *Am J Psychiatr* 157:148–149, 2000.
95. Chandavasu O, Chatkupt S: Central nervous system depression from chlorpromazine poisoning: successful treatment with naloxone. *J Pediatr* 106:515–516, 1985.
96. Kawamura T, Kodama I, Toyama J, et al: Combined application of class I antiarrhythmic drugs causes "additive," "reductive," or "synergistic" sodium channel block in cardiac muscles. *Cardiovasc Res* 24:925–931, 1990.
97. Lumpkin J, Watanabe AS, Rumack BH, et al: Phenothiazine-induced ventricular tachycardia following acute overdose. *JACEP* 8:476–478, 1979.
98. Turner-Lawrence DE, Kerns II W: Intravenous fat emulsion: a potential novel antidote. *J Med Toxicol* 4:109–114, 2008.
99. Finn SDH, Uncles DR, Willers J, et al: Early treatment of a quetiapine and sertraline overdose with Intralipid. *Anaesthesia* 64:191–194, 2009.
100. Kulig K, Bar-Or D, Cantrill SV, et al: Management of acutely poisoned patients without gastric emptying. *Ann Emerg Med* 14:562–567, 1985.
101. Koppel C, Schirop T, Ibe K, et al: Hemoperfusion in chlorprothixene overdose. *Intensive Care Med* 13:358–360, 1987.
102. Donlon PT, Tupin JP: Successful suicides with thioridazine and mesoridazine. *Arch Gen Psychiatry* 34:955–957, 1977.
103. Hals PA, Jacobsen D: Resin hemoperfusion in levomepromazine poisoning: evaluation of effect on plasma drug and metabolite levels. *Hum Toxicol* 3:497–503, 1984.
104. Bailie GR, Nelson MV, Krenzelok EP, et al: Unusual treatment response of a severe dystonia to diphenhydramine. *Ann Emerg Med* 16:705–708, 1987.
105. Merck and Company, Inc: Cogentin, in *Physicians' Desk Reference*. Montvale, NJ, Medical Economics, 2002 pp 2055–2056.

Chapter 106 ▪ Beta-Blocker Poisoning

SHAN YIN • JAVIER C. WAKSMAN

Since 1958, when dichloroisoprenaline, the first β-adrenergic blocker, was synthesized, more than a dozen β-blockers have been introduced into the international pharmaceutical markets. Originally developed for the treatment of angina pectoris and dysrhythmias, β-blockers are now used in a wide variety of disorders. Intoxication may result from oral, parenteral, and even ophthalmic use.

PHARMACOLOGY

β-Blockers act by competitively inhibiting the binding of epinephrine and norepinephrine to β-adrenergic neuroreceptors in the heart (β_1), blood vessels, bronchioles (β_2), and other organs (Table 106.1). Binding to the β receptor (a G-protein–coupled receptor) activates phosphodiesterase and increases cytoplasmic cyclic adenosine monophosphate (cAMP). This in turn leads to modification of cellular processes and changes in ionic channel conductance. By reducing the activity of β receptors, the production of cAMP is decreased and β effect is diminished [1].

β-Blockers are usually rapidly absorbed after oral administration. The β-blocker dose required to produce a toxic effect is variable, depending on the sympathetic tone and metabolic capacity of the person and the pharmacologic properties of the particular β-blocker [1]. The first signs of toxicity may appear 20 minutes after ingestion, with peak effects typically occurring 1 to 2 hours after an immediate-release preparation overdose. Absorption of modified-release formulations may be erratic after an overdose, however, and clinical toxicity may be significantly delayed. The duration of toxicity may be several days [1].

The pharmacologic and pharmacokinetic properties of β-blockers are variable (Table 106.2). Cardioselectivity tends to be lost at high doses, and membrane-stabilizing effects, which are minimal at therapeutic doses, assume a more important role

TABLE 106.1

Distribution and Function of β-Receptors

Receptor Subtype	Location	Response to Stimulation
β_1	Eye	Aqueous humor production
	Heart	Increased automaticity, conduction velocity, contractility, and refractory period
β_2	Kidney	Renin production
	Blood vessels	Smooth muscle contraction
	Bronchioles	Smooth muscle contraction
	Fat	Lipolysis
	Liver	Gluconeogenesis, glycogenolysis
	Pancreas	Insulin release
	Skeletal muscle	Increased tone, potassium uptake
	Uterus	Smooth muscle relaxation

TABLE 106.2

Pharmacologic and Pharmacokinetic Properties of β-Adrenergic Blocking Agents

Agent	Adrenergic Receptor-Blocking Activity	Intrinsic Sympathomimetic Activity	Lipid Solubility	Extent of Absorption (%)	Absolute Oral Bioavailability (%)	Half-life (h)	Protein Binding (%)	Metabolism/Excretion
Acebutolol	β_1^a	+	Low	90	20–60	3–4	26	Hepatic, renal excretion 30%–40%, nonrenal 50%–60%
Atenolol	β_1^a	0	Low	≈50	≈50	5–8	<5	≈75% excreted unchanged in urine and feces
Betaxolol	β_1^a	0	Low	100	89	14–22	≈50	Hepatic; >80% recovered in urine
Bisoprolol	β_1^a	0	Low	≥90	80	9–12	≈30	≈50% excreted unchanged in urine, remainder as inactive metabolites
Esmolol	β_1^a	0	Moderate	NA	NA	0.15	55	Rapid metabolism by esterases in cytosol of red blood cells
Metoprolol, long-acting	β_1^a	0	Moderate	95	40–50	3–7	12	Hepatic, renal excretion, <5% unchanged
Carteolol	β_1, β_2	++	Low	80	85	6	23–30	50%–70% unchanged in urine
Nadolol	β_1, β_2	0	Low	30	30–50	20–24	30	Urine, unchanged
Penbutolol	β_1, β_2	+	High	≈100	≈100	5	80–98	Hepatic (conjugation and oxidation); renal excretion of metabolites
Pindolol	β_1, β_2	+++	Moderate	95	≈100	3–4[b]	40	Urinary excretion of metabolites (60%–74%) and unchanged drug (35%–40%)
Propranolol, long-acting	β_1, β_2	0	High	90	30	3–5	90	Hepatic; <1% excreted unchanged in urine
Sotalol	β_1, β_2	0	Low	No data	90–100	12	0	Not metabolized; excreted unchanged in urine
Timolol	β_1, β_2	0	Low to moderate	90	75	4	10	Hepatic; urinary excretion of metabolites and unchanged drug
Carvedilol	$\beta_1, \beta_2, \alpha_1$	0	High	NA	25–35	6–10	95–98	Hepatic (aromatic ring oxidation and conjugation), 16% renal excretion
Labetalol	β_1, α_1	0	Moderate	100	30–40	5.0–5.8	50	55%–60% excreted in urine as conjugates or unchanged drug

0, none; +, low; ++, moderate; +++, high; NA, not applicable (available intravenously only).

[a]Inhibits β_2 receptors (bronchial and vascular) at higher doses.

[b]In elderly hypertensive patients with normal renal function, $t_{1/2}$ is variable (7–15 h).

Reprinted from Olin BR, Hebel SK (eds): *Drug Facts and Comparisons*. St. Louis, MO, Facts and Comparisons, Inc, 1997; Hardman J, Limbird L, Molinoff P, et al. (eds): *Goodman and Gilman's Pharmacological Basis of Therapeutics*. 9th ed. New York, NY, McGraw-Hill, 1996.

[1]. Membrane dysfunction may account for many of the central nervous system (CNS) and myocardial depressant effects in patients poisoned by membrane-active drugs such as propranolol. The half-life may be significantly prolonged in patients with decreased hepatic and renal perfusion [1]. Intrinsic heart, kidney, and liver disease as well as the concomitant use of drugs with similar activity increase the risk of toxicity.

CLINICAL TOXICITY

The major manifestations relate to the cardiovascular system and CNS. Respiratory, peripheral vascular, and metabolic (hypoglycemic and hyperkalemic) effects have been infrequently reported [1,2].

Patients with severe poisoning frequently present with hypotension and bradycardia. Tachycardia and hypertension have been reported with agents possessing intrinsic sympathomimetic activity, particularly pindolol [1]. Congestive heart failure and pulmonary edema have infrequently been reported and mainly occur in patients with underlying heart disease [3]. Electrocardiographic manifestations may include prolonged PR interval, intraventricular conduction delay, progressive atrioventricular heart block, nonspecific ST-segment and T-wave changes, early repolarization, prolonged QTc, and asystole [4–6]. Sotalol poisoning may result in ventricular tachycardia, torsade de pointes, ventricular fibrillation, and multifocal ventricular extrasystoles [7]. Labetalol, which also has mild β-receptor–blocking properties, may cause profound hypotension, possibly from decreased peripheral resistance.

Depression of the level of consciousness, ranging from drowsiness to coma with seizures, is another common feature of β-blocker poisoning. Significant CNS depression has been reported in the absence of cardiovascular compromise [1] or hypoglycemia and may be due to direct membrane effects [8]. Cerebral hypoperfusion, hypoxia, and metabolic or respiratory acidosis frequently contribute to CNS toxicity. β-Blockers with high lipid solubility (e.g., propranolol, penbutolol, metoprolol) appear more likely to cause CNS effects than those with low lipid solubility (e.g., atenolol) [9].

Bronchospasm is a relatively rare consequence of β-blocker poisoning and usually occurs among patients with preexisting reactive airway disease. In most instances, respiratory depression appears to be secondary to a CNS effect [10–11].

Although it does occur, hypoglycemia is not a common complication of β-blocker poisoning. It appears to be more common in diabetics, children, and uremic patients, and it is the consequence of impaired glycogenolysis and hepatic gluconeogenesis [12]. A blunted tachycardic response to hypoglycemia may occur among patients with β-blocker toxicity, although other symptoms of hypoglycemia appear unaffected.

DIAGNOSTIC EVALUATION

The history should include the time, amount, and formulation of drugs ingested; the circumstances involved; time of onset and nature of any symptoms; and treatments rendered before arrival, as well as underlying health problems. β-Blocker poisoning may be difficult to recognize, especially when multiple drugs have been ingested [1]. β-Blocker poisoning should be suspected in a patient in whom hypotension or seizures suddenly develop or who has bradycardia resistant to the usual doses of chronotropic drugs. Evaluation of patients with suspected β-blocker poisoning should begin with a complete set of vital signs, continuous cardiac rhythm monitoring, and a 12-lead electrocardiogram. Physical examination should focus on the cardiovascular, pulmonary, and neurologic systems. Vital signs and physical examination should be frequently repeated.

Serum drug levels may help confirm the diagnosis but are rarely available quickly enough to be clinically useful. In addition, differences in individual patient metabolism and sympathetic tone may make interpretation of blood levels difficult [1,2]. A serum and urine specimen can be saved for later analysis for forensic cases. Continuous cardiac rhythm monitoring, interpretation of 12-lead electrocardiograms, and measurement of oxygen saturation should be routine. Laboratory evaluation of symptomatic patients should include electrolytes, blood urea nitrogen, creatinine, bicarbonate, and glucose. Arterial blood gas and a chest film should be obtained as clinically indicated. Serum acetaminophen and aspirin levels should be obtained in patients with suicidal ideation.

The differential diagnosis of β-blocker toxicity includes antidysrhythmic drugs, calcium channel blockers, cholinergic agents, clonidine, digitalis, narcotics, sedative hypnotics, and tricyclic antidepressants. Anaphylactic, cardiogenic, hypovolemic, and septic shock should also be considered.

MANAGEMENT

Treatment is primarily supportive. This may include prompt endotracheal intubation and mechanical ventilation and management of life-threatening bradydysrhythmias, hypotension, bronchospasm, and seizures. These attempts should precede any measures (as described later) used to prevent or reduce drug absorption. A bedside glucose measure or, alternatively, an intravenous bolus of glucose (50 mL of $D_{50}W$ in adults; 5 mL per kg of $D_{10}W$ in children) as well as naloxone (2 mg in adults and children) should be considered for patients with altered mental status.

Activated charcoal is the preferred method for gastrointestinal decontamination. Gastric lavage has not been shown to improve outcomes after poisoning and should not be used routinely, but could be considered for recent life-threatening ingestions in patients who have not already vomited [13]. Whole-bowel irrigation with polyethylene glycol at a rate of 2 L per hour until the rectal effluent is clear may be considered for gastrointestinal decontamination in modified-release preparation overdoses.

Hypotension should be first treated with judicious intravenous crystalloid fluids. Because hypotension seldom responds solely to this treatment and because administration of high volumes (greater than 2 L) of intravenous fluids may pose a risk of developing pulmonary edema, the prompt use of inotropic drugs such as dopamine, dobutamine, epinephrine, norepinephrine, or phenylephrine is usually required [14]. Bradycardia from β-adrenergic antagonist poisoning seldom responds to atropine.

Calcium

The goal of calcium therapy is to increase extracellular calcium concentrations, thus increasing calcium influx through any unblocked calcium channels. Calcium has demonstrated effectiveness in animal models [15] and improvement has been reported for human cases [16]. However, responses are variable and often short-lived, and patients with significant toxicity usually fail to improve with calcium alone. Conduction disturbances, contractility, and blood pressure may be improved, but generally there is no increase in heart rate.

Calcium chloride compared to calcium gluconate contains three times the amount of elemental calcium on a milliequivalent basis (10% calcium chloride: 272 mg elemental calcium or 13.6 mEq per 1 g ampule; 10% calcium gluconate: 90 mg elemental calcium or 4.5 mEq per 1 g ampule). However, it is recommended to only give calcium chloride via a central venous catheter. Calcium gluconate can be given via a peripheral line.

Optimum calcium dosing is not well established. Initial doses are generally given as boluses (10 to 20 mL of 10% calcium chloride, or 30 to 60 mL of 10% calcium gluconate). Additional boluses may be given every 10 to 20 minutes. Boluses should be given over a 5-minute period in conjunction with cardiac monitoring as rapid infusions have resulted in hypotension, atrioventricular dissociation, and ventricular fibrillation. The effects of boluses may be transient, and a constant infusion may be required. Infusions can be started at 0.4 mL/kg/h for calcium chloride and 1.2 mL/kg/h for calcium gluconate and titrated to effect. Additional boluses can be given as needed. Calcium levels should be monitored. Raising serum ionized calcium to 2 to 3 mEq per L improves canine cardiac performance in verapamil poisoning, and is a reasonable goal to attain. It may be necessary to continue therapy despite high serum calcium levels if the patient is only responding to calcium administration. Hypercalcemia can lead to renal failure and limb or mesenteric ischemia. It is recommended to stop calcium infusions if no beneficial effect is observed.

Glucagon

Although there are no controlled trials of glucagon for βblocker overdose in humans, glucagon has served as an effective agent for reversing hypotension and bradycardia in multiple case reports [17,18] and has a long history of use. Glucagon is typically given as an initial bolus of 3 to 5 mg for adults and 0.05 mg per kg for children. If there is no response to the initial bolus, a second bolus of 6 to 10 mg (0.10 mg per kg in children) can be given. Glucagon has a half-life of 20 minutes, so a continuous intravenous infusion of 1 to 10 mg per hour is recommended if the bolus is successful for improving hemodynamic parameters. The continuous infusion rate is set at the successful bolus rate (i.e., if a 5 mg bolus was successful, the infusion would be 5 mg per hour). Large total doses may be required. The dose should be tapered once the patient's clinical condition improves. The mechanism by which glucagon produces positive inotropic and chronotropic effects on the heart is believed to be activation of the adenyl cyclase pathway, which converts adenosine triphosphate to cAMP through an independent receptor, changing membrane ion conductivity, altering calcium influx, and augmenting contractility even in the presence of complete β-adrenergic blockade [17].

Phosphodiesterase Inhibitors

The simultaneous use of multiple agents may be effective when a single agent fails. Although theoretically promising, phosphodiesterase inhibitors such as amrinone and milrinone, which inhibit the breakdown of cAMP to AMP, have not proven to be superior to glucagon for reversing the hemodynamic effects of β-blocker overdose in a canine model [19]. It has been suggested that phosphodiesterase inhibitors might be used in cases of β-blocker poisoning when adequate doses of glucagon are not available [19]. The phosphodiesterase inhibitor enoximone has been successfully used in cases of β-blocker overdoses [20].

Sodium Bicarbonate

A number of β-blockers (propranolol, carvedilol, pindolol, and acebutolol) also affect cardiac sodium channels producing membrane-stabilizing effects which may result in quinidine-like dysrhythmias (e.g., wide QRS complexes). This effect may respond to intravenous boluses of sodium bicarbonate, albeit in a canine model sodium bicarbonate was ineffective for treating propranolol toxicity that resulted in bradycardia, hypotension, and wide QRS intervals [21]. In a case report, sodium bicarbonate appeared to reverse QRS widening following an acebutolol overdose [22]. The recommended dose is 1 to 2 mEq per kg given as a rapid infusion over several minutes.

Hyperinsulin Euglycemia Treatment

High-dose insulin while maintaining euglycemia has been proposed as an antidote for β-blocker poisoning. Insulin is an inotropic agent, which may enhance response to catecholamines and reverse metabolic acidosis. Although results in animals remain encouraging [23,24], further studies are needed in humans. There are several human case reports where high-dose insulin resulted in improvements in hemodynamic parameters for isolated βblocker overdoses [25,26]. The general recommended starting dose is a 1.0 U per kg bolus followed by a continuous infusion of 0.5 to 1.0 U/kg/h. This rate can be titrated up to effect. A second intravenous infusion of $D_{10}W$ or $D_{25}W$ containing potassium chloride should be simultaneously administered to the insulin infusion at a rate sufficient to maintain the serum glucose and potassium concentrations in the normal range.

Vasopressin

The use of vasopressin for βblocker toxicity has been suggested. In one animal trial which compared vasopressin with glucagon as the treatment for β-blocker toxicity; vasopressin neither increased survival nor had a significant effect on any of the cardiac parameters tested compared to glucagon [27]. High-dose insulin treatment also improved survival when compared to vasopressin with epinephrine in a swine model [24].

Lipid Emulsion

The use of lipid emulsion has been suggested for the treatment of the cardiotoxic effects of local anesthetics. Various animal models of bupivacaine toxicity have demonstrated faster return of spontaneous circulation following treatment with lipid emulsion therapy [28,29] as well as improved cardiodynamic parameters when compared with epinephrine [30]. In a rabbit model, lipid emulsion successfully improved hypotension induced by propranolol when compared with placebo [31]. In a separate study of rats, pretreatment with lipid emulsion resulted in a significant reduction in QRS duration and a nonsignificant improvement in bradycardia induced by propranolol when compared with placebo [32]. Positive outcomes with the use of lipid emulsion were described for human case reports of bupivacaine [33,34], bupropion and lamotrigine [35], and quetiapine and sertraline overdoses [36]. There are no controlled trials of humans but in a number of case reports there was dramatic improvement [25,37]. The mechanism of how lipid emulsion may be beneficial is not completely understood. Possible explanations include the creation of lipid sink for fat-soluble drugs, augmentation of cardiac energy substrates, or the improvement in mycocardial function by increasing intracellular calcium [37]. No standard dosing regimen exists. However, a loading dose of 1.5 mL per kg administered over 1 minute, repeated 1 to 2 times every 3 to 5 minutes as needed, is often used. If hemodynamic improvement is noted, the loading dose should be followed by a continuous infusion at a rate of 0.25 to 0.5 mL/kg/min. Further information can be found at www.lipidrescue.org.

Extracorporeal Removal

Although the efficacy of hemodialysis for acute β-blocker poisoning has not been studied in controlled clinical trials, it is theoretically useful for removing β-blockers that have a low volume of distribution, are not significantly protein bound, and are hydrophilic. This would include acebutolol, atenolol, nadolol, sotalol, and timolol. Hemodialysis appeared to be clinically useful in a number of case reports involving various β blockers [38,39]. Continuous Veno-Venous Hemo-Dia-Filtration (CVVHDF) was also successfully used for the treatment of a combined atenolol/nifedipine overdose [40].

Other Interventions

Transient blood pressure elevations caused by pindolol usually require no specific treatment. Short-acting agents such as nitroprusside should be used if marked blood pressure elevation occurs, especially if it is accompanied by organ ischemia. Ventricular dysrhythmias induced by sotalol have been treated with lidocaine, isoproterenol, magnesium, and cardioversion defibrillation [5]. Electrical cardiac pacing may be needed if bradycardia, hypotension, and heart block fail to respond to pharmacologic therapy [1], or if ventricular tachydysrhythmias associated with a prolonged QTc interval are difficult to control [5]. For severe overdoses, a pacemaker may not capture. If capture occurs, the increased heart rate may not increase blood pressure. Heart rates greater than 90 to 100 beats per minute significantly decrease diastolic filling time and may adversely affect inotropy. Intraaortic balloon pump counterpulsation and extracorporeal circulation [41] have been successfully used for cardiovascular support.

Patients with β-blocker overdose who have abnormal vital signs, altered mental status, or dysrhythmias on presentation should be admitted to an intensive care unit. If vital signs can be supported, complete recovery should be expected within 24 to 48 hours. Patients may be discharged after at least 6 hours of emergency department observation if they have ingested an immediate-release product, present with mild to absent toxicity and remain or become asymptomatic, have normal vital signs on discharge, and have received activated charcoal. These patients should be referred for psychiatric evaluation in the event of an intentional overdose or discharged in the care of a reliable observer after an accidental overdose. Any other symptoms mandate longer observation or admission. Because of the potential for delayed toxicity, prolonged observation is recommended after modified-release preparation overdose.

References

1. Frishman W, Jacob H, Eisenberg E, et al: Clinical pharmacology of the new beta-adrenergic blocking drugs. Part 8. Self-poisoning with beta-adrenoceptor blocking agents: recognition and management. *Am Heart J* 98:798–811, 1979.
2. Prichard BN, Battersby LA, Cruickshank JM: Overdosage with beta-adrenergic blocking agents. *Adverse Drug React Acute Poisoning Rev* 3:91–111, 1984.
3. Richards DA, Prichard BN: Self-poisoning with beta-blockers. *Br Med J* 1:1623–1624, 1978.
4. Lagerfelt J, Matell G: Attempted suicide with 5.1 g of propranolol. A case report. *Acta Med Scand* 199:517–518, 1976.
5. Khan A, Muscat-Baron JM: Fatal oxprenolol poisoning. *Br Med J* 1:552, 1977.
6. Gwinup GR: Propranolol toxicity presenting with early repolarization, ST segment elevation, and peaked T waves on the ECG. *Ann Emerg Med* 17:171–174, 1988.
7. Baliga BG: Beta-blocker poisoning: prolongation of Q-T interval and inversion of T wave. *J Indian Med Assoc* 83:165, 1985.
8. Frishman W, Kostis J, Strom J, et al: Clinical pharmacology of the new beta-adrenergic blocking drugs. Part 6. A comparison of pindolol and propranolol in treatment of patients with angina pectoris. The role of intrinsic sympathomimetic activity. *Am Heart J* 98:526–535, 1979.
9. Buiumsohn A, Eisenberg ES, Jacob H, et al: Seizures and intraventricular conduction defect in propranolol poisoning. A report of two cases. *Ann Intern Med* 91:860–862, 1979.
10. Wallin CJ, Hulting J: Massive metoprolol poisoning treated with prenalterol. *Acta Med Scand* 214:253–255, 1983.
11. Weinstein RS, Cole S, Knaster HB, et al: Beta blocker overdose with propranolol and with atenolol. *Ann Emerg Med* 14:161–163, 1985.
12. Bressler P, DeFronzo RA: Drugs and diabetes. *Diabetes Rev* 2:53–84, 1994.
13. Benson BE, Hoppu K, Troutman WG, et al: Position paper update: gastric lavage for gastrointestinal decontamination. *Clin Toxicol* 51:140–146, 2013.
14. Critchley JA, Ungar A: The management of acute poisoning due to beta-adrenoceptor antagonists. *Med Toxicol Adverse Drug Exp* 4:32–45, 1989.
15. Vick JA, Kandil A, Herman EH, et al: Reversal of propranolol and verapamil toxicity by calcium. *Vet Hum Toxicol* 25:8–10, 1983.
16. O'Grady J, Anderson S, Pringle D: Successful treatment of severe atenolol overdose with calcium chloride. *CJEM* 3:224–227, 2001.
17. Illingworth RN: Glucagon for beta-blocker poisoning. *Practitioner* 223:683–685, 1979.
18. Robson RH: Glucagon for beta-blocker poisoning. *Lancet* 1:1357–1358, 1980.
19. Love JN, Leasure JA, Mundt DJ, et al: A comparison of amrinone and glucagon therapy for cardiovascular depression associated with propranolol toxicity in a canine model. *J Toxicol Clin Toxicol* 30:399–412, 1992.
20. Hoeper MM, Boeker KH: Overdose of metoprolol treated with enoximone. *N Engl J Med* 335:1538, 1996.
21. Love JN, Howell JM, Newsome JT, et al: The effect of sodium bicarbonate on propranolol-induced cardiovascular toxicity in a canine model. *J Toxicol Clin Toxicol* 38:421–428, 2000.
22. Donovan KD, Gerace RV, Dreyer JF: Acebutolol-induced ventricular tachycardia reversed with sodium bicarbonate. *J Toxicol Clin Toxicol* 37:481–484, 1999.
23. Kerns W, Schroeder D, Williams C, et al: Insulin improves survival in a canine model of acute beta-blocker toxicity. *Ann Emerg Med* 29:748–757, 1997.
24. Holger JS, Engebretsen KM, Fritzlar SJ, et al: Insulin versus vasopressin and epinephrine to treat beta-blocker toxicity. *Clin Toxicol (Phila)* 45:396–401, 2007.
25. Stellpflug SJ, Harris CR, Engebretsen KM, et al: Intentional overdose with cardiac arrest treated with intravenous fat emulsion and high dose insulin. *Clin Toxicol* 48:227–229, 2010.
26. Page C, Hacket LP, Isbister GK: The use of high-dose insulin-glucose euglycemia in beta-blocker overdose:a case report. *J Med Toxicol* 5:139–143, 2009.
27. Holger JS, Engebretsen KM, Obetz CL, et al: A comparison of vasopressin and glucagon in beta-blocker induced toxicity. *Clin Toxicol (Phila)* 44:45–51, 2006.
28. Weinberg GL, VadeBoncouer T, Ramaraju GA, et al: Pretreatment or resuscitation with a lipid infusion shifts the dose-response to bupivacaine-induced asystole in rats. *Anesthesiology* 88:1071–1075, 1998.
29. Weinberg G, Ripper R, Feinstein DL, et al: Lipid emulsion infusion rescues dogs from bupivacaine-induced cardiac toxicity. *Reg Anesth Pain Med* 28:198–202, 2003.
30. Weinberg GL, Di Gregorio G, Ripper R, et al: Resuscitation with lipid versus epinephrine in a rat model of bupivacaine overdose. *Anesthesiology* 108:907–913, 2008.
31. Harvey MG, Cave GR: Intralipid infusion ameliorates propranolol-induced hypotension in rabbits. *J Med Toxicol* 4:71–76, 2008.
32. Cave G, Harvey MG, Castle CD: The role of fat emulsion therapy in a rodent model of propranolol toxicity: a preliminary study. *J Med Toxicol* 2:4–7, 2006.
33. Warren JA, Thoma RB, Georgescu A, et al: Intravenous lipid infusion in the successful resuscitation of local anesthetic-induced cardiovascular collapse after supraclavicular brachial plexus block. *Anesth Analg* 106:1578–1580, 2008.
34. Foxall G, McCahon R, Lamb J, et al: Levobupivacaine-induced seizures and cardiovascular collapse treated with Intralipid. *Anaesthesia* 62:516–518, 2007.
35. Sirianni AJ, Osterhoudt KC, Calello DP, et al: Use of lipid emulsion in the resuscitation of a patient with prolonged cardiovascular collapse after overdose of bupropion and lamotrigine. *Ann Emerg Med* 51:412–415, 415.e1.
36. Finn SDH, Uncles DR, Willers J, et al: Early treatment of a quetiapine and sertraline overdose with Intralipid. *Anaesthesia* 64:191–194, 2009.
37. Samuels RL, Uncles DR, Willers JW: Intravenous lipid emulsion treatment for propranolol toxicity: another piece in the lipid sink jigsaw fits. *Clin Toxicol* 49:769, 2011.
38. Snook CP, Sigvaldason K, Kristinsson J: Severe atenolol and diltiazem overdose. *J Toxicol Clin Toxicol* 38:661–665, 2000.
39. Rooney M, Massey KL, Jamali F, et al: Acebutolol overdose treated with hemodialysis and extracorporeal membrane oxygenation. *J Clin Pharmacol* 36:760–763, 1996.
40. Pfaender M, Casetti PG, Azzolini M, et al: Successful treatment of a massive atenolol and nifedipine overdose with CVVHDF. *Minerva Anestesiol* 74:97–100, 2008.
41. Rygnestad T, Moen S, Wahba A, et al: Severe poisoning with sotalol and verapamil. Recovery after 4 h of normothermic CPR followed by extra corporeal heart lung assist. *Acta Anaesthesiol Scand* 49:1378–1380, 2005.

Chapter 107 ■ Calcium Channel Antagonist Poisoning

CHRISTOPHER R. DEWITT

INTRODUCTION

Accidental and intentional overdoses of calcium channel antagonists (CCAs) can be life threatening. CCAs consistently top the list of cardiovascular medications with the greatest proportion of deaths per exposure. Severely poisoned patients demonstrate cardiovascular collapse, but also metabolic derangements that appear similar to diabetic acidosis. Cardiovascular instability is often refractory to typical cardiotonic therapies and medication doses. There is no antidote for CCAs, and no controlled clinical studies to guide therapy. Treatment recommendations are therefore based on case series, case reports, animal studies, and expert opinion. Simultaneous use of multiple therapies is often required, and should be tailored to the patient's cardiovascular and metabolic responses. Overall goals of treatment are to provide supportive care, optimize cardiovascular and metabolic function, and decrease drug absorption. If vital signs can be supported until the drug is metabolized or eliminated, most patients will survive without sequelae.

PHYSIOLOGY AND PATHOPHYSIOLOGY

Available CCAs antagonize calcium influx through L-type voltage-sensitive channels, a specific type of calcium channel found in the heart, vascular smooth muscle, and pancreatic β-islet cells. Multiple physiologic functions are dependent on calcium influx through these channels.

In the cardiovascular system, calcium influx through L-type channels is responsible for the spontaneous pacemaker activity of the sinoatrial (SA) node and depolarization of the atrioventricular (AV) node. Other myocardial cells rely on calcium entry via L-type channels during the plateau phase of the action potential. Calcium entry during the plateau phase signals the release of additional calcium from intracellular stores allowing contraction to occur. The magnitude and duration of myocardial contraction is proportional to the magnitude and duration of calcium entry via L-type channels. Vascular smooth muscle tone is also maintained by a similar mechanism. Thus, therapeutic clinical effects of CCAs arise from blockade of L-type channels resulting in decreased cytosolic calcium levels. Depending on the class of CCA administered (see "Pharmacology" section), the clinical result is depression of SA node automaticity, AV node conduction, myocardial contractility, and vasodilation. The pathophysiologic effects of CCA overdose are essentially an exaggeration of pharmacologic effects, which lead to cardiovascular shock.

In addition to cardiovascular effects, CCA poisoning also produces a diabetogenic effect of hyperglycemia and acidosis. Insulin secretion is dependent on calcium influx into pancreatic β-islet cells. Although generally not a concern at therapeutic doses, calcium channel blockers (CCBs) decrease insulin secretion [1]. In canine models of verapamil-induced shock, hyperglycemia occurs but systemic insulin levels fail to increase [2–4]. Verapamil toxicity also produces systemic [4] and myocardial [3] insulin resistance. The cause of this resistance may be multifactorial involving decreased substrate delivery from poor perfusion, interference with calcium-dependent cellular insulin responsiveness and glucose uptake, and inhibition of calcium-stimulated mitochondrial dehydrogenases (i.e., pyruvate dehydrogenase) and glucose catabolism [4]. More recent evidence suggests CCAs interfere with cellular signaling, specifically recruitment of glucose transporter proteins (GLUTs) from the intracellular space to cell membranes [5,6]. These GLUTs are responsible for normal cellular uptake of glucose.

Verapamil toxicity also produces a state of hyperlacticacidemia because of a combination of tissue hypoperfusion and probably a defect in carbohydrate metabolism [4]. In stressed states such as CCA toxicity, the heart switches from preferentially using free fatty acids to carbohydrates (glucose and lactate) for energy production [2,3,7]. Although there is an abundance of circulating carbohydrates (e.g., glucose and lactate), they are essentially unavailable for use because of decreased insulin availability and systemic insulin resistance.

In essence, CCAs decrease cytosolic calcium levels resulting in desirable cardiovascular effects at therapeutic doses, and at toxic doses an exaggeration of those effects. Additionally, toxicity produces a vicious cycle where the myocardium is preferentially metabolizing carbohydrates, yet carbohydrate utilization is hindered by impaired insulin release and systemic insulin resistance.

PHARMACOLOGY

Clinically available CCAs fall into one of three classes: phenylalkylamine (verapamil), benzothiazepine (diltiazem), and dihydropyridines (nifedipine and all other agents). At therapeutic doses, each class has differing affinities for myocardial tissues and vascular smooth muscle. Verapamil and diltiazem are potent inhibitors of SA node automaticity, AV node conduction, myocardial contractility, and cause modest vasodilation [8]. Verapamil affects the SA node, contractility, and vasodilation more than diltiazem [8]. This is probably why toxic ingestion of verapamil generally causes more deaths than other CCAs. Dihydropyridines are far more selective for vascular smooth muscle, and at therapeutic doses have very little effect on cardiac pacemaker cells or contractility [8]. In significant poisoning, this selectivity is however lost.

Pharmacologic properties of CCAs make extracorporeal removal of limited or no value. However, plasmapheresis was believed to be beneficial in several cases [9–11] and recently albumin dialysis with the Molecular Adsorbent Recirculating System was used successfully in three severe CCA poisonings [12]. Therapeutic half-lives of CCBs are variable, but in overdose can be prolonged [13]. The duration of toxicity for most cases is less than 24 hours, but has been reported to last 48 hours with sustained-release (SR) verapamil [14] and for more than 5 days with amlodipine [15].

Verapamil, diltiazem, nifedipine, and several of the newer dihydropyridines are available in both immediate-release (IR) and SR formulations. This information becomes important when considering how long to observe asymptomatic patients after an overdose. IR preparations produce signs or symptoms of toxicity within 6 hours of ingestion, whereas toxicity with SR products may be delayed 6 to 12 hours [16] or rarely longer [17]. Amlodopine, a dihydropyridine, has unique pharmacokinetics however. It is not a SR product, but has a late onset of peak effect and long half-life allowing for delayed and prolonged toxicity.

There is no accurate definition of a toxic dose. Patients have demonstrated significantly different effects at similar doses. Unintentional overdoses are common, but uncommonly result in significant effect. However, several adult patients have developed toxicity and death at doses less than maximum recommended daily doses [18]. Factors that could have contributed to this are advanced age, underlying medical conditions, additional medications, and chewing and swallowing SR preparations—essentially changing the pharmacokinetics into an IR formulation [18]. Generally, the most significant poisonings are large intentional ingestions, but patients with significant underlying medical diseases or advanced age are prone to effects at lower doses.

CLINICAL MANIFESTATIONS

Cardiovascular effects are the primary manifestation of CCA poisoning. Alterations in mental status without significant hypotension should not be attributed to CCA ingestion. Minimally intoxicated patients, or those who present soon after ingestion, may demonstrate no signs of toxicity. All CCAs can cause hypotension in the setting of an overdose. However, the causes of the hypotension are typically an extension of the drugs' therapeutic effects (i.e., dihydropyridines causing significant vasodilation with reflex tachycardia where verapamil and diltiazem slow SA and AV node conduction, decrease contractility, and cause vasodilation). Thus, for overdose, normal sinus rhythm or reflex tachycardia is commonly seen early in nifedipine poisonings, where sinus bradycardia, AV nodal blocks, and junctional rhythm are common with verapamil and diltiazem ingestions [16]. This selectivity may be lost in large overdoses such that dihydropyridine poisoning results in bradycardia and/or impaired cardiac conduction [15,16,19–21]. Although overdose experience with dihydropyridines other than nifedipine is limited [15,20–22], they would be expected to have effects similar to nifedipine. The exception may be amlodipine where toxic effects may be delayed [21].

Severe poisoning is characterized by hypotension and bradycardia [16,23–25], hyperglycemia [19–21,23,26–32], and metabolic acidosis [2,15,19,21,27,32,33]. Hyperglycemia is caused by the aforementioned alterations in insulin and carbohydrate homeostasis (see "Physiology and Pathophysiology" section). In fact, in a recent review of 40 CCA overdoses, the degree of hyperglycemia was the best predictor of composite end points of death, pacemaker requirement, or vasopressor requirement [34]. Dysfunctional carbohydrate metabolism and tissue hypoperfusion can result in hyperlacticacidemia. Additionally, tissue hypoperfusion can result in cerebrovascular accidents, seizures, renal failure, myocardial infarction, and noncardiogenic pulmonary edema [35].

DIFFERENTIAL DIAGNOSIS

CCA poisoning should be considered for any patient presenting with hypotension and bradycardia. Suspicions that the patient is poisoned with a CCA should be raised even further if there is associated hyperglycemia and acidosis. However, the differential diagnosis of a patient with hypotension and bradycardia includes other toxicologic causes such as β-blockers, digoxin and other cardiac glycosides, antidysrhythmics, and clonidine. However, nontoxicologic causes such as myocardial disease, hyperkalemia, sepsis, and hypothyroidism should also be considered.

MANAGEMENT

General

Management of a patient with CCA poisoning begins with airway management and maintenance of vital signs. Vascular access should be obtained, and continuous blood pressure and cardiac monitoring initiated. Preemptive intubation should strongly be considered for patients with significant ingestions or signs of toxicity because of the potential for rapid deterioration. Among bradycardic patients, administration of atropine before intubation may prevent vagal responses from laryngoscopy. An electrocardiogram (ECG) should be obtained. The presence of dysrhythmias or conduction disturbances, which may be as subtle as PR prolongation for some patients, should be noted. Measurements of renal function, electrolytes, complete blood counts, liver function tests, arterial blood gases, and acetaminophen, salicylate, and digoxin levels should be guided by the clinical picture and medical history.

Serum CCA levels are not routinely available and do not help with patient management, but may be necessary for confirmation of the diagnosis. For patients with severe or refractory hypotension, urinary and central venous catheterization are recommended to guide fluid and vasopressor therapy. Finally, early consultation with a medical toxicologist regarding medical therapy, and a cardiologist regarding pacemaker or intraaortic balloon pump placement, is recommended.

Gastrointestinal Decontamination

Definitive data regarding the utility of gastrointestinal decontamination for CCA overdoses are lacking, and all forms of decontamination carry potential risks. However, CCA overdoses can result in serious morbidity and mortality, such that potential benefits of decontamination may outweigh the risks. Risks and benefits should be considered on a case by case basis, and interventions necessary to maintain vital signs take precedence over decontamination. Aspiration is one of the main risks associated with decontamination. Thus, assurance of airway control prior to decontamination is necessary.

Activated charcoal should be administered to all significant ingestions. The greatest benefit of charcoal administration occurs within the first 2 hours after ingestion [36]. However, it may hold benefit, especially for SR preparations, up to 4 hours after ingestion [36]. Gastric lavage should not be used routinely, but considered for recent life-threatening ingestions in patients who have not vomited [37]. Like laryngoscopy, lavage may theoretically increase vagal tone and exacerbate bradydysrhythmias. Administration of atropine prior to insertion of the lavage tube may ameliorate these effects.

Large ingestions of SR preparations may provide a gastrointestinal depot of drug causing recurrent cardiovascular compromise, or rise in serum drug levels up to 18 hours after initial decontamination [17,24,27,30,38,39]. A rise in serum amlodipine levels has been demonstrated 24.5 hours after ingestion—approximately 22 hours after decontamination [40]. Therefore, repeat charcoal doses or whole-bowel irrigation (WBI) with polyethylene glycol should be considered for large ingestions of SR products in patients with functioning gastrointestinal tracts [35]. Repeat charcoal dosing has also been recommended for large overdoses of IR products [13]. One or two additional doses of activated charcoal (0.5 g per kg without cathartic) separated by 2 to 4 hours may be sufficient. Because of the large volumes necessary, polyethylene glycol WBI should be administered via a nasogastric tube (0.5 L per hour for small children and 1 to 2 L per hour for adults). However, it may be prudent to withhold WBI in patients with hemodynamic compromise [41].

Cardiovascular Support

Hypotension should initially be treated with intravenous crystalloids with close monitoring for fluid overload. Although usually ineffective for severe poisoning [16,17,23,30], atropine should be given for symptomatic bradycardia. Treatment beyond general supportive care, intravenous fluids, and atropine will depend on the clinical situation. Seriously poisoned patients may require rapid simultaneous administration of multiple therapies. Transvenous pacing may be attempted, but in significant poisoning there may be failure to capture, and blood pressure may not improve despite an increase in heart rate [16,17].

Vasopressors

The exact sequence of pharmacologic therapies has not been studied. However, health care providers generally have the greatest familiarity with dosing and administration of vasopressor agents. Thus, these agents can often be initiated rapidly and may improve cardiovascular instability. Ideally, an agent with both α-1 and β-agonist effects should be instituted. Improvements have been noted with dopamine, dobutamine, norepinephrine, isoproterenol, and epinephrine. However, no specific agent has demonstrated superiority, so it is reasonable for clinicians to start with the agent they are most familiar with. There is scant information regarding vasopressin utility in CCA poisoning, but based on available data, it should not be used as monotherapy in CCA poisoning. Animal models have demonstrated either no improvement in mean arterial pressure [42] or decreased survival [43] with vasopressin compared to saline controls. However, there was improvement in systemic vascular resistance and blood pressure after vasopressin was administered to two patients unresponsive to multiple other therapies [44].

Multiple simultaneous vasoactive agents may be required depending on the hemodynamic response, and require doses much higher advanced cardiac life support (than ACLS) -based doses [45]. Because vasopressors can result in tachydysrhythmias, increased myocardial oxygen consumption and vasospastic events, these agents should be the first to be weaned from a patient who has stabilized.

Hyperinsulinemic Euglycemia

Hyperinsulinemic euglycemia (HIE) refers to the administration of high-dose regular insulin while maintaining normal serum glucose levels. HIE is thought to overcome the CCA-induced compromise of cardiovascular carbohydrate uptake, thus improving hemodynamic embarrassment. The exact mechanisms underlying these actions still remain controversial [46], but may be best described in the following animal studies.

Four animal studies (mongrel dogs) of HIE in verapamil poisoning [2,3,7,47] have been rated as very good to excellent quality by an expert panel [45]. Where survival from poisoning was measured, 100% of animals treated with insulin survived [47]. However, survival with epinephrine [2,47], glucagon [2,47], and calcium [2] was 33%, 0%, and 17%, respectively. Insulin also increased the mean lethal dose of verapamil and time to death compared to epinephrine and glucagon [7]. In these studies, HIE improved and sustained cardiac contractility, systolic and diastolic function, and systemic and cardiac blood flow compared to calcium, glucagon, and epinephrine [2,3,7,47]. Insulin improved myocardial metabolism and function without increasing myocardial oxygen consumption [3,7]. Epinephrine, glucagon, and calcium however contribute to oxygen wasting [2].

The first report of HIE therapy, published in 1999, included five CCA poisoned patients who failed to respond to other therapies [22]. The benefit of HIE was striking. Insulin dosing included a 10 to 20 IU bolus with a 25 g bolus of glucose followed by an infusion of insulin 0.1 to 1.0 IU/kg/h (mean 0.5 IU/kg/h) and dextrose 10 to 75 g per hour (mean 28.4 g per hour). One patient had failed to improve with respiratory support, crystalloids, atropine, calcium, and glucagon. After initiation of HIE, blood pressure improved, complete heart block resolved, and ejection fraction increased from 10% to 30%. Many other cases have been published and the clinical data supporting HIE have been reviewed [46,48]. The data provide multiple examples of CCA poisoned patients improving with HIE therapy after failing treatments such as atropine, pacing, vasopressors, calcium, glucagon, and phosphodiesterase inhibitors (PDI).

Clinical improvement from HIE is gradual and may take 30 minutes or more. However, one patient who failed to respond to dopamine, norepinephrine, calcium, and glucagon showed a dramatic response within 15 minutes of receiving a 10-fold dosing error of insulin (1,000 IU) [49]. Patients responding to insulin therapy demonstrate improved blood pressure, myocardial contractility, and metabolic acidosis, whereas effects on bradycardia and cardiac conduction are variable [46].

Failures of HIE therapy have also been reported. Our lack of knowledge regarding optimum dosing of insulin has been suggested as a reason for failures with HIE [50]. Canine studies of verapamil toxicity employed insulin doses of up to 16 IU/kg/h, but a dose-response relationship for insulin has not been determined [50]. The timing of HIE administration may also be a consideration. In several failures HIE was initiated multiple hours after ingestion when significant hemodynamic compromise was already present. This suggests a threshold point in CCA poisoning where there may be no beneficial intervention once that threshold is crossed. Therefore, HIE should be instituted as soon as hemodynamic abnormalities occur and well before profound shock supervenes. Although an optimal dosing scheme has yet to be established, a rational starting point is an initial insulin bolus of 1 IU per kg with 25 g of dextrose, followed by an infusion at 1 U/kg/h and 0.5 g/kg/h of dextrose [35,46]. It is believed supraphysiologic insulin doses are required to overcome CCA inhibition of insulin responsive GLUTs (see "Physiology and Pathophysiology" section) [5]. Increasing the insulin dose may be of benefit if response is insufficient. Doses up to 10 IU/kg/h have been recommended by some authors [51]. Serum glucose should be monitored closely and dextrose infusions adjusted to maintain normal ranges.

Hypoglycemia and hypokalemia, expected adverse effects of HIE, can be easily detected and treated. The safety of HIE therapy was demonstrated in a prospective observational study [52]. Serum glucose and potassium were monitored every 30 minutes until stable and then 1 to 2 hourly thereafter. Out of seven patients, only one episode of hypoglycemia (43.5 mg per dL) occurred (occurring 33.5 hours after ingestion when the maximal effects of CCA-induced insulin resistance would be waning). Hypokalemia (2.5 to 3.5 mmol per L) occurred in two patients without any clinical significance. Mild hypokalemia may actually provide a beneficial effect in CCA poisoning [22,32].

The effects of insulin may last for hours after discontinuing an infusion. Thus, ongoing glucose monitoring is necessary even after insulin is discontinued. Aggressive correction of insulin-induced hypokalemia is unnecessary unless the patient is symptomatic or potassium falls below an arbitrarily suggested level of 2.5 mEq per L [22].

Calcium

The goal of calcium therapy is to increase extracellular calcium concentrations thereby increasing calcium influx through any unblocked calcium channels. Calcium has demonstrated effectiveness in animal models [53], and improvement has been reported in human cases [17,54]. However, responses are variable and often short-lived, and patients with significant toxicity often fail to improve with calcium alone [16,23]. Conduction disturbances, contractility, and blood pressure may be improved, but generally there is no increase in heart rate [16,23,30]. Optimum dosing has yet to be established, and 4.5 to 95.3 mEq were used in one case series without an identifiable dose–response [16].

Calcium chloride contains three times the amount of elemental calcium of calcium gluconate (10% calcium chloride: 272 mg elemental calcium or 13.6 mEq per 1 g ampule; 10% calcium gluconate: 90 mg elemental calcium or 4.5 mEq per 1 g ampule). The higher elemental calcium content in calcium chloride also poses a greater risk for tissue injury should extravasation occur. Thus, calcium chloride administration via central venous access is generally preferred.

Optimum calcium dosing is not well established. Initial doses are generally given as boluses (10 to 20 mL of 10% calcium chloride or 30 to 60 mL of 10% calcium gluconate). Additional boluses may be given every 10 to 20 minutes. Some authors suggest more aggressive dosing of 1 g every 2 to 3 minutes until clinical response is seen [31]. Boluses should be given over a 5-minute period in conjunction with cardiac monitoring as rapid infusions have resulted in hypotension, AV dissociation, and ventricular fibrillation. The effects of boluses may be transient, and a constant infusion required [21,31]. Infusions can be started at 0.4 mL/kg/h for calcium chloride and 1.2 mL/kg/h for calcium gluconate and titrated to effect. Additional boluses can be given as needed. Calcium levels should be monitored. One author recommends maintaining serum ionized calcium levels approximately twice normal [55]. Raising serum ionized calcium to 2 to 3 mEq per L improves canine cardiac performance in verapamil poisoning [2,53], and is a reasonable goal to attain. It may be necessary to continue therapy despite high serum calcium levels if the patient is only responding to calcium administration. Significantly poisoned patients have tolerated high serum calcium levels without untoward effect [39,54], including one patient who obtained a peak serum calcium level of 23.8 mg per dL [17]. However, a patient in another report achieved a peak calcium level of 32.3 mg per dL and developed auric renal failure and eventually died [56]. Repeated calcium dosing or infusions should be discontinued if no beneficial effect is observed.

Glucagon

Glucagon possesses both inotropic and chronotropic effects, and experimentally increases heart rate, cardiac output, and reverses AV nodal blocks in CCA poisoning [57]. Several case reports noted improvement with glucagon therapy [26,38], but failures are also reported [30,32]. Five to 10 mg (150 μg per kg) given intravenously over 1 to 2 minutes is a typical starting dose [57]. Cardiovascular effects of glucagon last only 10 to 15 minutes [58], so repeat boluses may be required every 5 to 10 minutes followed by a continuous infusion of 2 to 10 mg per hour (50 to 100 μg/kg/h) [57]. Glucagon is a potent emetic [58], so airway control should be ensured before administration. Hyperglycemia and hypokalemia may also be observed with glucagon administration [58].

Phosphodiesterase Inhibitors

PDI such as inamrinone (amrinone) and milrinone increase cytosolic calcium and improve inotropy. PDI have been used in combination with other therapies to treat CCA poisoned patients [28,29], and appear to be effective in animal models [59,60]. However, they can be difficult to titrate and cause vasodilation and hypotension so are not generally recommended.

RESCUE AND EXPERIMENTAL THERAPIES

Nonpharmacologic Therapies

If available, intraaortic balloon counterpulsation, extracorporeal membrane oxygenation (ECMO), or cardiopulmonary bypass [30] may provide a bridge to survival in patients unresponsive to other therapies.

Pharmacologic Therapies

4-Aminopyridine

4-Aminopyridine is an orphan drug used to treat spinal cord injury and multiple sclerosis. It improves contractility by indirectly increasing intracellular calcium levels and has shown benefit in animal studies of verapamil toxicity [61,62] and in one human case report [63]. Unfortunately, it causes seizures and has a narrow therapeutic index. It may be considered if all other treatments are failing.

Methylene Blue

Methylene blue inhibits the nitric oxide–cyclic guanosine monophosphate pathway and has been used to treat vasodilatory shock such as in sepsis and anaphylaxis. A recent case report demonstrated hemodynamic improvement after methylene blue administration in a patient with vasodilatory shock from amlodipine poisoning who was failing HIE, dopamine, and norepinephrine [64]. The dose used was 2 mg per kg over 20 minutes followed by 1 mg/kg/h. Response to methylene blue may be specific to amlodipine as it is reported to have effects on the nitric oxide pathway, but in another recent amlodipine ingestion, there was no notable response to methylene blue administration [65]. A recent animal model of amlodipine poisoning did not show a survival benefit from methylene blue compared to saline [64]. However, mean arterial pressure, heart rate, and time to death were increased in animals receiving methylene blue. Therefore, its use may be considered in CCA poisoned patients with vasodilatory shock who are failing other therapies with the understanding that adverse effects such as hemolysis as potentiation of serotonin syndrome can occur [66].

Intravenous Lipid Emulsion

Perhaps the most novel therapy for CCA poisoning is intravenous lipid emulsion (ILE). Intravenous lipids have traditionally been used as a source of free fatty acids in parenteral nutrition. A chance observation led to the finding that ILE is beneficial in the treatment of local anesthetic-induced cardiac arrest [67]. Multiple animal studies followed demonstrating dramatic results with ILE for local anesthetic toxicity. This led to the incorporation of ILE into anesthesiology guidelines for the treatment of local anesthetic cardiotoxicity, but ILE has now been used to treat poisoning from over 30 different agents including CCAs [68]. Animal studies have demonstrated prolonged survival with ILE in CCA poisoning [69–71]. In a case series of severely ill overdoses, ILE was thought to have facilitated survival in 55% of patients who, they believe, would otherwise have died [72]. Six of the nine patients in this series were poisoned with CCAs. Three of those six survived.

Proposed mechanisms of ILE therapy include creation of a "lipid sink" where lipid soluble toxins are sequestered, augmenting cardiac energy supplies, and increasing intracellular calcium in cardiac myocytes [73].

Lipemic serum is an obvious adverse effect of ILE which interferes with many laboratory results and may interfere with ECMO [74] and renal replacement circuits [75]. Although not definitively causative, more significant adverse effects, such as acute respiratory distress syndrome and pancreatitis [76,77], and even cardiac arrest [78], have been temporally related to ILE administration.

Clinical evidence supporting ILE for CCA poisoning is currently limited and likely suffers from reporting bias. However, it still should be considered for patients who are failing adequate doses of other more traditional therapies. Optimum ILE dosing has not been established but one of the most commonly used regimens can be found at www.lipidrescue.org.

DISPOSITION

Patients with signs or symptoms of toxicity require intensive care unit admission. Disposition of asymptomatic patients depends on the formulation ingested. Patients with large or intentional ingestions of SR products or amlodipine should undergo appropriate decontamination and 24 hours of observation in a closely monitored setting. Patients with small unintentional ingestions of SR products may be medically cleared after appropriate decontamination if they remain asymptomatic with normal vital signs and ECGs for 8 to 12 hours. Close attention should be paid to subtle ECG signs of toxicity such as PR prolongation. Patients ingesting non-SR products may be cleared after 6 to 8 hours of observation if normal vital signs and ECGs are maintained.

References

1. Ohta M, Nelson J, Nelson D, et al: Effect of Ca++ channel blockers on energy level and stimulated insulin secretion in isolated rat islets of Langerhans. *J Pharmacol Exp Ther* 264(1):35–40, 1993.
2. Kline JA, Leonova E, Raymond RM: Beneficial myocardial metabolic effects of insulin during verapamil toxicity in the anesthetized canine. *Crit Care Med* 23(7):1251–1263, 1995.
3. Kline JA, Leonova E, Williams TC, et al: Myocardial metabolism during graded intraportal verapamil infusion in awake dogs. *J Cardiovasc Pharmacol* 27(5):719–726, 1996.
4. Kline JA, Raymond RM, Schroeder JD, et al: The diabetogenic effects of acute verapamil poisoning. *Toxicol Appl Pharmacol* 145(2):357–362, 1997.
5. Bechtel LK, Haverstick DM, Holstege CP: Verapamil toxicity dysregulates the phosphatidylinositol 3-kinase pathway. *Acad Emerg Med* 15(4):368–374, 2008.
6. Louters LL, Stehouwer N, Rekman J, et al: Verapamil inhibits the glucose transport activity of GLUT1. *J Med Toxicol* 6(2):100–105, 2010.
7. Kline JA, Raymond RM, Leonova ED, et al: Insulin improves heart function and metabolism during non-ischemic cardiogenic shock in awake canines. *Cardiovasc Res* 34(2):289–298, 1997.
8. Michel T, Hoffman BB: Chapter 27. Treatment of myocardial ischemia and hypertension, in Brunton LL, Chabner BA, Knollmann BC (eds): *Goodman & Gilman's The Pharmacological Basis of Therapeutics*. 12th ed. New York, NY, The McGraw-Hill Companies, 2011.
9. Kuhlmann U, Schoenemann H, Muller T, et al: Plasmapheresis in life-threatening verapamil intoxication. *Artif Cells Blood Substit Immobil Biotechnol* 28(5):429–440, 2000.
10. Ezidiegwu C, Spektor Z, Nasr MR, et al: A case report on the role of plasma exchange in the management of a massive amlodipine besylate intoxication. *Ther Apher Dial* 12(2):180–184, 2008.
11. Kolcz J, Pietrzyk J, Januszewska K, et al: Extracorporeal life support in severe propranolol and verapamil intoxication. *J Intensive Care Med* 22(6):381–385, 2007.
12. Pichon N, Dugard A, Clavel M, et al: Extracorporeal albumin dialysis in three cases of acute calcium channel blocker poisoning with life-threatening refractory cardiogenic shock. *Ann Emerg Med* 59(6):540–544, 2012.
13. Buckley CD, Aronson JK: Prolonged half-life of verapamil in a case of overdose: implications for therapy. *Br J Clin Pharmacol* 39(6):680–683, 1995.
14. Barrow PM, Houston PL, Wong DT: Overdose of sustained-release verapamil. *Br J Anaesth* 72(3):361–365, 1994.
15. Adams BD, Browne WT: Amlodipine overdose causes prolonged calcium channel blocker toxicity. *Am J Emerg Med* 16(5):527–528, 1998.
16. Ramoska EA, Spiller HA, Winter M, et al: A one-year evaluation of calcium channel blocker overdoses: toxicity and treatment. *Ann Emerg Med* 22(2):196–200, 1993.
17. Buckley N, Dawson AH, Howarth D, et al: Slow-release verapamil poisoning. Use of polyethylene glycol whole-bowel lavage and high-dose calcium. *Med J Aust* 158(3):202–204, 1993.
18. Olson KR, Erdman AR, Woolf AD, et al: Calcium channel blocker ingestion: an evidence-based consensus guideline for out-of-hospital management. *Clin Toxicol (Phila)* 43(7):797–822, 2005.
19. Herrington DM, Insley BM, Weinmann GG: Nifedipine overdose. *Am J Med* 81(2):344–346, 1986.
20. Boyer EW, Shannon M: Treatment of calcium-channel-blocker intoxication with insulin infusion [letter]. *N Eng J Med* 344(22):1721, 1722, 2001.
21. Rasmussen L, Husted SE, Johnsen SP: Severe intoxication after an intentional overdose of amlodipine. *Acta Anaesthesiol Scand* 47(8):1038–1040, 2003.
22. Yuan TH, Kerns WP, Tomaszewski CA, et al: Insulin-glucose as adjunctive therapy for severe calcium channel antagonist poisoning. *J Toxicol Clin Toxicol* 37(4):463, 474, 1999.
23. Ramoska EA, Spiller HA, Myers A: Calcium channel blocker toxicity. *Ann Emerg Med* 19(6):649–653, 1990.
24. Hofer CA, Smith JK, Tenholder MF: Verapamil intoxication: a literature review of overdoses and discussion of therapeutic options. *Am J Med* 95(4):431–438, 1993.
25. Ashraf M, Chaudhary K, Nelson J, et al: Massive overdose of sustained-release verapamil: a case report and review of literature. *Am J Med Sci* 310(6):258–263, 1995.
26. Walter FG, Frye G, Mullen JT, et al: Amelioration of nifedipine poisoning associated with glucagon therapy. *Ann Emerg Med* 22(7):1234–1237, 1993.
27. Isbister GK: Delayed asystolic cardiac arrest after diltiazem overdose; resuscitation with high dose intravenous calcium. *Emerg Med J* 19(4):355–357, 2002.
28. Goenen M, Col J, Compere A, et al: Treatment of severe verapamil poisoning with combined amrinone-isoproterenol therapy. *Am J Cardiol* 58(11):1142, 1143, 1986.
29. Wolf LR, Spadafora MP, Otten EJ: Use of amrinone and glucagon in a case of calcium channel blocker overdose. *Ann Emerg Med* 22(7):1225–1228, 1993.
30. Hendren WG, Schieber RS, Garrettson LK: Extracorporeal bypass for the treatment of verapamil poisoning. *Ann Emerg Med* 18(9):984–987, 1989.
31. Howarth DM, Dawson AH, Smith AJ, et al: Calcium channel blocking drug overdose: an Australian series. *Hum Exp Toxicol* 13(3):161–166, 1994.
32. Marques M, Gomes E, de Oliveira J: Treatment of calcium channel blocker intoxication with insulin infusion: case report and literature review. *Resuscitation* 57(2):211–213, 2003.
33. Erickson FC, Ling LJ, Grande GA, et al: Diltiazem overdose: case report and review. *J Emerg Med* 9(5):357–366, 1991.
34. Levine M, Boyer EW, Pozner CN, et al: Assessment of hyperglycemia after calcium channel blocker overdoses involving diltiazem or verapamil. *Crit Care Med* 35(9):2071–2075, 2007.
35. DeWitt CR, Waksman JC: Pharmacology, pathophysiology and management of calcium channel blocker and beta-blocker toxicity. *Toxicol Rev* 23(4):223–238, 2004.
36. Laine K, Kivisto KT, Neuvonen PJ: Effect of delayed administration of activated charcoal on the absorption of conventional and slow-release verapamil. *J Toxicol Clin Toxicol* 35(3):263–268, 1997.
37. Vale JA, Kulig K, American Academy of Clinical Toxicology, et al: Position paper: gastric lavage. *J Toxicol Clin Toxicol* 42(7):933–943, 2004.
38. Doyon S, Roberts JR: The use of glucagon in a case of calcium channel blocker overdose. *Ann Emerg Med* 22(7):1229–1233, 1993.
39. Luscher TF, Noll G, Sturmer T, et al: Calcium gluconate in severe verapamil intoxication. *N Engl J Med* 330(10):718–720, 1994.
40. Koch AR, Vogelaers DP, Decruyenaere JM, et al: Fatal intoxication with amlodipine. *J Toxicol Clin Toxicol* 33(3):253–256, 1995.
41. Cumpston K, Aks S, Sigg T, et al: Whole bowel irrigation and the hemodynamically unstable calcium channel blocker overdose: primum non nocere. *J Emerg Med* 38(2):171–174, 2010.
42. Sztajnkrycer MD, Bond GR, Johnson SB, et al: Use of vasopressin in a canine model of severe verapamil poisoning: a preliminary descriptive study. *Acad Emerg Med* 11(12):1253–1261, 2004.
43. Barry JD, Durkovich D, Cantrell L, et al: Vasopressin treatment of verapamil toxicity in the porcine model. *J Med Toxicol* 1(1):3–10, 2005.
44. Kanagarajan K, Marraffa JM, Bouchard NC, et al: The use of vasopressin in the setting of recalcitrant hypotension due to calcium channel blocker overdose. *Clin Toxicol (Phila)* 45(1):56–59, 2007.
45. Albertson TE, Dawson A, de Latorre F, et al: TOX-ACLS: toxicologic-oriented advanced cardiac life support. *Ann Emerg Med* 37[4 Suppl]:S78–S90, 2001.
46. Lheureux PE, Zahir S, Gris M, et al: Bench-to-bedside review: hyperinsulinaemia/euglycaemia therapy in the management of overdose of calcium-channel blockers. *Crit Care* 10(3):212, 2006.
47. Kline JA, Tomaszewski CA, Schroeder JD, et al: Insulin is a superior antidote for cardiovascular toxicity induced by verapamil in the anesthetized canine. *J Pharmacol Exp Ther* 267(2):744–750, 1993.
48. Mégarbane B, Karyo S, Baud FJ: The role of insulin and glucose (hyperinsulinaemia/euglycaemia) therapy in acute calcium channel antagonist and beta-blocker poisoning. *Toxicol Rev* 23(4):215–222, 2004.
49. Place R, Carlson A, Leiken J, et al: Hyperinsulin therapy in the treatment of verapamil overdose [abstract]. *J Toxicol Clin Toxicol* 38:576, 577, 2000.
50. Cumpston K, Mycyk M, Pallasch E, et al: Failure of hyperinsulinemia/euglucemia therapy in severe diltiazam overdose [abstract]. *J Toxicol Clin Toxicol* 40:618, 2002.
51. Engebretsen KM, Kaczmarek KM, Morgan J, et al: High-dose insulin therapy in beta-blocker and calcium channel-blocker poisoning. *Clin Toxicol (Phila)* 49(4):277–283, 2011.
52. Greene SL, Gawarammana I, Wood DM, et al: Relative safety of hyperinsulinaemia/euglycaemia therapy in the management of calcium channel blocker overdose: a prospective observational study. *Intensive Care Med* 33(11):2019–2024, 2007.
53. Hariman RJ, Mangiardi LM, McAllister RGJ, et al: Reversal of the cardiovascular effects of verapamil by calcium and sodium: differences between electrophysiologic and hemodynamic responses. *Circulation* 59(4):797–804, 1979.
54. Haddad LM: Resuscitation after nifedipine overdose exclusively with intravenous calcium chloride. *Am J Emerg Med* 14(6):602–603, 1996.
55. Kerns W: Management of beta-adrenergic blocker and calcium channel antagonist toxicity. *Emerg Med Clin North Am* 25(2):309–331, 2007, abstract viii.
56. Sim MT, Stevenson FT: A fatal case of iatrogenic hypercalcemia after calcium channel blocker overdose. *J Med Toxicol* 4(1):25–29, 2008.
57. Bailey B: Glucagon in beta-blocker and calcium channel blocker overdoses: a systematic review. *J Toxicol Clin Toxicol* 41(5):595–602, 2003.
58. Parmley WW: The role of glucagon in cardiac therapy. *N Engl J Med* 285(14):801, 802, 1971.
59. Alousi AA, Canter JM, Fort DJ: The beneficial effect of amrinone on acute drug-induced heart failure in the anaesthetised dog. *Cardiovasc Res* 19(8):483–494, 1985.

60. Koury SI, Stone CK, Thomas SH: Amrinone as an antidote in experimental verapamil overdose. *Acad Emerg Med* 3(8):762–767, 1996.
61. Agoston S, Maestrone E, van Hezik EJ, et al: Effective treatment of verapamil intoxication with 4-aminopyridine in the cat. *J Clin Invest* 73(5):1291–1296, 1984.
62. Tuncok Y, Apaydin S, Gelal A, et al: The effects of 4-aminopyridine and Bay K 8644 on verapamil-induced cardiovascular toxicity in anesthetized rats. *J Toxicol Clin Toxicol* 36(4):301–307, 1998.
63. ter Wee PM, Kremer Hovinga TK, Uges DR, et al: 4-Aminopyridine and haemodialysis in the treatment of verapamil intoxication. *Hum Toxicol* 4(3):327–329, 1985.
64. Jang DH, Nelson LS, Hoffman RS: Methylene blue in the treatment of refractory shock from an amlodipine overdose. *Ann Emerg Med* 58(6):565–567, 2011.
65. Bouchard N, Weinberg R, Burkart K, et al: Prolonged resuscitation for massive amlodipine overdose with maximal vasopressors, intralipids and Veno Arterial-Extracorporeal Membrane Oxygenation (VA ECMO). *Clin Toxicol* 48(6):613, 2010.
66. Jang DH, Donovan S, Nelson LS, et al: Efficacy of methylene blue in an experimental model of calcium channel blocker–induced shock. *Ann Emerg Med* 65(4):410–415, 2015.
67. Brent J: Poisoned patients are different--sometimes fat is a good thing. *Crit Care Med* 37(3):1157, 1158, 2009.
68. Waring WS: Intravenous lipid administration for drug-induced toxicity: a critical review of the existing data. *Expert Rev Clin Pharmacol* 5(4):437–444, 2012.
69. Tebbutt S, Harvey M, Nicholson T, et al: Intralipid prolongs survival in a rat model of verapamil toxicity. *Acad Emerg Med* 13(2):134–139, 2006.
70. Bania TC, Chu J, Perez E, et al: Hemodynamic effects of intravenous fat emulsion in an animal model of severe verapamil toxicity resuscitated with atropine, calcium, and saline. *Acad Emerg Med* 14(2):105–111, 2007.
71. Kang C, Kim DH, Kim SC, et al: The effects of intravenous lipid emulsion on prolongation of survival in a rat model of calcium channel blocker toxicity. *Clin Toxicol (Phila)* 53(6):540–544, 2015.
72. Geib A-J, Liebelt E, Manini AF, et al: Clinical experience with intravenous lipid emulsion for drug-induced cardiovascular collapse. *J Med Toxicol* 8(1):10–14, 2011.
73. Turner-Lawrence DE, Kerns Ii W: Intravenous fat emulsion: a potential novel antidote. *J Med Toxicol* 4(2):109–114, 2008.
74. Lee HMD, Archer JRH, Dargan PI, et al: What are the adverse effects associated with the combined use of intravenous lipid emulsion and extracorporeal membrane oxygenation in the poisoned patient? *Clin Toxicol (Phila)* 53(3):145–150, 2015.
75. Jeong J: Continuous renal replacement therapy circuit failure after antidote administration. *Clin Toxicol (Phila)* 52(10):1296, 1297, 2014.
76. Levine M, Skolnik AB, Ruha A-M, et al: Complications following antidotal use of intravenous lipid emulsion therapy. *J Med Toxicol* 10(1):10–14, 2013.
77. Sebe A, Dişel NR, Açıkalın Akpınar A, et al: Role of intravenous lipid emulsions in the management of calcium channel blocker and β-blocker overdose: 3 years experience of a university hospital. *Postgrad Med* 127(2):119–124, 2015.
78. Cole JB, Stellpflug SJ, Engebretsen KM: Asystole immediately following intravenous fat emulsion for overdose. *J Med Toxicol* 10(3):307–310, 2014.

Chapter 108 ▪ Cardiac Glycoside Poisoning

BRYAN S. JUDGE • MARK A. KIRK

Cardiac glycosides (CGs) are naturally occurring substances whose medicinal benefits have been recognized for centuries [1]. Digoxin is the major CG used for medicinal purposes today. Although its use throughout the United States has steadily declined in recent years, digoxin is still used in the treatment of congestive heart failure and atrial fibrillation [2]. Digoxin is responsible for most cases of CG poisoning; however, exposure to plant (i.e., dogbane, foxglove, lily of the valley, oleander, red squill, and Siberian ginseng), animal sources (i.e., *Bufo* toad species), and topical aphrodisiacs can also result in serious toxicity [3–5].

PHARMACOLOGY

Digoxin exerts a positive inotropic effect, thereby enhancing the force of myocardial contraction. Direct effects of digoxin include prolongation of the effective refractory period in the atria and the atrioventricular (AV) node, which diminishes the conduction velocity through those regions. CGs are readily absorbed through the gastrointestinal tract; digoxin has up to 80% bioavailability [6]. Digoxin has a volume of distribution (V_d) of 5.1 to 7.4 L per kg [7] and a half-life of 36 to 48 hours [8]. The generally accepted therapeutic serum concentration range for digoxin is 0.8 to 2.0 ng per mL for inotropic support in patients with left ventricular dysfunction. Higher concentrations (1.5 to 2.0 ng per mL) may be needed for ventricular rate control in patients with atrial dysrhythmias. Digoxin is primarily eliminated by renal excretion. In patients with renal dysfunction, digoxin clearance is reduced. Serum digoxin concentrations can be altered by numerous drug interactions [9–11].

Toxicity results from an exaggeration of therapeutic effects [6]. CGs bind to and inactivate the sodium–potassium adenosine triphosphatase pump (Na^+–K^+-ATPase) on cardiac cell membranes. This pump maintains the electrochemical membrane potential, vital to conduction tissues, by concentrating Na^+ extracellularly and K^+ intracellularly. When Na^+–K^+-ATPase is inhibited, the Na^+–calcium exchanger removes accumulated intracellular sodium in exchange for calcium. This exchange increases sarcoplasmic calcium and is the mechanism responsible for the positive inotropic effect of digitalis. Intracellular calcium overload causes delayed afterdepolarizations and gives rise to triggered dysrhythmias. Increased vagal tone and direct AV depression may produce conduction disturbances. The decreased refractory period of the myocardium increases automaticity.

CLINICAL PRESENTATION

Differences between the presentations of patients with CG poisoning due to a single acute ingestion and those with chronic toxicity resulting from excessive therapeutic doses are illustrated in Table 108.1. Diagnosing chronic CG toxicity is difficult because the presentation may mimic more common illnesses, such as influenza or gastroenteritis. Patients with chronic CG toxicity may present with constitutional, gastrointestinal, psychiatric, or visual complaints that may not be recognized as signs of digitalis toxicity. Symptoms most commonly reported include fatigue, weakness, nausea, anorexia, and dizziness [12]. Neuropsychiatric signs and symptoms include headache, weakness, vertigo, syncope, seizures, memory loss, confusion, disorientation, delirium, depression, and hallucinations [13]. The most frequently reported visual disturbances are cloudy or blurred vision, loss of vision, and yellow-green halos or everything appearing "washed in yellow" (xanthopsia) [14].

Cardiac manifestations of CG toxicity are common and potentially life threatening. An extremely wide variety of dysrhythmias has been reported [15,16]. Dysrhythmias frequently associated with CG toxicity include premature ventricular contractions, paroxysmal atrial tachycardia or atrial fibrillation with a conduction block, junctional tachycardia, sinus bradycardia, AV nodal blockade, ventricular tachycardia, and ventricular fibrillation. Atrial tachycardia (enhanced automaticity) with variable AV block (impaired conduction), atrial fibrillation with

TABLE 108.1

Characteristics of Acute and Chronic Cardiac Glycoside Toxicity

Clinical finding	Acute toxicity	Chronic toxicity
Gastrointestinal toxicity	Nausea, vomiting	Nausea, vomiting
Central nervous system toxicity	Headache, weakness, dizziness, confusion, and coma	Confusion, coma
Cardiac toxicity	Bradydysrhythmias, supraventricular dysrhythmias with AV block; ventricular dysrhythmias are uncommon	Virtually any dysrhythmia (ventricular or supraventricular dysrhythmias with or without AV block); ventricular dysrhythmias are common
Serum potassium	Elevated but may be normal (high concentrations correlated with toxicity)	Low or normal (hypokalemia secondary to concomitant diuretic use)
Serum digoxin concentration	Markedly elevated	May be within "therapeutic" range or minimally elevated

AV, atrioventricular.
Adapted and combined from references [1,12,13,15,29].

an accelerated or slow junctional rhythm (regularization of atrial fibrillation), and fascicular tachycardia are highly suggestive of CG toxicity [17,18]. Bidirectional ventricular tachycardia, a narrow-complex tachycardia with right bundle-branch morphology, is highly specific, but not pathognomonic, for digitalis toxicity [15].

Myocardial disease, myocardial ischemia, and metabolic [19] or electrolyte disturbances, such as hypokalemia, hypomagnesemia, and hypercalcemia [8], increase the risk of toxicity. The elderly are at increased risk, whereas renal impairment, hepatic disease, hypothyroidism, chronic obstructive pulmonary disease, and drug interactions alter sensitivity to CGs [1].

DIAGNOSTIC EVALUATION

Essential laboratory tests include serum digoxin concentrations, electrolytes, blood urea nitrogen, creatinine, calcium, magnesium, and an electrocardiogram. Additional laboratory tests should be obtained as clinically indicated. Serum digoxin concentrations can assist in the diagnosis of CG poisoning but must be interpreted carefully [18]. A therapeutic concentration does not exclude poisoning, as predisposing factors can cause an individual to become poisoned despite a concentration within the therapeutic range. Conversely, high serum digoxin concentrations after an acute ingestion do not always indicate toxicity [20]. Digoxin follows a two-compartment model of distribution, with relatively rapid absorption into the plasma compartment and then slow redistribution into the tissue compartment [8]. Serum digoxin concentrations most reliably correlate with toxicity when obtained after distribution is complete, which occurs 6 hours or more after oral or intravenous digoxin administration.

Naturally occurring digitalis glycosides from plants and animals can cross-react with the digoxin assay. The degree of cross-reactivity is unknown, and because the assays are not calibrated for nondigoxin glycosides, the measured value cannot be reliably interpreted [5]. A false-positive digoxin assay (usually a concentration below 3 ng per mL) may occur in neonates and patients with renal insufficiency, liver disease, and pregnancy because of endogenous digoxin-like immunoreactive factors [21–23].

Hyperkalemia may be a better indicator of end-organ toxicity than the serum digoxin concentration in the acutely poisoned patient [24]. In contrast, hypokalemia and hypomagnesemia are commonly seen in the chronically intoxicated patient, presumably as a result of concomitant diuretic use.

MANAGEMENT

The management of CG poisoning includes supportive care, prevention of further drug absorption, appropriate administration of digoxin antibody fragments, and safe disposition. Meticulous attention to supportive care and a search for easily correctable conditions, such as hypoxia, hypoventilation, hypovolemia, hypoglycemia, and electrolyte disturbances, are top priorities. All patients should have vascular access established and continuous cardiac monitoring. Patients with clinical toxicity or elevated serum digoxin concentrations in the setting of suspected overdose require close monitoring and often warrant intensive care unit (ICU) admission.

Prevention of further drug absorption should be addressed after life support measures have been initiated. Gastric lavage has little, if any, benefit in the management of digoxin toxicity. Activated charcoal effectively binds CGs, and multiple doses of activated charcoal enhance intestinal digoxin elimination after oral and intravenous digoxin administration [25].

Conventional treatment of bradydysrhythmia, including the use of atropine, isoproterenol, and cardiac pacing, may not be effective for bradycardia due to CG poisoning. Atropine has been used with variable success in patients with digitalis toxicity exhibiting AV block [26]. Although isoproterenol may increase ventricular ectopy and cardiac tissue may be unresponsive to electrical pacing, the fibrillation threshold may be lowered, and the pacing wire itself may induce ventricular fibrillation [27]. Digoxin-specific antibody fragments (Fab) are first-line therapy in patients with symptomatic bradycardia [28].

Digoxin-specific antibody Fab is also the treatment of choice for life-threatening ventricular dysrhythmias. If this therapy is not immediately available, phenytoin and lidocaine, which depress increased ventricular automaticity without slowing AV nodal conduction, should be the initial therapy [18,29]. Amiodarone was successful in two cases refractory to other antidysrhythmics [30,31]. Intravenous magnesium, 2 to 4 g (10 to 20 mL of a 20% solution) over 1 minute, may also be useful [32]. Quinidine and procainamide are contraindicated in digitalis toxicity because they depress AV nodal conduction and may worsen cardiac toxicity [1]. Electrical cardioversion of the digitalis-toxic patient should be performed with extreme caution and considered a last resort. A low-energy setting (e.g., 10 to 25 W per second) should be used and preparations made to treat potential ventricular fibrillation [29].

Hyperkalemia is common in patients with acute digoxin poisoning, and empiric administration of supplemental potassium should be avoided [33]. This increase in serum potassium concentration reflects a change in potassium distribution and not an increase in total body potassium stores. Significant hyperkalemia due to acute overdose is another indication for digoxin-specific antibody Fab. If digoxin-specific antibody Fab are not immediately available and the patient has hyperkalemia with associated electrocardiogram changes, intravenous glucose and insulin, sodium bicarbonate, continuous inhaled β agonists such as albuterol (if there is no tachydysrhythmia or ectopy), and sodium polystyrene sulfonate should be administered. The use of intravenous calcium to treat hyperkalemia in CG toxic patients remains controversial and has been previously avoided by many clinicians because additional calcium has been reported to enhance cardiac toxicity [19]. However, recently authors have questioned this dogma—citing animal studies and human case reports that document no untoward effects when calcium is administered in the setting of CG toxicity—and recommend the use of intravenous calcium in those patients with CG toxicity who have life-threatening hyperkalemia with significant changes on the electrocardiogram such as loss of P waves or widening of the QRS [34]. Hemodialysis may be of benefit in a CG-poisoned patient with renal failure and hyperkalemia.

Supplemental potassium may be beneficial in chronic digitalis toxicity when diuretic-induced hypokalemia is a factor. Potassium should be administered cautiously, as renal dysfunction may be the cause of digitalis toxicity. Hypomagnesemia is common in patients with chronic CG toxicity, and supplemental magnesium is recommended for such patients [35].

Digoxin-specific antibody Fab therapy is indicated for patients with dysrhythmias that threaten or result in hemodynamic compromise and patients with serum potassium greater than 5.0 to 5.5 mEq per L after acute CG overdose [36]. Chronically poisoned patients who are asymptomatic can often be managed with discontinuation of digoxin and close observation. However, the threshold for treatment with digoxin-specific antibody Fab should be lower in those patients with signs of cardiac toxicity (e.g., severe bradycardia with second- or third-degree AV block), or who have predisposing conditions such as chronic pulmonary disease, hypokalemia, hypothyroidism, renal dysfunction, or underlying cardiac disease [12,37]. Animal studies and case reports suggest digoxin-specific antibody Fab may be an effective treatment for patients poisoned by plant or animal sources of CG [3,5].

Digoxin-specific antibody Fab can reverse digitalis-induced dysrhythmias, conduction disturbances, myocardial depression, and hyperkalemia. In a multicenter study, 90% of patients with digoxin or digitoxin toxicity had a complete or partial response to digoxin-specific antibody Fab therapy [36]. Complete resolution of toxicity occurred in 80% of the patients, and partial response occurred in 10%. The time to initial response from end of digoxin-specific antibody Fab infusion was within 1 hour (mean 19 minutes), and the time to complete response was 0.5 to 6.0 hours (mean: 1.5 hours). However, the majority of these patients were acutely poisoned and it is possible that chronically poisoned patients may respond differently. Treatment failures have been attributed to inadequate or delayed dosing, moribund clinical state before digoxin-specific antibody Fab therapy, pacemaker-induced dysrhythmias, and incorrect diagnosis of digitalis toxicity [36,38].

Digoxin-specific antibody Fab dosage (number of vials) calculations are based on the serum digoxin concentration or estimated body load of digoxin. It is assumed that equimolar doses of antibody fragments are required to achieve neutralization [39]. A 40-mg dose of digoxin-specific antibody Fab (one vial) binds 0.6 mg of digoxin. The number of vials required can be calculated by dividing the total body burden by 0.6. The body burden can be estimated from the milligram amount of an acute ingestion or by multiplying the post-distribution serum digoxin concentration (ng per mL) by the volume of distribution of digoxin (= 5.6 L per kg times the body weight in kg) and dividing by 1,000.

In the largest prospective study of Fab for digoxin poisoning (n = 150, mean serum concentration of 8 ng per mL), the dose of Fab required to reverse digoxin toxicity was five vials with a range from 3 to 20 vials [36]. A severely toxic patient in whom the quantity ingested acutely is unknown should be given 5 to 10 vials at a time and the clinical response observed. If cardiac arrest is imminent or has occurred, the dose can be given as a bolus. Otherwise, it should be infused over 30 minutes. In contrast, patients with chronic therapeutic overdose often have only mildly elevated digoxin concentrations and respond to one to two vials of digoxin-specific antibody Fab. The recommended dose for a given patient can be determined using the tables in the package insert or by contacting a regional poison center or toxicology consultant.

The dose of digoxin-specific antibody Fab needed to treat nondigoxin CG poisoning is unknown but likely to be greater than that necessary for digoxin poisoning. Starting with 5 to 10 vials and repeating this dose as necessary is a reasonable approach.

Free digoxin concentrations are decreased to zero within 1 minute of digoxin-specific antibody Fab therapy, but total serum digoxin concentrations may be markedly increased [36,40]. Because most assay methods measure total (bound and free) digoxin, very high digoxin concentrations are seen after digoxin-specific antibody Fab treatment, but they have no correlation with toxicity [40]. Serum concentrations may be unreliable for several days after digoxin-specific antibody Fab therapy [41].

The digoxin–Fab complex is excreted in the urine and has a half-life of 16 to 20 hours [42]. In patients with renal failure, elimination of the digoxin–Fab complex is prolonged and free digoxin concentrations gradually increase over 2 to 4 days after digoxin-specific antibody Fab administration [43]. In one report of 28 patients with renal impairment given digoxin-specific antibody Fab, only one patient had recurrent toxicity, which occurred 10 days after digoxin-specific antibody Fab treatment and persisted for 10 days [44]. Monitoring of free digoxin concentrations may be beneficial for titrating effect in those patients reliant on the inotropic action of digoxin, detecting rebound toxicity in patients with renal impairment, assessing the need for further treatment with digoxin-specific antibody Fab, or in guiding the reinstitution of digoxin therapy [45]. Hemodialysis has not been reported to enhance digoxin–Fab complex elimination.

Digoxin-specific antibody Fab therapy has been associated with mild adverse drug events such as rash, flushing, and facial swelling [36,38]. However, neither acute anaphylaxis nor serum sickness has been described [38]. Before digoxin-specific antibody Fab administration, an asthma and allergy history should be obtained. Intradermal skin testing should be considered in high-risk patients. If a patient with a positive skin test is dying, however, the risk–benefit ratio obviously favors treatment [38]. A precipitous drop in the serum potassium, recurrence of supraventricular tachydysrhythmias previously controlled by digoxin, and development of cardiogenic shock in a patient dependent on digoxin for inotropic support have all been associated with digoxin-specific antibody Fab therapy [36]. Recurrent toxicity has been observed in 3% of patients [38]. In most, it was attributed to an inadequate initial dose of digoxin-specific antibody Fab dosing and reversed with a repeat dose.

Patients who receive digoxin-specific antibody Fab require continued monitoring in an ICU for at least 24 hours. Those with elevated drug concentrations resulting from chronic therapy who are hemodynamically stable can be observed on a telemetry unit. Discontinuing the use of digoxin or decreasing the dose, modifying predisposing factors, and closely monitoring subsequent therapy are necessary to avert further toxic episodes. Patients with suicidal ingestions should have a psychiatric evaluation before discharge.

References

1. Smith TW, Antman EM, Friedman PL, et al: Digitalis glycosides: mechanisms and manifestations. *Prog Cardiovasc Dis* 26:413–458, 1984.
2. Haynes K, Heitjan DF, Kanetsky PA, et al: Declining public health burden of digoxin toxicity from 1991 to 2004. *Clin Pharmacol Ther* 84:90–94, 2008.
3. Shumaik GM, Wu AW, Ping AC: Oleander poisoning: treatment with digoxin-specific Fab antibody fragments. *Ann Emerg Med* 17:732–735, 1988.
4. Rich SA, Libera JM, Locke RJ: Treatment of foxglove extract poisoning with digoxin-specific Fab fragments. *Ann Emerg Med* 22(12):1904–1907, 1993.
5. Brubacher JR, Ravikumar PR, Bania T, et al: Treatment of toad venom poisoning with digoxin-specific Fab Fragments. *Chest* 110(5):1282–1288, 1996.
6. Smith TW: Digitalis: mechanisms of action and clinical use. *N Engl J Med* 318:358–365, 1988.
7. Baselt RC: *Disposition of Toxic Drugs and Chemicals in Man.* 6th ed. Foster City, CA, Biomedical Publications, 2003, p 1146.
8. Smith TW: Pharmacokinetics, bioavailability and serum levels of cardiac glycosides. *J Am Coll Cardiol* 5:43A–50A, 1985.
9. Marcus FI: Pharmacokinetic interactions between digoxin and other drugs. *J Am Coll Cardiol* 5[Suppl A]:82A–90A, 1985.
10. Humphries TJ, Merritt GJ: Review article: drug interactions with agents used to treat acid-related diseases. *Aliment Pharmacol Ther* 13[Suppl 3]:18–26, 1999.
11. Izzo AA, Di Carlo G, Borrelli F, et al: Cardiovascular pharmacotherapy and herbal medicines: the risk of drug interaction. *Int J Cardiol* 98:1–14, 2005.
12. Wofford JL, Ettinger WH: Risk factors and manifestations of digoxin toxicity in the elderly. *Am J Emerg Med* 9:11–15, 1991.
13. Huffman JC, Stern T: Neuropsychiatric consequences of cardiovascular medications. *Dialogues Clin Neurosci* 9:29–45, 2007.
14. Piltz JR, Wertenbaker C, Lance SE, et al: Digoxin toxicity: recognizing the varied visual presentations. *J Clin Neuroophthalmol* 13:275–280, 1993.
15. Moorman JR, Pritchett EL: The arrhythmias of digitalis intoxication. *Arch Intern Med* 145:1289–1292, 1985.
16. Mahdyoon H, Battilana G, Rosman H, et al: The evolving pattern of digoxin intoxication: observations at a large urban hospital from 1980 to 1988. *Am Heart J* 120:1189–1194, 1990.
17. Marchlinski FE, Hook BG, Callans DJ: Which cardiac disturbances should be treated with digoxin immune Fab (Ovine) antibody? *Am J Emerg Med* 9:24–28, 1991.
18. Kelly RA, Smith TW: Recognition and management of digitalis toxicity. *Am J Cardiol* 69:108G–119G, 1992.
19. Akera T, Ng Y: Digitalis sensitivity of Na,K-ATPase, myocytes and the heart. *Life Sci* 48:97–106, 1991.
20. Offhaus JM, Judge BS: Massive unintentional digoxin ingestion successfully managed without the use of activated charcoal or digoxin-specific antibody fragments. *Clin Toxicol* 43:650, 2005.
21. Gervais A: Digoxin-like immunoreactive substance (DLIS) in liver disease: comparison of clinical and laboratory parameters in patients with and without DLIS. *Drug Intell Clin Pharm* 21:540, 1987.
22. Graves SW, Brown B, Valdes R: An endogenous digoxin-like substance in patients with renal impairment. *Ann Intern Med* 99:604–608, 1983.
23. Stone J, Bentur Y, Zalstein E, et al: Effect of endogenous digoxin-like substances on the interpretation of high concentrations of digoxin in children. *J Pediatr* 117:321–325, 1990.
24. Bismuth C, Gaultier M, Conso F, et al: Hyperkalemia in acute digitalis poisoning: prognostic significance and therapeutic implications. *Clin Toxicol (Phila)* 6:153–162, 1973.
25. Critchley JA, Critchley LA: Digoxin toxicity in chronic renal failure: treatment by multiple dose activated charcoal intestinal dialysis. *Hum Exp Toxicol* 16:733–735, 1997.
26. Duke M: Atrioventricular block due to accidental digoxin ingestion treated with atropine. *Am J Dis Child* 124:754–756, 1972.
27. Bismuth C, Motte G, Conso F, et al: Acute digitoxin intoxication treated by intracardiac pacemaker: experience in sixty-eight patients. *Clin Toxicol* 10:443–456, 1977.
28. Lapostolle F, Borron SW, Verdier C, et al: Digoxin-specific Fab fragments as single first-line therapy in digitalis poisoning. *Crit Care Med* 36:3014–3018, 2008.
29. Sharff JA, Bayer MJ: Acute and chronic digitalis toxicity: presentation and treatment. *Ann Emerg Med* 11:327–331, 1982.
30. Nicholls DP, Murtagh JG, Holt DW: Use of amiodarone and digoxin specific Fab antibodies in digoxin overdosage. *Br Med J* 53:462–464, 1985.
31. Maheswaran R, Bramble MG, Hardisty CA: Massive digoxin overdose—successful treatment with intravenous amiodarone. *Br Med J* 287:392–393, 1986.
32. French JH, Thomas RG, Siskind AP, et al: Magnesium therapy in massive digoxin intoxication. *Ann Emerg Med* 13:562–566, 1984.
33. Springer M, Olsen KR, Feaster W: Acute massive digoxin overdose: survival without use of digitalis-specific antibodies. *Am J Emerg Med* 4:364–368, 1986.
34. Erickson CP, Olson KR: Case files of the medical toxicology fellowship of the California poison control system—San Francisco: calcium plus digoxin—more taboo than toxic? *J Med Toxicol* 4:33–39, 2008.
35. Beller GA, Hood WB Jr, Smith TW, et al: Correlation of serum magnesium levels and cardiac digitalis intoxication. *Am J Cardiol* 33:225–229, 1974.
36. Antman EM, Wenger TL, Butler VP Jr, et al: Treatment of 150 cases of life-threatening digitalis intoxication with digoxin-specific Fab antibody fragments: final report of a multicenter study. *Circulation* 81:1744–1752, 1990.
37. Lapostolle F, Borrown SW, Verdier C, et al: Assessment of digoxin antibody use in patients with elevated serum digoxin following chronic or acute exposure. *Intensive Care Med* 34:1448–1453, 2008.
38. Hickey AR, Wenger TL, Carpenter VP, et al: Digoxin immune Fab therapy in the management of digitalis intoxication: safety and efficacy results of an observational surveillance study. *J Am Coll Cardiol* 17:590–598, 1991.
39. Smolarz A, Roesch E, Lenz H, et al: Digoxin specific antibody (Fab) fragments in 34 cases of severe digitalis intoxication. *Clin Tox* 23:327–340, 1985.
40. Smith TW, Haber E, Yeatman L, et al: Reversal of advanced digoxin intoxication with Fab fragments of digoxin-specific antibodies. *N Engl J Med* 294:797–800, 1976.
41. Gibbs I, Adams PC, Parnham AJ, et al: Plasma digoxin: assay anomalies in Fab-treated patients. *Br J Clin Pharmacol* 16:445–447, 1983.
42. Smith TW, Lloyd BL, Spicer N, et al: Immunogenicity and kinetics of distribution and elimination of sheep digoxin-specific IgG and Fab fragments in the rabbit and baboon. *Clin Exp Immunol* 36:384–396, 1979.
43. Allen NM, Dunham GD, Sailstad JM, et al: Clinical and pharmacokinetic profiles of digoxin immune Fab in four patients with renal impairment. *Drug Intell Clin Pharm* 25:1315–1320, 1991.
44. Wenger TL: Experience with digoxin immune Fab (Ovine) in patients with renal impairment. *Am J Emerg Med* 9:21–23, 1991.
45. Ujhelyi MR, Robert S: Pharmacokinetic aspects of digoxin-specific Fab therapy in the management of digitalis toxicity. *Clin Pharmacokinet* 28:483–493, 1995.

Chapter 109 ■ Cholinergic Poisoning

CYNTHIA K. AARON • ANDREW M. KING

Cholinergic (acetylcholinesterase [AChE] inhibitor) agents are used in medicine, as insecticides, and as "nerve agent" chemical weapons. Many poisonings result from accidental dermal contamination during agricultural use of pesticides [1]. The majority of suicide attempts are ingestions [2]. Food-borne exposures have produced epidemics such as "Ginger Jake paralysis" (delayed neuropathy) because of contamination of an alcoholic drink with triorthocresyl phosphate [3] and an epidemic affecting over 2,000 people with mild-to-moderate symptoms related to the use of aldicarb on watermelons; an insecticide that is no longer made in the United States and will no longer be available in 2018 [4].

PHARMACOLOGY

Cholinesterase inhibitors act primarily by blocking the active site of AChE. Organophosphates (OPs) form a covalent phosphate linkage at the enzyme active site. Enzyme regeneration occurs by either de novo synthesis, hydrolysis of the serine–organophosphorus bond, or oxime-aided reactivation. Over a period of time, in a process that is agent-dependent, the OP molecule "ages" on the enzyme and is resistant to reactivation by oxime therapy. Carbamates are reversible inhibitors of AChE, occupying but not modifying the catalytic region of the enzyme.

TABLE 109.1

Pharmacologic Effects of Cholinesterase Inhibition Receptor Type

Location	Effects
Muscarinic (increased stimulation)	
Pupils	Miosis (constriction)
Ciliary body	Blurred vision
Exocrine glands	Increased secretions
Lacrimal	Tearing
Salivary	Salivation
Respiratory	Bronchorrhea, rhinorrhea
Heart	Bradycardia
Smooth muscle	Contraction
Bronchial	Bronchoconstriction
Gastrointestinal	Nausea, vomiting, abdominal cramps, diarrhea
Bladder	Incontinence, frequency
Sphincter of Oddi	Pancreatitis
Central nervous system	Variable[a]
Nicotinic (stimulation; then depression)	
Skeletal muscle	Weakness, cramps, fasciculation, paralysis
Sympathetic ganglia	Tachycardia, hypertension; then hypotension
Central nervous system	Variable symptoms from anxiety and restlessness to confusion, obtundation, coma, and seizures[a]

[a]Relative contributions of nicotinic and muscarinic receptors to central nervous system effects are unclear.

AChE activity is restored when the carbamate spontaneously leaves the enzyme's active site [5]. Reversible AChE inhibitors such as tacrine, rivastigmine, donepezil, and galantamine have been used for the treatment of Alzheimer's dementia. The characteristics and treatment of exposure to these products are covered at the end of this chapter.

Inhibition of AChE allows the neurotransmitter acetylcholine to accumulate and remain active in the synapse, resulting in sustained depolarization of the postsynaptic neuron or effector organ. This effect occurs in the central nervous system (CNS) as well as at muscarinic sites in the peripheral nervous system, nicotinic sites in the sympathetic and parasympathetic ganglia, and nicotinic sites at the neuromuscular junction. In general, effects at muscarinic sites are sustained, whereas nicotinic sites are stimulated and then depressed (hyperpolarization block). Signs and symptoms of cholinergic toxicity typically appear when 60% to 80% of cholinesterase activity has been inhibited [6]. The pharmacologic and toxicologic effects of the AChE inhibitor are an extension of their mechanism of action (Table 109.1).

In addition to acute cholinergic effects, OPs cause two other toxic, non-muscarinic syndromes: intermediate syndrome (IMS) and organophosphorus-induced delayed peripheral neuropathy (OIDPN). IMS is a recurrence of weakness that occurs hours to days after a serious OP exposure [7]. Some authors have suggested that IMS is caused by inadequate oxime therapy when serum OP concentrations remain elevated because of redistribution, altered metabolism, or decreased clearance [8]. It is also possible that IMS is caused by desensitization block with downregulation and eventual decrease in the nicotinic receptor activity. As the nicotinic receptor has five subunits, there may be genetic variants that affect clinical responses [9].

The second noncholinergic syndrome is OIDPN. This is a delayed peripheral neuropathy which appears to be mediated by a membrane-bound specific "neuropathy target esterase." OPs that have been associated with OIDPN are aryl organophosphorus esters that contain either a pentavalent phosphorus atom (type I, including derivatives of phosphoric, phosphonic, and phosphoramidic acids, or phosphorofluoridates) or a trivalent phosphorus atom (type II or phosphorus acid derivatives). This neuropathy primarily involves motor fibers. Histologic analysis shows progressive neuronal degeneration, beginning with axonal swelling followed by demyelination, axonal degeneration, and neuronal cell body death and Wallerian degeneration or "dying back" phenomenon [10].

CLINICAL MANIFESTATIONS

Excessive acetylcholine produces symptoms of muscarinic and nicotinic excess. These clinical effects are outlined in Table 109.2. One mnemonic used to describe the muscarinic toxidrome is DUMBBBELS (*d*iarrhea, *u*rination, *m*iosis, *b*ronchospasm, *bronchorrhea*, *bradycardia*, *e*mesis, *l*acrimation, *s*alivation). A mnemonic to describe the nicotinic toxidrome is Monday-Tuesday-Wednesday-tHursday-Friday (mydriasis, tachycardia, weakness, hypertension, fasciculations). Either nicotinic or muscarinic effects may predominate and can lead to misdiagnosis [11]. Miosis may be the most sensitive marker for moderate or severe exposure to an AChE inhibitor [12]. Lacrimation, rhinorrhea, salivation, and profuse sweating are common in moderate to severe poisoning. Abdominal cramping, diarrhea, and vomiting are very common with severe poisoning. Fasciculations are typically observed in severe overdoses.

Respiratory failure is a common cause of death from AChE inhibitor poisoning [2]. Cholinergic excess has direct deleterious effects on the respiratory system: it causes bronchial muscle spasm and noncardiogenic pulmonary edema with exuberant mucus production, severe respiratory muscle impairment, and centrally mediated respiratory depression. Respiratory failure may be further complicated by aspiration.

Cardiac toxicity has been increasingly described as a complication of OP poisoning. There are three phases of reported toxicity including a brief period of intense sympathomimetic tone, a period of enhanced parasympathetic activity, and corrected QT (QTc) interval prolongation with potential for torsade de pointes. Prolongation of the QTc is a marker of severity, and patients with a QTc greater than 440 ms require higher doses of atropine and have a higher mortality than those with a QTc less than 440 ms [13]. Electrocardiographic abnormalities including nonspecific ST-T changes (including ST segment elevation), tachydysrhythmias, bradydysrhythmias, and polymorphic ventricular tachycardia (torsade de pointes) have been reported [14]. Autopsy examination of OP victims has demonstrated direct myocardial injury with myocardial interstitial edema, inflammation, and vascular congestion [15]. The effect on blood pressure is variable. Patients poisoned with dimethoate have an initial benign course but develop delayed refractory hypotension and cardiogenic shock within 36 to 48 hours [2].

The CNS effects of cholinergic poisoning include altered mental status, seizures, and coma [2]. Dystonias and choreoathetoid movements have also been observed [16]. Less severe acute manifestations include anxiety, agitation, emotional lability, headaches, insomnia, tremor, difficulty in concentrating, slurred speech, ataxia, and hyperreflexia or hyporeflexia. In some cases, acute OP poisoning may produce longer lasting neuropsychiatric sequelae [17]. This has been labeled the chronic organophosphorus-induced neuropsychiatric disorder. These

TABLE 109.2

Symptoms of Cholinergic Poisoning

Exposure only	Mild poisoning	Moderate poisoning	Severe poisoning
No symptoms	Can walk Fatigue Headache Dizzy Nausea Vomiting Numbness Sweating Salivation Chest tightness Abdominal cramps Diarrhea ChE 20%–50% of normal	Cannot walk Weakness Difficulty speaking Fasciculations Miosis ChE 10%–20% of normal	Unconscious Unreactive pupils Fasciculations Flaccid paralysis Secretions mouth/nose Moist rales Respiratory distress Seizures ChE <10% of normal

ChE, RBC cholinesterase.

problems seem most severe after serious acute intoxications and usually resolve within 1 year [17].

Cholinergic signs and symptoms typically begin minutes to hours after exposure [2]. Symptom onset is rarely more than 12 hours after exposure. Onset may be delayed for lipophilic compounds (e.g., fenthion, dichlofenthion, leptophos) [2] or compounds that require hepatic metabolism to a more toxic intermediate (e.g., parathion is metabolized to paraoxon) [18]. Dermal exposure may likewise lead to delayed systemic effects. Progressive or prolonged symptoms raise the suspicion of continued absorption of the poison and/or exposure to highly lipophilic compounds.

Life-threatening cholinergic symptoms from OP toxicity generally abate within 1 to 3 days, although many cases requiring weeks of intensive care are reported [19]. Symptoms usually resolve within 12 to 48 hours after exposure to carbamates and other reversible cholinesterase inhibitors [20].

The IMS is characterized by weakness of neck muscles, motor cranial nerves, proximal limb muscles, and respiratory muscles, but without prominent muscarinic findings. It usually begins 24 to 96 hours after the onset of poisoning and lasts 4 to 18 days. [8]. Clinical indications of this syndrome include the inability to lift one's heads up from his/her bed and a decrease in the pulmonary vital capacity [19].

Delayed neuropathy occurs 1 to 3 weeks after the acute cholinergic crises. Patients may initially recover then show progressive signs and symptoms of OIDPN. As this is a dying back axonopathy that usually spares the neuronal cell body, the peripheral neuropathy is characterized by both paresthesias and motor dysfunction occurring first in the longest skeletal nerves with development of foot drop and a high-stepping gait. Symptoms develop slowly and can be divided into three phases: progressive, stationary, and improvement. During the progressive phase, patients have a peripheral sensory neuropathy with complaints of burning, tightness, or pain in the legs and feet. This is followed by numbness and tingling. Subsequently, motor weakness develops, with weakness and loss of peroneal innervation causing foot drop. After approximately 1 week, the paresis may ascend symmetrically into the upper extremities. The sensory loss may occur in a stocking–glove distribution, and the patient loses proprioception. With time, a positive Romberg sign and loss of lower extremity deep tendon reflexes may develop. Flaccid paralysis may occur in severe cases. During the stationary phase, paresis and motor findings cease to progress. This may occur over 3 to 12 months. The improvement phase usually begins 6 to 18 months after exposure, though improvement may be seen as early as 2 to 9 weeks. Partial or complete motor function returns in reverse order of loss. During this phase, central cord or brain lesions may be unmasked and spasticity can develop [21].

DIAGNOSTIC EVALUATION

The diagnosis of the cholinergic poisoning is based on a history of exposure, clinical findings (toxidrome), and improvement after appropriate antidotal therapy. The primary laboratory studies for evaluating anticholinesterase poisoning are plasma cholinesterase (also known as butyrylcholinesterase or pseudocholinesterase) and red blood cell (RBC) AChE activity. Both may be used to confirm the clinical diagnosis. RBC AChE has a structure similar to synaptic AChE and has been validated as a surrogate for synaptic AChE [22]. These tests are not rapidly available in most hospital laboratories but portable Point of Care Testing kits with the ability to measure both plasma and erythrocyte cholinesterase are now available and are being used by the military [23] http://www.eqmresearch.com/.

Plasma cholinesterase is an acute phase reactant which is synthesized in the liver. It differs from RBC AChE in that it has a much more rapid response to inhibition and recovery. It is relatively insensitive to oxime therapy. Only transient decreases of RBC and plasma cholinesterase occur with carbamate poisoning because inactivated AChE spontaneously reactivates with plasma elimination half-lives of 1 to 2 hours [24].

In suspected cholinesterase inhibitor poisoning, plasma and RBC AChE levels should be sent for laboratory determination initially and repeated if the clinical course is atypical [25]. Blood for cholinesterase determination should be drawn into a fluoride-free tube as fluoride inactivates enzyme systems. Samples should be spun down and frozen for storage. The assaying laboratory should be contacted to obtain specific drawing and storing instructions.

Acute exposures are usually classified based on the degree of depression of RBC cholinesterase: mild (20% to 50% of baseline), moderate (10% to 20% of baseline), and severe (less than 10% of baseline) (see Table 109.2). An electromyography (EMG) using repetitive tetanic nerve stimulation can be done to characterize the block and to estimate the amount of enzyme inhibition [26]. As there is a wide variation in normal RBC cholinesterase level with substantial interindividual variation, a person's baseline should be established if the person will be return to working with pesticides [27]. Workers should be removed from exposure until RBC cholinesterase is at least 75% of their baseline values [28]. Workers who do not have an established RBC cholinesterase baseline should not return to work until their RBC cholinesterase values have reached a plateau.

Several OPs are metabolized to *p*-nitrophenol which is easily detected in the urine soon after poisoning [29]. OP concentrations can be measured in serum [30], but contribute little to patient management. These measurements can be useful in determining residual OP residue in a patient with prolonged signs of toxicity and thus can help guide further antidotal therapy. [26]. Supplemental studies include serum electrolytes, blood urea nitrogen, creatinine, glucose, calcium, magnesium, lipase, arterial blood gases, electrocardiography, and chest radiography.

The IMS is diagnosed by clinical findings associated with a reproducible EMG-nerve conduction study using repeated submaximal tetanic nerve stimulation and measuring compound muscle action potentials [31]. No specific laboratory studies are available for evaluating OIDPN. EMG may help to determine the extent of the peripheral neuropathy, and there are specific EMG findings associated with OIDPN [32].

Toxicologic differential diagnosis for cholinergic toxicity includes poisoning with nicotine, carbachol, methacholine, arecoline, bethanechol, pilocarpine, and *Inocybe* or *Clitocybe* mushrooms. Nontoxicologic diagnoses that may be mistaken for cholinergic toxicity include myasthenia gravis, Guillain–Barré, and Eaton–Lambert syndrome.

MANAGEMENT

Patients with all but the mildest symptoms should be admitted to an intensive care unit for careful observation and antidotal therapy as clinically indicated. The initial priorities are managing the patient's airway, breathing, and circulation. All personnel who are involved in the resuscitation and decontamination process should wear masks or respirators, aprons, and nitrile or butyl rubber gloves to avoid secondary contamination.

Clinical scoring systems are used in a variety of disease processes to predict mortality. A number of systems have been applied to the context of OP poisoning including the Acute Physiology and Chronic Health Evaluation (APACHE) II, the Peradeniya Organophosphorus Poisoning (POP) scale, the International Program on Chemical Safety Poison Severity Score (IPCS PSS), the Mortality Prediction Model (MPM), the Poisoning Severity Score (PSS), the Sequential Organ Failure Assessment (SOFA), the Glasgow Coma Score (GCS), and the Simplified Acute Physiology Score (SAPS) II. Numerous studies have been performed in different countries testing the relative performance of each scale with varying results [33–35]. Regardless, the value of clinical scoring systems likely resides in their ability to define a patient population that will require transfer to a higher level of care in under-resourced countries and/or can be used for implementation of treatment guidelines.

Most patients with severe cholinergic poisoning will require airway management and ventilatory assistance for respiratory failure. Succinylcholine should be used with caution to aid intubation because prolonged (hours to days) paralysis may result [36]. A reasonable alternative is to use a rapid-onset nondepolarizing neuromuscular blocker such as rocuronium. Airway and bronchial secretions are treated with atropine. The initial adult dose of atropine is 1 to 2 mg parenterally, which is doubled every 5 minutes (pediatric dose, 0.05 mg per kg) as needed until pulmonary secretions are controlled [37].

Initial resuscitation with intravenous (IV) fluids is needed because of significant fluid losses. Blood pressure support may require direct-acting pressors such as norepinephrine, phenylephrine, and epinephrine, and cardiac depression may require the use of inotropes such as dobutamine [2]. Patients should be treated with atropine until the systolic blood pressure is greater than 80 mm Hg and urine output exceeds 0.5 mL/kg/h in addition to biochemical signs of improved perfusion [37]. Electrical pacing is rarely needed to treat ventricular dysrhythmias. Potassium and magnesium should be normalized to minimize QTc prolongation.

Seizures should be treated with IV atropine and a benzodiazepine (diazepam, 0.2 to 0.4 mg per kg or an equivalent). Animal studies suggest that both atropine and benzodiazepine are effective [38]. Given the potential benefits of benzodiazepines in severe OP poisonings to mitigate neuropsychiatric sequelae, it is reasonable to administer a benzodiazepine even if seizures are not apparent. There is no evidence to support routine use of other anticonvulsants.

Decontamination can limit absorption and prevent reexposure. All of the patient's clothing should be removed, bagged in plastic and discarded, and the person should be thoroughly washed with mild soap and water. Dilute hypochlorite solution (household bleach) inactivates the organophosphorus ester and can be used to decontaminate equipment but should not be used on skin [39]. If an ingestion is recent, nasogastric suction can used to attempt to aspirate any product remaining in the stomach [40]. Although single and multidose charcoal did not change outcome in one trial [41], many of the subjects in this trial had long delays before treatment and it is possible that earlier treatment may limit toxicity.

Antimuscarinic antagonism is the mainstay of initial antidotal therapy. In fact, rapidly incremental atropine dosing regimens have demonstrated improvements in mortality [42]. Atropine is a competitive antagonist of acetylcholine at the muscarinic receptors but has no effect at the neuromuscular junction, so muscle weakness and paralysis are not affected and it does not affect the AChE regeneration rate. As noted previously, atropine is primarily indicated for control of pulmonary secretions and bronchospasm. It has a secondary role in helping to control seizures and CNS manifestations of poisoning [43]. A continuous atropine infusion may be necessary to stabilize the patient, after which the infusion can be titrated back under close observation. In a large Sri Lankan case series, most patients responded to 3 to 5 mg per hour [40]. In general, higher doses of atropine are required during the first 24 hours with OP pesticides than with nerve agents. Tachycardia is not a contraindication to atropine therapy and may reflect hypoxia or sympathetic stimulation. Mydriasis is an early response but is a poor marker for adequate atropinization. A common pitfall is inadequate atropine dosing during serious cholinergic agent overdoses. High doses of atropine are commonly needed for control of secretions. Daily doses in excess of 100 mg are occasionally required for several days [44]. Frequent clinical evaluation and reevaluation is necessary when titrating atropine to prevent atropine toxicity [40,42].

Glycopyrrolate is an antimuscarinic agent that does not penetrate the CNS and is unlikely to be effective in treating CNS effects such as seizures or coma. It can be substituted for atropine when isolated peripheral cholinergic toxicity is present. The recommended starting dose is 0.05 mg per kg. One study suggested that a combination of atropine and glycopyrrolate may improve outcomes [45]. Likewise, ipratropium may be considered for continued pulmonary secretions, although limited evidence exists.

Antidotal therapy with oximes such as pralidoxime (North America, India, and Asia) or obidoxime (Europe and Middle East) is considered a mainstay of treatment but is lacking robust evidence demonstrating improved outcome. Pralidoxime (2-PAM) and obidoxime are nucleophilic oximes that regenerate AChE at muscarinic and nicotinic synapses by reversing the AChE active site phosphorylation. Although pralidoxime does not enter the CNS well, rapid improvement in coma or termination of seizures has been observed after pralidoxime administration [46]. The antidotal effect of atropine and oximes is synergistic.

Although oximes remain a standard therapy for OP poisoning, recent studies have highlighted our limited understanding of their role. Available data are conflicting; one recent randomized controlled trial showed a dramatic treatment effect with pralidoxime [47], whereas a second trial found no benefit and a trend toward worse outcomes [48]. The most recent Cochrane review concluded "current evidence was insufficient to indicate whether oximes are harmful or beneficial" [49]. A more recent retrospective study found an association between mortality and the combination of delay in oxime administration, severity of poisoning, and duration of mechanical ventilation [50]. Another recent retrospective observational study found the use of "high-dose pralidoxime" was associated with decreased mortality (13% to 1.9%) [51].

There are several possible explanations for these discrepant results including differences in the OP lipophilicity, side chains (O′-dimethyl vs. O′-diethyl OPs), rate of aging, and interaction between inhibition/re-inhibition and spontaneous reactivation of the parent OP and oxime-bound compounds. Future studies will have to address these differences.

Although the optimal treatment protocol for pralidoxime is not known, there is consensus that many older protocols used insufficient doses [52]. Although earlier animal studies suggested maintaining a serum concentration of 4 mg/L [53], obtained by 1 to 2 g IV pralidoxime followed by 1 g every 6 to 12 hours [54,55], subsequent studies in poisoned patients have shown that the amount of circulating inhibitor (parent or metabolite of the original OP) actually determines the need for oxime dose [56]. Patients who have ingested massive amounts of an OP may have prolonged high levels of circulating inhibitor lasting for days after ingestion, and the pralidoxime blood level of 4 mg/L is too low to reactivate the AChE. Ideally, poisoned patients should be followed by serial evaluation of the ability to reactivate their cholinesterase in vitro [6]. As this is not feasible for most patients, the following suggestions can be made. The World Health Organization recommends an initial pralidoxime dose of 30 mg per kg IV followed by 8 mg/kg/h or alternatively, 30 mg per kg every 4 hours if a continuous infusion is not possible [52]. The appropriate dose of obidoxime 250 mg is initially followed by 750 mg over 24 hours [57]. In both cases, the dose is adjusted to effect. Muscle fasciculations and weakness should show a response within 60 minutes after dosing; the dose should be increased if the patient has breakthrough signs and symptoms. In mass casualty situations, the intramuscular route of administration may be more practical. The duration of therapy is based on clinical response and is usually 24 to 48 hours. Under ideal conditions, serum samples can be assayed for AChE reactivation and this can be used to guide oxime therapy [58]. Some patients may require continuous treatment for greater than 1 week, depending on the body burden and fat solubility of OP, and re-inhibition of reactivated AChE.

Although hemoperfusion can enhance the elimination of anticholinesterase agents [59], the availability of specific antidotes for OPs and the relatively short course of carbamate intoxications make this procedure unnecessary. There are no outcome studies using hemoperfusion.

Alternative therapies are under investigation. Administration of an enzyme that can scavenge, hydrolyze, and inactivate circulating OP has great theoretical appeal. Such hydrolases have been found in both bacteria and humans and are generically termed "OP hydrolases" [60]. These hydrolases can be genetically engineered to inactivate a wide variety of organophosphorus compounds [61]. Pretreatment studies in animals with hydrolases confer protection against various OPs, including nerve agents [62–65]. Data from animal studies, including nonhuman primates, show promise as rescue therapy [66–68]. It is unclear whether there will be a continued push toward clinical development.

Although other therapies including sodium bicarbonate [69], magnesium sulfate [70], β adrenergic agonists, and lipid emulsion therapies [71] have shown some promise, a lack of larger, randomized controlled trials in humans prevents them from being routinely recommended.

In general, carbamate poisonings have a good prognosis because the duration of serious signs and symptoms is limited. Severe OP poisonings may require prolonged respiratory support, with its attendant complications. Death from acute OP poisonings usually occurs within 24 hours in untreated cases. It should be noted that exposures to fenthion and dimethoate may be delayed beyond 72 hours even if treated [2]. Aggressive respiratory management, timely antidotal therapy, and intensive supportive care are expected to improve morbidity and mortality. Recovery from OIDPN may be gradual or not at all. CNS anoxic sequelae have the worse prognosis and are not specific to cholinesterase inhibitors but rather a consequence of prolonged hypoxia.

Toxicity of Acetylcholinesterase Inhibitors Used to Treat Alzheimer's Disease

With the increasing use of AChE inhibitors to treat dementia, there has been an increasing number of exposures to these medications. Symptoms can range from general weakness [72] to salivation and gastrointestinal effects [73] but are generally milder than pesticides. One case of deliberate ingestion of 288 mg of rivastigmine resulted in seizures, respiratory muscle weakness, and bronchial secretions [74]. Muscarinic effects should be treated with atropine and one report has suggested that isolated CNS effects without peripheral muscarinic symptoms can be treated with pralidoxime alone [75].

NERVE AGENTS USED IN WARFARE

Since the Persian Gulf War and in the aftermath of the terrorist attacks of September 11, 2001, there has been increasing concern about the potential use of G-series (GA [Tabun], GB [Sarin], GD [Soman]) V-series (VE, VG, VM, VX), and the Russian "Novichok" nerve agents. These chemicals are similar in structure and function to the OP insecticides but have a much greater potency. Please see Chapter 128 for a complete discussion of this topic.

References

1. Kahn E: Pesticide related illness in California farm workers. *J Occup Med* 18:693–696, 1976.
2. Eddleston M, Eyer P, Worek F, et al: Differences between organophosphorus insecticides in human self-poisoning: a prospective cohort study. *Lancet* 366:1452–1459, 2005.
3. Morgan JP: The Jamaica ginger paralysis. *JAMA* 248:1864–1867, 1982.
4. Centers for Disease Control (CDC): Aldicarb food poisoning from contaminated melons—California. *MMWR Morb Mortal Wkly Rep* 35:254–258, 1986.
5. Lotti M: Clinical toxicology of anticholinesterase agents in humans, in: Krieger R, (ed): *Handbook of Pesticide Toxicology Agents*. Vol 2. 2nd ed. San Diego, Academic Press, 2001, pp 1043–1085.
6. Thiermann H, Worek F, Eyer P, et al: Obidoxime in acute organophosphate poisoning. 2—PK/PD relationships. *Clin Toxicol (Phila)* 47:807–813, 2009.
7. Senanayake N, Karalliedde L: Neurotoxic effects of organophosphorus insecticides. An intermediate syndrome. *N Engl J Med* 316:761–763, 1987.
8. Senanayake N, Johnson MK: Acute polyneuropathy after poisoning by a new organophosphate insecticide. *N Engl J Med* 306:155–157, 1982.
9. Karalliedde L, Baker D, Marrs TC: Organophosphate-induced intermediate syndrome: aetiology and relationships with myopathy. *Toxicol Rev* 25:1–14, 2006.

10. Jokanovic M, Stukalov PV, Kosanovic M: Organophosphate induced delayed polyneuropathy. *Curr Drug Targets CNS Neurol Disord* 1:593–602, 2002.
11. Zwiener RJ, Ginsburg CM: Organophosphate and carbamate poisoning in infants and children. *Pediatrics* 81(1):121–126, 1988.
12. Okumura T, Takasu N, Ishimatsu S, et al: Report on 640 victims of the Tokyo subway sarin attack. *Ann Emerg Med* 28:129–135, 1996.
13. Shadnia S, Okazi A, Akhlaghi N, et al: Prognostic value of long QT interval in acute and severe organophosphate poisoning. *J Med Toxicol* 5:196–199, 2009.
14. Yurumez Y, Yavuz Y, Saglam H, et al: Electrocardiographic findings of acute organophosphate poisoning. *J Emerg Med* 36:39–42, 2009.
15. Anand S, Singh S, Nahar Saikia U, et al: Cardiac abnormalities in acute organophosphate poisoning. *Clin Toxicol (Phila)* 47(3):230–235, 2009.
16. Moody SB, Terp DK: Dystonic reaction possibly induced by cholinesterase inhibitor insecticides. *Drug Intell Clin Pharm* 22:311–312, 1988.
17. Rosenstock L, Keifer M, Daniell WE, et al: Chronic central nervous system effects of acute organophosphate pesticide intoxication. The Pesticide Health Effects Study Group. *Lancet* 338:223–227, 1991.
18. Buratti FM, Volpe MT, Meneguz A, et al: CYP-specific bioactivation of four organophosphorothioate pesticides by human liver microsomes. *Toxicol Appl Pharmacol* 186:143–154, 2003.
19. Eddleston M, Roberts D, Buckley N: Management of severe organophosphorus pesticide poisoning: *Crit Care* 6:259–259, 2002.
20. Lifshitz M, Shahak E, Bolotin A, et al: Carbamate poisoning in early childhood and in adults. *J Toxicol Clin Toxicol* 35:25–27, 1997.
21. Lotti M, Moretto A: Organophosphate-induced delayed polyneuropathy. *Toxicol Rev* 24:37–49, 2005.
22. Thiermann H, Szinicz L, Eyer P, et al: Correlation between red blood cell acetylcholinesterase activity and neuromuscular transmission in organophosphate poisoning. *Chem Biol Interact* 157–158:345–347, 2005.
23. Rajapakse BN, Thiermann H, Eyer P, et al: Evaluation of the Test-mate ChE (cholinesterase) field kit in acute organophosphorus poisoning. *Ann Emerg Med* 58(6):559–564.e6, 2011.
24. Lifshitz M, Rotenberg M, Sofer S, et al: Carbamate poisoning and oxime treatment in children: a clinical and laboratory study. *Pediatrics* 93:652–655, 1994.
25. Abdullat IM, Battah AH, Hadidi KA: The use of serial measurement of plasma cholinesterase in the management of acute poisoning with organophosphates and carbamates. *Forensic Sci Int* 162:126–130, 2006.
26. Thiermann H, Zilker T, Eyer F, et al: Monitoring of neuromuscular transmission in organophosphate pesticide-poisoned patients. *Toxicol Lett* 191:297–304, 2009.
27. Coye MJ, Lowe JA, Maddy KT: Biological monitoring of agricultural workers exposed to pesticides: I. Cholinesterase activity determinations. *J Occup Med* 28:619–627, 1986.
28. Agency Paetsooehhacep: Guidelines for physicians who supervise workers exposed to cholinesterase-inhibiting pesticides. Available at: http://www.oehha.ca.gov/pesticides/pdf/docguide2002.pdf. Accessed December 27, 2009.
29. Barr DB, Turner WE, DiPietro E, et al: Measurement of p-nitrophenol in the urine of residents whose homes were contaminated with methyl parathion. *Environ Health Perspect* 110[Suppl 6]:1085–1091, 2002.
30. Inoue S, Saito T, Mase H, et al: Rapid simultaneous determination for organophosphorus pesticides in human serum by LC-MS. *J Pharm Biomed Anal* 44:258–264, 2007.
31. Jayawardane P, Dawson AH, Weerasinghe V, et al: The spectrum of intermediate syndrome following acute organophosphate poisoning: a prospective cohort study from Sri Lanka. *PLoS Med* 5(7):e147, 2008.
32. Wadia RS, Chitra S, Amin RB, et al: Electrophysiological studies in acute organophosphate poisoning. *J Neurol Neurosurg Psychiatry* 50:1442–1448, 1987.
33. Peter JV, Thomas L, Graham PL, et al: Performance of clinical scoring systems in acute organophosphate poisoning. *Clin Toxicol (Phila)* 51(9):850–854, 2013.
34. Kim YH, Yeo JH, Kang MJ, et al: Performance assessment of the SOFA, APACHE II scoring system, and SAPS II in intensive care unit organophosphate poisoned patients. *J Korean Med Sci* 28(12):1822–1826, 2013.
35. Bilgin TE, Camdeviren H, Yapici D, et al: The comparison of the efficacy of scoring systems in organophosphate poisoning. *Toxicol Ind Health* 21(7–8):141–146, 2005.
36. Selden BS, Curry SC: Prolonged succinylcholine-induced paralysis in organophosphate insecticide poisoning. *Ann Emerg Med* 16:215–217, 1987.
37. Eddleston M, Buckley NA, Eyer P, et al: Management of acute organophosphorus pesticide poisoning: *Lancet* 371:597–607, 2008.
38. McDonough JH Jr, Jaax NK, Crowley RA, et al: Atropine and/or diazepam therapy protects against soman-induced neural and cardiac pathology. *Fundam Appl Toxicol* 13:256–276, 1989.
39. Holstege CP, Kirk M, Sidell FR: Chemical warfare. Nerve agent poisoning. *Crit Care Clin* 13:923–942, 1997.
40. Eddleston M, Dawson A, Karalliedde L, et al: Early management after self-poisoning with an organophosphorus or carbamate pesticide – a treatment protocol for junior doctors. *Crit Care* 8:R391–R397, 2004.
41. Eddleston M, Juszczak E, Buckley NA, et al: Multiple-dose activated charcoal in acute self-poisoning: a randomised controlled trial. *Lancet* 371:579–587, 2008.
42. Abedin MJ, Sayeed AA, Basher A, et al: Open-label randomized clinical trial of atropine bolus injection versus incremental boluses plus infusion for organophosphate poisoning in Bangladesh. *J Med Toxicol* 8(2):108–117, 2012.
43. Eddleston M, Singh S, Buckley N: Acute organophosphorus poisoning. *Clin Evid* 10:1652–1663, 2003.
44. Golsousidis H, Kokkas V: Use of 19 590 mg of atropine during 24 days of treatment, after a case of unusually severe parathion poisoning. *Hum Toxicol* 4:339–340, 1985.
45. Arendse R, Irusen E: An atropine and glycopyrrolate combination reduces mortality in organophosphate poisoning. *Hum Exp Toxicol* 28:715–720, 2009.
46. Lotti M, Becker CE: Treatment of acute organophosphate poisoning: evidence of a direct effect on central nervous system by 2-PAM (pyridine-2-aldoxime methyl chloride). *J Toxicol Clin Toxicol* 19:121–127, 1982.
47. Pawar KS, Bhoite RR, Pillay CP, et al: Continuous pralidoxime infusion versus repeated bolus injection to treat organophosphorus pesticide poisoning: a randomised controlled trial. *Lancet* 368:2136–2141, 2006.
48. Eddleston M, Eyer P, Worek F, et al: Pralidoxime in acute organophosphorus insecticide poisoning–a randomised controlled trial. *PLoS Med* 6:e1000104, 2009.
49. Buckley NA, Eddleston M, Li Y, et al: Oximes for acute organophosphate pesticide poisoning. *Cochrane Database Syst Rev* 16(2):CD005085, 2011.
50. Ahmed SM, Das B, Nadeem A, et al: Survival pattern in patients with acute organophosphate poisoning on mechanical ventilation: a retrospective intensive care unit-based study in a tertiary care teaching hospital. *Indian J Anaesth* 58(1):11–17, 2014.
51. Due P: Effectiveness of high dose pralidoxime for treatment of organophosphate poisoning. *Asian Pac J Med Toxicol* 3:97–103, 2014.
52. Buckley NA, Eddleston M, Szinicz L: Oximes for acute organophosphate pesticide poisoning. *Cochrane Database Syst Rev* CD005085, 2005. doi:10.1002/14651858.CD005085.
53. Sundwall A: Minimum concentrations of *N*-methylpyridinium-2-aldoxime methane sulphonate (P2 S) which reverse neuromuscular block. *Biochem Pharmacol* 8:413–417, 1961.
54. Medicis JJ, Stork CM, Howland MA, et al: Pharmacokinetics following a loading plus a continuous infusion of pralidoxime compared with the traditional short infusion regimen in human volunteers. *J Toxicol Clin Toxicol* 34:289–295, 1996.
55. Schexnayder S, James LP, Kearns GL, et al: The pharmacokinetics of continuous infusion pralidoxime in children with organophosphate poisoning. *J Toxicol Clin Toxicol* 36:549–555, 1998.
56. Eyer P, Worek F, Thiermann H, et al: Paradox findings may challenge orthodox reasoning in acute organophosphate poisoning. *Chem Biol Interact* 187(1–3):270–278, 2009.
57. Eyer F, Worek F, Eyer P, et al: Obidoxime in acute organophosphate poisoning: 1—clinical effectiveness. *Clin Toxicol (Phila)* 47:798–806, 2009.
58. Eyer P: The role of oximes in the management of organophosphorus pesticide poisoning. *Toxicol Rev* 22:165–190, 2003.
59. Peter JV, Moran JL, Pichamuthu K, et al: Adjuncts and alternatives to oxime therapy in organophosphate poisoning–is there evidence of benefit in human poisoning? A review. *Anaesth Intensive Care* 36:339–350, 2008.
60. Ceron JJ, Tecles F, Tvarijonaviciute A: Serum paraoxonase 1 (PON1) measurement: an update. *BMC Vet Res* 10:74, 2014.
61. Bird SB, Dawson A, Ollis D: Enzymes and bioscavengers for prophylaxis and treatment of organophosphate poisoning. *Front Biosci (Schol Ed)* 2:209–220, 2010.
62. Ashani Y, Rothschild N, Segall Y, et al: Prophylaxis against organophosphate poisoning by an enzyme hydrolysing organophosphorus compounds in mice. *Life Sci* 49(5):367–374, 1991.
63. Doctor BP, Raven L, Wolfe AD, et al: Enzymes as pretreatment drugs for organophosphate toxicity. *Neurosci Biobehav Rev* 15(1):123–128, 1991.
64. Raveh L, Segall Y, Leader H, et al: Protection against tabun toxicity in mice by prophylaxis with an enzyme hydrolyzing organophosphate esters. *Biochem Pharmacol* 44(2):397–400, 1992.
65. Ashani Y, Leader H, Rothschild N, et al: Combined effect of organophosphorus hydrolase and oxime on the reactivation rate of diethylphosphoryl-acetylcholinesterase conjugates. *Biochem Pharmacol* 55(2):159–168, 1998.
66. Gresham C, Rosenbaum C, Gaspari RJ, et al: Kinetics and efficacy of an organophosphorus hydrolase in a rodent model of methyl-parathion poisoning. *Acad Emerg Med* 17(7):736–740, 2010.
67. Jackson CJ, Carville A, Ward J, et al: Use of OpdA, an organophosphorus (OP) hydrolase, prevents lethality in an African green monkey model of acute OP poisoning. *Toxicology* 317:1–5, 2014.
68. Bird SB, Sutherland TD, Gresham C, et al: OpdA, a bacterial organophosphorus hydrolase, prevents lethality in rats after poisoning with highly toxic organophosphorus pesticides. *Toxicology* 247(2–3):88–92, 2008.
69. Roberts D, Buckley NA: Alkalinisation for organophosphorus pesticide poisoning. *Cochrane Database Syst Rev* (1):CD004897, 2005. doi:10.1002/14651858.CD004897.pub2.
70. Basher A, Rahman SH, Ghose A, et al: Phase II study of magnesium sulfate in acute organophosphate pesticide poisoning. *Clin Toxicol (Phila)* 51(1):35–40, 2013.
71. Dunn C, Bird SB, Gaspari R: Intralipid fat emulsion decreases respiratory failure in a rat model of parathion exposure. *Acad Emerg Med* 19(5):504–509, 2012.
72. Lai MW, Moen M, Ewald MB: Pesticide-like poisoning from a prescription drug. *N Engl J Med* 353:317–318, 2005.
73. Sener S, Ozsarac M: Case of the month: rivastigmine (Exelon) toxicity with evidence of respiratory depression. *Emerg Med J* 23:82–85, 2006.
74. Brvar M, Mozina M, Bunc M: Poisoning with rivastigmine. *Clin Toxicol (Phila)* 43:891–892, 2005.
75. Hoffman RS, Manini AF, Russell-Haders AL, et al: Use of pralidoxime without atropine in rivastigmine (carbamate) toxicity. *Hum Exp Toxicol* 28:599–602, 2009.

Chapter 110 ■ Cocaine Poisoning

RICHARD D. SHIH • STACEY FEINSTEIN • JUDD E. HOLLANDER

Cocaine (benzoylmethylecgonine) is an alkaloid compound derived from the South American plant *Erythroxylon coca*. Its use as an illicit drug of abuse has reached epidemic proportions. Thirty-four million US citizens have used cocaine at least once; 5.9 million have used cocaine in the past year; and 2.1 million have used cocaine in the past month [1]. Other than alcohol, cocaine is the most common cause of acute drug-related emergency department visits, accounting for 31% of all visits to the emergency department related to drug misuse or abuse [2].

PHARMACOLOGY

The pharmacologic effects of cocaine are complex, and they include direct blockade of the fast sodium channels, increase in norepinephrine release for the adrenergic nerve terminals, interference with neuronal catecholamine reuptake, and increase in excitatory amino acid concentration in the central nervous system (CNS). Blockade of the fast sodium channels stabilizes axonal membranes, producing a local anesthetic-like effect and a type I antidysrhythmic effect on the myocardium. The increase in catecholamine levels produces a sympathomimetic effect. The result of increased excitatory amino acid concentration in the CNS is increased extracellular dopamine concentration.

Cocaine is well absorbed through the mucosa of the respiratory, gastrointestinal, and genitourinary tracts, including less common routes of absorption such as the urethra, bladder, and vagina. The cocaine hydrochloride salt is the form most often abused nasally or parenterally. Crack cocaine and cocaine freebase are alkaloid forms of cocaine that are produced by an extraction process. These forms are heat stable, can be smoked, and are absorbed through the pulmonary system. When intravenously administered or inhaled, cocaine is rapidly distributed throughout the body and CNS, with peak effects in 3 to 5 minutes. With nasal insufflation, absorption peaks in 20 minutes.

Cocaine has a half-life of 0.5 to 1.5 hours. It is rapidly hydrolyzed to the inactive metabolites ecgonine methyl ester and benzoylecgonine, which account for 80% of cocaine metabolism. These compounds have half-lives of 4 to 8 hours and have some cardiovascular effects that are similar to the parent compound. Minor cocaine metabolites include ecgonine and norcocaine. Urinary toxicology screens for recreational drugs typically assess for the presence of benzoylecgonine, which is usually present for 48 to 72 hours after cocaine use [3].

Cocaine is frequently abused in combination with other drugs, particularly ethanol. This may be a popular combination because ethanol antagonizes the stimulatory effects of cocaine. The metabolism of cocaine in the presence of ethanol produces cocaethylene, which has additional cardiovascular and behavioral effects [4]. Cocaethylene and cocaine are similar with regard to behavioral effects. However, cocaethylene has been more likely to result in death in animal studies. Human studies demonstrate that cocaethylene produces milder subjective effects and similar hemodynamic effects when compared with cocaine. Cocaethylene also has a direct myocardial depressant effect [4,5].

Cocaine toxicity is due to an exaggeration of its pharmacologic effects, resulting in myriad consequences that have an impact on every organ system. The widespread effects of cocaine are related to its ability to stimulate the peripheral and central sympathetic nervous systems, in addition to local anesthetic-like effects. Cocaine-induced seizures are most likely due to excess catecholamine stimulation.

Cocaine causes vascular effects through multiple pathophysiologic mechanisms that have been best described in the heart [6–8]. These include arterial vasoconstriction, in situ thrombus formation, platelet activation, and inhibition of endogenous fibrinolysis. In addition, myocardial oxygen demand is increased by cocaine-induced tachycardia and hypertension [6–9]. The direct local anesthetic-like effect of cocaine or secondary cocaine-induced myocardial ischemia [6,10] may be responsible for cardiac conduction disturbances [10] and dysrhythmias.

CLINICAL PRESENTATION

Clinical manifestations of acute cocaine toxicity may occur in a number of different organ systems. Most severe cocaine-related toxicity and cocaine-related deaths are manifested by signs of sympathomimetic overdrive (e.g., tachycardia, hypertension, dilated pupils, and increased psychomotor activity). This increased psychomotor activity causes increased heat production and can lead to severe hyperthermia and rhabdomyolysis [11].

Cocaine-induced cardiovascular effects are common. Of cocaine-related emergency department visits, chest pain is the most common complaint. Although most of the patients do not have serious underlying etiology, myocardial infarction due to cocaine is a well-established entity and needs to be excluded [12,13]. It occurs in 6% of patients presenting with cocaine-associated chest pain [14]. The risk of myocardial infarction is increased 24-fold in the hour after cocaine use. In patients aged 18 to 45 years, 25% of myocardial infarctions is attributed to cocaine use [15]. Cocaine-associated myocardial infarction typically occurs in patients aged 18 to 60 years without apparent massive cocaine exposure or without evidence of cocaine toxicity. Patients with cocaine-associated myocardial infarctions frequently have atypical chest pain or chest pain that is delayed hours to days after their most recent cocaine use [6,12].

Cardiac conduction disturbances (e.g., prolonged QRS and QTc) and cardiac dysrhythmias (e.g., sinus tachycardia, atrial fibrillation/flutter, supraventricular tachycardias, idioventricular rhythms, ventricular tachycardia, torsade de pointes, and ventricular fibrillation) may occur after cocaine use [16–18]. Aortic dissection and endocarditis associated with cocaine abuse are uncommon [19].

The neurologic effects of cocaine may be manifested in a number of ways. Altered mental status and euphoria are typically short lived and without serious sequelae. The stimulatory effects of cocaine can lead to seizures, cerebral infarction, intracerebral bleeding, subarachnoid hemorrhage, transient ischemic attacks, migraine-type headache syndromes, cerebral vasculitis, anterior spinal artery syndrome, and psychiatric manifestations [20–24, 24a]. Cocaine is associated with a sevenfold increased risk of stroke in women [23].

Cocaine-induced seizures are typically single, brief, generalized, self-limited, and not associated with permanent neurologic deficit [24,24a]. These seizures may occur in the presence or absence of concurrent structural disease, such as infarction or hemorrhage. Multiple or focal seizures are usually associated with concomitant drug use or an underlying seizure disorder [20].

Cocaine has a number of direct and indirect effects on the lungs, and they are associated with how the drug is used [25].

These effects include asthma exacerbations, pneumothorax, pneumomediastinum, noncardiogenic pulmonary edema, alveolar hemorrhage, pulmonary infarction, pulmonary artery hypertrophy, and acute respiratory failure [26,27]. Asthma exacerbations are more common with crack cocaine usage, most likely due to particulate by-products of combustion [27]. Inhalation of cocaine is typically associated with deep Valsalva maneuvers to maximize drug delivery and can cause pneumothorax, pneumomediastinum, and noncardiogenic pulmonary edema.

The intestinal vascular system is particularly sensitive to cocaine effects because the intestinal walls have a wide distribution of α-adrenergic receptors. Acute intestinal infarction has been associated with all routes of cocaine administration [28].

The most deadly gastrointestinal manifestation of cocaine usage is seen in the patient who presents after ingesting packets filled with cocaine. These patients have been termed *body packers* or *body stuffers*. Body packers are patients who swallow carefully prepared condom or latex packets filled with large quantities of highly purified cocaine for the purposes of smuggling this drug into the country. In contrast, body stuffers are typically "street" drug dealers who swallow packets of cocaine while fleeing the police. These packets are generally prepared for distribution to individual customers and not to protect the body stuffer from absorbing cocaine. It was previously thought that cocaine ingested orally was metabolized in the gastrointestinal track and did not lead to systemic toxicity. This is clearly not the case and toxicity can develop in body stuffers and packers from cocaine leaking out of the swallowed packets. The dosage of cocaine exposure in body stuffers is generally substantially less than that of a body packer. However, toxicity is more likely to occur in the setting of body stuffers. Although massive exposure to leakage from a condom or latex-filled packet of a body packer can occur, most body packers identified by airport immigration officers do not develop clinical toxicity. However, any patient identified as a body packer who has developed any signs of systemic cocaine toxicity (tachycardia, hypertension, diaphoresis, etc.) can rapidly develop worsening symptoms including life-threatening ones. These patients, when identified, have a high potential for progressively worsening toxicity and mortality [29].

Premature atherosclerosis may develop in some chronic cocaine users. Further, cocaine-induced left ventricular dysfunction can lead to hypertrophy and eventually a dilated cardiomyopathy and congestive heart failure [6]. Cocaine-associated dilated cardiomyopathy appears to have a reversible component, and some patients have demonstrated improvement after cessation of cocaine use [6].

Chronic severe cocaine users can present with lethargy and a depressed mental status that is not attributable to any other etiology (diagnosis of exclusion), the "cocaine washout syndrome." This self-limited syndrome usually abates within 24 hours but can last for several days and is thought to result from excessive cocaine usage that depletes essential neurotransmitters [30].

Chronic inhalational use of cocaine does not appear to lead to long-term pulmonary effects. Spirometry and lung mechanics are typically normal even in heavy chronic users [31].

Chronic cocaine usage during pregnancy increases the chance of premature delivery and abruptio placentae [32]. Maternal cocaine usage is associated with low birth weight, small head circumference, developmental problems, and birth defects in the neonate [33–35]. Neonates exposed to cocaine in utero may develop cocaine withdrawal syndrome, which typically begins 24 to 48 hours after birth and is characterized by irritability, jitteriness, and poor eye contact.

In recent years, there has been an increased number of cases in which levamisole, an anthelmintic and immunomodulator, has been found as an adulterant in street cocaine. Although issues associated with levamisole are not directly caused by cocaine, the frequency with which levamisole is found as an adulterant makes this discussion relevant to cocaine toxicity. In addition, levamisole was withdrawn from the United States market by the FDA in 1999 due to concerns regarding agranulocytosis. In association with cocaine, levamisole has not only been implicated in cases of agranulocytosis, but has had multiple reports of cutaneous vasculitis. The purpose of adulterating street cocaine with levamisole is not known, but it is speculated to potentiate the effects of cocaine [36,37].

DIAGNOSTIC EVALUATION

Patients manifesting cocaine toxicity should have a complete evaluation focusing on the history of cocaine use, signs and symptoms of sympathetic nervous system excess, and evaluation of specific organ system complaints. It is of paramount importance to determine whether signs and symptoms are due to cocaine itself, underlying medical conditions, or cocaine-induced exacerbation of medical conditions.

When the history is clear and symptoms are mild, laboratory evaluation is usually unnecessary. In contrast, if the patient manifests moderate or severe toxicity, routine laboratory evaluation may include a complete blood cell count, serum electrolytes, glucose, blood urea nitrogen, creatinine, creatine kinase (CK), cardiac marker determinations, arterial blood gas analysis, electrocardiogram, and urinalysis. Sympathetic excess may result in hyperglycemia and hypokalemia. Elevated CK is associated with rhabdomyolysis. Cardiac markers are elevated in myocardial infarction. However, false elevations of CK–MB fraction are common [13]. Cardiac troponin is the preferred method to diagnose myocardial injury in cocaine users [13]. Urine drug testing may be helpful in establishing recent cocaine use.

Chest radiography and electrocardiography (ECG) should be obtained in patients with chest pain or cardiovascular complaints. The initial ECG is a less useful diagnostic tool than for patients with chest pain that is unrelated to cocaine. Many young cocaine-using patients have ST-segment elevation in the absence of acute myocardial infarction. This is due to early repolarization changes [16,17].

Observation for a 9- to 12-hour period is also a useful tool for the evaluation of patients presenting with cocaine-associated chest pain. Patients without new ischemic changes on ECG, a normal troponin test, and no cardiovascular complications during this observation (dysrhythmias, acute myocardial infarction, or recurrent symptoms) can safely be sent home with follow-up and planned outpatient workup [18,38]. The use of coronary computerized angiographic tomography might identify patients safe for discharge in a slightly more rapid time frame [39].

A brief seizure temporally related to cocaine use in an otherwise healthy person should be evaluated with a head computed tomography (CT). Further workup in an otherwise asymptomatic patient may not be necessary [20,24,24a]. Patients with concurrent headache, suspected subarachnoid hemorrhage, or other neurologic manifestations may necessitate lumbar puncture after head CT to rule out serious pathology. Patients who are suspected of body stuffing should be evaluated by abdominal radiographs and cavity searches (digital or visual examination of the rectum or vagina).

MANAGEMENT

The initial management of cocaine-toxic patients should focus on airway, breathing, and circulation. Treatments are directed at a specific sign, symptom, or organ system affected and are summarized in Table 110.1.

Patients who present with sympathetic excess and psychomotor agitation are at risk of hyperthermia and rhabdomyolysis. Management should focus on lowering core body temperature, halting further muscle damage and heat production, and ensuring good urinary output. The primary agents used for muscle relaxation are benzodiazepines [12].

TABLE 110.1

Treatment Summary for Cocaine-Related Medical Conditions

Medical condition	Treatments
Cardiovascular	
Dysrhythmias	
Sinus tachycardia	Observation
	Oxygen
	Diazepam or lorazepam
Supraventricular tachycardia	Oxygen
	Diazepam or lorazepam
	Consider diltiazem, verapamil or adenosine
	If hemodynamically unstable: cardioversion
Ventricular dysrhythmias	Oxygen
	Diazepam or lorazepam
	Consider sodium bicarbonate and/or lidocaine
	If hemodynamically unstable: defibrillation
Acute coronary syndrome	Oxygen
	Aspirin
	Diazepam or lorazepam
	Nitroglycerin
	Heparin
	For ST-segment elevation (STEMI): Percutaneous intervention (angioplasty and stent placement) preferred. Consider fibrinolytic therapy.
	Consider morphine sulfate, phentolamine, verapamil, or glycoprotein IIb/IIIa inhibitors
Hypertension	Observation
	Diazepam or lorazepam
	Consider nitroglycerin, phentolamine, and nitroprusside
Pulmonary edema	Furosemide
	Nitroglycerin
	Consider morphine sulfate or phentolamine
Hyperthermia	Diazepam or lorazepam
	Cooling methods
	If agitated, consider paralysis and intubation
Neuropsychiatric	
Anxiety and agitation	Diazepam or lorazepam
Seizures	Diazepam or lorazepam
	Consider phenobarbital
Intracranial hemorrhage	Surgical consultation
Rhabdomyolysis	Intravenous hydration
	Consider sodium bicarbonate or mannitol
	If in acute renal failure: hemodialysis
Cocaine washout syndrome	Supportive care
Body packers	Activated charcoal
	Whole-bowel irrigation
	Laparotomy or endoscopic retrieval

The use of antipsychotic agents for cocaine-induced neurobehavioral agitation is controversial [40]. In mild cases, antipsychotics may be useful. In cases of severe cocaine-induced agitation, few data exist on the safety and efficacy of antipsychotics. In these cases, benzodiazepines are preferred and supranormal cumulative doses may be necessary. Core body temperatures may be highly elevated. This should be treated aggressively with surface cooling devices. Some cases of severe muscle overactivity may require general anesthesia with nondepolarizing neuromuscular blockade. Succinylcholine, a depolarizing neuromuscular-blocking agent, may increase the risk of hyperkalemia in the setting of severe cocaine-induced rhabdomyolysis and should be avoided. In addition, plasma cholinesterase is responsible for the metabolism of both succinylcholine and cocaine. When these two agents are used simultaneously, prolonged clinical effects of either or both agents might result. Therefore, nondepolarizing agents are preferred.

Patients with severe hypertension can usually be safely treated with benzodiazepines. When benzodiazepines are not effective, nitroglycerin, nitroprusside, or phentolamine can be used. β-Blockers are contraindicated. Their use in this setting can lead to unopposed alpha stimulation with paradoxic exacerbation of hypertension and worsening coronary vasoconstriction [41].

Patients with chest pain and suspected cocaine-induced ischemia or myocardial infarction should be treated with aspirin, benzodiazepines, and nitroglycerin as first-line agents. Benzodiazepines decrease the central stimulatory effects of cocaine, thereby indirectly reducing its cardiovascular toxicity [12]. Benzodiazepines have been shown to have a comparable and possibly an additive effect to nitroglycerin with respect to chest pain resolution and hemodynamic and cardiac functional parameters (cardiac output) for patients with cocaine-associated chest pain [42,43] (Table 110.2). Weight-adjusted unfractionated heparin or enoxaparin would be reasonable to use in patients with documented ischemia. Patients who do not respond to these initial therapies can be treated with phentolamine or calcium channel blocking agents [44,45]. The International Guidelines for Emergency Cardiovascular Care recommend α-adrenergic antagonists (phentolamine) for the treatment of cocaine-associated acute coronary syndrome [46]. β-Blockers are contraindicated, as they can exacerbate cocaine-induced coronary artery vasoconstriction [41]. However, this recommendation has come under some scrutiny. Recent studies suggest that β-blocker usage in the setting of cocaine toxicity does not appear to obviously increase detrimental clinical outcomes [47,48]; however, the relatively low mortality associated with myocardial infarction due to the documented adverse effects of cocaine has resulted in the American College of Cardiology/American Health Association guidelines continuing to recommend against its use in cases of acute intoxication [13].

Primary reperfusion therapy is best done with percutaneous interventions, when available [49]. Fibrinolytic therapy in this setting is somewhat controversial. The mortality from cocaine-associated myocardial infarction is low. Patients with cocaine-associated chest pain have a high prevalence of "false-positive ST-segment elevations," up to 43% in one study [50]. Therefore, treatment of all patients with cocaine-associated chest pain who meet standard ECG thrombolysis in myocardial infarction criteria would result in fibrinolytic administration to more patients without acute myocardial infarction than with acute myocardial infarction.

Supraventricular dysrhythmias may be difficult to treat. Initially, benzodiazepines should be administered. Adenosine can be given, but its effects may be temporary. Use of calcium channel blockers in association with benzodiazepines appears to be most beneficial. β-Blockers should be avoided [41].

Ventricular dysrhythmias should be managed with benzodiazepines, lidocaine, or sodium bicarbonate [46]. Bicarbonate is preferred in patients with QRS widening and ventricular dysrhythmias that occur soon after cocaine use. In this setting,

TABLE 110.2

Summary of Recommendations Based on Randomized Controlled Clinical Trials

Reference	Population	Intervention	Control	Primary outcome	Design	Effect measure	Summary
[42]	40 patients with potential cocaine-associated acute coronary syndrome	Diazepam plus placebo nitroglycerin ($N = 12$), nitroglycerin and placebo diazepam ($N = 13$), or diazepam and nitroglycerin arms were used ($N = 15$). Diazepam was administered 5 mg intravenously every 5 min for a total dose of 15 mg. Nitroglycerin, 0.4 mg, was administered sublingually every 5 min for up to a total of 3 doses.	No patients received placebo diazepam and placebo nitroglycerin	Chest pain resolution, and changes in blood pressure, pulse rate, cardiac output, cardiac index, stroke volume, and stroke index over the 15-min treatment period.	Prospective, randomized, double-blind trial	Chest pain severity improved similarly in the 3 groups and there were no differences in the response of cardiac measures to the therapies administered.	No difference in treatment between diazepam only, nitroglycerin only, or combined therapy.
[43]	27 patients with cocaine-associated chest pain	Nitroglycerin (group I, $N = 15$) or nitroglycerin plus lorazepam (group II, $N = 12$) was utilized. The nitroglycerin was administered sublingually and the lorazepam was administered intravenously, 1 mg every 5 min for a total of 2 doses.	No patients received placebo	Chest pain score (0–10 scale) measured at 5 min after each medication administration.	Prospective, randomized, single-blind trial	5 min after initial treatment, there was no difference in the mean chest pain scores. 5 min after the second treatment, the mean scores were 4.6 and 1.5, respectively that was statistically significant.	Lorazepam with nitroglycerin appears to be more efficacious than nitroglycerin alone in the treatment of cocaine-associated chest pain

the dysrhythmias are presumably related to the sodium channel blocking effects of cocaine. Lidocaine or amiodarone can be used when dysrhythmias appear to be related to cocaine-induced ischemia [10,46].

Seizures should be treated with benzodiazepines and, phenobarbital or propofol. Phenytoin is not recommended in cases associated with cocaine. Although no studies have compared barbiturates to phenytoin or propofol for control of cocaine-induced seizures, barbiturates are theoretically preferable because they also produce CNS sedation and are generally more effective for toxin-induced convulsions. If these agents are not rapidly effective, nondepolarizing neuromuscular blockade and general anesthesia are indicated.

Patients with cerebrovascular complications or focal neurologic findings should be managed as usual. However, the utility of fibrinolytic agents in cocaine-associated cerebrovascular infarction is unknown.

Cocaine body stuffers who are asymptomatic should be given activated charcoal [51]. Whole-bowel irrigation with subsequent radiologic verification of passage of all drug-filled containers should be considered [29]. Body stuffers who manifest clinical signs of toxicity should be treated similar to other cocaine-intoxicated patients. Body packers who develop any signs of cocaine toxicity need to be identified as quickly as possible and treated very aggressively. These individuals have a high likelihood of developing worsening toxicity and life-threatening symptomatology. Initial use of activated charcoal and surgical removal of ruptured cocaine packets is warranted in almost all cases and can be life saving [29].

References

1. National Survey on Drug Use and Health, 2007. Available at http://www.samhsa.gov.
2. Schwartz BG, Rezkalla S, Kloner RA, et al: Cardiovascular effects of cocaine. *Circ* 122:2258, 2010.
3. Kolbrich EA, Barnes AJ, Gorelick DA, et al: Major and minor metabolites of cocaine in human plasma following controlled subcutaneous cocaine administration. *J Anal Toxicol* 30:501, 2006.
4. Patel MB, Opreanu M, Shah AJ, et al: Cocaine and alcohol: a potential lethal duo. *Am J Med* 122:e5, 2009.
5. Herbst ED, Harris DS, Everhart ET, et al: Cocaethylene formation following ethanol and cocaine administration by different rounts. *Exp Clin Psychopharmacol* 19:95, 2011.
6. Hollander JE: Management of cocaine associated myocardial ischemia. *N Engl J Med* 333:1267, 1995.
7. Lange RA, Hillis RD: Cardiovascular complications of cocaine use. *N Engl J Med* 345:351, 2001.
8. Pozner CN, Levine M, Zane R: The cardiovascular effects of cocaine. *J Emerg Med* 29:173, 2005.
9. Lange RA, Cigarroa RG, Yancy CW, et al: Cocaine-induced coronary-artery vasoconstriction. *N Engl J Med* 321:1557, 1989.
10. Shih RD, Hollander JE, Hoffman RS, et al: Clinical safety of lidocaine in cocaine associated myocardial infarction. *Ann Emerg Med* 26:702, 1995.
11. Singhal PC, Rubin RB, Peters A, et al: Rhabdomyolysis and acute renal failure associated with cocaine abuse. *J Toxicol Clin Toxicol* 28:321, 1990.
12. Hollander JE: Cocaine intoxication and hypertension. *Ann Emerg Med* 51:S18, 2008.
13. McCord J, Jneid H, Hollander JE, et al: Management of cocaine-associated chest pain and myocardial infarction: a scientific statement from the American Heart Association Acute Cardiac Care Committee of the Council on Clinical Cardiology. *Circulation* 117:1897, 2008.
14. Weber JE, Chudnofsky C, Wilkerson MD, et al: Cocaine associated chest pain: how common is myocardial infarction? *Acad Emerg Med* 7:873, 2000.
15. Qureshi AI, Suri FK, Guterman LR, et al: Cocaine use and the likelihood of nonfatal myocardial infarction and stroke. Data from the third National Health and Nutrition Examination Survey. *Circulation* 103:502, 2001.
16. Hollander JE, Lozano M Jr, Fairweather P, et al: "Abnormal" electrocardiograms in patients with cocaine-associated chest pain are due to "normal" variants. *J Emerg Med* 12:199, 1994.
17. Hamad A, Khan M: ST-segment elevation in patients with cocaine abuse and chest pain: is there a pattern? *Am J Cardiol* 86:1054, 2000.
18. Weber JE, Shofer FS, Larkin GL, et al: Validation of a brief observation period for patients with cocaine-associated chest pain. *N Engl J Med* 348:510, 2003.
19. Hsue PY, Salinas CL, Bolger AF, et al: Acute aortic dissection related to crack cocaine. *Circulation* 105:1592–1595, 2002.
20. Satel SL, Gawin FH: Migraine-like headache and cocaine use. *JAMA* 261:2995, 1989.
21. Bolla KI, Funderburk FR, Cadet JL: Differential effects of cocaine and cocaine alcohol on neurocognitive performance. *Neurology* 54:2285, 2000.
22. Kaye BR, Fainstat M: Cerebral vasculitis associated with cocaine abuse. *JAMA* 258:2104, 1987.
23. Petitti DB, Sidney S, Quesenberry C, et al: Stroke and cocaine or amphetamine use. *Epidemiology* 9:956, 1998.
24. Majlesi N, Shih RD, Fiesseler FW, et al: Cocaine-associated seizures and incidence of status epilepticus. *West J Emerg Med* 11:157, 2010.

24a. Wilson KC, Saukkonen JJ: Acute respiratory failure from abused substances. *J Intensive Care Med* 19:183, 2004.

25. Restrepo CS, Carrillo JA, Martínez S, et al: Pulmonary complications from cocaine and cocaine-based substances: imaging manifestations. *Radiographics* 27:941, 2007.
26. Wolff AJ, O'Donnell AE: Pulmonary effects of illicit drug use. *Clin Chest Med* 25:203, 2004.
27. Rome LA, Lippman ML, Dalsey WC, et al: Prevalence of cocaine use and its impact on asthma exacerbation in an urban population. *Chest* 117:1324, 2000.
28. Linder JD, Monkemuller KE, Raijman I, et al: Cocaine-associated ischemic colitis. *South Med J* 93:909, 2000.
29. Gill JR, Graham SM: Ten years of "body packers" in New York City: 50 deaths. *J Foren Sci* 47:843, 2002.
30. Sporer KA, Lesser M: Cocaine washed out syndrome. *Ann Emerg Med* 21: 112, 1992.
31. Kleerup EC, Koyal SN, Marques-Magallanes JA, et al: Chronic and acute effects of "crack" cocaine on diffusing capacity, membrane diffusion, and pulmonary capillary blood volume in the lung. *Chest* 122:629, 2002.
32. Dombrowski MP, Wolfe HM, Welch RA, et al: Cocaine abuse is associated with abruptio placentae and decreased birth weight, but not shorter labor. *Obstet Gynecol* 77:139, 1991.
33. Bada HS, Das A, Bauer CR, et al: Low birth weight and preterm births: Etiologic fraction attributable to prenatal drug exposure. *J Perinatol* 25:631, 2005.
34. Eyler FD, Behnke M, Conlon M, et al: Birth outcome from a prospective, matched study of prenatal crack/cocaine use: I. Interactive and dose effects on health and growth. *Pediatrics* 101:229, 1998.
35. Chavez GF, Mulinare J, Cordero JF: Maternal cocaine use during early pregnancy as a risk factor for congenital urogenital anomalies. *JAMA* 262:795, 1989.
36. Chang A, Osterloh J, Thomas J: Levamisole: a dangerous new cocaine adulterant. *Clin Pharm Ther* 88:408, 2010.
37. Vagi SJ, Sheikh S, Brackney M, et al: Passive multistate surveillance for neutropenia after use of cocaine or heroin possibly contaminated with levamisole. *Ann Emerg Med* 61:468, 2013.
38. Cunningham R, Walton MA, Weber JE, et al: One-Year medical outcomes and emergency department recidivism after emergency department observation for cocaine-associated chest pain. *Ann Emerg Med* 53:310, 2009.
39. Walsh KM, Chang AM, Perrone J, et al: Coronary computerized tomography angiography for rapid discharge of low risk patients with cocaine associated chest pain. *J Med Toxicol* 5:111, 2009.
40. Cleveland NJ, Dewitt CD, Heard K: Ziprasidone pretreatment attenuates the lethal effects of cocaine in a mouse model. *Acad Emerg Med* 12:385, 2005.
41. Lange RA, Cigarroa RG, Flores ED, et al: Potentiation of cocaine-induced coronary vasoconstriction by beta-adrenergic blockade. *Ann Intern Med* 112:897, 1990.
42. Baumann BM, Perrone J, Hornig SE, et al: Randomized controlled double blind placebo controlled trial of diazepam, nitroglycerin or both for treatment of patients with potential cocaine associated acute coronary syndromes. *Acad Emerg Med* 7:878, 2000.
43. Honderick T, Williams D, Seaberg D, et al: A prospective, randomized, controlled trial of benzodiazepines and nitroglycerine or nitroglycerine alone in the treatment of cocaine-associated acute coronary syndromes. *Am J Emerg Med* 21:39, 2003.
44. Chan GM, Sharma R, Price D, et al: Phentolamine therapy for cocaine-association acute coronary syndrome (CAACS). *J Med Toxicol* 2:108, 2006.
45. Negus BH, Willard JE, Hillis LD, et al: Alleviation of cocaine induced coronary vasoconstriction with intravenous verapamil. *Am J Cardiol* 73:510, 1994.
46. Albertson TE, Dawson A, de Latorre F, et al: TOX-ACLS: toxicologic-oriented advanced cardiac life support. *Ann Emerg Med* 37:S78, 2001.
47. Rangel C, Shu RG, Lazar LD, et al: Beta-blockers for chest pain associated with recent cocaine use. *Arch Int Med* 170:874, 2010.
48. Dattilo PB, Hailpern SM, Fearon K, et al: Beta-blockers are associated with reduced risk of myocardial infarction after cocaine use. *Ann Emerg Med* 51:117, 2008.
49. Hollander JE, Burstein JL, Shih RD, et al: Cocaine Associated Myocardial Infarction Study (CAMI) Group. Cocaine associated myocardial infarction: clinical safety of thrombolytic therapy. *Chest* 107:1237, 1995.
50. Gitter MJ, Goldsmith SR, Dunbar DN, et al: Cocaine and chest pain: clinical features and outcome of patients hospitalized to rule out myocardial infarction. *Ann Intern Med* 115:277, 1991.
51. Tomaszewski C, McKinney P, Phillips S, et al: Prevention of toxicity from oral cocaine by activated charcoal in mice. *Ann Emerg Med* 22:1804, 1993.

Chapter 111 ■ Corrosives Poisoning

ROBERT P. DOWSETT • KENNON HEARD

Initially referring to acids, the term *corrosives* is now used synonymously with *caustics*, a term originally applied to alkalis. In solution, acids and bases donate or accept a proton altering the hydrogen ion concentration. This is measured as pH, the negative logarithm of the H^+ ion concentration (mol/L). Water, at 25°C, has a pH of 7 and is considered neutral. Solutions with a pH of less than 2 or greater than 12 are considered strongly acidic or basic, respectively. The pH values of some common solutions are listed in Table 111.1.

Corrosives cause injury by reacting with organic molecules and disrupting cell membranes. They also cause thermal burns from the heat generated by dissolution and neutralization reactions. Reactions between strong acids and strong bases are usually highly exothermic. Metallic lithium, sodium, potassium, some aluminum and lithium salts, and titanium tetrachloride react violently when placed in water, producing large amounts of heat. Chlorine reacts with water in an exothermic reaction to form hydrochloric and hypochlorous acids, elemental chlorine, and free oxygen radicals. Similar reactions occur with bromine. Ammonia combines with water to form ammonium hydroxide in a reaction that liberates heat; the hydroxide formed is then responsible for the corrosive effects. Nitrogen dioxide reacts with water to release heat and produce nitric and nitrous acid. Hydrogen peroxide liberates oxygen on contact with water.

The mixing of chemicals can result in reactions that liberate caustic gases. Mixing ammonia with hypochlorite (household bleach) generates chloramine gases (NH_2Cl and $NHCl_2$), which are highly irritating to mucosal epithelia. Combining bleach with acid (acid toilet bowl or drain cleaners) produces chlorine gas. A number of metallic compounds react with acids, resulting in the liberation of potentially explosive hydrogen gas. The potential for unrecognized corrosives production can complicate the identification of the exposures, and diagnosis of caustic burn may need to be based on clinical presentation rather than on product identification.

During 2014, approximately 70,000 exposures to corrosive chemicals were reported to U.S. poison centers; actual exposures are estimated to be several times greater [1]. Although pediatic exposures are more common that adult exposures, adults often ingest larger amounts of corrosive [2]. Deaths most commonly result from intentional exposure to drain cleaners and acidic cleaners [1].

Concentrated lye (sodium or potassium hydroxide) solutions used for laundering and plumbing purposes caused most of the serious injuries due to corrosive ingestions before 1970 [2,3]. Currently available liquid lye drain cleaners are less concentrated (less than 10%) but are still responsible for the largest number of severe gastrointestinal injuries; however, acid bowl cleaners now account for almost as many deaths [1]. Severe alkali injuries can result from the ingestion of powdered automatic dishwasher detergents and oven cleaners [4]. Household ammonia and bleaches, and hydrogen peroxide solutions are, in general, much less potent than industrial ones but can cause significant injury if ingested in large amounts [4].

TABLE 111.1

Approximate pH of Common Solutions

Solution	pH
1.0 M hydrochloric acid	0
1 M hydrochloric acid solution	0
1 M nitric acid solution	0
0.1 M sulfuric acid	0.96
Battery acid (1% solution)	1.4
Gastric juice	1.2–3.0
Lemon juice	2
Domestic toilet cleaner (1%)	2.0
1 M acetic acid solution	2.37
1 M carbonic acid	5.7
Rain water	6.5
Water (pure, at 25°C)	7.0
Bleach (1% solution)	9.5–10.2
Automatic dishwasher detergents	10.4–13.0
Laundry detergents	11.6–12.6
Domestic ammonium cleaners	11.9–12.4
Ammonia 10%	12.5
Oven cleaner	13
Drain cleaner	13.3–14.0
1.0 M potassium hydroxide	14
1.0 M NaOH	14
Saturated ammonia solution	15

PATHOPHYSIOLOGY

Alkalis cause liquefaction necrosis, a process resulting from the saponification of fats, dissolution of proteins, and emulsification of lipid membranes. The resultant tissue softening and sloughing may allow the alkali to penetrate to deeper levels. Tissue injury progresses rapidly over the first few minutes but can continue for several hours [5]. Over the ensuing 4 days, bacterial infection and inflammation cause additional injury. Granulation tissue then develops, but collagen deposition may not begin until the second week. The tensile strength of healing tissue is lowest during the first 2 weeks. Epithelial repair may take weeks to months. Scar retraction begins in the 3rd week and continues for months.

Acid burns are characterized by coagulation necrosis. Protein is denatured, resulting in the formation of a firm eschar [6]. The release of heat is typically higher than for alkali reactions. Subsequent responses are similar to those seen with alkalis.

Hydrocarbons can produce injury by dissolving lipids in cell membranes and coagulating proteins. Significant damage may occur with ingestion or after prolonged dermal contact [7].

Alkaline solutions with a pH of greater than 12.5 are likely to cause mucosal ulceration, with deeper tissue necrosis resulting if the pH approaches 14 [8]. However, solutions with a pH of less than 12.5 can still cause significant injury, and solutions of different chemicals but the same pH produce different degrees of tissue damage [8].

The physical state of a chemical also influences its toxicity. Corrosives that are gases at room temperature primarily affect the skin, eyes, and airways. Saturated acid solutions may liberate significant amounts of acid fumes, particularly if heated. Solid compounds tend to produce highly concentrated solutions on contact with body fluids and cause more severe injuries [9]. Solutions with a high viscosity tend to cause deeper burns [8].

Most systemic effects that occur after exposure to corrosives are secondary to inflammation, acidosis, infection, and necrosis [10]. Fluid and electrolyte shifts occur, resulting in hypovolemia, acidosis, and organ failure. Some chemicals, such as phenol, hydrazine, and chromic acid, can be absorbed after dermal exposure or ingestion and cause systemic toxicity [11].

CLINICAL MANIFESTATIONS

Chemical burns to the eye range from irritation to severe and permanent damage [12]. Eye pain, blepharospasm, conjunctival hemorrhages, and chemosis are seen in all grades of injury. Decreased visual acuity may result from excessive tearing, corneal edema and ulceration, anterior chamber clouding, or lens opacities. Roper-Hall's classification of injury predicts severity of subsequent vision loss [13] (Table 111.2). Severe burns can result in increased intraocular pressure, anterior chamber clouding, lens opacities, and perforation of the globe [12]. Severity can be assessed by the extent of ischemia of conjunctival vessels at the limbus of the eye. If more than half of these vessels are obliterated, the prognosis is poor [13].

Significant differences exist between thermal and chemical burns of the skin. Although pain usually occurs immediately, it may be delayed several hours after corrosive exposure [14]. Assessing the depth of dermal injury can be difficult. Chemical burns rarely blister, and the affected skin is usually dark, insensate, and firmly attached regardless of the burn depth [15]. Healing usually takes longer than for thermal burns.

Some chemical warfare agents cause severe dermal injury. Sulfur mustard, the most commonly used antipersonnel agent, and lewisite (chlorovinylarsine dichloride) are potent alkylating agents, resulting in severe vesiculation of the skin 4 to 12 hours after exposure. Phosgene oxide has a similar action, but its effects are almost immediate. Respiratory burns are nearly always associated with sulfur mustard exposure [16]. White phosphorus is used in incendiary devices and in the manufacture of fertilizers and insecticides. It ignites spontaneously when exposed to air and can cause thermal burns.

Ingested corrosives typically injure the oropharynx, esophagus, and stomach but may cause damage as distal as the proximal jejunum [17,18]. Areas most commonly affected are those of anatomic narrowing: the cricopharyngeal area, diaphragmatic esophagus, and antrum and pylorus of the stomach [17]. Multiple sites are affected in up to 80% of patients [18]. Esophageal lesions are seen predominantly in the lower half, and gastric burns are usually most severe in the antrum [18]. Vomiting is associated with a higher incidence of severe esophageal injuries [19].

Ingestion of alkali is associated with a higher incidence and severity of esophageal lesions than ingestion of acid, which typically causes stomach injury although this is not a consistent finding [2,19]. Alkaline agents have little taste, but acids are extremely bitter and more likely to be expelled if accidentally ingested.

Alkaline solids may adhere to mucosa of the oropharynx and cause oral pain that limits the quantity swallowed, thus sparing the esophagus [20]. If alkaline solids are swallowed, severe upper esophageal burns are seen [21]. Shallow ulcers may result when tablets become lodged in the esophagus (pill esophagitis). Hemorrhage and stricture formation may occur after esophageal impaction of potassium chloride, iron, quinidine, etidronate, antibiotics, and anti-inflammatory agents [22].

Common symptoms from corrosive ingestion are oropharyngeal pain, dysphagia, abdominal pain, vomiting, and drooling [23]. Less commonly, stridor, hoarseness, hematemesis, and melena are seen. Patients who are asymptomatic are unlikely to have significant injuries, although this may be difficult to assess for children who may appear to have no or minimal symptoms [23]. Vomiting, drooling, and stridor appear to be predictive of more severe injuries [23], but the absence of burns in the oropharynx does not exclude burns further along the gastrointestinal tract, and it is not predictive of less severe distal injuries [23]. Patients with laryngeal burns have a greater incidence and severity of esophageal lesions [19].

Hemorrhage, perforation, and fistula formation may occur for patients with full-thickness esophageal necrosis [18]. Untreated, perforations rapidly progress to septic shock, organ failure, and death. Gastric perforations may become walled to form abscesses around the liver or in the lesser sac. Severe gastric burns may extend to adjacent organs [24]. Perforation of the anterior esophageal wall may lead to formation of a tracheoesophageal fistula and tracheobronchial necrosis [25]. Tracheoesophageal–aortic and aortoesophageal fistulas, rare and uniformly fatal complications, are suggested by hemoptysis or hematemesis, which develops into torrential bleeding.

Burns to the larynx occur in up to 50% of patients and are the most common cause of respiratory distress [19]. Typically, the epiglottis and aryepiglottic folds are edematous, ulcerated, or necrotic. The absence of respiratory symptoms on presentation does not exclude the presence of laryngeal burns that may eventually require intubation [19]. Respiratory distress may also be caused by the aspiration of corrosives [26].

Esophageal strictures develop in up to 70% of burns that result in deep ulceration, whether discrete or circumferential, and nearly all burns resulting in deep necrosis [18]. Strictures do not develop after superficial mucosal ulceration [26]. Strictures may become symptomatic as early as the end of the 2nd week; half develop during initial hospitalization, and 80% are evident within 2 months [27]. Those that develop early often progress rapidly and require urgent intervention. Gastric outlet strictures may also occur, but only 40% become symptomatic [18]. Strictures can develop in the mouth and pharynx [19]. Esophageal pseudodiverticulum may occur in patients with esophageal stricture as early as 1 week after corrosive ingestions. It appears to result from incomplete destruction of the esophageal wall and usually resolves with dilation of associated strictures [28].

Deaths that occur are in patients who have extensive necrosis in the upper gastrointestinal tract. Sepsis secondary to perforation is the most common cause of death; severe hemorrhage or aspiration may also contribute [18].

TABLE 111.2

Grading of Severity of Ocular Chemical Burns

Grade	Cornea	Limbal ischemia	Prognosis
I	Epithelial loss	None	Good
II	Stromal haze, iris details visible	<⅓ of vessels affected	Good
III	Total epithelial loss, iris details obscured	⅓–½ of vessels affected	Doubtful, vision reduced
IV	Opaque, no view of iris or pupil	>½ of vessels affected	Poor

Esophageal carcinoma, usually squamous cell, is a well-documented complication of alkali burns [29]. It occurs most commonly at the level of the tracheal bifurcation and is estimated to occur 1,000 times more frequently in patients who have had corrosive injuries than in the general population. Symptoms can develop more than 20 years after the initial insult.

Systemic toxicity has occurred with burns caused by arsenic and other heavy metals, cyanide, acetic acid, formic acid, fluoride, hydrazine, hydrochloric acid, nitrates, sulfuric acid, and phosphoric acid [11,30–34]. Severe acid burns may be accompanied by a metabolic acidosis and hypotension. The anion gap is usually elevated, although a hyperchloremic acidosis may be seen in hydrochloric acid and ammonium chloride ingestion. After hydrochloric acid ingestion, cardiovascular collapse is the most common cause of early death; myocardial infarction has occurred after large ingestions. Other findings associated with severe acid injuries include hemolysis, hemoglobinuria, nephrotoxicity, and pulmonary edema [31,32]. Vascular oxygen embolization can occur after the ingestion of concentrated hydrogen peroxide [35].

DIAGNOSTIC EVALUATION

Resuscitation and decontamination should take priority over completing a detailed history and physical examination. Medical staff should wear protective clothing to avoid becoming secondary casualties. The duration of exposure, symptoms, and details of prehospital treatment should be noted. Identification of the compounds involved and any measures required for their safe handling can be established by a number of means: Container labeling, material safety data sheets and safety officers in cases of workplace exposure, fire department hazardous materials units, and regional poison information centers. Measuring the pH of a product may be helpful.

If the exposure is the result of an industrial or transportation accident, the patient should be evaluated for traumatic injuries. Suicidal patients should be evaluated for other possible toxic exposures (e.g., ingestion of alcohol or medications).

After decontamination, assessment of eye exposures should include measurement of visual acuity and conjunctival pH and a slit-lamp examination. Chemosis, conjunctival hemorrhages, corneal epithelial defects, stromal opacification, and loss of limbic vessels should be noted. If injury to the anterior chamber is suspected, intraocular pressure should be measured.

Assessment of dermal injury is similar to that for thermal burns. Location, size, color, texture, and neurovascular status should be noted. If the affected area is greater than 15% of total body surface area or if systemic toxicity is possible, a complete physical examination with appropriate monitoring and laboratory testing should be performed.

With ingestions, the ability to swallow secretions and findings on examination of the oropharynx, neck, chest, and abdomen should be noted. Particular attention should be given to assessing the patency of the airway. Patients with signs and symptoms suggestive of significant injuries should have an electrocardiogram, arterial blood gas analysis, complete blood cell count, type and cross-match, coagulation profile, and biochemistry testing, including electrolytes, glucose, and liver and renal function testing. Radiologic studies should include a chest radiograph and an upright abdominal film. Upper gastrointestinal endoscopy should be performed in symptomatic patients or those with visible burns in the mouth or throat. Although the absence of symptoms or signs does not preclude the presence of gastrointestinal burns, in patients with accidental ingestions, such injuries are always of a minor nature and endoscopy is not necessary [17]. Minor symptoms or grade I visible burns following the accidental ingestion of substances shown to have low toxicity, such as sodium hypochlorite household bleach (less than 10% solution) and hair relaxer gel, do not necessarily require endoscopy, as significant injuries are rare in this setting [36]. However, endoscopy is still recommended if excessive drooling or dysphagia or significant mucosal burns occur after ingestion of these products or if there is doubt about the exact composition of the ingested substance [36]. In contrast, in those with ingestions of strong acids or bases, significant injuries may be present in the absence of clinical findings, and endoscopy is indicated. The optimal timing of endoscopy appears to be 6 to 24 hours after exposure. Because injuries may progress over several hours, endoscopy performed earlier may not detect the full extent of injury and therefore may need to be repeated. If performed later, the risk of perforation is increased.

In the past, it was recommended that the endoscope not be passed beyond the first circumferential or full-thickness lesion because of the risk of iatrogenic perforation. This complication was a significant problem in the days when rigid endoscopes were used. It is extremely rare with flexible endoscopy. Not examining beyond the first significant lesion results in failure to detect more distal lesions of the stomach or duodenum [37]. Flexible endoscopy, preferably using a small-diameter (e.g., pediatric) endoscope, of the entire upper gastrointestinal tract is safe and usually well tolerated [18]. The endoscope should be advanced across the cricopharynx under direct vision to assess for the presence of laryngeal burns [18]. If laryngeal edema or ulceration is noted, the airway should be intubated before endoscopy is continued. Examination should be done gently with minimal air insufflation, avoiding retroversion or retroflexion, and the procedure terminated if the endoscope cannot be easily passed through a narrowed area. Therapeutic dilation of the esophagus on initial endoscopy carries a high risk of perforation and should be avoided [17]. It should also be avoided during the subacute phase (5 to 15 days after ingestion), when the tensile strength of tissues is lowest [18].

A variety of systems for grading gastrointestinal burns have been proposed [17,18]. Some parallel grading systems used for thermal skin burns; others differentiate several levels of ulceration and necrosis (Table 111.3). The important findings are depth of ulceration and presence of necrosis. Injuries that consist only of mucosal inflammation or superficial ulceration and do not involve the muscularis are not at risk for stricture formation [18]. Patients with full-thickness circumferential burns and extensive necrosis are at high risk for perforation and stricture formation. Deep ulceration, whether transmural or not, and discrete areas of necrosis can sometimes lead to stricture formation.

TABLE 111.3

Examples of Classifications for Grading Severity of Gastrointestinal Corrosive Injury

Grade I	Mucosal inflammation
Grade II	A. Hemorrhages, erosions, and superficial ulceration
	B. Deep discrete or circumferential ulceration
Grade III	A. Small, scattered areas of necrosis
	B. Extensive necrosis involving the whole esophagus
First degree	Mucosal inflammation, edema, or superficial sloughing
Second degree	Damage extends to all layers of, but not through, the esophagus
Third degree	Ulceration through to periesophageal tissues

Contrast esophagography is less sensitive than endoscopy in visualizing ulceration but it has a role in the detection of suspected perforation [38]. A water-soluble contrast agent should be used. Cineesophagography can detect esophageal motility disorders, the pattern of which may predict the likelihood of stricture formation. Strictures can be expected to develop in all patients with an atonic dilated or rigid esophagus and in some individuals with abnormal, uncoordinated contractions [39]. Endoscopic ultrasonography can accurately grade corrosive injuries and predict complications [40]. Computed tomography may have a role in the evaluation of caustic injury, but current evidence suggests endoscopy is preferred [41]. Esophageal motility studies may predict the risk of stricture formation in those patients with no peristaltic response; these motility abnormalities persist for at least 3 months [42].

Evaluation of patients with symptoms and signs of systemic toxicity should include routine monitoring and ancillary testing. The extent and type of testing depend on the nature and severity of clinical abnormalities and the chemical involved. Patients with significant exposure to some phenols (e.g., nitrophenol and pentachlorophenol) and to hydrazine should have methemoglobin level determination.

MANAGEMENT

Advanced life support measures should be instituted as appropriate. Decontamination is the next priority; procedures are specific to the route of exposure. Treatment of systemic poisoning is primarily supportive; in some cases, antidotal therapy may also be necessary.

Irrigation should be performed immediately for eye exposures. The persistence of eye pain despite irrigation for at least 15 minutes indicates significant injury or incomplete decontamination. Failure to irrigate the eye adequately or remove particles after chemical exposure is associated with chronic complications [43]. Up to one-third of patients with lime burns still have particles present in the eye on presentation [43]. All cases in which injury is detected or symptoms persist require ophthalmologic evaluation. Management may consist of topical antibiotics, mydriatics, steroids, and eye patching. The role of neutralization of chemical burns is currently under investigation. Ascorbic acid had been used to treat alkali burns, but its effectiveness has not been well studied, and it cannot be recommended [12].

The initial treatment of dermal exposure is prompt irrigation with copious amounts of water for at least 15 minutes for acid exposures and 30 minutes for alkali. Longer irrigation is recommended for alkalis because they have detergent properties [13]. Although tissue neutralization occurs within 10 minutes with acids and within 1 hour with alkalis in experimental studies, delayed irrigation may be beneficial [44]. Clothes act as a reservoir, and failure to remove them may result in full-thickness burns developing from even mildly corrosive chemicals. Neutralization has been associated with good outcomes [45], but because systematic data on its efficacy are lacking, such therapy cannot be recommended.

In rare cases, water irrigation may be dangerous or ineffective. Metallic lithium, sodium, potassium and cesium, titanium tetrachloride, and organic salts of lithium and aluminum react violently with water; burns caused by these agents should be inspected closely and any particles removed and placed in an anhydrous solution (oil) before the area is irrigated. Alternatively, the area can be wiped with a dry cloth to remove particles and the skin then deluged with water to dissipate any heat. Phenol is not water soluble, and dilution with water may aid its penetration into tissues, increasing systemic absorption [22]. Soaking experimental phenol burns with isopropyl alcohol or polyethylene glycol in mineral oil is superior to rinsing with water [46]. Isopropyl alcohol and polyethylene glycol may be absorbed by burns, and their use should be followed by liberal washing with water. A report describes removing ready-mixed concrete from skin by soaking or irrigating with 50% dextrose in water [47].

Application of a copper sulfate solution has been suggested to assist in identification and neutralization of white phosphorus particles on the skin, but systemic absorption of copper sulfate can result in massive hemolysis with acute renal failure and death [48]. The use of a Wood's lamp to detect fluorescent phosphorus particles is safer. White phosphorous burns should be kept wet because phosphorus ignites in dry air. Because sulfur mustard is poorly water soluble, a mild detergent should be used for its removal. Military decontamination kits contain chloramine wipes, which inactivate sulfur mustard [49]. British antilewisite, or dimercaprol, is an effective chelator of lewisite and can be applied topically to the skin or eye [16].

Patients with second- or third-degree skin burns should be referred to a surgeon. Definitive management is the same as for thermal burns, although more aggressive use of early débridement and grafting has been suggested [15].

Despite the rapidity of tissue injury following ingestion, decontamination should be considered. Rinsing with water or saline is recommended for mouth exposures. Dilution by drinking up to 250 mL (120 mL for a child) water or milk is recommended for particulate ingestion, because the corrosive may adhere to the esophageal wall. Although this procedure exposes the stomach to the corrosive agent, it further dilutes the substance. Because the efficacy of dilution is greatest if performed within 5 minutes of exposure and declines rapidly thereafter, it is reasonable to use any drinkable beverage, except carbonated ones, if water or milk is not immediately available. The role of dilution for liquid ingestion is less clear, but it is usually recommended. It may, however, promote emesis and may not be effective in limiting tissue damage unless undertaken within minutes of injury. Emesis is contraindicated because of the risk of aspiration and its association with an increased severity of esophageal and laryngeal burns [19].

The administration of weak acids or bases can neutralize, as well as dilute, ingested corrosives [37]. Although weak acids are more effective than milk or water in neutralizing the pH, neutralization, which is accompanied by the production of heat, could lead to thermal injury in addition to corrosive effects. The heat generated by in vitro neutralization is small (less than 3°C) for liquid alkali but may be greater for solid forms [37]. The benefit of such therapy is unknown and not recommended.

Using a nasogastric tube for gastric aspiration, dilution, or lavage is another subject of debate [6]. Esophageal perforation is a potential complication, but no cases of nasogastric tube perforation have been reported. Placement of a gastric tube with fluoroscopic or endoscopic guidance has been suggested, but the blind, gentle introduction of a small-bore tube in a cooperative patient, particularly for a large acid ingestion, also appears to be safe [17]. If inserted, the tube should be firmly taped in place to avoid motion. Gastric contents should be aspirated. Dilution or lavage with small aliquots (120 to 250 mL) of water can then be performed.

Activated charcoal does not adsorb inorganic acids or alkali. In addition, because it interferes with endoscopic evaluation, unless a corrosive has a significant systemic toxicity and is known to be bound by activated charcoal, this agent should be avoided. Symptomatic patients should otherwise be given nothing by mouth before endoscopy.

Corticosteroids have been used to reduce the incidence and severity of esophageal strictures after alkali burns. Such therapy is based on studies showing a decrease in stricture formation in animals pretreated with steroids [50]. Because strictures do not develop in patients with first-degree esophageal burns, steroids are not indicated in those with such findings [51]. Similarly, steroids do not appear to influence the development of esophageal strictures after extensive deep ulceration or necrosis [51], and hence they are not recommended in patients with these injuries. Studies on the efficacy of steroids in patients with injuries of moderate severity have yielded conflicting results. Most have been retrospective and poorly controlled. There have been four prospective controlled studies comparing steroids to placebo for prevention of strictures. Two studies suggest no effect of steroids [52,53]. An older small study suggested a small decrease in the percentage of patients who will develop esophageal strictures [54]. A recent well-designed study found a 20% decrease in strictures and a decrease in the need for parenteral nutrition with high-dose methylprednisilone (1 g/1.73 m^2 IV per day for 3 days) in addition to ranitidine, ceftriaxone, and total parenteral nutrition [54]. One comparative study suggested a 30% absolute risk reduction in risk of stricture with dexamethasone (1 mg per kg per day) compared with prednisolone (2 mg per kg per day) [55]. A survey of emergency surgeons found that approximately half use steroids [56]. Overall, the data are inconclusive, and no definitive recommendations on the effectiveness of steroids can be provided.

If steroids are to be administered, it appears that patients with grade 2b esophageal injury (submucosal burns, ulcerations, and exudates that are circumferential) are the most likely to benefit [54]. Although prior recommendations suggested that therapy should be continued for at least 10 days [51], the most recent study suggests that 3 days of high-dose methlyprednisilone is effective.

The decision to administer steroids should be based on endoscopic evaluation. Patients with no injury or mucosal inflammation or small areas of superficial ulceration are not at risk for strictures or perforation and require supportive therapy only. Symptomatic relief can be provided with antacids, sucralfate, histamine-2–blockers (H_2-blockers), or analgesics. Patients with persistent symptoms or inconclusive findings on endoscopy should be admitted for observation. If symptoms persist, endoscopy should be repeated. Patients can commence oral fluids when they are able to swallow their own secretions. They can be discharged when tolerating oral fluids.

Prophylactic antibiotics have also been advocated for patients with significant gastrointestinal injuries. Their benefits have not been studied in humans, and opinions differ as to their value. Controlled animal experiments have shown a combination of steroids and antibiotics to give the best outcome with respect to stricture formation and mortality [57] and suggest that a broad-spectrum antibiotic (e.g., a second-generation cephalosporin) should be administered, particularly in those treated with steroids.

Patients with deep discrete ulcerations, circumferential or extensive superficial ulcerations, or small isolated areas of necrosis who are at risk for stricture formation should be given nothing by mouth. Fluids, analgesics, and H_2-blockers should be administered parenterally. Intravenous steroids and antibiotics should also be considered for those with alkali burns. Patients with deep transmural ulceration or necrosis are at risk for perforation as well as stricture formation. Although the use of steroids for this group is potentially hazardous and not recommended, antibiotics should be given along with other supportive measures. Nutritional support, either parenteral or by jejunostomy feeding tube, may be required.

Surgical exploration is indicated if perforation or penetration into surrounding tissues is suspected by findings such as fever, progressive abdominal or chest pain, hypotension, or signs of peritonitis or proved by endoscopic or radiographic findings. Tracheoesophageal fistulas are usually fatal unless recognized early and repaired, although one case reported successful conservative treatment [35]. Laparotomy and early excision have been suggested for patients with extensive full-thickness necrosis, but an advantage of this approach over more conservative treatment is not clear [58]. The mortality for patients who have major emergency surgery is 9% to 66% [58,59].

Stricture formation is usually treated with endoscopic dilatation beginning 3 to 4 weeks after ingestion. An average of eight sessions is required, and recurrence is common in the first 12 months [60]. In a group of 195 patients with corrosive-induced esophageal strictures, the risk of perforation for each dilatation session was 1.3%, but, because of the requirement for multiple dilations, the risk per patient was 17% [60]. Perforations were most likely to occur during the first three dilations. Features of perforation include dyspnea, malaise, tachycardia, fever, and subcutaneous crepitations. The majority are detected during the procedure or by the presence of pneumomediastinum, or pneumothorax or hydrothorax on chest radiograph, but occasionally contrast esophagography or esophagoscopy is required for confirmation. The death rate from perforation is 16% to 23% [60]. Early or prophylactic bougienage is of unclear benefit and has been associated with an increased risk of perforation. One study has shown a decrease in the number of dilatations required following interlesional steroid injection [61].

Placement of specialized nasogastric tubes or stents has lowered the rate of stricture formation in uncontrolled clinical trials and is superior to steroids in animal experiments [62]. An additional benefit of combining the use of a stent with systemic steroids has been suggested [62]. Sucrafate, H_2 histamine antagonists, and proton pump inhibitors are of unproven value.

If the patient has severe injury or perforation, surgical management may be required. Occasionally, resection and end-to-end anastomosis are possible, but usually extensive reconstruction, with colonic interposition, is necessary. The overall mortality from colonic replacement surgery is approximately 3% and commonly results from sepsis secondary to anastomosis leakage or colonic graft necrosis [63]. Gastrectomy or gastrojejunostomy may also be required if gastric outlet obstruction develops [64]. Early definitive surgery for gastric outlet obstruction appears to be more advantageous than staged surgery [65]. Endoscopic balloon dilation may be an acceptable alternative procedure [66]. Diode laser-assisted radiolysis using a rigid endoscope has also been used to treat strictures successfully [67].

Supportive management is the mainstay of treatment for systemic toxicity. Heavy metal, cyanide, and hydrogen sulfide poisoning may require antidotal therapy (see Chapter 125). Neurologic toxicity due to hydrazine may respond to intravenous pyridoxine, administered at an initial dose of 25 mg per kg repeated in several hours, if necessary [54] (see Chapter 125). Methemoglobinemia may require treatment with methylene blue (see Chapter 125).

References

1. Mowry JB, Spyker DA, Brooks DE, et al: 2014 Annual Report of the American Association of Poison Control Centers' National Poison Data System (NPDS): 32nd annual report. *Clin Toxicol (Philadelphia)* 53:962–1147, 2015.
2. Arevalo-Silva C, Eliashar R Wohlgelernter J, et al: Ingestion of caustic substances: a 15-year experience. *Laryngoscope* 116:1422–1426, 2006.
3. Leape LL, Ashcraft AW, Scarpelli DG, et al: Hazard to health: liquid lye. *N Engl J Med* 284:578–581, 1971.
4. Dogan Y, Erkan T, Çokugras FC, et al: Caustic gastroesophageal lesions in childhood: an analysis of 473 cases. *Clin Pediatr (Philadelphia)* 45:435–438, 2006.
5. Kirsh MM, Ritter F: Caustic ingestion and subsequent damage to the oropharyngeal and digestive passages. *Ann Thorac Surg* 21:74–82, 1976.
6. Ashcraft KW, Padula RT: The effect of dilute corrosives on the esophagus. *Pediatrics* 53:226–232, 1974.
7. Papini RP: Is all that's blistered burned? A case of kerosene contact burns. *Burns* 17:415–416, 1991.
8. Vancura EM, Clinton JE, Ruiz E, et al: Toxicity of alkaline solutions. *Ann Emerg Med* 9:118–122, 1980.
9. Crain EF, Gershel JC, Mezey AP: Caustic ingestions: symptoms as predictors of esophageal injury. *Am J Dis Child* 138:863–865, 1984.
10. Okonek S, Bierbach H, Atzpodien W: Unexpected metabolic acidosis in severe lye poisoning. *Clin Toxicol* 18:225–230, 1981.
11. Mozingo DW, Smith AA, McManus WF, et al: Chemical burns. *J Trauma-Injury Infect Crit Care* 28:642, 1988.
12. Beare JD: Eye injuries from assault with chemicals. *Br J Ophthalmol* 74:514–518, 1990.
13. Roper-Hall MJ: Thermal and chemical burns. *Trans Ophthalmol Soc U K* 85:631–653, 1965.

14. Wilson GR, Davidson PM: Full thickness burns from ready-mixed cement. *Burns Incl Therm Inj* 12:139–145, 1985.
15. Sawhney CP, Kaushish R: Acid and alkali burns: considerations in management. *Burns* 15:132–134, 1989.
16. Mellor SG, Rice P, Cooper GJ: Vesicant burns. *Br J Plast Surg* 44:434–437, 1991.
17. Sugawa C, Lucas CE: Caustic injury of the upper gastrointestinal tract in adults: a clinical and endoscopic study. *Surgery* 106:802–806, 1989.
18. Zargar SA, Kochhar R, Mehta S, et al: The role of fiberoptic endoscopy in the management of corrosive ingestion and modified endoscopic classification of burns. *Gastrointest Endosc* 37:165–169, 1991.
19. Vergauwen P, Moulin D, Buts JP, et al: Caustic burns of the upper digestive and respiratory tracts. *Eur J Pediatr* 150:700–703, 1991.
20. Madarikan BA, Lari J: Ingestion of dishwasher detergent by children. *Br J Clin Pract* 44:35–36, 1990.
21. Einhorn A, Horton L, Altieri M, et al: Serious respiratory consequences of detergent ingestions in children. *Pediatrics* 84:472–474, 1989.
22. Bott S, Prakash C, McCallum RW: Medication induced esophageal injury: survey of the literature. *Am J Gastroenterol* 82:758–763, 1987.
23. Gorman RL, Khin-Maung-Gyi MT, Klein-Schwartz W, et al: Initial symptoms as predictors of esophageal injury in alkaline corrosive ingestions. *Am J Emerg Med* 10:189–194, 1992.
24. Zargar SA, Kochhar R, Nagi B, et al: Ingestion of strong corrosive alkalis: spectrum of injury to upper gastrointestinal tract and natural history. *Am J Gastroenterol* 87:337, 1992.
25. Restrepo S, Mastrogiovanni L, Kaplan J, et al: Tracheoesophageal fistula caused by ingestion of a caustic substance. *Ear Nose Throat J* 82:349–350, 2003.
26. Cheng HT, Cheng CL, Lin CH, et al: Caustic ingestion in adults: the role of endoscopic classification in predicting outcome. *BMC Gastroenterol* 8:31, 2008.
27. Kikendall JW: Caustic ingestion injuries. *Gastroenterol Clin North Am* 20:847–857, 1991.
28. Kochhar R, Mehta SK, Nagi B, et al: Corrosive acid-induced esophageal intramural pseudodiverticulosis: a study of 14 patients. *J Clin Gastroenterol* 13:371–375, 1991.
29. Appelqvist P, Salmo M: Lye corrosion carcinoma of the esophagus: a review of 63 cases. *Cancer* 15:2655–2658, 1980.
30. Caravati EM: Metabolic abnormalities associated with phosphoric acid ingestion. *Ann Emerg Med* 16:904–906, 1987.
31. Greif F, Kaplan O: Acid ingestion: another cause of disseminated intravascular coagulation. *Crit Care Med* 14:990–991, 1986.
32. Jefferys DB, Wiseman HM: Formic acid poisoning. *Postgrad Med* 56:761–762, 1980.
33. Harati Y, Naikan E: Hydrazine toxicity, pyridoxine therapy, and peripheral neuropathy. *Ann Intern Med* 104:728–729, 1986.
34. Wang XW, Davies JWL, Sirvent RLZ, et al: Chromic acid burns and acute chromium poisonings. *Burns Incl Therm Inj* 11:181–184, 1985.
35. Pritchett S, Green D, Rossos P: Accidental ingestion of 35% hydrogen peroxide. *Can J Gastroenterol* 21:665–667, 2007.
36. Harley EH, Collins MD: Liquid household bleach ingestion in children: a retrospective review. *Laryngoscope* 107:122–125, 1997.
37. Homan CS, Singer AJ, Thomajan C, et al: Thermal characteristics of neutralization therapy and water dilution for strong acid ingestion: an in-vivo canine model. *Acad Emerg Med* 5:286–292, 1998.
38. Muhletaler CA, Gerlock AJ, de Soto L, et al: Acid corrosive esophagitis: radiographic findings. *Am J Roentgenol* 134:1137–1140, 1980.
39. Kuhn JR, Tunell WP: The role of initial cine-esophagography in caustic esophageal injury. *Am J Surg* 146:804–806, 1983.
40. Chiu HM, Lin JT, Huang SP, et al: Prediction of bleeding and stricture formation after corrosive ingestion by EUS concurrent with upper endoscopy. *Gastrointest Endosc* 60:827–833, 2004.
41. Bonnici KS, Wood DM, Dargan PI: Should computerised tomography replace endoscopy in the evaluation of symptomatic ingestion of corrosive substances? *Clin Toxicol (Phila)* 52:911–925, 2014.
42. Genc A, Mutaf O: Esophageal motility changes in acute and late periods of caustic esophageal burns and their relation to prognosis in children. *J Pediatr Surg Surg* 37:1526–1528, 2002.
43. Rozenbaum D, Baruchin AM, Dafna Z: Chemical burns of the eye with special reference to alkali burns. *Burns* 17:136–140, 1991.
44. Yano K, Hata Y, Matsuka K, et al: Experimental study on alkaline skin injuries: periodic changes in subcutaneous tissue pH and the effects exerted by washing. *Burns* 19:320–323, 1993.
45. Woodard D: Irrigation with acetic acid [letter]. *Ann Emerg Med* 18:911, 1989.
46. Hunter DM, Timerding BL, Leonard RB, et al: Effects of isopropyl alcohol, ethanol, and polyethylene glycol/industrial methylated spirits in the treatment of acute phenol burns. *Ann Emerg Med* 21:1303–1307, 1992.
47. Cuomo MD, Sobel RM: Concrete impaction of the external auditory canal. *Am J Emerg Med* 7:32–33, 1989.
48. Eldad A, Simon GA: The phosphorous burn: a preliminary comparative experimental study of various forms of treatment. *Burns* 17:198–200, 1991.
49. Borak J, Sidell FR: Agents of chemical warfare: sulfur mustard. *Ann Emerg Med* 21:303–308, 1992.
50. McNeil RA, Wellborn RB: Prevention of corrosive stricture of the esophagus of the rat. *J Laryngol* 80:346–358, 1966.
51. Fulton JA, Hoffman RS: Steroids in second degree caustic burns of the esophagus: a systematic pooled analysis of fifty years of human data: 1956–2006. *Clin Toxicol* 45:402–408, 2007.
52. Anderson KD, Rouse TM, Randolph JG: A controlled trial of corticosteroids in children with corrosive injury of the esophagus. *N Engl J Med* 323:637–640, 1990.
53. Dogan Y, Gulcan M, Urganci N, et al: The effect of steroid therapy on severe corrosive oesophageal burns in children; a multicentric prospective study [abstract]. *J Pediatr Gastroenterol Nutr* 40:656, 2005.
54. Hawkins DB, Demeter MJ, Barness TE: Caustic ingestions: controversies in management: a review of 214 cases. *Laryngoscope* 90:98–109, 1980.
55. Bautista A, Varela R, Villanueva A, et al: Effects of prednisolone and dexamethasone in children with alkali burns of the oesophagus. *Eur J Pediatr Surg* 6:198–203, 1996.
56. Kluger Y, Ishay OB, Sartelli M, et al: Caustic ingestion management: world society of emergency surgery preliminary survey of expert opinion. *World J Emerg Surg* 10:48, 2015.
57. Haller JR, Bachman K: The comparative effect of current therapy on caustic burns of the esophagus. *Pediatrics* 34:236–245, 1964.
58. Berthet B, Castellani P, Brioche MI, et al: Early operation for severe corrosive injury of the upper gastrointestinal tract. *Eur J Surg* 162:951–955, 1996.
59. Wu MH, Lai WW: Surgical management of extensive corrosive injuries of the alimentary tract. *Surg Gynecol Obstet* 177:12–16, 1993.
60. Karnak I, Tanyel FC, Buyukpamukcu N, et al: Esophageal perforations encountered during the dilation of caustic esophageal strictures. *J Cardiovasc Surg* 39:373–377, 1998.
61. Kochhar R, Makharia GK: Usefulness of intralesional triamcinolone in treatment of benign esophageal strictures. *Gastrointest Endosc* 56:829–834, 2002.
62. De Peppo F, Zaccara A, Dall'Oglio L, et al: Stenting for caustic strictures: esophageal replacement replaced. *J Pediatr Surg* 33:54–57, 1998.
63. Mutaf O, Ozok G, Avanoglu A: Oesophagoplasty in the treatment of caustic oesophageal strictures in children. *Br J Surg* 82:644–646, 1995.
64. Chaudhary A, Puri AS, Dhar P, et al: Elective surgery for corrosive-induced gastric injury. *World J Surg* 20:703–706, 1996.
65. Hwang TL, Chen MF: Surgical treatment of gastric outlet obstruction after corrosive injury—can definitive surgery be used instead of staged operation? *Int Surg* 81:119–121, 1996.
66. Kochhar R, Sethy PK, Nagi B, et al: Endoscopic balloon dilatation of benign gastric outlet obstruction. *J Gastroenterol Hepatol* 19:418–422, 2004.
67. Saetti R, Silvestrini M, Cutrone C, et al: Endoscopic treatment of upper airway and digestive tract lesions caused by caustic agents. *Ann Otol Rhinol Laryngol* 112:29–36, 2003.

Chapter 112 ■ Heavy Metal Poisoning

LUKE YIP

This chapter focuses on the aspects of acute poisoning by arsenic, lead, and mercury that are potentially life threatening or may lead to permanent organ damage and hence require immediate, usually intensive, medical care. Reviews of the evaluation and management of asymptomatic exposures and nonacute poisoning can be found elsewhere.

ARSENIC

Exposure to arsenic may come from natural sources, industrial processes, commercial products, food, or intentionally administered sources either with a benevolent (acute promyelocytic leukemia [APL] treatment, folk, or naturopathic remedies) or malevolent intent. Today, acute arsenic poisoning is most commonly the result of an accidental ingestion or the result of suicidal or homicidal intent.

Pharmacology

Arsenic compounds can be classified into three major groups: inorganic, organic, and arsine gas (AsH_3). The latter is discussed separately. Arsenic compounds can also be classified by their valence state. The three most common valence states are the metalloid (elemental [0] oxidation state), arsenite (trivalent [+3] state), and arsenate (pentavalent [+5] state). In general, the arsenic compounds can be arranged in order of decreasing toxicity: inorganic trivalent compounds, organic trivalent compounds, inorganic pentavalent compounds, organic pentavalent compounds, and elemental arsenic. Trivalent arsenic is generally two- to tenfold more toxic than pentavalent arsenic. The minimum oral lethal human dose of arsenic trioxide (trivalent) is probably between 10 and 300 mg. Some marine organisms and algae contain large amounts of organic arsenic in the form of arsenobetaine, a trimethylated arsenic compound, and arsenocholine. Arsenobetaine and arsenocholine are excreted unchanged in the urine, with total clearance in about 2 days, and exert no known toxic effects in humans.

The major routes of entry into the human body are ingestion and inhalation. Soluble forms of ingested arsenic are 60% to 90% absorbed from the gastrointestinal (GI) tract. The amount of arsenic absorbed by inhalation is also thought to be in this range. Toxic systemic effects have been reported from rare occupational accidents in which arsenic trichloride or arsenic acid was splashed on worker's skin.

After absorption, arsenic is bound to proteins in the blood and redistributed to the liver, spleen, kidneys, lungs, and GI tract within 24 hours. Clearance from these tissues is dose dependent. Two to 4 weeks after exposure ceases, most of the arsenic remaining in the body is found in keratin-rich tissues (e.g., skin, hair, nails).

Both forms of arsenic, arsenite and arsenate, undergo biomethylation in the liver to monomethylarsonic acid (MMA) and dimethylarsinic acid (DMA). The methylation process may represent detoxification because the metabolites exert less acute toxicity in experimental lethality studies. The liver's efficiency for methylation decreases with increasing arsenic dose. When the methylating capacity of the liver is exceeded, exposure to excess concentrations of inorganic arsenic results in increased retention of arsenic in soft tissues.

Arsenic is eliminated from the body primarily by renal excretion. Urinary arsenic excretion begins promptly after absorption, and depending on the amount of arsenic ingested, urinary arsenic excretion may remain elevated for 1 to 2 months. After acute intoxication by inorganic arsenic, arsenic is excreted in the urine as inorganic arsenic, MMA and DMA, but their proportion varies with time [1]. During the first 2 to 4 days after the intoxication, arsenic is mainly excreted in the inorganic form. This is followed by a progressive increase of the proportion excreted as MMA and DMA, reaching about 50% of the total arsenic excreted after 4 days and 90% between 6 and 9 days; mainly in the form of DMA. Pentavalent arsenic is cleared more rapidly than trivalent arsenic. Because arsenic is quickly cleared from the blood, blood concentrations may be normal, although urine concentrations remain markedly elevated. Renal dysfunction may be a major impediment to normal elimination of arsenic compounds.

Inorganic arsenic can cross the human placenta. This was evident by the high arsenic concentrations found in a neonate following acute maternal arsenic intoxication.

There are two major mechanisms by which arsenic compounds appear to produce injury involving multiorgan systems. It is believed that arsenic's overt toxicity is related to its reversible binding with sulfhydryl enzymes, leading to the inhibition of critical sulfhydryl-containing enzyme systems. Trivalent arsenite is particularly potent in this regard. The pyruvate and succinate oxidation pathways are particularly sensitive to arsenic inhibition. Dihydrolipoate, a sulfhydryl cofactor, appears to be a principal target. Normally, dihydrolipoate is oxidized to lipoate via a converting enzyme, dihydrolipoate dehydrogenase. Arsenic reacts with both dihydrolipoate and dihydrolipoate dehydrogenase, preventing the formation of lipoate. Lipoate is involved in the formation of key intermediates in the Krebs cycle. As a result of lipoate depletion, the Krebs cycle and oxidative phosphorylation are inhibited. Without oxidative phosphorylation, cellular energy stores (adenosine triphosphate [ATP]) are depleted, resulting in metabolic failure and cell death.

The other major mechanism by which arsenic is believed to produce cellular injury is termed *arsenolysis*. Pentavalent arsenate can competitively substitute for phosphate in biochemical reactions. During oxidative phosphorylation, energy is produced and stored in the form of ATP. The stable phosphate ester bond in ATP can be replaced by an arsenate ester bond. However, the high energy stored in the arsenate ester bond is wasted because it is unstable and rapidly hydrolyzed. Cellular respiration is stimulated in a futile attempt to restore this wasted energy. In effect, trivalent arsenic compounds inhibit critical enzymes in the Krebs cycle, leading to inhibition of oxidative phosphorylation, and pentavalent arsenic compounds uncouple oxidative phosphorylation by arsenolysis. This results in the disruption of cellular oxidative processes, leading to endothelial cellular damage. The fundamental lesion seen clinically is loss of capillary integrity, resulting in increased permeability of blood vessels and tissue hypoxia, leading to generalized vasodilation, transudation of plasma, hypovolemia, and shock.

In vitro, the effects of arsenic trioxide on repolarizing cardiac ion currents appear to be one of antagonism on both I_{Kr} and I_{Ks} as well as activation of $I_{K\text{-}ATP}$, which maintains normal repolarization [2]. In addition, arsenic trioxide increases cardiac calcium currents and reduces surface expression of the cardiac potassium channel human ether-a-go-go-related gene.

The variability in QTc interval prolongation and the onset of ventricular dysrhythmias during arsenic therapy may represent these competing effects.

Clinical Toxicity

The most prominent clinical findings associated with acute arsenic poisoning are related to the gastrointestinal (GI) tract. Some arsenicals are corrosive. Acute ingestion may lead to oral irritation and a burning sensation in the mouth and throat. A metallic taste and/or a garlicky odor to the breath have been described, but often are not present. Nausea, vomiting, and abdominal pain are common. The toxic effects of arsenic on the GI tract are manifested as increased peristalsis and profuse watery stools and bleeding. In serious cases, hemorrhagic gastroenteritis may ensue within minutes to hours after acute ingestion. Nausea, vomiting, and severe hemorrhagic gastroenteritis can all lead to profound intravascular volume loss, resulting in hypovolemia shock, which is the major cause of mortality and morbidity.

Noncardiogenic pulmonary edema may occur from increased capillary permeability, and cardiogenic pulmonary edema may occur from myocardial depression. Electrocardiogram (ECG) changes associated with arsenic poisoning consist of nonspecific ST- and T-wave changes, sometimes mimicking ischemia or hyperkalemia and QTc prolongation [3]. These ECG abnormalities are reported to occur in half the patients with arsenic poisoning, and these ECG changes may be evident from 4 to 30 hours postingestion, persisting for up to 8 weeks.

At least six cases of arsenic-induced polymorphic ventricular tachycardias consistent with torsades de pointes have been reported. In all these cases, QTc prolongation was evident on the admission ECG. Except in the case of the patient who presented with cyanosis and cardiorespiratory arrest, peripheral neuropathy was a prominent finding on physical examination at the time of hospital admission and the polymorphic ventricular tachydysrhythmias were ultimately self-limited. Although these cases were able to document as to when during the hospital course torsades de pointes were observed, the time between arsenic exposure and the onset of cardiac dysrhythmias can only be speculated.

Arsenicals have been used as part of traditional Chinese medicine for 2,400 years. They became a therapeutic mainstay for a variety of infectious and malignant diseases during the 18th, 19th, and early 20th centuries (e.g., Fowler's solution [potassium bicarbonate-based solution of arsenic trioxide] as treatment for chronic myeloid leukemia). Arsenic compounds fell into disuse in the 1930s with the advent of radiotherapy and cytotoxic chemotherapeutic agents and concerns about arsenic's toxicity and carcinogenicity. However, arsenic trioxide has attracted renewed attention as a treatment for APL on the basis of impressive results from clinical studies in China and the United States [2]. Arsenic trioxide is licensed for use in patients with relapsed or refractory APL. Arsenic trioxide is administered as an infusion 0.15 mg per kg until bone marrow remission or a cumulative maximum of 60 days or associated with adverse drug events (Table 112.1) [2]. Prolongation of the QTc was observed between 1 and 5 weeks after arsenic trioxide infusion, and then returned towards baseline by the end of 8 weeks.

Both acute and chronic arsenic poisoning may affect the hematopoietic system. A reversible bone marrow depression with pancytopenia, particularly leukopenia, may occur. However, it is the chronic form that is usually associated with severe hematopoietic derangements. A wide variety of hematologic abnormalities have been described with arsenic poisoning, including anemia, absolute neutropenia, thrombocytopenia, eosinophilia, and basophilic stippling [4]. Anemia is, in part, due to an increase in hemolysis and disturbed erythropoiesis/myelopoiesis with reticulocytosis and predominant normoblastic erythropoiesis. Accelerated pyknosis of the normoblast nucleus, karyorrhexis, is characteristic of arsenic poisoning, and the typical "cloverleaf" nuclei may be evident. Hematologic findings may appear within 4 days after acute arsenic ingestion, and in the absence of any specific therapy, erythrocytes, leukocytes, and thrombocytes were reported to return to normal values within 2 to 3 weeks after discontinuing arsenic exposure.

TABLE 112.1

Adverse Drug Events Associated with Arsenic Trioxide Induction Therapy

Cardiovascular	QTc prolongation ($\geq$500 ms), torsades de pointes, sudden death, tachycardia
Hematologic	Hyperleukocytosis (10,000–170,000 cells/μL)
Nervous system	Peripheral neuropathy, headache
Metabolic	Hypokalemia, hypomagnesemia, hyperglycemia
APLDS	Fever, pleural or pericardial effusion, pleural infiltrates, respiratory distress, weight gain, musculoskeletal pain
GI	Nausea, vomiting, diarrhea
Dermatologic	Skin rash

APLDS, acute promyelocytic leukemia differentiation syndrome; GI, gastrointestinal.

Neurologic manifestations of arsenic poisoning have included confusion, delirium, convulsions, encephalopathy, and coma [5]. Neuropathy is usually not the initial complaint associated with acute arsenic poisoning. Arsenic-induced polyneuropathy has traditionally been described as an axonal-loss sensorimotor polyneuropathy (low-amplitude/unelicitable sensory and motor conduction responses, often with preserved motor conduction velocities). The first symptoms of neuropathy have been reported to appear 1 to 3 weeks after the presumptive arsenic exposure [5]. Clinical manifestations span the spectrum from mild paresthesia with preserved ambulation to distal weakness, quadriplegia, and respiratory muscle insufficiency. Arsenic neuropathy is a symmetrical sensorimotor neuropathy, with the sensory component being more prominent in a "stocking-and-glove" distribution [6]. This polyneuropathy may progress in an ascending fashion to involve proximal arms and legs. Dysesthesias begin in the lower extremities, with severe painful burning sensation occurring in the soles of the feet. There is loss of vibration and positional sense, followed by the loss of pinprick, light touch, and temperature sensation. Motor dysfunction is characterized by the loss of deep tendon reflexes and muscle weakness. In severe poisoning, ascending weakness and paralysis may occur and involve the respiratory muscles, resulting in neuromuscular respiratory failure [7]. It has been reported that many of the patients with arsenic neuropathy were initially thought to have Guillain–Barré disease [5,7].

Because the fundamental lesion in arsenic toxicity is the loss of capillary integrity, increased glomerular capillary permeability may result in proteinuria. However, the kidneys are relatively spared from the direct toxic effects of arsenic. Hypovolemic shock associated with the prominent GI symptoms may lead to hypoperfusion of the kidneys, resulting in oliguria, acute tubular necrosis, and renal insufficiency or failure. The kidneys are the main route of excretion for arsenic compounds. Normal-functioning kidneys can excrete more than 75 mg of arsenic in the first 24 hours [8]. Because of shock and decreased glomerular filtration rate and depending on the dose of arsenic ingested, peak urinary arsenic excretion may often be delayed by 2 to 3 days. Hemodialysis contributes minimally to arsenic clearance compared with the normal-functioning kidneys. Accordingly, arsenic removal by hemodialysis has been reported to exceed its daily urinary excretion in patients with acute renal failure.

Dermal changes occurring most frequently in arsenic-exposed humans are hyperpigmentation, hyperkeratosis, and skin cancer [9]. The lesions usually appear 1 to 6 weeks after the onset of the illness. In most cases, a diffuse, branny desquamation develops over the trunk and extremities; it is dry, scaling, and nonpruritic. Patchy hyperpigmentation—dark-brown patches with scattered pale spots, sometimes described as "raindrops on a dusty road"—occurs particularly on the eyelids, temples, axillae, neck, nipples, and groin. Arsenic hyperkeratosis usually appears as cornlike elevations, less than 1 cm in diameter, occurring most frequently on the palms of the hands and on the soles of the feet. Most cases of arsenic keratoses remain morphologically benign for decades, and in other cases, marked atypia (precancerous) develops and appears indistinguishable from Bowen's disease—an in situ squamous cell carcinoma. Skin lesions take several years to manifest the characteristic pigmented changes and hyperkeratoses, whereas it may take up to 40 years before skin cancer becomes evident. Brittle nails with transverse white bands (leukonychia striata arsenicalis transversus), Reynolds–Aldrich–Mees lines, appearing on the nails have been associated with arsenic poisoning. It reflects transient disruption of nail plate growth during acute poisoning. Leukonychia striata arsenicalis transversus takes about 5 to 6 weeks to appear over the lunulae after an acute poisoning. Thinning of the hair and patchy or diffuse alopecia are also associated with arsenic poisoning.

Diagnostic Evaluation

The temporal sequence of organ system injury may suggest acute arsenic intoxication. After a delay of minutes to hours, severe hemorrhagic gastroenteritis becomes evident, which may be accompanied by cardiovascular collapse or death. Bone marrow depression with leukopenia may appear within 4 days of arsenic ingestion and usually reaches a nadir at 1 to 2 weeks. Encephalopathy, congestive cardiomyopathy, noncardiogenic pulmonary edema, and cardiac conduction abnormalities may occur several days after improvement from the initial GI manifestations. Sensorimotor peripheral neuropathy may become apparent several weeks after resolution of the initial signs (gastroenteritis or shock) of intoxication resulting from ingestion.

The differentiation between arsenic neuropathy and Landry–Guillain–Barré disease is based on clinical and laboratory findings in that arsenic neuropathy rarely involves the cranial nerves, sensory manifestations are more prominent, weakness in the distal portions of the extremities is more severe, and the cerebrospinal fluid protein concentrations are usually less than 100 mg per dL [5,6].

Laboratory investigation should include complete blood count with peripheral smear, electrolytes, liver enzymes, creatine phosphokinase, arterial blood gas, renal profile with urine analysis, electrocardiogram (ECG), chest radiograph, and blood and urine arsenic concentrations. Nerve conduction velocity studies may be indicated if peripheral neurologic symptoms are present. Some arsenic compounds, particularly those of low solubility, are radiopaque, and if ingested they may be visible on an abdominal radiograph.

The most important diagnostic test is urinary arsenic measurement. Urine arsenic concentrations may be measured as "spot," that is, the concentration in a single-voided urine specimen, reported in micrograms per liter. Urine arsenic concentrations may also be measured as a timed urine collection, or the concentration in urine collected during a 12- to 24-hour period, reported in micrograms per 12 or 24 hours. The quantitative 24-hour urine collection is considered the most reliable. In an emergency situation, the spot urine sample may be of value. Normal total urinary arsenic values are <50 μg per L or <25 μg per 24 hours. In the first 2 to 3 days following acute symptomatic intoxications, total 24-hour urinary arsenic excretion is typically in excess of several thousand micrograms, with spot urine concentration $>1,000$ mg per L, and depending on the severity, it may not return to background for weeks. Recent ingestion of seafood may markedly elevate urinary arsenic values for the next 2 days. Therefore, it is important to take a careful dietary history of the past 48 hours when only total urinary arsenic is measured. Speciation of the urinary arsenic can be performed in some laboratories. Otherwise, the urinary arsenic test should be repeated in 2 to 3 days. Whole blood arsenic, normally <1 μg per dL, may be elevated early on in acute intoxication. However, blood concentrations decline rapidly to normal values despite elevated urinary arsenic excretion and continuing symptoms. Elevated arsenic content in hair and nail segments, normally <1 part per million, may persist for months after urinary arsenic values have returned to background. However, caution should be exercised when interpreting the arsenic content obtained from hair and nails because the arsenic content of these specimens may be increased by external exposure.

Management

The management of acute arsenic poisoning relies on supportive care and chelation therapy. Treatment begins with eliminating further exposure to the toxin and providing basic and advanced life support. Anyone with arsenic intoxication necessitating hospitalization should initially be admitted to an intensive care unit (ICU).

Gastric lavage should be performed following an acute ingestion and should be considered if the ingestion has been within the past 24 hours because some arsenic compounds of low solubility may be retained in the stomach for a prolonged period. Frequently, seriously poisoned patients will have already vomited, evacuating some of their stomach contents. Activated charcoal and cathartics may be used, but their efficacy is unclear. When there is evidence of a heavy metal burden on an abdominal radiograph, whole-bowel irrigation (WBI) with a polyethylene glycol electrolyte solution may rapidly help clear the GI tract of the metallic load. However, the absence of radiopacities on the abdominal radiograph is nondiagnostic, and WBI should still be considered when there is a definite history that a poorly soluble arsenic compound has been ingested.

Intravascular volume depletion may require aggressive replacement with crystalloids, colloids, and blood products. Vasopressors are recommended for refractory hypotension. Invasive monitoring of the patient's hemodynamic status may be necessary.

For acute arsenic poisoning, extended cardiac monitoring for ventricular dysrhythmias is indicated for all patients who have prolonged QTc on their ECG. Electrolyte abnormalities—in particular, hypokalemia and hypomagnesemia—should be aggressively corrected, and concomitant QTc interval-prolonging drugs should be avoided. Serum potassium concentrations should be maintained at >4.0 mmol per L and serum magnesium concentrations at >0.74 mmol per L (1.8 mg per dL). There are no good data to indicate that suppression of ventricular dysrhythmias decreases mortality rates. If dysrhythmias occur, they should be treated according to current advanced cardiac life support guidelines. Type IA antidysrhythmic cardiac medications should be avoided because these drugs may themselves cause further QTc prolongation and worsen the polymorphic ventricular tachycardia. Lidocaine, magnesium, and isoproterenol have been used with limited success in the management of arsenic-induced torsades de pointes. A transvenous pacemaker for overdrive pacing may be necessary. Noncardiogenic and cardiogenic pulmonary edema should be managed according to current guidelines. In patients receiving arsenic trioxide induction therapy who develop prolonged QTc of more than 500 ms on ECG, the risk/benefits of continuing therapy should be considered.

Hematologic effects of arsenic poisoning should be managed symptomatically with blood component therapy and antibiotics as necessary for severe anemia, bleeding, or infections.

Patients with arsenic polyneuropathy should receive analgesics for pain and physical therapy for rehabilitation. Patients with polyneuropathy associated with severe arsenic poisoning should be observed closely for respiratory dysfunction. Neuromuscular respiratory failure may be delayed 1 to 2 months after the initial presentation. In cases in which there is progressive sensorimotor dysfunction, particularly ascending weakness, respiratory muscle function should be monitored carefully. When there is evidence of impending neuromuscular respiratory failure (e.g., negative inspiratory force <25 cm H_2O or vital capacity <20 mL per kg), aggressive supportive measures should be initiated in a timely fashion.

Patients with renal failure may benefit from hemodialysis. However, hemodialysis has limited use when normal renal function is present. Hemodialysis (initiated 24 to 96 hours postingestion) has been reported to remove about 4 mg of arsenic during a 4-hour period in patients with established renal failure. It should not be surprising that only small amounts of arsenic are removed by dialysis as minimal amounts of arsenic are left in the central compartment once tissue distribution and equilibration is complete.

The principle behind chelation therapy is to increase excretion of the metal and decrease the target organ's metal burden. A chelator is an organic compound that has a selective affinity for heavy metals. It competes with tissues and other compounds containing thiol groups for metal ions, removes metal ions that previously have been bound, and binds with the metal ion to form a stable complex (chelate), rendering the metal less reactive and less toxic. The metal–chelator complex is water soluble and can be excreted in the urine, bile, or both, and to some extent it can be removed by hemodialysis.

Dimercaprol (2,3-dimercapto-1-propanol [British anti-Lewisite, BAL]) is the traditional chelating agent that has been used clinically in arsenic poisoning. In humans and animal models, the antidotal efficacy of BAL has been shown to be most effective when it was promptly administered (i.e., minutes to hours) after acute arsenic exposure [10]. In cases of suspected acute symptomatic intoxication, treatment should not be delayed while waiting for specific laboratory confirmation. BAL is administered parenterally as a deep intramuscular (IM) injection. The initial dose is 3 to 5 mg per kg every 4 hours, gradually tapering to every 12 hours during the next several days. As the patient improves, this may be switched to 2,3-dimercaptosuccinic acid (DMSA; succimer) (see "Lead" section). In the United States, DMSA is available only in an oral formulation. This precludes its use in acute severe arsenic intoxication when shock, vomiting, gastroenteritis, and splanchnic edema limit GI absorption. For patients with stable GI and cardiovascular status, a dose regimen of 10 mg per kg every 8 hours for 5 days, reduced to every 12 hours for another 2 weeks, may be employed. D-Penicillamine has also been reported to be successful adjunct treatment in cases of acute pediatric arsenic toxicity [11]. Oral D-penicillamine, 25 mg per kg every 6 hours (maximum of 1 g per day), should be used if BAL or DMSA is unavailable or if the patient is unable to tolerate these medications. Disadvantages in using D-penicillamine include that it is administered only by the oral route, it is usually not well tolerated, it should be used with caution in patients who are allergic to penicillin, and it entails potential enhanced absorption of arsenic-chelate complex. Adverse drug events associated with long-term D-penicillamine treatment include fever, pruritus, leukopenia, thrombocytopenia, eosinophilia, and renal toxicity. A complete blood count and renal function tests should be monitored weekly during D-penicillamine therapy.

BAL and its metal chelate dissociate in an acid medium, and maintenance of an alkaline urine may protect the kidneys during chelation therapy. BAL should be administered with caution in patients with glucose-6-phosphate dehydrogenase deficiency because it may cause hemolysis. The adverse drug events of BAL appear to be dose dependent, with an incidence of >50% at a dose of 5 mg per kg [12]. The reported adverse drug events include pain at the injection site; systolic and diastolic hypertension with tachycardia; nausea; vomiting; headache; burning or constricting sensation in the mouth, throat, and eyes; lacrimation; salivation; rhinorrhea; muscle aches; tingling of the extremities; pain in the teeth; sense of constriction in the chest; abdominal pain; sterile or pyogenic abscesses at the site of injection; and a feeling of anxiety or unrest. In addition to these adverse drug events, a febrile reaction may occur in children. These signs and symptoms are most severe within 30 minutes after administration of BAL and usually dissipate within 1 to 1.5 hours. The adverse drug events may be lessened by the use of epinephrine or by pretreatment with antihistamine or ephedrine [12].

The therapeutic end points of chelation are poorly defined. Usually 24-hour urinary arsenic excretion is followed before, during, and after chelation with continued chelation therapy until the urinary arsenic excretion is <25 μg per 24 hours. Alternatively, when it can be demonstrated that >90% of the total arsenic excreted in the urine is in the form of MMA and DMA, endogenous biomethylation and detoxification may obviate the need for continued chelation [1]. This is likely to occur during the recovery period when urinary inorganic arsenic concentration has declined to less than 100 μg per 24 hours or total blood arsenic concentration is less than 200 μg per L [1].

Chelation therapy may not reverse neuropathy [5,6]. Early treatment may prevent incipient peripheral neuropathy in some, but not all, patients. However, the value of chelation in the treatment of an established arsenic neuropathy has not been demonstrated. In cases of chronic symptomatic arsenic intoxication with high urinary arsenic excretion, an empiric course of chelation may be warranted.

ARSINE GAS

Arsine (AsH_3) is a colorless, nonirritating, inflammable gas with a garlicky odor. It is considered to be the most toxic of the arsenic compounds. The garlic-like odor is not a reliable indicator of exposure because hazardous effects may occur below the odor threshold. Exposure usually occurs in industrial/occupational settings, such as smelting and refining of metals and ores, galvanizing, soldering, etching, lead plating, metallurgy, burning fossil fuels, and the microelectronic/semiconductor industry. (Computer chips made of gallium arsenide are etched with strong acids.)

Pharmacology

Arsine binds to red blood cells (RBCs), causing a rapid and severe Coombs' negative hemolytic anemia. The exact mechanism by which arsine is lytic to the RBC has not been definitively elucidated [13]. In vitro and animal studies indicate that hemolysis requires the presence of oxygen, there is a reduction in the RBCs' glutathione concentration, which is time and concentration dependent on arsine gas exposure, and there is an inverse correlation between the reduced glutathione concentration and the extent of hemolysis. These findings are consistent with a mechanism of oxidative stress-induced damages to the RBCs, resulting in hemolysis.

Toxic concentrations of arsine appear to have deleterious effect on the kidneys. Acute renal failure was often a common cause of death before advent of hemodialysis. Postulated mechanisms of arsine-induced renal failure include direct toxic effects of arsine on renal tubular cell respiration, hypoxia due to the hemolytic anemia, and the massive release of the "arsenic–hemoglobin–haptoglobin complex" precipitating in the tubular lumen, resulting in a toxic effect on the nephron [14]. Depending on the severity, renal failure may be evident by 72 hours from the time of exposure.

Clinical Toxicity

The severity and time to manifestation of arsine poisoning depend on the concentration and duration of the exposure. After an acute massive exposure, death may occur without the classic signs and symptoms of arsine poisoning. It is believed that after low-concentration exposures, arsine is rapidly and efficiently cleared from plasma into the RBCs. However, high concentrations of arsine may exceed the binding capacity of the erythrocytes, and the gas may directly damage vital organs. In cases in which signs and symptoms of arsine poisoning develop over time, the associated morbidity and mortality is partly related to the consequences of its hematologic and renal effects. In general, after a significant exposure to arsine, there is usually a delay of 2 to 24 hours before symptoms of arsine poisoning become apparent.

Initial complaints include dizziness, malaise, weakness, dyspnea, nausea, vomiting, diarrhea, headache, and abdominal pain. Dark-red discoloration of the urine, hemoglobinuria, and/or hematuria frequently appear 4 to 12 hours after inhalation of arsine. Depending on the severity of the exposure, reddish staining of the conjunctiva and duskily bronzed skin may become apparent within 12 to 48 hours [15]. However, the sensitivity of this sign is unclear. The conjunctival and skin discoloration is due to the presence of hemoglobin. This should be distinguished from true jaundice due to the presence of bilirubin. The triad of *abdominal pain*, *hematuria*, and *bronze-tinted skin* is recognized as a characteristic clinical feature of arsine poisoning [13].

In one study, ECG changes associated with arsine poisoning included peaked T waves, particularly in the precordial leads. The most pronounced T-wave changes occurred between the 2nd and the 12th day after exposure. The severity of illness did not correlate with the height of the T wave. There was no delay in atrioventricular or intraventricular conduction times. There was progressive normalization of the T-wave amplitude evident on the weekly follow-up ECG. The exact cause of the ECG change remains speculative.

Management

All patients hospitalized for arsine poisoning should be admitted in the ICU. The management of arsine poisoning should be directed at preventing further exposure to the gas, restoring the intravascular RBC concentration, monitoring the serum potassium, preventing further renal insult, and providing aggressive supportive care. In cases of acute and severe arsine poisoning, exchange transfusion or plasma exchange may be an efficient and effective means of management [13,16,17]. It is important to maintain good urine output (2 to 3 mL/kg/h) at all times. Alkalinization of the urine has been recommended to prevent deposition of RBC breakdown products in the kidneys. In situations in which there is evidence of renal insufficiency or failure, both exchange transfusion and hemodialysis may be required. There are practical and theoretic considerations for using exchange transfusion. It restores the intravascular RBC concentration and removes erythrocyte debris and arsenic–hemoglobin complexes. Hemolysis due to arsine poisoning can be a dynamic process; there is one report of ongoing hemolysis for at least 4 days in patients not selected for exchange transfusion. Theoretic support for the use of exchange transfusion came from animal studies where a large proportion of the fixed arsenic in the blood of animals poisoned with arsine was in a nondialyzable form, and adequate removal of arsine and its associated toxic complexes would be a problem with hemodialysis alone. It has been suggested that with early diagnosis of arsine poisoning and prompt institution of exchange transfusion, the incidence of renal damage and long-term renal insufficiency may be reduced.

The results of using BAL in the treatment of acute arsine poisoning have been disappointing [15,18]. BAL does not appear to afford protection against arsine-induced hemolysis. It remains speculative whether BAL would be of benefit in subacute or chronic arsine poisoning.

LEAD

The use of lead and its environmental contamination has increased dramatically since the beginning of the Industrial Revolution. However, for the past 20 years, environmental and occupational exposure to lead as well as the severity of lead poisoning have decreased because of government regulations and increased public health awareness of the problems associated with lead, especially at low-concentration exposures.

The major environmental sources of lead include vehicle exhaust, paint, food, and water. Combustion of leaded gasoline by motor vehicles produced lead in automobile emissions, which is the main source of airborne lead. Airborne lead can be inhaled directly or deposited in the environment (soil, water, and crops). The content of lead in residential paint was not regulated until 1977. More than half of the older residential and commercial structures built before 1960 have been painted with lead-based paints. With time, flaking, chipping, peeling, and chalking of the paint occurs—a potential source of lead exposure. Industrial use of corrosion-resistant lead paint continues. High-concentration exposure may result from renovation, sandblasting, torching, or demolition of older applications. Food may contain lead that has been deposited in the soil or water. Food may be contaminated with lead when it is harvested, transported, processed, packaged, and prepared. Lead exposure may occur from use of lead-glazed pottery or ceramic ware for cooking and eating as well as from the consumption of food from lead-soldered cans. Water from leaded pipes, soldered plumbing, and water coolers is also a potential source of lead exposure. Some traditional Hispanic, Asian, and Middle Eastern folk medicine has been shown to contain significant amounts of lead. Mexican folk remedies, "azarcon" and "greta," are prescribed by the local folk healers (curanderos) to treat nonspecific GI symptoms collectively known as "empacho." Azarcon is a bright-orange powder and greta is a fine yellowish powder. Other names such as alarcon, coral, liga, Maria Luisa, and rueda have been given to these lead-containing folk remedies. In Asian communities, lead-containing folk remedies include bali goli, chuifong tokuwan, ghasard, knadu, pay-loo-ah, and Po Ying Tan. Middle Eastern lead-containing folk medicines include alkohl, cebagin, kohl, saoott, and surma.

The most significant way in which children are exposed to lead is through inhalation and ingestion. Children can ingest chips from lead-painted surfaces, or by mouthing items contaminated with lead from dust, soil, or paint. Some children are given folk remedies containing large quantities of lead. Another potential source of lead exposure in children is the preparation of infant formulas in vessels with lead solder.

Aside from the environmental sources, lead exposure in adults primarily comes from the occupational setting, particularly for electricians; cable splicers; plumbers; lead, copper, zinc, and silver miners; printers; lead smelters and refiners; steel welders and cutters; painters; auto repairers (radiator repair mechanics); sandblasting, demolition, and construction workers; battery manufacturers; solderers; bricklayers; silversmiths; glass manufacturers; and ship builders. One source of lead exposure that is not often considered is retained lead bullets, especially those that are near synovial surfaces.

Hobbies and related activities such as home remodeling, target shooting at indoor firing ranges, stained glass making, glazed pottery making, lead soldering, and making illicitly distilled whiskey ("moonshine") can potentially subject adults and their families to high concentrations of lead.

Pharmacology

In adults, about 10% of an ingested dose is absorbed, whereas in children, up to 50% may be absorbed. GI absorption may be increased by iron or calcium deficiency and varies directly with the solubility of the lead compound ingested and inversely with particle size. The oral dose associated with the lowest observable effect level in humans is uncertain. Acute human ingestion of 15 g of lead oxide has resulted in fatality.

Inhalation of lead is a significant route of exposure as lead particles (e.g., dust) and fumes can potentially reach the alveoli, where absorption from the lower respiratory tract is nearly complete. Airborne lead particles are usually too large to enter the alveoli of small children. These particles (when inhaled) are returned to the posterior pharynx through ciliary action and swallowed. Dermal absorption of lead is rapid and extensive for alkyl lead compounds, but minimal for inorganic lead.

After absorption, almost all lead in the blood is located within the RBCs [19]. RBC lead has a half-life of 30 to 40 days and is circulated and distributed into soft tissues and bones. The half-life of lead in the soft tissues is about 40 days, whereas the half-life in bones is 20 to 30 years. Hence, blood lead concentration may be declining as the soft tissue and bone burdens are rising. Equilibration between bone and blood lead does occur. The major depot for lead in the body is the skeletal system, which contains more than 90% in adults and more than 70% in children, in terms of the total-body lead burden. The primary sources of lead that cause clinical and subclinical symptoms are the blood and soft tissues. Lead that is deposited and incorporated into the matrix of bone can be mobilized during pregnancy, lactation, osteoporosis, and prolonged immobilization. In addition, lead that is deposited in bone may have some toxic effects on bone growth and function.

The kidneys filter lead unchanged (with some active tubular transport at high concentrations), and the excretion rate depends on the glomerular filtration rate and renal blood flow. The kidneys account for about 75% of daily lead loss [19]. However, elimination of lead from the body is influenced by the relative concentration of lead in the various body compartments.

Common forms of inorganic lead are generally devoid of significant irritant or corrosive effects. However, alkyl lead compounds may be moderately irritating. The multisystemic toxicity of lead is mediated by at least two primary mechanisms: the inhibition of enzymatic processes, sometimes as a result of sulfhydryl group binding, and interaction with essential cations, in particular calcium, zinc, and ferrous iron. Pathologic alterations in cellular and mitochondrial membranes, neurotransmitter biosynthesis and function, heme biosynthesis, and nucleotide metabolism may also occur.

One of the principal toxic effects of lead is inhibition of enzymes along the heme biosynthesis pathway. Specifically, lead inhibits the enzymes δ-aminolevulinic acid (ALA) dehydrase and ferrochelatase. As a result, δ-ALA cannot be converted to porphobilinogen and iron cannot be incorporated into protoporphyrin IX. This is reflected by a measurable increase in serum ALA and protoporphyrin concentrations. The increase in protoporphyrin forms the basis of the erythrocyte protoporphyrin (EP) test, which has been used to screen for chronic lead exposure. Lead also inhibits the nonenzymatic mobilization of iron stores, which further contributes to the effect of anemia. Impaired heme biosynthesis may have widespread effects because of its impact on the cytochrome systems. In addition, lead appears to shorten erythrocyte survival time by interfering with the sodium–potassium–adenosine triphosphatase pump mechanism and by attaching to RBC membranes, causing increased mechanical fragility and cell lysis. Decreased heme synthesis and increased RBC destruction results in reticulocytosis. Inhibition of pyrimidine-5′-nucleotidase by lead results in accumulation of ribonucleic acid degradation products and aggregation of ribosomes in RBCs, which produce punctate basophilic stippling. However, neither anemia nor basophilic stippling is a sensitive or specific indicator of lead intoxication. Lead-induced anemia results from either a prolonged exposure or a concentrated short-term exposure with a latent period of several weeks.

Lead toxicity produces anatomic lesions in the proximal tubule and loops of Henle, which is characterized by round acidophilic intranuclear inclusion bodies. Most often, lead-induced renal injury is associated with prolonged exposure to large amounts of lead, resulting in progressive renal insufficiency.

The toxic effects of lead involve both the peripheral nervous system and the central nervous system (CNS). Peripheral nervous system toxicity is known as lead palsy and is due to the degenerative changes in the motoneurons and their axons, with secondary effects involving the myelin sheaths [20]. Lead palsy is usually a pure motor neuropathy and is the result of advanced chronic lead poisoning. Both adults and children can present with CNS dysfunction; however, acute encephalopathy is an unusual feature of adult lead intoxication. Although lead encephalopathy is rare today, it is the most serious consequence of lead poisoning and is probably due to inhibition of the intracellular enzyme systems within the CNS.

Clinical Toxicity

Poisoning is usually the result of continued exposure to small amounts of lead rather than a single acute event. However, acute ingestion can produce lead toxicity. Usually, the clinical presentation of acute lead toxicity appears to be associated with a sharp incremental rise in the concentration of lead in various soft tissues, and this often occurs against the background of chronic lead poisoning.

The multisystemic toxicity of lead presents a spectrum of clinical findings ranging from overt, life-threatening intoxication to subtle, subclinical deficits. Acute ingestion of very large quantities of lead (gram quantities) may cause abdominal pain, toxic hepatitis, and anemia (usually hemolytic).

Subacute or chronic exposure causes nonspecific constitutional symptoms such as fatigue, arthralgias, decreased libido, irritability, impotence, depression, anorexia, malaise, myalgias, weight loss, and insomnia [21]. Gastrointestinal symptoms include nausea, constipation or diarrhea, and intestinal spasm. The intestinal spasm, "lead colic," can cause severe, excruciating, paroxysmal, abdominal pain. Central nervous system findings range from impaired concentration, visual–motor coordination, and headache, to severe, life-threatening encephalopathy characterized by vomiting, tremors, hyperirritability, ataxia, confusion, delirium, lethargy, obtundation, convulsions, coma, and death. A peripheral motor neuropathy, predominantly affecting the upper extremities, may result in extensor weakness. In rare instances, severe cases may produce frank "wrist drop." Decreased intelligence, impaired neurobehavioral development, decreased stature or growth, and diminished auditory acuity may occur. Hematologic manifestations include normochromic or microcytic anemia. This may be accompanied by basophilic stippling of the erythrocytes. Nephrotoxic effects include overt reversible acute tubular dysfunction, in particular, Fanconi-like aminoaciduria in children, and chronic progressive renal interstitial fibrosis following heavy long-term exposure in lead workers. Sometimes hyperuricemia, with or without evidence of gout, may be associated with the renal insufficiency. An association between lead exposure and hypertension may exist in susceptible populations.

Repeated, intentional inhalation of leaded gasoline may result in ataxia, myoclonic jerking, hyperreflexia, delirium, and seizures.

Diagnostic Evaluation

Although encephalopathy and abdominal colic following a suspect activity may readily suggest the diagnosis of severe lead intoxication, the nonspecific nature of mild-to-moderate intoxication frequently presents a diagnostic challenge. Exposure is often not suspected, and symptoms are commonly attributed to a "nonspecific viral illness." Lead intoxication should be considered in patients presenting with multisystem findings including headache, abdominal pain, and anemia, and, less commonly, motor neuropathy, gout, and renal insufficiency. Lead encephalopathy should be considered in any child with delirium or seizures, and milder degrees of intoxication should be considered in children with neurobehavioral deficits or developmental delays. Lead encephalopathy has usually been associated with blood lead concentrations of 100 μg per dL or more [22]. Blood lead concentrations >80 μg per dL are occasionally associated with acute severe illness.

Whole blood lead concentration and EP are the two methods most commonly used in testing for lead intoxication. Whole blood lead concentration is the most useful screening and diagnostic test for acute or recent lead exposure. This test does not measure total-body lead burden, but it does reflect abrupt changes in lead exposure. Elevation in EP (>35 μg per dL) reflects lead-induced inhibition of heme biosynthesis. Because only actively forming erythrocytes are affected, elevations in EP will typically lag behind lead exposure by 2 to 6 weeks. EP value may help distinguish between recent and remote lead exposure. An extremely high whole blood lead concentration in the presence of a normal EP concentration would suggest a recent lead exposure. An elevated EP concentration is not specific for lead exposure and may also occur with iron deficiency. EP is not a sensitive screening tool for low-concentration (<30 μg per dL) lead poisoning. EP and blood lead concentrations should be used as complementary methods of testing for lead intoxication.

Erythrocyte protoporphyrin, free EP, and zinc EP measure the same basic process and have very similar interpretations, but are not identical. EP is the most precise terminology. Because lead blocks (ferrochelatase) the final step in heme biosynthesis, it was originally thought that "free" EP was formed. However, it was subsequently shown that other porphyrins were measured in minute amounts, and most protoporphyrin had nonenzymatically bound zinc and was therefore not "free."

Relationships between blood lead concentrations and clinical findings have generally been based on subacute and chronic exposure and not on transiently high values that may result immediately following exposure before tissue equilibration (Table 112.2). Interindividual variability in response is extensive.

Measurement of urinary lead excretion is not very useful in the diagnosis of lead exposure. Urinary lead excretion reflects the plasma lead concentration, which increases and decreases more rapidly than does blood lead concentration.

Nonspecific laboratory criteria consistent with lead toxicity include normochromic or microcytic anemia, basophilic stippling of RBC on peripheral smear, increased urinary ALA, and coproporphyrin. Liver transaminases may be elevated in acute intoxication. Low-molecular-weight proteinuria and enzymuria may precede elevations in serum creatinine. Radiopacities on abdominal radiograph may be evidence of lead in the GI tract following recent ingestion. This is especially true for lead-based ceramic glazes.

TABLE 112.2

Whole Blood Lead Concentration and Associated Clinical Findings

Whole blood lead concentration (μg/dL)	Associated clinical findings
<25	Decreased intelligence and impaired neurobehavioral development among children with in utero or early childhood exposure; generally without demonstrable toxic effects in adults
20–60	Mild overt effects such as headache, irritability, difficulty concentrating, slowed reaction time, impaired visual–motor coordination, and insomnia may emerge
	Anemia may begin to appear
	Reversible, subclinical slowing of motor nerve conduction velocity may be detected
60–80	Subclinical effects on renal function
	GI symptoms (e.g., anorexia, constipation, and/or diarrhea, and abdominal colic) may emerge
>80	Serious overt intoxication, including abdominal pain (colic), and nephropathy
>100	Encephalopathy and overt neuropathy

Management

Acute lead encephalopathy is a medical emergency that requires intensive care and monitoring of the patient. Prompt consultation with a toxicologist should be obtained to assist in the management. Because up to 25% of the children who survive an acute episode of encephalopathy sustain permanent CNS damage [22], medical treatment should be instituted before its onset. It has long been recommended that any child who is symptomatic from lead poisoning or has a whole blood lead concentration >80 μg per dL should be hospitalized immediately and treated as a medical emergency [22]. More recently, the Centers for Disease Control and Prevention has issued a statement that children with blood lead concentrations of 70 μg per dL or greater require immediate chelation therapy [23].

Although present-day recommendations for the treatment of lead encephalopathy were derived from experiences in managing children [22,24–26], they have been extrapolated to adults. The basic treatment plan consists of supportive measures and the use of chelating agents. As with any potential life-threatening emergency, assessment and aggressive management of the airway, breathing, and circulation should be paramount.

Gastrointestinal decontamination, beginning with gastric lavage, is indicated following acute ingestion of virtually any lead-containing substances because even small quantities of paint chip or a sip of lead-containing glaze may contain several hundred milligrams of lead. The use of activated charcoal has been suggested; however, its efficacy is unknown. Abdominal radiograph may reveal radiopaque foreign bodies in the GI tract following recent ingestion of lead-containing substances such as paint chips, lead weights, and lead-based ceramic glazes. Whole bowel irrigation with polyethylene glycol solution has been suggested as a means of decontaminating the GI tract when the presence of lead is evident on radiographic examination of the abdomen. The effectiveness of WBI can be followed by serial abdominal radiographs. Although it is important to eliminate the source of continued lead absorption, therapy should not be delayed by attempts at GI decontamination, especially in cases of encephalopathy. Ultimately, the chief priority is to identify and eradicate the source of lead exposure and institute control measures to prevent repeated intoxication. In addition, other possibly exposed persons should be promptly evaluated.

Lead-containing buckshot, shrapnel, or bullets in or adjacent to synovial spaces should be surgically removed if possible, especially if associated with evidence of systemic lead absorption.

In a child presenting with encephalopathy, immediate treatment should begin with establishing an adequate urine output [22]. This can be accomplished by intravenous (IV) infusion (10 to 20 mL per kg) of 10% dextrose in water during 1 to 2 hours. If this fails to produce a urine output, infusion of a 20% mannitol solution (1 to 2 g per kg) is recommended at 1 mL per minute. Once urine output has been established, IV fluids should be restricted to the calculated basal water and electrolyte requirements plus a careful assessment of continuing losses. An indwelling Foley catheter should be used to monitor the rate of urine formation. IV fluids should be adjusted hourly in order to maintain urine flow that is within the basal metabolic limits, which is 0.35 to 0.50 mL of urine secreted per calorie metabolized per 24 hours or 350 to 500 mL/m^2/24 hours. Such management is designed to avoid excessive fluid administration and prevent further development of cerebral edema. Severe lead encephalopathy can occur without cerebral edema [24]. However, when cerebral edema occurs in the presence of encephalopathy, there is further insult to the brain, and it may be the immediate cause of death. Children with encephalopathy may exhibit syndrome of inappropriate antidiuretic hormone [26].

If paralysis with sedation or general anesthesia is required for controlling seizure activities, a bedside electroencephalogram should be obtained to rule out electrical status. Because high doses of phenytoin and phenobarbital were often required to control the initial seizures in lead encephalopathy, paraldehyde was formerly used. However, barbiturates were recommended in the prevention of seizures during the early convalescent phase of lead encephalopathy. Repeated seizures and hypoxia can exacerbate cerebral edema, and so it was suggested that anticonvulsants be administered when there is evidence of increased muscle tone or muscle twitching; one should not wait for obvious seizure activity [22].

Computed tomography scan of the head should be performed in patients presenting with encephalopathy to screen for cerebral edema. If there is evidence of cerebral edema, intracranial pressure (ICP) monitoring may be indicated and neurosurgical consultation is recommended. Avoid performing a lumbar puncture when there is increased ICP associated with cerebral edema. Measures advocated to control cerebral edema and increased ICP include careful sedation and neuromuscular paralysis, elevation of the head of the bed, hyperventilation, restriction of fluid therapy, ventricular drainage, diuretics (e.g., mannitol or furosemide), and steroids. These measures are "borrowed" from the neurosurgical experience in managing increased ICP. Restriction of fluids, the use of mannitol, and hypertonic saline have been discussed previously. Maintaining the arterial partial pressure of carbon dioxide between 25 and 30 mm Hg by controlled hyperventilation has been shown to result in cerebral vasoconstriction and reduced ICP. The benefit of glucocorticoids for treating perifocal vasogenic edema due to an intrinsic intracranial mass lesion is well established. However, glucocorticoids have not been proved beneficial in models of intracellular cytotoxic edema, and neurologic outcome studies do not support the routine use of glucocorticoids following head injury, global brain ischemia, or cerebral vascular accidents [27]. If the cerebral edema associated with lead encephalopathy is believed to be vasogenic in origin, the empiric use of dexamethasone should be considered. Surgical attempts to relieve ICP by flap craniotomy have not been shown to be beneficial. However, ventricular drainage (via the intracranial bolt placed for ICP monitoring) may effectively reduce increased ICP.

Chelating agents have been shown to decrease blood lead concentrations and increase urinary lead excretion. Chelation has also been associated with improvement in symptoms and decreased mortality. However, controlled clinical trials demonstrating therapeutic efficacy is lacking, and treatment recommendations have been largely empiric. Although there appears to have been a sharp reduction in pediatric mortality due to acute lead encephalopathy with the advent of chelation treatment, there were concomitant advances in the management of elevated ICP, and the decline in mortality cannot necessarily be attributed to the use of chelation alone. BAL and calcium disodium edetate (CaEDTA) are the two chelators used in the treatment of lead encephalopathy. DMSA is used for less severe poisoning.

BAL increases both fecal and urinary excretion of lead. It is distributed widely throughout all body tissues, including the brain and RBCs. Because BAL is excreted in the urine and to some extent in the bile, patients with renal failure are not precluded from the use of BAL, whereas patients with hepatic insufficiency may have a lower tolerance to BAL [28]. Details regarding the use of this agent are discussed in the "Arsenic" section of this chapter. BAL and medicinal iron can form a toxic complex that is a potent emetic, and accordingly the treatment of anemia with iron should be delayed until BAL therapy has been completed. If severe anemia requires prompt intervention during chelation therapy, transfusion would be preferable.

CaEDTA enhances the elimination of lead and, to a lesser extent, the elimination of endogenous metals (e.g., zinc, manganese, iron, copper). Increased urinary lead excretion begins within 1 hour and is followed by a decrease in whole blood lead concentration over the course of treatment. CaEDTA diffuses rapidly and uniformly throughout the body, but it does not appear to enter RBCs and very slowly diffuses across the blood–brain barrier [29]. CaEDTA mobilizes lead (primarily) from soft tissues and from a fraction of the larger lead stores present in bone. CaEDTA is not metabolized; rather, it is cleared from the body by urinary excretion. It can be administered intravenously (IV) or intramuscularly (IM), with the former being the preferred and most effective route. Oral administration of CaEDTA has been shown to increase absorption of lead from the GI tract; therefore, it should not be given by this route. The principal toxic effect of CaEDTA is on the kidneys, which can result in renal tubular necrosis. The renal toxicity is dose related and reversible. Because CaEDTA increases renal excretion of lead and its accumulation increases the risk of nephrotoxicity, anuria would be a contraindication in its use. An adequate urine flow should be established before initiating CaEDTA therapy.

In the management of patients with lead encephalopathy, some clinicians advocate the use of BAL and CaEDTA beginning with a priming dose of BAL at the same time that an adequate urine output is being established. The priming dose of BAL is 75 mg per m^2 (3 to 5 mg per kg) IM and is administered every 4 hours. After 4 hours have elapsed since the priming dose of BAL, a continuous slow IV infusion of CaEDTA 1,500 mg/m^2/d (30 mg/kg/d) is started. For cases where there is evidence of cerebral edema and/or increased ICP associated with encephalopathy, CaEDTA (same dosage) should be given by deep IM injection in two to three divided doses every 8 to 12 hours. When the IM route is preferred, procaine (0.5%) should be given along with CaEDTA because IM administration of CaEDTA is extremely painful. BAL and CaEDTA are usually continued for 5 days. For patients with high body lead burdens, cessation of chelation is often followed by a rebound in blood lead concentrations as bone stores equilibrate with lower soft-tissue concentrations. A second course of chelation may be considered on the basis of whole blood lead concentration after 2 days of interruption of BAL and CaEDTA treatment, and the persistence or recurrence of symptoms. A third course may be required if the whole blood concentration rebounds to 50 mg per dL or greater within 48 hours after the second chelation treatment. If chelation is required for the third time, it should begin a week after the last dose of BAL and CaEDTA.

In the management of symptomatic patients with lead poisoning who are not overtly encephalopathic, most clinicians advocate the same course of treatment as for those with encephalopathy, but with lower doses of BAL and CaEDTA. The priming dose of BAL is 50 mg per m^2 (2 to 3 mg per kg) IM and is administered every 4 hours. After 4 hours have elapsed since the priming dose of BAL, a continuous slow IV infusion of CaEDTA 1,000 mg/m^2/d (20 to 30 mg/kg/d) is started. Alternatively, CaEDTA may be given in two to three divided doses every 8 to 12 hours by continuous infusion or deep IM injection. BAL and CaEDTA should be continued for 5 days with daily monitoring of whole blood lead concentrations. BAL may be discontinued any time during these 5 days if the whole blood lead concentration decreases to <50 μg per dL, but CaEDTA treatment should continue for 5 days. A second or third course of chelation may be considered on the basis of the same guidelines as discussed in the previous paragraph.

In the management of asymptomatic patients with whole blood lead concentrations 70 μg per dL or greater, some clinicians would advocate the use of BAL and CaEDTA in the same doses and with the same guidelines as for treatment of symptomatic lead poisoning without encephalopathy. A second course of chelation with CaEDTA alone may be necessary if the whole blood lead concentration rebounds to 50 μg per dL or more within 5 to 7 days after chelation has ceased; some clinicians prefer the use of DMSA.

A water-soluble analog of BAL, DMSA enhances the urinary excretion of lead, mercury, and arsenic. It has an insignificant effect on elimination of the endogenous minerals calcium, iron, and magnesium. Minor increases in zinc and copper excretion may occur. Oral DMSA is rapidly but variably absorbed, with peak blood concentrations occurring between 1 and 2 hours. The drug is predominantly cleared by the kidneys, with peak urinary elimination of the parent drug and its metabolites occurring between 1 and 4 hours. DMSA is approved for use for lead and mercury intoxications, in which it is associated with increased urinary excretion of the metals, and concurrent reversal of metal-induced enzyme inhibition. Oral DMSA is comparable to parenteral CaEDTA in decreasing whole blood lead concentration during treatment. Although treatment with DMSA has been associated with subjective clinical improvement, controlled clinical trials demonstrating therapeutic efficacy have not been reported. Reported adverse drug events of DMSA include GI disturbances (anorexia, nausea, vomiting, and diarrhea), mercaptan-like (sulfur) odor to the urine, rashes, mild-to-moderate neutropenia, and mild, reversible increases in hepatic transaminases.

Although DMSA is FDA approved for use only in children with whole blood concentration in excess of 45 μg per dL, it has similar ability to lower whole blood lead concentration in adults. Treatment is initiated at an oral dose of 10 mg per kg (350 mg per m^2) every 8 hours for 5 days. Treatment is then continued at the same dose every 12 hours for an additional 2 weeks. An additional course of treatment may be considered on the basis of posttreatment whole blood lead concentrations and the persistence or recurrence of symptoms. Whole blood lead concentration may decline by more than 50% during treatment, but patients with large body burdens may experience rebound to within 20% of pretreatment concentrations as bone body stores reequilibrate with tissue concentrations. An interval of two or more weeks may be indicated to assess the extent of posttreatment rebound in whole blood lead concentration. Experience with oral DMSA in severe lead intoxication (e.g., lead encephalopathy or lead colic) is very limited, and consideration should be given to parenteral chelation therapy in such cases.

MERCURY

Mercury (Hg) is a naturally occurring metal that is mined chiefly as mercuric sulfate (HgS) in cinnabar ore. It is converted into three primary forms, each with a distinct toxicology: elemental (Hg^0) mercury, inorganic (mercurous [Hg^{+1}] and mercuric [Hg^{2+}]) mercury salts, and organic (alkyl and phenyl) mercury. The pattern and severity of toxicity are highly dependent on the form of mercury and route of exposure, mostly because of different pharmacokinetic profiles.

Elemental Mercury

Elemental mercury is the only metal that exists in liquid form at standard temperature and pressure. As such, metallic mercury can evaporate slowly at room temperature or rapidly when heated, and can contribute to the partial pressure of the ambient air that is breathed. A small spill in an enclosed space (e.g., a bedroom) can also produce high concentrations of mercury in the air because of its high vapor pressure. Various instruments contain elemental mercury including thermometers, manometers, barometers, switches, pumps, and special surgical tubes (such as Miller–Abbott, Canter, and Kaslow). Dental amalgam is prepared with elemental mercury and contains approximately 50% elemental mercury by weight.

Personnel in occupational settings who are potentially exposed include chlor-alkali mercury cell operation workers, electroplaters, explosives manufacturers, laboratory personnel, pesticide/fungicide production and application workers, manufacturers of batteries or mercury vapor lamps, metallurgists, and miners and processors of cinnabar, gold, silver, copper, and zinc. Exposure to mercury vapor from elemental mercury spill, work hazard, home gold ore purification, accidental heating of metallic mercury, and vacuum cleanup of a mercury spill have also been reported [30].

Pharmacology

When ingested, elemental mercury is poorly absorbed (<0.01%) from the healthy, intact, and normal-functioning GI tract. In contrast, inhaled mercury vapor is believed to cross the alveolar membranes rapidly because of its high diffusibility and high lipid solubility. About 75% of the inhaled dose is retained [31]. The absorbed elemental mercury vapor rapidly diffuses into the RBCs, where it undergoes oxidation to the mercuric ion and binds to ligands in the RBC. However, a certain amount of the dissolved vapor persists in the plasma to reach the blood–brain barrier, which it crosses readily. Once in the brain tissue, the dissolved mercury vapor is oxidized to mercuric ion, trapping it within the CNS, where it is available for binding tissue ligands. Elemental mercury vapor is also easily transported across the placenta.

Elemental mercury vapor is eliminated from the body mainly as mercuric ion by urinary and fecal routes. Exhalation of mercury vapor and secretion of mercuric ions in saliva and sweat do occur and contribute to the elimination process. The rate of excretion is dose dependent. Elemental mercury follows a biphasic elimination rate, initially rapid and then slow, with a biologic half-life in humans of about 60 days.

Mercuric ion has an affinity to bind and react with sulfhydryl moieties of proteins, leading to nonspecific inhibition of enzyme systems and pathologic alteration of cellular membranes.

The pulmonary and central nervous systems bear the brunt of the insult for elemental mercury vapor poisoning. Damage to the respiratory system results from acute inhalation exposure to high concentrations of elemental mercury vapor, which acts as a direct airway irritant and a cellular poison [30,32]. Pulmonary toxicity is characterized by exudative alveolar and interstitial edema, erosive bronchitis and bronchiolitis with interstitial pneumonitis, and desquamation of the bronchial epithelium. The ensuing obstruction can result in alveolar dilatation, interstitial emphysema, pneumatocele formation, pneumothorax, and mediastinal emphysema.

In the CNS, a cumulative toxic effect occurs as the inhaled elemental mercury vapor is oxidized to mercuric ion, leading to progressive CNS dysfunction. As would be expected, CNS toxicity is typically the result of chronic elemental mercury vapor exposure.

Clinical Toxicity

The ingestion of elemental mercury usually causes no adverse effects. However, systemic absorption of mercury is possible in the presence of any bowel abnormality affecting mucosal integrity or impeding normal motility and transit. In addition, inflammatory bowel disease or enteric fistula allowing for prolonged elemental mercury exposure and the conversion of metallic mercury to an inorganic ion has been reported. Elemental mercury that is retained in the appendix can result in local inflammation, perforation, and the consequent possibility of systemic mercury intoxication. Signs of appendiceal inflammation or systemic mercury absorption and toxicity should be appropriately monitored and treated. Prophylactic appendectomy in the absence of signs and symptoms of appendicitis should be avoided because of the risk of mercury extravasation through the surgical anastomosis and intra-abdominal suppurative complications [33].

Subcutaneous injection of elemental mercury may cause a local fibrous reaction, local abscess, granuloma formation, and systemic embolization, and systemic absorption with toxic manifestations.

Intravenously injected elemental mercury has been reported to cause pulmonary and systemic mercury embolization, associated with an elevated blood mercury concentration, and sequelae may include tremor, lower extremity weakness, and reduced carbon monoxide diffusing capacity. Mercury extravasation at the injection site can produce a severe local inflammatory reaction. Granuloma formation with fibrosis and inflammation with systemic mercury absorption has also been reported.

Acute intense inhalation of mercury vapor in a confined or poorly ventilated space may result in death. Initial symptoms usually occur within several hours following exposure and include fever, chills, headache, dyspnea, gingivostomatitis, nausea, vomiting, metallic taste in the mouth, paroxysmal cough, tachypnea, chest tightness, diarrhea, and abdominal cramping [32]. These symptoms may subside or, in severe cases, may progress to interstitial pneumonitis, bilateral infiltrates, atelectasis, noncardiogenic pulmonary edema, interstitial pulmonary fibrosis, and death. In addition, complications such as subcutaneous emphysema, pneumomediastinum, and pneumothorax may occur. Children younger than 30 months seem to be particularly susceptible to such exposures.

Although aspiration of elemental mercury may cause no acute respiratory symptoms, it may cause cough and mild dyspnea, acute pneumonitis, or progressive cough with copious amounts of frankly bloody sputum production, leading to respiratory compromise and death [34]. Most patients remain asymptomatic or recover without any significant sequelae. In two cases, systemic absorption of the aspirated elemental mercury was suggested by elevations in the 24-hour urinary mercury concentrations, but neither patient became symptomatic. Elemental mercury was consistently evident on chest radiographs obtained on follow-up examination, which varied from 1 month to 20 years. One case with postmortem findings from the lungs 22 years later included globules of elemental mercury surrounded by extensive fibrosis and granuloma formation. Subclinical changes in peripheral nerve function and renal function have been reported, but symptomatic neuropathy and nephropathy are rare.

Diagnostic Evaluation

Diagnosis depends on integration of characteristic findings with a history of known or potential exposure, and the presence of elevated whole blood mercury concentration and urinary mercury excretion. Abdominal radiographs may be used to document the extent of the GI contamination following elemental mercury ingestion. Radiographs of the injection site may help to define the extent of the infiltrated mercury. Chest radiograph and computed axial tomography scan may be useful in determining the location of systemic embolization.

Whole blood and urinary mercury concentrations are useful in confirming exposure. In most people without occupational exposure, whole blood mercury concentration is less than 2 μg per dL and "spot" or single-voided urine mercury concentration is less than 10 μg per L. A quantitative 24-hour urinary mercury excretion, usually less than 50 μg per 24 hours, is probably the most useful tool in diagnosing acute exposure (Table 112.3).

Management

Any patient requiring hospitalization because of acute elemental mercury inhalation or aspiration should be admitted to the ICU. As with any potential life-threatening emergency, assessment and aggressive management of the airway, breathing, and circulation should be paramount. Treatment is primarily supportive. Another priority is to identify and eradicate the source of elemental mercury exposure and to identify and evaluate other possibly exposed persons.

In cases for which elemental mercury ingestion has been documented, WBI with polyethylene glycol electrolyte solution or surgical removal may be necessary, depending on radiographic

TABLE 112.3

Elemental Mercury Vapor Exposure

Urine mercury concentration (μg/L)	Associated clinical findings
30–50	Subclinical neuropsychiatric effects
50–100	Early subclinical tremor
>100	Overt neuropsychiatric disturbances
>200	True tremors

evidence of mercury retention, elevated blood urine mercury concentrations, and the patient's clinical status. Repeat abdominal radiographs may be used to document the effectiveness of WBI or to follow the progress of the ingested metallic mercury.

Aggressive local wound management of the injection site(s) should include prompt excision of all readily accessible subcutaneous areas in which metallic mercury is demonstrated, copious saline irrigation to remove metallic mercury droplets, and suction removal of the mercury [35]. Surgical excision of mercury granulomas has also been recommended. Injection of BAL into the wound is not recommended as it may delay wound healing.

Patients acutely exposed to elemental mercury vapor should be monitored closely for respiratory symptoms. Chest radiographs, arterial blood gases, and pulmonary function should be followed in symptomatic patients. Oxygen and bronchodilators should be administered as needed. Progressive deterioration of respiratory function may require aggressive airway management with tracheal intubation, mechanical ventilation, and positive end-expiratory pressure. Early treatment with corticosteroids has been used in an attempt to reduce the complication of pulmonary fibrosis. However, neither corticosteroids nor prophylactic antibiotics have proved to be beneficial in the management of elemental mercury vapor–induced pulmonary complications.

Patients who have aspirated elemental mercury should be managed in a similar fashion. Vigorous suctioning, postural drainage, and good pulmonary toilet may assist the patient in expectorating some of the aspirated mercury. In addition, bronchoscopy may be indicated.

Chelating agents that are commercially available in the United States for use in the treatment of mercury poisoning include BAL, DMSA, and D-penicillamine (see the "Arsenic" and "Lead" sections). The choice of chelator depends on the form of mercury involved and the presenting signs and symptoms of the patient. DMSA and D-penicillamine may facilitate the absorption of mercury from the GI tract and should not be given when there is evidence of mercury present in the gut. Because animal studies show that BAL may redistribute mercury to the brain from other tissue sites [36–38] and the brain is a target organ in elemental mercury poisoning, it would seem prudent not to use BAL for the treatment of inhalational exposures. DMSA appears to be associated with fewer adverse events and more efficient mercury excretion when compared with D-penicillamine and is preferred for mercury vapor poisoning. DMSA may enhance urinary mercury excretion and reduce nephrotoxicity after GI absorption of elemental mercury. The initial recommended dose of DMSA is 10 mg per kg every 8 hours, tapering to every 12 hours during the next several days. DMSA can be administered via nasogastric tube in severe poisoning cases in which endotracheal intubation is required.

The therapeutic end points of chelation are poorly defined. Probably the only objectively measurable effectiveness of chelation therapy is enhanced urinary excretion of mercury. A potential end point for chelation may be when the patient's urinary mercury concentration approaches normal. Although the use of chelators is recommended to increase excretion and relieve target organs of metal burden, the use of BAL has not been proved to affect the course of elemental mercury–induced respiratory failure, and the effect of DMSA on clinical outcome has not yet been fully studied.

There does not appear to be a role for multiple-dose activated charcoal, hemoperfusion, or hemodialysis in removing elemental mercury.

Inorganic Mercury

Acute inorganic mercury poisoning is usually the result of intentional or accidental ingestion. Most of the literature on inorganic mercury poisoning deals with mercuric chloride (mercuric bichloride [$HgCl_2$]), with the lethal adult dose estimated to be between 1 and 4 g.

Mercurials are available in medications (antiparasitic, antihelminthic, vermifuge, antiseptic, antipruritic, and disinfectant), paints, stool fixatives, permanent-wave solutions, teething powder, button batteries, fungicides/biocides, folk remedies (Mexican American treatments for "empacho," a chronic stomach ailment; Asian, particularly Chinese, herbal or patent medications), and occult practices (Latin American and Caribbean natives). Although mercurial medications have largely been replaced by less toxic drugs, topical antiseptics containing mercury are still being used.

Pharmacology

Absorption of inorganic mercury salt from the GI tract is probably dose dependent. After absorption, the salt dissociates into the ionic form and is initially distributed between RBCs and plasma. Distribution of mercury within the body and within the organs varies widely. It has been demonstrated by animal autoradiographic study that mercuric ion is accumulated predominantly in the renal cortex. Mercury ions do not appear to significantly cross the blood–brain barrier or the placental barrier. However, on the basis of the autoradiographic study, the brain does take up mercury slowly and retains it for a relatively longer period of time [39]. Mercury ions are eliminated from the body mainly by the urinary and fecal routes. The rate of excretion is dose dependent. Inorganic mercury follows a biphasic elimination rate, initially rapid and then slow, with a biologic half-life of about 60 days in humans.

Mercury ions have an affinity to bind and react with sulfhydryl moieties of proteins, leading to nonspecific inhibition of enzyme systems and pathologic alteration of cellular membranes. In addition, inorganic mercurials are highly corrosive substances.

The target organs of inorganic mercury poisoning are the GI tract and kidneys. The caustic property of the inorganic mercurials could potentially cause damage throughout GI tract, including corrosive stomatitis, necrotizing esophagitis, gastritis, and ulcerative colitis. A report of postmortem examination of patients who died within 48 hours postingestion showed severe hemorrhagic necrosis of the upper GI wall. Acute oliguric renal failure and uremia may result from acute tubular necrosis of the distal portions of the proximal convoluted tubules [40,41]. The CNS is usually spared because only small amounts of mercuric ion can cross the blood–brain barrier. However, cases of CNS toxicity have been described with chronic mercury ingestion.

Clinical Toxicity

The clinical effects of acute inorganic mercury poisoning can be divided into the initial local corrosive effect on the GI tract, followed by the injury that occurs at the site of excretion, which are the kidneys.

Inorganic mercury is a highly caustic substance. Depending on the amount ingested, the GI symptoms that follow may vary from mild gastritis to severe necrotizing ulceration of the intestinal mucosa, which can be fatal within a few hours. Ingestion of 100 mg of inorganic mercury has been reported to be associated with a bitter metallic taste in the mouth, a sense of constriction about the throat, substernal burning, gastritis, abdominal pains, nausea, and vomiting. Abrupt onset of hematemesis, hemorrhagic gastroenteritis, and abdominal pain are expected following a serious acute ingestion, and intestinal necrosis may ensue. In addition, massive bleeding from the colon has been reported as late as 8 to 9 days postingestion. Most of the bleeding came from the rectum, which was the most severely involved section of the colon. Such injuries to the GI tract can lead to massive fluid, electrolyte, and blood loss, resulting in shock and death.

Acute inorganic mercury ingestion may lead to acute oliguric renal failure. Invariably, those patients who develop renal involvement initially have severe GI symptoms. Typically, oliguric renal failure occurs within 72 hours postingestion, and, as such, the initial GI symptoms may be resolving although renal toxicity ensues. Spontaneous resolution of acute toxic anuria with renal tubular regeneration may be expected to occur between 8 and 12 days [42], with clinical recovery (if it occurs) between 9 and 14 days. Chronic exposure may result in CNS toxicity.

Diagnostic Evaluation

Diagnosis depends on integration of characteristic findings with a history of known or potential exposure and presence of elevated whole blood mercury concentration and urinary mercury excretion. Inorganic mercury may be visualized on an abdominal radiograph as radiopaque foreign bodies in the GI tract. A positive radiograph would support the diagnosis, but a negative one would not exclude it.

Whole blood and urinary mercury concentrations (see "Elemental Mercury" section) are useful in confirming exposure. Whole blood mercury concentration >50 μg per dL in acute inorganic mercury poisoning is often associated with gastroenteritis and acute renal tubular necrosis.

Management

General management considerations are the same as for elemental mercury poisoning. In patients with acute ingestion, GI decontamination should be performed as soon as possible to minimize absorption and decrease the corrosive effect of the ingested inorganic salt. As with the ingestion of any corrosive substance, inducing emesis is to be discouraged. Elective tracheal intubation may be prudent before attempting GI decontamination. Gastric lavage should be performed with caution as the GI tract may have already been severely damaged. Endoscopy is recommended if corrosive injury (drooling, dysphagia, and abdominal pain) is suspected. Although theoretically reasonable but not rigorously studied, the use of a protein gastric lavage solution (1 pint of skim milk with 50 g of glucose, 20 g of sodium bicarbonate, and 3 eggs beaten into a mixture) to bind the mercury has been suggested, along with rinsing the stomach with egg white or concentrated human albumin after the lavage [41]. Activated charcoal may be considered as 1 g of charcoal is capable of binding 850 mg of mercuric chloride.

In cases in which there is radiographic evidence of radiopaque foreign bodies in the GI tract and if there is no evidence of gastroenteritis, WBI with polyethylene glycol electrolyte solution should be considered. Repeat abdominal radiographs may be used to document the effectiveness of WBI.

Gastrointestinal injury may result in severe fluid, electrolyte, and blood loss, and attention should be given to monitoring the patient's volume status. Replace intravascular and GI losses by the appropriate administration of crystalloids, colloids, and blood products. An indwelling Foley catheter should be placed to carefully monitor the urine output, which should be maintained at 2 to 3 mL/kg/h. It is important to distinguish between oliguria due to inadequate volume resuscitation and oliguria due to toxic nephropathy resulting in renal failure. Invasive hemodynamic monitoring may be necessary.

It should be remembered that inorganic mercury is a highly corrosive substance. Aggressive surgical intervention may be required in cases in which there is severe gastric necrosis or when hemorrhagic ulcerative colitis becomes life threatening. It has been suggested that the rectum should be resected at the time of colectomy when it is indicated for controlling hemorrhage from the colon [40].

British anti-Lewisite and DMSA (see "Arsenic" and "Lead" sections) are the chelating agents of choice. The effectiveness of BAL depends on the promptness of its administration and the administration of an adequate dose. BAL is most effective if given within 4 hours of ingestion [43]. Prompt intervention is paramount in reducing renal injury, and so expedient chelation therapy would be prudent in suspected cases of acute inorganic mercury poisoning. Chelation should not be withheld while waiting for laboratory confirmation of mercury poisoning. DMSA is also effective, but the capacity of the GI tract to absorb orally administered DMSA may be very much impaired in cases of severe inorganic mercury poisoning when hemorrhagic gastroenteritis, hemodynamic instability, and splanchnic edema are present. Once the GI and cardiovascular status has been stabilized, chelation with DMSA may be substituted for BAL.

Once renal damage has occurred from inorganic mercury poisoning, therapy should be directed at the acute renal failure that may ensue. Hemodialysis should be used to support the patient through the oliguric or anuric renal failure period. A potential problem arises with continued BAL therapy in patients who develop renal insufficiency because the kidneys are one of the main routes by which BAL-Hg is eliminated. In such circumstances, BAL therapy may be judiciously continued as there is some evidence from animal studies that a significant fraction of BAL-Hg is also excreted in the bile. Some studies suggest hemodialysis may contribute to the elimination of BAL-Hg in patients with renal failure. For a patient who has renal failure but is otherwise stable and has a functional GI tract, DMSA is an alternative to BAL.

Organic Mercury

The organomercurials are compounds in which the mercury atom is joined to a carbon atom via a covalent bond. It is the relative stability of this covalent bond that determines the toxicology of the organic mercury compounds. The organomercurials can be classified as short-chain alkyl (methyl-, ethyl-, and propylmercury), long-chain alkyl, and aryl (phenyl) mercury compounds. In general, the short-chain alkyl group, particularly methylmercury, is considered the most toxic. Acute ingestion of 10 to 60 mg per kg of methylmercury may be lethal, and chronic daily ingestion of 10 μg per kg may be associated with adverse neurologic and reproductive effects.

Potential sources of exposure to organic mercury include herbicide, fungicide, germicide, and timber preservative. In the general population, the major source of exposure to methylmercury is through the consumption of predacious fish (e.g., pike, tuna, swordfish). Major incidents of human poisoning with methylmercury have occurred (Minamata and Iraq epidemics) with devastating outcomes.

Pharmacology

Organic mercury antiseptics undergo limited skin penetration; however, in rare cases, such as topical application to an infected omphalocele, dermal absorption can occur.

Methylmercury is well absorbed after inhalation, ingestion, and probably dermal exposure. It is widely distributed throughout the body. In the blood, more than 90% is found in the RBCs, with whole blood–to–plasma ratios of 200:1 to 300:1 [44]. Methylmercury is present in the body as water-soluble complexes mainly attached to thiol ligands and is highly mobile. It enters the endothelial cells of the blood–brain barrier as a specific complex with L-cysteine. This L-cysteine complex is structurally similar to the large neutral amino acid L-methionine and is carried across the cell membrane on the large neutral amino acid carrier [45]. Methylmercury is transported out of mammalian cells as a complex with reduced glutathione and is secreted into bile as a glutathione complex. The glutathione moiety is degraded in the bile duct and gallbladder and finally to the L-cysteine complex. It is reabsorbed and returned to the liver, thereby completing the enterohepatic cycle [46]. In humans, about 10% of the body's methylmercury burden is in the CNS and the biologic half-life of methylmercury is 45 to 70 days. Methylmercury readily passes the blood–brain barrier as well as the placenta barrier. In animal studies, the dissociation between the carbon and mercury bond of methylmercury is very slow [44], and phenylmercury undergoes rapid breakdown to inorganic mercury within 24 hours. In humans, the major route of excretion of methylmercury is in the feces, with less than 10% appearing in the urine. Extensive enterohepatic recirculation in the GI tract has been demonstrated to occur with methylmercury [47].

Mercury has an affinity to bind and react with sulfhydryl moieties of proteins, leading to nonspecific inhibition of enzyme systems and pathologic alteration of cellular membranes. The CNS is particularly vulnerable to the toxic effects of methylmercury and is a potent teratogen and reproductive toxin. Methylmercury has been shown to alter brain ornithine decarboxylase, an enzyme associated with cellular maturity, and neurotransmitter uptake at the pre- and postsynaptic adrenergic receptor sites.

Clinical Toxicity

Most of the detailed information regarding toxicity has been derived from methylmercury poisoning cases. Methylmercury is a cumulative poison, primarily affecting the CNS. There does not appear to be a distinct difference between acute and chronic methylmercury poisoning. Following acute methylmercury intoxication, symptoms are usually delayed for several weeks or months. The classic triad of methylmercury poisoning is *dysarthria*, *ataxia*, and *constricted visual fields* [48]. Other signs and symptoms include paresthesias, hearing impairment, progressive incoordination, loss of voluntary movement, and mental retardation. Perinatal exposure to methylmercury has caused mental retardation and a cerebral palsy type of syndrome in offspring. Ethylmercury compounds may also cause gastroenteritis. Phenylmercury compounds produce a pattern of toxicity intermediate between alkyl and inorganic mercury.

Diagnostic Evaluation

Diagnosis depends on integration of characteristic findings with a history of known or potential exposure, and presence of elevated whole blood mercury concentration, which may reflect recent exposure. Whole blood mercury concentrations greater than 20 μg per dL have been associated with symptoms. Hair concentrations have been used to document remote exposure. Urinary mercury concentrations are not useful.

Management

General management considerations are the same as for elemental mercury poisoning. Following acute ingestion of organic mercurials, gastric lavage should be performed. Administration of activated charcoal may be of benefit. A successful way to increase the rate of methylmercury excretion is to introduce a nonabsorbable mercury-binding substance (polythiol resin) into the GI tract so as to interrupt the enterohepatic recirculation of methylmercury [49,50]. Repeated oral administration of a polythiol resin in methylmercury intoxication may be beneficial.

Limited data suggest that oral neostigmine may improve motor strength in patients with moderate-to-severe chronic methylmercury intoxication. DMSA is the preferred chelating agent. BAL appears to be ineffective in treating neurologic signs and symptoms of methylmercury poisoning. In addition, animal studies show that BAL may redistribute mercury to the brain from other tissue sites [36–38]. In contrast, DMSA was effective in reducing the brain concentration of methylmercury, and DMSA prevented the development of cerebellar damage in methylmercury-poisoned animals [51]. However, in humans, the effect of DMSA on clinical outcome has not yet been fully studied.

Hemodialysis is of little value because methylmercury has a large volume of distribution, and a considerable amount of methylmercury resides within the RBCs.

References

1. Mahieu P, Buchet JP, Roels HA, et al: The metabolism of arsenic in humans acutely intoxicated by As_2O_3. Its significance for the duration of BAL therapy. *Clin Toxicol* 18:1067, 1981.
2. Au WY, Kwong YL: Arsenic trioxide: safety issues and their management. *Acta Pharmacol Sin* 29:296–304, 2008.
3. Beckman KJ, Bauman JL, Pimental PA, et al: Arsenic-induced torsade de pointes. *Crit Care Med* 19:290, 1991.
4. Kyle RA, Pease GL: Hematologic aspects of arsenic intoxication. *N Engl J Med* 273:18, 1965.
5. Heyman A, Pfeiffer JB, Willett RW, et al: Peripheral neuropathy caused by arsenical intoxication. *N Engl J Med* 254:401, 1956.
6. Jenkins RB: Inorganic arsenic and the nervous system. *Brain* 89:479, 1966.
7. Donofrio PD, Wilbourn AJ, Albers JW, et al: Acute arsenic intoxication presenting as Guillain-Barre-like syndrome. *Muscle Nerve* 10:114, 1987.
8. Fesmire FM, Schauben JL, Roberge RJ: Survival following massive arsenic ingestion. *Am J Emerg Med* 6:602, 1988.
9. Shannon RL, Strayer DS: Arsenic-induced skin toxicity. *Hum Toxicol* 8:99, 1989.
10. Eagle M, Magnuson HJ: The systemic treatment of 227 cases of arsenic poisoning (encephalitis, dermatitis, blood dyscrasias, jaundice, fever) with 2,3 dimercaptopropanol (BAL). *Am J Syph Gonor Ven Dis* 30:420, 1946.
11. Peterson RG, Rumack BH: D-penicillamine therapy of acute arsenic poisoning. *J Pediatr* 91:661, 1977.
12. Tye M, Siegel JM: Prevention of reaction to BAL. *JAMA* 134:1477, 1947.
13. Fowler BA, Weissberg JB: Arsine poisoning. *N Engl J Med* 291:1171, 1974.
14. Muehrcke RC, Pirani CL: Arsine-induced anuria: a correlative clinicopathological study with electron microscopic observations. *Ann Intern Med* 68:853, 1968.
15. Macaulay DB, Stanley DA: Arsine poisoning. *Br J Ind Med* 13:217, 1956.
16. Hesdorffer CS, Milne FJ, Terblanche J, et al: Arsine gas poisoning: the importance of exchange transfusions in severe cases. *Br J Ind Med* 43:353, 1986.
17. Song Y, Wang D, Li H, et al: Severe acute arsine poisoning treated by plasma exchange. *Clin Toxicol (Phila)* 45:721–727, 2007.
18. Pino SS, Petronella SJ, Johns DR, et al: Arsine poisoning: a study of thirteen cases. *Arch Ind Hyg Occup Med* 1:437, 1950.
19. Rabinowitz MB, Wetherill GW, Kopple JD: Kinetic analysis of lead metabolism in healthy humans. *J Clin Invest* 58:260, 1976.
20. Thomson RM, Parry GJ: Neuropathies associated with excessive exposure to lead. *Muscle Nerve* 33:732–741, 2006.
21. Cullen MR, Robins JM, Eskenazi B: Adult inorganic lead intoxication: presentation of 31 new cases and a review of recent advances in the literature. *Medicine (Baltimore)* 62:221, 1983.
22. Chisolm JJ Jr: Treatment of lead poisoning. *Mod Treat* 8:593, 1971.
23. Centers for Disease Control and Prevention (CDC): *Managing Elevated Blood Lead Levels Among Young Children: Recommendations from the Advisory Committee on Childhood Lead Poisoning Prevention. March 2002*. Atlanta, GA, CDC. Available at: http://www.cdc.gov/nceh/lead/casemanagement/managingEBLLs.pdf. Accessed December 4, 2015.
24. Coffin R, Phillips JL, Staples WI, et al: Treatment of lead encephalopathy in children. *J Pediatr* 69:198, 1966.
25. Chisolm JJ Jr: The use of chelating agents in the treatment of acute and chronic lead intoxication in childhood. *J Pediatr* 73:1, 1968.
26. Chisolm JJ Jr, Kaplan E: Lead poisoning in childhood-comprehensive management and prevention. *J Pediatr* 73:942, 1968.
27. Jastremski M, Sutton-Tyrrell K, Vaagenes P, et al: Glucocorticoid treatment does not improve neurological recovery following cardiac arrest. *JAMA* 262:3427, 1989.
28. Stocken LA, Thompson RM: Reactions of British anti-lewisite with arsenic and other metals in living systems. *Physiol Rev* 29:168, 1949.
29. Foreman H, Trujillo TT: The metabolism of C^{14}-labeled ethylenediaminetetraacetic acid in human beings. *J Lab Clin Med* 43:566, 1954.
30. Clarkson TW, Magos L: The toxicology of mercury and its chemical compounds. *Crit Rev Toxicol* 36(8):609–662, 2006.
31. Cherian MG, Hursh JB, Clarkson TW, et al: Radioactive mercury distribution in biological fluids and excretion in human subjects after inhalation of mercury vapor. *Arch Environ Health* 33:109, 1978.
32. Asano S, Eto K, Kurisaki E, et al: Acute inorganic mercury vapor inhalation poisoning. *Pathol Int* 50:169–174, 2000.
33. Rusyniak DE, Nanagas KA: Conservative management of elemental mercury retained in the appendix. *Clin Toxicol* 46(9):831–833, 2008.

34. Janus C, Klein B: Aspiration of metallic mercury: clinical significance. *Br J Radiol* 55:675, 1982.
35. Bleach N, McLean LM: The accidental self-injection of mercury: a hazard for glass-blowers. *Arch Emerg Med* 4:53, 1987.
36. Berlin M, Ullrebg S: Increased uptake of mercury in mouse brain caused by 2,3-dimercaptopropanol. *Nature* 197:84, 1963.
37. Berlin M, Lewander T: Increased brain uptake of mercury caused by 2,3-dimercaptopropanol (BAL) in mice given mercuric chloride. *Acta Pharmacol* 22:1, 1965.
38. Canty AJ, Kishimoto R: British anti-lewisite and organomercury poisoning. *Nature* 253:123, 1972.
39. Berlin M, Ullrebg S: Accumulation and retention of mercury in the mouse. *Arch Environ Health* 6:589, 1963.
40. Sanchez-Sicilia L, Seto DS, Nakamoto S, et al: Acute mercurial intoxication treated by hemodialysis. *Ann Intern Med* 59:692, 1963.
41. Schreiner GE, Maher JF: Toxic nephropathy. *Am J Med* 38:409, 1965.
42. Fishman AP, Kroop IG, Leiter HE, et al: A management of anuria in acute mercurial intoxication. *N Y State J Med* 48:2363, 1948.
43. Longcope WT, Luetscher JA Jr, Calkins E, et al: Clinical uses of 2,3 dimercaptopropanol (BAL). *J Clin Invest* 25:557, 1946.
44. Norseth T, Clarkson TW: Studies on the biotransformation of 203 Hg-labeled methyl mercury chloride in rats. *Arch Environ Health* 21:717, 1970.
45. Kerper LE, Ballatori N, Clarkson TW: Methylmercury transport across the blood-brain barrier by an amino acid carrier. *Am J Physiol* 262:R761, 1992.
46. Dutczak WJ, Ballatori N: γ-Glutamyl transferase dependent biliary-hepatic recycling of methyl mercury in the guinea pig. *J Pharmacol Exp Ther* 262:619, 1992.
47. Norseth T, Clarkson TW: Intestinal transport of 203 Hg-labeled methylmercury chloride. *Arch Environ Health* 22:568, 1971.
48. Hunter D, Bonford RR, Russell DS: Poisoning by methylmercury compounds. *Q J Med* 9:193, 1940.
49. Clarkson TW, Small H, Norseth T: The effect of a thiol containing resin on the gastrointestinal absorption and fecal excretion of methylmercury compounds in experimental animals. *Fed Proc* 30:543, 1971.
50. Bakir F, Damluji SF, Amin-Zaki L, et al: Methylmercury poisoning in Iraq. An interuniversity report. *Science* 181:230, 1973.
51. Magos L, Peristianis GC, Snowden RT: Postexposure preventive treatment of methylmercury intoxication in rats with dimercaptosuccinic acid. *Toxicol Appl Pharmacol* 45:463, 1978.

Chapter 113 ■ Hydrocarbon Poisoning

WILLIAM J. LEWANDER • ALFRED ALEGUAS, JR

Hydrocarbons are a group of organic compounds composed primarily of hydrogen and carbon. Although often mixtures, hydrocarbons may be divided into four basic types: aliphatic, halogenated, aromatic, and terpene.

Hydrocarbon exposures are frequent and account for an inordinate number of health care visits and hospital admissions. The American Association of Poison Control Centers reported 32,551 hydrocarbon exposures in 2015 [1]. Twenty-five percent were seen in a health care facility, and there were 18 deaths. Nearly 30% of total exposures occurred in children younger than 6 years of age and involved ingestions, and most of these were accidental. Almost 5% of the fatalities in this age group were related to hydrocarbons during the year of this report [1].

Storage in unmarked, readily accessible containers and an attractive color or aroma account for the high percentage of exposures in young children. In adolescents and adults, poisoning generally results from inhalational abuse, occupational exposure, intentional ingestion, or accidental aspiration during the siphoning of fuels. Cutaneous and even intravenous exposures have also been described. Intentional ingestions by adults usually involve larger volumes, and there is a much greater likelihood of other coingested drugs or toxins. The majority of deaths are caused by intentional inhalational abuse.

ALIPHATIC HYDROCARBONS

Aliphatic hydrocarbons, known as petroleum distillates, are straight-chain compounds produced from the fractional distillation of natural petroleum (Table 113.1). They are the most common cause of hydrocarbon poisoning.

After ingestion, the major toxicity of petroleum distillates is their potential to cause a fulminant, and sometimes fatal, chemical pneumonitis. Aspiration of even small amounts may produce severe pulmonary toxicity. Although vomiting often precedes and precipitates aspiration, lack of vomiting does not preclude the possibility that aspiration has occurred. Little or no systemic toxicity occurs even with intragastric administration of large doses (12 to 18 mL per kg) [2].

The risk of aspiration increases with lower viscosity, lower surface tension, and higher volatility. Viscosity, the tendency to resist flow, is the most important property determining aspiration potential [3]. Substances with low viscosity (e.g., gasoline, mineral seal oil, and kerosene) have a high aspiration potential, whereas those with high viscosity (e.g., mineral oil and fuel oil) have a lower potential for aspiration. Reduced surface tension may also allow a substance to spread rapidly from the upper gastrointestinal (GI) tract to the trachea. High volatility (tendency of a liquid to become a gas) increases the likelihood of pulmonary absorption.

Aspirated petroleum distillates inhibit the function of surfactant, resulting in alveolar collapse, ventilation–perfusion mismatch, and subsequent hypoxemia. In addition, bronchospasm and

TABLE 113.1

Common Petroleum Distillates

Product	Synonym	Main use
Gasoline	Petroleum spirits	Fuel
Petroleum naphtha fluid	Ligroin	Cigarette lighter
VM and P naphtha thinner	Varnish naphtha	Paint or varnish
Mineral spirits	Painter's naphtha	Dry cleaner
	Stoddard solvent	Solvent
	White spirits	Paint thinner
	Varsol	
	Mineral turpentine	
	Petroleum spirits	
Kerosene fluid	Coal oil	Charcoal lighter
		Solvent
		Fuel for stoves, lamps
Fuel oil	Home heating oil	Fuel
Diesel oil	Gas oil	Furniture polish

direct capillary damage lead to a chemical pneumonitis and hemorrhagic bronchitis–alveolitis [3,4]. In animals exposed to kerosene, acute alveolitis peaked at 3 days and resolved by 10 days [4]. Histologically, a chronic proliferative process occurred, peaking at 10 days and resolving over several weeks. When highly viscous petroleum distillates are aspirated, a less inflammatory, more localized, and indolent lipoid pneumonia may occur [5].

Following ingestion of aliphatic hydrocarbons, central nervous system (CNS) manifestations result principally from hypoxia and acidosis caused by pulmonary toxicity [6]. Although systemic toxicity is uncommon, it may be seen if the petroleum distillate is a vehicle for more toxic substances (e.g., heavy metal and pesticide), if it contains additives, or if a concomitant or massive ingestion has occurred [7]. Cardiovascular, hepatic, renal, and hematologic toxicities depend on the specific toxic substance involved.

Use of aliphatic hydrocarbons as volatile substances of abuse (VSA) is a serious and growing problem. It is most often seen in adolescents who use VSA as an easily available, legal, and affordable substitute for other intoxicants [8]. The most common aliphatic VSA are *n*-hexane, *n*-butane, isobutane, and propane—seen in adhesives, aerosols, liquefied petroleum gas (i.e., cigarette lighter refills and camp stoves), and gasoline. Inhalation may involve sniffing, "huffing" (spraying the solvent onto a cloth held to the mouth and nose), "bagging" (spraying the solvent into a paper or plastic bag and repeatedly inhaling the vapors), or a variant of these techniques [8]. These highly lipid-soluble substances are rapidly absorbed through the lungs and distributed to the CNS and fatty tissues [9]. The onset of symptoms occurs in seconds to minutes, with peak effects occurring somewhat later owing to slower diffusion into tissues. Elimination of aliphatic hydrocarbon VSA is primarily by pulmonary excretion, and successive oxidation and metabolism by hepatic cytochrome P450 mixed-function oxidases [9].

Aliphatic VSA toxicity includes acute and chronic neurologic dysfunction; asphyxia; cardiovascular abnormalities; and pulmonary, GI, and cutaneous irritation. CNS toxicity ranges from stimulation at initial or low doses to a depressant effect, with general inhibition of cortical function at high doses [10]. Peripheral neuropathy and irreversible CNS damage have been reported [11,12]. Inhaled aliphatic hydrocarbons are asphyxiants (as well as pulmonary irritants) and may cause hypoxemia by decreasing the concentration of oxygen in inspired air. Their arrhythmogenic effects are thought to be owing to their potentiation of endogenous catecholamines (cardiac sensitization), which may promote dysrhythmias (e.g., ventricular tachycardia or fibrillation) [13]. Additional factors such as hypoxia, acidosis, electrolyte abnormalities, and underlying cardiac conditions may contribute to arrhythmias. Dermal and mucosal irritation is due to their ability to dissolve lipids after prolonged or high-dose exposure [14]. Deaths associated with inhalational abuse may result from coma with respiratory depression, aspiration, or injuries incurred while intoxicated as well as from cardiac arrhythmias [15].

Clinical Manifestations

The clinical course after the ingestion of petroleum distillates primarily depends on the presence or absence of concomitant aspiration and its severity. The patients who aspirate generally demonstrate symptoms within 30 minutes; those who do not have symptoms within 6 hours will remain asymptomatic [16]. Presenting signs and symptoms usually involve three main organ systems: pulmonary, CNS, and GI. Cardiovascular, renal, hematologic, and cutaneous toxicity have also been reported [16,17]. In most cases, symptoms resolve during the next 2 to 5 days with supportive care [16,17].

Initial coughing, gasping, and choking may progress and peak during the first 24 to 48 hours to tachypnea with grunting respirations, nasal flaring, retractions, and cyanosis [7,16]. The odor of petroleum distillates may be apparent on the breath. Wheezing, rhonchi, and rales may be heard on auscultation. In severe cases, pulmonary edema and hemoptysis occur. Arterial blood gases may demonstrate hypoxemia from ventilation–perfusion mismatch and early hypocarbia, which progresses to hypercarbia and acidosis. Abnormalities on chest radiographs occur in up to 75% of hospitalized patients, appearing within 2 hours in 88% of the patients and 12 hours in 98% [7,16], but may be delayed up to 72 hours. Early radiographic abnormalities include unilateral, but more commonly bilateral, basilar infiltrates and fine punctate perihilar densities. Localized areas of atelectasis are often present, whereas pleural effusions, pneumatoceles, and pneumothoraces occur infrequently [18]. Pneumatoceles generally occur 3 to 15 days after ingestion and resolve during 15 days to 21 months [19]. Radiographic findings correlate poorly with clinical symptoms and may persist for several days to weeks after symptoms have resolved [18,19]. Asymptomatic patients may have abnormal chest radiographs, whereas symptomatic patients may have minimal or no radiographic abnormalities early in the course [7].

Within the first 24 to 48 hours, fever (38°C to 39°C) and leukocytosis are common [16]. The persistence of fever beyond 48 hours suggests bacterial superinfection.

CNS involvement may occur in those with aspiration-induced hypoxemia, large intentional ingestions, or ingestions of mixtures that contain other toxic agents (e.g., aromatic hydrocarbons). Symptoms range from dizziness and lethargy (91%) to somnolence (5%) and, rarely, coma (3%) and convulsions (1%) [7]. The severity of CNS dysfunction often correlates with the severity of aspiration.

GI symptoms, such as local irritation of the oropharynx (e.g., burning), nausea, vomiting, and abdominal pain, are commonly reported. Hematemesis and melena occur rarely [7]. Vomiting appears to increase the likelihood of aspiration [20]. Cardiovascular toxicity is uncommon, but dysrhythmias and sudden death after gasoline siphoning have been reported [13,14].

Inhalation abuse may result in a range of acute CNS manifestations, including dizziness, incoordination, restlessness, excitement, euphoria, confusion, hallucinations, slurred speech, and coma with respiratory depression [10,11]. Peripheral neuropathy has been reported after chronic exposure [11]. Pulmonary toxicity may present as respiratory distress with cyanosis, or syncope with tachycardia or bradycardia. GI irritation may cause nausea, vomiting, and abdominal pain. Dermatologic manifestations range from perioral frost or pigmentation (after direct inhalation from a container) to local skin irritation [7].

Cases of acute renal tubular necrosis [21], hemoglobinuria secondary to intravascular hemolysis [22], severe burns after prolonged immersion in gasoline [23], and supraglottitis [24] have been reported. Aliphatic hydrocarbons are highly flammable, especially gasoline, and accidental thermal burns may occur during recreational use [25]. Therefore, the patients with unexplained burns should be questioned regarding possible inhalation abuse. Chronic leaded gasoline inhalation may also be accompanied by organolead poisoning [26]. Parenteral administration of petroleum distillates has caused local cellulitis, thrombophlebitis, and necrotizing myositis, with resultant compartment syndromes. Associated systemic effects include febrile reactions, hemorrhagic pneumonitis, pulmonary edema, seizures, and CNS depression [27,28].

Diagnostic Evaluation

After ingestion, diagnostic evaluation includes a thorough history (e.g., identity, amount, and concentration of toxin; time of ingestion; and symptoms before presentation at health care facility) and a physical examination (focusing on vital signs and the respiratory, CNS, and GI systems). Pulse oximetry should be monitored and a chest radiograph obtained in all symptomatic patients and in cases in which aspiration is suspected. In symptomatic patients or those who have ingested concomitant toxins or toxic additives, laboratory evaluation should include an arterial blood gas determination; complete blood cell count; electrolyte, blood urea nitrogen, creatinine, and glucose measurements; liver function tests; and a urinalysis.

Management

The patients with ingestions who remain or become asymptomatic with a normal chest radiograph (obtained 2 hours or more after exposure) may be discharged after 6 hours of observation. All symptomatic patients, those with abnormal chest radiographs, arterial blood gases, or pulse oximetry, and the patients with suicidal intent should be hospitalized. Gastric decontamination is not recommended in petroleum distillate ingestion because absorption and systemic toxicity are minimal, and spontaneous or induced vomiting increases the risk of aspiration and pneumonitis [29]. Gastric decontamination is recommended only if potentially toxic amounts of aromatic or halogenated hydrocarbons, pesticides, heavy metals, or other substances have been ingested within 1 to 2 hours or if time of ingestion is unknown and there are no contradictions. Ipecac syrup is not recommended for GI decontamination. The patients who are unconscious, unable to protect the airway (e.g., poor or absent gag reflex), or deteriorating should be intubated with a cuffed endotracheal tube and then have gastric aspiration or lavage performed. Activated charcoal and cathartic are indicated only if a toxic additive is present or concomitant ingestion has occurred. If cutaneous exposure has occurred, contaminated clothing should be removed cautiously and the skin thoroughly washed with soap and water [7].

All patients with respiratory symptoms should be given oxygen, placed on a cardiac monitor, and have intravenous access established. An arterial blood gas determination and chest radiograph should be obtained. The need for intubation should be based on clinical assessment of respiratory distress and objective data from arterial blood gases or pulse oximetry. Chest radiographs do not always correlate with clinical status and should not be used as the sole determinant for respiratory interventions. Noninvasive ventilation may be helpful for maintaining oxygenation, and the patient should be carefully monitored for the development of a pneumothorax. Bronchospasm should be treated with β_2-agonist bronchodilators [13].

Supportive care of pneumonitis includes careful monitoring of acid–base, fluid, and electrolyte balance (e.g., cautious hydration to avoid pulmonary edema), serial arterial blood gases or pulse oximetry, and chest radiograph evaluation. Complete blood cell counts with differential, sputum, or tracheal aspirate Grams stains and cultures can assist in determining if bacterial superinfection has occurred. Baseline renal and liver function studies and a toxic screen should be obtained if toxic additives or concomitant ingestion is suspected. Animal and clinical investigations have failed to demonstrate any beneficial effect of steroid treatment [30]. Two animal studies indicate that they may be harmful [31,32]. In addition, prophylactic antibiotics have not been shown to be helpful [31]. Fever and leukocytosis secondary to chemical pneumonitis are common during the first 24 to 48 hours in the absence of superimposed bacterial pneumonia [7]. Antibiotics should be given only to patients with documented bacterial pneumonias (based on Gram stain with culture of sputum or tracheal aspirate results) or worsening chest radiograph, leukocytosis, and fever after the first 40 hours [7]. Successful use of high-frequency percussive ventilation and extracorporeal membrane oxygenation for the treatment of respiratory failure has been reported [33–35]. Other measures such as cardiopulmonary bypass, partial liquid fluorocarbon ventilation, and exogenous surfactant have been suggested for refractory cases, but the data to support their use are limited [36].

Most patients with petroleum distillate poisoning recover fully with supportive care. Because minor pulmonary function abnormalities have been detected in as many as 82% of the patients with aspiration pneumonitis who subsequently become asymptomatic [37], follow-up care with pulmonary function testing should be considered. When appropriate, the patient should receive psychiatric evaluation and poison-prevention education before final disposition.

HALOGENATED HYDROCARBONS

Halogenated hydrocarbons are aliphatic and aromatic derivatives that contain one or more atoms of chlorine, bromine, fluorine, or iodine. Although dozens of halogenated hydrocarbons are currently recognized, relatively few account for the majority of the toxic exposures. Like the aliphatic agents, halogenated hydrocarbons pose an aspiration risk. However, they are more readily absorbed from the GI tract and can cause systemic toxicity, most notably of the CNS, cardiovascular system, and hepatic and renal systems.

Halogenated hydrocarbons are used in the household and industry. They are frequently used as solvents, degreasers, dry-cleaning agents, refrigerants, aerosol propellants, and fumigants. Toxic exposures occur most commonly through inhalation, and several halogenated hydrocarbons (e.g., trichloroethylene, methylene chloride, and fluorocarbons) are intentionally inhaled for recreational purposes [11]. Bagging and huffing have been associated with a number of solvent-abuse deaths.

After absorption from the GI tract and occasionally through the skin, halogenated hydrocarbons are concentrated in adipose tissue, liver, and kidney. Metabolism and elimination vary according to the individual substance, with most undergoing at least some excretion through the lungs as unchanged parent compound and nearly all undergoing some degree of metabolism in the liver, with subsequent excretion of metabolites by the lungs and/or kidneys. Carbon tetrachloride (CCl_4), methylene chloride, and trichloroethane are prototypes of this class.

Carbon Tetrachloride

Previously used as a dry-cleaning agent and antihelminthic, CCl_4 is now restricted to industrial use, primarily in the production of refrigerants, aerosol propellants, and solvents. It is well absorbed through the skin [38], lungs, and GI tract, and it is concentrated in adipose tissue [39]. Approximately 50% of an absorbed dose is excreted unchanged by the lungs. Most of the remainder is metabolized by the liver to reactive intermediates or free radicals, or both, which covalently bind to proteins and induce lipid peroxidation, resulting in hepatocellular damage [40]. Ethanol, methanol, and isopropyl alcohol all increase CCl_4 hepatotoxicity, presumably through enzyme induction [41]. At lower doses, fatty degeneration of the liver occurs; at higher concentrations, centrilobular necrosis results [42]. In addition to hepatic damage, CCl_4 produces acute tubular necrosis of the kidney, affecting the proximal tubules and Henle's loop. Although a direct nephrotoxic effect is likely [43], volume contraction may contribute to renal failure in some patients [44].

Inhalation exposure to CCl_4 may produce symptoms ranging from mild CNS depression to coma and death [45]. Although the estimated lethal dose of orally ingested CCl_4 is 90 to 100 mL, deaths have occasionally been reported after much smaller doses.

Nausea, vomiting, abdominal pain, diarrhea, drowsiness, and light-headedness usually occur within a few hours of exposure, regardless of route of exposure. Although liver enzymes may start to rise on the first day after exposure, clinical hepatotoxicity generally occurs on Days 2 to 4, with fever, liver tenderness and enlargement, and jaundice [45]. Decline in renal function may occur concomitantly with hepatic dysfunction, although renal failure occasionally appears in the absence of hepatic failure [46]. Rarely, CCl_4 toxicity is accompanied by coma, convulsions, or myocarditis.

Early fatalities are a result of respiratory depression or cardiac dysrhythmias caused by cardiac sensitization to circulating catecholamines. Later deaths occur as the result of hepatic or renal failure, generally within the first week. In nonfatal cases, liver function tests generally return to normal within 2 weeks; recovery is usually complete.

Treatment initially involves stabilization and monitoring for respiratory depression and cardiac dysrhythmias. Exposure should be interrupted by removing victims of inhalation from the exposure site; in dermal exposures, contaminated clothing should be removed and the skin washed thoroughly. The patients who ingest more than 0.3 mL per kg should undergo gastric aspiration or lavage, preferably within 3 to 4 hours of ingestion [47]. Abdominal radiographs may be helpful in confirming suspected ingestions because CCl_4 is radiopaque [48]. There is no evidence regarding the use of activated charcoal in adsorbing CCl_4. Laboratory evaluation should include a complete blood cell count, routine serum chemistries, liver function tests, and urinalysis. The patients with respiratory symptoms or altered mental status should also be evaluated for possible aspiration pneumonitis, as described for aliphatic hydrocarbon exposures. Although CCl_4 appears not to be well removed by hemodialysis, dialysis may be required in cases of renal failure [49].

Animal studies suggest that hyperbaric oxygen may increase survival after intragastric administration of CCl_4 [50], although little human data exist on this topic [51]. Additional experimental work is being conducted to examine the utility of *N*-acetylcysteine in the reduction of CCl_4-induced hepatotoxicity. Because toxic intermediates of hepatic P450 are thought to be responsible for CCl_4 toxicity, it is thought that *N*-acetylcysteine may help prevent the development of liver failure [52]. Although human experience with this therapy is extremely limited in this setting and still considered experimental, a dosage schedule identical to that for acetaminophen is generally used.

Methylene Chloride

Methylene chloride is a colorless, volatile liquid commonly used as a solvent in aerosol products and as a degreaser and paint remover. It is well absorbed through the lungs and GI tract, but absorption through intact skin appears to be minimal. The majority of a dose is metabolized by the liver to carbon dioxide and carbon monoxide with small amounts exhaled unchanged [53].

The main toxicity of methylene chloride is CNS depression, which results from direct effects and from cellular asphyxia due to elevated levels of carboxyhemoglobin [54]. An 8-hour exposure to 250 ppm of methylene chloride resulted in carboxyhemoglobin fractions greater than 8% [55], and with large exposures, carboxyhemoglobin fractions up to 50% have been reported. In the few cases of methylene chloride ingestion that have been reported, CNS depression, tachypnea, and corrosive injury to the GI tract were the most common findings [56]. When the carboxyhemoglobin fraction is elevated, signs and symptoms of carbon monoxide poisoning may also be evident [57]. Nephrotoxicity and hepatotoxicity have also been reported [58,59].

Treatment involves stabilization, evaluation, and monitoring for aspiration, CNS and cardiovascular depression, dysrhythmias, corrosive injury, carbon monoxide poisoning, and hepatic and renal dysfunction. The patient should be removed from the source of inhalation exposure, and contaminated clothing should be removed. Exposed skin should be washed with soap and water. In cases of ingestion, gastric aspiration, or lavage should be considered. The role of activated charcoal in methylene chloride ingestions is unclear [60]. In all cases, the carboxyhemoglobin fraction as well as complete blood cell count, routine serum chemistries, liver function tests, and urinalysis should be determined and supplemental oxygen provided.

Hyperbaric oxygen is controversial for carbon monoxide poisoning and its role in methylene chloride toxicity is even less clear [61]. It is reasonable to institute hyperbaric therapy when elevated carboxyhemoglobin levels and symptoms of carbon monoxide toxicity are present. Management is otherwise supportive.

Trichloroethane

1,1,1-Trichloroethane has been widely marketed as a safer alternative to CCl_4 for use as a cleaning agent and degreaser. It is also present in typewriter correction fluid and aerosol hairsprays, water repellents, and furniture polishes. In spite of its relative safety, death can occur, usually as a result of occupational or recreational inhalation exposure [62,63].

Trichloroethane is rapidly absorbed through the lungs and GI tract. Under most circumstances, significant cutaneous absorption is unlikely. Distribution is greatest to tissues with a high concentration of lipid, including the CNS. Most of an absorbed dose is excreted unchanged through the lungs, with smaller quantities metabolized in the liver and excreted by the kidneys [7,9].

Toxicity primarily involves the CNS, with signs and symptoms ranging from dizziness, headache, fatigue, and ataxia with mild-to-moderate exposures to seizures, coma, apnea, and death at higher vapor concentrations [64].

As with the aliphatic hydrocarbons, trichloroethane-induced cardiac sensitization to the effects of circulating catecholamines is thought to be responsible for sudden death associated with inhalational exposure [65]. Premature ventricular contractions and ST depression have been observed after acute inhalation [66], and myocarditis has been reported after chronic inhalation abuse [67]. Hepatic and renal toxicities are rare.

Management involves the evaluation and treatment for aspiration, CNS and cardiovascular depression, and dysrhythmias. Decontamination measures may also be appropriate. In the absence of sudden death, recovery is generally rapid and complete.

AROMATIC HYDROCARBONS

Aromatic hydrocarbons contain one or more benzene rings. They include benzene, toluene, xylene, diphenyl, phenol, and styrene. Aromatic hydrocarbons are common constituents of glues, paints, paint removers, lacquers, degreasers, and adhesives. Although the aromatic hydrocarbons have aspiration risks similar to those of the other hydrocarbons, they also exhibit potentially severe systemic toxicity. Exposure is primarily through inhalation (occupational or abuse) or from ingestion. Benzene, toluene, and xylene are the three most commonly encountered agents.

Benzene

Benzene is a colorless liquid used widely in the chemical industry and less commonly as a solvent. It is well absorbed through the lungs and GI tract, but absorption through the skin is limited [68]. The lungs excrete up to 50% of an absorbed dose unchanged, whereas most of the remaining amount is metabolized by hepatic P450 enzymes to potentially cytotoxic metabolites,

[69]. Elimination of the parent compound and its metabolites generally occurs within 48 hours.

Benzene has acute and chronic toxicity. Acute exposure primarily causes CNS depression [70]. Initial euphoria is rapidly followed by nausea, dizziness, and headache; subsequent progression to ataxia, seizures, and coma may occur. Persistent symptoms may include insomnia, anorexia, and headache.

Inhalation of high concentrations may lead to development of pulmonary edema; as with other hydrocarbons, aspiration, and cardiac dysrhythmias may develop. Long-term exposure to benzene may result in a depression of bone marrow elements, which may progress to aplastic anemia [71]. Epidemiologic studies also suggest an increased risk of acute myelocytic and monocytic leukemia in workers with prolonged exposure to benzene [72].

Management should focus on stabilizing the patients, and evaluation and monitoring for aspiration, CNS and cardiovascular depression, and dysrhythmias. It is generally agreed that amounts in excess of 1 to 2 mL per kg should be removed from the GI tract (via gastric aspiration or lavage), although some sources recommend removal of virtually any amount. The role of activated charcoal in this setting is unproven [7]. Subsequent therapy is supportive.

Toluene

Toluene is a colorless, volatile, and sweet-smelling liquid that is a common ingredient in paints, paint thinners, lacquers, and glues (e.g., airplane model glue). Although toxicity may occur accidentally in industry or in the household, toluene is one of the most commonly abused solvents [73]. It is highly lipid soluble, and peak blood concentrations occur within 15 to 30 minutes with inhalation [45]. Animal studies suggest that ingested toluene is well absorbed from the GI tract, within 1 to 2 hours after exposure. Absorption through intact skin is slow.

Approximately 20% of an absorbed dose is exhaled unchanged. Most of the remainder is metabolized by the liver's cytochrome P450 system. Elimination is biphasic, with an initial α-phase having a half-life of 4 to 5 hours [74] and representing exhalation combined with distribution to fatty tissues [9]. The β-phase has an apparent half-life of 15 to 20 hours and represents hepatic metabolism.

Toxic effects involve the CNS and peripheral nervous system as well as the kidney and heart [75]. Electrolyte and metabolic disturbances may also result. Acute exposure to toluene has variable effects on the CNS, depending on the concentration and duration of exposure [73]. Initially, toluene causes intoxication, which can progress to coma with prolonged exposure to high concentrations. Chronic abuse may also lead to persistent signs and symptoms of acute toxicity, including neuropsychiatric symptoms, weakness, nausea, vomiting, peripheral neuropathy, rhabdomyolysis [73], and abdominal pain [8]. Toluene toxicity is associated with a high incidence of renal dysfunction, particularly renal tubular acidosis (i.e., bicarbonate wasting) [73,76]. Laboratory findings include metabolic acidosis (generally without an increased anion gap), electrolyte disturbances (e.g., hypokalemia, hypocalcemia, hypophosphatemia, and hyperchloremia), and hematuria, proteinuria, and pyuria [76]. These abnormalities are the result of tubulointerstitial damage and are generally reversible on cessation of exposure. As with other hydrocarbons, acute toluene inhalation has also been associated with sudden cardiorespiratory arrest [77].

The diagnosis of toluene poisoning is generally made on the basis of the history, with known exposure or solvent abuse the prominent features. Toluene toxicity should also be considered in any individual with altered mental status and metabolic acidosis of unclear cause [78]. Management includes evaluation and treatment for aspiration; CNS and cardiovascular depression; dysrhythmias; renal dysfunction; fluid, electrolyte, and acid–base disturbances; and rhabdomyolysis. Laboratory testing should include calcium and phosphate levels. Gastric aspiration or lavage may be appropriate in cases of ingestion (with recognition of the aspiration risk).

Xylene

Xylene is a clear liquid that is widely used as a solvent in paints and lacquers, degreasers, adhesives, cleaning agents, and aviation fuel. It is rapidly absorbed by the pulmonary and GI systems and, to some extent, through the skin. The highest concentrations are found in the adrenal gland, bone marrow, spleen, brain, and blood [45]. Small amounts are excreted unchanged through the lungs; most of the remainder is metabolized in the liver and metabolites excreted in the urine. Ethanol consumption causes delays to metabolic clearance of xylene.

Xylene primarily affects the CNS [79]. As with other hydrocarbons, inhalation has been associated with sudden death, presumably secondary to cardiac dysrhythmia [80]. At low doses, headache, nausea, light-headedness, and ataxia may develop; at higher doses, confusion, coma, and respiratory depression may develop. Hepatic damage, Fanconi syndrome, and pulmonary edema have also been described [80,81]. The evaluation and treatment of xylene exposure are similar to that described for other aromatic hydrocarbons.

TERPENES

Terpenes are aliphatic cyclic hydrocarbons. They include turpentine, pine oil, and camphor. Camphor is discussed elsewhere [7,82]. As its name suggests, pine oil is the product of pine trees and composed primarily of terpene alcohols. It is a component in household cleaners (e.g., Pine-Sol, Clorox Company, Oakland, CA), normally present in concentrations of 20% to 35%, but occasionally in concentrations exceeding 60%. Turpentine is a pine tree distillate commonly used as a solvent for paint and varnish.

Toxicity almost always results from ingestion. The aspiration risk appears to be somewhat less than that of other aliphatic hydrocarbons, presumably because of the lower volatility of terpenes; CNS and GI effects are more pronounced, however. Ingestions of more than 2 mL per kg of turpentine are considered potentially toxic [83]. Although 60 to 120 g of pine oil is commonly cited as the lethal dose in adults, survival has been reported after ingestion of 400 to 500 g [84]. The minimal lethal dose of pine oil reported in children is 14 g [85].

Turpentine is well absorbed through the lungs and GI tract [83] and distributed throughout the body, with highest concentrations in the liver, spleen, brain, and kidney [83]. Although the specifics of its metabolism are unclear, turpentine or its metabolites are largely excreted through the kidney. Pine oil is also well absorbed from the GI tract, and after absorption, it is metabolized by the epoxide pathway and excreted in the urine [84]. Although the volume of distribution is unknown, it is thought to be large, with high concentrations in the brain, kidney, and lung.

Manifestations of toxicity include nausea, vomiting, diarrhea, weakness, somnolence, or agitation. In severe cases, stupor or coma may result, although seizures appear to be uncommon [86]. Systemic toxicity, when it occurs, usually develops within 2 to 3 hours of ingestion. In mild and moderate cases, GI and CNS symptoms generally resolve within 12 hours. Turpentine ingestion has been associated with hemorrhagic cystitis, with dysuria and hematuria occurring 12 hours to 3 days after exposure [87].

Management includes the evaluation and treatment for aspiration, gastroenteritis, and CNS depression. The distinctive odors of turpentine and pine oil may provide a clue to diagnosis.

Gastric aspiration or lavage is recommended for patients who present within 2 hours of ingesting greater than 2 mL per kg of turpentine or 5 mL of pure pine oil [88]. Because of the risk of aspiration, airway protection should be considered in all but the most alert patients.

The patients who remain asymptomatic or have only mild GI or CNS symptoms 6 hours after ingestion are unlikely to develop serious complications. The patients with pulmonary complications or severe CNS depression require intensive care unit admission and often require ventilatory support.

References

1. Mowry JB, Spyker DA, Brooks DE, et al: 2015 Annual Report of the American Association of Poison Control Centers' National Poison Data System (NPDS): 33rd Annual Report. *Clin Tox* 54:924–1109, 2016.
2. Wolfe B, Brodeur A, Shields J: The role of gastrointestinal absorption of kerosene in producing pneumonitis in dogs. *Pediatrics* 76:867, 1970.
3. Gerarde HW: Toxicologic studies on hydrocarbons IX. The aspiration hazard and toxicity of hydrocarbons and hydrocarbon mixtures. *Arch Environ Health* 6:329, 1963.
4. Gross P, McNemey JM, Babyale MA: Kerosene pneumonitis: an experimental study with small doses. *Am Rev Respir Dis* 88:656, 1963.
5. Beermann B, Christensson T, Moller P, et al: Lipoid pneumonia: an occupational hazard of fire-eaters. *Br Med J* 289:1728, 1984.
6. Wolfsdorf J: Kerosene intoxication: an experimental approach to the etiology of the CNS manifestations in primates. *J Pediatr* 88:1037, 1976.
7. Shannon MW, Borron SW, Burns MJ: *Haddad and Winchester's Clinical Management of Poisoning and Drug Overdose, Petroleum Distillates*. 4th ed. Philadelphia, PA, Saunders Elsevier, 2007, pp 1343–1346.
8. Williams JF, Storck M: Inhalant abuse. *Pediatrics* 119:1009–1017, 2007.
9. Baselt RC, Caravey RH: *Disposition of Toxic Drugs and Chemicals in Man*. 5th ed. Foster City, CA, Chemical Toxicology Institute, 1995, p 235.
10. Sandmeyer EE: Aliphatic hydrocarbons, in Clayton GD, Clayton FE (eds): *Patty's Industrial Hygiene and Toxicology*. 5th ed. New York, NY, John Wiley and Sons, 2000, p 3175.
11. Kurtzmann TL, Otsuka KN, Wahl RA: Inhalant abuse by adolescents. *J Adolesc Health* 28:170–180, 2001
12. Hormes J, Filley C, Rosenberg N: Neurologic sequelae of chronic solvent vapor abuse. *Neurology* 36:698, 1986.
13. Brock WJ, Rusch WJ, Trochimowitz HJ: Cardiac sensitization: methodology and interpretation in risk assessment. *Regul Toxicol Pharmacol* 38:78–90, 2003.
14. Fortenberry JD: Gasoline sniffing. *Am J Med* 79:740, 1985.
15. Anderson HR, Dick B, MacNair RS, et al: An investigation of 140 deaths associated with volatile substance abuse in the United Kingdom (1971–1981). *Hum Toxicol* 1:207, 1982.
16. Anas N, Namasonthia V, Ginsburg CM: Criteria for hospitalizing children who have ingested products containing hydrocarbons. *JAMA* 246:840, 1981.
17. Anene O, Castello FV: Myocardial dysfunction after hydrocarbon ingestion. *Crit Care Med* 22:528, 1994.
18. Eade NR, Taussig LM, Marks MI: Hydrocarbon pneumonitis. *Pediatrics* 54:351, 1974.
19. Bergeson PS, Hales SW, Lustgarten MD, et al: Pneumatoceles following hydrocarbon ingestion. *Am J Dis Child* 129:49, 1975.
20. Bratton L, Haddow JE: Ingestion of charcoal lighter fluid. *J Pediatr* 87:633, 1974.
21. Battle DC, Sabatini S, Kurzman NA: On the mechanism of toluene-induced renal tubular acidosis. *Nephron* 49:210–218, 1988.
22. Adler R, Robinson RG, Bindin NJ: Intravascular hemolysis: an unusual complication of hydrocarbon ingestion. *J Pediatr* 89:679, 1976.
23. Walsh WA, Scarpa FJ, Brown RS, et al: Gasoline immersion burn case report. *N Engl J Med* 291:830, 1974.
24. Grufferman S, Walker FW: Supraglottitis following gasoline ingestion. *Ann Emerg Med* 11:368, 1982.
25. Cole M, Herndon HN, Desai MH, et al: Gasoline explosions, gasoline sniffing: an epidemic in young adolescents. *J Burn Care Rehabil* 7:532, 1986.
26. Chessare JD, Wodarcyk K: Gasoline sniffing and lead poisoning in a child. *Am Fam Physician* 38:181, 1988.
27. Neeld EM, Limacher MC: Chemical pneumonitis after the intravenous injection of hydrocarbons. *Radiology* 129:36, 1978.
28. Tenenbein M: Pediatric toxicology: current controversies and recent advances. *Curr Probl Pediatr* 16:185, 1986.
29. Litovitz T, Green AE: Health implications of petroleum distillate ingestion. *Occup Med* 3:555, 1988.
30. Steele RW, Conklin RH, Mark HM: Corticosteroids and antibiotics for the treatment of fulminant hydrocarbon aspiration. *JAMA* 219:1424, 1972.
31. Brown J, Burke B, Dajani AS: Experimental kerosene pneumonia: evaluation of some therapeutic regimens. *J Pediatr* 84:396, 1974.
32. Marks MI, Chicoine L, Legere G, et al: Adrenocorticosteroid treatment of hydrocarbon pneumonia in children. A cooperative study. *J Pediatr* 81:366, 1972.
33. Liebelt EI, DeAngelis CD: Evolving trends and treatment advances in pediatric poisoning. *JAMA* 282:1113, 1999.
34. Mabe TG, Honecutt T, Cairns BA, et al: High frequency percussive ventilation in a pediatric patient with hydrocarbon aspiration. *Ped Crit Care* 8:383–385, 2007.
35. Chyka PA: Benefits of extracorporeal membrane oxygenation for hydrocarbon pneumonitis. *J Toxicol Clin Toxicol* 34:357, 1996.
36. Willson DF, Thomas NJ, Markovitz BP, et al: Effect of exogenous surfactant (Calfactant) in pediatric acute lung injury: a randomized controlled trial. *JAMA* 293(4):470–476, 2005.
37. Gurwitz D, Kattan M, Levison H, et al: Pulmonary function abnormalities in asymptomatic children after hydrocarbon pneumonitis. *Pediatrics* 62:789, 1978.
38. Javier Perez A, Courel M, Sobrado J, et al: Acute renal failure after topical application of carbon tetrachloride. *Lancet* 1:515, 1987.
39. Sanzgiri UY, Srivatsan V, Muralidhara S, et al: Uptake, distribution, and elimination of carbon tetrachloride in rat tissues following inhalation and ingestion exposures. *Toxicol Appl Pharmacol* 143:120, 1997.
40. Castro GD, Diaz Gomez MI, Castro JA: DNA bases attack by reactive metabolites produced during carbon tetrachloride biotransformation and promotion of liver microsomal lipid peroxidation. *Res Commun Mol Pathol Pharmacol* 95:253, 1997.
41. Cornish HH, Adefuin J: Potentiation of carbon tetrachloride toxicity by aliphatic alcohols. *Arch Environ Health* 14:447, 1967.
42. Plaa GL: Chlorinated methanes and liver injury: highlights of the past 50 years. *Annu Rev Pharmacol Toxicol* 40:42, 2000.
43. Koren G: The nephrotoxic potential of drugs and chemicals. Pharmacological basis and clinical relevance. *Med Toxicol Adverse Drug Exp* 4:59, 1989.
44. Sinicrope RA, Gordon JA, Little JR, et al: Carbon tetrachloride nephrotoxicity: a reassessment of pathophysiology based upon the urinary diagnostic indices. *Am J Kidney Dis* 3:362, 1984.
45. Bergman K: Application and results of whole-body autoradiography in distribution studies of organic solvents. *Crit Rev Toxicol* 12:59, 1983.
46. Alston WC: Hepatic and renal complications arising from accidental carbon tetrachloride poisoning in the human subject. *Clin Pathol* 23:249, 1970.
47. Fogel RP, Davidman M, Poleski MH, et al: Carbon tetrachloride poisoning treated with hemodialysis and total parenteral nutrition. *Can Med Assoc J* 128:560, 1983.
48. McGuigan MA: Carbon tetrachloride. *Clin Toxicol Rev* 9:1, 1987.
49. Spiegel SM, Hyams BB: Radiographic demonstration of a toxic agent. *J Can Assoc Radiol* 34:204, 1984.
50. Burk RF, Reiter R, Lane JM: Hyperbaric oxygen protection against carbon tetrachloride hepatotoxicity in rats: association with altered metabolism. *Gastroenterology* 90:812, 1986.
51. Burkhart KK, Hall AH, Gerace R, et al: Hyperbaric oxygen treatment for carbon tetrachloride poisoning. *Drug Saf* 6:332, 1991.
52. Simko V, Michael S, Katz J, et al: Protective effect of oral acetylcysteine against the hepatorenal toxicity of carbon tetrachloride potentiated by ethyl alcohol. *Alcohol Clin Exp Res* 16:795, 1992.
53. Jonsson F, Bois F, Johanson G: Physiologically based pharmacokinetic modeling of inhalation exposure of humans to dichloromethane during moderate to heavy exercise. *Toxicol Sci* 59:209, 2001.
54. Dhillon S, Von Burg R: Methylene chloride. *J Appl Toxicol* 15:329, 1995.
55. Lawwerys RR: *Industrial Chemical Exposure:Guidelines for Biological Monitoring*. Davis, CA, Biomedical, 1983, p 83.
56. Chang YL, Yang CC, Deng JF, et al: Diverse manifestations of oral methylene chloride poisoning: report of 6 cases. *J Toxicol Clin Toxicol* 37:497, 1999.
57. Agency for Toxic Substances and Disease Registry: Methylene chloride toxicity. *Am Fam Physician* 47:1159, 1993.
58. Miller L, Pateras V, Friederici H, et al: Acute tubular necrosis after inhalation exposure to methylene chloride. *Arch Intern Med* 145:145, 1985.
59. Kim H: A case of acute toxic hepatitis after suicidal chloroform and dichloromethane ingestion. *Am J Emerg Med* 26(9):1073.e3–1073.e6, 2008.
60. Soslow A: Methylene chloride. *Clin Toxicol Rev* 9:1, 1987.
61. Rudge FW: Treatment of methylene chloride induced carbon monoxide poisoning with hyperbaric oxygenation. *Mil Med* 155:570, 1990.
62. King GS, Smialek JE, Troutman WG: Sudden death in adolescents resulting from the inhalation of typewriter correction fluid. *JAMA* 253:1604, 1985.
63. Jones RD, Winters DP: Two case reports of deaths on industrial premises attributed to 1,1,1-trichloroethane. *Arch Environ Health* 38:59, 1983.
64. Laine A, Seppalainen AM, Savolainen K, et al: Acute effects of 1,1,1-trichloroethane inhalation on the human central nervous system. *Int Arch Occup Environ Health* 69:53, 1996.
65. Adgey AA, Johnston PW, McMechan S: Sudden cardiac death and substance abuse. *Resuscitation* 29:219, 1995.
66. Herd PA, Lipsky M, Martin HF: Cardiovascular effects of 1,1,1-trichloroethane. *Arch Environ Health* 28:227, 1974.
67. McLeod AA, Margot R, Monaghan MJ, et al: Chronic cardiac toxicity after inhalation of 1,1,1-trichloroethane. *BMJ* 294:727, 1987.
68. Susten AS, Dames BL, Burg JR, et al: Percutaneous penetration of benzene in hairless mice: an estimate of dermal absorption during tire-building operations. *Am J Ind Med* 7:323, 1985.
69. Lovern MR, Cole CE, Schlosser PM: A review of quantitative studies of benzene metabolism. *Crit Rev Toxicol* 31:285, 2001.
70. Snyder R: Overview of the toxicology of benzene. *J Toxicol Environ Health A* 61:339, 2000.
71. Smith MT: Overview of benzene-induced aplastic anaemia. *Eur J Haematol Suppl* 60:107, 1996.

72. Ireland B, Collins JJ, Buckley CF, et al: Cancer mortality among workers with benzene exposure. *Epidemiology* 8:318, 1997.
73. Flanagan RJ, Ruprah M, Meredith TJ, et al: An introduction to the clinical toxicology of volatile substances. *Drug Saf* 5:359, 1990.
74. Von Burg R: Toluene. *J Appl Toxicol* 13:441, 1993.
75. Greenberg MM: The central nervous system and exposure to toluene: a risk characterization. *Environ Res* 72:1, 1997.
76. Fischman CM, Oster JR: Toxic effects of toluene. A new cause of high anion gap metabolic acidosis. *JAMA* 241:1713, 1979.
77. Carder JR, Fuerst RS: Myocardial infarction after toluene inhalation. *Pediatr Emerg Care* 13:117, 1997.
78. Fay M, Eisenmann C, Diwan S, et al: ATSDR evaluation of health effects of chemicals. V. Xylenes: health effects, toxicokinetics, human exposure, and environmental fate. *Toxicol Ind Health* 14:571, 1998.
79. Morley R, Eccleston DW, Douglas CP, et al: Xylene poisoning: a report of one fatal case and two cases of recovery after prolonged unconsciousness. *BMJ* 3:442, 1970.
80. Rastogi SP, Gold RM, Arruda JAL: Fanconi's syndrome associated with carburetor fluid intoxication. *Am J Clin Pathol* 82:124, 1984.
81. Abu Al Ragheb S, Salhab AS, Amr SS: Suicide by xylene ingestion: a case report and review of literature. *Am J Forensic Med Pathol* 7:327, 1986.
82. McGuigan MA: Turpentine. *Clin Toxicol Rev* 8:1, 1985.
83. Koppel C, Tenczer J, Tennesmann U, et al: Acute poisoning with pine oil: metabolism of monoterpenes. *Arch Toxicol* 49:73, 1981.
84. Hill RM, Barer J, Hill LL, et al: An investigation of recurrent pine oil poisoning in an infant by the use of gas chromatographic-mass spectrometric methods. *J Pediatr* 87:115, 1975.
85. Troulakis G, Tsatsakis AM, Tzatzarakis M, et al: Acute intoxication and recovery following massive turpentine ingestion: clinical and toxicological data. *Vet Hum Toxicol* 39:155, 1997.
86. Klein FA, Hackler RH: Hemorrhagic cystitis associated with turpentine ingestion. *Urology* 16:187, 1980.
87. Brook MP, McCarron MM, Mueller JA: Pine oil cleaner ingestion. *Ann Emerg Med* 18:391, 1989.
88. Scalzo AJ, Weber TR, Jaeger RW, et al: Extracorporeal membrane oxygenation for hydrocarbon aspiration. *Am J Dis Child* 144:867, 1990.

Chapter 114 ■ Hydrofluoric Acid Poisoning

KENNON HEARD

INTRODUCTION

Hydrofluoric acid (HF) is a commonly encountered industrial reagent that is available in the concentrations from 6% to 90%. It is used for the production of fluorocarbons, etching glass, and silicone, and as a household rust-removal agent. Sodium fluoride is used as a rodenticide and also as a preservative in blood collection tubes. A related compound, ammonium bifluoride is used in rust removers, commonly found in commercial car washes.

MECHANISM OF ACTION

HF ($pK_a = 3.8$) is a weak acid. Hence, compared with other acids, it is relatively less ionized at any given pH. This allows HF to penetrate more deeply into tissue and to be more readily absorbed into the systemic circulation than other acids. Once absorbed, it disassociates and the fluoride anion binds to divalent cations, forming insoluble salts (primarily calcium fluoride, fluorapatite, and magnesium fluoride). This results in tissue and systemic hypocalcemia and hypomagnesemia. Fluoride also directly poisons several enzymes and cellular transport proteins. High-concentration HF exposures result in rapid onset of local pain and tissue injury with or without systemic toxicity, whereas low-concentration exposures can result in life-threatening hypocalcemia and hypomagnesemia, with minimal or absent local corrosive effect.

DERMAL EXPOSURE

Clinical Manifestations

Although most dermal exposures will result in minor symptoms or superficial chemical burns, systemic toxicity may occur following dermal exposure. Symptoms may be delayed for 24 hours or more following low-concentration (<20% HF) exposure, and there is often severe pain with minimal skin abnormalities. Symptoms can develop within several hours of exposure to medium concentrations (20% to 50% HF). Although the initial injury is not always visible, the patients exposed to medium-concentration products often go on to have erythema, blanching, or necrosis of the involved area. High-concentration (>50% HF) exposures result in the immediate injury expected after exposure to concentrated acids. The patients may develop full- or partial-thickness injury that includes tissue necrosis and eschar formation [1].

Evaluation and Treatment

Laboratory studies are not indicated for small, low-concentration dermal exposures. However, exposure to products containing more than 50% HF that involve more than 1% of the skin or exposure to any HF product that affects more than 5% of the skin can cause hypocalcemia, so the patients with these burns should have serum calcium levels monitored, as described in the 'Systemic Toxicity' section [2].

The most important step in the treatment is decontamination by irrigating the affected area for at least 15 minutes as quickly as possible. In one large case series of exposures, many of which involved concentrations of greater than 40% HF, immediate irrigation produced excellent outcome in the majority of the patients [3]. Hexafluoride, an irrigating solution developed to bind fluoride, does not appear to offer any improvement over water irrigation [4].

After irrigation, apply a 2.3% to 2.5% calcium gluconate preparation in a water-soluble gel to the exposed areas for at least 30 minutes or until symptoms resolve [5]. This treatment often remains effective, if it is delayed several hours after symptoms develop [6]. The role of topical therapy following high-concentration exposures is less well defined, but it is recommended [7].

If pain is not relieved by topical therapy, regional intra-arterial or intravenous calcium perfusion should be initiated. The major drawback of intra-arterial perfusion is the requirement for arterial catheterization. Brachial, radial, and femoral catheterization have all been described. Following cannulation, monitor arterial waveform to assure that the catheter remains patent and properly placed within the artery. If there is any question as to adequate placement, performs arteriography prior to infusing calcium. Flushing the catheter with heparin may help keep the catheter patent [2]. The largest case series reported infusion of

50 mL of 2.5% calcium gluconate in saline over 4 hours [2]. It is not uncommon to have to repeat the dose several times over a 12- to 24-hour period.

Regional perfusion using a Bier block may allow treatment without arterial cannulization. Some clinicians advocate this technique before proceeding to intra-arterial administration. This technique requires venous cannulation in the affected extremity. The extremity is exsanguinated by elevation and compression with an Esmarch bandage. The blood pressure cuff should be inflated to a pressure of 100 mm Hg above systolic pressure and remain up for 15 to 20 minutes following calcium administration. The usual dose is 40 mL of a 2.5% calcium gluconate solution [8]. The cuff is then gradually deflated over 5 minutes. Pain is usually relieved within minutes of the calcium administration.

If the affected area is not an extremity, calcium can be directly injected into the burn. The most common method is injection of 0.3 to 0.5 mL per cm^2 of 2.5% calcium gluconate. Calcium chloride should not be used, because it can cause tissue injury. Excision of exposed tissue is not recommended.

OCULAR EXPOSURE

Clinical Manifestations

Although most human reports describe good outcomes following ocular HF exposure, animal studies have demonstrated that severe injury is possible. Although most patients have rapid onset of pain, HF can penetrate the eye and cause severe and delayed injury.

Evaluation and Treatment

Immediate irrigation is the most important treatment. Irrigation with calcium salts appears to offer no benefit over saline in animal models, and may increase the incidence of ulceration [9]. Following irrigation, the pH should be measured and a fluorescein examination should be performed. All patients with persistent symptoms or obvious corneal damage should have immediate evaluation by an ophthalmologist. Some will require admission for continuous irrigation. The patients who are asymptomatic after irrigation should have next-day follow-up with an ophthalmologist. Routine therapy for corneal burns from HF has included mydriatics, topical antibiotics, and steroids [10–12]. Treatment of these burns with calcium gluconate eyedrops has been suggested, but systematic human studies have not been reported [12].

INHALATION

Clinical Manifestations

Inhalation of HF may result in the severe airway injury, pulmonary injury, and systemic fluoride poisoning. The patients may present with severe or minimal symptoms and go on to develop complications over time [13]. Although systemic fluoride poisoning may occur [14], the major mechanism of pulmonary injury is acute lung injury.

Evaluation and Treatment

Following inhalation of HF, the patients should have chest radiographs, evaluation of oxygenation, and monitoring for hypocalcemia. Treatment is supportive, and early airway intervention may be required for the patients with symptoms of upper airway obstruction. There are several uncontrolled reports of good outcomes following treatment with nebulized calcium gluconate solution (2.5% to 5.0%) [15,16].

INGESTION

Clinical Manifestations

Oropharyngeal burns are rarely noted, even in fatal poisonings [17]. Although gastrointestinal symptoms such as nausea, vomiting, and gastritis may occur, the primary manifestation of oral HF exposures is systemic fluoride toxicity (see below). Following accidental sip ingestions, the patients who are able to swallow should be given 30 to 60 mL of water to drink to dilute any HF still in contact with the esophageal mucosa. Although it is commonly recommended to administer calcium or magnesium antacids, animals studies have found that very high doses are required to affect mortality [18,19]. The patients with accidental ingestion of products containing more than 7% HF or deliberate ingestion of any HF or ammonium fluoride product are at risk for systemic poisoning and require continuous cardiac monitoring, reliable vascular access, and close monitoring of serum calcium levels, as described in the next section.

Systemic Toxicity

Systemic fluoride toxicity may occur following inhalation, dermal, or oral exposure to HF-containing products. Although the exact mechanism of fluoride toxicity requires continued research [20], human cases of fatal HF toxicity consistently demonstrate profound hypocalcemia [21]. Other manifestations include hypomagnesemia, acidosis, and hyperkalemia. Minimally symptomatic patients may progress rapidly to cardiovascular collapse [22].

Because successful resuscitation from cardiac arrest following systemic fluoride poisoning is rare, treatment should be started early to prevent cardiac dysrhythmias and arrest. The patients should have continuous cardiac monitoring, reliable vascular access, and frequent measurement of serum calcium and magnesium levels. If the history suggests that there has been a significant exposure, prophylactic calcium should be initiated at a rate of 1 g over 30 minutes [20]. The patients who have normal vital signs and remain stable should have serum calcium levels monitored every 30 minutes for the first 2 to 3 hours. Calcium chloride 1-g boluses should be repeated as needed to maintain the serum calcium in the high normal range. The patients with hypocalcemia, dysrhythmias, or hypotension should receive 2 to 3 g of calcium every 15 minutes, and central venous access should be obtained. Successful treatment of cardiac arrest has generally been associated with administration of large doses (>10 g) of calcium. Intravenous magnesium sulfate 2 to 6 g over 30 minutes followed by a continuous 1- to 4-g infusion has also been suggested.

Beyond calcium and magnesium administration, fluoride-poisoned patients require aggressive supportive care. The patients with symptoms of airway involvement should be intubated. Similarly, ventilation and oxygenation problems are rare but should be treated promptly when present. Successful electrical cardioversion for dysrhythmias following calcium and magnesium therapy has been reported [23].

A therapy that is unproven but has theoretical benefit is serum and urine alkalinization. One animal study showed that systemic alkalosis increased the fatal fluoride dose in rats [24]. Although this study has obvious limitations, serum alkalinization should be considered in critically ill patients. However, over alkalinization may worsen hypocalcemia; therefore, serum pH should be maintained between 7.4 and 7.5. Although fluoride is cleared by hemodialysis, the patients with severe poisoning may be too unstable to tolerate dialysis.

References

1. Division of Industrial Hygiene: National Institute of Health hydrofluoric acid burns. *Ind Med* 12:634, 1943.
2. Siegel DC, Heard JM: Intra-arterial calcium infusion for hydrofluoric acid burns. *Aviat Space Environ Med* 63(3):206–211, 1992.
3. Hamilton M: OH Congress. Hydrofluoric acid burns. *Occup Health (Lond)* 27(11):468–470, 1975.
4. Hojer J, Personne M, Hulten P, et al: Topical treatments for hydrofluoric acid burns: a blind controlled experimental study. *J Toxicol Clin Toxicol* 40(7):861–866, 2002.
5. Trevino MA, Herrmann GH, Sprout WL: Treatment of severe hydrofluoric acid exposures. *J Occup Med* 25(12):861–863, 1983.
6. El Saadi MS, Hall AH, Hall PK, et al: Hydrofluoric acid dermal exposure. *Vet Hum Toxicol* 31(3):243–247, 1989.
7. Sadove R, Hainsworth D, Van Meter W: Total body immersion in hydrofluoric acid. *South Med J* 83(6):698–700, 1990.
8. Graudins A, Burns MJ, Aaron CK: Regional intravenous infusion of calcium gluconate for hydrofluoric acid burns of the upper extremity [see comments]. *Ann Emerg Med* 30(5):604–607, 1997.
9. Beiran I, Miller B, Bentur Y: The efficacy of calcium gluconate in ocular hydrofluoric acid burns. *Hum Exp Toxicol* 16(4):223–228, 1997.
10. McCulley JP, Whiting DW, Petitt MG, et al: Hydrofluoric acid burns of the eye. *J Occup Med* 25(6):447–450, 1983.
11. McCulley JP: Ocular hydrofluoric acid burns: animal model, mechanism of injury and therapy. *Trans Am Ophthalmol Soc* 88(1):649–684, 1990.
12. Rubinfeld RS, Silbert DI, Arentsen JJ, et al: Ocular hydrofluoric acid burns. *Am J Ophthalmol* 114(4):420–423, 1992.
13. Kirkpatrick JJ, Enion DS, Burd DA: Hydrofluoric acid burns: a review. *Burns* 21(7):483–493, 1995.
14. Watson AA, Oliver JS, Thorpe JW: Accidental death due to inhalation of hydrofluoric acid. *Med Sci Law* 13(4):277–279, 1973.
15. Lee DC, Wiley JF II, Synder JW II, et al: Treatment of inhalational exposure to hydrofluoric acid with nebulized calcium gluconate. *J Occup Med* 35(5):470, 1993.
16. Kono K, Watanabe T, Dote T, et al: Successful treatments of lung injury and skin burn due to hydrofluoric acid exposure. *Int Arch Occup Environ Health* 73[Suppl]:S93–S97, 2000.
17. Bost RO, Springfield A: Fatal hydrofluoric acid ingestion: a suicide case report. *J Anal Toxicol* 19(6):535–536, 1995.
18. Kao WF, Deng JF, ChiangSC, et al: A simple, safe, and efficient way to treat severe fluoride poisoning—oral calcium or magnesium. *J Toxicol Clin Toxicol* 42(1):33–40, 2004.
19. Heard K, Delgado J: Oral decontamination with calcium or magnesium salts does not improve survival following hydrofluoric acid ingestion. *J Toxicol Clin Toxicol* 41(7):789–792, 2003.
20. McIvor ME: Acute fluoride toxicity: pathophysiology and management. *Drug Saf* 5(2):79–85, 1990.
21. Rabinowitch IM: Acute fluoride poisoning. *Can Med Assoc J* 52(2):345–349, 1945.
22. Kao WF, Dart RC, Kuffner E, et al: Ingestion of low-concentration hydrofluoric acid: an insidious and potentially fatal poisoning. *Ann Emerg Med* 34(1):35–41, 1999.
23. Stremski ES, Grande GA, Ling LJ: Survival following hydrofluoric acid ingestion. *Ann Emerg Med* 21(11):1396–1399, 1992.
24. Reynolds KE, Whitford GM, Pashley DH: Acute fluoride toxicity: the influence of acid-base status. *Toxicol Appl Pharmacol* 45(2):415–427, 1978.

Chapter 115 ■ Iron Poisoning

MILTON TENENBEIN

Historically, iron poisoning is the most common cause of poisoning death in children younger than 6 years [1]; however, morbidity and mortality have decreased secondary to unit-dose packaging of iron supplements [2]. Notably, a clinically important proportion of iron overdoses is purposeful, involving adolescents and adults, and resulting in significant morbidity and mortality [3].

Iron occurs naturally in the body. It is highly reactive, and there are complex mechanisms for its absorption, transport, and storage. The capacity of these systems to cope with an acute overdose is unknown; it likely varies from individual to individual and with the state of iron stores. Incomplete understanding of iron toxicokinetics is primarily responsible for controversies regarding (a) toxic dose; (b) gastrointestinal decontamination; (c) efficacy of intragastric complexation therapies; and (d) the indications, dose, duration, and efficacy of deferoxamine therapy.

PHARMACOLOGY

Iron is readily available as ferrous salts, either alone or in combination with other minerals and vitamins. Its common salts are ferrous gluconate, sulfate, fumarate, and succinate, which are 12%, 20%, 33%, and 35% elemental iron, respectively. These fractions are important because toxicity is related to the amount of elemental iron ingested. Carbonyl iron is a highly purified form of metallic iron. It is uncharged and not a salt [4].

Iron absorption, transport, and storage are well reviewed elsewhere [5]. Because there is no endogenous mechanism for iron excretion, total body iron is a function of the absorptive process. Absorption occurs in the proximal small bowel, with approximately 10% of the ingested dose absorbed, but with 10-fold variations, depending on iron stores and the amount ingested. The actual mechanism of iron absorption is not well understood, but it is believed to be an active process. Even after massive overdose, a relatively small amount (15%) is actually absorbed [6].

Peak serum iron concentrations occur within 4 to 6 hours after overdose. The half-life after therapeutic dosing is approximately 6 hours [5], with rapid decline because of tissue distribution. In plasma, iron is bound to transferrin, a specific β_1-globulin responsible for iron transport throughout the body. In iron overdose, transferrin-binding capacity is exceeded, but free plasma iron does not truly exist. Iron complexes with other plasma proteins and organic ligands and is referred to as *nontransferrin-bound plasma iron* [7]. However, it is only loosely bound and is quite available to produce tissue damage and organ dysfunction.

There are two typical overdose scenarios: innocent overdose by young children and purposeful overdose by adolescents and adults. Serious iron overdose in young children frequently involves the ingestion of a product intended for adults, typically a prenatal iron supplement. Ingestion of pediatric preparations, such as multivitamin plus iron tablets, is more common [8]; such preparations are unlikely to result in significant toxicity because of their low elemental iron content (as little as 4 mg per tablet). Although liquid iron preparations are often found in homes with infants and toddlers, there are no published cases of clinically important iron poisoning from these products. Iron overdose is less common among teenagers and adults, but when it occurs, it is typically more severe. Of particular note is the high incidence of deliberate iron overdose in pregnant women [9].

Iron exerts both local and systemic effects. The local irritant effect on the gastrointestinal tract results in nausea, vomiting, abdominal cramps, and diarrhea. These symptoms are produced by relatively small doses (20 mg per kg of elemental iron). The extent of systemic toxicity is dose related. Because most published data are anecdotal, specific values have not been established. In the pediatric literature, more than 60 mg per kg of elemental iron produces significant systemic toxicity [10], with a lethal dose being 200 to 250 mg per kg [10]. Both the figures are likely overestimates; more realistic figures are probably half as much. The lowest reported lethal dose for a toddler is approximately 75 mg per kg of elemental iron [11]. The author's own experience and that of others [12] suggests that the toxic dose in adults is similar to that in children. An ingestion of 1.5 g of elemental iron by an adult should be cause for concern. Adults have died after ingestion of as little as 2 g [13] and 5 g [12] of elemental iron; the former patient had significant hepatic disease, and the latter ingested 70 mg per kg. There have been no published reports of serious or fatal poisoning from the ingestion of carbonyl iron products [4]. Although its bioavailability after therapeutic dosing is similar to that of ferrous salts, its absorption is limited after an overdose. Single doses of 10 g (140 mg per kg) have been tolerated in humans.

Poor, unpredictable absorption of iron and its unknown capacity for binding by ferritin and as hemosiderin contribute to uncertainty regarding the toxic dose. As reflected by serum iron concentrations, which are measured in micrograms per deciliter, the size of the potentially toxic iron pool is likely to be small—on the order of milligrams—even after gram quantities of iron have been ingested. That the body burden of iron is relatively small after an overdose is not well appreciated, but it has important implications for the dose and duration of deferoxamine therapy.

Iron itself is neither caustic nor corrosive. It is a potent catalyst of free radical formation, which results in highly reactive species that attack intracellular molecules [14]. Iron-generated free radical formation is thought to contribute to acute iron toxicity [15] and to be responsible for much of the damage and dysfunction of chronic iron overload [7].

Free radicals produce damage at their site of origin. Because of local protective mechanisms, a significant concentration of free radicals is required to cause damage. Sites exposed to high iron concentrations are most susceptible to injury. One such area is the gastrointestinal tract. Gastrointestinal mucosal necrosis and bleeding [16] may occur without systemic toxicity. Notably, gut toxicity can occur distally with proximal sparing [16] and may be absent in the face of fatal systemic poisoning [6].

Systemic toxicity results when the absorbed iron is transported to target organs, such as the liver and heart. Nontransferrin-bound iron is rapidly cleared by the liver [17], putting this organ at risk for toxicity [18].

CLINICAL TOXICITY

Traditionally, acute iron intoxication is divided into five clinical stages [19]: gastrointestinal toxicity, relative stability, circulatory shock, hepatic necrosis, and gastrointestinal scarring. An orderly progression through all these stages may not occur. Fatalities are possible without significant gastrointestinal involvement [6], and hepatotoxicity may be absent in otherwise severe poisoning. Presenting symptoms and signs depend on the time since ingestion.

The most common time of presentation is during the first stage (gastrointestinal toxicity), when abdominal pain, vomiting, diarrhea, hematemesis, and hematochezia can be seen. Gastrointestinal toxicity usually occurs within the first few hours of overdose. The severity of this stage is variable. Life-threatening hypovolemic shock may occur, especially if initial symptoms were severe or ignored. Occasionally, segmental intestinal infarction may occur, necessitating bowel resection [16]. Isolated hepatotoxicity or gastrointestinal obstruction would be an unlikely presentation of iron poisoning.

The second stage, a period of relative stability, follows initial gastrointestinal symptoms. Apparent improvement in the patient's clinical status should not lead to complacency. Patients are not completely asymptomatic; careful assessment and repeated monitoring typically shows some degree of hypovolemia, hypoperfusion, and acidosis.

The third stage, circulatory shock, can occur within several hours of iron overdose and may persist up to 48 to 72 hours. Its pathogenesis is complex and poorly understood and is based on the results of limited experimental animal data [20–23]. Circulatory shock may be hypovolemic, distributive, or cardiogenic. The time of onset can be somewhat helpful in elucidating its cause, but there is considerable overlap. Shock occurring within a few hours of the overdose suggests hypovolemia secondary to fluid and, rarely, blood loss from the gastrointestinal tract. Hyperferremia-associated coagulopathy may contribute to bleeding [24]. Distributive shock depends on iron absorption and begins within the first 24 hours. Suggested mechanisms include direct effects of iron or ferritin or an effect mediated by release of vasoactive substances, resulting in decreased vascular tone or increased vascular permeability [22]. Cardiogenic shock usually occurs 1 to 3 days after overdose [25].

The occurrence of metabolic acidosis in iron poisoning usually precedes circulatory shock. Acidosis is a direct toxic effect of iron that occurs after the plasma's capacity to bind the absorbed ferric ion has been exceeded. When this occurs, the ferric ion becomes hydrated and protons are released [$Fe^{3+} + 3H_2O \rightarrow Fe(OH)_3 + 3H^+$]. Thus, each unbound ferric ion generates three protons. The acidosis can be quite profound, requiring large amounts of bicarbonate for treatment [23]. Other factors contributing to acidosis include the generation of organic acids resulting from iron's interference with intracellular oxidative metabolism and lactate production secondary to shock.

The fourth stage, hepatotoxicity, is second only to shock as a cause of death [18]. It may occur any time during the first 48 hours after overdose. The pathogenesis of hepatic necrosis is believed to be iron-catalyzed free radical production and subsequent lipid peroxidation of hepatic mitochondrial membranes [15].

The fifth stage, gastrointestinal scarring, is the consequence of iron's local action on the gut and usually occurs 2 to 4 weeks after overdose. Ongoing and protracted abdominal pain during the first week is associated with the later development of this complication [16]. Most cases involve the gastric outlet, but isolated strictures of the distal intestine have been reported [16].

The consequences of iron poisoning in pregnant women are no different from those in other patients, but because transplacental iron passage is an energy-requiring saturable process, the fetus is relatively protected [26]. Although deferoxamine in animals is associated with potential harm to the fetus, its risk in humans is overemphasized [26]. The health of the fetus depends on its mother, and treatment should be no different from that given to a nonpregnant woman.

DIAGNOSTIC EVALUATION

Essential laboratory tests include abdominal radiographs, serum iron and bicarbonate concentrations, and blood gas determinations. Because iron tablets are radiopaque, an abdominal radiograph can be used to verify an overdose and quantify the amount ingested [27–29]. However, iron tablets may not be visible if they have dissolved or been chewed, a liquid preparation has been ingested, or there is only a small amount of iron in each tablet (e.g., pediatric iron-containing multivitamins) [30].

If tablets are visible, serial abdominal radiographs may be used to judge the effectiveness of gastrointestinal decontamination.

Serum iron concentration is the single most important test. It verifies the ingestion, guides management, and provides prognostic information. A peak serum concentration of less than 500 μg per dL (90 μmol per L) is usually associated with negligible-to-mild systemic toxicity; however, there may be significant gastrointestinal symptoms. Moderate systemic toxicity is expected with a peak concentration of 500 to 1,000 μg per dL (90 to 180 μmol per L). A peak serum concentration greater than 1,000 μg per dL (180 μmol per L) is associated with severe toxicity, such as profound acidosis, shock, hepatotoxicity, coma, and death. Mortality approaches 100% when serum concentration is greater than 10,000 μg per dL (1,800 μmol per L). The time of blood sampling to estimate peak serum iron concentration should be 4 to 6 hours after an overdose. Serial serum iron concentration determinations are recommended during the early hours after overdose, especially when the first value is 300 to 500 μg per dL (55 to 90 μmol per L). Determinations should be obtained every 2 hours until a definite downward trend is established. A concurrent abdominal radiograph may be helpful. If many tablets are visible, the subsequent serum iron concentration will likely be higher. However, a negative radiograph does not guarantee that peak serum iron concentration has occurred. It is desirable to obtain blood specimens before initiating deferoxamine therapy because it can confound the laboratory determination of serum iron concentration, resulting in falsely lower values [31]. When clinically indicated, deferoxamine therapy should not be delayed because of blood sampling issues.

Blood gas or serum bicarbonate determinations should be done early because acidosis is an early objective indicator of systemic toxicity. Frequency of blood gas determinations is guided by previous values, the need for bicarbonate therapy, and clinical course. A pH of less than 7.30 indicates significant toxicity.

Recommended laboratory tests include blood coagulation, hepatic, and renal panels. Coagulation studies should be done early and repeated throughout the first few days in patients with significant toxicity because a biphasic coagulopathy may develop [24]. Blood should be typed and cross-matched as clinically indicated. Hepatic panels should be monitored daily during the first 72 hours and longer if values remain significantly abnormal. Renal panels should be obtained regularly, especially during deferoxamine therapy, because of the risk for acute renal failure [32].

The total iron-binding capacity (TIBC) is not recommended in the assessment or management of patients with iron overdose because it is unreliable during hyperferremic states and it does not predict iron toxicity [33]. It is difficult to accurately predict outcomes because the published literature chiefly consists of anecdotal reports. Survival is expected with peak serum iron concentrations of less than 1,000 μg per dL (180 μmol per L) and appropriate supportive care. The chief causes of death are shock and hepatic failure. Acute renal failure may result from shock or deferoxamine therapy without adequate volume replacement [32]. *Yersinia septicemia* has been reported in patients treated with deferoxamine [27,34].

Differential diagnosis becomes an issue only when the history of iron overdose is unknown. In such situations, diagnosis can be quite challenging because of the multiple and varied clinical features at presentation (e.g., abdominal pain, gastrointestinal hemorrhage, shock, and coma). From the poisoning perspective, corrosive ingestion and acute heavy metal poisoning are the main considerations.

MANAGEMENT

The initial management of a patient with an iron overdose presents a challenge because the patient often presents before maximal clinical toxicity. Many patients, especially young children, may be asymptomatic or only mildly ill. The challenge lies in identifying those who are destined to suffer significant toxicity in order to place them in an appropriate setting for the required level of care. The decision for the iron-overdosed critically ill patient is straightforward. Table 115.1 provides guidelines for intensive care unit admission for those patients who are not critically ill.

Because activated charcoal does not adsorb iron [28], whole-bowel irrigation (WBI) (Fig. 115.1) is recommended as the decontamination procedure of choice for the iron-overdose patient [29]. WBI should be considered when there is radiographic documentation of iron ingestion and when there is a history of elemental iron ingestion greater than 60 mg per kg in children and 1.5 g per kg in adults. If emesis hampers effective WBI, consider metoclopramide (1 mg per kg intravenously in adults and 0.1 mg per kg in children) or ondansetron (8 mg per kg intravenously in adults or 0.1 to 0.2 mg per kg in children).

Iron can become adherent to the gastrointestinal mucosa or may form tablet bezoars [35]. Radiographs in three planes (flat, upright, and decubitus) should identify these two situations. A computed tomographic (CT) scan is another consideration. Barium studies are unlikely to be helpful because of the anticipated lack of contrast between barium and iron. If WBI is ineffective, removal of iron via gastrotomy should be considered [35,36]. For surgical intervention to be effective, it should be done before the iron is absorbed, and most tablets must be in a localized area rather than scattered throughout the gastrointestinal tract. A

TABLE 115.1

Suggested Criteria for Admission of the Noncritically Ill Iron-Overdosed Patient to an Intensive Care Unit

	Admit to ICU	Strongly consider admission to ICU
Amount of elemental iron ingested		
Child (<6 y)	>60 mg/kg	45–60 mg/kg
Adult (all others)	>3.0 g	2.0–3.0 g
Tablets seen in radiograph[a]		
Child (<6 y)	1/kg	0.75–1.00/kg
Adult (all others)	>50	33–50
Peak serum iron concentrations	>1,000 μg/dL (>180 μmol/L)	750–1,000 μg/dL (135–180 μmol/L)
Arterial pH	<7.30	7.30–7.35

Not all criteria need to be present.
[a]Assuming 60-mg elemental iron/tablet.

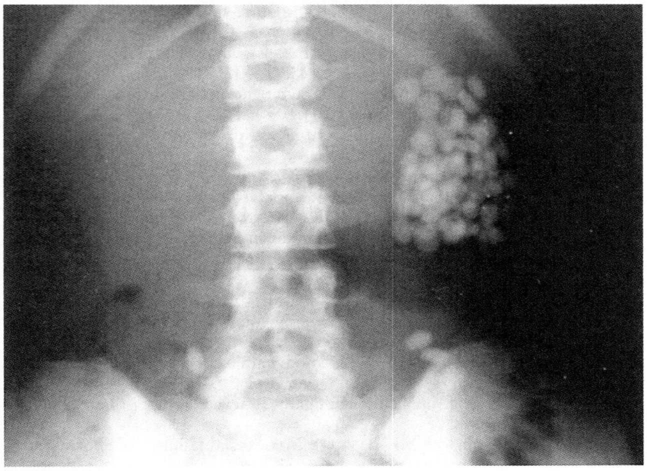

FIGURE 115.1 Abdominal radiograph of a 16-year-old girl with a potentially lethal iron overdose after syrup of ipecac-induced emesis and gastric lavage. Gastroscopy ruled out adherence of iron to the stomach wall and medication concretion. She subsequently underwent whole-bowel irrigation. Her peak serum iron concentration was 253 μg per dL (46 μmol per L), and she was not treated with deferoxamine.

combined approach of gastrotomy for tablet retrieval followed by WBI after surgery has been described [36]. The former removed the iron from the stomach, and the latter removed it from the intestinal tract. Endoscopic removal of an iron bezoar from the stomach has been reported [37].

The oral administration of bicarbonate, phosphate, or deferoxamine is not recommended. These agents have been advocated as a way to decrease iron absorption by precipitating it as an insoluble salt or by chelating it. In vitro [38] and animal [39] studies do not support bicarbonate or phosphate administration, and the latter therapy has resulted in hypocalcemia and hypovolemia in iron-overdosed patients [40]. Oral deferoxamine is not recommended. It is neither appreciably toxic nor absorbed from the gastrointestinal tract, but the same is not true of its chelate, ferrioxamine [19,21,41]. The latter has been shown to be lethal in animals [21,42].

Supportive care should be provided concurrently with gastrointestinal decontamination. In patients with severe poisoning, two intravenous (IV) lines are required: one for fluid resuscitation and bicarbonate administration and the other for deferoxamine therapy. Very large amounts of crystalloid and bicarbonate may be required [23], and occasionally, colloid or blood may be necessary. Because of the complex nature of shock in iron poisoning, assessment of cardiac output or myocadial contractility by ultrasound may be helpful. Early shock should respond to vigorous volume resuscitation; occasionally, pressor therapy may be needed. Late shock usually requires inotropic support. An arterial catheter for frequent blood gas determinations and a Foley catheter for monitoring urine output are essential in all critically ill patients.

Parameters requiring serial monitoring include arterial blood gas; hematocrit; serum electrolytes; and renal, hepatic, and blood coagulation panels. The frequency of these determinations depends on previous results and the patient's clinical condition and response to therapy.

Acute hepatic failure is managed by standard protocols. Acute renal failure may be a consequence of shock or deferoxamine therapy in the setting of hypovolemia [32]. Hemodialysis may be required in such situations, especially if deferoxamine therapy is continued, to remove the toxic chelate, ferrioxamine. Coagulopathy during the first few hours after overdose is related to serum iron concentration and is transient. Specific therapy is unnecessary. Deferoxamine lowers the serum iron concentration and may hasten its resolution [24]. Coagulopathy occurring many hours to a few days after overdose is a manifestation of hepatic failure. Administration of fresh-frozen plasma is recommended, because vitamin K_1 is unlikely to be helpful.

Hemodialysis or hemoperfusion is not recommended for iron removal because of the rapid extravascular distribution of the iron and its binding to plasma proteins as non–transferrin-bound iron [7]. However, hemodialysis is indicated for patients with renal failure.

Deferoxamine, the specific treatment of choice for acute iron poisoning [15,19], is a naturally occurring siderophore isolated from *Streptomyces pilosus*. Its pharmacology was described in the early 1960s [43,44]. Its binding constant for ferric iron is 10^{31}, which compares with 10^{27} to 10^{29} for transferrin. It is capable of removing iron from ferritin and hemosiderin and, to a very minor degree, from transferrin, but not at all from cytochromes, hemoglobin, or myoglobin.

Although deferoxamine is regarded as the treatment of choice, its effectiveness has been questioned because it has limited chelating capacity and only small amounts of iron are recovered in the urine after its administration to iron-poisoned patients [45]. The manufacturer's recommended daily deferoxamine dosage of 6 g is capable of chelating 510 mg of iron or 8.5 ferrous sulfate tablets. Although this would seem to be insignificant in the patient who has ingested 50 tablets, the poor absorption of iron and the body's large storage capacity for it result in only a relatively small amount being responsible for toxicity. Therefore, the chelation of small amounts of iron may be beneficial. Alternatively, 510 mg of iron is approximately 10% of the total amount of iron and approximately 35% of the nonheme iron in a 70-kg man [46].

Historically, therapy was based on the deferoxamine chelation challenge test and relied on visual detection of a change in urine color to rusty orange (vin rosé) caused by the presence of ferrioxamine after intramuscular administration of deferoxamine. This test has never been validated and is not recommended.

Traditional indications for deferoxamine therapy have been based on the peak serum iron concentration, the serum iron concentration relative to the TIBC, the results of a chelation challenge test, and the patient's clinical condition. The therapy has been recommended for those with peak serum iron concentrations ranging from 300 to 500 μg per dL (55 to 90 μmol per L) [47]. Significant morbidity is unlikely with peak concentrations of less than 500 μg per dL (90 μmol per L). Hence, a serum iron concentration of 500 μg per dL (90 μmol per L) or greater is recommended as an indication for deferoxamine therapy in an otherwise asymptomatic patient. Deferoxamine therapy is indicated when symptoms and signs of severe iron poisoning are present, regardless of the serum iron concentration. These include acidosis, shock, and decreased level of consciousness or coma. Although some toxicologists also advocate deferoxamine therapy for those with recurrent vomiting or diarrhea, these symptoms can be seen in patients who do not develop systemic toxicity.

Deferoxamine should be administered intravenously. The patient should be fluid resuscitated prior to IV deferoxamine therapy, which should be initiated slowly and gradually increased to 15 mg per kg per hour for 20 to 30 minutes. Continuous IV infusion is the recommended method for administering deferoxamine. This is based on studies in patients with transfusion-induced iron overload, demonstrating that IV deferoxamine results in greater urinary iron elimination, higher peak and more stable serum deferoxamine concentrations [48].

The optimal dose of deferoxamine is uncertain. The manufacturer recommends a daily maximum dose of 6 g given in divided doses. A continuous infusion protocol of 15 mg per kg per hour until 24 hours after the urine returns to its normal color has also been recommended [15]. The latter protocol exceeds the manufacturer's guidelines for patients heavier than 17 kg. Neither recommendation is evidence based. Only two patients treated with 15 mg per kg per hour over a prolonged course have been well described in the literature [49,50]. Furthermore, continuous IV deferoxamine therapy in patients with acute iron poisoning for longer than 24 to 48 hours has been associated with the development of adult respiratory distress syndrome [51]. Four patients with mild-to-moderate iron poisoning without evidence of shock, acidosis, or sepsis who received 15 mg per kg per hour of deferoxamine intravenously for 2 to 3 days died of noncardiogenic pulmonary edema [51]. Continuous IV deferoxamine therapy should not routinely exceed the first 24 hours. If prolonged chelation therapy is deemed necessary, interrupting therapy for 12 of every 24 hours to allow excretion of ferrioxamine can be considered. Careful monitoring of pulmonary status is required during prolonged therapy.

Indications for discontinuing deferoxamine therapy include resolution of the symptoms and signs of systemic iron toxicity and correction of acidosis. Deferoxamine therapy is rarely needed beyond 24 hours and should be used with caution for periods longer than this.

Adverse drug events from short-term deferoxamine therapy are few, but significant. Rapid IV administration is associated with tachycardia, hypotension, shock, a generalized beet-red flushing of the skin, blotchy erythema, and urticaria. Acute renal failure can result when deferoxamine is administered to patients with hypovolemia [32]. Pulmonary toxicity and acute respiratory distress syndrome are associated with continuous IV therapy over several days [51]. Patients receiving deferoxamine may be at increased risk for *Yersinia* infections [27,34].

Before discharge, a psychiatric assessment is indicated for all patients with purposeful ingestions. Those who have required deferoxamine therapy should have a follow-up visit approximately 1 month after discharge. At this time, the patient's iron status and gastrointestinal tract should be assessed. He or she should also be advised of the symptoms of gastrointestinal obstruction and to return immediately if they occur. Chronic hepatic or cardiac dysfunction has not been reported after acute iron overdose.

References

1. Litovitz T, Manoguerra A: Comparison of pediatric poisoning hazards: an analysis of 38 million exposure incidents. A report from the American Association of Poison Control Centers. *Pediatrics* 89:999–1006, 1992.
2. Tenenbein M: Unit-dose packaging of iron supplements and reduction of iron poisoning in young children. *Arch Pediatr Adolesc Med* 159:557–560, 2005.
3. Mowry JB, Spyker DA, Cantilena LR Jr, et al: 2013 Annual report of the American association of poison control centers' national poison data system. *Clin Toxicol* 52:1032–1283, 2014.
4. Madiwale T, Liebelt E: Iron: not a benign therapeutic drug. *Curr Opin Pediatr* 18:174–179, 2006.
5. Harju E: Clinical pharmacokinetics of iron preparations. *Clin Pharmacokinet* 17:69–89, 1989.
6. Reissman KR, Coleman TJ, Budai BS, et al: Acute intestinal iron intoxication. I. Iron absorption, serum iron and autopsy findings. *Blood* 10:35–45, 1955.
7. Hershko C, Peto TE: Non-transferrin plasma iron. *Br J Haematol* 66:149–151, 1987.
8. Krenzelok EP, Hoff JV: Accidental childhood iron poisoning: a problem of marketing and labeling. *Pediatrics* 63:591–596, 1979.
9. Rayburn W, Aronow R, DeLancey B, et al: Drug overdose during pregnancy: an overview from a metropolitan poison control center. *Obstet Gynecol* 64:611–614, 1984.
10. Henretig FM, Temple AR: Acute iron poisoning in children. *Emerg Med Clin North Am* 2:121–132, 1984.
11. Smith RP, Jones CW, Cochran EW: Ferrous sulfate toxicity. *N Engl J Med* 243:641–645, 1950.
12. Olenmark M, Biber B, Dottori O, et al: Fatal iron intoxication in late pregnancy. *J Toxicol Clin Toxicol* 25:347–359, 1987.
13. Lavender S, Bell SA: Iron intoxication in an adult. *BMJ* 2:406, 1970.
14. Halliwell B, Gutteridge JMC: Oxygen free radicals and iron in relation to biology and medicine: some problems and concepts. *Arch Biochem Biophys* 246:501–514, 1986.
15. Robotham JL, Lietman PS: Acute iron poisoning. *Am J Dis Child* 134:875–879, 1980.
16. Tenenbein M, Littman C, Stimpson RE: Gastrointestinal pathology in adult iron overdose. *J Toxicol Clin Toxicol* 28:311–320, 1990.
17. Wright TL, Brissot P, Ma W, et al: Characterization of non-transferrin-bound iron clearance by rat. *J Biol Chem* 261:10909–10914, 1986.
18. Robertson A, Tenenbein M: Hepatotoxicity in acute iron poisoning. *Hum Exp Toxicol* 24:559–562, 2005.
19. Banner W Jr, Tong TG: Iron poisoning. *Pediatr Clin North Am* 33:393–409, 1986.
20. Reissmann KR, Coleman TJ: Acute intestinal iron intoxication. II. Metabolic, respiratory and circulatory effects of absorbed iron salts. *Blood* 10:46–51, 1955.
21. Whitten CF, Chen Y, Gibson GW: Studies in acute iron poisoning: further observations on desferrioxamine in the treatment of acute experimental iron poisoning. *Pediatrics* 38:102–110, 1966.
22. Whitten CF, Chen YC, Gibson GW: Studies in acute iron poisoning: the hemodynamic alterations in acute experimental iron poisoning. *Pediatr Res* 2:479–485, 1968.
23. Vernon DD, Banner W, Dean JM: Hemodynamic effects of experimental iron poisoning. *Ann Emerg Med* 18:863–866, 1989.
24. Tenenbein M, Israels SJ: Early coagulopathy in severe iron poisoning. *J Pediatr* 113:695–697, 1988.
25. Tenenbein M, Kopelow ML, deSa DJ: Myocardial failure and shock in iron poisoning. *Hum Toxicol* 7:281–284, 1988.
26. Tenenbein M: Poisoning in pregnancy, in Koren G (ed): *Maternal-Fetal Toxicology: A Clinician's Guide*. New York, NY, Marcel Dekker Inc, 1990, p 89.
27. Mofenson HC, Caraccio TR, Sharieff N: Iron sepsis. Yersinia enterocolitica septicemia possibly caused by an overdose of iron. *N Engl J Med* 316:1092–1093, 1987.
28. Decker WJ, Combs HF, Corby DG: Adsorption of drugs and poisons by activated charcoal. *Toxicol Appl Pharmacol* 13:454–460, 1968.
29. Thanacoody R, Caravati EM, Troutman B, et al: Position paper update: whole bowel irrigation for gastrointestinal decontamination of overdose patients. *Clin Toxicol (Phila)* 53:5–12, 2015.
30. Everson GW, Oudjhane K, Young LW, et al: Effectiveness of abdominal radiographs in visualizing chewable iron supplements following overdose. *Am J Emerg Med* 7:459–463, 1989.
31. Gevirtz NR, Wasserman LR: The measurement of iron and iron-binding capacity in plasma containing deferoxamine. *J Pediatr* 68:802–804, 1966.
32. Koren G, Bentur Y, Strong D, et al: Acute changes in renal function associated with deferoxamine therapy. *Am J Dis Child* 143:1077–1080, 1989.
33. Tenenbein M, Yatscoff RW: The TIBC in iron poisoning: is it useful? *Am J Dis Child* 145:437–439, 1990.
34. Melby K, Slordahl S, Gutteberg TJ, et al: Septicemia due to Yersinia enterocolitica after oral overdoses of iron. *BMJ* 285:467–468, 1982.
35. Foxford R, Goldfrank L: Gastrotomy: a surgical approach to iron overdose. *Ann Emerg Med* 14:1223–1226, 1985.
36. Tenenbein M, Wiseman N, Yatscoff RW: Gastrotomy and whole bowel irrigation in iron poisoning. *Pediatr Emerg Care* 7:286–288, 1991.
37. Ng HW, Tse ML, Lau FL, et al: Endoscopic removal of iron bezoar following acute overdose. *Clin Toxicol* 46:913–915, 2008.
38. Czajka PA, Konrad JD, Duffy JP: Iron poisoning: an in vitro comparison of bicarbonate and phosphate lavage solutions. *J Pediatr* 98:491–494, 1981.
39. Dean BS, Krenzelok EP: In vivo effectiveness of oral complexation agents in the management of iron poisoning. *J Toxicol Clin Toxicol* 25:221–230, 1987.
40. Bachrach L, Correa A, Levin R, et al: Iron poisoning: complications of hypertonic phosphate lavage therapy. *J Pediatr* 94:147–149, 1979.
41. Whitten CF, Gibson GW, Good MH, et al: Studies in acute iron poisoning. I. Deferoxamine in the treatment of acute iron poisoning: clinical observations, experimental studies and theoretical considerations. *Pediatrics* 36:322–335, 1965.
42. Adamson IY, Sienko A, Tenenbein M: Pulmonary toxicity of deferoxamine in iron-poisoned mice. *Toxicol Appl Pharmacol* 120:13–19, 1993.
43. Moeschlin S, Schnider U: Treatment of primary and secondary hemochromatosis and acute iron poisoning with a new potent iron-eliminating agent (desferrioxamine B). *N Engl J Med* 269:57–66, 1963.
44. Keberle H: The biochemistry of desferrioxamine and its relation to iron metabolism. *Ann N Y Acad Sci* 119:758–768, 1964.
45. Proudfoot AT, Simpson D, Dyson EH: Management of acute iron poisoning. *Med Toxicol* 1:83–100, 1986.
46. Worwood M: The clinical biochemistry of iron. *Semin Hematol* 14:3, 1977.
47. Bosse GM: Conservative management of patients with moderately elevated serum iron levels. *J Toxicol Clin Toxicol* 33:135–140, 1995.
48. Propper RD, Shurin SB, Nathan DG: Reassessment of the use of desferrioxamine B in iron overload. *N Engl J Med* 294:1421–1423, 1976.
49. Peck MG, Rogers JF, Rivenbark JF: Use of high doses of deferoxamine (Desferal) in an adult patient with acute iron overdosage. *J Toxicol Clin Toxicol* 19:865–869, 1982.
50. Henretig FM, Karl SR, Weintraub WH: Severe iron poisoning treated with enteral and intravenous deferoxamine. *Ann Emerg Med* 12:306–309, 1983.
51. Tenenbein M, Kowalski S, Sienko A, et al: Pulmonary toxic effects of continuous desferrioxamine administration in acute iron poisoning. *Lancet* 339:699–701, 1992.

Chapter 116 ■ Isoniazid Poisoning

JAMES B. MOWRY • R. BRENT FURBEE

Isoniazid (isonicotinic acid hydrazide [INH]) is the cornerstone of treatment and prevention of tuberculosis. It is available under a variety of brand names as 50-, 100-, and 300-mg tablets; as an oral syrup (50 mg per 5 mL); as an injectable solution (100 mg per mL); and in powder form. It is also available in combination with rifampin, pyridoxine, and other antitubercular drugs.

In 2013, the American Association of Poison Control Centers reported 149 cases with exposure to INH, including 104 single exposures; 44% of the cases involved adults or adolescents, with 21% being intentional. No deaths were reported, but 21% of the cases exhibited moderate-to-severe toxicity.

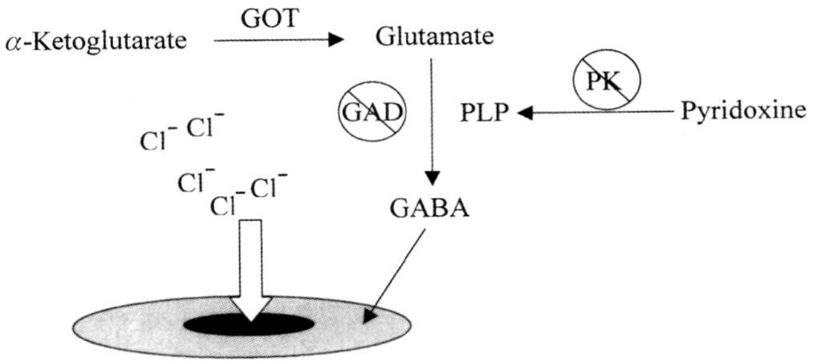

FIGURE 116.1 Role of isoniazid in the reduction of γ-aminobutyric acid (GABA) concentration. Cl^-, chloride ions; GAD, glutamic acid decarboxylase; GOT, glutamic oxaloacetic transaminase; PK, pyridoxine kinase; PLP, pyridoxal 5′-phosphate; circled division slash inhibited by isoniazid.

PHARMACOLOGY

As a bactericidal agent, INH interferes with lipid and nucleic acid biosynthesis in the growing *Mycobacterium* organism. It is rapidly and almost completely absorbed after oral administration, with peak plasma concentrations occurring within 1 to 2 hours [1]. The rate and extent of absorption are decreased by food. The volume of distribution of INH approximates total body water (0.67 ± 0.15 L per kg), with cerebrospinal fluid concentrations 90% of those of serum [2]. INH passes into breast milk and through the placental barrier. There is little protein binding.

Between 75% and 95% of an INH dose is acetylated in the liver within 24 hours by N-acetyltransferase 2 (NAT2) to acetylisoniazid and by hydrolysis to isonicotinic acid and hydrazine [1]. In addition, variable amounts of both INH and acetylisoniazid are oxidized by CYP2E1 to hepatotoxic intermediaries [3]. Genetic variation of the enzymes responsible for its metabolism causes significant variations of plasma concentration, elimination half-life, and toxicity. The elimination half-life in rapid acetylators (e.g., Asians, Eskimos, and American Indians) is 0.5 to 1.5 hours, whereas it is 2 to 4 hours in slow acetylators (e.g., people of African descent and Caucasians) [4]. The elimination half-life can be prolonged in people with liver disease. Rapid acetylators excrete 2.5% of INH as unchanged drug, compared with 10% in slow acetylators [1]. In addition, slow acetylators may have a higher percentage of the dose metabolized to hydrazine, a potential hepatotoxin [5]. INH exhibits dose-dependent inhibition of the mixed-function oxidases CYP2C19 and CYP3A, increasing the risk of adverse drug reactions in slow acetylators during the coadministration of drugs metabolized by these enzymes (e.g., phenytoin, carbamazepine, and diazepam).

Acute ingestion of 1.5 to 3.0 g in adults may be toxic, with 6 to 10 g uniformly associated with severe toxicity and significant mortality [6]. In patients with preexisting seizure disorders, convulsions have occurred with therapeutic dosing at doses as low as 14 mg/kg/d; 19 mg/kg/d resulted in seizures in a 7-year-old child [6].

Daily therapeutic INH doses produce peak serum concentrations between 1 and 7 μg per mL. Intermittent INH therapy may produce concentrations between 16 and 32 μg per mL. Serum INH concentrations in acute ingestions have ranged from 20 μg per mL to more than 710 μg per mL, with little correlation to severity of intoxication [7–10].

The central nervous system toxicity of INH and its metabolites is believed to be due to a decrease in the concentration of γ-aminobutyric acid (GABA), an inhibitory neurotransmitter that suppresses neuronal depolarization by opening chloride ionophores (Fig. 116.1). INH combines with pyridoxine (vitamin B_6) and is excreted in the urine as pyridoxal isonicotinylhydrazine [11]. It also competes with pyridoxine for pyridoxine kinase, the enzyme that converts pyridoxine to pyridoxal 5′-phosphate, the cofactor for glutamic acid decarboxylase–mediated conversion of glutamate to GABA [12]. In addition, INH inhibits glutamic acid decarboxylase activity. Its metabolism results in metabolites such as hydrazides and hydrazones, which inhibit pyridoxal 5′-phosphate and pyridoxine kinase, respectively [13].

INH causes a peripheral neuropathy that may be responsive to pyridoxine supplementation [14]. Wallerian degeneration of the myelin sheath and axon with blockade of fast axoplasmic transport is noted, with sensory nerves affected more than motor nerves. Peripheral neuropathy is most commonly associated with chronic INH use in slow acetylators but may occur after acute massive overdose [15,16].

The mechanism of INH-induced hepatic injury is not completely understood. Hepatitis occurs in 0.1% to 1.1% of patients receiving INH, especially those with advanced age and alcohol consumption [17–20]. Concurrent rifampin therapy increases the incidence of hepatitis to 2.7% in adults and 6.9% in children [17–21]. It is unclear whether this effect is due to an influence of rifampin on INH metabolism, or to the additive effect of two hepatotoxic drugs [19]. The histopathologic pattern of hepatic injury closely resembles viral hepatitis. Hypersensitivity seems unlikely, as rechallenge often fails to produce recurrence. Hepatic damage may be due to hydrazine metabolites of INH that covalently bind to liver macromolecules resulting in necrosis [22]. The severity of hepatotoxicity may be related to high-activity genotypes of CYP2E1 producing increased concentrations of reactive metabolites [3]. Recent work suggests that slow acetylators are more susceptible to antitubercular drug–induced hepatitis and may develop more severe hepatotoxicity than do rapid acetylators [3]. Additional risk factors may include homozygous null mutations in GSTM112 or GSTT113, the absence of HLA-DQA1*0102, and the presence of HLA-DQB1*0201 alleles [3].

The severe metabolic acidosis seen in acute INH intoxication is almost entirely due to seizure activity [23]. Although INH may interfere with nicotinamide adenine dinucleotide (NAD)–mediated conversion of lactate to pyruvate, acidosis was not observed in animal studies until seizures occurred with lactic acidosis resolving within 2 hours of cessation of seizures [23]. β-hydroxybutyric acid production has also been reported following INH overdose, but does not appear responsible for INH-induced acidosis.

Hyperglycemia may result from disruptions of the Krebs cycle that require NAD and from stimulation of glucagon secretion [9].

CLINICAL PRESENTATION

Signs and symptoms usually appear within 30 minutes to 2 hours following an acute INH overdose. Nausea, vomiting, dizziness, slurred speech, blurred vision, and visual hallucinations (e.g., bright colors, spots, and strange designs) are among the first manifestations [6,7]. Stupor and coma can develop rapidly, followed by intractable tonic–clonic generalized or localized seizures, hyperreflexia or areflexia, and cyanosis [6,7]. In severe cases, cardiovascular and respiratory collapse results in death. Oliguria progressing to anuria has been reported [6]. The metabolic alterations are striking and include severe metabolic acidosis, hyperglycemia, glycosuria, ketonuria, and hyperkalemia [6,7,9]. The triad of seizures refractory to anticonvulsants, metabolic acidosis refractory to sodium bicarbonate therapy, and coma suggests INH toxicity.

Hepatotoxicity usually presents as elevated serum aspartate aminotransferase values within the first few months of therapy. Fatalities from INH-induced hepatitis during chemoprophylaxis are between 4.2 and 7.0 per 100,000 persons [24]. When peripheral neuropathy occurs, it is within 3 to 35 weeks of initiating the therapy [25]. Other chronic effects include dysarthria, irritability, seizures, dysphoria, and inability to concentrate [17]. Optic neuritis and optic atrophy have also been reported, but their occurrence is often associated with the administration of ethambutol as well.

Psychosis has been reported as early as 1957. The patients were usually taking therapeutic doses at the time of onset. Symptoms include irritability, disorientation, visual and auditory hallucinations, paranoid delusions, and suicidal ideation. INH-associated psychosis has been reported in patients on multiple and mono drug therapies, with and without a previous psychiatric history, and therapy with and without pyridoxine [26].

Pellegra is a syndrome of dermatitis, diarrhea, and dementia, which is potentially fatal. Its rare association with isoniazid was first reported in 1956 in a patient also taking prophylactic pyridoxine. It is thought that isoniazid and perhaps pyridoxine as well, competitively inhibit nicotinamide-adenine dinucleotide (NAD) and nicotinamide-adenine dinucleotide phosphate (NADP) production in genetically susceptible individuals. This causes a decreased ability to repair cellular damage in tissues with high cellular turnover rates, such as skin and gastrointestinal mucosa, resulting in photosensitivity and gastrointestinal cell damage [27].

DIAGNOSTIC EVALUATION

Initial laboratory evaluation should include serum electrolytes, blood urea nitrogen, creatinine, glucose, calcium, and magnesium levels. Laboratory workup for anion-gap metabolic acidosis (e.g., serum methanol, ethylene glycol, salicylate, and acetaminophen levels) should also be considered. Arterial blood gases, electrocardiogram, chest radiograph, head computed tomography, and lumbar puncture should be obtained as clinically indicated.

Qualitative INH identification in urine using reagent-impregnated paper strips or a point-of-care testing device sensitive to INH metabolites and quantitative serum INH identification are not widely available to be clinically useful in real time.

Acute INH intoxication should be considered in the differential diagnosis of any patient presenting with unexplained intractable seizure activity, metabolic acidosis, or coma [6,10]. See Table 116.1 for some conditions that may resemble INH toxicity and/or cause anion-gap metabolic acidosis.

TABLE 116.1

Differential Diagnosis: INH Intoxication

Clinical presentation	Anion-gap metabolic acidosis
Central nervous system tumors and infections	Alcoholic ketoacidosis
Electrolyte abnormalities	Diabetic ketoacidosis
Hypoglycemia	Diethylene glycol
Thyroid dysfunction	Ethylene glycol
Poisonings	Iron
Antihistamines	Lactic acidosis
Carbon monoxide	Metformin
Cholinergics	Methanol
Cyanide	Propylene glycol
Meperidine (normeperidine)	Salicylates
Organophosphates	Starvation
Propoxyphene (norpropoxyphene)	Uremia
Sympathomimetics	
Theophylline	
Tricyclic antidepressants (e.g., amoxapine)	

Ingestion of rifampin–INH combination products may produce, in addition to the symptoms of INH poisoning, (a) a striking red-orange discoloration of the skin, urine, sclera, and mucus membranes; (b) periorbital or facial edema; (c) pruritus; and (d) nausea, vomiting, or diffuse abdominal tenderness [28]. Transient elevations in total bilirubin and alkaline phosphatase, indicating cholestasis, may also be noted.

MANAGEMENT

The initial management of a patient with acute INH overdose focuses on protection of airway, support of respiration, treatment of seizures, correction of metabolic acidosis, minimization of drug absorption, and in selected cases, enhancement of INH elimination.

Gastrointestinal decontamination, if performed, should consist of the administration of activated charcoal. Gastric lavage followed by activated charcoal should be considered in severely ill patients who have been intubated. Emesis is contraindicated because of the potential for rapid and unpredictable onset of seizures and coma.

Patients who have ingested a potentially toxic INH dose should be observed for at least 6 hours [6]; those who remain asymptomatic after gastrointestinal decontamination may be referred for psychiatric evaluation. All symptomatic patients should be admitted to an intensive care setting.

Seizures are often refractory to most conventional anticonvulsants [29]. Pyridoxine has dose-related effectiveness against convulsions and prevents lethality at doses from 75 to 300 mg per kg in canine models of INH toxicity [30]. In animal studies, when single-anticonvulsant regimens of pyridoxine, phenobarbital, pentobarbital, phenytoin, and diazepam were compared to the latter four anticonvulsants in combination with pyridoxine, pyridoxine was the only single agent that reduced the severity of convulsions and prevented death [29,30]. The combination of each of the other anticonvulsants with pyridoxine also prevented both convulsions and death. Therefore, pyridoxine, in conjunction with a benzodiazepine such as diazepam or lorazepam, is the preferred treatment for neurologic toxicity. Pyridoxine restores GABA production so that GABA agonists such as benzodiazepines or barbiturates can enhance GABA receptor activity. If pyridoxine is unavailable, diazepam appears to be the most effective single anticonvulsant, but its effectiveness may be limited and large doses may be required. Barbiturates are also effective, but may be more sedating than benzodiazepines.

Intravenous pyridoxine therapy should be administered at the first sign of neurologic toxicity in doses equal to the amount of INH ingested [6,7,31]. In patients actively convulsing, 1 g of pyridoxine should be administered for each gram of isoniazid ingested at a rate of 1 g per minute. INH-overdosed patients treated with such pyridoxine doses exhibited no recurrent seizure activity, a decreased duration of coma, and prompt resolution of their metabolic acidosis [10]. If the amount of INH ingested is unknown, at least 5 g of pyridoxine should be administered [6,7]. In patients without seizures, the pyridoxine dose may be administered over 30 to 60 minutes. In those with seizure activity, it may be given as a bolus during 3 to 5 minutes. The pyridoxine dose should be repeated if seizures persist or recur. Intravenous diazepam or lorazepam should also be given in conjunction with pyridoxine [6,29]. As there may be inadequate intravenous stores of pyridoxine in treating facilities, oral high-dose pyridoxine may be tried in the same doses as intravenous pyridoxine [32]. To accomplish this, pyridoxine tablets may be crushed, mixed with fluid, and administered via nasogastric tube. Seizures refractory to pyridoxine and diazepam have been successfully treated with thiopental-induced coma. Reversal of prolonged INH-induced coma has been temporally associated with pyridoxine therapy [33].

Treatment of metabolic acidosis should be guided by arterial blood gas and electrolyte measurements. In most cases, intravenous sodium bicarbonate will not correct acid–base abnormalities until seizure activity is terminated [10]. Bicarbonate should be considered if the serum pH is lower than 7.2 or if the acidosis does not rapidly resolve after seizure control.

Konigshausen et al. [34] reported two patients with apparent high-dose INH ingestions who presented with seizure and coma. One patient was treated with hemodialysis over 9 hours. His clearance rate was determined by arteriovenous differences as 76 mL per minute. The second patient was treated with pyridoxine and charcoal hemoperfusion. They reported that the initial CSF concentration fell from 25.6 to 4.1 μg per mL. The apparent half-life of 3.4 hours was within the reported normal elimination half-life for INH. The patient also underwent forced diuresis during that time. Both patients recovered fully. However, while hemodialysis and charcoal hemoperfusion can increase the clearance of INH and decrease its half-life by 50%, they have not been reported to remove significant quantities of INH (90 to 340 mg) [34–36].

Though exchange transfusion has been used in the treatment of isoniazid poisoning, there is no current application for its use [37]. The role of forced diuresis in the management of INH overdose is unproved. While large amounts of INH were recovered in the urine of some patients (43% to 58% of ingested doses), they are offset by those reporting minimal recovery (6 to 144 mg) [8,34,38]. Peritoneal dialysis is somewhat effective but inefficient [38]. One case using continuous veno-venous hemodiafiltration (CVVHDF) reported a fourfold increase over endogenous clearance, but did not quantitate the amount removed [39].

Considering the rapid elimination half-life of INH and the efficacy of pyridoxine and benzodiazepine therapy, measures to enhance INH elimination are of limited use in the routine management of INH toxicity. However, patients with intractable acid–base disturbances, persistent seizures, liver or renal dysfunction, or coma may be considered candidates for hemodialysis or charcoal hemoperfusion [36].Unless the patient has experienced significant anoxia as a result of coma or seizures, neurologic recovery may be expected within 24 to 48 hours.

Prevention of peripheral neuropathy during chronic INH therapy can be accomplished by the administration of pyridoxine, 15 to 50 mg per day, in high-risk patients. Peripheral neuropathy that develops during INH therapy is generally reversible on withdrawal of INH and treatment with high-dose pyridoxine (100 to 200 mg per day). However, the neuropathy may take months to a year or more to resolve, and in some cases, it may be permanent.

The management of INH-induced hepatotoxicity includes supportive care and cessation or reduction of INH administration. It is recommended that INH be discontinued in patients whose transaminase concentrations have risen to three times the upper limit of normal in the presence of jaundice or hepatitis symptoms or greater than five times the upper limit of normal if asymptomatic [18,40].

Psychosis usually responds to pyridoxine administration and patients may also benefit from antipsychotic medications such as risperidone or quetiapine [26].

The rare complication of pellagra responds to discontinuation of INH and institution of nicotinamide therapy [27].

References

1. Ellard G, Gammon P: Pharmacokinetics of isoniazid metabolism in man. *J Pharmacokinet Biopharm* 4:83–113, 1976.
2. Thummel KE, Shen DD, Isoherranen N: Appendix II. Design and optimization of dosage regimens: pharmacokinetic data, in Brunton LL, Chabner BA, Knollmann BC (eds): *Goodman & Gilman's the Pharmacological Basis of Therapeutics*. 12th ed. New York, NY, McGraw-Hill, 2011, p 1943.
3. Metushi IG, Cai P, Zhu X, et al: A fresh look at the mechanism of isoniazid-induced hepatotoxicity. *Clin Pharmacol Ther* 89:911–914, 2011.
4. Jeanes C, Schaefer O, Eidus L: Inactivation of isoniazid by Canadian Eskimos and Indians. *Can Med Assoc J* 106:331–335, 1972.
5. Sarma G, Immanuel C, Kailasam S, et al: Rifampin-induced release of hydrazine from isoniazid: a possible cause of hepatitis during treatment of tuberculosis with regimens containing isoniazid and rifampin. *Am Rev Respir Dis* 133:1072–1075, 1986.
6. Sievers ML, Kerrier RN: Treatment of acute isoniazid toxicity. *Am J Hosp Pharm* 32:202–206, 1975.
7. Brown C: Acute isoniazid poisoning. *Am Rev Respir Dis* 105:206–216, 1972.
8. Sitprija V, Holmes J: Isoniazid intoxication. *Am Rev Respir Dis* 90:248–254, 1964.
9. Terman D, Teitelbaum D: Isoniazid self-poisoning. *Neurology* 20:299–304, 1970.
10. Wason S, Lacouture P, Lovejoy F: Single high-dose pyridoxine treatment for isoniazid overdose. *JAMA* 246:1102–1104, 1981.
11. Sah P: Nicotinyl and isonicotinyl hydrazones of pyridoxal. *J Am Chem Soc* 76:300, 1954.
12. Williams H, Killah M, Jenny E: Convulsant effects of isoniazid. *JAMA* 152:1317–1321, 1953.
13. Biehl J, Vilter R: Effects of isoniazid on pyridoxine metabolism. *JAMA 156:1549-1552,*
14. Schröder JM: Isoniazid, in Spencer PS, Schaumberg HH (eds): *Experimental and Clinical Neurotoxicology*. 2nd ed. New York, NY, Oxford University Press, 2000, p 690-697.
15. Gurnani A, Chawla R, Kundra P, et al: Acute isoniazid poisoning. *Anaesthesia* 47:781–783, 1992.
16. Yamamoto M, Sobue G, Mukoyama M, et al: Demonstration of slow acetylator genotype of N-acetyltransferase in isoniazid neuropathy using an archival hematoxylin and eosin section of a sural nerve biopsy specimen. *J Neurol Sci* 135:51–54, 1996.
17. Blumberg H, Burman W, Chaisson R, et al: American Thoracic Society/Centers for Disease Control and Prevention/Infectious Diseases Society of America: treatment of tuberculosis. *Am J Respir Crit Care Med* 167:603–662, 2003.
18. Dickinson D, Bailey W, Hirschowitz B, et al: Risk factors for isoniazid (INH)-induced liver dysfunction. *J Clin Gastroenterol* 3:271–279, 1981.
19. Steele MA, Burk RF, DesPrez RM: Toxic hepatitis with isoniazid and rifampin. A meta-analysis. *Chest* 99:465–471, 1991.
20. Tostmann A, Boeree M, Aarnoutse R, et al: Antituberculosis drug-induced hepatotoxicity: concise up-to-date review. *J Gastroenterol Hepatol* 23:192–202, 2008.
21. O'Brien R, Long M, Cross F, et al: Hepatotoxicity from isoniazid and rifampin among children treated for tuberculosis. *Pediatrics* 72:491–499, 1983.
22. Timbrell J, Mitchell J, Snodgrass W, et al: Isoniazid hepatotoxicity: the relationship between covalent binding and metabolism in vivo. *J Pharmacol Exp Ther* 213:364–369, 1980.
23. Chin L, Sievers M, Herrier R, et al: Convulsions as the etiology of lactic acidosis in acute isoniazid toxicity in dogs. *Toxicol Appl Pharmacol* 49:377–384, 1979.
24. Millard P, Wilcosky T, Reade-Christopher S, et al: Isoniazid-related fatal hepatitis. *West J Med* 164:486–491, 1996.

25. Ochoa J: Isoniazid neuropathy in man: quantitative electron microscope study. *Brain* 93:831–850, 1970.
26. Witkowski AE, Manabat CG, Bourgeois JA: Isoniazid-associated psychosis. *Gen Hosp Psychiatry* 29:85–86, 2007.
27. Darvay A, Basarab T, McGregor JM, et al: Isoniazid induced pellagra despite pyridoxine supplementation. *Clin Exp Dermatol* 24:167–169, 1999.
28. Holdiness M: A review of the Redman syndrome and rifampin overdosage. *Med Toxicol Adverse Drug Exp* 4:444–451, 1989.
29. Chin L, Sievers M, Herrier R, et al: Potentiation of pyridoxine by depressants and anticonvulsants in the treatment of acute isoniazid intoxication in dogs. *Toxicol Appl Pharmacol* 58:504–509, 1981.
30. Chin L, Sievers M, Laird H, et al: Evaluation of diazepam and pyridoxine as antidotes to isoniazid intoxication in rats and dogs. *Toxicol Appl Pharmacol* 45:713–722, 1978.
31. Wood J, Peesker S: The effect on GABA metabolism in brain of isonicotinic acid hydrazide and pyridoxine as a function of time after administration. *J Neurochem* 190:1527–1537, 1972.
32. Hira HS, Ajmani A, Jain SK, et al: Acute isoniazid poisoning: role of single high oral dose of pyridoxine. *J Assoc Physicians India* 35:792–793, 1987.
33. Brent J, Vo N, Kulig K, et al: Reversal of prolonged isoniazid-induced coma by pyridoxine. *Arch Intern Med* 150:1751–1753, 1990.
34. Konigshausen T, Altrogge G, Hein D, et al: Hemodialysis and hemoperfusion in the treatment of most severe INH poisoning. *Vet Hum Toxicol* 21[Suppl]:12–15, 1979.
35. Jorgensen HE, Wieth JO: Dialysable poisons: hemodialysis in the treatment of acute poisoning. *Lancet* 1:81–84, 1963.
36. Orlowski JP, Paganini EP, Pippenger CE: Treatment of a potentially lethal dose isoniazid ingestion. *Ann Emerg Med* 17:73–76, 1988.
37. Katz BE, Carver MW: Acute poisoning with isoniazid treated by exchange transfusion. *Pediatrics* 18:72–76, 1956.
38. Cocco A, Pazourek L: Acute isoniazid intoxication: management by peritoneal dialysis. *N Engl J Med* 269:852–853, 1963.
39. Skinner K, Saiao A, Mostafa A, et al: Isoniazid poisoning: pharmacokinetics and effect of hemodialysis in a massive ingestion. *Hemodial Int* 19:E37–E40, 2015. doi: 10.1111/hdi.12293:1.
40. Saukkonen JJ, Cohn DL, Jasmer RM, et al: An official ATS statement: hepatotoxicity of antituberculosis therapy. *Am J Respir Crit Care Med* 174:935–952, 2006.

Chapter 117 ▪ Lithium Poisoning

THANJIRA JIRANANTAKAN • KENT R. OLSON

Lithium was introduced in the 19th century for the treatment of gout. Toxicity was rarely encountered because of low recommended doses. In the 1940s, lithium chloride was briefly marketed as a salt substitute, but was withdrawn after several cases of serious intoxication and death resulted from its use. In 1949, its antimanic properties were reported, and lithium has found increasingly wide psychiatric use since its approval by the U.S. Food and Drug Administration (FDA) in 1970 [1]. Lithium treatment in psychiatric diseases has been modified over five decades, but it remains a cornerstone "mood stabilizer" that is used worldwide [2].

Many studies have shown the benefits of lithium as a treatment for bipolar disorder, acute mania, and bipolar depression; however, recommendations concerning its clinical use vary among international guidelines. Lithium is recommended as monotherapy, as first-line treatment, or in combination with other antidepressive or antipsychotic agents based on different clinical scenarios and various guidelines [3].

Lithium induces neutrophilia (up to 1.5 to 2.0 times the reference leukocyte counts) by enhanced production of granulocyte colony-stimulating factor and stimulation of pluripotent stem cell production. Lithium has been prescribed for patients with various causes of neutropenia. Lithium has not been widely used in patients with thrombocytopenia despite evidence of megakaryocytopoiesis and thrombopoiesis demonstrated in a few studies [4,5].

Lithium is available in conventional tablets or capsules containing 150 mg, 300 mg, and 600 mg (4.06, 8.12, and 16.24 mmol, respectively) of lithium carbonate or in modified-release preparations containing 300 mg and 450 mg (8.12 and 12.18 mmol, respectively) of lithium carbonate. Liquid solutions of lithium citrate containing 8 mmol per 5 mL are also available. It is important to note that although lithium carbonate and lithium citrate are the commonly prescribed forms, other lithium salts (lithium acetate, lithium gluconate, lithium orotate, and lithium sulphate) are also available in some countries [6].

PHARMACOLOGY

Lithium is the lightest alkali metal (74 Da), occupying the same column in the periodic table as sodium and potassium, elements with which it shares some properties. Lithium forms a single-charged cation (Li^+) that is associated with various salts. Lithium has no known normal physiologic role in the human body. The exact mechanism of its therapeutic and toxic effects remains poorly elucidated. Lithium is known to suppress inositol signaling, which may be the mechanism for mood stabilization. It inhibits glycogen synthase kinase-3, a component of diverse signaling pathways responsible for energy metabolism, neuroprotection, and neuroplasticity. Lithium decreases the release of norepinephrine and dopamine from terminal nerve endings and may temporarily increase the release of serotonin. Lithium affects ion transport and cell membrane potential by competing with sodium and potassium and possibly other cations. However, unlike sodium and potassium, lithium does not produce a large distribution gradient and, therefore, cannot maintain a significant membrane potential [6,7].

Lithium is readily absorbed from the gastrointestinal tract. The bioavailability of conventional tablets and capsules and the liquid solution is 95% to 100%; bioavailability is not affected by food. Normally, absorption is complete within 6 hours; peak levels are reached in 1 to 2 hours. Modified-release preparations are less predictably absorbed (60% to 90%), and peak levels may be lower than with the conventional form and may be delayed by more than 4 to 12 hours [6–8]. Overdose has resulted in delayed peak levels or secondary peak levels as long as 148 hours following ingestion [8].

Lithium initially occupies an apparent volume of distribution of 0.3 to 0.4 L per kg, but further distribution into various intracellular tissue compartments occurs over 6 to 10 hours, with a final volume of distribution of 0.7 to 1.0 L per kg. This explains why initial serum lithium levels may be very high, with few or no signs of toxicity. After a single dose, the equilibrium (postdistributional) serum lithium concentration can be expected to increase by 1.0 to 1.5 mmol per L for each 1.0 mmol of lithium per kilogram of body weight. Steady-state tissue levels are achieved after 3 to 4 days of therapy. Tissue distribution is uneven; whereas the cerebrospinal fluid lithium concentration is only 50% to 80% that of plasma, the bile concentration may be two times greater than that of plasma. Lithium is not bound to serum proteins. It freely crosses the placenta [6]. One animal study demonstrated that brain lithium accumulation is prominent in acute-on-chronically poisoned rats compared with acutely poisoned rats. Moreover, brain lithium distribution is increased in chronically poisoned rats compared with acute-on-chronically poisoned rats [9].

Lithium is not metabolized. More than 95% of absorbed lithium is excreted by the kidneys, with 4% to 5% eliminated in sweat and 1% in the feces. It is also excreted in breast milk. Eighty percent of renally filtered lithium is reabsorbed in the proximal tubule (60%) and the thick ascending limb of the loop of Henle and collecting duct (20%) against a concentration gradient that does not distinguish lithium from sodium. Sodium depletion can result in as much as a 50% increase in lithium reabsorption. The usual renal clearance is 15 to 30 mL per minute, but it may be 10 to 15 mL per minute or less in the elderly and in patients with renal dysfunction or dehydration [6].The lithium excretion rate may vary in different types of renal failure. One study demonstrated increased fractional excretion of lithium in patients with prerenal failure, but decreased fractional excretion in acute tubular necrosis renal failure [10]. The elimination half-life averages 16 to 30 hours; in patients with chronic intoxication, it may be as long as 58 hours [7,11].

Therapeutic levels are achieved by administration of 600 to 1,200 mg (16 to 32 mmol) of lithium carbonate per day in adults. Therapeutic serum lithium concentrations are usually considered to be 0.60 to 1.20 mmol per L; prophylaxis against recurrent manic-depressive illness may be achieved with levels of 0.75 to 1.00 mmol per L. Drug levels should be drawn at least 12 hours after the last dose to allow for complete tissue distribution. Onset of therapeutic effects usually requires 5 to 21 days after initiation of daily drug administration. Careful monitoring of lithium levels is essential because of its low toxic-to-therapeutic ratio or so-called narrow therapeutic index [2,3,12].

Lithium intoxication primarily involves the central nervous system (CNS) and kidneys, although a variety of other organ systems are also affected (Table 117.1). Lithium intoxication may follow an acute overdose, an increase in the daily therapeutic dose, or a decrease in lithium elimination by the kidneys. Most serious toxicity occurs in patients with chronic intoxication, especially in older patients and patients with renal insufficiency [11].

Acute ingestion of at least 40 mg per kg (1 mmol per kg) of lithium carbonate in a lithium-naive person would be required to produce a potentially toxic serum lithium level. The acute toxic dose in a patient already taking lithium ("acute-on-chronic" overdose) depends on the existing serum lithium level ("tissue soaking"). The dose required to produce chronic intoxication depends on the individual's rate of renal lithium elimination.

TABLE 117.1

Common Features of Lithium Intoxication

Feature	Number	Percentage of total
Confusion	19[a]	68
Agitation	17	61
Drowsiness	16[a]	57
Mutism	5	18
Coma (grades III–IV)	1	4
Convulsions	4	14
Hyperreflexia	22	79
Increased tone	16	57
Ankle clonus	4	14
Extensor plantar responses	3	11
Tremor	18	64
Ataxia	14	50
Dysarthria	10	36
Myoclonus	7	25
Vomiting	7	25
Diarrhea	4	14
Acute diabetes insipidus	3	11
Acute renal failure	2	7

[a]Excludes one patient who also took temazepam in overdose.
Reprinted from Dyson EH, Simpson D, Prescott LF, et al: Self-poisoning and therapeutic intoxication with lithium. *Hum Toxicol* 6:325, 1987, with permission.

CLINICAL MANIFESTATIONS

There are three clinical patterns of lithium intoxication: *acute* lithium poisoning in a lithium-naive individual who takes an acute overdose; *acute-on-chronic* lithium poisoning (a previously treated patient who takes an acute overdose); and *chronic* lithium poisoning in a previously treated patient who gradually accumulates lithium without taking an acute overdose [7]. Classification for severity of lithium intoxication may be based on serum lithium concentration: *mild* (1.5 to 2.5 mmol per L), *serious* (2.5 to 3.5 mmol per L), and *life-threatening* (>3.5 mmol per L). However, there does not appear to be a clear-cut relationship between serum concentrations and severity of toxicity, and decisions for treatment should be based on clinical parameters [13].

Symptoms and signs of mild lithium intoxication include nausea, vomiting, lethargy, fatigue, memory impairment, and fine tremor. Moderate signs and symptoms of toxicity include confusion, agitation, delirium, coarse tremor, hyperreflexia, hypertension, tachycardia, dysarthria, nystagmus, ataxia, muscle fasciculations, extrapyramidal syndromes, and choreoathetoid movements. Patients with severe toxicity may also exhibit bradycardia, complete heart block, coma, seizures, nonconvulsive status epilepticus (which may clinically resemble a nonictal encephalopathy), hyperthermia, neuroleptic malignant syndrome, serotonin syndrome, and hypotension [14]. Permanent sequelae include choreoathetosis, tardive dystonia, tremor, peripheral neuropathy, scanning speech, dysarthria, muscle rigidity, cognitive deficits, nystagmus, and ataxia [15].

Neurotoxic effects of lithium usually develop gradually and may become progressively severe over several days. Neurologic manifestations may worsen even as serum lithium levels are falling and may persist for days to weeks after cessation of the therapy, in part because of slow movement of lithium into and out of intracellular brain sites and possibly brain damage, such as demyelination caused by lithium. Lithium can cause persistent neurologic deficits longer than 2 months after cessation of lithium, also known as "Syndrome of Irreversible Lithium-Effectuated Neurotoxicity" or "SILENT." The most common sequela of this syndrome appears to be persistent cerebellar dysfunction, but extrapyramidal, cognitive, and brainstem dysfunctions were also evident [15]. Reduced brain volume was demonstrated in one patient who suffered from SILENT [16]. Risk factors for SILENT include high serum lithium levels during acute intoxication, presence of fever, concomitant use of other drugs such as antipsychotics, tricyclic antidepressants, and anticonvulsive drugs. It is important to note that SILENT can occur in patients with low or normal serum lithium levels [15].

Cardiovascular manifestations due to lithium intoxication are nonspecific and can be delayed owing to progressive equilibrium between intracellular and extracellular compartments. Abnormalities in the electrocardiogram (ECG) are often similar to those seen with hypokalemia and may result from displacement of intracellular potassium by lithium; U waves and flattened, biphasic, or inverted T waves can be seen with therapeutic doses and mild overdoses. Sinus and junctional bradycardia, sinoatrial and first-degree atrioventricular (AV) block, and QRS and QTc interval prolongation may be seen with severe intoxication [17]. Life-threatening dysrhythmias are rare but may result in death. Patients with complete heart block during lithium treatment have been reported [14,18]. This is more common in patients older than 65 years with baseline ECG abnormalities, conduction abnormalities, use of renal toxic medications, and concomitant use of AV nodal–blocking agents [18]. Lithium cardiotoxicity can mimic ischemia. A case of lithium intoxication with ECG findings of ST elevation and of a lithium-intoxicated patient who developed Takotsubo cardiomyopathy has been reported [19,20]. Pulse and blood pressure abnormalities may be seen in moderate or severe poisoning, but they are usually not pronounced. Hypotension is more often caused by dehydration, which can be a cause and a complication of lithium intoxication, rather than direct cardiotoxicity [17].

Effects on renal function in chronic lithium therapy include impaired urinary concentrating ability, nephrogenic diabetes insipidus (NDI), and a sodium-losing nephritis [2]. NDI is the most common renal side effect of lithium intoxication [21]. Clinically, this manifests as polyuria and polydipsia. Risk factors include lithium duration, dose, serum level, slow release form, and clinical nonresponse. These effects appear to be dose related and usually correct within several weeks of discontinuing the therapy [17]. Excessive water and sodium loss lead to increased proximal tubular reabsorption of lithium by transport mechanisms designed for sodium reabsorption. The accumulation of lithium may be enhanced by illnesses that result in decreased glomerular filtration rate, such as fever with sweating, gastroenteritis, and heart failure, or by diuretic drugs that enhance sodium and fluid loss. Rising lithium levels may further aggravate nephrotoxicity. A stable patient on a constant daily lithium dose with a therapeutic serum lithium concentration for years may suddenly develop life-threatening intoxication.

Metabolic abnormalities associated with lithium use include hypercalcemia, hypermagnesemia, nonketotic hyperglycemia, transient diabetic ketoacidosis, and goiter. Hypothyroidism or hyperthyroidism due to lithium intoxication is rarely reported [2,17].

Lithium is classified as FDA pregnancy category D. It is teratogenic in rats, mice, and rabbits. Ebstein's anomaly, hypothyroid, and "floppy-baby syndrome" have been reported in infants born to mothers on lithium therapy [2].

Several drugs may interact with lithium to alter its pharmacokinetics or directly enhance its toxicity. Diuretics may promote fluid and sodium depletion, leading to enhanced tubular lithium reabsorption. This effect appears to be much less apparent with furosemide than with thiazide diuretics. Aminophylline, urea, bicarbonate, and acetazolamide may decrease serum lithium levels by increasing the glomerular filtration rate. Nonsteroidal anti-inflammatory drugs, including the selective cyclooxygenase-2 inhibitor rofecoxib, may decrease the glomerular filtration rate and lithium elimination. Antipsychotic medications may have additive CNS depressant effects; in addition, lithium may enhance their dopamine-blocking and serotonergic effects and induce or aggravate rigidity and hyperthermia, possibly inducing neuroleptic malignant syndrome and serotonin syndrome [17]. Angiotensin-converting enzyme inhibitors have been reported to increase steady-state lithium concentrations by 36.1% and reduce lithium clearance by 25.5%, resulting in lithium toxicity [22].

DIAGNOSTIC EVALUATION

The history should include the type of lithium preparation ingested, the amount(s) and time(s) of ingestion, and the nature of the symptoms. It is important to differentiate patients with acute lithium overdose from those with chronic intoxication resulting from excessive daily doses or impaired renal elimination given that patients with chronic lithium intoxication can manifest greater toxicity despite lower serum lithium levels compared with acute overdose.

The physical examination should focus on the vital signs, neurologic function, and cardiovascular status. All patients should have an ECG and laboratory evaluation, including serum electrolytes, glucose, blood urea nitrogen, creatinine, and serum lithium level. Lithium levels should be obtained at least 12 hours after the last lithium dose and repeated at intervals of 4 to 6 hours after acute overdose until peak levels are observed. If the levels are elevated, they should be repeated until they are in the therapeutic range and the patient becomes asymptomatic [12]. Blood for thyroid function testing and calcium and magnesium levels may be warranted in some cases [2]. Electroencephalography (EEG) should be considered in patients who present with coma, altered or depressed mental status to rule out nonconvulsive status epilepticus. The EEG may demonstrate triphasic waves, commonly seen in metabolic encephalopathy, or bihemispheric slowing (4- to 5-Hz theta range) with bilateral periodic triphasic waves of 1- to 2-Hz frequency, which have also been found in a patient with Creutzfeldt–Jakob disease [23].

Patients with chronic lithium overdose are typically brought to medical attention by a family member or therapist because of gradual onset of neurologic symptoms. There is usually a recent history of excessive fluid loss caused by gastroenteritis, other infective illness, renal insufficiency, or the addition of new drugs such as diuretics and nonsteroidal anti-inflammatory agents [12].

After acute lithium overdose, the predominant initial symptoms are nausea, vomiting, abdominal pain, or diarrhea [2]. Patients do not usually have significant neurologic manifestations despite high serum lithium levels during the first 12 hours or more after ingestion because lithium is taken up slowly by the brain and other tissues [11]. Serum lithium concentrations as high as 10.6 mmol per L without significant toxicity have been reported after acute overdose [24]. However, toxicity may develop during the subsequent 24 to 48 hours, even as serum levels fall [15,17]. There does not appear to be any clinical variable that accurately predicts which patients will deteriorate. The use of cerebrospinal fluid levels to estimate brain levels more closely has been advocated. However, cerebrospinal fluid levels do not reflect intracellular brain tissue levels or predict the level of coma [6,9].

Patients with acute-on-chronic lithium overdose have a clinical course similar to those following an acute overdose. However, a smaller total dose may produce severe intoxication, depending on the preoverdose serum lithium level.

Elevated blood urea nitrogen and creatinine reflect renal insufficiency and suggest that intoxication results from gradual accumulation of lithium rather than acute ingestion. Elevated creatinine may also be caused by cross-reactivity of the assay with creatinine from muscle destruction and should prompt the measurement of serum creatinine phosphokinase and urinalysis for myoglobinuria.

Patients with lithium-induced NDI usually have dilute urine with a low measured osmolality relative to serum. Hypernatremia can be observed. The diagnosis of NDI is confirmed by lack of urinary concentration in response to administered vasopressin [21].

Leukocytosis may be evident in patients on lithium therapy. It is a nonspecific finding and does not reflect severity of intoxication. A reduced or absent anion gap may occur with severe lithium carbonate intoxication, probably because the carbonate anion (but not the lithium cation) is measured and used in calculating the anion gap [25].

Plain abdomen imaging may or may not reveal radiopaque lithium tablets after acute ingestion. A negative radiograph should not be used to rule out an acute ingestion [26].

Differential diagnosis of patients with lithium poisoning includes hypoxia, hypoglycemia, hypothermia or hyperthermia, electrolyte disturbances, CNS infection, head trauma, and intracranial bleeding. In a patient with hyperthermia and rigidity who is also taking antipsychotic medications, neuroleptic malignant syndrome and serotonin syndrome should be considered. Other drug intoxications should be considered, especially if CNS symptoms appear shortly after an acute overdose.

MANAGEMENT

Initial management of patients with altered mental status should include assessment and stabilization of the airway; administration of oxygen and assisted ventilation, if needed; vascular access and continuous ECG monitoring; and administration of drugs (e.g., dextrose, naloxone, and thiamine) if appropriate. Benzodiazepines or barbiturates should be administered to patients with seizures. The EEG should be used to confirm the resolution of seizure activity in patients with nonconvulsive status epilepticus. If hyperthermia is present, cooling measures should be instituted, including evaporative cooling, tepid sponging, and fanning. Neuromuscular paralysis and endotracheal intubation, a reliable approach to rapidly lower body temperature, can be considered as needed. Hypovolemia, if present, should be treated with intravenous crystalloids. Cardiac dysrhythmias do not usually require treatment, but should respond to the current recommended pharmacologic treatment of dysrhythmias.

Gastrointestinal tract decontamination should be considered after acute ingestion to prevent continued absorption of lithium. Ipecac-induced emesis is not recommended. Gastric lavage may be of benefit in selected clinical situations (e.g., symptomatic patient following a massive overdose) [27]. Activated charcoal does not effectively bind lithium and should be given only if coingestion of another drug is suspected [28]. Whole-bowel irrigation (see Chapter 97) has been recommended for large ingestions, especially if they involve modified-release tablets [29]. If a tablet mass or concretion is suspected because of sustained high levels after 2 to 3 days, contrast imaging studies, ultrasound, or gastroduodenal endoscopy and endoscopic removal should be considered [30]. Preliminary evidence in animals and human volunteers suggests that the cation exchange resin sodium polystyrene sulfonate (Kayexalate) binds lithium and may enhance its elimination [31–33]. One case report describes its use in a patient with acute-on-chronic lithium overdose. Treatment emergent adverse events include constipation and mild hypokalemia. The clinical effectiveness of sodium polystyrene sulfonate treatment in lithium overdose remains to be determined.

Observation in asymptomatic patients following an acute or acute-on-chronic overdose of lithium in conventional formulation should be for a minimum of 6 hours, and observation for a minimum of 24 hours following an overdose of lithium in modified-release formulation [6–8]. Serial lithium levels should be obtained to confirm lack of significant absorption. Patients with mild overdoses can often be monitored and treated in the emergency department. Symptomatic patients, patients with a massive acute ingestion, and those whose levels continue to rise beyond 6 hours after ingestion should be admitted to an intensive care setting.

Delayed clinical manifestations and peak serum lithium concentrations may occur in patients who overdose on modified-release formulations of lithium. Serial serum lithium concentrations should be obtained (e.g., every 4 to 6 hours) until serum lithium concentrations have decreased to the therapeutic range.

Lithium-induced NDI does not respond to vasopressin, but it has been reported to improve with hydrochlorothiazide, amiloride, carbamazepine, and indomethacin [17]. However, the gradual onset and the duration required of hydrochlorothiazide, carbamazepine, and amiloride therapy would limit their clinical usefulness. One case report suggests indomethacin may be acutely effective in treating lithium-induced NDI [34].

Intravenous fluid therapy is effective in restoring glomerular filtration rate and maintaining renal elimination of lithium in most patients with mild or moderate intoxication. A crystalloid solution (half-normal or normal saline) aiming for urine output of 1 to 3 mL/kg/h should be administered after an initial saline bolus (10 to 20 mL per kg), depending on the degree of dehydration. Serum electrolytes should be followed closely because hypernatremia may occur.

A crude estimate of renal lithium clearance can be calculated from simultaneous urine and serum lithium levels and urine flow rate: Renal lithium clearance = urine flow rate (mL per minute) × urine lithium (mmol per L)/serum lithium (mmol per L). Normal lithium clearance is 15 to 30 mL per minute. If the clearance is below normal in a patient without underlying cardiac or renal dysfunction, the rate of fluid administration should be increased because this suggests low renal perfusion secondary to dehydration. In human studies, water loading, furosemide, thiazide, ethacrynic acid, ammonium chloride, and spironolactone did not increase lithium clearance.

Hemodialysis is the most efficient method for removing lithium, achieving clearance rates of up to 170 to 180 mL per minute [7,35,36]. However, lithium is only slowly removed from intracellular tissue compartments, especially the brain, and rebound increases of serum lithium levels often occur within several hours after dialysis. Hemodialysis should be repeated frequently until the serum level drawn 6 to 8 hours after the last dialysis is 1 mmol per L or less [7,12,36]. However, despite repeated dialyses, patients with significant neurologic toxicity do not promptly improve. Recovery, if it occurs, may be protracted.

The indications for hemodialysis are not well established, and hence recommendations for management of lithium poisoning vary widely, as demonstrated in a survey of 163 health care professionals from 33 countries [37]. It is generally agreed that patients with severe clinical toxicity and those with renal dysfunction should undergo dialysis. Asymptomatic patients or those with mild-to-moderate intoxication who are otherwise healthy may be managed with intravenous fluids as long as they remain clinically stable or are improving with satisfactory lithium clearance (>15 to 20 mL per minute). Renal replacement therapy (e.g., venovenous or arteriovenous hemodiafiltration) has been reported to successfully remove lithium without the need for hemodialysis [38]. In one case, 14 hours of continuous arteriovenous hemodiafiltration was estimated to achieve lithium elimination equivalent to 5.75 hours of hemodialysis [39]. In another case report, clearances of up to 38 mL per minute were achieved with continuous venovenous hemodiafiltration [40]. However, in the acute setting, *hemodialysis* is most effective for quickly reducing the serum lithium concentration, and it can be followed by continuous renal replacement therapy to maintain a slow but continuous removal of lithium, thus mitigating a rebound in the central compartment lithium concentration.

A systematic review and consensus recommendations were published in 2015 by the Extracorporeal Treatments in Poisoning (EXTRIP) Workgroup, an international panel of reviewers from a broad range of medical specialties and representing diverse professional societies. The systematic review indicated there is a very low quality of evidence for all recommendations, because most publications were case reports. The panel's recommendation for extracorporeal treatment based on history taking, physical examination, ECG findings, and serum lithium levels were based largely on opinion [7]. Recommendations by the EXTRIP Workgroup are summarized in Figure 117.1.

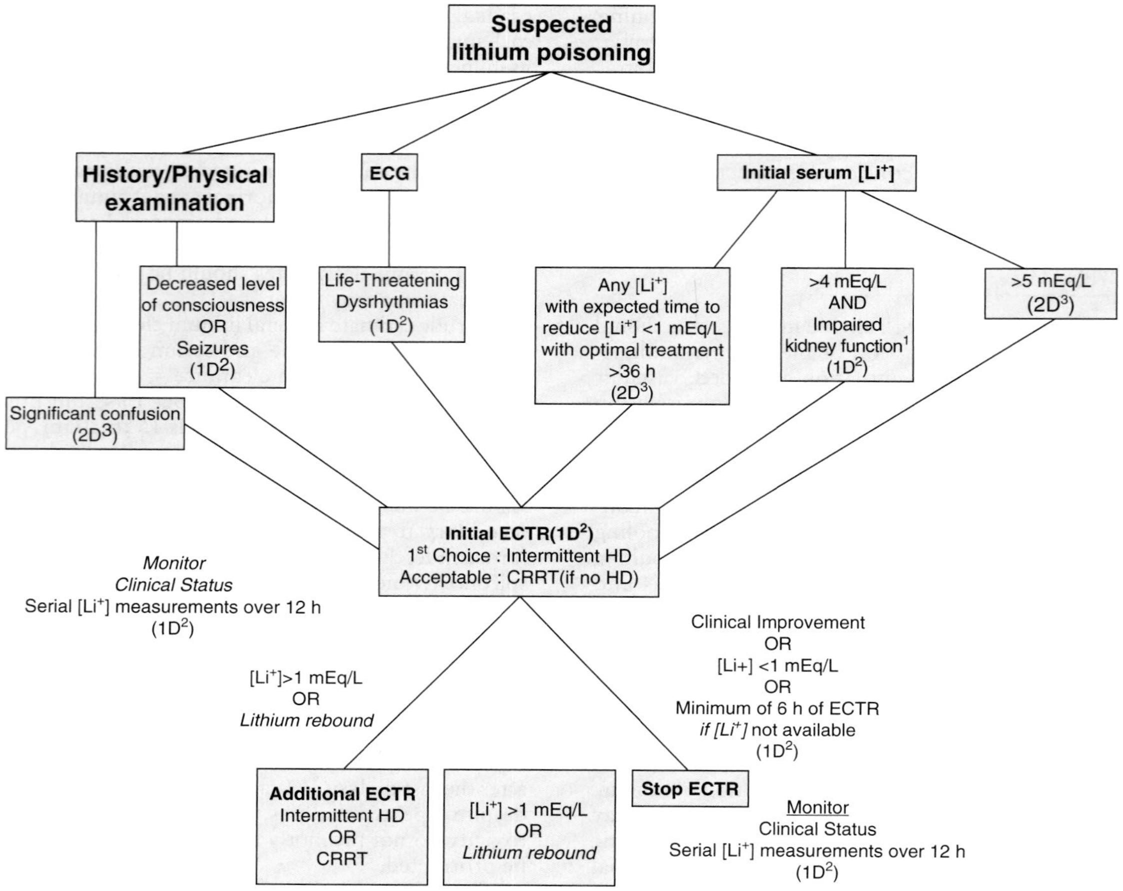

FIGURE 117.1 Extracorporeal Treatment (ECTR) for lithium poisoning; Recommendation from the Extracorporeal Treatments in Poisoning (EXTRIP) Workgroup (2015). [1]Impaired kidney function defined as (1) stage 3B, 4 or 5 CKD (i.e., eGFR <45 mL/min per 1.73 m^2; (2) Kidney Disease Improving Global Outcomes stage 2 or 3 AKI; (3) If no baseline creatinine, Serum Cr 2 mg/dL (176 μmol/L) in adults and 1.5 mg/dL (132 μmol/L) in elderly/low-muscle mass patients; and (4) If no baseline creatinine, Serum Cr > 2 times the upper limit of normal for age and sex in children, the presence of oligo/anuria should raise awareness of impaired kidney function. $1D^2$: Strong recommendation, very low evidence, $2D^3$: Weak recommendation, very low evidence.

References

1. Shorter E: The history of lithium therapy. *Bipolar Disord* 11[Suppl 2]:4–9, 2009.
2. Grandjean EM, Aubry JM: Lithium: updated human knowledge using an evidence-based approach: part III: clinical safety. *CNS Drugs* 23(5):397–418, 2009.
3. Yatham LN, Kennedy SH, Parikh SV, et al: Canadian Network for Mood and Anxiety Treatments (CANMAT) and International Society for Bipolar Disorders (ISBD) collaborative update of CANMAT guidelines for the management of patients with bipolar disorder: update 2013. *Bipolar Disord* 15(1):1–44, 2013.
4. Young W: Review of lithium effects on brain and blood. *Cell Transplant* 18(9):951–975, 2009.
5. Focosi D, Azzara A, Kast RE, et al: Lithium and hematology: established and proposed uses. *J Leukoc Biol* 85(1):20–28, 2009.
6. Grandjean EM, Aubry JM: Lithium: updated human knowledge using an evidence-based approach. Part II: Clinical pharmacology and therapeutic monitoring. *CNS Drugs* 23(4):331–349, 2009.
7. Decker BS, Goldfarb DS, Dargan PI, et al: Extracorporeal treatment for lithium poisoning: systematic review and recommendations from the EXTRIP Workgroup. *Clin J Am Soc Nephrol* 10(5):875–887, 2015.
8. Friedberg RC, Spyker DA, Herold DA: Massive overdoses with sustained-release lithium carbonate preparations: pharmacokinetic model based on two case studies. *Clin Chem* 37(7):1205–1209, 1991.
9. Hanak AS, Chevillard L, El Balkhi S, et al: Study of blood and brain lithium pharmacokinetics in the rat according to three different modalities of poisoning. *Toxicol Sci* 143(1):185–195, 2015.
10. Steinhauslin F, Burnier M, Magnin JL, et al: Fractional excretion of trace lithium and uric acid in acute renal failure. *J Am Soc Nephrol* 4(7):1429–1437, 1994.
11. Dyson EH, Simpson D, Prescott LF, et al: Self-poisoning and therapeutic intoxication with lithium. *Hum Toxicol* 6(4):325–329, 1987.
12. Sadosty AT, Groleau GA, Atcherson MM: The use of lithium levels in the emergency department. *J Emerg Med* 17(5):887–891, 1999.
13. Hansen HE, Amdisen A: Lithium intoxication (Report of 23 cases and review of 100 cases from the literature). *Q J Med* 47(186):123–144, 1978.
14. Shiraki T, Kohno K, Saito D, et al: Complete atrioventricular block secondary to lithium therapy. *Circ J* 72(5):847–849, 2008.
15. Adityanjee, Munshi KR, Thampy A: The syndrome of irreversible lithium-effectuated neurotoxicity. *Clin Neuropharmacol* 28(1):38–49, 2005.
16. Ikeda Y, Kameyama M, Narita K, et al: Total and regional brain volume reductions due to the Syndrome of Irreversible Lithium-Effectuated Neurotoxicity (SILENT): a voxel-based morphometric study. *Prog Neuropsychopharmacol Biol Psychiatry* 34(1):244–246, 2010.
17. Simard M, Gumbiner B, Lee A, et al: Lithium carbonate intoxication. A case report and review of the literature. *Arch Intern Med* 149(1):36–46, 1989.
18. Serinken M, Karcioglu O, Korkmaz A: Rarely seen cardiotoxicity of lithium overdose: complete heart block. *Int J Cardiol* 20;132(2):276–278, 2009.
19. Puhr J, Hack J, Early J, et al: Lithium overdose with electrocardiogram changes suggesting ischemia. *J Med Toxicol* 4(3):170–172, 2008.
20. Kitami M, Oizumi H, Kish SJ, et al: Takotsubo cardiomyopathy associated with lithium intoxication in bipolar disorder: a case report. *J Clin Psychopharmacol* 34(3):410–411, 2014.
21. Erden A, Karagoz H, Basak M, et al: Lithium intoxication and nephrogenic diabetes insipidus: a case report and review of literature. *Int J Gen Med* 6:535–539, 2013.
22. Finley PR, O'Brien JG, Coleman RW: Lithium and angiotensin-converting enzyme inhibitors: evaluation of a potential interaction. *J Clin Psychopharmacol* 16(1):68–71, 1996.
23. Kaplan PW, Birbeck G: Lithium-induced confusional states: nonconvulsive status epilepticus or triphasic encephalopathy? *Epilepsia* 47(12):2071–2074, 2006.
24. Nagappan R, Parkin WG, Holdsworth SR: Acute lithium intoxication. *Anaesth Intensive Care* 30(1):90–92, 2002.
25. Leon M, Graeber C: Absence of high anion gap metabolic acidosis in severe ethylene glycol poisoning: a potential effect of simultaneous lithium carbonate ingestion. *Am J Kidney Dis* 23(2):313–316, 1994.
26. Savitt DL, Hawkins HH, Roberts JR: The radiopacity of ingested medications. *Ann Emerg Med* 16(3):331–339, 1987.

27. Teece S, Crawford I: Best evidence topic report: no clinical evidence for gastric lavage in lithium overdose. *Emerg Med J* 22(1):43–44, 2005.
28. Favin FD, Klein-Schwartz W, Oderda GM, et al: In vitro study of lithium carbonate adsorption by activated charcoal. *J Toxicol Clin Toxicol* 26(7):443–450, 1988.
29. Smith SW, Ling LJ, Halstenson CE: Whole-bowel irrigation as a treatment for acute lithium overdose. *Ann Emerg Med* 20(5):536–539, 1991.
30. Thornley-Brown D, Galla JH, Williams PD, et al: Lithium toxicity associated with a trichobezoar. *Ann Intern Med* 1;116(9):739–740, 1992.
31. Ghannoum M, Lavergne V, Yue CS, et al: Successful treatment of lithium toxicity with sodium polystyrene sulfonate: a retrospective cohort study. *Clin Toxicol* 48(1):34–41, 2010.
32. Tomaszewski C, Musso C, Pearson JR, et al: Lithium absorption prevented by sodium polystyrene sulfonate in volunteers. *Ann Emerg Med* 21(11):1308–1311, 1992.
33. Gehrke JC, Watling SM, Gehrke CW, et al: In-vivo binding of lithium using the cation exchange resin sodium polystyrene sulfonate. *Am J Emerg Med* 14(1):37–38, 1996.
34. Martinez EJ, Sinnott JT, Rodriguez-Paz G, et al: Lithium-induced nephrogenic diabetes insipidus treated with indomethacin. *South Med J* 86(8):971–973, 1993.
35. Okusa MD, Crystal LJ: Clinical manifestations and management of acute lithium intoxication. *Am J Med* 97(4):383–389, 1994.
36. Meertens JH, Jagernath DR, Eleveld DJ, et al: Haemodialysis followed by continuous veno-venous haemodiafiltration in lithium intoxication; a model and a case. *Eur J Intern Med* 20(3):e70–e73, 2009.
37. Roberts DM, Gosselin S: Variability in the management of lithium poisoning. *Sem Dial* 27(4):390–394, 2014.
38. Beckmann U, Oakley PW, Dawson AH, et al: Efficacy of continuous venovenous hemodialysis in the treatment of severe lithium toxicity. *J Toxicol Clin Toxicol* 39(4):393–397, 2001.
39. Bellomo R, Kearly Y, Parkin G, et al: Treatment of life-threatening lithium toxicity with continuous arterio-venous hemodiafiltration. *Crit Care Med* 19(6):836–837, 1991.
40. van Bommel EF, Kalmeijer MD, Ponssen HH: Treatment of life-threatening lithium toxicity with high-volume continuous venovenous hemofiltration. *Am J Nephrol* 20(5):408–411, 2000.

Chapter 118 ■ Methylxanthine Poisoning

JANETTA L. IWANICKI

The methylxanthines most commonly used in the clinical setting are theophylline and its ethylenediamine salt, aminophylline. Until recently, theophylline was used exclusively as a bronchodilator for the management of reversible obstructive pulmonary diseases and as a respiratory stimulant for the treatment of apnea of prematurity in neonates. During the 1980s, its use fell dramatically as more effective therapies for recurrent bronchospasm became available [1]. However, there has been renewed interest in theophylline as the scope of its pharmacologic benefits broadens. Potential uses for theophylline now include preconditioning of cardiac ischemia [2], treatment of bradycardia [3], amelioration of perinatal asphyxia [4], and protection from contrast-induced nephropathy [5]. Recent clinical trials of theophylline for asthma have demonstrated substantial benefit, restoring interest in the drug for this indication [6,7]. Despite its renewed popularity, theophylline, with its potent pharmacologic actions, variable metabolic disposition in humans, and narrow therapeutic-to-toxic ratio, is a common cause of intoxication [1,8].

Caffeine and theobromine are other widely used methylxanthines. Caffeine is found in beverages such as coffee and tea, energy drinks (e.g., sodas or water) or dietary energy supplements (e.g., guarana or kola), energy foods such as mints and gum, and pharmaceutical preparations (e.g., antisleep drugs). Although severe toxicity from caffeine ingestion is uncommon, case reports of serious poisoning in children and adults are well documented [9]. Because caffeine and other xanthine derivatives are structurally similar to theophylline, signs and symptoms of toxicity resemble those seen in theophylline intoxication, and the approach to management should be similar.

Three clinical circumstances account for most cases of theophylline poisoning: unintentional ingestions by children, intentional ingestions (suicide attempts) by adolescents or adults, and medication errors (miscalculation of dose, change in frequency of administration, lack of serum drug level monitoring, or an unrecognized drug–drug or drug–disease interaction) [1,10,11]. Most cases of theophylline intoxication result from chronic, unintentional overmedication.

PHARMACOLOGY

Theophylline is available commercially as a liquid, tablet, sustained-release capsule, or solution for intravenous administration. Overdose of sustained-release theophylline can lead to a marked delay in complete absorption, with peak serum theophylline concentrations occurring as long as 15 to 24 hours after ingestion [12]. Therapeutic serum theophylline concentrations range from 10 to 20 μg per mL.

A loading dose of 5 to 6 mg per kg of intravenous aminophylline should produce a serum theophylline level of 10 μg per mL in patients not currently taking theophylline. Maintenance dosages vary with age and underlying conditions (Table 118.1). For patients taking theophylline regularly, a loading dose increases the steady-state serum theophylline level. Typically, administration of 1 mg per kg of theophylline raises the serum drug concentration by 2 μg per mL. This relationship can also be used to predict the theophylline concentration after an overdose; the maximum possible drug concentration (in μg per mL) should be no more than twice the ingested or administered dose (in mg per kg).

Theophylline has a volume of distribution of 0.4 L per kg and is 40% to 65% bound to plasma proteins [13]. Its metabolism is almost exclusively by hepatic cytochrome P450 system; it is oxidized or demethylate in the liver by at least two isoenzymes (CYP1A2 and CYP3A4) [13]. Less than 15% of the drug is excreted unchanged in urine. At therapeutic doses, hepatic

TABLE 118.1

Intravenous Aminophylline Maintenance Doses

Age group	Infusion rate (mg/kg/h)
Newborn	0.3–0.4
1–6 mo	0.5–0.6
6 mo–9 y	1.0–1.2
9–16 y	0.9–1.1
Smoker age 12–50 y	1.0
Nonsmoker age 16–50 y	0.5–0.7
Older than 50 y	0.4–0.6
Cor pulmonale	0.3–0.5
Liver failure	0.1–0.5
Congestive heart failure	0.1–0.5

TABLE 118.2

Factors Affecting Serum Theophylline Concentrations

Drugs that *increase* theophylline clearance
Barbiturates
Carbamazepine
Cigarette smoke
Phenytoin
Rifampin
Drugs that *decrease* theophylline clearance
Cimetidine
Ciprofloxacin
Clarithromycin
Fluvoxamine
Erythromycin
Norfloxacin
Ofloxacin
Zafirlukast
Conditions that *increase* theophylline clearance
Cigarette smoking
Cystic fibrosis
Hyperthyroidism
Conditions that *decrease* theophylline clearance
Hepatitis/cirrhosis
Congestive heart failure
Some viral infections

metabolism generally occurs by first-order elimination kinetics [14]. The drug exhibits saturable (Michaelis–Menten) kinetics in overdose leading to prolonged, unpredictable elimination rates. The elimination half-life of theophylline also varies widely with age: typical half-lives are 20 to 30 hours in premature infants, 4 to 7 hours in newborns, 3 to 4 hours in children 6 months to 18 years of age, and 8 to 9 hours in adults [13,14]. Many xenobiotics, chemicals, and medical conditions affect the steady-state serum concentration and elimination half-life of theophylline (Table 118.2). The xenobiotics that inhibit theophylline clearance are those that inhibit CYP1A2 and CYP3A4, including erythromycin, clarithromycin, ciprofloxacin, and cimetidine [13,15]. Xenobiotics that increase theophylline clearance include barbiturates, carbamazepine, and the polyaromatic hydrocarbons of cigarette smoke (including passive smoke inhalation) [16]. Enzyme induction by these xenobiotics can be temporary; in patients who smoke quit abruptly, theophylline clearance can fall to normal within days, leading to inadvertent theophylline intoxication unless dose is adjusted accordingly. Several disease states are also associated with a reduction in theophylline clearance, including heart failure and liver disease [13]. Both hyperthyroidism and cystic fibrosis are associated with increased elimination of theophylline [17].

Theophylline has a variety of physiologic effects at therapeutic doses (Table 118.3). These effects include smooth muscle relaxation, mild central nervous system (CNS) excitation, and diuresis. Intoxication is associated with an array of other metabolic and clinical consequences. Although the effects of theophylline have been well characterized, their pharmacologic and pathophysiologic mechanisms remain poorly understood. Three primary cellular mechanisms of theophylline action have been theorized: inhibition of cyclic guanosine monophosphate or cyclic adenosine monophosphate (cAMP) activity, adenosine receptor antagonism, and adrenergic hyperstimulation (particularly at the β-receptor) secondary to elevated levels of circulating plasma catecholamines [18,19]. Inhibition of calcium translocation and leukotriene production have also been postulated as additional mechanisms.

TABLE 118.3

Physiologic Effects of Theophylline

Central nervous system
Stimulation of cortical centers
Stimulation of medullary respiratory center
Nausea and emesis
Cerebral vasoconstriction and decreased cerebral blood flow
Cardiovascular
Positive inotropic and chronotropic effects
Vascular smooth muscle relaxation
Pulmonary
Bronchial smooth muscle relaxation
Increased ventilation
Stimulation of diaphragmatic and intercostal muscles
Gastrointestinal
Increased gastric acid and pepsin secretion
Relaxation of esophageal smooth muscle and possible reflux
Renal
Increased blood flow and glomerular filtration rate
Increased diuresis (<48 h)
Endocrine
Increased plasma catecholamines
Augmented dopamine β-hydroxylase and rennin
Metabolic
Lipolysis
Gluconeogenesis and glycogenolysis
Musculoskeletal
Augmented contractility
Disturbances in depolarization (e.g., tremor)

The physiologic changes seen with therapeutic doses of theophylline, including tachycardia, diuresis, bronchodilation, and CNS excitation, were thought to result from theophylline's inhibition of phosphodiesterase, the intracellular enzyme that inactivates cAMP, an important "second messenger" [20]. Such enzyme inhibition would lead to elevated intracellular cAMP concentrations, affecting a broad range of physiologic responses. However, this theory has been brought into question; in vitro data suggest phosphodiesterase inhibition does not occur at therapeutic serum concentrations of theophylline and that increased cAMP activity is not a major mechanism of its therapeutic effects [21]. Whether the increased theophylline concentrations seen in the intoxicated patient are sufficient to inhibit phosphodiesterase activity is unclear.

Investigation has also been directed at the role of adenosine receptor antagonism as a mechanism of theophylline action. Adenosine is a nucleoside that promotes smooth muscle constriction, slows cardiac conduction, and acts as an endogenous anticonvulsant. With the structure of theophylline being similar to that of adenosine and with the drug having opposite physiologic actions, theophylline may be a simple competitive antagonist at bronchial and vascular smooth muscle, cardiac, and CNS sites. However, adenosine antagonism alone does not provide a complete explanation for theophylline's pharmacologic effects [22].

Additional data suggest that many of theophylline's actions can be accounted for by its stimulation of plasma catecholamine release [17]. Plasma concentrations of epinephrine, norepinephrine, and dopamine all rise significantly after theophylline administration. With therapeutic doses, plasma catecholamine activity typically increases four- to sixfold. After theophylline intoxication, plasma catecholamine activity may rise to 30-fold

[18,19]. Increased plasma catecholamines provide a ready explanation for many of the effects of theophylline seen after therapeutic doses and potentially mediate many of the effects of theophylline intoxication. In all probability, the combined effects of adenosine receptor antagonism and catecholamine release are responsible for most features of theophylline intoxication.

Plasma catecholamines, particularly epinephrine, are capable of inducing hypokalemia, hyperglycemia, and metabolic acidosis. Epinephrine-induced hypokalemia appears to result from β_2-adrenergic receptor–linked stimulation of Na^+/K^+ adenosine triphosphatase. This leads to increased intracellular transport of potassium with preservation of total body potassium content [23]. Consistent with the theories of plasma catecholamine activity is the observation that theophylline-induced hypokalemia can be inhibited by pretreatment with propranolol or reversed by propranolol administration [24].

The CNS effects of theophylline intoxication include respiratory stimulation, vomiting, and seizures. These may result from disturbances in CNS cyclic guanosine monophosphate activity, adenosine antagonism, or adrenergic excess. Changes in neuronal transmembrane potentials by any of these mechanisms would lower excitation thresholds. In addition, there are theories that theophylline inhibits CNS γ-aminobutyric acid receptor activity and stimulates *N*-methyl-D-aspartate and other excitatory neurotransmitter production. Theophylline administration has been associated with an abnormal electroencephalogram pattern in 34% of children and 12% of adults [25]. Cerebral vascular effects are also significant with theophylline and other methylxanthines because they are potent cerebral vasoconstrictors. This is the presumed mechanism of the efficacy of caffeine in the treatment of migraine headache. However, decreases in cerebral blood flow can be extreme, particularly during inhalational anesthetic administration [26].

CLINICAL TOXICITY

Manifestations of theophylline intoxication can be classified into five categories: cardiac, CNS, gastrointestinal, musculoskeletal, and metabolic [1,8]. The cardiovascular effects of theophylline intoxication consist of rhythm and vascular disturbances. The hallmark (and first sign) of theophylline poisoning is sinus tachycardia, which occurs in more than 95% of cases. With more severe intoxication, unstable supraventricular tachydysrhythmias and ventricular dysrhythmias may occur. A common cause of death with severe theophylline intoxication is intractable ventricular dysrhythmias.

Blood pressure disturbances are also common. At lower ranges of intoxication, a mildly elevated blood pressure may be present, although severe hypertension is unusual in isolated theophylline poisoning. In severe cases of theophylline poisoning, hypotension with a widened pulse pressure is seen in the face of an increased cardiac index. Hypotension is caused by a marked fall in systemic vascular resistance.

The CNS effects of theophylline poisoning become prominent for those with severe overdose. The stimulatory actions of theophylline first produce hyperventilation with mild respiratory alkalosis. Significantly intoxicated patients develop agitation and anxiety. Vomiting, which can be severe, results partly from stimulation of the vomiting center of the medullary chemoreceptor trigger zone.

The most severe CNS manifestation of theophylline intoxication is seizures; these are a poor prognostic sign. Theophylline-induced seizures are typically tonic–clonic in nature and may be focal; they may be single, but are commonly multiple and typically resistant to conventional anticonvulsants. Seizures after theophylline intoxication are associated with a high frequency of adverse neurologic outcomes and a mortality that approaches 50% among elderly patients [27].

The gastrointestinal effects of theophylline poisoning consist of vomiting, diarrhea, and hematemesis. Vomiting results in part from hypersecretion of gastric acid and the enzymes gastrin and pepsin [28]. These acids and digestive enzymes are gastric irritants that can produce mucosal hemorrhage with hematemesis. Finally, theophylline is a potent relaxer of lower esophageal sphincter resting tone; this action facilitates the reflux of gastric contents.

Skeletal muscle tremor is a common feature of theophylline poisoning. These tremors are coarse; myoclonic jerks may also be present. Muscular hypertonicity also appears to be linked to theophylline's actions as a β_2-adrenoreceptor; this is evidenced by a similar syndrome occurring after excess administration of potent β_2-agonists (e.g., terbutaline).

A number of metabolic disturbances accompany theophylline intoxication: metabolic acidosis, hypokalemia, hyperglycemia, hypophosphatemia, hypomagnesemia, and hypercalcemia [29,30]. Metabolic acidosis may appear late and is typically modest; acidemia may not occur because of a superimposed respiratory alkalosis. Hypokalemia and hyperglycemia correlate strongly with the degree of intoxication after acute theophylline poisoning [31]. However, there are no obvious clinical consequences of hypokalemia. Hypercalcemia and hypophosphatemia are common, but not invariable, disturbances. Their cause is unclear, although theophylline (and epinephrine) has been shown to increase concentrations of parathyroid hormone, and correction of theophylline-induced hypercalcemia has been reported after propranolol administration [32].

Several studies have suggested that the metabolic and clinical consequences of theophylline intoxication vary, depending on whether the poisoning occurs through a single ingestion (or single intravenous overdose), chronic overmedication, or acute-on-therapeutic intoxication, in which the patient has maintained serum theophylline concentrations in the therapeutic range but then received a single toxic dose [11]. With *acute theophylline intoxication*, the patient ingests a single toxic dose of theophylline or inadvertently receives a toxic dose of intravenous aminophylline. The clinical course of acute theophylline intoxication strongly correlates with serum theophylline concentration. Serum theophylline concentrations of 20 to 40 μg per mL are associated with nausea, vomiting, and tachycardia. When theophylline concentrations are 40 to 70 μg per mL, premature ventricular contractions, agitation, and tremor appear. At theophylline concentrations greater than 80 μg per mL, life-threatening events, including severe cardiac dysrhythmias and intractable seizures, may occur (Table 118.4) [33]. Hypokalemia can be profound after acute intoxication, with serum potassium concentrations falling to as low as 2.1 mEq per L. Serum glucose can be as high as 300 to 350 mg per dL.

In *chronic theophylline overmedication*, the patient ingests theophylline for at least 24 hours in doses or under conditions that exceed theophylline clearance. The result is a relatively slow rise in body "theophylline burden" to toxic concentrations. Victims of chronic overmedication are more likely to be neonates or elderly patients who have underlying cardiac disease or are

TABLE 118.4

Signs and Symptoms Associated with Acute Theophylline Toxicity

Serum theophylline concentration (μg/mL)	Signs and symptoms
20–40	Nausea, vomiting, tachycardia
40–70	Premature ventricular contractions, agitation, tremor
>80	Life-threatening events, severe cardiac dysrhythmias, seizures, status epilepticus

taking/receiving medications that inhibit theophylline metabolism. These factors contribute to greater morbidity and mortality after chronic theophylline overmedication [1]. Signs of severe intoxication may occur with steady-state serum theophylline concentrations as low as 20 to 30 μg per mL. Seizures have occurred in patients with concentrations as low as 17 μg per mL. Patients with chronic theophylline overmedication are also less likely to have hypokalemia and hyperglycemia. The most striking feature of chronic theophylline overmedication is that there is *no significant correlation* between serum theophylline concentration and the appearance of life-threatening events [1,11,34]. Seizures and dysrhythmias may appear with serum theophylline concentrations in the therapeutic or mildly toxic range [11,34]. As a result, serum theophylline concentration *should not be used* to predict the appearance of these events.

Patients who are chronically receiving theophylline in appropriate doses and then take or receive an acute overdose of theophylline develop *acute-on-therapeutic theophylline intoxication*. In these patients, clinical and metabolic consequences have features that are intermediate between those found with acute intoxication and chronic overmedication. Clinical manifestations are somewhat predicted by peak serum theophylline concentration, with life-threatening events usually not appearing until serum theophylline concentrations exceed 60 μg per mL. Metabolic disturbances are not as severe and have little or no correlation with serum theophylline concentration [1,10,11].

Patient age appears to be a significant risk factor for the development of life-threatening events after theophylline intoxication for those at extremes of age (i.e., neonates and elderly patients) [1]. For example, after chronic overmedication, patients older than 75 years have an almost 10-fold greater risk of a life-threatening event than do adolescents with comparable serum theophylline concentration [1]. There is evidence that for patients with chronic theophylline intoxication, age is a better predictor of major toxicity than serum theophylline concentration. Potential explanations for this observation include the differing pharmacokinetics found at extremes of age or the higher prevalence of significant underlying multisystem disease and use of multiple drugs in these patients.

DIAGNOSTIC EVALUATION

Essential laboratory studies to obtain in the patient with theophylline intoxication include serum theophylline concentration, serum electrolytes, blood urea nitrogen, creatinine, glucose, calcium, magnesium, phosphorus, liver function panel, and creatinine phosphokinase. Urine should be frequently evaluated for evidence of myoglobinuria. An electrocardiogram should be obtained; all patients with theophylline intoxication should be placed on continuous electrocardiogram monitoring. Arterial blood gas and complete blood cell count should be obtained as clinically indicated.

Sequential serum theophylline concentrations should be obtained every 1 to 2 hours until a plateau and subsequent substantive decline have been documented because delayed peaks in serum theophylline concentration may occur after an overdose. All abnormal laboratory studies should be serially monitored until all values have returned to baseline.

MANAGEMENT

The management of theophylline intoxication consists of stabilization, decreasing absorption, and enhancing elimination. After acute ingestion, decreasing absorption is a primary concern. Treatment of chronic intoxication or intoxication after intravenous administration of theophylline generally focuses more on enhancing elimination.

Airway protection is paramount, and the threshold for tracheal intubation in the patient with seizures or other alterations in consciousness should be low. Assisted ventilation may be necessary if there is coingestion of a CNS depressant or if medications that depress respiratory drive, such as diazepam for seizures, are required for management.

If hypotension does not respond to an initial intravenous fluid bolus, propranolol may have a positive effect on blood pressure stabilization. If a vasopressor is also required, α-adrenergic agents such as phenylephrine or norepinephrine may be more efficacious; dopamine, which has some vasodilating properties at low doses, may be relatively ineffective.

Although no controlled clinical studies are available, there have been reports of success in treating tachydysrhythmias, particularly supraventricular tachycardias, with β-adrenergic antagonists, such as propranolol. Propranolol counters tachycardia, restores coronary blood flow, and interrupts the reentry phenomena that often underlie theophylline-induced dysrhythmias [18]. A potential hazard of propranolol administration is drug-induced bronchospasm; therefore, it should be used cautiously, if at all, in patients with significant reactive airways disease. Esmolol, an ultrashort-acting β_1-selective antagonist, has also been shown to be effective for select theophylline-induced tachydysrhythmias [35].

The antidysrhythmic agent adenosine has become the treatment of choice for supraventricular tachycardias and may be an important therapeutic addition in the management of theophylline-induced tachyarrhythmias. Having a significant effect on atrioventricular node conduction, adenosine can promptly reverse supraventricular tachycardias. Moreover, because of the evidence that adenosine and theophylline compete for the same receptor, adenosine may be a specific antidote for theophylline-induced supraventricular tachycardia. However, published clinical data in this regard are limited [36,37]. Amiodarone or lidocaine is the recommended treatment of ventricular irritability associated with hemodynamic compromise.

Seizures should be treated aggressively. High-dose benzodiazepine may be necessary for seizure termination. Phenytoin may be ineffective for theophylline-induced seizures [38], and in animal studies, it appears to contribute to theophylline-induced seizures. If seizures become prolonged, a rapid-acting barbiturate, such as thiopental or pentobarbital, may be necessary. Neuromuscular blockade and general anesthesia should be considered for seizures that are unresponsive to these modalities, because significant morbidity may result from the rhabdomyolysis, hyperthermia, and acidosis of status epilepticus. There is some evidence that propranolol may help prevent or control theophylline-induced seizures [39].

Vomiting can be treated with the H_2-antagonist ranitidine, which reduces gastric acid hypersecretion [40]. Cimetidine administration is relatively contraindicated in theophylline poisoning because it inhibits theophylline metabolism. The dose of ranitidine is 50 to 100 mg per kg given intravenously for adults and 0.1 to 0.5 mg per kg for children. Doses can be repeated every 6 to 8 hours. Metoclopramide also is an effective antiemetic that stimulates upper gastrointestinal motility and increases lower esophageal tone, without affecting theophylline clearance. The initial dose of metoclopramide is 0.5 to 1.0 mg per kg given intravenously for adults or 0.1 mg per kg for children (maximum, 1.0 mg per kg) and is associated with dystonic reactions. Ondansetron is an alternative antiemetic, offering the advantage of effective antiemesis with no alterations in mental status and no risk of dystonic reaction. The phenothiazine antiemetics prochlorperazine and promethazine can lower seizure threshold and should not be administered.

Treatment of metabolic acidosis is aimed at maintaining a normal serum pH. For hypokalemia, it is important to emphasize that because hypokalemia's origin is predominantly the intracellular shift of potassium with minimal losses of total body potassium content through urine or vomitus, reversal of hypokalemia is best accomplished by lowering the theophylline concentration. Aggressive replacement of potassium may result in "overshoot" hyperkalemia [41]. Intravenous infusions of potassium chloride or potassium phosphate at 40 mEq per L in a saline solution should be adequate; intravenous boluses are usually not indicated. Hypophosphatemia, hypomagnesemia, hypercalcemia, and hyperglycemia rarely require correction.

Because vomiting is such a prominent feature of theophylline intoxication, there is rarely a need to perform gastric emptying. However, activated charcoal (see Chapter 97) is highly effective in reducing the absorption of theophylline and should be administered to all patients with recent ingestions. Whole-bowel irrigation (see Chapter 97) may be effective, particularly for sustained-release formulations, but its role in the treatment of theophylline intoxication remains undefined.

The repeated administration of activated charcoal (multiple-dose activated charcoal [MDAC]; see Chapter 97) is a valuable therapeutic measure for enhancing theophylline elimination [42,43]. Moreover, because MDAC acts through the principle of "gastrointestinal dialysis," it is effective even if theophylline intoxication occurs after intravenous administration of aminophylline. MDAC is potentially as effective as hemodialysis in accelerating theophylline clearance [44]. However, it is not a substitute for hemodialysis in situations where rapid reduction in body theophylline burden is essential. All patients with significant theophylline intoxication should receive MDAC until the theophylline level is less than 15 μg per mL. Typical dosing is 1 g per kg charcoal every 4 hours (maximum, 50 g per dose). An effective alternative is 20 g every 2 hours [43]. Another alternative to bolus serial charcoal is administration via continuous nasogastric infusion at a rate of 0.25 to 0.50 g/kg/h. Repeated vomiting, present in up to 80% of patients with theophylline intoxication [45], may delay or prevent successful MDAC administration. Aggressive antiemetic therapy is usually necessary.

In severely intoxicated patients or patients with moderate toxicity who are unable to tolerate MDAC, rapid removal of theophylline is essential. This is best accomplished by hemodialysis or hemoperfusion. If the need for extracorporeal drug removal is anticipated, a nephrologist should be involved early in management. Because of the time and personnel required to initiate extracorporeal drug removal, early notification can expedite the process once the decision has been made. Morbidity and mortality may be significantly lower if these procedures are undertaken before the onset of life-threatening disturbances. Indications for extracorporeal drug removal include hemodynamic instability or repeated seizures (regardless of serum theophylline concentration) and acute intoxication with a serum theophylline concentration greater than 80 μg per mL. Extracorporeal measures should be considered in patients younger than 6 months or older than 60 years with chronic intoxication *and* a theophylline concentration greater than 30 μg per mL (Table 118.5).

Charcoal hemoperfusion has traditionally been considered the extracorporeal drug-removal method of choice for theophylline intoxication [46]. It reduces the elimination half-life of theophylline to as low as 0.7 to 2.1 hours [44], increasing clearance four- to sixfold [46]. However, hemoperfusion has significant risks, including hypotension, thrombocytopenia, red cell destruction, bleeding diathesis, and hypocalcemia. Also, there are few medical centers with the equipment and personnel needed to perform this procedure. The combination of scarce access to the procedure, increasing efficiency of hemodialysis, and the comparable efficacy of the two procedures has made hemodialysis the preferred procedure for treatment of severe theophylline intoxication [47].

Hemodialysis has many advantages over hemoperfusion. First, it is a technique that is widely available and relatively simple to perform. The need for administration of blood products is considerably less with hemodialysis. Dialysis can also increase theophylline clearance substantially, depending on the blood flow rates achieved by the device. Also, hemodialysis does not require the same degree of anticoagulation required by hemoperfusion, which lowers the risk of bleeding diathesis. Finally, the overall rate of complications is lower for hemodialysis than for hemoperfusion.

Peritoneal dialysis is an ineffective mode of drug removal in theophylline intoxication and is not recommended. Exchange transfusion, formerly thought to have no role in theophylline poisoning, has been used successfully in neonates with severe intoxication [48]. Other extracorporeal drug-removal methods, such as hemofiltration and plasmapheresis, have not been sufficiently evaluated, although there are case reports that these procedures have therapeutic value [49]. Hemofiltration, because it is a slow, passive, cardiac output–dependent technique, is unlikely to effect the rapid removal of theophylline that is necessary in severe intoxications.

TABLE 118.5

Considerations for Extracorporeal Enhanced Elimination of Theophylline

Hemodynamic instability (e.g., persistent cardiac dysrhythmias and hypotension)
Seizures (e.g., status epilepticus or recurrent seizures)
Acute intoxication: Serum theophylline level >80 μg/mL
Chronic intoxication: Age <6 mo or >60 y *and* theophylline level >30 μg/mL

CAFFEINE

Caffeine is a component of the three most popular beverages in the world: coffee, tea, and carbonated soft drinks. It is also used therapeutically as an antisleep aid and in many headache medications. Having a wide margin of safety and a relatively short elimination half-life—3 hours in adults, but 1 to 6 days in neonates—caffeine can be ingested daily in amounts as high as 1 g [50]. However, daily doses in this range are associated with adverse events such as anxiety, jitteriness, and tachycardia. The U.S. Food and Drug Administration considers caffeine in cola-type beverages to be generally regarded as safe [51].

The pharmacokinetic profile of caffeine resembles theophylline, with an important exception: whereas metabolism of theophylline (1,3-dimethylxanthine) produces inactive metabolites, caffeine (1,3,7-trimethylxanthine) undergoes 7-demethylation to form theophylline. Therefore, caffeine ingestion is invariably associated with measurable serum theophylline concentrations. After caffeine intoxication, serum theophylline concentration is a useful measure of toxicity. Many of the clinical manifestations of caffeine intoxication may in fact result from the effects of theophylline at its susceptible end organs.

The single ingestion of more than 1.5 g of caffeine (30 to 50 mg per kg in children) can produce serious adverse effects with the same manifestations found in acute theophylline intoxication [52]. Ingestions of more than 100 to 200 mg per kg are potentially lethal [50]. The five major disturbances occurring after caffeine intoxication are gastrointestinal, neurologic, metabolic, cardiac, and musculoskeletal [9]. Nausea and vomiting, with occasional hematemesis, predominate. CNS excitation may be manifested by anxiety, agitation, and seizures in severe cases. The same hypokalemia, hyperglycemia, and metabolic acidosis that appear after severe acute theophylline intoxication occur with caffeine poisoning. The most common cause of death after caffeine intoxication is intractable cardiac dysrhythmias [53]; severe acute overdoses have led to myocardial infarction. Musculoskeletal effects can be prominent with caffeine intoxication; one feature is the appearance of severe rhabdomyolysis. Life-threatening events after acute caffeine intoxication are associated with serum concentrations of more than 100 to 150 μg per mL. However, seizures after caffeine intoxication have occurred at serum concentrations as low as 50 μg per mL. Death has been reported with serum concentrations as low as 80 μg per mL. However, serum caffeine concentrations as high as 385 μg per mL have been associated with survival [54].

In recent years, the growing popularity of "energy" drinks and foods containing caffeine, taurine, and guarana has led to increased concerns regarding caffeine toxicity. The amount of caffeine contained in these drinks and foods is highly variable, and the reported amounts often do not take into account guarana and other additives. Rising use of energy drinks and foods has led to increased emergency department visits due to caffeine toxicity, with symptoms ranging from palpitations and tremor to ventricular dysrhythmias and seizures. In addition, several deaths have occurred in conjunction with energy drink use [55]. The combined use of energy drinks with alcohol is of particular concern, with some evidence to show that the combination leads to decreased fatigue from alcohol intoxication and an increased desire to continue drinking with potential for increased risky behaviors [56].

Management of caffeine intoxication follows the same principles as theophylline intoxication. Patient stabilization includes treatment of life-threatening seizures and cardiac dysrhythmias. Activated charcoal should be administered as soon as possible to provide gastrointestinal decontamination. Aggressive antiemetic therapy should be administered. MDAC is presumed to be equally effective for caffeine intoxication. Caffeine can be eliminated via hemodialysis; this procedure should be considered in those with seizures, cardiac dysrhythmias, or serum caffeine concentrations in excess of 100 μg per mL.

ACKNOWLEDGMENT

Michael W Shannon, MD (deceased), contributed to this chapter in a previous edition.

References

1. Shannon M: Life-threatening events after theophylline overdose. A 10-year prospective analysis. *Arch Intern Med* 159:989, 1999.
2. Schaefer S, Correa SD, Valente RJ, et al: Blockade of adenosine receptors with aminophylline limits ischemic preconditioning in human beings. *Am Heart J* 142:E4, 2001.
3. Cawley M, Al-Jazairi A, Stone E: Intravenous theophylline—an alternative to temporary pacing in the management of bradycardia secondary to AV nodal block. *Ann Pharmacother* 35:303, 2001.
4. Jenik A, Ceriani Cernadas JM, Gorenstein A, et al: A randomized double-blind, placebo-controlled trial of the effects of prophylactic theophylline on renal function in term neonates with perinatal asphyxia. *Pediatrics* 105:E45, 2000.
5. Bagshaw S, Ghali W: Theophylline for prevention of contrast-induced nephropathy: a systematic review and meta-analysis. *Arch Intern Med* 165:1087, 2005.
6. Kawai M, Kato M: Theophylline for the treatment of bronchial asthma: present status. *Methods Find Exp Clin Pharmacol* 22:309, 2000.
7. Wheeler D, Jacobs BR, Kenreigh CA, et al: Theophylline versus terbutaline in treating critically ill children with status asthmaticus—a prospective, randomized, controlled trial. *Pediatr Crit Care Med* 6:237, 2005.
8. Adinoff A: Life-threatening events after theophylline overdose: a 10-year prospective analysis. *Pediatrics* 106:467, 2000.
9. Zimmerman P, Pulliam J, Schwengels J, et al: Caffeine intoxication: a near fatality. *Ann Emerg Med* 14:1227, 1985.
10. Shannon M, Lovejoy F: Effect of acute versus chronic intoxication on clinical features of theophylline poisoning in children. *J Pediatr* 121:125, 1992.
11. Shannon M: Predictors of major toxicity after theophylline overdose. *Ann Intern Med* 119:1161, 1993.
12. Robertson NJ: Fatal overdose from a sustained-release theophylline preparation. *Ann Emerg Med* 14:154, 1985.
13. Hendeles L, Jenkins J, Temple R: Revised FDA labeling guidelines for theophylline oral dosage forms. *Pharmacotherapy* 15:409, 1995.
14. Gaudreault P, Guay J: Theophylline poisoning—pharmacological considerations and clinical management. *Med Toxicol* 1:169, 1986.
15. Faber MS, Jetter A, Fuhr U: Assessment of CYP1A2 activity in clinical practice: why, how, and when? *Basic Clin Pharmacol Toxicol* 97(3):125–134, 2005.
16. Khan MI, Khan S: Smoking causes an upwards shift of the narrow therapeutic window of xanthine derivatives, theophylline (XD, T), resulting in an underestimation of its effective therapeutic dose, and may result in treatment failure. *Chest* 122:83S, 2002.
17. Self T, Chafin C, Soberman J: Effect of disease states on theophylline serum concentrations: are we still vigilant? *Am J Med Sci* 319:177, 2000.
18. Curry SC, Vance MV, Requa R, et al: The effects of toxic concentrations of theophylline on oxygen consumption, ventricular work, acid base balance and plasma catecholamine levels in the dog. *Ann Emerg Med* 14:554, 1985.
19. Shannon M: Hypokalemia, hyperglycemia and plasma catecholamine activity after severe theophylline intoxication. *Clin Toxicol (Phila)* 32:41, 1991.
20. Lipworth B: Phosphodiesterase type inhibitors for asthma: a real breakthrough or just expensive theophylline? *Ann Allergy Asthma Immunol* 96:640, 2006.
21. Polson JB, Kranowski JJ, Goldman AL, et al: Inhibition of human pulmonary phosphodiesterase activity by therapeutic levels of theophylline. *Clin Exp Pharmacol Physiol* 5:535, 1978.
22. Li H, Henry J: Adenosine receptor blockade reveals *N*-methyl-D-aspartate receptor- and voltage-sensitive dendritic spikes in rat hippocampal CA1 pyramidal cells in vitro. *Neuroscience* 100:21, 2000.
23. DeFronzo RA, Bia M, Birkhead G: Epinephrine and potassium homeostasis. *Kidney Int* 20:83, 1981.
24. Amin DN, Henry JA: Propranolol administration in theophylline overdose. *Lancet* 1:520, 1985.
25. Richards W, Church JA, Brent DK: Theophylline-associated seizures in children. *Ann Allergy* 54:276, 1985.
26. Muhling J, Dehne MG, Sablotzki A, et al: Effects of theophylline on human cerebral blood flow velocity during halothane and isoflurane anaesthesia. *Eur J Anaesthesiol* 16:380, 1999.
27. Nakada T, Kwee IL, Lerner AM, et al: Theophylline-induced seizures: clinical and pathophysiologic aspects. *West J Med* 138:371, 1983.
28. Fredholm BB: On the mechanism of action of theophylline and caffeine. *Acta Med Scand* 217:149, 1985.
29. Charytan D, Jansen K: Severe metabolic complications from theophylline intoxication. *Nephrology* 8:239, 2003.
30. Shannon M, Lovejoy F: Hypokalemia after theophylline intoxication. The effects of acute vs. chronic poisoning. *Arch Intern Med* 149:2725, 1989.
31. Shannon MW, Lovejoy FH, Woolf A: Prediction of serum theophylline concentration after acute theophylline intoxication [abstract]. *Ann Emerg Med* 19:627, 1990.
32. McPherson ML, Prince SR, Atamer ER, et al: Theophylline-induced hypercalcemia. *Ann Intern Med* 105:52, 1986.
33. Baker MD: Theophylline toxicity in children. *J Pediatr* 109:538, 1986.
34. Bertino JS, Walker JW: Reassessment of theophylline toxicity-serum concentrations, clinical course, and treatment. *Arch Intern Med* 147:757, 1987.
35. Gaar GG, Banner W, Laddu AR: The effects of esmolol on the hemodynamics of acute theophylline toxicity. *Ann Emerg Med* 16:1334, 1987.
36. Biery JC, Kauflin MJ, Mauro VF: Adenosine in acute theophylline intoxication. *Ann Pharmacother* 29:1285–1288, 1995.
37. Giagounidis AA, Schäfer S, Klein RM, et al: Adenosine is worth trying in patients with paroxysmal supraventricular tachycardia on chronic theophylline medication. *Eur J Med Res* 3(8):380–382, 1998.
38. Blake KV, Massey KL, Hendeles L, et al: Relative efficacy of phenytoin and phenobarbital for the prevention of theophylline-induced seizures in mice. *Ann Emerg Med* 17:1024, 1988.
39. Schneider SM, Zea B, Michelson EA: Beta-blockade for acute theophylline-induced seizures. *Vet Hum Toxicol* 29:451, 1987.
40. Amitai Y, Yeung AC, Moye J, et al: Repetitive oral activated charcoal and control of emesis in severe theophylline toxicity. *Ann Intern Med* 105:386, 1986.
41. D'Angio R, Sabatelli F: Management considerations in treating metabolic abnormalities associated with theophylline overdose. *Arch Intern Med* 147:1837, 1987.
42. Kulig KW, Bar-Or D, Rumack BH: Intravenous theophylline poisoning and multiple-dose charcoal in an animal model. *Ann Emerg Med* 16:842, 1987.
43. Park GD, Radomski L, Goldberg MJ, et al: Effect of size and frequency of oral doses of charcoal on theophylline clearance. *Clin Pharmacol Ther* 34:663, 1983.
44. Heath A, Knudsen K: Role of extracorporeal drug removal in acute theophylline poisoning—a review. *Med Toxicol Adverse Drug Exp* 2:294, 1987.
45. Paloucek FP, Rodvold KA: Evaluation of theophylline overdoses and toxicities. *Ann Emerg Med* 17:135, 1988.
46. Russo ME: Management of theophylline intoxication with charcoal-column hemoperfusion. *N Engl J Med* 300:24, 1979.
47. Shannon M: Comparative efficacy of hemodialysis and hemoperfusion in severe theophylline intoxication. *Acad Emerg Med* 4:674, 1997.
48. Shannon M, Wernovsky B, Morris C: Exchange transfusion in the treatment of severe theophylline poisoning. *Pediatrics* 89:145, 1992.
49. Okada S, Teramoto S, Matsuoka R: Recovery from theophylline toxicity by continuous hemodialysis with filtration. *Ann Intern Med* 133:922, 2000.
50. Dalvi RR: Acute and chronic toxicity of caffeine: a review. *Vet Hum Toxicol* 28:144, 1986.
51. US Food and Drug Administration: Caffeine. *Code of Federal Regulations* Title 21, Vol 3, Sec 182.1180. Revised April 1, 2015.
52. Benowitz N, Osterloh J, Goldschlager N: Massive catecholamine release from caffeine poisoning. *JAMA* 248:1097, 1982.
53. Strubelt O, Diederich KW: Experimental treatment of the acute cardiovascular toxicity of caffeine. *Clin Toxicol (Phila)* 37:29, 1999.
54. Dietrich AM, Mortensen M: Presentation and management of an acute caffeine overdose. *Pediatr Emerg Care* 6:296, 1990.
55. Jabbar SB, Hanly MG: Fatal caffeine overdose: a case report and review of literature. *Am J Forensic Med Pathol* 34:321, 2013.
56. McKetin R, Coen A, Kaye S: A comprehensive review of the effects of mixing caffeinated energy drinks with alcohol. *Drug Alcohol Depend* 151:15, 2015.

Chapter 119 ■ Opioid Poisoning

LUKE YIP • ROBERT P. DOWSETT

Natural opioids (e.g., morphine and codeine) are harvested from the seedpods of the poppy plant *Papaver somniferum*. Semisynthetic opioids (e.g., dextromethorphan, heroin, hydrocodone, hydromorphone, oxycodone, and oxymorphone) are derivatives of morphine, whereas synthetic opioids (e.g., buprenorphine, butorphanol, diphenoxylate, fentanyl, meperidine, methadone, nalbuphine, pentazocine, propoxyphene, and tramadol) are not.

Clandestine laboratories have produced potent opioids as new manufacturing methods have been developed to circumvent the use of controlled or unavailable precursor compounds. Because these xenobiotics may contain a wide variety of active ingredients, adulterants, and contaminants, the clinical syndromes seen in the abuser may be only partly related to the opioid component.

PHARMACOLOGY

Opioids interact with central nervous system (CNS) receptors to produce their analgesic, euphoric, and sedative effects. Historically, on the basis of animal studies, three major opioid receptors designated as *mu*, *kappa*, and *sigma* have been proposed. The *sigma* receptor is no longer considered an opioid subtype, because it is insensitive to naloxone, has dextrorotatory stereochemistry binding, and has no endogenous ligand. The International Union on Receptor Nomenclature recommends a change from the Greek alphabet to one similar to other neurotransmitter systems; receptors are denoted by their endogenous ligand (opiates peptides) with a subscript denoting their order of discovery: *delta* to OP_1, *kappa* to OP_2, and *mu* to OP_3 (Table 119.1).

Most opioid analgesics are well absorbed after parenteral administration, from the pulmonary capillaries and mucosal sites. Analgesia is promptly achieved after parenteral administration and within 15 to 30 minutes after oral dosing. Peak plasma levels are generally attained within 1 to 2 hours after therapeutic oral doses. However, acute overdose may produce decreased intestinal peristalsis, resulting in delayed and prolonged absorption. Therapeutic and toxic serum xenobiotic concentrations are not well established.

All opioids undergo hepatic biotransformation, including hydroxylation, demethylation, and glucuronide conjugation. Considerable first-pass metabolism accounts for the wide variations in oral bioavailability noted with xenobiotics such as morphine and pentazocine. Only small fractions of the parent xenobiotic are excreted unchanged in the urine. Active metabolites can contribute to the toxicologic profile of specific xenobiotics.

All opioids elicit the same overall physiologic effects as morphine, the prototype of this group. A typical morphine dose (5 to 10 mg) usually produces analgesia without altering mood or mental status in a patient. Sometimes dysphoria rather than euphoria is manifest, resulting in mild anxiety or a fear reaction. Nausea is frequently encountered, and vomiting is occasionally observed. Morphine and most of its congeners cause miosis in humans. This effect is exacerbated after an overdose, resulting in profound pupillary constriction, predominantly a central effect. Cerebral circulation does not appear to be altered by therapeutic doses of morphine unless respiratory depression and carbon dioxide retention result in cerebral vasodilation.

Respiratory failure is the most serious consequence of opiate overdose. Opioid agonists reduce the sensitivity of the medullary chemoreceptors in the respiratory centers to an increase in carbon dioxide tension and depress the ventilatory response to hypoxia. Even small doses of morphine depress respiration, decreasing minute, and alveolar ventilation. The peak respiratory-depressant effect is usually noted within 7 minutes of intravenous (IV) morphine administration, but may be delayed up to 30 minutes if the drug is intramuscularly administered. Normal carbon dioxide sensitivity and minute volume usually return 5 to 6 hours after a therapeutic dose.

Therapeutic opiate doses cause arteriolar and venous dilation, and may result in a mild decrease in blood pressure. This change in blood pressure is clinically insignificant while the patient is supine, but significant orthostatic changes are common. Hypotension appears to be mediated by histamine release. Myocardial damage in opiate overdose associated with prolonged hypoxic coma may be mediated by cellular components released during rhabdomyolysis, direct toxic effects, or hypersensitivity to the opioids or adulterants.

Heroin (diacetylmorphine) has two to five times the analgesic potency of morphine. Virtually all street heroin in the United States is produced in clandestine laboratories and adulterated before distribution (Table 119.2). The purity of street heroin is between 5% and 90%. Physiologically, the effects of heroin are identical to those described for morphine. Heroin can be administered intravenously, intranasally, or inhaled as a volatile vapor, and can be mixed with other drugs of abuse, typically amphetamine or cocaine (speed ball). The plasma half-life of heroin is 5 to 15 minutes. Heroin is initially deacetylated, in the liver and plasma, into 6-monoacetyl-morphine (6-MAM) and subsequently into morphine [1]. Morphine is mostly metabolized in both liver and brain by enzymatic-dependent glucuronidation activities that produce morphine-3-glucuronide (M3G) and morphine-6-glucuronide (M6G). An individual variation in sensitivity and tolerance makes correlation of serum levels with clinical symptoms difficult.

TABLE 119.1

Opiate Receptor System and Clinical Effects

OP1 (delta [δ])	OP2 (kappa [κ])	OP3 (mu [μ])
Supraspinal/spinal analgesia	Supraspinal/spinal analgesia	Supraspinal/spinal analgesia
Modulation of OP_3 function	Dysphoria	Peripheral analgesia
Respiratory depression	Psychotomimesis	Sedation
	Diuresis	Euphoria
	Miosis	Respiratory depression
		Miosis
		Constipation
		Pruritus
		Bradycardia
		Prolactin release
		Growth hormone release
		Physical dependence

TABLE 119.2

Heroin Adulterants

Mannitol	Antipyrine
Dextrose	Boric acid
Lactose	Mercurous salts
Talc	Animal manure
Sodium bicarbonate	Cocaine
Quinine	Amphetamine
Strychnine	Methamphetamine
Caffeine	Barbiturates
Phenacetin	Flour
Procaine	Magnesium sulfate
Lidocaine	Antihistamines
Benzocaine	Phencyclidine
Tetracaine	Scopolamine

The initial heroin "rush" is owing to its high lipid solubility, rapid penetration into the CNS, and its rapid conversion to 6-MAM. The majority of its lasting effects are attributed to its metabolite morphine, and in patients with acute kidney failure the lasting effects appear to be derived from M6G. M3G has virtually no affinity for OP_3 receptors, and its accumulation is believed to be related to neurotoxic effect of long-term morphine use (e.g., myoclonus and neuroexcitatory behavior).

Codeine (methylmorphine) is formulated as a sole ingredient and in combination with aspirin or acetaminophen. Codeine is rapidly absorbed by the oral route, producing a peak plasma level within 1 hour of a therapeutic dose. Usually 10% of codeine is metabolized to morphine by CYP2D6; this may be greatly increased in patients with duplicated or amplified CYP2D6 genes, resulting in opioid toxicity [2]. Clearance of codeine by CYP3A4 may be inhibited by clarithromycin and voriconazole. Codeine and morphine appear in the urine within 24 to 72 hours. However, only morphine is detected in the urine at 96 hours. The effect of codeine on the CNS is comparable with, but less pronounced than that of, morphine. Fatal ingestions with codeine alone are rare.

Fentanyl, a phenylpiperidine derivative, has a potency 200 times that of morphine. Legitimate use is limited to anesthesia, and it is known to be commonly abused by hospital personnel. Rapid IV administration may result in acute muscular rigidity primarily involving the trunk and chest wall, which impairs respiration. Although motor activity resembling seizures have been associated with fentanyl use, simultaneous electroencephalogram recording during fentanyl induction of general anesthesia failed to show epileptiform activity [3]. This suggests a myoclonic rather than epileptic nature of the observed muscle activity.

Fentanyl is available as a transdermal delivery system that establishes a depot of drug in the upper skin layers, where it is available for systemic absorption. After removal of the patch, serum fentanyl concentrations gradually decline; 50% in 20 to 27 hours. Continued absorption of fentanyl from the skin accounts for a slower disappearance of the drug from the serum than is seen after an IV infusion, where the apparent half-life is 7 hours (range 3 to 12).

By manipulating the chemical structure of fentanyl, α-methylfentanyl (China white), 3-methylfentanyl, and para-fluoro-fentanyl has been produced and distributed on the street as heroin substitutes. They are 200 to 3,000 times more potent than heroin. α-Methyl-acetyl-fentanyl, α-methyl-fentanyl acrylate, and benzylfentanyl are 6,000 times more potent than morphine.

Meperidine, another phenylpiperidine derivative, is less than half as effective when given orally as compared to the parenteral route. Peak plasma levels occur 30 minutes after intramuscular administration, and 1 to 2 hours after an oral dose. The duration of action is 2 to 4 hours. Meperidine is metabolized primarily by *N*-demethylation to normeperidine, an active metabolite with half the analgesic and euphoric potency of its parent and twice the convulsant property. Excretion is primarily through the kidneys as conjugated metabolites. Typical values of the elimination half-lives of meperidine and normeperidine are 3 to 4 hours and 15 to 30 hours, respectively. Prolonged meperidine administration may lead to normeperidine accumulation, especially in the presence of renal impairment. The neuroexcitatory effects of meperidine toxicity (e.g., agitation, tremors, myoclonus, and seizures) have been attributed to the accumulation of normeperidine [4].

A synthetic meperidine analog, methyl-phenyl-propionoxy-piperidine, a contaminant produced during the clandestine synthesis of this agent, led to an epidemic of Parkinsonism among IV drug abusers within days of repeated injections [5].

Diphenoxylate is structurally similar to meperidine. Diphenoxylate (2.5 mg) is formulated with 0.025 mg atropine sulfate (Lomotil) and used in the treatment of diarrhea. In therapeutic doses, the drug has no significant CNS effects. Signs and symptoms arising from a toxic ingestion, primarily reported in pediatric patients, may be delayed because of decreased gastrointestinal (GI) motility and accumulation of the hepatic metabolite difenoxin, a potent opioid with a long serum half-life [6].

Methadone is used for chronic pain conditions and maintenance of opiate addicts. It is well absorbed orally, producing a peak plasma level within 2 to 4 hours. It has a prolonged but variable serum half-life with mean estimates between 15 and 55 hours, and is usually assumed to be 24 hours, but may have a median elimination half-life of 48 hours in patients on long-term maintenance therapy [7]. The principle enzyme system responsible for methadone metabolism is CYP3A4; other main enzymes responsible are CYP2D6 and CYP1A2. Xenobiotics that interact with these enzyme systems may precipitate withdrawal (e.g., CYP3A4 induction, rifampicin, and fluconazole) or enhance the risk of overdose (e.g., CYP3A4 substrates or inhibitors, fluoxetine, and fluvoxamine). A protracted clinical course is expected following an overdose.

Propoxyphene is structurally related to methadone. It is available alone or in combination with aspirin or acetaminophen. Oral administration is followed by rapid absorption, with peak serum levels occurring in 1 hour. The plasma half-life of propoxyphene and its main active metabolite, norpropoxyphene, is 6 to 12 hours and 37 hours, respectively. Norpropoxyphene is the primary metabolite excreted in the urine [8]. It is believed to play a role in the prolonged clinical course after an overdose.

Pentazocine is a synthetic analgesic in the benzomorphan class and has been involved in the drug abuse trade. It has agonist as well as weak antagonist activity at the opioid receptors. It has one-third the analgesic potency of morphine. When orally administered, pentazocine achieves peak plasma levels within 1 hour and is extensively metabolized in the liver with the parent compound and metabolites detectable in either urine or plasma [9]. Pentazocine, in combination with the antihistamine tripelennamine, is known on the street as *T's and Blues* and is used as a heroin substitute [10]. In an attempt to curtail pentazocine abuse, the oral preparation was reformulated to contain 0.5 mg naloxone. When it is parenterally administered, the effects of pentazocine are antagonized by naloxone, which has precipitated withdrawal in opiate-dependent individuals. Because the duration of action of pentazocine exceeds that of naloxone, delayed respiratory depression may occur.

Dextromethorphan, an analog of codeine, is found in a large number of nonprescription cough and cold remedies. It is available as a single ingredient but usually formulated in combination with sympathomimetic and antihistamine xenobiotics.

Dextromethorphan is well absorbed from the GI tract, with peak plasma levels occurring 2.5 and 6.0 hours after ingestion of regular and sustained-release preparations, respectively. Dextromethorphan is rapidly metabolized to dextrorphan by hepatic CYP2D6 with a plasma half-life of 2 to 4 hours, and the level of dextrorphan may be highly variable depending on a person's CYP2D6 genotype [11]. Both dextromethorphan and dextrorphan are noncompetitive antagonists of the *N*-methyl-D-aspartate (NMDA) receptor as well as serotonin reuptake inhibitors. Animal data suggest the physical effects of dextromethorphan and its abuse potential are caused by dextrorphan [12]. Within the therapeutic dose, dextromethorphan lacks analgesic, euphoric, and physical dependence properties.

Hydromorphone and oxycodone are orally administered opioids used in the treatment of chronic pain conditions. A number of sustained-release formulations are available, and can result in prolonged poisoning in overdose. The sustained-release properties of some formulations of oxycodone can be circumvented by crushing or dissolving the tablet, resulting in fatal narcotic overdoses among drug abusers [13].

Tramadol is structurally similar to morphine. It is a centrally acting analgesic with moderate affinity for OP_3 receptors. The metabolite, *O*-demethyl-tramadol, appears to have a higher affinity than the parent compound. Most of the analgesic effects are attributed to nonopioid properties of the drug, probably by blocking the reuptake of biogenic amines (e.g., norepinephrine and serotonin) at synapses in the descending neural pathways, which inhibits pain responses in the spinal cord [14].

Buprenorphine is a partial agonist activity with high affinity to, and slow dissociation from, the OP_3 receptor. It displaces other opioids and its dose–response curve has a ceiling effect, resulting in less respiratory depression in overdose, although apnea may still occur [15,16]. It has poor oral bioavailability and is administered sublingually. It is also formulated with naloxone that is active only if intravenously administered. Other partial agonists include butorphanol and nalbuphine. They can precipitate opioid withdrawal (see Chapter 126) in those taking other opioids.

CLINICAL PRESENTATION

Miosis, respiratory depression, and coma are the hallmarks of opiate intoxication, with the magnitude and duration of toxicity dependent on the dose and degree of tolerance. The clinical effects of an overdose with any one of the agents in this class are similar. However, there are important differences between certain xenobiotics. Overdoses resulting in toxicity often have a prolonged clinical course, in part because of opiate-induced decreased GI motility when taken orally and prolonged half-life of the xenobiotic or its active metabolite(s). Miosis is considered a pathognomonic finding in opiate poisoning, with the exception of meperidine, propoxyphene, pentazocine, and dextromethorphan use, in the case of a mixed overdose with an anticholinergic or sympathomimetic drug, or when severe acidemia, hypoxemia, hypotension, or CNS structural disorder is present.

CNS depression occurs in most severely intoxicated patients. However, codeine, meperidine, and dextromethorphan intoxications are remarkable for CNS hyperirritability, resulting in a mixed syndrome of stupor and delirium. In addition, the patients with meperidine toxicity may also have tachypnea, dysphoric and hallucinogenic episodes, tremors, muscular twitching, and spasticity, whereas the patients with dextromethorphan toxicity may also manifest restlessness, nystagmus, and clonus [17].

Pulmonary edema may complicate the clinical course of opioid overdose and appear more prevalent with heroin, morphine, codeine, methadone, and propoxyphene. Pulmonary edema has occurred in postoperative patients who received naloxone and after naloxone therapy in overdose patients [18,19]. Typically, the patient has a depressed consciousness and respiration. After naloxone administration, the patient awakens and over minutes to hours is noted to become hypoxic and develop pulmonary edema. Acute naloxone-induced withdrawal has been associated with massive CNS sympathetic discharge, which may be a precipitating factor in the development of neurogenic pulmonary edema [18]. It appears the acute lung injury is at the alveolar–capillary membrane, resulting in manifestations consistent with acute respiratory distress syndrome.

The patients with heroin-induced pulmonary edema typically have normal capillary wedge pressures and elevated pulmonary arterial pressures [20]. In contrast, elevated systemic, pulmonary arterial, and pulmonary capillary wedge pressures and total systemic vascular resistance are seen with pentazocine dosing [21]. This effect is believed to result from transient endogenous catecholamine release. Adulterants in street drugs are potential pulmonary irritants and toxins, and may cause dyspnea, hypoxemia, and the presence of multiple reticulonodular infiltrates on chest radiograph. A summary of the potential pulmonary complications associated with opioid abuse is provided in Table 119.3.

Heroin toxicity may be associated with cardiac conduction abnormalities and dysrhythmias, which may be the result of metabolic derangements associated with hypoxia, a direct effect of the abused agent, or adulterants (e.g., quinine) in street drugs [22].

Leukoencephalopathy associated with inhalational abuse of heroin (chasing the dragon) typically progresses for several weeks. Initially, cerebellar ataxia and motor restlessness may be followed by the development of pyramidal tract lesions, pseudobulbar reflexes, spastic paresis, myoclonic jerks, and choreoathetoid movements. A quarter of patients may progress to hypotonic paresis, akinetic mutism, and death [23].

Seizures and focal neurologic signs are usually absent with opioid intoxication unless it is complicated by events such as severe hypoxia and an intracranial process (e.g., brain abscess and subarachnoid hemorrhage), when proconvulsive adulterants or when opioids such as meperidine, propoxyphene, pentazocine (*T's and Blues*), and tramadol are involved [10,24–26]. Meperidine- and propoxyphene-related seizures may become more frequent in chronic drug abusers with renal insufficiency.

Disabling myoclonus has been reported after several days of fentanyl therapy by the transdermal delivery system [27].

The clinical course after propoxyphene overdose may be severe and rapidly progressive and include seizures, respiratory failure, cardiac dysrhythmias, and circulatory collapse [28]. Propoxyphene appears to be responsible for CNS toxicity (e.g., respiratory depression and seizures) as well as cardiac toxicity (e.g., QRS prolongation and dysrhythmias), whereas norpropoxyphene contributed only to the cardiotoxicity [29]. Cardiotoxicity may be exacerbated by hypoxia or adulterants (e.g., quinine) in street drugs.

Anxiety, dysphoria, and hallucinations are more common with pentazocine than with other opiate derivatives [9]. Acute toxicity in combination with tripelennamine (*T's and Blues*)

TABLE 119.3

Pulmonary Complications Associated with Opiate Abuse

Pulmonary edema	Lung abscess
Pulmonary arteritis (cotton)	Bacterial pneumonia
Pulmonary thrombosis (talc)	Aspiration pneumonitis
Pulmonary hypertension (talc)	Atelectasis
Pulmonary granulomatosis (talc)	Bronchiectasis
Pulmonary fibrosis (talc)	Pneumomediastinum
Septic emboli	Respiratory arrest

results in the typical opiate intoxication syndrome as well as dyspnea, hyperirritability, hypertension, and seizures. It is believed that these effects may be directly related to tripelennamine [10].

Hypotension may occur after opiate overdose, although pentazocine intoxication may result in hypertension [10]. Electrocardiographic abnormalities associated with heroin overdose include nonspecific ST-segment and T-wave changes, sinus tachycardia, atrial fibrillation, and ventricular tachycardia, and may be related to hypoxemia, direct effects of heroin, its metabolites, or adulterants (e.g., quinine) in street drugs [22].

CNS manifestations are the primary presenting symptoms of patients acutely intoxicated on dextromethorphan and include euphoria, altered mental status (ranging from somnolence to hyperexcitability), dissociative stupor, depersonalization, disorientation, paranoia, dyskinesia, ataxia, nystagmus, disordered speech, vivid auditory, and visual hallucinations [11,12]. These effects appear to be dose-related. Respiratory depression, tachycardia, hypertension, seizures, and death may result from severe acute dextromethorphan intoxication, whereas chronic dexthromethorphn abuse is associated with frank psychosis. Dextromethorphan abuse may be associated with a psychologic as well as physiologic dependence syndrome. Chronic dextromethorphan hydrobromide abuse can also cause bromide poisoning [12]. Typical symptoms of bromide toxicity include impaired CNS function including behavioral changes, headache, apathy, irritation, weight loss, acneiform rash, slurred speech, psychosis, tremulousness, ataxia, hallucinations, and coma.

Methadone can produce bradycardia, QTc prolongation, and torsades de pointes. QTc prolongation and torsades de pointes have been associated with mean daily methadone dose 397 ± 238 mg; mean QTc interval on presentation was 615 ± 77 ms. In one case series, the majority of patients were receiving a potentially QT-prolonging xenobiotic, 41% of the patients had hypokalemia, and 18% of the patients were found to have structural heart disease [30]. A proposed mechanism is inhibition of the cardiac potassium channel by the nontherapeutic (*S*)-methadone isomer [31]. This isomer is metabolized by CYP2B6; 6% of the population are slow metabolizers, resulting in elevated levels of (*S*)-methadone and increased QTc intervals [31,32].

The onset of anticholinergic and opioid effects may be significantly delayed after a diphenoxylate overdose [6]. Atropine effects (e.g., CNS excitement, hypertension, fever, and flushed dry skin) may occur before, during, or after opioid effects. However, opioid effects (e.g., CNS and respiratory depression with miosis) may predominate or occur without signs of atropinism.

Following a tramadol overdose, the patients may present with signs and symptoms that include tachycardia, hypertension, respiratory depression, lethargy, agitation, seizures, coma, and metabolic acidosis [26]. Tramadol-associated seizures are reported to be self-limited.

Interaction between meperidine and monoamine oxidase inhibitors (MAOIs), dextromethorphan and MAOIs, and tramadol and selective serotonin reuptake inhibitors may result in the serotonin syndrome [33,34]. The patients with severe serotonin syndrome exhibit rapid onset of altered mental status, muscle rigidity, hyperthermia, autonomic dysfunction, coma, seizures, and death.

Rhabdomyolysis, hyperkalemia, myoglobinuria, and acute renal failure may complicate the clinical course of an acute opioid overdose [35]. Acute renal failure may be owing to direct insult by the abused substance, adulterants in street drugs, and prolonged coma. Chronic parenteral drug use may result in glomerulonephritis and renal amyloidosis and has been associated with concurrent bacterial infections [36]. Potential lethal acute infections have been associated with clostridia contamination [37].

Body packers or "mules" are people who transport large number of concentrated heroin packets in their GI tract from one country to another. If one of these packets ruptures, the amount of drug released may cause severe and prolonged toxicity [38]. They may also develop features of intestinal obstruction, intestinal perforation, and peritonitis [39].

DIAGNOSTIC EVALUATION

Laboratory studies such as complete blood cell count, serum electrolytes, blood urea nitrogen, creatinine and creatine phosphokinase, urinalysis, arterial blood gas, electrocardiography, chest and abdominal radiography, head computed tomography, and lumbar puncture should be obtained as clinically indicated. Arterial blood gas usually reflects hypoventilation, respiratory acidosis, and metabolic acidosis [40]. If pulmonary edema develops, chest radiographs typically reveal bilateral fluffy alveolar infiltrates, occasionally unilateral in nature, and echocardiograms show normal cardiac function [41]. A negative anion gap with hyperchloremia should raise the suspicion of bromide poisoning from chronic dextromethorphan use, and can be confirmed by a serum bromide level [12]. Chest radiographic findings of pulmonary edema usually resolve within 24 to 48 hours.

It is recommended that an ECG be obtained prior to commencing methadone therapy and within 30 days of commencement and then yearly to monitor the QTc interval [42].

Leukoencephalopathy associated with inhalational abuse of heroin appears as hypoattenuation in the affected white matter, although this may not be apparent until late in the disease. Magnetic resonance imaging typically demonstrates white matter hyperintensity on T2-weighted sequences. The affected areas are initially the occipital and cerebellar white matter, followed by involvement of the parietal, temporal, and frontal lobes. The cerebellar peduncles, splenium of the corpus callosum, posterior limb of the internal capsules, corticospinal tract, medial lemniscus, and tractus solitarius may also be involved [23].

Quantitative serum opiate levels do not contribute to patient management. A urine toxicology screen may confirm the diagnosis, but is rarely necessary for acute patient management. Commercial opioid assays are unlikely to detect synthetic opioids. The metabolites of naloxone are chemically related to oxymorphone, but naloxone is not known to give false-positive immunoassay urine screens for opioid substances [43]. False-positive serology tests for syphilis have been reported among drug addicts [44]. Laboratory investigation should also include tests for infection in patients with fever (Table 119.4).

MANAGEMENT

A diagnosis of opioid poisoning should be considered in all comatose patients. However, the classic triad of opiate toxicity

TABLE 119.4

Infectious Complications in Intravenous Drug Abusers

Endocarditis	Lymphadenitis
Aspergillosis	Epidural abscess
Bacterial meningitis	Phlebitis
Cutaneous abscess	Viral hepatitis
Mycotic aneurysm	Wound botulism
Cellulitis	Tetanus
Brain abscess	Osteomyelitis
Lymphangitis	Septicemia
Subdural abscess	HIV/AIDS

AIDS, acquired immunodeficiency syndrome; HIV, human immunodeficiency virus.

(coma, miosis, and respiratory depression) may not be apparent after a mixed overdose. Respiratory support is paramount in the management of patients with opioid toxicity; one should secure the airway and ventilate with 100% oxygen. Vascular access should be established. The patient should be placed on continuous pulse oximetry and cardiac monitoring. Vital signs should be monitored frequently.

Naloxone is a specific opiate receptor antagonist and can reverse the analgesia, respiratory depression, miosis, hyporeflexia, and cardiovascular effects of opiate toxicity [45]. The goal of naloxone therapy is to re-establish adequate spontaneous ventilation. The initial IV naloxone dose should be 0.1 mg if the patient is possibly opioid dependent; larger doses may precipitate acute opioid-withdrawal syndrome. Otherwise, an initial 2 mg dose can be administered. If there is history of an opiate exposure, a strong suspicion based on presenting signs and symptoms, or a partial response to the initial naloxone dose, repeated IV naloxone boluses up to 10 mg should be administered because methadone, pentazocine, propoxyphene, diphenoxylate, and sustained-release preparations of oxycodone and hydromorphone may not respond to the usual naloxone doses [46]. Despite its strong affinity to OP_3 receptors, buprenorphine overdose can be treated effectively with usual doses of naloxone [16].

Intramuscular, intralingual, endotracheal, intraosseous, and intranasal routes of naloxone administration are acceptable alternatives when IV access is not readily available [47–49]. Repeat naloxone boluses may be required every 20 to 60 minutes because of its short elimination half-life (60 to 90 minutes). A continuous naloxone infusion may be considered for patients who have a positive response but require repeated bolus doses because of recurrent respiratory depression [50]. A therapeutic continuous naloxone infusion can be made by administering two third of the effective naloxone bolus dose per hour (see Chapter 125-Antidotes). The infusion is titrated to maintain adequate spontaneous ventilation without precipitating acute opioid withdrawal and empirically continued for 12 to 24 hours. The patient should be admitted to an intensive care or high-dependency setting for continuous monitoring. After the naloxone therapy is discontinued, the patient should be carefully observed for 4 hours for recurrent respiratory depression.

Nebulized naloxone, 2 mg mixed with 3 mL normal saline delivered by a nebulizer face mask with the side ports partially occluded with tape to prevent excessive loss of medication, appears to be a safe and effective treatment of suspected opioid overdose in patients with a minimum respiratory rate of 6 breaths per minute [51].

Naloxone is effective in reversing diphenoxylate-induced opioid toxicity. However, recurrence of respiratory and CNS depression is common [6]. All patients with significant diphenoxylate overdose should be observed in an intensive care setting for at least 24 hours. The value of naloxone use for dextromethorphan toxicity is debatable [12].

Hypotension may respond to naloxone therapy but may require fluid resuscitation and vasopressors. Overzealous fluid resuscitation should be avoided because of the risk of pulmonary edema.

The management of seizures should follow current treatment guidelines and include benzodiazepines or barbiturates. Adjunct naloxone therapy may be effective in propoxyphene, but not in meperidine- or tramadol-related seizures [52]. Seizures have been reported after naloxone administration for tramadol overdose [26].

The patients with significant CNS signs or symptoms from bromide toxicity may require urgent hemodialysis for bromide removal.

The management of serotonin syndrome is primarily supportive (see Chapters 104 and 185); and in severe toxicity ICU admission, intubation and neuromuscular paralysis, active cooling, and 5-HT_{2A} antagonists treatment may be necessary (e.g., cyproheptadine 12 mg orally or by nasogastric tube, followed by 4 to 8 mg every 6 hours or chlorpromazine 12.5 to 25 mg IV, followed by 25 mg every 6 hours) [53].

GI decontamination should be considered for orally administered opioids after vital signs have been stabilized. The clinical benefits of multiple oral doses of activated charcoal are unproven, but it is potentially beneficial because of the prolonged absorption phase that is typically encountered with opiate overdoses. Repeat charcoal doses should not be used in the absence of active bowel sounds.

The management of pulmonary edema should include adequate ventilation, oxygenation, and low tidal volume positive-pressure ventilation as needed [54]. Inotropic agents and diuretics appear to be of little value.

Bradycardia secondary to methadone administration responds to ceasing the drug; atropine has not been utilized. If the patients receiving methadone develop a QTc interval of more than 500 milliseconds, consideration should be given to reducing the dose or discontinuing the drug [42].

Asymptomatic body packers should be conservatively managed when the condition of packaging does not appear to be compromised. One proposed guideline involves the oral administration of a water-soluble contrast solution followed by serial abdominal radiographs (Table 119.5) [55]. Whole-bowel irrigation (WBI) with polyethylene glycol electrolyte lavage solution (PEG-ELS) has also been advocated on the basis of case reports [56].

Pruritus is a common opioid adverse event. It may be localized or general, and ranges from mild to severe. Antihistamines are usually ineffective, but naloxone has frequently been found to offer relief. Ondansetron has been reported to provide relief in refractory cases [57].

Leukoencephalopathy associated with inhalational abuse of heroin has been reported to improve following the antioxidant ubiquinone (coenzyme Q10) administration in doses of 30 to 300 mg QID [58].

Nalmefene is also effective for the reversal of opioid-induced CNS effects and can be administered orally or intravenously. Its half-life and dose-dependent duration of action are 4 to 8 hours after IV administration [59]. The initial adult dose is 0.5 mg for those who are not opioid dependent and 0.1 mg for those suspected of having opioid dependency. If there is an incomplete response or no response, additional doses can be given at 2- to 5-minute intervals. A total dose of 1.5 mg may be necessary to exclude the possibility of opioid poisoning. The principal advantage over naloxone is its considerably longer duration of antagonistic action. However, withdrawal syndromes precipitated by nalmefene use would also be prolonged.

Naltrexone is a potent, long-acting pure opiate antagonist that is effective orally. Its use is primarily limited as adjunctive

TABLE 119.5

Medical Management for Asymptomatic Body Packers

1. Administer an oral dose of water-soluble contrast (e.g., Gastrografin): 1 mL/kg[a]
2. Perform abdominal radiographs (supine and upright) at least 5 h after oral contrast administration
3. If radiographs are positive, perform daily abdominal radiographs, and after a spontaneous bowel movement
4. All bowel movements are checked for drug packets
5. The patient may be discharged after passage of two packet-free bowel movements *and* negative abdominal radiographs

[a]The patients are permitted to feed normally, and vascular access should be maintained.

therapy for opioid detoxification. Naltrexone may induce a withdrawal syndrome that lasts up to 72 hours.

References

1. Anton B, Salazar A, Flores A, et al: Vaccines against morphine/heroin and its use as effective medication for preventing relapse to opiate addictive behaviors. *Hum Vaccin* 5:214, 2009.
2. Gasche Y, Daali Y, Fathi M, et al: Codeine intoxication associated with ultrarapid CYP2D6 metabolism. *N Engl J Med* 351:2827, 2004.
3. Smith NT, Benthuysen JL, Bickford RG, et al: Seizures during opioid anesthetic induction—are they opioid-induced rigidity? *Anesthesiology* 71:852, 1989.
4. Hershley LA: Meperidine and central neurotoxicity. *Ann Intern Med* 98:548, 1983.
5. Langston JW, Irwin I, Langston EB, et al: Chronic Parkinsonism in humans due to a product of meperidine-analog synthesis. *Science* 219:979, 1983.
6. McCarron MM, Challoner KR, Thompson GA: Diphenoxylate-atropine (Lomotil) overdose in children: an update (report of eight cases and review of the literature). *Pediatrics* 87:694, 1991.
7. Corkery JM, Schifano F, Ghodse AH, et al: The effects of methadone and its role in fatalities. *Hum Psychopharmacol* 19:565, 2004.
8. Verbely K, Inturrisi CE: Disposition of propoxyphene and norpropoxyphene in man after a single oral dose. *Clin Pharmacol Ther* 15:302, 1973.
9. Brogden RN, Speight TM, Avery GS: Pentazocine: a review of its pharmacological properties, therapeutic efficacy and dependence liability. *Drugs* 5:6, 1973.
10. Debard ML, Jagger JA: "T's and B's:" Midwestern heroin substitute. *Clin Toxicol* 18:1117, 1981.
11. Linn KA, Long MT, Pagel PS: "Robo-Tripping:" dextromethorphan abuse and its anesthetic implications. *Anesth Pain Med* 4:e20990, 2014.
12. Wolfe TR, Caravati EM: Massive dextromethorphan ingestion and abuse. *Am J Emerg Med* 13:174, 1995.
13. Charatan F: Time-release analgesic drug causes fatal overdoses in United States. *West J Med* 175:82, 2001.
14. Raffa RB, Friderichs E, Reimann W, et al: Opioid and nonopioid components independently contribute to the mechanism of action of tramadol, an "atypical" opioid analgesic. *J Pharmacol Exp Ther* 260:275, 1992.
15. Carrieri MP, Amass L, Lucas GM, et al: Buprenorphine use: the international experience. *Clin Infect Dis* 15:S197, 2006.
16. Boyd J, Randell T, Luurila H, et al: Serious overdoses involving buprenorphine in Helsinki. *Acta Anaesthesiol Scand* 47:1031, 2003.
17. Pender ES, Parks BR: Toxicity with dextromethorphan-containing preparations: a literature review and report of two additional cases. *Pediatr Emerg Care* 7:163, 1991.
18. Pallasch TJ, Gill CJ: Naloxone-associated morbidity and mortality. *Oral Surg* 52:602, 1981.
19. Schwartz JA, Koenigsberg MD: Naloxone-induced pulmonary edema. *Ann Emerg Med* 16:1294, 1987.
20. Gopinathan K, Saroja D, Spears R, et al: Hemodynamic studies in heroin-induced acute pulmonary edema. *Circulation* III-44:61, 1970.
21. Lee G, DeMaria AN, Amsterdam EA, et al: Comparative effects of morphine, meperidine and pentazocine on cardiocirculatory dynamics in patients with acute myocardial infarction. *Am J Med* 60:949, 1976.
22. Glauser FL, Downie RL, Smith WR: Electrocardiographic abnormalities in acute heroin overdosage. *Bull Narc* 29:85, 1977.
23. Hagel J, Andrews G, Vertinsky T, et al: "Chasing the dragon"—imaging of heroin inhalation leukoencephalopathy. *Can Assoc Radiol J* 56:199, 2005.
24. Tennant FS: Complication of propoxyphene abuse. *Arch Intern Med* 132:191, 1973.
25. Amine ARL: Neurosurgical complications of heroin addiction: brain abscess and mycotic aneurysm. *Surg Neurol* 7:385, 1977.
26. Spiller HA, Gorman SE, Villalobos D, et al: Prospective multicenter evaluation of tramadol exposure. *J Toxicol Clin Toxicol* 35:361, 1997.
27. Hibbs J, Perper J, Winek CL: An outbreak of designer drug-related deaths in Pennsylvania. *JAMA* 265:1011, 1991.
28. Sloth Madsen P, Strom J, Reiz S, et al: Acute propoxyphene self-poisoning in 222 consecutive patients. *Acta Anaesthesiol Scand* 28:661, 1984.
29. Afshari R, Maxwell S, Dawson A, et al: ECG abnormalities in co-proxamol (paracetamol/dextropropoxyphene) poisoning. *Clin Toxicol* 43:255, 2005.
30. Krantz MJ, Lewkowiez L, Hays H, et al: Torsade de pointes associated with very-high-dose methadone. *Ann Intern Med* 137:501, 2002.
31. Eap CB, Crettol S, Rougier JS, et al: Stereoselective block of hERG channel by (S)-methadone and QT interval prolongation in CYP2B6 slow metabolizers. *Clin Pharmacol Ther* 81:719, 2007.
32. Crettol S, Deglon JJ, Besson J, et al: ABCB1 and cytochrome P450 genotypes and phenotypes: influence on methadone plasma levels and response to treatment. *Clin Pharmacol Ther* 80:668, 2006.
33. Gillman PK: Monoamine oxidase inhibitors, opioid analgesics and serotonin toxicity. *Br J Anaesth* 95:434, 2005.
34. Nelson EM, Philbrick AM: Avoiding serotonin syndrome: the nature of the interaction between tramadol and selective serotonin reuptake inhibitors. *Ann Pharmacother* 46:1712, 2012.
35. Schwatzfarb D, Singh G, Marcus D: Heroin-associated rhabdomyolysis with cardiac involvement. *Arch Intern Med* 137:1255, 1977.
36. Dubrow A, Mittman N, Ghali V, et al: The changing spectrum of heroin-associated nephropathy. *Am J Kidney Dis* 5:36, 1985.
37. Finn SP, Leen E, English L, et al: Autopsy findings in an outbreak of severe systemic illness in heroin users following injection site inflammation: an effect of Clostridium novyi exotoxin? *Arch Pathol Lab Med* 127:1465, 2003.
38. Utecht MJ, Stone AF, McCarron MM: Heroin body packers. *J Emerg Med* 11:33, 1993.
39. Hutchins KD, Pierre-Louis PJ, Zaretski L, et al: Heroin body packing: three fatal cases of intestinal perforation. *J Forensic Sci* 45:42, 2000.
40. Duberstein JL, Kaufman DM: A clinical study of an epidemic of heroin intoxication and heroin-induced pulmonary edema. *Am J Med* 51:704, 1971.
41. Jaffe RB, Koschmann EB: Intravenous drug abuse: pulmonary, cardiac and vascular complications. *Am J Roentgenol Radium Ther Nucl Med* 109:107, 1970.
42. Krantz MJ, Martin J, Stimmel B, et al: QTc interval screening in methadone treatment. *Ann Intern Med* 150:387, 2009.
43. Storrow AB, Wians FH, Mikkelsen SL, et al: Does naloxone cause a positive urine opiate screen? *Ann Emerg Med* 24:1151, 1994.
44. Cushman P Jr, Sherman C: Biologic false-positive reactions in serologic tests for syphilis in narcotic addiction. Reduced incidence during methadone maintenance treatment. *Am J Clin Pathol* 61:346, 1974.
45. Handal KA, Schauben JL, Salamone FR: Naloxone. *Ann Emerg Med* 12:438, 1983.
46. Schneir AB, Vadeboncoeur TF, Offerman SR, et al: Massive OxyContin ingestion refractory to naloxone therapy. *Ann Emerg Med* 40:425, 2002.
47. Maio RF, Gaukel B, Freeman B: Intralingual naloxone injection for narcotic-induced respiratory depression. *Ann Emerg Med* 16:572, 1987.
48. Tandberg D, Abercrombie D: Treatment of heroin overdose with endotracheal naloxone. *Ann Emerg Med* 11:443, 1982.
49. Kelly AM, Kerr D, Dietze P, et al: Randomised trial of intranasal versus intramuscular naloxone in prehospital treatment for suspected opioid overdose. *Med J Aust* 182:24, 2005.
50. Goldfrank LR, Weisman RS, Errick JK, et al: A dosing nomogram for continuous infusion intravenous naloxone. *Ann Emerg Med* 15:566, 1986.
51. Baumann BM, Patterson RA, Parone DA, et al: Use and efficacy of nebulized naloxone in patients with suspected opioid intoxication. *Am J Emerg Med* 31:585, 2013.
52. Fiut RE, Picchioni AL, Chin L: Antagonism of convulsive and lethal effects induced by propoxyphene. *J Pharm Sci* 55:1085, 1966.
53. Gillman PK: The serotonin syndrome and its treatment. *J Psychopharmacol* 13:100, 1999.
54. Sporer KA, Dorn E: Heroin-related noncardiogenic pulmonary edema: a case series. *Chest* 120:1628, 2001.
55. Marc B, Baud FJ, Aelion MJ, et al: The cocaine body-packer syndrome: evaluation of a method of contrast study of the bowel. *J Forensic Sci* 35:345, 1990.
56. Traub SJ, Hoffman RS, Nelson LS: Body packing—the internal concealment of illicit drugs. *N Engl J Med* 349:2519, 2003.
57. Larijani GE, Goldberg ME, Rogers KH: Treatment of opioid-induced pruritus with ondansetron: report of four patients. *Pharmacotherapy* 16:958, 1996.
58. Gacouin A, Lavoue S, Signouret T, et al: Reversible spongiform leucoencephalopathy after inhalation of heated heroin. *Intensive Care Med* 29:1012, 2003.
59. Gal TJ, Difazio CA: Prolonged antagonism of opioid action with intravenous nalmefene in man. *Anesthesiology* 64:175, 1986.

Chapter 120 ■ Pesticide—Herbicide Poisoning

WILLIAM K. CHIANG • RICHARD Y. WANG

A pesticide is as an agent intended for killing, preventing, repelling, or mitigating any pest. Despite their inherit toxicity, pesticide usage continues to increase; environmental contamination and reports of epidemic pesticide poisoning are inevitable. The health consequences from the long-term and low-level exposure to these chemicals, such as carcinogenesis, teratogenicity, reproductive disorders, and neurologic sequelae, may be significant and difficult to measure. In many countries in which there are limited regulations on pesticide usage, pesticide ingestion is one of the leading forms of suicide, and pesticide exposure is a major occupational risk. Even in the United States, pesticide exposures remain a major public health problem. Worldwide statistics on pesticides poisonings are limited because of gross under reporting in developing countries. Conservative estimates for suicides from pesticides worldwide exceeded 250,000 deaths annually [1].

This chapter focuses on selected pesticides that are most clinically important. Some of the common pesticides are provided in Table 120.1. Organophosphate insecticides are covered in Chapter 109. Further information on the identification and toxicity of pesticide products may be obtained from sources such as material data safety sheets, *Hayes' Handbook of Pesticide Toxicology, Farm Chemicals Handbook*, and the pesticide label database (http://www.cdpr.ca.gov/docs/label/labelque.htm).

ORGANOCHLORINES

Organochlorine compounds are commonly used as insecticides, soil fumigants, solvents, and herbicides. Human toxicity can result from either acute or chronic exposure. Contamination typically occurs during production or application of these agents. Infants and toddlers are at risk for toxicity from bioaccumulation in foodstuffs and excretion in breast milk. Maternal exposure is important because these compounds can be concentrated in fetal tissues. These toxicants can cause a variety of systemic manifestations, but are most notable for their central nervous system (CNS) effects. Organochlorines can be divided into four structural categories: dichlorodiphenyltrichloroethane (DDT) and related agents, hexachlorocyclohexanes, cyclodienes, and toxaphenes. Chlordane, chlordecone (Kepone), DDT, dieldrin, endrin, heptachlor, kevelan, methoxychlor, and mirex are no longer being used or registered for use in the United States.

Pharmacology

The organochlorines are well absorbed from the gastrointestinal (GI) tract. For example, death can occur within 2 hours of intentionally ingesting endosulfan, and most deaths associated with chlordane have been from oral exposures by children. The serum half-lives of these chemicals are long, varying from days to months, because of their high lipid solubility. This allows these agents to be stored in fatty tissues (e.g., brain) with the resultant delays in clearance. The organochlorines are known to concentrate in breast milk and fetal tissues. At delivery, it has been shown that fetal blood and tissue had higher concentrations of lindane (γ-hexachlorocyclohexane, Kwell) than maternal samples [2,3]. However, teratogenic effects have not been demonstrated in the limited number of animal studies performed [4].

Organochlorines are metabolized by the hepatic cytochrome P450 (CYP) enzymes in the liver. Toxaphene, chlordane, DDT, and lindane can induce CYP activity and affect not only their own metabolism but also the effects of coadministered medications [5].

Chlordane has several metabolites, such as heptachlor, oxychlordane, and heptachlor epoxide. Most of the available information on chlordane and metabolite tissue distribution is from case reports of unintentional and suicidal exposures. Depending on the source, the elimination half-life of chlordane varies from 21 to 88 days [6,7]. Most of the chlordane and metabolites are excreted by the biliary system. On absorption into the body, aldrin is rapidly metabolized to the epoxide derivative, dieldrin. Because very little of aldrin remains, its toxicity is attributed to dieldrin. Dieldrin is stored in fatty tissues, and its elimination half-life in humans is approximately 369 days [8]. Endrin, an isomer of dieldrin, is rapidly metabolized in both humans and animals, with an elimination half-life of 2 to 6 days [9].

Organochlorines have several mechanisms of action. They alter sodium and potassium channel activity and ion movement across the neuronal membranes and can be toxic to axons. For example, DDT facilitates sodium ion transport and inhibits potassium transport. This can result in spontaneous firing and prolongation of action potentials and repetitive firing after a stimulus. DDT also inhibits Na^+/K^+ adenosine triphosphatase and calmodulin activities, which can reduce the rate of neuronal repolarization. This may account for some of the neurologic manifestations such as paresthesias, thought disturbances, myoclonus, and seizures. Cyclodienes, hexachlorocyclohexanes, and toxaphene manifest neurotoxicity by inhibiting γ-aminobutyric acid receptor function in the CNS. In the limbic system, lindane can directly excite neurons and result in agitation and seizures [10]. Abnormalities in respiratory rate patterns can result from direct medullary toxicity or pulmonary aspiration. The level of toxicity of the various organochlorines can be categorized into high, moderate, and low (Table 120.2).

Clinical Toxicity

Poisoning can result from ingestion, dermal absorption, or inhalation. Inadvertent human exposures to aldrin and dieldrin have resulted from pesticide spraying and mixing which causes dermal and inhalational absorption. The use of lindane in home vaporizers has resulted in significant inhalation toxicity. Agents such as dieldrin, lindane, and Kepone have good dermal penetration. As little as two total body applications on two successive days of 1% lindane (Kwell), a common scabicide, resulted in seizures in an 18-month-old child [11]. The peak concentration of lindane occurs 6 hours after dermal application; thus, delayed and prolonged manifestations of toxicity may occur from dermal absorption. Workers who directly handled lindane had health complaints of headaches, paresthesias, tremors, confusion, and memory impairment [12]. Also, seizures have been reported by occupational surveys among sprayers and applicators of aldrin and dieldrin [13]. Dermatitis can occur from the topical exposure dicofol and methoxychlor. Intradermal and subcutaneous injections of these agents can result in chemical dermatitis and sterile abscesses [14]. Dicofol and methoxychlor have minimal toxicity.

Seizures are the most prominent CNS effect of these agents. The seizures occur soon after exposure, may present without a

TABLE 120.1

Common Pesticides

- Inorganic and organometal pesticides
  - Aluminum phosphide
  - Antimony potassium tartrate
  - Arsenical pesticides
  - Barium carbonate
  - Boric acid
  - Calcium chloride
  - Copper sulfate
  - Elemental mercury
  - Elemental sulfur
  - Lead arsenate
  - Mercuric chloride
  - Methylmercury
  - Phosphorus
  - Sodium chlorate
  - Sodium dichromate
  - Thallium sulfate
  - Zinc chloride
  - Zinc phosphide
- Pyrethrins, pyrethroids, and plant-derived pesticides
  - Anabasine
  - Barthrin
  - Blasticidin S
  - Cartap
  - Chlordecone
  - Cyfluthrin
  - Cyfluthrinate
  - Cyhalothrin
  - Cypermethrin
  - Decamethrin
  - Deltamethrin
  - Fluvalerate
  - Fluvalinate
  - Nicotine
  - Phenothrin
  - Pyrethrins
  - Resmethrin
  - Ricin
  - Rotenone
  - Sabadilla
  - Strychnine
  - Tralocythrin
  - Tralomethrin
- Fumigants and nematocides
  - Acrylonitrile
  - Aluminum phosphide
  - Boron trifluoride
  - Carbon disulfide
  - Carbon tetrachloride
  - Chloropicrin
  - 1,2-Dibromoethane
  - 1,2-Dichloroethane
  - *p*-Dichlorobenzene
  - 1,2-Dichloropropane
  - 1,3-Dichloropropene
  - Epoxyethane
  - Hydrogen cyanide
  - Methylbromide
  - Naphthalene
  - 1,1,1-Trichloroethane
  - Trichloroethylene
- Synthetic organic rodenticides
  - ANTU
  - Brodifacoum
  - Chloralose
  - Difenacoum
  - Diphacinone
  - Fluoroacetamide
  - Fluoroethanol
  - Norbormide
  - Pyriminil
  - Sodium fluoroacetate
  - Warfarin
- Herbicides
  - Amitrole
  - Atrazine
  - Bromoxynil
  - Cycloate
  - Dicamba
  - Dichlobenil
  - 2,4-Dichlorophenoxyacetic acid
  - Diquat
  - Diuron
  - Ioxynil
  - MCPA
  - Mecoprop
  - Molinate
  - Phenmedipham
  - Paraquat
  - Propanil
  - Propazine
  - Pyrazon
  - Silvex
  - Simazine
  - TCA
  - 2,3,5-Trichlorophenoxyacetic acid
- Fungicides and biocides
  - Benomyl
  - Captafol
  - Captan
  - 1-Chloro dinitrobenzene
  - Dichloran
  - Diphenyl
  - Maneb
  - Organotins (tributyltin)
  - Quintozene
  - Tetrachlorophthalide
  - Thiabendazole
  - Thiram
  - Thiophanate-methyl
  - Zineb
  - Ziram
- Organochlorine insecticides
  - Aldrin
  - Chlordane
  - Chlorobenzilate
  - Chlordecone
  - DDT
  - Dicofol
  - Dieldrin
  - Endrin
  - Endosulfan
  - Ethylan
  - Heptachlor
  - Hexachlorobenzene
  - Isobenzan
  - Kelevan
  - Kelthane
  - Lindane (γ-hexachlorocyclohexane)
  - Mirex
  - Methoxychlor
  - TDE
  - Toxaphene
- Organophosphate insecticides
  - Azinphos-methyl
  - Carbophenothion
  - Carejin
  - Chlorfenvinphos
  - Chlorphoxim
  - Chlorpyrifos
  - Demeton
  - Demeton-methyl
  - Dialifos
  - Diazinon
  - Dicapthon
  - Dichlofenthion
  - Dichlorvos
  - Dicrotophos
  - Dimefox
  - Dioxathion
  - Edifenphos
  - Endothion
  - Fenitrothion
  - Fensulfothion
  - Fenthion
  - Fonofos
  - Formothion
  - Jodfenphos
  - Leptophos
  - Malathion
  - Merphos
  - Methidathion
  - Mevinphos
  - Mipafox
  - Monocrotophos
  - Naled
  - Oxydemeton-methyl
  - Parathion
  - Parathion-methyl
  - Phenthoate
  - Phorate
  - Phosalone
  - Phosphamidon
  - Phoxim
  - Pirimiphos-methyl
  - Schradan
  - Temephos
  - Thiometon
  - Trichlorfon
- Carbamates
  - Aldicarb
  - Bendiocarb

(continued)

TABLE 120.1

Common Pesticides (*continued*)

4-Benxiothielyn-*N*-methylcarbamate	Phencyclocarb	Metaldehyde
Bufencarb	Promecarb	Methotrexate
Carbaryl	Propoxur	Porfiromycin
Carbofuran	Miscellaneous pesticides	Propargite
Dioxacarb	Azoxybenzene	Thiotepa
Isolan	Busulfan	Nitro compounds and related phenolic pesticides
3-Isopropyl phenyl-*N*-methylcarbamate	Chlorambucil	Binapacryl
Landrin	Chlordimeform	Dinocap
Methomyl	Chlorfenxon	2,4-Dinitrophenol
Mexacarbate	DEET	Dinoseb
Oxamyl	5-Fluorouracil	Pentachlorophenol
	Hexamethylmelamine	

ANTU, α-naphthylthiourea; DDT, dichlorodiphenyltrichloroethane; DEET, *N-N*-diethyl-*m*-toluamide; MCPA, 4-chloro-2-methylphenoxyacetic acid; TCA, trichloroacetic acid; TDE, 1,1-dichloro-2,2-bis(4-chlorophenyl)ethane.
Classifications adapted from Hayes WJ Jr, Laws ER (eds): *Handbook of Pesticide Toxicology.* San Diego, Academic, 1991.

TABLE 120.2

Organochlorine Levels of Toxicity

High	Endrin, dieldrin, aldrin, and endosulfan
Moderate	Chlordecone, heptachlor, chlordane, toxaphene, dichlorodiphenyltrichloroethane, and hexachlorobenzene
Low	Methoxychlor, perthane, kelthane, chlorobenzilate, and mirex

prodrome, and can be protracted in frequency [9]. Late-onset seizures may result from delayed GI or dermal absorption. Acute exposures to DDT present initially with tremors, nausea, vomiting, muscle weakness, and confusion, which may progress to seizures [15]. Among the organochlorines, both psychomotor agitation and CNS depression have been described. Chlordecone, mirex, and endosulfan are more likely to cause tremors and agitation than seizures. Kelthane, perthane, methoxychlor, and lindane are more likely to cause CNS sedation than excitation. Endrin is considered one of the most toxic of the cyclodienes, with reports of hyperthermia and decerebrate posturing [9]. In 1984, an outbreak of endrin toxicity from contaminated foodstuffs occurred in Pakistan, where seizures resulted in a 10% mortality rate [16].

Neurologic symptoms resolve quickly because of rapid distribution of the organochlorines from blood to lipid stores. Because redistribution back into the blood pool can occur at a later time, continual observation of the patient for delayed toxicity may be warranted. Some of the long-term CNS effects (i.e., thought disturbances) after significant exposures may be owing to direct chemical toxicity or anoxic encephalopathy from sustained seizures. Chlordecone is a recognized neurotoxin, causing peripheral neuropathies [17].

Nausea, vomiting, and diarrhea may occur after ingestions, especially if petroleum distillates are part of the preparation. Pulmonary aspiration of these agents can cause tachypnea and significant respiratory distress, with resultant pulmonary edema. When dicofol is heated or comes in contact with an acid, it decomposes to hydrogen chloride, which causes respiratory irritation [9]. Hypersensitivity pneumonitis may result from inhalational exposures when the organochlorine is mixed with pyrethrins.

Hypotension with decreased cardiac output and a prolonged QT interval have been reported from endosulfan poisoning [18].

Significant elevations of liver enzymes were reported in a group of 19 workers with a 10-year exposure to lindane [19]. Acute oral exposures to lindane in animals may cause fatty degeneration and necrosis of the liver. From the few reports of human exposures to chlordane, there is little evidence of hepatotoxicity from this agent [20]. Microsomal enzyme induction has been demonstrated in animals that were orally administered chlordane. Long-term exposure among 233 workers with aldrin, dieldrin, endrin, and kelodrin for 4 to 12 years was not associated with any significant elevation of hepatic enzymes or hepatic enzyme induction.

Hematologic dyscrasias, including aplastic anemia, leukopenia, leukocytosis, granulocytopenia, granulocytosis, eosinophilia, thrombocytopenia, and pancytopenia, have been reported after repeated lindane exposures [21]. However, all of the involved preparations also contained benzene, which can account for such findings. Megaloblastic anemia and bone marrow depression have been associated with chlordane exposures. DDT and toxaphene are suspected human carcinogens [22]. The risks for aldrin and dieldrin as human carcinogens could not be determined by IARC (International Agency for Research on Cancer) because of insufficient human and animal data.

Diagnostic Evaluation

Serum concentrations of these organochlorines are commonly measured by gas chromatography/mass spectrometry. In an obvious exposure to these agents, these measurements are academic and would not alter clinical management. There are no correlations between concentrations in body tissues and specific health effects. If the diagnosis is in doubt, these measurements can at least confirm or rule out the exposure to the insecticide. Although blood is commonly sampled for the detection of these chemicals, adipose tissue, or human milk may be used as well. The laboratory should be consulted regarding the availability of analytical methods for biologic specimens other than blood. An acute exposure can be determined by a quantitative comparison of parent compound to metabolite. Because DDT and aldrin are rapidly metabolized upon systemic absorption, their elevated concentrations in the blood would support a recent exposure.

Chlorinated hydrocarbons are radiopaque, and their radiopacity is directly related to the number of chlorine atoms per molecule. Thus, radiographs can assist in demonstrating aspiration pneumonia and gut burden.

Management

Rescue workers and health care providers must use proper equipment, such as gloves and gowns, to prevent unnecessary exposure to these chemicals when providing assistance to these patients. Initial treatment of organochlorine exposure involves limiting further chemical absorption by the patient. The patient should be removed from the scene, disrobed, and thoroughly and repeatedly washed with soap and water. Washing should include hair and fingernails. The patient's clothing and leather goods must be placed in a plastic bag and discarded because of the tenacious binding of these agents to leather. All wash water should be contained and discarded as hazardous waste by qualified personnel.

The role of gastric decontamination depends on the clinical presentation. Immediately after an intentional ingestion and in asymptomatic patients without spontaneous emesis, gastric aspiration should be carefully performed with a small nasogastric tube. Activated charcoal should be administered soon after ingestion (preferably within 1 hour) because it can limit further gut absorption [23]. Also, cholestyramine may interrupt enteric circulation and enhance elimination. Chlordecone and chlordane undergo enterohepatic circulation, and cholestyramine is indicated in symptomatic patients. In a controlled trial, cholestyramine was administered as 16 g per day to symptomatic factory workers exposed to chlordecone. After 5 months, chlordecone fecal elimination was shown to increase by 3.3 to 17.8 times, with neurologic symptoms improving as concentrations declined [24]. Milk- and oil-based cathartics should be avoided because their high lipid solubility can enhance gut absorption. Hemodialysis is not effective in enhancing elimination of these chemicals because of their high volume of distribution and protein binding [25]. Hemoperfusion is probably of no benefit [25].

Organochlorine-induced seizures are managed with benzodiazepines and barbiturates. Phenytoin has not been demonstrated to be more effective as an anticonvulsant than barbiturates and it may actually increase the incidence of these seizures [26]. For uncontrolled status epilepticus, muscle paralysis, and general anesthesia may be necessary. Aggressive seizure control is warranted to limit further development of CNS damage, metabolic acidosis, hyperthermia, rhabdomyolysis, and myoglobinuric renal failure.

Respiratory distress caused by bronchospasm is managed with humidified oxygen and nebulized bronchodilators. Parenteral administration of adrenergic amines is not recommended because it may potentiate myocardial irritability. Early administration of steroids and prophylactic use of antibiotics for pulmonary aspiration has not been demonstrated to improve patients' outcomes. The early use of antibiotics may predispose to the selective growth of resistant bacterial organisms.

After appropriate decontamination, asymptomatic patients with an oral exposure can be observed for 6 hours and then discharged if their clinical status remains unchanged. The patients presenting with cardiovascular, CNS, or persistent respiratory manifestations should be admitted for further therapy and observation.

PYRETHROIDS

Pyrethrum is a collection of naturally occurring insecticide esters from the chrysanthemum flower. The pyrethrin I ester has the greatest insecticidal activity and is subject to rapid environmental degradation. To enhance their effectiveness in commercial use, synthetic alternatives known as pyrethroids were developed that are more resistant to decay. These compounds are present in consumer products, from flea and tick removers for pets to topical pediculicides.

Pharmacology

Pyrethroids can be separated into two classes based on their chemical structures. For example, Type II pyrethroids have a cyano group at the alpha carbon, such as deltamethrin. The pyrethroids (including pyrethrins) delay closure of the sodium channel during the end of depolarization, with resultant insect paralysis. Type I pyrethroids maintain the sodium channel in the open position for a shorter period than Type II pyrethroids. In addition, Type II pyrethroids antagonize inhibitory chloride channels and alter calcium ion transients, but the contribution of these findings to clinical toxicity is unclear. Piperonyl butoxide is commonly added to commercial preparations to inhibit insects' ability to metabolize the pyrethroid and prolong activity. In mammals, these agents are relatively nontoxic because of the low concentrations and the rapid mammalian metabolism of these chemicals. However, people who are allergic to ragweed may have hypersensitivity reactions to pyrethroids. The degree of this cross-sensitization has been reported to be as high as 46%. Pyrethroids have no effects on cholinesterase activity, and atropine and pralidoxime are not indicated in therapy.

Pyrethroids are readily absorbed from the GI tract. Dermal absorption varies depending on the type of agent and additive organic solvents. Systemic absorption is enhanced in the presence of petroleum distillates. These compounds are highly lipid-soluble and largely metabolized by the mixed-function oxidase enzymes in the liver.

Clinical Toxicity

Poisoning from pyrethroids can result from inhalational, dermal, or oral exposures. Nausea, vomiting, and diarrhea may occur after ingestion [27,28]. Neurologic manifestations and hypersensitivity reactions, including anaphylaxis, are the most common forms of systemic toxicity. Neurologic findings depend on the type and concentration of the pyrethroid and include paresthesias, muscle fasciculations, coma, and seizures [27,28]. For example, poisoned patients tend to present with tremors from Type I pyrethroids and with choreoathetosis and salivation from Type II pyrethroids. The patients with an intentional ingestion of a mixture containing an organophosphate and a pyrethroid can present with predominant cholinergic manifestations.

Management

Treatment is very similar to that described for organochlorines (see previous discussion). GI decontamination may be appropriate but there is no role for repeat-dose–activated charcoal and cholestyramine therapy because enterohepatic circulation has not been demonstrated for the pyrethroids. Hypersensitivity reactions, including anaphylaxis, should be managed with epinephrine, steroids, antihistamines, bronchodilators, and vasopressors, as indicated.

Asymptomatic patients with oral exposures can be observed for 6 hours and medically cleared of toxicity if their clinical status remains unchanged. The patients presenting with cardiovascular, CNS, or persistent respiratory manifestations should be admitted for further therapy and observation. The patients presenting with cholinergic manifestations after a mixed ingestion of pesticides should be treated for organophosphate toxicity (see Chapter 109), which includes pralidoxime and an appropriate amount of atropine to dry secretions.

ANTICOAGULANTS

Bishydroxycoumarin (dicumarol), the first anticoagulant, was isolated as the hemorrhagic agent in *sweet clover disease*, a bleeding disorder that resulted from the ingestion of spoiled clover silage. Numerous congeners, such as warfarin (3-α-acetonylbenzyl-4-hydroxycoumarin), have since been synthesized and used as rodenticides. Typically, for the bait to be effective, the rodent must consume it for 3 to 10 days; however, continuous feeding for 21 days may be necessary to achieve 100% mortality. As rodents became increasingly resistant, warfarin derivatives were introduced and have supplanted warfarin. These "superwarfarins," or long-acting anticoagulants, including brodifacoum, difenacoum, and indanedione derivatives, have longer lipophilic phenyl side chains that increase their potency (approximately 100 times more potent than warfarin) and their half-life and duration of action [29]. Most anticoagulant rodenticide is packaged with cereal or other food products as bait, with the amount of rodenticide in the product varying from 0.005% to 0.025% per weight. Acute accidental or suicidal ingestion of a minimal amount of bait containing long-acting anticoagulants is unlikely to cause toxicity [30]. However, a "mouthful" of a long-acting anticoagulant ingestion in an adult human has been reported to cause significant coagulopathy.

Pharmacology

Warfarin and its derivatives are oxidized by CYP hepatic microsomal enzymes into inactive metabolites in the liver. More specifically, warfarin and its enantiomers are metabolized by CYP 2D6, 3A4, and 2C9 [31]. The plasma half-life of warfarin is 42 hours, with duration of action of 2 to 5 days. The long-acting anticoagulants are concentrated in the liver and have extremely long half-lives; brodifacoum has a half-life of 120 days in dogs, 61 hours in rabbits, and 156 hours in rats [32,33]. The half-life of long-acting anticoagulants may be affected by the dose. The exact half-life of long-acting anticoagulants in humans is unknown. Case reports in human exposures have reported half-lives of 6 to 23 days for chlorophacinone and 16 to 39 days for brodifacoum [29,34–36]. Clinical coagulopathy may persist as long as 42 to 300 days [29,34–36].

These anticoagulants inhibit vitamin K 2,3-epoxide reductase and, to a lesser extent, vitamin K reductase. These enzymes are responsible for the cyclic regeneration of vitamin K [37]. Vitamin K is the active coenzyme responsible for activation of clotting factors II, VII, IX, and X, as well as anticoagulant factors protein C and protein S, by hepatic γ-carboxylation of the *N*-terminal glutamate residual of these proteins [37]. Once activated, vitamin K–dependent clotting factors can interact with calcium and phospholipids in the coagulation cascade. Inhibition of vitamin K 2,3-epoxide reductase and vitamin K reductase depletes vitamin K and vitamin K–dependent clotting factors, resulting in coagulopathy and bleeding. The half-lives of vitamin K–dependent clotting factors are 7 hours for factor VII, 24 hours for factor IX, 36 hours for factor X, and 50 hours for factor II [35]. Because factor VII has the shortest half-life of the vitamin K–dependent clotting factors, increases in prothrombin time or international normalized ratio (INR) are not seen until 50% to 70% of factor VII is depleted. In a healthy person, this change occurs 24 to 48 hours after ingestion [29,30]. Clinical coagulopathy may not be evident for several days when the other vitamin K–dependent factors are also depleted, however.

Clinical Toxicity

The primary manifestation of poisoning is coagulopathy. The most common signs are cutaneous bleeding, soft-tissue ecchymosis, gingival bleeding, epistaxis, hematuria, and increased menstrual bleeding [29,34]. Gross hematuria, GI bleeding, hemoptysis, and peritoneal and diffuse alveolar bleeding may occur in patients with more serious poisoning [29,38]. Fatalities are uncommon and usually result from complications of intracranial hemorrhage [29,39].

Management

Gastric decontamination with activated charcoal should be initiated for acute ingestions. The most important laboratory studies are the prothrombin time and INR. Soon after an acute ingestion, values are expected to be normal; assays must be repeated at least 48 hours after exposure because of delayed coagulopathy. Prophylactic vitamin K therapy can delay the onset of coagulopathy, and is not recommended as it may obscure the diagnosis and mandate prolonged coagulation profile monitoring, which might otherwise be unnecessary. Clotting factor analysis, particularly for factor VII, is a more sensitive and earlier indicator of coagulopathy. Factor analysis does not offer more useful information in most patients with minimal ingestions, however. Occasionally, serum detection for warfarin and its derivatives has demonstrated unsuspected exposures in patients with coagulopathy of unknown cause. In patients with coagulopathy, serial monitoring of warfarin derivative concentrations can assist in predicting the duration of coagulopathy and therapy [35].

The primary treatment of anticoagulant toxicity is vitamin K replacement, which is indicated in patients with evidence of coagulopathy. Warfarin and its congeners have much less effect on human than on rat vitamin K reductase, thus allowing vitamin K rescue therapy for anticoagulant toxicity in humans. Because a single dose of vitamin K therapy cannot affect the prolonged toxicity of the long-acting anticoagulants, empiric vitamin K therapy is not recommended unless the patient has a coagulopathy. Vitamin K is not immediately effective in reversing coagulopathy; four-factor prothrombin factor concentrates (PCC) are indicated in patients with significant bleeding diathesis (Table 120.3) [40]. Four-factor PCC are preferred over three-factor PCC, which lack factor VII, and activated factor VII [40,41]. PCC are also preferable to fresh frozen plasma (FFP) because of less fluid load, lower infection risk, and more rapid correction of the INR in

TABLE 120.3

Treatment Guidelines for Coagulopathy from Long-Acting Anticoagulant Rodenticides in Patients with no Underlying Risks for Thromboembolism

Active bleeding, major, and life threatening

1. Clotting factors replacement:
   4-Factor prothrombin complex concentrates (50 units/kg)[a]
   and
2. Vitamin K_1 intravenous (adult 10 mg, pediatrics 100 μg/kg by slow infusion)
3. Packed red blood cells for significant bleeding (i.e., anemia and hypotension)

No active bleeding and international normalized ratio (INR) ≥4.0

1. Oral vitamin K_1, start at 50 mg 3–4 times daily until coagulopathy is reversed (1–2 d), then maintain at 100 mg daily, with continue monitoring of INR, factor VII, and long-acting anticoagulant rodenticide level to determine vitamin K dosing and duration of therapy

[a]Second line therapy: fresh-frozen plasma (15 mL/kg).

patients with a coagulopathy from warfarin toxicity [40,41]. PCC contain heparin and may be contraindicated in patients with heparin-induced thrombocytopenia.

Only vitamin K_1 (phytonadione) should be used because the other forms (K_2, K_3, and K_4) are ineffective in the treatment of anticoagulant toxicity. Vitamin K_1 can be administered orally, subcutaneously, intramuscularly, and intravenously. Intravenous administration has been associated with anaphylactoid reactions and death [42]; slow intravenous administration (10 mg over 30 to 60 minutes) is recommended for those with acute bleeding diathesis. Intramuscular injection may cause hematoma formation in patients with coagulopathy. Subcutaneous administration of vitamin K_1 is safe and may be less effective than the oral route [43]. Treatment should be switched to oral vitamin K_1 once bleeding is controlled and the patient's GI tract deemed intact for oral absorption. The half-life of oral vitamin K_1 is approximately 6 hours [35]. The oral vitamin K_1 dose required to reverse coagulopathy is variable, but typically ranges from 100 to 300 mg per day, divided three to four times per day [29,35]. Once coagulopathy is reversed, the most common maintenance dose for oral vitamin K_1 is 100 mg (range 20 to 300 mg) daily, but can also be divided into two doses daily [29]. The amount of vitamin K therapy must be titrated to clinical response, however. The duration of vitamin K therapy and coagulopathy is also highly variable, ranging from 40 to 300 days [29]. When the patient's INR has remained normal for several days after stopping the treatment, vitamin K therapy can be discontinued. The trend of the patient's concentration of clotting factors during this period may assist the determination of this clinical endpoint. Various methods have been proposed to decrease the duration of coagulopathy, including administration of hepatic enzyme inducers such as phenobarbital. There is no good evidence to support any of these therapies, however.

STRYCHNINE

The use of strychnine as a pesticide dates back to the 16th century, when an extract of the Filipino St. Ignatius bean (*Strychnos ignatii*) was introduced as a rodenticide in Europe. Strychnine was used as a tonic, cathartic, and aphrodisiac as late as 1970, and resulted in numerous deaths [44]. It is also found as an adulterant in illicit drugs, such as cocaine and heroin. The only "legitimate" uses of strychnine today are as a pesticide and in research study of neural transmission.

Pharmacology

Strychnine is rapidly absorbed through the nasal mucosa and orally in the small intestine. It undergoes hepatic oxidative transformation to unknown metabolites, and only 10% to 20% is excreted unchanged in the urine within 24 hours. The half-life of strychnine in humans is 10 to 16 hours, and the volume of distribution is 13 L per kg [45,46].

Strychnine competitively antagonizes postsynaptic glycine receptors at the spinal cord and, to a lesser degree, at the brain stem, cerebral cortex, and hippocampus [44]. Strychnine-binding sites overlap, but are distinct from glycine-binding sites at the glycine receptor [47]. Glycine receptors at the cerebral cortex and hippocampus are of a subtype insensitive to strychnine and are minimally affected [44]. The action of glycine is similar to that of γ-aminobutyric acid in that it enhances chloride ionic channel conduction, resulting in hyperpolarization of postsynaptic membrane and an increased threshold for neurologic transmission [48]. The highest concentration of glycine receptors is found at the ventral horn motor neurons in the spinal cord [48]. Glycine antagonism reduces neuromuscular inhibition, including reciprocal inhibition between antagonistic muscles, resulting in contraction of both flexor and extensor muscle groups [49]. The pharmacologic effect of strychnine is similar to that of tetanus toxin, which inhibits the release of glycine at postsynaptic neurons in the spinal cord [48].

Clinical Toxicity

The onset of toxicity is usually within 15 to 30 minutes of exposure. The lethal dose in adults is typically 50 to 100 mg, but it may be as little as 5 to 10 mg in children. Diffuse muscle contractions and spasms are the primary manifestations of strychnine toxicity. Facial muscle spasms result in risus sardonicus (the "sardonic smile") and trismus. Opisthotonos, abdominal muscle contractions, and tonic movements of the extremities may resemble convulsions. Because glycine has limited effects in the higher CNS centers, seizures are unlikely and mental status is normally preserved until the patient is hypoxic or moribund [49]. The extensor muscles appear to be more affected than the flexor muscles because they are the antigravity muscles and generally stronger. Muscle contractions can be triggered or amplified by any stimulations, including auditory, tactile, and visual stimuli, and may lead to lactic acidosis, rhabdomyolysis, and hyperthermia [49,50]. Respiratory depression results from sustained chest and diaphragmatic muscle contractions and brain-stem depression. Death is related to respiratory depression, anoxia, hyperthermia, and complications from significant muscle contractions [45]. The clinical manifestations of strychnine toxicity differ from tetanus infection in that the onset of symptoms of tetanus infection is more gradual and the duration of illness is more prolonged.

Management

Securing the airway, assisting breathing, and maintaining the circulatory system are the immediate goals in symptomatic patients. Electrolytes, acid–base changes, oxygenation saturation, renal function, urine output, and temperature should be monitored carefully in symptomatic patients. GI decontamination should be performed in any case of suspected strychnine ingestion. Enhanced elimination by urinary manipulation has no effect because of minimal renal elimination. Hemodialysis or charcoal hemoperfusion is ineffective because of the large volume of distribution.

Termination of muscle contractions prevents or reverses lactic acidosis, rhabdomyolysis, hyperthermia, and respiratory depression. Benzodiazepines are the initial agents of choice in attenuating musculoskeletal signs and symptoms [50,51]. Benzodiazepines enhance γ-aminobutyric acid effects in the spinal cord and may displace strychnine binding to glycine receptors [47,48]. Barbiturates also are reported to be useful in the treatment of strychnine toxicity. These agents may not be completely effective in patients with severe strychnine poisoning, however, and other agents such as propofol and adjunct nondepolarizing neuromuscular blockade may be required [47,51]. Strychnine toxicity usually resolves within 12 to 24 hours [44,51]. Supportive therapy should be continued until the patient is asymptomatic.

SODIUM MONOFLUOROACETATE

Sodium monofluoroacetate is frequently referred to as "compound 1080," the number assigned to the compound during its initial development. It is the primary toxic constituent in the South African gifblaar (*Dichapetalum cymosum*), but it is also present in other plants in South America and Australia. Fluoroacetate is highly toxic to all mammals, and its use was banned in the United States in 1972 because of human fatalities and indiscriminate extermination of non-targeted species. The congener sodium fluoroacetamide (compound 1081), also used as a pesticide, has mechanisms and effects similar to those of fluoroacetate. Since 1985, fluroacetate was re-introduced but restricted to livestock protection collars (tubular collars filled with 1% sodium fluroroacetate solution, which is released when bitten by predators). In Australia and New Zealand, fluoroacetate is still use as a pesticide for control of invasive mammals, such as rabbits, foxes, feral pigs, wild dogs, and possums.

Pharmacology

Fluoroacetate appears to be minimally absorbed through skin but rapidly absorbed from the GI tract. It is metabolized to fluorocitrate in the tricarboxylic acid (TCA) cycle, with 12% of the ingested dose excreted in the urine [52]. In animals with relative resistance to monofluoroacetate, a hepatic defluorination system cleaves the carbon–fluoride bond to detoxify the compound.

Fluoroacetate is structurally similar to acetate and is incorporated into the TCA cycle with the assistance of acetyl coenzyme A. Fluoroacetate combines with citrate to form fluorocitrate in the TCA cycle [53]. Fluorocitrate inhibits aconitase and succinate dehydrogenase and disrupts the TCA cycle, halting cellular respiration and causing cell death [53]. Organs with high metabolic demands, such as the brain and heart, are immediately affected [53]. The lethal dose of sodium monofluoroacetate is 2 to 10 mg per kg.

Clinical Toxicity

The onset of poisoning occurs within 1 to 2 hours of exposure. Nausea and vomiting are followed by CNS and cardiovascular manifestations, which are the primary toxicities in humans [53,54]. The patient may present with agitation, lethargy, seizures, and coma [54–56]. Cardiovascular manifestations include tachycardia, premature ventricular contractions, ST-segment abnormalities, hypotension, ventricular tachycardia, and ventricular fibrillation [53]. Acute renal failure may be related to hypotension, rhabdomyolysis, and the direct toxic effects of monofluoroacetate on kidney function [54]. Fatality is related to CNS and cardiovascular toxicities [53,55]. Laboratory abnormalities include significant metabolic acidosis and hypocalcemia from the fluoride, citrate, and fluoroacetate ions [53].

Management

General supportive measures are paramount and aimed at maintaining the airway, breathing, and circulation. Activated charcoal should be administered in all suspected oral exposures presenting within 1 to 2 hours after ingestion. Seizures should be treated with benzodiazepines, barbiturates, or propofol. Hypocalcemia and prolonged QTc intervals may require calcium and magnesium supplementation. Various treatments have been tested in animals [57]. The most useful agent appears to be glyceryl monoacetate, which provides excess acetate as a substrate for the TCA cycle [53,57]. The clinical use of glyceryl monoacetate remains unproven, however.

ALUMINUM AND ZINC PHOSPHIDES

Aluminum and zinc phosphides (AlP and Zn_3P_2) are highly toxic insecticides and rodenticides commonly used as solid fumigants and grain preservatives. They are considered to be ideal pesticides for grain preservation because of the simplicity of application, low cost, and high efficacy without grain contamination. Although highly restricted in the United States, aluminum phosphide is widely available and commonly used for home grain storage in Asia and the Middle East, often sold as "Rice Tablet." Typically, each pellet contains 3 g of 56% aluminum phosphide. Aluminum phosphide has become one of the most common suicidal agents in rural India and parts of the Middle East. As little as 0.5 g can be fatal to an adult. Phosphides are widely used by grain freighters and have emerged as the major maritime occupational health hazard. Phosphine (PH_3) is slowly liberated when phosphides react with moisture in the environment.

Pharmacology

Phosphides react with water to form phosphine; the reaction is exothermic and it may be accelerated in the acidic environment of the stomach [58]. Phosphine is then readily absorbed in the stomach. Phosphine itself can also be absorbed through the lungs. There is limited information on the pharmacokinetics and metabolism of phosphine, although it is known to be partly eliminated through the lungs.

The exact mechanisms of toxicity have not been completely elucidated but likely multi-factorial. The most cited mechanism is related to non-competitive inhibition of cytochrome C oxidase (complex IV in the mitochondria) but this inhibition may be incomplete [59,60]. Other important mechanisms include the inhibition of catalase and peroxidase, causing increases in the production of superoxide dismutase and lipid peroxidation [59–61]. As a cellular toxin, phosphine has deleterious effects on multiple organ systems, particularly organs with high metabolic demands.

Clinical Toxicity

Inhalation of phosphine gas results in immediate eye and mucus membrane irritation and early onset of pulmonary symptoms [58]. Oral ingestion of phosphides causes profound GI symptoms, including nausea, vomiting, and abdominal pain [58]. In these instances, esophageal lesions, such as ulcers, perforations, and strictures, can occur and they are typically associated with the ingestion of undiluted pellets [58]. The diagnosis may be suggested from a decaying fish odor released by substituted phosphines and diphosphines. Silver nitrate–impregnated paper blackens in the presence of phosphine in the gastric fluid [60]. Respiratory symptoms include cough, dyspnea, and chest tightness. Pulmonary edema and respiratory failure may be delayed for several hours after oral exposure to phosphides [62]. Hypotension and shock are expected within 6 hours in serious exposures. Fatalities are related to cardiovascular collapse from vasodilation and myocardial damage [60,63–65]. Cardiac hypokinesis and decreased left ventricular ejection fractions have been demonstrated by echocardiography [60]. Various electrocardiographic changes have been reported, including ST-segment elevation and depression, QRS prolongation, bundle-branch blocks, atrioventricular nodal blockade, and supraventricular and ventricular tachycardia [63–65]. CNS symptoms may include headache, drowsiness, paresthesia, and tremor, but encephalopathy is uncommon unless the patient is in shock [60]. Other manifestations include severe metabolic acidosis, hepatitis, and renal failure [60,66]. Mortality rates vary from 38% to 77% in suicidal ingestions.

Management

The patient should be immediately removed from the contaminated environment after the rescuer is adequately protected. Airway, breathing, and circulatory support are important in the immediate management. Even though there is no reported secondary toxicity to health care providers, the resuscitation area should be well ventilated. Activated charcoal should be mixed with sorbitol or magnesium citrate, rather than plain water, to reduce further liberation of phosphine in the GI tract. Other suggestions including careful lavage with sodium bicarbonate, antacid, potassium permanganate, or coconut oil but has not been adequately studied and cannot be recommended currently.

Cardiac monitoring and electrocardiography should be performed in suspected phosphine toxicity. Respiratory status should be monitored by continued clinical evaluation. Hypo- and hypermagnesemia have been reported with aluminum phosphide poisoning [63,64]. Chest radiography, pulse oximetry, and arterial blood gases should be obtained as clinically indicated.

There is no antidote for phosphine poisoning. The mainstay of therapy is supportive care and expected mortality is high. Although intravenous magnesium therapy has been successful in treating various dysrhythmias, current studies results are contradictory [64,66]. Magnesium therapy in phosphide poisoning should be considered in patients with dysrhythmias or hypomagnesemia.

METHYL BROMIDE

Methyl bromide (Bromomethane, CH_3Br) is a colorless halogenated hydrocarbon gas primarily used as a fumigant for the control of nematodes, insects, rodents, fungi, and weeds. Methyl bromide was one of the most widely used pesticides in the United States and worldwide since the abandonment of chlordane and acrylonitrile as fumigants. Because methyl bromide causes ozone depletion in the stratosphere, the Montreal Protocol restricted its use in most developed countries since 2005. The United Nations proposed complete elimination of methyl bromide use worldwide by 2015. However, methyl bromide is still in use many countries and in the United States at least until 2017 under critical use exemptions. Methyl bromide was particularly popular in the food industry because it is extremely effective, is able to diffuse into any empty spaces, and does not leave any residues after proper ventilation. Space fumigation of fruits and tobacco can be performed in an airtight (fumigation) chamber. For soil fumigation, methyl bromide can be applied underground and sealed with an overlying tent or polyethylene cover. For structural fumigation, gas-proof tarpaulins are applied over the structure before the application of methyl bromide. Methyl bromide is still used for the manufacture of chemicals such as aniline dyes. It has a musty and chloroform-like odor at high concentrations, but it is odorless at lower, but still very toxic, concentrations. Because methyl bromide is heavier than air, it is particularly dangerous in an enclosed environment. Inadvertent exposures from accidents or inadequate ventilation have caused significant toxicities and fatalities [67–69].

Pharmacology

Methyl bromide is primarily absorbed through the lungs. Cutaneous absorption is minimal. Methyl bromide easily penetrates and is retained in cloth, rubber, and leather. It is eliminated unchanged in the lungs, but a small proportion is metabolized to 5-methylcysteine and inorganic bromide; these are excreted in the urine [70].

Because of the low electronegativity of bromide, methyl bromide is a highly reactive chemical [68]. The mechanism of toxicity is probably related to the methylation of sulfhydryl groups in different intracellular enzymes and depletion of glutathione [68]. Methyl bromide can readily penetrate through lipid cell membranes [68]. Low concentrations of bromide may be detected in the serum after significant exposure to methyl bromide, but they do not correlate well with toxicity [67]. The symptoms of methyl bromide toxicity are distinctly different from those of bromide salt toxicity [71].

Toxic effects primarily involve the central nervous and pulmonary systems [68]. Although exposures to concentrations of 2,000 ppm or greater may produce immediate CNS depression and respiratory failure, symptoms may be delayed for 1 to 6 hours or longer with exposure to lower concentrations. The current occupational exposure limits for methyl bromide are a California/Division of Occupational Safety and Health (Cal/OSHA) permissible exposure limit of 1 ppm with an 8-hour time weighted average and an American Conference of Governmental Industrial Hygienists (ACGIH) threshold limit value of 1 ppm [72].

Clinical Toxicity

The patients with mild toxicity may manifest dizziness, headache, confusion, weakness, nausea, vomiting, and dyspnea [68]. Initial or mild symptoms are frequently dismissed as viral symptoms. Skin irritation and burns commonly underlie clothes and rubber gloves, where the methyl bromide gas is trapped. After a significant exposure, the patient may present with tremor, myoclonus, and behavioral changes [67,73]. Severe toxicity may result in bronchitis, pulmonary edema, convulsions, and coma [67]. Fatality is related to pulmonary and CNS toxicities, although damage to different internal organs has been demonstrated [67,71]. Prolonged exposure to low concentrations of methyl bromide may cause subacute neurologic effects, such as headaches, confusion, behavioral changes, visual disturbance, and motor and sensory deficits [73–75]. Residual neurologic deficits may remain after significant acute or chronic exposure [71,75].

The essential laboratory studies for patients with methyl bromide intoxication are arterial blood gas or pulse oximetry monitoring. Chest radiography is useful in evaluating the patients with pulmonary symptoms. Serum bromide concentrations may suggest exposure, but do not correlate with the severity of exposure. Serum bromide concentrations varied from 4.0 to 65.6 mg per dL in methyl bromide fatalities [67,71,76]. When the serum bromide concentration is significantly elevated, an elevated chloride concentration may be observed with older chemistry analyzers [75].

Management

Treatment consists of supportive therapy, particularly of the airway, breathing, and circulation. Because methyl bromide is a gas, GI decontamination is not relevant. Clothing should be completely removed and the skin washed with soap and water to eliminate potential methyl bromide residues. Various compounds with sulfhydryl groups, such as dimercaprol and *N*-acetylcysteine, have been suggested as potential antidotes, but have not been demonstrated to be effective.

N,N-DIETHYL-*m*-TOLUAMIDE

N,N-Diethyl-*m*-toluamide (diethyltoluamide, or DEET) was initially synthesized in 1954 and marketed as an insect repellent. Currently, DEET is the most effective and one of the most widely used insect repellents. Use of DEET continues to increase with increasing public concern with arthropod-borne diseases, including Lyme disease, Dengue, and West Nile virus infections. The concentration of DEET in the various products varies from 5% to 100%.

Pharmacology

DEET is well absorbed through the skin, with 48% of the applied dose absorbed within 6 hours. The plasma concentration peaks 1 hour after dermal application [77]. DEET is primarily metabolized in the liver by several cytochrome P450 enzymes (CYPs), and 70% of the absorbed dose is excreted as metabolites within the first 24 hours. Another 10% to 15% is excreted unchanged in the urine [77,78]. DEET and its metabolites may accumulate in the fatty tissue, particularly after repeated applications.

The mechanism of DEET toxicity remains to be elucidated. Animals develop CNS symptoms similar to those reported in humans. Most reports of human poisoning involve children, likely because children absorb a higher ratio of DEET relative to their body weight. The initial theory suggested that the patients with ornithine-carbamoyltransferase deficiency might be particularly susceptible to DEET toxicity. However, this theory has not been substantiated.

Clinical Toxicity

Toxicity from DEET is primarily related to dermal exposures. Given the ubiquitous use of DEET, the overall reported adverse events are uncommon [78,79]. DEET may cause toxicity that is limited to skin irritation, contact dermatitis, skin necrosis, and urticaria [78]. Anaphylactic reactions have occasionally been reported with cutaneous application [80]. Manifestations of systemic poisoning vary from anxiety to behavioral changes, tremors, lethargy, ataxia, confusion, seizures, and coma [79,81,82]. Almost all of these case reports are related to application of concentrated DEET preparations or repeated application of lower concentration preparations [78,79]. Oral exposures to DEET are uncommon, but can result in rapid onset of confusion, opisthotonus, and seizures even with small ingestions [83].

Management

Treatment is largely supportive. The patients with dermal exposure should have their skin washed with soap and water to prevent further systemic absorption. Activated charcoal may be considered for oral ingestion within 1 hour of presentation. Seizures may be treated with benzodiazepines, barbiturates, or propofol. Neurologic workup may be required in many patients. The symptoms of DEET toxicity should be distinguished from those of Reye syndrome. There is no antidote, and extracorporeal removal procedures are not helpful. Measures to prevent DEET toxicity may be the most important treatment. These include avoidance of concentrated DEET preparations. Products containing 20% to 30% DEET are adequate and safer than those with higher concentrations; concentrations of 10% or less are recommended for children. DEET should be applied only to exposed skin. An additional agent, such as permethrin, can be applied to clothing and may decrease the need of DEET. The skin should be washed with soap when the insect repellent is no longer required, and the number of repeat applications should be limited.

PENTACHLOROPHENOL

Pentachlorophenol was first synthesized in 1841 and first used as a pesticide in 1936. It is primarily used as a wood preservative, however. Unlike other types of pesticide toxicity in adults, pentachlorophenol poisoning usually results from occupational exposure. Occupational exposures to pentachlorophenol at wood-treating facilities frequently result from improper ventilation and inadequate engineering controls. Low-concentration, prolonged exposures to pentachlorophenol have been reported in log home residents from pentachlorophenol-treated wood. Epidemics of infant poisoning have resulted from diapers improperly laundered with pentachlorophenol-containing antimicrobial soaps.

Pharmacology

Pentachlorophenol can be absorbed by the respiratory, oral, and dermal routes, although pulmonary absorption is the most efficient route. The volume of distribution is 0.35 L per kg and the pK_a is 5.0 [84]. Pentachlorophenol is primarily (74%) eliminated unchanged in the urine. A small proportion is oxidized to chlorohydroquinone, which is then eliminated in the urine. After a single oral exposure, the plasma half-life of pentachlorophenol is 27 to 35 hours [84]. Because of the low pK_a and significant renal elimination, pentachlorophenol elimination can be enhanced by urinary alkalinization [85].

The mechanism of toxicity of pentachlorophenol is similar to that of dinitrophenol: these agents uncouple oxidative phosphorylation by altering the mitochondrial membrane and function as chemical ionophores to transport protons without linking them to ATP synthesis [86]. The shift in the proton electrochemical gradient resulted in potential energy dissipation as heat instead of ATP production, leading to altered thermohomeostasis and hyperthermia.

Clinical Toxicity

Acute exposure results in headache, diaphoresis, nausea, vomiting, weakness, abdominal pain, and fever. With severe toxicity, significant hyperthermia (up to 108°F or 42.2°C), coma, convulsions, cerebral edema, and cardiovascular collapse may occur [87,88]. Laboratory studies may reveal a respiratory alkalosis and metabolic acidosis from significant exposures. Chronic exposures to pentachlorophenol have been reported to cause aplastic anemia, intravascular hemolysis, and pancreatitis [89–91]. Chloracne has also been reported from these exposures because of dioxin contamination in the product.

Management

Initial treatment includes oxygen supplementation, airway support, fluid resuscitation, and cardiac monitoring. Glucose should be monitored for hypoglycemia. Core temperature should be frequently monitored, and external cooling should be initiated immediately for significant hyperthermia. Seizures should be treated with benzodiazepines, barbiturates, or propofol to prevent further temperature increase and rhabdomyolysis. Fluid administration should be adequate to maintain a urine output of 1 to 2 mL per minute. Gastric decontamination (see Chapter 97) should be performed for oral exposure. The skin should be decontaminated with soap and water. Urinary alkalinization should be considered in patients with significant pentachlorophenol toxicity, although its clinical efficacy remains unproven [85].

PARAQUAT

Paraquat (1,1-dimethyl,4,4-bipyridyl dichloride) was developed in 1882 and for many years was used as an oxidation–reduction indicator. An electron donation to the compound forms a blue free radical; hence, paraquat was commonly called *methyl viologen*. The herbicidal properties of paraquat were discovered in 1955, and it was marketed as an herbicide in 1962. Today, paraquat is most commonly used as a nonselective contact herbicide in many countries. Paraquat can be applied safely when used according to the manufacturer's guidelines. Typically, it is available as a 10% to 30% concentrated solution for agricultural use or as a 5% powder for domestic use. A new and safer formulation Inteon (contains an alginate that gels in acidic milieu, an emetic, and the osmotic cathartic magnesium sulfate) is designed to slow gastric absorption of paraquat, and increase vomiting and intestinal transit, but these effects have not been substantiated. Once diluted, paraquat has limited absorption through the skin [92] and by aerosolization into the respiratory system [93]. Paraquat is naturally inactivated in the soil and leaves little active residue in the environment. Despite its many desirable properties, however, the consequences of ingesting concentrated paraquat products are deadly. The median lethal dose of paraquat is 3 to 5 g in adults. As little as a mouthful (10 to 15 mL) of a 20% solution of paraquat is fatal. Paraquat ingestion is a prevalent method of suicide in countries in the Asia-Pacific region and the West Indies [1].

Pharmacology

Although oral exposure to paraquat is the most common route of toxicity, less than 5% of the ingested amount is actually absorbed. Any recent food ingestion may decrease the amount of systemic absorption. The peak plasma and lung concentration are reached within 1 to 2 hours and 5 to 7 hours after ingestion, respectively [94]. Plasma paraquat concentrations decline rapidly after peak absorption because of tissue distribution. Paraquat is particularly sequestered in the lungs, kidneys, and muscles [94,95]. The volume of distribution of paraquat is approximately 1.2 to 1.6 L per kg, but follows a multicompartment distribution model [95,96]. Paraquat is eliminated unchanged by the kidneys, with 90% of the ingested dose within 12 to 24 hours [95]. The terminal plasma half-life of paraquat is 12 hours with normal renal function, but it may be as long as 120 hours as renal function deteriorates [95].

Dermal absorption of paraquat is minimal unless the exposure is prolonged with concentrated solutions [92]. Aerosolized paraquat particles have a diameter greater than 5 μm and do not reach the lower respiratory tree [93]. Concern about paraquat absorption from smoking marijuana is unfounded because much of the paraquat is pyrolyzed during the smoking process [97]. Paraquat toxicity from marijuana smoking has not been reported.

The primary organ of toxicity is the lung because of selective accumulation of paraquat. Paraquat is actively transported into type I and II alveolar cells through an existing transport system for endogenous polyamines. Paraquat and polyamines share a common structural property: they have two positively charged quaternary nitrogen atoms separated by a distance of 6 to 7 nm [98]. Diquat, another related herbicide with different structural features, is not selectively taken up and does not appear to cause pulmonary toxicity. Inside the cell, paraquat undergoes redox recycling, where a single-electron reduction into paraquat free radical by NADPH. This free radical reacts (oxidizes by) with oxygen to form superoxide free radicals and recycles back to react with NADPH. This reaction depletes NADPH. The superoxide free radicals deplete glutathione, cause lipid peroxidation and cellular apoptosis [99,100]. This mechanism of action is also responsible for the phytotoxic property of paraquat. There is also evidence for direct inhibition of electron chain transfers in mitochondria [99].

Clinical Toxicity

The onset and severity of poisoning are largely determined by the amount of exposure. The patients who ingest more than 40 mg per kg usually die within hours to a few days. These patients experience multiple organ failure, including acute lung injury, cerebral edema, myocardial necrosis, and hepatic and renal failure [99,100]. Death can be dramatic and may occur even before the development of significant chest radiographic abnormalities [99]. The patients who ingest 20 to 40 mg per kg of paraquat are most likely to die from pulmonary fibrosis, which progresses after a few days to a few weeks [99]. Ingestion of less than 20 mg per kg may lead to mild toxicity.

Paraquat is extremely corrosive to mucous membranes, and the patients frequently complain of pain in the mouth, throat, esophagus, and abdomen [99]. The absence of significant ulcerations in the esophagus or stomach within the first 24 hours of exposure may be a good prognostic indicator. The development of renal failure is a poor prognostic indicator [100]. This phenomenon cannot be fully explained by the decreased elimination of paraquat in the body because most of the paraquat dose is eliminated within the first 24 hours, even in the setting of renal failure [94]. Conversely, renal failure may signify a large paraquat exposure. Almost all patients with renal failure from paraquat have significant pulmonary toxicity, but there are occasional reports of renal failure without significant pulmonary toxicity [101]. The prognosis for a patient with paraquat ingestion can be best determined by the measurement of plasma paraquat concentration and its relation to time of ingestion. The nomogram initially was presented by Proudfoot et al. [102] and subsequently refined by Hart et al. [103]. The severity index of paraquat poisoning (SIPP) can also be calculated based on the paraquat serum concentration in mg per L multiply the time of ingestion in hours. A SIPP of 10 to 50 predicts death from respiratory failure and greater than 50 predicts death from circulatory failure [104]. The availability of paraquat measurements depends on regional practice because this laboratory analysis is not routine. Sodium dithionite test is readily available can be applied to the urine or plasma for prognosis [105]. Although it is generally accepted that paraquat is not absorbed through the skin, it can be corrosive to the skin and nails. Occasionally, dermal absorption and systemic toxicity may occur from prolonged exposure or exposure to concentrated products [92].

Management

It is critical to prevent systemic absorption of paraquat. Once ingested, it is rapidly absorbed and sequestered, frequently leading to death. GI decontamination should be performed in any suspected paraquat ingestion. Orogastric lavage should be performed if the ingestion is within 1 to 2 hours and if the patient did not have any vomiting. Fuller earth (1 to 2 g per kg) or activated charcoal should be administered with a cathartic agent as soon as possible to bind any residual paraquat in the GI tract [106]. Multiple doses of oral adsorbents should be continued until there is evidence of adsorbent in the stool. This is done to prevent desorption of the paraquat. Any dermal exposure should be thoroughly washed with soap and water. Plasma and urine analytical methods to detect paraquat are useful to confirm the diagnosis and assess the prognosis. A rapid qualitative screen for paraquat exposure may be performed by the addition of sodium dithionite to urine under alkaline condition. A change in color to blue confirms exposure to paraquat [99]. Furthermore, prognosis may be predicted by the degree of color change: dark blue for poor prognosis and light blue for moderate-to-severe poisoning [105].

The treatment of paraquat toxicity consists of supportive care, particularly for circulatory monitoring and support. Palliative care should be considered and discussed with the patients and their family in those determined to have poor prognosis. Oxygen supplementation should be avoided because it may increase the formation of paraquat free radicals and worsen pulmonary toxicity [99,107]. Supplemental oxygen should be administered only when it is necessary and should maintained pulse oximetry no higher than 90% saturation, even though the prognosis is grave in this group of the patients.

Experimental therapies for paraquat toxicity have been formulated using various strategies. Forced diuresis does not have significant effects on paraquat elimination. Hemodialysis and charcoal hemoperfusion are similar to endogenous renal clearance of paraquat but may increase elimination in those with renal dysfunction. In an animal model, the institution of charcoal hemoperfusion within 2 hours after paraquat ingestion decreased the fatality rate, and institution of hemoperfusion 2 hours after paraquat administration did not alter the paraquat concentration in the central compartment [96]. Clinically, hemodialysis, charcoal hemoperfusion, and continuous arteriovenous hemofiltration have not altered mortality rates but may be necessary in patients with renal failure. There are significant limitations in applying extracorporeal procedures. Because of the relatively large volume of distribution, rapid sequestration into tissue compartments, and good endogenous clearance, extracorporeal removal must be performed during peak absorption (within 2 hours after ingestion) to significantly decrease the paraquat load in the central compartments [96]. Because most patients present a number of hours after ingestion and the logistics of extracorporeal removal typically translate into an additional 1- to 2-hour delay, the amount of paraquat removed in most instances is insignificant.

Immunotherapy with monoclonal antibody fragments (Fab, Fv) against paraquat or against the active transport mechanism in the cells is intriguing [108]. More research is required to assess the value of this therapy, however. Various agents such as putrescine and spermidine and β-adrenergic receptor blockers have been demonstrated to prevent active transport of paraquat into lung tissues but failed to provide any benefits in vivo [99].

Various antioxidants and free radical scavengers, such as vitamins C and E, deferoxamine, superoxide dismutase, clofibrate, selenium, glutathione peroxide, and *N*-acetylcysteine, have been tested against paraquat toxicity. To date, there has been no or insignificant improvement in animal models [99]. A recent study using inhaled nitric oxide in rats demonstrated benefits in preventing pulmonary injuries and survival [99]. The most controversial treatment is related to the use of pulse-dose methylprednisolone and cyclophosphamide therapy, to limit acute inflammatory response. Corticosteroid also activates p-glycoprotein to increase efflux and decrease the intracellular concentration of paraquat [109]. Several studies have demonstrated increased patient survival with corticosteroids and cyclophosphamide therapy (Table 120.4) [109–111]. Meta-analysis of the three prospective randomized controlled studies with the use of methylprednisolone and cyclophosphamide in 164 patients appears to decrease mortality (RR 0.72, 95% CI 0.59 to 0.89) in patients with moderate-to-severe poisoning from ingested paraquat [112]. All patients received GI decontamination and two sessions of charcoal hemoperfusion within 24 hours of hospitalization, which were completed prior to the initiation of the pulse-dose therapy. Cyclophosphamide can cause a transient leukopenia (WBC < 3,000 per μL) in patients treated with the protocol [110]. The largest prospective randomized controlled study of 298 patients, was terminated early because the sale of paraquat was banned in Sri Lanka and it demonstrated no difference in mortality, 71% in the placebo group versus 68% in the treatment group [113]. These results have only been published in abstract format so far. The effectiveness of methylprednisolone and cyclophosphamide will be further determined by the publication of these results and the meta-analysis of all prospective controlled study data.

TABLE 120.4

Treatment Guidelines for Pulse-Dose Methylprednisolone and Cyclophosphamide in Patients with Paraquat Toxicity [110]

Initial pulse-dose therapy
Cyclophosphamide 15 mg/kg/d administered as an infusion in 200 mL D5NS over 2 h for 2 d
Methylprednisolone 1 g/d administered as an infusion in 200 mL D5NS over 2 h for 3 d
After initial pulse-dose therapy
Dexamethasone 5 mg IV every 6 h until $PaO_2 \geq 80$ mm Hg or death
If $PaO_2 < 60$ mm Hg after initial pulse therapy, repeat pulse-dose therapy with
Methylprednisolone 1 g/d administered as an infusion in 200 mL D5NS over 2 h for 3 d, and
If WBC > 3,000 per μL at >2 wk after initial pulse-dose therapy, add
Cyclophosphamide 15 mg/kg/d administered as an infusion in 200 mL D5NS over 2 h for 1 d

Initiated after gastrointestinal decontamination and two sessions of charcoal hemoperfusion within 24 h of ingesting paraquat in patients with moderate-to-severe toxicity.

Other agents that may alter pulmonary fibrosis, such as colchicine, nonsteroidal anti-inflammatory agents, collagen synthesis inhibitors, and angiotensin-converting enzyme inhibitors, also require further study. Lysine and sodium acetylsalicylates modulate inflammation and apoptosis, chelate paraquat, may have potential effects in animals but require further investigation. Niacin, which increases nicotinamide adenine dinucleotide phosphate synthesis, has some protective effects in rats, but it is unclear if it is applicable to human toxicity [99].

Early lung transplantation has been unsuccessful because of toxicity to the transplanted lung when paraquat is redistributed from tissue stores [114,115]. A successful case of lung transplantation was performed in a patient 44 days after paraquat poisoning, however [116]. Extracorporeal membrane oxygenation should be investigated in the future as a potential bridge to delayed pulmonary transplant [117].

DIQUAT

Diquat (1,1′-ethylene-2,2′-dipyridylium ion) is a contact herbicide with action and structure similar to that of paraquat. Diquat and paraquat liberate hydrogen peroxide and oxygen free radicals, resulting in toxicity to plants and animals [118]. The use of diquat is more limited and hence results in fewer intoxications than paraquat. Diquat is often formulated with paraquat.

Pharmacology

The kinetics of diquat are unknown in humans. In animal models, less than 10% of the oral dose is absorbed. More than 90% of the absorbed dose is eliminated unchanged by the kidneys [119]. There are no known metabolites of diquat.

Although diquat is less toxic than paraquat, human fatalities have been reported with ingestion of 20 to 50 mL of a 20% solution [120]. Similar to paraquat, diquat causes multiple organ damage. Diquat normally spares the pulmonary system, however [120]. This is because diquat is not actively transported to and concentrated in the alveolar cells of the lungs [98].

Clinical Toxicity

Symptoms of diquat toxicity may be delayed several hours to 2 days [120]. Vomiting, abdominal pain, GI tract erosions, and paralytic ileus are common manifestations of toxicity [120,121]. Acute renal failure may be related to hypovolemia and the direct toxic effects. The effects of diquat on the CNS may result in lethargy, seizures, and coma [121]. Brain-stem infarctions may be specific to diquat toxicity. All patients who die have significant CNS manifestations before cardiovascular collapse [121,122]. Topical exposure to diquat can occasionally result in severe skin burn [123].

Management

Treatment is largely supportive and similar to that for paraquat. Gastric lavage should be performed for any potential diquat ingestion within 1 hour if the patient has not vomited. Fuller's earth or activated charcoal should be administered as soon as possible. Hemodialysis or hemoperfusion has not been demonstrated to be effective for the treatment of diquat toxicity but may be necessary in patients with renal failure [122,124].

CHLOROPHENOXY HERBICIDES

Chlorophenoxy herbicides are used to control broad-leaf weeds and woody plants. They exert their effects by mimicking the action of auxins (plant growth hormones) and cause overstimulation of plant growth. Numerous derivatives are available for agricultural and domestic use [125]. The most commonly used agents include 2,4-dichlorophenoxyacetic acid (2,4-D), 2,4,5-trichlorophenoxyacetic acid (2,4,5-T), and 2-methyl-4-chlorophenoxypropionic acid. Many preparations contain more than one chlorophenoxy herbicide or other types of herbicides. Despite extensive use of these agents, fatality and significant toxicity are limited. The chlorophenoxy herbicides are notorious because of dioxin contamination in Agent Orange, a 1-to-1 mixture of 2,4-D and 2,4,5-T used extensively in the Vietnam War, so named for the color of the drums used to store it. Agent Orange contained dioxin (2,3,7,9-tetrachlorodibenzodioxin), a contaminant in the synthesis of chlorophenoxy compounds and a potent teratogen in animals [126,127].

Pharmacology

In general, chlorophenoxy herbicides are well absorbed orally. Inhalation absorption from occupational exposure can be significant with associated systemic toxicity. They have small volumes of distribution, large renal excretion, and a low pK_a [128]. 2,4-D has a volume of distribution of 0.1 to 0.3 L per kg and a pK_a of 2.6 to 3.5 [149]. Oral doses of 5 mg per kg in human volunteers produce no ill effects. The peak serum concentration is achieved within 4 to 12 hours [129], 80% of the absorbed dose is eliminated unchanged in the urine, and 13% is eliminated as acid-labile conjugates. The plasma half-life is 18 to 40 hours and varies with urine pH; it may range from 4 to 220 hours [130]. The volume of distribution of 2,4,5-T is 6.1 L per kg. It is exclusively excreted unchanged in the urine, and the plasma half-life is 11 to 23 hours [131].

Various mechanisms of toxicity in humans are postulated. Uncoupling of oxidative phosphorylation has been demonstrated in vitro and may be responsible for a mild heat exhaustion syndrome [132,133]. Chlorophenoxy herbicides can interfere with the TCA cycle and cellular metabolism by forming analogues with acetyl coenzyme A [131,132]. There may be other direct toxic effects on skeletal muscles and peripheral nerves [134].

Clinical Toxicity

GI symptoms are common, and the patients frequently experience nausea, vomiting, diarrhea, and abdominal pain [135,136]. Ulcerations may occur at the mouth and pharynx, but are uncommon elsewhere in the GI tract [132]. A mild heat exhaustion syndrome consisting of fever, diaphoresis, and hyperventilation can be seen [135]. The CNS is particularly affected, and the patients may present with confusion, lethargy, convulsions, and coma [135,137]. Prolonged coma (up to 4 days) has been reported with 2,4-D toxicity [138]. Myotonia, rhabdomyolysis, and chronic muscle weakness are also reported [136]. Renal complications may result from rhabdomyolysis and myoglobinuria [139]. Hypocalcemia may occasionally be seen as a result of rhabdomyolysis and hyperphosphatemia [137]. Fatality is uncommon, and the cause of death remains unclear [130,140,141]. Chlorophenoxy assays are not widely available and do not correlate well with clinical toxicity, even though a total chlorophenoxy herbicide concentration of greater than 0.5 g per L was purported to be associated with severe toxicity [133,134].

Management

Gastric decontamination with lavage may be considered within 1 hour of ingestion in patients without vomiting. Activated charcoal should be administered. Skin should be decontaminated with soap and water. Basic supportive therapies include the maintenance of good urine output (1 to 2 mL/kg/h) with fluid resuscitation and external cooling for hyperthermia. Because of the low pK_a and renal elimination of chlorophenoxy herbicides, urinary alkalinization can significantly enhance renal excretion and decrease the plasma half-life of various chlorophenoxy herbicides [135]. Thus, it should be initiated in patients with significant toxicity by using a sodium bicarbonate infusion to titrate the urinary pH to 7.50 to 8.0. The patient's fluid status should be closely monitored because renal dysfunction may develop from chlorophenoxy herbicide toxicity. Although the utility of extracorporeal elimination of chlorophenoxy herbicides in poisoned patients has not been studied, hemodialysis may be useful for 2,4-D because of its small volume of distribution. In severe cases and in patients with renal insufficiency, hemodialysis may be preferred because it produces good herbicide clearance, without the need for pH manipulation and administration of large amount of intravenous fluid.

CHLORATE SALTS

Chlorate salts (sodium chlorate [$NaClO_3$] and potassium chlorate [$KClO_3$]) are nonspecific herbicides. They are also used in the manufacture of explosives, dyestuffs, tanning agents, and matches.

Pharmacology

Chlorates are strong oxidizing agents that result in methemoglobinemia and hemolysis. They have direct toxic effects on the kidneys and indirect nephrotoxicity from hemoglobinuria. Because chlorates are primarily eliminated by the kidneys, nephrotoxicity further enhances their toxicity. The acute lethal dose is 25 to 35 g [142].

Clinical Toxicity

GI symptoms are prominent within hours after an acute exposure and include nausea, vomiting, diarrhea, and abdominal pain [142–144]. Methemoglobinemia and hemolytic anemia result from the oxidizing effects. Both entities may result in a significantly decreased oxygen-carrying capacity and cellular hypoxia [143,145]. Cyanosis may be evident with significant methemoglobinemia. Acute renal failure typically develops within 48 hours after exposure [144,146]. Significant hyperkalemia from hemolysis is another potential fatal complication.

Management

Initial supportive care should be directed at the airway, breathing, and maintenance of circulation. Continuous cardiac monitoring should be initiated. Gastric decontamination should be performed within 2 hours after ingestion unless the patient already has significant vomiting. Laboratory studies should include hemoglobin, serum electrolytes, blood urea nitrogen, creatinine, and methemoglobin concentrations. Electrocardiogram and arterial blood gas should be obtained as clinically indicated. Intravenous or oral sodium thiosulfate (2 to 5 g in 200 mL of 5% sodium bicarbonate solution) has been advocated to inactivate the chlorate ion, but its efficacy has not been clinically proven [147]. Methylene blue should be administered for clinically significant methemoglobinemia, but it may not be effective in the setting of significant hemolysis because intact intracellular enzymes are required for its therapeutic effect [148]. Methylene blue is indicated in patients with a methemoglobin concentration of more than 20% or at a lower value in symptomatic patients with anemia. The initial dose is 1 to 2 mg per kg administered intravenously over 5 minutes and a response is anticipated within 30 minutes. Subsequent doses of methylene blue can be administered if there is an initial success, but it is withheld if no response is observed. Exchange transfusion may be required for refractory methemoglobinemia or significant hemolysis. Hemodialysis can remove chlorates and is recommended for patients with associated renal dysfunction [142,147].

ACKNOWLEDGMENTS

The findings and conclusions in this report are those of the author(s) and do not necessarily represent the official position of the Centers for Disease Control and Prevention.

References

1. Gunnell D, Eddleston M, Phillips MR, et al: The global distribution of fatal pesticide self-poisoning: systemic review. *BMC Public Health* 7:357, 2007.
2. Roncevic N, Pavkov S, Galetin-Smith R et al: Serum concentrations of organochlorine compounds during pregnancy and the newborn. *Bull Environ Contam Toxicol* 38:117–124, 1987.
3. Saxena MC, Siddiqui MK, Agarwal V, et al: A comparison of organochlorine insecticide contents in specimens of maternal blood, placenta, and umbilical-cord blood from stillborn and live-born cases. *J Toxicol Environ Health* 11:71–79, 1983.
4. Palmer AK, Cozens DD, Spicer EJ, et al: Effects of lindane upon reproductive function in a 3-generation study in rats. *Toxicology* 10:45–54, 1978.
5. Conney AH, Welch RM, Kuntzman R, et al: Effects of pesticides on drug and steroid metabolism. *Clin Pharmacol Ther* 8:2–10, 1967.
6. Kutz FW, Strassman SC, Sperling JF, et al: A fatal chlordane poisoning. *J Toxicol Clin Toxicol* 20:167–174, 1983.
7. Olanoff LS, Bristow WJ, Colcolough J Jr, et al: Acute chlordane intoxication. *J Toxicol Clin Toxicol* 20:291–306, 1983.
8. Hunter CG, Robinson J, Roberts M: Pharmacodynamics of dieldrin (HEOD). Ingestion by human subjects for 18 to 24 months, and postexposure for eight months. *Arch Environ Health* 18:12–21, 1969.
9. Hayes W: Chlorinated hydrocarbon insecticides, in Hayes WJ (ed): *Pesticides Studied in Man*. Baltimore, Williams & Wilkins, 1982, p 172.
10. Shankland DL: Neurotoxic action of chlorinated hydrocarbon insecticides. *Neurobehav Toxicol Teratol* 4:805–811, 1982.
11. Telch J, Jarvis DA: Acute intoxication with lindane. *Can Med Assoc J* 127:821, 1982.
12. Nigma SK, Karnik AB, Majumber SK, et al: Serum hexachlorocyclohexane residues in workers engaged at a HCH manufacturing plant. *Int Arch Occup Environ Health* 57:315, 1986.
13. Kazantzis G, McLaughlin AI, Prior PF: Poisoning in Industrial Workers by the Insecticide Aldrin. *Br J Ind Med* 21:46–51, 1964.
14. Goldberg LH, Shupp D, Weitz HH, et al: Injection of household spray insecticide. *Ann Emerg Med* 11:626–629, 1982.
15. Ozucelik DN, Karcioglu O, Topacoglu H, et al: Toxicity following unintentional DDT ingestion. *J Toxicol Clin Toxicol* 42:299–303, 2004.
16. Rowley DL, Rab MA, Hardjotanojo W, et al: Convulsions caused by endrin poisoning in Pakistan. *Pediatrics* 79:928–934, 1987.
17. Taylor JR: Neurological manifestations in humans exposed to chlordecone: follow-up results. *Neurotoxicology* 6:231–236, 1985.
18. Blanco-Coronado JL, Repetto M, Ginestal RJ, et al: Acute intoxication by endosulfan. *J Toxicol Clin Toxicol* 30: 575–583, 1992.
19. Kashyap SK: Health surveillance and biological monitoring of pesticide formulators in India. *Toxicol Lett* 33:107–114, 1986.
20. Barnes R: Poisoning by the insecticide chlordane. *Med J Aust* 1:972–973, 1967.
21. Berry DH, Brewster MA, Watson R, et al: Untoward effects associated with lindane abuse. *Am J Dis Child* 141:125–126, 1987.
22. National Toxicology Program: Report on carcinogens. 14th ed. Research Triangle Park, U.S. Dept. of Health and Human Services, Public Health Service, 2014. https://ntp.niehs.nih.gov/pubhealth/roc/index-1.html. December 14, 2016.
23. Kassner JT, Maher TJ, Hull KM, et al: Cholestyramine as an adsorbent in acute lindane poisoning: a murine model. *Ann Emerg Med* 22: 1392–1397, 1993.
24. Cohn WJ, Boylan JJ, Blanke RV, et al: Treatment of chlordecone (kepone) toxicity with cholestyramine. Results of a controlled clinical trial. *N Engl J Med* 298;243–248, 1978.
25. Daerr W, Kaukel E, Schmoldt A: Hemoperfusion—a therapeutic alternative to early treatment of acute lindane poisoning [in German]. *Dtsch Med Wochenschr* 110:1253–1255, 1985.
26. Tilson HA, Hong JS, Mactutus CF: Effects of 5,5-diphenylhydantoin (phenytoin) on neurobehavioral toxicity of organochlorine insecticides and permethrin. *J Pharmacol Exp Ther* 233:285–289, 1985.
27. He F, Wang S, Liu L, et al: Clinical manifestations and diagnosis of acute pyrethroid poisoning. *Arch Toxicol* 63:54–58, 1989.
28. Yang PY, Lin JL, Hall AH, et al: Acute ingestion poisoning with insecticide formulations containing the pyrethroid permethrin, xylene, and surfactant: a review of 48 cases. *J Toxicol Clin Toxicol* 40:107–113, 2002.
29. King N, Tran MH: Long-acting anticoagulant rodenticide (superwarfarin) poisoning: a review of its historical development, epidemiology, and clinical management. *Transfusion Med Rev* 29:250–258, 2015.
30. Smolinske SC, Scherger DL, Kearns PS, et al: Superwarfarin poisoning in children: a prospective study. *Pediatrics* 84:490–494, 1989.
31. Stehle S, Kircheiner J, Lazar A, et al: Pharmacogenetics of oral anticoagulants. A basis for dose individualization. *Clin Pharmacokinet* 47:566–594, 2008.
32. Bachmann KA, Sullivan TJ: Dispositional and pharmacodynamic characteristics of brodifacoum in warfarin-sensitive rats. *Pharmacology* 27:281–288, 1983.
33. Breckenridge AM, Cholerton S, Hart JA, et al: A study of the relationship between the pharmacokinetics and the pharmacodynamics of the 4-hydroxycoumarin anticoagulants warfarin, difenacoum and brodifacoum in the rabbit. *Br J Pharmacol* 84:81–91, 1985.
34. Burucoa C, Mura P, Robert R, et al: Chlorophacinone intoxication. A biological and toxicological study. *J Toxicol Clin Toxicol* 27:79–89, 1989.
35. Bruno GR, Howland MA, McMeeking A, et al: Long-acting anticoagulant overdose: brodifacoum kinetics and optimal vitamin K dosing. *Ann Emerg Med* 36:262–267, 2000.
36. Hollinger BR, Pastoor TP: Case management and plasma half-life in a case of brodifacoum poisoning. *Arch Intern Med* 153:1925–1928, 1993.
37. Furie B, Furie BC: Molecular basis of vitamin K-dependent gamma-carboxylation. *Blood* 75:1753–1762, 1990.
38. Barnett VT, Bergmann F, Humphrey H, et al: Diffuse alveolar hemorrhage secondary to superwarfarin ingestion. *Chest* 102:1301–1302, 1992.
39. Kruse JA, Carlson RW: Fatal rodenticide poisoning with brodifacoum. *Ann Emerg Med* 21:331–336, 1992.
40. Guyatt GH, Akl EA, Crowther M, et al: Executive summary: antithrombotic therapy and prevention of thrombosis, 9th ed: American College of Chest Physicians evidence-based clinical practice guidelines.*Chest* 141:7S–47S, 2012.
41. Kinard TN, Sarode R: Four factor prothrombin complex concentrate (human): review of the pharmacology and clinical application for vitamin K antagonist reversal. *Expert Rev Cardiovasc* 12:417–427, 2014.
42. Rich EC, Drage CW: Severe complications of intravenous phytonadione therapy. Two cases, with one fatality. *Postgrad Med* 72:303–306, 1982.
43. Crowther MA, Douketis JD, Schnurr T, et al: Oral vitamin K lowers the international normalized ratio more rapidly than subcutaneous vitamin K in the treatment of warfarin-associated coagulopathy. A randomized, controlled trial. *Ann Intern Med* 137:251–254, 2002.
44. Hayes WJ, Laws ER: Botanical rodenticides, in Hayes WJ, Laws ER (eds): *Handbook of Pesticide Toxicology*. San Diego, Academic Press, 1991, p 615.
45. Heiser JM, Daya MR, Magnussen AR, et al: Massive strychnine intoxication: serial blood levels in a fatal case. *J Toxicol Clin Toxicol* 30:269–283, 1992.
46. Palatnick W, Meatherall R, Sitar D, et al: Toxicokinetics of acute strychnine poisoning. *J Toxicol Clin Toxicol* 35:617–620, 1997.

47. O'Connor V, Phelan PP, Fry JP: Interactions of glycine and strychnine with their receptor recognition sites in mouse spinal cord. *Neurochem Int* 29:423–434, 1996.
48. Westfall TC, Westfall DP: Neurotransmission: the autonomic and somatic motor nervous systems, in Goodman LS, Gilman A, Brunton LL, Lazo JS, et al (eds): *Goodman & Gilman's the Pharmacological Basis of Therapeutics.* 11th ed. New York, NY, McGraw-Hill, 2006, p 267.
49. Boyd RE, Brennan PT, Deng JF, et al: Strychnine poisoning. Recovery from profound lactic acidosis, hyperthermia, and rhabdomyolysis. *Am J Med* 74:507–512, 1983.
50. Yamarick W, Walson P, DiTraglia J: Strychnine poisoning in an adolescent. *J Toxicol Clin Toxicol* 30:141–148, 1992.
51. O'Callaghan WG, Joyce N, Counihan HE, et al: Unusual strychnine poisoning and its treatment: report of eight cases. *Br Med J (Clin Res Ed)* 285:478, 1982.
52. Baselt RC: Fluoroacetate, in Baselt RC (ed): *Disposition of Toxic Drugs and Chemicals in Man.* 7th ed. Foster City, Biomedical Publications, 2004, p 470.
53. Proudfoot AT, Bradberry SM, Vale JA: Sodium fluoroacetate poisoning. *Toxicol Rev* 25:213–219, 2006.
54. Chung HM: Acute renal failure caused by acute monofluoroacetate poisoning. *Vet Hum Toxicol* 26[Suppl 2]:29–32, 1984.
55. Brockmann JL, McDowell AV, Leeds WG: Fatal poisoning with sodium fluoroacetate; report of a case. *J Am Med Assoc* 159:1529–1532, 1955.
56. Gajdusek DC, Luther G: Fluoroacetate poisoning a review and report of a case. *Am J Dis Child* 79:310–320, 1950.
57. Omara F, Sisodia CS: Evaluation of potential antidotes for sodium fluoroacetate in mice. *Vet Hum Toxicol* 32:427–431, 1990.
58. Siwach SB, Yadav DR, Arora B, et al: Acute aluminum phosphide poisoning—an epidemiological, clinical and histo-pathological study. *J Assoc Physicians India* 36:594–596, 1988.
59. Anand R, Sharma DR, Verma D, et al: Mitochondrial electron transport chain complexes, catalase and markers of oxidase stress in platelets of patients with severe aluminum phosphide poisoning. *Hum Exp Toxicol* 32:807–816, 2013.
60. Anand R, Binukumar BK, Gill KD: Aluminum phosphide poisoning: an unsolved riddle. *J Appl Toxicol* 31:499–505, 2011.
61. Hsu CH, Chi BC, Liu MY, et al: Phosphine-induced oxidative damage in rats: role of glutathione. *Toxicology* 179:1–8, 2002.
62. Chugh SN, Ram S, Mehta LK, et al: Adult respiratory distress syndrome following aluminium phosphide ingestion. Report of 4 cases. *J Assoc Physicians India* 37:271–272, 1989.
63. Chugh SN, Jaggal KL, Sharma A, et al: Magnesium levels in acute cardiotoxicity due to aluminium phosphide poisoning. *Indian J Med Res* 94:437–439, 1991.
64. Katria R, Eihence GP, Mehrotta ML: A study of aluminium phosphide poisoning with special references to electrocardiographic changes. *J Assoc Physicians India* 38:471, 1990.
65. Singh S, Singh D, Wig N, et al: Aluminum phosphide ingestion—a clinico-pathologic study. *J Toxicol Clin Toxicol* 34:703–706, 1996.
66. Siwach SB, Singh P, Ahlawat S, et al: Serum & tissue magnesium content in patients of aluminium phosphide poisoning and critical evaluation of high dose magnesium sulphate therapy in reducing mortality. *J Assoc Physicians India* 42:107–110, 1994.
67. Marraccini JV, Thomas GE, Ongley JP, et al: Death and injury caused by methyl bromide, an insecticide fumigant. *J Forensic Sci* 28:601–607, 1983.
68. Bulathsingala AT, Shaw IC: Toxic chemistry of methyl bromide. *Hum Exp Toxicol* 33:81–91, 2014.
69. Goldman LR, Mengle D, Epstein DM, et al: Acute symptoms in persons residing near a field treated with the soil fumigants methyl bromide and chloropicrin. *West J Med* 147:95–98, 1987.
70. Baselt RC: Methyl bromide, in Baselt RC (ed): *Disposition of Toxic Drugs and Chemicals in Man.* 7th ed. Foster City, Biomedical Publications, 2004, p 711.
71. Hine CH: Methyl bromide poisoning. A review of ten cases. *J Occup Med* 11:1–10, 1969.
72. Occupational Safety and Health Administration (OSHA) Permissible exposure limits-annotated table Z-1. Washington, D.C., U.S. Dept. of Labor, 2013. https://www.osha.gov/dsg/annotated-pels/tablez-1.html. December 3, 2015.
73. Shield LK, Coleman TL, Markesbery WR: Methyl bromide intoxication: neurologic features, including simulation of Reye syndrome. *Neurology* 27:959–962, 1977.
74. Chavez CT, Hepler RS, Straatsma BR: Methyl bromide optic atrophy. *Am J Ophthalmol* 99:715–719, 1985.
75. Zatuchni J, Hong K: Methyl bromide poisoning seen initially as psychosis. *Arch Neurol* 38:529–530, 1981.
76. Behrens RH, Dukes DC: Fatal methyl bromide poisoning. *Br J Ind Med* 43:561–562, 1986.
77. Lur'e AA, Gleiberman SE, Tsizin Iu S: Pharmacokinetics of insect repellent, N,N-diethyltoluamide. *Med Parazitol (Mosk)* 47:72–77, 1978.
78. Sudakin DL, Trevathan WR: DEET: a review and update of safety and risk in the general population. *J Toxicol Clin Toxicol* 41:831–839, 2003.
79. Centers for Disease Control and Prevention: Seizures temporally associated with use of DEET insect repellent—New York and Connecticut. *MMWR Morb Mortal Wkly Rep* 38:678–680, 1989.
80. Miller JD: Anaphylaxis associated with insect repellant. *N Engl J Med* 307:1341–1342,1982.
81. Roland EH, Jan JE, Rigg JM: Toxic encephalopathy in a child after brief exposure to insect repellents. *Can Med Assoc J* 132:155–156, 1985.
82. Edwards DL, Johnson CE: Insect-repellent-induced toxic encephalopathy in a child. *Clin Pharm* 6:496–498, 1987.
83. Petrucci N, Sardini S: Severe neurotoxic reaction associated with oral ingestion of low dose diethyltoluamide-containing insect repellent in a child. *Ped Emerg Care* 16:341–342, 2000.
84. Baselt RC: Pentachlorophenol, in Baselt RC (ed): *Disposition of Toxic Drugs and Chemicals in Man.* 7th ed. Foster City, Biomedical Publications, 2004, p 855.
85. Uhl S, Schmid P, Schlatter C: Pharmacokinetics of pentachlorophenol in man. *Arch Toxicol* 58:182–186, 1986.
86. Harper JA, Dickinson K, Brand MD: Mitochrondrial uncoupling as a target for drug development for the treatment of obesity. *Obes Rev* 2:255–265, 2001.
87. Exon JH: A review of chlorinated phenols. *Vet Hum Toxicol* 26:508–520, 1984.
88. Gray RE, Gilliland RD, Smith EE, et al: Pentachlorophenol intoxication: report of a fatal case, with comments on the clinical course and pathologic anatomy. *Arch Environ Health* 40:161–164, 1985.
89. Roberts HJ: Aplastic anemia due to pentachlorophenol. *N Engl J Med* 305:1650–1651, 1981.
90. Cooper RG, Macauley MB: Pentachlorophenol pancreatitis. *Lancet* 1:517, 1982.
91. Hassan AB, Seligmann H, Bassan HM: Intravascular haemolysis induced by pentachlorophenol. *Br Med J (Clin Res Ed)* 291:21–22, 1985.
92. Smith JG: Paraquat poisoning by skin absorption: a review. *Hum Toxicol* 7:15–19, 1988.
93. Chester G, Ward RJ: Occupational exposure and drift hazard during aerial application of paraquat to cotton. *Arch Environ Contam Toxicol* 13:551–563, 1984.
94. Houze P, Baud FJ, Mouy R, et al: Toxicokinetic of paraquat in humans. *Hum Exp Toxicol* 9:5–12, 1990.
95. Bismuth C, Scherrmann JM, Garnier R, et al: Elimination of paraquat. *Hum Toxicol* 6:63–67, 1987.
96. Pond SM, Rivory LP, Hampson E, et al: Kinetics of toxic doses of paraquat and the effects of hemoperfusion in the dog. *Clin Toxicol* 31:229–246, 1993.
97. Landrigan PJ, Powell KE, James LM, et al: Paraquat and marijuana: epidemiologic risk assessment. *Am J Public Health* 73:784–788, 1983.
98. Rose MS, Smith LL: Tissue uptake of paraquat and diquat. *Gen Pharmacol* 8:173–176, 1977.
99. Gawarammana IB, Buckley NA: Medical management of paraquat ingestion. *Br J Clin Pharmacol* 72:745–757, 2011.
100. Bismuth C, Garnier R, Dally S, et al: Prognosis and treatment of paraquat poisoning: a review of 28 cases. *J Toxicol Clin Toxicol* 19:461–474, 1982.
101. Florkowski CM, Bradberry SM, Ching GW, et al: Acute renal failure in a case of paraquat poisoning with relative absence of pulmonary toxicity. *Postgrad Med J* 68:660–662, 1992.
102. Proudfoot AT, Stewart MS, Levitt T, et al: Paraquat poisoning: significance of plasma-paraquat concentrations. *Lancet* 2:330–332, 1979.
103. Hart TB, Nevitt A, Whitehead A: A new statistical approach to the prognostic significance of plasma paraquat concentrations. *Lancet* 2:1222–1223, 1984.
104. Sawada Y, Yamamoto I, Hirokane T, et al: Severity index of paraquat poisoning. *Lancet* 1:1333, 1988.
105. Koo JR, Yoon JW, Han SJ, et al: Rapid analysis of plasma paraquat using sodium dithionite as a predictor of outcome in acute paraquat poisoning. *Am J Med Sci* 338:373–377, 2009.
106. Meredith TJ, Vale JA: Treatment of paraquat poisoning in man: methods to prevent absorption. *Hum Toxicol* 6:49–55, 1987.
107. Keeling PL, Pratt IS, Aldridge WN, et al: The enhancement of paraquat toxicity in rats by 85% oxygen: lethality and cell-specific lung damage. *Br J Exp Pathol* 62:643–654, 1981.
108. Pond SM, Chen N, Bowles MR: Prevention of paraquat toxicity in alveolar type II cells by paraquat-specific antibodies [abstract]. *Vet Hum Toxicol* 35:332, 1993.
109. Lin JL, Leu ML, Liu YC, et al: A prospective clinical trial of pulse therapy with glucocorticoid and cyclophosphamide in moderate to severe paraquat-poisoned patients. *Am J Respir Crit Care Med* 159:357–360, 1999.
110. Lin JL, Lin-Tan DT, Chen KH, et al: Repeated pulse of methylprednisolone and cyclophosphamide with continuous dexamethasone therapy for patients with severe paraquat poisoning. *Crit Care Med* 34:368–373, 2006.
111. Afzali S, Gholyaf M: The effectiveness of combined treatment with methylprednisolone and cyclophosphamide in oral paraquat poisoning. *Arch Iran Med* 11:387–391, 2008.
112. Li LR, Sydenham E, Chaudhary B, et al: Glucocorticoid with cyclophosphamide for paraquat-induced lung fibrosis. *Cochrane Database Syst Rev* 8:008084, 2014.
113. Gawarammana I, Buckey NA, Mohammed F, et al: A randomised controlled trial of high-dose immunosuppression in paraquat poisoning. *Clin Toxicol* 50:278, 2012.
114. Kamholz S, Veith FJ, Mollenkopf F, et al: Single lung transplantation in paraquat intoxication. *N Y State J Med* 84:82–84, 1984.
115. Toronto Lung Transplant group: sequential bilateral lung transplantation for paraquat poisoning. *J Thorac Cardiovasc Surg* 89:734–742, 1985.
116. Walder B, Brundler MA, Spiliopoulos A, et al: Successful single-lung transplantation after paraquat intoxication. *Transplantation* 64:789–791, 1997.
117. Bertram A, Haenel SS, Hadem J, et al: Tissue concentration of paraquat on day 32 after intoxication and failed bridge to transplantation by extracorporeal membrane oxygenation therapy. *BMC Pharmacol Toxicol* 14:45–50, 2013.
118. Stancliffe TC, Pirie A: The production of superoxide radicals in reactions of the herbicide diquat. *FEBS Lett* 17:297–299, 1971.
119. Baselt RC: Diquat, in Baselt RC (ed): *Disposition of Toxic Drugs and Chemicals in Man.* 7th ed. Foster City, Biomedical Publications, 2004, p 368.

120. Vanholder R, Colardyn F, De Reuck J, et al: Diquat intoxication: report of two cases and review of the literature. *Am J Med* 70:1267–1271, 1981.
121. McCarthy LG, Speth CP: Diquat intoxication. *Ann Emerg Med* 12:394–396, 1983.
122. Powell D, Pond SM, Allen TB, et al: Hemoperfusion in a child who ingested diquat and died from pontine infarction and hemorrhage. *J Toxicol Clin Toxicol* 20:405–420, 1983.
123. Manoguerra AS: Full thickness skin burns secondary to an unusual exposure to diquat dibromide. *J Toxicol Clin Toxicol* 28:107–110, 1990.
124. Okonek S, Hofmann A: On the question of extracorporeal hemodialysis in diquat intoxication. *Arch Toxicol* 33:251–257, 1975.
125. Arnold EK, Beasley VR: The pharmacokinetics of chlorinated phenoxy acid herbicides: a literature review. *Vet Hum Toxicol* 31:121–125, 1989.
126. Klaassen CD: Toxic effects of pesticides, in Casarett LJ, Doull J, Klaassen CD (eds): *Casarett and Doull's Toxicology: the Basic Science of Poisons*. 6th ed. New York, McGraw-Hill Medical Pub. Division, 2001, p 791.
127. Centers for Disease Control and Prevention: Serum 2,3,7, 8-tetrachlorodibenzo-p-dioxin levels in US Army Vietnam-era veterans. The Centers for Disease Control Veterans Health Studies. *JAMA* 260:1249–1254, 1988.
128. Baselt RC: 2,4-Dichlorophenoxyacetic acid, in Baselt RC (ed): *Disposition of Toxic Drugs and Chemicals in Man*. 7th ed. Foster City, Biomedical Publications, 2004, p 323.
129. Kohli JD, Khanna RN, Gupta BN, et al: Absorption and excretion of 2,4-dichlorophenoxyacetic acid in man. *Xenobiotica* 4:97–100, 1974.
130. Dudley AW Jr, Thapar NT: Fatal human ingestion of 2,4-D, a common herbicide. *Arch Pathol* 94:270–275, 1972.
131. Baselt RC: 2,4,5-Trichlorophenoxyacetic acid, in Baselt RC (ed): *Disposition of Toxic Drugs and Chemicals in Man*. 7th ed. Foster City, Biomedical Publications, 2004, p 1147.
132. Dickey W, McAleer JJ, Callender ME: Delayed sudden death after ingestion of MCPP and ioxynil: an unusual presentation of hormonal weedkiller intoxication. *Postgrad Med J* 64:681–682, 1988.
133. Flanagan RJ, Meredith TJ, Ruprah M, et al: Alkaline diuresis for acute poisoning with chlorophenoxy herbicides and ioxynil. *Lancet* 335:454–458, 1990.
134. Friesen EG, Jones GR, Vaughan D: Clinical presentation and management of acute 2,4-D oral ingestion. *Drug Saf* 5:155–159, 1990.
135. Prescott LF, Park J, Darrien I: Treatment of severe 2,4-D and mecoprop intoxication with alkaline diuresis. *Br J Clin Pharmacol* 7:111–116, 1979.
136. Roberts DM, Seneviratne R, Mohammed F, et al: Intentional self-poisoning with the chlorophenoxy herbicide 4-chloro-2-methylphenoxyacetic acid (MCPA). *Ann Emerg Med* 46:275–284, 2005.
137. Meulenbelt J, Zwaveling JH, van Zoonen P, et al: Acute MCPP intoxication: report of two cases. *Hum Toxicol* 7:289–292, 1988.
138. O'Reilly JF: Prolonged coma and delayed peripheral neuropathy after ingestion of phenoxyacetic acid weed killers. *Postgrad Med J* 60:76–77, 1984.
139. Berwick P: 2,4-dichlorophenoxyacetic acid poisoning in man. Some interesting clinical and laboratory findings. *JAMA* 214:1114–1117, 1970.
140. Fraser AD, Isner AF, Perry RA: Toxicologic studies in a fatal overdose of 2,4-D, mecoprop, and dicamba. *J Forensic Sci* 29:1237–1241, 1984.
141. Osterloh J, Lotti M, Pond SM: Toxicologic studies in a fatal overdose of 2,4-D, MCPP, and chlorpyrifos. *J Anal Toxicol* 7:125–129, 1983.
142. Jackson RC, Elder WJ, Mc DH: Sodium-chlorate poisoning complicated by acute renal failure. *Lancet* 2:1381–1383, 1961.
143. Jansen H, Zeldenrust J: Homicidal chronic sodium chlorate poisoning. *Forensic Sci* 1:103–105, 1972.
144. Stavrou A, Butcher R, Sakula A: Accidental self-poisoning by sodium chlorate weed-killer. *Practitioner* 221:397–399, 1978.
145. Cunningham NE: Chlorate poisoning—two cases diagnosed at autopsy. *Med Sci Law* 22:281–282, 1982.
146. Steffen C, Wetzel E: Pathologic aspects of chlorate poisoning. *Hum Toxicol* 4:541, 1985.
147. Helliwell M, Nunn J: Mortality in sodium chlorate poisoning. *Br Med J* 1:1119, 1979.
148. Curry S: Methemoglobinemia. *Ann Emerg Med* 11:214–221, 1982.
149. Baselt RC: 2,4-Dichlorophenoxyacetic acid, in Baselt RC (ed): *Disposition of Toxic Drugs and Chemicals in Man*. 7th ed. Foster City, Biomedical Publications, 2004, p 323.

Chapter 121 ■ Phencyclidine and Hallucinogen Poisoning

JENNIE A. BUCHANAN • LUKE YIP

PHENCYCLIDINE

Phencyclidine (phenyl-cyclohexyl-piperidine, or PCP) is a dissociative anesthetic chemically related to ketamine. PCP is a synthetic compound developed in the 1950s as a general anesthetic (Sernyl). It was associated with an unacceptably high incidence of postoperative hallucinations, delirium, and mania. In 1967, PCP was reintroduced and marketed as a veterinary anesthetic (Sernylan). Currently, PCP is a Schedule II substance in the United States; ketamine is a Schedule III agent. As an illicit drug, PCP is available as a white crystalline powder (angel dust), tablet (PeaCe Pill), crystals, and liquid (whack); it can be snorted, smoked, ingested, or injected. Tables 121.1 and 121.2 display some of the common slang, or street names, for both PCP and ketamine.

TABLE 121.1

Slang Terms (Street Names) for Phencyclidine

Angel dust	KJ
Cyclone	Lovely
DOA	Mist
Elephant tranquilizer	Ozone
Embalming fluid	PeaCe pill
Goon	Rocket fuel
Hog	Scuffle
Horse tranquilizer	Whack

TABLE 121.2

Slang Terms (Street Names) for Ketamine

Green	Special K
Jet	Special LA coke
K	Super acid
Mauve	Super C
Purple	

Pharmacology

There are two forms of PCP, acid and base. Both are odorless, nonvolatile, and sold as "angel dust," and may be ingested or injected. PCP acid is a white crystalline substance sold as or incorporated into tablets. It deteriorates when heated and is not suitable for smoking. PCP base is a grayish-white amorphous powder that can be smoked after incorporation into marijuana (e.g., supergrass, superweed) or tobacco (e.g., clickers, primos) cigarettes. More often, the base is dissolved in a liquid hydrocarbon and applied to the wrapper of a tobacco cigarette. The ether-like or formaldehyde odor surrounding some patients who have used PCP is from the volatile hydrocarbon used to dissolve PCP base.

Several analogs of PCP are occasionally used as street drugs (Table 121.3). Their pharmacologic actions are similar to those of PCP and cannot be clinically distinguished. In addition, street PCP samples may be contaminated with

TABLE 121.3

Phencyclidine Analogs Used as Street Drugs

PCE (cyclohexamine)
PCPP (phenylcyclopentylpiperidine)
PHP (phenylcyclohexylpyrrolidine)
TCP (thienylcyclohexylpiperidine)

1-piperidinocyclohexane-carbonitrile, a precursor of PCP that is more potent than PCP and capable of generating cyanide, although the clinical significance of this is unknown.

PCP has multiple mechanisms of action (Table 121.4), which helps to explain the varied signs and symptoms associated with PCP intoxication [1–11]. It is well absorbed from the gastrointestinal (GI) and respiratory tracts. PCP is a weak base (pK_a 8.5), has a volume of distribution 6.2 L per kg, and is extensively protein-bound (65%) [12]. PCP concentrates in the brain, lungs, adipose tissue, and liver. The average serum half-life in controlled studies is 17 hours. PCP is metabolized by the liver and excreted predominantly as inactive compounds. Small amounts of PCP are excreted in perspiration, saliva, and gastric juice. PCP has been detected in umbilical and infant blood, amniotic fluid, and breast milk.

Clinical Toxicity

Drinking PCP, intravenous PCP, or swallowing remnants of PCP-soaked cigarettes have resulted in severe intoxication within 1 hour. Clinical experience with PCP intoxication is derived from case reports and clinical series [13–20]. The characteristics of PCP intoxication are nystagmus and hypertension. Nystagmus may be horizontal, vertical, or rotary. The patients may have systolic or diastolic hypertension. Hypertension usually resolves within 4 hours, but a significant number of patients may remain hypertensive for more than 24 hours.

Tachycardia is common. However, heart rates greater than 120 per minute are unusual. Hypothermia (<36.7°C), hyperthermia (>38.9°C), respiratory compromise, tachypnea, hypotension, and cardiac arrest have been reported.

The patients may present with delirium or normal sensorium. Lethargy, stupor, and unconsciousness are uncommon presentations. The most common behavioral effects are violent and agitated behavior, which may predispose patients to traumatic injuries. The patients may exhibit bizarre behaviors such as driving less than 10 mph on the freeway, "playing bumper cars" on the freeway, sleeping on top of cars that are blocking traffic, lying down in a busy street, and wandering or acting wildly in public. Approximately 20% of PCP users report hallucinations or delusions. The visual hallucinations are typically concrete and realistic (e.g., blue fish). The patients may appear mute or have a "blank stare" appearance.

The most common neuromuscular finding is rigidity of all extremities. It is often associated with jerky or thrashing movements, tremors, or twitching. Other musculoskeletal disturbances include oculogyric crisis, trismus, facial grimacing, circumoral muscle twitching, lip smacking or chewing movements, torticollis, tongue spasms, opisthotonos, and catalepsy. The patients may exhibit self-limited slow, writhing movements of the extremities or body. Athetosis and muscle stiffness may simultaneously appear. Intermittent athetoid movements may last for more than 10 hours. Rhabdomyolysis may occur, even in calm-appearing patients. Grand mal seizures and status epilepticus are uncommon.

The major autonomic effects are profuse diaphoresis, copious oral or pulmonary secretions, and urinary retention. Bronchospasm has been reported in patients who smoked or sniffed or snorted PCP. Pupillary size is usually normal, but miosis or mydriasis has been described.

Clinically, acute PCP intoxication can be divided into major and minor clinical syndromes [19]. Major syndromes, representing moderate-to-severe PCP intoxication, are delirium, toxic psychosis, catatonic syndrome, and coma. They may include any of the previously discussed effects. Minor syndromes are lethargy or stupor, bizarre behavior, violent behavior, agitation, and euphoria. They represent mild PCP intoxication, and complications are rare.

Delirium is the most common presentation of PCP intoxication. The patients may be found wandering in traffic or appear intoxicated with ethanol. The patients may exhibit slurred, bizarre, or repetitive speech; ataxia; disorientation; confusion; poor judgment; inappropriate affect; amnesia of recent events; bizarre behavior; agitation; and violence. The duration of this syndrome often lasts for a few hours and rarely lasts more than 3 days, but has been reported to persist for 1 to 3 weeks.

Psychosis may appear in some patients following PCP use and may last for days or weeks despite abstinence; typically symptoms become more severe during the first few days of its

TABLE 121.4

Phencyclidine Pharmacology

Sites	Actions
N-Methyl-D-aspartate receptor	Glutamate antagonist
D_2 dopamine receptor	Blocks dopamine reuptake
	Interferes with dopamine release
Serotonergic receptor	Antagonist
Cholinesterase	Antagonist
Nicotinic receptor	Antagonist
Muscarinic receptor	Anticholinergic effects (e.g., tachycardia, mydriasis, and urinary)
	Cholinergic effects (e.g., miosis, salivation, and diaphoresis)
	Binds to receptors in the heart
Na^+ and K^+ channels	Antagonist
Presynaptic brain neurons	Increase catecholamine release

Data from Refs. [1–11].

course. PCP psychosis may be defined as a schizophreniform psychosis. Characteristically, there is autistic and delusional thinking, commonly including global paranoia, delusions of superhuman strength and invulnerability, as well as delusions of persecution and grandiosity. Affect is generally blunted, with periods of suspiciousness often alternating with extreme anger or terror. These patients are ambivalent and their behavior is unpredictable even toward their friends and relatives. They may be reluctantly cooperative one minute and violently aggressive the next. Some carry lethal weapons to protect themselves from their imagined persecutors. Bystanders have been unexpectedly, furiously, and unremittingly attacked without provocation. Hallucinations may be auditory or visual, or both, and may involve seeing brilliantly colored objects, but objects are not distorted and there are no kaleidoscopic effects. The patients may be preoccupied with religious thoughts or have religious delusions. It is common for patients to have pressured speech, scream, or make animal sounds. In the initial phase of PCP psychosis, the patients may be an immediate danger to themselves on the basis of impaired judgment and being unable to care for themselves. Their violent and threatening behavior may provoke lethal countermeasures by those around them. These patients may also be a danger to others because of their misperceptions, paranoia, and hostility, compounded by their confusion, tendency towards violence, and the unpredictability of behavior. This initial phase will gradually transition to a phase characterized by intermittent periods of gross paranoia, agitation, terror, and hyperactivity alternating with quiet paranoid watchfulness over the course of a week. Affect may remain constricted. The patients may explode in an unexpected flurry of violence when inappropriate demands are not immediately met. A third phase begins on an average of 10th day of hospitalization, and is characterized by rapid reintegration of premorbid personality, development of insight into the events leading to the hospitalization. There is often amnesia from the early events of the psychosis.

The catatonic syndrome manifests primarily as a combination of signs: posturing, catalepsy, rigidity, mutism, staring, negativism, nudism, impulsiveness, agitation, violence, and stupor. Stereotypies, mannerisms, grimacing, and verbigeration may also be present. The patients are typically mute, staring blankly, motionless, stiff, standing with extremities or head in bizarre positions, and unresponsive to noxious stimuli. Most catatonic syndromes usually do not persist for more than 24 hours (range 2 to 6 days), and most patients recover within 4 to 6 hours. The patients may emerge from catatonic syndrome with agitation or combativeness, delirium, lethargy, psychosis, bizarre behavior, or normal sensorium.

Violent, agitated, and euphoric patients typically have a clear sensorium. The patients with euphoria may report a sense of "well being" or feeling "spaced out," "freaked out," or "tingling all over." The patients with delirium and violent or bizarre behavior may subsequently lapse into coma. Coma may also occur abruptly and may last up to 6 days. The patients emerging from coma may exhibit delirium, catatonic syndrome, toxic psychosis, stupor, agitation, violence, bizarre behavior, or normal sensorium. The duration of the emergent phenomenon is variable.

Neonatal jitteriness, hypertonicity, and vomiting have been associated with maternal PCP use. Chronic PCP intoxication has not been described, and there is no documentation of PCP flashbacks. Common clinical effects are summarized in Table 121.5

TABLE 121.5

Common Phencyclidine Effects

Hypertension, tachycardia
Nystagmus
Delirium or normal sensorium
Violent or agitated, bizarre behaviour
Rigid extremities
Athetoid movements
Rhabdomyolysis
Diaphoresis, copious oral or pulmonary secretions, urinary retention

Diagnostic Evaluation

PCP intoxication is a clinical diagnosis. It is based on a history of possible PCP exposure associated with clinical findings consistent with PCP intoxication and the exclusion of other neuropsychiatric or behavioral disorders. Drug history should include type of product, method of use, time of exposure, circumstances surrounding intoxication, and description of effects witnessed by others or experienced by the patient. Particular attention should be paid to abnormal behavior that may have resulted in occult trauma (e.g., jumps or falls).

The physical examination should focus on vital signs, sensorium, behavior, and musculoskeletal, autonomic, and neurologic findings. A thorough examination should be performed to exclude occult trauma. Explosions in clandestine laboratories may have consequences of smoke or chemical inhalation, thermal or chemical burns, and blunt or penetrating trauma.

Laboratory tests should include complete blood cell count, serum electrolytes, blood urea nitrogen, creatinine, glucose, creatinine phosphokinase (CPK), liver function tests, and urine analysis to include myoglobin. Common abnormal test results associated with PCP intoxication include hypoglycemia, elevated white blood cell count, serum CPK, liver function tests, and uric acid. Chest radiograph, electrocardiogram, arterial blood gas, computed tomography of the head, and lumbar puncture should be obtained as clinically indicated.

Serum or urine PCP levels can confirm the diagnosis of PCP intoxication, but neither contributes to patient management nor correlates with severity of intoxication. Rapid urine qualitative drug screens that detect PCP should be interpreted with caution. Diphenhyramine, ketamine, lamotrigine, thioriadizine, tramadol, ibuprofen, imipramine, meperdine, mesoridizine, venlafaxine, and *o*-desmethylvenlafaxine may cause false-positive PCP results on urine qualitative drug screens. Diphenhydramine may interfere with PCP determination by gas–liquid chromatography.

Management

The immediate management is to assess and treat acute threats to the airway, breathing, and circulation. Close monitoring of the patient in a quiet area with limited stimuli may reduce the need for physical restraint or sedation and provide a safe environment for the patient, attending staff, and other patients. Routine gastric decontamination is not recommended.

The patients with major PCP intoxication syndrome or complicated minor PCP intoxication syndrome should be managed in an intensive care unit. These patients should receive supplemental oxygen, secure vascular access, and have their vital signs and cardiac rhythm continuously monitored. A core temperature should be obtained for all patients.

Hemodynamic effects of PCP usually do not require specific treatment. Abnormal vital signs should be managed in the context of the overall clinical status of the patient. Mild sinus tachycardia or hypertension not associated with psychomotor agitation or evidence of end organ damage usually does not require pharmacologic treatment. Treatment of psychomotor agitation using benzodiazepine sedation often results in improvement or resolution of sinus tachycardia and hypertension. Persistent significant hypertension despite resolution of psychomotor agitation, or if there is evidence of end organ damage, should be treated with intravenous nitroprusside or nitroglycerin titrated to effect. The use of β-adrenergic antagonists to treat drugs of abuse-induced tachycardia or hypertension is not routinely recommended and may have deleterious effects (e.g., unopposed α-adrenergic effects).

The patients with hypotension should receive fluid resuscitation while alternative causes are being investigated (e.g., occult trauma). Persistent hypotension refractory to fluids necessitates a vasopressor such as norepinephrine or epinephrine. Pulmonary artery catheter hemodynamic monitoring may provide important data to guide pharmacologic intervention. Cardiac dysrhythmias should be managed according to current Advanced Cardiac Life Support guidelines.

Core temperature approaching or exceeding 104°F (40°C) is immediately life-threatening and warrants aggressive management. Rapid-sequence induction (sedation and paralysis), intubation, and ventilation may be required. Completely undress the patient, begin continuous monitoring of the patient's core temperature, and initiate active cooling measures. Active cooling should be terminated when the patient's core temperature approaches 101°F (38.3°C). Antipyretics (e.g., acetaminophen, aspirin, and nonsteroidal anti-inflammatory drugs) are not useful, and there is no good evidence that dantrolene, bromocriptine, or amantadine enhances the cooling process in patients with life-threatening hyperthermia.

The initial management of a patient with altered mental status should include assessment and treatment of all readily reversible causes such as hypoxia, hypoglycemia, opioid toxicity, and thiamine deficiency. Imaging studies of the head should be performed for patients with persistent altered mental status, followed by lumbar puncture as clinically indicated. Antibiotic and antiviral medications should be administered as soon as the diagnosis of meningitis or encephalitis is entertained.

Mild psychomotor agitation usually does not require active intervention. However, aggressive treatment of PCP psychosis is critical to prevent injury to the patient or others. The patient should be isolated in a secured bare seclusion room with frequent, but unobtrusive observation; seclusion safeguards staff and other patients, calms the patient through reduction of stimuli. Haloperidol and chlorpromazine (after excluding acute PCP and anticholinergic toxicity) have been reported to be safe and effective treatment of PCP psychosis [17,21], and benzodiazepines may be preferred for patients because they lack anticholinergic and extrapyramidal side effects, do not lower seizure threshold, and have not been associated with hyperthermia or neuroleptic malignant syndrome. The dose of benzodiazepine should be titrated to achieve moderate sedation to obviate physical restraints. Occasionally, large doses (e.g., >100 mg of diazepam) may be necessary to achieve safe gentle sedation. The patient's ability to protect the airway should be carefully monitored. Intubation and ventilation are rarely necessary.

Seizures should be treated with intravenous benzodiazepines. Cumulative high-dose benzodiazepines may be required. If seizure activity is not rapidly controlled, intravenous propofol or phenobarbital is indicated. Seizures refractory to sedative hypnotic drugs should be managed with nondepolarizing neuromuscular blockade and general anesthesia, along with continuous electroencephalogram monitoring.

Fluid management should address electrolyte and acid–base abnormalities. Management of rhabdomyolysis should include treatment of psychomotor agitation and generous intravenous crystalloid fluids to maintain urine output of at least 2 to 3 mL/kg/h to maximize glomerular filtration rate. Because serum myoglobin levels are not usually rapidly available, serum CPK may be monitored noting that the clinically important myoglobin serum peak may precede the CPK peak by several hours. Care should be taken to prevent dependent muscle injury.

Although urinary acidification can increase renal PCP excretion, the risks associated with urinary acidification outweigh potential benefits. Hemodialysis is not indicated for enhanced drug elimination but may be necessary in patients with acute renal failure.

The patients with suicidal ideation or persistent psychosis should be referred to the psychiatric service.

HALLUCINOGENS

The term "hallucinogen" has come to describe lysergic acid (LSD, or "acid"), and related compounds based on their reported hallucinogenic effect. However, it has been argued that common recreational doses rarely produce frank hallucinations. Other designations for this class of drugs include psychedelics, psychotomimetics, and entheogens. Hallucinogens are primarily composed of synthetic indolamines (derivatives of tryptamine), phenethylamines (derivatives of amphetamine, see Chapter 100), and botanical products. The psychedelic experience may precipitate homicidal acts, self-destructive behavior, accidental injuries, and acute or chronic psychosis. Physiologic effects vary from mild flushing to life-threatening alterations in vital signs, coma, seizures, and coagulopathy.

Pharmacology

Synthetic hallucinogens are sold as liquid, powder, tablets, capsules, microdots (dried drug residue) on printed paper, liquid-impregnated blotter paper, and as windowpanes (translucent 3 × 3 mm gelatin squares).

The routes of administration are oral, intranasal, sublingual, conjunctival, smoking, or intravenous injection. Blotter paper is chewed and swallowed, whereas microdot paper is usually licked. Windowpanes are usually placed under the tongue or in the conjunctival sac, and may also be swallowed.

The mechanisms of action for hallucinogens are presumed to involve various neurotransmitters in the central nervous system. Hallucinogenic effects on thought and perception appear to primarily involve serotonin (5-hydroxytryptamine, or 5HT) neurotransmission. Serotonin modulates psychologic and physiologic processes such as affect, mood, personality, sexual activity, appetite, motor function, pain perception, sleep induction, and temperature regulation. Tryptamine, derivatives from the tryptophan metabolism, has been shown to be a sigma-1 receptor agonist and their hallucinogenic effects are believed to be primarily mediated by the 5-HT_{2A} receptor [22].

Hallucinogens are readily absorbed from the GI tract, metabolized by the liver, and excreted predominately as pharmacologically inactive compounds. The clinical effects produced by different agents are very similar.

LSD, the most widely abused tryptamine derivative, was originally synthesized from an ergot alkaloid. The structural similarity between tryptamines and serotonin engenders significant activity at serotonergic receptors across this chemical class. LSD has the highest affinity for the 5-HT_{2A} receptor and the highest potency for hallucinogenic effects in humans [23]. Experimentally, the stimulus effects of LSD are completely antagonistic by acting as a highly selective 5-HT_{2A} antagonist. The usual street form is a 1 cm^2 piece of blotter paper (tabs). At doses of 100 μg, LSD produces perceptual distortions and hallucinations.

Morning glory (*Ipomoea* and *Rivea* genera) seeds contain LSD derivatives that are one-tenth as potent as LSD. Users report that to achieve the desired hallucinogenic effect requires ingestion of 200 to 300 macerated seeds.

Psilocybin and psilocin are tryptamine derivatives found in *Psilocybe* and other hallucinogenic fungi (magic mushrooms). It is usually sold in the form of dried mushroom, capsules, or paper packets of brown powder. Pure psilocybin is available in capsules of white powder. The effective psilocybin dose is 5 to 15 mg, which is equivalent to ingestion of one to five large mushrooms. However, the clinical effects are dependent on a number of factors, including dose, method of preparation, and individual patient factors.

The toads of the genus *Bufo* secrete venom from their parotid glands onto their skin. This venom contains bufodienolides, which is a mixture of purported hallucinogenic tryptamine derivatives (e.g., 5-hydroxy-*N*,*N*-dimethyltryptamine, 5-OH-DMT, also known as bufotenine) and cardioactive compounds (e.g., bufogenin and bufotoxin); see Chapter 100 [24]. *Bufoalvarius* possesses an unusual enzyme, *O*-methyl transferase that converts bufotenine to a potent hallucinogen 5-methoxy-*N*,*N*-dimethyltryptamine (5-MeO-DMT). 5-OH-DMT is reported to be a constituent of hallucinogenic snuffs from northwest South America, derived from the leguminaceous tree, *Anadenanthera peregrine*. 5-MeO-DMT accounts for much of the psychoactivity of South American snuffs derived from *Anadenantheraperegrina* as well as those derived from species of *Virola*, a genus of trees in the nutmeg family. Hence, toad licking has been popularized by the belief that hallucinogenic effects may be achieved by licking the skin of live toads.

Dimethyltryptamine (DMT), a tryptamine derivative, is an endogenous hallucinogen in some plant species (e.g., *Virolacalophylla*, *Phalarisaquatica*, *Acacia maidenii*, *Acacia phlebophylla* and *Acacia obtusifolia*) and is a trace amine that is endogenously synthesized from tryptophan in mammals. DMT is rapidly and extensively metabolized to 3-indoleacetic acid by MAO-A, which may explain the reported lack of psychoactive effects following DMT ingestion and its significant psychotropic activity when smoked, injected, or insufflated [22]. However, the psychoactive activity of DMT is preserved when ingested in combination with a MAOI (e.g., "ayahuasca," a DMT, and β-carboline plant decoction). Street DMT is available as a liquid or yellow-tan powder that it is sprinkled on tobacco, marijuana, or parsley and smoked. Smoking is the preferred route of exposure, and is claimed to produce potent psychospiritual effects.

Mescaline, another amphetamine congener, is the psychedelic constituent of peyote (North American dumping cactus, *Lophophora williamsii*) and other cacti. Small segments of the crown of the cactus, known as "buttons" or "moons," may be swallowed whole or chopped into small pieces. Ground peyote may be smoked. The hallucinogenic dose of mescaline is approximately 300 mg, corresponding to 6 to 12 buttons.

Clinical Toxicity

Acute psychedelic effects (trip or tripping) are characterized by changes in sensory perception. They include euphoria or dysphoria; an increase in the intensity of sensory perception; distortions of time, place, and body image; visual hallucinations; synesthesias (i.e., seeing sounds and hearing colors); illusions; loss of spatial sense; and feelings of unreality. The visual hallucinations are characteristically nebulous, rapidly changing, and unreal (e.g., streaks and blobs of color or kaleidoscopic, multicolored shifting patterns). Visions and mystical experiences have been described. Hallucinogenic drug effects may be variable, even in the same individual on different occasions. The person is usually awake and may appear hyperalert, but is often quiet, calm, withdrawn, depressed, uncommunicative, and oblivious to surroundings or preoccupied with internal stimuli. For some people, the psychedelic experience may be frightening or terrifying, which results in anxiety, agitation, violence, or panic (e.g., a bad trip or bummer). In general, tryptamine, amphetamine derivatives, and mescaline have clinical effects similar to those of LSD. The most common presentation is acute panic reactions. The patients typically present with anxiety, apprehension, a sense of loss of self-control, and frightening illusions.

The subjective effects of LSD (e.g., alterations of mood, perceptual changes, and cognitive impairment) typically begin within 30 to 60 minutes, peak at 2 to 4 hours, and return to baseline within 12 hours. Although LSD may induce profound perceptual changes, there is a lack of good data to suggest adverse physical events as a direct consequence of LSD administration. There does not appear to be a documented case of LSD overdose death. However, massive LSD overdose has resulted in severe autonomic effects such as coma, toxic psychosis, hyperventilation, respiratory arrest, hypertension, hyperthermia, tachycardia, athetosis, dystonic movements, and coagulopathy [25,26]. LSD use has been associated with Serotonin syndrome. An adverse consequence attributed to LSD use that is recognized in DSM-V is "Hallucinogen Persisting Perception Disorder" or "flashbacks," a condition in which a person re-experiences, following the cessation of hallucinogen exposure, perceptual symptoms that were experienced while intoxicated with the hallucinogen [27]. "Flashbacks" can be triggered by stress, illness, and exercise. Persistent LSD effects may include prolonged psychotic reactions, depression, and exacerbation of pre-existing psychiatric illness.

The initial effects of morning glory seeds are listlessness, apathy, and irritability, followed by mild LSD-type effects. Severe psychedelic reactions as well as "flashbacks" have been reported [28].

The effects of "magic mushrooms" may include mydriasis, tachycardia, hypertension, hyperreftexia, facial or truncal flushing, behavior, emotional or mood alterations (e.g., dysphoria and frightening experiences or "bad trips"), perceptual disorders (e.g., visual distortions, hallucinations, distortions of body image or depersonalization, and paraesthesias), and panic attacks [29]. The experience of serious negative effects (e.g., bad trip) is probably a reason for seeking medical care. In these cases, the individuals may be severely agitated, confused, extremely anxious, disoriented with impaired concentration and judgment (e.g., walking beside a railway line), and acutely psychotic experiencing bizarre and frightening images, severe paranoia, and total loss of reality with consequent accidents, self-injury or suicide attempts. A "bad trip" is usually followed by faintness, sadness and depression and paranoid interpretations, which may persist for months. Some of these symptoms may be associated with concomitant use of other illicit substances. For some individuals, the use of "magic mushrooms" may exacerbate underlying personality disorders and psychosis-like states. Flashbacks have been reported following psilocybin intoxication [30]. Intravenous injection of *Psilocybe* mushroom extract has resulted in systemic autonomic effects that include nausea, protracted vomiting, diarrhea, rigors, hyperpyrexia, arthralgias, severe myalgias, loin pain, headache, and skin eruptions. Laboratory results included hypoxemia, leukocytosis with a left shift, elevated renal and liver function studies, and mild methemoglobinemia.

The purported hallucinogenic effects that may be derived from licking the skin of live toads of the genus *Bufo* may be clinically inconsequential compared with the serious effects of the cardioactive compounds (e.g., cardiac dysrhythmias and death); see Chapter 100.

DMT effects include colorful visualhallucinations (e.g., rapidly moving, multidimensional, kaleidoscopic display of intensely colored abstract and representational images), auditory effects that were not frank hallucinations, dissociation of awareness from the physical body, transient anxiety, a dream-like state, euphoria, and feelings of alternating heat and cold, which usually peaks after a few minutes and resolve within 30 minutes [31].

Peyote can have strong emetic effects, and has been reported to cause profound nausea and vomiting preceding hallucinations.

Diagnostic Evaluation

Hallucinogen intoxication is a clinical diagnosis. It is based on a history of possible hallucinogen exposure associated with clinical findings consistent with hallucinogenic effects. The history should include a prior drug abuse and psychiatric illness. Often, the name of the drug is not given but the route of intoxication and dosage form are described (e.g., ate a paper, chewed a button, put acid in my eye). Sometimes the only history is "on a trip."

Physical examination should focus on eliciting signs of autonomic disturbances, synesthesias, illusions, hallucinations, delusions, and abnormal behavior. Laboratory tests should include serum electrolytes, blood urea nitrogen, creatinine, glucose, CPK, and urinalysis. Urine toxicology screen may confirm the diagnosis of psychedelic hallucinogen intoxication and may be useful in patients with unexplained hallucinations. Quantitative hallucinogen drug levels are not clinically useful and do not contribute to patient management. Although laboratory tests are available for LSD and its metabolite, it is not part of most standard drug abuse screens. Electrocardiogram, arterial blood gas, imaging studies, and lumbar puncture should be obtained as clinically indicated.

Management

Management of hallucinogenic tryptamine is similar to that for PCP exposure. The patients should be placed in a quiet area with limited stimuli accompanied by a patient advocate. The advocate should provide reality testing and reassure the patient that it is a drug-induced experience and the adverse drug event will resolve within a few hours. This approach may not be practical or effective for severely disturbed or uncommunicative patients, and liberal intravenous benzodiazepine doses should be administered to control anxiety. Depressed or withdrawn patients are unpredictable and should be kept under close observation. GI decontamination is unlikely to benefit a symptomatic patient and is not indicated. In patients exhibiting serotonin syndrome, treatment with chlorpromazine or cyproheptadine may be considered (see Chapter 125). The patients are expected to completely recover within 24 hours. Persistent signs and symptoms may be caused by a psychiatric condition precipitated by the hallucinogenic drug, and the patient should be referred to the psychiatric service for evaluation.

References

1. Boyorh MA, Zukowska-Grojec Z, Palkovits M, et al: Effect of phencyclidine (PCP) on blood pressure and catecholamine levels in discrete brain nuclei. *Brain Res* 321:315, 1984.
2. Fosset M, Renaud JF, Lenoie MC, et al: Interaction of molecules of phencyclidine series with cardiac cells: association with the muscarinic receptor. *FEBS Lett* 103:133, 1979.
3. Haring R, Kloog Y, Sokolovsky M: Localization of phencyclidine binding sites on alpha and beta subunits of the nicotinic acetylcholine receptor from Torpedo ocellata electric organ using azido phencyclidine. *J Neurosci* 4:627, 1984.
4. Johnson SW, Haroldsen PE, Hoffer BJ, et al: Presynaptic dopaminergic activity of phencyclidine in rat caudate. *J Pharmacol Exp Ther* 229:322, 1984.
5. Paster Z, Maayani S, Weinstein H, et al: Cholinolytic action of phencyclidine derivatives. *Eur J Pharmacol* 25:270, 1974.
6. Quirion R, Hammer RP, Herkenham M, et al: Phencyclidine (angel dust) sigma opiate receptor: visualization by tritium-sensitive film. *Proc Natl Acad Sci USA* 78:5881, 1981.
7. Smith RC, Meltzer HY, Arora RC, et al: Effects of phencyclidine on catecholamines and serotonin uptake in synaptosomal preparations from rat brain. *Biochem Pharmacol* 26:1436, 1977.
8. Tourneur Y, Romey G, Lazdunski M: Phencyclidine blockade of sodium and potassium channels in neuroblastoma cells. *Brain Res* 245:154, 1982.
9. Vincent JP, Cavey D, Kamenk JM, et al: Interaction of phencyclidines with the muscarinic and opiate receptors in the central nervous system. *Brain Res* 152:176, 1978.
10. Vincent JP, Vignon J, Kartalovski B, et al: Compared properties of central and peripheral binding sites for phencyclidine. *Eur J Pharmacol* 68:79, 1980.
11. Wong EHF, Kemp JA: Sites for antagonism of N-methyl-D-aspartate receptor channel complex. *Annu Rev Pharmacol Toxicol* 31:401, 1991.
12. Cook CE, Brine DR, Jeffcoat AR, et al: Phencyclidine disposition after intravenous and oral doses. *Clin Pharmacol Ther* 31:625, 1982.
13. Burns RS, Lerner SE: Perspectives: acute phencyclidine intoxication. *Clin Toxicol* 9:477, 1976.
14. Burns RS, Lerner SE: Phencyclidine deaths. *JACEP* 7:135, 1978.
15. Barton CH, Sterling ML, Vaziri ND: Phencyclidine intoxication: clinical experience in 27 cases confirmed by urine assay. *Ann Emerg Med* 10:243, 1981.
16. Liden CB, Lovejoy FH, Costello CE: Phencyclidine: nine cases of poisoning. *JAMA* 234:513, 1975.
17. Luisada PV: The phencyclidine psychosis, phenomenology and treatment, in Peterson RC, Stillman RC (eds): *Phencyclidine (PCP) Abuse: An Appraisal.* Washington, DC, NIDA Research Monograph 21, 1978, p 241.
18. McCarron MM, Schulze BW, Thompson GA, et al: Acute phencyclidine intoxication: incidence of clinical findings in 1,000 cases. *Ann Emerg Med* 10:237, 1981.
19. McCarron MM, Schulze BW, Thompson GA, et al: Acute phencyclidine intoxication: clinical patterns, complications, and treatment. *Ann Emerg Med* 10:290, 1981.
20. Cravey RH, Reed D, Ragle JL: Phencyclidine-related deaths: a report of nine fatal cases. *J Anal Toxicol* 3:199, 1979.
21. Giannini AJ, Nageotte C, Loiselle RH, et al: Comparison of chlorpromazine, haloperidol and pimozide in the treatment of phencyclidine psychosis: DA-2 receptor specificity. *J Toxicol Clin Toxicol* 22:573, 1984–1985.
22. Araújo AM, Carvalho F, Bastos ML: The hallucinogenic world of tryptamines: an updated review. *Arch Toxicol* 89:1151–1173, 2015.
23. Fantegrossi WE, Murnane KS, Reissig CJ: The behavioral pharmacology of hallucinogens. *Biochem Pharmacol* 75:17, 2008.
24. Weil AT, Davis W: Bufoalvarius: a potent hallucinogen of animal origin. *J Ethnopharmacol* 41:1, 1994.
25. Friedman SA, Hirsch SE: Extreme hyperthermia after LSD ingestion. *JAMA* 217:1549, 1971.
26. Klock JC, Boerner U, Becker CE: Coma, hyperthermia and bleeding associated with massive LSD overdose. *West J Med* 120:183, 1974.
27. Halpern JH, Pope HG: Hallucinogen persisting perception disorder: what do we know after 50 years? *Drug Alcohol Depend* 69:109, 2003.
28. Fink PJ, Goldman MJ, Lyons I: Morning glory seed psychosis. *Arch Gen Psychiatry* 15:209, 1966.
29. Peden NR, Bissett AF, Macaulay KE, et al: Clinical toxicology of "magic mushroom" ingestion. *Postgrad Med J* 57(671):543–545, 1981.
30. Dewhurst K: Psilocybin intoxication. *Br J Psychiatry* 137:303, 1980.
31. Strassman RJ: Human psychopharmacology of N,N-dimethyltryptamine. *Behav Brain Res* 73:12, 1996.

Chapter 122 ▪ Salicylate and Other Nonsteroidal Anti-inflammatory Drug Poisoning

MARCO L.A. SIVILOTTI • CHRISTOPHER H. LINDEN

Nonsteroidal anti-inflammatory drugs (NSAIDs) include aspirin, related salicylates (Table 122.1), and a variety of other drugs (e.g., ibuprofen, indomethacin, phenylbutazone, and ketorolac), which modulate inflammation by inhibiting cyclooxygenase (COX). In clinical use for 100 years, aspirin still enjoys widespread popularity in the adult population, both by self-medication and by physician-recommended usage.

While the institution of child-resistant packaging and concerns about Reye's syndrome resulted in a dramatic decline in pediatric overdose, aspirin remains a leading cause of death due to pharmaceutical overdose [1–3]. Reducing the amount of aspirin available over the counter was associated with fewer overdose deaths in the United Kingdom [4]. Nevertheless, vigilance remains necessary because chronic salicylate intoxication, particularly in the elderly, is commonly unrecognized or mistaken for other conditions, such as sepsis, dehydration, dementia, and multiorgan failure. In contrast, most other NSAIDs have a substantially greater safety margin than aspirin in overdose. Although availability without prescription has resulted in increased use and frequency of overdose, significant acute toxicity is uncommon [1,5,6].

PHARMACOLOGY

All NSAIDs have analgesic and antipyretic as well as anti-inflammatory activities. These effects are due to inhibition of COX, also known as *prostaglandin G/H synthase*, the enzyme responsible for the conversion of arachidonic acid to prostaglandins and thromboxanes [7]. The analgesic dose of most NSAIDs is approximately one-half the anti-inflammatory dose. For some NSAIDs, such as aspirin, ibuprofen, and fenoprofen, this gap is larger, whereas the converse is true for sulindac and piroxicam. Antipyretic effects appear to be due to decreased pyrogen production peripherally as well as to a central hypothalamic effect. The existence of central nervous system (CNS) sites of action mediating analgesic activity has been postulated [8].

Two isoforms of COX have been characterized: COX-1, constitutionally present in platelets, endothelium, gastric mucosa, and the kidneys; and COX-2, induced by a variety of inflammatory mediators (e.g., cytokines, endotoxin, growth factors, hormones, and tumor promoters) but suppressed by glucocorticoids [7]. The anti-inflammatory and analgesic properties of NSAIDs appear to be primarily due to the inhibition of COX-2. Their adverse effects on gastric mucosa (e.g., hemorrhage, ulceration, and perforation) and kidney function (e.g., decreased renal blood flow and glomerular filtration rate), and their effects on platelet function appear to be mediated primarily by COX-1 [7,9,10].

NSAIDs can be classified on the basis of their selectivity for COX-2. In particular, the coxibs rofecoxib, valdecoxib, and celecoxib were developed specifically for their COX-2 selectivity and the promise of improved safety. However, an increased risk of myocardial infarction and stroke was identified in clinical trials and led to regulatory restrictions [11,12]. These adverse cardiovascular effects appear to be due to a relative excess of COX-1–generated thromboxane A_2, which is vasoconstrictive and platelet-activating (i.e., prothrombic), and a relative lack of COX-2–generated prostaglandin I_2 (prostacyclin), which is vasodilatory and platelet inhibitory (i.e., antithrombotic) [7,11]. It is important to note that traditional NSAIDS diclofenac, meloxicam, and nabumetone exhibit partial COX-2 selectivity, and that other traditional, nonselective NSAIDs may also contribute to adverse cardiovascular events. Thus, selectivity is relative, and all NSAIDs inhibit both COX isoforms in a dose-dependent manner. Inhibition of COX-1 may result in increased lipoxygenation of arachidonic acid to leukotrienes. This alternate metabolic pathway seems to be responsible for the sometimes fatal allergic reactions to NSAIDs especially prevalent in adults with asthma and nasal polyps [13,14].

Aspirin (acetylsalicylic acid) is unique in that it acetylates a serine residue near the active site of COX, thereby irreversibly inhibiting its catalytic function. In contrast, the inhibition of COX by other NSAIDs is reversible and transient. This difference in activity is most notable in platelets, in which thromboxane A_2 is essential for normal function [15]. Even in low doses (80 mg), aspirin inhibits platelet aggregation and prolongs the bleeding time for up to 1 week (pending the production of new platelets), whereas other NSAIDs do not have clinically significant effects on platelets [16].

In high doses, aspirin and other salicylates also inhibit the hepatic synthesis of clotting factor VII and, to some degree, factors IX and X, thereby prolonging the prothrombin time. This effect appears to be due to interference with the activity of vitamin K and can be reversed by administration of phytonadione (vitamin K_1). In contrast, other NSAIDs have insignificant effects on clotting-factor synthesis [16].

Salicylates

Salicylates are available in oral, rectal, and topical formulations. Enteric-coated and sustained-release aspirin tablets are also marketed. Aspirin preparations frequently contain other drugs such as anticholinergics, antihistamines, barbiturates, caffeine, decongestants, muscle relaxants, and opioids. The recommended pediatric dose of aspirin is 10 to 20 mg per kg of body weight every 6 hours, up to 60 mg/kg/d; for adults, the recommended dose is 1,000 mg initially, followed by 650 mg every 4 hours for anti-inflammatory effect. Multiple formulations of other salicylate salts exist with various indications, and may contain very high concentrations of salicylate (see Table 122.1). After a single oral dose of aspirin, therapeutic effects begin within 30 minutes, peak in 1 to 2 hours, and last approximately 4 hours.

Being a weak acid (pK_a, 3.5), aspirin is predominantly nonionized at gastric pH and, therefore, theoretically well absorbed in the stomach. However, gastric acidity slows the dissolution of tablets. Hence, most absorption actually occurs in the small intestine, probably because of its much larger surface area and despite its higher pH. Peak serum salicylate levels of 10 to 20 mg per dL (0.7 to 1.4 mmol per L) occur 1 to 2 hours after ingestion of a single therapeutic dose. Levels up to 30 mg per dL can occur with long-term therapy and may be targeted for maximal anti-inflammatory effects in some patients. Absorption is delayed or prolonged after ingestion of enteric-coated or sustained-release preparations and suppository use [17]. With overdose, slow pill dissolution, and delayed gastric emptying due to aspirin-induced pylorospasm may lead to absorption continuing for 24 hours or longer after ingestion [18,19].

TABLE 122.1

Salicylate Preparations

Compound	Common/trade names	Percentage salicylate
Acetylsalicylic acid	Aspirin	75
Bismuth subsalicylate	In Pepto-Bismol	37
Choline salicylate	Arthropan	56
Choline and magnesium salicylate	Trilisate	76
Difluorophenyl salicylic acid	—	—
Diflunisal	Dolobid	—[a]
Homomenthyl salicylate	In sunscreens	51
Magnesium salicylate	Doan's Caplets, Magan	90
Methyl salicylate	Oil of wintergreen	89
Salicylic acid	In topical keratolytics	100
Salicylsalicylic acid	Salsalate, Disalcid	96
Sodium salicylate	Pabalate	84
Trolamine salicylate	Aspercreme	48

[a]Not hydrolyzed to salicylic acid but may cause screening tests for salicylate to be falsely positive.

During absorption, aspirin is rapidly hydrolyzed to its active metabolite, salicylic acid. At physiologic pH, salicylic acid (pK_a, 3.0) is more than 99.9% ionized to salicylate, which, in contrast to nonionized salicylic acid, diffuses poorly across cell membranes. The drug may become sequestered preferentially in inflamed tissue due to this pH-dependent ionization.

The apparent volume of distribution of salicylate at pH 7.4 is only 0.15 L per kg at therapeutic doses, in part due to its extensive protein binding. Only free (i.e., unbound) salicylate is pharmacologically active. However, salicylate is somewhat unique in that its apparent volume of distribution is not constant. Higher drug levels as a result of chronic therapeutic dosing or acute overdose, low albumin levels, and the presence of other drugs that bind to albumin increase the amount and fraction of free drug. When this occurs, the apparent volume of distribution may increase to 0.60 L per kg [20]. Acidemia, as a consequence of either concomitant illness or severe poisoning, may further increase the fraction of nonionized, diffusible drug, promote its tissue penetration, and increase the apparent volume of distribution even more.

After single therapeutic doses, salicylate is metabolized in the liver to the inactive metabolites salicyluric acid (the glycine conjugate; 75% of the dose), salicylphenolic glucuronide (10%), salicylacyl glucuronide (5%), and gentisic acid (less than 1%). The remaining 10% of the dose is excreted unchanged in the urine. When serum concentrations exceed 20 mg per dL, the two main pathways of metabolism become saturated, and elimination changes from first order (i.e., proportional to the serum level) to zero order (constant), as described by Michaelis–Menton kinetics. Hence, the apparent half-life of salicylate is 2 to 3 hours after a single therapeutic dose, 6 to 12 hours with chronic therapeutic dosing (i.e., serum levels of 20 to 30 mg per dL), and 20 to 40 hours with overdose (i.e., when levels exceed 30 mg per dL) [21]. Because of saturable metabolism, a small increase in the daily dose can lead to a large increase in serum drug levels, with the potential for unintentional poisoning [22]. Depletion of glycine stores may reduce the capacity of the salicyluric acid pathway and further slow elimination in overdose [23].

Renal excretion of salicylate becomes the most important route of elimination when hepatic transformation becomes saturated. The rate of excretion is determined by the glomerular filtration, active proximal tubular secretion of salicylate, and passive distal tubular reabsorption of salicylic acid. Alkalinization of the urine decreases the passive reabsorption of salicylic acid by converting it to ionized, nondiffusible salicylate and thereby increases drug excretion. Similarly, increasing the rate of urine flow increases drug clearance by increasing the glomerular filtration and decreasing the distal tubular reabsorption of salicylic acid (by diluting its concentration in the tubular lumen). Combined alkalinization and diuresis can augment the renal elimination of salicylate by 20-fold or more [24,25]. Conversely, dehydration and aciduria perhaps due to preexisting illness or to salicylate poisoning itself decrease salicylate excretion, and increase the duration of toxicity once it develops.

Salicylates readily cross the placenta and enter breast milk. Salicylate elimination in the fetus or infant may be prolonged because of immature metabolic pathways and renal function [26]. It may also be prolonged in patients with liver or renal disease.

The pathophysiology of salicylate poisoning is multifactorial [27–30]. Initially and in mild poisoning, direct stimulation of the respiratory center in the medulla by toxic salicylate concentrations results in a respiratory alkalosis, unless blunted by concomitant ingestion of CNS depressants [28]. Direct stimulation of the medullary chemoreceptor zone and irritant effects on the gastrointestinal tract are responsible for nausea and vomiting. Exaggerated antipyretic effects involving the hypothalamus may cause vasodilation and sweating [31]. Dehydration results from gastrointestinal, skin, and insensible fluid losses. The osmotic diuresis that occurs as bicarbonate is excreted in response to alkalemia also contributes to dehydration. Sodium and potassium depletion result from excretion of these electrolytes along with bicarbonate (in exchange for hydrogen ion reabsorption). A functional hypocalcemia (decreased ionized calcium) may accompany alkalemia and cause or contribute to cardiac arrhythmias, tetany, and seizures.

Subsequently, in moderate poisoning, the accumulation of salicylate in cells causes uncoupling of mitochondrial oxidative phosphorylation, inhibition of the Krebs cycle and amino acid metabolism, and stimulation of gluconeogenesis, glycolysis, and lipid metabolism [32]. These derangements result in increased but ineffective metabolism, with increased glucose, lipid, and oxygen consumption and increased amino acid, carbon dioxide, glucose, ketoacid, lactic acid, and pyruvic acid production. High serum levels of organic acids contribute to an increased anion-gap metabolic acidosis, and the renal excretion of these acids results in aciduria. However, increased carbon dioxide production further stimulates the respiratory center, and the respiratory alkalosis persists, resulting in alkalemia with paradoxical aciduria.

In severe poisoning, progressive dehydration and impaired cellular metabolism cause multisystem organ dysfunction. Metabolic acidosis with acidemia becomes the dominant acid–base disturbance. Respiratory acidosis, lactic acidosis, and impaired renal excretion of organic acids due to dehydration and acute tubular necrosis contribute to the acidemia. Acidemia increases the fraction of nonionized salicylate in serum, thereby promoting its tissue penetration and toxicity, and precipitous clinical deterioration may ensue with increasing brain salicylate levels. Impaired cellular metabolism can cause increased capillary permeability leading to cerebral edema and noncardiogenic pulmonary edema or acute respiratory distress syndrome. Coma, hyperthermia, and seizures may result from impaired cellular metabolism, cardiovascular depression, cerebral edema, acidemia, hypoglycemia, and acute white matter damage due to myelin disintegration and activation of glial caspase-3 [33,34]. Respiratory alkalosis may be replaced by respiratory acidosis if coma or seizures cause respiratory depression. Tissue hypoxia resulting from pulmonary edema, impaired perfusion, or seizures may lead to anaerobic metabolism and concomitant lactic acidosis.

Hemorrhagic diathesis may result from increased capillary fragility, decreased platelet adhesiveness, thrombocytopenia, and coagulopathy secondary to liver dysfunction. It occurs primarily in patients with chronic poisoning.

Other Nonsteroidal Anti-inflammatory Drugs

Despite their structural diversity, the pharmacokinetics of traditional NSAIDs are quite similar. Like aspirin, they are weak acids, with pK_a ranging from 3.5 to 5.6 and pH-dependent ionization being the major determinant of tissue distribution and sequestration. They are rapidly absorbed after ingestion, have small volumes of distribution (0.08 to 0.20 L per kg), and are 90% to 99% protein bound (principally to albumin). Most have half-lives of less than 8 hours, with low non–flow-dependent hepatic clearance, primarily by the CYP2C subfamily of cytochrome P450 enzymes, to inactive metabolites that are then conjugated, mostly with glucuronic acid, and excreted in the urine. Sulindac is one exception in that its sulfide metabolite is the active form of the drug and has a half-life of 16 hours [35]. Nabumetone is also a prodrug, and its active metabolite, 6-methoxy-2-naphthylacetic acid, has a half-life of more than 20 hours (and even longer in the elderly) [36]. Phenylbutazone, oxyphenbutazone, and piroxicam are notable for half-lives of longer than 30 hours. Diflunisal, like aspirin, has a dose-dependent half-life of 5 to 20 hours. Indomethacin, sulindac, etodolac, piroxicam, carprofen, and meloxicam undergo enterohepatic recirculation [35,37,38]. Small amounts (less than 10%) of nonsalicylate NSAIDs are excreted unchanged in the urine, limiting the effect of urine pH on clearance. The coxibs are nonacidic drugs [10], highly protein bound and primarily metabolized in the liver.

In contrast to salicylates, the metabolism of most nonsalicylate NSAIDs is not saturable or prolonged in overdose, and elimination follows first-order kinetics. An exception is phenylbutazone, whose elimination may follow Michaelis–Menton kinetics.

Toxic effects of NSAIDs appear to be primarily due to exaggerated pharmacologic effects, with gastric irritation and renal dysfunction resulting from the inhibition of prostaglandin synthesis. In contrast to salicylate poisoning, the acidosis that sometimes occurs with large overdoses of these agents appears to be due to high levels of parent drug and metabolites rather than to disruption of metabolism [39].

CLINICAL TOXICITY

Salicylates

Salicylate poisoning may occur with acute as well as chronic overdose [27–30,40–46]. It most commonly results from ingestion, but poisoning due to topical use [47] and rectal self-administration [48] has been reported. The ingestion of topical preparations of methyl salicylate (oil of wintergreen, also present in Chinese propriety medicines) can result in rapid-onset poisoning, due to its concentration, rapid absorption kinetics, and higher lipid solubility. Infants may become poisoned by ingesting the breast milk of women chronically taking therapeutic doses of salicylate [49]. Intrauterine fetal demise resulting from poisoning during pregnancy [50] and neonatal poisoning resulting from the transplacental diffusion of therapeutic doses of salicylate taken before delivery [51] have also been described. Delays to presentation, diagnosis, and chronicity increase the severity and mortality [42,52,53]. With severe poisoning, the fatality rate may be as high as 50% [43,46].

Regardless of whether poisoning is acute or chronic, it can be characterized as mild, moderate, or severe on the basis of the serum pH and underlying acid–base disturbance (Table 122.2). This approach was first described in the classic papers by Done [40,54], who also developed a nomogram that attempted to correlate the severity of poisoning with a timed salicylate level after acute ingestion. Although Done's nomogram has subsequently been shown to have poor predictive value [41,52], his observation that the clinical severity of poisoning correlates with acid–base status remains undisputed.

Mild poisoning is characterized by alkalemia (serum pH greater than 7.45) and a pure respiratory alkalosis. It may develop 2 to 8 hours after acute ingestion of 150 to 300 mg per kg of aspirin [40,54] or any time during chronic therapy. Associated signs and symptoms include nausea, vomiting, abdominal pain, headache, tinnitus, tachypnea (or subtle hyperpnea), ataxia, dizziness, agitation, and lethargy. The anion gap (see Chapter 198) is normal until late in this stage, when compensatory renal bicarbonate excretion eventually lowers the serum bicarbonate level. Serum glucose, potassium, and sodium values may be high, low, or normal. Despite total body fluid and electrolyte depletion and clinical dehydration, laboratory evidence of dehydration (e.g., hemoconcentration, increased serum blood urea nitrogen [BUN] and creatinine, increased urine specific gravity) may be absent.

Moderate poisoning is characterized by a near normal serum pH (7.35 to 7.45) with an underlying metabolic acidosis as well as respiratory alkalosis. It can occur 4 to 12 hours after an acute overdose of 300 to 500 mg per kg of aspirin [40,54]. It may also occur in patients with chronic ingestion who delay seeking medical care for symptoms of mild poisoning and continue to take salicylate. Electrolyte analysis demonstrates a low serum bicarbonate value with an increased anion gap. Gastrointestinal and neurologic symptoms are more pronounced. There may be agitation, asterixis, diaphoresis, deafness, pallor, confusion, slurred speech, disorientation, hallucinations, tachycardia, tachypnea, and orthostatic hypotension. Leukocytosis, thrombocytopenia, increased or decreased serum glucose and sodium

TABLE 122.2

Severity of Salicylate Poisoning

Severity grade	Serum pH	Underlying acid-base abnormality
Mild	>7.45	Respiratory alkalosis
Moderate	7.35–7.45	Combined respiratory alkalosis and metabolic acidosis; paradoxical aciduria
Severe	<7.35	Metabolic acidosis with or without respiratory acidosis

values, hypokalemia, and increased serum BUN, creatinine, and ketones may be present.

Severe poisoning is defined by the presence of acidemia (serum pH less than 7.35) with underlying metabolic acidosis and a high anion gap. It can occur 6 to 24 hours or more after the acute ingestion of more than 500 mg per kg of aspirin [40,54] or in unrecognized or untreated chronic poisoning. Severe dehydration and marked sinus tachycardia are often present. Other findings may include coma, seizures, papilledema, hypotension, dysrhythmias, congestive heart failure, oliguria, hypothermia or hyperthermia, rhabdomyolysis, and multiple organ failure [46,53,55]. Hypoglycemia, pulmonary edema, and cerebral edema or hemorrhage may be present [45]. Asystole is the most common terminal dysrhythmia, but ventricular tachycardia and ventricular fibrillation can also occur [45,46,56,57]. When cardiac arrest occurs, death appears to be inevitable. Successful resuscitation in this situation has yet to be reported [57].

Although an increased anion-gap metabolic acidosis is often said to be a hallmark of salicylate poisoning, in reality a variety of acid–base disturbances may be seen depending on the delay to presentation and severity of poisoning. As noted earlier, the anion gap may be normal and acidosis absent in early or mild intoxication. In addition, the anion gap is rarely above 20 mEq per L, even in advanced poisoning [28]. In adults, combined respiratory alkalosis and metabolic acidosis is the most common finding (50% to 61%), followed by pure respiratory alkalosis (20% to 25%), pure metabolic acidosis (15% to 20%), and a combined respiratory and metabolic acidosis (5%) [28,46]. Metabolic acidosis is more common and respiratory alkalosis more often absent in children than in adults [42,46] suggesting that children progress more rapidly from mild to severe poisoning, perhaps because of more rapid and extensive tissue distribution of drug [58]. Metabolic acidosis is also more common in patients with large acute ingestions, chronic intoxication, and delayed presentation or treatment [28,42,43,46,59]. The onset and progression of toxicity may be delayed after overdose with enteric-coated or sustained-release formulations [17].

Potential complications of both therapeutic and toxic doses of salicylate include gastrointestinal tract bleeding, increased prothrombin time, hepatic toxicity, pancreatitis, proteinuria, and abnormal urinary sediment. Significant bleeding, gastrointestinal tract perforation, blindness, and inappropriate secretion of antidiuretic hormone are rare complications of acute poisoning.

Other Nonsteroidal Anti-inflammatory Drugs

With the exception of mefenamic acid and phenylbutazone, significant toxicity from acute overdose is unusual and occurs following massive ingestion. Manifestations typically include nausea, vomiting, abdominal pain, headache, confusion, tinnitus, drowsiness, and hyperventilation [5,60,61]. Glycosuria, hematuria, and proteinuria are also common. Occasionally, acute renal failure (acute tubular necrosis or interstitial nephritis) can develop. Symptoms rarely last more than several hours, and acute renal toxicity is almost always reversible over a period of a few days to weeks. Experience with selective COX-2 inhibitor overdose is limited, but acute toxicity appears to be similar to nonselective NSAIDS [62].

Muscle twitching and grand mal seizures have been reported in 30% of mefenamic acid overdoses [63]. Apnea, coma, and cardiac arrest can also occur [63]. Metabolic acidosis, coma, seizures, hepatic dysfunction, hypotension, and cardiovascular collapse are relatively frequent after phenylbutazone overdose [60,61,64–66]. Uncommonly, coma, hyperactivity, hypothermia, seizures, metabolic acidosis, acute renal insufficiency, thrombocytopenia, acute respiratory distress syndrome, upper gastrointestinal tract bleeding, and respiratory depression are seen in ibuprofen poisoning [39,66–69]. Death from ibuprofen alone is extremely rare [1,5,6]. Seizures and metabolic acidosis have also been reported in ketoprofen and naproxen poisoning [70,71].

Minimum toxic and lethal doses are not well defined. Little correlation was found between the amount of ibuprofen reportedly ingested and symptoms in adults [65]. In the pediatric population, however, the mean amount ingested was much greater in symptomatic patients (440 mg per kg) than asymptomatic ones (114 mg per kg) [67]. Elderly patients are at increased risk of developing toxicity with both therapeutic doses and overdoses. Even with severe poisoning, complete recovery usually occurs within 24 to 48 hours.

DIAGNOSTIC EVALUATION

The history should include the time or times of ingestion, the specific product and formulation, the amount ingested, and any concomitant ingestion or medication use. Physical examination should focus on vital signs, neurologic and cardiopulmonary function, and assessment of the state of hydration. Vital signs should include an accurate temperature and respiratory rate and, if possible, orthostatic measurements of pulse and blood pressure. The abdomen should be evaluated for peritoneal signs suggestive of perforation. The urine should be tested for pH, ketones, and occult blood.

Salicylates

Laboratory evaluation of patients with salicylate poisoning should include arterial or venous blood gases, complete blood cell count, serum electrolyte, glucose, BUN, creatinine, and salicylate levels, and urinalysis. Patients with moderate-to-severe salicylate poisoning should also have serum calcium, magnesium, and ketones, liver function tests, coagulation profile, electrocardiogram, and chest radiograph. Because patients often confuse aspirin and acetaminophen, testing should be performed for both.

The ferric chloride spot test can be used to rapidly detect the presence of salicylate in urine or commercial products [72]. Several drops of 10% ferric chloride turn urine purple if salicylate is present. A positive urine test indicates exposure but not overdose, because positive results are seen with therapeutic dosing. False-positive reactions may be caused by acetoacetic acid, phenylpyruvic acid, phenothiazines, and phenylbutazone. Diflunisal may result in falsely elevated serum salicylate levels when measured by fluorescence polarization immunoassay or the Trinder colorimetric assay [73].

Serum salicylate concentrations must be interpreted with respect to the duration (i.e., acute vs. chronic overdose), time of ingestion, and the serum pH. At similar salicylate concentrations, patients with chronic poisoning tend to be more ill than those with acute poisoning [29,45,46]. Soon after an acute overdose, concentrations can be quite high (e.g., greater than 60 mg per dL) in the absence of significant toxicity. Conversely, with chronic overdosage and late in the course of an acute overdose, moderate or severe toxicity may be present despite serum salicylate concentrations in or just above the high therapeutic range. At similar salicylate concentrations, children, the elderly, and those with underlying disease tend to be more ill than otherwise healthy adults [29,44,58,74]. Poisoning in such patients, particularly if chronic, can occasionally be seen with therapeutic salicylate levels. Acidemia facilitates passage of drug into the brain, worsening toxicity. Hence, as noted previously, the severity of poisoning is ultimately determined by acid–base status and clinical findings.

Serial salicylate levels are necessary for confirming the diagnosis and monitoring the efficacy of treatment, but do not obviate the need for continued clinical and metabolic monitoring. Depending on the severity and course of poisoning, drug levels and other laboratory tests should initially be repeated at 2-hour intervals. Because of delayed and erratic absorption, it is imperative to demonstrate a falling and near-zero salicylate concentration to exclude significant ongoing absorption after overdose, which generally requires at least 12 hours even in mild overdoses [19].

Historically, approximately 1 in 4 patients with chronic salicylate poisoning are initially undiagnosed [28,43,59]. These patients are typically elderly, have a variety of presenting complaints and underlying illnesses, and have been taking aspirin with therapeutic intent. To avoid missing the diagnosis, all patients should be asked specifically about the use of nonprescription drugs. Asking about tinnitus or hearing distortion, which occurs with salicylate levels in the high end of the therapeutic range (i.e., 20 to 30 mg per dL), may also suggest the diagnosis in patients with unknown ingestions or unexplained complaints. Occult salicylate poisoning should be considered in any patient with an unexplained acid–base disturbance, altered mental status, hyperthermia, diaphoresis, dyspnea, vomiting, or pulmonary edema [28,59].

The differential diagnosis of salicylate poisoning includes infection, CNS trauma and tumors, congestive heart failure, chronic obstructive pulmonary disease, poisoning with carbon monoxide, isoniazid, lithium, and valproate, and other causes of an elevated anion-gap acidosis, particularly methanol and ethylene glycol (see Chapter 198). Hemodynamic, autonomic, and laboratory manifestations of severe poisoning resemble the systemic inflammatory response syndrome and may be mistaken for sepsis [51,55,75]. Salicylate poisoning has also been misdiagnosed as alcohol intoxication, alcohol withdrawal, dementia, diabetic ketoacidosis, impending myocardial infarction, hepatic encephalopathy, and viral encephalitis.

In infants and children, salicylate poisoning may be confused with inborn errors of metabolism. It may be particularly difficult to distinguish from Reye's syndrome, because they are not only similar in presentation but appear to be interrelated [76,77]. Fatty infiltration of the liver on pathologic examination of a biopsy specimen, low (i.e., subtherapeutic) cerebrospinal fluid salicylate levels, and high alanine, glutamine, and lysine levels indicate Reye's syndrome rather than salicylate poisoning. Radiopaque densities in the stomach on abdominal radiograph suggest the possibility of an enteric-coated or sustained-release formulation or a magnesium or bismuth salt of salicylate.

Other Nonsteroidal Anti-inflammatory Drugs

The initial evaluation of patients with nonsalicylate-NSAID overdose is similar to that for salicylates. Evaluation of acid–base, electrolyte, and renal parameters is particularly important. Additional ancillary testing is dictated by clinical severity. Quantitative serum levels of nonsalicylate NSAIDs are neither routinely available nor necessary for treatment.

Many medical conditions and other intoxications cause signs and symptoms similar to those seen in nonsalicylate NSAID poisoning. In the absence of a history of ingestion, the diagnosis is made by exclusion of other etiologies.

MANAGEMENT

Salicylates

Supportive care, limiting drug absorption, and enhancing drug elimination are the goals of therapy. Resuscitative measures should be instituted when necessary. It is critically important to remember that, should endotracheal intubation be necessary, hyperventilation must be accomplished before, during, and after this procedure to prevent worsening acidemia, which increases the fraction of nonionized salicylic acid available for tissue distribution, thereby enhancing toxicity. The administration of respiratory depressants or failure to adequately hyperventilate unconscious or paralyzed patients can result in rapid deterioration and death of severely poisoned patients [52,56,78]. Because an increase in the partial pressure of carbon dioxide (PCO_2) is almost inevitable following intubation and mechanical ventilation, it is recommended that patients with arterial PCO_2 values below 20 mm Hg be given an intravenous bolus of 1 to 2 mEq per kg sodium bicarbonate at the time of intubation. Arterial blood gases should always be checked after intubation and after bicarbonate therapy.

Because CNS hypoglycemia may occur despite a normal serum glucose value [79], 50 mL of 50% dextrose in water should be given intravenously to any patient with an altered mental status whose capillary glucose concentration is not elevated [41]. Anticonvulsants (e.g., benzodiazepines, propofol, or barbiturates) as well as supplemental glucose should be given to patients with seizures. It is also prudent to administer sodium bicarbonate to patients who have seizures, as acidemia is likely to worsen. Hyperthermia should be treated with cooling blankets, ice packs, and evaporative methods (see Chapter 185).

Central venous pressure monitoring may be necessary for optimal treatment of hypotension, especially if there is evidence of heart failure or pulmonary edema. Patients with noncardiac pulmonary edema should be treated with positive pressure ventilation rather than diuretics. Again, maintaining hyperventilation and reducing acidemia are critical in patients with compromised pulmonary function.

Additional supportive measures are directed at correction of dehydration and metabolic derangements. The degree of dehydration parallels the severity of poisoning [54], but it is often unappreciated, underestimated, or undertreated. Patients with mild, moderate, or severe poisoning typically have volume deficits of 1 to 2, 3 to 4, or 5 to 6 L (20, 40, and 60 mL per kg in children), respectively. In the presence of acidemia, hypokalemia is more severe than indicated by the serum potassium level (by approximately 0.6 mEq per L for each 0.1 unit of decrease in pH) and should be treated accordingly.

Acidemia should also be treated aggressively with intravenous $NaHCO_3$. Since the respiratory alkalosis is a concomitant primary acid–base disturbance and not just a compensatory response, the administration of bicarbonate is unlikely to blunt the respiratory drive and increase the PCO_2, which might otherwise limit the change in serum pH. In addition, the goal of therapy is to limit the tissue distribution of salicylates by increasing the serum pH. The dose of bicarbonate needed may be substantial, and is typically 200 to 300 mEq in an adult with severe poisoning.

As with repleting volume, at least half of the $NaHCO_3$ deficit should be given during the first hour either by continuous infusion or by 0.5 to 1.0 mEq per kg boluses every 10 minutes. Arterial blood gases should be reevaluated during and after such therapy. Potential complications of $NaHCO_3$ administration include excessive alkalemia, hypokalemia, hypocalcemia, hypernatremia, and fluid overload. Relative contraindications to hypertonic $NaHCO_3$ include oliguric renal failure, congestive heart failure, and cerebral or pulmonary edema.

Tetany should be treated with intravenous calcium chloride or calcium gluconate (10 mL of a 10% solution over 5 to 10 minutes). Fresh-frozen plasma, red blood cell, and platelet transfusions may be required for patients with active bleeding or significant blood loss. Asymptomatic increases in international normalized ratio can be treated with subcutaneous vitamin K.

Gastrointestinal decontamination should be performed in all patients with intentional overdoses and those with accidental ingestions of greater than 150 mg per kg. Because of delayed absorption, decontamination may be effective for as long as 24 hours after overdose, even in patients with spontaneous vomiting [18]. Considerable diversity of opinion exists, however, regarding the optimal method of decontamination [80].

Activated charcoal is effective in preventing salicylate absorption and, therefore, it is recommended for all significant ingestions, regardless of delay in presentation. Multiple oral doses of charcoal [81] or gastric lavage preceded and followed by activated charcoal may be even more effective for preventing the absorption of large overdoses [82]. Many grams of aspirin have been recovered by lavage up to 24 hours after ingestion [18]. Repeated doses of activated charcoal or whole-bowel irrigation may be effective for patients who have ingested enteric-coated or sustained-release formulations and those with serum drug levels that continue to rise despite other decontamination measures [83].

The efficacy of multiple-dose charcoal therapy in enhancing salicylate elimination may depend on the formulation. Increases in serum salicylate elimination reported using an effervescent preparation containing bicarbonate [84] could not be replicated with multiple doses of noneffervescent charcoal in simulated overdose (i.e., less than 3 g) in humans [85–88]. Oral charcoal did not substantially accelerate the elimination of intravenously administered salicylic acid, discounting the role of gut dialysis or enterohepatic circulation [89]. If multiple-dose charcoal is used, sorbitol should not be included with the subsequent doses [90,91].

Salicylate elimination can be enhanced by urine alkalinization and diuresis [24,25,29,92], extracorporeal removal [93], and perhaps by glycine administration [44]. It should be emphasized that alkalinizing the serum and urine, and establishing a urine output of 1 to 2 mL/kg/h are critically important goals in the management of patients with salicylate toxicity [30,94]. Moreover, alkalinization of the urine is difficult to achieve in patients with acidemia and aciduria (i.e., severe clinical toxicity) [54]. Theoretical concerns regarding pulmonary or cerebral edema should not preclude aggressive fluid therapy, as administering only maintenance fluids intravenously is insufficient treatment for a patient with salicylate poisoning.

Indications for urine alkalinization and alkaline diuresis include acid–base abnormalities and systemic symptoms with a salicylate level that is greater than 30 mg per dL after an acute overdose. Patients with chronic overdoses may be symptomatic and require treatment at lower salicylate levels. The goal is to achieve a urine pH of 7.5 or greater. All patients treated with alkaline diuresis need close monitoring in an intensive care unit or step down setting. Bladder catheterization is essential in those with moderate or severe poisoning, as hourly monitoring of urine output and pH is required. Arterial or venous blood gases, electrolytes, BUN, creatinine, glucose, and salicylate concentrations should initially be rechecked at 2-hour intervals, depending on the severity of poisoning, the results of previous testing, and the response to therapy. Cardiac monitoring and frequent reevaluations of vital signs, mental status, and pulmonary function are also necessary during alkaline diuresis [94].

Alkalinization of the urine may be impossible to achieve in the presence of either dehydration or hypokalemia, because hydrogen ions are excreted in exchange for reabsorbed sodium and potassium, respectively [52]. Therefore, correction of fluid and potassium deficits is critical.

The amount of bicarbonate and supplementary potassium necessary to achieve and maintain an alkaline urine depends on the severity of poisoning (Table 122.2). For example, after 1 to 2 L of crystalloid by bolus, the initial intravenous fluids for a moderately poisoned adult could be 1 L over 2 hours of 5% dextrose in one-half normal saline to which 75 mEq of sodium bicarbonate (i.e., 1.5 ampules of 8.4% sodium bicarbonate) and 40 mEq of potassium chloride have been added. In severe poisoning, however, 150 mEq of sodium bicarbonate (i.e., 3 ampules of 8.4% sodium bicarbonate) and 60 mEq of potassium chloride should be added to each liter of 5% dextrose in water, and adjusted as necessary. In patients with hypernatremia, a more hypotonic solution should be used. Again, the use of a dextrose-containing solution is important because of the potential for occult CNS hypoglycemia. Although forced diuresis (e.g., 500 mL per hour urine output in adults) is no longer recommended [94,95], achieving a moderate diuresis (1 to 2 mL/kg/h) is recommended. While counterintuitive, even patients with mild poisoning (i.e., alkalemia) should be given bicarbonate (and fluids) to replace ongoing renal losses and prevent deterioration.

Carbonic anhydrase inhibitors (e.g., acetazolamide) should never be used to alkalinize the urine, because the resultant systemic acidosis may promote tissue distribution of salicylate and result in clinical deterioration [96,97]. Similarly, the use of tris-hydroxymethyl aminomethane, an organic H^+ buffer, to increase serum and urine pH is not recommended. Although tris-hydroxymethyl aminomethane has been suggested for the treatment of acidemia and aciduria refractory to bicarbonate administration, it has not been studied in human salicylate poisoning and has a number of potential adverse effects (e.g., hypoglycemia, extravasation necrosis, phlebitis, respiratory depression, and increased intracellular pH leading to decreased pH gradients with increased tissue distribution and intracellular trapping of salicylate) [98].

The complications of alkaline diuresis include excessive alkalemia, hypokalemia, hypocalcemia, hypernatremia, and fluid overload [44,94,95]. Young children, the elderly, and those with severe poisoning are most susceptible to such complications. Alkaline diuresis is contraindicated in patients with oliguric renal failure, congestive heart failure, and cerebral or pulmonary edema. Such therapy should be withheld or discontinued if the serum pH exceeds 7.55.

Hemodialysis is indicated in patients with severe poisoning and those with moderate poisoning who fail to improve with alkaline diuresis [30,31,43,44,52,93]. Hemodialysis is essential in patients with coma, seizures, cerebral or pulmonary edema, and renal failure [31,46]. Hemodialysis should also be strongly considered when patients demonstrate any impairment in the level of consciousness, rather than waiting for unresponsiveness or coma [93]. Acidemia and temperature greater than 38°C are associated with high mortality [46] and should also be considered potential indications for hemodialysis, particularly if the patient is resistant to bicarbonate and fluid therapy. Similarly, patients with moderate poisoning who have liver dysfunction and, hence, impaired ability to eliminate salicylate may also benefit from hemodialysis.

A high salicylate level is often cited as a stand-alone indication for hemodialysis but recommendations vary widely, with cutoffs ranging from 40 to 200 mg per dL (100 mg per dL being the most common) for acute ingestions and 60 to 80 mg per dL for chronic exposures [98]. A recent international multidisciplinary group "recommended" extracorporeal treatment when concentrations exceed 100 mg per dL, and "suggested" it for concentrations over 90 mg per dL, based on "very weak" evidence [93]. In one study [43], salicylate levels in fatal cases ranged from 34 to 193 mg per dL and in another [45], some patients died with drug levels in the therapeutic range. Moreover, drug levels do not discriminate patients who die from survivors [45,46]. Clearly, the salicylate level should not be used as the sole indication for hemodialysis. Instead, the severity of poisoning is determined by clinical findings, which reflect *tissue* drug concentration, and do not necessarily correspond to blood levels, especially when acidemia is present [96]. Moreover, a serum salicylate concentration should be interpreted in the context of a simultaneous measurement of serum pH. Hence, hemodialysis is appropriate for patients with high drug levels who have severe clinical toxicity (particularly acidemia), but it may not be necessary in those without such manifestations [46]. Conversely, patients with low salicylate levels, particularly those with significant underlying cardiorespiratory disease, should be treated with hemodialysis if they exhibit clinical or laboratory manifestations of severe toxicity. Because of delays inherent in the turnaround time for measuring salicylate and in preparing for hemodialysis, the projected clinical course should also be considered. Waiting for the salicylate level to reach some predetermined level before initiating hemodialysis in patients who are severely poisoned or deteriorating despite other treatments is ill-advised.

Hemodialysis is preferred over continuous renal replacement therapy or hemoperfusion due to the rapid clearances and correction of fluid, electrolyte, and acid–base abnormalities achieved [93,99]. Peritoneal dialysis and exchange transfusion are also less effective [100]. A high-bicarbonate (e.g., up to 40 mEq per L) dialysate solution (bath) should be used, and potassium should usually be added to the dialysate solution. Hemodialysis should be performed for at least 4 to 6 hours, and salicylate concentrations are below 20 mg per dL [93].

Failure to adequately correct fluid deficits prior to initiating hemodialysis can result in disastrous consequences. In contrast to the typical dialysis (i.e., renal failure) patient who is fluid overloaded, those with salicylate poisoning are typically hypovolemic. Uncorrected or occult hypovolemia can result in cardiovascular decompensation with hemodynamic instability, and even cardiac arrest, when dialysis is started because of the acute decrease in intravascular volume that can occur at the beginning of dialysis. This complication can be prevented or minimized by ensuring adequate volume resuscitation, and priming the tubing and pump with saline (rather than blood) prior to initiating dialysis.

Oral administration of glycine or *N*-glycylglycine has been used in overdose patients to promote drug clearance [23,101]. Because the conjugation of salicylic acid with glycine to form salicyluric acid becomes saturated and glycine levels decrease in overdose patients, supplemental glycine can enhance the formation and excretion of this metabolite. To date, clinical experience with this therapy is limited, its comparative efficacy is unknown, and the side effects of nausea and vomiting with glycine have been problematic. Doses used ranged from 8 g dissolved in water initially, followed by 4 g every 4 hours for 16 hours, to 20 g followed by 10 g every 2 hours for 10 hours for glycine. The dose for *N*-glycylglycine was 8 g dissolved in water followed by 2 to 4 g every 2 hours for 16 hours.

Other Nonsteroidal Anti-inflammatory Drugs

The treatment of nonsalicylate NSAID poisoning is supportive and symptomatic, and most patients require only observation. However, airway protection and mechanical ventilation, fluid resuscitation, anticonvulsants for seizures, bicarbonate for acidosis, and blood products for gastrointestinal tract bleeding may occasionally be required. Renal function should be monitored carefully in patients with abnormal urinalysis, underlying renal disease, or advanced age. Liver function tests should be followed in patients with severe phenylbutazone and piroxicam poisoning [66].

Gastrointestinal decontamination with activated charcoal should be considered for patients who present soon after a significant ingestion, defined as greater than ten therapeutic doses in adults and more than five adult doses in children [60,61]. Although charcoal hemoperfusion has been used to treat a patient with severe phenylbutazone poisoning who had impaired renal and hepatic function [64], extracorporeal elimination measures are unlikely to be effective because of the high-protein binding and rapid intrinsic elimination of these agents. Multiple-dose charcoal therapy enhances the elimination of therapeutic doses of phenylbutazone by 30% [102] and may be similarly effective for other agents, but the clinical benefit of such therapy after overdose is likely to be limited.

References

1. Mowry JB, Spyker DA, Cantilena LR Jr, et al: 2013 annual report of the American Association of Poison Control Centers' National Poison Data System (NPDS): 31st annual report. *Clin Toxicol (Phila)* 52:1032, 2014.
2. Brigden M, Smith RE: Acetylsalicylic-acid-containing drugs and nonsteroidal anti-inflammatory drugs available in Canada. *CMAJ* 156:1025, 1997.
3. McLoone P, Crombie IK: Hospitalisation for deliberate self-poisoning in Scotland from 1981 to 1993: trends in rates and types of drugs used. *Br J Psychiatry* 169:81, 1996.
4. Hawton K, Simkin S, Deeks J, et al: UK legislation on analgesic packs: before and after study of long term effect on poisonings. *BMJ* 329:1076–1081, 2004.
5. Smolinske SC, Hall AH, Vandenberg SA, et al: Toxic effects of nonsteroidal anti-inflammatory drugs in overdose: an overview of recent evidence on clinical effects and dose-response relationships. *Drug Saf* 5:252, 1990.
6. Veltri JC, Rollins DE: A comparison of the frequency and severity of poisoning cases for ingestion of acetaminophen, aspirin, and ibuprofen. *Am J Emerg Med* 6:104, 1988.
7. Patrono C, Garcia Rodriguez LA, Landolfi R, et al: Low-dose aspirin for the prevention of atherothrombosis. *N Engl J Med* 353:2373, 2005.
8. Bannwarth B, Demotes-Mainard F, Schaeverbeke T: Central analgesic effects of aspirin-like drugs. *Fundam Clin Pharmacol* 9:1, 1995.
9. Jouzeau J-Y, Terlain B, Abid A, et al: Cyclooxygenase isoenzymes. *Drugs* 53:563, 1997.
10. FitzGerald GA, Patrono C: The coxibs, selective inhibitors of cyclooxygenase-2. *N Engl J Med* 345:433, 2001.
11. Fitzgerald GA: Coxibs and cardiovascular disease. *N Engl J Med* 351:1709, 2004.
12. Cairns JA: The coxibs and traditional nonsteroidal anti-inflammatory drugs: a current perspective on cardiovascular risks. *Can J Cardiol* 23:125–131, 2007.
13. Arm JP, Auten KF: Leukotriene receptor and aspirin sensitivity. *N Engl J Med* 347:1524, 2002.
14. Gollapaudi RR, Teirstein PS, Stevenson DD, et al: Aspirin sensitivity: implications for patients with coronary artery disease. *JAMA* 292:3017, 2004.
15. Buchanan MR: Biological basis and clinical implications of acetylsalicylic acid resistance. *Can J Cardiol* 22:149–151, 2006.
16. Romsing J, Walther-Larsen S: Peri-operative use of nonsteroidal anti-inflammatory drugs in children: analgesic efficacy and bleeding. *Anaesthesia* 52:673, 1997.
17. Wortzman DJ, Grunfeld A: Delay absorption following enteric-coated aspirin overdose. *Ann Emerg Med* 16:434, 1987.
18. Matthew H, Mackintosh TF, Tompsett SL, et al: Gastric aspiration and lavage in acute poisoning. *Br Med J* 1:1333, 1966.
19. Drummond R, Kadri N, St-Cyr J: Delayed salicylate toxicity following enteric-coated acetylsalicylic acid overdose: a case report and review of the literature. *CJEM* 3:44, 2001.
20. Rubin GM, Tozer TN, Oie S: Concentration-dependence of salicylate distribution. *J Pharm Pharmacol* 35:115, 1983.
21. Snodgrass W, Rumack BH, Peterson RG, et al: Salicylate toxicity following therapeutic doses in young children. *Clin Toxicol* 18:247, 1981.
22. Levy G, Tsuchiya T: Salicylate accumulation kinetics in man. *N Engl J Med* 287:430, 1972.
23. Patel DK, Ogunbona A, Notarianni LJ, et al: Depletion of plasma glycine and effect of glycine by mouth on salicylate metabolism during aspirin overdose. *Hum Exp Toxicol* 9:389, 1990.
24. Morgan AG, Polak A: The excretion of salicylate in salicylate poisoning. *Clin Sci* 41:475, 1971.
25. Levy G: Pharmacokinetics of salicylate in man. *Drug Metab Rev* 9:3, 1979.
26. Garretson LK, Procknal JA, Levy G: Fetal acquisition and neonatal elimination of a large amount of salicylate. *Clin Pharmacol Ther* 17:98, 1975.
27. Segar WE, Holliday MA: Physiologic abnormalities of salicylate intoxication. *N Engl J Med* 259:1191, 1958.
28. Gabow PA, Anderson RJ, Potts DE, et al: Acid base disturbances in the salicylate intoxicated adult. *Arch Intern Med* 138:1481, 1978.
29. Temple AR: Acute and chronic effects of aspirin toxicity and their treatment. *Arch Intern Med* 141:364, 1981.
30. O'Malley GF: Emergency department management of the salicylate-poisoned patient. *Emerg Med Clin North Am* 25(2):333–346, 2007.
31. Lovejoy F: Aspirin and acetaminophen: a comparative view of their antipyretic and analgesic activity. *Pediatrics* 62[Suppl]:904, 1978.
32. Smith M: The metabolic basis of the major symptoms in acute salicylate intoxication. *Clin Toxicol (Phila)* 1:387, 1968.
33. Kuzak N, Brubacher JR, Kennedy JR: Reversal of salicylate-induced euglycemic delirium with dextrose. *Clin Toxicol (Phila)* 45:526–529, 2007.
34. Rauschka H, Aboul-Enein F, Bauer J, et al: Acute white matter damage in lethal salicylate intoxication. *Neurotoxicology* 28:33–37, 2007.
35. Davies NM, Watson MS: Clinical pharmacokinetics of sulindac: a dynamic old drug. *Clin Pharmacokinet* 32:437, 1997.
36. Roth SH: Nabumetone: a new NSAID for rheumatoid arthritis and osteoarthritis. *Orthop Rev* 21:223, 1992.
37. Laufen H, Leitold M: The effect of activated charcoal on the bioavailability of piroxicam in man. *Int J Clin Pharmacol Ther Toxicol* 24:48, 1986.
38. Turck D, Roth W, Busch U: A review of the clinical pharmacokinetics of meloxicam. *Br J Rheumatol* 35[Suppl 1]:13, 1996.
39. Linden CH, Townsend PL: Metabolic acidosis after acute ibuprofen overdosage. *J Pediatr* 111:922, 1987.
40. Done AK: Salicylate intoxication: significance of measurements of salicylates in blood in cases of acute ingestion. *Pediatrics* 26:800, 1960.
41. Dugandzic RM, Tierney MG, Dickinson GE, et al: Evaluation of the validity of the Done nomogram in the management of acute salicylate intoxication. *Ann Emerg Med* 18:1186, 1989.
42. Goudrealt P, Temple AR, Lovejoy FH: The relative severity of acute versus chronic salicylate poisonings in children: a clinical comparison. *Pediatrics* 70:566, 1982.

43. McGuigan MA: A two-year review of salicylate deaths in Ontario. *Arch Intern Med* 147:510, 1987.
44. Notarianni L: A reassessment of the treatment of salicylate poisoning. *Drug Saf* 7:292, 1992.
45. Thisted B, Krantz T, Shrom J, et al: Acute salicylate poisoning in 177 consecutive patients treated in ICU. *Acta Anaesthesiol Scand* 31:312, 1987.
46. Chapman BJ, Proudfoot AT: Adult salicylate poisoning: deaths and outcome in patients with high plasma salicylate concentrations. *Q J Med* 72:699, 1989.
47. Brubacher JR, Hoffman RS: Salicylism from topical salicylate: review of the literature. *J Toxicol Clin Toxicol* 34:431, 1996.
48. Watson JE, Tagupa ET: Suicide attempt by means of aspirin enema. *Ann Pharmacother* 28:467, 1994.
49. Clark JH, Wilson WG: A 16-day-old breast-fed infant with metabolic acidosis caused by salicylate. *Clin Pediatr (Phila)* 20:53, 1981.
50. Palatnick W, Tenebein M: Aspirin poisoning during pregnancy: increased fetal sensitivity. *Am J Perinatol* 15:39, 1998.
51. Buck ML, Grebe TA, Bond GR: Toxic reaction to salicylate in a newborn infant: similarities to neonatal sepsis. *J Pediatr* 122:955, 1993.
52. Yip L, Dart RC, Gabow PA: Concepts and controversies in salicylate toxicity. *Emerg Med Clin North Am* 12:351, 1994.
53. Leventhal LJ, Kuritsky L, Ginsberg R, et al: Salicylate-induced rhabdomyolysis. *Am J Emerg Med* 7:409, 1989.
54. Done AK: Aspirin overdosage: incidence, diagnosis and management. *Pediatrics* 62[Suppl]:890, 1978.
55. Montgomery H, Porter JC, Bradley RD: Salicylate intoxication causing a severe systemic inflammatory response and rhabdomyolysis. *Am J Emerg Med* 12:531, 1994.
56. Berk WA, Anderson JC: Salicylate-associated asystole: report of two cases. *Am J Med* 86:505, 1989.
57. Kent K, Ganetsky M, Cohen J, et al: Non-fatal ventricular dysrhythmias associated with severe salicylate toxicity. *Clin Toxicol (Phila)* 46:297–299, 2008.
58. Nigogi SK, Rieders R: Salicylate poisoning: differences in tissue levels and distribution between children and adults. *Eur J Toxicol* 2:234, 1969.
59. Anderson RJ, Potts DE, Gabow PA: Unrecognized adult salicylate intoxication. *Ann Intern Med* 85:745, 1976.
60. Vale JA, Meredith TS: Acute poisoning due to non-steroidal anti-inflammatory drugs: clinical features and management. *Med Toxicol* 1:12, 1986.
61. Court H, Volans GN: Poisoning after overdose with nonsteroidal anti-inflammatory drugs. *Adverse Drug React Acute Poisoning Rev* 3:1, 1984.
62. Forrester MB: Celecoxib exposures reported to Texas poison control centres from 1999 to 2004. *Hum Exp Toxicol* 25:261–266, 2006.
63. Balali-Mood M, Proudfoot AT, Critchley JA, et al: Mefenamic acid overdose. *Lancet* 1:1354, 1981.
64. Berlinger WG, Spector R, Flanigan MJ: Hemoperfusion for phenylbutazone poisoning. *Ann Intern Med* 96:334, 1982.
65. Strong JE, Wilson J, Douglas JF, et al: Phenylbutazone self-poisoning treated by charcoal haemoperfusion. *Anaesthesia* 34:1038, 1979.
66. Virji MA, Venkataraman SK, Lower DR, et al: Role of laboratory in the management of phenylbutazone poisoning. *J Toxicol Clin Toxicol* 41:1013–1024, 2003.
67. Hall AH, Smolinske SC, Conrad FL, et al: Ibuprofen overdose: 126 cases. *Ann Emerg Med* 15:1308, 1986.
68. Oker EE, Hermann L, Baum CR, et al: Serious toxicity in a young child due to ibuprofen. *Acad Emerg Med* 7:821, 2000.
69. Seifert SA, Brownstein AC, McGuire T: Massive ibuprofen ingestion with survival. *Clin Toxicol (Phila)* 38:55, 2000.
70. Bond GR, Curry SC, Arnold-Capell PA, et al: Generalized seizures and metabolic acidosis after ketoprofen overdose. *Vet Hum Toxicol* 31:369, 1989.
71. Martinez R, Smith DW, Frankel LR: Severe metabolic acidosis after acute naproxen sodium ingestion. *Ann Emerg Med* 18:1102, 1989.
72. Hoffman RJ, Nelson LS, Hoffman RS: Use of ferric chloride to identify salicylate-containing products. *J Toxicol Clin Toxicol* 40:547, 2002.
73. Duffens KR, Smilkstein MJ, Bessen HA, et al: Falsely elevated salicylate levels due to diflunisal overdose. *J Emerg Med* 5:499, 1987.
74. Bailey RB, Jones SR: Chronic salicylate intoxication: a common cause of morbidity in the elderly. *J Am Geriatr Soc* 37:556, 1989.
75. Chalasani N, Roman J, Jurado RL: Systemic inflammatory response syndrome caused by chronic salicylate intoxication. *South Med J* 89:479, 1996.
76. Quint PA, Allman FD: Differentiation of chronic salicylism for Reye's syndrome. *Pediatrics* 74:1117, 1984.
77. Osterloh J, Cunningham W, Dixon A, et al: Biochemical relationships between Reye's and Reye's-like metabolic and toxicological syndromes. *Med Toxicol Adverse Drug Exp* 4:272, 1989.
78. Greenberg MI, Hendrickson RG, Hoffman M: Deleterious effects of endotracheal intubation in salicylate poisoning. *Ann Emerg Med* 41:583, 2003.
79. Thurston J, Pollock PG, Warren SK, et al: Reduced brain glucose with normal plasma glucose in salicylate poisoning. *J Clin Invest* 49:2130, 1970.
80. Juurlink DN, McGuigan MA: Gastrointestinal decontamination for enteric-coated aspirin overdose: what to do depends on who you ask. *J Toxicol Clin Toxicol* 38:465, 2000.
81. Filippone G, Fish SS, Laconture PG, et al: Reversible adsorption (desorption) of aspirin from activated charcoal. *Arch Intern Med* 147:1390, 1987.
82. Burton GT, Bayer MJ, Barron L, et al: Comparison of activated charcoal and gastric lavage in the prevention of aspirin absorption. *J Emerg Med* 1:411, 1984.
83. Kirshenbaum LA, Mathews SC, Sitar DS, et al: Whole-bowel irrigation versus activated charcoal for the ingestion of modified-release pharmaceuticals. *Clin Pharmacol Ther* 46:264, 1989.
84. Hillman RJ, Prescott LF: Treatment of salicylate poisoning with repeated activated charcoal. *Br Med J (Clin Res Ed)* 291:1472, 1985.
85. Ho JL, Tierney MG, Dickinson GE: An elevation of the effect of repeated doses of oral activated charcoal on salicylate elimination. *J Clin Pharmacol* 29:366, 1989.
86. Kirshenbaum LA, Matthew SC, Sitar DS, et al: Does multiple-dose charcoal therapy enhance salicylate excretion? *Arch Intern Med* 150:1281, 1990.
87. Mayer AL, Sitar DS, Tenenbein M: Multiple-dose charcoal and whole bowel irrigation do not increase clearance of absorbed salicylate. *Arch Intern Med* 152:393, 1992.
88. Barone JA, Raia JJ, Huang YC: Evaluation of the effects of multiple-dose activated charcoal on the absorption of orally administered salicylate in a simulated toxic ingestion model. *Ann Emerg Med* 17:34, 1988.
89. Johnson D, Eppler J, Giesbrecht E, et al: Effect of multiple-dose activated charcoal on the clearance of high-dose intravenous aspirin in a porcine model. *Ann Emerg Med* 26:569, 1995.
90. Keller RE, Schwab RA, Krenzelok EP: Contribution of sorbitol combined with activated charcoal in prevention of salicylate absorption. *Ann Emerg Med* 19:654, 1990.
91. Gren J, Woolf A: Hypermagnesemia associated with catharsis in a salicylate-intoxicated patient with anorexia nervosa. *Ann Emerg Med* 18:200, 1989.
92. Prescott LF, Balali-Mood M, Critchley JA, et al: Diuresis or urinary alkalinization for salicylate poisoning? *Br Med J (Clin Res Ed)* 285:1383, 1982.
93. Juurlink DN, Gosselin S, Kielstien JT, et al: Extracorporeal treatment for salicylate poisoning: systematic review and recommendations from the EXTRIP workgroup. *Ann Emerg Med* 66:165, 2015.
94. Proudfoot AT, Krenzelok EP, Vale JA: Position paper on urine alkalinization. *J Toxicol Clin Toxicol* 42:1, 2004.
95. Lawson AA, Proudfoot AT, Brown SS, et al: Forced diuresis in the treatment of acute salicylate poisoning in adults. *Q J Med* 38:31, 1969.
96. Hill JB: Experimental salicylate poisoning: observations on the effects of altering blood pH on tissue and plasma salicylate concentrations. *Pediatrics* 47:658, 1971.
97. Sweeney K, Chapron D, Brandt L, et al: Toxic interaction between acetazolamide and salicylate: case reports and a pharmacokinetic explanation. *Clin Pharmacol Ther* 40:518, 1986.
98. Yip L, Jastremski MS, Dart RD: Salicylate intoxication. *J Intensive Care Med* 12:66, 1997.
99. Goodman JW, Goldfarb DS: The role of continuous renal replacement therapy in the treatment of poisoning. *Semin Dial* 19:402–407, 2006.
100. Schlegel RJ, Altstatt LB, Canales L, et al: Peritoneal dialysis for severe salicylism: an evaluation of indications and results. *J Pediatr* 69:553, 1966.
101. Muhlebach S, Steger P, Conen D, et al: Successful therapy of salicylate poisoning using glycine and activated charcoal. *Schweizer Med Wochenschr* 126:2127, 1996.
102. Neuvonen PJ, Elonen E: Effect of activated charcoal on absorption and elimination of phenobarbitone, carbamazepine, and phenylbutazone in man. *Eur J Clin Pharmacol* 17:51, 1980.

Chapter 123 ■ Sedative-Hypnotic Agent Poisoning

ANDIS GRAUDINS • DINO DRUDA

Sedative-hypnotics include benzodiazepines (BZDs), barbiturates, non-BZD/nonbarbiturate agents (NBNBs). In the 1960s, NBNBs, such as meprobamate, were introduced and became popular. NBNBs have been mostly supplanted by BZDs, which have greater efficacy and a larger therapeutic ratio, and are currently one of the most widely prescribed classes of drug (Table 123.1). BZDs and their derivatives are used to treat anxiety, depression, panic disorders, insomnia, musculoskeletal disorders, seizures, and alcohol withdrawal, and are used as adjuncts for anesthesia and procedural sedation. The chronic use of all sedative-hypnotics can result in physical tolerance, addiction, misuse, and withdrawal syndromes on abrupt cessation of therapy. Withdrawal syndromes are discussed in Chapter 126.

TABLE 123.1

Sedative-Hypnotic Agents

Benzodiazepines
Alprazolam
Bromazepam
Brotizolam
Chlordiazepoxide
Clobazam
Clorazepate
Diazepam
Estazolam
Flunitrazepam
Flurazepam
Halazepam
Lorazepam
Midazolam
Nitrazepam
Oxazepam
Quazepam
Triazolam
Barbiturates
Amobarbital
Aprobarbital
Butalbital
Mephobarbital
Pentobarbital
Phenobarbital
Secobarbital
Thiopental
Nonbenzodiazepine nonbarbiturates
Alpidem
Baclofen
Buspirone
Chloral hydrate
Chlormethiazole
Ethinamate
Ethchlorvynol
Glutethimide
Meprobamate
Methaqualone
Methyprylon
Paraldehyde
Zolpidem

BENZODIAZEPINES

Pharmacology

BZDs exert their therapeutic effect at specific BZD receptor sites in the central nervous system (CNS). The BZD receptor is located within the γ-aminobutyric acid-A (GABA-A) receptor supra-molecular complex (GRSMC). Binding of GABA or GABA plus a BZD causes an allosteric change in the GRSMC. This results in an increase in the frequency of chloride channel opening, with a resultant increase in chloride flux and hyperpolarization. Activation of GRSMC by a BZD potentiates synaptic GABA-mediated inhibition [1]. These GRSMCs are located throughout the brain and spinal cord. GABA is an inhibitory neurotransmitter, and activation of GABA neurons leads primarily to inhibition of dopamine release, although norepinephrine and acetylcholine are also affected. The effect on serotonin release is minimal.

BZD absorption from the gastrointestinal (GI) tract depends on the properties and pharmaceutical formulation of each drug. Peak serum concentration commonly results within 3 hours post-ingestion; intramuscular absorption varies from agent to agent but can be erratic and delayed. Duration of action is dependent on the lipophilicity of each compound: the more lipophilic, the shorter the duration of action. BZDs are highly protein-bound (85% to 99%). Their volume of distribution depends on lipid solubility and varies from 0.26 to 0.58 L per kg for chlordiazepoxide to 0.95 to 2.00 L per kg for diazepam. BZDs are primarily metabolized in the liver by CYP3A4 and then glucuronidated. Metabolism may be reduced by CYP3A4 inhibitors such as fluoxetine [2]. BZDs can be classified on the basis of elimination half-life (Table 123.2).

Fatality from pure BZD overdose is rare. Toxicity is dose-dependent and may vary between individual agents. Alprazolam overdose, in particular, results in more frequent intensive care unit admission, mechanical ventilation, and flumazenil use than other BZDs [3]. A retrospective review of 1,239 overdoses from one medical examiner's office revealed only two deaths solely related to diazepam overdose [4]. For chronic abusers, rapid clinical recovery after BZD overdose results from adaptation or tolerance to the depressant effects [5].

Clinical Presentation

Overdose commonly occurs as a part of multidrug and or ethanol ingestion. BZDs alone produce slurred speech, lethargy, ataxia, amnesia, nystagmus, and coma. Loss of deep tendon reflexes and apnea are unusual except with a massive overdose. Complications such as pulmonary aspiration, hypoxic cardiac arrest, and acute lung injury are also possible, but are more likely to occur in mixed sedative ingestions.

Diagnostic Evaluation

Recommended laboratory studies include serum electrolytes, creatinine, and glucose. Because BZDs may be involved in a

TABLE 123.2

Duration of Action and Elimination Half-Life (t½) of Benzodiazepines

Agent	Duration (h)	Elimination t½(h)	Peak effect (h)	Active metabolites
Ultra-short–acting	<10			
Midazolam (Versed)		2–5	0.3–0.8	–
Temazepam (Restoril)		10	2–3	–
Triazolam (Halcion)		1.7–3.0	0.5–1.5	+
Brotizolam		5	1	–
Short-acting	10–24			
Alprazolam (Xanax)		11–14	0.7–1.6	+
Lorazepam (Ativan)		10–20	2	–
Oxazepam (Serax)		3–21	1–2	–
Bromazepam		8–20	1–2	–
Flunitrazepam		20–30	2–8	+
Estazolam		10–24	1	–
Long-acting	>24	5–30	2–4	+
Chlordiazepoxide (Librium)		36–200	1.0–2.5	+
Clorazepate (Tranxene)		10–50	1–4	–
Clonazepam (Klonopin)		20–50	1–2	+
Diazepam (Valium)		50–100	3–6	+
Flurazepam (Dalmane)		26–200	6	+
Quazepam		11–77	1–3	+
Clobazam		14	1–3	+
Halazepam		Metabolites: 50–100		+
Prazepam (Centrax)		25–41 Metabolites: 40–114	6	+

multidrug overdose, serum acetaminophen concentration and a 12-lead electrocardiogram should also be obtained. Qualitative urine drug screening using immunoassay techniques has limitations in detecting the presence of certain BZDs. Immunoassay technologies are based upon competitive binding between an antibody and antigen. The antibodies used are usually sensitive and specific for a certain drug, which for BZD immunoassays is commonly oxazepam. However, many BZDs do not form oxazepam or similar metabolites during metabolism and may be missed by screening [6]. As a result, it is important to know what screening immunoassay a laboratory uses for urine drug screening, as this will list which agents can and cannot be detected. Quantitative serum BZD concentration estimation is not useful in the clinical management of overdose.

Management

The most important aspect of BZD overdose management is supportive care. Airway management should precede all interventions, and intubation is indicated if the patient cannot adequately maintain spontaneous ventilation or protect the airway. Vascular access should be established. The patient should be placed on continuous pulse oximetry and cardiac monitoring. Activated charcoal (1 g per kg) administration in simple BZD intoxication is unlikely to be of benefit and may be harmful in patients who are initially awake and subsequently become sedated if the airway is unprotected. The risks of charcoal administration to a sedated patient with isolated BZD ingestion must be weighed against the low risk of morbidity and mortality seen with this poisoning. There is no evidence that repeat-dose charcoal enhances BZD elimination [7].

Flumazenil (Romazicon, Anexate) is a BZD antagonist that binds to the GRSMC competitively inhibiting BZD binding and thereby reversing BZD sedative and anxiolytic effects [8]. The effect on BZD-induced respiratory depression is less predictable and it cannot be relied upon to maintain adequate respiratory effort. Flumazenil does not fully reverse the amnestic effects of BZDs. Patients may appear awake and alert, but subsequent recall (e.g., of instructions) may be poor.

For most patients with pure BZD poisoning, supportive care with attention to airway and ventilatory status is all that is required to manage their overdose. It is uncommon for patients to require administration of flumazenil to treat sedation alone. This agent should never be considered in place of airway intervention in compromised patients. As BZDs are most commonly part of multidrug ingestions, flumazenil use is rarely indicated. Adverse drug events associated with flumazenil use include anxiety, nausea, agitation, and crying. It should particularly be avoided in patients suspected to be BZD-tolerant [9]. Flumazenil may precipitate an abrupt withdrawal syndrome with potential for seizures in these patients. This may occur after short-term use of BZDs [10]. Flumazenil should also be avoided in patients with suspected multidrug ingestion where reversal of BZD effect may unmask the epileptogenic effects of the other drugs (e.g., cyclic antidepressants, isoniazid, or cocaine). Flumazenil is especially contraindicated in patients with electrocardiographic evidence of sodium channel blockade (e.g., cyclic antidepressant poisoning) with prolonged QRS duration. Flumazenil has been suggested as a diagnostic tool for undifferentiated coma and after iatrogenic toxicity. Despite this, its role and indications remain unclear in the management of the BZD-poisoned patient. Flumazenil use does not reduce hospital length of stay or the need for high-dependency monitoring. The response to flumazenil is titratable. If administering flumazenil, the initial dose should be small (0.05 to 0.1 mg). This can be repeated at 30-second intervals. In general, if there is no response after a total dose of 1 mg, the diagnosis of BZD poisoning is unlikely. The aim of therapy is to give enough to have the patient moderately drowsy and easily aroused and *not* to have the patient awake, alert, and keen to self-discharge from hospital. Flumazenil has a short half-life (approximately 50 minutes); it may be administered as an infusion in severe BZD poisoning, in a fashion similar to naloxone in severe opioid poisoning. Seizures that result from flumazenil therapy may require large doses of BZDs or barbiturates such as thiopental or phenobarbital.

BARBITURATES

Since the development of BZDs and other newer sedative-hypnotics, the prescription of barbiturates and the incidence of severe poisoning has declined. However, as recently as 2011, barbiturates were still in the top 20 most common classes of drugs associated with fatality in the United States [11]. The recommendation that pentobarbital is a good drug for euthanasia in pro-euthanasia resources may also be leading to an increase in self-poisonings with barbiturates obtained illicitly for this purpose [12].

Pharmacology

Barbiturates depress the activity of all excitable tissues. They enhance GABA post-excitatory inhibition and have a binding site on the GABA-A receptor complex, leading to increased chloride flux by increasing the duration of chloride channel opening.

Barbiturates are available in all forms and are classified according to their duration of action. Ultra-short–acting barbiturates are highly lipid soluble and rapidly partition into the CNS, with subsequent redistribution to all tissues. When parenterally administered, they have rapid onset with less than 1-hour duration of effect; their predominant role is for induction of anesthesia. Short- and intermediate-acting barbiturates are intermediate in lipid solubility and are used as anxiolytics and sedatives. Long-acting barbiturates have relatively low lipid solubility and are mainly used as anticonvulsants. Systemic toxicity tends to be a function of the drug's elimination half-life (Table 123.3).

Barbiturates are well absorbed from the GI tract; serum concentration and symptoms are detectable within 30 minutes, and their peak effect occurs by 4 hours. Barbiturates are variably metabolized by the liver. Most of the highly lipid-soluble metabolites are renally excreted after glucuronidation. Barbiturates induce microsomal enzymes and increase the metabolism of medications that are CYP substrates. This includes barbiturates themselves resulting in auto-induction of metabolism, which contributes to tolerance. The longer acting barbiturates rely more on urinary excretion for elimination (phenobarbital, 25% to 33%; barbital, 95%; primidone, 15% to 42%; phenylethylmalonamide a metabolite of primidone, 95%). Renal elimination can be enhanced by urinary alkalinization as they are weak acids. The kinetics of barbiturate elimination are mixed: first order at low concentrations and zero order at high ones [13]. Therapeutic serum drug concentration is between 10 and 40 μg per mL for phenobarbital and 1 to 5 μg per mL for the short-acting barbiturates. Toxic dose is in the range of 6 to 10 g for the long-acting barbiturates and 3 to 6 g for the

TABLE 123.3

Duration of Action and Elimination Half-Life (t½) of Barbiturates

Barbiturate	Duration (h)	Elimination t½ (h)
Ultra-short–acting	<½	
Thiopental (Pentothal)		6–46
Thiamylal (Surital)		NA
Methohexital (Brevital)		1–2
Short-acting	3	
Hexobarbital (Sombulex)		3–7
Pentobarbital (Nembutal)		15–48
Secobarbital (Seconal)		19–34
Intermediate-acting	3–6	
Amobarbital (Amytal)		8–42
Aprobarbital (Alurate)		14–34
Butabarbital (Butisol)		34–42
Butalbital (Fiorinal, Esgic)		NA
Long-acting	6–12	
Barbital		48
Mephobarbital (Mebaral)		48–52
Phenobarbital (Luminal)		24–144
Primidone (Mysoline)		10–12

NA, not available.
Adapted from: Harves SC: Hypnotics and sedatives, in Goodman L, Gilman A (eds): *The Pharmacological Basis of Therapeutics.* 8th ed. New York, NY, Macmillan, 1990, p 357.

short-acting ones. Most patients demonstrate some degree of sedation after ingestion of more than 8 mg per kg. Tolerance rapidly develops, and chronic users may require 5 to 10 times the normal dose for sedation. Depending on the degree of tolerance, the drug concentration associated with coma ranges from 80 to 120 μg per mL for phenobarbital and 15 to 50 μg per mL for short-acting agents. Other sedative drug ingestions can have an additive effect and result in toxicity at lower doses and blood concentrations [14].

Clinical Manifestations

The most common toxic scenario results from accidental or intentional oral barbiturate overdose. When barbiturates are combined with other sedative medications or alcohol, additive CNS and respiratory depressive effects make overdose more serious. The primary effect is on the CNS, with onset of sedation within 30 minutes. This rapidly progresses to respiratory depression and coma in larger overdoses. Barbiturates suppress the medullary respiratory center and produce respiratory depression [15]. Cardiovascular toxicity can occur after large overdoses. It is caused by direct depression of the medullary centers, direct myocardial suppression, and peripheral vasodilatation. These combine to cause hypotension and cardiovascular collapse. Cardiac dysrhythmias are rare. Hypothermia may result from loss of autonomic function and decrease in overall muscle activity. The gut becomes atonic. Bullous skin lesions (known as "barb blisters") can occur over pressure points in up to 6% of patients [16]. These are tense bullous lesions containing acellular fluid with detectable amounts of barbiturate. Bullae formation, although common for severe barbiturate poisoning, is not pathognomonic for this poisoning. Bullae formation is also reported in cases of poisoning from other toxicants including carbon monoxide,

BZDs, tricyclic antidepressants, phenothiazines, and opioids [17]. Crystalluria is reported following primidone overdose.

Diagnostic Evaluation

Serum phenobarbital concentrations should be measured in poisoning with phenobarbital or primidone. Assay results for detection of other serum barbiturate concentrations are not usually available in a clinically useful timeframe. Other recommended investigations include complete blood cell count, serum electrolytes, renal function studies, creatinine phosphokinase, glucose and liver function tests. An ECG should also be obtained. As barbiturates may be involved in multidrug overdoses, and reliable history may not be available in the case of an unconscious patient, a serum acetaminophen concentration should be measured to exclude occult ingestion. Urinalysis, blood gas analysis, imaging, and lumbar puncture should be considered as clinically indicated.

Management

The mainstay of management following barbiturate overdose is supportive care. Early attention to airway management and ventilation is imperative as up to 40% of patients can develop pulmonary aspiration. Frequent monitoring of vital signs, including temperature, is indicated. Vascular access should be obtained, and the patient should be placed on continuous pulse oximetry and cardiac monitoring. GI decontamination with a dose of activated charcoal (1 g per kg) should be considered in large ingestions in patients with airway protection. Hypotension is initially treated with intravenous crystalloid loading. Because of the multifactorial nature of hypotension, vasopressors or inotropes may be required to treat hypotension unresponsive to fluid challenge. Bedside echocardiography or invasive hemodynamic monitoring can guide choice of vasoactive medications. Hypothermic patients require rewarming.

There is no specific antidote for barbiturate overdose. However, treatments that enhance the elimination of barbiturates should be considered in severe poisoning, with the aim of reducing the duration of coma, requirement for ventilatory support, and reduce cardiovascular instability.

Urinary alkalinization and multidose activated charcoal (MDAC) enhance the elimination of phenobarbital and possibly other barbiturates. In a human volunteer study, MDAC alone was more effective than urinary alkalinization or a combination of the two treatments in decreasing plasma phenobarbital concentrations and reducing plasma half-life. This was associated with greater total body clearance than seen with no treatment [18]. In a joint position statement from the American and European toxicology associations, it was determined that urinary alkalinization could not be recommended as first-line treatment for phenobarbital ingestions as MDAC is more effective [19]. In a position statement regarding MDAC, the same organizations recommend that this should be administered when a life-threatening amount of phenobarbital is ingested [7].

Other options for enhanced elimination of barbiturates are extracorporeal methods. In a systematic review of enhanced elimination techniques in barbiturate poisoning, primidone was amenable to enhanced elimination by MDAC. However, despite extracorporeal removal increasing the clearance of short-acting barbiturates to some degree, the clinical utility is limited [20]. The EXTRIP group recommends that extracorporeal treatments be considered for severe long-acting barbiturate poisoning (e.g., phenobarbital) when life-threatening toxicity is present [15]. However, extracorporeal treatments are not as effective in short-acting barbiturate poisoning. The recommended modality is intermittent hemodialysis. If this is not available, then hemoperfusion or continuous renal replacement therapy is the acceptable alternative. Suggested indications for dialysis include prolonged coma, persistent shock despite fluid resuscitation, ongoing toxicity despite MDAC, rising barbiturate concentrations despite MDAC, and if respiratory depression necessitating mechanical ventilation is present. Dialysis should be ceased when there is evidence of clinical improvement. Treating clinicians should be aware of the potential for rebound toxicity, and for precipitation of withdrawal after dialysis in barbiturate-dependent patients [20].

Importantly, following barbiturate poisoning, there is potential for full recovery with good supportive care, despite the presence of prolonged coma, and an isoelectric EEG. Any decision to withdraw care should involve a multidisciplinary approach with input from neurology and toxicology services as available and confirmation that the serum barbiturate concentration is undetectable.

NONBENZODIAZEPINE, NONBARBITURATE SEDATIVE-HYPNOTICS

NBNB sedative-hypnotics include glutethimide (Doriden), ethchlorvynol (Placidyl), meprobamate (Miltown), chloral hydrate (Noctec), and the antispasmodic muscle relaxants carisoprodol (Soma) and baclofen (Lioresal). Toxic effects can be seen from legitimate and illicit use. Newer agents have also been introduced that vary in their toxicity in overdose. These include buspirone, which binds to 5-hydroxytryptamine receptors; zopiclone, a cyclopyrrolone with sedative-hypnotic activity; and zolpidem, which is an imidazopyridine sedative-hypnotic and anxiolytic agent. All of these medications have a high abuse potential secondary to their ability to induce tolerance and dependence.

Chloral Hydrate

Chloral hydrate has been used as a sedative-hypnotic drug since the mid to late nineteenth century. It is still used in pediatric patients for procedural sedation, often in outpatient settings, with ongoing incidence of toxicity and fatality [21]. Chloral hydrate is rapidly absorbed from the GI tract, with onset of action within 30 minutes. It is rapidly metabolized in the liver by alcohol dehydrogenase to the active metabolite trichloroethanol (TCE), which is primarily responsible for its sedative properties. However, alcohol dehydrogenase is inhibited by fomepizole. Increased sedation is seen when chloral hydrate is administered in animal studies suggesting that the parent compound is more sedative than TCE [22]. Chloral hydrate and ethanol influence each other's metabolism in a number of ways. Chloral hydrate competes with ethanol for alcohol dehydrogenase, thereby prolonging the effect of ethanol. Also, the metabolism of ethanol generates nicotinamide adenine dinucleotide (NADH), which is needed as a cofactor to metabolize chloral hydrate to TCE [23]. TCE is further metabolized, either by glucuronidation to inactive urocholic acid, or by oxidation to trichloroacetic acid, which is also inactive. The elimination half-life of TCE is 4 to 12 hours. Metabolism of TCE changes with age, primarily due to the immaturity of the glucuronidation pathway in neonates. The elimination half-life of TCE is three to four times longer in neonates and infants than it is in older children [23]. This has clinical implications for neonates, especially if chloral hydrate is administered in a multiple dose regimen. It is thought that the metabolism of TCE is saturable at high doses, prolonging elimination further [24].

The usual dose of chloral hydrate in children is 25 to 100 mg per kg. Significant toxicity in children is reported with doses of 1.5 g and survival reported with doses as high as 38 g. For adults, toxicity is seen after more than 2 g, with serious toxicity and death possible with doses greater than 10 g [24]. Survival is reported in adults following ingestion of as much as 70 g, with significant toxicity requiring intensive care support and extracorporeal elimination [25].

Clinical features of toxicity from chloral hydrate overdose develop rapidly following ingestion. Patients may exhibit a characteristic pear-like odor. CNS effects of poisoning manifest as drowsiness, coma, hypothermia and respiratory depression. Pupils may initially be small, but in deep coma, may become dilated. GI effects from mucosal irritation can lead to gastritis, nausea and vomiting with risk of pulmonary aspiration. The most serious manifestation of toxicity is cardiovascular instability. Resistant ventricular tachyarrhythmias are seen and frequently result in death following overdose [24]. Chloral hydrate shortens the refractory period and depresses contractility of the myocardium. There is also an increased sensitivity of the myocardium to catecholamines, a property common to other halogenated hydrocarbons. Dysrhythmias reported include multifocal premature ventricular ectopic beats, supraventricular dysrhythmias, and ventricular dysrhythmias [24,26].

The treatment of chloral hydrate overdose is primarily supportive. All patients with a suspected ingestion should have intravenous access, continuous pulse oximetry, and cardiac monitoring. Hypothermia can be treated with passive rewarming. Activated charcoal (1g per kg) should be administered to patients with significant ingestions and appropriate airway protection. Chloral hydrate is radiopaque, and large ingested amounts may be seen on abdominal radiographs. Airway support and ventilation should be instituted as clinically indicated. Cardiac arrhythmias may not respond to standard antiarrhythmic agents such as lidocaine. β-Blockers, such as propranolol, have been used to successfully terminate refractory arrhythmias [24,27]. A suggested dosage regimen is an intravenous loading dose of 1 to 2 mg propranolol followed by an infusion of 1 to 2 mg per hour [24,27]. Alternatively, in situations/countries where parenteral propranolol is no longer available, a shorter acting agent such as esmolol can be considered. In cases of massive overdose with ongoing coma, refractory arrhythmias, or hypotension, enhanced elimination with hemodialysis and hemoperfusion have been used to clear TCE in particular [25].

Ethchlorvynol

Ethchlorvynol is a hypnotic with muscle relaxant and anticonvulsant activities. Clinical effects are apparent within 15 to 30 minutes, and peak serum concentration is seen in 1 to 2 hours. Ethchlorvynol is highly lipid soluble and is stored in adipose tissue and the brain. It has a unique half-life, being 10 to 25 hours with therapeutic ingestion but up to 100 hours in very large overdoses. Ninety percent of the drug is metabolized by the liver. The patient presents with an altered sensorium ranging from dizziness to facial tingling, giddiness, excitement, dysarthria, ataxia, mydriasis, nystagmus, or areflexia after smaller doses. Severe overdose is characterized by profound and prolonged coma (more than 1 week), hypothermia, respiratory depression, hypotension, and bradycardia. Comatose patients may have an isoelectric electroencephalogram. Seizures are also reported after acute ethchlorvynol ingestion. A sometimes diagnostically useful property of ethchlorvynol is its aromatic and quite pungent odor, described as similar to that of a new car or plastic shower curtain. This may be detected on the patient's breath.

Overdose treatment is supportive. Hemoperfusion effectively clears the drug. However, redistribution to lipid stores means that repeated hemoperfusion may be necessary because of post-dialysis rebound in serum concentrations.

Glutethimide

The toxic dose of glutethimide is more than 3.0 g, with a usual fatal dose being 10 to 20 g. Glutethimide is highly lipid soluble and displays two-compartment kinetics, with rapid uptake to the brain, followed by systemic distribution. GI glutethimide absorption is erratic, and onset of action is 20 to 30 minutes. Glutethimide is metabolized in the liver to an active metabolite, 4-hydroxy-2-ethyl-2-phenylglutarimide [28], which has a longer duration of action and is more potent than the parent compound [29]. It also stimulates induction of CYP2D6 and has considerable anticholinergic activity.

Signs of acute glutethimide overdose are similar to those seen with barbiturate poisoning. Profound and prolonged coma may result. A unique aspect of acute glutethimide intoxication is a fluctuating level of consciousness [29]. The reason for this is unclear, but theories include enterohepatic recirculation of the parent drug and its metabolites, prolonged absorption of the parent compound from anticholinergic-induced paralytic ileus, and redistribution from adipose stores. Increased intracranial pressure, seizures, areflexia, and muscular twitching may be evident. Hypotension, hypothermia, persistent acidosis, and cardiac arrest have all been reported [29]. The chronic use of glutethimide leads to tolerance and addiction. The mainstay of treatment for glutethimide poisoning is supportive care. Because there may be a significant anticholinergic-induced delay in gastric emptying, late administration of activated charcoal may be effective. Treatment with MDAC may increase glutethimide and 4-hydroxy-2-ethyl-2-phenylglutarimide elimination because of enterohepatic circulation. Case reports suggest that charcoal hemoperfusion may hasten recovery from coma, but this has never been examined in a controlled fashion [30].

Carisoprodol and Meprobamate

Carisoprodol (Soma, Rela) is a congener of meprobamate used as a muscle relaxant. Carisoprodol is metabolized in the liver and excreted in the urine, with an elimination half-life of 4 to 6 hours. Some of the ingested dose is metabolized to meprobamate by CYP2C19. The predominant side effect of the drug is drowsiness. Rarely seen idiosyncratic reactions include asthenia, transient quadriplegia, dizziness, ataxia, diplopia, agitation, confusion, and disorientation. Its toxicity and treatment are otherwise similar to those of meprobamate [31].

Meprobamate (e.g., Equanil, Miltown) is an unusual member of this class of medication. It has antianxiety and muscle-relaxant effects in addition to sedative properties. Meprobamate is available in regular and sustained-release formulations. Toxicity is seen after ingestion of as little as 2 g and fatalities with as little as 12 g [32]. Survival is reported with doses as high as 40 g.

Meprobamate is rapidly and completely absorbed after an oral dose [32]. Peak effect is seen in 3 hours, with a half-life of 10 hours. Most patients feel an effect for up to 36 hours. The drug is largely metabolized in the liver by CYP3A4 and its inactive metabolites are excreted in the urine. Very little of the drug is plasma protein-bound.

The clinical picture of meprobamate poisoning is similar to that of the other medications in this class, with predominately CNS and respiratory function impairment [32]. Hypotension is mediated by a fall in systemic vascular resistance. A persistently elevated serum concentration indicates ongoing drug absorption from bezoar formation. A concentration greater than 2.05 mg per L is associated with CNS depression and coma. Treatment of meprobamate poisoning is similar to that for the other medications in this class. MDAC may be of value after large ingestions because of potential for gastric concretion formation [33]. Hemoperfusion hastens drug clearance and should be considered in patients with cardiovascular compromise or failure to improve despite aggressive supportive treatment.

Baclofen

Although usually not considered a sedative or hypnotic drug, baclofen (Lioresal) toxicity mimics that of sedative-hypnotics, and treatment is similar. Baclofen is a synthetic analogue of GABA, and acts as a potent inhibitor of GABA-B neurons, especially in the spine; this has led to it being widely used as an antispasmodic agent to treat various neurologic conditions. Recently, baclofen is increasingly used for the management of alcohol misuse disorders. Baclofen can be administered either orally or intrathecally via programmable implanted infusion pumps, which avoids unwanted systemic side effects.

Following oral ingestion, baclofen is well absorbed from the GI tract, with peak plasma concentration reached within 2 hours. Baclofen is renally eliminated, with only a small portion hepatically transformed. Elimination is by first-order elimination kinetics, with a half-life of 2 to 6 hours after therapeutic dosing.

Baclofen toxicity following intrathecal delivery is predominantly associated with the refilling process, pump programming errors, or problems with dose titration. Overdosing resulting from pump malfunction is less common [34].

Clinical features of toxicity are similar following oral or intrathecal overdose, apart from a latent period following oral ingestion as plasma concentrations reach their peak. Signs include seizures, myoclonus, delirium, altered conscious state, coma, apnea, and hypothermia. Hypotension and hypertension are both reported [35]. Cardiac effects including prolongation of PR and QT intervals, blocked premature atrial contractions, and junctional escape beats may also occur [36]. Bradycardia or tachycardia can occur. Coma can be deep and prolonged for up to a week, with unreactive pupils and near-absent brainstem reflexes, mimicking brain death. Ingested doses of greater than 200 mg are associated with a higher incidence of delirium and coma requiring mechanical ventilation as well as increased hospital length of stay [37].

Management of baclofen toxicity is supportive. It is reasonable to consider the early use of a single dose of 50 g activated charcoal in patients with a protected airway, especially if more than 200 mg baclofen was ingested. Hypotension may respond to intravenous crystalloid bolus. BZDs should be used to control seizures or myoclonus, while being aware that they will contribute to further respiratory or CNS depression. In toxicity caused by intrathecal baclofen misadventure, specific steps may help reduce the drug burden. The specialist physician monitoring the therapy should be alerted as soon as possible, and the pump should be stopped and programming interrogated for errors. Cerebrospinal fluid can be drained, either via lumbar puncture or through the pump reservoir. Physostigmine has been used as an antidote for coma in cases of intrathecal baclofen toxicity. Reports of efficacy are mixed and it is not routinely recommended [34]. The baclofen infusion should not be ceased for more than 48 hours, as this may cause damage to the pump system and lead to a withdrawal syndrome [34].

Mechanical ventilation may be required for several days in deeply comatose patients and baclofen intoxication can mimic brain death [37].

Buspirone

Buspirone is an anxiolytic drug, which is a partial agonist at serotonin receptors (5-HT_{1A}). It also has moderate antagonist effects at central dopamine receptors [38]. It also has central acetylcholine and norepinephrine-mediated effects. The mechanism of action is not completely understood. At low doses, it is predominately anxiolytic, although it may take several weeks to reach this effect. At high doses, it can cause sedation similar to that seen with BZDs (20 mg per day). However, the sedation is much less than that seen with an equivalent dose of the BZD. It is well absorbed orally, and peak serum concentration is seen within an hour. It is hepatically metabolized, undergoing oxidative dealkylation by CYP3A4, with an elimination half-life of 2 to 3 hours.

Adverse drug events reported during therapeutic dosing include weakness, GI distress, dysphoria, headache, and dizziness. It may cause a withdrawal syndrome after prolonged use but does not cross-react with BZDs in treating BZD withdrawal. Flumazenil does not reverse buspirone effect.

Buspirone is not commonly seen in the overdose setting. Serotonin toxicity has rarely been reported when buspirone has been added to therapy in patients prescribed other serotonergic medications [38]. Supportive care is the mainstay of therapy after an overdose.

Z-drugs

Zopiclone and Eszopiclone

Zopiclone (Imovane) has a cyclopyrrolone structure, structurally unrelated to BZDs or other sedative-hypnotics. It is available as a racemic mixture of two stereoisomers, one of which, the S-isomer, is marketed in the United States as eszopiclone (Lunesta).

Zopiclone binds to the BZ1 receptor, preferentially acting at the subunits associated with sedation and amnesia. Eszopiclone differs from the racemic mixture in that it has less activity at the receptor subunits responsible for sedation and amnesia, and more affinity for those involved in sleep regulation and anxiolysis [39]. Both zopiclone and eszopiclone are well absorbed orally, reaching maximal concentration within 1 to 2 hours. They undergo extensive metabolism, primarily by CYP3A4, with active metabolites that are excreted renally. Elimination half-life of zopiclone is 5 to 6 hours [39].

Adverse effects after therapeutic dosing include a bitter taste in the mouth and hangover sedation into the next day, with potential adverse influences on psychomotor performance.

Isolated zopiclone poisoning commonly follows a benign course, with sedation being the predominant feature. Patients with concurrent ethanol or other sedative medication ingestion may develop greater sedation. A report of a series of eszopiclone ingestions reported that the commonest effect was drowsiness, with agitation, ataxia, and tachycardia also occurring [40]. Methemoglobinemia has been noted following overdose of zopiclone. This may be related to oxidative stress caused by an N-oxide metabolite of the parent drug [41].

Management of zopiclone and eszopiclone poisoning is supportive, with attention to airway and respiratory support. In view of the rapid absorption and sedative effects, decontamination with activated charcoal is not indicated. Sedation from zopiclone poisoning may respond to flumazenil [42]. If methemoglobinemia occurs, it should be managed along conventional lines, with administration of supplemental oxygen, and methylene blue if symptoms are significant or methemoglobin concentration is greater than 20%.

Zolpidem

Zolpidem is an imidazopyridine drug and exerts its effects at the BZ1 receptor. It is a potent sedative-hypnotic, with minimal anxiolysis [39]. It is available as both an immediate (IR) and a controlled-release (CR) preparation. After ingestion, the time to maximum concentration is 1 to 2 hours for the IR preparation and 1.5 to 2.5 hours for the CR preparation. It is highly protein bound and metabolized in the liver, predominantly by CYP3A4 to inactive metabolites. Elimination half-life is 2.5 to 3 hours. Zolpidem has displayed zero-order kinetics following overdose in a pediatric patient [43]. Adverse events associated with zolpidem are similar to zopiclone, and include anxiety, dizziness, headache, drowsiness, GI upset, and hangover effects with residual impairment of psychomotor performance after wakening.

Following zolpidem overdose, the most common clinical feature of intoxication is drowsiness. Significant coma and respiratory depression are unusual [39]. Commonly, symptoms improve within a few hours. Other reported effects include tachycardia, ataxia, slurred speech, vomiting, and hallucinations [44]. The reported effects of poisoning with IR and CR preparations are similar. However, the CR formulation was less likely to cause drowsiness and hallucinations and more likely to result in ataxia [44]. Deaths are reported following overdose of zolpidem in combination with other CNS depressants.

Management of zolpidem intoxication is similar to that of zopiclone and treatment is predominantly supportive. Flumazenil has been used to reverse sedation from zolpidem overdose in adult and pediatric patients [43].

γ-Hydroxybutyrate

γ-Hydroxybutyrate (GHB) was initially trialed as an anesthetic induction agent in the 1960s and 1970s. Its adverse effect profile, narrow therapeutic index, and lack of analgesic effects meant that it never gained widespread clinical use [45]. GHB was subsequently found to be a naturally occurring GABA precursor and metabolite in the CNS. It acts as a neuromodulator in the GABA system, and interacts with specific GHB receptors. It has effects on dopamine neurotransmission, and modulates the serotonin and opioid systems. Exogenous sources of GHB can act as a partial agonist at GABA-B receptors and are metabolized to form GABA [46].

GHB is used as a recreational drug. Colloquially it is known as "G," "Liquid ecstasy," or "Fantasy," and became popular for its euphoric, relaxant, and sexual effects. It is also implicated in drug-facilitated sexual assault. Because of rescheduling of GHB in various countries, there has been increasing use of precursor chemicals such as γ-butyrolactone (GBL) and 1,4 butanediol (1,4-BD), which are solvents obtainable from industrial sources. Both are rapidly metabolized to GHB and have similar clinical effects. In a worldwide case of commercial GHB toxicity, children accidentally ingested a brand of toy beads ("Bindeez" or "Aquadots") that were contaminated with 1,4-BD rather than the intended 1,5-pentanediol. This led to an international recall of the products [47]. The sodium salt of GHB, sodium oxybate (Xyrem), is approved as a treatment for cataplexy associated with narcolepsy in the United States and other countries.

Following oral administration, GHB and its precursors are rapidly absorbed, reaching peak concentration within 30 minutes. GBL is rapidly converted to GHB by serum lactonase. 1,4-BD is metabolized hepatically by alcohol dehydrogenase, then aldehyde dehydrogenase to GHB. This reaction can be inhibited by ethanol and fomepizole [46]. GHB is metabolized in the liver by succinate semialdehyde to succinate, which then enters the Krebs cycle, and is ultimately metabolized to carbon dioxide and water. Metabolism is saturable at high doses leading to zero-order kinetics initially. A small amount of GHB (2% to 5%) is eliminated unchanged in the urine.

Clinical effects of GHB poisoning occur rapidly after ingestion, and may be potentiated by the effects of alcohol or other drugs. Drowsiness, euphoria, hallucinations, delirium, nausea, vomiting, and mild hypothermia are seen. Myoclonic jerks and seizure-like activity may occur. Pupils are commonly small. Doses of greater than 50 mg per kg lead to coma and respiratory depression [46]. Cardiovascular effects include bradycardia and hypotension. Recovery from coma is typically rapid, with return of conscious state occurring within a few hours of ingestion. Deaths have been reported, either due to drug ingestion itself or occurring as a result of misadventure while intoxicated, both with GHB in isolation, or in combination with other drugs of abuse. In a series of GHB-related deaths, the most common cause of death was prehospital cardiorespiratory arrest [45]. Chronic use can lead to tolerance and physical dependence, and there is a well-documented withdrawal syndrome comprising anxiety, agitation, hallucinations, paranoia, tachycardia, and hypertension. This can occur rapidly following abstinence from the last dose, even within a matter of hours [46].

Management of GHB overdose is supportive. Airway protection and ventilatory support are the mainstays of treatment. Prolonged sedation may indicate co-ingestion of other sedative drugs. Because of the expected short period of unconsciousness and expected rapid recovery, practice regarding the necessity of intubation is variable, depending on experience within centers. In a study comparing conservative airway management to intubation between two tertiary referral hospitals in the same city, it was found that intubation was associated with a greater emergency department length of stay and increased likelihood of hospital admission [48]. Because GHB is usually ingested in liquid form, and rapid deterioration in conscious state can be expected, GI decontamination with activated charcoal is not indicated. There is no specific antidote for GHB poisoning, but various agents have been investigated. Physostigmine, flumazenil, and naloxone do not reverse sedation following GHB use in humans, and are not recommended [46].

Hemodialysis has been used to successfully treat severe acidemia in a patient following a massive (600 mL) GBL ingestion [49]. It is theorized that the rapid metabolism of large quantities GBL to GHB by plasma lactonase resulted in dissociation of the GHB (pK_a 4.72) to its anion and hydrogen ions, producing the severe acidosis in this case. In most cases, the ingested dose is not as large as in this one and rapid endogenous clearance results in a short duration of symptoms. Importantly, hemodialysis was not used to enhance GBL or GHB elimination in this case, only to treat the marked acidemia.

References

1. Dennis TDA, Benavides J, Scatton B: Distribution of central omega 1 (benzodiazepine1) and omega 2 (benzodiazepine2) receptor subtypes in the monkey and human brain: An autoradiographic study with [3H] flunitriazepam and the omega 1 selective ligand [3H] zolpidem. *J Pharmacol Exp Ther* 247:309–322, 1988.
2. Chouinard G, Lefko-Singh K, Teboul E: Metabolism of anxiolytics and hypnotics: benzodiazepines, buspirone, zoplicone, and zolpidem. *Cell Mol Neurobiol* 19:533–552, 1999.
3. Isbister GK, O'Regan L, Sibbritt D, et al: Alprazolam is relatively more toxic than other benzodiazepines in overdose. *Br J Clin Pharmacol* 8:88–95, 2004.
4. Finkle BS, McCloskey KL, Goodman LS, et al: Diazepam and drug associated deaths: a survey in the United States and Canada. *JAMA* 242:429–434, 1979.
5. Olson KR, Yin L, Osterloh J, et al: Coma caused by trivial triazolam overdose. *Am J Emerg Med* 3:210–211, 1985.
6. Tenore PL: Advanced urine toxicology testing. *J Addict Dis* 29:436–448, 2010.
7. Anonymous: Position statement and practice guidelines on the use of multi-dose activated charcoal in the treatment of acute poisoning. American Academy of Clinical Toxicology; European Association of Poisons Centres and Clinical Toxicologists. *J Toxicol Clin Toxicol* 37:731–751, 1999.
8. Benavides J, Peny B, Durand A, et al: Comparative in vivo and in vitro regional selectivity of central omega (benzodiazepine) site ligands in inhibiting [3H] flumazenil binding in the rat central nervous system. *J Pharmacol Exp Ther* 263: 884–896, 1992.
9. Seger DL: Flumazenil-treatment or toxin? *J Toxicol Clin Toxicol* 42:209–216, 2004.
10. Mintzer MZ, Griffiths RR: Flumazenil-precipitated withdrawal in healthy volunteers following repeated diazepam exposure. *Psychopharmacology (Berl)* 178:259–267, 2005.
11. Bronstein AC, Spyker DA, Cantilena LR, et al: 2011 Annual report of the American Association of Poison Control Centers' National Poison Data System (NPDS): 29th annual report. *Clin Toxicol* 50:911–1164, 2012.
12. Cantrell FL, Nordt S, McIntyre I, et al: Death on the doorstep of a border community—intentional self-poisoning with veterinary pentobarbital. *Clin Toxicol (Phila)* 48:849–850, 2010.
13. Sumner DJ, Kalk J, Whiting B: Metabolism of barbiturate after over-dosage. *BMJ* 1:335, 1975.

14. McCarron MM, Schulze BW, Walberg CB, et al: Short acting barbiturate overdosage. *JAMA* 248:55–61, 1982.
15. Mactier R, Laliberté M, Mardini J, et al: Extracorporeal treatment for barbiturate poisoning: recommendations from the EXTRIP Workgroup. *Am J Kidney Dis* 64:347–358, 2014.
16. Beveridge GW, Lawson AAH: Occurrence of bullous lesions in acute barbiturate poisoning. *BMJ* 1:835–837, 1965.
17. Waring WS, Sandilands EA: Coma blisters. *Clin Toxicol* 45:808–809, 2007.
18. Ebid A, Hana'a M: Pharmacokinetics of phenobarbital during certain enhanced elimination modalities to evaluate their clinical efficacy in management of drug overdose. *Ther Drug Monit* 23:209–216, 2001.
19. Proudfoot AT, Krenzelok EP, Vale JA: Position Paper on urine alkalinization. *J Toxicol Clin Toxicol* 42:1–26, 2004.
20. Roberts DM, Buckley NA: Enhanced elimination in acute barbiturate poisoning—a systematic review. *Clin Toxicol (Phila)* 49:2–12, 2011.
21. Nordt SP, Rangan C, Hardmaslani M, et al: Pediatric chloral hydrate poisonings and death following outpatient procedural sedation. *J Med Toxicol* 10:219–222, 2014.
22. Hung O, Kaplan J, Hoffman R, et al: Improved understanding of the ethanol-chloral hydrate interaction using 4-MP. *J Toxicol Clin Toxicol* 35:507, 1997.
23. Pershad J, Palmisano P, Nichols M: Chloral hydrate: the good and the bad. *Pediatr Emerg Care* 15:432–435, 1999.
24. Graham SR, Day RO, Lee R, et al: Overdose with chloral hydrate: a pharmacological and therapeutic review. *Med J Aust* 149:686–688, 1988.
25. Ludwigs U, Divino Filho JC, Magnusson A, et al: Suicidal chloral hydrate poisoning. *J Toxicol Clin Toxicol* 34:97–99, 1996.
26. Bowyer K, Glasser SP: Chloral hydrate overdose and cardiac arrhythmias. *Chest* 77:232–235, 1980.
27. Zahedi A, Grant MH, Wong DT: Successful treatment of chloral hydrate cardiac toxicity with propranolol. *Am J Emerg Med* 17:490–491, 1999.
28. Crow JW, Lain P, Bochner F, et al: Glutethimide and pharmacokinetics in man. *Clin Pharmacol Ther* 22:458, 1977.
29. Hansen AR, Kennedy KA, Ambre JJ, et al: Glutethimide poisoning. A metabolite contributes to morbidity and mortality. *N Engl J Med* 292:250–252, 1975.
30. Vale JA, Rees AJ, Widdop B, et al: Use of charcoal haemoperfusion in the management of severely poisoned patients. *BMJ* 1:5–9, 1975.
31. Siddiqi M, Jennings CA: A near-fatal overdose of carisoprodol (SOMA): case report. *J Toxicol Clin Toxicol* 42:239–240, 2004.
32. Bailey DN: The present status of meprobamate ingestion: a five year review of cases with serum concentrations and clinical findings. *Am J Clin Pathol* 75:102–106, 1981.
33. Hassen E: Treatment of meprobamate overdose with repeated oral doses of activated charcoal. *Ann Emer Med* 15:73–76, 1986.
34. Watve SV, Sivan M, Raza WA, et al: Management of acute overdose or withdrawal state in intrathecal baclofen therapy. *Spinal Cord* 50:107–111, 2012.
35. Pommier P, Debaty G, Bartoli M, et al: Severity of deliberate acute baclofen poisoning: a nonconcurrent cohort study. *Basic Clin Pharmacol Toxicol* 114:360–364, 2013.
36. Nugent S, Katz MD, Little TE: Baclofen overdose with cardiac conduction abnormalities: Case report and review of the literature. *J Toxicol Clin Toxicol* 24:321–328, 1986.
37. Leung NY, Whyte IM, Isbister GK: Baclofen overdose: defining the spectrum of toxicity. *Emerg Med Australis* 18:77–82, 2006.
38. Manos GH: Possible serotonin syndrome associated with buspirone added to fluoxetine. *Ann Pharmacother* 34:871–874, 2000.
39. Gunja N: The clinical and forensic toxicology of Z-drugs. *J Med Toxicol* 9:155–162, 2013.
40. Forrester MB: Eszopiclone ingestions reported to Texas poison control centers, 2005–2006. *Hum Exp Toxicol* 26:795–800, 2007.
41. Fung HT, Lai CH, Wong OF, et al: Two cases of methemoglobinemia following zopiclone ingestion. *J Toxicol Clin Toxicol* 46:167–170, 2008.
42. Cienki JJ, Burkhart KK, Donovan JW: Zopiclone overdose responsive to flumazenil. *Clin Toxicol* 43:385–386, 2005.
43. Thornton SL, Negus E, Carstairs SD: Pediatric zolpidem ingestion demonstrating zero-order kinetics treated with flumazenil. *Pediatr Emerg Care* 29:1204–1206, 2013.
44. Forrester MB: Immediate- and controlled-release zolpidem ingestions reported to Texas poison centers. *Hum Exp Toxicol* 28:505–509, 2009.
45. Zvosec DL, Smith SW, Porrata T, et al: Case series of 226 γ-hydroxybutyrate-associated deaths: lethal toxicity and trauma. *Am J Emerg Med* 29:319–332, 2011.
46. Schep LJ, Knudsen K, Slaughter RJ, et al: The clinical toxicology of γ-hydroxybutyrate, γ-butyrolactone and 1,4-butanediol. *Clin Toxicol (Phila)* 50:458–470, 2012.
47. Gunja N, Doyle E, Carpenter K, et al: Gamma-hydroxybutyrate poisoning from toy beads. *Med J Aust* 188:54–55, 2008.
48. Dietze P, Horyniak D, Agius P, et al: Effect of intubation for gamma-hydroxybutyric acid overdose on emergency department length of stay and hospital admission. *Acad Emerg Med* 21:1226–1231, 2014.
49. Roberts DM, Smith MWH, Gopalakrishnan M, et al: Extreme γ-butyrolactone overdose with severe metabolic acidosis requiring hemodialysis. *Ann Emer Med* 58:83–85, 2011.

Chapter 124 ■ Terrestrial Envenomations

ROBERT LEE NORRIS

Few topics in medicine are as steeped in controversy and anecdotal treatment recommendations as the field of toxicology. Fortunately, the toll of human suffering that venomous creatures exact in developed countries is relatively low. In developing nations, however, life-threatening encounters with venomous snakes and scorpions are more common. This chapter offers guidance for the evaluation and management of bites and stings of venomous snakes, spiders, and scorpions indigenous to North America (Table 124.1). Although the general principles of management of envenomations outlined here may be applicable to other regions of the world, specific approaches, such as indications for and types and doses of antivenoms, vary by region, and local experts should be consulted for advice.

SNAKE ENVENOMATION

All of the terrestrial American venomous snakes belong to one of two families: Viperidae (subfamily Crotalinae, or pit vipers) and Elapidae (or coral snakes). Venomous snakes are native to every state of the United States except Alaska, Hawaii, Maine, and Rhode Island.

Pit Viper Envenomation

The vast majority of venomous snakebites in North America are inflicted by pit vipers, which include the rattlesnakes (genera *Crotalus* and *Sistrurus*), and the cottonmouth water moccasins, copperheads, and cantils (*Agkistrodon* spp). These snakes possess paired, pitlike heat receptors (foveal organs) on the anterolateral aspects of the head. These receptors aid the snake in aiming its strike and determining the quantity of venom to be injected [1].

Pit viper venoms contain numerous enzymatic components and a number of nonenzymatic, low-molecular-weight polypeptides. Venom compositions vary not only from species to species, but from snake to snake within a species, and even in an individual snake depending on its age, size, health, and other factors [1]. In general, the most serious envenomations in North America are caused by the rattlesnakes (particularly *Crotalus* spp), with cottonmouth water moccasin (*Agkistrodon piscivorus* spp) bites being less severe and copperhead (*A. contortrix* spp) bites causing predominantly local findings with little serious systemic toxicity.

The major enzymes in pit viper venoms include hyaluronidase (spreading factor), phospholipase A (responsible for cell membrane disruption), and various proteases (causing local tissue destruction) [1]. Venom metalloproteinases, termed *disintegrins*, result in disruption of vascular integrity [2]. Despite the impressive toxicity of such enzymes, the nonenzymatic, low-molecular-weight polypeptide fractions appear to be up to 20 times more lethal, on a weight-for-weight basis, than crude venom [3]. The toxicity of pit viper venom is enhanced by release of various autopharmacologic compounds from damaged tissue (e.g., histamine, bradykinin, and serotonin) [1].

Clinical Manifestations

Envenomated patients typically experience moderate-to-severe pain at the bite site within 5 to 10 minutes. The pain is often described as burning and may radiate along the bitten extremity. Swelling at the bite site, often associated with ecchymosis, soon follows and may progress along the entire extremity within hours. Rapid lymphatic absorption of venom may lead to impressive, early lymphangitis and regional adenopathy.

Within the first 24 to 36 hours, vesicles and hemorrhagic bullae may develop at the bite site and along the bitten extremity. These are less common in bites treated early with adequate amounts of antivenom [1,3]. Petechiae or purpura may also be present.

Systemic manifestations of pit viper envenomation can involve virtually any organ system. Nausea and vomiting are common and may appear early with severe bites [3]. Weakness, diaphoresis, fever and chills, dizziness, and syncope may also occur [1]. Some patients experience a minty, rubbery, or metallic taste in their mouth [1,3]. Muscle fasciculations (myokymia) or paresthesias of the scalp, face, tongue, or digits indicate a moderate-to-severe envenomation. Systemic coagulopathy can lead to bleeding at any anatomic site, including the gastrointestinal, respiratory, genitourinary, and central nervous systems, although clinically significant bleeding is uncommon following bites in North America [3].

Alterations in heart rate and blood pressure may occur. Early hypotension is usually caused by pooling of blood in the pulmonary and splanchnic vascular beds, whereas delayed shock results from blood loss, third spacing of intravascular volume, and hemolysis [1,4]. Pulmonary edema can occur in severe envenomations, and is secondary to disruption of pulmonary vasculature intimal linings and pooling of pulmonary blood [5].

Multifactorial renal failure may occur, but is uncommon. Contributing factors include hypotension; hemoglobin, myoglobin, and fibrin deposition in renal tubules; and direct venom nephrotoxicity [3].

Muscle weakness may be seen after bites by some rattlesnakes such as the eastern diamondback rattlesnake (*Crotalus adamanteus*) and some specimens of the Mohave rattlesnake (*Crotalus scutulatus*) [5,6] that possess phospholipase A_2 neurotoxins in their venoms. Although neuromuscular respiratory failure is rare, it can occur in severe bites. Respiratory distress may also occur because of respiratory muscle fasciculations and incoordination, pulmonary edema, or anaphylactic reactions to venom or antivenom [3].

Snake venoms do not appear to cross the blood–brain barrier to any significant extent, and rare findings such as seizures and coma are secondary to hypotension, hypoxia, or intracranial bleeding. In rare cases, prothrombotic venom components can cause cerebral infarcts [7].

Diagnostic Evaluation

Important aspects of the history include details of the incident (such as type and size of snake if known, time and number of bites, and methods of first aid applied) and the patient's medical history (including any prior snakebites, medications, allergies, and tetanus immunization status).

Pit viper envenomation is a true medical emergency with potential for multisystem involvement, and the treating clinician must maintain vigilance for onset or progression of signs and symptoms. Although approximately 20% of bites by US pit vipers result in no envenomation ("dry bites") [8], in some cases where envenomation has occurred, onset of toxicity may be delayed for hours and severity can then progress rapidly. Consultation with an authority in the area of toxicology such as a regional poison control center specialist is prudent.

Puncture-wound patterns can be misleading in the diagnosis of snakebite. Occasionally, there is only a single puncture wound or many tiny punctures [9]. A dry bite may or may not have fang puncture marks, but there is no more pain than would be expected from simple puncture wounds. Envenomation is confirmed by the presence of local tissue effects (particularly progressive swelling as assessed by serial measurements of limb circumference; see Table 124.1), systemic effects, and/or laboratory abnormalities.

Essential laboratory studies include a complete blood cell count, serum electrolytes, blood urea nitrogen, creatinine, creatine phosphokinase, prothrombin time or international normalized ratio, fibrinogen, fibrin degradation products, and urine analysis. Blood for type and screening should also be sent for evaluation as soon as possible because direct venom effects and antivenom effects may interfere with this process later. Obtain a chest radiograph, an arterial blood gas, and an electrocardiogram as clinically indicated.

Occasionally, the history and diagnosis may be unclear, especially in children. When patients present without having seen a snake and have no findings other than puncture wounds and mild pain, the differential diagnosis includes a dry bite, bite by other animal or arthropod (e.g., nonvenomous snake, centipede, or spider), and mechanical puncture wounds (e.g., cactus spines). Persistent oozing of blood that should have coagulated from puncture wounds suggests the presence of coagulopathy and should heighten suspicion of pit viper bite in this clinical context.

Management

First-aid efforts are best limited to reassuring the victim, immobilizing and splinting the extremity at the level of the heart, and transporting as quickly as possible to a hospital. Previously recommended first-aid measures including incision, suction, constriction bands, pressure immobilization, tourniquets, packing of the extremity in ice, or application of electric shocks should be avoided because they are ineffective and may result in further complications [9,10,11].

Initial management should focus on any derangements of the patient's airway, breathing, or circulation. Cardiac, blood pressure, and pulse oximetry monitoring should be in place. Two large-bore intravenous (IV) lines infusing normal saline are started, preferably in sites other than the bitten extremity, and blood work is sent to the laboratory. Any devices applied in the field in an attempt to limit venom spread should be temporarily left in place until an IV line is established.

Management of significant pit viper envenomation centers on the judicious use of an appropriate antivenom. In North America, antivenom therapy is indicated for victims with progressive local tissue findings or systemic abnormalities (significant systemic symptoms or signs, or laboratory abnormalities [e.g., paresthesias, hypotension, prolongation of prothrombin time or international normalized ratio, hypofibrinogenemia, or thrombocytopenia]) (see Fig. 124.1). Controversy exists, however, on the use of antivenom for copperhead (*A. contortrix*) bites presenting with progressive soft-tissue swelling in the absence of systemic abnormalities. Given that most such bites do well with conservative therapy alone, the risk versus benefit of giving antivenom in these cases is currently unclear and is being investigated [12]. Again, consultation with a toxicology expert is prudent in such cases.

TABLE 124.1

Summary of Hospital Management Guidelines for Envenomations in North America

Syndrome	Management
Pit viper	
Rattlesnake (*Crotalus* or *Sistrurus* spp), cottonmouth water moccasin, or copperhead (*Agkistrodon* spp)	• ABCs, O_2, cardiac/pulse oximetry monitoring, two large-bore IV lines, physiologic saline infusion • Mark & measure extremity circumferences every 15 min during acute phase • Laboratory assessment (see text) • Update tetanus immunization status as needed • No evidence of envenomation—monitor for a minimum of 8 h • Mild envenomation without evidence of progression—no antivenom, admit for monitoring • Mild envenomation with progression OR moderate-to-severe envenomation (evidence of systemic toxicity [systemic signs or symptoms, or laboratory abnormalities])—administer antivenom (see text) • Shock management includes IV physiologic saline boluses (10–20 mL/kg) and high-dose antivenom; if refractory, consider albumin and, as last resort, vasopressors • Blood products uncommonly required after administration of adequate antivenom (always give antivenom first) • Opioids as needed for pain control • If concerned re: compartment syndrome, measure intracompartmental pressures (see text); fasciotomy only for documented increase in pressures unresponsive to elevation of the extremity and antivenom (with or without a trial of mannitol) • Antibiotics only for evidence of secondary infection (uncommon)
Coral snake	
Texas or Eastern coral snake (*Micrurus* spp)	• ABCs, O_2, cardiac/pulse oximetry monitoring, at least one large-bore IV line, physiologic saline infusion • Early intubation and respiratory support if any evidence of difficulty with breathing or handling secretions • Update tetanus immunization status as needed • No evidence of envenomation—admit for monitoring (minimum of 24 h) • Evidence of neurotoxicity—administer antivenom if available (see text); if no antivenom available, supportive care only; admit for monitoring until recovered
Sonoran coral snake (*Micruroides euryxanthus*)	• ABCs, O_2, cardiac/pulse oximetry monitoring, at least one large-bore IV line, physiologic saline infusion • Update tetanus immunization status as needed • No evidence of envenomation—admit for monitoring (minimum of 24 h) • Evidence of neurotoxicity—admit for monitoring until recovered, supportive care only
Widow spider (*Latrodectus* spp)	• ABCs, O_2, cardiac/pulse oximetry monitoring, at least one large-bore IV line, physiologic saline infusion • Update tetanus immunization status as needed • No evidence of envenomation—monitor for 6–8 h • Evidence of envenomation Mild: analgesics and muscle relaxants (narcotics and benzodiazepines) More severe or high-risk patient (see text): consider antivenom administration with informed consent (see text)
Recluse spider (*Loxosceles* spp)	• Laboratory assessment (see text) • Conservative wound care (cleansing, splinting, debride only clearly necrotic tissue) • Update tetanus immunization status as needed • Any evidence of infection: broad-spectrum antibiotics (include MRSA coverage) • Daily wound checks until progressive healing • Delay any required skin grafts for 6–8 wk (see text) • If evidence of systemic toxicity: admit, IV fluids, steroids (see text); blood product transfusion, and dialysis for renal failure as needed
Scorpion	
Bark scorpion (*Centruroides sculpturatus*)	• ABCs (secure the airway as needed), O_2, cardiac/pulse oximetry monitoring, at least one large-bore IV line, physiologic saline infusion • Cautious opioids for pain, benzodiazepines for agitation • Antivenom (see text) • Update tetanus immunization status as needed
Nonneurotoxic scorpion	• Analgesics as needed • Update tetanus immunization status as needed

These are guidelines only and do not replace individual physician judgment. Consultation with an expert toxicologist or poison control center specialist may be helpful.

ABCs, airway, breathing, circulation assessment and management as needed; O_2, oxygen; IV, intravenous; MRSA, methicillin-resistant *Staphylococcus aureus*.

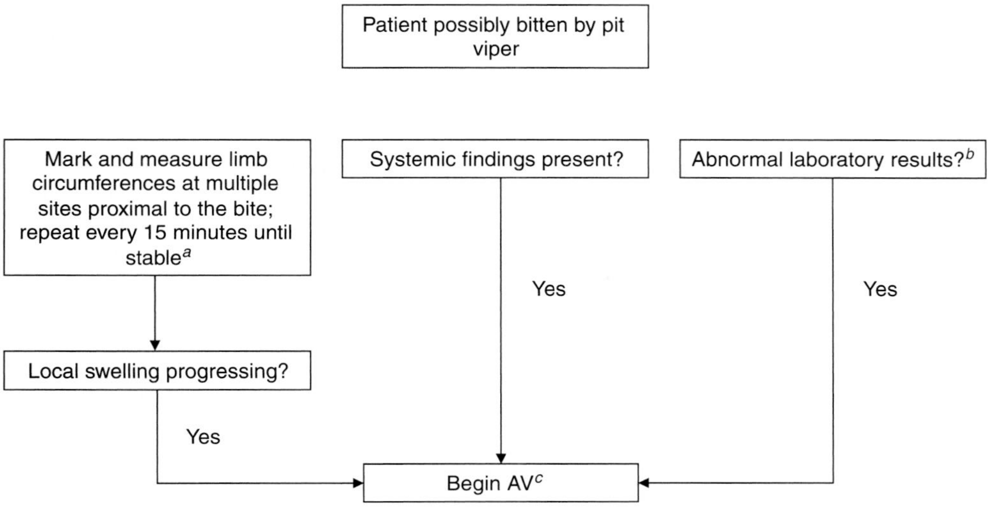

FIGURE 124.1 Guidelines for beginning antivenom therapy for victims of pit viper bite in the United States (see text for details). [a]Keep extremity at heart level, being careful to differentiate redistribution of edema (with changing limb position) from progression of severity of swelling. [b]Repeat normal lab work every hour for 4 to 6 hours until AV is started or the decision is made that AV is not necessary (i.e., the bite resulted in no envenomation or a mild, nonprogressive envenomation). [c]Abnormal coagulation studies may not return to normal for 4 to 6 hours after antivenom administration—time necessary for the body to replete coagulation factors after neutralization of venom. AV, antivenom.

Antivenom Administration

If possible, informed consent should be obtained before antivenom administration. Antivenom should be administered in a closely monitored setting. Epinephrine and endotracheal intubation equipment should be immediately available at the bedside during initial antivenom administration, and a physician should be available to manage any acute adverse drug effects that may develop.

In the United States, at the time of this writing, there is currently a single commercially available antivenom for pit viper bites—CroFab Crotalidae Polyvalent Immune Fab, Ovine (BTG International Inc., West Conshohocken, PA) (FabAV). This antiserum contains pooled, purified Fab immunoglobulin fragments from sheep immunized with one of four different pit viper venoms. It comes in a lyophilized state and is effective against all North American pit vipers.

Antivenom should be started as soon as possible after the indication for administration is apparent. Although there are no defined end points in terms of time or dosage for when to withhold antivenom, antivenom is beneficial for treating only findings directly related to continued presence of unbound, circulating venom (e.g., ongoing coagulopathy). It is ineffective in reversing end-organ damage that has resulted from prior venom effects (e.g., renal failure). The efficacy of antivenom in preventing local wound necrosis is limited, because it cannot reverse local cellular damage once it has been initiated by rapidly acting venom enzymes and nonenzymatic polypeptides [13]. Any ability to reduce necrosis depends on early administration.

Dosing of FabAV is based not on age or size of the patient, but rather on the potential venom load delivered to the victim. As children generally receive similar quantities of venom in a bite as adults do, pediatric dosing is the same as for adults. The starting dose is four to six vials for patients with signs or symptoms of systemic toxicity or evidence of progressive local venom effects. In victims with hypotension or severe bleeding, the starting dose should be increased to 8 to 12 vials [14]. Each vial should be reconstituted with 18 to 25 mL of warm sterile water or saline and the vials gently agitated (vigorous shaking of the vials may cause development of foam, resulting in less delivered protective antibody fragments). The total dose to be administered is diluted in 250 mL of normal saline and infused over 1 hour (starting slowly at the onset of infusion and gradually increasing the rate). During the first hour after the dose is completed, the patient is monitored for further progression of local effects and systemic symptoms, and laboratory studies are rechecked. The starting dose of FabAV is repeated if venom effects continue to progress. This pattern is continued until the patient stabilizes. Coagulation studies may not normalize after the initial dose, because time is required for repletion of coagulation factors after venom neutralization, but there should be evidence of improvement [15,16]. After stabilization, two vials of FabAV are administered every 6 hours for three additional doses to prevent recurrence of venom toxicity. Further doses may be needed at the physician's discretion depending on the patient's clinical picture.

Adverse effects of antivenoms, as heterologous serum products, are divided into three major groups: acute allergic and nonallergic anaphylaxis, and delayed serum sickness. Acute reactions most commonly manifest with urticaria, although bronchospasm, hypotension, and angioedema can also occur [17]. Serum sickness is characterized by pruritus, fever, arthralgias, lymphadenopathy, and malaise, which can occur 1 to 2 weeks after antivenom therapy [18]. The incidence of acute reactions to CroFab is approximately 8%, and serum sickness occurs in approximately 13% of patients [19]. Management of acute reactions centers on rapid diagnosis, temporarily halting the infusion and treating with epinephrine, antihistamines, and steroids (see Chapter 69). Generally, once the reaction is controlled, the antivenom infusion can be restarted, possibly in a more dilute state and at a slower rate. Serum sickness is relatively benign and easily treated with steroids, antihistamines, and nonsteroidal anti-inflammatory drugs until symptoms resolve. Most cases do well with oral prednisone (1 to 2 mg/kg/d) until symptoms resolve, followed by a taper over another week.

Supportive Measures

Venom-induced hypotension should be treated with antivenom and volume expansion. If organ perfusion fails to respond promptly with crystalloid infusion (1 to 2 L in an adult and 20 to 40 mL per kg in a child), administration of albumin may be considered [1,7]. Vasoactive amines may be required after adequate volume resuscitation of refractory cases [1].

Although pit viper envenomation can result in significant coagulopathies, the incidence of clinically significant bleeding in the United States is low [20]. Management of coagulopathy in patients with evidence of major bleeding may require administration of packed red blood cells, platelets, fresh-frozen plasma, and/or cryoprecipitate [1,21]. There is limited experience using recombinant factor VIIa for severe coagulopathy following rattlesnake bite [22]. It is important to begin antivenom therapy before the infusion of such products to avoid augmenting the consumptive coagulopathy.

Therapy to prevent acute renal failure includes ensuring adequate hydration and monitoring urinary output. If renal failure occurs, dialysis may be required, although it does not remove circulating venom components [1,3].

Although steroids are useful in the management of adverse reactions to antivenom (see previous discussion), there is no role for them in the primary management of snake envenomation.

Wound Care and Surgery

Wound care begins with cleaning the bite site with a suitable germicidal solution and covering it with a dry, sterile dressing. As soon as antivenom, if indicated, has been started, the extremity should be elevated in a well-padded splint in a position of function with cotton between the digits [1]. Antibiotics are unnecessary unless field management involved incisions into the bite site [23] or the wound appears clinically infected. Tetanus immunization status should be updated as necessary.

Intact hemorrhagic blebs and bullae should be protected. If ruptured, they should be unroofed after any attendant coagulopathy has been reversed, and managed with wet to dry dressings [3]. Wound debridement may be necessary if there is significant tissue necrosis. The use of hyperbaric oxygen therapy to treat these wounds has yet to be fully studied [1,24]. Physical therapy is an important part of the care plan for returning the extremity to its pre-envenomation functional capacity.

The role of surgery in the primary management of pit viper envenomation is very limited. The speed with which snake venom is absorbed makes routine excision of the bite site fruitless, and routine exploration of the site does little to mitigate systemic effects of venom, may worsen the overall outcome by adding surgical trauma, and can prolong hospitalization [1].

The incidence of compartment syndrome after snake envenomation appears low despite the frequently impressive local findings of bitten extremities [25]. Myonecrosis that occurs is usually caused by direct venom effects and rarely vascular compromise from elevated intracompartmental pressures [25]. In combined series of nearly 2,000 victims of pit viper envenomation, only four patients required fasciotomy; each of these patients received inappropriate ice treatment or inadequate antivenom therapy [25]. If there is concern about an impending compartment syndrome, intracompartmental pressures should be checked using any standard technique. If pressures exceed 30 to 40 mm Hg and remain elevated for more than 1 hour despite treatment with antivenom, limb elevation, and possibly mannitol infusion (1 to 2 g per kg in a normotensive patient), fasciotomy may be required [26]. While some evidence suggests that fasciotomy may actually worsen local myonecrosis [27], unabated elevation of intracompartmental pressures can have disastrous effects, such as debilitating neuropathy [28], and fasciotomy may still be required. Whenever possible, informed consent should be obtained before proceeding with fasciotomy.

Disposition and Outcome

Patients with apparent dry bites can be discharged from the emergency department if they remain asymptomatic with normal laboratory values (repeated prior to discharge) and vital signs after 8 hours of observation [29]. The envenomated patient can be discharged from the hospital when all venom effects have begun to resolve and when antivenom therapy is complete, which is usually within 48 hours after admission. At the time of discharge, every patient should have appropriate follow-up arranged for continued wound care and physical therapy, and should be warned about the symptoms of serum sickness. If such symptoms occur, the patient should seek medical care promptly.

Venom-induced coagulopathy and thrombocytopenia may recur anytime up to 14 days after the last dose of antivenom [30], and fatal intracranial bleeding and other cases of major delayed bleeding have been reported [31,32]. Patients should be followed closely after discharge from the hospital with repeat complete blood count and coagulation studies at 2 to 3 days and 3 to 5 days after the last dose of FabAV, and they should be warned to avoid elective procedures and risky activities (such as contact sports) for at least 2 weeks [14]. If on follow-up there is evidence of clinically significant bleeding, if the laboratory coagulopathy is worsening or severe (i.e., platelet count $<25,000$ per mm^3, INR >3, aPTT >50 seconds, fibrinogen <50 mg per dL, or multicomponent coagulopathy), or if the patient has an underlying condition that makes him prone to bleeding or engages in activities that make him prone to trauma, additional antivenom can be considered, although its efficacy at reversing delayed recurrence of coagulopathy is reduced [15,16,30,33].

The historical mortality rate for patients treated with antivenom in the United States was 0.28%, compared with 2.61% for patients not receiving antivenom [34]. The impact of FabAV on mortality rates remains to be determined. Death after pit viper poisoning is most likely to occur 6 to 48 hours after envenomation [34]. Fewer than 17% of deaths occur within 6 hours and fewer than 4% within 1 hour [34]. The major reasons for poor outcomes in pit viper envenomation are delay in presentation, inadequate fluid resuscitation, inappropriate use of vasopressors, and delay in administration or inadequate dosing of antivenom [35]. The incidence of upper-extremity functional disability after pit viper envenomation is at least 32% [36], and may be higher when careful, objective functional measurements are obtained [37].

Coral Snake Envenomation

There are fewer than 100 coral snake bites reported in the United States each year [38]. The US coral snakes include the eastern coral snake (*Micrurus fulvius*), the Texas coral snake (*Micrurus tener*), and the Sonoran coral snake (*Micruroides euryxanthus*). Mexico boasts 15 *Micrurus* species as well as the Sonoran coral snake [39]. Coral snakes lack the foveal organs of pit vipers. Owing to their much less effective venom-delivery mechanism (small fangs fixed in an upright position on the anterior maxillae), only approximately 40% of coral snake bites result in envenomation [1,40], although it has been estimated that one large coral snake is capable of delivering enough venom to kill four to five humans [41]. In the United States, it appears that the severity of envenomation tends to be greatest with the eastern coral snake (*M. fulvius*), less with the Texas coral snake (*M. tener*), and least with the Sonoran coral snake (*Micruroides euryxanthus*) [1,42].

Clinical Manifestations

Coral snake venoms are primarily neurotoxic. Low-molecular-weight polypeptides in the venom are capable of inducing nondepolarizing, postsynaptic blockade at neuromuscular junctions [43]. There are few local findings at the bite site, and the onset of systemic symptoms may be delayed for many hours [40,44]. Fang marks may be small and difficult to detect [45], with variable pain and little swelling at the site [44]. The patient may experience local paresthesias that may radiate proximally and be associated with muscle fasciculations [44]. The earliest systemic findings may include alteration of mental status [46]. Nausea and vomiting may occur, along with increased salivation [40]. Bulbar-type paralysis can occur as early as 90 minutes after the bite and progress to peripheral paralysis [1]. Findings may include extraocular muscle paresis, ptosis, pinpoint pupils, dysphagia, dysphonia, slurred speech, and laryngeal spasm [40,44]. Death from coral snake envenomation has been reported because of respiratory failure or cardiovascular collapse [1].

Diagnostic Evaluation

The important history is similar to that obtained from victims of pit viper bites. In areas where coral snakes coexist with harmless coral snake mimics, such as milk snakes (*Lampropeltis* spp), it is helpful if the color pattern of the offending snake can be reliably obtained or, better yet, if the victim can produce a digital photo of the offending reptile. The differential diagnosis of coral snake envenomation is usually limited to bites by other brightly colored, nonvenomous snakes. Native US coral snakes can be identified by a characteristic red, yellow, and black banding pattern, with the red and yellow bands contiguous ("red on yellow, kill a fellow; red on black, venom lack") and the bands completely encircling the body. In the harmless coral snake mimics, the red and yellow bands are separated by black bands, and the bands do not completely encircle the body. This color pattern does not, however, reliably identify coral snakes south of Mexico City [47]. The remainder of the differential diagnosis is the same as for pit vipers.

Management

Rapid transportation to a hospital is of utmost priority following coral snake bites. In Australia, where all native venomous snakes are elapid relatives of the coral snake, a potentially beneficial first-aid intervention is use of a pressure-immobilization wrap. In this technique, the entire bitten extremity is firmly wrapped with an elastic or crepe bandage and splinted [48]. The wrap is applied snuggly—as tightly as for a sprained ankle [48]—and it is important that the extremity be kept as immobile as possible and the patient carried to medical care [49]. One small animal study has demonstrated apparent benefit of the technique in prolonging survival following coral snake venom injection [50].

As with pit viper bites, attention is initially directed to the patient's airway, breathing, and circulatory status. Supplemental oxygen should be administered, cardiac and pulse oximetry monitoring established, and at least one IV line should be started. Impending respiratory failure is suggested by cyanosis, trismus, laryngeal or pharyngeal spasm, increased salivation, or any sign of cranial nerve paralysis [44]. If any of these findings is present, prophylactic intubation is indicated to prevent aspiration. Once the airway and respiratory status are addressed, a more complete physical examination is performed. Any swelling should be documented and observed for progression.

Antivenom Therapy

As with most venomous snakebites, definitive management of significant *Micrurus* bites should center on the use of appropriate antivenom. Production of the only Food and Drug Administration (FDA)–approved antivenom for coral snake bites in the United States, Antivenin (*Micrurus fulvius*) (Wyeth Laboratories Inc., Marietta, PA), has been discontinued by the manufacturer. At the time of this writing, the FDA has extended the expiration date on the single remaining lot of this antivenom until January 31, 2018. It is possible that Pfizer, Inc. may resume coral snake antivenom production for the United States at some point or that ongoing research into the use of an alternative foreign-produced antivenom for US coral snake bites may lead to approval of another product. (Updates on this topic can be obtained by contacting regional poison control centers.) If an effective coral snake antivenom is available, it should be administered in a monitored setting (with epinephrine available), in consultation with an expert in snake venom poisoning, and with informed consent if possible. Administer antivenom to any patient clearly bitten by an eastern coral snake (*Micrurus fulvius*) specimen, even in the absence of signs or symptoms, because once signs or symptoms appear, it may be difficult to reverse or halt their progression [40,44]. This is likely unnecessary if the offending snake was a Texas coral snake (*M. tener*) [42]. There is no antivenom for the Sonoran coral snake (*Micruroides euryxanthus*), but the venom of this snake is much less toxic, and there have been no reported deaths after its bite [1,46]. Management of any coral snake bite, in the absence of available antivenom, is entirely supportive. Airway protection and ventilatory support may be required for days following *Micrurus* bites [44], but with modern intensive care, the prognosis should be good.

Wound Care

The wounds from a coral snake bite should be washed with a germicidal solution and tetanus prophylaxis updated as necessary. Prophylactic antibiotics are not indicated.

Disposition and Outcome

All patients with potential coral snake bites should be admitted to an intensive care unit for at least 24 hours for close monitoring regardless of symptoms or antivenom requirement [51]. The projected case-fatality rate in untreated cases is up to 10% [40]. Total resolution of all signs or symptoms (e.g., weakness) may take several weeks [44].

Exotic (Imported) Snake Envenomation

Exotic venomous snakes are commonly kept in zoos, museums, and sometimes by private individuals in "underground zoos." Occasionally, they may be inadvertently found in imported goods and produce. If a patient has been bitten by an exotic venomous snake, every effort should be made to definitively identify the reptile. This can be done by contacting available zoo personnel or herpetologists. The treating physician should then call a regional poison control center for assistance (1-800-222-1222). These centers have access to a national listing of available sources of exotic antivenoms in stock in the United States. Antivenoms tend to be quite specific for the species against which they protect, and should be used only if there is clear evidence of their efficacy against the offending species. Sound supportive care, combined with an appropriate antivenom when available, should offer the best chances of an optimal outcome.

SPIDER ENVENOMATION

Although many spiders are capable of biting humans, only two types in North America are medically significant in that they have the potential to cause significant sequelae and possibly death: the widow spiders (*Latrodectus* spp) and the recluse spiders (*Loxosceles* spp).

Widow Spider Envenomation

Of five known species of widow spider in the United States, the black widows (*Latrodectus mactans*, *L. hesperus*, and *L. variolus*) are the best known [52]. The female black widow is dark black and oval shaped, with a characteristic, typically hourglass-shaped, ventral red, orange, or yellow marking on the abdomen. The body is approximately 1.5 cm long with a leg span up to 4 cm. The other two species in the United States are the red-legged widow or red widow (*L. bishopi*) and the brown widow (*L. geometricus*) [52]. Widow spiders are found in all of the 48 contiguous states and Hawaii [53], and are responsible for most of the exceedingly rare spider-related deaths in North

America. Only the female is dangerous to humans; the male, a nondescript and much smaller brown spider, is incapable of delivering a bite through human skin.

The venom of all species of widow spiders is similar in composition and toxic effects. The most deleterious venom component is alpha-latrotoxin, a potent neurotoxin that acts primarily at the neuromuscular junction [54]. The venom initially stimulates the release of neurotransmitters (acetylcholine, epinephrine, and norepinephrine) and then blocks neurotransmission by depleting synaptic vesicles [55,56]. It does not cause dermonecrosis or hemolysis [57].

Clinical Manifestations

The widow spider's bite may be unnoticed by the patient or may be felt as a sharp sting [55]. The bite site may be visible, with tiny fang marks approximately 1 mm apart, and the area may be slightly warm and blanched with a surrounding erythematous, indurated zone [58]. Swelling is minimal [59].

Significant symptoms usually appear 10 minutes to 2 hours after envenomation [58]. The most prominent symptom is pain. It begins at the bite site as a dull ache and spreads first to local muscle groups and then to larger regional muscle groups of the abdomen, back, chest, pelvis, and lower extremities. Muscle spasms and rigidity are classically present [58,60,61]. Spasms of abdominal musculature can mimic an acute abdomen, although rebound tenderness is absent. Chest muscle rigidity may produce respiratory distress [60,61]. The respiratory rate increases, and there may be associated tachycardia and hypertension. Pain severity typically peaks after several hours [62]. In patients at risk, the hypertension can lead to cerebrovascular accidents, exacerbation of congestive heart failure, and myocardial ischemia [55]. Cardiac dysrhythmias and priapism have been reported, and there are extremely rare cases of myocarditis [58,63].

Associated signs or symptoms include diaphoresis (local or diffuse; possibly asymmetrical), fever, headache, nausea and vomiting, restlessness and anxiety, periorbital edema, and skin rash [58,60,64]. Deep tendon reflexes may be increased [61].

Diagnostic Evaluation

The history surrounding a widow spider bite is confusing if a spider was not seen. A high index of suspicion should be maintained in patients presenting with compatible complaints. It is important to obtain a medical history, such as hypertension, pregnancy status, allergies, and tetanus immunization status. The physical examination entails a general screening with particular attention to the vital signs, which should be checked at frequent intervals. Close examination for a bite site may be productive.

There are no diagnostic changes in routine laboratory tests in widow spider envenomation. An elevation in white blood cell count and serum creatine phosphokinase values may be seen [65], and proteinuria has been reported [66]. An electrocardiogram and chest radiograph should be obtained as clinically indicated. A pregnancy test should be obtained in women of childbearing age because widow spider venom is a potent abortifacient.

The differential diagnosis includes envenomations by other arthropods, such as neurotoxic scorpions (see "Scorpion Envenomation" section), and systemic disorders, such as sympathomimetic overdose, acute rhabdomyolysis, heat cramps, heat stroke, neuroleptic malignant syndrome, tetanus, and strychnine poisoning. Other causes of abdominal pain and rigidity should be considered.

Management

Although there are no specific first-aid measures effective in widow spider bites, temporary application of ice to the bite site may reduce pain. Adequate airway, respiration, and circulatory status should be ensured. After instituting oxygen, cardiac and pulse oximetry monitoring, and starting an IV line, attention should be directed to alleviating painful muscle spasms using a cautious combination of benzodiazepines and opioids [52], although analgesia may prove difficult to achieve [67]. Calcium gluconate and other muscle relaxants such as methocarbamol are not consistently effective.

Hypertension usually responds to bed rest, muscle relaxants, analgesics, and sedation [54]. Specific antihypertensive agents can be used if necessary [54].

Antivenom

A specific, equine, whole-immunoglobulin widow spider antivenom available in the United States, Antivenin (*Latrodectus mactans*) (Black Widow Spider Antivenin) (manufactured by Merck & Co., Inc., West Point, PA), appears, in vitro, to be able to bind all *Latrodectus* venoms, regardless of species [68]. Indications for antivenom use in *Latrodectus* envenomations remain controversial, however, given recent evidence that questions its efficacy in relieving pain or reversing systemic toxicity [67] as well as its small but real risk of adverse reactions (see below). Antivenom might be considered in patients who are severely envenomated, pregnant, or in labor, or in those who have a history of cardiovascular disease or other major medical problems and evidence of significant envenomation despite benzodiazepine and opioid therapy [58,61,62]. Assistance from an expert toxicologist or poison center is helpful in making the decision about whether to administer antivenom.

If antivenom is to be given, informed consent should be obtained, and the patient should be in a monitored setting with epinephrine available at the bedside. Consideration can be given to premedicating with IV antihistamines (H_1 and H_2 blockers), although the benefit of such an approach is unproven. The antivenom can be given intravenously (one reconstituted vial further diluted in 50 to 100 mL of normal saline, administered over 30 minutes) or intramuscularly (IM) (one reconstituted vial in the anterolateral thigh) [69], with the physician in immediate attendance to observe for any sign of adverse drug events. Although studies suggest that there is no clinical benefit to administering *Latrodectus* antivenom IV over IM [68], the IV route may be best if the patient is in shock or younger than 12 years old [69]. The dosage is the same for children [54,60]. One vial is generally given initially, but a second vial can be administered if deemed necessary [60,62]. Signs or symptoms should completely resolve within a few hours of antivenom administration [60,62].

The types of adverse drug events seen with widow spider antivenom are the same as for snake antivenoms, with acute reactions occurring in approximately 2% and serum sickness in approximately 10% [64]. Deaths due to acute reactions have occurred following administration of widow spider antivenom [65,70]; this, plus questions of efficacy should limit its use to cases that are truly severe and potentially life threatening. It is hoped that ongoing research into a new $F(ab')_2$ widow spider antivenom might demonstrate improved efficacy with less risk, resulting in a safe, clearly effective antivenom use for widow spider bites in North America [71].

The clinical course of most patients with widow spider envenomation is benign [58,72], but significant pain and spasms can persist for 2 to 3 days [62]. Most healthy adults do well with supportive measures and adequate administration of parenteral benzodiazepines and opioids [58].

Disposition and Outcome

Patients can be discharged from the hospital when signs or symptoms of envenomation have been significantly controlled, although it may be best to admit and observe younger children. Patients should be given analgesics and muscle relaxants, prescribed bed rest, and instructed to return if they worsen. The mortality rate from widow spider envenomation in the United States is much less than 1% [55,58], and it is debatable if there are truly deaths from envenomation. Recovery from widow spider envenomation may sometimes be slow, with weakness, fatigue, paresthesias, headache, and insomnia persisting for several months [54].

Recluse Spider Envenomation

Of the approximately 13 species of recluse spider (*Loxosceles* spp) found in the United States [73], the brown recluse (*Loxosceles reclusa*) is best known [74]. All species are characterized by a violin-shaped marking on the dorsal aspect of the cephalothorax (though this may be hard to see in some specimens) and three pairs of eyes, in contrast to the four pairs found in most spiders. The adult body is 10 to 15 mm long and the legs span 2 to 3 cm. Both the male and female spiders are dangerous [62].

The brown recluse is found throughout the southern, south-central, and midwestern United States; other species are found in the western part of the country [52]. While recluse spiders may cause severe dermonecrosis (necrotic arachnidism), the majority of bites actually result in insignificant lesions [75].

The venoms of the different species of recluse spider have similar toxic effects [76]. They contain a number of different proteins, most of which demonstrate enzymatic activity [77]. Sphingomyelinase D is likely responsible for the venom's cytotoxic and hemolytic effects [78,79]. Venom activation of the complement cascade induces a series of autopharmacologic changes that amplify toxicity to a variable degree in victims [80].

The cutaneous changes seen after a recluse spider bite are initiated by venom-induced endothelial damage in small dermal vessels that become occluded with microthrombi, producing vascular stasis and infarction [81]. Polymorphonuclear leukocytes are attracted to the site via a chemotactic response and propagate the inflammatory, necrotic reaction [81,82]. Accumulation of polymorphonuclear leukocytes at the site appears to be a vital component of the dermonecrotic response and is related to complement activation [82].

Clinical Manifestations

The clinical course of recluse spider envenomation varies from a mild temporary irritation at the bite site to a rare, severe, potentially fatal outcome [74]. The bite is occasionally felt as a mild stinging sensation, although it may go completely unnoticed. During the next several hours, there may be pruritus, tingling, mild swelling, and redness or blanching at the bite site [83]. Variable degrees of local pain and tenderness due to local vasospasm and ischemia occur within 2 to 8 hours [83,84]. At 12 to 18 hours, a small central vesicle (clear or hemorrhagic) often develops at the site and is surrounded by an irregular zone of erythema or ecchymosis and edema, which may have a distinct gravitational distribution around the central lesion [85]. The vesicle ruptures, and the erythema gives way to violaceous discoloration [84]. In 5 to 7 days, the bite site undergoes aseptic necrosis (i.e., dry, gangrenous slough), with the center becoming depressed below the normal level of the skin, and a black eschar forms. The eschar later sloughs, leaving an open ulcer that heals in weeks to months [84]. Bites to fatty regions of the body tend to be more severe, with undermining of the skin and more extensive scarring [84]. Necrosis rarely involves deeper structures such as nerves, muscles, tendons, or ligaments [86]. Lesions destined to develop significant necrosis usually demonstrate early evidence of local ischemia [83].

Systemic (viscerocutaneous) loxoscelism is rare, but can be rapidly progressive and severe, particularly in children [62]. Systemic symptoms generally start 24 to 72 hours after the bite and occasionally occur before cutaneous findings become impressive [87]. Symptoms are often flulike, with fever, chills, headache, malaise, weakness, nausea and vomiting, myalgias, and arthralgias [84]. Hemolytic anemia with hemoglobinemia, hemoglobinuria, jaundice, thrombocytopenia, disseminated intravascular coagulation, acute renal failure, seizures, and coma have been reported [62]. The severity of systemic symptoms is directly related to the quantity of venom deposited, but does not necessarily correlate with the severity of cutaneous changes [85].

Diagnostic Evaluation

It is uncommon for a victim of a *Loxosceles* bite to see the offending spider because the bite is relatively painless, and, given that the spider is nocturnal, a large percentage of bites occur while the victim is asleep [75]. As the spider is rarely available for identification, determining the cause of early lesions is difficult [85], and the diagnosis of spider bite is usually presumptive. The working diagnosis should be cutaneous necrosis if the precise cause is unknown and necrotic arachnidism if a biting spider was seen but not identified.

An examination for evidence of systemic loxoscelism should be performed. The severity of any lesion present should be assessed and any evidence of secondary infection noted. There are no characteristic changes in routine laboratory tests in recluse spider envenomation. In patients with severe envenomation, laboratory studies should include a complete blood cell count and urinalysis [84]. If there is any evidence of consumptive coagulopathy, hemolysis, or hemoglobinuria, further studies should include prothrombin time and partial thromboplastin time, electrolytes, blood urea nitrogen, and creatinine, and a specimen should be sent for blood typing and screening. The white blood cell count may be as high as 20,000 to 30,000 per mm^3, and the hemoglobin may fall to as low as 4 g per dL [57,62,84]. Serial complete blood cell counts and urinalyses should be obtained in patients with significant lesions or systemic loxoscelism [84].

There is no commercially available test to definitively diagnose recluse spider envenomation. The differential diagnosis for *Loxosceles* envenomation includes bites or stings by other arthropods (e.g., other spiders, ticks, scorpions, ants, fleas, kissing bugs, bedbugs, and biting flies), superficial skin infections (especially methicillin-resistant *Staphylococcus aureus*), cutaneous anthrax, diabetic ulcers, plant puncture wounds, sporotrichosis, toxic epidermal necrolysis, pyoderma gangrenosum, erythema nodosum, erythema migrans, herpes zoster, herpes simplex, erythema multiforme, purpura fulminans, and contact dermatitis.

Management

No commercial antivenoms exist for *Loxosceles* bites in the United States. The majority of cases require only local wound care, including cleansing of the bite site, application of a sterile dressing, immobilization with a well-padded splint, and tetanus prophylaxis as necessary [57]. Frequent local application of ice or cold packs during the first 72 hours to reduce sphingomyelinase D activity may be beneficial [74]. If an ulcer develops, it should be cleaned several times each day with hydrogen peroxide or povidone–iodine solution [84]. Pruritus can be treated with antihistamines. Antibiotics to prevent secondary cellulitis can be considered [74] and should include coverage for methicillin-resistant *S. aureus* when evidence of secondary infection is present [88].

It is important to emphasize to patients that nothing has been proven to decrease the extent of dermonecrosis after these bites and that most lesions heal quite satisfactorily with conservative management alone [57,84]. Controversial modalities for managing the wound include the use of steroids, dapsone, colchicine, surgery, hyperbaric oxygen therapy, and topical nitroglycerine application [77,89–92]. Routine use of these agents should be avoided until prospective controlled studies prove that benefits outweigh risks.

Early excision of the wound site is contraindicated because it is impossible to predict the ultimate extent and severity of the lesion [77]. Severe-appearing lesions commonly involute and regress spontaneously to leave minimal defects [93]. Surgical procedures that might be required, such as skin grafting, should be postponed at least 6 to 8 weeks to ensure that the necrotic process has been completed and to improve chances of healing [77]. Hyperbaric oxygen therapy may be useful in particularly severe wounds if it is easily and readily available, but this remains unproven [77].

Initial management of systemic loxoscelism includes adequate hydration, maintaining electrolyte balance, and administering nonsalicylate antipyretics and analgesics [57,84]. Although the use of systemic corticosteroids to stabilize red blood cell membranes has yet to be studied in a controlled fashion, an early, short course of therapy may be beneficial in patients with hemolysis. The recommended dose is 1 mg/kg/d of prednisone orally for 2 to 4 days [57]. Blood products are used as indicated to treat anemia or thrombocytopenia [57]. If hemoglobinuria occurs, hydration becomes critically important, and urine output should be maintained at 2 to 3 mL/kg/h [84]. If renal failure develops, dialysis may be indicated [57,84], and dialysis does not remove venom or hemoglobin from the circulation [84]. Therapeutic plasma exchange may have a role in refractory hemolysis [94,95].

Disposition and Outcome

Any patient with suspected systemic loxoscelism should be admitted to the hospital and have frequent (every 1 to 6 hour) hemoglobin measurements to detect the onset of any hemolysis. Young children who cannot tolerate frequent blood draws should have their urine monitored for free hemoglobin [96]. Patients with isolated cutaneous involvement should have frequent outpatient wound checks until the wound is clearly healing.

Occasionally wounds caused by recluse spiders can be disfiguring and debilitating, requiring surgical repair and revision, but most heal well with conservative therapy alone. Although there have been no reports of deaths in patients bitten by positively identified recluse spiders in the United States [62,84], there is potential for death from systemic loxoscelism, especially in children.

SCORPION ENVENOMATION

Although there are at least 40 species of scorpions found in the United States, only one, the bark scorpion (*Centruroides sculpturatus* [formerly *C. exilicauda*]), is sufficiently toxic to be medically significant [97]. All other US species cause only mild, local envenomation without neurotoxicity. The bark scorpion is found throughout Arizona with isolated colonies located in surrounding counties of bordering states (Nevada, Texas, New Mexico, and California). Other closely related *Centruroides* scorpions of medical importance are found in Mexico. The bark scorpion is 13 to 75 mm long and yellow-brown in color, with variable striping on the dorsum [98], and has a small subaculear tubercle at the base of the stinger.

The venom of *C. sculpturatus* is complex. It contains at least five distinct neurotoxins that cause release of neurotransmitters from the autonomic nervous system and adrenal medulla and stimulate depolarization of neuromuscular junctions [99,100]. Its venom contains no major enzymatic components [101].

Clinical Manifestations

Although most *C. sculpturatus* stings are minor, envenomation may be severe, especially in children. In the largest series of bark scorpion stings in children, the mean onset of symptoms was 20 minutes (range 0 to 130 minutes) [102]. There is usually intense pain, which may extend beyond the site and be associated with paresthesias. Local signs, such as swelling or bruising, are uncommon following bark scorpion stings [101].

Systemic findings may include fever, motor hyperactivity, opsoclonus, tachycardia, hypersalivation, hypertension, vomiting, respiratory distress, hypoxemia, stridor and diaphoresis, and, in patients treated without antivenom, almost one-fourth will require intubation and mechanical ventilation [102].

Clinical findings after envenomation by other US scorpions (nonneurotoxic) consist of immediate, brief, intense pain, mild soft-tissue swelling, and mild ecchymosis [103]. Systemic manifestations are uncommon, and allergic reactions are rare [104].

Diagnostic Evaluation

Adults and older children stung by scorpions frequently see the offending organism and can give a reliable history. In younger children, the history may be unclear, and the clinical picture after a bark scorpion sting may be confused with another diagnosis such as central nervous system infection, widow spider envenomation, tetanus, dystonic drug reaction, intoxication (e.g., pesticides, anticholinergics, sympathomimetics, xanthines, propoxyphene, and strychnine), drug withdrawal, anaphylaxis, or seizure disorder. A general medical history should be obtained, symptoms assessed, and prehospital treatments noted. Vital signs should be frequently monitored. The sting site should be inspected and the patient examined for signs of systemic toxicity. Table 124.2 is a useful grading scale for determining severity of bark scorpion stings [102].

There are currently no commercial laboratory tests of diagnostic benefit in patients suspected of *C. sculpturatus* envenomation. The white blood cell count and serum glucose may be elevated [99]. Increases in serum amylase, creatine phosphokinase, and renal function studies, mild abnormalities in coagulation parameters, and cerebral spinal fluid pleocytosis have been reported [102,105]. No labs are necessary for victims of nonneurotoxic scorpion stings.

Management

The majority of *C. sculpturatus* stings, particularly in adults, can be treated with cold compresses and analgesics, usually at home [99]. Adults with more severe envenomations and young children should be managed in a hospital. These patients should receive oxygen and have an IV line established, along with continuous cardiac and pulse oximetry monitoring. The key to managing signficant *C. sculpturatus* stings is the administration of antivenom (see below). The airway should be secured if there are signs of respiratory failure or inability to handle secretions

TABLE 124.2

Grading Scale for Bark Scorpion (*Centruroides sculpturatus*) Envenomation Severity

Mild Envenomation
- I: local pain &/or paresthesias at sting site
- II: pain &/or paresthesias remote from sting site

Severe Envenomation
- III: Either cranial nerve or neuromuscular dysfunction
- IV: Cranial nerve and neuromuscular dysfunction

Cranial nerve dysfunction: tongue fasciculations, hypersalivation, slurred speech, or opsoclonus

Neuromuscular dysfunction: involuntary shaking and jerking of the extremities.

[105]. Pain, anxiety, restlessness, muscular hyperactivity, and hypertension can initially be treated with parenteral opioids and benzodiazepines while antivenom is readied [102]. It is rare for specific antihypertensive agents to be required, especially after antivenom is given.

Antivenom

In 2011, the FDA approved the first antivenom (Anascorp; Instituto Bioclon, Mexico City, Mexico) for managing bark scorpion stings in children or adults [102]. Anascorp is an equine, $F(ab')_2$ product that has been shown to rapidly reverse systemic toxicity following *C. sculpturatus* envenomation. It is indicated in any patient with significant toxicity following bark scorpion sting. The starting dose (in children and adults) is 3 vials; however, it is reasonable to start with a single vial and repeat until symptoms are resolved. Each vial of lyophilized antiserum is reconstituted using 5 mL of normal saline, and the contents are placed in a 50 mL volume of normal saline. With the patient closely monitored, the entire dose is given intravenously over 10 minutes. The patient is then observed for 30 to 60 minutes. If symptoms fail to resolve, further antivenom is given in one vial aliquots (again diluted in 50 mL of normal saline and administered over 10 minutes). This sequence is repeated until symptoms improve. Most patients experience symptom resolution within 4 hours and can be discharged at that time [97].

Although bark scorpions historically caused more direct venom toxicity deaths in Arizona than any other venomous creatures [102], deaths are now exceptionally rare [98,99], but the potential for a fatal outcome should not be underestimated, especially in small children and the infirm.

CONCLUSION

The key to managing an envenomation victim, regardless of the offending organism, is to be alert for signs or symptoms suggesting worsening toxicity, and to be ready to intervene quickly when indicated. At times, that intervention may involve administration of a specific antidote such as antivenom, but more often it involves providing sound supportive care according to the tenets of critical care medicine.

References

1. Russell FE: *Snake Venom Poisoning*. 2nd ed. New York, Scholium, 1983.
2. Gutierrez JM, Rucavadoa R, Escalantea T, et al: Hemorrhage induced by snake venom metalloproteinases: biochemical and biophysical mechanisms involved in microvessel damage. *Toxicon* 45:997–1011, 2005.
3. Richardson WH, Goto CS, Gutglass DJ, et al: Rattlesnake envenomation with neurotoxicity refractory to treatment with crotaline Fab antivenom. *Clin Toxicol (Phila)* 45(5):472–475, 2007.
4. Schaeffer RC, Carlson RW, Puri VK, et al: The effects of colloidal and crystalloidal fluids on rattlesnake venom shock in the rat. *J Pharmacol Exp Ther* 206:687–695, 1978.
5. Bonilla CA, Fiero K, Frank LP: Isolation of a basic protein neurotoxin from *Crotalus adamanteus* venom. I. purification and biological properties. *Toxicon* 8:123, 1970.
6. Jansen PW, Perkin RM, Van Stralen D: Mojave rattlesnake envenomation: prolonged neurotoxicity and rhabdomyolysis. *Ann Emerg Med* 21:322–325, 1992.
7. Bush SP, Mooy GG, Phan TH: Catastrophic acute ischemic stroke after Crotalidae polyvalent immune Fab (ovine)-treated rattlesnake envenomation. *Wilderness Environ Med* 25(2):198–203, 2014.
8. Parrish HM, Goldner JC, Silberg SL: Poisonous snakebites causing no venenation. *Postgrad Med* 39:265–269, 1966.
9. Bucknall NC: Electrical treatment of venomous bites and stings. *Toxicon* 29:397–400, 1991.
10. Hardy DL: A review of first aid measures for pitviper bite in North America with an appraisal of Extractor suction and stun gun electroshock, in Campbell JA, Brodie ED (eds): *Biology of the Pitvipers*. Tyler, TX, Selva, 1992, p 405.
11. Bush SP, Hegewald KG, Green SM, et al: Effects of a negative pressure venom extraction device (Extractor) on local tissue injury after artificial rattlesnake envenomation in a porcine model. *Wilderness Environ Med* 11:180–188, 2000.
12. Gerardo CJ, Lavonas EJ, McKinney RE: Ethical considerations in design of a study to evaluate a US Food and Drug Administration-approved indication: antivenom versus placebo for copperhead envenomation. *Clin Trials* 11(5):560–564, 2014.
13. Dart RC, Seifert SA, Carroll L, et al: Affinity-purified, mixed monospecific crotalid antivenom ovine Fab for the treatment of crotalid venom poisoning. *Ann Emerg Med* 30:33–39, 1997.
14. Lavonas EJ, Ruha AM, Banner W, et al: Unified treatment algorithm for the management of crotaline snakebite in the United States: results of an evidence-informed consensus workshop. *BMC Emerg Med* 11:2, 2011.
15. Ruha A-M, Curry SC, Beuhler M, et al: Initial postmarketing experience with Crotalidae polyvalent immune Fab for treatment of rattlesnake envenomation. *Ann Emerg Med* 39:609–615, 2002.
16. Yip L: Rational use of Crotalidae polyvalent immune Fab (ovine) in the management of crotaline bite. *Ann Emerg Med* 39:648–650, 2002.
17. CroFab: CroFab Full Prescribing Information, 2012. Available at: http://www.crofab.com/documents/CroFab-Prescribing_Information.pdf. West Conshohocken, PA, BTG International Inc. Accessed August 15, 2015.
18. Russell FE, Carlson RW, Wainschel J, et al: Snake venom poisoning in the United States: experiences with 550 cases. *JAMA* 233:341–344, 1975.
19. Schaeffer TH, Khatri V, Reifler LM, et al: Incidence of immediate hypersensitivity reaction and serum sickness following administration of Crotalidae polyvalent immune Fab antivenom: a meta-analysis. *Acad Emerg Med* 19(2):121–131, 2012.
20. Van Mierop LH, Kitchens CS: Defibrination syndrome following bites by the Eastern diamondback rattlesnake. *J Fla Med Assoc* 67:21–27, 1980.
21. Burgess JL, Dart RC: Snake venom coagulopathy: use and abuse of blood products in the treatment of pit viper envenomation. *Ann Emerg Med* 20:795–801, 1991.
22. Ruha AM, Curry SC: Recombinant factor VIIa for treatment of gastrointestinal hemorrhage following rattlesnake envenomation. *Wilderness Environ Med* 20:156–160, 2009.
23. Clark RF, Selden BS, Furbee B: The incidence of wound infection following crotalid envenomation. *J Emerg Med* 11:583–586, 1993.
24. Stolpe MR, Norris RL, Chisholm CD, et al: Preliminary observations on the effects of hyperbaric oxygen therapy on western diamondback rattlesnake (*Crotalus atrox*) venom poisoning in the rabbit model. *Ann Emerg Med* 18:871–874, 1989.
25. Curry SC, Kraner JC, Kunkel DB, et al: Noninvasive vascular studies in management of rattlesnake envenomations to extremities. *Ann Emerg Med* 14:1081–1084, 1985.
26. Dart R, Russell FE: Animal poisoning, in Hall J, Schmidt G, Wood L (eds): *Principles of Critical Care.* New York, NY, McGraw-Hill, 1992, p 2163.
27. Tanen DA, Danish DC, Grice GA, et al: Fasciotomy worsens the amount of myonecrosis in a porcine model of crotaline envenomation. *Ann Emerg Med* 44:99–104, 2004.
28. Hardy DL, Zamudio KR: Compartment syndrome, fasciotomy and neuropathy after a rattlesnake envenomation: aspects of monitoring and diagnosis. *Wilderness Environ Med* 17:36–40, 2006.
29. Gomez HF, Dart RC: Clinical toxicology of snakebite in North America, in Meier J, White J (eds): *Handbook of Clinical Toxicology of Animal Venoms and Poisons*. Boca Raton, FL, CRC Press, 1995, p 619.
30. Boyer LV, Seifert SA, Clark RF, et al: Recurrent and persistent coagulopathy following pit viper envenomation. *Arch Intern Med* 159:706–710, 1999.
31. Kitchens C, Eskin T: Fatality in a case of envenomation by *Crotalus adamanteus* initially successfully treated with polyvalent ovine antivenom followed by recurrence of defibrinogenation syndrome. *J Med Toxicol* 4(3):180–183, 2008.
32. O'Brien NF, DeMott MC, Suchard JR, et al: Recurrent coagulopathy with delayed significant bleeding after crotaline envenomation. *Pediatr Emerg Care* 25(7):457–459, 2009.
33. Boyer LV, Seifert SA, Cain JS: Recurrence phenomena after immunoglobulin therapy for snake envenomations: part 2. Guidelines for clinical management with crotaline Fab antivenom. *Ann Emerg Med* 37(2):196–201, 2001.
34. Parrish HM: *Poisonous Snakebites in the United States*. New York, NY, Vantage Press, 1980.
35. Hardy DL: Fatal rattlesnake envenomation in Arizona: 1969–1984. *Clin Toxicol* 24:1–10, 1986.
36. Grace TG, Omer GE: The management of upper extremity pit viper wounds. *J Hand Surg Am* 5:168–177, 1980.
37. Simon TL, Grace TG: Envenomation coagulopathy from snake bites. *N Engl J Med* 305:1347–1348, 1981.
38. Mowry JB, Spyker DA, Cantilena LR Jr, et al: 2013 Annual Report of the American Association of Poison Control Centers' National Poison Data System (NPDS): 31st Annual Report. *Clin Toxicol (Phila)* 52(10):1032–1283, 2014.
39. Campbell JA, Lamar WW: *Venomous Reptiles of the Western Hemisphere*, Ithaca, NY, Cornell University Press, 2004, p 1.
40. Parrish HM, Khan MS: Bites by coral snakes: report of 11 representative cases. *Am J Med Sci* 253:561–568, 1967.
41. Fix JD: Venom yield of the North American coral snake and its clinical significance. *South Med J* 73:737–738, 1980.
42. Morgan DL, Borys DL, Stanford R, et al: Texas coral snake (*Micrurus tener*) bites. *South Med J* 100:152–156, 2007.
43. Lee CY: Elapid neurotoxins and their mode of action. *Clin Toxicol (Phila)* 3:457–472, 1970.
44. Kitchens CS, Van Mierop LHS: Envenomation by the Eastern coral snake (*Micrurus fulvius*): a study of 39 victims. *JAMA* 258:1615–1618, 1987.

45. Norris RL, Dart RC: Apparent coral snake envenomation in a patient without fang marks. *Am J Emerg Med* 7:402–405, 1989.
46. McCollough NC, Gennaro JF: Treatment of venomous snakebite in the United States. *Clin Toxicol (Phila)* 3:483–500, 1970.
47. Minton SA: Identification of poisonous snakes, in Minton SA (ed): *Snake Venoms and Envenomation*. New York, NY, Marcel Dekker Inc, 1971, p 1.
48. White J: Snakebite: an Australian perspective. *J Wilderness Med* 2:219–244, 1991.
49. Sutherland SK: Pressure immobilization for snakebite in southern Africa remains speculative. *S Afr Med J* 85:1039–1040, 1995.
50. German BT, Hack JB, Brewer K, et al: Pressure-immobilization bandages delay toxicity in a porcine model of eastern coral snake (*Micrurus fulvius fulvius*) envenomation. *Ann Emerg Med* 45:603–608, 2005.
51. Gaar GG: Assessment and management of coral and other exotic snake envenomations. *J Fla Med Assoc* 83:178–182, 1996.
52. Russell FE, Madon NB: New names for the brown recluse and the black widow. *Postgrad Med* 70:31, 1981.
53. Brown KS, Necaise JS, Goddard J: Additions to the known U.S. distribution of *Latrodectus geometricus* (Araneae: Theridiidae). *J Med Entomol* 45:959–962, 2008.
54. Kobernick M: Black widow spider bite. *Am Fam Physician* 29:241–245, 1984.
55. Maretic Z: Latrodectism: variations in clinical manifestations provoked by *Latrodectus* species of spiders. *Toxicon* 21:457–466, 1983.
56. Baba A, Cooper JR: The action of black widow spider venom on cholinergic mechanisms in synaptosomes. *J Neurochem* 34:1369–1379, 1980.
57. Anderson PC: Necrotizing spider bites. *Am Fam Physician* 26:198–203, 1982.
58. Moss HS, Binder LS: A retrospective review of black widow spider envenomation. *Ann Emerg Med* 16:188–191, 1987.
59. Reeves JA, Allison EJ, Goodman PE: Black widow spider bite in a child. *Am J Emerg Med* 14:469–471, 1996.
60. Russell FE: Muscle relaxants in black widow spider (*Latrodectus mactans*) poisoning. *Am J Med Sci* 243:159–161, 1962.
61. Russell FE, Marcus P, Streng JA: Black widow spider envenomation during pregnancy: report of a case. *Toxicon* 17:188,189, 1979.
62. Wong RC, Hughes SE, Voorhees JJ: Spider bites. *Arch Dermatol* 123:98–104, 1987.
63. Levine M, Canning J, Chase R, et al: Cardiomyopathy following *Latrodectus* envenomation. *West J Emerg Med* 11(5):521–523, 2010.
64. Isbister GK, Fan HW: Spider bite. *Lancet* 378(9808):2039–2047, 2011.
65. Clark RF, Wethern-Kestner S, Vance MV, et al: Clinical presentation and treatment of black widow spider envenomation: a review of 163 cases. *Ann Emerg Med* 21:782–787, 1992.
66. Sherman RP, Groll JM, Gonzalez DI, et al: Black widow spider (*Latrodectus mactans*) envenomation in a term pregnancy. *Curr Surg* 57:346–348, 2000.
67. Isbister GK, Page CB, Buckley NA, et al: Randomized controlled trial of intravenous antivenom versus placebo for latrodectism: the second Redback Antivenom Evaluation (RAVE-II) study. *Ann Emerg Med* 64(6):620–628, 2014.
68. Isbister GK, Graudins A, White J, et al: Antivenom treatment in arachnidism. *J Toxicol Clin Toxicol* 41(3):291–300, 2003.
69. Merck & Co, Inc: Antivenin (*Latrodectus mactans*) (Black Widow Spider Antivenin) Equine Origin. Merck & Co, Inc, Whitehouse Station, NJ. 2015. Available at: http://www.merck.com/product/usa/pi_circulars/a/antivenin/antivenin_pi.pdf. Accessed August 28, 2015.
70. Murphy CM, Hong JJ, Beuhler MC: Anaphylaxis with *Latrodectus* antivenin resulting in cardiac arrest. *J Med Toxicol* 7(4):317–321, 2011.
71. Monte AA: Black widow spider (*Latrodectus mactans*) antivenom in clinical practice. *Curr Pharm Biotechnol* 13(10):1935–1939, 2012.
72. Monte AA, Bucher-Bartelson B, Heard KJ: A US perspective of symptomatic *Latrodectus* spp. envenomation and treatment: a National Poison Data System review. *Ann Pharmacother* 45(12):1491–1498, 2011.
73. Gertsch WJ, Ennik F: The spider genus *Loxosceles* in North America, Central America, and the West Indes, Aranie (Loxoscelidae). *Bull Am Museum Nat Hist* 175:264–360, 1983.
74. Wilson DC, King LE: Spiders and spider bites. *Dermatol Clin* 8:277–286, 1990.
75. Berger RS, Millikan LE, Conway F: An *in vitro* test for *Loxosceles reclusa* spider bites. *Toxicon* 11:465–470, 1973.
76. Smith CW, Micks DW: A comparative study of the venom and other components of three species of *Loxosceles*. *Am J Trop Med Hyg* 17:651–656, 1968.
77. Wasserman GS: Wound care of spider and snake envenomations. *Ann Emerg Med* 17:1331–1335, 1988.
78. Rees RS, Nanney LB, Yates RA, et al: Interaction of brown recluse spider venom on cell membranes: the inciting mechanism? *J Invest Dermatol* 83:270–275, 1984.
79. Kurpiewski G, Forrester LJ, Barrett JT, et al: Platelet aggregation and sphingomyelinase D activity of a purified toxin from the venom of *Loxosceles reclusa*. *Biochim Biophys Acta* 678:467–476, 1981.
80. Jansen GT, Morgan PN, McQueen JN, et al: The brown recluse spider bite: controlled evaluation of treatment using the white rabbit as a model. *South Med J* 64:1194–1202, 1971.
81. Berger RS, Adelstein EH, Anderson PC: Intravascular coagulation: the cause of necrotic arachnidism. *J Invest Dermatol* 61:142–150, 1973.
82. Smith CW, Micks DW: The role of polymorphonuclear leukocytes in the lesion caused by the venom of the brown spider, *Loxosceles reclusa*. *Lab Invest* 22:90–93, 1970.
83. Rees R, Campbell D, Rieger E, et al: The diagnosis and treatment of brown recluse spider bites. *Ann Emerg Med* 16:945–949, 1987.
84. Wasserman GS, Anderson PC: Loxoscelism and necrotic arachnidism. *J Toxicol Clin Toxicol* 21:451–472, 1983–1984.
85. Arnold RE: Brown recluse spider bites: five cases with a review of the literature. *JACEP* 5:262–264, 1976.
86. Fardon DW, Wingo CW, Robinson DW, et al: The treatment of brown spider bite. *Plast Reconstr Surg* 40:482–488, 1967.
87. Dillaha CJ, Jansen GT, Honeycutt WM, et al: North American loxoscelism. *JAMA* 188:153–156, 1964.
88. Frithsen IL, Vetter RS, Stocks IC: Reports of envenomation by brown recluse spiders exceed verified specimens of *Loxosceles* spiders in South Carolina. *J Am Board Fam Med* 20:483–488, 2007.
89. Berger RS: A critical look at therapy for the brown recluse spider bite. *Arch Dermatol* 107:298, 1973.
90. Hansen RC, Russell FE: Dapsone use for *Loxosceles* envenomation treatment. *Vet Hum Toxicol* 26:260, 1984.
91. Burton KG: Nitroglycerine patches for brown recluse spider bites. *Am Fam Physician* 51:1401, 1995.
92. Lowry BP, Bradfield JF, Carroll RG, et al: A controlled trial of topical nitroglycerine in a New Zealand white rabbit model of brown recluse spider envenomation. *Ann Emerg Med* 37:161–165, 2001.
93. Anderson PC: What's new in loxoscelism 1978? *Mo Med* 74:549–552, 1977.
94. Said A, Hmiel P, Goldsmith M, et al: Successful use of plasma exchange for profound hemolysis in a child with loxoscelism. *Pediatrics* 134(5):e1464–e1467, 2014.
95. Abraham M, Tilzer L, Hoehn KS, et al: Therapeutic plasma exchange for refractory hemolysis after brown recluse spider (*Loxosceles reclusa*) Envenomation. *J Med Toxicol* 11(3):364–367, 2015.
96. Gehrie EA, Nian H, Young PP: Brown recluse spider bite mediated hemolysis: clinical features, a possible role for complement inhibitor therapy, and reduced RBC surface glycophorin A as a potential biomarker of venom exposure. *PLoS One* 27;8(9):e76558, 2013.
97. Rare Disease Therapeutics, Inc: *Anascorp Expanded Brochure*. Available at: http://www.anascorp-us.com/resources/Expanded_Brochure.pdf. Accessed July 17, 2015.
98. Likes K, Banner W, Chavez M: *Centruroides exilicauda* envenomation in Arizona. *West J Med* 141:634–637, 1984.
99. Rachesky IJ, Banner W, Dansky J, et al: Treatments for *Centruroides exilicauda* envenomation. *Am J Dis Child* 138:1136–1139, 1984.
100. Simard JM, Watt DD: Venoms and toxins, in Polis GA (ed): *The Biology of Scorpions*. Stanford, CA, Stanford University Press, 1990, p 414.
101. Curry SC, Vance MV, Ryan PJ, et al: Envenomation by the scorpion *Centruroides sculpturatus*. *J Toxicol Clin Toxicol* 21:417–419, 1983–1984.
102. O'Connor A, Ruha AM: Clinical course of bark scorpion envenomation managed without antivenom. *J Med Toxicol* 8(3):258–262, 2012.
103. Ellis MD: *Dangerous Plants, Snakes, Arthropods and Marine Life of Texas*. Washington DC, U.S. Department of Health, Education, and Welfare, Public Health Service, U.S. Government Printing Office, 1975.
104. King LE, Rees RS: Spider bites and scorpion stings, in Rakel RE (ed): *Conn's Current Therapy*. 39th ed. Philadelphia, PA, WB Saunders, 1987, p 970.
105. Berg RA, Tarantino MD: Envenomation by the scorpion *Centruroides exilicauda* (*C. sculpturatus*): severe and unusual manifestations. *Pediatrics* 87:930–933, 1991.

Chapter 125 ■ Therapeutic Agents for Overdoses and Poisonings

LUKE YIP • SUSAN E. GORMAN* • JERRY D. THOMAS* • IAN M. BALL

This is a list of therapeutic agents that are used in medical toxicology, and has been organized into a Table format to facilitate rapid access to concise information guiding indication and dosing of a therapeutic agent. The table is divided into four columns. The first column is alphabetically organized in terms of a specific agent; individual agents appear alphabetically in the Index. The second column focuses on indications and uses in medical toxicology. The third column provides guidelines for dosing of the therapeutic agent. The fourth column highlights caveats and potential complications. The content of this table is not intended to be a comprehensive list of therapeutic agents and is not a substitute for reference textbooks in medical toxicology (e.g., Goldfrank Toxicologic Emergencies and Medical Toxicology) and does not address envenomations by exotic venomous creatures or envenomations outside the United States. Some of the listed therapeutic agents may not be available to every clinician, and it may be prudent to be familiar with the therapeutic agents that are available in the respective clinician's practice.

*The findings and conclusions in this study are those of the authors and do not necessarily represent the views of the U.S. Department of Health and Human Services, or the U.S. Centers for Disease Control and Prevention. Use of trade names and commercial sources is for identification only and does not constitute endorsement by the U.S. Department of Health and Human Services, or the U.S. Centers for Disease Control and Prevention.

Therapeutic agent	Uses	Dosing	Caveat Complication
Activated charcoal	GI decontamination • Multiple dose consideration: carbamazepine, dapsone, methotrexate, phenobarbital, quinine, theophylline.	Oral/nasogastric single dose: 1–2 g/kg Oral/nasogastric multiple doses: Hourly, every 2 h, *or* every 4 h at a dose equivalent to 12.5 g/h for 12–24 h.	Ensure adequate airway protection prior to activated charcoal therapy. Should not be administered in patients with decreased bowel sounds/ileus. Co-administration of cathartics (e.g., magnesium, sorbitol) may result in hypernatremia, hypokalemia, hypermagnesemia, and metabolic acidosis.
	Theophylline poisoning	Activated charcoal 1–2 g/kg followed by hourly, every 2 h, *or* every 4 h at a dose equivalent to 12.5 g/h (Peds: 10–25 g) until serum theophylline <15 μg/mL; alternatively, 0.25–0.5 g/kg/h via continuous nasogastric infusion; not in patients with decreased bowel sounds/ileus.	
Antivenom	Known or suspected elapidae (e.g., coral snake) envenomation	Elapidae • IV coral snake antivenom 4–6 vials, each vial diluted in 50–100 mL of normal saline and administered over 1 h; if signs/symptoms appear or progress, administer 4–6 more vials of antivenom.	Precaution: Be prepared to treat acute anaphylactic (shock) and anaphylactoid reactions. May be effective in late presenters. Serum sickness: May occur 7–21 days following therapy.
	Viperidae (subfamily Crotalinae: pitvipers, e.g., rattle snake)	Viperidae • IV CroFab (Protherics, Inc., London): administer 4–6 vials; carefully monitor for further progression of local effects and systemic symptoms; repeat laboratory studies (i.e., CBC, PT/INR, fibrin, fibrin degradation products) 1 h after completing antivenom infusion; administer additional 4–6 vials antivenom if initial control (i.e., reversal or marked attenuation of all venom effects) not achieved; continue with additional 4–6 vials antivenom until control is evident then administer 2 vials of CroFab every 6 h for three additional doses; most cases 8–12 vials to establish initial control. • Reconstitute each CroFab vial with normal saline 10 mL and roll vials between hands; dilute total dose to be administered in normal saline 250 mL and infuse over 1 h.	Precaution: See **Elapidae**. Antivenom: Ovine origin; most effective within 24 h of envenomating, may be beneficial in late presenters with severe findings (e.g., coagulopathy); limited effectiveness in preventing wound necrosis or reversing cellular damage; thrombocytopenia may be resistant to antivenom therapy. Serum sickness: See **Elapidae**.
	Known or suspected widow spider (*Latrodectus* sp., e.g., black widow) envenomation	*Lactrodectus* • IV antivenom (preferable) 1 reconstituted vial further diluted in normal saline 50–100 mL over 30 min or IM antivenom 1 reconstituted vial in the anterolateral thigh; signs/symptoms should completely resolve within few hours; a second vial can be administered if necessary.	Precaution: See **Elapidae**. Antivenom: Equine origin; most effective in acute setting, may be beneficial in late presenters (e.g., 96 h) with prolonged symptoms. Serum sickness: See **Elapidae**.

Antivenom	Known or suspected scorpion (*Centruroides* sp.) envenomation	*Centruroides* • IV Anascorp: Administer 3 vials (adults or pediatrics); closely monitor for resolution of clinically important signs of envenoming during and up to 60 min following antivenom infusion; administer additional antivenom, if needed, one vial every 30–60 min and monitor for resolution of clinically important signs of envenomating during and up to 60 min following antivenom infusion. • Reconstitute each Anascorp vial with normal saline 5 mL and mix by continuous gentle swirling; dilute total dose to be administered in normal saline 50 mL and infuse over 10 min.	Precaution: See **Elapidae.** Antivenom: Equine origin; most effective in acute setting, may be beneficial in late presenters with prolonged symptoms. Serum sickness: See **Elapidae.**
Atropine	Cholinesterase inhibitors (e.g., organophosphorus agents, nerve agents)	IV atropine 1–4 mg (Peds: 0.05 mg/kg), double the dose every 5–10 min as needed until pulmonary secretions are controlled (tachycardia *not* a contraindication to atropine); once stabilized start atropine infusion (10%–20% of total dose for stabilization per hour); restart atropine at the first signs of cholinergic excess; administer with pralidoxime (see **Pralidoxime**).	Carbamates and other reversible cholinesterase inhibitors: Atropine *and* pralidoxime are used to treat acutely ill patients unless carbaryl (Sevin) is known to be involved, then just atropine and supportive care. Atropine requirement in severe organophosphorus agent toxicity may be hundreds of mg whereas in nerve agent poisoning may be significantly less. Atropine has no effect on muscle weakness or paralysis and will not affect acetylcholinesterase regeneration rate.
Botulism antitoxin heptavalent (A, B, C, D, E, F, G)—BAT	Botulism	BAT, equine-derived antibody to seven known botulinum toxin types (A–G), treatment of naturally occurring *noninfant* botulism is available from state/local health department or Centers for Disease Control and Prevention (CDC); additional emergency consultation available from CDC botulism duty officer via CDC Emergency Operations Center, telephone, 770-488-7100; additional information regarding CDC's botulism treatment program is available at http://www.bt.cdc.gov/agent/botulism.	Respiratory support is mainstay of therapy. Be prepared to treat acute anaphylactic (shock) and anaphylactoid reactions. Administer antitoxin as soon as possible; lethality of botulinum toxin outweighs risk of adverse events from antitoxin treatment, and treatment is considered acceptable for anyone with presumed illness or potential exposure to the toxin. Antitoxin does not reverse paralysis but stops its progression. Serum sickness may occur 7–21 d following therapy. Report suspected botulism cases immediately to their state health department; all states maintain 24-h telephone services for reporting botulism and other public health emergencies.
	Infant botulism types A and B	BabyBIG (botulism immune globulin) available through the California Infant Botulism Treatment and Prevention Program, www.infantbotulism.org for further instructions to obtain BabyBIG.	Cases of infant botulism have been treated with BAT.

(*continued*)

Therapeutic agent	Uses	Dosing	Caveat Complication
Calcium	Calcium channel antagonist poisoning	IV calcium chloride (10%) 0.2 mL/kg followed by continuous calcium chloride infusion 0.2–0.5 mL/kg/h, titrate infusion to cardiac output; follow ionized calcium levels every 30 min initially and then every 2 h, maintain ionized calcium twice normal; if using IV calcium gluconate (10%) 0.6 mL/kg bolus over 5–10 min followed by continuous calcium gluconate infusion (10%) 0.6–1.5 mL/kg/h.	Threefold difference in calcium cation between calcium chloride (13.6 mEq/6.8 mmol Ca^{+2}/g) and calcium gluconate (4.7 mEq/2.4 mmol Ca^{2+}/g); calcium 2+ valence, mEq equals two times mmol. Primarily inotropic effect; mixed clinical experience (disappointing at times). May not be effective as sole therapy (see **Euglycemic clamp** and **Lipid emulsion therapy**).
	Hydrofluoric acid • Digital exposure and pain	Apply a 2.3%–2.5% calcium gluconate preparation in a water-soluble gel to exposed area(s) ≥30 min or until symptoms resolve. Pain unrelieved by gel therapy • Regional intra-arterial: Place catheter in direction of blood flow by Seldinger technique, continuously monitor arterial waveform (arteriography if concern as to adequate placement), infuse 50 mL of 2.5% calcium gluconate in normal saline over 4 h; repeated doses may be required over 12–24 h. OR • Administer 40 mL of a 2.5% calcium gluconate solution by Bier block technique (i.e., catheterize a distal vein and exsangunate extremity by elevation and compression with an esmarch bandage, inflate blood pressure cuff to 100 mm Hg above systolic pressure and maintain for 15–20 min following calcium administration, gradually deflate cuff over 5 min).	
	• Symptomatic inhalation exposure	Nebulized calcium gluconate (e.g., 4 mL of 2.5% solution in normal saline) treatment may improve symptoms following mild exposure.	
	• History suggestive of a substantive dermal or oral exposure that may lead to systemic toxicity	Oral calcium or magnesium containing antacids 30–60 mL. IV calcium chloride 1 g over 30 min; patients with normal vital signs and hemodynamic stability should be monitored with serum calcium levels every 30 min for the first 2–3 h; IV calcium chloride 1 g boluses to maintain serum calcium concentration in the high normal laboratory reference range, repeat as needed; a fall in serum calcium concentration below the normal range, dysrhythmias or a fall in blood pressure is treated with IV calcium chloride 2–3 g boluses every 15 min *or* IV magnesium sulfate (see **Magnesium**).	

Carboxypeptidase-G2 (glucarpidase)	Methotrexate (MTX) overdose or serum MTX concentration >1 μmol/L with delayed MTX clearance due to renal dysfunction.	(**2 h after leucovorin administration**) IV carboxypeptidase (CPDG2) 50 U/kg over 5 min; a second 50 U/kg dose may be administered 48 h later; **do not administer** leucovorin within 2 h before or after a CPDG2 dose; leucovorin is a CPDG2 substrate (see **Folinic acid** and **Sodium bicarbonate**). IntrathecalCPDG2 2,000 U in 12 mL normal saline over 5 min.	CPDG2 acts only on extracellular MTX and MTX redistribution may occur; second CPDG2 dose at 48 h. MTX metabolite may cross-react with commercial MTX immunoassays, and HPLC is preferred for measuring MTX ≤48 h of CPDG2.
Carnitine	Valproic acid overdose • Coma, symptomatic hyperammonemia, symptomatic hepatotoxicity, or rising serum ammonia levels • Acute overdose without hepatic enzyme abnormalities or hyperammonemia	IV L-carnitine 100 mg/kg (max 6 g) over 30 min followed by 15 mg/kg (over 10–30 min) every 4 h until clinical improvement; consider treatment for patients with serum VPA >450 μg/mL. Consider oral L-carnitine 100 mg/kg/d (max 3 g) divided every 6 h.	
Chelators • Dimercaprol (BAL, British Anti-Lewisite) • Edetate calcium disodium ($CaNa_2EDTA$, calcium disodium versenate) • Deferoximine (DFO) • Diethylenetriaminepentaacetate (DTPA) • Prussian blue (ferric hexacyanoferrate) • 2,3-Dimercaptosuccinic acid (DMSA, Succimer)	Arsenic (As): suspected acute symptomatic As poisoning	IM BAL 3–5 mg/kg every 4 h, gradually tapering to every 12 h over several days; switch to DMSA 10 mg/kg every 8 h for 5 d, reduced to every 12 h for another 2 wks; additional course of treatment may be considered based on post-treatment results: 24-h urinary As excretion is followed before, during, and after chelation with continued chelation therapy until the urinary As excretion <25 μg/24 h *or* during the recovery period when urinary inorganic As concentration <100 μg/24 h *or* total blood As <200 μg/L.	
	Lead (Pb) • Symptomatic Pb encephalopathy	IM BAL 75 mg/m^2 (3–5 mg/kg) every 4 h. After 4 h have elapsed since the priming dose of BAL start IV $CaNa_2EDTA$ 1,500 mg/m^2/d (30 mg/kg/d). In cases of cerebral edema and or increased intracranial pressure associated with encephalopathy, administer $CaNa_2EDTA$ (same dosage) by deep IM injection (extremely painful) along with procaine 0.5% in two to three divided doses every 8–12 h. Continue BAL and $CaNa_2EDTA$ 5 days. Cessation of chelation is often followed by a rebound in blood Pb concentration, a second chelation course may be considered based on whole blood Pb concentration after 2 days' interruption of BAL and $CaNa_2EDTA$ treatment and the persistence or recurrence of symptoms. A third course may be required if the whole blood concentration rebounds ≥50 μg/dL within 48 h after second chelation treatment. If chelation is required for the third time, it should begin a week after the last dose of BAL and $CaNa_2EDTA$.	

(*continued*)

Therapeutic agent	Uses	Dosing	Caveat Complication
Chelators	• Symptomatic patients who are not overtly encephalopathic	IM BAL 50 mg/m^2 (2–3 mg/kg) every 4 h. After 4 h have elapsed since the priming dose of BAL, start IV $CaNa_2EDTA$ 1,000 mg/m^2/d (20–30 mg/kg/d) or in 2–3 divided doses every 8–12 h. BAL and $CaNa_2EDTA$ should be continued for 5 d with daily monitoring of whole blood Pb concentrations. BAL may be discontinued any time during these 5 d if the whole blood Pb level <50 μg/dL, but $CaNa_2EDTA$ treatment should continue for 5 d. A second or third course of chelation may be considered based on same guidelines in previous paragraph.	
	• Asymptomatic patients with whole blood Pb levels ≥70 μg/dL	BAL and $CaNa_2EDTA$ same doses and same guidelines as for symptomatic Pb poisoning without encephalopathy. Second course of $CaNa_2EDTA$ chelation alone may be necessary if whole blood Pb concentration rebounds ≥50 μg/dL within 5–7 d after chelation has ceased. Alternative: Oral DMSA 10 mg/kg (350 mg/m^2) every 8 h for 5 d then every 12 h for 2 wks. Consider additional course of treatment based on post-treatment whole blood Pb concentrations and persistence or recurrence of symptoms. An interval ≥2 wks may be indicated to assess extent of post-treatment rebound in whole blood Pb concentration.	
	Mercury (Hg) • Elemental Hg poisoning	Oral DMSA (10 mg/kg every 8 h, tapering to every 12 h over the next several days and continued until urinary Hg concentration approaches background) may enhance urinary Hg excretion and reduce nephrotoxicity after GI absorption of elemental Hg.	Chelation not proven to improve clinical outcomes. BAL may redistribute Hg to the brain. Confirming elemental Hg exposure: 24-h urinary Hg excretion <50 μg/24 h most useful tool in diagnosing acute exposure (normal whole blood mercury concentration <2 μg/dL and "spot" urine mercury Hg concentration <10 μg/L).
	• Suspected acute inorganic Hg poisoning	BAL and DMSA (see **Arsenic**).	BAL most effective within 4 h of ingestion. Confirming Hg exposure: See **Elemental Hg**; whole blood Hg concentrations >50 μg/dL in acute poisoning associated with gastroenteritis and acute renal tubular necrosis.
	• Organic Hg poisoning	DMSA appears promising in animal studies (see **Elemental Hg**).	Chelation not proven to improve clinical outcomes. Confirmatory Hg exposure: Whole blood Hg concentrations >20 μg/dL associated with symptoms; urinary Hg concentration not useful.

Chelators	Iron (Fe) poisoning: symptomatic patient (e.g., recurrent vomiting or diarrhea, acidosis, shock and decreased level of consciousness or coma) regardless of serum Fe concentration or asymptomatic patient with serum Fe concentration ≥500 μg/dL (90 μmol/L).	IV DFO initiated slowly and gradually increased to 15 mg/kg/h over 20–30 min and continued for 24 h; continuous IV DFO therapy >24 h (rarely needed) is interrupted for 12 of every 24 h; treatment endpoints include resolution of systemic signs/symptoms, correction of acidosis, and return of urine color to normal (if the patient developed vin rosé colored urine during therapy).	Rapid infusion associated with tachycardia, hypotension, shock, generalized beet red flushing of the skin, blotchy erythema, and urticaria. Acute renal failure can result when deferoxamine is administered to hypovolemic patients. Pulmonary toxicity associated with continuous infusion therapy over days. Deferoxamine therapy may increase risk for *Yersinia* bacteremia.
	Known or suspected internal contamination with radioactive cesium (Cs) or radioactive/nonradioactive thallium (Tl).	Adults/adolescents: Oral Prussian blue 3 g t.i.d., Peds (2–12 yrs): 1 g t.i.d.; treatment for 30 d minimum and reassess patient for residual whole body radioactivity, treatment duration guided by level of contamination and clinical judgment.	Administer Prussian blue as soon as possible after suspected contamination; verify contamination as soon as possible. Prussian blue does not treat the complications of radiation exposure. Obtain quantitative baseline of internalized radioactive contamination by whole-body counting and/or bioassay (e.g., Biodosimetry) or feces/urine sample. Obtain weekly radioactivity counts in urine and fecal samples to monitor radioactive elimination rate. Prussian blue capsules can be opened and mixed with food or drinks. Complications of Prussian blue treatment include constipation, hypokalemia, blue-colored stools, and blue discoloration of mouth/teeth.
	Known or suspected internal contamination with plutonium, americium, or curium.	Day 1: IV calcium-DTPA (CaDTPA) 1 g (Peds 14 mg/kg, max 1 g) in 5 mL over 3–4 min *or* in 100–250 mL D5W, normal saline, or LR over 30 min. Day 2: IV zinc-DTPA (ZnDTPA) 1 g (Peds 14 mg/kg, max 1 g) in 5 mL over 3–4 min *or* in 100–250 mL D5W, normal saline, or LR over 30 min every day (continue with daily CaDTPA dosing if ZnDTPA not available); treatment duration based on individual response and weekly radioactivity in blood, urine, and fecal samples.	Administer DTPA as soon as possible after suspected contamination; verify contamination as soon as possible. ZnDTPA should be used for any further chelation after the first dose of CaDTPA; monitor CBC with differential, BUN, serum chemistries and electrolytes, and urinalysis regularly; if using more than one CaDTPA dose, monitor these laboratory tests carefully and consider mineral supplementation containing zinc as appropriate.
	Internal plutonium, americium, or curium contamination by inhalation.	Day 1: Nebulize diluted CaDTPA 1 g (Peds 14 mg/kg, max 1 g) at a 1:1 ratio with sterile water or saline. Day 2: Nebulize diluted ZnDTPA 1 g (Peds 14 mg/kg, max 1 g) at a 1:1 ratio with sterile water or saline; after nebulization, encourage individuals not to swallow any expectorant; treatment duration based on individual response and weekly radioactivity in blood, urine, and fecal samples.	Obtain quantitative baseline of internalized radioactive contamination by whole-body counting and/or bioassay (e.g., Biodosimetry) or feces/urine sample. Obtain weekly radioactivity counts in blood, urine and fecal samples to monitor radioactive contaminant elimination rate. Nebulized therapy may exacerbate asthma or precipitate respiratory adverse events.

(continued)

Therapeutic agent	Uses	Dosing	Caveat Complication
Coagulation factors • Prothrombin complex concentrate (PCC) • FEIBA or activated PCC • Fresh frozen plasma (FFP) • Recombinant activated factor VII (rFVIIa)	Patients with or suspected major vitamin K antagonist (e.g., warfarin or superwarfarin [e.g., brodifacoum]) anticoagulant-related hemorrhage.	Patients with or suspected major vitamin K antagonist-related hemorrhage or INR >20 • IV PCC 50 U/kg *or* IV FEIBA 80 IU/kg *or* IV FFP 10–20 mL/kg *or* IV rFVIIa 15–90 μg/kg. AND • IV vitamin K_1 (see **Vitamin K_1**). Excessive INR with and without bleeding in patients on warfarin • INR <5.0: Lower dose *or* omit next warfarin dose. • INR 5.0–9.0: Discontinue warfarin for several doses, high risk (e.g., age, recent hemorrhage, alcoholism, hepatic or renal impairment, and NSAID use) omit next warfarin dose *and* administer oral vitamin K_1 1.0–2.5 mg *or* IV vitamin K_1 0.5–1.0 mg. • INR 9.0–20.0: Oral vitamin K_1 3.0–5.0 mg • INR >20.0: IV vitamin K_1 10 mg and PCC *or* FFP *or* rFVIIa *and* repeat vitamin K_1 doses every 12 h as needed.	PCC: Contraindicated in disseminated intravascular coagulation and uncompensated liver disease; adverse drug events include thrombosis, disseminated intravascular coagulation, blood-borne pathogens transmission, allergic reactions. rFVIIa: Unlikelihood of blood-borne pathogens transmission, obviate volume constraints of FFP administration, reduces time for administration and achieving adequate hemostasis.
	Idarucizumab unavailable for suspected major dabigatran-related hemorrhage *or* patients on dabigatran to undergo emergency surgery/urgent procedures.	IV PCC 50 U/kg *or* IV FEIBA 80 IU/kg *or* FFP 10–20 mL/kg.	
	ACE inhibitor associated angioedema.	IV FFP 2–4 U.	Priority airway management.
Complement 1 (C1) esterase inhibitor concentrate	ACE inhibitor associated angioedema.	IV C1 esterase inhibitor concentrates 20 IU/kg.	Priority airway management.
Cyanide "antidote" • Dicobalt edetate • Hydroxocobalamin • Sodium nitrite and sodium thiosulfate (i.e., Nithiodote) • 4-Dimethylaminophenol (4-DMAP)	Known or suspected CN toxicity (e.g., fire in an enclosed space), severe and unexplainable anion gap metabolic acidosis (i.e., plasma lactate ≥8.0 mmol/L).	IV hydroxocobalamin 5 g over 15 min, repeat 1–2 doses base on clinical response; transient pink discoloration of mucous membranes, skin, urine; may interfere with colorimetric determinations of serum iron, bilirubin, creatinine concentration, OR	

<table>
<tr><td>Cyanide “antidote”</td><td></td><td>IV sodium nitrite 300 mg (10 mL of a 3% solution at 2.5–5 mL/min) (Peds: 0.2 mL/kg of a 3% solution [6 mg/kg or 6–8 mL/m^2 BSA] at 2.5–5 mL/min, max 10 mL [300 mg]) and IV sodium thiosulfate 12.5 g (50 mL of a 25% solution immediately following sodium nitrite) (Peds: 1 mL/kg [250 mg/kg or 30–40 mL/m^2 BSA], max 12.5 g [50 mL]); reduce sodium nitrite dosage proportionately to Hgb concentration in patients with known anemia; repeat treatment using one-half original dose of sodium nitrite and sodium thiosulfate if signs of poisoning reappear; if diagnosis uncertain, administer IV sodium thiosulfate alone.

OR</td><td>Nitrites should be cautiously used in cases of suspected concomitant carbon monoxide exposure (e.g., house fires).
Nitrite dosing based on Hgb concentration:
<table>
<tr><th>Hgb (g/dL)</th><th>Sodium nitrite (3%) (mL/kg)</th></tr>
<tr><td>7.0</td><td>0.19</td></tr>
<tr><td>8.0</td><td>0.22</td></tr>
<tr><td>9.0</td><td>0.25</td></tr>
<tr><td>10.0</td><td>0.27</td></tr>
<tr><td>11.0</td><td>0.30</td></tr>
<tr><td>12.0</td><td>0.33</td></tr>
<tr><td>13.0</td><td>0.36</td></tr>
<tr><td>14.0</td><td>0.39</td></tr>
</table></td></tr>
<tr><td></td><td></td><td>IV 4-DMAP 3–5 mg/kg.

OR</td><td>4-DMAP: Precise extent of induced methemoglobinemia may not be predictable.</td></tr>
<tr><td></td><td></td><td>IV dicobalt edetate 300 mg (Peds: 10 mg/kg) over 1–5 min if certain of the diagnosis particularly when patient is unconscious with deteriorating vital signs; repeat 1–2 dose base on clinical response.</td><td>Adverse events of dicobalt edetate include hypotension, cardiac dysrhythmias, and angioedema.</td></tr>
<tr><td>Dextrose</td><td>Hypoglycemia</td><td>Bolus
• Adult: IV dextrose 0.5–1.0 g/kg (D50W 1.0–2.0 mL/kg).
• Child: IV dextrose 0.5 g/kg (D25W 2 mL/kg).
• Infant: IV dextrose 0.5 g/kg (D10W 5 mL/kg).</td><td>Repeat bolus(es) may be indicated depending on clinical response.

Continuous infusion of D5W or D10W in patients requiring multiple boluses (e.g., sulfonylurea overdose) (see Octreotide).</td></tr>
<tr><td>Digoxin-specific antibody fragments</td><td>Digoxin overdose: Symptomatic patients, cardiac dysrhythmias that threaten or result in hemodynamic compromise, serum potassium >5.0 mmol/L, serum digoxin concentration >10.0 ng/mL (12.8 nmol/L) 6 h after overdose or >15 ng/mL (19.2 nmol/L) at any time.</td><td>DigiFab dosing:
• From dose ingested: One vial DigiFab (40 mg) binds 0.6 mg digoxin; Example: Ingestion of 3 mg of digoxin (bioavailability 80% [0.8]) requires 4 vials.
• From serum digoxin concentration: see Box 125.1.
• By titration: Administer 4–6 vials of DigiFab and repeat depending on clinical effect.
• Empiric therapy (e.g., malignant dysrhythmia): 10–20 vials (adult or pediatric).</td><td>Box 125.1: Digoxin antibody (DigiFab) dosing calculator allows neutralizing fractional serum digoxin concentration in patients on digoxin therapy; neutralize enough digoxin to stabilize patient.

May be effective treatment following naturally occurring cardioactive steroid (e.g., plants or animals origin) poisoning.

DigiFab (1,200 mg) is safe and effective treatment for yellow oleander induced cardiac dysrhythmias (e.g., bradycardia, <40 per min), sinus arrest or block, atrial tachydysrhythmias, second or third degree atrioventricular block.</td></tr>
</table>

(continued)

Therapeutic agent	Uses	Dosing	Caveat Complication
Ethanol	Toxic alcohol (e.g., methanol, ethylene glycol) poisoning.	IV ethanol (10% solution in D5W) 10 mL/kg over 1 h followed by 1.5 mL/kg/h, target serum ethanol 100 mg/dL until toxic alcohol is undetectable and clear clinical–biochemical recovery. Hemodialysis consideration: Increase ethanol infusion to 3.0 mL/kg/h at time of hemodialysis and decrease to 1.5 mL/kg/h after hemodialysis; continue ethanol treatment until undetectable serum toxic alcohol level (significant toxic alcohol may rebound following hemodialysis).	Adverse events include hypoglycemia, fluid overload, inebriation. Frequent serum ethanol and glucose concentration monitoring to help adjust ethanol dosing to maintain serum EtOH ≥100 mg/dL and avoid hypoglycemia. Ethanol only *inhibits* metabolism of toxic alcohols. Consider fomepizole therapy (see **Fomepizole**).
	Known, suspected, or symptomatic monofluoroacetate exposure.	Oral ethanol (96%) 40–60 mL, followed by IV ethanol (10% solution in D5W) 10 mL/kg over 1 h and 1.5 mL/kg/h for next 6–8 h.	Ethanol treatment of monofluoracetate exposure is unproven in humans.
Euglycemic clamp	Calcium channel and β-adrenergic antagonist poisoning with hypodynamic myocardium.	IV regular insulin 1 IU/kg bolus followed by infusion 0.5 IU/kg/h titrated every 30 min to desired effect on contractility or blood pressure (echocardiography for measuring myocardial response); euglycemia = serum glucose 100–250 mg/dL (5.5–14 mmol/L) is maintained by IV dextrose 25 g bolus with initial insulin bolus (unless serum glucose >400 mg/dL [22 mmol/L]) followed by dextrose infusion 0.5 g/kg/h titrated based on bedside glucose monitoring every 20–30 min until serum glucose is stable and then every 1–2 h.	Clinical response not immediate; increase chance of benefit with early detection (e.g., echocardiography) of hypodynamic myocardium and early initiation of therapy. Adverse events include numerical hypoglycemia, hypokalemia, hypophosphatemia, and hypomagnesemia; replace potassium if <2.5 mmol/L *and* a source of potassium loss.
Flumazenil	*Diagnostic* aid in assessing benzodiazepine (BZD) poisoning.	IV flumazenil 0.1–0.2 mg followed by 0.1–0.2 mg every minute (max 2 mg) until awake, failure to respond makes BZD unlikely cause.	Not a treatment for BZD poisoning. Use in patients on chronic BZD therapy or in tricyclic/BZD overdose may result in status epilepticus. Reverses sedative/anxiolytic effects; inconsistent in reversing BZD-induced respiratory depression.
Folinic acid (leucovorin)	Methotrexate (MTX) overdose (see **Carboxypepdidase-G2** and **Sodium bicarbonate**)		Leucovorin is active form of folic acid, which is not and cannot be a substitute for folinic acid.
	• Known amount of MTX ingested or administered	Initial IV leucovorin dose (mg) ≥ estimated ingested MTX dose, repeat the folinic acid dose 3–6 h until serum MTX concentration $<1 \times 10^{-7}$ molar.	Leucovorin most beneficial ≤1 h of exposure, and given as soon as possible after excessive MTX exposure.
	• Unknown MTX dose	IV leucovorin 10 mg/m^2.	Leucovorin infusion rate should be <160 mg/min.
	• Leucovorin dosing based on serum MTX drug concentration.	MTX $\geq 1 \times 10^{-5}$ M: IV leucovorin 1,000 mg/m^2 every 6 h. MTX 5×10^{-6}–1×10^{-5} M: IV leucovorin 100 mg/m^2 every 3 h. MTX 5×10^{-7}–5×10^{-6} M: IV leucovorin 10 mg/m^2 every 3 h *or* 30 mg/m^2 every 6 h. MTX 1×10^{-7}–5×10^{-7} M: Oral leucovorin 10 mg/m^2 every 6 h until MTX $<1 \times 10^{-7}$ M.	**Do not administer** leucovorin within 2 h before or after a dose of CPDG2; leucovorin is a CPDG2 substrate. Monitor serum MTX concentrations at 12, 24, and 48 h postexposure and adjust leucovorin dosage accordingly.

Folinic acid (leucovorin)	Methanol and ethylene glycol poisoning	IV leucovorin 2 mg/kg every 4–6 h until toxic alcohol is undetectable, clear clinical–biochemical recovery; if leucovorin not available IV folic acid 50–70 mg every 4 h; leucovorin preferred over folic acid. Hemodialysis consideration: Administer additional leucovorin dose at end of hemodialysis.	Continue leucovorin until serum MTX concentration <0.1 μmol/L in patients undergoing chemotherapy or <0.01 μmol/L in patients without cancer; continued therapy until marrow recovery in severe cases even when serum MTX becomes undetectable.
Fomepizole (4-methylpyrazole, 4MP)	Toxic alcohol (e.g., methanol, ethylene glycol)	IV 4MP 15 mg/kg followed by 10 mg/kg every 12 h × 4 doses, then 15 mg/kg every 12 h thereafter until toxic alcohol is undetectable and clear clinical–biochemical recovery; all infusions over 30 min. Hemodialysis consideration: Administer next scheduled 4MP dose if ≥6 h since last dose; during hemodialysis dosing is every 4 h; end of dialysis and time of last dose 1–3 h: administer half of next scheduled dose, >3 h: administer next scheduled dose. Continue 4MP treatment until undetectable serum toxic alcohol level (significant toxic alcohol may rebound following hemodialysis).	4MP only *inhibits* metabolism of toxic alcohols. 4MP extends elimination half-life of toxic alcohols; consider concurrent hemodialysis (*not* renal replacement therapy or hemofiltration).
Glucagon	Calcium channel and β-adrenergic antagonist poisoning with associated bradycardia.	IV glucagon 5 mg bolus, titrate to heart rate by doubling the bolus dose every 5–10 min; if effective dose is achieved start an infusion to deliver the effective bolus dose each hour (e.g., heart rate increased after two successive 5 mg boluses, then administer 10 mg/h).	Vomiting and aspiration: Pretreatment with anti-emetic and active airway management. More of a chronotropic than ionotropic effect.
Icatibant	ACE inhibitor associated angioedema.	Subcutaneous icatibant 30 mg injected into abdominal area.	Priority airway management.
Idarucizumab	Patients with serious bleeding or requiring emergency surgery/urgent invasive procedures while on dabigatran therapy.	IV idarucizumab 5 g (2 vials, each contains 2.5 g) either as bolus injection by consecutively injecting both vials *or* as two consecutive infusions *and* blood component therapy (e.g., PRBC, PCC, FEIBA, FFP); additional idarucizumab dosing based on at least 12 hourly coagulation profile (e.g., ECT, TT, aPTT, INR or PT), 6-8 hourly in renal failure.	Normalization of coagulation profile precedes clinical hemostasis by hours. Blood component therapy bridges the time between normalization of coagulation profile and establishment of clinical hemostasis. Serious idarucizumab adverse reaction risk in patients with hereditary fructose intolerance due to sorbitol excipient; adverse events include headache, hypokalemia, delirium, constipation, fever, and pneumonia. The need to establish clinical hemostasis outweights the risk of developing thrombotic adverse events in patient with uncontrolled hemorrhage.

(*continued*)

Therapeutic agent	Uses	Dosing	Caveat Complication
Lipid emulsion therapy (LET)	Local anesthetic (e.g., bupivacaine) toxicity	IV lipid emulsion (e.g., Intralipid, Liposyn III 20%, 500 mL bottle) • 1–2 mL/kg over 1 min and infusion 0.25 mL/kg/min • Repeat bolus at 3–5 min intervals 2–3× if circulation not been restored • After another 5 min increase infusion rate to 0.5 mL/kg/min if circulation not been restored • Continue infusion until hemodynamic recovery (>8 mL/kg unlikely to be effective?)	Laboratory data and clinical experiences with bupivacaine, levobupivacaine, mepivacaine, prilocaine, and ropivacaine toxicity suggest early LET attenuate progression of local anesthetic toxic syndrome. Consider LET in patients with severe lipophilic xenobiotic toxicity (e.g., bupropion, haloperidol, lamotrigine, nebivolol, quetiapine, sertraline, verapamil). Adverse events include pancreatitis, acute lung injury, and lipemia-induced laboratory interference.
Magnesium	Hydrofluoric acid • Oral exposure • History suggestive of substantive exposure that may lead to systemic toxicity	Oral calcium or magnesium containing antacids 30–60 mL. IV magnesium sulfate 2–6 g over 30 min follow by an infusion 1–4 g/h; additional magnesium boluses as indicated by careful clinical assessments and laboratory investigations *or* IV calcium chloride (see **Calcium**).	Assess patella reflexes frequently for sign of magnesium toxicity.
Methylene blue (1% solution)	Symptomatic methemoglobinemia or methemoglobin >20%	IV methylene blue 1–2 mg/kg over 5 min, repeat doses may be needed; onset of action ≤30 min; effectiveness may be limited in chlorate (inactivates glucose-6-phosphate dehydrogenase) methemoglobinemia and may need to proceed with hemodialysis.	Repetitive or continuous methylene blue dosing and GI decontamination may be needed when there is continued absorption or slow elimination of an agent producing methemoglobinemia: IV methylene blue 0.05% (in normal saline) 0.1 mg/kg/h *or* 3–7 mg/h has been suggested.
***N*-Acetylcysteine** (NAC)	Acetaminophen (APAP) Other causes of liver failure (e.g., essential oil toxicity)	Oral: 140 mg/kg followed by 70 mg/kg every 4 h (dilute 3:1 with carbonated/fruit beverage for palatability); repeat the same oral dose if vomiting occurs within 1 h. OR IV: 150 mg/kg in 200 mL D5W over 1 h followed by 50 mg/kg in 500 mL D5W over 4 h followed by 100 mg/kg in 1 L D5W over 16 h (6.25 mg/kg/h).	Oral NAC: IV antiemetic (e.g., ondansetron 8 mg; Peds: 0.2 mg/kg, max 8 mg) for associated nausea/vomiting. Duration of 72 hours. Anaphylactoid reaction: Asthmatics may be more sensitive; consider reducing NAC infusion rate by 50% or changing to oral NAC. Mindful of infusion volume in pediatrics.
Naloxone	Opioid overdose with respiratory, CNS, or cardiovascular compromise.	IV naloxone 0.04–0.1 mg if opioid dependent otherwise 2 mg; 10–20 mg may be required for high potency opioids (e.g., methadone, pentazocine, propoxyphene, diphenoxylate); repeat IV naloxone boluses may be required every 20–60 min Therapeutic IV naloxone infusion: Multiply effective naloxone bolus dose by 6.6, adding that quantity to 1 L normal saline, infuse solution at 100 mL/h, titrated to maintain adequate spontaneous ventilation without precipitating opioid withdrawal, empirically continued for 12–24 h; carefully observed for 2–4 h for recurrent respiratory depression after discontinuing naloxone infusion; allow naloxone to abate in acute iatrogenic opioid withdrawal.	Rapid reversal of opioid may lead to vomiting in semi-conscious patient; aspiration risk. Goal: Re-establish adequate spontaneous ventilation. Intralingual/endotracheal/intraosseous administration acceptable if no immediate IV access; IM/SC less desirable in urgent situation. May be effective following clonidine overdose.

Octreotide	Sulfonurea-induced hypoglycemia	IV octreotide 50 μg/h *or* IM octreotide 100 μg.	Acute hypoglycemia should be treated with IV dextrose (see **Dextrose**).
Physostigmine	Physostigmine *diagnostic* aid: selective use in anticholinergic agitation and delirium resulting from unknown ingestion; a positive response (e.g., patient awakens, provides history consistent with anticholinergic toxicity) obviates additional testing (e.g., cranial computed tomography and lumbar puncture).	IV physostigmine 0.5–2 mg at ≤0.5 mg/min (Peds: 0.02 mg/kg at 0.5 mg/min), if no reversal of anticholinergic effect within 10–20 min administer an additional 1–2 mg.	Contraindications include early (<6 h) cyclic antidepressant overdose, overdose with cardiac conduction delay, cyclic antidepressant poisoning with high-dose/drug-level phenomena (e.g., hypotension, coma, seizures, cardiac conduction delays, and dysrhythmias, bronchospasm, mechanical intestinal or urogenital tract obstruction).
Polyethylene glycol electrolyte (PEG) solution	Whole bowel irrigation (WBI) for gastrointestinal decontamination following oral ingestion/overdose (e.g., modified-release drug formulation, heavy metal).	See **Box 125.2.**	WBI: After patient stablization, patient is able to tolerate charcoal/WBI, and precautionary measures to minimize aspiration.
Pralidoxime	Cholinesterase inhibitors (e.g., organophosphorus agents, nerve agents, physostigmine) poisoning.	IV pralidoxime 30 mg/kg over 30 min followed by a continuous infusion 8–10 mg/kg/h with empiric dose adjustment based on clinical response, continue until atropine has not been required for 24–48 h and patient extubated; restart pralidoxime if recurrent signs/symptoms.	To be administered with atropine following organophosphorous or nerve agent poisoning (see **Atropine**).
Protamine	Heparin • Known amount administered	IV protamine dose (1 mg of protamine sulfate neutralizes 100 U (1 mg) of heparin) is calculated from the dose of heparin administered and heparin's approximate half-life (i.e., 60–90 min), such that the amount of protamine does not exceed the expected intravascular amount of heparin at the time of infusion. Slowly administer protamine over 15 min.	Be prepared to treat acute anaphylactic (shock) and anaphylactoid reactions. Protamine administered in the absence of heparin or in an amount exceeding that necessary for heparin neutralization can act as an anticoagulant and may inhibit platelet function with a resultant weaker clot.
	• Patient is believed to have been overdosed with an unknown quantity, decision to use protamine is based on a correct clinical setting and a prolonged partial thromboplastin time (PTT) and persistent bleeding. Empiric protamine dosing based on activated coagulation time (ACT).	ACT 200–300 s: IV protamine 0.6 mg/kg ACT 300–400 s: IV protamine 1.2 mg/kg Repeat ACT 5–15 min following protamine dose and in 2–8 h to evaluate heparin rebound, further dosing based on these values. ACT not available: IV protamine 25–50 mg (adult) and adjusted accordingly. Repeat dosing in several hours may be necessary if heparin rebound occurs.	*Incomplete neutralization of low-molecular-weight heparins.*

(continued)

Therapeutic agent	Uses	Dosing	Caveat Complication
Pyridoxine	Ethylene glycol poisoning	IV Pyridoxine 3–5 mg/kg/d *or* 50 mg every 6 h until toxic alcohol is undetectable and acidemia resolved.	
	Isoniazid (INH) overdoses • First sign of neurotoxicity	IV benzodiazepine *and* pyridoxine in milligram doses equal to the amount of INH ingested *or* 5 g in cases of unknown amount of ingestion administered over 30–60 min.	Required doses often exceed hospital and/or regional supplies.
	• Seizing patients	IV benzodiazepine *and* pyridoxine in milligram doses equal to the amount of INH ingested *or* 5 g in cases of unknown amount of ingestion at 500 mg/min until seizures terminate and remainder of dose infused over next few hours; repeat pyridoxine dose if seizures persist or recur.	
Silibinin	Amanita mushroom poisoning	Open-label clinical trial using an *investigational new drug*, IV silibinin, in treatment of suspected-mushroom poisoning is available in the United States, call Legalon SIL hotline: 866-520-4412; http://sites.google.com/site/legalonsil/home	
Sodium bicarbonate	Ethylene glycol and methanol poisoning	IV sodium bicarbonate 1–2 mmol/kg boluses, target blood pH 7.40 and urine pH 7.0–8.0.	Large doses may be needed to treat metabolic acidosis and may produce hypocalcemia. Potassium replacement/supplement.
	Type I antidysrhythmic drug toxicity (sodium channel antagonist effect e.g., tricyclic antidepressants, quinidine)	ECG (maximal limb-lead) QRS ≥120 ms *or* RaVR ≥3 mm *or* R/SaVR ≥0.7: IV sodium bicarbonate 1–2 mmol/kg bolus × 2; repeat ECG every 3–5 min; IV sodium bicarbonate 1–2 mmol/kg bolus until QRS duration stabilized.	
	Salicylate poisoning	Urine alkalinization: IV sodium bicarbonate 1–2 mmol/kg bolus followed by continuous infusion of sodium bicarbonate 150 mmol mixed in 1 L D5W starting at 1.5–2.0 times maintenance rate, adjusted to maintain urinary pH 8.0 and arterial pH <7.55; assess clinical status/laboratory parameters (e.g., electrolytes, acid–base, urine pH) hourly; terminate when clear clinical–biochemical recovery and serial decline in serum ASA concentration towards therapeutic range.	
	Methotrexate (see **Carboxypeptidase-G2** and **Folinic Acid**) and chlorpropamide overdoses, symptomatic chlorphenoxyherbicide poisoning, known or symptomatic pentachlorophenol poisoning	Urine alkalinization: See **Salicylate poisoning**; reassess clinical status/laboratory parameters (e.g., electrolytes, acid–base, urine pH) hourly; terminate when clear clinical–biochemical recovery.	

Thiamine	Ethylene glycol poisoning	IV thiamine 100 mg/d *or* every 6 h until toxic alcohol is undetectable and acidemia resolved.	
Vitamin K_1	Patients with or suspected major vitamin K antagonist (e.g., warfarin and superwarfarin [e.g., brodifacoum]) anticoagulant-related hemorrhage or INR >20.	IV vitamin K_1 10 mg (diluted with 5% dextrose, 0.9% sodium chloride, *or* 5% dextrose in 0.9% sodium chloride; administered at ≤1 mg/min; be preparing to treat anaphylaxis) *or* oral/nasogastric vitamin K_1 7 mg/kg/d divided every 6 h. Endpoint of vitamin K_1 therapy: Discontinue therapy at an arbitrary time and obtain serial INR/PT, restart vitamin K_1 when INR/PT is elevated *or* monitor serum factor VII concentration when vitamin K_1 therapy is withheld, restart vitamin K_1 when a progressive decrease in factor VII levels to 30% of normal *or* serum brodifacoum concentration <10 ng/mL, *or* when serum vitamin K 2,3-epoxide concentration begins to fall.	IV vitamin K is associated with anaphylaxis. Life-threatening hemorrhage: *Concurrently* administered IV prothrombin complex concentrate (PCC) 50 U/kg *or* IV fresh frozen plasma (FFP) 10–20 mL/kg *or* IV recombinant activated factor VII (rFVIIa) 15–90 μg/kg with vitamin K_1.

ACE, angiotensin-converting enzyme; aPTT, activated partial thromboplastin time; D50W, dextrose 50% water; D25W, dextrose 25% water; D10W, dextrose 10% water; ECT, ecarin clotting time; h, hours; IM, intramuscular; IV, intravenous; LR, Lactated Ringer; max, maximum; NS, normal saline, Peds, Pediatrics; RaVR, terminal R wave in lead aVR; R/SaVR, R-wave/S-wave ratio in lead aVR; TT, thrombin time; wks, weeks.

BOX 125.1

Digoxin Antibody (DigiFab) Dosing Calculator

$$\text{Number of vials} = \frac{(\text{Digoxin body burden to be neutralized in ng/mL (nmol/L} \times 1.28) \times \text{weight (kg)} \times \text{volume of distribution } (V_d))}{(1{,}000 \times 0.6 \text{ mg/vial})}$$

V_d: adults 8 L/kg, children 2–10 yrs 13 L/kg, infants 2–24 mo 16 L/kg, neonates 10 L/kg.

BOX 125.2

Polyethylene Glycol Solution (PEG) Whole Bowel Irrigation

Insert nasogastric/oral tube and administer PEG solution at 2 L/h for 5 h and clear rectal effluent is evident (small children: 500 mL/h); doubtful patients would be cooperative or tolerate oral PEG.

Chapter 126 ■ Withdrawal Syndromes

PAUL M. WAX • ASHLEY HAYNES

As many as 20% of hospitalized adult patients in most medical settings may have a history of an alcohol-related condition [1]. In recent surveys, as many as 14% of Americans experience an alcohol use disorder during their lifetime [2]. Anticipation and recognition of early signs of sedative–hypnotic withdrawal of the sedative–hypnotic abuser allow timely treatment and prevent the development of serious withdrawal consequences, such as seizures, hyperthermia, delirium, and death. The management of withdrawal syndromes from γ-hydroxybutyrate (GHB) and baclofen may be particularly challenging. Recognition and treatment of the less life-threatening signs and symptoms of opioid withdrawal avoid unnecessary investigation of the frequently severe gastrointestinal symptoms and make the patient more comfortable and able to cooperate. Because ethanol and other sedative–hypnotic withdrawal may have life-threatening consequences, the patients with signs of significant withdrawal should be admitted to the intensive care unit (ICU) for the stabilization and monitoring. In addition, drug-dependent patients admitted to the ICU for the management of other serious medical or surgical problems may subsequently enter withdrawal in this substance-free environment [3].

Clinical withdrawal implies the presence of physical tolerance and dependency. Factors contributing to the development of dependency include dose of the drug, duration of effect, frequency of administration, and duration of abuse. Shorter-acting drugs require more frequent administration to produce dependency and are associated with more acute and severe withdrawal symptoms than longer-acting drugs. *Tolerance* is defined as a decreased physiologic response elicited by a given dose of the drug. The patient who chronically ingests a large amount of ethanol may not be sedated by a dose that would render a nondrinker comatose. A heroin abuser who has been drug-free during a year's imprisonment may suffer fatal respiratory depression from a dose of heroin that previously would have provided only mild sedation. This physiologic tolerance to drug effect that occurs with chronic use may arise from changes in drug metabolism, such as induction of one or cytochrome P450 enzymes and changes in drug affect at the cellular level. Cross-tolerance occurs when the chronic ingestion of one substance decreases the response to a second substance. Cross-dependency allows one drug to be substituted for another to alleviate or prevent withdrawal symptoms. Ethanol, barbiturates, and nonbarbiturate sedative–hypnotic agents are cross-tolerant and cross-dependent with one another but not with other sedating drugs such as opioids, neuroleptics, or antihistamines. These factors have important therapeutic implications.

ETHANOL WITHDRAWAL

Pathophysiology

Ethanol produces its toxic effects (relaxation, euphoria, disinhibition, slurred speech, ataxia, sedation, stupor, coma, and respiratory depression (see Chapter 99); through modulation of a variety of neuroreceptors and ion channels [4]. It acts, in part, by interacting with the γ-aminobutyric acid ($GABA_A$) receptor complex, potentiating inhibitory GABA-ergic receptor function by inducing chloride flux through the chloride channels of the receptor complex. Ethanol also inhibits excitatory *N*-methyl-D-aspartate (NMDA) glutamate receptor function, contributing to impaired cognition and blackouts associated with chronic ethanol use [5]. Inhibition of NMDA receptor function changes intracellular calcium levels and, as a result, affects cell-signaling cascades, including phosphorylation [5]. Other neurotransmitter systems affected by ethanol include dopamine and serotonin [6]. Ethanol has been found to affect 5-hydroxytryptamine receptor function by increasing the potency with which agonists bind this receptor [4]. Ethanol consumption may also result in an increase in endogenous opiates, particularly with respect to ligands for the kappa opioid receptor, contributing to its euphoric effect [7]. Although it was not recognized until the 1950s that delirium was a manifestation of ethanol withdrawal rather than toxicity, the hallmarks of ethanol and other sedative–hypnotic intoxication are distinctly different from the manifestations of withdrawal from these agents [8,9].

Ethanol withdrawal produces a hyperadrenergic state characterized by intense sympathetic nervous system activation. This may be due in part to compensatory central nervous system (CNS) mechanisms that counteract the depressant effects of ethanol intoxication. During withdrawal, these compensatory mechanisms are unopposed, resulting in increased neural stimulation [10]. In support of this theory, elevated levels of plasma and urinary catecholamines have been associated with tachycardia, elevated blood pressure, and tremors observed in withdrawing patients. A decrease in the inhibitory activity of presynaptic α_2-receptors has been demonstrated and may explain, in part, the increase in norepinephrine levels. In addition, an increase in β-adrenergic receptors during withdrawal has been demonstrated. One study showed an increase in plasma levels of the dopamine metabolite homovanillic acid in patients presenting with delirium tremens [11].

Compensatory changes in number and function of inhibitory $GABA_A$ receptors and excitatory NMDA glutamate receptors during chronic ethanol use may contribute to the CNS stimulation brought on by the cessation of ethanol. The abrupt withdrawal of the GABA-potentiating effects of ethanol leads to a disinhibition of neural pathways in the CNS [6]. During withdrawal, ethanol's enhancing effect on chloride flux is lost, resulting in a decrease in GABA-ergic function. Tachycardia, diaphoresis, tremors, anxiety, and seizures have been associated with this reduction in GABA-induced chloride flux [6]. Upregulation in NMDA glutamate receptors and changes in their receptor subunit composition increases calcium flux through these receptors [12]. This likely contributes to the excitotoxic neuronal cell death associated with ethanol withdrawal [13]. Repeated episodes of withdrawal increase the propensity for ethanol withdrawal seizures through altered $GABA_A$ and NMDA receptor function [6]. Because NMDA receptors mediate dopaminergic transmission, the increased NMDA receptor function that occurs during withdrawal may also lead to decreased dopaminergic and serotonergic transmission, contributing to alcohol craving [5].

Ethanol withdrawal occurs when a dependent patient suddenly stops drinking or drinks at a slower rate than previously. In either case, a significant drop in the serum ethanol level occurs. In chronic alcoholics, signs of withdrawal are commonly present even when their serum ethanol concentrations are higher than 100 mg per dL [14]. The patients admitted to the ICU with ethanol withdrawal often have a significant underlying disease that has led to an inability to maintain an ethanol intake adequate to prevent withdrawal. Alcoholic gastritis, hepatitis, pancreatitis, and pneumonia commonly precipitate decreased ethanol use and withdrawal. These patients typically present to the hospital after 24 to 48 hours of abdominal pain or fever and may be tremulous or have had a withdrawal seizure. Another type of ICU patient prone to withdrawal is one who has continued to imbibe ethanol nearly to the moment of arrival at the hospital. Intoxicated patients are prone to experience traumatic events and arrive in the operating room, recovery room, or ICU still intoxicated. A history of ethanol abuse or previous withdrawal may not be available in the postoperative or intubated patient when initial signs of withdrawal occur. Failure to recognize ethanol withdrawal in the seriously ill or injured patient may lead to prolonged complications [2,15].

Clinical Manifestations

Ethanol withdrawal results in a variety of signs and symptoms that vary in severity and duration. In their landmark article, Victor and Adams [9] described withdrawal as a tremulous–hallucinating–epileptic–delirious state. Although this description is often used to divide ethanol withdrawal syndrome into four stages, it is important to remember that the various manifestations of ethanol withdrawal form a progressive continuum of severity. The patient in ethanol withdrawal may exhibit one or more of these manifestations. The sequence of clinical events may be inconsistent. The severity of the withdrawal is often dose-dependent, with more severe reactions associated with heavier and longer periods of drinking [14].

Tremulousness and seizures are the most common clinical manifestations of ethanol withdrawal. They tend to occur early and are generally considered mild-to-moderate ethanol withdrawal symptoms. Delirium tremens is a late manifestation of ethanol withdrawal and constitutes the most serious clinical presentation. Although dramatic and life-threatening, delirium tremens is but one aspect of ethanol withdrawal and affects 5% of withdrawal patients [1,6].

Mild ethanol withdrawal is usually characterized by a period of acute tremulousness (the "shakes"). It begins 6 to 8 hours after a reduction in ethanol intake [1,6,16]. The patients usually complain of tremulousness, nausea, vomiting, anorexia, anxiety, and insomnia. Physical examination reveals an evidence of mild CNS and autonomic hyperactivity, which includes tachycardia, mild hypertension, hyperreflexia, irritability, and a resting tremor. Occasionally, significant tremor may not be appreciated despite the patient's complaint of feeling "shaky inside." Despite the fact that the patients in delirium tremens have evidence of significant disorientation, this milder form of withdrawal is characterized by a clear sensorium, although the patient may have a minor disorientation to time. Symptoms of mild ethanol withdrawal usually peak between 24 and 36 hours, and 75% to 80% of these patients recover uneventfully in a few days. Approximately 20% to 25% of the patients presenting with mild ethanol withdrawal progress to serious withdrawal manifestations, which include seizures, hallucinations, or delirium tremens. A few studies have attempted to identify predictors of deterioration, and a correlation with the amount of regular alcohol consumption, elevated blood alcohol concentration at the time of admission, and an age over 40 years has been demonstrated, at least in a trauma population [17]. Additionally, thrombocytopenia, hypokalemia, and elevated homocysteine levels may indicate increased risk for the development of delirium tremens, though they may represent markers of the degree of regular alcohol consumption rather than independent determining factors [2,18]. It remains impossible to reliably predict which the patients will deteriorate [14].

Seizures that occur among alcoholics may or may not be due to ethanol withdrawal. Although ethanol withdrawal accounts for many of these seizures, other common causes include pre-existing idiopathic and post-traumatic epilepsy [8,9,18]. Other complications of ethanol abuse not necessarily associated with withdrawal, such as hypoglycemia, hypomagnesemia, and hyponatremia, may also precipitate seizure activity [18]. Ethanol intoxication itself is not thought to be proconvulsant. Alcoholic patients with a history of epilepsy appear to have a greater incidence of seizures than those without a pre-existing seizure disorder. Failure to comply with anticonvulsant regimens may, in part, account for this. Brief abstinence (even overnight) may also lower the seizure threshold sufficiently to provoke seizures in susceptible patients. Because management strategies differ depending on whether the patient has a history of seizure disorder unrelated to ethanol withdrawal, differentiating between them becomes important [19].

Early studies showed that as many as 25% to 33% of the patients with ethanol withdrawal demonstrate seizure activity [8,9]. Most ethanol withdrawal seizures (rum fits) occur between 6 and 48 hours after cessation or relative abstinence from drinking [6,16]. Mild-to-moderate signs of withdrawal may precede the seizures, or the seizure may herald the onset of ethanol withdrawal. They are short, generalized, tonic–clonic seizures, 40% of which are limited to a single isolated event. Often a short burst of two to six seizures with normal sensorium between seizures occurs over a few hours. The patients with ethanol withdrawal seizures usually have normal baseline electroencephalograms, in contrast to those with underlying seizure disorders. Status epilepticus or recurrent seizure activity lasting longer than 6 hours is distinctly uncommon in ethanol withdrawal and suggests another diagnosis.

Ethanol-related seizures may foreshadow the development of delirium tremens. In one series of the patients with ethanol withdrawal seizures, delirium tremens developed in 35% [18]. In some patients, postictal confusion blends imperceptibly into delirium tremens. As many as 40% of the patients in whom delirium tremens subsequently developed exhibited an initial clearing of their postictal state followed by the onset of delirium tremens 12 hours to 5 days later [16].

Disordered perceptions characterized by hallucinations and nightmares were noted in 25% of tremulous patients in early withdrawal by Victor and Adams [9]. The hallucinations were predominantly visual in nature, auditory only in 20% of the cases, and rarely tactile or olfactory. Commonly described visual phenomena in this setting may include the graphic depiction of bugs crawling on the walls or bed.

A subset of hallucinating patients does not demonstrate tremulousness or other signs of sympathetic hyperactivity, known as *acute alcoholic hallucinosis*, this uncommon clinical presentation (occurring in 2% of the patients of Victor and Adams) is a distinct manifestation of ethanol withdrawal that usually begins within 8 to 48 hours of cessation of drinking [9]. It is characterized by disabling auditory hallucinations, often of a persecutory nature. These patients display no evidence of formal thought disorder, have no personal or family history of schizophrenia, and are usually oriented to person and place. In most cases, symptoms last for 1 to 6 days, although they may persist for months and come to resemble chronic paranoid schizophrenia. These symptoms usually respond to therapy with cross-tolerant agents such as benzodiazepines.

Delirium tremens is characterized by a significant alteration of sensorium associated with dramatic autonomic and CNS hyperactivity. Only 5% of the patients who exhibit any of the previously discussed manifestations of ethanol withdrawal progress to delirium tremens. Delirium tremens appears to be more common among the patients with a history of significant withdrawal and a long history of ethanol use. The patients for whom delirium tremens develops may not have demonstrated earlier signs of withdrawal. Other patients who have had ethanol withdrawal seizures or hallucinations may deceptively improve before the onset of delirium tremens, which is rarely seen before 48 to 72 hours after cessation or reduction in drinking and may be delayed for as long as 5 to 14 days [6,9]. These patients are truly delirious, exhibiting disorientation, global confusion, hallucinations, and delusions. Speech is unintelligible. Psychomotor disturbances, such as picking at bedclothes, significant restlessness, and agitation, are common and often require the use of physical restraints. Autonomic disturbances, such as tachycardia, hypertension, tachypnea, hyperpyrexia, diaphoresis, and mydriasis, are present. Cardiac dysrhythmias may also occur [20]. Seizures rarely occur during delirium tremens. Concomitant illness, trauma, seizures, or therapeutic drugs may mask or modify the typical presentation.

Mortality for delirium tremens varies with the presence of underlying disease. Higher mortality is associated with superimposed pneumonia, meningitis, pancreatitis, gastrointestinal bleeding, or major trauma [17,20]. For the untreated patient without serious coexisting medical disease, mortality usually is a consequence of severe dehydration or hyperthermia, or both, precipitating cardiovascular collapse [20,21]. Before adequate therapeutic agents were available, a mortality rate of 24% to 35% was cited in the literature [22]. This has been steadily decreasing over time, and with the use of benzodiazepines, intensive supportive care, and earlier recognition of withdrawal has approached 0% to 2% in more recent studies [17,23,24].

Diagnostic Evaluation

The differential diagnosis of ethanol withdrawal includes other causes of a hyperadrenergic state. Most importantly, ethanol-related hypoglycemia needs to be differentiated from withdrawal. Clinically, these two conditions may appear remarkably similar, although only hypoglycemia rapidly improves after intravenous (IV) glucose administration.

Intoxication with sympathomimetic agents such as cocaine or amphetamine shares many features with ethanol withdrawal, including signs and symptoms of adrenergic excess. Overdose of monoamine oxidase inhibitors, phencyclidine, anticholinergic agents, and lithium, as well as neuroleptic malignant syndrome and serotonin syndrome may all demonstrate marked agitation and confusion. For the elderly patient, almost any therapeutic drug may be associated with delirium, with opioids, benzodiazepines, anticholinergics, and antidepressants being of particular concern [25]. Withdrawal from other sedative–hypnotics, such as benzodiazepines, barbiturates, GHB, and baclofen, may precipitate a delirium-tremens-like state (see following discussion).

Significant underlying metabolic, traumatic, and infectious disorders should be excluded for the patient with altered mental status associated with ethanol withdrawal. Differentiation may require lumbar puncture, laboratory tests, and computed tomographic scan of the head. These include CNS emergencies, such as intracranial bleeds, meningitis, and encephalitis; metabolic causes, including hypoxia, hypercarbia, sepsis, thiamine deficiency, and sodium and calcium abnormalities; and endocrine disturbances, such as thyroid storm and pheochromocytoma. Distinguishing between delirium tremens and hepatic encephalopathy may be difficult, especially because these conditions often coexist.

Management

A successful strategy for treating ethanol withdrawal must address several key goals: alleviation of symptoms, prevention of progression of withdrawal to a more serious stage, avoidance of complications, treatment of coexisting medical problems, and planning for long-term rehabilitation and drug independence [6]. Initial management involves securing the airway, breathing, and circulation. The patients with an altered level of consciousness require oxygen and IV administration of at least 100 mg thiamine and 50 g glucose. The latter two substrates are particularly important, as Wernicke encephalopathy and hypoglycemia may be confused or coexist with ethanol withdrawal. Severely agitated patients may initially require physical restraints to prevent injury and facilitate sedation. Prolonged use of physical restraints without adequate sedation, however, may be detrimental because agitated patients often continue to struggle against their restraints. Such activity perpetuates the risk for hyperthermia, muscle destruction, and resultant myoglobinuric renal failure. One retrospective review of 35 deaths in delirium tremens found that mortality correlated with the use of restraints and hyperthermia [26].

Volume resuscitation, correction of electrolyte abnormalities, and vigilance in the diagnosis and treatment of coexisting medical and surgical disorders are vital for reducing morbidity and mortality of the patient with delirium tremens [6,16].

Achievement of adequate sedation is the cornerstone of successful treatment of ethanol withdrawal [27]. Sedation alleviates the excitatory manifestations of withdrawal, prevents progression to delirium tremens, and prevents common complications of agitation, including trauma, rhabdomyolysis, and hyperthermia. Although many agents have been used over the years, benzodiazepines have proved the most effective [1,6,16,27,28]. Benzodiazepines, unlike the neuroleptics, are cross-tolerant with ethanol and function as a replacement drug for the short-acting ethanol, increasing the affinity of GABA for the $GABA_A$ receptor [6].

Diazepam (Valium), chlordiazepoxide (Librium), and lorazepam (Ativan) are the most commonly used parenteral agents. All three drugs can easily be given intravenously to facilitate rapid sedation and titration of effect. Of these agents, only lorazepam has reliable intramuscular (IM) absorption [6,14]. Diazepam and chlordiazepoxide are long-acting agents with active metabolites that prolong their therapeutic effect, avoiding the need for frequent dosing that is associated with shorter-acting agents. Lorazepam, a shorter-acting agent, has no active metabolite and is better tolerated in the elderly and in patients with hepatic dysfunction, producing less sedation. Prolonged therapy (e.g., >1 month) with high-dose IV lorazepam, however, has also been associated with acute tubular necrosis secondary to the polyethylene glycol used as the lorazepam diluent. Continuous IV infusion of midazolam, a short-acting agent, has also been recommended in the treatment of delirium tremens. However, this approach requires more vigilant monitoring and does not provide the advantages of a long-acting benzodiazepine that is gradually eliminated over several days. Midazolam infusion is also considerably more expensive than therapy with longer-acting agents [27].

The benzodiazepine of choice in the treatment of ethanol withdrawal remains controversial [29]. Currently, the literature does not support the efficacy of one benzodiazepine over another [6,27,28,30]. Although some investigators have suggested that lorazepam may be the preferred agent [31], long-acting benzodiazepines such as diazepam may be more effective in preventing ethanol withdrawal seizures and contributing to smoother withdrawal with less breakthrough or rebound symptoms [32].

Symptom-triggered benzodiazepine treatment for alcohol withdrawal is strongly encouraged [24,33]. The Clinical Institute Withdrawal Assessment for Alcohol (CIWA-A) scale is a reliable, validated scale to assess severity of alcohol withdrawal, so treatment can be appropriately titrated and individualized. It includes subjective parameters such as anxiety, auditory and visual disturbances, headache, and nausea as well as objective parameters such as tremor, sweating, agitation, and clouding of sensorium. A score >18 indicates the patient is considered severe and at risk for complications if not treated. In severely agitated or intubated patients, subjective parameters may be difficult to evaluate, and a tool such as the Richmond Agitation-Sedation Scale may be used instead [6]. The dose of benzodiazepines needed to achieve adequate sedation varies considerably depending on the patient's tolerance. Although oral therapy may be appropriate in patients with mild withdrawal, those with significant signs of withdrawal require IV treatment. Therapy with an IV benzodiazepine is titrated to the patient's needs by the use of frequent boluses until withdrawal symptoms subside. Using such a front-loading technique helps avoid undertreatment or excessive sedation. For example, 5 to 20 mg of diazepam can be administered to the patient every 5 minutes until he/she is quietly asleep but can be easily awakened. Initial safe titration of benzodiazepines requires continual reevaluation by an observer at the bedside. In patients with moderate withdrawal symptoms, a study showed that using a symptom-triggered approach, instead of a fixed-schedule approach, resulted in the administration of less total medication and fewer hours of medication (9 hours vs. 68 hours) [34]. A 2003 study in a surgical ICU demonstrated that this symptom-orientated bolus-titrated approach decreases the severity and duration of alcohol withdrawal symptoms, resulting in reduced medication requirements, fewer days of ventilation, lower incidence of pneumonia, and shorter ICU stay [35].

Failure to obtain adequate sedation with standard doses of the chosen agent should not prompt a switch to an alternative benzodiazepine. Some patients require very high doses to achieve sedation; cases of the patients receiving up to 2,000 mg of diazepam during the first 2 days have been reported [1]. Recent research into GABA receptor physiology suggests that resistance to large doses of benzodiazepines in some patients with alcohol withdrawal may be due to alterations in $GABA_A$ receptor subunit expression [36]. In two studies of alcoholics, increased levels of $GABA_A$ receptor α_1 subunit mRNA was noted in the prefrontal cortex with no change in the expression of α_2, α_3, or α_4 mRNA. The total concentration of α subunits also appears to be increased. If the patient with severe alcohol withdrawal does not respond to large doses of a benzodiazepine, such as 200 mg of diazepam or 40 mg of lorazepam over 3 to 4 hours, the administration of an alternative agent may be warranted [6]. Cases requiring greater than 40 mg of diazepam in the first hour are often considered resistant alcohol withdrawal. The sequential addition of other agents may be necessary. A barbiturate, which acts on the $GABA_A$ receptor regardless of its specific α subunit composition, is often the next agent added [15].

Barbiturates, particularly intermediate and long-acting agents such as pentobarbital and phenobarbital, are cross-tolerant sedative–hypnotic agents that can be used in the treatment of ethanol withdrawal, either alone or as an adjunct for resistant alcohol withdrawal [10,15]. Dosing of phenobarbital may require up to 1,500 to 2,000 mg orally or intravenously on Day 1 in patients with delirium [1]. Although excess sedation and a greater tendency to produce respiratory depression may be more of a concern with barbiturates as compared with benzodiazepines, the drugs are still titrated until the patient is quietly asleep but easily awakened [6,37]. Withdrawal patients with idiopathic or post-traumatic epilepsy who require maintenance anticonvulsant levels may particularly benefit from this alternative strategy.

Recent research also suggests that changes in NMDA glutamate receptor physiology may be important in both clinical signs and symptoms of ethanol withdrawal and the excitotoxic neuronal cell death that may occur. In animal studies, NMDA receptor antagonists may attenuate the development of ethanol dependence if administered concomitantly, and may prevent withdrawal seizures and neuronal excitotoxicity if given during periods of withdrawal [12]. The patients who are refractory to high dose $GABA_A$ agonists may potentially benefit from addressing the glutaminergic as well as the GABA-ergic manifestations of ethanol withdrawal.

Options in the setting of refractory ethanol withdrawal are limited, but drugs such as propofol, which possess both GABA agonist and NMDA antagonist properties, may be particularly helpful. Although it maintains cross-tolerance with GABA receptors, the effect is less than benzodiazepines and does not preclude the use of benzodiazepines [38]. Propofol, a sedative–hypnotic agent used for induction and maintenance of anesthesia, has been used successfully for treatment of severe ethanol withdrawal that is resistant to large doses of benzodiazepines (>1,000 mg per day) [6,38,39]. Like ethanol, it acts as an agonist at the $GABA_A$ receptor and also inhibits the NMDA receptor. Its onset of action is rapid, it is easily titratable, and sedative effects wear off quickly after short-term use (<72 hours). The fact that it addresses the glutaminergic as well as the GABA-ergic aspects of ethanol withdrawal may be one reason for its increased apparent effectiveness in patients resistant to standard therapy with benzodiazepines. Disadvantages of its use include prolonged sedation and the potential for propofol infusion syndrome when it is used for extended periods [39]. A recent retrospective cohort of the patients treated with benzodiazepine monotherapy compared to those with added propofol demonstrated similar length of alcohol withdrawal, length of stays, and mechanical ventilation with fewer benzodiazepine boluses in the propofol group [40]. Another retrospective study suggested longer and more complicated hospital stays in those receiving propofol as part of their regimen [41].

Ketamine is another agent with NMDA antagonistic properties that has been used for the treatment of alcohol withdrawal. Unlike propofol, it has no GABA effects. One retrospective review has demonstrated a reduction in benzodiazepine requirements, but additional data are still required before ketamine can be recommended [42].

Since 2008, reports of successful use of dexmedetomidine, an α_2-receptor agonist, have been emerging [43]. This agent was designed from clonidine to maximize sedation. It has anesthetic, anxiolytic, analgesic, and sympatholytic effects and is indicated for sedation, but does not cause significant respiratory depression [44]. Recent studies have shown its use can decrease the amount of benzodiazepine used in the first 24 hours, though may not reduce long-term benzodiazepine use in alcohol withdrawal

[45]. When compared with propofol, it seems to produce less hypotension, lower intubation rates, decreased ICU length of stays, and comparable benzodiazepine use [46]. Bradycardia may occur more frequently. Because dexmedetomidine has no GABA agonistic properties, its use does not obviate the need for benzodiazepines but may be beneficial in controlling the hyperadrenergic picture that occurs during withdrawal.

Other central adrenergic agonists, such as the α_2-receptor agonists clonidine and lofexidine, have been promoted as primary agents and adjuncts to sedative–hypnotic treatment in the treatment of alcohol withdrawal. Clonidine acts centrally to attenuate sympathetic outflow from the locus ceruleus [14]. Although α_2 agonists may help relieve mild withdrawal symptoms such as tremor, diaphoresis, and tachycardia, there is no evidence that they prevent delirium tremens [6]. A double-blind study comparing oral benzodiazepines (diazepam or alprazolam) to clonidine in the treatment of mild ethanol withdrawal showed that the benzodiazepines were significantly more efficacious in decreasing withdrawal symptoms [47]. β-Blockers have also been used as agents in the treatment of ethanol withdrawal. These agents do not prevent agitation, hallucinations, confusion, and seizures and should be used only as adjunctive treatment [6].

IV and oral ethanol have been used to suppress withdrawal and continue to be used by some medical practitioners, especially surgeons [48]. However, IV ethanol intensifies the biochemical abnormalities associated with ethanol metabolism, shifting energy production toward lactate and ketogenesis [49]. The use of ethanol in the treatment of ethanol withdrawal is not recommended [50].

Baclofen is a $GABA_B$ agonist that appears to have a role in the treatment of alcohol withdrawal. In a randomized, controlled trial, it was comparable to benzodiazepines in relieving symptoms of moderate alcohol withdrawal in an outpatient setting [51]. It has also been shown to be more effective than placebo in controlling craving and in inducing abstinence from alcohol [52]. The mechanism for this effect may be due to the influence of $GABA_B$ agonist on the mesolimbic dopamine pathway. Baclofen has not been studied for use in the treatment of alcohol withdrawal in the intensive care setting and a recent COCHRANE review suggested additional data were needed to draw conclusions about its role in alcohol withdrawal [53].

Sodium oxybate, the sodium salt of γ-hydroxybutyric acid (GHB), is another $GABA_B$ agonist which recent research has suggested may have a role in the treatment of alcohol withdrawal. It is currently approved for use in some European countries. In randomized, controlled trials, it was comparable to benzodiazepines and clomethiazole in relieving symptoms of moderate alcohol withdrawal in an outpatient setting. Transient vertigo was the most commonly reported side effect, but also occurred with clomethiazole and benzodiazepine treatment. GHB may resolve withdrawal-associated symptoms of anxiety, agitation, and depression more quickly than benzodiazepines, possibly due to its action on dopaminergic and serotonergic neurotransmitter systems. This method of treatment is not commonly used, and further study is warranted.

The use of phenothiazines and butyrophenones to treat ethanol withdrawal has been associated with excessive fatalities [27,49]. These agents have been shown to lower the seizure threshold, induce hypotension, impair thermoregulation, prolong the QT interval, and precipitate dystonic reactions [6]. These drugs have no role in the management of sedative–hypnotic withdrawal.

Magnesium sulfate has been suggested as a potential therapy for alcohol withdrawal, but studies have been concerning for biases and limited in scope. Currently, too little data are available to confirm that magnesium supplementation helps alleviate signs or symptoms of alcohol withdrawal, either in normomagnesemic or in hypomagnesemic patients [54].

Valproate has been suggested as an alternative or adjunctive treatment for ethanol withdrawal. It appears to potentiate GABA-ergic neural transmission through a variety of mechanisms, including activation of glutamic acid decarboxylase. Although there is evidence that valproate may be effective in alleviating withdrawal symptoms, further research is needed before it can be recommended for use in ethanol withdrawal [55].

Adequate sedation of the patient with early signs of withdrawal prevents the development of ethanol withdrawal seizures and progression to delirium tremens. The patients who have had an ethanol withdrawal seizure are at risk for progression to delirium tremens and should be sedated with benzodiazepines or barbiturates, as previously discussed. A randomized, controlled trial evaluating patients presenting to the emergency department with ethanol withdrawal seizures and lacking other signs of moderate alcohol withdrawal showed that a one-time dose of lorazepam, 2 mg IV, was more effective than placebo in preventing recurrent ethanol withdrawal seizures [56]. No evidence has been shown to prove that phenytoin is efficacious in the treatment or prevention of ethanol withdrawal seizures [6,57]. Clinical studies failed to show any significant benefit of IV phenytoin when compared with placebo in the prevention of subsequent ethanol withdrawal seizures [57].

The use of anticonvulsants to prevent or treat ethanol withdrawal seizures should be limited to the patients with an underlying seizure disorder who require maintenance anticonvulsant therapy [6]. These patients often seize at the onset of mild withdrawal secondary to poor compliance with their anticonvulsant regimen and require restoration of adequate serum levels with an anticonvulsant such as phenytoin. The patients who present with an apparent ethanol withdrawal seizure but do not have a history of either underlying seizure disorder or previous ethanol withdrawal seizures require a full seizure workup. For those rare patients in ethanol withdrawal in whom status epilepticus develops, aggressive anticonvulsant treatment is indicated with phenobarbital in addition to benzodiazepines. Because status epilepticus and seizures during delirium tremens are rare sequelae of ethanol withdrawal, their occurrence requires a search for underlying traumatic injuries and infection, regardless of any previous history of ethanol withdrawal seizures.

Adequate early treatment with benzodiazepines usually suppresses significant manifestations of withdrawal and prevents progression to delirium tremens. If delirium tremens is already manifest, sedation with a benzodiazepine does not completely reverse mental status abnormalities. This may be a consequence of the incomplete cross-tolerance of benzodiazepine with ethanol or perhaps the lack of immediate reversibility of some of the CNS effects of withdrawal.

BENZODIAZEPINE WITHDRAWAL

Since their introduction in the early 1960s, benzodiazepines have replaced the barbiturates as the most widely prescribed sedative–hypnotic agents. Initially, these newer agents were not thought to have the same serious withdrawal problems associated with the barbiturates [58]. Subsequent experience has shown that withdrawal from benzodiazepines may be as severe as withdrawal from barbiturates or ethanol. It is estimated that 5% to 10% of the adults in the United States use benzodiazepines on a regular basis [59]. The early signs of withdrawal from benzodiazepines are the same as those of ethanol withdrawal. Differences include delayed time of onset, depending on the duration of action of the agent involved, and the presence or absence of active metabolites. When delayed tachycardia, hypertension, and irritability develop in a hospitalized patient, prior benzodiazepine abuse should be suspected.

Pathophysiology

Signs and symptoms of benzodiazepine withdrawal occur when tolerant patients experience a decline in brain benzodiazepine levels. Individuals who have not developed tolerance do not experience symptoms of withdrawal. The patients who have taken therapeutic amounts of these drugs over an extended period may experience withdrawal (therapeutic dose withdrawal) [58], although more commonly it occurs in those who have been regularly taking higher than recommended antianxiety doses [60]. A high daily dose and long duration of benzodiazepine use correlate with a greater risk of developing a moderate-to-severe withdrawal syndrome [61]. Although withdrawal usually occurs after abrupt discontinuation of these medications, it may occur to a lesser extent during drug tapering [62]. Iatrogenic benzodiazepine withdrawal has also been described for the patients following discontinuation of midazolam-induced sedation in the ICU [63].

The mechanisms for benzodiazepine tolerance and withdrawal involve modulation of $GABA_A$ receptor conformations and subunits, similar to those that occur with chronic ethanol use, may be responsible [64]. Ultimately, a decrease in the availability of exogenous benzodiazepine results in unopposed nervous system stimulation and an increase in agitation and anxiety.

Variability in the time course and severity of withdrawal among the various benzodiazepines can be explained by their differing pharmacokinetics [58]. Drug half-life and the presence of active metabolites correlate with the onset, frequency, and severity of withdrawal symptoms. The onset of withdrawal from shorter-acting agents without active metabolites, such as lorazepam or alprazolam, may be precipitous, with marked symptoms as early as 24 hours after cessation of the drug. Signs of withdrawal from longer-acting agents, such as diazepam, which have a long elimination half-life in addition to active metabolites, may be delayed for 8 days or longer. Withdrawal symptoms from long-acting benzodiazepines may persist for months [58]. Concurrent use of other cross-tolerant sedative–hypnotic substances, such as ethanol, barbiturates, chloral hydrate, glutethimide, ethchlorvynol, or meprobamate, along with benzodiazepines increases the probability of developing withdrawal on abrupt discontinuation of these substances.

The administration of the competitive benzodiazepine antagonist flumazenil can result in iatrogenic benzodiazepine withdrawal. Flumazenil is sometimes used to reverse sedation in the settings of benzodiazepine overdose, IV conscious sedation, and general anesthesia. However, it may not fully reverse respiratory depression associated with benzodiazepine toxicity [60]. A history of benzodiazepine use and dependence may not be available when unconscious patients are admitted to the ICU, and benzodiazepine withdrawal with seizures and death has been reported after the use of flumazenil. Recently, safety was reported in a very small study of flumazenil use in the emergency department [65]. Flumazenil should be used with caution (see Chapters 123 and 125).

Clinical Manifestations

Benzodiazepine withdrawal is characterized by CNS excitation and autonomic hyperactivity. Mild early manifestations of withdrawal include psychological symptoms such as anxiety, apprehension, irritability, mood swings, dysphoria, and insomnia. Somatic complaints commonly include nausea, palpitations, tremor, diaphoresis, and muscle twitching.

More severe signs of withdrawal include vomiting, cramps, tachycardia, postural hypotension, and hyperthermia. Significant neuromuscular hyperactivity may be manifested as fasciculations, myoclonic jerks, and seizures [16,58]. Agitated delirium accompanied by hallucinations and paranoid delusions, and catatonia, have been described [66].

For the patients taking clonazepam, withdrawal symptoms may develop 3 to 4 days after cessation of therapy. Clonazepam withdrawal may be precipitated or accentuated, or both, by concomitant neuroleptic therapy [67].

Diagnostic Evaluation

Benzodiazepine withdrawal may be difficult to distinguish from an underlying anxiety disorder [58,60]. The time course of the symptoms helps distinguish these two diagnoses. Withdrawal symptoms often worsen rapidly in the early period, followed by gradual improvement and resolution. Unmasked anxiety disorders tend not to deteriorate significantly and persist with time. Perceptual disturbances, not generally associated with underlying anxiety disorders, are commonly found during early withdrawal and may also help distinguish withdrawal from the return of anxiety. These disturbances include paresthesias, tinnitus, visual abnormalities, vertigo, metallic taste, depersonalization, and derealization [16,58].

Management

Treatment strategies for benzodiazepine withdrawal are similar to those used for ethanol withdrawal with the exception that reintroduction of the drug is often warranted for benzodiazepine withdrawal. Reinstitution of the drug at a dose that relieves withdrawal symptoms followed by slow withdrawal during 2 to 4 weeks minimizes symptoms and affects the desired decrease in CNS tolerance. Alternatively, a similar cross-tolerant agent can be used. A long-acting benzodiazepine such as diazepam or chlordiazepoxide is preferred in severe withdrawal. Short-acting agents may be disadvantageous because maintenance of therapeutic serum drug levels requires frequent drug administration. In patients with moderate-to-severe symptoms (e.g., seizures and delirium), small IV boluses, such as 5 mg of diazepam, should be given until adequate sedation is achieved. The patients experiencing milder symptoms can be treated by the oral route. Barbiturates such as pentobarbital and phenobarbital can also be used in the treatment of benzodiazepine withdrawal [60].

β-Blockers and clonidine have also been used for the treatment of benzodiazepine withdrawal. Propranolol (10 to 40 mg every 6 hours) may help ameliorate tremor, muscle twitching, tachycardia, and hypertension. However, it has little effect on anxiety, agitation, and dysphoria. Clonidine use has also been advocated, although its efficacy in modulating the intensity, severity, and duration of withdrawal has been questioned. As with ethanol withdrawal, it is important to realize that treating peripheral manifestations of withdrawal may obscure early signs of impending delirium and impedes the assessment of adequate sedation. Phenothiazines and butyrophenones exhibit no cross-tolerance to the benzodiazepines and do not have a role in the treatment of benzodiazepine withdrawal, for the same reasons seen in ethanol withdrawal.

Limited data are available on the treatment of flumazenil-induced benzodiazepine withdrawal. Because flumazenil has a relatively short half-life (approximately 1 hour), supportive care should be sufficient in the treatment of mild withdrawal symptoms. The precipitation of seizure activity may require treatment with a benzodiazepine or barbiturate. Owing to flumazenil blockade of benzodiazepine binding site, higher doses of GABA-ergic agonists may be required [58,60].

γ-HYDROXYBUTYRATE WITHDRAWAL

Withdrawal from the commonly abused street drugs GHB or its congeners γ-butyrolactone and 1,4-butanediol (see Chapter 121) may be dramatic and potentially life-threatening [68]. The pathophysiology is similar to that for benzodiazepine withdrawal. Heavy users of these chemicals report using multiple daily doses (as frequent as every 1 to 3 hours) around the clock [69]. GHB acts as an agonist at GHB and $GABA_B$ receptors. Withdrawal symptoms may include agitation, mental status changes, hypertension, and tachycardia. Other findings are tremulousness, diaphoresis, tachypnea, rigidity, irritability, paranoia, insomnia, and auditory and visual hallucinations [68]. High-frequency users appear to be at greatest risk for developing withdrawal delirium after abrupt discontinuation of these agents. Onset of symptoms may begin as early as 1 to 6 hours after the last dose [70]. Severe withdrawal symptoms may persist from 5 to 15 days onward and require prolonged ICU care. Many of these patients require physical restraints and heavy sedation. The use of IV benzodiazepine and other cross-tolerant agents is recommended in the management of these patients, although some patients may be refractory to large doses of benzodiazepines. Successful treatment of this subset of the patients with propofol, barbiturates and baclofen have been reported, but rigorous prospective clinical trials have yet to be conducted [68]. Barbiturates such as pentobarbital may be helpful because unlike benzodiazepines, they are capable of opening $GABA_A$ chloride channels independently of GABA's presence. Pentobarbital dosages used in case series were 1 to 2 mg per kg IV every 30 to 60 minutes, titrated to improvement in vital signs and altered sensorium [71]. Baclofen's usefulness may stem from the fact that like GHB, it is an agonist at $GABA_B$ receptors, whereas benzodiazepines act only on the $GABA_A$ receptor. One case report describes dosing of 10 mg orally three times daily successfully prevented seizures which occurred every time GHB was withdrawn from a dependent patient [72].

BACLOFEN WITHDRAWAL

Baclofen is a $GABA_B$ receptor agonist used to treat spasticity resulting from multiple sclerosis or CNS injury. It can be taken orally or delivered by an intrathecal pump, which allows higher CNS levels without the side effects associated with large oral doses. An abrupt discontinuation or decrease in either oral or intrathecal baclofen dose may result in a withdrawal syndrome [73]. The pathophysiology is similar to that for benzodiazepine withdrawal. There are many scenarios in which an intrathecal drug delivery system may fail, including errors in programming the pump or filling the reservoir, the development of kinks or occlusions in the tubing, and battery failure.

Onset of withdrawal symptoms may occur within a few hours to a few days after a decrease in baclofen dose or sudden intrathecal pump failure [74,75]. Mild-to-moderate withdrawal symptoms may include increased spasticity, tachycardia, hypertension, fever, neuromuscular rigidity, hyperreflexia, psychosis, and delirium. Severe withdrawal may result in coma, seizures, rhabdomyolysis, hyperthermia, disseminated intravascular coagulation, circulatory failure, delirium, and coma. The features of withdrawal from oral and intrathecal baclofen are similar with onset at similar times following last administration, though some reports indicate hallucinations may be more frequent in those withdrawing from oral baclofen. The mechanism for this is not entirely known. Occasionally, the patients may develop a reversible cardiomyopathy. In the most severe cases, multiorgan failure and death may occur [73,76]. The delirium observed with baclofen withdrawal may resemble the altered mental status caused by baclofen intoxication, and baclofen intoxication should always be considered along with withdrawal in the differential diagnosis of delirium in the patient on baclofen. The severe withdrawal syndrome may also mimic other conditions such as infection, serotonin syndrome, and neuroleptic malignant syndrome. In cases such as these, the diagnosis may be easy to miss, and evaluation for pump failure should always be considered. Any reason for pump failure should be identified and remedied, with the previous intrathecal baclofen dose reinstituted [77]. Pump integrity and function may be assessed by plain films, dye studies, nuclear medicine flow studies, port aspirations, or if necessary, operative exploration. Cautiously administering a bolus of baclofen by the pump, by way of lumbar puncture, or by a lumbar drain, and assessing for improvement in 30 to 60 minutes may help confirm the diagnosis. Oral baclofen may also be used, though large doses may be needed and clinical improvement may be delayed by several hours [78].

In addition to supportive care, the most important step in the management of baclofen withdrawal is the replacement of the baclofen. The patients who were receiving oral therapy may have the drug administered by nasogastric tube if they are unable to take it by mouth secondary to their withdrawal symptoms. The patients withdrawing from intrathecal baclofen may require high doses of oral baclofen, or may not respond to oral replacement therapy [77]. Replacement oral baclofen doses for intrathecal baclofen withdrawal often range between 10 and 30 mg orally, every 4 to 8 hours [78]. If there is any delay in administering baclofen intrathecally in these patients, other sedative medications such as benzodiazepines, barbiturates, or propofol should be provided intravenously. As with oral baclofen dosing and with benzodiazepine treatment of severe ethanol withdrawal, large doses of these agents may be necessary to control severe symptoms, with attention to airway support if the patient is not already intubated. Cyproheptadine (4 to 8 mg orally every 6 to 8 hours) has been suggested as a useful adjunctive therapy in patients with intrathecal baclofen withdrawal who are well enough to take oral medications. More study is needed before this can be definitively recommended.

OPIOID WITHDRAWAL

Opioid withdrawal occurs when a tolerant individual experiences a decline in CNS levels of a chronically used opioid. Unlike withdrawal from sedative–hypnotic agents, the manifestations of opioid withdrawal are not usually life-threatening [16]. Recognition of the problem facilitates optimal management of the critically ill patient.

Pathophysiology

Opioid receptors in the locus ceruleus bind exogenous opioids, such as heroin, methadone, or codeine, as well as endogenous opioid-like substances known as *endorphins* and *enkephalins*. Stimulation of opioid receptors reduces the firing rate of locus ceruleus noradrenergic neurons, resulting in the inhibition of catecholamine release. The stimulation of inhibitory adrenergic receptors, also found in the locus ceruleus, causes a similar reduction in sympathetic outflow. Chronic opioid use may produce an increase or upregulation of these adrenergic receptors. Subsequent withdrawal of opioids results in increased sympathetic discharge and noradrenergic hyperactivity.

The time course of the withdrawal syndrome depends on pharmacokinetic parameters of the individual opioids. Withdrawal symptoms usually appear about the time of the next expected dose [16,79]. Withdrawal from heroin, which has a short half-life, begins 4 to 8 hours after the last dose, whereas withdrawal from methadone, with a long half-life, is delayed until 36 to 72 hours after the last dose. Withdrawal symptoms are more intense if the opioid has a shorter half-life, whereas symptoms are less dramatic but often more prolonged if the abused opioid has a longer half-life. Methadone withdrawal may not peak until the 6th day of abstinence and may persist for weeks. Because prolonged opioid use may be required to facilitate ventilator management in intensive care patients, iatrogenic opioid withdrawal may complicate ventilator weaning [80].

Clinical Manifestations

Early signs of opioid withdrawal include mydriasis, lacrimation, rhinorrhea, diaphoresis, yawning, piloerection, anxiety, and restlessness [16,79]. With time, these symptoms may worsen and be accompanied by mild elevation in pulse, blood pressure, and respiratory rate. Myalgias, vomiting, diarrhea, anorexia, abdominal pain, and dehydration accompany more severe withdrawal. Although these patients may become extremely restless, fever and central agitation such as seizures (except in cases of neonatal withdrawal) and mental status alteration are not part of opioid withdrawal. An intense craving for the drug accompanies withdrawal. Recognition of these signs and symptoms in the ICU patient obviates the need for extensive evaluation of the gastrointestinal symptoms and puts clinically puzzling pain complaints in perspective. Appropriate therapy alleviates the patient's discomfort and facilitates the management of more pressing ICU problems. After the resolution of most of the objective signs of withdrawal, subjective symptoms, especially dysphoria, may persist for weeks.

Opioid withdrawal may occur suddenly in the opioid-dependent patient given naloxone [81]. This iatrogenic withdrawal often occurs after naloxone is given to the patient who is lethargic or comatose and has unrecognized opioid dependency. Naloxone-induced withdrawal may also occur in dependent patients after use of naloxone to reverse the effects of an opioid used during procedural sedation. Vomiting and subsequent aspiration of the unconscious patient are the major complications arising from this problem, an important concern in the setting of mixed sedative intoxications. This abstinence syndrome is of brief duration due to the short half-life of naloxone, lasting 20 to 60 minutes, and treatment with opioids to reverse the unwarranted effects of naloxone is not indicated. Naloxone, if required, should not be withheld in the dependent patient. A starting dose of 0.04 to 0.10 mg should be used and titrated until the desired effect is achieved or mild signs of withdrawal occur. Coma or hypoventilation that persists after the onset of withdrawal signs is not reversed by the administration of additional naloxone. This suggests another contributing substance or cause for coma [82].

Naltrexone, an orally active opioid antagonist, induces withdrawal symptoms for up to 48 hours. Nalmefene, another opioid antagonist, may also cause prolonged withdrawal symptoms in the opioid-tolerant patient. A less commonly recognized cause of opioid withdrawal is the use of agonist–antagonist in the opioid-dependent person. Drugs with agonist–antagonist activity include pentazocine (Talwin), nalbuphine (Nubain), butorphanol (Stadol), and buprenorphine (Subutex).

Management

Treatment of opioid withdrawal is a two-tier approach, using cross-tolerant opioid replacement or sympatholytic therapy (e.g., clonidine), or both. The benzodiazepines are not cross-tolerant with opioids. Their role is limited to the management of significant anxiety associated with opioid withdrawal.

Substitution of long-acting methadone for heroin has played a prominent role in the management of opioid addiction. First used in the 1960s for the treatment of heroin addiction, methadone was chosen for its chemical similarity to heroin, oral availability, and long half-life (24 to 36 hours). Although the use of methadone for the outpatient treatment of opioid dependence is tightly regulated, physicians do not need special licensing to prescribe methadone to hospitalized patients. Methadone administered by nasogastric tube or subcutaneously has been successfully used to treat iatrogenic opioid withdrawal symptoms as well. The use of methadone may shorten the phase of ventilator weaning in these patients [83].

Methadone may be useful for treating the uncomfortable symptoms in patients who depend on any opioid. The dose should be judiciously titrated to relieve symptoms but avoid oversedation. A safe initial dose is 20 mg orally or 10 mg IM. The IM route guarantees absorption in the vomiting patient [79]. Relief of symptoms usually occurs within 30 to 60 minutes when the drug is given parenterally and longer when it is given orally. A second 10 mg IM dose can be given if significant relief is not achieved 1 hour after the first IM dose. Administering 10 to 20 mg by IM route blocks most manifestations of physiologic withdrawal, although some patients may require 20 to 40 mg daily or divided twice per day to avoid psychological withdrawal. In general, dosing to prevent withdrawal symptoms requires considerably less drug than dosing for methadone maintenance. Although withdrawal from opioids should not be attempted during an acute medical illness, once they are medically stabilized, heroin-dependent patients can be tapered with methadone over 1 week [84].

Methadone-dependent patients require 4 weeks or more of gradually decreasing dosages [84]. Notable drugs that interact with methadone, lowering its plasma concentration and potentially precipitating opioid withdrawal, include rifampin and phenytoin.

For those patients enrolled in methadone maintenance programs, considerably larger doses of methadone are often employed. Some of these patients, particularly early in treatment, may continue to abuse heroin. Higher methadone doses, as much as 150 mg a day or more, have been recommended as a means to reduce concurrent heroin use and retain patients in treatment programs [85]. Some community clinics use doses as high as 200 to over 300 mg per day in selected patients.

The treatment of pain in patients receiving methadone may require the use of additional opioid analgesia, such as morphine, codeine, or oxycodone. In patients on methadone maintenance, the established maintenance dose may not provide adequate analgesia because of tolerance to the analgesic effects of methadone. Successful pain relief requires the continuation of the methadone maintenance dose supplemented by additional analgesics [86].

Every attempt should be made to minimize significant withdrawal manifestations for the opioid-dependent pregnant patient. Withdrawal in these patients may adversely affect the developing fetus, causing fetal distress and even intrauterine death. Oral methadone maintenance is more compatible with maternal and fetal well-being than continued heroin abuse and would likely also decrease the risk of intrauterine acquisition of acquired immunodeficiency syndrome [87]. Cautious treatment of these patients with sufficient methadone to avoid withdrawal may avert these additional complications. After delivery, the neonate must be hospitalized and withdrawn from the drug. In selected pregnancies, lowering the maternal methadone dosage may lead to decreased incidence and severity of neonatal withdrawal [88].

Although methadone has been extensively used for decades to help opiate addicted patients circumvent the health problems associated with illicit IV drug abuse, there are valid concerns about its safety as well. Methadone is known to cause dose-related respiratory depression and sleep apnea, which varies greatly based on an individual patient's underlying tolerance. The risk of apnea increases when methadone is combined with other depressant drugs [89]. Other concerns have increasingly come to light in recent years. Disproportionate numbers of the patients on methadone were found to have suffered sudden cardiac death, often without underlying structural heart disease [89]. Though the majority of methadone associated sudden deaths are likely due to respiratory depression, it was also discovered that methadone is a potent potassium channel blocker, especially at higher doses. This prolongs cardiac repolarization (lengthening the QTc interval and predisposing to Torsades de Pointe). Although it is unknown how clinically significant this finding may be, some experts suggest that QTc intervals be checked prior to initiating methadone therapy and be followed during chronic therapy to watch for lengthening of the QTc [90].

In recent years, buprenorphine, a partial mu-opioid agonist and K-opioid antagonist, has been increasingly advocated as an alternative to methadone for both maintenance, short-term management of opioid detoxification and opioid withdrawal during concurrent medical illness [91,92]. Buprenorphine can be given orally, sublingually, intramuscularly, or intravenously. Because of its partial agonist activity, it causes less CNS and respiratory depression and has a ceiling effect, so is less likely to be dangerous in overdose than methadone (though respiratory depression may still occasionally be seen, especially at higher doses, and deaths have been reported). This characteristic also renders it able to block the euphoric effects of heroin and morphine. It produces only a mild withdrawal syndrome when treatment is ceased, but care should be taken when initiating therapy in opioid-dependent patients as it may precipitate withdrawal. Of interest, one case of deliberate buprenorphine overdose resulted not in respiratory depression but severe opioid withdrawal lasting 4 days [93]. Opioid withdrawal symptoms may resolve more quickly with buprenorphine than with methadone but the effectiveness for maintenance treatment of heroin dependence is similar between the two agents [94]. Buprenorphine does not seem to have the same propensity to prolong the QT interval as methadone [90]. Buprenorphine has an even longer half-life than methadone of approximately 40 hours, so an additional benefit is that it may be administered every other day or even three times a week as maintenance therapy for opioid addicted patients. Special training and licensing are required for physicians who wish to prescribe buprenorphine or methadone (when used as treatment for opioid dependence) on an outpatient basis.

Sublingual buprenorphine tablets and solution are available as monotherapies as well as in combination with naloxone in a 4:1 (buprenorphine:naloxone) ratio (Suboxone). The naloxone is poorly absorbed sublingually and therefore does not interfere with buprenorphine's effects when taken as directed. Naloxone is added to the buprenorphine to block buprenorphine's euphorigenic effects if an attempt is made to divert the drug for illicit IV use (crushing and dissolving tablets, among others).

Sublingual dosing of buprenorphine for opioid dependence maintenance therapy starts with an introductory dose of 4 to 8 mg, based on the patient's degree of neuroadaptation to opioids. Current recommendations are for the use of buprenorphine–naloxone therapy (Suboxone). Dosing may be advanced by 4 mg per day on subsequent induction days as necessary to control withdrawal symptoms up to a total dose of 32 mg per day. Symptomatic management should be undertaken for additional withdrawal symptoms. Because buprenorphine binds more tightly to the mu-opioid receptor than does heroin or methadone, it displaces any residual drug from the receptor and blocks its agonist effects since buprenorphine itself is only a partial agonist. Ideally buprenorphine induction is done when the patient is exhibiting early signs of withdrawal, such as yawning and rhinorrhea, which lowers the chance of precipitating further withdrawal as buprenorphine will not be displacing a more potent opioid. This is usually at least 6 hours after the last heroin use. If the patient is on methadone, the dose of methadone should be tapered to no more than 30 mg per day for at least 1 week prior to transitioning medications. This minimizes risk of withdrawal and improves success; starting on too high a dose increases the risk of precipitated withdrawal. The first dose of buprenorphine should be given at least 24 hours after the last dose of methadone. In this instance, Suboxone monotherapy is preferred with transition to combined therapy with naloxone on Day 2. Precipitated withdrawal symptoms usually start 1 to 4 hours after the buprenorphine dose and last about 12 hours. These symptoms are worst during the first day, but the patients transitioning to buprenorphine from methadone may experience mild discomfort and dysphoria for up to 1 to 2 weeks, depending on how much methadone they were using previously. Symptomatic treatment with medication such as clonidine may be employed during this period as needed.

In addition to maintenance therapy, various tapering opioid detoxification regimens using buprenorphine exist, with starting doses ranging from 1 to 8 mg daily. Therapy may be tapered over 5 to 14 days [95].

Clonidine, a central α_2-adrenergic agonist that binds to the α_2-receptors in the locus ceruleus, is also used to treat opioid withdrawal [96]. Stimulation of central α_2-receptors results in feedback inhibition of the norepinephrine activity, decreasing the firing rate of the noradrenergic neurons. These noradrenergic neurons also possess opioid receptors whose stimulation produces a similar reduction in sympathetic activity through the same intracellular messenger system. Clonidine used without the addition of a replacement opioid has been found to be as effective as methadone in preventing opioid withdrawal symptoms in medically ill hospitalized patients. Clonidine may be administered in doses of 0.1 to 0.2 mg every 4 to 6 hours. Treatment is often continued for 5 to 10 days and then slowly tapered by 0.2 mg per day. Clonidine transdermal patches provide steady-state clonidine levels and may also be useful. Tachyphylaxis to the effects of clonidine may develop by 10 to 14 days. The most concerning side effect of clonidine is hypotension, especially with the first dose. This requires close monitoring. In more recent studies, the patients administered buprenorphine–naloxone were more likely to complete short-term detoxification programs and report fewer withdrawal and craving symptoms than those treated with clonidine [97]. Although buprenorphine–naloxone seems to be more efficient than clonidine in reducing opioid withdrawal symptoms during the initial course of detoxification differences may wane after a few days [98]. The long-term success of this approach is unclear.

Combination therapy with clonidine and naltrexone has also been used for rapid opioid detoxification. Proponents of this approach emphasize the shortened period of withdrawal associated with the addition of naltrexone. Continuing naltrexone as deterrent therapy after opioid withdrawal (akin to the use of disulfiram with alcoholics) has also been advocated, but this approach has a high attrition rate. Delirium has been reported during rapid opioid detoxification of methadone maintenance patients.

Administering high doses of opioid antagonists to addicted individuals while under anesthesia has been suggested as a method of achieving detoxification from opiates within 24 to 48 hours. This method, known as ultrarapid detoxification, has been associated with pulmonary and renal failure as well as other complications, including death. Additionally, long-term follow-up has demonstrated relapse of drug abuse in many of these patients [99]. This approach is not recommended.

NICOTINE WITHDRAWAL

In the United States, 18% of the population continues to smoke tobacco cigarettes [100]. Tobacco exposure is a major risk factor for multiple respiratory, cardiovascular and infectious diseases, as well as carcinogenic. Nicotine binds nicotinic acetylcholine receptors and induces their upregulation. Nicotine withdrawal has been identified as a risk factor for agitation and delirium in the ICU [101]. Cessation of smoking has been associated with sweating, drowsiness and bradycardia [16]. Symptoms generally begin 1 to 2 days after last use, peak within the first week, and persist for 2 to 4 weeks or longer with cravings lasting up to 6 weeks [101]. Supportive care is often used. Nicotine replacement can be used to prevent withdrawal or alleviate symptoms with transdermal nicotine patches to reduce symptoms. Gums and lozenges containing nicotine are also available but their use is often limited in the ICU. Recent studies have evaluated mortality in association with nicotine replacement but are limited by their small size. The only prospective evaluation demonstrated no difference in mortality, length of stay or ventilator use in smokers receiving nicotine replacement versus those not receiving replacement therapy [102]. Additional evidence is necessary before a formal conclusion can be made. Bupropion, a long-acting serotonin and norepinephrine reuptake inhibitor, may be used at low doses alone or in combination with nicotine replacement to assist with smoking cessation. Varenicline is a $\alpha4\beta2$ nicotinic receptor partial agonist that has also been used for smoking cessation. Clinical studies regarding the roles of bupropion and varenicline for critically ill adults are lacking [101].

References

1. Schuckit MA: Recognition and management of withdrawal delirium (delirium tremens). *N Engl J Med* 371:2109–2113, 2014.
2. Goodson CM, Clark BJ, Douglas IS: Predictors of severe alcohol withdrawal syndrome: a systematic review and meta-analysis. *Alcohol Clin Exp Res* 38:2664–2677, 2014.
3. Fruensgaard K: Withdrawal psychosis: a study of 30 consecutive cases. *Acta Psychiatr Scand* 53:105–118, 1976.
4. Narahashi T, Kuriyama K, Illes P, et al: Neuroreceptors and ion channels as targets of alcohol. *Alcohol Clin Exp Res* 25:182S–188S, 2001.
5. Davis KM, Wu JY: Role of glutamatergic and GABAergic systems in alcoholism. *J Biomed Sci* 8:7–19, 2001.
6. Perry EC: Inpatient management of acute alcohol withdrawal syndrome. *CNS Drugs* 28:401–410, 2014.
7. Walker BM, Valdez GR, McLaughlin JP, et al: Targeting dynorphin/kappa opioid receptor systems to treat alcohol abuse and dependence. *Alcohol* 46:359–370, 2012.
8. Isbell H, Fraser HF, Wikler A, et al: An experimental study of the etiology of rum fits and delirium tremens. *Q J Stud Alcohol* 16:1–33, 1955.
9. Victor M, Adams RD: The effect of alcohol on the nervous system. *Res Publ Assoc Res Nerv Ment Dis* 32:526–573, 1953.
10. Carlson RW, Kumar NN, Wong-Mckinstry E, et al: Alcohol withdrawal syndrome. *Crit Care Clin* 28:549–585, 2012.
11. Sano H, Suzuki Y, Ohara K, et al: Circadian variation in plasma homovanillic acid level during and after alcohol withdrawal in alcoholic patients. *Alcohol Clin Exp Res* 16:1047–1051, 1992.
12. Nagy J, Kolok S, Boros A, et al: Role of altered structure and function of NMDA receptors in development of alcohol dependence. *Curr Neuropharmacol* 3:281–297, 2005.
13. Dodd P: Neural mechanisms of adaptation in chronic ethanol exposure and alcoholism. *Alcohol Clin Exp Res* 20[8 Suppl]:151A–156A, 1996.
14. Mendelson JH, Mello NK: Medical progress. Biologic concomitants of alcoholism. *N Engl J Med* 301:912–921, 1979.
15. Wong A, Benedict NJ, Kane-Gill SL: Multicenter evaluation of pharmacologic management and outcomes associated with severe resistant alcohol withdrawal. *J Crit Care* 30:405–409, 2015.
16. Tetrault JM, O'Connor PG: Substance abuse and withdrawal in the critical care setting. *Crit Care Clin* 24:767–788, 2008.
17. Lukan JK, Reed DN Jr, Looney SW, et al: Risk factors for delirium tremens in trauma patients. *J Trauma* 53:901–906, 2002.
18. Kim DW, Kim HK, Bae EK, et al: Clinical predictors for delirium tremens in patients with alcohol withdrawal seizures. *Am J Emerg Med* 33:701–704, 2015.
19. Simon RP: Alcohol and seizures. *N Engl J Med* 319:715–716, 1988.
20. Monte R, Rabunal R, Casariego E, et al: Analysis of the factors determining survival of alcoholic withdrawal syndrome patients in a general hospital. *Alcohol Alcohol* 45:151–158, 2010.
21. Tavel ME, Davidson W, Batterton TD: A critical analysis of mortality associated with delirium tremens. Review of 39 fatalities in a 9-year period. *Am J Med Sci* 242:18–29, 1961.
22. Moore M, Gray MG: Delirium Tremens: a study of cases at the Boston City Hospital 1915–1936. *N Engl J Med* 220:953, 1939.
23. Lee JH, Jang MK, Lee JY, et al: Clinical predictors for delirium tremens in alcohol dependence. *J Gastroenterol Hepatol* 20:1833–1837, 2005.
24. Jaeger TM, Lohr RH, Pankratz VS: Symptom-triggered therapy for alcohol withdrawal syndrome in medical inpatients. *Mayo Clin Proc* 76:695–701, 2001.
25. Catic AG: Identification and management of in-hospital drug-induced delirium in older patients. *Drugs Aging* 28:737–748, 2011.
26. Khan A, Levy P, DeHorn S, et al: Predictors of mortality in patients with delirium tremens. *Acad Emerg Med* 15:788–790, 2008.
27. Mayo-Smith MF, Beecher LH, Fischer TL, et al: Management of alcohol withdrawal delirium. An evidence-based practice guideline. *Arch Intern Med* 164:1405–1412, 2004.
28. Amato L, Minozzi S, Vecchi S, et al: Benzodiazepines for alcohol withdrawal. *Cochrane Database Syst Rev* 3:CD005063, 2010.
29. Bird RD, Makela EH: Alcohol withdrawal: what is the benzodiazepine of choice? *Ann Pharmacother* 28:67–71, 1994.
30. Ramanujam R, L P, G S, et al: A comparative study of the clinical efficacy and safety of Lorazepam and chlordiazepoxide in alcohol dependence syndrome. *J Clin Diagn Res* 9:FC10–FC13, 2015.
31. Miller WC Jr, McCurdy L: A double-blind comparison of the efficacy and safety of lorazepam and diazepam in the treatment of the acute alcohol withdrawal syndrome. *Clin Ther* 6:364–371, 1984.
32. Mayo-Smith MF: Pharmacological management of alcohol withdrawal. A meta-analysis and evidence-based practice guideline. American Society of Addiction Medicine Working Group on Pharmacological Management of Alcohol Withdrawal. *JAMA* 278:144–151, 1997.
33. Daeppen JB, Gache P, Landry U, et al: Symptom-triggered vs fixed-schedule doses of benzodiazepine for alcohol withdrawal: a randomized treatment trial. *Arch Intern Med* 162:1117–1121, 2002.
34. Saitz R, Mayo-Smith MF, Roberts MS, et al: Individualized treatment for alcohol withdrawal. A randomized double-blind controlled trial. *JAMA* 272:519–523, 1994.
35. Spies CD, Otter HE, Huske B, et al: Alcohol withdrawal severity is decreased by symptom-orientated adjusted bolus therapy in the ICU. *Intensive Care Med* 29:2230–2238, 2003.
36. Enoch MA: The role of GABA(A) receptors in the development of alcoholism. *Pharmacol Biochem Behav* 90:95–104, 2008.
37. Gold JA, Rimal B, Nolan A, et al: A strategy of escalating doses of benzodiazepines and phenobarbital administration reduces the need for mechanical ventilation in delirium tremens. *Crit Care Med* 35:724–730, 2007.
38. McCowan C, Marik P: Refractory delirium tremens treated with propofol: a case series. *Crit Care Med* 28:1781–1784, 2000.
39. Barr J, Egan TD, Sandoval NF, et al: Propofol dosing regimens for ICU sedation based upon an integrated pharmacokinetic-pharmacodynamic model. *Anesthesiology* 95:324–333, 2001.
40. Sohraby R, Attridge RL, Hughes DW: Use of propofol-containing versus benzodiazepine regimens for alcohol withdrawal requiring mechanical ventilation. *Ann Pharmacother* 48:456–461, 2014.
41. Wong A, Benedict NJ, Lohr BR, et al: Management of benzodiazepine-resistant alcohol withdrawal across a healthcare system: Benzodiazepine dose-escalation with or without propofol. *Drug Alcohol Depend* 154:296–299, 2015.
42. Wong A, Benedict NJ, Armahizer MJ, et al: Evaluation of adjunctive ketamine to benzodiazepines for management of alcohol withdrawal syndrome. *Ann Pharmacother* 49:14–19, 2015.
43. Darrouj J, Puri N, Prince E, et al: Dexmedetomidine infusion as adjunctive therapy to benzodiazepines for acute alcohol withdrawal. *Ann Pharmacother* 42:1703–1705, 2008.
44. DeMuro JP, Botros DG, Wirkowski E, et al: Use of dexmedetomidine for the treatment of alcohol withdrawal syndrome in critically ill patients: a retrospective case series. *J Anesth* 26:601–605, 2012.
45. Mueller SW, Preslaski CR, Kiser TH, et al: A randomized, double-blind, placebo-controlled dose range study of dexmedetomidine as adjunctive therapy for alcohol withdrawal. *Crit Care Med* 42:1131–1139, 2014.
46. Lizotte RJ, Kappes JA, Bartel BJ, et al: Evaluating the effects of dexmedetomidine compared to propofol as adjunctive therapy in patients with alcohol withdrawal. *Clin Pharmacol* 6:171–177, 2014.
47. Adinoff B: Double-blind study of alprazolam, diazepam, clonidine, and placebo in the alcohol withdrawal syndrome: preliminary findings. *Alcohol Clin Exp Res* 18:873–878, 1994.
48. Rosenbaum M, McCarty T: Alcohol prescription by surgeons in the prevention and treatment of delirium tremens: historic and current practice. *Gen Hosp Psychiatry* 24:257–259, 2002.
49. Golbert TM, Sanz CJ, Rose HD, et al: Comparative evaluation of treatments of alcohol withdrawal syndromes. *JAMA* 201:99–102, 1967.
50. Hodges B, Mazur JE: Intravenous ethanol for the treatment of alcohol withdrawal syndrome in critically ill patients. *Pharmacotherapy* 24:1578–1585, 2004.
51. Addolorato G, Leggio L, Abenavoli L, et al: Baclofen in the treatment of alcohol withdrawal syndrome: a comparative study vs diazepam. *Am J Med* 119:276.e213–278.e213, 2006.
52. Imbert B, Alvarez JC, Simon N: Anticraving effect of baclofen in alcohol-dependent patients. *Alcohol Clin Exp Res* 39:1602–1608, 2015.
53. Liu J, Wang LN: Baclofen for alcohol withdrawal. *Cochrane Database Syst Rev* 4:CD008502, 2015.
54. Sarai M, Tejani AM, Chan AH, et al: Magnesium for alcohol withdrawal. *Cochrane Database Syst Rev* 6:CD008358, 2013.
55. Harris JT, Roache JD, Thornton JE: A role for valproate in the treatment of sedative-hypnotic withdrawal and for relapse prevention. *Alcohol Alcohol* 35:319–323, 2000.
56. D'Onofrio G, Rathlev NK, Ulrich AS, et al: Lorazepam for the prevention of recurrent seizures related to alcohol. *N Engl J Med* 340:915–919, 1999.
57. Rathlev NK, D'Onofrio G, Fish SS, et al: The lack of efficacy of phenytoin in the prevention of recurrent alcohol-related seizures. *Ann Emerg Med* 23:513–518, 1994.
58. Ashton H: The diagnosis and management of benzodiazepine dependence. *Curr Opin Psychiatry* 18:249–255, 2005.
59. Olfson M, King M, Schoenbaum M: Benzodiazepine use in the United States. *JAMA Psychiatry*72:136–142, 2015.
60. Weaver MF: Prescription Sedative Misuse and Abuse. *Yale J Biol Med* 88:247–256, 2015.
61. O'Brien CP: Benzodiazepine use, abuse, and dependence. *J Clin Psychiatry* 66[Suppl 2]:28–33, 2005.
62. Lader M: Benzodiazepine harm: how can it be reduced? *Br J Clin Pharmacol* 77:295–301, 2014.
63. Best KM, Boullata JI, Curley MA: Risk factors associated with iatrogenic opioid and benzodiazepine withdrawal in critically ill pediatric patients: a systematic review and conceptual model. *Pediatr Crit Care Med* 16:175–183, 2015.
64. Gielen MC, Lumb MJ, Smart TG: Benzodiazepines modulate GABAA receptors by regulating the preactivation step after GABA binding. *J Neurosci* 32:5707–5715, 2012.

65. Nguyen TT, Troendle M, Cumpston K, et al: Lack of adverse effects from flumazenil administration: an ED observational study. *Am J Emerg Med* 33:1677–1679, 2015.
66. Rosebush PI, Mazurek MF: Catatonia after benzodiazepine withdrawal. *J Clin Psychopharmacol* 16:315–319, 1996.
67. Jaffe R, Gibson E: Clonazepam withdrawal psychosis. *J Clin Psychopharmacol* 6:193, 1986.
68. Schep LJ, Knudsen K, Slaughter RJ, et al: The clinical toxicology of gamma-hydroxybutyrate, gamma-butyrolactone and 1,4-butanediol. *Clin Toxicol* 50:458–470, 2012.
69. Miotto K, Darakjian J, Basch J, et al: Gamma-hydroxybutyric acid: patterns of use, effects and withdrawal. *Am J Addict* 10:232–241, 2001.
70. Wojtowicz JM, Yarema MC, Wax PM: Withdrawal from gamma-hydroxybutyrate, 1,4-butanediol and gamma-butyrolactone: a case report and systematic review. *CJEM* 10:69–74, 2008.
71. Sivilotti ML, Burns MJ, Aaron CK, et al: Pentobarbital for severe gamma-butyrolactone withdrawal. *Ann Emerg Med* 38:660–665, 2001.
72. LeTourneau JL, Hagg DS, Smith SM: Baclofen and gamma-hydroxybutyrate withdrawal. *Neurocrit Care* 8:430–433, 2008.
73. Kao LW, Amin Y, Kirk MA, et al: Intrathecal baclofen withdrawal mimicking sepsis. *J Emerg Med* 24:423–427, 2003.
74. Stetkarova I, Brabec K, Vasko P, et al: Intrathecal baclofen in spinal spasticity: frequency and severity of withdrawal syndrome. *Pain Physician*18:E633–E641, 2015.
75. Watve SV, Sivan M, Raza WA, et al: Management of acute overdose or withdrawal state in intrathecal baclofen therapy. *Spinal Cord* 50:107–111, 2012.
76. Turner MR, Gainsborough N: Neuroleptic malignant-like syndrome after abrupt withdrawal of baclofen. *J Psychopharmacol* 15:61–63, 2001.
77. Greenberg MI, Hendrickson RG: Baclofen withdrawal following removal of an intrathecal baclofen pump despite oral baclofen replacement. *J Toxicol Clin Toxicol* 41:83–85, 2003.
78. Zuckerbraun NS, Ferson SS, Albright AL, et al: Intrathecal baclofen withdrawal: emergent recognition and management. *Pediatr Emerg Care* 20:759–764, 2004.
79. Haber PS, Demirkol A, Lange K, et al: Management of injecting drug users admitted to hospital. *Lancet* 374:1284–1293, 2009.
80. Zapantis A, Leung S: Tolerance and withdrawal issues with sedation. *Crit Care Nurs Clin North Am* 17:211–223, 2005.
81. Kim HK, Nelson LS: Reducing the harm of opioid overdose with the safe use of naloxone: a pharmacologic review. *Expert Opin Drug Saf* 14:1137–1146, 2015.
82. Jones JD, Mogali S, Comer SD: Polydrug abuse: a review of opioid and benzodiazepine combination use. *Drug Alcohol Depend* 125:8–18, 2012.
83. Devlin JW, Roberts RJ: Pharmacology of commonly used analgesics and sedatives in the ICU: benzodiazepines, propofol, and opioids. *Crit Care Clin* 25:431–449, vii, 2009.
84. Amato L, Davoli M, Minozzi S, et al: Methadone at tapered doses for the management of opioid withdrawal. *Cochrane Database Syst Rev* 2:CD003409, 2013.
85. Faggiano F, Vigna-Taglianti F, Versino E, et al: Methadone maintenance at different dosages for opioid dependence. *Cochrane Database Syst Rev* 3:CD002208, 2003.
86. Alford DP, Compton P, Samet JH: Acute pain management for patients receiving maintenance methadone or buprenorphine therapy. *Ann Intern Med* 144:127–134, 2006.
87. Stimmel B, Adamsons K: Narcotic dependency in pregnancy. Methadone maintenance compared to use of street drugs. *JAMA* 235:1121–1124, 1976.
88. Dashe JS, Sheffield JS, Olscher DA, et al: Relationship between maternal methadone dosage and neonatal withdrawal. *Obstet Gynecol* 100:1244–1249, 2002.
89. Chugh SS, Socoteanu C, Reinier K, et al: A community-based evaluation of sudden death associated with therapeutic levels of methadone. *Am J Med* 121:66–71, 2008.
90. Anchersen K, Clausen T, Gossop M, et al: Prevalence and clinical relevance of corrected QT interval prolongation during methadone and buprenorphine treatment: a mortality assessment study. *Addiction* 104:993–999, 2009.
91. Lintzeris N, Bell J, Bammer G, et al: A randomized controlled trial of buprenorphine in the management of short-term ambulatory heroin withdrawal. *Addiction* 97:1395–1404, 2002.
92. Welsh CJ, Suman M, Cohen A, et al: The use of intravenous buprenorphine for the treatment of opioid withdrawal in medically ill hospitalized patients. *Am J Addict* 11:135–140, 2002.
93. Clark NC, Lintzeris N, Muhleisen PJ: Severe opiate withdrawal in a heroin user precipitated by a massive buprenorphine dose. *Med J Aust* 176:166–167, 2002.
94. Mattick RP, Breen C, Kimber J, et al: Buprenorphine maintenance versus placebo or methadone maintenance for opioid dependence. *Cochrane Database Syst Rev* 2:CD002207, 2014.
95. Robinson SE: Buprenorphine-containing treatments: place in the management of opioid addiction. *CNS Drugs* 20:697–712, 2006.
96. Gold MS, Redmond DE Jr, Kleber HD: Clonidine blocks acute opiate-withdrawal symptoms. *Lancet* 2:599–602, 1978.
97. Ling W, Amass L, Shoptaw S, et al: A multi-center randomized trial of buprenorphine-naloxone versus clonidine for opioid detoxification: findings from the National Institute on Drug Abuse Clinical Trials Network. *Addiction* 1008:1090–1100, 2005.
98. Hussain SS, Farhat S, Rather YH, et al: Comparative trial to study the effectiveness of clonidine hydrochloride and buprenorphine-naloxone in opioid withdrawal—a hospital based study. *J Clin Diagn Res* 91:FC01–FC04, 2015.
99. Gowing L, Ali R, White JM: Opioid antagonists under heavy sedation or anaesthesia for opioid withdrawal. *Cochrane Database Syst Rev* 1:CD002022, 2010.
100. Agaku IT, King BA, Dube SR; Centers for Disease Control and Prevention (CDC): Current cigarette smoking among adults—United States, 2005–2012. *MMWR Morb Mortal Wkly Rep* 63:29–34, 2014.
101. Awissi DK, Lebrun G, Fagnan M, et al; Regroupement de Soins Critiques, Respiratoires, Québec: Alcohol, nicotine, and iatrogenic withdrawals in the ICU. *Crit Care Med* 41[9 Suppl 1]:S57–S68, 2013.
102. Cartin-Ceba R, Warner DO, Hays JT, et al: Nicotine replacement therapy in critically ill patients: a prospective observational cohort study. *Crit Care Med*.39:1635–1640, 2011.

Section 11
CRITICAL CARE CONSEQUENCES OF WEAPONS (OR AGENTS) OF MASS DESTRUCTION

LAWRENCE C. MOHR JR

Chapter 127 ■ Planning and Organization for Emergency Mass Critical Care

RYAN C. MAVES • MARY A. KING • LAWRENCE C. MOHR JR • JAMES GEILING

HOSPITAL AND COMMUNITY DISASTER RESPONSE

The Importance of Hospitals for Disaster Response

Disasters are, by definition, unplanned occurrences. Large-scale catastrophes can strike communities and their hospitals without warning, with events ranging from sudden traumatic events, such as an earthquake or explosion, to sustained pandemics such as H1N1 influenza or the severe acute respiratory syndrome (SARS). Hospitals are a major source of a community's medical care, particularly during acute emergencies. In the setting of a large-scale disaster, ambulances will routinely transport critically ill or injured patients to the nearest hospital, often independently of a given hospital's stated capabilities. It is especially difficult to provide critical care outside of the hospital setting during such a disaster. Although it may be possible to provide medical care in a building of opportunity, such as a school gymnasium, for low-acuity patients, the provision of critical care in such a setting requires significant amounts of medical equipment, supplies, and trained staff.

In order to maintain its capability to care for the most critically ill patients during a disaster, the hospital must be part of a community-based health care response system that can be efficiently mobilized during a catastrophic event. Hospitals which are accredited by the Joint Commission or other accrediting agencies must meet specific requirements for disaster preparedness. These requirements include continuity-of-operations plans, an internal operations center with an incident command structure, and the planning and conduct of disaster response exercises in coordination with the neighboring community [1]. The Centers for Medicare and Medicaid Services (CMS) published updated emergency preparedness requirements for both health care providers and suppliers on September 16, 2016. The primary goal of the updated CMS regulations is to maintain access to health care services during emergencies. Requirements are broken down into four elements: (1) emergency planning, (2) policies and procedures, (3) communication, and (4) training and testing. In order to continue to receive CMS funding, hospitals have until November 15, 2017 to comply with these new emergency preparedness regulations [2]. (https://www.federalregister.gov/documents/2016/09/16/2016-21404/medicare-and-medicaid-programs-emergency-preparedness-requirements-for-medicare-and-medicaid).

The large numbers of the patients requiring care immediately after a disaster, the continued flow of patients during a prolonged disaster, and the loss of hospital infrastructure as a result of a disaster all have the potential to overwhelm hospital resources. A hospital's *surge capacity* refers to "the ability to provide adequate medical evaluation and care during events that exceed the limits of the normal medical infrastructure of an affected community [3]." To provide adequate surge capacity and maintain medical system resiliency during disasters, hospitals, and communities must have medical preparedness plans, as well as carefully planned command and control systems that efficiently manage the medical responses.

Local Community Medical Response

Incident Command Systems

In the United States, the National Incident Management Systems (NIMS) provides a framework for disaster response by hospitals and local governments [4]. This includes the requirement that both hospitals and communities have an Incident Command System (ICS) [5]. In general, ICS uses a modular system with a single incident commander (IC) who directly supervises a variable number of subsections. A typical ICS includes five principal components:

1. *Leadership*—This is the command section, chaired by the leader of the response effort (the IC). The IC is supported by special staff, such as public affairs, safety, legal counsel, and others as needed.
2. *Operations*—This section oversees and coordinates the immediate response and ongoing operational activities. This tends to be the most active section during a disaster.
3. *Planning*—This section assesses the potential for future events, develops contingency plans for future events, and plans timelines for the deployment of critical resources. These planning activities permit the operations branch to focus on managing the response to active events.
4. *Logistics*—This section focuses on the logistical support that every event requires, including equipment, personnel, supply, and infrastructure support.
5. *Finance*—This section accounts for and manages all money that is spent during the response to a disaster. Although immediate costs and purchases during a disaster may be supported by affected communities and hospitals, accurate purchasing records, inventory records, personnel costs, and transportation costs must be carefully managed in order to recoup costs after the event insofar as possible.

The Hospital Incident Command System (HICS) manages the response within the hospital and coordinates the hospital's efforts with the overall community response. Similar to the community IC, the HICS is also led by hospital IC from within the hospital's existing leadership structure. The hospital's IC and the community IC communicate with each other directly or via liaison personnel. The organization and leadership of the HICS are usually different than the organizational structure and leadership of day-to-day hospital operations [6]. Hospitals, including their intensive care units (ICUs), must assign personnel to specific HICS positions as part of their disaster preparedness planning. Each individual assigned to an HICS position has specific duties that must be performed prior to, during, and following the disaster response. It is imperative that all HICS personnel be fully trained for the duties they are required to perform.

During day-to-day hospital operations, different ICUs often function as individual, independent silos. During a disaster scenario with limited resources, these ICUs must coordinate patient movement and resource utilization, and do it quickly often without typical infrastructure in place. The American College of Chest Physicians (ACCP) Taskforce for Mass Critical Care recommended in their 2014 guideline document the specific inclusion of a new HICS position to lead this ICU coordination: the Critical Care Team Leader (CCTL). The primary role of the CCTL would be to facilitate horizontal coordination across all ICUs and between ICUs and other areas of the hospital. The CCTL should communicate directly with hospital IC and all ICUs, as well as with inflow/outflow points such as the ED, OR, and wards. The CCTL is critical to create a coordinated emergency mass critical care response.

Surge Capacity

Surge capacity refers to the ability of a hospital or other health care system to expand its normal operating capacity in the setting of an emergency. The key aspects of surge capacity can be summarized as "stuff, staff, and space." Inadequacy in any of these three categories will reduce a hospital's ability to surge optimally in a disaster. The American College of Chest Physicians (ACCP) Task Force for Mass Critical Care (henceforth referred to as "the ACCP Task Force") provides a classification system for differing levels of surge response in their 2014 guidelines on the management of the critically ill during disasters and pandemics [7]:

- *Conventional capacity*: In this category of surge response, the hospital should be able to increase its critical care capacity by approximately 20% above its normal limitations. This level would be implemented during major mass-casualty incidents that trigger activation of the hospital emergency operations plan. Most facilities should be able to achieve this level of response using existing staffing and resources, including strategies such as cancellation of elective procedures and transferring of appropriate patients out of ICUs [8].
- *Contingency capacity*: This level would be used temporarily during a major mass-casualty incident, or on a longer-term basis during a disaster whose medical demands exceeded routine hospital and community resources. This level of response implies the need to increase a hospital's critical care capacity by 100% and may require the use of alternate hospital resources for the provision of critical care, for example, the use of postanesthesia care unit spaces and staff [9]. In general, the level of medical care provided at this degree of surge response would be within the usual community standards.
- *Crisis capacity*: This level would be implemented during catastrophic situations that result in a significant impact on the standard of medical care that can be provided. Examples of such an event, which implies a 200% increase of the critical care demand on a hospital, include a prolonged pandemic, a natural disaster with extensive destruction of infrastructure, a large-scale terrorist attack, or a prolonged violent conflict. Severe limitations of space, staff, and supplies would not allow hospitals to provide the usual standard of medical care. At the crisis level, institutions will need to consider triage principles, rationing of care, and other potential ethical challenges while maximizing their ability to provide the best possible care to the greatest number of the patients.

Hospitals and their critical care units should develop disaster preparedness plans that contain specific criteria for each level of surge capacity. Identical disasters might have very different effects on different hospitals, depending on an institution's size and mission. For example, an eight-victim automobile crash may require a conventional level of surge capacity for a large hospital that includes a level 1 trauma center, but could require a contingency or crisis level of surge capacity for a small community hospital.

During contigency and crisis capacity scenarios, a hospital may need to optimize its resources in order to maximize its ability to care for those patients in greatest need. Several state and local governments in the United States, in collaboration with the Office of Public Health Preparedness and Response at the CDC, have developed plans based on the Modular Emergency Medical System (MEMS) framework. MEMS provides a method for a community to manage a surge of patients who require screening, triage, antibiotic treatment, immunizations, prophylaxis, or noncritical inpatient care. By providing temporary facilities for noncritical care, hospitals can redirect resources towards higher-acuity patients.

The major MEMS components are Neighborhood Emergency Help Centers (NEHC) and Acute Care Centers (ACC). Both types of centers can provide screening and triage. The NEHC provides routine, nonurgent outpatient care. The ACC can provide inpatient care to acutely ill noncritical patients. The ACC can receive patients directly from an incident or permit hospitals can offload stable inpatients in order to free up hospital critical care bed space during overwhelming events. Local or regional authorities can open an NEHC or an ACC under two scenarios: (a) when a federal public health incident or a federal disaster is declared or (b) when the state governor has issued a state of emergency. Both types of temporary facilities will operate under the command and control of the local community ICS with support from a Regional Multiagency Command [10]. A carefully executed MEMS plan allows hospitals to offload stable patients to an ACC, preventing the hospital from being overwhelmed during a disaster and allowing the hospital to expand its critical care capabilities by utilizing non-ICU hospital beds for critical care, when necessary.

CRITICAL CARE DURING DISASTERS

During a major disaster, nothing will challenge hospitals more than attempting to provide high-quality critical care with limited resources. The Hospital Preparedness Program (HPP) of the U.S. Department of Health and Human Services spends approximately $255 million per year, or over $4 billion since 2002, in grant support to local institutions to enhance their ability to respond to disasters, including improvements of surge capacity [11]. A 2008 report by the U.S. Government Accountability Office indicated that many states were not adequately prepared to respond to a major catastrophe, such as an influenza pandemic [12]. A follow-up report in 2013 indicated that US hospitals receiving HPP funds have made some improvements of their disaster planning, but shortcomings still persist in the number of emergency medical volunteers, decontamination systems available, and hospital bed count notification to coordinating authorities [13].

Disasters requiring critical care resources include massive trauma events, such as natural disasters, transportation-related accidents, or violent trauma such as deliberate explosions or mass shootings. Since the 2003 SARS outbreak in Toronto and the 2009 to 2010 H1N1 influenza pandemic, greater attention has been paid to disease outbreaks as a form of disaster for hospitals, especially for their long-term impact on critical care. Lastly, disasters may affect hospitals through destruction of the hospital infrastructure itself, such as during a hurricane or earthquake, or by illness or injury that afflict the hospital staff; in both scenarios, the mission of the hospital can be impaired at a time when it is needed most.

These three categories of disaster (trauma, epidemic, and degradation of hospital functions) can and do co-exist. The 2010 earthquake in Haiti led to the immediate death of 230,000 people, but the mass trauma was followed by a cholera epidemic that affected 352,033 during 2011 alone. The devastation to Haiti's medical system, already fragile before the quake, further impaired that country's ability to cope with the other two disasters [14]. Conversely, it is estimated that the case-fatality rate of the 2003 SARS epidemic was reduced from a predicted 20% to the actual rate of 6.5%, despite some shortcomings noted by advance planning efforts [15,16].

As of 2010, there were an estimated 103,900 critical care beds in the United States, a 17.8% increase from 2000 despite a 2.2% decrease in the total number of staffed hospital beds [17]. The bulk of this growth has occurred in academic medical centers and other large hospitals, suggesting that potential surge capacity may be limited at smaller, nonteaching hospitals [18]. Mean ICU bed occupancy in the US was 68.2%, and on average 39.5% of the patients in US ICUs required mechanical ventilation at any given time [19]. The ratio of ICU beds to population (approximately 20 beds/100,000 residents) is relatively high in the US; the Canadian Critical Care Trials Group in 2014 identified 3,170 ICU beds and 4,982 mechanical ventilators available for patients in Canada, with a ratio of 9.5 beds/100,000 residents [20]. Among other developed countries, Australia, New Zealand, and the United Kingdom maintain bed ratios comparable to that of Canada, while Taiwan, Belgium and Germany exceed the US in their numbers of beds per population [21–23].

Of special note, a disproportionate paucity of pediatric critical care resources would exist should we become resource limited during a disaster. In 2010, there were only 4,044 PICU beds in the United States (3.9% of all 103,900 critical care beds listed above), yet 24% of the population was pediatric (0 to 17 years old). This relative scarcity of pediatric critical care resources may present unequal access to care for children as compared to adults during disasters, a time when children often are disproportionately affected. Creative problem-solving, such as sending adolescents and large grade-school children to adult ICUs with just-in-time training and simple color-coding tools for adult providers or repurposing some of the 20,000 NICU beds that exist in the United States for disaster-affected infants 0 to 12 months old, could be two potential ways to improve access to pediatric critical care during disasters, but such changes would require system-wide coordination [21–23].

Overall, these data suggest that hospitals of developed countries have a consistent, although uneven, ability to expand their critical care capacity during a disaster. However, even with normal excess capacity, there may not be a sufficient number of critical care beds to meet the demands of a pandemic that might affect the entire nation at the same time. Critically ill patients who are not admitted to an ICU have a three- to fivefold greater mortality rate compared with those who are cared for in an ICU [24]. Thus, if critical care capabilities become overwhelmed by large numbers of critically ill or injured patients during a disaster, high mortality rates will likely occur.

Surging Assets to Optimize Critical Care Capability

When planning for surge capacity during disasters, hospitals need to prepare for events that have a sudden impact and are of relatively short duration, such as transportation accidents and explosions, as well as more prolonged events, such as natural disasters and pandemics [3,5]. The ACCP Task Force identifies three key elements of planning critical care surge capacity [7,25]:

- *Stuff*: the medical supplies and equipment necessary for providing critical care.
- *Staff*: the availability of trained critical care providers and support personnel.
- *Space*: the physical space within (or rarely outside of) the hospital that can be used to provide critical care to a large number of critically ill or injured patients.

Stuff

Patients are generally admitted to ICUs because of monitoring needs, the need for intensive-care nursing, or the need for treatments with special equipment or medications. The provision of mechanical ventilation is the most common requirement needed to manage critically ill patients with respiratory compromise. The main challenge of providing this important therapeutic modality during a disaster is the availability of mechanical ventilators.

During a major influenza pandemic, demand for mechanical ventilators in the United States could increase by 60,000, assuming a 30% attack rate and a high case-fatality rate of 0.25% to 0.5% [26]. The United States has approximately 62,000 full-feature ventilators, or 20 of these per 100,000 residents, plus an additional 100,000 ventilators with fewer features but which could be used during a disaster [27]. Of these 100,000 "extra" ventilators, however, it is estimated that the US could utilize no more than 56,000 additional ventilators due to limitations of the numbers of trained respiratory therapists [28]. Thus, in preparing to provide mechanical ventilation to a large number of critically ill disaster casualties, planners need to consider other options, such as high-flow nasal cannula oxygenation or noninvasive positive-pressure ventilation for selected patients. Anesthesia machines and transport ventilators could serve as additional options, although these could be similarly limited by the number of trained personnel and have disadvantages with regard to infection control [29–32].

The provision of critical care during a disaster will also require that a large quantity of supplies and pharmaceuticals be on hand and readily available to critical care providers. The Joint Commission currently requires that accredited hospitals plan for 96 hours of autonomous function, without external resupply, in the event of disaster (although 96 hours of supplies and the ability to function at full capacity are not required). In 2005, during the Hurricane Katrina disaster in New Orleans, the lack of available supplies, pharmaceuticals, and operational equipment forced the dedicated staff at Charity Hospital to improvise critical care practices and deviate from the usual standards of care prior to final evacuation of the hospital [33]. Hospitals in areas affected by the Great East Japan Earthquake and subsequent tsunami of 2011 and by Hurricane Sandy in 2012 showed comparable experiences. In Miyagi Prefecture in Japan, for example, six out of 14 of hospitals had less than 1 day of food on hand at the time of the quake, and another six hospitals had less than 1 day of medical supplies. Just-in-time supply practices at New York City hospitals produced some similar shortages, offset in part by supplies available from elsewhere in the city [34,35].

Figure 127.1 provides recommendations from the ACCP Task Force on means to conserve supplies at differing levels of surge response.

Staff

A significant challenge of maintaining critical care capability during a disaster will be the availability of a sufficient number of trained personnel. Shortages of intensivists, critical care nurses, respiratory therapists, critical care pharmacists, and other specially trained personnel may be a limiting factor in caring for large numbers of critically ill patients. In infectious outbreaks or natural disasters, hospital staff may themselves be victims, further decreasing the institution's ability to respond [36,37]. The ACCP Task Force's 2014 consensus statement endorsed prior recommendations on the surging of staff [25,38]. These recommendations state that experienced providers should perform direct patient care, when feasible. Those providers not normally operating in critical care settings should be cross-trained, or retrained, on essential bedside skills in the ICU as part of a hospital's disaster preparedness program. Finally, systematic procedures (such as protocols) should be instituted and understood

	Definition	Conventional	Contingency	Crisis
Prepare	Cache materials, maintain adequate par levels	✓	✓	✓
Conserve	Restricting use to maintain supply may play a significant role at all stages of response, for example, conserving oxygen to maintain saturations > 90% in contingency or only using antivirals for selected high-risk patients in contingency or crisis (depending on the risk of a poor outcome without the therapy) or medication dose titration where applicable	✓	✓	✓
Substitute	Using one resource instead of another for the same function; class/class substitutions of benzodiazepines would be a conventional example, and antibiotic substitutions of varying efficacy could span the spectrum to crisis	✓	✓	✓
Adapt	Repurposing supplies or equipment; for example, using the heart rate alarms on oxygen saturation monitors to detect tachydysrhythmias and bradydysrhythmias or using anesthesia machines for mechanical ventilation		✓	✓
Reuse	Reuse in contingency would present minimal risk (supplies requiring disinfection, eg, cervical collars, nasogastric tubes); reuse of sterile supplies would enter into crisis care		✓	✓
Reallocate	Taking treatments from one patient to give to another; this is restricted to crisis care and usually applied to mechanical ventilation and other life-preserving, binary treatments (that cannot be titrated)			✓

FIGURE 127.1 Methods for optimizing available supplies in differing degrees of surge response during disasters. (From Hick JL, Einav S, Hanfling D, et al: Surge capacity principles: care of the critically ill and injured during pandemics and disasters: CHEST consensus statement. *Chest* 146:e1S–e16S, 2014.)

by all critical care providers, in order to standardize processes, maximize good outcomes, and maximize safety to patients and staff during a disaster.

During contigency and crisis surge conditions, intensivists will need to focus part of their effort on supervising cross-trained physicians from other specialties. Nonintensivist physicians who are skilled in proving hands-on care, such as hospitalists, emergency physicians, general surgeons, or anesthesiologists, could be assigned six patients each (assuming that other urgent clinical duties do not take precedence). Intensivists could supervise four to eight such providers, thereby extending their critical care coverage to almost 50 patients.

Comparable models have been proposed for critical care nurses supervising non-CCRNs, critical care pharmacists supervising other pharmacists, and so forth. During a crisis surge scenario, standard patient ratios may not be achievable. ICU charge nurses could match several non-ICU nurses to appropriate patients, leaving only the most complex patients under the sole care of other ICU nurses. Specific bedside care procedures could be assigned to non-ICU nurses (bathing, vital signs, catheter management, medication delivery, among others), thereby permitting ICU nurses to oversee the provision of specific critical nursing care to several patients. Respiratory therapists usually provide care to four to six ICU patients, but surge requirements may mandate a higher ratio of patients per therapist, ICU therapists supervising outpatient or non-ICU therapists, or even ICU therapists directing nontherapists in basic care. Finally, oncology, outpatient, or other non-ICU pharmacists may similarly be asked to support operations under the tutelage of critical care pharmacists. Training for such processes will become necessary for prolonged events that will severely strain staff resources during a major disaster [25,38].

Space

It is important to remember that critical care is a concept, not a location. During a major disaster, space limitations may require that critical care be provided in other areas of a hospital [24,39]. When it becomes necessary to provide critical care outside of an ICU during a major disaster, it should be provided in those areas of a hospital that are most analogous to an ICU in medical function.

In the initial phases of a surge requirement, hospitals should be able to accommodate up to a 20% increase of critically ill patients with minimal impact, assuming that supplies and staff are available and the hospital is not at maximum capacity. Stable ICU patients requiring minimal care or monitoring can be transferred to step-down units, telemetry areas, postanesthesia care units, or other settings as appropriate. Total hospital bed space should be decompressed by transferring stable ward patients to home care, to skilled nursing facilities, or to alternate community facilities such as an ACC. As an emergency mass critical care event progresses, formal critical care space will need to expand into other areas of the hospital, with the hospital continuing to make room for critically ill patients by transferring the most stable inpatients elsewhere.

An alternative to expanding internal ICU capability is for communities to develop and deploy "field" ICUs. Critical care has been provided in such settings before, with recent experience in New York City following the damage to Bellevue Hospital by Hurricane Sandy as well as during humanitarian international missions or military operations [25,40,41]. However, because of the logistical requirements for specialized equipment, infection control support, and the relocation of trained personnel, critical care should only be provided in "field" settings as a last resort. For most major disaster situations, such facilities can be best used for the management of noncritically ill patients who are transferred from hospitals in order to free up space for the management of the critically ill. The 2014 ACCP Task Force recommends using alternate sites for patients requiring less-intensive management, thus permitting the expansion of critical care services within the hospital; deployable, "field"-style ICUs are to be used for critical care as a temporizing measure pending transfer to safer locations [25].

RESOURCE ALLOCATION AND TRIAGE DURING TIMES OF OVERWHELMING DEMAND

The Greatest Good for the Greatest Number

The goal of surging critical care resources during a disaster is to provide the greatest good for the greatest number of event victims. Critical care providers and institutions should strive to manage resources within their own facility and region with the goal of providing usual critical care practices to the extent possible. However, in a major disaster, because resources become increasingly limited, health care providers and leaders must have a plan in place to change the focus of critical care from the needs of the individual to the needs of the population as a whole. This requires a defined triage plan to be developed, communicated, and implemented fairly.

Ethical and Legal Principles

Utilitarian principles guide the theory of the "greatest good for the greatest number." In times of overwhelming resource constraints, limited capabilities should be targeted to those with the greatest likelihood of benefiting from the care. Those who are unlikely to recover or improve with the available care are not abandoned, but are provided with appropriate palliative care. This fundamental principle guides the implementation of a mass-casualty triage system during major disasters [42,43].

The ACCP Task Force supports the concept that when surge measures do not meet demand, then individual autonomy may be limited. It mandates a fair and just rationing of resources, based on objective information and decision-making, in order to benefit the population as a whole, rather than individual patients. Such a shift in health care priorities requires active community involvement and an open, transparent decision-making processes. Ideally, plans for the fair and just rationing of critical care resources during periods of overwhelming demand should be developed prior to the disaster.

Importantly, in order to implement such processes, providers must feel secure in their legal protection. Hence, providers should be legally protected from local and state law if there is a need to deviate from the usual standards of care during periods of scarce resources. The ACCP Task Force recommends that uniformly accepted, predetermined algorithms be developed for triaging critically ill patients during a disaster, with adherence to these algorithms being sufficient to provide necessary legal protection to providers and other decision-makers [42]. The need for such legal protection was poignantly highlighted in New Orleans during the Hurricane Katrina disaster, as palliative care was provided to some patients as evacuation attempts were repeatedly delayed and hospital capabilities were overwhelmed [44]. In response to these events, New York State has developed ventilator allocation guidelines for pandemics and other mass-casualty events, with other states now following its lead [45]. Notably, critical care providers should not implement triage and resource allocation processes without the direction and support of their hospital administration through HICS.

Critical Care Triage

There remains debate about the preferred method of triage during a major disaster where patient needs have exceeded critical care resources. It would be difficult to develop a single uniform triage method for all potential scenarios. In the specific setting of ventilator allocation for pandemic influenza, controversy persists regarding the most equitable form of patient selection, including first-come-first-serve, the use of PaO_2/FiO_2 ratios, or the Simple Triage Scoring System (STSS) [46–48]. Although each of these concepts has its merits; none have been prospectively evaluated in a disaster setting.

The ACCP Task Force recommends that planning for the triage of critically ill patients during a major disaster should include well-defined "triggers" that promptly alert hospital and community leadership to the fact that critical care resources are being overwhelmed and there is a need to direct the use of a triage process. Such triggers would include a lack of critical equipment or medical supplies, inadequate critical care spaces, inadequate staff, and inadequate capability to transfer noncritically ill patients to other facilities.

Once the requirement to triage care has been directed, critical care providers must determine which patients should receive critical care and which patients should not. This process needs to be carefully planned and evaluated with community involvement prior to a catastrophic event. If, for example, a health care system or region proposes to exclude critical care to the very elderly during a major disaster, then community representatives from the elderly population would need to be included in such decisions. That is, the elderly would participate in advance planning with providers on how to triage the elderly during future mass-casualty emergencies.

Several severity-of-illness models have been developed for the ICU setting that may be applied to the triage process. However, all have similar limitations in that they have not been rigorously evaluated in emergency mass critical care scenarios. The Task Force and other groups have advocated the use of the Sequential Organ Failure Assessment (SOFA) score because of its demonstrated effectiveness for the ongoing assessment of critically ill patients and the ease with which it can be calculated with minimal laboratory requirements [42].

The ACCP Task Force recommends that hospitals establish a triage system in advance of a disaster, with either a designated triage officer or triage team who will make decisions based on predetermined guidelines. A triage team, consisting of an experienced intensivist and another acute care physician, may be preferable to a single triage officer, given the emotional burden and the utility of a second "set of eyes" during a crisis. This group, operating independently from the bedside clinicians, would gather periodic patient data to determine the severity of illness and document improvement, stability, or deterioration of critically ill patients over time. The patients who deteriorate or fail to improve over time would have their critical care resources reallocated to other patients (Fig. 127.2). The ACCP Task Force proposes that the patients with a predicted mortality of >90% not be offered critical care; a prior recommendation to withhold critical care from patients with SOFA scores >11 has since been revised due to conflicting data about the significance of such a score during pandemic influenza [42,49]. The availability of an experienced critical care triage team has the advantage of removing the burden of triage decisions from busy clinicians who are providing critical care at the bedside. This team also removes some of the inherent bias that providers may have when making decisions for patients personally known to them. In the HICS, the critical care triage team should operate under the command of the Hospital Operations Section Chief.

In order to assure compliance and integrity of the triage process, a review committee should be established to oversee triage plans and operations. This committee, distinct from the triage team, would:

- Work with regional planners and maintain situational awareness of the community and state, regarding the ongoing use and need of triage protocols.
- Review the implementation of the local triage protocol, to ensure compliance and integrity of triage operations.
- Serve as a forum for appeals by patients, families, and staff regarding the accurate and ethical implementation of the triage tool.

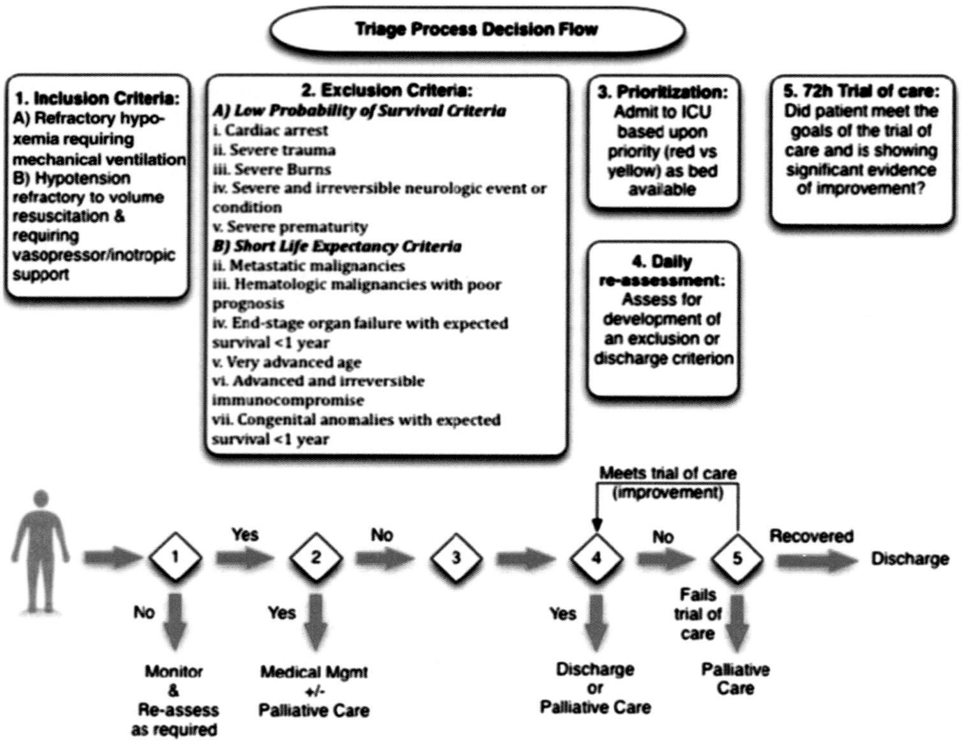

FIGURE 127.2 Critical care triage algorithm. (From Christian MD, Sprung CL, King MA, et al: Triage: care of the critically ill and injured during pandemics and disasters: CHEST consensus statement. *Chest* 146:e61S–e74S, 2014.)

- Participate in the real-time epidemiological evaluation of the catastrophic event, to help public health and other officials determine the ongoing validity of SOFA scoring as a triage tool for critically ill patients.

SUMMARY

Preparing ICUs for disasters requires a methodical approach within a defined organizational structure in order to optimize care for large numbers of critically ill patients. Ideally, hospitals are the optimal setting to provide critical care for severely ill and injured patients. During major disasters, hospitals should coordinate with community medical response systems to offload patients with minor injuries or illnesses so that hospital resources can be focused on the care of critically ill patients.

Predisaster planning and training are essential for mitigating the adverse effects of an overwhelming disaster on hospitals and their communities. Carefully developed plans for surging critical care resources will facilitate continuation of usual hospital processes for the largest number of the patients. However, when surge procedures fail to meet the critical care demands of an overwhelming patient influx, processes to triage and alter the usual standards of critical care must be implemented. These planning concepts and guidelines can help guide critical care practitioners to care for their patients under the challenging conditions of a catastrophic disaster.

DISCLAIMER

One of the authors (RM) is a United States military service member and another (JG) employee of the Department of Veterans Affairs. This work was prepared as part of their official duties. Title 17 U.S.C. §105 provides that "Copyright protection under this title is not available for any work of the United States Government." Title 17 U.S.C. §101 defines a U.S. Government work as a work prepared by a military service member or employee of the U.S. Government as part of that person's official duties. The opinions and assertions contained herein are those of the authors and do not necessarily reflect the views or position of the Department of the Navy, Department of Defense, Department of Veterans Affairs, the United States Government, nor of the academic institutions with which the authors are affiliated.

References

1. Byrne Ke: 2016 Hospital Accreditation Standards: The Joint Commission, 2015.
2. Medicare and Medicaid Programs: Emergency Preparedness Requirements for Medicare and Medicaid Participating Providers and Suppliers. 2016. Available at http://www.federalregister.gov/documents/2016/09/16/2016-21404/medicare-and-medicaid-programs-emergency-preparedness-requirements-for-medicare-and-medicaid. Accessed October 19, 2016.
3. United States Department of Health and Human Services Medical Surge Capacity Handbook. Available at http://www.phe.gov/Preparedness/planning/mscc/handbook/Pages/default.aspx. Accessed September 15, 2016.
4. National Incident Management System (NIMS). Available at http://www.fema.gov/national-incident-management-system. Accessed September 15, 2016.
5. NIMS Implementation Activities for Hospitals and Healthcare Systems. Available at http://www.fema.gov/pdf/emergency/nims/imp_hos.pdf. Accessed September 15, 2016.
6. California Emergency Medical Services Authority: Hospital Incident Command System Guidebook (5th ed). Available at http://www.emsa.ca.gov/media/default/HICS/HICS_Guidebook_2014_11.pdf. Accessed September 15, 2016.
7. Hick JL, Einav S, Hanfling D, et al: Surge capacity principles: care of the critically ill and injured during pandemics and disasters: CHEST consensus statement. *Chest* 146:e1S–e16S, 2014.
8. Soremekun OA, Zane RD, Walls A, et al: Cancellation of scheduled procedures as a mechanism to generate hospital bed surge capacity-a pilot study. *Prehosp Disaster Med* 26:224–229, 2011.
9. Bala M, Willner D, Keidar A, et al: Indicators of the need for ICU admission following suicide bombing attacks. *Scand J Trauma Resusc Emerg Med* 20:19, 2012.
10. Office of Public Health Preparedness and Response, Centers for Disease Control and Prevention. Available at http://www.cdc.gov/phpr/healthcare/essentialhc.htm. Accessed September 15, 2016.
11. Department of Health and Human Services. Fiscal Year 2016 Public Health and Social Services Emergency Fund—Justification of Estimates for Appropriations Committees. Available at http://www.hhs.gov/sites/default/files/budget/

fy2016/fy2016-public-health-social-services-emergency-budget-justification.pdf. Accessed September 16, 2016.
12. GAO Report on Emergency Preparedness, June 2008. Available at http://www.gao.gov/new.items/d08668.pdf. Accessed September 16, 2016.
13. GAO Report on National Preparedness, March 2013. Available at http://www.gao.gov/assets/660/653259.pdf. Accessed September 16, 2016.
14. Domercant JW, Guillaume FD, Marston BJ, et al; Centers for Disease Control and Prevention: Update on progress in selected public health programs after the 2010 earthquake and cholera epidemic—Haiti, 2014. *MMWR Morb Mortal Wkly Rep* 64:137–140, 2015.
15. Booth CM, Matukas LM, Tomlinson GA, et al: Clinical features and short-term outcomes of 144 patients with SARS in the greater Toronto area. *JAMA* 289:2801–2809, 2003.
16. Booth CM, Stewart TE: Severe acute respiratory syndrome and critical care medicine: the Toronto experience. *Crit Care Med* 33:S53–S60, 2005.
17. Halpern NA, Goldman DA, Tan KS, et al: Trends in critical care beds and use among population groups and medicare and medicaid beneficiaries in the United States: 2000–2010. *Crit Care Med* 44:1490–1499, 2016.
18. Wallace DJ, Seymour CW, Kahn JM: Hospital-level changes in adult ICU bed supply in the United States. *Crit Care Med* 45:e67–e76, 2017.
19. Wunsch H, Wagner J, Herlim M, et al: ICU occupancy and mechanical ventilator use in the United States. *Crit Care Med* 41:2712–2719, 2013.
20. Fowler RA, Abdelmalik P, Wood G, et al: Critical care capacity in Canada: results of a national cross-sectional study. *Crit Care* 19:133, 2015.
21. Martin JM, Hart GK, Hicks P: A unique snapshot of intensive care resources in Australia and New Zealand. *Anaesth Intensive Care* 38:149–158, 2010.
22. Wunsch H, Angus DC, Harrison DA, et al: Variation in critical care services across North America and Western Europe. *Crit Care Med* 36:2787–2793, e1–e9, 2008.
23. Cheng KC, Lu CL, Chung YC, et al: ICU service in Taiwan. *J Intensive Care* 2:8, 2014.
24. Simchen E, Sprung CL, Galai N, et al: Survival of critically ill patients hospitalized in and out of intensive care. *Crit Care Med* 35:449–457, 2007.
25. Einav S, Hick JL, Hanfling D, et al: Surge capacity logistics: care of the critically ill and injured during pandemics and disasters: CHEST consensus statement. *Chest* 146:e17S–e43S, 2014.
26. Meltzer MI, Patel A, Ajao A, et al: Estimates of the demand for mechanical ventilation in the United States during an influenza pandemic. *Clin Infect Dis* 60 Suppl 1:S52–S57, 2015.
27. Rubinson L, Vaughn F, Nelson S, et al: Mechanical ventilators in US acute care hospitals. *Disaster Med Public Health Prep* 4:199–206, 2010.
28. Ajao A, Nystrom SV, Koonin LM, et al: Assessing the capacity of the US Health Care System to use additional mechanical ventilators during a large-scale public health emergency. *Disaster Med Public Health Prep* 9:634–641, 2015.
29. *Infection Prevention and Control of Epidemic- and Pandemic-Prone Acute Respiratory Infections in Health Care*. Geneva, World Health Organization, 2014.
30. Papazian L, Corley A, Hess D, et al: Use of high-flow nasal cannula oxygenation in ICU adults: a narrative review. *Intensive Care Med* 42:1336–1349, 2016.
31. Rubinson L, Branson RD, Pesik N, et al: Positive-pressure ventilation equipment for mass casualty respiratory failure. *Biosecur Bioterror* 4:183–194, 2006.
32. Daugherty EL, Carlson AL, Perl TM: Planning for the inevitable: preparing for epidemic and pandemic respiratory illness in the shadow of H1N1 influenza. *Clin Infect Dis* 50:1145–1154, 2010.
33. deBoisblanc BP: Black Hawk, please come down: reflections on a hospital's struggle to survive in the wake of Hurricane Katrina. *Am J Respir Crit Care Med* 172:1239–1240, 2005.
34. Abramson DM, Redlener I: Hurricane sandy: lessons learned, again. *Disaster Med Public Health Prep* 6:328–329, 2012.
35. Kudo D, Furukawa H, Nakagawa A, et al: Resources for business continuity in disaster-based hospitals in the great East Japan earthquake: survey of Miyagi Prefecture disaster base hospitals and the prefectural disaster medicine headquarters. *Disaster Med Public Health Prep* 7:461–466, 2013.
36. Morris AM, Ricci KA, Griffin AR, et al: Personal and professional challenges confronted by hospital staff following hurricane sandy: a qualitative assessment of management perspectives. *BMC Emerg Med* 16:18, 2016.
37. Suwantarat N, Apisarnthanarak A: Risks to healthcare workers with emerging diseases: lessons from MERS-CoV, Ebola, SARS, and avian flu. *Curr Opin Infect Dis* 28:349–361, 2015.
38. Rubinson L, Nuzzo JB, Talmor DS, et al: Augmentation of hospital critical care capacity after bioterrorist attacks or epidemics: recommendations of the Working Group on Emergency Mass Critical Care. *Crit Care Med* 33:2393–2403, 2005.
39. Smith SW, Jamin CT, Malik S, et al: Freestanding emergency critical care during the aftermath of hurricane sandy: implications for disaster preparedness and response. *Disaster Med Public Health Prep* 10:496–502, 2016.
40. Dulski TM, Basavaraju SV, Hotz GA, et al: Factors associated with inpatient mortality in a field hospital following the Haiti earthquake, January–May 2010. *Am J Disaster Med* 6:275–284, 2011.
41. Jawa RS, Heir JS, Cancelada D, et al: A quick primer for setting up and maintaining surgical intensive care in an austere environment: practical tips from volunteers in a mass disaster. *Am J Disaster Med* 7:223–229, 2012.
42. Christian MD, Sprung CL, King MA, et al: Triage: care of the critically ill and injured during pandemics and disasters: CHEST consensus statement. *Chest* 146:e61S–e74S, 2014.
43. Biddison LD, Berkowitz KA, Courtney B, et al: Ethical considerations: care of the critically ill and injured during pandemics and disasters: CHEST consensus statement. *Chest* 146:e145S–e155S, 2014.
44. Strained by Katrina, a Hospital Faced Deadly Choices. New York Times Magazine August 30, 2009.
45. New York State Task Force on Life and the Law, New York State Department of Health. Ventilator Allocation Guidelines. November 2015.
46. Morton B, Tang L, Gale R, et al: Performance of influenza-specific triage tools in an H1N1-positive cohort: P/F ratio better predicts the need for mechanical ventilation and critical care admission. *Br J Anaesth* 114:927–933, 2015.
47. Adeniji KA, Cusack R: The Simple Triage Scoring System (STSS) successfully predicts mortality and critical care resource utilization in H1N1 pandemic flu: a retrospective analysis. *Crit Care* 15:R39, 2011.
48. Winsor S, Bensimon CM, Sibbald R, et al: Identifying prioritization criteria to supplement critical care triage protocols for the allocation of ventilators during a pandemic influenza. *Healthc Q* 17:44–51, 2014.
49. Shahpori R, Stelfox HT, Doig CJ, et al: Sequential Organ Failure Assessment in H1N1 pandemic planning. *Crit Care Med* 39:827–832, 2011.

Chapter 128 ■ Chemical Agents of Mass Destruction

JAMES GEILING • RANDY WAX • LAWRENCE C. MOHR JR

If supposedly civilized nations confined their warfare to attacks on the enemy's troops, the matter of defense against warfare chemicals would be purely a military problem, and therefore is beyond the scope of this study. But such is far from the case. In these days of total warfare, the civilians, including women and children, are subject to attack at all times [1,2].

Chemical agents of terror have moved to the forefront of concern for health care providers as weapons of mass destruction (WMD) have become readily available to both domestic and international terrorists. Critical care physicians must be familiar with these agents, their impact on patients, and the potential dangers these compounds can cause to health care workers.

Although terrorists have traditionally focused their efforts on the use of conventional explosives, chemical agents have emerged as attractive weapons of terrorism for a variety of reasons:

- Raw materials for their production are readily available throughout the world.
- Raw materials are inexpensive.
- A chemical weapon of mass destruction can be produced with relatively small amounts of raw materials.
- They may be odorless, colorless, and tasteless.
- They are difficult to detect.
- They do not destroy infrastructure.

- They possess a latency period between the time of exposure and the development of clinical symptoms.
- Their use produces a mass media response [3].

The events of September 11, 2001, and subsequent terrorist threats have changed the nature of physician training and preparation requirements. Whereas most physicians have prepared for mass casualty events from multisystem trauma, as in transportation accidents, they now must know how to provide mass care to victims following a WMD event. This chapter focuses on the recognition and management of patients exposed to common chemical agents of mass destruction.

HISTORY

Chemical agents of mass destruction are gaseous, liquid, or solid substances that are employed against a population because of their direct toxic effects. Virtually any toxic substance can be used as an agent of mass destruction. However, those that have been successfully weaponized are characterized by ease of production, ease of handling during weapon assembly, dispersion properties, and ability to cause injury and death at relatively low concentrations [4].

Although the first reported use of chemical agents dates back to 1000 BC when Chinese forces used arsenical smokes, the use of chemical agents for warfare began in earnest during World War I when German forces seeking a breakout from the stalemate of trench warfare released 150 tons of chlorine gas on April 15, 1915, near Ypres, Belgium, resulting in 800 deaths and the retreat of 15,000 Allied troops, largely because of the psychologic terror produced by the attack.

The next major use of chemical weapons took place more than 2 years later, on July 12, 1917, again near Ypres, when German forces attacked Allied troops with artillery shells containing sulfur mustard. Although many of the 20,000 casualties had debilitating injuries, less than 5% of the troops died as a result of the chemical attack. Persistent and nonvolatile, sulfur mustard caused a host of new problems for Allied forces, including a latency period before the effects appeared and the need for men, and their horses, to wear protective overgarments [5].

The Geneva Convention of 1925 banned the use of chemical warfare agents because of the physical and psychologic trauma they imposed on their victims.

Nerve agents appeared in the 1930s when the German industrial chemist, Dr. Gerhard Schrader, began research into the development of stronger insecticides, the first two of which were tabun and sarin. German forces stockpiled these for use in World War II, but never used them.

Chemical agents were used sporadically in the second half of the twentieth century. The United States used defoliants and riot-controlled agents in Vietnam. Iraq used mustard, tabun, and eventually sarin against Iran in the Iran–Iraq war of the 1980s. Later in the 1980s, reports implicated Iraq in the use of cyanide against the Kurdish population of northern Iraq [6].

The Aum Shinrikyo religious cult released sarin gas on two occasions in Japan in the 1990s. The first took place on June 27, 1994, in Matsumoto and resulted in 600 persons exposed, 58 admitted to the hospital, and seven deaths [7]. The more famous and larger event took place the following year, on March 20, 1995, when they released sarin gas in the Tokyo subway system during rush hour. The subway system attack resulted in the deaths of 11 commuters and the medical evaluation of approximately 5,000 individuals [8].

In 2002, Chechan separatists overtook a Moscow theater, taking over 800 hostages. Four days later Russian Special Forces fumigated the building with a derivative of the narcotic fentanyl. Although this method broke the siege, all but two of the 41 terrorists and 129 hostages died from opiate toxicity [9].

The most recent use of chemical weapons occurred in the early morning hours of August 21, 2013 in the Ein Tarma and Zamalka suburbs of Damascus, Syria. Social media reports and videos as well as satellite imagery demonstrated large numbers of sick adults and children with no visible trauma; medical personnel described the symptoms as most consistent with exposure to a nerve agent [10]. Three Damascus hospitals received over 3,000 casualties where the principle antidote atropine was in short supply and exposure to contaminated patients at one hospital resulted in 41 staff members, including 10 doctors, becoming contaminated [11]. The attack killed approximately 1,429 people, including 426 children [12].

In 1993, the Chemical Weapons Convention (CWC) went into effect as an international treaty that bans the use, development, production, acquisition, transfer, stockpiling, and retention of chemical weapons by signatory nations. At the time of this writing, the CWC was ratified by 192 nations, including the USA; North Korea and Egypt have not done it. The CWC is administered by the Organisation for the Prohibition of Chemical Weapons, which conducts regular inspections and monitors compliance with provisions of the treaty [13].

DETECTION AND DECONTAMINATION

Initial steps for the management of chemical agent casualties include detection of the chemical agent used during the attack and the decontamination of casualties. Detailed discussions on detection and decontamination are beyond the scope of this chapter. However, hospital-based critical care physicians should understand basic concepts of these topics to better care for their patients and protect themselves and their facilities from potential harm.

The most important tool for detecting the use of these agents is accurate and timely intelligence from military or law enforcement agencies. Unfortunately, hospitals are not usually in the information-sharing and decision-making circles with these groups. As a result, initial awareness of a chemical agent attack typically occurs with the first patient presenting to the emergency department. Hospitals and physicians can improve their preparedness for the management of chemical agent casualties by actively participating in disaster-planning activities at their respective communities.

Various types of sensing devices can be used for the detection of chemical agents in the environment. At the present time, all commercially available detection equipment uses point source technology; that is, proximity to the substance is required. The handheld Chemical Agent Monitor uses ion mobility spectrometry to detect mustard and nerve agents. Chemical agent detection papers, such as the M8 and M9 papers (Anachemia, Lachine, Quebec, Canada), can be used to detect mustard and nerve agents. The M256 Detection Kit (Anachemia, Lachine, Quebec, Canada) can detect mustard, nerve agents, phosgene, and cyanide. Standoff capability, that is, detecting agents from as far away as 5 km, has been developed to detect contaminated areas without being exposed [14]. Many of the readily available detection strategies cannot detect lower levels of chemical agent, thus being less useful to confirm successful decontamination or detect chemical agents remotely from the site of exposure. Most hospitals will not have capability to confirm exposure or nature of chemical agents used in a timely manner to influence patient care or protect their facilities.

As health care providers, use of samples from patients rather than environmental sampling may be helpful for clinical and forensic purposes. For example, dilute traces of chemical agent metabolites of sulfur mustard (HD), sarin (GB), soman (GD), VX, and Russian VX (RVX) can be detected in urine samples from exposed patients using fast liquid chromatography–tandem mass spectrometry [15]. Sulfur mustard exposure can also be determined from hair analysis of patients with suspected exposure [16]. Further development of rapid, easy, and affordable technology to help hospitals detect and identify chemical weapon agents is expected to make new technologies available.

Ideally, the decontamination of chemical agent casualties should be accomplished by first responders or hazardous material personnel prior to evacuation or transport to a medical facility. Unfortunately, most disaster victims bypass emergency medical system transport and arrive unannounced at the closest hospital. As a result, hospitals must be prepared to decontaminate chemical agent casualties prior to admission. Facilities and protocols to decontaminate such casualties should be developed by all hospitals. Such processes are needed to protect the victims from further exposure and to prevent the spread of chemical agents within the hospital and among health care providers.

Critical care physicians, nurses, and support personnel may be called on to help develop decontamination protocols and assist in the decontamination process. It is imperative that all individuals designated to serve on decontamination teams be thoroughly trained in the procedures, precautions, and protective clothing required by the decontamination process. Attempting to provide help in a contaminated environment without prior training puts the health care provider at risk of being exposed to a chemical agent and could impede the delivery of effective medical care for the victims of a chemical attack. One common (and potential fatal) error made by health care providers is to rely on personal protective equipment effective for protection from biologic hazards (such as N95 respirators) which provide insufficient protection during decontamination or care of contaminated chemical agent exposed casualties.

The sarin gas release in Tokyo provides a clear example of the need for preparation and training prior to a chemical attack. Of the 1,364 emergency personnel who responded to the attack, 135 (9.9%) became symptomatic and required medical support themselves. None of the first responders wore protective clothing or face masks and off-gassing of the chemical agent from clothing of victims played a significant role in their complaints. These effects were evident among hospital staff as well first responders. It was reported that 23% of the staff at the hospital that received the patients also experienced symptoms [17].

The Occupational Safety and Health Administration (OSHA) mandates that all health care providers be trained to perform their duties without jeopardizing the health and safety of themselves or coworkers. It provides guidance for the use of personal protective equipment and requires that written plans be developed for hospitals to train teams for the use of personal protective equipment to receive contaminated victims [18]. Most medical facilities prepare their decontamination teams to operate in OSHA personal protective equipment Level C; that is, full-face mask with an air-purifying canister respirator and chemical-resistant clothing. Recurrent training and drills in the use of available and appropriate personal protective equipment by hospital staff is recommended to ensure readiness in the event of a chemical agent event.

Decontamination strategies for chemical exposure can include mechanical removal of agents (e.g., washing or wiping), chemical deactivation, or a combination of both approaches. Mechanical removal without deactivation may result in spread of some agents at the decontamination area and create contaminated waste. Chemical deactivation may be generic or specific for certain agents. For most situations, effective chemical decontamination can be performed by carefully removing the victim's clothing and thoroughly washing the victim with soap and water. It has been reported that removing contaminated clothing alone can eliminate 85% to 90% of chemical contaminants [19]. Use of specific solutions to facilitate decontamination, such as 0.5% hypochlorite solutions, may be less useful than water/soap strategies given the potential delay of preparing and deploying specialized solutions.

The M291 Skin Decontamination Kit has been in use by the military for many years, and can facilitate mechanical removal and partial deactivation of some agents. Newer technology, such as Reactive Skin Decontamination Lotion (RSDL) (O'Dell Engineering Ltd/E-Z-EM Canada Inc., Canada) may be superior [20]. It is not used for prophylactic protection or total body decontamination, but, if applied early following exposure, is effective for neutralizing chemical warfare agents and T2 mycotoxins [21]. However, during exposures associated with trauma, RSDL may interfere with normal wound healing [22].

In addition to skin and wound decontamination products, other strategies may be used to decontaminate personal protective equipment and external surfaces. For example, FAST-ACT (TIMILON Technology Acquisitions, Fort Myers, Florida) acts as a nanosorbent to adsorb and neutralize chemical agents and is available in a spray powder, pressure bottles, and on the surface of a glove for easy wiping. EasyDECON (Envirofoam Technologies, Huntsville, Alabama) can be used to decontaminate exposed environmental surfaces. Normally employed as a foam, it effectively neutralizes a variety of chemical agents including nerve gases and mustard [23]. A recent study from the Czech Republic provides an excellent example of a comparative approach to chemical agent decontamination strategies, taking into consideration multiple factors relevant to different operating environments and expected exposures [24].

Finally, medical facilities must consider environmental variables such as wind direction, wind velocity, temperature, and water runoff when setting up decontamination areas. These environmental considerations are important for protecting patients and employees from exposure to chemical agents, as well as minimizing the risk of contaminating buildings and equipment during the patient decontamination process.

CLASSIFICATION OF CHEMICAL AGENTS

Chemical agents are normally classified into broad categories based on their mechanisms of action and physiologic effects. The most common classification scheme divides them into the following categories:

- Nerve agents
- Vesicants
- Cyanide agents or "blood" agents
- Pulmonary agents or "choking" agents
- Nonlethal incapacitating agents

Nerve Agents

Because they are the most toxic, nerve agents are the most feared of chemical agents. All nerve agents are organophosphorus compounds, which inhibit butyrylcholinesterase in the plasma, acetylcholinesterase in the red blood cell (RBC), and acetylcholinesterase at cholinergic receptor sites in the central and peripheral nervous systems. The chemical bond between nerve agent molecules and acetylcholinesterase is irreversible, its activity returning only with new acetylcholinesterase synthesis or RBC turnover (1% per day) [25]. The decrease of acetylcholinesterase activity results in the accumulation of acetylcholine at both muscarinic and nicotinic receptors in the central nervous system and neuromuscular junctions of the peripheral nervous system. Cholinergic overstimulation resulting from the accumulation of excess acetylcholine at these sites is responsible for the clinical manifestations of nerve agent toxicity [26].

After an acute exposure to nerve agents, RBC acetylcholinesterase reflects nervous system acetylcholinesterase activity better than the activity of butyrylcholinesterase in the plasma. The measurement of RBC acetylcholinesterase activity can now be confirmed with commercially available point-of-care testing, assuming that the devices are present and personnel are trained on their usage [27]. However, its measurement is not common at most clinical laboratories.

Several different nerve agents currently exist, each characterized by a unique molecular structure that irreversibly inhibits acetylcholinesterase. Compounds that were originally developed in Germany have been designated as the "G" series of nerves agents. The "V" series of agents are better absorbed through the skin than the "G" agents and are so designated because they are more "venomous." The most common nerve agents include:

- GA (tabun): ethyl N,N-dimethylphosphoramidocyanidate
- GB (sarin): isopropyl methyl phosphonofluoridate
- GD (soman): pinacolyl methyl phosphonofluoridate
- GF: O-cyclohexyl-methylphosphonofluoridate
- VX: O-ethyl S-(2-(diisopropylaminoethyl) methyl phosphonothiolate

The "G" agents are volatile, whereas VX is a persistent, oily substance with better percutaneous absorption. Each of these agents can be dispersed through a variety of weapons and munitions.

Inhalation of nerve gas is the most effective means of producing clinical effects, although it can also be ingested. High doses of persistent nerve agents, such as VX, can be absorbed through the skin. The clinical effects of nerve agent toxicity occur as a result of acetylcholine accumulating at both nicotinic sites (autonomic ganglia and skeletal muscle) as well as muscarinic sites (including postganglionic parasympathetic fibers, glands, and pulmonary and gastrointestinal smooth muscles). Nicotinic receptors appear to be most sensitive to the effects of nerve agents, with inactivation of acetylcholinesterase in autonomic ganglia and the neuromuscular junction of skeletal muscle responsible for many symptoms and signs of nerve agent exposure. The typical clinical manifestations of nerve agent toxicity are similar to those produced by organophosphate insecticides, although nerve agents are up to 1,000 times more toxic [26].

The basic clinical syndrome produced by nerve agents can be remembered by the acronym "SLUDGE": salivation, lacrimation, urination, defecation, gastric distress, and emesis. Alternatively, "DUMBELS" (diarrhea, urination, miosis, bradycardia/bronchorrhea/bronchospasm, emesis, lacrimation, salivation/secretion/sweating) provides a more detailed tool to remember the muscarinic signs and symptoms [28]. Specific signs and symptoms of various organ systems depend on the dose of nerve agent received. Inhalation of a nerve agent usually produces immediate effects that occur within seconds to minutes after exposure. Dermal absorption usually produces delayed effects that can develop at any time between 10 minutes and 18 hours after skin exposure, depending on the dose. Common signs and symptoms for each organ system are summarized here.

Inhalation of a nerve agent results in the development of rhinorrhea, bronchorrhea, and bronchoconstriction soon after exposure. Dyspnea and chest tightness are common early symptoms. Coughing and wheezing may occur. The volume of airway secretions, the magnitude of bronchoconstriction, and the severity of airway symptoms all increase with higher exposure doses. High-dose or prolonged exposure may result in diaphragmatic weakness and centrally mediated apnea, which can result in ventilatory failure [25,26].

Although vagally mediated bradycardia is the expected heart rate response from cholinergic overstimulation of muscarinic receptors, this is commonly overridden by tachycardia resulting from nicotinic-mediated adrenergic stimulation and hypoxia. First-, second-, and third-degree heart block may occur [25,26]. Prolongation of the QTc interval can precipitate torsade de pointes and has a poor prognosis [29]. Although hypertension may occur as a result of nicotinic-mediated adrenergic stimulation, blood pressure usually remains normal. A decline of blood pressure is typically a sign of impending death [5].

Muscarinic and nicotinic stimulation of the peripheral nervous system results in muscle fasciculations and profuse sweating, respectively. Muscle weakness and muscle paralysis may occur following high-dose exposures. Seizures can develop suddenly. The seizures may resolve spontaneously, but can be prolonged with status epilepticus [25,26]. Smaller-exposure doses typically result in nonspecific neurologic findings including an inability to concentrate, insomnia, irritability, and depression. A variety of psychologic and behavioral changes, ranging from mild confusion to severe anxiety, can also occur [23]. Hallucinations or complete disorientation do not appear. Mild exposure also may result in a slight decline of memory function, as observed in first responders in the Tokyo sarin gas release of 1995 [30]. In the decade since that event, those exposed continue to have mild cerebellar effects and posttraumatic stress disorder [31].

Direct contact of the eyes with nerve agent vapor causes miosis that is usually associated with intense ocular pain. Patients also complain of blurred or dim vision and typically have injected conjunctivae with significant lacrimation.

Nausea and vomiting may be among the first signs of nerve agent toxicity. Abdominal cramping and diarrhea may also occur [25,26].

Unfortunately, few of the clinical signs or symptoms listed here may appear following exposure to a high dose of nerve agent. This is due to the fact that the range of exposure of doses, which produce clinical symptoms, is only slightly less than those which cause death. Therefore, central nervous system collapse with seizures, loss of consciousness, and central apnea may be the first signs of nerve agent toxicity following a high-dose exposure [25].

Management of all nerve agent casualties begins with the traditional "ABCs" of resuscitation: airway, breathing, and circulation support. Contaminated patients should be managed in the following order:

- Airway management
- Breathing support
- Circulation and hemorrhage control
- Antidote administration
- Decontamination
- Wound dressing
- Evacuation to a noncontaminated treatment location [32]

Ventilatory failure is the primary cause of death following nerve agent exposure [33]. As a result, airway management and breathing support are extremely important for the management of nerve agent casualties. The nausea and vomiting that these patients typically experience must be considered during their airway management. In this regard, all patients should be considered to have a full stomach. Endotracheal intubation and assisted ventilation are required for the management of ventilatory failure. High airway resistance necessitating the need of pressures up to 50 to 70 cm of water may complicate ventilatory support [26]. Because of high airway pressures, if a cuffed endotracheal tube cannot be placed, a double-lumen Combitube (Tyco Healthcare, Pleasanton, CA) is preferable to a laryngeal mask airway [34]. Once an effective airway has been established, ventilatory assistance can be provided by manual ventilation using a bag-valve device or by mechanical ventilation. Nebulized ipratropium can be used for the treatment of bronchospasm that may, in turn, result in decreased airway resistance [25]. Frequent suctioning is necessary to remove the copious airway secretions associated with nerve agent exposure. The use of depolarizing neuromuscular blocking agents during ventilatory assistance should be avoided [35].

The principal antidote for nerve agents is atropine. Atropine is an anticholinergic drug that blocks acetylcholine receptor sites. As a result, atropine blocks the pathophysiologic effects of the excess acetylcholine that accumulates as a result of nerve gas exposure; it is most effective at muscarinic sites. Atropine is primarily used for the purpose of drying up the copious airway secretions that patients develop following nerve agent exposure. The standard adult dosing regimen is 2 mg, administered intramuscularly, every 5 to 10 minutes, titrated to the patient's secretions. The recommended pediatric dose is 0.05 mg/kg, with a minimum dose of 0.1 mg, administered intravenously every 2 to 5 minutes, titrated to effect [26,33]. Among severe cases, adult patients may require 10 to 20 mg of atropine in the first hour to control secretions. The administration of atropine to a hypoxemic patient could precipitate the development of ventricular fibrillation. Therefore, oxygen should be administered and hypoxemia corrected before atropine is given [32,36]. Miosis will not respond to parenteral atropine. Topical tropicamide is effective for the treatment of miosis and the relief of ocular pain [33]. Atropine alone may not be an effective treatment for terminating seizures or reversing ventilatory failure [26,36]. Bulk atropine is available for reconstitution and may be required in the setting of mass nerve agent casualties.

Pralidoxime chloride is the other major antidote for nerve agents. It functions by "prying off" the nerve agent molecule from acetylcholinesterase, thereby rendering the enzyme active again. Unfortunately, it must be given early, before the agent–enzyme bond matures or "ages" which occurs in as little as 2 minutes for soman but takes 3 to 4 hours for sarin. Once the agent–enzyme bond completely ages, the bond is irreversible and pralidoxime chloride has no therapeutic effect. Pralidoxime chloride is only effective at nicotinic sites and, therefore, helps to increase muscle strength. The standard adult dose is 15 to 25 mg/kg or 1 g, given intravenously (in 100 to 250 mL of 0.9% saline) during 20 to 30 minutes. The initial dose may be followed by an infusion of 200 to 500 mg per hour, if necessary. Higher dosing with a 2 g load followed by 1 g per hour for 48 hours has been shown to significantly decrease atropine requirements and the duration of mechanical ventilation for patients poisoned by organophosphate pesticides [37]. The recommended pediatric dose is 15 to 25 mg/kg administered intravenously during 30 to 40 minutes. Severe hypertension is a potential side effect of pralidoxime chloride, and this can be rapidly reversed by a 5-mg intravenous infusion of phentolamine [33].

Atropine and pralidoxime chloride come packaged as two autoinjectors in commercially available kits, called MARK-I Nerve Agent Antidote Kits (Meridian Medical Technologies, Columbia, MD). Each kit contains one AtroPen autoinjector containing 2 mg of atropine and one pralidoxime chloride autoinjector containing 600 mg of pralidoxime chloride. The same company also now produces Antidote Treatment Nerve Agent, Autoinjector (ATNAA), a single autoinjector 2.1 mg of atropine and 600 mg of pralidoxime chloride [38].

Historically, diazepam has been the anticonvulsant recommended for the management of seizures associated with nerve agent exposure. In the hospital setting, diazepam may be given intravenously. The adult intravenous dose is 5 to 10 mg every 10 to 20 minutes until seizures resolve, but not to exceed 30 mg in an 8-hour period. The pediatric dose is 15 to 25 mg/kg [33]. Autoinjectors that contain 10 mg of diazepam (CANA—Convulsant Antidote for Nerve Agent) are available for use in the field (Meridian Medical Technologies). In both hospital and prehospital settings, health care providers must carefully monitor patients for signs of ventilatory failure following the administration of diazepam. Lorazepam and midazolam that are typically used in a critical care environment are also effective in controlling seizures following nerve agent exposure [39,40]. The use of phenytoin is not recommended [41].

Newer therapies with bioscavengers are currently being investigated as an additional means of mitigating or treating the effects of nerve agents; they can be stoichiometric (cholinesterases) or catalytic (paraoxonase, phosphotriesterase). These enzymes sequester the agent before they reach the cholinesterase targets, thus preventing any "downstream" clinical effects once the esterase has been inhibited. This therapeutic modality may prove most useful for slow-release VX [42,43].

Moderately poisoned patients with systemic signs and symptoms of exposure required 2.5 hospitalization days following the Tokyo sarin gas attack, whereas those on mechanical ventilation stayed over 8 days. Length of stay from the clinical effects of the persistent VX may be mitigated by titrating the need ongoing oxime therapy based upon red blood cell AchE activity [27].

Decontamination remains a key step during the treatment of nerve agent casualties because minimizing exposure to the agent decreases the severity of toxic effects. Removal of all clothing, rinsing the eyes with water or normal saline for 10 minutes, and washing the entire body once with soap and water should suffice. Decontamination should be conducted as soon as possible after ventilatory and circulatory support has been initiated and antidotes have been administered. Rapid decontamination is especially important for nerve agents that can be absorbed through the skin. It is important for health care providers to wear protective clothing and face masks prior to and during contamination of nerve agent casualties [17,25].

Vesicants

The two principal vesicants or "blister agents" are sulfur mustard and lewisite. This section focuses on the more notable sulfur mustard (bis-[2-chloroethyl] sulfide) that is commonly referred to as mustard. Lewisite has similar health effects except for the immediacy of its action in comparison to mustard. It normally takes several hours between contact with mustard and the onset of signs and symptoms, with the specific latency period depending on the exposure dose. In general, the higher the exposure dose, the shorter the latency period. Mustard is an oily liquid that ranges from clear to pale yellow to dark brown in color. It classically smells like onion, garlic, or mustard, which is allegedly how it got its name. At temperate conditions, it is a persistent liquid that volatilizes slowly. At temperatures greater than 100°F, however, mustard evaporates and mustard vapor becomes a major hazard. As a weapon, mustard will most likely be employed as a contact agent [44].

On entering living cells, mustard alkylates and cross-links DNA causing DNA strand breaks and eventually leading to cell death. Mustard damages any skin that it contacts, resulting in vesicle or bullae formation within 4 to 24 hours after exposure. Vesicle formation typically peaks within several days after contact with the skin; the bullae fluid is not toxic and is therefore not a threat to providers. As the most sensitive organ to low dosage exposures, contact with the eyes may result in painful irritation, conjunctivitis, blepharospasm, and corneal opacity related to edema and pannus formation. Blindness can occur if the corneal pannus is severe and covers the visual axis. Eyelid burns may be first or second degree.

Mild-to-severe airway damage can occur following mustard inhalation with most effects occurring in the upper airways. However, the extent and severity of airway damage is dose-dependent, with lower doses primarily affecting the upper airways and higher doses affecting both upper and lower airways. High inhalational doses can cause a severe inflammatory exudate, pulmonary edema with hemorrhage, necrosis of mucous membranes, mucosal sloughing, parenchymal tissue destruction, and pseudomembrane formation. Sloughed mucosal tissue and pseudomembranes can cause obstruction of the lower airways and serve as a nidus for respiratory tract infections, principally *Pseudomonas*. Other pulmonary problems include asthma, laryngospasm, acute bronchitis, chronic bronchitis, bronchiectasis, tracheobronchial stenosis, pulmonary fibrosis, bronchiolitis obliterans, and pleural thickening [45–47]. Hypoxia and hypercarbia may occur as a result of ventilation–perfusion mismatching caused by airway mucosal sloughing and hyperreactive or bronchitic airways. Severe gastrointestinal side effects and bone marrow suppression can occur following ingestion of high doses of mustard. Leukopenia with a cell count less than 200 cells/mm^3 portends a poor prognosis. Sepsis may occur as a result of leukopenia and the breakdown of skin, respiratory epithelium, and gastrointestinal mucosa [48].

Decontamination is a critical component of the management of mustard casualties. Indeed, decontamination within 1 to 2 minutes after exposure is the most effective means of reducing serious skin and tissue damage from mustard. Because of its persistence, removal of mustard from casualties must occur before admission to a medical treatment facility so health care workers do not become contaminated. In general, the medical care of mustard casualties is supportive. Areas of denuded skin should be treated like burns and liberally covered with silver sulfadiazine ointment [19]. Calamine lotion and topical steroids may soothe mild burning and itching in erythematous areas of skin. Nonsteroidal anti-inflammatory drugs may help to mitigate pain associated with cutaneous inflammation. Cooling the skin to 15°C and applying deferoxamine or zinc oxide may also be beneficial [49,50]. Skin healing following mustard exposure takes longer than skin healing following thermal burns. Some patients may require skin grafts and reconstructive surgery.

Respiratory care is mostly supportive. Bronchodilators may be useful for the treatment of asthma-like symptoms related to hyperreactive airways. N acetyl-cysteine may not only treat bronchial lesions, but also prevent further injury from oxidative stress. Corticosteroids may also be helpful, but should be used with caution because of the risk of superinfection [51]. Intubation and ventilatory support may be necessary for the management of severe laryngospasm or respiratory failure following high doses of inhaled mustard. Outpatient noninvasive ventilation may mitigate hospital admissions for those with chronic lung disease [52]. Bronchoscopy may be necessary to remove pseudomembrane fragments from the airway. Chronic, progressive tracheobronchial stenosis has been reported following mustard inhalation, and may require periodic bronchoscopy with bougienage or balloon dilation, or laser photoresection to maintain airway patency [53].

For systemic toxicity, early treatment with nonsteroidal anti-inflammatory agents may be useful. Thiosulfate decreases toxicity for animals; also in animal models, granulocyte colony stimulating factor has been shown to reduce the duration of neutropenia by approximately half [54].

In summary, acute mortality is relatively low, but morbidity is high following exposure to a vesicant. The severity and duration of illness and injuries are directly related to the exposure dose and routes of exposure. Because of the persistence of mustard, decontamination is critically important in the management of mustard casualties and for protecting health care workers from being exposed. Victims will consume significant health care resources in the management of their acute care needs and some will require prolonged periods of treatment and rehabilitation for chronic sequelae.

Cyanide

Cyanide can exist either as gas or as a colorless, volatile liquid that easily vaporizes. In both physical states, it typically has the smell of bitter almonds, although 40% to 60% of the population is unable to detect this odor. It is a chemical asphyxiant of the type that is historically classified as a "blood" agent. Cyanide can be used as an agent of mass destruction in two chemical forms: hydrogen cyanide and cyanogen chloride. Although very lethal in high doses, the volatility of cyanide makes it difficult to weaponize, and it ranks among the least lethal of the common chemical agents of mass destruction. Cyanide produces its pathologic effects by binding to iron-containing sites on mitochondrial cytochrome a_3, a key enzyme of the cytochrome oxidase system involved in aerobic metabolism. The binding of cyanide to cytochrome a_3 can occur very rapidly, effectively stopping cellular respiration and forcing affected cells into anaerobic metabolism. Cyanide also has an increased affinity for the ferric ion of methemoglobin that is a property exploited for treatment of cyanide poisoning [55].

The clinical manifestations of cyanide poisoning result from the inability of cells to extract and use oxygen. The onset of signs and symptoms occurs rapidly following inhalation (within 15 seconds), whereas a delayed response of up to 30 minutes follows ingestion. Metabolic acidosis develops as a consequence of increased lactate production from anaerobic metabolism. Compensatory mechanisms to increase oxygen delivery to tissues include tachycardia and increased minute ventilation, which are the earliest clinical signs. Dyspnea may occur as a result of the hyperpnea. Other signs include agitation, anxiety, vertigo, headache, muscle weakness, and trembling. Diaphoresis and flushing sometimes occur. Seizures have been reported. Dilated, unresponsive pupils and coma are late signs of cyanide poisoning and portend a poor prognosis. Without treatment, cyanide victims eventually develop apnea and cardiac dysrhythmias, followed by death from cardiac arrest [55].

Both the administration of specific antidotes and supportive care must be given as soon as possible after exposure to cyanide. Sodium nitrite and sodium thiosulfate are the traditional antidotes used to treat cyanide poisoning. This treatment focuses on detoxifying and excreting the cyanide, as well as on preventing its reentry into the cell. One ampule containing 300 mg of sodium nitrite in 10 mL of diluent (30 mg/mL) is administered intravenously for 2 to 4 minutes to form methemoglobin. The pediatric dose of sodium nitrite is 0.33 mL/kg of a 3% solution given intravenously for 2 to 4 minutes, not to exceed 10 mL. Cyanide binds more effectively and preferentially to the ferric ion site on methemoglobin in comparison to cytochrome a_3. Therefore, the methemoglobin generated by sodium nitrite removes cyanide from cytochrome a_3-binding sites and frees the enzyme to once again participate in the processes of cellular respiration and aerobic metabolism. Following sodium nitrite administration, 12.5 g of sodium thiosulfate in 50 mL of diluent is administered intravenously at a rate of 3 to 5 mL per minute. The pediatric dose of sodium thiosulfate is 412.5 mg/kg (1.65 mL/kg), given intravenously at a rate of 3 to 5 mL per minute. Sodium thiosulfate acts as substrate for rhodanese, converting the cyanide to thiocyanate that is then excreted in the urine. Sodium nitrite and sodium thiosulfate are very effective antidotes for the treatment of cyanide poisoning when they are given before the cessation of cardiac activity [55,56].

A specific challenge during the management of these patients is in the prehospital environment, specifically in hypoxia environments such as fires or smoke, inhalation where decreased oxygen-carrying capacity can be exacerbated by the induction of methemoglobinemia. Hydroxocobalamin, a precursor of vitamin B_{12}, provides an alternative treatment option for both pre- and in-hospital management. Cyanokit (Dey L.P., Napa CA., www.cyanokit.com) contains two vials of 2.5 g of lyophilized hydroxocobalamin that is reconstituted in 100 cc saline for administration. The standard initial adult dose is 5 g infused over 15 minutes with an additional 5 g given depending on the patient's condition. Hydroxocobalamin binds with cyanide to form cyanocobalamin that is then excreted in the urine. It is well tolerated with no known major toxicities. Of note, this red molecule results in red mucous membranes, skin, and urine [57]. A major impediment to widespread use of this modality is its cost which is over twice as expensive as the sodium nitrite/sodium thiosulfate kit [58].

Unfortunately, these therapies require intravenous antidote administration and several minutes time before becoming effective. These factors impede their application to large numbers of victims. Thus research efforts have recently focused on developing quick acting, intramuscular antidotes. Sulfanegen, a dimer prodrug of 3-mercaptopyruvate, serves as a sulfur donor via 3-mercaptopyruvate sulfur transferase to cyanide, producing thiocyanate and pyruvate. In addition to its stability for IM injection, it also exerts its effects within 3 minutes [59,60].

Supportive care for cyanide poisoning includes the administration of oxygen that has been shown to be effective for managing hypoxia, even though the poor cellular uptake and utilization of oxygen found with cyanide toxicity would suggest supplemental oxygen to be of little efficacy. Hyperbaric oxygen may also be beneficial for selected severely ill patients, though this therapy would be difficult to institute in a mass casualty setting [19]. Ventilatory support should be provided when needed. Consideration should be given to the administration of sodium bicarbonate for the treatment of severe lactic acidosis in patients who are unconscious or hemodynamically unstable. Arterial blood gas analysis is used to guide the need for repeat doses of sodium bicarbonate to ensure that a metabolic alkalosis does not develop. In most cases of cyanide poisoning, appropriate supportive care in conjunction with the administration of sodium nitrite and sodium thiosulfate, or hydroxocobalamin before cardiac arrest can result in a complete recovery over a period of several days [55,57,61].

Pulmonary or "Choking" Agents

Pulmonary or "choking" agents cause acute lung injury after inhalation. The acute lung injury produced by these agents typically results in the development of pulmonary edema. Phosgene and chlorine are the two most common chemical agents in this category. Both were used as chemical warfare agents in World War I. Their effects relate, in part, to their water solubility. Highly water-soluble gases like ammonia, hydrogen chloride, and sulfur dioxide affect primarily the eyes and upper airway mucous membranes. Chlorine, a moderately water-soluble gas, affects the upper airway less but also damages the lower airway. Finally, slightly water-soluble gases like phosgene affect primarily the lower airways.

Phosgene is a colorless gas at room temperature, but becomes a volatile liquid on cooling or compression. The gaseous form has an odor of green corn or freshly mown hay. The gas is denser than air and accumulates in low-lying areas. On exposure to water, phosgene hydrolyzes to form carbon dioxide and hydrochloric acid. These hydrolysis products may cause phosgene gas to appear as a white cloud when it comes into contact with water vapor in the air [62].

Initial symptoms of phosgene poisoning are primarily related to inflammatory irritation of the eyes and mucous membranes of the oronasopharynx. The irritation is caused by the hydrochloric acid that is formed when phosgene reacts with tissue water. Initial symptoms occur shortly after exposure and include burning sensation in eyes, conjunctival erythema, increased lacrimation, soreness of the throat and nasal membranes, rhinorrhea, coughing, choking, and tightness in the chest. Nausea, occasional vomiting, and headache have also been reported to occur shortly after phosgene exposure. These may be the only symptoms that occur following a low-concentration exposure. However, a life-threatening illness, characterized by noncardiogenic pulmonary edema and respiratory failure, can develop after exposure to higher concentrations.

Inhaled phosgene causes the formation of hydrochloric acid in the airways and alveoli that causes direct inflammatory injury to epithelial cells and endothelial cells of pulmonary capillaries. In addition, phosgene causes an acylation reaction with amino, hydroxyl, and sulfhydryl groups on cellular macromolecules, resulting in changes to surfactant structure and function and the development of reactive oxygen and nitrogen species. In addition, phosgene stimulates neuronal Ca^{2+} channels, resulting in neurotransmitter release, and can induce vasoconstriction [63]. It also stimulates the synthesis of lipoxygenase-derived leukotrienes that results in the chemotactic attraction of neutrophils and their accumulation in the lung. In the lung, the damaged alveolar-capillary membrane leads to pulmonary edema. This effect only occurs through direct inhalation.

As noted earlier, inhaled phosgene affects primarily the lower respiratory tract, causing diffuse bronchoalveolar injury, bronchospasm, and noncardiogenic pulmonary edema. Exertion tends to decrease the latency period between phosgene inhalation and the development of pulmonary symptoms, as well as exacerbate pulmonary symptoms once they occur. Phosgene-produced pulmonary edema may begin as early as 2 to 6 hours after inhalation. Although the pulmonary edema may appear to be mild at first, it can become extensive and life threatening. Normal pulmonary lymphatic drainage may be overwhelmed by increasing pulmonary edema that leads to the development of the acute respiratory distress syndrome (ARDS) in some individuals. The onset of ARDS may be delayed for up to 48 hours after phosgene inhalation [64].

Chlorine is a greenish-yellow, noncombustible gas at room temperature and normal atmospheric pressure. It is heavier than air and gravitates to low-lying areas if released in the environment. Chlorine has a strong, pungent odor similar to bleach that is usually detectable by smell, even in low concentrations. It is a highly reactive element and, like phosgene, forms hydrochloric acid on contact with water [62].

Symptoms of chlorine exposure are similar to those following exposure to phosgene. Initial symptoms occur within minutes after exposure and include burning of the eyes; redness of the conjunctivae; increased lacrimation; soreness of the throat and nasal membranes; rhinorrhea; coughing; choking; and tightness in the chest. Burning and blistering of the skin can occur shortly after contact of chlorine with exposed areas [65].

Inhalation of chlorine, even in low concentrations, causes immediate coughing and choking that can be severe. The coughing and choking tend to prevent some of the inhaled chlorine from reaching the peripheral airways and lung tissue. Thus, inhaled chlorine typically affects the upper airway primarily, causing laryngeal edema, laryngospasm, and bronchospasm. Hoarseness and aphonia may occur. Dyspnea is the first sign of upper airway involvement, followed by copious secretions, productive cough, and chest tightness. Wheezing typically occurs with bronchospasm. Individuals with a history of asthma or airway hyperactivity may have particularly severe bronchospasm. Severe bronchospasm may cause mediastinal and subcutaneous emphysema secondary to air trapping. Inhalation of high concentrations of chlorine may produce laryngospasm that is severe enough to cause sudden death [62]. Chlorine exposure also may result in long-term neurocognitive deficits, including choice reaction time, balance, visual field changes, and verbal recall [66].

Noncardiogenic pulmonary edema can occur within 2 to 4 hours following the inhalation of chlorine, especially at high concentrations [67]. Frothy sputum and rales may be the first clinical signs of pulmonary edema. Radiographic signs of pulmonary edema typically lag behind the development of clinical symptoms [68]. The development of ARDS with hypoxemic respiratory failure may eventually occur. The fluid losses associated with severe pulmonary edema and ARDS can be so profound that hypovolemic shock develops.

Management of individuals exposed to inhaled phosgene and chlorine is essentially supportive with no specific antidote available for either agent. For all cases, the patient must be removed from the contaminated environment and decontaminated as soon as possible by washing the patient with soap and copious amounts of water for 3 to 5 minutes. The eyes should be flushed with normal saline. Exertion should be minimized during transport and hospitalization.

Aggressive bronchodilator therapy with a nebulized β_2 agonist is the mainstay of therapy for bronchospasm. Nebulized ipratropium may be added if the β_2 agonist alone is ineffective. Systemic corticosteroids may be useful for the treatment of severe bronchospasm, particularly among individuals who have a history of asthma or airway hyperreactivity. Animal studies have shown that inhaled corticosteroids improve oxygenation and attenuate the development of acute lung injury, especially when given in conjunction with an inhaled bronchodilator [69]; this has not, however, been validated for humans. The combination of steroids with nebulized sodium bicarbonate was efficacious in the treatment of 25 soldiers who were exposed to acute chlorine gas inhalation [70]. Thus, although systemic corticosteroids are recommended for life-threatening situations, there is no definitive clinical evidence for their efficacy in reducing the severity of acute lung injury or pulmonary edema.

Bacterial superinfection of the airways can lead to the development of severe tracheobronchitis and pneumonia 3 to 5 days after toxic irritant exposure. The presence of persistent fever, elevated white blood, or the production of thick, purulent sputum should prompt the physician to obtain cultures of sputum, blood, and any pleural fluid that is evident on chest radiograph. Empiric antibiotics should be given in accordance with the guidelines for intensive care unit patients with community-acquired pneumonia [62].

Intubation and mechanical ventilation may be required for severe bronchospasm, laryngospasm, and pulmonary edema. They are usually required for the management of ARDS and respiratory failure. Given the rapidity with which these problems can develop, preparations for intubation and mechanical ventilation should take place during the latency period, before serious respiratory problems develop. Nasotracheal intubation should not be performed because of nasal inflammation. Orotracheal intubation with visualization of the airways is the recommended technique. During mechanical ventilation, an appropriate amount of positive end-expiratory pressure, typically in the range of 5 to 10 cm H_2O, and other rescue therapies may be needed to improve oxygenation for patients with pulmonary edema or ARDS (see Chapters 163 and 166). Using animal models, protective ventilation strategies with 6 mL/kg tidal volumes improve oxygenation, are thought to decrease shunt fraction, and improve mortality [71].

Careful attention must be given to fluid balance and the administration of intravenous fluids in patients with pulmonary edema and ARDS. Vasopressors may be required for the treatment of hypovolemic shock. Both ibuprofen and acetylcysteine aerosol have demonstrated some efficacy for preventing phosgene-induced lung injury of animal models, although there are no human clinical trials regarding their use [72,73].

Pulmonary edema that appears within 4 hours after phosgene or chlorine exposure is a poor prognostic sign. Some individuals may develop the reactive airways dysfunction syndrome (RADS) following phosgene or chlorine inhalation [74,75]. This disorder is characterized by chronic, nonspecific airway hyperreactivity that persists after the patient has recovered from the effects of an acute exposure. Patients who develop RADS should receive prompt treatment with oral prednisone (40 to 80 mg daily for 10 to 15 days) followed by treatment with a high dose of an inhaled corticosteroid, such as beclomethasone (2,000 μg per day). RADS patients should be followed closely with serial methacholine bronchial challenge testing, and the dose of oral corticosteroid should be tapered in accordance with improvements of airway hyperresponsiveness. It may take years for some individuals with RADS to show significant improvement in airway hyperresponsiveness [76]. However, most individuals who survive phosgene or chlorine exposure will recover completely with no long-term effects [62].

With increased understanding of the mechanisms of cellular damage, newer therapies are being investigated. These may include neuromodulators that interrupt signalling pathways, phosphodiesterase inhibitors, angiotensin, and endothelin [64]. Approaches to upregulate repair to damaged alveolar membranes with keratinocyte growth factor, epithelial growth factor, and basic fibroblast growth factor are being explored in the management of ARDS that results from inhalation [77]. Several stem cell lines could also prove useful in the future in mitigating the long-term effects of inhalation injury such as asthma, COPD, pulmonary fibrosis, and lung cancer [78].

Nonlethal Incapacitating Agents

Chemical agents that cause temporary incapacitation are commonly classified as nonlethal agents. These chemical agents, although potentially lethal in high concentrations, are typically employed at doses that cause temporary injury. They are commonly used to incapacitate unruly individuals or groups in riot control situations. However, they could also be used by terrorists during an attack. In this regard, they could be used alone, they could be used prior to an attack with conventional weapons, or they could be used in conjunction with other chemical, biologic, or radiologic agents of mass destruction.

The most common incapacitating agent is BZ (QNB; 3-quinuclidinyl benzilate), a competitive inhibitor of acetylcholine at postsynaptic and postjunctional muscarinic receptors. BZ is a stable, odorless, persistent crystalline solid. It is usually dispersed as a fine solid powder, although it can be dissolved in a liquid substrate and dispersed as a liquid aerosol. Both the powder and aerosolized forms can be readily ingested or inhaled. Ingestion and inhalation of BZ particles that are 1 μm in size result in bioavailabilities that are approximately 80% and 50% of a parenteral dose, respectively [79].

The clinical effects of BZ are similar to those of atropine, although BZ is approximately 25 times more potent and has a much longer duration of action. Symptoms of exposure include mydriasis; blurred vision; dry mouth; indistinct speech; dry skin; increased deep tendon reflexes; poor coordination; decreased level of concentration; illusions; and short-term memory deficits. The most prominent central nervous system effects of BZ are related to the so-called "anticholinergic delirium." The delirium typically occurs after high-dose exposure and has been described as a "walking dream," a syndrome characterized by periods of staring, unintelligible muttering, occasional shouting, and bizarre hallucinations. The degree of delirium can fluctuate frequently from minute to minute, with periods of lucidity and appropriate responses interspersed among periods of severely altered mental status [5,79].

The intensity and duration of anticholinergic symptoms associated with BZ exposure are dose-dependent, with higher doses causing more severe symptoms and a longer durations of effects. Incapacitating symptoms typically appear within 1 hour after exposure, peak at approximately 8 hours after exposure, and subside gradually during the next 48 to 72 hours. All individuals exposed to BZ should be decontaminated by washing the entire body with soap and water. Medical therapy is mostly supportive, to include control of the patient for the prevention of accidents, removal of dangerous objects from the patient's environment to prevent self-inflicted harm during delirium, moist swabs or hard candy for dryness of the mouth, keeping the room temperature at 75°F or below to prevent the development of hyperthermia, and the use of topical antibiotics and sterile dressings for abrasions of dry, parched skin. Severe signs and symptoms of BZ exposure can be treated with physostigmine which temporarily raises acetylcholine concentrations by binding reversibly to anticholinesterase on postsynaptic or postjunctional membranes. Physostigmine can be administered either intravenously or intramuscularly. The recommended intravenous dose is 0.5 to 1.0 mg by slow infusion at a rate over 2 to

5 minutes for adults and 0.01 mg/kg for children. The patient should be evaluated every hour for improvement in signs and symptoms, with physostigmine readministered periodically at a dose and time interval that is titrated to the severity of clinical signs. Physostigmine can cause a precipitous decrease in heart rate and patients should be carefully monitored during its administration. It should not be administered to any patient with cardiopulmonary instability, hypoxemia, electrolyte imbalance, or acid–base disturbances that predispose to cardiac dysrhythmias and seizures. An intravenous test dose of 1 mg should be administered to adults if the diagnosis of BZ exposure is in doubt. If slight improvement is noted and there are no adverse effects within 1 hour, the full dose can be given [5,79].

Riot control agents are intended to produce unpleasant but nonpersistent medical effects. They are sometimes referred to as *irritants*. The two riot control agents most commonly used are 2-chloro-1-phenylethanone (CN or MACE; MACE Security International, Cleveland, OH) and 2-chlorobenzalmalononitrile (CS or tear gas). Another product used for riot control or security is oleoresin capsaicin (OC or pepper spray). All riot control agents cause significant irritation to the eyes, upper airways, and skin. In addition to burning of the eyes and increased lacrimation, exposed individuals may experience temporary blepharospasm with transient blindness. Upper airway symptoms include rhinorrhea, sneezing, salivation, and tightness of the chest. Exposed individuals with preexisting reactive airway disease may develop bronchospasm, which can progress to respiratory failure [80]. Because riot control agents are dispersed as a solid powder, decontamination consists of getting the victims out of any confined spaces and into fresh air, removing their clothing, and irrigating their eyes and mucous membranes with normal saline. Treatment is nonspecific and supportive. The latency period for most symptoms is hours to several weeks, and most resolve in 15 to 30 minutes though they can last several days; exacerbation of reactive airway disease may last many months. Episodes of acute bronchospasm in susceptible individuals should be treated with a short-acting β_2 agonist administered by nebulizer [81,82]. Providers must be aware that exposure to agents in a patient's oropharynx may produce symptoms in the provider during endotracheal or nasogastric intubations.

Finally, a variety of other readily available compounds can be aerosolized and need to be considered as potential incapacitating agents. Nausea-producing agents such as diphenylaminearsine (DM or "adamsite") can produce incapacitating gastrointestinal symptoms. Psychedelic drugs, such as 3,4-methylenedioxymethamphetamine and phencyclidine, are easily obtained and could be used as aerosolized incapacitating agents. In October 2002, carfentanil, a potent aerosolized derivative of fentanyl, was probably employed in combination with halothane in an attempt by Russian authorities to release more than 800 hostages held by terrorists in Moscow's Dubrovka Theater. Unfortunately, 127 hostages in the theater died, and more than 650 were hospitalized after being exposed to the chemicals that were used in the rescue attempt [83]. This is a good example of how readily available pharmaceutical agents can be used to incapacitate, or even kill, a large number of individuals.

SUMMARY

Chemical agents pose a significant threat to populations throughout the world, whether accidentally released from an industrial or transportation accident, or released intentionally as part of a crime or terrorist event. Regardless of the cause of release, they have the potential to produce a large number of casualties in a short period of time. However, the terminology *weapons of mass destruction* does not entirely reflect the impact that a terrorist attack with such agents could have on the general population. Even a relatively small number of casualties from a terrorist attack would be likely to cause significant psychologic trauma, resulting in anxiety and behavioral changes among large numbers of "worried well." Such psychologic trauma could significantly disrupt healthy business and community activities for a long period of time. Instilling widespread fear and anxiety in the general population is a primary goal of terrorism and, unfortunately, the use of chemical agents is an efficient method of achieving that goal.

Critical care providers must be prepared to deal with the recognition, decontamination, transport, medical treatment, and psychologic trauma of casualties resulting from chemical agents. They must also be prepared to protect themselves and colleagues from contamination with chemical agents during the course of patient care. Training in the medical management of chemical agent casualties and planning for mass casualty situations are essential to ensure that the best possible care is provided to the victims of a chemical exposure or chemical attack.

DECLARATION

The opinions and assertions contained herein are those of the authors and do not necessarily reflect the views or position of the Department of Veterans Affairs, The Geisel School of Medicine at Dartmouth, or the Medical University of South Carolina.

References

1. Colonel Edgar Erskine Hume, Medical Corps, U.S. Army, 1943.
2. Hume EE: *Victories of Army Medicine*. Philadelphia, PA, JB Lippincott, 1943, p 10.
3. Cieslak TJ: *Biological Warfare and Terrorism*. USA, Fort Detrick, Frederick, MD, U.S. Army Medical Research Institute of Infectious Diseases, 2000.
4. White SM: Chemical and biological weapons. Implications for anaesthesia and intensive care. *Br J Anaesth* 89:306, 2002.
5. U.S. Army Medical Research Institute of Chemical Defense: *Medical Management of Chemical Casualties Handbook*. 3rd ed. Aberdeen Proving Ground, MD, U.S. Army Medical Research Institute of Chemical Defense, 2000.
6. Smart JK: History of chemical and biological warfare: an American perspective, in Sidell FR, Takafuji ET, Franz DR (eds): *Medical Aspects of Chemical and Biological Warfare*, in Zajtchuk R, Bellamy RF (eds): *Textbook of Military Medicine, Part I: Warfare, Weaponry and the Casualty*. Washington, DC, United States Department of the Army, Office of the Surgeon General and Borden Institute, 1997, p 9.
7. Okudera H, Morita H, Iwashita T, et al: Unexpected nerve gas exposure in the city of Matsumoto; report of rescue activity in the first sarin gas terrorism. *Am J Emerg Med* 15:527, 1997.
8. Okumura T, Takasu N, Ishmatsu S, et al: Report on 640 victims of the Tokyo subway sarin attack. *Ann Emerg Med* 28:129, 1996.
9. Wax PM, Becker CE, Curry SC: Unexpected "gas" casualties in Moscow: a medical toxicology perspective. *Ann Emerg Med* 41(5):700–705, 2003.
10. BBC News: Syria chemical attack: what we know. September 24, 2013. Available at: http://bbc.com/news/world-middle-east-23927399/. Accessed July 26, 2016.
11. Gulland A: Lack of atropine in Syria hampers treatment after gas attacks. *BMJ* 347:f5413, 2013.
12. Plumer B: Everything you need to know about Syria's chemical weapons. The Washington Post September 5, 2013. Available at http://washingtonpost.com/. Accessed July 26, 2016.
13. Convention on the Prohibition of the Development, Production, Stockpiling and Use of Chemical Weapons and on their Destruction (Chemical Weapons Convention). Available at: http://www.opcw.org/chemical-weapons-convention/. Accessed September 2, 2016.
14. Mobile Chemical Agent Detector: Available at: http://www.northropgrumman.com/Capabilities/MCAD/Pages/default.aspx. Accessed November 9, 2016.
15. Rodin I, Braun A, Stavrianidi A, et al: 'Dilute-and-shoot' RSLC-MS-MS method for fast detection of nerve and vesicant chemical warfare agent metabolites in urine. *J Anal Toxicol* 39(1):69–74, 2015. doi: 10.1093/jat/bku119. Epub 2014 Oct 17.
16. Spiandore M, Piram A, Lacoste A, et al: Hair analysis as a useful procedure for detection of vapour exposure to chemical warfare agents: simulation of sulphur mustard with methyl salicylate. *Drug Test Anal* 6 Suppl 1:67–73, 2014. doi: 10.1002/dta.1659.
17. Okamura T, Suzuki K, Fukuda A, et al: The Tokyo subway sarin attack: disaster management, Part 2: hospital response. *Acad Emerg Med* 5:618, 1998.
18. Horton D, Berkowitz Z, Kaye WE: Secondary contamination of ED personnel from hazardous materials events, 1995–2001. *Am J Emerg Med* 21:199, 2003.

19. Kales SN, Christiani DC: Acute chemical emergencies. *N Engl J Med* 350:800, 2004.
20. Schwartz MD, Hurst CG, Kirk MA, et al: Reactive skin decontamination lotion (RSDL) for the decontamination of chemical warfare agent (CWA) dermal exposure. *Curr Pharm Biotechnol.* 13(10):1971–1979, 2012.
21. RSDL Skin Decontamination Product: Available at: http://www.rsdecon.com/. Accessed November 9, 2016.
22. Walters T, Kauvar D, Reeder J, et al: Effect of reactive skin decontamination lotion on skin wound healing in laboratory rats. *Mil Med* 172:318, 2007.
23. Lindsey J: Amazing terrorism tool: new foam could revolutionize decon. *JEMS* 28:84, 2003.
24. Capoun T, Krykorkova J: Comparison of selected methods for individual decontamination of chemical warfare agents. *Toxics* 2:307–326, 2014. doi:10.3390/toxics2020307.
25. Leikin JB, Thomas RG, Walter FG, et al: A review of nerve agent exposure for the critical care physician. *Crit Care Med* 30:2346, 2002.
26. Sidell FR: Nerve agents, in Sidell FR, Takafuji ET, Franz DR (eds): *Medical Aspects of Chemical and Biological Warfare*, in Zajtchuk R, Bellamy RF (eds): *Textbook of Military Medicine, Part I: Warfare, Weaponry and the Casualty*. Washington, DC, United States Department of the Army, Office of the Surgeon General and Borden Institute, 1997, p 129.
27. Thierman H, Worek F, Kehe K: Limitations and challenges in the treatment of acute chemical warfare agent poisoning. *Chemical-Biological Interactions* 206:435,2013.
28. Thomas RG: Chemoterrorism: nerve agents, in Walter FB, Klein R, Thomas RG (eds): *Advanced Hazmat Life Support Provider Manual*. 3rd ed. Tucson, AZ, University of Arizona Board of Regents, 2003, p 302.
29. Chuang FR, Jang SW, Lin JL, et al: QTc prolongation indicates a poor prognosis in patients with organophosphate poisoning. *Am J Emerg Med* 14:451, 1996.
30. Nishiwaki Y, Maekawa K, Ogawa Y, et al: Effects of sarin on the nervous system in rescue team staff members and police officers 3 years after the Tokyo sarin attack. *Environ Health Perspect* 109:1169, 2001.
31. Hoffman A, Eisenkraft A, Finkelstein A, et al: A decade after Tokyo sarin attack: a review of neurological follow-up of the victims. *Mil Med* 172:607, 2007.
32. Berkenstadt H, Marganitt B, Atsmon J: Combined chemical and conventional injuries—pathophysiological, diagnostic, and therapeutic aspects. *Isr J Med Sci* 27:623, 1991.
33. Lee EC: Clinical manifestations of sarin nerve gas exposure. *JAMA* 290:659, 2003.
34. De Jong RH: Nerve gas terrorism: a grim challenge to anesthesiologists. *Anesth Analg* 96:819, 2003.
35. Cosar A, Kenar L: An anesthesiological approach to nerve agent victims. *Mil Med* 171:7, 2006.
36. Marik P, Bowles S: Management of patients exposed to biological and chemical warfare agents. *J Int Care Med* 17:147, 2002.
37. Pawar K, Bhoite R, Pillay C, et al: Continuous pralidoxime infusion versus repeated bolus injection to treat organophosphorus pesticide poisoning: a randomized controlled trial. *Lancet* 368:2136, 2006.
38. DuoDote Auto-Injector: Available at: http://www.meridianmeds.com/products/duodote. Accessed November 9, 2016.
39. Wiener SW, Hoffman RS: Nerve agents: a comprehensive review. *J Intensive Care Med* 19:22, 2004.
40. McDonough J, McMonagle J, Copeland T, et al: Comparative evaluation of benzodiazepines for control of soman-induced seizures. *Arch Toxicol* 73:473, 1999.
41. Anderson P: Emergency management of chemical weapons injuries. *J Pharm Pract* 25(1):61–68, 2012.
42. Kuca K, Jun D, Musilek K, et al: Prophylaxis and post-exposure treatment of intoxications caused by nerve agent and organophosphorus pesticides. *Mini Rev Med Chem* 13:1, 2013.
43. Rice H, Mann T, Armstrong S, et al: The potential role of bioscavengers in the medical management of nerve-agent poisoned casualties. *Chem Biol Interact* 259:1, 2016.
44. Sidell FR, Urbanetti JS, Smith WJ, et al: Vesicants, in Sidell FR, Takafuji ET, Franz DR (eds): *Medical Aspects of Chemical and Biological Warfare*, in Zajtchuk R, Bellamy RF (eds): *Textbook of Military Medicine, Part I: Warfare, Weaponry and the Casualty*. Washington, DC, United States Department of the Army, Office of the Surgeon General and Borden Institute, 1997, p 197.
45. Emad A, Rezaian GR: The diversity of the effects of sulfur mustard gas inhalation on respiratory system 10 years after a single, heavy exposure: analysis of 197 cases. *Chest* 112:734, 1997.
46. Thomason JW, Rice TW, Milstone AP: Bronchiolitis obliterans in a survivor of a chemical weapons attack. *JAMA* 290:598, 2003.
47. Khazdair M, Boskabady M, Ghorani V: Respiratory effects of sulfur mustard exposure, similarities and differences with asthma and COPD. *Inhal Toxicol* 27:731–744, 2015.
48. Wattana M, Bey T: Mustard gas or sulfur mustard: an old chemical agent as a new terrorist threat. *Prehosp Disaster Med* 24:19, 2009.
49. Karayilanoglu T, Gunhan O, Kenar L, et al: The protective and therapeutic effects of zinc chloride and desferrioxamine on skin exposed to nitrogen mustard. *Mil Med* 168:614, 2003.
50. Poursaleh Z, Ghanei M, Babamahmoodi F, et al: Pathogenesis and treatment of skin lesions caused by sulfur mustard. *Cutan Ocul Toxicol* 31:241–249, 2012.
51. Poursaleh Z, Harandy A, Vahedi E, et al: Treatment for sulfur mustard lung injuries; new therapeutic approaches from acute to chronic phase. *DARU* 20:27–37, 2012.
52. Aliannejad A, Peyman M, Ghanei M: Noninvasive ventilation in mustard airway diseases. *Respir Care* 60:1324–1329, 2015.
53. Freitag L, Firusian N, Stamatis G, et al: The role of bronchoscopy in pulmonary complications due to mustard gas inhalation. *Chest* 100:1436, 1991.
54. Anderson D, Holmes W, Lee R, et al: Sulfur mustard-induced neutropenia: treatment with granulocyte colony-stimulating factor. *Mil Med* 171:448, 2006.
55. Baskin SI, Brewer TG: Cyanide poisoning, in Sidell FR, Takafuji ET, Franz DR (eds): *Medical Aspects of Chemical and Biological Warfare*, in Zajtchuk R, Bellamy RF (eds): *Textbook of Military Medicine, Part I: Warfare, Weaponry and the Casualty*. Washington, DC, United States Department of the Army, Office of the Surgeon General and Borden Institute, 1997, p 271.
56. Berlin CM: The treatment of cyanide poisoning in children. *Pediatrics* 6:793, 1970.
57. Guidotti T: Acute cyanide poisoning in prehospital care: new challenges, new tools for intervention. *Prehosp Disaster Med* 21:s40, 2005.
58. BoundTree Medical: Available at: www.boundtree.com. Accessed November 9, 2016.
59. Petrikovics I, Budai M, Kovacs K, et al: Past, present and future of cyanided antagonism research: from the early remidies to current therapies. *World J Methodol* 5(2):88–100, 2015.
60. Patterson S, Moeller B, Nagasawa H, et al: Development of sulfanegen for mass cyanide casualties. *Ann NY Acad of Sci* 1374:202–209, 2016.
61. Brivet F, Delfraissy JF, Bertrand P, et al: Acute cyanide poisoning: recovery with non-specific supportive therapy. *Intensive Care Med* 9:33, 1983.
62. Urbanetti JS: Toxic inhalational injury, in Sidell FR, Takafuji ET, Franz DR (eds): *Medical Aspects of Chemical and Biological Warfare,* in Zajtchuk R, Bellamy RF (eds): *Textbook of Military Medicine, Part I: Warfare, Weaponry and the Casualty*. Washington, DC, United States Department of the Army, Office of the Surgeon General and Borden Institute, 1997, p 247.
63. Holmes W, Keyser B, Paradiso D, et al: Conceptual approaches for treatmentt of phosgene inhalation-induced lung injury. *Toxicol Lett* 244:8–20, 2016.
64. Prevention and treatment of injury from chemical warfare agents. *Med Lett Drugs Ther* 44:1, 2002.
65. Kaufman J, Burkons D: Clinical, roentgenological and physiological effects of acute chlorine exposure. *Arch Environ Health* 23:29, 1971.
66. Kilburn K: Effects of chlorine and its cresylate byproducts on brain and lung performance. *Arch Env Health* 58:746–755, 2003.
67. Das R, Blanc PD: Chlorine gas exposure and the lung. *Toxicol Ind Health* 9:439, 1993.
68. Bunting H: The pathology of chlorine gas poisoning, in *Fasciculus on Chemical Warfare Medicine*. Washington, DC, Committee on Treatment of Gas Casualties, National Research Council, 1945, p 24 (vol 2).
69. Wang J, Winskog E, Walther SM: Inhaled and intravenous corticosteroids both attenuate chlorine gas-induced lung injury in pigs. *Acta Anaesthesiol Scand* 49:183, 2005.
70. Cevik Y, Onay M, Akmaz I, et al: Mass casualties from acute inhalation of chlorine gap. *Southern Med J* 102(12):129-1213, 2009.
71. Parkhouse D, Brown R, Jugg B, et al: Protective ventilation strategies in the management of phosgene-induced acute lung injury. *Mil Med* 172:295, 2007.
72. Sciuto AM, Strickland PT, Kennedy TP, et al: Protective effects of N-acetylcysteine treatment after phosgene exposure in rabbits. *Am J Respir Crit Care Med* 151:768, 1995.
73. Sciuto AM, Hurt HH: Therapeutic treatments of phosgene-induced lung injury. *Inhal Toxicol* 16:565, 2004.
74. Currie GP, Ayres JG: Assessment of bronchial responsiveness following exposure to inhaled occupational and environmental agents. *Toxicol Rev* 23:75, 2004.
75. Evans RB: Chlorine: state of the art. *Lung* 183:151, 2004.
76. Lemière C, Boulet L, Cartier A: Reactive airways dysfunction syndrome and irritant induced asthma. Up To Date February 2, 2016, update. Available at: www.uptodate.com. Accessed November 9, 2016.
77. Holmes WW, Keyser BM, Paradiso DC, et al: Conceptual approaches for treatment of phosgene inhalation-induced lung injury. *Toxicol Lett* 244:8–20, 2016.
78. Angelini D, Dorsey R, Willis K, et al: Chemical warfare agent and biological toxin-induced pulmonary toxicity: could stem cells provide potential therapies? *Inhal Toxicol* 25(1):37–62, 2013.
79. Ketchum JS, Sidell FR: Incapacitating agents, in Sidell FR, Takafuji ET, Franz DR (eds): *Medical Aspects of Chemical and Biological Warfare,* in Zajtchuk R, Bellamy RF (eds): *Textbook of Military Medicine, Part I: Warfare, Weaponry and the Casualty*. Washington, DC, United States Department of the Army, Office of the Surgeon General and Borden Institute, 1997, p 287.
80. Thomas R, Smith P: Riot control agents, in Roy MJ (ed): *Physician's Guide to a Terrorist Attack*. Totowa, NJ, Human Press, 2004, p 325.
81. Sidell FR: Riot control agents, in Sidell FR, Takafuji ET, Franz DR (eds): *Medical Aspects of Chemical and Biological Warfare,* in Zajtchuk R, Bellamy RF (eds): *Textbook of Military Medicine, Part I: Warfare, Weaponry and the Casualty*. Washington, DC, United States Department of the Army, Office of the Surgeon General and Borden Institute, 1997, p 307.
82. Dimitroglou Y, Rachiotis G, Hadjichristodoulou C: Exposure to the riot control agent CA and potential health effects: a systematic review of the literature. *Int J Environ Res Public Heatlh* 12:1397–1411, 2015.
83. Wax PM, Becker CE, Curry SC: Unexpected "gas" casualties in Moscow: a medical toxicology perspective. *Ann Emerg Med* 41:700, 2003.

Chapter 129 ■ The Management of Acute Radiation Casualties

ARVIND K. SUNDARAM • MARY JANE REED • JOHN SCOTT PARRISH • JAMES GEILING • LAWRENCE C. MOHR, JR

INTRODUCTION

The objective of this chapter is to become familiar with the medical consequences and casualty management considerations following a radiologic or nuclear incident.

TYPES OF RADIATION EMERGENCIES

Radiation emergencies may result from a number of accidental or deliberate events. Radiologic dispersion devices (RDDs), or "dirty bombs," are devices that cause intentional dissemination of radioactive material without a nuclear detonation. The radioactive material is released and dispersed by the detonation of the high-explosive charge. It is important to note that dirty bombs are not nuclear weapons and are not weapons of mass destruction. "Dirty bombs" may cause internal radiation exposure through the inhalation or ingestion of contaminated materials in the food chain and external radiation exposure through surface contamination [1,2]. The adverse health effects depend on the type and amount of explosive and radioactive material used and atmospheric conditions at the time of detonation. Most injuries from a dirty bomb will come from the blast effects of the conventional explosion [1,2]. Acute and delayed health effects caused by radiation are unlikely. Delayed health effects, such as the development of cancers, following an RDD attack, are related to the radiation exposure dose and to the amount of internal radiation that results from the inhalation, ingestion, and absorption of radioactive material through the skin or open wounds. An RDD can cause significant impact on the short- and long-term social, psychologic health of the masses [2,3].

Radiologic exposure devices (REDs) are radioactive nuclear materials that are covertly placed with the intention of exposing victims to harmful radiation without their knowledge [1]. The dangers of an RED depend upon the type and amount of radioactive material used, the duration of exposure, the proximity of the source, and the part of the body exposed. Unexplained burns, cytopenias, or the development of other symptoms consistent with the acute radiation syndrome (ARS) can alert providers to the possible presence of an RDD. Some radioactive materials of concern used as RDDs are the americium-241, californium-252, cobalt-60, caesium-137, iridium-192, and strontium-90 [2].

A nuclear explosion results from nuclear fission or from thermonuclear fusion, during which a tremendous amount of energy is suddenly released in the form of heat, blast, and radiation. Human injury is caused by exposure to a combination of these three forms of energy following a nuclear detonation. The energy released from a nuclear explosion can be very intense and lead to a life-threatening ARS, radiation burns, thermal burns, and blast injuries. Radiation exposure can result in the development of various types of cancer and leukemia over a period of many years if an individual survives the initial short-term effects of a nuclear explosion. These radiation effects on the human body can be classified into two categories: deterministic effects and stochastic effects. Deterministic effects are dose-dependent, and their effects are absent below certain threshold; they are responsible for organ damage and infertility. Stochastic effects are dose-independent, and the effects are not proportional to the dose of radiation; they are responsible for cancer and genetic damage [3].

Nuclear power plant accidents are another potential source of radiation exposure. The Chernobyl nuclear accident, Three Mile Island event, and the recent Fukushima Daiichi Nuclear Power Plant accident are the most notable examples in recent times.

Nuclear power plant accidents differ from nuclear weapon detonations, in that nuclear weapons use enriched uranium or plutonium in higher concentrations and configurations than those used by power plants. Reactor accidents can release various radioisotopes that have different effects on humans. Radioisotopes with very short or very long half-lives and gaseous forms that are released in small quantities may not produce significant internal or external radiation injuries, whereas iodine-131 isotope can contaminate the environment with long-term effects [4]. The accident at the Fukushima Daiichi Nuclear Power Plant in Japan in March 2011 resulted in the environmental release of radioactive substances, predominantly iodine-131, caesium-134, xenon-133, and strontium-90. Most of the radioactivity was released during a period of approximately 40 days with traces of radioisotopes detected globally. No acute radiation injuries were reported from the Fukushima Daiichi Nuclear Power Plant disaster. Based on the published data, the maximum estimated lifetime cancer mortality and morbidity from Fukushima Daiichi Nuclear Power Plant, however, are increased for the exposed population [4–6].

Accidental exposure during the transportation, industrial use, or medical use of radioactive materials has also led to a wide range of radiation injuries.

ARS is a deterministic effect that may develop among radiation-exposed individuals following a radiologic incident. The pathophysiology behind the cell damage from ionizing radiation is owing to the radiosensitivity of certain cell lines. ARS consists of a continuum of complex and unique medical subsyndromes that involve the hematopoietic, gastrointestinal, and central nervous systems in a dose-related fashion. Patients who develop any of the acute radiation subsyndromes require prompt assessment and critical care management to minimize loss of life. The ARS and its associated subsyndromes are discussed in detail later in the chapter.

BASIC RADIATION PHYSICS

Radiation is defined as energy that is transmitted through space. The transmitted energy may be in the form of high-speed particles or electromagnetic waves. There are two general types of radiation: ionizing radiation and nonionizing radiation. Ionizing radiation has enough energy to remove tightly bound electrons from their orbits and cause an atom to become charged. Nonionizing radiation does not have enough energy to remove electrons from their orbits. Ionizing radiation is more harmful to humans than nonionizing radiation and is the type of radiation that would be expected to be released by a radiologic or nuclear attack.

Ionizing radiation can take four forms: alpha, beta, gamma, and neutron. Alpha radiation consists of the emission of a helium nucleus from a parent nucleus, such as uranium-235; it is a particle that has an atomic mass of four and a charge of plus one. Beta radiation is the emission of a small negatively charged particle from a parent nucleus, such as potassium-40. Beta particles have a mass that is almost undetectable and a charge of minus one, similar to that of an electron. Gamma radiation is the emission of high-energy electromagnetic waves from a parent nucleus, such as cobalt-60. Gamma rays have no mass and no charge and frequently accompany the emission of alpha or beta particles. Neutrons are very high-energy particles emitted from parent nuclei, such as uranium-235 and plutonium-239 during a nuclear chain reaction. Nuclear chain reactions can be controlled, such as the kind found in a nuclear reactor, or they can be uncontrolled, such as the type that causes a nuclear explosion. Neutrons can induce severe damage to human cells and tissues [8,9].

Each specific type of ionizing radiation has a different penetrating distance on inert material and human tissues. Alpha particles will not penetrate paper or intact human skin. However, if alpha particles are ingested, inhaled, or internalized through a break in the skin, they can do a tremendous amount of internal damage to human cells and tissues [8,9].

Beta radiation will penetrate paper, thin layers of skin, and the conjunctiva of the eye but will not penetrate thin layers of plastic or aluminum foil. Beta particles travel relatively short distances and will be stopped by most clothing. As with alpha particles, beta radiation can induce severe damage to human tissues when inhaled or ingested [8,9].

Gamma rays can travel significant distances and are a highly penetrating type of ionizing radiation. They readily penetrate skin and clothing. Gamma radiation can cause considerable damage to human cells and tissues after penetration. Several inches of lead or several feet of concrete are required to stop gamma rays [8,9].

Neutrons are high-energy nuclear particles that have no charge. Neutron radiation easily penetrates skin and clothing and can cause significant damage to internal tissues and organs. Neutrons primarily cause biologic damage by colliding with other particles. They transfer the most energy when they collide with particles that are about the same size, especially protons. These high-energy, subatomic collisions result in the dislodgement of both protons and tightly bound electrons from atoms that are bombarded by neutrons, with ionization of atoms in surrounding cells and tissues. Neutron radiation is extremely harmful to humans. It cannot be stopped by plastic, glass, or lead; it can only be stopped by several feet of concrete [8,9].

Ionizing radiation causes damages to human cells and tissues through two biologic mechanisms: (1) direct high-energy damage to deoxyribonucleic acid (DNA) molecules and (2) the generation of free radicals, which secondarily damage DNA molecules by superoxide radicals generated from ionized water. The fate of irradiated human cells is dependent on the dose of radiation received. Low-dose exposures are characterized by DNA and cellular repair. Moderate-dose exposures are characterized by permanently damaged DNA and significantly altered cells, which may be eliminated by apoptosis or may be reproduced abnormally and eventually leading to the development of a cancer. High-dose radiation exposures typically result in cell death, which causes several serious ARSs that can result in the death of the organism [10,11].

Human radiation exposure can be categorized as either external or internal. External exposure may occur in either whole body or partial body depending on the surface area exposed to radiation. Internal exposure may occur from the inhalation, ingestion, or transdermal penetration of radioactive material. Combined radiation injuries may also occur among cases where radiation exposure and trauma occur concurrently. During combined radiation injuries, radioactive material can be introduced through open wounds.

RADIATION DOSES

There are two units of radiation doses that physicians must be familiar with: the rad and the gray (Gy). It is not essential for clinicians to understand the physics that underlie the determination of these doses, but it is important for them to know that these are the units that are used to express the amount of radiation that is absorbed by human tissues. The Rad is the traditional unit of radiation-absorbed dose. The Gy is the newer Standard International unit of radiation exposure. One Gy (100 centigrays or 100 cGy) is equal to 100 rads [12].

Radiation doses can be measured by using several techniques. Radiation detection, indication, and computation (RADIAC) devices such as the Geiger–Muller counters can help by detecting radiation exposures at a given time compared with dosimeters that measure the total dose accumulated. There are many different types of radiac meters, each of which may be more sensitive to specific types of radiation, such as alpha, gamma, or neutrons, than to other types of radiation. It is important, therefore, to know both the capabilities and limitations of any radiac meter that one uses to determine radiation doses. Useful clinical indicators of whole body radiation dose are time to vomiting and total lymphocyte count at 24 to 48 hours postexposure [13]. The dose range in Gy and the estimated lethality associated with each dose range are illustrated in Table 129.1.

Chromosomal aberrations and translocations in lymphocytes can also provide a useful estimate of both the type of radiation that one has been exposed to as well as the radiation dose. One such method called the dicentric chromosomal assay is considered the gold standard in the estimation of absorbed dose of the exposed radiation and is very sensitive to ionizing radiation [14,15]. These methods require considerable expertise in fluorescent in situ hybridization techniques as well as expertise in the interpretation of the chromosomal abnormalities.

TABLE 129.1

Prognosis at 48 Hours based on Lymphocyte Count Depression after Acute Whole Body Exposure

Minimal lymphocyte count absorbed 48 hours after exposure	Approximate absorbed dose (Gy)	Prognosis
1,000–3,000/mm^3 (normal range)	0–0.5	No significant injury
·1,000–1,500/mm^3	1–2	Significant but probably nonlethal injury, good prognosis.
500–1,000/mm^3	2–4	Severe injury, fair prognosis
100–500/mm^3	4–8	Very severe injury poor prognosis
<100/mm^3	>8	High incidence of lethality Even with hematopoietic stimulation

From Flynn DF and Goans RE: Triage and treatment of radiation and combined-injury mass casualties. Textbooks of military medicine: medical consequences of radiological and nuclear weapons. Borden Institute, Office of The Surgeon General, AMEDD center and school, p. 23, 2013. Available at http://www.cs.amedd.army.mil/borden/FileDownloadpublic.aspx?docid=b3d9d96a-a8b8-499c-bddf-e27791466b77. Accessed September 28, 2017.

OVERVIEW OF RADIATION CASUALTIES

Radiation casualties are of two general types: an ARS and delayed illnesses that may occur many years after radiation exposure. ARS is a life-threatening condition consisting of a continuum of dose-related subsyndromes that occur shortly after a high-dose radiation exposure, such as those that occur following the detonation of a nuclear weapon. Delayed illnesses include malignancies such as leukemia, lymphoma, and various solid tumors; late organ damage includes thyroid dysfunction; fibrotic changes of organs including the skin, blood vessels, and lymphatics; pregnancy loss; and genetic abnormalities of progeny. Delayed illness caused by radiation is likely from exposure that is lower than that is needed for the ARS. In general, the higher the radiation dose, the more severe the acute effects of radiation exposure, the greater the probability of delayed illnesses, and the higher the mortality rate [3,7].

In considering the human dose–response to radiation exposure, the measurement LD (lethal dose)$_{50/60}$ is commonly used. The $LD_{50/60}$ is the radiation dose that causes a 50% mortality rate in an exposed population within 60 days following exposure. For whole body radiation exposure, the $LD_{50/60}$, with no treatment, is 3 to 4 Gy. Therefore, 50% of a population that receives a radiation dose of 3 to 4 Gy will die within 60 days unless they receive treatment. With appropriate treatment including antibiotics and transfusions following radiation exposure, the $LD_{50/60}$ can be calculated as 4 to 5 Gy [7].

ACUTE RADIATION SYNDROME AND SUBSYNDROMES

ARS is a continuum of dose-related organ system subsyndromes that develop after an acute radiation exposure of greater than 1 Gy. There are three main subsyndromes that occur: the hematopoietic subsyndrome, the gastrointestinal subsyndrome, and the central nervous system subsyndrome. Each of these subsyndromes occurs in a dose-dependent manner. The hematopoietic subsyndrome occurs with radiation exposures greater than 1 Gy. The gastrointestinal subsyndrome occurs in addition to the hematopoietic subsyndrome at radiation exposures greater than 6 Gy. The central nervous system subsyndrome occurs in addition to the hematopoietic and gastrointestinal subsyndromes at radiation exposures greater than or equal to 20 Gy.

All acute radiation subsyndromes begin with a *prodromal phase* of nausea, vomiting, diarrhea, and fatigue that last for minutes to days. The higher the radiation dose, the more rapid the onset and the more severe the symptoms of the prodromal phase. After this phase, the patient enters a *latent phase*, in which he or she appears to recover and is often asymptomatic. The latent phase may last for several days to 1 month, with the period inversely proportional to the radiation exposure dose; that is, the higher the dose, the shorter this phase. After the asymptomatic latent phase, the patient enters the *manifest illness phase*. This phase of acute radiation illness lasts from several days to several weeks and is characterized by the manifestation of the hematopoietic, gastrointestinal, and central nervous system subsyndromes, according to the exposure dose that the patient received [16].

Some individuals may develop radiation-associated multiple organ dysfunction syndromes (MODSs) in association with the organ-specific clinical syndromes mentioned above. Multiple organ system dysfunction typically occurs in the manifest illness phase but may also occur early after a sublethal radiation exposure. Many patients with hematopoietic, gastrointestinal, central nervous system and MODSs will require management in an intensive care unit [17].

The Hematopoietic Subsyndrome

The hematopoietic subsyndrome typically occurs with a radiation dose of greater than 1 Gy. It is characterized by bone marrow suppression resulting from the radiation-induced destruction of hematopoietic stem cells within the bone marrow. Hematopoietic stem cell destruction results in a progressive decrease in lymphocytes, neutrophils, and platelets in the peripheral blood. Both the magnitude and the time course of the pancytopenia are related to the radiation dose. In general, the higher the radiation dose, the more profound and the quicker the pancytopenia occurs [7].

Lymphocytic stem cells are exquisitely sensitive to radiation, and circulating lymphocytes decrease rapidly following radiation exposure (see Table 129.1). Erythrocytic stem cells, on the other hand, seem to be more resistant to radiation than lymphocytic, neutrophilic, and thrombocytic stem cells. Therefore, the red blood cell count and hemoglobin concentration typically do not decrease to the same extent as lymphocytes, neutrophils, or platelets following radiation exposure [13].

As shown in Table 129.1, the hematologic effects of acute radiation exposure are dependent on the radiation dose. A radiation exposure of 3 Gy or more results in more significant hematologic effects than a radiation exposure of 1 Gy. Lymphocytes will decrease very rapidly following a radiation exposure of 3 Gy, and they will stay low for a relatively long period. Typically, it takes approximately 90 days before lymphocytes begin to recover from a 3-Gy radiation exposure. Neutrophils, after an initial period of intravascular demargination, will also begin to decline fairly rapidly following a 3-Gy exposure. Neutrophils do not fall as rapidly as lymphocytes, but between 3 and 5 days following exposure, such patients will be significantly neutropenic. Platelets also decrease steadily following a 3-Gy exposure, and patients will become significantly thrombocytopenic at 2 to 3 weeks. Both platelets and neutrophils will reach a nadir, with values close to zero, at approximately 30 days following a 3-Gy exposure. Platelets and neutrophils then recover gradually during the next 30 to 40 days. Lymphocytes remain low for a longer period, however, and typically do not begin to recover for at least 90 days following a 3-Gy exposure. Thus, there is a period of about a month following a 3-Gy exposure when patients will be significantly lymphopenic, neutropenic, and thrombocytopenic. Such patients are susceptible to developing serious infections and serious bleeding problems during that time [13,18].

The Gastrointestinal Subsyndrome

The gastrointestinal subsyndrome typically occurs following an acute radiation dose of greater than 6 Gy. It develops as a result of radiation damage to intestinal epithelial cells. The loss of epithelial cells results in denudation of the intestinal mucosa. Following the asymptomatic latent phase, patients will develop a manifest illness phase characterized by fever, vomiting, and severe diarrhea. Malabsorption, severe fluid losses, and severe electrolyte derangements will follow. Most patients will have severe pancytopenia as a result of a coexisting hematopoietic subsyndrome. Mucosal translocation of pathogens, sepsis, and opportunistic infections commonly occur. The resulting sepsis can be very severe and typically involves enteric organisms that migrate into the systemic circulation through damaged and denuded gastrointestinal mucosa. Approximately 10 days after the onset of the manifest illness phase, these patients typically develop fulminant bloody diarrhea that usually results in shock and subsequent death [7,16,19].

The Central Nervous System Subsyndrome

The central nervous system subsyndrome is seen with radiation doses greater than or equal to 20 Gy, although cognitive dysfunction can be seen with radiation doses greater than 10 Gy. The latent period is very short, lasting from several hours to 3 days. Following the asymptomatic latent period, patients typically develop nausea, vomiting, diarrhea, and confusion. Microvascular leaks in the cerebral circulation result in cerebral edema. Elevated intracranial pressure and cerebral anoxia may develop rapidly. Mental status changes develop early in the manifest illness phase, and the patient eventually becomes comatose. Seizures and burning dysesthesia may occur. Patients typically die within hours to several days after onset of the manifest illness phase of the central nervous system subsyndrome [1,7,20,21].

Multiple Organ Dysfunction Syndrome

Some patients may develop multiple organ system dysfunction following exposure to ionizing radiation. This syndrome was first reported following the September 30, 1999, Tokaimura nuclear accident [22]. Radiation-induced multiorgan involvement or multiple organ failure (MOF) is defined as a progressive dysfunction of greater than two organs over time [17]. They are not limited to the four-organ system included in the ARS. Prominent organs involved are the lungs, liver, kidney, and the cardiovascular system. There is no well-defined dose–effect relationship that has been associated with its development. The pathophysiology behind the development of MODSs and MOF is still not well construed, though it may be a consequence of a "two-hit phenomenon" where the initial insult is considered a consequence of irradiation-induced radiolysis of cells, inflammation, increased prooxidative metabolic reactions, injury to hematopoietic, lymphoid tissues, intestinal mucosa, or vascular endothelium. The injury to gut mucosa leads to bacterial translocation and spread of the bacterial pathogens and proinflammatory agents through the vascular system leading to septic inflammatory and metabolic responses [7,17,23–25]. Such patients will require prompt supportive care and treatment in an intensive care unit to maximize their potential for survival [17].

Prognosis

The prognosis of patients who develop acute radiation subsyndromes depends on the radiation dose to which they were acutely exposed and whether they have concomitant trauma. Nearly all patients exposed to 1 to 2 Gy will survive. Survival is possible for patients exposed to doses of 2 to 6 Gy, but many of these patients will require prompt treatment and intensive care to survive. Survival is possible, but improbable, for patients exposed to doses of 6 to 8 Gy. In addition to prolonged critical care support, these patients may require stem cell transplantation. Even with the most aggressive treatment, survival is extremely rare following exposure doses above 10 Gy and has not been reported following doses greater than 20 Gy [29].

Management

Initial medical care for all casualties of a radiologic event will include triage, resuscitation and first aid, medical stabilization, decontamination, and treatment of minor injuries. All patients with significant acute radiation exposure will receive supportive care. This consists of fluids and electrolyte replacement, antiemetic agents to manage vomiting, antidiarrheal agents to manage diarrhea, proton pump inhibitors for gastrointestinal ulcer prophylaxis, pain management, psychologic support, and palliative care when death is imminent. The main objective of management for ARS is to prevent neutropenia that can lead to sepsis. Care should be taken to prevent the development of infection or bleeding by avoiding unnecessary instrumentation particularly involving the gastrointestinal tract.

Hematopoietic growth factors or colony-stimulating factors (CSFs) are endogenous glycoproteins that stimulate the bone marrow stem cells to mature into blood cell types. The basis to use CSFs for patients exposed to radiation is derived from studies that followed cancer patients, among a small cohort of radiation-exposed victims, and several prospective trials of canines and nonhuman primates exposed to radiation. Granulocyte CSF (G-CSF), although not approved by US Food and Drug Administration for hematopoietic ARS, is used off-label for the management of ARS [7]. Growth factor therapies should be prophylactically initiated for early recovery of hematopoiesis preferably within 2 to 4 days for those exposed to a significant level of whole body radiation particularly greater than 3 Gy. Multiple studies have demonstrated the role of G-CSFs for reducing the duration of radiation-induced neutropenia, enhancing neutrophil recovery, and providing survival benefits. For radiologic events involving <100 casualties, growth factor therapy can be considered for patients exposed to radiation of 2 to 6 Gy when there is no significant burn or trauma. If the exposure is between 2 and 6 Gy and the patients have burns or trauma, growth factor therapy is still warranted. The therapy is usually continued until the absolute neutrophil count is more than 1,000 per mm^3 [29]. If the exposure is greater than 6 Gy without trauma, it is prudent to consider stem cell transplant [30].

Various types of G-CSFs can be given: G-CSF (filgrastim), pegylated G-CSF (pegfilgrastim), or GM-CSF (sargramostim) and recently added tbo-filgrastim. These are all commercially available preparations and used for the management of hematopoietic subsyndromes. The recommended doses of the various cytokines for the treatment of acute radiation subsyndromes in adults are summarized in Table 129.2 [29]. The role of antibiotics for the management of ARS depends on the patient's absorbed radiation dose, absolute neutrophil counts, and potential sources of infection. No antibiotic prophylaxis is recommended for patients who received radiation <2 Gy. For patients exposed to a moderate amount of radiation ranging from 2 to 6 Gy, antibacterials are initiated for febrile neutropenia along with possible antiviral and antifungal prophylaxis. Antibacterials are considered when focal infections are identified in patients who are afebrile, but neutropenic. For severe cases of radiation exposure to 5 to 10 Gy, early antiviral, antifungal, and antibiotics are started for anticipated significant immune suppression fluoroquinolones with or without amoxicillin/penicillin for streptococcal coverage, which is the preferred prophylactic regimen in these patients. The preferred antifungal and antiviral are fluconazole and acyclovir, respectively. Prophylactic antibacterials are continued until treatment failure or development of neutropenic fever or when the absolute neutrophil count is greater than 500/mm^3. In such cases, fluoroquinolones are discontinued, and antibacterials with antipseudomonal coverage are introduced. Gram-positive coverage is initiated as per the hospital sensitivity biogram. The Infectious Diseases Society of America guidelines for neutropenic fever management are recommended for febrile neutropenic patients [13,30].

Blood transfusions are indicated for patients with an acute radiation subsyndrome who have severe bone marrow damage

TABLE 129.2

Available Colony-Stimulating Factors (CSFs)

Growth factor/CSF	Dose
Filgrastim	2.5–5 μg/kg/d qd subcutaneously (SC) or the equivalent (100–200 μg/m^2/d)
Sargramostim (GM-CSF)	5–10 μg/kg/d qd SC or (200–400 μg/m^2/d)
Pegfilgrastim (pegylated G-CSF)	6 mg once SC
Tbo-filgrastim	5 μg/kg/d administered as an SC.

or who require concurrent trauma resuscitation. Transfusion requirements do not rise until 2 to 4 weeks after exposure unless the patient needs replacement of blood products for concurrent trauma. The purpose of blood transfusions for such patients is to provide erythrocytes for the improvement of oxygen-carrying capacity, blood volume to improve hemodynamic parameters, and platelets to help prevent bleeding. All cellular products in the blood to be transfused should be leukoreduced and irradiated to 25 Gy to prevent transfusion-related graft-versus-host reaction among immunocompromised patients [30].

Stem cell transplantation should be considered for certain patients with acute radiation illness. Allogeneic stem cell transplantation is indicated for individuals who have a radiation exposure dose of 7 to 10 Gy [30].

ACUTE RADIATION ILLNESS AND TRAUMA

The blast from a nuclear detonation can produce significant trauma along with the associated radiation injuries. The injuries from these blasts arise from the high pressures and wind, flash from the nuclear detonation, thermal pulses, and secondary fires.

The management of combined radiation injuries and trauma presents special challenges to the physician. There is a significant increase in mortality among patients who have this combination of an ARS and an injury. These patients require prompt medical and surgical care to survive. They should receive the treatments for ARSs, as described earlier in the subsyndrome sections. They are also very susceptible to operative and postoperative infections as a result of decreased neutrophil and lymphocyte counts and require 2 to 3 months for their bone marrow to recover from the acute radiation exposure. For a patient with a combination of an ARS and trauma requiring surgery, the surgery must be performed 36 to 48 hours after the initial radiation exposure because of high risk of radiation-induced cell damage and resultant poor healing. If surgery is not performed in this "window of opportunity" following acute radiation exposure, it may have to be postponed for up to 2 months until full hematopoietic recovery happens [13,30].

ACUTE RADIATION DERMATITIS

An acute radiation dermatitis may occur in conjunction with acute radiation illness. The symptoms and signs of acute radiation dermatitis typically appear several days *after* an acute radiation exposure. Although acute radiation dermatitis is essentially a radiation burn, it is different from the thermal burns that may occur immediately after exposure of the skin to a nuclear explosion. The Centers for Disease Control and Prevention has classified cutaneous radiation injury into three grades based on the extent of exposure to radiation. Exposure of the skin to radiation doses greater than 2 Gy causes epilation and typically occurs 14 to 21 days postexposure. On exposure to 6 Gy, erythema develops secondary to arteriolar constriction with capillary dilation and local edema. At 10 to 15 Gy radiation, dry desquamation occurs because of the involvement of the germinal layer of the epidermis. This leads to thinning of the epidermis and desquamation of skin. Wet desquamation occurs when the skin is exposed to 10 to 25 Gy of radiation to the development of intracellular edema progressing to macroscopic bullae. For patients exposed to greater than 25 Gy of radiation, radionecrosis and ulceration of skin occur. The two main approaches for managing acute radiation skin injury are operative and nonoperative treatment. Nonoperative treatments include infection control and pain and wound care management. Operative treatments include superficial debridement to prevent septic foci and skin grafting when this is required. Topical antibiotics with dressings are used for blistering phase, and silver sulfadiazine cream with nonadherent dressings is preferred for wet desquamation. Systemic antibiotics are used for selected cases. Radiation-induced skin ulcers, nonhealing wounds, and skin ulcers with intractable pain need surgical interventions. Tissue grafts may be required at necrotic sites involving large dermal area [13,30].

INTERNAL CONTAMINATION

Internal contamination is contamination within the body and can occur by the inhalation, ingestion, injection, or the transdermal penetration of radioactive materials. Contamination enters via a variety of portals, such as the nose, the mouth, and a wound, or with a large enough dose, by the penetration of gamma rays or neutrons directly through intact skin. Internal organs commonly affected by internal radiation contamination are the thyroid, the lung, the liver, adipose tissue, and bone. Leukemia and various types of cancers can develop in these organs many years after an acute radiation exposure with internal contamination.

Assessment of Potential Internal Radiation Contamination

The patient history is crucial to determining whether they may have experienced internal contamination. Any history that suggests that a patient may have inhaled, ingested, or internalized radioactive material through open wounds should prompt further evaluation for internal contamination. This assessment should attempt to identify both the radiation dose received and, if possible, the specific isotopes that caused the internal contamination. An initial survey of the patient should be performed with a radiac meter, especially around the mouth, nose, and wounds, to give some idea of the extent of any possible internal exposure. The diction of radioactive isotopes on nasal swabs can be very helpful to determine whether a patient has been exposed internally. If it is suspected that a person has inhaled a significant amount of radioactive material, bronchoalveolar lavage can be considered for identifying inhaled radioactive isotopes as well as for removing residual contaminated materials from the lungs. Bronchoalveolar lavage has been shown to be effective for removing inhaled material contaminated with radioactive isotopes from the lungs of animals. The collection and analysis of stool and urine samples can be very helpful for determining both the type and the amount of internal radiation that an individual might have received. Chest and whole body radiation counts can also be helpful for determining the extent of internal radiation contamination. Unfortunately, however, most medical institutions do not have the capability to do either chest or whole body radiation counts. The analysis of nasal swabs, stool samples, and urine samples is the most practical method for determining the type and extent of internal radiation contamination that is used by hospital-based physicians [13].

Treatment of Internal Radiation Contamination

Patients who have experienced internal radiation contamination should be promptly treated to reduce the absorbed radiation dose and prevent the development of future health problems. The goals of treatment are to reduce absorption and enhance elimination of the internal radionuclide contaminant. There are three main categories of agents that are used to treat internal radiation contamination: purgative agents, blocking agents, and chelation agents. Specific agents are used to treat internal contamination by specific radioactive isotopes. Such treatment is most effective when given as soon as possible after the radiation exposure. Gastric lavage can be used to empty the stomach completely after the potential ingestion of radionuclides. When promptly performed, it can decrease the concentration of radionuclides in the gastrointestinal tract. This could result in a decrease in the absorbed radiation dose. In deciding whether to treat a patient for internal radiation contamination, the physician should treat potentially exposed individuals empirically based on the information that is available [1,13,26,30].

Purgative Agents

Purgative agents help to remove radionuclides from the gastrointestinal tract. The most common purgatives are laxatives and enemas, which are helpful for reducing the residence time of radionuclides in the colon. Prussian blue (ferric ferrocyanide) is an ion exchange resin that binds cesium-137 in the gastrointestinal tract and facilitates its secretion. Patients who have experienced internal cesium-137 should be treated with oral Prussian blue (3 g, three times daily) for at least 3 weeks. Aluminum phosphate binds strontium-90 in the gastrointestinal tract. A single, 100 mL oral dose of aluminum phosphate gel will reduce the gastrointestinal absorption of strontium-90 by 85%. Oral aluminum phosphate should be used if internal contamination with strontium-90 is expected [1,13,26-30].

Blocking Agents

Blocking agents block both the uptake and bioavailability of internal radionuclide contaminants. The most important blocking agent is potassium iodide, which is used for the treatment of internal contamination with iodine-125/131. Potassium iodide blocks the uptake of radioactive iodine by increasing the uptake of the nonradioactive isotope. Because the thyroid gland is very sensitive to the effects of internal contamination with iodine-125/131, potassium iodine should be given as soon as possible after radioactive iodine exposure. It is recommended that patients take 300 mg of potassium iodide per day for 7 to 14 days following a potential iodine-125/131 exposure. Potassium iodide can also be taken prophylactically if there is sufficient warning of a potential iodine-125/131 exposure. The standard prophylactic regimen is a single 130 mg dose of potassium.

Chelation Agents

Chelation agents are the mainstay of treatment for internal radiation contamination. Chelation agents are substances that bind strongly with certain metals to form a stable, soluble complex that can be excreted by the kidneys. Diethylenetriaminepentaacetic acid (DTPA) is the most effective and commonly recommended chelation agent for the treatment of internal radiation contamination. DTPA complexes are very stable and water-soluble and are unlikely to release bound radionuclides before renal excretion. DTPA chelation therapy is especially effective for the treatment of internal radiation contamination with curium, americium, and plutonium. DTPA is administered as an intravenous solution of 1 g dissolved in 250 mL of saline or 5% glucose, infused over 1 hour per day for up to 5 days. The use of DTPA is contraindicated for the treatment of uranium-238/235 contamination because of an increased risk of renal damage. It is recommended that internal contamination with uranium-238/235 be treated with oral sodium bicarbonate, with the dose regulated to maintain an alkaline urine pH. Excretion of uranium-238/235 can be enhanced with the addition of a diuretic, such as furosemide [1,13].

Dimercaprol is a chelation agent that is particularly useful for the treatment of internal contamination with polonium-210. Dimercaprol is a chelation agent for mercury poisoning. For polonium-210 contamination, 5 mg per kg of dimercaprol should be given initially, followed by 2.5 mg per kg two times daily for 10 days. Dimercaprol should be given by deep intramuscular injection only; it should not be given intravenously. Dimercaprol is very nephrotoxic and should always be used with caution. It is recommended that oral sodium bicarbonate be given to maintain an alkaline urine pH, which decreases the risk of nephrotoxicity by preventing the dissociation of the dimercaprol–polonium-210 complex in the urine. Serum creatinine and urine pH should be carefully monitored during treatment with dimercaprol [1,13,26-30].

Need for Rapid Treatment

To be most effective, treatment for internal contamination should begin within hours after the radiation exposure. Early information on the history of a radiation exposure incident may or may not identify the major isotopes involved. Patients will likely present with no clinical symptoms other than conventional trauma. Therefore, critical decisions regarding the initial, empirical treatment of potential internal radiation contamination may have to be based on the historical information that is provided. It is imperative that physicians who could be involved in the management of radiation casualties be familiar with the agents used for the treatment of the most likely internal radiation contaminants. These agents are summarized in Table 129.3.

DECONTAMINATION

To prevent contamination of other patients and medical staff, radiation casualties must be decontaminated before admission into a hospital. However, life-saving emergency medical care should be performed as soon as possible and before decontamination takes place. Therefore, a special emergency treatment area, where potentially contaminated patients can be treated and stabilized, will have to be set up outside the hospital. Once a patient has been stabilized, decontamination can occur in another specially designated area that is also outside the hospital. It is recommended

TABLE 129.3

Agents Used to Treat Common Internal Radiation Contaminants

Radionuclide	Primary toxicity	Treatment	Agent category	Route
Americium-241	Bone and liver	Diethylenetriaminepentaacetic acid (DTPA)	Chelation	Intravenous (IV) infusion
Cesium-137	Total body	Prussian blue	Purgative	Oral
Cobalt-60	Total body	DTPA	Chelation	IV infusion
Iodine-125/131	Thyroid	Potassium iodide blocking	Oral	
Plutonium-239	Bone and lung	DTPA	Chelation	IV infusion
Polonium-210	Lung and kidney	Dimercaprol	Chelation	Intramuscular injection
Strontium-90	Bone	Aluminum phosphate	Purgative	Oral
Uranium-238/235	Kidney	$NaHCO_3$ and diuretic	Chelation	Oral

that the designated decontamination area be at least 50 yards downwind from the hospital or another treatment area.

All health care workers should protect themselves with scrubs, gowns, masks, double gloves, and shoe covers during the treatment and decontamination of radiation casualties. These measures provide sufficient protection from most radioactive isotopes that could be contaminating a patient. It is recommended that health care workers continue to observe these measures after decontamination of a radiation casualty because it is possible that the decontamination could be incomplete, and residual radioactive material could remain on or in the patient. It is best to assume that every patient near a radiation exposure event has been contaminated, even if no radiation is detected by a radiac meter. Such patients should be decontaminated as usual, and members of the decontamination team and medical treatment staff should wear protective clothing.

The decontamination process is quite simple. All of the patient's clothing must be removed and discarded into a clearly labeled and secure container so that it does not further contaminate people and surroundings after removal. If the clothing needs to be cut off the patient, the scissors should be washed with soap and water between each cut to avoid spreading contamination on subsequent cuts. After all the clothing has been removed, the patient is thoroughly washed with soap and water. This simple soap-and-water process has been shown to be effective in removing more than 95% of external residual radioactive material from radiation-exposed patients [1,13,26-30].

Once a radiation-exposed patient has been stabilized and decontaminated, he or she should be admitted into the hospital or another treatment facility for definitive care. Again, it is best to assume that hospitalized radiation-exposed patients may still be contaminated, even after the decontamination process has been completed. It is recommended that all radiation casualties be admitted to specially designated areas of the hospital and that the staff of these areas should wear appropriate protective clothing, as described earlier.

Patients exposed to potentially life-threatening doses of radiation will require critical care management during the manifest illness phase of an acute radiation subsyndrome. To reduce the potential for radioactive contamination, it is recommended that such patients be cared for in specially designated areas of intensive care units or in a designated hospital area that has been converted to an intensive care unit for the management of radiation casualties.

References

1. Oak Ridge Institute for Science and Education: Introduction and radiation basics in the medical aspects of radiation incidents. Revised ed. Oak Ridge, TN, Radiation Emergency Assistance Center/Training site REAC/TS 18, p 3–4, 2013. Available at https://orise.orau.gov/reacts/documents/medical-aspects-of-radiation-incidents.pdf. Accessed September 25, 2017.
2. Responding to an RDD/RED Emergency: the HHS Playbook, guidance for executive decision makers within the Department of Health and Human Services (HHS) in the event of an actual radiological terrorist attack in a U.S. city. (HHS/ASPR, April 2010).
3. Miller AC, Satyamitra M, Kulkarni S, et al: Late and low-level effects of ionizing radiation: medical consequences of radiological and nuclear warfare. Textbooks of military medicine: medical consequences of radiological and nuclear weapons. Borden Institute, Office of The Surgeon General, AMEDD center and school, 2013, p 197–198. Available at http://www.cs.amedd.army.mil/borden/FileDownloadpublic.aspx?docid=6a01adbd-9f6d-411d-9b18-05e0fc73cd65. Accessed July 22, 2016.
4. Christodouleas JP, Forrest RD, Ainsley CG, et al: Short-term and long-term health risks of nuclear-power-plant accidents. *N Engl J Med* 364(24):2334–2341, 2011.
5. William AB, José S, Catherine O'Hara, et al: 5 years after Fukushima—insights from current research. Amsterdam, Netherland, Elsevier online publishing, March 10, 2016.
6. Anzai K, Ban N, Ozawa T, et al: Fukushima Daiichi Nuclear Power Plant accident: facts, environmental contamination, possible biological effects, and countermeasures. *J Clin Biochem Nutr* 50(1):2–8, 2012. doi:10.3164/jcbn.D-11-00021.
7. Goans RE, Flynn DF: Acute radiation syndrome in humans. Medical Consequences of Nuclear Warfare, Textbooks of military medicine: medical consequences of radiological and nuclear weapons. Borden Institute, Office of The Surgeon General, AMEDD center and school, 2013, p 19–21, 25–26. Available at http://www.cs.amedd.army.mil/borden/FileDownloadpublic.aspx?docid=423f63d0-dc11-4ab1-99f2-31a5b47cc5ca. Accessed July 22, 2016.
8. Armed Forces Radiobiology Research Institute: Types of radiation, in Medical Management of Radiological Casualties. 4th ed. Bethesda, MD, Armed Forces Radiobiology Research Institute, p 8. Available at https://www.usuhs.edu/sites/default/files/media/afrri/pdf/4edmmrchandbook.pdf. Accessed July 22, 2016.
9. Shepherd G: Type of radiation: basic theory explained for the NonPhysicist, in *Medical Response to Terrorism: Preparedness and Clinical Practice*, 2005, p 138.
10. Hall EJ: Physics and chemistry of radiation absorption, in *Radiobiology of the Radiologist*. 7th ed. Philadelphia, PA, Lippincott, Williams and Wilkins, 2012.
11. Sedelnikova OA, Redon CE, Dickey JS, et al: Role of oxidatively induced DNA lesions in human pathogenesis. *Mutat Res* 704:152, 2010.
12. Armed Forces Radiobiology Research Institute: Units of radiation, in Medical Management of Radiological Casualties. 4th ed. Bethesda, MD, Armed Forces Radiobiology Research Institute, 2033, p 8, 9. Available at https://www.usuhs.edu/sites/default/files/media/afrri/pdf/4edmmrchandbook.pdf. Accessed July 22, 2016.
13. Flynn DF, Goans RE: Triage and treatment of radiation and combined-injury mass casualties. Textbooks of military medicine: medical consequences of radiological and nuclear weapons. Borden Institute, Office of The Surgeon General, AMEDD center and school, 2013, p 43–44, 61. Available at http://www.ncf-net.org/radiation/MedicalConsequencesOfNuclearWarfare3.pdf. Accessed September 28, 2017.
14. Sullivan JM, Prasanna PG, Grace MB, et al: Assessment of biodosimetry methods for a mass-casualty radiological incident: medical response and management considerations. *Health Phys* 105(6):540–554, 2013.
15. Woodruff CR Jr, et al: Radiological events and their consequences. Textbooks of military medicine: medical consequences of radiological and nuclear weapons. Borden Institute, Office of The Surgeon General, AMEDD center and school, 2013, p14. Available at http://www.cs.amedd.army.mil/borden/FileDownloadpublic.aspx?docid=45c8dcd5-8221-42b4-9dcc-e2ff0a5a4d9f. Accessed on July 22, 2016.
16. Dainiak N, Gent RN, Carr Z, et al: Literature review and global consensus on management of acute radiation syndrome affecting non-hematopoietic organ systems. *Disaster Med Public Health Prep* 5:183–201, 2011.
17. Radiation effect on blood counts (Illustration). Available at https://www.remm.nlm.gov/rad_bloodcounts.htm. Updated on January 12, 2016. Accessed on July 22, 2016.
18. Armed Forces Radiobiology Research Institute: Gastrointestinal syndrome. Medical Management of Radiological Casualties. 4th ed. Bethesda, MD, Armed Forces Radiobiology Research Institute, 2033, p 14. Available at https://www.usuhs.edu/sites/default/files/media/afrri/pdf/4edmmrchandbook.pdf. Accessed July 22, 2016.
19. Centers for Disease Control and Prevention: Acute Radiation Syndrome: A Fact Sheet for Physicians. Available at http://emergency.cdc.gov/radiation/arsphysicianfactsheet.asp. Accessed July 22, 2016.
20. Heslet L, Bay C, Nepper-Christensen S: Acute radiation syndrome (ARS)—treatment of the reduced host defense. *Int J Gen Med* 5:105–115, 2012.
21. Ishii T, Futami S, Nishida M, et al: Brief note and evaluation of acute-radiation syndrome and treatment of a Tokai-mura criticality accident patient. *J Radiat Res* 42(Suppl):167, 2001.
22. Radiation Emergency Medical Management: Multi-organ Injury, Multi-organ Dysfunction Syndrome, Multi-organ Failure: A New Hypothesis of Whole Body Radiation Effects. Available at https://www.remm.nlm.gov/multiorganinjury.htm. Accessed July 22, 2016.
23. Fliedner TM, Dörr HD, Meineke V: Multi-organ involvement as a pathogenetic principle of the radiation syndromes: a study involving 110 case histories documented in SEARCH and classified as the bases of haematopoietic indicators of effect. *Br J Radiol* (2005), 2014. (Suppl 27):1–8. doi:10.1259/bjr/77700378
24. Gorbunov NV, Sharma P: Protracted oxidative alterations in the mechanism of hematopoietic acute radiation syndrome. *Antioxidants (Basel)* 4(1):134–152, 2015.
25. Flynn DF, Goans RE: Triage and treatment of radiation and combined-injury mass casualties. Textbooks of military medicine: medical consequences of radiological and nuclear weapons. Borden Institute, Office of The Surgeon General, AMEDD center and school.2013, p 19, 24. Available at http://www.cs.amedd.army.mil/borden/FileDownloadpublic.aspx?docid=b3d9d96a-a8b8-499c-bddf-e27791466b77. Accessed July 22, 2016.
26. Singh VK, Romaine PL, Newman VL: Biologics as countermeasures for acute radiation syndrome: where are we now? *Expert Opin Biol Ther* 15(4):465–471, 2015.
27. Armed Forces Radiobiology Research Institute: Other injuries from nuclear weapon, in Medical Management of Radiological Casualties. 4th ed. Bethesda, MD, Armed Forces Radiobiology Research Institute, 2033, p 24, 36–37. Available at https://www.usuhs.edu/sites/default/files/media/afrri/pdf/4edmmrchandbook.pdf. Accessed July 22, 2016.
28. Armed Forces Radiobiology Research Institute: Medical management of internally deposited radionuclides. Medical Management of Radiological Casualties. 4th ed. Bethesda, MD, Armed Forces Radiobiology Research Institute, 2033, p 29–36. Available at https://www.usuhs.edu/sites/default/files/media/afrri/pdf/4edmmrchandbook.pdf. Accessed July 22, 2016.
29. Kalinich JF: Treatment of Internal radionuclide contamination. Medical consequences of radiological and nuclear weapons. p 75–78, 2012.
30. Armed Forces Radiobiology Research Institute: Medical Management of Radiological Casualties. 4th ed. Bethesda, MD, Armed Forces Radiobiology Research Institute, 2033, p 44–46. Available at https://www.usuhs.edu/sites/default/files/media/afrri/pdf/4edmmrchandbook.pdf. Accessed July 22, 2016.

Chapter 130 ■ Critical Care Consequences of Weapons (or Agents) of Mass Destruction—Biological Agents of Mass Destruction

RYAN C. MAVES • KONRAD L. DAVIS • CHARLES G. VOLK • ASHA V. DEVEREAUX

OVERVIEW

Ancient use of contaminated water, animal carcasses, and toxins used as tools against enemy forces date as early as prehistoric times and the first evidence of mass use was in 184 BCE when Hannibal ordered serpent-filled pots to be hurled onto enemy decks in the naval battle of Eurymedon. The pots shattered, and the ensuing chaos gave victory to the Carthaginians. During the French and Indian War in 1763, British Captain Ecuyer used "two Blankets and a Handkerchief from the Smallpox Hospital" intentionally as a biologic agent to weaken Native Americans supportive of the French, leading to outbreaks of smallpox among tribes in the Ohio region [1]. German, Japanese, British, and American forces all evaluated the potential use of bioweapons during World War I. Bioterrorism remains an active concern today owing to discoveries of Al-Qaeda laboratories for biologic weapons in Iraq and sporadic criminal events such as the October 2001 anthrax attacks in the US mail, leading to 22 cases of anthrax and five deaths [2,3]. These attacks demonstrate the need for clinicians to be prepared to deal with bioterrorism attacks in their respective communities. Additionally, the concept of "biocrime" is important for clinicians to distinguish, where there is a malevolent motivation to use a biologic agent against an individual person [4].

The Center for Disease Control (CDC) categorizes potential bioterrorism agents based on their severity, availability, and potential for widespread harm in the event of release. The agents in each category are summarized in Table 130.1. *Category A* agents have the greatest potential for the production of mass casualties and a major adverse public health impact. *Category B* agents have some potential for large-scale dissemination and mass casualties, but would be expected to cause less illness and death than Category A agents. *Category* C agents are those that do not pose a high bioterrorism threat at the present time but could emerge as a future threat. This chapter focuses on Category A agents that have the greatest ability to cause mass casualties and significant loss of life. However, some Category B agents, such as ricin, are also discussed because of their potential to be used as clandestine agents of terrorism [5,6]. Table 130.2 provides the clinician some useful Emergency Response Phone Numbers in case there is suspicion of an incident.

SMALLPOX

The last case of endemic smallpox occurred in Somalia in 1977. In 1980, the World Health Organization (WHO) declared that the disease was eradicated. However, in recent years there has been renewed concern about the variola virus, the causative agent of smallpox, primarily owing to the potential of the variola virus to be used as a biologic weapon of mass destruction. As a result of this concern, the WHO has restricted the number of laboratories officially authorized to serve as repositories for the variola virus to two: the CDC in Atlanta, Georgia, and the Vektor Institute in Novosibirsk, Russia [7,8].

Although smallpox has been officially declared to be eradicated, there is a possibility for its reemergence. Live smallpox virus has been inadvertently stored in laboratories from past experiments, leading to the potential for accidental release [9]. There is historical evidence of smallpox virus survival in interred and exhumed individuals from the 18th century [10].

The US military began vaccination of deploying forces against smallpox on December 13, 2002 [11]. Much has been learned regarding the indications, contraindications, and efficacy of the vaccine since this mass immunization process began. Considerable thought has also been given to the dire consequences of a smallpox attack and the preparations necessary to manage a

TABLE 130.1

Bioterrorism Risk Categories

Category A	Category B	Category C
Bacillus anthracis (anthrax)	*Coxiella burnetii* (Q fever)	Nipah virus
Yersinia pestis (plague)	Brucella spp. (brucellosis)	Hantavirus
Variola major (smallpox)	*Burkholderia mallei* (Glanders)	Tickborne hemorrhagic fever viruses
Clostridium botulinum (botulism)	Ricin	Tickborne encephalitis viruses
Francisella tularensis (tularemia)	*Clostridium perfringens*	Yellow fever
Viral hemorrhagic fevers	Epsilon toxin	Multidrug-resistant tuberculosis
	Staphylococcal enterotoxin B	

Adapted from CDC.gov; Christian MD: Biowarfare and bioterrorism. Crit Care Clin 29:717–756, 2013.

TABLE 130.2

Emergency Response Phone Numbers

USAMRIID Emergency Response Line	888-872-7443
United States Army Chemical Materials Activity Operations Center Line	410-436-4484
(CDC) Emergency Response Line	770-488-7100
FEMA Center for Domestic Preparedness Line	866-213-9553

CDC, Center for Disease Control; FEMA, Federal Emergency Management Agency; USAMRIID, United States Army Medical Research Institute of Infectious Diseases.

large-scale epidemic resulting from such an attack [12,13]. This section focuses on those aspects of smallpox infection that are most relevant to the critical care physician.

Virology

The causative agent of smallpox, the variola virus, is a member of the Poxviridae family, subfamily Chordopoxvirinae, and genus Orthopoxvirus. This genus also includes vaccinia (used in the smallpox vaccine), monkey pox virus, camel pox, and cowpox. The variola virus, like other members of the Poxviridae family, is a large, enveloped, deoxyribonucleic acid (DNA) virus. Poxviridae are the only viruses that can replicate in the cytoplasm of cells without involvement of the cell nucleus. The variola virus has a brick-shaped morphology, measures 260 by 150 nm, and has one of the largest viral genomes known. Its large genome makes it difficult to genetically engineer or synthesize the virus in the laboratory. Humans are the only known reservoir for the variola virus, although monkeys are susceptible to infection [14]. The variola virus is very stable and maintains infectivity for long periods of time outside the human host [15]. There are two strains of variola, variola major and variola minor. Variola major is more virulent with a mortality rate between 20% and 50% in infected individuals. Variola minor causes a similar illness, but the mortality is less than 1% [16].

Transmission and Pathogenesis

Transmission of variola occurs from person to person by the dispersion of respiratory droplet nuclei. Transmission is enhanced by infected individuals who have a cough, however, detailed dispersal and pathogenic mechanisms are unclear owing to limited technologic tools available when smallpox was an endemic human disease [17]. Although infrequent, infection has also been known to occur following contact with infected clothing, bedding, or other contaminated fomites [18].

Following inhalation, the variola virus seeds the mucus membranes of the upper and lower respiratory tract and then migrates to regional lymph nodes, where viral replication occurs. Viral replication in regional lymph nodes leads to viremia, which results in systemic dissemination of the virus to other organs including the liver, spleen, skin, lung, brain, and bone marrow, where it continues to replicate. Clinical symptoms typically develop after an incubation period of 7 to 17 days. Following the initial infection period of 1 to 4 days in which viremia occurs, the clinical manifestations of smallpox appear in a series of distinct phases. These phases are uniquely characteristic of smallpox and are summarized in Table 130.3.

Unlike varicella, the skin lesions of smallpox are mostly of the same type and same stage of development throughout each clinical phase (Figs. 130.1 and 130.2). In contrast, the skin lesions associated with varicella are greatest on the trunk, spare the hands and soles, and are at multiple stages at any given time, with papules, vesicles, and crusts all present simultaneously.

The mortality rate from the usual variety of smallpox is 3% in vaccinated individuals and 30% in the unvaccinated. Death from smallpox is presumed to be secondary to overwhelming quantities of immune complexes and soluble variola antigen. This smallpox-associated systemic inflammatory response results in severe hypotension during the second week of illness. Respiratory complications, such as pneumonia, and secondary bacteremia are common. Severe intravascular volume and electrolyte imbalances may occur, along with associated acute kidney injury. Rare secondary manifestations include encephalitis, arthritis, and orchitis [16].

Two atypical manifestations of smallpox have very high mortality rates. Hemorrhagic smallpox occurs in less than 3% of infected individuals. The hemorrhagic form is characterized by a short incubation period and an erythematous skin eruption that later becomes petechial and hemorrhagic, similar to the lesions seen in meningococcemia. Most individuals with the hemorrhagic form of smallpox die in 5 to 6 days after onset of the rash. The malignant form, or "flat smallpox," is characterized by a fine-grained, reddish, nonpustular, and confluent rash, occasionally with hemorrhage. The malignant form occurs in 2% to 5% of infected individuals. Affected patients have severe systemic illness and most die within several days. Pulmonary edema occurs frequently in both hemorrhagic and malignant smallpox, contributing to the high mortality rates [16,18].

The primary long-term sequela of smallpox is the "pockmarks" that affect the skin. These are pitted lesions that permanently scar the face owing to involvement of sebaceous glands. Panophthalmitis, viral keratitis, and corneal ulcers can cause permanent blindness in 1% of infected individuals. Infection with smallpox results in lifelong immunity [19].

Diagnosis

The differential diagnosis of papulovesicular lesions that can be confused with smallpox includes chickenpox (varicella), shingles (herpes zoster), disseminated herpes simplex, monkeypox, drug eruptions, generalized vaccinia, eczema vaccinatum, impetigo, bullous pemphigoid, erythema multiforme, molluscum contagiosum, and secondary syphilis. Severe varicella is the most common eruption that can be confused with smallpox. Table 130.4 delineates clinical features that can help to distinguish varicella from smallpox.

Confirmation of smallpox can be performed by the analysis of skin scrapings, vesicular fluid, or oropharyngeal swabs. Specimens should be collected using respiratory and contact isolation procedures, ideally by previously vaccinated personnel. Specimen collection techniques and guidelines are available from public health departments, the CDC, and the WHO [20]. https://www.cdc.gov/smallpox/lab-personnel/specimen-collection/specimen-collection-procedures.html.

The brick-shaped variola virus is distinguished from varicella-zoster by electron microscopy. However, polymerase chain reaction (PCR) assays are the mainstay of diagnosis at the present time. Serologic testing is not useful for differentiating the variola virus from other orthopoxviruses. Laboratory specimens should only be manipulated and processed at laboratories with Biosafety Level 4 facilities [12]. If smallpox is suspected, the local public health department must be notified immediately. Public health departments can provide valuable assistance in collecting specimens and getting them to an appropriate laboratory for analysis.

Infection Control

Although the primary transmission of smallpox is via respiratory droplet nuclei, infected clothing and bedding can also transmit

TABLE 130.3

Smallpox Disease	Smallpox Signs and Symptoms
Incubation period (Duration: 7 to 17 d) *Not contagious*	**Exposure to the virus** is followed by an incubation period during which people do not have any symptoms and may feel fine. This incubation period averages about 12 to 14 d but can range from 7 to 17 d. During this time, people are not contagious.
Initial symptoms *(Prodrome)* (Duration: 2 to 4 d) *Sometimes contagious*[a]	The **first symptoms** of smallpox include fever, malaise, head and body aches, and sometimes vomiting. The fever is usually high, in the range of 101 to 104°F. At this time, people are usually too sick to carry on their normal activities. This is called the *prodrome* phase and may last for 2 to 4 d.
Early rash (Duration: about 4 d) *Most contagious*	A **rash emerges** first as small red spots on the tongue and in the mouth. These spots develop into sores that break open and spread large amounts of the virus into the mouth and throat. At this time, the person becomes **most contagious**.
Rash distribution: View enlarged image.	Around the time the sores in the mouth break down, a rash appears on the skin, starting on the face and spreading to the arms and legs and then to the hands and feet. Usually the rash spreads to all parts of the body within 24 h. As the rash appears, the fever usually falls and the person may start to feel better. By the third day of the rash, the rash becomes raised bumps. By the fourth day, the bumps fill with a thick, opaque fluid and often have a depression in the center that looks like a bellybutton. (This is a major distinguishing characteristic of smallpox.) Fever often will rise again at this time and remain high until scabs form over the bumps.
Pustular rash (Duration: about 5 d) *Contagious*	The bumps become **pustules**—sharply raised, usually round and firm to the touch as if there's a small round object under the skin. People often say the bumps feel like BB pellets embedded in the skin.
Pustules and scabs (Duration: about 5 d) *Contagious*	The pustules begin to form a crust and then **scab**. By the end of the second week after the rash appears, most of the sores have scabbed over.
Resolving scabs (Duration: about 6 d) *Contagious*	The scabs begin to fall off, leaving marks on the skin that eventually become pitted **scars**. Most scabs will have fallen off 3 wks after the rash appears. The person is contagious to others until all of the scabs have fallen off.
Scabs resolved *Not contagious*	Scabs have fallen off. Person is no longer contagious.

[a]Smallpox may be contagious during the *prodrome* phase, but is most infectious during the first 7 to 10 d following rash onset.
From https://www.cdc.gov/smallpox/symptoms/index.html. Accessed September 17, 2016; https://upload.wikimedia.org/wikipedia/commons/6/6a/Smallpox_%28variola_orthopox_virus_%29_Early_Rash_vs_chickenpox.gif.

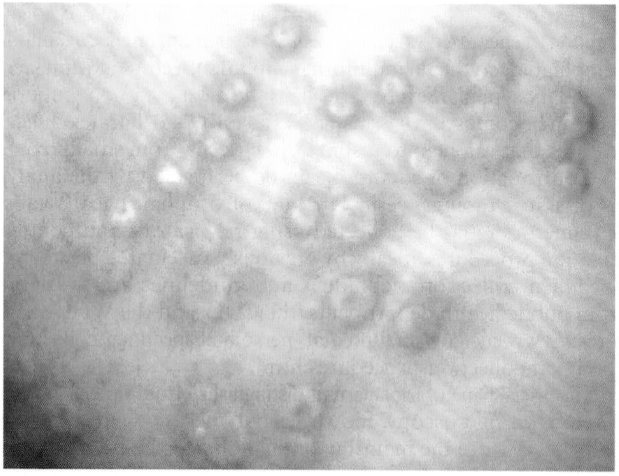

FIGURE 130.1 Smallpox pustular phase umbilicated lesions (Picture from "Quick Bio-Agents Guide, First Edition, 2012. Available for download at http://www.usamriid.army.mil/education/instruct.htm. Accessed September 21, 2016).

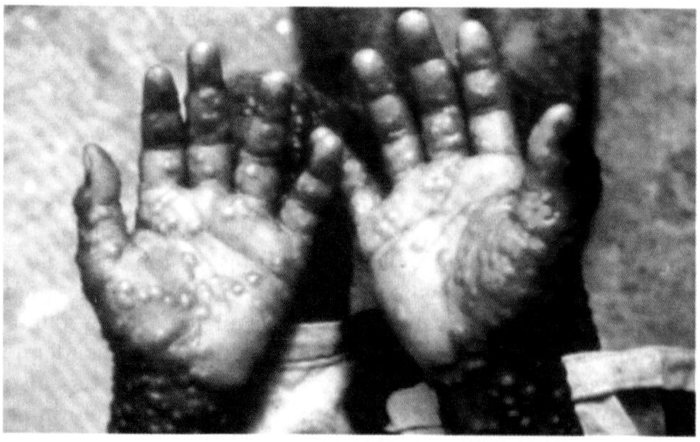

FIGURE 130.2 Smallpox pustular lesions of the hands (Picture from "Quick Bio-Agents Guide, First Edition, 2012. Available for download at http://www.usamriid.army.mil/education/instruct.htm Accessed September 21, 2016).

disease [10]. Individuals with smallpox are most infectious within the first 7 to 10 days of the rash, but the disease is contagious until all crusted lesions have fallen off [16]. Secondary cases occur in family members or health care workers who are exposed to an infectious individual. It is estimated that the rate of transmission may be as high as six new cases for every infected person among unvaccinated contacts [21]. All individuals who have direct contact with the index case should be quarantined for 17 days in respiratory isolation. Home quarantine will be necessary during mass casualty situations. Health care workers caring for infected individuals should be vaccinated and use strict airborne and contact isolation procedures. Infected patients should be placed in respiratory and contact precautions and managed in a negative-pressure isolation room. Patients should remain under precautions until all crusted lesions have fallen off. Patients and exposed personnel should also be vaccinated if the disease is in the early stage. If performed early, vaccination may significantly decrease the severity of smallpox symptoms [19,22].

TABLE 130.4

Distinguishing Characteristics Between Smallpox and Chickenpox

	Smallpox	Chickenpox
Prodrome	2–4 d of high fever, headache backache, vomiting, abdominal pain	Absent-to-mild, 1 d
Rash	Starts in oral mucosa, spreads to face, and expands centripetally	Starts on trunk and expands centrifugally
Palms/soles	Common	Rare
Timing	Lesions appear and progress at same time	Lesions occur in crops; lesions at varied stages of maturation
Pain	May be painful	Often pruritic
Depth	Pitting and deep scars	Superficial; does not scar

Treatment

Cidofovir is an antiviral drug, currently approved in the US for use in cytomegalovirus retinitis. This agent has broad-spectrum in vitro activity against numerous DNA viruses, including orthopoxviruses in animal models. Cidofovir is a long-acting nucleotide analogue that must be administered intravenously and carries a high risk of nephrotoxicity, requiring coadministration with oral probenecid to minimize this risk. Cidofovir given at the time of, or immediately following, exposure has the potential to prevent cowpox, vaccinia, and monkeypox. Aerosolized cidofovir has been shown to protect mice against intranasal challenge with the cowpox virus [23] and against rabbits undergoing rabbitpox challenge [24].

Other investigational agents with evidence of activity against variola include tecovirimat (ST-246), a novel inhibitor of orthopoxvirus egress from infected mammalian cells, and brincidofovir (CMX001), an oral lipid conjugate of cidofovir [25] (Table 130.5). Anti-vaccinia immune globulin decreases pulmonary viral loads and pneumonitis in animals with vaccinia or cowpox, but its benefit in smallpox is unproven [24,26–33].

Immunization

Smallpox vaccination is based on the principle of cross-immunity between variola and vaccinia, a derivative of the closely related cowpox virus (and the ultimate source of the word "vaccine"). Vaccination continues to be the mainstay of smallpox prevention. First-generation live virus vaccines (Dryvax, Aventis Pasteur Smallpox Vaccine [APSV], Lancy-Vaxina, and L-IVP) were effective, but at the cost of numerous side effects, reactions, and contraindications. Newer-generation vaccines include replication-competent vaccines such as ACAM2000 (Sanofi Pasteur) and the APSV (Aventis Pasteur), which are capable of replication in human cells, and Imvamune (Bavarian Nordic), a highly attenuated vaccinia strain which is incapable of replication in mammalian cells and is recommended for use in immunocompromised persons for whom ACAM2000 and APSV would be contraindicated. There has been considerable discussion regarding the efficacy of preexposure mass vaccination to protect the public against smallpox in the event of a bioterrorism attack. The CDC maintains three smallpox vaccines in the national stockpile: ACAM2000, Aventis Pasteur Smallpox Vaccine (APSV), and Imvamune [19]. Table 130.6 provides recommended usage.

The WHO and CDC instructions for the administration of smallpox vaccine are as follows:

- *Site of vaccination*: Outer aspect of upper arm over the insertion of the deltoid muscle.
- *Preparation of skin*: None, unless the site is obviously dirty. Use water to cleanse the site because the use of a disinfectant can kill the virus.
- *Withdrawal of vaccine from the ampule*: A cool, sterile bifurcated needle is inserted into the reconstituted vaccine ampule. A droplet is sufficient for vaccination and is contained within the fork of the needle. Never dip the same needle back into the ampule to avoid contamination.
- *Application*: The needle is held at 90 degrees perpendicular to the skin; the needle then touches the skin to release the droplet. For primary vaccination, three strokes are made in a 5-mm area. For revaccination, 15 up/down, perpendicular strokes of the needle are rapidly made in the area of 5 mm diameter (through the drop of vaccine deposited on the skin). The strokes should be sufficiently vigorous so that a trace of blood appears at the site. If blood does not appear, the procedure (three strokes) should be repeated with the same needle.
- *Dressing*: Although the WHO does not recommend a dressing, the CDC recommends a loose sterile gauze dressing covered by a semipermeable dressing to prevent transmission of the

TABLE 130.5

Investigational Agents in the Treatment of Smallpox

Agent	Mechanism and response
Cidofovir	Long-acting nucleotide analogue that selectively inhibits viral DNA polymerase. Intravenous, nephrotoxic; must be coadministered with probenecid. Investigational inhaled form (NanoFOVIR, Nanotherapeutics Corp., Florida, USA) under investigation for postexposure prophylaxis in rabbit model of poxvirus infection.
Brincidofovir (CMX001)	Lipid-conjugated form of cidofovir; may be administered orally. Available under investigational new drug protocol via manufacturer (Chimerix).
Tecovirimat (ST-246)	Inhibits poxvirus egress from infected host cells, with reductions in dermal lesion counts, oropharyngeal virus shedding, and viral DNA circulating in the blood of nonhuman primates. Resistance has been described when used in treatment of human disseminated vaccinia.
VIG	Utilized in the treatment of disseminated vaccinia with experience during monkeypox outbreaks. No human data on efficacy against smallpox. Must be obtained from CDC Strategic National Stockpile via state public health departments.

Derived from Smee DF: "Orthopoxvirus inhibitors that are active in animal models: an update from 2008 to 2012." Future Virol 8:891–901, 2013.
DNA, deoxyribonucleic acid; CDC, Center for Disease Control; VIG, vaccinia immune globulin.

TABLE 130.6

Summary of CDC Recommendations for Smallpox Vaccine Use During a Postevent Vaccination Program, by Population and Risk

Population	Exposed to smallpox virus	High risk for smallpox infection without known exposure to smallpox virus
Persons without severe immunodeficiency or relative contraindications	Recommended with ACAM2000	Recommended with ACAM2000
Severely immunodeficient persons who are not expected to benefit from smallpox vaccine include those with: • HIV CD4 cell count <50 cells/μL • bone marrow transplant (<4 mo) • SCID • complete DiGeorge syndrome • other immunocompromised states requiring isolation	Not recommended but reasonable to consider Imvamune when antivirals are not immediately available	Not recommended
Persons with other immunocompromised states (i.e., solid organ transplant recipients within 3 mo of transplantation, bone marrow transplant recipients during the 4–24 mo time period following transplantation, transplant recipients with active graft-versus-host disease, and individuals receiving immunosuppressive therapies)	Recommended with ACAM2000	Recommended with Imvamune if vaccine is available and regulatory mechanism in place
Atopic dermatitis	Recommended with ACAM2000	Recommended with Imvamune but ACAM2000 preferred for persons with history of smallpox vaccination without complications
HIV CD4 cell count 50–199 cells/μL	Recommended with ACAM2000	Recommended with Imvamune
HIV CD4 cell count ≥200 cells/μL	Recommended with ACAM2000	Recommended with ACAM2000
Allergy to vaccine or vaccine component	*Previous dose:* Recommended with ACAM2000 in facility capable of treating an anaphylactic reaction *Vaccine component of ACAM2000:* Recommended with APSV, but if unavailable, administer ACAM2000 in facility capable of treating an anaphylactic reaction	If available, use vaccine that does not contain the known allergen (vaccine strain or component). If such a vaccine is unavailable, the person should be offered vaccination with any available smallpox vaccine in a facility capable of treating an anaphylactic reaction
Pregnant and breastfeeding women[a]	Recommended with ACAM2000	Recommended with ACAM2000
Age: pediatric and geriatric[a]	Recommended with ACAM2000	Recommended with ACAM2000
Known heart disease or cardiac risk factors[a]	Recommended with ACAM2000	Recommended with ACAM2000
Health-care workers[a]	Recommended with ACAM2000	Recommended with ACAM2000
Persons who cannot be vaccinated for any reason (e.g., medical conditions, resource constraints, or otherwise)	Provide clear information about prodromal and disease-specific manifestations, how to self-assess for these symptoms, and when and where to seek care if these symptoms occur. Monitor for signs and symptoms suggestive of smallpox, including fever and prostration	

[a]Persons with a relative contraindication should be classified on the basis of the relative contraindication rather than on their pregnancy, breastfeeding, age, cardiac, or health-care worker status.
CD4, cluster of differentiation 4; CDC, Center for Disease Control; HIV, human immune deficiency virus; SCID, severe combined immunodeficiency.
From Petersen BW DI, Pertowski CA: Clinical guidance for smallpox vaccine use in a postevent vaccination program. MMWR 64:1–30, 2015.

virus. Absorb the excess blood and vaccine with gauze, and dispose the gauze in a biohazard receptacle.

- *Unused vaccine*: Unused vaccine is good for 90 days after reconstitution and should be refrigerated without any special light precautions.

The most common adverse reactions following smallpox vaccination are tenderness and erythema at the injection site and secondary bacterial infections [34]. Inadvertent autoinoculation of another body site, generalized vaccinia (vesicles or pustules appearing on normal skin distant from the vaccination site), eczema vaccinatum, vaccinia keratitis, encephalitis, and progressive vaccinia have been reported in primary vaccinations. A review of approximately 39,000 people vaccinated against smallpox (36% primary vaccinations and 64% revaccinations) reported the following adverse reactions: encephalitis in one individual, myopericarditis in 21 individuals, generalized vaccinia in two individuals, inadvertent inoculation in seven individuals, and ocular vaccinia in three individuals [35].

Myopericarditis was reported for 200 cases from a prior US military vaccination program, at a rate of 117 cases per million vaccines [11,36]. This postvaccination myopericarditis is likely to be immunologically mediated and not the result of direct viral infection of the myocardium. The reported rate of cardiac mortality is 1.1 deaths per million primary vaccines. Routine vaccination is not recommended for persons with known cardiac disease or three or more risk factors for coronary artery disease, but vaccination is recommended for persons following a known exposure or at high risk for exposure [19].

Contraindications to smallpox vaccination are infants less than 1 year of age; immune suppression; eczema; exfoliative skin conditions; pemphigus; cardiac disease as previously described; allergy to any component of the vaccine; and pregnant or breastfeeding women. Individuals who are taking high-dose corticosteroids should not be vaccinated within 1 month of completing corticosteroid therapy. Although testing for human immunodeficiency virus (HIV) is not mandatory prior to smallpox vaccination, HIV testing should be readily available to all individuals considering smallpox vaccination [37,38]. Individuals with a contraindication to vaccination should avoid people who have been recently vaccinated, owing to possible transmission of vaccinia from viral shedding at the vaccination site. A small number of deaths (12/68) in the 1960s were attributed to unvaccinated persons exposed to recently vaccinated friends or family members [35].

Health care workers must be aware of the possibility for the nosocomial transmission of vaccinia during the hospitalization of a recently vaccinated patient. Nosocomial infection can result in mortality up to 11% [39,40]. Direct carriage of the virus on the hands, nasal mucosa, fomites, contaminated equipment, and laundry has been implicated in the transmission of vaccinia. Risk of the nosocomial transmission can be mitigated by several simple precautions. Semipermeable dressings should be applied to the site of a recent vaccination and changed frequently if there is evidence of the accumulation of purulent material. Gloves must be worn during dressing changes and meticulous handwashing with antimicrobial soap must be performed by all health care providers, both before and after contact with a recently vaccinated patient. Contaminated dressings should be disposed of in a biohazard container. Care should be taken to avoid contact of the vaccination site with material or equipment that could transmit the virus to other individuals. Clothing, towels, and other cloth materials that have contact with the site can be decontaminated by routine laundering with hot water. If at all possible, health care workers who are responsible for dressing changes should be vaccinated against smallpox, but nonvaccinated individuals are acceptable as long as appropriate precautions are observed [19,37].

Treatment of adverse effects following smallpox vaccination include supportive therapy, administration of vaccinia immune globulin, cidofovir, and an antiviral ophthalmic ointment, such as trifluridine or vidarabine, for eye involvement. Vaccinia immune globulin is available from the CDC, although the supply is limited. Cidofovir is available at no cost from the CDC under investigational use if a patient fails to respond to VIG, the patient is near death, or all inventories of VIG are depleted. The dose of cidofovir is 5 mg per kg, given intravenously, over 60 minutes as a single dose [41]. More recently, the oral prodrug of cidofovir, brincidofovir (CMX001), has been used in patients with disseminated vaccinia in combination with VIG and tecovirimat (ST-246) with reasonable outcomes [42]. Based on this limited human experience as well as animal data [26], it appears that combination therapy with VIG and either cidofovir or brincidofovir represents the best available therapy for disseminated vaccinia, and possibly for smallpox, at this time.

ACAM2000, a cell culture-derived smallpox vaccine that has demonstrated 94% efficacy in phase II clinical trials, was licensed by the Federal Drug Administration (FDA) for administration to people at high risk of smallpox or other orthopoxvirus diseases in 2007. Over 200 million doses of the vaccine have been purchased by the US Strategic National Stockpile (covering approximately 62% of the population), but it is not available for commercial use. Clinical trials show similar efficacy and side effects profile to the older Dryvax vaccination, but ACAM200 cannot be diluted [43].

In the event of an intentional release of variola virus, the priority of vaccination (Table 130.6) is as follows [19]:

- *Group 1*: Individuals directly exposed to the release.
- *Group 2*: Individuals with face-to-face household contact with a directly exposed individual.
- *Group 3*: Personnel directly involved in the evaluation, care, or transport of infected patients.
- *Group 4*: Laboratory personnel responsible for handling and processing specimens, and others who may be exposed to infectious materials.

ANTHRAX

In the fall of 2001, 22 cases of anthrax with five deaths occurred in the USA as a result of anthrax spores in envelopes sent through the US mail. Early recognition and treatment of anthrax by astute clinicians was responsible for preventing additional deaths [2,3]. Identification of a single case should prompt notification of local, state, and national public health authorities. The CDC and US military have rapid response teams with specialized expertise, training, and equipment that can be deployed immediately to assist local authorities in the event of a bioterrorism attack [44]. Cases of endemic anthrax occur in developing countries worldwide, with sporadic cases occurring in industrialized countries owing to occupational exposure or illegal drug abuse.

Microbiology

Bacillus anthracis is a large, gram-positive, aerobic, spore-forming, nonmotile bacillus as shown in Figure 130.3. The endospore form of *B. anthracis* is found in the soil of many regions of the world. Its virulence is determined by two plasmids. One plasmid involves the synthesis of a poly-D-glutamic acid capsule that inhibits phagocytosis of vegetative bacilli and the other contains genes for the synthesis of exotoxins. The exotoxins are known as *protective antigen*, *edema factor*, and *lethal factor*. The *protective antigen* is a binding protein that is necessary for entry into the host cell and combines with both edema factor and lethal factor to produce "edema toxin" and "lethal toxin" [45]. Edema toxin converts adenosine triphosphate to cyclic adenosine monophosphate (cAMP), resulting in high intracellular cAMP levels that impair water homeostasis and thereby cause cellular edema. Lethal toxin stimulates the overproduction of cytokines, primarily tumor necrosis factor-α and interleukin-1-β that cause macrophage lysis. The sudden release of inflammatory mediators appears to be responsible for the marked clinical toxicity of the bacteremic form of anthrax [46].

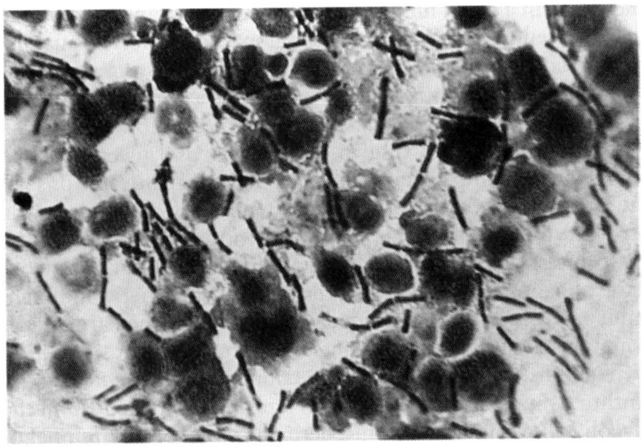

FIGURE 130.3 *Bacillus anthracis* (This photomicrograph reveals numerous rod-shaped *Bacillus anthracis* bacteria, demonstrating typical large, rectangular-appearing gram-positive bacilli in chains with classic "box-car" morphology. Public Health Image Library, Centers for Disease Control and Prevention, http://phil.cdc.gov.)

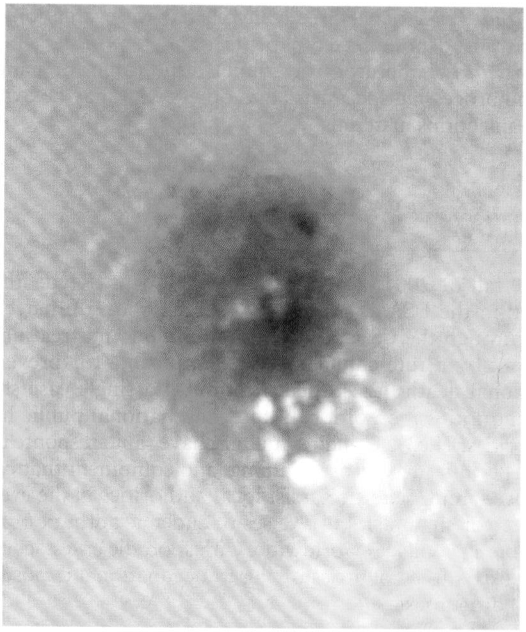

FIGURE 130.4 Cutaneous anthrax papule. (Picture from "Quick Bio-Agents Guide, First Edition, 2012. Available for download at http://www.usamriid.army.mil/education/instruct.htm).

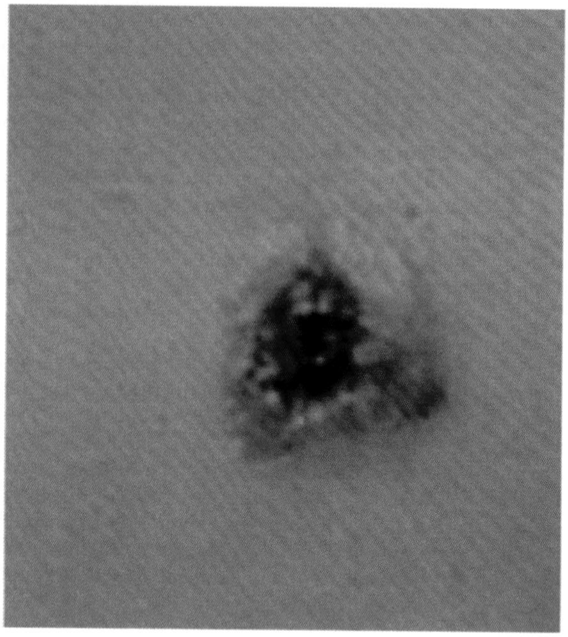

FIGURE 130.5 Cutaneous anthrax eschar (Picture from "Quick Bio-Agents Guide, First Edition, 2012. Available for download at http://www.usamriid.army.mil/education/instruct.htm).

Clinical Manifestations

There are three major forms of anthrax infection. The clinical characteristics of each form are determined by the route of entry of the anthrax spores. *Cutaneous anthrax* is the most common naturally occurring form, comprising approximately 95% of cases. Spores enter the body through breaks in the skin and germinate within days, resulting in soft tissue or mucosal edema and localized necrosis. Initially, a painless, pruritic papule appears as in Figure 130.4, followed by vesiculation, ulceration, and a black, "coal-like" painless eschar as shown in Figure 130.5, thereby demonstrating the origin or the name, anthrax (*anthrax* is the Greek term for coal). A surrounding rim of nonpitting edema may distinguish the eschar of anthrax from other diseases, such as typhus. The eschar sloughs within 2 to 3 weeks of onset [47]. Abscess formation occurs only with superinfection. Painful proximal lymphadenopathy and lymphangitis may accompany the primary lesion. Cutaneous anthrax may spread hematogenously with significant morbidity and death in a small number of individuals. Cutaneous anthrax has been reported to cause microangiopathic hemolytic anemia, renal dysfunction, and coagulopathy [48]. *Gastrointestinal* and *oropharyngeal anthrax* usually occur following the ingestion of contaminated meat. This is a rare manifestation of anthrax, with most cases occurring in Africa. Mucosal ulcers, edema, and regional lymphadenopathy are initial manifestations. In the oropharyngeal form, pseudomembranes are seen in the oropharynx and upper airway obstruction can develop. In the gastrointestinal form, a necrotizing infection progresses from the esophagus to the cecum. Fever, nausea, vomiting, abdominal pain, gastrointestinal bleeding, and bloody diarrhea are typical symptoms. Death results from intestinal perforation or sepsis [45].

The third form of anthrax infection is *inhalational anthrax*. Anthrax spores are 1 to 1.5 μm in size and easily deposit in the alveoli following inhalation. There, the endospores are phagocytosed by the pulmonary macrophages and transported via lymphatics to the mediastinal lymph nodes, where they may remain dormant as "vegetative cells" for approximately 10 to 60 days or longer. Once germination in the lymph nodes is complete, bacterial replication occurs. The replicating bacteria release edema and lethal toxins that produce a hemorrhagic mediastinitis.

Inhalational anthrax may present as a biphasic illness, with the initial syndrome resembling an upper respiratory tract infection to include fever, chills, fatigue, nonproductive cough, nausea, dyspnea, chest pain, and myalgias (Table 130.7). These symptoms typically last for 2 to 3 days and then progress to a more severe, fulminant illness. Meningitis should be considered early in the evaluation, because its presence may warrant more aggressive therapy [44]. Almost 50% of patients with inhalational anthrax develop hemorrhagic meningitis as a result of the hematogenous spread of *B. anthracis*. Dyspnea and shock characterize the fulminant phase of inhalational anthrax, although the severity of presentation may vary based on inoculum size and underlying host factors [49]. Chest radiographs show mediastinal widening and pleural effusions that may be massive. *B. anthracis* bacilli, bacillary fragments, and anthrax antigens can be identified by immunohistochemistry testing of the pleural fluid [50]. Although parenchymal infiltrates are not prominent, a focal hemorrhagic necrotizing pneumonitis was noted in 11 of 42 autopsy patients from the accidental release of anthrax in Sverdlovsk, USSR, in 1979. Massive bacteremia causes overwhelming septic shock and death within hours after the onset of symptoms [51]. The lethal dose to kill 50% of persons exposed (LD_{50}) to weapons-grade anthrax is reported as 2,500 to 55,000 spores, but as few as one to three spores may be sufficient to cause infection and estimates vary [45,52].

Diagnosis

A high index of suspicion is necessary to make the diagnosis of anthrax. Laboratory findings from the US outbreak in 2001 showed that patients had a mild neutrophil-predominant leukocytosis, in the range of 7,500 to 13,300 per μL. Peak white blood cell count during illness ranged from 11,900 to 49,600 per μL. Elevated transaminases, hyponatremia, and hypoxemia were also noted [53,54]. All of these patients had abnormal chest radiographs with mediastinal widening, pleural effusions, consolidation, and infiltrates predominating. When present,

TABLE 130.7

Number and Percentage of Symptoms, Signs, and Diagnostic Findings at Hospital Admission for Patients in the USA with Inhalational Anthrax, 2001–2011

Characteristic	No.	%
Symptom		
Fever/Chills	12/13	92
Fatigue/Malaise	12/13	92
Cough	11/13	85
Nausea/Vomiting	9/13	69
Diaphoresis	8/13	62
Chest pain	7/13	54
Myalgia	6/13	46
Confusion	5/13	38
Headache	4/13	31
Sign		
Heart rate >90 beats/min	13/13	100
Abnormal core temperature fever >38.0°C or hypothermia <36.0°C)	8/13	62
Hypoxemia (PaO_2 <85 mm Hg)	3/9	33
Tachypnea (>20 breaths/min)	2/13	15
Abnormal laboratory value		
Elevated transaminases (ALT or AST above normal limits)	9/11	82
Leukocytosis (WBC $>12 \times 10^3/\mu L$)	2/13	15
Radiographic finding		
Pleural effusion	9/13	69
Infiltrate	8/13	62
Mediastinal widening	5/13	38

Bower WA, Hendricks K, Pillai S, et al: Centers for disease control and prevention, clinical framework and medical countermeasure use during an anthrax mass-casualty incident, CDC recommendations. MMWR Recomm Rep 64:4, 2015; http://www.cdc.gov/mmwr/indrr_2015.html.
ALT, alanine transaminase; AST, aspartate transaminase; WBC, white blood cells

mediastinal widening should be considered diagnostic of anthrax until proven otherwise, although computed tomography may be necessary to confirm its presence [54,55]. Hemorrhagic necrotizing lymphadenitis and mediastinitis are pathognomonic of anthrax but are typically only noted on autopsy. *B. anthracis* is easily cultured from blood, cerebral spinal fluid, ascites, and vesicular fluid with standard microbiology techniques. The laboratory must be notified when the diagnosis of anthrax is being considered, because many hospital laboratories will not further characterize *Bacillus* species unless requested. Biosafety Level 2 conditions apply for workers handling specimens, because most clinical specimens have spores in the vegetative state that are not easily transmitted. The presence of large gram-positive rods in short chains that are positive on India ink staining is considered presumptive of *B. anthracis* until the results of cultures and other confirmatory tests are obtained. Confirmatory testing can be performed by the CDC Laboratory Response Network. Rapid detection tests based on immunohistochemistry and PCR techniques are available via the Laboratory Response Network [56]. Nasal swabs are only useful for determining exposure in large groups of exposed persons; they have no role in individual diagnosis. In June 2004, the FDA approved the Anthrax Quick ELISA test (Immunetics, Inc., Boston, MA) that detects antibodies to the protective antigen of *B. anthracis* exotoxin. The test can be completed in less than 1 hour and is available to hospital and commercial laboratories by the manufacturer [56].

Treatment

Owing to the fulminant course of systemic anthrax, prompt initiation of therapy is essential for survival. Meningitis is a common complication of systemic anthrax and must be either excluded by lumbar puncture or treated empirically [57].

Systemic anthrax should be divided into meningeal and nonmeningeal disease for purposes of initial therapy. Current guidelines for the management of anthrax recommend the combination of an intravenous fluoroquinolone (ciprofloxacin, levofloxacin, or moxifloxacin) with a carbapenem (meropenem or imipenem) and either a protein-synthesis inhibitor (clindamycin or linezolid) or rifampin (an RNA polymerase inhibitor with similar efficacy as the traditional protein-synthesis inhibitors). Once meningitis has been excluded, either a quinolone or a carbapenem may be used; combination therapy is not necessary in that setting. Carbapenems may be replaced with intravenous penicillin G or ampicillin once penicillin susceptibility has been confirmed. Doxycycline may be used in lieu of clindamycin or linezolid in less-severe, nonmeningeal disease. Tables 130.8 and 130.9 provide dosage summaries.

TABLE 130.8

Intravenous Treatment for Systemic Anthrax with Possible/Confirmed Meningitis

Bactericidal agent (fluoroquinolone)
Ciprofloxacin, 400 mg every 8 h
Or
Levofloxacin, 750 mg every 24 h
Or
Moxifloxacin, 400 mg every 24 h
Plus
Bactericidal agent (β-lactam)
For all strains, regardless of penicillin susceptibility or if susceptibility is unknown
Meropenem, 2 g every 8 h
Or
Imipenem, 1 g every 6 h[a]
Alternatives for penicillin-susceptible strains only
Penicillin G, 4 million units every 4 h
Or
Ampicillin, 3 g every 6 h
Plus
Protein synthesis inhibitor
Linezolid, 600 mg every 12 h[b]
Or
Clindamycin, 900 mg every 8 h
Or
Rifampin, 600 mg every 12 h[c]
Or
Chloramphenicol, 1 g every 6–8 h[d]

Duration of treatment: ≥2–3 wks until clinical criteria for stability are met (see text). Patients exposed to aerosolized spores will require prophylaxis to complete an antimicrobial drug course of 60 d from onset of illness. Systemic anthrax includes anthrax meningitis; inhalation, injection, and gastrointestinal anthrax; and cutaneous anthrax with systemic involvement, extensive edema, or lesions of the head or neck. Preferred drugs are indicated in boldface.
[a]Increased risk for seizures associated with imipenem/cilastatin treatment.
[b]Linezolid should be used with caution in patients with thrombocytopenia. Linezolid use for >14 d has additional hematopoietic toxicity.
[c]Rifampin is not a protein synthesis inhibitor. However, it may be used in combination with other antimicrobial drugs on the basis of its in vitro synergy.
[d]Should only be used if other options are not available because of toxicity concerns.
Recommendations derived from Hendricks KA, Wright ME, Shadomy SV, et al: Centers for disease control and prevention expert panel meetings on prevention and treatment of anthrax in adults. Emerg Infect Dis 20:e130687, 2014.

TABLE 130.9

Intravenous Therapy for Systemic Anthrax When Meningitis Has Been Excluded

Bactericidal drug
For all strains, regardless of penicillin susceptibility or if susceptibility is unknown
Ciprofloxacin, 400 mg every 8 h
Or
Levofloxacin, 750 mg every 24 h
Or
Moxifloxacin, 400 mg every 24 h
Or
Meropenem, 2 g every 8 h
Or
Imipenem, 1 g every 6 h†
Or
Vancomycin, 60 mg/kg/d intravenous divided every 8 h (maintain serum trough concentrations of 15–20 μg/mL)
Alternatives for penicillin-susceptible strains
Penicillin G, 4 million units every 4 h
Or
Ampicillin, 3 g every 6 h
Plus
Protein synthesis inhibitor
Clindamycin, 900 mg every 8 h
Or
Linezolid, 600 mg every 12 h‡
Or
Doxycycline, 200 mg initially, then 100 mg every 12 h§
Or
Rifampin, 600 mg every 12h

Duration of treatment: for 2 wks until clinical criteria for stability are met. Patients exposed to aerosolized spores will require prophylaxis to complete an antimicrobial drug course of 60 d from onset of illness. Systemic anthrax includes anthrax meningitis; inhalation, injection, and gastrointestinal anthrax; and cutaneous anthrax with systemic involvement, extensive edema, or lesions of the head or neck. Preferred drugs are indicated in *boldface*.
[a]Increased risk for seizures associated with imipenem/cilastatin treatment.
[b]Linezolid should be used with caution in patients with thrombocytopenia because it might exacerbate it. Linezolid use for >14 d has additional hematopoietic toxicity.
[c]A single 10–14 d course of doxycycline is not routinely associated with tooth staining.
[d]Rifampin is not a protein synthesis inhibitor. However, it may be used in combination with other antimicrobials drugs on the basis of its in vitro synergy
Recommendations derived from Hendricks KA, Wright ME, Shadomy SV, et al: Centers for disease control and prevention expert panel meetings on prevention and treatment of anthrax in adults. *Emerg Infect Dis* 20:e130687, 2014.

There are limited data regarding treatment of pregnant women for anthrax, but anthrax infection is associated with both maternal and fetal death. Patients who are pregnant, postpartum, or lactating should therefore receive the same treatment as nonpregnant adults with only a few exceptions. Fluoroquinolones (ciprofloxacin, levofloxacin, or moxifloxacin) should be given to pregnant women for both postexposure prophylaxis and treatment unless otherwise contraindicated. Doxycycline is relatively contraindicated in pregnancy and should only be considered if ciprofloxacin is unavailable or absolutely contraindicated. For systemic anthrax infection with possible or confirmed meningitis, a carbapenem (meropenem, imipenem, or doripenem) and protein synthesis inhibitor with good CNS penetration (linezolid, clindamycin, and rifampin) should be added to fluoroquinolone treatment. Therapy should continue for 60 days. Patients can be switched to oral therapy once stable. The use of systemic corticosteroids has been suggested for meningitis, severe edema, and airway compromise [58].

Cutaneous anthrax with systemic involvement; significant edema; and lesions of the head and neck should be treated similarly. Uncomplicated cutaneous anthrax can be treated with oral ciprofloxacin or doxycycline for 7 to 10 days; however, owing to the possibility of concomitant inhalational exposure, a 60-day course is recommended [59,60].

A review of anthrax cases in adults from 1900 to 2004 noted that fulminant inhalational anthrax is often fatal despite advances in medical care. Early diagnosis, initiation of therapy and drainage of all effusions, improved survival and is pivotal for decreasing mortality in inhalational anthrax [54]. Similarly, a review of anthrax cases in children from 1900 to 2005 shows that early diagnosis and treatment of all forms of anthrax are critical for improved survival of children [61]. In the setting of a mass event, resources may become overwhelmed. In December 2015, the CDC Working Group for Anthrax Countermeasures proposed a "Clinical Framework and Medical Countermeasure Use During an Anthrax Mass-Casualty Incident" to be implemented only if triggered by local/state/federal authority [44]. Figure 130.6 shows the proposed triage algorithm (also see Chapter 127).

Prophylaxis

All patients exposed to anthrax should receive prophylaxis with oral ciprofloxacin (500 mg twice daily), levofloxacin (500 mg daily), or doxycycline (100 mg twice daily) for 60 days, regardless of laboratory test results. Nasal swabs can confirm exposure to anthrax, but cannot exclude it. High-dose penicillin or ampicillin may be an acceptable alternative for 60 days in patients who are allergic or intolerant to the recommended antibiotics [56]. More than 5,000 people received postexposure prophylaxis following the 2001 US outbreak, but only about half completed the 60-day course. The main reasons for discontinuing therapy were gastrointestinal or neurologic side effects (75%) or a low perceived risk (25%).

The anthrax vaccine (AVA-Biothrax) manufactured by BioPort Corporation in Lansing, Michigan, is the only licensed human anthrax vaccine in the USA. The vaccine consists of supernatant material from cultures of a toxigenic, nonencapsulated strain of *B. anthracis*. A six-dose series has been used by the US military. The anthrax vaccine is not available to the general public at the present time. Approximately 95% of vaccinated individuals seroconvert after the third dose of vaccine. There has been no conclusive evidence of lasting harm in over 1 million doses of anthrax vaccine given by the US military program, and the vaccine is generally considered to be safe by the FDA. A review by the US Army Medical Research Institute of Infectious Diseases reported a 1% (101/10,722) incidence of systemic symptoms, most commonly headache. Local or injection site reactions occurred in 3.6% [60]. A study comparing four subcutaneous injections of anthrax vaccine adsorbed (AVA) with three and four intramuscular injections of AVA showed similar immunoprotection at 7 months with fewer adverse effects at the injection site. Following an aerosolized *B. anthracis* attack, postexposure prophylactic vaccination and antibiotic therapy remain the most effective and least expensive strategies [56,62].

Adjunctive immunotherapy is available in the event of suspected or confirmed anthrax exposure. There are currently three products available, to be given in combination with antibacterial therapy: raxibacumab, a recombinant monoclonal antibody directed against the *B. anthracis* protective antigen (PA) [63,64]; obiltoxaximab, a humanized chimeric monoclonal antibody also directed against PA [65,66]; and Anthrax Immune Globulin Intravenous (AIGIV), which is a purified polyclonal preparation of anti-anthrax immunoglobulin derived from vaccinated human donors [67]. There are no head-to-head trials comparing these three products (and nor do any such trials appear likely),

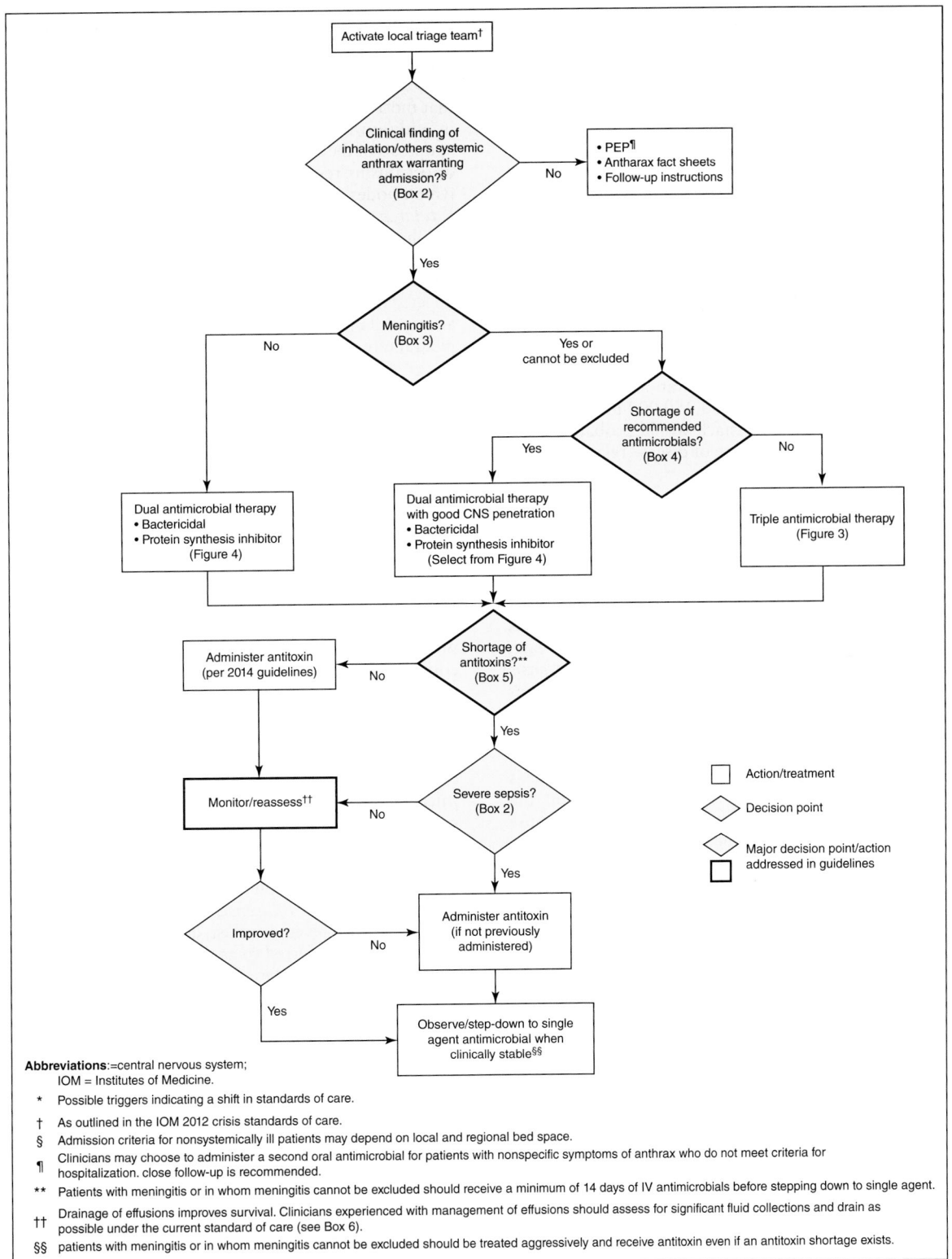

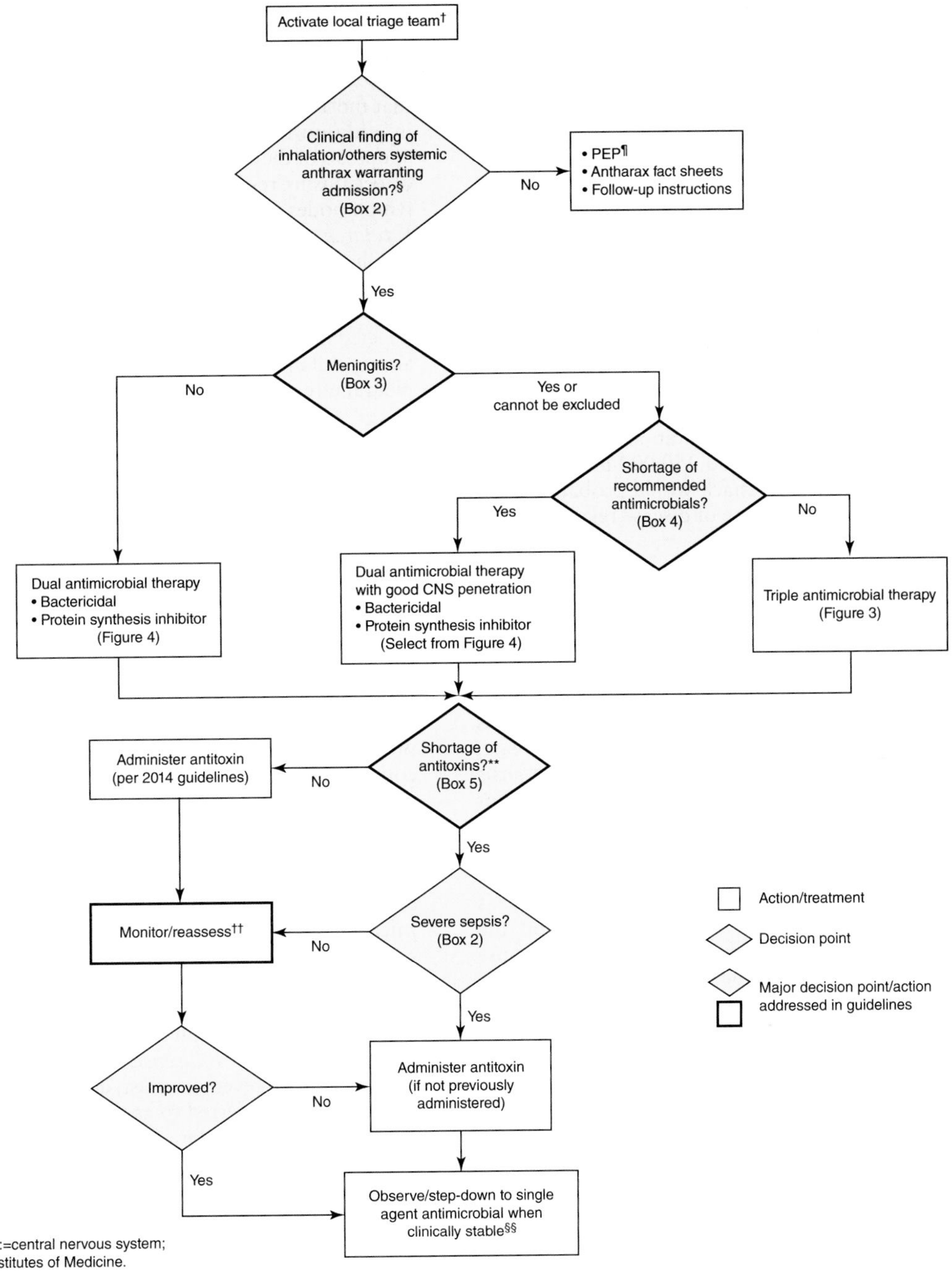

Abbreviations:=central nervous system;
IOM = Institutes of Medicine.

* Possible triggers indicating a shift in standards of care.

† As outlined in the IOM 2012 crisis standards of care.

§ Admission criteria for nonsystemically ill patients may depend on local and regional bed space.

¶ Clinicians may choose to administer a second oral antimicrobial for patients with nonspecific symptoms of anthrax who do not meet criteria for hospitalization. close follow-up is recommended.

** Patients with meningitis or in whom meningitis cannot be excluded should receive a minimum of 14 days of IV antimicrobials before stepping down to single agent.

†† Drainage of effusions improves survival. Clinicians experienced with management of effusions should assess for significant fluid collections and drain as possible under the current standard of care (see Box 6).

§§ patients with meningitis or in whom meningitis cannot be excluded should be treated aggressively and receive antitoxin even if an antitoxin shortage exists.

FIGURE 130.6 Crisis standards of care* framework for medical countermeasure prioritization among hospitalized persons with known or potential exposure to anthrax. The clinical algorithm addresses four decision points where resource limitations might impact clinical management during an anthrax mass-casualty incident. The first decision point involves diagnostic evaluation of anthrax meningitis, which is necessary to determine optimal antimicrobial therapy. The second decision point involves treatment regimens of combination intravenous antimicrobial therapy. The third decision point involves administration of antitoxins, as an adjunctive therapy. The fourth decision point involves the identification and drainage of fluid collections, which have been associated with a survival benefit. Local triage teams should be activated as outlined in the *IOM 2012 Crisis Standards of Care. Admission criteria for nonsystemically ill patients may depend on local and regional bed space. Clinicians may choose to administer a second oral antimicrobial for patients with nonspecific symptoms of anthrax who do not meet criteria for hospitalization. Close follow-up is recommended. Patients with meningitis or in whom meningitis cannot be excluded should be treated aggressively and receive antitoxin even if an antitoxin shortage exists. Drainage of effusions improves survival. Clinicians experienced with management of effusions should assess for significant fluid collections and drain as possible under the current standard of care. Patients with meningitis or in whom meningitis cannot be excluded should receive a minimum of 14 days of IV antimicrobials before stepping down to single agent.

but all three have been recently approved by the FDA and are reasonable adjuncts to antimicrobial therapy and aggressive critical care in the treatment of anthrax.

TULAREMIA

Tularemia is a zoonosis caused by *Francisella tularensis*, an intracellular, nonspore-forming, aerobic gram-negative coccobacillus. Its primary reservoirs in nature are small mammals, such as rodents and rabbits. In the mid-20th century, both the USA and the former Soviet Union developed biologic weapons that could disperse *F. Tularensis* [68]. Although biologic weapons have now been banned, there remains concern that *F. tularensis* could be used as an agent of bioterrorism and has been speculated to have been used by Serbia against Kosovo in the 1990s [69,70]. In a 1970 report, the WHO estimated that 50 kg of aerosolized *F. tularensis* dispersed over a metropolitan area of 5 million people could cause 19,000 deaths and 250,000 incapacitating illnesses. The impact of such an attack would probably linger for several weeks to months because of disease relapses [71].

Microbiology

F. tularensis is a hardy organism that can survive in moist soil, water, and animal carcasses for many weeks. Chlorination of water prevents its spread through water contamination. *F. tularensis* can be aerosolized, and inhalation of aerosolized organisms poses a threat to those exposed. The most common isolate, and the most virulent form, is *F. tularensis* biovar *tularensis* (Group A). Inoculation or inhalation of as few as 10 organisms may cause clinical disease [70]. Transmission of *F. tularensis* to humans occurs predominantly through tick and fleabites, handling of infected animals, ingestion of contaminated food and water, and inhalation of the aerosolized organism. There is no human-to-human transmission. As a biologic weapon, the organism would most likely be dispersed as an aerosol, and cause mass casualties from an acute febrile illness that may progress to severe pneumonia [46,72].

Epidemiology

Tularemia occurs throughout the northern hemisphere, with highest incidence in Russia and Scandinavian countries. In the USA, tularemia cases are reported most often from the south-central and western states (Arkansas, Illinois, Missouri, Oklahoma, Tennessee, Texas, Utah, Virginia, and Wyoming). The predominant mode of transmission to humans in the USA is by tick bites, most often in spring and summer. Hunters and trappers exposed to animal reservoirs are at high risk for exposure [73]. In Europe and Japan, mosquito bites and the handling of infected animals appear to cause the disease. A large outbreak of tularemia in 2003 along with small summer outbreaks between 1995 and 2005 in Sweden suggests environmental sources clustering around recreational areas [74]. An outbreak of tularemia on Martha's Vineyard, Massachusetts, during the summer of 2000 was associated with lawn mowing and brush cutting [75]. A water-borne outbreak resulting in 21 cases of oropharyngeal and five cases of glandular tularemia was reported in the Republic of Georgia [76].

Pathogenesis

F. tularensis enters the human host via the eye, respiratory tract, gastrointestinal tract, or a break in the skin. The virulence of the organism depends on its ability to replicate within the macrophage. On initial entry into the macrophage, *F. tularensis* uses a bacterial acid phosphatase, AcpA, to inhibit the bactericidal respiratory burst response of the macrophage and continues to replicate in the host macrophage using IglC, a 23-kDa protein that most likely affects Toll-like receptor-4 signal transduction in addition to other factors yet to be identified. Eventually, apoptosis of the macrophage occurs with the subsequent release of organisms resulting in secondary involvement of the local lymph nodes and bacteremia [70]. Once bacteremia develops, *F. tularensis* infects the lungs, pleura, spleen, liver, and kidney. The host defense against *F. tularensis* is T-cell independent in the first 3 days and T-cell dependent after 3 days of infection. On histopathology, granulomata with necrosis may be seen in infected organs. Following inhalational exposure, hemorrhagic airway inflammation may progress to pneumonia, pleuritis, and pleural effusion. The role of humoral immunity is uncertain.

Clinical Features

The clinical manifestations of tularemia depend on the site of entry, exposure dose, virulence of the strain, and host immune factors. Hematogenous spread may occur from any of the initial clinical presentations. Syndromes associated with tularemia are classified as primary pneumonic, typhoidal, ulceroglandular, oculoglandular, oropharyngeal, and septic. The *ulceroglandular form* is the most common naturally occurring form of tularemia. After an incubation period of 3 to 6 days (range, 1 to 25 days) following a vector bite or animal contact, patients present with high fevers (85%), chills (52%), headache (45%), cough (38%), and myalgias (31%). They may also have malaise, chest pain, abdominal pain, nausea, vomiting, and diarrhea. A pulse-temperature dissociation (Faget's sign) is often seen. At the site of inoculation, a tender papule develops that later becomes a pustule and ulcerates as shown in Figure 130.7. Lymph nodes draining the inoculation site become enlarged and painful (85%). Infected lymph nodes may become suppurative, ulcerate, and remain enlarged for a long period of time. Exudative pharyngitis and tonsillitis may develop following ingestion of contaminated food or inhalation of the aerosolized organism. Pharyngeal ulceration and regional lymphadenopathy may be present. Systemic illness caused by *F. tularensis* without lymphadenopathy and presenting with fever, diarrhea, dehydration, hypotension, and meningismus is referred to as the *typhoidal form*.

The *pneumonic form* of tularemia may occur as a primary pleuropneumonia following the inhalation of aerosolized organisms. The pneumonic form may also occur as a result of hematogenous spread from other sites of infection or following

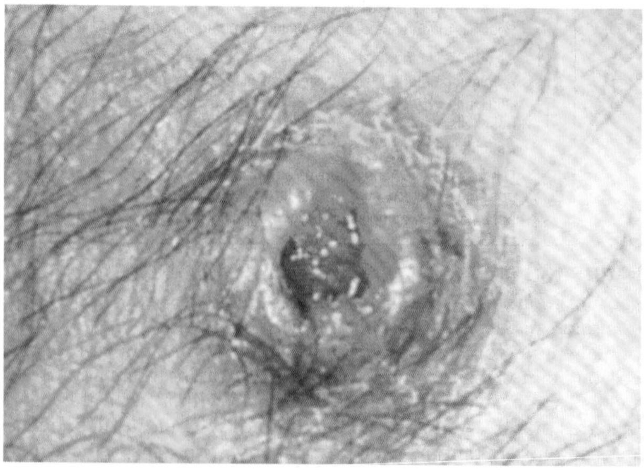

FIGURE 130.7 Tularemia cutaneous ulcer with heaped up edges (Picture from "Quick Bio-Agents Guide, First Edition, 2012. Available for download at http://www.usamriid.army.mil/education/instruct.htm.)

oropharyngeal tularemia. After inhalational exposure, constitutional symptoms, such as fever and chills, typically precede the onset of respiratory symptoms. The respiratory symptoms include a dry or minimally productive cough, pleuritic chest pain, shortness of breath, and hemoptysis. Pleural effusions, either unilateral or bilateral, can occur. Pneumonic tularemia can rapidly progress to respiratory failure with acute respiratory distress syndrome, multiorgan failure, disseminated intravascular coagulation, rhabdomyolysis, renal failure, and hepatitis [46,70]. Rarely, peritonitis, pericarditis, appendicitis, osteomyelitis, erythema nodosum, and meningitis have been reported to occur. Delays in diagnosis and failure to institute prompt aminoglycoside therapy result in higher morbidity and mortality. The mortality rate of untreated pneumonic tularemia is 60%, but with proper antibiotic therapy the mortality rate is significantly reduced to 1% to 2.5% [70,77].

Laboratory and Radiographic Findings

A high index of suspicion is needed in order to make an early diagnosis of tularemia. Lack of response to conventional treatment for skin ulcers or community-acquired pneumonia, along with a history of exposure to animals, may serve as diagnostic clues. Routine laboratory tests, such as a complete blood count and serum chemistry panels, are generally nondiagnostic. A complete blood count may show a leukocytosis with a normal differential or mild lymphocytosis. Mild elevations of lactic dehydrogenase, transaminases, and alkaline phosphatase may be seen on a serum chemistry panel. If rhabdomyolysis is present, an elevated serum creatine kinase concentration and urine myoglobin may be seen. Sterile pyuria has been reported. Mild abnormalities in cerebrospinal fluid cell counts, protein, and glucose have also been reported [70,77].

Tularemia can present with multiple abnormalities on a chest radiograph (Fig. 130.8). A report of the chest radiographic findings in 50 patients who had a confirmed diagnosis of tularemia showed the following abnormalities: patchy airspace opacities (74%, unilateral in 54%); hilar adenopathy (32%, unilateral in 22%); pleural effusion (30%, unilateral in 20%); unilateral lobar or segmental opacities (18%); cavitation (16%); oval opacities (8%); and cardiomegaly with a pulmonary edema pattern (6%). Rare findings such as apical infiltrates, empyema with bronchopleural fistula, miliary pattern, residual cyst, and residual calcification have been reported in less than 5% of patients [78].

Diagnosis

It is possible to isolate *F. tularensis* from sputum, blood, and other body fluids, but the organism can be difficult to culture on conventional media; cysteine or sulfhydryl compounds are required for *F. tularensis* to grow. Notification of laboratory personnel that tularemia is suspected is mandatory, both to enhance the yield of culture and to ensure that appropriate biosafety procedures are observed. Routine diagnostic procedures can be performed in Biosafety Level 2 conditions. Examination of cultures in which *F. tularensis* is suspected may be done in a biologic safety cabinet, but procedures that might produce aerosols or droplets must be conducted under Biosafety Level 3 conditions [77].

Owing to the high infectivity and difficulty with cultures, serologic evaluation is often employed. Examination of secretions and biopsy specimens with direct fluorescent antibody or immunochemical stains may help to identify the organism. The diagnosis is often made through serologic testing using enzyme-linked immunosorbent assay (ELISA). Serologic titers may not be elevated early in the course of disease. A fourfold rise is typically seen during the course of illness. A single tularemia antibody titer of 1:160 or greater is supportive of the diagnosis [70,79]. Antibodies to *F. tularensis* may cross-react with other bacteria, such as *Brucella*, *Proteus*, and *Yersinia* species because of their particular variant of endotoxin (a lipooligosaccharide), which decreases the specificity of serology-based assays. Antibiotic therapy can blunt the serologic response, which could mask the convalescent rise in titer needed to confirm the diagnosis. Antibody levels against *F. tularensis* can persist for years, so distinguishing between acute and remote infection also may be difficult.

The combined use of ELISA and confirmatory Western blot analysis was found to be the most suitable approach to the serologic diagnosis of tularemia [80,81]. Other diagnostic methods include antigen detection assays and PCR. A multitarget

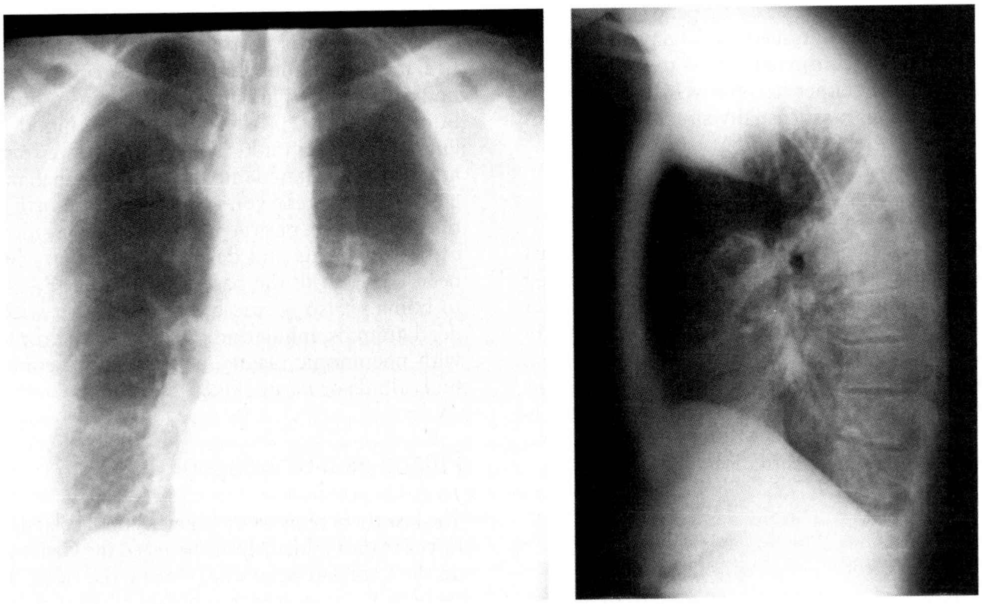

FIGURE 130.8 Tularemia pneumonia. Chest radiograph from a 27-year-old man who contracted tularemic pneumonia after skinning a rabbit that he had hunted (Courtesy of Angeline A. Lazarus, MD.).

real-time TaqMan PCR assay (Applied Biosystems, Foster City, CA) has been reported to have high sensitivity and specificity for the diagnosis of tularemia and may be a valuable tool for the analysis of clinical specimens and field samples following a bioterrorism attack [82,83].

Treatment

The traditional treatment of choice for tularemia in adults is streptomycin, 10 to 15 mg per kg, given intramuscularly (IM) or intravenously (IV) twice daily. Gentamicin, 5 mg per kg, given IM or intravenously (IV) once daily, is an acceptable alternative. For children, the preferred antibiotics are streptomycin, 15 mg per kg, given IM twice daily (not to exceed 2 g per day) or gentamicin, 2.5 mg per kg, given IM or IV thrice daily. Alternate choices for adults with milder disease are doxycycline, 100 mg IV twice daily; chloramphenicol, 15 mg per kg, given IV four times daily; or ciprofloxacin, 400 mg, given IV or PO twice daily. For children, alternate choices are doxycycline, 100 mg, given IV twice daily if the child weighs 45 kg or more, and doxycycline, 2.2 mg per kg, given IV twice daily for children weighing less than 45 kg. Chloramphenicol and ciprofloxacin can also be used as alternate antibiotics for children. The ciprofloxacin dose for children should not exceed 1 g per day. Gentamicin is preferred over streptomycin for treatment during pregnancy and chloramphenicol should not be given to pregnant patients. Treatment with streptomycin, gentamicin, or ciprofloxacin should be continued for 10 days. Treatment with doxycycline or chloramphenicol should be continued for 14 to 21 days. Patients beginning treatment with doxycycline, chloramphenicol, or ciprofloxacin can be switched to oral antibiotics when clinically appropriate. β-Lactams and macrolides are not recommended for treatment of tularemia, but there has been two isolated case reports of glandular/abscess forms treated with a 6 week courses of cefuroxime or amoxicillin/clavulanic acid in pregnant women who refused first-line treatments [84].

In a mass casualty setting caused by tularemia, the preferred antibiotic for adults and pregnant women is doxycycline, 100 mg, taken orally twice daily, or ciprofloxacin 500 mg, taken orally twice daily. For children, the preferred choices are doxycycline, 100 mg, taken orally twice daily if the child weighs 45 kg or more; doxycycline, 2.2 mg per kg, taken orally twice daily if the child weighs less than 45 kg; or ciprofloxacin, 15 mg per kg, taken orally twice daily and not to exceed 1 g per day. Treatment with ciprofloxacin should be continued for 10 days; treatment with doxycycline should be continued for 14 to 21 days. For immunosuppressed patients, either streptomycin or gentamicin is the preferred antibiotic in mass casualty situations [70].

Prophylaxis

Individuals exposed to *F. tularensis* may be protected against systemic infection if they receive prophylactic antibiotics during the incubation period. For postexposure prophylaxis, either doxycycline 100 mg, taken orally twice daily, or ciprofloxacin 500 mg, taken orally twice daily for 14 days, is recommended. Both doxycycline and ciprofloxacin can be taken by pregnant women for postexposure prophylaxis, but ciprofloxacin is preferred. Postexposure prophylaxis for children is the same as treatment during mass casualty situations [77].

Immunization

In Russia, a live attenuated vaccine has been used to offer protection to those living in tularemia-endemic areas and transferred to the USA in 1956. It is currently the only vaccine available under FDA Investigational New Drug Status and has been administered to hundreds since the 1950s by the US Army Medical Research Institute of Infectious Diseases (USAMRIID). Very few side effects from the scarification (similar to smallpox vaccine) occur and partial high-dose respiratory protection against the Type A strain has been shown. Novel investigational vaccines remain under development but are not yet available for clinical use owing to the difficulty of targeting a T-cell epitope against the intracellular *F. tularensis* pathogen [71,85].

PLAGUE

Few infectious diseases have had the same impact on human history and human biology as the plague. Similar to tularemia, plague is a zoonosis with a natural reservoir in rodents for which humans are incidental hosts. Multiple pandemics of plague are believed to have occurred since the 6th century CE, with the "Black Death" of the 14th century taking the lives of over 40 million people while leaving deep impressions in European and Asian culture, religion, and art [86]. The causative organism, *Yersinia pestis*, was identified by and ultimately named for French physician Alexandre Yersin during the 1894 plague epidemic in Hong Kong [87]. In recent years, the highly contagious nature of plague has raised concerns about its possible use as an agent of bioterrorism.

Microbiology

Plague is caused by *Yersinia pestis*, a gram-negative, nonmotile coccobacillus of the family Enterobacteriaceae, closely related to *Escherichia*, *Klebsiella*, and other enteric gram-negative organisms and sharing their typical bipolar "safety pin" staining appearance under Wright–Giemsa stains (Fig. 130.9). In common with other gram-negative bacilli, *Y. pestis* has a lipopolysaccharide endotoxin that mediates much of the exuberant host inflammatory response, with resulting sepsis, acute respiratory distress syndrome, and multiorgan failure [86,88]. In addition, *Y. pestis* carries three distinct plasmids responsible for much of its virulence: pYV/pCD1, which encodes for a secretion apparatus that permits the delivery of cytotoxins into mammalian host cells; pFra/pMT1, which encodes for the anti-phagocytic fimbrial antigen F1; and pPst/pPCP/pPla, which encodes for a plasminogen activator and other exotoxins permitting invasion of host tissues [89–91].

Y. pestis is naturally transmitted by the bite of a plague-infected flea, most commonly *Xenopsylla cheopis*, although the human body louse may play a role in human-to-human transmission in epidemics [92]. After ingestion of blood from an infected animal, bacteria multiply in the digestive tract of the flea and are then regurgitated into the next mammalian victim following a bite. Major reservoirs of plague in North America include the deer mouse, prairie dog and ground squirrel, but infections of domestic cats and dogs with secondary human cases have been reported in the past two decades [93–96]. Transmission to humans also occurs by direct contact with infected live or dead animals, inhalation of respiratory droplets from patients with pneumonic plague, or from direct contact with infected body fluids or tissue [86,89,97,98].

Plague as a Bioweapon

The history of biowarfare begins with the plague. In 1346, Mongol forces of the Golden Horde besieged the Genoese enclave of Kaffa on the Crimean peninsula. During the siege, the Golden Horde reportedly catapulted the corpses of plague victims into the city, an event which may have led to the introduction of plague to Western Europe and ultimately to the Black Death [99]. In more

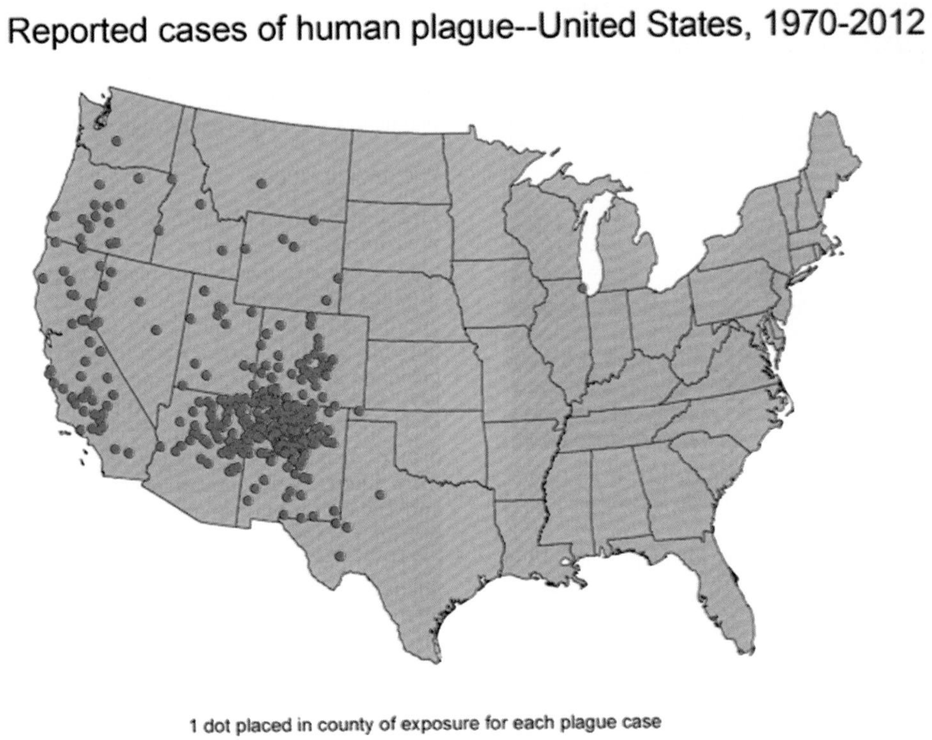

Reported cases of human plague--United States, 1970-2012
1 dot placed in county of exposure for each plague case

FIGURE 130.9 Reported cases of human plague—USA, 1970–2012 (CDC website, September 2015; https://www.cdc.gov/plague/maps/.)

recent years, plague was developed as a bioweapon by the former Soviet Union, Imperial Japan, and the USA before the destruction of the US biologic weapon stockpile in the early 1970s [100].

When used as a bioweapon, *Y. pestis* may produce differing syndromes depending on the mode of dispersal. Aerosol spread would be expected to produce pneumonic plague, whereas the release of infected fleas should lead to bubonic or septicemic plague [5,97,100]. Due the highly contagious nature of pneumonic plague, the WHO estimates that 50 kg of *Yersinia pestis* aerosolized over a population of 5 million people could result in 150,000 infections and 36,000 deaths from primary infections and secondary transmission [101]. The CDC currently classifies plague as a tier 1 threat agent, indicating a pathogen or toxin with maximum potential risk to public health in the event of release.

Epidemiology

Plague exists worldwide, with most of the 3,248 human cases reported to the WHO between 2010 and 2015 occurring in developing countries of Africa and Asia [102]. Since 2001, there have been a median of three human plague cases per year in the USA, with a mortality rate of 16% with appropriate antimicrobial and supportive treatments [103,104]. The majority of plague cases in the USA come from the states of Arizona, New Mexico, California, and Colorado, with rare cases from Texas and Oregon as shown in Figure 130.10. In the pre-antibiotic era, the plague mortality rate for the USA was approximately 66%, with increased mortality seen among ethnic minorities (91%) compared with non-Latino whites (53%). Since the advent of effective antibiotic therapy, no gender- or racial-associated differences in US plague mortality have been noted, however [104].

Pathogenesis

Human plague occurs in *bubonic, septicemic*, and *primary pneumonic* forms. After entering the body through a flea bite,

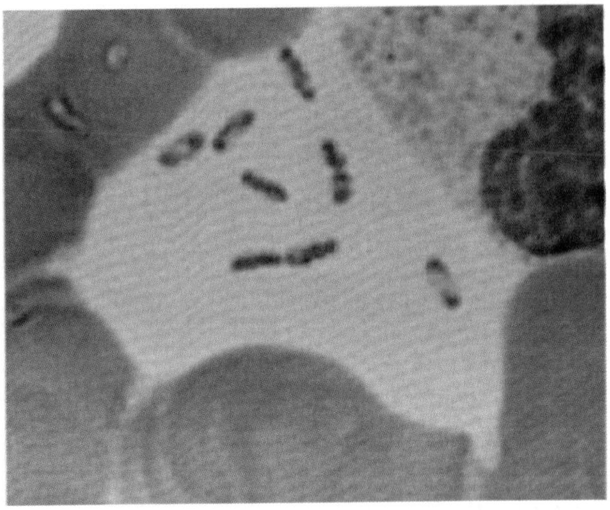

FIGURE 130.10 Wright–Giemsa stain of blood showing nonmotile, encapsulated, aerobic rod with "safety pin" appearance of *Yersinia pestis* (Picture from "Quick Bio-Agents Guide, First Edition, 2012. Available for download at http://www.usamriid.army.mil/education/instruct.htm.)

bacteria migrate via cutaneous lymphatics to the regional lymph nodes and are subjected to phagocytosis. *Y. pestis* is taken up by host neutrophils and macrophages but evades destruction by phagocytosis through plasmid-encoded proteins such as Yops and F1 fimbrial antigen [105,106]. Surviving bacteria then proliferate intracellularly, with secondary spread through host lymphatics and ultimately progress to bacteremia and sepsis. Host tissue invasion is enhanced by the production of procoagulant and anticoagulant enzymes by the bacterium, including plasminogen activators [91,107]. The initial infection causes lymphadenitis and local swelling that is referred to as the "bubo" (hence, the name "bubonic plague") (Fig. 130.11). These buboes contain dense concentrates of *Yersinia* bacilli along with necrosis.

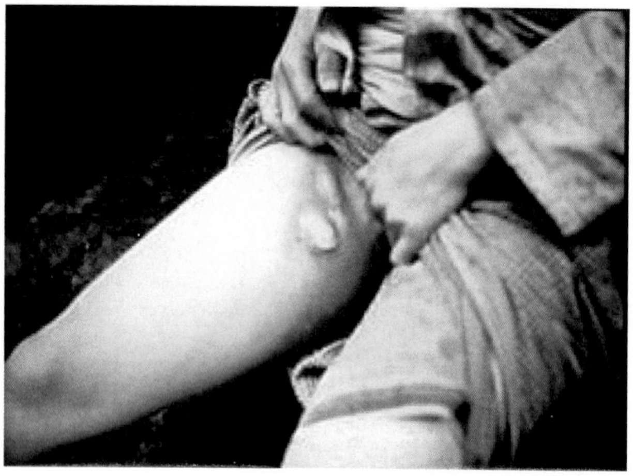

FIGURE 130.11 Bubonic plague with characteristic bubo (From: CDC Web Site: http://www.cdc.gov/ncidod/dvbid/plague/diagnosis.).

Bacterial modification of lipopolysaccharide helps evade host innate immunity by blunting the sensitivity of Toll-like receptor 4 to endotoxin, further facilitating bacterial proliferation and spread [108]. In the absence of therapy, bacteremia, sepsis, and death usually follow [86,90,97].

In a minority of cases, primary **pneumonic plague** results from the inhalation of infected droplets, either from another infected host or from the aerosolization of a draining bubo. Human pneumonic plague resulting from transmission from infected animals has been reported [93,109]. Following inhalation, *Y. pestis* bacilli are engulfed preferentially by pulmonary macrophages before neutrophil recruitment takes place [110]. They are then transported to the lymphatic system and regional lymph nodes, with secondary bacteremia and seeding of the spleen, liver, skin, mucous membranes, and other organs [93,97,110]. **Primary septicemic plague** results from the direct inoculation of *Y. pestis* bacilli into the bloodstream, which presents with nonspecific signs similar to other acute febrile illnesses with sepsis. It is important to note that these entities may overlap; pneumonic and bubonic plague can and often do progress to septicemia. Rare forms of plague are *plague meningitis* and *plague pharyngitis*. Plague meningitis occurs following the hematogenous spread of *Y. pestis* bacilli to the meninges. Plague pharyngitis may occur following the ingestion or inhalation of *Y. pestis* bacilli [5].

Clinical Presentation

The incubation period and clinical manifestations of plague vary according to mode of transmission. 80% to 85% of plague cases diagnosed in the USA are bubonic, 10% to 12% are primary septicemic, and roughly 3% are primary pneumonic plague [103]. Bubonic plague may progress to septicemic or pneumonic plague in 23% and 9% of cases, respectively. The clinical presentation of plague of children is similar to that of adults, although secondary progression to plague meningitis appears to be more common in children [86,92,103]. There is little data regarding unique manifestations of plague in pregnant women [111].

Septicemic Plague

A minority of patients exposed to *Y. pestis* develop septicemic plague, either as a primary form (without buboes) or secondary to the hematogenous spread of bubonic or primary pneumonic plague. Presenting features of septicemic plague are nonspecific and difficult to distinguish from other undifferentiated febrile syndromes, with fever, delirium, nausea, and hypotension being typical. Abdominal pain, hepatosplenomegaly, disseminated intravascular coagulation, and purpura fulminans have been reported, along with distal gangrene of the nose and digits, similar in appearance to meningococcemia. Without rapid treatment, the disease progresses to septic shock, anuria, and the acute respiratory distress syndrome. The untreated mortality rate of septicemic plague has been reported as high as 93% to 100% [86,104].

Pneumonic Plague

Plague is highly contagious by the airborne route, and droplet precautions are mandatory for any patient suspected of having plague. Primary pneumonic plague occurs by inhaling infected droplets, which may result from respiratory transmission from another patient with pneumonic plague as well as from a draining bubo, and is characterized by a severe, rapidly progressive pneumonia and sepsis that is rapidly fatal if not treated promptly [97]. Buboes may develop in the cervical area. Acute respiratory failure requiring mechanical ventilation is common. Strict droplet isolation is mandatory. Chest radiographs most often show bilateral alveolar airspace opacities, although effusions and cavitation may occur [92,97,112]. Alveolar opacities in secondary pneumonic plague may have a nodular appearance consistent with hematogenous spread. Anterior mediastinal adenopathy is very rare in primary pneumonic plague, but hilar node enlargement is often present, a feature which may distinguish pneumonic plague from inhalational anthrax [5]. Similar to septicemic plague, the untreated mortality rate of primary pneumonic plague is 100% [97,104].

Secondary pneumonic plague occurs among approximately 12% of individuals with bubonic plague or primary septicemic plague following the hematogenous spread of *Y. pestis* bacilli to the lungs. It typically presents as a severe bronchopneumonia with cough, dyspnea, chest pain, and hemoptysis. Chest radiographs show bilateral, patchy alveolar infiltrates that may progress to consolidation. In contrast to primary pneumonic plague, mediastinal, cervical, and hilar adenopathy may occur (Fig. 130.12) [86,97,112].

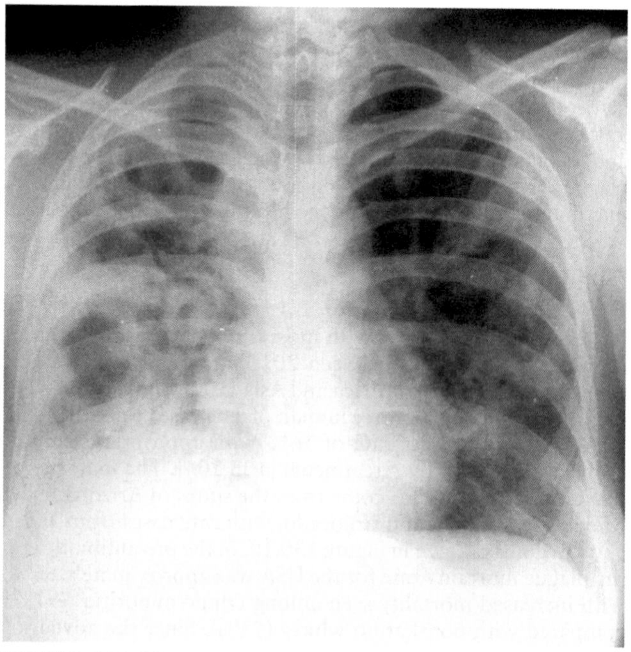

FIGURE 130.12 A 38-year-old man from Himachal Pradesh was admitted with complaints of fever, cough, hemoptysis, and dyspnea. There is endemic pneumonic plague owing to the prevalent custom of hunting wild rats and rodents. Sputum examination was positive for *Yersinia pestis*. The patient was successfully treated with antibiotics (Chest radiograph courtesy of Sanjay Jain, MD, Department of Internal Medicine, and Surinder K. Jindal, MD, Professor of Medicine, Postgraduate Institute of Medical Education and Research, Chandigarh, India.).

Diagnosis

The presence of a bubo in an ill patient should serve as an adequate clue for the majority of clinicians to the possibility of plague. Similar lesions and clinical syndromes may be seen with ulceroglandular tularemia (which raises similar concerns in regards to bioterrorism and is managed with comparable antimicrobial agents), epidemic typhus, suppurative infections (e.g., *Staphylococcus aureus*), and bartonellosis. The lesions of chancroid, lymphogranuloma venereum, syphilitic lymphadenitis, and mycobacterial disease may be grossly similar but present in a more subacute manner and generally without the severe illness and prostration seen with plague.

Conversely, the diagnosis of pneumonic and septicemic plague can be markedly more difficult given the absence of distinctive clinical findings. The radiographic findings of pneumonic plague are nonspecific, although the absence of mediastinal widening may help distinguish it from inhalational anthrax. The presence of the characteristic gram-negative rods in the sputum of an immunocompetent patient, particularly with a suitable exposure history, must raise the concern for plague. Primary septicemic plague's high mortality is related in part to delays of diagnosis. Exposure history, purpura fulminans, septic shock, and acral gangrene are all consistent but strongly resemble the syndromes seen with meningococcemia; rickettsioses; and pneumococcal and pseudomonal sepsis [5,86,89,97,104,112].

Laboratory Diagnosis

A mild-to-moderate leukocytosis with neutrophil predominance and toxic granulations are seen in all forms of plague. In severe cases, elevated transaminases, azotemia, and coagulopathy with disseminated intravascular coagulation are seen. Gram stains of sputum; blood; or lymph node aspirates may show typical enteric gram-negative bacilli with bipolar staining, similar to *Escherichia coli*, *Klebsiella*, and other Enterobacteriaceae. Microscopic examination of a sputum specimen prepared with Wright–Giemsa stain will show the characteristic bipolar staining pattern more clearly (Fig. 130.10) [93].

Y. pestis will grow rapidly on conventional bacteriologic media. However, misidentification of *Y. pestis* has been described with automated bacterial identification devices [113]. With the increasing availability of mass spectrometry (matrix-assisted laser desorption/ionization time-of-flight, or MALDI-TOF) in clinical laboratories, these errors should be less frequent [114]. Rapid diagnostic tests such as immunoglobulin-M immunoassay, direct fluorescent antibody testing, and PCR are available through the CDC, Department of Defense laboratories (including the US Army Research Institute for Infectious Diseases), and state public health laboratories. Rapid plague detection through the use of multiplex PCR panels (which also often include primers for multiple potential bioterror agents) are available and are highly sensitive [115]. Direct fluorescent antibody staining for *Yersinia pestis* (Fig. 130.13) and dipstick antigen detection tests are highly specific and are available at some centers. Rapid diagnostic assays using monoclonal antibodies to the F1 capsular antigen show promise for the early on-site diagnosis of plague [116,117], as do monoclonal antibodies directed at detection of *Y. pestis* lipopolysaccharide [118]. Additional tests for detection and confirmation that are available through the Laboratory Response Network include PCR assays; molecular-based subtyping; and immunohistochemistry on formalin-fixed tissues.

Plague should be suspected among persons with symptoms of fever and lymphadenopathy if they reside in, or have recently travelled to, a plague-endemic area and if gram-negative and/or bipolar-staining coccobacilli are seen on a smear taken from affected tissues. The diagnosis of plague should be presumed if immunofluorescence staining of smear or material is positive for the presence of *Y. pestis* F1 antigen and/or a single serum specimen shows the anti-F1 antigen in a titer of greater than 1:10 by agglutination. A diagnosis of plague is confirmed if one or more of the following criteria are met: isolation of *Y. pestis* from a clinical specimen, a single *Y. pestis* antibody titer of more than 1:128 dilution, a fourfold rise in paired sera antibody titer to *Yersinia pestis* F1 antigen (with the second assay obtained 6 to 8 weeks after convalescence), or if PCR-based testing of body fluids or tissues is positive for *Y. pestis*. Antibody susceptibility testing should be performed at a reference laboratory.

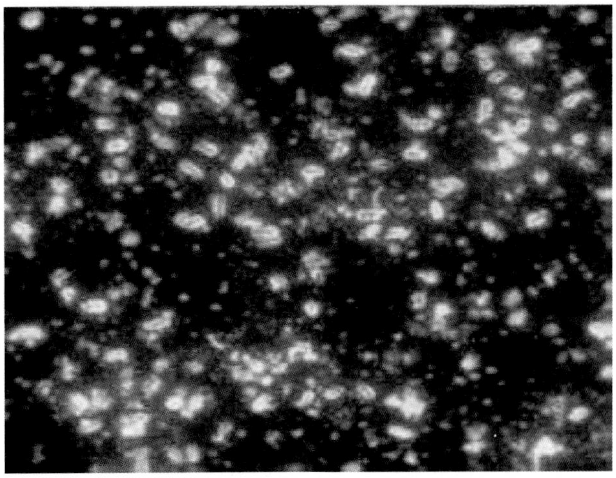

FIGURE 130.13 Fluorescence antibody positivity for *Yersinia pestis* is seen as bright, intense green staining around the bacterial cell (From CDC Web site: http://www.cdc.gov/ncidod/dvbid/plague/bacterium.htm.).

Plague as a bioterrorism agent should be suspected when multiple cases of severe and rapidly progressive pneumonic plague cases are seen with fulminant systemic symptoms and hemoptysis. Although pretreatment specimens should be obtained when possible, treatment of suspected plague should not be delayed while awaiting confirmatory results.

Treatment

Traditionally, streptomycin or gentamicin has been the mainstays of therapy for *Yersinia pestis*. Other acceptable antibiotics are ciprofloxacin, tetracycline, doxycycline, and chloramphenicol [5,86]. Methylprednisolone and imipenem have shown evidence of efficacy in murine models of plague but lack supporting human data at this time [119,120]. Antimicrobial resistance among *Y. pestis* has been reported but appears to be rare, with the great majority of clinical isolates maintaining susceptibility to the recommended agents [121–124]. The recommendations of the Working Group on Civilian Biodefense from the year 2000 remain the basis of current CDC guidance (Tables 130.10 and Click here to enter text. 130.11). For adult patients with plague in a small, contained casualty setting, recommended regimens include streptomycin 1 g IM, given twice daily; gentamicin, 5 mg per kg IM or IV, once daily; or a 2 mg per kg loading dose of gentamicin followed by 1.7 mg per kg IM or IV every 8 hours. The dosing of aminoglycosides must include adjustment for renal function. The duration of treatment is 10 to 14 days. Oral therapy may be initiated once a patient demonstrates clinical stabilization and improvement. Alternate therapy with fluoroquinolones can be used in either setting, although initial therapy should be intravenous. For breastfeeding mothers and infants, treatment with gentamicin is recommended, but tetracyclines and fluoroquinolones may be used if gentamicin is unavailable or otherwise inappropriate [125].

TABLE 130.10

Plague Treatment

Adults	Antibiotic	Dose	Route of administration	Notes
	Streptomycin	1 g twice daily	IM	Not widely available in the USA
	Gentamicin	5 mg/kg once daily, or 2 mg/kg loading dose followed by 1.7 mg/kg every 8 hours	IM or IV	Not FDA approved but considered an effective alternative to streptomycin.[a] Owing to poor abscess penetration, consider alternative or dual therapy for patients with bubonic disease.
	Levofloxacin	500 mg once daily	IV or PO	Bactericidal. FDA approved based on animal studies but limited clinical experience treating human plague. A higher dose (750 mg) may be used if clinically indicated.
	Ciprofloxacin	400 mg every 8–12 hours	IV	Bactericidal. FDA approved based on animal studies but limited clinical experience treating human plague.
		500–750 mg twice daily	PO	
	Doxycycline	100 mg twice daily or 200 mg once daily	IV or PO	Bacteriostatic, but effective in a randomized trial when compared to gentamicin.[b]
	Moxifloxacin	400 mg once daily	IV or PO	
	Chloramphenicol	25 mg/kg every 6 h	IV	Not widely available in the USA

[a]Boulanger LL, Ettestad P, Fogarty JD, et al: Gentamicin and tetracyclines for the treatment of human plague: review of 75 cases in New Mexico, 1985–1999. *Clin Infect Dis.* 2004 38(5):663–669.
[b]Mwengee W, Butler T, Mgema S, et al: Treatment of plague with gentamicin or doxycycline in a randomized clinical trial in Tanzania. *Clin Infect Dis.* 2006 42(5):614–621.
FDA, Federal Drug Administration; IM, intramuscular; IV, intravenous; PO, oral.
Adapted from https://www.cdc.gov/plague/healthcare/clinicians.html Accessed September 23, 2016.

Mass Casualty Treatment and Prophylaxis

In a mass casualty situation from the intentional release of plague, the urgency to initiate prompt treatment of infected individuals, as well as prophylaxis for those exposed but uninfected, may cause a significant stress on health care capabilities. The ability to administer prompt parenteral streptomycin or gentamicin for symptomatic individuals is ideal, but may be limited. The Working Group on Civilian Biodefense recommends the use of ciprofloxacin 500 mg, taken orally twice daily or doxycycline 100 mg, taken orally twice daily for adults and pregnant women, both for treatment and postexposure prophylaxis. All individuals who come within 2 meters of a patient with pneumonic plague should receive postexposure prophylaxis. The recommendations of Table 130.12 are consensus-based for treating plague following an intentional release or bioterrorism attack and may not reflect FDA-approved use or indications [126].

Immunization

There is no approved vaccine available in the USA at present. A killed, whole-cell vaccine against plague was available until 1999 for those at high risk for exposure, but this vaccine was not effective against pneumonic plague and was unlikely to provide adequate protection in a biowarfare setting. Current vaccines in development include adenovirus and *Salmonella* vectors encoding for *Yersinia* epitopes [126,127], oral subunit vaccines comprising F1 and rV antigens [128,129], and attenuated strains of the closely related but less virulent *Yersinia pseudotuberculosis* [130,131].

Infection Control

Patients suspected of plague should be placed immediately into respiratory droplet precaution isolation, with access to the patient room restricted to essential staff. Gowns, gloves, surgical masks, and eye protection should be worn by all staff. Aerosolizing procedures should be kept to an absolute minimum and avoided if possible. Negative pressure isolation or N95 masks are not necessary for plague, although infections that may present similarly to pneumonic plague (e.g., SARS-associated coronvairus) may require negative pressure rooms or PAPRs, thus requiring a higher level of protection while diagnostic testing is underway. Following 48 hours of therapy with appropriate antibiotics and with clear clinical improvement, patients with both nonpneumonic plague and pneumonic plague may be removed from isolation [132]. Laboratory workers must be warned of potential plague infection owing to the risk of laboratory-acquired plague [98].

BOTULINUM TOXIN

Botulinum is an extremely potent neurotoxin that inhibits acetylcholine release and is produced by *Clostridium botulinum*, an anaerobic, spore-forming gram-positive bacterium present in the soil. Botulinum toxin can be inactivated by temperatures above 85°C for 5 minutes, but *Clostridium* spores can survive temperatures of 105°C for up to 4 hours, although they are readily destroyed by chlorine. Spores may remain viable for over 30 years in a dry state and are resistant to ultraviolet light exposure [133]. The botulinum toxin is among the most poisonous substances known. It can cause a serious, life-threatening paralytic illness among exposed individuals, is easily produced in a laboratory, and can be easily transported. In view of these properties, botulinum toxin has been designated as a Category A bioterrorism threat by the CDC [5,8]. There are reports that several countries may have stockpiled or are developing botulinum toxin for use as a bioweapon [133]. The general features and management of botulism are presented in Chapter 86 (ref 8th ed. Rippe), but the implications of botulism as a bioterrorist weapon are discussed here.

TABLE 130.11

Plague Treatment, Children

	Antibiotic	Dose	Route of administration	Notes
Children[a]	Streptomycin	15 mg/kg twice daily (maximum 2 g/d)	IM	Not widely available in the USA
	Gentamicin	2.5 mg/kg/dose every 8 hours	IM or IV	Not FDA approved but considered an effective alternative to streptomycin.[1] Owing to poor abscess penetration, consider alternative or dual therapy for patients with bubonic disease.
	Levofloxacin	10 mg/kg/dose (maximum 500 mg/dose)	IV or PO	Bactericidal, FDA approved based on animal studies but limited clinical experience treating human plague.
	Ciprofloxacin	15 mg/kg/dose every 12 hours (maximum 400 mg/dose)	IV	Bactericidal. FDA approved based on animal studies but limited clinical experience treating human plague.
		20 mg/kg/dose every 12 hours (maximum 500 mg/dose)	PO	
	Doxycycline	Weight <45 kg: 2.2 mg/kg twice daily (maximum 100 mg/dose) Weight ≥45 kg: same as adult dose	IV or PO	Bacteriostatic, but FDA approved and effective in a randomized trial when compared to gentamicin.[2] No tooth staining after multiple short courses.[b]
	Chloramphenicol (for children >2 years)	25 mg/kg every 6 h (maximum daily dose, 4 g)	IV	Not widely available in the USA
Pregnant women[a]	Gentamicin	Same as adult dose	IM or IV	See notes above
	Doxycycline	Same as adult dose	IV	See notes above
	Ciprofloxacin	Same as adult dose	IV	See notes above

[a]All recommended antibiotics for plague have relative contraindications for use in children and pregnant women; however, use is justified in life-threatening situations.
[b]Todd SR, Dahlgren FS, Traeger MS, et al: No visible dental staining in children treated with doxycycline for suspected Rocky Mountain spotted fever. *J Pediatr* 166(5):1246–1251, 2015.
FDA, Federal Drug Administration; IM, intramuscular; IV, intravenous; PO, oral.
https://www.cdc.gov/plague/healthcare/clinicians.html (Accessed September 23, 2016).

Botulinum Toxin as an Agent of Bioterrorism

There are three forms of naturally occurring botulism: *foodborne botulism*, *wound botulism*, and *intestinal (infant and adult) botulism*. All forms of botulism can produce a serious paralytic illness that can lead to respiratory failure and death.

Botulinum toxin solution is a colorless, odorless, tasteless liquid that is easily inactivated by heating at a temperature greater than 85°C for 5 minutes. There are seven different antigenic types: botulinum A, B, C, D, E, F, and G. Given its extreme potency, botulinum toxin could produce devastating effects and mass casualties, if intentionally dispersed by aerosol or used to contaminate the water supply [5,133]. Botulinum toxin types A, B, E, and F have been associated with naturally occurring foodborne botulism. Types C and D botulinum toxin cause natural disease in birds and cattle. Type G botulinum toxin is found in South America, but it has not been associated with foodborne botulism. Inhalational challenge studies with aerosolized botulinum toxin of primates have demonstrated the development of illness following exposure to all seven toxins. Researchers suspect that humans are also susceptible to these types [134].

The intentional use of botulinum toxin can be either inhalational or foodborne. In the 1930s, the Japanese reportedly executed a number of Manchurian prisoners by feeding them cultures of *Clostridium botulinum*. Botulinum toxin was produced by the USA for use as a bioweapon from World War II to the early 1970s when the bioweapon program was terminated. Following the 1972 Convention on the Prohibition of the Development and Stockpiling of Biological and Toxin Weapons, both the former Soviet Union and Iraq continued to develop botulinum toxin as a biowarfare agent. After the 1991 Persian Gulf War, Iraq admitted to UN weapons inspectors that it had produced and stockpiled biologic weapons containing botulinum toxin [134].

There remains considerable concern about the potential use of botulinum toxin as bioweapon. Contamination of either a food or a beverage source with botulinum toxin could result in mass casualties, overwhelming hospitals and intensive care units,

TABLE 130.12

Mass Casualty Exposure Treatment and Prophylaxis for Plague

Adults	Doxycycline 100 mg PO BID	or	Ciprofloxacin 500 mg PO BID	or	Chloramphenicol 25 mg/kg IV q6h (not to exceed 4 g/d, and should not be given to children under age 2)	Duration of treatment is 7 d.
Children > 45 kg			Ciprofloxacin 20 mg/kg PO BID			
Children < 45 kg	Doxycycline 2.2 mg/kg PO BID					
Pregnant women	Doxycycline 100 mg PO BID		Ciprofloxacin 500 mg PO BID			

BID, twice a day; IV, intravenous; PO, oral.
Adapted from Inglesby TV, Dennis DT, Henderson DA, et al: Plague as a biological weapon: medical and public health management. Working Group on Civilian Biodefense. *JAMA* 283:2281–2290, 2000 [125].

and creating significant anxiety among the general population [134]. It has been estimated that 1 g of botulinum toxin added to milk that is commercially distributed and consumed by 568,000 individuals can result in 100,000 cases of botulism [135]. It has also been estimated that 1 g of aerosolized botulinum toxin could potentially kill more than 1 million people [133,134].

Pathogenesis

Inhalational and foodborne exposures typically have a 12 to 36 hour incubation period, however symptoms have been reported within 6 hours and as late as 10 days following exposure [136]. Following exposure, the toxin enters the circulation, and the heavy chain of the toxin binds to the neuronal membrane on the presynaptic side of the neuromuscular junction. The toxin enters the neuronal cell, after which the light chain of the toxin cleaves the synaptic proteins that form the synaptic fusion complex. See Figure 130.14 for structure of botulinum toxin A. Disruption of the synaptic fusion complex prevents release of acetylcholine release into the synaptic cleft, leading to paralysis that may last for several months. Death from botulism is most often caused by respiratory muscle paralysis. The central nervous system is unaffected, because botulism toxin does not cross the blood–brain barrier. A prospective, observational cohort study of 91 botulism patients in Thailand showed that those individuals presenting with dyspnea; moderate-to-severe ptosis; and pupillary changes were likely to progress to respiratory failure, whereas a long incubation period before symptoms appeared was associated with a more favorable prognosis [137].

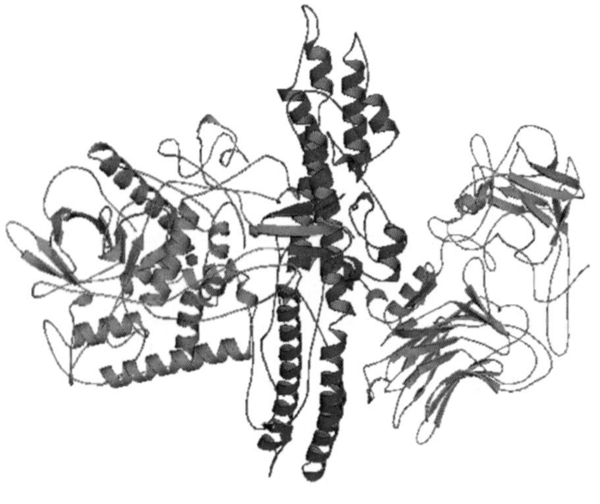

FIGURE 130.14 Botulinum neurotoxin-a is composed of an ~50 Kda light chain (red) linked by a single disulfide bond to the ~100 Kda heavy chain. The light chain functions as a zinc-dependent endopeptidase. The heavy chain has two components (blue and purple). (Original work by Lacy DB, Tepp W, Cohen AC, et al: Crystal structure of botulinum neurotoxin type A and implications for toxicity. *Nat Struct Biol* 5:898–902, 1998. Reproduced from the Chapter 16, Botulinum Toxin, Medical Agents of Biologic Warfare, USAMRIID, 10th edition, 2012 [open source].)

Treatment

The treatment of botulism includes supportive care, mechanical ventilation if necessary, and the administration of botulinum antitoxin. In severe cases, 2 to 8 weeks of ventilator support may be required prior to recovery. In an outbreak following an intentional release, the health care demands may rapidly overwhelm current capabilities, especially with regard to the availability of mechanical ventilators and critical care providers. There is a supply of mechanical ventilators in the Strategic National Stockpile (SNS) and in some state caches that can be deployed in the event of a mass casualty. The request must be coordinated via the local-state-national Incident Command System.

Rega et al. suggest an algorithm and triage tool to assess the severity of botulism cases that may be helpful during mass casualty situations [138,139]. Specific therapy for botulism involves the administration of botulinum antitoxin. Early suspicion of botulism and the prompt administration of botulinum antitoxin can reduce nerve damage and disease severity. The goal of antitoxin therapy is to prevent further paralysis by neutralizing unbound botulinum toxin in the circulation. A new heptavalent botulinum antitoxin (HBAT) approved by the FDA replaced the former trivalent botulinum antitoxin in 2013 [140]. This heptavalent antitoxin contains equine-derived antibody to all seven botulinum toxins from A to G. If a case of botulism is suspected, prompt diagnosis is essential. If botulism is confirmed, the CDC will provide heptavalent antitoxin and detailed instructions for its intravenous administration (contact the local health department or if unavailable, the CDC at 770-488-7100) [133,141]. Additional doses of botulinum antitoxin will be needed when multiple cases of botulism occur after an intentional release. Following the initial administration of botulinum antitoxin, patients should be carefully assessed for refractory symptoms, such as rapidly progressing paralysis, severe airway obstruction, or

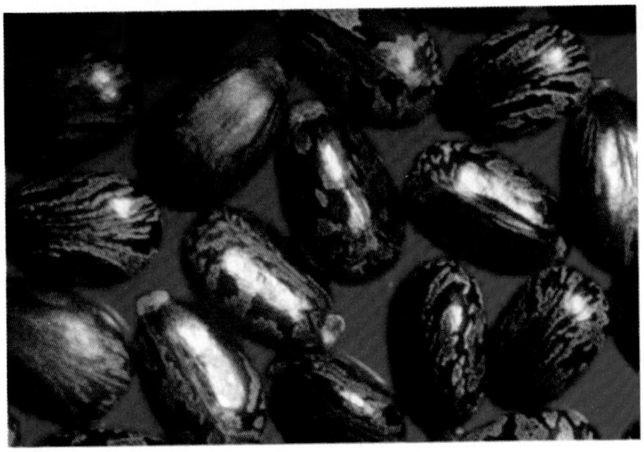

FIGURE 130.15 Castor beans (*Ricinus communis*) (Picture from "Quick Bio-Agents Guide, First Edition, 2012. Available for download at http://www.usamriid.army.mil/education/instruct.htm).

overwhelming respiratory tract secretions, which may indicate the need for an additional dose.

Hypersensitivity reactions to botulinum antitoxin may occur. These include anaphylaxis, serum sickness, chills, fever, dyspnea, cutaneous erythema, and edema of the tongue. The incidence of hypersensitivity with the recommended one-vial dose is about 1%. A small dose can be given initially to screen for hypersensitivity, but this may be impractical in a mass casualty situation [133,134,142,143].

Human-derived anti–botulinum toxin immunoglobulin (BabyBIG-IV) is available as an orphan drug for the treatment of infant botulism, but it has not been tested for adults and is currently only available for infants under one year of age [144].

Prophylaxis

In the USA, a pentavalent botulinum toxoid vaccine was previously available from the CDC for the immunization of laboratory workers and military personnel at risk for botulinum toxin exposure, but this vaccine is no longer available as of 2011 owing to evidence of decreasing immunogenicity from the source strain. At the present time, there is no generally recommended prophylactic therapy for the prevention of botulism. High-risk exposures may receive HBAT on a case-by-case basis, in consultation with CDC [145].

RICIN

Ricin is a potent toxin belonging to the broad family of ribosome-inhibiting proteins and is easily extracted from seeds contained in the bean (Fig. 130.15) of the castor plant, *Ricinis communis* [146]. The castor plant, a native plant of Africa, is a common outdoor plant in warm climates and is also used for ornamental purposes. Castor bean seeds, castor oil, and the castor plant have been used for many centuries for their medicinal, lubricant, and decorative properties. Castor bean seeds contain high concentrations of ricin, and ingestion of as few as three seeds can be fatal. Ricin is an immunotoxin, allergen, and toxic enzyme that inhibits protein synthesis. As a result of its biochemical properties, ricin has antitumor effects and has undergone phase I and phase II clinical trials as a chemotherapeutic agent. Ricin can be inactivated by heating to 175°F for 10 minutes. It is odorless and tasteless and can be produced in liquid, crystalline, or dry powder forms. Both the liquid and powder forms have the potential to be aerosolized [72,146].

Toxicology

Ricin is 66-kd globular protein consisting of two sulfide-linked polypeptide chains, A and B. The B-chain binds to the cell surface at galactose-containing sites and facilitates entry of the A-chain into the cell [147,148]. The A-chain then enters the cytosol of a cell; inactivates the 28S ribosomal subunits; inhibits protein synthesis; and causes cell death. Both the toxicity and the lethality of ricin depend on the exposure dose and the route of administration. In murine models, the LD50 and time of death are 3 to 5 μg per kg and 60 hours by inhalation, 5 μg per kg and 90 hours by intravenous injection, and 20 mg per kg and 85 hours by intra-gastric administration. The lethal doses of ricin for humans are estimated to be 5 to 10 μg per kg by inhalation and 1 to 10 μg per kg by injection [149]. On exposure to lethal doses of ricin by inhalation, rats develop a necrotizing tracheobronchitis and pneumonia with parenchymal inflammation and pulmonary edema [150]. In nonhuman primates, inhalation of ricin leads to death within 48 hours of exposure, and autopsy shows diffuse necrosis of airways, severe pulmonary edema, severe fibrinopurulent pneumonia, and mediastinal lymphadenitis [148].

Ricin as an Agent of Bioterrorism

The high toxicity, relative ease of production, ease of dissemination, and stability of ricin in ambient conditions make it a potential agent of bioterrorism. Ricin can be dispersed as an aerosol or as a contaminant of food and beverages for the purpose of causing multiple casualties. Ricin may be an ideal agent for small-scale bioterrorism attacks against high-value targets, because the large quantities needed for a large-scale attack are thought be logistically difficult [146].

There have been several reports of the use or intended use of ricin in terrorist activities. In 1978, a Bulgarian diplomat named Georgi Markov, was killed in London by a ricin-containing pellet fired from an umbrella-based weapon [151,152] as shown in Figure 130.16. In January 2003, British authorities arrested 10 individuals from North Africa who were residing in a London apartment where ricin was found. In October 2003, ricin was identified in an envelope at a Greenville, South Carolina, post office [147]. In November 2003, an envelope addressed to the White House was reportedly intercepted by the Secret Service and was found to contain ricin. In February 2004, ricin was reportedly detected in the Dirksen Senate Office Building [146]. These events highlight the need for clinicians to be familiar with the recognition and management of ricin poisoning.

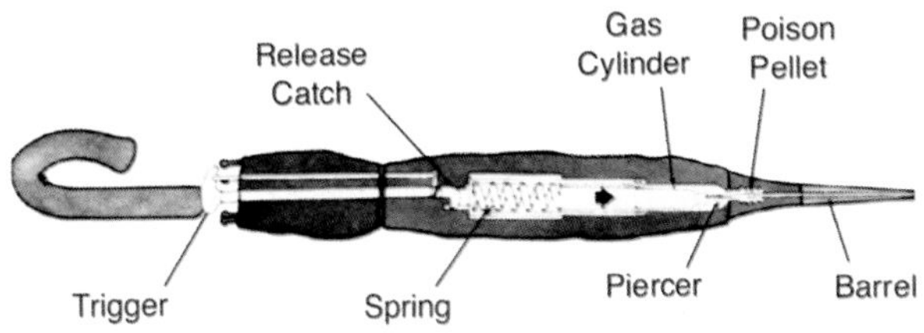

FIGURE 130.16 Diagram of "umbrella gun" clandestine weapon used to assassinate Bulgarian exile Georgi Markov in London in 1978. The poison projectile was propelled through the hollow tip by the pressure released from a carbon dioxide cartridge. (Original work van Keuren RT: Chemical and Biological Warfare, An Investigative Guide. Washington, DC, Office of Enforcement, Strategic Investigations Division, US Customs Service, 1990 [89]. Reproduced from the Chapter 1, History of Biological Weapons: From Poisoned Darts to Intentional Epidemics, Medical Agents of Biologic Warfare, USAMRIID, 10th edition, 2012.)

Ricin Toxicity in Humans

The pathologic changes and clinical symptoms caused by ricin exposure depend on the exposure dose and the route of exposure. The clinical effects of ricin for humans have been described following cases of castor seed ingestion and parenteral use in chemotherapeutic clinical trials. The clinical findings observed in animal models after the oral or parenteral administration of ricin appear to correlate with the clinical findings of humans exposed to oral or parenteral ricin. Human data on inhalational exposure to ricin is very limited. The findings from animals following inhalational exposure are presumed to be similar to those that would be experienced by humans following ricin inhalation. Leukocytosis appears to be a consistent finding, regardless of the route of exposure. Ricin toxicity by any route of exposure can produce a flu-like illness with fevers, myalgias, and arthralgias, as well as hallucinations and seizures [72].

Gastrointestinal Route

Compared to other routes of ricin exposure, the gastrointestinal route is the least toxic, and severity can vary based on the amount of ricin ingested. A review of 880 cases of mostly accidental castor seed ingestions reported symptoms consisting of nausea, vomiting, and abdominal cramping within a few hours after ingestion, followed by diarrhea that may become bloody and lead to volume depletion, hypotension, severe electrolyte loss, tachypnea, tachycardia, and delirium with hallucinations. Case fatality rates of 1.5% were reported [146,147,153].

Parenteral Route

In cases of ricin toxicity produced by parenteral administration, pain at the site of injection, fatigue, malaise, headache, rigors, and fever were noted in the first 24 hours. Patients also showed local necrotic lymphadenopathy. Ricin, when used as a chemotherapeutic agent at a dose of 18 to 20 μg per kg, caused nausea, vomiting, myalgia, and fatigue. More serious adverse effects may include pulmonary edema, hypoalbuminemia, cardiac failure, hypotension, hypovolemic shock, acute hepatic and renal failure, gastrointestinal bleeding, thrombocytopenia, and bleeding diathesis [146,148].

Inhalational Route

Patients with inhalational exposure of ricin may develop symptoms within 3 to 24 hours. In nonhuman primate models, aerosolized ricin given in lethal doses produces severe diffuse, necrotizing bronchiolitis, massive alveolar edema with hemorrhage, and hemorrhagic tracheobronchial lymphadenitis, with death occurring in as little as 36 hours after exposure [154]. Sublethal exposure appears to produce a chronic pulmonary fibrosis in surviving animals [155]. The only information regarding human inhalational exposure is related to castor seed dust. Reported symptoms from dust inhalation include itchy eyes, nasal and bronchial congestion, urticaria, chest tightness, and bronchospasm, all suggestive of an allergic syndrome [146].

Ricin as an Allergen

Type I and IV hypersensitivity syndromes have been reported following dermal exposure to castor seeds and castor seed dust, including an anaphylactic-type reaction in a woman when a seed from her castor-bean necklace disintegrated in her fingers. The woman experienced rhinitis, sneezing, periorbital edema, and facial urticaria, requiring a subcutaneous injection of epinephrine [156]. Although the incidence of ricin-associated allergic reactions is unknown, they may be relatively frequent among exposed individuals because of the immunogenic properties of the ricin molecule.

Diagnosis

The diagnosis of ricin toxicity is challenging. The differential diagnosis includes exposure to staphylococcal enterotoxin, phosgene, oxides of nitrogen, and organohalides. If a bioterrorism attack is suspected, anthrax, plague, and tularemia should also be considered. Ricin intoxication by the inhalational route can be confirmed by ELISA analysis of nasal mucosal swabs taken within 24 hours of exposure. Specific ricin antigen testing or immunochemical staining of serum and respiratory secretions can also be performed [157]. Serum and respiratory samples may also be sent for PCR evaluation [158]. Because ricin is an immunogenic toxin, a significant increase of the anti-ricin antibody titer 2 weeks after exposure may also be helpful for confirming the diagnosis. It is recommended that acute and convalescent antibody titers be obtained for all individuals suspected of ricin intoxication. However, anti-ricin antibodies are rapidly metabolized and excreted, so the absence of a significant increase in titer does not exclude the diagnosis [147]. Urine testing for the ricin biomarker ricinine is under investigation [159,160].

Neutrophilic leukocytosis is usually present in peripheral blood. Pleural effusions and bilateral alveolar infiltrates, indicative of pulmonary edema, may be seen on chest radiographs. Arterial blood gases should be monitored to assess oxygenation, the adequacy of ventilation, and acid–base status. Myocardial ischemia, cardiac dysrhythmias, and cardiac conduction abnormalities may occur and should be evaluated through routine electrocardiography and echocardiography [146,148].

Treatment

The management of ricin intoxication is largely supportive, regardless of the route of exposure. All patients suspected of ricin intoxication should be decontaminated by removing all clothing and washing the skin with soap and water. Careful attention to fluid and electrolyte balance is essential, especially in patients with pulmonary edema. Vasopressors may be needed for the management of severe hypotension. If ricin ingestion has occurred, gastric lavage may be helpful for removing ricin from the gastrointestinal tract. If the patient is alert, activated charcoal can be given.

If inhalation is the route of exposure, effective airway management is essential. Bronchospasm should be treated with a nebulized bronchodilator. Patients with severe pulmonary edema will require intubation and mechanical ventilation. Oxygen should be administered at a concentration sufficient to keep the arterial oxygen tension (PaO_2) between 60 and 100 mm Hg. Myocardial infarction, myocardial ischemia, cardiac dysrhythmias, and cardiac conduction abnormalities should be treated as appropriate. Mild allergic reactions can be treated with an antihistamine. Epinephrine should be given for anaphylaxis. A nonsteroidal anti-inflammatory drug can be given for arthralgias and myalgias [146].

There is no specific therapy for ricin. Chimeric and monoclonal antibodies directed against the A chain of ricin toxin have demonstrated benefits in animal models; however, human clinical data is presently lacking [161–163]. Some reported case series have described a positive experience with early plasma exchange of children following castor bean ingestion with symptoms of ricin intoxication [164,165]. Most patients with ricin intoxication should survive the acute effects if appropriate supportive care is given promptly after exposure. However, because the clinical effects of ricin intoxication are dose-related, individuals exposed to high concentrations may die from cardiopulmonary arrest in spite of the best supportive care [166].

TABLE 130.13

Summary of Common Clinical Syndromes Caused by Agents of Bioterrorism

Condition	Pathogen or source	Clinical syndrome(s)	Contagious	Incubation period	Vaccine available	Empiric therapy	Mortality
Anthrax	*Bacillus anthracis*	Cutaneous, inhalational, GI	No	1–6 d	Yes	Isolated cutaneous Cutaneous: ciprofloxacin 500 mg PO twice daily	Inhalational: 46%–94% GI: 25%–60% Cutaneous: 5%–20%
Botulism	*Clostridium botulinum*	Inhalational or gastrointestinal	No	½–5 d	No	Botulinum antitoxin	3%–5%
Plague	*Yersinia pestis*	Bubonic, septicemic, pneumonic	Yes	1–7 d (usually 2–3 d)	No	Streptomycin or gentamicin 5 mg/kg IV q24h	Bubonic: 10%–20% Septicemic: 10%–22% Pneumonic: 50%–100%
Ricin toxin	*Ricinus communis*	Gastrointestinal, parenteral, inhalational	No	18–24 h	No	Supportive	Not known
Smallpox	Variola virus	Classic, hemorrhagic	Yes	7–17 d (average 12 d)	Yes	Supportive; consider cidofovir, brincidofovir, tecovirimat, anti-vaccinia IgG	Classic: 10%–60% Hemorrhagic: >95%
Tularemia	*Francisella tularensis*	Ulceroglandular, oculoglandular, pneumonic, typhoidal	No	1–21 d (average 3–6 d)	No	Streptomycin or gentamicin 5 mg/kg IV q24h	5%–35%

GI, gastrointestinal; IV, intravenous; PO, oral.
Derived from Adalja AA, Toner E, Inglesbey TV: Clinical management of potential bioterrorism-related conditions. N Engl J Med 372:954–962, 2015, and from Christian MD: Biowarfare and bioterrorism. Crit Care Clin 717–756, 2013.

Immunization

RiVax/Alum (Soliginex, Princeton, New Jersey) and RVEc (USAMRIID, Fort Detrick, Maryland) are recombinant inactivated ricin A-chain toxoid vaccines that have been shown to be immunogenic and safe in small phase 1 human trials [167,168]. These vaccines appear to be comparably immunogenic when compared in a murine model [169]. The use of these agents in cases of a human outbreak or attack remains to be determined.

Table 130.13 provides a useful summary table of biologic agents, clinical features, and initial treatment.

References

1. Dembek ZF: *Medical Aspects of Biological Warfare*. Washington, DC, Falls Church, Va. Fort Sam Houston, Tex., Borden Institute & Office of the Surgeon General United States Army, 2007.
2. Bush LM, Abrams BH, Beall A, et al: Index case of fatal inhalational anthrax due to bioterrorism in the United States. *NEJM* 345:1607, 2001.
3. Hughes J, Gerberding JL: Anthrax bioterrorism: lessons learned and future directions. *Emerg Infect Dis* 8(10):1013, 2002.
4. Martin JW, Christopher GW, Eitzen EM: History of biological weapons: from poisoned darts to intentional epidemics, in *Textbook of Military Medicine*. Falls Church, VA, Borden Institute and US Army Office of the Surgeon General, 2007.
5. Christian MD: Biowarfare and bioterrorism. *Crit Care Clin* 29:717–756, 2013.
6. Rotz LD, Khan AS, Lillibridge SR, et al: Public health assessment of potential biological terrorism agents. *Emerg Infect Dis* 8:225, 2002.
7. Weisfeld J, Henderson DA, Millar D, et al: Smallpox Eradication: Memories and Milestones, 2007. http://scott.library.emory.edu/ghcexportfiles/emory1dpk8.pdf. Accessed September 18, 2016.
8. McFadden G: Killing a killer. *PLoS Pathog* 29(6), 2010.
9. McCarthy M: Smallpox samples are found in FDA storage room in Maryland. *BMJ* 349:g4545, 2014.
10. Ambrose C: Osler and the infected letter. *Emerg Infect Dis* 11:689, 2005.
11. Grabenstein JD, Winkenwerder W: U.S. military smallpox vaccination program experience. *JAMA* 289:3278, 2003.
12. Henderson DA, Inglesby TV, Bartlett JG, et al: Smallpox as a biological weapon: medical and public health management. *JAMA* 281(22):2127–2137, 1999.
13. Henderson DA: Smallpox epidemic models and response strategies. *Biosecur Bioterror* 11(1):73–74, 2013.
14. Horgan ES, Ali HM: Cross immunity experiments in monkey between variola, alastrim and vaccinia. *J Hyg* 39:615, 1939.
15. Noble J, Rich JA: Transmission of smallpox by contact and by aerosol routes in Macaca irus. *Bull World Health Organ* 40:279, 1969.
16. Breman JG, Henderson DA: Diagnosis and management of smallpox. *N Engl J Med* 346:1300, 2002.

17. Cann JA, Jahrling PB, Hensley LE, et al: Comparative pathology of smallpox and monkeypox in man and macaques. *J Comp Pathol* 148(1):6–21, 2013.
18. Jahrling PB, Huggins JW, Ibrahim MS, et al: Smallpox and related orthopoxviruses, in Dembek ZSE (ed): *Medical Aspects of Biological Warfare*. Falls Church, Va., 2007.
19. Petersen BW, Damon IK, Pertowski CA: Clinical guidance for smallpox vaccine use in a postevent vaccination program. *MMWR* 64(2):1–30, 2015.
20. CDC: SMALLPOX FACT SHEET—Information for Lab Workers. 2013. Available at https://www.cdc.gov/smallpox/lab-personnel/index.html. Accessed September 20, 2016.
21. Gani R, Leach S: Transmission potential of smallpox in contemporary populations. *Nature* 414:748–751, 2001.
22. Belongia EA, Naleway AL: Smallpox vaccine: the good, the bad, and the ugly. *Clin Med Res* 1(2):87–92, 2003.
23. Bray M, Martinez M, Smee DF, et al: Cidofovir protects mice against lethal aerosol or intranasal cowpox viral challenge. *J Infect Dis* 181(10), 2000.
24. Verreault D, Sivasubramani SK, Talton JD, et al: Evaluation of inhaled cidofovir as postexposure prophylactic in an aerosol rabbitpox model. *Antiviral Res* 93:204–208, 2012.
25. Jahrling PB, Fritz EA, Hensley LE: Countermeasures to the bioterrorist threat of smallpox. *Curr Mol Med* 5:817–826, 2005.
26. Smee DF, Dagley A, Downs B, et al: Enhanced efficacy of cidofovir combined with vaccinia immune globulin in treating progressive cutaneous vaccinia virus infections in immunosuppressed hairless mice. *Antimicrob Agents Chemother* 59(1):520–526, 2015.
27. Israely T, Paran N, Lustig S, et al: A single cidofovir treatment rescues animals at progressive stages of lethal orthopoxvirus disease. *Virol J* 9(119):1–12, 2012.
28. Trost LC, Rose ML, Khouri J, et al: The efficacy and pharmacokinetics of brincidofovir for the treatment of lethal rabbitpox virus infection: a model of smallpox disease. *Antiviral Res* 117:115–121, 2015.
29. Olson VA, Smith SK, Foster S, et al: In vitro efficacy of brincidofovir against variola virus. *Antimicrob Agents Chemother* 58(9):5570–5571, 2014.
30. Mucker EM, Goff AJ, Shamblin JD, et al: Efficacy of tecovirimat (ST-246) in nonhuman primates infected with variola virus (smallpox). *Antimicrob Agents Chemother* 57(12):6246–6253, 2013.
31. Berhanu A, Prigge JT, Silvera PM, et al: Treatment with the smallpox antiviral tecovirimat (ST-246) alone or in combination with ACAM2000 vaccination is effective as a postsymptomatic therapy for monkeypox virus infection. *Antimicrob Agents Chemother* 59(7):4296–4300, 2015.
32. Guimaraes AP, de Souza FR, Oliveira AA, et al: Design of inhibitors of thymidylate kinase from Variola virus as new selective drugs against smallpox. *Eur J Med Chem* 91:72–90, 2015.
33. Maxurkov OY, Kabanov AS, Shishkina LN, et al: New effective chemically synthesized anti-smallpox compound NIOCH-14. *J Gen Virol* 97:1229–1239, 2016.
34. Frey SE, Couch RB, Tacket CO, et al: Clinical responses to undiluted and diluted smallpox vaccine. *NEJM* 346(17):1265–1274, 2002.
35. Fulginiti VA: Risks of smallpox vaccination. *JAMA* 290(11):1452, 2003.
36. Neff J, Modlin J, Birkhead GS, et al: Monitoring the safety of a smallpox vaccination program in the United States: report of the joint Smallpox Vaccine Safety Working Group of the Advisory Committee on Immunization Practices and the Armed Forces Epidemiological Board. *Clin Infect Dis* 46 Suppl 3:S258–S270, 2008.
37. Wharton M, Strikas RA, Harpaz R, et al: Recommendations for using smallpox vaccine in a pre-event vaccination program. Supplemental recommendations of the Advisory Committee on Immunization Practices (ACIP) and the Healthcare Infection Control Practices Advisory Committee (HICPAC). *MMWR Recomm Rep* 52:1–16, 2003.
38. Bartlett J, del Rio C, DeMaria A Jr, et al: Smallpox vaccination and the HIV-infected patient: a Roundtable. *AIDS Clin Care* 15(7):61–63, 2003.
39. Jerek Z, Szczenioski M, Paluku KM, et al: Human monkeypox: clinical features of 282 patients. *J Infect Dis* 156:293–298, 1987.
40. Weber DJ, Rutala WA: Risks and prevention of nosocomial transmission of rare zoonotic diseases. *Clin Infect Dis* 32:446–456, 2001.
41. Chimerix Inc: *CMX001 for the Treatment of Smallpox*. Durham, North Carolina, Chimerix, pp 1–48.
42. Lederman ER, Davidson W, Groff HL, et al: Progressive vaccinia: case description and laboratory-guided therapy with vaccinia immune globulin, ST-246, and CMX001. *J Infect Dis* 206(9):1372–1385, 2012.
43. Handley L, Buller RM, Frey SE, et al: The new ACAM2000 vaccine and other therapies to control orthopoxvirus outbreaks and bioterror attacks. *Expert Rev Vaccines* 8:841, 2009.
44. Bower WA, Hendricks K, Pillai S, et al: Clinical framework and medical countermeasure use during an anthrax mass-casualty incident-CDC recommendations. *MMWR* 64(4):26, 2015.
45. Purcell BK, Worsham PL, Friedlander AM: Anthrax, in Dembek Z Sr (ed): *Medical Aspects of Biological Warfare*. Falls Church, VA, Borden Institute and US Army Office of the Surgeon General, 2007.
46. Adalja AA, Toner E, Inglesby TV: Clinical management of potential bioterrorism-related conditions. *N Engl J Med* 372(10):954–962, 2015.
47. Shafazand S: When bioterrorism strikes: diagnosis and management of inhalational anthrax. *Semin Respir Infect* 18(3):134–145, 2003.
48. Freedman A, Afonja O, Chang MW, et al: Cutaneous anthrax associated with microangiopathic hemolytic anemia and coagulopathy in a 7-month-old infant. *JAMA* 287(7):869–874, 2002.
49. Barakat LA, Quentzel HL, Jernigan JA, et al: Fatal inhalational anthrax in a 94-year-old Connecticut woman. *JAMA* 287(7):863–868, 2002.
50. Guarner J, Jernigan JA, Shieh WJ, et al: Pathology and pathogenesis of bioterrorism-related inhalational anthrax. *Am J Pathol* 163(2):701–709, 2003.
51. Walker D: Sverdlovsk revisited: pulmonary pathology of inhalational anthrax versus anthraxlike Bacillus cereus pneumonia. *Arch Pathol Lab Med* 136(3):235–236, 2012.
52. Toth DJ, Gundlapalli AV, Schell WA, et al: Quantitative models of the dose-response and time course of inhalational anthrax in humans. *PLoS Pathog* 9(8):e1003555, 2013.
53. Mayer TA, Bersoff-Matcha S, Murphy C, et al: Clinical presentation of inhalational anthrax following bioterrorism exposure: report of 2 surviving patients. *JAMA* 286(20):2549–2553, 2001.
54. Holty JE, Bravata DM, Liu H, et al: Systematic review: a century of inhalational anthrax cases from 1900 to 2005. *Ann Intern Med* 144(4):270–280, 2006.
55. Holty JE, Kim RY, Bravata DM: Anthrax: a systematic review of atypical presentations. *Ann Emerg Med* 48(2):200–211, 2006.
56. Hendricks KA, Wright ME, Shadomy SV, et al: Centers for disease control and prevention expert panel meetings on prevention and treatment of anthrax in adults. *Emerg Infect Dis* 20(2), 2014.
57. Katharios-Lanwermeyer S, Holty JE, Person M, et al: Identifying meningitis during an anthrax mass casualty incident: systematic review of systemic anthrax since 1880. *Clin Infect Dis* 62(12):1537–1545, 2016.
58. Meaney-Delman D, Zotti ME, Creanga AA, et al: Special considerations for prophylaxis for and treatment of anthrax in pregnant and postpartum women. *Emerg Infec Dis* 20(2):1–7, 2014.
59. Bartlett JG, Inglesby TV Jr, Borio L: Management of anthrax. *Clin Infec Dis* 35(7):851–858, 2002.
60. Inglesby TV, O'Toole T, Henderson DA, et al: Anthrax as a biological weapon, 2002: updated recommendations for management. *JAMA* 287(17):2236–2252, 2002.
61. Bravata DM, Holty JE, Wang E, et al: Inhalational, gastrointestinal, and cutaneous anthrax in children: a systematic review of cases: 1900 to 2005. *Arch Pediatr Adolesc Med* 161(9):896–905, 2007.
62. Kaur M, Bhatnagar R: Recent progress in the development of anthrax vaccines. *Recent Pat Biotechnol* 5(3):148–159, 2011.
63. Kummerfeldt CE: Raxibacumab: potential role in the treatment of inhalational anthrax. *Infect Drug Resist* 7:101–109, 2014.
64. Migone TS, Bolmer S, Zhong J, et al: Added benefit of raxibacumab to antibiotic treatment of inhalational anthrax. *Antimicrob Agents Chemother* 59(2):1145–1151, 2015.
65. Yamamoto BJ, Shadiack AM, Carpenter S, et al: Obiltoxaximab prevents disseminated bacillus anthracis infection and improves survival during pre- and post-exposure prophylaxis in animal models of inhalational anthrax. *Antimicrob Agents Chemother* 60:5796–5805, 2016. doi: 10.1128/AAC.01102-16.
66. Yamamoto BJ, Shadiack AM, Carpenter S, et al: Obiltoxaximab for inhalational anthrax: efficacy projection across a range of disease severity. *Antimicrob Agents Chemother* 60(10):5787–5795, 2016. doi: 10.1128/AAC.00972-16.
67. Kammanadiminti S, Patnaikuni RK, Comer J, et al: Combination therapy with antibiotics and anthrax immune globulin intravenous (AIGIV) is potentially more effective than antibiotics alone in rabbit model of inhalational anthrax. *PLoS One* 9:e106393, 2014.
68. Christopher GW, Cieslak TJ, Pavlin JA, et al: Biological warfare. A historical perspective. *JAMA* 278(5):412–417, 1997.
69. Reintjes R, Dedushaj I, Gjini A, et al: Tularemia outbreak investigation in Kosovo: case control and environmental studies. *Emerg Infect Dis* 8(1):69–73, 2002.
70. Hepburn MJ, Friedlander AM, Dembek ZF: Tularemia, in *Medical Aspects of Biological Warfare*. Falls Church, VA, Borden Institute and US Army Office of the Surgeon General, 2007.
71. Putzova D, Senitkova I, Stulik J: Tularemia vaccines. *Folia Microbiol* 61:495–504, 2016.
72. Balali-Mood M, Moshiri M, Etemad L: Medical aspects of bio-terrorism. *Toxicon* 69:131–142, 2013.
73. Sjostedt A: Tularemia: history, epidemiology, pathogen physiology, and clinical manifestations. *Ann N Y Acad Sci* 1105:1–29, 2007.
74. Desvars A, Furberg M, Hjertqvist M, et al: Epidemiology and ecology of tularemia in Sweden, 1984–2012. *Emerg Infect Dis* 21(1):32–39, 2015.
75. Feldman KA, Stiles-Enos D, Julian K, et al: Tularemia on Martha's Vineyard: seroprevalence and occupational risk. *Emerg Infect Dis* 9(3):350–354, 2003.
76. Chitadze N, Kuchuloria T, Clark DV, et al: Water-borne outbreak of oropharyngeal and glandular tularemia in Georgia: investigation and follow-up. *Infection* 37(6):514–521, 2009.
77. Dennis DT, Inglesby TV, Henderson DA, et al: Tularemia as a biological weapon: medical and public health management. *JAMA* 285(21):2763–2773, 2001.
78. Rubin SA: Radiographic spectrum of pleuropulmonary tularemia. *Am J Roentgenol* 131(2):277–281, 1978.
79. Weant KA, Bailey AM, Fleishaker EL, et al: Being prepared: bioterrorism and mass prophylaxis: part I. *Adv Emerg Nurs J* 36(3):226–238, 2014.
80. Chaignat V, Djordjevic-Spasic M, Ruettger A, et al: Performance of seven serological assays for diagnosing tularemia. *BMC Infect Dis* 14(234):1–6, 2014.
81. Kilic S, Celebi B, Yesilyurt M: Evaluation of a commercial immunochromatographic assay for the serologic diagnosis of tularemia. *Diagn Microbiol Infect Dis* 74(1):1–5, 2012.
82. Gunnell MK, Lovelace CD, Satterfield BA, et al: A multiplex real-time PCR assay for the detection and differentiation of Francisella tularensis subspecies. *J Med Microbiol* 61(11):1525–1531, 2012.
83. Yapar D, Erenler AK, Terzi O, et al: Predicting tularemia with clinical, laboratory and demographical findings in the ED. *Am J Emerg Med* 34(2):218–221, 2016.

84. Kosker M, Celik T, Yuksel D: Treatment of Tularemia during pregnancy. *J Infect Dev Ctries* 9(1):118–119, 2015.
85. Mahawar M, Rabadi SM, Banik S, et al: Identification of a live attenuated vaccine candidate for tularemia prophylaxis. *PLoS One* 8(4):e61539, 2013.
86. Worsham PL, McGovern TW, Vietri NJ, et al: Plague, in Demberk ZF (ed): *Medical Aspects of Biological Warfare*. Washington, DC, Borden Institute, 2007.
87. Butler T: Plague history: Yersin's discovery of the causative bacterium in 1894 enabled, in the subsequent century, scientific progress in understanding the disease and the development of treatments and vaccines. *Clin Microbiol Infect* 20(3):202–209, 2014.
88. Sun W, Six DA, Reynolds CM, et al: Pathogenicity of Yersinia pestis synthesis of 1-dephosphorylated lipid A. *Infect Immun* 81(4):1172–1185, 2013.
89. Williamson ED, Oyston PC: The natural history and incidence of Yersinia pestis and prospects for vaccination. *J Med Microbiol* 61(7):911–918, 2012.
90. Atkinson S, Williams P: Yersinia virulence factors—a sophisticated arsenal for combating host defences. *F1000Res* 5, 2016.
91. Korhonen TK, Haiko J, Laakkonen L, et al: Fibrinolytic and coagulative activities of Yersinia pestis. *Front Cell Infect Microbiol* 3:35, 2013.
92. Raoult D, Mouffok N, Bitam I, et al: Plague: history and contemporary analysis. *J Infect* 66(1):18–26, 2013.
93. Runfola JK, House J, Miller L, et al: Outbreak of human pneumonic plague with dog-to-human and possible human-to-human transmission—Colorado, June–July 2014. *MMWR* 64(16):429–434, 2015.
94. Nichols MC, Ettestad PJ, Vinhatton ES, et al: Yersinia pestis infection in dogs: 62 cases (2003–2011). *J Am Vet Med Assoc* 244(10):1176–1180, 2014.
95. Walsh M, Haseeb MA: Modeling the ecologic niche of plague in sylvan and domestic animal hosts to delineate sources of human exposure in the western United States. *PeerJ* 3:e1493, 2015.
96. Gerhold RW, Jessup DA: Zoonotic diseases associated with free-roaming cats. *Zoonoses Public Health* 60(3):189–195, 2013.
97. Pechous RD, Sivaraman V, Stasulli NM, et al: Pneumonic plague: the darker side of Yersinia pestis. *Trends Microbiol* 24(3):190–197, 2016.
98. Silver S: Laboratory-acquired lethal infections by potential bioweapons pathogens including Ebola in 2014. *FEMS Microbiol Lett* 362(1):1–6, 2015.
99. Wheelis M: Biological warfare at the 1346 siege of Caffa. *Emerg Infect Dis* 8(9):971–975, 2002.
100. Carus WS: The history of biological weapons use: what we know and what we don't. *Health Secur* 13(4):219–255, 2015.
101. Center for Infectious Disease Research and Policy: Plague. University of Minnesota. 2013. Available at http://www.cidrap.umn.edu/infectious-disease-topics/plague#overview. Accessed September 21, 2016.
102. WHO: WHO weekly epidemiologic record. *GEI* 91(8):89–104, 2016.
103. Kwit N, Nelson C, Kugeler K, et al: Human Plague—United States, 2015. *MMWR* 64(33):918–919, 2015.
104. Kugeler KJ, Staples JE, Hinckley AF, et al: Epidemiology of human plague in the United States, 1900–2012. *Emerg Infect Dis* 21(1):16–22, 2015.
105. Spinner JL, Winfree S, Starr T, et al.:Yersinia pestis survival and replication within human neutrophil phagosomes and uptake of infected neutrophils by macrophages. *J Leukoc Biol* 95(3):389–398, 2014.
106. Ke Y, Chen Z, Yang R: Yersinia pestis: mechanisms of entry into and resistance to the host cell. *Front Cell Infect Microbiol* 3:106, 2013.
107. Jarvinen HM, Laakkonen L, Haiko J, et al: Human single-chain urokinase is activated by the omptins PgtE of Salmonella enterica and Pla of Yersinia pestis despite mutations of active site residues. *Mol Microbiol* 89(3):507–517, 2013.
108. Hajjar AM, Ernst RK, Fortuno ES, et al: Humanized TLR4/MD-2 mice reveal LPS recognition differentially impacts susceptibility to Yersinia pestis and Salmonella enterica. *PLoS Path* 8(10):e1002963, 2012.
109. Bosch SA, Musgrave K, Wong D: Zoonotic disease risk and prevention practices among biologists and other wildlife workers—results from a national survey, US National Park Service, 2009. *J Wildl Dis* 49(3):475–585, 2013.
110. Pechous RD, Sivaraman V, Price PA, et al: Early host cell targets of Yersinia pestis during primary pneumonic plague. *PLoS Path* 9(10):e1003679, 2013.
111. Dotters-Katz SK, Kuller J, Heine RP: Arthropod-borne bacterial diseases in pregnancy. *Obstet Gynecol Surv* 68(9):635–649, 2013.
112. Alsofrom DJ, Mettler FA Jr, Mann JM: Radiographic manifestations of plague in New Mexico, 1975–1980. A review of 42 proved cases. *Radiology* 139(3):561–565, 1981.
113. Tourdjman M, Ibraheem M, Brett M, et al: Misidentification of Yersinia pestis by automated systems, resulting in delayed diagnoses of human plague infections—Oregon and New Mexico, 2010–2011. *Clin Infect Dis* 55(7):e58–e60, 2012.
114. Ayyadurai S, Flaudrops C, Raoult D, et al: Rapid identification and typing of Yersinia pestis and other Yersinia species by matrix-assisted laser desorption/ionization time-of-flight (MALDI-TOF) mass spectrometry. *BMC Microbiol* 10:285, 2010.
115. Euler M, Wang Y, Heidenreich D, et al: Development of a panel of recombinase polymerase amplification assays for detection of biothreat agents. *J Clin Microbiol* 51(4):1110–1117, 2013.
116. Simon S, Demeure C, Lamourette P, et al: Fast and simple detection of Yersinia pestis applicable to field investigation of plague foci. *PLoS One* 8(1):e54947, 2013.
117. Tsui PY, Tsai HP, Chiao DJ, et al: Rapid detection of Yersinia pestis recombinant fraction 1 capsular antigen. *Appl Microbiol Biotechnol* 99(18):7781–7789, 2015.
118. Anish C, Guo X, Wahlbrink A, et al: Plague detection by anti-carbohydrate antibodies. *Angew Chem Int Ed Engl* 52(36):9524–9528, 2013.
119. Levy Y, Vagima Y, Tidhar A, et al: Adjunctive corticosteroid treatment against Yersinia pestis improves bacterial clearance, immunopathology, and survival in the mouse model of bubonic plague. *J Infect Dis* 214(6):970–977, 2016.
120. Heine HS, Louie A, Adamovicz JJ, et al: Evaluation of imipenem for prophylaxis and therapy of Yersinia pestis delivered by aerosol in a mouse model of pneumonic plague. *Antimicrob Agents Chemother* 58(6):3276–3284, 2014.
121. Urich SK, Chalcraft L, Schriefer ME, et al: Lack of antimicrobial resistance in Yersinia pestis isolates from 17 countries in the Americas, Africa, and Asia. *Antimicrob Agents Chemother* 56(1):555–558, 2012.
122. Heine HS, Hershfield J, Marchand C, et al: In vitro antibiotic susceptibilities of Yersinia pestis determined by broth microdilution following CLSI methods. *Antimicrob Agents Chemother* 59(4):1919–21, 2015.
123. Galimand M, Guiyoule A, Gerbaud G, et al: Multidrug resistance in Yersinia pestis mediated by a transferable plasmid. *N Engl J Med* 337(10):677–680, 1997.
124. Welch TJ, Fricke WF, McDermott PF, et al: Multiple antimicrobial resistance in plague: an emerging public health risk. *PLoS One* 2(3):e309, 2007.
125. Inglesby TV, Dennis DT, Henderson DA, et al: Plague as a biological weapon: medical and public health management. Working Group on Civilian Biodefense. *JAMA* 283(17):2281–2290, 2000.
126. Sanapala S, Rahav H, Patel H, et al: Multiple antigens of Yersinia pestis delivered by live recombinant attenuated Salmonella vaccine strains elicit protective immunity against plague. *Vaccine* 34(21):2410–2416, 2016.
127. Sha J, Kirtley ML, Klages C, et al: A replication-defective human type 5 adenovirus-based trivalent vaccine confers complete protection against plague in mice and nonhuman primates. *Clin Vaccine Immunol* 23(7):586–600, 2016.
128. Chu K, Hu J, Meng F, et al: Immunogenicity and safety of subunit plague vaccine: a randomized phase 2a clinical trial. *Human Vaccin Immunother* 12(9):2334–2340, 2016.
129. Derbise A, Hanada Y, Khalife M, et al: Complete protection against pneumonic and bubonic plague after a single oral vaccination. *PLoS Negl Tropical Dis* 9(10):e0004162, 2015.
130. Sun W, Sanapala S, Rahav H, et al: Oral administration of a recombinant attenuated Yersinia pseudotuberculosis strain elicits protective immunity against plague. *Vaccine* 33(48):6727–6735, 2015.
131. Demeure CE, Derbise A, Carniel E: Oral vaccination against plague using Yersinia pseudotuberculosis. *Chem Biol Interact* 267:89–95, 2017. doi: 10.1016/j.cbi.2016.03.030.
132. Siegel JD, Rhinehart E, Jackson M, et al: *2007 Guideline for Isolation Precautions: Preventing Transmission of Infectious Agents in Healthcare Settings*. Atlanta, Georgia, Centers for Disease Control and Prevention, 2007.
133. Dembek ZF, Smith LA, Rusnak JM: Botulinum toxin, in Dembek Z Sr (ed): *Medical Aspects of Biological Warfare Chapter 16, Textbook of Military Medicine*. Falls Church, VA, Borden Institute and the US Army Office of the Surgeon General, 2007.
134. Arnon SS, Schechter R, Inglesby TV, et al: Botulinum toxin as a biological weapon: medical and public health management. *JAMA* 285(8):1059–1070, 2001.
135. Wein LM, Liu Y: Analyzing a bioterror attack on the food supply: the case of botulinum toxin in milk. *Proc Natl Acad Sci USA* 102(28):9984–9989, 2005.
136. CDC: Botulism/Clinicians. 2016. Available at https://www.cdc.gov/botulism/health-professional.html. Accessed Septemeber 21, 2016.
137. Witoonpanich R, Vichayanrat E, Tantisiriwit K, et al: Survival analysis for respiratory failure in patients with food-borne botulism. *Clin Toxicol (Phila)* 48(3):177–183, 2010.
138. Rega P, Burkholder-Allen K, Bork C: An algorithm for the evaluation and management of red, yellow, and green zone patients during a botulism mass casualty incident. *Am J Disaster Med* 4(4):192–198, 2009.
139. Rega PP, Bork CE, Burkholder-Allen K, et al: Single-Breath-Count Test: an important adjunct in the triaging of patients in a mass-casualty incident due to botulism. *Prehosp Disaster Med* 25(3):219–222, 2010.
140. Federal Drug Administration: FDA. 2013.
141. Cangene Corporation: *BAT, Botulism Antitoxin Heptavalent (A, B, C, D, E, F, G)-Package Insert*, 21, 2013.
142. Dembek ZF, Smith LA, Rusnak JM: Botulism: cause, effects, diagnosis, clinical and laboratory identification, and treatment modalities. *Disaster Med Public Health Prep* 1(2):122–134, 2007.
143. Black RE, Gunn RA: Hypersensitivity reactions associated with botulinal antitoxin. *Am J Med* 69(4):567–570, 1980.
144. Arnon SS, Schechter R, Maslanka SE, et al: Human botulism immune globulin for the treatment of infant botulism. *N Engl J Med* 354(5):462–471, 2006.
145. CDC: Notice of CDC's Discontinuation of Investigational Pentavalent (ABCDE) botulinum toxoid vaccine for workers at risk for occupational exposure to botulinum toxins. *MMWR* 60(42):1454–1455, 2011.
146. Poli MA, Roy C, Huebner KD et al: Ricin, in Dembek Z (ed): *Medical Aspects of Biological Warfare*. Falls Church, VA, Borden Institute and the US Army Office of the Surgeon General, 2007.
147. Audi J, Belson M, Patel M, et al: Ricin poisoning: a comprehensive review. *JAMA* 294(18):2342–2351, 2005.
148. Spivak L, Hendrickson RG: Ricin. *Crit Care Clin* 21(4):815–824, 2005.
149. Griffiths GD: Understanding ricin from a defensive viewpoint. *Toxins* 3:1373–1392, 2011.
150. Alipour M, Pucaj K, Smith MG, et al: Toxicity of ricin toxin A chain in rats. *Drug Chem Toxicol* 36(2):224–230, 2013.
151. Crompton R, Gall D: Georgi Markov—death in a pellet. *Med Leg J* 48(2):51–62, 1980.
152. Papaloucas M, Papaloucas C, Stergioulas A: Ricin and the assassination of Georgi Markov. *Pak J Biol Sci* 11(19):2370–2371, 2008.

153. Worbs S, Kohler K, Pauly D, et al: Ricinus communis intoxications in human and veterinary medicine-a summary of real cases. *Toxins* 3(10):1332–1372, 2011.
154. Bhaskaran M, Didier PJ, Sivasubramani SK, et al: Pathology of lethal and sublethal doses of aerosolized ricin in rhesus macaques. *Toxicol Pathol* 42(3):573–581, 2014.
155. Pincus SH, Bhaskaran M, Brey RN, et al: Clinical and pathological findings associated with aerosol exposure of macaques to ricin toxin. *Toxins* 7(6):2121–2133, 2015.
156. Lockey SD Jr, Dunkelberger L: Anaphylaxis from an Indian necklace. *JAMA* 206(13):2900–2901, 1968.
157. Diakite ML RJ, Jary D, et al: Point-of-care diagnostics for ricin exposure. *Lab Chip* 15:2308–2317, 2015.
158. Yin HQ, Jia MX, Shi LJ, et al: Evaluation of a novel ultra-sensitive nanoparticle probe-based assay for ricin detection. *J Immunotoxicol* 11(3):291–295, 2014.
159. Pittman CT, Guido JM, Hamelin EI, et al: Analysis of a ricin biomarker, ricinine, in 989 individual human urine samples. *J Anal Toxicol* 37(4):237–240, 2013.
160. Hamelin EI, Johnson RC, Osterloh JD, et al: Evaluation of ricinine, a ricin biomarker, from a non-lethal castor bean ingestion. *J Anal Toxicol* 36(9):660–662, 2012.
161. Sully EK, Whaley KJ, Bohorova N, et al: Chimeric plantibody passively protects mice against aerosolized ricin challenge. *Clin Vaccine Immunol* 21(5):777–782, 2014.
162. Zhang T, Yang H, Kang L, et al: Strong protection against ricin challenge induced by a novel modified ricin A-chain protein in mouse model. *Hum Vaccin Immunother* 11(7):1779–1787, 2015.
163. Van Slyke G, Sully EK, Bohorova N, et al: Humanized monoclonal antibody that passively protects mice against systemic and intranasal ricin toxin challenge. *Clin Vaccine Immunol* 23(9):795–799, 2016.
164. Wang CF, Nie XJ, Chen GM, et al: Early plasma exchange for treating ricin toxicity in children after castor bean ingestion. *J Clin Apher* 30(3):141–146, 2015.
165. Chen GM, Yu ZH, Nie XJ, et al: Plasma exchange parameter selection and safety observation of children with severe ricinism. *Genet Mol Res* 14(2):4169–4176, 2015.
166. Lazarus AA, Devereaux AV, Mohr LC: Biological agents of mass destruction, in *Irwin and Rippe's Intensive Care Medicine.* 7th ed. Baltimore, MD, Lippincott Williams & Wilkins, 2011.
167. Vitetta ES, Smallshaw JE, Schindler J: Pilot phase IB clinical trial of an alhydrogel-adsorbed recombinant ricin vaccine. *Clin Vaccine Immunol* 19(10):1697–1699, 2012.
168. Pittman PR, Reisler RB, Lindsey CY, et al: Safety and immunogenicity of ricin vaccine, RVEc, in a Phase 1 clinical trial. *Vaccine* 33(51):7299–7306, 2015.
169. O'Hara JM, Brey RN, Mantis NJ: Comparative efficacy of two leading candidate ricin toxin a subunit vaccines in mice. *Clin Vaccine Immunol* 20(6):789–794, 2013.

Section 12 ICU DESIGN, ORGANIZATION, OPERATION, AND OUTCOME MEASURES

NEIL A. HALPERN

Chapter 131 ■ Intensive Care Unit Design: Current Standards and Future Trends

DIANA C. ANDERSON • NEIL A. HALPERN

INTRODUCTION

In 2010, there were approximately 6,100 intensive care units (ICUs) with over 104,000 beds in the 3,100 acute care hospitals in the USA [1]. Periodically, these ICUs need to be renovated or new ICUs built [2].Thus, hospital-based intensivist administrators at some point in their careers may be asked to participate in designing new or renovating existing ICUs. For simplicity of presentation, we have divided this chapter into five sections: the ICU design process; the ICU patient room; central clinical, visitor and staff support, and administrative areas; ICU informatics; and future trends. Although we classify these areas separately, they are indeed interrelated.

THE ICU DESIGN PROCESS

Health care and design are complex processes that must accommodate and address continuously evolving guidelines and regulatory standards [3]. Several core principles should guide ICU-specific design [4]. First, an ICU is a semiautonomous mini-hospital. Second, new or renovated ICU locations should be harmonized with other ICUs and hospital support services. Third, the design must balance innovation and functionality, space and physical limitations, costs, and security and healing. Fourth, ICU design should account for long-term functionality, because the ICU design must last a decade or more. Finally, ICU design should embrace the growing field of Evidence-Based Design (EBD) [3,5–7]. In EBD, design decisions about the built environment are predicated upon credible research to achieve the best possible results. Thus, facility design and positive health care outcomes are linked to produce workforce safety, satisfaction, productivity, cost savings, and energy efficiency [2,3,8–11].

The design should also accommodate evolving perspectives for the number of ICU beds per unit and differences between critical care delivery models for large and small hospitals. The average number of ICU beds per unit has increased between 1993 and 2012. Adult ICUs are now bigger by almost six beds, or 29% [12]. Additionally, there are usually a high percentage of hospital beds dedicated to critical care in larger than smaller hospitals [13]. Moreover, within the large academic medical centers there are multiple specialty ICUs (i.e., medical, surgical, coronary care, cardiothoracic, neurosurgical, pediatric, and neonatal), whereas, one large multipurpose adult ICU may suffice in smaller community hospitals. Additionally in large academic Emergency Departments (ED), an ICU may be incorporated into the ED.

ICU Design Team

ICU design can succeed only if common goals for design, space, purpose, and funding are shared between the critical care medicine team and the hospital administration [4]. Because critical care is multidisciplinary, the ICU design process benefits from being inclusive and collaborative [3,4,8]. Therefore, the ICU design team should include a variety of disciplines including hospital administration; the ICU clinical team (physicians, nurses, and pharmacists); allied health care support (infection control specialists, respiratory therapy, nutrition support, care coordination, and social work); and the technical groups (architects, engineers, equipment, and informatics). Ideally, architects and engineers with a prior track record of successful ICU design experience should be engaged. It is also important to include end users (patient and family representatives), because these groups can offer unique insights [9].

Initial Vision & Benchmarking

The 40,000 foot perspective articulating the vision for the new ICU precedes design specific deliberations [4,14]. This perspective includes the location of the unit, the number of beds, the apportionment of space between patient and supportive areas, and the logistics of unit function (centralized or decentralized). The vision for the new ICU should reflect the desired atmosphere and approach to patient and family care, workflow, technology, and the ICU's physical and logistical relationships with the remainder of the hospital. Developing the vision may be helped by benchmarking their ideas with visits to select ICUs and meeting with their staffs.

Design Guidelines & Regulatory Standards

The design process should be initiated by utilizing existing evidence-based guidelines, recommendations and expert opinions to gather core knowledge of ICU design [4,5,14–19]. An early understanding and integration of ICU guidelines and standards allows the team to develop the broad strokes of a functional program and a roadmap which will define the character, services, scope, and space requirements in sufficient detail for subsequent design.

Two primary sources include the *Guidelines for Design and Construction of Hospitals and Outpatient Facilities*, published by the Facility Guidelines Institute (FGI) [19] and *The Guidelines for Intensive Care Unit Design* published by the Society of Critical Care Medicine (SCCM) [15]. The FGI and SCCM guidelines are periodically updated. FGI focuses on minimum standards for design and construction (space; risk assessment; architectural detail; surface and furnishing needs; and engineering). The SCCM guidelines describe universal functions that should be accommodated in the modern ICU. Interestingly, both codes and guidelines have expanded their recommendations to include the social, psychologic, and/or cultural aspects of facility performance, thus responding to the need for a more comprehensive approach to health facility design [2]. SCCM also maintains a digest of the ICU design award winners and includes architectural design drawings, pictures, and videos of outstanding ICUs from throughout the world [20].

Design Timeline & Mock-Ups

The ICU design process may take several years from initial design vision to initial occupancy [4]. Design committee meetings that are regularly scheduled and provide continuously updated schematics and computerized renderings of the various architectural concepts generated by the team speed the process along. Full-scale prototypes or "mock-ups" of the patient rooms are now standard practice and allow for an experiential rather than an observational understanding. Moreover, mock-ups permit staff to gain a sense of how the space and size of the room will accommodate patient care and workflow of the design. The mock-ups can range from simple tape on the floor to indicate room outlines and components, to the use of cardboard walls and spaces with devices and finishings [8,21].

Renovation versus New Construction

Both renovations and new construction are heavily regulated by building codes. Renovations are mandated to update existing space as much as possible to current building codes. In contrast, in new construction, the design begins with a clean slate and is built to current code. Renovations of existing ICUs are usually limited in scope and may range from a cosmetic upgrade to a total overhaul. Renovations are often more complicated than new build because of the restrictions of building in an older space (i.e., existing floor-to-ceiling heights; structural depths; and presence of elevators and staircases). Renovations also need to include planned phasing in order to minimize disruption to existing patient services. Phasing plans should include considerations of noise and vibration control that result from construction activities [19].

Occupancy Phase and Post-Occupancy Evaluation

Preoccupancy preparations including moving day simulations can diminish moving day anxiety and mistakes. Non-ICU staff and the family members of current ICU patients should be made aware of the moving date in order to minimize their angst.

A post-occupancy evaluation (POE) process has been developed to identify major issues and unanticipated problems and plan for short- and long-term fixes. POEs tend to focus on end-user impressions after occupying the facility, but not necessarily on clinical performance measures [2]. When implemented in health care design, research findings demonstrate that POEs can positively impact patient and visitor experiences and satisfaction; create supportive work environments for staff and caregivers; and help achieve organizational objectives [22].

THE ICU PATIENT ROOM

ICU Layout

Before discussing the patient room, we must think about the ICU layout, arguably the most important design feature that affects all aspects of intensive care services including patient privacy; comfort and safety; staff working conditions; throughput; logistical support; and family integration [23,24]. Layout determines the location of different spaces and/or functions within an ICU, the relationship of internal and external spaces, and how their functions relate. Within the physical limitations of the space, designers have applied various types and combinations of layouts (Fig. 131.1) to solve throughput and circulation challenges for patients, staff and visitors, clean and used supplies and equipment [12].

The ICU layout choices are usually dictated by the physical configuration of the facility and the location of fixed components (i.e., windows, staircases, elevators, and plumbing). Layout decisions may also be guided by considerations that address safety versus efficiency; support versus function; and revenue-generation (patient rooms) versus logistical spaces [12]. The racetrack (patient beds around the perimeter with services in the center and a loop corridor space in between) appears to be the most dominant unit layout among award-winning adult ICUs [23].

ICU Patient Room

The central point of the ICU experience is the patient room [5,14–17,21]. Guidelines advise single bed [15,19] rather than multibed rooms in order to enhance patient safety and privacy. Each room should be equipped to function as an autonomous area with the necessary space for procedures and associated staff [25]. Each patient room should offer a healing environment; support infection prevention measures; and have access to outdoor views through windows. Concomitantly, the rooms should be fully interwoven into the ICU and hospital workflow and social fabric.

Patient Room Standardization

Ideally, all ICU patients' rooms should be standardized for layout. The patient rooms can be designed identically (same-handed) or as mirror images of each other [26]. Room standardization may save design and construction time and costs and improve patient safety [21,27]. Importantly, patient room standardization allows staff to move in and out of each room efficiently because the staff members always know where devices are installed and supplies stored and placed. Layout standardization is commonly restricted by plumbing conduits for bathrooms.

Additionally, the rooms should be standardized for size. At a baseline, minimal patient room size requirements are guided by the FGI and state-based rules [19]. However, the consistency of space availability depends upon the existing physical layout; this is particularly limiting in ICU renovations. Additionally, some care environments, notably surgical specialty ICUs, may purposefully build a few rooms larger than others as large spaces are needed for some supportive technologies. The build of at least one large bariatric room per ICU should be considered as obesity rates are increasing, reflecting a trend in the general population.

Patient Room Zones

ICU patient rooms can be subdivided, physically or virtually, into four zones: patient, caregiver (work), family (visitor), and entry way (Fig. 131.2) [15,17]. The room's focal point is the patient bed. Optimally, all medical equipment should be installed on a medical utility distribution system; this approach clears the floor and facilitates ready access to the patient by visitors and staff. The caregiver zone includes work areas and space for medication preparation and procedures, as well as computers, displays, and storage areas. The design of the caregiver physical environment should not hinder the interplay between critically ill patients and their families [28]. The family zone

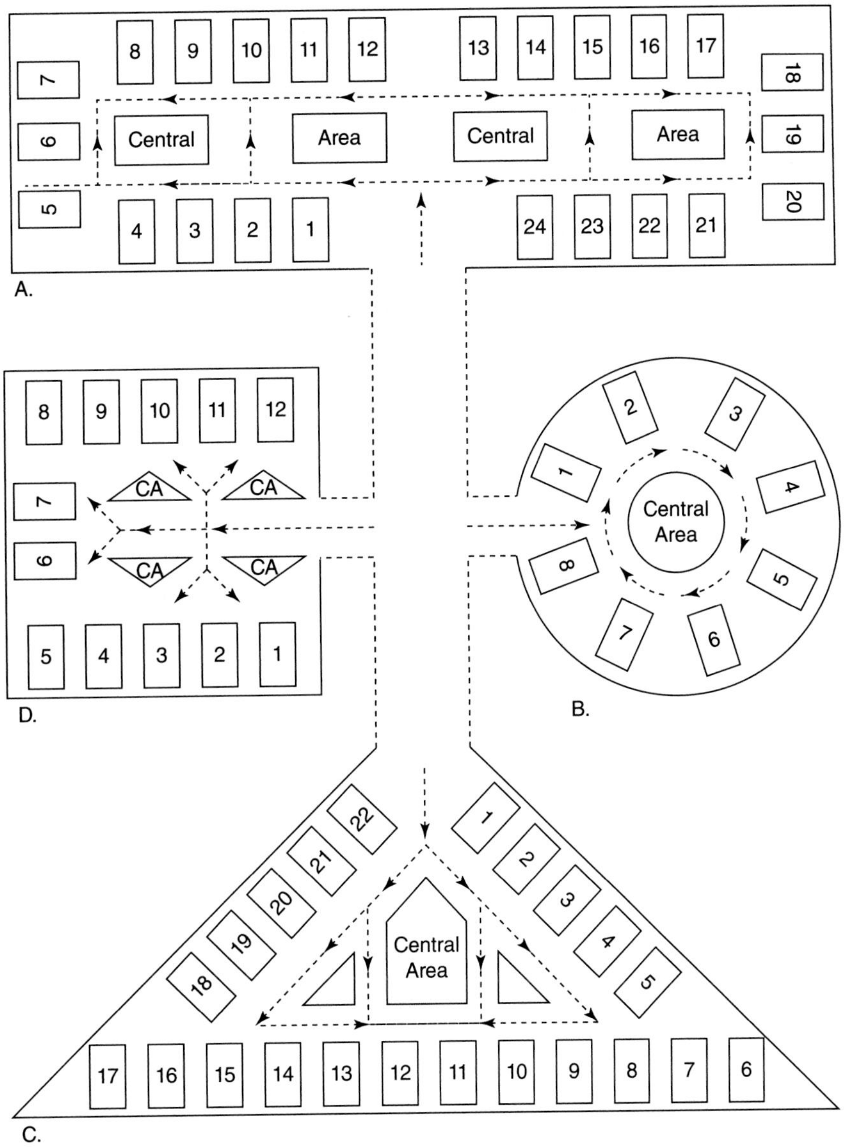

FIGURE 131.1 ICU configurations: rectangular (**A**), circular (**B**), triangular (**C**), and square (**D**). The "racetrack" (A) with patient beds around the perimeter and nursing stations and supportive services in the CA is most common in current ICUs. Corridors cut through the central areas to facilitate staff movement.
CA, center area; ICU, intensive care unit.

should incorporate comfortable chairs; power outlets; wireless access; and, if space permits, a long-term visiting alcove with a chair–sofa–bed, table, light, sink, locker, and refrigerator. The entry way for each patient room may open directly onto the hallway or be set back from the hallway (Fig. 131.3). Opening directly to the hall provides the largest possible patient room; however, setting the room back may provide a staging area that incorporates a decentralized workstation; handwashing system; storage space; coat hangers; and identification and informational display systems. A hybrid design that incorporates both direct hallway access and a setback may provide the best of both worlds (Fig. 131.3C).

Medical Utility Distribution Systems

The primary decision that guides the room's utilization involves the selection of the medical utility distribution systems [29]. This system brings the hospital's supportive infrastructure (medical gases, vacuum, plumbing, electrical and data jacks) to the patient and provides the venue for installing medical devices (physiologic monitors, mechanical ventilators, infusion pumps), and communications and entertainment systems. The choices are divided between fixed headwalls or floor mounted columns versus mobile articulating columns (booms) mounted to the ceilings or walls (Fig. 131.4). The stationary systems are less expensive than the mobile systems; however, the mobile booms offer greater flexibility, patient access and bed movement.

Bedside Medical Technologies

Core ICU room medical devices ideally include the ICU bed; physiologic monitor; mechanical ventilator; infusion and feeding pumps; pneumatic compression devices; patient lift; computers; chairs for the patient and visitors; overbed tables, laboratory-specimen label printer; nurse-call intercom station; webcam; entertainment system; storage areas; and waste disposal bins. The design team should also address point-of-care testing

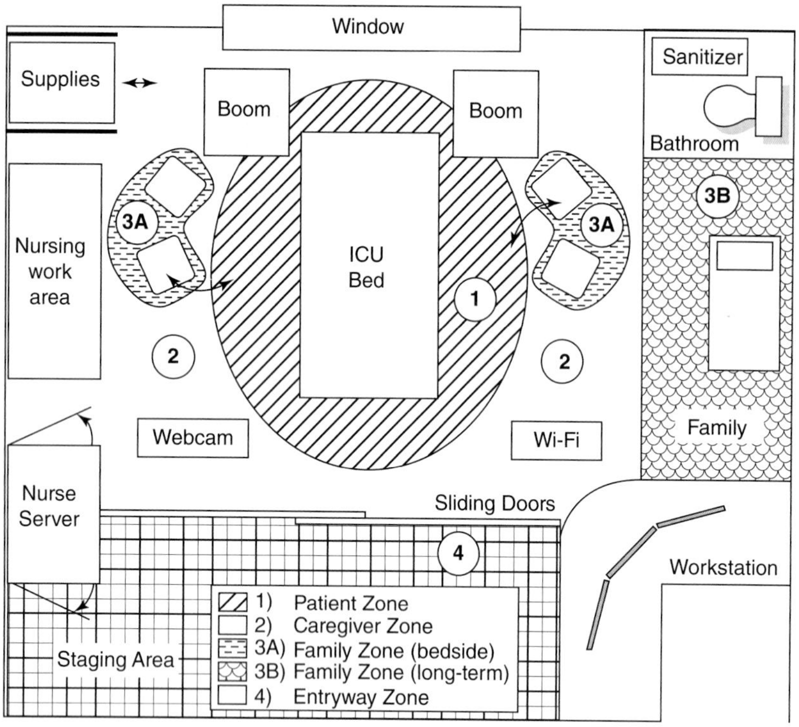

FIGURE 131.2 The ICU patient room is divided into four zones: patient (*1*), caregiver (2), family (bedside—*3A* or long term—*3B*) and entryway (*4*). This figure also demonstrates a nurse server with bidirectional access, work area, supply space, mobile articulating arms (booms), bathroom, webcam, Wi-Fi transmitter, and a workstation and a staging area immediately outside the room.
ICU, intensive care unit.

(POCT) and ultrasonography and whether these devices should be placed in each room or positioned centrally.

Patient Room Logistics and Waste Management Systems

Adequate storage spaces for supplies, medications, linens, and waste management systems should be incorporated into each patient room. Storage is achieved through a mix of permanently based secured and nonsecured drawers and cabinets, and/or mobile carts. Nurse servers (cabinets with bidirectional and secure access from both outside and inside the room) may be a good solution (Fig. 131.2) to improve privacy and infection control by stocking the room from the outside.

ICU patient rooms must now have direct access to separate enclosed bathrooms [19]. Therefore, the design must determine the optimal bathroom location (i.e., front of room, back of room, or front and back of adjacent rooms) (Fig. 131.5). These decisions will probably be based upon the availability of plumbing; nevertheless the impact on patient visualization, window availability or workflow is quite important. Patient bathrooms should have either sanitizers to clean reusable bedpans or macerators to destroy single-use bed pans.

Front of ICU Room and Decentralized Workstations

The front of the ICU patient room is the interface of the room with the ICU hallway and ICU central areas. This space controls room entry; patient privacy; sound transmission; control of infection; and impedance of smoke, and allows for patient observation and monitoring. Options for front-of-room privacy include curtains; clear glass doors and curtains; and glass doors with integrated privacy solutions (manually or electronically controlled integral blinds or electronic glass [Liquid Crystal Devices (LCD) or e-glass]). Curtains are more economical to install than glass systems; however, the curtains are not efficacious controllers of sound, infectious agents, or smoke. Glass systems are also easier to clean.

The front of each room also provides a ready location for patient observation and monitoring through the incorporation of a clinical workstation (decentralized). These workstations facilitate the deployment of staff close to the patient [6]. Such workstations are generally designed as one per room or one per two rooms depending on space considerations and room build (Fig. 131.3B and C). The workstations should have ready digital access to all bedside physiologic data (mirrored on displays or web-based) and to the electronic medical record.

The Room as a Healing Environment

Although the exact design features that transform ICUs into healing environments are not definitively identified, it is well known that the physical environment affects the physiology, psychology, and social behaviors of all those who experience it [7,30]. Thus, it makes good sense that the patient room environment promote healing and serenity by addressing sound, light, temperature, visuals, and entertainment aspects [31,32].

Sound control positively influences patient outcomes by lowering physiologic stress, sleep disturbance, and feelings of fear [33,34]. The highest noise levels in the ICU have been shown to be related to staff conversation and the use of advanced technical equipment. Acoustic control within the ICU is generally achieved through the integration of sound minimizers (sound-absorbent finishings and ceiling tiles, acoustic baffling in the walls, soundproofed windows, and sound attenuators in the HVAC system), patient level sound mitigaters (sound cancelling headphones or sound masking) and systems that control bedside alarm volume and communication broadcasts.

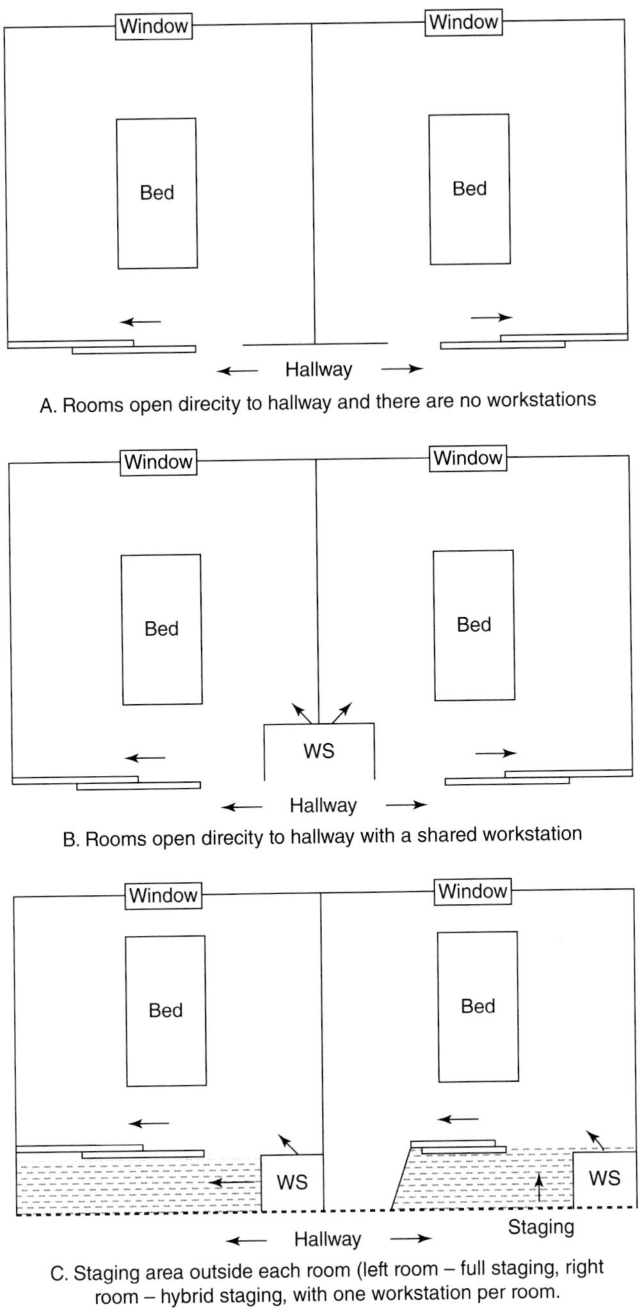

FIGURE 131.3 Patient rooms may open directly into the hallway without any workstations (WS) (**A**) or with a shared workstation for the two rooms (**B**). Alternatively, the rooms can be set back to provide a staging area (C—left room—full staging or right room—partial or hybrid staging) in front of each room with one workstation per room.

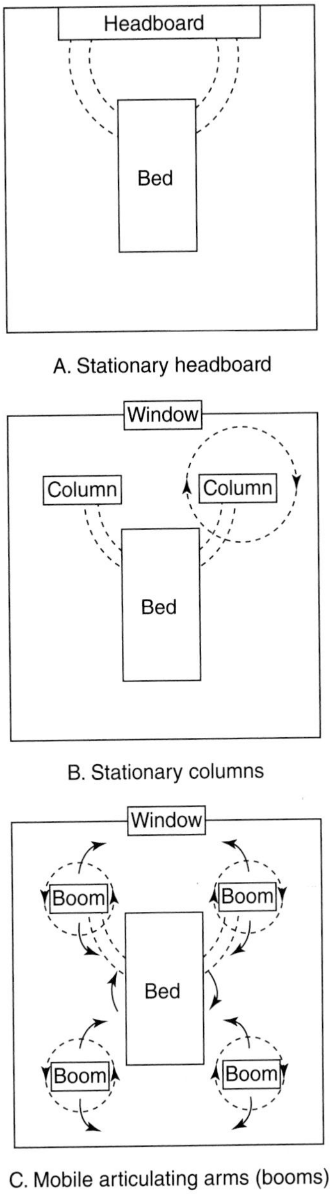

FIGURE 131.4 Utilities and devices are mounted on a stationary headboard (**A**), stationary (**left**) or rotating (**right**) columns (**B**), or mobile articulating columns (booms) (**C**). The booms can be attached to the walls or ceiling, at any corner of the bed and swivel and move horizontally or vertically.

Natural light is essential to the well-being of patients and staff. Thus, ICU patient rooms are now all required to have windows [15,19,32]. However, the associated glare should be controlled with antiglare glass as well as sunlight reducing shades, preferably with electronic controllers. The room itself should have multiple lighting arrangements to accommodate patient and staff needs, including multifunction LED lights (with low energy or heat producing bulbs) and procedure lighting.

Artwork can be mounted on the ICU walls, embedded in privacy curtains and ceiling tiles, electronically projected on video displays, or integrated into monitors or television/computers. Entertainment may also be provided through visor-based video displays. A "low-tech" white board should also be available in each room for the display of positive messages, get-well cards, and family pictures.

Electronic and computer-based integration of the environmental (light, shades, temperature, and artwork) and entertainment systems into remote handsets (pillow speaker) or wall based computer switches facilitates efficient patient and staff centered control of the room. Environmental profiles can then be tailored to day and night, procedures or no procedures, and individual patient preferences. Multiparameter sensors that monitor temperature, humidity, light, sound and provide alerts for uncomfortable environmental circumstances also help track and maintain the healing environment.

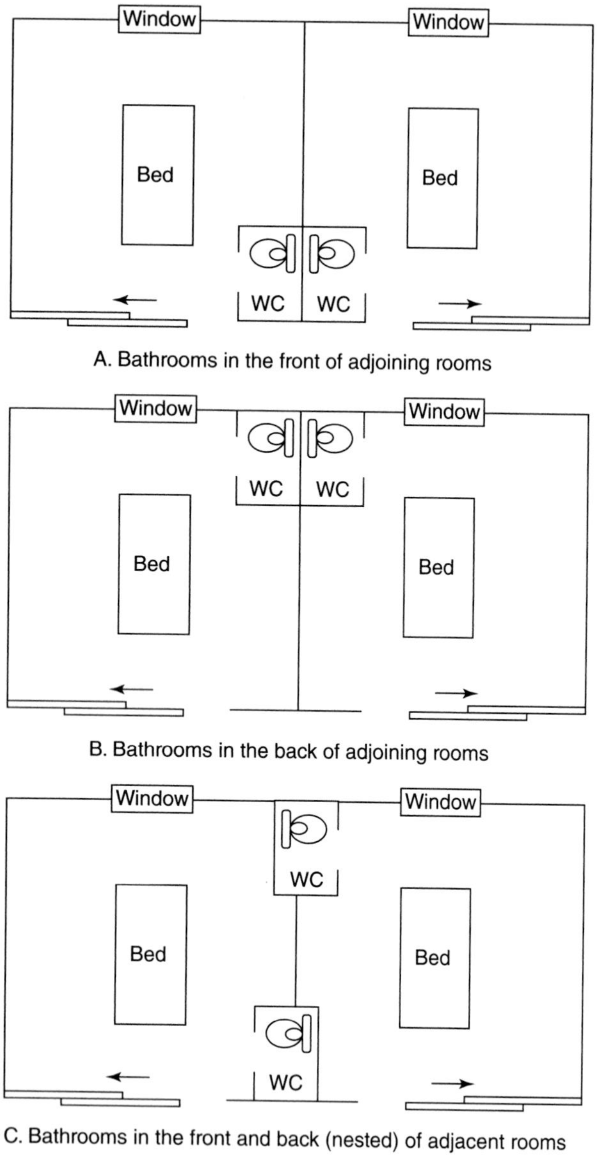

FIGURE 131.5 The ICU patient room bathroom (WC) can be located in front of the room (**A**) ("inboard"), back of room ("outboard") (**B**) and in the front of one room and the back of the adjacent room ("nested") (**C**). The impact on patient visualization from the hallway, window availability and workflow should be considered by the design team. ICU, intensive care unit.

CENTRAL CLINICAL, VISITOR AND STAFF, AND ADMINISTRATIVE SUPPORT AREAS

The central stations and corridors unite all the patient rooms as well as other supportive areas and can create unit cohesiveness. The goals of all central areas are to support bedside care, offer a welcoming and warm atmosphere, and provide access to logistical support areas. Design of these areas is governed by the hospital's and ICU's approaches to centralized or decentralized care and logistics and space availability.

Central Care Stations

The composition of the central care stations includes greeting desks; areas for quiet work and conferencing; as well as offices and restrooms. Technologies usually include nurse-call communication stations; telephones; communications boards; computers; high-definition image review stations; laboratory-specimen label printers; pneumatic tube stations; nourishment stations; emergency alerts; and cut-off switches for ICU utilities.

In a small ICU, one centrally located station may suffice; in contrast, multiple central stations may be needed for a large ICU with several bed pods. The layout of these areas is primarily affected by the bed configurations (Fig. 131.1). Optimally, unobstructed views of the ICU beds should be available from the central care stations. Studies have suggested that decreased visibility may negatively affect clinical outcomes for severely ill patients assigned to rooms that are poorly visualized by staff [35,36]. In reality, unimpeded views are commonly precluded by the ICU layout. However, visibility from central areas can be enhanced electronically through the use of webcams in each room and central displays of bedside devices.

Corridors

ICU corridors provide pathways for transit and promote physical and social unity. However, physical barriers (staircases, elevators, supportive conduits, and closets) can limit optimal corridor design. If possible, separate hallways should be designated for patients or supplies to enhance patient privacy and decrease visitor distractions. Corridor design may also have to support access to permanent imaging and procedural suites as well as passageways for large mobile imaging technologies (i.e., mobile CT scanners).

Corridors are fixed spaces that provide access to permanent rooms; however, the corridor design should be more expansive and include access to transport systems (i.e., elevators and helicopters) and the design plan can also address the transport systems themselves. For example, in a new build, transport elevators should not only be large enough to accommodate the patient bed, staff, and other care devices, but should be equipped with utility panels that provide power, oxygen and suction. The outdoor passageways, or pre- or post-helipad areas should likewise include supportive utilities.

The corridors through their finishings, artwork, sound control, and lighting set the emotional tone for the ICU. These considerations are relevant, because hallways are commonly used to conduct rounds, impromptu clinical consultations, and family meetings. Moreover, the corridors may also impact the patient psyche as patients frequently walk through the corridors within the context of early mobility programs [37].

ICU Storage Spaces, Supplies, and Medical Devices

Right-sizing and properly positioning the storage areas (central and bedside) requires a sound understanding of the logistical approaches (centralized and/or decentralized) that the hospital and ICU deploy. Right-sizing the storage space also requires correct assumptions of ICU supply utilization of consumables. Outfitted storage units and expensive supplies and equipment with electronic tags promote inventory management and permit the use of real-time locating systems/solutions (RTLS) [38].

Storage spaces may include traditional supply rooms (with stationary or track-based shelving; closed supply cabinets; or rolling exchange carts) as well as alcoves along the ICU hallways. Storage spaces should be accessible to transport or cargo elevators and be fairly close to the patient care areas. Central storage spaces must also be able to handle and charge supplementary medical devices (i.e., infusion pumps; ventilators; and specialty monitoring or imaging devices).

Pharmacy

Hospitals may have centralized or decentralized pharmacy and medication distribution systems and staffing models. Therefore, ICU pharmacy systems must be coordinated with the hospital's pharmacy and ICU bedsides. Options include a fully equipped satellite ICU pharmacy versus a pharmacy area with minimal resources. Both alternatives commonly utilize decentralized self-contained and secure automated medication disposing units. Medications may also be stored in secured cabinets at the ICU bedside.

ICU Laboratory and POCT

Many ICUs utilize laboratory testing from a centralized lab. However, if point-of-care testing (POCT) will be incorporated, the design must accommodate POCT systems.

POCT focuses primarily on whole blood analyses using either large devices placed in defined ICU locations (ICU stat laboratory or central station) or on carts, or smaller devices amenable for positioning at each ICU bedside [39]. A combination of POCT modalities and locations may be used depending on the ICU workflow, required testing, and available space and resources. Pneumatic tube stations are still required to transport specimens to laboratories outside the ICU area as POCT is currently not a complete replacement for the central laboratory.

Infection Control and Prevention

Effective infection control requires an ICU culture that is responsive to infection deterrence and an ICU infrastructure designed to support infection prevention measures. Core infrastructure elements include systems that provide clean air and water, and waste sequestration and elimination. Nonporous, well-sealed, and easy-to-clean surfaces and finishings throughout the patient rooms; and ubiquitous, visible, and accessible hand sanitizers and fluid dispensers are critical to infection control. Advanced modalities include electronic handwashing surveillance; self-cleaning copper or silver surfaces; surface surveillance monitors; and the use of environmental decontamination systems (i.e., ultraviolet light, hydrogen peroxide dispersion, and continuous air disinfection) [17].

Unfortunately, even in the setting of optimal infection control design, serious infections will likely remain an ICU problem. Therefore, ICUs may have to maintain duplicate devices to be used primarily with highly infectious patients (i.e., bronchoscopy towers and disposable bronchoscopes) and may even have to develop "super" isolation zones that group highly infectious patients together with designated ICU traffic patterns.

Visitor and Staff Support

It is well recognized that family support is a significant factor in patient recovery. Concomitantly, family members and visitors can become emotionally depleted when their loved one is an ICU patient. With these factors in mind, it is important to build family "waiting" areas to promote visitor wellness [40,41].

ICU visitors need a healing environment in close proximity to the ICU to recharge between visits with their loved ones. Soft lighting, warm colors, large windows, nature-themed artwork (either real or electronic), and quiet background entertainment set a serene tone. Privacy should be provided using small groups of comfortable chairs that are separated by dividers. Informatics support may include wireless Internet access; computers; and smartphone charging stations. Nourishment areas as well as bathrooms, lockers, and coat hangers should be the norm. Long-term sleeping accommodations, if possible, provide a space for visitors who prefer to remain nearby. The inclusion of consultation rooms and social work offices near the waiting areas and the addition of respite areas for ICU visitors within the ICU hallways also helps promote family meetings and social and emotional support.

Areas for Staff Respite and Meetings

Similar to the ICU visitors, ICU clinicians regularly face extreme stress. Therefore, the ICU design must address the impact of staff spaces. Well-designed staff lounges (break rooms) and on-call suites located within the ICU provide a private place adjacent to patient care areas for staff relaxation. The lounges should be tastefully decorated with outside lighting; comfortable seating; tables and access to computers; ICU communications; and entertainment. Bathrooms; changing areas; lockers and scrub dispensers; napping alcoves; and nourishing stations complete the lounge furnishings. In ICUs that maintain 24/7 clinician availability, sleeping accommodations (on-call suites) with bathrooms and showers should also be provided.

Conference Rooms

Staff meetings, educational programs, and family meetings are sustained through the construction of multipurpose conference rooms within the ICU environment. The seating capacities of these rooms should be based upon predicted usage. Furnishings should include comfortable seating; conference tables with built-in informatics access; audiovisual video systems; wireless access; smart boards; electronic attendance and scheduling systems; food preparation; and storage areas.

Staff Communications

Telephones, smart phones, nurse-call intercom systems, pagers, and bidirectional transmitters are integral to the ICU communications environment. These devices may all be integrated into one platform (i.e., within a nurse call system, a primary communication platform, or an alarm system). Functionalities include point-to-point and global messaging, telephone and alarm communications, and real-time locating of staff. Even in these advanced settings, land-line telephones and overhead speakers continue to be of value in providing reliable ICU communications. Panic buttons can be installed in commonly used work areas in order to ensure staff safety or incorporated into communications gear.

Signage and Wayfinding

In addition to a well-designed ICU layout, good signage is necessary for efficient wayfinding. Directional signs should be clear in their message and easily visible. Destination signs should identify each room. Signs at the ICU entrance provide information about the ICU and can include the ICU designation (i.e., surgical ICU), management names (i.e., ICU director and nurse leader), and visiting hours.

Security and Fire Safety

Security and fire safety is crucial in the ICU setting. Electronic identification card–coded access should be used for staff at all secure doorways. The ICU entrance optimally should be staffed by dedicated clerks. However, staffing limitations commonly preclude full-time greeters; therefore, other systems for visitor identification (i.e., closed-circuit televisions with electronic buzzers) should be installed at ICU entrances.

Beyond the basic fire safety devices (smoke detectors, automated sprinklers, fire extinguishers) and fire and smoke alerting systems (fire alarm pull-stations, sound or light alerts and overhead speakers), four design elements help ensure the safety of the ICU in the settings of fire or smoke. The first involves selection of products and furnishings with a low fire load and minimal release of heat and toxic smoke. The second addresses the construct of compartments that are fire and smoke-rated. The third is the use of protective technologies within the HVAC systems to prevent the spread of smoke and other products of combustion from one area to another. The last is the integration of experienced fire safety officers into the ICU design process [17].

ADVANCED INFORMATICS

The deployment of advanced informatics into an ICU, thus creating a "smart" ICU, certainly provides enormous positive potential for unit operations [18]. However, designing the informatics infrastructure requires a different skill set than the standard build and therefore, requires a team trained in the intricacies of informatics. The primary objective of advanced informatics systems should be to electronically integrate the patient and staff with all aspects of care. The second goal is to transform patient-related data into actionable information. The biggest challenges in this endeavour are harmonizing the technologies of multiple vendors into an operational platform that will meet the ICU needs and be fully synchronized with hospital informatics systems.

Building the Smart ICU

The smart ICU infrastructure requires a connectivity envelope (Fig. 131.6) around the patient. This envelope encompasses the patient, medical devices, health care staff, as well as pharmacologic and other care elements [18]. The core components include a robust wired and wireless infrastructure at each bedside, connectivity hardware within the patient room to connect and communicate with data sources, identification tags on data sources for tracking purposes, transmitters on medical devices to transmit their data, and middleware (the software that connects, provides interoperability and other applications between medical devices and the hospital's operating systems) on hospital and ICU networks.

The Food and Drug Administration (FDA) classifies middleware as either Class 1 medical device data systems (MDDS) or Class 2 devices. MDDS devices maintain data storage and data transfer, and also convert proprietary device languages into interoperability-standardized formats. Class 2 applications additionally offer active patient monitoring and alarms and therefore,

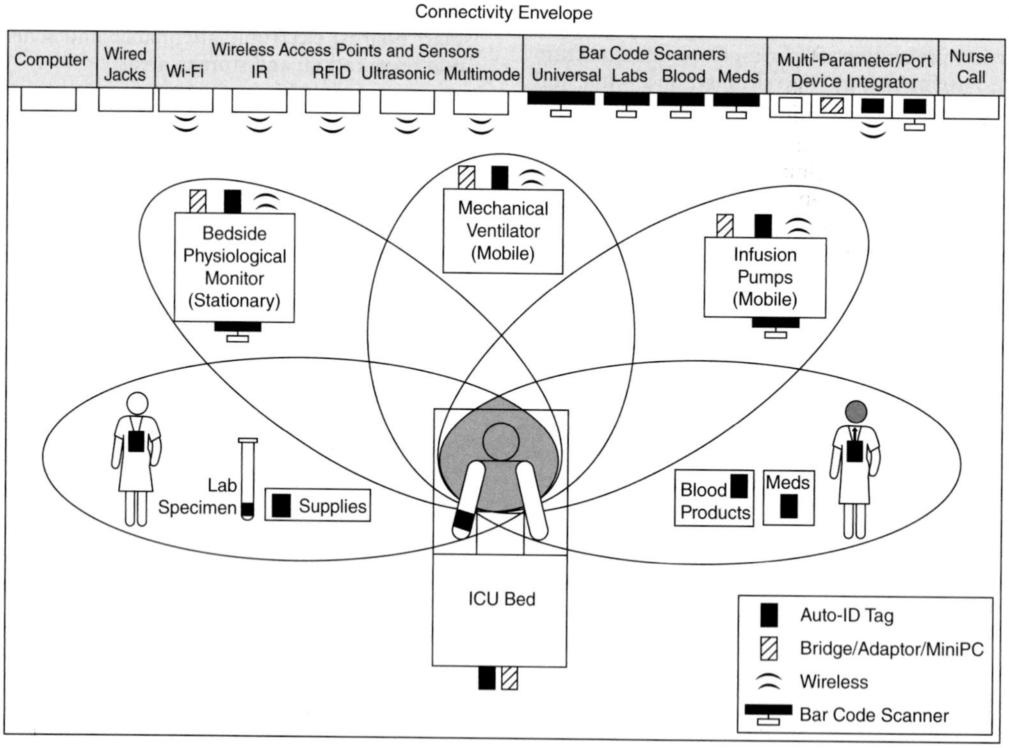

FIGURE 131.6 Data from bedside devices (stationary or mobile) including physiologic monitors; mechanical ventilators and infusion pumps; clinical and other support staff; supplies and medical applications (lab samples, blood products, and medications) must be associated (linked) with the patient. Each data source must have its own Auto-Identifier (Auto-ID tag) for tracking purposes or be used with RTLS. Medical devices also require Bridge/Adaptor/MiniPCs to identify the devices, and transmit information about the devices and data generated by the devices. The Auto-ID tags and the Bridge/Adaptor/MiniPCs are tracked by the room's connectivity envelope [wired jacks; wireless access points and sensors; bar code scanners (device or application specific or universal); multiparameter device integrators; and nurse call]. Devices themselves can have their own on-board connectivity solutions (i.e., Wi-Fi transmitters or bar code scanners). Devices may also be linked to the connectivity envelope indirectly through Nurse Call system rather than directly to the network.
RTLS, real-time locating systems.

receive enhanced FDA scrutiny. Applications inherent in ICU middleware include transforming hospital and ICU data and alarms into actionable information, managing devices, applying RTLS, creating smart displays, providing decision support, and facilitating telemedicine programs. The hospital's bed management system should be interfaced with the ICU middleware to automatically populate the ICU middleware with the ICU census. ICU middleware should also be compliant with hospital privacy protocols and lastly should have off-site backup systems.

Advanced ICU Informatics Concepts

Integral to advanced informatics are four concepts. The first is the linkage or association (location or patient centric) of the patient with the medical devices and the data generated by those devices (Fig. 131.6). The location-centric approach uses the patient's location for data linkage, whereas the patient-centric approach uses the patient's unique medical identification number. The location-centric solution is simpler to implement than the patient-centric method; however, the latter solution always attaches the data to the patient, regardless of patient movement within the hospital. The second concept is the application of interoperability between systems. Interoperability aligns the proprietary data output languages of the medical devices with the recipient middleware. Interoperability allows the data generated by one device to be clearly understood by the receiving middleware. Without interoperability, the data produced by the medical device may not be integrated into the electronic medical record even though the devices are connected to the hospital network. The third concept addresses time synchronization between all medical devices, middleware and the hospital network. Time synchronization helps create a correctly time-stamped medical record for all data from all sources. The fourth concept equates medical devices with informatics platforms. All new medical devices are actually advanced computers and consistently changing software versions and occasional hardware upgrades. Thus, informatics purchases should be carefully assessed in simulation laboratories to best evaluate their proposed informatics capabilities. As for all informatics platforms, the costs of annual software upgrades and licensing agreements should be prospectively budgeted.

Alarm Systems

Alarm middleware transforms select alarms from medical devices into relevant and actionable information. Such middleware can deliver the alarms to designated providers in real-time in a variety of formats and displays. The most sophisticated of these systems can process and create customized alarms based upon combinations of alarms and other data (i.e., multiple physiologic and laboratory values) as well as create personalized patient alarms from streaming raw device data.

Virtual Device Communities

Stand-alone medical devices (i.e., mechanical ventilators) are commonly linked to an individual patient. Alternatively, all ventilators can be linked together through device middleware to generate a "virtual" device community. In this setting, one can view all ventilators (settings, data and alarms) in the facility simultaneously. Additionally, such systems provide data storage, alarm transmission, report generation, remote viewing capabilities, and a portal for software upgrades and device monitoring by the vendor.

Real-Time Locating Systems

RTLS middleware offers solutions to improve workflow efficiencies of all assets (staff, patients, equipment, consumables, and patient rooms) [38]. RTLS to date are used primarily to locate tagged devices (mobile asset tracking) and to provide notification if devices leave designated areas. RTLS can also track the usage of consumable-tagged supplies to monitor inventory and directly link supplies to patient utilization. Within the ICU, RTLS can be integrated into nurse call systems and used to monitor patient and staff movements, compliance with hand washing protocols, and the environment.

Data Integration, Smart Displays, and Decision Support

Middleware applications can integrate, transmit and display data from a host of data sources (i.e., EMR, bedside devices, bed management systems, RTLS, imaging servers, webcams, and decision support systems). Such data can then be displayed imaginatively in a variety of formats and devices. Other middleware systems provide real-time intelligent algorithms and decisions support to monitor and sniff (automated systems that search for preselected data elements) for clinical abnormalities that may not be detected by traditional monitoring systems.

Telemedicine

The ICU informatics design also provides the framework for telemedicine through the use of interfaces and bidirectional communications systems. These technologies transmit data, clinician orders, video and voice between the various ICU areas and the hospitals' telemedicine support center. This allows the remote intensivists to identify signals of potential physiologic instability and communicate actionable intelligence to bedside caregivers. Such solutions are applicable whether the hospital outsources telemedicine to a third party at either an on- or off-site location, or internally to the hospital's own telemedicine team. Alternatively, the hospital can install web-based middleware that interfaces with hospital systems and allows dedicated members of the critical care team to respond in real time to integrated information from hospital (laboratory, imaging studies, and reports from consultants) and ICU systems using various handheld platforms.

THE FUTURE OF ICU DESIGN

ICU design of the future will likely incorporate the cost-savings possibilities derived from evolving trends in critical care models. Thus, larger units with more ICU beds per unit may become the norm, as hospitals look for the efficiencies thought to be associated with building and managing units with economies of scale. Larger units may also become multispecialty units, subdivided into smaller groupings of beds supported by a balance of centralized and decentralized work stations, and logistical support areas.

Standardization may become the norm for ICU design with identical vender-based technologies and systems in multiple units within one medical center. ICUs will likely be located in close proximity to each other especially in new facilities. Core areas adjacent to or within these units may include shared multiuse diagnostic and treatment technologies; administrative, educational, and/or research spaces; and family areas. Patient- and family-centered care will be encouraged through the build of larger patient rooms that are better able to accommodate family and required bathroom space. Ceiling mounted life support systems will replace fixed models and wirelessly integrated devices will allow for improved documentation, communication, and patient access. Segregation of public/visitor and patient/support circulation types will be pursued.

CONCLUSION

The goal of intensive care is to provide the highest-quality treatment in order to achieve the best outcomes for critically ill patients. Research supporting the impact of the built environment has exerted a strong influence on multidisciplinary design teams, as they seek solutions to maximize operational efficiency and create supportive healing environments for patients, families, and clinical staff. The ICU is an ever-changing and rapidly advancing environment. Future ICU designs will require planning for long-term flexibility by incorporating design decisions that accommodate changing care practices and information technology.

References

1. Halpern NA, Pastores SM: Critical care medicine beds, use, occupancy, and costs in the United States: a methodological review. *Crit Care Med* 43(11):2452–2459, 2015.
2. Ferri M, Zygun DA, Harrison A, et al: A study protocol for performance evaluation of a new academic intensive care unit facility: impact on patient care. *BMJ Open* 3(7), 2013.
3. Taylor E, Levin D: Patient protection, affordable care, and accountable design. *Front Health Serv Manage* 31(1):39–46, 2014.
4. Halpern NA: Innovative designs for the smart ICU: Part 1: from initial thoughts to occupancy. *Chest* 145(2):399–403, 2014.
5. Hamilton DK, Shepley MM: *Design for Critical Care: An Evidence-Based Approach*. Burlington, MA: Elsevier Ltd., 2010.
6. Stroupe JM: Design for safety in the critical care environment: an evidence-based approach: considering the caregiver-patient-family experiences. *Crit Care Nurs Q* 37(1):103–114, 2014.
7. Ferri M, Zygun DA, Harrison A, et al: Evidence-based design in an intensive care unit: end-user perceptions. *BMC Anesthesiol* 15:57, 2015.
8. Redden PH, Evans J: It takes teamwork... the role of nurses in ICU design. *Crit Care Nurs Q* 37(1):41–52, 2014.
9. Braun D, Barnhardt K: Critical thinking: optimal outcomes through end user involvement in the design of critical care areas. *Crit Care Nurs Q* 37(1):33–40, 2014.
10. Ulrich RS, Zimring C, Barch XZ, et al: A review of the research literature on evidence-based healthcare design. *HERD* 1(3):61–125, 2008.
11. Sadler BL, Dubose J, Zimring C: The business case for building better hospitals through evidence-based design. *HERD* 1(3):22–39, 2008.
12. Rashid M: Two decades (1993–2012) of adult intensive care unit design: a comparative study of the physical design features of the best practice examples. *Crit Care Nurs Q* 37(1):3–32, 2014.
13. Halpern NA, Pastores SM, Thaler HT, et al: Changes in critical care beds and occupancy in the United States 1985–2000: differences attributable to hospital size. *Crit Care Med* 34(8):2105–2112, 2006.
14. Kesecioglu J, Schneider MM, van der Kooi AW, et al: Structure and function: planning a new ICU to optimize patient care. *Curr Opin Crit Care* 18(6):688–692, 2012.
15. Thompson DR, Hamilton DK, Cadenhead CD, et al: Guidelines for intensive care unit design. *Crit Care Med* 40(5):1586–1600, 2012.
16. Valentin A, Ferdinande P: Recommendations on basic requirements for intensive care units: structural and organizational aspects. *Intensive Care Med* 37(10):1575–1587, 2011.
17. Halpern NA: Innovative designs for the smart ICU: Part 2: the ICU. *Chest* 145(3):646–658, 2014.
18. Halpern NA: Innovative designs for the smart ICU: Part 3: advanced ICU informatics. *Chest* 145(4):903–912, 2014.
19. *Guidelines for Design and Construction of Hospitals and Outpatient Facilities. 2014 Edition*. Dallas, TX, The Facilities Guidelines Institute, 2014.
20. Award Winning ICU Designs: How to build a better facility for patients and caregivers. www.sccm.org. Accessed Jun 2, 2017.
21. Evans J, Reyers E: Patient room considerations in the intensive care unit: caregiver, patient, family. *Crit Care Nurs Q* 37(1):83–92, 2014.
22. Pati D, Pati S: Methodological issues in conducting post-occupancy evaluations to support design decisions. *HERD* 6(3):157–163, 2013.
23. Cadenhead CD, Anderson DC: Critical Care Design: Trends in award winning designs. World Health Design 2009. Available from: http://www.worldhealthdesign.com/critical-care-design-trends-in-award-winning-designs.aspx. Accessed Jan 4, 2016.
24. Rashid M: A decade of adult intensive care unit design: a study of the physical design features of the best-practice examples. *Crit Care Nurs Q* 29(4):282–311, 2006.
25. Lavender SA, Sommerich CM, Patterson ES, et al: Hospital patient room design: the issues facing 23 occupational groups who work in medical/surgical patient rooms. *HERD* 8(4):98–114, 2015.
26. Maze C: Inboard, Outboard, or Nested? Healthcare Design Magazine 2009; (March 1, 2009). Available from: http://www.healthcaredesignmagazine.com/print/article/inboard-outboard-or-nested. Accessed Jan 4, 2016.
27. Reiling J, Hughes RG, Murphy MR: The impact of facility design on patient safety, in Hughes RG (ed). *Patient Safety and Quality: An Evidence-Based Handbook for Nurses. Ch 28*. Agency for Healthcare Research and Quality (US), 2008, pp 2-167–2-192.
28. Eriksson T, Lindahl B, Bergbom I: Visits in an intensive care unit—an observational hermeneutic study. *Intensive Crit Care Nurs* 26(1):51–517, 2010.
29. Pati D, Evans J, Waggener L, et al: An exploratory examination of medical gas booms versus traditional headwalls in intensive care unit design. *Crit Care Nurs Q* 31(4):340–356, 2008.
30. Drews FA: Human factors in critical care medical environments. Reviews of human factors and ergonomics, in *Reviews of Human Factors and Ergonomics*. Vol 8. Santa Monica, CA, Human Factors and Ergonomics Society, 2013, pp 103–148.
31. Lindahl B, Bergbom I: Bringing research into a closed and protected place: development and implementation of a complex clinical intervention project in an ICU. *Crit Care Nurs Q* 38(4):393–404, 2015.
32. Callahan CW, Repeta RJ Jr, Sherman SS: Evidence-based building design and organizational culture. *Front Health Serv Manage* 31(1):47–54, 2014.
33. Johansson L, Bergbom I, Lindahl B: Meanings of being critically ill in a sound-intensive ICU patient room—a phenomenological hermeneutical study. *Open Nurs J* 6:108–116, 2012.
34. Hagerman I, Rasmanis G, Blomkvist V, et al: Influence of intensive coronary care acoustics on the quality of care and physiological state of patients. *Int J Cardiol* 98(2):267–270, 2005.
35. Leaf DE, Homel P, Factor PH: Relationship between ICU design and mortality. *Chest* 137(5):1022–1027, 2010.
36. Lu Y, Ossmann MM, Leaf DE, et al: Patient visibility and ICU mortality: a conceptual replication. *HERD* 7(2):92–103, 2014.
37. Perme C, Chandrashekar R: Early mobility and walking program for patients in intensive care units: creating a standard of care. *Am J Crit Care* 18(3):212–221, 2009.
38. Kamel Boulos MN, Berry G: Real-time locating systems (RTLS) in healthcare: a condensed primer. *Int J Health Geogr* 11:25, 2012.
39. Halpern NA, Brentjens T: Point of care testing informatics. The critical care-hospital interface. *Crit Care Clin* 15(3):577–591, 1999.
40. Verhaeghe S, Defloor T, Van ZF, et al: The needs and experiences of family members of adult patients in an intensive care unit: a review of the literature. *J Clin Nurs* 14(4):501–509, 2005.
41. Sturdivant L, Warren NA: Perceived met and unmet needs of family members of patients in the pediatric intensive care unit. *Crit Care Nurs Q* 32(2):149–158, 2009.

Chapter 132 ■ Intensive Care Unit Organization and Management

THOMAS L. HIGGINS • JAY S. STEINGRUB

INTRODUCTION

Organization is the act of assembling elements into an orderly, functional whole. Management is the ongoing revision and renovation of that careful assembly to cope with change. The notion of organization is well known to intensive care unit (ICU) division and service chiefs and directors who have hospital or departmental responsibilities to deliver critical care services. The concept of "bedside management" is familiar to clinicians who titrate vasopressors or adjust ventilator settings. ICU management is itself a form of titration and continuous adjustment that addresses creating and implementing policies and procedures, arranging service and interprofessional rounds, preparing budgets, and complying with regulations. The successful ICU director must also have both organizational skills and leadership capabilities to relate to the rest of the hospital and innovate and facilitate change. Creativity is important in these processes, but perseverance may be the most essential character trait because of the many ways a typical organization will resist change. Table 132.1 outlines the strategic (leadership) and tactical (managerial) responsibilities of an ICU director.

Knowing how to navigate the obvious and the subtle impediments to change is a key skill for ICU leaders, beginning with the nurse manager and physician medical director and extending through a hospital's or system's leadership hierarchy. The contemporary trend toward increasing requests for ICU admissions and shrinking reimbursement for services rendered will require ever more sophisticated organization and experienced ICU managers. Although organizational reporting has historically been based on traditional departmental structure (e.g., medicine, surgery, and pediatrics), there is an emerging trend in North America toward Critical Care Organizations (CCOs) [1] that supervise and govern the delivery of critical care services across departments and increasingly across entities of a health delivery network.

The conceptual frameworks [2] and business skills for successful ICU leadership must be acquired, whether in business school or on the job [3]. Important characteristics of leaders include self-awareness, self-regulation, motivation, empathy, and social skills [4]. The American Association for Physician Leadership is an organization that provides guidance on how to prepare for and succeed in medical management [5] ranging from journals to seminars to master's degree preparation. A formal Masters of Business Administration program will typically include courses on accounting, data analysis, ethics, financial analysis, human resource management, information systems, marketing, production/operation management, organizational behavior, organizational planning and strategy, quality improvement (QI), teambuilding, and leadership. Many physician practice groups now offer training and business career development. This chapter will focus on the most relevant subset of ICU organization patterns, human resource issues, the roles of the ICU director, methods for monitoring clinical ICU care, and ancillary management issues.

ICU ORGANIZATION: GOVERNANCE

ICUs were initially developed to facilitate nursing efficiency by permitting higher nurse to patient ratios in a geographically constrained area and also to accommodate then-unfamiliar technologies such as telemetry and mechanical ventilation. Early units were typically converted contiguous double-bed patient rooms or hospital wards, with purpose-built facilities becoming more common after the 1960s. Many hospitals organized specialty-specific units (e.g., Medical ICU, Surgical ICU, and Pediatric ICU) governed as critical care services or divisions within existing departments of medicine, surgery, or pediatrics. Larger and academic medical centers additionally developed a variety of highly specialized units (e.g., trauma, burn, neurosurgery, and cardiac

TABLE 132.1

Strategic (Leadership) Versus Tactical (Management) Duties of the Intensive Care Unit (ICU) Director

Strategic goals/leadership	Tactical interventions/management
Creating ICU vision and mission statement	Communicating vision, onboarding new team members
Creating a healthy culture and work environment	Conflict resolution, adherence to policy and regulations, culture of safety
Evaluating and improving quality of care	Daily use of care "bundles" and protocols
Matching physician, nursing, and ancillary capacity to patient demand	Hiring new staff; creating call schedules, dealing with coverage emergencies, reassigning tasks
Fostering interdisciplinary relationships	Supporting interdisciplinary rounds and joint conferences with time and effort
Planning for the future	Creating budget requests for space and equipment
Delivering value	Specific cost containment initiatives such as length-of-stay reduction
Economic self-sufficiency of hospital (Part A) and physician (Part B) practice	Monthly review of financial statements, on-going salary, and variable compensation adjustments
Developing professional capabilities	Physician and nursing education, fundamentals of critical care training
Efficient resource management	Written policies for bed management, triage, insertion and removal of devices, and technology
Exploiting advanced technology	Improving electronic medical records, situational awareness monitors, bar code scanning

surgery) reporting through existing departments or subspecialty service lines. Smaller hospitals might have a single shared unit caring for all critically ill patients, but separately directed by medical, surgical, cardiology, or pediatric services. Although some hospitals created hospital-wide critical care practice committees to coordinate bed management, purchasing, common protocols, or "Code Blue" responses, units were more often silos within specialty service lines rather than highly coordinated.

The concept of a "CCO" within a hospital is a more recent development. With the consolidation of individual hospitals into integrated health care delivery networks, enterprise-wide committees seek to standardize practices. Many institutions have transitioned from traditional academic departments (e.g., medicine, surgery, and pediatrics) to service lines, centers, or institutes (e.g., neurosciences, heart and vascular, and digestive diseases) that employ physicians and other providers from multiple departments and thus require matrix reporting arrangements. Critical care may be structured as a support service for the entire organization (e.g., one or more multidisciplinary ICUs caring for both medical and surgical patients) or embedded within a service line (e.g., a Neuro ICU within neurosciences, a cardiac care unit within heart and vascular). Either way, system-wide coordination is essential on matters of triage, training of nurses and support personnel, protocols and order sets in the electronic medical record (EMR), standardization of equipment, equipment and operating budgets, recruitment, quality assurance, education, and research.

A number of operational models exist, ranging from a simple coordinating committee to a formal CCO that oversees all the different ICUs and/or step-down units within a medical center or network. Additionally even without a CCO, some hospitals have created a position called an associate chief of staff, associate chief medical officer, or an associate physician in chief who is responsible for all critical care operations. These programs are in line with the changes nurses have made for years putting all the ICUs under one umbrella. The evolution of critical care services or divisions to enterprise-wide CCOs has only rarely been studied [1]; potential benefits include system budgetary support for critical care, sharing of resources, protocols and best practices, group purchasing, plus physician and nursing cross-coverage in person or via telemedicine.

ICU ORGANIZATION: PHYSICIAN PRIVILEGES AND CARE MODELS

Although for the majority of countries worldwide the critically ill population is cared for in "closed" ICUs, the controversy around the "closed" versus "open" model of care continues to exist in the United States. In broad terms, there are three common models for ICU organization:

- **Open ICU:** Traditionally, in an open ICU model unit, a primary physician with hospital privileges may admit and care for patients in any appropriate bed, including the ICU. Patient care decisions are made by the admitting physician, often with the input of consultants. Admission and discharge (triage) decisions fall to the ICU director only in the event of a bed or staffing shortage. Elective consultation with intensivists (when available) may be ordered at the discretion of the admitting physician. The major perceived benefit of this model is the continuity of care, although arguably less so when the admitting physician is a hospitalist rather than the patient's primary care provider. By necessity, the open model remains prevalent in the United States, with greater than 50% of ICUs (typically in smaller hospitals) lacking daytime intensivist coverage [6].
- **Closed ICU:** All patients are managed by a team of intensivists (physicians with specialty training in intensive care medicine) or in partnership with an admitting primary attending service for the duration of the ICU stay. Depending on local institutional tradition, the admitting physician may remain closely involved or collaborate from a distance. Theoretical benefits of this model include more timely patient assessment and treatment initiation; use of clinical protocols and checklists; and attention to evidence-based critical care with reductions in mortality, complications, resource use, and ICU and hospital length of stay (LOS). This model is most common in Europe, Latin America [7], Australia, and New Zealand but continues to gain acceptance in the United States, based on research findings and response to external pressure from the Leapfrog Group [8] and payers.

  Intensivist staffing contributes to a hospital's overall safety score, and smaller hospitals without full-time intensivists may find it difficult to achieve a Leapfrog Safety Score [8] of "A," unless telemedicine is employed. Of interest, among the center participants in the Extended Prevalence of Infection in Intensive Care Study trial, 83% of them were a closed staff model worldwide versus 63% in North America [9]. Closed ICU units are frequently unworkable in smaller community hospitals where it would be financially prohibitive to support a full-time intensivist in a 4- to 6-bed ICU on net practice service revenue alone, especially with a poor payer mix. Although ample evidence suggests that on-site intensivists improve processes of care and staff satisfaction and decrease ICU complications and hospital LOS [10], other studies have found no difference in mortality with high-intensity daytime physician staffing [11]. There are little data documenting exactly what elements of the closed ICU organizational models are responsible for improvement of care.
- **Transitional (Semi-closed or Hybrid) ICU:** Patients are referred for ICU admission to an intensivist, who reviews all admissions for appropriateness (gatekeeping). Final decisions regarding admission, discharge, and triage rest with the physician unit director or his/her designee. The intensivist may be responsible for some patients but not others and via specific consultation may participate in some or all of the patients' care in conjunction with the patients attending physician. The intensivist's role may be limited to triage functions and emergency response but more often encompasses hemodynamic, respiratory, fluid, nutritional, preventive care, and safety management. This model is seen in the transition phase between open and closed structures and remains common among surgical practices where the attending surgeon addresses overall supervision and the specific operative aspects of a patient's care (e.g., wound care and transplant immunosuppressive regimens) while delegating emergency resuscitation, physiologic monitoring, organ system support, and ICU safety issues to the intensivist. Arguably, ICU telemedicine (discussed later) is becoming the dominant form of the semi-closed unit.

Pronovost et al. [12] conducted a systematic review of articles examining physician staffing patterns and clinical outcomes published through 2001. The model of care in each of 17 studies was classified as low-intensity staffing (a model other than closed or mandatory consult) or high-intensity staffing (closed ICU model or mandatory critical care consultation model). The high-intensity model was associated with lower ICU mortality (pooled mortality risk estimate = 0.61) and lower hospital mortality (pooled mortality risk estimate = 0.71). Although the literature overwhelmingly favors intensivist staffing models, a retrospective analysis of the Project IMPACT database by Levy et al. [11] demonstrated higher odds for hospital mortality for patients managed by critical care physicians. These counterintuitive findings have been challenged as being caused by differences between studies in ICU administration, team composition and function, and unmeasured confounders including case-mix differences [9] and the role of trainees and part-time academic faculty [13]. The higher risk-adjusted mortality of teaching hospitals where more invasive interventions are performed [14] may also obscure beneficial effects of full-time intensivists.

Case–control studies, where outcomes have been examined before and after implementing a closed model, offer additional insight into the value of intensivists. Patients admitted to closed units tend to be sicker [15,16], as might be expected with tighter triage criteria. Nursing confidence in physician clinical judgment improves [17], because a closed system allows the nurse to contact one managing physician rather than having to call the pulmonologist for ventilator changes, the nephrologist for fluid and electrolyte issues, and the cardiologist for arrhythmias. These efficiencies are generally reflected in shorter ICU and hospital LOS [18]. The effect of dedicated intensivist staffing on ICU LOS remains significant after case-mix is adjusted for risk factors such as patient age, admission severity of illness, pre-ICU LOS, and percentage of patients requiring mechanical ventilation [19]. Moreover, the closed ICU model may decrease resource use by allowing the intensivist to reduce inappropriate admissions, lessen complications that may impact duration of stay, and enhance opportunities for more timely discharge from the ICU.

ICU PROVIDER STAFFING

Providing around-the-clock (24 hours × 7 days, or 24/7) intensivist coverage requires substantially more physician hours and thus costs more than the traditional model where intensivists may make daily or twice-daily rounds and are otherwise available if paged to return. Despite intuition that more intensivist hours in ICUs might provide better outcomes, there is no difference in risk-adjusted mortality or family satisfaction metrics with 24/7 staffing of ICUs in the presence of high-intensity daytime intensivists [20]. Additional data suggest that there are no differences, independent of severity of illness, in mortality, ICU and hospital LOS, or duration of mechanical ventilation when nighttime coverage of the ICU is provided by nonintensivists or trainees [17]. A single center trial found no differences of mortality or ICU LOS for a night shift intensivist compared to having an intensivist on call from home via phone contact [18]. Perhaps the nonsuperiority of a 24/7 model of care may simply indicate that protocolized ICU care set up and driven by intensivists during the day effectively reduces the need for intensivist presence at night. Although outcome differences can be demonstrated as a function of ICU admission time and day of week [21–25], at the hospital level, there is no statistically significant mortality difference based on the time of admission for most (77%) diagnoses [26], including acute myocardial infarction, congestive heart failure, pneumonia, stroke, gastrointestinal bleeding, and many surgical conditions. Mortality was higher, though, among patients with ruptured abdominal aortic aneurysms, acute epiglottitis, and pulmonary embolism, when these patients presented on a weekend rather than a weekday. Practically speaking, in-house 24/7 intensivist coverage is impractical for more than half of US hospitals, and efforts are now underway to properly educate the hospitalist workforce for this task [27].

A survey of CCOs from 23 academic medical centers (104 ICUs) revealed ICU models of care comprising full-time intensivists (33%), shift-work intensivists (28%), and a hybrid model of full-time and shift-work intensivists (26%). Physician extenders provided care in 36% of the ICUs with hospitalist involvement in 21% of medical centers. Fourteen percent of these academic centers provided ICU telemedicine services [1].

ICU TELEMEDICINE

In ICU telemedicine, critical care physicians, physician extenders, and nurses provide a team-based real-time support to multiple critical care units (CCUs) from a centralized location. Remote intensive care with ICU telemedicine has emerged as a partial solution to the shortage of intensivists. ICU telemedicine has grown from 0.9% of total US ICU beds in 2003 to 7.9% in 2010 [28]. Using intensivists and physician extenders to provide supplemental monitoring and management of ICU patients between noon and 7 AM, Breslow et al. were able to demonstrate reductions in hospital mortality (relative risk = 0.73), ICU LOS (3.63 vs. 4.35 days), and lower variable costs per case [29]. Given the critical shortage of intensivists, tele-ICU systems can potentially permit these specialists to monitor more patients including those who otherwise might not have access to an intensivist. Thus far, hospitals adopting ICU telemedicine have tended to be larger, urban, covered by residents, and located in large metropolitan areas [28], while a pressing need remains in small, rural hospitals without house staff.

There are numerous models of ICU telemedicine. These range from total 24/7 coverage by an intensivist at the control center with hospitalists or advanced practitioners on site to episodic night or weekend coverage with on-site intensivists conducting rounds and weekday coverage, or any variation of the above. Research is needed to determine how local hospital operating factors (i.e., level and experience of physician and nursing staffing, sophistication of the EMR and order sets, protocols, and local culture) affect the design of the telemedicine coverage [30].

Despite the shortage of data, the Leapfrog Group and the University Health System Consortium have encouraged the application of tele-ICU [31]. A major methodological limitation of "before and after" study design is the inability to control for other temporal changes in case-mix, staffing, and use of decision-support tools or new electronic medical software introduced at the same time. Potential benefits of ICU telemedicine include better adherence to evidence-based practice, continuous availability of critical care expertise, and better survival [32]. These must be balanced against costs, reimbursement, privacy and medicolegal issues, the potential for downtimes and malfunctions, and depersonalization of the patient–physician relationship inherent in introducing a layer of technology [31].

Additionally, there are many costs to implementing telemedicine that are in part determined by the sophistication of any existing EMR and ICU systems. Full telemedicine requires cameras and bidirectional communication systems in each ICU room as well as the waiting room or conference room, interfaces for the ICU bedside devices as well as the EMR, and ongoing licensing fees. Installation can be turnkey, or built with "off the shelf" technology [33]. Thus, the capital costs of implementing and ongoing costs of maintaining telemedicine support can be substantial; more research is needed to determine whether cost-effectiveness is limited to certain circumstances or is more universal. Yoo et al. conducted a simulation analysis assuming per-patient per-hospital-stay ICU cost and hospital mortality based on published literature. Additional costs for tele-ICU were estimated at $909 to $1,057 per patient, and the mortality reduction from tele-ICU was to be 23.7% (range 18.5% to 28.9%). In this simulation, ICU telemedicine was cost-effective in most cases (considering a threshold of $100,000 per additional quality-adjusted life year), and cost-saving in some circumstances [34].

PHYSICIAN HUMAN RESOURCE ISSUES

Hiring full-time critical care specialists is already a challenge with the growing shortage of intensivists [35]. Critical care workforce needs have not been adequately addressed by public policy; the current reimbursement at Medicare/Medicaid rates is frequently insufficient to cover physician salary and benefits. Angus et al. predicted in 2000 that serious shortfalls would occur by 2020 [36], and these predictions still are on track, especially given differences between the number of Critical Care Medicine (CCM)-certified individuals and those actually practicing critical care [37]. Intensivists previously willing to work 66 hour/weeks and 10- to 12-hour shifts are finding nonbedside care alternatives as they age [38]. It is unclear that the next generation of intensivists will continue to work at this level of intensity or that critical care will even be a viable career choice when remuneration is better for specialties with shorter working hours and less stress. Typical schedules for emergency medicine physicians (three 12-hour shifts for 46 weeks or 1,656 annual clinical hours) or hospitalists (typically 1,760 hours per year) are already more attractive than standard critical care jobs, and it is likely that a reduced annual critical care workload will become a cost of doing business as older physicians retire.

Current Leapfrog Group standards call for *in-house* intensivist staffing for a minimum of 8 hours, 7 days per week [13,39], or > 2,920 hours per year to cover one ICU, with requirements for off-hours coverage met by an intensivist on beeper call, plus a Fundamentals of Critical Care Support–certified physician or physician extender immediately available in-house. Hospitalists have both potential value and limitations acknowledged in a joint position paper from the Society of Hospital Medicine and the Society of Critical Care Medicine (SCCM) [27].

It is helpful to consider the concept of a clinical full-time equivalent (FTE) to represent the amount of work done by one individual working only on direct patient care tasks in the ICU. In reality, some ICU clinicians will also allocate professional time to research, administration, or education; choose to work part-time; or spend part of their clinical time on the trauma team, in the pulmonary or sleep clinic, or in administering anesthesia. A full-time physician working only in the ICU might have grant funding for 0.25 FTE stipend and another 0.25 stipend for administrative and educational activities, leaving 0.5 FTE for ICU clinical activity.

How many hours will one FTE work in a year? Respondents to an SCCM survey reported annual work hours from less than 1,000 to more than 4,000, but most commonly 2,000 to 2,500 hours [40]. Because attractive jobs currently offer at least 4 weeks' vacation, about 10 paid holidays and at least 5 days of professional meeting time, for arguments sake, we will consider annual work to be 45 weeks with 10-hour days, yielding approximately 2,250 hours, within the range reported in the SCCM survey. If in-house coverage for the ICU is around-the-clock 365 days per year, with 30-minutes overlap for sign-out at the beginning and end of 12-hour shifts, then annual hours to be covered are 8,760; 8,760/2,250 implies 3.9 FTEs would be required to cover the workload, edging closer to 5.0 FTE if additional overlap hours are required or if annual clinical hours are reduced closer to hospitalist norms. Additional nonclinical time would be needed for administrative, educational, and quality assurance activities. In an academic medical center, clinical care time for full-timers is frequently set at 80% to 90% of paid hours (0.8 to 0.9 clinical FTE) to allow for teaching or administrative activities.

The ICU medical director will need significant administrative time (0.2 to 0.5 FTE, depending on the size of the ICU and the number of physicians and advanced practitioners supervised). If coverage is only during the daytime (3,650 hours per year), then fewer FTEs would be required; on-call hours must still be staffed, unless tele-ICU coverage provides full support [1]. In one survey of 152 ICUs at 24 academic hospitals, intensivists were in-house in 49%, with off-hours in house coverage provided by advanced practitioners (63%), hospitalists (21%), and via telemedicine (14%) [41].

Staffing calculations must consider intensivist-to-patient staffing ratios, which are not well defined. In England and Wales, where intensivists staff 80% of ICUs, the average 6-bed general ICU has three consultants committed to the unit and another three consultants participating in the on-call rotation [42]. A retrospective study from the Mayo Clinic [37] did not find differences in severity-adjusted mortality rates at daytime intensivist-to-bed ratios between 1:7.5 and 1:15 although ICU LOS increased at the higher extreme. Larger hospitals with closed units may take advantage of cross-coverage between units, providing daytime care at intensivist-to-patient ratios of 1:8 to 1:12 and increasing the ratio during off-hours when there are fewer acute interventions or procedures to be performed.

The number of critical care physicians is not increasing as fast as the number, size, and occupancy rates of ICUs, leading to a potential intensivist shortage [43]. A recent SCCM taskforce has made a number of recommendations for "closed" ICUs where intensivists control triage and patient care. Although they could not advocate a specific maximum number of patients under one physician's care, the taskforce concluded that proper staffing affects care, large caseloads should not preclude timely rounding, staffing levels should consider surge capacity, and regular institutional reassessment of staffing levels is necessary. In addition, high turnover rates or deteriorating quality indicators may be markers of overload, and telemedicine may be useful to alleviate overburden but needs more study. In teaching institutions, faculty and trainee feedback may illuminate the effects of understaffing on medical education, and there is some evidence that intensivist- to-patient ratios less favorable than 1:14 negatively impact patient care, education, and staff well-being [44].

MULTIDISCIPLINARY MODELS: ADVANCED PRACTITIONERS

Strategies suggested to offset the shortage of intensivists in the United States include the use of advanced practitioners to fill out 24/7 ICU coverage. Driving forces that have accelerated the employment of advanced practitioners include cutbacks of federal funding for residency training and Accreditation Council for Graduate Medical Education standards placing duty hour limitations at teaching hospitals for medical trainees [37]. Advanced practitioner is a broad term covering health care providers such as nurse practitioners (NPs), certified registered nurse anesthetists, certified nurse midwives, and physician assistants (PAs). An NP is a registered nurse who has completed substantial advanced training and will typically be independently licensed in the state where practicing. Following state licensure, NPs may seek national certification from professional nursing boards and/or pursue specialty certification. NPs have more latitude to practice independently, although scope of practice laws varies by state. PAs must complete an accredited education program, usually 2 years in duration, but typically requiring prior college and health care experience. PAs must pass a national examination to obtain a license and always work under a physician's supervision. It is vital for the intensivist team to recognize that NPs and PAs directly out of school may have minimal CCM experience. Therefore, intense onboarding and ongoing education is required in order for expectations of critical care excellence from advanced practitioners to be satisfied.

NPs and PAs are increasingly involved in critical care. Surveys suggest that PAs provide care in approximately 25% and NPs in >50% of adult ICUs in academic medical centers in the United States [40]. A comparison of house staff–covered medical ICU care to that staffed by NPs and PAs functioning simultaneously in a single academic center showed no differences of mortality, readmission rates, or ICU LOS [45]. A prospective cohort study (2011 to 2013) comparing 90-day survival and ICU and hospital mortality and LOSs found comparable outcomes for critically ill patients cared for by advanced practitioner nurses and residents [46]. Nonphysician providers have been shown to improve patient satisfaction, LOS, mortality, and duration of mechanical ventilation [41]. NP and PA responsibilities may be focused on procedures or implementation of protocolized bundles of care [47], freeing the intensivists to deal with difficult diagnoses or the most complex management.

Introduction of NP/intensivist team–based care can be beneficial to patient outcomes, financial outcomes, LOS, and patient satisfaction [48]. An attending physician/NP team can safely manage former ICU patients admitted to a subacute unit, therefore allowing the intensivist/fellow team time to care for higher acuity ICU patients [44]. Decreased overall LOS and ICU

LOS, lower rates of urinary tract infection and skin breakdown, and a shorter time to mobilization have been documented after the introduction of an NP team to neuroscience ICUs [49]. NP participation with weaning protocols for mechanical ventilation has been associated with greater reductions of mechanical ventilation days, ICU LOS, and hospital LOS when compared to pre-NP participation [50]. NPs and physicians in training had equivalent efficacies for performing the required tasks, but residents spend more time in nonunit activities (e.g., lectures and rounds) and NPs spend more time monitoring patients, talking to families, and collaborating with other health team members [44].

Sharing the Care

As health care financing transitions from fee-for-service (FFS) to global payments, it becomes economically viable to transfer tasks to other providers, so that each provider is working at the "top of their license" [51]. Figure 132.1 suggests an approach to sharing the care in the ICU environment. The universe of patient presentations can be plotted on the y-axis of "certain versus uncertain," and the x-axis of "simple versus complex." In an accountable care environment, critical care physicians can concentrate on efforts where confidence in the diagnosis is low, or physiology is unstable. Tactical comprehensive care (where the diagnosis is known) can be delegated to advanced practitioners. The lower left corner of the graph represents protocol-driven care that could be delivered by respiratory therapists and nurses (supervised by physicians), and advances in artificial intelligence may allow highly automated care. The goal is to redistribute the workload with limited intensivist resources to create capacity for additional uncertain or highly complex patients.

A team-oriented culture characterized by timely communication is associated with a shorter ICU LOS, greater ability to accommodate the needs of patient families, and a higher quality of technical care [52]. Including PAs on house staff–directed ICU teams does not appear to affect the rates of occupancy, mortality, or complications for ICUs with well-established protocols for common ICU diagnoses [53].

Intensive care services are among the most urgent and costly aspects of health care in the United States, and national surveys indicate the need to accommodate between 50,000 and 68,000 patients per day [37,43]. Professional societies are projecting an inability to meet this demand with intensivists; therefore, the role of advanced practitioners, respiratory therapists, dieticians, pharmacists, and other professionals will become a major component of the health care delivery model for critically ill patients.

ROLE OF THE ICU DIRECTOR, DIVISION OR SECTION CHIEF, OR SERVICE LEADER

The Joint Commission requires that an individual be designated as the ICU director, but actual job descriptions vary [41]. At one end of the spectrum, the medical director may simply approve critical care policies and serve as a resource for questions that cannot be solved by nursing administration. He or she may triage only in times of high census and may have very little role in the bedside delivery of critical care, other than to his or her own patients. At the other extreme, the medical director may lead the team of intensivists and other professionals that assumes total responsibility for all patients occupying ICU beds. Associated tasks might include management of multiple units, patient flow management, fellowship training programs, development of advanced practitioner programs, billing, recruitment and retention of staff, QI, research, and representing and marketing critical care to the greater hospital community. These responsibilities may apply at a local traditional CCM service or division within a department or at the level of CCO. Typically, the local ICU director will have a close working relationship with the unit's nursing manager/leader and interact extensively with other professionals (e.g., pharmacists, dieticians, social workers, clergy, and utilization management specialists). Essential character traits of the successful ICU director include willingness to collaborate, ability to delegate, trust in colleagues, and excellent communication skills.

Nonclinical duties for physician managers may consume more work effort than clinical responsibilities when committee membership, administrative tasks, budget preparation, educational activities, and the business of running the ICU physician practice are included. ICU occupancy rates and the number of patients misallocated to ICU beds decline with involved physician management [54]. Executive resolution of chronic process issues also impacts transitions of care (including ICU readmissions) by addressing policies to avoid postdischarge medical deterioration, improper triage, or administrative problems [55]. Knowledge of case management rules (and consultation with the physician advisor to hospital case management) can improve ICU performance relative to standards for levels of care.

Tasks performed by the ICU director can best be divided into strategic versus tactical (see Table 132.1). Strategic tasks involve the "big picture" including data analysis, recognition of patterns and trends, setting priorities, considering alternatives, and implementing change. The ICU director is often the champion for process improvement projects. Areas deserving of strategic

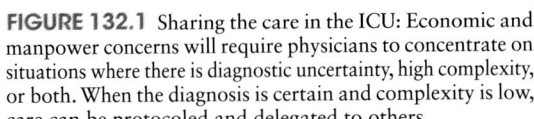

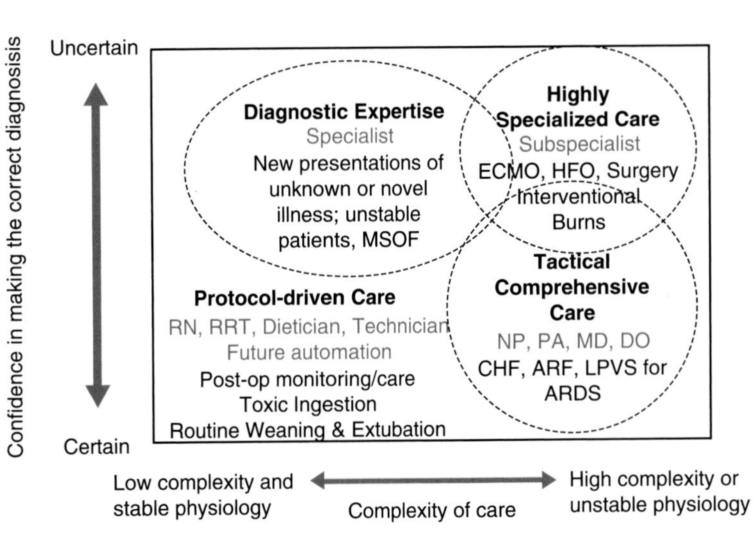

FIGURE 132.1 Sharing the care in the ICU: Economic and manpower concerns will require physicians to concentrate on situations where there is diagnostic uncertainty, high complexity, or both. When the diagnosis is certain and complexity is low, care can be protocoled and delegated to others.
ARDS, acute respiratory distress syndrome; ARF, acute renal failure; CHF, congestive heart failure; DO, doctor of osteopathy; ECMO, extracorporeal membrane oxygenation; HFO, high frequency oscillation; LPVS, lung protective ventilatory strategy; MD, medical doctor; MSOF, multiple systems organ failure; NP, nurse practitioner; PA, physician assistant; RN, registered nurse; RRT, respiratory therapist.

consideration include cost containment; the overall culture of the ICU; QI efforts; education of physicians, nurses, and other health professionals; optimizing the implementation of electronic medical systems; and coping with change driven by ICU, hospital, and external factors [56]. Developing a strategic vision, communicating it well, and leading by example are essential.

Tactical chores consist of the day-to-day, "hands-on" running of the unit. Leaving aside patient care, which in itself can fill the day, there are human resource issues, scheduling concerns, patient triage, bed allocation, and conflict resolution [57]. The ICU director may be granted by hospital policy the authority to intervene in any patient's care and may also be charged with evaluating issues and complaints that originate from family members, nursing staff, other physicians, or hospital administration. Tools to assist with the tactical aspects of patient care include checklists [58] and electronic support systems. The danger is that tactical chores multiply to occupy all available time, leaving little time for strategic direction. Implementation of computerized order sets, therapist-directed protocols, and other "bundles" of care helps to minimize the individual, routine tactical decisions and leave more time for strategic thinking.

The difference between strategy and tactics reflects the difference between leading and managing. Applied to academic teaching rounds as an example, the attending physician or ICU fellow should be leading (strategizing), not getting lost in the details, but rather planning at a higher level exactly what broad changes and interventions will be required to get the patient recovered and discharged from the unit. In contrast, the residents or advanced practitioners should be patient managers (tacticians) who respond to the information flow of physical examination findings, laboratory tests, and radiology reports. They collect and analyze these data and develop a daily or even hourly plan. It is difficult to concentrate on both strategy and tactics at the same time, which argues for dividing the effort with a team approach. However, the strategic leader should not be isolated from patient contact, for it is the experienced interpretation of clues and subtleties that define the expert clinician [59].

The job responsibilities of the ICU director (and by delegation, the triage physician of the day) create an inherent conflict of interest. A treating physician's fiduciary responsibility is to advocate for an individual patient's best interest. As the ICU manager, however, there is a responsibility to do the most good for the greatest number of patients. The essence of triage is to maximize benefits for the group, even at the expense of an individual. In times of bed shortages, the ethical principle of beneficence ("do good") may conflict with the ethical principle of social justice. The reader is referred to Chapter 34 for a more comprehensive discussion of ethical issues in the ICU, but it is important for the ICU director to recognize these conflicts and preemptively construct ICU and hospital policy to address how such conflicts should be resolved.

BUDGET AND PROFESSIONAL REIMBURSEMENT ISSUES

The ICU director may be responsible for managing the budget of the entire CCU, including the nursing and respiratory therapy components, but more typically will be particularly concerned primarily with revenue from physician professional activity. In the United States, critical care revenue is generated by billing critical care codes (Current Procedural Terminology (CPT) codes 99291 and 99292) when the patient qualifies for time-based bedside critical care or otherwise for evaluation and management (E&M) codes (typically CPT code 99232-33 for subsequent hospital care and 99251-53 inpatient consultation) [60,61]. Various procedures have specific codes, and each code is associated with relative value units (RVUs) that form the basis for eventual payment. The connection between RVU generation and clinical effort in the ICU setting, however, is tenuous at best, in part due to the difficulty of documenting and billing the multitude of small tasks accomplished over the course of the day.

The majority of billable services may occur during the normal business day. Thirty-one to seventy-four minutes of bedside attention to one patient will justify a single CPT code 99291. Additional services rendered to that patient throughout a 24-hour period would have to exceed 74 total minutes to additionally bill CPT 99292. As a result, off-hours interventions may generate less income than what it costs to staff those hours, although revenue will depend on the number of patients seen, their severity of illness, and the reimbursement rate for a particular locale. In many institutions, revenue received may be 50% or less of what was actually billed, owing to low Medicaid rates and negotiated contractual agreements with insurers. Thus, under systems of reimbursement used in the United States, it may not be possible for a critical care physician group to be self-funding on patient care revenue alone especially when providing extended hours of in-house coverage. The landscape of billing and coding is constantly changing, and the 2015 Medicare Access and CHIP Reauthorization Act [62] encourages a transition from FFS billing to population health where global "per member per month" payments cover all medical care. Current information on CPT coding is available at the American Medical Association website [63] and through the SCCM [64].

The ICU director plays an increasingly important role for managing the business aspects of the critical care practice. It is helpful to have a tracking system to ensure that each physician is submitting his or her patient care charges in a timely manner and that the billing service is properly submitting and capturing these charges. On a monthly basis, patient care volume, charges submitted, and RVUs should be reviewed for each provider and compared with budgeted amounts and past trends. Thus, individual physician performance by billing code should be tracked, not only for productivity, but also to ensure that codes are being used appropriately and consistent with a typical specialty profile. It would be unusual for all patients to qualify for critical care codes; some percentage of patients may only qualify for E&M billing, with or without additional procedures. Of note, for ICUs with advanced practitioners, the billing must account for the use of the CCM codes within a 24-hour period for all members of the CCM team that may include both attending physicians and the advanced practitioners.

Most US institutions perform periodic internal audits that help to confirm physician compliance with Medicare and insurer billing rules; it is easier and less costly to identify and rectify any issues internally. The alternative may be an external audit, where any errors detected in a small sample of charts will be applied proportionately over a multiyear period to demand a large retrospective repayment for billing errors. A provision in the American Recovery and Reinvestment Act of 2009 mandates annual fraud and abuse training for health care providers.

The Centers for Medicare and Medicaid Services (CMS) implemented a Recovery Audit Contractor program to review billing and identify over- and underpayment [65]. Regional auditing firms are paid on a contingency basis to review medical record documentation, especially the diagnostic specificity of admitting and discharge diagnoses, listings of comorbidities, and evidence of medical necessity as patients' transition from care environments (e.g., operating room, recovery room, emergency department, inpatient vs. observation status). The coding of diagnosis-related groups (DRGs) comes under particular scrutiny, as does location of service (ICU, ward admission, or observation). DRGs likely to trigger review include many common ICU conditions including sepsis (vs. infection alone), acute respiratory failure (vs. acute systolic or diastolic heart failure), pneumonia, chest pain, and stroke (vs. transient ischemic attack). "Pay for performance" initiatives are increasingly tracking adherence to diagnosis-specific bundles of care; failure to document that elements of care have been completed can reduce hospital reimbursement.

MONITORING CLINICAL CARE

Good structure (attributes of the setting in which care occurs) facilitates good process (what is actually done), which hopefully promotes good outcomes (or results) [66]. Although the Joint Commission historically focused on structural elements such as medical staff organization, available equipment, and human resources, their emphasis has now shifted to analyses of process and outcome [67]. Most benchmarking currently takes place by outcome assessment, commonly using mortality and resource utilization as end points. Because patients present with different levels of disease and physiologic reserve, raw outcome measures such as mortality must be adjusted for severity of illness [68]. For the ICU, tools include the Acute Physiology and Chronic Health Evaluation (APACHE) system [69–71], the Mortality Probability Models (MPM) [72,73]; the Simplified Acute Physiology Score (SAPS) [74,75], and the Intensive Care National Audit and Research Centre (ICNARC) model [76]. These systems are based on large databases, report acceptable discrimination, and calibration and have been extensively examined in the peer-reviewed literature. However, only a minority of hospitals consistently collect this type of data. Although APACHE and MPM are generally used in North America, SAPS in Europe and South America, and ICNARC in Great Britain, models can be employed in any location as long as the model is recalibrated for the local environment [77].

ICU severity models facilitate comparisons between ICUs and are most useful for retrospective analysis of performance, with limited but improving utility for real-time management. Careful definition of data elements and outcomes to be collected enables comparison of local outcomes with national data.

An APACHE IV score is comprised of the Acute Physiology Score ("APS" see below), age, and chronic health items. The APS is generated by summing point values based on physiologic derangement in 17 variables and then adding points for age and chronic health status [78]. The APS is interpreted in light of the main patient diagnosis, patient location, and duration of hospital stay prior to admission to the ICU. Mechanical ventilation during the first ICU day and emergency surgical status also influence an individual's predicted mortality. Although the error bars around the mortality estimate are large for any individual patient, the APACHE system has been shown to be quite reliable at assessing mortality outcome for sufficiently large groups of patients. APACHE IV is also useful for assessing ICU LOS (resource consumption) in groups of patients even though utility is limited for individuals [79].

The MPM-III model was developed and validated using Project IMPACT data (an initiative of the SCCM) from 55,459 patients at 103 participating ICUs in North America [78]. With the acquisition of Project IMPACT by Cerner, the APACHE system and Project IMPACT have been consolidated into a single critical care information system that takes advantage of the ease and immediacy of the MPM score (generated on admission) with the more detailed, disease-specific predictions of the APACHE system at 24 hours and beyond. Plans call to extend the APACHE system beyond the ICU to a new product called APACHE Outcomes Across Venues [80].

Specialized scoring systems are more appropriate for pediatric [81], trauma [82,83], or cardiac surgical units [84]. Pediatric scoring (e.g., Pediatric Risk of Mortality) differs from adult scoring because of expected differences in normal physiologic ranges. Cardiac surgical systems downplay acute physiology, which is deliberately controlled by the operating room team, and emphasize variables such as left ventricular function, intra-aortic balloon pump use, and cardiopulmonary bypass time that might not be available or clinically relevant in other patient groups. Performance of the general severity models deteriorates when case-mix in an ICU becomes skewed [85]. APACHE-IV accommodates case-mix differences by including disease-specific coefficients. MPM-III provides subgroup models for use when an individual ICU's case-mix is skewed from average [86], although the general model is essentially as good as specialized models for identifying performance outliers.

The primary clinical limitation of all outcome adjustment models is that they apply to the analysis of outcome in groups of patients, but not when making individual therapeutic decisions. At best, the prognostic estimates for an individual patient may be used in a probabilistic manner to predict bed or other resource utilization but could be inaccurate if applied as a prediction for application or denial of individual medical therapy, because of the uncertainty of individual estimates. A patient's risk will change over time, making it problematic, for example, to use the admission severity score to determine eligibility for later therapy. In fact, ICU physicians discriminate between survivors and nonsurvivors more accurately than scoring systems, at least in the initial 24 hours of care [87].

ICU performance can be ascertained by generating predicted mortality rates for groups of patients using APACHE, ICNARC, MPM ,or SAPS as a tool and then comparing observed actual results (numerator) to that prediction (denominator). The ratio of observed mortality to predicted mortality is called the standardized mortality ratio (SMR). An ICU with an SMR close to 1.0 would be exhibiting expected performance for its case-mix of patients. SMRs significantly greater than 1 indicate a higher than expected mortality, whereas SMRs less than 1 suggest outcomes better than expected. The sample size and distribution of patient acuities will determine exactly how far from 1.0 (in either direction) the SMR becomes significant.

Events and therapy prior to ICU admission that alters physiology at admission create a "lead time" bias that has a measurable effect on outcome [88]. Because the SMR will be affected by differing use of postacute facilities and the percentage of patients with DNR orders, it may not always be valid in interhospital comparisons, unless applied to similar types of hospitals with similar policies [89].

Both clinical performance and cost-effectiveness should be considered when defining high-quality ICU care [90]. Rapoport and Teres initially described a method, since updated [91] that graphically displays both severity-adjusted clinical outcome and cost-effectiveness, using weighted hospital days as a proxy for cost. With this method, normalized severity-adjusted mortality is displayed on the x-axis and normalized weighted hospital days on the y-axis (Figure 132.2). Standard deviations of the normalized scale are displayed relative to the group mean at the origin (0,0). Units performing significantly better than predicted for both dimensions of care will chart in the right upper quadrant of the graph.

Individual hospitals may participate with proprietary organizations that assess quality at groups of member hospitals. In this setting, each hospital submits all of its clinical and cost data to the large hospital consortium which in turn crosswalks these data into a large universal hospital data set. Thus, the ICU data (i.e., admission rate, infection rate, occupancy rate, and mortality rate) of the individual participant hospital can be compared with other ICUs of similar hospitals and ICUs for benchmarking purposes [92].

CRITICAL CARE OUTREACH SERVICE AND EARLY WARNING SYSTEMS (EWS)

Illness is commonly heralded by a constellation of quantifiable changes in physiologic and biochemical measurements. Abnormal values of selected physiologic measurements are useful as an objective indication of a patient's risk level (as with severity scores) but may also be used "real time" to predict subsequent clinical deterioration on hospital wards. In theory, if hospital staff were to identify and provide interventions to these patients at an earlier stage, outcomes could improve, in terms of reduced intensive care admissions and LOS. Given that a number of studies have observed clinical signs of physiologic deterioration hours prior

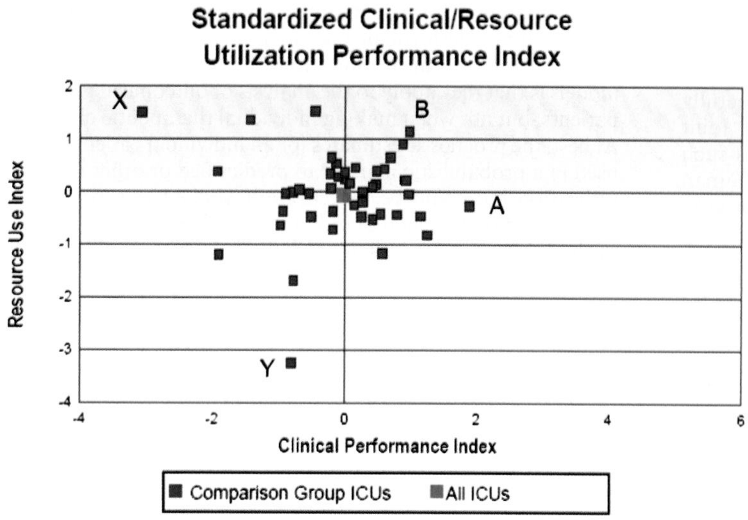

FIGURE 132.2 Standardized clinical/resource utilization performance index (Rapoport-Teres plot). Hospital A has superior risk-adjusted mortality, while hospital B has a superior risk-adjusted length of stay. Hospital X has a short length of stay, but risk-adjusted mortality worse than predicted. Hospital Y has length-of-stay issues, while remaining within the expected severity-adjusted mortality range (risk-adjusted index of −1 to +1).

to a cardiorespiratory arrest, many hospitals have introduced a rapid response team (RRT) program and/or an EWS to facilitate the diagnosis and early treatment of patients with nascent clinical deterioration. The organization of RRTs varies among institutions with most hospitals offering some combination of a critical care nurse, respiratory therapist hospitalist, PA, resident, or fellow and smaller hospitals only having a single nurse.

Real-time surveillance of EMR data using EWS can be utilized to automatically activate an RRT team, but depending on sensitivity and specificity could potentially result in overutilization of the RRT without adequate benefits. At our organization, the EMR automatically flags patients with physiologic deterioration. Patient deterioration results in a notification on the nurse's task list along with an e-mail message to the attending physician but does not automatically trigger the RRT response. Although the RRT *could* be summoned electronically, many systems have opted for nurse or physician notification to avoid overuse of the RRT.

Analysis postimplementation of an RRT model of care (also called medical emergency team) on hospital wards demonstrates 17% to 50% fewer cardiorespiratory arrests [93]. Few studies to date have shown any significant decline in the rate of unintended ICU admissions or overall hospital mortality with the introduction of an RRT model of care delivery. A 2010 meta-analysis by Chan et al. involving over 1.3 million patient admissions concluded that evidence supporting the effectiveness for RRT programs to reduce hospital mortality was lacking although there was a reduction in rates of cardiopulmonary arrest outside the ICU [94]. Clinical trial results have suffered from methodological limitations, varying staffing models, and limited number of randomized control trials. It is possible that the RRT involvement may boost end-of-life discussions and delivery of comfort care for patients on the wards that might otherwise not have taken place, thus avoiding cardiopulmonary resuscitation and consequently not changing hospital mortality rates. Because EWS and RRT deployment will affect ICU resource utilization, ICU leaders need to be involved in planning, implementing, and maintaining these systems [95].

OPERATIONAL ISSUES

Nursing staffing levels are now subject to public scrutiny [96]. Excessive nursing workload has been shown to correlate with increased mortality [97], longer hospital LOS, increased complications [65,66], and the spread of resistant bacterial organisms in the ICU [98]. Adverse events have been reported to occur in about 20% of critically ill patients, with roughly half reportedly being preventable [99]. The most common cause of an adverse event is failure to carry out intended treatment correctly, often because of miscommunication or poor coordination of care [100]. Some hospitals have explored crew resource management training, adapted from the aviation industry, to improve team collaboration and coordination and ultimately improve patient safety. The medical director, in conjunction with the nurse manager and other professionals, will play a major role for defining and maintaining the organizational culture of the ICU. Disruptive physician behavior adversely affects nursing retention [101] and occasionally will require the intervention of the medical director, perhaps with the assistance of the hospital's Physician Health or Medical Staff Health committee. Effective teamwork is essential, and team leadership is vital for promoting team interaction and coordination. Interdisciplinary communication is fostered by a number of formal and informal efforts. At a basic level, the format for daily interprofessional ICU rounds should encourage all members of the team to contribute information, ask questions, and make suggestions for the direction of care. Formal multidisciplinary rounds for long-stay patients, often held weekly, are useful when discussing the trajectory of care with the opportunity to collect additional insight from allied health professionals, social service, and clergy. Conferences, journal club, lectures, and research projects offer opportunities for beneficial interdisciplinary interaction.

QUALITY IMPROVEMENT INITIATIVES

ICU quality checklists are tools increasingly applied to ensure that basic issues (e.g., safety protocols, nutrition, and catheter removal) are not inadvertently forgotten during the inevitable "crisis mode" in a typical ICU day. Pronovost et al. showed that a combination of a checklist and a listing of daily goals reduced central line–associated blood stream infection rates [102].

As discussed earlier, ICU directors should be tracking severity-adjusted mortality, complications, and resource utilization (LOS). Increasingly, a balanced scorecard approach will also track patient satisfaction, typically via postdischarge surveys of patients through the Hospital Consumer Assessment of Healthcare Providers and Systems (HCAHPS) program [103] administered by the CMS. Although ICUs are not specifically tracked by HCAHPS, the ICU stay is part of the patient's hospital experience and can contribute to patient impressions. Items such as nurse responsiveness, physician explanations, and the ICU environment are considered in the questionnaire. Patient families deserve special consideration, especially because the family is likely to notice and appreciate the operational efficiencies and communication style that reflects the ICU's culture. A multicenter evaluation of a scoring system for family satisfaction [104] identifies the key components for family satisfaction as assurance (the need to feel hope for a desired outcome), proximity (the need for personal contact and to be physically and emotionally near the patient), information (which should be consistent, realistic, and timely), personal comfort, and support (resources, support systems, and ventilation). Written materials (e.g., booklets and information sheets) can help meet family informational needs, especially with older, better educated patients and their relatives [105].

SUMMARY

Economic considerations continue to drive the agenda for hospitals and ICUs, and with the wave of "baby boomers" reaching retirement; increasing incidence of obesity, diabetes, and vascular disease in the population; and sporadic emergence of new threats, such as newer viral pathogens (e.g., Ebola, Zika, pandemic strains of the Influenza A virus), we can expect further changes. With a sicker, more chronic disease burdened population, hospitals have become places for the hyper-acutely ill, with much of recovery and recuperation outsourced to other facilities. Thus, intensive care will continue to consume an ever-greater proportion of total hospital costs, even as this growth becomes constrained by economics, bed shortages, and most importantly, insufficient numbers of nurses and physicians specializing in critical care. For many hospitals, what was once the province of the ICU has migrated to step-down and specialty units, leaving the ICU populated by the "sickest of the sick." The advent of hospitalists and RRTs are but two manifestations of this continuing evolution in how care is delivered—the "ICU without walls." These changes have forced a reevaluation of ICU organizational practices (increasing the value of "closed" units), human resource needs, a more management-oriented role for the ICU director, and critical care management approaches that involve shared decision-making by professionals from more than one ICU [106]. Benchmarking critical care outcome becomes essential for managing the increasingly complex world of the ICU, and we are on the threshold of having computerized real-time systems to automate some of the tactical decisions that occupy better applied professional time. Telemedicine, increased automation, use of physician extenders, and protocol supported care are all potential solutions to the impending crisis in critical care delivery. Continued change emphasizes the need for clinically and managerially competent physicians to organize and manage the increasingly complex world of critical care [107].

References

1. Pastores SM, Halpern NA, Oropello JM, et al: Critical care organizations in academic medical center in North America: a descriptive report. *Crit Care Med* 43:2239–2244, 2015.
2. Bekes CE, Dellinger RP, Brooks D, et al: Critical care medicine as a distinct product line with substantial financial profitability: the role of business planning. *Crit Care Med* 32:1207–1214, 2004.
3. St Andre A: The formation, elements of success, and challenges in managing a critical care program: Part I. *Crit Care Med* 43:874–879, 2015.
4. Goleman D: What makes a leader? *Harv Bus Rev* 76:93–102, 1998.
5. American Association for Physician Leadership: http://www.physicianleaders.org/. Accessed October 30, 2015.
6. Costa DK, Wallace DJ, Kahn JM: The association between daytime intensivist physician staffing and mortality in the context of other ICU organizational practices: a multicenter cohort study. *Crit Care Med* 43:2275–2282, 2015.
7. Sakr Y, Moreira CL, Rhodes A, et al: The impact of hospital and ICU organizational factors on outcome in critically ill patients: results from the extended prevalence of infection in intensive care study. *Crit Care Med*, 2015. doi: 10.1097/CCM.0000000000000754.
8. Leapfrog Group: http://www.leapfroggroup.org. Accessed October 30, 2015.
9. Gajic O, Afessa B, Hanson AC, et al: Effect of 24-hour mandatory versus on-demand critical care specialist presence on quality of care and family and provider satisfaction in the intensive care unit of a teaching hospital. *Crit Care Med* 36:36–44, 2008.
10. Pronovost PJ, Angus DC, Dorman TD, et al: Physician staffing patterns and clinical outcomes in critically ill patients: a systematic review. *JAMA* 288:2151–2162, 2002.
11. Levy MM, Rapoport J, Lemeshow S, et al: Association between critical care physician management and patient mortality in the intensive care unit. *Ann Intern Med* 148:801–809, 2008.
12. Higgins TL, Nathanson B, Teres D: What conclusions should be drawn between critical care physician management and patient mortality in the ICU? *Ann Intern Med* 149:767, 2008.
13. Marik P, Myburgh J, Annane D, et al: What conclusions should be drawn between critical care physician management and patient mortality in the ICU? *Ann Intern Med* 149:770–771, 2008.
14. Metnitz PG, Reiter A, Jordan B, et al: More interventions do not necessarily improve outcome in critically ill patients. *Intensive Care Med* 30:1586–1593, 2004.
15. Topeli A, Laghi F, Tobin MJ: Effect of closed unit policy and appointing an intensivist in a developing country. *Crit Care Med* 33:299–306, 2005.
16. Carson SS, Stocking C, Podsadecki T, et al: Effect of organizational change in the medical intensive care unit of a teaching hospital: a comparison of "open" and "closed" formats. *JAMA* 276:322–328, 1996.
17. Higgins TL, McGee WT, Steingrub JS, et al: Early indicators of prolonged intensive care unit stay: impact of illness severity, physician staffing, and pre-intensive care unit length of stay. *Crit Care Med* 31:45–51, 2003.
18. Wallace DJ, Andus DC, Barnato AE, et al: Nighttime intensivist staffing and mortality among critically ill patients. *N Engl J Med* 366(22):2093–101, 2012.
19. Wise KR, Akopov VA, Williams BR Jr, et al: Hospitalists and intensivists in the medical ICU: a prospective observational study comparing mortality and length of stay between two staffing models. *J Hosp Med* 7(3):183–189, 2012.
20. Kerlin MP, Small DS, Cooney E, et al: A randomized trial of nighttime physician staffing in an intensive care unit. *N Engl J Med* 368(23):2201–2209, 2013.
21. Barnett MJ, Kaboli PJ, Sirio CA, et al: Day of the week of intensive care admission and patient outcomes: a multisite regional evaluation. *Med Care* 40:530–539, 2002.
22. Uusaro A, Kari A, Ruokonen E: The effects of ICU admission and discharge times on mortality in Finland. *Intensive Care Med* 29:2144–2148, 2003.
23. Wunsch H, Mapstone J, Brady T, et al: Hospital mortality associated with day and time of admission to intensive care units. *Intensive Care Med* 30:895–901, 2004.
24. Morales IJ, Peters SG, Afessa B: Hospital mortality rate and length of stay in patients admitted at night to the intensive care unit. *Crit Care Med* 31:858–863, 2003.
25. Ensminger SA, Morales IJ, Peters SG, et al: The hospital mortality of patients admitted to the ICU on weekends. *Chest* 126:1292–1298, 2004.
26. Bell CM, Redelmeier DA: Mortality among patients admitted to hospitals on weekends as compared with weekdays. *N Eng J Med* 345:663–668, 2001.
27. Siegal EM, Dressler DD, Dichter JR, et al: Training a hospitalist workforce to address the intensivist shortage in American hospitals: a position paper from the Society of Hospital Medicine and the Society of Critical Care Medicine. *Crit Care Med* 40:1952–1956, 2012.
28. Kahn JM, Cicero BD, Wallance DJ, et al: Adoption of ICU telemedicine in the United States. *Crit Care Med* 42(2):362–368, 2014.
29. Breslow MJU, Rosenfeld BA, Doerfler M, et al: Effect of a multiple site intensive care unit telemedicine program on clinical and economic outcomes: an alternative paradigm for intensivist staffing. *Crit Care Med* 32:31–38, 2004.
30. Kahn JM, Hill NS, Lilly CM, et al: The research agenda in ICU telemedicine: a statement from the critical care societies collaborative. *Chest* 140:230–238, 2011.
31. Factsheet: ICU Physician Staffing (IPS). The Leapfrog Group. Available at http://www.leapfroggroup.org/media/file/ICUPhysicianStaffing.pdf. Accessed October 30, 2015.
32. Nguyen YL, Kahn JM, Angus DC: Reorganizing adult critical care delivery. The role of regionalization, telemedicine and community outreach. *Am J Respir Crit Care Med* 181:1164–1169, 2010.
33. Fortis S, Weintert C, Bushinski R, et al: A health system-based critical care program with a novel tele-ICU: implementation, cost and structure details. *J Am Coll Surg* 219:676–683, 2014.
34. Yoo B, Kim K, Sasaki T, et al: Economic evaluation of telemedicine for patients in the ICU. *Crit Care Med* 44:265–274, 2016.
35. Halpern NA, Pastores SM, Oropello JM, et al: Critical care medicine in the United States: addressing the intensivist shortage and image of the specialty. *Crit Care Med* 41:2754–2761, 2013.
36. Angus DC, Kelley MA, Schmitz RJ, et al: Current and projected workforce requirements for car of the critically ill and patients with pulmonary disease: can we meet the requirements of an aging population. *JAMA* 284:2762–2770, 2000.
37. Society of Critical Care Medicine: *Compensation of Critical Care Professionals*. Des Plains, IL, 2005, p 9.
38. Manthous, CA: Leapfrog and critical care: evidence and reality based intensive care for the 21st century. *Am J Med* 115:188–193, 2004.
39. Audit Commission: *Critical to Success: The Place of Efficient and Effective Critical Care Services Within the Acute Hospital*. London, England: Audit Commission, 1999.
40. Dara SI, Afesso B: Intensivist-to-bed ratio. Association with outcomes in the medical ICU. *Chest* 128:567–572, 2005.
41. Ward NS, Afessa B, Kleinpell R, et al; Members of Society of Critical Care Medicine Taskforce on ICU Staffing. Intensivist/Patient ratios in closed ICUs: a statement from the Society of Critical Care Medicine Taskforce on ICU staffing. *Crit Care Med* 41(2):638–645, 2013. doi: 10.1097/CCM.0b013e3182741478.
42. Gershengorn HB, Johnson MP, Factor P: The use of nonphysician providers in adult intensive care units. *Am J Respir Crit Care Med* 185(6):600–605, 2012. doi: 10.1164/rccm.201107-1261CP.
43. Gershengorn HB, Wunsch H, Wahab R, et al: Impact of non-physician staffing on outcomes in a medical ICU. *Chest* 139(6):1347–1353, 2011.

44. Landsperger JS, Semler MW, Wang L, et al: Outcomes of nurse practitioner-delivered critical care: a prospective cohort study. *Chest* 149(5):1146–1154, 2016. doi: 10.1016/j.chest.2015.12.0.
45. Gershengorn HB, Johnson MP, Factor P: The use of nonphysician providers in adult intensive care units. *Am J Respir Crit Care Med* 185(6):600–605, 2012.
46. Hoffman LA, Tasota FJ, Scharfenverg C, et al: Management of patients in the intensive care unit: comparison via work sampling analysis of an acute care nurse practitioner and physicians in training. *Am J Crit Care* 12(5):436–443, 2003.
47. Rudy EB, Davidson LJ, Daly B, et al: Care activities and outcomes of patients cared for by acute nurse practitioners, physician assistants, and resident physicians: a comparison. *Am J Crit Care* 7:267–281, 1998.
48. Hoffman LA, Tasota FJ, Zullo TG, et al: Outcomes of care managed by an acute care nurse practitioner/attending physician team in a subacute medical intensive care unit. *Am J Crit Care* 14:121–132, 2005.
49. Russell D, VorderBruegge M, Burns SM: Effect of an outcomes-managed approach to care of neuroscience patients by acute care nurse practitioners. *Am J Crit Care* 11:353–362, 2002.
50. Burns SM, Earven S: Improving outcomes for mechanically ventilated medical intensive care unit patients using advanced practice nurses: a 6-year experience. *Crit Care Med Clin North Am* 14:231–243, 2002.
51. Higgins TL, Hodnicki D, Artenstein A: Sharing care in an ACO Environment. *Am J Accountable Care* 9(14):27–30, 2014.
52. Hoffman LA, Happ MB, Scharfenberg C, et al: Perceptions of physicians, nurses and respiratory therapists about the role of acute care nurse practitioners. *Am J Crit Care* 13:480–488, 2004.
53. Dubayo B, Samson M, Carlson R: The role of physician assistants in critical care units. *Chest* 99:89–91, 1991.
54. Mallick R, Strosberg M, Lambrinos J, et al: The intensive care unit medical director as manager: impact on performance. *Med Care* 33:611–624, 1995.
55. Levin PD, Worner TM, Sviri S, et al: Intensive care outflow limitation—frequency, etiology and impact. *J Crit Care* 18:206–211, 2003.
56. Higgins TL, Teres D: External forces shaping critical care, in Irwin RS, Rippe JM (eds): *Intensive Care Medicine* .5th ed. Lippincott Williams and Wilkins, Philadelphia, PA, 2003, pp 2224–2231.
57. Leape LL, Fromson JA: Problem doctors: is there a system-level solution? *Ann Intern Med* 144:107–115, 2006.
58. Pronovost P, Berenholt S, Dorman T, et al: Improving communication in the ICU using daily goals. *J Crit Care* 18:71–75, 2003.
59. Klein G: Power to see the invisible, in *Sources of Power. How People Make Decisions*. The MIT Press, Cambridge, Massachusetts, 1999, pp 147–175.
60. McLain T: Tackling four common myths about critical care service codes. *Today's Hospitalist* 4-5, 2004.
61. Dorman T, Loeb L, Sample G: Evaluation and management codes: from current procedural terminology through relative update commission to Center for Medicare and Medicaid Services. *Crit Care Med* 34:S71–S77, 2006.
62. MACRA Act: Congress.gov. Available at https://www.congress.gov/bill/114th-congress/house-bill/2. Accessed October 31, 2015.
63. AMA CPT Code: Available at http://www.ama-assn.org/ama/pub/physician-resources/solutions-managing-your-practice/coding-billing-insurance/cpt.page. Accessed October 31, 2015.
64. Coding and Billing website; Society of Critical Care Medicine. Available at http://www.sccm.org/Education-Center/Administration/Pages/Coding-and-Billing.aspx Accessed October 31, 2015.
65. Centers for Medicare and Medicaid Services, RAC website. https://www.cms.gov/Research-Statistics-Data-and-Systems/Monitoring-Programs/Medicare-FFS-Compliance-Programs/Recovery-Audit-Program/Recent_Updates.html. Accessed October 31, 2015.
66. Donabedian A: The quality of care. How can it be assessed? *JAMA* 260:1743–1748, 1988.
67. Joint Commission National Hospital Quality Measures—ICU. Available at http://www.jointcommission.org/national_hospital_quality_measures_-_icu/ Accessed October 31, 2015.
68. Nathanson BH, Higgins TL: An introduction to statistical methods used in binary outcome modeling. *Semin Cardiothorac Vasc Anesth* 12:153–166, 2008.
69. Knaus WA, Draper EA, Wagner DP, et al: APACHE II: a severity of disease classification system. *Crit Care Med* 13:818–829, 1985.
70. Knaus WA, Wagner DP, Draper EA, et al: The APACHE III prognostic system. Risk prediction of hospital mortality for critically ill hospitalized adults. *Chest* 100:1619–1636, 2005.
71. Zimmerman JE, Kramer AA, McNair DS, et al: Acute physiology and chronic health evaluation (APACHE) IV: hospital mortality assessment for today's critically ill patients. *Crit Care Med* 34:2674–2676, 2006.
72. Lemeshow S, Teres D, Klar J, et al: Mortality probability models (MPM II) based on an international cohort of intensive care unit patients. *JAMA* 270:2478–2486, 1993.
73. Higgins TL, Teres D, Copes W, et al: Assessing contemporary intensive care unit outcome: an updated Mortality Probability Model—MPM_0-III. *Crit Care Med* 35:827–835, 2007.
74. Le Gall J-R, Lemeshow S, Saulnier F: A new simplified acute physiology score (SAPS II) based on a European/North American multicenter study. *JAMA* 270:2957–2963, 1993.
75. Moreno RP, Metnitz PGH, Almeida E, et al: SAPS 3—from evaluation of the patient to evaluation of the intensive care unit. Part 2: Development of a prognostic model for hospital mortality at ICU admission. *Intensive Care Med* 31:1345–1355, 2005.
76. Harrison DA, Parry GJ, Carpenter JR, et al: A new risk prediction model for critical care: The Intensive Care National Audit & Research Centre (ICNARC) model. *Crit Care Med* 35:1091–1098, 2007.
77. Harrison DA, Brady AR, Parry GJ, et al: Recalibration of risk prediction models in a large multicenter cohort of admissions to adult, general critical care units in the United Kingdom. *Crit Care Med* 34:1378–1388, 2006.
78. Zimmerman JE, Kramer AA, McNair DS, et al: Intensive care unit length of stay: benchmarking based on acute physiology and chronic health evaluation (APACHE) IV. *Crit Care Med* 34:2517–2529, 2006.
79. Higgins TL, Kramer AA, Nathanson BH, et al: Prospective validation of the intensive care unit admission Mortality Probability Model (MPM_0-III). *Crit Care Med* 37:1619–1623, 2009.
80. APACHE Outcomes website. Available at http://www.cernerworks.com/Solutions/Hospitals_and_Health_Systems/Critical_Care/APACHE_Outcomes/. Accessed October 31, 2015.
81. Pollack MM, Ruttimann UE, Getson PR: Pediatric risk of mortality (PRISM) score. *Crit Care Med* 16:1110–1116, 1988.
82. Baker SP, O'Neil B, Haddon W, et al: The injury severity score: a method for describing patients with multiple injuries and evaluating emergency care. *J Trauma* 14:187–196, 1974.
83. Champion HR, Sacco WJ, Copes WS, et al: A revision of the trauma score. *J Trauma* 33:417–423, 1992.
84. Higgins TL, Estafanous FG, Loop FD, et al: Stratification of morbidity and mortality outcome of preoperative risk factors in coronary artery bypass patients. *JAMA* 267:2344–2348, 1992.
85. Murphy-Filkins RL, Teres D, Lemeshow S, et al: Effect of changing patient mix on the performance of an intensive care unit severity-of-illness model: how to distinguish a general from a specialty intensive care unit. *Crit Care Med* 24:1968–1973, 1996.
86. Nathanson B, Higgins TL, Kramer AA, et al: Subgroup mortality probability models: are they necessary for specialized intensive care units? *Crit Care Med* 37:2375–2386, 2009.
87. Sinuff T, Adhikari NK, Cook DJ, et al: Mortality predictions in the intensive care unit: comparing physicians with scoring systems. *Crit Care Med* 34:878–885, 2006.
88. McQuillan P, Pilkington S, Allan A, et al: Confidential inquiry into quality of care before admission to intensive care. *BMJ* 316:1853–1858, 1998.
89. Teres D, Higgins TL, Steingrub JS, et al: Defining a high-performance ICU system for the 21st century: a position paper. *J Intensive Care Med* 13:195–205, 1998.
90. Rapoport J, Teres D, Lemeshow S, et al: A method for assessing the clinical performance and cost effectiveness of intensive care units: a multi-center inception cohort study. *Crit Care Med* 22:1385, 1994.
91. Nathanson BH, Higgins TL, Teres D, et al: A revised method to assess intensive care unit clinical performance and resource utilization. *Crit Care Med* 35:1853–1862, 2007.
92. Kramer A, Higgins T, Zimmerman J: Comparing observed and predicted mortality among ICUs using different prognostic systems: why do performance assessments differ? *Crit Care Med* 43:261–269, 2015.
93. Buist MD, Moore GE, Bernard SA, et al: Effects of a medical emergency team on reduction of incidence of and mortality from unexpected cardiac arrests in hospital: preliminary study. *BMJ* 324:387–390, 2002.
94. Chan PS, Khalid A, Longmore LS, et al: Hospital-wide code rates and mortality before and after implementation of a rapid response team. *JAMA* 300:2506–2513, 2008.
95. Harrison A, Gajic O, Pickering B, et al: Development and implementation of Sepsis alert systems. *Clin Chest Med* 37:219–229, 2016.
96. Debate renewed on nurse staffing: Agency's proposal on ICUs criticized. Boston Globe, 6/9/15. Available at https://www.bostonglobe.com/business/2015/06/09/state-poised-mandate-nurse-staffing-levels/nDThJn7CmpiUTu6asY0cYP/story.html. Accessed October 31, 2015.
97. Tarnow-Mordi WO, Hau C, Warden A, et al: Hospital mortality in relation to staff workload: a 4-year study in an adult intensive care unit. *Lancet* 356:185–189, 2000.
98. Vicca AF: Nursing staff workload as a determinant of methicillin-resistant Staphylococcus aureus spread in an adult intensive therapy unit. *J Hosp Infect* 43:109–113, 1999.
99. Rothschild JM, Landrigan CP, Cronin JW, et al: The critical care safety study: the incidence and nature of adverse events and serious medical erros in intensive care. *Crit Care Med* 33:1694–1700, 2005.
100. Baggs JG, Schmitt MH, Mushlin AI, et al: Association between nurse-physician collaboration and patient outcomes in three intensive care units. *Crit Care Med* 27:1991–1996, 1999.
101. Rosenstein A: Nurse-physician relationships: impact on nurse satisfaction and retention. *Amer J Nursing* 102:26–34, 2002.
102. Pronovost P, Needham D, Berenholtz S, et al: An intervention to decrease catheter-related bloodstream infections in the ICU. *N Engl J Med* 355(26):2725–2732, 2006.
103. HCAHPS information webpage. http://www.hcahpsonline.org/home.aspx. Accessed January 1, 2016.
104. Wasser T, Matchett S, Ray D, et al: Validation of a total score for the critical care family satisfaction survey. *JCOM* 11:502–507, 2004.
105. Soltner C, Lassalle V, Galienne-Bouygues S, et al: Written information that relatives of adult intensive care unit patients would like to received—a comparison to published recommendations and opinion of staff members. *Crit Care Med* 37:2197–2202, 2009.
106. Ganz F, Endelberg R, Torres N, et al: Development of a model of interprofessional shared clinical decision making in the ICU: a mixed methods study. *Crit Care Med* 44:680–689, 2016.
107. Gershengorn H, Kocher R, Factor P: Management strategies to effect change in intensive care unites: lessons from the world of business. *Ann Am Thorac Soc* 11(3):444–453, 2014.

Chapter 133 ■ Critical Care Information Systems: Structure, Function, and Future

JOSEPH J. FRASSICA • VITALY HERASEVICH • MYRON MICHAEL SHABOT

INTRODUCTION

In over 5 decades since the first implementation of the electronic health record (EHR) in the USA, there has been the rise, definition, and establishment of critical care medicine as a specialty and important force in health care both in research and practice.

Although technology has played an essential role for the creation of the specialty (e.g., ventilators and cardiovascular monitoring), the implementation of the EHR in US hospitals and intensive care units (ICUs) remained a meager 1.5% until the 2009 passage of the American Recovery and Reinvestment Act (ARRA), which included Health Information Technology for Economic and Clinical Health (HITECH) Act [1]. The HITECH Act stimulated the implementation of EHRs at US hospitals, owing to bonuses for achievement of "meaningful use" of information technology (IT), and penalties for failure of achievement. This represents the broadest single transformation ever undertaken of the clinical information infrastructure of US health care.

This chapter reviews a number of key components of IT in the modern ICU. The reader is introduced to some of the most important innovative technologies that have influenced the safe, effective, and efficient delivery of critical care services.

General information about the electronic medical record, departmental information systems, and coding and billing information systems is extensively documented thus we assume that the reader has a working knowledge of these basic components of the modern health care information infrastructure. Herein, we address the ICU-specific IT functionality of greatest interest to the practicing critical care physician. In 2016, within the USA, core functionality for ICU record-keeping is primarily delivered through a core EMR system. The diagram below details a view of systems that sits adjacent to and above this core record keeping function that in many instances delivers ICU-specific functionalities, enhancing the value of the core record-keeping EMR system. In many cases these enhanced functions are delivered through the User Interface (UI) of the EMR and in some circumstances the workflow of the clinician or information content dictates that the knowledge be delivered through UI's that are adjacent or delivered in other formats such as mobile devices, or within the UI's of bedside devices that monitor and deliver therapeutic care. In other parts of the developed and developing world, core record keeping functionality primarily resides within location-specific departmental systems that deliver workflow, decision support, and other functionalities listed in the diagram below either directly or in concert with supporting systems. Outside of the USA, the penetration of core EMR systems is currently limited but growing.

A schematic relationship between IT elements is outlined in Figure 133.1.

In this chapter, we address (a) telemedicine in the ICU, (b) clinical decision support (CDS) systems, and (c) information systems for prediction of outcomes.

The most mature implementation of critical care clinical information systems consists of tools which largely meet the needs of the hands-on caregivers. Historically, massive amounts of data documenting an ICU patient's clinical status and treatment were recorded on large double-sided paper flow sheets, which were plagued with problems of legibility; inaccurate calculations; and use restricted to a single person at a time. By replacing this document with computer screens, each customized to a specific purpose, those problems have been improved dramatically.

Going beyond simple replacement of paper documents provides an opportunity to present information such that patterns are more easily recognized. For example, correlation of measures of physiological stability; clinical status (such as urinary output and body weight); and administration of medications can facilitate clinical analyses by juxtaposing interdependent variables. With these tools, physiological trends occurring over longer periods of time can be easily displayed, whereas in the past, these were laboriously drawn by hand.

Optimal use of clinical information systems should also guide the hands-on caregivers to provide care using evidence-based protocols. For example, simply creating a place to document the position of head of the bed underscores that this is an important issue to be managed in prevention of ventilator-associated pneumonia (VAP). Explanatory information can also be provided on a just-in-time basis to encourage protocol compliance. Computer provider order entry prompts and order sets can also facilitate standardization of care.

Collecting and displaying information electronically, in a coded, computable form makes these data available for continuous analysis, and enables detection of patterns of possible clinical deterioration. Collecting this information electronically also allows scrutiny of vastly larger datasets than can be retained and analyzed by the human brain. These analyses can also occur continuously and simultaneously for every patient providing a safety net early warning system that can notify clinicans of potential deterioration that may otherwise go unnoticed until significantly advanced.

Finally, computable information that describes in detail both the patient's status and treatment can be used to analyze adherence to protocols for optimal care, resource utilization, and outcomes. Monitoring on a near real-time basis provides timely feedback and is an opportunity to intervene to improve ongoing care.

Critical Care—Specific Technologies

The Electronic Flowsheet

On the most basic level, Critical Care Information Systems (CCIS) put an end to juggling awkwardly large multi-page flow sheets. Like CPOE, they eliminate the confusion and potential errors that can result from illegible handwriting and other issues that arise in a highly dynamic environment like the ICU. The truly significant contributions CCIS makes to patient safety are in the areas of care processes and medical decision-making. First among these is the ease of access to data. Access to a paper record can be problematic in the ICU, where multiple clinicians need to assess the patient's clinical condition and response to treatment. Electronic records allow multiple caregivers to view the data at the same time, without waiting to access the one-and-only paper chart. Clinicians not in the ICU can also check on a patient's status without physically having to be in the unit, allowing them

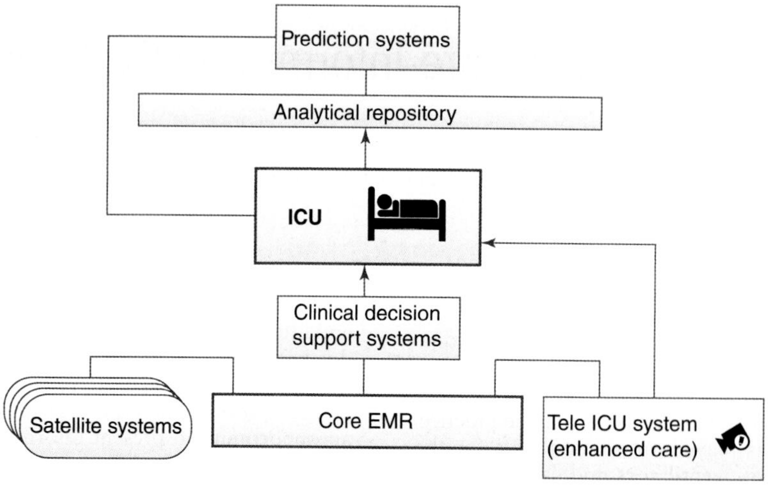

FIGURE 133.1 Typical components of modern IT infrastructre in Critical Care.

to be consulted at the very moment their expertise is needed. When timeliness is critical, access is a critical enabler.

The impact of access on patient safety is enhanced when clinicians have confidence that the data provided are accurate and timely. By automating bedside data acquisition, CCIS ensures that relatively simple measures such as input/output and more complicated and time consuming calculations such as hemodynamic calculations are presented. Once validated by a clinician, automated data becomes a part of the legal patient record. In addition, CCIS can automatically acquire data directly from monitoring equipment and ventilators, eliminating delays and errors of data gathering. Such automated data gathering provides today's decision support systems with access to up to the minute data for surveillance and prediction. Today, the automated acquisition and utilization of real-time data is aided by advances of analytics and machine learning that allow systems to filter out outlier and erroneous data.

Unlike the paper flow sheet, with its fixed format, CCIS offer the potenital for multiple displays of data. Each display may provide a problem-oriented view suitable for problem oriented analyses.

CCIS further supports the clinician by easing trend recognition. Specific displays can establish the correlation of events over time. Other displays provide multiday views, which are critical for measures like fluid balance and fever curves, surpassing the paper flow sheet's view of only 1 day at a time. The displays in CCIS integrate multiple data elements that stood in isolation on the paper flow sheet. By combining vital signs, laboratory results, ventilator settings, medication drips, and medication administration, the CCIS enables clinicians to address the complicated clinical scenarios characteristic of critically ill patients in ICUs. This integrated record also assures attention to details that might be lost in a frenetic setting; for example, by issuing a warning that a medication is overdue or being dosed earlier than appropriate per orders [2].

Real-Time Clinical Decision Support

CDS has been defined as a system that uses two or more items of patient data to generate case-specific advice [3]. In practical terms, CDS includes a wide range of functions, including predefined rules, alerts, reminders, workflow, and collaboration tools—and associated content—for improved medical decision-making [4–6].

Based on functionality CDS could be divided to six broad caregories:

1. Alerting
2. Interpretation
3. Assisting
4. Critiquing
5. Diagnosing
6. Managing

CDS is often intended to facilitate the introduction of and conformance to evolving evidence-based medical protocols and standards of care while enabling appropriate individual physician discretion (such as during order entry). Basic CDS is frequently driven by rules which are built on IF/THEN logic statements. Rule-based CDS systems create recommendations that are often easily converted into human-readable form allowing clinicians to understand the logic underlying the CDS recommendations. Recent advances of machine learning and the availability of large-scale data with high-resolution physiological parameters have enabled the development of more advanced and complex CDS tools. Such complex CDS must also provide a means for clinicians to understand the underlying calculations and/or input parameters that lead to treatment recommendations.

Over the past decade, the primary user experience of CDS has been the alert message. A growing number of studies have revealed the critical limitation of alerts that, by design, interrupt the clinician's workflow, in particular, during order entry [7,8]. The primary reason for this limitation lies in the fact that these CDS systems were designed mainly to alert post hoc—after the clinician has requested a particular item (e.g., drug, dose or test).

CDS has the potential to provide special value in settings like the ICU owing to the density of data routinely presented to the busy critical care physician and the ability of computers to combine, synthesize, and correlate these data and then create more complex rules and information interpretation displays [6]. Studies have demonstrated that critical care rounds may challenge the physician with 20 times more data elements than the human brain can simultaneously process [7]. In the past, we have relied on the team approach to cope with this data overload. However, in the current practice reality of competing priorities for intensivist time and numerous handoffs among providers, there is a growing need for IT solutions to take more of a primary role in caring for the patient and unburdening the ICU clinician. Emerging developments in the areas of visual design and complex rules and algorithms aimed at addressing these needs for more automation to handle the massive amount of ICU data as described later in this chapter.

Early Warning Systems

In the ICU and throughout the hospital, specialized tools can address "failure to rescue," which has been identified by the

Agency for Healthcare Research and Quality (AHRQ) as accounting for the majority of patient-safety Medicare deaths. These tools provide proactive clinical surveillance, interpret patient data (which are collected by the CCIS), and act as early warning systems (EWS). EWS helps caregivers recognize critical data among the numerous data elements on every patient and may even provide early warnings for the Systemic Inflammatory Response Syndrome (SIRS), severe sepsis and other adverse conditions.

In failure to rescue, the patient experiences clinical decompensation over a period of hours, without intervention by caregivers. This error of omission occurs for any of several reasons. The changes of the patient's condition may be subtle; for example, a physiological value may be decreased, but not alarmingly so unless viewed as part of a trend. In other cases, changes may not be appreciated for what they signify. Clinicians may lack the necessary expertise to discern such changes or may be overwhelmed with other tasks. Indeed, according to the AHRQ, there is strong evidence that level of staffing and the nursing skill-mix are both factors in this type of delay.

Delays for detecting changes are of grave concern for a simple reason: the earlier the intervention, the greater the likelihood for a better clinical outcome. Intervening at the first signs of decompensation may make it possible to avert cardiorespiratory and renal failure or address a more treatable complications. Studies of clinical instability suggest that patients experience symptoms before critical events like cardiac arrest. In one study, 70% showed evidence of respiratory deterioration within 8 hours of arrest; in another, 66% of patients showed abnormal signs and symptoms within 6 hours [9].

Proactive clinical surveillance systems highlight trends and out-of-bounds values and conditions for further scrutiny. They provide displays—"dashboards"—that integrate different data elements to optimize evaluation of clinical problems. An additional feature offers severity scoring for the purpose of early detection of decompensation, issuing modified early warning scores to alert clinicians, especially on hospital wards, of developing but unrecognized problems.

Although early knowledge of patient deterioration is an important step for improving safety, a complete approach requires a mechanism to respond to patient deterioration as well. One approach is to create rapid response teams (RRT) or medical emergency teams [10,11]. The RRT consists of clinicians and nurses with critical care expertise that can be called anywhere in the hospital when a patient experiences acute physiological conditions.

Concurrent Process Monitoring

Concurrent process monitoring is also provided by CCIS and electronically monitors the details that define how adherence rates to a clinical care process. When data are captured and stored as discrete data elements, they are available for analysis. When analyses are concurrent (e.g., performed as care is delivered), this data allows managers and caregivers to have visibility into global processes of care. In the ICU, concurrent process monitoring allows evaluation of whether a particular practice is actually being implemented and whether it is affecting outcomes, such as elevation of the head of the bed to reduce the likelihood of VAP, or documenting the central line insertion bundle to decrease the likelihood of a Central Line Associated Blood Stream Infection (CLABSI).

Historically, organizations are good at creating policies and procedures, but much less effective in deploying them. Although it is easy to sit in a conference room and discuss policies and procedures it is much more difficult to get people to follow them. If data are extracted and tabulated manually, it is laborious to determine whether a particular practice is being implemented. Additionally, the reporting is retrospective long after the events being studied have occurred. In such cases, caregivers may believe "It used to be that bad, but now we're better." In contrast, concurrent process analyses allow the implementation of evidence-based practices by identifying and reinforcing practice patterns as they occur. Moreover, concurrent monitoring takes advantage of data already being gathered in the course of care, eliminating the need for duplicate data entry or chart abstraction.

AUTOMATED ICU PERFORMANCE MEASUREMENT AND MANAGEMENT

Since the Institute of Medicine published its 1999 "exposé" on patient safety [12], the ICU has received increased national attention as an important target for medical error reduction and improved quality. Both the Leapfrog Group collaborative of large employers and the Centers for Medicare and Medicaid Services have focused on developing national performance measurement metrics for ICU and Acute Care [13,14]. Information Technology can be used to more easily gather patient, process, and outcomes data that support reporting solutions that facilitate improvement. Performance measures are typically categorized as structural (how care is organized), process (what is done), or outcomes (including medical/functional, such as death or the ability to perform specific functions of daily life); experiential, which covers both patients/families and providers; and financial, which includes both cost/resource use and profitability perspectives.

Structure and process measures are used on the presumption that their variance causes a specific significant variance in one or more outcomes. Popular examples of structural ICU measurable processes include intensivist coverage [14] and nurse staffing levels. Head-of-bed elevation for mechanically ventilated patients to prevent nosocomial pneumonia and associated increased mortality are examples of contemporary measurable processes.

One of the most significant challenges in quality improvement efforts is the lack of trust or alignment that can exist among clinicians, hospital administrators, insurance companies, and government over the motivation behind measurement. Clinicians believe that the purpose of measurement should be to understand and improve—although they too often, and too often rightly, assume payers' and overseers' plan to use metrics only to judge and to penalize—not to reward superior performance or improve patient care but only to drive down costs.

Given this environment, without standardized measures of meaningful medical outcomes that are defined, understood, and accepted by the relevant clinical community, making significant progress is difficult. Business intelligence systems, including performance dashboard techniques, that combine clinical data from computer-based patient records with financial data for analysis and reporting solutions are predicted to be an area of increased interest. As this evolution occurs, critical care leaders will want to assure that their unique information needs are met in these systems and that appropriate attention is given to elements like risk adjustment and critical care-specific process analysis. Niche ICU analytical systems such as the Virtual Pediatric Intensive Care Unit (PICU) Performance System/National Association of Children's Hospitals and Related Institutions, the Vermont-Oxford Network for neonatal intensive care, and Cerner Corporation's Acute Physiology, Age, Chronic Health Evaluation (APACHE) prognostic, concurrent, and retrospective decision support system focused on adult ICU patients are also available [15].

RISK ADJUSTMENT MODELS FOR COMPARING ICU OUTCOMES

Risk adjustment, severity adjustment, or case-mix adjustment are terms used to describe mathematical models derived from large datasets of a particular population whose purpose is to represent the relative risks individual patients bring at the entry point to care process. Patient risk factors impact which care processes and resources are required to produce similar outcomes and what the best realistically achievable outcomes are. Modeling research needs to define three elements: (a) the binary or continuous outcome variable(s) to be modeled (e.g., lived/died, length of stay), (b) the beginning and end points in time (e.g., at admission to the ICU, at discharge from the hospital, at a specific time point like 100 days), and (c) the specific risk factors to be included (e.g., age/gestational age, weight/birth weight, diagnosis, physiology). Because many hospital patient records are still paper-based, the most viable data source developing risk adjustment has been those using administrative (claims) data, examples being APR-DRGs (all patient refined diagnosis-related groups) and disease staging. Model developers juggle the collection cost versus the desirability of capturing specific data, but unequivocally more detailed patient data than that included in claims databases are required to adequately represent patient-risk variance in the ICU population. Model developers also struggle with defining reasonable end points for capturing outcomes. They also need to consider and factor in relationships among institutions and settings, potentially "gaming" the system. A report card that inadequately adjusts for patient risk might under value hospitals and physicians who take on the highest risk patients, or encourage entities to transfer dying patients to reduce their mortality [15]. As Iezonni [16] notes, "developing risk adjusters de novo is complicated and often frustrating." Risk models for adult, pediatric, and neonatal ICU populations have been sufficiently vetted and have sufficiently evolved to serve as the foundation for nationally standardized outcomes measurement in an increasingly automated hospital environment. Risk models need to be reevaluated periodically to assure that they remain consistent with current patient factors, care process improvements, and outcomes experience. They should also be evaluated for their appropriateness at geographies not included in their modeling datasets.

There are multiple risk-adjustment models in current use. Representative examples of ICU risk-adjustment models based primarily on US patient data include:

1. APACHE IV (Acute Physiology, Age, Chronic Health Evaluation, 4th version) [15,17]
2. PRISM (Pediatric Risk of Mortality) [18]
3. SNAP/SNAPPE (Score for Neonatal Acute Physiology) [19]
4. Neonatal Risk Models of the Vermont-Oxford Network

EVALUATING RISK-ADJUSTED OUTCOMES INFORMATION

Because risk-adjusted assessments are based on mathematical models, taking an objective approach to understanding the causes of variance data is logical. For example, there are four main causes of variance, and sequentially evaluating them helps clinicians gain familiarity with the models and acceptance of variance between actual and predicted results. These models include (a) data randomness (small sample), (b) existence of patient risk factors not incorporated or (c) adequately weighted in the particular model, and (d) variance likely attributable to differences in care.

EMERGING INFORMATICS TRENDS

Telemedicine

The realities of the critical care environment are such that patients may be critically ill and yet not be in a setting where their care needs can be expeditiously met. For example, a patient might be in a small or distant hospital where intensivist coverage is not available. Or, even in a tertiary or quarternary medical center, patients may decompensate outside the ICU and, indeed, even in the ICU after hours, an intensivist might not be physically present or able to respond.

Two technological approaches (on-demand consultative medicine and vigilance telemedicine remote monitoring) to dealing with this problem have been developed. Each is dependent on the availability of a suitably trained intensivist at a remote location equipped with a microphone and speaker and a high-bandwidth Internet connection, one or more high-resolution cameras (which may be controlled by the remote physician) and communication systems to speak with caregivers, patients and family who are in or near the patient's room. Medical devices such as stethoscopes can be connected as well. Connectivity of the telemedicine system and the hospital varies according to institutional capabilities and can incldue access to the real-time physiological monitoring system; clinical information system; image archiving and communication systems; webcams, etc. [3]. Evaluations are still limited in that hands-on physician diagnostic and therapeutic maneuvers that can not be performed by available non physicians are not available when the physician is off-site.

On-demand/Consultative Telemedicine

On-Demand or Consultative Telemedicine technology allows a remote caregiver to provide expert consultation from a location remote from the patient. This capability allows for distributed systems of care to effectively deal with relatively low frequency events such as effectively triaging suspected stroke patients to necessary levels of care or the treatment and safe transport of severely ill children who present for emergency care to institutions without the immediate availability of pediatric specialists and to guide pre-transfer resuscitation and stabilization.

A form of technology that is particularly well suited for the interaction with an individual patient is a mobile robot, offering what is referred to as "robotic telepresence." One form of this device can actually be driven remotely by the physician from its storage location to the patient's location in the appropriately equipped facility. Using wireless connectivity, the robot establishes a similar connection to that which exists in rooms that have been specifically wired for these capabilities. As the costs of connectivity have decreased, institutions that formerly limited installations to those fixed in ICUs have been able to deploy telemedicine more widely across the hospital. It is clear that patients in other patient care locations can decompensate and may need to be monitored. Robots may provide a lower cost means to augment the expertise of rapid response teams.

Human-human interaction is a large part of succesful implementation of Telemedicine systems. Interactions may be initiated by the caregiving staff from any care location. In such circumstances acceptance has been generally very favorable as nurses feel that trained physicians with access to patient data are available to help them and their patients at all hours.

Vigilance Telemedicine/Remote Monitoring

In institutions where multiple ICUs have been equipped with cameras in each room and connectivity to clinical information systems and other clinical data sources has been established, a team may be established at a central monitoring location which may be distant from the ICUs and hospital(s). Automated analyses and alerts of data from bedside monitors, mechanical ventilators and laboratory tests inform off-site providers to perform patient assessments. Alternatively, bedside providers can request evaluation and off-site management. Interventions, including the ordering of diagnostic tests, medications or consultations, or the manipulation of life support devices can be done by off-site providers or by their linked on-site providers.

Thus, a single patient interaction may be initiated by the off-site physician as well as by hands-on caregivers. Like any team endeavor, effectiveness is determined in part by communication timeliness and dynamics of trust and responsibility among the bedside and off-site team members.

The primary responsibilities of the remote monitoring team are identification of unfavorable trends and to intervene to enhance best practice adherence, perform care plan reviews for patients admitted after day time hours and provide ICU pharmacist [20] and review of after hours medications orders which provides an additional safety net for patients in the ICU [20,21].

An important capability of remote monitoring is the opportunity to perform virtual rounds on the sickest patients. The acuity status is used to identify which patients might most benefit from closer observation. In this way, the remote physician can perform virtual rounds at intervals customized to the patient condition to judge the effects of medications that may have been administered or support technologies and to determine whether physiological responses are improving or deteriorating. This surveillance can be an important complement to bedside care.

An additional role played by a central monitoring team is to identify when patients who are eligible for a protocol are not being mannged according to an established protocol. It is important to recognize that clinical care protocols active at US hospitals require local hospital approval, which may include formal approval by an appropraite administartive body such as a physician Medical Executive Committee. For best alignment, protocolized care management by the remote monitoring team needs to conform to local hospital protocols.

Modern smartphones and small tablets have replaced many medical pagers and also provide the means to deliver high-resolution bedside monitoring device (BMDI) data, as well as complete access to the electronic medical record and highly automated decision support systems from any location at any time. Although telemedicine has enabled new health care structures, as noted earlier, these new technologies delivered to the individual practitioner are likely to transform medicine and the practice of telemedicine in the coming years in ways that are similar to their impact in the business world [22].

Predictive Analytics

Predictive analytics enable an organization to estimate or anticipate the risk of future events, and are used increasingly in other industries, such as for predicting consumer behavior. In health care, these techniques are often applied for planning demand for health care services and facilities; for identification of at-risk populations; and for actuarial projection of health care utilization or life span. Multiple Mathematical modeling and Machine Learning methods can be used for creation of models (Fig. 133.2).

CDS systems of the future will take more advantage of larger databases composed of increasingly granular patient data to drive pattern recognition engines that will help clinicians predict physiologic deterioration progressively earlier in the ICU course. Examples of predictive models in use today include the individual patient predictions components of the APACHE IV ICU models referenced previously [17], and the Northern New England Cardiovascular Disease Study Group's preoperative mortality risk and cerebrovascular accident and risk of vascular complication models [23]. In addition, clinical registries for cardiac surgery, invasive cardiology, general surgery, and stroke, among others, can provide expected risk, complication and mortality models for a specific populations of patients. Not intended to replace but to support physician judgment, predictive models to date have focused on evaluating the appropriateness of ICU admission and readiness for discharge, assessing patient progress and effectiveness of current therapies, building care team consensus around

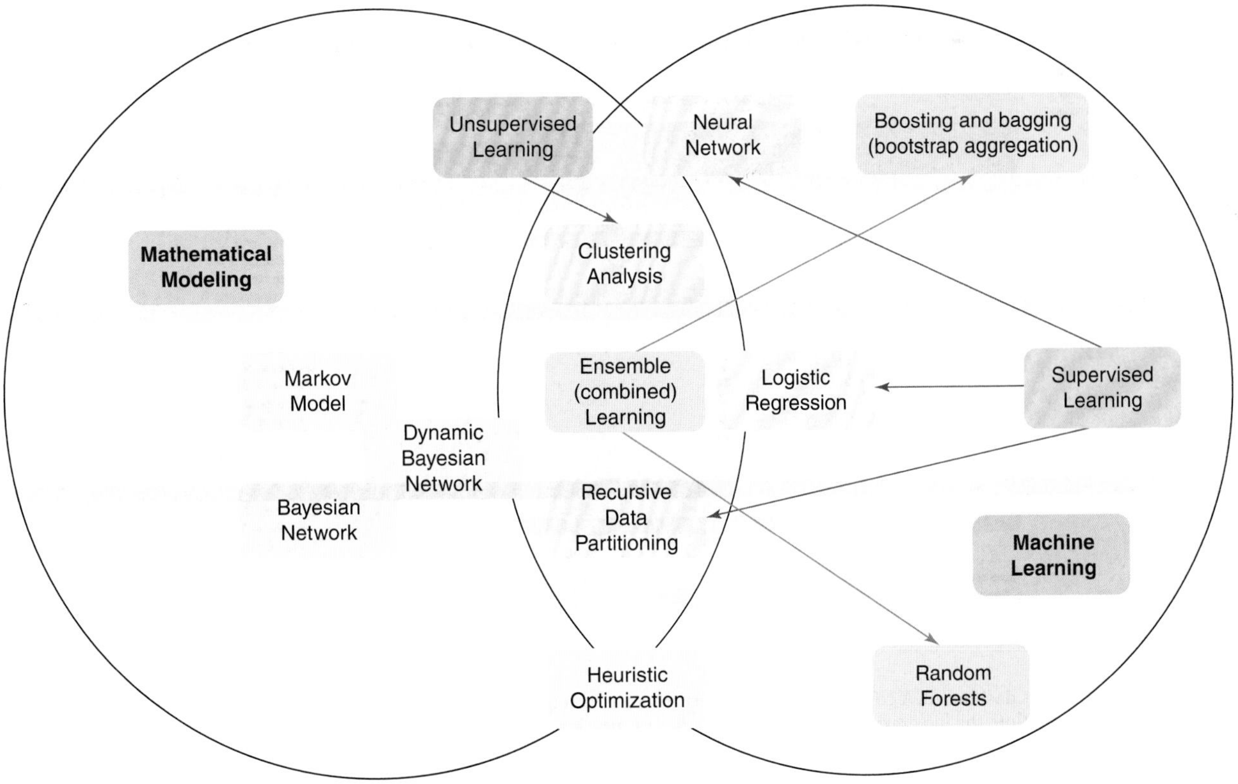

FIGURE 133.2 Predicitive analytical methods that can be used for building clinical models.

prognosis and care strategies, identifying patients for palliative care assessments, and improving communications and setting realistic expectations with patients and families. Additional efforts now underway include a database being developed at the Mayo Clinic that incorporates clinical patient data along with genomic and expression data. The expectation is that powerful prediction models will result from analysis of this large-scale aggregated patient history, outcomes, and genomic dataset [24].

Another large-scale database is currently being collected and analyzed by a collaborative of industrial, medical, and academic partners (MIT, Philips Healthcare, and the Beth Israel Deaconess Medical Center) [25]. To date analysis of this dataset (MIMIC II) has resulted in several prediction models that provide "early warning systems" for several specific types of physiological deterioration. One such model consists of a rule set that, when applied to near real-time patient physiological data, is capable of predicting hemodynamic deterioration hours before its occurrence [26,27]. Early warning alerts from advanced CDS systems hold the promise of improving response times to patient events. Although it seems to logically follow that such early identification of physiological deterioration would allow earlier intervention and prevention of patient crises, the effects of these interventions on patient outcomes are yet to be determined. Another example of a multidimentional near–real-time database is the ICU datamart of the Mayo Clinic. This data system includes laboratory, radiology, medication, fluids, physicians' notes, nurses' flow sheet data as well as CPOE. It contains over 250,000 ICU visits over 13 years [28].

ADVANCES OF DATA VISUALIZATION

Although many organizations have successfully applied performance metrics, severity scores, and predictive risk models for improved quality and decision-making, data collection/calculation and integrated display is likely to expand more in the next decade than in all previous ones. Designers have much work to do to accomplish meaningful display of the most important patient, process, alerting, and predictive information without overloading the clinician's ability to absorb and respond. Three examples of the application of modern data visualization techniques are represented in Figures 133.3 to 133.5.

MEMORIAL HERMANN
Breakthroughs every day

ICU Clinical Performance Metrics Report **January 2016**

Unit Name	[illegible] - Intensive Care
Unit Abbreviation	[illegible]-ICU ([illegible])
Medical Director	[illegible], MD
Nursing Director	[illegible], RN

[illegible] - Intensive Care

	January	December	November	6 Month Avg	12 Month Avg	Current vs 12 mo Trend	Notes
Operating Beds	22.0	22.0	22.0	22.0	22.0		
Discharges	104.0	103.0	89.0	97.0	98.2	Increase of 5.8	
Occupancy	66.9 %	70.8 %	66.6 %	65.8 %	64.3 %	Increase of 2.6%	
Average ICU Length of Stay (days)	4.39	4.69	4.94	4.48	4.32	Increase of 0.07	
Average Hospital Length of Stay (days)	11.88	12.44	8.73	10.08	9.55	Increase of 2.33	
% IMU/Routine Room Charges	58.3 %	51.3 %	48.2 %	53.9 %	53.2 %	Increase of 5.1%	
ICU Glucose Monitoring							
Bedside glucose measurements per day	8.25	7.14	7.15	7.33	6.92	Increase of 1.33	All measurements
% 1 or more hypoglycemic episodes	23.8 %	23.8 %	26.5 %	21.7 %	20.5 %	Increase of 3.3%	
Hypoglycemia <60 mg/dL	0.8 %	1.7 %	1.2 %	1.5 %	1.5 %	Decrease of 0.7%	Exlcudes first 24 hrs
Hyperglycemia >200 mg/dL	12.4 %	4.6 %	6.3 %	8.8 %	10.9 %	Increase of 1.5%	Exlcudes first 24 hrs
ICU HAI Bundle Compliance							
VAE Bundle Compliance – MD	90.7 %	94.7 %	92.4 %	94.0 %	95.3 %	Decrease of 4.6%	
VAE Bundle Compliance – Nursing	95.4 %	96.5 %	99.2 %	95.8 %	96.5 %	Decrease of 1.1%	
CLABSI Insertion Bundle Compliance	96.4 %	93.9 %	100.0 %	96.9 %	96.7 %	Decrease of 0.3%	
CLABSI Line Maintenance Compliance	87.7 %	82.3 %	89.5 %	88.4 %	88.9 %	Decrease of 1.2%	
CLABSI Count	0	0	0	0	0.3	Decrease of 0.3	
CAUTI Count	0	0	0	0	0	No Change (<1%)	6 & 12 month sum
Ultrasound Use	100.0 %	100.0 %	100.0 %	99.1 %	99.2 %	Increase of 0.8%	
ICU Utilization							
% App pts w/enteral nutrition <48hrs	100.0 %	95.8 %	92.6 %	93.4 %	90.4 %	Increase of 9.6%	
Antibiotics cost per day	$26.72	$20.60	$21.87	$29.66	$27.34	Decrease of $0.62	
Average # Ventilator Days	4.20	4.52	4.60	4.27	3.96	Increase of 0.24	For ventilated patients only
# Unplanned Extubations (/100 Vent Days)	0 (0.00)	5 (1.81)	4 (1.36)	3 (1.04)	3 (1.18)	Decrease of 3	
# Reintubations	2	4	3	4	3	Decrease of 1	
% Avoidable ICU Days	14.9 %	7.9 %	3.2 %	5.8 %	6.2 %	Increase of 8.7%	Subject to reporting revision
ICU Costs & Margin							
Total Indirect cost per patient day	$ [illegible]	$ [illegible]	$ [illegible]	$ [illegible]	$ [illegible]	Decrease of $70	
Total Direct cost per Patient day	$[illegible]	$[illegible]	$ [illegible]	$[illegible]	$[illegible]	Decrease of $205	
Laboratory	$178	$209	$247	$230	$234	Decrease of $56	
Chargeable Supplies	$212	$223	$256	$224	$228	Decrease of $16	
Pharmacy	$347	$335	$345	$382	$378	Decrease of $31	
Radiology	$45	$41	$47	$45	$45	Decrease of $0	
Respiratory	$181	$193	$180	$188	$179	Increase of $2	
Room & Other	$ [illegible]	$ [illegible]	$ [illegible]	$ [illegible]	$ [illegible]	Decrease of $106	
Contribution Margin per ICU Case[1]	$[illegible]	$ [illegible]	$ [illegible]	$ [illegible]	$[illegible]	Increase of $1384	
ICU Outcomes							
% Readmissions	3.1 %	6.8 %	2.2 %	4.1 %	4.0 %	Decrease of 0.9%	
Within 48 hrs leaving ICU	1.0 %	2.9 %	0.0 %	1.2 %	1.1 %	Decrease of 0.1%	
After 48 hrs leaving ICU	2.0 %	3.9 %	2.2 %	2.9 %	2.9 %	Decrease of 0.9%	
% Mortality ICU (Hospital)	13.46% (0.66%)	15.53% (0.67%)	8.99% (0.64%)	12.20% (0.60%)	10.28% (0.56%)	Increase of 3.18%	
High Risk[2] (APR-DRG)	Delayed 1 month	15.5 %	9.0 %	11.3 %	9.8 %	Increase of 5.7%	APR-DRG ROM = 3 or 4
Low Risk[2] (APR-DRG)	Delayed 1 month	0.0 %	0.0 %	0.2 %	0.1 %	Decrease of 0.1%	APR-DRG ROM = 1 or 2

1. Contribution Margin based on Blended Payments minus Direct costs
2. % will not sum to total mortality due to cases not yet fully coded
3. Ranges shown are preliminary targets defined by ICU metrics taskforce. Detail files will be available monthly in CO - Quality & Patient Safety

Distinguished	Target	Commendable	Concern

FIGURE 133.3 ICU metrics dashboard. A comprehensive ICU performance management dashboard, as used by the Memorial Hermann Healthcare System in Houston, Texas. Note the integration of different categories of metrics, such as census; occupancy; glycemic control; infection prevention bundle compliance; medication and ventilator utilization; financial data; and patient outcomes. This is a fully automated monthly report that is electronically distributed to ICU and executive management across the health system. Courtesy of Memorial Hermann Healthcare System, Houston, Texas.

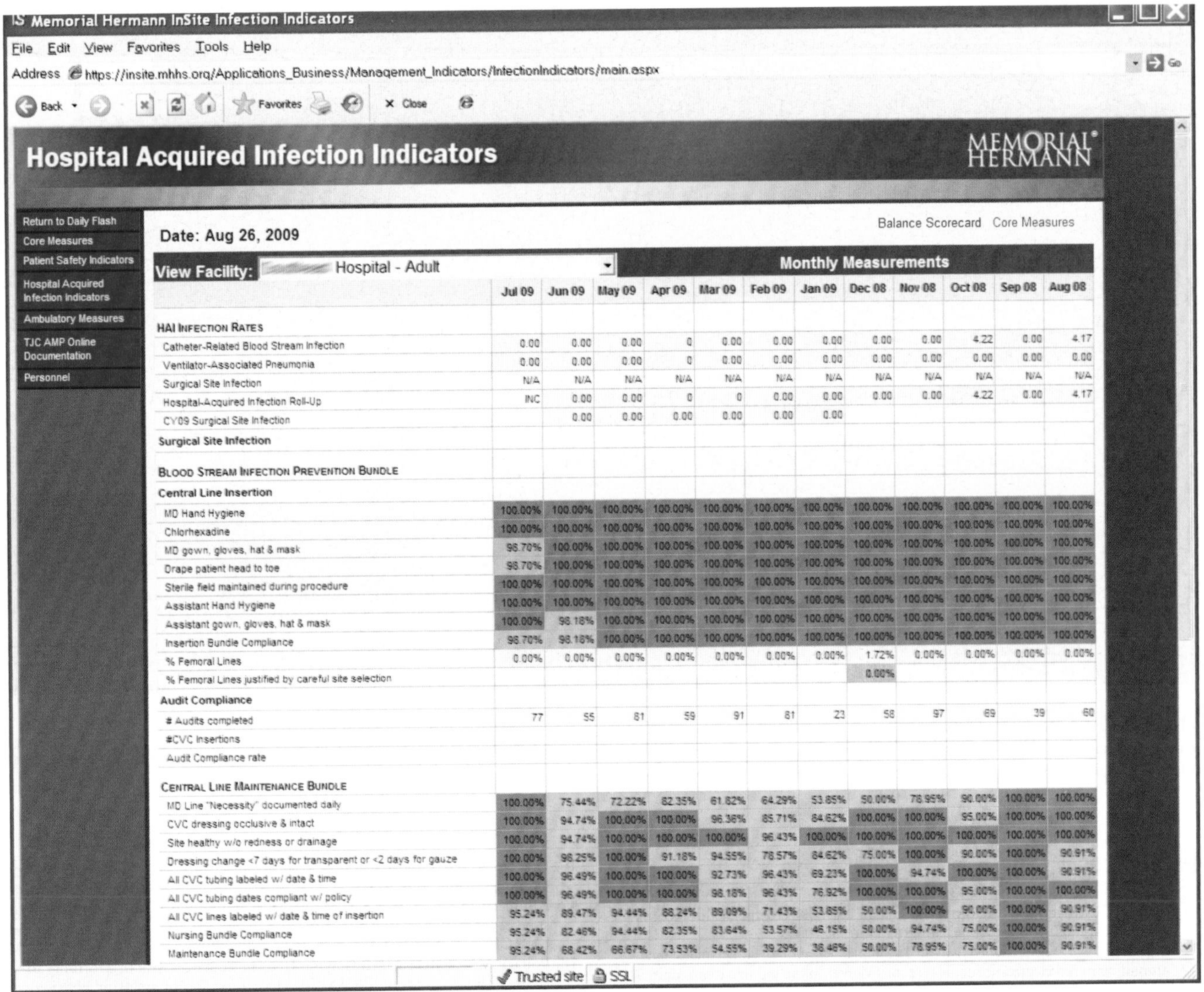

Memorial Hermann InSite Infection Indicators

File Edit View Favorites Tools Help

Address https://insite.mhhs.org/Applications_Business/Management_Indicators/InfectionIndicators/main.aspx

Hospital Acquired Infection Indicators

MEMORIAL HERMANN

Return to Daily Flash
Core Measures
Patient Safety Indicators
Hospital Acquired Infection Indicators
Ambulatory Measures
TJC AMP Online Documentation
Personnel

Date: Aug 26, 2009

Balance Scorecard Core Measures

View Facility: Hospital - Adult

Monthly Measurements

	Jul 09	Jun 09	May 09	Apr 09	Mar 09	Feb 09	Jan 09	Dec 08	Nov 08	Oct 08	Sep 08	Aug 08
HAI INFECTION RATES												
Catheter-Related Blood Stream Infection	0.00	0.00	0.00	0	0.00	0.00	0.00	0.00	0.00	4.22	0.00	4.17
Ventilator-Associated Pneumonia	0.00	0.00	0.00	0	0.00	0.00	0.00	0.00	0.00	0.00	0.00	0.00
Surgical Site Infection	N/A	N/A	N/A	N/A	N/A	N/A	N/A	N/A	N/A	N/A	N/A	N/A
Hospital-Acquired Infection Roll-Up	INC	0.00	0.00	0	0	0.00	0.00	0.00	0.00	4.22	0.00	4.17
CY09 Surgical Site Infection		0.00	0.00	0.00	0.00	0.00	0.00					
Surgical Site Infection												
BLOOD STREAM INFECTION PREVENTION BUNDLE												
Central Line Insertion												
MD Hand Hygiene	100.00%	100.00%	100.00%	100.00%	100.00%	100.00%	100.00%	100.00%	100.00%	100.00%	100.00%	100.00%
Chlorhexadine	100.00%	100.00%	100.00%	100.00%	100.00%	100.00%	100.00%	100.00%	100.00%	100.00%	100.00%	100.00%
MD gown, gloves, hat & mask	98.70%	100.00%	100.00%	100.00%	100.00%	100.00%	100.00%	100.00%	100.00%	100.00%	100.00%	100.00%
Drape patient head to toe	98.70%	100.00%	100.00%	100.00%	100.00%	100.00%	100.00%	100.00%	100.00%	100.00%	100.00%	100.00%
Sterile field maintained during procedure	100.00%	100.00%	100.00%	100.00%	100.00%	100.00%	100.00%	100.00%	100.00%	100.00%	100.00%	100.00%
Assistant Hand Hygiene	100.00%	100.00%	100.00%	100.00%	100.00%	100.00%	100.00%	100.00%	100.00%	100.00%	100.00%	100.00%
Assistant gown, gloves, hat & mask	100.00%	98.18%	100.00%	100.00%	100.00%	100.00%	100.00%	100.00%	100.00%	100.00%	100.00%	100.00%
Insertion Bundle Compliance	98.70%	98.18%	100.00%	100.00%	100.00%	100.00%	100.00%	100.00%	100.00%	100.00%	100.00%	100.00%
% Femoral Lines	0.00%	0.00%	0.00%	0.00%	0.00%	0.00%	0.00%	1.72%	0.00%	0.00%	0.00%	0.00%
% Femoral Lines justified by careful site selection								0.00%				
Audit Compliance												
# Audits completed	77	55	81	59	91	81	23	58	97	69	39	60
#CVC Insertions												
Audit Compliance rate												
CENTRAL LINE MAINTENANCE BUNDLE												
MD Line "Necessity" documented daily	100.00%	75.44%	72.22%	82.35%	61.82%	64.29%	53.85%	50.00%	78.95%	90.00%	100.00%	100.00%
CVC dressing occlusive & intact	100.00%	94.74%	100.00%	100.00%	96.36%	85.71%	84.62%	100.00%	100.00%	95.00%	100.00%	100.00%
Site healthy w/o redness or drainage	100.00%	94.74%	100.00%	100.00%	100.00%	96.43%	100.00%	100.00%	100.00%	100.00%	100.00%	100.00%
Dressing change <7 days for transparent or <2 days for gauze	100.00%	98.25%	100.00%	91.18%	94.55%	78.57%	84.62%	75.00%	100.00%	90.00%	100.00%	90.91%
All CVC tubing labeled w/ date & time	100.00%	96.49%	100.00%	100.00%	92.73%	96.43%	69.23%	100.00%	94.74%	100.00%	100.00%	90.91%
All CVC tubing dates compliant w/ policy	100.00%	96.49%	100.00%	100.00%	98.18%	96.43%	76.92%	100.00%	100.00%	95.00%	100.00%	100.00%
All CVC lines labeled w/ date & time of insertion	95.24%	89.47%	94.44%	88.24%	89.09%	71.43%	53.85%	50.00%	100.00%	90.00%	100.00%	90.91%
Nursing Bundle Compliance	95.24%	82.46%	94.44%	82.35%	83.64%	53.57%	46.15%	50.00%	94.74%	75.00%	100.00%	90.91%
Maintenance Bundle Compliance	95.24%	68.42%	66.67%	73.53%	54.55%	39.29%	38.46%	50.00%	78.95%	75.00%	100.00%	90.91%

Trusted site SSL

FIGURE 133.4 Hospital-acquired infection indicators dashboard. A comprehensive real-time ICU hospital-acquired infection (HAI) dashboard, including HAI rates and detailed bundle compliance results for prevention of catheter-related blood stream infection and VAP. This is a live intranet web display that is updated constantly. Both reports are widely available within the Memorial Hermann system and have helped drive performance excellence. Near real-time availability of bundle compliance and hand hygiene data have driven the incidence of CLABSI and VAP to zero or near zero levels across the Memorial Hermann system [29]. Courtesy of Memorial Hermann Healthcare System, Houston, Texas.

In conclusion, the modern CCIS is a dynamic information instrument or set of functionalities delivered by a core EMR that extends the capabilities of the intensive care physician and staff in ways that would be considered science fiction only a generation ago. The rapid adoption of these new information tools is now anticipated, as the complexity of medical care, particularly in the ICU setting, becomes increasingly demanding and evidence-based decision-making moves from a goal to an expectation of acute medical care. The most citical element, to taking advantage of these new possibilities, is that senior medical executives, ICU directors, and clinicians must "own" responsibility for localizing and embracing performance metrics and the advancing base of evidence-based decision support being made available by these new tools.

ACKNOLWEDGMENTS

The authors would like to thank the previous authors of this chapter who provided an excellent basis for this edition. We are very grateful to William F. Bria, MD, Richard M. Kremsdorf, MD, and Violet L. Shaffer for their foundational work on this topic—much of which remains within this chapter.

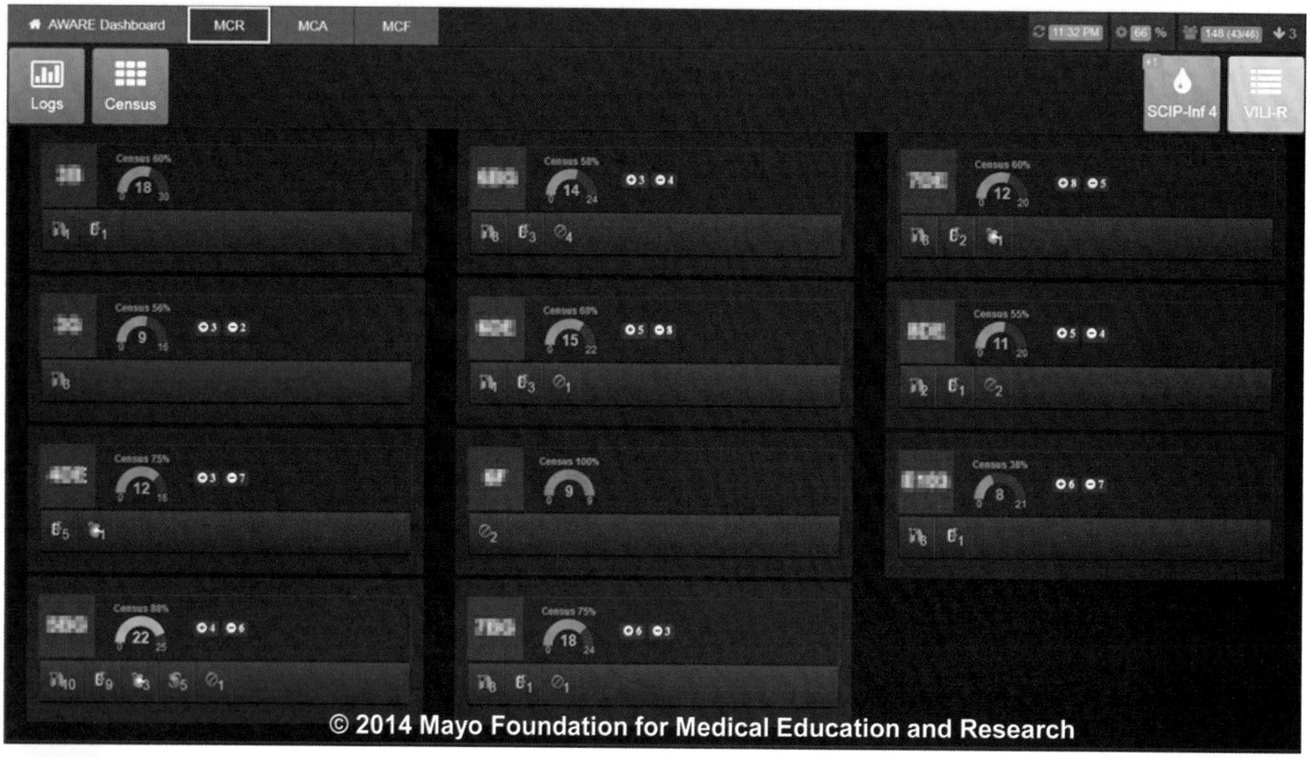

FIGURE 133.5 Real-time electronic "cockpit" for ICU resource utilization in Mayo Clinic ICUs.
Automatic resource utilization "cockpit" at Mayo Clinic ICUs. It shows in real time the number of current patients, admissions, discharges, ventilator utilizations, ECMO machines, Do-not-resuscitate patients; and patients with organ support like dialysis and vasopressors

References

1. Jha AK, DesRoches CM, Campbell EG, et al: Use of electronic health records in U.S. hospitals. *N Engl J Med* 360:1628–1638, 2009.
2. Pickering BW, Dong Y, Ahmed A, et al: The implementation of clinician designed, human-centered electronic medical record viewer in the intensive care unit: a pilot step-wedge cluster randomized trial. *Int J Med Inf* 84:299–307, 2015.
3. Berenson RA, Grossman JM, November EA: Does telemonitoring of patients—the eICU—improve intensive care? *Health Aff (Millwood)* 28:w937–w947, 2009.
4. Ries M: Tele-ICU: a new paradigm in critical care. *Int Anesthesiol Clin* 47:153–170, 2009.
5. Morris A: *Principles and Practice of Intensive Care Monitoring*. McGraw-Hill, 1998, pp 1355–1381.
6. Breslow MJ: Remote ICU care programs: current status. *J Crit Care* 22:66–76, 2007.
7. Miller GA: The magical number seven plus or minus two: some limits on our capacity for processing information. *Psychol Rev* 63:81–97, 1956.
8. Han YY: Unexpected increased mortality after implementation of a commercially sold computerized physician order entry system. *Pediatrics* 116:1506–1512, 2005.
9. Rosenfeld BA, Dorman T, Breslow MJ, et al: Intensive care unit telemedicine: alternate paradigm for providing continuous intensivist care. *Crit Care Med* 28:3925–3931, 2000.
10. Institute for Healthcare Improvement: Building Rapid Response Teams. Available at: http://www.ihi.org/resources/Pages/ImprovementStories/BuildingRapidResponseTeams.aspx. Accessed September 2, 2016.
11. Bellomo R, Goldsmith D, Uchino S, et al. Prospective controlled trial of effect of medical emergency team on postoperative morbidity and mortality rates. *Crit Care Med* 32:916–921, 2004.
12. Homsted L: Institute of Medicine report: to err is human: building a safer health care system. *Fla Nurse* 48:6, 2000.
13. Centers for Medicare and Medicaid Services. CMS Measures Inventory. 2016. Available at: https://www.cms.gov/Medicare/Quality-Initiatives-Patient-Assessment-Instruments/QualityMeasures/CMS-Measures-Inventory.html. Accessed September 2, 2016.
14. The Leapfrog Group: The Leapfrog Group. 2016. Available at: http://www.leapfroggroup.org/. Accessed September 2, 2016.
15. Knaus WA, Wagner DP, Draper EA, et al. The APACHE III prognostic system. Risk prediction of hospital mortality for critically ill hospitalized adults. *Chest* 100:1619–1636, 1991.
16. Lezzoni L: *Risk Adjustment for Measuring Healthcare Outcomes*. Health Administration Press, 2003.
17. Zimmerman JE, Kramer AA, McNair DS, et al: Intensive care unit length of stay: benchmarking based on Acute Physiology and Chronic Health Evaluation (APACHE) IV. *Crit Care Med* 34:2517–2529, 2006.
18. Pollack MM, Patel KM, Ruttimann UE: The Pediatric Risk of Mortality III—Acute Physiology Score (PRISM III-APS): a method of assessing physiologic instability for pediatric intensive care unit patients. *J Pediatr* 131, 575–581, 1997.
19. Zupancic JA, Richardson DK, Horbar JD, et al: Revalidation of the score for neonatal acute physiology in the Vermont Oxford Network. *Pediatrics* 119:e156–e163, 2007.
20. Forni A, Skehan N, Hartman CA, et al: Evaluation of the impact of a tele-ICU pharmacist on the management of sedation in critically ill mechanically ventilated patients. *Ann Pharmacother* 44:432–438, 2010.
21. Lilly CM: Hospital mortality, length of stay, and preventable complications among critically ill patients before and after tele-ICU reengineering of critical care processes. *JAMA* 305:2175, 2011.
22. Thomas EJ: Association of telemedicine for remote monitoring of intensive care patients with mortality, complications, and length of stay. *JAMA* 302:2671, 2009.
23. O'Connor GT, Plume SK, Olmstead EM, et al: Multivariate prediction of in-hospital mortality associated with coronary artery bypass graft surgery. Northern New England Cardiovascular Disease Study Group. *Circulation* 85:2110–2118, 1992.
24. IBM: Mayo Clinic, IBM Aim to Drive Medical Breakthroughs. Available at: https://www-03.ibm.com/press/us/en/pressrelease/7255.wss. Accessed September 2, 2016.
25. Saeed M, Lieu C, Raber G et al: MIMIC II: a massive temporal ICU patient database to support research in intelligent patient monitoring. *Comput Cardiol* 29:641–644, 2002.
26. Eshelman LJ, et al: Development and evaluation of predictive alerts for hemodynamic instability in ICU patients. *AMIA Annu Symp Proc* 379–383, 2008.
27. Potes C, Conroy B, Xu M, et al: 1010: an automated algorithm for the early detection of hemodynamic instability in the PICU. *Crit Care Med* 43:254, 2015.
28. Herasevich V, Pickering BW, Dong Y, et al: Informatics infrastructure for syndrome surveillance, decision support, reporting, and modeling of critical illness. *Mayo Clin Proc* 85:247–254, 2010.
29. Shabot MM, Chassin MR, France AC, et al: Using the targeted solutions tool to improve hand hygiene compliance is associated with decreased health care-associated infections. *Jt Comm J Qual Patient Saf* 42:6–17, 2016.

Chapter 134 ■ Defining and Measuring Patient Safety in the Critical Care Unit

HAYLEY B. GERSHENGORN • STEVEN Y. CHANG • DAVID E. OST • KELLY L. CERVELLIONE • ALAN M. FEIN

Patient safety has become a major concern of the general public, policy makers, and local, state, and national governments. Frequent news coverage has been devoted to victims of serious medical errors. In the 1999 publication of the Institute of Medicine (IOM), "To Err Is Human: Building a Safer Health Care System" [1], the substantial risks of American medical care were highlighted, particularly the nearly 100,000 deaths per year that could be attributed to medical errors.

The importance of a safety culture in the high-risk environment of the intensive care unit (ICU) is becoming increasingly recognized and promoted [2]. In order to be effective, the development of a culture of safety must represent a central structure that promotes patient well-being through the use of coordinated intra- and interdisciplinary networks. Such a culture emerges from the presence of leaders who are committed to safety. Of equal importance is staff who understand that errors are inevitable, acknowledge that errors are to be reported, dedicate time to learn about new risks and hazards, support teamwork and open communication, and upgrade procedures and implement safeguards on a continuing basis [3]. Organizational characteristics of safe programs with low accident rates include successful safety programs with strong management commitment, safety training as part of new employee's training, frequent open contacts between workers and management, general environmental control and good housekeeping, a stable workforce, and positive reinforcement for good safety practices. Similar to other areas of the hospital environment, the ICU benefits from integrated systems that identify patient safety problems and report them to providers so they can improve performance.

On a broad scale, ICU patient safety reporting systems identify trends and patterns, allowing healthcare organizations, governmental agencies, and private accreditation organizations to monitor the quality and safety of healthcare delivery [4]. Patient safety reporting systems also have the potential to create large data repositories that inform the development of strategies to reduce the risk of preventable medical incidents [5,6]. In the 2003 report, "Patient Safety: Achieving a New Standard of Care," the IOM emphasized the importance of standardizing information on patient safety to improve outcomes of care [5], including the development of a common taxonomy of patient safety terms. Standardized terminology permits healthcare providers to capture and describe events in consolidated reports [1,7,8]. To date, governmental and private sector accrediting bodies have not coordinated their efforts to develop actionable, integrated, validated, and reliable systems to measure and report medical errors and patient safety [9]. A recent trend involves more direct regulation by government agencies like Centers for Medicare and Medicaid Services (CMS) and state health departments. In some cases, mandated reporting and specific treatment algorithms have been recommended for critical illness like sepsis and ventilator-associated pneumonia. This chapter will explore the elements of patient safety in the ICU, related definitions, culture, education, and trends in the regulatory environment.

SAFETY LESSONS FROM OTHER INDUSTRIES

Safety and error prevention in the healthcare setting compares unfavorably with that of aviation, banking, chemical manufacturing, and peacetime military services. Approaches to safety used by these industries include well-defined strategies to protect workers and customers. Technology-based approaches are part of this strategy, but organizational and psychological factors contribute as well. For example, developing a culture of safety has been identified as one important method of improving safety. The aviation industry has focused on the importance of teamwork in reinforcing a safety culture.

Although technical, organizational, and psychological interventions have been effective for other industries, it is also worth noting the limits of these methods. Persistence of fatalities for the aviation and auto transportation industries suggests that safety efforts may be counterbalanced by other competing risk factors such as high volumes, greater complexity of the product, cost pressure, and rapidly changing designs. These risk factors are particularly relevant to healthcare because the patient population is changing (with greater numbers of very old, immunocompromised, and high-risk patients), and technology is evolving at very rapid rates [10]. Thus, there is likely an upper limit in terms of cost-effective healthcare safety that can be reached. However, this level has yet to be attained, or even identified. Health services are being encouraged by the IOM report to aim for an error rate of less than 3.4 per million, that is, "six-sigma quality." The discipline of anesthesiology in particular has made substantial contributions through its development of a safety culture and equipment manufacturing standardization, resulting in a reduction in anesthesia-related deaths to 4.4 per million, that is, "five-sigma standard."

To achieve the six sigma level for ICU patients, there must be precise definitions of the terms needed to study patient safety, their methods of measurement, and the applications of these methods to the special problems of ICU organization within government regulations. Specialized physician training and development of a culture of safety will also be essential in order to achieve such an excellent level of safety in the setting of intensive care.

DEFINITIONS

The basic terms in common use to define concepts of patient safety are listed in Table 134.1, along with the working definitions of these terms that have entered into the lexicon of the patient safety industry [11]. Healthcare quality is defined by the IOM as "the degree to which health services for individuals and populations increase the likelihood of desired health outcomes and are consistent with current professional knowledge" [3,12]. The IOM has also listed several attributes of quality care that define quality care as being safe, patient-centered, timely, effective, efficient, and equitable [13]. Thus, patient safety is one domain within the broader concept of quality.

Patient safety has been defined by the Agency for Health Care Research and Quality (AHRQ) as "the absence of the potential for, or the occurrence of, healthcare associated injury to patients created by avoiding medical errors as well as taking action to prevent errors from causing injury" [14] and "freedom from accidental or preventable injuries produced by medical care" [15].

Within this context of safety, medical errors are defined as "mistakes made in the process of care that result in or have

TABLE 134.1

General Terms Used in Patient Safety

Quality:	The degree to which health services for individuals and populations increase the likelihood of desired health outcomes and are consistent with current professional knowledge
Patient safety:	The absence of the potential for, or the occurrence of, healthcare-associated injury to patients created by avoiding medical errors as well as taking action to prevent errors from causing injury. Freedom from accidental or preventable injuries produced by medical care
Medical errors:	Mistakes made in the process of care that result in or have the potential to result in harm to patients. Mistakes include the failure of a planned action to be completed as intended or the use of a wrong plan to achieve an aim. These can be the result of an action that is taken (error of commission) or an action that is not taken (error of omission)
Active errors:	Errors that occur at the interface between a human provider and a care delivery system (e.g., mechanical ventilator, intravenous pump) and typically involve readily apparent actions (e.g., adjusting a dial incorrectly)
Latent errors:	Less obvious failures of a healthcare organization or structure that contributed to errors or allowed the errors to harm patients. An example of a latent error would be understaffing of nurses in an intensive care unit
Serious medical errors:	A medical error that causes harm (or injury) or has the potential to cause harm. Includes preventable adverse events, intercepted serious errors, and nonintercepted serious errors. Does not include trivial errors with little or no potential for harm or nonpreventable adverse events
Intercepted serious error:	A serious medical error that is caught before reaching the patient
Nonintercepted serious error:	A serious medical error that is not caught and therefore reaches the patient but because of good fortune or because the patient had sufficient reserves to buffer the error, it did not cause clinically detectable harm
Nonpreventable adverse event:	Unavoidable injury due to appropriate medical care
Preventable adverse event:	Injury due to a nonintercepted serious error in medical care
Slips:	Failures of automatic behaviors or lapses in concentration (e.g., forgetting to perform a routine task due to a lapse in memory) and often occur from fatigue or distractions in the workplace
Mistakes:	Incorrect choices, such as choosing the wrong drug, a clinical condition and typically result from inexperience or lack of knowledge or training
Incident:	An event or circumstance that could have, or did lead to, unintended and/or unnecessary harm to a person
Harm:	Death, injury, suffering, dissatisfaction, or disability experienced by a person
Near miss:	Any incident that could potentially lead to patient harm
Adverse event:	Any injury due to medical management, rather than the underlying disease

Adapted from references [11,12,14–18].

the potential to result in harm to patients. Mistakes include the failure of a planned action to be completed as intended or the use of a wrong plan to achieve an aim. These can be the result of an action that is taken (error of commission) or an action that is not taken (error of omission)" [14]. Errors of commission (e.g., ordering an incorrect drug dose) are more readily noted than errors of omission (e.g., failure to order heparin for venous thromboembolism prophylaxis). Errors are further classified as active or latent [16,17]. Active errors occur at the interface between a human provider and a care delivery system (e.g., mechanical ventilator, intravenous pump), and typically involve readily apparent actions (e.g., adjusting a dial incorrectly). Latent errors define a less obvious failure of a healthcare organization or structure that have contributed to errors or allowed the errors to harm patients. An example of a latent error is understaffing of nurses in an ICU. Other typologies include domains that ascribe characteristics of preventability, seriousness, and whether the error was intercepted before affecting a patient [18] (Table 134.1). The concept of medical error has become increasingly elastic because government regulation has further encroached on medical decision-making, as in the case of "ICU bundles."

Errors have also been classified as slips or mistakes. Slips are failures of automatic behaviors or lapses in concentration (e.g., forgetting to perform a routine task due to a lapse in memory), and often occur from fatigue or distractions in the workplace. Mistakes represent incorrect choices, such as choosing the wrong drug for a clinical condition, and typically result from inexperience or lack of knowledge or training. The remedies for these two types of errors differ; slips are more responsive to removing distractions from the workplace or automating monotonous tasks, whereas mistakes respond to increased training or supervision.

Incidents are defined as unexpected or unanticipated events or circumstances not consistent with the routine care of a particular patient, which could have or did lead to an unintended or unnecessary harm to a person, or to a complaint, loss, or damage. Adverse events are different than incidents and are defined as an "untoward and usually unanticipated outcome that occurs in association with health care" [14] or in the broader terms of the IOM as "an injury resulting from a medical intervention" [1]. The Critical Care Safety Study defines adverse events as "Any injury due to medical management, rather than the underlying disease" [18]. An adverse event does not necessarily mean that the event was related to poor quality care [19]. As an example, if proper procedures are followed for central line placement but the patient develops a pneumothorax, this would constitute an adverse event. Errors of diagnosis have been less studied but are emerging as equally important causes of unsafe patient management in the ICU [20]. As the safety and quality movement has progressed, it is increasingly difficult to look at one aspect isolated from the other. Although it may be useful for research purposes to identify issues as either safety related or quality related, on a day-to-day basis the distinction between safety and quality issues is increasingly nominal.

MEASUREMENT OF SAFETY IN THE INTENSIVE CARE UNIT

Patient safety analysis can be viewed from the perspective of whether the measure identifies a structure, process, or outcome related to safety. Structure is defined by the physical environment and plant (buildings, equipment, information technology resources). Process and outcome can sometimes be conflated but in fact are distinct. Process refers to the way healthcare is delivered, i.e., how the system of care works. Outcomes are the downstream measures of health status. The most concrete outcome is mortality; the term can also include quality of life measures, specific morbidities, exercise capacity, and others. An additional dimension worth considering is the context in which care is delivered, also called "safety culture." This reflects the attitudes and beliefs of local healthcare providers as well as the medical community at large. Measurement of this dimension, while difficult, may be worthwhile as there is some evidence that variations in culture are linked to clinical outcomes [21]. The primary methods of measuring safety culture include incident reporting, targeted monitoring, use of discharge data sets, process of care measurement, trigger tools, ICU audits, and direct observation [18].

Incident Reporting

In terms of collecting safety measurement data, traditional methods based on incident reporting of specific adverse events have been largely ineffective for several reasons [22]. First, reports have been generated in a punitive environment that focuses on the provider who committed an error rather than on systems of care, and thus discourages self-reporting of errors [5]. Second, each report of an error represents a "numerator" value that does not give insight into the denominator pool of patients at risk of similar errors. In the absence of these values, the incidence of errors and the overall safety of an ICU cannot be assessed. Third, definitions of errors used by incident reporting systems vary, which impedes data synthesis, analysis, collaborative work, and evaluation of the impact of changes in healthcare delivery [23]. And fourth, appropriate functional data spanning the domains of structure, process, and outcome are not collected, which impedes the ability to "deconstruct" an error to understand its root causes and patient impact.

Recent advances in incident reporting have enhanced the detection and analysis of errors. Internet-based systems allow anonymous reporting of errors, encouraging providers who have either committed an error or have knowledge of an error to enter related information into a central data repository [24]. The Intensive Care Unit Safety Reporting System (ICUSRS) is an anonymous reporting system that focuses on "systems factors" rather than "person factors" and provides expert analysis with feedback and guidance to improve processes of care and prevent error recurrences [11,25]. The University Health Systems Consortium's Safety Net reporting system can generate consolidated reports with application to the ICU [24].

Institutional commitment to a "culture of safety" has a motivational effect on error reporting because healthcare providers recognize that "someone is listening." The mere fact that errors are reported and there is accountability can generate improved quality of care if the system works properly. This culture requires several essential process elements to enhance error reporting: A team (a) convenes to develop preventative solutions to a reported error, (b) generates plans to improve the care, and (c) has a method for implementing and measuring the impact of their plan [23]. However, problems remain with the taxonomy used to describe errors and adverse events. The Joint Commission (JC) published a patient safety event taxonomy and classification scheme for near misses, errors, and adverse events [11]. The taxonomy used was designed to conform to an analytical framework and common word usages to promote its use and the understanding of its output. Data entered allows classification of a patient safety event within five complementary primary groups: impact—the outcome or effects of medical error and systems failure, commonly referred to as harm to the patient; type—the implied or visible processes that were faulty or failed; domain—the characteristics of the setting in which an incident occurred and the type of individuals involved; cause—the factors and agents that led to an incident; and prevention and mitigation—the measures taken or proposed to reduce incidence and effects of adverse occurrences.

The ICUSRS reporting platform uses a similar framework for evaluating factors that contribute to an incident [11]. Both the JC and ICUSRS systems recognize that errors are multifactorial and therefore include multiple variables along the three domains of structure, process, and outcomes, such as caregiver performance, systems of care, resource availability, functioning of teams, and the environment of care. These systems describe events with a multidimensional taxonomy to facilitate the comprehensive description and full deconstruction of errors to determine their root causes [9]. However, even if the taxonomy issues of incidence reporting are improved, the problem of determining the true incidence rate remains. A comprehensively described and deconstructed incident only gives insight into the numerator; it does not provide information on the number of patients at risk and does not allow determination of true incidence rates.

Targeted Monitoring

A complementary approach to incident reporting is targeted monitoring. ICUs can measure their patient safety outcomes by monitoring a specific indicator, such as the incidence of *Clostridium difficile* infection in the ICU or ventilator-associated pneumonia. In so doing, ICUs are challenged to define their denominators and select indicators that can be readily detected and counted to provide an accurate numerator. The denominators are especially difficult to determine because these measurements have major impacts on interpretation [11]; for instance, *C. difficile* infection rates can be described per ICU patient, patient ICU days, or at-risk patient ICU days. The numerator data are equally challenging because of the time and expense of chart extraction needed for their collection. If the characteristics of the patient population change over time, then these factors must be accounted for as well. For example, if the patient population changes or new services such as transplantation are offered by a given hospital, then the patient mix will change and adjusted hazard rates will be needed. Thus, for this approach to be effective, a multidisciplinary team that includes people with ICU training, organizational skills, database management, and epidemiology is needed.

Discharge Data

Discharge data represents a potential source of information to allow the retrospective collection of quality and safety indicators to profile ICU performance [26–28]. Recently, AHRQ has developed empiric measures of quality and safety from multistate discharge data in a redesign of the original Healthcare Cost and Utilization Project Quality Indicators [29]. The Patient Safety Indicators are relevant to ICU safety of care. Although most of these indicators relate to surgical patients, newer indicators are being designed to measure the safety of care for medical patients with critical illnesses, such as myocardial infarction, stroke, and congestive heart failure.

Although this method is powerful and can be quite useful, it is important to also recognize its limitations. Discharge data analysis gives insight into outcomes, but little information on structure or process. Large data sets such as these also have limited data quality for clinically relevant covariates, so controlling for confounders is difficult. Because all of the clinically relevant covariates are not included, the problem of residual confounding is always a problem and caution should be exercised when interpreting results. Making interinstitutional comparisons is therefore difficult, and even when trending data over time, results must be analyzed with caution. When patient populations and their problems are relatively homogenous and stable over time (e.g., surgical patients), this is a good system. When there is marked heterogeneity in terms of clinical problems and rapid changes in process of care over time, this approach will face difficulties. Having said this, discharge data sets can be an important tool for hypothesis generation so that ICU leaders can then launch more systematic studies of particular problems.

Process of Care Measurement

Safety can also be measured through determination of the proportion of patients who receive certain processes of care that have a strong evidentiary base for improving clinical outcomes. However, it may be difficult to isolate and ascertain the contributory effect of influential factors, such as adherence to best practice by the caregiving team, the role of complications, or level of care. Physicians and other clinicians often have a stronger sense of accountability toward a process measure than an outcome measure because the process measure can be more strongly linked to a particular care provider or team behaviors [30]. Physicians may also believe that outcomes can be overly influenced by severity of disease and prove resistant to quality improvement efforts. To serve as an accurate measure of safety and to influence quality improvement, process measures must have a causal relationship with the outcome they intend to represent.

Examples of process measures include approaches to ordering therapy in the ICU. Medication errors and adverse drug events occur commonly in the ICU [31] and can be limited by the use of formatted or electronic drug-ordering forms [32]. Computerized physician order entry (order-sets) for drugs has the potential to decrease the rate of serious medication errors [33] and to improve clinical outcomes when applied to antibiotic prescribing [34]. Additional care processes that should be in place to support patient safety can be constructed by adding allergy or drug–drug interaction monitoring and reviewing evidence-based clinical practice guidelines [35], such as standardizing orders for ventilator management in the ICU [36].

Process of care measurement is often very effective for certain types of problems (like computerized order entry), but it is important to recognize some of the limitations and difficulties inherent in this system when applied to more complex problems. When strong evidence-based clinical practice guidelines are available, it is a feasible strategy, but often this is not the case. In addition, properly identifying those patients eligible for a particular protocol during the appropriate time period is critical. Examples include the use of thrombolytics for myocardial infarction and stroke. Determining the numerator for such process of care measures is fairly easy (who actually received the drug), but determining the denominator can be more difficult and can be costly because of the time and expense needed for data collection (e.g., reviewing every chart in the emergency department of patients presenting with angina or suspected myocardial infarction). In addition, chart abstraction in such cases usually requires a high level of expert judgment, which makes it variable, difficult, and costly. Thus, process of care measurement, because of cost and time considerations, may be a suitable approach to improving safety for those problems in which there is a strong evidence base and for which the costs of identifying the patient population (both numerator and denominator) are sustainable and warranted by the value of information obtained.

Intensive Care Unit Audits

An audit of the existing structure of an ICU can also measure patient safety. Evidence supports improved outcomes in ICUs staffed by sufficient numbers of board-certified intensivists [37,38]. Additional structure measures of safety include the presence of resources to establish ongoing competency of medical staff and residents [39], adequate nurse staffing and skill sets [40,41], and appropriate technology resources, such as smart pumps and bar coding [42]. Surveys exist that allow ICU directors to assess the status of their units' culture of safety [43–46]. Pronovost and Sexton [45] recommend measuring the entire hospital annually with the full Safety Attitudes Questionnaire that has construct validity and sufficient reliability for measuring the single construct of safety culture. Once measured, the culture of safety can be improved with focused interventions geared toward any low-scoring hospital areas, such as an ICU.

Trigger Tools

Trigger tools refer to techniques used to detect organizational signals for adverse events. For instance, orders for flumazenil may identify patients who were given an overdose of a benzodiazepine drug. The flumazenil order, therefore, would serve as a trigger to perform a chart review. A trigger or set of triggers can be used to identify medical records for retrospective review to assess organizational safety, or used in "real time" as a tool to identify a specific patient at risk of an adverse outcome. Trigger tools for the ICU have been shown to be a practical approach to enhancing detection of adverse events among critically ill patients [47].

Limitations of Existing Metrics and Their Applications

Currently, the majority of data collected to measure safety is process oriented. However, there is only limited evidence that the use of current process measures translates into better outcomes [48,49]. Quality metrics that include patient outcomes would provide better information to inform benchmarking and to assist in policy development, but proper assessment of ICU outcomes often requires extensive abstraction of clinical data, which can be prohibitively costly. In addition, risk adjustment to facilitate valid comparisons increases the amount and complexity of data abstraction required, further increasing costs. Sometimes the benefits of such safety programs warrant their costs. This is especially true when events are rare, which is usually the case with safety. In such instances, proper measures require collecting information on a very large population, which constitutes the denominator of the rates being measured.

It is also very important to consider carefully the attributes of performance measures and how the measures are arrived at. To be valid, measures usually have to be rates, defined as an event per person time at risk. This is different than a proportion, which has events per case, with no measure of time at risk. Most "rates" reported in the patient safety literature are actually proportions. For some outcomes, such as pneumothorax following lung biopsy, a proportion may be suitable. But for many other outcomes, person time at risk is relevant (e.g., ventilator-associated pneumonia), and a proportion will not suffice. In addition, the magnitude and direction of bias for reporting can be greater than the true variation of outcomes. This is because most reporting systems, such as the Patient Safety Reporting System, provide data from a non-randomly selected sample and the population at risk is not known. When interpreting safety metrics, careful attention must be paid, bias must be considered, and all results should be viewed with caution.

An additional area to consider is which indicators should be used. There are a variety of endorsed quality and safety measures currently available, some with a stronger evidence base than others, but which ones are best is not clear and will depend largely on local factors. The cost-effectiveness of even the best evidence-based measures and interventions is difficult to prove, and the potential benefits of implementation are likely to vary depending on the local context. The National Quality Forum measures for quality in intensive care serve to highlight some of the difficulties encountered. As of October 2015, The National Quality Forum had endorsed various quality measures for intensive care, including ICU length of stay, venous thromboembolism prophylaxis, in-hospital mortality, catheter-associated urinary tract infection, and *C. difficile* infection [50]. However, it is informative to note the measures that were previously sanctioned but are no longer authorized.

These include severity-standardized average length of stay, the ventilator bundle, central line bundle compliance, and measures of glycemic control with intravenous insulin. Investigators have tried through survey, expert panels, and literature reviews to identify the most useful indicators for measurement in ICUs, often with varying results [51,52].

Currently, there is no single common safety score card that is appropriate for universal use. As such, the choice of safety and quality metrics for a given ICU needs to be driven by local factors. The selection process should take into account whether the measures are valid rates, whether proportions are sufficient, whether the outcomes being measured are truly preventable with intervention, potential sources of bias, costs of implementation, and the strength of the evidence supporting a given intervention.

INTENSIVE CARE UNIT ORGANIZATION

Providing safe and high-quality critical care has a significant impact on patient safety and quality. Although the vast majority of the literature supports the value of intensivist-based critical care, a landmark study by Angus et al. in 2000 found that more than three-fifths of critically ill patients in the United States are not seen by an intensivist. Moreover, it was estimated that this gap between supply and demand will only widen in the coming decades [53]. On the other hand, many patients in U.S. ICUs are not critically ill and, therefore, are not in need of an intensivist-led care team [54].

Current controversies in this area include: (1) whether round-the-clock intensivist staffing is required for quality care, (2) how many patients an intensivist should oversee care for, (3) whether an intensivist's role extends beyond the walls of the ICU, (4) whether to employ nonphysician providers and non-intensivist physicians in the ICU, and (5) whether regional intensive care centers and/or telemedicine are useful, safe, and effective.

24/7 Coverage by an Intensivist

Patients become critically ill 24 hours a day, 7 days a week. For this reason, having an intensivist present throughout the night hours is commonplace in Germany (81% of ICUs [55]); however, this staffing strategy is less frequently employed elsewhere around the world (3% of ICUs in the United Kingdom [56], 8% to 15% of ICUs in the U.S. [57–59], and 50% of ICUs in Thailand [60]). The evidence base is still incomplete and when taken together, shows that having an intensivist onsite overnight is not associated with improvements in patient outcomes. Before–after studies of onsite coverage overnight produced conflicting results—one found improvements in standardized mortality ratios whereas the other showed no difference in survival (albeit improvements in complications and ICU length of stay) [61–64]. However, for some, but not others, addition of such providers improved mortality for units with low daytime staffing intensity. A meta-analysis supported this lack of association of nighttime intensivists and meaningful patient outcomes [65]. Other studies found no association with the shiftwork model (including overnight onsite intensivist) and any measured patient outcome [66,67].

Intensivist-to-Patient Ratios

Higher staffing ratios, whether nursing or physician, should theoretically improve quality of care as care providers have more time to spend with each patient. But does the existing evidence support this idea?

In 2005, Dara et al. published a single-center observational study in an academic medical ICU in which the number of patients cared for by each intensivist changed over time from 2001 to 2003. In comparing intensivist-to-patient ratios of 1:7.5, 1:9.5, 1:12, and 1:15, there was no difference in hospital or ICU mortality, although a higher ICU length of stay was seen in patients whose intensivist cared for 15 people [38]. A survey conducted in 2012 by Ward et al. of U.S. Pulmonary and Critical Care Medicine fellowship directors revealed that the median number of patients each intensivist cared for in his/her unit was 13 (interquartile range: 10 to 16), with respondents reporting increased time constraints, stress, and difficulties teaching trainees as patient load increased [68]. Finally, in 2015, Neuraz et al. published a prospective observational study of eight ICUs in which they found that the relative risk of death for ICU patients was 2.0 (95% confidence interval: 1.3 to 3.2) for shifts in which an intensivist cared for >14 patients compared with one in which he/she cared for fewer [69].

In 2013, the Society of Critical Care Medicine concluded that "advocating a specific maximum number of patients cared for is unrealistic," yet cautioned that care must be taken to recognize the impact of staffing ratios on direct patient care, efficiency of ICU rounds, non-patient care–related activities, and trainee education.

Intensivists Outside the Walls of the ICU

When discussing a safe culture of critical care, it is important to remember that critically ill patients exist outside the walls of the ICU [70–72]. At times these patients are at the onset of their critical illness and, at others, they are awaiting transfer to an ICU—a situation known to be associated with poor outcomes [73,74]. Having an intensivist at the non-ICU bedside of these critically ill patients is a topic which has gained interest of late.

A common form of intensivist outreach is the rapid response or medical emergency team and consultation, which is called when a patient clinically deteriorates outside of the ICU [75]. Although staffing of these teams is inconsistent, many include an intensivist [76–78]. Notably, such teams are being employed more and more frequently in U.S. hospitals [79]. Data about these teams' impact on patient safety and outcomes are inconsistent [80–83], but, interestingly, satisfaction of ward staff is improved when they are available [84–86].

Non-intensivist Providers in the ICU

As safety demands consideration of drawing the intensivist out of the ICU, it also mandates consideration of whether it is safe to staff ICUs with providers other than traditionally-conceived-of intensivists.

Physician assistants and nurse practitioners have been increasingly involved in the care of ICU patients over the past two decades [58,87,88]. Although trained in vastly different manners, it is now possible for both types of providers to specialize in critical care (residency in critical care medicine for physician assistants [89]; acute care track for nurse practitioners [90]), and both providers can assume similar roles in the ICU. Several staffing paradigms have been explored, but a seemingly common one (and one examined in published studies) is the substitution of a nonphysician provider into a role traditionally assumed by house staff of academic ICUs. In several studies comparing a medical ICU staffed with nonphysician providers to one staffed with residents, there was no difference in outcomes, including mortality, length of stay, and discharge destination for survivors [91–93].

More recently, interest has risen in the United States about the use of non-intensivist attending physicians who demonstrate interest and receive training in critical care. In a joint position paper by the Society of Critical Care Medicine and the Society of Hospitalist Medicine, the potential merits of an expedited educational track for practicing hospitalists interested in critical care was detailed [94–97]. Finally, there are now pathways established through the American Board of Internal Medicine, the American Board of Surgery, and the American Board of Anesthesiology for emergency medicine residency graduates who complete a critical care fellowship to sit for the Critical Care Medicine board examinations [98]. Although relatively new, these initiatives designed to train a broader group of attending physicians in critical care will assuredly lead to the provision of safer care to more patients.

Alternative Strategies for Delivering Critical Care

Trained intensivists very likely improve the outcomes of critically ill patients [63,99], so there are pressures from various stakeholders to increase critical care physician coverage of ICUs. For instance, hospitals wanting to meet the standards of the Leapfrog Group (www.leapfroggroup.org) are required to have intensivists who manage or comanage ICU patients. These intensivists need to be: (1) present during daytime hours and exclusively providing care in the ICU, and (2) able to return pages at least 95% of the time within 5 minutes when not on site; or be available via telemedicine and arrange for an intensivist or physician extender to be available within 5 minutes. There is, however, a shortage of critical care physicians; thus, not all ICUs can be staffed to these standards [53,57,100].

One potential solution to the critical care workforce shortage is the regionalization of intensive care services in which high-risk patients can be transferred to centers of excellence [101–103]. Such regionalization has already occurred in the care of trauma patients and neonates [104].

It has been shown that the hospital volume of non-surgically mechanically ventilated patients correlates with improved outcomes (i.e., a positive volume–outcome relationship) [105]. Likewise, it may make sense to centralize aggressive life support therapies such as extracorporeal membrane oxygenation (ECMO). Data for widespread use of ECMO as a therapy for severe acute respiratory failure are lacking despite the positive results seen in the CESAR trial, a study in which patients were either randomized to transfer to a single site for possible ECMO or to conventional care at their originating center [106]. The call for ECMO to be studied and regionalized is supported by mixed results using ECMO during the 2009 H1N1 pandemic and a recent meta-analysis demonstrating a positive volume–outcome relationship [107–110]. Although it has been shown that the most critically ill, including those on ECMO, can be safely transported, it is not clear that regionalization is the best solution [111]. Strong data do not yet exist to show mortality benefit for regionalization of ICU services [112].

Intuitively, ICU telemedicine is appealing, and it makes sense that it should improve the outcomes of critically ill patients, but like regionalization, it requires further study [113]. At present, there are some data to suggest that ICU telemedicine improves outcomes in a variety of settings, whereas no data exist to show worsened outcomes [114–117]. Even in a well-staffed critical care system, the addition of a supplementary layer of telemedicine monitoring improved hospital, ICU mortality and length of stay, and adherence to critical care "best practices." [115]. Despite its theoretical and demonstrated advantages, ICU telemedicine has not been widely adopted. Between 2003 and 2010, the number of U.S. hospitals employing this strategy increased from 0.4% to 4.6%. Most of the expansion was in the first 4 years (101% growth), after which growth plateaued at 8.1% per year [118].

PHYSICIAN TRAINING AND DEVELOPMENT OF A CULTURE OF SAFETY

It is during residency training that physicians acquire not only their clinical knowledge, but also their familiarity with system-based practice attitudes toward patient safety. Because developing a culture of safety is one of the elements of solving patient safety issues, resident training is central to developing long-term solutions to patient safety problems. However, the ICU experience can be one in which residents themselves become a safety issue. Residents need to acquire the body of knowledge, skills, and experience necessary to function as attending physicians, and as part of this training they need to develop a culture of safety. Yet, lack of supervision, experience, and resident fatigue can adversely affect patient safety, especially in the ICU setting. It is thus useful to separate the issues of safety into those related to proper resident training, which affects the culture of safety in the long term, and those related to resident performance, which impacts patient safety in the short term.

Optimal resident performance requires adequate rest, supervision, and sufficient training to perform increasingly complicated problem-solving tasks. Each of these areas can contribute to safety as they represent potentially latent medical errors (errors due to the design of the educational system as well as the healthcare delivery system).

Fatigue has been associated with altered moods, depression, anxiety, confusion, anger, and most recently, impairment of clinical performance [119,120]. However, extended work hours and exhaustion among trainees were long-standing traditions in medical education and had often been the hallmarks of "excellence" in educational programs. In the past, workweeks of 120 hours and on-call shifts of 48 hours were not uncommon. Fatigue and long hours were likely some of the factors involved in the death of Libby Zion in New York City (http://www.washingtonpost.com/wp-dyn/content/article/2006/11/24/AR2006112400985.html; [121]). Because of this case, New York State instituted duty hour restrictions in 1989, based on the Bell Commission's recommendations that trainees could not work more than 80 hours per week, or more than 24 consecutive hours. Additionally, new requirements mandated that more senior physicians be present in the hospital 24/7. Responding primarily to public pressure and outside forces and with little high-level evidence, the Accreditation Council for Graduate Medical Education (ACGME) instituted standards which were similar to those of the Bell Commission in 2003, with further restrictions in 2011 [122,123]. Assumptions were made that patient safety and medical education would benefit from well-rested house staff.

Much of the existing research literature with regard to the effects of work hour restrictions has resulted from the changes implemented by the ACGME, rather than vice versa. A 2004 study found that medical interns made more serious errors in the critical care setting when working a "traditional" work schedule when compared with a work schedule in which extended shifts were eliminated and the number of hours worked per week was shortened [124]. There were concerns, however, about the need for attending physicians to make decisions based on second-hand information provided by covering residents, the need for attending hypervigilance, and compromised house staff education [125,126]. Other studies have either shown no benefit or worse outcomes with institution of the ACGME restrictions [127–129]. A systematic review by the ACGME was inconclusive and called for further high-quality research into the benefits and harms of work hour restrictions [130]. A survey of ICU Directors and Critical Care program directors (Medicine, Surgery, Anesthesiology, and Pediatrics) showed that there was a feeling that the mandated work hour restrictions adversely limited trainee education, professionalism, and patient care [131].

A prospective multicenter trial examining the effects of the ACGME work hour restrictions on surgical outcomes (Flexibility in Duty Hour Requirements for Surgical Trainees [FIRST] trial) demonstrated no variation in death rate or complications between hospitals with strict versus flexible adherence to ACGME rules, as long as total work hour limits were maintained [132].

Even when trainees have sufficient rest, they still require adequate training and supervision. The question becomes how to acquire sufficient experience while minimizing patient risks. Previous paradigms of critical care education have emphasized knowledge acquisition over performance. The most common educational tools in the ICU are teaching at the bedside and formal lectures. Although senior physicians are willing to change their approach to teaching, there are real barriers to innovative education. Clinical workload for attending physicians has increased, whereas resident availability for teaching has decreased, partly because of ACGME-mandated changes, and there is a lack of funding to offset lost clinical revenue for time spent teaching. On this front, attending physicians seem most open to incorporating web-based learning modules and simulations (computer-based and/or with a mannequin) [131].

Simulation can be used to train physicians in the cognitive, procedural, and problem-solving aspects of critical care. Simulation has been increasingly used as an effective tool for training in medical settings [120]. First pioneered by Edward Leap, who designed a flight simulator for pilots in the 1920s, simulators are used today by all commercial airlines, by astronauts, the military, and the nuclear power industry. Medical simulators today frequently incorporate computers and virtual reality, but it is important to recognize that simulation training does not necessarily imply use of a computer. Simulators have traditionally focused on cardiopulmonary resuscitation models and normal/abnormal heart sounds, but many forms of simulation training are becoming available. Other simulators relevant to the ICU include mechanical models of the airway to teach basic bronchoscopy as well as newer bronchoscopy simulators with virtual reality augmentation [133]. The type of simulator (computer driven, mechanical, or a combination) depends upon the task being learned. For critical care, tasks can be broadly grouped into cognitive tasks (e.g., management of acute respiratory failure and hemodynamic compromise [134], conflict resolution [135], mechanical procedural tasks (e.g., bag-valve mask ventilation [136], intubation [137,138], bronchoscopy [133], central line placement [139]), and team performance tasks (e.g., respiratory failure using the Anesthesia Crisis Resource Management [ACRM] course [140], Advanced Cardiac Life Support (ACLS) [141]). Simulation has been applied to all three areas.

The incremental benefit of simulation training as compared with standard teaching methods on real-life performance has been demonstrated in only a few studies [132,138,142]. However, there is a much larger body of evidence in which surrogate outcomes (not real-life performance per se) have been used to demonstrate the positive effects of simulation training. Surrogate outcomes from these cases have included measures of student confidence [138] or performance on a model [136–138,141]. On balance, although the current evidence base is still incomplete with only a few randomized trials documenting superior real-life performance after simulation training, it is reasonable to conclude that simulation training will play an increasingly important role in critical care education.

The advantages hypothesized for simulation include safety, efficiency, and availability. Intricate elements and potential complications of difficult procedures, as well as the response to equipment malfunction, can be selectively and repeatedly rehearsed. The ability to provide immediate feedback and team training is also enhanced. Employing simulation models may positively impact direct and indirect costs associated with training and educating personnel through reduced use of operating rooms, and may potentially reduce malpractice claims. It is anticipated that as the expense of such equipment diminishes, simulators will be increasingly adopted by medical school curricula and for residency training. The American Thoracic Society Skills-based Working Group has formalized recommendations for using simulation as an adjunct to traditional training [143].

The Agency for Health Care Quality and Research has made development of simulation devices and protocols an important priority. At the present time, there is only limited clinical evidence supporting the efficacy of simulators on improving patient-based outcomes such as length of stay and mortality.

REGULATION AND GOVERNMENT IMPACT ON PATIENT SAFETY

The role of governmental and nongovernmental regulation has increased during the past decade and has taken on an international scope. As the public has become more aware of the need for patient safety and quality improvement within healthcare, there have been many new regulatory and reimbursement initiatives originating from the public sector (federal and state governments and agencies [e.g., www.ahrq.com]), state and county health departments, purchasers, nongovernmental organizations (e.g., JC, ACGME), and international organizations (e.g., World Health Organization [WHO]). The hypothesis that significant mortality can be attributed to medical errors has facilitated the implementation of rules and guidelines. Regulatory efforts encompass rules and regulations, but also accreditation of organizations, certification of providers, and reimbursement programs based on patient safety processes and outcomes.

The CMS has adopted pay-for-performance reimbursement models [144] and non-reimbursement strategies for complications of care-related to specific "never events" [145]. Appropriate levels of regulatory oversight of patient safety research that ensures patient protection must be balanced against the need to acquire new knowledge necessary to improve patient care in the ICU [146]. Many regulatory initiatives seek to improve outcomes, but others may risk causing confusion and malaise for healthcare providers as they attempt to comply with conflicting rules, mandates, and guidelines, and thus may actually become impediments to patient safety. For example, national guidelines for sepsis management were recently incorporated into the CMS inpatient quality reporting requirements (posted QualityNet April, 2015). This spurred significant comment from the critical care and emergency medicine communities, given the rapid adjustment of guideline recommendations. As has been suggested, protocols that mandate certain physician behaviors may adversely affect diagnosis, antibiotic choices, utilization of invasive procedures, and consumption of critical care resources [147,148]. Two important trends are greater collaboration for developing safety efforts between relevant organizations and the emergence of international partnerships among regulatory organizations. These efforts may result in improved harmonization of standards and regulations.

In regard to physician-related accreditation and certification, the ACGME has included patient safety concerns in its resident program accreditation process, both when mandating duty hour limitations and for requiring the inclusion of patient safety in educational curricula. Likewise, the American Board of Medical Specialties requires evidence of practice improvement efforts for maintenance of certification. Regarding organizational-level regulations, the JC publishes an annual update of its national patient safety goals in support of their standards for accreditation, which include ICU-related processes of care [149]. In 2005, the JC and Joint Commission International were designated by the WHO as the first members of the WHO Collaborating Centre for Patient Safety Solutions. The Collaborating Centre has organized an international network to identify, evaluate, adapt, and disseminate patient safety solutions (http://www.ccforpatientsafety

.org/WHO-Collaborating-Centre-for-Patient-Safety-Solutions-continued/). This effort demonstrates the international intent to create links between key organizations and individuals with expertise in patient safety (accrediting bodies, national patient safety agencies, professional societies, and others).

Independent, not-for-profit organizations, such as the Institute for Healthcare Improvement (IHI), develop programs to accelerate improvement by promoting cultures for change, stimulating promising concepts for improving quality and safety, and assisting healthcare organizations to implement these new concepts. The IHI has had considerable influence on regulatory organizations with respect to adoption of IHI initiatives, such as ventilator bundles, central line bundles, sepsis bundles, intensivist staffing models, and rapid response teams (http://www.ihi.org/IHI/Topics/CriticalCare/IntensiveCare/Changes/IntensiveCareChangesIndex.htm). Because of the emphasis on swift promotion of promising new interventions, such organizations have occasionally endorsed interventions (such as tight glycemic control) prematurely, ahead of supporting evidence.

Other proposed areas of regulation include minimum nursing staffing ratios to meet workload demands [150] for Medicare-participating hospitals and limitations of excessive work hours for nurses and residents. Hospitals have been required to implement specific improvements and to develop a program for quality assessment. The IHI has also suggested that a patient safety officer needs to be an important component of all large healthcare organizations [151].

Safety is an increasingly pressing concern in the high-risk environment of the ICU. There is ongoing implementation of integrated and coordinated systems that identify patient safety problems and report them back to providers. Such systems can improve performance of the ICU as well as "their structure, processes and outcomes of care." ICU reporting systems identify trends and patterns that facilitate healthcare improvement and reduction in preventable medical incidents. Because safety and error prevention in the healthcare setting compares unfavorably with those of other industries, a major thrust has been to adopt strategies and technologies that have proved successful in other settings and to apply them to the ICU. Continuing to establish common definitions of healthcare-related safety concepts as well as systems for safety monitoring and reporting will improve individual and group capabilities, thus improving patient safety. Approaches that have been implemented to some extent in the ICU community include incident reporting, targeted monitoring of process of care and discharges, trigger tools and ICU audits. Integration of electronic ICU patient data—such as hospital admissions information, laboratory results, progress notes, imaging, and authentication data—with non-ICU patient data across a hospital's computerized medical record is a prerequisite for promoting patient safety. ICU organization and staffing models [152], team training efforts [153], and programs in critical care telemedicine all impact safety for the ICU and continue to be studied. Hospital and ICU designs, emphasizing patient and staff safety, as well as a focus on ICU location within the hospital (i.e., placement of the ICU adjacent to emergency departments and surgical suites to facilitate rapid transfer of unstable patients), and new informatics systems that electronically distribute filtered and targeted smart alarms will come under increasing review. Although regulation by public sector agencies will impact the safety of the critical care environment, developing a culture of safety through graduate and postgraduate medical education may prove to be even more important in achieving substantive and long-lasting quality improvement for critical care.

References

1. Kohn L, Corrigan J, Donaldson MS (eds): *To Err is Human: Building a Safer Health System*. Washington, DC, National Academies Press, 2000.
2. Berwick DM: Health for life 6 keys to safer hospitals. *Newsweek*, December 12, 2005, p 76.
3. Donabedian G: A evaluating the quality of medical care. *Milbank Mem Fund Q* 44[Suppl]:166, 1966.
4. Centers for Medicare and Medicaid Services: Hospital Quality Information Initiative. Available at: http://cms.hhs.gov/quality/hospital/hqii.asp. Accessed December 29, 2005.
5. Institute of Medicine: *Patient Safety: Achieving a New Standard of Care*. Washington, DC, National Academies Press, 2003.
6. Needham DM, Sinopoli DJ, Thompson DA, et al: A system factors analysis of "line, tube, and drain" incidents in the intensive care unit. *Crit Care Med* 33:1701, 2005.
7. Hofer TP, Kerr EA, Hayward RA: What is an error? *Eff Clin Pract* 3:261, 2000.
8. Runciman WB, Webb RK, Helps SC, et al: A comparison of iatrogenic injury studies in Australia and the USA. II: reviewer behavior and quality of care. *Int J Qual Health Care* 12:379, 2000.
9. Chang A, Schyve PM, Croteau RJ, et al: The JCAHO patient safety event taxonomy: a standardized terminology and classification schema for near misses and adverse events. *Int J Qual Health Care* 17:95, 2005.
10. Guarnieri M: Landmarks in the history of safety. *J Saf Res* 23:151, 1992.
11. Pronovost PJ, Thompson DA, Holzmueller CG, et al: Defining and measuring patient safety. *Crit Care Clin* 21:1, 2005.
12. Lohr KN, Schroeder SA: A strategy for quality assurance in medicare. *N Engl J Med* 322:707, 1990.
13. Institute of Medicine: *Crossing the Quality Chasm: A New Health System for the 21st Century*. Washington, DC, National Academies Press, 2001.
14. AHRQ: AHRQ's Patient safety initiative: building foundations, reducing risks. Interim Report to the Senate Committee on Appropriations. AHRQ Publications 04-RG005, 2003.
15. PSNet Patient Safety Net: Glossary. Available at: http://psnet.ahrq.gov/glossary.aspx. Accessed June 19, 2009.
16. Reason J: *Human Error*. New York, Cambridge University Press, 1990.
17. Reason J: Human error: models and management. *BMJ* 320:768, 2000.
18. Rothschild JM, Landrigan CP, Cronin JW, et al: The Critical Care Safety Study: the incidence and nature of adverse events and serious medical errors in intensive care. *Crit Care Med* 33:1694–1700, 2005.
19. Sax HC, Browne P, Mayewski RJ: Can aviation-based team training elicit sustainable behavioral change? *JAMA* 303(2):159–161, 2010.
20. Newman-Toker DE, Pronovost PJ: Diagnostic errors—the next frontier for patient safety. *JAMA* 301:1060–1062, 2009.
21. Pronovost P, Holzmueller CG, Needham DM, et al: How will we know patients are safer? An organization-wide approach to measuring and improving safety. *Crit Care Med* 34:1988–1995, 2006
22. Garland A: Improving the ICU: part 2. *Chest* 127:2165–2179, 2005.
23. Kaplan HS, Battles JB, Van der Schaaf TW, et al: Identification and classification of the causes of events in transfusion medicine. *Transfusion* 38:1071, 1998.
24. Heavner J, Siner J: Adverse event reporting and quality improvement in the intensive care unit. *Clin Chest Med* 36(3) 461–467 2015.
25. Needham DM, Thompson DA, Holzmueller CG, et al: A system factors analysis of airway events from the Intensive Care Unit Safety Reporting System (ICUSRS). *Crit Care Med* 32:2227, 2004.
26. Poniatowski L, Stanley S, Youngberg B: Using information to empower nurse managers to become champions for patient safety. *Nurs Adm Q* 29:72, 2005.
27. Romano PS, Geppert JJ, Davies S, et al: A national profile of patient safety in U.S. hospitals. *Health Aff (Millwood)* 22:154, 2003.
28. Zhan C, Miller MR: Excess length of stay, charges, and mortality attributable to medical injuries during hospitalization. *JAMA* 290:1868, 2003.
29. Agency for Healthcare Research and Quality: AHRQ Quality Indicators. Available at: http://www.qualityindicators.ahrq.gov/. Accessed June 19, 2009.
30. Rubin HR, Pronovost P, Diette GB: The advantages and disadvantages of process-based measures of health care quality. *Int J Qual Health Care* 13:469, 2001.
31. Leape LL, Cullen DJ, Clapp MD, et al: Pharmacist participation on physician rounds and adverse drug events in the intensive care unit. *JAMA* 282:267, 1999.
32. Wasserfallen JB, Butschi AJ, Muff P, et al: Format of medical order sheet improves security of antibiotics prescription: the experience of an intensive care unit. *Crit Care Med* 32:655, 2004.
33. Bates DW, Leape LL, Cullen DJ, et al: Effect of computerized physician order entry and a team intervention on prevention of serious medication errors. *JAMA* 280:1311, 1998.
34. Pestotnik SL, Classen DC, Evans RS, et al: Implementing antibiotic practice guidelines through computer-assisted decision support: clinical and financial outcomes. *Ann Intern Med* 124:884, 1996.
35. Pronovost PJ, Berenholtz SM, Ngo K, et al: Developing and pilot testing quality indicators in the intensive care unit. *J Crit Care* 18:145, 2003.
36. Krimsky WS, Mroz IB, McIlwaine JK, et al: A model for increasing patient safety in the intensive care unit: increasing the implementation rates of proven safety measures. *Qual Saf Health Care* 18:74–80, 2009.
37. Carson SS, Stocking C, Podsadecki T, et al: Effects of organizational change in the medical intensive care unit of a teaching hospital: a comparison of "open" and "closed" formats. *JAMA* 276:322, 1996.
38. Dara SI, Afessa B: Intensivist-to-bed ratio: association with outcomes in the medical ICU. *Chest* 128:567, 2005.
39. Sherertz RJ, Ely EW, Westbrook DM, et al: Education of physicians-in-training can decrease the risk for vascular catheter infection. *Ann Intern Med* 132:641, 2000.

40. Carayon P, Gurses AP: A human factors engineering conceptual framework of nursing workload and patient safety in intensive care units. *Intensive Crit Care Nurs* 21:284, 2005.
41. Tibby SM, Correa-West J, Durward A, et al: Adverse events in a paediatric intensive care unit: relationship to workload, skill mix and staff supervision. *Intensive Care Med* 30:1160, 2004.
42. Husch M, Sullivan C, Rooney D, et al: Insights from the sharp end of intravenous medication errors: implications for infusion pump technology. *Qual Saf Health Care* 14:80, 2005.
43. Zohar D: Safety climate in industrial organizations: theoretical and applied implications. *J Appl Psychol* 65:96, 1980.
44. Pronovost PJ, Weast B, Holzmueller CG, et al: Evaluation of the culture of safety: survey of clinicians and managers in an academic medical center. *Qual Saf Health Care* 12:405, 2003.
45. Pronovost P, Sexton B: Assessing safety culture: guidelines and recommendations. *Qual Saf Health Care* 14:231, 2005.
46. Kho ME, Carbone JM, Lucas J, et al: Safety climate survey: reliability of results from a multicenter ICU survey. *Qual Saf Health Care* 14:273, 2005.
47. Resar RK, Rozich JD, Simmonds T, et al: A trigger tool to identify adverse events in the intensive care unit. *Jt Comm J Qual Patient Saf* 32:585–590, 2006.
48. Lee GM, Kleinman K, Soumerai SB, et al: Effect of nonpayment for preventable infections in U.S. hospitals. *N Engl J Med* 367:1428–1437, 2012.
49. Pronovost PJ, Miller MR, Wachter RM: Tracking progress in patient safety: an elusive target. *JAMA* 296:696–699, 2006.
50. National Quality Forum: National Quality Forum - Intensive Care Endorsed Measures. Available at: http://www.qualityforum.org/home.aspx. Accessed February 28, 2017.
51. de Vos M, Graafmans W, Keesman E, et al: Quality measurement at intensive care units: which indicators should we use? *J Crit Care* 22:267–274, 2007.
52. Rhodes A, Moreno RP, Azoulay E, et al: Prospectively defined indicators to improve the safety and quality of care for critically ill patients: a report from the Task Force on Safety and Quality of the European Society of Intensive Care Medicine (ESICM). *Intensive Care Med* 38:598–605, 2012.
53. Angus DC, Kelley MA, Schmitz RJ, et al: Caring for the critically ill patient. Current and projected workforce requirements for care of the critically ill and patients with pulmonary disease: can we meet the requirements of an aging population? *JAMA* 284(21):2762–2770, 2000.
54. Kahn JM, Rubenfeld GD: The myth of the workforce crisis. Why the United States does not need more intensivist physicians. *Am J Respir Crit Care Med* 191(2):128–134, 2015.
55. Graf J, Reinhold A, Brunkhorst FM, et al: Variability of structures in German intensive care units – a representative, nationwide analysis. *Wien Klin Wochenschr* 122:572–578, 2010.
56. Wilcox ME, Harrison DA, Short A et al. Comparing mortality among adult, general intensive care units in England with varying consultant cover patterns: retrospective cohort study. *Crit Care* 18:491, 2014.
57. Angus DC, Shorr AF, White A, et al: Critical care delivery in the United States: distribution of services and compliance with Leapfrog recommendations. *Crit Care Med* 34:1016–1024, 2006.
58. Hyzy RC, Flanders SA, Pronovost PJ, et al: Characteristics of intensive care units in Michigan: not an open and closed case. *J Hosp Med* 5:4–9, 2010.
59. Parshuram CS, Kirpalani H, Mehta S, et al: In-house, overnight physician staffing: a cross-sectional survey of Canadian adult and pediatric intensive care units. *Crit Care Med* 34:1674–1678, 2006.
60. Chittawatanarat K, Bhurayanontachai R, Thongchai C, et al: Characters of physician and nurse staffing in Thai intensive care units (ICU-Resource I study). *J Med Assoc Thai* 97[Suppl 1]:S38–S44, 2014.
61. Blunt MC, Burchett KR: Out-of-hours consultant cover and case-mix-adjusted mortality in intensive care. *Lancet* 356:735–736, 2000.
62. Gajic O, Afessa B, Hanson AC, et al: Effect of 24-hour mandatory versus on-demand critical care specialist presence on quality of care and family and provider satisfaction in the intensive care unit of a teaching hospital. *Crit Care Med* 36:36–44, 2008.
63. Wallace DJ, Angus DC, Barnato AE, et al: Nighttime intensivist staffing and mortality in critically ill patients. *N Eng J Med* 366:2093–2101, 2012.
64. Kerlin MP, Harhay MO, Kahn JM, et al: Nighttime intensivist staffing, mortality, and limits on life support: a retrospective cohort study. *Chest* 147:951–958, 2015.
65. Wilcox ME, Chong CA, Niven DJ et al. Do intensivist staffing patterns influence hospital mortality following ICU admission? A systematic review and meta-analyses. *Crit Care Med* 41:2253–2274, 2013.
66. Garland A, Roberts D, Graff L: 24 hour intensivist presence: a pilot study of effects on ICU patients, families, doctors and nurses. *Am J Respir Crit Care Med* 185:738–743, 2012.
67. Kerlin MP, Small DS, Cooney E, et al: A randomized trial of nighttime physician staffing in an intensive care unit. *N Eng J Med* 368:2201–2209, 2013.
68. Ward NS, Read R, Afessa B, et al: Perceived effects of attending physician workload in academic medical intensive care units: a national survey of training program directors. *Crit Care Med* 40(2):400–405, 2012.
69. Neuraz A, Guerin C, Payet C, et al: Patient mortality is associated with staff resources and workload in the ICU: a multicenter observational study. *Crit Care Med* 43(8):1587–1594, 2015.
70. Durand M, Hutchings A, Black N, et al: 'Not quite Jericho, but more doors than there used to be'. Staff views of the impact of 'modernization' on boundaries around adult critical care services in England. *J Health Serv Res Policy* 15:229–235, 2010.
71. Halpern NA, Pastores SM, Oropello JM, et al: Critical care medicine in the United States: addressing the intensivist shortage and image of the specialty*. *Crit Care Med* 41:2754–2761, 2013.
72. Abella Álvarez A, Torrejón Pérez I, Enciso Calderón V, et al: ICU without walls project. Effect of the early detection of patients at risk. *Med Intensiva* 37:12–18, 2013.
73. Cardoso LT, Grion CM, Matsuo T, et al: Impact of delayed admission to intensive care units on mortality of critically ill patients: a cohort study. *Crit Care* 15(1):R28, 2011.
74. Harris S, Singer M, Rowan K, et al: Delay to admission to critical care and mortality among deteriorating ward patients in UK hospitals: a multicentre, prospective, observational cohort study. *Lancet* 385[Suppl 1]:S40, 2015.
75. Cretikos MA, Parr MJ: The Medical Emergency Team: 21st century critical care. *Minerva Anestesiol* 71:259–263, 2005.
76. Morris DS, Schweickert W, Holena D, et al: Differences in outcomes between ICU attending and senior resident physician led medical emergency team responses. *Resuscitation* 83:1434–1437, 2012.
77. Rothberg MB, Belforti R, Fitzgerald J, et al: Four years' experience with a hospitalist-led medical emergency team: an interrupted time series. *J Hosp Med* 7:98–103, 2012.
78. Repasky TM, Pfeil C: Experienced critical care nurse-led rapid response teams rescue patients on in-patient units. *J Emerg Nurs* 31:376–379, 2005.
79. Agency for Healthcare Research and Quality: Patient Safety Primers—Rapid Response Systems. https://psnet.ahrq.gov/primers/primer/4/rapid-response-systems.
80. McNeill G, Bryden D: Do either early warning systems or emergency response teams improve hospital patient survival? A systematic review. *Resuscitation* 84:1652–1667, 2013.
81. McGaughey J, Alderdice F, Fowler R, et al: Outreach and Early Warning Systems (EWS) for the prevention of Intensive Care admission and death of critically ill adult patients on general hospital wards (review). *Cochrane Database Syst Rev* 18:CD005529, 2007.
82. Laurens NH, Dwyer TA: The effect of medical emergency teams on patient outcome: a review of the literature. *Int J Nurs Pract* 16:533–544, 2010.
83. Winters BD, Weaver SJ, Pfoh ER, et al: Rapid-response systems as a patient safety strategy: a systematic review. *Ann Intern Med* 158:417–425, 2013.
84. Jones D, Baldwin I, McIntyre T, et al: Nurses' attitudes to a medical emergency team service in a teaching hospital. *Qual Saf Health Care* 15:427–432, 2006.
85. Bagshaw SM, Mondor EE, Scouten C, et al: A survey of nurses' beliefs about the medical emergency team system in a Canadian tertiary hospital. *Am J Crit Care* 19:74–83, 2010.
86. Niven DJ, Bastos JF, Stelfox HT: Critical care transition programs and the risk of readmission or death after discharge from an ICU: a systematic review and meta-analysis*. *Crit Care Med* 42:179–187, 2014.
87. Moote M, Krsek C, Kleinpell R, et al: Physician assistant and nurse practitioner utilization in academic medical centers. *Am J Med Qual* 26(6):452–460, 2011.
88. Riportella-Muller R, Libby D, Kindig D: The substitution of physician assistants and nurse practitioners for physician-residents in teaching hospitals. *Health Aff (Millwood)* 14(2):181–191, 1995.
89. Gonzales P: Physician Assistant Residencies. http://doseofpa.blogspot.com/2014/03/physician-assistant-residencies.html. Updated March 26, 2011. Accessed March 1, 2017
90. American Association of Critical-Care Nurses: Schools with Curriculums Verified for ACNPC-AG Certification. http://www.aacn.org/wd/certifications/content/aprn-approved-programs-adult-gero-np.pcms?menu=certification. Accessed February 28, 2017.
91. Dubaybo BA, Samson MK, Carlson RW: The role of physician assistants in critical care units. *Chest* 99(1):89–91, 1991.
92. Gershengorn HB, Wunsch H, Wahab R, et al: Impact of non-physician staffing on outcomes in a medical ICU. *Chest* 139(6):1347–1353, 2011.
93. Kawar E, DiGiovine B: MICU care delivered by PAs versus residents: do PAs measure up? *JAAPA* 24(1):36–41, 2011.
94. Siegal EM, Dressler DD, Dichter JR, et al: Training a hospitalist workforce to address the intensivist shortage in American hospitals: a position paper from the Society of Hospital Medicine and the Society of Critical Care Medicine. *Crit Care Med* 40:1952–1956, 2012.
95. Siegal EM, Dressler DD, Dichter JR, et al: Training a hospitalist workforce to address the intensivist shortage in American hospitals: a position paper from the Society of Hospital Medicine and the Society of Critical Care Medicine. *J Hosp Med* 7:359–364, 2012.
96. Pisitsak C, Champunot R, Morakul S: The role of the hospitalists in the workforce to address the shortages of intensivists in hospitals here in Thailand. *J Med Assoc Thai* 97[Suppl 1]:S132–S136, 2014.
97. Wise KR, Akopov VA, Williams BR Jr, et al: Hospitalists and intensivists in the medical ICU: a prospective observational study comparing mortality and length of stay between two staffing models. *J Hosp Med* 7(3):183–189, 2012.
98. Emergency Medicine Resident's Association: Critical Care Division. http://www.emra.org/committees-divisions/critical-care-division/. Accessed February 28, 2016.
99. Pronovost PJ, Angus DC, Dorman T, et al: Physician staffing patterns and clinical outcomes in critically ill patients: a systematic review. *JAMA* 288:2151–2162, 2002.
100. Milbrandt EB, Kersten A, Rahim MT, et al: Growth of intensive care unit resource use and its estimated cost in Medicare. *Crit Care Med* 36:2504–2510, 2008.
101. Ewart GW, Marcus L, Gaba MM, et al: The critical care medicine crisis: a call for federal action: a white paper from the critical care professional societies. *Chest* 125:1518–1521, 2004.

102. Nguyen YL, Kahn JM, Angus DC: Reorganizing adult critical care delivery: the role of regionalization, telemedicine, and community outreach. *Am J Respir Crit Care Med* 181:1164–1169, 2010.
103. Thompson DR, Clemmer TP, Applefeld JJ, et al: Regionalization of critical care medicine: task force report of the American College of Critical Care Medicine. *Crit Care Med* 22:1306–1313, 1994.
104. Kahn JM, Linde-Zwirble WT, Wunsch H, et al: Potential value of regionalized intensive care for mechanically ventilated medical patients. *Am J Respir Crit Care Med* 177:285–291, 2008.
105. Kahn JM, Goss CH, Heagerty PJ, et al: Hospital volume and the outcomes of mechanical ventilation. *N Engl J Med* 355:41–50, 2006.
106. Peek GJ, Mugford M, Tiruvoipati R, et al: Efficacy and economic assessment of conventional ventilatory support versus extracorporeal membrane oxygenation for severe adult respiratory failure (CESAR): a multicentre randomised controlled trial. *Lancet* 374:1351–1363, 2009.
107. Barbaro RP, Odetola FO, Kidwell KM, et al: Association of hospital-level volume of extracorporeal membrane oxygenation cases and mortality. Analysis of the extracorporeal life support organization registry. *Am J Respir Crit Care Med* 191:894–901, 2015.
108. Combes A, Brodie D, Bartlett R, et al: Position paper for the organization of extracorporeal membrane oxygenation programs for acute respiratory failure in adult patients. *Am J Respir Crit Care Med* 190:488–496, 2014.
109. Noah MA, Peek GJ, Finney SJ, et al: Referral to an extracorporeal membrane oxygenation center and mortality among patients with severe 2009 influenza A(H1N1). *JAMA* 306:1659–1668, 2011.
110. Pham T, Combes A, Roze H, et al: Extracorporeal membrane oxygenation for pandemic influenza A(H1N1)-induced acute respiratory distress syndrome: a cohort study and propensity-matched analysis. *Am J Respir Crit Care Med* 187:276–285, 2013.
111. Javidfar J, Brodie D, Takayama H, et al: Safe transport of critically ill adult patients on extracorporeal membrane oxygenation support to a regional extracorporeal membrane oxygenation center. *ASAIO J* 57:421–425, 2011.
112. Barnato AE, Kahn JM, Rubenfeld GD, et al: Prioritizing the organization and management of intensive care services in the United States: the PrOMIS Conference. *Crit Care Med* 35:1003–1011, 2007.
113. Kahn JM, Hill NS, Lilly CM, et al: The research agenda in ICU telemedicine: a statement from the Critical Care Societies Collaborative. *Chest* 140:230–238, 2011.
114. Breslow MJ, Rosenfeld BA, Doerfler M, et al: Effect of a multiple-site intensive care unit telemedicine program on clinical and economic outcomes: an alternative paradigm for intensivist staffing. *Crit Care Med* 32:31–38, 2004.
115. Lilly CM, Cody S, Zhao H, et al: Hospital mortality, length of stay, and preventable complications among critically ill patients before and after tele-ICU reengineering of critical care processes. *JAMA* 305:2175–2183, 2011.
116. Lilly CM, McLaughlin JM, Zhao H, et al: A multicenter study of ICU telemedicine reengineering of adult critical care. *Chest* 145:500–507, 2014.
117. Willmitch B, Golembeski S, Kim SS, et al: Clinical outcomes after telemedicine intensive care unit implementation. *Crit Care Med* 40:450–454, 2012.
118. Kahn JM, Cicero BD, Wallace DJ, et al: Adoption of ICU telemedicine in the United States. *Crit Care Med* 42:362–368, 2014.
119. Buysse DJ, Barzansky B, Dinges D, et al: Sleep, fatigue, and medical training: setting an agenda for optimal learning and patient care. *Sleep* 26:218–225, 2003.
120. Grenvik A, Schaefer JJ 3rd, DeVita MA, et al: New aspects on critical care medicine training. *Curr Opin Crit Care* 10:233–237, 2004.
121. Robins NS: *The Girl Who Died Twice: Every Patient's Nightmare: The Libby Zion Case and The Hidden Hazards of Hospitals*. New York, NY, Delacorte Press, 1995.
122. Nasca TJ, Day SH, Amis ES Jr, et al: The new recommendations on duty hours from the ACGME Task Force. *N Engl J Med* 363:e3, 2010.
123. Philibert I, Friedmann P, Williams WT, et al: New requirements for resident duty hours. *JAMA* 288:1112–1114, 2002.
124. Landrigan CP, Rothschild JM, Cronin JW, et al: Effect of reducing interns' work hours on serious medical errors in intensive care units. *N Engl J Med* 351:1838–1848, 2004.
125. Drazen JM: Awake and informed. *N Engl J Med* 351:1884, 2004.
126. Pennell NA, Liu JF, Mazzini MJ: Interns' work hours. *N Engl J Med* 352:726–728, 2005; author reply 726–728.
127. Frankel HL, Foley A, Norway C, et al: Amelioration of increased intensive care unit service readmission rate after implementation of work-hour restrictions. *J Trauma* 61:116–121, 2006.
128. Landrigan CP, Fahrenkopf AM, Lewin D, et al: Effects of the accreditation council for graduate medical education duty hour limits on sleep, work hours, and safety. *Pediatrics* 122:250–258, 2008.
129. McCoy CP, Halvorsen AJ, Loftus CG, et al: Effect of 16-hour duty periods on patient care and resident education. *Mayo Clin Proc* 86:192–196, 2011.
130. Philibert I, Nasca T, Brigham T, et al: Duty-hour limits and patient care and resident outcomes: can high-quality studies offer insight into complex relationships? *Annu Rev Med* 64:467–483, 2013.
131. Chudgar SM, Cox CE, Que LG, et al: Current teaching and evaluation methods in critical care medicine: has the Accreditation Council for Graduate Medical Education affected how we practice and teach in the intensive care unit? *Crit Care Med* 37:49–60, 2009.
132. Bilimoria KY, Chung JW, Hedges LV, et al: National cluster-randomized trial of duty-hour flexibility in surgical training. *N Engl J Med* 25:713–727, 2016.
133. Ost D, DeRosiers A, Britt EJ, et al: Assessment of a bronchoscopy simulator. *Am J Respir Crit Care Med* 164:2248–2255, 2001.
134. Schroedl CJ, Corbridge TC, Cohen ER, et al: Use of simulation-based education to improve resident learning and patient care in the medical intensive care unit: a randomized trial. *J Crit Care* 27:219 e7–219 e13, 2012.
135. Chiarchiaro J, Schuster RA, Ernecoff NC, et al: Developing a simulation to study conflict in intensive care units. *Ann Am Thorac Soc* 12:526–532, 2015.
136. Kory PD, Eisen LA, Adachi M, et al: Initial airway management skills of senior residents: simulation training compared with traditional training. *Chest* 132:1927–1931, 2007.
137. Kovacs G, Bullock G, Ackroyd-Stolarz S, et al: A randomized controlled trial on the effect of educational interventions in promoting airway management skill maintenance. *Ann Emerg Med* 36:301–309, 2000.
138. Lim TJ, Lim Y, Liu EH: Evaluation of ease of intubation with the GlideScope or Macintosh laryngoscope by anaesthetists in simulated easy and difficult laryngoscopy. *Anaesthesia* 60:180–183, 2005.
139. Britt RC, Novosel TJ, Britt LD, et al: The impact of central line simulation before the ICU experience. *Am J Surg* 197:533–536, 2009.
140. Lighthall GK, Barr J, Howard SK, et al: Use of a fully simulated intensive care unit environment for critical event management training for internal medicine residents. *Crit Care Med* 31:2437–2443, 2003.
141. Wayne DB, Butter J, Siddall VJ, et al: Simulation-based training of internal medicine residents in advanced cardiac life support protocols: a randomized trial. *Teach Learn Med* 17:210–216, 2005.
142. Crabtree NA, Chandra DB, Weiss ID, et al: Fibreoptic airway training: correlation of simulator performance and clinical skill. *Can J Anaesth* 55:100–104, 2008.
143. McSparron JI, Michaud GC, Gordan PL, et al: Simulation for skills-based education in pulmonary and critical care medicine. *Ann Am Thorac Soc* 12:579–586, 2015.
144. Rosenthal MB: Beyond pay for performance—emerging models of provider-payment reform. *N Engl J Med* 359:1197–1200, 2008.
145. Milstein A: Ending extra payment for "never events"—stronger incentives for patients' safety. *N Engl J Med* 360:2388–2390, 2009.
146. ARISE Investigators; Anzics Clinical Trials Group; Peake SL, et al: Goal-directed resuscitation for patients with early septic shock. *N Engl J Med* 371:1496–1506, 2014.
147. ProCESS Investigators; Yealy DM, Kellum JA, et al: A randomized trial of protocol-based care for early septic shock. *N Engl J Med* 370:1683–1693, 2014.
148. Kass N, Pronovost PJ, Sugarman J, et al: Controversy and quality improvement: lingering questions about ethics, oversight, and patient safety research. *Jt Comm J Qual Patient Saf* 34:349–353, 2008.
149. The Joint Commission: National Patient Safety Goals. Oak Brook, IL, The Joint Commission, 2009. Available at: http://www.JointCommission.org /PatientSafety/NationalPatientSafetyGoals/. Accessed June 18, 2009.
150. Carayon P, Alvarado CJ: Workload and patient safety among critical care nurses. *Crit Care Nurs Clin North Am* 19:121–129, 2007.
151. Institute of Healthcare Improvement: Patient Safety Officer Executive Development Program. Available at: http://www.ihi.org/IHI/Programs /ProfessionalDevelopment/PatientSafetyOfficerTraining. Accessed June 19, 2009.
152. Gajic O, Afessa B: Physician staffing models and patient safety in the ICU. *Chest* 135:1038–1044, 2009.
153. Dunn EJ, Mills PD, Neily J, et al: Medical team training: applying crew resource management in the veterans health administration. *Jt Comm J Qual Patient Saf* 33:317–325, 2007.

Chapter 135 ■ Assessing the Value and Impact of Critical Care in an Era of Limited Resources: Outcomes Research in the ICU

ANDREW F. SHORR • MARYA D. ZILBERBERG • DEREK C. ANGUS

During the last four decades, critical care has matured to a distinct medical specialty. Sepsis, respiratory failure, and the care of the complicated postoperative patients are now perceived as the purview of the intensivist. Concomitant with this evolution of critical care medicine has been a growing focus on health care outcomes. This emphasis on the end points and effects of medical care generally, and critical care specifically, reflects the realization that critically ill subjects face a high risk of death and that many interventions applied in the intensive care unit (ICU) are expensive. Some older studies estimate that nearly 1% of the gross national product of the United States is consumed in the ICU and, relative to days spent on hospital wards, others suggest that ICU costs are nearly three times greater [1,2]. More recent investigations suggest that less of the GNP is spent on ICU care, but concerns with the expense of ICU care continue [3].

Whether it is mechanical ventilation (MV), extensive nursing care, or acute dialysis, many of the technologies and medications used in the ICU are associated with substantial economic costs. In addition, some believe that ICU interventions only delay mortality rather than prevent mortality, or that mortality reduction in the ICU comes only at the price of significant morbidity. Thus, there is increasing pressure to carefully evaluate and to understand the results of ICU care. This pressure becomes even more evident when one considers that ICU outcomes must be evaluated from both patient and societal perspectives. In other words, the emphasis on outcomes in the ICU reflects an underlying question about value. In that vein, outcomes research reflects a systematic effort to address these issues and concerns. According to a position statement on outcomes research in critical care, "Outcomes research is employed to formulate clinical practice guidelines, to evaluate the quality of care, and to inform health policy decisions" [4]. Like clinical critical care, outcomes research draws on many different tools and expertise in multiple disciplines.

More than only an issue of economics, outcomes research requires expertise in psychology and anthropology (to understand patient and physician behavior), epidemiology (to identify disease patterns and burdens), and health services research (to appreciate process) [4]. Use of a term like *outcomes*, though, presupposes a question: Outcomes for whom? At the bedside, the clinician or the investigator focuses on pathophysiology of a sole patient. Outcomes research also addresses broader issues. Rather than being either centered on a particular disease or a physiologic measure, outcomes research deals with the overall results of care for the patient, for the family, and for society. Also in distinction to traditional clinical research, outcomes research has clear policy aspects as well; it attempts to facilitate debates about competing plans for resource allocation, research priorities, and national health policy. As an example, a randomized clinical trial deals with issues of efficacy (Does intervention "*x*" in a controlled environment have an independent impact?) and outcomes research is more concerned with effectiveness (What are the implications of intervention "*x*" applied outside a controlled setting and in the "real world" for the patient and society?). Traditional clinical research, moreover, often employs the experimental approaches, and observational methods that are routinely used in outcomes research.

In short, outcomes research attempts to use methods from the social sciences to augment the understanding of health care as opposed to using only methods from conventional "hard" sciences. As a recent summary regarding outcomes research for sepsis indicated, the outcomes researcher seeks to answer a question separate from traditional research [5]. The clinical investigator essentially asks, "Does this work?" and outcomes researchers deal with the concern, "Does it help?" [5]. Readers should note that outcomes research is now a key component of the biomedical enterprise. It is no longer seen as an option or an add-on. It fits with mechanistic and clinical work in building the triumvirate of information needed to translate research findings into clinical practice. The absence of outcomes studies can lead to the failure to adopt what otherwise might be useful interventions. The most recent policy example of the import of outcomes research in the United States is the efforts by the Centers for Medicare and Medicaid Services (CMS) to drive quality by altering hospital and physician reimbursements. This initiative, known as Value Based Purchasing, is a broad effort to enhance quality throughout the hospital. However, many of its components deal with issues directly related to ICU care. Concurrently, the federal government has now funded the Patient Centered Outcomes Research Institute (PCORI). PCORI was created as part of the Patient Protection and Affordable Care Act to help fund and lead research into comparative-effectiveness so that patients and clinicians can make better choices.

METHODS IN OUTCOMES RESEARCH

Outcomes research relies on multiple methods for exploring patient-centered concerns. Generally, researchers employ both qualitative and quantitative methods [4]. Qualitative approaches offer insight into complex processes that do not easily lend themselves to standard hypothesis testing. As such, qualitative work often results in the generation of important hypotheses for more formal testing. In other words, qualitative works, such as surveys of patient preferences, can form the foundation for quantitative modeling. Quantitative methods are more standard for outcomes research in critical care and have two general aspects. First, they use some tool to measure a particular outcome (e.g., mortality, quality of life, functional status, costs). Second, quantitative techniques then seek to compare the outcome of interest between at least two alternatives. Unlike the controlled environment of the bench laboratory or even the randomized controlled trial (RCT), outcomes research is necessarily exposed to multiple potential confounders that can and do affect the primary measure of interest. Because critical care outcomes research remains patient-centered, it is important to acknowledge that these subjects bring with them complexities that may alter their mortality, quality of life, and function. Moreover, the impact of these preceding factors may affect a researcher's end point of interest in ways that have little to do with the intervention under study. Similarly, after any intervention in the ICU, many post-ICU variables come into play that might affect the results of an outcomes study.

To address these complexities requires adoption of various techniques, all of which must be rigorous and reproducible. Therefore, outcomes research has relied on more than RCTs. RCTs are well suited for deciding if specific interventions or agents can alter an easily ascertainable end point such as mortality. For example, use of large sample sizes combined with both block randomization techniques and protocols for patient care help to ensure that the potential confounders previously noted are minimized and, in turn, allows one to explore questions such as how low tidal volume MV affects mortality at day 28. But if the policy or research query deals with the functional status or total cost of care for survivors of acute respiratory distress syndrome (ARDS) more than a year after their hospital discharge, one may require additional approaches. In any event, critical care outcomes research begins by defining a particular question. The investigator can subsequently determine which approach is most appropriate. In fact, sometimes outcomes research requires entirely separate study designs and major modifications to traditional models of clinical research or a combination of approaches. In other cases, more traditional models of investigation can be expanded to incorporate outcomes measures. This generally requires building these measures into the trial during the study inception phase. Currently, this is often done so that data needed for understanding the costs or societal implications of an intervention are gleaned at the same time as a primary trial is underway. This approach also facilitates the collection of information desired and often required by payers prior to decisions about coverage and reimbursement for novel therapies. Hence, outcomes research represents an extension and complement to standard research practices.

The advent and diffusion of electronic health records (EHRs) has fostered outcomes research generally. EHRs represent a rich source of data that can be examined as part of many research efforts, irrespective of methodology. The data captured in EHR can allow investigators to track patients, their resource use, and their outcomes across many transitions of care, while also providing information about multiple components of that care. The increasing reliance on EHRs also makes it simpler for investigators to amass significant amounts of data on larger cohorts of patients with relative ease. The larger sample sizes and more extensive data that one can glean from EHRs have made the EHR a major resource in outcomes research.

Observational Studies

Of the various types of observational studies (e.g., case series, case–control, cross-sectional, and cohort), two are particularly important in critical care outcomes. A cross-sectional design has the advantage of looking at one precise time or over a short period of time at a specific disease or practice. This snapshot-in-time approach can provide important insight into both epidemiology and aid health services research. For example, a recent 1-day international survey of respiratory failure in the ICU demonstrated the burden of this syndrome relative to other diseases treated in the ICU and also documented the wide range in practice style with respect to the use of MV [6]. The Sepsis Occurrence in Acutely Ill Patients (SOAP) study, a European sepsis registry using an essentially cross-sectional design (it covered a set 2-week period) confirmed the burden of sepsis in the ICU and underscored the variability in the use of various medical therapies in the care of these patients [7]. Hence, these cross-sectional analyses generated important information about the current state of affairs and therefore provided a potential benchmark for use in future comparisons. Cross-sectional studies also serve to provide important benchmark data so that changes over time can be more easily assessed. As an example, Esteban and coworkers [8] completed a similar point prevalence survey regarding the need for MV and were able to show how outcomes were improving over time via a cross-sectional study design.

In addition, cohort studies are valuable components of outcomes research. With this strategy, subjects are selected based on some common exposure (e.g., a diagnosis, a risk factor) and then observed [9]. Thus, cohort analyses may have the advantage of being prospective as compared to cross-sectional analyses. Cohort studies also specify a set starting time for the observations (e.g., time zero) from which observations proceed forward. Researchers can then look at the interplay of certain predefined risk factors or interventions and the characteristics that defined the cohorts to see how these affect the outcome. Often a cohort design is used either to describe the natural history of a disease, to assess quality of life, or to capture the real world outcomes associated with certain interventions/therapies (as opposed to what might be gleaned in the strictly controlled environment of a randomized trial). Although theoretically straightforward, cohort studies pose important challenges for the researcher. Selection bias and the inherent heterogeneity of critically ill patients can confound efforts to create a homogeneous cohort. Similarly, one needs to ensure means for capturing multiple potential exposure variables and acknowledge or model interaction between risk factors, exposures, and time which is complex when there are multiple confounders.

As Needham et al. [9] and Dowdy et al. [10] indicate in a review of methodologic issues associated with cohort studies, this study design has three key components: subjects, outcomes and exposures, and time. Subjects must be carefully identified, but the cohort study gives the researcher flexibility to define the population as sharing particular characteristics, such as common diagnoses, or risk factors. Alternatively, cohorts can be developed such that two groups emerge: individuals exposed to a particular event or variable and those not exposed. As a result, one can, using this technique, begin to draw conclusions about causal relationships. Generally, because the cohort shares some common time of designation (e.g., time zero) by observing the population one can evaluate the strength of the relationship between the given exposure and the outcome. Unlike the rigidity of an RCT, in which randomization works to ensure study groups are similar except for the intervention in question, a cohort design provides the researcher the opportunity to explore multiple exposures simultaneously, and how they interact with each other. To the point, in an RCT of a novel treatment for sepsis, any differences seen in outcomes should be a function of the particular intervention experimentally introduced, provided that randomization worked. The ICU organization, pre-ICU care, and posthospital events should not affect the outcome because randomization should ensure that the impact of these variables is equalized between the active and comparator groups.

The purpose of a cohort study is to enhance the RCT by providing information that cannot, by definition, be gleaned from the RCT. The caveat, of course, is that cohort studies are prone to confounding and may lack generalizability. Nonetheless, expanded adoption of cohort studies can also facilitate better understanding of natural history by shifting the focus back to a time prior to ICU admission. Without some initial work via a cohort approach, we face challenges when addressing significant questions relating to what determines which patients get admitted to the ICU, who most likely benefits from ICU care, and the outcomes for those never admitted to the ICU. Most importantly, cohort studies allow researchers to identify potential patterns and relationships which can suggest causal connections, and, which in turn, can serve as the foundation for future randomized trials. As an example, the initial work on the impact of delirium on ICU outcomes all derived from cohort work and then became the foundation for multiple subsequent interventional trials [11].

INTERVENTIONS AND END POINTS IN CRITICAL CARE OUTCOMES RESEARCH

Unlike traditional biomedical research, which looks at either novel technologic interventions (new drugs, new devices) or perhaps management strategies, the interventions studied in outcomes research are more diverse. Certain clinical measures have significant outcomes implications for the patient and society. However, managerial and organizational changes may be equally important. The issue of management and organization of critical care services is particularly acute at present, given current (and conflicting) data suggesting that the model of ICU administration affects both mortality and cost [12,13]. The question of organization and management is broader than simply whether one uses a closed, full-time intensivist model or a more traditional open ICU model. Under the rubric of organization and management are questions of nurse-to-patient ratios, the role for respiratory therapy, assessments of the impact of a dedicated critical care pharmacists, and the significance of and adherence to protocols and bundles in the care of the ICU patient. Measuring how these types of potential features of the ICU work and whether they help patients and society is perhaps as important a question as if a new molecule for sepsis alters mortality. Issues of management and organization can provide feedback to affect the conduct of traditional research. Whether it is studies of resuscitation strategies or rapid response teams, these types of interventions include service, delivery, and organizational aspects. If any one of these components of the trial collapses, the entire venture may be jeopardized.

Mortality

With respect to end points, mortality remains the center of investigative efforts because it has tangible meaning to the patient, to health care institutions, and to society. When outcomes research addresses mortality, it tries to do it in an appropriate context. In other words, the question of mortality begs the question of when? Is the appropriate timeframe survival to ICU discharge or to hospital discharge? Are these time points too myopic? Altering long-term mortality (e.g., 2 years after ICU admission) would be an admirable goal. Historically, 28-day all-cause mortality has served as the primary end point for trials in critical care. However, after some period of time it seems reasonable to postulate that occurrences and interventions in the ICU diminish in their impact while the patient's age [14] and health state prior to his or her ICU admission become the main drivers of outcomes. Thus, the issue revolves around the timeframe chosen for measurement and its likely mechanistic link to the intervention under evaluation [15].

It is important to be cautious, though, since one can artificially alter ICU mortality by early use of certain interventions (e.g., tracheotomy in order to facilitate transfer to a chronic ventilator care facility). Likewise, decisions about when to suggest withdrawal of care can alter the apparent timing of death in the ICU. The central limitation is that with all time-dependent end points, there can be confounding by multiple factors. As the recent American Thoracic Society position statement on outcomes research appropriately observes, "The 'correct' mortality endpoint depends on the specific research question, the mechanisms and timing of the disease and/or treatment under study, and the study design" [4]. In addition, if a disease state is not associated with significant mortality, use of this measure may simply fail to capture the value of a particular intervention. Finally, mortality as the sole end point of any research ignores the entire concern about morbidity and the tradeoff between mortality and morbidity. Focusing only on mortality fails to address the quality of life of the survivor and misses the potential for survival to be rated by some as even worse than death.

Mortality, moreover, has limitations as a tool for comparing outcomes across different ICUs. Although recorded and tracked nearly uniformly among ICUs throughout the world, ICU mortality is a relatively uninformative measure of ICU performance. Extensive variability exists in not only the types of patients admitted to different ICUs but also in admission and discharge policies [15]. Some ICUs serve as major referral centers for and receive multiple transfers from other hospitals. These patients tend to be sicker or in need of specialized care. Hence, the mortality rates of the ICUs that send these persons elsewhere may be artificially low compared to the ICUs that accept such high-risk cases. Similarly, ICUs with intermediate-care facilities can transition individuals out of the ICU at different rates than ICUs lacking access to these resources. This fact can alter apparent ICU mortality rates because one might essentially be able to transition patients receiving comfort care only out of the ICU so that when they die the death is not captured as an ICU-related event.

One could correct for these possible variables by employing a definition of ICU mortality (for benchmarking performance) that removed transfers from both the numerator and denominator of the crude mortality rate. Adjusting for differences for availability of "stepdown" wards can be made by limiting comparisons to like-sized hospitals. However, even these efforts would be insufficient for purposes of performance and quality assessments because issues of case-mix remain unaddressed. Case-mix as a concept tries to capture that different ICUs admit different types of patients with differing severity of illnesses. It is important to note that case-mix as a concept describes more than differences in disease severity [16]. Case-mix adjusting tries to balance issues with underlying diagnosis, comorbidity, age, and severity of illness [16]. To illustrate the breadth of the aspects related to case-mix, one need only consider an ICU that cared for only postoperative cardiothoracic patients should report low mortality rates and an ICU that admitted mainly immunocompromised persons would certainly describe different outcomes, even after one adjusted for severity of illness. As a corollary, comparing mortality between similar types of ICUs that admit similar types of patients, after controlling for disease severity, can prove helpful and identify potential outliers which require further investigation [16].

Severity of Illness Tools

To address disease severity, multiple tools exist. They differ with respect to the variables they measure, when they measure these variables, and if they try to describe ICU mortality or hospital mortality. The Acute Physiology and Chronic Health Evaluation (APACHE) score is commonly used in the United States and the Simplified Acute Physiology Score (SAPS) system is more regularly employed in Europe [17–19]. Severity of illness scores has been developed for application to specific types of patients (e.g., pediatrics, trauma) and others try to deal with a broader range of subjects. Other modeling systems include the Sequential Organ Failure Assessment (SOFA) score and the Multiple Organ Dysfunction Score [20,21]. A major limitation of all scoring systems is that they are developed and validated on large patient populations. Therefore, predicted mortality estimates for individual patients cannot and should not be translated into decisions at the bedside as to whether, based solely on predicted mortality, one should withhold or offer aggressive care. This is also true with severity of illness and prognostication tools developed for use in specific disease states that may require care in the ICU, such as the Pulmonary Embolism Severity Index (PESI) or scores developed to examine outcomes after ARDS [22,23].

Another concern with severity of illness tools as they relate to mortality is that some were initially created many years ago. Over time, new interventions and technologies have altered patient care and mortality. Hence, older iterations of certain models may no longer apply and no longer have adequate calibration to be informative. Like many scales, they require recalibration. As an example, the APACHE system is now on its fourth revision, and with APACHE II versus APACHE IVa, there are significant differences in terms of the explanatory power [24]. Nonetheless, in critical care research, many have adopted the APACHE II and III approach as its equations are published and free available (APACHE IVa remains proprietary and subject to purchase). Researchers and administrators need therefore be cautious when assuming that similar scores computed by an older rubric necessarily translate into similar predicted mortalities among populations or across ICUs. APACHE generally functions by exploring historical cohorts of patients and creating prediction scores based on this "control" population. Alternatively, one can also use the acuity measures used for these instruments to derive from predictions that are specific for the population of interest or under study.

Calculations of the actual scores for patients can also be prone to error. Several studies document significant interobserver variability among even trained researchers as to the calculation of severity of illness scores [25]. With APACHE II, one project revealed that the interrater agreement was strikingly poor ($\kappa = 0.20$) [26]. The main sources of variability appeared to be in assessment of the Glasgow Coma Score, but variability was evident even for the determination of the blood pressure. Changes in practice can also have unpredicted effects on severity of illness scores. Nearly all scoring systems rest on measurement of physiologic parameters such as blood pressure, platelet count, and hemoglobin. The more extreme the actual value from the "normal" range, the greater the negative impact of this factor on the individual's composite severity of illness score. As an example, low hemoglobin in the first 24 hours after ICU admission is associated with more APACHE II points than normal hemoglobin. Clinicians, though, may now be more tolerant of lower hemoglobin than they were when APACHE II was created. In fact, a restrictive transfusion strategy that necessarily allows the hemoglobin to drift lower may improve outcomes [27]. Consequently, APACHE II scores among ICU patients could rise over time, owing to changes in practice. This increase in APACHE II-predicted mortality when actual mortality might improve because of a change in clinical practice based on a large randomized trial underscores a significant assumption and limitation of severity of illness scoring classifications.

Severity of Illness and Performance Assessment

Mortality prediction equations can also result in calculation of a standardized mortality ratio (SMR) [15]. This ratio compares observed mortality to predicted mortality. Conceptually, the SMR can be calculated irrespective of the severity of illness system used to determine the predicted mortality. Ratios greater than 1 suggest excess mortality and those less than 1 imply enhanced survivorship. Implicitly, an SMR greater than 1 indicates an ICU with inferior outcomes after adjusting for severity of illness case-mix. Alternatively, though, differences in SMR can reflect more than quality. First, scoring systems may be generally imprecise (see previous discussion) and may not capture some aspects of disease severity or other case-mix issues. Second, the SMR can be affected by the quality of data collection and by the sample size. If the data collected is biased, then the calculations of predicted mortality may be incorrect. Likewise, if the sample size is small, the estimated confidence intervals around the SMR may be so wide as to reinforce the notion that the ICU in question is performing as predicted when there is a great likelihood that it is not. There is also discordance in the published literature exploring if and how well the SMR correlates with other markers of ICU quality. Some investigators suggest that the SMR sufficiently captures aspects of quality and others conclude that the relationship between other markers of quality and the SMR is less clear [15]. It is likely that no one SMR calculation method accurately reflects quality. Therefore, as policy makers, third-party payers, and patients demand simple report cards that allegedly capture quality, it is important that the intensivist resist the urge to simply publish SMRs without references to case-mix. Some more recent scoring systems address this (i.e., APACHE IVa) but still may be imprecise as they derive from periodically updated historical cohorts. We need to encourage the use of multiple measures beyond the SMR to describe qualitative differences in ICUs given these limitations of the SMR.

Nevertheless, the SMR can be used over time to assess interventions within an ICU or group of relatively homogenous ICUs [15]. Although one may not be able to conclude that SMR differences across institutions reflect true differences in quality and performance, when used as a benchmarking tool the SMR can be insightful. If one ICU has historical data about its case-mix and performance, it can then track over time how the SMR varies in response to interventions. Conversely, an increasing SMR can suggest the presence of some change in practice or structure that is adversely of positively affecting mortality. By identifying these trends and investigating them, ICU staff and administrators can elucidate potentially harmful or helpful changes that have transpired and attempt to address them.

The key limitation relating to the use of the SMR rests on the endpoint chosen. Is mortality to be measured at the ICU level or at hospital discharge? Again, as noted above, various models are calibrated for different time points. Calculating the SMR for the entire hospitalization with a tool designed only to look at ICU mortality can lead one to reach faulty conclusions. Several investigators have documented that if one looks at an SMR for only ICU events as opposed to all in-hospital deaths, one can reach vastly different conclusions about the relative quality of various ICUs [28-30].

Organ Failures

One effort to move beyond mortality as the primary outcome measure for critical care has been the evolution of the concept of organ failure-free days [3]. The free-day paradigm recognizes that reducing mortality in the ICU may not always reduce morbidity. In fact, reductions in mortality may only increase morbidity by keeping alive for several additional days patients who otherwise would have died but then, nonetheless, succumb to the acute illness. From a different vantage, some interventions may appear attractive on a superficial level because they decrease the duration of either MV or vasopressor support. However, a shorter duration of MV in one population may only reflect a higher death rate in that cohort. In other words, there is a competing impact of mortality in the assessment of such time-to-event (e.g., liberation from MV) phenomena.

These two facts promoted the development of the "failure-free" day paradigm. As a consensus conference on sepsis stated, this concept evolved out of a need to evaluate "the net effects of therapy" and to try to "integrate mortality with morbidity" [3]. Failure-free days are computed so that each day alive free of the organ failure in question is counted during the specified observation period. If a patient dies before the study termination or requires support beyond this time point, he or she is assigned 0 failure-free days. Historically, failure-free days are measured up to day 28 following the start of an investigation. The 28-day cutpoint, however, is arbitrary and reflects that most trials in critical care use the 28-day mark as the final date for ascertaining vital status. One could follow subjects out further if there were a biologically plausible reason to believe that the intervention under analysis could have an impact to that time point. As an example, if one were interested in MV-free days accrued during the 28 days following a patient's enrollment in a study and the patient died on day 7 while still on MV, he or she would be credited with no ventilation-free days. If the individual required 7 days of ventilation and was alive at day 28, he or she would have earned 21 MV-free days. If remaining on the ventilator for all 28 days, no ventilator-free days would accrue.

The failure-free-day approach has the potential advantage of capturing morbidity that transpires outside the ICU, such as the need for continued dialysis, as it is organ system–specific rather than defined purely based on the subject's location of care. It can further account for shifts in a patient's clinical status that might not be measured accurately if a researcher only recorded mortality. A patient with chronic obstructive pulmonary disease, for instance, might require 2 days of ventilatory support initially, be liberated from MV, but then several days later deteriorate and need to be placed back on ventilatory support. This waxing and waning clinical status can potentially be accurately described from an outcomes perspective with the use of ventilator-free days.

Is it appropriate to pool death with requiring 28 days of MV but still surviving? The fundamental struggle in this question illustrates why organ failure-free days can only be used as an adjunct to other measures of outcomes in critical care. It is certainly not clear that organ failures correlate with meaningful clinical outcomes or if surviving 28 days on a ventilator with a respiratory organ failure is comparable with death. On the other hand, the concept of organ failure-free days allows one to examine if and how a novel approach or therapy might accelerate recovery. In turn, it lays the foundation for the use of pooled end points in clinical trials in critical care. If mortality remains the only primary end point for studies in critical care, then investigators may fail to pursue options that may prove valuable in other ways. The organ failure-free-day concept also allows one to capture the effect of interventions on markers of resource utilization and cost. Differences in the use of ventilation, dialysis, and vasopressors have important implications for patients. Simultaneously, because of the costs associated with these interventions, decreasing organ failures and morbidity has ramifications for health care institutions, third-party payers, and policy makers. Future work in this area may in fact move beyond organ failure and try to develop metrics that incorporate this with mortality into a form of quality-adjusted survival measure. At present, the concept of the organ failure-free day is often recorded as a secondary endpoint in trials of dealing with sepsis, pneumonia, and respiratory failure. However, because of the issues noted above, it generally is not considered sufficiently robust to serve as a primary endpoint.

Health Status

From the patient's perspective, surviving the ICU raises many issues. Most patients will require some additional time for further recovery along with the potential need for rehabilitation. Moreover, some physical impairment persists after ICU care, and this impairment can affect functional status, mental health, and quality of life. Globally, each of these concepts (functional state, mental health, quality of life) all attempt to capture the concept of health status. The need for adequate assessments of health status is made more acute given the limitations of a sole focus on mortality.

Readers should note that, although the concepts are intertwined, functional status (either physical or mental) is distinct from quality of life. Functional status depicts the subject's capacities; in contrast, quality of life attempts to gauge an individual's satisfaction and state of well-being. As a result of this subtle distinction, someone who has a major functional limitation may rate his or her quality of life as high while another patient with relatively minor limitations might describe his or her quality of life as poor. Moreover, quality of life essentially relies on using the individual as his or her own control even if the plan is to eventually compare quality of life between patients. Persons are asked to rate their quality of life relative to what they perceive it was prior to needing ICU therapy. Functional status, on the other hand, generally measures capabilities relative to a fixed scale of performance that is set irrespective of what the person's prior functional status might have been. As such, functional status tends to be more objective. Quality of life, alternatively, is influenced by a person's values, perceptions, and preferences [31]. Quality of life is also measured in a social context. Assessing an ARDS survivor's lung function provides no insight into how having physical limitations after surviving ARDS alters one's interactions with their family and friends.

Functional status captures physiologic assessments of impairment along with global and mental/neuropsychologic performance. Early outcomes studies after critical care and functional status explored the long-term pulmonary complications of ARDS [32]. Researchers examined how gas exchange and radiographs varied over time in ARDS survivors. Other investigators have used general measures of functional status to describe survivors of ICU care [32]. Often-used tools for this include the 6-minute walk test and the activities of daily living (ADL) system. ADL assessments as a tool have the advantage of being widely familiar to clinicians and easy to implement. Some, though, question their applicability to critical care outcomes [32]. ADLs may be of limited value because they were developed specifically for the elderly. Young survivors of critical illness may recover to a state of function beyond what the ADLs generally capture. The information that does exist indicates that severe functional impairment results following ICU care and that it may resolve slowly. For example, Herridge et al. [32], in a prospective observational analysis of ARDS survivors, noted that only 50% had returned to work by 1 year and many reported persistent limitations of their ADLs.

Evaluation of cognitive impairment complements appraisals of functional status. Again, because of the difficulty in assembling cohorts of critical care survivors, the heterogeneity of these patients, and the lack of validated tests appropriate for ICU survivors, limited information exists regarding this as an outcome parameter. In a comprehensive review of this issue, Hopkins and Brett [33] reported that at 1 year, nearly a third of ARDS patients had cognitive limitations. A more recent study of a cohort of 51 ICU subjects suggested that 35% of these subjects scored at or below a level similar to the lowest fifth percentile of a normal population [34]. However, over time, 95% had experienced significant improvements of cognitive function [34].

The implications of persistent cognitive impairment are significant because they may portend difficulties with future employment and return to work. Hence, improved evaluations of cognitive recovery after critical illness in clinical trials, and the time course of that recovery, may help identify interventions that can have major implications for our patients. Again, if not incorporated into outcomes research, one cannot determine if and how ICU care affects this variable. Likewise, it seems that different approaches to care in the ICU can alter neuropsychologic recovery from critical illness. Specifically, posttraumatic stress disorder (PTSD) is an emerging concern in outcomes research. The incidence of PTSD following an ICU course is unknown, but some survivors report disturbing memories and meet the clinical criteria for PTSD. Outcomes researchers have linked the development of PTSD to previous delusional memories while hospitalized, suggesting that our approach to sedation during the acute phase of a subject's illness can affect the rates of PTSD [35]. Confirming this, Kress et al. [36] observed that the incidence of PTSD approached 33% in persons randomized to standard sedation practices in the ICU and there was no PTSD in those allocated to a strategy relying on a daily interruption of sedation. The strongest evidence documents the significance of PTSD on patients, and thus ICU outcomes, derives from work that describes the "post-sepsis syndrome (PSS)." PSS describes a range of various impairments neurocognitive and other impairments that substantially affect post-ICU recovery and functioning. For example, beyond PTSD, many patients may suffer from cognitive impairments which specifically relate to higher-order thinking and executive functions. Depression and anxiety also are prevalent among ICU survivors [36].

Quality of Life

In distinction to functional parameters such as the 6-minute walk distance or even cognitive function, estimating quality of life poses several unique challenges. Determining both the validity and reliability of quality-of-life measures, for example, is difficult. In addition, quality-of-life evaluations represent an intersection of clinical science with social science because many of the tools for rating quality of life rely on psychometrics for their theoretical foundations. Furthermore, the results of quality-of-life determinations can be affected by who is asking the questions and how they are asked. Research documents clearly that a patient and his spouse may score the patient's quality of life differently.

In general, quality-of-life tests attempt to score this on some form of a scale, which may be either continuous or categorical. The survey tool itself is often composed of select items that ask about certain aspects of life, functionality, quality, and so forth [37]. Items that inquire about certain, specific categories or aspects of quality of life are considered to fall within the same domain. Examples of domains routinely used to classify quality of life include pain and impairment, functional status, social role, satisfaction, and death (as death may be viewed by some as worse than surviving). In reporting the results of quality-of-life testing, both aggregate scores and scores within a certain domain may be reported. The aggregate score often gives a sense of the overall health-related quality of life. Breaking out scores across the various dimensions can presents a profile of how an illness impacts different aspects of quality of life. In addition, two distinct types of quality-of-life data are regularly collected: health profiles and utility measures [37].

In contrast to quality of life measures, utility measures represent the preferences of groups of individuals who share certain common characteristics, such as exposure to like treatments or similar underlying disease states. Quality-of-life scales may be either generic or disease-specific. Generic scales, such as the Sickness Impact Profile (SIP) or the Short-Form 36 (SF-36), have been developed in large diverse populations so that normal values are available [37]. Using these types of instruments allows comparisons across multiple disease states and various populations. Disease-specific instruments, such as the St. George's Respiratory Disease Questionnaire, may be better calibrated to detect changes over time as they focus on only one disease state or organ system [37]. These disease-specific measures are also focused on aspects of quality of life that may be of most concern to that specific group of patients. In other words, there is a tradeoff among rubrics between generalizability and resolution. Therefore, understanding critical care outcomes and ICU care's impact on quality of life necessitates studies using both approaches. Examples of various quality-of-life measures are shown in Table 135.1.

Despite using differing tools, examination of different types of patient cohorts, and issues with follow-up evaluation, most quality-of-life research indicates that this is substantially impaired initially in ICU survivors. For example, Tian and Miranda [38] evaluated more than 3,500 ICU patients 1 year after initial admission. Employing the SIP, they observed that scores were substantially reduced among survivors. The main source of the impairment in quality-of-life assessment arose in the area of physical functioning. Interestingly, there was no correlation between the extent of the limitation of quality of life and either severity of illness at ICU admission or the duration of stay in the ICU. Others have confirmed this observation that severity of illness does not explain the limited quality of life reported by some persons. In a cohort of elderly survivors of prolonged MV, Chelluri et al. [39] observed that initial severity of illness as measured by the APACHE III score failed to explain both subsequent functional limitations and lower quality-of-life scores during the year following ICU discharge. Using the SF-36 rather than the SIP, Heyland et al. [40] concentrated on sepsis survivors. Compared to the general U.S. population, scores were significantly lower for nearly all domains. Both physical functioning and social functioning were rated at approximately two-thirds the level noted in a general U.S. sample. However, when analyzed against a cohort of subjects with chronic disease such as either chronic obstructive pulmonary disease or congestive heart failure, the self-reported quality of life of sepsis survivors was similar.

More recent studies have explored how quality of life changes over time after ICU discharge. Most surveys of quality of life represent cross-sectional efforts measuring this at only one time point and therefore provide little information about rates of change in quality of life or how pre-ICU quality of life affects quality of life after discharge. Addressing these limitations, Cuthbertson and coworkers [41] prospectively followed 300

TABLE 135.1

Examples of Quality-of-Life Measures

Name	Goal	Description	Concepts assessed
Sickness Impact Profile (SIP)	To assess health-related dysfunction	36 items in 12 domains	Physical, psychosocial, other (e.g., sleep, rest)
Short-Form 36 (SF-36)	Survey of general health status	36 items in eight domains and a summary score	Physical, mental
Nottingham Health Profile	To determine perceived physical, social, and emotional health	Initial part of 38 items and second section of seven items	Physical mobility, energy, pain, social isolation, emotional
Euroquol	To measure health state and to determine preferences for 14 hypothetical health states	Five items measured at three levels	Physical and mental functioning

Adapted from Chaboyer W, Elliot D: Health-related quality of life in ICU survivors: review of the literature. *Intensive Crit Care Nurs* 16:88–97, 2000.

consecutive patients admitted to their ICU. They measured quality of life using two different tools at 3, 6, and 12 months after ICU discharge. At 3 months, quality of life was substantially reduced compared to the subjects' premorbid states. During the ensuing year, quality of life improved and approached the pre-ICU level. Unfortunately, at 1 year, the quality of life of survivors still remained lower than that reported for a general population. Among 109 persons with ARDS, Herridge et al. [32] reported similar patterns in the recovery of quality of life. During 12 months, scores on the SF-36 for physical functioning doubled and those for social functioning rose by 75%.

Several general themes appear in the quality-of-life literature relating to ICU care. First, quality of life is substantially impaired in ICU survivors, but this improves with time after ICU discharge. Second, despite changes in quality of life, this may not return to preadmission levels and the time course of recovery may be slow. Third, it is unclear what factors contribute to the quality of life of ICU survivors and how interventions in the ICU can affect subsequent quality of life.

Hence, many issues remain unresolved in this area of critical care outcomes research. Plaguing efforts to better comprehend this important patient-centered measure are multiple methodologic issues. As one systematic review of quality-of-life studies concluded: "There is no agreement as to the optimal instrument and (that) differences between studies preclude meaningful comparisons or pooling of results" [41]. These concerns explain why there has been a paucity of work in this area and why one group of investigators observed that fewer than 2% of all articles dealing with general critical care published from 1992 to 1995 dealt with this topic [37]. Despite all these concerns, an expert panel on surviving sepsis endorsed the SF-36 as best suited for outcomes research for sepsis patients who received critical care [4].

More recent work with SF-36 among ICU survivors provides some striking observations about survivors relative to population controls. Orweilus et al. examined quality of life among nearly 800 ICU survivors of different ICUs. Compared to nearly 7,000 controls matched for age, gender, and comorbidities, the authors found no significant difference in quality of life between the groups. On the one hand, this is encouraging news. Alternatively, given the prevalence of PTSD and post-sepsis syndrome, the conclusion that ICU survivors pay no quality-of-life penalty lacks face validity for some. Hence, the issue may be that the SF-36 fails to capture important aspects of HRQL that are unique to survivors of critical illness [42].

In an effort to address this and to simultaneously deal with issues related to quality of life while hospitalized in the ICU, some researches have attempted to design and validate tools for use in the ICU. These tools are specifically targeted for application during critical illness and may even be completed for mechanically ventilated patients. As an example, Pandian and colleagues [43] created such a tool and found that it correlated well with other accepted quality-of-life assessment measures.

ECONOMIC OUTCOMES

A final aspect of critical care outcomes deals with economic and financial issues. The ICU remains a major focus for concerns relating to cost. Part of this arises from the fact that many expensive technologies are applied in the ICU. Simultaneously, ICU bed days are disproportionately expensive compared with costs related to general ward bed days. Adding to increased costs is a growing demand for ICU care. With the aging of the population, the need for critical care resources will escalate. For example, during the next several decades, the incidence of severe sepsis and septic shock has been projected to rise by 30% [44].

Relative to the entire U.S. economy, it was estimated that, approximately two decades ago, ICU costs accounted for nearly 1% of the nation's gross national product [1]. In a similar analysis, total critical care costs by the year 2000 had nearly tripled from 1984 and now exceeded $55.5 billion annually [3]. As a function of the national economy, however, the proportion of the gross domestic product devoted to the ICU had decreased to 0.56% [3]. Despite this relative fall in the resources consumed by critical care, which essentially reflects the faster growth of the overall U.S. economy compared to ICU expenditures, the ICU now accounts for one in seven dollars spent on hospital care in the United States [3]. On a per-day basis, the most recent analyses indicate that costs for the initial day of MV in the ICU exceed $10,000 and fall to $4,000 per day by ICU day 3 when most subjects are clinically stable [2]. In short, from any perspective, whether societal or local, critical care remains exceedingly expensive.

Although the amounts cited above describe estimated costs generally, it may be that costs vary by admitting diagnosis. This is most clear in the case of ARDS. Bice et al., [45] in a review of costs and outcomes related to ARDS, convincingly document that direct health care costs related to ARDS (to include both fixed and variable costs) are higher than those for other patients needing mechanical ventilation in the ICU.

As a result of this economic pressure, patients, physicians, third-party payers, and policy makers are all demanding improved efficiency and optimization of resource allocation. In the United Kingdom, formal cost analyses have become the purview of regulatory agencies, and recommendations from these authorities influence the adoption of new therapies. In the United States, legislation to require formal economic analyses for the approval of new pharmaceuticals is under consideration. Critical care practitioners, therefore, require an appreciation of economics and finance in order to advocate for their patients and the resources they need to care for the critically ill. The need to appreciate the financial and economic aspects of care is even more acute now in the United States since CMS has continued to expand its value-based purchasing program.

A Primer on Economic Analysis

Economic analysis represents a means for understanding and appreciating value in order to facilitate the efficient allocation of limited resources in light of competing claims for those resources. In many scenarios, the criteria employed to determine how to spend limited dollars may not be evident or may be filled with assumptions and biases. The essential goal of economic analyses is to make explicit both the means and criteria used for decision-making. Reflecting the growing significance of economic issues, multiple formal position statements now exist describing both the means to conduct and the implications of financial studies for health care [46,47].

There are several basic varieties of economic analyses in health care: cost-minimization, cost-benefit, cost-effectiveness, and cost-utility. Cost-minimization presupposes that the outcome of interest is fixed and competing approaches are equally efficacious. The main issue, therefore, is which alternative costs less. In critical care, though, few interventions achieve similar results, so a more complex means for comparing options is required. When both costs and outcomes differ, it is necessary to assign the distinct options a value in some common schema (such as dollars). After converting potential results of interventions into dollars, one can proceed with cost-benefit analyses. Cost-benefit analyses are rarely used in health care because many end points are not easily converted into dollar values (e.g., the dollar value of a life) and because cost-benefit approaches may inadvertently assign more value to those who have higher earning potential. Cost-effectiveness acknowledges the limitations of cost-benefit and thus leaves the outcome (or denominator) in clinical terms such that one is now comparing costs per common measure of effectiveness. Often-used examples of this for critical care explore costs per year of life saved or per ICU days avoided. Cost-utility analysis builds on cost-effectiveness analysis by adjusting the clinical outcome for the quality that results from the intervention.

The standard denominator for these types of studies is the quality-adjusted life-year (QALY). The QALY concept acknowledges that a year of life spent in a long-term ventilator facility is not viewed by the patient as being of the same quality as a year lived being fully independent. Although arbitrary, most consider cost-effective interventions that yield a price per QALY saved of between $50,000 and $100,000.

One source of confusion and controversy in economic analyses is estimation of costs. Given the market structure of health care, charges rarely reflect costs. In fact, formal means exist to convert charges to costs based on published cost-to-charge ratios. Analytically, costs can be computed through microcosting, in which the unique costs for each component of care are determined and then summed. Costs can also be estimated based on average bed-day costs. Both approaches have limitations: Microcosting may underestimate the fixed costs associated with care delivery and a bed-day approach assumes that costs remain similar despite the intensity of care the patient requires.

Any conversation about cost, though, has an underlying central question: Cost to whom? This issue of perspective is key in all economic analyses. Some intervention may appear cost-effective to an institution because it shifts costs to a third-party payer. For the payer, though, the intervention will be seen as less than optimal. To address this fact, formal recommendations for the conduct of cost-effectiveness analyses encourage adoption of a societal perspective [46,47]. Utilization of a common societal perspective can also facilitate comparisons across alternatives. However, in critical care, a societal perspective poses specific challenges. As one review notes: "The societal perspective forces consideration of outcomes and costs not usually considered in critical care studies and a time horizon longer than most critical care studies" [47].

Uncertainty represents a final aspect of cost-effectiveness and outcomes that merits mention. All estimates for any study's inputs are bracketed by assumptions and uncertainty. The issue then becomes how one's conclusions are affected by this inherent uncertainty. If the costs of an ICU day are half what one assumes, does it alter the outcome of an analysis? Determining the impact of this uncertainty is best done through sensitivity analyses. Sensitivity analysis is a tool for varying a model's inputs across a range of assumptions and seeing if and how the results vary in response to this. If introducing such variability fails to affect the conclusions, one can be more confident as to the strength of the outcomes.

Disease-Specific Costs

Multiple studies in the last several years have attempted to gauge the costs of various diseases commonly encountered in the ICU. These reports help provide estimates of disease-state costs, which can be then used for cost-effectiveness analyses of preventive interventions or be relied on for budget planning.

With respect to nosocomial infection, Warren et al. [48] calculated the attributable cost of a catheter-related blood stream infection (CRBSI) to be nearly $12,000 per event. Their study prospectively followed a cohort of critically ill subjects and compared those developing CRBSIs to those not suffering this complication. In addition, they controlled for multiple potential confounders such as severity of illness, use of MV, and need for dialysis. Blot et al. [49], in a retrospective case-controlled study in Europe, reached similar conclusions. They reported that a CRBSI significantly prolonged the duration of MV and ICU length of stay and resulted in net excess costs totaling €14,000 [49].

Reflecting these high costs, multiple preventive strategies have been shown to be cost-effective. In an analysis of a multifaceted educational intervention emphasizing the pathogenesis, implications, and prevention of CRBSI, researchers from Washington University demonstrated that their efforts saved approximately $500,000 during the course of a year [50]. Likewise, use of chlorhexidine rather than povidone, adherence to the need for full barrier drapes, and adoption of antibiotic-impregnated catheters have been shown to yield net savings despite their initially high acquisition costs.

Ventilator-associated pneumonia also represents a common and costly ICU-acquired infection. Rello and coworkers [51] observed that the costs of this disease exceeded $40,000 per case. This analysis, though, was limited because it was a retrospective assessment of a large administrative database such that the definition of pneumonia employed might have led to selection bias. Alternatively, Warren et al. [52], in a prospective study of a community ICU, suggested that the costs of ventilator-associated pneumonia were similar to those reported by Rello et al. Hence, two distinct studies using different approaches reached similar conclusions.

For non-ICU acquired processes, community-acquired pneumonia (CAP) represents a major driver of national health care expenditures by the U.S. government. Describing outcomes in a cohort of patients with severe CAP, Angus et al. [53] suggested that persons with CAP needing ICU care generated total hospital costs in excess of $21,000. Strikingly, this amount was more than three times greater than the costs for inpatient CAP not needing ICU admission. From a societal perspective, Kaplan et al. [54] reviewed data from Medicare and calculated that national ICU costs for CAP surpassed $2.1 billion. The financial implications of sepsis are also staggering. Multiple reports document hospital costs per case at approximately $30,000 to $40,000 [55,56]. An analysis by Shorr and coworkers [57] suggested that the costs per case for severe sepsis exceeded $30,000 per case with survivorship being associated with lower per-patient costs. Costs in Europe were seen to be somewhat lower than those noted in the United States. For example, Adrie et al. [58] prospectively recorded costs for sepsis in six French ICUs. The mean cost of severe sepsis equaled €22,800. They further described that sepsis costs varied based on whether the infection was community-acquired or evolved while the subject was hospitalized. In attempting to determine cost drivers in sepsis, Burchardi and Schneider [59] reviewed multiple costing reports and concluded that direct costs account for only 20% to 30% of overall costs in sepsis.

Cost-Effectiveness Studies in Critical Care

Coincident with the growing interest in cost-containment in critical care has been a rise in the number of formal cost-effectiveness analyses published in this field. Examples of such analyses have explored multiple resource-intense processes such as the use of MV in ARDS, and reliance on renal replacement therapies (RRT) for acute renal failure in the ICU. In ARDS, Hamel et al. [60] used information from the Study to Understand the Prognoses and Preferences for Outcomes and Risks of Treatments (SUPPORT) to investigate the value of MV. They estimated that ventilatory support was a cost-effective strategy overall, but that the cost-effectiveness ratio varied from $29,000 per QALY saved to $110,000 per QALY based on the subject's initial risk of death. Their analysis was insensitive to patient age as the cost-effectiveness ratio in subjects younger than 65 years was $32,000 versus $46,000 per QALY in those older than 75 years. One strength of this analysis was its close follow-up of patients, and thus the ability to more precisely account for postdischarge health care utilization. Cooke and coworkers conducted a similar analysis focusing on the cost-effectiveness of low tidal volumes in ARDS. Not surprisingly, given the few costs related to implementing a low-tidal-volume approach along with the substantial mortality benefit related to this, low-tidal-volume use is a dominant economic strategy [61].

Also using similar techniques, Korkeila et al. [62] investigated RRT. They tracked patients needing RRT and calculated that the costs per 6-month survivor were $80,000. In a comparable study to the one by Hamel et al., [63] the SUPPORT investigators reported that the cost per QALY saved by initiating dialysis and continuing aggressive care was $128,000. Again, underlying prognosis, not surprisingly, affected the cost-effectiveness ratio. In the best prognosis group, cost per QALY approached $68,000. In the worse prognosis group, it measured $274,000 per QALY saved. The authors concluded that, except in those with exceedingly good prognoses, this approach was not cost-effective. Readers should note that these cost estimates are from nearly a decade ago, and if updated to reflect health care inflation would only reinforce the impression that acute RRT has substantial financial implications for society.

Although not a definitive review of the many cost-effectiveness analyses performed in critical care outcomes research, these three examples illustrate that this approach can be used successfully to inform both professional and policy dialogue. They also help to demonstrate the value of ICU care despite its seemingly expensive implications for third-party payers and national governments. Uniformly, these reports illustrate that it is possible to measure proxies for cost rather easily and hence should become routine in the conduct of clinical research. Cost researchers, alternatively, need to be cautious as the time period they choose to study (e.g., short term, intermediate term, and long term) can affect their results and conclusions. Short-term costs may be saved with a novel intervention. Over the longer term, though, what might have appeared attractive economically could result in major costs to society.

CONCLUSIONS

Outcomes research remains an emerging field in critical care. As appreciation of patient-centered issues expands along with improved understanding of the diseases treated in the ICU, the need for more extensive and refined outcomes research will grow. Outcomes research, fortunately, encompasses a wide area of interest, and patient-centered outcomes can now be better folded into end points of clinical trials. Although methodologic issues continue to exist and further refinement in analytical techniques is required, the practicing intensivist benefits from an understanding of the issues central to outcomes research.

References

1. Berenson RA: *Intensive Care Units: Clinical Outcome, Costs, and Decision Making (Health Technology Case Study 28)*. Washington, DC, Prepared for the Office of Technology Assessment, US Congress, OTA_HCS_28, 1984.
2. Dasta JF, McLaughlin TP, Mody SH, et al: Daily cost of an intensive care unit day: the contribution of mechanical ventilation. *Crit Care Med* 33:1266–1271, 2005.
3. Halpern NA, Pastores SM: Critical care medicine in the United States 2000–2005: an analysis of bed numbers, occupancy rates, payer mix, and costs. *Crit Care Med* 38:65–71, 2010.
4. Rubenfeld GD, Angus DC, Pinsky MR, et al: Outcomes research in critical care: results of the American Thoracic Society Critical Care Assembly workshop on outcomes research. The Members of the Outcomes Research Workshop. *Am J Respir Crit Care Med* 160:358–367, 1999.
5. Marshall JC, Vincent JL, Guyatt G, et al: Outcome measures for clinical research in sepsis: a report of the 2nd Cambridge Colloquium of the International Sepsis Forum. *Crit Care Med* 33:1708–1716, 2005.
6. Esteban A, Anzueto A, Frutos F, et al: Characteristics and outcomes in adult patients receiving mechanical ventilation: a 28-day international study. *JAMA* 287:345–355, 2002.
7. Vincent JL, Sakr Y, Reinhart K, et al: Is albumin administration in the acutely ill associated with increased mortality? Results of the SOAP study. *Crit Care* 9:R745–R754, 2005.
8. Esteban Y, Frutos-Vivar A, Muriel A, et al: Evolution of mortality over time in patients receiving mechanical ventilation. *Am J Respir Crit Care Med* 188:220–230, 2013.
9. Needham DM, Dowdy DW, Mendez-Tellez PA, et al: Studying outcomes of intensive care unit survivors: measuring exposures and outcomes. *Intensive Care Med* 31:1153–1160, 2005.
10. Dowdy DW, Needham DM, Mendez-Tellez PA, et al: Studying outcomes of intensive care unit survivors: the role of the cohort study. *Intensive Care Med* 31:914–921, 2005.
11. Ely EW, Shintani A, Truman B, et al: Delirium as a predictor of mortality in mechanically ventilated patients in the intensive care unit. *JAMA* 291:1753–1762, 2004.
12. Pronovost PJ, Angus DC, Dorman T, et al: Physician staffing patterns and clinical outcomes in critically ill patients: a systematic review. *JAMA* 288:2151–2162, 2002.
13. Levy MM, Rapoport J, Lemeshow S, et al: Association between critical care physician management and patient mortality in the intensive care unit. *Ann Intern Med* 148:801–809, 2008.
14. Feng Y, Amoateng-Adjepong Y, Kaufman D, et al: Age, duration of mechanical ventilation, and outcomes of patients who are critically ill. *Chest* 136:759–764, 2009.
15. Beck D: Mortality probabilities and case-mix adjustment by prognostic models, in Ridley S (ed): *Outcomes in Critical Care*. Oxford, Reed Elsevier, 1992.
16. Boyd O: Case-mix adjustment and prediction of mortality—the problems with interpretation, in Ridley S (ed): *Outcomes in Critical Care*. Oxford, Reed Elsevier, 1992.
17. Knaus WA, Draper EA, Wagner DP, et al: APACHE II: a severity of disease classification system. *Crit Care Med* 13:818–829, 1985.
18. Zimmerman JE, Kramer AA: Outcome prediction in critical care: the Acute Physiology and Chronic Health Evaluation models. *Curr Opin Crit Care* 14:491–497, 2008.
19. Le Gall JR, Loirat P, Alperovitch A, et al: A simplified acute physiology score for ICU patients. *Crit Care Med* 12:975–977, 1984.
20. Vincent JL, Moreno R, Takala J, et al: The SOFA (Sepsis-related Organ Failure Assessment) score to describe organ dysfunction/failure. On behalf of the Working Group on Sepsis-Related Problems of the European Society of Intensive Care Medicine. *Intensive Care Med* 22:707–710, 1996.
21. Marshall JC, Cook DJ, Christou NV, et al: Multiple organ dysfunction score: a reliable descriptor of a complex clinical outcome. *Crit Care Med* 23:1638–1652, 1995.
22. Chan CM, Woods CJ, Shorr AF: Comparing the pulmonary embolism severity index and the prognosis in pulmonary embolism scores as risk stratification tools. *J Hosp Med* 7:22–27, 2012
23. Schmidt M, Zogheib E, Rozé H, et al: The PRESERVE mortality risk score and analysis of long-term outcomes after extracorporeal membrane oxygenation for severe acute respiratory distress syndrome. *Intensive Care Med* 2013 39:1704–1713, 2013
24. Zimmerman JE, Kramer AA, Douglas S, et al: Acute Physiology and Chronic Health Evaluation (APACHE) IV ICU length of stay benchmarks for today's critically ill patients. *Chest* 128[Suppl 1]:297S, 2005.
25. Ledoux D, Finfer S, McKinley S: Impact of operator expertise on collection of the APACHE II score and on the derived risk of death and standardized mortality ratio. *Anaesth Intensive Care* 33:585–590, 2005.
26. Booth FV, Short M, Shorr AF, et al: Application of a population-based severity scoring system to individual patients results in frequent misclassification. *Crit Care* 9(5):R522–R529, 2005.
27. Hebert PC, Wells G, Blajchman MA, et al: A multicenter, randomized, controlled clinical trial of transfusion requirements in critical care. Transfusion requirements in critical care investigators, Canadian Critical Care Trials Group. *N Engl J Med* 340:409–417, 1999.
28. Ridley S: Non-mortality outcomes measures, in Ridley S (ed): *Outcomes in Critical Care*. Oxford, Reed Elsevier, 1992.
29. Koutsogiannis DJ, Noseworthy T: Quality of life after critical care, in Ridley S (ed): *Outcomes in Critical Care*. Oxford, Reed Elsevier, 1992.
30. Siegel T, Adamski J, Nowakowski P, et al: Prospective assessment of standardized mortality ratio (SMR) as a measure of quality of care in intensive care unit–a single-centre study. *Anaesthesiol Intensive Ther* 47:328–332, 2015.
31. Herridge MS: Long-term outcomes after critical illness. *Curr Opin Crit Care* 8:331–336, 2002.
32. Herridge MS, Cheung AM, Tansey CM, et al: One-year outcomes in survivors of the acute respiratory distress syndrome. *N Engl J Med* 348:683–693, 2003.
33. Hopkins RO, Brett S: Chronic neurocognitive effects of critical illness. *Curr Opin Crit Care* 11:369–375, 2005.
34. Jackson JC, Gordon SM, Ely EW, et al: Research issues in the evaluation of cognitive impairment in intensive care unit survivors. *Intensive Care Med* 30:2009–2016, 2004.
35. Nickel M, Leiberich P, Nickel C, et al: The occurrence of posttraumatic stress disorder in patients following intensive care treatment: a cross-sectional study in a random sample. *J Intensive Care Med* 19:285–290, 2004.
36. Kress JP, Gehlbach B, Lacy M, et al: The long-term psychological effects of daily sedative interruption on critically ill patients. *Am J Respir Crit Care Med* 168:1457–1461, 2003.
37. Chaboyer W, Elliott D: Health-related quality of life of ICU survivors: review of the literature. *Intensive Crit Care Nurs* 16:88–97, 2000.
38. Tian ZM, Miranda DR: Quality of life after intensive care with the sickness impact profile. *Intensive Care Med* 21:422–428, 1995.

39. Chelluri L, Pinsky MR, Donahoe MP, et al: Long-term outcome of critically ill elderly patients requiring intensive care. *JAMA* 269:3119–3123, 1993.
40. Heyland DK, Hopman W, Coo H, et al: Long-term health-related quality of life in survivors of sepsis. Short Form 36: a valid and reliable measure of health-related quality of life. *Crit Care Med* 28:3599–3605, 2000.
41. Cuthbertson BH, Scott J, Strachan M, et al: Quality of life before and after intensive care. *Anaesthesia* 60:332–339, 2005.
42. Heyland DK, Guyatt G, Cook DJ, et al: Frequency and methodologic rigor of quality-of-life assessments in the critical care literature. *Crit Care Med* 26:591–598, 1998.
43. Pandian V, Thompson CB, Feller-Kopman DJ, et al: Development and validation of a quality-of-life questionnaire for mechanically ventilated ICU patients. *Crit Care Med* 43:142–148, 2015.
44. Angus DC, Linde-Zwirble WT, Lidicker J, et al: Epidemiology of severe sepsis in the United States: analysis of incidence, outcome, and associated costs of care. *Crit Care Med* 29:1303–1310, 2001.
45. Bice T, Cox CE, Carson SS: Cost and health care utilization in ARDS–different from other critical illness? *Semin Respir Crit Care Med* 34:529–536, 2013.
46. Siegel JE, Weinstein MC, Russell LB, et al: Recommendations for reporting cost-effectiveness analyses. Panel on cost-effectiveness in health and medicine. *JAMA* 276:1339–1341, 1996.
47. Understanding costs and cost-effectiveness in critical care: report from the Second American Thoracic Society Workshop on Outcomes Research. *Am J Respir Crit Care Med* 165:540–550, 2002.
48. Warren DK, Zack JE, Elward AM, et al: Nosocomial primary bloodstream infections in intensive care unit patients in a nonteaching community medical center: a 21-month prospective study. *Clin Infect Dis* 33:1329–1335, 2001.
49. Blot SI, Depuydt P, Annemans L, et al: Clinical and economic outcomes in critically ill patients with nosocomial catheter-related bloodstream infections. *Clin Infect Dis* 41:1591–1598, 2005.
50. Warren DK, Zack JE, Mayfield JL, et al: The effect of an education program on the incidence of central venous catheter-associated bloodstream infection in a medical ICU. *Chest* 126:1612–1618, 2004.
51. Rello J, Ollendorf DA, Oster G, et al: Epidemiology and outcomes of ventilator-associated pneumonia in a large US database. *Chest* 122:2115–2121, 2002.
52. Warren DK, Shukla SJ, Olsen MA, et al: Outcome and attributable cost of ventilator-associated pneumonia among intensive care unit patients in a suburban medical center. *Crit Care Med* 31(5):1312–1317, 2003.
53. Angus DC, Marrie TJ, Obrosky DS, et al: Severe community-acquired pneumonia: use of intensive care services and evaluation of American and British Thoracic Society diagnostic criteria. *Am J Respir Crit Care Med* 166:717–723, 2002.
54. Kaplan V, Angus DC, Griffin MF, et al: Hospitalized community-acquired pneumonia in the elderly: age- and sex-related patterns of care and outcome in the United States. *Am J Respir Crit Care Med* 165:766, 2002.
55. Wood KA, Angus DC: Pharmacoeconomic implications of new therapies in sepsis. *Pharmacoeconomics* 22:895–906, 2004.
56. Piacevoli Q, Palazzo F, Azzeri F: Cost evaluation of patients with severe sepsis in intensive care units. *Minerva Anestesiol* 70:453–471, 2004.
57. Shorr AF, Micek ST, Jackson WL Jr, et al: Economic implications of an evidence-based sepsis protocol: can we improve outcomes and lower costs? *Crit Care Med* 35:1257–1262, 2007
58. Adrie C, Alberti C, Chaix-Couturier C, et al: Epidemiology and economic evaluation of severe sepsis in France: age, severity, infection site, and place of acquisition (community, hospital, or intensive care unit). *J Crit Care* 20:46–58, 2005.
59. Burchardi H, Schneider H: Economic aspects of severe sepsis: a review of intensive care unit costs, cost of illness and cost effectiveness of therapy. *Pharmacoeconomics* 22:793–813, 2004.
60. Hamel MB, Phillips RS, Davis RB, et al: Outcomes and cost-effectiveness of ventilator support and aggressive care for patients with acute respiratory failure due to pneumonia or acute respiratory distress syndrome. *Am J Med* 109(8):614–620, 2000.
61. Cooke CR, Kahn JM, Watkins TR, et al: Cost-effectiveness of implementing low-tidal volume ventilation in patients with acute lung injury. *Chest* 136:79–88, 2009.
62. Korkeila M, Ruokonen E, Takala J: Costs of care, long-term prognosis and quality of life in patients requiring renal replacement therapy during intensive care. *Intensive Care Med* 26(12):1824–1831, 2000.
63. Hamel MB, Phillips RS, Davis RB, et al: Outcomes and cost-effectiveness of initiating dialysis and continuing aggressive care in seriously ill hospitalized adults. SUPPORT Investigators. Study to understand prognoses and preferences for outcomes and risks of treatments. *Ann Intern Med* 127:195–202, 1997.

Section 13
ENDOCRINE PROBLEMS IN THE INTENSIVE CARE UNIT

NEIL ARONIN • DAVID M. HARLAN

Chapter 136 ■ Management of Hyperglycemia in Critically Ill Patients

MICHAEL J. THOMPSON • DAVID M. HARLAN • SAMIR MALKANI • JOHN P. MORDES

INTRODUCTION

Hyperglycemia is a common problem that complicates the delivery of intensive care. By 2014 estimates, 29.1 million people, or 9.3% of the U.S. population, have diabetes [1]. On the basis of 2000 to 2011 National Health Interview Survey data, the lifetime risk of diabetes for a 20-year-old in the United States is estimated at approximately 40% [2]. In addition, the growing worldwide prevalence of obesity is increasing the prevalence of diabetes for many nations [3]. The global prevalence of diabetes among adults is predicted to be 7.7%, or 439 million adults, by 2030 [4]. Epidemiology alone would make diabetes a common problem in the intensive care unit (ICU), but poorly controlled diabetes also predisposes to cardiovascular [5,6], renal [7–9], and infectious [10–16] complications that often require intensive surgical and medical care. In addition, hyperglycemia frequently occurs among severely ill ICU patients who have no prior history of diabetes [17,18].

Whatever the primary problem, hyperglycemia amplifies the challenges of intensive care. Often, preexisting diabetes itself is the primary problem, as in ketoacidosis and hyperosmolar coma. These conditions are discussed in Chapter 137.

ETIOLOGY AND PATHOPHYSIOLOGY

Metabolic Homeostasis

Individuals with normal glucose tolerance maintain their blood glucose concentration between 60 and 120 mg per dL. Maintenance of glucose within this narrow range is controlled by the degree of tissue insulinization (Fig. 136.1) [19]. This is a function of the amount of insulin available and the responsiveness of

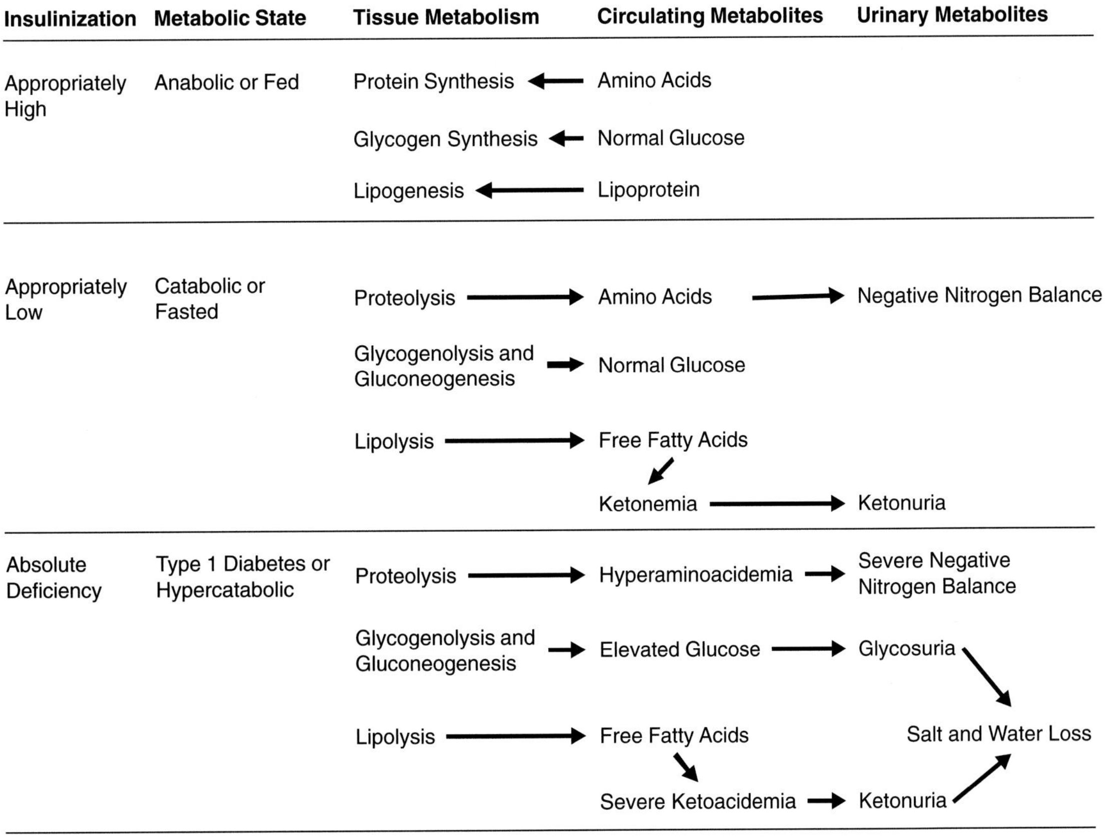
Insulinization
Metabolic State
Tissue Metabolism
Circulating Metabolites
Urinary Metabolites
Appropriately High
Anabolic or Fed
Protein Synthesis
Amino Acids
Glycogen Synthesis
Normal Glucose
Lipogenesis
Lipoprotein
Appropriately Low
Catabolic or Fasted
Proteolysis
Amino Acids
Negative Nitrogen Balance
Glycogenolysis and Gluconeogenesis
Normal Glucose
Lipolysis
Free Fatty Acids
Ketonemia
Ketonuria
Absolute Deficiency
Type 1 Diabetes or Hypercatabolic
Proteolysis
Hyperaminoacidemia
Severe Negative Nitrogen Balance
Glycogenolysis and Gluconeogenesis
Elevated Glucose
Glycosuria
Lipolysis
Free Fatty Acids
Salt and Water Loss
Severe Ketoacidemia
Ketonuria

FIGURE 136.1 Metabolic effects of insulin in normal and diabetic states. **Upper:** entries illustrate the anabolic, storage-promoting effects of insulin that occur with eating. **Middle:** entries illustrate the controlled catabolic effects that occur during fasting. **Bottom:** entries illustrate the *uncontrolled catabolism that ensues from absolute deficiency of insulin in type 1 diabetes.*

target tissues. After eating, blood glucose concentration rises but remains within the normal range as a result of increased insulin secretion. Insulin first promotes the transport of glucose into cells and the repletion of glycogen and protein stores. It then mediates the storage of excess glucose as triglycerides. When absorption of nutrients is complete, the concentrations of all metabolites and hormones return to basal levels.

In the fasting state, two mechanisms keep blood glucose concentration in the normal range, glycogenolysis and gluconeogenesis. Initially, hepatic glycogen is mobilized. If fasting persists longer than 12 to 18 hours, peripheral tissues begin to use free fatty acids for fuel, thereby sparing glucose. A low level of circulating insulin is permissive to the lipolytic release of these fatty acids. At the same time, gluconeogenesis supplies glucose for obligate glycolytic tissues, most notably the central nervous system.

When starvation continues for more than 72 hours, the brain begins to use ketone bodies as an alternative fuel, further sparing glucose utilization [19]. At this stage, a progressive decrease in hepatic gluconeogenesis occurs as a consequence of decreased amino acid release in the periphery. As starvation continues, lactate, pyruvate, and glycerol become the main gluconeogenic precursors in place of amino acids. At all times, a low level of circulating insulin regulates the rate of lipolysis, glucose transport, and gluconeogenesis. Healthy humans always have detectable and appropriate levels of insulin (i.e., adequate insulinization).

TABLE 136.1

Classification of Diabetic Syndromes [20]

Type 1 diabetes (β-cell destruction) autoimmune (Type 1A) and idiopathic (Type 1B)
Type 2 diabetes (insulin resistance with variable insulin secretory defect)
Other specific types
Genetic defects of β-cell function (e.g., MODY, mitochondrial DNA)
Genetic defects in insulin action (e.g., lipoatrophic diabetes)
Diseases of the exocrine pancreas (see Table 136.2)
Endocrinopathies (see Table 136.2)
Drug or chemical induced (see Table 136.2)
Infections (e.g., congenital rubella)
Uncommon forms of immune-mediated diabetes (e.g., stiff-man syndrome)
Other genetic syndromes associated with diabetes
Gestational diabetes mellitus

MODY, maturity-onset diabetes of the young.

Metabolic Stress

Major surgery and critical illness are physiologically stressful events that provoke complex metabolic responses. Tissue hypoxia and hypoxemia adversely affect normal oxidative phosphorylation, and counterregulatory hormones are secreted. These hormones include epinephrine, norepinephrine, cortisol, growth hormone, glucagon, and various cytokines (e.g., tumor necrosis factor-α). They raise blood glucose concentration, mobilize alternative fuels, and increase peripheral resistance to the effects of insulin. For the ICU patient, their effects may be further amplified by the concurrent administration of exogenous vasopressors, glucocorticoids, and other drugs that can affect intermediary metabolism.

Stress and the Diabetic State

Stress-induced changes in metabolism normally lead to increased insulin release. This in turn enhances peripheral glucose utilization and inhibits alternative fuel mobilization. In this way, the body resists stress without losing control of the biochemical machinery. Among patients with decreased insulin reserves (i.e., diabetes mellitus), failure of this feedback loop produces hyperglycemia and related metabolic complications. To preclude these complications, careful management of insulin, fluid, and electrolytes is necessary.

Classification of Diabetes

Diabetes is not one disease but rather a family of syndromes that have in common hyperglycemia resulting from inadequate insulinization. These syndromes vary with respect to genetics, pathophysiology, and appropriate treatment modalities. Table 136.1 outlines the American Diabetes Association's classification system [20].

Type 1 Diabetes

In type 1 diabetes, the insulin-producing β cells of the pancreatic islets are destroyed, resulting in near total deficiency of insulin [19,21]. Hyperglycemia develops rapidly, most commonly during childhood and adolescence. Most cases of type 1 diabetes are autoimmune in origin [21]. About 5% of persons with diabetes have this form of the disorder [1].

Patients with type 1 diabetes require exogenous insulin for survival (Fig.136.1). The insulin can be given either as a continuous insulin infusion or as conventional subcutaneous injections. The key ICU issue is continuity of treatment. Inappropriate discontinuation of insulin treatment, even for relatively brief intervals, can lead to serious metabolic complications.

Patients with type 1 diabetes who are not given insulin can neither store nor use glucose, and unregulated gluconeogenesis and lipolysis occur (Fig. 136.1). In this hypercatabolic state, accelerating amino acid and fat mobilization produce hyperglycemia, hyperlipidemia, and ketosis. The excess glucose produced by uncontrolled gluconeogenesis remains in the circulation, because there is no insulin to stimulate glucose transport into cells. The osmotic diuresis of glucose and the buffering of ketoacids produce secondary fluid and electrolyte shifts. Ultimately, diabetic ketoacidosis occurs. This disorder is discussed in Chapter 137.

Type 2 Diabetes

Type 2 diabetes is characterized by relative, rather than absolute, deficiency of insulin. It involves defects in both insulin action and insulin secretion. Impaired response to insulin of peripheral tissues is often the dominant feature [22–25]. It develops insidiously, most commonly among obese individuals more than 40 years old, although it is now increasingly diagnosed at younger ages. It may go undetected for years, only to be discovered serendipitously or during the stress of surgery or other illness.

Many patients with type 2 diabetes can be treated with diet, exercise, and oral hypoglycemic agents. Some patients, especially those who are not obese, need insulin to control their hyperglycemia. This is done to prevent symptoms (e.g., polyuria) and long-term complications. Even when type 2 diabetes is untreated, there is usually enough insulin present to control lipid mobilization and prevent ketoacidosis when the patient is otherwise well. They can, however, develop diabetic ketoacidosis (DKA) in the presence of sufficient intercurrent stress.

In the ICU, patients with type 2 diabetes whose diabetes is uncontrolled should be treated with insulin. Keys to management include attention to both blood glucose concentration and acid–base balance. Infection, metabolic stress, and many medications commonly used for ICU patients can exacerbate type 2 diabetes and lead to ketoacidosis [26], hyperosmolar coma, or lactic acidosis. These disorders are discussed in Chapter 137.

Other Types of Diabetes

Additional forms of diabetes involve specific genetic defects or are secondary to intercurrent diseases, infections, medications, or a combination of these [27]. The broad categories into which these other specific types of diabetes fall are given in Table 136.1. A partial listing of the other types of diabetes and precipitants of secondary diabetes is given in Table 136.2.

ICU patients with any form of uncontrolled hyperglycemia require insulin to control hyperglycemia and prevent short-term metabolic complications. Patients who have undergone total pancreatectomy have absolute insulin deficiency, are ketosis prone, and are insulin dependent. Patients with other diseases of the exocrine pancreas (e.g., pancreatitis) can develop variable degrees of insulin deficiency and, while in the ICU, should be considered at risk for ketoacidosis. Gestational diabetes of an ICU patient should also be treated with insulin.

DIAGNOSIS OF HYPERGLYCEMIA FOR THE INTENSIVE CARE UNIT PATIENT

Diagnostic Criteria

All acutely ill patients should have their blood glucose level measured at entry into the ICU and at regular intervals throughout their stay. In the outpatient setting, diabetes is diagnosed by a fasting blood glucose level over 126 mg per dL, or a glucose level greater than or equal to 200 mg per dL measured 2 hours after a 75-g oral glucose tolerance test. A formal diagnosis of new onset diabetes should be made tentatively during the stress of an ICU admission as hyperglycemia may subsequently resolve. Hyperglycemic ICU patients with no prior history of diabetes should be evaluated for persistence of impaired glucose tolerance after recovery.

The majority of seriously ill patients with hyperglycemia do not have a preexisting diagnosis of diabetes. In one study of 1,200 subjects treated in a medical ICU, 70% of individuals at some time experienced a plasma glucose concentration of more than 215 mg per dL, and only about 17% of these patients had a prior history of diabetes [28].

TABLE 136.2

Some Causes of "Secondary" Diabetes

Type	Examples	Type	Examples
Drug-induced	Thiazide diuretics Loop diuretics (e.g., furosemide, ethacrynic acid, metolazone) Antihypertensive agents (e.g., β-adrenergic blockers, calcium channel blockers, clonidine, diazoxide) HIV protease inhibitors Hormones (e.g., glucocorticoids, oral contraceptives, α-adrenergic agents, glucagon, growth hormone) Interferon-α Sympathomimetic drugs Antineoplastic agents (e.g., asparaginase, mithramycin, streptozocin, 5-fluorouracil) Phenytoin (Dilantin) Theophylline Niacin Cyclosporine Phenothiazines Lithium Isoniazid Pentamidine Olanzapine (Zyprexa) Gatifloxacin	Other endocrine disorders	Cushing's syndrome Pheochromocytoma and paraganglionoma Acromegaly Primary hyperaldosteronism Hyperthyroidism Polyendocrine autoimmune syndromes POEMS syndrome (e.g., polyneuropathy, organomegaly, endocrinopathy, monoclonal gammopathy, skin changes) Somatostatinoma Glucagonoma
		Other genetic syndromes	Down syndrome Kleinfelter syndrome Turner syndrome Wolfram syndrome Friedreich ataxia Huntington disease Lawrence–Moon–Bardet–Biedl syndrome Myotonic dystrophy Prader–Willi–Labhardt syndrome Porphyria Glycogen storage disease type III
Pancreatic diseases	Hemochromatosis Pancreatic cancer Pancreatitis Cystic fibrosis Fibrocalculous pancreatopathy Abdominal trauma		

Partial listing of causes of secondary diabetes [20,88]. Additional possible causes have been published as isolated case reports.

Assessment of Severity

Whenever the glucose concentration of any patient is greater than about 250 mg per dL, actual or impending ketoacidosis and hyperosmolality must be considered. Ketoacidosis can be diagnosed on the basis of history, physical findings, and the presence of an anion-gap acidosis and ketonemia. Osmolality can be measured by the laboratory or calculated from the serum concentrations of glucose, blood urea nitrogen, sodium, and potassium (Table 137.1 of the comas Chapter 137). Hyperosmolar states in the setting of diabetes are usually associated with severe dehydration, obtundation, and extreme hyperglycemia. Diabetic ketoacidosis and hyperosmolar coma require urgent treatment (see Chapter 137). In this chapter, we describe the goals, methods, and pitfalls of treating intercurrent diabetes mellitus in the ICU when neither ketoacidosis nor hyperosmolar coma is the primary disease process.

TREATMENT OF CRITICALLY ILL PATIENTS WITH PREEXISTING DIABETES

Initial Evaluation

Physicians caring for patients with diabetes in an ICU should attempt to determine the type of diabetes, its duration, the presence of diabetic complications, and the degree of previous glycemic control. Patients with type 1 diabetes require insulin treatment at all times; those with type 2 diabetes may or may not require insulin. Patients with diabetes that is secondary to some other disorder (Table 136.2) require diagnosis and treatment of the precipitating factors.

Long-standing diabetes is associated with complications that tend to be more severe for patients with glycemia that is poorly controlled [29,30]. These sequelae of diabetes complicate the management of critical illnesses. Diabetes is a leading cause of cardiovascular and peripheral vascular disease. Assessments of both cardiac function and peripheral circulation are advisable for all patients with diabetes. Diabetic neuropathy can affect the autonomic nervous system, with implications for managing blood pressure, heart rate, and voiding. Autonomic neuropathy should be suspected in patients with an abnormal pupillary response to light or absence of heart rate response (R-R interval change in the electrocardiogram) during a Valsalva maneuver. Assessment of kidney function should include a urinalysis for protein; albuminuria precedes abnormalities of blood urea nitrogen and creatinine levels. Diabetic eye disease is not a contraindication to anticoagulation, but its severity should be documented before instituting therapy.

A history of poor glycemic control should alert the clinician to other potential problems. Poorly controlled diabetes is associated with poor nutrition. This has important implications for resistance to infections and for wound healing; nutritional assessment and vitamin repletion may be helpful. Thiamine, in particular, is a critical cofactor in carbohydrate metabolism, and patients with uncontrolled diabetes may be thiamine deficient. Occult infections to which individuals with diabetes are particularly susceptible include osteomyelitis, cellulitis, tuberculosis, cholecystitis, gingivitis, sinusitis, cystitis, and pyelonephritis [11,12,31,32]. Patients with type 2 diabetes frequently have hypertriglyceridemia and may develop pancreatitis because of high levels of triglycerides [33].

Hospital-grade bedside blood glucose monitoring systems for point-of-care glucose determinations are accurate [34,35], but can be influenced by hematocrit, creatinine concentration, plasma protein concentration, and PO_2, all of which can be abnormal among ICU patients [36–38]. Extremely elevated blood glucose concentrations may be outside the range accurately measured by the bedside monitor and should be verified with a serum sample sent to the laboratory [39]. In general, however, therapy should not be delayed by waiting for confirmatory results of laboratory glucose concentration in the proper clinical setting.

Promising new technology for continuous glucose monitoring (CGM) has the potential to improve detection and prevention of hypoglycemia in ICU [40]. CGM devices that measure subcutaneous glucose readings may be less accurate in patients with impaired microperfusion such as occurs during extracorporeal ventricular assist therapy [41]. Invasive indwelling intravascular sensors that measure blood glucose directly are also under development and have the potential for increased accuracy for critically ill patients [42]. The ultimate goal is to couple CGM devices to intravenous insulin infusions as a closed-loop artificial pancreas system [43].

Why Control Hyperglycemia during critical illness?

Hyperglycemia among the Critically Ill Predicts Adverse Outcomes

It is intuitively plausible to assume that glucose concentration should always be in the normal range, and studies show that hyperglycemia among critically ill patients is associated with adverse outcomes. Even minimal hyperglycemia, plasma glucose concentration >110 mg per dL, has been shown to predict increased in-hospital mortality and the risk of congestive heart failure among patients with acute myocardial infarction [44]. Hyperglycemic patients also have an increased risk of wound infection as well as overall mortality following cardiac surgery [45,46]. Hyperglycemia is also associated with poor outcomes among patients with stroke [47]. Patients in whom diabetes is diagnosed for the first time during an ICU admission reportedly have an 18-fold increase in their risk of in-hospital mortality [48].

How Does Hyperglycemia Adversely Affect Outcomes?

Hyperglycemia predisposes to disturbances in sodium, potassium, and phosphate concentrations. Because uncontrolled hyperglycemia also provokes an osmotic diuresis, symptomatic hyponatremia can result. Hypokalemia predisposes to arrhythmia, and hypophosphatemia may interfere with platelet function and white cell motility. Control of glycemia prevents these problems and the need for compensatory correction. The susceptibility of patients with diabetes to infections is well recognized [11,12,31]. Uncontrolled glycemia appears to impair innate immunity (cytokine, pathogen recognition pathways, and phagocytic capacity), granulocyte function (chemotaxis, phagocytosis, and killing), and, possibly, lymphocyte function and adaptive immune function, including antibody formation [49–52]. Some microorganisms express more virulence factors in a high-glucose environment [49]. Endothelial functions may also be impaired by hyperglycemia [53]. In general, better regulation of blood glucose leads to improvement of these parameters.

What Is the Evidence That Control of Blood Glucose Concentration Alters Clinical Outcomes for Intensive Care Unit Patients?

Recognizing that hyperglycemia is a risk factor for adverse outcomes is not the same as saying that tight control of hyperglycemia for critically ill patients, with the attendant risk of hypoglycemia, is beneficial. Hyperglycemia, hypoglycemia, and increased glycemic variability are all independently associated with mortality of critically ill patients [54].

In 2001, a widely discussed study of surgical ICU patients by Van den Berghe et al. [55] reported that intensive insulin therapy with a "near-normal" target plasma glucose concentration <110 mg per dL reduced in-hospital mortality by 34%, septicemia by 46%, acute renal failure by 41%, and critical-illness polyneuropathy by 44%. This study, together with the results of other single-institution reports and retrospective studies [46,56,57], generated widespread acceptance of the concept that intensive glycemic control is important for critically ill patients. This then led to implementation of intensive glycemic control protocols in a majority of academic ICU programs [58].

A subsequent report from the Van den Berghe group [28] as well as two large multicenter randomized controlled trials of blood glucose management of heterogeneous ICU populations failed to show benefits for near-normal diabetes control in the ICU. The GLUControl trial randomized 3,000 medical and surgical ICU patients in several centers in Europe to two regimens of insulin therapy targeted to achieve a plasma glucose concentration of either 80 to 110 mg per dL or 140 to 180 mg per dL [59]. The trial was stopped early because of an increased frequency of hypoglycemia together with lack of clinical benefit in the intensive insulin therapy cohort. The NICE-SUGAR (Normoglycemia in Intensive Care Evaluation and Survival Using Glucose Algorithm Regulation) trial randomized 5,000 medical and surgical ICU patients at multiple centers in Australia, New Zealand, and Canada to intensive (81 to 108 mg per dL) or conventional (≤180 mg per dL) management [60]. The investigators reported that intensive glucose control increased mortality and the rate of hypoglycemia compared with the conventional target cohort.

A number of trials have now highlighted the importance of avoiding hypoglycemia of the critically ill patient [61]. Among critically ill patients, an association exists between even mild or moderate hypoglycemia and mortality [62,63] (See also Chapter 138). Preexisting diabetes increases the risk of mortality from hypoglycemia; the higher the glucose level before admission to the ICU, the higher the mortality risk when patients experienced hypoglycemia [64]. It has been suggested that patients with diabetes may benefit from higher glucose target ranges than will those without diabetes [54,64]. The preponderance of available evidence suggests that intensive management of hyperglycemia to within the normal range for critically ill adults is not beneficial, although the precise ideal target is still controversial [65,66].

Recommended Glycemic Targets

The American Diabetes Association (ADA) recommends a glycemic target of 140 to 180 mg per dL in the ICU setting, noting that greater benefit may be realized at the lower end of this range [67]. Table 136.3 summarizes our recommendations. Glucose concentrations of less than 80 mg per dL should be stringently avoided because they pose the hazard of hypoglycemia and might contribute to mortality [55,62,63]. An intensive insulin treatment program to achieve the American Association of Clinical Endocrinologists (AACE)/ADA targets requires a strong institutional commitment. It is a team effort requiring participation of physicians, nursing, and pharmacy staff.

TABLE 136.3

Diabetes Treatment Goals in Critically Ill and Surgical Patients[a]

Zone	Target blood glucose (mg/dL)
Too low for safety	<120
Goal	140–180
Hyperglycemia	181–300
Severe hyperglycemia	>300
Surgical Range	140–200

[a]At our institutions, we recommend that all intensive care unit patients with blood glucose concentrations >140 mg/dL be treated with a continuous intravenous infusion of regular insulin with a target as close as possible to 140 [67]. A less stringent target range may be preferred during the perioperative period and whenever staffing or training constraints prevent the implementation of more intensive therapy. Patients with type 1 diabetes must be treated with insulin at all times.

Treatment of Hyperglycemia for the Critically Ill

The majority of ICU patients will require treatment for hyperglycemia, and we recommend that they be treated with a continuous intravenous infusion of regular insulin. This is irrespective of prior history of diabetes or previous treatment modalities. Patients known to have type 1 diabetes are absolutely insulin dependent, and they must be treated with exogenous insulin at all times. Oral hypoglycemic agents should not be used in the ICU for many reasons. Their absorption, metabolism, and excretion cannot be adequately predicted for the individual critically ill patient. Sulfonylureas can cause severe hypoglycemia [68] (See Chapter 138). Metformin should be discontinued because it can cause lactic acidosis in the setting of renal failure [69]. SGLT-2 inhibitors can lead to dehydration and euglycemic DKA [70,71].

Our recommendations for the management of patients with ketoacidosis or hyperosmolar syndrome are given elsewhere (see Chapter 137). For patients whose primary ICU diagnosis is not diabetic ketoacidosis or hyperosmolar hyperglycemic syndrome, we recommend the treatment program advocated by the AACE and ADA [67].

Insulin Therapy

Although optimal glycemic targets are now agreed to, insulin infusion algorithms to achieve those targets need to be individualized by the responsible multidisciplinary teams. Every protocol will require development of guidelines for adjustment of the insulin infusion rate in response to both the absolute value and the rate of change in the glucose concentration. Glucose concentration should be checked hourly until it is consistently in the target range of 140 to 180 mg per dL, and every 2 to 4 hours thereafter. During the initial period, adjustments to the insulin infusion rate will depend on the patient's sensitivity to insulin (see below) and the observed response to therapy, which cannot be exactly predicted. Concurrent glucose infusions or parenteral or enteral feeding will also affect the dose required. Tight glycemic control has been associated with a high incidence of hypoglycemia and an increased risk of death in patients not receiving parenteral nutrition [72]. A list of currently available insulin preparations is given in Table 138.2 in Chapter 138.

Diluted insulin solutions prepared from continuous insulin infusions have a limited storage life because insulin adheres to the plastic infusion bag. There is no advantage to the use of rapid-acting semisynthetic insulin for this purpose, but it can be used when regular insulin is unavailable. It should be stressed that it is entirely appropriate to infuse insulin at low rates (e.g., 0.5 U per hour). A low rate of insulin infusion is often all that is needed to prevent ketoacidosis among patients with type 1 diabetes.

Adjustment of the Insulin Infusion Rate

The amount of insulin required by a given ICU patient will depend in large part on the degree of insulin resistance induced by the primary illness, the agents used in its treatment, and the patient's body mass index. It will also depend on the type and amount of nutritional support being given. An escalating insulin infusion requirement is a sensitive indicator of increasing insulin resistance and requires careful reevaluation of the patient's overall metabolic status. Stressors that increase insulin resistance include sepsis, occult infections, heart disease, tissue ischemia, hypoxemia, and various medications. The most common offending medications are glucocorticoids and vasopressors.

In otherwise stable patients, instituting or increasing enteral or parenteral nutrition typically increases insulin requirements. Insulin-mediated glucose disposal is impaired among stressed patients with hyperglycemia, and even extremely high insulin infusion rates cannot prevent hyperglycemia due to unmanageable carbohydrate loads. To control hyperglycemia among the critically ill, a choice must sometimes be made between increasing insulin infusion rates and reducing carbohydrate feeding. We recommend that insulin infusion rates not be increased beyond 20 units per hour (480 units per day) without first decreasing any exogenous carbohydrate loads, especially for patients who are obese. This suggestion is based on the fact that maximal insulin effects are achieved when only some of the available insulin receptors are occupied [73,74]. High concentrations of insulin, such as those achieved during continuous intravenous infusions at high rates, desensitize target tissues at both the receptor and postreceptor levels, paradoxically enhancing insulin resistance [75].

Factors that increase insulin sensitivity among critically ill patients include improvement of intercurrent illnesses, changes in medications, and reductions of enteral or parenteral feeding. Occasionally, hepatic failure, renal failure, or adrenal insufficiency leads to decreased insulin requirements.

When plasma glucose concentration is lower than 140 mg per dL, a common response is to discontinue insulin completely. For patients with type 1 diabetes, this is *always inappropriate* because it can precipitate hyperglycemia and ketosis within hours. The proper response is to reduce the insulin infusion rate to 1 or even 0.5 units per hour and, if necessary, to give glucose in the form of 5% or 10% dextrose in water. We recommend the same strategy for most other hyperglycemic ICU patients as well. Unless their primary disease state has improved dramatically, they frequently experience recurrent hyperglycemia. Critically ill patients with hyperglycemia should receive continuous intravenous insulin until they demonstrate clear improvement of overall clinical status and stability of glycemic control that extends over several blood glucose determinations.

Transition to Other Forms of Therapy

When the condition of a critically ill patient with hyperglycemia has improved to such an extent that continuous insulin infusion is no longer needed, subsequent therapy will depend on the cause of the hyperglycemia. Patients with "secondary diabetes" (e.g., catecholamine- or steroid-induced) may need no further treatment for glucose control after the offending drug is stopped. In contrast, all patients with type 1 and most with type 2 diabetes will continue to require insulin. This should include intermediate- or long-acting insulin, e.g., neutral protamine Hagedorn (NPH), glargine, or detemir (See Table 138.2 in Chapter 138 for details). We recommend against the use of insulin degludec for inpatients since its duration of action of up to 42 hours limits options for daily adjustment.

It is not uncommon for glycemic control to deteriorate during the transition from intravenous insulin therapy to subcutaneous insulin therapy. It is essential that the intravenous infusion of regular insulin be continued for 2 to 3 hours after the first subcutaneous injection of insulin is given. The initial dose of subcutaneous insulin should be estimated from a review of the preceding intravenous insulin requirements. Presumably at the time the patient is ready to transition to subcutaneous therapy, he or she will have had reasonably stable insulin requirements. We recommend basing this dose on the average hourly insulin requirement during the 6 hours prior to discontinuation of the insulin drip using the following procedure:

Calculating the Starting Intermediate (NPH) or Long-acting (Glargine or Detemir) Insulin Dose

1. The average hourly insulin drip rate for the last 6 hours is ___units per hour.
2. Multiply by 24 to give a daily usage rate: ___units per day.
3. Multiply by 70% to 85% to estimate the first day's total insulin dose: ___units.
4. All can be administered in divided doses twice daily; glargine and detemir can be given once daily. Dose adjustment may be necessary after first dose given. Review daily thereafter.

When patients are able to eat, a rapid-acting insulin (e.g., lispro, aspart, or glulisine) should be given before each meal. Some stable patients with type 2 diabetes can be managed with oral hypoglycemic agents (Chapter 138, Table 138.3) or diet alone, but that therapeutic decision is best made after discharge from the ICU on a regimen of subcutaneous insulin.

SURGERY IN THE CRITICALLY ILL PATIENT WITH DIABETES

Critically ill patients frequently require invasive procedures, surgery, and intensive postoperative care. In such situations, the treatment of intercurrent diabetes is obviously of importance. The possibility of diabetes must be considered during all surgical emergencies, and both glucose and electrolytes must be measured immediately. A critically ill patient with diabetes, even when previously undiagnosed, can rapidly develop metabolic derangements.

It is generally accepted that good perioperative control of glucose is desirable, but the target levels of glucose and the ideal method of insulin delivery during surgery need to be individualized [76]. Perioperative control of blood pressure and vascular responses may be as important as glucose control for prevention of adverse perioperative events.

Abdominal pain accompanied by guarding and rebound tenderness is a common symptom of diabetic ketoacidosis. The diagnosis of diabetic ketoacidosis has on occasion been made at laparotomy, and this disorder must be excluded in every patient being evaluated for an abdominal surgery. The patient with trauma being prepared for surgery should also be evaluated for diabetes, regardless of mental status. The stress of major trauma and shock is less likely to be survived if ketoacidosis or hyperosmolality is present or allowed to develop. Severe trauma causes the release of counterregulatory hormones, cytokines, and other unidentified factors that can rapidly induce a state of severe insulin resistance.

Transfers from the Intensive Care Unit to the Operating Room

The ICU patient with diabetes who requires surgery should be sent to the operating room or procedure suite with infusions of both insulin and 5% dextrose in half-normal saline.

Management During Emergency Surgery

Treatment of hyperglycemia of diabetic patients being prepared for urgent major surgery is also best achieved with an intravenous insulin infusion. Frequent monitoring of blood glucose levels is essential. Proper fluid and electrolyte balance must accompany the proper degree of insulinization; the amount and the type of fluid administered must be assessed on an individual basis.

In general, premedication of patients with diabetes should be kept to a minimum. With respect to the type and the route of anesthesia, the regional and local are preferred if possible. Inhalant and parenteral anesthetics affect carbohydrate metabolism either directly through impairment of insulin secretion or indirectly through interference with the peripheral action of insulin on glucose utilization [76–78]. Volatile anesthetics including halothane and isoflurane inhibit insulin release, and nitrous oxide, promote sympathetic stimulation and catecholamine release. Barbiturates share some of these effects and also block the removal of glucose and perhaps free fatty acids from the circulation. Some anesthetic agents, including halothane, have also been associated with hypoglycemia (see Chapter 138, Table 138.4).

Management After Emergency Procedures

Patients managed with an insulin infusion must either be maintained on the infusion or switched to subcutaneous intermediate-acting insulin. Those kept on the infusion must have frequent blood glucose testing. Patients no longer critically ill who are able to resume oral feedings can generally resume their usual insulin regimen. The most important point is that insulin should not be abruptly discontinued, because severe hyperglycemia and ketosis may ensue. Patients who remain critically ill should remain on a continuous intravenous insulin infusion.

Postoperative recovery in the ICU may be accompanied by reduced levels of counterregulatory hormones and cytokines and may require reduced insulin doses. An increase in insulin requirements during the postoperative period may signify increasing insulin resistance and should prompt the search for infection or another complication.

Hyperalimentation and Diabetes

If blood glucose rises above 140 mg per dL for a severely ill patient on hyperalimentation, an insulin infusion should be administered. The hyperalimentation should be continuous. The admixture of insulin with parenteral nutrition formulations, although a common practice, can be problematic. There is too much variability among severely ill patients to rely on a fixed ratio of insulin to carbohydrate. If insulin is added to parenteral nutrition formulations, the dose should be limited to less than 50% of the individual's total insulin requirement, with the residual administered by intravenous insulin infusion or subcutaneous injection. This allows rapid adjustment of the insulin dose for changing metabolic needs. If an obese patient receiving hyperalimentation develops severe hyperglycemia and a large insulin requirement, consideration should be given to reducing the amount of carbohydrate administered [79,80]. ICU physicians should be aware that infusions of fructose, sorbitol, and other total parenteral nutrition formulations have occasionally led to lactic acidosis [81].

PITFALLS IN THE CARE OF THE CRITICALLY ILL PATIENT WITH HYPERGLYCEMIA

Sliding Scales

We cannot overstate the need to obtain frequent blood glucose specimens for evaluating glucose control. During critical illness, these should be used to guide adjustments of the rate of insulin

TABLE 136.4

Advances in Management of Diabetes in Critically Ill Patients

Recommendation	Comments
Anticipate hyperglycemia at any time during an ICU admission.	New onset of hyperglycemia due to stress is very common [28,89]. We recommend treating diabetes in all patients whose plasma glucose concentration is >140 mg/dL [67]. ICU patients with newly recognized hyperglycemia should be evaluated for persistence of impaired glucose tolerance after recovery.
Avoid hyperglycemia in the ICU because it is associated with poor outcome.	Observational studies have documented an adverse association of hyperglycemia with wound infection, congestive heart failure, recovery from stroke, and overall mortality [44,45,47,48].
Avoid hypoglycemia in the ICU because it is associated with increased mortality	Two recent clinical studies document increased mortality in critically ill patients who experience hypoglycemia during hospitalization [62,63].
With current technology it is not safe to seek to lower glucose concentration to <110 mg/dL in ICU patients	Five large randomized clinical trials have demonstrated either no reduction [28,59,61,90] or an increase in ICU mortality [60] associated with intensive insulin treatment. All showed increased risk of hypoglycemia. Only one of these showed reduced morbidity [28].
Be alert to the presence of type 1 diabetes.	Patients with type 1 diabetes are absolutely insulin dependent, and they must be treated with insulin at all times.
Treatment of diabetes using only "sliding scale" boluses of insulin, whether intravenous or subcutaneous, should be avoided.	Sliding scale prescriptions given only after hyperglycemia has occurred amplify the risk of hypoglycemia, recurrent hyperglycemia, and even ketoacidosis. There is no role for them in the ICU [82] and their use is actively discouraged [83]. Continuous insulin infusion is the treatment of choice for diabetes in the ICU.
Oral hypoglycemic agents should not be used in the ICU.	Insulin is the only acceptable agent for control of diabetes in the ICU. The absorption, metabolism, distribution, and excretion of oral agents cannot be predicted in the critically ill patient. As a result, for example, sulfonylureas can cause persistent hypoglycemia [68], and metformin can cause lactic acidosis in the setting of renal failure [69].

infusion. There is no role for intermittent insulin boluses that are given only after hyperglycemia has occurred [82]; the use of "sliding scales" should be actively discouraged [83]. Patients with type 1 diabetes whose insulin is withheld until hyperglycemia occurs can quickly become ketoacidotic.

A patient who has begun taking insulin should continue to receive it daily until the need has unequivocally disappeared. A previously normoglycemic patient who develops hyperglycemia in the course of a severe illness should be treated continuously with insulin until the stress of the illness has been reduced to the point at which an independent assessment of the need for insulin can be made.

Sporadic Insulin Administration

Unfortunately, some patients are treated with regular insulin injections on an intermittent schedule, whenever a very high blood glucose concentration is noticed. This disorganized approach to the management of hyperglycemia leads to erratic glycemic control and potentially serious shifts in fluids and electrolytes. The best way to avoid these problems is to maintain ICU patients with hyperglycemia on a continuous infusion of regular insulin.

Hypoglycemia due to Sensitivity to Short-Acting Insulin

Unusual sensitivity to insulin can be observed in two situations. The first is in some patients presenting with hyperosmolar hyperglycemic syndrome. When treated with short-acting insulin, their glucose concentrations may decline very rapidly. This problem is discussed in Chapter 138. The second situation occurs in patients with long-standing type 1 diabetes. They sometimes develop extreme sensitivity to the glucose-lowering effects of short-acting insulin. The reason is unclear, but this sensitivity frequently contributes to increased risk of hypoglycemia. This is principally a problem for outpatient management and should rarely complicate insulin infusion therapy. However, among insulin-dependent patients with long-standing diabetes, the initial use of short-acting insulin should be approached with some caution. Hypoglycemia can result from the use of as little as 5 to 10 units given either subcutaneously or intravenously. When short-acting insulin is needed for patients who are suspected to be sensitive, the initial doses should be small (2 to 4 units) and the response monitored by bedside blood glucose determinations. This is particularly important because these patients may have intercurrent hypoglycemia–associated autonomic failure with hypoglycemia unawareness and defective counterregulatory hormone responses [84].

The Diabetic Kidney and Radiographic Contrast Agents

Acute hyperglycemia appears to be an independent risk factor for the development of contrast-induced nephropathy (CIN). The risk of CIN is even greater for the diabetic patient with preexisting renal insufficiency, hypotension, congestive heart failure, or anemia. Mehran et al. [85] have developed a scoring system that can be used to quantify the risk of CIN. Consensus guidelines recommend adequate intravenous volume expansion with isotonic crystalloid (1.0 to 1.5 mL/kg/h) for 3 to 12 hours before the procedure and continued for 6 to 24 hours afterward to lessen the probability of CIN in patients at risk [86]. Data regarding the use of bicarbonate and *N*-acetylcysteine remain equivocal [87].

CONCLUSIONS

The key to successful care of the very ill patient with diabetes is careful monitoring of glycemia and fastidious treatment with a continuous infusion of insulin. These patients have defects of normal metabolic regulation, and only attentive treatment can compensate for the diabetes during the metabolic stress of critical illness or surgery. Careful monitoring of blood glucose followed by adjustment of insulin infusion rates minimizes swings to either hyperglycemia or hypoglycemia. Point-of-care glucose determinations make this intensive metabolic care possible not only during an ICU stay but also in the operating room, recovery room, emergency department, and procedural suite. Evidence-based glycemic targets have been developed. Advances in therapy, based on randomized controlled trials or meta-analyses of such trials, are summarized in Table 136.4. Although achieving recommended targets demands time and attention, achieving them will minimize the special risks faced by patients with hyperglycemia complicating the stress of severe illness or surgery.

References

1. Centers for Disease Control and Prevention National Diabetes Statistics Report: Estimates of Diabetes and Its Burden in the United States, 2014. http://www.cdc.gov/diabetes/data/statistics/2014statisticsreport.html. 2014. Accessed March 3, 2017.
2. Gregg EW, Zhuo X, Cheng YJ, et al: Trends in lifetime risk and years of life lost due to diabetes in the USA, 1985–2011: a modelling study. *Lancet Diabetes Endocrinol* 2(11):867–874, 2014.
3. Hossain P, Kawar B, El Nahas M: Obesity and diabetes in the developing world–a growing challenge. *N Engl J Med* 356(3):213–215, 2007.
4. Shaw JE, Sicree RA, Zimmet PZ: Global estimates of the prevalence of diabetes for 2010 and 2030. *Diabetes Res Clin Pract* 87(1):4–14, 2010.
5. Nesto RW: Correlation between cardiovascular disease and diabetes mellitus: current concepts. *Am J Med* 116:11–22, 2004.
6. Sobel BE, Schneider DJ: Cardiovascular complications in diabetes mellitus. *Curr Opin Pharmacol* 5(2):143–148, 2005.
7. Gruden G, Gnudi L, Viberti G: Pathogenesis of diabetic nephropathy, in LeRoith D, Taylor SI, Olefsky JM, (eds): *Diabetes Mellitus. A Fundamental and Clinical Text.* 3rd ed. Philadelphia, PA, Lippincott Williams & Wilkins, 2004, pp 1315–1330.
8. Molitch ME, DeFronzo RA, Franz MJ, et al; American Diabetes Association. Diabetic nephrology. *Diabetes Care* 23:S69–S72, 2000.
9. Balakumar P, Arora MK, Ganti SS, et al: Recent advances in pharmacotherapy for diabetic nephropathy: current perspectives and future directions. *Pharmacol Res* 60(1):24–32, 2009.
10. Casqueiro J, Casqueiro J, Alves C: Infections in patients with diabetes mellitus: a review of pathogenesis. *Indian J Endocrinol Metab* 16[Suppl 1]:S27–S36, 2012.
11. Shah BR, Hux JE: Quantifying the risk of infectious diseases for people with diabetes. *Diabetes Care* 26(2):510–513, 2003.
12. Joshi N, Caputo GM, Weitekamp MR, et al: Infections in patients with diabetes mellitus. *N Engl J Med* 341:1906–1912, 1999.
13. Shilling AM, Raphael J: Diabetes, hyperglycemia, and infections. *Best Pract Res Clin Anaesthesiol* 22(3):519–535, 2008.
14. Jeffcoate WJ, Lipsky BA, Berendt AR, et al: Unresolved issues in the management of ulcers of the foot in diabetes. *Diabet Med* 25(12):1380–1389, 2008.
15. Samaras K: Prevalence and pathogenesis of diabetes mellitus in HIV-1 infection treated with combined antiretroviral therapy. *J Acquir Immune Defic Syndr* 50(5):499–505, 2009.
16. Dooley KE, Chaisson RE: Tuberculosis and diabetes mellitus: convergence of two epidemics. *Lancet Infect Dis* 9(12):737–746, 2009.
17. Cely CM, Arora P, Quartin AA, et al: Relationship of baseline glucose homeostasis to hyperglycemia during medical critical illness. *Chest* 126(3):879–887, 2004.
18. Dungan KM, Braithwaite SS, Preiser JC: Stress hyperglycaemia. *Lancet* 373(9677):1798–1807, 2009.
19. Flakoll PJ, Jensen MD, Cherrington AD: Physiologic action of insulin, in LeRoith D, Taylor SI, Olefsky JM, (eds): *Diabetes Mellitus. A Fundamental and Clinical Text.* 3rd ed. Philadelphia, PA, Lippincott Williams & Wilkins, 2004, pp 165–181.
20. American Diabetes Association: Classification and diagnosis of diabetes. *Diabetes Care* 39[Suppl 1]:S13–S22, 2016.
21. Barker JM, Eisenbarth GS: The natural history of autoimmunity in type 1A diabetes mellitus, in LeRoith D, Taylor SI, Olefsky JM, (eds): *Diabetes Mellitus. A Fundamental and Clinical Text.* 3rd ed. Philadelphia, PA, Lippincott Williams & Wilkins, 2004, pp 471–482.
22. LeRoith D: Beta-cell dysfunction and insulin resistance in type 2 diabetes: role of metabolic and genetic abnormalities. *Am J Med* 113:3S–11S, 2002.
23. Petersen KF, Shulman GI: Etiology of insulin resistance. *Am J Med* 119[5 Suppl 1]:S10–S16, 2006.

24. Reaven GM: Insulin resistance and its consequences: type 2 diabees mellitus and the insulin resistance syndrome, in LeRoith D, Taylor SI, Olefsky JM, (eds): *Diabetes Mellitus. A Fundamental and Clinical Text*. 3rd ed. Philadelphia, PA, Lippincott Williams & Wilkins, 2004, pp 899–916.
25. Samuel VT, Shulman GI: Mechanisms for insulin resistance: common threads and missing links. *Cell* 148(5):852–871, 2012.
26. Westphal SA: Occurrence of diabetic ketoacidosis in non-insulin-dependent diabetes and newly diagnosed diabetic adults. *Am J Med* 101:19–24, 1996.
27. American Diabetes Association: Diagnosis and classification of diabetes mellitus. *Diabetes Care* 33[Suppl 1]:S62–S69, 2010.
28. Van den Berghe G, Wilmer A, Hermans G, et al: Intensive insulin therapy in the medical ICU. *N Engl J Med* 354(5):449–461, 2006.
29. Diabetes Control and Complications Trial Research Group: The effect of intensive treatment of diabetes on the development and progression of long-term complications in insulin-dependent diabetes mellitus. *N Engl J Med* 329:977–986, 1993.
30. Genuth S, Eastman R, Kahn R, et al; American Diabetes Association: Implications of the United Kingdom prospective diabetes study. *Diabetes Care* 22:S27–S31, 1999.
31. Boyko EJ, Lipsky BA: Infection and diabetes, in National Diabetes Data Group, (ed): Diabetes in America. 2nd ed. Bethesda, MD, National Institutes of Health, 1995, pp 485–499.
32. Nicolle LE: Urinary tract infection in diabetes. *Curr Opin Infect Dis* 18(1):49–53, 2005.
33. Goldberg IJ: Clinical review 124—diabetic dyslipidemia: causes and consequences. *J Clin Endocrinol Metab* 86:965–971, 2001.
34. Lacara T, Domagtoy C, Lickliter D, et al: Comparison of point-of-care and laboratory glucose analysis in critically ill patients. *Am J Crit Care* 16(4):336–346, 2007.
35. Goldstein DE, Little RR, Lorenz RA, et al: Tests of glycemia in diabetes. *Diabetes Care* 27(7):1761–1773, 2004.
36. Kurahashi K, Maruta H, Usuda Y, et al: Influence of blood sample oxygen tension on blood glucose concentration measured using an enzyme-electrode method. *Crit Care Med* 25(2):231–235, 1997.
37. Desachy A, Vuagnat AC, Ghazali AD, et al: Accuracy of bedside glucometry in critically ill patients: influence of clinical characteristics and perfusion index. *Mayo Clin Proc* 83(4):400–405, 2008.
38. Eastham JH, Mason D, Barnes DL, et al: Prevalence of interfering substances with point-of-care glucose testing in a community hospital. *Am J Health Syst Pharm* 66(2):167–170, 2009.
39. Kanji S, Buffie J, Hutton B, et al: Reliability of point-of-care testing for glucose measurement in critically ill adults. *Crit Care Med* 33(12):2778–2785, 2005.
40. Rodbard D: Continuous glucose monitoring: a review of successes, challenges, and opportunities. *Diabetes Technol Ther* 18[Suppl 2]:S23–S213, 2016.
41. Gottschalk A, Welp HA, Leser L, et al: Continuous glucose monitoring in patients undergoing extracorporeal ventricular assist therapy. *PLoS One* 11(3):e0148778, 2016.
42. Crane BC, Barwell NP, Gopal P, et al: The development of a continuous intravascular glucose monitoring sensor. *J Diabetes Sci Technol* 9(4):751–761, 2015.
43. El-Khatib FH, Russell SJ, Nathan DM, et al: A bihormonal closed-loop artificial pancreas for type 1 diabetes. *Sci Transl Med* 2(27):27ra27, 2010.
44. Capes SE, Hunt D, Malmberg K, et al: Stress hyperglycaemia and increased risk of death after myocardial infarction in patients with and without diabetes: a systematic overview. *Lancet* 355(9206):773–778, 2000.
45. Furnary AP, Zerr KJ, Grunkemeier GL, et al: Continuous intravenous insulin infusion reduces the incidence of deep sternal wound infection in diabetic patients after cardiac surgical procedures. *Ann Thorac Surg* 67:352–360, 1999.
46. Furnary AP, Gao G, Grunkemeier GL, et al: Continuous insulin infusion reduces mortality in patients with diabetes undergoing coronary artery bypass grafting. *J Thorac Cardiovasc Surg* 125(5):1007–1021, 2003.
47. Capes SE, Hunt D, Malmberg K, et al: Stress hyperglycemia and prognosis of stroke in nondiabetic and diabetic patients: a systematic overview. *Stroke* 32(10):2426–2432, 2001.
48. Umpierrez GE, Isaacs SD, Bazargan N, et al: Hyperglycemia: an independent marker of in-hospital mortality in patients with undiagnosed diabetes. *J Clin Endocrinol Metab* 87(3):978–982, 2002.
49. Geerlings SE, Hoepelman AIM: Immune dysfunction in patients with diabetes mellitus (DM). *FEMS Immunol Med Microbiol* 26:259–265, 1999.
50. Alexiewicz JM, Kumar D, Smogorzewski M, et al: Polymorphonuclear leukocytes in non-insulin-dependent diabetes mellitus: abnormalities in metabolism and function. *Ann Intern Med* 123:919–924, 1995.
51. McMahon MM, Bistrian BR: Host defenses and susceptibility to infection in patients with diabetes mellitus. *Infect Dis Clin North Am* 9(1):1–9, 1995.
52. Abrass CK: Fc receptor-mediated phagocytosis: abnormalities associated with diabetes mellitus. *Clin Immunol Immunopathol* 58:1–17, 1991.
53. Langouche L, Vanhorebeek I, Vlasselaers D, et al: Intensive insulin therapy protects the endothelium of critically ill patients. *J Clin Invest* 115(8):2277–2286, 2005.
54. Krinsley JS, Egi M, Kiss A, et al: Diabetic status and the relation of the three domains of glycemic control to mortality in critically ill patients: an international multicenter cohort study. *Crit Care* 17(2):R37, 2013.
55. Van den Berghe G, Wouters P, Weekers F, et al: Intensive insulin therapy in critically ill patients. *N Engl J Med* 345(19):1359–1367, 2001.
56. Krinsley JS: Effect of an intensive glucose management protocol on the mortality of critically ill adult patients. *Mayo Clin Proc* 79(8):992–1000, 2004.
57. Kanji S, Singh A, Tierney M, et al: Standardization of intravenous insulin therapy improves the efficiency and safety of blood glucose control in critically ill adults. *Intensive Care Med* 30(5):804–810, 2004.
58. Niven DJ, Rubenfeld GD, Kramer AA, et al: Effect of published scientific evidence on glycemic control in adult intensive care units. *JAMA Intern Med* 175(5):801–809, 2015.
59. Preiser JC, Devos P, Ruiz-Santana S, et al: A prospective randomised multi-centre controlled trial on tight glucose control by intensive insulin therapy in adult intensive care units: the Glucontrol study. *Intensive Care Med* 35(10):1738–1748, 2009.
60. Finfer S, Chittock DR, Su SY, et al: Intensive versus conventional glucose control in critically ill patients. *N Engl J Med* 360(13):1283–1297, 2009.
61. Annane D, Cariou A, Maxime V, et al: Corticosteroid treatment and intensive insulin therapy for septic shock in adults: a randomized controlled trial. *JAMA* 303(4):341–348, 2010.
62. Egi M, Bellomo R, Stachowski E, et al: Hypoglycemia and outcome in critically ill patients. *Mayo Clin Proc* 85(3):217–224, 2010.
63. Hermanides J, Bosman RJ, Vriesendorp TM, et al: Hypoglycemia is associated with intensive care unit mortality. *Crit Care Med* 38(6):1430–1434, 2010.
64. Egi M, Krinsley JS, Maurer P, et al: Pre-morbid glycemic control modifies the interaction between acute hypoglycemia and mortality. *Intensive Care Med* 42(4):562–571, 2016.
65. Krinsley JS, Preiser JC: Time in blood glucose range 70 to 140 mg/dl >80% is strongly associated with increased survival in non-diabetic critically ill adults. *Crit Care* 19:179, 2015.
66. Umpierrez G, Cardona S, Pasquel F, et al: Randomized controlled trial of intensive versus conservative glucose control in patients undergoing coronary artery bypass graft surgery: GLUCO-CABG trial. *Diabetes Care* 38(9):1665–1672, 2015.
67. Moghissi ES, Korytkowski MT, DiNardo M, et al: American Association of Clinical Endocrinologists and American Diabetes Association consensus statement on inpatient glycemic control. *Diabetes Care* 32(6):1119–1131, 2009.
68. Kagansky N, Levy S, Rimon E, et al: Hypoglycemia as a predictor of mortality in hospitalized elderly patients. *Arch Intern Med* 163(15):1825–1829, 2003.
69. Luft FC: Lactic acidosis update for critical care clinicians. *J Am Soc Nephrol* 12:S15–S19, 2001.
70. Peters AL, Henry RR, Thakkar P, et al: Diabetic ketoacidosis with canagliflozin, a sodium-glucose cotransporter 2 inhibitor, in patients with type 1 diabetes. *Diabetes Care* 39:532–538, 2016.
71. Peters AL, Buschur EO, Buse JB, et al: Euglycemic diabetic ketoacidosis: a potential complication of treatment with sodium-glucose cotransporter 2 inhibition. *Diabetes Care* 38(9):1687–1693, 2015.
72. Marik PE, Preiser JC: Toward understanding tight glycemic control in the ICU: a systematic review and metaanalysis. *Chest* 137(3):544–551, 2010.
73. Shulman GI: Cellular mechanisms of insulin resistance. *J Clin Invest* 106:171–176, 2000.
74. Shepherd PR, Kahn BB: Mechanisms of disease—glucose transporters and insulin action—implications for insulin resistance and diabetes mellitus. *N Engl J Med* 341:248–257, 1999.
75. Olefsky JM, Nolan JJ: Insulin resistance and non-insulin-dependent diabetes mellitus: cellular and molecular mechanisms. *Am J Clin Nutr* 61[Suppl]:980S–986S, 1995.
76. Dierdorf SF: Anesthesia for patients with diabetes mellitus. *Curr Opin Anaesthesiol* 15(3):351–357, 2002.
77. Tanaka K, Kawano T, Tomino T, et al: Mechanisms of impaired glucose tolerance and insulin secretion during isoflurane anesthesia. *Anesthesiology* 111(5):1044–1051, 2009.
78. Tuttnauer A, Levin PD: Diabetes mellitus and anesthesia. *Anesthesiol Clin* 24(3):579–597, 2006.
79. Choban PS, Burge JC, Scales D, et al: Hypoenergetic nutrition support in hospitalized obese patients: a simplified method for clinical application. *Am J Clin Nutr* 66:546–550, 1997.
80. Shikora SA, Jensen GL: Hypoenergetic nutrition support in hospitalized obese patients. *Am J Clin Nutr* 66:679–680, 1997.
81. Cohen RD, Woods HF: Lactic acidosis revisited. *Diabetes* 32:181–191, 1983.
82. Queale WS, Seidler AJ, Brancati FL: Glycemic control and sliding scale insulin use in medical inpatients with diabetes mellitus. *Arch Intern Med* 157:545–552, 1997.
83. Baldwin D, Villanueva G, McNutt R, et al: Eliminating inpatient sliding-scale insulin: a reeducation project with medical house staff. *Diabetes Care* 28(5):1008–1011, 2005.
84. Cryer PE: Mechanisms of hypoglycemia-associated autonomic failure in diabetes. *N Engl J Med* 369(4):362–372, 2013.
85. Mehran R, Aymong ED, Nikolsky E, et al: A simple risk score for prediction of contrast-induced nephropathy after percutaneous coronary intervention: development and initial validation. *J Am Coll Cardiol* 44(7):1393–1399, 2004.
86. McCullough PA, Stacul F, Becker CR, Adam A, Lameire N, Tumlin JA, Davidson CJ; CIN Consensus Working Panel: Contrast-induced nephropathy (CIN) consensus working panel: executive summary. *Rev Cardiovasc Med* 7(4):177–197, 2006.
87. Subramaniam RM, Suarez-Cuervo C, Wilson RF, et al: Effectiveness of prevention strategies for contrast-induced nephropathy: a systematic review and meta-analysis. *Ann Intern Med* 164(6):406–416, 2016.
88. Ganda OP: Prevalence and incidence of secondary and other types of diabetes, in National Diabetes Data Group, (ed): *Diabetes in America*. 2nd ed. Bethesda, MD, National Institutes of Health, 1995, pp 69–84.
89. Conner TM, Flesner-Gurley KR, Barner JC: Hyperglycemia in the hospital setting: the case for improved control among non-diabetics. *Ann Pharmacother* 39(3):492–501, 2005.
90. Brunkhorst FM, Engel C, Bloos F, et al: Intensive insulin therapy and pentastarch resuscitation in severe sepsis. *N Engl J Med* 358(2):125–139, 2008.

Chapter 137 ■ Diabetic Comas: Ketoacidosis and Hyperosmolar Hyperglycemic State

SAMIR MALKANI • DAVID M. HARLAN • MICHAEL J. THOMPSON • JOHN P. MORDES

INTRODUCTION

The Acute Metabolic Complications of Diabetes: The Overlap Concept

The most urgent metabolic complications of diabetes are the four diabetic comas: hypoglycemia, diabetic ketoacidosis (DKA), hyperglycemic hyperosmolar syndrome (HHS), and alcoholic ketoacidosis (ethanol-induced hypoglycemia). These diagnostic possibilities must be considered for any lethargic or comatose patient. In addition to being life-threatening conditions, they account for thousands of hospitalizations and substantial costs [1]. Recognition of these diabetic comas is particularly important because these conditions are reversible with appropriate treatment. We use diabetic coma as a generic term that encompasses both frank coma and the milder metabolic abnormalities that precede loss of consciousness. This chapter considers the hyperglycemic crises; hypoglycemia and alcoholic ketoacidosis are discussed in Chapter 138.

Although DKA and HHS are discussed separately, it is important to recognize that metabolic decompensation related to hyperglycemia can take many forms depending on the severity of insulin deficiency, underlying genetic predispositions, and intercurrent illnesses. There is frequent overlap of the clinical phenotypes, and clinicians should be aware of this concept [1,2]. DKA can occur for a patient with type 2 diabetes; up to a third of patients with HHS have no prior history of diabetes; both DKA and HHS can be complicated by lactic, uremic, or other form of metabolic acidosis, and ketoacidosis itself can occur in the setting of profound hypoglycemia [3]. These metabolic disturbances can overlap to yield both classical DKA and nonclassical presentations of HHS and other ketotic and acidotic states.

For a comatose patient with a blood glucose concentration of less than 50 mg per dL or if for any reason the blood glucose cannot be measured rapidly, the first diagnostic and therapeutic step should be the infusion of 50 mL of a 50% dextrose solution, or when intravenous is not available, injection of 1 mg glucagon intramuscularly or subcutaneously. The hypoglycemic patient who awakens is resuscitated; coma of any other origin is not adversely affected.

DIABETIC KETOACIDOSIS

DKA is comprised of the triad of hyperglycemia, metabolic acidosis, and ketonemia. Any person with diabetes can develop DKA [1], but it most often occurs in those with type 1 diabetes. Before the discovery of insulin, most patients with type 1 diabetes died during an episode of DKA. With current intensive care, overall mortality from DKA has fallen to less than 1%, but is higher among the elderly and those with concomitant major illness [4]. Deaths are associated with intercurrent heart disease or infection of older patients and cerebral edema of younger patients.

Pathophysiology and Etiology

Normal Glucose Homeostasis

After a meal, pancreatic islet β cells release insulin into the circulation, enabling fuels to enter cells and activating enzymes for their storage or metabolism. Glucose enters most tissues only in the presence of insulin; erythrocytes, heart, and brain are exceptions. Glucose is stored in liver and muscle cells as glycogen. Some glucose is metabolized; some is converted into triglycerides.

In adipose tissue, insulin activates lipoprotein lipase, which clears lipoproteins from the circulation, and stores the triglycerides intracellularly. Insulin also inhibits the breakdown and release of previously stored fat. Insulin has similar effects on skeletal muscle, permitting both amino acids and glucose to enter cells for oxidation or storage [5,6].

During starvation, insulin concentrations decrease, catabolic pathways are activated, and stored fuels (glucose, amino acids, and fats) are mobilized to meet energy needs. Liver glycogen provides glucose for only several hours. Muscle glycogen is not directly available due to lack of glucose-6-phosphatase in muscle cells because glucose-6-phosphate cannot cross the plasma membrane. To support plasma glucose, muscle glycogen undergoes anaerobic glycolysis, generating lactate which can cross the plasma membrane and be converted into glucose in the liver. After glycogen stores are exhausted, the liver synthesizes glucose from muscle-derived amino acids through the process of gluconeogenesis [7]. To conserve muscle mass during starvation, glucose consumption is reduced and fatty acids released from adipose tissue become the principal fuel source. Some fatty acids are transformed by the liver into ketoacids [8].

The rate of catabolism is regulated by insulin. As circulating glucose concentration decreases, insulin concentration also decreases—but never to zero. Low insulin levels permit lipolysis and proteolysis while stimulating gluconeogenesis, all to maintain normal glucose concentrations. Increased glucose concentration stimulates insulin secretion, which in turn reduces or halts catabolism. Precise regulation of insulin secretion, even in the absence of food intake, achieves continuous control of carbohydrate metabolism.

Abnormal Glucose Homeostasis

DKA can be viewed as a "super-fasted" state that occurs when there is insufficient insulin available to regulate carbohydrate metabolism [6]. Without insulin, glucose no longer enters most cells and is neither stored nor metabolized. Glucagon secretion is increased and hepatic glucose production increases without restraint. When the renal threshold for glucose is exceeded (180 to 200 mg per dL), an osmotic diuresis ensues and water and electrolytes are lost. If insulin deficiency persists, the stress-response hormones cortisol, epinephrine, norepinephrine, glucagon, and growth hormone are released and accelerate catabolism. Glucagon excess is responsible for the oxidation of fatty acids to ketone bodies by the liver. When the rate of hepatic ketoacid generation exceeds peripheral utilization, DKA ensues with the life-threatening combination of hyperglycemia, acidemia, ketonemia, loss of free water, and depletion of electrolytes.

The cause of ketoacidosis is insulin deficiency. New-onset type 1 diabetes commonly presents as ketoacidosis, but most cases occur among individuals known to have diabetes. Dietary indiscretion of a person with known treated diabetes may produce classic hyperglycemia, polydipsia, and polyuria but not ketosis. Ketonuria with any hyperglycemic diabetic patient should suggest the presence of DKA. Such patients must be carefully evaluated for the presence of acidemia. Ketoacidosis occurs most often among patients who have omitted their insulin or who have an intercurrent infection [9].

Infection and other stressors produce a state of insulin resistance, in part because of the presence of high inflammatory cytokine levels (in particular, tumor necrosis factor α); infection may be the most common trigger of DKA patients admitted to an intensive care unit (ICU) [10]. Severe stress occasionally causes ketosis among patients with type 2 diabetes [4]. African Americans with type 2 diabetes may be particularly susceptible to the development of ketosis [11,12]. Other factors that can precipitate ketosis include acute myocardial infarction, emotional stress, cancer, drugs that interfere with insulin release or action, pregnancy, menstruation, and various endocrinopathies. The use of sodium-glucose cotransporter-2 (SGLT-2) inhibitors (see Chapter 138 on Hypoglycemia) appears to increase the risk of DKA [9,13]. Among those using insulin pumps, catheter site problems resulting in leakage or nondelivery of insulin can precipitate DKA [9]. Occasionally, no precipitating factor can be identified.

Clinical Manifestations

Most patients with DKA are lethargic; about 10% are comatose [14]. They have typically lost large quantities of fluid; their skin, lips, and tongue are dry; and their eyes are soft to palpation. Postural hypotension is common, but shock is rare [15].

Patients with DKA have rapid deep respiration (called Kussmaul), and their breath has a sweet fruity odor. Some patients with new-onset DKA have been misdiagnosed as having psychological hyperventilation [16]. If a patient with DKA is not tachypneic, the physician should suspect that severe acidosis (pH <7.1) may be depressing the respiratory drive [17].

It is important to measure the temperature accurately. Because the patient is hyperventilating, rectal or tympanic temperature should be measured. Patients with DKA do not have fever unless an intercurrent process, usually infection, is present. Similarly, the rare cases of hypothermia in DKA are associated with sepsis [18].

Abdominal pain is common and may be accompanied by a tender guarded abdomen with diminished or absent bowel sounds. DKA should always be excluded when evaluating abdominal pain [19]. What may appear to be a surgical condition will resolve with correction of the acidosis.

Patients with DKA may be nauseous and vomit guaiac-positive coffee grounds–like material. This is probably due to gastric atony, distention, and rupture of mucosal blood vessels. Pleuritic chest pain may also be present. The cause is unknown, but it resolves with treatment of the DKA.

The nose and sinuses of all patients with DKA should be examined. Acute sinusitis and a black intranasal eschar should suggest mucormycosis, an opportunistic fungal infection that disseminates rapidly in acidotic patients. Mucormycosis is often fatal; survival requires prompt diagnosis [20]. DKA as a complication of pregnancy can occur at lower glucose concentrations and progress rapidly. During pregnancy, rates of fetal loss can be high when DKA occurs with new-onset diabetes, when it is due to poor adherence to insulin therapy in preexisting diabetes, or when pregnancy is complicated by infection [21].

Laboratory Diagnosis

Hyperglycemia, acidemia, and ketosis in the appropriate clinical setting are the criteria for the diagnosis of DKA.

Blood Glucose. Normal plasma glucose concentration is 60 to 120 mg per dL (3.3 to 6.7 mmol). Whole blood glucose concentrations are 15% to 20% lower. Fingerstick blood glucose determinations are performed on whole capillary blood, and most meters correct for this offset. Calibrated glucose meters suitable for use in the ICU are accurate over a wide range of concentrations, but accuracy is reduced by very high and low glucose concentrations and acidemia; when these conditions are present, results should be confirmed by a clinical laboratory measurement [22]. Meters intended for home use may give less reproducibly accurate results.

Among patients with DKA, blood glucose concentrations of 400 to 800 mg per dL are typical. As many as 15% of cases of DKA present with blood glucose concentrations less than 300 mg per dL [23], and in rare situations, patients present with blood glucose below 180 mg per dL and ketoacidosis [24]. This has been described as euglycemic DKA. Typically, these are younger patients with a high glomerular filtration rate (GFR). Administration of insulin prior to presentation, antecedent food restrictions, and use of SGLT-2 inhibitors can also lower plasma glucose at presentation [4]. More often, the solute diuresis causes dehydration, decreases the GFR, and further increases circulating blood glucose concentration.

Electrolytes

Sodium. Serum sodium concentration is quite variable in DKA and must be interpreted in the context of serum glucose and lipid concentrations. If extremely abnormal, it needs special attention during management. Large amounts of sodium are lost during the osmotic diuresis of DKA, and the serum concentration does not necessarily reflect this loss. Because sodium resides principally in the extracellular fluid space, elevated sodium concentration may simply reflect the degree of free water loss.

Abnormally low sodium concentrations may be due to the osmotic effect of large amounts of extracellular glucose. The osmotic activity of glucose, drawing free water from the intracellular to the extracellular space, produces a fall of 1.6 mEq per L of sodium for every increase of 100 mg per dL in blood glucose concentration more than 100 mg per dL [25]. The "corrected" serum sodium of a patient with a measured concentration of 135 mEq per L and a glucose concentration of 600 mg per dL is $[1.6 \times (6 - 1) + 135]$, or 143 mEq per L. The patient presenting with an elevated serum sodium concentration despite hyperglycemia has a severe total body free water deficit.

It is also important to be certain that abnormally low serum sodium concentrations of DKA patients are not factitious. Sodium resides only in the aqueous phase of plasma and when the nonaqueous constituents such as triglycerides increase substantially, the reported concentration of sodium will be spuriously low with older testing methods. Current technology using "ion-specific" electrodes is unaffected by this problem.

Chloride. Chloride concentrations are usually not helpful for the diagnosis of DKA, although they may provide useful information. Hyperchloremia may sometimes represent a more chronic ketoacidotic state [26] and may be associated with slower recovery [27]. Extremely low levels of chloride may result from vomiting [28]. Hyperchloremic acidosis can also occur during recovery from DKA as a consequence of urinary losses of neutralized ketone body salts [29].

Potassium. Potassium is the electrolyte that must be watched most carefully and often during therapy. All patients with DKA are at risk of life-threatening hypokalemia during treatment, despite the fact that the serum potassium concentration is usually elevated at presentation [27,30]. This elevation is due to catabolism of tissue, dehydration, and shifts in potassium from the intracellular to the extracellular space as hydrogen ions are buffered. An initially elevated serum potassium concentration should never obscure the fact that total body potassium loss (in the range of 200 to 700 mEq) occurs with ketoacidosis. The greatest potassium loss accompanies the osmotic diuresis of glucose. Additional losses are due to the excretion of ketone bodies as potassium salts, dehydration-induced secondary hyperaldosteronism, and vomiting. Potassium replacement is virtually always necessary early in the course of DKA therapy. It should be started as soon as the potassium concentration is at the upper end of the normal range because continued insulin therapy will invariably cause the potassium concentration to fall further. Normal or low concentrations of potassium early in ketoacidosis reflect a very severe potassium deficit.

Magnesium. Like potassium, serum magnesium concentrations among patients with untreated DKA tend to be elevated initially, but they fall with subsequent hydration.

Bicarbonate. Serum bicarbonate concentrations are low with ketoacidosis [17] because of neutralization of ketone bodies, which are acids. Bicarbonate buffer in the extracellular compartment represents the first line of defense in acid–base homeostasis. The process is summarized in Figure 137.1. Hydrogen ion (H^+) from ketoacids is neutralized by bicarbonate, producing carbonic acid, water, and CO_2. As CO_2 is cleared through the lungs, the neutralized salts of the ketone bodies are excreted in the urine. Among patients with established DKA, the serum bicarbonate concentration is typically less than 15 mEq per L, and can be much lower.

Phosphorous. Elevated serum phosphate concentrations are common with untreated DKA; the mechanism is not clear. After

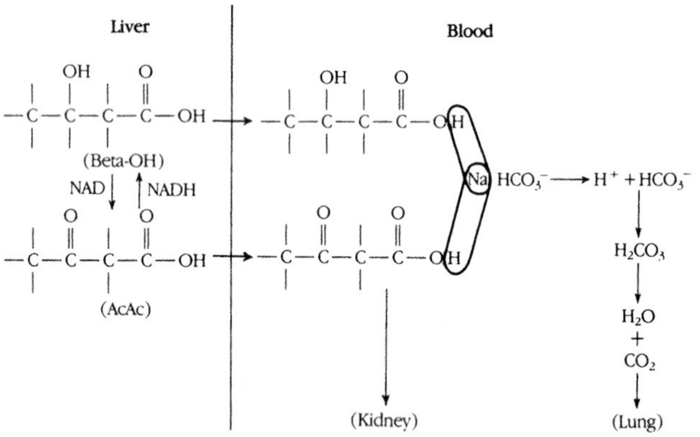

FIGURE 137.1 Neutralization of ketoacids. Hydrogen ion from ketoacids is neutralized by bicarbonate, producing carbonic acid that then decomposes to H_2O and CO_2. The latter is expelled by the lungs. The neutralized salts of ketone bodies are excreted in the urine. NAD, nicotinamide adenine dinucleotide; NADH, reduced form of NAD; AcAc, acetoacetate; Beta-OH, β-hydroxybutyrate.

TABLE 137.1

Calculations

Anion gap[a]	Anion Gap = $Na^+ - (Cl^- + HCO_3^-)$
Osmolality[b]	$2(Na^+ + K^+)$ + Glucose/18 + BUN/2.8

[a]Normal Anion Gap is less than 12 mEq per L for most laboratories. Refer to your lab normal range.
[b]Normal osmolality: 285 to 295 mOsm per kg. BUN, blood urea nitrogen.

therapy, there is a precipitous decline to subnormal levels. It has been estimated that as much as 1 mmol per kg of phosphate is lost during DKA. Hypophosphatemia of less than 0.5 mmol per L has been described for both DKA and HHS [31].

Acidosis. Arterial blood gas and pH measurements are essential for the management of all but the mildest cases of DKA. The arterial pH in DKA is almost always less than 7.3. If arterial samples cannot be obtained, venous or capillary samples may be used, although they provide less information [32]. DKA classically presents as an anion gap acidosis. The anion gap should be calculated for all acidemic patients (Table 137.1). In addition to confirming the diagnosis of DKA, the anion gap can be used together with plasma ketone measurements to obtain important additional insight into the nature and severity of a given case [33]. More chronic ketoacidotic states may be associated with hyperchloremic rather than anion gap acidosis [26], probably as a consequence of the loss of neutralized ketone body salts [29]. Rare cases of DKA are complicated by intercurrent metabolic alkalosis, most often from severe vomiting [28,34].

Plasma Ketones and β-Hydroxybutyrate

Plasma ketones should be measured for all patients with diabetes who appear critically ill or exhibit signs of dehydration at the time of presentation. When the nitroprusside test is used, the results are usually expressed as the highest dilution of serum that gives a positive reaction. This test is always positive (>1:2 dilution) during DKA, but its result may not reflect the full extent of ketogenesis. This is because the test measures only acetoacetate (AcAc) and acetone. It does not measure β-hydroxybutyrate (BOHB), which, although a "ketone body," is a hydroxyl acid and not a ketone (Fig. 137.2). Normally, the BOHB-to-AcAc ratio is 3:1, but acidosis increases the ratio to 6:1 or even 12:1 as pH decreases. The BOHB-to-AcAc ratio at pH 7.1 is at least 6:1.

BOHB can be measured directly, and the test is available from many hospital laboratories. Measurement of BOHB concentration, if the result is available rapidly, can also be used to establish the diagnosis of DKA. The advantage of BOHB measurement derives from the fact that it is the major ketone body and its concentration is a better indicator of the severity of ketoacidosis.

The results of plasma ketone, BOHB, anion gap, and arterial pH measurements can be used to determine whether a pure or mixed anion gap acidosis is present. The highest positive

FIGURE 137.2 Biochemical interrelationships of the ketone bodies. Acetoacetate and acetone are ketones, whereas β-hydroxybutyrate, although a "ketone body," is β-hydroxy carboxylic acid and not a ketone. NAD^+, nicotine adenine dinucleotide; NADH, reduced form of NAD.

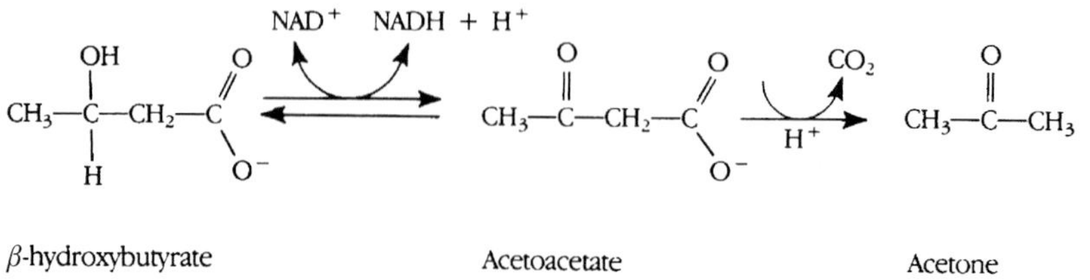

ketone dilution is multiplied by 0.1 mmol per L to obtain an estimate of AcAc concentration; the BOHB can be measured directly. If a patient's anion gap as calculated in Table 137.1 is greater than the estimated contribution of ketone bodies (AcAc plus BOHB), the presence of an additional unmeasured anion should be considered (e.g., lactate, salicylate, uremic compounds, methanol, or ethylene glycol; see Chapter 198).

Ketone body measurements are also useful for monitoring the resolution of DKA. During severe acidosis, ketones as measured by the nitroprusside reaction initially rise rather than fall as the acidosis improves. This is due to conversion of BOHB back to AcAc. Clearance of ketone bodies occurs slowly; frequent measurement of ketones and BOHB is generally unnecessary.

It is worth noting that certain home blood monitors have the capacity to measure not only glucose but also "ketones." These meters measure BOHB rather than AcAc using strips distinct from those used to measure glucose. They can warn patients of impending or established ketoacidosis prior to hospital presentation.

Blood Urea Nitrogen and Creatinine. The blood urea nitrogen (BUN) of patients with DKA is typically elevated to values between 25 and 50 mg per dL due not only to prerenal azotemia from volume depletion but also from increased ureagenesis. Patients with DKA are in a state of uncontrolled gluconeogenesis; the large quantities of amino acids released from muscle for conversion to glucose produce hyperaminoacidemia. These amino acids increase substrate availability for ureagenesis. Although the serum creatinine concentration usually reflects the degree of dehydration and prerenal azotemia during DKA accurately [35], spurious elevations occasionally occur because AcAc interferes with some older creatinine assays [36].

Complete Blood Count. Hematocrit and hemoglobin during DKA are usually high and in proportion to the degree of dehydration. Low values suggest preexisting anemia or acute blood loss. A characteristic hematologic finding during DKA is leukocytosis. The white cell count can be elevated to 20,000 or more with a shift to the left in the absence of infection, but concurrent infection should be actively sought whenever the white count is significantly elevated [14,37].

Triglycerides. Insulin deficiency impairs clearance of lipid from the circulation and accelerates hepatic production of very low-density lipoprotein [5]. During DKA, there is marked elevation of serum triglyceride concentrations that may be clinically obvious in the form of lactescent serum. With insulin therapy, this biochemical derangement reverses. If a patient can eat during the onset of DKA, hyperchylomicronemia may also be present.

Urine. Urinary glucose and acetone should be measured. If pyuria is present, a urine specimen should be sent for culture and sensitivity. Catheterization should be avoided unless the patient is comatose or anuric. A pregnancy test should be performed for women of childbearing age, as pregnancy can precipitate DKA.

Serum Amylase and Lipase. Serum amylase and lipase concentrations are sometimes elevated during acute ketoacidosis, but they do not necessarily imply exocrine pancreatic disease [38,39]. For some cases, the amylase may be of salivary gland origin.

Other Laboratory Findings. Uric acid concentrations may be elevated during acute DKA [40] as a result of impaired renal function or competition from ketone bodies at sites of tubular secretion. Hepatic enlargement with fatty infiltration of parenchymal cells may occur during acute DKA. Increased levels of C-reactive protein and interleukin-6 may be indicative of underlying infection precipitating DKA [41].

Treatment

Patients with severe DKA should be hospitalized in an ICU. Delaying intensive care greatly increases morbidity, and detaining patients in the emergency room long after the diagnosis is established should be avoided. Some hospitals are able to treat DKA outside the ICU with protocols involving close monitoring, and report good outcomes [42]. Treatment should be directed at three main problems—fluid deficits, electrolyte abnormalities, and insulin deficiency—in that order [43]. Table 137.2 highlights the key components of therapy.

Recording of Data

The comprehensive flow sheet of vital signs, laboratory data, and treatment that is part of the modern electronic ICU greatly enhances management. In the absence of electronic records, a comprehensive paper flow sheet is essential to follow the responses to therapy. Standardized protocols may improve efficiency of care.

Fluid Replacement

Fluid and electrolyte therapy always takes precedence over insulin administration during the treatment of DKA. As described later in the "Complications" section of this chapter, insulin administration before volume and potassium repletion can cause shock and arrhythmias [44].

The free water deficits of adults with DKA generally range between 5 and 11 L, typically about 100 mL per kg, and is due primarily to the osmotic diuresis of hyperglycemia [43,45]. Vomiting and hyperventilation may also contribute to water losses. Initial fluid resuscitation should be an infusion of 0.9% saline. Approximately 2 L or 25 mL per kg should be given during the first hour to restore blood volume, stabilize blood pressure, and reestablish urine flow. Another liter of 0.9% saline can typically be given during the next 2 hours. The subsequent rate of fluid replacement depends on individual clinical circumstances. During the first 24 hours, 75% of the estimated total water deficit should be replaced. Urine flow should be maintained at approximately 30 to 60 mL or 0.5 mL/kg/h. Fluid replacement after the first 2 L may be changed to hypotonic 0.45% saline when hypernatremia is present [46].

Electrolytes

Sodium, Chloride, and Potassium. Sodium and chloride are replaced together with free water as just described. Potassium must be added to the saline. Because serum potassium concentration does not accurately reflect total body potassium, replacement should be initiated early during treatment. Until the serum potassium concentration is known, replacement should be carried out cautiously. The recommended initial repletion rate is 20 mEq per hour as KCl or K_3PO_4. When the serum value is known, the rate of potassium administration can be adjusted. If a nasogastric tube is in place, electrolyte losses due to gastric suctioning must also be considered. Typical potassium deficits in DKA are 3 to 5 mEq per kg, but if hypokalemia or normokalemia is present at the time of admission, the deficit may be much higher, up to 10 mEq per kg.

Potassium concentration often falls precipitously after starting therapy. K^+ shifts from the extracellular to the intracellular space in the presence of glucose and insulin. As acidemia resolves, buffered intracellular H^+ is exchanged for extracellular K^+, further lowering the serum potassium concentration. A sudden reduction in serum potassium concentration can cause flaccid paralysis, respiratory failure, and life-threatening cardiac arrhythmias. If a patient in mild DKA is alert and able to tolerate liquids, potassium should be given orally.

Phosphate. Depletion of phosphate occurs with DKA. Initially, the concentration of phosphate is elevated, but levels may decrease to less than 1 mmol per L within 4 to 6 hours of starting insulin treatment. Persistent severe hypophosphatemia can cause neurologic disturbances, arthralgias, muscle weakness with respiratory impairment, rhabdomyolysis, and liver dysfunction [47].

Except when hypophosphatemia is severe (≤1.0 mg per dL), however, the need for phosphate replacement during treatment of DKA may be more theoretical than real. No studies have demonstrated that replacement of phosphate affects the course or outcome from ketoacidosis [48,49].

For treating severe hypophosphatemia, potassium phosphate (20 mEq K^+; 16 mmol PO_4^{3-}) can be added to replacement fluids in place of KCl. Because phosphate deficits during DKA average only 1.0 mmol per kg, it is rarely necessary to administer more than one 5-mL ampule of potassium phosphate. Thereafter, potassium should be replaced as KCl. The hazards of parenteral phosphate administration include hypomagnesemia, hypocalcemia, and metastatic calcification [50]. If a patient with DKA can tolerate oral medication, phosphate-containing antacids (e.g., Neutra Phos) can be given.

Bicarbonate. Despite the presence of a low serum bicarbonate concentration and severe acidemia, most authorities now concur that there is no need for the routine use of bicarbonate therapy for DKA [51–55]. Neutralization is intuitively appealing, but fluid and electrolyte replacement alone will ameliorate the acidosis, and bicarbonate therapy may produce adverse effects. These include severe acute hypokalemia [56], late alkalosis due to paradoxical cerebrospinal fluid acidosis [57], a shift in the oxygen dissociation curve to the left that results in tissue hypoxia and lactic acidosis [58], and increased hepatic ketogenesis [53]. Among children, bicarbonate therapy may increase the risk of cerebral edema [59]. Bicarbonate replacement during DKA should be used only when hypotensive shock is unresponsive to rapid fluid replacement [60], buffering capability is completely exhausted, respiratory responses are maximal, and acidemia is worsening [43], or for those with advanced preexisting renal dysfunction [61]. Even in these circumstances, bicarbonate can only "buy time" until metabolic treatment reverses the acidosis. On those rare occasions when it may possibly be beneficial, two ampules of sodium bicarbonate (100 mEq total) in 400 mL of sterile water with 20 mEq KCL should be infused over 2 hours [4,61].

Magnesium. Hypermagnesemia may occur early in the course of DKA [62], but serum Mg^{2+} concentrations generally return to normal without specific treatment. For some patients, Mg^{2+} stores may be depleted, and hypomagnesemia may rarely lead to cardiac arrest [63]. Dysrhythmia should alert the physician to the possible need for magnesium supplementation.

Insulin

Insulin therapy for DKA is essential but should be instituted only after fluid and electrolyte resuscitation is underway [43]. Continuous low-dose infusion after an intravenous loading dose is the preferred method [64]. For adults, we recommend a bolus of 10 U of short-acting insulin followed by a continuous intravenous infusion starting at 5 to 10 U per hour. For children, the recommended initial bolus is 0.1 U per kg of body weight and the infusion rate is 0.1 U/kg/h [65–67]. If for some reason a continuous infusion cannot be given, an initial intravenous bolus of 10 units of short-acting insulin followed by repeated subcutaneous or intramuscular short-acting insulin injections can be used. Regular (crystalline) insulin is typically used for intravenous infusions; semisynthetic rapid-acting insulins approved for intravenous administration offer no advantage by this route. The onset of action of intravenous regular insulin occurs within minutes; bolus doses peak within 30 minutes, and the duration of action is 2 to 3 hours.

When DKA is treated with frequent subcutaneous insulin injections, very short-acting analogues may be advantageous because of their rapid onset of action. Their shorter duration of action may, however, require more frequent monitoring of blood glucose concentration. The safety and efficacy of repeated subcutaneous injections of rapid-acting insulin analogues every 1 to 2 hours for the treatment of uncomplicated DKA is well documented [68].

Insulin for infusion should be added to 0.45% saline (at a concentration of 0.5 U per mL), and the container swirled before use. Blood glucose concentration should be measured every 1 to 2 hours after starting the infusion. If the glucose concentration has not decreased by 50 to 75 mg/dL/h, the insulin infusion rate should be doubled. When the glucose concentration has fallen by more than 150 mg per dL, the infusion rate should be decreased by 50%, but it should never be stopped.

Once the plasma glucose concentration approaches 200 mg per dL, glucose infusion (D5W) or D5 1/2NS should be started, and the insulin infusion rate should be adjusted to ≈ 1.0 U per hour to maintain insulinization and inhibit ketogenesis. Following this, the goal should be to maintain the blood glucose concentration between 150 and 200 mg per dL, by adjusting the glucose infusion and insulin infusion rates until DKA resolves. Insulin should never be stopped entirely during the treatment of DKA, even if the infusion rate is reduced to only 0.5 U per hour or less. This is particularly important for children with DKA because their high GFR and high rate of urinary glucose excretion can lead to a low blood glucose concentration before ketone production has been reversed by insulin administration.

As noted above, resolving DKA is often accompanied by an increase in plasma ketones (principally AcAc) as BOHB is reoxidized. Total ketone bodies (AcAc plus BOHB) slowly fall throughout treatment, and the increase in measured ketones is transient. An increase in conventionally measured "plasma ketones" during the early hours of DKA treatment does not necessarily mean that treatment is inadequate and that more insulin is needed. The entire clinical picture must be assessed, and when the acidosis and hyperglycemia are resolving, the rise in ketones should be interpreted as a sign of improvement.

Complications

The morbidity and mortality associated with DKA are proportional to the severity of coma and acidemia at the time of presentation. Many complications can occur despite appropriate therapy.

Hypotension and Shock

Hypotension is an important complication of DKA. It is usually caused by volume depletion, and normally fluid replacement alone will reverse it [69]. Persistent hypotension should prompt consideration of fluid shifts, bleeding, severe acidosis, hypokalemia, arrhythmia, myocardial infarction, sepsis, and adrenal insufficiency.

When insulin is administered to a patient with DKA, both glucose and water move to the intracellular space. Blood pressure may then fall as extracellular and intravascular volumes decrease. Increasing the rate of fluid replacement can usually reverse this.

If shock persists despite fluid replacement, occult blood loss should be considered. Patients with gastric ulcer, colitis, or hemorrhagic pancreatitis can bleed into the gut lumen or peritoneum. Physical examination and an inappropriately low hematocrit in the face of dehydration are clues to this complication.

A shift in K^+ from the extracellular to the intracellular fluid space after insulin administration can lower serum potassium concentration and cause cardiac arrhythmias.

Patients with hypotension and increased central venous pressure should be evaluated for heart disease. Myocardial infarction is the most common finding, but other conditions such as cardiac tamponade and diastolic cardiac dysfunction can occur. Myocardial infarction is a common complication of long-standing diabetes, and its classic symptoms may be less obvious in the diabetic population. Patients in DKA who have had a myocardial infarction have a poorer prognosis [70].

Gram-negative sepsis is another cause of shock in ketoacidosis [60]. Pyelonephritis and pneumonia are common among such cases and must be treated appropriately when encountered. Ketoacidosis per se does not cause fever.

It is not uncommon for patients with type 1 diabetes to have other autoimmune diseases, and adrenal insufficiency should be considered among cases of ketoacidosis with refractory shock. The stress of DKA may uncover a state of partial adrenal insufficiency requiring glucocorticoid replacement.

The initial approach to the patient in shock is additional fluid replacement. (See Chapters 39 and 37 for a detailed discussion of the subsequent management of this problem.) Thereafter, further diagnostic procedures are necessary. Cardiac rhythm, respiratory, and hemodynamic monitoring is recommended.

Thrombosis

The dehydration and intravascular volume contraction common with DKA may activate coagulation factors [71]. Thrombosis of cerebral vessels and stroke are recognized complications of DKA. Some authorities suggest the routine use of low-dose heparin during the management of DKA, but there are no controlled studies to document its efficacy [72].

Cerebral Edema

Subclinical brain edema may be common during DKA [73], but clinically important cerebral edema is a rare complication among adults. It occurs more commonly among children [66], with a reported frequency of 0.3% to 0.5% in pediatric cases of DKA [65,74]. Cerebral edema has been associated with very high mortality (24%) [74], but a recent retrospective analysis shows current mortality rates are less than 10% [75]. It usually occurs a few hours after the initiation of therapy. Children who develop cerebral edema during treatment for DKA may initially have a relatively normal serum osmolality and then experience a progressive decline in serum sodium concentration [76]. Treatment with bicarbonate increases the risk of cerebral edema among children with DKA who present with azotemia and a low PCO_2 [59]. Greater baseline acidosis, higher potassium and urea concentrations, and large volumes of administered fluids are also risk factors for cerebral edema [77].

The exact mechanism of cerebral edema is unknown, but it may involve a combination of fluid shifts, thrombosis of intracerebral vessels, and effects on ion exchange mechanisms [61,78]. The most effective treatment for cerebral edema is probably mannitol [75,79], although hypertonic saline is being used with increasing frequency [75,80]. Steroids are not recommended [81,82]. Unfortunately, even when diagnosed early, cerebral edema may cause permanent neurologic damage or death.

Renal Failure

Hyperglycemic patients given intravenous fluids should have brisk urine flow. Patients with DKA who do not void within a few hours of therapy should be considered oliguric. A common cause of oliguria is postrenal obstruction and bladder scanning is recommended. A dilated atonic bladder is common in comatose patients and even more common in diabetic patients with severe neuropathy and DKA. Occasionally, patients with DKA precipitated by pyelonephritis develop acute tubular necrosis. Acute renal failure in the absence of infection is an uncommon complication of DKA [83].

Recurrent Diabetic Ketoacidosis

If ketoacidosis reappears for a patient who has received adequate amounts of insulin, infection or a severe contra-insulin state (e.g., Cushing's syndrome) should be suspected. More commonly, the problem is iatrogenic. The physician treating DKA notes that the blood glucose concentration has fallen, mistakenly assumes the condition has been cured, and discontinues insulin treatment. Because the duration of action of intravenous insulin is brief and these patients make no insulin, ketone production resumes and ketosis soon recurs [2]. Insulin infusions should be continued, if only at 0.5 to 1 U per hour, until the patient is well enough to be switched to subcutaneous injections of long-acting insulin. The intravenous infusion of insulin should be continued for 2 to 3 hours *after* the first subcutaneous injection of intermediate-acting or long-acting insulin is given so that the subcutaneous insulin has time to appear in the bloodstream. Cases of insulin-resistant DKA with recurrent hyperglycemia that respond to treatment with insulin-like growth factor I have been described [84], but these are extremely uncommon.

Low Blood Glucose Concentration

The blood glucose concentrations during DKA usually decrease rapidly as a result of renal excretion as soon as fluid is administered and urine flow is established [69]. After insulin is given, glucose is metabolized as well as excreted, and blood glucose concentrations may fall rapidly. The physician must be alert to the possibility of precipitous reductions in glycemia and frequent monitoring of blood glucose is recommended. To avoid cerebral edema, the goal of the first 24 hours of DKA treatment is a blood glucose concentration not less than 200 mg per dL.

When the blood glucose concentration falls to 200 mg per dL, a D5 containing intravenous fluid should be administered together with insulin [85]. Dual therapy inhibits ketone production while precluding hypoglycemia. For the first 24 hours of treatment, continuous intravenous infusion of insulin is recommended.

Follow-up Care of Diabetic Ketoacidosis

After a patient has recovered from DKA, the physician's goal should be the prevention of further episodes [86]. This requires the identification of any precipitating factors. Any lack of education regarding diabetes should be remedied.

HYPERGLYCEMIC HYPEROSMOLAR SYNDROME

Severe hyperglycemia, dehydration, and coma have long been known to occur in the absence of significant acidosis or ketonemia among older patients with diabetes [87]. This syndrome is designated as HHS. Mortality with HHS has historically been high, on the order of approximately 50%, but increasing recognition and improved ICU-based treatment have substantially improved this figure; mortality more recently is on the order of 15% [70,88]. With optimal care, HHS managed in an ICU setting can carry a relatively favorable prognosis. Of note is the fact that, with the increasing prevalence of obesity and type 2 diabetes among children, a similar disorder is being reported for the pediatric population [89,90]. The syndrome can be the initial presentation of type 2 diabetes and, in the United States, may occur with disproportionate frequency among African American youth.

Pathophysiology and Etiology

The pathophysiology that gives rise to HHS requires that three interrelated elements be present: insulin deficiency, renal impairment, and cognitive impairment.

Insulin Deficiency

Relative lack of insulin is the fundamental defect in HHS. Patients have sufficient insulin to inhibit ketone body formation but not enough to prevent hyperglucagonemia, glycogenolysis, and gluconeogenesis [91]. The resulting hyperglycemia induces an osmotic diuresis, with resultant fluid and electrolyte losses.

Paradoxically, venous insulin concentration levels of patients with HHS are comparable with those sometimes observed in DKA [92]. Animals with experimentally induced HHS have portal insulin concentrations higher than those of animals with experimental ketoacidosis [93]. The data suggest that partial insulinization of the liver with HHS enables affected patients to metabolize free fatty acids and thereby avoid ketogenesis in the face of severe hyperglycemia. Additional data indicate, however, that hepatic insulinization alone cannot account for the absence of ketosis in HHS. Ketone bodies can be induced when medium-chain triglycerides (precursors of fatty acids) are administered to animals with an experimental HHS syndrome [94]. The result suggests that patients with HHS would produce ketones despite hepatic insulinization if enough substrate in the form of free fatty acids were present. Their resistance to ketosis must therefore depend on limited availability of circulating free fatty acids [95].

The low concentrations of free fatty acids during HHS may be due to relatively low concentrations of lipolytic hormones [96] including growth hormone and cortisol, concentrations of which are lower in HHS than in DKA. Another explanation is that hyperosmolality itself inhibits the release of free fatty acids [97]. Additional unidentified factors may play a role.

Renal Impairment

Some degree of renal impairment accompanies all cases of HHS. Younger patients with diabetes have a normal GFR and, even in the event of DKA, filter enough glucose into the urine to prevent extreme hyperglycemia. In contrast, typical patients with HHS are older. Their renal blood flow and GFR are reduced, and they cannot readily excrete a glucose load. When they become hyperglycemic, the glucose is neither metabolized nor excreted. It remains in the extracellular fluid space. The resulting increase in osmolality, together with the decreased GFR, causes still less glucose to be excreted (Fig. 137.3). It has been suggested that, among children with baseline normal renal function, extreme hyperglycemia may be precipitated by intake of large amounts of sugary drinks to compensate for urinary fluid losses [89].

The underlying renal abnormality of HHS may be prerenal, renal, or postrenal. The common result is that affected patients are unable to compensate for the hyperglycemia with an osmotic diuresis. The result is an extremely high glucose concentration. Severe hyperglycemia itself can cause prerenal azotemia because glycosuria causes a hypotonic osmotic diuresis resulting in urinary loss of free water. If not replaced orally, this loss causes reductions in intravascular volume and renal perfusion.

Cerebral Impairment

Hyperglycemia leading to hyperosmolality normally activates thirst. The combination of mild diabetes and azotemia does not lead to HHS unless the affected individual does not drink sufficient water to prevent hyperosmolality. Invariably, HHS involves acute or chronic impairment of cerebral function. A common history involves an elderly patient with impaired cognitive function due to cerebrovascular disease, dementia, or central nervous system–depressant medications. This impairment may involve either concurrent impairment of the normal thirst mechanism or an inability to respond to thirst due to speech or motor deficits. Patients with trauma or burns have large insensible water losses, are often unable to drink, and are also susceptible to HHS in the absence of adequate parenteral fluids.

Animal studies confirm that fluid restriction is necessary to produce an HHS-like disorder. Diabetic rats do not develop HHS unless they are deprived of water [98]. Decreased thirst leads to increased dehydration, increased stupor, and further decreases in fluid intake. Other factors, such as angiotensin, may also be involved [99].

Interrelationships

To summarize, three interrelated factors are required for HHS. Insulin deficiency leads to hyperglycemia and glycosuria. Impaired renal function exaggerates the hyperglycemia and leads to hyperosmolality. Decreased free water intake precludes dilutional compensation and further exacerbates prerenal azotemia. Together, these three factors produce dehydration and the hyperosmolar hyperglycemic state (Fig. 137.4).

The severe dehydration that occurs with this syndrome is due to the osmotic diuresis of glucose in the absence of compensatory free water intake. Dehydration, in turn, leads to hemoconcentration, setting the stage for severe prerenal azotemia, thrombosis, and shock. As glucose and osmolality rise, cerebral function is progressively compromised. Coma ensues when the serum

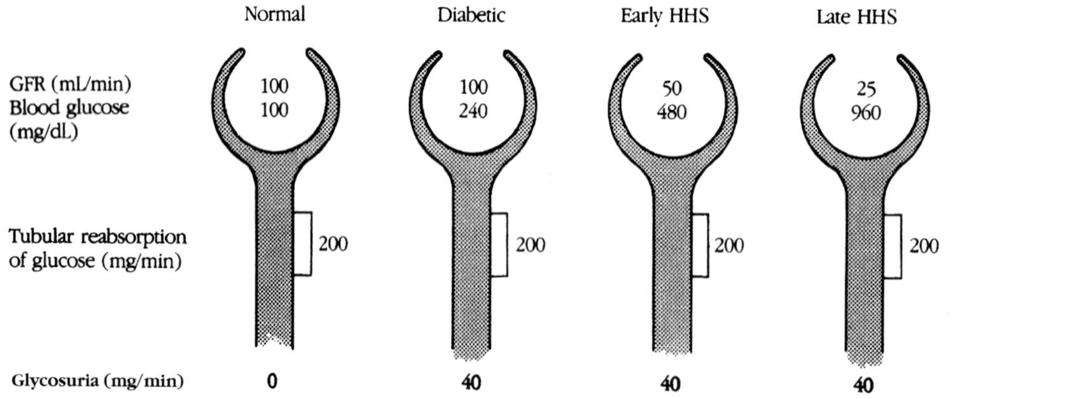

FIGURE 137.3 Interrelationship of blood glucose concentration, glomerular filtration rate (GFR), and renal excretion of glucose. This diagram illustrates the importance of dehydration and diminished GFR in the development of extreme hyperglycemia in hyperglycemic hyperosmolar syndrome (HHS). The normal individual, with normal GFR and normoglycemia, is never glycosuric. A diabetic individual with normal renal function and normal thirst response may become hyperglycemic if glycemic control is poor, but the high GFR leads to glycosuria, and severe hyperglycemia does not usually develop. In a patient with HHS, in contrast, osmotic diuresis and impairment of thirst response lead to progressive deterioration in GFR. The kidney's ability to excrete glucose declines and extreme hyperglycemia develops.

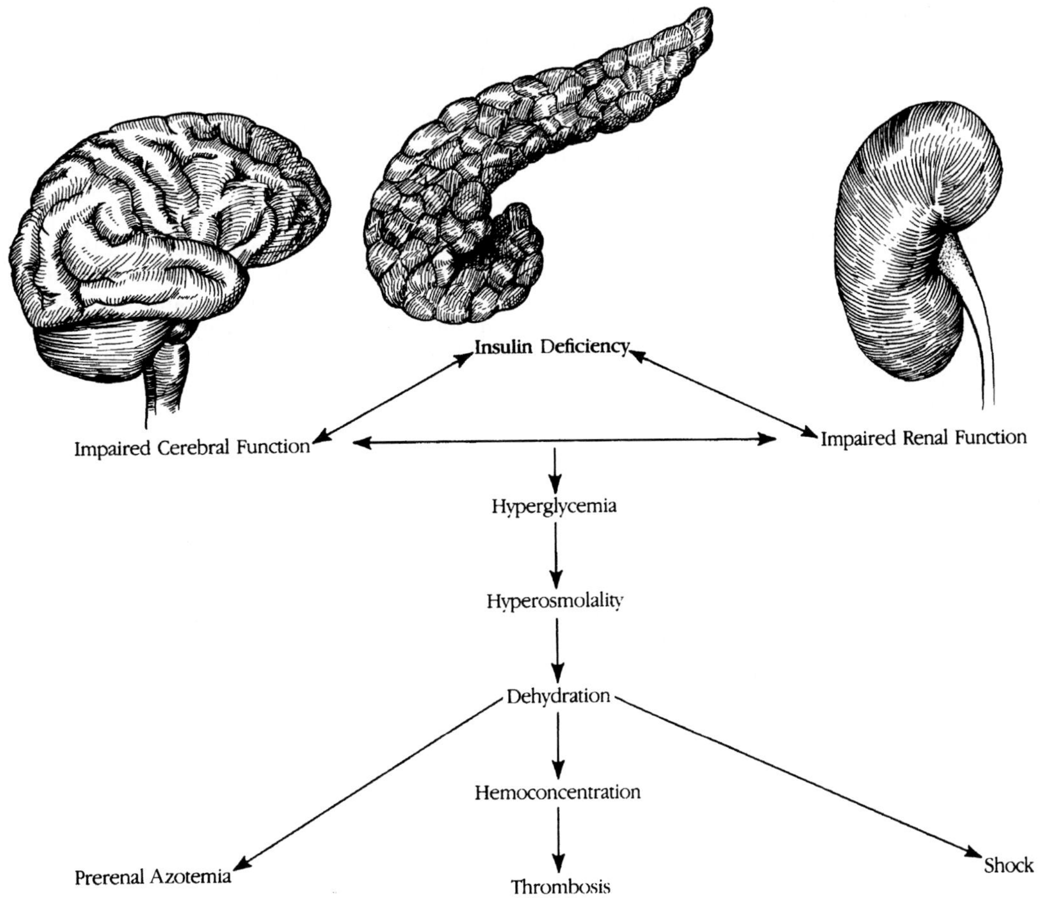

FIGURE 137.4 Pathogenesis of hyperglycemic hyperosmolar syndrome (HHS). Three interrelated factors give rise to HHS: insufficient insulin leads to hyperglycemia and glycosuria, impaired renal function exaggerates the hyperglycemia and hyperosmolality, and impaired cognition leads to decreased free water intake. Together, these factors lead to dehydration and the hyperosmolar hyperglycemic state.

osmolality is 350 mOsm per kg [100]. Severe HHS may take several days to develop.

Clinical Findings in Hyperglycemic Hyperosmolar Syndrome

Patients who develop HHS are typically middle aged or elderly [101,102]. The syndrome occurs less commonly among younger patients and rarely among infants [90] and may represent an overlap with DKA [2]. Patients often have a history of type 2 diabetes treated with diet and/or oral hypoglycemic agents. There may be a prodrome of progressive polyuria and polydipsia and, occasionally, polyphagia lasting days to several weeks.

Most patients have underlying diseases. Renal and cardiovascular disorders are the most common. Other intercurrent problems include infection, myocardial infarction, stroke, hemorrhage, and trauma [102]. Additional predisposing factors include dialysis [103], hyperalimentation [104], and medications. Diazoxide [105], phenytoin [106], propranolol [107], immunosuppressive agents [108], cimetidine [109], and the antipsychotic drugs clozapine and olanzapine [110,111] all impair insulin secretion or action and have been implicated as causes of HHS. The disorder has also been associated with treatment of HIV with the nucleoside analogue didanosine [112] and lithium-induced diabetes insipidus [113,114].

Fever is a common finding during HHS even in the absence of infection, but infection must be rigorously excluded for all cases. Patients may have hypotension and tachycardia due to dehydration, and they frequently hyperventilate. Neurologic manifestations include tremors and fasciculations. Mental status ranges from mild disorientation to obtundation and coma depending on the degree of abnormalities in osmolality and perfusion [115]. Up to a third of patients with HHS may seize [116], and many in this group are misdiagnosed as having primary intracerebral disease. Once treatment has been instituted, neurologic symptoms may clear rapidly. The hyperventilation may reflect lactic acidosis, a common complication of severe dehydration and hypotension. Rapid respiration of a hyperglycemic patient does not always imply ketoacidosis.

Diagnosis

The key to the diagnosis of HHS is the demonstration of hyperglycemia and hyperosmolality without significant ketosis in the appropriate clinical setting.

Blood Glucose Concentration

Blood glucose concentrations in HHS are generally higher than in DKA, usually greater than 600 mg per dL. Values as high as 2,000 mg per dL occur.

Acetone

Most patients in HHS are not ketonemic. Serum acetone levels are usually normal or only slightly elevated, seldom exceeding a dilution of 1:2. Occasionally, patients with HHS develop a severe intercurrent metabolic acidosis. In these very ill patients, a severe hyperosmolar state may overlap with ketoacidosis. Such cases are uncommon.

Osmolality

Serum osmolality of comatose patients is usually more than 350 mOsm per kg. It can be measured directly in the laboratory but is easily and quickly approximated from BUN, sodium, potassium, and glucose concentrations as shown in Table 137.1.

Acid–Base Balance

Most patients with HHS are only mildly acidotic. Serum bicarbonate concentration and arterial pH are usually close to normal. The average pH is about 7.25 before treatment, and HCO_3 is typically ≥15 mEq per L. The acidemia most often represents either mild lactic acidosis or uremic acidosis. When a significant anion gap is present (see Table 137.1), other causes of acidosis should be considered. These include salicylate, methanol, and ethylene glycol ingestions.

Renal Function

As outlined above, renal function is always impaired among patients with HHS. In addition to any preexisting renal disease, dehydration induces prerenal azotemia, and the ratio of BUN to creatinine is usually greater than 30:1. BUN and creatinine should be repeated after treatment to determine the degree of intrinsic renal impairment.

Electrolytes

The serum sodium concentration during early HHS is highly variable, ranging between 100 and 180 mEq per L. Hyponatremia may result from the dilutional effect of osmotically active glucose among patients with high free water intake in the face of impaired renal function. As mentioned previously, for each 100 mg per dL increase in blood glucose in excess of 100 mg per dL, serum sodium concentration falls approximately 1.6 mEq per L. When severe hypotonic fluid losses occur in the later stages of HHS, patients may become hypernatremic. Because sodium remains in the extracellular fluid compartment, this electrolyte should be followed to assess the state of hydration. Frequent calculations of the corrected sodium need to be done to properly guide the choice of fluids and rates for rehydration [117].

Serum potassium concentration during HHS syndrome is also variable. It may range from 2.2 to 7.8 mEq per L. Hypokalemia requires immediate potassium replacement. As mentioned later, serum potassium concentrations decrease after treatment with insulin is begun. Hyperkalemia often responds to fluid replacement and improvement in urinary output. Patients with HHS, like those with DKA, lose substantial quantities of electrolytes.

Treatment

Overview

The best treatment for HHS is prevention. The condition can be avoided by periodic attention to blood glucose control and mental status. Susceptible individuals are those with mildly impaired glucose metabolism. They are often the elderly who live alone. They may be hospitalized in patients who have experienced trauma, undergone extensive surgery, or been placed on hyperalimentation regimens. They may also be residents of nursing homes, although improvements in care appear to have reduced this risk [102]. Individuals in all of these settings can be at risk of hyperglycemia and hyperosmolality. When HHS does occur, continuous vigilance for monitoring the details of the patient's clinical progress at the bedside is the key to achieving a successful outcome.

Fluid Replacement

Patients with HHS are, without exception, profoundly dehydrated. Within the first 2 hours, 1 to 2 L of 0.9% saline should be given. Normal saline is recommended, even if hypernatremia is present, to expand the extracellular fluid compartment rapidly. After initial volume expansion and restoration of normotension, subsequent treatment for dehydration in this syndrome emphasizes free water replacement. The osmotic diuresis of glucose produces free water loss in excess of solute loss. The initial infusion of normal saline must never be overlooked, however, because it rapidly expands the extracellular compartment and helps reestablish adequate perfusion (see Table 137.2). The corrected serum sodium can be used to help decide when the switch from 0.9% saline to 0.45% saline should be made.

The typical HHS patient requires 6 to 8 L of fluids (100 to 200 mL per kg) during the first 12 hours of treatment. The rate of fluid administration must be adjusted as appropriate to the patient's clinical status. Elderly patients with cardiovascular impairment may require less aggressive replacement.

Electrolytes

As soon as adequate urine flow has been established and the degree of hypokalemia estimated, potassium supplementation should be added to intravenous fluids. During the initial phases of therapy, serum potassium concentration should be checked frequently and the electrocardiogram monitored for changes in morphology and rhythm. A sudden fall in serum potassium concentration frequently accompanies the initiation of insulin therapy [95]. Cardiac arrhythmias induced by hypokalemia may be irreversible, particularly among the elderly. The potassium deficit of HHS can be ≥5 mEq per kg, but generally, the magnitude of the loss is not as great as that encountered during DKA [118].

Insulin

Most patients with HHS are more sensitive to insulin than are patients with DKA [95]. In addition, blood glucose concentration in HHS can fall rapidly when urine output is reestablished after volume expansion with saline. The combination of insulin sensitivity and glucose diuresis puts patients with HHS at risk of sudden unexpected hypoglycemia. Treatment with insulin is essential but should be instituted with careful monitoring and only after fluid and electrolyte resuscitation is underway.

Only short-acting insulin should be used. Continuous infusion is now standard but must be used with great caution. We do not recommend an initial intravenous insulin bolus. For the infusion, we recommend a starting dose of 1 to 5 U per hour, depending on individual circumstances. This dose is sufficient to insulinize the patient and is usually not high enough to cause severe hypoglycemia. If continuous insulin infusion therapy is not possible, treatment should be with boluses of intravenous regular insulin. The initial dose should not exceed 10 to 30 U. Boluses should be given every 2 to 4 hours, with dose adjusted on the basis of blood glucose determinations.

As emphasized repeatedly, normalization of glucose is not the primary goal of treatment; fluid and electrolyte resuscitation take precedence and often improve glycemia substantially before any insulin is given. An attempt should be made to maintain blood glucose concentration near 250 mg per dL for the first 24 hours. Rapid fall in blood glucose concentration correlates with the development of cerebral edema [100,119].

TABLE 137.2

Evidentiary Basis of Management

Recommendation	Comments
Begin fluid resuscitation of DKA and HHS before insulin therapy.	Studies have shown that hydration lowers plasma glucose by improvement in glomerular filtration and increase in net urinary glucose loss. There is partial correction of pH and plasma bicarbonate with hydration [43].
Low dose (0.1 unit/kg/h) infusion of rapid-acting insulin is recommended.	Randomized controlled trials have shown lower rates of insulin infusion to be as effective as higher rates. Lower insulin rates confer reduced risk of hypokalemia and hypoglycemia [64].
Potassium replacement should begin early.	Studies have shown that insulin administration before volume and potassium repletion can cause shock and arrhythmias [27,30].
Bicarbonate replacement is not recommended in managing DKA.	Trials have shown no benefit of bicarbonate use in patients with pH >6.9 with respect to resolution of ketonemia, acidosis, or hyperglycemia [51–55]. No trials of bicarbonate use in patients with pH <6.9 have been reported.
Phosphate replacement has not been shown to be of benefit in DKA.	Randomized trials have not demonstrated clinical benefit from the routine use of phosphate replacement in DKA [48–50].
Intravenous insulin infusion is preferred for moderate to severe DKA, whereas repeated doses of subcutaneous insulin may be used instead in mild DKA.	Trials comparing intravenous insulin infusion to subcutaneous insulin injections showed similar eventual outcomes, but quicker resolution of ketosis and hyperglycemia with intravenous insulin. In patients with mild DKA, trials show subcutaneous injections of fast-acting insulin every 1–2 h to be as effective as intravenous infusion of regular insulin [68].

Treatment of the diabetic comas has evolved incrementally over many decades. This table summarizes the validation of key components of therapy. DKA, diabetic ketoacidosis; HHS, hyperglycemic hyperosmolar syndrome.

Complications

Hypotension

When insulin is administered to patients with HHS syndrome, glucose shifts from the extracellular to the intracellular compartment. Because glucose is osmotically active, the movement of glucose intracellularly draws free water from the extracellular compartment. The rapid intracellular movement of free water compromises intravascular volume and may precipitate hypotension and shock [120]. The use of normal (0.9%) saline for initial volume replacement helps prevent hypotension. The higher osmolality of normal (308 mOsm per L) compared with half-normal (154 mOsm per L) saline reduces the osmotic effect of the glucose shifts that follow insulin administration [121].

The magnitude of the fluid shifts that can be induced by insulin was illustrated in a dramatic case report. A patient with congestive heart failure and preexisting renal disease was found to have severe hyperglycemia. Because fluid replacement was contraindicated, the patient was treated with insulin alone. The insulin treatment resulted in a shift in fluid from the extracellular to the intracellular compartment sufficient to ameliorate the congestive heart failure [122].

Cerebral Edema

Blood glucose concentrations should never be reduced precipitously. Rapid reduction is a major contributor to the development of cerebral edema and a fatal outcome in HHS. The exact cause of cerebral edema in HHS is unknown, but animal studies suggest that neuronal intracellular osmolality increases in HHS. The osmotically active solute has not been identified. The term idiogenic osmoles is used to describe these uncharacterized, osmotically active, nondiffusible substances [123]. They draw water into neurons when the extracellular osmolality drops as a result of the intracellular movement of glucose. This is followed by severe edema, increased intracranial pressure, and disturbed hypothalamic function.

Thrombosis

Large vessel thromboembolic events are an important cause of mortality from HHS. Severe dehydration and hyperosmolality lead to reduced cardiac output and hyperviscosity, predisposing to venous and arterial thrombosis. Use of low-dose heparin prophylaxis is recommended for high-risk patients [124].

CONCLUSIONS

The diabetic comas are often described as discrete entities, but they frequently present as overlapping disorders [2]. Patients with DKA often have concurrent mild lactic acidosis and may also develop hyperosmolality. Initial treatment of all diabetic comas must always emphasize fluid resuscitation and electrolyte repletion. DKA and HHS also require careful management of insulin therapy. Physicians must obtain the relevant history, perform a thorough physical examination, classify the disorder, and treat appropriately. The approach to treatment is summarized in Fig. 137.5. With care, nearly all patients with DKA and most with HHS can survive.

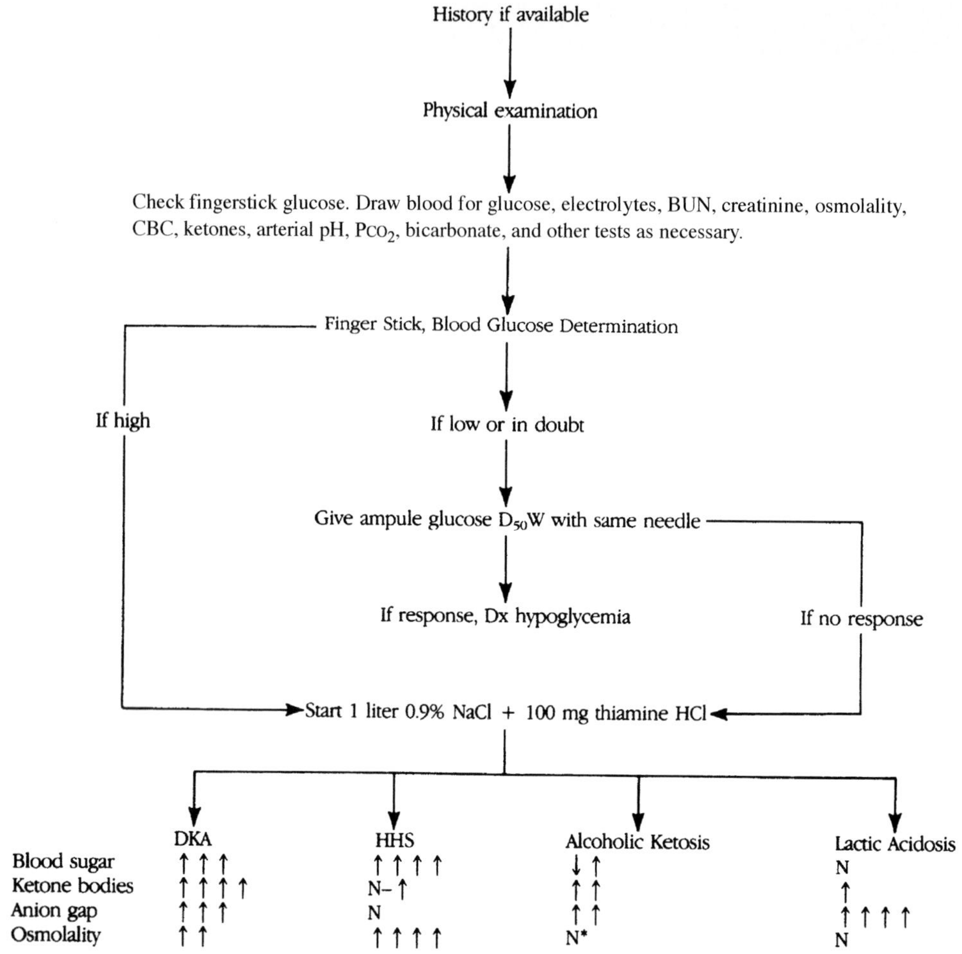

FIGURE 137.5 Algorithm for the diagnosis of diabetic coma. Measured osmolality is greater than predicted; result in freezing point depression test is increased by 1 mOsm/5 mg% EtOH. CBC, complete blood count; N, normal; ↑, mildly elevated; ↓, mildly depressed; ↑, moderately elevated; ↑↑↑, severely elevated; ↑↑↑, extremely elevated. BUN, blood urea nitrogen. (Adapted from Lindsey CA, Faloon GR, Unger RH: Plasma glucagon in hyperosmolar coma. *JAMA* 229:1771, 1974, with permission. Illustration by Albert Miller.)

References

1. Maletovic J, Drexler A: Diabetic ketoacidosis and hyperglycemic hyperosmolar state. *Endocrinol Metab Clin North Am* 42:677, 2013.
2. Hare JW, Rossini AA: Diabetic comas: the overlap concept. *Hosp Pract* 14:95:1028, 1979.
3. McGuire LC, Cruickshank AM, Munro PT: Alcoholic ketoacidosis. *Emerg Med J* 23:417, 2006.
4. Kitabchi AE, Umpierrez GE, Miles JM, et al: American Diabetes Association: hyperglycemic crises in patients with diabetes mellitus. *Diabetes Care* 32:1335, 2009.
5. Flakoll PJ, Jensen MD, Cherrington AD: Physiologic action of insulin, in LeRoith D, Taylor SI, Olefsky JM (eds): *Diabetes Mellitus. A Fundamental and Clinical Text.* 3rd ed. Philadelphia, PA, Lippincott Williams & Wilkins, 2003, pp 165–182.
6. Cahill GF Jr: The Banting Memorial Lecture 1971. Physiology of insulin in man. *Diabetes* 20:785, 1971.
7. Cherrington AD: Banting Lecture 1997. Control of glucose uptake and release by the liver in vivo. *Diabetes* 48:1198, 1999.
8. Beylot M: Regulation of in vivo ketogenesis: role of free fatty acids and control by epinephrine, thyroid hormones, insulin and glucagon. *Diabetes Metab* 22:299, 1996.
9. Nyenwe EA, Kitabchi AE: The evolution of diabetic ketoacidosis: an update of its etiology, pathogenesis and management. *Metabolism* 65:507, 2016
10. Azoulay E, Chevret S, Didier J, et al: Infection as a trigger of diabetic ketoacidosis in intensive care-unit patients. *Clin Infect Dis* 32:30, 2001.
11. Umpierrez GE, Kelly JP, Navarrete JE, et al: Hyperglycemic crises in urban blacks. *Arch Intern Med* 157:669, 1997.
12. Banerji MA, Chaiken RL, Huey H, et al: GAD antibody negative NIDDM in adult black subjects with diabetic ketoacidosis and increased frequency of human leukocyte antigen DR3 and DR4: flatbush diabetes. *Diabetes* 43:741, 1994.
13. Peters AL, Buschur EO, Buse JB, et al: Euglycemic diabetic ketoacidosis: a potential complication of treatment with sodium-glucose cotransporter 2 inhibition. *Diabetes Care* 38:1687, 2015
14. Snorgaard O, Eskildsen PC, Vadstrup S, et al: Diabetic ketoacidosis in Denmark: epidemiology, incidence rates, precipitating factors and mortality rates. *J Intern Med* 226:223, 1989.
15. Beigelman PM: Severe diabetic ketoacidosis (diabetic "coma"). 482 episodes in 257 patients: experience of three years. *Diabetes* 20:490, 1971.
16. Treasure RA, Fowler PB, Millington HT, et al: Misdiagnosis of diabetic ketoacidosis as hyperventilation syndrome. *Br Med J (Clin Res Ed)* 294:630, 1987.
17. Verdon F, van Melle G, Perret C: Respiratory response to acute metabolic acidosis. *Bull Eur Physiopathol Respir* 17:223, 1981.
18. Guerin JM, Meyer P, Segrestaa JM: Hypothermia in diabetic ketoacidosis. *Diabetes Care* 10:801, 1987.
19. Campbell IW, Duncan LJ, Innes JA, et al: Abdominal pain in diabetic metabolic decompensation. Clinical significance. *JAMA* 233:166, 1975.
20. Sugar AM: Mucormycosis. *Clin Infect Dis* 14[Suppl 1]:S126–S129, 1992.
21. Sibai BM, Viteri OA: Diabetic ketoacidosis in pregnancy. *Obstet Gynecol* 123:167, 2014.
22. Corl DE, Yin TS, Mills ME, et al: Evaluation of point-of-care blood glucose measurements in patients with diabetic ketoacidosis or hyperglycemic hyperosmolar syndrome admitted to a critical care unit. *J Diabetes Sci Technol* 7:1265, 2013.
23. Munro JF, Campbell IW, McCuish AC, et al: Euglycaemic diabetic ketoacidosis. *Br Med J* 2:578, 1973.
24. Jenkins D, Close CF, Krentz AJ, et al: Euglycaemic diabetic ketoacidosis: does it exist? *Acta Diabetol* 30:251, 1993.
25. Katz MA: Hyperglycemia-induced hyponatremia—calculation of expected serum sodium depression. *N Engl J Med* 289:843, 1973.
26. Halperin ML, Bear RA, Hannaford MC, et al: Selected aspects of the pathophysiology of metabolic acidosis in diabetes mellitus. *Diabetes* 30:781, 1981.
27. Adrogué HJ, Wilson H, Boyd AE III, et al: Plasma acid-base patterns in diabetic ketoacidosis. *N Engl J Med* 307:1603, 1982.

28. Elisaf MS, Tsatsoulis AA, Katopodis KP, et al: Acid-base and electrolyte disturbances in patients with diabetic ketoacidosis. *Diabetes Res Clin Pract* 34:23, 1996.
29. Oh MS, Carroll HJ, Uribarri J: Mechanism of normochloremic and hyperchloremic acidosis in diabetic ketoacidosis. *Nephron* 54:1, 1990.
30. Fulop M: Hyperkalemia in diabetic ketoacidosis. *Am J Med Sci* 299:164, 1990.
31. Bohannon NJ: Large phosphate shifts with treatment for hyperglycemia. *Arch Intern Med* 149:1423, 1989.
32. Hale PJ, Nattrass M: A comparison of arterial and non-arterialized capillary blood gases in diabetic ketoacidosis. *Diabet Med* 5:76, 1988.
33. Emmett M, Narins RG: Clinical use of the anion gap. *Medicine (Baltimore)* 56:38, 1977.
34. Zonszein J, Baylor P: Diabetic ketoacidosis with alkalemia—a review. *West J Med* 149:217, 1988.
35. Owen OE, Licht JH, Sapir DG: Renal function and effects of partial rehydration during diabetic ketoacidosis. *Diabetes* 30:510, 1981.
36. Molitch ME, Rodman E, Hirsch CA, et al: Spurious serum creatinine elevations in ketoacidosis. *Ann Intern Med* 93:280, 1980.
37. Slovis CM, Mork VG, Slovis RJ, et al: Diabetic ketoacidosis and infection: leukocyte count and differential as early predictors of serious infection. *Am J Emerg Med* 5:1, 1987.
38. Vinicor F, Lehrner LM, Karn RC, et al: Hyperamylasemia in diabetic ketoacidosis: sources and significance. *Ann Intern Med* 91:200, 1979.
39. Nsien EE, Steinberg WM, Borum M, et al: Marked hyperlipasemia in diabetic ketoacidosis. A report of three cases. *J Clin Gastroenterol* 15:117, 1992.
40. Goldberg LH: Hyperuricemia, diabetes mellitus, and diabetic ketoacidosis. *Pa Med* 79:40, 1976.
41. Gogos CA, Giali S, Paliogianni F, et al: Interleukin-6 and C-reactive protein as early markers of sepsis in patients with diabetic ketoacidosis or hyperosmosis. *Diabetologia* 44:1011, 2001.
42. Gershengorn HB, Iwashyna TJ, Cooke CR, et al: Variation in use of intensive care for adults with diabetic ketoacidosis. *Crit Care Med* 40:2009–2015, 2012.
43. DeFronzo RA, Matsuda M, Barrett EJ: Diabetic ketoacidosis: a combined metabolic-nephrologic approach to therapy. *Diabetes Rev* 2:209, 1994.
44. Soler NG, Bennet MA, Dixon K, et al: Potassium balance during treatment of diabetic ketoacidosis with special reference to the use of bicarbonate. *Lancet* 2:665, 1972.
45. Lang F: Osmotic diuresis. *Ren Physiol* 10:160, 1987.
46. Foster DW, McGarry JD: The metabolic derangements and treatment of diabetic ketoacidosis. *N Engl J Med* 309:159, 1983.
47. Subramanian R, Khardori R: Severe hypophosphatemia. Pathophysiologic implications, clinical presentations, and treatment. *Medicine (Baltimore)* 79:1, 2000.
48. Fisher JN, Kitabchi AE: A randomized study of phosphate therapy in the treatment of diabetic ketoacidosis. *J Clin Endocrinol Metab* 57:177, 1983.
49. Wilson HK, Keuer SP, Lea AS, et al: Phosphate therapy in diabetic ketoacidosis. *Arch Intern Med* 142:517, 1982.
50. Zipf WB, Bacon GE, Spencer ML, et al: Hypocalcemia, hypomagnesemia, and transient hypoparathyroidism during therapy with potassium phosphate in diabetic ketoacidosis. *Diabetes Care* 2:265, 1979.
51. Morris LR, Murphy MB, Kitabchi AE: Bicarbonate therapy in severe diabetic ketoacidosis. *Ann Intern Med* 105:836, 1986.
52. Green SM, Rothrock SG, Ho JD, et al: Failure of adjunctive bicarbonate to improve outcome in severe pediatric diabetic ketoacidosis. *Ann Emerg Med* 31:41, 1998.
53. Okuda Y, Adrogue HJ, Field JB, et al: Counterproductive effects of sodium bicarbonate in diabetic ketoacidosis. *J Clin Endocrinol Metab* 81:314, 1996.
54. Gamba G, Oseguera J, Castrejon M, et al: Bicarbonate therapy in severe diabetic ketoacidosis. A double blind, randomized, placebo controlled trial. *Rev Invest Clin* 43:234, 1991.
55. Chua HR, Schneider A, Bellomo R: Bicarbonate in diabetic ketoacidosis - a systematic review. *Ann Intensive Care* 1:23, 2011.
56. Schade DS, Eaton RP: Dose response to insulin in man: differential effects on glucose and ketone body regulation. *J Clin Endocrinol Metab* 44:1038, 1977.
57. Bureau MA, Begin R, Berthiaume Y, et al: Cerebral hypoxia from bicarbonate infusion in diabetic acidosis. *J Pediatr* 96:968, 1980.
58. Bellingham AJ, Detter JC, Lenfant C: The role of hemoglobin affinity for oxygen and red-cell 2,3-diphosphoglycerate in the management of diabetic ketoacidosis. *Trans Assoc Am Physicians* 83:113, 1970.
59. Glaser N, Barnett P, McCaslin I, et al: Risk factors for cerebral edema in children with diabetic ketoacidosis. *N Engl J Med* 344:264, 2001.
60. Clements RS Jr, Vourganti B: Fatal diabetic ketoacidosis: major causes and approaches to their prevention. *Diabetes Care* 1:314, 1978.
61. Kamel SK, Halperin ML: Acid base problems in diabetic ketoacidosis. *N Engl J Med* 372:546, 2015.
62. Mordes JP, Wacker WE: Excess magnesium. *Pharmacol Rev* 29:273, 1977.
63. McMullen JK: Asystole and hypomagnesaemia during recovery from diabetic ketoacidosis. *Br Med J* 1:690, 1977.
64. Kitabchi AE: Low-dose insulin therapy in diabetic ketoacidosis: fact or fiction? *Diabetes Metab Rev* 5:337, 1989.
65. Felner EI, White PC: Improving management of diabetic ketoacidosis in children. *Pediatrics* 108:735, 2001.
66. White NH: Diabetic ketoacidosis in children. *Endocrinol Metab Clin North Am* 29:657, 2000.
67. Kecskes SA: Diabetic ketoacidosis. *Pediatr Clin North Am* 40:355, 1993.
68. Umpierrez GE, Cuervo R, Karabell A, et al: Treatment of diabetic ketoacidosis with subcutaneous insulin aspart. *Diabetes Care* 27:1873, 2004.
69. Waldhausl W, Kleinberger G, Korn A, et al: Severe hyperglycemia: effects of rehydration on endocrine derangements and blood glucose concentration. *Diabetes* 28:577, 1979.
70. Hamblin PS, Topliss DJ, Chosich N, et al: Deaths associated with diabetic ketoacidosis and hyperosmolar coma 1973–1988. *Med J Aust* 151:439, 441, 444, 1989.
71. Paton RC: Haemostatic changes in diabetic coma. *Diabetologia* 21:172, 1981.
72. Lebovitz HE: Diabetic ketoacidosis. *Lancet* 345:767, 1995.
73. Krane EJ, Rockoff MA, Wallman JK, et al: Subclinical brain swelling in children during treatment of diabetic ketoacidosis. *N Engl J Med* 312:1147, 1985.
74. Edge JA, Hawkins MM, Winter DL, et al: The risk and outcome of cerebral oedema developing during diabetic ketoacidosis. *Arch Dis Child* 85:16, 2001.
75. Decourcey DD, Steil GM, Wypij D, et al: Increasing use of hypertonic saline over mannitol in the treatment of symptomatic cerebral edema in pediatric diabetic ketoacidosis: an 11-year retrospect analysis of mortality. *Pediatr Crit Care Med* 14:694, 2013.
76. Hale PM, Rezvani I, Braunstein AW, et al: Factors predicting cerebral edema in young children with diabetic ketoacidosis and new onset type I diabetes. *Acta Paediatr* 86:626, 1997.
77. Edge JA, Jakes RW, Roy Y, et al: The UK case-control study of cerebral oedema complicating diabetic ketoacidosis in children. *Diabetologia* 49:2002, 2006.
78. Silver SM, Clark EC, Schroeder BM, et al: Pathogenesis of cerebral edema after treatment of diabetic ketoacidosis. *Kidney Int* 51:1237, 1997.
79. Rosenbloom AL, Hanas R: Diabetic ketoacidosis (DKA): treatment guidelines. *Clin Pediatr (Phila)* 35:261, 1996.
80. Dunger DB, Sperling MA, Acerini CL, et al: ESPE/LWPES consensus statement on diabetic ketoacidosis in children and adolescents. *Arch Dis Child* 89:188, 2004.
81. Strachan MW, Nimmo GR, Noyes K, et al: Management of cerebral oedema in diabetes. *Diabetes Metab Res Rev* 19:241, 2003.
82. Levin DL: Cerebral edema in diabetic ketoacidosis. *Pediatr Crit Care Med* 9:320, 2008.
83. Murdoch IA, Pryor D, Haycock GB, et al: Acute renal failure complicating diabetic ketoacidosis. *Acta Paediatr* 82:498, 1993.
84. Usala A-L, Madigan T, Burguera B, et al: Brief report: treatment of insulin-resistant diabetic ketoacidosis with insulin-like growth factor I in an adolescent with insulin-dependent diabetes. *N Engl J Med* 327:853, 1992.
85. Krentz AJ, Hale PJ, Singh BM, et al: The effect of glucose and insulin infusion on the fall of ketone bodies during treatment of diabetic ketoacidosis. *Diabet Med* 6:31, 1989.
86. Flexner CW, Weiner JP, Saudek CD, et al: Repeated hospitalization for diabetic ketoacidosis. *Am J Med* 76:691, 1984.
87. Pasquel FJ, Umpierrez GE: Hyperosmolar hyperglycemic state: a historic review of the clinical presentation, diagnosis and treatment. *Diabetes Care* 37:3124, 2014.
88. Pinies JA, Cairo G, Gaztambide S, et al: Course and prognosis of 132 patients with diabetic non ketotic hyperosmolar state. *Diabete Metab* 20:43, 1994.
89. Zeitler P, Haqq A, Rosenbloom A, et al: Hyperglycemic hyperosmolar syndrome in children: pathophysiological considerations and suggested guidelines for treatment. *J Pediatr* 158:9, 2011.
90. Rosenbloom AL: Hyperglycemic hyperosmolar state: an emerging pediatric problem *J Pediatr* 156:180, 2010.
91. Lindsey CA, Faloona GR, Unger RH: Plasma glucagon in nonketotic hyperosmolar coma. *JAMA* 229:1771, 1974.
92. Henry DP II, Bressler R: Serum insulin levels in non-ketotic hyperosmotic diabetes mellitus. *Am J Med Sci* 256:150, 1968.
93. Joffe BI, Seftel HC, Goldberg R, et al: Factors in the pathogenesis of experimental nonketotic and ketoacidotic diabetic stupor. *Diabetes* 22:653, 1973.
94. Wilson HK, Keuer SP, Lea AS, et al: Experimental hyperosmolar diabetic syndrome. Ketogenic response to medium-chain triglycerides. *Diabetes* 24:301, 1975.
95. Gerich JE, Martin MM, Recant L: Clinical and metabolic characteristics of hyperosmolar nonketotic coma. *Diabetes* 20:228, 1971.
96. Turpin BP, Duckworth WC, Solomon SS: Simulated hyperglycemic hyperosmolar syndrome. Impaired insulin and epinephrine effects upon lipolysis in the isolated rat fat cell. *J Clin Invest* 63:403, 1979.
97. Gerich J, Penhos JC, Gutman RA, et al: Effect of dehydration and hyperosmolarity on glucose, free fatty acid and ketone body metabolism in the rat. *Diabetes* 22:264, 1973.
98. Bavli S, Gordon EE: Experimental diabetic hyperosmolar syndrome in rats. *Diabetes* 20:92, 1971.
99. Malvin RL, Mouw D, Vander AJ: Angiotensin: physiological role in water-deprivation-induced thirst of rats. *Science* 197:171, 1977.
100. Arieff AI, Carroll HJ: Cerebral edema and depression of sensorium in nonketotic hyperosmolar coma. *Diabetes* 23:525, 1974.
101. Cahill GF Jr: Hyperglycemic hyperosmolar coma: a syndrome almost unique to the elderly. *J Am Geriatr Soc* 31:103, 1983.
102. Wachtel TJ, Silliman RA, Lamberton P: Predisposing factors for the diabetic hyperosmolar state. *Arch Intern Med* 147:499, 1987.
103. Emder PJ, Howard NJ, Rosenberg AR: Non-ketotic hyperosmolar diabetic pre-coma due to pancreatitis in a boy on continuous ambulatory peritoneal dialysis. *Nephron* 44:355, 1986.
104. Sypniewski E Jr, Mirtallo JM, Schneider PJ: Hyperosmolar, hyperglycemic, nonketotic coma in a patient receiving home total parenteral nutrient therapy. *Clin Pharm* 6:69, 1987.
105. Balsam MJ, Baker L, Kaye R: Hyperosmolar nonketotic coma associated with diazoxide therapy for hypoglycemia. *J Pediatr* 78:523, 1971.

106. Gharib H, Munoz JM: Endocrine manifestations of diphenylhydantoin therapy. *Metabolism* 23:515, 1974.
107. Podolsky S, Pattavina CG: Hyperosmolar nonketotic diabetic coma: a complication of propranolol therapy. *Metabolism* 22:685, 1973.
108. Woods JE, Zincke H, Palumbo PJ, et al: Hyperosmolar nonketotic syndrome and steroid diabetes. Occurrence after renal transplantation. *JAMA* 231:1261, 1975.
109. Pomare EW: Hyperosmolar non-ketotic diabetes and cimetidine [letter]. *Lancet* 1:1202, 1978.
110. Nugent BW: Hyperosmolar hyperglycemic state. *Emerg Med Clin North Am* 23:629, 2005.
111. Newcomer JW: Second-generation (atypical) antipsychotics and metabolic effects: a comprehensive literature review. *CNS Drugs* 19[Suppl 1]:1, 2005.
112. Munshi MN, Martin RE, Fonseca VA: Hyperosmolar nonketotic diabetic syndrome following treatment of human immunodeficiency virus infection with didanosine. *Diabetes Care* 17:316, 1994.
113. MacGregor D, Baker AM, Appel RG, et al: Hyperosmolar coma due to lithium-induced diabetes insipidus. *Lancet* 346:413, 1995.
114. Azam H, Newton RW, Morris AD, et al: Hyperosmolar nonketotic coma precipitated by lithium-induced nephrogenic diabetes insipidus. *Postgrad Med J* 74:39, 1998.
115. Maccario M: Neurological dysfunction associated with nonketotic hyperglycemia. *Arch Neurol* 19:525, 1968.
116. Daniels JC, Chokroverty S, Barron KD: Anacidotic hyperglycemia and focal seizures. *Arch Intern Med* 124:701, 1969.
117. Palmer BF, Clegg DJ: Electrolyte and acid base disturbances in patients with diabetes mellitus. *N Engl J Med* 373:548, 2015.
118. Walsh CH, Soler NG, James H, et al: Studies on whole-body potassium in non-ketoacidotic diabetics before and after treatment. *Br Med J* 4:738, 1974.
119. Maccario M, Messis CP: Cerebral oedema complicating treated non-ketotic hyperglycaemia. *Lancet* 2:352, 1969.
120. Brown RH, Rossini AA, Callaway CW, et al: Caveat on fluid replacement in hyperglycemic, hyperosmolar, nonketotic coma. *Diabetes Care* 1:305, 1978.
121. Feig PU, McCurdy DK: The hypertonic state. *N Engl J Med* 297:1444, 1977.
122. Axelrod L: Response of congestive heart failure to correction of hyperglycemia in the presence of diabetic nephropathy. *N Engl J Med* 293:1243, 1975.
123. Arieff AI, Kleeman CR: Cerebral edema in diabetic comas. II. Effects of hyperosmolality, hyperglycemia and insulin in diabetic rabbits. *J Clin Endocrinol Metab* 38:1057, 1974.
124. Kian K, Eiger G: Anticoagulant therapy in hyperosmolar non-ketotic diabetic coma. *Diabet Med* 20:603, 2003.

Chapter 138 ■ Hypoglycemia

JOHN P. MORDES • MICHAEL J. THOMPSON • DAVID M. HARLAN • SAMIR MALKANI

Hypoglycemia occurs often in the intensive care unit (ICU) setting as both an admission diagnosis and a complication of therapy. Many factors predispose to it [1,2]. In a study of intensive insulin therapy from a surgical ICU population, hypoglycemia occurred among up to 5.1% of patients [3]. Another study of more than 2,200 ICU patients reported that nearly 7% experienced at least one episode of hypoglycemia [4]. Estimates of prevalence range as high as 25% [5]. Severe, prolonged hypoglycemia can cause permanent neurologic and cardiovascular damage [6–8]. Hypoglycemia is a consistent marker of poor outcomes including increased mortality among hospitalized patients in general [9–13], and in particular among critically ill adults [14–16] and children [17], irrespective of the presence or absence of a previous diabetes diagnosis [16].

DEFINITION OF HYPOGLYCEMIA

No specific blood glucose concentration defines hypoglycemia [7]. "Whipple's triad" [18] defines hypoglycemia as (a) documentation of a low blood glucose concentration, (b) concurrent symptoms of hypoglycemia, and (c) resolution of symptoms after administration of glucose. Typically, this concentration in serum is <50 mg per dL (2.8 mmol). For persons with known diabetes, the American Diabetes Association advocates the definitions given in Table 138.1 [19]. The physiologic definition is a blood glucose concentration low enough to cause the release of counterregulatory hormones (e.g., catecholamines) and impair the function of the central nervous system (CNS). That blood glucose threshold can be quite variable.

TABLE 138.1

Classification of Hypoglycemia in Persons with Known Diabetes

Severe	Requires assistance; recovery with CHO; with or without measured glucose
Documented symptomatic	Typical symptoms; glucose <70 mg/dL
Asymptomatic	Glucose <70 mg/dL; no symptoms
Probable asymptomatic	Symptoms with no measured glucose
Relative or pseudohypoglycemia	Symptoms with measured glucose >70 mg/dL

Definitions of hypoglycemia in diabetes proposed by a workgroup of the American Diabetes Association and the Endocrine Society [19]. CHO, carbohydrate.

SYMPTOMS AND SIGNS OF HYPOGLYCEMIA

Counterregulatory hormones released in response to low glucose concentrations cause sympathoadrenal symptoms and signs. Prominent symptoms include hunger, tingling, shakiness, weakness, palpitations, and anxiety [20]. Corresponding signs include diaphoresis, tachycardia, peripheral vasoconstriction, and widening of the pulse pressure. These findings may be absent among patients receiving sympatholytic drugs (e.g., β-blockers) and among patients with diabetes who have autonomic neuropathy. Hypoglycemia-associated autonomic failure (HAAF) compromises awareness of, and responses to, low glucose and is a major contributor to the development of severe and recurrent hypoglycemia in patients with type 1 or advanced type 2 [21].

Early symptoms and signs of neuroglycopenia include altered vision, difficulty thinking and sensations of warmth, weakness, and fatigue. These may be followed by confusion, slurred speech, and other nonspecific behavioral changes [20]. Severe neuroglycopenia can cause disturbances of integrative function, obtundation, seizures, coma, and, rarely, a permanent vegetative state.

Hypoglycemia can be associated with acute pulmonary edema [22], supraventricular and ventricular tachycardias, atrial fibrillation, and junctional dysrhythmias [23–25]. Electrocardiographic abnormalities associated with hypoglycemia include T-wave flattening, increased Q-T interval, ST segment depression, and repolarization abnormalities [26–28]. Bradycardias have also been attributed to hypoglycemia, but only rarely [29]. Prolonged hypoglycemia can be associated with hypothermia

[30–32], respiratory failure [33], hypokalemia, and hypophosphatemia [34]. Mortality rates attributable to hypoglycemia reportedly remain elevated for weeks after discharge from the ICU, but the causal relationship of that association, if any, is not understood [16].

NORMAL GLUCOSE REGULATORY PHYSIOLOGY

Glucose Utilization

Plasma glucose concentration is maintained in a narrow range (~60 to ~120 mg per dL; ~3.3 to ~6.7 mmol). The organ most dependent on glucose is the brain, which consumes ~150 g per day. Unlike fat or muscle, the CNS does not require insulin for glucose transport. During starvation, the brain uses ketone bodies as a substitute fuel (see Chapter 137 on diabetic Coma), but acquisition of the capability to use this alternate substrate requires hours to days. Even during prolonged starvation, the brain still needs ~44 g per day of glucose. Other tissues with obligate glucose needs include erythrocytes (~36 g per day) and renal medulla (~25 g per day).

Sources of Plasma Glucose

There are two sources of blood glucose: endogenously produced and ingested carbohydrate. In the postprandial state, the concentration of circulating insulin rises in response to the increase in glucose concentration and, to a lesser extent, other stimuli. Insulin promotes (a) transport of glucose into skeletal muscle for immediate use or storage as muscle glycogen and (b) hepatic storage of glucose in the form of liver glycogen. When all other metabolic demands for glucose are being met, some excess glucose is used for synthesis of triglycerides.

During brief starvation, such as when asleep, the principal source of glucose is hepatic glycogen. During prolonged starvation, glucose is derived principally from conversion of muscle-derived amino acids. Smaller contributions to gluconeogenesis are made by (a) glycerol derived from fat and (b) lactate produced by anaerobic glycolysis. When euglycemia is maintained by glycogenolysis or gluconeogenesis, insulin levels are low but never zero.

The liver stores only 60 to 80 g of glycogen, a supply that is exhausted by an overnight fast. Muscle glycogen stores are ~120 g, but this glycogen is not directly available for the maintenance of systemic glucose concentrations due to the lack of glucose-6-phosphatase in muscle. Muscle glycogen contributes to plasma glucose only via anaerobic glycolysis leading to the production of lactate, which is transported to the liver and converted into glucose. The shuttling of glucose to muscle and lactate to the liver comprises the Cori cycle. Muscle can also amidate pyruvate to form alanine, which is then exported to the liver and converted to glucose. Gluconeogenesis occurs principally in the liver, and to a lesser extent in the renal cortex, using amino acids, glycerol, and lactate as substrates. The enzymes and pathways required for gluconeogenesis are presented in Figure 138.1.

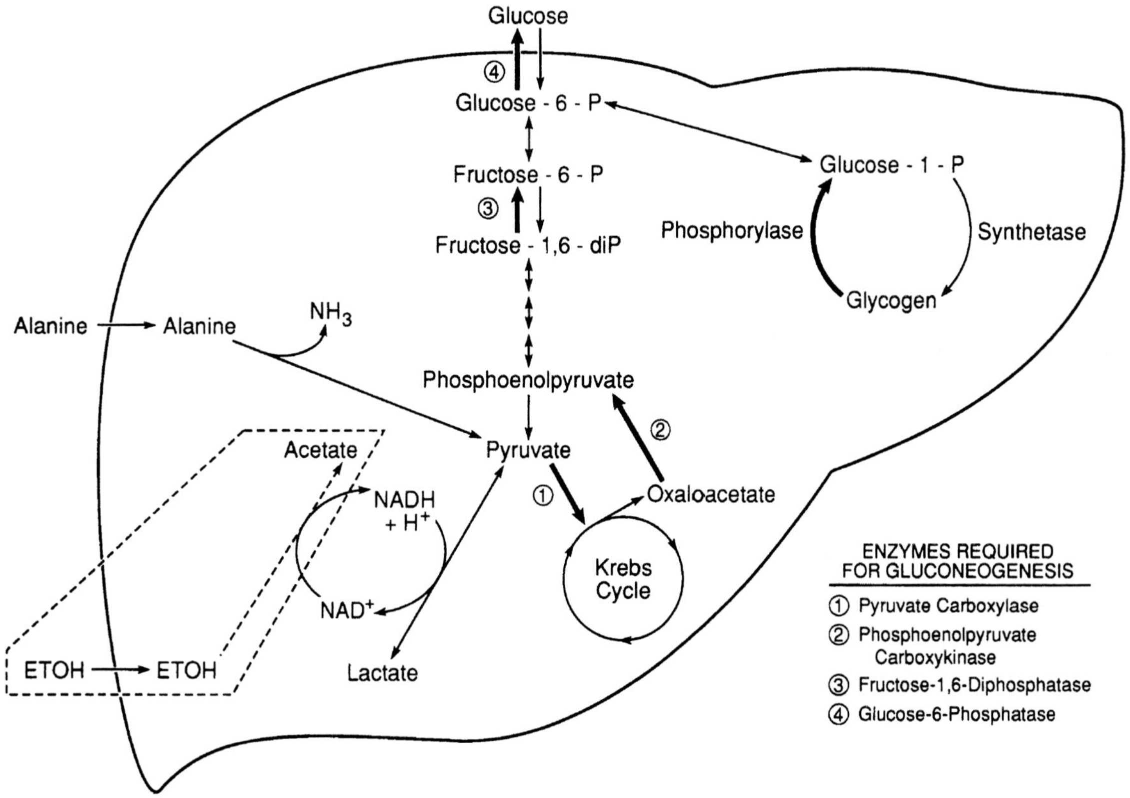

FIGURE 138.1 Metabolic pathways important in the response to hypoglycemia. The *thick, annotated arrows* indicate the key steps in glycogen breakdown and gluconeogenesis. In the presence of low circulating insulin concentrations, phosphorylase activity is increased, leading to the release of glucose-1-phosphate, which is then converted to glucose-6-phosphate and finally to glucose through the action of glucose-6-phosphatase. Glucose is also generated from three carbon precursors by gluconeogenesis. This process essentially reverses glycolysis and is controlled by four enzymes: (*1*) pyruvate carboxylase, (*2*) phosphoenolpyruvate carboxykinase, (*3*) fructose-1,6-diphosphatase, and (*4*) glucose-6-phosphatase. Within the box delimited by *dotted lines*, the metabolic effects of ethanol ingestion are indicated. Ethanol is converted to acetaldehyde and then to acetate, producing reduced nicotinamide adenine dinucleotide (NADH). The high concentration of NADH favors the generation of lactate from pyruvate, decreasing the concentration of the latter. As the availability of pyruvate as a gluconeogenic precursor declines, glucose production via gluconeogenesis also declines, and hypoglycemia can ensue.

Hormonal Regulation of Plasma Glucose Concentration

Insulin is the most important regulator of glycemia, promoting glucose uptake and storage in the fed state, and regulating glycogenolysis, gluconeogenesis, and lipolysis in the fasted state. Glucagon, glucocorticoids, catecholamines, growth hormone, and, to a lesser degree, thyroxine promote the formation of glucose in the fasted state and in general counteract the actions of insulin. Foremost among these "counterregulatory" hormones is glucagon, which is secreted in response to low glucose. It promotes both glycogenolysis (an immediate effect) and gluconeogenesis (a delayed but more enduring effect). Glucocorticoids antagonize the action of insulin, stimulating gluconeogenesis and inhibiting extrahepatic glucose utilization. Catecholamines also promote glycogenolysis and gluconeogenesis. The mechanism by which growth hormone promotes blood glucose elevation is not fully understood. The influence of thyroxine on blood glucose concentration is probably indirect. Fasting glucose tends to be elevated and decreased among hyperthyroid and hypothyroid patients, respectively.

CLASSIFICATION OF HYPOGLYCEMIA

Hypoglycemia can be classified as fasting (or postabsorptive) or postprandial (or "reactive"). The former always represents a major health problem that requires further evaluation. Hypoglycemia that occurs only after eating can be difficult to assess. It is usually minimally symptomatic and is attributed variously to an exaggerated insulin response, renal glycosuria, defects of glucagon responses, and/or high insulin sensitivity [35,36]. Some cases of postprandial hypoglycemia, however, are severe and associated with health issues including mutations of the insulin receptor [37], autoantibodies against insulin [38], gastric "dumping" after bypass surgery, and nesidioblastosis, all of which are described below. Postprandial hypoglycemia generally does not require intensive care.

DIFFERENTIAL DIAGNOSIS OF HYPOGLYCEMIA

Hypoglycemia that fulfills Whipple's triad always implies a major disturbance in glucose homeostasis, which is dependent on three factors: (a) the hormonal milieu, (b) the viability of organs responsible for gluconeogenesis, and (c) availability of substrate for conversion to glucose [7]. The differential diagnosis of medically important hypoglycemia subsumes three corresponding categories: (a) states of hormonal imbalance, principally excess insulin, (b) states of impaired endogenous glucose production, and (c) states in which gluconeogenic substrates are unavailable.

Hypoglycemia due to Hormonal Imbalance

Insulin

Insulin Overdoses in Diabetic Patients. Insulin overdose is the most common cause of hypoglycemia. In an outpatient setting, it is frequently the result of a missed meal or increased exercise and less often the result of inadvertent injection of short-acting in place of long-acting insulin. Occasionally, an overdose is intentional, particularly among adolescents. Rarely, overdoses represent attempts at suicide and homicide [39]. The rapidity of onset [40] and duration of hypoglycemia [41] depend on the type of insulin (see Table 138.2).

Hypoglycemia is often more severe among patients with long-standing type 1 diabetes and advanced type 2 diabetes due to intercurrent HAAF [21]. This is characterized by defective counterregulatory responses and hypoglycemia unawareness. Impaired glucagon and epinephrine responses are common, resulting in the abrupt development of severe hypoglycemia [42]. When counterregulation is impaired, adrenergic warning signals like tremor, diaphoresis, and tachycardia may not occur and neuroglycopenic symptoms can develop rapidly. Inadequate counterregulatory responses can also delay recovery from hypoglycemia.

Hypoglycemia among ICU patients can result from rapid changes in clinical status, medications that impair counterregulation (e.g., high-dose β-adrenergic blockers), and the presence

TABLE 138.2

Insulin Preparations

Class	Preparation	Onset of action	Peak	Duration
Short-acting	Aspart (NovoLog)[a]	15 min	45–90 min	3–5 h
	Glulisine (Apidra)[a]	15 min	50–60 min	~4 h
	Lispro (Humalog)[a]	15–30 min	30 min–2.5 h	3–6 h
	Regular (Humulin R, Novolin R)[b]	30–60 min	2–4 h	5–7 h
Intermediate-acting	NPH (Humulin N, Novolin N)	1–2 h	4–14 h	16–24 h
Long- and ultra–long-acting	Glargine (Lantus)[a]	1.5–5 h	No peak	18 to >24 h[c]
	Detemir (Levemir)[a]	1 h	No peak	Up to 24 h
	Regular U500 (Humulin R U-500)	30–60 min	2–4 h	Up to 24 h
	Degludec (Tresiba)[a]	1 h	No peak	Up to 42 h
Combinations	70% NPH, 30% Regular (Humulin 70/30, Novolin 70/30)	30 min	4–8 h	24 h
	75% protamine lispro, 25% lispro[a]	15 min	1.5 h	10–16 h
	70% protamine aspart, 30% aspart[a]	15 min	1.5 h	10–16 h
	50% protamine lispro, 50% lispro[a]	15 min	1.5 h	10–16 h

Data are for recombinant human insulin or semisynthetic insulin administered subcutaneously. Protamine lispro and protamine aspart insulins are available only in fixed ratio combinations.
[a]Semi-synthetic insulin.
[b]Humulin is available in U100 and U500 concentrations.
[c]Study ended at 24 hour. Trade names are given in parentheses. Additional semisynthetic insulins are under development.

of intercurrent disease processes. Although insulin-induced hypoglycemia is easily diagnosed in the ICU, it is crucial to determine exactly why it occurred. Vigilance is critical.

Intensive insulin management is demanding [43] and hypoglycemia can occur frequently [4,5]. Occasionally, insulin is administered either in the wrong dose or in response to a factitiously elevated blood glucose measurement or to the wrong patient. Even the most careful attempts to lower blood glucose in the ICU to levels <110 mg per dL, can frequently be associated with hypoglycemia [44–48]. The occurrence of hypoglycemia is more closely associated with excessive rates of insulin infusion than with the cumulative dose [49]. Failure to adjust insulin infusion rate after decreasing nutritional support is common, for example after interruption of enteral or parenteral for some reason [4]. Total parenteral nutrition solutions containing insulin can produce hypoglycemia [5], particularly if improvement in a patient's underlying condition restores peripheral insulin sensitivity. Insulin-induced hypoglycemia in the ICU can be related to adrenal insufficiency, renal failure, sepsis, or drug toxicities, continuous venovenous hemofiltration with bicarbonate replacement fluid, and need for inotropic support [5].

Intentional Insulin and Oral Hypoglycemic Agent Overdoses among Nondiabetic Patients. "Factitious" hypoglycemia should be suspected for anyone with access to insulin or oral hypoglycemic agents, including health care workers and relatives of persons with diabetes. The diagnosis can be difficult. These patients are trying to frustrate rather than facilitate a diagnosis, and they may devise ingenious methods to conceal their actions. Insulin intended for surreptitious injection has been found hidden in electronic devices and body cavities. Surreptitious use of oral hypoglycemic agents, which act by increasing endogenous insulin secretion, can be particularly problematic to diagnose [50,51]. Factitious hypoglycemia can represent malingering, attempted suicide or homicide, Münchausen syndrome, and Münchausen-by-proxy syndrome [39]. It has also been reported to result from adulteration of herbal and counterfeit prescription drugs with oral agents [52,53].

Insulinoma. Insulinomas are insulin-secreting pancreatic islet tumors. They are uncommon but do represent the most common form of pancreatic islet neoplasm. Most (>90%) are nonmalignant. They are typically small and difficult to visualize radiographically. Endocrine Society guidelines specify the critical diagnostic findings as: plasma insulin concentrations of at least 3 μU per mL (18 pmol per L), plasma C-peptide concentrations of at least 0.6 ng per mL (0.2 nmol per L), and plasma proinsulin concentrations of at least 5.0 pmol per L when the fasting plasma glucose concentrations are below 55 mg per dL (3.0 mmol per L) [54]. For some cases, a modification of these criteria may be of use [55].

It can be difficult to differentiate among insulinoma, factitious hypoglycemia due to self-administration of insulin, and abuse of oral hypoglycemic agents. When intentional insulin overdose is suspected, insulin measurements are of limited value. Patients with factitious hypoglycemia may have circulating antiinsulin antibodies that interfere with the radioimmunoassay for insulin. This is true even when human insulin is injected. These patients may appear to have elevated levels of insulin, just as would patients with an insulinoma. In this circumstance, simultaneous glucose, insulin, and C-peptide concentrations are helpful. Insulin and C-peptide are normally co-secreted by the pancreas in equimolar quantities, but C-peptide is not present in insulin for injection. Absence of C-peptide in a patient with unexplained fasting hypoglycemia strengthens the possibility of surreptitious insulin use. If oral hypoglycemic agent abuse is suspected, both serum and urine should be screened.

Non-islet Tumors that Secrete Insulin. Rarely, complex endocrine tumors may secrete both insulin and other hormones [56–58]. Hypoglycemia due to ectopic secretion of insulin by non-endocrine tumors is rare [59–61].

Nesidioblastosis or Persistent Hyperinsulinemic Hypoglycemia (PHH). Nesidioblastosis (nonmalignant islet cell hyperplasia) is a rare form of nonmalignant islet cell adenomatosis that leads to insulin-mediated hypoglycemia. Among infants, nesidioblastosis is typically characterized by islet hyperplasia, βcell hypertrophy, and increased βcell mass. It can be either diffuse or focal and is sometimes termed PHH of infancy [62–65]. Rapid diagnosis of the childhood form is crucial to avoid hypoglycemic damage to the maturing CNS. Several different genetic mutations have been associated with the disorder cases [63,64,66–69]. Special cases of hyperinsulinemic hypoglycemia of infancy include Costello syndrome [70] and the Beckwith–Wiedemann syndrome, which is due to defects in pancreatic βcell potassium channels [71].

A few cases of adult nesidioblastosis have been reported [63,72,73]. The pathologic findings are less consistent than for infants [74], and the cause is unknown. Additional cases of PHH have been diagnosed in adults who had previously undergone Roux-en-Y gastric bypass surgery for weight reduction [75,76]. Whether these cases represent nesidioblastosis [75,77], "dumping syndrome," or a reactive process leading to or unmasking a defect in β cell function [78] is unclear, perhaps in part because the pathologic diagnosis of nesidioblastosis is difficult [74]. The initial approach to patients with post-gastric bypass hypoglycemia should focus on avoidance of high carbohydrate content meals. Should that fail, other treatment options include diazoxide, streptozocin, calcium channel blockade [79], α-glucosidase inhibition [79], octreotide (discussed below), percutaneous gastrostomy into the remnant stomach [80], as well as partial pancreatectomy [77].

Antibody-Mediated ("Autoimmune") Hypoglycemia. Autoimmune hypoglycemia can result from autoantibodies directed against insulin itself or autoantibodies directed against the insulin receptor [81]. Both can occur in either insulin-treated [82] or nondiabetic individuals, and both types of autoantibody can be found in the same patient [83]. About 90% of cases have been reported from Japan [84]. Serum insulin concentrations typically are extremely high, usually higher than those produced by insulinomas. It is assumed that for these cases, glucose administration causes an excessive insulin response because the antibodies buffer most of the insulin secreted [85].

Endogenous antibodies that bind to and activate the insulin receptor can also cause hypoglycemia [86]. Some, but not all, cases are associated with other autoimmune disorders [87–89], and a few have occurred among patients with myeloma [90]. Previous exposure to exogenous insulin is not necessary, but some patients may have an abnormal insulin molecule [91]. Metformin may be helpful in management [92]. Some cases respond to immunosuppressive therapy [86]. The natural history of this syndrome is that the anti-receptor antibodies disappear and the syndrome resolves over months to years [38].

Pancreas and Islet Transplantation. Hypoglycemia after pancreas and islet transplantation can occur [93], but it is generally not a significant clinical problem [94,95]. Islet transplantation has been reported to resolve hypoglycemia unawareness [96]. There is a report of nesidioblastosis-like transformation of a successful pancreas allograft [97].

Non-islet Tumors with Insulin-like Activity. Certain tumors not of pancreatic islet origin are associated with fasting hypoglycemia clinically indistinguishable from that caused by islet cell neoplasms. Whereas insulinomas are typically quite small, non-pancreatic neoplasms associated with hypoglycemia tend to be large mesenchymal tumors. The large size initially suggested that excessive glucose utilization by the tumor was the cause of the hypoglycemia, but subsequent studies suggest that most cases result from secretion of high-molecular-weight insulin-like growth factor II (pro-IGF-II or "big IGF-II") [98–100]. Pro-IGF-II levels decrease significantly and hypoglycemia resolves after successful tumor resection [101–106]. Abnormal processing of the IGF-II molecule may play a role for some cases [102,104,107]. Non-islet cell neoplasms associated with hypoglycemia include gastrointestinal stromal cell tumors [108], hemangiopericytoma [109–111], hepatoma [112,113], uterine tumors [114], renal tumors [115], mesenteric sarcomas [116], colorectal cancer [117], gastric cancer [118], adrenocortical carcinoma, Hodgkin's lymphoma [119], poorly differentiated thyroid cancer [120], somatostatinoma [121], phyllodes tumor [122], and leukemia [123]. Multiple myeloma may also cause hypoglycemia via an antibody-mediated mechanism described below [89].

The diagnosis of hypoglycemia due to production of pro-IGF-II by non-islet cell tumors requires the exclusion of insulinoma. As noted above, this can be done by obtaining simultaneous insulin and glucose measurements during hypoglycemia. The observation of increased blood glucose concentration after intravenous administration of glucagon, an index of adequate glycogen stores, may also help discriminate between insulin and IGF-secreting tumors [124]. Methods have been developed for measuring serum pro-IGF-II directly [99]. Hypoglycemia associated with high levels of IGF-I has rarely been reported [125].

Hypoglycemia due to Non-insulin Hypoglycemic Agents

Pharmaceuticals other than insulin that are used to treat type 2 diabetes fall into two classes. "Hypoglycemic agents" enhance insulin secretion and can cause hyperinsulinemic hypoglycemia. The sulfonylureas and meglitinides belong to this class; all are taken orally. The second class is "antidiabetic agents." These promote normoglycemia through mechanisms other than enhancement of insulin secretion; they include both oral and injectable agents. When given as monotherapy they do not cause hypoglycemia, but they can amplify the glucose-lower activity of insulin and the oral hypoglycemic agents. The thiazolidinediones (TZDs), biguanides, α-glucosidase inhibitors, SGLT-2 inhibitors, gliptins, and bromocriptine mesylate are oral antidiabetic agents. Exenatide, liraglutide, and pramlintide, among others, are injectable antidiabetic agents. As discussed below, many drugs not used for the treatment of diabetes can also amplify the glucose-lowering activity of oral hypoglycemic agents, and a complete medication history can be critical for the diagnosis of hypoglycemia.

Sulfonylureas. After insulin, these are the most common cause of hypoglycemia [126]. Sulfonylureas reduce serum glucose by increasing insulin secretion, which also inhibits inhibiting glycogenolysis and gluconeogenesis, enhancing the response of target tissues to the effects of insulin [127]. Three "second-generation" sulfonylureas are in use in the United States, glipizide, glyburide, and glimepiride (Table 138.3). Severe hypoglycemia is not common with appropriate administration of these drugs [128], but it can be observed in several contexts [129]. In all age groups the condition is most often observed in the context of decreased carbohydrate intake. Maternal treatment of diabetes with glyburide can lead to postpartum hypoglycemia of their neonates [130]. Among patients between the ages of 11 and 30 years, a substantial number of hypoglycemic comas is due to sulfonylurea agents [51]. Half of these cases are suicide attempts [126]. Among patients with type 2 diabetes older than 60 years, sulfonylurea-induced hypoglycemia is a frequent complication [129,131]. Reported risk of hypoglycemia with glimepiride is 0.9% to 1.7%, with glipizide 3%, and with glyburide 21.3% [6,8]. When combined with metformin or a TZD, the risk increases 7% to 37% [6,8].

Liver disease decreases the clearance of glipizide, glyburide, and glimepiride (Table 138.3). Metabolites of sulfonylureas are excreted in urine with one exception; 50% of glyburide metabolites is excreted in the bile. Accordingly, sulfonylurea-induced hypoglycemia is often observed among older individuals in the setting of acute or chronic starvation superimposed on mild to moderate liver or renal failure.

The half-life of some sulfonylureas is >24 hours and the duration of action is often even longer (Table 138.3). Hepatic and renal insufficiency can extend their half-lives. Patients with sulfonylurea-induced hypoglycemia should therefore be hospitalized after initial resuscitation with glucose. They require continued treatment with oral and intravenous glucose for a minimum of 18 to 24 hours.

When oral agent overdose is suspected, serum and urine should be screened for sulfonylurea compounds. Sulfonylurea drugs circulate bound to proteins, and drugs of several classes can displace sulfonylureas and enhance their hypoglycemic effect (Table 138.3). The constellation of insulin concentration ≥3.9 μU per mL, C-peptide ≥1.4 ng per mL, and glucose <49 mg per dL may be helpful in diagnosing sulfonylurea-induced hypoglycemia [50].

Repaglinide and Nateglinide. Repaglinide (Prandin) and nateglinide (Starlix), like the sulfonylureas, increase endogenous insulin secretion but do so by a different mechanism. The risk of hypoglycemia from repaglinide is 16% to 31% and from nateglinide 1.3% to 3% [6,8]. Both are rapidly eliminated. Surreptitious use of repaglinide has been reported [132].

Antidiabetic Agents. Biguanides, when given as monotherapy, induce hypoglycemia much less frequently than do sulfonylureas

TABLE 138.3

Oral Hypoglycemic Agents

Sulfonylureas	Usual total daily dose (mg)	Half-life (h)	Duration of action (h)
Glimepiride (Amaryl)	1–4	2–8	12–24
Glipizide (Glucotrol)	10–20	1.1–3.7	12–24
Glyburide (DiaBeta, Glynase, Micronase)	3–20	0.7–3.0	12–24
Other insulin secretagogues			
Nateglinide (Starlix)	180–360	1.5	<4
Repaglinide (Prandin)	1.5–16	1	4

Oral hypoglycemic agents available in the United States. Glipizide is also known as glibenclamide. Gliclazide and gliquidone are second-generation sulfonylureas available outside of the United States. Overdoses with any of these drugs can cause hypoglycemia. Some trade names are given in parentheses. "First-generation" sulfonylureas are no longer used and have been omitted.

[133,134], probably by inhibiting gluconeogenesis. Metformin is the only biguanide currently available in the United States. It is also available in combination with the oral hypoglycemic agents glyburide (Glucovance), glipizide (Metaglip), and repaglinide (Prandimet); overdosage with these combination drugs can cause severe hypoglycemia. TZDs, and gliptins are also available in fixed ratio combinations with metformin; some of these have been associated with hypoglycemia.

Drugs of the TZD class, including pioglitazone (Actos) and rosiglitazone (Avandia), do not cause hypoglycemia when used as monotherapy but can potentiate hypoglycemia caused by insulin or sulfonylureas. They act by increasing insulin sensitivity.

Acarbose (Precose) and miglitol (Glyset) are α-glucosidase inhibitors that inhibit the digestion of complex carbohydrates; they have not been reported to cause hypoglycemia when used as monotherapy. Patients treated with insulin or sulfonylureas in addition to acarbose who experience hypoglycemia may not respond to the oral administration of complex sugars, but should respond to monomeric glucose.

Exenatide (Byetta), dulaglutide (Trulicity), albiglutide (Tanzeum), lixisenatide (Lyxumia), and liraglutide (Victoza) are injectable mimetics of gut incretins [135,136]. They augment glucose-dependent insulin secretion and reduce postprandial glucagon secretion. When given as monotherapy they rarely cause hypoglycemia but the risk increases with concurrent sulfonylurea use.

Gliptins are inhibitors of the enzyme dipeptidyl peptidase-4. They inhibit the degradation of endogenous gut incretins and have glucose-lowering effects and hypoglycemia risks similar to those of the gut incretins. Drugs in this class include sitagliptin (Januvia), linagliptin (Tradjenta), alogliptin (Nesina), and saxagliptin (Onglyza).

Pramlintide (Symlin) is a mimetic of the islet hormone amylin [136]. It suppresses post-meal glucagon secretion and delays gastric emptying. It is targeted at controlling post-meal hyperglycemia in diabetic patients who are also taking insulin. Like exenatide, it has been associated with hypoglycemia.

Gliflozins are inhibitors of the sodium-glucose transport protein 2 (SGLT2) in the kidney. They reduce blood glucose by reducing reabsorption of glucose by the kidney and as monotherapy do not cause hypoglycemia [6]. Available SGLT2 inhibitors include canagliflozin (Invokana), empagliflozin (Jardiance) and dapagliflozin (Farxiga). All are available in combination with metformin or a gliptin and these combination products can sometimes cause hypoglycemia. Bromocriptine is an oral dopamine agonist that is used in the treatment of pituitary tumors and Parkinson's disease. A micronized formulation (Cycloset) is approved for treating type 2 diabetes [137]. Its mechanism of action is unclear. It has not been reported to cause hypoglycemia, but experience with the drug is limited.

Medication Errors. Severe hypoglycemia can result from inadvertent substitution of an oral hypoglycemic agent for a different medication. Medication errors due to phonetic similarity in name are exemplified by cases in which chlorpropamide or chloroquine has been prescribed but chlorpropamine (an older sulfonylurea) inadvertently dispensed [126,138].

Other Drugs and Poisons that Cause Hypoglycemia

Hundreds of drugs and toxins have been reported to cause or predispose to hypoglycemia (Table 138.4). For some, like ethanol, the association is well documented and the mechanism well understood. For most, however, the evidence supporting an association is poor and the mechanism of action is unknown. Some are based only on a single case report. In some instances, drug–drug interactions may be amplifying the hypoglycemic effect of concurrently administered oral hypoglycemic agents. In other instances, the data are contaminated by intercurrent sepsis or other disease. Few re-challenge data to support the association are available. An analysis of the quality of the evidence implicating many drugs as the cause hypoglycemia is available [139] as is a review of mechanisms and relative risk [8]. Some drugs with stronger supporting evidence are indicated in Table 138.4.

Ethanol-Induced Hypoglycemia (Alcoholic Ketoacidosis)

Ethanol-induced hypoglycemia is most often observed among children and chronic alcohol abusers. The most common history is binge drinking in the setting of poor intake of other dietary carbohydrates. Patients usually present in a stuporous or comatose state; nausea, vomiting, and abdominal pain are common. Ethanol concentration is typically low, and alcoholic hypoglycemia can occur up to 30 hours after the ingestion of alcoholic beverages. Blood glucose as low as 5 mg per dL has been recorded. Ketonuria and ketonemia are frequently present and reflect the appropriately low circulating insulin concentration [140].

Ethanol causes hypoglycemia by suppressing hepatic gluconeogenesis. Glycogenolysis is not affected. When ethanol is oxidized to acetaldehyde and acetate, NAD^+ is reduced to nicotinamide adenine dinucleotide (NADH). The reduced NAD^+:NADH ratio produces an unfavorable intracellular environment for the oxidation of substrates of gluconeogenesis such as lactate and glutamate to pyruvate and α-ketoglutarate, respectively (Fig. 138.1). As a result, intracellular levels of pyruvate are below the Michaelis constant (*Km*) of pyruvate carboxylase, one of the rate-limiting steps for gluconeogenesis. Ethanol also inhibits hepatic uptake of the gluconeogenic precursors glycerol, alanine, and lactate, and inhibits the release of alanine from muscle [141].

Management consists of rehydration with intravenous fluids and glucose to correct hypoglycemia. Parenteral thiamine (100 mg) should be given to prevent Wernicke's encephalopathy. Treatment with glucose and fluids rapidly reverses the condition and sodium bicarbonate is generally unnecessary.

β-Adrenergic Receptor Antagonists

The nonselective β-blockers propranolol, pindolol, and nadolol reportedly predispose to hypoglycemia in diverse clinical settings, often by synergizing with another agent or delaying recovery. Both diabetic and nondiabetic patients undergoing hemodialysis are susceptible. Neonates may also have hypoglycemia during their first 24 hours of life as a result of propranolol treatment of the mother for cardiac arrhythmias, hypertension, or thyrotoxicosis. Hypoglycemia of infants treated with propranolol for congenital hemangiomas, cyanotic heart disease, and neonatal thyrotoxicosis has also been reported. Hypoglycemia is a documented complication of β blockade among pediatric ICU patients [142]. These drugs increase the risk of hypoglycemia among patients who are undernourished or who have liver disease [141] and occasionally when administered prior to cardiac surgery [126,143].

Antiarrhythmic Agents

Quinidine can enhance insulin secretion and produce hypoglycemia in ill, fasting patients [144]. Hypoglycemia has been reported in patients treated with diisopyramide, an antiarrhythmic agent with pharmacologic properties similar to those of quinidine [145,146]. In neither case is supporting evidence strong. The investigational antiarrhythmic cibenzoline is more convincingly associated with hypoglycemia [147].

Antibiotics

There is evidence [139] that pentamidine, used to treat *Pneumocystis jiroveci* infection, can be toxic to pancreatic β cells, causing

TABLE 138.4

Drugs and Toxins Associated with Hypoglycemia

Agents that increase circulating insulin	Agents that impair gluconeogenesis	Uncertain or other mechanisms of action	
Direct stimulants of insulin secretion	*Hepatotoxins*	ACE Inhibitors Acetazolamide (Diamox)	Haloperidol [255]
Oral hypoglycemic agents (Table 138.3)	Acetaminophen (Tylenol, Tempra)	Aspirin	Halothane
β-2 adrenergic agonists (e.g., Albuterol [247])	***Propoxyphene (Darvon)***	Aluminum hydroxide (Dialume)	Herbal extracts
Calcium	Amanita toxin	Anabolic steroids	Imatinib (Gleevec) [256]
Chloroquine (Aralen)	*Inhibition of gluconeogenesis*	Azapropazone	***Indomethacin***
Cibenzoline	Akee fruit	Chlorpromazine (Thorazine)	Interferon-α
Diisopyramide (Norpace)	Ethanol	Cimetidine	Isoxsuprine
Quinidine	Metformin	***Ciprofloxacin, gatifloxacin, clinafloxacin***	Lidocaine
Quinine	Metoprolol (Lopressor)	Clofibrate	***Lithium***
Ritodrine (Yutopar)	Nadolol (Corgard)	Dandelions [249]	Mefloquin
Terbutaline	Phenformin	Dexmedetomidine [250]	Nefazodone
Trimethoprim/sulfamethoxazole (Bactrim) [158,159]	Pindolol (Visken)	Diphenhydramine	NSAIDs
Destruction of β cells with insulin release	Propranolol (Inderal)	Doxepin (Sinequan, Adapin)	Orphenadrine
Pentamidine (Pentam)		'Ecstasy' (MDMA) [251]	Oxytetracycline
Streptozocin		Enflurane Formestane	Para-aminobenzoic acid
Agents that enhance the action of oral agents		Ethylenediaminetetraacetic acid (Versene)	Para-aminosalicylic acid
Clarithromycin [248]		Etanercept [252,253]	Perhexiline
Imipramine (Tofranil)		Etomidate [254]	Phenytoin (Dilantin)
NSAIDs		Fenoterol	Rantidine (Zantac)
Phenylbutazone (Butazolidin)		Fluoxetine	Salicylates
Salicylates			Selegiline
Sulfonamides			Sulfadiazine
Warfarin (Coumadin)			Sulfisoxazole (Gantrisin)
			Sunatinib [257]
			Valproate

Adapted from [39,100,126,139]. A sampling of common trade names is shown in parenthesis; the enumeration of trade names is not exhaustive. Data for some listed agents are very limited or anecdotal or involved treatment with more than one drug. Drugs for which better documentation is available are indicated in bold italic. MDMA: 3,4-methylenedioxymethamphetamine
ACE, angiotensin-converting enzyme.

transient hypoglycemia due to the release of stored insulin. It eventually results in diabetes in some patients [126]. Similarly, quinine, chemically related to quinidine, is known to elevate insulin concentrations of patients being treated for malaria [148,149]. Those with cerebral malaria are most prone to hypoglycemia, possibly due to the high intake of glucose by malarial parasites, coupled with the increased insulin release. Quinine may rarely cause hypoglycemia among normal individuals [150].

Gatifloxacin (Tequin) [151–154], levofloxacin (Levaquin) [151,155], ciprofloxacin (Cipro) [156,157], and other fluoroquinolones reportedly cause hypoglycemia, particularly when administered to patients who are also receiving sulfonylureas. Gatifloxacin may carry the highest risk of hypoglycemia, yet paradoxically some patients treated with this drug also experience new-onset hyperglycemia [151]. Trimethoprim/sulfamethoxazole has also been reported to cause hyperinsulinemic hypoglycemia in the setting of malnutrition and infection, renal failure [158], and oral hypoglycemic therapy [159].

Salicylates

Salicylate intoxication reportedly causes hypoglycemia occasionally among children but only very rarely in adults [126,160]. Among children, it may be a component of aspirin-associated Reyes syndrome [161]. The frequency of salicylate-induced hypoglycemia is difficult to ascertain due to intercurrent acidosis and renal or hepatic impairment for many cases of intoxication.

Angiotensin-Converting Enzyme Inhibitors

Cases of hypoglycemia associated with angiotensin-converting enzyme (ACE) inhibitors have been reported among persons with both types 1 and 2 diabetes [162–165], but the quality of the evidence is low [139]. No mechanism for the effect has been identified, and a retrospective analysis of nearly 14,000 persons with diabetes failed to identify an increased risk of hypoglycemia associated with this class of drugs [166].

Poisons

Several plant substances can cause hypoglycemia. Hypoglycin A toxin is found in akee fruit, a staple of the Jamaican diet. The ripe fruit is edible, but immature fruit causes vomiting a few days after ingestion. Affected patients have severe hypoglycemia due to inhibition of hepatic gluconeogenesis by hypoglycin [167]. Amanita toxins produced by the mushroom *Amanita phalloides* are inhibitors of RNA polymerase and cause hepatocellular necrosis. Fatal hypoglycemia can result from the ensuing complete depletion of hepatic glycogen and decreased capacity for gluconeogenesis [141].

Hypoglycemia Associated with Deficiencies of Counterregulatory Hormones

Glucocorticoid insufficiency can cause hypoglycemia among children by decreasing glycogenolysis and gluconeogenesis. In adults, it causes hypoglycemia uncommonly [168]. Malnutrition may contribute to the development of hypoglycemia in these cases. Patients with panhypopituitarism are prone to hypoglycemia and have increased sensitivity to insulin [168]. Although catecholamines play a significant role in preventing and reversing hypoglycemia, their absence does not commonly predispose to hypoglycemia. Adrenalectomized patients with sympathetic denervation due to spinal cord transection maintain euglycemia. Glucagon deficiency, as in persons with post-pancreatectomy diabetes, can contribute to hypoglycemia.

Fasting Hypoglycemia due to Inadequate Production of Endogenous Glucose

Liver Damage

About 90% of gluconeogenesis occurs in the liver, and the remainder in the renal cortex. Hepatic injury can cause hypoglycemia but only when the insult is very severe; only about 20% of normal liver biosynthetic capability is needed to maintain normal glucose homeostasis [169]. Hypoglycemia seldom occurs in the setting of isolated, limited hepatic failure and is not the cause of hepatic coma [141]. Hypoglycemia due to toxic or infectious hepatitis is rare but does occur when the disorder is fulminant. Hepatotoxins that can impair gluconeogenesis and cause hypoglycemia include carbon tetrachloride, the *A. phalloides* mushroom toxin, and urethane. Drugs that cause hypoglycemia by inducing hepatocellular necrosis include acetaminophen, isoniazid, sodium valproate, methyldopa, tetracycline, and halothane [141]. Neither tests of hepatocellular integrity (e.g., transaminases) nor tests of hepatic function (e.g., bilirubin concentration) nor the presence of structural damage (e.g., cirrhosis, chronic active hepatitis, metastatic liver disease) correlate well with the capability of the liver to maintain normoglycemia.

Congestive heart failure (CHF) from any cause can lead to hepatic congestion and hypoglycemia among adults and children. Patients with this syndrome usually have severe failure with cardiac cachexia, malnutrition, and muscle wasting. The mechanism by which CHF leads to hypoglycemia is not completely understood. Changes in hepatic blood flow may alter the delivery of gluconeogenic precursors or changes in intracellular redox state may decrease the gluconeogenic capacity of the hepatocyte. Hypoglycemia in this setting resolves with successful treatment of the CHF [141]. Hypoglycemia in association with CHF due to thyrotoxicosis [170] and rewarming from severe hypothermia [171] have been reported.

Renal Damage

Some patients with diabetes develop improved glucose tolerance with the onset of renal failure. A decrease in insulin requirements and more frequent episodes of hypoglycemia may also occur [172]. There is no correlation between degree of renal failure and severity of hypoglycemia for these patients, and the underlying mechanisms are not completely understood. Investigators variously implicate delayed insulin clearance, deficiencies of the delivery of gluconeogenic substrate [168], and hepatic insufficiency secondary to uremia [173].

Symptomatic hypoglycemia occurs among many diabetic patients receiving either hemodialysis or ambulatory peritoneal dialysis [174,175]. Any dialysis patient who experiences a change in mental status should be evaluated for hypoglycemia. The symptoms and signs of neuroglycopenia resemble those of the dialysis disequilibrium syndrome commonly induced by fluid shifts. These include fatigue, confusion, lethargy, and even coma. Post-dialysis hypoglycemia in diabetic patients, if prolonged, can be fatal [176].

Spontaneous fasting hypoglycemia has also been reported to occur among nondiabetic patients with end-stage renal disease [177–179]. It is not clear, however, whether these rare cases represent a distinct clinical entity [180] or instances of renal failure enhancing intercurrent disorders that predispose to hypoglycemia [181]. These might include drug ingestion, liver disease, and adrenal or pituitary insufficiency.

Fasting Hypoglycemia due to the Unavailability of Gluconeogenic Substrate

Substrate deficiency leads to hypoglycemia in ketotic hypoglycemia of childhood [182]. Patients with this condition, a variant of the normal response to starvation, are usually diagnosed between 18 months and 5 years of age. The hallmark of the condition is a low basal concentration of the gluconeogenic precursor alanine, and the hypoglycemia can be corrected with either glucose or alanine.

Other Causes of Hypoglycemia

Sepsis

Sepsis has occasionally been implicated as a cause of hypoglycemia [183–186]. Shock and liver failure were intercurrent problems in some cases [184]. Under conditions of decreased hepatic reserve, the combination of circulatory failure and impairment of gluconeogenesis by endotoxin may lead to hypoglycemia. Septic hypoglycemic patients are often acidotic, and the fatality rate is high [183,184]. In one report, only 1 of 15 such patients survived 1 month after onset of hypoglycemia and hypotension [184].

Congenital Disorders

The most common cause of neonatal hypoglycemia is maternal diabetes [187]. Congenital enzyme deficiencies and other abnormalities of the function of specific enzymes typically produce hypoglycemia in the context of glycogen storage disease, impaired hepatic gluconeogenesis, or respiratory chain defects [188]. Mutations of the sulfonylurea receptor can also cause this disorder [67]. These uncommon conditions usually present as hypoglycemia during infancy, but they can rarely present as unexplained persistent hypoglycemia of a critically ill adult [83,189]. The pediatric disorders are reviewed elsewhere [64,65,190].

Exercise-induced Hypoglycemia

Exercise-induced hyperinsulinemic hypoglycemia is an autosomal-dominant hyperinsulinemia syndrome [191]. The cause appears to be to failure of β cell–specific transcriptional silencing of a gene, monocarboxylate transporter 1, important for pyruvate-stimulated insulin release [192].

LABORATORY DIAGNOSIS OF HYPOGLYCEMIA

Normal Blood Glucose Concentration

Normal plasma glucose is 60 to 120 mg per dL (3.3 to 6.7 mmol). Whole blood glucose concentrations are 15% to 20% lower. Fingerstick blood glucose determinations are performed on whole capillary blood, and most meters reflect this offset. Symptoms of hypoglycemia generally occur when plasma glucose is <50 mg per dL (2.8 mmol) or the whole blood glucose concentration is <40 mg per dL (2.2 mmol), but for any given individual (especially in individuals with long-standing hyperglycemia), it may occur at higher glucose concentrations (Table 138.1). Calibrated hospital-quality glucose meter technology is accurate over a wide range of concentrations; values between 40 and 350 mg per dL generally agree well with values obtained using standard laboratory methods. Glucose meters for home use can be less accurate [193]. Because fingerstick blood glucose determinations can be less accurate at the lower end of their scale, they may require confirmation by a clinical laboratory. Interpretation of fingerstick glucose should take into account the clinical context, symptoms, and response to glucose administration. Fingerstick glucose can be particularly misleading among patients who are hypoperfused [194,195], in shock [196], or undergoing cardiopulmonary resuscitation [197]. Certain meter technologies are inaccurate in the presence of various interfering substances [198,199]. Newer point of care glucose meters that are FDA approved for use in critically ill patients are recommended over older ones for use in the ICU [200]. Nevertheless, in patients who are hypoperfused or with anasarca, the accuracy of fingerstick glucose values should be confirmed by whole blood glucose values before relying on fingerstick obtained specimens.

There are several physiologic exceptions to guideline values for diagnosing hypoglycemia in very ill patients. After about 48 hours of starvation, many individuals, particularly women, have a plasma glucose concentration less than 50 mg per dL (2.8 mmol). After 72 hours of fasting, the plasma glucose may approach 40 mg per dL (2.2 mmol). Starved individuals are nonetheless asymptomatic, do not fulfill Whipple's triad, and are not physiologically or clinically hypoglycemic. The absence of symptoms is due to the shift to ketones for CNS metabolism. Comparably low plasma glucose, 60 mg per dL (3.3 mmol) or less, can also be encountered during pregnancy. Again, there are no symptoms of hypoglycemia per se in these cases. Finally, rare individuals may have an anomalously low "set point" for blood glucose concentration, and such individuals appear asymptomatic in the face of persistent glycemia in the range of 35 to 45 mg per dL [201].

Spurious Hypoglycemia

This term applies to glucose concentrations that are reported to be low but come from a normoglycemic patient. This most commonly occurs as a result of storing blood samples at room temperature for long periods before laboratory analysis. As a result of anaerobic glycolysis by blood elements, the actual glucose concentration in the test tube may decline. The effect is enhanced if large numbers of white blood cells are present in the sample as the result of severe leukocytosis or leukemia [202]. Perhaps surprisingly, even a laboratory glucose determination can be spurious because plasma glucose concentration remains difficult to assay with consistent accuracy [203].

Spurious Hyperglycemia Leading to Insulin Overdose

Falsely elevated glucose readings can lead to inappropriate insulin administration and hypoglycemia. The commonest cause of spurious hyperglycemia in the ICU is measurement of glucose of blood obtained from an extremity into which glucose is being infused. An uncommon cause of hypoglycemia in the ICU results from a "drug–device interaction" affecting patients receiving parenteral nutrition products containing maltose or galactose. These products cause certain monitoring systems to give falsely elevated glucose readings leading to inappropriate insulin treatment [198].

Testing for Ketonuria

Urinary ketone testing can facilitate the differential diagnosis of hypoglycemia. Normally, fasting is associated with low circulating insulin that promotes gluconeogenesis and lipolysis. Hypoglycemia in association with ketonuria enhances the likelihood that the cause is not excess insulin.

Other Studies

In addition to glucose and urinary ketones, additional tests should be ordered as appropriate to the patient's underlying medical condition. In general, these should always include studies of hepatic and renal function. Obtain additional serum and plasma samples from any comatose, hypoglycemic patient when they are first seen. This permits assays for medications, insulin/glucose ratios, proinsulin, and C-peptide to be performed later, if indicated. Testing for oral hypoglycemic agents requires sophisticated laboratory methods, and it is recommended that laboratory personnel be consulted to insure that appropriate specimens (urine, blood, or both) are ordered. A cosyntropin (Cortrosyn) test should be performed when adrenal insufficiency is suspected.

MANAGEMENT OF HYPOGLYCEMIA

Initial Management with Glucose

When symptomatic hypoglycemia is suspected, remember Whipple's triad. After fingerstick glucose determination, the treatment is glucose administration, and the diagnostic outcome is resolution of symptoms. It is important to document the presence of hypoglycemia before giving glucose. Most patients with depressed mental status are not hypoglycemic [204].

The practice of giving intravenous glucose empirically assumes that it could be useful and is always harmless [205]. This belief has been called into question. In cases of stroke, in particular ischemic stroke, hyperglycemia may be predictive of poor outcome [206,207], and empiric use of hypertonic dextrose has been discouraged by many authors [197,204,208,209]. In addition, even for those cases in which empiric glucose appears to be resuscitative, there is no way to back-calculate what might have been the antecedent glucose concentration [210]. In the hospital, treatment of hypoglycemia is with intravenous D-glucose (dextrose) if a patient is unresponsive or might aspirate, but if a patient is alert and cooperative, oral carbohydrate (e.g., sucrose in orange juice or glucose tablets or gel) is preferable.

In general, all comatose patients, including trauma patients, should undergo fingerstick glucose determination, and the threshold for administration of intravenous glucose in addition to standard life-support measures should be low. Treatment with glucose is lifesaving in the presence of hypoglycemic coma. Early responders recognize that altered mental status due to hypoglycemia is sometimes the root cause of an accident [211].

The initial treatment of hypoglycemia for the patient with stupor or coma has traditionally consisted of the intravenous injection of 50 mL of 50% dextrose in water ($D_{50}W$) over 3 to 5 minutes. Care must be taken to avoid subcutaneous extravasation; the solution is hypertonic and can cause local tissue damage and severe pain. Alternatively, 10% dextrose delivered in 5 g (50 mL) aliquots can be equally efficacious and results in lower posttreatment blood glucose levels [212]. If hypoglycemia is present, treatment with glucose usually leads to improved mental status within minutes. It is difficult, however, to predict the magnitude of the glucose response to a bolus of intravenous glucose [209], and elderly patients and patients with very prolonged hypoglycemia may have a delayed response.

Subsequent Management

Glucose

The prompt improvement that usually occurs in hypoglycemic patients treated with intravenous glucose can be misleading. When hypoglycemia occurs in a diabetic patient taking insulin, no additional treatment may be needed, but there are many other causes of hypoglycemia. The initial bolus of glucose treats the symptoms of hypoglycemia but *not their cause*. The most common error of the management of hypoglycemia is inadequate treatment leading to recurrent symptoms.

After the first bolus of $D_{50}W$, an infusion of D_5W or $D_{10}W$ glucose should be started in any patient whose hypoglycemic episode is not clearly due simply to excess short- or intermediate-acting insulin. The choice of D_5W or $D_{10}W$ glucose depends on the severity of the initial hypoglycemia. This infusion allows the critical care physician to evaluate the cause of the hypoglycemic episode while protecting the patient from recurrence. An appropriate target glucose concentration is 100 mg per dL (5.6 mmol). It is advisable not to overtreat with glucose, especially for oral hypoglycemic agent poisoning. Extremely high serum glucose may stimulate endogenous insulin secretion, causing rebound hyperinsulinemia and recurrent hypoglycemia [213].

Hypoglycemia due to Long-acting Insulin

When a long-acting insulin (Table 138.2) might have caused the hypoglycemic episode, continuation of the glucose infusion, fingerstick blood glucose testing, and periodic adjustment of the infusion rate may be required. The duration of therapy depends on the particular insulin preparation and the dose taken. Massive insulin overdose (2,500 units of NPH) has been associated with persistent hypoglycemia for up to 6 days [211].

Hypoglycemia due to Sulfonylureas

When the cause of hypoglycemia is sulfonylurea ingestion (Table 138.3), the patient should usually be admitted to hospital because of the prolonged duration of action of most members of this class of drugs. Efforts to prevent drug absorption and increase elimination should be considered. Activated charcoal adsorbs sulfonylureas, and urinary alkalinization may enhance excretion [214,215]. Charcoal hemoperfusion is probably not indicated except in the setting of renal failure and massive overdose [216]. Continuous intravenous glucose is mandatory. Oral carbohydrate should be provided when the patient can eat. It is particularly important that the glucose infusion be continued while the patient recovering from a sulfonylurea overdose is asleep. Cases of persistent sulfonylurea-induced hypoglycemia requiring up to 27 days of intravenous glucose have been reported [217]. The typical patient with this condition requires 2 to 3 days of intravenous glucose therapy [126,218]. As discussed below, octreotide and diazoxide may be helpful adjuvant therapies for some cases.

Refractory Hypoglycemia

If the history and physical examination do not immediately establish the underlying cause of hypoglycemia, continuation of the infusion and glycemia monitoring are required. Persistent severe hypoglycemia requires intensive monitoring. Blood glucose should be measured every 1 to 3 hours and the serum glucose concentration maintained at a target level of 100 mg per dL (5.6 mmol per L). Diagnostic studies can be obtained as appropriate during continuous glucose infusion.

Intravenous glucose should continue until normoglycemia is achieved. To determine whether parenteral glucose is no longer needed, the infusion should be discontinued and blood glucose concentration measured every 15 minutes. If blood glucose falls to <50 mg per dL or if the patient becomes symptomatic, glucose infusion is resumed. Depending on the etiology of the hypoglycemia, parenteral glucose infusion may be required for many days and the use of additional drugs should be considered (see below). When hypoglycemia is due to impaired gluconeogenesis in the setting of liver disease, renal disease, or CHF, only treatment of the underlying condition will prevent recurrence. When a tumor is the course of hypoglycemia, surgery is the definitive therapy.

Drugs Other than Glucose for the Management of Hypoglycemia

Most cases of hypoglycemia in the ICU can be treated with glucose alone. When recurrent severe hypoglycemia or volume management are problems, intensivists may wish to consider the addition of adjunctive therapies. Particularly when hypoglycemia is due to an insulinoma, nesidioblastosis, or other tumor, it may be necessary to supplement the glucose infusion with drugs that inhibit insulin secretion.

Glucocorticoids

Parenteral adrenocortical steroids can increase gluconeogenic substrates and inhibit insulin action in the periphery. Hydrocortisone sodium succinate can be given at a dose of 100 mg per L of glucose infused. This therapy is beneficial for patients whose hypoglycemia is in the context of adrenocortical insufficiency; one case report describes utility for hemangiopericytoma-associated hypoglycemia [110]. It is not helpful for sulfonylurea poisoning [219].

Octreotide (Sandostatin)

Somatostatin is produced in pancreatic islet delta cells and inhibits insulin secretion. The long-acting analog octreotide can inhibit sulfonylurea-induced insulin secretion, and it has been used as supplemental therapy for insulinomas [220], oral agent-induced hypoglycemia [221–228], quinine-induced hypoglycemia in with the treatment of malaria [149], and reportedly in insulin glargine overdose where the mechanism of action is obscure [229]. The dose is 1 to 2 units per kg every 8 hours [224].

Diazoxide (Hyperstat)

Diazoxide is a benzothiadiazine non-diuretic antihypertensive agent that blocks the secretion of insulin from both normal and neoplastic β cells. To treat hypoglycemia, diazoxide is infused at a dose of 300 mg (1 to 3 mg per kg in children) in D_5W over 30 minutes every 4 hours, or as a constant infusion of 1 mg/kg/h. It has been reported to be effective in reversing severe, refractory hypoglycemia due to sulfonylurea poisoning [219], noninsulinoma pancreatogenous hypoglycemia syndrome (NIPHS) [230], and neonatal hyperinsulinemic hypoglycemia due to certain gene mutations [231].

Glucagon

The primary action of exogenous glucagon in the treatment of hypoglycemia is the promotion of glycogenolysis. It is most effective in patients with ample liver glycogen stores. Glucagon is a useful drug for out-of-hospital treatment of hypoglycemia due to excess insulin of known diabetic patients. It is good practice to teach family members of diabetic patients to administer parenteral glucagon. In the intensive care setting, however, there is seldom need to administer glucagon unless vascular access cannot be maintained. In addition, glucagon can stimulate insulin secretion and promote recurrent hypoglycemia [232]. It has also been associated with hypoglycemia when used as premedication for endoscopy [233].

Rapamycin (Sirolimus)

In one case report, rapamycin was effective in controlling intractable hypoglycemia in a patient with metastatic insulinoma [234]. The drug was thought to act both by reducing the malignant β cell proliferation and by inhibiting insulin production. In another case report it was used to treat hyperinsulinemic hypoglycemia of infancy [235].

PREVENTION OF HYPOGLYCEMIA IN THE ICU

With reported prevalence rates of 5% and higher [3–5], prevention of hypoglycemia is central to the metabolic management of the ICU patient. In general, oral antidiabetic agents like sulfonylureas should be discontinued for seriously ill patients [236]. Insulin infusions require meticulous management. Several studies have demonstrated that hypoglycemia can be avoided while achieving glycemic control by using structured insulin orders and management algorithms [237,238]. Such protocols are discussed in detail in Chapter 136. Up to a third of patients admitted to an emergency department with severe hypoglycemia may experience recurrent hypoglycemia in the hospital [239]. Strategies for preventing recurrent hypoglycemia have been outlined above.

Finally, it is becoming clear that promising new technology for continuous monitoring of glucose concentration has the potential to prevent hypoglycemia in the ICU [240]. Initial reports suggest that this technology enhances the detection of hypoglycemia in neonates [241] and reduces the frequency of hypoglycemic events in the adult ICU [242–244], though newer studies have not confirmed this [245]. It may not be useful in certain circumstances [245]. How this technology will affect glycemic control [242] or the management of neonatal hypoglycemia [241] or ICU outcomes remains to be determined but is potentially transformative, especially as closed-loop artificial pancreas systems are perfected [246].

TABLE 138.5

Hypoglycemia: Diagnosis, Management, Evidence

Recommendation	Comments
Suspect hypoglycemia in all cases of altered mental status	Hypoglycemia is a very common reversible cause of altered mental status
Be aware that intensive therapy with insulin infusions carries a risk of hypoglycemia	Attempting to lower blood glucose in the ICU to levels <110 mg/dL is frequently associated with hypoglycemia [44–48]. (See Chapter 137 on Diabetes Management)
Always determine blood glucose concentration before administering glucose	Most patients with altered mental status are not hypoglycemic [204] and empiric glucose administration should not be assumed to be completely risk free [197,204,206–208]
Consider 10% dextrose rather than 50% dextrose.	$D_{10}W$ can be as efficacious as $D_{50}W$ while lessening the risk of subsequent hyperglycemia [212]
Fingerstick glucose concentrations can at times be misleading	Measurements from an extremity in which glucose is being infused or in the setting of shock [196], CPR [197], and parenteral nutrition products containing maltose or galactose [258] may be inaccurate
Suspect overdose of an antidiabetic medication when unexplained hypoglycemia is encountered in the ICU	Medication errors are common in hospitals [259]. Hypoglycemia is commonly caused by overdosage with exogenous insulin and overdosage with oral hypoglycemic agents that enhance endogenous insulin secretion
If hypoglycemia is thought to be due to a drug not used to treat diabetes, evaluate the case thoughtfully	Many medications reportedly cause hypoglycemia (Table 138.4), but evidence supporting the association is often poor [139]. Hypoglycemia may be due to a drug–drug interaction, and discontinuation of a suspect medication may not always be appropriate
When treating refractory hypoglycemia always exclude adrenal insufficiency	Cortisol is an important glucose-counterregulatory hormone and renal insufficiency predisposes to hypoglycemia in persons being treated for diabetes
The role of continuous glucose monitoring in the ICU is promising but still investigational	Continuous monitoring of glucose concentration holds out the promise enhanced detection and reduced frequency of hypoglycemia in the ICU setting. How this technology will affect glycemic control [242] or the management of neonatal hypoglycemia [241] remains to be determined, and studies to validate its use in the setting of intercurrent illness are at an early stage [243]

Key elements in the diagnosis and management of hypoglycemia in the ICU.
ICU, intensive care unit; CPR, cardiopulmonary resuscitation.

CONCLUSIONS

Hypoglycemia is a serious problem for any hospitalized patient and a predictor of mortality for the critically ill [14,15]. It must be considered for all cases of stupor and coma. Diagnosis is based on Whipple's triad, and evaluation should take no more than a few minutes. After initial therapy with glucose, remember that only the symptoms and not the cause have been treated. The most common cause of hypoglycemia is insulin overdosage among individuals with diabetes; in the ICU this can be a complication of strict glucose control protocols. Hypoglycemia due to intercurrent medical conditions requires correction of the underlying disorder. Patients with sulfonylurea- or insulinoma-induced hypoglycemia may require aggressive treatment of hypoglycemia with parenteral glucose for many days. Key points are summarized in Table 138.5.

References

1. Mahmoodpoor A, Hamishehkar H, Beigmohammadi M, et al: Predisposing factors for hypoglycemia and its relation with mortality in critically ill patients undergoing insulin therapy in an intensive care unit. *Anesth Pain Med* 6(1):e33849, 2016.
2. Giakoumidakis K, Eltheni R, Patelarou E, et al: Effects of intensive glycemic control on outcomes of cardiac surgery. *Heart Lung* 42(2):146–151, 2013.
3. Van den Berghe G, Wouters P, Weekers F, et al: Intensive insulin therapy in critically ill patients. *N Engl J Med* 345(19):1359–1367, 2001.
4. Vriesendorp TM, van Santen S, DeVries JH, et al: Predisposing factors for hypoglycemia in the intensive care unit. *Crit Care Med* 34(1):96–101, 2006.
5. Mechanick JI, Handelsman Y, Bloomgarden ZT: Hypoglycemia in the intensive care unit. *Curr Opin Clin Nutr Metab Care* 10(2):193–196, 2007.
6. Scheen AJ: SGLT2 inhibition: efficacy and safety in type 2 diabetes treatment. *Expert Opin Drug Saf* 14(12):1879–1904, 2015.
7. Alsahli M, Gerich JE: Hypoglycemia. *Endocrinol Metab Clin North Am* 42(4):657–676, 2013.
8. Vue MH, Setter SM: Drug-induced glucose alterations Part 1: drug-induced hypoglycemia. *Diab Spectr* 24(3):171–177, 2011.
9. Mendoza A, Kim YN, Chernoff A: Hypoglycemia in hospitalized adult patients without diabetes. *Endocr Pract* 11(2):91–96, 2005.
10. Kagansky N, Levy S, Rimon E, et al: Hypoglycemia as a predictor of mortality in hospitalized elderly patients. *Arch Intern Med* 163(15):1825–1829, 2003.
11. Mortensen EM, Garcia S, Leykum L, et al: Association of hypoglycemia with mortality for subjects hospitalized with pneumonia. *Am J Med Sci* 339(3):239–243, 2010.
12. Garg R, Hurwitz S, Turchin A, et al: Hypoglycemia, with or without insulin therapy, is associated with increased mortality among hospitalized patients. *Diabetes Care* 36(5):1107–1110, 2013.
13. Brutsaert E, Carey M, Zonszein J: The clinical impact of inpatient hypoglycemia. *J Diabetes Complications* 28(4):565–572, 2014.
14. Egi M, Bellomo R, Stachowski E, et al: Hypoglycemia and outcome in critically ill patients. *Mayo Clin Proc* 85(3):217–224, 2010.
15. Hermanides J, Bosman RJ, Vriesendorp TM, et al: Hypoglycemia is associated with intensive care unit mortality. *Crit Care Med* 38(6):1430–1434, 2010.
16. Finfer S, Liu B, Chittock DR, et al: Hypoglycemia and risk of death in critically ill patients. *N Engl J Med* 367(12):1108–1118, 2012.
17. Jeschke MG, Pinto R, Herndon DN, et al: Hypoglycemia is associated with increased postburn morbidity and mortality in pediatric patients. *Crit Care Med* 42(5):1221–1231, 2014.
18. Whipple AO: The surgical therapy of hyperinsulinism. *J Int Chir* 3:237–276, 1938.
19. Seaquist ER, Anderson J, Childs B, et al: Hypoglycemia and diabetes: a report of a workgroup of the American Diabetes Association and the Endocrine Society. *Diabetes Care* 36(5):1384–1395, 2013.
20. Cryer PE: Symptoms of hypoglycemia, thresholds for their occurrence, and hypoglycemia unawareness. *Endocrinol Metab Clin North Am* 28:495–500, 1999.
21. Cryer PE: Mechanisms of hypoglycemia-associated autonomic failure in diabetes. *N Engl J Med* 369(4):362–372, 2013.
22. Margulescu AD, Sisu RC, Cinteza M, et al: Noncardiogenic acute pulmonary edema due to severe hypoglycemia—an old but ignored cause. *Am J Emerg Med* 26(7):839–836, 2008.
23. Navarro-Gutierrez S, Gonzalez-Martinez F, Fernandez-Perez MT, et al: Bradycardia related to hypoglycaemia. *Eur J Emerg Med* 10(4):331–333, 2003.
24. Chelliah YR: Ventricular arrhythmias associated with hypoglycaemia. *Anaesth Intensive Care* 28(6):698–700, 2000.
25. Odeh M, Oliven A, Bassan H: Transient atrial fibrillation precipitated by hypoglycemia. *Ann Emerg Med* 19(5):565–567, 1990.
26. Shimada R, Nakashima T, Nunoi K, et al: Arrhythmia during insulin-induced hypoglycemia in a diabetic patient. *Arch Intern Med* 144(5):1068–1069, 1984.
27. Lindstrom T, Jorfeldt L, Tegler L, et al: Hypoglycaemia and cardiac arrhythmias in patients with type 2 diabetes mellitus. *Diabet Med* 9(6):536–541, 1992.
28. Marques JL, George E, Peacey SR, et al: Altered ventricular repolarization during hypoglycaemia in patients with diabetes. *Diabet Med* 14(8):648–654, 1997.
29. Pollock G, Brady WJ Jr, Hargarten S, et al: Hypoglycemia manifested by sinus bradycardia: a report of three cases. *Acad Emerg Med* 3(7):700–707, 1996.
30. Hillson RM: Hypoglycemia and hypothermia. *Diabetes Care* 6(2):211, 1983.
31. Kedes LH, Field JB: Hypothermia: a clue to the diagnosis of hypoglycemia. *N Engl J Med* 271:785–786, 1964.
32. Passias TC, Meneilly GS, Mekjavic IB: Effect of hypoglycemia on thermoregulatory responses. *J Appl Physiol* 80(3):1021–1032, 1996.
33. Arem R, Zoghbi W: Insulin overdose in eight patients: insulin pharmacokinetics and review of the literature. *Medicine (Baltimore)* 64(5):323–332, 1985.
34. Matsumura M, Nakashima A, Tofuku Y: Electrolyte disorders following massive insulin overdose in a patient with type 2 diabetes. *Intern Med* 39(1):55–57, 2000.
35. Brun JF, Fedou C, Mercier J: Postprandial reactive hypoglycemia. *Diabetes Metab* 26(5):337–351, 2000.
36. Hofeldt FD: Reactive hypoglycemia. *Endocrinol Metab Clin North Am* 18(1):185–201, 1989.
37. Hojlund K, Hansen T, Lajer M, et al: A novel syndrome of autosomal-dominant hyperinsulinemic hypoglycemia linked to a mutation in the human insulin receptor gene. *Diabetes* 53(6):1592–1598, 2004.
38. Taylor SI, Barbetti F, Accili D, et al: Syndromes of autoimmunity and hypoglycemia. Autoantibodies directed against insulin and its receptor. *Endocrinol Metab Clin North Am* 18:123–143, 1989.
39. Marks V, Teale JD: Drug-induced hypoglycemia. *Endocrinol Metab Clin North Am* 28:555–577, 1999.
40. Stapczynski JS, Haskell RJ: Duration of hypoglycemia and need for intravenous glucose following intentional overdoses of insulin. *Ann Emerg Med* 13(7):505–511, 1984.
41. Samuels MH, Eckel RH: Massive insulin overdose: detailed studies of free insulin levels and glucose requirements. *J Toxicol Clin Toxicol* 1989;27(3):157–168.
42. Cryer PE: Hypoglycemia: still the limiting factor in the glycemic management of diabetes. *Endocr Pract* 14(6):750–756, 2008.
43. Sauer P, Van Horn ER: Impact of intravenous insulin protocols on hypoglycemia, patient safety, and nursing workload. *Dimens Crit Care Nurs* 28(3):95–101, 2009.
44. Finfer S, Chittock DR, Su SY, et al: Intensive versus conventional glucose control in critically ill patients. *N Engl J Med* 360(13):1283–1297, 2009.
45. Annane D, Cariou A, Maxime V, et al: Corticosteroid treatment and intensive insulin therapy for septic shock in adults: a randomized controlled trial. *JAMA* 303(4):341–348, 2010.
46. Van den Berghe G, Wilmer A, Hermans G, et al: Intensive insulin therapy in the medical ICU. *N Engl J Med* 354(5):449–461, 2006.
47. Preiser JC, Devos P, Ruiz-Santana S, et al: A prospective randomised multi-centre controlled trial on tight glucose control by intensive insulin therapy in adult intensive care units: the Glucontrol study. *Intensive Care Med* 35(10):1738–1748, 2009.
48. Brunkhorst FM, Engel C, Bloos F, et al: Intensive insulin therapy and pentastarch resuscitation in severe sepsis. *N Engl J Med* 358(2):125–139, 2008.
49. Radosevich JJ, Patanwala AE, Frey PD, et al: Higher insulin infusion rate but not 24-h insulin consumption is associated with hypoglycemia in critically ill patients. *Diabetes Res Clin Pract* 110(3):322–327, 2015.
50. DeWitt CR, Heard K, Waksman JC: Insulin and C-peptide levels in sulfonylurea-induced hypoglycemia: a systematic review. *J Med Toxicol* 3(3):107–118, 2007.
51. Klonoff DC, Barrett BJ, Nolte MS, et al: Hypoglycemia following inadvertent and factitious sulfonylurea overdosages. *Diabetes Care* 18:563–567, 1995.
52. Kao SL, Chan CL, Tan B, et al: An unusual outbreak of hypoglycemia. *N Engl J Med* 360(7):734–736, 2009.
53. Dalan R, Leow MK, George J, et al: Neuroglycopenia and adrenergic responses to hypoglycaemia: insights from a local epidemic of serendipitous massive overdose of glibenclamide. *Diabet Med* 26(1):105–109, 2009.
54. Cryer PE, Axelrod L, Grossman AB, et al: Evaluation and management of adult hypoglycemic disorders: an Endocrine Society Clinical Practice Guideline. *J Clin Endocrinol Metab* 94(3):709–728, 2009.
55. Nauck MA, Meier JJ: Diagnostic accuracy of an "amended" insulin-glucose ratio for the biochemical diagnosis of insulinomas. *Ann Intern Med* 157(11):767–775, 2012.
56. Furrer J, Hättenschwiler A, Komminoth P, et al: Carcinoid syndrome, acromegaly, and hypoglycemia due to an insulin-secreting neuroendocrine tumor of the liver. *J Clin Endocrinol Metab* 86:2227–2230, 2001.
57. Morken NH, Majak B, Kahn JA: Insulin producing primary ovarian carcinoid tumor. *Acta Obstet Gynecol Scand* 86(4):500, 501, 2007.
58. Morgello S, Schwartz E, Horwith M, et al: Ectopic insulin production by a primary ovarian carcinoid. *Cancer* 61(4):800–805, 1988.
59. Seckl MJ, Mulholland PJ, Bishop AE, et al: Hypoglycemia due to an insulin-secreting small-cell carcinoma of the cervix. *N Engl J Med* 341:733–736, 1999.
60. Shetty MR, Boghossian HM, Duffell D, et al: Tumor-induced hypoglycemia: a result of ectopic insulin production. *Cancer* 49(9):1920–1923, 1982.
61. Uysal M, Temiz S, Gul N, et al: Hypoglycemia due to ectopic release of insulin from a paraganglioma. *Horm Res* 67(6):292–295, 2007.
62. Raffel A, Krausch MM, Anlauf M, et al: Diffuse nesidioblastosis as a cause of hyperinsulinemic hypoglycemia in adults: a diagnostic and therapeutic challenge. *Surgery* 141(2):179–184, 2007.
63. Kaczirek K, Niederle B: Nesidioblastosis: an old term and a new understanding. *World J Surg* 28(12):1227–1230, 2004.

64. Sperling MA, Menon RK: Differential diagnosis and management of neonatal hypoglycemia. *Pediatr Clin North Am* 51(3):703–723, 2004.
65. Straussman S, Levitsky LL: Neonatal hypoglycemia. *Curr Opin Endocrinol Diabetes Obes* 17(1):20–24, 2010.
66. Thompson GB, Service FJ, Andrews JC, et al: Noninsulinoma pancreatogenous hypoglycemia syndrome: an update in 10 surgically treated patients. *Surgery* 128:937–944, 2000.
67. Magge SN, Shyng SL, MacMullen C, et al: Familial leucine-sensitive hypoglycemia of infancy due to a dominant mutation of the b-cell sulfonylurea receptor. *J Clin Endocrinol Metab* 89(9):4450–4456, 2004.
68. Sperling MA, Menon RK: Hyperinsulinemic hypoglycemia of infancy. Recent insights into ATP-sensitive potassium channels, sulfonylurea receptors, molecular mechanisms, and treatment. *Endocrinol Metab Clin North Am* 28:695–708, 1999.
69. Otonkoski T, Ämmälä C, Huopio H, et al: A point mutation inactivating the sulfonylurea receptor causes the severe form of persistent hyperinsulinemic hypoglycemia of infancy in Finland. *Diabetes* 48:408–415, 1999.
70. Alexander S, Ramadan D, Alkhayyat H, et al: Costello syndrome and hyperinsulinemic hypoglycemia. *Am J Med Genet A* 139(3):227–230, 2005.
71. Hussain K, Cosgrove KE, Shepherd RM, et al: Hyperinsulinemic hypoglycemia in Beckwith-Wiedemann syndrome due to defects in the function of pancreatic beta-cell adenosine triphosphate-sensitive potassium channels. *J Clin Endocrinol Metab* 90(7):4376–4382, 2005.
72. Rinker RD, Friday K, Aydin F, et al: Adult nesidioblastosis: a case report and review of the literature. *Dig Dis Sci* 43:1784–1790, 1998.
73. Anlauf M, Wieben D, Perren A, et al: Persistent hyperinsulinemic hypoglycemia in 15 adults with diffuse nesidioblastosis: diagnostic criteria, incidence, and characterization of b-cell changes. *Am J Surg Pathol* 29(4):524–533, 2005.
74. Klöppel G, Anlauf M, Raffel A, et al: Adult diffuse nesidioblastosis: genetically or environmentally induced? *Hum Pathol* 39(1):3–8, 2008.
75. Service GJ, Thompson GB, Service FJ, et al: Hyperinsulinemic hypoglycemia with nesidioblastosis after gastric-bypass surgery. *N Engl J Med* 353(3):249–254, 2005.
76. Rariy CM, Rometo D, Korytkowski M: Post-gastric bypass hypoglycemia. *Curr Diab Rep* 16(2):19, 2016.
77. Patti ME, McMahon G, Mun EC, et al: Severe hypoglycaemia post-gastric bypass requiring partial pancreatectomy: evidence for inappropriate insulin secretion and pancreatic islet hyperplasia. *Diabetologia* 48(11):2236–2240, 2005.
78. Meier JJ, Butler AE, Galasso R, et al: Hyperinsulinemic hypoglycemia after gastric bypass surgery is not accompanied by islet hyperplasia or increased beta-cell turnover. *Diabetes Care* 29(7):1554–1559, 2006.
79. Mordes JP, Alonso LC: Evaluation, medical therapy, and course of adult persistent hyperinsulinemic hypoglycemia after Roux-En-Y Gastric Bypass Surgery: a case series. *Endocr Pract* 21:237–242, 2015.
80. McLaughlin T, Peck M, Holst J, et al: Reversible hyperinsulinemic hypoglycemia after gastric bypass: a consequence of altered nutrient delivery. *J Clin Endocrinol Metab* 95(4):1851–1855, 2010.
81. Lupsa BC, Chong AY, Cochran EK, et al: Autoimmune forms of hypoglycemia. *Medicine (Baltimore)* 88(3):141–153, 2009.
82. Koyama R, Nakanishi K, Kato M, et al: Hypoglycemia and hyperglycemia due to insulin antibodies against therapeutic human insulin: treatment with double filtration plasmapheresis and prednisolone. *Am J Med Sci* 329(5):259–264, 2005.
83. Kim CH, Park JH, Park TS, et al: Autoimmune hypoglycemia in a type 2 diabetic patient with anti-insulin and insulin receptor antibodies. *Diabetes Care* 27(1):288, 289, 2004.
84. Burch HB, Clement S, Sokol MS, et al: Reactive hypoglycemic coma due to insulin autoimmune syndrome: case report and literature review. *Am J Med* 92:681–685, 1992.
85. Vogeser M, Parhofer KG, Furst H, et al: Autoimmune hypoglycemia presenting as seizure one week after surgery. *Clin Chem* 47(4):795–6, 2001.
86. Redmon JB, Nuttall FQ: Autoimmune hypoglycemia. *Endocrinol Metab Clin North Am* 28:603–618, 1999.
87. Varga J, Lopatin M, Boden G: Hypoglycemia due to antiinsulin receptor antibodies in systemic lupus erythematosus. *J Rheumatol* 17:1226–1229, 1990.
88. Uchigata Y, Takayama-Hasumi S, Kawanishi K, et al: Inducement of antibody that mimics insulin action on insulin receptor by insulin autoantibody directed at determinant at asparagine site on human insulin B chain. *Diabetes* 40:966–970, 1991.
89. Selinger S, Tsai J, Pulini M, et al: Autoimmune thrombocytopenia and primary biliary cirrhosis with hypoglycemia and insulin receptor autoantibodies. A case report. *Ann Intern Med* 107:686–688, 1987.
90. Redmon B, Pyzdrowski KL, Elson MK, et al: Hypoglycemia due to a monoclonal insulin-binding antibody in multiple myeloma. *N Engl J Med* 326:994–998, 1992.
91. Seino S, Fu ZZ, Marks W, et al: Characterization of circulating insulin in insulin autoimmune syndrome. *J Clin Endocrinol Metab* 62:64–69, 1986.
92. Miranda-Garduno LM, Gomez-Perez FJ, Rull JA: Improvement of autoimmune hypoglycemia by decreasing circulating free insulin concentrations with metformin. *Endocr Pract* 14(4):511–513, 2008.
93. Shen J, Gaglia J: Hypoglycemia following pancreas transplantation. *Curr Diab Rep* 8(4):317–323, 2008.
94. Redmon JB, Teuscher AU, Robertson RP: Hypoglycemia after pancreas transplantation. *Diabetes Care* 21:1944–1950, 1998.
95. Stagner JI, Mokshagundam SP, Samols E: Induction of mild hypoglycemia by islet transplantation to the pancreas. *Transplant Proc* 30:635, 636, 1998.
96. Leitao CB, Tharavanij T, Cure P, et al: Restoration of hypoglycemia awareness after islet transplantation. *Diabetes Care* 31(11):2113–2115, 2008.
97. Semakula C, Pambuccian S, Gruessner R, et al: Clinical case seminar: hypoglycemia after pancreas transplantation: association with allograft nesidiodysplasia and expression of islet neogenesis-associated peptide. *J Clin Endocrinol Metab* 87(8):3548–3554, 2002.
98. Christofilis MA, Remacle-Bonnet M, Atlan-Gepner C, et al: Study of serum big-insulin-like growth factor (IGF)-II and IGF binding proteins in two patients with extrapancreatic tumor hypoglycemia, using a combination of Western blotting methods. *Eur J Endocrinol* 139:317–322, 1998.
99. Miraki-Moud F, Grossman AB, Besser M, et al: A rapid method for analyzing serum pro-insulin-like growth factor-II in patients with non-islet cell tumor hypoglycemia. *J Clin Endocrinol Metab* 90(7):3819–3823, 2005.
100. Fang C, Fan CW, Yu YY, et al: Severe hypoglycemia caused by recurrent sarcomatoid carcinoma in the pelvic cavity: a case report. *Medicine (Baltimore)* 94(42):e1577, 2015.
101. Daughaday WH, Trivedi B: Measurement of derivatives of proinsulin-like growth factor- II in serum by a radioimmunoassay directed against the E-domain in normal subjects and patients with nonislet cell tumor hypoglycemia. *J Clin Endocrinol Metab* 75:110–115, 1992.
102. Daughaday WH, Trivedi B, Baxter RC: Serum "big insulin-like growth factor II" from patients with tumor hypoglycemia lacks normal E-domain O-linked glycosylation, a possible determinant of normal propeptide processing. *Proc Natl Acad Sci USA* 90:5823–5827, 1993.
103. Daughaday WH, Emanuele MA, Brooks MH, et al: Synthesis and secretion of insulin-like growth factor II by a leiomyosarcoma with associated hypoglycemia. *N Engl J Med* 319(22):1434–1440, 1988.
104. Daughaday WH, Wu JC, Lee SD, et al: Abnormal processing of pro-IGF-II in patients with hepatoma and in some hepatitis B virus antibody-positive asymptomatic individuals. *J Lab Clin Med* 116(4):555–562, 1990.
105. Cotterill AM, Holly JM, Davies SC, et al: The insulin-like growth factors and their binding proteins in a case of non-islet-cell tumour-associated hypoglycaemia. *J Endocrinol* 131(2):303–311, 1991.
106. Trivedi N, Mithal A, Sharma AK, et al: Non-islet cell tumour induced hypoglycaemia with acromegaloid facial and acral swelling. *Clin Endocrinol (Oxf)* 42(4):433–435, 1995.
107. Baxter RC, Daughaday WH: Impaired formation of the ternary insulin-like growth factor-binding protein complex in patients with hypoglycemia due to nonislet cell tumors. *J Clin Endocrinol Metab* 73(4):696–702, 1991.
108. Escobar GA, Robinson WA, Nydam TL, et al: Severe paraneoplastic hypoglycemia in a patient with a gastrointestinal stromal tumor with an exon 9 mutation: a case report. *BMC Cancer* 7:13, 2007.
109. Lawson EA, Zhang X, Crocker JT, et al: Hypoglycemia from IGF2 overexpression associated with activation of fetal promoters and loss of imprinting in a metastatic hemangiopericytoma. *J Clin Endocrinol Metab* 94(7):2226–2231, 2009.
110. Anaforoglu I, Simsek A, Turan T, et al: Hemangiopericytoma-associated hypoglycemia improved by glucocorticoid therapy: a case report. *Endocrine* 36(1):151–154, 2009.
111. Adams J, Lodge JPA, Parker D: Liver transplantation for metastatic hemangiopericytoma associated with hypoglycemia. *Transplantation* 67:488, 489, 1999.
112. Saigal S, Nandeesh HP, Malhotra V, et al: A case of hepatocellular carcinoma associated with troublesome hypoglycemia: management by cytoreduction using percutaneous ethanol injection. *Am J Gastroenterol* 93:1380, 1381, 1998.
113. Atiq M, Safa M: Recurrent hypoglycemia associated with poorly differentiated carcinoma of the liver. *Am J Clin Oncol* 30(2):213, 214, 2007.
114. Wakami K, Tateyama H, Kawashima H, et al: Solitary fibrous tumor of the uterus producing high-molecular-weight insulin-like growth factor II and associated with hypoglycemia. *Int J Gynecol Pathol* 24(1):79–84, 2005.
115. Korn E, Van Hoff J, Buckley P, et al: Secretion of a large molecular-weight form of insulin-like growth factor by a primary renal tumor. *Med Pediatr Oncol* 24(6):392–396, 1995.
116. Sato R, Tsujino M, Nishida K, et al: High molecular weight form insulin-like growth factor II-producing mesenteric sarcoma causing hypoglycemia. *Intern Med* 43(10):967–971, 2004.
117. Ko AH, Bergsland EK, Lee GA: Tumor-associated hypoglycemia from metastatic colorectal adenocarcinoma: case report and review of the literature. *Dig Dis Sci* 48(1):192–196, 2003.
118. Kato A, Bando E, Shinozaki S, et al: Severe hypoglycemia and hypokalemia in association with liver metastases of gastric cancer. *Intern Med* 43(9):824–828, 2004.
119. Lim HC, Munshi LB, Sharon D: Persistent hypoglycemia in patient with Hodgkin's disease. *Case Rep Oncol Med* 2015:820286, 2015.
120. Rosario PW, Furtado MS, Castro AF, et al: Non-islet cell tumor hypoglycemia in a patient with poorly differentiated thyroid cancer. *Thyroid* 17(1):84, 85, 2007.
121. He X, Wang J, Wu X, et al: Pancreatic somatostatinoma manifested as severe hypoglycemia. *J Gastrointestin Liver Dis* 18(2):221–224, 2009.
122. Hino N, Nakagawa Y, Ikushima Y, et al: A case of a giant phyllodes tumor of the breast with hypoglycemia caused by high-molecular-weight insulin-like growth factor II. *Breast Cancer* 17(2):142–145, 2010.
123. Daughaday WH: Hypoglycemia in patients with non-islet cell tumors. *Endocrinol Metab Clin North Am* 18:91–101, 1989.
124. Hoff AO, Vassilopoulou-Sellin R: The role of glucagon administration in the diagnosis and treatment of patients with tumor hypoglycemia. *Cancer* 82:1585–1592, 1998.

125. Ogiwara Y, Mori S, Iwama M, et al: Hypoglycemia due to ectopic secretion of insulin-like growth factor-I in a patient with an isolated sarcoidosis of the spleen. *Endocr J* 57(4):325–330, 2010.
126. Seltzer HS: Drug-induced hypoglycemia. A review of 1418 cases. *Endocrinol Metab Clin North Am* 18:163–183, 1989.
127. Gerich JE: Oral hypoglycemic agents. *N Engl J Med* 321:1231–1245, 1989.
128. Aldhahi W, Armstrong J, Bouche C, et al: b-Cell insulin secretory response to oral hypoglycemic agents is blunted in humans *in vivo* during moderate hypoglycemia. *J Clin Endocrinol Metab* 89(9):4553–4557, 2004.
129. Shorr RI, Ray WA, Daugherty JR, et al: Individual sulfonylureas and serious hypoglycemia in older people. *J Am Geriatr Soc* 44:751–755, 1996.
130. Langer O, Conway DL, Berkus MD, et al: A comparison of glyburide and insulin in women with gestational diabetes mellitus. *N Engl J Med* 343:1134–1138, 2000.
131. Ben-Ami H, Nagachandran P, Mendelson A, et al: Drug-induced hypoglycemic coma in 102 diabetic patients. *Arch Intern Med* 159:281–284, 1999.
132. Hirshberg B, Skarulis MC, Pucino F, et al: Repaglinide-induced factitious hypoglycemia. *J Clin Endocrinol Metab* 86:475–477, 2001.
133. Bodmer M, Meier C, Krahenbuhl S, et al: Metformin, sulfonylureas, or other antidiabetes drugs and the risk of lactic acidosis or hypoglycemia: a nested case-control analysis. *Diabetes Care* 31(11):2086–2091, 2008.
134. Bailey CJ, Turner RC: Metformin. *N Engl J Med* 334:574–579, 1996.
135. DeFronzo RA, Ratner RE, Han J, et al: Effects of exenatide (exendin-4) on glycemic control and weight over 30 weeks in metformin-treated patients with type 2 diabetes. *Diabetes Care* 28(5):1092–1100, 2005.
136. Kendall DM, Riddle MC, Rosenstock J, et al: Effects of exenatide (exendin-4) on glycemic control over 30 weeks in patients with type 2 diabetes treated with metformin and a sulfonylurea. *Diabetes Care* 28(5):1083–1091, 2005.
137. Pijl H, Ohashi S, Matsuda M, et al: Bromocriptine—a novel approach to the treatment of type 2 diabetes. *Diabetes Care* 23:1154–1161, 2000.
138. Hargett NA, Ritch R, Mardirossian J, et al: Inadvertent substitution of acetohexamide for acetozolamide. *Am J Ophthalmol* 84:580–583, 1977.
139. Murad MH, Coto-Yglesias F, Wang AT, et al: Clinical review: drug-induced hypoglycemia: a systematic review. *J Clin Endocrinol Metab* 94(3):741–745, 2009.
140. McGuire LC, Cruickshank AM, Munro PT: Alcoholic ketoacidosis. *Emerg Med J* 23(6):417–420, 2006.
141. Arky RA: Hypoglycemia associated with liver disease and ethanol. *Endocrinol Metab Clin North Am* 18:75–90, 1989.
142. Britt J, Moffett BS, Bronicki RA, et al: Incidence of adverse events requiring intervention after initiation of oral beta-blocker in pediatric cardiac intensive care patients. *Pediatr Cardiol* 35(6):1062–1066, 2014.
143. Brown DR, Brown MJ: Hypoglycemia associated with preoperative metoprolol administration. *Anesth Analg* 99(5):1427–1428, 2004.
144. Phillips RE, Looareesuwan S, White NJ, et al: Hypoglycaemia and antimalarial drugs: quinidine and release of insulin. *Br Med J* 292:1319–1321, 1986.
145. Goldberg IJ, Brown LK, Rayfield EJ: Disopyramide (Norpace)-induced hypoglycemia. *Am J Med* 69:463–466, 1980.
146. Nappi JM, Dhanani S, Lovejoy JR, et al: Severe hypoglycemia associated with disopyramide. *West J Med* 138:95–97, 1983.
147. Takada M, Fujita S, Katayama Y, et al: The relationship between risk of hypoglycemia and use of cibenzoline and disopyramide. *Eur J Clin Pharmacol* 56(4):335–342, 2000.
148. White NJ, Warrell DA, Chanthavanich P, et al: Severe hypoglycemia and hyperinsulinemia in falciparum malaria. *N Engl J Med* 309:61–66, 1983.
149. Phillips RE, Looareesuwan S, Molyneux ME, et al: Hypoglycaemia and counterregulatory hormone responses in severe falciparum malaria: treatment with Sandostatin. *Q J Med* 86:233–240, 1993.
150. Limburg PJ, Katz H, Grant CS, et al: Quinine-induced hypoglycemia. *Ann Intern Med* 119:218, 219, 1993.
151. Park-Wyllie LY, Juurlink DN, Kopp A, et al: Outpatient gatifloxacin therapy and dysglycemia in older adults. *N Engl J Med* 354(13):1352–1361, 2006.
152. Khovidhunkit W, Sunthornyothin S: Hypoglycemia, hyperglycemia, and gatifloxacin. *Ann Intern Med* 141(12):969, 2004.
153. Brogan SE, Cahalan MK: Gatifloxacin as a possible cause of serious postoperative hypoglycemia. *Anesth Analg* 101(3):635–636, 2005, table.
154. Menzies DJ, Dorsainvil PA, Cunha BA, et al: Severe and persistent hypoglycemia due to gatifloxacin interaction with oral hypoglycemic agents. *Am J Med* 113(3):232–234, 2002.
155. Bansal N, Manocha D, Madhira B: Life-threatening metabolic coma caused by levofloxacin. *Am J Ther* 22(2):e48–e51, 2015.
156. Lin G, Hays DP, Spillane L: Refractory hypoglycemia from ciprofloxacin and glyburide interaction. *J Toxicol Clin Toxicol* 42(3):295–297, 2004.
157. Kelesidis T, Canseco E: Quinolone-induced hypoglycemia: a life-threatening but potentially reversible side effect. *Am J Med* 123(2):e5, e6, 2010.
158. Strevel EL, Kuper A, Gold WL: Severe and protracted hypoglycaemia associated with co-trimoxazole use. *Lancet Infect Dis* 6(3):178–182, 2006.
159. Roustit M, Blondel E, Villier C, et al: Symptomatic hypoglycemia associated with trimethoprim/sulfamethoxazole and repaglinide in a diabetic patient. *Ann Pharmacother* 44(4):764–767, 2010.
160. Raschke R, Arnold-Capell PA, Richeson R, et al: Refractory hypoglycemia secondary to topical salicylate intoxication. *Arch Intern Med* 151:591–593, 1991.
161. Maheady DC: Reye's syndrome: review and update. *J Pediatr Health Care* 3(5):246–250, 1989.
162. Arauz-Pacheco C, Ramirez LC, Rios JM, et al: Hypoglycemia induced by angiotensin-converting enzyme inhibitors in patients with non-insulin-dependent diabetes receiving sulfonylurea therapy. *Am J Med* 89:811–813, 1990.
163. Buller GK, Perazella M: ACE inhibitor-induced hypoglycemia. *Am J Med* 91:104, 105, 1991.
164. Herings RMC, De Boer A, Stricker BHC, et al: Hypoglycaemia associated with use of inhibitors of angiotensin converting enzyme. *Lancet* 345:1195–1198, 1995.
165. Morris AD, Boyle DIR, McMahon AD, et al: ACE inhibitor use is associated with hospitalization for severe hypoglycemia in patients with diabetes. *Diabetes Care* 20:1363–1367, 1997.
166. Shorr RI, Ray WA, Daugherty JR, et al: Antihypertensives and the risk of serious hypoglycemia in older persons using insulin or sulfonylureas. *JAMA* 278:40–43, 1997.
167. Billington D, Osmundsen H, Sherratt HS: The biochemical basis of Jamaican akee poisoning. *N Engl J Med* 296:1482, 1976.
168. Arky RA: Hypoglycemia, in DeGroot LJ, Cahill GF Jr, Martini L, et al, (eds): *Endocrinology*. New York, Grune and Stratton, 1979, pp 1099–1123.
169. Marks V: Hepatogenous and nephrogenic hypoglycemia, in Marks V, Rose FC, (eds): *Hypoglycemia*. 2nd ed. Oxford, Blackwell Scientific, 1981, pp 216–226.
170. Nakatani Y, Monden T, Sato M, et al: Severe hypoglycemia accompanied with thyroid crisis. *Case Rep Endocrinol* 2012:168565, 2012.
171. Strapazzon G, Nardin M, Zanon P, et al: Respiratory failure and spontaneous hypoglycemia during noninvasive rewarming from 24.7 degrees C (76.5 degrees F) core body temperature after prolonged avalanche burial. *Ann Emerg Med* 60(2):193–196, 2012.
172. Muhlhauser I, Toth G, Sawicki PT, et al: Severe hypoglycemia in type I diabetic patients with impaired kidney function. *Diabetes Care* 14:344–346, 1991.
173. Garber AJ, Bier DM, Cryer PE, et al: Hypoglycemia in compensated chronic renal insufficiency. Substrate limitation of gluconeogenesis. *Diabetes* 23:982–986, 1974.
174. Comty CM, Leonard A, Shapiro FL: Nutritional and metabolic problems in the dialyzed patient with diabetes mellitus. *Kidney Int Suppl* 1974;1:51–57.
175. Tzamaloukas AH, Murata GH, Eisenberg B, et al: Hypoglycemia in diabetics on dialysis with poor glycemic control: hemodialysis versus continuous ambulatory peritoneal dialysis. *Int J Artif Organs* 15:390–392, 1992.
176. Greenblatt DJ: Insulin sensitivity in renal failure. Fatal hypoglycemia following dialysis. *N Y State J Med* 74:1040,1041, 1974.
177. Rutsky EA, McDaniel HG, Tharpe DL, et al: Spontaneous hypoglycemia in chronic renal failure. *Arch Intern Med* 138:1364–1368, 1978.
178. Avram MM, Wolf RE, Gan A, et al: Uremic hypoglycemia. A preventable life-threatening complication. *N Y State J Med* 84:593–596, 1984.
179. Bansal VK, Brooks MH, York JC, et al: Intractable hypoglycemia in a patient with renal failure. *Arch Intern Med* 139:101, 102, 1979.
180. Pun KK: Hypoglycaemia and insulin resistance in uraemia associated with insulin fragments. *Med Hypotheses* 17:243–248, 1985.
181. Toth EL, Lee DW: 'Spontaneous'/uremic hypoglycemia is not a distinct entity: substantiation from a literature review. *Nephron* 58:325–329, 1991.
182. Pagliara AS, Kari IE, De Vivo DC, et al: Hypoalaninemia: a concomitant of ketotic hypoglycemia. *J Clin Invest* 51(6):1440–1449, 1972.
183. Miller SI, Wallace RJ Jr, Musher DM, et al: Hypoglycemia as a manifestation of sepsis. *Am J Med* 68:649–654, 1980.
184. Nouel O, Bernuau J, Rueff B, et al: Hypoglycemia. A common complication of septicemia in cirrhosis. *Arch Intern Med* 141:1477, 1478, 1981.
185. Scheetz A: Hypoglycemia and sepsis in two elderly diabetics. *J Am Geriatr Soc* 38:492, 1990.
186. Romijn JA, Godfried MH, Wortel C, et al: Hypoglycemia, hormones and cytokines in fatal meningococcal septicemia. *J Endocrinol Invest* 13:743–747, 1990.
187. Maayan-Metzger A, Lubin D, Kuint J: Hypoglycemia rates in the first days of life among term infants born to diabetic mothers. *Neonatology* 96(2):80–85, 2009.
188. Mochel F, Slama A, Touati G, et al: Respiratory chain defects may present only with hypoglycemia. *J Clin Endocrinol Metab* 90(6):3780–3785, 2005.
189. Kluge S, Kühnelt P, Block A, et al: A young woman with persistent hypoglycemia, rhabdomyolysis, and coma: recognizing fatty acid oxidation defects in adults. *Crit Care Med* 31(4):1273–1276, 2003.
190. Stanley CA: Perspective on the genetics and diagnosis of congenital hyperinsulinism disorders. *J Clin Endocrinol Metab* 101(3):815–826, 2016.
191. Otonkoski T, Kaminen N, Ustinov J, et al: Physical exercise-induced hyperinsulinemic hypoglycemia is an autosomal-dominant trait characterized by abnormal pyruvate-induced insulin release. *Diabetes* 52(1):199–204, 2003.
192. Otonkoski T, Jiao H, Kaminen-Ahola N, et al: Physical exercise-induced hypoglycemia caused by failed silencing of monocarboxylate transporter 1 in pancreatic beta cells. *Am J Hum Genet* 81(3):467–474, 2007.
193. Kimberly MM, Vesper HW, Caudill SP, et al: Variability among five over-the-counter blood glucose monitors. *Clin Chim Acta* 364(1–2):292–297, 2006.
194. Kulkarni A, Saxena M, Price G, et al: Analysis of blood glucose measurements using capillary and arterial blood samples in intensive care patients. *Intensive Care Med* 31(1):142–145, 2005.
195. Desachy A, Vuagnat AC, Ghazali AD, et al: Accuracy of bedside glucometry in critically ill patients: influence of clinical characteristics and perfusion index. *Mayo Clin Proc* 83(4):400–405, 2008.
196. Atkin SH, Dasmahapatra A, Jaker MA, et al: Fingerstick glucose determination in shock. *Ann Intern Med* 114(12):1020–1024, 1991.
197. Thomas SH, Gough JE, Benson N, et al: Accuracy of fingerstick glucose determination in patients receiving CPR. *South Med J* 87(11):1072–1075, 1994.

198. Kirrane BM, Duthie EA, Nelson LS: Unrecognized hypoglycemia due to maltodextrin interference with bedside glucometry. *J Med Toxicol* 5(1):20–23, 2009.
199. Eastham JH, Mason D, Barnes DL, et al: Prevalence of interfering substances with point-of-care glucose testing in a community hospital. *Am J Health Syst Pharm* 66(2):167–170, 2009.
200. Karon BS, Blanshan CT, Deobald GR, et al: Retrospective evaluation of the accuracy of Roche AccuChek Inform and Nova StatStrip glucose meters when used on critically ill patients. *Diabetes Technol Ther* 16(12):828–832, 2014.
201. Sood V, Costello BA, Burge MR: How low can you go? Chronic hypoglycemia versus normal glucose homeostasis. *J Invest Med* 49:205–209, 2001.
202. Astles JR, Petros WP, Peters WP, et al: Artifactual hypoglycemia associated with hematopoietic cytokines. *Arch Pathol Lab Med* 119:713–716, 1995.
203. Gambino R: Glucose: a simple molecule that is not simple to quantify. *Clin Chem* 53(12):2040, 2041, 2007.
204. Hoffman JR, Schriger DL, Votey SR, et al: The empiric use of hypertonic dextrose in patients with altered mental status: a reappraisal. *Ann Emerg Med* 21(1):20–24, 1992.
205. Plum F, Posner JB: *The Diagnosis of Stupor and Coma*. 3rd ed. Philadelphia, F.A. Davis, Co, 1982.
206. Candelise L, Landi G, Orazio EN, et al: Prognostic significance of hyperglycemia in acute stroke. *Arch Neurol* 42(7):661–663, 1985.
207. Pulsinelli WA, Levy DE, Sigsbee B, et al: Increased damage after ischemic stroke in patients with hyperglycemia with or without established diabetes mellitus. *Am J Med* 74(4):540–544, 1983.
208. Browning RG, Olson DW, Stueven HA, et al: 50% dextrose: antidote or toxin? *Ann Emerg Med* 19(6):683–687, 1990.
209. MacLeod DB, Montoya DR, Fick GH, et al: The effect of 25 grams i.v. glucose on serum inorganic phosphate levels. *Ann Emerg Med* 23(3):524–528, 1994.
210. Balentine JR, Gaeta TJ, Kessler D, et al: Effect of 50 milliliters of 50% dextrose in water administration on the blood sugar of euglycemic volunteers. *Acad Emerg Med* 5(7):691–694, 1998.
211. Luber SD, Brady WJ, Brand A, et al: Acute hypoglycemia masquerading as head trauma: a report of four cases. *Am J Emerg Med* 14(6):543–547, 1996.
212. Moore C, Woollard M: Dextrose 10% or 50% in the treatment of hypoglycaemia out of hospital? A randomised controlled trial. *Emerg Med J* 22(7):512–515, 2005.
213. Losek JD: Hypoglycemia and the ABC'S (sugar) of pediatric resuscitation. *Ann Emerg Med* 35(1):43–46, 2000.
214. Neuvonen PJ, Karkkainen S: Effects of charcoal, sodium bicarbonate, and ammonium chloride on chlorpropamide kinetics. *Clin Pharmacol Ther* 33(3):386–393, 1983.
215. Kannisto H, Neuvonen PJ: Adsorption of sulfonylureas onto activated charcoal in vitro. *J Pharm Sci* 73(2):253–256, 1984.
216. Ludwig SM, McKenzie J, Faiman C: Chlorpropamide overdose in renal failure: management with charcoal hemoperfusion. *Am J Kidney Dis* 10(6):457–460, 1987.
217. Ciechanowski K, Borowiak KS, Potocka BA, et al: Chlorpropamide toxicity with survival despite 27-day hypoglycemia. *J Toxicol Clin Toxicol* 37(7):869–871, 1999.
218. Sills MN, Ogu CC, Maxa J: Prolonged hypoglycemic crisis associated with glyburide. *Pharmacotherapy* 17(6):1338–1340, 1997.
219. Palatnick W, Meatherall RC, Tenenbein M: Clinical spectrum of sulfonylurea overdose and experience with diazoxide therapy. *Arch Intern Med* 151(9):1859–1862, 1991.
220. Viola KV, Sosa JA: Current advances in the diagnosis and treatment of pancreatic endocrine tumors. *Curr Opin Oncol* 17(1):24–27, 2005.
221. Boyle PJ, Justice K, Krentz AJ, et al: Octreotide reverses hyperinsulinemia and prevents hypoglycemia induced by sulfonylurea overdoses. *J Clin Endocrinol Metab* 76:752–756, 1993.
222. Green RS, Palatnick W: Effectiveness of octreotide in a case of refractory sulfonylurea-induced hypoglycemia. *J Emerg Med* 25(3):283–287, 2003.
223. Crawford BA, Perera C: Octreotide treatment for sulfonylurea-induced hypoglycaemia. *Med J Aust* 180(10):540, 541, 2004.
224. McLaughlin SA, Crandall CS, McKinney PE: Octreotide: an antidote for sulfonylurea-induced hypoglycemia. *Ann Emerg Med* 36(2):133–138, 2000.
225. Gonzalez RR, Zweig S, Rao J, et al: Octreotide therapy for recurrent refractory hypoglycemia due to sulfonylurea in diabetes-related kidney failure. *Endocr Pract* 13(4):417–423, 2007.
226. Sherk DK, Bryant SM: Octreotide therapy for nateglinide-induced hypoglycemia. *Ann Emerg Med* 50(6):745–746, 2007.
227. Vallurupalli S: Safety of subcutaneous octreotide in patients with sulfonylurea-induced hypoglycemia and congestive heart failure. *Ann Pharmacother* 44(2):387–390, 2010.
228. Yamaguchi S, Ikejima M, Furukawa A, et al: Octreotide for hypoglycemia caused by sulfonylurea and DPP-4 inhibitor. *Diabetes Res Clin Pract* 109(2):e8–e10, 2015.
229. Groth CM, Banzon ER: Octreotide for the treatment of hypoglycemia after insulin glargine overdose. *J Emerg Med* 45(2):194–198, 2013.
230. Fountoulakis S, Malliopoulos D, Papanastasiou L, et al: Reversal of impaired counterregulatory cortisol response following diazoxide treatment in a patient with non insulinoma pancreatogenous hypoglycemia syndrome: case report and overview of pathogenetic mechanisms. *Hormones (Athens)* 14(2):305–311, 2015.
231. Flanagan SE, Kapoor RR, Mali G, et al: Diazoxide-responsive hyperinsulinemic hypoglycemia caused by HNF4A gene mutations. *Eur J Endocrinol* 162(5):987–992, 2010.
232. Thoma ME, Glauser J, Genuth S: Persistent hypoglycemia and hyperinsulinemia: caution in using glucagon. *Am J Emerg Med* 14(1):99–101, 1996.
233. Hashimoto T, Adachi K, Ishimura N, et al: Safety and efficacy of glucagon as a premedication for upper gastrointestinal endoscopy--a comparative study with butyl scopolamine bromide. *Aliment Pharmacol Ther* 16(1):111–118, 2002.
234. Bourcier ME, Sherrod A, DiGuardo M, et al: Successful control of intractable hypoglycemia using rapamycin in an 86-year-old man with a pancreatic insulin-secreting islet cell tumor and metastases. *J Clin Endocrinol Metab* 94(9):3157–3162, 2009.
235. Meder U, Bokodi G, Balogh L, et al: Severe Hyperinsulinemic hypoglycemia in a neonate: response to sirolimus therapy. *Pediatrics* 136(5):e1369–e1372, 2015.
236. Varghese P, Gleason V, Sorokin R, et al: Hypoglycemia in hospitalized patients treated with antihyperglycemic agents. *J Hosp Med* 2(4):234–240, 2007.
237. Maynard G, Lee J, Phillips G, et al: Improved inpatient use of basal insulin, reduced hypoglycemia, and improved glycemic control: effect of structured subcutaneous insulin orders and an insulin management algorithm. *J Hosp Med* 4(1):3–15, 2009.
238. Kaukonen KM, Rantala M, Pettila V, et al: Severe hypoglycemia during intensive insulin therapy. *Acta Anaesthesiol Scand* 53(1):61–65, 2009.
239. Lin YY, Hsu CW, Sheu WH, et al: Risk factors for recurrent hypoglycemia in hospitalized diabetic patients admitted for severe hypoglycemia. *Yonsei Med J* 51(3):367–374, 2010.
240. Rodbard D: Continuous glucose monitoring: a review of successes, challenges, and opportunities. *Diabetes Technol Ther* 18[Suppl 2]:S23-S213, 2016.
241. Harris DL, Battin MR, Weston PJ, et al: Continuous glucose monitoring in newborn babies at risk of hypoglycemia. *J Pediatr* 157(2):198–202, 2010.
242. Holzinger U, Warszawska J, Kitzberger R, et al: Real-time continuous glucose monitoring in critically ill patients: a prospective randomized trial. *Diabetes Care* 33(3):467–472, 2010.
243. Holzinger U, Warszawska J, Kitzberger R, et al: Impact of shock requiring norepinephrine on the accuracy and reliability of subcutaneous continuous glucose monitoring. *Intensive Care Med* 35(8):1383–1389, 2009.
244. Boom DT, Sechterberger MK, Rijkenberg S, et al: Insulin treatment guided by subcutaneous continuous glucose monitoring compared to frequent point-of-care measurement in critically ill patients: a randomized controlled trial. *Crit Care* 18(4):453, 2014.
245. Gottschalk A, Welp HA, Leser L, et al: Continuous glucose monitoring in patients undergoing extracorporeal ventricular assist therapy. *PLoS One* 11(3):e0148778, 2016.
246. El-Khatib FH, Russell SJ, Nathan DM, et al: A bihormonal closed-loop artificial pancreas for type 1 diabetes. *Sci Transl Med* 2(27):27ra27, 2010.
247. Ozdemir D, Yilmaz E, Duman M, et al: Hypoglycemia after albuterol overdose in a pediatric patient. *Pediatr Emerg Care* 20(7):464, 465, 2004.
248. Khamaisi M, Leitersdorf E: Severe hypoglycemia from clarithromycin-repaglinide drug interaction. *Pharmacotherapy* 28(5):682–684, 2008.
249. Goksu E, Eken C, Karadeniz O, et al: First report of hypoglycemia secondary to dandelion (Taraxacum officinale) ingestion. *Am J Emerg Med* 28(1):111, 112, 2010.
250. Bernard PA, Makin CE, Werner HA: Hypoglycemia associated with dexmedetomidine overdose in a child? *J Clin Anesth* 21(1):50–53, 2009.
251. Montgomery H, Myerson S: 3,4-methylenedioxymethamphetamine (MDMA, or "ecstasy") and associated hypoglycemia. *Am J Emerg Med* 15(2):218, 1997.
252. Wambier CG, Foss-Freitas MC, Paschoal RS, et al: Severe hypoglycemia after initiation of anti-tumor necrosis factor therapy with etanercept in a patient with generalized pustular psoriasis and type 2 diabetes mellitus. *J Am Acad Dermatol* 60(5):883–885, 2009.
253. Cheung D, Bryer-Ash M: Persistent hypoglycemia in a patient with diabetes taking etanercept for the treatment of psoriasis. *J Am Acad Dermatol* 60(6):1032–1036, 2009.
254. Banerjee A, Rhoden WE: Etomidate-induced hypoglycaemia. *Postgrad Med J* 72(850):510, 2009.
255. Walter RB, Hoofnagle AN, Lanum SA, et al: Acute, life-threatening hypoglycemia associated with haloperidol in a hematopoietic stem cell transplant recipient. *Bone Marrow Transplant* 37(1):109–110, 2006.
256. Haap M, Gallwitz B, Thamer C, et al: Symptomatic hypoglycemia during imatinib mesylate in a non-diabetic female patient with gastrointestinal stromal tumor. *J Endocrinol Invest* 30(8):688–692, 2007.
257. Fountas A, Tigas S, Giotaki Z, et al: Severe resistant hypoglycemia in a patient with a pancreatic neuroendocrine tumor on sunitinib treatment. *Hormones (Athens)* 14(3):438–441, 2015.
258. U.S.Food and Drug Administration: Important safety information on interference with blood glucose measurement following use of parenteral maltose/parenteral galactose/oral xylose-containing products, 2005. https://wayback.archive-it.org/7993/20170112171028/http://www.fda.gov/Safety/MedWatch/SafetyInformation/SafetyAlertsforHumanMedicalProducts/ucm153046.htm
259. Dean-Franklin B, Vincent C, Schachter M, et al: The incidence of prescribing errors in hospital inpatients: an overview of the research methods. *Drug Saf* 28(10):891–900, 2005.

Chapter 139 ■ Hypoadrenal Crisis and the Stress Management of the Patient on Chronic Steroid Therapy

HEATHER ELIAS • NEIL ARONIN

The adrenal glands secrete five types of hormones, but two are critical in the intensive care unit (ICU) setting. Mineralocorticoids (primarily aldosterone) regulate electrolyte balance. Glucocorticoids (primarily cortisol) promote gluconeogenesis and have many other actions. Aldosterone and cortisol are life sustaining; deficiency of either can result in hypoadrenal crisis. The other three adrenal hormones (dehydroepiandrosterone and its sulfate, estrone, and catecholamines) do not play a major role in the acute care settings.

Hypoadrenal crisis can occur as an acute event in individuals lacking a prior history of adrenal disorders. A high index of suspicion arises for patients who have inadequate responses to initial therapies. Patients treated with glucocorticoids have a heightened risk for inadequate cortisol response to stress. Diagnosis of cortisol deficiency can be elusive; conditions that contribute to ICU admission (e.g., sepsis and acute respiratory failure) might interfere with traditional tests of adrenal function.

The uncertainty of biochemical diagnosis of adrenal hypofunction invokes the use of clinical judgment for starting therapy. Recent studies indicate that varied diseases among ICU patients do not allow a unified algorithm for treatment. Because excess glucocorticoids are beset with side effects and exacerbation of illness, it is prudent to use them only when clinically necessary.

ETIOLOGY

The most common cause of primary adrenal failure is Addison's disease, an autoimmune disease that is frequently known before ICU admission. Addison's disease often coexists with other autoimmune endocrinopathies, such as Hashimoto thyroiditis. Other causes of adrenal insufficiency present a difficult diagnosis in the ICU: overwhelming sepsis, hemorrhage secondary to trauma, circulating anticoagulants or anticoagulant therapy, tuberculosis, fungal diseases, amyloidosis, acquired immune deficiency syndrome, antiphospholipid syndrome, adrenal infarction, irradiation, metastatic disease, and drugs [1–3]. Therefore, critical illness can cause or unmask adrenal insufficiency. Waterhouse-Frideichson syndrome is one of adrenal hemorrhage and is associated with meningococcemia. Petechiae have been reported in 50% of patients. There have been other infectious etiologies that have been associated with adrenal hemorrhage and sepsis as well.

The most common cause of secondary adrenal insufficiency is suppression of corticotrophin (adrenocorticotrophic hormone [ACTH]) release by prior glucocorticoid therapy. ACTH regulates the maintenance of cells in the zona fasciculata and the synthesis and release of cortisol from these cells. Glucocorticoid therapy suppresses ACTH, thereby causing involution of the cortisol-producing cells. The anterior pituitary regains its ability to respond to stress before normal adrenal function is restored. There are no cut-offs on duration of glucocorticoid therapy, its route of administration, and its dosage that can cause adrenal cortical atrophy (zona fasciculata) and inadequate cortisol reserve. Adrenal suppression may even occur in patients without obvious clinical signs of Cushing syndrome. Symptoms of withdrawal mimic those of Addison disease, such as weakness, lethargy, abdominal discomfort, arthralgias, myalgias, and weight loss. After short-term glucocorticoid treatment, symptoms may arise despite an intact hypothalamic–pituitary–adrenal axis by standard tests of adrenal reserve. These findings underscore the widespread and differential action of glucocorticoids among individual patients.

Pituitary dysfunction can also result in cortisol but not aldosterone insufficiency. Noteworthy causes of impaired pituitary function are tumors in the region of the sella turcica and irradiation of the pituitary or hypothalamus. Pituitary apoplexy is a rare cause of adrenal crisis. Patients usually have sudden symptoms due to cortisol deficiency such as shock. Patients with infarction of a large tumor usually have a severe headache and may have acute visual loss or decrease in visual fields.

Actions of Aldosterone and Cortisol

The adrenal cortex secretes aldosterone from the zona glomerulosa and cortisol from the zona fasciculata. Aldosterone promotes the reabsorption of sodium and the secretion of potassium and hydrogen in the renal tubule [4]. This mineralocorticoid is controlled mainly by the renin–angiotensin system; regulation of blood pressure is coordinated in the short term (angiotensin action on a membrane-bound receptor) and in the longer term (aldosterone, nuclear action on gene expression). Glucocorticoid suppression of ACTH, or primary ACTH loss, does not suppress aldosterone in the zona glomerulosa. Glucocorticoids promote gluconeogenesis and protein wasting and increase the secretion of free water by the kidney [5]. In large doses, cortisol binds to aldosterone receptors in the kidney, thereby increasing sodium reabsorption and potassium and hydrogen ion excretion. Glucocorticoids act on numerous tissues, including the central nervous system, and affect the sense of well-being, appetite, and mood. They inhibit ACTH release through hypothalamic and pituitary actions. Glucocorticoids have direct effects on the cardiovascular system and maintain blood pressure, although mechanisms are not established.

Excess glucocorticoid therapy causes lymphopenia, leukocytosis, and eosinopenia [6]. It can lead to osteoporosis and reduction of hypercalcemia [7] and can impair host defenses to infectious diseases. These possible adverse effects should be considered in the decision to treat ICU patients with glucocorticoids.

Aldosterone deficiency results in sodium wasting, with concomitant loss of water and an increase in renal reabsorption of potassium. A decrease in plasma volume and dehydration occurs, with subsequent increases in blood urea nitrogen and plasma renin activity.

Reduction of circulating cortisol levels causes a marked increase in circulating levels of ACTH and a corresponding increase in β-lipotropin, from which melanocyte-stimulating hormone activity increases. In longstanding primary adrenal insufficiency, the skin (especially creases and scars) develops hyperpigmentation [8]. Orthostatic hypotension can progress to frank shock in a crisis. Hypoglycemia and an increase in sensitivity to insulin are commonplace. Hyponatremia is a hallmark of aldosterone deficiency, but may also be found in cortisol deficiency. The mechanism for the latter may invoke increased sensitivity to vasopressin [9]; serum potassium levels would be normal.

DIAGNOSIS

Clinical manifestations that suggest adrenal insufficiency include a nonspecific history of progressive weakness, lassitude, fatigue, anorexia, vomiting, and constipation. A patient in adrenal crisis is volume depleted and hypotensive or in frank shock [10,11]. He or she often has a fever or is in a stupor or coma. In a precipitous event (adrenal hemorrhage, overwhelming infection, anticoagulant therapy, trauma, and surgery), adrenal crisis lacks hyperpigmentation. In one study, flank pain was observed in 86% of patients who had adrenal hemorrhage or infection as the cause of their adrenal insufficiency. Nausea was also reported in the same case report of 20 patients to be present in 47% of patients.

Severely ill patients are often suspected of developing absolute adrenal hypofunction, but actual incidence is about 3%. To further complicate recognition of adrenal dysfunction, glucocorticoid resistance has been postulated in critical illness.

Among critically ill patients, the diagnosis of adrenal hypofunction is less apparent than it is for ambulatory outpatients. Severe illness can interfere with the adrenal response to ACTH, making difficult interpretation of cortisol reserve and adrenal function. Lack of ACTH shares symptoms of primary glucocorticoid deficiency, in particular hypoglycemia. ACTH deficiency due to pituitary disease generally occurs after deficiency of other pituitary hormones; deficits of overall pituitary secretion can lead to signs of other endocrine gland dysfunctions. These patients do not have hyperpigmentation as their ACTH is not elevated as in primary adrenal insufficiency.

In primary adrenal insufficiency, plasma concentrations of cortisol are usually low or in the low normal range. Response to ACTH stimulation is inadequate and is the definitive test for a diagnosis of adrenal hypofunction. After administering 250 μg of cosyntropin (Cortrosyn; synthetic ACTH 1–24) intravenously to the patient, an adequate adrenal response shows a 10 μg increase of cortisol over baseline at 30 or 60 minutes, or a stimulated cortisol level of 18-20 μg per dL.

The altered adrenal response to ACTH of critically ill patients limits interpretation of standard stimulation tests. Recognition of the complexity of adrenal hypofunction has led to reconsideration of its diagnosis in the ICU. Serum-free cortisol measurement is shown to be more accurate than total serum cortisol in determining cortisol adequacy [12]. ICU patients often have hypoproteinemia. Most circulating cortisol is bound to protein. Changes in protein abundance or dynamics therefore affect interpretation of total cortisol measurements. A serum-free cortisol of <9 μg per dL is sufficient to initiate glucocorticoid replacement [13]. However, measurement of free cortisol is unavailable in most hospitals. A random total cortisol of <10 μg per dL is useful as a threshold for glucocorticoid therapy. It is a practical guideline, but not supported by extensive clinical study. The American College of Critical Care considers this recommendation to be weak with moderate quality of evidence [11]. The concept of situational adrenal insufficiency is an idea inchoate, but a threshold concentration of total cortisol provides a mark for intervention. The term *critical illness-related corticosteroid insufficiency* is preferred for assessing adrenal function among the severely ill, because of the uncertainties of diagnosis.

Other diagnostic clues are useful in the diagnosis of adrenal crisis in ICU patients. Computed tomography scan can reveal adrenal hemorrhage or infiltration. Electrolytes vary, but hyponatremia is found in primary adrenal failure with hyperkalemia (sometimes not to a major degree) and in secondary adrenal failure without hyperkalemia. Hypoglycemia, elevated blood urea nitrogen, hypercalcemia, eosinophilia, lymphocytosis, and a normocytic, normochromic anemia are frequently present.

TREATMENT

The management of the hypoadrenalism has been vetted by a committee of international experts and the American College of Critical Care Medicine [11]. Recommendations have been provided as guidelines for the usefulness of glucocorticoid therapy in hypoadrenal function and critical illness (Table 139.1). There is agreement that hypoadrenalism needs to be treated as soon as it is raised as a possible problem. Diagnostic tests for ACTH and cortisol should be tested before administering glucocorticoids if possible to aid in the diagnosis.

For critical illness in which primary adrenal function is suspected (e.g., evidence of hemorrhage), a bolus of 100 mg of hydrocortisone should be administered intravenously and then 100 mg over the next 24 hours. The patient ought to receive isotonic saline to maintain volume. After the initial therapy and stabilization of the patient, hydrocortisone can be decreased by 50% each day. Maintenance is 20 to 30 mg per day. Fludrocortisone 0.1 mg per day is started at the time of the maintenance glucocorticoid dose. In the corticosteriods and intensive therapy for septic shock trial, patients in shock were randomly assigned to high-dose hydrocortisone or high-dose hydrocortisone plus fludrocortisone. There was no difference in clinical outcomes. This trial supports the theory that hydrocortisone alone has sufficient mineralocorticoid effect.

Dexamethasone can be used in place of hydrocortisone therapy if adrenal reserve of cortisol needs to be studied. Dexamethasone does not interfere with cortisol testing. Isotonic saline infusion is necessary with glucocorticoid administration and will maintain circulating volume. Fludrocortisone (because its main activity is regulation of gene transcription) does not act quickly. Fludrocortisone would need to be given with dexamethasone because dexamethasone does not have mineralocorticoid properties.

TABLE 139.1

Summary of Advances in Managing Hypoadrenal Crisis

- Primary adrenal hypofunction in crisis (glucocorticoid and aldosterone insufficiency) presents with hypotension, fever, volume depletion, and often stupor and coma [9,21].
- The most common cause of secondary adrenal failure is glucocorticoid suppression, which can occur in as few as 5 d after prednisone treatment and last up to 1 y after chronic glucocorticoid withdrawal [22–24].
- Because cortisol is bound to corticosteroid-binding globulin and albumin, which is often reduced in critical care patients, interpretation of the cosyntropin stimulation test should consider the serum albumin concentration [12].
- Supplementation with glucocorticoid and mineralocorticoid improves survival in a subset of critically ill patients (renal failure, hypotension with poor response to pressor agents, lactic acidosis) who have documented inadequate cortisol response to cosyntropin [25].
- In patients with functional adrenals, use of glucocorticoids has not been established with high-quality data. Use of glucocorticoids early in severe shock might be useful [11,14].

Based on data from three small trials and the French trial, patients in septic shock who received hydrocortisone had a 10% absolute reduction in mortality compared with patients who had not received hydrocortisone. However, in the trials Corticus and Hypress, there was not a significant decrease in mortality in those patients who received hydrocortisone over those who did not. A meta-analysis of all the trials concludes that there is improvement in early shock reversal with glucocorticoids. This is a weak recommendation based on weak or moderate quality evidence. Intravenous hydrocortisone (50 mg q6h) has been advocated for patients with septic shock [14]. Of note, those patients with secondary adrenal insufficiency should have evaluation and replacement of other pituitary hormone deficiencies. Replacement of thyroid hormone without replacement of glucocorticoids can bring about acute adrenal crisis.

GLUCOCORTICOID USE FOR STRESSED PATIENTS ON GLUCOCORTICOID TREATMENT

General Principles

For healthy subjects, the secretion rate of cortisol increases from 10 mg per day to 50 to 150 mg per day during surgical procedures, but rarely exceeds 200 mg per day [18]. The degree of response depends, in part, on the extent and duration of surgery.

Historically, the withdrawal of chronic glucocorticoid therapy (and adrenal suppression) has been linked to the development of shock. Although in theory glucocorticoid withdrawal could lead to hypotension, documentation is sparse. Shock among acutely ill or surgical patients on steroid therapy (or within 1 year of withdrawal) should not be attributed solely to decreased adrenal responsiveness. Adrenal glucocorticoids should be administered, but other causes of hypotension should be sought. Suppression of the hypothalamic–pituitary–adrenal axis can occur after only 5 days of glucocorticoid treatment. After their long-term administration, the hypothalamic–pituitary–adrenal axis may respond inadequately to appropriate stimulation up to 1 year after glucocorticoid withdrawal. Adrenal suppression cannot be predicted based on glucocorticoid dosage and duration, or the measurement of a normal serum cortisol [19].

Diagnosis and Treatment

The patients with high risk for adrenal suppression are those who have taken pharmacologic or replacement doses of glucocorticoids for at least 4 weeks or stopped this treatment within the prior year. The cosyntropin test provides an assessment of adrenal cortisol reserve and estimates the adequacy of a stress response. A subnormal response predicts the need for supplemental glucocorticoids.

For minor surgical procedures, the patient's usual dose of glucocorticoid is often sufficient, but a single dose of 25 mg hydrocortisone or its equivalent can be given. For moderate surgery, divided IV doses of hydrocortisone 50 to 75 mg are recommended on the day of surgery and the first postoperative day and then returning to the usual dose if the patient is hemodynamically stable. For major surgery, 100 to 150 mg hydrocortisone are recommended given in divided doses for 2 to 3 days and then returning to the usual dose if possible. Excessive glucocorticoid dosing can have untoward effects [20]; more is not necessarily better.

References

1. Rusnak RA: Adrenal and pituitary emergencies. *Emerg Med Clin North Am* 7:903–925, 1989.
2. Vella A, Nippoldt TB, Morris JC III: Adrenal hemorrhage: a 25-year experience at the Mayo Clinic. *Mayo Clin Proc* 76:161–168, 2001.
3. Xarli VP, Steele AA, Davis PJ, et al: Adrenal hemorrhage in the adult. *Medicine (Baltimore)* 57:211–221, 1978.
4. Loffing J, Zecevic M, Feraille E, et al: Aldosterone induces rapid apical translocation of ENaC in early portion of renal collecting system: possible role of SGK. *Am J Physiol Renal Physiol* 280:F675–F682, 2001.
5. Boykin J, DeTorrente A, Erickson A, et al: Role of plasma vasopressin in impaired water excretion of glucocorticoid deficiency. *J Clin Invest* 62:738–744, 1978.
6. Ilfeld DN, Krakauer RS, Blaese RM: Suppression of the human autologous mixed lymphocyte reaction by physiologic concentrations of hydrocortisone. *J Immunol* 119:428–434, 1977.
7. Lukert BP, Raisz LG: Glucocorticoid-induced osteoporosis: pathogenesis and management. *Ann Intern Med* 112:352–364, 1990.
8. Krieger DT, Liotta AS, Brownstein MJ, et al: ACTH, beta-lipotropin, and related peptides in brain, pituitary, and blood. *Recent Prog Horm Res* 36:277–344, 1980.
9. Oelkers W: Adrenal insufficiency. *N Engl J Med* 335:1206–1212, 1996.
10. Annane D, Bellissant E, Bollaert PE, et al: Corticosteroids in the treatment of severe sepsis and septic shock in adults: a systematic review. *JAMA* 301:2362–2375, 2009.
11. Marik PE, Pastores SM, Annane D, et al: Recommendations for the diagnosis and management of corticosteroid insufficiency in critically ill adult patients: consensus statements from an international task force by the American College of Critical Care Medicine. *Crit Care Med* 36:1937–1949, 2008.
12. Hamrahian AH, Oseni TS, Arafah BM: Measurements of serum free cortisol in critically ill patients. *N Engl J Med* 350:1629–1638, 2004.
13. Siraux V, De Backer D, Yalavatti G, et al: Relative adrenal insufficiency in patients with septic shock: comparison of low-dose and conventional corticotropin tests. *Crit Care Med* 33:2479–2486, 2005.
14. Annane D, Sebille V, Charpentier C, et al: Effect of treatment with low doses of hydrocortisone and fludrocortisone on mortality in patients with septic shock. *JAMA* 288:862–871, 2002.
15. Sprung CL, Annane D, Keh D, et al: Hydrocortisone therapy for patients with septic shock. *N Engl J Med* 358:111–124, 2008.
16. Annane D, Bellissant E, Bollaert PE, et al: Corticosteroids for treating sepsis. *Cochrane Database Syst Rev* 12:CD002243, 2015.
17. Siemieniuk RA, Meade MO, Alonso-Coello P, et al: Corticosteroid therapy for patients hospitalized with community-acquired pneumonia: a systematic review and meta-analysis. *Ann Intern Med* 163:519–528, 2015.
18. Lamberts SW, Bruining HA, de Jong FH: Corticosteroid therapy in severe illness. *N Engl J Med* 337:1285–1292, 1997.
19. Henzen C, Suter A, Lerch E, et al: Suppression and recovery of adrenal response after short-term, high-dose glucocorticoid treatment. *Lancet* 355:542–545, 2000.
20. Udelsman R, Ramp J, Gallucci WT, et al: Adaptation during surgical stress. A reevaluation of the role of glucocorticoids. *J Clin Invest* 77:1377–1381, 1986.
21. Malchoff CD, Carey RM: Adrenal insufficiency. *Curr Ther Endocrinol Metab* 6:142–147, 1997.
22. Streck WF, Lockwood DH: Pituitary adrenal recovery following short-term suppression with corticosteroids. *Am J Med* 66:910–914, 1979.
23. Graber AL, Ney RL, Nicholson WE, et al: Natural history of pituitary-adrenal recovery following long-term suppression with corticosteroids. *J Clin Endocrinol Metab* 25:11–16, 1965.
24. Schlaghecke R, Kornely E, Santen RT, et al: The effect of long-term glucocorticoid therapy on pituitary-adrenal responses to exogenous corticotropin-releasing hormone. *N Engl J Med* 326:226–230, 1992.
25. Loriaux L: Glucocorticoid therapy in the intensive care unit. *N Engl J Med* 350:1601–1602, 2004.

Chapter 140 ■ Disorders of Mineral Metabolism

SETH M. ARUM

Disorders of mineral metabolism, although common, are rarely the primary cause of admission to an intensive care unit (ICU). However, these disorders frequently exacerbate life-threatening injuries and illness. Calcium, magnesium, and phosphorus are the main, clinically relevant minerals that can have an important impact on general health and on the course of a critical illness. Calcium ions regulate membrane potentials, the coagulation cascade, neurotransmitter release, hormone–receptor interactions, and intercellular communication through channels and ion exchange. Magnesium is necessary for parathyroid hormone (PTH) secretion and maintenance of serum calcium, neuromuscular function, and membrane sodium-potassium adenosine triphosphatase (ATPase) activity. Phosphate, the major intracellular anion, is also instrumental for normal cellular function. It is a component of nucleic acids, phospholipids, and high-energy nucleotides, and is necessary for oxidative metabolic pathway function. Phosphorus can also bind calcium in the body, and thus, phosphorus metabolism is related to calcium and magnesium homeostasis. Therefore, symptoms of abnormal phosphorus metabolism often reflect the abnormalities in circulating calcium and magnesium. Calcium, magnesium, and phosphate balance are controlled through the interactions of PTH, 1α,25-dihydroxyvitamin D (1,25 D), calcitonin, and fibroblast growth factor 23 (FGF-23).

CALCIUM DISORDERS

Calcium Physiology

Ninety-eight percent of total body calcium is stored in bone, whereas about 1% is located in extracellular fluids [1]. Approximately half of the calcium in the extracellular fluids is bound to albumin or other anions with the remaining free/ionized calcium being biologically active [2]. Acid–base balance affects the binding of calcium to albumin [3]. Hyperventilation, and the resultant respiratory alkalosis, enhances the binding of calcium to albumin, thereby acutely decreasing the ionized calcium and causing symptoms of hypocalcemia despite unchanged levels of total calcium. Similarly, changes in serum protein levels affect total serum calcium. The measured total calcium level in the serum can be corrected to account for changes in serum proteins by using the following formula:

Corrected total calcium (mg/dL) = Measured total calcium (mg/dL) + (0.8 × [4 − measured albumin (g/dL)]) [4]

Although the formula takes into account changes in serum proteins, it does not consider the impact of alterations in pH that frequently occur during acute illness. Measuring the ionized calcium directly is another option that should not be affected by either the serum proteins or the pH.

Calcium homeostasis is a function of absorption from the intestine (primarily the small intestine by active transport and facilitated diffusion), bone resorption/formation, and urinary excretion. The average diet contains 500 to 1,500 mg of calcium per day. For young individuals, the efficiency of intestinal absorption varies inversely with the amount of calcium ingested. Approximately 300 mg of calcium is exchanged daily between plasma and bone. Serum calcium is in equilibrium with intracellular calcium and calcium in bone and is filtered through the kidney. Urinary calcium excretion (normally 100 to 300 mg of calcium per day) depends on the glomerular filtration rate and the tubular sodium reabsorption. Loop diuretics enhance urinary calcium excretion in conjunction with their effect on sodium excretion.

Hormonal Regulation of Calcium

Calcium absorption, excretion, and bone resorption/formation are in large part regulated by three hormones: PTH, 1,25 D, and calcitonin.

Parathyroid Hormone

PTH is an 84-amino acid polypeptide produced and secreted by the chief cells of the parathyroid gland [5]. Secretion of PTH is suppressed by the calcium-sensing receptor, thereby stimulated by low levels of serum calcium. The rapid release of PTH in response to hypocalcemia is essential for calcium homeostasis. The target organs for PTH are bone and kidneys. Chronic PTH secretion stimulates osteoclasts via the production of receptor activator of nuclear factor kappa ligand (RANKL) from osteoblasts [6]. This results in bone resorption and dissolution of hydroxyapatite crystals resulting in the release of calcium and phosphate. The renal effects of PTH include decreased proximal tubular reabsorption of phosphate (phosphate wasting), enhanced distal tubular calcium reabsorption (calcium retention), and increased renal 1α-hydroxylase activity (enhanced 1,25 D production). It is through the increased production of 1,25 D that PTH indirectly increases intestinal absorption of calcium.

As opposed to the catabolic effects that PTH can have on bone through stimulating RANKL production, anabolic effects occur with intermittent administration of low-dose PTH. Intermittent administration of PTH does not impact RANKL as it does with constant administration, likely explaining the differing effects on bone mass [6]. In fact, daily subcutaneous injections of PTH derivatives have been shown to increase bone mineral density and decrease fracture risk in various populations [7,8].

Magnesium is mandatory for PTH secretion and end-organ response. Studies have shown that hypomagnesemia impairs PTH secretion and the renal response to PTH administration. Much of this is often reversible with magnesium repletion [9]. Clinically, correction of the hypocalcemia can often only be achieved after correcting hypomagnesemia.

Vitamin D

Vitamin D is a steroid hormone that is essential for calcium balance and is also likely important in numerous other cellular functions [10]. Activation of vitamin D requires 25-hydroxylation in the liver and 1-hydroxylation in the kidney to form the active hormone 1,25 D. Negative feedback is exerted by 1,25 D on its own production by suppressing 1α-hydroxylase activity and stimulating the enzyme 24-hydroxylase to produce the biologically inactive steroids $24,25(OH)_2D$ and $1,24,25(OH)_3D$. FGF-23 also suppresses 1,25 D synthesis [11], though this is discussed in more detail as part of its role in phosphorus physiology.

The effects of 1,25 D are exerted through interactions with nuclear receptors located in a variety of cells, including enterocytes, parathyroid chief cells, osteoblasts, and renal tubular cells. 1,25 D increases intestinal absorption of calcium and phosphate. It has also been shown to suppress PTH gene expression as a negative feedback mechanism [11].

Calcitonin

Calcitonin is a 32-amino acid polypeptide produced by the C-cells of the thyroid [12]. It is secreted in response to elevations in serum calcium. It can also be stimulated by certain gastrointestinal (GI) tract hormones (e.g., gastrin). The primary physiologic function of calcitonin in humans remains unclear. Medullary carcinoma of the thyroid is a malignant neoplasm of the C-cells and is characterized by elevated calcitonin levels. However, calcium, phosphate, and PTH levels remain normal. Also, patients can have undetectable levels of calcitonin after a thyroidectomy with no clear detrimental systemic effects.

Despite the lack of clinical consequences from endogenous calcitonin excess or deficiency, exogenous calcitonin is a potent inhibitor of bone resorption. It also acts on the kidneys to enhance excretion of calcium, phosphate, magnesium, and sodium [12]. Both of these mechanisms make calcitonin useful in the treatment of hypercalcemia. The effect of calcitonin on bone resorption is lost over time due to tachyphylaxis [12]. This phenomenon, possibly due to downregulation of calcitonin receptors, is of clinical importance when treating patients with hypercalcemia. The excellent short-term effects of calcitonin to lower serum calcium (within 12 to 48 hours) allows the institution of therapies that require several days to attain maximal effectiveness (e.g., bisphosphonates).

Calcitonin can also be used for the treatment of osteoporosis. The administration of a salmon calcitonin nasal spray has been shown to decrease markers of bone turnover, increase bone mineral density at the spine, and decrease the risk of vertebral fractures in postmenopausal women with osteoporosis [13].

Hypercalcemia

Hypercalcemia is an abnormality of the balance between different body compartments and can result from increased bone resorption, decreased renal excretion, increased GI absorption, or any combination of these mechanisms.

The signs and symptoms of hypercalcemia are protean and can be divided into four groups: (a) mental, (b) neurologic and musculoskeletal, (c) GI and urologic, and (d) cardiovascular. The mental manifestations of hypercalcemia include stupor, obtundation, apathy, lethargy, confusion, disorientation, and coma. In general, for a given level of hypercalcemia, older patients exhibit more of the mental signs than younger patients. The neurologic and musculoskeletal effects of hypercalcemia are reduced muscle tone and strength, myalgias, and decreased deep tendon reflexes. The GI and urologic signs are vomiting, constipation, polyuria, and polydipsia. The major cardiovascular effect of hypercalcemia, which the intensive care physician must address, is shortening of the QT interval. In the presence of ventricular ectopic beats, calcium-induced shortening of the QT interval increases the potential for fatal arrhythmias or asystole.

Differential Diagnosis

Elevated serum calcium measurements have been reported in approximately 1% of the general population [14]. The causes of hypercalcemia can be differentiated into two broad groups defined by whether or not the process is driven by abnormal parathyroid tissue. Hence, the groups are termed: (a) PTH-independent hypercalcemia; and (b) PTH-dependent hypercalcemia. In PTH-independent hypercalcemia, the hypercalcemia is not mediated by abnormal parathyroid tissue, and the PTH level should be appropriately suppressed. In PTH-dependent hypercalcemia, the process is driven by dysregulated parathyroid tissue, and the PTH level should be elevated, or inappropriately normal.

PTH-independent hypercalcemia is more common among hospitalized patients. Hypercalcemia of malignancy is the most common cause of PTH-independent hypercalcemia. The malignancies most often associated with hypercalcemia include lung (35%), breast (25%), hematologic (myeloma and lymphoma [14%]), head and neck (6%), and renal (3%) [15]. The hypercalcemia can be mediated by secretion of parathyroid hormone–related peptide (PTHrP), most commonly seen in squamous cell carcinomas (often lung or head and neck tumors); autonomous activation of 1,25 D (occasionally seen with lymphomas); or by lytic bone lesions/metastases [16]. See Chapter 95 for a complete discussion of the hypercalcemia of malignancy.

Other possible causes of PTH-independent hypercalcemia include granulomatous diseases, immobilization, milk-alkali syndrome, thyrotoxicosis, vitamin D or vitamin A intoxication, or Addison's disease.

Granulomatous diseases such as sarcoidosis, tuberculosis, etc., can cause hypercalcemia due to autonomous 1,25 D production by the granulomas (similar to certain lymphomas). These patients have increased intestinal calcium absorption and sensitivity to vitamin D intake. Hypercalcemia occurs in 10% of patients, though hypercalciuria has been documented in as many as 20% [17].

Immobilization causes hypercalcemia as a result of decreased bone formation and persistent bone resorption. Hypercalcemia in the immobilized individual occurs most commonly among patients with high bone turnover (e.g., adolescents during the growth spurt or individuals with Paget's disease or thyrotoxicosis).

PTH-dependent hypercalcemia is much more common among outpatients, although these patients can be hospitalized due to other issues. PTH-dependent hypercalcemia can be caused by primary or tertiary hyperparathyroidism. Another possible cause is familial hypocalciuric hypercalcemia (FHH). The routine measurement of serum calcium has altered the clinical presentation of hyperparathyroidism with most patients presenting with asymptomatic hypercalcemia.

Primary or tertiary hyperparathyroidism results from autonomous secretion of PTH despite elevated serum calcium levels. The latter occurs typically after chronic secondary hyperparathyroidism in the setting of end-stage renal failure. Hypercalcemia develops due to increased bone resorption, increased intestinal calcium absorption from stimulation of 1,25 D production, and increased renal tubular calcium reabsorption. The patient can be hypophosphatemic due to the phosphaturic effect of PTH. The hormone also induces renal bicarbonate wasting, resulting in a mild hyperchloremic acidosis. In primary hyperparathyroidism, a single adenoma is present in 80% to 85% of cases, whereas four-gland hyperplasia occurs in 10% to 15% of cases [18]. Parathyroid cancer is present among less than 1% of these patients and typically presents with much higher serum calcium levels [19].

Parathyroid hyperplasia or adenomas can also occur as part of the multiple endocrine neoplasia (MEN) syndromes. Type I MEN involves tumors of the pituitary, pancreas, and parathyroids (usually hyperplasia), whereas type II is associated with pheochromocytoma, medullary cancer of the thyroid, and primary hyperparathyroidism (hyperplasia or adenoma) [20].

FHH is an autosomal dominant disorder characterized by hypercalcemia with inappropriately normal or elevated PTH levels. It is usually caused by an inactivating mutation in the calcium-sensing receptor gene [21], thereby requiring higher serum calcium levels to suppress secretion of PTH (i.e., an increased set point of serum calcium). In contrast to primary hyperparathyroidism, patients with FHH have relative hypocalciuria (fractional excretion of calcium <0.01), do not seem to be at increased risk of nephrolithiasis or bone disease, and cannot be cured surgically, unless rendered hypocalcemic by removal of all parathyroid tissue [22].

Several medications can induce hypercalcemia as well. Hypercalcemia associated with the use of thiazide diuretics is often an indicator of underlying primary hyperparathyroidism. Vitamin D and vitamin A intoxication can also cause hypercalcemia. Lithium may also affect parathyroid function and is associated with hypercalcemia and either elevated, or inappropriately normal, PTH levels (PTH-dependent hypercalcemia) [23].

Laboratory Evaluation

Hypercalcemia should always be considered for the patient with altered mental status. A total serum calcium level alone usually makes the diagnosis. However, altered binding of calcium to proteins, as can occur with hypoalbuminemia or with abnormal proteins (e.g., myeloma), or an acid–base imbalance may affect the free calcium level. Ionized calcium levels should not be affected by these issues. Because of the interrelationships of calcium, magnesium, and phosphorus, the latter two minerals should be measured in all cases involving altered calcium metabolism. An electrocardiogram to determine the QT interval is very important to assess the severity and urgency of the patient's hypercalcemia.

The differential diagnosis of the hypercalcemia can be narrowed down with a serum intact PTH measurement. If PTH levels are physiologically suppressed by the hypercalcemia, then PTH-independent sources should be sought, with malignancy being the most common. If malignancy is suspected, obtaining PTHrP and 1,25 D levels can provide useful clues. In the absence of PTH, elevated 1,25 D levels imply autonomous production, most commonly associated with lymphomas and granulomatous diseases [16,17]. A bone scan may identify a metastatic process. Because myeloma is characterized by bone resorption with little bone formation, the bone scan is usually negative, but a skeletal survey may find lytic lesions. The diagnosis would then be confirmed by urine immunoelectrophoresis, serum protein electrophoresis, and bone marrow examination.

The diagnosis of milk-alkali syndrome is made by the patient's history, often revealing large quantities of calcium carbonate ingestion. In this instance, the patient should also be alkalotic with an elevated bicarbonate level. Thyrotoxicosis and Addison's disease can be ruled out with thyroid function tests and a cosyntropin stimulation test, respectively (see Chapter 139 for a discussion about evaluating adrenal function in the critically ill). Vitamin D intoxication is quite rare, but the possibility can be eliminated by measuring 25-hydroxyvitamin D levels. Vitamin A levels can be measured if the diagnosis remains unclear.

If PTH-dependent hypercalcemia is confirmed with elevated or inappropriately normal PTH levels, a 24-hour urine for a fractional excretion of calcium can be done to differentiate primary or tertiary hyperparathyroidism from FHH, though this test may be altered by renal failure or the use of various diuretics.

Management

The aim of treatment of hypercalcemia is to minimize its effects on central nervous system (CNS), renal, and cardiovascular function. Appropriate treatment of hypercalcemia depends, in part, on the cause. General concepts in the management involve attempts to (a) increase renal calcium clearance, (b) decrease bone resorption, and (c) decrease intestinal calcium absorption. To this end, it is critical that the pathophysiology of the disease process be understood. If, for example, the hypercalcemia in a patient with myeloma is due to a combination of increased bone resorption plus decreased renal calcium clearance, successful management of the hypercalcemia requires that both processes be treated. Specific measures directed toward the pathophysiology of the hypercalcemia are discussed.

Hydration and Diuresis. Saline hydration creates a diuresis that increases renal calcium excretion by decreasing calcium reabsorption in the proximal tubule. Hydration plays a critical role in the initial management of hypercalcemia because the onset of the therapeutic response is rapid. The aim of therapy is to achieve a urine output >75 mL per hour. This often requires the administration of 200 to 500 mL per hour of normal saline [16,24]. Because a potential complication of administration of this amount of saline is congestive heart failure, extreme care must be taken in treating the patient with underlying cardiac disease or renal insufficiency. The concomitant administration of a loop diuretic helps prevent volume overload and further increases renal calcium excretion by inhibiting distal tubular calcium reabsorption. Although the clinical benefits of using this routinely are debated [16,25], furosemide 20 to 40 mg administered by the intravenous (IV) route has been used historically once rehydration has been achieved [24], especially if volume overload develops. Measurement of serum electrolytes, phosphorus, and magnesium is mandatory during saline hydration to replace adequately the quantities lost in the urine. If renal or cardiac failure precludes the use of saline hydration, dialysis with a calcium-free dialysate is an effective alternative.

Calcitonin. Calcitonin reduces the resorption of calcium from bone by inhibiting osteoclasts. It also exerts transient effects to increase the renal excretion of calcium, along with sodium, potassium, magnesium, and phosphate. The benefits of calcitonin for the treatment of hypercalcemia include (a) rapid onset within 2 hours, (b) maximal effect within 24 to 48 hours, and (c) low toxicity [12]. It can be used safely in patients with renal failure, and its side effects are limited to transient nausea, facial flushing, and occasional hypersensitivity at the injection site. The dose is 4 to 8 IU per kg body weight subcutaneously or intramuscularly every 12 hours [16]. Usually calcitonin is effective for only 4 to 7 days [12], but it is still used for the rapid response, as bisphosphonates often require several days to attain maximal effectiveness.

Bisphosphonates. Bisphosphonates are synthetic analogues of pyrophosphate that are potent inhibitors of bone resorption through inhibition of osteoclastic activity and survival [16]. Because of the delay of reduction in serum calcium with bisphosphonates, these agents are often used in conjunction with other therapies. Pamidronate can be infused intravenously as 60 or 90 mg over 2 to 6 hours [16]. Zoledronic acid at a dose of 4 mg intravenously over not less than 15 minutes has been shown to be more effective at normalizing serum calcium in patients with hypercalcemia of malignancy [26]. Renal function must be monitored, and the doses of either medication may be repeated after a minimum of 7 days to allow a full response to the initial dose [16]. With long-term use, there is an increased risk of developing osteonecrosis of the jaw [27].

Denosumab. Denosumab is a monoclonal antibody directed against RANKL, preventing the binding of RANKL to osteoclasts, thereby inhibiting their development/activity and decreasing bone resorption. This agent is approved for the treatment of postmenopausal women with osteoporosis and has been shown to reduce the incidence of vertebral, non-vertebral, and hip fractures [28]. It has also been approved for the prevention of skeletal-related events in patients with bone metastases from solid tumors [29]. Recently, a single-arm study of 33 patients with hypercalcemia of malignancy refractory to bisphosphonates showed that 64% of subjects had a complete response to a dose of 120 mg subcutaneously on days 1, 8, 15, 29, and every 4 weeks for a median of 8 weeks [30]. The short-term adverse events were worsening hypercalcemia and dyspnea, but like bisphosphonates, long-term use is associated with an increased risk of developing osteonecrosis of the jaw [27]. This study prompted FDA approval in December 2014 for patients with hypercalcemia of malignancy refractory to bisphosphonates [16].

Cinacalcet. Cinacalcet is an agonist of the calcium-sensing receptor (also called a calcimimetic). In PTH-dependent hypercalcemia, it will suppress PTH secretion and lower serum calcium levels [31]. It has been approved for the chronic treatment of severe hypercalcemia in patients with primary hyperparathyroidism who are unable to undergo parathyroidectomy, but it has no role in the treatment of acute hypercalcemia and so will not be discussed further.

Hypocalcemia

Hypocalcemia is frequently encountered among critically ill patients. Although low serum albumin concentrations may explain some hypocalcemia, up to 18% of hospitalized patients and 85% of patients in ICUs were found to have hypocalcemia [32]. The symptoms of hypocalcemia can range from paresthesias and tetany, to seizures or fatal laryngospasm. A positive Chvostek's sign (muscle spasm in response to tapping the facial nerve) is suggestive, but not diagnostic, of hypocalcemia. Trousseau's sign (carpal spasm precipitated by inflation of a blood pressure cuff above the systolic blood pressure) is more sensitive and specific [32]. In contrast to the QT interval shortening in hypercalcemia, hypocalcemia is attended by an increase in the QT interval on the electrocardiogram, predisposing patients to cardiac arrhythmias. Chronic hypocalcemia is associated with basal ganglia calcification and cataract formation [4].

Differential Diagnosis

Risk factors for the development of hypocalcemia among hospitalized patients include alkalosis, renal failure, and multiple transfusions. Although pancreatitis is associated with hypocalcemia, the mechanism is unclear. Hyperphosphatemia is the suspected cause of hypocalcemia attending tumor lysis and rhabdomyolysis.

Inadequate, or absent, PTH secretion is a cause of hypocalcemia. Hypoparathyroidism is most common after neck surgery for thyroid or parathyroid disease, but it can also rarely be seen with neck irradiation, as a result of iron deposition in hemochromatosis or thalassemia, or in severe magnesium deficiency [4]. Idiopathic hypoparathyroidism can be familial or sporadic. An autoimmune phenomenon may explain the idiopathic variety and may be found together with other autoimmune endocrine dysfunction. Target tissue unresponsiveness due to a defect in the cell membrane G protein is characterized by hypocalcemia and hyperphosphatemia in the presence of elevated PTH levels. This is commonly known as pseudohypoparathyroidism, and can be associated with Albright's hereditary osteodystrophy (short, stocky habitus; round facies; and short metacarpals, metatarsals, or both) [33].

Hypocalcemia can also signify vitamin D deficiency. Although nutritional rickets is rare in the United States, vitamin D deficiency is not [11]. Vitamin D deficiency may be the result of liver or renal failure with impaired hydroxylation of the parent compound, but is most often caused by inadequate sun exposure or malabsorption.

Laboratory Evaluation

A low corrected serum calcium or ionized calcium level confirms the diagnosis. Studies to discern the cause may include creatinine, phosphate, amylase, and magnesium levels; liver function tests; and 25-hydroxyvitamin D and PTH levels. In hypoparathyroidism due to the absence of PTH or target tissue unresponsiveness, serum phosphate levels tend to be high as a result of absence of the phosphaturic effect of PTH.

Management

Treatment of hypocalcemia depends on its severity and chronicity. Symptomatic patients should be treated with IV calcium. A 10-mL vial of 10% calcium gluconate provides 93 mg of elemental calcium. One or two 10-mL vials should be administered in 100 mL 5% dextrose in water over 10 minutes [32]. Calcium to be administered intravenously should always be diluted because concentrated solutions are very irritating to veins. Electrocardiographic monitoring during calcium supplementation is recommended as arrhythmias can occur from overcorrection. Often, the initial bolus needs to be followed by a continuous infusion which can be started with 10 vials of calcium gluconate in 1 L of 5% dextrose in water running at 50 mL per hour. This can then be adjusted to maintain the serum calcium levels in the lower portion of the normal range [32]. Hypocalcemia may mask digitalis toxicity. In these situations, a slower rate of calcium administration is recommended to prevent cardiac arrhythmias.

Oral supplementation should be instituted concurrently to provide 500 to 1,000 mg of elemental calcium three times daily. If calcium supplementation alone cannot maintain serum calcium levels, vitamin D preparations may be administered. Ergocalciferol (vitamin D_2) has a wide safety margin and relatively low cost. The usual dose is 25,000 to 100,000 IU daily. This preparation has a slow onset of action because it must be 25-hydroxylated in the liver and 1α-hydroxylated in the kidney. The preparation has a long half-life because it is stored in fat. Activated vitamin D preparations that act more rapidly are also available. Calcitriol is 1,25 D_3 and can be given as 0.25 to 1.0 μg, once or twice daily. This has a shorter half-life than vitamin D but is more potent. It can be used for long-term management but has a narrower therapeutic window [4].

Up until recently, there was no approved hormone replacement for hypoparathyroidism. In 2013, a phase 3 trial of recombinant human PTH (1-84) showed that 53% of subjects with hypoparathyroidism were able to reduce their calcium and active vitamin D doses by >50% [34]. This prompted FDA approval of this medication in 2015 for patients with hypoparathyroidism who are not well controlled on standard treatment with calcium and active vitamin D [35].

The goal of treating hypocalcemia is to prevent symptoms attributable to low calcium and to avoid hypercalciuria and hypercalcemia. In the hypoparathyroid patient, total serum calcium should be maintained between 8.0 and 8.5 mg per dL. In the absence of PTH, circulating calcium levels greater than 9.0 mg per dL are often attended by hypercalciuria and an increased risk of nephrolithiasis or nephrocalcinosis. If hypercalciuria occurs despite lower serum calcium concentrations, thiazide diuretics can be used to try and enhance tubular reabsorption of calcium [4]. This could be less of an issue if injectable PTH is used in the treatment regimen [35].

MAGNESIUM DISORDERS

Magnesium Physiology

Magnesium is the major intracellular divalent cation. Two-thirds of the total body content of magnesium is found in bone and only 2% is found in the extracellular space. Muscle and liver are the soft tissues that contain the greatest amount of magnesium. Thirty percent of extracellular magnesium circulates bound to protein [5]. Therefore, as with circulating calcium levels, the serum albumin concentration must be known to interpret total magnesium levels. Magnesium absorption occurs throughout the small intestine. Like calcium, magnesium is reabsorbed in the kidney tubules.

Magnesium is necessary for normal sodium- and potassium-activated ATPase, PTH secretion, and neuromuscular function. Decreased sodium- and potassium-activated ATPase due to hypomagnesemia can result in intracellular potassium depletion. Magnesium-induced decreases in PTH secretion result in hypocalcemia that can only be corrected by magnesium replacement.

Hypomagnesemia is often attended by CNS hyperexcitability, whereas hypermagnesemia results in CNS depression. This can be independent of changes in serum calcium concentration [36].

Hypermagnesemia

Hypermagnesemia is often attended by a loss of deep tendon reflexes and CNS depression. Flaccid paralysis, hypotension, confusion, and coma may result from magnesium levels greater than 6 mg per dL [36]. The most common cause of hypermagnesemia in the hospitalized patient is renal failure. The hypermagnesemia may be aggravated by the administration of magnesium-containing antacids. Diabetic ketoacidosis is usually attended by hypermagnesemia, but this typically reflects dehydration, which masks the total body magnesium depletion resulting from the glucose-induced osmotic diuresis.

Management

The actions of magnesium on neuromuscular function are antagonized by calcium. Emergency treatment of the magnesium-induced CNS depression includes IV administration of one to two 10-mL vials of calcium gluconate diluted in 100 mL 5% dextrose in water over 5 to 10 minutes to prevent venous irritation [36]. The dose may be repeated as necessary. Total serum calcium must be monitored and not allowed to exceed 11 mg per dL.

Definitive treatment of the hypermagnesemia requires increasing renal magnesium excretion. In the presence of normal renal function, increased magnesium excretion can be achieved by IV administration of furosemide, 20 to 40 mg IV, every 1 to 2 hours, along with fluid hydration, though there is little literature to support its use [36]. Serum electrolytes, particularly potassium, must be closely monitored. Dialysis is the treatment of choice when kidney function is impaired and the patient is symptomatic from hypermagnesemia.

Hypomagnesemia

Hypomagnesemia is much more common than hypermagnesemia among hospitalized patients [5]. The increased CNS excitability in the patient with hypomagnesemia is partly due to the accompanying hypocalcemia, which results from impaired PTH secretion and decreased peripheral tissue responsiveness to PTH. The intracellular potassium depletion seen with hypomagnesemia can also exacerbate digitalis toxicity.

Hypomagnesemia may result from decreased intestinal absorption (e.g., steatorrhea), or more commonly from increased renal excretion due to an osmotic diuresis (e.g., hyperglycemia), or drugs (e.g., ethanol, aminoglycosides, or cisplatin). Dietary deficiency alone is rarely the explanation for hypomagnesemia. The exceptions are starvation or prolonged parenteral feeding [36].

The drugs that most commonly increase renal magnesium excretion are alcohol and diuretics. Hypomagnesemia in the alcohol abuser may also be partly attributable to dietary deficiency. Hypomagnesemia is encountered in 30% of alcoholics [36].

Management

Magnesium may be administered orally or parenterally. If serum magnesium levels are below 1.2 mg per dL, or if the patient is symptomatic, parenteral treatment is indicated. Because magnesium is predominately intracellular, the serum levels typically underestimate the deficit. Therefore, it is recommended to give 8 to 12 g of magnesium sulfate over the first 24 hours followed by 4 to 6 g per day for 3 to 4 days to replete body stores [36]. Serum magnesium and calcium levels should be monitored. The dose should be reduced by 75% in patients with renal failure.

In the patient with mild magnesium deficiency, oral therapy is usually satisfactory. Magnesium oxide 400 mg (241 mg of elemental magnesium) can be given as one to two tablets daily. Diarrhea is the most common side effect. As with all magnesium supplementation, levels must be monitored closely in the patient with renal insufficiency.

PHOSPHORUS DISORDERS

Phosphorus Physiology

Eighty-five percent of total body phosphorus is found in bone. Extracellular phosphate accounts for only 1% of total body phosphorus [5]. Phosphorus is a component of nucleic acids and phospholipids and is a cofactor for a number of enzymes. Because of shifts in phosphate between intracellular and extracellular compartments, serum phosphate levels often do not accurately reflect total body stores. For example, because acidosis causes a shift in phosphate from within cells to the extracellular compartment, serum phosphate levels may be normal in the acidotic patient despite depletion of total body stores [3]. As the acidosis is corrected, serum phosphate levels may fall.

Phosphorus is also regulated by PTH and 1,25 D, as well as FGF-23. PTH stimulates phosphate excretion by the kidneys, similar to FGF-23 secreted by the osteocytes (classifying it as a "phosphatonin") [5]. In addition, FGF-23 directly suppresses 1α-hydroxylase activity. Therefore, phosphate retention (as in renal failure) leads to an increase in FGF-23, thereby suppressing 1,25 D production and inhibiting phosphorus absorption in the intestine. In the setting of normal renal function, excess FGF-23 (as in X-linked hypophosphatemic rickets or tumor-induced osteomalacia) leads to excess phosphaturia, hypophosphatemia, and mineralization defects in bone [37].

Hyperphosphatemia

Increased phosphate levels are most often encountered among patients with renal failure or hypoparathyroidism. Both of these conditions result in impaired phosphate excretion. Hyperphosphatemia can also be seen from cellular leaks as in hemolysis, rhabdomyolysis, or the tumor lysis syndrome. The hyperphosphatemia, along with diminished renal 1,25 D production from increased FGF-23, results in hypocalcemia. The symptoms are usually attributable to the accompanying hypocalcemia, and not the hyperphosphatemia per se [38]. Therefore, in the symptomatic patient, therapy should be directed at correction of the hypocalcemia.

Chronic management of hyperphosphatemia can be accomplished with limiting phosphate intake as well as using phosphate binders, such as calcium acetate 667 mg, two tablets with meals, sevelamer 800 mg, one to two tablets with meals, or lanthanum carbonate 500 to 1,000 mg with meals [3,38].

Hypophosphatemia

Hypophosphatemia can be seen in up to 3% of hospitalized patients or 34% of patients in the ICU [39]. It can result from impaired intestinal phosphate absorption or increased renal phosphate excretion. The cause of hypophosphatemia in alcoholics is often multifactorial but most likely reflects malnutrition and the accompanying vomiting. When taken in excess, phosphate-binding antacids impair phosphate absorption. The resulting hypophosphatemia can stimulate 1,25 D production and cause hypercalcemia, which has been confused with hyperparathyroidism.

Renal phosphate excretion is increased in hyperparathyroidism, vitamin D deficiency, and with osmotic diuresis. There are also rare genetic and paraneoplastic conditions that cause increased phosphate excretion through excess FGF-23 levels [37]. PTH inhibits renal tubular phosphate reabsorption, resulting in hypophosphatemia when secreted in excess. Serum phosphate levels are reduced in vitamin D deficiency due to impaired intestinal phosphate absorption and increased renal phosphate excretion (the result of secondary hyperparathyroidism in response to the associated hypocalcemia). The patient in diabetic ketoacidosis has a total body phosphorus deficit, despite normal serum phosphorus levels. In the early stages of the illness, the rising serum glucose levels cause an osmotic diuresis with increased renal phosphate loss. However, the developing acidosis causes a shift in phosphorus from the intracellular to the extracellular compartment. This shift, along with the accompanying volume depletion, tends to normalize the serum phosphorus levels. Rehydration and insulin treatment with resolution of the acidosis may cause a rapid fall in serum phosphorus levels.

The potential consequences of severe hypophosphatemia are impaired oxygen delivery to the tissues due to decreased 2,3-diphosphoglycerate levels, muscle weakness, and rhabdomyolysis. The latter is most likely to occur when severe hypophosphatemia occurs after prolonged mild hypophosphatemia (e.g., in the hospitalized alcoholic in whom phosphate falls precipitously during carbohydrate administration).

Management

Severe hypophosphatemia (<1.5 mg per dL) requires parenteral therapy [3]. Potassium phosphate or sodium phosphate can be used depending on the patient's potassium level. 15 mmol may be added to 5% dextrose in water and given intravenously over 2 hours [39]. Further treatment depends on the serum phosphate levels and clinical condition. The dose may be repeated up to three times in the first 24 hours until phosphate levels normalize.

Parenteral therapy should be limited for the patient with renal failure or hypocalcemia. In the patient with renal failure, IV therapy can cause hyperphosphatemia, worsen hypocalcemia, and cause metastatic calcification, primarily in the kidney. The latter can occur if the patient is hypercalcemic or if the phosphate is administered too rapidly. Initial doses should be 50% lower if the patient is in renal failure or hypercalcemic [3].

Oral preparations of potassium phosphate (K-Phos Neutral) can be used for milder hypophosphatemia or for chronic management. The usual oral dose is 1 to 4 g per day in divided doses. The most common side effect is diarrhea.

References

1. Bushinksy DA, Monk RD: Electrolyte quintet: calcium. *Lancet* 352:306–311, 1998.
2. Fong J, Khan A: Hypocalcemia: updates in diagnosis and management for primary care. *Can Fam Physician* 58:158–162, 2012.
3. Kraft MD, Btaiche IF, Sacks GS, et al: Treatment of electrolyte disorders in adult patients in the intensive care unit. *Am J Health Syst Pharm* 62:1663–1682, 2005.
4. Shoback D: Hypoparathyroidism. *N Engl J Med* 359:391–403, 2008.
5. Moe SM: Disorders involving calcium, phosphorus, and magnesium. *Prim Care* 35:215–237, v–vi, 2008.
6. Khosla S: Minireview: The OPG/RANKL/RANK system. *Endocrinology* 142:5050–5055, 2001.
7. Neer RM, Arnaud CD, Zanchetta JR, et al: Effect of parathyroid hormone (1-34) on fractures and bone mineral density in postmenopausal women with osteoporosis. *N Engl J Med* 344:1434–1441, 2001.
8. Saag KG, Shane E, Boonen S, et al: Teriparitide or alendronate in glucocorticoid-induced osteoporosis. *N Engl J Med* 357:2028–2039, 2007.
9. Rude RK, Oldham SB, Singer FR: Functional hypoparathyroidism and parathyroid hormone end-organ resistance in human magnesium deficiency. *Clin Endocrinol (Oxf)* 5:209–224, 1976.
10. Nagpal S, Na S, Rathnachalam R: Noncalcemic actions of vitamin d receptor ligands. *Endocr Rev* 26:662–687, 2005.
11. Holick MF: Vitamin D deficiency. *N Engl J Med* 357:266–281, 2007.
12. Wisneski LA: Salmon calcitonin in the acute management of hypercalcemia. *Calcif Tissue Int* 46:S26–S30, 1990.
13. Chesnut CH III, Silverman S, Andriano K, et al: A randomized trial of nasal spray salmon calcitonin in postmenopausal women with established osteoporosis: the prevent recurrence of osteoporotic fractures study. *Am J Med* 109:267–276, 2000.
14. Palmer M, Jakobsson S, Akerstrom G, et al: Prevalence of hypercalcaemia in a health survey: a 14-year follow-up study of serum calcium values. *Eur J Clin Invest* 18:39–46, 1988.
15. Mundy GR, Martin TJ: The hypercalcemia of malignancy: pathogenesis and management. *Metabolism* 31:1247–1277, 1982.
16. Thosani S, Hu MI: Denosumab: a new agent in the management of hypercalcemia of malignancy. *Future Oncol* 11:2865–2871, 2015.
17. Horwitz MJ, Hodak SP, Stewart AF: Non-parathyroid hypercalcemia, in Rosen CJ, (ed): *Primer on the Metabolic Bone Diseases and Disorders of Mineral Metabolism*. 8th ed. Washington DC, ASBMR/Wiley-Blackwell, 2013, p 562.
18. Marcocci C, Cetani F: Clinical practice. Primary hyperparathyroidism. *N Engl J Med* 365:2389–2397, 2011.
19. Rodgers SE, Perrier ND: Parathyroid carcinoma. *Curr Opin Oncol* 18:16–22, 2006.
20. Brandi ML, Gagel RF, Angeli A, et al: Guidelines for diagnosis and therapy of MEN type 1 and type 2. *J Clin Endocrinol Metab* 86:5658–5671, 2001.
21. Pollak MR, Brown EM, Chou YHW, et al: Mutations in the human Ca^{2+}-sensing receptor gene cause familial hypocalciuric hypercalcemia and neonatal severe hyperparathyroidism. *Cell* 75:1297–1303, 1993.
22. Marx SJ, Spiegel AM, Brown EM, et al: Divalent cation metabolism: familial hypocalciuric hypercalcemia versus typical primary hyperparathyroidism. *Am J Med* 65:235–242, 1978.
23. Saunders BD, Saunders EFH, Gauger PG: Lithium therapy and hyperparathyroidism: an evidenced-based assessment. *World J Surg* 33:2314–2323, 2009.
24. Stewart AF: Clinical practice. Hypercalcemia associated with cancer. *N Engl J Med* 352:373–379, 2005.
25. LeGrand SB, Leskuski D, Zama I: Narrative review: furosemide for hypercalcemia: an unproven yet common practice. *Ann Intern Med* 149:259–263, 2008.
26. Major P, Lortholary A, Hon J, et al: Zoledronic acid is superior to pamidronate in the treatment of hypercalcemia of malignancy: a pooled analysis of two randomized, controlled, clinical trials. *J Clin Oncol* 19:558–567, 2001.
27. Khan AA, Morrison A, Hanley DA, et al; International Task Force on Osteonecrosis of the Jaw: Diagnosis and management of osteonecrosis of the jaw: a systematic review and international consensus. *J Bone Miner Res* 30:3–23, 2015.
28. Cummings SR, San Martin J, McClung MR, et al: Denosumab for prevention of fractures in postmenopausal women with osteoporosis. *N Engl J Med* 361:756–765, 2009.
29. Body JJ, Lipton A, Gralow J, et al: Effects of denosumab in patients with bone metastases, with and without previous bisphosphonate exposure. *J Bone Miner Res* 25:440–446, 2010.
30. Hu MI, Glezerman IG, Leboulleux S, et al: Denosumab for treatment of hypercalcemia of malignancy. *J Clin Endocrinol Metab* 99:3144–3152, 2014.
31. Peacock M, Bolognese MA, Borofsky M, et al: Cinacalcet treatment of primary hyperparathyroidism: biochemical and bone densitometric outcomes in a five-year study. *J Clin Endocrinol Metab* 94:4860–4867, 2009.
32. Cooper MS, Gittoes NJL: Diagnosis and management of hypocalcemia. *BMJ* 336:1298–1302, 2008.
33. Lemos MC, Thakker RV: GNAS mutations in pseudohypoparathyroidism type 1a and related disorders. *Hum Mutat* 36:11–19, 2015.
34. Mannstadt M, Clark BL, Vokes T, et al: Efficacy and safety of recombinant human parathyroid hormone (1-84) in hypoparathyroidism (REPLACE): a double-blind, placebo-controlled, randomized phase 3 study. *Lancet Diabetes Endocrinol* 1:275–283, 2013.
35. Stack BC Jr, Bimston DN, Bodenner DL, et al: Postoperative hypoparathyroidism – definitions and management. *Endocr Pract* 21:674–685, 2015.
36. Topf JM, Murray PT: Hypomagnesemia and hypermagnesemia. *Rev Endocr Metab Disord* 4:195–206, 2003.
37. Carpenter TO, Imel EA, Holm IA, et al: A clinician's guide to X-linked hypophosphatemia. *J Bone Miner Res* 26:1381–1388, 2011.
38. Malberti F: Hyperphosphatemia: treatment options. *Drugs* 73:673–688, 2013.
39. Brunelli SM, Goldfarb S: Hypophosphatemia: clinical consequences and management. *J Am Soc Nephrol* 18:1999–2003, 2007.

Chapter 141 ■ Severe Hyperthyroidism

MARJORIE S. SAFRAN

Patients with thyrotoxicosis rarely need hospitalization. However, some patients with severe thyrotoxicosis develop a decompensated clinical presentation called *thyroid storm.* It is characterized by hyperpyrexia, tachycardia, and delirium [1] and generally occurs among patients with severe thyrotoxicosis, who then experience a physiological insult. The cause of this rapid decompensation is unknown, but it may be partly because of a sudden inhibition in thyroid hormone binding to plasma proteins, resulting in a rise in the already elevated free hormone pool [2]. Thyroid storm accounts for no more than 2% of hospital admissions for all forms and complications of thyrotoxicosis, and the diagnosis is often difficult to make because there is a fine line between severe thyrotoxicosis and thyroid storm. Even when properly treated, thyroid storm has a mortality rate of 7% to 30% [3].

ETIOLOGY

Before the preoperative use of iodides and the antithyroid drugs propylthiouracil (PTU) and methimazole (MMI; Tapazole), thyroid storm was most frequently seen during and after subtotal thyroidectomy. Because these agents are used to restore euthyroidism before surgery, thyroid storm is rarely seen in this context. Thyroid storm now occurs most commonly among patients with severe underlying thyrotoxicosis, frequently undiagnosed, who become ill for other reasons, such as infections, trauma, labor, diabetic ketoacidosis, or pulmonary and cardiovascular disorders. It can occur during or after nonthyroid surgery, and has been reported after external beam radiation to the neck [4], ingestion of sympathomimetic drugs (such as pseudoephedrine) in a thyrotoxic patient [5], and rarely with intentional or accidental overdoses [6,7]. Thyroid storm may rarely occur approximately 10 to 14 days after the administration of iodine 131 in patients with large goiters who have not been adequately pretreated with PTU or MMI to deplete the gland of stored thyroxine (T_4) and triiodothyronine (T_3) [8]. β-blockers are used to decrease symptoms of excess thyroid hormone release, but *may not* prevent thyroid storm.

CLINICAL MANIFESTATIONS

There is no absolute level of circulating thyroid hormones indicative of thyroid storm, and the diagnosis is made on a clinical basis [3]. Patients with thyroid storm are almost always febrile (temperature usually higher than 100°F) and have rapid sinus tachycardia and tachyarrhythmias (especially atrial fibrillation in elderly patients) out of proportion to the degree of fever that can frequently result in congestive heart failure. Patients are often agitated, delirious, and tremulous, with hot, flushed skin due to vasodilation. The skin may be moist or dry, depending on the state of hydration. Diarrhea occurs frequently and contributes to dehydration and hypovolemia. Vascular collapse and shock, which are poor prognostic signs, may occur. Hepatomegaly with abnormal liver enzymes and splenomegaly can be present; jaundice portends a poor prognosis.

Most patients display the classic signs of thyrotoxic Graves' disease, including ophthalmopathy, or toxic uninodular or multinodular goiter. However, in elderly patients, apathy, severe myopathy, profound weight loss, and congestive heart failure may be the predominant findings. As thyroid storm progresses, coma, hypotension, vascular collapse, and death may ensue unless active therapy is instituted.

DIAGNOSIS AND DIFFERENTIAL DIAGNOSIS

The diagnosis of thyroid storm is made on clinical grounds. Thyroid function tests do not differentiate between severe thyrotoxicosis and thyroid storm. Serum T_4 concentrations are usually similar, although it has been suggested that the serum-free T_4 concentration is significantly higher in patients with thyroid storm [2], which might partially explain their more severe symptoms. On the other hand, the serum T_3 concentrations are not higher and in fact may be less elevated or even normal in these patients when the precipitating cause is an intercurrent illness or surgery, because peripheral T_3 production from T_4 is markedly impaired in a wide variety of acute and chronic systemic illnesses. Liver function tests are frequently abnormal, especially in elderly patients with congestive heart failure. Elevations in total and free serum calcium concentrations may occur.

The differential diagnosis for a patient presenting with hyperpyrexia, delirium, and tachycardia includes severe infection, malignant hyperthermia [9], neuroleptic malignant syndrome, and acute mania with life-threatening catatonia. Thyroid storm can be distinguished from these disorders clinically by a history of thyroid disease, thyroid hormone, or iodine ingestion, and the presence on physical examination of a goiter or the stigmata of Graves' disease, including ophthalmopathy, onycholysis, and pretibial myxedema. However, any of the disorders mentioned in the differential diagnosis can coexist with thyroid storm since they may precipitate decompensation for a patient with preexisting hyperthyroidism.

TREATMENT

Treatment of thyroid storm is directed toward therapy of the underlying illness, supportive care, blocking peripheral effects of thyroid hormone, and inhibition of thyroid hormone synthesis and release (Table 141.1).

Underlying Illness

Nonthyroidal illness and surgery in previously undiagnosed or only partially treated patients with hyperthyroidism are the most common causes of thyroid storm. Thus, the precipitating disease should be vigorously treated. Cardiac arrhythmias and congestive heart failure require approximately twice the dose of digoxin needed in euthyroid patients or alternative management, and refractory arrhythmias should alert the physician to the presence of thyrotoxicosis. Patients may also have peripheral resistance to heparin and insulin, and higher doses may be required. It is evident that these patients must receive adequate antibiotic therapy; careful fluid, electrolyte, and vitamin supplementation; vigorous pulmonary therapy; and careful pre- and postoperative care. If emergency surgery is required for a thyrotoxic patient, propranolol, PTU or MMI, iodides, and perhaps corticosteroids should be given before, during, and after surgery.

TABLE 141.1

Treatment of Thyroid Storm

Therapy of underlying intercurrent illness	
Digoxin, diuretics, antibiotics, IV fluid supplemented with B-complex vitamins, and insulin for diabetic ketoacidosis	
Supportive care	
Cooling blanket, antipyretics (*not* aspirin), or both for hyperpyrexia	
Block peripheral effects of thyroid hormone	
β-Adrenergic blocking drugs	
Propranolol (β_1- and β_2-blocker)	1 mg IV/min for a total of 2–10 mg 40–120 mg PO q4–6h
Metoprolol (β_1-blocker)	100–400 mg PO q12h
Atenolol (β_1-blocker)	50–100 mg PO daily
Esmolol (β_1-blocker)	500 μg/kg over 1 min, then 50–100 μg/kg/min
Deplete catecholamines	
Reserpine	Test dose of 0.25 mg IM, then initial dose of 1–5 mg 1.0–2.5 mg IM q4–6h
Guanethidine	1–2 mg/kg PO q4–6h
Inhibition of synthesis of thyroid hormones	
Propylthiouracil (PTU)	~800 mg PO stat and 200–300 mg q8h 600 mg in 90 mL of water by rectum, as a retention enema, followed by 250 mg q4h
Methimazole (MMI)	~80 mg PO stat and 40 mg PO q12h 40 mg dissolved in aqueous solution by rectum q6h
Block release of thyroid hormone from thyroid gland	
Saturated solution of potassium iodide	5 drops PO q8h
Lugol's solution	10 drops PO q8h
Lithium	300 mg q6h, adjust to serum lithium level ~1 mEq/L
Inhibition of peripheral 5′-monodeiodination of thyroxine (T_4) to triiodothyronine (T_3)	
Corticosteroids	Equivalent to 300–400 mg hydrocortisone daily, especially dexamethasone, 2 mg q6h
Propranolol, metoprolol, atenolol, and possibly esmolol	
Propylthiouracil	
Remove thyroid hormones from the circulation	
Plasmapheresis	
Charcoal hemoperfusion	
Cholestyramine	4 g PO q6h

IM, intramuscularly; IV, intravenous; PO, oral.

Supportive Care

A cooling blanket can be used if the temperature rises above 101°F, but the shivering response that results from central cooling should be decreased by using drugs that block the central thermoregulatory centers, such as chlorpromazine or meperidine, 25 to 50 mg every 4 to 6 hours. Antipyretics other than salicylates may also be given. Salicylates should be avoided because they displace thyroid hormones from serum-binding proteins and can increase the free hormone concentrations [10]. Dehydration is frequently present and should be treated with intravenous fluid while monitoring for congestive heart failure.

Blockade of Peripheral Effects of Thyroid Hormone

Many of the clinical manifestations of hyperthyroidism can be alleviated by the administration of drugs that deplete or block the peripheral action of the catecholamines. β-adrenergic blocking agents are currently the drugs of choice in alleviating the catecholamine-dependent signs and symptoms of thyrotoxicosis and thyroid storm. The widest experience has been achieved with propranolol, which also has the advantage of decreasing T_4 to T_3 conversion (see later). Tachycardia and tremors can be improved within minutes of intravenous administration. Oral doses in the range of 60 to 120 mg every 6 hours may be required [11].

Because propranolol may be contraindicated for patients with congestive heart failure, it is frequently debated whether to use β-blockers for patients with severe thyrotoxicosis or thyroid storm. However, tachycardia and tachyarrhythmias are major contributing factors to the congestive failure in many of these patients, so β-blockers may be used cautiously along with digoxin and other cardiotropic drugs and diuretics. Rarely, hypotension and cardiac arrest occur after intravenous administration of β-blockers among patients with severe congestive failure and severe thyrotoxicosis [12]. For patients with asthma, the more selective β_1-blocking drugs, such as metoprolol and atenolol, may be used. A short-acting β_1-blocker, esmolol [13], and diltiazem can also be used to control the tachyarrhythmias associated with thyrotoxicosis [14].

Inhibition of Thyroid Hormone Synthesis

The antithyroid drugs, PTU and MMI, are potent inhibitors of the synthesis of both T_4 and T_3. Although the onset of action is rapid, PTU and MMI only partially block thyroid hormone synthesis. Weeks are required to deplete the thyroid of stored hormone and observe clinical effects of these drugs. Intravenous MMI is available in Europe, but in the United States, administration by either nasogastric tube or by rectum may be used [15]. PTU has the added advantage of partially blocking the peripheral conversion of T_4 to T_3 and therefore may be the drug of choice, although a recent retrospective study showed no difference in mortality or disease severity in patients treated with MMI versus PTU [16]. These drugs are not effective if thyroid storm is caused by excess ingestion of thyroid hormone (see the section Thyrotoxicosis Factitia) or painful or silent thyroiditis because they affect the synthesis of thyroid hormone and do not affect its release or peripheral activity.

Blockade of Thyroid Hormone Release

Iodide administration plays a major role in the treatment of thyroid storm because of its rapid inhibition of thyroid hormone release from the gland. This effect occurs almost immediately after oral or intravenous administration. Some inhibition of hormone synthesis may also occur in the hyperfunctioning gland. As with PTU and MMI, iodide therapy is not useful in thyroid storm caused by ingestion of excess amounts of thyroid hormone (thyrotoxicosis factitia) because it affects the synthesis and release of endogenously synthesized thyroid hormone.

Lugol's solution or saturated solution of potassium iodide can be given orally or as a potassium iodide enema, 1 g in 60 mL of water, followed by 500 mg of potassium iodide in 20 mL of water every 6 hours, given rectally in a patient who is unable to receive oral medication. Iodide therapy results in dramatic improvement and should be maintained until the serum T_4 and T_3 concentrations are normal or near normal. However, iodides can exacerbate hyperthyroidism when the patient is not pretreated with PTU or MMI and also delay the option of radioactive iodine for subsequent, definitive treatment. Escape from the iodide effect often occurs when PTU or MMI is not concomitantly used [17]. In patients allergic to iodine, lithium has been used to inhibit thyroid hormone release and partially inhibit thyroid hormone synthesis [18].

Inhibition of Peripheral Generation of Triiodothyronine

It is generally believed that the major bioactive hormone is T_3, that the major source of circulating T_3 is derived from T_4, and that most, if not all, of the metabolic effects of T_4 result from the intracellular generation of T_3 from T_4. A variety of drugs impair the outer-ring monodeiodination of T_4 to T_3, thus decreasing the peripheral generation of T_3. Propranolol, some selective β_1-blocking drugs [19], and PTU are relatively weak inhibitors of T_4 to T_3 conversion. The corticosteroids, especially dexamethasone, are potent inhibitors when administered at high doses and also have an inhibitory effect on thyroid hormone hypersecretion. Their importance for treating thyroid storm has been well documented; the survival rate for thyroid storm was improved when corticosteroids were added to the treatment regimen. Because relative adrenal insufficiency may be present in patients with thyroid storm, glucocorticoid therapy would also correct this possibility. Indeed, combination therapy of severe hyperthyroidism with PTU, iodides, and dexamethasone has resulted in a marked reduction of serum T_3 concentration within 24 hours.

The gallbladder dyes, iopanoic acid (Telepaque), and ipodate (Oragrafin), are potent inhibitors of T_4 to T_3 conversion and succesfully used in treatment of thyroid storm [20], but are no longer available in the United States. Similarly, amiodarone also decreases T_3 levels. In addition, it is rich in iodine, and may also block entrance of T_4 into the cell. Although this drug has been used in the short-term (2 weeks) treatment of thyrotoxicosis, it should not be used in the treatment of thyroid storm because its long half-life and high iodide content can cause persistent, severe hyperthyroidism [21].

Removal of Thyroid Hormone from the Circulation

Direct removal of thyroid hormone from the circulation is occasionally required in patients who do not respond to conventional medical treatment. There are case reports of successful use of plasmapheresis [22] and charcoal plasma perfusion [23]. Cholestyramine, which binds T_3 and T_4 in the gut and decreases serum T_3 and T_4 concentrations by increasing the fecal excretion of these hormones [24], may also be useful, particularly if used early in a patient with an overdose.

Thyrotoxicosis Factitia

The inadvertent ingestion of excess amounts of thyroid hormone most commonly occurs in children, although adults may also ingest excess hormone for weight reduction or as a suicide attempt [6,7,25]. Gastric lavage or emesis induction should be performed as soon as possible after ingestion. Occasionally, oral charcoal administration can be useful. As previously mentioned, this form of thyrotoxicosis is not caused by endogenous production of thyroid hormone; therefore, drugs that inhibit the synthesis of T_4 and T_3 or those that block thyroid hormone release are not helpful. Therapy should focus on preventing the peripheral effects of excessive thyroid hormone with β-adrenergic blocking drugs and possibly corticosteroids. Cholestyramine may also be useful to decrease serum thyroid hormone levels, as above.

CONCLUSIONS

It is evident that each patient must be treated individually and that a set protocol cannot be advised for all patients. Specific therapy should be directed toward inhibiting the synthesis and release of T_4 and T_3 from the thyroid, blocking the peripheral conversion of T_4 to T_3, relieving the catecholamine-mediated effects by β-adrenergic blockade, and treating the possibility of decreased adrenal reserve with corticosteroids. Associated and precipitating diseases should, of course, be vigorously treated. Iodine often works quickly to improve thyroid hormone levels, but will delay the use of radioactive iodine treatment of hyperthyroidism and thus should be saved for patients with thyroid storm, not just severe thyrotoxicosis.

References

1. Abend SL, Braverman LE: Acute thyroid disorders, in May HL (ed): *Emergency Medicine.* 2nd ed. Boston, Little, Brown and Company, 1992, p 1274.
2. Brooks MH, Waldstein SS: Free thyroxine concentration in thyroid storm. *Ann Intern Med* 93:694–697, 1980.
3. Burch HB, Wartofsky L: Life-threatening thyrotoxicosis. Thyroid storm. *Endocrinol Metab Clin North Am* 22:263–277, 1993.
4. Diaz R, Blakey MD, Murphy PB, et al: Thyroid storm after intensity-modulated radiation therapy: a case report and discussion. *Oncologist* 14:233–239, 2009.
5. Wilson BE, Hobbs WN: Case report: pseudoephedrine-associated thyroid storm: thyroid hormone-catecholamine interactions. *Am Med Sci* 306:317–319, 1993.
6. Bhasin S, Wallace W, Lawrence JB, et al: Sudden death associated with thyroid hormone abuse. *Am J Med* 71:887–890, 1981.
7. Hartung B, Schott M, Daldrup T, et al: Lethal thyroid storm after uncontrolled intake of liothyronine in order to lose weight. *Int J Legal Med* 124(6):637–640, 2010.
8. Kadmon PM, Noto RB, Boney CM, et al: Thyroid storm in a child following radioactive iodine (RAI) therapy: a consequence of RAI versus withdrawal of antithyroid medication. *J Clin Endocrinol Metab* 86:1865–1867, 2001.

9. Nishiyama K, Kitahara A, Natsume H, et al: Malignant hyperthermia in a patient with Graves' disease during subtotal thyroidectomy. *Endocr J* 48:227–232, 2001.
10. Larsen PR: Salicylate-induced increases in free triiodothyronine in human serum. *J Clin Invest* 51:1125–1134, 1972.
11. Ringel MD: Management of hypothyroidism and hyperthyroidism in the intensive care unit. *Crit Care Clin* 17:59–74, 2001.
12. Dalan R, Leow MK: Cardiovascular collapse associated with beta blockade in thyroid storm. *Exp Clin Endocrinol Diabetes* 115(6):392–396, 2007.
13. Vijayakumar HR, Thomas WO, Ferrara JJ: Peri-operative management of severe thyrotoxicosis with esmolol. *Anaesthesia* 44:406–408, 1989.
14. Roti E, Montermini M, Roti S, et al: The effect of diltiazem, a calcium channel-blocking drug, on cardiac rate and rhythm in hyperthyroid patients. *Arch Intern Med* 148:1919–1921, 1988.
15. Alfadhli E, Gianoukakis, AG: Management of severe thyrotoxicosis when the gastrointestinal tract is compromised. *Thyroid* 21: 215–220, 2011.
16. Isozaki O, Satoh T, Wakino S, et al: Treatment and management of thyroid storm: analysis of the nationwide surveys. *Clin Endocrinol*, 2015. doi: 10.1111/cen.12949.
17. Emerson CH, Anderson AJ, Howard WJ, et al: Serum thyroxine and triiodothyronine concentrations during iodide treatment of hyperthyroidism. *J Clin Endocrinol Metab* 40:33–36, 1975.
18. Nayak B, Burman K: Thyrotoxicosis and thyroid storm. *Endocrinol Metab Clin North Am* 35:663–686, 2006.
19. Perrild H, Hansen JM, Skovsted L, et al: Different effects of propranolol, alprenolol, sotalol, atenolol and metoprolol on serum T_3 and serum rT_3 in hyperthyroidism. *Clin Endocrinol* 18:139–142, 1983.
20. Tyer NM, Kim TY, Martinez DS: Review of oral cholecystographic agents for the management of hyperthyroidism. *Endocr Pract* 20:1084–1092, 2014.
21. Bogazzi F, Bartalena L, Martino E: Approach to the patient with amiodarone-induced thyrotoxicosis. *J Clin Endocrinol Metab* 95:2529–2535, 2010.
22. Vyas A, Vyas P, Vijayakrishnan R, et al: Successful treatment of thyroid storm with plasmapheresis in methimazole-induced agranulocytosis. *Endocr Pract* 16:673–676, 2010.
23. Kreisner E, Lutzky M, Gross JL: Charcoal hemoperfusion in the treatment of levothyroxine intoxication. *Thyroid* 20:209–212, 2010.
24. Solomon B, Wartofsky L, Burman KD: Adjunctive cholestyramine therapy for thyrotoxicosis. *Clin Endocrinol (Oxf)* 38:39–43, 1993.
25. Cohen JH III, Ingbar SH, Braverman LE: Thyrotoxicosis due to ingestion of excess thyroid hormone. *Endocr Rev* 10:113–124, 1989.

Chapter 142 ■ Myxedema Coma

MIRA SOFIA TORRES • CHARLES H. EMERSON

Myxedema coma is a syndrome that occurs in advanced untreated hypothyroidism [1–5]. It is defined by a group of characteristic clinical features and not by laboratory evidence of severe hypothyroidism (Table 142.1). Myxedema coma is generally preceded by increasingly severe signs and symptoms of thyroid insufficiency. Fortunately, it is quite rare. Hypothyroid patients who are neglectful or whose contact with family and friends is limited are most vulnerable. Despite early and intensive treatment, mortality from myxedema coma is still as high as 30% to 50% [2,4,6,7].

ETIOLOGY AND PATHOPHYSIOLOGY

By definition, myxedema coma does not occur in the absence of hypothyroidism. If hypothyroidism is due to hypothalamic or pituitary insufficiency, the condition is even more serious because it is also accompanied by adrenal failure. Pituitary tumors are the major cause of central hypothyroidism in the United States. In regions with poor access to health care, postpartum pituitary necrosis is quite prevalent and is therefore another important cause of secondary hypothyroidism.

More than 95% of patients with hypothyroidism have primary thyroid disease. Most patients with primary hypothyroidism have either autoimmune thyroid failure or hypothyroidism secondary to ablative procedures on the thyroid. These include radioactive iodine and surgery for hyperthyroidism, thyroid resection for thyroid cancer, and external thyroid irradiation for head and neck tumors. Certain drugs, such as lithium carbonate and amiodarone, can cause hypothyroidism but are only rarely associated with myxedema coma.

Myxedema coma is distinguished from uncomplicated hypothyroidism by a variety of features that relate to central nervous system (CNS) dysfunction. The pathophysiology of myxedema coma will become clearer when there is a better understanding of the effects of thyroid hormone on the brain. Narcotics and hypnotics should be used with caution in hypothyroid patients because these patients are very sensitive to their sedative effects. These agents, alone or in combination with other factors, may precipitate myxedema coma in hypothyroid patients. Other precipitating factors are trauma, surgery, and severe infection [1–9]. The most important factor in temperate climates, however, is cold stress. In one series, 9 of 11 patients with myxedema coma were admitted in the late fall or winter [2].

TABLE 142.1

Clinical Features of Myxedema Coma

Mental obtundation
Course, dry skin
Myxedema facies
Hypothermia
Hypoglycemia
Bradycardia and hypotension
Electrocardiographic changes
Atonic gastrointestinal tract
Atonic bladder
Pleural, pericardial, and peritoneal effusions

CLINICAL MANIFESTATIONS

Patients are partially or completely obtunded. Therefore, the history must often be obtained from other sources. Friends, relatives, and acquaintances might have noted increasing lethargy, complaints of cold intolerance, and changes in the voice. An outdated container of L-thyroxine discovered with the patient's belongings suggests that he or she has been remiss in taking medication. The medical record may also indicate that the patient was taking thyroid hormone or may refer to previous treatment with radioactive iodine. A thyroidectomy scar suggests the possibility of hypothyroidism. Other than coma itself, the cardinal manifestations are hypothermia and hypotension. Hypotonia of the gastrointestinal tract is common and often so severe as to suggest an obstructive lesion. Urinary retention due to a hypotonic bladder is related but less frequently observed. Most patients have the physical features of severe hypothyroidism, including bradycardia and slow relaxation of the deep tendon reflexes. A myxedematous facies (Fig. 142.1) results from the dry puffy skin, pallor, hypercarotenemia, periorbital edema, and patchy hair loss.

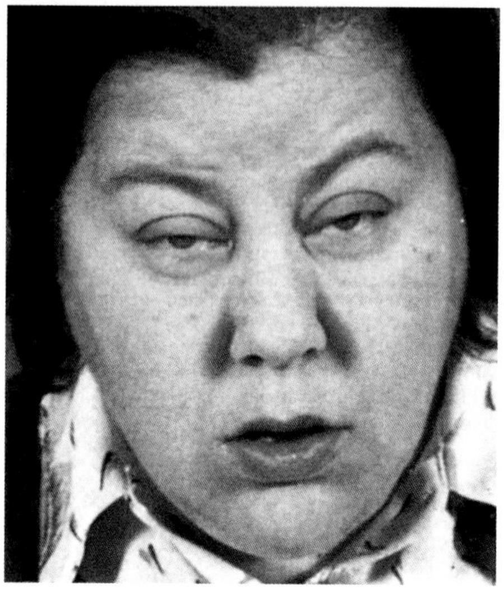

FIGURE 142.1 Characteristic facies of severe hypothyroidism. Note the facial and periorbital puffiness and the dull, lethargic expression.

DIAGNOSIS AND DIFFERENTIAL DIAGNOSIS

The diagnosis of myxedema coma is based on the presence of the characteristic clinical syndrome in a patient with hypothyroidism. The laboratory's role is to confirm that the patient is hypothyroid and determine whether there are treatable complications of myxedema coma, such as hypoventilation, hypoglycemia, and hyponatremia. Because of the gravity of myxedema coma, treatment must be instituted before laboratory tests confirm the diagnosis.

The diagnostic laboratory features of primary hypothyroidism are a subnormal serum-free thyroxine index or serum-free thyroxine (T_4) concentration and an elevated serum thyroid-stimulating hormone (TSH) concentration. The serum-free thyroxine index or free T_4 is also low in severely ill patients with a wide variety of conditions. This is the so-called "sick euthyroid syndrome" or nonthyroidal illness. Unlike patients with myxedema coma, however, serum TSH concentrations are not elevated among patients with the sick euthyroid syndrome, except in a small percentage, and usually as they are clearly recovering from their severe illness. Distinction between hypothyroidism secondary to pituitary or hypothalamic disease (i.e., central hypothyroidism) and the sick euthyroid syndrome is difficult because serum TSH concentrations are low or, when TSH bioactivity is reduced as in secondary hypothyroidism, only mildly elevated in patients with central hypothyroidism. It is important to measure TSH as well as the serum-free thyroxine or free thyroxine index for patients presenting with myxedema coma. In central hypothyroidism, the typical clinical presentation of the myxedematous patient would help establish the diagnosis. The sick euthyroid syndrome is discussed in Chapter 143. The measurement of the total serum triiodothyronine (T_3) concentration is of no value for the diagnosis of hypothyroidism or myxedema coma. It lacks sensitivity for the diagnosis of hypothyroidism and is depressed not only by illness but also by fasting.

Alone, few of the signs and symptoms described in this chapter are unique to myxedema coma. For example, the differential diagnosis of hypothermia (see Chapter 184) includes numerous conditions, such as malnutrition, sepsis, hypoglycemia, multisystem trauma, prolonged cardiac arrest, and exposure to alcohol and certain drugs or toxins [10,11]. Hypotension and hypoventilation, other cardinal features of myxedema coma, occur in other disease states. What distinguishes myxedema coma from other disorders is laboratory evidence of hypothyroidism, characteristic myxedema facies with periorbital puffiness, skin changes, obtundation, and, frequently, a constellation of other physical signs characteristic of severe hypothyroidism. Recently, two scoring systems have been proposed for the diagnosis of myxedema coma, based on clinical features and laboratory or imaging findings. However, these are both based on small groups of patients, and their utility has not been well validated [12,13].

TREATMENT

As noted earlier, for most patients with myxedema coma, hypothyroidism is due to primary thyroid disease. The initial management of myxedema coma due either to primary thyroid disease or central (pituitary or hypothalamic) disease is similar, since glucocorticoids are recommended in all patients. The only proviso is that in patients with central hypothyroidism, additional evaluation of the CNS for the presence of space-occupying lesions is warranted. Therefore, the management team must be alert for evidence of space-occupying lesions within or in the region of the pituitary for all patients with myxedema coma.

Treatment of myxedema coma consists of management of hypoglycemia, respiratory depression, hyponatremia, hypothermia, hypotension, and administration of thyroid hormone (Table 142.2). All patients require continuous monitoring of the electrocardiogram and an intravenous line to administer fluids and drugs. Baseline thyroid function tests, serum cortisol, complete blood count, blood urea nitrogen, creatinine, plasma glucose, and electrolytes are mandatory. Pneumonia commonly develops or may be the precipitating factor and must be treated promptly (see Chapter 181). Hypothyroidism and myxedema coma are also associated with hemostatic abnormalities, particularly capillary bleeding and cerebral hemorrhage [2,14,15]. Although bleeding should be anticipated in some patients, few strategies have evolved to counter this disorder.

Hypoglycemia

Because hypoglycemia is not unusual in myxedema coma, 50 mL of 50% glucose should immediately be administered intravenously when point of care glucose testing is not available to avoid any delay in treatment of this serious complicaton. Chapter 138 details the management of hypoglycemia.

Hypoventilation

Respiratory center depression is common in severe hypothyroidism and myxedema coma. Arterial blood gases should be routinely

TABLE 142.2

Treatment of Myxedema Coma

Assisted ventilation for hypoventilation
Intravenous glucose for hypoglycemia
Water restriction or hypertonic saline for severe hyponatremia
Passive rewarming for hypothermia
Administration of T_4 or T_3 IV[a]
Administration of hydrocortisone[a]
Treatment of underlying infection and other illnesses, if present
Avoidance of all sedatives, hypnotics, and narcotics

[a]Dosage must be individualized (see text).
IV, intravenously; T_3, triiodothyronine; T_4, thyroxine.

obtained, therefore, to rule out hypoventilation. If respiratory center depression is clinically obvious, assisted ventilation with oxygen supplementation must be started without delay, taking care not to correct chronic hypercapnia too rapidly (see Chapters 165, 166, 167).

Hyponatremia

Hyponatremia, which results from impaired free water clearance, is most deleterious to CNS function when it develops rapidly. Although hyponatremia is present in some patients, it is usually not the cause of coma because its onset tends to be gradual. A limiting factor is that water intake decreases as myxedema coma develops, offsetting the tendency toward hyponatremia. Treatment consists of restriction of free water. If the serum sodium concentration is less than 110 mEq per L, hypertonic saline and, in some cases, furosemide should be administered (see Chapter 199).

Hypothermia

Hypothermia is one of the hallmarks of myxedema coma. It can be overlooked or its severity underestimated, however, if an out-of-date or poorly calibrated thermometer is used. Regardless of the cause, hypothermia is associated with a decrease in the basal metabolic rate, myocardial irritability, and blood pressure alterations. Blood pressure initially rises and then gradually falls. Changes in the cardiovascular status are accompanied by electrocardiographic changes. First, there is sinus bradycardia, then T wave inversion, and finally the development of a J wave [10]. At core temperatures below 28°C, ventricular fibrillation is a major threat to life.

Despite its gravity, the management of the hypothermia of myxedema coma differs from the treatment of exposure-induced hypothermia in euthyroid subjects. In myxedema coma, the patient should be kept in a warm room and covered with blankets. Active rewarming should be avoided, because it increases oxygen consumption and promotes peripheral vasodilation and circulatory collapse. Active rewarming is recommended only for situations of severe hypothermia in which ventricular fibrillation is an immediate threat.

Hypotension

Hypotension is another ominous feature of myxedema coma. Hypothermia and thyroid hormone deficiency per se are the two most important causes of hypotension, but bleeding and, perhaps in some cases, decreased adrenal reserve may also play a role. Because hypothermia itself produces hypotension, some improvement in blood pressure can be expected if passive measures to restore body temperature are successful. Intravenous fluids should be administered carefully as patients undergo rewarming. Anemia is common in hypothyroidism and has a multifactorial basis. In patients in whom anemia is severe or there appears to be active bleeding, a case can be made for transfusion. If this course is chosen, it must be done with great caution because patients with myxedema coma are extremely prone to circulatory collapse. Sympathomimetic vasoconstrictors or inotropic agents have very limited use in myxedema coma. The response to these drugs is poor, and myxedematous patients are very sensitive to their toxic effects.

Glucocorticoid Therapy

Although there is little evidence that hypotension in myxedema coma results from adrenal insufficiency, there are at least theoretical reasons for considering that these patients have decreased adrenal reserve. Furthermore, it is sometimes unclear whether the myxedema coma is due to primary or pituitary-hypothalamic hypothyroidism. Therefore, one of the immediate measures in treating myxedema coma is to administer 300 mg hydrocortisone intravenously in three divided doses during the first 24 hours. Gradually decreasing doses of hydrocortisone should be administered over the next few days, depending on the patient's response, or until adrenal insufficiency has been excluded. This protocol is recommended even in the absence of hypotension.

Sepsis

Infections, especially pneumonia and urosepsis, are precipitants or comorbidities in up to 80% of patients with myxedema coma, and sepsis is an important cause of death for these patients [2,4,6–8]. Some signs of sepsis such as tachycardia and fever may be absent in the initial presentation of patients with myxedema. A careful evaluation for underlying infections should be conducted for each patient. When suspected, such infections should be treated aggressively. The management of sepsis is discussed in detail in Chapter 39.

Thyroid Hormone

Administration of thyroid hormone is the definitive treatment of myxedema coma and is essential for reversing hypotension, hypothermia, and depressed consciousness. The sensorium may be improved for a few patients when glucose is given or hypoventilation corrected, but deterioration recurs if thyroid hormone is not given. The gastrointestinal absorption of thyroid hormone is often markedly reduced in myxedema coma. Therefore, thyroid hormone must be given by the intravenous route. To ensure proper dosing, synthetic preparations should be used.

There are no large controlled studies of the optimum form of thyroid hormone for myxedema coma or, for that matter, any aspect of the treatment of myxedema coma. Both T_4 and T_3 have been used with varying degrees of success, and each has its theoretical advantages. T_4 is advantageous because most thyroid hormone is secreted in the form of T_4. For this and other reasons, plasma and intracellular T_4 and T_3 profiles are more stable and representative of the normal condition if T_4 rather than T_3 is administered. Conversely, T_3 is advantageous because it has a more rapid onset of action than T_4.

The best doses for treating myxedema coma have not been studied in a rigorous fashion. As is the case when deciding between T_4 and T_3, the choice is not straightforward. In patients with long-standing untreated hypothyroidism, thyroid hormone treatment is usually initiated at low doses. These patients frequently have underlying arteriosclerotic cardiovascular disease, and initial therapy with full replacement doses of thyroid hormone can precipitate angina or myocardial infarction. On the other hand, in near-terminal patients with myxedema coma, the need for thyroid hormone is urgent. In this setting, the blood pressure and body temperature can increase within hours after thyroid hormone is started.

We and others [16] prefer T_4 in all but the most severe cases of myxedema coma. Except in elderly patients, the initial intravenous dose of T_4 should be between 0.2 and 0.4 mg, with the larger doses in this range used for more comatose patients, those with more severe hypotension or hypothermia, and those with large body mass. In the elderly patient or those with a history of heart disease, the initial T_4 dose should probably not exceed 0.4 mg. Doses exceeding 0.5 mg per day may be associated with higher mortality [6]. If there is no improvement in the state of consciousness, blood pressure, or core temperature in the first 6 to 12 hours after the initial dose, T_4 should again be administered to bring the total dose during the first 24 hours to 0.4 mg. Thyroid hormone should then be given again 24 hours later and every 24 hours thereafter. After the first 24 hours, the subsequent doses should range from 0.05 to 0.2 mg daily, depending on the clinical response. If the treatment is not maintained, coma may recur. One prospective study randomly assigned 11 patients to two groups: one received a loading dose of 0.5 mg of T_4 intravenously followed by a daily maintenance dose of 0.1 mg intravenously ("high-dose" group); the other group received only the maintenance dose of 0.1 mg daily ("low-dose" group). Four of eleven patients died, but only one of them was in the "high-dose" group. The mortality rate was lower in the" high-dose" group, but did not reach statistical significance. However, the sample size was small. Based on this information, it was suggested that patients who receive a loading dose fared better than those on less vigorous regimens [8]. A smaller dose in comatose patients is probably indicated in very elderly patients [6], or in patients who are normotensive and euthermic and have another explanation for their comatose state, such as CNS trauma or recent sedative ingestion. Another situation that calls for lower doses is the patient who has had an acute myocardial infarction and whose hypotension appears to be secondary to the myocardial infarction, which is a major contributor to the patient's depressed sensorium. In these cases, ventilatory support should be given and intravenous doses of as little as 0.05 to 0.1 mg of T_4 administered in the first 24 hours. Care must be taken when making the diagnosis of myocardial infarction, however, since creatine kinase-MB activity is increased in the absence of myocardial infarction in a few patients with myxedema coma [17,18]. Troponin levels are more specific markers of cardiac injury, and are probably affected to a lesser degree, although there have also been reports of troponin elevations in hypothyroidism in the absence of cardiac disease [19–23].

For severe cases of myxedema coma where there is a poor initial response to levothyroxine, addition of intravenous T_3 may be considered [16]. If T_3 is used, however, greater caution must be exercised to avoid overstimulation of the cardiovascular system [2] and too rapid an increase in oxygen consumption. It is clear that T_3 has been lifesaving in some patients, but high doses of administered T_3 and high calculated plasma T_3 concentrations have also been associated with increased mortality [2,6]. Although doses as high as 0.2 mg of T_3 in the first 24 hours have been used, as little as 0.0025 mg has been reported to increase cardiac output, heart rate, ventricular stroke work, oxygen consumption, and oxygen delivery in myxedema coma [24]. Based on recent American Thyroid Association (ATA) recommendations, a loading dose 5 to 20 μg of T_3 can given intravenously, in addition to levothyroxine. This can be followed by a dose of 2.5 to 10 μg of T_3 every 8 hours [16]. If signs of myocardial ischemia develop, the dose of T_3 should be reduced. Particularly worrisome would be a decrease in blood pressure in the face of an increase in body temperature, suggesting that cardiovascular decompensation is occurring in the face of increased oxygen demands. If there is gradual improvement of metabolic parameters, the T_3 can be tapered and T_4 treatment continued. When the patient stabilizes and is fully conscious, T_4 can be given by the oral instead of the intravenous route. T_4 therapy must be closely monitored, however, as T_4 malabsorption can be a serious problem in a variety of clinical settings. If the clinical response to oral T_4 is not maintained or serum T_4 concentrations fall, the patient should be switched back to intravenous T_4 therapy.

Although myxedema coma is associated with a high mortality, many patients survive by using judicious therapy aimed at correcting the secondary metabolic disturbances and reversing the hypothyroid state. This must be done in a sustained but gradual fashion, however, because an effort to correct hypothyroidism too rapidly may completely negate the beneficial effects of the initial treatment.

TABLE 142.3

Pertinent Clinical Studies of Myxedema Coma

- Myxedema coma has a high mortality rate and is often the first manifestation of thyroid disease [2,5–8]
- Old age is associated with increased mortality in myxedema coma [2,6].
- Sepsis and infection are important contributors to mortality [2,4,6–8].
- Higher doses of T4 ($\geq$0.5 mg/d) combined with T_3 ($\geq$75 μg/d) have been associated with worse outcome. It is not known this association is due to patients with more severe forms of myxedema coma being treated with higher doses of thyroid hormone [2,6].

Pertinent clinical studies of myxedema coma are listed in Table 142.3.

References

1. Pereira VG, Haron ES, Lima-Neto N, et al: Management of myxedema coma: report on three successfully treated cases with nasogastric or intravenous administration of triiodothyronine. *J Endocrinol Invest* 5(5):331–334, 1982.
2. Hylander B, Rosenqvist U: Treatment of myxoedema coma–factors associated with fatal outcome. *Acta Endocrinol (Copenh)* 108(1):65–71, 1985.
3. Nicoloff JT, LoPresti JS: Myxedema coma. A form of decompensated hypothyroidism. *Endocrinol Metab Clin North Am* 22(2):279–290, 1993.
4. Jordan RM: Myxedema coma. Pathophysiology, therapy, and factors affecting prognosis. *Med Clin North Am* 79(1):185–194, 1995.
5. Reinhardt W, Mann K: Incidence, clinical picture and treatment of hypothyroid coma. Results of a survey. *Med Klin (Munich)* 92(9):521–524, 1997.
6. Yamamoto T, Fukuyama J, Fujiyoshi A: Factors associated with mortality of myxedema coma: report of eight cases and literature survey. *Thyroid* 9(12):1167–1174, 1999.
7. Dutta P, Bhansali A, Masoodi SR, et al: Predictors of outcome in myxoedema coma: a study from a tertiary care centre. *Crit Care* 12(1):R1, 2008.
8. Rodriguez I, Fluiters E, Perez-Mendez LF, et al: Factors associated with mortality of patients with myxoedema coma: prospective study in 11 cases treated in a single institution. *J Endocrinol* 180(2):347–350, 2004.
9. Ragaller M, Quintel M, Bender HJ, et al: Myxedema coma as a rare postoperative complication. *Anaesthesist* 42(3):179–183, 1993.
10. Reuler JB: Hypothermia: pathophysiology, clinical settings, and management. *Ann Intern Med* 89(4):519–527, 1978.
11. Aslam AF, Aslam AK, Vasavada BC, et al: Hypothermia: evaluation, electrocardiographic manifestations, and management. *Am J Med* 119(4):297–301, 2006.
12. Chiong YV, Bammerlin E, Mariash CN: Development of an objective tool for the diagnosis of myxedema coma. *Transl Res* 166(3):233–243, 2015.
13. Popoveniuc G, Chandra T, Sud A, et al: A diagnostic scoring system for myxedema coma. *Endocr Pract* 20(8):808–817, 2014.
14. Squizzato A, Romualdi E, Buller HR, et al: Clinical review: thyroid dysfunction and effects on coagulation and fibrinolysis: a systematic review. *J Clin Endocrinol Metab* 92(7):2415–2420, 2007.
15. ORR FR: Haemorrhage in myxoedema coma. *Lancet* 2(7264):1012–1015, 1962.
16. Jonklaas J, Bianco AC, Bauer AJ, et al: Guidelines for the treatment of hypothyroidism: prepared by the american thyroid association task force on thyroid hormone replacement. *Thyroid* 24(12):1670–1751, 2014.
17. Hickman PE, Silvester W, Musk AA, et al: Cardiac enzyme changes in myxedema coma. *Clin Chem* 33(4):622–624, 1987.
18. Nee PA, Scane AC, Lavelle PH, et al: Hypothermic myxedema coma erroneously diagnosed as myocardial infarction because of increased creatine kinase MB. *Clin Chem* 33(6):1083–1084, 1987.
19. Ness-Abramof R, Nabriski DA, Shapiro MS, et al: Cardiac troponin T is not increased in patients with hypothyroidism. *Intern Med J* 39(2):117–120, 2009.
20. Buschmann IR, Bondke A, Elgeti T, et al: Positive cardiac troponin I and T and chest pain in a patient with iatrogenic hypothyroidism and no coronary artery disease. *Int J Cardiol* 115(2):e83–e85, 2007.
21. Cohen LF, Mohabeer AJ, Keffer JH, et al: Troponin I in hypothyroidism. *Clin Chem* 42(9):1494–1495, 1996.
22. Gunduz H, Arinc H, Yolcu M, et al: A case of hypothyroidism mimicking acute coronary syndrome. *Int J Cardiovasc Imaging* 22(2):141–145, 2006.
23. Khan IA, Tun A, Wattanasauwan N, et al: Elevation of serum cardiac troponin I in noncardiac and cardiac diseases other than acute coronary syndromes. *Am J Emerg Med* 17(3):225–229, 1999.
24. McCulloch W, Price P, Hinds CJ, et al: Effects of low dose oral triiodothyronine in myxoedema coma. *Intensive Care Med* 11(5):259–262, 1985.

Chapter 143 ■ Nonthyroidal Illness Syndrome (Sick Euthyroid Syndrome) in the Intensive Care Unit

SHIRIN HADDADY • ALAN P. FARWELL

INTRODUCTION

Critical illness causes multiple alterations in thyroid hormone concentrations among patients who have no previously diagnosed intrinsic thyroid disease [1–8]. These effects are nonspecific and relate to the severity of the illness. The most common alterations of thyroid hormone parameters seen among these cases includes low triiodothyronine (T_3) levels, normal thyroid stimulating hormone (TSH) levels, and increased reverse triiodothyronine (rT_3) levels. Despite abnormalities of serum thyroid hormone parameters, there is little evidence that these patients have clinically significant thyroid dysfunction. The changes in serum thyroid function associated with a wide variety of acute illness have been termed "sick euthyroid syndrome," "nonthyroidal illness syndrome," or "low T_3 syndrome." The changes in thyroid hormone parameters seen with the sick euthyroid syndrome are thought to be a response to systemic illness through a variety of different pathways. These changes are rarely isolated and often are associated with alterations in other endocrine systems, such as reductions in serum gonadotropin and sex hormone concentrations [9] and increases in serum corticotropin and cortisol levels [10]. Similar changes in endocrine function have been shown experimentally by the administration of cytokines from the interleukin (IL) and interferon families as well as tumor necrosis factor-α (TNF-α) [11]. One theory postulates that euthyroid sick syndrome may be a compensatory mechanism in response to the oxidative stress of acute illness. Thus, the sick euthyroid syndrome should not be viewed as an isolated pathologic event but as part of a coordinated systemic reaction to illness that involves both the immune and endocrine systems.

The differentiation between patients with the sick euthyroid syndrome and those with intrinsic thyroid disease is a frequent diagnostic problem for intensive care unit (ICU) physicians. This chapter will first review normal thyroid physiology and discuss the changes in thyroid hormone metabolism seen with critical illness. Management of these patients and the identification of those with intrinsic thyroid disease will then be discussed. Finally, the use of thyroid hormone replacement in the sick euthyroid syndrome will be reviewed.

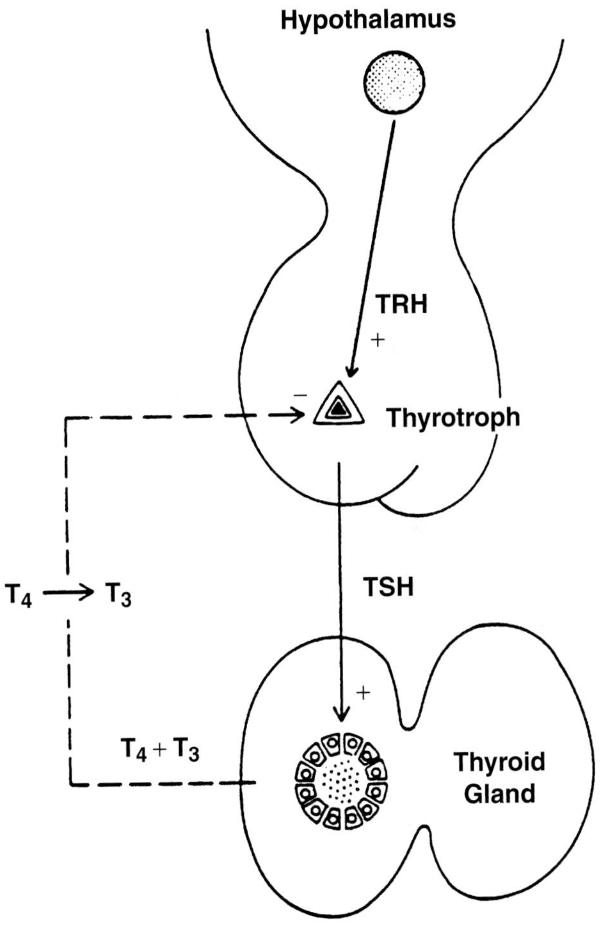

FIGURE 143.1 Diagram of the hypothalamic–pituitary–thyroid axis. The inhibitory effect of T_4 and T_3 on thyrotropin (TSH) secretion is shown by the dashed line and minus sign, and the stimulatory effects of thyrotropin-releasing hormone (TRH) on TSH secretion and TSH on thyroid secretion are shown by the solid lines and plus signs. T_4 and T_3 may also have an inhibitory effect on TRH secretion. (From Toft AD: Thyrotropin: assay, secretory physiology, and testing of regulation, in Braverman LE, Utiger RD (eds): *The Thyroid: A Fundamental and Clinical Text*. Philadelphia, JB Lippincott, 1991, with permission.)

NORMAL THYROID HORMONE ECONOMY

Regulation

The synthesis and secretion of thyroid hormone is under the control of the anterior pituitary hormone, thyrotropin (TSH). In a classic negative feedback system, TSH secretion increases when serum thyroid hormone levels fall and decreases when they rise (Fig. 143.1). TSH secretion is also under the regulation of the hypothalamic hormone, thyrotropin-releasing hormone (TRH). The negative feedback of thyroid hormone is targeted mainly at the pituitary level but likely affects TRH release from the hypothalamus as well. In addition, input from higher cortical centers can affect hypothalamic TRH secretion.

Under the influence of TSH, the thyroid gland synthesizes and releases thyroid hormone. Thyroxine (T_4, 65% iodine by weight) is the principal secretory product of the thyroid gland, comprising ~90% of secreted thyroid hormone under normal conditions [12]. Although T_4 may have direct actions in some tissues, T_4 primarily functions as a hormone precursor that is metabolized in peripheral tissues to the transcriptionally active 3,5,3′-triiodothyronine (T_3, 59% iodine by weight).

Metabolic Pathways

The major pathway of metabolism of T_4 is by sequential monodeiodination [13] (Fig. 143.2). At least three deiodinases, each with its unique expression in different organs, catalyze the deiodination reactions involved in the metabolism of T_4. Removal of the

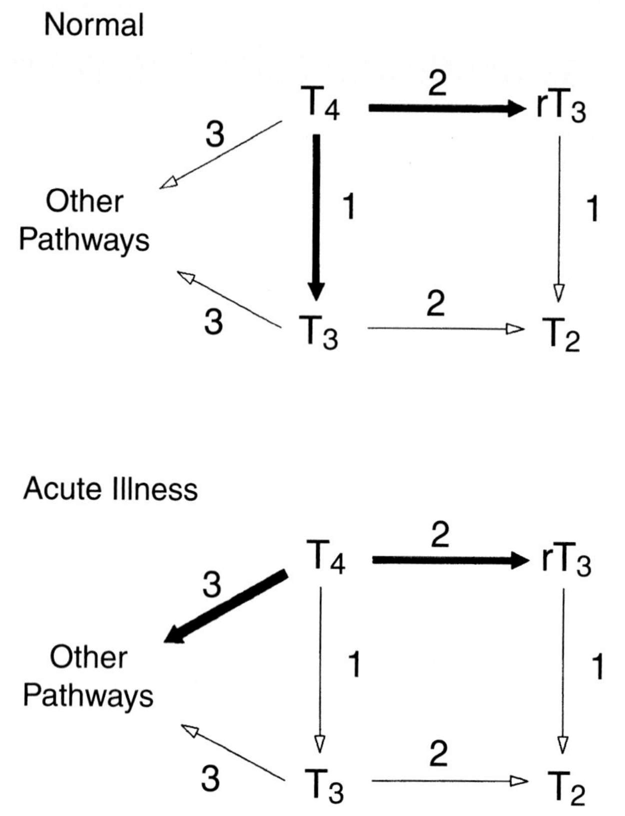

FIGURE 143.2 Pathways of thyroid hormone metabolism. Thyroid hormones are metabolized by outer ring deiodination (*1*, type 1 and type 2 5′-deiodinase), inner ring deiodination (*2*, type 3 5-deiodinase), or by nondeiodinative pathways (*3*). Deiodination is the major route of T_4 metabolism in healthy individuals, and nondeiodinative pathways of metabolism assume a greater role in critically ill patients.

5′-, or outer ring, iodine by type 1 iodothyronine 5′-deiodinase (type 1 deiodinase, D1) is the "activating" metabolic pathway, leading to the formation of T_3. Removal of the inner ring, or 5-, iodine by type 3 iodothyronine deiodinase (type 3 deiodinase, D3) is the "inactivating" pathway, producing the metabolically inactive hormone, 3,3′,5′-triiodothyronine (reverse T_3, rT_3). Type 1 deiodinase (D1) is found most abundantly in the liver, kidneys, and thyroid. It is upregulated in hyperthyroidism and downregulated in hypothyroidism. Type 3 deiodinase is expressed primarily in the brain, in skin, and in placental and chorionic membranes. The actions of D3 also include the inactivation of T_3 to form T_2, another inactive metabolite. Under normal conditions, ~41% of T_4 is converted to T_3, ~38% is converted to rT_3, and ~21% is metabolized via other pathways, such as conjugation in the liver and excretion in the bile [4,5].

T_3 is the metabolically active thyroid hormone and exerts its actions via binding to chromatin-bound nuclear receptors and regulating gene transcription in responsive tissues [14]. Important for understanding of the alterations of circulating thyroid hormone levels seen with critical illness is the fact that only ~10% of circulating T_3 is secreted directly by the thyroid gland, whereas >80% of T_3 is derived from conversion of T_4 in peripheral tissues [12,13]. Thus, factors that affect peripheral T_4 to T_3 conversion will have significant effects on circulating T_3 levels. Serum levels of T_3 are approximately 100-fold less than those of T_4, and, like T_4, T_3 is metabolized by deiodination to form diiodothyronine (T_2) and by conjugation in the liver. The half-lives of circulating T_4 and T_3 are 5 to 8 days and 1.3 to 3 days, respectively [15].

Serum-Binding Proteins

Both T_4 and T_3 circulate in the serum as bound hormones to several proteins synthesized by the liver [16]. Thyroxine-binding globulin (TBG) is the predominant transport protein and binds ~80% of the circulating serum thyroid hormones. The affinity of T_4 for TBG is approximately 10-fold greater than that of T_3 and is part of the reason that circulating T_4 levels are higher than T_3 levels. Other serum-binding proteins include transthyretin [17], which binds ~15% of T_4 but little, if any T_3, and albumin, which has a low affinity but a very large binding capacity for T_4 and T_3. Overall, 99.97% of circulating T_4 and 99.7% of circulating T_3 is bound to plasma proteins.

Free Hormone Concept

Essential to the understanding of the regulation of thyroid function and the alterations of circulating thyroid hormones seen with critical illness is the "free hormone" concept, which is that only the unbound hormone has any metabolic activity. Under the regulation by the pituitary, overall thyroid function is affected when there are any changes in free hormone concentrations. Changes in either the concentrations of binding proteins or the binding affinity of thyroid hormone to the serum-binding proteins have significant effects on the total serum hormone levels because of the high degree of binding of T_4 and T_3 to these proteins. Despite these changes, this does not necessarily translate into thyroid dysfunction.

THYROID HORMONE ECONOMY WITH CRITICAL ILLNESS

The widespread changes in thyroid hormone economy of the critically ill patient occurs as a result of: (a) alterations of the peripheral metabolism of the thyroid hormones, (b) alterations of TSH regulation, (c) alterations of the binding of thyroid hormone to TBG, (d) alterations of thyroid hormone transporters, and (e) alterations of nuclear thyroid hormone receptors [7].

Alterations of Metabolic Pathways

The acute decrease in T_3 and increase in rT_3 early in the euthyroid sick syndrome initially was thought to result solely from the acute inhibition of D1 in liver and kidneys by a variety of factors (Table 143.1) [13]. However, increased D3 activity in

TABLE 143.1

Factors That Inhibit Type 1 5′-Deiodinase Activity

Acute and chronic illness
Caloric deprivation
Malnutrition
Glucocorticoids
β-Adrenergic blocking drugs (e.g., propranolol)
Oral cholecystographic agents (e.g., iopanoic acid, sodium ipodate)
Amiodarone
Propylthiouracil
Fatty acids
Fetal/neonatal period
Selenium deficiency
Cytokines (interleukins 1 and 6)
Hepatic disease

liver and inflammatory cells has been reported in both animal models of tissue injury and hospitalized patients with acute illnesses [18]. Studies of human tissues obtained from patients who died during acute illness showed a decrease in D1 activity and an increase in D3 activity, whereas there was no change or absent D2 activities in liver and skeletal muscles [19–21]. In addition, increases in nondeiodinative pathways such as sulfoconjugation [22] and alanine side chain deamination/decarboxylation [1] have been reported to be increased with the euthyroid sick syndrome. Thus, it has become clear that there are many pathways that all serve to drive down T_3 levels early in the euthyroid sick syndrome.

An extensive review of thyroid hormone metabolism with inflammation and infection by Boelen et al. [23] described different alterations of deiodinase activity in different tissues during acute illness, as summarized in Table 143.2. In a rodent model of acute inflammation, liver D1 expression is decreased, presumably as a result of regulation through thyroid hormone receptor $\beta 1$ (TR$\beta 1$) [23]. Changes in deiodinase expression have also been seen in a pig model of septic shock induced by bacterial endotoxin, lipopolysaccharide (LPS), with decreases in liver and kidney D1 expression and activity and increases in hypothalamic, thyroidal, and liver D3 activity [24].

In the hypothalamus, D2 is thought to be the major contributor of hypothalamic T_3 production. In the rodent model of acute illness, there is an increase in D2 mRNA expression and activity seen in the hypothalamus [25], which is also seen in the mouse model of chronic inflammation [8,23] and among rabbits with chronic illness [26]. The mechanism of this increase of D2 expression and activity is unclear at this time, but it appears independent of change in serum T_3 levels, and the activation of nuclear factor-κB pathway may be involved [23]. On the other hand, hypothalamic D3 activity is unaltered among rabbits with chronic illness [26] and decreased for mice models of both acute and chronic inflammation [23]. The subsequent increase in local hypothalamic T_3 levels may contribute to the decrease in hypothalamic TRH mRNA expression seen with acute illness.

Data from the deiodinase knockout mice model have raised questions regarding the clinical significance of the changes in deiodinase activity with the euthyroid sick syndrome. The illness-induced changes in serum T_4 and T_3 levels were not significantly different between wild-type and TR$\beta 1$ knockout mice, despite differences seen for liver D1 mRNA expression and activity [27]. Similar findings were reported for alterations of liver D3 expression and activity in mouse models [23]. The relative lack of effects of changes in deiodinase expression and activity on serum thyroid hormone levels have also been shown in various deiodinase knockout mice models, as serum T_3 appears preserved even though rT_3 levels are undetectable [27,28].

Alterations of Thyroid Stimulating Hormone Secretion

Serum TSH levels usually remain normal during early phases of acute illness. However, with illness progression, TSH steadily decreases as a result of multiple factors (Table 143.3). These include several medications used for treatment of critical illness, such as dopamine and glucocorticoids, that have a direct inhibitory effect on TSH secretion [29,30]. Elevated endogenous cortisol also plays a role in suppressing TSH, especially during fasting and undernutrition [31]. In addition, D2 activity has been reported to be increased in the pituitary with the euthyroid sick syndrome, increasing local production of T_3 and decreasing TSH synthesis [32–34]. Further, increased production of thyroid hormone metabolites such as 3,5,3′-triiodothyroacetic acid (Triac) during acute illnesses also has a direct inhibitory effect on TSH synthesis.

There is ample evidence of decreased TRH production and secretion leading to a decrease in TSH in the euthyroid sick syndrome [1,23]. Leptin, a hormone encoded by the *ob* gene and secreted by adipocytes, plays a role in balancing energy intake and expenditure. Leptin has been reported to directly regulate TRH production, and leptin and TSH levels are directly related [35,36]. Serum leptin levels decrease during fasting as well as among elderly patients with the euthyroid sick syndrome, leading to subsequent decreases in TSH levels [37]. These changes likely serve as an adaptive mechanism to reduce catabolic process and energy expenditure in the setting of acute illness [37–39]. Increased hypothalamic D2 activity

TABLE 143.2

Tissue-Specific Alterations in Iodothyronine Deiodinases in Illness [14]

Organ	Model	Alterations in deiodinases
Hypothalamus		
Rodent—acute illness		Increased D2 mRNA expression and activity
Mouse—acute inflammation		Decreased D3 activity
Mouse—chronic inflammation		Increased D2 expression; decreased D3 activity
Rabbit—critical illness		Increased D2 expression; unchanged D3 activity
Liver		
Rodent—acute inflammation		Decreased D1 expression; decreased D3 expression
Rodent—chronic inflammation		D1 mRNA expression unaffected; decreased D3 mRNA expression and activity
Muscle		
Rodent—acute inflammation		Increased D2 expression; decreased D3 expression
Mice—chronic inflammation		Increased D2 and D3 mRNA expression and activity
Humans and mice—bacterial sepsis		Decreased D2 expression; unchanged or increased D3 expression
Adipose tissue		
Humans—bacterial sepsis		No change in D1 or D3 activities

TABLE 143.3

Factors That Alter TSH Secretion

Increase	Decrease
Chlorpromazine	Acute and chronic illness
Cimetidine	Adrenergic agonists
Domperidone	Caloric restriction
Dopamine antagonists	Carbamazepine
Haloperidol	Clofibrate
Iodide	Cyproheptadine
Lithium	Dopamine and dopamine agonists
Metoclopramide	Endogenous depression
Sulfapyridine	Glucocorticoids
Radiographic contrast agents	Insulin-like growth factor-1
	Metergoline
	Methysergide
	Opiates
	Phenytoin
	Phentolamine
	Pimozide
	Somatostatin
	Serotonin
	Surgical stress
	Thyroid hormone metabolites

TSH, thyroid stimulating hormone.

as well as increased Triac production also has been reported to directly decrease TSH production, similar to that observed in the pituitary [23].

Some investigators have hypothesized a central role for decreased TRH production in the euthyroid sick syndrome [40]. Further, TRH therapy has been postulated as a therapeutic intervention. Indeed, a trial of exogenous TRH administration in conjunction with growth hormone-releasing petide-2 in 14 patients with prolonged critical illness has been shown to restore the alterations seen in serum thyroid hormone parameters, with subsequent improvement for some of the cardiometabolic parameters such as protein degradation [40].

Alterations of Serum Thyroid Hormone-Binding Proteins

The majority of thyroid hormone is bound to various binding proteins in plasma, primarily TBG as well as transthyretin and albumin. As both acute and prolonged illness are typically accompanied by malnutrition and high catabolic state, serum levels of binding protein are frequently reduced [16]. A rapid decrease in TBG levels has also been seen among postcardiac bypass patients, which may also contribute to the decrease in serum T_3 shortly after cardiac surgery [41].

In addition to decreases in the serum levels of binding proteins, binding of T_4 to TBG is frequently decreased by a variety of factors present with critical illness (Table 143.4) [1]. Certain medications (heparin, furosemide, anti-seizure medications, salicylates) have been implicated in this decrease in binding. In addition, a factor that has the characteristics of unsaturated nonesterified fatty acids has been reported to interfere with TBG binding as well as inhibit T_4 to T_3 conversion [8] and block transport of T_4 into tissue in the euthyroid sick syndrome [8,42,43].

TABLE 143.4

Factors That Alter Binding of T_4 to TBG

Increase binding	Decrease binding
Estrogens	**Drugs**
Methadone	Glucocorticoids
Clofibrate	Androgens
5-Fluorouracil	L-Asparaginase
Heroin	Salicylates
Tamoxifen	Mefenamic acid
Liver disease	Antiseizure medications (phenytoin, Tegretol), raloxifene
Porphyria	Furosemide
HIV infection	Heparin
Inherited	**Systemic factors**
	Inherited
	Acute illness
	Nonesterified free fatty acids

HIV, human immunodeficiency virus.

Alterations of Thyroid Hormone Transporters

Thyroid hormones are transported across the plasma membrane by specific thyroid hormone transporters, most notably those of the monocarboxylate transporter (MCT) and organic anion-transporting polypeptide (OATP) families [44,45]. Of these, MCT8, MCT10, and OATP1C1 have been extensively studied. OATP1C1 has been characterized in rat brain and found to have significant action for transporting T_4 across the blood–brain barrier. It is also found to be regulated, in part, by thyroid hormone levels in the brain [46]. MCT8 is found in cortical regions, striatum, cerebellum, and hypothalamus, and transports both T_4 and T_3, whereas MCT10 preferentially transports T_3 and is expressed in liver, kidney, and muscle [45,47].

There is impaired transport of T_4 into peripheral tissues such as liver and kidney seen with the euthyroid sick syndrome and with starvation, thereby decreasing the availability of substrate for T_3 production in these tissues [48]. Consistent with these observations, liver and muscle MCT8 mRNA expression is decreased among patients with acute illness or acute surgical stress, although MCT10 mRNA expression was not affected. However, there are conflicting data from animal studies showing increased OATP1C1 and MCT10 mRNA expression, while MCT8 mRNA expression did not change in a rabbit model of prolonged illness, contrary to what would be expected given findings seen with the euthyroid sick syndrome and starvation [26]. On the other hand, a more recent study using a pig model of septic shock showed decreases in pituitary, liver, and kidney MCT8 expression [24]. Further studies are needed to better elucidate the underlying mechanisms of altered thyroid hormone transport with the euthyroid sick syndrome.

Alterations of Nuclear Thyroid Hormone Receptors

Thyroid hormone activity is mediated by binding to TRs, with two main isoforms: TRα and TRβ. TRs are ligand-bound transcription factors that regulate transcription of a variety of target genes in various tissues [49]. Concentrations of the receptor isoforms vary by tissues, with TRα predominating in brain, TRβ in liver, and both in cardiac muscles. Animal studies have shown conflicting data regarding changes in TRs with the euthyroid sick syndrome. In a mouse model of acute illness induced by bacterial endotoxin, LPS, a rapid decrease in mRNA for both TRα and TRβ as well as coactivator expression was seen in cardiac tissue [50]. This decrease in TRβ mRNA expression was also seen in heart, liver, and kidney with a LPS-induced pig model of acute septic shock [24]. On the other hand, there was no significant change in the levels of either TRα or TRβ among rabbits in a prolonged illness model [26]. Human studies of patients with liver and renal failure showed increased TRα and TRβ expression in mononuclear cells [51]. These findings were different from that seen for humans with chronic liver disease, where no change in TR expression in hepatic tissues was seen [23]. Meanwhile, adipose tissue from patients with septic shock showed decreased levels of transcription factors for TRβ1, with no significant change in expression for TRα1 and other coactivators or corepressors [23]. The mechanisms for these alterations in TRs remain unclear.

Role of Cytokines for the Pathogenesis of the Sick Euthyroid Syndrome

Cytokines are medium-sized polypeptide hormones secreted by mononuclear cells of the lymphoid system in response to a variety of stimuli, including infection by foreign organisms, invasion by foreign cells, metabolic derangements, and organ system dysfunction [52]. Cytokines have an array of systemic and local actions characteristic of illness, such as fever, prostration, inflammation, and the initiation of wound repair. Cytokine production by lymphoid cells is essential for the development and maintenance of immunity. The actions of cytokines include both autocrine and paracrine effects on cell proliferation and differentiation and on induction of other cytokines. Classes of cytokines include the ILs (1 to 12), interferons (α, β, and γ), TNFs (α and β), and other assorted growth factors. Of these cytokines, TNF-α and several ILs (IL-1, 6, and 10) have been extensively studied for their role in the pathogenesis of the sick euthyroid syndrome [5,11], 53.

TNF-α, IL-1, and IL-6 concentrations are increased with systemic illness and are implicated as mediators of endotoxemia-induced shock, fever, and metabolic acidosis. TNF-α and IL-1 both induce the production of IL-6 and TNF-α also induces IL-1 production [54] and activates nuclear factor-kappa B (NF-κB), which has been shown to inhibit hepatic type 1 5′-deiodinase activity [55]. Serum concentrations of these cytokines have shown to be inversely proportional to serum T_3 concentrations in children (IL-6 and TNF-α [56]); postoperative patients (IL-6 [57]); hospitalized patients, including those with acute myocardial infarction (IL-6 [58–60]); after bone marrow transplantation (IL-6 and TNF-α [61]); and among nursing home patients (TNF-α [62]). However, there have been reports of a lack of correlation between IL-6 and TNF-α after abdominal surgery [63] and with rheumatoid arthritis [64]. The administration of cytokines to animals produces an acute fall in serum T_3 concentrations among rats (TNF-α [65], IL-1 [66,67], IL-6 [68]) and mice (IL-1 [69,70], IL-6 [71]) and shows a direct inhibitory effect on thyroid cells in culture (TNF-α [65,72,73] and IL-1 [73–75]). Variable effects on deiodinase enzymes have been reported, including an inhibition of type 1 5′-deiodinase (IL-1β [76], NF-κB [55]) and inhibition (TNF-α, IL-1, and IL-6 [77]) and induction of type 2 5′-deiodinase (response to LPS [32]).

The administration of TNF-α [78] or IL-6 [79] to healthy human volunteers as well as isolated limb perfusion of cancer patients with TNF-α [80] also produced an acute decrease in both serum T_3 and TSH concentrations and a rise in serum rT_3 concentrations, whereas the administration of an IL-1α receptor antagonist failed to alter the decrease in serum thyroid hormone concentrations observed after infusion of endotoxin in healthy males [81]. In addition, recovery from these changes in thyroid hormone parameters was associated with a rise in TSH [80], similar to the recovery phase of the sick euthyroid syndrome (see later).

Other cytokines have been variably investigated as to their role in the pathogenesis of the sick euthyroid syndrome. Interferon α causes a decrease in serum T_3 and TSH and a rise in serum rT_3 concentrations in both humans [82] and mice [74], and has been shown to directly inhibit thyroidal type 1 5′-deiodinase activity [72,73], whereas interferon γ appears to have no effect on thyroid hormone parameters [83]. An increase in TSH has been observed among patients treated with IL-2 [84]. Soluble cytokine receptors may play a regulatory role for the cytokine cascade by functioning as either carrier proteins or cytokine inhibitors [52,54], and serum T_3 levels were found to be inversely proportional to soluble receptors for TNF-α, IL-1, and IL-2 among hospitalized patients [74].

Oxidative stress, whether or not mediated via cytokines, also may play a role in the development of the sick euthyroid syndrome. *N*-acetylcysteine (a potent intracellular antioxidant) administration to patients with acute myocardial infarction has been shown to prevent changes in T_3 and rT_3 seen during the acute phase of sick euthyroid syndrome, without altering the increased levels of IL-6 [85]. This observation may hint that oxidative stress due to increased reactive oxygen species seen with many disorders may play a role in disruption of deiodinases.

From the data discussed earlier, it is likely that cytokines play a role in the alterations of thyroid hormone metabolism that occur during systemic illness. Although all cytokines examined to date can produce the sick euthyroid syndrome in either humans or rodents when administered at pharmacologic doses, no one cytokine can be singled out as the primary mediator of the syndrome. This is not unexpected, given the diverse interrelationships and cascade nature of the cytokine network. Whether the sick euthyroid syndrome results from activation of the cytokine network or simply represents an endocrine response to systemic illness resulting from the same mediators that trigger the cytokine cascade remains to be determined.

Stages of the Sick Euthyroid Syndrome

As discussed earlier, critical illness causes multiple nonspecific alterations of thyroid hormone concentrations among patients without intrinsic thyroid dysfunction that relate to the severity of the illness [3,86,87]. One author has postulated that sick euthyroid syndrome may be a compensatory mechanism in response to the oxidative stress of acute illness [88]. Irrespective of the underlying cause, these alterations of thyroid hormone parameters represent a continuum of changes that depend on the severity of the illness and that can be categorized into several distinct stages (Fig. 143.3) [1]. The wide spectrum of changes observed often results from the differing points in the course of the illness that the thyroid function tests were obtained. Importantly, these changes are rarely isolated and often associated with alterations of other endocrine systems, such as decreases in serum gonadotropin and sex hormone concentrations [89] and increases in serum adrenocorticotropic hormone and cortisol levels [90]. Thus, the sick euthyroid syndrome should not be viewed as an isolated pathologic event but as part of a coordinated systemic reaction to illness involving both the immune and endocrine systems.

Low T_3 State

Common to all of the abnormalities of thyroid hormone concentrations seen among critically ill patients is a substantial depression of serum T_3 levels, which can occur as early as 24 hours after the onset of illness. Over half of the patients admitted to the medical service will demonstrate depressed serum T_3 concentrations [91,92]. The development of the low T_3 state

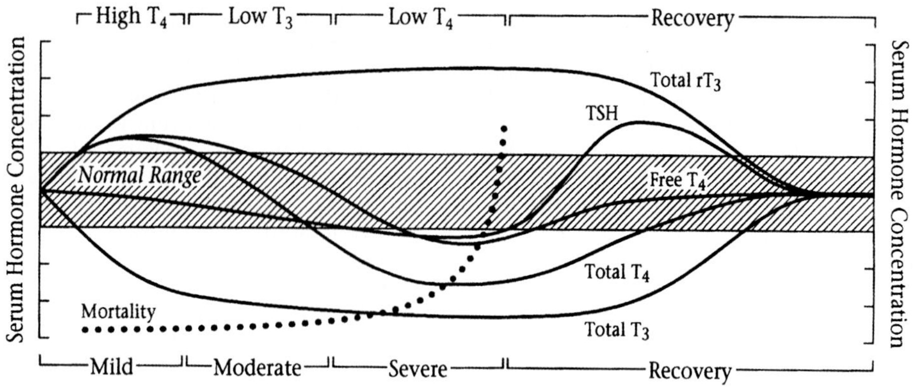

FIGURE 143.3 Alterations in thyroid hormone concentrations with critical illness. Schematic representation of the continuum of changes in serum thyroid hormone levels in patients with nonthyroidal illness. These alterations become more pronounced with increasing severity of the illness and return to the normal range as the illness subsides and the patient recovers. A rapidly rising mortality accompanies the fall in total and free T_4 levels.

arises from the impairment of peripheral T_4 to T_3 conversion through the inhibition of type 1 deiodinase (discussed earlier). This results in the marked reduction in T_3 production and rT_3 degradation [93], thereby leading to the reciprocal changes in serum T_3 and serum rT_3 concentrations. Low T_3 levels are also found in the peripheral tissues [19]. Previously, it was thought that the inhibition of type 1 deiodinase was the sole cause of the low T_3 syndrome by decreasing T_3 production. Recent studies suggest that increased type 3 deiodinase with critical illness increases T_3 disposal, adding to the decrease in serum T_3 levels [18,19]. TR expression is also decreased with acute nonthyroidal illnesses [94], possibly in response to the decrease in tissue T_3 levels.

High T_4 State

Serum T_4 levels may be elevated early in acute illness because of either the acute inhibition of type 1 deiodinase or increased TBG levels. This is seen most often among the elderly and among patients with psychiatric disorders. As the duration of illness increases, nondeiodinative pathways of T_4 degradation increase serum T_4 levels to the normal range [91].

Low T_4 State

As the severity and the duration of the illness increase, serum total T_4 levels decrease into the subnormal range. Contributors to this decrease in serum T_4 levels are (a) a decrease in the binding of T_4 to serum carrier proteins, (b) a decrease in serum TSH levels leading to decreased thyroidal production of T_4, and (c) an increase in nondeiodinative pathways of T_4 metabolism. The decline of serum T_4 levels correlates with prognosis in the ICU, with mortality increasing as serum T_4 levels drop below 4 μg per dL and approaching 80% for patients with serum T_4 levels below 2 μg per dL [95–97]. Despite marked decreases in serum total T_4 and T_3 levels among critically ill patients, their free hormone levels have been reported to be normal or even elevated [98,99], providing a possible explanation for why most patients appear euthyroid despite thyroid hormone levels in the hypothyroid range. Thus, the low T_4 state is unlikely to be a result of a hormone-deficient state and is probably more of a marker of multisystem failure of these critically ill patients.

Recovery State

As acute illness resolves, so do the alterations in thyroid hormone concentrations. This stage may be prolonged and is characterized by modest increases in serum TSH levels [100]. Full recovery, with restoration of thyroid hormone levels to the normal range, may require several weeks [101] or months after hospital discharge [92]. One study reported that 35 of 40 patients with nonthyroidal illness after coronary artery bypass grafting (CABG) were able to regain normal thyroid function within 6 months after surgery [102].

ALTERATIONS OF THYROID FUNCTION IN SPECIFIC CRITICAL ILLNESSES

Caloric Deprivation

Most, if not all, nonthyroidal illness is associated with decreased caloric intake, catabolism, and/or malnutrition. Caloric deprivation is the most common inhibitory factor of type 1 5′-deiodinase [13,103,104]. Serum T_3 levels decrease and rT_3 levels increase within 24 hours of the onset of a fast. The decrease in serum T_3 levels may possibly be an adaptive response in order to preserve the total body protein stores. Indeed, restoring the serum T_3 to normal during starvation results in a marked increase in urinary nitrogen excretion [105]. Thus, the inhibition of T_4 to T_3 conversion during starvation can be viewed as a condition of adaptive hypothyroidism. Further support for the role of caloric deprivation during the development of the sick euthyroid syndrome is the demonstration that early nutritional support for postoperative patients can prevent development of the euthyroid sick syndrome [106]. On the other hand, early feeding within 24 hours of hospitalized burn patients with evidence of the euthyroid sick syndrome, compared to delayed feeding after more than 48 hours, was associated with prevention of the euthyroid sick syndrome development as well as decreased length of stay (Table 143.5) [107]. Recently, a large randomized clinical trial suggested that parenteral nutrition postponed to 1 week after ICU admission had beneficial effects on the rates of complications as well as timing of recovery [108]. Comparison of critically ill patients who received early parenteral nutrition to patients who received parenteral nutrition after 1 week showed a lower level of T_3 and T_3/rT_3 and a higher level of rT_3 in the latter group.

HIV Infection

A unique pattern of changes in circulating thyroid hormone levels is seen among patients with human immunodeficiency virus (HIV) infection and in those with acquired immune deficiency syndrome (AIDS) [109]. A progressive increase in TBG levels is commonly observed, and T_4 levels rarely

TABLE 143.5

Summary of Clinical Trials on the Effects of Treatment of the Sick Euthyroid Syndrome with Thyroid Hormone

Illness	Results of trial
Starvation/undernutrition	Treatment with T_3 results in increased protein breakdown and increased nitrogen excretion in fasting normal and obese patients [105,195,196]
General intensive care unit patients	No benefit of L-T_4 on general medical patients [140], patients with acute renal failure [141], or those undergoing renal transplantation [142] No benefit of T_3 in burn patients [143]
Premature infants	No benefit of L-T_4 on developmental indices of premature infants at 26–28 wk's gestation [155] Possible beneficial effect of L-T_4 on infants of 25–26 wk's gestation but possible deleterious effects on infants of 27–30 wk's gestation [156] No benefit of T_3 [160] Meta-analysis shows no significant effects of thyroid hormone treatment in premature infants [161]
Patients undergoing cardiac surgical procedures	Small studies suggest improved hemodynamic variables with T_3 [171,172] Large trials show no benefit of T_3 in patients undergoing cardiac bypass [173,175,197] Possible improvement in hemodynamic variables and hospital stay with T_3 in children undergoing cardiac surgical procedures [176,177]
Cardiac donors	Variable results—helpful [179,180], no benefit [178,181]—of the effects of T_3 in preserving function of normal hearts in brain dead cardiac donors before transplantation Possible benefits of T_3 in improving function of impaired hearts before transplantation, potentially increasing the pool of organs available for transplantation [178,182] Consensus conferences recommend the use of T_3 as part of the hormonal resuscitation in donors whose cardiac ejection fraction is <45% [180]
Congestive heart failure	Small uncontrolled study suggested that short-term L-T_4 therapy increased cardiac output and functional capacity and decreased systemic vascular resistance [189] Improved hemodynamic variables and neurohumoral profiles with short-term intravenous T_3 infusion, possibly necessitating supraphysiologic concentrations [190,191]

T_3, triiodothyronine; L-T_4, levothyroxine.
Adapted from Sun L, Farwell AP: Euthyroid sick syndrome. *Compr Physiol* 6(2):1071–1080, 2016.

decrease below the normal range. Serum rT_3 levels fail to rise with advancing infections and are only modestly increased in preterminal AIDS patients. Most striking is the observation that serum T_3 levels remain in the normal range despite progression of the HIV infection and are only mildly decreased among critically ill AIDS patients, suggesting that these "inappropriately normal" T_3 levels play a role in the wasting and weight loss seen in the terminal phases of this disease. In contrast to T_4 levels of the sick euthyroid syndrome, it is the decreased serum T_3 levels in AIDS patients admitted to the ICU with *Pneumocystis jirovecii* infections that correlates with increased mortality [110].

Liver Disease

In contrast to the decrease in thyroid hormone levels seen in critically ill patients, individuals suffering from acute and chronic hepatocellular dysfunction often have marked elevations of total T_4 levels similar to those seen in patients with thyrotoxicosis [111]. T_3 levels are also higher than expected with illness and tend to fall late in the course of terminal liver disease. The etiology of these increased thyroid hormone concentrations is the increased discharge of TBG following destruction of hepatocytes. Free hormone measurements remain in the normal range. As with other illnesses, the low T_4 syndrome can be seen among patients with cirrhosis and is associated with increased mortality [112].

Cardiac Disease

Thyroid hormones have profound effects on the cardiovascular system [113]. Cardiac contractility, systolic time intervals, and heart rate are all increased in thyrotoxicosis and decreased in hypothyroidism. Multiple cardiac genes are either positively or negatively altered by thyroid hormone [114,115]. Serum T_4 and T_3 levels fall acutely following myocardial infarction [116], cardiac arrest [117–119], and CABG with and without cardiopulmonary bypass [102,120–123]. A significant inverse relationship between free T_3 and global oxygen consumption has been demonstrated after CABG with and without cardiopulmonary bypass [123]. Nonthyroidal illness syndrome has also been found with a prevalence of 62.2% among patients with stress cardiomyopathy [124]. In contrast to other medical illnesses where serum T_4 levels are correlated with prognosis, serum T_3 concentrations are a negative prognostic factor for patients with congestive heart failure [125,126] and with coronary artery disease [127], raising a question as to what, if any, role thyroid hormones play in acute cardiac injury.

MANAGEMENT OF THE CRITICALLY ILL PATIENT WITH ABNORMAL THYROID FUNCTION TESTS

Evaluation

The identification of the critically ill patient with intrinsic thyroid disease is often difficult and always a diagnostic challenge. The routine screening of an ICU population for the presence of thyroid dysfunction is not recommended because of the high prevalence of abnormal thyroid function tests and low prevalence of true thyroid dysfunction. Whenever possible, it is best to defer evaluation of the thyroid–pituitary axis until the patient has recovered from his or her acute illness. In principle, when thyroid function tests are ordered for a hospitalized patient, it should be with a high clinical index of suspicion for the presence of thyroid dysfunction. For example, thyroid function should be evaluated for the patient admitted to the ICU with tachyarrhythmias when that patient also has a goiter, proptosis, and a tremor. Similarly, the patient with a large pericardial effusion, hypothermia, a goiter, and "hung-up" deep tendon reflexes should suggest the diagnosis of hypothyroidism. In practice, however, thyroid function tests are ordered in the patient with less-specific clinical findings and often present a diagnostic dilemma. Because every test of thyroid hormone function can be altered in the critically ill patient, no single test can definitively rule in or rule out the presence of intrinsic thyroid dysfunction.

Primary Tests

Sensitive Thyrotropin Assays

The development of the sensitive TSH assay has both helped and hindered the evaluation of thyroid function among the critically ill. These new assays have greatly expanded the lower range of the TSH assay, so the typical sensitive TSH assay has a lower limit of detection of 0.01 to 0.03 mU per L, which is 20- to 30-fold lower than the lower limit of the normal range. With this improved sensitivity has come the recognition of an increased frequency of subnormal TSH values among hospitalized patients, indicating that transient abnormalities of TSH secretion are commonplace among those with acute illness. To what degree this TSH dysregulation represents clinically significant alterations of thyroid function is uncertain.

Abnormal thyroid function tests have been reported in 20% to 40% of acutely ill patients, of which >80% have no intrinsic thyroid dysfunction after the resolution of the illness [91,92,128]. In a study of 1,580 hospitalized patients, only 24% of patients with suppressed TSH values (TSH <assay limit of detection) and 50% of patients with TSH values >20 mU per L were found to have thyroid disease [91,92]. More importantly, none of the patients with subnormal but detectable TSH values and only 14% of patients with elevated TSH values <20 mU per L were subsequently diagnosed with intrinsic thyroid dysfunction. The development of sensitive third-generation TSH assays has led to small improvements in discerning between overt hyperthyroidism and nonthyroidal illness [92]. Overall, however, while a normal TSH level has a high predictive value for normal thyroid function, an abnormal TSH value alone is not helpful for the evaluation of thyroid function in the critically ill patient.

Serum T_4 Assays

Measurement of free thyroid hormone concentrations in the patient with nonthyroidal illness is fraught with difficulty [99]. The gold standard of the determination of free hormone levels is by equilibrium dialysis. However, this technique is labor intensive and time consuming and, thus, is rarely used. The most commonly available laboratory tests of thyroid hormone concentrations, the free T_4 index, free T_4, and free T_3, are measured by analog methods, which represent estimates of the free hormone concentration and are therefore subject to inaccuracies [98].

The free T_4 index is determined by multiplying the total T_4 concentration by the T_3- or T_4-resin uptake, which is an inverse estimate of serum TBG concentrations [129]. Recent developments have allowed the measurement of free T_4 levels by the analog method, a less expensive alternative to the free T_4 index [130], but the two tests are likely comparably accurate [131]. In a healthy population, there is a close correlation between the free T_4 index and free T_4 levels. Among critically ill patients, this association is no longer seen, mainly due to difficulties in estimating TBG binding with resin uptake tests. In spite of this, the sensitivity of the free T_4 index in a large study of hospitalized patients was 92.3%, as compared to 90.7% for the sensitive TSH test [92].

Secondary Tests

Serum T_3 and rT_3 Assays

As previously discussed, serum T_3 concentrations are affected to the greatest degree by the alterations in thyroid hormone economy resulting from acute illness. Therefore, there is no indication for the routine measurement of serum T_3 levels in the initial evaluation of thyroid function in the critically ill patient. This test should only be obtained if thyrotoxicosis is clinically suspected in the presence of a suppressed sensitive TSH value and an elevated or high normal free T_4 index or free T_4 determination. Thus, in patients with an elevated free T_4 index or free T_4 and a suppressed TSH, the finding of an elevated serum T_3 concentration will differentiate between thyrotoxicosis and the high T_4 state of the sick euthyroid syndrome. The total T_3 assay is preferable to the free T_3 (analog) assay because of the variability between laboratories with the latter test [129].

Although some investigators have reported that serum rT_3 levels are a significant prognostic indicator of mortality in the ICU [132], rT_3 levels are generally unreliable and should not be used to distinguish between intrinsic thyroid dysfunction and nonthyroidal illness [133].

Serum Thyroid Autoantibodies

Autoantibodies to thyroglobulin and thyroid peroxidase, two intrinsic thyroid proteins, are commonly ordered tests [129]. Although significant titers of either or both of these antibodies indicate the presence of autoimmune thyroid disease, the presence of thyroid autoantibodies alone does not necessarily indicate thyroid dysfunction, as they are present among approximately 12% to 26% of the general population [134]. Thyroid autoantibodies do, however, add to the sensitivity of abnormal TSH and free thyroxine index values for diagnosing known intrinsic thyroid disease [91,92].

Imaging Studies

Imaging studies are rarely essential for the diagnosis of thyroid disorders of the critically ill patient. Occasionally, functional analysis of the thyroid gland using the radioisotope ^{123}I may be useful for the patient with suspected thyrotoxicosis and equivocal laboratory tests. However, these studies are labor intensive and the management of the underlying acute illness often overshadows the benefits of obtaining these studies. Although anatomic studies such as ultrasound, isotopic imaging, computed tomography, and magnetic resonance imaging are useful in the evaluation of thyroid nodules and goiter, these conditions rarely are the cause of acute illness; as such, these studies are not usually helpful for the critically ill patient.

Diagnosis

As indicated, the diagnostic significance of a single abnormal thyroid function test is low. The best single test to screen for thyroid dysfunction is either the free T_4 index or the free T_4, realizing that subtle changes in thyroid function will be missed. However, a reasonable approach to the initial evaluation of the thyroid function in the critically ill patient is to obtain either free T_4 index or free T_4 and TSH measurements in patients with a high clinical suspicion for intrinsic thyroid dysfunction. Assessment of these values in the context of the duration, severity, and stage of illness of the patient will allow the correct diagnosis for most patients. For example, a mildly elevated TSH coupled with a low free T_4 index or free T_4 is more likely to indicate primary hypothyroidism early in an acute illness as opposed to the same values obtained during the recovery phase of the illness. Similarly, the combination of an elevated TSH and low normal free T_4 index or free T_4 is more likely to indicate thyroid dysfunction in the hypothermic, bradycardic patient than the tachycardic, normothermic individual. A rise in TSH during worsening stages of critical illness is likely to be due to thyroid hormone deficiency, so attention should be given to thyroid hormone replacement or titration of thyroid hormone dose in a patient who is already on treatment [135]. If both the free T_4 index or free T_4 and TSH are normal, thyroid dysfunction is effectively eliminated as a significant contributing factor to the clinical picture. If the diagnosis is still unclear, measurement of thyroid antibodies is helpful as a marker of intrinsic thyroid disease and increases the sensitivity of both the free T_4 index or free T_4 and the TSH. Only in the case of a suppressed TSH and a mid-to-high normal free T_4 index or free T_4 is measurement of serum T_3 levels indicated.

Prognosis

Both serum T_4 and serum T_3 concentrations have been associated as negative indicators of prognosis when they are low. As mentioned previously, a direct relationship exists between low serum T_4 levels and poor outcomes among critically ill patients [128]. In acutely ill older patients with nonthyroidal illness syndrome, mortality rate was significantly higher, with an inverse relationship between free T_3 values and death rates [136]. The same relationship was found for burn patients, with free T_3 and TSH levels lower in non-survivors compared to survivors [137]. Among patients on mechanical ventilation, patients with low free T_3 had higher mortality rate and longer duration of mechanical ventilation and ICU length of stay [138]. Addition of free T_3 level to the APACHE II (Acute Physiology and Chronic Health Evaluation II) score has been suggested by some investigators to improve the ability to predict mortality of critically ill adults [139]. In different types of cardiac diseases the prognostic value of low T_3 has been shown, including coronary artery disease and chronic heart failure [125–127]. Whether this is a causal association or simply reflecting multiorgan failure is unclear.

TREATMENT OF THE SICK EUTHYROID SYNDROME WITH THYROID HORMONE

Thyroid Hormone Therapy of General ICU Patients

There are only a few studies examining the use of supplemental thyroid hormone therapy for the critically ill general medical patient. The initial study of medical ICU patients by Brent and Hershman examined the effect of thyroid hormone therapy for patients with serum T_4 levels <5 μg per dL but with no evidence of intrinsic thyroid dysfunction [140]. Either T_4 or placebo was given intravenously on a daily basis, with subsequent normalization of serum T_4 levels by day 5 in the T_4-treated group. There was no difference in mortality between the two groups and the elevation of TSH and serum T_3 concentrations seen during the recovery phase of acute illness was delayed for the T_4-treated group, suggesting that T_4 replacement was detrimental to the restoration of normal pituitary–thyroid regulation. A double-blind study with T_4 for patients with acute renal failure [141] showed that the mortality in the non–T_4-treated control group was significantly less than in the T_4-treated group; however, the mortality of the T_4-treated group was similar to that institution's experience and in historical controls, so a specific deleterious effect of T_4 could not be proved. A follow-up double-blind study with T_4 for patients after renal transplantation by the same group [142] also failed to find any benefit.

One could argue that L-T_4 therapy for the sick euthyroid syndrome would be unlikely to have any effect because of the marked inhibition of T_4 to T_3 conversion, preventing significant increases in serum T_3 concentrations. Addressing this issue, Becker et al. [143] examined the effect of treatment with T_3 among 36 patients with acute burn injuries. Treatment with L-T_3 200 μg daily in four divided doses orally normalized serum T_3 concentrations but resulted in no change in either mortality or basal metabolic rate. Thus, despite the poor prognosis of the general ICU patients with the sick euthyroid syndrome [128], it does not appear that treatment with either L-T_4 or L-T_3 provides significant benefit to these patients.

Thyroid Hormone Therapy in Premature Infants

Fetal thyroid function begins between 8 and 10 weeks' gestation and continues to mature throughout pregnancy [144,145]. Serum T_4 concentrations remain low throughout most of the second trimester and then steadily increase, with a twofold rise occurring between 24 and 34 weeks, at which time serum T_4 levels plateau [146]. There has been a remarkable increase in the number of surviving premature infants, especially in those <30 weeks' gestation. All premature infants have some degree of transient hypothyroxinemia, with serum T_4 concentrations varying directly with gestational age [147]. Approximately 50% of infants born <30 weeks' gestation have serum T_4 concentrations <6.5 μg per dL [146,148,149]. Superimposed on this physiologic hypothyroxinemia often are concurrent illnesses such as respiratory distress syndrome, infections, and malnutrition that contribute to the development of the sick euthyroid syndrome. Severe hypothyroxinemia with concentrations <4 μg per dL were seen in 21% of preterm babies, ranging from 40% at 23 weeks' gestation to 10.2% at 29 weeks [147]. Unlike adults, among whom most abnormalities resulting from clinical hypothyroxinemia are reversible, untreated congenital hypothyroxinemia can potentially have a devastating effect on brain development of the neonate [150-152].

Reuss et al. [153] showed that severe hypothyroxinemia of premature infants of <33 weeks' gestation correlated with a fourfold increase in a diagnosis cerebral palsy. In the study with the longest follow-up, hypothyroxinemia in premature infants of <32 weeks' gestation was associated with a 30% increase in school failure, poor school performance, and need for special education by 9 years of age [154].

The initial double-blind study of T_4 treatment of 23 premature infants of gestational age 26 to 28 weeks with hypothyroxinemia showed no differences between the groups in developmental indices at 1 year of age [155]. In the largest study to date, 200 infants born at 25 to 30 weeks' gestation received either thyroxine or placebo for 6 weeks and neurologic development was assessed periodically up to 24 months [156]. Although there appeared to be a beneficial effect for thyroxine in the very young (25 to 26 weeks' gestation), there also appeared to be a deleterious effect on the infants of 27 to 30 weeks' gestation.

This study group was reevaluated 3 years later at early school age and reported a trend toward a benefit of T_4 supplementation on IQ and behavioral issues at 24/25 weeks' gestation but a significant deleterious effect on IQ and no effect on behavioral issues in those treated at 29 weeks' gestation [157]. Three other studies, two using T_4 [158,159] and one using T_3 [160], failed to show any significant effects of thyroid hormone treatment. Finally, an extensive meta-analysis and review of the literature concluded that thyroid hormone treatment failed to reduce neonatal mortality, improve neurodevelopmental outcome, or reduce the severity of the respiratory distress syndrome [161]. Thus, there is no indication currently for the use of thyroid hormone treatment for premature infants.

Thyroid Hormone Therapy in Cardiac Surgery

Within 15 to 30 minutes after placing the patient on bypass, serum T_4 and T_3 levels fall and serum rT_3 levels increase [162]. These alterations may persist for several days postoperatively [102,120]. These changes also have been observed in off-pump cardiopulmonary bypass [122]. Alterations of thyroid hormone parameters during and after cardiopulmonary bypass have been confirmed by multiple human and animal studies [102,120,121,163-166]. The etiology of these rapid changes in thyroid hormone concentrations remains unclear; one proposal suggests that these alterations may result from enhanced degradation of TBG [41]. Experimental studies of animals have shown that T_3 replacement after cardiopulmonary bypass significantly improves cardiac contractility and left ventricular function and decreases systemic vascular resistance [167-170]. Initial studies on the use of T_3 for humans undergoing cardiac surgery suggested that hormone-treated patients may require less ionotropic support [171] and have improved hemodynamic parameters [172]. However, the clearly demonstrable benefit of T_3 repletion in animals has not been translated into similar benefits for humans undergoing coronary artery bypass in controlled clinical trials.

A large placebo-controlled trial [173] found no effect of T_3 on any postoperative hemodynamic parameters, although a follow-up report of this same patient group suggested a lower incidence in atrial fibrillation for the T_3-treated group after the first postoperative day [174]. However, a lack of effect for T_3 was shown conclusively in a double-blind, placebo-controlled trial [175], as there were no significant differences in the incidence of arrhythmia or the need for ionotropic support or vasodilator drugs in the 24 hours following surgery or in perioperative mortality or morbidity between the T_3 and the placebo groups. Somewhat more promising results have been reported for children undergoing cardiac surgery with improved hemodynamic parameters and a suggestion that the need for intensive postoperative care is decreased with intravenous L-T_3 [176,177]. Further studies may be indicated in this population. However, despite the promise of animal studies, there is no indication for the routine use of T_3 in adult patients undergoing cardiac surgery.

T_3 for Brain-Dead Potential Heart Donors

After brain death occurs, there is a progressive reduction in cardiac contractility, depletion of high-energy phosphates, and accumulation of tissue lactate [178,179]. These changes coincide with a rapid decline in serum T_3 concentrations and an increase in serum rT_3 concentrations within minutes to hours. An initial study of human heart donors [179] showed that T_3 treatment in human heart donors results in hemodynamic stability, a decrease in ionotropic support, and preservation of cardiac function prior to transplantation. At least four other groups have subsequent beneficial effects of T_3 therapy in conjunction with other hormones for organ donors, especially those that are unstable [180]. Two other groups found no significant clinical effects of T_3 over placebo on human donor cardiac function [178,181], provided there was no antecedent cardiac dysfunction of the donor. Another study examined the use of T_3 to resuscitate impaired donor hearts with lower ejection fractions, higher filling pressures, and increased ionotropic support prior to transplantation [178,182]. Subsequently, several consensus conferences held in the United States and Canada have recommended the use of hormonal resuscitation consisting of T_3 (4 μg bolus followed by a 3 μg per hour infusion), vasopressin, methylprednisolone, and insulin for donors whose cardiac ejection fraction is less than 45% in an effort to increase the suitability of hearts for transplantation [180,183]. Thus, T_3 may be beneficial to stabilize or improve cardiac function of donors prior to cardiac transplantation.

Thyroid Hormone Therapy in Congestive Heart Failure

When T_3 and thyroid hormone analogs were initially studied as adjuncts to the treatment of heart failure [184,185], the rationale for the use of these hormones had been as pharmacologic agents for their potential ionotropic properties and interactions with the adrenergic system rather than as hormonal replacement therapy to correct abnormal serum thyroid hormone concentrations. Recently, more attention has been paid to the interactions between the heart and the thyroid hormones for cardiac disease states. For both cardiac failure and hypothyroidism, cardiac output and cardiac contractility is decreased. Decreased serum T_3 concentrations typical of the sick euthyroid syndrome are often observed among patients with congestive heart failure, whereas serum T_4 concentrations remain normal [186–188]. Importantly, the T_3 found in cardiac myocytes appears to come from the circulating T_3 pool rather than from local deiodination of T_4, indicating that the heart may be more responsive to changes in circulating serum T_3 concentrations [114,115]. Consistent with this observation, similar decreases in cardiac genes, including α-myosin heavy chain, SR calcium ATPase, and β_1 adrenergic receptors, have been observed for both hypothyroidism and in heart failure [114,115]. Finally, low T_3 levels have been determined to be a strong predictor of mortality for patients with congestive heart failure [125,126]. These observations have led several investigators to examine the role of thyroid hormone treatment for patients with congestive heart failure.

An initial uncontrolled study examined the effect of oral T_4 therapy on 20 patients with dilated cardiomyopathy [189]. Cardiac output and functional capacity was increased and systemic vascular resistance decreased. Hamilton et al. [190] examined the effect of a supraphysiologic intravenous infusion of T_3 on cardiac function for patients with New York Heart Association (NYHA) Class III or IV heart failure. Cardiac output increased and systemic vascular resistance decreased without any untoward effects. More recently, Pingitore et al. [191] randomized 20 patients with NYHA Class III or less heart failure to a 3-day intravenous infusion of T_3 or placebo. During the first day of the T_3 infusion, serum T_3 levels were supraphysiologic and then declined to the high normal range on day 2 and 3. The T_3 infusion produced a significant improvement in the neurohumoral profile, with a decrease in serum noradrenaline, N-terminal pro-B-type natriuretic peptide, and aldosterone concentrations, and an increase in left ventricular end diastolic volume. As above normal serum T_3 concentrations were achieved during all or part of these two studies, there is a question of whether the beneficial effects of T_3 are a pharmacologic effect rather than a physiologic one. There are currently no studies on the long-term use of T_3 for the treatment of congestive heart failure. However, as with children undergoing cardiac surgery, more studies may be indicated in this patient population.

Thyroid Hormone Therapy for the Hypothyroid Patient in the Intensive Care Unit

This chapter has discussed the evaluation and management of patients without intrinsic thyroid dysfunction who present with abnormal thyroid hormone parameters as a result of nonthyroidal illness. However, thyroid hormone therapy is needed when the hypothyroid patient presents to the ICU. By definition, the nonthyroidal illness syndrome excludes patients with intrinsic thyroid dysfunction; however, all of the changes in TSH secretion, thyroid hormone metabolism, and thyroid-binding proteins discussed earlier also occur in the hypothyroid patient. As such, the same caveats toward measuring thyroid hormone parameters exist. Most importantly, an admission to the ICU is not the time to determine the adequacy of thyroid hormone replacement in a hypothyroid patient on a previously stable outpatient regimen.

Hypothyroid patients should be continued on their outpatient L-T_4 dose. Oral L-T_4 is the preferred method for replacing thyroid hormone in a hypothyroid patient. Because of the long half-life of about 7 days of L-T_4, the L-T_4 dose can be held for 1 to 2 days if the oral route is unavailable. If oral therapy cannot be resumed within 3 days, intravenous L-T_4 should be administered. Because less than 75% of an oral dose of L-T_4 is absorbed, the intravenous L-T_4 dose should be ~75% less than the oral dose. Neither oral nor intravenous L-T_3 is indicated in the hypothyroid patient in the absence of myxedema coma.

If hypothyroidism is diagnosed in the ICU setting and initiation of thyroid hormone replacement is required, special consideration should be given to patients with coronary artery disease. In patients with significant preexisting coronary artery disease, starting thyroid hormone may aggravate angina. It is recommended that the initial dose of L-T_4 should not exceed 25 μg for those with known ischemic heart disease and 50 μg for patients aged 65 years or older without such a preexisting diagnosis.

The oral dose of L-T_4 may differ in the ICU setting due to pharmacologic agents or gastrointestinal conditions that may decrease the absorption of L-T_4. Patients with jejunoileal bypass surgery, bowel resection, malabsorptive disorders (like celiac disease), and conditions that impair gastric acidity may need adjustment in the dose of L-T_4. L-T_4 should not be administered within 2 to 3 hours of calcium carbonate, bile acid sequestrants, ferrous sulfate, phosphate binders, sucralfate, and aluminum-containing antacids as they may interfere with the absorption of L-T_4. Also by their effect of decreasing gastric acidity, proton pump inhibitors, if given for a long period, may decrease the absorption of L-T_4.

SUMMARY

In summary, the spectrum of alterations of thyroid hormone concentrations and regulation seen among critically ill patients is the result of a coordinated systemic reaction to illness. The question of whether the sick euthyroid syndrome of critically ill patients represents pathologic alterations of thyroid function that negatively impacts these patients or simply reflects multisystem failure (i.e., respiratory, cardiac, renal, hepatic failure) that occurs among critically ill patients is still debatable [86,192–194]. The interpretation of thyroid function tests of the ICU patient and the identification of patients with intrinsic thyroid dysfunction is often difficult and must take into consideration both the clinical assessment of the patient and the duration and severity of the illness. Whenever possible, it is best to defer the evaluation of thyroid function until the patient has recovered from the critical illness. Thyroid hormone replacement therapy has not been shown to be of benefit in the vast majority of these patients in the published studies to date (Table 143.4 [86]). At the present time, in the absence of any clinical evidence of hypothyroidism, there does not appear to be any compelling evidence for the use of thyroid hormone therapy for any patient with decreased thyroid hormone parameters due to the sick euthyroid syndrome.

References

1. Haddady S, Farwell AP: Sick euthyroid syndrome in the intensive care unit, in Irwin RS, Rippe JM (eds): *Intensive Care Medicine.* Philadelphia, PA, Lippincott Williams & Wilkins, 2012, pp 1182–1194.
2. Mebis L, Debaveye Y, Visser TJ, et al: Changes within the thyroid axis during the course of critical illness. *Endocrinol Metab Clin North Am* 35(4):807–821, 2006.
3. Burman KD, Wartofsky L: Thyroid function in the intensive care unit setting. *Crit Care Clin* 17(1):43–57, 2001.
4. DeGroot LJ: "Non-thyroidal illness syndrome" is functional central hypothyroidism, and if severe, hormone replacement is appropriate in light of present knowledge. *J Endocrinol Invest* 26(12):1163–1170, 2003.
5. Farwell AP: Sick euthyroid syndrome. *J Intensive Care Med* 12:249–260, 1997.
6. Langton JE, Brent GA: Nonthyroidal illness syndrome: evaluation of thyroid function in sick patients. *Endocrinol Metab Clin North Am* 31(1):159–172, 2002.
7. Sun L, Farwell AP: Euthyroid sick syndrome. *Compr Physiol* 6(2):1071–1080, 2016.
8. Farwell AP: Nonthyroidal illness syndrome. *Curr Opin Endocrinol Diabetes Obes* 20:478–484, 2013.
9. Brierre S, Kumari R, Deboisblanc B: The endocrine system during sepsis. *Am J Med Sci* 328(4):238–247, 2004.
10. Hamrahian AH, Oseni TS, Arafah BM: Measurements of serum free cortisol in critically ill patients. *N Engl J Med* 350(16):1629–1638, 2004.
11. Papanicolaou DA: Euthyroid sick syndrome and the role of cytokines. *Rev Endocr Metab Disord* 1(1–2):43–48, 2000.
12. Larsen PR, Silva JE, Kaplan MM: Relationships between circulating and intracellular thyroid hormones: physiological and clinical implications. *Endocr Rev* 2(1):87–102, 1981.
13. Bianco AC, Larsen PR: Intracellular pathways of iodothyronine metabolism, in Braverman LE, Utiger RD (eds): *Werner and Ingbar's The Thyroid.* Philadelphia, PA, Lippincott Williams and Wilkins, 2013, pp 103–126.
14. Yen PM: Physiological and molecular basis of thyroid hormone action. *Physiol Rev* 81(3):1097–1142, 2001.
15. Zimmermann MB: Iodine deficiency. *Endocr Rev* 30(4):376–408, 2009.
16. Benvenga S: Thyroid hormone transport proteins and the physiology of hormone binding, in Braverman LE, Utiger RD (eds): *Werner and Ingbar's The Thyroid: A Fundamental and Clinical Text.* Philadelphia, PA, Lippincott Williams & Wilkins, 2013, pp 93–102.
17. Palha JA: Transthyretin as a thyroid hormone carrier: function revisited. *Clin Chem Lab Med* 40(12):1292–1300, 2002.
18. Huang SA, Bianco AC: Reawakened interest in type III iodothyronine deiodinase in critical illness and injury. *Nat Clin Pract Endocrinol Metab* 4(3):148–155, 2008.
19. Peeters RP, van der Geyten S, Wouters PJ, et al: Tissue thyroid hormone levels in critical illness. *J Clin Endocrinol Metab* 90(12):6498–6507, 2005.
20. Mebis L, Langouche L, Visser TJ, et al: The type II iodothyronine deiodinase is up-regulated in skeletal muscle during prolonged critical illness. *J Clin Endocrinol Metab* 92(8):3330–3333, 2007.
21. Heemstra KA, Soeters MR, Fliers E, et al: Type 2 iodothyronine deiodinases in skeletal muscle: effects of hypothyroidism and fasting. *J Clin Endocrinol Metab* 94:2144–2150, 2009.
22. Chopra IJ, Santini F, Wu SY, et al: The role of sulfation and de-sulfation in thyroid hormone metabolism, in Wu S, Visser TS, (eds): *Thyroid Hormone Metabolism: Molecular Biology and Alternate Pathways.* Moca Raton, CRC Press, 1994, pp 119–138.
23. Boelen A, Kwakkel J, Fliers E: Beyond low plasma T3: local thyroid hormone metabolism during inflammation and infection. *Endocr Rev* 32:670–693, 2011.
24. Castro I, Quisenberry L, Calvo R-M, et al: Septic shock non-thyroidal illness syndrome causes hypothyroidism and conditions for reduced sensitivity to thyroid hormone. *J Mol Endocrinol* 50:255–266, 2013.
25. Coppola A, Liu Z-W, Andrews ZB, et al: A central Thermogenic-like mechanism in feeding regulation: an interplay between arcuate nucleus T3 and UCP2. *Cell Metab* 5:21–33, 2007.
26. Mebis L, Debaveye Y, Ellger B, et al: Changes in the central component of the hypothalamus-pituitary-thyroid axis in a rabbit model of prolonged critical illness. *Crit Care* 13(5):R147, 2009.
27. Galton VA, Schneider MJ, Clark AS, et al: Life without thyroxine to 3,5,3'-triiodothyronine conversion: studies in mice devoid of the 5'-deiodinases. *Endocrinology* 150:2957–2963, 2009.
28. St Germain DL, Galton VA, Hernandez A: Minireview: defining the roles of the iodothyronine deiodinases: current concepts and challenges. *Endocrinology* 150:1097–1107, 2009.
29. Van den Berghe G, de Zegher F, Lauwers P, et al: Dopamine and the sick euthyroid syndrome in critical illness. *Clin Endocrinol* 41:731–737, 1994.
30. Boonen E, Van den Berghe G: Endocrine responses to critical illness: novel insights and therapeutic implications. *J Clin Endocrinol Metab* 99:1569–1582, 2014.
31. Samuels MH, McDaniel PA: Thyrotropin levels during hydrocortisone infusions that mimic fasting-induced conrtisol elevations: a clinical research center study. *J Clin Endocrinol Metab* 82(11):3700–3704, 1997.

32. Fekete C, Gereben B, Doleschall M, et al: Lipopolysaccharide induces type 2 iodothyronine deiodinase in the mediobasal hypothalamus: implications for the nonthyroidal illness syndrome. *Endocrinology* 145:1649–1655, 2004.
33. Fekete C, Lechan RM: Negative feedback regulation of hypophysiotropic thyrotropin-releasing hormone (TRH) synthesizing neurons: role of neuronal afferents and type 2 deiodinase. *Front Neuroendocrinol* 28:97–114, 2007.
34. Lechan RM, Fekete C: Role of thyroid hormone deiodination in the hypothalamus. *Thyroid* 15:883–897, 2005.
35. Boelen A, Wiersinga WM, Fliers E: Fasting-induced changes in the hypothalamus-pituitary-thyroid axis. *Thyroid* 18:123–129, 2008.
36. Mullur R, Liu Y-Y, Brent GA: Thyroid hormone regulation of metabolism. *Physiol Rev* 94:355–382, 2014.
37. Corsonello A, Buemi M, Artemisia A, et al: Plasma leptin concentrations in relation to sick euthyroid syndrome in elderly patients with nonthyroidal illnesses. *Gerontology* 46(2):64–70, 2000.
38. Warner MH, Beckett GJ: Mechanisms behind the non-thyroidal illness syndrome: an update. *J Endocrinol* 205(1):1–13, 2010.
39. Van der Berghe G: Non-thyroidal illness in the ICU: a syndrome with different faces. *Thyroid* 24:1456–1465, 2014.
40. Van den Berghe G, Wouters P, Weekers F, et al: Reactivation of pituitary hormone release and metabolic improvement by infusion of growth hormone-releasing peptide and thyrotropin-releasing hormone in patients with protracted critical illness. *J Clin Endocrinol Metab* 84:1311–1323, 1999.
41. Afandi B, Schussler GC, Arafeh AH, et al: Selective consumption of thyroxine-binding globulin during cardiac bypass surgery. *Metabolism* 49(2):270–274, 2000.
42. Lim CF, Docter R, Visser TJ, et al: Inhibition of thyroxine transport into cultured rat hepatocytes by serum of nonuremic critically ill patients: effects of bilirubin and non-esterified fatty acids. *J Clin Endocrinol Metab* 76:1165–1172, 1993.
43. Stockigt JR, Lim CF: Medications that distort in vitro tests of thyroid function, with particular reference to estimates of serum free thyroxine. *Best Pract Res Clin Endocrinol Metab* 23(6):753–767, 2009.
44. Van der Deure WM, Peeters RP, Visser TJ: Molecular aspects of thyroid hormone transporters, including MCT8, MCT10, and OATPs, and the effects of genetic variation in these transporters. *J Mol Endocrinol* 44:1–11, 2010.
45. Visser WE, Friesema EC, Visser TJ: Minireviewe: thyroid hormone transporters: the knowns and the unknowns. *Mol Endocrinol* 25:1–14, 2011.
46. Sugiyama D, Kusahara H, Taniguchi H, et al: Functional characterization of rat brain-specific organic anion transporter (Oatp14) at the blood-brain barrier high affinity transporter for thyroxine. *J Biol Chem* 278:43489–43495, 2003.
47. Heuer H, Maier MK, Iden S, et al: The monocarboxylate transporter 8 linked to human psychomotor retardation is highly expressed in thyroid hormone-sensitive neuron populations. *Endocrinology* 146:1701–1706, 2005.
48. Hennemann G, Krenning EP: The kinetics of thyroid hormone transporters and their role in non-thyroidal illness and starvation. *Best Pract Res Clin Endocrinol Metab* 21(2):323–338, 2007.
49. Oetting A, Yen PM: New insights into thyroid hormone action. *Best Pract Res Clin Endocrinol Metab* 21:193–208, 2007.
50. Feingold K, Kim MS, Shigenaga J, et al: Altered expression of nuclear hormone receptors and coactivators in mouse heart during the acute-phase response. *Am J Physiol Endocrinol Metab* 286:E201–E207, 2007.
51. Williams GR, Franklyn JA, Neuberger JM, et al: Thyroid hormone receptor expression in the "sick euthyroid" syndrome. *Lancet* 2:1477–1481, 1989.
52. Charo IF, Ransohoff RM: The many roles of chemokines and chemokine receptors in inflammation. *N Engl J Med* 354(6):610–621, 2006.
53. Nylen ES, Seam N, Khosla R, et al: Endocrine markers of severity and prognosis in critical illness. *Crit Care Clin* 22(1):161–179, viii, 2006.
54. Rees RC: Cytokines as biological response modifiers. *Clin Pathol* 45:93–98, 1992.
55. Nagaya T, Fujieda M, Otsuka G, et al: A potential role of activated NF-kappa B in the pathogenesis of euthyroid sick syndrome. *J Clin Invest* 106(3):393–402, 2000.
56. Hashimoto H, Igarashi N, Yachie A, et al: The relationship between serum levels of interleukin-6 and thyroid hormone in children with acute respiratory infection. *J Clin Endocrinol Metab* 78:288–291, 1994.
57. Murai H, Murakami S, Ishida K, et al: Elevated serum interleukin-6 and decreased thyroid hormone levels in postoperative patients and effects of Il-6 on thyroid cell function in vitro. *Thyroid* 6:601–606, 1996.
58. Boelen A, Platvoet-Ter Schiphorst MC, Wiersinga WM: Association between serum interleukin-6 and serum 3,5,3'-triiodothyronine in non-thyroidal illness. *J Clin Endocrinol Metab* 77:1695–1699, 1993.
59. Kimura T, Kanda T, Kotajima N, et al: Involvement of circulating interleukin-6 and its receptor in the development of euthyroid sick syndrome in patients with acute myocardial infarction. *Eur J Endocrinol* 143(2):179–184, 2000.
60. Kimur T, Kotajima N, Kanda T, et al: Correlation of circulating interleukin-10 with thyroid hormone in acute myocardial infarction. *Res Commun Mol Pathol Pharmacol* 110(1–2):53–58, 2001.
61. Lee WY, Kang MI, Oh KW, et al: Relationship between circulating cytokine levels and thyroid function following bone marrow transplantation. *Bone Marrow Transplant* 33(1):93–98, 2004.
62. Mooradian AD, Reed RL, Osterweil D, et al: Decreased serum triiodothyronine is associated with increased concentrations of tumor necrosis factor. *J Clin Endocrinol Metab* 71:1239–1242, 1990
63. Michalaki M, Vagenakis AG, Makri M, et al: Dissociation of the early decline in serum T_3 concentration and serum IL-6 rise and TNFalpha in nonthyroidal illness syndrome induced by abdominal surgery. *J Clin Endocrinol Metab* 86(9):4198–4205, 2001.
64. Wellby ML, Kennedy JA, Pile K, et al: Serum interleukin-6 and thyroid hormones in rheumatoid arthritis. *Metabolism* 50(4):463–467, 2001.
65. Pang X-P, Hershman JM, Mirell CJ, et al: Impairment of hypothalamic-thyroid function in rats treated with human recombinant tumor necrosis factor a. *Endocrinology* 125:76–84, 1989.
66. Dubuis JM, Dayer JM, Siegrist-Kaiser CA, et al: Human recombinant interleukin-1b decreases plasma thyroid hormone and thyroid stimulating hormone levels in rats. *Endocrinology* 123:2175–2181, 1988.
67. Hermus RM, Sweep CG, van der Meet MJ, et al: Continuous infusion of interleukin-1b induces an nonthyroidal illness syndrome in the rat. *Endocrinology* 131:2139–2146, 1992.
68. Bartalena L, Grasso L, Brogioni S, et al: Interleukin 6 effects on the pituitary-thyroid axis in the rat. *Eur J Endocrinol* 131:302–306, 1994.
69. Enomoto T, Sugawa H, Kosugi S, et al: Prolonged effects of recombinant human interleukin-1 a on mouse thyroid function. *Endocrinology* 127:2322–2327, 1990.
70. Fujii T, Sato K, Ozawa M, et al: Effect of Interleukin-1 (Il-1) on thyroid hormone metabolism in mice: stimulation by Il-1 of iodothyronine 5'-deiodinating activity (type I) in the liver. *Endocrinology* 124:167–174, 1989.
71. Boelen A, Platvoet MC, Wiersinga WM: Systemic and local illness in interleukin-6 knock-out mice: the role of Il-6 in the sick euthyroid syndrome. *J Endocrinol Invest* 19:S79, 1996.
72. Tang K-T, Braverman LE, De Vito WJ: Tumor necrosis factor-a and interferon-g modulate gene expression of type I 5′-deiodinase, thyroid peroxidase and thyroglobulin in FRTL-5 rat thyroid cells. *Endocrinology* 136:881–888, 1995.
73. Pekary AE, Berg L, Santini F, et al: Cytokines modulate type I iodothyronine deiodinase mRNA levels and enzyme activity in FRTL-5 rat thyroid cells. *Mol Cell Endocrinol* 101:R31–R35, 1994.
74. Boelen A, Platvoet-ter Schiphorst MC, Bakker O, et al: The role of cytokines in the lipopolysaccharide-induced sick euthyroid syndrome in mice. *J Endocrinol* 146:475–483, 1995.
75. Rasmussen AK, Bendtzen K, Feldt-Rasmussen U: Thyrocyte-interleukin-1 interactions. *Exp Clin Endocrinol Diabetes* 108(2):67–71, 2000.
76. Jakobs TC, Mentrup B, Schmutzler C, et al: Proinflammatory cytokines inhibit the expression and function of human type I 5′-deiodinase in HepG2 hepatocarcinoma cells. *Eur J Endocrinol* 146(4):559–566, 2002.
77. Molnar I, Czirjak L: Euthyroid sick syndrome and inhibitory effect of sera on the activity of thyroid 5'-deiodinase in systemic sclerosis. *Clin Exp Rheumatol* 18(6):719–724, 2000.
78. van der Poll F, Romijn JA, Endert E, et al: Tumor necrosis factor: a putative mediator of the sick euthyroid syndrome in man. *J Clin Endocrinol Metab* 71:1567–1572, 1990.
79. Stouthard JM, van der Poll T, Endert E, et al: Effects of acute and chronic interleukin-6 administration on thyroid hormone metabolism in humans. *J Clin Endocrinol Metab* 79:1342–1346, 1994.
80. Feelders RA, Swaak AJ, Romijn JA, et al: Characteristics of recovery from the euthyroid sick syndrome induced by tumor necrosis factor alpha in cancer patients. *Metabolism* 48(3):324–329, 1999.
81. van der Poll T, Van Zee KJ, Endert E, et al: Interleukin-1 receptor blockade does not affect endotoxin-induced changes in plasma thyroid hormone and thyrotropin concentrations in man. *J Clin Endocrinol Metab* 80:1341–1346, 1995.
82. Corssmit EP, Heyligenberg R, Endert E, et al: Acute effects of interferon-a administration on thyroid hormone metabolism in healthy men. *J Clin Endocrinol Metab* 80:3140–3144, 1995.
83. de Metz J, Romijn JA, Endert E, et al: Administration of interferon-gamma in healthy subjects does not modulate thyroid hormone metabolism. *Thyroid* 10(1):87–91, 2000.
84. Witzke O, Winterhagen T, Saller B, et al: Transient stimulatory effects on pituitary-thyroid axis in patients treated with interleukin-2. *Thyroid* 11(7):665–670, 2001.
85. Vidart J, Wajner SM, Leite RS, et al: N-Acetylcystein administration prevents nonthyroidal illness syndrome in patients with acute myocardial infarction: a randomized clinical trial. *J Clin Endocrinol Metab* 99(12):4537–4545, 2014.
86. Farwell A: Thyroid hormone therapy is not indicated in the majority of patients with the sick euthyroid syndrome. *Endocr Pract* 14:1180–1187, 2008.
87. DeGroot LJ: Dangerous dogmas in medicine: the nonthyroidal illness syndrome. *J Clin Endocrinol Metab* 84(1):151–164, 1999.
88. Selvaraj N, Bobby Z, Sridhar MG: Is euthyroid sick syndrome a defensive mechanism against oxidative stress? *Med Hypotheses* 71(3):404–405, 2008.
89. Woolf PD, Hamill RW, McDonald JV, et al: Transient hypogonadism caused by critical illness. *J Clin Endocrinol Metab* 60(3):444–450, 1985.
90. Parker LN, Levin ER, Lifrak ET: Evidence for adrenocortical adaptation to severe illness. *J Clin Endocrinol Metab* 60(5):947–952, 1985.
91. Spencer CA: Clinical utility and cost-effectiveness of sensitive thyrotropin assays in ambulatory and hospitalized patients. *Mayo Clin Proc* 63(12):1214–1222, 1988.
92. Spencer C, Elgen A, Shen D, et al: Specificity of sensitive assays of thyrotropin (TSH) used to screen for thyroid disease in hospitalized patients. *Clin Chem* 33(8):1391–1396, 1987.
93. Rodriguez-Perez A, Palos-Paz F, Kaptein E, et al: Identification of molecular mechanisms related to nonthyroidal illness syndrome in skeletal muscle and adipose tissue from patients with septic shock. *Clin Endocrinol (Oxf)* 68(5):821–827, 2008.
94. Beigneux AP, Moser AH, Shigenaga JK, et al: Sick euthyroid syndrome is associated with decreased TR expression and DNA binding in mouse liver. *Am J Physiol Endocrinol Metab* 284(1):E228–E236, 2003.

95. Kaptein EM, Weiner JM, Robinson WJ, et al: Relationship of altered thyroid hormone indices to survival in nonthyroidal illness. *Clin Endocrinol (Oxf)* 16:565–574, 1982.
96. Slag MF, Morley JE, Elson MK, et al: Hypothyroxinemia in critically ill patients as a predictor of high mortality. *JAMA* 245:43–45, 1981.
97. Maldonado LS, Murata GH, Hershman JM, et al: Do thyroid function tests independently predict survival in the critically ill? *Thyroid* 2(2):119–123, 1992.
98. Nelson JC, Weiss RM: The effect of serum dilution on free thyroxine concentration in the low T_4 syndrome of nonthyroidal illness. *J Clin Endocrinol Metab* 61:239–246, 1985.
99. Chopra IJ: Simultaneous measurement of free thyroxine and free 3,5,3'-triiodothyronine in undiluted serum by direct equilibrium dialysis/radioimmunoassay: evidence that free triiodothyronine and free thyroxine are normal in many patients with the low triiodothyronine syndrome. *Thyroid* 8(3):249–257, 1998.
100. Hamblin S, Dyer SA, Mohr VS, et al: Relationship between thyrotropin and thyroxine changes during recovery from severe hypothyroxinemia of critical illness. *J Clin Endocrinol Metab* 62:717–722, 1986.
101. Iglesias P, Munoz A, Prado F, et al: Alterations in thyroid function tests in aged hospitalized patients: prevalence, aetiology and clinical outcome. *Clin Endocrinol (Oxf)* 70(6):961–967, 2009.
102. Cerillo AG, Storti S, Mariani M, et al: The non-thyroidal illness syndrome after coronary artery bypass grafting: a 6-month follow-up study. *Clin Chem Lab Med* 43(3):289–293, 2005.
103. Douyon L, Schteingart DE: Effect of obesity and starvation on thyroid hormone, growth hormone, and cortisol secretion. *Endocrinol Metab Clin North Am* 31(1):173–189, 2002.
104. Visser TJ, Lamberts SW, Wilson JH, et al: Serum thyroid hormone concentrations during prolonged reduction of dietary intake. *Metabolism* 27(4):405–409, 1978.
105. Gardner DF, Kaplan MM, Stanley CA, et al: Effect of tri-iodothyronine replacement on the metabolic and pituitary responses to starvation. *N Engl J Med* 300(11):579–584, 1979.
106. Richmond DA, Molitch ME, O'Donnell TF: Altered thyroid hormone levels in bacterial sepsis: the role of nutritional adequacy. *Metabolism* 29:936–942, 1980.
107. Perez-Guisado J, De Haro-Padilla JM, Rioja LF, et al: The potential association of later initiation of oral/enteral nutrition on euthyroid sick syndrome in burn patients. *Int J Endocrinol* 707360, 2013, 2013.
108. Langouche L, Vander Perre S, Marques M, et al: Impact of early nutrition restriction during critical illness on the non-thyroidal illness syndrome and its releation with outcome: a randomized, controlled clinical study. *J Clin Endocrinol Metab* 98(3):1006–1013, 2013.
109. Koutkia P, Mylonakis E, Lewis RM: Human immunodeficiency virus infection and the thyroid. *Thyroid* 12(7):577–582, 2002.
110. Fried JC, LoPresti JS, Micon M, et al: Serum triiodothyronine values: prognostic indicators of acute mortality due to *Pneumocystis carinii* pneumonia associated with the acquired immunodeficiency syndrome. *Arch Intern Med* 150:406–409, 1990.
111. Yamanaka T, Ido K, Kimura K, et al: Serum levels of thyroid hormones in liver diseases. *Clinica Chim Acta* 101:45–55, 1980.
112. Caregaro L, Alberino F, Amodio P, et al: Nutritional and prognostic significance of serum hypothyroxinemia in hospitalized patients with liver cirrhosis. *J Hepatol* 28(1):115–121, 1998.
113. Klein I, Danzi S: Thyroid disease and the heart. *Circulation* 116(15):1725–1735, 2007.
114. Danzi S, Klein I: Thyroid hormone-regulated cardiac gene expression and cardiovascular disease. *Thyroid* 12(6):467–472, 2002.
115. Klein I, Ojamaa K: Thyroid hormone and the cardiovascular system. *N Engl J Med* 344(7):501–509, 2001.
116. Wiersinga WM, Lie KI, Touber JL: Thyroid hormones in acute myocardial infarction. *Clin Endocrinol (Oxf)* 14:367–374, 1984.
117. Worstman J, Premachandra BN, Chopra IJ, et al: Hypothyroxinemia in cardiac arrest. *Arch Intern Med* 147:245–248, 1987.
118. Longstreth WT Jr, Manowitz NR, DeGroot LJ, et al: Plasma thyroid hormone profiles immediately following out-of-hospital cardiac arrest. *Thyroid* 6:649–653, 1996.
119. Iltumur K, Olmez G, Ariturk Z, et al: Clinical investigation: thyroid function test abnormalities in cardiac arrest associated with acute coronary syndrome. *Crit Care* 9(4):R416–R424, 2005.
120. Reinhardt W, Mocker V, Jockenhovel F, et al: Influence of coronary artery bypass surgery on thyroid hormone parameters. *Horm Res* 47:1–8, 1997.
121. Holland FW, Brown PS, Weintraub BD, et al: Cardiopulmonary bypass and thyroid function: a euthyroid sick syndrome. *Ann Thorac Surg* 52:46–50, 1991.
122. Cerillo AG, Sabatino L, Bevilacqua S, et al: Nonthyroidal illness syndrome in off-pump coronary artery bypass grafting. *Ann Thorac Surg* 75(1):82–87, 2003.
123. Velissaris T, Tang AT, Wood PJ, et al: Thyroid function during coronary surgery with and without cardiopulmonary bypass. *Eur J Cardiothorac Surg* 36(1):148–154, 2009.
124. Lee SJ, Kang JG, Ryu OH, et al: The relationship of thyroid hormone status with myocardial function in stress cardiomyopathy. *Eur J Endocrinol* 160(5):799–806, 2009.
125. Iervasi G, Pingitore A, Landi P, et al: Low-T_3 syndrome: a strong prognostic predictor of death in patients with heart disease. *Circulation* 107(5):708–713, 2003.
126. Pingitore A, Landi P, Taddei MC, et al: Triiodothyronine levels for risk stratification of patients with chronic heart failure. *Am J Med* 118(2):132–136, 2005.
127. Coceani M, Iervasi G, et al: Thyroid hormone and coronary artery disease: from clinical correlations to prognostic implications. *Clin Cardiol* 32(7):380–385, 2009.
128. Plikat K, Langgartner J, Buettner R, et al: Frequency and outcome of patients with nonthyroidal illness syndrome in a medical intensive care unit. *Metabolism* 56(2):239–244, 2007.
129. Baloch Z, Carayon P, Conte-Devolx B, et al: Laboratory medicine practice guidelines. Laboratory support for the diagnosis and monitoring of thyroid disease. *Thyroid* 13(1):3–126, 2003.
130. Midgley JE: Direct and indirect free thyroxine assay methods: theory and practice. *Clin Chem* 47(8):1353–1363, 2001.
131. Liewendahl K, Mahonen H, Tikanoja S, et al: Performance of direct equilibrium dialysis and analogue-type free thyroid hormone assays, and an immunoradiometric TSH method in patients with thyroid dysfunction. *Scand J Clin Lab Invest* 47(5):421–428, 1987.
132. Peeters RP, Wouters PJ, van Toor H, et al: Serum 3,3',5'-triiodothyronine (rT_3) and 3,5,3'-triiodothyronine/rT_3 are prognostic markers in critically ill patients and are associated with postmortem tissue deiodinase activities. *J Clin Endocrinol Metab* 90(8):4559–4565, 2005.
133. Burmeister LA: Reverse T_3 does not reliably differentiate hypothyroid sick syndrome from euthyroid sick syndrome. *Thyroid* 5(6):435–441, 1995.
134. Prummel MF, Wiersinga WM: Thyroid peroxidase autoantibodies in euthyroid subjects. *Best Pract Res Clin Endocrinol Metab* 19(1):1–15, 2005.
135. Jonklaas J, Bianco AC, Bauer AJ, et al: Guidelines for treatment of hypothyroidism. *Thyroid* 24(12):1670–1750, 2014.
136. Tognini S, Marchini F, Dardano A, et al: Non-thyroidal illness syndrome and short-term survival in a hospitalised older population. *Age Ageing* 39(1):46–50, 2010.
137. Gangemi EN, Garino F, Berchialla P, et al: Low triiodothyronine serum levels as a predictor of poor prognosis in burn patients. *Burns* 34(6):817–824, 2008.
138. Bello G, Pennisi MA, Montini L, et al: Nonthyroidal illness syndrome and prolonged mechanical ventilation in patients admitted to the ICU. *Chest* 135(6):1448–1454, 2009.
139. Wang F, Pan W, Wang H, et al: Relationship between thyroid function and ICU mortality: a prospective observation study. *Crit Care* 16:R11, 2012.
140. Brent GA, Hershman JM: Thyroxine therapy in patients with severe nonthyroidal illnesses and low thyroxine concentration. *J Clin Endocrinol Metab* 63(1):1–8, 1986.
141. Acker CG, Singh AR, Flick RP, et al: A trial of thyroxine in acute renal failure. *Kidney Int* 57(1):293–298, 2000.
142. Acker CG, Flick R, Shapiro R, et al: Thyroid hormone in the treatment of post-transplant acute tubular necrosis (ATN). *Am J Transplant* 2(1):57–61, 2002.
143. Becker RA, Vaughan GM, Ziegler MG, et al: Hypermetabolic low triiodothyronine syndrome of burn injury. *Crit Care Med* 10(12):870–875, 1982.
144. Obregon MJ, Calvo RM, Del Rey FE, et al: Ontogenesis of thyroid function and interactions with maternal function. *Endocr Dev* 10:86–98, 2007.
145. Burrow GN, Fisher DA, Larsen PR: Maternal and fetal thyroid function. *N Engl J Med* 331:1072–1078, 1994.
146. Fisher DA: Euthyroid low thyroxine and triiodothyronine states in prematures and sick neonates. *Pediatr Clin North Am* 37:1297–1312, 1990.
147. Reuss ML, Leviton A, Paneth N, et al: Thyroxine values from newborn screening of 919 infants born before 29 weeks' gestation. *Am J Public Health* 87(10):1693–1697, 1997.
148. Uhrmann S, Marks KH, Maisels MJ, et al: Frequency of transient hypothyroxinemia in low birthweight infants. *Arch Dis Child* 56:214–217, 1981.
149. Frank JE, Faix JE, Hermos RJ, et al: Thyroid function in very low birth weight infants: effects on neonatal hypothyroidism screening. *J Pediatr* 128:548–554, 1996.
150. Bernal J: Thyroid hormones and brain development. *Vitam Horm* 71:95–122, 2005.
151. Rovet J, Daneman D: Congenital hypothyroidism: a review of current diagnostic and treatment practices in relation to neuropsychologic outcome. *Paediatr Drugs* 5(3):141–149, 2003.
152. Anderson GW: Thyroid hormones and the brain. *Front Neuroendocrinol* 22(1):1–17, 2001.
153. Reuss ML, Paneth N, Pinto-Martin JA, et al: The relationship of transient hypothyroxinemia in preterm infants to neurologic development at two years of age. *N Engl J Med* 334:821–827, 1996.
154. Den Ouden AL, Kok JH, Verkerk PH, et al: The relation between neonatal thyroxine levels and neurodevelopmental outcome at age 5 and 9 years in a national cohort of very preterm and/or very low birth weight infants. *Pediatr Res* 39:142–145, 1996.
155. Chowdhry P, Scanlon JW, Auerbach R, et al: Results of controlled double-blind study of thyroid replacement in very-low-birth-weight premature infants with hypothyroxinemia. *Pediatrics* 73:301–305, 1984.
156. van Wassenaer AG, Kok JH, de Vijlder JJ, et al: Effects of thyroxine supplementation on neurologic development in infants born at less than 30 weeks' gestation. *N Engl J Med* 336(1):21–26, 1997.
157. Briet JM, van Wassenaer AG, Dekkar FW, et al: Neonatal thyroxine supplementation in very preterm children: developmental outcome evaluated at early school age. *Pediatrics* 107(4):712–718, 2001.
158. Smith LM, Leake RD, Berman N, et al: Postnatal thyroxine supplementation in infants less than 32 weeks' gestation: effects on pulmonary morbidity. *J Perinatol* 20(7):427–431, 2000.
159. Vanhole C, Aerssens P, Naulaers G, et al: L-thyroxine treatment of preterm newborns: clinical and endocrine effects. *Pediatr Res* 42(1):87–92, 1997.
160. Amato M, Guggisberg C, Schneider H: Postnatal triiodothyronine replacement and respiratory distress syndrome of the preterm infant. *Horm Res* 32(5–6):213–217, 1989.

161. Osborn DA: Thyroid hormones for preventing neurodevelopmental impairment in preterm infants. *Cochrane Database Syst Rev* (4):CD001070, 2001. doi:10.1002/14651858.CD001070.
162. Bremner WF, Taylor KM, Baird S, et al: Hypothalamo-pituitary-thyroid axis during cardiopulmonary bypass. *J Thorac Cardiovasc Surg* 75:392–399, 1978.
163. Chu SH, Huang TS, Hsu RB, et al: Thyroid hormone changes after cardiovascular surgery and clinical implications. *Ann Thorac Surg* 52:791–796, 1991.
164. Robuschi G, Medici D, Fesani F, et al: Cardiopulmonary bypass: "a low T_4 and T_3 syndrome" with blunted thyrotropin response to thyrotropin-releasing hormone. *Horm Res* 23:151–158, 1986.
165. Clark RE: Cardiopulmonary bypass and thyroid hormone metabolism. *Ann Thorac Surg* 56:S35–S42, 1993.
166. Broderick TJ, Wechsler AS: Triiodothyronine in cardiac surgery. *Thyroid* 7:133–137, 1997.
167. Novitzky D, Human PA, Cooper DK, et al: Ionotropic effect of triiodothyronine following myocardial ischemia and cardiopulmonary bypass: an experimental study in pigs. *Ann Thorac Surg* 45:50–55, 1988.
168. Novitzky D, Human PA, Cooper DK, et al: Effect of triiodothyronine on myocardial high energy phosphates and lactate after ischemia and cardiopulmonary bypass. *J Thorac Cardiovasc Surg* 96:600–607, 1988.
169. Novitzky D, Matthews N, Shawley D, et al: Triiodothyronine replacement on the recovery of stunned myocardium in dogs. *Ann Thorac Surg* 51:10–17, 1991.
170. Kazmierczak P, Polak A, Mussur M: Influence of preischemic short-term triiodothyronine administration on hemodynamic function and metabolism of reperfused isolated rat heart. *Med Sci Monit* 10(10):BR381–BR387, 2004.
171. Novitzky D, Cooper DK, Swanepoel A, et al: Inotropic effect of triiodothyronine following myocardial ischemia and cardiopulmonary bypass: an initial experience in patients undergoing open-heart surgery. *Eur J Cardiothorac Surg* 3:140–145, 1989.
172. Novitzky D, Cooper DK, Barton CI, et al: Triiodothyronine as an ionotropic agent after open-heart surgery. *J Thorac Cardiovasc Surg* 98:972–978, 1989.
173. Klemperer JD, Klein I, Gomez M, et al: Thyroid hormone treatment after coronary-artery bypass surgery. *N Engl J Med* 333(23):1522–1527, 1995.
174. Klemperer JD, Klein IL, Ojamaa K, et al: Triiodothyronine therapy lowers the incidence of atrial fibrillation after cardiac operations. *Ann Thorac Surg* 61(5):1323–1327; discussion 1328–1329, 1996.
175. Bennett-Guerrero E, Jimenez JL, White WD, et al: Cardiovascular effects of intravenous triiodothyronine in patients undergoing coronary artery bypass surgery. A randomized, double-blind, placebo-controlled trial. *JAMA* 275:687–692, 1996.
176. Bettendorf M, Schmidt KG, Grulich-Henn J, et al: Tri-iodothyronine treatment in children after cardiac surgery: a double-blind, randomised, placebo-controlled study. *Lancet* 356(9229):529–534, 2000.
177. Chowdhury D, Ojamaa K, Parnell VA, et al: A prospective randomized clinical study of thyroid hormone treatment after operations for complex congenital heart disease. *J Thorac Cardiovasc Surg* 122(5):1023–1025, 2001.
178. Jeevanandam V: Triiodothyronine: spectrum of use in heart transplantation. *Thyroid* 7:139–145, 1997.
179. Novitzky D: Novel actions of thyroid hormone: the role of triiodothyronine in cardiac transplantation. *Thyroid* 6:531–536, 1996.
180. Novitzky D, Cooper DK, Rosendale J, et al: Hormonal therapy of the brain-dead organ donor: experimental and clinical studies. *Transplantation* 82(11):1396–1401, 2006.
181. Goarin J-P, Cohen S, Riou B, et al: The effects of triiodothyronine on hemodynamic status and cardiac function in potential heart donors. *Anesth Anal* 83:41–47, 1996.
182. Jeevanandam V, Todd B, Regillo T, et al: Reversal of donor myocardial dysfunction by triiodothyronine replacement therapy. *J Heart Lung Transplant* 13:681–687, 1994.
183. Zaroff JG, Rosengard BR, Armstrong WF, et al: Consensus conference report: maximizing use of organs recovered from the cadaver donor: cardiac recommendations, March 28–29, 2001, Crystal City, Va. *Circulation* 106(7):836–841, 2002.
184. Morkin E, Pennock GD, Raya TE, et al: Studies on the use of thyroid hormone and a thyroid hormone analogue in the treatment of congestive heart failure. *Ann Thorac Surg* 56:S54–S60, 1993.
185. Tielens ET, Forder JR, Chatham JC, et al: Acute L-triiodothyronine administration potentiates ionotropic responses to beta-adrenergic stimulation in the isolated perfused rat heart. *Cardiovasc Res* 32:306–310, 1996.
186. Hamilton MA: Prevalence and clinical implications of abnormal thyroid hormone metabolism in advanced heart failure. *Ann Thorac* 56:S48–S53, 1993.
187. Gomberg-Maitland M, Frishman WH: Thyroid hormone and cardiovascular disease. *Am Heart J* 135(2, Pt 1):187–196, 1998.
188. Shanoudy H, Soliman A, Moe S, et al: Early manifestations of "sick euthyroid" syndrome in patients with compensated chronic heart failure. *J Card Fail* 7(2):146–152, 2001.
189. Moruzzi P, Doria E, Agostoni PG: Medium-term effectiveness of L-thyroxine treatment in idiopathic dilated cardiomyopathy. *Am J Med* 101(5):461–467, 1996.
190. Hamilton MA, Stevenson LW, Fonarow GC, et al: Safety and hemodynamic effects of intravenous triiodothyronine in advanced congestive heart failure. *Am J Cardiol* 81(4):443–447, 1998.
191. Pingitore A, Galli E, Barison A, et al: Acute effects of triiodothyronine (T3) replacement therapy in patients with chronic heart failure and low-t3 syndrome: a randomized, placebo-controlled study. *J Clin Endocrinol Metab* 93(4):1351–1358, 2008.
192. Bello G, Paliani G, Annetta MG, et al: Treating nonthyroidal illness syndrome in the critically ill patient: still a matter of controversy. *Curr Drug Targets* 10(8):778–787, 2009.
193. Lechan RM: The dilemma of the nonthyroidal illness syndrome. *Acta Biomed* 79(3):165–171, 2008.
194. De Groot LJ: Non-thyroidal illness syndrome is a manifestation of hypothalamic-pituitary dysfunction, and in view of current evidence, should be treated with appropriate replacement therapies. *Crit Care Clin* 22(1):57–86, vi, 2006.
195. Byerley LO, Heber D: Metabolic effects of triiodothyronine replacement during fasting in obese subjects. *J Clin Endocrinol Metab* 81:968–976, 1996.
196. Koppeschaar HP, Meinders AE, Schwartz F: Metabolic responses in grossly obese subjects treated with a very low-calorie diet with and without triiodothyronine treatment *Int J Obes* 7:133–141, 1983.
197. Teiger E, Menasche P, Mansier P, et al: Triiodothyronine therapy in open-heart surgery: from hope to disappointment. *Eur Heart J* 14:629–633, 1993.

Section 14 NEUROLOGIC PROBLEMS IN THE INTENSIVE CARE UNIT

DAVID A. DRACHMAN • DAVID PAYDARFAR

Chapter 144 ■ An Approach to Neurologic Problems in the Intensive Care Unit

DAVID A. DRACHMAN

Neurologic problems present in the intensive care unit (ICU) in two modes: (a) primary neurologic problems, usually under the care of a neurologist or neurosurgeon, and (b) secondary neurologic complications, occurring in patients with other medical or surgical disorders. Only a handful of common clinical situations bring neurologists and patients together in the ICU, although they may be caused by myriad disease states [1]. These situations include:

1. Depressed state of consciousness; coma
2. Altered mental function
3. Required support of respirations or other vital functions
4. Monitoring of increased intracranial pressure (ICP), respirations, state of consciousness
5. Determination of brain death
6. Prevention of further damage to the central nervous system
7. Management of seizures or status epilepticus
8. Evaluation of a neurologic disease that occurs in the course of a severe medical disease
9. Management of a severe medical disease that develops in the course of a neurologic illness

Patients with primary neurologic problems most commonly have conditions with an identified cause, such as stroke, seizures, infectious or immune meningoencephalitis, Guillain–Barré syndrome, head trauma, or myasthenia gravis. Such patients are admitted to the ICU for close observation and management of vital functions, such as respiration, control of ICP, or arrest of seizure activity. These patients represent the minority of neurologic problems seen in the ICU. Far more frequently the neurologist is called on to evaluate the neurologic complications of medical disease: impairment of consciousness in a patient who has undergone cardiopulmonary resuscitation, development of delirium in an elderly individual with a serious infection, or occurrence of focal neurologic deficits in a patient with a ponderous medical record that reveals long-standing diabetes, renal failure, hypertension, and pulmonary disease.

The questions posed to the neurologic consultant are often imperfectly framed. Background observations regarding the origin, onset, and course of the neurologic abnormality may be unavoidably sparse and the history unavailable. The classic neurologic methodology, which involves a comprehensive history and meticulous examination, is rarely possible in patients encumbered with endotracheal tubes, cardiac monitors, and indwelling arterial and venous lines. For these reasons, neurologists must adopt special strategies to function effectively in the ICU, focusing sharply on the specific question with which they are dealing.

INDICATIONS FOR NEUROLOGIC CONSULTATION IN THE INTENSIVE CARE UNIT

Depressed State of Consciousness

The patient with the most common of ICU neurologic problems—a depressed state of consciousness, ranging from lethargy to coma—raises a host of questions. Does the patient have a focal brainstem lesion or diffuse cerebral involvement? Is there an anatomic lesion or a metabolic disorder? Have vital brainstem functions been impaired? Is ICP increased?

The most common primary neurologic causes of depressed consciousness include head trauma, intracranial hemorrhage, post cardiac arrest anoxia–ischemia, and less commonly, inapparent seizures. The secondary conditions seen most often are metabolic, such as anoxia, drug intoxication, or diabetic ketoacidosis. Sometimes the diagnosis is evident, as in head trauma; at other times, determination of the cause of depressed consciousness may present a diagnostic challenge, demanding a race against the clock to avoid irreversible changes. In every case, it is crucial to establish whether depressed consciousness is due to intrinsic brainstem damage, increased ICP, toxins, widespread anoxia or ischemia, or some other less common cause. It is particularly important to sort out rapidly the component(s) that may be treatable.

Examination of the patient with depressed consciousness exemplifies some of the difficulties of neurologic care in the ICU. Details of this examination are described elsewhere [2]. Like the standard neurologic examination, however, it includes evaluation of mental status, cranial nerve functions, motor functions and coordination, reflexes, sensation, and vascular integrity. The observations made must be used to answer the questions posed above, supplemented by appropriate laboratory studies when possible.

A detailed evaluation of memory and cognitive function is rarely possible for patients who are lethargic, and never possible in those who are stuporous or comatose. Instead, the physician must estimate the patient's responsiveness. Can the patient say any words or respond to commands? Does the patient open his or her eyes? Does the patient groan in response to a painful stimulus or attempt to remove it in a purposeful way? What is the status of the vital functions? Is the respiratory pattern disturbed? The Glasgow Coma Scale score is a simple, but useful, way to document the patient's sensorium [3].

Cranial nerve evaluations include determination of vision, done by observing how the patient follows a large object or a light, gazes toward right and left visual fields, or blinks to a visual threat. Pupillary size, equality, and responsiveness to light are assessed. Corneal reflexes, cough, and vibrissal (nasal) reflexes are evaluated. "Doll's eyes" (vestibuloocular) responses are determined by rotation of the head from side to side; if they are absent, ice water caloric testing can be carried out. Facial movements are assessed in response to painful supraorbital stimuli; the gag reflex is tested in the usual fashion.

Motor function is evaluated as completely as possible. All limbs are observed for spontaneous movement and symmetry as well as tremor or other adventitious movements. If no spontaneous movements take place, a pinch or other noxious stimulus can be used to observe purposeful defensive movements. Decerebrate (i.e., four-limb extensor) and decorticate (i.e., upper limbs flexor, lower limbs extensor) rigidity are observed. Tone is assessed passively for spasticity or rigidity. Deep tendon reflexes are checked in the usual way, working around restraints and intravenous tubing. Grasp, suck, snout, and plantar reflexes are evaluated.

Pain is often the only sensory modality that can be tested. The physician must determine whether withdrawal from pinch or pinprick is appropriately defensive or (in the lower extremities) merely part of an exaggerated extensor–plantar response with triple flexion (flexion at hip, knee, and great toe), which may be mistaken for purposeful withdrawal. Finally, the vascular status is evaluated by listening for bruits over the carotid and subclavian arteries, the vertebral arteries, and the orbits.

Such an examination reveals the patient's state of consciousness, the integrity of brainstem reflexes, and the presence or absence of lateralizing or focal neurologic deficits. The value of the systematic (if limited) neurologic examination cannot be overestimated. For example, in a comatose patient, the finding of decerebrate rigidity that points to significant damage at the level of the pons may be more valuable than many laboratory studies, and unilateral weakness of limbs with ipsilateral hyperreflexia indicates a focal brain disorder rather than a diffuse metabolic problem.

Neurodiagnostic studies are often critical in the analysis of comatose patients in the ICU, but the patient's immobility and dependence on life support systems present special difficulties. A neuroradiology suite that is distant from the ICU presents additional obstacles. It is frequently difficult to obtain an MRI (magnetic resonance imaging) or CT (computed tomographic) brain scan, or arteriogram on a patient who is dependent on a respirator. Paradoxically, in patients with the most urgent problems, it is often least convenient to obtain the maximum amount of neurodiagnostic information. The decision that a patient is too sick to have the crucial study performed is often incorrect. In such desperate cases, risks must be taken to obtain lifesaving information.

Management of the patient with depressed consciousness depends largely on the cause. Techniques for eliminating toxins, reducing ICP, and maintaining vital functions must be applied, depending on the diagnostic context (see Chapter 145).

Altered Mental Function

In patients who remain relatively alert, other organic disorders may affect mental function, producing an often perplexing variety of clinical patterns. These include confusion, delirium, aphasia, and isolated memory impairment. The first question for the physician is whether the patient's abnormal mental function represents a recent change that is part of the present illness, or instead is part of a long-standing problem. It is also critical to note whether the change developed abruptly (e.g., after surgery or cardiac arrest) or if there is no known precipitating event; and whether it is improving, worsening, or stable.

Confusion and delirium are commonly reversible and generally result from metabolic and toxic disorders (see Chapters 145 and 157). Persistent aphasia and isolated memory impairment suggest focal damage to the brain, and an anatomic lesion should be sought. Dementia—cognitive and memory impairment—cannot be accurately evaluated in patients who have a depressed state of consciousness or the other mental changes indicated above. When dementia occurs de novo in a patient with a clear sensorium, it may indicate either reversible conditions (e.g., drug-induced, depression-related) or irreversible damage (e.g., diffuse anoxia or ischemia; see Chapter 145).

Any recent change in mental status in a patient in the ICU requires *prompt* investigation. Whether it signals worsening of the underlying medical disorder or direct involvement of the brain, the change should be assessed by an experienced neurologist as early in its evolution as possible, before it is complicated by the passage of time, advance of disease, and effects of additional treatments.

Support of Respiration and Other Vital Functions

Respiratory support is needed for neurologic patients in two circumstances: loss of brainstem reflex control of respiration and impairment of effective transmission of reflex impulses to functioning respiratory muscles. Ischemia, anoxia, compression, hemorrhage, and toxic depression may alter brainstem control of respirations, producing characteristic respiratory patterns that depend on the site of damage [2], such as central neurogenic hyperventilation, Cheyne–Stokes or periodic breathing, or apnea. The intensivist and neurologist should be familiar with the use of positive end-expiratory pressure and other ventilatory regimens, operation and interpreting readout of the hospital's respirators, and the endotracheal intubation equipment. Further, the neurologist must understand the neurologic significance of different respiratory patterns, which are as much a part of the ICU neurologic examination as is reflex testing.

Effective transmission of respiratory impulses may be impaired at the cervical spinal cord, anterior horn cells, peripheral nerves, neuromuscular junctions, or muscles of respiration. Cervical traumatic injuries, amyotrophic lateral sclerosis, Guillain–Barré syndrome, myasthenia gravis, and muscular dystrophy may interfere with breathing at the respective levels noted. Some of these conditions are transitory (e.g., Guillain–Barré syndrome) or treatable (e.g., myasthenia gravis), with complete recovery depending largely on the success of maintaining respiration. Even in incurable conditions (e.g., amyotrophic lateral sclerosis), sustaining respiration during periods of decompensation, such as respiratory infections, can prolong life significantly.

Monitoring of Intracranial Pressure and State of Consciousness

In a number of neurologic disorders, extremely close observation is needed to avoid the development of dangerous, often irreversible, further damage to the brain. The most common disorder requiring such monitoring is head trauma. The lethargic patient must be carefully observed for evidence of increasing ICP due to cerebral edema, intracranial (subdural, epidural, intracerebral) hemorrhage, or both [4].

The need for prompt recognition and early treatment of significantly increased ICP cannot be overemphasized. Once uncal or tonsillar herniation with brainstem compression and development of Duret hemorrhages has occurred, the consequences of this secondary effect of brain injury may far outweigh the initial damage. (The methods for monitoring ICP with pressure-detecting catheters or bolts and assessing consciousness and brainstem functions with the Glasgow Coma Scale are described in Chapters 31 and 41.)

Determination of Brain Death

With the recognition that death of the brain and brainstem is equivalent to death of the patient, even though the heart continues to beat and respirations are sustained by artificial ventilation, the need to ascertain brain death has become more critical [5]. Early identification of brain death has three important justifications: (a) the use of viable donor organs for transplantation; (b) the termination of the hopeless vigil of a distraught family; and (c) the freeing of ICU beds for patients who may be helped. When one or more of these conditions prevails, it is important to determine the occurrence of brain death promptly. When none of the conditions is present, there is no urgency in declaring the patient brain dead.

It should be emphasized that brain death is specifically a determination that the brain and the brainstem are already dead—not a prediction that useful recovery is unlikely. It is also true that the longer one waits in even marginally uncertain cases, the clearer the evidence of brain death becomes. (The criteria for brain death are discussed extensively in Chapters 56 and 145.) The "CADRE" mnemonic may be useful in recalling the established criteria for brain death, in the absence of sedative drugs: *C*oma; *A*pnea; *D*ilated, fixed pupils; *R*eflex (brainstem) absence; and *E*lectroencephalographic silence.

Prevention of Further Damage to the Central Nervous System

A variety of neurologic disorders have the potential to cause further damage to the central nervous system. Acute strokes, or stroke in evolution, for example, may be arrested by thrombolytic treatment [6], endovascular clot removal [7] or angioplasty, and stenting. These modalities may limit or even reverse the underlying ischemic process; and neuroprotective agents may, in the foreseeable future, prevent further damage. Coma following cardiac arrest should be promptly treated with hypothermia to preserve neurologic function [8]. Spinal cord compression by metastatic tumor urgently requires surgical decompression followed by radiation therapy to avoid irreversible complete cord transection [9]. Among the infectious diseases of the nervous system, bacterial meningitis and certain treatable encephalitides (e.g., herpes simplex) require the immediate institution of antibiotic or antiviral therapy; spinal epidural abscess requires prompt surgical decompression as well. Although much of neurologic practice involves disorders for which progress is measured in months or years, cerebral anoxia, ischemia, hemorrhage, increased ICP, spinal cord compression, infectious diseases, and other acute disorders require prompt institution of treatment to avoid extension of the initial process. It is useful to remember that, as a largely postmitotic structure, the brain has a limited capability for regeneration, and its ability to survive without a continuing supply of nutrients is measured in minutes. Only in the ICU, with its facilities for careful monitoring and adjustment of therapy, can many of these treatments be successfully carried out.

Management of Status Epilepticus

Unlike simple, brief seizures, status epilepticus threatens lasting deficits or death if not controlled (see Chapter 151). Any patient whose sequential seizures cannot be arrested promptly with routine management (e.g., intravenous benzodiazepines, phenytoin) must be observed in the ICU, where therapy ranging up to general anesthesia with artificial ventilation may be required.

Evaluation of Neurologic Disease Accompanying Severe Medical Disease

Neurologic signs or symptoms develop in many patients admitted to the ICU for myocardial infarction, subacute bacterial endocarditis, cardiac arrhythmia, pneumonia, acute respiratory distress syndrome, septic shock, renal disease, hepatic failure, and other similar disorders while they are under treatment for the primary medical problem. Numerous questions are raised: Is the neurologic finding a consequence of the underlying disease, or is it coincidental? Does it demand further investigation at once, or can it wait? Should therapy be changed, or should new therapy be started? These issues demand the attention of the neurologist.

Management of Severe Medical Disease Accompanying Neurologic Illness

For patients with severe medical disease accompanying neurologic illness, unrelated medical illness most often develops in the setting of a chronic neurologic disorder. The demented patient may experience a myocardial infarction, or septicemia may develop in the patient with multiple sclerosis. Indirect relationships should be sought. Does the demented patient have multiple cerebral emboli from underlying cardiac disease? Is the patient with multiple sclerosis septicemic from a bladder infection due to impaired urinary control? Early recognition of a change in the seriousness of the neurologic patient's condition is often difficult, but it may be critical to a successful outcome.

PROGNOSTIC AND ETHICAL CONSIDERATIONS

When severe damage involves the brain, either as a separate neurologic condition or as a secondary consequence of other medical disease, the physician who requested neurologic consultation and the family often need guidance regarding the probable outcome. There are three critical questions: Will the patient survive? Has irreversible brain damage occurred? What is the likely degree of residual disability?

There are few simple rules that can be applied infallibly to determine the prognosis in, for example, comatose patients, especially early in the course. The most important consideration is often whether irreversible damage has affected crucial areas of the brain, rather than the depth of impairment of consciousness. The patient with glutethimide poisoning, for example, may show no evidence of any neurologic function yet can recover fully if vital functions are maintained. In contrast, the comatose patient with head trauma resulting in pontine hemorrhage and decerebrate rigidity may have a far worse prognosis. The probability of neurologic recovery generally declines with advancing age, size and location of the lesion, and duration of deficit. A number of studies have provided statistical guidelines that are of value in gauging the probability of recovery [10,11]. Guidelines for the evaluation of prognosis following cardiac arrest and resuscitation are particularly well documented, and the absence of pupillary and corneal reflexes or motor response to pain, the occurrence of myoclonic status epilepticus, absence of somatosensory evoked potentials (N20), and elevated neuron-specific enolase are particularly useful in early determination of poor prognosis [10].

Early in the course of coma, the physician should not be hasty in abandoning hope and vigorous medical efforts to maintain survival and to limit neurologic damage. Late in the course, or as poor prognostic signs accumulate, it is important to recognize the outer limits of possible recovery and to assess the value of continuing life support accordingly. The patient's wishes, expressed in a living will or durable power of attorney for health care and as interpreted by close, responsible family members ("substituted judgment"), should combine with the physician's prognostic judgment to help determine a medical course of action. Although management in the ICU usually entails the unstinting use of every available means of life support and treatment, there must eventually be a transition either to recovery or to a permanent state of dependence, and the nature and extent of continued treatment should be adjusted accordingly. The technical means of maintaining survival almost indefinitely by the use of extraordinary measures is now available. It is important for the physician and the patient's family to consider whether, in the case of a patient with irreversible and severe neurologic damage, they are extending life or prolonging the process of dying [12].

It is clear that neurologic problems abound in the ICU. A successful approach to these disorders requires the physician to recognize the nature of the clinical situation prompting neurologic consultation or admission to the ICU. An analysis of which of the nine types of neurologic clinical situations is being encountered often guides the physician initially in diagnosis and management. The following chapters discuss some of the more common neurologic problems encountered in the ICU, with specific attention to management in the ICU and a broader view of the neurologic conditions in general.

References

1. Ropper AH, Gress DR, Mayer S, et al: *Neurological and Neurosurgical Intensive Care*. 4th ed. Philadelphia, PA, Lippincott Williams & Wilkins, 2004.
2. Posner JB, Saper CB, Schiff ND, et al: *Plum and Posner's Diagnosis of Stupor and Coma*. 4th ed. New York, NY, Oxford University Press, 2007.
3. Teasdale G, Jennett B: Assessment of coma and impaired consciousness. A practical scale. *Lancet* 2:81–84, 1974.
4. Jennett B, Teasdale G: *Management of Head Injury*. Philadelphia, PA, FA Davis, 1981.
5. Wijdicks EF: The diagnosis of brain death. *N Engl J Med* 344(16):1215–1221, 2001.
6. Cronin CA: Intravenous tissue plasminogen activator for stroke: a review of the ECASS III results in relation to prior clinical trials. *J. Emergency Med* 38(1): 99–105, 2010.
7. Berkhemer OA, Fransen PS, Beumer D, et al: A randomized trial of intraarterial treatment for acute ischemic stroke. *N Engl J Med* 372:11–20, 2015.
8. Arrich J, Holzer M, Herkner H, et al: Hypothermia for neuroprotection in adults after cardiopulmonary resuscitation. *Cochrane Database Syst Rev* 4: CD004128, 2009.
9. Patchell RA, Tibbs PA, Regine WF, et al: Direct decompressive surgical resection in the treatment of spinal cord compression caused by metastatic cancer: a randomised trial. *Lancet* 366:643–648, 2005.
10. Wijdicks EFM, Hijdra A, Young GB, et al: Practice parameter: prediction of outcome in comatose survivors after cardiopulmonary resuscitation (an evidence-based review). *Neurology* 67:203–210, 2006.
11. Zandbergen EG, Hijdra A, Koelman JHTM, et al; For the PROPAC Study Group: Prediction of poor outcome within the first three days of postanoxic coma. *Neurology* 66:62–68, 2006.
12. Wanzer SH, Federman DD, Adelstein SJ, et al: The physician's responsibility toward hopelessly ill patients: a second look. *N Engl J Med* 320:844–849, 1989.

Chapter 145 ■ Evaluating the Patient with Altered Consciousness in the Intensive Care Unit

RAPHAEL A. CARANDANG • LAWRENCE J. HAYWARD • DAVID A. DRACHMAN

The spectrum of disease that leads to acute impairment of consciousness is broad; the disorders are varied and potentially life-threatening and may be treatable if recognized early. The clinician evaluating the patient with an altered level of consciousness must do so in a systematic and efficient fashion. The approach consists of (a) rapidly determining the type of mental status change, (b) administering life-support measures where urgently needed, (c) obtaining a detailed history and physical examination directed at determining more precisely the cause(s) of the nervous system disorder, (d) selecting appropriate and informative diagnostic and laboratory studies, and (e) initiating more definitive treatment based on this assessment.

As a practical matter, *consciousness* refers to a state of awareness of self and environment that depends on intact arousal and content [1,2]. Arousal is the level of attentive wakefulness and readiness to respond to relevant sensory information. Alerting stimuli activate the ascending reticular activating system (ARAS), which extends from the superior pons to the thalamus and projects to multiple cortical areas. Diminished arousal implies dysfunction of either the ARAS or both cerebral hemispheres; lesions of the brainstem sparing the ARAS (e.g., of the medulla) or of only one hemisphere do not affect wakefulness. This chapter defines altered states of consciousness and presents a systematic approach to bedside evaluation and prognostication of the comatose patient.

ALTERED STATES OF CONSCIOUSNESS

Neurologists are frequently consulted for evaluation of patients who appear unconscious, confused, or awake and alert but noncommunicative.

Patient Who Appears Unconscious

Patients who appear unconscious lie mostly motionless, usually with the eyes closed and seemingly unaware of their environment. The causes of this condition include normal sleep, depressed consciousness, psychogenic coma, locked-in state, vegetative states, minimally conscious state, and brain death.

Sleep

The normal unconsciousness of sleep is characterized by prompt reversibility on threshold sensory stimulation, and maintenance of wakefulness following arousal. The degree of stimulation required depends on the stage of sleep (stage IV non–rapid eye movement sleep is the deepest), and the sensory stimulation used.

TABLE 145.1

Differential Diagnosis of Depressed Consciousness

I. Depressed consciousness with lateralizing signs of brain disease: brain tumor, cerebral hemorrhage, cerebral thrombosis, cerebral embolism, contusion, subdural or epidural hemorrhage, brain abscess, hypertensive encephalopathy

II. Depressed consciousness with signs of meningeal irritation: meningitis, subarachnoid hemorrhage, leptomeningeal carcinoma, or lymphoma

III. Depressed consciousness without lateralizing or meningeal signs: alcohol, barbiturate, or opiate intoxication: carbon monoxide poisoning, neuroleptic malignant syndrome, anoxia, hyponatremia, hypoglycemia, diabetic coma, uremia, hepatic coma, hypercapnia, nonconvulsive status epilepticus, infectious encephalitis, acute hydrocephalus, concussion, diffuse axonal injury, hypothermia

Adapted from Adams RD, Victor M: *Principles of Neurology*. 4th ed. New York, McGraw-Hill, 1989.

Depressed Consciousness

Consciousness is deemed depressed when suprathreshold sensory stimulation is required for arousal and wakefulness cannot be maintained unless the stimulation is continuous [1,2]. Responsible specific lesions involve the ARAS, or both cerebral hemispheres. Brainstem damage may be direct, or due to indirect compression by masses situated in other compartments. Bilateral cerebral hemispheric damage may be due to multifocal insults, or to large unilateral lesions with resulting major mass effect. In addition, a wide array of metabolic derangements, toxins, or diffuse injuries may depress consciousness by affecting the ARAS, the cerebral hemispheres, or both. The spectrum of depressed states—lethargy, hypersomnolence, obtundation, stupor, and coma—is defined by the level of consciousness observed on examination. The etiologies are diverse (Table 145.1), with the degree of depression dependent on the nature of the insult, its duration, and the location and extent of involvement of the brain.

The first signs of brain dysfunction may be mild and barely noticeable. The patient may be described initially as confused or drowsy before progressing to *lethargy* or *hypersomnolence* and eventually to a more depressed state. Hypersomnolent patients maintain arousal only with vigorous and continuous sensory stimulation; while awake, however, they may be oriented and make appropriate responses. The most common cause of hypersomnolence in the hospital is sleep deprivation, mostly iatrogenic, especially in the around-the-clock care setting of the intensive care unit (ICU). Patients with discrete diencephalic or midbrain tegmentum lesions may also present with hypersomnolence [3,4]. Because these lesions affect the ARAS and spare the cerebral hemispheres, cognitive content is usually preserved. Rostral extension of a midline lesion may involve thalamic structures (especially the dorsomedial nuclei) and cause difficulties with the ability to store new memories. Other mesencephalic structures may be affected and cause abnormalities of pupillary function, internuclear ophthalmoplegia, and third nerve dysfunction.

Obtunded patients usually can be aroused by light stimuli but are mentally dulled and unable to maintain wakefulness. *Stuporous* patients can be aroused only with vigorous noxious stimulation. While awake, neither obtunded nor stuporous patients demonstrate a normal content of consciousness, but both may display purposeful movements, attempting to ward off painful stimuli or to remove catheters, endotracheal tubes, or intravenous lines.

Patients in *coma* are unresponsive to suprathreshold sensory stimulation, including noxious stimulation that is strong enough to arouse a deeply sleeping patient but not strong enough to cause physical injury. Although the patient usually lies motionless, movements such as stereotyped, inappropriate postures (decerebration and decortication) and spinal cord reflexes (triple flexion and Babinski responses) may occur. Irrespective of the etiology, the duration of coma is typically no longer than 2 to 4 weeks, after which one of the three conditions supervenes: arousal to full or partial recovery, a vegetative state, or death.

Most of the literature on prognosis of comatose patients comes from nontraumatic coma, largely anoxic–ischemic brain injury. A landmark paper by Levy, Plum, and associates from 1981 established the neurologic examination—particularly absence of brainstem reflexes including pupillary, corneal, and oculocephalic reflexes—as important predictors of poor outcome in nontraumatic coma [5]. Multiple studies followed which confirmed the importance of motor responses in addition to brainstem examination, and some diagnostic tests were established as useful in predicting outcomes; these are well summarized in the American Academy of Neurology Practice Parameter on post-cardiopulmonary resuscitation by Wijdicks et al., published in 2006 [6]. Given the life-or-death responsibility of the physician providing a prognosis, only clinical indicators or diagnostic tests that are highly specific with a near-zero false-positive rate are utilized. A poor outcome is predicted by the absence of pupillary and corneal reflexes, absent or extensor motor responses, absent responses to caloric testing of the oculovestibular reflex at day 3 post-arrest, and the presence of myoclonic status epilepticus on day 1 post-arrest. The absence of N20 responses on somatosensory evoked potential (SSEP) testing, and the finding of serum neuron-specific enolase levels more than 33 μg per L on days 1 to 3 post-arrest also indicate a poor prognosis (Fig. 145.1). Prognostication must include consideration of the etiology of the disease process, the clinical examination findings, and radiologic evidence of damage to the upper pons, midbrain, diencephalon, and other vital structures for arousal.

Psychogenic Coma

Patients in psychogenic coma appear comatose but have clinical and laboratory evidence of wakefulness [1]. Psychogenic unresponsiveness may be suggested by active resistance or rapid closure of the eyelids, pupillary constriction to visual threat, fast phase of nystagmus (i.e., a saccade) on oculovestibular or optokinetic testing, and avoidance of self-injury (e.g., by averting an arm dropped toward the patient's face) or annoying stimulation such as a nasal tickle (moving head away from stimulus). Caloric testing with ice water irrigation of the ear will elicit a normal nystagmoid response with the fast phase directed away

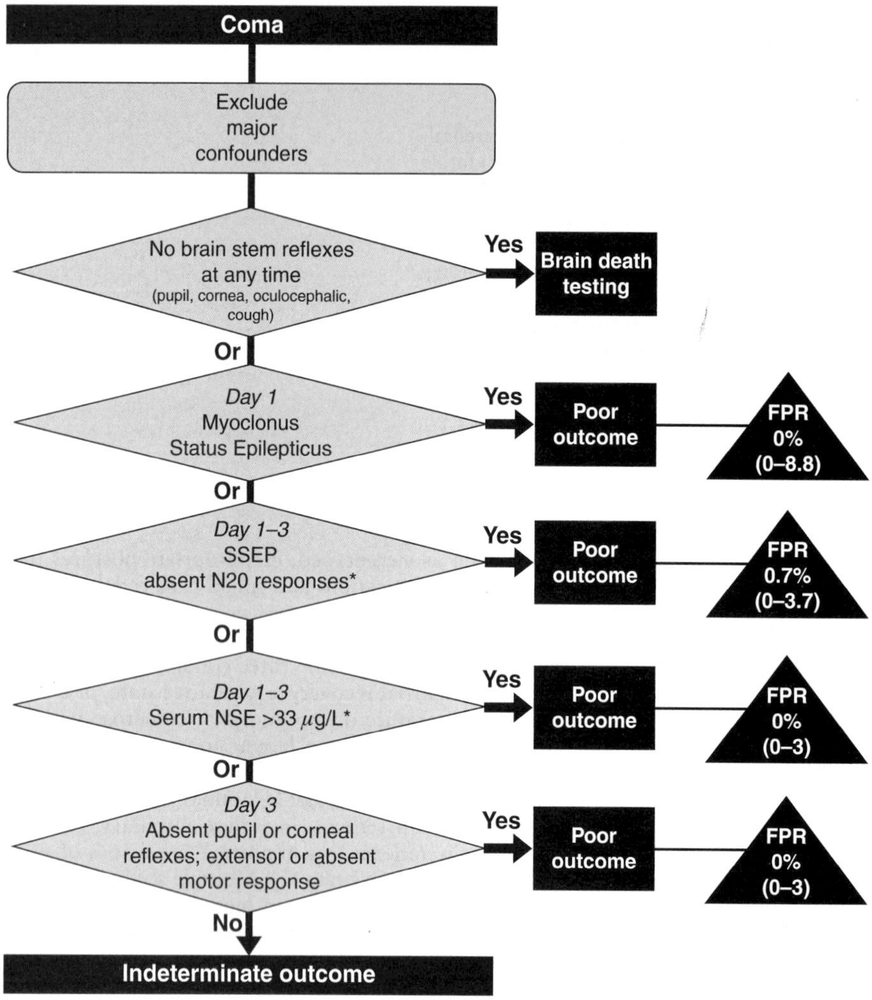

*These test results may not be available on a timely basis. Serum NSE testing may not be sufficiently standardized.

FIGURE 145.1 Algorithm for predicting outcome in comatose patients after cardiopulmonary arrest. FPR, false-positive rate; NSE, neuron-specific enolase; SSEP, somatosensory evoked potential. (From Wijdicks EF: The diagnosis of brain death. *N Engl J Med* 344:1215, 2001.)

from the irrigated ear, and possibly some nausea and vomiting. Deep tendon reflex examination is often normal but can be voluntarily suppressed. Electroencephalogram (EEG) α waves that attenuate with eye opening are inconsistent with coma or sleep. Most diagnostic tests will be unrevealing. Psychiatric conditions that may be associated with psychogenic coma are conversion reactions secondary to hysterical personality, severe depression, or acute situational reaction, catatonic schizophrenia, dissociative or fugue states, severe psychotic depression, and malingering.

Locked-in State

The locked-in state is a nearly total paralysis without loss of consciousness [7,8]. Because the most common cause of this state is destruction of the base of the pons, the patient is completely paralyzed except for muscles subserved by midbrain structures (i.e., vertical eye movements and blinking). Consciousness is preserved because the ARAS is located in the tegmentum of the pons, dorsal to the damaged area. The most frequent cause is cerebrovascular such as cerebral infarction from a basilar thromboembolism, or pontine hemorrhage from uncontrolled hypertension; less frequent etiologies of the syndrome are acute polyneuropathy (Guillain–Barré syndrome), acute poliomyelitis, or toxins that block transmission at the neuromuscular junction. It is important to note that locked-in patients are capable of hearing, seeing, and feeling external stimuli and pain. Adequate analgesia and anxiolysis should be provided despite the absence of external signs of pain and anxiety. A 5- to 10-year survival has been reported in as high as 80% of patients in some series and a surprising 58% of patients surveyed reported satisfaction with life despite their disability in a small case series [8].

Brain Death

The term *brain death* refers to a determination of physical death by brain-based, rather than cardiopulmonary-based, criteria [9]. Brain death is the irreversible destruction of the brain, with the resulting total absence of all cortical and brainstem function, although spinal cord reflexes may remain [10,11]. It is not to be confused with severe but incomplete brain damage with a poor prognosis or with a vegetative state, conditions in which some function of vital brain centers still remains. In brain death, support of other organs is futile for the patient, whereas when there is some residual brain or brainstem function, or a vegetative state, decisions regarding ongoing life support clearly depend on the wishes of the patient or his or her proxy.

In brain death, pupils are midposition and round (not oval), and apnea persists even when arterial carbon dioxide tension (PCO_2) is raised to levels that should stimulate respiration. Table 145.2 summarizes the guidelines used in the United States. Brain death may be simulated by drug intoxications and *cannot*

TABLE 145.2

Criteria for Brain Death

Prerequisites

1. Clinical or neuroimaging evidence of an acute CNS catastrophe compatible with the clinical diagnosis of brain death
2. Exclusion of complicating medical conditions that may confound clinical assessment (no severe electrolyte, acid–base, or endocrine disturbance)
3. No drug intoxication or poisoning
4. Core temperature = 32°C (90°F)

Criteria

1. Cerebral functions are absent.
   - Coma, and absence of motor responses including decerebrate posturing, although spinal reflexes may be seen
2. Brainstem functions are absent.
   - Absence of pupillary responses to light; pupils at midposition and dilated
   - Absent corneal reflexes, caloric reflexes, gag reflex, cough in response to tracheal suctioning, sucking and rooting reflexes
   - Absence of respiratory drive at $PaCO_2$ 60 mm Hg, or 20 mm Hg above normal baseline values
   - Interval between two separate examinations varies depending on the age of the patient if pediatric, but for adults is usually at least 6 h
3. Ancillary diagnostic tests:
   - EEG showing electrocerebral silence
   - Technetium (99mTc) hexametazime nuclear scan showing absence of activity in brain
   - Cerebral angiography showing absence of blood flow in cerebral vessels
   - Transcranial Doppler showing lack of diastolic or reverberating flow and small systolic peaks in early systole

CNS, central nervous system.
Revised table from AAN Practice Guidelines. A Report of the Quality Standards Subcommittee of the American Academy of Neurology 1994; and Wijdicks EF: The diagnosis of brain death. *N Engl J Med* 344:1215, 2001.

be evaluated when toxic drugs are present; depending on preserved renal and hepatic function, most such toxic effects do not persist longer than 36 hours. Hypothermia also precludes a diagnosis of brain death, and the patient must be brought to normal temperature prior to declaring death. Brain death is a clinical diagnosis, but ancillary tests such as an EEG and blood flow studies (transcranial Doppler, technetium-99m scan, or conventional cerebral angiography) may be useful where the clinical examination is compromised by sedating medications. Unresponsiveness that can mimic brain death may occur with extensive brainstem destruction, for example, after basilar artery thrombosis. Despite absent brainstem reflexes, continued cortical activity on the EEG and persistent cerebral blood flow would demonstrate that the patient is not brain dead.

The American Academy of Neurology has published practice parameters for the determination of brain death. The criteria take into account etiology, performance of two separate clinical examinations 6 hours apart, and include the method of apnea testing with preoxygenation and oxygen [11]. As criteria for brain death vary from state to state, and procedures to determine brain death differ among institutions, it is important to be familiar with the guidelines in your institution [12]. The occurrence of brain death provides the opportunity for organ donation, and most institutions have a protocol that includes informing organ bank organizations to facilitate this.

Patient Who Appears Confused

Confusion is a general term used for patients who do not think with customary speed, clarity, or coherence. The causes of this condition include among others an acute confusional state, toxic encephalopathies, dementia, inapparent seizures, and receptive aphasia.

Acute Confusional State

When the cerebral hemispheres are negatively affected by toxic, metabolic, anoxic, structural, or infectious processes, the patient may appear acutely confused [13,14]. Poor arousal and an abnormal content of consciousness may contribute to the clinical presentation, and the etiologies are legion (Table 145.3). Patients with clouded consciousness are easily distracted or startled by environmental stimuli. Their processing of information is slow and effortful, state of consciousness fluctuates from drowsiness to hyperexcitability, attention span is poor, and recall and recent memory are impaired. If sensorial clouding becomes more advanced, sensory input is increasingly misinterpreted, daytime drowsiness alternates with nocturnal agitation, disorientation for place and time becomes apparent, and repeated prompting is required for a response to even the simplest commands.

Delirious patients typically manifest acutely fluctuating confusion, with psychomotor overactivity, agitation, autonomic instability, and often visual hallucinations. Clinical observations frequently suggest that the disturbance of cognition or perception is directly related to a potentially reversible general medical condition rather than to an evolving dementia. Hyperexcitability may alternate with periods of drowsiness or relative lucidity. Signs of autonomic overactivity include pupillary dilatation, diaphoresis, tachycardia, and hypertension. Patients with delirium may not sleep, sometimes for periods of several days; the success of treatment can be judged by the development of normal sleep. Delirium tremens, the most serious consequence of ethanol withdrawal, is perhaps the best-known example of this state. Because the routine Mini-Mental State Examination often cannot be administered to unstable, intubated patients, alternative screening tools have been developed for early detection and monitoring of delirium in the ICU [15,16]. Validated tools such as the Confusion Assessment Method, or CAM-ICU scale, have the advantage of being simple and easy to administer, highly reliable and applicable in patients who are intubated. Systematic screening may help detect early delirium and allow prompt, cost-effective treatment. Delirium has been linked to prolonged ICU stay and ventilator days, and is associated with postdischarge cognitive dysfunction and worse 6-month mortality outcomes [16,17]. The use of interventions that reduce delirium in the ICU include reduction and intermittent use of sedatives, or spontaneous awakening trials, as well as sedation with α adrenergic medications such as dexmedetomidine [18,19].

In beclouded dementia, confusion is superimposed on an underlying subacute or chronic cognitive disorder. The preexisting cerebral dysfunction may be mental retardation, dementia, or the deficits from a vascular, neoplastic, or demyelinative process. In some cases, the underlying disorder is not diagnosed until the confusion appears during an intercurrent illness (e.g., sepsis or infection, congestive heart failure, surgical procedures, anemia, drug overdose, or intolerance).

Dementia

Patients with dementia have subacute or chronic intellectual dysfunction unaccompanied by a reduction in arousal [20].

TABLE 145.3

Classification of Acute Confusional States

- ACS not associated with focal or lateralizing neurologic signs and normal CSF
  - Metabolic disorders
    - Hepatic encephalopathy
    - Uremia
    - Hypercapnia
    - Hypoglycemia
    - Diabetic ketotic coma
    - Porphyria
    - Hypercalcemia
  - Infectious disorders
    - Septicemia[a]
    - Pneumonia[a]
    - Typhoid fever[a]
    - Rheumatic fever[a]
  - Drug intoxication
    - Opiates
    - Barbiturates
    - Tricyclic antidepressants
    - Other sedatives
    - Amphetamines[a]
    - Anticholinergic medications[a]
  - Abstinence states (i.e., withdrawal states)
    - Alcohol (delirium tremens)[a]
    - Barbiturates[a]
    - Benzodiazepines[a]
  - States that reduce cerebral blood flow or oxygen content
    - Hypoxic encephalopathy
    - Congestive heart failure
    - Cardiac arrhythmias
  - Situational psychoses (diagnoses)
    - Postoperative psychosis[a]
    - Posttraumatic psychosis[a]
    - Puerperal psychosis[a]
    - Intensive care unit psychosisa
- ACS associated with focal or lateralizing neurologic signs and/or abnormal CSF
  - Cerebrovascular disease or space-occupying lesions (especially of the right parietal, inferofrontal, and temporal lobes)
    - Ischemic infarct[a]
    - Neoplasm[a]
    - Abscess[a]
    - Hemorrhage (intraparenchymal, subdural, epidural)[a]
    - Granuloma
  - Infectious disorders
    - Meningitis[a]
    - Encephalitis[a]
  - Subarachnoid hemorrhage[a]
  - Cerebral contusion and laceration[a]
- ACS sometimes associated with focal or lateralizing neurologic signs
  - Postconvulsive delirium[a]
  - Acute hydrocephalus
  - Nonconvulsive status epilepticus
  - Nonketotic diabetic coma

[a]These disorders may be associated with signs of psychomotor overactivity or delirium.

ACS, acute confusional state; CSF, cerebrospinal fluid.

Adapted from Adams RD, Victor M: *Principles of Neurology*. 4th ed. New York, McGraw-Hill, 1989.

The patient exhibits a decline in multiple cognitive functions, including memory, language, spatial orientation, personality, abstract thinking, and insight. The ability to carry out testing requires relative preservation of attention and language comprehension. The causes of dementia include degenerative processes (Alzheimer's disease, frontotemporal degeneration, Lewy body dementia, Huntington's disease), metabolic and nutritional disorders (Wernicke–Korsakoff's syndrome with thiamine deficiency, hypothyroidism, pellagra, vitamin B_{12} deficiency), infectious diseases (subacute spongiform encephalopathy [Creutzfeldt–Jakob disease, CJD], acquired immunodeficiency syndrome, dementia, neurosyphilis, Lyme encephalitis, chronic meningitis, progressive multifocal leukoencephalopathy), cerebrovascular disorders (multiinfarct dementia, anoxia-ischemia), hydrocephalus with normal or increased intracranial pressure, and multiple toxins.

Inapparent Seizures

Patients with nonconvulsive status epilepticus may appear disoriented, episodically unresponsive, or alternately lucid and confused; the EEG shows continuous or frequent epileptiform discharges [21,22]. Careful observation may alert the clinician to seizure phenomena, such as episodic staring, eye deviation or nystagmoid jerks, facial or hand clonic activity, and automatisms. The syndrome may be the result of a generalized (absence) status or a complex partial status. Complex partial status is the more common form seen in the ICU and may not be preceded by a history of complex partial seizures. The origin of the abnormal focal discharge may be from the temporal, frontal, or occipital lobes, and the EEG pattern during the ictus is variable. Inapparent seizures may occur in as many as 19% of all patients in the ICU, and 56% of patients who are comatose at the time of monitoring. The yield of EEG monitoring is increased by continuous monitoring for 24 hours [23]. Nonconvulsive status epilepticus should be considered, and is the cause of otherwise unexplained coma in as many as 8% of patients [24]. A benzodiazepine, such as diazepam or lorazepam, or an anticonvulsant drug may eliminate the discharge and improve the patient's state of consciousness.

Receptive Aphasia

Patients with receptive aphasia often appear confused because they have a disorder of language comprehension [14]. The patient is awake and alert but unable to comprehend written or verbal commands despite voluminous (fluent) spontaneous speech. Paraphasias may be present (especially when the patient is asked to name objects) and consist of either inappropriately substituted words or nonsensical jargon. The responsible lesions are located in the dominant temporoparietal cortex and are often associated with subtle focal neurologic signs, including mild pronator drift of the right hand, right homonymous hemianopsia or superior quadrantanopsia, and right-sided sensory loss; gross hemiparesis is usually not found, as the frontal motor cortex is not affected.

Patient Who Appears Awake and Alert but Noncommunicative

Although sensory stimulation may arouse these patients, they seem unable or unwilling to speak. The causes of this condition include mutism, akinetic mutism, and the persistent vegetative state.

Mutism

Mutism is a manifestation of many clinical conditions, including aphonia, anarthria, oral-lingual apraxia, and aphasia. Only in aphasia, however, is written expression also impaired (i.e., agraphia).

Aphonia due to paralysis of the vocal cords and anarthria due to paralysis of the articulatory muscles are usually evident clinically in patients who are unable to make sounds but who mouth words appropriately. Oral-lingual (facial) apraxia is a disorder of learned mouth movements (e.g., speaking, blowing kisses, sucking through a straw, protruding the tongue to command) seen with isolated and discrete lesions involving the facial area of the dominant motor cortex [14,25].

Patients with expressive aphasia are unable to communicate normally by verbal or written language [1,13,14]. Nonfluent (Broca's) aphasia with diminished "telegraphic" output is usually intensely frustrating to the patient; occasionally, singing his or her words, rather than merely saying them, improves speech. Lesion location differs depending on whether comprehension is also affected or whether comprehension and repetition of words are relatively preserved or lost. At the least, the dominant frontal cortex is involved, and some degree of right hemiparesis is usually present.

Abulia

Patients with abulia "lack will" and are apathetic with slow to no responses to verbal stimuli and do not initiate any activity or conversations. When adequately stimulated, these patients appear to be cognitively intact. In contrast to the obtunded or stuporous patient, they are fully, alertly awake [1]. Abulic patients often have bilateral frontal lobe disease. Specific regions implicated include the anterior cingulate cortex but also been described in other subcortical lesions.

Akinetic Mutism

Patients with akinetic mutism appear alert and exhibit sleep–wake cycles, but they show little evidence of cognitive function and do not meaningfully interact with the environment [1,14]. Brainstem function is intact, and patients may open their eyes to verbal stimuli or track moving objects. They have a paucity of movement even to noxious stimulation, despite little evidence of corticospinal or corticobulbar damage. Akinetic mutism is a more severe form of abulia and is associated with large bilateral lesions of the basomedial frontal lobes, small lesions of the paramedian reticular formation in the posterior diencephalon and midbrain, and subacute communicating hydrocephalus.

Persistent Vegetative State

Patients in a persistent vegetative state are also akinetic and mute but lack outward manifestations of any significant brain activity other than reflex responses [1,14]. These may include decerebrate or decorticate posturing, deep tendon reflexes, Babinski or triple flexion reflexes, yawning, and so on. The term is usually reserved for the patient who has recovered only to this extent from coma due to a severe anoxic, metabolic, or traumatic brain injury, and has been in this condition for over a month. Neuropathologic findings in anoxic encephalopathy may include cortical pseudolaminar necrosis, cerebellar Purkinje cell loss, and necrosis of hippocampal cortex but relative sparing of brainstem structures [26]. Persistent vegetative state is considered permanent if the patient has been in this state for 3 months after nontraumatic or anoxic brain injury, and more than 12 months after traumatic brain injury [27].

Minimally Conscious State

These are patients who, similar to those in the vegetative state, have severely impaired consciousness, also manifest the posturing, reflexes, and diurnal cycles, but in addition show evidence of self and environmental awareness. They may follow simple commands, give gestural yes or no responses, verbalize intelligibly, and do other purposeful behaviors and visual tracking [1,13,14]. This is considered to be a transitional phase of recovery from coma after persistent vegetative state (PVS), and patients with traumatic brain injury who are in a minimally conscious state have significantly better outcomes at 1 year than PVS patients. Many publicized reports of late recoveries from vegetative states were actually patients in minimally conscious state (MCS).

BEDSIDE EVALUATION OF THE COMATOSE PATIENT

Coma in the ICU is a medical emergency. The goal of each evaluation is to identify and treat promptly (if applicable) the cause of the comatose state; even if no definitive treatment is available, general medical and neurologic support is necessary. A neurologic consultation should be obtained early; the practice of obtaining imaging studies before a careful and systematic examination is often counterproductive when it delays focused evaluation and treatment. The proper approach requires (a) immediate administration of life-support measures, (b) completion of a general physical examination, (c) performance and interpretation of the neurologic examination, (d) selection of ancillary tests, and (e) institution of definitive treatment, based on the above observations.

Initial Measures

As in all emergencies, vital signs, respiration, and circulation are first stabilized and monitored; the comatose patient often requires an endotracheal tube for respiratory support and airway protection. A large-bore intravenous line is started, and the blood is drawn for a complete blood cell count, glucose, electrolytes (including Ca^{2+}), blood urea nitrogen, creatinine, liver transaminases, and a toxicology screen. Arterial blood is obtained for determination of oxygen tension, PCO_2, and pH. If there is any doubt about the etiology of coma, 100 mg thiamine, 50 g glucose, and 0.4 mg naloxone are administered intravenously.

General Physical Examination

In addition to the usual complete examination, several points warrant special attention [1,2,13]. Severe hypothermia (rectal temperature less than or equal to 32°C or 89.6°F) may cause coma (as in elderly patients exposed to the cold) or provide clues to other etiologies (e.g., overwhelming sepsis, drug or alcohol intoxication, hypothyroidism, hypoglycemia, Wernicke's encephalopathy) [28]. Severe hyperthermia may result from intracranial causes, including infection and anterior hypothalamic or pontine destruction. Meningeal signs (e.g., nuchal rigidity) may be absent in deeply comatose patients, even in the presence of overwhelming bacterial meningitis. This sign should never be sought if cervical spine fracture or dislocation is suspected.

The skin should be thoroughly inspected for signs of trauma. Basilar skull fractures may be signaled by blood behind the ear (Battle's sign), cerebrospinal fluid rhinorrhea, or otorrhea. Orbital fractures may cause bleeding into periorbital tissues ("raccoon eyes").

The breath odor may suggest metabolic derangement or intoxication. The spoiled fruit odor of diabetic coma, the uriniferous odor of uremia, and the musty fetor of hepatic encephalopathy sometimes can be recognized. Although the odor of alcohol is usually noted, its presence does not rule out superimposed structural causes of coma (e.g., subdural hematoma), and its absence does not rule out intoxication with odorless spirits (e.g., vodka).

Respiratory patterns in comatose patients are distinctive [1,13,14]. Bilateral hemispheric or diencephalic disturbances as well as systemic disorders may lead to periodic breathing in which increasing and then decreasing breaths (crescendo–decrescendo) alternate with apnea (Cheyne–Stokes respirations). Lesions of the midbrain-pontine tegmentum may give rise to tachypnea and a respiratory alkalosis unresponsive to oxygen (central neurogenic hyperventilation), but this is much less common than hyperpnea due to low oxygen tension, metabolic acidosis, or a primary respiratory alkalosis (e.g., salicylate poisoning). Lesions of the inferior pons may be associated with 2- to 3-second pauses following full inspiration (apneustic breathing). Compressive or intrinsic lesions of the medulla may cause chaotic breathing of varying rate and depth (Biot's breathing). Complete brainstem destruction results in apnea that is unresponsive to elevated PCO_2.

Neurologic Examination

The goal of the neurologic examination in the comatose patient is to determine the location of the lesion (ARAS or bilateral cerebral hemispheres) and its etiology (structural, causing destruction or compression of brain substance; toxic, metabolic, anoxic, or traumatic, affecting the nervous system in a diffuse or multifocal manner; subarachnoid blood or infection; or nonconvulsive status epilepticus). A critical part of this determination is the medical history, and heroic efforts to locate family members, witnesses, and medication lists are almost always rewarded. For example, truly sudden coma in a healthy person suggests drug intoxication, intracranial hemorrhage, meningoencephalitis, or an unwitnessed seizure.

Often an intubated patient with altered mental status will be on pharmacologic sedation or anxiolysis for management of respiration, or safety in agitated or combative patients. Neurologic examination should be performed after discontinuing any sedating medication that may alter the patient's responsiveness and significantly alter the examination findings.

Neurologic assessment must include a description of the level of consciousness, examination of the pupils, direct ophthalmoscopy, observation of spontaneous and induced ocular movements, elicitation of the corneal reflex, and tests of motor system function (including spontaneous and induced limb movements and asymmetries of tone), deep tendon reflexes, pathologic reflexes, and response to sensory stimulation—often pain. The importance of repeat examinations to document the temporal course of the patient's condition cannot be overemphasized.

Level of Consciousness

The level of consciousness is determined first by observing the patient undisturbed for several minutes. Any spontaneous (e.g., yawning, sneezing) or responsive (e.g., to ventilator noise) movements or postures are noted. A battery of graduated sensory stimuli is applied (whispered names, shouted names, loud noise, visual threat, noxious stimulation by supraorbital compression, vibrissal [nasal hair] stimulation, sternal rub, nail bed compression, or medial thigh pinch) and the response recorded (e.g., opens eyes, squeezes eyes shut, blinks symmetrically to visual threat, nods, turns head, groans, grimaces, purposefully withdraws, displays stereotyped posturing). Initially using centrally located noxious stimulation such as a sternal rub is important in order to tell if the patient is localizing or merely withdrawing. Such careful documentation allows serial assessments of subtle changes over time by multiple examiners.

Serial documentation and accurate and reliable communication of findings can be facilitated by the use of standardized scales such as the Glasgow Coma Scale. Although originally intended for use in traumatic brain injury, the Glasgow Coma Scale has become widely used and has been found to be predictive of outcomes, particularly in traumatic brain injury (Table 145.4). Because of its limitations, a more comprehensive coma scale called the Full Outline of Unresponsiveness, or FOUR score, incorporates brainstem reflexes and respiration [1,13,14,29] (Table 145.4). These grading scales are helpful to standardize assessment, improve communication and serial monitoring, but are limited and cannot be substituted for a detailed bedside neurologic examination.

TABLE 145.4

Coma Grading Scales

Glasgow Coma Scale
Eye response
4 = eyes open spontaneously
3 = eye opening to verbal command
2 = eye opening to pain
1 = no eye opening
Motor response
6 = obeys commands
5 = localizing pain
4 = withdrawal from pain
3 = flexion response
2 = extension response
1 = no motor response
Verbal response
5 = oriented
4 = confused
3 = inappropriate words
2 = incomprehensible words
1 = no verbal response

FOUR score
Eye response
4 = eyelids open or opened, tracking, or blinking to command
3 = eyelids open but not tracking
2 = eyelids closed but open to loud voice
1 = eyelids closed but open to pain
0 = eyelids remained closed with pain
Motor response
4 = thumbs up, fist, or peace sign
3 = localizing to pain
2 = flexion response to pain
1 = extension response to pain
0 = no response to pain or generalized myoclonus
Brainstem reflexes
4 = pupils and corneals intact
3 = one pupil wide and fixed
2 = pupil or corneal absent
1 = pupil and corneal absent
0 = absent pupil, corneal, and cough reflex
Respiration
4 = not intubated, regular breathing pattern
3 = not intubated, Cheyne–Stokes breathing
2 = not intubated, irregular breathing
1 = breathes above ventilator rate
0 = breathes at ventilator rate or apnea

Pupils

The pupils are examined for size, equality, and reactivity to light. Normal pupils confirm the integrity of a circuit involving the retina, optic nerve, midbrain, third cranial nerve, and pupillary constrictors. A strong flashlight and magnifying glass, or an ophthalmoscope, are usually necessary, and darkening the room is helpful. In difficult cases, sometimes pupillometry can be employed.

Symmetrically small, light-reactive pupils (miosis) are normally seen in elderly and sleeping patients. Opiates, organophosphates, pilocarpine, phenothiazines, and barbiturates produce small pupils that may appear to be unreactive to light, whereas a large lesion of the pons (i.e., hemorrhage) characteristically produces tiny pinpoint pupils. Symmetrically large pupils (mydriasis) that do not react to light suggest midbrain damage, but they may also be seen following resuscitation when atropine has been used (in this case, the pupils do not constrict to 1% pilocarpine) [30], in cases of anoxia, following pressor doses of dopamine [31], and often in amphetamine or cocaine intoxication. Bilaterally fixed and midposition pupils indicate absent midbrain function, although severe hypothermia [28], hypotension, or intoxication with succinylcholine [32] or glutethimide [33] must be ruled out.

Pupillary asymmetry (anisocoria) suggests neurologic dysfunction if it is of recent onset, the inequality is more than 1 mm, and the degree of anisocoria changes with ambient lighting [34]. When the larger pupil is sluggishly reactive or fixed to light (but the contralateral consensual response is spared), uncal herniation due to an ipsilateral hemispheric mass compressing the third cranial nerve against the petroclinoid ligament must be considered. Unilateral pupillary dilatation may also indicate a mass in the cavernous sinus, aneurysm of the posterior communicating artery, focal seizure, or topical atropine-like drugs (e.g., used for ophthalmoscopic examination). On the other hand, with Horner's syndrome, the affected pupil is smaller. In this condition, the pupillary asymmetry is increased in darkness and the smaller pupil is associated with partial ptosis of the upper eyelid, straightening of the lower eyelid, and facial anhidrosis. It may be caused by damage to descending sympathetic fibers anywhere from the hypothalamus to the upper thoracic cord, or to ascending sympathetic fibers in the cervical sympathetic chain, the superior cervical ganglion, the carotid artery, or the cavernous sinus.

Measuring the neurologic pupil index (NPI) with a pupillometer can facilitate assessment in situations when pupil assessment is clinically difficult and changes in the NPI can be an early indicator of increased intracranial pressure [35].

Direct Ophthalmoscopy

Direct ophthalmoscopy may be limited by miosis or cataracts, but the pupils should never be pharmacologically dilated without clear documentation (with a large sign taped to the patient's bed), or if the patient's condition is uncertain or unstable. Obscuration of the disk margins, absent venous pulsations, and flame-shaped hemorrhages suggest early papilledema from an intracranial mass or systemic hypertension [36]. Subhyaloid and vitreous hemorrhages may be observed in the patient with subarachnoid hemorrhage or suddenly increased intracranial pressure.

Ocular Movements

Assessment of ocular movements begins by observing for tonic deviation of the eyes at rest [1]. The eyes may deviate toward the side of a lesion in the motor cortex (a gaze preference—away from the hemiparetic limbs) but usually can be induced to cross the midline. The eyes deviate away from the side of a pontine lesion (toward the hemiparetic limbs) and cannot be moved across the midline (a gaze paralysis). A seizure focus in the frontal (area 8) or supplementary motor (area 6) cortex can drive the eyes or cause nystagmoid jerks contralaterally (toward the side of the convulsing limbs) [37]. Tonic upward eye deviation may be seen after anoxia [38], and tonic downward deviation may be seen in thalamic hemorrhage, midbrain compression, and hepatic encephalopathy.

Spontaneous eye movements may have a localizing value. Roving eye movements (slow and random, usually conjugate and horizontal) and periodic alternating ("Ping-Pong") gaze (cyclic, conjugate excursions to the extremes of lateral gaze every 2 to 3 seconds) [39] are found in patients with intact brainstem function. Ocular bobbing consists of a rapid conjugate downward jerk followed by a slow upward drift (rate and rhythm are variable) and suggests a lesion in the pons or posterior fossa, especially if horizontal eye movements are impaired [40]. The reverse movement, ocular dipping (slow downward, fast upward), can also be seen less reliably in pontine lesions but also after anoxia and in status epilepticus [41]. Conjugate spasmodic eye movements, rotating the eyes upward for minutes or longer (oculogyric crisis), in some patients may be an untoward effect of neuroleptic medications.

If spontaneous eye movements are absent or restricted to a particular direction, reflex movements should be tested by oculocephalic ("doll's eyes") and oculovestibular (caloric) stimulation [1,17,18,42]. Full eye movements induced by these maneuvers confirm the integrity of the brainstem tegmentum from the medullary–pontine junction to the midbrain. Oculocephalic testing is never done in patients with suspected cervical spine fracture or dislocation. The maneuver is performed by holding the patient's eyelids open and briskly rotating the head from one side to the other (for horizontal eye movements) and from flexion to extension (for vertical eye movements). In comatose patients with an intact brainstem, the eyes deviate to the side opposite the direction of head movement. If the oculocephalic response is not obtained or the movements are limited or asymmetric, the oculovestibular reflex should be tested. This is never done until the tympanic membrane is examined and seen to be intact. The patient's head is elevated to 30 degrees above horizontal, and up to 120 mL ice water is instilled slowly in the external auditory meatus with a large syringe and attached Teflon catheter. Each ear is tested separately for horizontal eye movements, with a 5-minute interval between right and left ears. In awake patients (or those in psychogenic coma), nystagmus with the fast phase away from the irrigated ear is induced. In comatose patients with an intact brainstem, a tonic conjugate eye deviation toward the irrigated ear is seen; a defective response implies brainstem damage. Vertical eye movements can be induced by irrigating both ears simultaneously with cold water (eyes deviate downward) and with warm (44°C) water (eyes deviate upward). Absent or deranged responses can be caused, in addition to various brainstem lesions, by previous vestibular (labyrinthine end-organ) lesions, vestibulosuppressant drugs (e.g., benzodiazepines, antihistamines, anticholinergics), hepatic encephalopathy, and neuromuscular blockers (e.g., succinylcholine). An ophthalmoplegia after intravenous phenytoin is well known [43].

Corneal Reflex

The corneal reflex is obtained by lightly touching the limbus of the cornea with a fine material (wisp of cotton, rolled corner of tissue paper, or a squirt of air or saline). Both eyes should blink to unilateral stimulation, confirming the integrity of a circuit involving the fifth cranial nerve, trigeminal sensory and facial motor nuclei in the pons, and both seventh cranial nerves. A blunted corneal response is commonly seen in chronic contact lens wearers. An absent blink on the stimulated side with an intact contralateral (consensual) response indicates ipsilateral motor damage.

Motor System

The examination of the motor system identifies whether limb movements are appropriate and purposeful or inappropriate and stereotyped. Left–right asymmetries or worsening of the motor response over time must be carefully noted. Appropriate movements include spontaneous turning in bed, drawing up the sheets, crossing the legs modestly, or rapid withdrawal (especially abduction) from noxious stimulation. Applying noxious stimuli centrally such as a sternal rub or pinching the proximal area of an arm or leg will allow distinction between localization which is purposeful and indicates intact awareness at a cortical level versus mere withdrawal which can be a brainstem reflex and this can have prognostic implications. Inappropriate movements include spontaneous or induced flexion–internal rotation of the arms with extension of the legs (decorticate posturing) or extension-adduction of all limbs (decerebrate posturing); whether flexor or extensor postures are induced depends partly on the position of the limbs [44]. These responses may occur occasionally in toxic-metabolic coma [45,46] but are more common with anatomic brainstem lesions. Facial grimaces or groans despite absent motor responses suggest that sensory pathways are grossly intact. Flexion of the leg at the hip, knee, and ankle (triple flexion response) is a spinally mediated exaggerated Babinski reflex that may persist in brain death.

Other spontaneous movements of the limbs and trunk have been observed in brain dead patients and are all forms of spinal reflexes, including myokymia, trunk flexion, and the Lazarus sign, wherein the patient actually extends and pronates his or her arms forward and then crosses them over the chest [1,17,18,47]. These signs are easily misinterpreted by family members as well as medical practitioners who are not versed in the neurologic examination.

INTERPRETATION OF THE NEUROLOGIC EXAMINATION

In general, focal neurologic signs suggest a structural cause of coma. Nevertheless, focal weakness is not unknown in hypoglycemia, hyperglycemia, hyponatremia, hyperkalemia, and rarely hepatic and uremic encephalopathies [48,49]; and continuous focal motor seizures (epilepsia partialis continua) may be a presenting sign of the hyperglycemic nonketotic hyperosmolar state [50]. Focal signs due to preexisting deficits may deceive even the ablest clinician. For example, if generalized seizures from a new metabolic imbalance develop in a patient with an old hemiplegia due to a cerebral infarction, apparently focal convulsions of the nonplegic limbs might falsely suggest a structural lesion of the intact cerebral hemisphere contralateral to the previously infarcted one. Other false localizing signs include sixth nerve palsies (due to transmitted increased intracranial pressure), visual field cuts (due to compression of the posterior cerebral artery), and hemiparesis ipsilateral to a third nerve palsy (due to compression of the contralateral cerebral peduncle against the tentorium [Kernohan's notch]).

Conversely, a nonfocal examination does not invariably indicate toxic-metabolic coma. Symmetric neurologic dysfunction may be caused by meningoencephalitis, subarachnoid hemorrhage, bilateral subdural hematomas, or thrombosis of the superior sagittal sinus. Multifocal seizures, myoclonus, asterixis, or fluctuation of the examination suggests a toxic or metabolic etiology, although periodic increases in intracranial pressure (plateau waves) and nonconvulsive seizures may lead to a waxing and waning mental status.

A preserved pupillary light reflex even in deep coma with absent oculovestibular and motor responses suggests a toxic or metabolic etiology. It is important to note that the pupils may be unreactive to light in severe hypothermia, deep barbiturate coma (the patient is usually apneic and hypotensive if the pupils are fixed), and glutethimide overdose. In addition, an expanding posterior fossa mass (e.g., cerebellar hemorrhage) may present with early signs of pontine compression and small, light-reactive pupils [51].

A useful rule is that toxic-metabolic coma usually has incomplete but symmetric dysfunction of neural systems affecting many levels of the neuraxis simultaneously while retaining the integrity of other functions at the same levels. Structural coma is characterized by regionally restricted anatomic defects [1,13,14]. For example, toxic-metabolic coma might present with intact pupillary reactivity and corneal reflexes but an absence of horizontal (pontine) and vertical (midbrain) reflex eye movements to oculovestibular testing. Such a presentation would be inconsistent with coma from a structural cause.

ANCILLARY TESTS

Imaging studies are often necessary and always informative in the patient with altered consciousness to shed light on the etiology or structural contributors to the patient's clinical presentation, but require interpretation specific to the patient's clinical data and examination. Neuroanatomic correlation of imaging and examination are essential in their use and also provide useful prognostic information. A computed tomographic (CT) scan can be considered the initial brain imaging study in patients with coma if lesions that require emergent surgical intervention, such as acute cerebellar hemorrhage, are considered [1,13,14]. A CT scan without contrast infusion can reliably demonstrate intracranial bleeding such as intraparenchymal, epidural or subdural hematoma, or intraventricular hemorrhage. CT scans can reveal hydrocephalus; and may show anoxic–ischemic brain injury, with loss of gray–white differentiation, border-zone infarction from hypoperfusion, and diffuse cerebral edema (Fig. 145.2). Other coma-inducing lesions shown by CT scan include massive middle cerebral infarction, uncal herniation, and midline shift from large mass lesions with cerebral edema. Contrast enhancement may be required for suspected infectious or neoplastic masses. The CT scan does not reliably rule out inflammation, infection, subarachnoid blood, or early ischemia. CT angiography can be helpful in showing large vessel occlusion or dissection but has limited sensitivity and specificity.

Magnetic resonance imaging (MRI) is clearly superior to CT scan in resolution, and special sequences are highly sensitive to acute ischemia and encephalitis. MRI is superior for anatomic detail and can produce excellent images of the posterior fossa, brainstem, and craniocervical junction. Diffusion weighted MRI studies, and particularly whole brain median apparent diffusion coefficient imaging, is useful in assessing prognosis following anoxic–ischemic coma [52–54]. Although it is not always logistically possible to perform MRI imaging on patients in the ICU, whenever possible it provides important information.

New developments and research using functional magnetic resonance imaging (fMRI) are not only shedding light on the importance of specific structures to consciousness, and other clinical states such as abulia, but are also furthering our understanding of the importance of connectivity [55] and specific circuits to coma. (Fig.145.3). Numerous studies in patients with persistent vegetative and minimally conscious states show activation in the primary auditory cortex and higher order temporal lobe areas when their names are spoken to them by familiar voices. Other speech comprehension tasks in which the level of activation is highest in patients who improved from PVS to MCS suggest the possibility of a new frontier in clinical understanding of coma, and clinical utility in prognostication [56,57].

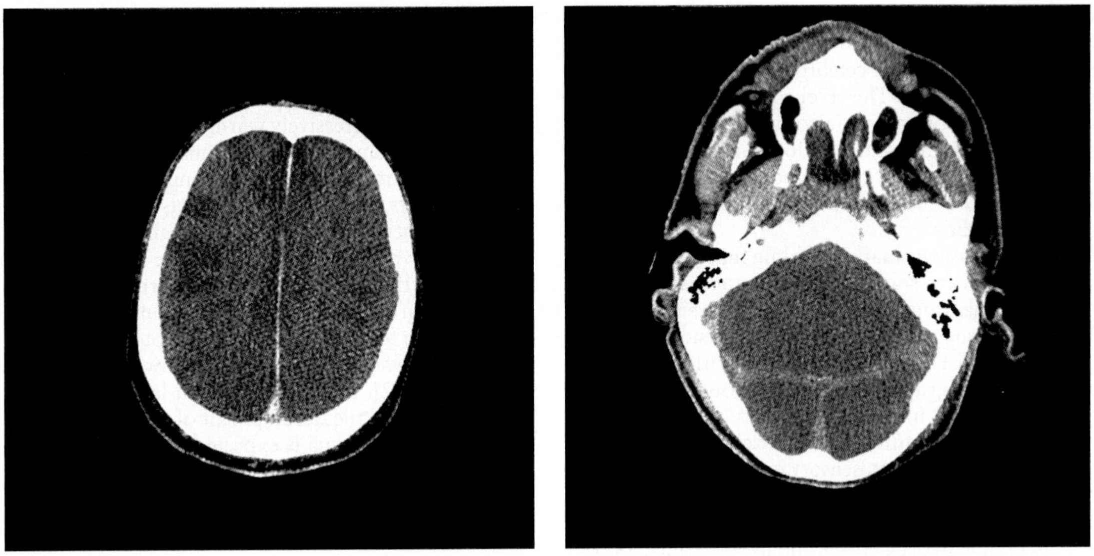

FIGURE 145.2 Noncontrast CT scan of patient with anoxic brain injury. Diffuse cerebral edema with loss of gray–white differentiation, obliteration of basal cisterns, multiple areas of hypodensity suggestive of anoxic–ischemic injury, and venous stasis with hyperdensity of the venous sinuses. This patient was brain dead clinically and by apnea testing.

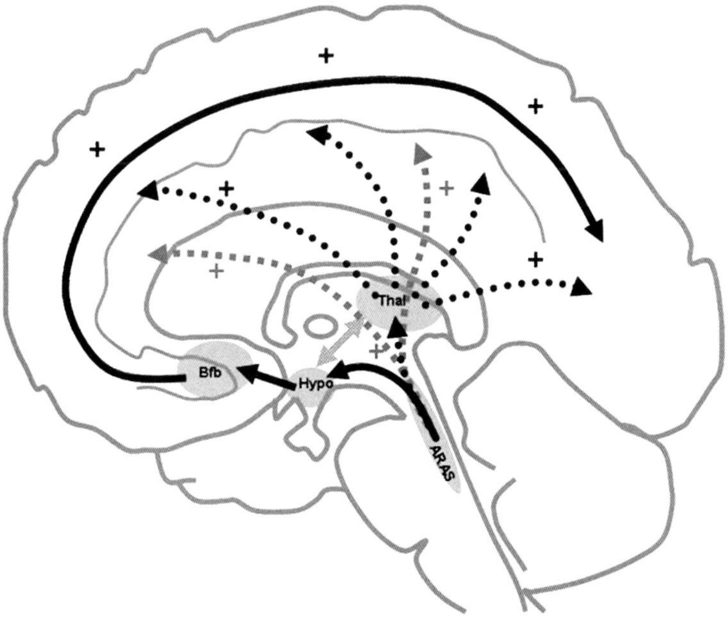

FIGURE 145.3 Anatomic substrates of arousal and awareness. Consciousness involves two main components: arousal and awareness of oneself and of the environment. Awareness is dependent on the integrity of specific anatomic regions. The ascending reticular activating system (ARAS), the primary arousal structure, is located in the upper pons and lower midbrain in the posterior part of the upper two-thirds of the brainstem. A ventral pathway (*black solid arrows*) projects to the hypothalamus (hypo) and basal forebrain (Bfb); a dorsal pathway (*black dashed arrows*) projects to the reticular nuclei of the thalamus (thal); and a third pathway (*light gray arrows*) projects directly into the cortical regions. From the basal forebrain, two main bundles project diffusely to several cortical areas. The reticular nuclei of the thalamus connect to other nuclei in the thalamus. They are involved in a thalamocortical circuit that controls cortical activity. Some regions of the cerebral cortex may also make specific contributions to consciousness. (From Weiss N, Galanaud D, Carpentier A, et al: Clinical review: prognostic value of magnetic resonance imaging in acute brain injury and coma. *Crit Care* 11:230, 2007. doi:10.1186/cc6107.).

The cerebrospinal fluid must be examined if meningoencephalitis is suspected or if subarachnoid blood is not visualized on the CT scan. Occasionally, a sterile cerebrospinal fluid pleocytosis follows status epilepticus [58]. The cerebrospinal fluid sent for protein 14-3-3, or tau protein, may also be useful in the diagnosis of CJD. Cytology and vascular endothelial growth factor levels can confirm the diagnosis of carcinomatous meningitis; and antibodies can be evaluated in paraneoplastic syndromes such as limbic encephalitis.

EEG provides a physiologic marker of brain function and may be helpful in nonconvulsive status epilepticus and psychogenic coma, and for documenting (but not primarily establishing) brain death by the presence of electrocerebral silence. Current research correlates EEG background patterns with fMRI and positron emission tomography scans in response to speech comprehension tasks, and investigates the utility of EEG for prognostication in patients with altered consciousness [59].

In unresponsive patients, somatosensory or brainstem auditory evoked potentials may be very useful in evaluating the integrity of spinal, brainstem, or cortical pathways and, compared to EEG, are much less susceptible to drug effects and hypothermia. SSEPs are useful in prognostication of recovery from anoxic–ischemic coma during the first few days after cardiac arrest.

INITIATION OF EMERGENCY TREATMENT

Definitive treatment of altered consciousness depends on the underlying pathophysiologic process, but urgent therapeutic interventions may be required in life-threatening conditions or to prevent further central nervous system insult. Meticulous nursing care (fluid replacement, oxygenation and prevention of aspiration, nutrition, corneal protection, and conscientious skin, bowel, and bladder care) is essential. *Unnecessary sedation should be avoided*—it obscures evaluation of the patient's state of consciousness and makes assessment of any changes in the sensorium or cognition inaccessible to testing.

Recent and ongoing clinical trials are continuing to validate acute therapies that may protect the brain after insults such as cardiac arrest, traumatic brain injury, and stroke. For example, the induction of mild hypothermia (33°C for 12 to 24 hours) in comatose survivors of cardiac arrest improved the neurologic outcome in two randomized clinical trials [60,61]. Based on these studies, the American Heart Association and the International Liaison Committee on Resuscitation advised therapeutic mild hypothermia for unconscious victims of cardiac arrest [62]. Hypothermia appeared ineffective as an acute treatment for traumatic brain injury in one large randomized controlled trial [63] but may have been related to the delay in achieving goal temperature, duration of cooling, as well as other factors. A recent systematic review of 12 randomized controlled trials that pooled 1,069 patients concluded that clinical mortality and outcome benefit may be derived from cooling patients with traumatic brain injury to a temperature of 32°C to 33°C for 48 hours and slowly rewarming them 24 hours after discontinuation of therapy [64]. A multicenter trial of early induced hypothermia for severe traumatic brain injury for 48 hours failed to show benefit, but was terminated prematurely and was confounded by intracranial hypertension during rewarming [65].

A more recent clinical trial of therapeutic hypothermia (33°C) versus normothermia (36.5°C) in children who remained unconscious after out-of-hospital cardiac arrest again showed no benefit in survival with good functional outcome at 1 year [66]. Despite several failed clinical trials, there remains a physiologic basis for its use, and there is still some interest in hypothermia and its effects on edema and intracranial pressure. However, the challenges of achieving therapeutic hypothermia and multiple complications including cardiac arrhythmia, coagulopathy, and infection, as well as complications of rewarming have hindered significant progress in its utility [67,68]. Many guidelines are now adapting a more conservative targeted temperature management protocol which includes an option for goal temperature of 36°C rather than the previous 32°C to 34°C [69,70]. If patients sustaining a neurologic insult are hypothermic upon admission to the ICU, it may be prudent to avoid aggressively warming them to normothermic levels. The benefit from mild hypothermia likely involves more complex biochemical mechanisms than simple reduction in oxygenation requirements. The deleterious effects of fever in brain injury are well documented in the laboratory and clinical outcome studies in a variety of diseases [71]. No large studies have prospectively addressed the effects of induced normothermia on outcomes. Comparison of endovascular and standard normothermia protocols to achieve a temperature of 36.5°C found no increase of adverse events, but was underpowered to show any benefit on neurologic outcomes [72]. Further study in a larger sample of patients is warranted, and the development of protocols to control fever or induce normothermia is expected to benefit these patients.

CONCLUSION

Altered consciousness is common in patients in the ICU. A systematic and efficient approach is required to determine the location of the responsible lesion(s) or the cause(s) of impaired consciousness, both to allow institution of definitive therapies and to assess the prognosis accurately.

References

1. Posner JB, Saper CB, Schiff ND, et al: *Plum and Posner's Diagnosis of Stupor and Coma*. 4th ed. New York, NY, Oxford University Press, 2007.
2. Fisher CM: The neurological examination of the comatose patient. *Acta Neurol Scand* 45[Suppl 36]:1, 1969.
3. Caplan LR: Top of the basilar syndrome. *Neurology* 30:72, 1980.
4. Bogousslvsky J, Regli F, Uske A: Thalamic infarcts: clinical syndromes, etiology, and prognosis. *Neurology* 38:837, 1988.
5. Levy DE, Bates D, Corona JJ, et al: Prognosis in non-traumatic coma. *Ann Intern Med* 94:293–301, 1981.
6. Wijdicks EF, Hijdra A, Young GB, et al: Practice parameter: prediction of outcome in comatose survivors after cardiopulmonary resuscitation (an evidence-based review): report of the Quality Standards Subcommittee of the American Academy of Neurology. *Neurology* 67:203, 2006.
7. Patterson JR, Grabois M: Locked-in syndrome: a review of 139 cases. *Stroke* 17:758, 1986.
8. Doble JE, Haig AJ, Anderson C, et al: Impairment, activity, participation, life satisfaction and survival in persons with locked-in syndrome for over a decade: follow up on a previously reported cohort. *J Head Trauma Rehabil* 18:435–444, 2003.
9. President's Commission for the Study of Ethical Problems in Medicine and Biomedical and Behavioral Research: *Defining Death: Medical, Legal, and Ethical Issues in the Determination of Death*. Washington, DC, US Government Printing Office, 1981.
10. Wijdicks EF: The diagnosis of brain death. *N Engl J Med* 344:1215, 2001.
11. Quality Standards Subcommittee of the American Academy of Neurology: Practice parameters for determining brain death in adults [summary statement]. *Neurology* 45:1012, 1995.
12. Greer DM, Varelas PN, Haque S, et al: Variability of brain death determination guidelines in leading US neurologic institutions. *Neurology* 70:284–289, 2008.
13. Ropper AH, Gress DR, Diringer MN, (eds) et al: *Neurological and Neurosurgical Intensive Care*. 4th ed. Philadelphia, PA, Lippincott Williams & Wilkins, 2004.
14. Ropper AH, Samuels MA: *Adams and Victor's Principles of Neurology*. 9th ed. New York, NY, McGraw-Hill, 2009.
15. Bergeron N, Dubois MJ, Dumont M, et al: Intensive care delirium screening checklist: evaluation of a new screening tool. *Intensive Care Med* 27:859, 2001.
16. Ely EW, Inouye SK, Bernard G, et al: Delirium in mechanically ventilated patients: validity and reliability of the confusion assessment method for the intensive care unit (CAM-ICU). *JAMA* 286:2703–2710, 2001.
17. Ely EW, Shintani A, Truman B, et al: Delirium as a predictor of mortality in mechanically ventilated patients in the intensive care unit. *JAMA* 291:1753–1762, 2004.
18. Girard TD, Kress JP, Fuchs BD, et al: Efficacy and safety of a paired sedation and ventilator weaning protocol for mechanically ventilated patients in intensive care (Awakening and Breathing Controlled trial): a randomised controlled trial. *Lancet* 371:126–134, 2008.
19. Riker RR, Shehabi Y, Bokesch PM, et al; for the SEDCOM (Safety and Efficacy of Dexmedetomidine Compared With Midazolam) Study Group: Dexmedetomidine vs midazolam for sedation of critically ill patients: a randomized trial. *JAMA* 301(5):489–499, 2009.

20. Strub RL, Black FW: *Neurobehavioral Disorders: A Clinical Approach*. Philadelphia, PA, FA Davis, 1988.
21. Cascino GD: Nonconvulsive status epilepticus in adults and children. *Epilepsia* 34[Suppl 1]:S21, 1993.
22. Tomson T, Svangorg E, Wedlund JE: Nonconvulsive status epilepticus: high incidence of complex partial status. *Epilepsia* 27:276, 1986.
23. Claassen J, Mayer SA, Kowalski RG, et al: Detection of electrographic seizures with continuous EEG monitoring in critically ill patients. *Neurology* 62:1743–1748, 2004.
24. Towne AR, Waterhouse EJ, Boggs JG, et al: Prevalence of nonconvulsive status epilepticus in comatose patients. *Neurology* 54:340, 2000.
25. Geschwind N: The apraxias: neural mechanisms of disorders of learned movement. *Am Sci* 63:188, 1975.
26. Kinney HC, Samuels MA: Neuropathology of the persistent vegetative state: a review. *J Neuropath Exp Neurol* 53:548, 1994.
27. Multi-Society Task Force on PVS: Medical aspects of the persistent vegetative state. *N Engl J Med* 330:1499–508, 1994.
28. Fischbeck KH, Simon RP: Neurological manifestations of accidental hypothermia. *Ann Neurol* 10:384, 1981.
29. Wijdicks EF, Bamler WR, Maramattom BV, et al: Validation of a new coma scale: the FOUR score. *Ann Neurol.* 58:585–593, 2005
30. Thompson HS, Newsome DA, Loewenfeld IE: The fixed dilated pupils: sudden iridoplegia or mydriatic drops? A simple diagnostic test. *Arch Ophthalmol* 86:21, 1971.
31. Ong GL, Bruning HA: Dilated fixed pupils due to administration of high doses of dopamine hydrochloride. *Crit Care Med* 9:658, 1981.
32. Tyson RN: Simulation of cerebral death by succinylcholine sensitivity. *Arch Neurol* 30:409, 1974.
33. Brown DG, Hammill JF: Glutethimide poisoning: unilateral pupillary abnormalities. *N Engl J Med* 285:806, 1971.
34. Glaser JS: *Neuro-Ophthalmology*. Philadelphia, PA, Lippincott Williams & Wilkins, 1999.
35. Chen JW, Gombart ZJ, Rogers S, et al: Pupillary reactivity as an early indicator of increased intracranial pressure: the introduction of the neurological pupil index. *Surg Neurol Int* 2:82, 2011. doi:10.4103/2152-7806.82248.
36. Neetens A, Smets RM: Papilledema. *Neuro-Ophthalmology* 9:81, 1989.
37. Wyllie E, Ludes H, Morris HH, et al: The lateralizing significance of versive head and eye movements during epileptic seizures. *Neurology* 36:606, 1986.
38. Keane JR: Sustained upgaze in coma. *Ann Neurol* 9:409, 1981.
39. Stewart JD, Kirkham TH, Mathieson G: Periodic alternating gaze. *Neurology* 29:222, 1979.
40. Mehler MF: The clinical spectrum of ocular bobbing and ocular dipping. *J Neurol Neurosurg Psychiatry* 51:725, 1988.
41. Ropper AH: Ocular dipping in anoxic coma. *Arch Neurol* 28:297, 1981.
42. Leigh RJ, Hanley DF, Munschauer FE, et al: Eye movements induced by head rotation in unresponsive patients. *Ann Neurol* 15:465, 1984.
43. Spector RH, Davidoff RA, Schwartzman RJ: Phenytoin-induced ophthalmoplegia. *Neurology* 26:1031, 1976.
44. Barolet-Romana G, Larson SJ: Influence of stimulus location and limb position on motor responses in the comatose patient. *J Neurosurg* 61:725, 1984.
45. Greenberg DA, Simon RP: Flexor and extensor postures in sedative drug-induced coma. *Neurology* 32:448, 1982.
46. Seibert DG: Reversible decerebrate posturing secondary to hypoglycemia. *Am J Med* 78:1036, 1985.
47. Saposnik G, Basile VS, Young GB: Movements in brain death: a systematic review. *Can J Neurol Sci* 36:154–160, 2009.
48. Cadranel JF, Lebiez E, Di Martino, et al: Focal neurological signs in hepatic encephalopathy in cirrhotic patients: an underestimated entity? *Am J Gastroenterol* 96:515–518, 2001.
49. Palmer CA: Neurologic manifestations of renal disease. *Neurol Clin* 20:23–34, 2002.
50. Singh BM, Strobos RJ: Epilepsia partialis continua associated with nonketotic hyperglycemia: clinical and biochemical profile of 21 patients. *Ann Neurol* 8:155, 1980.
51. Cuneo RA, Caronna JJ, Pitts L, et al: Upward transtentorial herniation. *Arch Neurol* 36:618, 1979.
52. Weiss N, Galanaud D, Carpentier A, et al: Prognostic value of magnetic resonance imaging in acute brain injury and coma. *Crit Care* 11:230, 2007.
53. Wijdicks EF, Campeau NG, Miller GM: MR imaging in comatose survivors of cardiac resuscitation. *Am J Neuroradiol* 22:1561–1565, 2001.
54. Wu O, Sorensen AG, Brenner T, et al: Comatose patients with cardiac arrest: predicting clinical outcome with diffusion weighted MRI imaging. *Radiology* 252:173–181, 2009.
55. Siegel JS, Snyder AZ, Metcalf NV, et al: The circuitry of abulia: insights from functional connectivity MRI. *Neuroimage Clin* 6:320–326, 2014.
56. Owen AM, Schiff ND, Laureys S: A new era of coma and consciousness science. *Prog Brain Res* 177:399–411, 2009.
57. Laureys S, Schiff ND: Coma and consciousness: paradigms (re)framed by Neuroimaging. *Neuroimage* 61:478–491, 2012.
58. Devinsky O, Nadi NS, Theodore WH, et al: Cerebrospinal fluid pleocytosis following simple, complex partial, and generalized tonic-clonic seizures. *Ann Neurol* 23:402, 1988.
59. Forgacs PB, Conte MM, Fridman EA, et al: EEG Background is useful in assessing patients with impaire consciousness after brain injury. *Ann Neurol* 76:869–879, 2014.
60. Hypothermia after Cardiac Arrest Study Group: Mild therapeutic hypothermia to improve the neurologic outcome after cardiac arrest. *N Engl J Med* 346:549, 2002.
61. Bernard SA, Gray TW, Buist MD, et al: Treatment of comatose survivors of out-of-hospital cardiac arrest with induced hypothermia. *N Engl J Med* 346:557, 2002.
62. Nolan JP, Morley PT, Vanden Hoek TL, et al: Therapeutic hypothermia after cardiac arrest: an advisory statement by the advanced life support task force of the International Liaison Committee on Resuscitation. *Circulation* 108:118, 2003.
63. Clifton GL, Miller ER, Choi SC, et al: Lack of effect of induction of hypothermia after acute brain injury. *N Engl J Med* 344:556, 2001.
64. McIntyre LA, Fergusson DA, Hebert PC, et al: Prolonged therapeutic hypothermia after traumatic brain injury in adults: a systematic review. *JAMA* 289:2992–2999, 2003.
65. Clifton GL, Valadka A, Zygun D, et al: Very early hypothermia induction in patients with severe brain injury. (the National Acute Brain Injury Study: Hypothermia II) A randomized trial. *Lancet Neurol* 10:131–139, 2011.
66. Moler FW, Silverstein FS, Holubkov R, et al; for the THAPCA Trial Investigators: Therapeutic hypothermia after out-of-hospital cardiac arrest in children. *N Eng J Med* 372:1898–1908, 2015.
67. Polderman KH: Application of therapeutic hypothermia in the ICU: opportunities and pitfalls of a promising treatment modality—Part 1: indications and evidence. *Intensive Care Med* 30:556, 2004.
68. Polderman KH: Application of therapeutic hypothermia in the ICU: opportunities and pitfalls of a promising treatment modality—Part 2: practical aspects and side effects. *Intensive Care Med* 30:757, 2004.
69. Monsieurs KG, Nolan JP, Bossaert L, et al; for the ERC Guidelines 2015 Writing Group: European resuscitation council guidelines for resuscitation 2015. *Resuscitation* 95:1–80, 2015.
70. Rittenberger JC, Friess S, Polderman KH: Emergency neurological life support: resuscitation following cardiac arrest. *Neurocrit Care*, 2015. doi:10.1007/s12028-015-0171-4.
71. Badjatia N: Hyperthermia and fever control in brain injury. *Crit Care Med* 37(7):S250–S257, 2009.
72. Broessner G, Beer R, Lackner P, et al: Prophylactic endovascularly based long-term normothermia in ICU patients with severe cerebrovascular disease: bicenter, prospective randomized trial. *Stroke* 40:e657–e665, 2009.

Chapter 146 ▪ Metabolic Encephalopathy

PAULA D. RAVIN • ABDUL MIKATI • SUSANNE MUEHLSCHLEGEL

Metabolic encephalopathy is a general term used to describe any process that affects global cortical function by altering the biochemical function of the brain. It is the most common cause of altered mental status in the intensive care unit (ICU) setting, either medical or surgical, and is also one of the most treatable. Early recognition of metabolic encephalopathy, therefore, is critical to the management of the ICU patient. The patients who are most at risk for development of a metabolic encephalopathy are those with single or multiple organ failure, the elderly (>60 years of age), those receiving multiple drugs with central nervous system (CNS) toxicity, and those with severe nutritional deficiencies such as cancer patients and alcoholics. Other risk factors include infection, temperature dysregulation (hypothermia or fever), chronic degenerative neurologic or psychiatric diseases such as dementia or schizophrenia, and endocrine disorders. Metabolic encephalopathy is always suspected when there is an altered cognitive status in the absence of focal neurologic signs or an obvious anatomic lesion such as an acute cerebrovascular accident or head injury. A patient may progress over days from intermittent agitation into depressed consciousness or quickly into coma without any antecedent signs (e.g., with hypoglycemia). In mild cases, it is easily mistaken for fatigue or psychogenic depression, whereas more severe cases may develop into coma and are life-threatening.

The altered mental status observed can start as mild confusion with intermittent disorientation to person, time, or place and difficulty attending to questions or tasks at hand. Delirium is a further change toward heightened arousal alternating with somnolence, often worse at night and fluctuating throughout the day. Finally, progression to lethargy, a state of sleepiness in which the person is difficult to arouse by vigorous stimulation, can lead into stupor or coma as impaired consciousness ensues. This sequence of events is often punctuated by focal or generalized tonic–clonic seizures and postictal somnolence as part of the overall clinical picture (Table 146.1).

TABLE 146.1

Patient Profile in Metabolic Encephalopathy

Gradual onset over hours
Progressive if untreated
Waxing and waning level of consciousness
Patient treated with multiple CNS-acting drugs
Patient with organ failure, postoperative state, electrolyte disturbance, endocrine disease
No evidence of brain tumor or stroke on neurologic examination—usually nonfocal (except hypoglycemia or focal seizures)
Sometimes heralded by seizures—focal or generalized
Increased spontaneous motor activity—restlessness, asterixis, myoclonus, tremors, rigidity, and so forth
Abnormal blood chemistries, blood gases, anemia
Usually normal CNS imaging studies
Generalized electroencephalographic abnormalities—slowing, triphasic waves
Gradual recovery once treatment is initiated

CNS, central nervous system.

Disorders that can be confused with metabolic encephalopathy include brain tumors, encephalitis, meningitis, closed head trauma, and brainstem cerebrovascular events. Brain tumors are usually recognizable because they produce focal neurologic deficits such as hemiplegia or hemianopsia, as do traumatic lesions of the brain and cortical strokes. Hypoglycemia can also present focally and is discussed further in the section on Hypoglycemic Encephalopathy. Brainstem stroke due to thrombosis of the basilar artery can be deceptive because there may be a gradual progression of signs and symptoms over several hours rather than a sudden presentation. Table 146.2 outlines some of the cardinal differences between brainstem stroke and metabolic encephalopathy.

EVALUATION

Clinical Examination

Initial observation of the patient's level of arousal, posture in bed, breathing pattern, vital signs, and behavioral fluctuations is highly suggestive of a metabolic disturbance in many cases. Waxing and waning levels of activity are the hallmark of metabolic encephalopathy and may occur over hours to days. Often signs of sympathetic overactivity (tachycardia, elevated blood pressure, tremulousness) and abnormal sleep patterns or "sun-downing" are present.

Mild *behavioral changes* are the earliest manifestations, such as lack of attentiveness to surroundings or a paucity of spontaneous speech, which may give the patient an apathetic or withdrawn appearance. The Mini-Mental State Examination easily reveals mild confusion and can be used to grade the patient's level of cognitive performance sequentially [1]. When there is impaired consciousness, however, this test is unreliable.

The *cranial nerve examination* is focused on pupillary responses, oculomotor function, and respiratory patterns (Table 146.3). As a rule, pupils are small, symmetric, and responsive to light in metabolic causes of obtundation or coma. Noteworthy exceptions to this are anticholinergic poisoning (e.g., atropine, scopolamine), which produces dilated sluggish pupils, and glutethimide (Doriden) poisoning, which results in mid- to large-sized sluggish or fixed pupils [2]. Ocular movements are usually unaffected initially, with eyes in midline position or slightly deviated outward and upward at rest (Bell's phenomenon). Doll's eye maneuvers produce conjugate deviation of the eyes opposite to the direction of head rotation. As the level of brainstem suppression progresses to coma, these responses may disappear completely, especially with an overdose of sedative drugs. In the face of hyperpnea and decerebrate rigidity, the preservation of doll's eyes is a useful sign pointing to a metabolic, rather than anatomic, cause of coma.

Changes in the respiratory pattern are the next most important finding for the diagnosis of metabolic encephalopathy, also providing a clue as to its etiology. In the mildly confused patient, breathing may be normal, but lethargic or mildly obtunded patients tend to hyperventilate, with brief spells of apnea. This is due to transient lowering of the partial pressure of carbon dioxide (PCO_2) below 15 mm Hg without the appropriate CNS drive to breathe more rapidly at a lower tidal volume. After 12 to 30 seconds of apnea, the cycle of hyperventilation appears

TABLE 146.2

Signs and Symptoms of Brainstem Cerebrovascular Accident (CVA) and Metabolic Encephalopathy

	Brainstem CVA	Metabolic encephalopathy
Patient profile	Known vascular disease Hypercoagulable state Acute onset (<8 h), usually >50 y	Organ failure Subacute onset (>8 h) except in hypoglycemia Any age, often >60 y
Motor involvement	Hemiplegic or paraplegic	Moving all limbs except for hypoglycemia
Sensory involvement	Unilateral facial sensory change, or hemianesthesia	No sensory symptoms
Mental status	Obtunded or agitated	Waxing and waning
Pupils	May have Horner's; may have fixed, dilated pupil	Small, normoactive
Eye movements	Disconjugate, skew deviation, cr N. III, IV, VI paresis	Conjugate, midline
Respirations	Apneustic, central hyperpnea, ataxic	Normal, hyperpneic + brief apnea

TABLE 146.3

Evaluation for Metabolic Encephalopathy

- Neurologic examination
  - Mental status
  - Pupillary responses
  - Oculomotor responses
  - Respiratory pattern
  - Motor activity, strength
  - Deep tendon reflexes, plantar responses
- Initial laboratory tests
  - Blood sugar, electrolytes, lactate dehydrogenase, serum glutamic oxaloacetic transaminase, serum glutamic pyruvic transaminase, ammonia, blood urea nitrogen, creatinine, white blood cell count/differential, hemoglobin, hematocrit, blood gases
- Electroencephalography
- Neuroimaging
  - Head computed tomography or magnetic resonance imaging
  - ±Lumbar puncture, toxicity screens, serum and urine osmolality, psychiatric examination

again, resulting in a pattern of "periodic respirations" [3]. Hypoventilation is usually seen with depressant drug overdoses, chronic pulmonary failure, and metabolic alkalosis of any cause. Cheyne–Stokes respiration, a rhythmic cycle of waxing and waning hyperpnea/apnea, is another pattern that is occasionally seen in metabolic encephalopathy caused by uremia or hypoxia, but more commonly this indicates bilateral structural lesions of the cortex. Other neurogenic respiratory patterns, such as constant or "central" neurogenic hyperventilation, cluster breathing, and ataxic breathing, are signs of brainstem dysfunction due to structural damage or suppression by barbiturates. These changes are seen only when the patient is stuporous or comatose.

Abnormal motor activity is characteristic of many metabolic encephalopathies and is quite varied in appearance; tremors, myoclonus, asterixis, rigidity, and choreoathetosis may be seen. Tremors are rhythmic, involuntary oscillatory movements seen in all limbs and often exaggerated during voluntary movement. Tremors occur most often in early hypoglycemic encephalopathy, thyrotoxicosis, acute uremia, chronic dialysis encephalopathy, hypercapnia, and drug intoxication, especially with sympathomimetic agents.

Myoclonus is multifocal, appearing as brief shock-like contractions of large muscle groups. Synchronous myoclonic jerks in all limbs can be seen in any patient who is slipping in and out of a drowsy sleep—also known as *sleep-onset myoclonus*. This is often seen in patients who are receiving large doses of narcotics. Multifocal myoclonus, in contrast, is seen in hypoxic–ischemic encephalopathy, chronic hepatic failure of all types, uremia, pulmonary failure, and intoxication with methaqualone and psychedelic agents [4].

Asterixis is a flapping movement produced by unsustained muscle contractions against gravity. Rhythmic extension and flexion of the outstretched limb is present, which disappears at rest. The most common setting for this is in hepatic encephalopathy of any cause, frequently with flapping of the hands, feet, jaw, and tongue. Subacute uremia and pulmonary failure produce asterixis accompanied by myoclonus, which presents a picture of almost constant muscular jerking movements.

Rigidity or generalized muscle spasms are states of constant muscle contraction that are seen when the degree of metabolic encephalopathy is more severe and leads to stupor or coma. This can be the result of end-stage hepatic failure, hypoglycemia (<25 mg glucose per dL) lasting more than a few minutes, acute renal failure, hyperthermia, and hypothermia below 92°F rectally. Rigidity with dystonic posturing is a clue to amphetamine or phenothiazine poisoning. Choreoathetosis, on the other hand, occurs in chronic hepatic failure, subacute bacterial endocarditis, posthypoxic insult, Reye's syndrome, chronic dialysis, chronic hypoglycemia, and chronic hyperparathyroidism, appearing as a nonpatterned sequence of twisting or dance-like limb movements.

The *reflex examination* often reveals diffuse hyperreflexia, symmetric except in limbs that were previously affected by a structural lesion. Plantar responses, also known as the Babinski reflex, are typically extensor in both feet and can be elicited easily. In contrast, the sensory examination is usually not affected, but is unreliable if the patient is agitated or obtunded. Response to pinprick, painful pinch/pressure, or a cold stimulus on the limbs is the most useful in demonstrating a grossly intact sensory arc.

Abnormal autonomic responses in metabolic encephalopathy may demand intervention and can cause significant morbidity and mortality. Hypotension, unresponsive to volume expansion, points to intoxication with barbiturates or opiates, myxedema, or Addisonian crisis. In this setting, occult sepsis must always be ruled out before treating for specific metabolic derangements. Fever and leukocytosis may be absent in very debilitated patients. Examination of urine, blood cell counts and coagulation factors, blood and sputum cultures, chest x-ray, and a lumbar puncture are essential to rule out infection. If there remains any doubt about the cause of hypotension, empiric antibiotics, naloxone hydrochloride (Narcan) for possible opiate overdose, intravenous (IV) glucose (one ampoule), and vasopressor should be added to other supportive measures acutely while the cause is being investigated.

Seizures are another significant symptom of metabolic encephalopathy, especially in uremia, hypoglycemia, pancreatic failure, and various types of metabolic acidosis (e.g., ethylene glycol, salicylates, and so forth). They occur most often at the onset of the metabolic disturbance, for example, as the blood urea nitrogen (BUN) is climbing acutely, and as a preterminal expression of severe neuronal injury in a comatose patient. Management of the seizures is typically ineffective until the underlying cause is corrected. In renal failure, however, one-third to half of the standard loading doses of phenytoin or phenobarbital may be all that is needed to control seizures. The interictal electroencephalogram (EEG) serves as a guideline to the need for continued treatment once the encephalopathy has cleared or has become chronic and stable. A persistent focus of epileptiform activity on the recording warrants further investigation and anticonvulsant therapy.

The *laboratory investigation* of patients with delirium or coma is crucial in defining the cause of a metabolic encephalopathy. Blood tests for glucose, electrolytes, and blood gases should be drawn immediately along with a panel of hepatic function tests (ratio of serum alanine aminotransferase to serum aspartate aminotransferase, lactate dehydrogenase, ammonia [NH_4^+]), BUN, and creatinine. Serum and urine osmolality, cerebrospinal fluid (CSF) analysis, serum magnesium and phosphate levels, and specific hormone levels may be needed to define the cause of encephalopathy further. Careful review of all medications taken before and during hospitalization may direct attention to toxicology screens of blood and urine. The general toxicology screen should be sensitive to opiates, benzodiazepines, caffeine and salicylates, theophylline, barbiturates, and alcohol. Additional drug levels should be ordered if their use is known or suspected (e.g., digoxin, cocaine, phenytoin, and so forth). If there has been a sudden change in mental status, a bolus of 25 g glucose should be administered intravenously without hesitation to avoid prolonged hypoglycemia.

Pharmacogenomic studies have revealed that there are 58 genetic variants in metabolic pathways that play a significant role in drug metabolism and activity at target sites, thus influencing toxicity. The most significant of these are Cytochrome P450 (CYP) 3A9 and CYP2D6 which can be overexpressed (ultrarapid metabolizers), underexpressed (poor metabolizers), or normal. Many selective serotonin reuptake inhibitors and cardiovascular agents are metabolized by these two classes of enzymes and the aforementioned variants may cause drug levels to be too high or to be converted to active forms so quickly that peak levels are higher than expected, contributing to the adverse effect profiles. Poor metabolizers may also have more drug–drug interactions because of competitive inhibition of clearance of one drug versus the other when coadministered. Reference lists for problematic pharmacogenomic effects are updated regularly and widely available on websites for pharmacologists and toxicologists. General availability of testing for cytochrome P (CYP) variants is limited currently but may become important in the near future in screening for drug-induced encephalopathy as the technology becomes less expensive and quicker.

In general, the EEG in metabolic encephalopathy is abnormal; background slowing is the most common pattern found (<9 Hz) [5]. Other patterns can also be useful in identifying or corroborating the cause of the encephalopathy. Slow activity that is prominent frontally, with deep triphasic waves (in the 2- to 4-Hz range), is characteristic of hepatic encephalopathy but can be seen in renal failure too [6]. This has also been reported in levetiracetam toxicity [7], hyperammonemic states due to gastroplasty [8] and ureterosigmoidostomy [9], and rare metabolic disorders such as ornithine transcarbamylase deficiency [10]. Spreading of the slow activity toward the occipital leads is a sign of deepening coma in this setting. Bursts of high voltage activity amidst normal background frequencies are also a sign of diffuse metabolic disturbance. More importantly, the EEG in a patient with an acute encephalopathy of unknown cause may reveal subclinical (electrical, non-convulsive) status epilepticus, warranting urgent and aggressive anticonvulsant treatment. This is particularly common in the case of alcoholics and diabetics, who are at risk of multiple CNS insults.

Neuroimaging (computed tomography [CT] or magnetic resonance imaging [MRI]) scans are often crucial in situations in which there is rapid deterioration of mental status without focal signs or an obvious metabolic cause such as hypoglycemia. Most mass lesions, such as subdural hematomas or brain tumors, are evidenced clinically by a rostrocaudal progression of neurologic signs. The initial picture may be nonfocal with obtundation, but this is followed sequentially by flexor or extensor posturing on one or both sides and then the loss of pupillary or caloric responses. Later, medullary respiratory patterns or bradycardia appear. A noncontrast head CT or MRI is definitive in many cases but does not always distinguish a brainstem stroke. Early consultation by a neurologist is crucial, especially when the cause of impaired consciousness is not clearly due to a metabolic disorder. Transient changes in vascular permeability associated with Wernicke's encephalopathy can manifest as vasogenic edema in the brainstem periaqueductal and fourth ventricular areas along with contrast enhancement of the mammillary bodies [11] on brain MRI.

Lumbar puncture is also indicated when there is a rapid onset of encephalopathy, especially with a fever, headache, or meningismus. Occult subarachnoid hemorrhage, infection, or elevated intracranial pressure may be found in the absence of funduscopic changes or clear-cut clinical history. Ideally, the lumbar puncture should be performed atraumatically with a small (22-gauge) spinal needle and a simultaneous sample of serum obtained to compare glucose and protein levels in the blood and CSF.

ETIOLOGY

Hepatic Failure

The clinical onset of *hepatic encephalopathy* may be subtle, with a blunting of affect and lethargy, or dramatic in 10% to 20%, with mania or an agitated delirium [12]. It is easy to recognize hepatic encephalopathy in an individual with the obvious stigmata of chronic liver disease, such as ascites, varices, or jaundice. In those without apparent liver disease, the mental changes may only appear after an additional metabolic demand on the liver. Such stressors are a high-protein meal, gastrointestinal bleeding with increased blood absorption from the gut, or hepatically metabolized drugs [13]. Sedatives and acetazolamide are particularly offensive in this situation.

Asterixis is the next most common clinical sign, appearing in all limbs, the jaw, and the tongue. As the patient progresses into a coma, asterixis may be replaced by muscle spasticity and decorticate or decerebrate posturing to stimulation. The Babinski responses are present (extensor plantar reflexes), and gaze-evoked ocular movements are variable at this stage; pupillary responses are always preserved. Oculocephalic and vestibuloocular (caloric) responses remain until the patient is moribund. Hyperventilation is another consistent sign of hepatic encephalopathy and results in respiratory alkalosis. The ocular, pupillary, and respiratory patterns above help to distinguish severe hepatic encephalopathy from space-occupying lesions of the cortex and brainstem.

The pathophysiology of hepatic coma is not certain, but it is thought to be caused by portacaval shunting of neurotoxic substances. These putative toxins include excess ammonia, large molecules normally excluded by the blood–brain barrier [14], increased water, and the "false" neurotransmitter octopamine [15]. Hypoglycemia, as a result of decreased glycogen stores in the liver, may complicate the CNS picture.

The serum transaminases are usually elevated two- to threefold, and serum ammonia is at least in the high normal range once the patient is lethargic—with a linear correlation thereafter between higher laboratory values and lower cognitive state. The CSF remains normal until the serum bilirubin exceeds approximately 5 mg per dL, which tints the fluid yellow. The EEG characteristically shows progressive slowing from the frontal to the occipital leads as coma deepens. Triphasic waves are seen in most cases but are not pathognomonic.

Therapy for hepatic encephalopathy is directed toward decreasing the amount of toxic substances that are being shunted to the brain. Neomycin and lactulose help to sterilize and flush the gut. A protein-restricted diet and the exclusion of hepatically cleared drugs decrease the metabolic load, and IV glucose effectively maintains the serum glucose level. Neurologic recovery then depends on the capacity of the liver to regenerate at least 25% of its full function. With prolonged or repeated bouts of hepatic coma, there may be persistent, irreversible signs of basal ganglia dysfunction evidenced by chorea, postural tremors, or a parkinsonian picture (acquired hepatocerebral degeneration) [16].

Reye's Syndrome

Reye's syndrome is a unique and quite morbid form of acute hepatic encephalopathy seen in children, usually between ages 1 and 10 years. It occurs in the clinical setting of an acute viral infection, for example, chickenpox or influenza A or B, plus aspirin therapy [17]. Approximately 4 to 7 days after the viral symptoms start, the child becomes irritable, with vomiting and sometimes with headache or blurred vision. An agitated delirium, combativeness, and progressive obtundation rapidly ensue over hours, followed by hyperventilation, pupillary dilatation, and generalized seizures. Later in the course, decerebrate rigidity, Babinski responses, and papilledema may develop as well.

The pathology of Reye's syndrome includes infiltration of the liver and other visceral organs with small fat droplets and diffuse cerebral edema. In cases that are complicated by severe hypoglycemia and seizures, anoxic damage with laminar necrosis of the cerebral cortex is also found. The cause of these changes is presumed to be mitochondrial poisoning, but the pathogenic agent has not yet been identified. Acetylsalicylic acid has consistently been implicated in this cellular damage. This has led to the standard practice of prescribing acetaminophen instead of aspirin for viral symptoms in children, notably reducing the incidence of Reye's syndrome [17].

The differential diagnosis relies on measurement of liver function and a high index of suspicion in the appropriate setting. The serum transaminases rise three- to fivefold in the first 48 hours, and the serum ammonia is dramatically increased, sometimes into the 200 μmol per L range. Hypoglycemia is also an early sign, aggravating the lactic acidosis and respiratory alkalosis that are seen later in the course.

Treatment for Reye's syndrome is directed toward diminishing the cerebral edema, controlling seizures, and providing adequate electrolytes and glucose for support while the liver is effectively shut down with respect to oxidative metabolism. This is best achieved in an ICU with a standard protocol for Reye's disease using intracranial pressure monitoring and mannitol or glycerol for reduction of intracranial pressure [18].

The prognosis in recent years has improved markedly; mortality and morbidity are now 10% to 20%, as opposed to 40% to 50% two decades ago. Factors that contribute to a poor outcome are age less than 1 year, serum ammonia levels more than five times normal at their peak, and a prothrombin time more than 20 seconds. Other negative prognostic indicators are renal failure and a very rapid progression of liver failure in the first 48 hours. Early intervention is the key to a good outcome neurologically and systemically.

Renal Failure

Uremic encephalopathy may develop acutely, be superimposed on chronic renal insufficiency, or occur as a consequence of chronic dialysis. It is often a complication of systemic diseases that independently affect the kidneys and the CNS such as collagen vascular disease, malignant hypertension, drug overdoses, diabetes, or bacterial sepsis. The clinical picture is initially variable and does not correlate directly with measures of renal failure such as BUN and creatinine.

The first sign of encephalopathy in uremia is delirium or a decrease in the level of consciousness; hyperventilation and increased motor activity follow as the patient becomes obtunded. Also, there is a high frequency of generalized convulsions at the outset and a metabolic acidosis with low serum bicarbonate. The motor component is prominent in many patients with multifocal myoclonus, hypertonus or asterixis, and tremors, together producing a picture of "tic convulsif"—as if the patient has fasciculations [19]. Oculomotor function and pupillary responses are normal, but deep tendon reflexes may be asymmetric, and focal weakness often occurs, with shifting hemiparesis during a single period of encephalopathy. The variability of focal motor signs helps to rule out a structural lesion but does not obviate the need to look for multifocal seizures in a patient with overt twitching and depressed consciousness.

Studies of the effect of uremia on neuronal function have not been able to demonstrate a direct correlation between the cognitive state and levels of BUN or with any other biochemical or electrolyte markers. The EEG, although becoming slower with higher levels of BUN, also does not correlate with mental status changes, especially in chronic uremia [20]. Hence, the pathophysiology of uremic encephalopathy is not known.

The major diagnostic differential to consider is between a hypertensive crisis and uremic encephalopathy, because malignant hypertension often leads rapidly to renal failure and neurologic signs. Evidence of papilledema, retinal vasospasm, and cortical blindness or aphasia, with a diastolic blood pressure of more than 120 mm Hg, argues strongly for a hypertensive crisis. In contrast, a sudden rise of BUN alone is most consistent with uremic encephalopathy.

Two variants of this disorder are seen in patients on peritoneal dialysis or hemodialysis. The *acute dialysis disequilibrium syndrome* is seen in children more often than in adults undergoing hemodialysis with large exchanges of dialysate. A sudden shift of solutes out of the vascular compartment produces a hyperosmolar state in the brain and subsequent water resorption intracerebrally. This results in water intoxication, with florid encephalopathy within 30 to 60 minutes. Slower dialysis obviates the problem in general [21].

Dialysis dementia is insidious by comparison and is evidenced by postdialysis lethargy, asterixis, myoclonus, dysphasia, and progressive loss of cognitive abilities over years. This disorder has been linked to increased amounts of aluminum in the dialysate augmented by aluminum-containing antacids in the diet [21]. Although the brains of patients with this disorder do not contain excess aluminum compared to those of other dialysis patients, elimination of aluminum from these sources helps reverse the symptoms in the early stages. This syndrome is now relatively rare.

The body's response to sepsis and its pathophysiologic response to infection can include encephalopathy ranging from decreased attention, to disorientation and even to coma [22]. Sepsis-associated encephalopathy (SAE) is a transient and reversible brain dysfunction, occurring when the source of sepsis is outside the central nervous system [23]. Defining SAE must logically exclude patients with CNS insults such as TBI, CNS infection, or stroke, to name a few [22]. Some argue it is important to distinguish between altered consciousness due to shock or hypoxemia also caused by sepsis; however, it can also be argued that this is one of the mechanisms sepsis can cause encephalopathy, thus including it in the definition of SAE [24]. Inflammatory signals reach the brain via the vagal nerves stimulating medullary autonomic nuclei and the circumventricular organs that allow transport of inflammatory mediators into the brain. Thus, different areas, ranging from the brainstem to the frontal cortex, can be affected. Three major processes are thought to occur centrally. The first is neuroinflammation mediated by microglia as well as astrocytes. It is thought that this inflammation can lead to oxidative stress and mitochondrial dysfunction. Furthermore, it can cause a second process, which is the buildup of glutamate secondary to decreased removal by astrocytes. This causes apoptosis due to excitotoxicity. The third process is thought to be ischemic in nature. It is thought that sepsis and inflammation leads to macro- and microcirculatory dysfunction as well as neurovascular uncoupling, which lead to ischemia. SAE can have EEG findings ranging from theta rhythm to delta rhythms to triphasic waves or even burst suppression. Imaging with MRI can be normal or show focal findings such as white matter hyperintensity or ischemic stroke [23]. The incidence of SAE varies widely between studies and can occur at any time during the illness. One study by Feng et al. found 42.3% incidence among patients in the ICU with sepsis. They also found higher early mortality among septic patients with SAE and higher 28-day and 1-year mortality with an RR of 2.868 (95% CI, 1.73 to 4.754). SAE was found to be correlated with *E. coli* sepsis, higher lactate, higher AST, lower WBC, and lower PaO_2/FiO_2. Interestingly, there was no difference in quality-of-life indicators among sepsis survivors with or without SAE [22].

Pulmonary Failure

A combination of *hypoxemia* and *hypercarbia* can produce typical changes of a metabolic encephalopathy in patients with underlying pulmonary failure. Individuals with chronic obstructive pulmonary disease, for example, tolerate a PCO_2 of 50 to 60 mm Hg without mental status changes. However, a sudden increase of PCO_2 of up to 65 to 70 mm Hg due to hypoventilation, or impaired oxygen exchange, can lead to lethargy, headaches, and a rise in intracranial pressure. Associated signs are papilledema or retinal vein congestion, extensor Babinski signs, asterixis, myoclonus, and often, generalized tremors. Seizures are rarely seen, and pupillary and oculomotor functions are preserved unless there is a concomitant hypoxic–ischemic insult [25].

This course of events may be precipitated by systemic infection with fatigue of ventilatory muscles, paralysis of these muscles by neuromuscular disease or Guillain–Barré syndrome, and sedative drugs with their depressant effect on the medullary respiratory center. In the well-compensated hypercarbic individual, oxygen therapy may be counterproductive by decreasing respiratory drive from the medulla. Rapid correction of hypercarbia by artificial ventilation exacerbates the compensatory chronic metabolic alkalosis that these patients have, possibly resulting in a further depression of mental status plus seizures [26].

The critical factor in the development of pulmonary encephalopathy is a rapid increase in serum PCO_2. This may be complicated by the presence of sedatives, hypoxemia, cardiac failure, and renal hypoperfusion. Treatment is directed toward slow correction of hypercarbia while maintaining an adequate PO_2 and good cerebral blood flow. Prognosis for full neurologic recovery is good if the patient is not subjected to cerebral ischemia as well.

Hypoglycemic Encephalopathy

Hypoglycemia can occur as an isolated problem or as a complication of liver failure, of tumors producing insulin-like substances, or of urea cycle defects. The most common case is that of a diabetic with an accidental or deliberate overdose of insulin or oral hypoglycemic agents. An initial insulin reaction occurs when the serum glucose drops below approximately 40 mg per dL, producing flushing, sweating, faintness, palpitations, nausea, and anxiety. This persists for several minutes before the patient becomes confused and either agitated or drowsy [27]. Focal neurologic signs such as hemiparesis, cortical blindness, or dysphasia may appear at this point, mimicking an acute stroke [28]. If the serum glucose drops precipitously below 30 mg per dL, generalized convulsions may occur in flurries followed by a postictal coma. Prompt correction of the hypoglycemia at this point leads to reversal of the neurologic deficits, but repeated episodes can result in a subtle dementia evolving over many years [29].

When severe hypoglycemia is sustained for more than 10 minutes, stepwise progression of neurologic signs occurs. The first step is motor restlessness with frontal release signs such as sucking, grasping, and a tonic jaw jerk. Next, diffuse muscle spasms appear and sometimes myoclonic jerks. Finally, decerebrate rigidity is seen before the so-called medullary phase of hypoglycemia. The *medullary phase* describes a state of deep coma with dilated pupils, bradycardia, hypoventilation, and generalized flaccidity, much like hypoxic–ischemic coma. The pathologic changes associated with bouts of hypoglycemic encephalopathy are also similar to hypoxic–ischemic insults, although the cerebellum is relatively spared [30].

Differentiating hypoglycemic coma from a seizure disorder, a cerebrovascular accident, or a drug overdose is not possible at the outset unless stat serum glucose is obtained before IV fluids are administered. One should not delay treatment with a bolus of 50 mL 50% glucose (one ampoule) if there is doubt about the cause of a rapidly evolving coma, because hypoglycemic encephalopathy can result in permanent neurologic deficits if not reversed in 20 minutes or less. The first bolus of glucose must be followed by close monitoring of blood glucose levels, because most agents that lead to symptomatic hypoglycemia are long acting [31].

Hyperglycemic Encephalopathy

Hyperglycemia that is severe enough to produce mental status changes rarely occurs in isolation from other metabolic disturbances. Hypokalemia and hypophosphatemia, hyperosmolality and ketoacidosis, or lactic acidosis often accompanies serum glucose levels more than 300 mg per dL. In contrast, acidosis may be absent in nonketotic hyperglycemic hyperosmolar states, whereas the serum osmolality is often more than 350 mOsm per kg and serum glucose more than 800 mg per dL. The neurologic changes in any case appear to correlate best with abnormalities of serum osmolality and the rate at which it is corrected [32]. In juvenile or "brittle" diabetics, ketoacidosis develops after a dose of insulin is missed or an occult infection occurs. The first changes are mild confusion, lethargy, and deep regular inspirations (Kussmaul's breathing) in addition to signs of dehydration. Elderly patients are more prone to nonketotic hyperglycemia, especially when they have an inadequate diet, take medications that interfere with insulin metabolism (e.g., phenytoin [Dilantin], steroids), or take oral hypoglycemic agents [33]. Lactic acidosis may be present, in particular, with phenformin. These patients also tend to have focal or generalized seizures and transient or shifting hemiplegia as the level of coma deepens. The preservation of pupillary and oculocephalic responses helps to identify the clinical picture in such cases as being metabolic rather than structural.

The hyperosmolality occurring with hyperglycemia of any type causes a shift of water from the intracerebral to intravascular space with resulting brain shrinkage [34]. How this produces the neurologic changes observed is not known. More importantly, rapid correction of hyperosmolality by IV hydration and insulin results in cerebral water intoxication and signs of increased intracranial pressure. This is exemplified by the patient who begins to awaken from a hyperglycemic coma during IV therapy but later develops a headache and recurrent lethargy and seems to drift back into the previous state. Significant morbidity and mortality follow if these fluctuations are not observed and the IV treatment is modified appropriately [35]. Other details of the management of diabetic coma are addressed in Chapter 137.

Other Electrolyte Disturbances

Acute hyponatremia and *hypernatremia* cause fluid shifts and critical changes in serum osmolality, with the same effects on cerebral dysfunction as those described above. Mild to moderate acute *hyponatremia* (120 to 130 mEq per L) is evidenced by confusion or delirium with asterixis and multifocal myoclonus. If the serum sodium goes below 110 mEq per L, or drops at a rate more than 5 mEq/L/h to 120 mEq per L and below, seizures and coma are likely to follow. This course of events portends permanent neurologic damage even after careful therapy [36]. Common causes of hyponatremia are (a) the syndrome of inappropriate antidiuretic hormone secretion, with myriad etiologies; (b) excess volume expansion with hypotonic IV solutions; and (c) renal failure with a decreased glomerular filtration rate [37]. Other less common causes include psychogenic polydipsia, severe congestive heart failure, and Addison's disease.

The neurologic signs of hyponatremia are nonspecific, and the general approach to evaluation of an encephalopathy often identifies the problem. Treatment is directed toward the underlying cause with fluid restriction in mild cases, unless total body sodium is depleted. In moderate cases (i.e., a serum sodium of 105 to 115 mEq per L), per os (PO) sodium supplementation may be needed as well. A serum sodium below 100 mEq per L is life-threatening. Correction of hyponatremia requires ICU monitoring and calculated sodium replacement (see Chapter 199). Excessively rapid correction of severe hyponatremia, especially in alcoholic or malnourished individuals, can be associated with another rare but serious neurologic complication known as *central pontine myelinolysis (CPM)* [38]. CPM starts with a flaccid quadriparesis and inability to chew, swallow, or talk, or "locked-in syndrome" developing over a period of days. Patients who recover from the underlying systemic disorder may be left with a spastic paraparesis and pseudobulbar speech; almost half may improve significantly over several months.

Hypernatremia is not seen very often outside the hospital setting except in children with severe diarrhea and inadequate PO fluid intake. Excess diuretic therapy, hyperosmolar tube feedings, and restricted access to PO fluids are reflected in a serum sodium of more than 155 mEq per L usually seen in institutionalized patients. Clinically, one sees progressive confusion and obtundation in subacute cases. With levels of sodium more than 170 mEq per L developing acutely, the brain may shrink, and subdural hematomas can occur as a result of stretching of the dural vessels. These patients may complain of headache, develop seizures, or simply drift into a stupor. Catastrophic complications such as venous sinus thrombosis and irreversible coma are seen with a serum sodium level of more than 180 mEq per L due to the marked hyperosmolality that accompanies it.

The cause of profound hypernatremia is often diabetes insipidus, which may be secondary to head trauma or other structural lesions of the hypothalamic stalk. Impaired thirst mechanisms or depressed consciousness interfere with the polydipsia that is pathognomonic of diabetes insipidus [39]. The treatment of symptomatic hypernatremia depends on its cause: dehydration alone or complicated by additional sodium depletion due to hyperosmolar diuresis or excessive sweating. Fluid replacement is accomplished with 5% dextrose and water at a rate dependent on the total body water deficit—half of the water needed being administered IV in the first 12 to 24 hours and no faster (see Chapter 199). Saline solutions of half normal strength (0.45%) are used in most other cases. The exception is hyperosmolar diabetic coma, in which insulin and normal saline are both necessary to correct the severe serum hypertonicity.

Metabolic acidosis by itself produces only mild delirium or confusion [40] but may be accompanied by organ failure, direct CNS toxicity from drug metabolites, or volume depletion. The first sign of an encephalopathy caused by metabolic acidosis is hyperpnea followed by mental status changes and mild muscular rigidity. Ingestion of toxic doses of poisons such as methanol, ethylene glycol, and salicylates results in encephalopathy along with low serum bicarbonate levels (less than 15 mEq per L) [41]. Therapy must be directed toward vigorous correction of the metabolic acidosis while the specific cause is being elucidated.

Pancreatic Failure

Acute pancreatitis rarely leads to mental status changes during the initial bout. When recurrent or chronic, symptoms of encephalopathy may prominently wax and wane [42]. The clinical presentation is abdominal pain followed over 2 to 5 days by hallucinosis, delirium, focal or generalized seizures, and bilateral extensor Babinski responses. As the serum amylase continues to rise, the patient may lapse into a coma as a result of secondary hyperglycemia, hypocalcemia, and hypotension. The exact cause of the encephalopathy is unknown; the prognosis and treatment depend on the underlying cause and severity of the pancreatitis [43].

Endocrine Disorders

Adrenal disorders are an important consideration in acute encephalopathy, because hypo- and hyperadrenalism produce alterations in CNS function.

Addison's disease or *secondary adrenocortical deficiency* occurs acutely in the setting of septicemia, surgery, and, most frequently, sudden withdrawal of chronically administered steroids. In the latter, one does not see the stigmata of chronic adrenocorticotropic hormone deficiency but rather hypotension, a mild hyponatremia, hypoglycemia, and hyperkalemia, together with a delirium or stupor that fluctuates erratically [44]. The electrolyte disturbances in most cases are not severe enough to explain the encephalopathy; other pathologic mechanisms such as cerebral hypoperfusion or water intoxication have been suggested. Unlike many metabolic encephalopathies, adrenocortical insufficiency is associated with *decreased* muscle tone and deep tendon reflexes. Seizures and papilledema may appear when the patient has a profound adrenocorticotropic hormone deficiency and coma. The neurologic picture does not clear until cortisone replacement is given along with treatment of the electrolyte imbalances. These patients are also particularly sensitive to sedative medications and may lapse into coma with small doses of narcotics or barbiturates [45].

Excess steroids produce different forms of encephalopathy depending on whether the source is endogenous or exogenous. In Cushing's disease, psychomotor depression and lethargy are the norm, whereas high doses of prednisone usually cause elation, delirium, or frank psychosis [46]. The latter is not uncommon in the ICU setting due to the administration of stress levels of steroids and multiple other CNS toxins. The behavioral changes are key to recognizing this problem because there are no specific metabolic markers [47]. Treatment consists of withdrawal of the steroids and sometimes temporary use of tranquilizers or lithium for the psychiatric features as well. Full neurologic recovery may lag behind the treatment by several days to weeks.

Hypothyroidism is now a rare cause of encephalopathy and coma. It may be confused initially with other causes of hypotension, hypoventilation, and hyponatremia, such as septic shock, brainstem infarcts, or an overdose of sedatives. The diagnosis should be considered in any patient with hypothermia, pretibial edema, pseudomyotonic stretch reflexes (e.g., delayed relaxation of the knee jerk), and coarse hair or facies. Muscle enzymes, serum cholesterol, and lipids may be elevated along with the thyroid-stimulating hormone (TSH) level [48]. Diagnostic confirmation is often delayed pending results of thyroid function tests, but replacement therapy should be initiated early with IV triiodothyronine or thyroxine. The constitutional symptoms may take several weeks to respond, but the neurologic picture clears promptly with proper treatment. Another form of hypothyroid-associated encephalopathy is seen in Hashimoto's thyroiditis with a subacute subtle change in personality, memory deficits, and cerebellar ataxia accompanied by cerebellar atrophy on imaging studies. Confirmation of the diagnosis requires specific tests for antithyroglobulin and antithyroperoxidase antibodies along with an elevated TSH. Treatment with thyroid replacement therapy often results in recovery over a few months.

Thyrotoxicosis is more difficult to recognize because it can present in an apathetic form, as a thyroid storm, or in a subacute form. Elderly patients are more likely to appear depressed or stuporous and without evidence of hypermetabolism [49]. The key to the diagnosis in such cases is evidence of recent weight loss and atrial fibrillation, often with congestive heart failure and a proximal myopathy. In a thyroid storm, the patient with indolent hyperthyroidism may be stressed by an infection or surgery and responds with marked signs of hypermetabolism: tachycardia, fever, profuse sweating, and pulmonary or congestive heart failure. Neurologically, the individual becomes acutely agitated and delirious and then progresses into a stupor [50]. The subacute picture that precedes this is one of mild irritability, nervousness, tremors, and hyperactivity, and is often misconstrued as an affective disorder rather than endocrine in origin. Ophthalmologic signs such as proptosis, chemosis, and periorbital edema are useful in identifying this form of thyrotoxicosis.

Therapy for thyrotoxic encephalopathy is aimed at ablation of the gland, but supportive care may require β-blockers, digoxin, diuretics, and sometimes dexamethasone and sedatives for the associated hypermetabolic state. Encephalopathy is also seen in disorders of the pituitary gland and parathyroid gland, although rarely as a primary process. *Hypopituitarism* may result from radiation or surgery to the area of the sella and can present as a chronic encephalopathy with features of thyroid or adrenal insufficiency, or both. An acute coma due to infarction or hemorrhage of the pituitary gland, known as *pituitary apoplexy*, can be seen in acromegalics with large adenomas or in patients with postpartum hemorrhage and hypotension (Sheehan's syndrome) [51]. Subarachnoid blood and ocular abnormalities plus signs of increased intracranial pressure help to identify the pituitary lesion in such cases. Encephalopathy from *hyperpituitarism* reflects the specific neurohumoral substance that is being released in excess and does not represent a unique syndrome.

Hyperparathyroidism may be manifest neurologically with asthenia or a vague change in personality. The patient is mildly depressed, lacks energy, and fatigues easily. A serum calcium more than 12 mg per dL and elevated parathormone levels are important diagnostic findings. Occasionally, psychiatric symptoms predominate, starting with delirium and psychosis, or obtundation and coma when the serum calcium exceeds 15 mg per dL. Hypercalcemia caused by metastatic bone lesions, paraneoplastic parathormone-like substances, sarcoidosis, primary bone diseases, and renal failure are associated with a subacute or chronic encephalopathy similar to hyperparathyroidism. Treatment in these cases must be directed toward the underlying disease rather than addressing the hypercalcemia alone. Primary hyperparathyroidism is effectively managed by ablation of the overactive gland. This is not always possible, because the glands often are ectopic and may escape discovery on selective angiography or exploratory surgery.

Hypocalcemia due to *hypoparathyroidism* produces an encephalopathy that parallels the depression of serum calcium levels. At less than 4.0 mEq per L calcium, a blunted effect and seizures are common and may be confused with a dementing process or epilepsy. The motor signs of hypocalcemia, that is, tetany or neuromuscular irritability, should make one suspicious of a metabolic disturbance [39]. Another diagnostic dilemma is the occasional presentation of hypocalcemia with papilledema and headache. The opening pressure on lumbar puncture is elevated to the same degree as in pseudotumor cerebri, but a head CT is likely to show basal ganglia calcifications [48]. Furthermore, the presence of cataracts and mental dullness in a previously normal individual should lead one to check the serum calcium and parathormone levels.

The mechanism by which hypocalcemia and hypoparathyroidism produce these varied neurologic symptoms is not known. Replacement of serum calcium by dietary means is usually inadequate to correct the CNS disorder. Supplementation with vitamin D and calcitriol enhances the absorption and utilization of oral calcium.

Other Causes of Encephalopathy

The list of causes of diffuse or metabolic encephalopathies is so lengthy that the problem of diagnosis must be resolved by a process of elimination. Drugs and toxins lead all other possible causes, with a frequency of approximately 50% (see Chapters 97 through 126). Hepatic, renal, or pulmonary failure is causative in another 12% and endocrine or electrolyte disturbances in approximately 8%. Other less common etiologies include thiamine deficiency (Wernicke's encephalopathy), cardiac bypass surgery, subacute bacterial endocarditis, and hyperthermia. All of these disorders produce microembolic or microhemorrhagic/petechial lesions in specific areas of the brain.

Wernicke's encephalopathy develops acutely in the clinical setting of an alcoholic or a malnourished individual, especially when IV glucose solutions without vitamin supplementation are given. Because thiamine is a cofactor in the utilization of cerebral glucose, it is depleted by the IV infusion [52,53]; confusion, obtundation, and loss of short-term memory rapidly ensue. The hallmark of this entity is a striking impairment of ocular movements, causing an external ophthalmoplegia, nystagmus, and diminished oculocephalic responses. Prompt IV and PO administration of 100 mg thiamine restores ocular function completely. The cerebral symptoms resolve slowly with the addition of 100 mg PO thiamine daily for 3 days or more. If untreated, the patient may lapse into a coma due to autonomic failure with accompanying shock and hypothermia and often death. Repeated or untreated episodes of Wernicke's disease may result in a chronic Korsakoff's psychosis with profound memory impairment [49].

More recently, recognition of autoantibodies to potassium channels (VGKC-Ab) and *N*-methyl-D-aspartate receptors presenting with a subacute limbic-type encephalopathy has led to exciting research into the role of channel blockade in reversible mental status changes. In many cases, there is no evidence of an occult cancer (e.g., testicular or ovarian in young people) and the prognosis with immunoglobulin or steroid therapy is good [54].

Hyperthermia due to heat stroke also has a characteristic clinical setting—young individuals experiencing excessive sweating caused by overactivity and elderly people receiving anticholinergics who are exposed to a hot environment [51]. In both cases, neurologic changes occur when the core body temperature reaches 42°C (107.6°F). The patient may become agitated and confused with intermittent generalized seizures or may immediately lapse into a coma as if due to a stroke. The presence of tachycardia, hot and dry skin, and diffuse hypertonus occurring in the appropriate circumstances identifies the likely etiology. Normal pupillary size and reflexes (except with anticholinergics) and oculocephalic responses, and the absence of focal motor signs also point to a nonstructural lesion. However, if the core body temperature is not lowered early in the course, the patient may be left with sequelae similar to those seen in hypoxic–ischemic encephalopathy. Other causes of temperature more than 42°C are rare and are not discussed here [55].

Up to 20% of patients with *bacterial or marantic endocarditis* can present with a subacute encephalopathy manifested by confusion and hyperpnea with or without fever [56]. It should be suspected in any patient with gram-negative sepsis [56]; ovarian cancer; malignant melanoma; adenocarcinoma of the lung, breast, prostate, or pancreas; and an immunocompromised state. Definitive diagnosis rests on the blood culture results and an echocardiogram showing vegetations. Treatment is directed toward reducing or removing the cardiac source.

CONCLUSIONS

Metabolic encephalopathy is one of the most frequently seen neurologic disorders in the ICU. It is also one of the most diverse in its clinical presentations and requires a systematic approach to define the etiology and to institute effective treatment. The features that distinguish most metabolic encephalopathies from structural lesions are (a) a nonfocal neurologic examination, (b) increased motor activity, (c) intact ocular and pupillary reflexes, and (d) laboratory abnormalities that support the clinical picture. Additional tests such as an EEG, head CT, or toxicology screen are useful in ruling out other possible causes.

One should keep in mind that many patients in the ICU have an underlying chronic encephalopathy due to long-standing illness. Therefore, they are more susceptible to minor metabolic perturbations induced by small doses of drugs, slight shifts of fluid balance, or worsening organ failure. Early recognition and correction of such factors improve the patient's prognosis for a full neurologic recovery. Toward this end, it is prudent to consult the neurologist before the complications of multiple treatments and further changes confound the clinical course.

References

1. Folstein MF, Folstein SE, McHugh PR: Mini-mental state: a practical method for grading the cognitive state of patients for the clinician. *J Psycholinguist Res* 12:189–198, 1975.
2. Cohen PJ: Signs and stages of anesthesia, in Goodman LS, Gilman A (eds): *The Pharmacologic Basis of Therapeutics*. 5th ed. New York, NY, Macmillan, 1975, p 60.
3. Posner JB, Saper CB, Schiff ND, et al: Examination of the comatose patient, in *Plum and Posner's Diagnosis of Stupor and Coma*. 4th ed. New York, NY, Oxford University Press, 2007, pp 46–53.
4. Celesia GG, Grigg MM, Ross E: Generalized status myoclonus in acute anoxic and toxic-metabolic encephalopathies. *Arch Neurol* 45(7):781–784, 1988.
5. Kaplan PW: The EEG in metabolic encephalopathy and coma. *J Clin Neurophys* 21(5):307–318, 2004.
6. Leonard JV: Acute metabolic encephalopathy: an introduction. *J Inherit Metab Dis* 28(3):403–406, 2005.
7. Vulliemoz S, Iwanowski P, Landis T, et al: Levetiracetam accumulation in renal failure causing myoclonic encephalopathy with triphasic waves. *Seizure* 18(5):376–378, 2009.
8. Cirignotta F, Manconi M, Mondini S, et al: Wernicke-Korsakoff encephalopathy and polyneuropathy after gastroplasty for morbid obesity: report of a case. *Arch Neurol* 49:653–656, 1992.
9. Edwards RH: Hyperammonemic encephalopathy related to ureterosigmoidostomy. *Arch Neurol* 41:1211–1212, 1984.
10. Hu W, Kantarci O: Ornithine transcarbamylase deficiency presenting as encephalopathy during adulthood following bariatric surgery. *Arch Neurol* 64:126–128, 2007.
11. Breningstall GN: Neurologic syndrome in hyperammonemic disorders. *Pediatr Neurol* 2(5):253–262, 1986.
12. Christensen E, Krintel JJ, Hansen SM, et al: Prognosis after the first episode of gastrointestinal bleeding or coma in cirrhosis. Survival and prognostic factors. *Scand J Gastroenterol* 24(8):999–1006, 1989.
13. Laursen H, Westergaard G: Enhanced permeability to horseradish peroxidase across cerebral vessels in the rat after portacaval anastomosis. *Neuropathol Appl Neurobiol* 3:29–43, 1979.
14. James JH, Escourroule J, Fisher JE: Blood-brain neutral amino-acid transport activity is increased after portacaval anastomoses. *Science* 200:1395–1397, 1978.
15. Klos KJ, Ahlskog J, Josephs JE, et al: Neurologic spectrum of chronic liver failure and basal ganglia T1 hyperintensity on magnetic resonance imaging: probable manganese neurotoxicity. *Arch Neurol* 62(9):1385–1390, 2005.
16. Hurwitz ES: Reye's syndrome. *Epidemiol Rev* 11:249–253, 1989.
17. Arrowsmith JB, Kennedy DL, Kuritsky JN, et al: National patterns of aspirin use and Reye syndrome reporting, United States, 1980–1985. *Pediatrics* 79(6):858–863, 1987.
18. Fishman RA: Brain edema and disorders of intracranial pressure, in Rowland LP (ed): *Merritt's Textbook of Neurology*. 8th ed. Philadelphia, PA, Lea & Febiger, 1989, p 262.
19. Chadwick D, French AT: Uremic myoclonus: an example of reticular reflex myoclonus? *J Neurol Neurosurg Psychiatry* 42:52–55, 1979.
20. Hagstam KE: EEG frequency content related to clinical blood parameters in chronic uremia. *Scand J Urol Nephrol* 19[Suppl 7]:1–56, 1971.
21. Alfrey AC: Dialysis encephalopathy syndrome. *Annu Rev Med* 29:93–98, 1978.
22. Feng Q, Ai YH, Gong H, et al: Characterization of sepsis and sepsis-associated encephalopathy. *J Intensive Care Med* 885066617719750, 2017. doi:10.1177/0885066617719750.
23. Heming N, Mazeraud A, Verdonk F, et al: Neuroanatomy of sepsis-associated encephalopathy. *Crit Care* 21(1):65, 2017. doi:10.1186/s13054-017-1643-z.
24. Yamaga S, Shime N, Sonneville R, et al: Risk factors for sepsis-associated encephalopathy. *Intensive Care Med* 2017. doi:10.1007/s00134-017-4875-0.
25. Glaser G, Pincus JH: Neurologic complications of internal disease, in Baker AB, Baker LH (eds): *Clinical Neurology*. Vol 4. Philadelphia, PA, Harper & Row, 1983, p 17.
26. Rotherman EB, Safar P, Robin ED: CNS disorder during mechanical ventilation in chronic pulmonary disease. *JAMA* 189:993–996, 1964.
27. Fishbain DA, Rotundo D: Frequency of hypoglycemic delirium in a psychiatric emergency service. *Psychosomatics* 29(3):346–348, 1988.
28. Garty BZ, Dinari G, Nitzan M: Transient acute cortical blindness associated with hypoglycemia. *Pediatr Neurol* 3(3):169–170, 1987.
29. Malouf R, Brust JCM: Hypoglycemia: causes, neurological manifestations and outcome. *Ann Neurol* 17:421–430, 1985.
30. Foster JW, Hart RG: Hypoglycemic hemiplegia: two cases and a clinical review. *Stroke* 18(5):944–946, 1987.
31. Kitabchi EA, Goodman RC: Hypoglycemia, pathophysiology and diagnosis. *Hosp Pract* 22(11A):45–56, 59–60, 1987.
32. Wachtel TS, Silliman RA, Lamberton P: Predisposing factors for the diabetic hyperosmolar state. *Arch Intern Med* 147(3):499–501, 1987.
33. Arieff AI, Carroll HJ: Cerebral edema and depression of sensorium in nonketotic hyperosmolar coma. *Diabetes* 23:525–531, 1974.
34. Ryner MM, Fishman RA: Protective adaptation of brain to water intoxication. *Arch Neurol* 28:49–54, 1973.
35. Posner JB, Saper CB, Schiff ND, et al: Multifocal, diffuse and metabolic brain diseases causing stupor and coma, in *Plum and Posner's Diagnosis of Stupor and Coma*. 4th ed. New York, NY, Oxford University Press, 2007, pp 179–296.
36. Ayus JC, Krothapalli RK, Arieff AI: Treatment of symptomatic hyponatremia and its relation to brain damage. A prospective study. *N Engl J Med* 317(19):1190–1195, 1987.
37. Streeton DH, Moses AM, Miller M: Disorders of the neurohypophysis, in Braunwald E, Isselbacher K, Petersdorf R, et al (eds): *Harrison's Principles of Internal Medicine*. 11th ed. New York, NY, McGraw-Hill, 1987, p 1729.
38. Hattori S, Mochio S, Isogai Y, et al: Central pontine myelinolysis followed by frequent hyperglycemia and hypoglycemia—report of an autopsy case. *Brain Nerve* 41(8):795–798, 1989.
39. Adams RD, Victor M: Hypothalamic pituitary syndromes: diabetes insipidus, in Adams RD (ed): *Principles of Neurology*. 4th ed. New York, NY, McGraw-Hill, 1989, p 448.
40. Levinsky N: Fluids and electrolytes: metabolic acidosis, in Braunwald E, Isselbacher K, Petersdorf R, et al (eds): *Harrison's Textbook of Internal Medicine*. 11th ed. New York, NY, McGraw-Hill, 1987, p 210.
41. Perry S: Substance-induced organic mental disorders, in Hales RE, Yudofsky SC (eds): *Textbook of Neuropsychiatry*. Washington, DC, The American Psychiatric Press, 1987, p 214.
42. Sjaastad O, Gjessing L, Ritland S, et al: Chronic relapsing pancreatitis, encephalopathy with disturbance of consciousness and CSF amino acid aberration. *J Neurol* 220:83–94, 1979.
43. Johnson DA, Tong NT: Pancreatic encephalopathy. *South Med J* 70:165–167, 1977.
44. Kaminski HJ, Ruff RL: Neurologic complications of endocrine diseases. *Neurol Clin* 7(3):489–508, 1989.
45. Posner JB, Saper CB, Schiff ND, et al: Addison's disease, in *Plum and Posner's Diagnosis of Stupor and Coma*. 4th ed. New York, NY, Oxford University Press, 2007, pp 234–235.
46. Whybrow P, Hurwitz TI: Psychological disturbances associated with endocrine disease and hormone therapy, in Sachar EJ (ed): *Hormones, Behavior and Pathophysiology*. New York, NY, Raven Press, 1976.
47. Boston Collaborative Drug Surveillance Program: Acute adverse reactions to prednisone in relation to dosage. *Clin Pharmacol Ther* 13:694–698, 1997.
48. Greene R: The thyroid gland: its relationship to neurology, in Vinken PJ, Bruyn GW (eds): *The Handbook of Clinical Neurology*. Vol 27, Pt 1. New York, NY, Elsevier North-Holland, 1976, p 253.
49. Nemeroff CB: Clinical significance of psychoneuroendocrinology in psychiatry: focus on the thyroid and adrenal. *J Clin Psychiatry* 50[Suppl]:13–21, 1989.
50. Leypoldt F, Armangue T, Dalmau J: Autoimmune encephalopathies. *Ann N Y Acad Sci* 1338:94–114, 2015. doi: 10.1111/nyas.12553.
51. Tsementzis SA, Loizou LA: Pituitary apoplexy. *Neurochirurgie* 29(3):90, 1986.
52. Goto I, Nagara H, Tateishi J, et al: Thiamine-deficient encephalopathy in rats: effects of deficiencies of thiamine and magnesium. *Brain Res* 372(1):31–36, 1986.
53. Victor M: Neurologic disorders due to alcoholism and malnutrition, in Baker AB, Baker LH (eds): *Clinical Neurology*. Vol 4. Philadelphia, PA, Harper & Row, 1983, p 57.
54. da Silva IR, Frontera JA: Neurologic complications of acute environmental injuries. *Handb Clin Neurol* 141:685–704, 2017. doi:10.1016/B978-0-444-63599-0.00037-5.
55. Delplace PO, Wery D, Lemort M, et al: A case of multiple brain calcifications associated with hypoparathyroidism (in French). *J Belge Radiol* 72(4):263–266, 1989.
56. Terpenning MS, Guggy BP, Kauffman CA: Infective endocarditis: clinical features in young and elderly patients. *Am J Med* 83:626–634, 1987.

Chapter 147 ■ Mental Status Dysfunction in the Intensive Care Unit: Postoperative Cognitive Impairment

JOAN M. SWEARER • ELIZABETH R. DEGRUSH

Cognitive dysfunction following major surgery is one of the common reasons neurologists are asked to see postoperative patients in the intensive care unit (ICU): patients whose memory and intellectual abilities seem impaired when they otherwise appear to have recovered physically from the immediate effects of surgery. Cognitive dysfunction is not the same as delirium or encephalopathy, nor is it the same as an altered state of consciousness. It is a major concern for the family, the patient, and the physician when a patient is found not to be intellectually the same on awakening following surgery as he or she was before. Most patients will return to their preoperative levels of cognitive functioning within 1 to 3 months of surgery [1,2], but a percentage of patients will have persistent changes for months and even years later, and the precise pathophysiologic mechanisms for this have yet to be elucidated.

There has been extensive research on cognitive changes following major cardiac and major noncardiac surgeries. It is, however, difficult to compare the studies in literature reviews and meta-analyses directly because of differences in the methods used, including patient sampling, specific tests used, testing intervals, definition of cognitive decline, variable consideration of comorbid factors, and lack of comparison groups [1,3]. Despite these differences, increased age and risk factors for cerebrovascular disease have been the most consistent factors associated with postoperative cognitive dysfunction [2,4].

MENTAL STATUS EXAMINATION IN THE INTENSIVE CARE UNIT

The primary objectives of a mental status evaluation in the ICU are to screen for the presence of postoperative cognitive decline, delirium, or neurologic events such as stroke or transient ischemic attack. Examiners analyze the nature and extent of the impairment, and change over time. Cognitive changes may be obvious when there are gross deficits in learning, memory, attention, or concentration. The decline can also be subtle, with problems in initiative or planning.

Many mental status screening tests are available [e.g., 5–10]. The Confusion Assessment Method for the ICU (CAM-ICU [10]) was designed and validated in the ICU, and can be used on intubated and nonverbal patients. A brief screening test may provide a general impression of the patient's mental status, but the clinician must be able to assess areas of relative strength and weakness in greater depth. The following is offered as an outline for a mental status evaluation in the ICU [11–13].

Behavioral Observation and Patient Variables

Visual observation of the patient in the ICU is an extremely useful part of the mental status examination. Many details can be gathered from the moment the examiner enters the room, including the patient's alertness, the use of sedating medications or mechanical ventilation and their level of mental acuity. Determining the patient's level of arousal and attention is the essential first step in a mental status examination. Arousal may range from unresponsiveness to noxious stimuli, minimally responsive to voice or touch, normal alertness, hyper-alertness, or even manic states. Attention is the patient's ability to maintain sustained focus on a task. Mental status examination depends greatly on arousal level and attention, and it is difficult to interpret higher cognitive functions when these are not adequate.

A patient who is easily distractible will perform poorly on most cognitive tests. Lack of motivation and effort during testing can have deleterious effects on test performance, and may lead to an overestimation of cognitive impairment. Abnormalities in mood and affect, and behavioral disturbances such as psychosis, disinhibition, hyperactivity, or impulsivity will also negatively impact the patient's test performance. Test performance is compromised by postoperative pain, use of analgesic and sedating medications, limitations in strength and mobility, and possible sensory loss. Regardless, limitations of testing give the examiner useful information about the patient's current status and ability to interact with his or her surroundings.

Other patient factors that can influence test performance include demographic variables such as premorbid cognitive abilities, age, gender, education, cultural background; and medical and psychosocial history including psychiatric history, social history, and present life circumstances. A history from family members is extremely useful in defining these variables.

Attention

The patient's level of attention can be assessed at the bedside using digit span, which also depends on immediate verbal recall. Repetition of digits both forward and backward should be evaluated. Both tests consist of increasingly longer strings of random number sequences that are presented aloud to the patient. Seven digits forward (plus or minus two) is the average score obtained by adults. Digits backward normally does not differ from forward span by more than two digits. If preferred, spelling WORLD forward and then backward or alphabetizing the word EARTH can be alternatives to using digit span [7,14].

Perseverance or the ability to sustain behavioral output can be measured at the bedside by mental tracking tests. Reciting the alphabet or days of the week forward requires minimal perseverance. Examples of more discriminating attention tests include serial subtraction of 7s from 100 to 65 [7] or reciting the months of the year backward.

Resistance to interference and response inhibition are examples of executive functioning and can easily be observed during testing informally. Patients who struggle with task switching, perseverate on previous tasks, and who answer impulsively or intrusively show poor executive functioning. This can be tested formally with motor sequencing tasks. Examples include the "go-no-go" test (when the examiner taps once, the patient taps twice, but when the examiner taps twice the patient does not tap [15]); or the patient listens to a list of letters and taps his or her hand when they hear the identified letter [8]. Vigilance can also be tested by writing alternating sequences (e.g., copying a sequence of script such as m n m n m n [16]). Patients with impaired attention may perseverate on one element of the task rather than alternating between the sequences. A useful test of attention is having the patient do a verbal alpha-numeric sequence—alternating letters and numbers through the alphabet (A-1, B-2, C-3. . .to Z-26).

Speech and Language Functions

Speech output should be assessed for fluency (rate and effort of speech), articulation (normal or dysarthric), phrase length, prosody (melody, rhythm, inflection), content (semantics and syntax), and paraphasias (substitutions of rhyming alteration of words). Output can be observed in verbal responses to open-ended questions or by having the patient verbally describe a complex visual scene, such as a photograph ("propositional speech") or the Cookie Theft Picture [17]. The patient can be asked to tell someone who has never seen one, "what is a dog?; or "what is a box?" Disorders of repetition can be elicited by having the patient repeat phrases that vary in grammatical complexity (e.g., "Today is a sunny day" vs. "no ifs, ands, or buts").

Auditory comprehension can be assessed at the bedside in a number of ways. Examples include pointing to named objects, such as body-part identification (e.g., "Point to your left thumb," "show me two fingers on your right hand," "point to the ceiling after pointing to the floor," "point your way out of this room") and following multistage oral commands. Speech comprehension can also be assessed by asking "yes/no" questions such as "Do cows fly?"

Common objects (e.g., watch, pen, eyeglasses) can be used to test naming to confrontation. Component parts (e.g., lens, frame) may detect more subtle naming deficits. Oral reading can be done at bedside by having the patient read a brief passage from a newspaper, and then asked "yes-no" questions about its content.

Asking the patient to write a sentence of their own or copy from dictation are excellent screening tests for aphasic writing deficits. Comprehension can also be assessed by having the patient follow written directions (e.g., "Point to the ceiling" or "close your eyes" [7]). Word-list generation by specific category (e.g., animals, items found in supermarket or hardware store) and by specific initial letter are sensitive to both language and attention disorders.

Memory Functions

Memory functions include immediate memory span, learning capacity and retention, and retrieval of previously learned information (recent and remote). Immediate memory span is commonly assessed with a digit span forward test (described previously). Learning capacity can be investigated in a number of ways. For example, three or four unrelated words are presented and the patient is instructed to remember them. After 5 minutes of other testing, the patient is asked to recall the words. Nonverbal learning can be assessed in a similar fashion using line drawings of simple geometric figures or by pointing to three or four objects in the room and asking the patient to recall them a few minutes later.

Remote memory can be tested by asking questions about political figures (e.g., naming the three previous Presidents), dates or details of major world events, and personal history (e.g., name of high school attended).

Visuospatial and Visuoconstructive Abilities

Visuoconstructive ability is tested by having the patient copy simple figures (e.g., cube, daisy, interlocking pentagons). Spatial planning can be assessed with clock drawing. The patient is asked to draw the face of a clock and to fill in all the numbers. Left-sided visual inattention or hemispatial neglect is suggested if the patient places all the numerals on one side of the clock, or omits all numerals normally on one side. Capacity to process number/time relationships can be tested by having the patient "Set the time to 10 minutes past 11 o'clock."

Executive Functions and Other Cognitive Abilities

Executive functioning status is gathered throughout the examination as described above, monitoring for ability to switch tasks and inhibit responses when needed. Abstract thought can be assessed by asking how word pairs are alike. An example of an easy similarity test pair is "broccoli–cauliflower"; a more difficult pair is "fish–dandelion." Mental arithmetic problems (e.g., "How many quarters are in $1.50?") test reasoning ability as well as immediate memory and concentration. Insight and judgment can be approximated when discussing the patient's recent medical care, their understanding of their status; and their ability to manipulate data, make and maintain a decision regarding the next steps. Unfortunately, there are no reliable tests of judgment. Patients may be able to describe an appropriate response to how they would handle a scenario (e.g., a small emergency), but may not behave so in a real situation.

MENTAL STATUS DYSFUNCTION IN THE INTENSIVE CARE UNIT

Acute Confusional State (Delirium)

Delirium is a very common cause of mental dysfunction in postoperative patients in the ICU. The hallmark features of delirium are inattentiveness, confusion, and psychomotor agitation, as well as sleep–wake alterations, and in many patients hyper-alertness, with hallucinations or visual misinterpretation of common objects. Hypoactive delirium with alterations in arousal is often under-recognized. Fever, sepsis, metabolic and endocrine disturbances, as well as medication use or withdrawal are among the causes of delirium; this is discussed in more detail in Chapters 145 and 157.

Focal Syndromes

Stroke is another adverse neurologic outcome from surgery—especially cardiac surgery [2] or endovascular procedures, such as angioplasty—and is usually recognized by the presence of focal or lateralizing deficits of sudden onset with motor weakness or sensory deficits (see Chapters 149 and 150). Focal cognitive deficits indicative of cortical dysfunction include aphasia, apraxia, and agnosia. These can be discovered by a careful and thorough mental status examination.

Postoperative Cognitive Decline/Dysfunction

As previously noted, changes in memory and concentration are often seen in the ICU in the initial postoperative period. These changes can, however, persist beyond the immediate postoperative period when the effects of anesthesia and analgesia directly affecting cognitive functions have clearly worn off. Most mental status changes improve, but in some cases may continue following discharge, even weeks, months, and years later with associated impaired quality of life and increased mortality [4,18].

Elderly patients undergoing major cardiac (e.g., coronary artery bypass grafting, thoracic vascular surgery) and major noncardiac (e.g., orthopedic, abdominal) surgery are at the greatest risk for postoperative cognitive decline. Other individual features that increase the risk of mental status dysfunction include previous cerebrovascular disease, previous and undetected cognitive impairment or dementia, and cardiovascular risk factors such as hypertension, diabetes, and peripheral vascular disease [2,19–23].

Intraoperative risk factors include surgical technique (e.g., duration of cardiopulmonary bypass, duration of aortic cross-clamping), hypotension, manipulation of diseased aorta, and the effects of general anesthesia and hypothermia. To assess these factors requires close scrutiny of the operative record, and of the anesthesia chart. Atherothromboembolic phenomena (microemboli) and hypoxia with watershed area injury secondary to hypoperfusion are possible causative mechanisms of postoperative cognitive dysfunction due to intraoperative events during surgery [2].

A number of postoperative factors can also affect cognitive status in the ICU, including the use of analgesics, degree of physical discomfort, and depression [3,24]. These factors may produce short-term but self-limited cognitive change. Nevertheless, they should be taken into account when assessing the mental status of a patient in the ICU.

SUMMARY

Testing for mental status dysfunction of a patient in the ICU can be a complex and difficult task. Interpretation of test results can be confounded by premorbid patient characteristics (e.g., presence of a dementing illness presurgically) and the patient's current status (e.g., drowsiness in the context of high-dose analgesics, sedatives, and other medications). Mental status testing should not be attempted when arousal is abnormal or if the patient is too ill. The approach to testing should be flexible and targeted to the individual patient's complaints and level of functioning. Postoperative cognitive changes can range from obvious deficits in concentration and memory to subtle deficits in executive functions. Evidence of abnormality during a screening evaluation warrants a thorough neurologic evaluation.

References

1. Nadelson MR, Sanders RD, Avidan MS: Perioperative cognitive trajectory in adults. *Br J Anesth* 112(3):440–451, 2014.
2. Selnes OA, Gottesman RF, Grega MA, et al: Cognitive and neurological outcomes after coronary-artery bypass surgery. *N Engl J Med* 366(3):250–257, 2012.
3. Rudolph KA, Schreiber DJ, Culley RE, et al: Measurement of post-operative cognitive dysfunction after cardiac surgery: a systematic review. *Acta Anaestesiol Scand* 54:663–677, 2010.
4. Monk TG, Weldon BC, Garvan CW, et al: Predictors of cognitive dysfunction after major noncardiac surgery. *Anesthesiology* 108(1):18–30, 2008.
5. Solomon PR, Hirschoff A, Kelly B, et al: A 7 minute neurocognitive screening battery highly sensitive to Alzheimer's disease. *Arch Neurol* 55(3):349–355, 1998.
6. Drachman DA, Swearer JM, Kane K, et al: The Cognitive Assessment Screening Test (CAST) for dementia. *Neurology* 9(4):200–208, 1996.
7. Folstein M, Folstein S, McHugh PR: Mini-mental state: a practical method for grading the cognitive state of patients for the clinician. *J Psychiatric Res* 12(3):189–198, 1975.
8. Nasreddine ZS: The Montreal Cognitive Assessment Test. www.mocatest.org. 2015. Accessed March 7, 2017.
9. Fong TG, Jones RN, Rudolph JL, et al: Development and validation of a brief cognitive assessment tool: The Sweet 16. *Arch Intern Med* 171(5):432–437, 2011.
10. Ely EW: Confusion Assessment Method for the ICU (CAM-ICU): The Complete Training Manual. www.icudelirium.org. 2014. Accessed March 7, 2017.
11. Mendez MF, Cummings JL: *Dementia: A Clinical Approach*. 3rd ed. Philadelphia, PA, Butterworth-Heinemann, 2003.
12. Lezak MD, Howienson DB, Bigler ED, et al: *Neuropsychological Assessment*. 5th ed. New York, NY, Oxford University Press, 2012.
13. Weintraub S: Neuropsychological assessment of mental state, in Mesulam MM (ed): *Principles of Behavioral and Cognitive Neurology*. 2nd ed. Oxford, Oxford University Press, 2000.
14. Benjamin S, Lauterbach M: The Brain Card. www.thebraincard.com. 2010. Accessed March 7, 2017.
15. Drewe EA: Go no-go learning after frontal lobe lesions in humans. *Cortex* 11(1):8–16, 1975.
16. Luria A: *Human Brain and Psychological Processes*. New York, NY, Harper & Row, 1966.
17. Goodglass H, Kaplan E, Barresi B: *The Assessment of Aphasia and Related Disorders*. 3rd ed. Austin, TX, Pro-Ed, 2001.
18. Steinmetz J, Christensen KB, Lund T, et al: Long-term consequences of postoperative cognitive dysfunction. *Anesthesiology* 110(3):548–555, 2009.
19. Krenk L, Ramussen LS, Kehlet H: New insights into the pathophysiology of postoperative cognitive dysfunction. *Acta Anaesthesiol Scand* 54(8):951–956, 2010.
20. Kozora E, Kongs S, Collins JF, et al: Cognitive outcomes after on- versus off-pump coronary artery bypass surgery. *Ann Thorac Surg* 90(4):1134–1141, 2010.
21. Yocum GT, Gaudet JG, Teverbaugh LA, et al: Neurocognitive performance in hypertensive patients after spine surgery. *Anesthesiology* 110(2):254–261, 2009.
22. Price CC, Tanner JJ, Schmalfuss I, et al: A pilot study evaluating presurgery neuroanatomical biomarkers for postoperative cognitive decline after total knee arthroplasty in older adults. *Anesthesiology* 120(3):601–613, 2014.
23. Silbert B, Evered L, Scott DA, et al: Preexisting cognitive impairment is associated with postoperative cognitive impairment after hip joint replacement therapy. *Anesthesiology* 122(6):1224–1234, 2015.
24. Zywiel MG, Prabhu A, Perruccio AV, et al: The influence of anesthesia and pain management on cognitive dysfunction after joint arthroplasty. *Clin Orthop Relat Res* 472(5):1453–1466, 2014.

Chapter 148 ■ Generalized Anoxia/Ischemia of the Nervous System

BANU SUNDAR • CAROL F. LIPPA • MAJAZ MOONIS

Anoxic brain injury results from inadequate oxygen supply to the brain. The clinical picture ranges from mild confusion to deep coma with loss of brainstem responses. Anoxic damage can be caused by circulatory collapse; respiratory failure; or inadequate hemoglobin or its ability to bind and release oxygen. Prognosis and management of the anoxic patient depend in part on which of these mechanisms has caused the injury.

PATHOGENESIS

The brain is unique in that it uses almost exclusively aerobic metabolism of glucose. The continuous availability of oxygen is secured by the cerebral vasculature's autoregulatory mechanisms [1], which control the rate of blood flow over a wide range of blood pressures. If blood pressure drops too low for autoregulatory mechanisms to operate, oxygen extraction from the blood increases. Failure of this compensatory mechanism results in a changeover from aerobic to anaerobic metabolism.

In cardiac arrest (CA), depletion of brain oxygen reserves occurs within 10 seconds, thereby eliminating the major source of neuronal energy from ATP (adenosine triphosphate) and phosphokinase. Excessive glutamate release and reduced reuptake lead to activation of the NMDA (*N*-methyl-D-aspartate) receptors and consequent ischemic cascade. The resulting intracellular (cytotoxic) edema leads to increased intracranial pressure. The changeover to anaerobic metabolism results in neuronal catabolism. In cardiovascular collapse, loss of venous outflow leads to the accumulation of lactic acid and pyruvate, the end products of anaerobic metabolism. Buildup of these catabolites potentiates neuronal damage.

DIAGNOSIS

The first question to address when evaluating a comatose or obtunded patient with a possible hypoxic insult is whether the impaired consciousness is the result of a metabolic insult or a structural brain lesion. Coma caused by a mass lesion is usually associated with focal neurologic signs. Computed axial tomography (CT) or magnetic resonance imaging (MRI) scans usually reveal focal lesions in this setting. Metabolic causes, including anoxic encephalopathy, should be suspected when patients with impaired consciousness present with a nonfocal examination.

The diagnosis is often suggested by the clinical setting (e.g., CA in patients with arrhythmias or myocardial infarctions, or severe episodes of intraoperative hypotension). Arterial blood gas determination, if obtained during the causal event, can confirm the diagnosis. Acute decrease in the partial pressure of oxygen to less than 40 mm Hg causes confusion, and to less than 30 mm Hg results in coma [2]. Associated abnormalities that potentiate anoxic damage include anemia, acidosis, hypercapnia, hyperthermia, and hypotension.

The internist or neurologist is often consulted to evaluate the patient who has impaired consciousness after well-documented cerebral hypoperfusion event that has occurred during surgical operations requiring the use of extracorporeal circulation. The neurological examination is usually nonfocal. Because surgical patients with such a history often have preexisting illnesses (vascular disease, borderline renal function, hepatic impairment, and diabetes), it is the obligation of the intensive care physician to determine whether the new deficits are caused by anoxic encephalopathy, or by other treatable conditions secondary to metabolic, infectious, or iatrogenic factors such as sedating medications. Intracerebral hemorrhage and subdural hematomas should also be sought, because they can occur spontaneously in the perioperative period, especially in anticoagulated patients.

CLINICAL COURSE AND PROGNOSIS

The clinical outcomes for patients with anoxic injuries depend on the degree and duration of oxygen deprivation to the brain as well as the maintenance of blood flow. With complete cessation of blood flow to the brain, consciousness is lost after several seconds. If anoxia is moderately prolonged, the patient awakens but may have residual deficits, such as cognitive impairment, or later sequelae, including extrapyramidal movement disorders or seizures, which may not develop for days to weeks.

A delayed postanoxic syndrome may occur rarely in patients with anoxic insults after the initial coma. Three to 30 days following the initial anoxic insult, after the patient has regained consciousness and cognitive function, there is a secondary decline characterized by irritability, confusion, lethargy, clumsiness, and increased muscle tone; patients may become comatose again and die. This uncommon condition occurs most often in cases of carbon monoxide poisoning. Pathologically, widespread demyelination is seen without gray matter changes. The cause is unknown, but it may be caused by alteration of enzymatic processes; edema; or damage to small blood vessels [2,3].

The overall prognosis for a meaningful recovery in patients with nontraumatic coma is guarded; the longer patients are in coma, the worse the outcome [4–6]. Maximal improvement usually occurs within the first 30 days. Non-anoxic metabolic coma carries the best prognosis, whereas anoxic coma has a better prognosis than coma resulting from structural lesions. A good outcome is seen in 50% of patients who awaken within 24 hours. Although infrequent seizures or myoclonus do not affect prognosis, myoclonic or nonconvulsive status epilepticus is a grave prognostic sign and is associated with poor recovery [4,7].

If consciousness is maintained during a hypoxic event, there is rarely permanent brain damage. Irreversible damage is rarely seen in healthy individuals if the duration of anoxia is less than 4 minutes, although it may occur for individuals with preexisting cerebrovascular disease in shorter periods.

In cases of nontraumatic coma, the most valuable prognostic information is obtained from the physical examination. Favorable prognostic indicators include the following:

1. Recovery of multiple brainstem responses within 48 hours (pupillary, oculocephalic, and corneal) [4].
2. Return of purposeful responses to painful stimuli by 24 hours.
3. Primary pulmonary event leading to coma.
4. Hypothermia at the time of the anoxic event may be protective.
5. Younger age [8].

Poor prognostic indicators in persistent coma include the following:

1. Absence of pupillary and corneal responses, and withdrawal response to pain in 24 hours [9].

2. The loss of vestibulo-ocular responses at 12 hours; presence of decerebrate or decorticate posturing at 24 hours; and absent motor response to pain by the third day [5,8,10].
3. Electroencephalogram (EEG) within 24 hours after CA showing unfavorable patterns such as isoelectric, low-voltage, and burst suppression with identical bursts [11].
4. Bilateral absences of the N20 of the somatosensory evoked potentials (SSEPs) of at least 24 hours' duration [12].
5. Noncontrast CT scan shows lower gray–white matter ratio in comatose patients after CA [13].
6. Extensive abnormalities on diffusion-weighted imaging [14,15].
7. Myoclonus or status epilepticus the first day.

SSEPs are not abolished in reversible coma owing to metabolic or toxic causes, sedative or anesthetic administration, nor even in barbiturate coma, which makes its absence potentially useful in the diagnosis of brain death [16].

A recent Academy of Neurology Practice Parameter evidence-based review for predicting the outcome in survivors of cardiopulmonary resuscitation (CPR) suggests the following as poor prognosticators of outcome: Absence of pupillary light reflex, corneal reflexes, and motor response to pain; occurrence of myoclonus or status epilepticus. Serum neuron-specific enolase (NSE), and SSEP studies can assist in accurately predicting poor outcome in comatose patients after CPR for CA [17]. When prognosticating by the clinical criteria alone, one must be careful that no sedative, anesthetic, or anticonvulsant is being used, because these agents can suppress brainstem reflexes.

Generalized cerebral anoxia due to respiratory insufficiency, with maintained circulation, carries a better prognosis. A low partial pressure of oxygen does not necessarily convey a bad prognosis in cases of isolated hypoxia, if circulation is carefully maintained [18,19]. Conversely, the presence of metabolic abnormalities, such as lactic acidosis, worsens prognosis.

In cases of out-of-hospital CA (OHCA), survival depends on the total time required to establish effective cerebral blood flow. The arrest time (AT) and the CPR time to effective cardiac function represent a continuum from absence of cerebral blood flow to effective circulation, and together represent the total duration of ineffective cerebral blood flow. Short AT is compatible with good outcomes even after longer periods of CPR, whereas increasing lengths of AT reduce the time window for successful CPR. If AT is less than 6 minutes, prognosis for recovery is related to CPR time; over half of patients on whom CPR is successful within 30 minutes make a good neurologic recovery. When CPR time is longer, prognosis for neurologic recovery drops significantly. If AT exceeds 6 minutes, and CPR time 5 minutes or less 50% recovered neurologic function. If CPR time was between 6 and 15 minutes 19% recovered neurologic function, and no patients recovered good neurologic function if CPR time was over 15 minutes [20]. The OHCA outcome differed by time to first CPR and first documented rhythm; shortening of time to first CPR is crucial for improving the OHCA outcome [21]. Unsuccessful CPR before arrival at the emergency room predicts a poor prognosis [22]. Emergency crew–witnessed arrests; consciousness level on admission; and requirement for ventilation are independently useful to predict in-hospital outcome and mortality [23].

Magnetic resonance spectroscopy demonstrating elevated lactate and reduced *N*-acetyl aspartate peaks is associated with a poor prognosis [24,25].

Cerebrospinal fluid (CSF) lactate levels, NSE, and brain-type creatine kinase isoenzyme levels, may have predictive value 24 hours after CA [26,27]. Patients with either serum NSE more than 33 μg per L at 24 hours, or CSF brain-type creatine kinase isoenzyme more than 50 U per L at 48 to 72 hours, had a poor outcome [12,28]. S-100 protein, an astroglial marker, is elevated in anoxic arrest. Values more than 0.2 mmol/L on Day 2 are associated with 100% mortality, whereas lower values are associated with a nearly 90% survival.

After OHCA, the overall probability of awakening is roughly 50% [29]. Much of this depends on the duration of the coma. The longer a patient survived without awakening, the smaller the probability of awakening without deficits [30,31]. In cases of OHCA, patients who are comatose on admission, but who awake to follow commands within 2 days, have an 80% probability of good neurologic function on discharge or later [29].

TREATMENT

Treatment approaches for CA and perioperative hypoxic encephalopathy are similar. Optimal therapy is directed at preventing the recurrence of hypoxia. To ensure that the oxygen-carrying capacity of the blood is restored, excess oxygen administration is suggested for several hours after anoxic events. Blood pressure is maintained at normotensive or mildly elevated levels. Mean arterial pressure should be 90 to 110 mm Hg in patients who are usually normotensive. The partial pressure of oxygen should be more than 100 mm Hg. The partial pressure of carbon dioxide is kept at the patient's baseline (usually 40 mm Hg), unless there are active signs of cerebral herniation; if herniation is suspected, the patient should be hyperventilated. Mild hypovolemia and elevation of the head of the bed to 30 degrees reduce intracranial pressure. Vital signs, hematocrit, electrolytes, blood sugar, and serum osmolality should be maintained in the normal range. In all cases, a head CT or MRI scan and complete metabolic studies should be obtained to exclude structural and other functional causes. When any uncertainties exist, a neurologist should be consulted.

Seizures occur in 25% of patients in anoxic coma [4]. They are treated with loading and then maintenance doses of fosphenytoin (loading dose, 15 to 20 mg phenytoin equivalents per kg, rate not to exceed 100 mg phenytoin equivalents per minute; maintenance dose, 5 mg phenytoin equivalents per kg per day). Alternatively, intravenous phenytoin can be used (loading dose, 18 to 20 mg per kg; rate, 50 mg per minute; maintenance dose, 5 mg per kg). Other newer intravenous medications have the advantage of less drug interaction but no proven efficacy over the known medications. Their indiscriminate use can lead to escalation in health care cost without known non-inferiority or superiority. Patients with cardiac conduction abnormalities need to be carefully monitored while being loaded with fosphenytoin or phenytoin. Phenobarbital is usually avoided because of its sedative effects. If necessary, loading doses in adults are up to 500 mg intravenously, and maintenance doses are 2 to 4 mg/kg/d [32]. Because status epilepticus or frequent untreated seizures can further damage the brain, an EEG should be obtained if there is any question of subclinical epileptiform activity [9]. Some postanoxic patients develop delayed intention myoclonus. This can be distinguished from seizure activity because the latter is accompanied by an epileptiform discharge on the EEG, whereas myoclonus is not.

Steroids, mannitol, and glycerol are ineffective and result in elevated serum blood glucose, which increase production of lactic acid, possibly potentiating preexisting damage.

There is strong evidence that mild or moderate hypothermia may improve outcome after CA [33,34]. The 2010 American Heart Association (AHA) guidelines recommend cooling between 32 and 34 degrees in comatose adult patients with Return of Spontaneous Circulation (ROSC) after out-of-hospital ventricular fibrillation (VF) CA, for 12 to 24 hours [35]. Also induced hypothermia (IH) may be considered after in-hospital CA with any initial rhythm; or after OHCA with an initial rhythm of pulseless electrical activity or asystole [35]. A recent international trial of unconscious survivors in OHCA patients did not show a difference in neurological outcome following targeted body temperature of 33°C compared with a targeted body temperature of 36°C [36]. The authors raised the question of whether the observed benefit of hypothermia following CA is caused by prevention of fever, or a specific result of brain protection. This study does not alter the AHA guidelines to lower the temperature of patients following CA.

TABLE 148.1

Effect of Induced Hypothermia on Neurological Outcomes and Survival among Adults with Cardiac Arrest

Setting of IH	Outcome on patients surviving CA
OHCA	Moderate hypothermia appears to improve outcome [34]
CA due to VF	Therapeutic mild hypothermia increased the rate of favorable neurological outcome and reduced mortality [33]
Prehospital cooling immediately after ROSC in CA survivors	Did not improve survival or neurological status [39]
OHCA assigned either 33 or 36 degrees	No difference between two groups on mortality or neurological function [36]

Select RCT included.
CA, cardiac arrest; IH, induced hypothermia; OHCA, out-of-hospital cardiac arrest; ROSC, return of spontaneous circulation; VF, ventricular fibrillation.

Summary of selected large randomized controlled trials (RCT) on the outcomes after IH on surviving patients with witnessed CA is outlined in Table 148.1.

Contraindications for therapeutic hypothermia (TH) include [37]:

1. Patients demonstrating rapid and complete neurological recovery.
2. Patients with Do-not-Resuscitate (DNR) orders.
3. Patients with active bleeding or those at high risk of bleeding.

SUMMARY

The effects of oxygen deprivation depend on many factors; the degree and duration of hypoxia are the most important. In cases of CA, brain damage is proportional to the amount of time without perfusion. The patient's age, underlying medical conditions, infection, and other metabolic imbalances also play a role in the body's ability to withstand oxygen deprivation.

Treatment strategies for the acute phase focus on supportive care. Elevation of the head of the bed; maintaining a relatively hypovolemic state; and avoidance of hypotension may be of benefit. A vigorous search should be made for concurrent metabolic abnormalities. Administration of steroids, osmotic agents, neuroprotective agents, and prophylactic anticonvulsants is ineffective and may worsen the prognosis.

Prognosis is best determined by the early return of brainstem and cranial nerve function. Absence of brainstem functions 72 hours after the event is associated with poor outcome [17]. Other poor prognostic signs include BAER showing no cortical waves 8 hours after the circulatory arrest; absence of cortical SSEP; and a CT scan demonstrating diffuse edema, loss of gray–white matter distinction, or watershed infarcts. The overall functional recovery rate is approximately 13%. If a patient has not regained consciousness by 6 hours after the onset of coma, the chance of survival for 1 year is 10%, and many of these survivors remain in a vegetative state.

IH improves outcome in CA survivors. Numerous studies have shown that TH can be applied safely with minimal side effects. More studies will be required to determine the optimal duration of TH, and identification of patients who might benefit from deeper or more prolonged hypothermia [38]. It might be possible that even less severely injured patients might benefit more from TH, aiding in better functional recovery—a possibility that can be explored in future studies.

References

1. Dewey RC, Hunt WE: Cerebral hemodynamic crisis. Physiology, pathophysiology, and approach to therapy. *Am J Surg* 131:338, 1976.
2. Posner JB, Saper CB, Schiff ND, et al: *Plum and Posner's Diagnosis of Stupor and Coma*. 4th ed. Oxford, Oxford University Press, 2007.
3. Plum F, Posner JB, Hain RF: Delayed neurological deterioration after anoxia. *Arch Intern Med* 110:56, 1962.
4. Levy DE, Bates D, Caronna JJ, et al: Prognosis in nontraumatic coma. *Ann Intern Med* 94:293, 1981.
5. Snyder BD, Ramirez-Lassepas M, Lippert DM: Neurologic status and prognosis after cardiopulmonary arrest: I. A retrospective study. *Neurology* 27:807, 1977.
6. Edgren E, Hedstrand U, Kelsy S, et al: Assessment of neurological prognosis in comatose survivors of cardiac arrest. BRCT1 study group. *Lancet* 343(8905):1055, 1994.
7. Wijdicks EF, Parisi JE, Sharbrough FW: Prognostic value of myoclonus in comatose survivors of cardiac arrest. *Ann Neurol* 38(4):697, 1994.
8. Dickey W, Adgey AAJ: Resuscitation: mortality within hospital after resuscitation from ventricular fibrillation outside hospital. *Br Heart J* 67:334, 1992.
9. Mellion ML: Neurologic consequences of cardiac arrest and preventive strategies. *Med Health R I* 88:382, 2005.
10. Zandbergen EGJ, de Haan RJ, Stoutenbeek CP, et al: Systematic review of early predictors of poor outcome in anoxic-ischemic coma. *Lancet* 352:1808, 1998.
11. Hofmeijer J, Beernink TMJ, Bosch FH, et al: Early EEG contributes to multimodal outcome prediction of pastanoxic coma. *Neurology* 85:1, 2015.
12. Zandbergen EG, Hijdra A, Koelman JH, et al: Prediction of poor outcome within the first 3 days of postanoxic coma. *Neurology* 66:62–68, 2006.
13. Torbey MT, Selim M, Knorr J, et al: Quantitative analysis of the loss of distinction between gray and white matter in comatose patients after cardiac arrest. *Stroke* 31:2163–2167, 2000.
14. Arbelaez A: Diffusion weighted MR imaging of global cerebral anoxia. *AJNR Am J Neuroradiol* 20(6):999, 1999.
15. Wijdicks EFM, Campeau NG, Miller GM: MR Imaging in comatose survivors of cardiac resuscitation. *AJNR Am J Neuroradiol* 22:1561–1565, 2001.
16. Facco E, Liviero MC, Munari M, et al: Short latency evoked potentials: new criteria for brain death? *J Neurol Neurosurg Psychiatry* 3:351, 1990.
17. Wijdicks EF, Hijdra A, Young GB, et al: Practice parameter: prediction of outcome in comatose survivors after cardiopulmonary resuscitation (an evidence-based review): report of the Quality Standards Subcommittee of the American Academy of Neurology. *Neurology* 67:203, 2006.
18. Safar P, Bleyaert A, Nemoto EM, et al: Resuscitation after global brain ischemia-anoxia. *Crit Care Med* 6:215, 1978.
19. Pfeifer R, Borner A, Krack A, et al: Outcome after cardiac arrest: predictive values and limitations of the neuroproteins neuron-specific enolase and protein S-100 and the Glasgow Coma Scale. *Resuscitation* 65:49, 2005.
20. Abramson NS, Safar P, Detre KM: Neurologic recovery after cardiac arrest: effect of duration of ischemia. *Crit Care Med* 14:930, 1985.
21. Hara M, Hayashi K, Hikoso S: Different impacts of time from collapse to first cardiopulmonary resuscitation on outcomes after witnessed out-of-hospital cardiac arrest in adults. *Circ Cardiovasc Qual Outcomes* 8:277–284, 2015.
22. Gray WA, Capone RJ, Most AS: Unsuccessful emergency medical resuscitation: are continued efforts in the emergency department justified? *N Engl J Med* 325:1393, 1991.
23. Grubb NR, Elton RA, Fox KA: In hospital mortality after out of hospital cardiac arrest. *Lancet* 346:417, 1995.
24. Lechleitner P, Felber S, Birbamer G, et al: Proton magnetic resonance spectroscopy of brain after cardiac resuscitation. *Lancet* 340:913, 1992.
25. Moonis M, Fisher M: Imaging of acute stroke. *Cerebrovasc Dis* 11:143, 2001.
26. Roine RO, Somer H, Kaste M, et al: Neurologic outcome after out-of-hospital cardiac arrest: prediction by cerebrospinal fluid enzyme analysis. *Arch Neurol* 46:753, 1989.
27. Edgren E, Headstrand U, Nordin M, et al: Prediction of outcome after cardiac arrest. *Crit Care Med* 15:820, 1987.
28. Schoerkhuber W, Kittler H, Sterz F, et al: Time course of neuron-specific enolase. A predictor of neurological outcome after cardiac arrest. *Stroke* 30:1598, 1999.
29. Earnest MP, Yarnell PR, Merrill SL, et al: Long-term survival and neurologic status after resuscitation from out-of-hospital cardiac arrest. *Neurology* 30:1298, 1980.
30. Tweed WA, Thomassen A, Wernberg M: Prognosis after cardiac arrest based on age and duration of coma. *Can Med Assoc J* 126:1058, 1982.
31. Longstreth WT, Inui TS, Cobb LA, et al: Neurologic recovery after out-of-hospital c arrest. *Ann Intern Med* 98:588, 1983.
32. Simon RP, Aminoff MJ: Electrographic status epilepticus in fatal anoxic coma. *Ann Neurol* 20:351, 1986.
33. The Hypothermia after Cardiac Arrest Study Group: Mild therapeutic hypothermia to improve the neurologic outcome after cardiac arrest. *N Engl J Med* 346:549, 2002.
34. Bernard SA, Gray TW, Buist MD, et al: Treatment of comatose survivors of out-of-hospital cardiac arrest with induced hypothermia. *N Engl J Med* 346:557, 2002.
35. Peberdy MA, Callaway CW, Neumar RW, et al: Part 9: post-cardiac arrest care. *Circulation* S768–S786, 2010.
36. Kim F, Nichol G, Maynard C, et al: Effect of prehospital induction of mild hypothermia on survival and neurological status among adults with cardiac arrest. *JAMA* 311(1):45–52, 2014.
37. Nielsen N, Wetterslev J, Cronberg T, et al: Targeted temperature management at 33°C versus 36°C. after cardiac arrest. *N Engl J Med* 369:23, 2013.
38. Rittenberger JC, Polderman KH, Smith WS, et al: Emergency neurological life support: resuscitation following cardiac arrest. *Neurocrit Care* 2012, 17:S21.
39. Polderman KH, Varon J: How low should we go? Hypothermia or strict normothermia after cardiac arrest? *Circulation* 131:669, 2015.

Chapter 149 ■ Cerebrovascular Diseases

RICHARD P. GODDEAU, JR • JOHN P. WEAVER • MAJAZ MOONIS

Cerebrovascular diseases encompass ischemic stroke from thrombosis or embolism, and hemorrhagic stroke including intracerebral hemorrhage (ICH) and subarachnoid hemorrhage. Many patients require management in the intensive care unit (ICU) owing to the severity of disease or for monitoring after acute thrombolytic therapy. This chapter reviews the basic concepts of pathogenesis, diagnosis, evaluation, and management for patients with ischemic cerebrovascular disease (ICVD) and ICH. Subarachnoid hemorrhage is discussed in Chapter 150.

ISCHEMIC CEREBROVASCULAR DISEASE

ICVD includes transient ischemic attack (TIA) and ischemic stroke and comprises 87% of all strokes; it is the most common neurologic problem that leads to acute hospitalization [1]. To facilitate accurate diagnosis and appropriate therapy, ICVD can be categorized along three axes: acuity, anatomic territory, and underlying mechanism.

Acuity

Stroke is a paroxysmal disorder, most frequently occurring suddenly and without warning. However, in the thrombolytic era, accompanying an increased understanding of the neuronal and vascular pathophysiology of ICVD, it has become increasingly important to conceptualize a stroke that "is happening" rather than one that "has happened." This distinction reflects the circumstances when an opportunity to intervene to attenuate, prevent recurrence, or reverse the deficits related to ICVD exists and includes both TIAs and hyperacute stroke.

TIAs are brief episodes of neurologic dysfunction resulting from cerebral ischemia not resulting in cerebral infarction [2]. Classically, symptoms last for a few to 15 minutes but occasionally may persist for hours. Risk of recurrent TIA or stroke is highest in the ensuing few days [3]. By contrast, patients with transient symptoms and evidence of infarction by imaging are properly diagnosed with stroke. Both acute circumstances represent unstable cerebrovascular conditions for which prompt evaluation and treatment is required.

Acute stroke, or sometimes "hyperacute" stroke, refers to the first several hours after a stroke has occurred, when thrombolytic therapy may be indicated. (Table 149.1). Labeling presently suggests the use of rt'PA in applicable patients within 3 hours, but this has recently been expanded to within 4.5 hours and is supported by approbation from the American Heart Association [4]. Beyond this period, and extending typically for the next 1 to 3 days, is the acute period in which care directed at minimizing worsening or recurrence is paramount. The subacute period extends through two weeks after the event and is often characterized by attention to rehabilitative efforts. Beyond this point—the chronic period—rehabilitative efforts continue, and the focus on optimizing long-term secondary preventive therapy is critical.

Anatomic Territory

Two broad clinical anatomic categories of ICVD syndromes are recognized, based on division of the cerebrovascular supply into those areas supplied by the carotid system (anterior circulation) and those supplied by the vertebral-basilar system (posterior circulation).

Symptoms commonly encountered in carotid system disease include aphasia; monoparesis or hemiparesis; monoparesthesias or hemiparesthesias; binocular visual field disturbance (hemianopia); or monocular visual loss. Symptoms that may be seen in vertebral-basilar system disease include hemianopia; cortical blindness; diplopia; vertigo; dysarthria; ataxia; and limb paresis or paresthesias, frequently with ipsilateral involvement of cranial nerve functions, and contralateral body involvement. Loss of consciousness or isolated vertigo rarely occurs without other vertebral-basilar symptoms (less than 5%). Other isolated symptoms, such as diplopia, amnesia, dysarthria, and light-headedness, usually do not serve as a basis for the diagnosis of vertebral-basilar disease; however, association with other brainstem symptoms may support this diagnosis [5].

Underlying Mechanism

Acute ICVD can be categorized as being owing to *large vessel thrombosis*; *small vessel thrombosis*, *cardioembolism*; *other known etiology*; or *stroke of undetermined etiology*. Large vessel atherothrombotic occlusion is caused by atherosclerosis in the carotid or vertebral-basilar arteries, and is a common cause of acute ICVD. The pattern and severity of the neurologic deficit depend on the arterial territory; completeness of occlusion; and extent of collateral flow [5]. Small vessel occlusion occurs frequently owing to lipohyalinosis of the lenticulostriate arteries or basilar penetrators, and results in a small area of cerebral infarction called a *lacune* (Fig. 149.1). If a lacune occurs in the internal capsule, thalamus, or basis pontis, substantial neurologic deficits may occur even with a small lesion. The most common lacunar syndromes are pure motor hemiparesis, pure sensory loss, ataxic hemiparesis, and dysarthria-clumsy hand syndrome [6].

The typical presentation of a cardioembolic stroke is with maximal deficit at onset, although a small minority may have a stuttering clinical course. Diagnosis may be difficult if the patient has coexistent large arterial lesions; as many as one-third of patients with a cardiac embolic source have another potential explanation for their strokes [7]. The most common cardiac sources associated with cerebral embolic events are outlined in Table 149.2. Nonvalvular embolic source with atrial fibrillation is associated with an annual stroke risk between 2.2% and 15% according to associated risk factors [8]. Transmyocardial infarction, atrial fibrillation, and mechanical valves are associated with a high risk, whereas the risk is lower for patients with bioprosthetic valves. Patent right-to-left cardiac shunts have been recognized by contrast echocardiography with increasing frequency among younger stroke patients. In the absence of a hypercoagulable state or atrial septal aneurysm, a patent foramen ovale (PFO) is not considered a significant risk factor for cardioembolic stroke, because up to 25% of the healthy population have a small PFO [9].

The aggregated category of "other known" etiology includes rarer causes distinct from the other categories. This includes traumatic or spontaneous extracranial or intracranial arterial dissection, an important cause of stroke in patients under age 50. Thrombophilias, whether congenital or acquired, are more likely to impact the venous system but may be an unusual cause of artery occlusion including ischemic stroke. Border-zone infarction

TABLE 149.1

IV rt-PA Inclusion/Exclusion Criteria

Inclusion criteria
Diagnosis of ischemic stroke causing measurable neurologic deficit
Onset of symptoms <3 h before beginning treatment
Age ≥18 y
For patients presenting between 3 and 4.5 h, additional including criteria:
Age <80 y
Absent combined history of prior stroke and diabetes
Absent use of anticoagulants (irrespective of INR)
Informed consent obtained from patient/representative
Exclusion criteria
Significant head trauma or prior stroke in previous 3 mo
Symptoms suggest subarachnoid hemorrhage
Arterial puncture at noncompressible site in previous 7 d
History of previous intracranial hemorrhage
Intracranial neoplasm, arteriovenous malformation, or aneurysm
Recent intracranial or intraspinal surgery
Elevated blood pressure (systolic >185 mm Hg or diastolic >110 mm Hg)
Blood glucose concentration <50 mg/dL (2.7 mmol/L)
Active internal bleeding
Acute bleeding diathesis, including but not limited to:
Platelet count <100,000/mm^3
Heparin received within 48 hours, resulting in abnormally elevated aPTT greater than the upper limit of normal
Current use of anticoagulant with INR >1.7 or PT >15 s
Current use of direct thrombin inhibitors or direct factor Xa inhibitors with elevated sensitive laboratory tests (such as aPTT, INR, platelet count, and ECT; TT; or appropriate factor Xa activity assays)
CT demonstrates multilobar infarction (hypodensity >1/3 cerebral hemisphere) Relative exclusion criteria
Relative Contraindications
(Recent experience suggests that under some circumstances—with careful consideration and weighting of risk to benefit—patients may receive fibrinolytic therapy despite one or more relative contraindications. Consider risk to benefit of IV rt-PA administration carefully if any of these relative contraindications are present)
Only minor or rapidly improving stroke symptoms (clearing spontaneously)
Pregnancy
Seizure at onset with postictal residual neurologic impairments
Major surgery or serious trauma within previous 14 d
Recent gastrointestinal or urinary tract hemorrhage (within previous 21 d)
Recent acute myocardial infarction (within previous 3 mo)

aPTT, activated partial thromboplastin time; ECT;ecarin clotting time; INR, international normalized ratio; IV rt-PA, intravenous recombinant tissue plasminogen activator; PT, prothrombin time; TT, thrombin time.

is caused by globally diminished cerebral blood flow resulting from cardiac arrest or systemic hypotension, often associated with cerebral arterial stenosis, resulting in focal infarction and deficits occurring in well-described patterns in the endarterial distribution between major vessels [10] (Fig. 149.2). In the carotid circulation, border-zone infarcts occur between the distribution of the middle cerebral artery (MCA) and either the anterior or posterior cerebral arteries.

Stroke of undetermined etiology, or cryptogenic, is assessed after full evaluation for other known causes has been unrevealing. This nosologic entity is associated with better outcome than stroke of other categories and requires the treating clinicians to do a comprensive evaluation when the cause of the stroke is not apparent.

Differential Diagnosis

Symptoms suggestive of ICVD may mimic the symptoms of other neurologic entities. An important distinction is between ICH and ICVD. Symptoms considered classic for ICH such as early obtundation, coma, seizures, headache, and vomiting are known to be insufficiently reliable to make that diagnosis, because a similar presentation may be seen with ischemic stroke. Conditions other than cerebrovascular events can occasionally cause acute focal neurologic deficits and must be also be considered. Primary or metastatic brain tumors with hemorrhage into the tumor may resemble a stroke (Fig. 149.3). Subdural hematomas may rarely present with acute focal neurologic

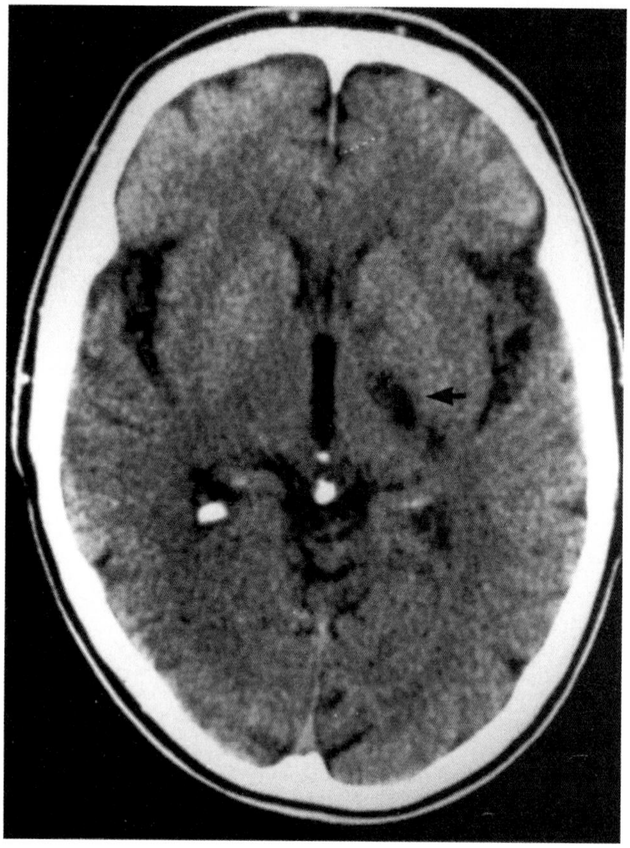

FIGURE 149.1 Lacunar infarct involving the left internal capsule seen on a computed tomography scan.

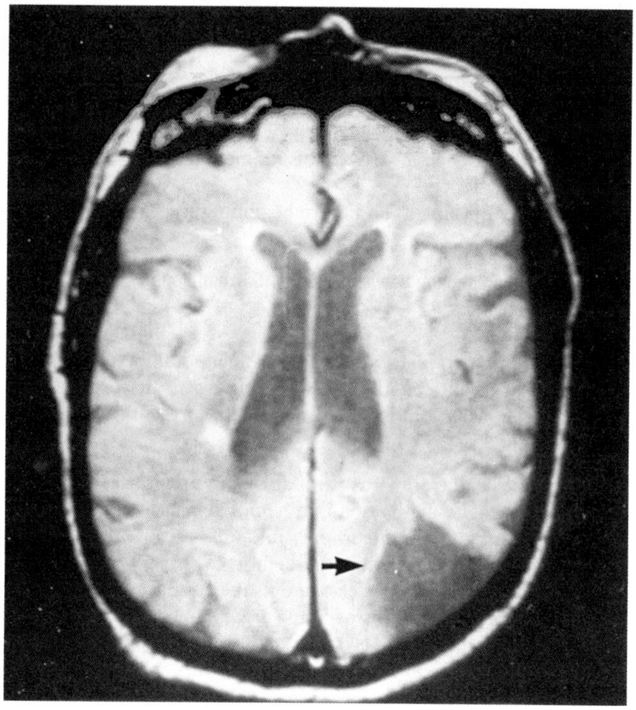

FIGURE 149.2 T1-weighted magnetic resonance imaging scan demonstrating a watershed infarction (*arrow*) in the border zone between the middle and posterior cerebral arteries.

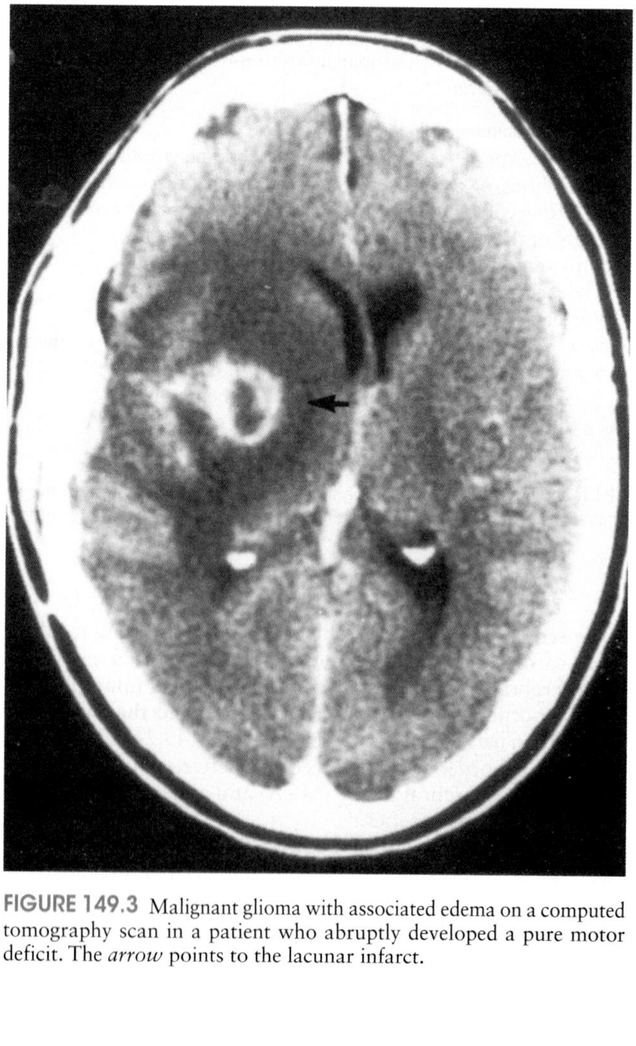

FIGURE 149.3 Malignant glioma with associated edema on a computed tomography scan in a patient who abruptly developed a pure motor deficit. The *arrow* points to the lacunar infarct.

TABLE 149.2

Cardiac Sources for Cerebral Emboli

Common
- Nonvalvular atrial fibrillation
- Acute anterior wall myocardial infarction
- Ventricular aneurysms and dyskinetic segments
- Rheumatic valvular disease
- Prosthetic cardiac valves
- Right-to-left shunts
- Bacterial endocarditis

Less common
- Mitral valve prolapse
- Cardiomyopathy
- Bicuspid aortic valve
- Atrial myxoma
- Nonbacterial endocarditis
- Mitral annulus calcification
- Idiopathic hypertrophic subaortic stenosis
- Atrial septal aneurysm

deficits and must be considered in elderly patients, even without a history of head trauma. Patients with migraine headaches sometimes develop focal neurologic symptoms either before or during the early phase of the headache. Rarely, these deficits may occur in the absence of a headache (acephalgic migraine) or may persist (migrainous infarction). Patients with focal seizures may develop sensory, motor, and aphasic symptoms that can mimic ICVD, although they are usually stereotypical and transient. Occasionally, focal neurologic deficits may follow seizures and persist for 24 hours or longer (Todd's paralysis). Diffusion-weighted magnetic resonance imaging (MRI), abnormal in acute stroke, is most often normal in patients with Todd's paralysis. An important, uncommon, and reversible cause of acute focal neurologic deficits is hypoglycemia, which should always be assessed before any aggressive treatment is initiated for a presumed ischemic stroke. Similarly, in young patients or patients with a psychiatric history, objective neurologic signs, or corroborative radiologic evidence must be established to avoid treating a functional paralysis with relatively aggressive therapy. Finally, worsening of an old deficit should prompt a metabolic/infectious evaluation, because the damaged lesion may act as a *locus minoris resistentiae*, with focal clinical worsening of a chronic deficit.

Laboratory and Radiologic Evaluation

A comprehensive workup to determine stroke subtype and severity, and to identify possible multiple risk factors is important to determine effective treatment options. Urgent imaging should remain the goal for all potential stroke patients presenting acutely, with or without demonstration of a worsening neurologic status. Imaging also helps in the differential diagnosis and is key in protocols for therapeutic intervention with recombinant tissue plasminogen activator (rt-PA). Both CT and CT angiogram and MRI studies (brain MRI, MR angiogram) are reliable and sensitive means of differentiating between ICVD, hemorrhage, and other mass lesions as well as defining the vascular territory involved. CT Perfusion or MR Perfusion studies can help guide the intravenous or endovascular therapy for equivocal or uncertain cases. MRI is more sensitive than CT for the identification of brain tumors and MRI can identify infarction at an earlier stage (after several minutes of ischemia). MRI based diffusion-weighted imaging (DWI) has important bearing on acute stroke diagnosis and treatment [11]. Selected cases of suspected intracranial hemorrhage with equivocal or negative findings on CT, MRI may detect subarachnoid, subdural, and intraparenchymal hemorrhage [12].

An electrocardiogram should be obtained to assess possible underlying or concurrent cardiac rhythm or ischemic changes. Confusion may arise because T-wave, ST-segment, QRS complex changes, and rhythm disturbances may occur secondary to the cerebral ischemic event. Two-dimensional transthoracic, or transesophageal echocardiography, and telemetry/Holter monitoring should be done routinely because patients often have more than one potential underlying pathophysiology, and a cardiac structural or rhythm abnormality may change the treatment approach (Fig. 149.4). For patients with cryptogenic stroke, prolonged ambulatory telemetry, or loop monitoring, may identify additional patients with hitherto occult atrial fibrillation [13]. A transesophageal echocardiogram should especially be considered in younger patients, patients with an enlarged left atrium, and for cryptogenic stroke victims of all ages [14,15].

A study of the cervical and cranial vascular status is important to identify the location of the lesion; confirm the thrombotic etiology of the symptoms; provide important information regarding the risk of recurrence or deterioration; and help to identify relevant findings in patients appropriate for endovascular catheter-based thrombolytic therapies. MR-based or CT-based angiography can be used. CT angiography allows a more rapid triage than MRI, because every minute wasted before thrombolysis is initiated results in a progressive reduction of salvageable tissue. If a coronary CT angiography (CTA) or magnetic resonance angiography (MRA) cannot be obtained to image the craniocervical vasculature, carotid artery ultrasound—a fast, reliable, and noninvasive technique—should be employed for suspected ischemic stroke of the carotid system as well as small vessel stroke, because of a high incidence of coexisting large vessel atherosclerotic stenosis. Furthermore, transcranial Doppler ultrasound (TCD) can provide additional information about the status of the intracranial vessels, both in the carotid and vertebral-basilar arterial territories [16,17].

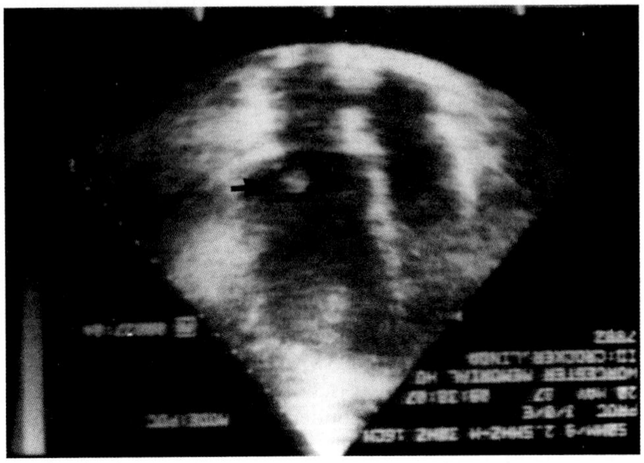

FIGURE 149.4 Echocardiogram in a patient with cardioembolic stroke, demonstrating a large thrombus (*arrow*) attached to the left mitral valve.

Complete blood count, partial thromboplastin time (PTT), prothrombin time (PT), comprehensive blood chemistry, chest radiograph, erythrocyte sedimentation rate, syphilis serology, and urinalysis should be obtained on day 1. Of these, if thrombolytic therapy is being contemplated, the blood glucose, PTT, PT, and platelet count should be obtained immediately as point-of-care tests. Fasting lipid profile, homocysteine, and C-reactive protein can be obtained by day 2. Other blood studies, including anticardiolipin antibodies, hypercoagulable testing (protein S, protein C, antithrombin 3, factor V Leiden, and prothrombin-2 gene mutation), serum viscosity, serum protein electrophoresis, and fibrinogen, should be performed for younger patients and for patients with a history of cancer, recurrent deep vein thrombosis, or a family history suggestive of an autosomal-dominant pattern of stroke. A lumbar puncture should be performed only when meningitis is suspected, for suspected vasculitis of the nervous system, or when diagnosis of subarachnoid hemorrhage is a consideration, despite a negative result in a brain imaging study (non-contrast computerized tomography [NCCT] or MRI). Electroencephalography may be helpful when associated seizure activity is suspected.

Treatment

The treatment of ICVD can be divided into three major categories: prevention, supportive therapy, and acute interventions.

Stroke Prevention

Stroke prevention has improved, as risk factors have been identified and treatments developed [18]. Adherence to a diet rich in fruits and vegetables and a regimen including routine aerobic exercise are important for cerebrovascular health. The treatment of hypertension and smoking cessation are helpful for the prevention of stroke. Systolic blood pressure reduction by 5 to 10 mm Hg may reduce relative risk of ischemic stroke by 20% to 25%. Angiotensin-converting enzyme inhibitors and angiotensin receptor blockers may offer additional protection against first or recurrent ischemic stroke. Patients with hyperglycemia should be aggressively treated to maintain euglycemic control. Use of HMG CoA reductase inhibitors (statins) reduces the risk of ischemic stroke by 16% to 30% for patients with or without underlying ischemic heart disease, and possibly improves the outcome after ICVD. The American College of Chest Physicians and American Stroke Association guidelines recommend starting all inpatients with hyperlipidemia (low-density lipoprotein [LDL] greater than 100 mg per dL) on a statin. More recent trials of statins suggest that reducing LDL cholesterol to 70 mg per dL is safe and may have a plaque stabilization effect [19]. Patients with *symptomatic* carotid artery stenosis of greater than 70% benefit from carotid endarterectomy, provided the combined mortality and morbidity of the surgical procedure in the treating institution is less than 5.65% [20]. For nonsurgical TIA or stroke patients, antiplatelet therapy with aspirin; aspirin and extended-release dipyridamole (25/200 mg) twice daily; clopidogrel 75 mg once daily; or ticlopidine 250 mg twice daily is beneficial [21,22]. Atrial fibrillation with or without valvular heart disease is associated with a high risk of stroke. Anticoagulation using warfarin reduces the absolute recurrent stroke relative risk by 8% in patients with nonvalvular atrial fibrillation. The annual risk of symptomatic hemorrhage is 1%, which can be minimized by keeping the international normalized ratio (INR) between 2 and 3 [15]. Several newer anticoagulants have shown benefit in reducing the risk of cardioembolic stroke [23–26] (Fig. 149.3). They have the notable advantage over warfarin at not requiring routine blood monitoring or dietary restrictions. However, the experience with these drugs is comparatively modest regarding their safety in elderly patients and with nonvalvular atrial fibrillation. In addition, reversal agents are not yet available for all of these agents (Table 149.3).

Supportive Therapy

Supportive therapy for ICVD patients should begin upon hospitalization. Elevated blood pressure should not be treated in the first 24 hours of an ischemic stroke unless malignant hypertension (>220 mm Hg systolic, 120 mm Hg diastolic) is present or other end-organ failure becomes evident (e.g., congestive heart failure, renal failure, and hypertensive encephalopathy). The blood pressure typically autoregulates spontaneously with bed rest; if it remains substantially elevated, it should be carefully lowered daily up to 20% of the mean arterial pressure. Subcutaneous heparin or low molecular weight heparin therapy should be considered for immobilized ICVD patients to reduce the risk of deep venous thrombosis. As far as possible, indwelling urinary catheters and unneeded IV lines should be avoided, because they can serve as portals of entry for infections. Elevated temperature should be treated with antipyretics. Aspiration pneumonia can be avoided by delaying oral feedings until safe swallowing is demonstrated. Early mobilization and rehabilitation should be attempted.

Acute Treatment

Standard therapies for ICVD patients are directed at reversing the neurologic deficit and preventing progression. The National Institute of Neurological Disorders and Stroke (NINDS) trial demonstrated that patients treated with rt-PA within 3 hours of stroke onset had a 13% absolute greater chance of being free of disability or being left with minor disability at 3 months. The benefit was greatest for those treated within the first 90 minutes of stroke onset compared to those treated between 90 and 180 minutes. There was a 5.8% greater incidence of ICH in treated patients, as compared to placebo (6.4% vs. 0.6%). However, overall mortality at 3 months was comparable in the rt-PA and placebo groups. Predictors of ICH include large hemispheric infarcts, National Institutes of Health Stroke Scale (NIHSS) score greater than 23, and the presence of associated severe hypertension [27]. Subsequently, based on prospective trial (ECASS III) results, it is possible to extend the time window

TABLE 149.3

Newer Anticoagulants for Cardioembolic Stroke Prevention

Trial	RE-LY (Dabigatran)	ROCKET-AF (Rivaroxaban)	ARISTOTLE (Apixaban)	ENGAGE-AF (Edoxaban)
N	18113	14264	18201	21105
CHADS2>1	67%	100%	66%	100%
% therapeutic warfarin time	64%	55%	62%	68%
Stroke/year	**1.0% vs. 1.6%**	1.7% vs. 2.0%	**1.2% vs. 1.5%**	1.5% vs. 1.7%
Ischemic stroke/year	**0.9% vs. 1.2%**	1.3% vs. 1.4%	1.0% vs. 1.1%	1.3% vs. 1.3%
Hemorrhage/year	3.1% vs. 3.4%	5.6% vs. 5.4%	**4.1% vs. 6.0%**	**2.8% vs. 3.3%**
ICH/year	**0.3% vs. 0.7%**	**0.8% vs. 1.2%**	**0.3% vs. 0.8%**	**0.4% vs. 0.9%**

Comparative results are listed as "study drug vs. warfarin."
Bold denotes significant difference within study.
ICH = intracerebral + subdural + epidural + subarachnoid bleeding.
Hemorrhage = symptomatic bleeding or drop hgb 2g/L or transfusion.
RE-LY and ENGAGE-AF values reported in reference to higher dosing regimens used.

of intravenous rt-PA up to 4.5 hours. The absolute benefits, although significant, were, as expected, less in this extended time window (absolute risk reduction [ARR] of 7%). Although the study excluded patients over age 80; those on anticoagulation (irrespective of the INR or PTT); and those with diabetes mellitus and stroke, the validity of these exclusions has not been substantiated, and individual management should be decided for individuals based on the physician's judgment [28]. The total dose of IV t-PA for stroke is 0.9 mg per kg, given as a 60-minute IV infusion, with 10% of the total dose given as an initial bolus. After rt-PA infusion, patients need to be admitted to the ICU or to a dedicated stroke unit. Blood pressure and neurologic status need to be carefully assessed at specified frequent time periods. Systolic blood pressure above 185 mm or mean blood pressure over 130 mm are treated with intravenous labetalol/nicardipine or dose-titrated intravenous sodium nitroprusside. Neurologic worsening should prompt an urgent CT scan to look for possible hemorrhagic conversion of the infarct. Anticoagulants and antiplatelet agents are avoided in the first 24 hours. IV access and invasive procedures should be kept to a minimum in the first 24 hours after rt-PA administration.

Patients presenting within 4.5 hours or selected patients beyond 4.5 hours with large artery occlusion (basilar artery, internal carotid artery, and proximal MCA) may benefit from intra-arterial interventions. The results of several contemporary trials each showed clear benefit of the use of intra-arterial thrombectomy in selected patients beyond the standard of intravenous tissue plasminogen activator (IV tPA) therapy alone. These trials were undertaken after the development of stent-retriever thrombectomy devices, favored over earlier device iterations in both efficacy and safety. Each of these trials was terminated early when interim analyses showed significant efficacy of the endovascular treatment arms (Table 149.4). Consistent with the expected target population, most treated patients had occlusion in the proximal MCA, had severe stroke scores (NIHSS 16 to 17), and were treated with endovascular therapy in addition to IV rt-PA. The majority of patients were treated within 6 hours of symptom onset and had relatively subtle findings of ischemia on head CT. Favorable functional outcome at 90 days were significantly more frequent for the treatment arms of the trials; symptomatic ICH was not significantly higher than in the control groups.

Anticoagulation with heparin or low–molecular weight heparin has been used traditionally without any proof of efficacy. Likewise, there is no evidence that supports the use of IV heparin anticoagulation to improve stroke outcome in progressive stroke. Furthermore, the risk of recurrent stroke is low (2% to 3%) in the first few weeks after an acute ischemic stroke (AIS) [29,30]. Cardioembolic stroke patients have a higher risk of recurrence (4.5% to 8.0%) within 2 weeks of the initial event, especially with associated intracardiac thrombi. Heparin therapy may reduce this risk and may be considered within 24 to 48 hours of the initial stroke [29]. Patients with large infarcts should not receive heparin, because they have a higher risk of bleeding into the area of infarction [19,29]. An alternative and safer approach is to begin warfarin, as soon as the patient can safely swallow, leading to adequate anticoagulation within 4 to 14 days of stroke onset [31].

Aspirin may reduce the risk of stroke recurrence after TIA or established stroke and is widely used for this indication [20]. Combined aspirin and extended-release dipyridamole therapy may be more effective than aspirin alone in reducing stroke recurrence [21]. In aspirin-allergic patients, clopidogrel or ticlopidine can be used. The incidence of serious side effects is greater with ticlopidine, which may cause neutropenia and thrombotic thrombocytopenic purpura. Because thrombotic thrombocytopenic purpura has been reported with both drugs, weekly complete blood count and liver function tests should be done in the first 4 to 6 weeks of initiating therapy [32].

Cerebral edema among ICVD patients is maximal between 48 and 72 hours after onset, but may extend up to 5 days after onset for infarcts in the brainstem and cerebellum. Corticosteroids are not effective for ICVD [33]. Osmotic diuretics, such as mannitol, are of potential value for cerebral edema with mass effect associated with ICVD; we consider using pulse doses (1 g per kg, then 0.5 g per kg every 6 hours) if massive edema begins to develop. Intracranial pressure (ICP) monitoring to guide therapy should also be considered. Controlled hyperventilation is perhaps the fastest and most effective temporizing measure to reduce cerebral edema, but its effects are transient, and regional cerebral ischemia may worsen owing to vasoconstriction. Patients with large ischemic infarctions in the MCA territory are at risk of massive cerebral edema and herniation (malignancy MCA syndrome). Timely decompressive hemicraniectomy reduces the risk of death by 50% (1 in 2 patients) and improves the outcome by 25% (1 in 4 patients). Interestingly enough, the outcomes of this trial were independent of the site of infarction or the presence or absence of aphasia [33].

TABLE 149.4

Contemporary Endovascular Ischemic Stroke Treatment Trials

Variable	MR CLEAN	ESCAPE	EXTEND-IA	REVASCAT	SWIFT-PRIME
N	500	316	70	206	196
NIHSS (median)	17 vs. 18	16 vs. 17	17 vs. 13	17 vs. 17	17 vs. 17
Age (mean)	65	71	70	66	66
Active treatment	IA (any) + IV tPA (87%)	IA + IV tPA (73%)	IA (Solitaire device) + IV tPA (100%)	IA (Solitaire device) + IV tPA (68%)	IA (Solitaire device) + IV tPA (100%)
Control treatment	IV tPA (90%)	IV tPA (79%)	IV tPA (100%)	IV tPA (77%)	IV tPA (100%)
90day good outcome	**33% vs. 19%**	**53% vs. 29%**	**71% vs. 40%**	**45% vs. 28%**	**60% vs. 35%**
ICH rate	7.7% vs. 6.4%	3.6% vs. 2.7%	0% vs. 6%	1.9% vs. 1.9%	0% vs. 3%

Comparative results are listed as combined treatment (IV rt-PA + IA stent retriever clot removal) vs. IV rt-PA alone.
Bold denotes significant difference within study in favor of combined IV and endovascular therapy (14% to 31%).
IA, intra-arterial; IV tPA, intravenous tissue plasminogen activator

Summary

Advances are being made in the treatment of ICVD. It is clear that successful therapy requires early appropriate intervention, directed by the CT/CTA/±CTP protocol. In large vessel occlusion with a viable penumbra, IV, rt-PA should be initiated and rapid transfer of the patient to a site where intra-arterial intervention is available should be the goal. Physicians should not wait for IV rt-PA to finish, but should initiate a transfer for possible thrombectomy as soon as practical. For all other situations, start IV rt-PA and transfer patients to a neuro-ICU for completion and post rt-PA management. Treatment of TIA has undergone a dramatic change since we recognized that the risk of a full-blown ischemic stroke is 10.5% after a cursory ER visit, and that this risk can be reduced by 80% with acute inpatient management for 1 to 2 days, as demonstrated by the Oxfordshire study and the 2009 stroke guidelines on management of TIA [2]. The recognition that acute high-dose statins reduce the risk of stroke and improve outcomes irrespective of the LDL levels is an important addendum to our management strategy within the acute period after an ischemic stroke. In the future, it is probable that a combination of treatments directed at the multiple metabolic and perfusion abnormalities associated with ICVD will be required [34].

Decompressive hemicraniectomy with duraplasty is highly effective in reducing death or disability related to large MCA infarcts, with 50% absolute survival rate and 25% improved chances of a good outcome. Finally, stroke prevention is the most effective means of reducing the first or recurrent stroke. Aggressive use of statins for patients with either hyperlipidemia or elevated C-reactive protein reduces the risk of progression of atherosclerotic small and large vessel disease and may have a cardioprotective role (Table 149.5).

INTRACEREBRAL HEMORRHAGE

Nontraumatic ICH occurs less frequently than ICVD, but carries a higher morbidity and often requires management in the ICU. The majority of these cases are caused by spontaneous (primary) ICH, defined as bleeding within the brain parenchyma without an underlying cause, such as neoplasm, vasculitis, bleeding disorder, prior embolic infarction, aneurysm, vascular malformation, or trauma. One-half of primary ICH cases result from longstanding hypertension. Owing to the aggressive control of hypertension, the incidence of ICH has decreased since the mid-1960s. Nonetheless, ICH accounts for 4% to 11% of all stroke cases in the USA and 16% to 26% of all stroke-related deaths [35].

Pathophysiology

Primary ICH is believed to be caused by extravasation of arterial blood from ruptured microaneurysms along the walls of small intracerebral arterioles. Microaneurysms known as *Charcot–Bouchard or miliary aneurysms* tend to form on vessels at the usual sites of ICH and develop at sites of vascular branching where mechanical stress is maximal. The aneurysm wall lacks normal vascular histology and is composed mainly of connective tissue layers, which represent a weak point in the arterial system. The formation of these aneurysms is favored by the processes of

TABLE 149.5

Summary of Recommendations Based on Randomized Controlled Clinical Trials

Ischemic & hemorrhagic stroke management

- TIA: High incidence of stroke early and up to 30 d; early inpatient treatment reduces the risk of ischemic stroke by 80%.
- ICVD:
    - Combined treatment (IV rt-PA + IA thrombectomy) improves absolute outcome by 18%–31% in selected patients with large vessel stroke.
    - In hyperacute ischemic stroke, early high-dose statins are associated with reduced recurrence and improved survival.
    - In malignant MCA syndrome, early DHC increases survival by 50% and improves outcome by 25% in malignant MCA syndrome.
    - Stroke prevention stategies: BP <140/90 (ACEI/ARB preferred); lipid reduction of LDL <70 mg/dL with statins; aggressive DM control, HBA1c <7%; and low-dose aspirin are highly effective in reducing the risk of first or recurrrent stroke.
- ICH
    - Early reduction of SBP to 140 improves survival.
    - Rapid reversal of anticoagulation to INR <1.4 may improve survival.
    - Intraventricular shunts may be helpful in improving survival in patients with ICH and IVH.
    - Surgical decompression in cerebellar hemorrhage >3 cm diameter or with brainstem compression and obstructive hydrocephaus improves neurologic outcome and survival.
    - Hematoma evacuation or decompressive hemicraniectomy after ICH are of unproven benefit.

ACEI, angiotensin-converting enzyme inhibitor; ARB, angiotensin receptor blocker; BP, blood pressure; DHC, decompressive hemicraniectomy; DM, diabetes mellitus; HBA1c, glycated haemoglobin; IA, intra-arterial; ICH, intracerebral hemorrhage; ICVD, ischemic cerebrovascular disease; INR, international normalized ratio; IVH, intraventricular hemorrhage; IV rt-PA,intravenous recombinant tissue plasminogen activator; LDL, low-density lipoprotein; MCA, middle cerebral artery; SBP, systolic blood pressure; TIA, transient ischemic attack.

lipohyalinosis and fibrinoid necrosis, which weaken the walls of arterioles, and are accelerated by chronic hypertension. Although Charcot–Bouchard aneurysms also appear in the normotensive aging brain, their frequency is notably increased in hypertensive patients. They are commonly observed along the lenticulostriate arteries, thalamoperforate arteries, and paramedian branches of the basilar artery. Although this distribution corresponds to the common sites of ICH, it is impossible to prove that these aneurysms are always the cause of bleeding, and the concept of arteriolar microdissection has been raised as an alternative explanation [35].

In elderly patients, particularly those with a history of cogntive impairment or dementia, lobar ICH related to amyloid angiopathy is an important underlying mechanism [36]. Five to ten percent of cases of spontaneous ICH result from amyloid angiopathy, making it second to hypertension as an etiology for ICH [37]. Age-related deposition of β-amyloid along the small arterials is thought to increase vessel wall fragility through decreased elasticity and render the artery susceptible to spontaneous rupture [38]. Diagnosis of this mechanism is often presumptive as proof of amyloid deposition via brain biopsy can be prohibitively invasive, particularly as therapy is supportive and an imaging signature showing multiple lobar areas of microhemorrhage is diagnostically supportive [39].

Continued extravasations of blood result in the formation of a hematoma with secondary accumulation of cerebral edema. The lesion may become massive enough to cause midline shift of cerebral structures followed by transtentorial herniation, which leads to secondary brainstem hemorrhages known as *Duret hemorrhages*. These linear lesions in the midbrain and upper pons are generally multiple and bilateral. Progression of this process results in brainstem dysfunction and death. Depending on the size and location of the ICH, intraventricular extension can occur and lead to the development of acute obstructive hydrocephalus or the later development of a chronic communicating hydrocephalus from impaired cerebrospinal fluid resorption. Some cases of thromboembolic stroke may be misclassified as ICH, because blood may extravasate and accumulate into large hematomas in areas of infarction. This secondary hemorrhage may be mislabeled if an early imaging study is not performed.

Clinical Manifestations

The clinical presentation of ICH is distinctive. In most cases, the onset is during the waking state when the patient is active; it is unusual for ICH to occur during sleep. The onset is abrupt, and the development of neurologic deficits occurs progressively over minutes to hours. This contrasts with the fluctuating or stepwise progression of deficits commonly seen in atherothrombotic infarcts, and with the appearance of maximal deficits at onset of cardioembolic strokes. In addition, prior TIA is rare with ICH and relatively common with ischemic stroke. The average age of onset of ICH, 50 to 70 years, is younger than that of other types of stroke. Patients may report lateralized headache; vomiting is common and nuchal rigidity may be present. Seizures are seen more frequently at the onset of ICH (17%) than in ICVD and are more likely to occur if the bleeding involves the cerebral cortex [40]. When first seen by a physician, 44% to 72% of patients are comatose.

The clinical presentation of ICH is monophasic, with symptoms rapidly progressing to maximum. Subsequent clinical deterioration is usually because of the effects of cerebral edema [41]; however, secondary bleeding and subsequent deterioration may also occur. It was recently suggested that thalamic hemorrhages may bleed further in patients whose hypertension is not adequately controlled [42].

Diagnosis

The diagnosis of ICH can be made by CT scan, which provides accurate information about the size and site of the hematoma as well as the midline shift, and development of cerebral edema. Typically, the hemorrhage is hyperdense on CT scan during the acute phase, although severe anemia or ongoing hemorrhage may make the appearance more isodense or hypodense. The appearance of blood on the MRI scan varies because signal intensity is related to the state of degradation of the hemoglobin. This state changes with time; therefore, MRI is not the study of choice for initial imaging of ICH. In summary, deoxyhemoglobin is found in the first 3 days after ICH and is not well visualized on T1-weighted images but appears as an area of reduced signal intensity on T2-weighted images. Days 3 to 10 after ICH, methemoglobin appears as increased signal intensity of T1-weighted images, but the intracellular portion has reduced signal intensity on T2-weighted images. In the chronic state, the ICH has broken down to hemosiderin, which is poorly visualized on T1-weighted images but appears as reduced signal intensity on T2-weighted images. Magnetic resonance or conventional angiography should be considered for selected cases when an underlying aneurysm or arteriovenous malformation is suspected.

Lumbar puncture is contraindicated in acute ICH because of the risk of herniation from mass effect. Testing on admission for ICH should include coagulation profile and platelet counts for all patients, as well as bleeding time, if the patient is on aspirin.

Differential Diagnosis

Although the majority of ICH is from hypertensive or amyloid pathologies, other etiologies should always be considered. Ruptured arteriovenous malformation is an important cause of ICH, particularly for younger patients or those without risk factors for more typical causes. Secondary cerebral hemorrhage may occur after embolic infarction as the lodged embolus fragments and ischemic distal vessels may rupture with reperfusion. This is more common for patients with large embolic infarcts, in patients who are anticoagulated, and in patients with poorly controlled hypertension. ICH secondary to reperfusion may also occur after carotid endarterectomy.

ICH accounts for 0.5% to 1.5% of all bleeding events related to the use of oral anticoagulants. Oral anticoagulation increases the risk of ICH 8 to 11fold, compared to unanticoagulated patients. Compared with patients with spontaneous ICH, there is a trend toward larger hematomas and a higher mortality rate in patients on anticoagulants [43]. Cerebellar hemorrhage is relatively common among anticoagulated patients, and mortality for these cases may be as high as 65%. Therefore among anticoagulated patients, the onset of focal neurologic signs, even if slowly progressive, necessitates CT scan to rule out ICH [44].

The use of fibrinolytic therapy, such as rt-PA, for coronary artery occlusion has also been associated with ICH, especially when adjunctive anticoagulant therapy is used. These cases have shown a predilection for the subcortical white matter and lobar areas, generally having a poor prognosis [45].

ICH associated with the presence of primary or secondary brain tumors is infrequent, accounting for only 2% of all cases of ICH. Higher-grade malignancies, such as glioblastoma multiforme, are more likely to bleed. The presence of thin-walled vessels in areas of neovascularization is thought to be the underlying reason for these hemorrhages. Metastatic lesions with the tendency to bleed include bronchogenic carcinoma, melanoma, renal cell carcinoma, and choriocarcinoma. ICH is frequent in hematologic disorders such as leukemia and reflects both the underlying thrombocytopenia and disseminated intravascular coagulopathy. When disseminated intravascular coagulopathy is caused by other organ failures, it can also lead to ICH.

Sympathomimetic drugs, such as methamphetamine, pseudoephedrine, and phenylpropanolamine, have caused ICH in the subcortical white matter. These agents are suspected of inducing vasculopathy with vasospasm or sometime a vasculitis. Cocaine, which blocks dopamine and norepinephrine reuptake, has been associated with ICH. Cocaine, especially crack cocaine, appears to incite cerebral vasospasm rather than a vasculitis. The secondary hypertension related to sympathetic stimulation may also cause ICH from any of these agents. This may explain the lack of abnormal angiographic findings among some of these cases [46,47], although recently cerebral vasospasm was demonstrated with MRA after acute cocaine administration [48]. Acute elevation of blood pressure in otherwise normotensive people, such as that which may follow migraine, is postulated to result at times in ICH.

Specific Syndromes of Intracerebral Hemorrhage

Hypertension related ICH tends to occur in stereotyped locations. In order of descending frequency, these locations are the putamen (30% to 50%), subcortical white matter (15%), thalamus (10%), pons (10%), and cerebellum (10%) [49].

ICH in the putamen is caused by bleeding from a lenticulostriate vessel. Clinically it is manifested by development of flaccid hemiplegia, hemisensory disturbances of all primary modalities, homonymous hemianopia, paralysis of conjugate gaze to the side opposite the lesion, and early alteration in level of consciousness. Subcortical aphasia may occur when a putamen hemorrhage involves the dominant hemisphere, and a hemineglect syndrome when it is on the nondominant side.

Thalamic ICH is characterized by a unilateral sensorimotor deficit in which sensory findings predominate. A variety of eye signs occur: Parinaud's syndrome; forced disconjugate down-gaze deviation medially on the side opposite the lesion; pseudoabducens paresis; and up-gaze paresis. The most specific localizing sign is inferomedial disconjugate gaze paresis contralateral to the side of the lesion. A permanent skew deviation, with vertical separation of images, may leave the patient with persistent diplopia. Owing to the location, thalamic ICH may rupture into the ventricular system.

Pontine ICH has the highest mortality. Quadriplegia, brainstem dysfunction, and small, unreactive pupils are seen at presentation and many patients rapidly develop coma. Bleeding typically arises from a paramedian branch of the basilar artery and almost always extends into the fourth ventricle. Cases of unilateral pontine ICH have a better outcome [50].

Cerebellar ICH most commonly involves the dentate nucleus (see Fig. 149.5). Alteration of consciousness is unusual at onset, but progressive deterioration with drowsiness typically occurs. The majority of patients initially manifest two of the following: (a) gait, truncal, or limb ataxia; (b) lower motor neuron facial paresis; and (c) an ipsilateral gaze palsy. Other common presenting signs and symptoms are headache, nausea, vomiting, vertigo, nystagmus, and limb ataxia [51]. Early surgical intervention is indicated for lesions larger than 3 cm or in smaller lesions with clinical progression, because cerebellar hemorrhage causes death in up to 60% of cases. Neurologic deterioration due to hemorrhage, causing obstructive hydrocephalus at the level of the fourth ventricle, is not uncommon. Surgical mortality is lower for patients who are still awake before operation; therefore, early intervention is indicated [51].

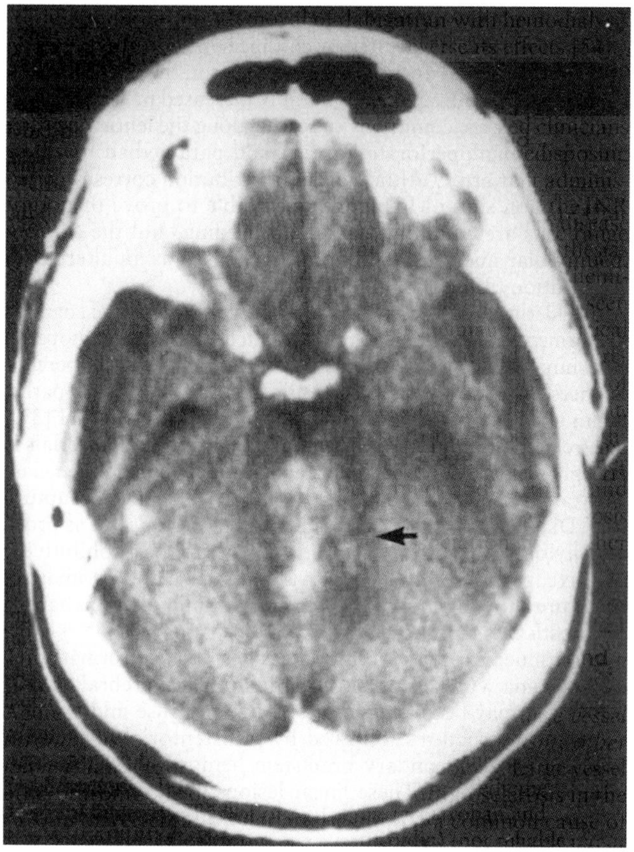

FIGURE 149.5 Midline cerebellar hemorrhage (*arrow*) seen on a computed tomography scan.

Approximately 3% of cases of ICH are primarily intraventricular in location. These events have minimal focal signs, but there may be loss of consciousness at onset. Hydrocephalus is a major complication [52].

Treatment

The acute medical management of ICH is aimed at correction of any predisposing systemic factors to prevent further clinical deterioration. Following ICH, there is a hematoma growth of 22% within the first 24 hours and hypertension is a major management problem in these cases. In response to the acute elevation of ICP caused by the hematoma, systemic blood pressure rises to maintain adequate cerebral perfusion pressure. This response, known as *Cushing's reflex*, serves to protect the brain against ischemia, but autoregulation of cerebral blood flow can be impaired after ICH or infarction. In patients with underlying chronic hypertension, the result may be excessively high blood pressure. The best management of this dilemma remains controversial. In chronic hypertension, the lower limit of cerebral autoregulation is shifted toward higher blood pressure; and acute lowering of systolic blood pressure is known to result in unfavorable decreases in cerebral perfusion pressure. Sustained hypertension in the acute phase of ICH, however, can lead to further bleeding or rapid accumulation of cerebral edema [49]. The recommended goal of systolic blood pressure in the acute phase of ICH is between 140 and 160 mm Hg [53]. Blood pressure should be lowered gently, and β-blockers are the

TABLE 149.6

ICH Score

Age 80+			Yes = 1 No = 0			
GCS at presentation			3–4 = 2 5–12 = 1 13–15 = 0			
ICH volume 30+ mL			Yes = 1 No = 0			
Intraventricular blood			Yes = 1 No = 0			
Infratentorial origin of ICH			Yes = 1 No = 0			
SCORE (30 d mortality)	0 = 0%	1 = 13%	2 = 26%	3 = 72%	4 = 97%	5–6 = 100%

ICH, intracerebral hemorrhage; GCS, Glasgow Coma Scale.

agents of choice. Alternatively, a calcium channel blocker such as intravenous nicardipine may be useful because it does not elevate ICP like other vasodilators [49].

If the hematoma and associated cerebral edema raise ICP, clinical deterioration typically occurs. Acutely, hyperventilation effectively lowers ICP, but only for a matter of hours. Hyperosmolar agents, such as mannitol, sorbitol, and glycerol, can provide more sustained reductions in ICP. Their utility remains unclear and the osmotic diuresis induced by these agents can lead to dehydration, electrolyte imbalances, and pulmonary edema if the patient is not actively managed. Treatment of ICH with steroids can be detrimental to overall outcomes, so they are not routinely administered [54]. The value of ICP monitoring in these situations remains controversial. Elevation of ICP owing to hydrocephalus is treated with ventricular cerebrospinal fluid diversion.

Anticonvulsants are not routinely used in ICH. If seizures are not present at onset, patients are generally at low risk for developing seizures, but hemorrhage into the cortex, regardless of site of origin, predisposes to seizures. Subarachnoid or intraventricular extension of bleeding does not increase the risk of seizures. Seizures have been noted with hemorrhages in the caudate but not with putaminal or thalamic events. Although the incidence of chronic epilepsy from ICH is low (6.5% to 13.0%), any seizures usually begin within the first 2 years after the event [55]. Prophylaxis against peripheral venous thrombosis should be accomplished with pneumatic boots.

After the patient is acutely stabilized, angiography may be performed if there is no history of hypertension or the bleeding is in an atypical location. This is particularly important or pertinent for younger patients, in whom a larger percentage of cases of ICH are caused by underlying vascular lesions, such as arteriovenous malformation or aneurysm. At present, surgery may be indicated for lobar ICH in which the patient continues to deteriorate, and for cerebellar ICH. Emergency ventriculostomy to relieve hydrocephalus should be considered if this condition develops acutely. Surgical intervention for putaminal ICH remains controversial; it is inappropriate for thalamic and pontine hemorrhages.

The prognosis for ICH is worse for larger lesions. By location, pontine ICH has the highest mortality, followed by cerebellar and then basal ganglia lesions. Lobar ICH carries the most favorable outlook for survival and functional recovery [43]. Clinical scoring systems can provide insight into mortality and disability risk, important considerations for clinicians and patients with their families alike [56,57]. The ICH score estimates risk of death by 30 days and is predicated on patient age, admission Glasgow Coma Scale (GCS) score, hemorrhage size, intraventricular extension, and infratentorial origin of bleeding (Table 149.6).

Summary

ICH can be neurologically devastating. Patients with ICH often require an ICU setting because of the severity of disease, particularly when it is complicated by markedly increased ICP. Treatments remain supportive, directed at attenuating complications and promoting recovery. Although ICH is more severe than ICVD, many patients have significant recovery with expert supportive care, and restorative and rehabilitative efforts (Table 149.5).

References

1. Mozaffarian D, Benjamin EJ, Go AS, et al: Heart disease and stroke statistics—2015 update. *Circulation* 131:e29, 2015.
2. Easton D, Saver JL, Albers G, et al: Definition and evaluation of transient ischemic attack: a scientific statement for healthcare professionals from the American Heart Association/American Stroke Association Stroke Council; Council on Cardiovascular Surgery and Anesthesia; Council on Cardiovascular Radiology and Intervention; Council on Cardiovascular Nursing; and the Interdisciplinary Council on Peripheral Vascular Disease: The American Academy of Neurology affirms the value of this statement as an educational tool for neurologists. *Stroke* 40:2273–2296, 2009.
3. Rothwell PM, Giles MF, Flossmann E, et al: A simple score (ABCD) to identify individuals at high early risk of stroke after transient ischaemic attack. *Lancet* 366:29, 2005.
4. Jauch EC, Saver JL, Adams HP Jr, et al: Guidelines for the early management of patients with acute ischemic stroke: a guideline for healthcare professionals from the American Heart Association/American Stroke Association. *Stroke* 44:870, 2013.
5. Cerebrovascular diseases, in Ropper AH, Samuels MA, Klein JP (eds): *Adams and Victor's Principles of Neurology*. 10th ed. New York, NY, McGraw-Hill, 2014, pp 778–885.
6. Sacco S, Marini C, Totaro R, et al: A population-based study of the incidence and prognosis of lacunar stroke. *Neurology* 66:1335, 2006.
7. Bogousslavsky J, Hachinski VC, Boughner DR, et al: Cardiac and arterial lesions in carotid transient ischemic attacks. *Arch Neurol* 43:223, 1988.
8. Lip GY, Nieuwlaat R, Pisters R, et al: Refining clinical risk stratification for predicting stroke and thromboembolism in atrial fibrillation using a novel risk factor-based approach: the euro heart survey on atrial fibrillation. *Chest* 137:263, 2010.
9. Messe SR, Silverman IE, Kizer JR, et al: Practice parameter: recurrent stroke with patent foramen ovale and atrial septal aneurysm: report of the Quality Standards Subcommittee of the American Academy of Neurology. *Neurology* 62(7):1042, 2004.
10. Bogousslavsky J, Regli F: Unilateral watershed cerebral infarcts. *Neurology* 36:372, 1988.
11. Moonis M, Fisher M: Imaging of acute stroke. *Cerebrovasc Dis* 11(3):143, 2001.
12. Rivers CS, Wardlaw JM, Armitage PA, et al: Do acute diffusion-and perfusion-weighted MRI lesions identify final infarct volume in ischemic stroke? *Stroke* 37:98, 2006.

13. Flint AC, Banki NM, Ren X, et al: Detection of paroxysmal atrial fibrillation by 30-day event monitoring in cryptogenic ischemic stroke: the Stroke Monitoring for PAF in Real Time (SMART) Registry. *Stroke* 43:2788, 2012.
14. Parsons MW, Barber PA, Chalk J, et al: Diagnostic impact and prognostic relevance of early contrast-enhanced transcranial color-coded duplex sonography in acute stroke. *Stroke* 29:955, 1998.
15. Tegler CH, Burke GL, Dalley GM, et al: Carotid emboli predict poor outcome in stroke. *Stroke* 24:186, 1993.
16. Cerebral Embolism Task Force: Cardiogenic brain embolism. The second report of the Cerebral Embolism Task Force [published erratum appears in *Arch Neurol* 46(10):1079, 1989] [see comments]. *Arch Neurol* 46(7):727, 1989.
17. Dewitt LD, Wechsler LR: Transcranial doppler. *Stroke* 19:915, 1988.
18. Sacco RL, Adams R, Albers G, et al: Guidelines for prevention of stroke in patients with ischemic stroke or transient ischemic attack: a statement for healthcare professionals from the American Heart Association/American Stroke Association Council on Stroke: co-sponsored by the Council on Cardiovascular Radiology and Intervention: the American Academy of Neurology affirms the value of this guideline. *Circulation* 113:409, 2006.
19. Moonis M, Fisher M: HMG CoA reductase inhibitors (statins): use in stroke prevention and outcome after stroke. *Expert Rev Neurother* 4(2):241, 2004.
20. North American Symptomatic Carotid Endarterectomy Trial Collaborators: Beneficial effects of carotid endarterectomy in symptomatic patients with high grade carotid stenosis. *N Engl J Med* 325:445, 1991.
21. The European Stroke Prevention Study (ESPS): Principal endpoints. The ESPS Group. *Lancet* 2:1351, 1987.
22. Gent M, Blakely JA, Easton JD, et al: The Canadian American Ticlopidine Study (CATS) in thromboembolic stroke. *Lancet* 1:1215, 1989.
23. Connolly SJ, Ezekowitz MD, Yusuf S, et al: Dabigatran versus warfarin in patients with atrial fibrillation. *N Engl J Med* 361:1139, 2009.
24. Granger CB, Alexander JH, McMurray JJ, et al: Apixaban versus warfarin in patients with atrial fibrillation. *N Engl J Med* 365:981, 2011.
25. Patel MR, Mahaffrey KW, Garg J, et al: Rivaroxaban versus warfarin in nonvalvular atrial fibrillation *N Engl J Med* 365;883, 2011.
26. Giugliano RP, Ruff CT, Braunwald E, et al: Edoxaban versus warfarin in patients with atrial fibrillation. *N Engl J Med* 369:2093, 2013.
27. The National Institute of Neurological Disorders and Stroke rt-PA Stroke Study Group: Tissue plasminogen activator for acute ischemic stroke. *N Engl J Med* 333:1581, 1995.
28. Hacke W, Kaste M, Bluhmki E: Thrombolysis with Alteplase 3 to 4.5 hours after acute ischemic stroke. *N Engl J Med* 359:1317–1329, 2008.
29. Moonis M, Fisher M: Considering the role of heparin and low-molecular-weight heparins in acute ischemic stroke. *Stroke* 33(7):1927, 2002.
30. Moonis M, Wingard E, Selveraj N, et al: Factors predisposing to secondary hemorrhagic conversion in acute ischemic stroke. *Ann Neurol* 48:497, 2000.
31. Paciaroni M, Agnelli G, Falocci N, et al: Early recurrence and cerebral bleeding in patients with acute ischemic stroke and atrial fibrillation: effect of anticoagulation and its timing: the RAF study. *Stroke* 46:26130094, 2015.
32. Hankey GJ: Clopidogrel and thrombotic thrombocytopenic purpura. *Lancet* 356(9226):269, 2000.
33. Vahedi K, Hofmeijer J, Juettler C, et al: Early decompressive surgery in malignant infarction of the middle cerebral artery: a pooled analysis of three randomized controlled trials. *Lancet* 6:215–222, 2007.
34. Moonis M: Intraarterial thrombolysis within the first three hours after acute ischemic stroke in selected patients. *Stroke* 40:2611–2622, 2009.
35. Mimatsu K, Yamaguchi T: Management of intracerebral hemorrhage, in Fisher M (ed): *Stroke Therapy*. Boston, Butterworth Heinemann, 2001, p 287.
36. Knudsen KA, Rosand J, Karluk D, et al: Clinical diagnosis of cerebral amyloid angiopathy: validation of the Boston Criteria. *Neurology* 56;537, 2001.
37. Izumihara A, Suzuki M, Ishihara T: Recurrence and extension of lobar hemorrhage related to cerebral amyloid angiopathy: multivariate analysis of clinical risk factors. *Surg Neurol* 64:160, 2005.
38. Viswanathan A, Greenberg SM: Cerebral amyloid angiopathy in the elderly. *Ann Neurol* 70:871, 2011.
39. Vernooij MW, van der Lugt A, Ikram MA, et al: Prevalance and risk factors of cerebral microbleeds: the Rotterdam Scan Study. *Neurology* 70:1208, 2008.
40. Berger AR, Lipton RB, Lesser ML, et al: Early seizures following intracerebral hemorrhage: implications for therapy. *Neurology* 38:1363, 1988.
41. Fisher CM: Clinical syndromes in cerebral hemorrhage, in Fields WS (ed): *Pathogenesis and Treatment of Cerebrovascular Disease*. Springfield, IL, Charles C Thomas, 1961, p 318.
42. Chen ST, Chen SD, Hsu CY, et al: Progression of hypertensive intracerebral hemorrhage. *Neurology* 39:1509, 1989.
43. Radberg JA, Olson JE, Radberg CT: Prognostic parameters in spontaneous hematomas with special reference to anticoagulation treatment. *Stroke* 22:571, 1991.
44. Kase CS, Robinson RK, Stein RW, et al: Anticoagulant-related intracerebral hemorrhage. *Neurology* 35:943, 1983.
45. Kase CS, O'Neil AM, Fisher M, et al: Intracranial hemorrhage after use of tissue plasminogen activator. *Ann Intern Med* 112:17, 1990.
46. ISIS-3 Collaborative Group: A random trial of streptokinase vs tissue plasminogen activator vs anistreplase. *Lancet* 339:753, 1992.
47. Toffol GJ, Biller J, Adams HP: Nontraumatic intracerebral hemorrhage in young adults. *Arch Neurol* 44:483, 1987.
48. Kaufman MJ, Levin JM, Ross MH, et al: Cocaine-induced cerebral vasoconstriction detected in humans with magnetic resonance angiography. *JAMA* 279:376, 1998.
49. Duff TA, Ayeni S, Louim AB, et al: Neurosurgical management of spontaneous intracerebral hematomas. *Barrow Neurol Inst Q* 1:29, 1985.
50. Chung CS, Park CM: Primary pontine hemorrhage: a new CT classification. *Neurology* 42:830, 1992.
51. Jensen MB, St Louis EK: Management of acute cerebellar stroke. *Arch Neurol* 62:537, 2005.
52. Darby DG, Donnan GA, Saling MA, et al: Primary intraventricular hemorrhage: clinical and neuropsychological findings in a prospective stroke series. *Neurology* 38:68, 1988.
53. Borges LF: Management of nontraumatic brain hemorrhage, in Ropper AM, Kennedy SF (eds): *Neurological and Neurosurgical Intensive Care*. Rockville, MD, Aspen, 1988, p 209.
54. Poungvarin N, Bhoopat W, Viniarejakul A, et al: Effects of dexamethasone in primary supratentorial intracerebral hemorrhage. *N Engl J Med* 316:1229, 1987.
55. Faught E, Peters D, Bartolucci A, et al: Seizures after primary intracerebral hemorrhage. *Neurology* 39:1089, 1989.
56. Hemphill JC 3rd, Bonovich DC, Besmertis L, et al: The ICH Score: a simple, reliable grading scale for intracerebral hemorrhage. *Stroke* 32:891, 2001.
57. Rost NS, Smith EE, Chang Y, et al: Prediction of functional outcome in patients with primary intracerebral hemorrhage: the FUNC score. *Stroke* 39:2304, 2008.

Chapter 150 ■ Subarachnoid Hemorrhage

RIBAL BASSIL • SUSANNE MUEHLSCHLEGEL

INTRODUCTION

Subarachnoid hemorrhage (SAH) results from bleeding into the cerebrospinal fluid (CSF)-filled cisterns between the arachnoid and pia mater (Fig. 150.1). The treatment, complications, and prognosis vary according to the underlying cause of the hemorrhage. A ruptured cerebral aneurysm is the most common and best-studied form of SAH, accounting for 3% of all strokes [1]. SAH is a neurologic emergency requiring urgent management and intensive care unit (ICU) level of monitoring. Improvements in functional outcomes are owing to early recognition, intervention, and intensive care management to limit the risks of rebleeding, consequences of cerebral vasospasm (cVSP), and medical complications.

EPIDEMIOLOGY

SAH incidence and mortality are lower for Caucasians than other racial groups [1]. The overall incidence is 9 per 100,000 person per year and progressively increases with age up to 31 per 100,000 person per year after the age of 85 for all types of SAH combined. The median age of the most common form of SAH, the aneurysmal type, is 53 years [1]. SAH is a female-predominant disease, with two-thirds of SAH patients being women [2]. Mortality rate from a ruptured aneurysmal subarachnoid hemorrhage (aSAH) varies between 32% and 44%, with early rebleeding carrying the highest risk of mortality [3].

PATHOGENESIS

Saccular (berry) aneurysms lack the normal muscular media and elastic lamina layers, making it more vulnerable to rupture. Eighty-five percent of saccular aneurysms are located in the anterior circulation and 15% are in the posterior circulation [4]. Common sites for aneurysms are at the junction of the anterior cerebral and anterior communicating arteries, the origin of the posterior communicating artery, the middle cerebral artery trifurcation, and at the top of the basilar artery. 20% to 30% of patients have multiple aneurysms. Several connective tissue diseases such as polycystic kidney disease, Marfan syndrome, Ehlers–Danlos syndrome type IV, Neurofibromatosis Type 1, fibromuscular dysplasia, and coarctation of the aorta are associated with an increased incidence of intracerebral aneurysms [4,5]. Seven to 20% of patients with aSAH have first- or second-degree relatives with intracranial aneurysms [4]. Familial intracranial aneurysms, as well as the increased frequency of other familial syndromes, lend support to the congenital theory. Using modern genomic analysis, multiple genetic loci associated with the presence of cerebral aneurysms have been and continue to be identified [6]. Important risk factors include later age of onset, hypertension, cigarette smoking, alcohol consumption, amphetamine, or cocaine use. These factors may contribute to aneurysmal formation and expansion through degenerative processes [4].

Non-aSAH is determined based on the failure to illustrate an aneurysm on initial as well as repeat imaging studies, or when another etiology has been identified (Fig. 150.2). Common causes include vascular malformation, traumatic SAH, cerebral amyloid angiopathy, and Reversible Cerebral Vasoconstriction Syndrome (RCVS) [7]. The clinical presentation is often similar to that of aneurysmal SAH.

Perimesencephalic SAH refers to the collection of blood in the subarachnoid space centered on the basal and suprasellar cisterns around the pons and the midbrain (Fig. 150.3). When a ruptured aneurysm cannot be identified as the cause of the bleed, this distribution of subarachnoid blood is thus known as nonaneurysmal perimesencephalic SAH. It represents 5.8%

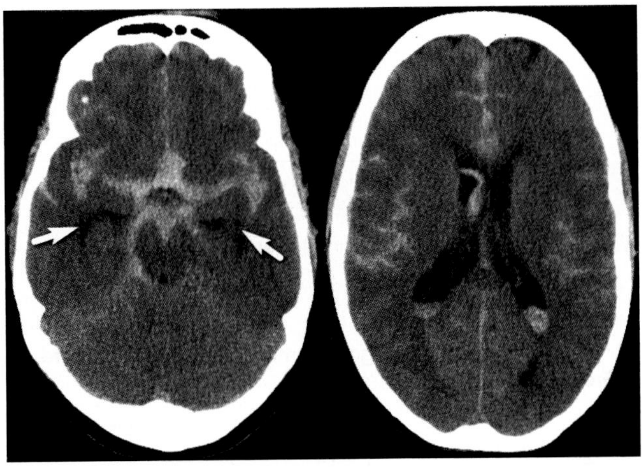

FIGURE 150.1 Shown is the noncontrast head CT of a large SAH from a ruptured berry aneurysm, resulting in blood in all major cisterns, interhemispheric and sylvian fissures, and both ventricles. Mild obstructive hydrocephalus is also present, as visible by the slightly dilated temporal horns (*white arrows*).

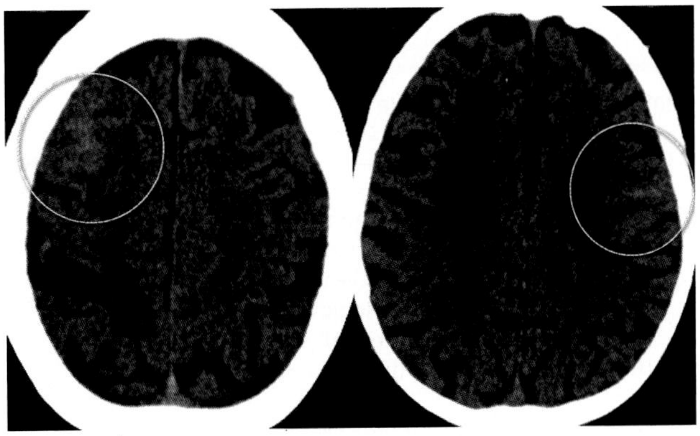

FIGURE 150.2 These noncontrast head CT from two different patients show high frontal–parietal nonaneurysmal SAH filling the sulci in a localized area (*circles*). Both SAH were spontaneous, and repeat cerebral angiography was negative in both cases. Some nonaneurysmal SAH can be subtle (as in these two patients); therefore, the head CT must be reviewed carefully, especially when there is a convincing clinical history of a sudden onset of headache.

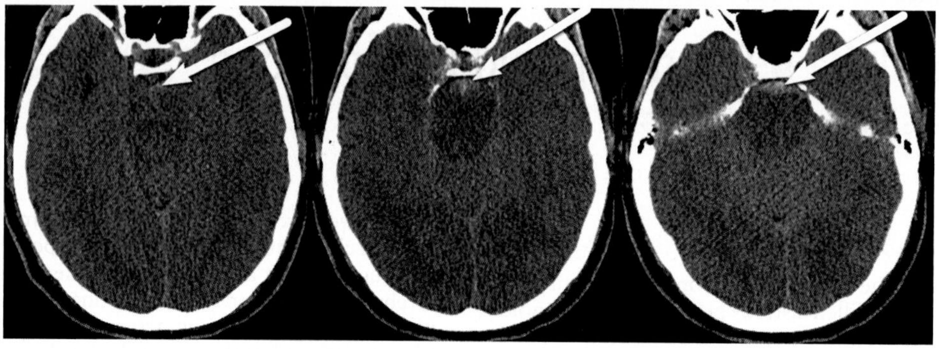

FIGURE 150.3 This noncontrast head CT from a single patient with perimesencephalic SAH reveals blood in the perimesencephalic and prepontine cisterns (*white arrows*) only. This patient's cerebral angiogram was repeated twice, and never revealed any source of bleeding.

of all SAH, often lacks identification of a specific cause and commonly follows a rather benign course [7,8].

CLINICAL PRESENTATION

A "sentinel" (warning) hemorrhage occurs among approximately 20% of patients and is characterized by headache or meningismus that lasts at least 48 hours in 70% of cases. The event is misdiagnosed in 20% to 40% as tension headache, migraine, sinusitis, viral syndrome, aseptic meningitis, or malingering [9]. Evidence of a warning leak must be treated with a high index of suspicion because such events precede major hemorrhage. Neurologic and functional outcomes are greatly improved if the patient is treated while neurologically intact before a major rehemorrhage [10].

SAH produces severe headache (maximum at onset, "worst headache of life"), neck pain, nausea and vomiting, dizziness, diplopia, photophobia, and lethargy. At the time of rupture, 45% of patients lose consciousness and may demonstrate abducens nerve palsies, reflecting the acute rise in intracranial pressure (ICP) that may transiently equal or exceed mean arterial pressure [11]. Early seizures after SAH (8% to 11%) reflect a rise in ICP but are not indicative of the site or severity of rupture [12,13].

CLINICAL AND RADIOLOGIC GRADING

Several clinical grading scales have been developed to assess the severity and prognosis based on the initial presentation. The grading scale developed by Hunt and Hess [14] is useful in correlating the patient's clinical status with prognosis (Table 150.1). Grades I and II at presentation have a relatively good prognosis, grade III has an intermediate prognosis, and grades IV and V have a poor prognosis. The Hunt and Hess scale, however, is clinically used only in the United States, although the rest of the world has adopted the World Federation of Neurological Surgeons scale (WFNS) [15]. The WFNS uses the combined Glasgow Coma Scale along with clinical motor deficit to estimate the likelihood of poor outcome (Table 150.2).

The radiologic Fisher Score was developed in 1981 using first-generation head CT to estimate the risk of symptomatic vasospasm based on the blood distribution pattern on the initial CT [16]. Major disadvantages of the original Fisher Score were its nonordinal increase in the vasospasm risk, making it nonintuitive to use at the bedside, as well as that it was difficult to incorporate into statistical models used in the research. Therefore, the score has been revised and validated using modern-technology head CT in a much larger number of patients, and is now known and routinely used as the Revised Fisher Score [17]. Its linear increase in vasospasm risk based on SAH clot thickness and the presence or absence of intraventricular hemorrhage (IVH) makes it the preferred radiologic score in current use (Table 150.3).

TABLE 150.1

Hunt and Hess Grading Scale

Grade	Symptoms	Mortality
I	Asymptomatic, or minimal headache and slight nuchal rigidity	11%
II	Moderate-to-severe headache, nuchal rigidity, no neurologic deficit other than cranial nerve palsy	26%
III	Drowsiness, confusion, or mild focal deficit	37%
IV	Stupor, moderate-to-severe hemiparesis	71%
V	Deep coma, decerebrate rigidity, moribund appearance	100%

Serious systemic disease such as hypertension, diabetes, severe arteriosclerosis, chronic pulmonary disease, and severe vasospasm seen on arteriography, result in placement of the patient in the next less favorable category.

TABLE 150.2

World Federation of Neurologic Surgeons Grading Scale

Grade	Motor deficit	Glasgow coma scale	Risk of severe disability, vegetative state or death
1	–	15	13%
2	–	13–14	20%
3	+	13–14	42%
4	– or +	7–12	51%
5	– or +	3–6	68%

TABLE 150.3

Modified Fisher Scale

Grade	IVH	SAH characteristics on admission CT head scan	Risk of symptomatic vasospasm
1	−	Localized thin or diffuse thin	24%
2	+	Absent or localized thin or diffuse thin	33%
3	−	Localized thick or diffuse thick	33%
4	+	Localized thick or diffuse thick	40%

SAH, subarachnoid hemorrhage; IVH, intraventricular hemorrhage.

DIAGNOSTIC EVALUATION

When SAH is suspected, an urgent noncontrast head CT should be obtained to identify, localize, and quantify the hemorrhage. The sensitivity of a noncontrast CT head reaches almost 100% in the first 6 to 12 hours and remains over 90% sensitive at 24 hours when interpreted by an experienced physician [18,19]. The sensitivity progressively declines with time to around 50% at 5 days. When a noncontrast CT head is nondiagnostic and the clinical suspicion of SAH remains high, an urgent lumbar puncture is indicated. The diagnostic finding is xanthochromia, a yellowish appearance of the CSF following centrifugation. This is the result of blood product degradation that is detected ≥2 hours after the onset of SAH and remains detectable in the CSF for up to 2 weeks. Protein may be elevated and glucose may be very slightly depressed. Opening pressure at the time of lumbar puncture may reflect the elevation of ICP.

CT-angiogram is the preferred noninvasive study to identify an aneurysm in the emergent setting with sensitivities and specificities nearing over 98% [20,21]. Magnetic resonance angiogram (MRA) can be particularly helpful to diagnose SAH several days after symptom onset when a head CT may be negative. MRI, however, is less readily available and more time consuming [22].

Four-vessel cerebral angiography remains the gold standard and is necessary to localize the lesion, assess vasospasm, and the possible presence of multiple aneurysms (Fig. 150.4). It should be performed as soon as possible after initial hemorrhage, because endovascular treatment can commonly be provided simultaneously (Fig. 150.5). If angiography does not reveal an aneurysm, angiography may be repeated in 1 to 3 weeks; an intraluminal thrombus or extraluminal compression of a small aneurysm by subarachnoid clot can acutely interfere with angiographic visualization of aneurysms [23].

ANEURYSM MANAGEMENT

SAH is instantly fatal in 12% of cases [24] while the 28-day mortality is 35% [25]. In-hospital mortality is 18% [26]. The high mortality is due to further complications including rebleeding, delayed cVSP causing infarction, hydrocephalus, increased ICP, seizures, and medical complications such as myocardial infarction, stress cardiomyopathy, and neurogenic pulmonary edema [26].

After SAH, the initial goals of treatment are aimed at identification and early aneurysm treatment, by either coiling or clipping. The International Subarachnoid Aneurysm Trial (ISAT) concluded that patients receiving coiling were more likely to be alive and independent at 10 years compared to patients having undergone surgical clipping, albeit with a very low increased risk of rebleeding deemed not to outweigh the benefit [27]. One downside of coiling is the higher aneurysm recurrence rate on follow-up angiogram 6 months or longer after the initial coiling, sometimes requiring repeat coiling [27]. Based on ISAT, the endovascular treatment of intracranial aneurysms, rather than the surgical approach, is now the preferred treatment option [3].

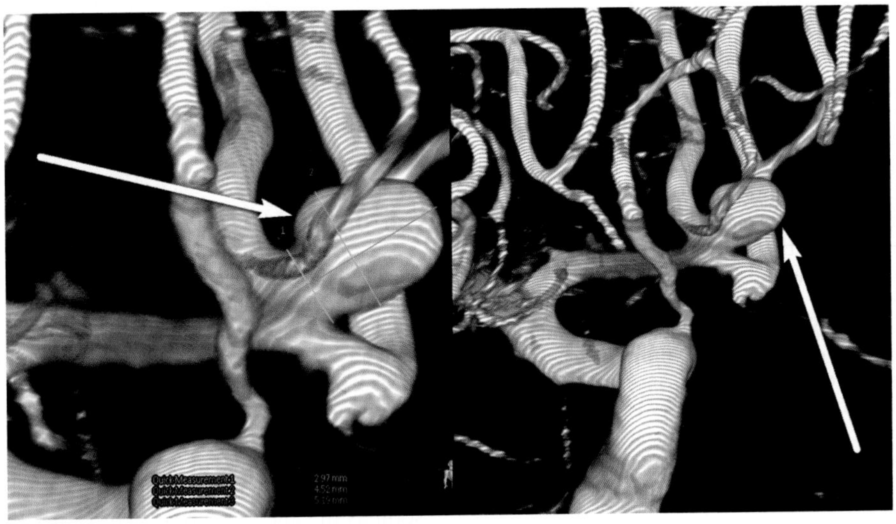

FIGURE 150.4 Shown is a 3D reconstruction of a large anterior communicating artery aneurysm (*arrows*). The advantage of 3D reconstruction techniques include a high-resolution view of the aneurysm to visualize smaller, penetrating arteries coming off the aneurysm versus parent vessel, as well as the ability to visualize smaller aneurysms and infundibulum-like outpouchings. Without 3D reconstructions, these could potentially be missed.

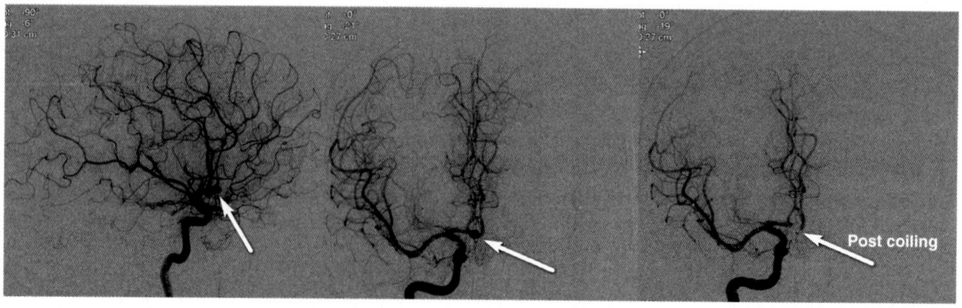

FIGURE 150.5 Shown is the cerebral angiography of the same patient from Figure 150.4, which reveals an anterior communicating artery aneurysm, precoil and postcoil (*arrows*). After coiling, the aneurysm no longer fills. Although it appears that there may be a filling defect, it is merely the coil mass overlying the parent vessel in the anterior–posterior 2D view.

NEUROLOGIC COMPLICATIONS

Rebleeding

Rebleeding is a serious and frequent complication of SAH. The rebleeding risk is 5.8% in the first 24 hours after aSAH and carries a 57% mortality [28]. Clinical symptoms include sudden increase in headache, seizure, nausea, vomiting, depressed level of consciousness, and new neurologic deficits. A well-recognized risk factor for rebleeding is hypertension and the fluctuation of blood pressures. Although a relatively elevated blood pressure could promote rebleeding, low blood pressure may diminish cerebral perfusion, especially in the setting of high ICP. Prior to securing the aneurysm, systolic blood pressure < 160 mm Hg has been recommended [29], with the necessity to titrate on a case-by-case basis factoring in any signs of cerebral hypoperfusion. The blood pressure should be lowered gently and is best managed with short acting agents such as nicardipine or labetalol [30].

cVSP and Delayed Cerebral Ischemia

cVSP and subsequent delayed cerebral ischemia (DCI) are a major cause of morbidity and mortality post-SAH. Only symptomatic, but not angiographic or transcranial Doppler (TCD)-detected cVSP, has been associated with DCI, and therefore considered the clinically meaningful type of cVSP [31].

cVSP is evident on TCD for 71% of patients and by angiogram for 60% of patients [32], but it causes clinically evident symptoms in only 36% [33]. This difference probably reflects the adequacy of collateral circulation in the individual patient, the degree of vessel narrowing and the involvement of less critical brain structures. Unlike rebleeding, the clinical presentation of cVSP occurs progressively over a period of hours to days. It may be apparent as early as the third day after hemorrhage, with a peak between days 4 and 12, and rarely as long as 3 weeks after SAH [34].

Monitoring for cVSP includes frequent neurologic examinations, and daily or every-other-day TCD monitoring. Trends in the TCD from baseline early after SAH onset are clinically useful because an elevated blood flow velocity is often detected before the occurrence of symptomatic vasospasm. Disadvantages include diagnostic precision that is operator dependent, and much lower sensitivities for vessels other than the middle cerebral artery.

Although the calcium-channel blocker nimodipine has failed to prevent cVSP, it improves morbidity from vasospasm, and is the only therapeutic agent with level I evidence to support its use post-SAH [35]. The current standard of care is to administer prophylactically 60 mg of nimodipine orally every 4 hours for a 21-day course beginning at the onset of all aneurysmal SAH. The main adverse effect is mild transient hypotension.

"Triple H" (hypervolemic, hypertensive, and hemodilutional) therapy is no longer supported by guidelines, owing to the existing evidence of adverse associations with outcomes after the use of hemodilution [36]. Prior to the onset of symptomatic cVSP, maintaining a euvolemic state without prophylactically induced hypertension is now recommended [3]. Once symptomatic cVSP occurs, "HH-T" (hypertensive and hypervolemic therapy) is indicated. Elevation of systemic arterial pressure produces a significant increase in regional cerebral blood flow [37], while optimal increase in the amount of blood pressure, or the use of systolic versus mean arterial pressure thresholds are not known.

Intra-arterial infusion of vasodilators such as verapamil, nicardipine, and milrinone [38,39] or, in refractory cases, angioplasty, are other commonly used endovascular techniques for treatment of cVSP [40]. Patient selection criteria for treatment include the presence of clinically symptomatic cVSP without infarction in a patient with a repaired aneurysm.

The severity of cVSP and subsequent ischemia appears to relate to the amount of blood in the CSF space [41]. Thus, there is significant interest in the therapeutic drainage of bloody CSF. To achieve this, a ventriculostomy is commonly placed. In Europe, an additional lumbar drain is often placed [42,43], but due to the lack of large trials this practice has not been established as routine in the US. The experimental use of intrathecal or intraventricular urokinase or tissue plasminogen activator has suggested improved outcomes and a lower incidence of angiographic cVSP and infrequent complications [44], although the trials thus far have been underpowered.

Seizures

Seizures may increase ICP and may subsequently increase the risk for rebleeding. A middle cerebral artery aneurysm and a thick SAH blood clot may increase the risk of developing seizures, which is as high as 27%, and is the highest within the first day [45]. Use of prophylactic anticonvulsants such as phenytoin or levetiracetam is indicated prior to securing the aneurysm. Studies of the use of anticonvulsants, in particular phenytoin, have been implicated in worse neurologic recovery [46,47], and therefore guidelines recommend stopping the anticonvulsants as soon as the aneurysm has been secured, as long as the patient is not comatose and has a consistent neurologic examination to follow [3]. Continuation of anticonvulsants may be justified when the patient had seizures at SAH onset, or is thought to be at very high risk.

Hydrocephalus

Hydrocephalus can develop acutely within the first 24 hours after SAH because of impaired CSF resorption at the arachnoid granulations or the presence of an intraventricular clot obstructing CSF outflow [48]. Clinically significant hydrocephalus developing subacutely over a few days or weeks after SAH is manifested by impairment of vertical gaze and progressive lethargy. Ventricular CSF drainage is indicated when the clinical neurologic examination deteriorates. Although ventriculostomy or lumbar punctures should be performed with caution in patients with an unsecured aneurysm, it does not seem to be associated with a significant increased risk of rebleeding [49]. A delayed form of hydrocephalus manifested by cognitive changes and gait disorders may be observed several weeks after the SAH; in these cases, a ventriculoperitoneal shunt may be indicated [50].

Cardiac and Pulmonary Complications

Cardiac and pulmonary complications may be seen in high grade SAH in the first few days after aneurysm rupture [51,52]. Excessive sympathetic stimulation (sympathetic surge) at the time of aneurysm rupture leads to cardiac dysrhythmias in 28% of SAH cases [53]. The increased levels of circulating catecholamines influence the α-receptors of the myocardium and can result in prolonged myofibril contraction, eventually causing myofibrillar degeneration and necrosis. Elevated levels of serum troponin and brain natriuretic peptide levels are common, but not due to coronary artery plaque rupture with thrombocyte activation and adhesion. SAH is the most frequent neurologic cause for neurogenic electrocardiographic changes: large upright T waves, inverted T waves, prolonged QT intervals, prominent U waves and minor ST elevation or depression can occur. Despite ST–T changes, the incidence of myocardial ischemia remains low [53,54]. Pathologic Q waves are not common in SAH and suggest the need for further investigations for myocardial infarction.

The sympathetic surge also leads to stress cardiomyopathy and a global compromise in cardiac left ventricular (LV) function. This usually transient cardiomyopathy is characterized by global dysfunction not respecting the coronary arteries vascular territory and results in "apical ballooning," giving the cardiac silhouette the shape of a Japanese octopus fishing pot, hence the name "Takotsubo" cardiomyopathy. In rare instances, an intra-aortic balloon pump may be indicated during this transient cardiac dysfunction [55].

Neurogenic pulmonary edema is not uncommon with high grade SAH [52]. It is due to direct β-receptor stimulation in the lung during the sympathetic surge. This can lead to sudden and early massive increase in pulmonary lung water, with severe hypoxemia. Although the pulmonary edema is transient during the first 24 to 48 hours, early recognition and treatment with diuretics may be life saving [56].

GENERAL ICU MANAGEMENT

Once the aneurysm has been secured, general ICU management includes close neurologic and hemodynamic monitoring, head elevation to improve cerebral venous return and prevent increased ICP and good pulmonary toilet to avoid atelectasis and pneumonia.

Headache often persists for several weeks, even after securing the aneurysm, and is due to meningeal irritation (chemical meningitis) from the blood product breakdown. Pain control can be difficult, and narcotics are commonly required. In refractory pain, corticosteroids (dexamethasone) may help improve the meningitic symptoms.

Hyponatremia is found among 30% of SAH cases [57]. It is caused by hypothalamic dysfunction, sometimes causing the syndrome of inappropriate antidiuretic hormone (SIADH), but much more commonly cerebral salt wasting (CSW) owing to an increase in circulating brain natriuretic peptide levels. Serum sodium levels, osmolality as well as the volume status must be followed closely. The usual treatment for SIADH is fluid restriction; however, this is contraindicated in SAH, because it may exacerbated cVSP, and hypertonic saline should be used instead while maintaining euvolemia [58]. CSW is a hypovolemic hyponatremic state that responds to treatment with isotonic fluids and fludrocortisone [59].

Venous thromboembolism (VTE) prophylaxis should be started immediately on admission with the use of pneumatic compression boots. Although all antiplatelet and anticoagulation medication should be discontinued on admission, they should be restarted if still medically indicated along with subcutaneous fractionated or unfractionated heparin for VTE prophylaxis as soon as the aneurysm is secured. With decreasing platelet counts, one should have a high degree of clinical suspicion for heparin-induced thrombocytopenia type II, because it affects 6% of SAH patients [60].

Fever is a very common complication of SAH and it is associated with worse outcomes [61]. Although fever is, therefore, commonly treated with induced normothermia, one should note that no clinical trials have been conducted to show improved outcome by applying normothermia and suppressing fever. Anemia and hemoglobin concentration less than 9 g per dL have been associated with worse outcome as well; however, optimal hemoglobin goal levels are not known [62,63]. Hyperglycemia of >200 mg per dL is also associated with worse outcome but should be treated with strict avoidance of hypoglycemia [64].

HIGH-VOLUME SAH CENTERS

It is noteworthy that multiple studies have shown improved survival and overall outcomes when patients are treated in high-volume SAH treatment centers, defined as a yearly volume of >35 SAH patients per year [65,66]. Therefore, when feasible, direct admission, or transfer to a high-volume center with an experienced multidisciplinary team is strongly recommended [3].

Utility of Ultrasonography for Management of SAH

Neurogenic stunned myocardium (NSM) is a triad of transient LV dysfunction, elevation in cardiac enzymes, and electrocardiogram changes that may occur with SAH [67]. The intensivist who is competent in goal directed echocardiography (see chapter on critical care echocardiography) is able to establish the diagnosis at point of care.

Echocardiography Findings of NSM (Takotsubo Cardiomyopathy)

The usual pattern of abnormality is systolic wall motion abnormality that involves the apical LV segments with sparing of the mid and basal segments of the myocardium. The apical hypokinesis may be severe with akinesis or dyskinesis of the involved segments. Because the base of the heart continues to contract, the apical dyskinesia results in a pattern of apical ballooning during systole. Because the predominant abnormality is apical in position, the abnormality may not be apparent on the parasternal long axis view. The apical four-chamber and subcostal long axis views reveal the characteristic abnormality (Video 29.8 in Chapter 29 Echocardiography as a Monitoring Tool in the ICU).

Atypical patterns of NSM include segmental wall motion abnormalities involving the basal and mid ventricular myocardial segments resulting in an inverted Takosubo pattern where the apical segments exhibit normal contractility while the basal segments have reduced systolic function [68,69]. Abnormalities of right ventricular function have been described as well [70].

Echocardiography cannot distinguish between NSM and myocardial ischemia/infarction, as both entities result in segmental wall abnormalities. Echocardiographic findings support the diagnosis NSM, but clinical correlation is required for definitive diagnosis. Advanced echocardiographic measurements such as diastolic function, speckled tracking, and MRI/echocardiographic reveal characteristic abnormalities, but are not required for diagnosis [71–73]. Goal directed echocardiography examination is effective in identifying the characteristic features of NSM.

Summary of Recommendations

- Early identification and repair of the ruptured aneurysm by clipping, or preferably when feasible by coiling, is indicated to prevent rebleeding [27]
- ICU care should entail administration of enteral nimodipine for 21 d, euvolemia, normothermia, blood pressure management, and adequate oxygenation and ventilation [35]
- Only clinically symptomatic cVSP, but not TCD or angiographic cVSP, should be treated with hypertensive and hypervolemic therapies, as well as intra-arterial therapies [37]
- Prophylactic hypervolemia and hypertension before the onset of symptomatic cVSP are not indicated [3]
- Hemodilution is contraindicated after SAH [36]
- Hydrocephalus should be treated with ventricular or extraventricular CSF drainage [48,49]
- Anticonvulsants are only recommended prior to securing the aneurysms, and should be stopped as soon as possible thereafter [47,49]
- Cardiac and pulmonary complications can occur after high grade SAH; aggressive supportive care is warranted throughout the acute moribund phase, as they are usually reversible and transient [51–53]
- Admission to high-volume SAH centers (>35 SAH/y) is recommended as improved outcomes can be achieved compared to lower-volume centers [3,65,66]

ICU, intensive care unit; cVSP, cerebral vasospasm; TCD, transcranial Doppler; SAH, subarachnoid hemorrhage; CSF, cerebrospinal fluid.

References

1. Mozaffarian D, Benjamin EJ, Go AS, et al: Heart disease and stroke statistics—2015 update: a report from the American Heart Association. *Circulation* 131(4):e29–e322, 2015.
2. Go AS, Mozaffarian D, Roger VL, et al: Heart disease and stroke statistics—2014 update: a report from the American Heart Association. *Circulation* 129(3):e28–e292, 2014.
3. Connolly ES Jr, Rabinstein AA, Carhuapoma JR, et al: Guidelines for the management of aneurysmal subarachnoid hemorrhage: a guideline for healthcare professionals from the American Heart Association/american Stroke Association. *Stroke* 43(6):1711–1737, 2012.
4. Schievink WI: Intracranial aneurysms. *N Engl J Med* 336(1):28–40, 1997.
5. Schievink WI: Genetics of intracranial aneurysms. *Neurosurgery* 40(4):651–662, 1997; discussion 662-653.
6. Foroud T, Lai D, Koller D, et al: Genome-wide association study of intracranial aneurysm identifies a new association on chromosome 7. *Stroke* 45(11):3194–3199, 2014.
7. Schwartz TH, Solomon RA: Perimesencephalic nonaneurysmal subarachnoid hemorrhage: review of the literature. *Neurosurgery* 39(3):433–440, 1996; discussion 440.
8. Kapadia A, Schweizer TA, Spears J, et al: Nonaneurysmal perimesencephalic subarachnoid hemorrhage: diagnosis, pathophysiology, clinical characteristics, and long-term outcome. *World Neurosurg* 82(6):1131–1143, 2014.
9. Juvela S, Hillbom M, Numminen H, et al: Cigarette smoking and alcohol consumption as risk factors for aneurysmal subarachnoid hemorrhage. *Stroke* 24(5):639–646, 1993.
10. Jakobsson KE, Saveland H, Hillman J, et al: Warning leak and management outcome in aneurysmal subarachnoid hemorrhage. *J Neurosurg* 85(6):995–999, 1996.
11. Fisher CM: Clinical syndromes in cerebral thrombosis, hypertensive hemorrhage, and ruptured saccular aneurysm. *Clin Neurosurg* 22:117–147, 1975.
12. Lin CL, Dumont AS, Lieu AS, et al: Characterization of perioperative seizures and epilepsy following aneurysmal subarachnoid hemorrhage. *J Neurosurg* 99(6):978–985, 2003.
13. Byrne JV, Boardman P, Ioannidis I, et al: Seizures after aneurysmal subarachnoid hemorrhage treated with coil embolization. *Neurosurgery* 52(3):545–552, 2003; discussion 550-542.
14. Hunt WE, Hess RM: Surgical risk as related to time of intervention in the repair of intracranial aneurysms. *J Neurosurg* 28(1):14–20, 1968.
15. Teasdale GM, Drake CG, Hunt W, et al: A universal subarachnoid hemorrhage scale: report of a committee of the World Federation of Neurosurgical Societies. *J Neurol Neurosurg Psychiatry* 51(11):1457, 1988.
16. Fisher CM, Kistler JP, Davis JM: Relation of cerebral vasospasm to subarachnoid hemorrhage visualized by computerized tomographic scanning. *Neurosurgery* 6(1):1–9, 1980.
17. Frontera JA, Claassen J, Schmidt JM, et al: Prediction of symptomatic vasospasm after subarachnoid hemorrhage: the modified fisher scale. *Neurosurgery* 59(1):21–27, 2006; discussion 21-27.
18. Perry JJ, Stiell IG, Sivilotti ML, et al: Sensitivity of computed tomography performed within six hours of onset of headache for diagnosis of subarachnoid haemorrhage: prospective cohort study. *BMJ* 343:d4277, 2011.
19. Backes D, Rinkel GJ, Kemperman H, et al: Time-dependent test characteristics of head computed tomography in patients suspected of nontraumatic subarachnoid hemorrhage. *Stroke* 43(8):2115–2119, 2012.
20. Nijjar S, Patel B, McGinn G, et al: Computed tomographic angiography as the primary diagnostic study in spontaneous subarachnoid hemorrhage. *J Neuroimaging* 17(4):295–299, 2007.
21. Westerlaan HE, van Dijk JM, Jansen-van der Weide MC, et al: Intracranial aneurysms in patients with subarachnoid hemorrhage: CT angiography as a primary examination tool for diagnosis—systematic review and meta-analysis. *Radiology* 258(1):134–145, 2011.
22. Li MH, Cheng YS, Li YD, et al: Large-cohort comparison between three-dimensional time-of-flight magnetic resonance and rotational digital subtraction angiographies in intracranial aneurysm detection. *Stroke* 40(9):3127–3129, 2009.
23. Jung JY, Kim YB, Lee JW, et al: Spontaneous subarachnoid haemorrhage with negative initial angiography: a review of 143 cases. *J Clin Neurosci* 13(10):1011–1017, 2006.
24. Huang J, van Gelder JM: The probability of sudden death from rupture of intracranial aneurysms: a meta-analysis. *Neurosurgery* 51(5):1101–1105, 2002; discussion 1105-1107.
25. Stegmayr B, Eriksson M, Asplund K: Declining mortality from subarachnoid hemorrhage: changes in incidence and case fatality from 1985 through 2000. *Stroke* 35(9):2059–2063, 2004.
26. Lantigua H, Ortega-Gutierrez S, Schmidt JM, et al: Subarachnoid hemorrhage: who dies, and why? *Crit Care* 19:309, 2015.
27. Molyneux AJ, Birks J, Clarke A, et al: The durability of endovascular coiling versus neurosurgical clipping of ruptured cerebral aneurysms: 18 year follow-up of the UK cohort of the International Subarachnoid Aneurysm Trial (ISAT). *Lancet* 385(9969):691–697, 2015.
28. van Donkelaar CE, Bakker NA, Veeger NJ, et al: Predictive factors for rebleeding after aneurysmal subarachnoid hemorrhage: rebleeding aneurysmal subarachnoid hemorrhage study. *Stroke* 46(8):2100–2106, 2015.
29. Ohkuma H, Tsurutani H, Suzuki S: Incidence and significance of early aneurysmal rebleeding before neurosurgical or neurological management. *Stroke* 32(5):1176–1180, 2001.
30. Liu-Deryke X, Janisse J, Coplin WM, et al: A comparison of nicardipine and labetalol for acute hypertension management following stroke. *Neurocrit Care* 9(2):167–176, 2008.
31. Frontera JA, Fernandez A, Schmidt JM, et al: Defining vasospasm after subarachnoid hemorrhage: what is the most clinically relevant definition? *Stroke* 40(6):1963–1968, 2009.
32. Rabinstein AA, Friedman JA, Weigand SD, et al: Predictors of cerebral infarction in aneurysmal subarachnoid hemorrhage. *Stroke* 35(8):1862–1866, 2004.
33. Shimoda M, Takeuchi M, Tominaga J, et al: Asymptomatic versus symptomatic infarcts from vasospasm in patients with subarachnoid hemorrhage:

serial magnetic resonance imaging. *Neurosurgery* 49(6):1341–1348, 2001; discussion 1348-1350.
34. Hijdra A, Van Gijn J, Stefanko S, et al: Delayed cerebral ischemia after aneurysmal subarachnoid hemorrhage: clinicoanatomic correlations. *Neurology* 36(3):329–333, 1986.
35. Pickard JD, Murray GD, Illingworth R, et al: Effect of oral nimodipine on cerebral infarction and outcome after subarachnoid haemorrhage: British aneurysm nimodipine trial. *BMJ* 298(6674):636–642, 1989.
36. Naidech AM, Jovanovic B, Wartenberg KE, et al: Higher hemoglobin is associated with improved outcome after subarachnoid hemorrhage. *Crit Care Med* 35(10):2383–2389, 2007.
37. Dankbaar JW, Slooter AJ, Rinkel GJ, et al: Effect of different components of triple-H therapy on cerebral perfusion in patients with aneurysmal subarachnoid haemorrhage: a systematic review. *Crit Care* 14(1):R23, 2010.
38. Feng L, Fitzsimmons BF, Young WL, et al: Intraarterially administered verapamil as adjunct therapy for cerebral vasospasm: safety and 2-year experience. *AJNR Am J Neuroradiol* 23(8):1284–1290, 2002.
39. Ortega-Gutierrez S, Thomas J, Reccius A, et al: Effectiveness and safety of nicardipine and labetalol infusion for blood pressure management in patients with intracerebral and subarachnoid hemorrhage. *Neurocrit Care* 18(1):13–19, 2013.
40. Chalouhi N, Tjoumakaris S, Thakkar V, et al: Endovascular management of cerebral vasospasm following aneurysm rupture: outcomes and predictors in 116 patients.*Clin Neurol Neurosurg* 118:26–31, 2014.
41. Claassen J, Bernardini GL, Kreiter K, et al: Effect of cisternal and ventricular blood on risk of delayed cerebral ischemia after subarachnoid hemorrhage: the Fisher scale revisited. *Stroke* 32(9):2012–2020, 2001.
42. Nieuwkamp DJ, de Gans K, Rinkel GJ, et al: Treatment and outcome of severe intraventricular extension in patients with subarachnoid or intracerebral hemorrhage: a systematic review of the literature. *J Neurol* 247(2):117–121, 2000.
43. Al-Tamimi YZ, Bhargava D, Feltbower RG, et al: Lumbar drainage of cerebrospinal fluid after aneurysmal subarachnoid hemorrhage: a prospective, randomized, controlled trial (LUMAS). *Stroke* 43(3):677–682, 2012.
44. Kramer AH, Fletcher JJ: Locally-administered intrathecal thrombolytics following aneurysmal subarachnoid hemorrhage: a systematic review and meta-analysis. *Neurocrit Care* 14(3):489–499, 2011.
45. Rhoney DH, Tipps LB, Murry KR, et al: Anticonvulsant prophylaxis and timing of seizures after aneurysmal subarachnoid hemorrhage. *Neurology* 55(2):258–265, 2000.
46. Naidech AM, Kreiter KT, Janjua N, et al: Phenytoin exposure is associated with functional and cognitive disability after subarachnoid hemorrhage. *Stroke* 36(3):583–587, 2005.
47. Rosengart AJ, Huo JD, Tolentino J, et al: Outcome in patients with subarachnoid hemorrhage treated with antiepileptic drugs. *J Neurosurg* 107(2):253–260, 2007.
48. Suarez-Rivera O: Acute hydrocephalus after subarachnoid hemorrhage. *Surg Neurol* 49(5):563–565, 1998.
49. Hellingman CA, van den Bergh WM, Beijer IS, et al: Risk of rebleeding after treatment of acute hydrocephalus in patients with aneurysmal subarachnoid hemorrhage. *Stroke* 38(1):96–99, 2007.
50. Walcott BP, Iorgulescu JB, Stapleton CJ, et al: Incidence, timing, and predictors of delayed shunting for hydrocephalus after aneurysmal subarachnoid hemorrhage. *Neurocrit Care* 23(1):54–58, 2015.
51. van der Bilt IA, Hasan D, Vandertop WP, et al: Impact of cardiac complications on outcome after aneurysmal subarachnoid hemorrhage: a meta-analysis. *Neurology* 72(7):635–642, 2009.
52. Solenski NJ, Haley EC Jr, Kassell NF, et al: Medical complications of aneurysmal subarachnoid hemorrhage: a report of the multicenter, cooperative aneurysm study. Participants of the Multicenter Cooperative Aneurysm Study. *Crit Care Med* 23(6):1007–1017, 1995.
53. Coghlan LA, Hindman BJ, Bayman EO, et al: Independent associations between electrocardiographic abnormalities and outcomes in patients with aneurysmal subarachnoid hemorrhage: findings from the intraoperative hypothermia aneurysm surgery trial. *Stroke* 40(2):412–418, 2009.
54. Brouwers PJ, Wijdicks EF, Hasan D, et al: Serial electrocardiographic recording in aneurysmal subarachnoid hemorrhage. *Stroke* 20(9):1162–1167, 1989.
55. Lazaridis C, Pradilla G, Nyquist PA, et al: Intra-aortic balloon pump counterpulsation in the setting of subarachnoid hemorrhage, cerebral vasospasm, and neurogenic stress cardiomyopathy. Case report and review of the literature. *Neurocrit Care* 13(1):101–108, 2010.
56. Busl KM, Bleck TP: Neurogenic pulmonary edema. *Crit Care Med* 43(8):1710–1715, 2015.
57. Qureshi AI, Suri MF, Sung GY, et al: Prognostic significance of hypernatremia and hyponatremia among patients with aneurysmal subarachnoid hemorrhage. *Neurosurg* 50(4):749–755, 2002; discussion 755-746.
58. Woo CH, Rao VA, Sheridan W, et al: Performance characteristics of a sliding-scale hypertonic saline infusion protocol for the treatment of acute neurologic hyponatremia. *Neurocrit Care* 11(2):228–234, 2009.
59. Hasan D, Lindsay KW, Wijdicks EF, et al: Effect of fludrocortisone acetate in patients with subarachnoid hemorrhage. *Stroke* 20(9):1156–1161, 1989.
60. Alaraj A, Wallace A, Mander N, et al: Risk factors for heparin-induced thrombocytopenia type II in aneurysmal subarachnoid hemorrhage. *Neurosurgery* 69(5):1030–1036, 2011.
61. Fernandez A, Schmidt JM, Claassen J, et al: Fever after subarachnoid hemorrhage: risk factors and impact on outcome. *Neurology* 68(13):1013–1019, 2007.
62. Oddo M, Milby A, Chen I, et al: Hemoglobin concentration and cerebral metabolism in patients with aneurysmal subarachnoid hemorrhage. *Stroke* 40(4):1275–1281, 2009.
63. Naidech AM, Shaibani A, Garg RK, et al: Prospective, randomized trial of higher goal hemoglobin after subarachnoid hemorrhage. *Neurocrit Care* 13(3):313–320, 2010.
64. Frontera JA, Fernandez A, Claassen J, et al: Hyperglycemia after SAH: predictors, associated complications, and impact on outcome. *Stroke* 37(1):199–203, 2006.
65. Cross DT 3rd, Tirschwell DL, Clark MA, et al: Mortality rates after subarachnoid hemorrhage: variations according to hospital case volume in 18 states. *J Neurosurg* 99(5):810–817, 2003.
66. Berman MF, Solomon RA, Mayer SA, et al: Impact of hospital-related factors on outcome after treatment of cerebral aneurysms. *Stroke* 34(9):2200–2207, 2003.
67. Murthy SB, Shah S, Rao CP, et al: Neurogenic stunned myocardium following acute subarachnoid hemorrhage: pathophysiology and practical considerations. *J Intensive Care Med* 30:318–325, 2015.
68. Okura H: Echocardiographic assessment of takotsubo cardiomyopathy: beyond apical ballooning. *J Echocardiogr* 14:13–20, 2016.
69. Shoukat S, Awad A, Nam DK, et al: Cardiomyopathy with inverted tako-tsubo pattern in the setting of subarachnoid hemorrhage: a series of four cases. *Neurocrit Care* 18:257–260, 2013.
70. Rodrigues AC, Guimaraes L, Lira E, et al: Right ventricular abnormalities in Takotsubo cardiomyopathy. *Echocardiography* 30:1015–1021, 2013.
71. Haghi D, Fluechter S, Suselbeck T, et al: Cardiovascular magnetic resonance findings in typical versus atypical forms of the acute apical ballooning syndrome (Takotsubo cardiomyopathy). *Int J Cardiol* 120:205–211, 2007.
72. Abdelmoneim SS, Mankad SV, Bernier M, et al: Microvascular function in Takotsubo cardiomyopathy with contrast echocardiography: prospective evaluation and review of literature. *J Am SocEchocardiogr* 22:1249–1255, 2009.
73. Abdelmoneim SS, Wijdicks EF, Lee VH, et al: Real-time myocardial perfusion contrast echocardiography and regional wall motion abnormalities after aneurysmal subarachnoid hemorrhage. *J Neurosurg* 111:1023–1028, 2009.

Chapter 151 ■ Status Epilepticus

FELICIA C. CHU • CATHERINE A. PHILLIPS

DEFINITION AND CLASSIFICATION

Status epilepticus (SE) is a condition in which there is "failure of the 'normal' factors that serve to terminate a typical generalized tonic-clonic seizure" [1,2]. SE is defined as 5 minutes of continued seizure activity, or two or more seizures with incomplete recovery between. SE is usually divided into:

a. *convulsive SE*, where the patient does not regain consciousness between repeated generalized tonic–clonic attacks;
b. *focal SE* without altered cognition, behavior, or consciousness [3],characterized by continuous or repetitive focal seizures without loss of awareness [4]; and
c. *nonconvulsive SE* (NCSE), which includes generalized forms such as absence SE, and focal SE with behavioral features, (previously called complex partial SE).NCSE is also used to describe continued seizure activity in patients who are comatose, but have few other clinical signs.

Convulsive Status Epilepticus

Most generalized tonic–clonic SE consists of focal seizures that have generalized secondarily; genetic seizures uncommonly generalize [2,5]. Most patients do not convulse continuously, but a few minutes of seizures are followed by prolonged unconsciousness leading to the next seizure. During convulsive SE, massive autonomic discharge occurs with tachycardia and hypertension. Corneal and pupillary reflexes are lost and plantar reflexes may be extensor. As SE continues, the motor manifestations may evolve into more subtle activity such as focal twitching, nystagmus, eye deviation, or recurrent pupillary hippus [4]. Among patients who are very encephalopathic, SE may also present in this more subtle form, without initial convulsive activity; electroencephalography (EEG) is required to confirm the diagnosis. Myoclonic SE with repetitive, asynchronous myoclonus with variable clouding of consciousness is often classified as a form of convulsive SE and may evolve into generalized tonic–clonic SE. In adults, myoclonic syndromes are usually caused by toxic or metabolic encephalopathies, most commonly severe cerebral anoxia [6]. The patients are usually comatose, and the prognosis is poor.

Focal Status Epilepticus without Altered Cognition, Behavior, or Consciousness (Dyscognitive Features)

Focal SE without dyscognitive features is the second most common form of SE, after generalized tonic–clonic SE [4]. In focal motor SE, clonic activity is localized usually to the face or an extremity. This activity may spread, corresponding to the somatotopic organization of the motor cortex, known as a Jacksonian march. Alternatively, the focal motor seizures may be multifocal, often precipitated by metabolic disorders, such as hyperglycemia with a hyperosmolar nonketotic state [7]. *Epilepsia partialis continua* is a form of focal motor SE characterized by continuous, highly localized seizures that do not become generalized and in which consciousness is maintained.

Nonconvulsive Status Epilepticus

NCSE is an underrecognized cause of coma. In a recent study, NCSE was present in 8% of all comatose patients, without signs of seizure activity [8]. In other studies, a third of patients with unexplained altered mental status in intensive care units (ICUs) were in NCSE. NCSE is more likely to occur in the setting of acute medical problems, both systemic and neurologic [8–10].

NCSE includes absence SE and focal SE with dyscognitive features [4]. Clinically, both present with a prolonged period of altered behavior and can masquerade as a psychiatric fugue state. NCSE is defined as a prolonged confusional state of 30 minutes or longer, involving a variable level of altered consciousness [8]. Absence SE may be accompanied by subtle myoclonic movements of the face; eye blinking; and occasional automatisms of the face and hands. The EEG is diagnostic, revealing generalized spike/slow wave activity. Focal SE with dyscognitive features involves a series of focal seizures with staring, unresponsiveness, and motor automatisms, separated by a confusional state, or a more prolonged state of partial responsiveness and semipurposeful automatisms. The EEG usually shows more focal continuous epileptiform activity, but if an EEG shows rhythmical slowing with subtle clinical signs as described above, or there is an evolution of the EEG pattern, NCSE should be considered [11].

ETIOLOGY

Some of the major etiologies of SE are shown in Table151.1. Symptomatic SE, resulting from an acute or chronic neurologic or metabolic insult, is at least twice as common as idiopathic SE (presumed genetic etiology for the seizures in an otherwise neurologically normal person) [5]. In adults, a major cause of SE is stroke (up to 22% of cases) or decreasing antiepileptic drugs (AEDs) (up to 34% of cases) [2]. Other etiologies include autoimmune encephalitides—either limbic encephalitis or diffuse encephalitis—and may have a paraneoplastic or nonparaneoplastic cause [12]. New-onset refractory SE (NORSE) refers to bouts of refractory status epilepticus due to unknown causes, some of which were proven to be either infectious or autoimmune in etiology [13].

PROGNOSIS AND SEQUELAE OF STATUS EPILEPTICUS

Mortality for SE depends on the specific etiology; duration of the episode; and the age of the patient [2,5]. Anoxia has been associated with the highest mortality; and alcohol withdrawal and AED discontinuation with low mortality rates. Patients with idiopathic SE have a low mortality rate. The duration of SE longer than 30 minutes and age over 70 significantly increases mortality [5,14]. Despite improved medical care, convulsive SE still has an overall mortality rate of 20% [2,15]. The mortality of focal SE with dyscognitive features was 18% in one study [16]. Other adverse outcomes include intellectual deterioration, permanent neurologic deficits, and chronic epilepsy.

TABLE 151.1

Etiologies of Status Epilepticus

- Etiologies
  - Structural brain lesion
    - Brain trauma
    - Brain tumor
    - Stroke
    - Hemorrhage
  - Central nervous system infection (encephalitis or meningitis)
  - Autoimmune encephalitis
  - Systemic infection
  - Drugs
    - Toxic (e.g., theophylline, lidocaine, and penicillin)
    - Withdrawal state (e.g., alcohol and barbiturate)
    - AED
      - Errors in medication
      - Change in AED regimen
      - Altered drug absorption or drug–drug interaction
      - Noncompliance
  - Metabolic
    - Hypocalcemia
    - Hypomagnesemia
    - Hypoglycemia, hyperglycemia
    - Hyponatremia
    - Hyperosmolar state
    - Anoxia or hypoxia
    - Uremia
  - Idiopathic

AED, antiepileptic drug.

SE itself can produce profound neuronal damage. Neuropathologic studies of the brains of children and adults who died shortly after SE reveal ischemic neuronal changes in the hippocampus; middle layers of the cerebral cortex; cerebellum (Purkinje cells); basal ganglia; thalamus; and hypothalamus [17]. These changes mimic those of severe hypoxia or hypoglycemia. Hyperthermia during an episode of SE has also been shown to correlate closely with the degree of central nervous system (CNS) damage [18].

The perpetuation of SE is caused by an imbalance between excitotoxic (glutamate mediated) and inhibitory (γ-aminobutyric acid [GABA] mediated) mechanisms [15,16]. Downregulation of GABA receptors, or excitotoxic mechanisms involving glutamate receptors—both NMDA (*N*-methyl-D-aspartate) and non-NMDA receptors—are involved [2,15,19]. Calcium influx during excitation is a critical component of neuronal injury and cell death, with activation of proteases and lipases, leading to degradation of intracellular elements [19].

Abnormal neuronal activity alone can cause permanent neurologic injury; patients with focal dyscognitive or focal motor SE without concomitant hypotension, hypoxia, or hyperpyrexia can still have subsequent neurologic injury in the region of the brain associated with the seizure. Chronic memory impairment may follow focal dyscognitive SE [20], and focal neuronal necrosis (and edema) in the region of the brain involved with seizure activity has been found after focal motor status [21,22]. Focal magnetic resonance imaging (MRI) changes are seen after prolonged epileptic activity, particularly on diffusion-weighted and perfusion MRI, though these changes may dissipate over time [23]. Mortality in NCSE with preexisting epilepsy is lower compared to NCSE following an acute medical condition [8].

SYSTEMIC COMPLICATIONS

If convulsive SE is not terminated promptly, secondary metabolic and medical complications may occur (Table151.2). Hyperthermia

TABLE 151.2

Medical Complications of Status Epilepticus

Cardiovascular system

Hypertension, tachycardia, and arrhythmias may occur early owing to autonomic overactivity and be further complicated by shock due to lactic acidosis or by pharmacologic intervention for the status.

Respiratory system

Respiratory dysfunction may be caused by mechanical impairment from tonic muscle contraction, disturbed respiratory center function, and autonomic overactivity, producing increased bronchial constriction and secretions.Later complications include apnea, aspiration pneumonia, and neurogenic pulmonary edema.

Renal system

Renal impairment may occur from a combination of rhabdomyolysis with myoglobinuria and hypotension with poor renal perfusion. Later complications include uremia and acute tubular necrosis.

Metabolic

Increased lactate production from maximally exercised muscles results in metabolic acidosis within minutes after the start of SE, with a variable respiratory contribution to the acidosis from carbon dioxide retention.The degree of acidosis does not correlate with the extent of neuropathologic damage.After cessation of the seizure, lactate is rapidly metabolized, resulting in spontaneous resolution of the acidosis.

Systemically, hyperglycemia initially develops owing to catecholamine and glucagon release; later, hypoglycemia occurs due to increased plasma insulin, increased cerebral glucose consumption, and excessive muscle activity.

may follow excessive muscle activity and hypothalamic dysfunction, or may be caused by an underlying infection responsible for the initiation of SE. Both hyperthermia from an infection and that from SE can be accompanied by peripheral leukocytosis [17] due to demargination, with a white blood cell count in the range of 12,700 to 28,000 cells per μL. The differential may be normal or may show lymphocytic or polymorphonuclear predominance, but band forms are rarely present. A mild cerebrospinal fluid (CSF) pleocytosis can occur with SE [17]; the maximum cell count is usually less than 80 cells per mm^3, with an initial polymorphonuclear predominance that reverts to a lymphocytic predominance as the pleocytosis resolves over a few days. Mild transient elevations of CSF protein may also occur. Lowering of the CSF glucose level does not occur, and reduced CSF glucose immediately raises concern for an underlying infectious or inflammatory process.

DIAGNOSIS

SE is a medical emergency and must be treated immediately in a critical care setting. Pharmacologic intervention is more effective at an early stage of SE than after a delay [2,8,15,19,24,25]. Treatment must be fourfold: termination of seizures; prevention of recurrent seizures; identification of etiology; and treatment of complications.

The initial step is to confirm the diagnosis. A flurry of seizures separated by a normal level of consciousness does not constitute SE (although urgent treatment may still be required). NCSE may present clinically with a change in mental status only. As mentioned earlier, in this setting NCSE appears to be greatly underdiagnosed.

For diagnosis of NCSE, certain well-defined EEG criteria need to be met. These are (1) repetitive epileptiform activity at more than 2.5 per second or (2) repetitive epileptiform or rhythmic slow activity less than 2.5 per second and fulfilling secondary criteria, defined as (1) clear clinical and EEG improvement after intravenous (IV) antiepileptic medication; (2) associated subtle clinical ictal signs; or (3) evolution in frequency, morphology, or location of EEG activity [11].

INITIAL ASSESSMENT

Once a diagnosis of SE is made, it is important to perform a rapid initial assessment of medical stability and workup of potential etiologies (Table151.3). Obtain as much **history** as possible within the first few minutes, including any history of a preexisting chronic seizure disorder and AED use; alcohol or drug abuse; or any recent neurologic insult. The **examination** should focus on signs of systemic illness (e.g., uremia, hepatic disease, and infection); illicit drug use; evidence of trauma; or focal neurologic abnormalities. After appropriate **blood samples** have been obtained, **glucose administration** is recommended. Hypoglycemia is a rare but easily reversible cause of SE. Because glucose administration may precipitate Wernicke–Korsakoff syndrome in some individuals with marginal nutrition, **thiamine** should also be given. Subsequent IV infusions should consist of saline solution, because some AEDs precipitate in glucose solutions. The patient must be assessed for other metabolic consequences of status. **Hyperthermia** should be treated and **oxygenation** must be maintained. The metabolic acidosis that occurs does not adversely affect neurologic outcomes and does not need treatment with bicarbonate [26]. **Blood pressure** must be carefully monitored; the systemic hypertension and decreased cerebrovascular resistance of early SE provide adequate blood flow for the increased metabolic demand in the brain, but eventually hypotension may occur, making the brain vulnerable to inadequate perfusion. **Pharmacologic intervention** for the seizures can exacerbate any hypotension.

It is essential to determine whether a metabolic disorder is causing the SE; if this is the case, pharmacologic intervention for SE alone is not effective. Systemic and CNS infections must be excluded, and **lumbar puncture** is often necessary. A contrast-enhanced **head CT scan** can be useful after the patient has been medically stabilized. MRI is preferred for suspected small or subtle lesions but may not be practical in the emergent setting.

MEDICAL MANAGEMENT

Treatment of SE must proceed rapidly and deliberately. Table 151.3 outlines a management protocol. For generalized SE, the initial assessment and treatment should begin within 5 to 10 minutes of the onset of seizure activity. Dosing of drugs can be found in Tables 151.3 and 151.4, and pharmacologic properties and side effects in Table151.4.

IV benzodiazepines are the appropriate initial treatment. The Veterans Affairs Status Epilepticus Cooperative Study Group trial suggested that phenobarbital is also effective as initial therapy, but phenytoin alone without a benzodiazepine may be less effective [24,27]. Diazepam and lorazepam are both effective in treating generalized SE [28], but lorazepam has a longer duration of action (2 to 24 hours), compared to diazepam (10 to 25 minutes) [29], and does not have extensive peripheral tissue uptake, unlike diazepam. Although lorazepam has slower CNS penetration than diazepam, the onset of action of less than 3 minutes is acceptable. For these reasons, **lorazepam** is the recommended first-line agent for SE. Both these drugs have significant and essentially the same cardiac, respiratory, and CNS depressant side effects [25]. Respiratory depression and apnea, which are potentiated by age and previous administration of sedative drugs, may occur abruptly with doses as small as 1 mg. Hypotension, which occasionally occurs, may be partially caused by the propylene glycol solvent contained in the IV forms of diazepam and lorazepam.

In 2012, the RAMPART study showed that if IV access was not available, intramuscular midazolam was as effective as IV lorazepam for the prehospital treatment of SE by paramedics, and this was not associated with an increase in respiratory compromise or seizure recurrence [30]. Early administration of adequate doses of IV lorazepam remains the preferred first-line treatment for SE in the emergency room and other controlled clinical environments. Rectal diazepam (0.2mg per kg) has been successful in achieving rapid therapeutic levels and effectively terminating prolonged generalized seizures [31].Significant respiratory depression from rectal diazepam has not been reported [32]. IM administration of diazepam is unsuitable for the treatment of status owing to delayed peak levels [33]. Furthermore, the peak concentration after IM injection is much less than that after IV injection.

Phenytoin is usually given with benzodiazepines to control the SE and prevent recurrent seizures. A 20 mg per kg load is recommended, given at 50 mg per minute. If seizures continue, additional doses of up to another 10 mg per kg can be given. The serum level of phenytoin should be 15 to 30 mcg per mL. IM administration should not be used because it results in precipitation at the injection site and has slow, erratic absorption. Hypotension, electrocardiographic changes, and respiratory depression can occur and may be due partly to the propylene glycol diluent [2]. Simultaneous cardiac monitoring should be performed, and slower infusion rates (25 mg per minute) should be considered in patients who are elderly owing to increased susceptibility to cardiopulmonary adverse effects [34]. Intravenous infusion of phenytoin carries a risk of

TABLE 151.3

Management Guidelines for Generalized Status Epilepticus in Adults

0–9 min:
If diagnosis is uncertain, observe for: recurrence of generalized seizures without intervening recovery of consciousness; continuous seizure activity >5 min.
ABCs
Establish airway; pulse ox; administer 02; cardiac monitor.
Establish IV access (NS or saline lock), bedside rapid glucose determination. If hypoglycemic, give glucose (D50) 50–100 mL and thiamine 100 mg IV.
Labs: CBC/diff, electrolytes, BUN/Cr/Glu, anticonvulsant drug levels, toxicology screen, other labs as indicated by history/examination (including testing for pregnancy).
5–30 min:
Within 10 minutes:
Lorazepam 0.1 mg/kg IV (<2 mg/min), given 2 mg at a time or midazolam 10mg IM (or diazepam 0.1–0.2 mg/kg, up to 10 mg per dose, <2 mg/min).
Within 30 minutes:
Phenytoin 20 mg/kg IV at ≤50 mg/min (fosphenytoin150 mg PE[a]/min), slower rate in elderly or if hypotension or bradycardia develop. Draw blood for level 10 min after infusion complete.

- Cardiac monitoring; frequent BPs; careful observation of respiratory status; andoximetry.
- EEG monitoring, if possible.
- Consider additional 5 mg/kg boluses of phenytoin to a maximum dose 30 mg/kg if seizures persist.
- Lorazepam as needed for seizures during phenytoin load.

Alternatives for Phenytoin or if seizures continue:
Levetiracetam 20–60 mg/kg IV at 2–5 mg/kg/min IV.
Valproate sodium 20–30 mg/kg IV at 3–6 mg/kg/min, an additional 20 mg/kg may be given 10 min after loading infusion. Watch for hyperammonemia, pancreatitis, thrombocytopenia, and hepatotoxicity. Known teratogen.
Phenobarbital 20 mg/kg IV load, ≤100 mg/min. *Anticipate respiratory depression and need for intubation.* Consider for alcohol withdrawal.
Lacosamide 200–400 mg IV over 3–5 min. Adverse effects: prolonged PR interval; first degree AV block; and bradyarrhythmia.
31–90 min:
For persistent status: induce coma. Intubate if not previously done.
Continuous EEG to monitor for seizures and level of anesthesia.
Propofol 1–2 mg/kg IV bolus, 1–5 mg/kg/h infusion. Note: 5mg/kg/h = 83 mcg/kg/min. Monitor serum for lactate, triglycerides, CPK, and BUN/Cr.
OR
Midazolam 0.2 mg/kg IV bolus, infusion 0.1–2.0 mg/kg/h (tolerance after 72 h);
OR
Pentobarbital 5 mg/kg IV load (give over 20 min); repeat as needed to produce burst-suppression pattern on EEG. Complete EEG suppression may be needed if seizure activity persists during the bursts. Maintenance infusion 0.5–5 mg/kg/h. Monitor serum for lactate, osmolality, bicarb, and Cr for propylene glycol syndrome.
Once burst-suppression pattern is established on EEG, defined by 10 s of suppression with 1–2 s bursts of cerebral activity, continue for 24–48 h. If the bursts contain epileptiform activity, consider complete EEG suppression. Monitor EEG every 1–2 h. Adjust medication dose as needed.
Monitor for hypotension; ileus;propofol infusion syndrome; or propylene glycol syndrome (pentobarbital or IV lorazepam).
Continue maintenance doses of phenytoin, levetiracetam, valproic acid, lacosamide, or phenobarbital; monitor and maintain therapeutic levels.
Taper anesthetic medication at 24–48 h. If seizures recur, resume infusion for 24 h, then taper again. Continue this process as necessary.

[a]Fosphenytoin dosing in PE.
AV, atrioventricular block;BP, blood pressure; BUN, blood urea nitrogen; CBC, complete blood cell; Cr, creatine; CPK, creatine phosphokinase; D50, dextrose 50%; EEG, electroencephalogram; Glu, glucose; IV, intravenous; NS, normal saline; PE, phenytoin equivalents.

medication extravasation into adjacent tissue. Tissue necrosis can rarely occur [35].

Fosphenytoin, a water-soluble prodrug of phenytoin, is rapidly converted enzymatically to phenytoin. Rapid and complete absorption occurs after IM administration [36,37]. Therapeutic phenytoin concentrations are attained in most patients within 10 minutes of rapid IV infusion (150 mg per minute) and within 30 minutes of slower IV infusion or IM injection [36,37]. Dosing for fosphenytoin is the same as for phenytoin, but needs to be given in "phenytoin equivalents." **Cardiac monitoring** is required during IV infusions of fosphenytoin. Maintenance doses of phenytoin or fosphenytoin should be started within 24 hours of the loading dose, with levels maintained in the high therapeutic range (15 to 25 mcg per mL).

If there is contraindication to phenytoin or if seizures persist, levetiracetam, valproate sodium, phenobarbital, or lacosamide may be used instead as second line treatment of SE (See Table151.3) [2,38–40]. Intravenous valproate is well tolerated, with few

TABLE 151.4

Properties of Drugs Used to Treat Status Epilepticus

Drug	Route	Loading dose	Rate of administration	Time to enter brain	Time to peak brain concentration (min)	Minimum effective plasma concentration (μg/mL)	Side effects
Diazepam	IV, rectal	0.1–0.2 mg/kg, up to 20 mg	2 mg/min IV	<10 s	8	0.2–0.8	Respiratory depression/apnea (may be abrupt); hypotension; sedation, especially in combination with barbiturates
Lorazepam	IV	0.1 mg/kg (4–8mg)	2 mg/min	<2–3 min	23	0.03–0.10	Same as diazepam; amnesia
Phenytoin	IV	20 mg/kg	50 mg/min	1–3 min	3–6	15–30	Hypotension and electrocardiogram changes during acute administration; sedation at high doses
Phenobarbital	IV	20 mg/kg	50–100 mg/min	3 min	5–15	10–40	Respiratory depression and sedation common with increasing doses, especially when benzodiazepines used; hypotension
Valproate	IV	20–30 mg/kg, may go up to 60 mg/kg if needed	Up to 3–5 mg/kg/min;even higher bolus rates well tolerated [45]	10 min	60	70–140	Thrombocytopenia, hepatotoxicity, pancreatitis, hyperammonemic encephalopathy, rare hypotension

IV, intravenous.

adverse effects [41–46]. Valproate levels should be monitored. With phenobarbital infusions, respiratory depression can occur, especially if benzodiazepines have been used.

SE persisting after this time is considered **refractory SE** (RSE). Treatment from this point on may vary. For drug-induced coma, all patients must be intubated. Agents commonly used for RSE include midazolam, propofol, or pentobarbital (see Table151.3) [2,34]. All are extremely effective for suppressing clinical and electrographic seizures. Simultaneous EEG monitoring is mandatory during induction of coma. Phenobarbital is not used for this purpose, because it can result in very prolonged coma.

Propofol, a GABA agonist, is a potent antiepileptic agent [2,47,48]. Propofol has the advantage of rapid induction and elimination, but slow downward titration is important to avoid recurrent seizures [49]. One significant disadvantage of this drug is the propofol infusion syndrome. This consists of profound hypotension, rhabdomyolysis, hyperlipidemia, cardiac arrhythmias, and metabolic acidosis.

Midazolam is comparably well tolerated and effective. Compared to pentobarbital, patients on midazolam have less cardiac depression and regain consciousness more rapidly after discontinuation [50,51]. Midazolam can be used in combination with propofol to decrease risk propofol infusion syndrome. Tolerance to the antiepileptic effects of midazolam can develop after 36 to 48 hours, which can lead to escalating dose requirements. Because of this, if SE is not terminated within 72 hours of midazolam treatment, changing to an alternative infusion such as propofol or pentobarbital is recommended.

Pentobarbital infusion may result in cardiac depression, and careful hemodynamic monitoring is required. Vasopressors are frequently needed, and ileus is also common. Propylene glycol toxicity has been reported in patients treated with barbiturate coma for refractory SE. These patients can develop hypotension and hepatic and renal failure. Treatment may include hemodialysis [52].

There is relatively little prospective data to suggest that propofol, midazolam, or pentobarbital are dramatically different in efficacy for SE. Several studies seem to indicate that patients treated with pentobarbital have fewer treatment failures and breakthrough seizures, but more frequent episodes of hypotension. There is no clear difference in mortality among the three agents [53].

The dose of propofol, midazolam or pentobarbital must be sufficient to terminate any seizure activity seen on the EEG. In many cases, the goal is to produce a burst-suppression EEG pattern, characterized by a flat background of at least 10 seconds punctuated by bursts of mixed-frequency activity lasting 1 to 2 seconds in duration. If the bursts contain electrographic seizure activity, the coma should be deepened, at times to virtual electrocerebral silence. During this time of drug-induced coma, it is essential to maintain high therapeutic levels of all antiepileptic medications to avoid recurrence of SE upon tapering of anesthetic agents. Phenobarbital may be used as a bridge if initial weaning off pentobarbital results in recurrence of seizures.Temporary supratherapeutic levels of phenobarbital (i.e., 40 to 60 mcg per mL) may be needed in this situation.

NCSE must be treated quickly, although additional trials of antiepileptic medications are usually warranted prior to intubation and initiation of anesthetic agents. When needed, the medication doses are comparable to those used in generalized SE (see Table151.3).Both diazepam and lorazepam are effective in treating absence SE; focal motor SE; and focal dyscognitive SE. The response to benzodiazepines may be helpful for confirming the diagnosis if it is in question. The patient should also be started on antiepileptic medication appropriate for long-term management, given as a loading dose if appropriate. Valproate is very effective for treatment of absence SE as well as levetiracetam. Phenytoin is often ineffective at treating absence SE. Focal motor SE responds to phenytoin and other standard agents including levetiracetam, although epilepsia partialis continua can be notoriously resistant to treatment.

The ketogenic diet is an emerging nonpharmacologic treatment of superrefractory SE. The high-fat and low-protein/carbohydrate diet is administered via nasogastric tube which subsequently induces a metabolic shift toward acidosis, resulting in ketonuria, which can be present within a few days of initiation of the diet.Successful treatment of superrefractory NCSE with the ketogenic diet has been described [54].

CONCLUSION

SE is a true medical emergency and needs to be treated promptly and definitively. For convulsive SE, immediate termination of ongoing seizure activity; determination of underlying etiology; and medical stabilization of patients are essential. Lorazepam IV and more recently midazolam IM are medications for immediate short-term cessation of SE. A number of newer AEDs have been shown to be effective for the treatment of SE. There have been significant advances in ICU monitoring and management, as well as for the earlier identification of NCSE states. Physicians should be familiar with effective treatment protocols for SE, because prompt and appropriate therapy is essential for reducing morbidity and mortality.

References

1. Lowenstein DH, Bleck T, MacDonald RL: It's time to revise the definition of status epilepticus. *Epilepsia* 40:120, 1999.
2. Betjemann JP, Lowenstein DH: Status epilepticus in adults. *Lancet Neurol* 14(6):615–624, 2015.
3. Berg AT, Berkovic SF, Brodie MJ, et al: Revised terminology and concepts for organization of seizures and epilepsies: report of the ILAE Commission on Classification and Terminology, 2005–2009. *Epilepsia* 51(4):676–685, 2010.
4. Goodkin HP, Riviello JJ Jr: status epilepticus, in Wyllie E: *Treatment of Epilepsy: Principles and Practice*. 5th ed. Philadelphia, PA, Lippincott Williams & Wilkins, 2011, pp 469–470.
5. DeLorenzo RJ, Pellock JM, Towne AR, et al: Epidemiology of status epilepticus. *J ClinNeurophysiol* 12:316–325, 1995.
6. Hui AC, Cheng C, Lam A, et al: Prognosis following postanoxic myoclonus status epilepticus. *EurNeurol* 54(1):10, 2005.
7. Cokar O, Aydin B, Ozer F: Nonketotichyperglycemia presenting as epilepsia partialis continua. *Seizure* 13(4):264, 2004.
8. Meierkord H, Holtkamp M: Non-convulsive status epilepticus in adults: clinical forms and treatment. *Lancet Neurol* 6(4):329–339, 2007.
9. Claassen J, Mayer SA, Kowalski RG, et al: Detection of electrographic seizures with continuous EEG monitoring in critically ill patients. *Neurology* 62:1743–1748, 2004.
10. Shneker BF, Fountain NB: Assessment of acute morbidity and mortality in nonconvulsive status epilepticus. *Neurology* 61:1006, 2003.
11. Beniczky S, Hirsch LJ, Kaplan PW, et al: Unified EEG terminology and criteria for nonconvulsive status epilepticus. *Epilepsia* 54[Suppl 6]:28–29, 2013.
12. Davis R, Dalmau J: Autoimmunity, seizures, and status epilepticus. *Epilepsia* 54[Suppl 6]:46–49, 2013.
13. Gaspard N, Foreman BP, Alvarez V, et al; Critical Care EEG Monitoring Research Consortium (CCEMRC); Critical Care EEG Monitoring Research Consortium CCEMRC: New-onset refractory status epilepticus: etiology, clinical features, and outcome. *Neurology* 85(18):1604–1613, 2015.
14. DeLorenzo RJ, Garnett LK, Towne AR, et al: Comparison of status epilepticus with prolonged seizure episodes lasting from 10 to 29 minutes. *Epilepsia* 40(2):164–169, 1999.
15. Payne TA, Bleck TP: Status epilepticus. *Crit Care Clin* 13(1):17, 1997.
16. Simon RP: Physiologic consequences of status epilepticus. *Epilepsia* 26 [Suppl 1]:58, 1985.
17. Meldrum BS, Vigouroux RA, Brierley JB: Systemic factors and epileptic brain damage. *Arch Neurol* 29:82, 1973.
18. Alldredge BK, Lowenstein DH: Status epilepticus: new concepts. *Curr Opin Neurol* 12:183, 1999.
19. Lothman E: The biochemical basis and pathophysiology of status epilepticus. *Neurology* 40[Suppl 2]:13, 1990.
20. Krumholz A, Sung GY, Fisher RS, et al: Complex partial status epilepticus accompanied by serious morbidity and mortality. *Neurology* 45(8):1499, 1995.
21. Soffer D, Melamed E, Assaf Y, et al: Hemispheric brain damage in unilateral status epilepticus. *Ann Neurol* 20:737, 1986.
22. Fabene PF, Marzola P, Sbarbati A, et al: Magnetic resonance imaging of chages elicited by status epilepticus in the rat brain: diffusion-weighted and T2-weighted images, regional blood volume maps and direct correlation with tissue and cell damage. *Neuroimage* 18:375–389, 2003.
23. Szabo K, Poepel A, Pohlmann-Eden B, et al: Diffusion weighted and perfusion MRI demonstrate parenchymal changes in complex partial status epilepticus. *Brain* 128(6):1369, 2005.
24. Kaplan PW: Nonconvulsive status epilepticus. *SeminNeurol* 16:33–40, 1996.
25. Treiman DM, Meyers PD, Walton NY, et al: Veterans Affairs Status Epilepticus Cooperative Study Group: a comparison of four treatments for generalized convulsive status epilepticus. *N Engl J Med* 339(12):792, 1998.
26. Wijdicks EF, Hubmayr RD: Acute acid-base disorders associated with status epilepticus. *Mayo ClinProc* 69:1044, 1994.
27. Shaner DM, McCurdy SA, Herring MO, et al: Treatment of status epilepticus: a prospective comparison of diazepam and phenytoin versus phenobarbital and optional phenytoin. *Neurology* 38:202, 1988.
28. Treiman DM: Pharmacokinetics and clinical use of benzodiazepines in the management of status epilepticus. *Epilepsia* 30[Suppl 2]:S4, 1989.
29. Greenblatt DJ, Divoll M: Diazepam versus lorazepam: relationship of drug distribution to duration of clinical action, in Delgado-Escueta AV, Wasterlain CG, Treiman DM, et al (eds): *Advances in Neurology. Status Epilepticus*. Vol. 34. New York, NY, Raven Press, 1983, p 487.
30. Silbergleit R, Durkalski V, Lowenstein D, et al: Intramuscular versus intravenous therapy for prehospital status epilepticus. *N Engl J Med* 366(7): 591–600, 2012.
31. Cereghino JJ, Cloyd JC, Kuzniecky RI, et al: Rectal diazepam gel for treatment of acute repetitive seizures in adults. *Arch Neurol* 59(12):1915, 2002.
32. Pellock JM, Shinnar S: Respiratory adverse events associated with diazepam rectal gel. *Neurology* 64(10):1768, 2005.
33. Schmidt D: Benzodiazepines: diazepam, in Levy RH, Dreifuss FE, Mattson RH, et al (eds): *Antiepileptic Drugs*. New York, NY, Raven Press, 1989, p 735.
34. Manno EM: New management strategies in the treatment of status epilepticus. *Mayo ClinProc* 78:508, 2003.
35. O'Brien TJ, Cascino GD, So E, et al: Incidence and clinical consequence of the purple glove syndrome in patients receiving intravenous phenytoin. *Neurology* 51:1034, 1998.
36. Browne TR, Kugler AR, Eldon MA: Pharmacology and pharmacokinetics of fosphenytoin. *Neurology* 46[Suppl 1]:3, 1996.
37. DeToledo JC, Ramsay RE: Fosphenytoin and phenytoin in patients with status epilepticus. *Drug Saf* 22(6):459, 2000.
38. Knake S, Gruener J, Hattemer K, et al: Intravenous levetiracetam in the treatment of benzodiazepine refractory status epilepticus. *J Neurol Neurosurg Psychiatry* 79:588–589, 2008.
39. Yasiry Z. Shorvon SD: The relative effectiveness of five antiepileptic drugs in treatment of benzodiazepine-resistant convulsive status epilepticus: a meta-analysis of published studies. *Seizure* 23:167–174, 2014.
40. Hofler J, Unterberger I, Dobesberger J, et al: Intravenous lacosamide in status epilepticus and seizure clusters. *Epilepsia* 52:e148–e152, 2011.
41. Sinha S, Naritoku DK: Intravenous valproate is well tolerated in unstable patients with status epilepticus. *Neurology* 55(5):722, 2000.
42. Devinsky O, Leppik I, Willmore LJ, et al: Safety of intravenous valproate. *Ann Neurol* 38:670, 1995.
43. Venkataraman V, Wheless JW: Safety of rapid intravenous infusion of valproate loading doses in epilepsy patients. *Epilepsy Res* 35:147, 1999.
44. Limdi NA, Shimpi AV, Faught E, et al: Efficacy of rapid IV administration of valproic acid for status epilepticus. *Neurology* 64:353, 2005.
45. Whelass JW, Vazquez BR, Kanner AM, et al: Rapid infusion of valproate is well tolerated in patients with epilepsy. *Neurology* 63(8):1507–1508, 2004.
46. Peters CN, Pohlmann-Eden B: Intravenous valproate as an innovative therapy in seizure emergency situations including status epilepticus—experience in 102 adult patients. *Seizure* 14(3):164, 2005.
47. Rossetti A, Reichhart M, Schaller M, et al: Propofol treatment of refractory status epilepticus: a study of 31 episodes. *Epilepsia* 45(7):757, 2004.

48. Stecker MM, Kramer TH, Raps EC, et al: Treatment of refractory status epilepticus with propofol: clinical and pharmacokinetic findings. *Epilepsia* 39(1):18, 1998.
49. Kalviainen R, Eriksson K, Parviainen I: Refractory generalised convulsive status epilepticus: a guide to treatment. *CNS Drugs* 19(9):759, 2005.
50. Hanley DF, Kross JF: Use of midazolam in the treatment of refractory status epilepticus. *Clin Ther* 20(6):1093, 1998.
51. Koul RL, Raj Aithala G, Chacko A, et al: Continuous midazolam infusion as a treatment for status epilepticus. *Arch Dis Child* 76(5):445, 1997.
52. Bledsoe KA, Kramer AH: Propylene glycol toxicity in barbiturate coma. *Neurocrit Care* 9(1):122–124, 2008.
53. Claassen J, Hirsch LJ, Emerson RG, et al: Treatment of refractory status epilepticus with pentobarbital, propofol, or midazolam: a systematic review. *Epilepsia* 43(2):146, 2002.
54. Wusthoff CJ, Kranick SM, Morley JF, et al: The ketogenic diet in treatment of two adults with prolonged nonconvulsive status epilepticus. *Epilepsia* 51(6)1083–1085, 2010.

Chapter 152 ■ Guillain–Barré Syndrome

ISABELITA R. BELLA • DAVID A. CHAD

Guillain–Barré syndrome (GBS) was described by Guillain, Barré, and Strohl in 1916 as an acute flaccid paralysis with areflexia and elevated spinal fluid protein without pleocytosis [1]. It is the most common cause of rapidly progressive weakness due to peripheral nerve involvement, with an annual incidence of 0.6 to 2.0 cases per 100,000 population [2]. For decades, GBS has been viewed as an acute inflammatory *demyelinating* polyradiculoneuropathy (AIDP) affecting nerve roots and cranial and peripheral nerves of unknown cause that occurs at all ages. In the past 20 years, the recognition of primary *axonal* forms of GBS has broadened the spectrum of GBS to include the demyelinating form (AIDP) and axonal forms—acute motor axonal neuropathy (AMAN) and acute motor sensory axonal neuropathy (AMSAN), as well as the Miller Fisher syndrome. AIDP is the most common subtype in developed countries, whereas axonal forms are more common in northern China.

Because of the potential for the development of respiratory insufficiency and autonomic nervous system abnormalities [3], GBS is most appropriately recognized as a potential medical and neurologic emergency that typically requires intensive care, to treat and manage the potential complications of the illness [4].

DIAGNOSIS

Clinical Features in Acute Inflammatory Demyelinating Polyradiculoneuropathy

GBS often occurs 2 to 4 weeks after a flu-like or diarrheal illness caused by a variety of infectious agents [3], including cytomegalovirus; Epstein–Barr and herpes simplex viruses; mycoplasma; Chlamydia; and *Campylobacter jejuni* [5]. It can also be an early manifestation of human immunodeficiency virus (HIV) infection before the development of an immunosuppressed state [6]. Lyme disease may rarely produce a syndrome of polyradiculopathy reminiscent of GBS [7]. Other antecedent events include immunization; general surgery and renal transplantation; Hodgkin's disease; and systemic lupus erythematosus [2,3].

The illness is heralded by the presence of dysesthesias of the feet or hands, or both. The major feature is weakness that evolves rapidly (usually over days) and classically has been described as ascending from legs to arms and, in severe cases, to respiratory and bulbar muscles. Weakness may, however, start in the cranial nerves or arms and descend to the legs or start simultaneously in the arms and legs [2]. Proximal muscles are often involved early in the course of the disease. Approximately 50% of patients reach the nadir of their clinical course by 2 weeks into the illness, 80% by 3 weeks, and 90% by 1 month [8]. Progression of symptoms beyond 4 weeks but arresting within 8 weeks has been termed *subacute inflammatory demyelinating polyneuropathy* (SIDP) [9], whereas progression beyond 2 months is designated *chronic inflammatory demyelinating polyradiculoneuropathy* (CIDP), a disorder with a natural history different from GBS [10]. Up to 16% of patients with CIDP may present acutely as GBS; those that continue to progress to CIDP more often have pronounced sensory signs, and are less likely to have facial weakness, autonomic involvement, a preceding infectious illness, or require mechanical ventilation [11]. A small percentage of patients (up to 6%) have recurrent GBS; these patients are often younger than 30 years, have milder symptoms, and more often have Miller Fisher syndrome. Several years often pass between episodes, differentiating them from patients with treatment-related fluctuation, where worsening occurs within the first 8 weeks of disease onset after initial improvement/stabilization [12].

The extent and distribution of weakness in GBS are variable. Within a few days, a patient may become quadriparetic and become respirator dependent, or the illness may take a benign course and after progression for 3 weeks produce only mild weakness of the face and limbs.

Physical Findings

In a typical case of moderate severity, the physical examination discloses symmetric weakness in proximal and distal muscle groups with attenuation or loss of deep tendon reflexes (Table 152.1). In the early stage of the illness, there is no muscle wasting or fasciculation. If the attack is particularly severe and axons are interrupted, muscles undergo atrophy and scattered fasciculations may be seen after a number of months. Sensory loss is usually mild, although a variant of GBS is described in which sensory loss (involving large fiber modalities) is widespread, symmetric, and profound [8]. Respiratory muscles are often involved, and 10% to 25% of patients require ventilator assistance [13] within 18 days (mean of 10 days) after onset [14].

There is often mild to moderate bilateral facial weakness. Mild weakness of the tongue and the muscles of deglutition may

TABLE 152.1

Features of Guillain–Barré Syndrome

Clinical features	Laboratory features
Rapidly progressive weakness	Elevated cerebrospinal fluid protein
Loss of reflexes	Acellular cerebrospinal fluid
Mild dysesthesias (in AIDP)	Electromyogram:
Autonomic dysfunction	In AIDP: slow nerve conduction velocities, conduction block, and dispersed responses
Respiratory compromise	In axonal GBS: low motor amplitudes, normal conduction velocities, and normal sensory responses in AMAN

AIDP, acute inflammatory demyelinating polyradiculoneuropathy; AMAN, acute motor axonal neuropathy; GBS, Guillain–Barré syndrome.

also develop. Ophthalmoparesis from extraocular motor nerve involvement is unusual in the typical patient with GBS. In the Miller Fisher variant [15], however, ophthalmoplegia occurs in combination with ataxia and areflexia, with little limb weakness. Pupillary abnormalities have been noted in GBS [16] and in the Miller Fisher variant [17]. Papilledema is rare [18].

Autonomic nervous system disturbances occur in 50% of patients and are potentially lethal [3,4]. Autonomic dysfunction takes the form of excessive or inadequate activity of the sympathetic or parasympathetic nervous system, or both [19]. Common findings include cardiac arrhythmias (e.g., persistent sinus tachycardia, bradycardia, ventricular tachycardia, atrial flutter, atrial fibrillation, and asystole); orthostatic hypotension; and transient or persistent hypertension. Other changes include transient bladder paralysis; increased or decreased sweating; and paralytic ileus. The pathophysiology of these changes is not completely understood but may be caused by inflammation of the thinly myelinated and unmyelinated axons of the peripheral autonomic nervous system. A neuropathy predominantly affecting the peripheral autonomic nervous system has been described that may have a pathogenesis similar to that of GBS [20].

Clinical Features in Axonal Forms

Like AIDP, axonal forms present with rapidly progressive weakness, areflexia, and albuminocytological dissociation but differ in the following ways: (1) Patients with AMAN lack sensory abnormalities; (2) most often children and young adults in northern China, Mexico, or Japan develop AMAN during summer months; (3) Many have experienced an antecedent Campylobacter jejuni infection. Patients with AMAN also have a more rapid progression to their nadir, but recovery times are quicker [21] or similar [22] to AIDP in some, whereas other patients have a protracted recovery [21].

AMSAN is characterized by sensory and motor deficits, and a long time to recovery. In the series by Feasby et al. [23], these patients had a much shorter time to peak severity (1 week), had more severe symptoms with more than half requiring mechanical ventilation, and had inexcitable motor nerves; and most had a poor recovery.

Laboratory Features

The most characteristic laboratory features of GBS are an abnormal cerebrospinal fluid (CSF) profile with albuminocytologic dissociation (elevated protein without pleocytosis) and abnormal nerve conduction studies.

CSF examination is helpful in supporting the diagnosis of GBS. Although the CSF profile is usually normal during the first 48 hours after onset [8], by 1 week into the illness, the CSF protein is elevated in most patients, sometimes to levels as high as 1 g per dL. Rarely, even several weeks after onset of GBS, the CSF protein remains normal and the diagnosis must rest on the presence of otherwise typical clinical features [8]. The cell count may be slightly increased but rarely exceeds 10 cells per μL; the cells are mononuclear in nature. When GBS occurs as a manifestation of HIV infection or Lyme disease, the CSF white cell count is generally increased (25 to 50 cells per μL). The CSF glucose is expected to be normal.

Electrodiagnostic studies in AIDP typically show a non-length dependent, motor and sensory demyelinating polyneuropathy with slowing of motor nerve conduction velocities (less than 70% of the lower limit of normal); increases in distal motor latencies; and evidence of temporal dispersion and partial conduction block along motor fibers. F-waves are absent or have prolonged latencies; and sensory responses are reduced or absent [8,24]. The amplitude of the evoked motor responses may be reduced because of axon loss or distal nerve conduction block, and the responses are frequently dispersed because of differential slowing along still-conducting axons [8,24]. Because the pathologic process may be restricted to spinal nerve roots and proximal nerve segments, routine nerve conduction studies early in the course of the neuropathy may be normal initially. In such cases H-reflexes are often absent and F-responses are abnormal (absent or prolonged in latency).These abnormal late responses along with sural sparing (normal sural response), and reduced or absent median sensory response is characteristic of early GBS [25]. Early in the course of GBS, needle electrode examination of voluntary contraction of weak muscles demonstrates reduced motor unit potential recruitment (decreased numbers of normal appearing motor unit potentials firing rapidly) because of nerve conduction block. Several weeks later, needle examination of weak muscles reveals active denervation changes, with fibrillation potentials and positive sharp waves, reflecting the motor axon loss that is often part of AIDP, and central to the pathogenesis of AMAN and AMSAN.

In patients with the severe axonal form of GBS, AMSAN, motor and sensory nerves may be electrically inexcitable [23]. In AMAN, motor responses are low or absent, whereas conduction velocities and sensory responses are normal [26].The electrodiagnostic findings in the Miller Fisher syndrome are indicative of a sensory neuronopathy with reduced or absent sensory responses throughout despite normal motor studies.

Except for a mild increase in the erythrocyte sedimentation rate, hematologic studies are normal. Serum electrolytes may disclose hyponatremia [3], sometimes to a marked degree, because of inappropriate secretion of antidiuretic hormone (SIADH) caused by a disturbance of peripheral volume receptors. There may be evidence of previous viral or *mycoplasma* infection, such as lymphopenia or atypical lymphocytes. In some cases, evidence of recent viral infection may be sought by measuring antibody (immunoglobulin [Ig] M) titers against specific infectious agents, especially cytomegalovirus, Epstein–Barr virus, and *C. jejuni*. In selected cases, screening for HIV infection should be undertaken.

Approximately 90% of Miller Fisher syndrome patients have high titers of GQ1b antibodies, and their presence confirms the diagnosis of this disorder. Antibodies to GM1, GD1a,

GM1b, and GalNac-GD1a are associated with axonal forms of GBS. Anti-GM1 antibodies are reported in 10% to 42% of AMAN patients [27].

DIFFERENTIAL DIAGNOSIS

A number of well-defined conditions cause an acute or subacute onset of generalized weakness and must be differentiated from GBS (Table152.2). These are disorders of the motor unit affecting the neuromuscular junction (e.g., myasthenia gravis and botulism); peripheral nerve (e.g., tick paralysis, shellfish poisoning, toxic neuropathy, acute intermittent porphyria, and diphtheritic neuropathy); motor neuron (e.g., amyotrophic lateral sclerosis, poliomyelitis, and West Nile virus [WNV] neuroinvasive disease); and muscle (e.g., periodic paralysis, metabolic myopathies, and inflammatory myopathies). Other conditions characterized by severe generalized weakness are defined by the setting in which they are encountered—the intensive care unit (ICU)—and are designated *critical illness polyneuropathy* and the *myopathy of intensive care.*

Intensive Care Unit–Related Weakness

Unlike neuromuscular emergencies such as GBS, myasthenia gravis, or porphyria, in which rapidly progressive weakness develops before admission to the ICU, a number of conditions (polyneuropathy, myopathy, and neuromuscular junction disease) affect patients already in the ICU because of severe systemic illnesses. These conditions are discussed in more detail in Chapter 154. Critical illness polyneuropathy is an axonal sensory and motor polyneuropathy characterized by difficulty weaning from the ventilator, distal greater than proximal muscle weakness, and reduced or absent reflexes that develop in patients with sepsis and multiorgan failure [28]. The development of weakness in the midst of critical illness, as seen in critical illness polyneuropathy, helps differentiate this disorder from axonal GBS, in which weakness develops days to weeks after an infection [29]. A severe necrotizing myopathy can also be seen in critically ill patients [30]. An acute myopathy of intensive care initially described in patients treated with a combination of high-dose corticosteroids (equal to or greater than 1,000 mg methylprednisolone) and neuromuscular blocking agents (NMBAs) for status asthmaticus [31] may also be encountered in the setting of trauma, organ transplantation, burns, and critical illness. Patients have variable degrees of generalized weakness, including respiratory muscles, and this is often recognized when a patient has difficulty weaning from the ventilator. Prolonged neuromuscular blockade after use of the nondepolarizing NMBAs can be seen especially in patients with coexistent renal failure and metabolic acidosis. Presumably, the presence of an active metabolite accounts for the prolonged weakness [32].

Disorders of the Neuromuscular Junction

In patients with *myasthenia gravis*, limb weakness is predominant proximally and almost always associated with ocular and sometimes pharyngeal muscle weakness (see Table152.2; see Chapter 153). Muscular fatigability is a hallmark of the disease. Botulism may also cause acute weakness 6 to 36 hours after ingestion of the toxin formed by *Clostridium botulinum*. The condition is characterized by weakness of cranial nerve–innervated muscles, autonomic abnormalities (unreactive pupils and ileus), and occasional respiratory muscle weakness necessitating ventilator assistance. Electrodiagnostic findings of low compound motor action potential amplitudes with post-excercise facilitation are key in diagnosing this condition.

TABLE 152.2

Conditions That May Mimic Guillain–Barré Syndrome

Disorder	Major distinguishing features
Myasthenia gravis	Reflexes are spared Ocular weakness predominates Positive response to edrophonium EMG: decremental motor response
Botulism	Predominant bulbar involvement Autonomic abnormalities (pupils) EMG: normal velocities, low amplitudes, and incremental response (with high-frequency repetitive nerve stimulation)
Tick paralysis	Rapid progression (1–2 d) Tick present
Shellfish poisoning	Rapid onset (face, finger, and toe numbness) Follows consumption of mussels/clams
Toxic neuropathies	EMG: usually axon loss
Organophosphorus	Acute cholinergic reaction toxicity
Porphyric neuropathy	Mental disturbance Abdominal pain
Diphtheritic neuropathy	Prior pharyngitis Slower evolution Palatal/accommodation paralysis Myocarditis
Poliomyelitis	Weakness, pain, and tenderness Preserved sensation Cerebrospinal fluid: protein and cell count elevated
West Nile virus neuroinvasive disease	Associated fever, meningitis, or encephalitis Asymmetric weakness Cerebrospinal fluid: protein and cell count elevated
Periodic paralysis	Reflexes normal Cranial nerves and respiration spared Abnormal serum potassium concentration
Critical illness neuropathy	Sepsis and multiorgan failure >2 wk EMG: axon loss
Acute myopathy of intensive care	Tetraparesis and areflexia Follows prolonged treatment with neuromuscular-blocking agent and corticosteroids Trauma, status asthmaticus, and organ transplantation associated Clinical and EMG features of myopathy

EMG, electromyogram.

Disorders of Peripheral Nerve

Tick paralysis is produced by a toxin contained in the head of the tick *Dermacentor andersoni* or *D. vanabilis* that blocks nerve conduction in the fine terminal portions of motor and sensory nerves. Weakness associated with sensory impairment develops rapidly after the tick has embedded itself into the victim, usually over 1 to 2 days. *Shellfish poisoning* gives rise to symptoms immediately after contaminated mussels or clams are eaten. Patients complain of face, finger, and toe numbness and then note the development of rapidly progressive descending paralysis, which may involve respiratory muscles.

Toxic neuropathies may be caused by a number of heavy metals, including arsenic, thallium, and lead. These and other potential neurotoxins (e.g., nitrofurantoin) and industrial agents (e.g., hexacarbons) may produce a rapidly evolving peripheral neuropathy. Most acute toxic neuropathies are axon loss in character, but in the case of arsenic poisoning, electrodiagnostic features may simulate a demyelinating process identical to some forms of GBS [33]. Organophosphorus insecticide toxicity causes a short-lived acute cholinergic phase marked by miosis, salivation, sweating, and fasciculation followed in 2 to 3 weeks by an acute axon-loss polyneuropathy [34]. An intermediate syndrome occurring 24 to 96 hours after the cholinergic phase and characterized by multiple cranial nerve palsies and respiratory failure has also been described [35]. The latter probably results from a defect at the neuromuscular junction.

Acute intermittent porphyria causes an acute polyneuropathy clinically similar to GBS but differing by its association with mental disturbance and abdominal pain. Attacks of paralysis are precipitated by ingestion of a variety of drugs, including alcohol, barbiturates, estrogens, phenytoin, and sulfonamides. The diagnosis may be established by demonstrating increased levels of porphobilinogen and δ-aminolevulinic acid in the urine.

Diphtheritic neuropathy occurs 2 to 8 weeks after a throat infection. During the height of the infection, there is numbness of the lips and paralysis of pharyngeal and laryngeal muscles. At the time of the neuropathy, diphtheria organisms may be cultured from the throat. Other clues to the diagnosis are clinical and electrocardiographic features of myocarditis.

Disorders of Motor Neurons

Amyotrophic lateral sclerosis is a chronic disorder of the motor system that generally evolves over several years to produce a state of severe generalized muscle weakness, atrophy, and fasciculations. In most instances, respiratory muscle weakness occurs in the latter stages of the illness after the diagnosis has been established. Rarely, however, patients present with acute to subacute respiratory muscle weakness (ventilatory failure) as the first clinical manifestation of this disease. The examination of such patients often discloses some features of lower motor neuron loss (muscle atrophy and fasciculations) in limb and bulbar muscles. The presence of brisk deep tendon reflexes and preserved sensation helps to distinguish this disorder from the neuropathies that might cause acute ventilatory failure. Unlike the situation in GBS where a picture of albuminocytologic dissociation is found, the CSF findings in amyotrophic lateral sclerosis are normal.

Poliomyelitis is rarely seen today, but it has developed in close contacts of newborns immunized with the live attenuated oral vaccine, and individuals whose own immunity to the virus has become inadequate. The disease is characterized by weakness of rapid onset along with severe muscle pain and tenderness. Respiratory muscles are often involved. Deep tendon reflexes are depressed. The illness is distinguished from GBS clinically by the preservation of sensation and the CSF findings. Serum antibody studies may help identify the illness.

A poliomyelitis-like syndrome may also be seen with WNV neuroinvasive disease. Infection of the anterior horn cells by the WNV produces an acute flaccid paralysis, with asymmetric weakness of one or more limbs, particularly the legs, along with hyporeflexia or areflexia. Overt sensory loss is typically absent, whereas loss of bowel and bladder function may occur. Unlike GBS, there may be an associated meningitis, encephalitis, or fever, in addition to CSF pleocytosis and elevated CSF protein. Diagnosis depends on detection of WNV-specific antibodies in serum or CSF [36].

Disorders of Muscles

Periodic paralysis (hyperkalemic or hypokalemic) is a disorder of muscle usually inherited in an autosomal-dominant fashion. Patients develop generalized weakness over a period of hours (see Table152.2). Cranial nerve–supplied muscles are spared, there is generally no respiratory muscle involvement, reflexes are normal, and there is no sensory involvement. Serum potassium measurements aid in the diagnosis.

Rarely, metabolic myopathies may present with the sudden onset of muscle weakness. Patients with abnormalities of glycogen metabolism (e.g., phosphorylase deficiency) or lipid metabolism (e.g., carnitine palmityl transferase deficiency) may develop weakness associated with severe cramps and muscle fiber necrosis; the latter may result in creatine kinase elevations and myoglobinuria.

Dermatomyositis, an inflammatory myopathy, may present with the acute onset of proximal muscle (and, rarely, respiratory muscle) weakness. In contrast to the acute polyneuropathies, deep tendon reflexes are spared, cranial nerves are rarely involved, and serum creatine kinase is elevated.

PATHOGENESIS

AIDP is caused by immunologically mediated demyelination of the peripheral nervous system [3]. It is likely that humoral and cellular components of the immune system participate in macrophage-induced peripheral nerve demyelination [2,37]. Although the histological appearance of AIDP resembles experimental autoimmune neuritis, in which a predominantly T-cell–mediated immune response is directed against peripheral nerve myelin proteins, the role of T-cell–mediated immunity in AIDP remains unclear [37]. The finding of complement activation markers along the outer surface of the Schwann cell [38] have led to the speculation that complement-fixing antibodies directed toward as yet unidentified epitopes on the outer surface of the Schwann cell play a role in AIDP. Axonal degeneration may occur, especially in severe cases, as a "bystander" when there is intense inflammation [39,40].

In axonal subtypes, the immune response is targeted to a different portion of the peripheral nerve, the axon [41]. There is strong evidence that antibodies directed against ganglioside antigens on the axolemma target macrophages to invade the axon at the node of Ranvier [37]. The rapid decline and subsequent quick recovery in many AMAN patients suggests that severe axonal degeneration of the nerve roots is unlikely to be the pathological basis for this disorder; proposed mechanisms include physiological block of conduction or very distal degeneration and subsequent regeneration of the intramuscular motor nerve terminals [22].

The presence of antiganglioside antibodies (GM1, GD1a, GM1b, and GalNAcGD1a antibodies in axonal GBS and GQ1b in Miller Fisher syndrome), and the finding of ganglioside-like epitopes on some strains of *C. jejuni* have led to the concept of molecular mimicry [42], in which an immune attack occurs on the epitope shared by the nerve fiber and infectious organism [43], as a possible mechanism for GBS, especially *C. jejuni*–associated GBS. There is increasing evidence that anti-GM1 antibodies block sodium ion channels at the nodes of Ranvier, transiently producing conduction failure [27]. In addition, Koga et al. [44] found evidence that the genetic polymorphism of *C. jejuni* determines the production of specific autoantibodies and correlates with the clinical presentation of GBS, possibly through modification of the host-mimicking molecule.

PATHOLOGY

Pathological studies of nerves from patients dying with GBS have usually shown infiltration of the endoneurium by mononuclear cells, with a predilection for a perivenular distribution [39]. The inflammatory process occurs throughout the length of the nerve, from its origin at a root level to the distal ramifications of nerve twigs in the substance of muscle fibers. The brunt of the inflammatory process, however, occurs at more proximal levels (e.g., roots, spinal nerves, and major plexuses) and takes the form of discrete foci of inflammation. Macrophages invade intact myelin sheaths and denude the axons [37]. Patients with prominent axon loss are least likely to recover fully and may be left with functionally significant residual motor weakness.

In AMAN and AMSAN, there is evidence of Wallerian-like degeneration of nerve fibers, but only minimal inflammation or demyelination. Macrophages are seen within the periaxonal space especially at the nodes of Ranvier, displacing or surrounding the axon, and leaving the myelin sheath intact [26]. Abnormalities are seen in nerve roots and peripheral nerves; in those with AMSAN, motor and sensory fibers are affected, whereas only motor fibers are affected in AMAN, with sparing of sensory fibers.

NATURAL HISTORY

The natural history of GBS in the moderately to severely affected patient (i.e., a patient who is unable to walk or who has severe respiratory muscle weakness requiring a ventilator) is usually one of gradual improvement. The ability to walk unassisted returns, on average, in approximately 3 months; in the subset of respirator-dependent patients, the average time to recovery is 6 months [45].

MANAGEMENT

The three major treatment issues in GBS are controlling respiration and deciding when to intubate the patient, recognizing and managing autonomic dysfunction, and determining which patients are candidates for plasmapheresis or intravenous immunoglobulin (IVIG) (Table152.3).

Patients with GBS require excellent nursing care, medical management, and emotional support. Respiratory failure is one of the most serious complications of GBS. Need for a ventilator cannot be reliably predicted on the basis of extent of weakness; however, patients who are highly likely to require mechanical ventilation are those with rapid disease progression, bulbar weakness, autonomic dysfunction, and bilateral facial weakness [46]. Patients must be followed up carefully with measurements of maximum inspiratory pressure and forced vital capacity (FVC) (Fig. 152.1) until weakness has stopped progressing, so the respiratory insufficiency can be anticipated and managed appropriately. A normal FVC is 65 mL per kg; a level of 30 mL per kg is generally associated with a poor forced cough and requires careful observation and management with supplemental oxygen and chest physical therapy. At 25 mL per kg, the sigh mechanism is compromised and atelectasis occurs, leading to hypoxemia. Ropper and Kehne [47] suggest intubation if any one of the following criteria is met: mechanical ventilatory failure with reduced expiratory vital capacity (VC) of 12 to 15 mL per kg; oropharyngeal paresis with aspiration; falling VC over 4 to 6 hours; or clinical signs of respiratory fatigue at a VC of 15 mL per kg. Lawn et al. [46] found the following respiratory factors to be highly associated with progression to respiratory failure: VC less than 20 mL per kg; maximal inspiratory pressure (MIP) less than 30 cm H_2O; maximal expiratory pressure (MEP) less than 40 cm H_2O; or a reduction of more than 30% of VC, MIP, or MEP in 24 hours. Elective intubation may be considered in these patients at particularly high risk for progression to respiratory failure. Intubation should be accomplished with a soft-cuff low-pressure endotracheal tube. A decision to delay tracheostomy for 7 to 10 days is likely to avoid the operation in as many as one-third of patients who improve rapidly and can be extubated after the first few days [47]. Complications of intubation and ventilator assistance are described in Chapters 8 and 166.

TABLE 152.3

Management of Guillain–Barré Syndrome

General	Monitor respiratory parameters: VC, arterial blood gas
	Intubate if: VC <12–15 mL/kg Oropharyngeal paresis with aspiration Falling vital capacity over 4–6 h Respiratory fatigue with VC 15 mL/kg
	Use short-acting medications to control autonomic dysfunction
	Nursing care: frequent turns to avoid pressure sores
	Place pads at elbows and fibular head to avoid compression neuropathies
	Physical therapy
	Subcutaneous heparin
Treatment:	
Plasmapheresis	Exchange a total of 200 mL plasma/kg body weight over 7–14 d (40–50 mL/kg for 3–5 sessions)[a]
	Albumin is used as replacement solution, not fresh-frozen plasma
	During plasmapheresis, monitor blood pressure and pulse every 30 min
	Obtain complete blood cell count (baseline and before each exchange to calculate plasma volume)
	Obtain immunoglobulin levels before first exchange and after last exchange; if immunoglobulin G <200 mg/dL after last plasma exchange, infuse 400 mg/kg IVIG
IVIG	2 g/kg divided over 5 consecutive d[b] (0.4 g/kg/d for 5 d)

[a]This is the authors' approach, following the Guillain–Barré Syndrome Study Group guidelines [44]. Other published guidelines recommend two sessions (exchanging 40 mL/kg per session) for ambulatory patients and four sessions (exchanging 40 mL/kg per session) for nonambulatory patients [53].
[b]The authors adhere to the protocol published by the Dutch Guillain–Barré Study Group [54].
IVIG, intravenous immunoglobulin; VC, vital capacity.

The nursing and medical team must also be aware of the many autonomic nervous system disturbances that can occur [19]. Fluctuating blood pressure with transient hypertensive episodes, sometimes associated with extreme degrees of agitation, may be present. Other manifestations of sympathetic nervous system overactivity include sudden diaphoresis, general

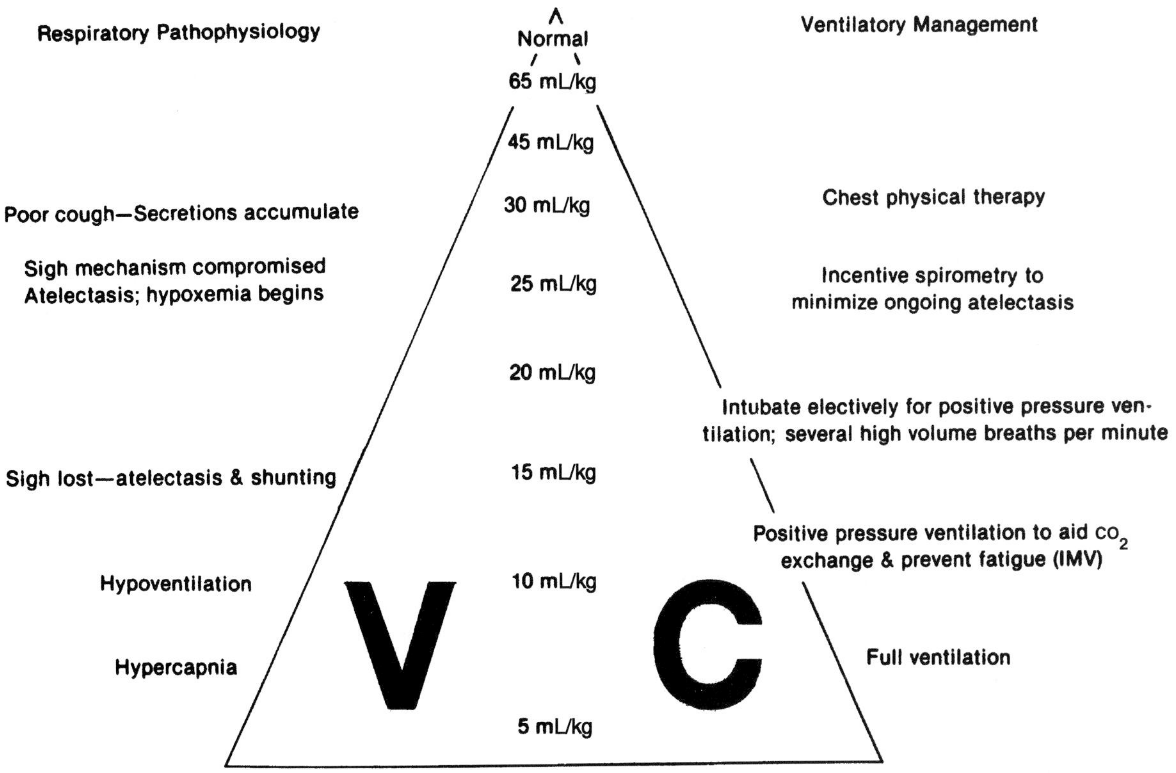

FIGURE 152.1 Relations between vital capacity (VC), pathophysiology of lung function, and suggested therapy in mechanical ventilatory failure. IMV, intermittent mandatory ventilation. (From Ropper AH: Guillain-Barré syndrome, in Ropper AH, Kennedy SK, Zervas NT (eds): *Neurological and Neurosurgical Intensive Care*. Baltimore, University Park Press, 1983, with permission.)

vasoconstriction, and sinus tachycardia. Evidence of underactivity of the sympathetic nervous system includes presence of marked postural hypotension and heightened sensitivity to dehydration and sedative–hypnotic agents. Excessive parasympathetic nervous system activity is reflected in facial flushing associated with a feeling of generalized warmth and bradycardia. Electrocardiographic changes, consisting of ST-and T-wave changes, also occur. Therefore, careful monitoring of blood pressure, fluid status, and cardiac rhythm is absolutely essential to manage the GBS patient. Hypertension may be managed with short-acting α-adrenergic blocking agents, hypotension with fluids, and bradyarrhythmias with atropine [19]. As noted earlier, hyponatremia may occur and is probably best managed by free water restriction.

The bedridden patient needs to be turned frequently to avoid the development of pressure sores. Paralyzed limbs require the attention of the physiotherapist so that passive limb movements can be carried out and contractures prevented. The ICU team needs to be aware of the potential for development of compression neuropathies (most commonly of the ulnar and peroneal nerves), and insulating pads should be placed over the usual susceptible sites (the elbow and the head of the fibula). Pain may be treated with standard doses of analgesic agents, but they do not often provide adequate relief. Gabapentin or carbamazepine is particularly helpful in treating the pain in the acute phase [48] and, when disabling, epidural morphine may be necessary [49]. Deep venous thrombosis and pulmonary embolism are ever-present dangers in the bedridden patient with immobilized limbs; for these patients, in addition to physical therapy, subcutaneous heparin (5,000 U twice per day) and support stockings are recommended [48].

A number of multicenter studies [45,50,51] showed that plasmapheresis has a beneficial effect on the course of the illness, even in those patients with several poor prognostic signs [52]. Patients treated with plasmapheresis are able to walk, on average, 1 month earlier than untreated patients; respirator-dependent patients so treated walk 3 months sooner than those who do not receive plasma exchange [45]. The GBS study group guidelines recommend exchanging 200 to 250 mL plasma per kg body weight over 7 to 14 days in three to five treatments [45]. Five percent salt-poor albumin is used as replacement fluid (fresh-frozen plasma should be avoided because of risks of hepatitis, HIV, and occasionally pulmonary edema). It is important to keep in mind, however, that there are also risks with albumin, including bleeding, thrombosis, and infection (owing to loss of coagulating factors and γ-globulins during plasma exchange, which are not present in the albumin replacement fluid). After each exchange, γ-globulin can be infused to prevent infection.

Plasmapheresis, in general, is recommended for patients who have reached or are approaching the inability to walk unaided, who require intubation or demonstrate a falling VC, and who have weakness of the bulbar musculature leading to dysphagia and aspiration [53]. The French Cooperative Group on Plasma Exchange in Guillain–Barré Syndrome [54] also showed that treatment of patients with mild GBS (i.e., those who are still ambulatory) is beneficial; two plasma exchanges were more beneficial than none in time to onset of motor recovery in patients with mild GBS. Patients with moderate (not ambulatory) or severe (mechanically ventilated) GBS benefited from four exchanges; those with severe GBS did not benefit any further with the addition of two more exchanges. Because of its potential for inducing hypotension, patients who have compromise of their cardiovascular system or autonomic dysfunction may not tolerate this procedure. Plasmapheresis is safe in pregnant women and children [4]. Plasmapheresis is generally not used in patients who are no longer progressing 21 days or more after the onset of GBS.

For many years, plasmapheresis was the gold standard for the treatment of GBS. In 1992, a large randomized trial performed by

Dutch investigators demonstrated that treatment with IVIG was at least as effective as plasmapheresis and might be superior [55]. A subsequent large randomized controlled trial (the Plasma Exchange/Sandoglobulin Guillain–Barré Syndrome Trial Group) confirmed the equivalence of IVIG and plasma exchange; in addition, there was no substantial benefit of using a combination of plasma exchange followed by IVIG [56]. In light of these studies, plasma exchange or IVIG may be used to treat GBS. Although both treatments are equally efficacious, IVIG has become the preferred treatment because of its relative ease of administration (plasmapheresis is not available in all centers, and it requires good venous access and a stable cardiovascular system). In 3% to 12% of patients given IVIG, side effects may occur that range from minor reactions such as flulike symptoms, headache, nausea, and malaise to more severe side effects, including anaphylactic reactions in IgA-deficient persons, transmission of hepatitis C, aseptic meningitis, and acute renal failure in those with renal insufficiency. Absolute contraindications to IVIG are unusual, however. For example, patients with IgA deficiency may be given an IgA-poor preparation with very careful monitoring and precautions (pretreatment with corticosteroids, diphenhydramine, and acetaminophen); individuals with renal insufficiency must be given an IVIG sucrose-poor preparation with very close monitoring of their renal status and consultation with a specialist in Nephrology before infusion.

A recent American Academy of Neurology practice parameter recommends treatment of GBS patients who are unable to walk with either plasmapheresis or IVIG; treatment is beneficial if given within 4 weeks of onset of neuropathic symptoms for plasmapheresis and within 2 weeks (and possibly 4 weeks) of onset for IVIG [57]. For those patients who are still ambulatory, plasmapheresis may also be considered if given within 2 weeks of onset. Treatment with plasmapheresis followed by IVIG is not recommended.

In a small number of patients (5%), spontaneous relapse occurs within days to weeks after treatment with IVIG or plasmapheresis, often in those treated early in their illness. Relapse rates are similar in frequency between IVIG and plasmapheresis [58]. Although retreatment with the same therapy is commonly practiced [59], evidence-based literature is lacking regarding the efficacy of repeat treatment [58]. Retreatment with the same therapy has also been suggested in those patients who are severely affected and unresponsive to treatment.

Although it seems intuitively obvious that treatment of GBS with corticosteroids should be beneficial, corticosteroids are ineffective and are not recommended in the treatment of GBS.

Finally, it is most important to address the emotional needs of the patient with GBS, who will almost certainly be anxious, fearful, and depressed. The strong likelihood of a good outcome, even in ventilated patients, is noted later in this chapter. Sometimes, it is helpful for the patient to speak with a person who has recovered from GBS.

OUTCOME AND PROGNOSTIC FACTORS

In most patients recovery occurs over weeks or months, but in some patients, muscle strength may take 1.5 to 2.0 years to reach its best state with an intensive rehabilitation program [2]. Recovery is not always complete; only 60% of patients recover full motor strength at 1 year, whereas 14% have severe motor problems. About 80% are able to walk independently at 6 months, improving to 84% by 1 year [60]. Although patients who are restored to nearly normal function can resume work and leisure activities, some degree of ankle dorsiflexor weakness or numbness of the feet is commonly encountered. About 5% to 10% have a protracted course, are ventilator dependent for several months, and do not fully recover [61]. Despite close monitoring in the ICU, deaths from GBS do occur, with mortality in the range of 3% to 8% [4]. Causes of fatal outcomes include dysautonomia, sepsis, acute respiratory distress syndrome, and pulmonary emboli [4].

Poor prognostic factors include older age (≥50 years); severe disease at nadir (bedbound or requiring mechanical ventilation); rapid onset of disease; preceding diarrheal illness; and evidence of axonal loss (reflected on electrodiagnostic studies) [27,37,60,62]. More recently, elevated CSF neurofilament levels predicted poor outcome, presumably reflecting axonal damage of the proximal motor nerve root [63]. A clinical prognostic scoring system has been developed to help predict the risk of respiratory failure during the first week along with the risk of being unable to walk at 6 months using several of the above prognostic factors [64,65]; it is available online at https://gbstools.erasmusmc.nl/prognosis-tool.

SUMMARY

Careful attention to the patient's history and thorough examination usually point to the diagnosis of GBS, which may be corroborated by the CSF findings (i.e., albuminocytologic dissociation) and results of electrophysiologic testing (i.e., acquired demyelinating or axon-loss polyneuropathy). The mainstay of treatment is excellent nursing and medical care, with close attention to respiratory and autonomic function. Although 10% of patients

TABLE 152.4

Advances in Management Based on Major Controlled Clinical Trials of Plasmapheresis and Intravenous Immunoglobulin in Guillain–BarréSyndrome

References	Purpose	Results
[44]	Compared PE with supportive care	PE showed beneficial effect in time to improve one clinical grade, time to independent walking, and outcome.
[53]	Compared various PE treatment schedules in three severity groups	Mild group: Two PEs more effective than none. Moderate group: Four PEs more effective than two PEs. Severe group: Six PEs not more beneficial than four PEs.
[50]	(a) To determine effect of PE initiated within 17 d onset and (b) to compare albumin and FFP as replacement fluids	PE beneficial when administered early. No significant difference between albumin and FFP but albumin preferred owing to less risks.
[54]	To determine whether IVIG is as effective as PE	IVIG is as effective as PE and may be superior.
[55]	Compared IVIG with PE, and combined regimen of PE followed by IVIG	PE and IVIG are equivalent in efficacy when treatment is given within the first 2 weeks of symptoms. The combination of PE followed by IVIG was not more beneficial.

IVIG, intravenous immunoglobulin; FFP, fresh-frozen plasma; PE, plasmapheresis.

with GBS are left with substantial residual neurologic deficits, the majority improve and resume their premorbid lifestyles; plasmapheresis and IVIG have been shown to enhance recovery.

Advances in the management of GBS, based on randomized controlled trials or meta-analyses of such trials, are summarized in Table 152.4.

References

1. Guillain G, Barré JA, Strohl A: Sur un syndrome de radiculo-nevrite avec hyperalbuminose du liquidecephalo-rachidien sans reaction cellulaire: remarquessur les characterescliniques et graphiques des reflexes tendineux. *Bull Mem Soc Med Hop Paris* 40:1462, 1916.
2. Ropper AH, Wijdicks EFM, Truax BT: *Guillain-Barré Syndrome*. Philadelphia, PA, FA Davis, 1991.
3. Arnason BGW: Acute inflammatory demyelinating polyradiculoneuropathy, in Dyck PJ, Thomas PK, Griffin JW, et al (eds): *Peripheral Neuropathy*. Philadelphia, PA, WB Saunders, 1993, p 1437.
4. Ropper AH: The Guillain–Barré syndrome. *N Engl J Med* 326:1130, 1992.
5. Ropper AH: Campylobacter diarrhea and Guillain–Barré syndrome. *Arch Neurol* 45:655, 1988.
6. Cornblath DR, McArthur JC, Kennedy PGE, et al: Inflammatory demyelinating peripheral neuropathies associated with human T-cell lymphotropic virus type III infection. *Ann Neurol* 21:32, 1987.
7. Pachner AR, Steere AC: The triad of neurologic manifestations of Lyme disease: meningitis, cranial neuritis, and radiculoneuritis. *Neurology* 35:47, 1985.
8. Asbury AK, Cornblath DR: Assessment of current diagnostic criteria for Guillain–Barré syndrome. *Ann Neurol* 27[Suppl]:S21, 1990.
9. Oh SJ, Kurokawa K, De Almeida DF, et al: Subacute inflammatory demyelinating polyneuropathy. *Neurology* 61:1507, 2003.
10. Barohn R, Kissel J, Warmolts J, et al: Chronic inflammatory polyradiculoneuropathy. Clinical characteristics, course, and recommendations for diagnostic criteria. *Arch Neurol* 46:878, 1989.
11. Dionne A, Nicolle MW, Hahn AF: Clinical and electrophysiological parameters distinguishing acute-onset chronic inflammatory demyelinating polyneuropathy from acute inflammatory demeylinating polyneuropathy. *Muscle Nerve* 41:202, 2010.
12. Kuitwaard K, van Koningsveld R, Ruts L, et al: Recurrent Guillain-Barré syndrome. *J Neurol Neurosurg Psychiatry* 80:56, 2009.
13. Hahn A: The challenge of respiratory dysfunction in Guillain–Barré syndrome. *Arch Neurol* 58:871, 2001.
14. Andersonn T, Siden A: A clinical study of the Guillain–Barré syndrome. *Acta Neurol Scand* 66:316, 1982.
15. Fisher CM: Unusual variant of acute idiopathic polyneuritis (syndrome of ophthalmoplegia, ataxia and areflexia). *N Engl J Med* 255:57, 1956.
16. Anzai T, Uematsu D, Takahashi K, et al: Guillain–Barré syndrome with bilateral tonic pupils. *Int Med* 33:248, 1994.
17. Mori M, Kuwabara S, Fukutake T, et al: Clinical features and prognosis of Miller Fisher syndrome. *Neurology* 56:1104, 2001.
18. Ersahin Y, Mutluer S, Yurtseven T: Hydrocephalus in Guillain–Barré syndrome. *Clin Neurol Neurosurg* 97:253, 1995.
19. Lichtenfeld P: Autonomic dysfunction in the Guillain–Barré syndrome. *Am J Med* 50:772, 1971.
20. Suarez GA, Fealey RD, Camilleri M, et al: Idiopathic autonomic neuropathy: clinical, neurophysiologic, and follow-up studies on 27 patients. *Neurology* 44:1675, 1994.
21. Hiraga A, Mori M, Ogawara K, et al: Recovery patterns and long term prognosis for axonal Guillain–Barré syndrome. *J NeurolNeurosurg Psychiatry* 76:719, 2005.
22. Ho TW, Li CY, Cornblath DR, et al: Patterns of recovery in the Guillain–Barré syndromes. *Neurology* 48:695, 1997.
23. Feasby TE, Gilbert JJ, Brown WF, et al: An acute axonal form of Guillain–Barré polyneuropathy. *Brain* 109:1115, 1986.
24. Albers JW: AAEM Case report #4: Guillain–Barré syndrome. *Muscle Nerve* 12:705, 1989.
25. Gordon PH, Wilbourn AJ: Early electrodiagnostic findings in Guillain–Barré syndrome. *Arch Neurol* 58:913, 2001.
26. Griffin JW, Li CY, Ho TW, et al: Guillain–Barré syndrome in northern China: the spectrum of neuropathological changes in clinically defined cases. *Brain* 118:577, 1995.
27. Vucic S, Kiernan MC, Cornblath DR: Guillain-Barré syndrome: an update. *J Clin Neurosc* 16:733, 2009.
28. Zochodne DW, Bolton CF, Wells GA, et al: Critical illness polyneuropathy: a complication of sepsis and multiple organ failure. *Brain* 110:819, 1987.
29. Bolton CF: Critical illness polyneuropathy, in Asbury AK, Thomas PK (eds): *Peripheral Nerve Disorders 2*. Boston, Butterworth–Heinemann, 1995, p 262.
30. Helliwell TR, Coakley JH, Wagenmakers AJM, et al: Necrotizing myopathy in critically-ill patients. *J Pathol* 164:307, 1991.
31. Lacomis D, Giuliani MJ, Cott AV, et al: Acute myopathy of intensive care: clinical, electromyographic, and pathological aspects. *Ann Neurol* 40:645, 1996.
32. Segredo V, Caldwell JE, Matthay MA, et al: Persistent paralysis in critically ill patients after long-term administration of vecuronium. *N Engl J Med* 327:524, 1992.
33. Donofrio PD, Wilbourn AJ, Albers JW, et al: Acute arsenic intoxication presenting as Guillain–Barré syndrome. *Muscle Nerve* 10:114, 1987.
34. Senanayake N, Johnson MK: Acute polyneuropathy after poisoning by a new organophosphate insecticide. *N Engl J Med* 306:155, 1982.
35. Senanayake N, Karalliedde L: Neurotoxic effects of organophosphorus insecticides: an intermediate syndrome. *N Engl J Med* 316:761, 1987.
36. Davis LE, DeBiasi R, Goade DE, et al: West Nile virus neuroinvasive disease. *Ann Neurol* 60:286, 2006.
37. Hughes RA, Cornblath DR: Guillain–Barré syndrome. *Lancet* 366:1653, 2005.
38. Hafer-Macko CE, Sheikh KA, Li CY, et al: Immune attack on the Schwann cell surface in acute inflammatory demyelinating polyneuropathy. *Ann Neurol* 39:625, 1996.
39. Asbury AK, Arnason BG, Adams RD: The inflammatory lesion in idiopathic polyneuritis: its role in pathogenesis. *Medicine* 489:173, 1969.
40. Powell HC, Myers RR: The axon in Guillain–Barré syndrome: immune target or innocent bystander? *Ann Neurol* 39:4, 1996.
41. Hafer-Macko C, Hsieh S, Li CY, et al: Acute motor axonal neuropathy: an antibody-mediated attack on axolemma. *Ann Neurol* 40:635, 1996.
42. Willison HJ: The immunobiology of Guillain–Barré syndromes. *J Peripher Nerv Syst* 10:94, 2005.
43. Sheikh KA, Ho TW, Nachamkin I, et al: Molecular mimicry in Guillain–Barré syndrome. *Ann N Y Acad Sci* 845:307, 1998.
44. Koga M, Takahashi M, Masuda M, et al: Campylobacter gene polymorphism as a determinant of clinical features of Guillain–Barré syndrome. *Neurology* 65:1376, 2005.
45. The Guillain–Barré Syndrome Study Group: Plasmapheresis and acute Guillain–Barré syndrome. *Neurology* 35:1096, 1985.
46. Lawn ND, Fletcher DD, Henderson RD, et al: Anticipating mechanical ventilation in Guillain–Barré syndrome. *Arch Neurol* 58:893, 2001.
47. Ropper AH, Kehne SM: Guillain–Barré syndrome: management of respiratory failure. *Neurology* 35:1662, 1985.
48. Hughes RAC, Wijdicks EFM, Benson E, et al: Supportive care for patients with Guillain–Barré syndrome. *Arch Neurol* 62:1194, 2005.
49. Rosenfeld B, Borel C, Henley D: Epidural morphine treatment of pain in the Guillain–Barré syndrome. *Arch Neurol* 43:1194, 1986.
50. Dyck PJ, Kurtzke JF: Plasmapheresis in Guillain–Barré syndrome. *Neurology* 35:1105, 1985.
51. The French Cooperative Group on Plasma Exchange in Guillain–Barré Syndrome: Efficiency of plasma exchange in Guillain–Barré syndrome: role of replacement fluids. *Ann Neurol* 22:753, 1987.
52. McKhann GM, Griffin JW, Cornblath DR, et al: Plasmapheresis and Guillain–Barré syndrome: analysis of prognostic factors and the effect of plasmapheresis. *Ann Neurol* 23:347, 1988.
53. McKhann GM, Griffin JW: Plasmapheresis and the Guillain–Barré syndrome. *Ann Neurol* 22:762, 1987.
54. The French Cooperative Group on Plasma Exchange in Guillain–Barré Syndrome: Appropriate number of plasma exchanges in Guillain–Barré Syndrome. *Ann Neurol* 41:298, 1997.
55. Van der Meche FGA, Schmitz PIM; Dutch Guillain–Barré Study Group: A randomized trial comparing intravenous immune globulin and plasma exchange in Guillain–Barré syndrome. *N Engl J Med* 326:1123, 1992.
56. Plasma Exchange/Sandoglobulin Guillain–Barré Syndrome Trial Group: Randomised trial of plasma exchange, intravenous immunoglobulin, and combined treatments in Guillain–Barré syndrome. *Lancet* 349:225, 1997.
57. Hughes RAC, Widjicks EFM, Barohn R, et al: Practice parameter: immunotherapy for Guillain–Barré syndrome. Report of the Quality Standards Subcommittee of the American Academy of Neurology. *Neurology* 61:736, 2003.
58. Donofrio PD, Berger A, Brannagan TH, et al: Consensus statement: the use of intravenous immunoglobulin in the treatment of neuromuscular conditions. Report of the AANEM ad hoc committee. *Muscle Nerve* 40(5):890–900, 2009.
59. Hughes RAC, Swan AV, Raphaél JC, et al: Immunotherapy for Guillain–Barré syndrome: a systematic review. *Brain* 130:2245, 2007.
60. Rajabally YA, Uncini A: Outcome and its predictors in Guillain-Barré syndrome. *J Neurol Neurosurg Psyciatry* 83:711, 2012.
61. Kissel JT, Cornblath DR, Mendell JR: Guillain-Barré syndrome, in *Diagnosis and Management of Peripheral Nerve Disorders*. New York, NY, Oxford University Press, 2001.
62. Chió A, Cocito D, Leone M, et al: Guillain–Barré syndrome: a prospective, population-based incidence and outcome survey. *Neurology* 60:1146, 2003.
63. Petzold A, Brettschenider J, Kin K, et al: CSF protein biomarkers for proximal axonal damage improve prognostic accuracy in the acute phase of Guillain–Barré syndrome. *Muscle Nerve* 40:42, 2009.
64. Walgaard C, Lingsma HF, Ruts L, et al: Prediction of respiratory insufficiency in Guillain-Barré syndrome. *Ann Neurol* 67(6):781, 2010.
65. Walgaard C, Lingsma HF, Ruts L, et al: Early recognition of poor prognosis in Guillain-Barré syndrome. *Neurology* 76:968, 2011.

Chapter 153 ■ Myasthenia Gravis in the Intensive Care Unit

ISABELITA R. BELLA • JOHNNY S. SALAMEH

Few physicians have more than a passing acquaintance with myasthenia gravis, although it is by no means rare. The key to handling the emergent problems associated with myasthenia is simply the management of airway and ventilatory support with the same care as in any other instance of respiratory failure (see Chapters 8, 65, and 166). With respiration under control, the treatment of the underlying disease can be unhurried and orderly, and it is successful in most patients. This chapter reviews briefly the pathogenesis, clinical spectrum, and diagnosis of myasthenia gravis and focuses on the intensive care setting, including management of the patient in crisis or in the perioperative period.

PATHOGENESIS

Myasthenia gravis is an autoimmune disorder of neuromuscular transmission [1]. Circulating antibodies react with components of acetylcholine receptors (AChRs) within postsynaptic muscle membrane and activate complement-mediated lysis of the muscle membrane, accelerate receptor degradation, and impair receptor activation (i.e., interfere with normal receptor activation by acetylcholine) [2]. The result is fewer receptors that can be activated at affected neuromuscular junctions, causing weaker muscular contraction. Electrophysiologic study of myasthenic neuromuscular junctions discloses end-plate potentials that are diminished in amplitude [3]. These observations have been clearly linked to the receptor alterations and an altered postsynaptic response to normal quantal transmitter release from the presynaptic nerve terminals. Understanding of this underlying pathophysiology has, in turn, enabled rational approaches to treatment. Various immunosuppressive therapies and acetylcholinesterase inhibitors are primary therapeutic options in managing myasthenia gravis (see later).

EPIDEMIOLOGY

Myasthenia gravis is not rare; its prevalence in Western populations is approximately 1 in 20,000 [4]. The overall female to male ratio is approximately 3:2, although there are two distinct sex-specific incidence peaks, with the incidence among women peaking in the third decade and that among men in the fifth to sixth decades. A mild familial predisposition has been noted, although Mendelian inheritance does not apply.

CLINICAL SPECTRUM

The clinical spectrum of myasthenia gravis is characterized as much by its diversity as it is by its common themes. It may range from a mild and relatively inconsequential disease over a normal lifetime to a fulminant incapacitating disorder. The course of a given patient may also vary widely. The clinical hallmarks of the disease are weakness and exaggerated muscle fatigue. The specific muscles involved and the severity of weakness are highly variable, between individuals and within the same individual over time.

Ocular muscles are most frequently involved; diplopia is common, and various patterns of ophthalmoparesis are seen. Bulbar muscles are also frequently affected, leading to varying combinations of facial paresis, dysarthria, and dysphagia. Ptosis is common, but the pupils are never affected. Limb muscle involvement may vary from very isolated weakness to generalized (usually proximal) weakness and fatigability. Respiratory muscle weakness is unfortunately not rare, and respiratory insufficiency and the inability to handle oral and upper airway secretions are the critical problems that bring myasthenics to the intensive care setting. Myasthenia should also be considered in any patient who cannot be weaned from ventilator support after an otherwise uncomplicated surgical procedure.

Approximately 15% to 20% of myasthenics have only ocular and eyelid involvement. Longitudinal studies indicate that if an individual manifests only oculomotor weakness for more than 2 years, there is little chance of later limb or respiratory weakness. Although several clinical classification schemes have been devised for categorizing myasthenics according to the distribution and severity of their disease, it is preferable to emphasize the fact that myasthenics often fluctuate over time, with variability rather than constancy being the norm. Some factors contributing to fluctuations of strength are recognizable (see later); many fluctuations appear to occur at random.

DIAGNOSTIC STUDIES

The diagnosis of myasthenia gravis is clinically suggested in patients who present with chronic ocular, bulbar, or appendicular weakness, variable over time, with preservation of normal sensation and reflexes. More restricted presentations require a much broader differential diagnosis. Myasthenia gravis should always be considered in the differential diagnosis of isolated ocular or bulbar weakness. Again, prominent muscular fatigability and temporal fluctuation are key features of the disease. Normal pupils, normal sensation, and normal reflexes are to be expected and are helpful in diagnosing myasthenia gravis when coincident with an acute or subacute paralytic illness.

Once the diagnosis of myasthenia gravis is suggested, confirmation rests on the exclusion of other diseases and supporting clinical and laboratory studies. It is important to stress that although abnormal tests may be diagnostic, normal test results do not exclude the diagnosis.

Edrophonium Test

Edrophonium hydrochloride (Enlon; formerly "Tensilon") is a fast, short-acting parenteral cholinesterase inhibitor. It reaches peak effect within 1 minute after intravenous injection and persists to some extent for at least 10 minutes. Myasthenic weakness typically improves transiently after administration of 4 to 10 mg (0.4 to 1.0 mL). The edrophonium test may be blinded, with drug or normal saline being injected. Whether drug or placebo, a 0.2-mL test dose is given to screen for excessive cholinergic side effects, such as cardiac arrhythmia, gastrointestinal hyperactivity, or diaphoresis. A resuscitation cart should always be available, and patients with known cardiac disease and elderly patients warrant electrocardiographic monitoring. The remaining 0.8 mL is given after 1 minute. Interpretation of the test depends on identifying and observing an unequivocal baseline muscular deficit that can be improved following the injection of edrophonium.

Ptosis and ophthalmoparesis, if present, are semiquantifiable and well suited; if respiratory compromise is present, monitoring maximum inspiratory pressure (MIP) or vital capacity is useful. As a general rule, positive responses are dramatic; if there is any doubt about the positivity of the test, it should be considered negative. False-positive edrophonium tests are quite rare; false negatives are common. In children, the appropriate test dose is 0.03 mg per kg, one-fifth of which may be given as a test dose.

Neostigmine is a longer-acting parenteral cholinesterase inhibitor that sometimes effects a more obvious clinical response. It is also typically associated with more obvious autonomic side effects. The 1.5-mg test dose (0.04 mg per kg in children) should therefore be preceded by 0.5 mg of atropine; both may be given subcutaneously.

Serologic Testing

Recognition of the immune nature of myasthenia gravis has provided a relatively sensitive and highly specific diagnostic study. Approximately 85% of myasthenics have detectable serum antibodies, which bind to AChRs [5]. The sensitivity drops to 70% in those with purely ocular myasthenia [6]. The antibodies themselves constitute a heterogeneous group, reacting against various receptor subunits. Although the actual antibody titer is of little significance, correlating poorly with the severity of disease or clinical response to therapy, the presence of antibodies is a strong indication of the disease. A normal test does not exclude the diagnosis, especially in the patient presenting with predominantly ocular symptoms and signs. Of note, these antibodies have also been found in a small percentage of patients with Lambert–Eaton myasthenic syndrome;patients with autoimmune liver disease; and patients with lung cancer without neurologic disease [6].

Among seronegative myasthenic patients, from 30% to 70% may be found to have antibodies directed against muscle-specific tyrosine kinase [MuSK], an enzyme that catalyzes AChR aggregation in the formation of neuromuscular junctions [7]. Animal models have also recently shown that MuSK antibodies may reduce AChR clustering and thus impair neuromuscular transmission [8]. Patients who have antibodies to MuSK are often young women (onset of symptoms before 40 years of age) with prominent bulbar involvement [9] and neck or respiratory muscle weakness [7]. They tend to have more severe disease requiring aggressive immunosuppressive treatment [9] and have a higher frequency of respiratory crisis compared to seronegative or AChR-positive myasthenics [10]. Unlike patients with antibodies to AChR, there appears to be a correlation between MuSK antibody levels and disease severity, with antibody levels often decreasing after various immunosuppressive treatments except thymectomy [11].

About 10% of patients with generalized myasthenia gravis do not have detectable antibodies to AChR or muscle specific kinase: double seronegative myasthenia. The presence of anti-low density lipoprotein receptor–related protein 4 antibodies (LRP4 Abs) has recently been reported in a variable proportion of double seronegative cases [12].

Striated muscle antibodies that react with muscle proteins titin and ryanodine receptor have also been found, mainly in patients with thymoma and in those with late onset myasthenia (onset of symptoms >50 years of age). Thus, they may be helpful in the detection or recurrence of thymoma. In addition, they tend to be associated with more severe disease, and therefore may aid in prognosis [13].

Myasthenics also have an increased incidence of other autoantibodies, including antithyroid antibodies, antiparietal cell antibodies, and antinuclear antibodies, although routine screening for these is not part of the diagnostic evaluation for suspected myasthenia gravis.

Electromyographic Studies

The electromyographic hallmark of myasthenia gravis is a decrement in the amplitude of the muscle potential seen after exercise or slow repetitive nerve stimulation. The decrement should be at least 10% and preferably 15% or more. Routine motor and sensory conduction studies are normal, as is the conventional needle examination. The more severely affected patient is more likely to show a decremental response; responses are most consistently elicited from facial and proximal muscles. If a significant decrement is observed, exercising the muscle briefly for 10 seconds transiently reverses the decrement [14]. Single-fiber electromyography is highly sensitive, documenting increased jitter [15]—variability in the temporal coupling of single fibers within the same motor unit. Increased jitter, however, is far from specific; most peripheral neurogenic diseases also lead to increased jitter.

MISCELLANEOUS STUDIES

Myasthenia gravis may be associated with either malignant thymoma or thymic hyperplasia. Once a diagnosis is established, chest imaging should be obtained. Because there is also a significant association with thyroid and other autoimmune diseases, appropriate screening studies are indicated in the newly diagnosed myasthenic. Muscle biopsy has no role in the evaluation of myasthenia, unless there is a strong consideration of neurogenic or inflammatory weakness.

CRITICAL CARE OF THE MYASTHENIC PATIENT

Patient in Crisis

Crisis refers to threatened or actual respiratory compromise in a myasthenic patient. It may reflect respiratory muscle insufficiency or inability to handle secretions and oral intake, but it is typically a combination of both. With currently available treatments, myasthenic crisis is not common. An occasional patient presents with fulminating disease; crisis management then coincides with initial evaluation and institution of therapy. Otherwise, crisis may be precipitated by other illnesses, such as influenza or other infections, or by surgery.

General Measures

The respiratory function of any acutely deteriorating or severely weak myasthenic should be monitored compulsively. When the weakening myasthenic reaches a point at which increased respiratory effort is required, fatigue often prevents the effective use of secondary muscles, and respiratory failure rapidly ensues. Arterial blood gas values and even oxygen saturation are poor indicators of incipient failure in the face of respiratory muscle compromise. Forced vital capacity (FVC) and MIP are better indices and should be serially charted. The FVC should be assessed with the patient both sitting and supine, because diaphragmatic paresis may be accentuated in the supine position. MIP measurement requires special care if the patient also has significant facial weakness. An FVC less than 20 mL per kg or an MIP greater than (i.e., not as negative as) −40 cm H_2O suggests impending failure and usually warrants intubation. If a downward trend is noted (greater than 30% decrease) [16], elective intubation should be considered even sooner, unless there is a realistic expectation of rapid reversal.

Acute deterioration in a myasthenic always warrants consideration of contributing circumstances or concurrent illness

TABLE 153.1

Conditions That May Underlie Interim Deterioration in Myasthenic Patients

Intercurrent infection; occult infection should be excluded
Electrolyte imbalance (Na, K, Ca, P, and Mg)
Cholinergic crisis: if any doubt, discontinue cholinesterase inhibitors
Thyrotoxicosis, hypothyroidism
Medication effects (see Table 153.2)

that may accentuate the underlying defect in neuromuscular transmission. The major considerations are listed in Table 153.1 and discussed later.

The possibility of cholinergic crisis in patients receiving anticholinesterase drugs (e.g., pyridostigmine), albeit rare, should not be overlooked. The presence of fasciculations, diaphoresis, or diarrhea should alert the clinician to this possibility. In the past, the importance of differentiating between myasthenic crisis and cholinergic crisis was stressed. Edrophonium testing was used to differentiate between the two; abrupt deterioration after a conventional 10-mg test dose indicated overdosage with cholinesterase inhibitors. One had to be adequately prepared for deterioration and increased respiratory secretions. Because oftentimes it is very difficult to determine the response and because of the potential side effects with overdosage of anticholinesterase drugs of increased pulmonary secretions, many authors now recommend discontinuation of cholinesterase inhibitors at the time of crisis [2,17,18] and reinstituting them when patients are stronger. This assumes that adequate respiratory monitoring and support are in effect. A brief holiday from cholinesterase inhibition also often results in an enhanced response to therapy when reinstituted.

Intercurrent infection is often associated with increased weakness in the myasthenic patient. There should be a comprehensive search for systemic infection in the deteriorating patient, particularly the patient receiving immunosuppressive therapy. Any infections should be treated aggressively. Both hypothyroid and hyperthyroid states are often associated with increased weakness. Again, there is an increased association between thyrotoxicosis and myasthenia gravis. The manifestations of electrolyte imbalance may be enhanced in myasthenic patients. Otherwise, insignificant electrolyte effects on transmitter release or muscle membrane excitability may be amplified at the myasthenic neuromuscular junction. Potassium, calcium, phosphate, and magnesium alterations should be corrected. Myasthenia gravis may also impart enhanced sensitivity to a number of medications that have only minimal effects on neuromuscular function in normal individuals. Aminoglycoside and fluoroquinolone antibiotics, β-blockers, and many cardiac antiarrhythmics may have adverse effects. Anticholinergics, respiratory depressants, and sedatives of any kind should be avoided or used only with great caution. *Neuromuscular-blocking agents should never be administered to myasthenic patients in the intensive care unit (ICU) setting*, because they often have profound and prolonged effects. This increased sensitivity occasionally results in postoperative failure to wean in an undiagnosed mild myasthenic patient who has undergone surgery for an unrelated problem. Table 153.2 provides a comprehensive listing of medications that may further impair neuromuscular transmission in myasthenic patients.

Some attention should also be given to the general environment in which the myasthenic is managed. The typical noisy, brightly illuminated ICU is not conducive to rest and sleep, which is crucial for the myasthenic patient in whom fatigue may be critical.

Special consideration must be given to respiratory care of the myasthenic. Incentive spirometry should be avoided, because muscular fatigue outweighs any potential benefit, even in the postoperative patient. Careful attention to efficient clearance of respiratory secretions is key and can be complicated by cholinesterase inhibitors, which increase respiratory secretions. Atropine may be used to minimize this effect, but its other autonomic side effects, such as ileus, constipation, and delirium, may limit longer-term use.

THERAPY IN MYASTHENIC CRISIS

Therapeutic agents used in the critical care setting parallel those available to the patient with milder myasthenia gravis. Immunosuppressive therapies are the major considerations. Any myasthenic patient in crisis, if not already receiving immunosuppressive

TABLE 153.2

Medications That May Accentuate Weakness in Myasthenic Patients

Antibiotics	Neuromuscular blockers and muscle relaxants	Antiarrhythmics and antihypertensives	Antirheumatics	Antipsychotics	Others
Amikacin	Anectine (succinylcholine)	Lidocaine	Chloroquine	Lithium	Opiate analgesics
Clindamycin	Norcuron (vecuronium)	Quinidine	D-Penicillamine	Phenothiazines	Oral contraceptives
Colistin	Pavulon (pancuronium)	Procainamide		Antidepressants	Antihistamines
Fluoroquinolones					
Gentamicin	Tracrium (atracurium)	β-blockers			Anticholinergics
Kanamycin	Benzodiazepines	Calcium blockers			
Lincomycin	Curare				
Neomycin	Dantrium (dantrolene)				
Polymyxin	Flexeril (cyclobenzaprine)				
Streptomycin	Lioresal (baclofen)				
Tobramycin	Robaxin (methocarbamol)				
Tetracyclines	Soma (carisoprodol)				
Trimethoprim/sulfamethoxazole	Quinamm (quinine sulfate)				

therapy, requires it. Symptomatic therapy with cholinesterase inhibitors is now primarily used on a shorter-term basis, pending response to immunomodulating therapies. Plasmapheresis; intravenous human immune globulin; corticosteroids; and longer-term immunosuppressants and cholinesterase inhibitors are discussed individually.

Plasmapheresis

Recognition of the role of immunoglobulins in the pathogenesis of myasthenia gravis stimulated early, uncontrolled clinical trials of plasmapheresis as soon as efficient pheresis technology became available [19]. The results have been quite favorable, prompting the National Institutes of Health Consensus Conference to support its use despite the lack of controlled trials [20]. Most patients demonstrate a significant clinical response within 48 hours of initiation of plasmapheresis, although the response is short lived unless therapy is continued on an intermittent basis. The rapid response from plasmapheresis can be crucial in the face of crisis, providing a short-term reprieve during which alternative therapy can be initiated or any intercurrent medical problems resolved. Approximately 50 mL per kg should be exchanged per session [21], approximating 60% to 70% of total plasma volume. Plasma removed is replaced by an equal volume of normal saline and 5% albumin, adjusted to maintain physiologic concentrations of potassium, calcium, and magnesium. The usual course of treatment includes three to seven pheresis sessions at 24-to 48-hour intervals. Many patients develop increased sensitivity to cholinesterase inhibitors after plasmapheresis; dosage should be correspondingly reduced. The major potential complications of plasmapheresis include hypotension; arrhythmia; and hypercoagulability due to hemoconcentration. Coincident cardiovascular disease is a relative contraindication to plasmapheresis. Although plasmapheresis is too invasive to be used for long-term therapy in the majority of patients, periodic plasmapheresis has been beneficial in some patients with moderate to severe myasthenia refractory to immunosuppressive agents [22]. Selective removal of AChR antibodies using immunoadsorption columns may also be a promising alternative to plasmapheresis, but further clinical studies are required [23].

Intravenous Immunoglobulin (IVIG)

Intravenous human immune globulin also frequently leads to rapid yet transient improvement in myasthenic patients [24]. Intravenous immunoglobulin (IVIG) is a therapeutic option in the event of crisis or in the perioperative period, particularly if the patient's cardiovascular status limits plasmapheresis. Although IVIG and plasmapheresis were found to be equally efficacious in some trials [25,26], others have reported that plasmapheresis was more efficacious than IVIG; however, complications occurred more often with plasmapheresis [27]. The customary dose is 400 mg/kg/d for 5 consecutive days. More recently, a total dose of 1 g per kg was reported to be equally efficacious to 2 g per kg, although there was a trend toward slight superiority of the higher dose [28]. Maximal improvement occurred by the second week after therapy, and the therapeutic response usually persists for several weeks. Patients should be pretreated with acetaminophen and diphenhydramine to prevent flu-like symptoms that commonly occur during infusion. In addition, adequate hydration will help reduce the potential complication of thrombosis. Renal function should be checked prior to initiation of therapy, because renal failure may occur in those with renal insufficiency. Likewise, an IgA level should be obtained,because patients with IgA deficiency may develop anaphylaxis.

Longer-Term Immunosuppression

Corticosteroids have proven to be an effective long-term therapy for almost all myasthenic patients whose clinical manifestations cannot be well managed with low doses of cholinesterase inhibitors. Despite potential side effects associated with corticosteroid therapy, a response rate of greater than 80% supports its use [29]. Side effects can be minimized with appropriate precautions. Carbohydrate metabolism, electrolytes, blood pressure, and diet should be closely monitored; bisphosphonates (e.g., alendronate sodium, 70 mg weekly), calcium (500 to 1,000 mg per day), and vitamin D supplementation (at least 800 to 1,000 IU per day) as well are prudent to minimize osteopenia. Screening for tuberculosis exposure with skin testing and chest radiographs should be done before initiation of therapy. Occult infection must be treated or excluded for the deteriorating myasthenic patients.

Recommendations regarding corticosteroid preparation, dose, and regimen vary. Approximately one-third of patients may become transiently weaker before they improve, if given high doses of prednisone initially [3]. Initiation with relatively low doses of prednisone and increasing in a stepwise manner has been advocated by some clinicians to minimize interim deterioration, especially if the patient is not intubated [17]. The authors prefer to begin with 15 to 25 mg of prednisone or its equivalent as a single daily dose, increasing the dose by 5 mg every second or third day until a dose of 1 mg/kg/d is reached. In the critical care setting, concurrent plasmapheresis or IVIG may offset initial steroid-related deterioration; high doses of corticosteroids (1 mg/kg/d) can be initiated in this situation, enabling a more rapid response. Oral corticosteroids are preferable,because there is a risk of developing acute steroid-induced myopathy in patients with myasthenia who are given high doses of intravenous corticosteroids [18,30].

Once maximal response is obtained, usually within 2 to 3 months, patients may be gradually shifted to alternate-day therapy by concurrently reducing the off-day dose and increasing the on-day dose, with a 10-mg shift made once each week. Some individuals note a definite off-day adverse effect; this can usually be countered with a 10-mg alternate-day dose. Once stabilized on alternate-day therapy, the on-day dose can be tapered by 5 mg per month. Many patients can be maintained in remission with as little as 20 to 25 mg of prednisone every other day (or alternating with 10 mg). Only rare patients remain in remission if therapy is discontinued, and overenthusiastic tapering of steroids is an all too common precipitant of unnecessary disability or even crisis. Myasthenia sometimes remits spontaneously, and if the patient has undergone thymectomy (see later), the probability of remission increases appreciably, making discontinuation of therapy a more realistic option.

Azathioprine is often used as an alternative agent for longer-term immunosuppression. It is effective in 70% to 90% of patients with myasthenia gravis [2] and is often initiated in patients with an insufficient response to corticosteroids, as a steroid-sparing agent, or in patients in whom corticosteroids are contraindicated [3]. Azathioprine is limited by a relatively long delay before its effects are clinically evident, up to 6 to 12 months, but its side-effect spectrum compares favorably with steroids over a time frame of many years. If a patient tolerates a 50-mg per day test dose, the daily dose can be increased by 50 mg each week up to 2 to 3 mg/kg/d. The dose is reduced if the white blood cell count is less than 3,000 per μL; an elevated mean corpuscular volume can also be used to assess adequate response [4,31]. In up to 10% of patients, an influenza-like reaction characterized by fever, malaise, and myalgias occurs within the first few weeks of therapy and resolves after discontinuing the drug [2,31]. Patients should be screened for thiopurine methyltransferase (TPMT) deficiency; those homozygous for

TPMT mutations cannot metabolize azathioprine and therefore should not receive the drug. Concurrent treatment with allopurinol should also be avoided,because it interferes with the degradation of azathioprine, thereby increasing the risk of bone marrow and liver toxicity [31].

Cyclosporine appears to be as effective as azathioprine in the treatment of myasthenia gravis [32] and is used mainly in patients who are intolerant or refractory to azathioprine. Onset of clinical improvement is quicker than with azathioprine, with most patients noticing improvement after 1 to 3 months, and becoming maximal around 7 months [33]. Its major limitations are renal toxicity and hypertension, which are seen in about one-quarter of patients. To minimize side effects, the starting dose of 5 mg/kg/d can be given in two divided doses 12 hours apart, followed by adjustments to maintain a predose trough level in the range of 100 to 150 ng per L. Subsequent adjustments can be made depending on creatinine levels and clinical improvement, with the aim to reduce the dose as much as possible, once maximal improvement is obtained [33]. Renal function (blood urea nitrogen and creatinine) must be continually monitored. Significant hypertension and preexisting renal disease are contraindications to the use of cyclosporine.

Another agent from the realm of transplant medicine, mycophenolate mofetil (CellCept), has also been used effectively for longer-term therapy. Several case series, retrospective analysis, and a small placebo-controlled, double-blind trial suggested that mycophenolate mofetil is beneficial in patients with myasthenia gravis [34–36]. Because it is better tolerated than other immunosuppressants, it has become widely used. Recently, however, two large double-blinded randomized controlled trials failed to show any benefit of mycophenolate mofetil over placebo in patients with myasthenia gravis [37,38]. One study showed that mycophenolate mofetil was not superior to placebo during a steroid taper [37], whereas the other study showed no benefit in taking mycophenolate mofetil with 20 mg prednisone compared to taking prednisone alone [38]. Several factors have been proposed to explain these surprisingly negative results including the short duration of the trials, selection of generally mildly affected patients, and the unexpected significant response to low-dose prednisone [2]. Further studies are warranted to establish the role of mycophenolate mofetil in myasthenia. Despite this, mycophenolate mofetil is still widely used in the treatment of myasthenia gravis. The standard dose is 1,000 mg twice a day, but doses up to 3,000 mg per day may be used. Monthly complete blood counts should be performed to monitor for any evidence of myelosuppression.

In refractory cases in which it has proven difficult to achieve or maintain remission, high-dose cyclophosphamide has proven effective [2]. However, it has significant side effects including bone marrow toxicity, hemorrhagic cystitis, teratogenicity, and increased risk of infections and malignancies. Oral dosage ranges from 1 to 5 mg/kg/d [17]. Recently, Drachman and colleagues reported dramatic clinical improvement by "rebooting the immune system" in patients with refractory myasthenia using high-dose cyclophosphamide 50 mg/kg/d for 4 days, followed by granulocyte colony-stimulating factor; clinical improvement lasted several years in some patients [39].

Several case series have reported a beneficial response of rituximab in patients with refractory myasthenia gravis and in those with MuSK myasthenia gravis [40]. Patients tolerated the treatment without significant side effects, making this a promising drug for the future.

Cholinesterase Inhibitors

Cholinesterase inhibition was the mainstay of pharmacotherapy for myasthenia gravis before the advent of immunosuppressive therapies and thymectomy. Many patients are now maintained in remission on corticosteroids or other immunosuppressive agents, whereas others, in particular, those with mild nonprogressive or purely ocular disease, require only treatment with an oral anticholinesterase drug, such as pyridostigmine (Mestinon). If an acutely deteriorating patient has been taking a cholinesterase inhibitor, the possibility of cholinergic crisis should be entertained. Overdosage of cholinesterase inhibitors may produce weakness accompanied by muscarinic symptoms such as increased pulmonary and gastric secretions; bradycardia; nausea; vomiting; diarrhea; and nicotinic symptoms such as fasciculations [2,18]. Many authors advocate discontinuing anticholinesterase therapy during myasthenic crisis to minimize secretions, avoid potential exacerbation of weakness due to overdosage of cholinergic medications, and allow for easier assessment of response to other therapies [17,18]. It is reasonable to reinstitute anticholinesterase therapy when patients are stronger, starting at a low dosage and gradually increasing the dose until there is clear benefit [17].

The use of intravenous anticholinesterase therapy is controversial. Infusion of intravenous pyridostigmine at 1 to 2 mg per hour during crisis was found in one small retrospective study to be comparable to plasmapheresis [41]. However, intravenous therapy carries the risk of dangerous side effects such as cardiac arrhythmias, myocardial infarction (due to coronary vasospasm), airway obstruction, and increased pulmonary secretions [18,42]. It is therefore more prudent to hold cholinergic drugs until the patient is able to take them orally or through a nasogastric tube [18]. If intravenous anticholinesterase therapy is deemed necessary, neostigmine and pyridostigmine preparations are available in parenteral forms. One mg of neostigmine given intravenously is roughly equivalent to 120 mg of pyridostigmine taken by mouth. Conversion of oral pyridostigmine to intravenous pyridostigmine is 30:1.

PERIOPERATIVE MANAGEMENT OF THE MYASTHENIC PATIENT

An intercurrent problem requiring surgical intervention was a common source of major morbidity and mortality for myasthenics before the 1960s. Subsequent developments in critical care techniques, especially respiratory care, and in therapy of the underlying disease have dramatically improved this situation. Perioperative management must be compulsive, yet myasthenia gravis should rarely preclude surgical treatment that is otherwise indicated.

Preoperative Considerations

Myasthenia gravis is a major variable in surgical management, whether the surgery is elective or emergent. A neurologist (preferably the neurologist who has been managing the patient) should be considered an integral member of the operative team. If the procedure is elective, the patient's myasthenic status should be optimized before anesthesia and surgery. Pulmonary function tests should be reviewed in detail; if respiratory or bulbar muscle function is compromised, therapy adjustments should be undertaken to improve respiratory muscle strength. All therapeutic options should be considered, with the possible exception of corticosteroids. If the patient is not receiving steroids, it is prudent to forego or delay this treatment until after surgery, because corticosteroids may increase the risk of infection and retard wound healing. If the patient is already receiving corticosteroids, therapy should be continued, with a short-term increment in dose to compensate for the added stress of anesthesia and surgery. Plasmapheresis or intravenous human immune globulin is often useful in the preoperative setting, providing a transient therapeutic benefit through the preoperative and postoperative periods. Once dose and regimen are optimized, cholinesterase inhibitors may be continued up to the time of surgery. They should then be discontinued because they stimulate respiratory secretions.

It is crucial that all physicians involved in perioperative management of the myasthenic are aware of the particular medications that may accentuate the underlying defect in neuromuscular transmission. It is appropriate to post a warning regarding specific medications on the patient's chart, in a manner analogous to that for medication allergies. Neuromuscular blockade should be avoided during surgery unless absolutely essential; if required, the shortest-acting agents should be used at minimal doses. Accentuated and prolonged effects should be anticipated. Aminoglycoside and fluoroquinolone antibiotics should be avoided when alternatives are available. There is no clear consensus in favor of any one halogenated anesthetic agent; ether adversely affects neuromuscular transmission. Again, close attention to metabolic homeostasis cannot be overemphasized.

Postoperative Care

Postoperative care of the myasthenic patient should not differ greatly from that of other patients, provided preoperative and intraoperative management has been successful. The patient's status before surgery is often the best indicator of the postoperative course. Intubation and mechanical ventilatory support must be continued until the patient is alert and responsive and demonstrates and maintains adequate pulmonary function. After extubation, serial pulmonary function testing is indicated. An FVC greater than 20 mL per kg and MIP less than (i.e., more negative than) −40 cm H_2O are threshold values when reintubation should be considered. If needed, cholinesterase inhibitors may be resumed as a continuous intravenous infusion until bowel function is restored and oral intake allowed. Increased sensitivity to cholinesterase inhibitors is expected after surgical procedures, especially thymectomy. Resumption at a rate of no more than one-half the preoperative equivalent is often sufficient. Subsequent adjustments should reflect clinical indices. The myasthenic whose neuromuscular function deteriorates during the postoperative period is the exception. In all probability, an intercurrent reversible factor underlies the deterioration. The spectrum of metabolic, infectious, and pharmacologic issues discussed previously should be reviewed.

Thymectomy

After several decades of controversy, there is a consensus that thymectomy favorably alters the natural history of myasthenia gravis, especially for younger patients, independent of the presence or degree of thymic hyperplasia [43]. Thymectomy should be considered early in the course of myasthenia, except in elderly, frail patients. Thymectomy remains an elective procedure, however. The myasthenic with marginal respiratory or bulbar function should be optimally treated before surgery. The perioperative management considerations discussed earlier apply to prethymectomy and postthymectomy management. Some controversy persists regarding the appropriate thymectomy procedure. Most centers favor the transsternal approach. Although more invasive, this approach facilitates recognition and removal of all thymus tissue and avoids postoperative respiratory compromise. There are some proponents of transcervical mediastinoscopic thymectomy; in experienced hands, this remains an alternative. Thymectomy by conventional thoracotomy has no place in the treatment of myasthenia.

CONCLUSION

Respiratory failure is no longer the source of major morbidity and mortality in myasthenia gravis that it once was. When it does occur, appropriate ventilatory support and airway protection provide time for resolution of any intercurrent problems and therapy of the underlying myasthenia. Plasmapheresis and immunosuppression are usually successful; extended intensive care stays should be rare occurrences. Treatment of myasthenia gravis with steroids, immunosuppressive agents, and thymectomy usually enables these patients to lead essentially normal lives.

References

1. Drachman DB, de Silva S, Ramsay D, et al: Humoral pathogenesis of myasthenia gravis, in Drachman DB (ed): *Myasthenia Gravis: Biology and Treatment*. New York, NY, Academy of Sciences, 1987, p 90.
2. Meriggioli MN, Sanders DB: Autoimmune myasthenia gravis: emerging clinical and biological heterogeneity. *Lancet Neurol* 8:475, 2009.
3. Drachman DB: Myasthenia Gravis. *N Engl J Med* 330:1797, 1994.
4. Keesey JC: Clinical evaluation and management of myasthenia gravis. *Muscle Nerve* 29:484, 2004.
5. Hughes BW, Moro De Casillas ML, Kaminski HJ: Pathophysiology of myasthenia gravis. *SeminNeurol* 24:21, 2004.
6. Lennon, VA: Serologic profile of myasthenia gravis and distinction from the Lambert–Eaton myasthenic syndrome. *Neurol* 48[Suppl5]:S23, 1997.
7. Vincent A, Leite MI: Neuromuscular junction autoimmune disease: muscle specific kinase antibodies and treatments for myasthenia gravis. *CurrOpinNeurol* 18:519, 2005.
8. Shigemoto K, Kubo S, Maruyama N, et al: Induction of myasthenia by immunization against muscle-specific kinase. *J Clin Invest* 116:1016, 2006.
9. Pasnoor M, Wolfe GI, Nations S, et al: Clinical findings in MuSK-antibody positive myasthenia gravis: a U.S. experience. *Muscle Nerve* 41(3):370–374, 2009.
10. Deymeer F, Bungor-Tuncer O, Yilmaz MS, et al: Clinical comparison of anti-MuSK-vs anti-AchR-positive and seronegative myasthenia gravis. *Neurology* 68:609, 2007.
11. Bartoccioni E, Scuderi F, Minicuci GM, et al: Anti-MuSK antibodies: correlation with myasthenia gravis severity. *Neurology* 67:505, 2006.
12. Zhang B, Tzartos JS, Belimezi M, et al: Autoantibodies to lipoprotein-related protein 4 in patients with double-seronegative myasthenia gravis. *Arch Neurol* 69:445–451, 2012.
13. Romi F, Skeie GO, Gilhus NE, et al: Striational antibodies in myasthenia gravis. *Arch Neurol* 62:442, 2005.
14. Jablecki CK: AAEM Case Report #3: myasthenia gravis. *Muscle Nerve* 14:391, 1991.
15. Sanders DB: Clinical impact of single-fiber electromyography. *Muscle Nerve Suppl* 11:515, 2002.
16. Thieben MJ, Blacker DJ, Liu PY, et al: Pulmonary function tests and blood gases in worsening myasthenia gravis. *Muscle Nerve* 32:664, 2005.
17. Ahmed S, Kirmani J, Janjua N, et al: An update on myasthenic crisis. *Curr Treat Opt Neurol* 7:129, 2005.
18. Lacomis D: Myasthenic crisis. *Neurocrit Care* 3:189, 2005.
19. Pinching AJ, Peters DK, Newson-Davis J: Remission of myasthenia gravis following plasma exchange. *Lancet* 2:1373, 1976.
20. NIH Consensus Conference: The utility of therapeutic plasmapheresis for neurological disorders. *JAMA* 256:1333, 1986.
21. Natarajan N, Weinstein R: Therapeutic apheresis in neurology critical care. *J Intensive Care Med* 20:212, 2005.
22. Triantafyllou NI, Grapsa EI, Kararizou E, et al: Periodic therapeutic plasma exchange in patients with moderate to severe chronic myasthenia gravis non-responders to immunosuppressive agents: an eight year follow-up. *TherApher Dial* 13:174, 2009.
23. Zisimopoulou P, Lagoumintzis G, Kostelidou K, et al: Towards antigen-specific apheresis of pathogenic autoantibodies as a further step in the treatment of myasthenia gravis by plasmapheresis. *J Neuroimmunol* 201–202:95, 2008.
24. Donofrio PD, Berger A, Brannagan TH III, et al: Consensus statement: the use of intravenous immunoglobulin in the treatment of neuromuscular conditions. Report of the AANEM Ad Hoc Committee. *Muscle Nerve* 40:890, 2009.
25. Gajdos P, Chevre S, Clair B, et al: Clinical trial of plasma exchange and high-dose intravenous immunoglobulin in myasthenia gravis. *Ann Neurol* 41:789, 1997.
26. Barth D, NabaviNouri M, Ng E, et al:Comparison of IVIg and PLEX in patients withmyasthenia gravis. *Neurology* 76:2017–2023, 2011.
27. Qureshi AI, Choundry MA, Akbar MS, et al: Plasma exchange versus intravenous immunoglobulin treatment in myasthenic crisis. *Neurology* 52:629, 1999.
28. Gajdos P, Tranchant C, Clair B, et al: Treatment of myasthenia gravis exacerbation with intravenous immunoglobulin: a randomized double-blind clinical trial. *Arch Neurol* 62:1689, 2005.
29. Johns TR: Long-term corticosteroid treatment of myasthenia gravis, in Drachman DB (ed): *Myasthenia Gravis: Biology and Treatment*. New York, NY, Academy of Sciences, 1987, p 568.

30. Panegyres PK, Squier M, Mills KR, et al: Acute myopathy associated with large parenteral dose of corticosteroid in myasthenia gravis. *J NeurolNeurosurg Psychiatry* 56:702, 1993.
31. Amato A, Russell J: Disorders of neuromuscular transmission, in Amato A, Russell J (eds): *Neuromuscular Disorders*. New York, NY, McGraw-Hill, 2008, p 457.
32. Schalke BCG, Kappos L, Rohrbach E, et al: Cyclosporine A vs. azathioprine in the treatment of myasthenia gravis: final results of a randomized, controlled double-blind clinical trial. *Neurology* 38[Suppl1]:135, 1988.
33. Ciafoloni E, Nikhar N, Massey JM, et al: Retrospective analysis of the use of cyclosporine in myasthenia gravis. *Neurology* 55:448, 2000.
34. Chaudhry V, Cornblath DR, Griffin JW, et al: Mycophenolatemofetil: a safe and promising immunosuppressant in neuromuscular diseases. *Neurology* 56:94, 2001.
35. Meriggioli MN, Ciafaloni E, Al-Hayk KA, et al: Mycophenolatemofetil for myasthenia gravis: avn analysis of efficacy, safety, and tolerability. *Neurology* 61:1438, 2003.
36. Meriggioli MN, Rowin J, Richman JG, et al: Mycophenolatemofetil for myasthenia gravis: a double-blind, placebo-controlled pilot study. *Ann N Y AcadSci* 998:494, 2003.
37. Sanders DB, Hart IK, Mantegazza R, et al: An international, phase III, randomized trial of mycophenolatemofetil in myasthenia gravis. *Neurology* 71:400, 2008.
38. The Muscle Study Group: A trial of mycophenolatemofetil with prednisone as initial immunotherapy in myasthenia gravis. *Neurology* 71:394, 2008.
39. Drachman DB, Adams RN, Hu R, et al: Rebooting the immune system with high-dose cyclophosphamide for treatment of refractory myasthenia gravis. *Ann N Y AcadSci* 1132:305, 2008.
40. Zebardast N, Patwa HS, Novella SP, et al: Rituximab in the management of refractory myasthenia gravis. *Muscle Nerve* 41(3):375–378, 2009.
41. Berrouschot J, Baumann I, Kalischewski P, et al: Therapy of myasthenic crisis. *Crit Care Med* 25:1228, 1997.
42. Chaudhuri A, Behan PO: Myasthenic crisis. *Q J Med*102:97, 2009.
43. Jaretzki A, Steinglass KM, Sonett JR: Thymectomy in the management of myasthenia gravis. *SeminNeurol* 24:49, 2004.

Chapter 154 ■ Newly Acquired Weakness in the Intensive Care Unit: Critical Illness Myopathy and Neuropathy

DAVID A. CHAD

Although preexisting neuromuscular disorders (such as myasthenia gravis and the Guillain–Barré syndrome) may cause severe weakness, leading to an intensive care unit (ICU) admission; two of the most common causes of *newly acquired weakness arising in the ICU setting*—also designated "intensive care unit acquired weakness" (ICUAW)—are critical illness myopathy (CIM) and critical illness polyneuropathy (CIP) [1–3]. CIM is probably the major contributor to severe ICUAW, causing most instances of failure to wean from a respirator in patients with severe systemic diseases in the ICU, whereas CIP affects 70% to 80% of patients with severe sepsis and multiorgan failure [4]. Even experienced clinicians have great difficulty distinguishing between the myopathy and the polyneuropathy of intensive care, especially because the two conditions often coexist in an individual patient [4–6]. In the sections that follow, we discuss each disorder and comment on the differential diagnosis of severe weakness arising in the ICU setting.

CRITICAL ILLNESS MYOPATHY

Diagnosis

The hallmark of CIM is weakness that is typically diffuse in distribution, affecting both limb and neck muscles [4,7]. As is typical of most myopathic disorders, weakness tends to have a proximal predominance in the limbs, but it may also involve distal muscles profoundly. Tendon reflexes tend to be depressed but present; however, on occasion they may be markedly attenuated or absent, possibly owing to a generalized reduction in membrane excitability that occurs with sepsis [4]. There may be facial muscle involvement, and rarely, extraocular muscles are affected [6]; other muscles supplied by cranial nerves are usually spared. A serious and common complication of the myopathy is failure to wean from a ventilator owing to marked weakness of the diaphragm. Although the majority of affected patients are adults, severe myopathic muscle weakness may occur in children who receive organ transplants [8], and also in critically ill children admitted to the Pediatric ICU [9].

Risk Factors

CIM develops in up to one-third of patients treated for status asthmaticus in the ICU; and in this population, intravenous corticosteroids and neuromuscular blocking agents are considered major risk factors [6]. Occasionally, the myopathy develops in patients who have received high-dose corticosteroids alone, without neuromuscular blocking agents, or in patients who have received neither corticosteroids nor neuromuscular blocking agents, but the latter group typically has severe systemic illness with multiorgan failure and sepsis [4]. Overall, CIM accounts for 42% of weakness among patients in the surgical and medical ICU setting [10].

Laboratory Studies

Serum creatine kinase (CK), electromyography (EMG), and muscle biopsy are the most important and revealing studies in the diagnosis of ICU-acquired muscle weakness. Although an elevated CK level usually helps to support the diagnosis of myopathy as the cause of weakness in an ICU patient, in CIM, the CK rise is only found in about 50% of affected patients, and occurs early in the course of the illness, peaks within a few days of onset, then declines back to the normal range [6,7].

EMG Studies

With nerve conduction studies, motor responses are typically low-amplitude or absent; and when responses can be elicited, the motor response durations are commonly increased substantially—an important clue to the presence of CIM. This is caused by slowing of muscle fiber conduction velocity and reduced excitability of the sarcolemmal membrane [6]. By contrast, sensory responses are relatively preserved, with amplitudes that are >80% of normal in two or more nerves (although they may be reduced when ICU polyneuropathy coexists with CIM). Sensory responses may also be reduced initially in association with sepsis and increase during clinical recovery [11]. Needle electrode examination shows fibrillation potential activity in resting muscle of some patients. On voluntary muscle activation, motor unit potentials are short in duration and polyphasic in form with early recruitment, but when there is severe weakness or encephalopathy the patient may be unable to contract muscles sufficiently to permit analysis of motor unit potentials. Patients with CIM demonstrated by direct muscle stimulation may have electrical inexcitability of the muscle membrane caused by myopathy [12,13]. In clinical practice, stimulation of the anterior tibial muscle and the peroneal nerve at the fibular head can be informative. In CIM the ratio of the amplitude of the muscle response to peroneal nerve stimulation is >0.5, and often nearly the same as with direct anterior tibial muscle stimulation-evoked response. When weakness is because of CIP, direct muscle excitability is normal, but the nerve-evoked response is less than half as large [6].

When there are any clinical or electrodiagnostic features that are atypical for CIM (e.g., prominent cranial nerve involvement as might be seen in myasthenia gravis, or autonomic dysfunction as in botulism) it is important to consider an alternative primary, or a coexisting, disorder of neuromuscular transmission. Repetitive nerve stimulation (2 to 3 Hz) studies for a decremental response as in myasthenia, and rapid rate (30 to 50 Hz) stimulation looking for evidence of post-synaptic facilitation as in botulism, may be helpful for the evaluation of the patient.

Muscle Biopsy

Muscle biopsy is usually not necessary to establish the diagnosis of ICU myopathy in patients with a stereotypical clinical presentation, and typical nerve conduction and needle examination findings of CIM. The muscle biopsy for CIM discloses muscle fiber atrophy, especially involving the type II fibers; a variable degree of muscle fiber necrosis, and the absence of any inflammatory cells. The hallmark of the disorder—loss of myosin—can be confirmed immunocytochemically or by electron microscopy as reduction in myosin–adenosine triphosphatase reactivity in nonnecrotic fibers [4,11]. Severity ranges from "cachectic myopathy"(a relatively mild myopathy without major structural damage) to a more severe myopathy with thick filament loss, and even the most severe myopathy with pronounced necrotizing features [14].

Pathophysiology

Myosin loss and muscle fiber necrosis contribute to persisting weakness. Myosin loss is characteristic of CIM; corticosteroids often cause the loss of myosin, but other agents that block the neuromuscular junction in ICU patients contribute as well [7,11]. Consistent with this hypothesis, patients with myasthenia can develop loss of myosin thick filaments after receiving high-dose corticosteroids [15]; and an animal model of dexamethasone plus denervation preferentially depletes thick filaments, with reduction in muscle fiber size [16]. Some systemically ill patients who are not exposed to corticosteroids or neuromuscular blocking agents, with metabolic acidosis and multiorgan failure, can also develop CIM. Acidosis may stimulate glucocorticoid production; increase muscle protein degradation; and trigger thick filament loss [7]; likewise, inflammation; immobilization; the endocrine stress response; mitochondrial dysfunction; nutritional deficits; and compromise in the microcirculation of muscle tissue can cause impaired protein synthesis [2,3,17,18].

Treatment

The treatment of CIM is symptomatic: treating the underlying systemic illness and discontinuing or minimizing corticosteroids and neuromuscular blocking agents to the extent possible. There is evidence from two large trials that intensive insulin therapy reduces electrophysiologic signs of CIM and CIP; and high quality evidence that it reduces duration of mechanical ventilation, ICU stay and 180-day mortality [19], but hypoglycemia remains a major concern [3].

Outcomes

When the patient survives their systemic illness, recovery occurs over weeks to months, depending on the severity of the myopathy [7].For patients whose disease severity was pronounced and for those with concomitant CIP, recovery is expected to take many months, along with the need for tracheostomy and long-term ventilatory support. In these patients some motor recovery ultimately occurs; but they will likely be left with residual long-term muscle weakness and atrophy, with compromise in daily functioning and ambulation. CIP is the main contributor to persistent disability; and in cases of CIM with coexisting CIP, it is CIP per se that impedes recovery [3]; CIM in isolation can be associated with complete recovery [4, 20].

CRITICAL ILLNESS POLYNEUROPATHY

Diagnosis

Patients with CIP develop a symmetrical, sensorimotor axon-loss polyneuropathy [4] most prominent in the lower extremities, with depressed or absent reflexes. Facial muscles are usually not affected helping to distinguish this disorder from the Guillain–Barré syndrome where bilateral facial paresis occurs in >50%.In most cases of CIP, distal muscles are affected more than proximal muscles, but when the disorder is severe there is generalized flaccid weakness and ventilatory failure. There is usually distal sensory loss of pain, temperature and vibration sense in patients alert enough to be tested [4]. Many patients with CIP have a concomitant encephalopathy from their underlying multiorgan system failure, sepsis, or both [4].

Risk Factors

Sepsis and multiorgan failure are the main risk factors for CIP [3].One prospective study that assessed patients clinically and electrophysiologically found that 70% of patients had evidence of an axonal polyneuropathy on average 28 days after onset of sepsis and multiorgan failure [21]. Approximately 50% of patients admitted to the ICU with sepsis and multiorgan failure for at least 2 weeks will have EMG evidence for an axon-loss polyneuropathy.

Laboratory Studies

EMG Studies

The most important diagnostic test for CIP is the EMG which shows an axonal polyneuropathy with reduced—and in severe cases, absent—sensory and motor responses. The nerves of the lower limbs are often more affected than those of the arms owing to the length-dependent distribution of pathology. Nerve conduction velocities are generally normal or only mildly reduced as is seen in axonal neuropathies[6]. Nerve conduction studies of the phrenic nerves will generally reveal reduced responses. In CIP the direct muscle stimulation-evoked response of the anterior tibial muscle is relatively higher than the response elicited by peroneal nerve stimulation; the ratio of the amplitude of nerve stimulation-evoked muscle response compared to direct muscle stimulation-evoked response is <0.5. Needle electrode examination reveals typical features of acute denervation—positive sharp waves and fibrillations—and reduced recruitment of motor unit potentials. More pronounced changes are seen in distal than in proximal muscles. Nerve biopsy is rarely indicated in evaluating a patient with suspected CIP, unless another treatable etiology is suspected. Nerve histology in CIP shows distal axonal degeneration of motor and sensory fibers; muscle shows atrophy of both type I and type II fibers [4].Skin biopsies show loss of intraepidermal nerve fibers and reduction in sweat gland innervation indicating small fiber pathology in the acute phase of critical illness [22,23].

Pathophysiology

The polyneuropathy is a complication of the systemic inflammatory response triggered by sepsis, severe trauma, or burns [4]. It may be caused by impaired microcirculation causing reduced nerve perfusion, edema, hypoxia, and breakdown in the blood–nerve barrier. The neuropathy may also be caused by damage from cytokines, or by insulin resistance causing hyperglycemia with damage to mitochondria [4]. Abnormal nerve excitability, caused by sodium channel inactivation may cause reversible weakness for some patients [3,24].

Treatment

Treatment is symptomatic and supportive, with stabilization of critical medical and surgical conditions and vigorous treatment of sepsis. No specific treatment reduces the incidence and severity of CIP (or CIM) [4]. Although intensive insulin treatment of hyperglycemia reduces the incidence of electrophysiologic signs of CIP and CIM, mortality is greater in patients treated to strict normoglycemia [3].

Outcome

Recovery of sensory and motor function occurs over weeks to months, depending on the severity of the neuropathy. In some instances of very slow recovery over months, long-term ventilatory support may be required, even after the underlying critical illness has resolved. Compared to patients with CIM, those with CIP tend to have a slower and less complete recovery. 88% of CIM patients recovered in 1 year compared with 55% of patients with CIP or CIP and CIM combined [20].Survivors of CIP may be left with painful dysesthesias from the small fiber neuropathy [22].

DIFFERENTIAL DIAGNOSIS

Other peripheral neuropathies, neuromuscular junction disorders, and myopathies may present with acutely evolving weakness and simulate CIM or CIP [6,25]. Among the acute and severe polyneuropathies, the most common acute and severe polyneuropathy is the Guillain–Barré syndrome (GBS) (see Chapter 152). Two-thirds of patients have had a preceding viral or bacterial syndrome, an inoculation or recent surgery. Most patients present with rapidly progressive areflexic paralysis beginning in the legs and spreading proximally; the diaphragm is involved in 25% of cases and the facial muscles in more than 50%. Most patients' EMGs reveal a demyelinating polyneuropathy with slowed nerve conduction velocity to <70% of normal, partial conduction block; prolonged distal motor latencies; and prolonged or absent late responses, distinguishing GBS from CIP. In most patients with GBS, the cerebrospinal fluid (CSF) examination shows an albuminocytologic dissociation (elevation in protein without pleocytosis) distinguishing GBS from CIP in which the CSF findings are normal. Guillain–Barré syndrome, an immune-mediated disorder, responds to intravenous γ-globulin or plasma exchange (unlike CIP or CIM which do not), making early recognition essential in an effort to start treatment early and reduce morbidity.

Peripheral neuropathy may be seen in some patients up to 30 days following a surgical procedure. Unlike CIM or CIP, these postsurgical axonal neuropathies are clinically heterogeneous, presenting as focal, multifocal, or diffuse (polyradiculoneuropathy) disorders [26]; and unlike CIM or CIP, magnetic resonance imaging (MRI) of nerves, roots, and plexuses shows inflammatory changes. These neuropathies often respond to immunotherapy.

The most important neuromuscular junction disorder causing acute weakness is myasthenia gravis (see Chapter 153). Most individuals present with ocular muscle weakness with ptosis and diplopia, and generalized weakness with a fatigable component. More than 90% of patients have antibodies to the acetylcholine receptor, and abnormal EMG findings, with a decremental motor response during repetitive nerve stimulation at 2 to 3 Hz.

Another neuromuscular junction disorder is prolonged neuromuscular blockade by muscle relaxants, nearly always seen in patients with renal or hepatic failure. It is often associated with elevated levels of the metabolite of vecuronium, and tends to improve after infusion of an acetylcholinesterase inhibitor.

Botulism is a presynaptic disorder characterized by rapidly progressive, diffuse, symmetrical weakness with a proximal predominance; dysarthria and dysphagia; respiratory involvement; and a prominent autonomic component (dilated pupils, bradyarrhythmia, ileus, orthostatic hypotension, and urinary retention). Management consists of supportive care and administration of trivalent antitoxin.

THE DIAGNOSTIC CHALLENGE: DISTINGUISHING CRITICAL ILLNESS MYOPATHY FROM CRITICAL ILLNESS POLYNEUROPATHY

Severe generalized weakness with failure to wean from mechanical ventilation; preserved reflexes and sensation; a transient rise in CK; and relatively preserved sensory responses on EMG suggests ICU myopathy rather than neuropathy [27]. With ICU polyneuropathy, sensory loss; areflexia; and the EMG findings of an acute neuropathic disorder are typical. Clinically, a polyneuropathy may easily be missed because in many patients detailed sensory examination is impossible in the ICU setting, especially if there is a coexisting encephalopathy. Further confounding the distinction, reflex loss can occur in both CIP and myopathy; fibrillation potentials may be found in both disorders, and motor unit potentials may not be elicitable owing to severe weakness or encephalopathy. In the final analysis, it may be difficult to distinguish one disorder from another in an individual case; and it is likely that in many patients *both* disorders are present in varying degrees [6,28], giving rise to a combined syndrome of CIM and CIP.

References

1. Fan E, Cheek F, Chlan L, et al: An official American Thoracic Society Clinical Practice Guideline: the diagnosis of intensive care unit—acquired weakness in adults. *Am J Resp Care Med* 190:1437–1436, 2015.
2. Kress JP, Hall JB: ICU acquired weakness and recovery from critical illness. *N Engl J Med* 370:1626–1635, 2014.
3. Hermans G, Van den Berghe G: Clinical review: intensive care unit acquired weakness. *Crit Care* 19:274, 2015.
4. Latronico N, Bolton CF: Critical illness polyneuropathy and myopathy: a major cause of muscle weakness and paralysis. *Lancet Neurology* 10:931–941, 2011.
5. De Jonghe B, Sharshar T, LeFaucheur JP, et al: Paresis acquired in the intensive care unit: a prospective multicenter study. *JAMA* 288:2859, 2002.
6. Lacomis D: Electrophysiology of neuromuscular disorders in critical illness. *Muscle Nerve* 47:452–463, 2013.

7. Lacomis D, Giuliani MJ, Van Cott A, et al: Acute myopathy of intensive care: clinical, electromyographic, and pathological aspects. *Ann Neurol* 40:645, 1996.
8. Banwell BL, Mildner RJ, Hassall AC, et al: Muscle weakness in critically ill children. *Neurology* 61:1779, 2003.
9. Kukreti V, Shamin M, Khilnani P: Intensive care unit acquired weakness in children: critical illness polyneuropathy and myopathy. *J Crit Care Med* 18:95–101, 2014.
10. Lacomis D, Petrella JT, Giuliani MJ: Causes of neuromuscular weakness in the intensive care unit: a study of ninety-two patients. *Muscle Nerve* 21:610, 1998.
11. Lacomis D, Zochodne DW, Bird S: Critical illness myopathy. *Muscle Nerve* 23:1785, 2000.
12. Rich MM, Bird SJ, Raps EC, et al: Direct muscle stimulation in acute quadriplegic myopathy. *Muscle Nerve* 20:665, 1997.
13. LeFaucheur JP, Nordine T, Rodriguez P, et al: Origin of ICU acquired paresis determined by direct muscle stimulation. *J Neurol Neurosurg Psychiatry* 77:500, 2006.
14. Pati S, Goodfellow JA, Iyadurai S, et al: Approach to critical illness polyneuropathy and myopathy. *Postgrad Med J* 84:354–360, 2008.
15. Panegyres PK, Squier M, Mills KR, et al: Acute myopathy associated with large parenteral doses of corticosteroids in myasthenia gravis. *J Neurol Neurosurg Psychiatry* 56:702, 1993.
16. Rouleau G, Karpati G, Carpenter S, et al: Glucocorticoid excess induces preferential depletion of myosin in denervated skeletal muscle fibers. *Muscle Nerve* 10:428, 1987.
17. Friedrich O, Reid MB, Van den Berghe G, et al: The sick and the weak: neuropathies/myopathies in the critically ill. *Physiol Rev* 95:1025, 2015.
18. Rich MM, Pinter MJ: Sodium channel inactivation in an animal model of acute quadriplegic myopathy. *Ann Neurol* 50:26, 2001.
19. Hermans G, De Jonghe B, Bruyninckx F, et al: Interventiona for preventing critical illness polyneuropathy and critical illness myopathy. *Cochrane Data base Syst Rev* 1:CD006832, 2014.
20. Koch S, Wollersheim T, Bierbrauer J, et al: Long-tern recovery in critical illness myopathy is complete, contrary to polyneuropathy. *Muscle Nerve* 50:431–436, 2014.
21. Intiso D, Amoruso L, Zarrelli M, et al: Long-term functional outcome and health status of patients with polyneuromyopathy. *Acta Neurol Scand* 123:211–219, 2011.
22. Latronico N, Filusto M, Figoni N, et al: Small nerve fiber pathology in critical illness. *PLoS One* 30:e75696, 2013.
23. Skorna M, Kopacik R, Vlckova E, et al: Small-nerve fiber pathology in critical illness documented by serial skin biopsies. *Muscle Nerve* 52:28–33, 2015.
24. Novak KR, Nardelli P, Cope TC, et al: Inactivation of sodium channels underlies reversible neuropathy during critical illness in rats. *J Clin Invest* 119:1150, 2009.
25. Gorson KC: Approach to neuromuscular disorders in the intensive care unit. *Neurocrit Care* 3:195, 2005.
26. Staff N, Engelstad J, Klein CJ, et al: Post-surgical inflammatory neuropathy. *Brain* 133:2866–2880, 2010.
27. Sander HW, Golden M, Danon MJ: Quadriplegic areflexic ICU illness: selective thick filament loss and normal nerve histology. *Muscle Nerve* 26:499, 2002.
28. Bird SJ, Rich MM: Critical illness myopathy and polyneuropathy. *Curr Neurol Neurosci Rep* 2:527, 2002.

Chapter 155 ■ Neuro-oncologic Problems in the Intensive Care Unit

NORMAN SCOTT LITOFSKY • YAW SARPONG

INTRODUCTION

Neuro-oncology encompasses the care of patients with neoplasms affecting the brain, spinal cord, and peripheral nervous system. These tumors may arise either within the nervous system itself or spread from systemic malignancies. Neuro-oncology patients may require care in an intensive care unit (ICU), following surgery—if they suffer catastrophic or near catastrophic neurologic decline; or if they are at high risk to suffer such a change. Lastly, neuro-oncology patients may also suffer from medical processes that require intensive care.

These issues include: elevated intracranial pressure (ICP); hydrocephalus; seizures; postoperative complications; spinal neoplastic disease; and medical systemic complications.

ELEVATED INTRACRANIAL PRESSURE

Elevated ICP frequently complicates the course of patients with both primary and metastatic cerebral neoplasms. Patients with aggressive brain tumors often succumb as a consequence of uncontrollable elevations in ICP.

Pathophysiology

Normal ICP ranges between 5 and 15 cm H_2O. This pressure is generated by the volumes of the various components contained in the "closed box" of the skull, including brain parenchyma; cerebrospinal fluid (CSF); extracellular water; and blood in vascular spaces. A perturbation of any of these components can increase ICP. Any additional tissue not normally present in the brain, such as a primary or metastatic tumor, or a hemorrhage associated with a tumor, can also increase intracranial pressure. Although the numerical value of the intracranial pressure cannot be ascertained by neuro-diagnostic images, some of the perturbations are evident on either computed tomography (CT) scan or magnetic resonance imaging (MRI).

Brain tumors can affect each intracranial component. In addition to the bulk owing to the neoplasm itself, cerebral neoplasms produce vasogenic edema [1], secondary to increased permeability of blood vessels within or adjacent to the tumor, thereby increasing extracellular fluid [2,3]. Radiographically, this edema results in hypodensity on CT or hyperintensity on T2-weighted MRI around the enhancing bulk of tumor. Tumor mass, or brain parenchyma displaced by tumor, may obstruct CSF pathways, causing hydrocephalus. Rarely, some brain tumors (choroid plexus papillomas and carcinomas) may produce excessive CSF which can cause hydrocephalus and thereby increase intracranial pressure [4] (Hydrocephalus is discussed in detail below). Intravascular blood volume also can increase in patients with tumors as a result of vasodilatation from hypoventilation. Hypoventilation can occur with seizure activity or ICP elevation, both of which can reduce respiratory drive. Hypoventilation increases pCO_2, causing arterial vasodilation, thereby increasing intravascular volume and intracranial pressure. This can cause a positive feedback loop by further reducing ventilatory drive.

Signs and Symptoms

Elevated intracranial pressure can cause variety of symptoms and signs, which do not necessarily correlate with the degree of elevated pressure, though generally the higher the intracranial pressure, the more severe the neurologic findings.

As ICP increases, compression of the reticular activating system depresses the patient's level of consciousness. This tends to occur sequentially, with the patient progressing from an awake and alert status to progressively more lethargic states and eventually to coma. Patients may develop varying degrees of cognitive changes including disorientation, short-term memory impairment, decreased fund of knowledge, and loss of insight and judgment.

As increasing ICP exceeds 19 mm H_2O, approaching the pressure of the central retinal vein, the patient usually loses spontaneous venous pulsations typically seen on routine funduscopic examination. Further elevation of ICP may cause swelling of the optic disks (papilledema). Papilledema usually occurs over several days. A patient with long-standing papilledema may have constriction of his/her visual fields and/or decreased visual acuity.

Brain masses causing elevated ICP can cause brain shifts from one intracranial compartment to another. Usually a brain shift, also known as a "herniation," is away from the mass causing the elevated ICP. Supratentorial masses may cause the brain to herniate inferiorly through the tentorial incisura. With a resulting central diencephalic herniation syndrome, the patient experiences simultaneous bilateral pupillary dilation from compression of the tectum, containing the Edinger–Westphal nucleus of the oculomotor nerve (CN III). A lateral cerebral mass, particularly in the temporal lobe, forces the uncus of the temporal lobe to herniate through the incisura, causing compression of CN III between the posterior cerebral artery and the superior cerebellar artery, with unilateral pupillary dilation. In both herniation syndromes, the constrictive phase of the light reflex can also cease to function (unreactive pupils). Usually, though not always, decrease in the patient's level of consciousness precedes pupillary dysfunction.

Patients can also have light-near dissociation. Pressure on the tectum can compress the retino-tectal fibers that are part of the afferent limb of the pupillary light reflex; the pupil does not constrict to light well. Fibers involved in the afferent limb of pupillary accommodation to near vision, which travel to the tectum through other pathways, are not affected, and pupils may constrict to accommodation but not to light if the patient is sufficiently alert. This finding is a very subtle sign of elevated intracranial pressure.

Double vision may be present. The abducens nerve (CN VI), which controls abduction of the eye, has the longest intracranial course of the cranial nerves and is at highest risk of dysfunction when ICP is elevated. Diplopia is usually more pronounced on lateral gaze, either unilaterally or bilaterally.

As the dura and blood vessels are stretched by elevated ICP, the patient may experience headache, frequently described as "band-like" or "pressure-like." It tends to occur more commonly in the early morning and may wake the patient from sleep. During sleep, the recumbent position decreases venous return to the heart, elevating ICP, and hypoventilation that occurs during sleep also elevates ICP, increasing the headache.

Not uncommonly, headache is associated with projectile vomiting owing to pressure on the area postrema.

Patients with elevated ICP often experience neurologic deficits from compression by the tumor mass on adjacent neural structures. These deficits can include hemiparesis; aphasia; visual field loss; hearing loss; ataxia (truncal or appendicular); and sensory loss. The presence of these findings is based on the size, location, and rapidity of growth of the mass. Slower growing tumors allow the brain to compensate; focal findings may not be evident until late in the patient's course.

Management

Mechanical and pharmacologic therapies are available to treat elevated ICP, with reduction or elimination of its manifestations. Some require very minimal intervention, whereas others are much more intensive or invasive.

Head elevation is perhaps the easiest treatment available, increasing venous drainage from the brain, and reducing intracranial blood volume. Head elevation poses minimal risk to the patient; although cerebral perfusion could be diminished, it is negligible in a patient with normal blood pressure.

Furosemide (Lasix), a loop diuretic, rapidly reduces systemic circulating volume. Extracellular and intracellular water in the brain are drawn into the vascular system and are redistributed. Lasix also promotes venous pooling, leading to similar redistribution of fluids. Lasix is generally used as an initial resuscitative dose of 1 mg per kg in patients with cerebral herniation. Risks are minimal in this setting, because electrolyte abnormalities are unlikely to occur with only a single dose. In a patient who has had frequent vomiting and is already dehydrated, Lasix can cause hypotension from loss of cardiac preload.

Mannitol, an osmotic diuretic, draws fluid out of the brain and into the vascular system by increasing serum osmolarity. From the vascular spaces, the fluid follows the mannitol as the kidney excretes it, reducing intracellular and extracellular water in the brain. Furthermore, mannitol improves blood flow, perfusing ischemic areas of brain adjacent to the tumor mass better [5]. Mannitol is frequently given as an initial resuscitative dose of 1 g per kg, followed by 0.25 g per kg every 4 to 6 hours to maintain the diuresis and control ICP. Mannitol is quite effective in lowering ICP and/or reversing early cerebral herniation. It may also be used if patients have significant mass effect identified on neuro-imaging studies to stabilize and improve their condition (Fig. 155.1). A number of potential risks are present with long-term mannitol use. Hypotension can occur in already hypovolemic patients. Patients can also become hyperosmolar and hypernatremic. Therefore, mannitol is usually withheld from the patient if serum osmolarity exceeds 320 mOsm per L.

Hypertonic saline (2% to 23.4% NaCl) can be used as an osmotic diuretic for increased ICP. Similar to mannitol, the infusion of saline in the intravascular space increases intravascular osmotic pressure, drawing fluid from the intracranial extracellular spaces into the vascular spaces, and decreasing intracranial pressure. Additionally, hypertonic saline increases arterial blood pressure; cerebral blood perfusion; blood flow; brain tissue oxygen (PbO_2), and brain tissue pH. Hypertonic saline may be better for decreasing ICP and may maintain its effects longer than mannitol [6]. Studies comparing the use of mannitol and hypertonic saline in patients undergoing brain tumor surgery show that hypertonic saline patients experience increased brain relaxation, need less fluid, and had normal to higher serum sodium [7,8]. Moreover, these studies suggest that hypertonic saline exerts its effect by reducing edema. Potential risks in the usage of hypertonic saline include cardiac arrhythmias, hypokalemia, acute hypotension with rapid infusion, and the neurologic side effects of rapid increase of serum sodium, including seizures; confusion; lethargy; and osmotic demyelination syndromes [9].

Glucocorticosteroids improve symptoms of elevated ICP and/or mass effect in patients with cerebral neoplasms by stabilizing cell membranes and reducing vasogenic edema [10,11]. Dexamethasone is the most commonly used glucocorticosteroid. An initial dose of 10 to 20 mg is followed by 4 to 6 mg every 4 to 6 hours, depending on the severity of the patient's clinical condition. Solu-Medrol (100 mg initially, and then 20 to 40 mg every 4 to 6 hours) is another option. Glucocorticosteroids are the medical mainstay of brain tumor care because their effects are sustained over time. A patient with vasogenic edema from tumor may require steroids for a significant period of time. Steroids can cause hyperglycemia and exacerbate diabetes mellitus, changing the patient's insulin requirements. Gastrointestinal hemorrhage or ulceration can occur; H_2 blockers such as Pepcid, Zantac, or Tagamet are frequently given prophylactically. The stimulatory effect of steroids frequently disrupts sleep. Long-term use of steroids may be associated with proximal

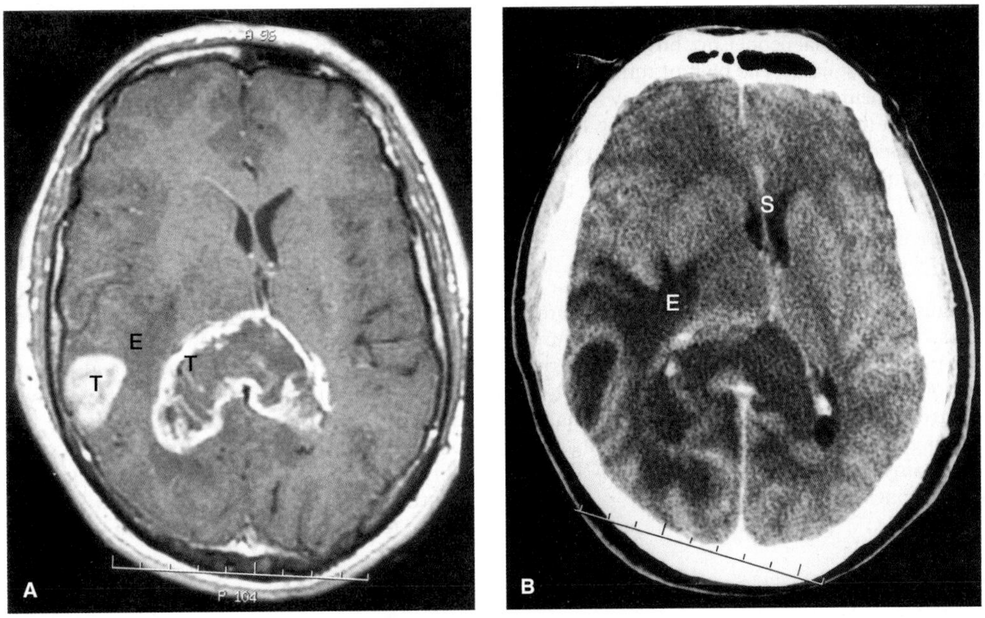

FIGURE 155.1 **A:** This MRI, performed on a patient presenting with headache and memory lapses, shows an enhancing mass (T) involving the corpus callosum and right parietal area, with surrounding edema (E). Stereotactic biopsy revealed glioblastoma multiforme. **B:** One week following biopsy, the patient was admitted to the ICU with obtundation and left hemiparesis. His CT shows increased edema (E) and right-to-left midline shift (S)—parafalcine herniation. He required mannitol; increased Decadron; and surgical decompression to improve. MRI, magnetic resonance imaging; ICU, intensive care unit; CT, computed tomography.

muscle weakness; avascular necrosis of the femoral head; easy bruising; and findings of Cushing's syndrome.

Hyperventilation, reducing blood pCO_2, causes cerebral vasoconstriction, which reduces the arterial intravascular blood volume within the brain. Hyperventilation can rapidly reduce intracranial pressure and reverse a cerebral herniation syndrome. Although initial hyperventilation can be performed with an AMBU bag, sustained hyperventilation requires endotracheal intubation and mechanical ventilation of the patient. Moderation of hyperventilation is necessary because at pCO_2 less than 25 torr, cerebral ischemia may result from profound vasoconstriction. A vasodilatory rebound from hyperventilation occurs after approximately 24 hours, thereby negating its positive effects if hyperventilation is used chronically [12].

One of the most effective means of rapidly reducing intracranial pressure is to drain CSF. Such a maneuver is effective whether or not the patient has hydrocephalus. In a patient with a brain tumor, the safest method of draining CSF is to place a ventriculostomy, a catheter usually passed into the frontal horn of the lateral ventricle via a small hole drilled through the skull. The procedure can be performed by a neurosurgeon at the bedside. After placement of a ventriculostomy, drainage of CSF into a bag at bedside can reduce ICP. The catheter can also be coupled to a pressure transducer so that ICP can be measured. Usually, CSF is drained if ICP exceeds 15 to 20 mm Hg. The risks of the procedure include hemorrhage and infection. Therefore, coagulation studies are appropriate before the procedure is done, especially in patients who have received recent chemotherapy. The longer the catheter remains in place, the higher the risk of infection. Sometimes, prophylactic antibiotics are used.

PbO_2 can also be monitored, using a device such as the Licox intracranial pressure monitor (Integra Neuroscience, Plainsboro, New Jersey) which monitors ICP and brain temperature, as well as PbO_2. The rationale behind this monitoring tool is to provide clinicians in the operating room (OR) or ICU information regarding oxygen supply and utilization in specific tissue beds [13], alerting clinicians to areas that are at increased risks for brain damage due to hypoxia. Tissue that might already be dead because of the tumor/its reactive changes can be differentiated from tissue that might be at risk from ischemia owing to the pressure exerted by the tumor mass and its associated edema. Combining this information with the measured ICP can assist in tailoring management of these patients in the neuro-critical care setting or the OR to detect and prevent secondary ischemic events promptly. One drawback of the device relates to concerns regarding its accuracy and reliability [14].

The best means of controlling ICP long-term is to remove or shrink the tumor when possible. Unfortunately, some tumors are unresectable. Gliomas or metastases of the thalamus or basal ganglia are generally not resected except in unusual circumstances. In these instances, medical management is necessary to control ICP until adjuvant therapy, such as radiation therapy, can shrink the tumor and reduce its edema producing capabilities. The same rationale applies in patients with multifocal cerebral masses; patients with more than one metastasis do not usually have multiple operations to resect each tumor, especially if symptoms are controllable with steroids. For patients with persistent hydrocephalus, CSF shunting can be performed as a permanent CSF diversion. In performing a shunt, a neurosurgeon can introduce a catheter into the ventricles and tunnel it subcutaneously into the abdomen or pleural space. Further, an adjustable valve is added to control the rate of CSF drainage. This drainage method decreases the risk of infection associated with prolonged usage of ventriculostomy. On the other hand, this procedure exposes the patient to risks associated with invasive surgical maneuvers, such as hemorrhage, stroke, device failure, infection, and pneumothorax [15].

If the tumor is resectable, its removal can relieve the brain of the extra mass, relieve obstruction to the flow of CSF, and reduce vasogenic edema. In addition to relieving the signs and symptoms of elevated ICP, tumor resection can also relieve the effects of compression on the surrounding brain, improving lateralizing findings. Some tumors can be removed completely. These include meningiomas, vestibular schwannomas, craniopharyngiomas, pituitary adenomas, and some metastatic tumors. Microscopic disease may still be present in the tumor bed, particularly in the case of metastases or craniopharyngioma, which may require adjuvant therapy, but ICP can be well controlled. Primary glial neoplasms, however, cannot be completely removed in most cases. The bulk of tumor can be resected, and postoperative neuro-diagnostic images may show no residual tumor, but most of these tumors have infiltrating fingers of tumor that are still present. Even so, debulking the tumor can alleviate elevated ICP, even if it is only partially removed.

HYDROCEPHALUS

Brain tumors often cause hydrocephalus, a situation in which the patient has an increased volume of CSF under increased pressure. Hydrocephalus is typically associated with enlargement of the ventricular system (or a portion thereof) and compression of the normal brain parenchyma. A patient with hydrocephalus may require urgent or emergent intensive care monitoring and treatment. Hydrocephalus is a special case of elevated ICP and warrants a unique approach.

Etiology

Hydrocephalus can occur from a variety of mechanisms in patients with brain tumors. The definitive treatment of hydrocephalus is often based on its specific mechanism of formation.

Carcinomatous meningitis, caused by leptomeningeal infiltration by tumor cells in the subarachnoid space, can prevent the absorption of CSF by the arachnoid granulations, either by occluding the granulations or preventing the flow of CSF from the outlet foramina of the fourth ventricle to the granulations. Metastatic tumors from the lung, breast, lymphoma, and leukemia are the most frequently involved systemic tumors; primary tumors behaving in this fashion include primitive neuroectodermal tumors (i.e., medulloblastoma), ependymoblastoma, and glioblastoma multiforme. A patient with carcinomatous meningitis will frequently have a stiff neck or cranial neuropathy in addition to symptoms and signs of elevated ICP.

Large extra-axial "benign" tumors, usually in the posterior fossa, can cause hydrocephalus (Fig. 155.2). These tumors include those in the cerebellopontine angle, such as meningioma or vestibular schwannoma. These tumors displace the cerebellar hemisphere and obstruct the fourth ventricle to prevent adequate circulation of CSF. Rarely, a choroid plexus papilloma can emerge from the Foramina of Luschka and similarly compress the cerebellar hemisphere. Meningiomas of the clivus or tentorium can also displace CSF pathways with resulting hydrocephalus.

Some tumors may originate in a ventricle or protrude into a ventricle and occlude CSF pathways, thus producing hydrocephalus. These tumors include medulloblastoma; ependymoma; choroid plexus papilloma; intraventricular meningioma; colloid cyst; central neurocytoma; giant cell astrocytoma of tuberous sclerosis; and pineal region tumors.

Parenchymal tumors often can occlude CSF pathways. Primary or metastatic tumors in the thalamus or basal ganglia can displace brain parenchyma and occlude the Foramina of Monro or the third ventricle [16,17]. Tumors in the pineal region may occlude the posterior third ventricle or cerebral aqueduct (Fig. 155.3). Brain stem gliomas or tumors in the cerebellar hemispheres can compress the fourth ventricle [18].

Symptoms and Signs

The clinical picture of a patient with hydrocephalus is frequently the same as that of a patient with elevated ICP. In fact, hydrocephalus must be considered in the differential diagnosis for causes of elevated ICP. Patients with midline masses or carcinomatous meningitis usually do not have lateralizing neurologic deficits such as hemiparesis. Patients with unilateral brain masses may develop lateralizing deficits from further compression of the previously marginally functioning brain by progressive hydrocephalus.

Evaluation

If hydrocephalus is suspected, evaluation should proceed promptly. Two questions must be answered—"Does the patient have hydrocephalus?" and "What is the cause of the hydrocephalus?" Either MRI or CT can answer these questions. MRI delineates anatomic definition of the brain, and more readily illustrates the relationship of the lesion to CSF pathways, so MRI with gadolinium is the preferred study. If the patient is too ill to obtain an MRI, or MRI is not readily available, a CT scan with intravenous (IV) contrast is sufficient. The purpose of the contrast agent with either study is to characterize the location of the lesion and its relationship to CSF pathways.

Management

Intervention for a patient with hydrocephalus depends on the cause of the hydrocephalus, the anatomic location of the obstruction to CSF flow, and the patient's clinical condition.

In patients experiencing rapidly progressive deterioration, such as cerebral herniation, emergent management with a ventriculostomy, to divert CSF temporarily, can improve the patient's clinical picture. Usually, the drainage chamber is set so that the system can be opened intermittently to drain CSF for ICP greater than 20 mm Hg. Some patients, however, require a lower ICP to achieve neurologic improvement, so the system can be opened for lower pressures. Alternatively the system can be set to drain CSF continuously at a particular pressure, for instance at 15 mm Hg. ICP is then recorded on an hourly basis. This technique of CSF drainage should be approached with some caution, because large volumes of CSF can drain if the patient strains or coughs, increasing intrathoracic pressure and therefore ICP temporarily. If too much CSF drains, patients can develop subdural or intraparenchymal hemorrhages.

A patient may have only mild hydrocephalus and not be significantly impaired clinically. Emergent intervention may not be necessary, and the patient can be stabilized with dexamethasone with or without mannitol. Resection of the tumor can provide long-term treatment of hydrocephalus by decompressing the CSF pathways, particularly with posterior fossa or pineal region tumors. Timely surgery is the best approach.

Occasionally hydrocephalus does not respond to surgical decompression alone, especially if not enough tumor can be resected to decompress the CSF pathways. Alternatively, absorptive capabilities may be compromised by inflammatory process from blood or tumor products. A permanent shunt is then necessary to treat the hydrocephalus. Although tumors with malignant cells in the CSF raise a concern that intraperitoneal spread of tumor may occur via the shunt, this complication is uncommon. Persistent symptomatic hydrocephalus dictates that the shunt be placed regardless of this concern.

In a patient with hydrocephalus who has been shunted, shunt malfunction may occur [19]. Cellular debris, proteinaceous material, or normal choroid plexus can occasionally occlude a shunt, manifested by recurrence of symptoms and signs of hydrocephalus and elevated ICP. Treatment requires operative revision of the occluded portion of the shunt, usually with replacement of the ventricular catheter or the valve.

Endoscopic third ventriculostomy (ETV) can be an alternative to a shunt in cases in which the outflow of the third ventricle

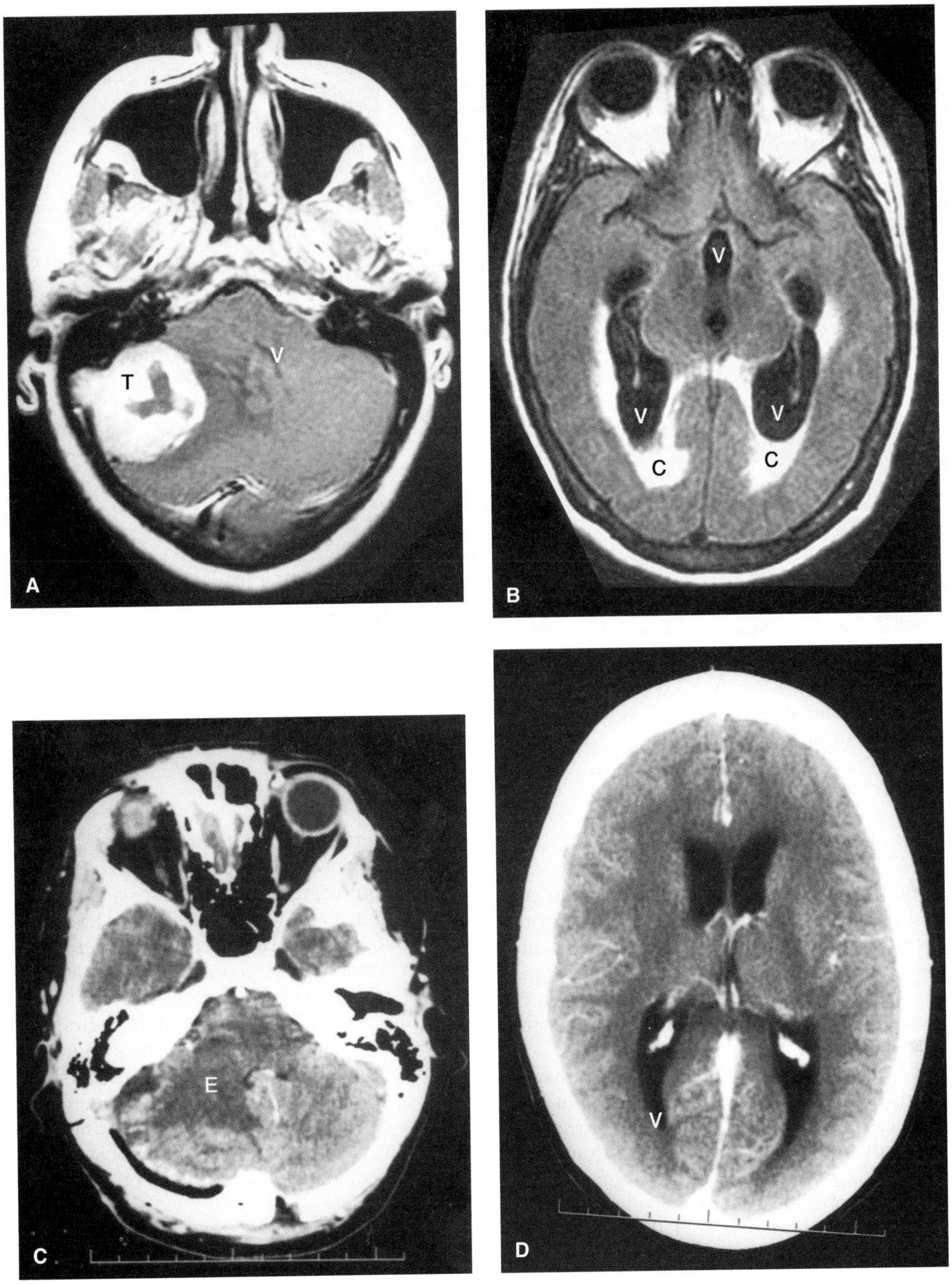

FIGURE 155.2 **A:** This MRI, performed on a patient presenting with headache and obtundation, shows an enhancing mass in the right cerebello-pontine angle (T) with displacement of the fourth ventricle (V) to the left. **B:** Additional views of the MRI show hydrocephalus, with enlarged, rounded ventricles (V) and transependymal spread of CSF (C). A ventriculostomy to drain CSF was placed to temporize the patient prior to surgery. **C:** After resection of the tumor, a meningioma, the fourth ventricle returns toward its normal position. Edema (E) in the cerebellar hemisphere is still present. **D:** Hydrocephalus has resolved, with the ventricle (V) returning to normal size and shape. MRI, magnetic resonance imaging; CSF, cerebrospinal fluid.

is obstructed if the patient has favorable anatomy. ETV is performed by using an endoscope to navigate through the lateral ventricle and the foramen of Monro to the third ventricular floor. A hole is made into the floor of the third ventricle between the infundibular recess and mammillary bodies to create a conduit into the subarachnoid space, provided that the distance between the clivus and basilar artery and the floor of the third ventricle is adequate, usually 3 to 5 mm [20,21]. Device failure is eliminated, but sometimes the ETV is not effective, and a shunt must subsequently be placed [20].

Hydrocephalus can be difficult to treat in a patient with a tumor adjacent to the third ventricle. In this uncommon situation, the lateral ventricles may not communicate with each other through the third ventricle, and in the most extreme case, the frontal horns of the lateral ventricles do not communicate with the occipital and temporal horns. A single shunt would be ineffective in relieving the CSF obstruction. A ventriculogram with intrathecal contrast placed into the lateral ventricle via a ventricular catheter can define the nature of the obstruction. The patient may require multiple ventricular catheters to drain CSF adequately. Tumors involving the medial septal structures of the brain, where this problem should be of concern, include craniopharyngioma, central neurocytoma, pilocytic astrocytoma of the hypothalamus, and glioblastoma.

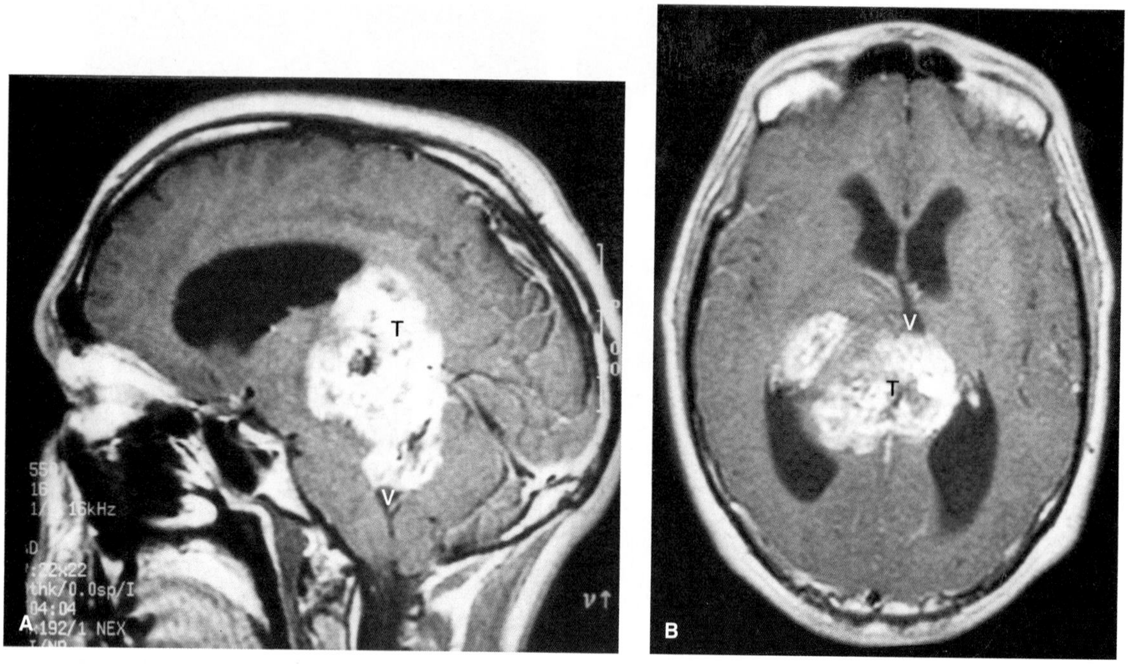

FIGURE 155.3 A: This sagittal MRI on a patient with headache, lethargy, and diffuse weakness shows an enhancing mass (T) extending from the pineal region to the fourth ventricle (V). B: Axial views show the tumor (T) compressing the third ventricle (V) with hydrocephalus. Despite an aggressive surgical resection of this glioblastoma multiforme, the patient subsequently developed recurrent hydrocephalus and required a ventriculo-peritoneal shunt. MRI, magnetic resonance imaging.

SEIZURES

Seizures are a common occurrence in patients with brain tumors. About 40% of patients with gliomas initially present to medical attention with seizure; about 55% of glioma patients have a seizure at some point in the course of their disease. Some low-grade gliomas, such as oligodendroglioma, have a very high likelihood of seizure. Approximately 20% of patients with metastatic tumors have a seizure at some time [22,23].

Seizures may be focal or generalized. A patient remains conscious during a focal seizure. The seizure may be a motor seizure in which the patient's mouth twitches or an extremity moves uncontrollably for a period of time. With a dominant hemisphere lesion, aphasia may occur. During a generalized seizure, the patient loses consciousness. Tonic–clonic movements may occur, and the patient may lose bladder control. A patient can also experience status epilepticus, a series of seizures occurring in rapid succession with the patient not regaining consciousness between seizures. Status epilepticus is a medical emergency that is addressed in Chapter 151. Occasionally a patient can have a seizure that is not witnessed or is subclinical in activity. The patient experiences a neurologic deficit, which subsequently improves, leaving health care providers puzzled as to the etiology of the transient deficit.

A seizure can occur in a patient with a known brain tumor if the patient's anticonvulsant medication level(s) is (are) subtherapeutic. Drug requirements may change as steroid requirements change; dexamethasone may interact with Dilantin to lower serum levels [24,25]. Serum drug levels are therefore essential. Other reasons for seizure include a change in the character of the tumor. The tumor may have grown in size [26] or a hemorrhage within the tumor may have occurred. A CT scan of the head without and with contrast helps to differentiate among these possibilities.

A less recognized seizure presentation in this patient population is nonconvulsive status epilepticus (NCSE), defined as seizure activity lasting greater than 30 minutes with the patient being alert or having a depressed (i.e., lethargic, obtunded, or comatose) level of consciousness [27]. NCSE can be diagnosed if EEG monitoring captures seizure spikes [28]. Commonly, these patients are in the ICU with depressed level of consciousness, often attributed to the presence of the intracranial mass, and thus are often mismanaged. According to recent estimates, approximately 10% of patients with depressed level of consciousness in these settings are experiencing NCSE [29]. Brain tumor patients with a depressed level of consciousness should undergo long-term continuous EEG monitoring to increase the ability of capturing the characteristic 3 Hz interictal spikes associated with these types of seizures [28,29]. Monitoring should be continued for 5 to 10 days to increase the yield of the study [29]. Once diagnosed, appropriate antiepileptic therapy should be started.

Treatment

Although a single generalized seizure usually does not have long-term consequences, such an event may precipitate rapid deterioration in a patient with elevated ICP. The associated hypercarbia from hypoventilation can increase ICP substantially; a stable patient can rapidly deteriorate even to the point of developing a herniation syndrome. Hypoxia can further compromise brain function by causing cerebral ischemia, especially in the area already affected by the tumor. Prompt intervention is therefore necessary.

Maintenance of an adequate airway and reestablishment of adequate ventilation is essential. Oxygen should be provided to the patient. Intubation and mechanical ventilation may be required if the patient experiences hypoventilation.

The best medication to stop seizure activity acutely in patients with status epilepticus is Ativan. The initial dose is 2 mg IV, and the dose is repeated every 5 minutes as needed, up to a total of 8 mg or until the seizure activity stops. Should 8 mg be required, mechanical ventilation will likely be required. Dilantin (15 mg per kg IV) or phenobarbital (15 mg per kg IV) must be used

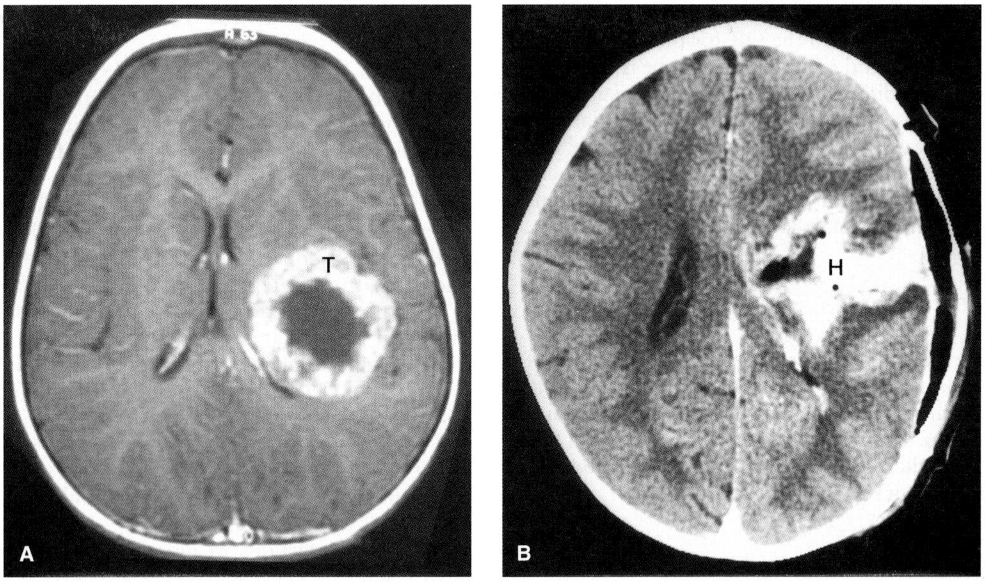

FIGURE 155.4 A: This MRI on a 2-year-old shows a large enhancing mass (T) in the left temporoparietal area. B: Immediately following surgery to remove the rhabdoid neuroepithelial tumor, the patient had sustained hypertension and awakened slowly from her anesthesia with a mild right hemiparesis. This CT scan shows hemorrhage (H) in the tumor bed. With blood pressure control and observation, the patient recovered to a normal level of consciousness with resolution of her hemiparesis over several days. MRI, magnetic resonance imaging; CT, computed tomography.

acutely in conjunction with Ativan, because the Ativan is only for short-term seizure control.

Prophylactic anticonvulsants administered without a seizure having occurred are rarely indicated unless the patient is going to surgery [30]. Following a seizure, the patient should be started on an anticonvulsant, such as Dilantin. The initial dose is 15 mg per kg intravenously, with oral maintenance dosing of 300 mg before bed or 200 mg twice a day. Phenobarbital, although more sedating than Dilantin, can also be used. Both Dilantin and phenobarbital are available in intravenous forms and be used if the patient is unable to take oral or enteral medications. Tegretol, on the other hand, is only available in an oral form, so it cannot be used in status epilepticus or in patients who cannot tolerate enteral intake.

POSTOPERATIVE COMPLICATIONS

One of the most common reasons for a patient with a neuro-oncologic illness to be admitted to an ICU is for observation following a neurosurgical procedure. This period of observation may just be overnight or it may be longer, as dictated by the patient's neurologic and/or medical condition. Although perioperative mortality is less than 2%, medical or neurologic complications may occur in up to 30% of cases; older patients and those with increased neurologic deficits are more likely to suffer these morbidities [31]. Therefore, a variety of intraoperative and postoperative complications must be recognized before the patient's neurologic or medical status is irreversibly compromised.

To anticipate potential complications, vital signs and neuro-checks are usually taken hourly by nurses in the ICU. One of the most important components of the neuro-checks is the patient's level of consciousness, usually denoted by the Glasgow Coma Scale (GCS) score [32,33] (See Chapter 145). Originally developed to document the level of consciousness in patients with head trauma, use of the GCS can readily, reliably, and reproducibly identify changes in the patient's level of consciousness—either deterioration or improvement. Other components of neuro-checks include pupillary light responses, orientation, and motor function. Any decrement in function warrants prompt evaluation. Such an evaluation should include a CT scan of the head, serum electrolytes, blood gases, and anticonvulsant level(s). Other tests may be required based on the patient's condition. Evaluation of the ICU patient for intracerebral hemorrhage or increased ventricular size can be performed at the patient's bedside with a mobile CT scanner, and allow for rapid diagnosis for patients with acute changes in mental status. Mobile CT scanning has also been utilized intraoperatively during resection of glial tumors which may allow for more complete resection of intracranial pathology [34].

Intracranial Hemorrhage

One of the most dramatic complications occurring in the postoperative period is intracranial hemorrhage. Significant hemorrhage usually becomes evident within 6 to 12 hours after the completion of surgery. A patient can bleed into the tumor bed (Fig. 155.4), or into the subdural or epidural spaces. Traction by the brain, slackened by tumor removal; mannitol; Lasix; hyperventilation; and CSF drainage, can tear or stretch draining veins, leading to blood accumulation in the subdural space. Because the dura is separated from the bone to perform the craniotomy, the epidural space is no longer just a potential space; rather, it is a real space into which blood can ooze from underneath the bone edges and accumulate. A patient who experiences significant hypertension or persistent coughing and "bucking" on emerging from anesthesia is at greater risk for developing a postoperative hemorrhage. Hypertension can cause bleeding from arterial-side vessels. The increase in intrathoracic pressure that occurs with coughing or bucking against the endotracheal tube can precipitate venous-side bleeding, as can thrombosis in a draining vein from manipulation.

Postoperative hemorrhage should be suspected in a patient who fails to emerge adequately from anesthesia. Intracranial hemorrhage should also be a concern if the patient deteriorates following emergence from anesthesia and develops progressive decline in level of consciousness, pupillary abnormalities or new motor deficits. Prompt evaluation with a CT scan is indicated. Coagulation deficits, particularly in patients who have had chemotherapy recently or who have liver disease, should be ruled out with laboratory testing for prothrombin time, partial thromboplastin time and platelet count.

Should a significant intracranial hemorrhage be identified, the patient may need to return to the OR for the hemorrhage to be evacuated. Mannitol and reintubation may be required to stabilize the patient's condition. Occasionally, if the neurologic deterioration is mild, observation or mannitol by itself may be sufficient intervention. As the blood degrades over time and edema subsides, the patient should improve clinically. Frequent follow-up CT scanning is necessary in nonoperative management to evaluate the status of the hemorrhage and surrounding brain.

Cerebral Edema

Manipulation of the tumor and adjacent brain can lead to cerebral edema. Clinical signs can appear quite similar to postoperative hemorrhage, although deficits from edema tend to occur in a more delayed fashion. Prompt treatment with mannitol and dexamethasone are indicated following a CT scan to confirm the etiology of the patient's neurologic change.

Endocrinopathy

Pituitary tumors may be associated with hypersecretory or hyposecretory states. Other tumors in the sella and parasellar areas may also be associated with endocrinopathy, usually hypopituitarism. Surgery for tumors in these locations can cause endocrine deficits, too. Most endocrinopathies encountered in the ICU are related to pituitary hypofunction.

The major neurologically related endocrinopathy evident in the ICU setting is diabetes insipidus, most commonly after craniopharyngioma or pituitary tumor resection. It usually occurs between 18 and 36 hours following surgery. Signs of diabetes insipidus include an increase in urine output greater than 200 mL per hour for 2 consecutive hours, a corresponding drop in urine specific gravity to less than 1.005, and an increase in serum sodium to greater than 147 mEq per L. A patient who is conscious usually experiences increased thirst. Hypotension can occur if the complication is not recognized early. Treatment with DDAVP 0.25 mL (1 μg) subcutaneously or intravenously is indicated when diabetes insipidus is recognized. DDAVP is usually given twice a day. One must be cautious that the patient is actually experiencing diabetes insipidus and is not just mobilizing surgical fluids. In a patient who has had a transsphenoidal resection of a pituitary tumor, increased thirst may be present only because the patient's nasal packs cause mouth-breathing. Diabetes insipidus is usually transient, resolving by about 72 hours postoperatively. For this reason, over the first several days, it is probably better to give the DDAVP only when the patient's findings indicate that treatment is appropriate. Occasionally, diabetes insipidus may be permanent. Intranasal DDAVP 0.2 mL at night is an effective dosing regimen for these patients in the subacute to chronic phases of diabetes insipidus.

Low serum cortisol is frequently not observed acutely in the ICU, because patients are usually on glucocorticosteroids. However, after abrupt cessation of steroid treatment, a patient may experience an Addisonian crisis. Hypotension, weakness, and fatigue are the major findings. Because the steroid depletion is acute, hyponatremia, hyperkalemia, and hyperpigmentation are not generally observed. Treatment should be instituted promptly with hydrocortisone 100 mg IV every 6 hours.

Hypothyroidism usually does not become evident for at least a week following surgical injury to the pituitary gland or hypothalamus. Fatigue, lethargy, and hyporeflexia may be present. Laboratory testing shows low T4 and free thyroxine uptake, as well as low thyroid stimulating hormone. For a patient with a sellar or parasellar tumor, preoperative recognition and treatment of hypothyroidism helps prevent this endocrinopathy from becoming bothersome postoperatively.

Postoperative Central Nervous System Infections

Infections of the central nervous system are uncommon in neuro-oncology patients. Perioperative antibiotics, such as cephalothin 1 g IV just prior to the skin incision and then for several doses following surgery, reduce infection rates [35,36]. The likelihood of a postoperative infection in the absence of CSF leak in a clean operative field (one which does not involve the paranasal or mastoid sinuses) is about 0.8% [37]. Should CSF leak occur or if operative time is extended, the risk of infection increases. Infection can occur in any of the operative spaces.

A patient may develop wound cellulitis. This superficial infection is associated with erythema, induration, and sometimes wound drainage or breakdown. The patient may have a fever and/or elevated white blood cell count. This complication usually occurs within the first week after surgery. It will usually respond to anti-staphylococcal antibiotics within several days. A 10-day course of antibiotics is usually sufficient. If drainage from the wound is present, then it should be cultured to tailor antibiotics appropriately.

Bone flap infections are more involved than simple postoperative cellulitis. They tend to occur in a delayed fashion. Drainage from a breakdown in the suture line or from the scalp near the bone flap will usually be present and should be cultured. White blood count and erythrocyte sedimentation rate are usually elevated. A CT scan of the head may show an epidural collection or a moth-eaten appearance of the bone. Parenteral antibiotics for several weeks are necessary, though usually insufficient by themselves. Because the bone flap is devascularized, removal of the infected bone flap is usually necessary to eradicate the infection. A cranioplasty can be performed 6 months after the infection has resolved to reconstitute the integrity of the skull.

Postoperative meningitis occurs infrequently, usually in the first week after surgery. Fever without another focus of infection, or a "stiff neck," are usually present. Lumbar puncture is essential to rule out meningitis. Usually a CT scan is performed first to rule out a structural cause of the change in level of consciousness that frequently accompanies the infection. The occurrence of meningitis often necessitates the return of the patient from the floor to the ICU. If meningitis is suspected, parenteral antibiotics should be instituted immediately after lumbar puncture. If cultures are positive, or the glucose is low in the presence of a neutrophil pleocytosis in the CSF, then a 14-day course of broad-spectrum antibiotics is appropriate [38]. When the cultures are negative, the antibiotics can be stopped.

A patient with cerebral empyema or abscess after surgery for a brain tumor typically experiences headache and other symptoms and signs of elevated intracranial pressure. Lateralizing neurologic deficits are often present. A CT scan with IV contrast is essential. In subdural or epidural empyema, the dura or arachnoid usually densely enhances with an adjacent low-density fluid collection. An abscess will show ring enhancement at the surgical site, which can look very similar to the original tumor in some cases. Suspicion of empyema or abscess necessitates an urgent return to the operating room to drain the collection of pus and obtain cultures. Six weeks of parenteral antibiotics are then necessary.

Radiation-related Complications

Most patients with high-grade primary brain tumors or metastatic tumors will receive external beam radiation as an adjuvant therapy to control tumor growth for as long as possible. Although such treatment is usually tolerated without difficulty, a patient may have worsening of his/her neurologic condition during treatment. This "early effect" worsening is usually related to cerebral edema. CT scan and MRI show an increase in low density/intensity signal around the tumor volume. The edema tends to be responsive to high dose glucocorticosteroids. Once the patient improves, steroids can be slowly tapered to usual maintenance doses.

Much more rarely, a patient may deteriorate in a delayed fashion. "Late effects" occur about 6 to 24 months after completing radiation therapy [39]. Imaging studies show intense enhancement in the area treated. It is often difficult to differentiate radiation necrosis from tumor recurrence solely on the basis of a contrast CT or gadolinium MRI as the two entities, particularly in the case of primary glioma, look similar. Single positron emitting computed tomography (SPECT) or MR spectroscopy can often be helpful in establishing the diagnosis; tumor tends to have high metabolic activity, whereas radiation necrosis is metabolically hypoactive. Sometimes, a stereotactic brain biopsy may be required to make a definitive diagnosis. High glucocorticosteroid doses are necessary to treat radiation necrosis. Mannitol may initially be required if the patient has significantly deteriorated in order to stabilize the patient and allow the steroids time to work. Occasionally, a craniotomy to remove the necrotic mass is required, as well.

Single fraction stereotactic radiosurgery is more likely to be associated with the development of symptomatic radiation necrosis than conventional external beam radiation. In radiosurgery, the patient receives a high dose of radiation to the tumor volume, sparing the surrounding normal brain. Even so, the radiation that the surrounding brain receives may exceed its tolerance if previous radiation therapy was also used. Treatment is as described above. Approximately 13% to 50% of gliomas and 10% of metastatic tumors treated with radiosurgery may require subsequent surgical decompression [40,41].

SPINAL TUMORS

Spinal tumors are much less common than intracranial tumors. Most patients with spine tumors do not require ICU treatment. Exceptions include patients with spinal tumors involving the cervical spine or those who have had transthoracic approaches to thoracic spinal neoplasms. A patient with a cervical spinal cord tumor may have compromise of intracostal musculature or decreased diaphragmatic function with resultant inability to maintain adequate ventilation, depending on the level of the tumor. Vital capacity should be assessed every 6 hours, because its decrement will usually be noted before respiratory insufficiency occurs. A decrease below 10 to 12 mL per kg usually requires semiurgent intubation and mechanical ventilation. Once oxygen desaturation is noted, the patient decompensates rapidly, and emergency resuscitative efforts may be required.

After spinal cord surgery, a patient may experience a temporary ileus. Bowel sounds may stop and the abdomen may become distended. Frequently the patient will need a nasogastric tube. No oral or enteral intake is appropriate until the ileus subsides. Medications will need to be given parenterally.

A spinal cord tumor is not infrequently associated with development of a neurogenic bladder. The patient often requires a Foley catheter to decompress the bladder; although such intervention is necessary, it can mask the findings. Attention to urinary retention following removal of the Foley is in order. Urinary tact infections are also not uncommon, either related to long-term Foley placement or suboptimal bladder emptying. A long-term intermittent catheterization program to maintain bladder volumes less than 500 mL is necessary if urinary retention persists.

SYSTEMIC COMPLICATIONS

Not infrequently patients with neuro-oncologic primary problems will experience systemic complications necessitating evaluation and treatment in the ICU.

Deep Venous Thrombosis and Pulmonary Embolism

Patients with brain and spinal cord tumors are at risk for development of deep venous thrombosis (DVT) and subsequent pulmonary embolism (PE). Factors such as prior history of DVT, female gender, older age, high-grade lesion, poor Karnofsky score, hypertension, and Caucasian background have been shown to increase the risk of thromboembolism in this patient population [42]. Further, tumor types such as oligodendroglioma, lymphoma, glioma, mixed tumor, and metastatic lesion increase the risk of DVT/PE development in patients [42,43] Precautions, including TED stockings or sequential leg compression boots, should be taken to prevent DVT from developing. Prophylaxis with subcutaneous heparin (5,000 units twice a day) could be started as early as postoperative day 1 [44]. However, most physicians advocate starting chemoprophylaxis at 3 to 5 days after surgery [45]. Venous duplex scanning can recognize DVT before it becomes symptomatic.

DVT should be suspected if the patient complains of leg pain or has a fever or elevated white count without a clear explanation. Venous duplex scanning of the bilateral lower extremities should be obtained to assess for development of DVT. PE usually presents with shortness of breath and chest pain. Blood gases show hypocarbia with mild to moderate hypoxia. Administration of oxygen is necessary and prompt evaluation with chest X-ray, $\dot{V}/\dot{Q}$ scan, and/or spiral CT of the chest is in order.

Once identified, treatment with anticoagulation may be problematic, especially in the immediate postoperative period because of fear of hemorrhage [46,47]. However, recent studies have shown that use of anticoagulation in the immediate post-op is safe and does not lead to increased risk of hemorrhage [42]. Alternatively, patients at high risk for PE can have placement of an inferior vena cava (Greenfield) filter to prevent PE until 2 weeks have transpired from surgery. After that time, the use of anticoagulation is much less risky and is the preferred treatment.

Cerebral Infarction

About 15% of cancer patients have significant cerebrovascular pathology noted at autopsy [48]. Patients with primary brain neoplasms are also at risk for cerebral infarction. This complication may be related to the hypercoagulable state present in patients with malignancies. Alternatively, because these patients may be older with premorbid atherosclerosis, they may suffer cerebral infarction. This event should be differentiated from hemorrhage into a tumor or progressive tumor enlargement. CT scan or MRI is essential. The issues regarding anticoagulation must be addressed as with DVT or PE. Daily aspirin is generally safe. Coumadin, if indicated, should be reserved for a patient who has not had hemorrhage into the tumor and who is at least 2 weeks post-op.

Systemic Infections

Systemic infections are not uncommon, and most often include pneumonia, urinary tract infections, or sepsis secondary to line placement. Their management does not differ in the neuro-oncology patient from any other patient in the ICU.

END-OF-LIFE IN THE ICU

Sadly, despite the variety of available therapies, almost all primary high-grade gliomas will progress and the patient harboring the tumor will succumb to the disease. A patient with metastatic brain disease may fail tumor treatments, as well. Hopefully, the patient's physicians have discussed these possibilities as the patient begins to show signs of decline. The patient and family may decide to limit the intensity of care, and treatment in the ICU is not an issue. However, a patient may deteriorate quickly from the illness and elevated ICP before limits on treatment can be discussed and defined. When these circumstances occur, the physicians in the ICU may need to discuss limiting inappropriate technologies with the patient and family. The most intensive interventions—surgery, ventriculostomy, and intubation for hyperventilation—may be most readily decided against. Other interventions, such as mannitol, may be withheld. Sometimes, a decision is made to stop all technologies and focus on comfort. Abrupt cessation of dexamethasone generally leads to a rapid demise of the patient.

On occasion, an aggressively treated patient will continue to deteriorate. Elevated ICP can cause cardiac arrhythmias in the end stage. Prior to the onset of such cardiac difficulties, however, the patient may progress to the point of "brain death." In the USA, the definition of brain death requires the patient be not hypotensive, not hypothermic, or on paralytic or sedative medications. The etiology of the patient's condition should be known. The clinical exam shows the patient to be comatose, without any brain stem reflexes, motor responses, or spontaneous respirations, and on no sedative medications. An apnea test is also necessary. In this test, the patient is provided flow-by oxygen at 100% to maintain adequate oxygenation. The patient is disconnected from the ventilator and observed for the absence of respirations for 10 minutes (until a pCO_2 of 60 mm Hg is reached). Confirmatory test, such as electrocerebral silence on an EEG, or absence of brain blood flow on a radionucleotide cerebral flow study, can also be helpful [49]. If these criteria are present, the patient should be declared brain dead and supportive technologies be discontinued. It is important and mandated by statute that the organ bank be contacted so the organ donation can be discussed with the family prior to discontinuing supportive technologies.

ACKNOWLEDGMENTS

The material presented in this chapter was derived in part from Litofsky NS, Muzinich MC: Neuro-oncologic problems in the intensive care unit, in Irwin RS, Cerra F, Rippe JM: *Irwin and Rippe's Intensive Care Medicine.* 7th ed. Philadelphia, PA, Lippincott Williams & Wilkins, 2012, pp 1787–1797.

References

1. Bartkowski H: Peritumoral edema. *Prog Exp Tumor Res* 27:179, 1984.
2. Bruce J, Criscuolo G, Merrill M, et al: Vascular permeability induced by protein product of malignant brain tumors: inhibition by dexamethasone. *J Neurosurg* 67:880, 1987.
3. Black KL, Hoff JT, McGillicuddy JE, et al: Increased leukotriene C4 and vasogenic edema surrounding brain tumors in humans. *Ann Neurol* 19:592, 1986.
4. Ellenbogen R, Scott MR: Choroid plexus tumors, in Kaye A, Laws E (eds): *Brain Tumors: Encyclopedic Approach*, 3rd ed. Boston, Elsevier, 450–461, 2012.
5. Muizelaar J, Wei E, Kontos H, et al: Mannitol causes compensatory cerebral vasoconstriction and vasodilation in response to blood viscosity changes. *J Neurosurg* 59:822, 1983.
6. Starke R, Dumont A: The role of hypertonic saline in neurosurgery. *World Neurosurg* 82:1040–1042, 2014.
7. Dostal P, Dostalova V, Schreiberova J, et al: A comparison of equivolume, equiosmolar solutions of hypertonic saline and mannitol for brain relaxation in patients undergoing elective intracranial tumor surgery: a randomized clinical trial. *J Neurosurg Anesthesiol* 27(1):51–56, 2015.
8. Kumar B, Bhagat H: A comparison of 3% saline and mannitol for brain relaxation during elective supratentorial brain tumor surgery. *Anesth Analg* 112(2):485, 2011.
9. Bhardwaj A, Ulatowski J: Cerebral edema: hypertonic saline solutions. *Curr Treat Options Neurol* 179–187, 1999.
10. Shapiro WR, Posner JB: Corticosteroid hormones: effects in an experimental brain tumor. *Arch Neurol* 30:217, 1974.
11. Yamada K, Ushio Y, Hayakawa T, et al: Effects of methylprednisolone on peritumoral brain edema: a quantitative autoradiography study. *J Neurosurg* 59:612, 1983.
12. Muizelaar JP, van der Poel HG, Li ZC, et al: Pial arteriolar vessel diameter and CO_2 reactivity during prolonged hyperventilation in the rabbit. *J Neurosurg* 69:923, 1988.
13. Mazzeo AT, Bullock R: Monitoring brain tissue oxymetry: will it change management of critically ill neurologic patients? *J Neurol Sci* 261(1–2):1–9, 2007.
14. Keddie S, Rohman L: Reviewing the reliability, effectiveness, and applications of Licox in traumatic brain injury. *Nurs Crit Care* 1478–5153, 2012.
15. Omarov AD, Kopachev DN, Sankidze AZ, et al: Ventriculoperitoneal and ventriculoatrial shunts in treatment of patients with brain tumors. *Zh Vopr Neirokhir Im N N Burdenko* 75:48, 2011.
16. Weaver D, Winn R, Jane J: Differential intracranial pressure in patients with unilateral mass lesions. *J Neurosurg* 55:660, 1982.
17. Johnson K, Ackerman LL, Douglas-Akinwande AC, et al: A foramen of Monro tumor. *Neuropathology* 31:658–661, 2011.
18. Raimondi A, Tomita T: Hydrocephalus and infratentorial tumors: incidence, clinical picture and treatment. *J Neurosurg* 55:174, 1981.
19. Sekhar L, Moossy J, Guthkelch N: Malfunctioning ventriculoperitoneal shunts: clinical and pathological features. *J Neurosurg* 56:411, 1982.
20. Jallo GI, Kothbauer KF, Abbott RI: Endoscopic third ventriculostomy. *Neurosurg Focus* 19:E11, 2005.
21. Aydin S, Yilmazlar S, Aker S, et al: Anatomy of the floor of the third ventricle in relation to endoscopic ventriculostomy. *Clin Anat* 22:916–924, 2009.
22. . Ketz E: Brain tumors and epilepsy, in Vinken JPJ, Bruyn GW (eds): *Handbook of Clinical Neurology.* Vol. 16. Amsterdam, Elsevier, 1974, p 254.
23. McKeran R, Thomas D: The clinical study of gliomas, in Thomas DGT, Graham DI (eds): *Brain Tumours: Scientific Basis, Clinical Investigation and Current Therapy.* London, Butterworths, 1980, p 194.
24. Chalk J, Ridgeway K, Brophy T, et al: Phenytoin impairs the bioavailability of dexamethasone in neurological and neurosurgical patients. *J Neurol Neurosurg Psychiatry* 47:1087, 1984.
25. Wong D, Longenecker RG, Liepman M, et al: Phenytoin-dexamethasone: a potential drug interaction. *JAMA* 254:2062, 1985.
26. Glantz M, Recht LD: Epilepsy in the cancer patient, in Vecht CJ: *Handbook of Clinical Neurology. Vol 25(69). Neuro-Oncology, Part III.* New York, NY, Elsevier, 1997, p 9.
27. Marcuse LV, Lancman G, Demopoulos A: Nonconvulsive status epilepticus in patients with brain tumors. *Seizure* 23(7):542–547, 2014.
28. Alroughani R, Javidan M, Qasem A et al: Non-convulsive status epilepticus; the rate of occurrence in a general hospital. *Seizure* 8(1):38–42, 2009.
29. Kennedy J, Schuele SU: Long-term monitoring of brain tumors: when is it necessary? *Epilepsia* 54 Suppl 9:50–55, 2013.
30. Cohen N, Stauss G, Lew R, et al: Should prophylactic anticonvulsants be administered to patients with newly-diagnosed cerebral metastases? A retrospective analysis. *J Clin Oncol* 6:1621, 1988.
31. Fadul C, Wood J, Thaler H, et al: Morbidity and mortality of craniotomy for excision of supratentorial gliomas. *Neurology* 38:1374, 1988.
32. Teasdale G, Jennett B: Assessment of coma and impaired conciousness. *Lancet* 2:81–84, 1974.
33. Jennett B, Teasdale G, Galbraith S, et al: Severe head injuries in three countries. *J Neurol Neurosurg Psychiatry* 40:291, 1977.
34. Gumprecht H, Lumenta CB: Intraoperative imaging using a mobile computed tomography scanner. *Minim Invasive Neurosurg* 46(6):317–322, 2003.
35. Haines S: Efficacy of antibiotic prophylaxis in clean neurosurgical operations. *Neurosurgery* 24:401, 1989.
36. Barker FG: Efficacy of prophylactic antibiotics for craniotomy: a meta-analysis. *Neurosurgery* 35:484, 1994.
37. Narotam PK, van Dellen JR, du Trevou MD, et al: Operative sepsis in neurosurgery: a method of classifying surgical cases. *Neurosurgery* 34:409, 1994.
38. Ross D, Rosegay H, Pons V: Differentiations of aseptic and bacterial meningitis in postoperative neurosurgical patients. *J Neurosurg* 69:669, 1988.
39. Leibel SA, Sheline GE: Radiation therapy for neoplasms of the brain. *J Neurosurg* 66:1, 1987.
40. McDermott MW, Chang SM, Keles GE, et al: Gamma knife radiosurgery for primary brain tumors, in Germano IM (ed): *LINAC and Gamma Knife Radiosurgery.* United States, American Association of Neurological Surgeons, 2000, p 189.
41. Alexander EA, Loeffler JS: Radiosurgery using a modified linear acclererator. *Neurosurg Clin North Am* 3:174,1992.
42. Smith TR, Nanney AD 3rd, Lall RR et al: Development of venous thromboembolism (VTE) in patients undergoing surgery for brain tumors: results from a single center over a 10 year period. *J Clin Neurosci* 22(3):519–525, 2015.
43. Chaichana KL, Pendleton C, Jackson C et al: Deep venous thrombosis and pulmonary embolisms in adult patients undergoing craniotomy for brain tumors. *Neurol Res* 35(2):206–211, 2013.
44. Scheller C, Rachinger J, Strauss C et al: Therapeutic anticoagulation after craniotomies: is the risk for secondary hemorrhage overestimated? *J Neurol Surg A Cent Eur Neurosurg* 75(1):2–6, 2013.
45. Lazio BE, Simard JM: Anticoagulation in neurosurgical patients. *Neurosurgery* 45:838, 1999.
46. Swann K, Black PM, Baker MF: Management of symptomatic deep venous thrombosis and pulmonary embolism on a neurosurgical service. *J Neurosurg* 64:563, 1986.
47. Choucair A, Silver P, Levin V: Risk of intracranial hemorrhage in glioma patients receiving anticoagulant therapy for venous thromboembolism. *J Neurosurg* 66:357, 1987
48. Graus F, Rogers L, Posner J: Cerebrovascular complications in patients with cancer. *Medicine* 64:16, 1985.
49. Wijdicks EFM: The diagnosis of brain death. *N Engl J Med* 344:1215, 2001.

Chapter 156 ■ Miscellaneous Neurologic Problems in the Intensive Care Unit

MAX MANDELBAUM • ANN L. MITCHELL

A wide variety of neurologic problems may confront the physician in the intensive care unit (ICU), including several important disorders for which basic information is not readily available. These include:

- Suicidal hanging, electrical shock, acute carbon monoxide poisoning, and decompression sickness, which present so blatantly that the diagnosis is rarely in question, yet the range of clinical manifestations and their management may be unanticipated.
- Cerebral fat embolism, which is often not initially suspected if other surgical or medical issues take precedence.
- Singultus (hiccups), which is an all too common secondary problem that may further weaken the severely ill patient.
- Compression neuropathies, which may complicate prolonged bed rest.

SUICIDAL HANGING

Hanging is the second most common means of committing suicide in the USA after self-inflicted gunshot wound [1]. Introduced in 5th-century England, hanging proceeded to become the official form of execution. Early on, there was no exact procedure, and most hangings resulted in slow strangulation [2]. Changes in techniques, with the victim dropped at least his height and the hangman's knot placed in the submental location, have produced a consistently fatal bilateral axis pedicle fracture, resulting in complete herniation of the disc and severance of the ligaments between C2 and C3 [3]. This injury causes almost immediate death by destroying the cardiac and respiratory centers, lacerating the carotid artery, and injuring the pharynx [2,3].

Suicidal hangings are rarely so expert, and death usually results from strangulation due to interruption of cerebral blood flow [4]. A minimal amount of compression occludes the jugular veins, whereas an increased force occludes the carotid arteries [5]. A much larger force is necessary to arrest blood flow in the vertebral arteries [5]. Pressure on the jugular veins from the noose results in venous obstruction and stagnation of cerebral blood flow, causing hypoxia and loss of consciousness [3]. Cervical muscle tone then decreases, allowing airway obstruction and arterial compression, further exacerbating hypoxia [3]. In addition, external compression of the carotid bodies or vagal sheath can increase parasympathetic tone, whereas pressure on the pericarotid area stimulates sympathetic tone; either can result in cardiac arrest [4,5]. The altered autonomic tone may also cause a release of catecholamines, resulting in neurogenic pulmonary edema, as well as affect the respiratory smooth muscle tone, causing respiratory acidosis and a further insult to cerebral oxygenation [3].

If blood flow is quickly restored, full recovery can often be expected. If the blood flow is interrupted for more than a few minutes, however, hypoxia causes cell death and cytotoxic and vasogenic edema, with increased intracranial pressure. There is selective vulnerability of the cerebral cortex (particularly the pyramidal cell layer), the globus pallidus, thalamus, hippocampus, and the cerebellar Purkinje cells to anoxia and ischemia.

Diagnosis

Although the diagnosis is rarely in doubt, the patient may show a range of findings, varying from rope burns to coma. In the immediate posthanging period, the patient most commonly shows evidence of an altered level of consciousness, ranging from restlessness, delirium, or violent agitation to lethargy, stupor, or coma. Seizures, and rarely status epilepticus, may occur [4,5]. Injury to the neck blood vessels occurs in 40% of patients, resulting in carotid dissection, thrombus formation, and distal ischemic infarcts [6]. Venous occlusion may lead to venous congestion, venous ischemia, and hemorrhage [7]. Development of the acute respiratory distress syndrome (ARDS) may result from central nervous system (CNS) catecholamine release, causing constriction of the pulmonary venules [3]. In incomplete hanging, the patient may also show signs of laryngeal and pharyngeal edema, resulting in hoarseness, dysphagia, and stridor [3,7]. Although infrequent in suicidal hangings, fracture of the odontoid and injury to the spinal cord may occur.

Careful neurologic examination should be performed, with particular attention to alterations in the level of consciousness and evidence of spinal cord injury, such as paraparesis, quadriparesis, or urinary retention. There should be frequent monitoring of vital signs for evidence of autonomic instability and stridor. Initial laboratory evaluations should include radiographs of the cervical spine; arterial blood gas determination; electrocardiogram (ECG); and cardiac monitoring. Computed tomography (CT) angiogram should also be considered if suspicious for dissection of the carotid artery [8].

Neuroimaging of the brain may be quite variable, from a normal head CT in many patients, to evidence of edema, hemorrhage, and ischemia. Owing to decreased blood flow and the resultant hypoxia, edema may be seen in the white matter tracts [9]. Subcortical and subarachnoid hemorrhages may result from venous occlusion, whereas ischemia may result from venous or arterial occlusion, particularly in the areas of greatest vulnerability: the basal ganglia, cortex, thalamus, and hippocampus [10].

Treatment

The patient may appear dead but might still be resuscitable. Patients quickly lose consciousness with hanging attempts, but may still have cardiac and respiratory function or can quickly regain these with prompt cardiopulmonary resuscitation (CPR). The goals of treatment are to maintain an adequate level of cerebral oxygenation, to decrease the raised intracranial pressure, and to monitor and treat any cardiac arrhythmias or respiratory distress that may develop. After hanging, the mechanical trauma induced by strangulation can also cause hemorrhage and edema in the paratracheal and laryngeal areas and result in delayed but significant airway obstruction at any time within the first 24 hours. Endotracheal intubation may be required if there is evidence of hypoxia due to ARDS, airway obstruction, or increased intracranial pressure [9].

Other concerns for victims of hangings include fractures and thrombi. A fracture of the odontoid requires immediate neurosurgical or orthopedic intervention to stabilize the cervical spine and protect the cord from injury. A carotid thrombus requires prompt vascular intervention to remove the clot and restore patency and blood flow. In addition, assessing the patient for other evidence of self-inflicted injuries and intoxications is also warranted, as is a complete psychiatric evaluation once the patient is able to cooperate.

Course

The prognosis for recovery is not immediately apparent with the first neurologic examination. Many patients have made a full recovery despite an initial Glasgow Coma Scale (GCS) score of 3 [4]. However, the fatality rate for suicidal hangings may range from 60% to 70% [11]. Indicators for a good recovery include a hanging time of less than 5 minutes, a heartbeat present at the scene or in the emergency room, CPR initiated at the scene, a GCS score greater than 3, and an incomplete circumferential ligature [4]. Predictors of a poorer prognosis include evidence of cardiopulmonary arrest, a spontaneous respiratory rate less than 4 per minute, need for intubation, and neurogenic pulmonary edema [5]. In patients who have cardiopulmonary arrest survival rate is less than 50%, with only about 12% of survivors having good neurologic outcome [12].

Other neurologic sequelae can become manifest either in the immediate posthanging period or after a relatively asymptomatic latent period. The individual may show evidence of a confusional state; a circumscribed retrograde amnesia; Korsakoff's syndrome; or even progressive dementia [7]. Transient hemiparesis; aphasia; abnormal movements; motor restlessness; and myoclonic jerks also can characterize this period [7]. Ear numbness may result from injury to the greater auricular nerve [13]. Most patients who survive the acute phase recover to variable degrees. Three more severe delayed outcomes have also been observed: (a) comatose state with minor neurologic improvement and death; (b) early neurologic recovery, followed by cerebral edema with uncontrollable uncal herniation and severe morbidity or mortality; and (c) complete neurologic recovery, followed by delayed encephalopathy and death [3].

ELECTRICAL INJURIES

Approximately 4,000 injuries and 1,000 deaths from electrical shock occur annually in the USA. Most fatalities occur in the workplace, but a third result from contact with household current [14]. Approximately 400 people per year are affected by lightning strikes, with one-third of victims dying owing to their exposure [15].

Pathophysiology

Electrical and lightning injuries are exceedingly variable and dependent on a number of factors. Current flowing between two potentials, or amperage, is equal to the voltage divided by the resistance to current flow ($I = V/R$). Current is generated by either an electrical source or a lightning strike. Current may be direct (DC), as with lightning, or alternating (AC), as with most household appliances. Alternating current has a tendency to produce tetanic contractions that prevent voluntary release from the current source, thus prolonging the electrical contact time and increasing the potential for injury. Higher voltages, such as those that occur with lightning or with contact with high-voltage conductors, produce more severe injuries than those caused by lower voltages. Wet skin and tissues high in water content provide low resistance to current flow and are at a higher risk for injury, whereas tissues high in fat and air, such as hollow organs, provide high resistance. Nerves and blood vessels have lower than expected resistances, and thus are more sensitive to electrical injury than their water content would suggest [16]. Other variables that affect the severity of damage include the current pathway (i.e., whether it involves the heart, diaphragm, spinal cord, or brain), the area of current contact and exit, and the duration of contact [16].

In addition, lightning injuries are classified according to the type of exposure [17]. "Direct strikes" involve direct contact between the lightning bolt and the highest point of the victim, often the head. "Side flash" involves the spread of electricity from the lightning bolt to a nearby object and then to the patient. Side flash victims are typically exposed to less voltage and current than with a direct strike. Finally, "stride current" involves the spread of electricity from the lightning bolt to the ground and then through contact points in the patient. Stride current patients are more likely to experience spinal cord injuries, because the current crosses through the spinal cord from one limb to another.

Neurologic Complications of Electrical and Lightning Injuries

Neurologic sequelae of electrical injuries affect both the central and peripheral nervous systems, with both immediate and long-term difficulties.

Immediate Effects

Immediate neurologic effects of electrical injuries are noted throughout the neuraxis. 10% to 50% of patients experience a brief loss of consciousness, as well as headache; retrograde amnesia; and confusion [18]. Patients with electrical and lightning injuries to the head may also suffer subarachnoid or parenchymal hemorrhages, particularly in the basal ganglia and brainstem [19]. In patients who suffer cardiac or respiratory arrest, posthypoxic encephalopathy may develop in "watershed" areas of the cerebral cortex. Less commonly, patients may present with cerebral infarction or a temporary cerebellar syndrome [19].

Catecholamine release may result in autonomic dysfunction, as evidenced by transitory hypertension; tachycardia; diaphoresis; vasoconstriction of the extremities; and fixed and dilated pupils [20]. Thus, lightning-strike victims should receive full resuscitative efforts despite pupillary changes, because these may not indicate permanent brainstem dysfunction. Lightning-strike victims may also suffer "keraunoparalysis," a self-limited paralysis more often involving the lower extremities, accompanied by a lack of peripheral pulses, pale and cold extremities, and variable paresthesias [19]. Keraunoparalysis is presumably caused by localized vasospasm from catecholamine release.

Acute spinal cord injuries are also seen, particularly with stride current injuries. The spectrum of spinal cord injuries includes paralysis, spasticity, autonomic dysfunction, and, later, chronic pain and pressure ulcers [19]. Acute neuropathies are typically not seen with lightning strikes, but may be seen with electrical injuries in association with compartment syndromes, local burns, or vascular injury [21]. Both electrical and lightning-strike victims are vulnerable to the subacute development of cataracts, whereas lightning-strike patients are peculiarly susceptible to tympanic membrane rupture; vertigo; and hearing loss [22,23].

Delayed Effects

Delayed effects of electrical and lightning injuries may also span the neuraxis. Recognized neuropsychiatric effects include depression; posttraumatic stress disorder; fatigue; irritability; and memory and concentration difficulties [24]. Movement disorders have also been described, such as transient dystonias, torticollis, and parkinsonism [19]. Delayed ophthalmologic and otologic consequences include cataracts, conductive and sensorineural hearing loss, and vertigo [22,23]. Delayed autonomic dysfunction may manifest as reflex sympathetic dystrophy, presenting as a limb with burning pain, cutaneous vasoconstriction, swelling, and sweating [20]. Prolonged and permanent spinal cord abnormalities may become manifest in the delayed development of a myelopathy or a motor neuronopathy [14,25]. Peripheral neuropathies may result from compression due to scarring and fibrosis from the original injury or delayed ischemia due to vascular occlusion [26]. Peripheral neuropathies are more likely to occur in areas directly involved by the electrical current, but may also occur in limbs that were not seemingly in the current path [27].

Evaluation

Initial evaluation of the electrical- or lightning-injured patient involves assessment of the scene and evaluation of safety. Disconnect electrical sources before evaluating the patient. Contrary to conventional mythology, lightning-strike victims are not electrically charged and may be examined immediately.

Assessment of cardiopulmonary status is essential, because many victims suffer cardiopulmonary arrest and may recover well if CPR is initiated promptly. Cardiac arrhythmias and asystole commonly accompany these injuries, as does respiratory arrest due to passage of current through the brainstem respiratory centers. Stabilization of the spine is also essential, owing to potential spinal cord injuries and fractures from falls.

Neurologic Examination

The neurologic examination should begin with assessment of the level of consciousness. Initially, many patients are comatose, but this is often brief and followed by a period of confusion and amnesia, lasting hours to days [28]. Seizures are uncommon. The cranial nerve examination may reveal fixed and dilated pupils; blindness; papilledema; partial hearing loss; and tinnitus. Rupture of the tympanic membranes may also be present with lightning injuries to the head. Evaluation of the motor system for focal weakness and reflex changes may indicate cerebral injuries, myelopathy, or neuropathy. Cerebral lesions, caused by hemorrhage or infarction, may result in contralateral hemiparesis. Spinal cord injuries are more common in the cervical region and produce paraparesis or quadriparesis. Peripheral nerve injuries in the immediate assessment are typically located in areas of extensive burns. Sensory loss is less frequent than motor deficits and is maximal in burned areas.

Laboratory Evaluation

Laboratory evaluations should be focused on the known complications of electrical and lightning injuries. Serial determinations of electrolytes, renal function, and hematocrit are essential for assessing adequate fluid replacement. Serum creatine kinase and urinary myoglobin are useful measures of muscle necrosis. Arterial blood gases may reveal a metabolic acidosis. ECG and cardiac monitoring are used in patients with cardiopulmonary arrest or with known current pathways through the thorax, because delayed cardiac arrhythmias may develop. Radiologic examinations of the long bones, spine, and skull are indicated when fractures or deep burns are suspected based on the history and physical examination. Magnetic resonance imaging (MRI) or myelography may be used to assess spinal cord damage if signs of myelopathy are present. Cranial imaging is indicated when there is prolonged alteration of consciousness and may reveal intracranial hemorrhages, cerebral edema, or the effect of diffuse cerebral hypoxia. The electroencephalogram (EEG) is also useful to rule out status epilepticus in patients with prolonged unconsciousness. The EEG background may remain slow even when the mental status has returned to baseline. Nerve conduction studies and electromyography may be useful in localizing and following axonal and demyelinating electrical injuries to the peripheral nerves and plexi, although they are not generally used in the acute evaluation.

Management

Evaluation and treatment of medical concerns are essential for good neurologic recovery. Efforts should focus on circulatory volume, hydration status, renal function, acidosis, and electrolyte balance. Because high-voltage electric shock victims usually have myoglobinuria secondary to burns and deep tissue injury, their fluid needs are similar to those of crush injuries. Ultrasonographic assessment of volume status can be helpful and urine output should be maintained at greater than 0.5 mL per kg hour. Alkalinization of the urine and osmotic diuresis with mannitol also help to prevent myoglobin nephropathy.

Extensive burns due to direct current or clothing ignition are best treated in specialized burn units. At times, skin grafts are required. Debridement of necrotic muscle and fasciotomy are sometimes necessary to prevent secondary ischemia from a compartment syndrome. Amputation might be required if there is significant necrosis. For these patients, arteriography may assist in identifying the level of viability. Tetanus prophylaxis and prevention of superinfection are also needed. Spine and long-bone fractures require stabilization.

Recurrent seizures are treated with phenytoin (18 to 20 mg per kg loading dose followed by 5 to 7 mg/kg/d). Other antiepileptics, such as levetiracetam, should also be considered. Because fluid restriction is contraindicated, patients with signs of increased intracranial pressure require osmotic diuresis with mannitol. Intracranial pressure monitoring may be useful in patients with cerebral edema. Specific treatment for electrical spinal cord injuries is not available, and early institution of physical therapy is recommended. In patients with cardiac arrest, the hypothermia protocol can be considered.

Prognosis

Prognosis is difficult to ascertain for electrical injuries to the nervous system. Patients with deficits at presentation might potentially recover fully, whereas those with delayed onset of neurologic deficits may have syndromes that progress over months to years.

CARBON MONOXIDE POISONING

Carbon monoxide is a colorless, tasteless, and odorless gas that gives no warning of its presence. It is normally present in the atmosphere in a concentration of less than 0.001%, but a concentration of 0.1% can be lethal [29]. Carbon monoxide is a byproduct of incomplete combustion and as such is found in automobile exhaust, fires, water heaters, charcoal-burning grills, methylene chloride, volcanic gas, and cigarette smoke. It is also endogenously formed from the degradation of hemoglobin, resulting in baseline carboxyhemoglobin saturation between 1% and 3% [29]. Smoking can raise the endogenous level to 6% to 7% saturation [29]. Carbon monoxide poisoning may occur in the acute and chronic setting. For further information on the pathogenesis, diagnosis, and treatment of carbon monoxide poisoning, see Chapter 178.

Diagnosis

It is important to consider carbon monoxide poisoning in the differential diagnosis of any individual who presents with an altered state of consciousness or headache, particularly in the setting of a long car ride or other exposure to poorly ventilated and incompletely combusted fuel. Of note, the carboxyhemoglobin levels are not indicative of the severity of toxicity and depend on factors such as duration of exposure, comorbid conditions, and ambient carbon monoxide concentration [30]. With mild intoxication, symptoms may include a mild headache; dyspnea on exertion; and fatigability [29]. With increasing levels of toxicity, more severe symptoms may include impaired motor dexterity; blurry vision; irritability; weakness; nausea; vomiting; and confusion [29]. At its most severe, carbon monoxide exposure may cause tachycardia; cardiac irritability; seizures; respiratory insufficiency; coma; and death [29]. In addition, there can be evidence of rhabdomyolysis, flame-shaped superficial retinal hemorrhages, and, occasionally, a cherry-red discoloration best appreciated in the lips, mucous membranes, and skin [29,31,32]. For mild carbon monoxide intoxication, in which there is no loss of consciousness and carboxyhemoglobin levels are less than 5% in nonsmokers or less than 10% in smokers, only headache and dizziness around the time of presentation were found to correlate with an increased incidence of delayed sequelae, including asthenia, headache, or decreased memory [33].

A head CT scan may be normal early on or show signs of cerebral edema as inferred from narrowed ventricles and effacement of the cerebral sulci. The degree of CT abnormalities does not predict the clinical course [34]. MRI findings may reveal diffuse, confluent diffusion-weighted imaging (DWI); FLAIR (fluid-attenuated inversion recovery); and T_2-weighted (time for 63% of transverse relaxation) hyperintensities bilaterally in the periventricular white matter, centrum semiovale [35,36], basal ganglia, particularly involving the globus pallidus, and the hippocampus [37]. The electroencephalogram usually demonstrates diffuse slowing but is generally of little prognostic value.

Treatment

The criteria for hospital admission include coma, loss of consciousness, or neurologic deficit at any time; any clinical or electrocardiographic signs of cardiac compromise; metabolic acidosis; abnormal chest radiograph; oxygen tension less than 60 mm Hg; and carboxyhemoglobin level greater than 10% in individuals with pregnancy, greater than 15% in those with cardiac disease, or greater than 25% in all other patients [31].

All patients should be treated with 100% oxygen as soon as the diagnosis of carbon monoxide poisoning is even considered. It should be administered through a tight-fitting nonrebreathing mask or after endotracheal intubation of severely sensorium-compromised patients. The administration of 100% oxygen can shorten the half-life of carbon monoxide from 4 to 5 hours to approximately 1 hour [30]. Oxygen should be administered until the carboxyhemoglobin level normalizes [29]. (See Chapters 169 and 178 for a discussion of hyperbaric oxygen therapy.) Traditionally, treatment with hyperbaric oxygen was considered for treatment of carbon monoxide poisoning; however, literature reviews have shown that although it washes out carbon monoxide more quickly, there is no additional clinical benefit to hyperbaric treatment, and there may even be increased risk of neurologic harm [32].

Course

The delayed appearance of neurologic sequelae found in many posthypoxic states occurs with particular frequency and severity after carbon monoxide poisoning. Up to 30% of patients may succumb to the initial exposure and 25% may develop a progressive encephalopathy resulting in a persistent vegetative state, with a 50% mortality rate [34]. Later sequelae may include seizures, cortical blindness, scotomas, Korsakoff's psychosis, irritability, hemiplegia, chorea, and peripheral neuropathy.

Between 10% and 30% of patients develop delayed neurologic sequelae, and there are no guidelines to indicate which patients are at greatest risk [31]. Although there seems to be a rough correlation between both duration of initial unconsciousness and increasing age with the development of delayed neurologic sequelae, even patients with mild toxicity can progress to develop the tardive signs [30]. Recently, some work has looked at markers in the blood to predict neurologic damange including neuron-specific enolase and S100B with some success [32]. The post–carbon monoxide syndrome begins 7 to 30 days after the initial insult and is characterized by gait disturbances, incontinence, and memory impairment, as well as signs of parkinsonism, mutism, and frontal lobe disinhibition [29,30,38]. The development of isolated cognitive impairment has considerable variability in the literature. Some report memory dysfunction, impaired attention, and affective disorders in moderate to severe carbon monoxide exposure, whereas other studies suggest that mildly exposed individuals have no cognitive impairments compared to matched controls in neuropsychiatric testing [30,39,40].

On average, 75% of affected individuals show recovery within a year of the insult, although 20% of these individuals continue to show evidence of mild to moderate impairment of memory and extrapyramidal function [41]. Although the specific cause of the delayed syndrome is unknown, it does correlate temporally with the pathologic findings of cerebral white matter demyelination found in the chronic stages of the illness, as opposed to the largely gray matter edema, ischemia, and hemorrhagic necrosis found in the acute stage [42]. There is no specific treatment for the delayed neuropsychiatric syndrome, although symptomatic treatment, including cognitive therapies and dopamine agonists, may be of benefit in the short term [41].

DECOMPRESSION SICKNESS

Decompression sickness ("the bends") occurs when gases dissolved in body fluids come out of solution, forming bubbles in tissues and venous blood. Situations in which decompression sickness arises include rapid ascent to the surface by tunnel workers or scuba divers, decompression or rapid ascent in an airplane, and high-altitude flying with inadequate cabin pressurization. In these situations, nitrogen and other inert gases that supersaturate the tissues under high pressure are released as bubbles under conditions of decreased pressure. As the bubbles coalesce, they may cause local tissue ischemia because of compression or venous obstruction. The microcirculation is further compromised by capillary endothelial edema; by activation of platelets, coagulation factors, and complement; and by hemoconcentration due to fluid extravasation [43,44]. Nitrogen, the largest component of inspired air, is lipophilic, and thus gas bubbles are more likely to form in the bone marrow, fat, and spinal cord. Additionally, gas bubbles may result in barotrauma to the pulmonary beds, releasing further air emboli into the venous circulation [43,44].

Symptoms of decompression sickness are variable. In most cases, the onset is within 6 hours of decompression, but may be seen later at 12 to 24 hours [43]. Fulminant cases present earlier. Any organ system can be affected, and symptoms range from a pruritic skin rash ("the creeps"), cough ("the chokes"), and joint pain to paraplegia, vertigo, altered level of consciousness, seizures, shock, and apnea.

Almost 80% of patients with decompression sickness have neurologic symptoms. The most frequent neurologic presentation is with paresthesias, which may be diffuse or focal, and result from gas bubble formation in the skin, joints, peripheral nerves, or spinal cord. Weakness, ranging from monoparesis to quadriplegia secondary to spinal cord involvement, may also occur. Cerebral symptoms are infrequent but can range from headache and lethargy to vertigo, visual disturbances, paralysis, and unconsciousness [43,44]. Vertigo, hearing loss, tinnitus, nausea, and vomiting are relatively common complaints, resulting from rupture of the cochlear and semicircular canal membranes.

Air embolism is a more serious decompression illness, and its onset is usually within 5 minutes of decompression. It probably results from tearing of the lung parenchyma secondary to overdistension, as the gases in the lungs expand during ascent [43]. The gas escapes into the pulmonary vein and may embolize into large vessels [43]. Venous gas bubbles are effectively filtered by the lungs, but arterial embolism may also result from gas passing through a patent foramen ovale. Based on their buoyancy, the emboli often produce neurologic symptoms by floating into and occluding cerebral arterioles. Unconsciousness and stupor are the most frequent symptoms. Death from cardiopulmonary arrest may also occur. In most patients, improvement in symptoms accompanies the redistribution of the gas emboli to the venous circulation [43].

Recompression is the definitive treatment for decompression diseases. The patient should be transported in a pressurized aircraft to the nearest decompression chamber with minimal delay. (See Chapter 61 for a more detailed discussion of the management and therapy for decompression syndrome.) The Divers Alert Network also maintains a 24-hour phone consultation service to assist with diving accidents, reached at (919) 684-9111.

Remarkable recovery may occur after recompression. Delay in treatment can limit its effectiveness, but recompression should be attempted even up to 2 weeks after the onset of symptoms. Relapses requiring repeated hyperbaric treatment may occur [45]. Patients with long-term sequelae from decompression illnesses should not be reexposed to conditions that allow their recurrence.

CEREBRAL FAT EMBOLISM SYNDROME

Fat embolism syndrome is characterized by diffuse pulmonary insufficiency with hypoxemia, neurologic dysfunction, and petechiae, occurring 12 to 48 hours after trauma [46,47]. At least subclinically, fat embolism is present after all fractures involving the long bones. It is clinically recognized in 0.5% to 2% of patients with long-bone fractures and in 5% to 10% of patients who have sustained multiple fractures [48,49]. There are also reports of fat embolism syndrome occurring in the setting of orthopedic procedures, such as hip arthroplasty, intramedullary rods, and leg lengthening procedures [48,50]. There is an increased risk associated with a patent foramen ovale [49].

Pathogenesis

The two main pathogenetic hypotheses of fat embolism syndrome are the mechanical and chemical theories. The mechanical theory posits that physical disruption of bone and blood vessels at the fracture site allows free fat globules to enter venous sinusoids and then to embolize to the lungs [46]. The chemical theory proposes that a trauma-induced catecholamine surge results in lipid mobilization from the fat stores or the coalescence of chylomicrons into fat globules [46,51]. The fat emboli in the circulation may then be broken down by lipases in the lungs or systemic circulation, generating free fatty acids [46,47,52]. The toxic fatty acids stimulate the release of inflammatory mediators, increasing permeability of capillaries, generating ARDS and cerebral vasogenic edema [46,47]. Furthermore, the inflammatory mediators may increase platelet adhesion and coagulation [52]. Fat emboli, in conjunction with increased platelet adhesion, may arrest blood flow, resulting in cerebral ischemia and hemorrhage [47,52].

Cerebral fat emboli and ischemia, rather than cerebral anoxia, produce the neurologic damage seen in this condition. The brain is edematous and shows a leptomeningeal inflammatory reaction and cortical surface petechiae. Microscopically, there are fat emboli and ball, ring, and perivascular hemorrhages. The fat emboli are more prevalent in the gray matter, but the hemorrhages are more common in the centrum semiovale; internal capsule; and cerebral and cerebellar white matter [53]. Electron microscopy reveals intravascular fat vacuoles; breakdown of endothelial walls; swollen neurons; and glia [53].

Diagnosis

Characteristically, there is a symptom-free interval of 12 to 48 hours between the inciting trauma and the onset of fat embolism syndrome [46]. Altered consciousness or development of neurologic deficits after a lucid interval following trauma should alert the physician to the possibility of fat embolism. The syndrome may present as a spectrum of disability, from subclinical presentations with only a decreased arterial partial pressure of oxygen (PaO_2), decreased platelets or hemoglobin, to a fulminant presentation. Gurd's diagnostic criteria for fat embolism syndrome include one or more major criteria (respiratory insufficiency, neurologic dysfunction, or petechial rash), four or more minor criteria (fever, tachycardia, retinal changes, jaundice, or renal changes), and one or more laboratory criteria (fat macroglobulinemia, decreased hemoglobin or platelets, or increased erythrocyte sedimentation rate) [47]. An alternative diagnostic scheme was proposed by Schonfeld [47], assigning a numerical score to similar criteria with a score of 5 or more suggestive of the diagnosis.

Sudden onset of fever, tachycardia, and tachypnea often herald onset of the syndrome. Respiratory distress and hypoxemia with an oxygen tension less than 60 mm Hg is common and may be the initial or only laboratory abnormality. The chest radiograph may be unremarkable for one-half of the cases, but fine stippling or hazy infiltrates of both lung fields should be sought, because they are consistent with fat embolism syndrome [51].

Petechiae are present in 50% to 60% of clinically recognized cases and are most often found on the lower palpebral conjunctivae; neck; anterior axillary folds; and anterior chest wall [47]. There is an associated thrombocytopenia, believed to be caused by the consumption of platelets with their aggregation around the embolic fat droplets, and a progressive anemia with hemoglobin levels commonly less than 9.5 g per 100 mL [51]. Retinal fat emboli and lipuria are each in evidence in more than 50% of patients [51]. The retinal emboli appear as small rosaries of microinfarcts surrounding the macula of both eyes, which over the course of the following 10 to 14 days evolve into yellowish, fatty plaques [51].

The CNS manifestations range from confusion to coma, and although they almost always accompany respiratory insufficiency, they can be the initial and sometimes only symptomatic manifestation of fat embolism syndrome [47]. Impaired consciousness is the earliest recognizable sign. The symptoms can begin with restlessness and confusion and may evolve gradually or abruptly to stupor and coma. Coma, especially if it develops abruptly, portends a poor prognosis [46]. Focal or generalized seizures can occur and may antedate the onset of coma [47]. Decerebrate rigidity is found in up to 15% of cases, and pyramidal signs of hyperreflexia and extensor plantar responses are found in 30% to 70%.

Focal neurologic signs, such as aphasia and hemiparesis, are usually restricted to patients with more severe disturbances of consciousness [47].

Neuroimaging of cerebral fat embolism syndrome reveals diffuse vasogenic and cytotoxic edema, as well as areas of hemorrhage and infarct, and these imaging findings are seen to evolve over time. The most common finding on head CT is evidence of diffuse brain edema, as shown by small ventricles and flattened sulci [54]. Brain MRI has been described to show five different patterns associated with cerebral fat emboli [55]. These range from acute findings of scattered embolic appearing ischemia to chronic changes with demyelinating changes and atrophy. Other changes include confluent cytotoxic edema, vasogenic edema, and petechial hemorrhages. The T_2 hyperintensities that appear as small subcortical foci in gray and white matter, indicative of vasogenic edema, are correlated with lower GCS scores [56].

Treatment

Rapid immobilization of fractures and their early definitive management decreases the likelihood of fat embolism syndrome [51]. Sequential clinical examinations, chest radiographs, and arterial blood gas determinations for patients believed to be at high risk may help identify early on those needing more aggressive care. These patients should have early and expedient replacement of fluids and blood and administration of 40% oxygen by mask [51].

The support of respiration and maintenance of arterial oxygen levels greater than 70 mm Hg sometimes requires intubation and mechanical ventilation. Steroids have been advocated as treatment to blunt the inflammatory response, to help preserve vascular integrity, and to minimize interstitial edema formation, but there are as yet no controlled trials demonstrating a consistent benefit. A brain CT or MRI is indicated to assess whether there are any direct cerebral traumatic injuries accounting for neurologic symptoms.

Prognosis

Mortality in fat embolism syndrome can reach 10% to 20%, but recent improvements in management have lessened this rate [57]. Twenty-five percent of patients experience permanent neurologic deficits [53]. A favorable prognosis is more likely with normal muscle tone, active deep tendon reflexes, and retention of appropriate pain response [47]. If patients survive the pulmonary insufficiency, neurologic dysfunction is often reversible [47]. A worse prognosis is portended by coma, severe ARDS, pneumonia, or congestive heart failure [46].

SINGULTUS (HICCUPS)

Hiccups are usually a benign and self-limited condition. Prolonged hiccups can produce fatigue, sleeplessness, weight loss, depression, difficulty in ventilation, and, in postoperative patients, wound dehiscence [58]. In intubated patients, persistent hiccups may result in hyperventilation and respiratory alkalosis [58].

Pathophysiology

Hiccups result from a sudden reflex contraction of the diaphragm, causing forceful inspiration, which is arrested almost immediately by glottic closure, producing the characteristic sound. Afferent pathways include the vagus and phrenic nerves and thoracic sympathetic fibers (T_6 to T_{12}). The efferent pathway includes the phrenic nerve to the diaphragm, the vagus nerve to the larynx, and the spinal nerves to the accessory muscles of inspiration. Although central control of this reflex is not well defined, it probably involves lower brainstem and upper cervical spinal levels, including the respiratory center, phrenic nerve nuclei, medullary reticular formation, and hypothalamus [59].

Etiology

Hiccups may result from a multitude of causes, owing to injury or irritation of the afferent or efferent pathways or disease within the central control mechanism. Hiccups most frequently result from irritation of the stomach wall or diaphragm, leading to impulses along the phrenic and vagus nerves. Abdominal disorders causing hiccups include gastric ulceration, gastric distention, gastroesophageal reflux, hiatus hernia, cholecystitis, peritonitis, subdiaphragmatic abscess, ileus, and bowel obstruction. Thoracic disorders that precipitate hiccups include esophagitis, pericarditis, myocardial infarction, pneumonia, and neoplasm. More proximally along the course of the nerves, neck masses, such as neoplasm and goiter, may also result in hiccups. Brainstem neoplasm or ischemia, multiple sclerosis, arteriovenous malformations, and meningoencephalitis are CNS causes [60]. Perioperative causes include neck extension, intubation, visceral traction, and intraoperative manipulation of efferent or afferent nerves [58]. Metabolic disorders, such as uremia, electrolyte abnormalities, alcohol intoxication, diabetes mellitus, and general anesthesia, have also been implicated [58,59]. Medications, most frequently corticosteroids and benzodiazepines, may also induce hiccups [61,62]. Hiccups have been reported in four patients with Parkinson's disease, and dopamine agonists appeared to play a causative role [63,64]. Some patients have idiopathic or psychogenic hiccups.

Evaluation

A history of gastrointestinal, cardiac, pulmonary, or CNS complaints or surgery may assist in determining the etiology of intractable hiccups. The physical examination should rule out inflammation or neoplasm in the thorax, abdomen, CNS, and neck. Chest and abdominal radiographs are obtained routinely, and fluoroscopic evaluation of the diaphragm is sometimes needed. Radiographic or endoscopic evaluation of the gastrointestinal tract is sometimes warranted. If the CNS is implicated, cranial CT or MRI may be useful. Electrocardiography (ECG) is required. Other investigations include determinations of electrolytes, renal function, glucose, creatine kinase (if myocardial infarction is suspected), and a toxicology screen for alcohol and barbiturates. Lumbar puncture is required if there is a suspicion of CNS infection. Electromyography may be useful if surgical therapy for hiccups is contemplated. Careful review of medications for potential causative agents is indicated.

Management

Initial management includes identification and treatment of disorders that may cause hiccups, such as inflammation, infection, or gastric dilatation. When this is unsuccessful, nonpharmacologic and pharmacologic treatments are available for intractable hiccups.

Nonpharmacologic therapies alter the reflex arc responsible for hiccups. Pharyngeal stimulation may resolve hiccups, either by nasogastric intubation, swallowing dry granulated sugar, or by the introduction of a red rubber catheter through the mouth or nares, followed by a jerky to-and-fro movement [58]. Pharyngeal stimulation tends to be a temporary measure. Counterstimulation of the vagus nerve by pressure on eyeballs, rectal massage, or irritating the tympanic membrane may also alleviate hiccups [59]. Breathing into a paper bag, gasping with fright, Valsalva maneuver, and supramaximal inspiration possibly abolish hiccups by interrupting the stimulus for respiration or increasing the carbon dioxide concentration [65]. If nonpharmacologic therapies are ineffective, drug therapy should be initiated. Baclofen 5 mg orally three times a day, increased to 10 mg three times a day, has been effective in decreasing and potentially eliminating hiccups [59]. Alternatively, chlorpromazine taken 25 to 50 mg orally or intramuscularly three or four times a day has also been effective. If this is ineffective in 2 to 3 days, then a slow intravenous infusion of chlorpromazine 25 to 50 mg in 500 to 1,000 mL of normal saline is indicated. Although hypotension may result from intravenous (IV) administration, chlorpromazine may be most effective by this route [60]. If IV chlorpromazine is ineffective, it should be discontinued and 10 mg of metoclopramide given orally four times per day. Other medications used in refractory patients include haloperidol (5 mg three times per day), anticonvulsants (e.g., gabapentin, phenytoin, carbamazepine, and valproic acid), amitriptyline, nifedipine, nimodipine, and amantadine [60].

Most patients respond to mechanical or drug therapy. In refractory cases, transcutaneous stimulation of the phrenic nerve, transesophageal diaphragmatic pacing, vagus nerve stimulation, phrenic nerve block or ablation, or microvascular decompression of the vagus nerve may be useful [60,66,67]. Because there are multiple efferent pathways involved, hiccups may remain even after phrenic nerve ablation.

COMPRESSION NEUROPATHIES

Compression neuropathies are common in the general population. In the ICU population, several nerves are particularly at risk, compression of which may result in delayed morbidity [68]. The ulnar nerve may be compressed in the condylar groove posterior to the medial epicondyle when the arms are positioned in a flexed, pronated, or semipronated fashion, or when the flexed elbows are used by the patient for repositioning. Ulnar nerve palsy causes weakness of the intrinsic muscles of the hand, and numbness of the fourth and fifth fingers. The peroneal nerve is also at risk where it courses around the fibular head. The everted immobile position of the leg in severely weak or paralyzed patients contributes to its vulnerability. Other compression neuropathies and brachial plexopathy may result from positions assumed during prolonged coma before hospitalization. Hematomas resulting from clotting disorders; anticoagulation; local injection; arterial puncture; or phlebotomy may also compress the peripheral nerves and plexi [69]. Evaluation of compression neuropathies includes an electromyography (EMG) to localize the lesion [68]. Proper positioning of the limbs to avoid compression of these nerves between the bed and bony prominences is key to prevention.

References

1. Kochanek KD, Murphy SL, Anderson RN, et al: Deaths: final data for 2002. *Natl Vital Stat Rep* 53(5):1–116, 2004.
2. McHugh TP, Stout M: Near-hanging injury. *Ann Emerg Med* 12:774–776, 1983.
3. Kaki A, Crosby ET, Lui ACP: Airway and respiratory management following non-lethal hanging. *Can J Anaesth* 44:445–450, 1997.
4. Matsuyama T, Okuchi K, Seki T, et al: Prognostic factors in hanging injuries. *Am J Emerg Med* 22:207–210, 2004.
5. Gunnell D, Bennewith O, Hawton K, et al: The epidemiology and prevention of suicide by hanging: a systematic review. *Int J Epidemiol* 34(2):433–442, 2005.
6. Nikolic S, Micic J, Atanasijevic T, et al: Analysis of neck injuries with hanging. *Am J Forensic Med Pathol* 24(2):179–182, 2003.
7. Vander KL, Wolfe R: The emergency department management of near-hanging victims. *J Emerg Med* 12:285–292, 1994.
8. Ikenaga T, Kajikawa M, Kajikawa H, et al: Unilateral dissection of the cervical portion of the internal carotid artery and ipsilateral multiple cerebral infarctions caused by suicidal hanging: a case report. *No Shinkei Geka* 24:853–858, 1996.
9. Ohkawa S, Yamadori A: CT in hanging. *Neuroradiology* 35:591, 1993.
10. Nakajo M, Onohara S, Shinmura K, et al: Computed tomography and magnetic resonance imaging findings of brain damage by hanging. *J Comput Assist Tomogr* 27:896–900, 2003.
11. Spicer RS, Miller TR: Suicide acts in 8 states: incidence and case fatality rates by demographics and method. *Am J Public Health* 90(12):1885–1891, 2000.
12. Wee JH, You YH, Lim H, et al: Outcomes of asphyxial cardiac arrest patients who were treated with therapeutic hypothermia: a multicenter retrospective cohort study. *Resuscitation* 89:81–86, 2015.
13. Arias M, Arias-Rivas S, Perez M, et al: Numb ears in resurrection: great auricular nerve injury in hanging attempt. *Neurology* 64:2153–2154, 2005.
14. Lammertse DP: Neurorehabilitation of spinal cord injuries following lightning and electrical trauma. *NeuroRehabilitation* 20:9–14, 2005.
15. Klein Schmidt-Demasters BK: Neuropathology of lightening-strike injuries. *Semin Neurol* 15(4):323–327, 1995.
16. Cooper MA: Emergent care of lightning and electrical injuries. *Semin Neurol* 15(3):268–278, 1995.
17. Cherington M: Central nervous system complications of lightning and electrical injuries. *Semin Neurol* 15(3):233–240, 1995.
18. Ten Duis HJ: Acute electrical burns. *Semin Neurol* 15(4):381–386, 1995.
19. Cherington M: Spectrum of neurologic complications of lightning injuries. *NeuroRehabilitation* 20:3–8, 2005.
20. Cohen JA: Autonomic nervous system disorders and reflex sympathetic dystrophy in lightning and electrical injuries. *Semin Neurol* 15(4):387–390, 1995.
21. Koumbourlis AC: Electrical injuries. *Crit Care Med* 30[Suppl 11]:S424–S430, 2002.
22. Norman ME, Albertson D, Younge BR: Ophthalmic manifestations of lightning strike. *Surv Ophthal* 46(1):19–24, 2001.
23. Ogren FP, Edmunds AL: Neuro-otologic findings in the lightning-injured patient. *Semin Neurol* 15(3):256–262, 1995.
24. Primeau M: Neurorehabilitation of behavioral disorders following lightning and electrical trauma. *NeuroRehabilitation* 20:25–33, 2005.
25. Johl HK, Olshansky A, Beydoun S, et al: Cervicothoracic spinal cord and potomedullary injury secondary to high-voltage electrocution: a case report. *J Med Case Rep* 23(6):1721–1723, 2014.
26. Wilbourn AJ: Peripheral nerve disorders in electrical and lightning injuries. *Semin Neurol* 15(3):241–254, 1995.
27. Smith MA, Muehlberger T, Dellon AL: Peripheral nerve compression associated with low-voltage electrical injury without associated significant cutaneous burn. *Plast Reconstr Surg* 109(1):137–144, 2002.
28. Primeau M, Engelstatter GH, Bares KK: Behavioral consequences of lightning and electrical injury. *Semin Neurol* 15(3):279–285, 1995.
29. Ernst A, Zibrak JD: Carbon monoxide poisoning. *N Engl J Med* 339(22): 1603–1608, 1998.
30. Weaver LK: Carbon monoxide poisoning. *Crit Care Clin* 15(2):297–317, 1999.
31. Dinerman N, Huber J: Inhalation injuries, in Rosen P (ed): *Emergency Medicine: Concepts and Clinical Practice*. 2nd ed. St. Louis, Mosby, 1988, p 585.
32. Chiew AL, Buckley, NA: Carbon monoxide poisoning in the 21st century. *Critical Care* 18(2):221–229, 2014.
33. Annane D, Chevret S, Jars-Guincestre C, et al: Prognostic factors in unintentional mild carbon monoxide poisoning. *Intensive Care Med* 27(11):1776–1781, 2001.
34. Lee MS, Marsden CD: Neurological sequelae following carbon monoxide poisoning clinical course and outcome according to the clinical types and brain computed tomography scan findings. *Mov Disord* 9(5):550–558, 1994.
35. Kim JH, Change KH, Song IC, et al: Delayed encephalopathy of acute carbon monoxide intoxication: diffusivity of cerebral white matter lesions. *Am J Neuroradiol* 24(8):1592–1597, 2003.
36. Chu K, Jung KH, Kim H-J, et al: Diffusion-weighted MRI and ^{99m}Tc-HMPAO SPECT in delayed relapsing type of carbon monoxide poisoning: evidence of delayed cytotoxic edema. *Eur Neurol* 51:98–103, 2004.
37. Hopkins RO, Fearing MA, Weaver LK, et al: Basal ganglia lesions following carbon monoxide poisoning. *Brain Inj* 20(3):273–281, 2006.
38. Choi IS: Parkinsonism after carbon monoxide poisoning. *Eur Neurol* 48(1):30–33, 2002.
39. Gale SD, Hopkins RO, Weaver LK, et al: MRI, quantitative MRI, SPECT, and neuropsychological findings following carbon monoxide poisoning. *Brain Inj* 13(4):229–243, 1999.
40. Deschamps D, Geraud C, Julien H, et al: Memory one month after acute carbon monoxide intoxication: a prospective study. *Occup Environ Med* 60:212–216, 2003.
41. Min SK: A brain syndrome associated with delayed neuropsychiatric sequelae following acute carbon monoxide intoxication. *Acta Psychiatr Scand* 73:80–86, 1986.
42. Garland H, Pearce J: Neurological complications of carbon monoxide poisoning. *Q J Med* 36:445–455, 1967.
43. Neuman TS: Arterial gas embolism and decompression sickness. *News Physiol Sci* 17:77–81, 2002.
44. Tetzlaff K, Shank ES, Muth CM: Evaluation and management of decompression illness—an intensivist's perspective. *Intensive Care Med* 29:2128–2136, 2003.
45. Leach RM, Rees PJ, Wilmshurst P: ABC of oxygen: hyperbaric oxygen therapy. *BMJ* 317:1140–1143, 1998.
46. Levy D: The fat embolism syndrome: a review. *Clin Ortho Relat Res* 261:281–286, 1990.
47. Johnson MJ, Lucas GL: Fat embolism syndrome. *Orthopedics* 19:41–49, 1996.
48. Kamano M, Honda Y, Kitaguchi M, et al: Cerebral fat embolism after a nondisplaced tibial fracture. *Clin Ortho Rel Res* 389:206–209, 2001.
49. Forteza AM, Rabinstein A, Koch S, et al: Endovascular closure of patent foramen ovale in the fat embolism syndrome. *Arch Neurol* 59:455–459, 2002.

50. Dive AM, Dubois PE, Ide C, et al: Paradoxical cerebral fat embolism: an unusual case of persistent unconsciousness after orthopedic surgery. *Anesthesiology* 96(4):1029–1031, 2002.
51. Peltier L: Fat embolism, in Schwartz G (ed): *Principles and Practice of Emergency Medicine*. Philadelphia, PA, WB Saunders, 1986, p 1589.
52. Muller C, Rahn BA, Pfister U, et al: The incidence, pathogenesis, diagnosis and treatment of fat embolism. *Orthop Rev* 23:107–117, 1994.
53. Kamenar E, Burger P: Cerebral fat embolism: a neuropathological study of a microembolic state. *Stroke* 11:477–484, 1980.
54. Ryu CW, Lee DH, Kim TK, et al: Cerebral fat embolism: diffusion-weighted MRI findings. *Acta Radiologica* 46:528–533, 2005.
55. Kuo KH, Pan YJ, Lan YJ, et al: Dynamic MR imaging patterns of cerebral fat embolism: A systemic review with illustrative cases. *AJNR Am J Neuroradiol* 35(6):1052–1057, 2014.
56. Parizel PM, Demey HE, Veeckmans G, et al: Early diagnosis of cerebral fat embolism syndrome by diffusion-weighted MRI. *Stroke* 32:2942–2944, 2001.
57. Guenter CA, Braun TE: Fat embolism syndrome. Changing prognosis. *Chest* 79:143–145, 1981.
58. Smith HS, Busracamowongs A: Management of hiccups in the palliative care population. *Am J Hosp Palliat Care* 20(2):149–154, 2003.
59. Friedman NL: Hiccups: a treatment review. *Pharmacotherapy* 16:986–995, 1996.
60. Chang FY, Chiang-Liang L: Hiccup: mystery, nature, and treatment: *J Neurogastroenterol Motil* 18(2):123–130, 2012.
61. Dickerman RD, Jaikumar S: The hiccup reflex arc and persistent hiccups with high-dose anabolic steroids: is the brainstem the steroid-responsive locus? *Clin Neuropharmacol* 24(1):62–64, 2001.
62. Thompson DF, Landry JP: Drug-induced hiccups. *Ann Pharmacother* 31:367–369, 1997.
63. Sharma P, Morgan JC, Sethi KD: Hiccups associated with dopamine agonists in Parkinson disease. *Neurology* 66:774, 2006.
64. Lester J, Beatriz Raina G, Uribe-Roca C, et al: Hiccup secondary to dopamine agonists in Parkinson's disease. *Mov Disord* 15:1667–1668, 2007.
65. Morris LG, Marti JL, Ziff DJ: Termination of idiopathic persistent singultus (hiccup) with supramaximal inspiration. *J Emerg Med* 27(4):416–417, 2004.
66. Johnson DL: Intractable hiccups: treatment by microvascular decompression of the vagus nerve. *J Neurosurg* 78:813–816, 1993.
67. Andres DW, Matthews TK: Transesophageal diaphragmatic pacing for treatment of persistent hiccups. *Anesthesiology* 102(2):483, 2005.
68. Angel MJ, Bril V, Shannon P, et al: Neuromuscular function in survivors of the acute respiratory distress syndrome. *Can J Neurol Sci* 34(04):427–432, 2007.
69. Nobel W, Marks SC, Kubik S: The anatomical basis for femoral neuropathy following iliacus hematoma. *J Neurosurg* 52(4):533–540, 1980.

Section 15

PSYCHIATRIC ISSUES IN INTENSIVE CARE

JOHN QUERQUES

Chapter 157 ■ Diagnosis and Treatment of Agitation and Delirium in the Intensive Care Unit Patient

JASON P. CAPLAN

> "... patients are attacked with insomnolency, so that the disease is not concocted; they become sorrowful, peevish, and delirious; there are flashes of light in their eyes, and noises in their ears; their extremities are cold, their urine unconcocted; the sputa thin, saltish, tinged with an intense color and smell; sweats about the neck, and anxiety; respiration, interrupted in the expulsion of the air, frequent and very large; expression of the eyelids dreadful; dangerous deliquia [syncope]; tossing of the bed-clothes from the breast; the hands trembling, and sometimes the lower lip agitated. These symptoms, appearing at the commencement, are indicative of strong delirium, and patients so affected generally die, or if they escape, it is with a deposit, hemorrhage from the nose, or the expectoration of thick matter, and not otherwise. Neither do I perceive that physicians are skilled in such things as these; how they ought to know such diseases as are connected with debility, and which are further weakened by abstinence from food, and those aggravated by some other irritation; those by pain, and from the acute nature of the disease, and what affections and various forms thereof our constitution and habit engender, although the knowledge or ignorance of such things brings safety or death to the patient."
>
> —*Hippocrates, 400 B.C.*

In *On Regimen in Acute Diseases*, Hippocrates identified agitation as a harbinger of severe illness and poor outcome [1]. His admonition that physicians understand the causes and treatments of agitation remains vital today, for the safety not only of patients but also of hospital staff attending to them. Nowhere is this more pertinent than in the intensive care unit (ICU) and its finely balanced environment of invasive and often delicate treatment modalities, interference with which is rarely as easily corrected as is "tossing of the bed-clothes." The sudden pulling of precisely placed central lines, intra-aortic balloon pumps, or endotracheal tubes can carry profound consequences for patients and those responsible for their care.

The term "ICU psychosis" has unfortunately entered common medical parlance in reference to agitation and confusion in the ICU patient [2]. This misnomer is inaccurate for several reasons. Classifying agitation as psychosis is usually diagnostically incorrect; moreover, drawing an etiologic connection between the patient's geographic location and the development of agitation is nonsensical. Historically, sensory deprivation and interruption of normal sleep patterns alone were thought to result in behavioral disturbances in the ICU, but modern research has not confirmed this relationship [2]. The causal attribution of mental status changes to the environment of the ICU is dangerous because it obviates the need for further diagnostic inquiry that could reveal a previously unidentified pathologic process. As with all new symptoms, careful diagnosis is the first step toward effective treatment.

This chapter reviews the causes, presentations, and treatments of common causes of agitation in the ICU patient, focusing on delirium.

DELIRIUM

Perhaps the most common cause of agitation in the general hospital as a whole, and the ICU in particular, delirium is a neuropsychiatric manifestation of a systemic disturbance (Table 157.1) [3]. As such, the paramount task in its treatment is the identification of its underlying cause(s).

Epidemiology

Prospective studies of all patients admitted to the ICU regardless of pathology have found incidence rates of delirium of 31% on admission [4] and 82% when limited to the population requiring intubation and mechanical ventilation [5].

A diagnosis of delirium exacts a profound toll on both the immediate and long-term well-being of patients and the economic resources required for their care. One study of mechanically ventilated patients in the ICU demonstrated significant increases in length of hospital stay and 6-month mortality, even after adjustment for age, severity of illness, comorbidities, coma, and medication exposure [5]. Another study of patients—limited to those who did not require mechanical ventilation—found that a diagnosis of delirium independently

TABLE 157.1

Diagnostic Criteria for Delirium

- Alteration of consciousness and attention
- Change in cognition (e.g., memory deficit, disorientation, language or perceptual disturbance) that is not due to dementia
- Development over hours to days
- Fluctuation during the course of the day
- Precipitation by a medical condition or its treatment

Adapted from American Psychiatric Association: *Diagnostic and Statistical Manual of Mental Disorders*. 5th ed. Washington, DC, American Psychiatric Publishing, 2013.

predicted longer hospital stay, even after correction for relevant covariates [6]. When framed in fiscal terms, delirium has been associated with 39% higher ICU costs and 31% higher hospital costs overall [7]. Delirium predicts greater hospital costs across multiple domains, including professional, technical, consultative, and nursing [8].

Disruptive behavior poses a grave risk of acute injury to the delirious ICU patient because of the extensive use of invasive technology in the ICU. This hazard has been specifically studied in patients who extubate themselves. Restlessness and agitation—two of the most frequent concomitants of delirium—independently predict self-extubation that can result in laryngeal and vocal cord trauma, emesis, aspiration, cardiac arrhythmia, respiratory arrest, and death [9].

Etiology

An exhaustive review of conditions that may precipitate delirium would likely cover the breadth of medical and surgical practice. Given the near limitless number of possible etiologies, when searching for a possible cause of delirium, it often proves useful to scan the clinical data searching for broad categories of pathology. The mnemonic "I WATCH DEATH" (Table 157.2) lists the processes most commonly related to delirium; the mnemonic "WWHHHHIMPS" (Table 157.3) aids recall of immediately life-threatening causes.

With complicated conditions requiring interventions on multiple fronts, patients in the ICU are often subjected to polypharmacy. A review of the patient's medication list with an eye toward certain categories of medications frequently causative of, or contributory to, delirium is warranted (Table 157.4). Particular offenders include anticholinergics, antihistamines, corticosteroids, opioids, and benzodiazepines [10,11].

TABLE 157.2

I WATCH DEATH: A Mnemonic for Common Causes of Delirium

*I*nfections	Pneumonia, urinary tract infection, encephalitis, meningitis, syphilis
*W*ithdrawal	Alcohol, sedative–hypnotics
*A*cute metabolic	Acidosis, alkalosis, electrolyte disturbances, hepatic or renal failure
*T*rauma	Heat stroke, burns, postoperative state
*C*entral nervous system pathology	Abscess, tumor, hemorrhage, seizure, stroke, vasculitis, normal pressure hydrocephalus
*H*ypoxia	Hypotension, pulmonary embolus, pulmonary or cardiac failure, anemia, carbon monoxide poisoning
*D*eficiencies	Vitamin B_{12}, niacin, thiamine
*E*ndocrinopathies	Hyper- or hypoglycemia, hyper- or hypoadrenalism, hyper- or hypothyroidism, hyper- or hypoparathyroidism
*A*cute vascular	Hypertensive encephalopathy, shock
*T*oxins or drugs	Medications, drugs of abuse, pesticides, solvents
*H*eavy metals	Lead, manganese, mercury

Adapted from Wise MG, Trzepacz PT: Delirium (confusional states), in Rundell JR, Wise MD (eds): *The American Psychiatric Press Textbook of Consultation-Liaison Psychiatry*. Washington, DC, American Psychiatric Press, 1996, pp 258–274.

TABLE 157.3

WWHHHHIMPS: A Mnemonic for Life-Threatening Causes of Delirium

*W*ithdrawal
*W*ernicke's encephalopathy
*H*ypoxia or hypoperfusion of the brain
*H*ypertensive crisis
*H*ypoglycemia
*H*yper- or hypothermia
*I*ntracranial hemorrhage or mass
*M*eningitis or encephalitis
*P*oisons (including medications)
*S*tatus epilepticus

Adapted from Wise MG, Trzepacz PT: Delirium (confusional states), in Rundell JR, Wise MD (eds): *The American Psychiatric Press Textbook of Consultation-Liaison Psychiatry*. Washington, DC, American Psychiatric Press, 1996, pp 258–274.

Pathology

Alertness is subserved by the ascending reticular activating system (RAS) and its bilateral thalamic projections; attention is mediated by neocortical and limbic inputs to this system [12]. Structural or neurochemical interference with these pathways could theoretically result in the deficits in alertness and attention that are the hallmarks of delirium. Because the primary neurotransmitter of the RAS is acetylcholine, the relative deficit of cholinergic reserve in the elderly (e.g., due to microvascular disease or atrophy) may be the neural basis of the heightened risk of delirium in the geriatric population. Medications with anticholinergic activity are likely to disrupt this system's functioning even further.

In the setting of impaired oxidative metabolism, dopaminergic neurons have been found to release excess amounts of dopamine; its subsequent reuptake and extracellular metabolism also are disrupted. Because, at high levels, dopamine is theorized to facilitate the excitatory effects of glutamate [13], this dopaminergic hypothesis constitutes a proposed mechanism for the agitation seen in delirium. In fact, oxidative dysfunction predicts increased risk of delirium [14].

Risk Factors and Detection

Risk factors for delirium can be divided into three broad categories: properties of the illness (acute physiologic), preexisting properties of the patient (chronic physiologic), and properties of the environment (iatrogenic) (Table 157.5) [15].

The majority of patients suffering from delirium present with the hypoactive subtype. Withdrawn and psychomotorically retarded, the patient with hypoactive delirium is frequently thought by caretakers and family to be depressed. Although these patients cause little disruption to the ICU environment and provoke less acute distress in their caregivers, they are no less subject to the adverse outcomes of an altered sensorium. Although the immediate threat to safety may be less apparent in these cases, hypoactive delirium can rapidly and unpredictably evolve into acute agitation as a result of unchecked, upsetting delusions. Moreover, the subjective experience of hypoactive delirium is as intense and distressing as the agitated variety [16].

Two delirium screening scales have been validated for use by nonpsychiatric personnel in the ICU. The Confusion Assessment Method for the ICU (CAM-ICU) features a four-domain assessment that can be administered in less than 1 minute [17]. Both

TABLE 157.4

Common ICU Drugs Associated with Delirium

Antiarrhythmics	β-Blockers
Disopyramide	Calcium channel blockers
Lidocaine	Digitalis preparations
Mexiletine	Diuretics
Procainamide	Acetazolamide
Quinidine	Dopamine agonists
Tocainide	Amantadine
Antibiotics	Bromocriptine
Aminoglycosides	Carbidopa
Amodiaquine	Levodopa
Amphotericin	Selegiline
Cephalosporins	H_2-Blockers
Fluoroquinolones	Immunosuppressants
Gentamicin	Azacitidine
Isoniazid	Chlorambucil
Metronidazole	Cyclosporine
Rifampin	Cytosine arabinoside
Sulfonamides	Dacarbazine
Tetracyclines	FK-506
Ticarcillin	5-Fluorouracil
Vancomycin	Hexamethylmelamine
Anticholinergics	Ifosfamide
Atropine	Interleukin-2
Benztropine	L-Asparaginase
Chlorpheniramine	Methotrexate
Diphenhydramine	Procarbazine
Eye and nose drops	Tamoxifen
Scopolamine	Vinblastine
Anticonvulsants	Vincristine
Phenytoin	Ketamine
Sodium valproate	Nonsteroidal anti-inflammatory drugs
Antidepressants	
Antiemetics	Ibuprofen
Promethazine	Indomethacin
Metoclopramide	Naproxen
Antiviral agents	Opioids
Acyclovir	Propylthiouracil
Efavirenz	Salicylates
Interferon	Steroids
Ganciclovir	Sympathomimetics
Nevirapine	Aminophylline
Baclofen	Theophylline
Barbiturates	Phenylpropanolamine
Benzodiazepines	Phenylephrine

Adapted from Cassem NH, Murray GB, Lafayette JM, et al: Delirious patients, in Stern TA, Fricchione GL, Cassem NH, et al (eds): *Massachusetts General Hospital Handbook of General Hospital Psychiatry*. 5th ed. Philadelphia, PA, Mosby, 2004, pp 119–134.

sensitivity and specificity are >90%, and it has been translated into several languages. The Intensive Care Delirium Screening Checklist (ICDSC) features eight items, each scored present or absent. Sensitivity and specificity of the ICDSC are 99% and 64%, respectively. The minimal time required to complete either of these scales allows for scoring several times daily, which is an important feature, given the waxing and waning nature of delirium. One comparison study of these scales found the CAM-ICU to be a superior predictor of increased length of stay and mortality [18]. Both scales are available at www.icudelirium.org. Careful screening and early detection can limit the sequelae of delirium and forestall the additional consequences attendant to the evolution of hypoactive delirium into agitation.

Diagnostic Evaluation

In ambiguous cases of delirium, an electroencephalogram (EEG) may provide objective data to aid diagnosis. Although the association of delirium and EEG changes was first described in the 1940s, no objective test since has demonstrated better performance in accurately detecting delirium. In their classic studies, Engel and Romano described three landmark electrographic findings in delirious patients: generalized slowing, consistency of this slowing despite wide-ranging underlying conditions, and resumption of a normal rhythm with treatment [19]. For all presentations of delirium, generalized slowing in the delta-theta range (delta: 0 to 4 Hz, theta: 4 to 8 Hz), poor organization of the background rhythm, and loss of reactive changes to eye opening and closing are considered diagnostic [20]. Recent studies have estimated the sensitivity of EEG in the diagnosis of delirium to be approximately 75%, with false–negative results likely a result of slowing not sizable enough to drop the patient's baseline rhythm from one range to the next.

EEG may also prove helpful in discerning the etiology of a delirium, since delirium tremens (DTs) as a result of alcohol or sedative–hypnotic withdrawal is associated with low-voltage fast activity superimposed on slow waves, while sedative–hypnotic toxicity is associated with fast beta activity (>12 Hz) [20]. EEG may also detect previously undiagnosed deliriogenic conditions, including nonconvulsive status epilepticus, complex partial seizures, or cerebral lesions that may act as seizure foci.

Once delirium is confirmed, the search for an underlying medical cause should commence. A careful step-by-step approach can help prune a near-endless list of possible etiologies. Although no evidence-based protocol of diagnostic studies most likely to identify a culprit exists, broad-based, relatively inexpensive, and noninvasive laboratory testing can often be informative (Table 157.6).

In most circumstances, psychiatric consultation can be beneficial to the patient and the consultee. A consultation psychiatrist's familiarity with delirium and its causes and treatments can speed diagnosis and intervention. Delay in psychiatric consultation has predicted lengthier hospitalization [21].

Pharmacologic Management

The definitive treatment of delirium is the identification and treatment of the underlying cause(s). In addition, numerous interventions may reduce its potentially harmful sequelae.

Cholinergic Agents

Given the hypocholinergic/hyperdopaminergic neurophysiological model of delirium, the intuitive goals of pharmacologic treatment are to increase cholinergic and decrease dopaminergic activities. By reversibly inhibiting metabolism of acetylcholine, the cholinesterase inhibitor physostigmine has been shown to reverse delirium resulting from multiple etiologies, but its clinical utility is limited by its brief duration of effect and a narrow therapeutic window. Therefore, physostigmine is usually used only when delirium is known (or highly suspected) to be caused by anticholinergic toxicity, for which it is considered the agent of choice [22].

Some small studies and case series of dementia-treating cholinesterase inhibitors have demonstrated possible delirioprotective effects [23,24], but these agents' utility in the acute setting is hampered by their long half-lives and subsequent extended interval before therapeutic serum levels are reached.

TABLE 157.5

Risk Factors for Delirium

Properties of environment/ treatment	Properties of illness (acute physiologic)	Properties of patient (chronic physiologic)
Hyper- or hyponatremia	Age >70 y	Administration of psychoactive medication
Hyper- or hypoglycemia	Transfer from a nursing home	Tube feeding
Hyper- or hypothyroidism	History of depression	Bladder catheter
Hyper- or hypothermia	History of dementia	Rectal catheter
BUN/creatinine ratio ≥18	History of stroke	Central venous catheter
Renal failure (creatinine >2 mg/dL)	History of seizure	Physical restraints
Liver disease (bilirubin >20 mg/dL)	Alcohol abuse within 1 mo	
Cardiogenic shock	Drug overdose or illicit use within 1 wk	
Septic shock	History of congestive heart failure	
Hypoxia	Human immunodeficiency virus infection	
	Malnutrition	

Adapted from Ely EW, Siegel MD, Inouye SK: Delirium in the intensive care unit: an under-recognized syndrome of organ dysfunction. *Semin Respir Crit Care Med* 22:115–126, 2001.

TABLE 157.6

Assessment of the Patient with Delirium

Basic laboratory tests—consider for all patients with delirium	Electrolytes
	Glucose
	Albumin
	Blood urea nitrogen
	Creatinine
	Aspartate aminotransferase
	Alanine aminotransferase
	Alkaline phosphatase
	Rapid plasma reagin
	Vitamin B_{12}
	Folate
	Thyroid stimulating hormone
	Arterial blood gases
	Complete blood count
	Electrocardiogram
	Chest radiograph
	Urinalysis
Additional laboratory tests—consider as clinically indicated	Heavy metal screen
	Lupus erythematosus preparation
	Antinuclear antibody
	Urine porphyrins
	Urine culture
	Urine drug screen
	Ammonia
	Human immunodeficiency virus antibody
	Venereal Disease Research Laboratory test
	Blood culture
	Serum medication levels (e.g., digoxin, theophylline, cyclosporine, phenobarbital, carbamazepine, FK-506)
	Lyme titer
	Cerebrospinal fluid analysis
	Brain computed tomography or magnetic resonance imaging
	Electroencephalogram

Adapted from American Psychiatric Association: Practice guideline for the treatment of patients with delirium. *Am J Psychiatry* 156[5, Suppl]: 1–20, 1999.

Two randomized, double-blind, placebo-controlled trials failed to demonstrate any benefit of donepezil in either preventing or treating postoperative delirium [25,26]. An additional randomized, placebo-controlled trial of rivastigmine for delirium prevention also failed to demonstrate any such benefit [27].

Haloperidol

As dopamine receptor antagonists, neuroleptics are theoretically suited to the task of dampening dopaminergic activity. Through decades of clinical experience and published data, haloperidol, a butyrophenone neuroleptic, has shown itself to be the agent of choice in the treatment of acute delirium [28,29]. It is ideal for use in the ICU since it can be administered by the oral, intramuscular (IM), or intravenous (IV) route. Although the U.S. Food and Drug Administration (FDA) has not approved the IV administration of haloperidol, FDA regulations permit the use of any approved drug for a non-approved indication or by an unsanctioned route in the context of innovative therapy. IV administration is preferable to the oral and IM routes for multiple reasons, including improved absorption; limitation of pain as a consequence of injection; minimization of apprehension on the part of the patient; and lower frequency of extrapyramidal side effects (EPS), including acute dystonia, parkinsonism, and akathisia [30]. Although there is no standard dosing regimen for the use of IV haloperidol, treatment is usually initiated with a bolus dose ranging from 0.5 mg (in the elderly) to 10 mg (for severe agitation). A 30-minute interval should be observed between doses to gauge the effect of the previously administered dose. If the initial dose does not achieve the desired effect, then the next dose can be effectively doubled until appropriate sedation is achieved (i.e., 1, 2, 5, 10 mg, and so on). Although a randomized, double-blind comparison trial did not support the use of benzodiazepines alone for the management of delirium (except when due to alcohol or sedative–hypnotic withdrawal), IV lorazepam in doses of 1 or 2 mg can be coadministered with haloperidol to achieve more rapid sedation [31]. The combination of haloperidol and lorazepam has been shown to allow for lower total doses of each drug [32] and to further reduce the frequency of EPS [33].

Complete absence of agitation should be targeted, and the regimen should be adjusted to achieve this goal. Once agitation is effectively quelled, haloperidol can be given two or three times daily, with additional doses provided as needed for breakthrough agitation. The total dose can be gradually decreased; it is usually wise to wean the evening dose last to provide prophylaxis for "sundowning."

Side Effects of Haloperidol. As with all pharmacologic interventions, the use of haloperidol is not without risk. Neurologic sequelae—EPS, seizures, neuroleptic malignant syndrome (discussed in detail in Chapter 185), and tardive dyskinesia—all have been associated with the chronic use of haloperidol. In practice, however, these are rare and are minimized by IV administration [30]. Of these neurologic symptoms, akathisia is often most problematic in the setting of delirium since the sense of having to be in motion at all times is noxious, tiring, and likely to exacerbate agitation. Treatment with β-blockade is often effective. In clinical practice, haloperidol's reported lowering of the seizure threshold appears negligible for those without seizures [34].

Hypotension, a rare complication, is easily detected by routine monitoring in the ICU. Haloperidol has been shown in some cases to prolong the QT interval, resulting in increased risk for torsade de pointes with increased risk for death [35,36]. An electrocardiogram should be ordered to measure the baseline corrected QT (QTc) interval, and serum potassium, magnesium, and calcium levels should be checked and monitored [28]. Once treatment begins, a QTc >500 ms or an increase >25% from baseline may warrant telemetry, cardiologic consultation, and reduction or discontinuation of haloperidol. In these cases, it is advisable to calculate the QTc manually, since the automated reading may overestimate the value and result in the needless interruption of necessary treatment. The minimization of other drugs with the potential to prolong the QTc also should be considered to allow the ongoing effective treatment of delirium. Other antipsychotics, including the newer agents, also have been associated with QT prolongation [37].

Other Dopamine Receptor Antagonists

Droperidol, the other member of the butyrophenone family of neuroleptics, had been used extensively for the treatment of delirium, but its use was constrained by the 2001 FDA-mandated black-box warning regarding QT prolongation, torsade de pointes, and death [38].

Phenothiazines, the other major class of so-called conventional or first-generation neuroleptic medications (e.g., chlorpromazine, fluphenazine, thioridazine, mesoridazine, perphenazine, and trifluoperazine), are poorly suited to the treatment of delirium due to sedation, anticholinergic effects, and α-adrenergic blockade.

Most of the so-called atypical or second-generation neuroleptic agents have been studied in the treatment of delirium. A variety of single case reports, case series, retrospective analyses, and open-label studies have found these medications to be safe, well tolerated, and effective. Randomized, controlled trials have demonstrated that risperidone, olanzapine, and quetiapine are effective for decreasing the severity of symptoms of delirium [39–44]. A randomized, controlled trial of ziprasidone did not show benefit in delirium, though this study was limited by measurement of delirium as a binary state (present or absent) rather than its severity [45].

Quetiapine may have a niche role in the treatment of delirium in patients with Parkinson's disease or Lewy body dementia, since its action at various subtypes of dopamine receptors is less likely to exacerbate these disorders [46]. Paliperidone may occupy a similar niche role in patients with hepatic compromise since it does not require significant hepatic metabolism [47]. The strict regulation of clozapine due to the risk of agranulocytosis precludes its routine use in delirium.

In 2005, the FDA required that a black-box warning be placed on all atypical neuroleptics indicating an increased risk of death when used to treat behavioral problems in elderly patients with dementia and, in 2008, broadened this warning to encompass conventional neuroleptics. In addition, risperidone, olanzapine, and aripiprazole carry warnings regarding a potential increased risk of cerebrovascular events in elderly patients with dementia-related psychosis. The benefits of neuroleptics in treating delirium often outweigh their risks.

Other Pharmacologic Interventions in Delirium

Dexmedetomidine is a selective α_2-adrenergic receptor agonist used as a sedative and analgesic in the ICU. A number of randomized, controlled trials have demonstrated a significantly lower incidence of delirium when ICU patients were sedated with dexmedetomidine compared with midazolam, lorazepam, or propofol [48–50]. An additional study comparing dexmedetomidine with morphine found a comparable incidence but a shorter duration of delirium with dexmedetomidine [51]. A randomized, open-label trial comparing dexmedetomidine infusion with IV haloperidol for the management of delirious intubated patients demonstrated significantly shortened time to extubation and length of ICU stay with dexmedetomidine [52]. Despite the relatively high cost of the drug, two studies have demonstrated it to be cost-effective due to the offset of time spent ventilated, time in the ICU, and the sparing of other expensive sedating agents [50,53].

The 5-HT-3 receptor antagonist ondansetron has been reported to be successful in managing symptoms of delirium in postcardiotomy patients [54]. The mechanism of this effect is uncertain, but 5-HT-3 receptors have been shown to play a role in cognition, and ondansetron has also demonstrated affinity for the opioid mu receptor and for sodium channels [55].

Randomized, Controlled Trials of Pharmacotherapy in Delirium

Randomized, controlled trials of pharmacotherapy in delirium are summarized in Table 157.7. Many of these interventions demonstrate efficacy in limiting, but not eliminating, symptoms of delirium. Since the definitive treatment of delirium requires identification and treatment of the underlying cause, it may not be reasonable to expect that a neuroleptic will completely eradicate all symptoms of a delirium to the point that it is undetectable. Rather, neuroleptics are intended to manage the symptoms of delirium and to reduce the likelihood of harm to the patient or ICU staff.

Prevention

A number of randomized, controlled trials have examined the use of medication in the prophylaxis of delirium. These are summarized in Table 157.8. A meta-analysis of five of these studies supported the use of neuroleptics as prophylaxis against delirium [64].

Specifically pertaining to postoperative delirium, one randomized, controlled trial of 921 elderly patients undergoing major noncardiac surgery found that operative anesthesia with bispectral index (BIS) monitoring reduced propofol delivery by 21%, volatile anesthetics by 30%, and postoperative delirium by 35% as compared to routine operative anesthesia [65].

A number of multicomponent non-pharmacological protocols have been established to formalize nursing and environmental approaches to delirium prevention. A meta-analysis of these studies concluded that they are effective in decreasing the incidence of delirium and preventing falls with a trend toward lowering length of stay [66].

OTHER CAUSES OF AGITATION

Dementia is a predisposing risk factor for the development of delirium. The demented patient, however, is also at risk of becoming agitated in the ICU as a result of unfamiliar surroundings

TABLE 157.7

Randomized, Controlled Trials of Pharmacotherapy in Delirium

Study	Agents compared	Total number of patients	Results
Breitbart et al. [31]	Haloperidol Chlorpromazine Lorazepam	30	Both neuroleptics significantly improved delirium. No improvement was seen with lorazepam. The lorazepam arm was terminated early due to adverse effects.
Han and Kim [39]	Haloperidol Risperidone	24	No significant difference was found in efficacy or response rate between haloperidol and risperidone.
Skrobik et al. [40]	Haloperidol Olanzapine	73	Clinical improvement was similar for both agents. Haloperidol was associated with extrapyramidal side effects not seen with olanzapine.
Devlin et al. [41]	Quetiapine Placebo	36	Scheduled quetiapine resulted in more rapid resolution of delirium, reduced agitation, and improved rates of transfer to home or a rehabilitation facility. Both groups received as-needed intravenous haloperidol.
Maneeton et al. [42]	Quetiapine Haloperidol	52	Both agents reduced the severity of delirium without a significant difference between the groups.
Grover et al. [43]	Haloperidol Risperidone Olanzapine	64	All three agents reduced the severity of delirium without a significant difference among the groups.
Kim et al. [44]	Risperidone Olanzapine	32	Both agents reduced the severity of delirium. Response to risperidone was poorer in patients older than 70 years.
Girard et al. [47]	Haloperidol Ziprasidone Placebo	101	All patients were mechanically ventilated. Neither neuroleptic significantly decreased duration of delirium.
Tagarakis et al. [54]	Ondansetron Intravenous haloperidol	80	Both agents reduced the severity of postcardiotomy delirium.
Page et al. [56]	Intravenous haloperidol Placebo	141	No significant difference was found in duration of delirium between the groups. A significantly higher number of patients in the placebo arm required open-label addition of neuroleptics due to symptoms of delirium.

TABLE 157.8

Randomized, Controlled Trials of Pharmacologic Prophylaxis of Delirium

Study	Agents compared	Total number of patients	Results
Kalisvaart et al. [57]	Haloperidol Placebo	430	Low-dose haloperidol did not reduce the incidence of postoperative delirium. It decreased severity and duration of delirium and length of stay.
Prakanrattana et al. [58]	Risperidone Placebo	126	Single-dose risperidone following cardiac surgery significantly reduced the incidence of postoperative delirium.
Wang et al. [59]	Intravenous haloperidol Placebo	457	Twelve-hour infusion of low-dose haloperidol after admission to the ICU decreased the incidence of postoperative delirium in elderly patients.
Larsen et al. [60]	Olanzapine Placebo	400	Perioperative administration of olanzapine decreased the incidence of delirium in elderly joint replacement patients.
Al-Aama at al. [61]	Melatonin Placebo	145	Nightly administration of melatonin 0.5 mg decreased the incidence of delirium.
de Jonghe et al. [62]	Melatonin Placebo	378	Nightly administration of melatonin 3 mg had no significant effect on the incidence of delirium.
Hatta et al. [63]	Ramelteon Placebo	67	Nightly administration of ramelteon decreased the incidence of delirium.
Papadopoulos et al. [55]	Ondansetron Placebo	106	Daily administration of ondansetron decreased both the incidence and the severity of delirium.

TABLE 157.9

Differential Diagnosis of Agitation

	Delirium	Dementia	Depression	Schizophrenia
Onset	Acute	Insidious[a]	Variable	Variable
Course	Fluctuating	Progressive[b]	Variable	Variable
Reversibility	Usually	Not usually	Usually	Not usually
Level of consciousness	Impaired	Unimpaired until late stages	Unimpaired	Unimpaired[c]
Attention and memory	Both poor	Poor memory without marked inattention	Attention usually intact, memory intact	Poor attention, memory intact
Hallucinations	Usually visual but can occur in any sensory modality	Visual or auditory	Usually auditory	Usually auditory
Delusions	Fleeting, fragmented, usually persecutory	Paranoid, often fixed	Complex and mood-congruent	Frequent, complex, systematized, and often paranoid

[a]Except when due to strokes, when the onset is acute.
[b]Lewy body dementia often presents with a waxing and waning course imposed on an overall progressive decline. Vascular dementia follows a stepwise pattern, worsening with each successive stroke.
[c]Except when complicated by catatonia.
Adapted from Trzepacz PT, Meagher DJ: Delirium, in Levenson JL (ed): *The American Psychiatric Publishing Textbook of Psychosomatic Medicine*. Washington, DC, American Psychiatric Publishing, 2005, pp 91–130.

and possible delusional beliefs. Behavioral measures should be employed to help the patient orient to the milieu. In cases of acute agitation, haloperidol is the treatment of choice; however, in cases of Lewy body dementia, quetiapine is less likely to exacerbate parkinsonian symptoms.

Similarly, the patient with preexisting schizophrenia may have difficulty in understanding and adapting to an ICU stay. Preemptive behavioral measures should be taken to make the ICU as familiar and comfortable as possible.

Inadequately controlled pain, panic-like anxiety, and a sense of hopelessness resulting from depression can also present with agitation. Anxiety and depression are discussed in Chapters 158 and 159, respectively. Once the trigger for agitation is understood, the appropriate course of treatment is often relatively straightforward. Table 157.9 compares and contrasts several diagnostic traits characteristic of different causes of agitation.

Various substance-withdrawal syndromes may present with agitation and delirium. These often require specific treatment (usually featuring replacement of the dependence-inducing agent and gradual taper) and are covered in Chapter 126.

NONPHARMACOLOGIC TREATMENT OF AGITATION

Despite all efforts to curtail agitated or disruptive behavior, some patients may ultimately require physical intervention to prevent injury to themselves or hospital staff. Interventions range from relatively unobtrusive (e.g., use of mitts to prevent interference with equipment or constant observation to minimize wandering) to more restrictive (e.g., soft limb restraints, Posey vests, four-point restraints) [28]. Most states and individual institutions have protocols governing the application and documentation of such procedures. Since the application of physical restraints can, in itself, be disquieting to the patient, such intervention should be accompanied by the administration of sedating medication.

LONG-TERM SEQUELAE

Patients diagnosed with delirium are at greater risk for a multitude of neuropsychiatric sequelae long after their discharge from the hospital. Multiple studies have demonstrated increased risk of longstanding cognitive impairment in delirious patients when compared to matched controls [67–69]; one study reported that a diagnosis of delirium resulted in an almost doubled risk of cognitive impairment at 2 years [70]. A review of the available literature by Jackson and colleagues concluded that the presence of delirium (regardless of severity or duration) predicts a greater risk of long-term cognitive impairment, including the development of dementia [71]. Posttraumatic stress disorder (PTSD) has been reported in up to 44% of patients admitted to the ICU [72]. While PTSD may result from the experience of actual physical experiences in the ICU, it has also been reported to occur as the sole result of frightening, hallucinatory, or delusional symptoms experienced in the context of delirium [73].

CONCLUSION

Agitation in the ICU patient jeopardizes the immediate safety of the patient and may signify a potentially unidentified pathologic process. Delirium is the most frequent cause of agitation and is associated with poorer outcomes across multiple facets of patient care. Careful evaluation of possible causes of delirium is vital, since its only definitive cure is identification and treatment of the responsible underlying condition. Management may involve both pharmacologic and environmental measures, with manipulation of the dopaminergic and cholinergic axes, the primary targets of pharmacologic intervention.

Agitation may also be a symptom of other psychiatric disorders. Preexisting diagnoses of dementia, depression, or psychosis do not rule out the presence of delirium; however, active delirium does rule out the possibility of being able to diagnose a new dementia, depression, or psychosis. Given this level of diagnostic primacy and its manifold associated deleterious sequelae, delirium should be at the cornerstone of any investigation of agitation in the ICU.

References

1. Hippocrates: On Regimen in Acute Diseases (Part 11), in Adams F (trans): *The Internet Classics Archive*. Available at: http://classics.mit.edu/Hippocrates/acutedis.html. Accessed February 3, 2010.
2. McGuire BE, Basten CJ, Ryan CJ, et al: Intensive care unit syndrome: a dangerous misnomer. *Arch Intern Med* 160:906–909, 2000.
3. American Psychiatric Association: *Diagnostic and Statistical Manual of Mental Disorders*. 5th ed. Washington, DC, American Psychiatric Publishing, 2013.
4. McNicoll L, Pisani MA, Zhang Y, et al: Delirium in the intensive care unit: occurrence and clinical course in older patients. *J Am Geriatr* Soc 51:591–598, 2003.
5. Ely EW, Shintani A, Truman B, et al: Delirium as a predictor of mortality in mechanically ventilated patients in the intensive care unit. *JAMA* 291:1753–1762, 2004.
6. Thomason JW, Shintani A, Peterson JF, et al: Intensive care unit delirium is an independent predictor of longer hospital stay: a prospective analysis of 261 non-ventilated patients. *Crit Care* 9:R375–R381, 2005.
7. Milbrandt EB, Deppen S, Harrison PL, et al: Costs associated with delirium in mechanically ventilated patients. *Crit Care Med* 32:955–962, 2004.
8. Franco K, Litaker D, Locala J, et al: The cost of delirium in the surgical patient. *Psychosomatics* 42:68–73, 2001.
9. Atkins PM, Mion LC, Mendelson W, et al: Characteristics and outcomes of patients who self-extubate from ventilatory support: a case-control study. *Chest* 112:1317–1323, 1997.
10. Tuma R, DeAngelis LM: Altered mental status in patients with cancer. *Arch Neurol* 57:1727–1731, 2000.
11. Gaudreau JD, Gagnon P, Harel F, et al: Psychoactive medications and risk of delirium in hospitalized cancer patients. *J Clin Oncol* 23:6712–6718, 2005.
12. Querques J: An approach to acute changes in mental status, in Stern TA (ed): *The Ten-Minute Guide to Psychiatric Diagnosis and Treatment*. New York, NY, Professional Publishing Group, 2005, pp 97–107.
13. Brown TM: Basic mechanisms in the pathogenesis of delirium, in Stoudemire A, Fogel BS, Greenberg D (eds): *Psychiatric Care of the Medical Patient*. 2nd ed. New York, NY, Oxford University Press, 2000, pp 571–580.
14. Seaman JS, Schillerstrom J, Carroll D, et al: Impaired oxidative metabolism precipitates delirium: a study of 101 ICU patients. *Psychosomatics* 47:56–61, 2006.
15. Ely EW, Siegel MD, Inouye SK: Delirium in the intensive care unit: an under-recognized syndrome of organ dysfunction. *Semin Respir Crit Care Med* 22:115–126, 2001.
16. Breitbart W, Gibson C, Tremblay A: The delirium experience: delirium recall and delirium-related distress in hospitalized patients with cancer, their spouses/caregivers, and their nurses. *Psychosomatics* 43:183–194, 2002.
17. Ely EW, Inouye SK, Bernard GR, et al: Delirium in mechanically ventilated patients: validity and reliability of the confusion assessment method for the intensive care unit (CAM-ICU). *JAMA* 286:2703–2710, 2001.
18. Tomasi CD, Grandi C, Salluh J, et al: Comparison of CAM-ICU and ICDSC for the detection of delirium in critically ill patients focusing on relevant clinical outcomes. *J Crit Care* 27:212–217, 2012.
19. Engel G, Romano J: Delirium, a syndrome of cerebral insufficiency. *J Chronic Dis* 9:260–277, 1959.
20. Jacobson S, Jerrier H: EEG in delirium. *Semin Clin Neuropsychiatry* 5:86–92, 2000.
21. Bourgeois JA, Wegelin JA: Lagtime in psychosomatic medicine consultations for cognitive-disorder patients: association with length of stay. *Psychosomatics* 50:622–625, 2009.
22. Burns MJ, Linden CH, Graudins A, et al: A comparison of physostigmine and benzodiazepines for the treatment of anticholinergic poisoning. *Ann Emerg Med* 35:374–381, 2000.
23. Dautzenberg PL, Wouters CJ, Oudejans I, et al: Rivastigmine in prevention of delirium in a 65 year old man with Parkinson's disease. *Int J Geriatr Psychiatry* 18:555–556, 2003.
24. Dautzenberg PL, Mulder LJ, Olde Rikkert MG, et al: Delirium in elderly hospitalized patients: protective effects of chronic rivastigmine usage. *Int J Geriatr Psychiatry* 19:641–644, 2004.
25. Liptzin B, Laki A, Garb JL, et al: Donepezil in the prevention and treatment of post-surgical delirium. *Am J Geriatr Psychiatry* 13:1100–1106, 2005.
26. Sampson EL, Raven PR, Ndhlovu PN, et al: A randomized, double-blind, placebo-controlled trial of donepezil hydrochloride (Aricept) for reducing the incidence of postoperative delirium after elective total hip replacement. *Int J Geriatr Psychiatry* 22:343–349, 2007.
27. Gamberini M, Bolliger D, Lurati Buse GA, et al: Rivastigmine for the prevention of postoperative delirium in elderly patients undergoing elective cardiac surgery—a randomized controlled trial. *Crit Care Med* 37:1762–1768, 2009.
28. American Psychiatric Association: Practice guideline for the treatment of patients with delirium. *Am J Psychiatry* 156[5, Suppl]:1–20, 1999.
29. Cassem NH, Murray GB, Lafayette JM, et al: Delirious patients, in Stern TA, Fricchione GL, Cassem NH, et al (eds): *Massachusetts General Hospital Handbook of General Hospital Psychiatry*. 5th ed. Philadelphia, PA, Mosby, 2004, pp 119–134.
30. Menza MA, Murray GB, Holmes VF, et al: Decreased extrapyramidal symptoms with intravenous haloperidol. *J Clin Psychiatry* 48:278–280, 1987.
31. Breitbart W, Marotta R, Platt MM, et al: A double-blind trial of haloperidol, chlorpromazine, and lorazepam in the treatment of delirium in hospitalized AIDS patients. *Am J Psychiatry* 153(2):231–237, 1996.
32. Adams F, Fernandez F, Andersson BS: Emergency pharmacotherapy of delirium in the critically ill cancer patient. *Psychosomatics* 27[1, Suppl]:33–38, 1986.
33. Menza MA, Murray GB, Holmes VF, et al: Controlled study of extrapyramidal reactions in the management of delirious, medically ill patients: haloperidol versus intravenous haloperidol plus benzodiazepines. *Heart Lung* 17:238–241, 1988.
34. Pisani F, Oteri G, Costa C, et al: Effects of psychotropic drugs on seizure threshold. *Drug Saf* 25:91–110, 2002.
35. Metzger E, Friedman R: Prolongation of the corrected QT and torsades de pointes cardiac arrhythmia associated with intravenous haloperidol in the medically ill. *J Clin Psychopharmacol* 13:128–132, 1993.
36. Hunt N, Stern TA: The association between intravenous haloperidol and torsades de pointes: three cases and a literature review. *Psychosomatics* 36:541–549, 1995.
37. Stöllberger C, Huber JO, Finsterer J: Antipsychotic drugs and QT prolongation. *Int Clin Psychopharmacol* 20:243–251, 2005.
38. Kao LW, Kirk MA, Evers SJ, et al: Droperidol, QT prolongation, and sudden death: what is the evidence? *Ann Emerg Med* 41:546–558, 2003.
39. Han CS, Kim YK: A double-blind trial of risperidone and haloperidol for the treatment of delirium. *Psychosomatics* 45:297–301, 2004.
40. Skrobik YK, Bergeron N, Dumont M, et al: Olanzapine vs haloperidol: treatment of delirium in the critical care setting. *Intensive Care Med* 30:444–449, 2004.
41. Devlin JW, Roberts RJ, Fong JJ, et al: Efficacy and safety of quetiapine in critically ill patients with delirium: a prospective, multicenter, randomized, double-blind, placebo-controlled pilot study. *Crit Care Med* 38:419–427, 2010.
42. Maneeton B, Manneton N, Srisurapanont M, et al: Quetiapine versus haloperidol in the treatment of delirium: a double-blind, randomized, controlled, trial. *Drug Des Devel Ther* 24:657–667, 2014.
43. Grover S, Kumar V, Chakrabati S: Comparitive efficacy study of haloperidol, olanzapine, and risperidone in delirium. *J Psychosom Res* 71:277–281, 2011.
44. Kim SW, Yoo JA, Lee, SY, et al: Risperidone versus olanzapine for the treatment of delirium. *Hum Psychopharmacol* 25:298–302, 2010.
45. Girard TD, Pandharipande PP, Carson SS, et al: Feasibility, efficacy, and safety of antipsychotics for intensive care unit delirium: the MIND randomized, placebo-controlled trial. *Crit Care Med* 38:428–437, 2010.
46. Lauterbach EC: The neuropsychiatry of Parkinson's disease and related disorders. *Psychiatr Clin North Am* 27:801–825, 2004.
47. Yoon HK, Kim YK, Han C, et al: Paliperidone in the treatment of delirium: results of a prospective open-label trial. *Acta Neuropsychiatr* 23:179–183, 2011.
48. Pandharipande PP, Pun BT, Herr DL, et al: Effect of sedation with dexmedetomidine vs lorazepam on acute brain dysfunction in mechanically ventilated patients: the MENDS randomized controlled trial. *JAMA* 298:2644–2653, 2007.
49. Riker RR, Shehabi Y, Bokesch PM, et al: Dexmedetomidine vs midazolam for sedation of critically ill patients: a randomized trial. *JAMA* 301:489–499, 2009.
50. Maldonado JR, Wysong A, van der Starre PJ, et al: Dexmedetomidine and the reduction of postoperative delirium after cardiac surgery. *Psychosomatics* 50:206–217, 2009.
51. Shehabi Y, Grant P, Wolfenden H, et al: Prevalence of delirium with dexmedetomidine compared with morphine based therapy after cardiac surgery: a randomized controlled trial (DEXmedetomidine COmpared to Morphine-DEXCOM Study). *Anesthesiology* 111:1075–1084, 2009.
52. Reade MC, O'Sullivan K, Bates S, et al: Dexmedetomidine vs. haloperidol in delirious, agitated, intubated patients: a randomised open-label trial. *Crit Care* 13:R75, 2009.
53. Dasta JF, Kane-Gill SL, Pencina M, et al: A cost-minimization analysis of dexmedetomidine compared with midazolam for long-term sedation in the intensive care unit. *Crit Care Med* 38:497–503, 2010.
54. Tagarakis GI, Voucharas C, Tsolaki F, et al: Ondansetron versus haloperidol for the treatment of postcardiotomy delirium: a prospective, randomized, double-blinded study. *J Cardiothorac Surg* 7:25, 2012.
55. Papadopoulos G, Pouangare M, Papathanakos G, et al: The effect of ondansetron on postoperative delirium and cognitive function in aged orthopaedic patients. *Minerva Anestesiol* 80:444–451, 2014.
56. Page VJ, Ely EW, Gates S, et al: Effect of intravenous haloperidol on the duration of delirium and coma in critically ill patients (Hope-ICU): a randomized, double-blind, placebo-controlled trial. *Lancet Respir Med* 1:515–523, 2013.
57. Kalisvaart KJ, de Jonghe JF, Bogaards MJ, et al: Haloperidol prophylaxis for elderly hip-surgery patients at risk for delirium: a randomized placebo-controlled study. *J Am Geriatr Soc* 53:1658–1666, 2005.
58. Prakanrattana U, Prapaitrakool S: Efficacy of risperidone for prevention of postoperative delirium in cardiac surgery. *Anaesth Intensive Care* 35:714–719, 2007.
59. Wang W, Li HL, Wang DX, et al: Haloperidol prophylaxis decreases delirium incidence in elderly patients after noncardiac surgery: a randomized controlled trial. *Crit Care Med* 40:731–739, 2012.
60. Larsen KA, Kelly SE, Stern TA, et al: Administration of olanzapine to prevent postoperative delirium in elderly joint-replacement patients: a randomized, controlled trial. *Psychosomatics* 51:409–418, 2010.
61. Al-Aama T, Brymer C, Gutmanis I, et al: Melatonin decreases delirium in elderly patients: a randomized, placebo-controlled trial. *Int J Geriatr Psychiatry* 26:687–694, 2011.
62. de Jonghe A, van Munster BC, Goslings JC, et al: Effect of melatonin on incidence of delirium among patients with hip fracture: a multicentre, double-blind, randomized controlled trial. *CMAJ* 186:E547–E556, 2014.

63. Hatta K, Kishi Y, Wada K, et al: Preventive effects of ramelteon on delirium: a randomized placebo-controlled trial. *JAMA Psychiatry* 71:397–403, 2014.
64. Teslyar P, Stock VM, Wilk CM, et al: Prophylaxis with antipsychotic medication reduces the risk of post-operative delirium in elderly patients: a meta-analysis. *Psychosomatics* 54:124-131, 2013.
65. Chan MTV, Cheng BC, Lee TM, et al: BIS-guided anesthesia decreases postoperative delirium and cognitive decline. *J Neurosurg Anesthesiol* 25:33-42, 2013.
66. Hshieh TT, Yue J, Oh E, et al: Effectiveness of multicomponent nonpharmacological delirium interventions: a meta-analysis. *JAMA Intern Med* 175:512–520, 2015.
67. Francis J, Kapoor WN: Prognosis after hospital discharge of older medical patients with delirium. *J Am Geriatr Soc* 40:601–606, 1992.
68. McCusker J, Cole M, Dendukuri N, et al: Delirium in older medical inpatients and subsequent cognitive and functional status: a prospective study. *CMAJ* 165:575–583, 2001.
69. Katz IR, Curyto KJ, TenHave T, et al: Validating the diagnosis of delirium and evaluating its association with deterioration over a one-year period. *Am J Geriatr Psychiatry* 9:148–159, 2001.
70. Dolan MM, Hawkes WG, Zimmerman SI, et al: Delirium on hospital admission in aged hip fracture patients: prediction of mortality and 2-year functional outcomes. *J Gerontol A Biol Sci Med Sci* 55:M527–M534, 2000.
71. Jackson JC, Gordon SM, Hart RP, et al: The association between delirium and cognitive decline: a review of the empirical literature. *Neuropsychol Rev* 14:87–98, 2004.
72. Kapfhammer HP, Rothenhausler HB, Krauseneck T, et al: Posttraumatic stress disorder and health-related quality of life in long-term survivors of acute respiratory distress syndrome. *Am J Psychiatry* 161:45–52, 2004.
73. DiMartini A, Dew MA, Kormos R, et al: Posttraumatic stress disorder caused by hallucinations and delusions experienced in delirium. *Psychosomatics* 48:436–439, 2007.

Chapter158 ■ Diagnosis and Treatment of Anxiety in the Intensive Care Unit Patient

SHELLEY A. HOLMER • ROBERT M. TIGHE

Anxiety is a normal, adaptive biological response to threat. It occurs when a person feels helpless and apprehensive about an uncertain future due to a perceived inability to predict or control a desired outcome. In contrast, *pathological anxiety* is normal anxiety run amok. It occurs spontaneously or amid usually benign circumstances, is excessive in intensity or duration, and impairs functioning and behavior. Anxiety manifests in a variety of ways, resulting in physical, affective, behavioral, and cognitive symptoms and signs (Table 158.1).

Patients admitted to the intensive care unit (ICU) commonly experience anxiety in response to pain, invasive procedures, an unfamiliar setting, and the fear of death. In moderation, anxiety can promote healthful behaviors, just as pain can lead to protection from future injury. In excess, however, anxiety can complicate diagnosis, interfere with treatment, and contribute to poor outcomes by increasing both morbidity and mortality. Anxiety can complicate the clinical picture, as symptoms and signs of many medical problems overlap with those of anxiety (e.g., chest pain, palpitations, tachycardia, diaphoresis, tremulousness). Overwrought patients may refuse tests or procedures they fear will cause pain or will lead to bad news. Patients with phobias of blood, needles, and confined spaces (e.g., computed tomography and magnetic resonance imaging machines) may forego necessary interventions. Pathological anxiety may contribute to the need for ICU admission.

This chapter reviews the physiological concomitants of anxiety, medical causes of anxiety, critical medical conditions particularly affected by anxiety, anxiety disorders specific to the ICU setting, and the treatment of anxiety.

TABLE 158.1

Symptoms and Signs of Anxiety

Physical	**Behavioral**
Tachycardia	Restlessness
Tachypnea	Agitation
Hypertension	Compulsiveness
Diaphoresis	Avoidance
Light-headedness	Noncompliance with diagnostic or therapeutic interventions
Tremulousness	Fidgetiness
Affective	**Cognitive**
Uneasiness	Apprehension
Edginess	Worry
Nervousness	Fear of emotional or bodily damage
Fright	Denial
Panic	Obsessiveness
Terror	Preoccupation with harm
	Thoughts about death

PHYSIOLOGICAL EXPRESSIONS OF ANXIETY

The physiological expressions of anxiety are myriad. By activating the *fight or flight response*, anxiety recruits the entire autonomic nervous system to respond to an unknown enemy. Multiple organ systems—cardiovascular, respiratory, gastrointestinal, musculoskeletal, endocrine, immune—are involved. Anxiety increases blood levels of cortisol, prolactin, and growth hormone [1]. A disquieted patient has enhanced gastric motility and gastric secretions, vasoconstriction of the splanchnic and cutaneous circulations, and vasodilation of striated muscle groups [2]. Anxiety also has direct effects on the immune system: a reduction in the chemotaxis of lymphocytes and neutrophils, a decrease in the phagocytic ability of neutrophils, and an increase in plasma levels of tumor necrosis factor α and superoxide anions [3]. This suggests complex physiological effects of anxiety for the critically ill.

The organ systems adversely affected by anxiety of most concern to the intensivist are the cardiovascular and respiratory systems. Anxiety affects the cardiovascular system by altering normal autonomic tone, manifested as increases in heart rate, blood pressure, cardiac output, and cardiac irritability. The stress of simply being hospitalized augments urinary excretion of catecholamines, which represents activation of the sympathetic nervous system and contributes to cardiac arrhythmias [4]. In the fight or flight response, augmentation of cardiac output prevents cardiovascular collapse, but, in heart failure and myocardial infarction (MI), excessive cardiac output can be detrimental. Anxiety increases respiratory rate, tidal volume, and airway resistance and can induce hyperventilation and syncope. These data suggest that anxiety, while exacting a psychological toll, also significantly alters cardiorespiratory physiology, especially in the critical care setting.

MEDICAL CAUSES OF ANXIETY

Because failure to identify and treat *organic* (i.e., *medical* or *secondary*) causes of anxiety can result in increased morbidity and mortality, the distinction between organic and *functional* (i.e., *psychiatric* or *primary*) causes is vitally important. The presence of an organic cause is suggested when anxiety occurs autonomously in the absence of an apparent psychologically charged situation or of a discrete physical event (e.g., acute pain or tachyarrhythmia). However, in any given patient, determination of what constitutes an appropriate or sufficient psychological precipitant for anxiety is difficult. Life history, cultural background, and prior behavioral conditioning are often unknown to clinicians in the fast-paced ICU setting. Therefore, when anxiety is present and no clear psychological or medical cause is obvious, a thorough search for an organic cause is indicated.

Anxiety is a symptom of hundreds of medical conditions; Table 158.2 provides a list of conditions common in the ICU. Two syndromes that are particularly difficult to distinguish from primary anxiety are delirium and substance withdrawal.

TABLE 158.2

Common Medical Causes of Anxiety

Neurologic
Delirium
Substance withdrawal syndromes
Complex partial seizures
Traumatic brain injury
Pain
Cardiac
Acute myocardial infarction
Shock
Paroxysmal tachycardia
Metabolic
Hypoglycemia
Hyperthyroidism
Pheochromocytoma
Cushing's syndrome
Addison's disease
Respiratory
Respiratory failure
Asthma
Hypoxia
Hyperventilation
Pneumothorax
Pulmonary edema
Pulmonary embolism
Toxic
Illicit drug intoxication
Anticholinergic intoxication
Prednisone
Isoniazid
Caffeine

Delirium

Treating the delirious patient solely with anxiolytics (e.g., benzodiazepines) can exacerbate confusion, so it is important to distinguish delirium from anxiety by doing a brief cognitive examination. In delirium, performance of tasks of attention, orientation, memory, and language is often impaired; rarely does an anxious patient have these deficits. By definition, delirium always has a medical cause; therefore, determination of its cause, rather than simply treating its symptoms, is vital. Recognition and management of delirium are discussed in Chapter 157.

Substance Withdrawal Syndromes

Because withdrawal from central nervous system depressants (e.g., opioids, benzodiazepines, alcohol) can be life-threatening, it should always be high on the differential diagnosis of anxiety. This diagnosis can be missed because patients either underreport their substance use or are unable to communicate. Patients can also withdraw from sedatives and opioids prescribed during a lengthy period of mechanical ventilation. Recognition and treatment of withdrawal syndromes are discussed in Chapter 126.

SCENARIOS IN WHICH ANXIETY SIGNIFICANTLY AFFECTS OUTCOMES OF MEDICAL ILLNESS

Acute Myocardial Infarction

As heart disease remains the leading cause of mortality in the United States, *acute coronary syndrome* (ACS) is a common reason for admission to the coronary care unit (CCU). Prevention and treatment have focused on awareness and alteration of traditional risk factors (e.g., hyperlipidemia, hypertension, family history). A developing literature supports consideration of psychosocial factors as well, most frequently, anxiety, depression, and personality traits [5].

Anxiety is a frequent occurrence in the CCU, both related to MI itself and as a premorbid condition contributing to the development of MI [5,6]. Anxiety occurs in 20% to 50% of patients after MI [7,8]. The stress of being cared for in an ICU, particularly the relinquishing of control and privacy, in addition to dealing with a potentially life-threatening disease, contribute to anxiety in this setting [9]. Anxiety in the CCU after MI rises rapidly and peaks within the first 12 hours; declines during the next 36 hours; and then increases again as patients face transfer out of the CCU and ultimately discharge from the hospital [10]. Physicians and nurses often under-recognize anxiety and underestimate its severity after MI [11]. Anxiolysis should be an early consideration in post-MI patients.

Physiologically, anxiety impacts the cardiovascular system through several mechanisms. Most generally, it activates the sympathetic nervous system, which directly causes vasoconstriction, tachycardia, increased blood pressure, platelet activation, and potential for arrhythmia [12,13]. Heart rate variability (HRV), the ability the sympathetic and parasympathetic nervous systems have to regulate the cardiac pacemaker, is decreased in many patients with anxiety [14]. Decreased HRV in patients following MI has been consistently associated with mortality [15]. Overall, these physiological changes may explain why anxiety—especially phobic anxiety—has been directly linked to an increased risk for sudden death [16].

Anxiety also appears to influence other physiological processes associated with ACS, including the inflammatory response [17,18], impaired coagulation [19], platelet activity [20], and endothelial dysfunction [21,22]. In addition to direct physiological effects, anxiety may lead to poor cardiac outcomes through its effects on important risk-reducing recommendations after MI, including stress reduction, greater socialization, smoking cessation, and improved diet [23].

Two groups have demonstrated that anxiety, independent of depressive symptoms, is associated with in-hospital complications after acute MI, including recurrent ischemia, re-infarction, congestive heart failure, and ventricular arrhythmias [9,24]. Further trials are required to determine whether the effect of anxiety is "dose"-dependent and whether effective anxiety treatment improves cardiac outcomes. In the setting of acute MI, benzodiazepines have been shown to reduce anxiety, pain, and cardiovascular activation. Their use leads to a reduction of circulating catecholamines and may also cause coronary vasodilatation, prevent dysrhythmias, and retard platelet aggregation [25].

The correlation between anxiety and post-MI outcomes in the long term is more complex. Some [5,6,26], but not all [27,28], prospective trials demonstrate that high levels of anxiety predict cardiac events (e.g., unstable angina, re-infarction) and/or mortality. Definitive study of the association between anxiety and cardiac events remains difficult due to confounding factors. For example, depression is a well-established independent risk factor for poor post-MI outcomes [29]; it is difficult to isolate anxious patients who do not also exhibit symptoms of depression. Additionally, anxiety can have either beneficial or detrimental effects on important cardiac outcomes (e.g., physical activity and compliance with medical treatment). It leads to activation in some and avoidance in others depending on level of anxiety and personality characteristics.

Despite uncertainty about the role anxiety plays as a prognostic factor in patients with ACS, several psychological and pharmacological interventions have been studied. Many have shown a positive effect on psychiatric symptoms and quality of life but equivocal effects on cardiac outcomes and mortality [30,31]. Firm links between anxiety and hard cardiac endpoints over the long term remain unproven, limiting development of definitive treatment guidelines.

Weaning from Mechanical Ventilation

Respiratory failure and consequent need for mechanical ventilation are common causes of admission to the ICU. Nearly three fourths of patients resume spontaneous, unassisted breathing with little difficulty. However, patients who require prolonged mechanical ventilation have longer hospital stays, face higher morbidity and mortality, and require lengthier rehabilitation. Therefore, the goal is to wean patients as soon as possible, as it is a central predictor of ICU survival.

Given the limitations of communication and easy fatigability in patients with critical illness, the evaluation of anxiety in this setting remains difficult. This difficulty extends to research efforts attempting to define the incidence of and factors leading to anxiety in the setting of ventilator weaning. Approximately 25% and 56% of patients experience symptoms of acute and chronic anxiety, respectively, related to mechanical ventilation [32]. The highest levels occur in patients intubated for primary respiratory disorders (e.g., chronic obstructive pulmonary disease [COPD]) and in those on prolonged (>22 days) artificial ventilation, the very groups who are most at risk for difficulty weaning from mechanical ventilation [33].

Although the physiological measures used to determine readiness to wean from the ventilator are well known and several of them have been studied closely in clinical trials, information about the effect of the patient's psychological state, specifically anxiety, on weaning from the ventilator is scant. Given the extensive overlap between physiological effects of anxiety and those of respiratory muscle fatigue, it can be difficult to separate ventilator weaning failure from anxiety. Anxiety may cause shortness of breath and a fear of death or abandonment, especially as ventilatory support is withdrawn. This can stimulate the sympathetic nervous system; cause bronchoconstriction; and increase airway resistance, work of breathing, and oxygen demand. This cascade can become a perpetuating cycle of anxiety, muscle fatigue, and thus weaning failure. Furthermore, the cascade of anxiety worsens with each additional ventilator weaning failure [34].

Anxiety should be considered for all patients during the weaning process, especially those who are intubated for primary respiratory causes and for a prolonged period. Given the paucity of data regarding the effect of anxiety on ventilator weaning, no clear treatment guidelines exist; however, it is well appreciated that weaning should be approached from a multidisciplinary standpoint. Treatment includes pharmacological, environmental, and educational approaches; it is enhanced when patient, family, physicians, and nurses are involved in the decision to wean and in the process of weaning.

Because anxiety and respiratory distress due to fatiguing respiratory muscles can produce similar cardiorespiratory manifestations, disentangling the two is critical. Only if one is convinced that anxiety is the cause should one consider pharmacotherapy for anxiety because pharmacotherapy with benzodiazepines can potentially prolong weaning due to suppression of respiratory drive. (see Chapter 168). Although this class of medications is associated with respiratory suppression and altered level of consciousness and may lead to drug-induced delirium, benzodiazepines can be quite effective when used judiciously in the correct setting. Neuroleptics are less associated with respiratory suppression and may be more beneficial than benzodiazepines, especially for patients whose weaning failure is due to fear or delirious agitation.

In addition to benzodiazepines and neuroleptics, dexmedetomidine, an α_2-adrenergic receptor agonist, is increasingly being used. This agent causes a rapid onset of sedation and analgesia but not respiratory suppression [35]. The lack of respiratory-suppressant effects allows patients to be extubated while remaining on dexmedetomidine, whereas benzodiazepines require discontinuation or reduction prior to extubation. Studies suggest that dexmedetomidine reduces both the length of ICU stay and time to extubation [36]. The greater success in extubation appears to be more pronounced in patients who had failed previous conventional extubation attempts [37]. Therefore, dexmedetomidine is a reasonable option for anxious patients who are at high risk for ventilator weaning failure.

Non-pharmacological efforts are critical to successful weaning. Nursing should remain as consistent as possible with an individual patient; during active weaning, a 1:1 nurse-to-patient ratio should be maintained. Weaning is more successful when patients are aware of their environment and engaged in discussions of the plan and process of weaning. Patients should be told and reminded that weaning without extubation does not represent a failure but is part of the process. Music therapy has been associated with decreased anxiety in ICU patients and reductions in both the frequency and the intensity of sedation and may facilitate weaning [38]. Finally, appropriate engagement of family members in the process of weaning should be considered.

ANXIETY DISORDERS SPECIFIC TO THE INTENSIVE CARE UNIT

Patients with a variety of anxiety disorders present to the ICU. Symptoms associated with these conditions can be exacerbated by the acute medical or surgical problem that led to the ICU admission. In addition, medications used to treat a pre-existing anxiety disorder may be discontinued on admission, or their bioavailability may be altered by interactions with newly prescribed medications. Both discontinuation and pharmacokinetic changes may significantly worsen pre-existing primary anxiety disorders. In addition to exacerbating established psychiatric illnesses, the experience of the ICU can lead to new, longstanding anxiety disorders. Anxiety disorders particularly relevant in the ICU include acute and posttraumatic stress disorders and panic disorder.

Acute and Posttraumatic Stress Disorders

The experience of treatment in the ICU—which includes frightening confusion, painful invasive procedures, and fear of death—can be traumatic for many patients. Often, especially in the surgical ICU, patients are admitted due to a traumatic event (e.g., motor vehicle collision, severe burn, and assault). These circumstances predispose patients to the development of acute stress disorder (ASD) and posttraumatic stress disorder (PTSD).

Diagnosis of both ASD and PTSD requires clinically significant distress following exposure to actual or threatened death, serious injury, or sexual violation. Symptoms are clustered into four categories: re-experiencing, avoidance, negative thoughts/mood, and arousal [39]. Re-experiencing manifests in dreams, intrusive memories, flashbacks, or intense distress when exposed to reminders of the event. Distressing memories, thoughts, feelings, or external reminders of the event may be avoided. Negative thoughts/mood may include a distorted sense of blame of self or others, diminished interest in activities, or an inability to remember key aspects of the event. Arousal symptoms can include aggressive, reckless, or self-destructive behavior; sleep disturbances; and hypervigilance. For a diagnosis of ASD, these symptoms must occur within the first month after the trauma; if symptoms persist beyond 1 month, a diagnosis of PTSD should be considered.

Some patients develop syndromes consistent with both ASD and PTSD consequent to events that occur in the ICU. One out of five patients exhibits clinically significant PTSD symptoms in the first 12 months after ICU discharge [40], significantly higher than the 3.5% prevalence of PTSD in the general population [41]. The risk of developing ASD and PTSD is presumed to be even higher in patients who are admitted to the ICU after a trauma.

ICU-related PTSD has been associated with worse health-related quality of life [42]. Specifically, PTSD secondary to acute coronary syndrome has been associated with a doubling of risk for death and recurrent cardiac events [43].

The most robust risks for ICU-related PTSD are pre-existing psychiatric conditions, greater ICU benzodiazepine administration, and early memories of in-ICU frightening experiences [40,44]. The positive correlation between benzodiazepine use and PTSD may be due to the need for higher doses of these medications in patients with pre-existing psychiatric conditions. Another possibility is that benzodiazepines can exacerbate delirium, which has been implicated as an independent risk factor for PTSD in some [45], but not all [46], studies. Delirium-associated delusions, hallucinations, and agitation requiring physical restraint may lead to both disturbing and false memories of the ICU stay, which have been correlated with higher rates of PTSD and worse health-related quality of life [47,48]. Therefore, interventions that target delirium, disorientation, and faulty reality testing may prevent PTSD.

Both behavioral and pharmacological interventions to prevent PTSD have been studied. Although there is a lack of randomized controlled trials to support their widespread adoption, both bedside psychological interventions (e.g., educational interventions, counselling, and stress management) and daily-event diaries to improve factual memory of time spent in intensive care have shown benefit in curtailing the development of PTSD [49–51].

Studies of psychopharmacological intervention for the prevention of PTSD have yielded mixed results. Several studies have demonstrated a decrease in the prevalence of PTSD for critically ill patients treated with stress doses of corticosteroids, which are thought to have an effect on traumatic-memory retrieval [52–54]. There is also evidence that treatment with β-receptor antagonists may protect against the development of PTSD, perhaps by blocking catecholamines, which enhance memory of emotionally arousing experiences [55,56]. However, this benefit was not seen in a randomized controlled trial of critically ill patients [57]. A recent meta-analysis of prophylactic treatment for PTSD in the general population showed no benefit with β-receptor antagonists and some potential benefit with corticosteroids [58].

In the ICU, acute trauma should be treated with supportive reassurance and symptom-targeted medications. Clinicians should identify and treat delirium, make efforts to reduce unnecessary sedation, and help orient patients to what is happening around them. A recent study identified other modifiable predictors of PTSD, including memories about pain, lack of control, and inability to express needs [59]. These can be addressed with appropriate pain assessment and management, allowing patients more choices in their care, and helping patients to communicate (e.g., using Passy-Muir valves in tracheostomized patients). Psychiatric consultation can be useful for both acute management and recommendations for outpatient treatment, especially in patients with pre-existing psychiatric illnesses.

Panic Disorder

Panic disorder is one of the most common psychiatric disorders in patients who are high users of medical services. The risk for development of panic disorder is higher in patients with migraine, mitral valve prolapse, asthma, and COPD [60]. As defined by the *Diagnostic and Statistical Manual of Mental Disorders* [39], a panic attack is a discrete period of fear or discomfort that develops suddenly, reaches a peak within 10 minutes, and is associated with the symptoms listed in Table 158.3. Panic

TABLE 158.3

Symptoms of a Panic Attack

Neurologic
Feeling dizzy, unsteady, light-headed, or faint
Feeling unreal or detached from oneself
Fear of losing control, going crazy, or dying
Paresthesias
Cardiovascular
Palpitations
Pounding heart
Tachycardia
Chest pain or discomfort
Respiratory
Dyspnea
Sensation of smothering
Feeling of choking
Gastrointestinal
Nausea
Abdominal distress
Miscellaneous
Diaphoresis
Trembling
Shaking
Chills
Hot flashes

Adapted from American Psychiatric Association: Diagnostic and Statistical Manual of Mental Disorders. 5th ed. Washington, DC, American Psychiatric Publishing, 2013.

disorder consists of recurrent panic attacks accompanied by persistent fear of having additional attacks, worry about the implications and consequences of the episodes, and a significant change in behavior related to the attacks. Many panic-disordered patients are hypervigilant to internal bodily stimuli, and some fear that their attacks indicate the presence of an undiagnosed, life-threatening illness. These concerns are assuaged only when the panic disorder is accurately diagnosed and effectively treated.

Risks for developing panic attacks include separation, disruption of important relationships, and medical illness—all endemic in the ICU. Timely diagnosis and treatment of panic disorder can circumvent unnecessary medical procedures and decrease morbidity and mortality. Because its presentation is similar to that of several medical conditions (e.g., stroke, MI, respiratory compromise, gastrointestinal conditions), especially in the ICU, panic disorder must be considered a diagnosis of exclusion. It is important to recognize panic attacks in the ICU setting not only to avoid misdiagnosis, but also because the physiological consequences of panic may exacerbate symptoms of pre-existing medical conditions and lead to more frequent medical hospitalizations. Emerging evidence also shows an association between panic disorder and post-ICU cardiovascular outcomes. Panic disorder is independently associated with incident coronary heart disease, MI, and major adverse cardiac events [61]. Panic disorder is also associated with an increased incidence of arrhythmias (e.g., atrial fibrillation), a frequent complication and reason for admission to the ICU [62]. The pathophysiology underlying these associations remains unknown.

Treatment for panic disorder includes psychotherapy and medication. Cognitive-behavioral techniques (e.g., psychoeducation, anxiety management skills, cognitive reframing, and exposure to somatic cues) have been well studied. Benzodiazepines and antidepressants—specifically the selective serotonin reuptake inhibitors (SSRIs)—are the standard of care for the psychopharmacological management of panic disorder.

TREATMENT OF ANXIETY IN THE INTENSIVE CARE UNIT

Treatments for anxiety in the ICU include both non-pharmacological and pharmacological options. Additionally, the stress placed on medical and nursing staff attending to anxious patients in an emotionally charged treatment setting where family members also experience poor sleep and anxiety must be acknowledged and addressed to improve the overall care of patients in the ICU [63].

Non-pharmacological methods that have been explored include education, environmental manipulation, muscle relaxation, and music therapy. As ICUs have become increasingly focused on providing patient-centered care to improve outcomes, these non-pharmacological modalities are more frequently utilized and studied. Additionally, non-pharmacological modalities have the added benefits of limiting adverse side effects related to sedative-hypnotics in critically ill patients. Patients should be made aware of their clinical situation and oriented to their

TABLE 158.4

Some Intravenous Medications for the Treatment of Anxiety

Drug	Typical dose	Onset (min)	Drug interactions	Side effects
Lorazepam	0.04 mg/kg	5–15	Fewer drug interactions than other benzodiazepines	Respiratory suppression, mixed in propylene glycol solution, venous irritation
Diazepam	0.1–0.2 mg/kg	1–3	Effects increased by cimetidine, erythromycin, isoniazid, ketoconazole, metoprolol, propranolol, valproate Effects decreased by rifampin and theophylline	Respiratory suppression, mixed in propylene glycol solution, venous irritation
Midazolam	0.025–0.35 mg/kg	1–3	Same as diazepam	Respiratory depression, accumulates with prolonged (>48 h) use, excessive sedation
Propofol	0.25–1 mg/kg (loading dose) then 1–6 mg/kg (continuous infusion)	<1	Minimal	Respiratory depression, vasodilation particularly with bolus dosing and in hemodynamically unstable patients
Haloperidol	1–5 mg	20–30	Effects decreased by rifampin Medications that widen QT interval	QT interval prolongation, neuroleptic malignant syndrome, EPS (less with IV than with oral use)
Dexmedetomidine	Initial recommended dose: 0.8 μg/kg/h titrated to a dose between 0.2 and 1.4 μg/kg/h	6	Minimal but has the potential to augment bradycardia induced by vagal stimuli or negative chronotropic drugs and may increase the effects of vasodilators	Hypotension, bradycardia

EPS, extrapyramidal symptoms; IV, intravenous.
Adapted from Marino PL (ed): *The ICU Book*. 2nd ed. Baltimore, Lippincott Williams & Wilkins, 1998; and Eisendrath SJ, Shim JJ: Management of psychiatric problems in critically ill patients. *Am J Med* 119:22, 2006.

environment. Provision of ambient light, a clock, and a calendar promotes accurate orientation and a normal sleep–wake cycle. In addition, to foster a sense of control and mastery of their situation, patients should be made an integral part of decision-making. In a randomized controlled trial of 41 CCU patients, those who were given choices about family visits, daily hygiene schedule, physical activity, and their room environment enjoyed significant improvement in anxiety and depression measures after 48 hours [64]. Additionally, research efforts have focused on measures to improve anxiety through audiovisual aids. Spiva et al. [65] demonstrated that use of guided imagery—60 minutes of images and voice recordings providing instructions on patient relaxation—was associated with reductions in Richmond Agitation-Sedation Scale (RASS) score, use of sedatives and analgesics, days requiring mechanical ventilation, and hospital length of stay. Music therapy also has been increasingly utilized. Chlan et al. [38] demonstrated a significant association between the use of music therapy and reductions in anxiety and frequency and intensity of sedation. Evaluation of multiple studies using music therapy clearly demonstrates a reduction in anxiety [66]. Studies also suggest that music therapy reduces respiratory rate and systolic blood pressure. Whether these physiological changes translate into reduced mortality or improved quality of life remains unknown.

Benzodiazepines represent the standard for anxiolysis in the ICU; of these, lorazepam is the most widely used. Available in an intravenous formulation, it undergoes little hepatic metabolism, has no active metabolites, and is more appropriate for use in patients with liver disease or with poor liver function. Lorazepam

TABLE 158.5

Randomized Trials of Anxiety Treatments in Critically Ill Patients

Study	Enrollment	Intervention	Results
Jones et al. [50]	126 ICU patients	Self-help rehabilitation manual vs. routine follow-up	Trend toward a lower rate of depression in intervention group. No differences in anxiety and PTSD symptoms between groups.
Knowles and Tarrier [51]	36 ICU patients	Prospective diary reviewed post discharge vs. standard of care	Improvement in both depression and anxiety symptoms in experimental group.
Kress et al. [32]	32 mechanically ventilated ICU patients	Daily sedation withdrawal vs. continuous sedation	Fewer PTSD symptoms in daily sedation withdrawal group.
Treggiari et al. [70]	137 mechanically ventilated ICU patients	Light vs. deep sedation	Fewer symptoms in the light sedation group at 4 weeks. No differences in anxiety and depression between groups.
Schelling et al. [52]	91 patients undergoing cardiac surgery, 48 followed up in 6 months	High-dose corticosteroids perioperatively vs. standard care	Reduced PTSD symptoms in the steroid group. No difference in traumatic memories between groups.
Weis et al. [71]	36 patients undergoing cardiac surgery	Stress-dose hydrocortisone vs. placebo	Reduced incidence of chronic stress symptoms and better health-related QoL in steroid group. No difference in traumatic memories between groups.
Schelling et al. [53]	20 patients with septic shock	Stress-dose hydrocortisone vs. placebo	Lower incidence of PTSD in intervention group. No difference in traumatic memories between groups.
Stein et al. [57]	48 patients admitted to a surgical trauma center	Propranolol vs. gabapentin vs. placebo	No differences in PTSD symptoms, depression, or ASD at 1, 4, and 8 months after injury.
Ziemann et al. [64]	41 CAD patients admitted to a CCU	Individualized contact with nurse vs. usual care	Significantly less anxiety, depression, and hostility in the experimental group.
Corbett et al. [67]	89 mechanically ventilated patients after non-emergent CABG	Propofol vs. dexmedetomidine	No differences in pain, anxiety, and sleep/rest between groups.
Chlan et al. [38]	373 mechanically ventilated patients for acute respiratory failure in 12 intensive care unites	Self-initiated patient-directed music (PDM) vs. noise-cancelling headphones (NCH) or usual care (UC)	PDM therapy resulted in greater reduction in anxiety than UC; reduced sedation frequency than NCH or UC; and a greater reduction in sedation intensity than UC.
Aghaie et al. [72]	120 patients who underwent coronary artery bypass surgery and were undergoing weaning from mechanical ventilation	Listening to nature-based sounds through headphones vs. wearing headphones with no sound	Listening to nature-based sounds resulted in a significant reduction in the levels of anxiety and agitation.

ASD, acute stress disorder; CABG, coronary artery bypass grafting; CAD, coronary artery disease; CCU, coronary care unit; ICU, intensive care unit; PTSD, posttraumatic stress disorder; QoL, quality of life.

is also useful for long-term sedation in ventilated patients as it is not associated with heart block (as is propofol) or with wide body storage (as is midazolam). However, intravenous formulations of lorazepam contain propylene glycol, and prolonged use of high doses can precipitate an osmolar-gap acidosis.

Another agent of recent interest and increasingly used in the ICU is dexmedetomidine, which inhibits the central and peripheral effects of norepinephrine and epinephrine, resulting in sedation and analgesia. While dexmedetomidine may cause bradycardia and hypotension, trial data suggest that clinically significant adverse hemodynamic changes are rare [35]. Dexmedetomidine and propofol performed equally in pain and anxiety reduction and sleep/rest promotion [67].

Other agents that may prove useful in the anxious patient are SSRIs, neuroleptic agents, and propofol. SSRIs have been shown to decrease the sense of dyspnea in anxious patients with COPD [68]. Neuroleptics are beneficial in patients who are fearful, delirious, or so anxious that they are nearly psychotic [69]. Use of neuroleptic agents is discussed in Chapter 157. Propofol continues to be the most commonly used medication for sedation in the ICU but is impractical for routine anxiolysis given its significant respiratory-depressant effects. Table 158.4 contrasts various agents commonly used to quell anxiety in critically ill patients. Table 158.5 presents a summary of randomized trials of anxiety treatments in critically ill patients.

CONCLUSION

Ubiquitous in the ICU, anxiety has a broad range of physiological and psychological consequences. Although it can be difficult to diagnose in the acutely ill, current evidence suggests that identification and treatment of anxiety enhance patient comfort and compliance and improve morbidity and mortality. Therefore, anxiety should be routinely assessed in critically ill patients. Psychiatric consultation should be considered whenever anxiety complicates the clinical course.

References

1. Gerra G, Zaimovic A, Mascetti GG, et al: Neuroendocrine responses to experimentally-induced psychological stress in healthy humans. *Psychoneuroendocrinology* 26:91, 2001.
2. Lader MH. Soma and psyche. *Br Med J (Clin Res Ed)* 287:1906, 1983.
3. Arranz L, Guayerbas N, De la Fuente M: Impairment of several immune functions in anxious women. *J Psychosom Res* 62:1, 2007.
4. Lown B, Verrier R, Corbalan R: Psychologic stress and threshold for repetitive ventricular response. *Science* 182:834, 1973.
5. Roest AM, Martens EJ, de Jonge P, et al: Anxiety and risk of incident coronary heart disease: a meta-analysis. *J Am Coll Cardiol* 56:38, 2010.
6. Roest AM, Martens EJ, Denollet J, et al: Prognostic association of anxiety post myocardial infarction with mortality and new cardiac events: a meta-analysis. *Psychosom Med* 72:563, 2010.
7. van Beek MH, Mingels M, Voshaar RC, et al: One-year follow up of cardiac anxiety after a myocardial infarction: a latent class analysis. *J Psychosom Res* 73:362, 2012.
8. Versteeg H, Roest AM, Denollet J: Persistent and fluctuating anxiety levels in the 18 months following acute myocardial infarction: the role of personality. *Gen Hosp Psychiatry* 37:1, 2015.
9. Moser DK, Riegel B, McKinley S, et al: Impact of anxiety and perceived control on in-hospital complications after acute myocardial infarction. *Psychosom Med* 69:10, 2007.
10. An K, De Jong MJ, Riegel BJ, et al: A cross-sectional examination of changes in anxiety early after acute myocardial infarction. *Heart Lung* 33:75, 2004.
11. Huffman JC, Smith FA, Blais MA, et al: Recognition and treatment of depression and anxiety in patients with acute myocardial infarction. *Am J Card* 98:319, 2006.
12. Anderson KP: Sympathetic nervous system activity and ventricular tachyarrhythmias: recent advances. *Ann Noninvasive Electrocardiol* 8:75, 2003.
13. Roth WT, Doberenz S, Dietel A, et al: Sympathetic activation in broadly defined generalized anxiety disorder. *J Psychiatr Res* 42:205, 2008.
14. Pittig A, Arch JJ, Lam CW, et al: Heart rate and heart rate variability in panic, social anxiety, obsessive-compulsive, and generalized anxiety disorders at baseline and in response to relaxation and hyperventilation. *Inter J Psychophysiol* 87:19, 2013.
15. Buccelletti E, Gilardi E, Scaini E, et al: Heart rate variability and myocardial infarction: systematic literature review and metanalysis. *Eur Rev Med Pharmacol Sci* 13:299, 2009.
16. Albert CM, Chae CU, Rexrode KM, et al: Phobic anxiety and risk of coronary heart disease and sudden cardiac death among women. *Circulation* 111:480, 2005.
17. Bankier B, Barajas J, Martinez-Rumayor A, et al: Association between anxiety and C-reactive protein levels in stable coronary heart disease patients. *Psychosomatics* 50:347, 2009.
18. Pitsavos C, Panagiotakos DB, Papageorgiou C, et al: Anxiety in relation to inflammation and coagulation markers among healthy adults: the ATTICA study. *Atherosclerosis* 185:320, 2006.
19. Geiser F, Meier C, Wegener I, et al: Association between anxiety and factors of coagulation and fibrinolysis. *Psychother Psychosom* 77:377, 2008.
20. Zafar MU, Paz-Yepes M, Shimbo D, et al: Anxiety is a better predictor of platelet reactivity in coronary artery disease patients than depression. *Eur Heart J* 31:1573, 2010.
21. Narita K, Murata T, Hamada T, et al: Interactions among higher trait anxiety, sympathetic activity, and endothelial function in the elderly. *J Psychiatr Res* 41:418, 2007.
22. Harris KF, Matthews KA, Sutton-Tyrrell K, et al: Associations between psychological traits and endothelial function in postmenopausal women. *Psychosom Med* 65:402, 2003.
23. Kuhl EA, Fauerbach JA, Bush DE, et al: Relation of anxiety and adherence to risk-reducing recommendations following myocardial infarction. *Am J Cardiol* 103:1629, 2009.
24. Huffman JC, Smith FA, Blais MA, et al: Anxiety, independent of depressive symptoms, is associated with in-hospital cardiac complications after acute myocardial infarction. *J Psychosom Res* 65:557, 2008.
25. Huffman JC, Stern TA: The use of benzodiazepines in the treatment of chest pain: a review of the literature. *J Emerg Med* 25:427, 2003.
26. Wrenn KC, Mostofsky E, Tofler GH, et al: Anxiety, anger, and mortality risk among survivors of myocardial infarction. *Am J Med* 126:1107, 2013.
27. Larsen KK, Christensen B, Nielsen TJ, et al: Post-myocardial infarction anxiety or depressive symptoms and risk of new cardiovascular events or death: a population-based longitudinal study. *Psychosom Med* 76:739, 2014.
28. Hosseini SH, Ghaemian A, Mehdizadeh E, et al: Levels of anxiety and depression as predictors of mortality following myocardial infarction: a 5-year follow-up. *Cardiol J* 21:370, 2014.
29. Meijer A, Conradi HJ, Bos EH, et al: Prognostic association of depression following myocardial infarction with mortality and cardiovascular events: a meta-analysis of 25 years of research. *Gen Hosp Psychiatry* 33:203, 2011.
30. Wu CK, Huang YT, Lee JK, et al: Anti-anxiety drugs use and cardiovascular outcomes in patients with myocardial infarction: a national wide assessment. *Atherosclerosis* 235:496, 2014.
31. Whalley B, Thompson DR, Taylor RS: Psychological interventions for coronary heart disease: cochrane systematic review and meta-analysis. *Int J Behav Med* 21:109, 2014.
32. Kress JP, Gehlbach B, Lacy M, et al: The long-term psychological effects of daily sedative interruption on critically ill patients. *Am J Respir Crit Care Med* 168:1457, 2003.
33. Chlan LL: Description of anxiety levels by individual differences and clinical factors in patients receiving mechanical ventilatory support. *Heart Lung* 32:275, 2003.
34. Chen YJ, Jacobs WJ, Quan SF, et al: Psychophysiological determinants of repeated ventilator weaning failure: an explanatory model. *Am J Crit Care* 20:292, 2011.
35. Riker RR, Shehabi Y, Bokesch PM, et al: Dexmedetomidine vs midazolam for sedation of critically ill patients: a randomized trial. *JAMA* 301:489, 2009.
36. Pasin L, Greco T, Feltracco P, et al: Dexmedetomidine as a sedative agent in critically ill patients: a meta-analysis of randomized controlled trials. *PLoS One* 8:e82913, 2013.
37. Shehabi Y, Nakae H, Hammond N, et al: The effect of dexmedetomidine on agitation during weaning of mechanical ventilation in critically ill patients. *Anaesth Intensive Care* 38:82, 2010.
38. Chlan LL, Weinert CR, Heiderscheit A, et al: Effects of patient-directed music intervention on anxiety and sedative exposure in critically ill patients receiving mechanical ventilatory support: a randomized clinical trial. *JAMA* 309:2335, 2013.
39. American Psychiatric Association: *Diagnostic and Statistical Manual of Mental Disorders*. 5th ed. Washington, DC, American Psychiatric Publishing, 2013.
40. Parker AM, Sricharoenchai T, Raparla S, et al: Posttraumatic stress disorder in critical illness survivors: a metaanalysis. *Crit Care Med* 43:1121, 2015.
41. Kessler RC, Chiu WT, Demler O, et al: Prevalence, severity, and comorbidity of 12-month DSM-IV disorders in the National Comorbidity Survey Replication. *Arch Gen Psychiatry* 62:617, 2005.
42. Svenningsen H: Associations between sedation, delirium and post-traumatic stress disorder and their impact on quality of life and memories following discharge from an intensive care unit. *Danish Med J* 60:B4630, 2013.
43. Edmondson D, Richardson S, Falzon L, et al: Posttraumatic stress disorder prevalence and risk of recurrence in acute coronary syndrome patients: a meta-analytic review. *PLoS One* 7:e38915, 2012.
44. Davydow DS, Gifford JM, Desai SV, et al: Posttraumatic stress disorder in general intensive care unit survivors: a systematic review. *Gen Hosp Psychiatry* 30:421, 2008.

45. Nelson BJ, Weinert CR, Bury CL, et al: Intensive care unit drug use and subsequent quality of life in acute lung injury patients. *Crit Care Med* 28:3626, 2000.
46. Davydow DS, Zatzick D, Hough CL, et al: A longitudinal investigation of posttraumatic stress and depressive symptoms over the course of the year following medical-surgical intensive care unit admission. *Gen Hosp Psychiatry* 35:226, 2013.
47. Jones C, Griffiths RD, Humphris G, et al: Memory, delusions, and the development of acute posttraumatic stress disorder-related symptoms after intensive care. *Crit Care Med* 29:573, 2001.
48. Ringdal M, Plos K, Ortenwall P, et al: Memories and health-related quality of life after intensive care: a follow-up study. *Crit Care Med* 38:38, 2010.
49. Peris A, Bonizzoli M, Iozzelli D, et al: Early intra-intensive care unit psychological intervention promotes recovery from post traumatic stress disorders, anxiety and depression symptoms in critically ill patients. *Crit Care* 15:R41, 2011.
50. Jones C, Skirrow P, Griffiths RD, et al: Rehabilitation after critical illness: a randomized, controlled trial. *Crit Care Med* 31:2456, 2003.
51. Knowles RE, Tarrier N: Evaluation of the effect of prospective patient diaries on emotional well-being in intensive care unit survivors: a randomized controlled trial. *Crit Care Med* 37:184, 2009.
52. Schelling G, Kilger E, Roozendaal B, et al: Stress doses of hydrocortisone, traumatic memories, and symptoms of posttraumatic stress disorder in patients after cardiac surgery: a randomized study. *Biol Psychiatry* 55:627, 2004.
53. Schelling G, Briegel J, Roozendaal B, et al: The effect of stress doses of hydrocortisone during septic shock on posttraumatic stress disorder in survivors. *Biol Psychiatry* 50:978, 2001.
54. Hauer D, Kaufmann I, Strewe C, et al: The role of glucocorticoids, catecholamines and endocannabinoids in the development of traumatic memories and posttraumatic stress symptoms in survivors of critical illness. *Neurobiol Learn Mem* 112:68, 2014.
55. Krauseneck T, Padberg F, Roozendaal B, et al: A beta-adrenergic antagonist reduces traumatic memories and PTSD symptoms in female but not in male patients after cardiac surgery. *Psychol Med* 40:861, 2010.
56. Gardner AJ, Griffiths J: Propranolol, post-traumatic stress disorder, and intensive care: incorporating new advances in psychiatry into the ICU. *Crit Care* 18:698, 2014.
57. Stein MB, Kerridge C, Dimsdale JE, et al: Pharmacotherapy to prevent PTSD: results from a randomized controlled proof-of-concept trial in physically injured patients. *J Trauma Stress* 20:923, 2007.
58. Sijbrandij M, Kleiboer A, Bisson JI, et al: Pharmacological prevention of post-traumatic stress disorder and acute stress disorder: a systematic review and meta-analysis. *Lancet Psychiatry* 2:413, 2015.
59. Myhren H, Toien K, Ekeberg O, et al: Patients' memory and psychological distress after ICU stay compared with expectations of the relatives. *Intensive Care Med* 35:2078, 2009.
60. Muller JE, Koen L, Stein DJ: Anxiety and medical disorders. *Curr Psychiatry Rep* 7:245, 2005.
61. Tully PJ, Turnbull DA, Beltrame J, et al: Panic disorder and incident coronary heart disease: a systematic review and meta-regression in 1,131,612 persons and 58,111 cardiac events. *Psychol Med* 45:2909, 2015.
62. Cheng YF, Leu HB, Su CC, et al: Association between panic disorder and risk of atrial fibrillation:a nationwide study. *Psychosom Med* 75:30, 2013.
63. Day A, Haj-Bakri S, Lubchansky S, et al: Sleep, anxiety and fatigue in family members of patients admitted to the intensive care unit: a questionnaire study. *Crit Care* 17:R91, 2013.
64. Ziemann KM, Dracup K: Patient-nurse contracts in critical care: a controlled trial. *Prog Cardiovasc Nurs* 5:98, 1990.
65. Spiva L, Hart PL, Gallagher E, et al: The effects of guided imagery on patients being weaned from mechanical ventilation. *Evid Based Complement Alternat Med* 2015:9, 2015.
66. Bradt J, Dileo C: Music interventions for mechanically ventilated patients. *Cochrane Database Syst Rev* 12:CD006902, 2014.
67. Corbett SM, Rebuck JA, Greene CM, et al: Dexmedetomidine does not improve patient satisfaction when compared with propofol during mechanical ventilation. *Crit Care Med* 33:940, 2005.
68. Smoller JW, Pollack MH, Systrom D, et al: Sertraline effects on dyspnea in patients with obstructive airways disease. *Psychosomatics* 39:24, 1998.
69. McDougle CJ, Epperson CN, Pelton GH, et al: A double-blind, placebo-controlled study of risperidone addition in serotonin reuptake inhibitor-refractory obsessive-compulsive disorder. *Arch Gen Psychiatry* 57:794, 2000.
70. Treggiari MM, Romand JA, Yanez ND, et al: Randomized trial of light versus deep sedation on mental health after critical illness. *Crit Care Med* 37:2527, 2009.
71. Weis F, Kilger E, Roozendaal B, et al: Stress doses of hydrocortisone reduce chronic stress symptoms and improve health-related quality of life in high-risk patients after cardiac surgery: a randomized study. *J Thorac Cardiovasc Surg* 131:277, 2006.
72. Aghaie B, Rejeh N, Heravi-Karimooi M, et al: Effect of nature-based sound therapy on agitation and anxiety in coronary artery bypass graft patients during the weaning of mechanical ventilation: a randomised clinical trial. *Int J Nurs Stud* 51:526, 2014.

Chapter 159 ■ Diagnosis and Treatment of Depression in the Intensive Care Unit Patient

EDITH S. GERINGER • JOHN QUERQUES • MEGHAN S. KOLODZIEJ • THEODORE A. STERN

In the intensive care unit (ICU), depression can be a psychologic reaction to an acute medical illness, a manifestation of a primary affective disorder, or a mood disorder associated with a specific organic disease or its treatment. For example, depression is associated with the development and the progression of, and with worse prognosis in, coronary heart disease (CHD) [1]. In fact, in 2014, the American Heart Association recommended that depression be considered a risk factor for adverse outcomes in patients with acute coronary syndrome (ACS) [2]. In addition, depression is a frequent complication after stroke and is associated with greater disability and mortality [3].

In this chapter, the term depression refers not to being transiently sad, discouraged, disappointed, despondent, or grief-stricken, but to major depressive disorder (MDD), defined in the 5th edition of the *Diagnostic and Statistical Manual of Mental Disorders* (DSM-5) [4] as a syndrome of distinct and persistent dysphoria associated with neurovegetative changes and functional impairment. Many physicians believe that depression is appropriate in the ICU because severe illness can be devastating to a person's life. However, we believe that whereas being dispirited may be an understandable response to critical illness, having a depressive disorder is not; therefore, it is always important to treat the latter. In fact, compelling evidence shows that untreated depression is associated with morbidity and mortality from cardiac and neurologic conditions and has detrimental effects on other, perhaps all, organ systems.

In this chapter, we focus on the links between depressive and medical conditions and the diagnosis, evaluation, and treatment of depression in critically ill patients.

DIAGNOSIS OF DEPRESSION

Important questions for the intensivist are "What is depression?" and "What does a patient experiencing depression look like in the ICU?" To qualify for a diagnosis of MDD according to the DSM-5, a patient must have five of the nine symptoms listed in Table 159.1, one of which must be either depressed mood or anhedonia, most of the day, nearly every day, for at least 2 weeks. The mnemonic—SIG: E CAPS (where SIG [abbreviation for the Latin, *signa*] refers to the instructions on a prescription, E refers to energy, and CAPS refers to capsules)—is a helpful guide to remember the eight neurovegetative symptoms associated with depressed mood. The mnemonic—ABCs of depression—portrays more richly the myriad affective, behavioral, and cognitive aspects of the condition (Table 159.2). Each symptom should be asked

TABLE 159.1

SIG: E CAPS—A Mnemonic for Diagnostic Criteria for Major Depressive Disorder

Depressed mood
*S*leep, increased or decreased
*I*nterest or pleasure in activities, markedly decreased (anhedonia)
*G*uilt or feelings of worthlessness
*E*nergy, decreased
*C*oncentration, decreased
*A*ppetite or weight, increased or decreased
*P*sychomotor agitation or retardation
*S*uicidal thinking

Adapted from American Psychiatric Association: *Diagnostic and Statistical Manual of Mental Disorders*. 5th ed. Washington, DC, American Psychiatric Publishing, 2013.

about, and questions about suicide should be raised directly. If a patient has thoughts of suicide, he or she should be asked whether there is a specific plan; the physician should then make a judgment about the likelihood of the patient's acting on the plan. If an active plan for suicide exists, psychiatric consultation is imperative (see Chapter 160). In medically ill patients, holding the cardinal symptoms of depressed mood and anhedonia to the strict requirement of presence most of the day, nearly every day, for at least 2 weeks is critical to avoid overdiagnosis of depression in medically ill patients.

Patients Who are Unable to Speak

It may be particularly difficult to diagnose depression in a patient who is being mechanically ventilated or has aphasia. Methods of assessing depression in these patients are summarized in Table 159.3. Some tracheostomized patients may be able to use a Passy-Muir valve. See Chapter 169 on Respiratory Adjunct Therapy for an indepth discussion of Passy-Muir valve use. Alternatively, electronic voice-output communication aids may be used. These devices pair prerecorded messages or synthesized speech with labeled icons; patients communicate messages by touching buttons on display screens or on touch-sensitive keyboards. Speech pathologists have knowledge of and access to such technology.

TABLE 159.3

Methods of Assessing Depression in Patients Who Cannot Speak

Watch facial expressions and body language
Read lips
Monitor changes in vital signs on monitors
Write questions and have patients write answers
Use letter or picture board
Observe whether facial expressions are consistent with content of discussion
Observe rate of change of affect
Ask about and observe neurovegetative features of depression
Ask about known sources of the patient's enjoyment (e.g., favorite hobby, grandchildren, and sports) and observe whether the patient takes pleasure in these things
Joke with the patient or tell a funny story and observe the patient's reaction
Ask the patient to draw a picture of himself or herself and what is wrong, then assess the pictures for a sense of demoralization or hopelessness
Make a fist and ask the patient, "What would you do if you had one of these?" and assess emotions in response to this maneuver

DIFFERENTIAL DIAGNOSIS OF DEPRESSION

Causes Related to Medical Conditions

A variety of medical illnesses can cause, contribute to, or worsen affective symptoms and disorders (Table 159.4). Clues that depression is due to a medical illness include older age at onset of symptoms; lower incidence of a family history of depression; and changes in personality and cognition. A thorough history (including a review of systems); physical (including neurologic) examination; and laboratory testing can distinguish between primary (i.e., due to a psychiatric condition) and secondary (i.e., due to a medical condition) causes of depression. For secondary causes, treatment of the underlying illness is usually more effective than is the use of psychotropic medications.

Perhaps the most important differential diagnosis to consider in a patient who appears to have MDD is hypoactive delirium. The key feature that distinguishes it from depression

TABLE 159.2

ABCs of Depression—Affective, Behavioral, and Cognitive Features

Affective	Behavioral	Cognitive
Depressed mood	Crying	Suicidal thinking
"Blue" mood	Increased or decreased sleep	Thoughts of death
Sadness	Increased or decreased appetite	Somatic preoccupation
Blunted affect	Decreased energy	Guilty rumination
Hopelessness	Psychomotor agitation or retardation	Confusion
Emptiness	Increased or intractable pain	Decreased concentration
Irritability	Deliberate self-injury	
Anger	Impulsivity	
Decreased interest	Poor eye contact	
	Noncompliance	

TABLE 159.4

Medical Conditions Associated with Depressive Symptoms

Cardiovascular
- Cardiac tumors
- Congestive heart failure
- Hypertensive encephalopathy

Collagen vascular
- Polyarteritis nodosa
- Systemic lupus erythematosus

Endocrine
- Diabetes mellitus
- Hyperadrenalism or hypoadrenalism
- Hyperparathyroidism or hypoparathyroidism
- Hyperthyroidism or hypothyroidism

Infectious
- Hepatitis
- Human immunodeficiency virus
- Mononucleosis
- Influenza

Metabolic
- Acid–base problems
- Hypokalemia
- Hypernatremia or hyponatremia
- Renal failure

Neoplastic
- Carcinoid
- Pancreatic carcinoma

Neurologic
- Brain tumor
- Multiple sclerosis
- Parkinson's disease (especially with on/off phenomenon)
- Temporal lobe epilepsy
- Stroke
- Subcortical dementia

Nutritional
- Vitamin B_{12} deficiency
- Wernicke's encephalopathy

is inattention (i.e., an inability to focus and sustain alertness on a given stimulus and to resist distraction by other stimuli). Delirium is discussed in Chapter 157.

Causes Related to Medical Treatments

The pharmacologic agents most often responsible for depression in the ICU are antihypertensives, β-blockers, antiarrhythmics, and steroids (Table 159.5). Some medications may cause depression only after several weeks or even months of continuous use. If a drug regimen or a dosage increase appears to be temporally related to the patient's depression, the dose should be lowered or the medication eliminated entirely. If the medication cannot be stopped without serious risk to the patient, the depression should be treated.

Steroids

Depression, mania, psychosis, and delirium are frequent side effects of corticosteroid therapy. Mood symptoms are dose-dependent and usually occur within the first 2 weeks of therapy, although they can arise on the first day. A practical rule of thumb holds that neuropsychiatric adverse effects are common with prednisone ≥80 mg per day (or equivalent), uncommon ≤30 mg per day, and not uncommon in between. Although it has been suggested that women are more likely to develop steroid-induced adverse effects, the apparent increased frequency may be due to the higher prevalence of rheumatologic diseases in women. Corticosteroid-induced mood disorders are generally reversible with dosage reduction or discontinuation of the medication.

TABLE 159.5

Drugs Associated with Depressive Symptoms

- Acyclovir (especially at high doses)
- Alcohol
- Amphetamine-like drugs (withdrawal): fenfluramine, phenmetrazine, and phenylpropanolamine
- Anabolic steroids: methandrostenolone and methyltestosterone
- Anticonvulsants (at high doses or plasma levels): carbamazepine, phenytoin, and primidone
- Antihypertensives: clonidine, hydralazine, methyldopa, reserpine, and thiazides
- Asparaginase
- Baclofen
- Barbiturates
- Benzodiazepines: alprazolam, clonazepam, clorazepate, diazepam, lorazepam, and triazolam
- β-blockers: atenolol, betaxolol, propranolol, and timolol
- Bromides
- Bromocriptine
- Cimetidine
- Cocaine (withdrawal)
- Oral contraceptives
- Corticosteroids
- Cycloserine
- Dapsone
- Digitalis (at high doses or in elderly patients)
- Diltiazem
- Disopyramide
- Ethionamide
- Halothane (postoperatively)
- Heavy metals
- Histamine-2 receptor antagonists: cimetidine and ranitidine
- Interferon α
- Isoniazid
- Isotretinoin
- Levodopa (especially in the elderly)
- Mefloquine
- Metoclopramide
- Metrizamide
- Metronidazole
- Nalidixic acid
- Narcotics: meperidine, methadone, morphine, pentazocine, and propoxyphene
- Nifedipine
- Nonsteroidal anti-inflammatory drugs
- Norfloxacin
- Phenylephrine
- Prazosin
- Procaine derivatives: lidocaine, penicillin G procaine, and procainamide
- Thyroid hormones
- Trimethoprim–sulfamethoxazole

TABLE 159.6

Laboratory Evaluation of Depression

Complete blood count with differential
Complete blood chemistries
Serum and urine toxicology
Urinalysis
Vitamin B_{12}
Folate
Rapid plasma reagin
Neuroimaging
Electroencephalogram
Cerebrospinal fluid analysis

LABORATORY EVALUATION OF DEPRESSION

Although the clinical interview and mental status examination are the most important components of psychiatric diagnosis, the use of laboratory tests is essential to exclude organic causes of depression. Although there is no consensus on the laboratory tests necessary in a patient with new-onset mood disorder, Table 159.6 lists those tests that should be considered. Thyroid-stimulating hormone is not on this list because many critically ill patients have abnormal thyroid biochemical profiles but do not have intrinsic thyroid disease. Syphilis and hypovitaminosis are rarely the sole causes of depression; tests for these conditions should be ordered only when there is a specific indication for them. Neuroimaging, electroencephalography, and cerebrospinal fluid analysis are relatively indicated in patients with new-onset psychiatric symptoms, altered cognition, new neurologic symptoms, seizures, and fever. The more of these features a patient has, the more important these additional tests become.

TREATMENT OF DEPRESSION

Patients who meet the criteria for MDD are usually treated with a somatic therapy (including pharmacotherapy and electroconvulsive therapy [ECT]), alone or in combination with psychotherapy (Table 159.7). In critical care units, somatic therapies are the most widely used treatments for depression. Pharmacotherapy may be used in critical care units also for patients who have an adjustment disorder with depressed mood, particularly when these patients have several neurovegetative symptoms. A patient who is neither eating nor sleeping and lacks the energy to participate in his or her rehabilitation may be helped considerably by antidepressants, especially psychostimulants.

Each type of pharmacotherapy has its own indications and contraindications. A useful guiding principle is to choose a medication with a side-effect profile that best fits a patient's needs. For instance, a patient who is having trouble sleeping will benefit from a sedating antidepressant. Conversely, a patient who has severe psychomotor retardation may benefit from a more stimulating antidepressant. With the exception of the psychostimulants, all antidepressants require approximately 4 to 6 weeks until full antidepressant effects are noted, although some response can occur in 1 to 2 weeks. Obviously, in critical care units, quicker effects are generally needed. Stimulants and ECT work more quickly, usually within several days. Patients with depression may also manifest considerable anxiety and may be helped by the use of an anxiolytic while awaiting response to an antidepressant. Depressed patients with psychosis (i.e., those with delusions or hallucinations) may need antipsychotics for symptom control.

Psychostimulants

Psychostimulants have been used to treat depressive symptoms since their development in the 1930s, but they fell into disrepute when they became known as drugs of abuse in the 1950s and 1960s. Since then, however, there have been numerous reports on the use of stimulants in the treatment of depressed patients, particularly apathetic and geriatric patients. Thought to be particularly effective in patients with cancer and stroke, their rapid onset is of great use in any setting where speed of recovery is crucial, including the ICU.

The psychostimulants most commonly used are dextroamphetamine (Dexedrine) and methylphenidate (Ritalin). Both appear to work through the direct neuronal release of dopamine and norepinephrine; dextroamphetamine blocks catecholamine reuptake and weakly inhibits monoamine oxidase. Both of these psychostimulants are predominantly excreted by the kidneys, although dextroamphetamine also undergoes a complex biotransformation.

The usual effects of stimulants are to increase motor behavior, increase arousal, and decrease appetite; however, in patients who are anorexic on the basis of depression, appetite is paradoxically increased, likely through dopaminergic stimulation of the nucleus accumbens. Their antidepressant effect is usually evident in the first 2 days of treatment, if not earlier. Stimulants do not have anticholinergic effects or cause orthostatic hypotension. They can increase heart rate and blood pressure and can cause coronary spasm and cardiac arrhythmias; however, these effects are rare (even with preexisting cardiac abnormalities) at the low doses (5 to 20 mg per day) usually used for the treatment of depression. In fact, stimulants have been used safely and effectively in a broad spectrum of patients, including those with critical illness, and have shown little potential for abuse or dependence. Contraindications to stimulant use include seizures, delirium, psychosis, significant hypertension, unstable angina, pregnancy, and the concurrent use of α-methyldopa (which becomes a sympathoamine when metabolized), monoamine oxidase inhibitors (MAOIs), or bronchodilators.

Psychostimulants should be the first consideration when treating depression for critically ill patients. Patients are started on 5 mg of methylphenidate or 2.5 to 5 mg of dextroamphetamine in the morning. The dose is increased by 5 mg per day (for methylphenidate) or 2.5 to 5 mg per day (for dextroamphetamine) until a therapeutic effect is detected or until a maximum dose of 20 mg has been reached. Heart rate and blood pressure should be monitored. Stimulants are usually given for at least 1 to 2 weeks after depressive symptoms have fully remitted. In most cases, after stimulants are stopped, depression does not recur.

Stimulants taken in overdose may cause seizures, coma, hallucinations, paranoia, hyperthermia, hypertension, cardiac arrhythmias, angina, and circulatory collapse. The major treatment for overdose is to acidify the urine (which enhances renal excretion) and to use supportive measures for all other abnormalities.

Modafinil (Provigil)—a wakefulness-promoting medication approved for narcolepsy, shift work sleep disorder, and obstructive sleep apnea/hypopnea syndrome—may be a beneficial alternative to the psychostimulants.

Selective Serotonin Reuptake Inhibitors

The selective serotonin reuptake inhibitors (SSRIs) cause a potent and selective blockade of serotonin reuptake. Since the introduction of fluoxetine (Prozac) in 1987, SSRIs have become the most widely prescribed class of antidepressants. Other SSRIs include sertraline (Zoloft), paroxetine (Paxil), fluvoxamine (Luvox), citalopram (Celexa), and escitalopram (Lexapro). They are far less anticholinergic, antihistaminergic, and anti-α_1-adrenergic than the older

TABLE 159.7

Comparative Properties of Some Antidepressants

Drug	Metabolism	ACh	Sedation	OH	Cardiac arrhythmia	Seizure risk	Target dose range (mg/d)	Drug interactions
Stimulants	Renal	0	0	0	Rare	Rare	5–20	
SSRIs								Risk of serotonin syndrome
Citalopram	Hepatic	+	+	+	Rare	Rare	20–60	Relatively few
Escitalopram	Hepatic	0–+	0–+	0–+	Rare	Rare	10–30	Relatively few
Fluoxetine	Hepatic	+	+	+	Rare	Rare	≥20	Increased levels of TCAs
Fluvoxamine	Hepatic	+	+	+	Rare	Rare	50–250	
Paroxetine	Hepatic	+	+	0	Rare	Rare	≥20	
Sertraline	Hepatic	0	0	0	Rare	Rare	50–200	
SNRIs								Risk of serotonin syndrome
Duloxetine	Hepatic	+	+	0–+	Rare	Rare	30–90	
Venlafaxine	Hepatic	0	0	0	Rare	Rare	150–300	
TCAs								
Amitriptyline	Hepatic	+++	+++	+++	Yes	Increased	≥150	
Amoxapine	Hepatic	+	++	+	Yes	Increased	≥200	
Desipramine	Hepatic	+	+	+++	Yes	Increased	≥150	
Doxepin	Hepatic	++	+++	++	Yes	Increased	≥200	
Imipramine	Hepatic	++	++	+++	Yes	Increased	≥200	
Maprotiline	Hepatic	+	+++	+	Yes	Increased	≥150	
Nortriptyline	Hepatic	++	++	+	Yes	Increased	≥100	
Protriptyline	Hepatic	+++	+	++	Yes	Increased	≥30	
MAOIs	Hepatic	0	+	+++	Rare	Rare	45–90	Hypertensive crisis with tyramine or sympathomimetics; avoid narcotics
Others								
Bupropion	Hepatic	+	0	0	Rare	Increased	IR, 200–300; SR/XL, 150–300	
Mirtazapine	Hepatic	+	+++	+	Rare	Rare	30–45	
Trazodone	Hepatic	0	+++	++	Yes	Increased	≥150	Digitalis toxicity

+, low; ++, moderate; +++, high; ACh, anticholinergic effects; IR, immediate release; MAOIs, monoamine oxidase inhibitors; OH, orthostatic hypotension; SNRIs, serotonin–norepinephrine reuptake inhibitors; SR, sustained release; SSRIs, selective serotonin reuptake inhibitors; TCAs, tricyclic antidepressants; XL, extended release.

Adapted, in part, from Mann JJ: The medical management of depression. *N Engl J Med* 353:1819, 2005.

tricyclic antidepressants (TCAs) and, therefore, are associated with far fewer side effects. They also have fewer cardiovascular effects and do not commonly cause orthostatic hypotension.

Pharmacokinetics

SSRIs are well absorbed from the gastrointestinal tract, and absorption is generally unaffected by food and antacids. They have a large volume of distribution and are highly protein-bound. They are extensively metabolized in the liver, where they are oxidized, methylated, and conjugated. The elimination half-lives of sertraline, paroxetine, fluvoxamine, and citalopram are approximately 1 day (although sertraline has a mildly active metabolite with a half-life of 66 hours); this allows once-a-day dosing. Fluoxetine has a half-life of 2 to 3 days and a highly active metabolite (norfluoxetine) with a mean half-life of 6.1 days. Fluoxetine takes a much longer time to reach steady state and, more importantly for drug overdoses, can take weeks to months to be fully cleared. Elimination half-lives are dose-dependent (i.e., higher doses and lengthier usage are associated with higher plasma levels and longer half-lives). SSRIs show wide inter-individual variation in pharmacokinetics and do not have a clearly established dose–response curve.

Metabolic Impairment

Fluoxetine, sertraline, fluvoxamine, and citalopram are unaffected by renal dysfunction. Paroxetine, although minimally excreted in the urine (like other SSRIs), shows increased plasma concentrations in the setting of renal disease. Fluoxetine, sertraline, paroxetine, and citalopram doses should be reduced by at least half in patients with liver disease. Fluvoxamine has been used in patients with cirrhosis and hepatic encephalopathy without adverse effects. The hepatic clearance, not the plasma concentration, of fluvoxamine is affected by cirrhosis. Therefore, the dosage frequency, rather than the total dosage, should be altered. In elderly individuals, fluoxetine does not have altered pharmacokinetics; in contrast, sertraline and paroxetine have increased plasma levels and slower clearance. Although citalopram has a

30% longer half-life in the elderly, the frequency and severity of side effects are not higher in this group.

Side Effects

SSRIs can cause tremulousness, agitation, irritability, insomnia, anorexia, nausea, vomiting, diarrhea, excess sweating, and sexual dysfunction (i.e., decreased libido, and erectile and orgasmic dysfunction). The syndrome of inappropriate antidiuretic hormone is an uncommon adverse effect reported with all of the SSRIs, especially in critically ill patients; other causes of hyponatremia should be sought before attributing the metabolic derangement to the SSRI. The SSRIs do not typically cause clinically significant changes in heart rate, blood pressure, or the electrocardiogram (ECG). Citalopram, however, has been associated with dysrhythmias, including torsade de pointes (especially in the setting of QT prolongation), and doses should generally not exceed 40 mg per day (20 mg per day in patients >60 years). There is also concern about escitalopram and dysrhythmias as well. Overdoses of SSRIs are discussed in Chapter 104.

Drug–Drug Interactions

The SSRIs are extensively metabolized by the cytochrome P450 system. All of them also inhibit various isoenzymes in this system and consequently raise the plasma levels of other drugs metabolized by those isoenzymes; sertraline, citalopram, and escitalopram do this the least. The interactions most likely to occur in an ICU are listed in Table 159.8. Attention to drug dosage can mitigate the harmful effects of these interactions.

Drug Discontinuation

The usually mild symptoms of the SSRI discontinuation syndrome (e.g., headache, dizziness, myalgias, and nausea) are generally eclipsed by more pressing issues in critically ill patients.

Serotonin–Norepinephrine Reuptake Inhibitors

Venlafaxine

Venlafaxine (Effexor) is a selective serotonin and norepinephrine reuptake inhibitor (SNRI). It is very similar to the SSRIs in most clinical and pharmacologic aspects. It has few anti-α_1-adrenergic, anticholinergic, and antihistaminergic side effects. Venlafaxine has a 6- to 8-hour half-life and must be given two to three times daily, but an extended-release preparation (Effexor XR) allows once-daily dosing. It causes a dose-dependent increase in systolic and diastolic blood pressure (up to 7.5 mm Hg), occurring in approximately 7% of patients taking daily doses between 200 and 300 mg and in up to 13% of patients taking >300 mg [5]. The major active metabolite of venlafaxine, desvenlafaxine, is now available as a primary compound (Pristiq); its advantages over its parent compound are uncertain.

Duloxetine

Another SNRI, duloxetine (Cymbalta) is indicated for MDD, generalized anxiety disorder, diabetic neuropathy, and fibromyalgia. Its half-life is 12 hours, and it can be given once or twice daily. Like venlafaxine, it has little effect on α_1-adrenergic, cholinergic, and histaminergic receptors. Any therapeutic advantage over venlafaxine, particularly for critically ill patients, has yet to be demonstrated.

Levomilnacipran

The latest SNRI to be approved, levomilnacipran (Fetzima) is the more active enantiomer of milnacipran. Levomilnacipran has an approximately twofold greater potency for norepinephrine relative to serotonin reuptake inhibition at low doses, although at higher doses, these potencies are the same [6]. It is not known to have affinity for adrenergic, muscarinic, or histaminergic receptors

TABLE 159.8

Selected Substrates and Inhibitors of Cytochrome P450 Isoenzymes

1A2	2C	2D6	3A3/4
		Substrates	
Acetaminophen	Barbiturates	Codeine	Amiodarone
Aminophylline	Diazepam	Encainide	Astemizole
Haloperidol	Mephenytoin	Flecainide	Calcium-channel blockers
TCAs	Omeprazole	Haloperidol	Cisapride
Theophylline	Phenytoin	Hydrocodone	Diazepam
	Propranolol	Metoprolol	Disopyramide
	TCAs	Propafenone	Lidocaine
		Propranolol	Loratadine
		TCAs	Macrolide antibiotics
		Timolol	Omeprazole
			Propafenone
			Quinidine
			Steroids
			Terfenadine
			TCAs
		Inhibitors	
Fluoxetine	Fluoxetine[a]	Fluoxetine[a]	Fluoxetine
Fluvoxamine[a]	Fluvoxamine[a]	Paroxetine[a]	Fluvoxamine[a]
Paroxetine	Sertraline	Sertraline	Nefazodone[a]
			Sertraline

[a]Strong inhibitor.
TCAs, tricyclic antidepressants.

[6]. Levomilnacipran is delivered in an extended-release capsule given once daily in a recommended dose range of 40 mg to 120 mg. Because levomilnacipran is metabolized by cytochrome P450 3A4, dose reduction is necessary when it is co-administered with CYP3A4 inhibitors. The half-life of the drug is approximately 12 hours. Elimination of levomilnacipran occurs renally. Dose reduction is recommended in patients with moderate to severe renal impairment; its use is not recommended for patients with end-stage renal disease [7]. Dose adjustment is not required in patients with hepatic insufficiency [8]. Adverse effects most commonly include hyperhidrosis, tachycardia, palpitations, nausea, vomiting, constipation, and erectile dysfunction. Levomilnacipran does not appear to prolong the QT interval, but it has been associated with orthostatic hypotension and minor increases in systolic and diastolic blood pressure.

Atypical Antidepressants

Vortioxetine

Approved in 2013, vortioxetine (Brintellix) is a serotonin reuptake inhibitor; a 5-HT_{1A} receptor full agonist; a 5-HT_{1B} receptor partial agonist; and a 5-HT_{1D}, 5-HT_{3A}, and 5-HT_7 receptor antagonist [9,10]. With a half-life of approximately 66 hours [11], it is dosed once daily between 5 mg and 20 mg. No dose adjustment is needed in patients with mild to moderate hepatic impairment or in patients with mild to end-stage renal impairment [11]. Vortioxetine is metabolized by multiple cytochrome P450 enzymes, primarily 2D6. It has no active metabolites [12].Vortioxetine has been found to be safe and effective in the geriatric population [13]. Its major side effects are nausea, vomiting, and constipation.

Vilazodone

Approved in 2011, vilazodone (Viibryd) is a serotonin reuptake inhibitor and 5-HT_{1A} partial agonist. Metabolized by the cytochrome P450 3A4 isozyme, vilazodone may need to be administered in lower dosages when combined with 3A4 inhibitors and in higher dosages when combined with 3A4 inducers [14]. No dose adjustment is recommended in patients with hepatic impairment [15]. Breakthrough seizures in a patient with a history of seizure disorder and seizure associated with serotonin syndrome in overdose have been reported with vilazodone [16,17]. Although few data exist, vilazodone has not been found to have an effect on heart rate or cardiac conduction [18]. The most common adverse effects are insomnia, nausea, vomiting, and diarrhea [19].

Bupropion

A monocyclic ketone antidepressant, bupropion (Wellbutrin) blocks norepinephrine and dopamine reuptake. As such, it can be activating and used in place of psychostimulants for patients who cannot tolerate these agents or in whom they are contraindicated. Its major side effects are agitation, insomnia, tremulousness, nausea, vomiting, and diarrhea. The immediate-release formulation is associated with an increased risk of seizures, but this risk in the sustained-release (SR) and extended-release (XL) preparations is comparable to that associated with other antidepressants. It carries a low risk of cardiac toxicity, though, in overdose, sinus tachycardia and intraventricular conduction delays have been reported [20]. Bupropion has gained widespread use as an aid in smoking cessation.

Mirtazapine

Mirtazapine (Remeron) is an analog of the tetracyclic antidepressant, mianserin. As an antagonist at presynaptic and postsynaptic α_2-adrenergic receptors and at postsynaptic 5-HT_2 and 5-HT_3 receptors, it enhances both norepinephrine and serotonin transmission. It has few anticholinergic and anti-α_1-adrenergic effects. Mirtazapine is a potent histamine blocker and can cause significant sedation, an increase in appetite, and weight gain—a side-effect profile that is often exploited to advantage in medically ill patients. Mirtazapine is devoid of significant effects on the cytochrome P450 system, making it less apt to cause drug–drug interactions.

Tricyclic Antidepressants

TCAs work by blocking reuptake of norepinephrine and serotonin at presynaptic sites. The most common side effects of TCAs are sedation, orthostatic hypotension, and anticholinergic effects (including confusion, blurred vision, dry mouth, constipation, and urinary hesitancy or retention). The tertiary-amine parent compounds, amitriptyline (Elavil) and imipramine (Tofranil), are more apt to produce these adverse effects than are their respective secondary-amine metabolites, nortriptyline (Pamelor) and desipramine (Norpramin).

Because of this extensive side-effect profile, including adverse effects on cardiac conduction and cardiac rhythm, the TCAs have largely been eclipsed in recent times by the SSRIs and other newer agents, which are safer and better tolerated. TCAs are relatively contraindicated in patients with cardiac disease and are not recommended in the acute post-MI period. In fact, some data even suggest that TCAs may precipitate arrhythmias and sudden death in cohorts other than just the post-MI population [21].

As a result, it is relatively unusual to see a patient on a TCA at an antidepressant dose in the ICU and highly unusual to start a TCA in an ICU patient. TCAs are still used with some regularity for neuropathic pain syndromes; when used in this situation, doses are much lower than those used in depression treatment. Overdoses with TCAs may be treated in the ICU and are discussed in Chapter 104.

Monoamine Oxidase Inhibitors

The MAOIs (isocarboxazid [Marplan], phenelzine [Nardil], and tranylcypromine [Parnate]) work by blocking the oxidative deamination of biogenic amines (e.g., norepinephrine and serotonin) and have been used for the treatment of depression since the 1950s. MAOIs may cause a profound hypertensive crisis when a patient taking MAOIs also takes a sympathomimetic medication (e.g., reserpine, guanethidine, pseudoephedrine, and ephedrine) or ingests tyramine-containing foods (e.g., aged cheeses, pickled foods, and yeast extracts). Coadministration with opioids, particularly meperidine, also may lead to hypertensive crises and to elevated blood levels of meperidine and its neurotoxic metabolite, normeperidine. The use of β-blockers with MAOIs may lead to unopposed α-adrenergic activity and also cause severe hypertension. For these reasons, similar to TCAs, MAOIs are infrequently used in recent times, even by psychiatrists, and it would be highly unusual to begin an MAOI in an ICU patient. Overdoses with MAOIs may be treated in the ICU and are discussed in Chapter 104.

Pharmacologic Treatment of Depression in Heart Disease

Table 159.9 summarizes the studies of the effect of antidepressant treatment on psychiatric or cardiovascular outcome or both in patients with heart disease [22–28].

The Sertraline Antidepressant Heart Attack Randomized Trial (SADHART) was designed to evaluate only the safety and efficacy of sertraline, not its effect on cardiac outcomes.

TABLE 159.9

Randomized, Controlled Trials of Depression Treatment in Patients with Cardiovascular Disease

Study	Enrollment	Intervention	Results
Glassman et al. (SADHART) [22]	369 patients with MDD and ACS (either MI or unstable angina)	Sertraline 50–200 mg/d vs. placebo for 24 wk	Sertraline had no significant effect on mean LVEF, increase in PVCs, QTc prolongation, and other cardiac measures. In cohorts with recurrent or severe MDD, depression scores were significantly lower in the sertraline group.
Berkman et al. (ENRICHD) [23]	2,481 patients with modified[a] DSM-IV major or minor depression and/or low perceived social support within 28 d after MI	Intervention (CBT ± sertraline 50–200 mg/d or other medication) vs. usual care for 6 mo	The intervention yielded a significant, though modest, improvement in depression and in social support after 6 mo. This effect was insignificant for depression after 30 mo and for social support after 42 mo. There was no significant difference between groups in death or nonfatal MI, all-cause mortality, cardiac mortality, or recurrent nonfatal MI after an average follow-up of 29 mo.
van Melle et al. (MIND-IT) [24]	331 patients with ICD-10 depression 3–12 mo after MI	Intervention (mirtazapine, citalopram, or nonpharmacologic treatment) vs. usual care for 6 mo	There was no difference between groups in mean BDI scores, presence of depression, and incidence of cardiac events at 18 mo.
Honig et al. (MIND-IT) [25]	91 patients with DSM-IV depression 3–12 mo after MI	Mirtazapine vs. placebo for 24 wk	Mirtazapine was superior to placebo on two of three depression scales at 8 and 24 wk. There was no assessment of effect on cardiac outcomes.
Lespérance et al. (CREATE) [26]	284 patients with DSM-IV MDD and CAD	Twelve weekly sessions of IPT with CM vs. CM alone, and citalopram 20–40 mg/d vs. placebo for 12 wk	The addition of IPT to clinical management conferred no therapeutic advantage. Citalopram was significantly more effective than placebo in reducing depression.
O'Connor et al. (SADHART-CHF) [27]	469 patients with DSM-IV MDD and LVEF ≤45%	Sertraline 50–200 mg/d vs. placebo for 12 wk	Sertraline was safe, but there was no significant difference between groups in reduction of depression or in improvement in cardiac status.
Rollman et al. (BtB) [28]	302 post-CABG patients with PHQ-9 score ≥10	Collaborative care vs. usual care for 8 mo	The intervention yielded greater improvements in mental health–related quality of life, physical functioning, and mood symptoms.

[a]Symptoms of ≥7 days' duration if there was ≥1 prior depressive episode, 14 days if not.
ACS, acute coronary syndrome; BDI, Beck Depression Inventory; CBT, cognitive-behavioral therapy; CM, clinical management; DSM-IV, *Diagnostic and Statistical Manual of Mental Disorders*, 4th edition; ICD-10, *International Classification of Diseases*, 10th edition; IPT, interpersonal therapy; LVEF, left ventricular ejection fraction; MDD, major depressive disorder; MI, myocardial infarction; PHQ, Patient Health Questionnaire; PVCs, premature ventricular contractions; QTc, QT interval corrected for heart rate; SSRI, selective serotonin reuptake inhibitor.

Nevertheless, the number of severe events (e.g., death, stroke, myocardial infarction [MI], recurrent angina, congestive heart failure [CHF]) was lower in patients treated with sertraline (14.5%) compared with those receiving placebo (22.4%) [22]. After a median follow-up of almost 7 years, baseline MDD severity and persistence of depression despite active or placebo treatment in the 6 months immediately after ACS independently predicted more than a doubling of mortality risk [29].

The Enhancing Recovery in Coronary Heart Disease Patients (ENRICHD) study was the first trial of the effect of depression treatment on mortality and reinfarction among post-MI patients [23]. The differential improvement of depression between the intervention and the usual-care groups was only modest and short-lived. Most notably, the intervention yielded no cardiac benefits. This negative result may have occurred because many of the patients in the usual-care arm received antidepressant medication, thus potentially obscuring any between-group differences. In fact, a secondary analysis found that patients exposed to SSRIs had a lower risk of death or recurrent MI and of all-cause mortality compared to patients who did not take SSRIs [30]. In addition, patients with mild, transient depressions likely to have improved on their own were included in the study, and the treatment duration of 6 months may have been too short to discern a salutary effect.

Carney et al. undertook a subgroup analysis of patients with full (rather than modified) criteria for MDD or minor depression, a baseline Beck Depression Inventory (BDI) score ≥10, and a history of at least one episode of MDD and completed the follow-up evaluation 6 months after enrollment (i.e., those patients who completed the intervention) [31]. Although the difference in the mean change in BDI score from baseline to 6 months between groups was higher in this narrowed sample than in the entire cohort, this enhanced improvement did not translate into a survival benefit. Although patients who responded to the intervention experienced a reduction in mortality, the authors recommended caution in evaluating this finding, because it was based on small numbers.

The Myocardial Infarction and Depression-Intervention Trial (MIND-IT) examined the effects of antidepressant treatment on cardiac prognosis and the long-term course of depression [24]. The active treatment arm included three possibilities: randomization to mirtazapine or placebo; open treatment with citalopram; or treatment at the discretion of the treating psychiatrist. Those randomized to mirtazapine or placebo were given the option to switch to unblinded citalopram if there was no response after 8 weeks. Similar to ENRICHD, no significant differences between active treatment and usual care were found in depressive or cardiac outcome. In a separate analysis of just the patients who received mirtazapine, this agent yielded a therapeutic advantage over placebo [25]. In a three-way comparison of responders and nonresponders to either antidepressant (mirtazapine or citalopram) and patients who received no treatment, responders had the least cardiac events, followed by the untreated patients and then the nonresponders, leading the authors to suggest that persistence of depression may be the crucial "cardiotoxic" attribute of depressive illness, for which treatment resistance may be a marker [32].

In an 8-year follow-up of MIND-IT participants, there remained no difference between intervention and usual-care groups in cardiovascular events and cardiac mortality [33]. However, those who received depression treatment, regardless of group assignment, experienced a reduction in all-cause mortality.

The Canadian Cardiac Randomized Evaluation of Antidepressant and Psychotherapy Efficacy (CREATE) trial, the first and only study designed to evaluate paired psychologic and pharmacologic interventions for depression treatment in CHD patients, failed to show a therapeutic advantage for interpersonal therapy, a manualized, short-term therapy focused on loss, grief, life transitions, interpersonal conflicts, and social isolation [26]. It demonstrated, however, that citalopram is an effective antidepressant in this population.

The lack of treatment benefit in the Sertraline Against Depression and Heart Disease in Chronic Heart Failure (SADHART-CHF) study may have been due to intervention and placebo groups both receiving nursing support, thus increasing the placebo response; the modest severity of depression; and the low average doses of sertraline used [27]. Secondary analyses showed that patients whose depression remitted had superior cardiac outcomes and greater improvement in physical and social function and quality of life [34,35].

In the Bypassing the Blues (BtB) study, the collaborative-care intervention involved a nurse care manager telephoning post-CABG patients to describe treatment options, including starting or adjusting antidepressant medications prescribed by their primary-care physicians [28]. A secondary analysis showed that the beneficial effect of the intervention was not because of adjustments in these medications [36], suggesting that other elements of the intervention (e.g., routine symptom monitoring, self-management of symptoms, psychiatric referral) may have been the active ingredients of collaborative care.

The first study of the prevention of depression in CHD patients, the Depression in Coronary Artery Disease (DECARD) trial randomized 240 patients with ACS, but without depression, to 1 year of escitalopram or placebo [37]. Two of 120 escitalopram-treated patients developed a depressive episode (ICD-10 criteria), whereas 10 of 119 (one randomized patient was ultimately excluded) placebo-treated patients did. The authors reported this as a statistically significant difference, but an accompanying editorial [38] suggested that the study was underpowered and raised concerns about its design, conduct, and reporting and about the cost and the prudence of exposing patients without depression to antidepressant medication.

Pharmacologic Treatment of Depression in Stroke

Tables 159.10 and 159.11 summarize findings from randomized, controlled trials of depression treatment and prevention, respectively, in patients with cerebrovascular disease [39–59]. Double-blind treatment trials have demonstrated the safety and efficacy of antidepressants in treating poststroke depression; SSRIs are typically preferred owing to their more favorable side-effect profile. Although concern has been raised about the risk of hemorrhagic stroke with SSRIs, given their impact on platelet activity, a large database-derived case–control study of nearly 400,000 patients showed no association [60].

Jorge et al. found that poststroke patients who received escitalopram showed more improvement in global cognitive functioning than did patients who received placebo or problem-solving therapy—independent of the antidepressant effect of the SSRI [61]. Similarly, in the Fluoxetine for Motor Recovery after Acute Ischemic Stroke (FLAME) trial, a randomized, double-blind, placebo-controlled study in patients with ischemic stroke and hemiplegia or hemiparesis, treatment with fluoxetine over 3 months was associated with improvement in motor recovery, independent of the antidepressant effect of fluoxetine [62].

Electroconvulsive Therapy

ECT is a safe and effective treatment that may be used in cases of severe or psychotic depression or when more conventional therapies cannot be used or are ineffective or intolerable to patients. Found to be particularly helpful for the depressive states accompanying stroke, Parkinson's disease, and dementia, ECT has become part of the standard of care for treatment of severe depression in the medically ill [63]. ECT is also used to treat catatonia.

There are no absolute contraindications to ECT, but patients with unstable cerebro- or cardiovascular disease or increased intracranial pressure warrant closer scrutiny [64–66]. The decision to proceed with ECT or not is made after a careful weighing of the risks of the treatment itself on any underlying physical morbidity against the risks of ongoing untreated depressive illness. This calculation is best done by a psychiatrist experienced in ECT in consultation with an anesthesiologist and other specialists. The latest research in this area has examined the memory impairment associated with ECT and the relationship of lead placement (e.g., bifrontal, bitemporal, and unilateral) to cognitive function [67–70].

Psychologic Management

Although pharmacologic treatments are the mainstay of treatment for depression in the ICU, psychologic remedies are also important. Patients often benefit from information, clarification, reassurance, and support. Psychologic therapies are most useful in cases of adjustment disorder with depressed mood, often as an adjunct to pharmacologic interventions. Brief psychotherapy at the bedside can facilitate increased resilience and hope.

When patients come to the ICU, they are often terrified about the outcome of the illness that brings them there. They frequently believe that the illness, no matter how well controlled in the ICU, will continue to be life-threatening after discharge. Some patients believe that their illness will necessitate a radical change in lifestyle. For example, many cardiac patients secretly believe that having had an MI means they will never be able to have sex again. One way to help patients with such concerns is to ask specific questions about how they believe their illness will affect daily life in the future. In this way, one will hear the patient's specific fears and be able to educate the patient about the realistic effects of the illness. Another example is the patient who is physically weak after an MI and thinks he or she is a cardiac cripple. The patient does not understand that the physical debility is the result of muscle wasting from prolonged bed rest. Education often reassures patients.

Another way to help patients cope with depression in the ICU involves learning about a patient's premorbid activities. Because patients in the ICU feel stripped of their identities and are demoralized, showing interest in who they are and what is important to them can remind them that they are respected and have lives outside the hospital. Families also can be helped

TABLE 159.10

Randomized, Controlled Trials of Depression Treatment in Patients with Cerebrovascular Disease

First author, year	Enrollment	Intervention	Results
Karaiskos, 2012 [39]	60 patients following acute ischemic stroke or intracerebral hemorrhage with DSM-IV depressive episode	Duloxetine 60–120 mg/d vs. citalopram 20–40 mg/d vs. sertraline 50–200 mg/d for 3 mo	All groups showed improvements in depression and anxiety but not fatigue. Duloxetine was well tolerated and more effective than the other two agents for anxiety.
Cravello, 2009 [40]	50 poststroke patients with depression	Venlafaxine SR 75–150 mg/d vs. fluoxetine 20–40 mg/d for 8 wk	Both agents yielded similar improvement in depressive symptoms. Venlafaxine showed more improvement on an alexithymia scale.
Choi-Kwon, 2008 [41]	152 patients 3–28 mo after stroke with depression, emotional incontinence, or anger proneness	Fluoxetine 20 mg/d vs. placebo for 3 mo	Fluoxetine produced significantly higher scores in the mental health, general health, and social functioning domains of QOL after 12 mo.
Li, 2008 [42]	150 poststroke patients with moderate to severe depression	FEWP[a] vs. fluoxetine vs. placebo for 8 wk	The active arms showed a higher clinical response than placebo, but no difference between FEWP and fluoxetine was discernible at the end of the study.
Robinson, 2008 [43]	159 patients with MDD 10 d to 3 mo after stroke	Nefiracetam[b] 600 or 900 mg/d vs. placebo	Both arms showed response rates >70% and remission rates >40%. Patients in the top quintile of HDRS scores showed a significant effect with 900 mg compared to 600 mg or placebo.
Williams, 2007 [44]	188 patients with poststroke depression	Patients received treatment through a medication algorithm with paroxetine, sertraline, venlafaxine or mirtazapine vs. usual care for 12 wk	Depression response and remission were more likely in the intervention group.
Choi-Kwon, 2006 [45]	152 poststroke patients with depression, emotional incontinence, or anger proneness	Fluoxetine 20 mg/d vs. placebo for 3 mo	Fluoxetine significantly improved emotional incontinence and anger proneness but not depression.
Murray, 2005 [46]	123 poststroke patients with MDD or minor depression	Sertraline 50–100 mg/d vs. placebo for 26 wk	Both groups improved substantially. There was no difference in depression between groups and significantly less emotional distress and better QOL in the treatment group.
Rampello, 2005 [47]	31 patients with "retarded" depression within 12 mo after stroke	Reboxetine[c] 4 mg twice daily vs. placebo for 16 wk	Reboxetine showed good efficacy, safety, and tolerability. There was a significant difference in change in HDRS and BDI scores between groups.
Rampello, 2004 [48]	74 poststroke patients with depression	Citalopram 20 mg/d vs. reboxetine 4 mg/d for 16 wk	Both agents showed good safety and tolerability. Citalopram showed a greater effect on anxious depression, reboxetine on retarded depression.
Fruehwald, 2003 [49]	50 poststroke patients with depression	Fluoxetine 20 mg/d vs. placebo for 3 mo	Both groups showed significant improvement, with no between-group difference, after 1 mo. At 18 mo, the fluoxetine group had significantly less depression.
Robinson, 2000 [50]	104 poststroke patients with and without depression	Nortriptyline 25–100 mg/d, fluoxetine 10–40 mg/d, or placebo for 12 wk	Nortriptyline resulted in a significantly higher response than fluoxetine or placebo in reversing depression, reducing anxiety, and improving functional status. Neither active treatment improved cognitive or social functioning in depressed or nondepressed patients.

(*continued*)

TABLE 159.10

Randomized, Controlled Trials of Depression Treatment in Patients with Cerebrovascular Disease (*continued*)

First author, year	Enrollment	Intervention	Results
Wiart, 2000 [51]	31 poststroke patients with MDD	Fluoxetine 20 mg/d vs. placebo for 6 wk	Fluoxetine produced a significant improvement in depression but not in motor, cognitive, or functional scores.
Grade, 1998 [52]	21 poststroke patients admitted to a rehabilitation facility	Methylphenidate 5–30 mg/d vs. placebo for 3 wk	Methylphenidate yielded lower HDRS and Zung[d] scores.
Andersen, 1994 [53]	66 patients with depression 2–52 wk after stroke	Citalopram 10–40 mg/d vs. placebo for 3 and 6 wk	Citalopram yielded greater improvement than placebo.

[a]A Chinese herbal antidepressant.
[b]A so-called cognitive enhancer used in patients with Alzheimer's disease.
[c]A norepinephrine reuptake inhibitor available in Europe.
[d]A depression rating scale.
BDI, Beck Depression Inventory; FEWP, Free and Easy Wanderer Plus; HDRS, Hamilton Depression Rating Scale; MDD, major depressive disorder; PSD, poststroke depression; QOL, quality of life; SR, sustained release.

TABLE 159.11

Randomized, Controlled Trials of Depression Prevention in Patients with Cerebrovascular Disease

First author, year	Enrollment	Intervention	Results
Tsai, 2011 [54]	92 patients following acute ischemic stroke	Milnacipran 50–100 mg/d for 12 mo	The milnacipran group had statistically significantly fewer cases of poststroke depression.
Robinson, 2008 [55]	176 patients without depression within 3 mo after stroke	Escitalopram vs. placebo vs. problem-solving therapy for 1 y for prophylaxis	Patients who received either escitalopram or therapy were significantly less likely to develop depression. In an intention-to-treat analysis, escitalopram, but not therapy, was significantly superior to placebo in depression prevention.
Almeida, 2006 [56]	111 patients without depression <2 wk after stroke	Sertraline 50 mg/d vs. placebo for 24 wk for prophylaxis	There was no significant difference in development of depressive symptoms.
Niedermaier, 2004 [57]	70 poststroke patients who were not depressed	Mirtazapine 30 mg/d vs. placebo for 1 y for prophylaxis and treatment	Significantly fewer patients in the treatment group developed depression. Fifteen out of 16 patients who developed depression were treated effectively with mirtazapine.
Rasmussen, 2003 [58]	137 poststroke patients who were not depressed at baseline	Sertraline 50–150 mg/d vs. placebo for 1 y for prophylaxis	Significantly fewer patients in the sertraline group developed depression compared to the placebo group.
Narushima, 2002 [59]	48 poststroke patients who were not depressed at baseline	Nortriptyline 25–100 mg/d, fluoxetine 10–40 mg/d, or placebo for 12 wk for prophylaxis	Significantly fewer depressive episodes occurred in the treatment groups. However, more nortriptyline-treated patients developed depression in the 6 months after treatment was stopped compared to the other two groups.

to have realistic expectations. Strategies to help patients and families cope effectively in the ICU are discussed in Chapter 161.

CONCLUSION

Treatment of depression in ICUs is multifaceted, and many difficulties are involved in treating depression in this setting. Nevertheless, aggressive treatment of depression in the ICU can drastically improve a patient's sense of well-being and transform a demoralized, hopeless patient into an active participant in treatment. In this chapter, we have outlined the recognition, differential diagnosis, and treatment of depression in ICUs. We strongly advocate that depression be treated as a serious illness; although a depressed mood is sometimes understandable, a depressive disorder is never appropriate.

References

1. Frasure-Smith N, Lespérance F: Depression and cardiac risk: present status and future directions. *Heart* 96:173, 2010.
2. Lichtman JH, Froelicher ES, Blumenthal JA, et al: Depression as a risk factor for poor prognosis among patients with acute coronary syndrome: systematic review and recommendations. *Circulation* 129:1350, 2014.
3. Robinson RG, Jorge RE. Post-stroke depression: a review. *Am J Psychiatry* 173:221–231, 2015.
4. American Psychiatric Association: *Diagnostic and Statistical Manual of Mental Disorders*. 5th ed. Washington, DC, American Psychiatric Publishing, 2013.
5. Thase ME: Effects of venlafaxine on blood pressure: a meta-analysis of original data from 3744 depressed patients. *J Clin Psychiatry* 59:502, 1998.
6. Auclair AL, Martel JC, Assie MG, et al: Levomilnacipran (F2695), a norepinephrine-preferring SNRI: profile in vitro and in models of depression and anxiety. *Neuropharmacology* 70:338, 2013.
7. Chen L, Greenberg WM, Brand-Schieber E, et al: Effect of renal impairment on the pharmacokinetics of levomilnacipran following a single oral dose of levomilnacipran extended-release capsule in humans. *Drug Des Devel Ther* 9:3293, 2015.

8. Chen L, Boinpally R, Greenberg WM, et al: Effect of hepatic impairment on the pharmacokinetics of levomilnacipran following a single oral dose of a levomilnacipran extended-release capsule in human participants. *Clin Drug Investig* 34:351, 2014.
9. Bang-Andersen B, Ruhland T, Jorgensen M, et al: Discovery of 1-[2-(2,4-dimethyl-phenylsulfanyl)phenyl]piperazine (Lu AA21004): a novel multimodal compound for the treatment of major depressive disorder. *J Med Chem* 54:3206, 2011.
10. Sanchez C, Asin KE, Artigas F: Vortioxetine, a novel antidepressant with multimodal activity: review of preclinical and clinical data. *Pharmacol Ther* 145:43, 2015.
11. Zhang J, Mathis MV, Sellers JW, et al: The US Food and Drug Administration's perspective on the new antidepressant vortioxetine. *J Clin Psychiatry* 76:8, 2015.
12. Areberg J, Sogaard B, Hojer AM: The clinical pharmacokinetics of Lu AA21004 and its major metabolite in health young volunteers. *Basic Clin Pharmacol Toxicol* 111:198, 2012.
13. Katona C, Hansen T, Olsen CK: A randomized, double-blind, placebo-controlled, duloxetine-referenced, fixed-dose study comparing the efficacy and safety of Lu AA21004 in elderly pateints with major depressive disorder. *Int Clin Psychopharmacol* 27:215, 2012.
14. Boinpally R, Gad N, Gupta S, et al: Influence of CYP3A4 induction/inhibition on the pharmacokinetics of vilazodone in health subjects. *Clin Ther* 36:1638, 2014.
15. Boinpally R, Henry D, Gupta S, et al: Pharmacokinetics and safety of vilazodone in hepatic impairment. *Am J Ther* 22:269, 2015.
16. McKean J, Watts H, Mokszycki R: Breakthrough seizures after starting vilazodone for depression. *Pharmacotherapy* 35:e6, 2015.
17. Acker EC, Sinclair EA, Beardsley AL, et al: Acute vilazodone toxicity in a pediatric patient. *J Emerg Med* 49:284, 2015.
18. Edwards J, Sperry V, Adams MH, et al: Vilazodone lacks proarrhythmogenic potential in healthy participants: a thorough ECG study. *Int J Clin Pharmacol Ther* 51:456, 2013.
19. Matthews M, Gommoll C, Chen D, et al: Efficacy and safety of vilazodone 20 and 40 mg in major depressive disorder: a randomized, double-blind, placebo-controlled trial. *Int Clin Psychopharmacol* 30:67, 2015.
20. Shrier M, Diaz J, Tsarouhas N: Cardiotoxicity associated with bupropion overdose [letter]. *Ann Emerg Med* 35:100, 2000.
21. Witchel HJ, Hancox JC, Nutt DJ: Psychotropic drugs, cardiac arrhythmias and sudden death. *J Clin Psychopharmacol* 23:58, 2003.
22. Glassman AH, O'Connor CM, Califf RM, et al: Sertraline treatment of major depression in patients with acute MI or unstable angina. *JAMA* 288:701, 2002.
23. Berkman LF, Blumenthal J, Burg M, et al: Effects of treating depression and low perceived social support on clinical events after myocardial infarction: the Enhancing Recovery in Coronary Heart Disease Patients (ENRICHD) Randomized Trial. *JAMA* 289:3106, 2003.
24. van Melle JP, de Jonge P, Honig A, et al: Effects of antidepressant treatment following myocardial infarction. *Br J Psychiatry* 190:460, 2007.
25. Honig A, Kuyper AMG, Schene AH, et al: Treatment of post-myocardial infarction depressive disorder: a randomized, placebo-controlled trial with mirtazapine. *Psychosom Med* 69:606, 2007.
26. Lespérance F, Frasure-Smith N, Koszycki D, et al: Effects of citalopram and interpersonal psychotherapy on depression in patients with coronary artery disease: the Canadian Cardiac Randomized Evaluation of Antidepressant and Psychotherapy Efficacy (CREATE) trial. *JAMA* 297:367, 2007.
27. O'Connor CM, Jiang W, Kuchibhatla M, et al: Safety and efficacy of sertraline for depression in patients with heart failure: results of the SADHART-CHF (Sertraline Against Depression and Heart Disease in Chronic Heart Failure) trial. *J Am Coll Cardiol* 56:692, 2010.
28. Rollman BL, Belnap BH, LeMenager MS, et al: Telephone-delivered collaborative care for treating post-CABG depression: a randomized controlled trial. *JAMA* 302:2095, 2009.
29. Glassman AH, Bigger JT, Gaffney M: Psychiatric characteristics associated with long-term mortality among 361 patients having an acute coronary syndrome and major depression: seven-year follow-up of SADHART participants. *Arch Gen Psychiatry* 66:1022, 2009.
30. Taylor CB, Youngblood ME, Catellier D, et al: Effects of antidepressant medication on morbidity and mortality in depressed patients after myocardial infarction. *Arch Gen Psychiatry* 62:792, 2005.
31. Carney RM, Blumenthal JA, Freedland KE, et al: Depression and late mortality after myocardial infarction in the Enhancing Recovery in Coronary Heart Disease (ENRICHD) study. *Psychosom Med* 66:466, 2004.
32. de Jonge P, Honig A, van Melle JP, et al: Nonresponse to treatment for depression following myocardial infarction: association with subsequent cardiac events. *Am J Psychiatry* 164:1371, 2007.
33. Zuidersma M, Conradi HJ, van Melle JP, et al: Depression treatment after myocardial infarction and long-term risk of subsequent cardiovascular events and mortality: a randomized controlled trial. *J Psychosom Res* 74:25, 2013.
34. Jiang W, Krishnan R, Kuchibhatla M, et al: Characteristics of depression remission and its relation with cardiovascular outcome among patients with chronic heart failure (from the SADHART-CHF study). *Am J Cardiol* 107:545, 2011.
35. Xiong GL, Fiuzat M, Kuchibhatla M, et al: Health status and depression remission in patients with chronic heart failure: patient-reported outcomes from the SADHART-CHF trial. *Circ Heart Fail* 5:688, 2012.
36. Meyer T, Belnap BH, Herrmann-Lingen C, et al: Benefits of collaborative care for post-CABG depression are not related to adjustments in antidepressant pharmacotherapy. *J Psychosom Res* 76:28, 2014.
37. Hansen BH, Hanash JA, Rasmussen A, et al: Effects of escitalopram in prevention of depression in patients with acute coronary syndrome (DECARD). *J Psychosom Res* 72:11, 2012.
38. Thombs BD, Ziegelstein RC: When prevention is a bad idea: problems with the DECARD trial and the premise behind it. *J Psychosom Res* 72:333, 2012.
39. Karaiskos D, Tzavellas E, Spengos K, et al: Duloxetine versus citalopram and sertraline in the treatment of poststroke depression, anxiety, and fatigue. *J Neuropsychiatry Clin Neurosci* 24:349, 2012.
40. Cravello L, Caltagirone C, Spalletta G: The SNRI venlafaxine improves emotional unawareness in patients with post-stroke depression. *Hum Psychopharmacol* 24:331, 2009.
41. Choi-Kwon S, Choi J, Kwon SU, et al: Fluoxetine improves the quality of life in patients with poststroke emotional disturbances. *Cerebrovasc Dis* 26:266, 2008.
42. Li L-T, Wang S-H, Ge H-Y, et al: The beneficial effects of the herbal medicine Free and Easy Wanderer Plus (FEWP) and fluoxetine on post-stroke depression. *J Altern Complement Med* 14:841, 2008.
43. Robinson RG, Jorge RE, Clarence-Smith K: Double-blind randomized treatment of poststroke depression using nefiracetam. *J Neuropsychiatry Clin Neurosci* 20:178, 2008.
44. Williams LS, Kroenke K, Bakas T, et al: Care management of poststroke depression: a randomized, controlled trial. *Stroke* 38:998, 2007.
45. Choi-Kwon S, Han SW, Kwon SU, et al: Fluoxetine treatment in poststroke depression, emotional incontinence, and anger proneness: a double-blind, placebo-controlled study. *Stroke* 37:156, 2006.
46. Murray V, von Arbin M, Bartfai A, et al: Double-blind comparison of sertraline and placebo in stroke patients with minor depression and less severe major depression. *J Clin Psychiatry* 66:708, 2005.
47. Rampello L, Alvano A, Chiechio S, et al: An evaluation of efficacy and safety of reboxetine in elderly patients affected by "retarded" post-stroke depression: a random, placebo-controlled study. *Arch Gerontol Geriatr* 40:275, 2005.
48. Rampello L, Chiechio S, Nicoletti G, et al: Prediction of the response to citalopram and reboxetine in post-stroke depressed patients. *Psychopharmacology* 173:73, 2004.
49. Fruehwald S, Gatterbauer E, Rehak P, et al: Early fluoxetine treatment of post-stroke depression: a three-month double-blind placebo-controlled study with an open-label long-term follow-up. *J Neurol* 250:347, 2003.
50. Robinson RG, Schultz SK, Castillo C, et al: Nortriptyline versus fluoxetine in the treatment of depression and in short-term recovery after stroke: a placebo-controlled, double-blind study. *Am J Psychiatry* 157:351, 2000.
51. Wiart L, Petit H, Joseph PA, et al: Fluoxetine in early poststroke depression: a double-blind placebo-controlled study. *Stroke* 31:1829, 2000.
52. Grade C, Redford B, Chrostowski J, et al: Methylphenidate in early poststroke recovery: a double-blind, placebo-controlled study. *Arch Phys Med Rehabil* 79:1047, 1998.
53. Andersen G, Vestergaard K, Lauritzen L: Effective treatment of poststroke depression with the selective serotonin reuptake inhibitor citalopram. *Stroke* 25:1099, 1994.
54. Tsai CS, Wu CL, Chou SY, et al: Prevention of poststroke depression with milnacipran in patients with acute ischemic stroke: a double-blind randomized placebo-controlled trial. *Int Clin Psychopharmacol* 26:263, 2011.
55. Robinson RG, Jorge RE, Moser DJ, et al: Escitalopram and problem-solving therapy for prevention of poststroke depression: a randomized controlled trial. *JAMA* 299:2391, 2008.
56. Almeida OP, Waterreus A, Hankey GJ: Preventing depression after stroke: results from a randomized placebo-controlled trial. *J Clin Psychiatry* 67:1104, 2006.
57. Niedermaier N, Bohrer E, Schulte K, et al: Prevention and treatment of poststroke depression with mirtazapine in patients with acute stroke. *J Clin Psychiatry* 65:1619, 2004.
58. Rasmussen A, Lunde M, Poulsen DL, et al: A double-blind, placebo-controlled study of sertraline in the prevention of depression in stroke patients. *Psychosomatics* 44:216, 2003.
59. Narushima K, Kosier JT, Robinson RG: Preventing poststroke depression: a 12-week double-blind randomized treatment trial and 21-month follow-up. *J Nerv Ment Dis* 190:296, 2002.
60. Douglas I, Smeeth L, Irvine D: The use of antidepressants and the risk of haemorrhagic stroke: a nested case control. *Br J Clin Pharmacol* 71:116, 2011.
61. Jorge RE, Acion L, Moser D, et al: Escitalopram and enhancement of cognitive recovery following stroke. *Arch Gen Psychiatry* 67:187, 2010.
62. Chollet F, Tardy J, Albucher JF, et al: Fluoxetine for motor recovery after stroke (FLAME): a randomized placebo-controlled trial. *Lancet Neurol* 10:123, 2011.
63. Christopher EJ: Electroconvulsive therapy in the medically ill. *Curr Psychiatry Rep* 5:225, 2003.
64. American Psychiatric Association: *The Practice of Electroconvulsive Therapy: Recommendations for Treatment, Training, and Privileging*. 2nd ed. Washington, DC, American Psychiatric Association, 2001.
65. Lisanby SH: Electroconvulsive therapy for depression. *N Engl J Med* 357:1939, 2007.
66. Tess AV, Smetana GW: Medical evaluation of patients undergoing electroconvulsive therapy. *N Engl J Med* 360:1437, 2009.
67. UK ECT Review Group: Efficacy and safety of electroconvulsive therapy in depressive disorders: a systematic review and meta-analysis. *Lancet* 361:799, 2003.
68. Kellner CH, Knapp R, Husain MM, et al: Bifrontal, bitemporal and right unilateral electrode placement in ECT: randomised trial. *Br J Psychiatry* 196:226, 2010.
69. Sienaert P, Vansteelandt K, Demyttenaere K, et al: Randomized comparison of ultra-brief bifrontal and unilateral electroconvulsive therapy for major depression: cognitive side-effects. *J Affect Disord* 122:60, 2010.
70. Smith GE, Rasmussen KG, Cullum CM, et al: A randomized controlled trial comparing the memory effects of continuation electroconvulsive therapy versus continuation pharmacotherapy: results from the Consortium for Research in ECT (CORE) study. *J Clin Psychiatry* 71:185, 2010.

Chapter 160 ■ Managing the Suicidal Patient in the Intensive Care Unit

SAORI A. MURAKAMI • CHRISTINA MASSEY

The assessment of the suicidal patient is a significant challenge for any intensive care team. Even when a psychiatrist is consulted to conduct an expert assessment of risk and to assist with the formulation of a treatment plan, the intensivist's ability to evaluate, manage, and safeguard the patient's safety is essential. The evaluation and management of a patient—whether contemplating suicide or recovering from a suicide attempt—require an understanding of risk factors, protective factors, the interplay among these various elements, and the relationship between the staff and the patient. In addition, the primary medical team should be aware of the necessity for ongoing psychiatric care during and after the stabilization of acute medical issues.

This chapter reviews the epidemiology of suicide, risk and protective factors, parasuicide, and intervention and management strategies for suicidal patients in the intensive care unit (ICU).

EPIDEMIOLOGY OF SUICIDE

Suicide is the 10th leading cause of death in the United States (7th in men and 14th in women) [1]. In 2013, suicide was responsible for 41,149 deaths, with higher rates among whites, men, and individuals between the ages of 45 and 64 years, with rates in this latter group increasing steadily over the last decade [1,2]. Also in 2013, 494,169 people presented to an emergency department for treatment of self-harm, and 224,811 people were hospitalized due to self-inflicted injuries [1].

RISK AND PROTECTIVE FACTORS

Although appraisals of suicide risk are incapable of absolute predictions of suicidal behavior, careful history-taking, detailed examination, and astute clinical judgment allow a comprehensive understanding and evaluation of risk factors, protective factors, and the interplay among them (Table 160.1).

The first set of factors is sociodemographic, including age, gender, race, marital status, and religion. In general, men are more likely to complete suicide, whereas women are more likely to make attempts [3,4]. White men are more likely to attempt suicide than nonwhites; among nonwhite populations, rates vary [1,3]. Suicide rates are higher for two distinct age distributions: late adolescence to young adulthood and older than age 70 years [4]; however, over the last several years, rates have been increasing among middle-aged individuals and slightly decreasing among the elderly. In general, the suicide rate is greatest among divorced and widowed people, followed by single individuals, and married people [4]. The combination of age, gender, and marital status also plays a role; young widowed men have a particularly high rate of suicide [4]. There is more recent evidence suggesting that sexual orientation and gender identity and expression are associated with suicide risk as those identifying with minority orientations appear to have a heightened risk [3–5].

Some evidence suggests that religious beliefs and the strength of one's religious convictions protect against suicide; however, for some, religion may increase suicide risk. For example, an individual who believes he will be reunited with his lost loved ones when he himself dies may be comforted by the idea of dying. Thus, the various meanings religion can have in different people's lives mandate careful exploration with the patient of the role of religion in death and suicide [4].

Psychiatric illness contributes significantly to the risk for suicide. Retrospective studies have identified one or more psychiatric

TABLE 160.1

Risk Factors for Suicide

- Sociodemographic factors
  - Age
  - Gender
  - Race, ethnicity, culture
  - Marital status
  - Religion
  - Sexual orientation
- Psychiatric history and present psychiatric conditions
  - Psychiatric disorders
  - Substance use disorders
  - History of suicide attempts
  - History of self-injurious behavior
  - History of homicidal, assaultive, or aggressive behavior
  - Impulsivity
  - History of physical or emotional trauma
  - Psychiatric treatment, both outpatient and inpatient
  - History of treatment adherence
  - Psychological factors
- Medical history and present medical conditions
  - Neurologic disorders
  - Head trauma, with or without cognitive and behavioral sequelae
  - Executive function deficits
  - Malignancies
  - Human immunodeficiency virus infection
  - Acquired immune deficiency syndrome
  - Peptic ulcer disease
  - Chronic inflammatory diseases
  - Hemodialysis-treated chronic renal failure
  - Heart disease
  - Chronic pulmonary disease
- Family history
  - Psychiatric illness
  - Substance use
  - History of completed suicide
- Psychosocial stressors
  - Family life
  - Work life
  - Relationships
  - Finances
  - Recent real or perceived loss

Adapted from American Psychiatric Association: *Practice Guideline for the Assessment and Treatment of Patients with Suicidal Behaviors*. Washington, DC, American Psychiatric Association, 2010. Available at http://psychiatry-online.org/pb/assets/raw/sitewide/practice_guidelines/guidelines/suicide.pdf. Accessed November 3, 2015.

disorders in individuals who have completed suicide or presented following a suicide attempt [3,4,6,7]. In addition, conditions that frequently occur with psychiatric illnesses (e.g., substance use disorders) increase suicide risk. Research indicates that risk may be particularly high when a mood disorder co-occurs with a disorder that results in increased distress level (e.g., anxiety disorder) or a disorder that is characterized by diminished restraint (e.g., conduct disorder or antisocial personality disorder) [3]. The presence of a past history of suicide attempts, suicidal thinking, feelings of hopelessness, self-injurious behavior, impulsivity, assaultiveness, and trauma (physical or emotional) is an important component of risk assessment. Whether a patient is in active outpatient psychiatric treatment—and compliant with it—is also a critical component of risk assessment. Psychological factors—coping skills, tolerance of emotions, personality traits, insight, and judgment—figure prominently in the estimation of how a patient handles stress.

The presence of a physical illness contributes to the risk for suicide [3,4,8]. Suicide risk is greater for patients with neurologic disorders (e.g., Huntington's disease, organic brain syndromes, multiple sclerosis, and spinal cord injuries), and suicide attempts are more common in patients with epilepsy and other chronic diseases [3,4]. In addition, head trauma is associated with an enhanced risk for suicide, particularly when behavioral or cognitive sequelae result. Executive function deficits due to delirium, dementia, or mental retardation also contribute to the risk for suicide [4,8]. Other illnesses of significance are listed in Table 160.1.

Psychosocial stressors—including states of family life, work life, relationships, and finances; legal difficulties; and losses—are important considerations when assessing risk. A family history of psychiatric disturbances, substance use, or completed suicide may indicate potential genetic vulnerabilities in the management of these stressors and response to interventions.

Protective factors include the presence of supports (e.g., family, friends, and faith), the ability to identify specific and important reasons for living, responsibility for young children or other family members, extraversion and optimism, effective coping and problem-solving skills, and the general absence of risk factors [3,4].

Risk and protective factors must be understood on a case-by-case basis [4,6]. Despite the significance of each factor, the weight to attribute to each element must be individualized, because the interaction among these features defines each patient's unique risk. For example, a 70-year-old unmarried white man with an incurable malignancy may be protected from suicide by his religion's prohibition against it and by his three grandchildren's frequent visits.

PARASUICIDE

Some physicians may differentiate "genuine" suicide attempts (in which the person's aim was to kill himself) from parasuicide, a deliberately self-harming but nonlethal act. Often, parasuicide or a so-called suicide gesture is not a failed attempt to kill oneself *per se*, but could be either a maladaptive way to cope with emotions or an effort to elicit a specific reaction from someone else, whether an emotional response (e.g., feeling hurt or sorry) or a behavioral one (e.g., forestalling abandonment or providing nurturance). As such, a physician may be tempted to construe parasuicide as less worrisome than an authentic attempt to end one's life. However, these individuals require equal attention and caution because parasuicide often recurs; when repeated often enough, such behavior may prove lethal, even if death is unintended. In addition, individuals can struggle to recognize in hindsight what their true intent or motive was, and there can be ambivalence as to the outcome of their suicide gesture. A history of parasuicide or suicide gestures may increase the subsequent risk for suicide, particularly as intent and lethality are not necessarily correlated and as increasing feelings of hopelessness and negative outcomes may influence intent [9,10]. For example, a man who commits parasuicide in an attempt to keep his wife from divorcing him may not recognize the potential lethality of his overdose, and he may later feel genuinely suicidal if his wife ends up leaving him.

TREATMENT OF THE SUICIDAL PATIENT

Nonpharmacologic Interventions

A patient's verbalization of intent to harm himself/herself poses a unique challenge for the ICU physician. Although such utterances can be variously motivated and belie different intentions, any such statement should be taken seriously and viewed as the patient's request for help and support. Suicidal statements may take the form of explicit declaration or implicit action (e.g., refusal to eat or to cooperate with care). The suicidal act can be impulsive or deliberate. Because accurate prediction of which statements will result in action is impossible, the ICU team must institute effective precautions whenever a patient avows suicide.

The ICU team should implement close monitoring, in the form of constant observation by a one-to-one sitter, video monitoring, or more frequent checks of the patient. Physical restraint of a patient at ongoing risk may be necessary when constant observation is not possible [8]. Staff should be aware of potential means by which patients may harm themselves. Any opportunity of jumping from windows or of hanging should be minimized, if not eliminated. All materials that a person may use to harm himself/herself (e.g., razors, scissors, needles, glass, medications, and eating utensils) must be removed and any personal belongings searched for these items. Staff should also be aware of items brought in by visitors. The team should review medications and consider decreasing or discontinuing medications that may heighten impulsivity or disinhibition. Estimations of safety should be made at least daily.

The primary team must also identify and address among themselves any negative feelings they have about the patient. Emotional reactions to dealing with psychological problems in the ICU can include helplessness, insecurity, fear, anxiety, guilt, and sympathy. People who repeatedly attempt suicide or whose motives have been deemed "manipulative" can engender frustration, anger, and exhaustion with demands for constant attention, thereby creating distance between the patient and the treatment team. It is important to understand these feelings and to prevent them from hampering patient care and clouding recognition of a potentially unsafe patient. For example, patients with borderline personality disorder can "split" the staff (i.e., behave well for one subset of the staff and badly for another) [11]. Regular communication among staff members and between the staff and the patient can minimize splitting and prevent team members from feeling defensive or apologetic in the face of a critical and demanding patient.

An empathic approach that seeks to understand what the patient feels can prevent these emotions from instigating counter-therapeutic responses. Even if a "suicide attempt" is an effort to elicit a particular response from others (rather than a genuine attempt to end one's life), the desperation required to put one's life at risk is nonetheless sobering. For people whose intent was to die, waking up from an unsuccessful suicide attempt can be accompanied by despair, shame, guilt, fear, anger, a sense of inferiority, or ambivalence about having survived. The physical discomfort of the life-sustaining measures employed in the ICU can compound such patients' pain.

Medications

The question of whether and when to restart psychiatric medications following a suicide attempt can be a difficult one, particularly if the person attempted to kill himself/herself by an overdose of these agents. The decision to resume outpatient medicines must be guided first and foremost by accurate psychiatric diagnosis. They should not be restarted reflexively just because they had been prescribed previously; they should be ordered only if the patient has a *bona fide* psychiatric condition. Psychiatric consultation can be beneficial when the diagnosis is uncertain.

The next consideration is the patient's physical condition and the medications' effects on organs that the suicidal act may have compromised. Medications that are potentially toxic to impaired organs should not be restarted. Attention should also be paid to the patient's level of arousal and the risks for seizures and arrhythmias because psychiatric medications may enhance these risks.

Anxiety is a potent risk factor for suicide and should be treated to prevent recurrence of suicidal behavior and intensification of suicidal thinking. Benzodiazepines can be particularly helpful in quelling anxiety, whereas neuroleptic medications—both conventional and atypical—are preferred when anxiety escalates into outright fear.

Psychiatric Consultation

Psychiatric consultation is strongly recommended whenever a patient's safety from self-harm is uncertain. The consultant will address psychiatric diagnoses, suicide risk, medications, and disposition. Consultation can also be helpful in understanding the psychological dynamics between patient and staff. The patient who may be thinking about, or at risk of, self-harm but has not articulated a specific thought also may benefit from expert consultation; elderly patients often do not report suicidal thoughts to caretakers [12].

When requesting a consultation, it is helpful to provide the consultant with as many details of the suicide attempt as possible (e.g., method, number of pills in cases of ingestion, and likelihood of rescue). The exact words used by a patient who makes a suicidal comment, as well as the context in which the statement was made, are critically important and should be included in the consultation request. Basic elements of the patient's mental status (e.g., level of wakefulness, affect, the presence of psychosis, and ongoing suicidal thinking) should be determined and relayed to the psychiatrist. Clear documentation from the nursing staff and physicians will help the consultant follow the patient's course and identify points of intervention.

Disposition

When medically and surgically stable, patients face two options for discharge—home or psychiatric facility. Patients who may benefit from or require continued treatment in a psychiatric facility are those whose risk factors outweigh their protective factors. This decision is usually made with the psychiatric consultant, who will also assist with placement, prior authorization (which is required by some insurance plans), and the handling of any legal matters (e.g., if the patient is unwilling to be hospitalized psychiatrically, and thus requires involuntary commitment).

CONCLUSION

Attempted suicide is a tragic consequence of mental and physical illness that represents a relatively small number of ICU admissions. Nonetheless, the care of a patient who is suicidal or has just attempted suicide requires attention to a number of details not usually considered in the management of a typical ICU patient. The ICU team must be cognizant of their emotional reactions to the patient and of patient–staff dynamics, vigilant for potentially dangerous objects in the physical environment, and knowledgeable about specific interventions, including constant observation of the potentially self-harming patient. Psychiatric consultation can be helpful in managing important aspects of care for this patient population, from diagnosis and safety assessment to medication management and disposition.

References

1. Centers for Disease Control and Prevention, National Center for Injury Prevention and Control: Web-based Injury Statistics Query and Reporting System (WISQARS). Available at: http://www.cdc.gov/injury/wisqars. Accessed November 3, 2015.
2. Kochanek KD, Murphy SL, Xu J: Deaths: final data for 2011. *Natl Vital Stat Rep* 63:1, 2015.
3. Tureki, G, Brent, DA: Suicide and suicidal behaviour. *The Lancet*: Advance online publication, 2015.
4. American Psychiatric Association: Practice Guideline for the Assessment and Treatment of Patients with Suicidal Behaviors. Washington, DC, American Psychiatric Association, 2010. Available at: http://psychiatryonline.org/pb/assets/raw/sitewide/practice_guidelines/guidelines/suicide.pdf. Accessed November 3, 2015.
5. Ploderl MD, Tremblay P: Mental health of sexual minorities. a systematic review. *International Review of Psychiatry* 27:367–385, 2015.
6. Moscicki EK: Suicidal behaviors among adults, in Nock MK (ed): *The Oxford Handbook of Suicide and Self-Injury*. New York, Oxford, 2014, p 92.
7. Dennis BB, Roshanov PS, Bawor M, et al: Re-examination of classic risk factors for suicidal behaviour in the psychiatric population. *Crisis* 36:231, 2015.
8. Perlis RH, Stern TA: Care of the suicidal patient, in Stern TA, Fricchione GL, Cassem NH, et al. (eds): *Massachusetts General Hospital Handbook of General Hospital Psychiatry*. 6th ed. Philadelphia, Saunders, 2010, p 541–554.
9. Heilbron N, Copmton J, Daniel S, et al: The problematic label of suicide gesture: alternatives for clinical research and practice. *Professional Psychology: Research and Practice* 41: 221–227, 2010.
10. Salman S, Idrees J, Hassan F, et al: Predictive factors of suicide attempt and non-suicidal self-harm in emergency department. *Emergency* 4:166–169, 2014.
11. American Psychiatric Association: *Diagnostic and Statistical Manual of Mental Disorders*. 5th ed. Washington, DC, American Psychiatric Association, 2013.
12. Duberstein PR, Conwell Y, Seidlitz L, et al: Age and suicidal ideation in older depressed inpatients. *Am J Geriatr Psychiatry* 7:289, 1999.

Chapter 161 ■ Problematic Behaviors of Patients, Family, and Staff in the Intensive Care Unit

CRAIGAN T. USHER

Nobody realizes that some people expend tremendous energy merely to be normal.

Albert Camus [1]

The intensive care unit (ICU) is a stressful environment for patients, family, and staff [2–8]. Under extreme medical and psychologic stress, *everyone* in the ICU—patients and physicians alike—may fail to work together.

In exploring difficult patient–staff interactions, though we may use terms like "the hateful patient" [7], the "angry attending," or the "problematic family member," such language erroneously locates problems as arising solely from one individual and risks eschewing dimensional thinking (the notion that most people borrow from a spectrum of problematic-to-healthful coping strategies and defense mechanisms) in favor of overly simplistic categorical distinction (a patient is healthy or not, hateful or loving). As such, although critical care team burnout and the conditions that contribute to systemic stress—staffing constraints, health care system financial structures—are extremely important, this chapter focuses largely on patient behavior and how best to meet the needs of indidivuals whose behavior may be perplexing or vexing. The chapter outlines a basic approach to problematic patient conduct in the ICU; details common patterns of exasperating behavior of critically ill patients and practical ways of meeting the individual's needs; and reviews operationalized modes of communication with families of patients in the ICU.

APPROACH TO PROBLEMATIC BEHAVIORS AND GUN VIOLENCE

Critically ill patients can behave in ways that jeopardize ICU activity. Some patients become child-like, crying or whimpering, turning away from care providers, refusing examinations. A number of patients grow demanding of nurses' and physicians' attention; they hurl insults when providers are not as attentive as they would like. Others may be violent in word or action, threatening staff and even punching and kicking caretakers.

Before deciding how to approach a disruptive patient or family member, one must first answer the question "Do I feel safe?" and then "Is the patient safe?" ICU personnel are often taught to override their fears as they perform procedures that demand brisk, decisive action. Unfortunately, such denial may lead physicians and nurses to fail to heed their internal sense of alarm and danger regarding patient behavior, resulting in injury to patients and staff. Particularly when negotiating very powerful emotions and holding life-and-death discussions with family members and those close to patients, some people may become extremely emotionally dysregulated.

Though many patients can become delirious and combative and family members discouraged and dysregulated in critical care settings, few grow violent or use firearms [8,9]. Still, given the overall growing problem of gun violence in the USA, a brief review of hospital-based shootings is timely. According to a study by Kelen and colleagues [10], there were 154 hospital-related shootings at 148 American hospitals between 2000 and 2011. Most shooters were men (91%) and the most frequent areas where shootings occurred included emergency departments (29%), parking lots (23%), and patient rooms (19%). Incidents typically involved a shooter targeting a particular individual, with motives including grudges (27%), suicide (21%), "euthanizing" an ill relative (14%), and prisoner escape (11%). A very low percentage of these incidents involved the targeting of nurses (5%) or physicians (3%).

Although hospital staff cannot readily influence the widespread availability of firearms, the relatively lax gun laws in the USA compared to other nations with far lower rates of gun violence [11], and the inadequacy of mental health services, there are things that medical personnel can do. First, though hospital shootings are very rare events, staff should be encouraged to err on the side of caution—summoning security or police if they fear that there is an imminent threat of confrontation or violence from family members, friends/visitors, or patients themselves. It is not a violation of the Health Insurance Portability and Accountability Act privacy rule to disclose information about a patient to law enforcement when a patient is considered to present a serious threat [12]. In addition, sufficient security cameras, strategic placement of panic buttons, and making certain employees are well trained in emergency procedures not only for traditional "code" situations but also for instances of gun violence are crucial interventions.

"Tuning into" a sense of alarm may involve administering calming medications, summoning security personnel if there is a risk of flight, and/or applying physical restraints in extreme situations [13,14]. Once the safety of the patient, other patients, and staff is assured, examination of the underlying causes of a patient's taxing behavior follows. Because irritability and emotional lability are the final common pathway of myriad medical and psychiatric conditions and of normal emotional responses, precise determination of the etiology of a patient's disruptive behavior is often vexing. Asking and answering the questions listed in Table 161.1 can be helpful in narrowing the vast differential diagnosis.

Delirium is a common source of troublesome patient behavior in the ICU. Patients who are hallucinating or harboring persecutory delusions that ICU staff are torturing them can be immensely problematic. Owing to its potentially lethal nature [15,16], delirium should be ruled out first as the driving force behind a patient's disruptiveness. A full discussion of delirium is provided in Chapter 157.

After delirium has been excluded, it is important to look for major psychiatric illnesses, which are frequently exacerbated by the chaos, vulnerability, and prolonged inner tension associated with being treated in the ICU [17]. The intensivist should discern if the patient has a history of psychotic disorder (e.g., schizophrenia), affective illness (e.g., bipolar or major depressive disorder), or anxiety disorder (e.g., posttraumatic stress or panic disorder), and should—if no contraindications such as drug–drug interactions exist—order any medications that have been effective in treating these conditions in the past. As part of this psychiatric workup, a substance use history also is imperative; data from collateral sources (e.g., family, friends, and therapists) may be necessary to confirm the patient's report. At any step in the process of assessing the roots of patients' problematic behaviors, psychiatric consultation may be useful in establishing and confirming diagnoses and in guiding treatment.

TABLE 161.1

Key Questions about Behavioral Problems in the ICU

Safety
- Is the patient's behavior dangerous? If so, how can I keep the patient and others safe?

Delirium
- Is the patient delirious? If so, am I effectively treating the underlying causes of delirium?

Psychiatric illness
- Does the patient have an anxiety, mood, or psychotic disorder or another psychiatric illness? If so, am I providing adequate treatment for these conditions?

Intoxication and withdrawal
- Is the patient intoxicated with or withdrawing from alcohol or another substance? Am I addressing the untoward effects of withdrawal?

Psychosocial stressors
- Can I reduce pain, sleeplessness, isolation, and other stressors related to being in the ICU?

Personality problems
- What is the patient's predominant mode of coping? How can I best manage this patient's uniquely taxing coping strategies?

While gathering data about psychiatric conditions and substance use, common sources of patient stress in the ICU—pain, sleeplessness, and isolation—should, as much as possible, be eliminated. Biancofiore and colleagues [18] showed that liver transplant recipients and patients who underwent major abdominal surgery identified "being unable to sleep, being in pain, having tubes in nose/mouth, missing husband/wife, and seeing family and friends only a few minutes a day as the major stressors." Provision of adequate analgesia, effective sleep aids, and uninterrupted interaction with individuals closest to a patient often significantly curtails problematic behaviors.

COMMON PATTERNS OF PROBLEMATIC BEHAVIOR

Critical illness leads many patients to feel lonely, dependent, or anxious about the prospect of death; as well, traumatic memories may be re-awakened. To keep these unpleasurable feelings and recollections at bay, ICU patients deploy a broad array of psychologic defenses.

Some patients' patterns of psychologic defense—that is, their personalities—are quite adaptive. By distracting themselves with television; enjoying the company of a loved one at their bedside; or engaging their caretakers with humor, forthrightness, and intellectualization, such patients contribute to ICU cohesion. On the other hand, some people lack the positive emotional backgrounds, reliable social supports, and ample psychologic armamentarium required to deal well with adversity. Such individuals may be said to have *poor psychologic resiliency* [19].

Patients with poor psychologic resiliency fall into two categories: (1) those with personality disorders who probably had difficulty navigating life even before becoming critically ill; and (2) those who have simply regressed and utilize primitive coping mechanisms [20] that, outside the ICU, would be less apparent. Because the focus in the ICU is on the here-and-now, distinguishing between these two categories is unnecessary. More important is recognition of the four pathologic personality styles [21] that frequently engender loathing in ICU personnel and require limit-setting and validation (Table 161.2).

TABLE 161.2

Common Problematic Coping Styles of Patients and Family Members in the ICU

Personality type	Core deficit	Characteristic behavior	Suggested response
Dependent	Hypersensitive to abandonment, inadequacy, and aloneness	• Craves attention • Demands special care • Child-like, easily cries and complains of abandonment and inadequate care	• Schedule exam and rounding times • Anticipate nursing staff changes, physician care shifts, transfer to floor • Validate patient's plight and offer to help within reason
Narcissistic	Hypersensitive to loss of control and stature and defended against looking weak	• Denies severity of illness • Shows bravado • Critical of ICU staff and care	• Acknowledge patient's stature • Enlist patient as active partner in care and decision-making
Obsessive	Hyperaware of loss of control and defended against looking weak	• Excessive focus on medical facts and minutiae • Restricted affect; not apt to "show emotional cards"	• Schedule patient and family meetings • Have a set amount of information to share with patient and family • Provide factual, opposed to nuanced, explanations of data • Avoid emotional commentary or inquiry
Dramatic	Difficulty feeling cared for or thought of except within emotionally extreme exchanges	• Engaging and charming to some staff, denigrating and caustic to others • May have multiple allergies and phobias • May "fire" some staff and take exceptions to rules	• Acknowledge patient's positive attributes • Validate patient's plight and offer to help within reason • Set limits as a team

Adapted from Kahana RJ, Bibring GL: Personality types in medical management, in Zinberg NE (ed): *Psychiatry and Medical Practice in a General Hospital.* New York, NY, International Universities Press, 1965, p 108.

Dependency

Dependent patients demand assistance in nearly every aspect of their ICU experience. Through urgent requests for spoon-feeding, bedpan assistance, pillow adjustment, analgesia, and better food, among sundry other entreaties, dependent patients drive nurses and house officers to distraction. Yet, when examined through an empathic lens, dependent patients are incredibly fearful and leverage demands for care to keep their nurses and doctors in sight, thus reducing their anxiety. In this way, demanding patients are like the toddler who, unable to hold onto the mental image of his mother, wails when she leaves the room. These patients are hypersensitive to being alone. To mitigate these fears, nurses and doctors should make extra efforts to inform them of the care plan, how to call for urgencies, when they plan to return, when rounds will take place, and when family will visit.

Still, for many dependent patients, basic information of this sort is insufficient to quiet their incessant demands for anxiety reduction. In these situations, validation of these patients' feelings, communication that their requests are understood, and explanation that the staff is unable to provide everything these patients want are key. These tasks are accomplished through "I wish" statements. For example, a particularly dependent and anxious patient in a busy ICU pled: "Doctor, I need you to check on me every hour, I am so scared!" The resident physician responded, "Your illness is very severe and frightening and while *I wish* I could visit you every hour, I have many people in the hospital to take care of, so I cannot be here quite so often. I promise, though, that I will visit you before I go home this evening at 5 o'clock and I will introduce you to the doctor who will be taking over." His fear and desire for attention validated, secure in the knowledge his physician would return, this patient became far less anxious and demanding.

Narcissism

Being critically ill in the ICU leads even the most psychologically healthy to feel infantilized; hence, for most patients, regaining a sense of control is extremely important [22]. For some patients, however, this need to regain control takes the form of demands and scathing critique. These patients often admonish nurses ("You're not doing that the right way!"); belittle their doctors (e.g., calling young house staff "Doogie Howser"); and name-drop ("Dr. Smith is an expert cardiologist I play golf with, and he would never allow that").

With such patients, it is best to appeal to, rather than to confront, their narcissism. When the narcissistic patient looks around the ICU, all he sees are his inadequacy, inability, and incapacity. The intravenous pump reminds him he cannot feed himself; the ventilator brings to mind that he cannot breathe unaided; the bedside commode or bedpan is a glaring reminder of his inability to move about nimbly. By using words that remind the patient that, despite his infirmities, he is still a valuable person, one then "joins" the patient and incurs less wrath and invective. Such "joining" can be done by respectfully calling patients "Mr.," "Ms.," and "Dr.," as appropriate. It is also helpful to ask them about their lives outside the hospital, promoting the notion that they are not frail and infantile but able-bodied adults endowed with personal agency but presently suffering critical illness.

The patient with substantial narcissistic needs appreciates any control he can be afforded. Even if this means only controlling the light switch, choosing the hour the physical therapist will arrive, or using patient-controlled analgesia, the narcissistic patient revels in feeling like a partner in his care. Finally, avoidance of power struggles and sharing of dilemmas are key to working with these patients effectively. For example, an astute medical intern said to a "very important person" (VIP) in the ICU: "While I realize the catheter may be uncomfortable, if I were to remove it right now, it is likely I would have to replace it tomorrow. I can do this if you'd like—it is your decision—but I am concerned that this would cause you even greater pain." Knowing he had a choice, the VIP felt greater self-agency and was thus able to defer to the doctor's educated opinion, electing to leave the catheter in for the time being.

Obsessionality

The obsessive patient is rules-based and acts much like a school-aged child clinging to the rules of a board game. Following the obsessive mantra "a place for everything and everything in its place," the obsessive patient wants to know what his X ray shows before it is taken. His day can rise and fall on laboratory minutiae. Like the narcissistic patient, the obsessive individual may feel his control slipping away at times of illness. However, rather than acting in a haughty manner to deny that illness is stripping him of his control, the obsessive patient attempts to attain mastery over his condition through excessive focus on detail. A master of "losing the forest for the trees," the obsessive patient gets lost in the fine points. He asks questions incessantly and wants to manage his own treatment. For example, one obsessive patient with myasthenia gravis saw an "L" next to her hematocrit and demanded to know why she wasn't being transfused when her hematocrit was 32.3%. When her nurse sat down at her bedside and provided a synopsis of her lab work and the team's rationale for management, the patient was soothed. For all patients, but particularly for obsessive ones, it is helpful to: (1) have in mind a set amount of information that the team wants to share with the patient, thus allowing the patient the mastery over illness he craves but without overwhelming him; (2) announce a regular time nurses and physicians will share a progress report; and (3) use scientific/deductive reasoning to explain each step in treatment.

Dramatic Behavior

Patients who are extremely dramatic may project their own thoughts and discomforts onto others or believe their own perceptions and ideas to be entirely accurate. For example, if they are feeling lonely, vulnerable, or inadequately validated, such patients may accuse staff of purposely ignoring them, belittling them, or being incompetent. Meanwhile, they may also project warm feelings and suddenly become overly intimate or familiar with some staff members. Dramatic invidiuals—many of whom meet criteria for borderline or histrionic personality disorder in the official psychiatric parlance [20]—engage their physicians and nurses in relationships that are intensely intimate or staggeringly conflictual. The dramatic patient thus seduces some staff members while alienating others; with some personnel, the dramatic patient acts charming and delightful, whereas with others the dramatic individual is devaluing, belligerent, and toxic. When clinicians who have had completely different experiences with a dramatic patient confer, they are at odds over how to handle the patient's demands. This discord creates tremendous tension, one that is relieved when clinicians acknowledge they have had contradictory emotional experiences with a patient. Once this "split" is named, the team can then strategize how best to set limits (Table 161.3).

Another feature of dramatic patients is their need to convey how much physical pain they are in (e.g., "Doctor, you don't understand the pain I'm going through. I can't possibly do physical therapy"). As with the dependent patient, communicating understanding of the patient's plight—in other words, validating their feelings—is important. Statements such as, "Given all that you've been through, I can only imagine how hard this is" can

TABLE 161.3

Principles of Establishing Limits and Negotiating Conflicts in the ICU

- Acknowledge the patient's real struggles.
- Explain limits in a clear and concise manner. Avoid jargon such as, "You are demonstrating unsafe behavior, sir. This is a non-smoking environment," and simply offer, "You can't smoke while you're in the unit."
- Before speaking with the patient, know what areas, if any, are flexible and make concessions to the patient in those areas.
- Determine consequences for transgressing limits in advance.
- Avoid long, drawn-out arguments, because they are rarely, if ever, useful. Leaving the patient's bedside in order to cool down, think of a new strategy, or consult a colleague is better than acting impulsively.

Adapted from Winnick JA, Wool CA, Geringer ES, et al: Problematic behavior of patients, family, and staff in the intensive care unit, in Irwin RS, Rippe JM (eds): *Irwin and Rippe's Intensive Care Medicine.* 5th ed. Philadelphia, PA, Lippincott Williams and Wilkins, 2003, p 2192.

be helpful. Further, even more than what is said, listening and eliciting the patient's experience is usually most beneficial: "I want to make sure I better understand what you are going through. If you are willing to share, I would be grateful."

> When people talk, listen completely. Don't be thinking what you're going to say.
>
> *Ernest Hemingway* [23]

COMMUNICATION WITH FAMILIES

Almost always for better, but occasionally for worse, family members are not mere visitors to the ICU [24]. Family members play an integral role in encouraging and comforting critically ill patients and informing distant loved ones of patients' progress or problems. With the exception of those patients who, prior to hospitalization, expressed their preferences for medical care, relatives are also responsible for learning about a patient's diagnosis and prognosis and making decisions for critically ill patients who lack the capacity to make medical choices for themselves.

It can be difficult to function in these roles, because the experience of having a family member in the ICU takes a psychologic toll. Family members of ICU patients suffer depression and anxiety; up to one-third of family members suffer posttraumatic stress symptoms 3 months after their family members are discharged from the ICU [5].

Adequate communication between ICU staff and family members of ICU patients is central to reducing family stress and dissatisfaction [25,26]; decreasing conflict around end-of-life decisions; limiting futile interventions [27]; and curtailing strife between families and ICU staff [28]. Some general principles of communication with families in the ICU include: providing clear and concise medical information; scheduling and keeping appointment times to meet with families; respecting the uniqueness of the family and the patient, listening for things that are special about both; and providing early diagnostic and prognostic information [29], even if this means saying, "I'm not sure" (Table 161.4).

Even with good communication, problems arise. Occasionally, before the physician can provide information regarding prognosis, family members will foreclose discussion and disagree with the

TABLE 161.4

CORE Principles of Communication with Families in the ICU

Clear

Provide family members with clear, concise descriptions of the patient's condition. Avoid jargon.

On Time

Schedule appointments for family conferences or treatment updates and try, as best as possible, to be on time. Send a representative if you must.

Respect the Patient's Uniqueness

These appointments are as much about what you say as how well you listen. Pay close attention to people's names and what makes the patient special.

Early Diagnosis and Prognosis

Even if it means saying, "I'm not sure," try to inform the family early in the ICU stay.

doctor or other family members about how much workup or end-of-life treatment to pursue. Some special situations related to the emotional life of family members bear examination in further detail. These include: the guilty family member; the family member compelled to preserve the dignity or "fighter status" of their loved one; and the vindictive family member. Physician interventions or "conversational reframes" in these situations are aimed, not at coercion, but at enhancement of doctor–family and family–family conversation about how best to proceed with a critically ill family member's care.

Occasionally, the sibling, parent, or child of an ICU patient—who has played little role in the ailing family member's life—attempts to rectify this estrangement by coming to the rescue at the eleventh hour. To assuage their guilt, these family members demand that "everything" be done for their relative, to the point of pushing for futile assessments and treatments. Reframing the dilemma for these family members, giving them a sense of authority, and explaining how they can be helpful can change the family–staff dialogue. For example, one intensivist told a particularly guilty son whose mother had suffered a severe stroke: "I know you've had to be away for several years and not been able to play a day-to-day role in your mother's care. However, this is a really big opportunity to help support your mother, who is dying, and your sister, who is struggling. You can help your sister come to a well thought-out decision about your mother's care." By educating this young person about how he might help in the here-and-now, while also indirectly addressing his guilt, the physician altered this family member's attitude.

When dealing with end-of-life care, some family members will demand that "everything" be done because they don't want their loved one to appear weak. "But he's a fighter," some relatives protest. In these situations, one should listen closely to why it is important that the patient's status as a "fighter" be maintained. Once this information is obtained, the ICU staff member can illustrate how the patient remains a "fighter" even when heroic measures are scaled back.

Some family members may be angry with the patient. Wasserman studied responses provided by relatives of patients who had attempted suicide and found that a family's request for "do not resuscitate" orders sometimes reflected anger toward the patient [30]. Eliciting these feelings during a family meeting may help family members acknowledge the hostile origins of their decisions and feel they have acted less impulsively and more thoughtfully about how to proceed with a loved one's care.

Communication between ICU staff and a patient's family may be disrupted when a family member does not want to make decisions on behalf of a loved one [31] or suffers symptoms of anxiety, depression, or another psychiatric illness. Such family members may derive great benefit from consultation with the ICU's social worker or an outpatient psychiatrist. Finally, in those situations where discussions over care reach a standstill and interventions stimulate little movement, referral to an ethics consultant or committee (particularly with regard to end-of-life care) or patient-rights advocate (regarding a family member's grievance) may be helpful in resolving conflict.

When an intensive care team faces the challenge of sharing with family members and patients "bad news" and having end-of-life care discussions, utilizing the SPIKES framework [32,33] for communicating with families may be particularly useful (Table 161.5). Utilizing this framework, practitioners pay special attention to Setting up the interview; eliciting patient's and family's Perceptions about their illness and treatment; Inviting patients and family members to be active participants in the process asking them about the quality (type) and quantity of information they would like; providing the patient and their supports with medical Knowledge; Empathically responding to the Emotions of those hearing bad news; and Summarizing and Sharing a Strategy for how best to proceed. Ultimately, no matter what protocol one utilizes, clinicians should remember that: (1) having a mindful framework versus "therapeutic winging it" is key; (2) there is great medical and psychologic *intensity* in this type of work and, as such, any kind of news (be it good or bad) is hard to deliver [34]; (3) even under the best circumstances, the most compassionate caregivers can sometimes come across as less empathic [35]; (4) problematic interactions can be an opportunity for self- and team reflection and improvement; and (5) learning to address the needs of families better requires an openness to reflection and whole-team commitment [36].

TABLE 161.5

Empathically Sharing "Bad News" and Collaborating with Families: The "SPIKES" Protocol

Setting

- Set up the communication space for privacy
- Have the *right* people there (people important to the patient and to his/her care)
- Have tissues ready
- Anticipate what questions might be asked/information might be desired and have this ready
- Set aside sufficient time to have a thorough discussion
- If an interpreter is needed for optimal communication, have that individual ready

Perceiving

- Listen and assess: "What questions do you have?" "What is your understanding of ___'s condition?" "What is your understanding of why we performed this test?"

Inviting

- Appreciate that some patients and families may want technical information, whereas others want a summary
- Ask questions like: "What is most important for us to cover?" "How much detail would you like me to go into regarding what we've learned or about the proposed treatment?"

Providing Knowledge

- Introduce ideas with sensitivity, beginning with phrases like: "I am sorry to say that . . ."
- Pause and ask for questions and ask for an invitation from the patient/family to continue
- Use lay language, avoiding jargon. Avoid the insensitivity of bluntness.

Being Emotionally-attuned and Empathic

- Observe patients'/families' emotions
- Consider that emotion and name it to oneself
- Identify the reason for this emotion (it may be coming as a surprise or confirm a worst fear)
- Connect the patient's affect and what you believe is driving it (e.g., "I had also hoped for a better result.")
- Assess that you have been accurately attuned

Summarizing and Outlining Strategy

- Summarize what has been discussed and reiterate the management strategy

Adapted from Baile WF, Buckman R, et al: SPIKES—a six-step protocol for delivering bad news: application to the patient with cancer. *Oncologist* 5:302, 2000.

CONCLUSIONS

Physicians, nurses, and other members of the critical care team are often confronted with patients and families whom they find unnerving, taxing, or even dangerous. Addressing difficult interactions and challenging personalities entails a commitment on the part of the practitioner to take an empathic stance, recognizing that behind the most troubling behavior is a person, someone in anguish whose words and actions represent his/her best attempts to cope with pain.

ICU staff should work to establish and maintain their and patients' safety; exclude causes of disruptive behavior that can be amenable to medical intervention; and examine patients' and family members' predominant mechanisms of defense (as well as their own). Patients and family members with traumatic pasts, poor coping strategies, and/or formal personality disorders often respond to limit-setting and validation of their distress, entailing a description of how they are expected to act and what they can expect from their caregivers. Family members and loved ones play a crucial role in critical care; ensuring that they are collaborative members of the ICU team involves providing clear and early diagnostic information; conveying respect for the uniqueness of patients and their familes; and providing regular, scheduled updates and clear, systematic team meetings regarding major decisions.

References

1. Camus A: Notebooks: 1942–1951 Vol. 2. Chicago, Ivan R Dee Publishers, 2010.
2. Myhren H, Ekeberg O, Stokland O: Job satisfaction and burnout among intensive care unit nurses and physicians. *Crit Care Res Pract* 2013:786176, 2013.
3. Le Gall JR, Azoulay E, Embriaco, et al: Burn out syndrome among critical care workers. *Bull Acad Natl Med* 195:389, 2011.
4. Rattray JE, Johnston M, Wildsmith JA: Predictors of emotional outcomes of intensive care. *Anaesthesia* 60:1085, 2005.
5. Azoulay E, Pochard F, Kentish-Barnes N, et al: Risk of post-traumatic stress symptoms in family members of intensive care unit patients. *Am J Respir Crit Care Med* 171:987, 2005.
6. Embriaco N, Hralech S, Azoulay E, et al: Symptoms of depression in ICUD physicians. *Ann Intensive Care* 2:34, 2012.
7. Groves JE: Taking care of the hateful patient. *N Engl J Med* 298:883, 1978.
8. Goralnick E, Walls R: An active shooter in our hospital. *Lancet* 385:1728, 2015.
9. Adashi EY, Gao H, Cohen G: Hospital-based active shooter incidents: sanctuary under fire. *JAMA* 313:1209, 2015.
10. Kelen GD, Catlett CL, Kubit JG, et al: Hospital-based shootings in the United States: 2000–2011. *Ann Emerg Med* 60:790, 2012.
11. Grinshteyn E, Hemenway D: Violent death rates: the US compared with other high-income OECD countries, 2010. *Am J Med* 129:266–273, 2015.
12. U.S. Department of Health and Human Services: Statement from HHS Secretary Sebelius on President's Sandy Hook response plan. http://www.hhs.gov/about/news/2013/01/16/statement-from-hhs-secretary-sebelius-on-presidents-sandy-hook-response-plan.html. Accessed December 31, 2015.

13. Rincon HG, Granados M, Unutzer J, et al: Prevalence, detection, and treatment of anxiety, depression, and delirium in the adult critical care unit. *Psychosomatics* 42:391, 2001.
14. Trenoweth S: Perceiving risk in dangerous situations: risk of violence among mental health inpatients. *J Adv Nurs* 42:278, 2003.
15. Shehabi Y, Riker RR, Bokesch PM, et al: Delirium duration and mortality in lightly sedated, mechanically ventilated intensive care patients. *Crit Care Med* 38:2311, 2010.
16. Ely EW, Shintani A, Truman B, et al: Delirium as a predictor of mortality in mechanically ventilated patients in the intensive care unit. *JAMA* 291:1753, 2004.
17. Whitehome K, Gaudine A, Meadus R, et al: Lived experience of the intensive care unit for patients who experienced delirium. *Am J Crit Care* 24:474, 2015.
18. Biancofiore G, Bindi ML, Romanelli AM, et al: Stress-inducing factors in ICUs: what liver transplant recipients experience and what caregivers perceive. *Liver Transpl* 11:967, 2005.
19. Karatsoreos IN, McEwan BS: The neurobiology and physiology of resilience and adaptation across the life course. *J Child Psychol Psychiatry* 54:337, 2013.
20. Vaillant GE: *Adapation to Life*. Boston, Little, Brown, 1977.
21. Bibring GL, Kahana RJ: *Lectures in Medical Psychology: An Introduction ot the Care of Patients*. New York, NY, International Universities Press, 1968.
22. American Psychiatric Association. *Diagnostic and Statistical Manual of Mental Disorders*. 5th ed. Washington, American Psychiatric Publishing, 2013.
23. Phillips LW (ed): *Ernest Hemingway on Writing*. New York, NY, Scribner, 1999.
24. Molter NC: Families are not visitors in the critical care unit. *Dimens Crit Care Nurs* 13:2, 1994.
25. Kodall S, Stametz RA, Bengier AC, et al: Family experience with intensive care unit care: association of self-reported family conferences and family satisfaction. *J Crit Care* 29:641, 2014.
26. Carlson EB, Spain DA, Mhutadie L, et al: Care and caring in the intensive care unit: family members distress and perceptions about staff skills, communication, and emotional support. *J Crit Care* 30(3):557–561, 2015.
27. Rivera S, Kim D, Garone S, et al: Motivating factors in futile clinical interventions. *Chest* 119:1944, 2001.
28. Fins JJ, Solomon MZ: Communication in intensive care settings:tThe challenge of futility disputes. *Crit Care Med* 29(2 Suppl):N10, 2001.
29. Leclaire MM, Oakes JM, Weinert CR: Communication of prognostic information for critically ill patients. *Chest* 128:1728, 2005.
30. Wasserman D: Passive euthanasia to attempted suicide: one form of aggressiveness of relatives. *Acta Psychiatr Scand* 79:460, 1989.
31. Azoulay E, Pochard F, Chevret S, et al: Half the family members of intensive care unit patients do not want to share in the decision-making process: a study in 78 French intensive care units. *Crit Care Med* 32:1832, 2004.
32. Baile WF, Buckman R, Lenzi R, et al: SPIKES—a six-step protocol for delivering bad news: application to the patient with cancer. *Oncologist* 5:302, 2000.
33. Kaplan M: SPIKES: a framework for breaking bad news to patients with cancer. *Clin J Oncol Nurs* 14:514, 2010.
34. Warraich HJ: Breaking good news can be as hard as breaking bad. *The New York Times*. September 10, 2015. Available at: http://well.blogs.nytimes.com/2015/09/10/breaking-good-news-can-be-as-hard-as-breaking-bad/?_r=0. Accessed November 11, 2015.
35. Tanco K, Rhondall W, Perez-Cruz P, et al: Patient perception of physician compassion after more optimistic vs a less optimistic message: a randomized clinical trial. *JAMA Oncol* 1:176, 2015.
36. Wessman BT, Sona C, Schallom M: Improving caregivers' perceptions regarding patient goals of care/end-of-life issues for the multidisciplinary critical care team. *J Intensive Care Med* 2015.

Chapter 162 ■ Recognition and Management of Staff Stress in the Intensive Care Unit

GUY MAYTAL

The intensive care unit (ICU) is a structurally, functionally, and socially complex entity with its own culture, personnel, protocols, and challenges [1]. Today, such units are frequently filled to capacity with complicated patients suffering from multiple life-threatening illnesses. As technology has advanced, patients with once terminal illnesses are surviving episodes of deterioration, raising ever more complicated ethical issues [2].

This environment can affect ICU staff adversely. The psychologic pressures on ICU personnel are myriad: increasingly sophisticated technologic advances; overwhelming amounts of data; burdensome demands on caretakers; long hours; nursing shortages; and trying ethical issues. Staff may not be prepared to handle their emotional reactions to these challenges while simultaneously tending to the technical and clinical aspects of intensive care.

This chapter reviews the general concepts of stress and burnout; the tensions associated with training and working as a physician or a nurse in an intensive care setting; and strategies for managing staff stress in the ICU.

STRESS

The physiologic, cognitive, and affective facets of stress are based on the seminal work of Selye [3] on the *general adaptation syndrome*. Selye defined stress as the nonspecific result of any demand on the body, and observed that different organisms and biologic systems respond to stress in a stereotyped and predictable three-part pattern. The initial alarm reaction (characterized by activation of the sympathetic nervous system and various hormonal, immunologic, and psychologic responses) is followed by the stage of resistance, during which the organism establishes a temporary homeostasis by marshalling various reserves to adapt to the new situation. However, the body's ability to adapt is finite, and, with continued exposure to the stressor, its reserves become depleted and the organism enters a stage of exhaustion.

Researchers in biology and sociology have expanded this work to encompass processes ranging from individual cellular responses to stress to the reactions of individuals and social systems to external and internal stressors. Over the past 50 years, the study of occupational stress (i.e., stress due to one's work situation) has consistently demonstrated the significant adverse impact of excessive occupational stress on physical health, mental health, and decision-making. Regardless of the field, low job satisfaction is often predicted by a small number of factors: little participation in decision-making, ambiguity about job security, poor use of skills, and lack of clarity about role. These stressors are consistent with the *demand–control model* of the effects of job demands on worker' well-being. This model predicts that the fewer demands and more control a worker has on the job, the less stress he will experience [4]. For example, the Return to Work Study found that subjects with low-demand, high-control jobs were substantially more likely to return to work after a period of medical disability [5].

Of the other well-recognized occupational stressors (including noise-related stress, nonstandard work hours, and excessive fatigue) [4], work overload and a poor social environment at work are the most significant determinants of work-related health problems. In particular, work overload and overall low job satisfaction are strongly associated with the development of psychiatric (particularly affective) problems. A meta-analysis of job satisfaction and health outcomes examined 485 studies (267,995 individuals) and concluded that poor job satisfaction was strongly associated with the development of depressive and other affective illnesses [6].

In addition to physical and mental health, decision-making also can be adversely affected by high levels of stress [7]. Awareness of one's limited knowledge and problem-solving capacities, fear that bad outcomes will occur regardless of which choice is made, worry about making a fool of oneself, and fear of loss of self-esteem if the decision is wrong can force decision-makers to come to "premature closure." Premature closure is a type of cognitive error in which the physician fails to consider reasonable alternatives after an initial diagnosis is made. It is a common cause of misdiagnosis. Such premature closure can lead to incorrect or even harmful decisions [8,9].

In a work environment, including the ICU, stressors (both work-related and non–work-related, both internal and external) affect each individual in a unique manner as mediated by a variety of factors. The interaction between stressors and mediating factors can lead the individual to experience either strain or job satisfaction [10]. When this interaction leads to strain that is chronic or particularly intense (or both), burnout can occur.

BURNOUT SYNDROME

Coined by the clinical psychologist Herbert Freudenberger [11] in 1974, *burnout syndrome* has been viewed as a behavioral or a psychologic condition, as well as a process or a syndrome [12]. Research during the past three decades (especially by Maslach and colleagues) has narrowed the current definition to encompass the spheres of emotional exhaustion, depersonalization (i.e., negative or cynical attitudes regarding work), and the absence of personal accomplishment—particularly among individuals who do "people work" (Table 162.1) [13]. Although emotional exhaustion is the key component of the syndrome, people with all three symptoms experience the greatest degree of burnout [14]. Ultimately, this definition describes a process whereby highly motivated and committed individuals lose their spirit; their motivation for creativity; and, in the ICU, their belief in their ability to help people [15,16].

Many have argued that the cause of burnout lies in our need to believe that our lives are meaningful and that what we do is useful and important [15]. Work takes on a central role in providing some people with this sense of meaning in their lives. In a supportive environment, highly motivated individuals reach their goals and achieve success, which leads to a sense of meaningfulness that itself increases the original motivation. However, in an unsupportive environment, these individuals cannot accomplish what they set out to do and consequently fail. For people who expect a sense of meaningfulness from work, such failure often leads to burnout.

Everyone experiences stress, but only those who start their careers with high levels of idealism, motivation, and commitment are at risk for burning out: "You cannot burn out unless you were 'on fire' initially" [15]. Burnout occurs almost exclusively among individuals who work with people, arising from the emotional stress that such interactions engender. ICU staff tend to be idealistic, committed, and driven—the very attributes that render them susceptible to burnout.

For the individual, burnout is characterized by physical, emotional, and attitudinal symptoms. Physical symptoms are nonspecific and include chronic fatigue, headaches, insomnia, weight changes, and worsening of chronic medical conditions. Burnout can lead to increased consumption of tobacco, alcohol, and illicit drugs. Emotional symptoms include despair, hopelessness, and depression. Relationships can become disrupted and the ability to work can be compromised [13].

On an organizational level, cynical attitudes toward work, colleagues, and patients can isolate coworkers and precipitate staff conflicts. At some hospitals, job dissatisfaction and burnout have led to absenteeism, accelerated staff turnover, and severe staff shortages, which may limit the number of ICU beds available for patient admissions [17].

STRESS AND BURNOUT IN HEALTH CARE PROFESSIONALS

Stress is a common aspect of medical practice for physicians, nurses, and trainees. Not surprisingly, studies have reported a high prevalence of burnout in health care professionals. Rates of burnout among physicians range from 25% to 60%, depending on working conditions and medical specialty [18–20]; burnout can develop at any stage of a physician's career. Shanafelt and colleagues surveyed 27,000 physicians and received 7,200 responses. They found that 45.8% of respondents had at least one symptom of burnout. In addition, physicians were more likely (than the general population) to have symptoms of burnout (37.9% vs. 27.8%) and to be dissatisfied with work–life balance (40.2% vs. 23.2%) [21]. Nurses also experience high levels of burnout. Studies of nurses indicate rates of 35% to 50%, depending on working conditions, clinical setting, and level of autonomy [14]. Multiple factors have been associated with burnout of health care professionals, but the best characterized include: heavy workload; stressful work environments (e.g., ICUs); severity of patients' illnesses; and conflicts with coworkers or patients [22,23].

Physicians who experience burnout suffer physical (e.g., anorexia, insomnia, tachycardia, and hypertension) and psychologic (e.g., irritability, frustration, apathy, indecision, and depression) symptoms. Burnout leads to increased nurse distress, decreased patient satisfaction, increased mortality in the ICU, and substance abuse [24,25].

Along with its professional impact, burnout also has a significant personal impact on physicians and medical trainees. Oreskovich and colleagues surveyed 7,288 American physicians regarding their substance use behavior and associated risk factors. They found that 12.9% of male respondents and 21.4% of female respondents met criteria for alcohol abuse or dependence [26]. They also found that burnout was independently associated with alcohol use or dependence. Other associated factors included depression, suicidal ideation, lower quality of life, and lower career satisfaction. Similarly, a national study of 4,402 US medical students found that burnout was independently associated with an increased risk of alcohol abuse or dependence [27].

Just as concerning are the effects of burnout on the personal lives of physicians. Physicians' personal relationships with spouses and children are damaged by burnout: "Being a physician is one of the few socially acceptable reasons for abandoning a family" [28]. Even more alarming is that burnout may be a contributing factor to increased suicidal ideation among physicians and physician trainees. A prospective study found that burnout at baseline was an independent predictor of suicidal ideation over the following year, whereas recovery from burnout has been shown to decrease the frequency of suicidal ideation [29]. Burnout clearly has a significant impact on the medical profession and on the public it serves.

STRESS AND ITS CONSEQUENCES IN PHYSICIAN TRAINING

Competitive, highly driven, and able to delay short-term gratification indefinitely, people attracted to medicine are more likely to have personalities that render them susceptible to the detrimental effects of stress and to burnout. As a rule, they are success-driven, tend to be "people-pleasers," and are unable to recognize their own limitations. Similarly, they do not often understand or attend to their own emotional and psychologic

TABLE 162.1

Three Components of Burnout

Emotional exhaustion	Reduced energy and job enthusiasm Emotional and cognitive distancing from the job
Depersonalization	Cynicism Lack of engagement and distancing from patients Treatment of patients as inanimate, unfeeling objects
Absence of personal accomplishment	A significantly diminished sense of efficacy, effectiveness, involvement, commitment, engagement, and capacity to innovate, change, and improve

Adapted from McManus IC, Keeling A, Paice E: Stress, burnout and doctors' attitudes to work are determined by personality and learning style: a twelve year longitudinal study of UK medical graduates. *BMC Med* 2:29, 2004.

health and, citing the need to be "strong," squelch their emotional reactions to stressful events [30,31].

Medical practice has changed dramatically over the past several decades, and many physicians who entered medicine to enhance their sense of control and mastery find themselves in a medical system that is increasingly out of their control [31]. Physicians have experienced a decline in status and autonomy alongside mounting work pressures. Under closer scrutiny by regulatory agencies and insurance companies, physicians have had to contend with ever growing amounts of paperwork. Owing to increased pressure to discharge patients, the acuity of patients in hospital settings has increased, "turnover" is more rapid, and interventions are more aggressive.

House officers, in particular, face a unique constellation of stressors. According to a review of burnout during residency training, the stressors faced by house officers are varied and include: burnout that is already present during medical school; intense time demands; lack of control over time management or planning; inherently difficult job situations; and strained interpersonal relationships [32]. All of these contribute to the risk of burnout in house officers.

In recent years, more quantitative evaluations of burnout have been undertaken at both the medical-student and resident level. A significant proportion of medical school graduates enter residency with high rates of burnout. One study of 1,428 fourth-year medical students found an overall prevalence of burnout of up to 49% [33]. Once in residency, this prevalence continues at about the same level or even increases to 60% [34]. Another study found the overall burnout rate in residency to range from 27% to 75% depending on specialty [35].

In an important longitudinal study that examined the impact of job stress on house officers, Tyssen and colleagues [36] followed 371 medical students from their last semester through the end of their internship. They found that 11% of these interns had mental health problems. The most important predictive factor was perceived job stress. Moreover, perceiving oneself as deficient in clinical skills or knowledge at the end of medical school was related to a mental health problem during internship. Importantly, gender, lack of sleep, and number of hours worked weekly were not linked to mental health problems.

More recently, Shapiro and colleagues [37] studied the relationship between loneliness and social connectedness in an urban academic medical center internal medicine residency program. They found a high rate of burnout among the residents (47%) and a dose-dependent correlation between how lonely a resident felt and the degree of burnout.

More worrisome, burnout has been clearly demonstrated to affect residents' clinical performance. Several studies have shown that patients cared for by residents with burnout are at increased risk of receiving suboptimal care and experiencing a medical error [38]. Burnout also impedes acquisition and assimilation of new knowledge, an essential purpose of residency. A study of nearly all US internal medicine residents found that those with burnout scored significantly lower on a national standardized examination of medical knowledge [39]. The differences in medical knowledge across the continuum of burnout were as large as the differences observed across an entire year of residency training.

Stress and burnout are associated not only with work hours but with a variety of internal and external factors; quality of teamwork, personality characteristics, and trouble with the work/home interface all contribute to the development of stress and burnout in house officers. A 12-year longitudinal study of medical school graduates found that specific personality traits (e.g., high neuroticism, low extraversion, and low conscientiousness) measured while in medical school strongly predicted the development of stress, burnout, and job satisfaction as a staff physician [40].

Despite work-hour restrictions, residents and fellows continue to shoulder stressful workloads that have a significant impact on their physiology and psychology. Gopal and coworkers [41] studied a single cohort of residents before (2003) and after (2004) restrictions on work hours were implemented. Residents in 2004 had less burnout, emotional exhaustion, sleep deprivation, and depression. However, the residents did not perceive any significant changes in their quality of life, and their learner satisfaction was significantly reduced.

STRESS AND BURNOUT AMONG INTENSIVISTS

Staff physicians—in particular those who work in ICUs—have a high prevalence of burnout syndrome. The protracted stress of working as a physician can lead to lower-quality patient care, disruptions in personal relationships, and even impairment of physical health [42]. Intensivists labor in an atmosphere of perpetual stress and often limited rewards. In addition, society often has unrealistic expectations of the physician not only as a professional but also as a spouse, parent, employer, and community member. Failure to live up to any of these can lead to a sense of failure [42].

Studies have attempted to quantify the way in which these stressors affect physicians who work in intensive care settings. Coomber and coworkers [42] surveyed all members of the Intensive Care Society in the UK (85% response rate, 758 respondents) to identify "distressed" doctors and to relate this state to "repeated and long-term exposure to job stressors." They found that nearly 30% of the physicians surveyed were distressed, 12% were depressed, and 3% had suicidal thoughts. These physicians reported that the most stressful aspects of their work were the feeling of being overstretched, the effect of work hours and stress on personal/family life, and the pressure to compromise standards when resources were limited.

In a survey of 978 French intensivists, Embriaco and colleagues [22] found that 46.5% had a high level of burnout syndrome. Risk factors included female sex, increased workload, and conflicts with coworkers. Workload (as measured by number of shifts per month and length of time from the last day off) was associated with higher rates of burnout. Similarly, in a survey of 6,000 American physicians, female physicians were 60% more likely to report burnout than their male counterparts [43]. Conflicts with coworkers are associated with higher levels of burnout, whereas good relationships with nurses are a protective factor [22,43].

More recently, van Mol and colleagues completed a systematic review of the literature on burnout among health care professionals in intensive care settings. Reviewing 40 studies (including a total of 14,770 respondents), they found the prevalence of burnout among ICU physicians to range from 14% (following a preventive intervention) to as high as 70.1% [44]. The authors concluded that working in an ICU correlates with a substantial risk of emotional distress.

STRESS AND BURNOUT AMONG INTENSIVE CARE UNIT NURSES

Although nurses and physicians work in the same physical environment, nurses have unique working conditions; emphasize different aspects of clinical care; and experience different stresses. Nurses usually work in the ICU indefinitely, compared to residents, and even critical care fellows and attendings, who rotate through different units in the hospital. Despite their relative permanence in the ICU, nurses do not generally accrue as much autonomy and stature as do physicians, which may lead to stress over career and organizational structure [45,46].

An important stressor that is frequently overlooked in the ICU is workplace violence. The ICU is often a setting of great emotional intensity for patients and their families. This can sometimes manifest as violent behavior. The ICU is also a setting where patients are delirious and agitated and can lash out physically against staff. Nursing staff in particular is vulnerable to physical violence by patients and families, with between 25% and 80% of acute-care nurses having reported patient violence in one form or another [47,48]. The short- or long-term exposure to any type of violence can result in negative consequences for nurses and adversely affect organizational climate. For nurses, there may be both physical consequences (e.g., injuries, temporary or permanent disability) and psychologic consequences (e.g., anger, fear, anxiety, posttraumatic stress disorder, reduced job satisfaction) [49,50].

There are also negative outcomes of workplace violence at the organizational level, including high staff turnover; decreased morale; nurse absenteeism; more frequent medical errors; more workplace injury claims; and increased costs due to disability leaves [51]. In Canada, 33% of workplace violence incidents occur in health-care and social-service settings, compared to 14% in accommodation or food services and 11% in educational services [52].

Multiple studies have found that nurses who work in critical care settings are at high risk of burnout (up to 30% to 40% of nurses surveyed) and higher risk of burnout compared to nurses in other settings [46,53]. Factors commonly found to be associated with burnout among critical care nurses include moral distress, emotional exhaustion, poor physical well-being, and limited autonomy regarding end-of-life situations [54].

MANAGEMENT OF STAFF STRESS AND BURNOUT IN THE INTENSIVE CARE UNIT

Given the deleterious effects of stress and burnout on ICU staff and patients, it is important to reduce and manage their impact. Various interventions for addressing this fall into several categories: enhancing a healthful lifestyle as a buffer against burnout; formal resilience training for ICU staff; and group-based interventions for managing stress and burnout. All have been shown to have efficacy in small trials or in descriptive papers; in addition, there is a growing number of studies demonstrating their statistical and clinical significance.

Lifestyle interventions aim to reduce staff stress and include relaxation training, time management, assertiveness training, team building, and meditation [13]. Strategies for coping, as proposed in the *Bulletin of the American College of Surgeons*, include maintaining healthful personal relationships and spiritual practices, seeking health care when needed, maintaining appropriate nutrition and physical fitness, and establishing work–life balance [55]. Having a peer network, supportive mentors, and institutional support are necessary for the success of these interventions.

Resilience refers to the ability of individuals to absorb life's challenges and to carry on and persevere in the face of adversity; it is an internal resource for mitigating the negative effects of stress and maintaining mental health [56,57]. In recent years, different resilience training programs have been developed and studied. A recent meta-analysis found that resilience training programs have a small to moderate effect on improving resilience and other mental health outcomes [58]. Several small studies indicate that resilience training for physicians and nurses can ameliorate or prevent the onset of burnout [59–61].

Groups and workshops have been reported as useful in managing stress [62]. Gunasingam and colleagues described a study where medical residents were randomized to four debriefing sessions over 2 months or no debriefing sessions [63]. Residents in the debriefing sessions found them to be a source of emotional and social support. McCue and Sachs [64] described the effectiveness of a stress management workshop for medical and pediatric residents; it cost little, was positively received, and demonstrated significant short-term improvement in stress and burnout scores.

On the organizational level, adequate staffing, shared decision-making, active review of unit policies and procedures, freeing up time for patient care or research, bolstering administrative support, and allowing flexibility to curtail work/home conflict may help reduce stress and increase job satisfaction [65].

CONCLUSION

Recognizing and attending to staff stress in the ICU are necessary to ensure the continued effectiveness and well-being of each individual and of the unit as a whole. Left unaddressed, staff stress and burnout can exact a heavy price. As Civetta [66] wrote:

> We must accentuate the positive qualities of human capabilities that are beyond technological advancement. . . . A smile, a touch, confidence and security are still beyond our programming capabilities. . . . We must focus on our distinct human qualities of insight and caring. In this way, the popular view that intensive care is a depersonalizing environment can be replaced by the recognition that human beings are caring for human beings.

References

1. Conway J, McMillan M: Exploring the culture of an ICU: the imperative for facilitative leadership. *Nurs Leadersh Forum* 6:117, 2002.
2. Flannery L, Ramjan LM, Peters K: End-of-life decisions in the Intensive Care Unit (ICU)—exploring the experiences of ICU nurses and doctors—a critical literature review. *Aust Crit Care* 2015; 29(2):97–103.
3. Selye H: History of the stress concept, in Goldberger L, Breznitz S (eds): *Handbook of Stress: Theoretical and Clinical Aspects*. 2nd ed. New York, Free Press, 1993, p 7.
4. Karasek R, Theorell T: *Healthy Work: Stress, Productivity and the Reconstruction of Working Life*. New York, Basic Books, 1990.
5. Haveraaen LA, Skarpaas LS, Berg JE, Aas RW: Do psychological job demands, decision control and social support predict return to work three months after the end of a return-to-work (RTW) programme? the rapid-RTW cohort study. *Work* 2015;53(1):61–71.
6. Faragher EB, Cass M, Cooper CL: The relationship between job satisfaction and health: a meta-analysis. *Occup Environ Med* 62:105, 2005.
7. Pottier P, Dejoie T, Hardouin JB, et al: Effect of stress on clinical reasoning during simulated ambulatory consultations. *Med Teach* 35:472, 2013.
8. Janis IL: Decision making under stress, in Goldberger L, Breznitz S (eds): *Handbook of Stress: Theoretical and Clinical Aspects*. 2nd ed. New York, Free Press, 1993, p 56.

9. Kumar B, Kanna B, Kumar S: The pitfalls of premature closure: clinical decision-making in a case of aortic dissection. *BMJ Case Rep* 2011. doi:10.1136/bcr.08.2011.4594.
10. Cooper CL, Sloan SJ, Williams S: *Occupational Stress Indicator: Management Guide*. Windsor, UK, NFER-Nelson, 1988.
11. Freudenberger HJ: Staff burnout. *J Soc Issues* 30:159, 1974.
12. Paine WS (ed): *Job Stress and Burnout*. Beverly Hills, CA, Sage Publications, 1982.
13. Maslach C, Schaufeli WB, Leiter MP: Job burnout. *Annu Rev Psychol* 52:397, 2001.
14. Embriaco N, Papazian L, Kentish-Barnes N, et al: Burnout syndrome among critical care healthcare workers. *Curr Opin Crit Care* 13:482, 2007.
15. Pines AM: Burnout, in Goldberger L, Breznitz S (eds): *Handbook of Stress, Theoretical and Clinical Aspects*. 2nd ed. New York, Free Press, 1993, p 386.
16. Marshall RE, Kasman C: Burnout in the neonatal intensive care unit. *Pediatrics* 65:1161, 1980.
17. Maslach C, Pines A: Burnout, the loss of human caring, in Pines A, Maslach C (eds): *Experiencing Social Psychology*. New York, Random House, 1979.
18. Grassi L, Magnani K: Psychiatric morbidity and burnout in the medical profession: an Italian study of general practitioners and hospital physicians. *Psychother Psychosom* 69:329, 2000.
19. van Mol MM, Kompanje EJ, Benoit DD, et al: The prevalence of compassion fatigue and burnout among healthcare professionals in intensive care units: a systematic review. *PLoS One* 10:e0136955, 2015.
20. Merlani P, Verdon M, Businger A, et al: Burnout in ICU caregivers: a multicenter study of factors associated to centers. *Am J Respir Crit Care Med* 184:1140, 2011.
21. Shanafelt TD, Boone S, Tan L, et al: Burnout and satisfaction with work-life balance among US physicians relative to the general US population. *Arch Intern Med* 172:1377, 2012.
22. Embriaco N, Azoulay E, Barrau K, et al: High level of burnout in intensivists: prevalence and associated factors. *Am J Respir Crit Care Med* 175:686, 2007.
23. Poncet MC, Toullic P, Papazian L, et al: Burnout syndrome in critical care nursing staff. *Am J Respir Crit Care Med* 175:698, 2007.
24. Linzer M, Visser MR, Oort FJ, et al: Predicting and preventing physician burnout: results from the United States and the Netherlands. *Am J Med* 111:170, 2001.
25. McCall SV: Chemically dependent health professionals. *West J Med* 174:50, 2001.
26. Oreskovich MR, Shanafelt T, Dyrbye LN, et al: The prevalence of substance use disorders in American physicians. *Am J Addict* 24:30, 2015.
27. Dyrbye L, Shanafelt T: A narrative review on burnout experienced by medical students and residents. *Med Educ* 50:132, 2016.
28. Colford JM, McPhee SJ: The ravelled sleeve of care: managing the stresses of residency training. *JAMA* 261:889, 1989.
29. Dyrbye LN, Thomas MR, Massie FS, et al. Burnout and suicidal ideation among US medical students. *Ann Intern Med* 149:334, 2008.
30. Gundersen L: Physician burnout. *Ann Intern Med* 125:125, 2001.
31. Tyssen R, Vaglum P, Gronvold NT, et al: The impact of job stress and working conditions on mental health problems among junior house officers: a nationwide Norwegian prospective cohort study. *Med Educ* 34:374, 2000.
32. Ishak WW, Lederer S, Mandili C, et al: Burnout during residency training: a literature review. *J Grad Med Educ* 1:236, 2009.
33. Dyrbye LN, Moutier C, Durning SJ, et al: The problems program directors inherit: medical student distress at the time of graduation. *Med Teach* 33:756, 2011.
34. Dyrbye LN, West CP, Satele D, et al: Burnout among US medical students, residents, and early career physicians relative to the general US population. *Acad Med* 89:443, 2014.
35. Pereira-Lima K, Loureiro SR: Burnout, anxiety, depression, and social skills in medical residents. *Psychol Health Med* 20:353, 2015.
36. Newbury-Birch D, Kamali F: Psychological stress, anxiety, depression, job satisfaction, and personality characteristics in preregistration house officers. *Postgrad Med J* 77:109, 2000.
37. Shapiro J, Zhang B, Warm EJ: Residency as a social network: burnout, loneliness, and social network centrality. *J Grad Med Educ* 7:617, 2015
38. Shanafelt TD, Bradley KA, Wipf JE, et al: Burnout and self-reported patient care in an internal medicine residency program. *Ann Intern Med* 136(5):358, 2002.
39. West, C. P., Shanafelt, T. D., & Kolars, J. C: Quality of life, burnout, educational debt, and medical knowledge among internal medicine residents. *JAMA* 306(9):952, 2011.
40. McManus IC, Keeling A, Paice E: Stress, burnout and doctors' attitudes to work are determined by personality and learning style: a twelve year longitudinal study of UK medical graduates. *BMC Med* 2:29, 2004.
41. Gopal R, Glasheen JJ, Miyoshi TJ, et al: Burnout and internal medicine resident work-hour restrictions. *Arch Intern Med* 165:2595, 2005.
42. Coomber S, Todd C, Park G, et al: Stress in UK intensive care unit doctors. *Br J Anaesth* 89:873, 2002.
43. McMurray JE, Linzer M, Konrad TR, et al: The work lives of women physicians results from the physician work life study. *J Gen Intern Med* 15:372, 2000.
44. van Mol MM, Kompanje EJ, Benoit DD, et al: The prevalence of compassion fatigue and burnout among healthcare professionals in intensive care units: a systematic review. *PLoS One* 10:e0136955, 2015.
45. Goodfellow A, Varnam R, Rees D, et al: Staff stress on the intensive care unit: a comparison of doctors and nurses. *Anaesthesia* 52:1037, 1997.
46. Rushton CH, Batcheller J, Schroeder K, et al: Burnout and resilience among nurses practicing in high-intensity settings. *Am J Crit Care* 24:412, 2015.
47. Arnetz JE, Hamblin L, Essenmacher L, et al: Understanding patient-to-worker violence in hospitals: a qualitative analysis of documented incident reports. *J Adv Nurs* 71:338, 2015.
48. Campbell JC, Messing JT, Kub J, et al: Workplace violence: prevalence and risk factors in the safe at work study. *J Occup Environ Med* 53:82, 2011.
49. Pai H, Lee S: Risk factors for workplace violence in clinical registered nurses in Taiwan. *J Clin Nurs* 20:1405, 2011.
50. Hesketh KL, Duncan SM, Estabrooks CA, et al: Workplace violence in Alberta and British Columbia hospitals. *Health Policy* 63:311, 2003.
51. Kisa S. Turkish nurses' experience of verbal abuse at work. *Arch Psychiatr Nurs* 22:200, 2008.
52. Léséleuc S. *Criminal Victimization in the Workplace*. Ottawa, Canadian Centre for Justice Statistics, 2004.
53. Gillespie M, Melby V: Burnout among nursing staff in accident and emergency and acute medicine: a comparative study. *J Clin Nurs* 12:842, 2015.
54. Shamali M, Shahriari M, Babaii A, et al: Comparative study of job burnout among critical care nurses with fixed and rotating shift schedules. *Nurs Midwifery Stud* 4:e27766, 2015.
55. Bittner JG, Khan Z, Babu M, et al: Stress, burnout, and maladaptive coping: strategies for surgeon well-being. *Bull Am Coll Surg* 96:17, 2011.
56. Earvolino-Ramirez M: Resilience: a concept analysis. *Nurs Forum* 42:73, 2007.
57. Lazarus RS, Folkman S: Transactional theory and research on emotions and coping. *Eur J Personal* 1:141, 1987.
58. Leppin AL, Bora PR, Tilburt JC, et al: The efficacy of resiliency training programs: a systematic review and meta-analysis of randomized trials. *PLoS One* 9:e111420, 2014.
59. Henderson J: The effect of hardiness education on hardiness and burnout on registered nurses. *Nurs Econ* 33:204, 2015.
60. Sood A, Sharma V, Schroeder DR, et al: Stress Management and Resiliency Training (SMART) program among Department of Radiology faculty: a pilot randomized clinical trial. *Explore* 10:358, 2014.
61. Mealer M, Conrad D, Evans J, et al: Feasibility and acceptability of a resilience training program for intensive care unit nurses. *Am J Crit Care* 23:e97, 2014.
62. Stern TA, Prager LM, Cremens MC: Autognosis rounds for medical housestaff. *Psychosomatics* 34:1, 1993.
63. Gunasingam N, Burns K, Edwards J, et al: Reducing stress and burnout in junior doctors: the impact of debriefing sessions. *Postgrad Med J* 91:182, 2015.
64. McCue JD, Sachs CL: A stress management workshop improves residents' coping skills. *Arch Intern Med* 151:2273, 1991.
65. Linzer M, Visser MR, Oort FJ, et al: Predicting and preventing physician burnout: results from the United States and the Netherlands. *Am J Med* 111:170, 2001.
66. Civetta JM: Beyond technology: intensive care in the 1980s. *Crit Care Med* 9:763, 1981.

Section 16
PULMONARY PROBLEMS IN THE INTENSIVE CARE UNIT

J. MARK MADISON • RICHARD S. IRWIN

Chapter 163 ■ Acute Respiratory Failure due to Acute Respiratory Distress Syndrome and Pulmonary Edema

GILMAN B. ALLEN • POLLY E. PARSONS

INTRODUCTION

Acute Respiratory Distress Syndrome (ARDS) is defined by noncardiogenic pulmonary edema and hypoxemia in the setting of direct or indirect lung injury. ARDS represents a common pathologic endpoint of various potential insults to the lung that almost invariably lead to hypoxemic respiratory failure, requiring support with mechanical ventilation. Despite the confirmed success of protective mechanical ventilation strategies for lowering mortality [1,2] and ongoing efforts to discover other effective interventions [3–8], treatment of this condition remains largely supportive, and ARDS continues to be a major source of morbidity and mortality in the intensive care unit (ICU) [9,10]. Fortunately, an enormous body of research already exists on the pathogenesis of this condition, and advances continue to develop with regard to our understanding of ARDS, its prognostic implications, and how to best manage the condition medically.

DEFINITION

ARDS was originally described in 1967 by Ashbaugh and Petty and defined somewhat arbitrarily, until an American and European Consensus Conference (AECC) definition was agreed upon in 1994 [11]. This definition was generally used clinically and epidemiologically, but it was limited by interpretations of timing for the onset of injury, poor interrater reliability of chest radiograph interpretations, and the influence of positive end-expiratory pressure (PEEP) on the P:F ratio [12,13]. To address these issues, the Berlin definition was established in 2012 [14]. ARDS is now defined as a diminished arterial oxygen pressure (PaO_2) to fractional inspired oxygen (FiO_2) ratio (P to F [P:F] ratio of less than 300), bilateral airspace disease on chest radiograph, and pulmonary edema from increased permeability, the latter defined by evidence of normal cardiac function [14]. The term "Acute Lung Injury (ALI)" has now fallen out of the definition in favor of a continuum of mild, moderate, and severe ARDS, in part to avoid the confusion that would frequently accompany the broad use of the term "ALI" when referring to generalized types of lung injury. Accordingly, in the Berlin definition, ARDS is now divided into three categories of severity based on the level of hypoxemia: mild (P:F ratio 300 to 201), moderate (P:F ratio 200 to 101), and severe (P:F ratio < or = to 100) [14]. However, because the P:F ratio can be effected by arbitrary ventilator settings [15], the new definition qualifies that the severity classifying P:F ratio be measured with PEEP of > or = to 5 cm H_2O. Several studies prior to the new Berlin definition had suggested that indices of oxygenation were not strongly predictive of outcome [16–18], but the cohort of patients used for this new definition demonstrated a link between increasing severity (by category) and both an increased risk of mortality and increased duration of mechanical ventilation among survivors [14].

Although the source of hypoxemia in ARDS is multifactorial, oxygenation is one of the most easily gauged markers of "lung injury" in the ICU and thus an important component of the definition. A more inclusive P:F ratio of less than 300 mm Hg can serve to identify patients earlier in their course, thus expediting the delivery of critical lifesaving interventions before progression to moderate or severe ARDS. For ARDS, the pulmonary edema is the result of capillary leak, a parameter that is difficult to measure in the clinical setting. Accordingly, non-cardiogenic pulmonary edema is defined using clinical parameters, which include the presence of "bilateral infiltrates" consistent with pulmonary edema on chest radiograph and either a pulmonary artery wedge pressure (PAWP) less than 18 mm Hg (when measured) or no clinical evidence of left atrial hypertension [14]. However, because the group recognized that ARDS does not always exist exclusively without heart failure, the consensus more explicitly defines ARDS as "a syndrome of inflammation and increased permeability that is associated with a constellation of clinical, radiologic, and physiologic abnormalities that cannot be explained by, but may coexist with, left atrial or pulmonary capillary hypertension"[11].

Despite the great lengths taken to clarify the current definition of ARDS, it is not without its shortcomings, particularly because it does not delineate the cause of hypoxemia (i.e., alveolar damage) or clearly establish the presence of increased permeability. Unfortunately, easily employed tests for microvascular permeability are not yet available at the bedside. It would also be impractical to base the clinical definition of ARDS upon histologic findings given the often critical condition of patients and their poor candidacy for biopsy by the time of clinical diagnosis. Nevertheless, when comparing prior clinical definitions to the gold standard definition of ARDS (histopathology from surgical lung biopsy or autopsy), the clinical definition has traditionally fallen short in recognizing all cases of ARDS [13,19].

HISTOPATHOLOGY

Despite having many different potential etiologies [20,21], the histologic findings of ARDS are fundamentally uniform and are collectively described by the term *diffuse alveolar damage* (DAD) [22]. DAD represents a continuum of changes that can be temporally divided into *exudative*, *proliferative*, and *fibrotic* phases [22], between which considerable overlap exists. The *exudative* phase of DAD is the earliest phase, during which clinical symptoms first develop and lung mechanical changes become manifest. This phase typically occupies the first week and is characterized by epithelial and endothelial cell death, neutrophil sequestration, platelet-fibrin thrombi, interstitial edema, and exudates within the airspaces, which consist of fluid, protein, and cellular debris [22]. These exudates compact into dense, protein-rich hyaline membranes that stain strongly with eosin and line the alveoli

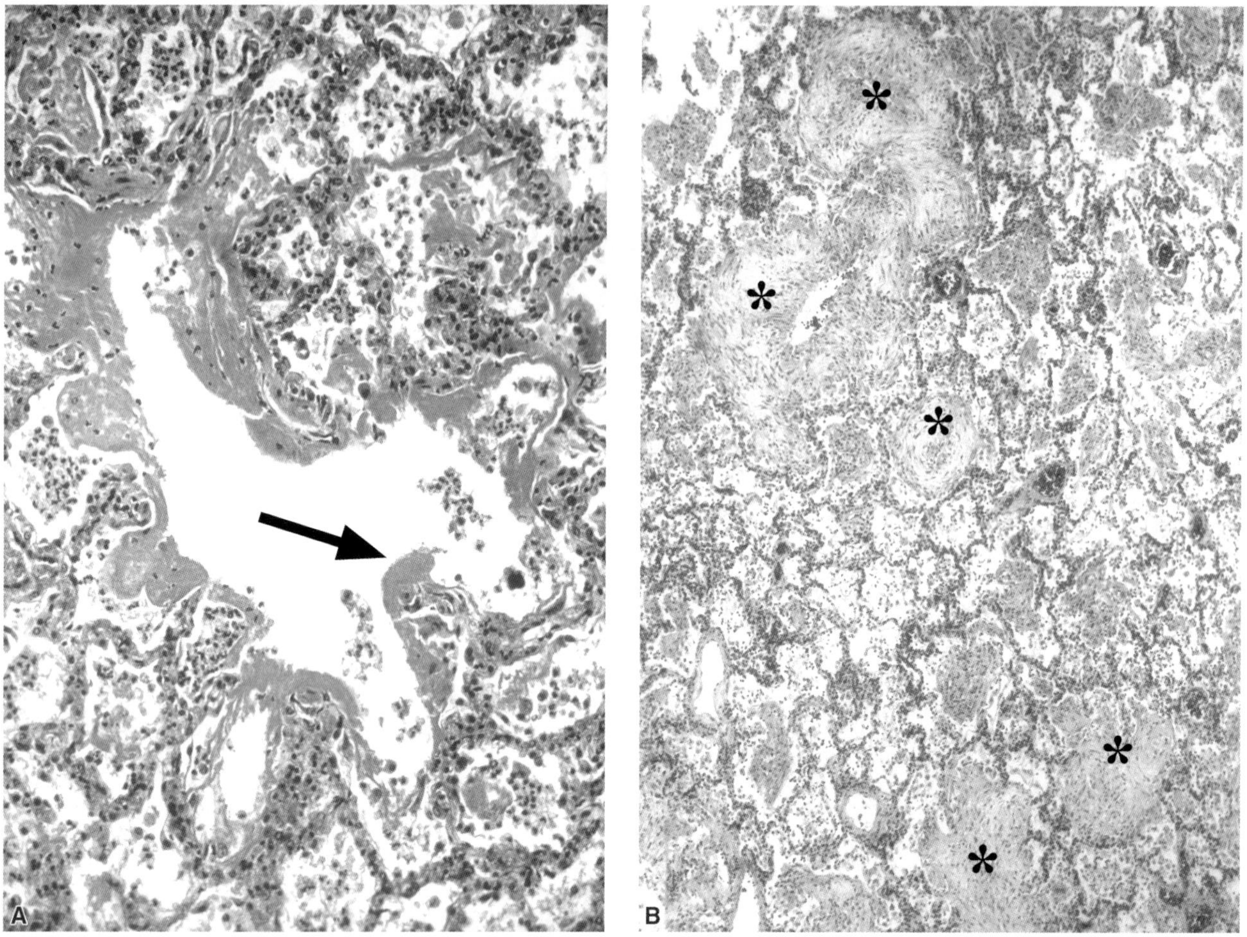

FIGURE 163.1 A: Histologic lung specimen from ARDS patient, showing red blood cells and neutrophils within the alveolar space and characteristic hyaline membranes (*arrow*) consistent with diagnosis of diffuse alveolar damage (DAD). B: Distal airspace granulation tissue (*asterisks*) consistent with organizing pneumonia (hematoxylin and eosin stained, 60X). Images were graciously provided by Dr. Martha Warnock.

and alveolar ducts (Fig. 163.1A). During protracted injury, the *proliferative* phase ensues and is characterized by organization of the intra-alveolar exudates and proliferation of type II alveolar cells, fibroblasts, and myofibroblasts. During this phase, it is common to find areas of squamous metaplasia and granulation tissue occluding alveolar ducts in a manner similar to that of organizing pneumonia (Fig.163.1B) [23].

The *fibrotic* phase has classically been considered the later phase of remodeling that occurs in patients whose disease course persists beyond 2 to 3 weeks [22], but studies suggest an increase in the *fibrotic* response to ARDS as early as 24 hours from presentation [24], and histologic evidence of fibrosis can be seen within days of presentation of some patients [25]. Because such overlap exists between the fibrotic and proliferative phases, the two are often described together as the *fibroproliferative* phase, and there is evidence that increased fibroproliferative signaling and fibrosis predict worse outcomes [24].

RADIOGRAPHIC FINDINGS

In the most recent Berlin definition of ARDS, the expert panel chose to retain the AECC criteria of bilateral airspace opacities consistent with pulmonary edema, but also allowed for this criteria to be recognized on computed tomography (CT) imaging, as well [14]. These infiltrates will often initially appear as heterogeneous opacities, but later become more homogeneous over hours to days [26] (see Fig. 163.2A). Although some have recommended using criteria such as cardiac silhouette size and vascular pedicle width to differentiate cardiogenic from noncardiogenic edema, this differentiation has proven to be frequently impossible [27]. Furthermore, the seemingly straightforward interpretation of bilateral infiltrates can be obscured by factors such as atelectasis, effusions, or isolated lower lobe involvement, all of which contribute to low interobserver agreement [12,28]. Therefore, the newer diagnostic criteria further require that the bilateral airspace opacities are not explained by effusion, lobar collapse, or nodules [13,14].

Prior to CT scanning, the pulmonary edema seen on chest radiograph was widely believed to be a diffuse process. However, CT imaging has demonstrated the distribution of ARDS to oftentimes be heterogeneous and patchy, with areas of normal-appearing, aerated lung interspersed among areas of mixed ground glass opacity and consolidation, the latter being concentrated in the more gravitationally dependent regions of the lung [27] (see Fig. 163.2B and C). Despite this pattern, a recent study using positron emission tomography (PET) to map cellular metabolic activity demonstrated that diffuse inflammatory change can be detected even in areas of the lung that appear spared radiographically [29]. Some investigators have also used PET imaging and magnetic resonance imaging (MRI) to estimate pulmonary microvascular leak and assist in the differentiation between high permeability and hydrostatic pulmonary edema [30,31], but these methods have yet to be adopted in clinical practice. One recent study demonstrated the clinical value of performing focused bedside thoracic and cardiac ultrasonography, using the presence or absence of B lines, left-sided pleural effusion, vena cava diameter, and left ventricular dysfunction to differentiate

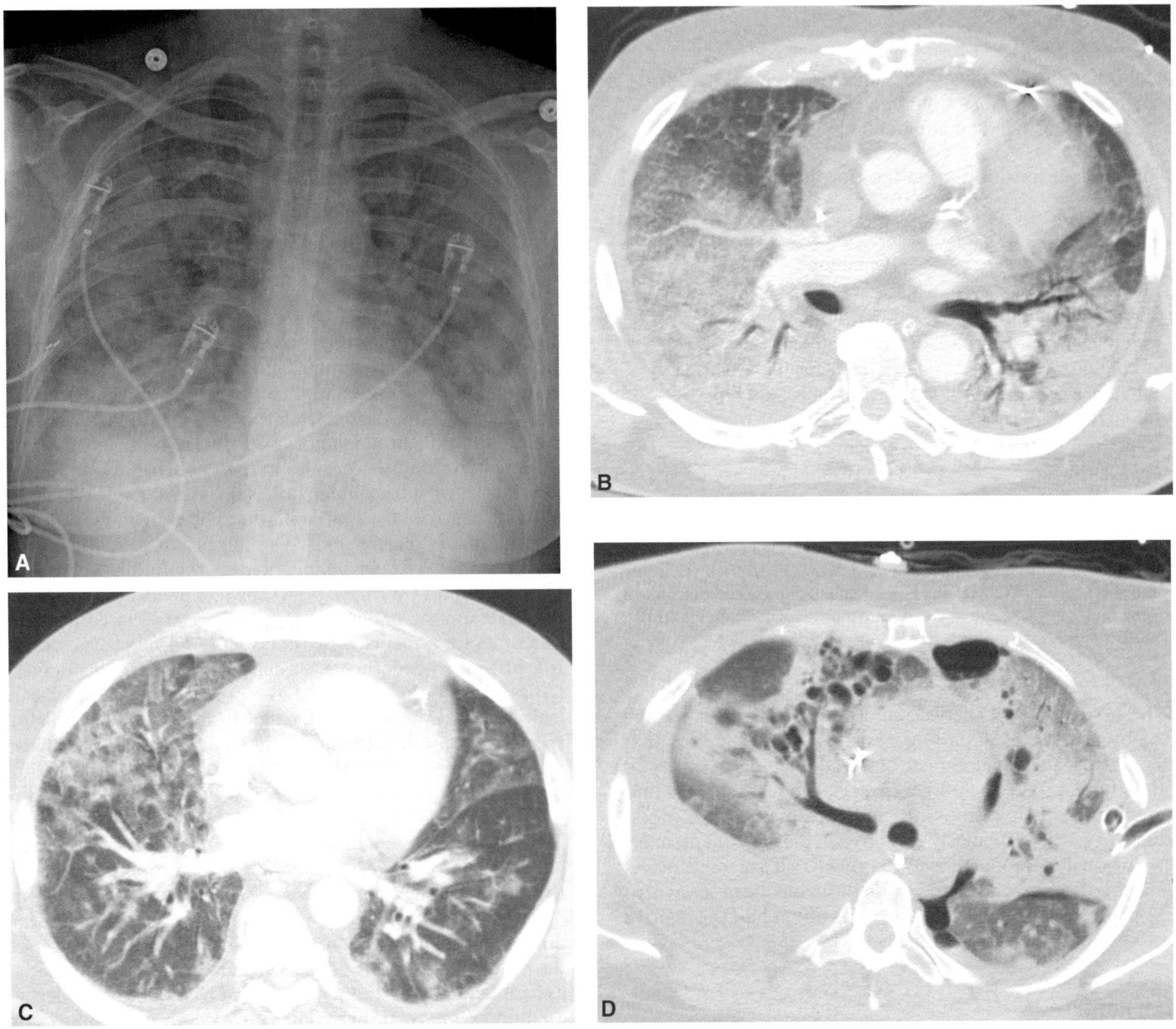

FIGURE 163.2 A plain chest radiograph from a patient with ARDS is shown in **A**. Computed tomography images of the chest from patients with ARDS are shown in **B**, **C**, and **D**. **B** and **C**: Diffuse patchy regions of consolidation with a predominance of ground glass infiltrates. **D**: More severe disease with a predominance of dense consolidation, a large right pleural effusion, and sequelae of barotrauma, with pneumatoceles throughout both lungs and a persistent pneumothorax on the left despite two chest tubes (one shown in cross section and one longitudinally).

cardiogenic pulmonary edema (CPE), ARDS, and miscellaneous causes of acute hypoxic respiratory failure from one another [32]. While the clinical utility of this tool is not widespread at this time, for those readers interested in learning more about the utility of point of care critical care ultrasonography or guidance in its use, a section has been added on its use at the end of this chapter.

EPIDEMIOLOGY

The estimated incidence of ARDS worldwide has been variable in the past because of its wide range of causes and previously nonuniform definition. The first estimate by the National Institutes of Health (NIH) projected an annual incidence of 75 cases per 100,000 in the US, but subsequent studies reported estimates between 1.3 and 22 per 100,000 person years, depending on population studied [33]. A much larger pool of prospective cases from the NHLBI-sponsored ARDS Network yielded a conservative estimate of 64.2 cases per 100,000 person years [33]. A more recent and significantly larger prospective cohort from King County in Washington State estimated an annual incidence of 78.9 cases per 100,000 person years, in keeping with the ARDS Network and original NIH estimates, and felt likely to be the most accurate estimate to date for incidence in the US [9]. This incidence, combined with a high morbidity, creates a substantial burden of cost to health care. ICU care accounts for approximately 13% of hospital costs in the US, and almost one-third of that is attributable to patients who require mechanical ventilation [34,35].

In patients at risk of developing ARDS, the onset is typically swift, with a median onset between 1 and 2 days [13,36]. Onset is less than 24 hours in just over half of patients with ARDS due to sepsis and in about one-third of patients with ARDS from trauma, and within 5 days of any insult in over 90% of all patients that develop ARDS [13]. The known causes and risk factors for the development of ARDS have been well characterized [20,21] (see Table 163.1) and can be categorized as ensuing from either direct or indirect injury to the lung [20,25]. This differentiation is justified by the observed physiologic differences between direct and indirect ARDS and the differing outcomes associated with each cause [9]. It is now well established that sepsis is the most commonly identified cause of ARDS and is associated with the worst outcomes overall [9,18], while trauma-related ARDS has a significantly lower mortality

TABLE 163.1

Clinical Disorders Associated with the Development of ARDS, Subcategorized into Those Commonly and Less Commonly Associated with Direct and Indirect Injury to the Lung

Clinical disorders leading to the development of ARDS	
Direct Injury	**Indirect Injury**
Common	Common
Pneumonia	Sepsis
Witnessed aspiration	Multisystem trauma
Pulmonary contusion	Less common
Less common	Transfusion of plasma
Pulmonary contusion	Products (and blood)
Inhalational injury	Acute pancreatitis
Reperfusion injury	Drug overdose
Near Drowning	Cardiopulmonary bypass
Fat emboli	Other surgeries

Lists compiled from Rubenfeld GD, Caldwell E, Peabody E, et al: Incidence and outcomes of acute lung injury. *N Engl J Med* 353:1685–1693, 2005; Brun-Buisson C, Minelli C, Bertolini G, et al: Epidemiology and outcome of acute lung injury in European intensive care units. Results from the ALIVE study. *Intensive Care Med* 30:51–61, 2004.

[9,37]. These differences between mortality rates may in part be caused by differences in pathogenesis [37]. Other factors that confer risk for the development of ARDS include a history of alcohol abuse, recent chemotherapy, delayed resuscitation and antimicrobial therapy, smoking, and transfusion with blood products [38,39], particularly fresh frozen plasma and platelets [40]. Curiously, among those at clinical risk for developing ARDS, the diagnosis of diabetes mellitus has been shown to confer protection from ARDS, providing about half the relative risk as that of nondiabetic patients [38].

PATHOGENESIS

In parallel with its predominant pathologic findings on histology, ARDS is, first and foremost, a condition triggered by injury to the alveolar epithelium and capillary endothelium. The insult can be initially isolated either to the epithelium, as in the case of aspiration, or to the endothelium, as in most forms of indirect ARDS, such as sepsis. However, injury is generally detected in both the endothelium and epithelium by the time of diagnosis [22]. This injury invariably leads to a leakage into the alveolar space of plasma proteins that in turn activate procoagulant and proinflammatory pathways, leading to the fibrinous and purulent exudates seen on histology. Through increased transcription and release of proinflammatory cytokines, and an increased expression of cell surface adhesion molecules, a profound acute inflammatory response ensues, with epithelial cell necrosis and a robust recruitment of neutrophils [25,39]. The increased expression of tissue factor (TF) and other procoagulant factors ultimately leads to coagulation within the microvasculature and airspaces, accompanied by a suppression of fibrinolysis, which helps perpetuate the microthrombi and fibrinous exudates that are pathognomonic for ARDS [25].

Injury to the alveolar epithelium plays a critical role for the pathogenesis of ARDS. One well-characterized marker of epithelial injury, the receptor of advanced glycosylation end-product (RAGE), found to be highly expressed on type I alveolar epithelial cells, can be detected in high abundance in the edema fluid and plasma of patients with ARDS [41]. In fact, elevated plasma levels of RAGE were shown to predict a longer ICU length of stay and duration of mechanical ventilation for patients at risk of ARDS following heart–lung transplantation [42]. Through epithelial cell necrosis and the loss of tight junctions and barrier function, plasma proteins and edema fluid seep into the alveolar space, leading to increased shunt fraction, higher alveolar surface tension, and a greater propensity for alveolar collapse. Clearance of both protein and fluid is crucial to the resolution of ARDS. Indeed, a greater alveolar fluid clearance (AFC) rate is associated with fewer days of mechanical ventilation and lower mortality among patients with ARDS [43]. On the other side of the alveolar capillary interface, injury to the endothelium results in increased permeability, release of inflammatory molecules, expression of cell adhesion molecules, and activation of procoagulant pathways. Increased microvascular permeability has been widely demonstrated among those with ARDS [41], but this may be caused more by a functional alteration or activation of intact endothelium than by actual cell lysis or necrosis. Conditions such as sepsis and bacteremia can activate endothelial cells to release von Willebrand factor (vWF), increase surface expression of potent adhesion molecules known as selectins, and increase expression of intracellular adhesion molecule-1, which helps to bind neutrophils and facilitate their transmigration across the endothelial barrier [41]. The important role of endothelial activation for ARDS is highlighted by the finding that elevated plasma levels of vWF have been shown to predict the development of ARDS among patients at risk and are associated with worse outcomes for patients with established ARDS [41]. Recently, the role of another endothelial cell activation marker, Angiopoietin-2 (Ang-2), has been recognized as a potential marker of capillary leak and ARDS severity. Released from endothelial cells in response to multiple activating insults, Ang-2 can lead to increased vascular permeability and adhesion of circulating neutrophils [41], and increased circulating levels have been correlated with an increased risk of developing and dying from ARDS [44,45].

The role of the neutrophil in ARDS pathogenesis has been widely accepted for years. Although the neutrophil is not essential for the development of ARDS, as evidenced by the development of ARDS in the setting of neutropenia, its course can often worsen during the recovery from neutropenia and after administration of the neutrophil growth and releasing factor, G-CSF [46]. Recently, experimental animal models have led to mounting evidence for a complex interplay between platelets and neutrophils during their adhesion to the endothelium, with both platelet depletion and pharmacologic inhibition of platelet function mitigating neutrophil recruitment and ARDS severity [47,48]. In support of these findings, one single center observational study has since demonstrated prehospital antiplatelet therapy to independently predict a reduced risk for the development of ARDS [49], but a secondary analysis of a separate cohort of patients failed to find the same association between prehospital aspirin use and development of ARDS [36,50]. Nevertheless, these findings have helped foster interest in a current ongoing multicenter trial investigating the role of aspirin in the prevention of ARDS (NCT01504867).

Activated leukocytes and endothelial cells also contribute to dysregulated intravascular and extravascular coagulation [25]. Extravascular alveolar fibrin arising from increased procoagulant activity and impaired fibrinolysis has been well described for ARDS [41]. Fibrin formation and clearance in the lung is in part governed by the differential activity of fibrinolysis promoters and inhibitors. At the point of coagulation and fibrin generation, TF has received notable attention because of its known interaction with factor VIIa and downstream generation of thrombin. TF expression is increased on the surface of alveolar epithelial cells and macrophages among patients with ARDS and is accompanied by increased procoagulant activity in the edema fluid [51], but TF has not been shown to be useful for diagnosis [41]. On the other hand, Plasminogen activator inhibitor-1 (PAI-1) can prevent fibrinolysis via direct binding and inhibition of plasminogen activators. Elevated plasma levels of PAI-1 and reduced plasma levels of the endogenous anticoagulant protein C have both been shown to discriminate between acute cardiogenic edema and ARDS and to be independent risk factors for mortality and adverse clinical outcomes [41,52]. Numerous additional pathways have been implicated in the pathogenesis of ALI, but an attempt to cover each in depth would extend beyond the intended breadth of this chapter.

PATHOPHYSIOLOGY

Because of the accumulation of extravascular lung water (i.e., pulmonary edema), the physiologic derangements of ALI invariably manifest as refractory hypoxemia, decreased respiratory compliance, and a propensity for alveolar closure [25]. As alveolar edema fluid and protein accumulate within the alveoli, physiologic shunt develops as blood flows through capillary units to alveoli that are either filled with fluid or have collapsed from increased surface tension (see Fig. 163.3A). Hypoxic vasoconstriction, the normal autoregulatory reflex that helps match ventilation and perfusion by shunting capillary blood flow away from poorly ventilated regions of the lung, is severely impaired within the diseased regions of the lung, leading to an imbalance and increased blood flow to poorly ventilated lung regions [53]. Increased vasoconstriction and scattered microthrombi within well-ventilated lung regions contribute to physiologic dead space or "wasted ventilation" via diminished blood flow to aerated lung [53] (see Fig. 163.3B). The combined effects of these derangements result in refractory hypoxemia and increased minute ventilation requirements, which explain the often challenging demands of managing these patients in the intensive care unit.

Overall, the average pulmonary vascular resistance is commonly elevated in patients with ARDS [25] likely because of a reduction in total luminal diameter of the vascular bed from vasoconstriction and thrombotic obstruction. This in turn leads to the common finding of pulmonary hypertension among these patients, which can alter right ventricular loading and function and predicts higher mortality in afflicted patients [54]. Because elevated pulmonary artery pressures could, in theory, contribute to increased pulmonary edema and right heart strain, it is unclear whether pulmonary hypertension is directly contributing to mortality or simply a marker of disease severity.

The mechanical characteristics of ARDS manifest primarily as a decrease of respiratory compliance. This is primarily caused by a decrease in compliance of the lung, particularly in the more direct forms of ARDS such as pneumonia. However, contribution from the chest wall and abdominal compartment can be significant under conditions such as trauma and peritonitis [55]. The reduction of lung compliance reflects the collective contribution of changes in the intrinsic elastic properties of the remaining aerated lung and a reduction in resting lung volume via alveolar flooding and collapse. The increased elastic properties of the aerated lung result from increased tissue stiffness due to interstitial edema and increased alveolar surface tension, the result of increased surface forces generated by a greater abundance of alveolar lining fluid and a decrease in surfactant activity [25]. This loss of surfactant activity is believed to result from inhibitory binding of surfactant by plasma proteins and cholesterol, and decreased production of functionally active surfactant by type II pneumocytes [56]. Furthermore, the biomechanical effects of mechanical ventilation alone can alter the structure and biophysical properties of surfactant [57].

Lower resting lung volumes in ARDS result from persistently fluid-filled or collapsed alveoli, leading to what has been colloquially referred to as "baby lung" [58]. The affected regions of the lungs are often so diseased that they may remain fluid filled or collapsed throughout each tidal inflation [59] and hence contribute negligibly to compliance. As a result, tidal volumes delivered to the heterogeneously fluid-filled and atelectatic lung are shunted preferentially to more compliant, aerated regions of the lung. This is one of the main postulated mechanisms through which mechanical ventilation can overdistend and injure the remaining regions of "normal lung" and lead to ventilator-induced lung injury (VILI) [60,61].

MANAGEMENT

Mechanical Ventilation

Mechanical Ventilation and Low Tidal Volumes

The early presentation of ARDS is chiefly characterized by hypoxemic respiratory failure and the almost invariable need for support with mechanical ventilation, but this may be changing in the wake of high-flow nasal cannula oxygen delivery [62]. Because the greatest danger posed to patients with ARDS is the development of multiorgan failure [63], establishing supportive ventilation modes that optimize hemodynamic function and oxygen delivery remains an important objective in the management of these patients. Prior to the late 1960s, endotracheal intubation and positive pressure mechanical ventilation were primarily used for supporting patients during general anesthesia. It was during this time that investigators first noted that larger tidal volumes could reduce the shunt associated with atelectasis during general anesthesia, and because many of the techniques used for the support of patients with acute respiratory failure were originally adopted from general anesthesia practice, employing

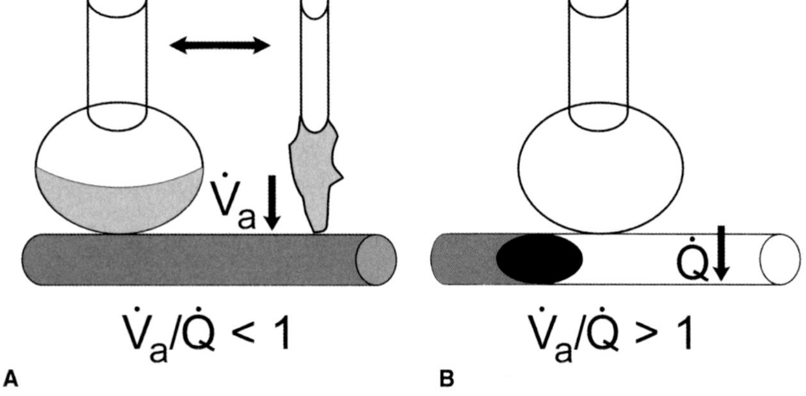

FIGURE 163.3 **A:** The edema-fluid-filled alveolus and a neighboring collapsed alveolus, both with unrestricted blood flow, contributing to physiologic shunt. *Double headed arrow* represents potential for fluid-filled alveolus to collapse and reexpand during normal tidal ventilation. **B:** The effect of a microthrombus (*black oval*) obstructing blood flow to a functioning alveolus, contributing to physiologic dead space.

tidal volumes of 10 to 15 mg per kg became the standard for improving oxygenation and ventilation for patients with ARDS [1,64]. We now know that idealized oxygenation and normal physiologic pH and $PaCO_2$ can come at a cost when employing higher tidal volumes in patients with ARDS. After the discovery that lung injury pathologically resembling ARDS could be induced de novo in animal models through lung overdistension with higher tidal volumes [25,60], small retrospective and prospective uncontrolled trials were completed that suggested a benefit from limiting tidal volume and peak airway pressures in patients with ARDS [25]. Numerous larger, randomized trials comparing traditional and lower tidal volumes have since been conducted, each trial differing in its methodology and results. The largest randomized, multicenter trial to date, conducted by the ARDS Network, ultimately demonstrated significantly lower mortality among those assigned to a tidal volume of 6 mL per kg of predicted ideal body weight and a target plateau pressure of 30 cm H_2O or less (mortality 31.0%) as opposed to a tidal volume of 12 mL per kg and a target plateau pressure less than 50 cm H_2O (mortality 39.8%) [1]. Following this landmark study, controversy arose regarding whether "artificially high" tidal volumes drove the benefits observed in the trial, but this assertion was not supported by data demonstrating consistent use of tidal volumes far in excess of 10 cc per kg in clinical practice prior to and long after the study was published [25,65,66]. Indeed, even years later, there was sufficient variation in practice among four hospitals in Baltimore to power a statistically significant 18% relative increase in observed mortality for each 1 mL per kg increase in average tidal volume delivered [67,68]. All this has led professional societies to recommend the use of lower tidal volumes at goal plateau pressures less than 30 cm H_2O in patients with established ARDS [69]. Going a step further, there is now evidence that the benefits of low tidal volumes are exclusive of simply maintaining a plateau pressure less than 30 cm H_2O, but added benefit is also gained by keeping plateau pressures substantially lower than 30 cm H_2O [70,71], leading some experts to suggest maintaining the lowest tidal volume and plateau pressure that can safely be achieved [67].

Because calculation of tidal volume based on total body weight may be partly responsible for the documented underuse of lower tidal volumes for patients with ARDS [65], the importance of using predicted ideal body weight (IBW), based upon measured height and sex, cannot be overstressed. IBW (in kg) for males is calculated as $50 + 0.91[(\text{height in cm}) - 152.4]$, and for females as $45.5 + 0.91[(\text{height in cm}) - 152.4]$ [1].

To achieve these practice guidelines, a strategy of "permissive hypercapnia" is often needed, in which a reduction in minute volume and an ensuing increase in $PaCO_2$ is tolerated in order to achieve lower target tidal volumes and airway pressures [72]. Numerous experimental animal models have actually demonstrated a protective effect of hypercapnic acidosis (HCA) that is abolished by buffering with bicarbonate solution [72], but other work suggests that HCA may worsen ARDS [73,74]. A recent secondary analysis of the ARDS Network study demonstrated a reduced 28-day mortality conferred by HCA in the 12 cc per kg group, but a similar benefit was not found for the 6 mL per kg group, suggesting that permissive hypercapnia is at the very least safe, and possibly beneficial [67,72,75]. These noted benefits, along with concerns that bicarbonate infusion may actually worsen intracellular acidosis, have led some experts to dissuade practitioners from buffering HCA with bicarbonate unless there is a clear rationale for doing so [67,72].

To better understand the protection conferred by low tidal volumes, investigators have studied how this strategy modulates the inflammatory cascades associated with ARDS and VILI. Evidence now exists to support the theory that low tidal volume ventilation improves outcomes at least in part through reduced activation of the inflammatory cascades associated with VILI and multiorgan failure. Among patients enrolled in the ARDS Network trial of low tidal volume, it was found that higher plasma levels of soluble receptors for tumor necrosis factor-α (TNF-α) were associated with higher mortality and fewer organ-failure–free days [76]. Furthermore, the lower tidal volume strategy was associated with lower levels of soluble TNF-α receptor I [76]. Elevated plasma levels of interleukin (IL)-6, 8, and 10 were also linked to increased mortality, while lower tidal volume was associated with a greater decline in IL-6 and IL-8 levels by day 3 of enrollment [77].

Currently, no firm guidelines exist regarding patients without established ARDS (with the exception of sepsis [69]), but there is now mounting clinical evidence that a low tidal volume strategy can help prevent progression to ARDS in patients at risk [78–80] and is also of clinical benefit in intermediate to high-risk patients undergoing major abdominal surgery [81]. Although data suggest that tidal volumes lower than 6 mL per kg may confer even greater protection from VILI [82], there is no general consensus regarding this practice. However, the authors note that in the original ARDS Network trial, the lower tidal volume assignment started with a goal of 6 mL per kg, but tidal volumes were oftentimes adjusted to as low as 4 mL per kg to maintain plateau pressures less than 30 cm H_2O [1], and some experts [67] argue that practitioners should target the lowest tidal volume and plateau pressures that can safely be achieved.

Recruitment

The physiologic abnormalities in ARDS can, for some patients, be reversed by a recruitment maneuver (RM), typically delivered as a sustained or stepwise deep inflation with the intention of reopening collapsed regions of the lung [67,83]. However, because of the unusually high surface tension within affected alveoli, the benefit is often transient, especially if not followed by sufficiently high levels of PEEP [84]. The rationale for using RMs is to recruit otherwise atelectatic lung to improve end-expiratory lung volume, and in turn mitigate the development of additional VILI accruing from atelectasis and cyclic alveolar reexpansion at end-expiration [61,83]. On the other hand, periodic RMs can promote hypotension by limiting venous preload return and cardiac output [83], and could conceivably even contribute to lung injury through excessive overdistension or repeated opening of collapsed lung [83,85].

Clinical studies have yielded highly variable results with regard to the impact of RMs on important outcomes. Although a trial from the Lung Open Ventilation Study (LOVS) group demonstrated a reduction in severe hypoxemia and need for rescue therapies with an "open lung" approach of combined RMs and higher PEEP, it did not demonstrate any reduction in all-cause mortality [86]. In a follow-up meta-analysis of 40 trials, which included the LOVS study and three other randomized controlled trials, authors found that, in general, ARDS patients receiving RMs exhibit a significant but short-lived improvement in oxygenation with often transient and self-limited hypotension and desaturation during the RM [83]. These mixed findings have led these and other experts to conclude that RMs can neither be recommended nor discouraged for all patients but can be considered on an individualized basis for patients with life-threatening hypoxemia [67,83,87].

Positive End-Expiratory Pressure

PEEP is the most widely employed strategy shown to retard alveolar derecruitment in the injured lung. Several studies have demonstrated the ability of PEEP to prevent or delay alveolar derecruitment and attenuate VILI [88,89]. However, the protective effect of higher PEEP was called into doubt after a multicenter randomized trial failed to demonstrate an improvement in outcomes using a higher PEEP strategy during low tidal volume ventilation in ALI patients [90]. In this trial, higher levels of PEEP were arbitrarily coupled to each stepwise increment in FiO_2

requirement during low tidal volume ventilation [90]. The study failed to demonstrate any benefit in mortality or ventilator-free days with higher PEEP [90], but potential underpowering of this study has left room for continued debate [91]. Additionally, since the amount of recruitable lung varies significantly among ARDS patients, some have suggested that setting PEEP levels without first determining the level of recruitable lung may offset the potential benefits of PEEP [88,89]. In another randomized trial from the Expiratory Pressure (ExPress) Study Group, where the selection of PEEP was more "patient directed" and set at a level required to maintain plateau pressures of 28 to 30 cm H_2O, the higher PEEP strategy again failed to demonstrate a reduction in mortality, but did demonstrate lasting improvements in oxygenation and compliance, an increase in ventilator-free and organ failure–free days, and a trend toward improved survival in more severe ARDS [92].

Since these trials, several post hoc analyses and meta-analyses have yielded a predominance of findings that suggest the use of higher PEEP to be of greater benefit in patients with moderate-to-severe ARDS, and of less benefit (or potential harm) in those with mild ARDS [89,93,94]. A larger meta-analysis by Briel and colleagues demonstrated a 10% relative risk reduction in in-hospital mortality with higher PEEP in moderate-to-severe ARDS but a trend toward increased mortality from higher PEEP in mild ARDS [93]. A subsequent meta-analysis concluded no benefit for mortality from higher PEEP [95], but experts have pointed out the failure of this analysis to stratify patients on the basis of disease severity [89,95]. A Cochrane review in 2013 also demonstrated no benefit with higher PEEP applied broadly, but a subgroup analysis supported the findings of Briel and colleagues favoring higher PEEP in moderate-to-severe ARDS [94]. Yet another secondary analysis of findings from the LOVS and ExPress trials found that among patients whose PEEP had been increased following randomization, a positive oxygenation response to PEEP (an increase of 25 mm Hg or greater in their P/F ratio) was associated with lower mortality, and the association was stronger in patients with more severe disease [96]. This could simply imply that patients with more "recruitable" lung have better outcomes, but these findings led the authors to speculate that this improved oxygenation response to PEEP may help better predict who will benefit from higher PEEP [96]. Alternatively, some experts have concluded that a more practical, bedside imaging modality for assessing lung recruitment from added PEEP is needed [88]. Others have shown that more directly targeting PEEP to transpulmonary pressure by measuring esophageal pressures may be a safer and more effective means of determining optimal PEEP [97], and a larger follow-up randomized trial of esophageal pressure–directed PEEP is currently enrolling patients with moderate-to-severe ARDS (clinicaltrials.gov NCT01681225) [89].

High-Frequency Ventilation and Extracorporal Membrane Oxygenation

With the data demonstrating a reduction in mortality with low tidal volumes, and animal studies showing that even lower tidal volumes offer additional protection [82], high frequency oscillation ventilation (HFOV), with tidal volumes equal to or less than dead space, would seem to be an ideal mechanical ventilation strategy for ARDS. Early investigations in the use of HFOV in adults with ARDS yielded mixed results [60,98], and a meta-analysis suggested that HFOV may provide a reduced risk of mortality when compared to conventional mechanical ventilation, but this benefit was mitigated when comparing HFOV to mandated low tidal volume ventilation [98]. However, two large randomized multicenter trials have since compared HFOV to a conventional low tidal volume strategy in adult patients with moderate-to-severe ARDS. One demonstrated no benefit in mortality or ventilator-free days from HFOV over conventional low tidal volume ventilation [99]. The other was terminated early on the basis of increased mortality in the HFOV group [100]. These results have led experts to clearly favor conventional low tidal volume ventilation over HFOV as first-line support for adult patients with ARDS [89], but they have not entirely excluded the option of turning to HFOV for patients failing conventional therapy in centers with expertise in safe HFOV delivery [60].

Extracorporeal membrane oxygenation (ECMO), used alone or in combination with protective ventilation, uses cardiopulmonary bypass to facilitate gas exchange while minimizing ventilation of the lung to limit barriers to healing. Despite demonstrated efficacy in neonates with severe respiratory distress syndrome, nonrandomized observational studies provided conflicting results regarding survival benefit of ECMO in adult ARDS, and earlier randomized trials were negative with high rates of mortality in both treatment assignments [89,101]. The largest randomized controlled trial to date in ECMO for severe adult ARDS demonstrated an improvement in 6-month survival without disability for the group that was transferred to an ECMO center for consideration of ECMO, when compared to the conventional treatment group [102]. However, only 76% of patients transferred to the specialized ECMO center actually received ECMO, and only 70% of patients assigned to the conventional treatment group received low tidal volume ventilation per protocol (vs. 93% in the ECMO group) [102]. This has led many experts to conclude that the study really only demonstrated a benefit in being transferred to a specialized ECMO-capable center [89,101].

Noninvasive and Partial Support Ventilation

Noninvasive ventilation (NIV) and partial support invasive ventilation modes, such as pressure support ventilation, allow for patient triggering and cycling of breaths, resulting in more spontaneous breathing. The potential advantages of spontaneous breathing over controlled mechanical ventilation include improved patient–ventilator synchrony, lower sedation requirements, and improved hemodynamics and ventilation/perfusion ($\dot{V}a/\dot{Q}$) matching [67]. Partial assist modes of ventilation can still effectively help unload respiratory workload, while helping to improve aeration and ventilation/perfusion matching within dependent lung regions, presumably because of more pronounced transpulmonary pressures generated within these regions by an actively moving diaphragm.

While many studies have demonstrated a high rate of success for preventing the need for intubation during hypoxemic respiratory failure, particularly in the setting of CPE, others have demonstrated high rates of NIV failure in patients with ARDS [103,104]. Furthermore, NIV failure has been associated with higher mortality rates (up to 64%) in patients with hypoxemic respiratory failure [105,106], leading many to urge the need for caution in using NIV in the support of patients with ARDS [67,103].

This high rate of NIV failure among patients with acute hypoxemic respiratory failure was once again demonstrated in a recent randomized trial comparing NIV to both standard and high-flow nasal cannula oxygen delivery [62]. The study demonstrated greater patient comfort for the high-flow nasal cannula group, but the reduced frequency of the need for intubation among this group (38%) only reached statistical significance in a post hoc analysis for patients with a P:F ratio of <200 mm Hg [62]. However, the hazard ratio for death was substantially higher for both the NIV (2.50) and standard nasal cannula (2.01) groups when compared to high-flow nasal cannula [62]. Regardless, these somewhat preliminary findings suggest that high-flow nasal cannula is a clearly safe means of potentially avoiding the need for intubation and perhaps safer than NIV with respect to long-term outcomes.

Prone-Positioning

Prone-positioning was shown to improve oxygenation for patients with hypoxic respiratory failure as early as the mid-1970s [89]. Proposed mechanisms have included recruitment and improved ventilation of the previously dependent dorsal lung, and improved ventilation–perfusion matching via redirection of the gravitationally distributed perfusion toward the newly dependent (better ventilated) lung. Contrary to earlier speculation, however, prone-positioning exerts limited gravitational effects on regional perfusion in either normal or injured lung [107], but it can improve ventilation within previously dependent dorsal lung regions [108] via regional changes in chest wall mechanics and reduced lung compression by the heart and mediastinum [89].

Despite these known physiologic benefits, most of the earlier clinical trials demonstrated improved oxygenation with prone-positioning, yet no reduction in mortality [109–111]. However, none of these earlier clinical trials were coupled to IBW-determined low tidal volume ventilation. Post hoc analysis of data from the first of these trials suggested an early survival advantage in the most severe subgroup of patients [109], a finding supported by subsequent studies [110]. Since these earlier negative trials were completed, the Proning Severe ARDS Patients (PROSEVA) study group concluded a multicenter randomized trial that demonstrated a significant reduction in mortality among patients with more severe (P:F ratio < 150) ARDS [4]. The protocol directed 16 consecutive hours of prone position for at least 28 days, was coupled with 6 mL per kg IBW tidal volumes, and a target plateau pressure less than 30 cm H_2O, and it demonstrated a significant reduction in 28-day mortality (hazard ratio for death 0.39) and 90-day mortality (hazard ratio 0.44) [4]. Since then, a meta-analysis examining combined data from these and other trials found a significant benefit from prone-positioning when examining patients with tidal volumes $<$8 mL per kg IBW, but not with tidal volumes $>$8 mL per kg [112], suggesting that the benefit of proning may extend beyond the most severe of ARDS patients when coupled to a low tidal volume strategy. Nevertheless, given the high reported rates of complications associated with prone-positioning [111,113], experts have concluded that prone-positioning should be limited to patients with severe hypoxemia and undertaken only in high expertise centers with experience in safe technique.

Fluid Management

Since pulmonary edema is the hallmark of ARDS, it seems reasonable to keep patients relatively "dry" in their total fluid volume. However, because the development of multiple organ dysfunction syndrome (MODS) increases mortality from ARDS, the critical maintenance of adequate peripheral perfusion may require liberal administration of intravenous fluid, at least initially. Earlier studies demonstrated an improvement of physiologic parameters with diuresis guided with and without vascular pressure measurement or by measurement of extravascular lung water [25]. Diuretic therapy with combined albumin and furosemide has been shown to improve oxygenation and hemodynamics in hypoproteinemic ARDS patients but did not reduce mortality [114]. The NHLBI ARDS Network trial of conservative versus liberal fluid management demonstrated no difference in 60-day mortality between the two different strategies [115]. However, subjects in the conservative strategy group had a lower 7-day cumulative fluid balance with improved lung function and a reduced duration of mechanical ventilation without an increase in nonpulmonary organ failure [115], providing some evidence to support the view that a conservatively lower fluid balance is safe and may provide more favorable outcomes. The caveats to these conclusions include barriers to generalizability of the findings in the setting of multiple exclusion factors (including renal failure and heart failure), and that all patients were allowed to receive a liberal fluid resuscitation strategy (if deemed clinically necessary), for on average up to the first 43 hours from their presentation, and most had optimized hemodynamics by the time of enrollment [116]. Further controversy exists in respect of what method should be used to guide fluid management. Whether the indwelling pulmonary artery (PA) catheter is vital to the management of ARDS depends on two important considerations. First, optimal fluid balance must be crucial to preventing the progression of lung injury. Evidence linking a more positive fluid balance to the development of ARDS [117] and evidence linking increased extravascular lung water to the development of MODS and ARDS [118,119] support this first requisite justification [120,121]. Second, however, PA catheters must provide a critical and unique understanding of this balance that sufficiently and appropriately modifies clinical practice, and this has yet to be proven. Most recent evidence from the ARDS Network trial of fluid management suggests that PA catheter–guided therapy does not improve survival in ARDS over therapy guided by simple central venous pressure (CVP) alone [122], but data supporting the use of CVP to guide therapy are also equally limited [121,123]. In fact, CVP has been repeatedly demonstrated to be an unreliable index of cardiac preload and fluid responsiveness [121,123]. Thus, with the wider adoption of bedside ultrasonography in critical care, numerous additional noninvasive bedside measurements have been used to predict fluid responsiveness during resuscitation [124], with the intent of avoiding overresuscitation in patients at risk for developing ARDS [125,126]. There are now multiple techniques currently being used to help guide resuscitation and limit volume overloading, including but not limited to echocardiographic measures of stroke volume variability and inferior vena cava distensibility, peripheral pulse pressure variation, and response to passive leg raise [124,125,127], all of which have demonstrated reasonably high sensitivity and specificity in predicting fluid responsiveness, but none of which have yet to contribute to a management strategy shown to improve outcomes.

Pharmacologic Interventions

As in any other medical disease or syndrome, it would seem that the "Holy Grail" among clinicians is the discovery of some novel agent that can either break the cycle of disease pathogenesis or help restore physiologic homeostasis and reduce disease severity and morbidity. The field of pharmacologic intervention has been exhaustively explored in the field of ALI, often yielding promising results in animal models and periodically demonstrating modest improvements in lung function and oxygenation in patients, but rarely translating into improved outcomes.

Pulmonary Vasodilators

Given the advanced endothelial injury, physiologic shunt, and commonly observed pulmonary hypertension in ARDS, therapeutic benefit of pharmacologic pulmonary vasodilation has been studied with a focus on inhaled nitric oxide, iNO. Unfortunately, despite several clinical trials demonstrating improvements of physiologic responses, including vasodilation and oxygenation, there has been no consistent improvement in mortality. In addition, adverse consequences, including dose-dependent methemoglobinemia, pulmonary hypertension, and renal impairment, have been identified [128–130], so iNO is not currently recommended for the treatment of ARDS, although it may still be used as a rescue therapy at some centers.

Surfactant Replacement

Not long after ALI was first described [131], investigators demonstrated a reduction in the amount of surfactant retrieved from the lung and a derangement in the retrieved surfactant's biophysical properties [132]. Since then, numerous studies have supported these findings. The fundamental rationale for surfactant replacement is to help restore the natural surfactant film and reduce surface tension at the air–liquid interface, thus reducing the tendency for alveolar collapse and improving oxygenation through a reduction in shunt. The evidence in support of surfactant replacement therapy for neonatal RDS is abundant, but results in adults with ARDS have been less promising [130,133]. Despite promising results of small trials, several larger randomized phase 3 trials in ARDS failed to demonstrate any reduction in mortality [56,134]. Some have speculated that the failure to demonstrate an improvement in mortality results from the lack of a direct relationship between mortality and severity of respiratory failure, the intricacies of surfactant administration, and/or its potential inactivation by plasma proteins following delivery [135].

Corticosteroids

Given the well-characterized acute inflammatory response of ARDS, considerable effort has been spent determining the therapeutic role of corticosteroid therapy for the early and late treatment of this condition. Numerous uncontrolled trials had initially suggested a potential benefit of corticosteroids, and the first randomized controlled trial of corticosteroids for late ARDS demonstrated improved lung injury scores and oxygenation, decreased multiorgan dysfunction scores, and reduced ICU and in-hospital mortality in the group receiving steroids [136], but this study drew criticism for its small size and baseline differences between the treatment groups. Subsequently, a significantly larger NHLBI-sponsored multicenter trial completed by the ARDS Network exploring the use of corticosteroids for late persistent ARDS demonstrated more ventilator-free days and improved oxygenation for the group treated with methylprednisolone compared to placebo, but no reduction in 60-day mortality [137]. There was, however, an increase in neuromuscular weakness, and a higher 60- and 180-day mortality was observed when steroid therapy was initiated after 14 days of onset, suggesting a serious risk from this therapy for late ARDS.

Initial studies of steroids for early ARDS did not demonstrate benefit, but a more recent study [138] suggested an improvement in ICU mortality. However, the study was small, and concerns were raised regarding imbalances among the treatment arms. Several meta-analyses of the effects of glucocorticoids on ARDS mortality have come to different conclusions, adding to the challenges in establishing guidelines [139–142].

Anticoagulation/Fibrinolysis

The importance of microvascular coagulation and thrombosis in ARDS is underscored by the physiologic dead space, or "wasted ventilation," observed in ARDS patients [143]. Minimizing microvascular thrombosis could conceivably improve oxygenation through improved ventilation–perfusion matching [144] and increase survival through prevention of multiorgan failure [145]. Despite promising results in a rat model [146], the most recent phase II clinical trial of the endogenous anticoagulant activated protein C (APC) in ARDS failed to demonstrate a reduction in ventilator-free days with the use of APC [147]. Critics expressed concern about the study's statistical power and a priori likelihood of success [148], but in a similar vein, despite promising animal studies [144,149], a multicenter phase II trial of tissue factor inhibitor (site-inactivated VIIa) in ARDS was terminated prematurely because of an increased risk of adverse bleeding and a higher projected mortality rate in the high-dose treatment arm [8]. Thus, it seems that the benefits of potent anticoagulation in ARDS may ultimately be outweighed by risks of adverse bleeding.

β-agonists

As discussed in the pathogenesis section, AFC often remains intact in the setting of injury. AFC can be directly increased by *β*-agonists in animal models [150,151], presumably through upregulated activity of Na, K-ATPase at the basolateral membrane [152]. *β*-agonists might thus promise to have significant potential for benefit in ARDS. In animal models and clinical studies, beta-agonists have been shown to increase AFC, decrease endothelial permeability, increase surfactant secretion, and decrease inflammation [130,153]. Early small clinical trials of *β*-agonists for ARDS were promising, but two large randomized multicenter clinical trials were disappointing. The Albuterol Treatment of Acute Lung Injury trial [6] was stopped for futility, and the *β*-agonist Lung Injury Trial 2 (BALTI-2) was stopped for safety concerns [5]. In the wake of findings, there is currently no support for the use of *β*-agonists in the treatment of ARDS.

However, both of these trials enrolled patients with existing lung injury, and it is possible that *β*-agonists could be more effective in promoting enhanced AFC if administered prior to epithelial barrier disruption. To test this hypothesis, there is currently a multicenter, placebo-controlled phase 2 trial, Lung Injury Prevention Study with Budesonide and *β* Agonist (LIPS-B), enrolling patients at risk for ARDS. Patients will be randomized to aerosolized budesonide/formoterol versus placebo for 5 days, and the primary outcome is improvement in oxygenation (clinicaltrials.gov NCT01783821).

Nutritional Supplementation

Over the past decade, enthusiasm has arisen over the use of nutritional supplements in sepsis and ALI, particularly with the use of omega-3 fatty acids and other natural antioxidants such as vitamin E. The rationale for supplementing patients with omega-3 fatty acids, such as eicosapentaenoic acid, in the setting of inflammatory disorders comes from the notion that they can directly suppress monocyte production of inflammatory cytokines and incorporate into cell membrane phospholipids to compete with omega-6 fatty acids to promote the production of more favorable profiles of prostaglandins and leukotrienes [154].

To further understand the effects of omega-3 fatty acids alone, a phase 2 trial of 90 patients was completed but showed no benefit [155]. The ARDS Network initiated a phase 3 trial of enteral administration of omega 3 fatty acid, linolenic acid, and antioxidants (OMEGA). The trial was stopped early in view of concerns over potential harm because the treatment group had significantly fewer ventilator-free, ICU-free, and organ failure–free days [156]. Of note, in tandem with the OMEGA trial, the ARDS Network randomized patients with ARDS to low-volume trophic enteral feeds versus full enteral feeds for 6 days. There were no significant differences in ventilator-free days, 60-day mortality, or infectious complications [157].

HMG-CoA Reductase Inhibitors (the "statins")

HMG-CoA Reductase Inhibitors (also called "statins"), a class of drugs originally developed for the treatment of dyslipidemia and now used widely for the prevention of atherosclerosis, seemed to have significant potential for the treatment of ARDS. These drugs decreased inflammation and prevented ARDS in animal models, and also decreased both systemic and pulmonary inflammation in a human model of LPS (bacterial lipopolysaccharide) inhalation lung injury [158,159]. Studies initially suggested that statin use was associated with a decreased risk for the development of sepsis and its associated complications, including death [160], and a decreased risk for the development of ARDS [161], but the largest observational study found no protective effect for the development of ARDS associated with previous or concurrent statin use [162]. Similarly, observational studies and meta-analyses had demonstrated that patients on statins prior to hospitalization for infection had decreased morbidity and mortality, although a more recent meta-analysis [163] did not confirm those findings.

Two large randomized trials of statins in ARDS also failed to demonstrate an improvement of clinical outcomes. The larger randomized trial of rosuvastatin for patients with sepsis-associated ARDS was stopped for futility [3]. It demonstrated no improvement in the primary clinical outcome, mortality before discharge or by day 60, or in secondary endpoints, including ventilator-free days and organ failure–free days, but there was also evidence of an increase in renal and hepatic dysfunction for the treatment group. The second smaller, phase 2 multicenter, double-blinded clinical trial of simvastatin in patients with ARDS also found no difference in the primary outcome of ventilator-free days, or in the secondary outcomes of days free of nonpulmonary organ failure and 28-day mortality, but also found no difference in adverse outcomes [164].

PROSPECTIVE FUTURE THERAPIES

Airway Pressure Release Ventilation (APRV)

"Airway pressure release ventilation" (APRV) is a mode of ventilation that utilizes sustained high airway pressures and spontaneous breathing to maximize lung recruitment, with brief periods of "pressure release" to facilitate ventilation while minimizing derecruitment during exhalation [165]. Proponents assert that the periods of pressure release are typically brief enough to avoid alveolar closure and reexpansion, and efficacy relies heavily on the presence of spontaneous ventilation, which is believed to generate regionally variable transpulmonary pressures that favor recruitment of dependent lung regions [166]. Another purported benefit is the potentially decreased sedation needs of patients receiving APRV, but some studies suggest this may not be the case [167]. Because a prolonged inflation pressure (i.e., P_{high}) is maintained between brief periods of pressure release, recruitment and gas exchange are often improved with typically lower maximal airway pressures than conventional ventilation [60]. However, the potential for added distension still exists while patients spontaneously breathe above the volume generated by P_{high} [60], and relatively high transpulmonary pressure swings and large expiratory tidal volumes can still occur during APRV [168] and conceivably contribute to VILI [67].

Thus far, most published experience with APRV for patients with ARDS has been in the surgical and trauma population [165,169,170]. One of the earliest randomized trials comparing APRV to synchronized intermittent mandatory ventilation (SIMV) demonstrated an improvement in physiologic outcomes but was stopped early for futility in demonstrating any improvement in mortality or ventilator-free days [171]. A retrospective study has since demonstrated an actual increase in ventilator days with APRV compared to conventional support in trauma patients with ARDS [172]. The most recent randomized control trial comparing APRV to a conventional low tidal volume strategy for adult trauma patients demonstrated equal safety profiles but also demonstrated a nonsignificant trend toward increased ventilator days and ICU length of stay in those assigned to APRV [170]. Taken together, these findings have led some experts to conclude that thus far there is insufficient evidence to support the routine use of APRV in management of ARDS [60]. On the other hand, others have been able to demonstrate that an appropriately extended duration of P_{high} (i.e., T_{high}) and an appropriately brief period of pressure release can minimize tissue strain, respectively, through stable alveolar recruitment (homogeneous ventilation) and avoidance of alveolar collapse during exhalation [173]. These authors propose a role for APRV as a preemptive intervention for preventing the progression to ARDS in those at risk [173]. Additional work is needed in the field before APRV can be recommended over conventional low tidal volume ventilation, and it may be that the choice of one over the other will need to be tailored to the patient's injury and lung mechanics [174].

Stem Cell Therapy

Recent attention has been given to the use of embryonic ("pluripotent") and adult-derived ("multipotent") stem cells and "progenitor" cells in their therapeutic potential for mitigating inflammation and enhancing tissue repair in ARDS [175]. Enthusiasm first came from findings suggesting a favorable rate of engraftment and epithelial differentiation of infused bone marrow–derived stem cells in the injured lungs of mice. More recent work suggests that the rates of stem cell engraftment and differentiation are not as robust as initially hoped [175]. The field has gained greater momentum with the discovery that the delivery of human bone marrow–derived mesenchymal stem/stromal cells (MSCs) attenuates lung injury in multiple animal models of ARDS [176], pneumonia [177,178], and VILI [179] and can even restore AFC in human lung explants [180]. As a result, there is currently an ongoing phase 2 randomized clinical trial recruiting patients to determine the safety and efficacy of a single infusion of human allogenic bone marrow–derived MSCs for ARDS (clinicaltirals.gov NCT02097641).

Keratinocyte Growth Factor

One group of investigators has demonstrated the protective effects of human bone marrow–derived MSCs to be, at least in part, related to their ability to release keratinocyte growth factor (KGF) [181], which may help promote healing through type II pneumocyte proliferation, enhanced AFC and surfactant production, and repair of oxidant injury [36]. A multicenter, placebo-controlled, phase 2 trial to determine the safety and efficacy of IV infused KGF in improving oxygenation in ARDS patients was recently completed, but the results are pending [36,182].

Neuromuscular Blockade

Clinical practice guidelines have long supported the use of neuromuscular blockade (NMB) as a means of controlling patient–ventilator synchrony, oxygenation, and ventilation [183], and studies have supported NMB for patients with ARDS as a means toward improving oxygenation [184]. A recent multicenter randomized controlled trial conducted by *the ARDS et Curarisation Sytematique* (ACURASYS) study group in France demonstrated a significant mortality benefit for severe ARDS from early NMB with cisatracurium [7]. The study demonstrated that NMB for 48 hours, within 48 hours of onset, in "severe" ARDS (P:F ratio < 150 mm Hg), led to a significant decrease in both 28- and 90-day mortality, without any concomitant increased risk of adverse neuromuscular weakness [7]. The benefits of NMB in ARDS, in theory, stem from a mitigation of VILI by preventing spontaneous breathing with larger than intended tidal volumes on inspiration and reduced alveolar collapse on forced exhalation [185,186]. A subsequent meta-analysis of three trials (including the ACURASYS trial) concluded that short-term NMB (48 hours cisatracurium infusion) in adult patients with ARDS reduces hospital mortality without increased risk of critical illness polyneuropathy (CIP) [187]. However, all three trials reviewed in this analysis came from the same group of investigators. Thus, some experts have urged caution in generalizing the use of NMB in all patients with ARDS [89], based upon inconsistently higher reported rates of CIP following NMB, the potential need for higher levels of sedation with NMB, and the undetermined dosing and benefit of other NMB agents.

Preemptive Intervention Protocols

The search for an effective pharmacologic intervention or management algorithm in ARDS has been extensive and has now spanned decades, but the benefits from most interventions have been limited to improvements in oxygenation or fewer days of mechanical ventilation. One important lesson from the work to date is that much of what we once thought was critical to the management of these patients, although grounded in sound rationale, is not only often ineffective but can be potentially harmful. We have, however, also become more aware of how sound basic principles of critical care, such as hand hygiene, prompt antimicrobial

TABLE 163.2

Table Summarizing All Positive Randomized Controlled Trials (RCTs) of Treatments and Management Strategies for Acute Respiratory Distress Syndrome Prior to 2000, and Most Positive and Negative RCTs Since 2000

Intervention	Year	Study	No. of patients	Findings	References
"Open-lung" approach (recruitment maneuver and "ideal PEEP"	1998	Phase 3 single center	53	Decreased 28-day but not in-hospital mortality	Amato et al. [2]
Glucocorticoids during late fibrosing alveolitis	1998	Phase 3	24	Decreased mortality, but study small	Meduri et al. [136]
Low tidal volumes (6 vs. 12 mL/kg)	2000	Phase 3, multicenter	861	Decreased mortality from 40% to 30%	NHLBI ARDS Network [1]
Prone-positioning during mechanical ventilation	2001	Phase 3, multicenter	304	Improved oxygenation, but no benefit in mortality	Gattinoni et al. [109]
Partial liquid ventilation	2002	Phase 3, multicenter	90	Lower progression to ARDS, but no benefit in mortality	Hirschl et al. [222]
Recombinant surfactant protein C-based surfactant	2004	Phase 3, multicenter	448	Improved oxygenation at 24 hours but no benefit in mortality	Spragg et al. [56]
Prone-positioning for hypoxemic acute respiratory failure	2004	Phase 3, multicenter	791	No benefit in 28- or 90-day mortality and some safety concerns	Guerin et al. [111]
Higher versus lower PEEP during low tidal volume ventilation	2004	Phase 3, multicenter	549	No benefit in mortality or days on the ventilator	Brower et al. [90]
Low and high dose partial liquid ventilation	2006	Phase 3, multicenter	311	No benefit in mortality and some safety concerns	Kacmerek et al. [223]
Glucocorticoids for late/persistent ARDS	2006	Phase 3, multicenter	180	No benefit in mortality; increased mortality if started after 2 weeks	NHLBI ARDS Network [137]
Conservative versus Liberal Fluid Management in ALI	2006	Phase 3, multicenter	1,000	No benefit in mortality; conservative strategy improved lung function and reduced ventilator days	NHLBI ARDS Network [115]
Prolonged prone-positioning for severe ALI	2006	Phase 3, multicenter	136	Nonsignificant reduction in mortality (43% vs. 58%, $p = 0.12$)	Mancebo et al. [110]
Low tidal volumes, recruitment maneuvers and high PEEP	2008	Phase 3, multicenter	983	No mortality benefit; less refractory hypoxemia and rescue therapy	Meade et al. [86]
Low tidal volumes with plateau pressure directed, high PEEP	2008	Phase 3, multicenter	767	No mortality benefit; higher organ failure–free and ventilator-free days and improved lung function	Mercat et al. [224]
Activated Protein C	2008	Phase 2, multicenter	75	No benefit in ventilator-free days or mortality; reduced dead space	Liu et al. [147]
L-2-oxothiazolidine-4-carboxylic acid	2008	Phase 2, multicenter	215	Terminated early due to higher 30-day mortality and reduced vent-free days	Morris et al. [189]
Early mobilization in ICU for patients with respiratory failure	2008	Multicenter prospective	330	Decreased intensive care unit and hospital length of stay in survivors	Morris et al. [189]
Early physical therapy in ICU for patients with respiratory failure	2009	Randomized, two centers	104	Decreased days on mechanical ventilation and ICU length of stay; increased functional independence at time of discharge	Schweickert et al. [190]
Site-inactivated factor VIIa	2009	Phase 2, multicenter	46	Terminated early due to higher 28-day mortality in high dose group and trend toward increased bleeding	Vincent et al. [8]

(continued)

TABLE 163.2

Table Summarizing All Positive Randomized Controlled Trials (RCTs) of Treatments and Management Strategies for Acute Respiratory Distress Syndrome Prior to 2000, and Most Positive and Negative RCTs Since 2000 (*continued*)

Intervention	Year	Study	No. of patients	Findings	References
ECMO versus conventional ventilatory support for severe adult respiratory failure	2009	Randomized multicenter	180	Reduced death or severe disability at 6 months	Peek et al. [102]
Exogenous natural surfactant for ALI and ARDS	2009	Phase 3, multicenter	418	No reduction in 28-day mortality and trend toward increased harm	Kesicioglu et al. [134]
Neuromuscular blockade in early severe ARDS	2010	Phase 3, multicenter	340	Decrease in 28-day and 90-day mortality	Papazian et al. [7]
Simvastatin for ARDS (HARP study)	2011	Phase 2, single center	60	Simvastatin safe and associated with improvement in nonpulmonary organ dysfunction	Craig et al. [158]
Aerosolized β-2 agonists for ALI (ALTA)	2011	Phase 2 and 3, multicenter	282	Terminated early for projected futility; no improvement in vent-free days	Matthay et al. [6]
Omega-3 fatty acids for treatment of ALI	2011	Phase 2 multicenter	90	No reduction in biomarkers of pulmonary or systemic inflammation	Stapleton et al. [155]
Omega-3 fatty acids supplementation for ALI (EDEN-Omega)	2011	Phase 3, multicenter	272	"Omega" arm terminated early due to project futility	Rice et al. [156]
Intravenous β-2 agonists for treatment of ARDS (BALTI-2)	2012	Phase 3, multicenter	325	Terminated early for safety concerns, no benefit, possibly harmful	Gao Smith et al. [5]
Initial trophic versus full enteral feeding in patients with ALI (EDEN)	2012	Phase 3, multicenter	1,000	No differences in vent-free days, 60-day mortality, or infectious complications	Rice et al. [157]
Prone-positioning for severe ARDS	2013	Phase 3, multicenter	466	Decrease in 28-day and 90-day mortality	Guerin et al. [4]
High-frequency oscillation for ARDS (OSCAR Study Group)	2013	Phase 3, multicenter	795	No reduction in 30-day mortality	Young et al. [99]
High-frequency oscillation in early ARDS (OSCILLATE trial)	2013	Phase 3, multicenter	548	Terminated early due to potential increase in mortality in treatment arm	Ferguson et al. [100]
Simvastatin in Acute Respiratory Distress Syndrome (HARP-2)	2014	Phase 3, multicenter	540	No reduction in mortality, vent-free days, or organ failure–free days	McAuley et al. [164]
Rosuvastatin for sepsis-associated ARDS (SAILS)	2014	Phase 3, multicenter	745	Terminated early for projected futility; no reduction in mortality or vent-free days	Truwit et al. [3]
High-flow nasal cannula oxygen for acute hypoxemic respiratory failure	2015	Randomized multicenter	310	Nonsignificant reduction in need for intubation, but increased vent-free days and reduced 90-day mortality	Frat et al. [62]

therapy, and protocols to prevent aspiration and nosocomial pneumonia, can substantially reduce overall morbidity in the ICU and likely contribute to the declining incidence of ARDS [36]. In fact, it has been shown that the downward trend in the incidence of ARDS over the past decade is most attributable to a decreasing incidence in hospital-acquired ARDS, with no change in the incidence of preadmission ARDS [188]. In keeping with the philosophy of preemptive intervention, other studies have demonstrated that not only is early intervention with physical therapy in mechanically ventilated patients safe and cost effective, but it can also reduce the duration of delirium, mechanical ventilation, ICU and hospital length of stay, and promote greater functional independence by the time of discharge [189,190]. Investigators have also discovered reductions of ARDS incidence following the enforcement of conservative transfusion policies and preemptive low tidal volume ventilation in the care of patients "at risk" for the development of ARDS [78,79]. In response to this wave of preemptive interventions, the Lung Injury Prevention Study group has since bundled all of these best practices into a Checklist for Lung Injury Prevention (CLIP) [191]. In addition, investigators have developed the Lung Injury Prediction Score (LIPS), a tool that can help stratify a patient's risk of developing ARDS and identify those most likely to benefit from preemptive intervention [192]. Although reasonably sensitive and specific, reliance on 22 different predisposing variables for calculation may limit the clinical feasibility of the LIPS, and this has helped foster interest in alternative prediction tools, such as the Early Acute Lung Injury Score, the latter being more simply based on oxygen requirement, respiratory rate, and presence/absence of immunosuppression [36,193].

PROGNOSIS AND OUTCOMES

Prognosis

While in-hospital and 28-day mortality rates can differ, depending on age, with substantially higher mortality among those over 85 years of age [9], the most currently reported mortality rates fall at around 30% [3,89]. Numerous clinical factors have been shown to predict a higher mortality rate in ARDS patients. These include male sex, African American race, advanced age, alcohol abuse, malignancy, liver disease, chronic steroid use, infection with human immunodeficiency virus, and ARDS secondary to sepsis or aspiration [18,194]. Curiously, although patients of advanced age, particularly >70 years of age, are at a significantly higher risk of death from ARDS, those who survive recover at the same rate as their younger counterparts [195,196]. Chronic alcohol abuse has been shown to increase the risk of developing not only ARDS in patients at risk, but also multiorgan dysfunction after the development of ARDS [197]. Body mass index (BMI) [198] exhibits a U-shaped distribution of relative risk for mortality in ARDS, with higher risk falling on both the low and high ends of the curve. In the case of BMI, although it is somewhat intuitive that patients with either an exceedingly low or excessively high BMI would be at greater risk of death, an unexpected finding was that of the lowest risk belonging to those considered "obese," with a BMI between 30 and 40 [198]. As the science of genomics has advanced, several candidate genes and genetic polymorphisms have been found to be associated with an increased susceptibility to the syndrome and to an increased risk of mortality [199,200]. Although no specific gene or polymorphism has been proven sensitive or specific enough for routine clinical screening, significant work has been done linking ARDS risk to genes affecting immune regulation, epithelial and endothelial function, and oxidative stress [200], and this area of research has increased our understanding of the pathogenesis of ARDS and is providing insight into potential new therapies [41,200].

Outcomes

Estimates of mortality from ARDS once ranged as high as 70% [63,201]. Despite a documented decline between the early 1980s and late 1990s [63,201], mortality from ARDS appears to have now plateaued between 30% and 40% for all patients [9,25]. As mortality has slowly improved for ARDS, there has been growing interest in the longer-reaching consequences of this condition [202,203]. In particular, ARDS survivors often suffer from an impairment in neurocognitive skills [204,205], and the perception of a poor quality of life [203,206]. By as far as 1 year from recovery, although many recover spirometric lung function, the majority of ARDS survivors have a diminished diffusing capacity and exercise tolerance lasting out to 5 years from discharge [203,207]. One report noted less than half of all ARDS survivors returning to work after 1 year and about three-quarters returning to work within 5 years [207]. Many survivors likewise suffer from depression and anxiety, with depression occurring in one-quarter to one-half of all ARDS survivors as far as 2 years out from recovery [203]. Rates of anxiety-related symptoms have been reported as high as 41%, remaining as high as 24% 1 to 2 years out from discharge [203]. Posttraumatic stress disorder (PTSD) is also a significant concern among ARDS survivors with psychiatrist-diagnosed PTSD rates of 44%, 25%, and 24% reported at discharge, 5, and 8 years later, respectively [208]. Of note, predictors of PTSD symptoms in this setting include higher benzodiazepine usage, and recall of delusional experiences from the ICU stay [203].

A regimented sedation protocol designed to promote daily sedation interruption and reduced total cumulative dosing in critically ill patients is associated with a decreased number of days in the ICU and fewer days on mechanical ventilation [209]. Furthermore, this strategy has been associated with lower rates of PTSD-related symptoms following recovery [210]. The feasibility and importance of establishing clear sedation goals and using validated tools for sedation assessment in critically ill patients have been firmly established, and this standard of care is now a part of established professional society guidelines for sedation in the ICU [211].

Utility of Ultrasonography for Diagnosis and Management of ARDS

A key differential point in the diagnosis of ARDS is whether the patient with bilateral lung infiltrates has primary lung injury, cardiac failure, or, on occasion, both ARDS and CPE. This is an important consideration when managing the patient who fulfills the Berlin criteria for ARDS, but where the question remains as to what extent cardiac failure may contribute to the process. Lung ultrasonography combined with echocardiography has utility in making this distinction.

Equipment Requirements and Scanning Technique

Equipment requirements and scanning technique are described in Chapter 11 Lung Ultrasonography. In addition to the standard phased array probe used for lung ultrasonography, the linear vascular probe has specific application for examination of pleural line morphology. Pleural line morphology is determined with the high-frequency linear probe, whereas B-line distribution is determined with the low-frequency phased array probe.

Diagnosis of ARDS

The characteristic findings of lung ultrasonography in ARDS include B lines and consolidation. The presence of multiple B lines indicates an alveolar interstitial syndrome (AIS) and correlates with an increase in extravascular lung water [212]. This may be caused by permeability failure, as in ARDS, or by elevation of left atrial pressure (LAP) with resulting CPE. The pattern of B-line distribution in ARDS is multifocal in association with irregularity of the visceral pleural surface (see Chapter 11 Lung Ultrasonography). The pattern of B-line distribution in CPE is typically more even, more distributed to the gravitationally dependent lung regions, and associated with a more smooth and regular pleural line (see Chapter 11 Lung Ultrasonography). The demonstration with ultrasonography of a nonhomogeneous AIS pattern with spared areas, pleural line irregularity, and lung consolidations is strongly predictive of ARDS (see Chapter 11 Lung Ultrasonography), whereas the finding of a homogeneous AIS pattern with smooth pleural line and no lung consolidations is strongly predictive of CPE [213].

Lung ultrasonography, chest radiography, and chest CT alone cannot make a diagnosis of ARDS or CPE, because there are other disease processes that can mimic these entities. The results of imaging can only support the diagnosis of ARDS, whereas other elements are required to meet the Berlin definition. Lung ultrasonography gives results that are superior to auscultation and standard radiography for detection of AIS and consolidation but provides utility similar to that of chest CT for the diagnosis of ARDS or CPE [214,215].

Similar to chest radiography and CT imaging, a limitation of lung ultrasonography is in the occasional patient who has both

ARDS and CPE, or in the patient who has preexisting lung disease with AIS and pleural irregularity with superimposed acute CPE. Categorization of acute hypoxemic respiratory failure between CPE, ARDS, and miscellaneous causes is aided by combining thoracic ultrasonography with basic echocardiography (see Chapter 16 on Critical Care Echocardiography). The combined findings of an abundance of B lines, the presence of reduced left ventricular function, a left-sided pleural effusion, and a dilated inferior vena cava can help support the diagnosis of CPE [32].

Echocardiography allows a semiquantitative estimate of LAP by application of a standard algorithm [216]. The examination requires training in advanced critical care echocardiography, because it utilizes Doppler measurements that are not part of the basic critical care–focused echocardiography examination. The operator applies an algorithm [217] that allows classification of LAP as normal or elevated, and this is useful for distinguishing ARDS from CPE. The primary measurement of interest is the ratio of the peak velocity of early mitral valve diastolic inflow (E), measured by pulse wave Doppler between the tips of the mitral valve leaflets, to the peak velocity of the early lateral mitral annulus diastolic movement (e′), the latter value obtained by tissue Doppler measurement (Video 163.1). These values are readily obtained in a large proportion of patients and are often useful, but they require advanced skills in tissue Doppler measurement technique, and they may yield an indeterminate result. If this is the case, the algorithm requires using a further series of measurements, the complexity of which precludes their regular use in the ICU [217].

Management of ARDS

The use of PEEP in ARDS results in recruitment of atelectatic and poorly aerated lung, which are detectable with lung ultrasonography. On ultrasound, atelectatic lung appears similar to that of consolidated lung, and poorly aerated lung is characterized by abundant B lines. Using a quantitative lung reaeration score, the application of PEEP in ARDS can result in lung recruitment detected by lung ultrasonography, which can be correlated with recruitment volumes interpolated from changes in the pressure volume curve [218]. The pressure at which lung recruitment is detected with lung ultrasonography correlates with the lower inflection point determined by a low-flow pressure–volume curve technique [219]. Although improvement of aeration pattern is observed during lung recruitment with PEEP, lung ultrasonography is not able to determine whether there is concomitant overdistension of some areas of the lung [218]. The utility of these results in routine practice is not yet well defined, but lung ultrasonography may offer a method of directly observing lung recruitment that is easily repeated at the bedside in serial fashion, making this technique potentially far more practical than serial chest CT imaging.

If lung ultrasonography and echocardiography indicate that CPE is the primary disease process, or that CPE is contributing to the severity of the ARDS, then the management strategy includes treatment directed toward CPE.

CONCLUSIONS

Since its first published description in 1967, our understanding of the pathogenesis and pathophysiology of ARDS has grown appreciably, and ongoing research efforts continue to provide hope for exciting new therapies in the future. Our improved understanding of this condition has already translated into improved outcomes for patients suffering from ARDS, but its still poor prognosis for those acutely afflicted in the hospital and for those fortunate enough to survive [203] has left room for ongoing progress in the management of these patients. Aside from the obvious importance of reducing mortality from this condition, a reduction of nonpulmonary organ failures, duration of mechanical ventilation, and ICU length of stay, as well as improved quality-of-life measures among survivors, all represent reasonable and tangible outcome goals, but researchers still face challenges in how to best measure and represent these outcomes [220]. Fortunately, there is no shortage of talented and passionately dedicated physicians and scientists searching for solutions to all of these yet unsolved issues.

References

1. ARDS-Network: Ventilation with lower tidal volumes as compared with traditional tidal volumes for acute lung injury and the acute respiratory distress syndrome. The Acute Respiratory Distress Syndrome Network. *N Engl J Med* 2000;342:1301–1308.
2. Amato MB, Barbas CS, Medeiros DM, et al: Effect of a protective-ventilation strategy on mortality in the acute respiratory distress syndrome. *N Engl J Med* 338:347–354, 1998.
3. Truwit JD, Bernard GR, Steingrub J, et al: Rosuvastatin for sepsis-associated acute respiratory distress syndrome. *N Engl J Med* 370:2191–2200, 2014.
4. Guerin C, Reignier J, Richard JC, et al: Prone positioning in severe acute respiratory distress syndrome. *N Engl J Med* 368:2159–2168, 2013.
5. Gao Smith F, Perkins GD, Gates S, et al: Effect of intravenous beta-2 agonist treatment on clinical outcomes in acute respiratory distress syndrome (BALTI-2): a multicentre, randomised controlled trial. *Lancet* 379:229–235, 2012.
6. Matthay MA, Brower RG, Carson S, et al: Randomized, placebo-controlled clinical trial of an aerosolized beta(2)-agonist for treatment of acute lung injury. *Am J Respir Crit Care Med* 184:561–568, 2011.
7. Papazian L, Forel JM, Gacouin A, et al: Neuromuscular blockers in early acute respiratory distress syndrome. *N Engl J Med* 363:1107–1116, 2010.
8. Vincent JL, Artigas A, Petersen LC, et al: A multicenter, randomized, double-blind, placebo-controlled, dose-escalation trial assessing safety and efficacy of active site inactivated recombinant factor VIIa in subjects with acute lung injury or acute respiratory distress syndrome. *Crit Care Med* 37:1874–1880, 2009.
9. Rubenfeld GD, Caldwell E, Peabody E, et al: Incidence and outcomes of acute lung injury. *N Engl J Med* 353:1685–1693, 2005.
10. Shah CV, Localio AR, Lanken PN, et al: The impact of development of acute lung injury on hospital mortality in critically ill trauma patients. *Crit Care Med* 36:2309–2315, 2008.
11. Bernard GR, Artigas A, Brigham KL, et al: The American-European Consensus Conference on ARDS. Definitions, mechanisms, relevant outcomes, and clinical trial coordination. *Am J Respir Crit Care Med* 149:818–824, 1994.
12. Meade MO, Cook RJ, Guyatt GH, et al: Interobserver variation in interpreting chest radiographs for the diagnosis of acute respiratory distress syndrome. *Am J Respir Crit Care Med* 161:85–90, 2000.
13. Thompson BT, Moss M: A new definition for the acute respiratory distress syndrome. *Semin Respir Crit Care Med* 34:441–447, 2013.
14. Ranieri VM, Rubenfeld GD, Thompson BT, et al: Acute respiratory distress syndrome: the Berlin Definition. *JAMA* 307:2526–2533, 2012.
15. Allardet-Servent J, Forel J-M, Roch A, et al: FIO_2 and acute respiratory distress syndrome definition during lung protective ventilation.[see comment]. *Crit Care Med* 37:202–207, 2009.
16. Doyle RL, Szaflarski N, Modin GW, et al: Identification of patients with acute lung injury. Predictors of mortality. *Am J Respir Crit Care Med* 152:1818–1824, 1995.
17. Monchi M, Bellenfant F, Cariou A, et al: Early predictive factors of survival in the acute respiratory distress syndrome. A multivariate analysis. *Am J Respir Crit Care Med* 158:1076–1081, 1998.
18. Zilberberg MD, Epstein SK: Acute lung injury in the medical ICU: comorbid conditions, age, etiology, and hospital outcome. *Am J Respir Crit Care Med* 157:1159–1164, 1998.
19. Ferguson ND, Frutos-Vivar F, Esteban A, et al: Acute respiratory distress syndrome: underrecognition by clinicians and diagnostic accuracy of three clinical definitions. *Crit Care Med* 33:2228–2234, 2005.
20. Ware LB, Matthay MA: The acute respiratory distress syndrome. *N Engl J Med* 342:1334–1349, 2000.
21. TenHoor T, Mannino DM, Moss M: Risk factors for ARDS in the United States: analysis of the 1993 National Mortality Followback Study. *Chest* 119:1179–1184, 2001.
22. Tomashefski JF Jr: Pulmonary pathology of acute respiratory distress syndrome. *Clin Chest Med* 21:435–466, 2000.
23. Cheung O, Leslie KO: Acute Lung Injury, in Leslie KO, Wick MW (eds): *Practical Pulmonary Pathology*. 1st ed. Philadelphia, PA, Churchill Livingstone, 2005, pp 71–95.
24. Marshall RP, Bellingan G, Webb S, et al: Fibroproliferation occurs early in the acute respiratory distress syndrome and impacts on outcome. *Am J Respir Crit Care Med* 162:1783–1788, 2000.
25. Wheeler AP, Bernard GR: Acute lung injury and the acute respiratory distress syndrome: a clinical review. *Lancet* 369:1553–1564, 2007.
26. Goodman PC, Quinones Maymi DM: Radiographic findings in ARDS, in Matthay MA, (ed). *Acute Respiratory Distress Syndrome*. New York, NY, Marcel Dekker, Inc., 2003, pp 55–73.
27. Desai SR: Acute respiratory distress syndrome: imaging of the injured lung. *Clin Radiol* 57:8–17, 2002.

28. Rubenfeld GD, Caldwell E, Granton J, et al: Interobserver variability in applying a radiographic definition for ARDS. *Chest* 116:1347–1353, 1999.
29. Bellani G, Messa C, Guerra L, et al: Lungs of patients with acute respiratory distress syndrome show diffuse inflammation in normally aerated regions: a [18F]-fluoro-2-deoxy-D-glucose PET/CT study. *Crit Care Med* 37:2216–2222, 2009.
30. Berthezene Y, Vexler V, Jerome H, et al: Differentiation of capillary leak and hydrostatic pulmonary edema with a macromolecular MR imaging contrast agent. *Radiology* 181:773–777, 1991.
31. Raijmakers PG, Groeneveld AB, Teule GJ, et al: Diagnostic value of the gallium-67 pulmonary leak index in pulmonary edema. *J Nucl Med* 37:1316–1322, 1996.
32. Sekiguchi H, Schenck LA, Horie R, et al: Critical care ultrasonography differentiates ARDS, pulmonary edema, and other causes in the early course of acute hypoxemic respiratory failure. *Chest* 148:912–918, 2015.
33. Goss CH, Brower RG, Hudson LD, et al: Incidence of acute lung injury in the United States. *Crit Care Med* 31:1607–1611, 2003.
34. Bice T, Cox CE, Carson SS: Cost and health care utilization in ARDS—different from other critical illness? *Semin Respir Crit Care Med* 34:529–536, 2013.
35. Dasta JF, McLaughlin TP, Mody SH, et al: Daily cost of an intensive care unit day: the contribution of mechanical ventilation. *Crit Care Med* 33:1266–1271, 2005.
36. Beitler JR, Schoenfeld DA, Thompson BT: Preventing ARDS: progress, promise, and pitfalls. *Chest* 146:1102–1113, 2014.
37. Calfee CS, Eisner MD, Ware LB, et al: Trauma-associated lung injury differs clinically and biologically from acute lung injury due to other clinical disorders [see comment]. *Crit Care Med* 35:2243–2250, 2007.
38. Iscimen R, Cartin-Ceba R, Yilmaz M, et al: Risk factors for the development of acute lung injury in patients with septic shock: an observational cohort study [see comment]. *Crit Care Med* 36:1518–1522, 2008.
39. Moazed F, Calfee CS: Environmental risk factors for acute respiratory distress syndrome. *Clin Chest Med* 35:625–637, 2014.
40. Khan H, Belsher J, Yilmaz M, et al: Fresh-frozen plasma and platelet transfusions are associated with development of acute lung injury in critically ill medical patients. *Chest* 131:1308–1314, 2007.
41. Janz DR, Ware LB: Biomarkers of ALI/ARDS: pathogenesis, discovery, and relevance to clinical trials. *Semin Respir Crit Care Med* 34:537–548, 2013.
42. Calfee CS, Budev MM, Matthay MA, et al: Plasma receptor for advanced glycation end-products predicts duration of ICU stay and mechanical ventilation in patients after lung transplantation. *J Heart Lung Transplant* 26:675–680, 2007.
43. Ware LB, Matthay MA: Alveolar fluid clearance is impaired in the majority of patients with acute lung injury and the acute respiratory distress syndrome. *Am J Respir Crit Care Med* 163:1376–1383, 2001.
44. Agrawal A, Matthay MA, Kangelaris KN, et al: Plasma angiopoietin-2 predicts the onset of acute lung injury in critically ill patients. *Am J Respir Crit Care Med* 187:736–742, 2013.
45. Calfee CS, Gallagher D, Abbott J, et al: Plasma angiopoietin-2 in clinical acute lung injury: prognostic and pathogenetic significance. *Crit Care Med* 40:1731–1737, 2012.
46. Azoulay E, Attalah H, Yang K, et al: Exacerbation with granulocyte colony-stimulating factor of prior acute lung injury during neutropenia recovery in rats. *Crit Care Med* 31:157–165, 2003.
47. Looney MR, Nguyen JX, Hu Y, et al: Platelet depletion and aspirin treatment protect mice in a two-event model of transfusion-related acute lung injury. *J Clin Invest* 119:3450–3461, 2009.
48. Zarbock A, Singbartl K, Ley K: Complete reversal of acid-induced acute lung injury by blocking of platelet-neutrophil aggregation. *J Clin Invest* 116:3211–3219, 2006.
49. Erlich JM, Talmor DS, Cartin-Ceba R, et al: Prehospitalization antiplatelet therapy is associated with a reduced incidence of acute lung injury: a population-based cohort study. *Chest* 139:289–295, 2011.
50. Kor DJ, Erlich J, Gong MN, et al: Association of prehospitalization aspirin therapy and acute lung injury: results of a multicenter international observational study of at-risk patients. *Crit Care Med* 39:2393–2400, 2011.
51. Bastarache JA, Wang L, Geiser T, et al: The alveolar epithelium can initiate the extrinsic coagulation cascade through expression of tissue factor. *Thorax* 62:608–616, 2007.
52. Ware LB, Matthay MA, Parsons PE, et al: Pathogenetic and prognostic significance of altered coagulation and fibrinolysis in acute lung injury/acute respiratory distress syndrome [see comment]. *Crit Care Med* 35:1821–1828, 2007.
53. Kaisers U, Busch T, Deja M, et al: Selective pulmonary vasodilation in acute respiratory distress syndrome. *Crit Care Med* 31:S337–S342, 2003.
54. Steltzer H, Krafft P, Fridrich P, et al: Right ventricular function and oxygen transport patterns in patients with acute respiratory distress syndrome. *Anaesthesia* 49:1039–1045, 1994.
55. Gattinoni L, Pelosi P, Suter PM, et al: Acute respiratory distress syndrome caused by pulmonary and extrapulmonary disease. Different syndromes? *Am J Respir Crit Care Med* 158:3–11, 1998.
56. Spragg RG, Lewis JF, Walmrath HD, et al: Effect of recombinant surfactant protein C-based surfactant on the acute respiratory distress syndrome. *N Engl J Med* 351:884–892, 2004.
57. Veldhuizen RA, Welk B, Harbottle R, et al: Mechanical ventilation of isolated rat lungs changes the structure and biophysical properties of surfactant. *J Appl Physiol* 92:1169–1175, 2002.
58. Gattinoni L, Caironi P, Pelosi P, et al: What has computed tomography taught us about the acute respiratory distress syndrome? *Am J Respir Crit Care Med* 164:1701–1711, 2001.
59. Hubmayr RD: Perspective on lung injury and recruitment: a skeptical look at the opening and collapse story. *Am J Respir Crit Care Med* 165:1647–1653, 2002.
60. Al-Hegelan M, MacIntyre NR: Novel modes of mechanical ventilation. *Semin Respir Crit Care Med* 34:499–507, 2013.
61. Saddy F, Sutherasan Y, Rocco PR, et al: Ventilator-associated lung injury during assisted mechanical ventilation. *Semin Respir Crit Care Med* 35:409–417, 2014.
62. Frat JP, Thille AW, Mercat A, et al: High-flow oxygen through nasal cannula in acute hypoxemic respiratory failure. *N Engl J Med* 372:2185–2196, 2015.
63. Stapleton RD, Wang BM, Hudson LD, et al: Causes and timing of death in patients with ARDS. *Chest* 128:525–532, 2005.
64. Petty TL: Acute respiratory distress syndrome (ARDS). *Dis Mon* 36:1–58, 1990.
65. Young MP, Manning HL, Wilson DL, et al: Ventilation of patients with acute lung injury and acute respiratory distress syndrome: has new evidence changed clinical practice? *Crit Care Med* 32:1260–1265, 2004.
66. Kalhan R, Mikkelsen M, Dedhiya P, et al: Underuse of lung protective ventilation: analysis of potential factors to explain physician behavior. *Crit Care Med* 34:300–306, 2006.
67. Hess DR: Ventilatory strategies in severe acute respiratory failure. *Semin Respir Crit Care Med* 35:418–430, 2014.
68. Needham DM, Colantuoni E, Mendez-Tellez PA, et al: Lung protective mechanical ventilation and two year survival in patients with acute lung injury: prospective cohort study. *BMJ* 344:e2124, 2012.
69. Dellinger RP, Levy MM, Rhodes A, et al: Surviving sepsis campaign: international guidelines for management of severe sepsis and septic shock: 2012. *Crit Care Med* 41:580–637, 2013.
70. Hager DN, Krishnan JA, Hayden D, et al: Tidal volume reduction in patients with acute lung inury when plateau pressures are not hig. *Am J Respir Crit Care Med* 172:1241–1245, 2005.
71. Terragni PP, Rosboch G, Tealdi A, et al: Tidal hyperinflation during low tidal volume ventilation in acute respiratory distress syndrome. *Am J Respir Crit Care Med* 175:160–166, 2007.
72. Laffey JG, O'Croinin D, McLoughlin P, et al: Permissive hypercapnia—role in protective lung ventilatory strategies. *Intensive Care Med* 30:347–356, 2004.
73. Lang JD, Figueroa M, Sanders KD, et al: Hypercapnia via reduced rate and tidal volume contributes to lipopolysaccharide-induced lung injury. *Am J Respir Crit Care Med* 171:147–157, 2005.
74. Doerr CH, Gajic O, Berrios JC, et al: Hypercapnic acidosis impairs plasma membrane wound resealing in ventilator-injured lungs. *Am J Respir Crit Care Med* 171:1371–1377, 2005.
75. Kregenow DA, Rubenfeld GD, Hudson LD, et al: Hypercapnic acidosis and mortality in acute lung injury. *Crit Care Med* 34:1–7, 2006.
76. Parsons PE, Matthay MA, Ware LB, et al: Elevated plasma levels of soluble TNF receptors are associated with morbidity and mortality in patients with acute lung injury. *Am J Physiol Lung Cell Mol Physiol* 288:L426–L431, 2005.
77. Parsons PE, Eisner MD, Thompson BT, et al: Lower tidal volume ventilation and plasma cytokine markers of inflammation in patients with acute lung injury. *Crit Care Med* 33:1–6; discussion 230–232, 2005.
78. Gajic O, Dara SI, Mendez JL, et al: Ventilator-associated lung injury in patients without acute lung injury at the onset of mechanical ventilation. *Crit Care Med* 32:1817–1824, 2004.
79. Yilmaz M, Keegan MT, Iscimen R, et al: Toward the prevention of acute lung injury: protocol-guided limitation of large tidal volume ventilation and inappropriate transfusion [see comment]. *Crit Care Med* 35:1660–1666; quiz 1667, 2007.
80. Determann RM, Royakkers A, Wolthuis EK, et al: Ventilation with lower tidal volumes as compared with conventional tidal volumes for patients without acute lung injury: a preventive randomized controlled trial. *Crit Care* 14:R1, 2010.
81. Futier E, Constantin JM, Paugam-Burtz C, et al: A trial of intraoperative low-tidal-volume ventilation in abdominal surgery. *N Engl J Med* 369:428–437, 2013.
82. Frank JA, Gutierrez JA, Jones KD, et al: Low tidal volume reduces epithelial and endothelial injury in acid-injured rat lungs. *Am J Respir Crit Care Med* 165:242–249, 2002.
83. Fan E, Wilcox ME, Brower RG, et al: Recruitment maneuvers for acute lung injury: a systematic review. *Am J Respir Crit Care Med* 178:1156–1163, 2008.
84. Tetenev K, Cloutier ME, von Reyn JA, et al: Synergy between acid and endotoxin in an experimental model of aspiration-related lung injury progression. *Am J Physiol Lung Cell Mol Physiol* 309:L1103–L1111, 2015.
85. Allen GB, Suratt BT, Rinaldi L, et al: Choosing the frequency of deep inflation in mice: balancing recruitment against ventilator-induced lung injury. *Am J Physiol Lung Cell Mol Physiol* 291:L710–L717, 2006.
86. Meade MO, Cook DJ, Guyatt GH, et al: Ventilation strategy using low tidal volumes, recruitment maneuvers, and high positive end-expiratory pressure for acute lung injury and acute respiratory distress syndrome: a randomized controlled trial [see comment]. *JAMA* 299:637–645, 2008.
87. Esan A, Hess DR, Raoof S, et al: Severe hypoxemic respiratory failure: part 1—ventilatory strategies. *Chest* 137:1203–1216, 2010.
88. Gattinoni L, Caironi P: Refining ventilatory treatment for acute lung injury and acute respiratory distress syndrome. *JAMA* 299:691–693, 2008.
89. O'Gara B, Fan E, Talmor DS: Controversies in the management of severe ARDS: optimal ventilator management and use of rescue therapies. *Semin Respir Crit Care Med* 36:823–834, 2015.

90. Brower RG, Lanken PN, MacIntyre N, et al: Higher versus lower positive end-expiratory pressures in patients with the acute respiratory distress syndrome. *N Engl J Med* 351:327–336, 2004.
91. Levy MM: PEEP in ARDS—How Much Is Enough? *N Engl J Med* 351:389–391, 2004.
92. Mercat A, Richard J-CM, Vielle B, et al: Positive end-expiratory pressure setting in adults with acute lung injury and acute respiratory distress syndrome: a randomized controlled trial [see comment]. *JAMA* 299:646–655, 2008.
93. Briel M, Meade M, Mercat A, et al: Higher vs lower positive end-expiratory pressure in patients with acute lung injury and acute respiratory distress syndrome: systematic review and meta-analysis. *JAMA* 303:865–873, 2010.
94. Santa Cruz R, Rojas JI, Nervi R, et al: High versus low positive end-expiratory pressure (PEEP) levels for mechanically ventilated adult patients with acute lung injury and acute respiratory distress syndrome. *Cochrane Database Syst Rev* 6:CD009098, 2013.
95. Dasenbrook EC, Needham DM, Brower RG, et al: Higher PEEP in patients with acute lung injury: a systematic review and meta-analysis. *Respir Care* 56:568–575, 2011.
96. Goligher EC, Kavanagh BP, Rubenfeld GD, et al: Oxygenation response to positive end-expiratory pressure predicts mortality in acute respiratory distress syndrome. A secondary analysis of the LOVS and ExPress trials. *Am J Respir Crit Care Med* 190:70–76, 2014.
97. Talmor D, Sarge T, Malhotra A, et al: Mechanical ventilation guided by esophageal pressure in acute lung injury [see comment]. *N Engl J Med* 359:2095–2104, 2008.
98. Sud S, Sud M, Friedrich JO, et al: High frequency oscillation in patients with acute lung injury and acute respiratory distress syndrome (ARDS): systematic review and meta-analysis. *BMJ* 340:c2327, 2010.
99. Young D, Lamb SE, Shah S, et al: High-frequency oscillation for acute respiratory distress syndrome. *N Engl J Med* 368:806–813, 2013.
100. Ferguson ND, Cook DJ, Guyatt GH, et al: High-frequency oscillation in early acute respiratory distress syndrome. *N Engl J Med* 368:795–805, 2013.
101. Abrams D, Brodie D: Extracorporeal circulatory approaches to treat acute respiratory distress syndrome. *Clin Chest Med* 35:765–779, 2014.
102. Peek GJ, Mugford M, Tiruvoipati R, et al: Efficacy and economic assessment of conventional ventilatory support versus extracorporeal membrane oxygenation for severe adult respiratory failure (CESAR): a multicentre randomised controlled trial. *Lancet* 374:1351–1363, 2009.
103. Agarwal R, Aggarwal AN, Gupta D: Role of noninvasive ventilation in acute lung injury/acute respiratory distress syndrome: a proportion meta-analysis. *Respir Care* 55:1653–1660, 2010.
104. Thille AW, Contou D, Fragnoli C, et al: Non-invasive ventilation for acute hypoxemic respiratory failure: intubation rate and risk factors. *Crit Care* 17:R269, 2013.
105. Carrillo A, Gonzalez-Diaz G, Ferrer M, et al: Non-invasive ventilation in community-acquired pneumonia and severe acute respiratory failure. *Intensive Care Med* 38:458–466, 2012.
106. Schettino G, Altobelli N, Kacmarek RM: Noninvasive positive-pressure ventilation in acute respiratory failure outside clinical trials: experience at the Massachusetts General Hospital. *Crit Care Med* 36:441–447, 2008.
107. Glenny RW, Lamm WJ, Albert RK, et al: Gravity is a minor determinant of pulmonary blood flow distribution. *J Appl Physiol* 71:620–629, 1991.
108. Lamm WJ, Graham MM, Albert RK: Mechanism by which the prone position improves oxygenation in acute lung injury. *Am J Respir Crit Care Med* 150:184–193, 1994.
109. Gattinoni L, Tognoni G, Pesenti A, et al: Effect of prone positioning on the survival of patients with acute respiratory failure. *N Engl J Med* 345:568–573, 2001.
110. Mancebo J, Fernandez R, Blanch L, et al: A multicenter trial of prolonged prone ventilation in severe acute respiratory distress syndrome. *Am J Respir Crit Care Med* 173:1233–1239, 2006.
111. Guerin C, Gaillard S, Lemasson S, et al: Effects of systematic prone positioning in hypoxemic acute respiratory failure: a randomized controlled trial. *JAMA* 292:2379–2387, 2004.
112. Beitler JR, Shaefi S, Montesi SB, et al: Prone positioning reduces mortality from acute respiratory distress syndrome in the low tidal volume era: a meta-analysis. *Intensive Care Med* 40:332–341, 2014.
113. Taccone P, Pesenti A, Latini R, et al: Prone positioning in patients with moderate and severe acute respiratory distress syndrome: a randomized controlled trial. *JAMA* 302:1977–1984, 2009.
114. Martin GS, Mangialardi RJ, Wheeler AP, et al: Albumin and furosemide therapy in hypoproteinemic patients with acute lung injury. *Crit Care Med* 30:2175–2182, 2002.
115. The National Heart Lung, and Blood Institute Acute Respiratory Distress Syndrome (ARDS) Clinical Trials Network: Comparison of two fluid-management strategies in acute lung injury. *N Engl J Med* 354:2564–2575, 2006. doi: 10.1056/NEJMoa062200.
116. Rivers EP: Fluid-management strategies in acute lung injury—liberal, conservative, or both? *N Engl J Med* 354:2598–2600, 2006.
117. Sakr Y, Vincent JL, Reinhart K, et al: High tidal volume and positive fluid balance are associated with worse outcome in acute lung injury. *Chest* 128:3098–3108, 2005.
118. Chung FT, Lin HC, Kuo CH, et al: Extravascular lung water correlates multiorgan dysfunction syndrome and mortality in sepsis. *PLoS One* 5:e15265, 2010.
119. LeTourneau JL, Pinney J, Phillips CR: Extravascular lung water predicts progression to acute lung injury in patients with increased risk. *Crit Care Med* 40:847–854, 2012.
120. Neamu RF, Martin GS: Fluid management in acute respiratory distress syndrome. *Curr Opin Crit Care* 19:24–30, 2013.
121. Martin GS: The role for invasive monitoring in acute lung injury. *Semin Respir Crit Care Med* 34:508–515, 2013.
122. The National Heart Lung, and Blood Institute Acute Respiratory Distress Syndrome (ARDS) Clinical Trials Network: Pulmonary-artery versus central venous catheter to guide treatment of acute lung injury. *N Engl J Med* 354:2213–2224, 2006. doi: 10.1056/NEJMoa061895.
123. Marik PE, Baram M, Vahid B: Does central venous pressure predict fluid responsiveness? A systematic review of the literature and the tale of seven mares. *Chest* 134:172–178, 2008.
124. Carsetti A, Cecconi M, Rhodes A: Fluid bolus therapy: monitoring and predicting fluid responsiveness. *Curr Opin Crit Care* 21:388–394, 2015.
125. Boyd JH, Forbes J, Nakada TA, et al: Fluid resuscitation in septic shock: a positive fluid balance and elevated central venous pressure are associated with increased mortality. *Crit Care Med* 39:259–265, 2011.
126. Boyd JH, Walley KR: The role of echocardiography in hemodynamic monitoring. *Curr Opin Crit Care* 15:239–243, 2009.
127. Marik PE, Monnet X, Teboul JL: Hemodynamic parameters to guide fluid therapy. *Ann Intensive Care* 1:1, 2011.
128. Adhikari NKJ, Burns KEA, Friedrich JO, et al: Effect of nitric oxide on oxygenation and mortality in acute lung injury: systematic review and meta-analysis [see comment]. *BMJ* 334:779, 2007.
129. Afshari A, Brok J, Moller AM, et al: Inhaled nitric oxide for acute respiratory distress syndrome and acute lung injury in adults and children: a systematic review with meta-analysis and trial sequential analysis. *Anesth Analg* 112:1411–1421, 2011.
130. Sweeney RM, Griffiths M, McAuley D: Treatment of acute lung injury: current and emerging pharmacological therapies. *Semin Respir Crit Care Med* 34:487–498, 2013.
131. Ashbaugh DG, Bigelow DB, Petty TL, et al: Acute respiratory distress in adults. *Lancet* 2:319–323, 1967.
132. Petty TL, Reiss OK, Paul GW, et al: Characteristics of pulmonary surfactant in adult respiratory distress syndrome associated with trauma and shock. *Am Rev Respir Dis* 115:531–536, 1977.
133. Davidson WJ, Dorscheid D, Spragg R, et al: Exogenous pulmonary surfactant for the treatment of adult patients with acute respiratory distress syndrome: results of a meta-analysis. *Crit Care* 10:R41, 2006.
134. Kesecioglu J, Beale R, Stewart TE, et al: Exogenous natural surfactant for treatment of acute lung injury and the acute respiratory distress syndrome. *Am J Respir Crit Care Med* 180:989–994, 2009.
135. Stevens TP, Sinkin RA: Surfactant replacement therapy. *Chest* 131:1577–1582, 2007.
136. Meduri GU, Headley AS, Golden E, et al: Effect of prolonged methylprednisolone therapy in unresolving acute respiratory distress syndrome: a randomized controlled trial. *JAMA* 280:159–165, 1998.
137. The National Heart Lung, and Blood Institute Acute Respiratory Distress Syndrome (ARDS) Clinical Trials Network: Efficacy and safety of corticosteroids for persistent acute respiratory distress syndrome. *N Engl J Med* 354:1671–1684, 2006.
138. Meduri GU, Golden E, Freire AX, et al: Methylprednisolone infusion in early severe ARDS: results of a randomized controlled trial [see comment]. *Chest* 131:954–963, 2007.
139. Agarwal R, Nath A, Aggarwal AN, et al: Do glucocorticoids decrease mortality in acute respiratory distress syndrome? A meta-analysis. *Respirology* 12:585–590, 2007.
140. Meduri GU, Bridges L, Shih MC, et al: Prolonged glucocorticoid treatment is associated with improved ARDS outcomes: analysis of individual patients' data from four randomized trials and trial-level meta-analysis of the updated literature. *Intensive Care Med* 42:829–840, 2016.
141. Peter JV, John P, Graham PL, et al: Corticosteroids in the prevention and treatment of acute respiratory distress syndrome (ARDS) in adults: meta-analysis. *BMJ* 336:1006–1009, 2008.
142. Tang BM, Craig JC, Eslick GD, et al: Use of corticosteroids in acute lung injury and acute respiratory distress syndrome: a systematic review and meta-analysis. *Crit Care Med* 37:1594–1603, 2009.
143. Nuckton TJ, Alonso JA, Kallet RH, et al: Pulmonary dead-space fraction as a risk factor for death in the acute respiratory distress syndrome. *N Engl J Med* 346:1281–1286, 2002.
144. Welty-Wolf KE, Carraway MS, Miller DL, et al: Coagulation blockade prevents sepsis-induced respiratory and renal failure in baboons. *Am J Respir Crit Care Med* 164:1988–1996, 2001.
145. Bernard GR, Vincent JL, Laterre PF, et al: Efficacy and safety of recombinant human activated protein C for severe sepsis. *N Engl J Med* 344:699–709, 2001.
146. Jian MY, Koizumi T, Tsushima K, et al: Activated protein C attenuates acid-aspiration lung injury in rats. *Pulm Pharmacol Ther* 18:291–296, 2005.
147. Liu KD, Levitt J, Zhuo H, et al: Randomized clinical trial of activated protein C for the treatment of acute lung injury [see comment]. *Am J Respir Crit Care Med* 178:618–623, 2008.
148. Rubenfeld GD, Abraham E: When is a negative phase II trial truly negative? *Am J Respir Crit Care Med* 178:554–555, 2008.
149. Miller DL, Welty-Wolf K, Carraway MS, et al: Extrinsic coagulation blockade attenuates lung injury and proinflammatory cytokine release after intratracheal lipopolysaccharide. *Am J Respir Cell Mol Biol* 26:650–658, 2002.

150. Frank JA, Wang Y, Osorio O, et al: Beta-adrenergic agonist therapy accelerates the resolution of hydrostatic pulmonary edema in sheep and rats. *J Appl Physiol* 89:1255–1265, 2000.
151. McAuley DF, Frank JA, Fang X, et al: Clinically relevant concentrations of beta2-adrenergic agonists stimulate maximal cyclic adenosine monophosphate-dependent airspace fluid clearance and decrease pulmonary edema in experimental acid-induced lung injury. *Crit Care Med* 32:1470–1476, 2004.
152. Barnard ML, Olivera WG, Rutschman DM, et al: Dopamine stimulates sodium transport and liquid clearance in rat lung epithelium. *Am J Respir Crit Care Med* 156:709–714, 1997.
153. Ortiz-Diaz E, Festic E, Gajic O, et al: Emerging pharmacological therapies for prevention and early treatment of acute lung injury. *Semin Respir Crit Care Med* 34:448–458, 2013.
154. Simopoulos AP: Omega-3 fatty acids in inflammation and autoimmune diseases. *J Am Coll Nutr* 21:495–505, 2002.
155. Stapleton RD, Martin TR, Weiss NS, et al: A phase II randomized placebo-controlled trial of omega-3 fatty acids for the treatment of acute lung injury. *Crit Care Med* 39:1655–1662, 2011.
156. Rice TW, Wheeler AP, Thompson BT, et al: Enteral omega-3 fatty acid, gamma-linolenic acid, and antioxidant supplementation in acute lung injury. *JAMA* 306:1574–1581, 2011.
157. Rice TW, Wheeler AP, Thompson BT, et al: Initial trophic vs full enteral feeding in patients with acute lung injury: the EDEN randomized trial. *JAMA* 307:795–803, 2012.
158. Craig TR, Duffy MJ, Shyamsundar M, et al: A randomized clinical trial of hydroxymethylglutaryl- coenzyme a reductase inhibition for acute lung injury (The HARP Study). *Am J Respir Crit Care Med* 183:620–626, 2011.
159. Shyamsundar M, McKeown ST, O'Kane CM, et al: Simvastatin decreases lipopolysaccharide-induced pulmonary inflammation in healthy volunteers. *Am J Respir Crit Care Med* 179:1107–1114, 2009.
160. Kouroumichakis I, Papanas N, Proikaki S, et al: Statins in prevention and treatment of severe sepsis and septic shock. *Eur J Intern Med* 22:125–133, 2011.
161. O'Neal HR Jr, Koyama T, Koehler EA, et al: Prehospital statin and aspirin use and the prevalence of severe sepsis and acute lung injury/acute respiratory distress syndrome. *Crit Care Med* 39:1343–1350, 2011.
162. Bajwa EK, Malhotra CK, Thompson BT, et al: Statin therapy as prevention against development of acute respiratory distress syndrome: an observational study. *Crit Care Med* 40:1470–1477, 2012.
163. Pasin L, Landoni G, Castro ML, et al: The effect of statins on mortality in septic patients: a meta-analysis of randomized controlled trials. *PLoS One* 8:e82775, 2013.
164. McAuley DF, Laffey JG, O'Kane CM, et al: Simvastatin in the acute respiratory distress syndrome. *N Engl J Med* 371:1695–1703, 2014.
165. Habashi NM: Other approaches to open-lung ventilation: airway pressure release ventilation. *Crit Care Med* 33:S228–S240, 2005.
166. Neumann P, Wrigge H, Zinserling J, et al: Spontaneous breathing affects the spatial ventilation and perfusion distribution during mechanical ventilatory support. *Crit Care Med* 33:1090–1095, 2005.
167. Gonzalez M, Arroliga AC, Frutos-Vivar F, et al: Airway pressure release ventilation versus assist-control ventilation: a comparative propensity score and international cohort study. *Intensive Care Med* 36:817–827, 2010.
168. Neumann P, Golisch W, Strohmeyer A, et al: Influence of different release times on spontaneous breathing pattern during airway pressure release ventilation. *Intensive Care Med* 28:1742–1749, 2002.
169. Dart BW, Maxwell RA, Richart CM, et al: Preliminary experience with airway pressure release ventilation in a trauma/surgical intensive care unit. *J Trauma* 59:71–76, 2005.
170. Maxwell RA, Green JM, Waldrop J, et al: A randomized prospective trial of airway pressure release ventilation and low tidal volume ventilation in adult trauma patients with acute respiratory failure. *J Trauma* 69:501–510; discussion 511, 2010.
171. Varpula T, Valta P, Niemi R, et al: Airway pressure release ventilation as a primary ventilatory mode in acute respiratory distress syndrome. *Acta Anaesthesiol Scand* 48:722–731, 2004.
172. Maung AA, Schuster KM, Kaplan LJ, et al: Compared to conventional ventilation, airway pressure release ventilation may increase ventilator days in trauma patients. *J Trauma Acute Care Surg* 73:507–510, 2012.
173. Nieman GF, Gatto LA, Bates JH, et al: Mechanical ventilation as a therapeutic tool to reduce ARDS incidence. *Chest* 148:1396–1404, 2015.
174. Smith BJ, Lundblad LK, Kollisch-Singule M, et al: Predicting the response of the injured lung to the mechanical breath profile. *J Appl Physiol (1985)* 118:932–940, 2015.
175. Horie S, Masterson C, Devaney J, et al: Stem cell therapy for acute respiratory distress syndrome: a promising future? *Curr Opin Crit Care* 22:14–20, 2016.
176. Rojas M, Cardenes N, Kocyildirim E, et al: Human adult bone marrow-derived stem cells decrease severity of lipopolysaccharide-induced acute respiratory distress syndrome in sheep. *Stem Cell Res Ther* 5:42, 2014.
177. Asmussen S, Ito H, Traber DL, et al: Human mesenchymal stem cells reduce the severity of acute lung injury in a sheep model of bacterial pneumonia. *Thorax* 69:819–825, 2014.
178. Devaney J, Horie S, Masterson C, et al: Human mesenchymal stromal cells decrease the severity of acute lung injury induced by E. coli in the rat. *Thorax* 70:625–635, 2015.
179. Hayes M, Masterson C, Devaney J, et al: Therapeutic efficacy of human mesenchymal stromal cells in the repair of established ventilator-induced lung injury in the rat. *Anesthesiology* 122:363–373, 2015.
180. McAuley DF, Curley GF, Hamid UI, et al: Clinical grade allogeneic human mesenchymal stem cells restore alveolar fluid clearance in human lungs rejected for transplantation. *Am J Physiol* 306:L809–L815, 2014.
181. Lee JW, Fang X, Gupta N, et al: Allogeneic human mesenchymal stem cells for treatment of E. coli endotoxin-induced acute lung injury in the ex vivo perfused human lung. *Proc Natl Acad Sci U S A* 106:16357–16362, 2009.
182. Cross LJ, O'Kane CM, McDowell C, et al: Keratinocyte growth factor in acute lung injury to reduce pulmonary dysfunction—a randomised placebo-controlled trial (KARE): study protocol. *Trials* 14:51, 2013.
183. Murray MJ, Cowen J, DeBlock H, et al: Clinical practice guidelines for sustained neuromuscular blockade in the adult critically ill patient. *Crit Care Med* 30:142–156, 2002.
184. Gainnier M, Roch A, Forel JM, et al: Effect of neuromuscular blocking agents on gas exchange in patients presenting with acute respiratory distress syndrome. *Crit Care Med* 32:113–119, 2004.
185. Hraiech S, Yoshida T, Papazian L: Balancing neuromuscular blockade versus preserved muscle activity. *Curr Opin Crit Care* 21:26–33, 2015.
186. Slutsky AS: Neuromuscular blocking agents in ARDS. *N Engl J Med* 363:1176–1180, 2010.
187. Alhazzani W, Alshahrani M, Jaeschke R, et al: Neuromuscular blocking agents in acute respiratory distress syndrome: a systematic review and meta-analysis of randomized controlled trials. *Crit Care* 17:R43, 2013.
188. Li G, Malinchoc M, Cartin-Ceba R, et al: Eight-year trend of acute respiratory distress syndrome: a population-based study in Olmsted County, Minnesota. *Am J Respir Crit Care Med* 183:59–66, 2011.
189. Morris PE, Goad A, Thompson C, et al: Early intensive care unit mobility therapy in the treatment of acute respiratory failure [see comment]. *Crit Care Med* 36:2238–2243, 2008.
190. Schweickert WD, Pohlman MC, Pohlman AS, et al: Early physical and occupational therapy in mechanically ventilated, critically ill patients: a randomised controlled trial. *Lancet* 373:1874–1882, 2009.
191. Kor DJ, Talmor DS, Banner-Goodspeed VM, et al: Lung Injury Prevention with Aspirin (LIPS-A): a protocol for a multicentre randomised clinical trial in medical patients at high risk of acute lung injury. *BMJ Open* 2, 2012.
192. Gajic O, Dabbagh O, Park PK, et al: Early identification of patients at risk of acute lung injury: evaluation of lung injury prediction score in a multicenter cohort study. *Am J Respir Crit Care Med* 183:462–470, 2011.
193. Levitt JE, Calfee CS, Goldstein BA, et al: Early acute lung injury: criteria for identifying lung injury prior to the need for positive pressure ventilation. *Crit Care Med* 41:1929–1937, 2013.
194. Moss M, Mannino DM: Race and gender differences in acute respiratory distress syndrome deaths in the United States: an analysis of multiple-cause mortality data (1979–1996). *Crit Care Med* 30:1679–1685, 2002.
195. Esteban A, Anzueto A, Frutos-Vivar F, et al: Outcome of older patients receiving mechanical ventilation. *Intensive Care Med* 30:639–646, 2004.
196. Ely EW, Wheeler AP, Thompson BT, et al: Recovery rate and prognosis in older persons who develop acute lung injury and the acute respiratory distress syndrome. *Ann Intern Med* 136:25–36, 2002.
197. Moss M, Parsons PE, Steinberg KP, et al: Chronic alcohol abuse is associated with an increased incidence of acute respiratory distress syndrome and severity of multiple organ dysfunction in patients with septic shock. *Crit Care Med* 31:869–877, 2003.
198. O'Brien JM Jr, Phillips GS, Ali NA, et al: Body mass index is independently associated with hospital mortality in mechanically ventilated adults with acute lung injury [see comment]. *Crit Care Med* 34:738–744, 2006.
199. Meyer NJ: Future clinical applications of genomics for acute respiratory distress syndrome. *Lancet Respir Med* 1:793–803, 2013.
200. Meyer NJ, Christie JD: Genetic heterogeneity and risk of acute respiratory distress syndrome. *Semin Respir Crit Care Med* 34:459–474, 2013.
201. Milberg JA, Davis DR, Steinberg KP, et al: Improved survival of patients with acute respiratory distress syndrome (ARDS): 1983–1993. *JAMA* 273:306–309, 1995.
202. Herridge M, Batt J, Santos CC, et al: Lung-injured patients do not need a specialized rehabilitation program: ICUAW as a case study. *Semin Respir Crit Care Med* 34:522–528, 2013.
203. Wilcox ME, Herridge MS: Long-term outcomes in patients surviving acute respiratory distress syndrome. *Semin Respir Crit Care Med* 31:55–65, 2010.
204. Hopkins RO, Weaver LK, Collingridge D, et al: Two-year cognitive, emotional, and quality-of-life outcomes in acute respiratory distress syndrome. *Am J Respir Crit Care Med* 171:340–347, 2005.
205. Mikkelsen ME, Shull WH, Biester RC, et al: Cognitive, mood and quality of life impairments in a select population of ARDS survivors. *Respirology* 14:76–82, 2009.
206. Dowdy DW, Eid MP, Dennison CR, et al: Quality of life after acute respiratory distress syndrome: a meta-analysis. *Intensive Care Med* 32:1115–1124, 2006.
207. Herridge MS, Tansey CM, Matte A, et al: Functional disability 5 years after acute respiratory distress syndrome. *N Engl J Med* 364:1293–1304, 2011.
208. Davydow DS, Desai SV, Needham DM, et al: Psychiatric morbidity in survivors of the acute respiratory distress syndrome: a systematic review. *Psychosom Med* 70:512–519, 2008.
209. Kress JP, Pohlman AS, O'Connor MF, et al: Daily interruption of sedative infusions in critically ill patients undergoing mechanical ventilation. *N Engl J Med* 342:1471–1477, 2000.
210. Kress JP, Gehlbach B, Lacy M, et al: The long-term psychological effects of daily sedative interruption on critically ill patients. *Am J Respir Crit Care Med* 168:1457–1461, 2003.

211. Barr J, Fraser GL, Puntillo K, et al: Clinical practice guidelines for the management of pain, agitation, and delirium in adult patients in the intensive care unit. *Crit Care Med* 41:263–306, 2013.
212. Picano E, Frassi F, Agricola E, et al: Ultrasound lung comets: a clinically useful sign of extravascular lung water. *J Am Soc Echocardiogr* 19:356–363, 2006.
213. Copetti R, Soldati G, Copetti P: Chest sonography: a useful tool to differentiate acute cardiogenic pulmonary edema from acute respiratory distress syndrome. *Cardiovasc Ultrasound* 6:16, 2008.
214. Lichtenstein D, Goldstein I, Mourgeon E, et al: Comparative diagnostic performances of auscultation, chest radiography, and lung ultrasonography in acute respiratory distress syndrome. *Anesthesiology* 100:9–15, 2004.
215. Xirouchaki N, Magkanas E, Vaporidi K, et al: Lung ultrasound in critically ill patients: comparison with bedside chest radiography. *Intensive Care Med* 37:1488–1493, 2011.
216. Nagueh SF, Appleton CP, Gillebert TC, et al: Recommendations for the evaluation of left ventricular diastolic function by echocardiography. *J Am Soc Echocardiogr* 22:107–133, 2009.
217. Narasimhan M, Koenig SJ, Mayo PH: Advanced echocardiography for the critical care physician: part 2. *Chest* 145:135–142, 2014.
218. Bouhemad B, Brisson H, Le-Guen M, et al: Bedside ultrasound assessment of positive end-expiratory pressure-induced lung recruitment. *Am J Respir Crit Care Med* 183:341–347, 2011.
219. Rode B, Vucic M, Siranovic M, et al: Positive end-expiratory pressure lung recruitment: comparison between lower inflection point and ultrasound assessment. *Wien Klin Wochenschr* 124:842–847, 2012.
220. Meade MO, Lamontagne F: Clinical trial design in acute lung injury—issues and controversies. *Semin Respir Crit Care Med* 34:516–521, 2013.
221. Brun-Buisson C, Minelli C, Bertolini G, et al: Epidemiology and outcome of acute lung injury in European intensive care units. Results from the ALIVE study. *Intensive Care Med* 30:51–61, 2004.
222. Hirschl RB, Croche M, Gore D, et al: Prospective, randomized, controlled pilot study of partial liquid ventilation in adult acute respiratory distress syndrome. *Am J Respir Crit Care Med* 165:781–787, 2002.
223. Kacmarek RM, Wiedemann HP, Lavin PT, et al: Partial liquid ventilation in adult patients with acute respiratory distress syndrome. *Am J Respir Crit Care Med* 173:882–889, 2006.
224. Mercat A, Richard JC, Vielle B, et al: Positive end-expiratory pressure setting in adults with acute lung injury and acute respiratory distress syndrome: a randomized controlled trial. *JAMA* 299:646–655, 2008.

Chapter 164 ▪ Acute Respiratory Failure in Pregnancy

CHRISTINE CAMPBELL-REARDON • HELEN M. HOLLINGSWORTH

The overall pregnancy-related maternal mortality ratio in the United States during 2006 to 2010 was 16 deaths per 100,000 live births [1]. Acute respiratory failure remains an important cause of maternal and fetal morbidity and mortality with 0.1% to 0.2% of pregnancies complicated by respiratory failure requiring mechanical ventilatory support [2]. Thromboembolism, amniotic fluid embolism (AFE), and venous air embolism together account for approximately 15% of maternal deaths [1].

This chapter focuses on the causes of acute respiratory failure that are increased in frequency during pregnancy, are unique to pregnancy, or present special management requirements during pregnancy. The spectrum of problems associated with eclampsia is discussed in Chapter 53. Management of the acute respiratory distress syndrome (ARDS) caused by sepsis, trauma, or other etiologies unrelated to pregnancy is discussed in Chapter 163. Table 164.1 lists the causes of acute respiratory failure in pregnancy.

TABLE 164.1

Causes of Acute Respiratory Failure in Pregnancy

Thromboembolism
Amniotic fluid embolism
Venous air embolism
Aspiration of gastric contents
Respiratory infections
Asthma
HELLP syndrome
β-Adrenergic tocolytic therapy
Pneumomediastinum and pneumothorax
Acute respiratory distress syndrome (see Chapter 47)
Cardiomyopathy

HELLP, *h*emolytic anemia, *e*levated *l*iver function tests, *l*ow *p*latelets.

NORMAL ALTERATIONS IN CARDIOPULMONARY PHYSIOLOGY DURING PREGNANCY

Pregnancy alters respiratory physiology by causing changes in lung volumes, mechanics of ventilation, and control of respiration. Despite airway mucosal changes of edema and hyperemia, spirometry studies reveal no significant changes in measurements of the forced expiratory volume in 1 second (FEV_1) during pregnancy, suggesting that airway function is maintained during pregnancy. Changes in lung volume associated with gestation are relatively small: total lung capacity decreases 4% to 6%, functional residual capacity (FRC) decreases approximately 15% to 25%, and residual volume remains constant. Despite the decrease in FRC, early airway closure has not been demonstrated and specific airway conductance remains constant [3,4]. Diffusing capacity is elevated during the first trimester but then declines, despite continued increases in cardiac output and plasma volume.

As gestation progresses, the resting level of the diaphragm rises, but diaphragmatic excursion with tidal breathing increases. An increased tidal volume (25% to 35%) accounts for much of the 20% to 40% increase in minute ventilation and the mild respiratory alkalosis that are characteristic of early-to-middle pregnancy. An increased respiratory rate also contributes to the increased minute ventilation late in pregnancy (Fig. 164.1).

Normal carbon dioxide tension ($PaCO_2$) during pregnancy is 27 to 34 mm Hg, suggesting chronic mild hyperventilation. The degree of hyperventilation has been found to be in excess of the amount needed to compensate for increased oxygen consumption; in fact, hyperventilation develops early in gestation, before any significant increase in oxygen consumption occurs. This has been attributed to elevation in levels of progesterone, which has known respiratory-stimulating effects. The exact mechanism by which it produces these effects is not known, but it is thought to include an increase in the central chemoreflex drive to breathe and to changes in acid–base balance such that central and plasma hydrogen ion concentration is increased for any given $PaCO_2$. In addition, pregnancy is associated with increased sensitivity to CO_2 as measured by CO_2 ventilatory

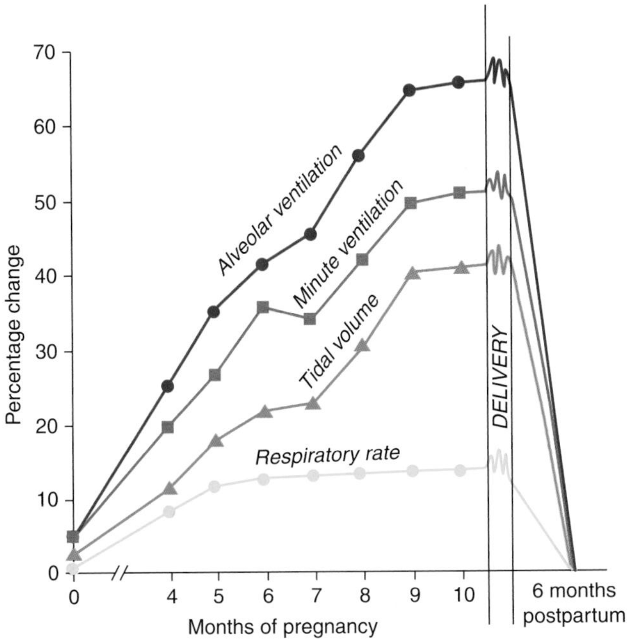

FIGURE 164.1 Changes in respiratory function during pregnancy. (Reprinted from Leontic EA: Respiratory disease in pregnancy. *Med Clin North Am* 61:111, 1977, with permission.)

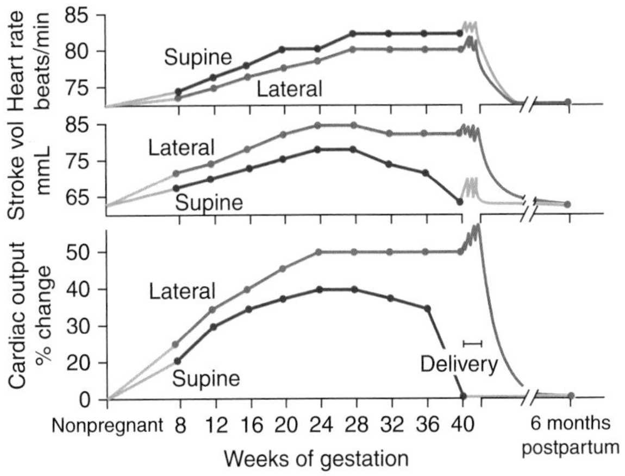

FIGURE 164.2 Changes in maternal heart rate, stroke volume, and output during pregnancy with the gravida in the supine and lateral positions. (Reprinted from Cheek TG, Gutsche BB: Maternal physiologic alterations during pregnancy, in Shnider SM, Levinson G (eds): *Anesthesia for Obstetrics*. Baltimore, MD, Williams & Wilkins, 1987, p 3, with permission.)

response curves, reflecting the new, lower set point in $PaCO_2$, possibly mediated by estrogen and progesterone. The respiratory alkalosis seen during pregnancy causes a compensatory renal excretion of bicarbonate to maintain an arterial pH between 7.40 and 7.45.

The normal arterial oxygen tension (PaO_2) in pregnant women ranges from 100 to 110 mm Hg. Oxygen consumption increases by 20% to 33% by the third trimester, secondary to both fetal and maternal demands. This increased rate of oxygen consumption and low oxygen reserve secondary to a reduced FRC place pregnant patients at risk for the rapid onset of hypoxia.

Circulatory changes occur during gestation to supply oxygen-rich blood to the placenta and to accommodate the stress of labor and delivery. Cardiac output begins to rise during the first trimester and peaks around the 20th week of gestation at 30% to 45% above resting, nonpregnant levels (Fig. 164.2). Thus, measured cardiac output during gestation that is in the normal range for a nonpregnant patient would represent significant hemodynamic compromise for the pregnant patient and, potentially, decreased oxygen delivery for the fetus. As pregnancy progresses, cardiac output becomes dependent on body position. In the supine position, cardiac output can be reduced by 25% to 30% because of compression of the inferior vena cava by the gravid uterus and a resultant decrease in venous return. Cardiac output is higher when the pregnant woman is in the left lateral decubitus position. Estimates of expected cardiac output during gestation should be revised upward for intercurrent stresses, such as fever, infection, and pain.

The gestation-related increase in cardiac output reflects a combination of increases in heart rate and stroke volume. Heart rate increases progressively throughout gestation, reaching a 20% increase over nonpregnant levels of approximately 15 beats per minute. Stroke volume increases more rapidly at first and then stabilizes. Left ventricular compliance must increase in pregnancy because the increased stroke volume appears to be related more to left ventricular enlargement than to increased emptying. The cardiac silhouette on chest radiography may appear enlarged as a result of mild normal left ventricular enlargement and lateral and upward displacement by the gravid uterus.

Further increases of cardiac output occur during labor; cardiac output increases up to 45% over third-trimester values, and, during uterine contraction, cardiac output transiently increases another 10% to 15% because of increased venous return from the contracting uterus. These "autotransfusions" may reach 500 mL when the uterus contracts after parturition. This effect, however, may be offset by blood loss at the time of delivery. In the first few minutes postpartum, cardiac output may increase as much as 80% over prelabor levels, then decrease to 40% to 50% over prelabor values by 1 hour postpartum, and finally return to nearly prepregnant levels by 1 to 2 weeks postpartum.

On the other hand, afterload may increase sharply during labor contractions because of inhibition of blood flow to the contracting uterine muscle. Because uterine blood flow at term accounts for a significant proportion of the cardiac output, marked increases in afterload can occur during contractions and immediately postpartum. These changes in afterload may be important in patients who are sensitive to afterload, such as patients with underlying cardiac disease.

Systemic vascular resistance is generally reduced during pregnancy because of vasodilatation and the low resistance of the uteroplacental vascular circuit. Possible factors leading to vasodilatation include a reduction in vascular responsiveness to norepinephrine and angiotensin II, increased endothelial prostacyclin production, and increased nitric oxide production. The mean blood pressure remains relatively constant despite increases in cardiac output. Pressures in the right ventricle, pulmonary artery, and pulmonary capillaries are no different from nonpregnant values.

During pregnancy, there is expansion of the extracellular fluid volume, with the plasma fluid volume increasing more than the interstitial volume. Maternal blood volume reaches its peak at 32 weeks and is 25% to 52% above prepregnancy levels. The erythrocyte mass increases by 20% to 30%. However, the plasma volume increases more than the erythrocyte volume, resulting in the physiologic anemia of pregnancy.

Colloid osmotic pressure measurements during gestation reveal a mean decrease of 5 mm Hg, which reaches a plateau at 26 weeks. This parallels a decrease in serum albumin concentrations from approximately 4.0 to 3.4 g per dL. A further decline in colloid osmotic pressure of roughly 4 mm Hg occurs immediately postpartum, probably as a result of a combination of factors, such as recumbency, crystalloid administration, and blood loss. These changes may be even more marked for patients with pregnancy-induced hypertension. Neither the absolute value of colloid osmotic pressure nor the colloid osmotic pressure–pulmonary capillary wedge pressure gradient is an accurate predictor of pulmonary edema because of the multiplicity of contributing variables. However, these trends of colloid osmotic pressure should be considered when interpreting pulmonary capillary wedge pressures, especially for patients who have received large amounts of crystalloid.

DETERMINANTS OF FETAL OXYGEN DELIVERY

Oxygen delivery to fetal tissues can be affected at many levels: maternal oxygen delivery to the placenta, placental transfer, and fetal oxygen transport from the placenta to fetal tissues. The major determinants of oxygen delivery to the placenta are the oxygen content of uterine artery blood, which is determined by maternal PaO_2; hemoglobin concentration and saturation; and uterine artery blood flow, which depends on maternal cardiac output. Thus, a decreased PaO_2 can be offset somewhat by increased blood hemoglobin concentration or by increased cardiac output. The combination of maternal hypoxemia and decreased cardiac output likely has a profoundly deleterious effect on fetal oxygenation.

Variations in maternal pH also influence oxygen delivery. Alkalosis causes vasoconstriction of the uterine artery, resulting in decreased fetal oxygen delivery. This effect is magnified by a leftward shift in the maternal oxyhemoglobin saturation curve, which increases oxygen affinity and, consequently, decreases oxygen transfer to the umbilical vein. Although mild maternal acidosis does not enhance uterine blood flow because the uterine vasculature is already maximally dilated, it shifts the maternal oxyhemoglobin saturation curve to the right, leading to decreased oxygen affinity and increased fetal oxygen delivery. Maternal hypotension and increased sympathetic stimulation (exogenous or endogenous) both cause uterine arterial vasoconstriction.

The importance of maternal cardiac output is supported by the observation that women with left ventricular outflow obstruction have an increased incidence of fetal death and surviving infants have an increased incidence of congenital heart disease. Data from a sheep model, however, suggests that a decrease in uterine blood flow up to 50% for brief periods does not appreciably decrease fetal and placental oxygen uptake. Chronically decreased maternal cardiac output may have other effects, perhaps on placental development, that explain the results in women with left ventricular outflow obstruction.

The interaction of maternal and fetal circulations in the placenta most likely follows a concurrent exchange mechanism. This is less efficient than a countercurrent exchange mechanism and partly explains why the PaO_2 in the fetal umbilical vein, which carries oxygenated blood to fetus, is in the range of 32 mm Hg, far lower than uterine vein PaO_2, and why increased maternal inspired oxygen increases uterine artery oxygen tension but does not cause major increases in umbilical vein PaO_2. Despite low umbilical vein PaO_2, fetal oxygen content is actually quite close to maternal oxygen content because of the shape of the oxyhemoglobin saturation curve for fetal hemoglobin (Fig. 164.3). This is one of the major protective mechanisms for fetal oxygenation. The fetal oxyhemoglobin saturation curve is relatively unaffected by changes in pH; although acidosis may decrease maternal oxygen affinity, fetal oxygen affinity remain unchanged.

Other placental factors that determine fetal oxygenation are the amount of intraplacental shunt, degree of matching of maternal and fetal blood flows, and the presence of any placental abnormalities, such as placental infarcts. There seem to be no placental autoregulatory mechanisms that increase blood flow in response to decreased maternal PaO_2.

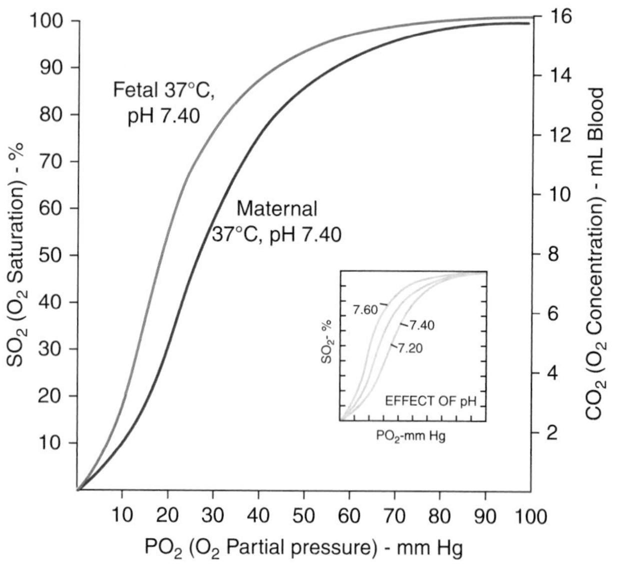

FIGURE 164.3 Oxygen dissociation (equilibrium) curves of human fetal and maternal blood. The effect of pH on the position of the curve (Bohr effect) is shown on the inset. The oxygen capacity of 16 mL per 100 mL blood on the right-hand ordinate refers to maternal blood. (Reprinted from Novy MJ, Edwards MJ: Respiratory problems in pregnancy. *Am J Obstet Gynecol* 99:1024, 1967, with permission.)

Mathematical models predicting the optimal apportionment of fetal cardiac output between umbilical (to collect oxygen) and systemic (to deliver oxygen) circulations have yielded values surprisingly close to those measured under normal physiologic conditions. This appears to be another compensation mechanism for the apparent inefficiency (concurrent exchange mechanism) of the placenta. One disadvantage in terms of oxygen delivery to fetal tissues is that oxygenated umbilical vein blood is mixed in the fetal inferior vena cava with deoxygenated systemic venous blood before delivery to the systemic circulation. Thus, fetal arterial blood has an even lower PaO_2 than umbilical vein blood. This is compensated for in part by a high fetal cardiac output relative to oxygen consumption, thus enhancing oxygen delivery to fetal tissues. The fetal circulation appears to have the ability to autoregulate in the face of hypoxemia to protect the brain, adrenal glands, and heart. How long this adaptation can be depended on safely before organ damage occurs is not known.

How well do the compensatory mechanisms that provide adequate oxygen supply to the fetus under normal conditions manage during maternal hypoxia? Calculation of oxygen stores in the term infant with 60% hemoglobin saturation yields a total oxygen content of 40 mL. Given an oxygen consumption of 6 mL/kg/min, or approximately 18 mL per minute at term, this reserve lasts barely 2 minutes when the maternal oxygen supply is completely interrupted. The shape of the fetal oxyhemoglobin dissociation curve places umbilical vein PaO_2 values below 30 mm Hg on the steep part of the curve, so small changes in maternal PaO_2 may cause significant changes in fetal oxygen content. A maternal PaO_2 greater than 70 mm Hg should be maintained to prevent adverse consequences to the fetus. Concern regarding the adequacy of fetal oxygen supply is further reduced if a normal maternal PaO_2 of 90 mm Hg or greater is achieved without too great a risk of maternal barotrauma or oxygen toxicity [5].

CAUSES OF ACUTE RESPIRATORY FAILURE

This section describes the more common causes of acute respiratory failure in pregnancy in terms of frequency, clinical presentation, pathophysiology, and diagnosis.

Thromboembolic Disease

Fatal pulmonary embolism (PE) is a rare complication in pregnancy, but it accounts for 9.3% of all pregnancy-related deaths in the United States [1]. Thromboembolic complications have been estimated to occur in 5 to 12 per 10,000 pregnancies [6]. The increased frequency of thromboembolic disease in pregnancy may be attributable to a hypercoagulable state along with venous stasis. During pregnancy, there is a progressive increase in coagulation factors I, II, VII, VIII, IX, and X. There is a decrease in protein S and a progressively increased resistance to activated protein C [7]. The activity of plasminogen activator inhibitor types 1 and 2, which are inhibitors of fibrinolysis, also increases [8]. Venous stasis may occur because of a hormonally induced dilation of capacitance veins and uterine pressure on the inferior vena cava [9]. Factors that further increase the risk of thromboembolic disease during pregnancy and the puerperium include (a) cesarean section, which has a 10 times greater risk of fatal PE than does vaginal delivery; (b) increased maternal age; (c) multiparity; (d) obesity, especially in association with bed rest; (e) personal or family history of thromboembolism; (f) suppression of lactation with estrogen; (g) surgical procedures during pregnancy and early puerperium; and (h) inherited thrombophilias such as deficiencies of protein C or S, the presence of antiphospholipid antibodies, the presence of factor V Leiden, and prothrombin gene mutations [9].

The appropriate diagnostic steps and treatment of venous thrombosis and PE in nonpregnant patients are reviewed in Chapter 92. This chapter focuses on the diagnosis and management of massive PE associated with severe respiratory and hemodynamic compromise during pregnancy. Respiratory failure may ensue in PE when extensive occlusion of the pulmonary vasculature or concomitant pulmonary edema occurs.

Although none of the symptoms, physical signs, or results of laboratory, radiographic, or electrocardiographic studies are specific for PE, these investigations can help rule out other diseases in the differential diagnosis. The usefulness of the serum D-dimer levels in diagnosing thromboembolic disease in pregnancy is limited because D-dimer levels are increased during normal pregnancy, with levels increasing as gestation progresses and peaking at delivery and in the early postpartum period [10].

The typical hemodynamic findings in nonpregnant patients with massive PE are delineated in Chapter 92. Although there are no data for pregnant patients with massive PE, similar findings would be anticipated because pregnancy does not significantly alter right heart and pulmonary artery pressures. Thus, in a pregnant patient with massive PE, pulmonary artery balloon occlusion pressure (i.e., pulmonary capillary wedge pressure) would be expected to be normal or low, mean pulmonary artery pressure moderately elevated ($\geq$35 mm Hg), and right atrial pressure moderately elevated ($>$8 mm Hg).

Recent guidelines have been published to aid in the diagnostic evaluation of pregnant patients suspected of having a PE [11]. In pregnant patients with suspected PE, with signs and symptoms of acute deep vein thrombosis (DVT), bilateral compression ultrasonography of the lower extremities should be performed. Further diagnostic evaluation is not required when a DVT is found in the legs, because the treatment for DVT and PE is the same. A negative compressive ultrasound of the lower extremities does not rule out the presence of PE, so further diagnostic investigation is required. In a pregnant patient with suspected PE, with no signs or symptoms of DVT, a chest X-ray should be performed with abdominal shielding. If the chest X-ray is normal, the next diagnostic test recommended is a ventilation–perfusion scan because this exposes the mother's breasts to less carcinogenic radiation than a computed tomography-pulmonary angiogram (CT-PA). A CT-PA is performed when the clinical suspicion for PE is high and the initial chest X-ray is abnormal or if the ventilation–perfusion scan is nondiagnostic [11]. In the nonpregnant patient population, CT-PA has become the study of choice for PE. Data from The Prospective Investigation of Pulmonary Embolism Diagnosis II Trial (PIOPED II) trail determined the sensitivity and specificity of CT-PA for detecting PE to be 83% and 96%, respectively [12]. Pregnancy was an exclusion criterion in this study, so there is a lack of prospective data assessing the sensitivity and specificity of CT-PAs in pregnancy.

Fetal exposure to radiation during imaging studies can be minimized by abdominal shielding and using brachial access. A CT-PA delivers slightly lower doses of radiation (0.003 to 0.131 mGy) to the fetus compared with ventilation–perfusion scanning (0.32 to 0.74 mGy) [13,14]. However, a CT-PA delivers higher radiation doses (7.3 mGy) to the mother compared with ventilation–perfusion scanning (0.9 mGy) [13–15].

Amniotic Fluid Embolism

AFE is a rare, but usually catastrophic, complication of pregnancy and delivery. The incidence of AFE is approximately 1.9 to 6.1 cases per 100,000 deliveries [16,17]. The mortality rates in patients presenting with the classic signs and symptoms of AFE exceed 60%. If AFE is complicated by cardiac arrest, fewer than 10% of these patients are discharged alive from the hospital [17]. Of the women who survive AFE, only 15% of them are neurologically intact as a result of hypoxic encephalopathy [16].

It is unknown why amniotic fluid enters the maternal circulation of some patients. Registry and cohort studies have been analyzed to determine potential predisposing risk factors for AFE. Suggested risk factors include older maternal age (mean, 32 years), multiparity (88% of cases), amniotomy, cesarean section, abruptio placentae, insertion of intrauterine fetal or pressure monitoring devices, and term pregnancy in the presence of an intrauterine device [16]. However, based upon the clinical evidence at this time, no specific demographic or clinical risk factor has been identified that could be intervened on to reduce the risk of AFE. AFE is considered unpredictable and unpreventable at this time [17].

Amniotic fluid enters the maternal circulation through one of three ports: endocervical veins, uterine tears (small tears may occur in the lower uterine segment as a part of normal labor), and uterine injury secondary to iatrogenic manipulation, such as cesarean section, insertion of monitoring devices, or membrane rupture. The two life-threatening consequences of AFE are cardiopulmonary collapse and disseminated intravascular coagulation (DIC). These may occur simultaneously or in sequence. The pathophysiologic process of cardiopulmonary collapse remains controversial. It is possible that amniotic fluid contains vasoactive substances or fetal antigens that provoke an abnormal hemodynamic and immunologic response in the mother that results in the AFE syndrome [17]. There may be a biphasic response to AFE with initial hypoxemia and acute pulmonary hypertension, followed by left ventricular failure. Elevation of the pulmonary capillary wedge pressure and reduction in cardiac output and left ventricular stroke work index have been documented [17].

Acute left heart failure contributes to the development of pulmonary edema, which leads to dyspnea, tachypnea, and cyanosis. Other factors potentially contributing to pulmonary edema include cardiodepressive humoral factors from the amniotic fluid, vigorous fluid resuscitation, increased permeability pulmonary edema, and hypoxia causing myocardial ischemia [18].

The other major consequence of AFE is coagulation failure. In 10% to 15% of patients, excessive bleeding, particularly uterine bleeding, may be the first sign of AFE. In all, 30% to 45% of women surviving the first 30 to 60 minutes of AFE will have clinical evidence of coagulopathy with severe bleeding. Bleeding from DIC may be seen within the first 10 to 30 minutes following AFE [18]. The factors that initiate DIC are not known.

The abrupt onset of severe dyspnea, tachypnea, and cyanosis during labor or the early puerperium is the classic presentation of AFE, characterizing more than one-half of cases. Shock, which is out of proportion to blood loss, is the first manifestation in another 10% to 15%. Seizure activity may be the presenting sign in 30% of cases. In addition, fetal bradycardia is seen in 17% of US registry cases. Bleeding is the forerunning sign in 10% to 15% of patients, and the longer the survival, the greater the likelihood that the patient will manifest respiratory failure, cardiovascular collapse, and DIC. Whatever the presenting symptom complex, 90% of cases occur before or during labor [18]. Other complications, such as acute renal failure and signs of central nervous system injury, are probably secondary to hypotension and hypoxemia. Prodromal symptoms, such as vomiting and shivering, are nonspecific and frequently associated with otherwise uneventful deliveries.

Diagnostic criteria for AFE previously rested on demonstration of fetal elements such as epithelial squamous cells from fetal skin, lanugo hairs, fat from the vernix caseosa, mucin from fetal gut, and bile-containing meconium in the maternal circulation. These elements are not pathognomonic for AFE, because these amniotic fluid components are found in the maternal circulation of healthy pregnant women without AFE [17]. Therefore, the antemortem diagnosis of AFE still rests predominantly on the clinical setting and the exclusion of other causes of acute respiratory failure. The role of echocardiography in the diagnosis of AFE is not yet known. Cardiac echo may show decreased left ventricular function or echodense material in the right atrium or right ventricular outflow tract [17]. Diagnostic biomarker assays are not currently available for clinical diagnosis of AFE.

Fetal outcome is also poor for AFE. The perinatal mortality from national registries ranges from 7% to 38%, with up to 50% of the surviving children experiencing permanent neurologic injury [18].

Venous Air Embolism

Venous air embolism is the entrainment of air into the venous system where it then travels to the right ventricle and the pulmonary circulation. Venous air embolism has been described during normal labor, delivery of patients with placenta previa, criminal abortions using air, and insufflation of the vagina during gynecologic procedures. Cases have also been reported of venous embolism occurring following orogenital sex [19]. Venous air embolism may account for as many as 1% of maternal deaths [1]. Presumably, the subplacental venous sinuses are the sites of air entry when antepartum or peripartum air embolism occurs.

The clinical presentation of venous air embolism varies according to the volume and speed of air entrainment into the vascular circulation. Venous air embolism can affect the cardiac, respiratory, and neurologic systems. Sudden, profound hypotension is the most common presenting sign of venous air embolism. Cough, dyspnea, dizziness, tachypnea, tachycardia, and diaphoresis may also be noted. Hypotension is usually followed quickly by respiratory arrest. The classic sign associated with air embolism is the mill wheel murmur, which is audible over the precordium [19]; a drum-like or bubbling sound may also be heard. Electrocardiographic evidence of ischemia, right heart strain, and arrhythmias have been described, and metabolic acidosis, presumably caused by lactic acid production, may be present [19] (see Chapter 198).

Neurologic symptoms develop as a consequence of cerebral hypoperfusion from cardiovascular collapse and from paradoxic embolization if a patent foramen ovale is present [19]. Transesophageal echocardiography (TEE) and transthoracic echocardiography have been utilized to identify air embolism, the route of the embolism, and the severity of the air embolism [19]. TEE is the most sensitive monitoring technique and is able to detect 0.02 mL per kg of air or bubbles measuring 5 to 10 microns [19]. Based on data from surgical procedures, precordial Doppler ultrasound can be used for surveillance of air embolism by detection of alterations in the ultrasonic pattern caused by the embolism and is able to detect as little as 0.05 mL per kg of air [20]. End-tidal carbon dioxide demonstrates a sudden increase in the level of end-tidal CO_2 during a venous air embolism event [19].

The volume of air that is likely to be lethal seems to vary with the rate of infusion and patient position. A bolus of 200 to 300 mL of air or 3 to 5 mL per kg has been reported to be the lethal dose in humans [19,20]. The mechanism by which air embolism leads to noncardiogenic pulmonary edema is not known. It is thought that entrapment of air bubbles in the pulmonary circulation leads to activation of complement, neutrophils, and platelets, resulting in mediator release, protease activation, oxidant stress, and endothelial injury [19]. This inflammatory response then precipitates noncardiogenic pulmonary edema [19].

Aspiration of Gastric Contents

Aspiration of acidic gastric contents into the tracheobronchial tree was first described in 1946 by Mendelson [21] in women during labor and delivery. Maternal deaths from pulmonary aspiration have been steadily declining as a result of changing anesthesia practices, including a shift to regional anesthesia from general anesthesia for delivery [22].

At term, several factors contribute to an increased risk of aspiration of stomach contents: (a) increased intragastric pressure caused by external compression by the gravid uterus, (b) progesterone-induced relaxation of the lower esophageal sphincter, (c) delayed gastric emptying during labor, (d) supine position, and (e) analgesia-induced decreased mental status and decreased vocal cord closure [23]. The pulmonary pathophysiologic consequences of gastric aspiration are a consequence of the acidity and the particulate content of the gastric contents and the risk of bacterial superinfection. Acid aspiration causes a direct injury to the airway resulting in desquamation and loss of ciliated and nonciliated cells, including the alveolar type II cells. An inflammatory response is also triggered by the acid aspiration, leading to an increase in alveolar permeability with a loss in lung compliance and a decrease in ventilation–perfusion matching [23]. Inhaled particulate matter may cause acute airway obstruction and immediate death.

The volume of acid aspiration determines, in part, the rapidity of symptom onset. Aspiration of smaller volumes may go unnoticed clinically until 6 to 8 hours later, when tachypnea, tachycardia, hypoxemia, hypotension, bronchospasm, and production of frothy, pink sputum are noted in association with diffuse opacities on chest radiography. Progression of chest radiographic findings may continue for up to 36 hours. The clinical course may follow one of three patterns: (a) rapid improvement during 4 to 5 days, (b) initial improvement followed by deterioration caused by supervening bacterial pneumonia, and (c) early death as a result of intractable hypoxia [23]. Predictors of poor outcome include low pH, large volume, and a greater amount of particulate content of the aspirate. The bacterial pathogens in this setting are usually oropharyngeal anaerobes, although the longer the patient is in the hospital before clinical development of pneumonia, the greater the likelihood of facultative, Gram-negative bacillary, and *Staphylococcus aureus* infections [23].

Respiratory Infections

The prevalence of pneumonia during pregnancy ranges from 0.78 to 2.7 cases per 1,000 deliveries. The maternal mortality rate from pneumonia has decreased from 20% to 3% since the advent of antibiotics [24]. The major factors in improving fetal and maternal outcome seem to have been earlier presentation and prompt institution of antibiotic therapy. Although pneumonia rarely progresses to respiratory failure, it is advisable to assess maternal oxygenation in all cases of maternal pneumonia. The spectrum of organisms to consider is similar to that in the nonpregnant population; the most common organisms are *Streptococcus pneumoniae*, *Haemophilus influenzae*, and *Mycoplasma pneumoniae*. *Legionella* pneumonia accounts for up to 22% of community-acquired pneumonia [25].

Certain other respiratory infections (e.g., influenza, varicella, coccidioidomycosis, tuberculosis [TB], listeriosis, and severe acute respiratory syndrome [SARS]) have been associated with increased maternal and fetal morbidity and mortality. These particular infections can be virulent in the pregnant patient because of alterations in the immune status. Specifically, during pregnancy, there is a decreased lymphocyte proliferative response, a decrease in the natural killer cell activity, and a decrease in the number of helper T4 cells [24]. Fortunately, the impairment in maternal immune response is mild, and the increase in maternal morbidity is small.

In the influenza pandemics of 1918, 1957, and 2009, an excess incidence of influenza pneumonia was noted among pregnant women. A 50% incidence of influenza pneumonia and an overall mortality of 27% for influenza in pregnancy were found in 1918 [26]. In the 1957 pandemic, several studies noted that 50% of deaths from influenza in women of childbearing age were in pregnant patients [26]. Autopsy reports noted that the cause of death in pregnant women was respiratory insufficiency caused by fulminant influenza pneumonia, rather than secondary bacterial infection, the more common cause of death in nonpregnant influenza patients. The pandemic in 2009 was attributed to influenza A(H1N1)pdm09 virus, and the Centers for Disease Control and Prevention data from 2009 to 2010 revealed that 12% of pregnancy-related deaths were attributed to influenza A(H1N1)pdm09 [27]. In addition, higher rates of miscarriage, preterm birth, and small for gestational age babies have been noted in mothers infected with influenza [26]. The typical symptoms of influenza include cough, fever, sore pharyngitis, rhinorrhea, diarrhea, headache, and myalgias [26].

The incidence of varicella infection during pregnancy is 1 to 5 cases per 10,000 pregnancies. The introduction of the varicella vaccine in 1995 has led to this lower incidence because of high rates of varicella-zoster virus seropositivity among adults in the United States [28]. Varicella pneumonia is estimated to complicate 10% to 20% of maternal infections, although a study of a large database cohort found the incidence of maternal varicella pneumonia to be 2.5% with no maternal deaths [28]. In this study, 13% of the patients required ventilatory support compared with 40% historically [28]. Furthermore, the mortality rate for maternal varicella pneumonia has declined significantly since the development of antiviral therapy and institution of varicella vaccination. Historically, the mortality rate for maternal varicella pneumonia was 41%, but, in the era of antiviral therapy and vaccination, the mortality rate is now estimated to be 3% to 14% [28]. Cigarette smoking appears to be an important risk factor in the progression of varicella into pneumonia [24].

Respiratory symptoms usually develop 2 days after the onset of fever, rash, and malaise. Typical symptoms are cough, dyspnea, hemoptysis, and chest pain [24]. Generalized varicella-zoster infections may also be associated with hepatitis, myocarditis, nephritis, thrombocytopenia, and adrenal hemorrhage [24]. Varicella during pregnancy can lead to intrauterine infection, which can result in prematurity, spontaneous abortion, and stillbirth [24]. In the absence of dissemination, herpes zoster does not appear to be associated with significant maternal morbidity or evidence of fetal infection [28].

SARS is an atypical pneumonia first described in 2002 that is caused by a coronavirus [24]. Symptoms of fever, chills, rigors, headache, malaise, and myalgias develop 2 to 7 days after exposure. A nonproductive cough or dyspnea may develop over 3 to 7 days. This may progress to hypoxemia and respiratory failure. The chest radiograph may show bilateral patchy interstitial opacities. The overall mortality rate for SARS is 3% [29]. One review of 12 cases of SARS during pregnancy demonstrated that 33% of pregnant women required mechanical ventilation, and the maternal mortality rate was 25% [24]. Pregnant patients with suspected or probable SARS should be placed on airborne precautions in a negative pressure isolation room [24].

Maternal *Coccidioidomycosis immitis* infections are rare, with less than 1 case in every 1,000 pregnancies. Historically, *Coccidioidomycosis* infection during pregnancy has been reported as having a 20.0% dissemination rate, compared with 0.2% in nonpregnant patients; infections contracted in the second or third trimester have a higher rate of dissemination [30]. Maternal mortality and fetal loss are preventable with appropriate treatment [30]. Case reports of cryptococcosis, blastomycosis, and sporotrichosis in pregnancy are rare enough to suggest that there may be no increased susceptibility to these infections [30].

Disseminated coccidioidal infection should be suspected in patients with primary or chronic progressive coccidioidal pneumonia in whom rapidly progressive respiratory failure and a clinical picture resembling miliary TB develop. Diagnosis is sometimes difficult because sputum is positive in less than 40% of cases, and complement fixation titers may be low [30]. Evaluation of these patients should include a careful search for extrapulmonary disease (e.g., lumbar puncture, urinalysis, culture of skin lesions) [30]. Peripheral blood eosinophilia is reported in 25% and may be a clue to the diagnosis.

Respiratory failure as a result of infection with *Mycobacterium tuberculosis* is rare. The prevalence of active TB in pregnant women living in low burden countries ranges from 0.06% to 0.25%. In high burden countries, the prevalence of active TB varies depending upon HIV status. In HIV-negative women, the incidence is 0.07% to 0.5% compared with 0.7% to 11% among women who are HIV positive [31]. Pregnancy does not alter the pathogenesis of tuberculous infection or increase the likelihood of latent TB infection progressing to active disease, although pregnant women who are HIV positive and have latent TB infection are more likely to progress to active TB disease [31]. Pregnancy does not alter the response to tuberculin skin testing, so all pregnant women from populations recommended for screening should have a skin or an interferon-γ release test performed if one has not been done previously [32].

In the United States, 24% of the HIV/AIDS cases occur in women [33]. Because the number of women infected with HIV grows, the spectrum of respiratory disease in pregnancy will include an increasing proportion of opportunistic infections and other respiratory complications related to AIDS. *Pneumocystis jiroveci* (formerly *Pneumocystis carinii*) pneumonia (PCP) is the most common cause of AIDS-related death in pregnant patients [24]. In a series of 22 patients with PCP in pregnancy, the rate of mechanical ventilation was 59% and the maternal mortality rate was 50%, compared with a mortality rate of 1% to 16% in nonpregnant patients [24]. Diagnostic evaluation follows the same protocol as in a nonpregnant patient with suspected PCP. Induced sputum should be examined for the presence of *P. jiroveci*; if this is negative, flexible bronchoscopy with bronchoalveolar lavage should be performed.

Listeria monocytogenes, a cause of meningitis and sepsis in immunocompromised hosts, also has a predilection for pregnant women, most commonly resulting in abortion or neonatal sepsis [34]. The incidence of *Listeria* infection among pregnant women is estimated at 3 per 100,000 compared with 0.29 per 100,000 in the general population [35]. The usual sporadic incidence is 1 to 3 cases for every 1 million of the population each year, but local outbreaks may occur as a result of ingestion of contaminated cheese, cabbage, or milk [35]. Diagnosis may be problematic because of difficulties with isolating the organism from respiratory tract secretions. When *L. monocytogenes* sepsis is suspected, cultures should be obtained from the blood, sputum, rectum, cervix, and amniotic fluid (at the time of delivery) [34]. Patients who develop sepsis or meningitis have been reported to have a case fatality rate of 20% to 30% [34].

Asthma

Asthma affects between 3.7% and 8.4% of pregnant women in the United States [36]. The scope of this section is limited to asthmatic exacerbations during pregnancy that lead to respiratory failure. Studies have shown that poor asthma control during pregnancy is associated with adverse fetal and maternal outcomes. Pregnant women with frequent or severe asthma attacks are more likely to have fetal complications, including growth retardation, preterm birth, low birth weight, neonatal hypoxia, and perinatal mortality. The maternal complications include preeclampsia, gestational hypertension, vaginal hemorrhage, hyperemesis, and complicated labor [36,37]. Women whose asthma is actively managed during pregnancy have no significant differences in maternal and fetal outcomes compared with those of healthy, nonasthmatic women [38,39].

The initial clinical assessment of a pregnant woman with asthma should include personal history (detailing etiologic factors and prior therapy), physical examination, and either peak expiratory flow rate or spirometric pulmonary function testing (see Chapter 172). Peak expiratory flow rates and spirometry do not change with pregnancy and advancing gestation. Therefore, peak expiratory flow rate and spirometry can be used as diagnostic and monitoring tools in the care of pregnant asthmatic women [36]. Although asthma may be the most common cause of airway obstruction during pregnancy, wheezing, shortness of breath, coughing, and sensation of chest tightness are nonspecific, and several other entities may mimic asthma (see Chapter 172).

Assuming the diagnosis of asthma is secure, certain findings taken together can be used to predict which patients are likely to require intensive care unit (ICU) admission. These include diaphoresis, use of accessory muscles, assumption of upright posture, altered level of consciousness, pulse rate greater than 120 beats per minute, respiratory rate greater than 30 breaths per minute, pulsus paradoxus greater than 18 mm Hg, peak expiratory flow rate less than 120 L per minute, or failure of the FEV_1 to increase at least 10% after inhaled bronchodilator therapy [40]. Peak flows have been used for the evaluation of nonpregnant patients with asthma to predict the need for arterial blood gas determination. Flows greater than 200 L per minute (50% of predicted) are virtually never associated with significant hypoxemia or hypercapnia (see Chapter 172). However, because alveolar–arterial oxygen tension gradients are known to be widened in pregnancy [3], it seems prudent to obtain arterial blood gas measurements in pregnant women with asthma who do not show a significant improvement (>20%) in peak expiratory flow rate after an initial inhaled bronchodilator treatment. Continuous oxygen saturation monitoring is also appropriate.

During acute asthma attacks, arterial blood gas measurements typically reveal mild hypocapnia ($PaCO_2$ of 35 mm Hg) and moderate hypoxemia. During pregnancy, as noted previously, the baseline $PaCO_2$ is usually already depressed [3] and probably decreases further with an acute asthma attack. The importance of this is twofold: (a) a $PaCO_2$ of 35 mm Hg during an acute attack may actually represent "pseudonormalization" caused by fatigue, inability to meet the increased work of breathing, and impending respiratory failure and (b) persistent hypocapnia with associated respiratory alkalosis (pH greater than 7.48) may result in uterine artery vasoconstriction and decreased fetal perfusion [5].

β-Adrenergic Tocolytic Therapy

Tocolytic therapy is administered to delay preterm delivery up to 48 hours so that systemic glucocorticoids can be given to optimize lung maturity with the aim of reducing neonatal morbidity and mortality. Many classes of medications are given for this purpose, including β-agonists, prostaglandin inhibitors, calcium channel blockers, magnesium sulfate, and oxytocin receptor blockers. These agents prevent preterm labor by inhibiting myometrial contractions [16]. The use of relatively β_2-selective agents, such as ritodrine and terbutaline, has diminished the frequency of unacceptable maternal tachycardia, but maternal pulmonary edema has remained a serious side effect. Pulmonary edema associated with tocolytic therapy appears to be unique to pregnancy because it has not been reported when these medications are used to treat asthma. Calcium channel blockers such as nifedipine and nicardipine have also been reported to cause pulmonary edema [41,42].

The typical symptoms and signs of β-adrenergic tocolytic-induced pulmonary edema are chest discomfort, dyspnea, tachypnea (24 to 40 breaths per minute), crackles, and pulmonary edema on chest radiography. Evidence of pulmonary edema develops relatively acutely, occasionally after only 24 hours but usually after 48 hours of β-adrenergic tocolytic therapy. A nonproductive cough is occasionally present. Wheezes, in addition to crackles, were noted in one case [43]. The size of the heart has been difficult to assess on radiographs because of the normal increase in cardiac diameter with pregnancy. The relatively rapid improvement that occurs with discontinuation of β-adrenergic tocolytic therapy (usually in less than 24 hours), the absence of hypotension and clotting abnormalities, and the lack of need for mechanical ventilation support the possibility that these cases represent a separate syndrome related to β-adrenergic tocolytic therapy.

The pathophysiologic mechanisms leading to the development of tocolytic-induced pulmonary edema are not well defined. Fluid overload is an important factor contributing to the pathogenesis. Augmented aldosterone secretion secondary to pregnancy and β-agonist stimulation causes salt and water retention. Tocolytic agents also stimulate antidiuretic hormone secretion, which increases water retention [43]. There are no compelling data to support the hypothesis of cardiac failure as the etiology of tocolytic-induced pulmonary edema. Echocardiography and hemodynamic assessment of affected patients have not revealed cardiac dysfunction [43]. The rapidity of improvement after diuresis is consistent with pulmonary edema caused by increased hydrostatic pressure, rather than an increase in capillary permeability [16].

Pneumomediastinum and Pneumothorax

Pneumomediastinum is another rare complication of pregnancy. Estimates of incidence range from 1 in 2,000 to 1 in 100,000 patients [44]. It occurs most commonly in the second stage of labor and is associated with chest or shoulder pain that radiates to the neck and arms, mild dyspnea, and subcutaneous emphysema of face and neck. Prolonged, dysfunctional labor, coughing, and severe emesis seem to be the predisposing factors. Air from ruptured alveoli tracks centrally along the perivascular sheath into the mediastinum and along fascial planes into the subcutaneous tissues. Very rarely, pneumomediastinum will cause cardiovascular collapse and require surgical decompression [44].

Spontaneous pneumothorax with tension may occur with or without associated pneumomediastinum. It occurs rarely during pregnancy with an incidence estimated at 1 per 10,000 deliveries, but it should be considered in the differential diagnosis of respiratory failure during pregnancy [45]. Risk factors for pneumothorax include asthma, cigarette smoking, crack cocaine use, and history of pneumothorax. Pneumothoraces usually occur during labor or in the immediate postpartum period. The occurrence of pneumothorax may be caused by rupture of subpleural blebs by the changes in intrapleural pressure caused by Valsalva maneuvers during labor [45]. Symptoms of pneumothorax include sudden pleuritic chest pain, dyspnea, and cough. Hypotension may develop if a tension pneumothorax develops. The clinical significance of pneumothorax during pregnancy relates to impaired ventilation and hypoxemia, which can lead to fetal hypoxemia.

Acute Respiratory Distress Syndrome

ARDS is a type of respiratory failure caused by an inflammatory injury to the alveolar–capillary interface that leads to alveolar edema and resultant hypoxemia. The diagnosis of ARDS in pregnant patients is the same for nonobstetric patients. The Berlin definition of acute respiratory distress syndrome (ARDS) states (a) onset of symptoms within 1 week of a known clinical insult or new or worsening respiratory symptoms, (b) chest imaging demonstrating bilateral opacities not fully explained by effusions, lobar/lung collapse, or nodules, (c) respiratory failure not fully explained by cardiac failure or fluid overload, and (d) oxygenation impairment while on positive end-expiratory pressure (PEEP) of 5 cm H_2O. The PaO_2 to FiO_2 ratio can be used to categorize the severity of ARDS. Mild ARDS is associated with PaO_2 to FiO_2 ratio of 201 to 299 mm Hg; moderate ARDS is present if the PaO_2 to FiO_2 ratio is 100 to 200 mm Hg; and severe ARDS is present if the PaO_2 to FiO_2 ratio is ≤ 100 mm Hg [46]. The pathogenesis of ARDS during pregnancy includes the same etiologies seen in the general population, such as sepsis, aspiration, pancreatitis, trauma, inhalational injury, drowning, and pneumonia. Unique entities of pregnancy that may lead to ARDS include AFE, eclampsia, HELLP syndrome, chorioamnionitis, and endometritis [6].

Published case series report maternal mortality rates between 23% and 39%, with multisystem organ failure as the most common cause of death [47]. Neonatal outcomes are not well studied, but the high rates of fetal death (23%) and spontaneous preterm labor have been reported. [4].

DIAGNOSTIC TESTING

Radiology

Evaluation of patients with respiratory failure usually requires at least one, if not sequential, chest radiograph. Potential adverse fetal effects include congenital malformation, intrauterine growth retardation, and increased risk of leukemia and other malignancies [13,14]. There is no evidence that there is an increased fetal risk of anomalies, growth retardation, or intellectual disability from radiation doses less than 0.05 Gy [13,14]. There may be a small increased risk of childhood leukemia, 1 in every 2,000 compared with a background rate of 1 in every 3,000 [13,14].

The National Council on Radiation Protection Handbook 54 established 5 rad (0.05 Gy or 5 cGy) as the embryonic exposure level not to exceed [14]. The estimated radiation exposures of selected procedures used in the evaluation of pregnant patients with respiratory failure are shown in Table 164.2 [13]. Portable chest radiographs performed daily for 2 weeks to assess location of endotracheal tubes and central venous catheters, as well as response of the underlying illness to treatment, would expose the fetus to approximately 7 mrad (0.07 Gy). A pregnant woman being evaluated for thromboembolic disease with a chest radiograph, ventilation–perfusion scan, and chest CT-PA would have a fetal exposure of less than 500 mrad (0.005 Gy or 0.5 cGy) [11].

TABLE 164.2

Fetal Radiation Dose

Diagnostic test	Dose mGy
Posteroanterior and lateral chest radiograph	<0.01
Helical chest CT scan	<0.06
Abdominal CT scan	8
Lung perfusion scan	0.06–0.12
Lung ventilation scan	0.01–0.19
Brachial pulmonary arteriogram	<0.50
Femoral pulmonary arteriogram	2.21–3.74

CT, computed tomography.
Adapted from Nguyen CP, Goodman LH: Fetal risk in diagnostic radiology. *Sem Ultrasound CT MRI* 33:4, 2012.

Magnetic resonance imaging (MRI) and ultrasonography are not known to be associated with adverse fetal outcomes [48]. The American College of Radiology has published guidelines in which MRI may be considered as a nonionizing imaging study during any trimester if the risk–benefit ratio to the mother is favorable [48]. Gadolinium crosses the placenta to the fetus, so the use of gadolinium-based contrast is not recommended unless the potential benefit to the mother outweighs the potential risk to the fetus [48].

Hemodynamic Monitoring

All pregnant women determined to be critically ill with respiratory failure require cardiopulmonary monitoring, including continuous monitoring of the patient's heart rate, cardiac rhythm, oxygen saturation, and respiratory rate. The blood pressure and temperature are also evaluated frequently. Pregnant women should also have fetal heart rate and uterine monitoring performed. The frequency of fetal monitoring is determined in consultation with the maternal–fetal medicine team and is dependent upon the gestational age of the fetus and the clinical status of the mother.

The potential indications for invasive hemodynamic monitoring with a pulmonary artery catheterization for obstetric patients include the diagnosis or management of septic shock, classes III and IV cardiac patients in labor, severe preeclampsia or eclampsia during labor, pulmonary hypertension, and severe ARDS. There are no reports of specific complications of pulmonary artery catheterization pertaining to obstetric patients, who are at equal risk as nonobstetric patients for complications such as hematoma or pneumothorax at the time of insertion, balloon rupture, catheter knotting, pulmonary infarct, pulmonary artery rupture, thrombosis, embolism, arrhythmias, right bundle-branch block, valvular damage, and infection (see Chapter 19).

In addition to increases of heart rate and cardiac output, several other changes occur in maternal hemodynamics during pregnancy, labor, and delivery [49]. Pulmonary artery catheterization of 10 healthy pregnant patients was done at term and repeated during the nonpregnant state to determine the hemodynamic changes of normal pregnancy. Significant decreases were noted in the systemic and pulmonary vascular resistances, colloid oncotic pressure, and the gradient between colloid oncotic pressure and pulmonary balloon occlusion pressure in the late third trimester. There was no significant change in central venous pressure, pulmonary balloon occlusion pressure, mean arterial pressure, or left ventricular stroke work index [49].

Because of the complications that may accompany pulmonary artery catheterization, the expense of the procedure, and the lack of formal demonstration of improved morbidity or mortality related to the technique, it has been suggested that caution be exercised when choosing to proceed with pulmonary artery catheterization [50]. Clinical assessment may be inadequate for obstetric patients to differentiate between cardiogenic and noncardiogenic pulmonary edema. Both increased permeability pulmonary edema and pulmonary edema caused by volume overload are common causes of respiratory failure in pregnancy. In addition, careful hemodynamic management is needed to maintain adequate uterine blood flow in compromised patients. Maintaining a good risk to benefit ratio depends on obtaining accurate information, interpreting this information in the context of the stage of pregnancy or labor, and determining the specific situations in which the information will contribute significantly to patient management.

Noninvasive hemodynamic monitoring techniques such as Doppler echocardiography, esophageal Doppler monitoring, thoracic electrical bioimpedance, arterial pressure waveform algorithms, pulse pressure variation, and stroke volume variation require further study in critically ill obstetric patients. Transthoracic echocardiography may assist in the differentiation of life-threatening hypotension of the critically ill pregnant patient. Cardiac echo is able to identify pericardial tamponade, right-sided heart failure or left-sided heart failure, intracardiac air, and enables the clinician to direct therapy appropriately [51].

Fetal Monitoring

Methods to assess antepartum fetal well-being include maternal assessment of fetal activity, cardiotocography, contraction stress testing, calculation of a biophysical profile, fetal Doppler ultrasound, and assessment of fetal lung maturity. When respiratory failure occurs early in gestation, before fetal viability is ensured, and when early delivery is not an option, the best course is to focus on optimizing care for the mother and not on minute-to-minute variations in fetal heart rate. However, it is reasonable to measure and record a daily fetal heart rate to document that the fetus is alive. When she is able, the mother can report whether fetal movement is present. Continuous external fetal heart rate monitoring via cardiotocography may be helpful during surgical procedures to alert the anesthesiologist to problems with maternal ventilation or cardiac output. If respiratory failure persists for several weeks, fetal growth measurement by ultrasound may be indicated. When gestation has progressed enough for delivery by cesarean section, amniocentesis may be helpful to determine fetal lung maturity [52].

TREATMENT

Supportive Therapy

Mechanical ventilation, nutritional support, and maintaining an adequate blood pressure are important considerations in respiratory insufficiency during pregnancy.

Mechanical Ventilation

The guidelines for intubation and mechanical ventilation are essentially the same for pregnant patients as for nonpregnant patients: (a) inability to maintain an adequate PaO_2 with supplemental oxygen, (b) uncompensated respiratory acidosis, and (c) inability to clear secretions or need to protect the airway because of altered mental status (see Chapters 8, 166, and 167). For nonpregnant patients, an adequate PaO_2 is considered to be 60 to 65 mm Hg, but, in pregnancy, a goal PaO_2 of 70 mm Hg or greater is preferred to provide better oxygenation for the fetus.

Pregnancy is associated with alterations in physiology that may make airway management more difficult compared with that of nonpregnant patients. Elevated estrogen levels and an increase in blood volume during pregnancy may contribute to mucosal edema [3]. Smaller endotracheal tubes sized 6 to 7 mm may be required to minimize the risk of upper airway trauma during intubation. The decreased FRC in pregnancy may lower the oxygen reserve such that, at the time of intubation, a short period of apnea may be associated with a precipitous decrease in PaO_2 [3]. Therefore, before any attempt at endotracheal intubation, 100% oxygen should be administered, either by mask when the patient is able to ventilate spontaneously or by hand resuscitation bag when the patient requires assisted ventilation. However, hyperventilation to increase the PaO_2 before intubation should be avoided because the associated respiratory alkalosis may actually decrease uterine blood flow. Multiple factors place a pregnant patient at an increase risk of aspiration during intubation. These include incompetence of the gastroesophageal junction caused by the position of the gravid uterus, delayed gastric emptying during labor, progesterone-mediated smooth muscle relaxation of the gastrointestinal mucosa, and decreased lower esophageal sphincter tone [3].

Initiating mechanical ventilation follows the same general principles for pregnant patients as for nonpregnant patients, although the goals of arterial blood gas are different in the pregnant patient. In general, the minute ventilation should be adjusted to aim for a $PaCO_2$ of 30 to 32 mm Hg, the normal level in pregnancy; marked respiratory alkalosis should be avoided because of the resultant decrease in uterine blood flow. Maternal permissive hypercapnia may also be deleterious to the fetus because of resultant fetal respiratory acidosis. The transfer of carbon dioxide across the placenta depends on the difference of 10 mm Hg between the fetal and maternal umbilical veins. Plateau pressure, which reflects transalveolar pressure, should be kept under 30 cm H_2O to minimize the risk of barotrauma. Adequate fetal oxygenation requires a maternal PaO_2 of 70 mm Hg or more which corresponds to an oxygen saturation of 95% [3].

Mechanical ventilation of a pregnant patient with ARDS should follow the guidelines of the ARDS Network Study using nonpregnant predicted body weight [53]. This study has shown the efficacy of delivering tidal volumes is based on ideal body weight. This strategy avoids overdistention of the lung and maintains a plateau pressure less than 30 cm H_2O. The initial setting for tidal volume is 6 to 8 mL per kg of ideal body weight. The respiratory rate is adjusted to maintain a maternal $PaCO_2$ between 28 and 32 mm Hg while monitoring for the development of intrinsic PEEP or dynamic hyperinflation. If the pregnant patient continues to have a respiratory acidosis despite a high respiratory rate, the tidal volume may be increased as long as the plateau pressure remains less than 30 cm H_2O. For most patients with ARDS, PEEP is initiated at 5 cm H_2O and adjusted upward depending on the required fraction of inspired oxygen (see Chapters 163 and 166). As in nonpregnant patients, the goals are to reduce the maternal inspired oxygen concentration to less than 50%, if possible, and to maintain adequate oxygen delivery without compromising cardiac output or risking further lung damage caused by excess intra-alveolar pressure. Strict monitoring of fluid status is necessary because the hypervolemia of pregnancy may contribute to the progression of respiratory failure.

Alternative ventilation strategies for patients failing conventional ventilation modes in ARDS have not been studied during pregnancy. The routine use of airway pressure-release ventilation, high-frequency oscillatory ventilation, lung recruitment maneuvers, prone positioning, and inhaled vasodilators during pregnancy need further study before they can be recommended. There have been several reports utilizing extracorporeal membrane oxygenation in pregnant patients with H1N1 influenza with severe refractory ARDS. The maternal and fetal mortality rates were reported to be 28% [54].

For patients with asthma, respiratory rate and tidal volume should be no greater than necessary to maintain oxygenation. Lower respiratory rates and tidal volumes help reduce airway pressures, thereby reducing volutrauma and barotrauma [53]. Inspiratory flow rates can be increased to allow adequate time for expiration. Increasing the inspiratory flow rate during volume-cycled mechanical ventilation decreases the inspiratory to expiratory ratio and mitigates air trapping (for further discussion of mechanical ventilatory support of the patient with asthma, see Chapters 166 and 172). Permissive hypercapnia is often necessary in patients with severe asthma to prevent volutrauma and hemodynamic compromise. There have been no reported cases of controlled hypoventilation during pregnancy, and the potential risk of fetal respiratory acidosis must be considered before instituting this therapy.

Lowering oxygen consumption by treating fever and suppressing spontaneous respiration is also helpful. The recommendations for sedation, analgesia, and muscle paralysis for pregnant women on mechanical ventilation are the same as those for all critically ill patients. Patients requiring sedation while on mechanical ventilation are managed using an assessment tool for agitation and sedation, with titration of sedation so that the patient is comfortable but easily aroused and able to follow simple commands. Patients are also assessed for delirium and pain while they are on mechanical ventilation. It is recommended that sedation be interrupted daily and coupled with a spontaneous breathing trial. Guidelines also recommended the use of analgesic medication as first-line therapy for patients requiring mechanical ventilation. Sedatives are then added only if management of analgesia is ineffective. Compliance with sedation monitoring, daily interruption of sedation, and a daily attempt at spontaneous breathing have resulted in fewer days on the ventilator and fewer days in the ICU [55]. Narcotics that may be used in pregnancy include morphine, fentanyl, and hydromorphone. Morphine is typically avoided in renal failure because of accumulation of active metabolites. These medications are not teratogenic, and appear to be without fetal effects except when used at the time of delivery or when used excessively, as in narcotic addiction [55]. The use of nonbenzodiazepines, rather than benzodiazepines, for patients requiring mechanical ventilation results in fewer days on mechanical ventilation, less delirium, and fewer days in the ICU. If a sedative is required for a mechanically ventilated patient, either propofol or dexmedetomidine is advised. Neither agent is teratogenic. Whether benzodiazepine use results in an increased risk of congenital malformations remains unclear, although the majority of studies are reassuring. Thus, this class of drugs is best avoided in the first trimester and used sparingly thereafter (see www.reprotox.org) [55].

Neuromuscular blockers may be required during mechanical ventilation in a pregnant patient with severe ARDS. These agents should be used at the lowest dose possible and for the minimal amount of time necessary. Patients should have paralytic dosing titrated based upon a train-of-four testing. It is also suggested that awareness based upon objective brain function testing be performed while being chemically paralyzed, such as the bispectral index to assist in sedation titration [55]. Cisatracurium has a pregnancy risk factor rating of B and is the agent of choice in patients with either liver or renal failure because its clearance is via Hofmann degradation. Vecuronium and pancuronium are risk factor C in pregnancy, with pancuronium accumulating in patients with hepatic dysfunction [55].

Although sitting is usually the most advantageous position for weaning nonpregnant patients from mechanical ventilation, it may result in inferior vena cava compression in patients near term, in which case the left lateral decubitus position is preferable. Weaning parameters for pregnant patients are not well established, but it seems reasonable to follow the same guidelines as for nonpregnant patients (see Chapter 168).

Reversal of Hypotension

A mean arterial pressure ([2 × diastolic + systolic]/3) of 65 mm Hg, or greater, is recommended to optimize tissue perfusion and oxygenation. Supine recumbency may cause a significant decrease in venous return in women in their second or third trimester. To counteract this, the right hip should be elevated 10 to 15 cm (15 degrees) to move the uterus off the inferior vena cava, or the left lateral decubitus position should be used. As a corollary to this, if patients in the second or third trimester become hypotensive, placing them in the Trendelenburg position is unlikely to help and may actually decrease venous return because of vena caval compression.

When hypotension does not respond to measures to reduce uterine pressure on the vena cava, the fluid status of the patient should be assessed. If fluid boluses with 250 to 500 mL of saline do not resolve hypotension and the patient appears to be euvolemic, vasopressors should be considered. The ideal vasopressor would restore maternal blood pressure without compromising uterine blood flow. Ephedrine, which has both α- and β-stimulating effects, tends to preserve uterine blood flow while reversing systemic hypotension related to epidural anesthesia [3]. Phenylephrine has been used alone or in combination with ephedrine to reverse maternal hypotension associated with epidural anesthesia [56]. The treatment guidelines for sepsis do not provide specific recommendations regarding vasopressors for pregnant women; however, following these guidelines for the management of maternal hypotension from septic shock is reasonable [57]. The latest recommendations suggest norepinephrine as the first-line vasopressor in patients who fail to respond to fluid resuscitation [57]. There is no good data regarding the use of vasopressin for septic shock in pregnant women, although theoretically its use could cause uterine contractions by binding to uterine V1a receptors. One should balance the maternal and fetal risks and benefits if vasopressin is considered [55].

Nutrition

The importance of adequate nutrition during gestation is well recognized in that maternal weight gain correlates with fetal weight gain and a successful outcome. Maternal body stores are generally protected at the expense of fetal growth during semistarvation. The duration of starvation or semistarvation that can be tolerated without ill effects on the fetus is unknown. In addition, maternal malnutrition has been shown to correlate in certain cases with intrauterine growth retardation and development of preeclampsia [58]. It is also well recognized that hospitalized patients who have experienced prolonged starvation have greater problems with wound healing and that diminished protein stores are associated with increased susceptibility to infection.

For critically ill obstetric patients, nutritional support is thought to be important for both maternal and fetal outcomes. As with nonobstetric patients, enteral nutrition is preferred over parenteral nutrition to avoid the risk of complications associated with central venous catheters, to reduce expense, and to minimize intestinal mucosal atrophy [59]. Pregnancy is associated with decreased lower esophageal sphincter tone and decreased gastric motility; therefore, nasoduodenal tubes are preferred over nasogastric tubes to decrease the likelihood of reflux and aspiration, although scientific evidence for this is lacking.

Total parenteral nutrition (TPN) can provide complete nutritional support during pregnancy with good fetal outcomes and low maternal morbidity [58]. Given the stress of respiratory failure and its underlying causes, it seems reasonable to extend this experience with TPN to patients with respiratory failure who are unable to eat for more than 48 hours and whose gastrointestinal system cannot be used. Blood glucose levels should be measured, along with serum electrolyte concentrations, acid–base status, and renal and hepatic function. Measurement of trace element concentrations is needed for prolonged TPN. Periodic nutritional assessment should include evaluation of nitrogen balance, lymphocyte counts, transferrin, maternal weight, and fetal growth by ultrasound. Micronutrient monitoring and adequate administration of vitamins A, vitamin D, vitamin K, zinc, and folic acid are recommended for pregnant patients who require TPN. Deficiencies of these vitamins may lead to fetal neural tube defects, eye abnormalities, and intracerebral hemorrhage [58]. If delivery occurs while the woman is receiving TPN, the neonate should be observed closely for hypoglycemia.

Specific Therapy

Thromboembolism

Recommendations for the treatment of venous thromboembolic disease of pregnancy have been published by the American College of Chest Physicians (ACCP) [60]. When massive PE is strongly suspected (>50% occlusion of pulmonary vascular bed or systemic hypotension), the major immediate goals of therapy are to (a) provide adequate oxygenation as dictated by arterial blood gas analysis, (b) treat hypotension and organ hypoperfusion by elevating right ventricular preload with colloid or crystalloid administration and vasopressor therapy if necessary, and (c) interrupt clot propagation by immediate anticoagulation with intravenous heparin. Anticoagulation should be instituted immediately in all patients without clear contraindications, such as active bleeding, rather than delaying therapy pending conclusive diagnostic studies. The therapeutic options available include subcutaneous low molecular weight heparin (LMWH), intravenous unfractionated heparin (UFH), or subcutaneous UFH. Heparin is not teratogenic because it does not cross the placenta. Subcutaneous LMWH is preferred because of its safety profile, ease of administration, and efficacy [60]. Meta-analysis data in nonpregnant patients has shown that patients treated with subcutaneous LMWH for PE had decreased mortality, a reduction in thrombus size, and were less likely to experience a major hemorrhage [61].

Intravenous UFH is recommended in pregnant patients who have persistent hypotension as a result of PE or who are considered to be at a high risk of bleeding. Intravenous UFH has a short half-life and can be reversed quickly upon discontinuation and administration of protamine [60]. UFH would also be recommended for pregnant patients with severe renal failure rather than LMWH [60]. The half-life of LMWH is decreased in pregnancy, which may lead to subtherapeutic anticoagulation levels [60]. Routine monitoring of anti-Xa levels in all patients is not necessary. Patients with extremes of weight <50 kg or >90 kg, should be considered for anti-Xa monitoring every 4 to 6 weeks, so that twice-daily regimens achieve anti-Xa levels of 0.6 to 1.0 U per mL 4 hours postinjection [62].

When hemodynamic and angiographic information confirms massive PE, placement of a retrievable inferior vena cava filter is usually indicated to provide immediate and reliable prophylaxis against recurrent thromboembolism. Placement of a retrievable inferior vena cava filter is also advised in pregnant patients with thromboembolic disease and a contraindication to anticoagulation or for those patients who suffer recurrent PE on therapeutic anticoagulation [61]. In the case of massive life-threatening PE in a pregnant patient, thrombolytic therapy, mechanical fragmentation of thrombus and catheter-directed thrombolysis, or surgical embolectomy may be indicated [61].

Thrombolysis is not indicated for submassive PE, because large studies have failed to document that thrombolytic therapy results in any significant improvement in mortality or morbidity compared with heparinization [61]. However, in massive PE, randomized trials in nonpregnant patients have shown thrombolytic therapy to be effective in resolving thrombosis and improving hemodynamics. The overall incidence of bleeding related to thrombolysis is 8% [61]. No controlled trials of the use of thrombolytics in pregnancy have been reported.

A recent review identified 189 pregnant women who received thrombolytics during pregnancy for venous thromboembolism. No maternal mortality was reported, and the risk of major bleeding was 2.6% [62]. In a review of 13 patients who received thrombolytic therapy for PE during pregnancy, there were no maternal deaths, four nonfatal maternal major bleeding complications, two fetal deaths, and five preterm deliveries. The authors concluded that the fetal deaths and preterm deliveries were a consequence primarily related to the PE rather than thrombolytic therapy [64].

Recombinant tissue plasminogen activator is the recommended agent for thrombolysis. Streptokinase does not cross the human placenta, but streptokinase antibodies do cross [61]. Tissue plasminogen activator does not cross the placenta, and the risk of allergic reactions is lower than that of streptokinase. If thrombolytic therapy is used during pregnancy, it seems reasonable to limit the duration of therapy to the time needed for restoration of acceptable hemodynamic function and to discontinue therapy at least 4 to 6 hours antepartum. Continuous uterine massage and methylergonovine maleate should be used postpartum if thrombolytic therapy was only recently discontinued. Aminocaproic acid crosses the placenta readily and is teratogenic, so this should not be used when rapid reversal of the lytic state is needed before delivery. Cryoprecipitate and fresh-frozen plasma are used to rapidly reverse the lytic state.

Laboratory monitoring of the lytic state during thrombolytic infusion is not recommended, because clot lysis and risk of bleeding do not correlate well with laboratory measurement of the lytic state [65]. Following completion of thrombolysis, heparin is administered once the activated partial thromboplastin time (aPTT) and thrombin time are less than twice the normal value [65]. If delivery is anticipated in the next 6 hours, initiation of heparin is delayed until after delivery.

Thrombolysis is contraindicated during delivery and the immediate postpartum state because of the bleeding risk. In these situations, surgical embolectomy may be a treatment option for massive PE when conventional therapy or thrombolytic therapy has failed, or if there is a contraindication for thrombolysis. There have been eight published cases in which pregnant women underwent surgical embolectomy for PE. There were no maternal deaths, although fetal death was reported in six cases and preterm delivery in four cases [64]. Surgical embolectomy should be reserved as a lifesaving measure for the mother because of the high incidence of fetal loss [64]. Catheter-directed therapy may include catheter-directed mechanical embolectomy and/or catheter-directed thrombolytic therapy. Among four cases using these techniques during pregnancy, one fetal death and one preterm delivery were reported [65].

Once the patient has stabilized, continuous intravenous heparin can be transitioned to subcutaneous therapy. This can be done with either LMWH or adjusted dose UFH to prolong the aPTT 1.5 to 2.5 times control. The patient should be anticoagulated for the remainder of the pregnancy and for at least 6 weeks postpartum [60]. If the PE occurs late in pregnancy or in the postpartum period, anticoagulant therapy should be continued for at least 6 months and, possibly, longer if persistent risk factors for a hypercoagulable state exist [60].

It is recommended that pregnant patients being treated with LMWH or UFH discontinue anticoagulation 24 hours prior to elective induction of labor [60]. If spontaneous labor occurs in a woman receiving adjusted doses of UFH, the aPTT should be monitored and corrected with protamine sulfate if delivery is near. Patients at high risk for recurrent thromboembolism during pregnancy should be placed on intravenous UFH, which can be discontinued 4 to 6 hours prior to expected delivery. This approach minimizes the period of time without therapeutic anticoagulation [60]. The timing of reinstitution of anticoagulation following delivery will vary depending upon the type of delivery, the presence of bleeding, and the presence of a neuraxial anesthesia catheter. As long as significant bleeding has not occurred, anticoagulation with a heparin may be resumed 6 hours after a vaginal birth or 12 hours after a cesarean section. However, after neuraxial anesthesia, therapeutic LMWH should be administered no earlier than 24 hours postoperatively [66].

The ACCP guidelines suggest limiting the use of fondaparinux and parenteral direct thrombin inhibitors in pregnant women to those with severe allergic reactions to heparin who cannot receive danaproid [60]. In addition, the ACCP guidelines recommend avoiding the use of oral direct thrombin inhibitor (dabigatran) and anti-Xa inhibitors (rivaroxaban and apixaban) during pregnancy [60].

Amniotic Fluid Embolism

Treatment of AFE is limited to supportive measures aimed at providing adequate ventilation and oxygenation, maintenance of left ventricular output, blood pressure support, and management of bleeding. Most patients require intubation and mechanical ventilation. PEEP is helpful for oxygenation in some patients. No particular drug regimen has been used with any clear success to reverse pulmonary hypertension. If pulmonary capillary wedge pressures are elevated, it seems reasonable to use a diuretic to reduce hydrostatic pressures across the injured capillary endothelium. Measurement of changes in cardiac output can be used to guide this. In addition to fluid resuscitation to reverse hypotension, vasopressor therapy is frequently required.

Treatment of coagulopathy and hemorrhage in AFE requires aggressive blood and component replacement most easily managed utilizing massive transfusion protocols. For active bleeding, transfusion with red blood cells, fresh-frozen plasma, cryoprecipitate, platelets, and factor replacement is indicated. Manual massage and uterotonic medications are used to reduce uterine bleeding after delivery. When uterine bleeding is refractory to these interventions, exploration for uterine tears or retained placenta should be considered. Hysterectomy may be required to control bleeding if all other medical interventions fail. There are case reports describing maternal survival from AFE following treatment with intra-aortic balloon counterpulsation, extracorporeal membrane oxygenation, and cardiopulmonary bypass [67]. In addition, one patient was treated successfully with inhaled nitric oxide, recombinant human factor VIIa, and a right ventricular assist device [68].

In the event of a maternal cardiac arrest from AFE, an emergent perimortem delivery is indicated to improve the likelihood of a good newborn outcome, if the fetus is of a viable gestational age [17].

Venous Air Embolism

The goals of treatment are to identify the source of air entry, prevent further air entrainment, restore circulation, and remove embolized air. Placing the patient in the left lateral decubitus position may restore forward blood flow by causing the bubble of air to migrate away from the right ventricular outflow tract to a nonobstructing position [19,29]. Closed-chest cardiac compression has also been reported to be helpful [20]. Aspiration of air from the right atrium, right ventricle, or pulmonary outflow tract can be attempted with a central venous or pulmonary artery catheter [19,20]. Air bubble resorption may be accelerated by ventilating the patient with 100% oxygen to facilitate diffusion of nitrogen from the embolus. When air embolism occurs during general anesthesia, nitrous oxide should be discontinued because it has a high solubility and tends to increase the size of air bubbles in the pulmonary vasculature [19,20].

Patients with continued evidence of neurologic deficits or cardiopulmonary compromise because of air embolism should be considered for hyperbaric oxygen therapy. Hyperbaric oxygen accelerates nitrogen resorption, decreases air bubble size, and increases the arterial oxygen content [19,20]. Use of anticoagulation with heparin has been suggested to treat fibrin microemboli, but has not been formally evaluated [19].

Aspiration of Gastric Contents

For patients with permeability pulmonary edema because of aspiration of gastric contents during labor and delivery, the main treatment is supportive care. Prophylactic antibiotics have not been found to be beneficial for aspiration pneumonitis [22]; therefore, antibiotics should be prescribed only when infection complicates the initial chemical pneumonitis. If the patient's clinical course suggests development of bacterial pneumonia, the choice of antibiotic should be guided by appropriate bacteriologic evaluation of respiratory secretions, pleural fluid (if present), and blood cultures. For patients who have been in the hospital for 48 hours or less, clindamycin or a β-lactam–β-lactamase inhibitor combination is a reasonable empiric choice to treat anaerobic organisms. Glucocorticoids are not recommended in the treatment of aspiration events because of a lack of benefit found by two large multicenter randomized trials [22].

Respiratory Infections

Antibacterial agents to treat pneumonia during pregnancy should be selected according to the same principles used for nonpregnant patients [4,24,25]. Drugs with the least risk to fetus and mother should be chosen whenever possible [6].

For community-acquired pneumonia in pregnancy, penicillins, ceftriaxone, azithromycin, and erythromycin (excluding the estolate, which is associated with an increased risk of cholestatic jaundice in pregnancy) are probably safe. Tetracycline is contraindicated because it is teratogenic and causes hepatic toxicity when administered intravenously in pregnancy. The aminoglycosides have the potential of causing eighth nerve toxicity in the fetus and should be used only when strong clinical indications exist. Serum drug levels should then be monitored closely. Sulfonamides are considered contraindicated at term because of the risk of neonatal kernicterus. Clindamycin has no reported adverse fetal effects, but experience is limited and it should be used with caution. Vancomycin hydrochloride may cause fetal renal and auditory toxicity and should be used with caution, with close monitoring of serum drug levels. Clarithromycin and levofloxacin are pregnancy risk factor class C and, therefore, should be used judiciously, weighing potential risks and benefits.

The predominant treatment of influenza pneumonia is supportive care, following the same practices as outlined for other causes of respiratory failure in pregnancy. The novel influenza A (H1N1) virus that appeared in 2009 is sensitive to the neuraminidase inhibitor antiviral medications such as oseltamivir and zanamivir, but it is resistant to the adamantine antiviral agents. It is recommended that pregnant women with a confirmed, probable, or suspected case of influenza A (H1N1) receive empiric institution of oseltamivir for a period of 5 or more days. Treatment should be started although results from testing are pending, because the maximal clinical benefit is seen when antiviral therapy is begun within 48 hours of the onset of symptoms [26,69]. Adamantanes are no longer recommended for influenza owing to concerns about antiviral resistance in the circulating influenza strains [69]. Fetal side effects have not been reported with either neuraminidase inhibitor, although experience with them is limited.

Intravenous acyclovir has been shown to decrease maternal mortality from varicella pneumonia. Acyclovir has not been shown to be teratogenic when used during human pregnancy. The recommended dosing is 10 mg per kg every 8 hours intravenously, with adjustments made for renal insufficiency. The recommended length of therapy is 7 days. Maintenance of a euvolemic fluid status minimizes renal impairment secondary to acyclovir. Initiation of acyclovir at the first evidence of respiratory system involvement in pregnant patients with cutaneous varicella infection optimizes the chances of a favorable outcome. Infants born to women in whom varicella infection developed within 4 days of delivery should receive varicella-zoster immune globulin within 72 hours of birth [70].

Amphotericin B is the drug of choice for severe disseminated coccidioidal infection during pregnancy [30]. Azoles are contraindicated during pregnancy: fluconazole exposure is teratogenic in the first trimester; and voriconazole is category D owing to documented fetal harm and teratogenicity. There is not enough safety data to recommend caspofungin during pregnancy. Amphotericin has been used with success in disseminated coccidioidal infection during pregnancy. It crosses the placenta and is present in umbilical cord serum at a concentration one-third of the maternal serum concentration. However, it does not appear to have an adverse effect on fetal development; normal, full-term infants have been born to women who received amphotericin B during the first trimester, as well as later in gestation. Because anemia and nephrotoxicity often occur during the course of amphotericin B therapy, blood cell counts and renal function should be monitored closely [30].

Active TB has been treated with modern chemotherapeutic agents with excellent maternal and fetal outcome. The initial treatment regimen should consist of isoniazid, rifampin, and ethambutol for a minimum of 9 months [32]. In the United States, pyrazinamide is not recommended for use during pregnancy [32]. Streptomycin has been associated with fetal hearing loss and vestibular dysfunction and should be avoided [32]. Ethionamide has been identified as a teratogen [32].

Treatment of PCP during pregnancy includes trimethoprim–sulfamethoxazole, with the addition of glucocorticoids for severe disease characterized by a PaO_2 less than 70 mm Hg or an alveolar–arterial oxygen gradient of more than 35 mm Hg [71]. For *L. monocytogenes*–associated pneumonia in pregnancy, high-dose ampicillin is the treatment of choice (2 g intravenously every 4 hours) for at least 14 days [72].

Asthma

The Working Group on Asthma and Pregnancy of the National Asthma Education Program has published a report summarizing the available data for asthma medications and management during pregnancy [73]. The first priority of therapy for pregnant women with asthma is to prevent or reverse the hypoxemia that, to some degree, accompanies virtually every exacerbation of asthma. Oxygen should be used in all asthmatic patients who present to the hospital with an exacerbation; the goal oxygen saturation is 95% or higher because hypoxemia may worsen initially with bronchodilator therapy, as a result of worsening ventilation–perfusion mismatch. Other therapies are directed at the rapid reversal of bronchoconstriction and airways inflammation (see Chapter 172).

Bronchoconstriction is managed with inhalation of selective rapid-onset β_2-agonist and anticholinergic agents, given at 20-minute intervals or continuously. Typically, nebulized medication is given prior to intubation and then switched to metered dose inhaler after intubation. The doses of albuterol and ipratropium are the same for both obstetric and nonobstetric patients presenting with status asthmaticus [73]. The effects of inhaled agents are predominantly local, which should decrease the amount of fetal exposure, and selective β_2-agonists do not adversely affect uterine blood flow. There has been no evidence of fetal injury from the use of either systemic or inhaled β-adrenergic agonists [73], although neonates exposed to systemic β-agonists just prior to delivery have demonstrated tachycardia, hypoglycemia, and tremor. These effects do not constitute a contraindication to the use of β-adrenergic agents.

Systemic glucocorticoids should be initiated promptly in all pregnant patients presenting with an acute asthma exacerbation who are not responding to one or two inhalational treatments with a β_2-agonist [73]. Institution of glucocorticoids helps to reverse airflow obstruction and, thereby, decrease the amount of high-dose β-adrenergic agonist therapy needed. The optimal dose of systemic glucocorticoid in this setting is not known. However, the same dose ranges are used in both obstetric and nonobstetric adults, prednisone or methylprednisolone 120 to 180 mg per day in three or four divided doses for the first 48 hours and then 40 to 60 mg a day until clinical improvement is significant and the peak expiratory flow has increased to 70% of predicted or personal best [73]. Further tapering is based on the response to treatment.

Prednisone and prednisolone cross the placenta poorly [73]. In rodents that were given glucocorticoids during gestation, an increased prevalence of spontaneous abortions, placental insufficiency, and cleft palate were found; it remains controversial whether a slight increase in risk of cleft palate pertains in humans [73]. Chronic maternal ingestion of systemic glucocorticoids has been associated with lower birth weight and increased incidence of premature deliveries [74].

In general, intravenous theophylline is not used during treatment of acute asthma exacerbations because of the lack of evidence of benefit [73]. However, for patients who normally take theophylline, the medication is normally continued during the hospitalization. If the patient is unable to take oral medication, intravenous theophylline is usually substituted, but without a loading dose. Because toxicity can develop in the fetus when theophylline is administered at the time of delivery [73], serum levels should be closely followed and kept below 15 mg per mL.

In patients with severe bronchoconstriction, who are refractory to inhaled nebulized albuterol sulfate, parenteral agents such as terbutaline sulfate, 0.3 mg, or epinephrine, 0.3 mL of a 1 to 1,000 solution, may rarely be given subcutaneously [73]. A major concern is that epinephrine may cause uterine artery vasoconstriction through its α-adrenergic effects; this potential risk would have to be balanced against the need to reverse refractory bronchoconstriction [73].

In the management of an acute exacerbation of asthma for a pregnant woman, monitoring of the respiratory rate and $PaCO_2$ levels is critical in the identification of impending respiratory failure. Normalization of the $PaCO_2$ in a pregnant patient may be the indication of respiratory muscle fatigue, and ventilatory support is indicated. Early intervention with noninvasive ventilation and/or intubation with ventilatory support should be seriously considered [4].

For patients who are extremely difficult to manage even with therapeutic levels of bronchodilators, high-dose glucocorticoids, and mechanical ventilation, a few less-studied therapeutic interventions such as intravenous magnesium sulfate and inhaled isoflurane [75] can be considered. None of these interventions have been studied in pregnancy, so their use should be limited to situations in which the woman's life is in danger and all other forms of therapy have failed (see Chapter 172, for a full discussion).

Once a pregnant woman reaches the point of life-threatening refractory asthma, emergent delivery of the fetus by cesarean section should be considered. There have been anecdotal reports of significant maternal improvement after delivery of the fetus [76]. The decision for urgent delivery is complicated and depends in part on the gestational age of the fetus and the clinical status of the mother [76].

Pneumomediastinum and Pneumothorax

The natural history of pneumomediastinum is spontaneous resolution within 3 to 14 days without permanent sequelae. Pneumomediastinum does not usually require drainage in adults because the air usually dissects out of the mediastinum into the subcutaneous tissues of the neck. Thus, treatment should be directed at improving any underlying predisposing cause, such as asthma, if present. Supplemental oxygen may promote reabsorption of the mediastinal air.

A spontaneous pneumothorax occupying less than 20% of the hemithorax in an asymptomatic patient not on mechanical ventilation can be monitored closely without immediate insertion of a chest tube. Supplemental oxygen should be administered to accelerate the resolution of the pneumothorax. In patients who are symptomatic, on mechanical ventilation, or have an enlarging pneumothorax, chest tube placement is mandatory. Patients whose pneumothorax develops as a complication of barotrauma during mechanical ventilation may also require adjustments in the ventilator settings to reduce airway pressures and further barotrauma.

Patients with an existing pneumothorax or history of one in the past are at increased risk of worsening or recurrence of pneumothorax during labor and delivery, particularly during the Valsalva maneuvers at parturition. Although formal evidence is lacking, use of epidural analgesia and assisted vaginal delivery is suggested to avoid prolonged Valsalva maneuvers [45]. For patients requiring cesarean section, analgesia with epidural anesthetic is preferred to general anesthesia with positive pressure ventilation.

The recurrence rate of ipsilateral spontaneous pneumothorax is 30% to 50% within 5 years without pleurodesis [45]. Pleurodesis with any tetracycline derivative through a chest tube is contraindicated in pregnancy because of possible fetal exposure. It is recommended that minimally invasive elective video-assisted thoracoscopic surgery (VATS) with bleb resection and mechanical pleurodesis be considered in the subsequent convalescent period to prevent a recurrent pneumothorax [45]. Thoracotomy or VATS with bleb resection and pleurodesis is indicated for pregnant patients with continued air leak and incomplete lung expansion [77]. Tocolytic therapy may be required to prevent preterm labor during this surgical intervention.

PREVENTION

Thromboembolic Disease

Preventing DVT is probably the most important intervention to reduce maternal mortality caused by PE. Patients who require bed rest or surgery during pregnancy should be treated prophylactically with an LMWH regimen such as dalteparin 5,000 U subcutaneously every 24 hours or enoxaparin 40 mg subcutaneously every 24 hours. In the setting of impaired creatinine clearance, UFH 5,000 U subcutaneously every 12 hours may be used [60]. Warfarin crosses the placenta and is teratogenic, so its use is contraindicated in pregnancy [60]. Patients who are receiving ongoing warfarin therapy for prior thromboembolic disease should be changed to subcutaneous heparin therapy before conception or at least before the sixth week of pregnancy. LMWH is recommended for prophylaxis and treatment because of the reduced risk of bone loss and heparin-induced thrombocytopenia as compared with UFH [60].

Pregnant women with a history of thromboembolic disease and/or hypercoagulable state should receive thromboembolic prophylaxis throughout pregnancy and for 4 to 6 weeks postpartum [60]. The ACCP guidelines recommend either prophylactic or intermediate-dose regimens of LMWH or UFH for these particular subgroups of pregnant patients (Table 164.3) [60]. Once adequate hemostasis has been accomplished postpartum, subcutaneous anticoagulation therapy can be resumed and continued until 6 weeks postpartum. Alternatively, warfarin can be added to subcutaneous heparin, and the heparin stopped when therapeutic prolongation of the International Normalized Ratio is achieved.

TABLE 164.3

Guidelines for Anticoagulation Regimens

Prophylactic LMWH: dalteparin 5,000 units subcutaneously every 24 hours or enoxaparin 40 mg subcutaneously every 24 hours
Intermediate-dose LMWH: dalteparin 5,000 units subcutaneously every 12 hours or enoxaparin 40 mg subcutaneously every 12 hours
Prophylactic UFH: UFH 5,000 units subcutaneously every 12 hours
Adjusted dose UFH: UFH subcutaneously every 12 hours adjusted to target an aPTT into therapeutic range

LMWH, low molecular weight heparin; UFH, unfractionated heparin; aPTT, activated thromboplastin time.

Adapted from Bates SM, Greer IA, Middeldorp S, et al: VTE, thrombophilia, antithrombotic therapy, and pregnancy: American College of Chest Physicians Evidence-Based Clinical Practice Guidelines (9th edition). *Chest* 141(2)[Suppl]:e691s, 2012.

Aspiration of Gastric Contents

Based on national surveys of obstetric practice, antacid administration, H_2 blockade, or proton pump inhibitors have been used for aspiration prophylaxis in pregnant women who require general anesthesia or analgesic therapy other than local or epidural anesthetics [22]. This is done despite the lack of complete protection achieved with gastric pH values greater than 2.5 and a recent meta-analysis that showed no evidence that any of these medications reduced the incidence of gastric aspiration [22,78]. Some authors recommend that all women in labor receive nothing by mouth except medications. This should probably be individualized, in view of the low risk of aspiration during spontaneous vaginal delivery in nonsedated patients and the small proportion of patients who require emergent general anesthesia.

RESPIRATORY INFECTIONS

Immunization is the most effective method to prevent influenza pneumonia. The Advisory Committee on Immunization Practices currently recommends the administration of the inactivated influenza vaccine for all pregnant women and also the intranasal flu vaccine should not be given to pregnant women because it contains a live-attenuated virus [79]. The parenteral influenza vaccine contains inactivated virus and is not associated with adverse pregnancy outcomes. Maternal vaccination will also protect newborn infants from influenza, which is important as infants <6 months are at increased risk of influenza-associated complications and are not eligible to receive influenza vaccination. In addition, influenza vaccination is recommended for all women who will be pregnant during the influenza season and should be administered between October and mid-November regardless of the trimester of pregnancy [79].

β-Adrenergic Tocolytic Therapy

The epidemiologic factors that place patients at increased risk for tocolytic-induced pulmonary edema include longer duration of intravenous β-adrenergic tocolytic therapy (24 to 48 hours), large volume of crystalloid infusion, multiple gestation, concomitant sepsis, and, possibly, preeclampsia [16]. If a β-adrenergic tocolytic agent must be used, limiting the intravenous phase of β-adrenergic therapy to less than 24 to 48 hours and adjusting the dose to keep the maternal heart rate under 120 beats per minute may reduce complications. The β-adrenergic agent should be discontinued immediately at the earliest sign of respiratory distress, such as chest pain, tachypnea, dyspnea, or reduced oxygen saturation. Careful fluid balance records should be maintained, and fluid restriction and, possibly, diuresis should be considered when intake exceeds output by greater than 500 mL. Sodium intake should be restricted to 4 to 6 g per day. If glucocorticoids are required to enhance fetal lung development, a formulation with the lowest mineralocorticoid potency should be used. Clinical improvement in tocolytic-induced pulmonary edema usually occurs within 12 hours after the drug is discontinued and diuresis is begun [16].

Patients with underlying cardiac disease, particularly structural defects causing outflow obstruction, should be excluded from β-adrenergic tocolytic therapy. Patients with severe preeclampsia would likely benefit more from early delivery than from combining the increased risks of tocolytic therapy with those of continuing pregnancy-induced hypertension.

Advances in management of pregnancy based upon randomized controlled clinical trials are summarized in Table 164.4.

TABLE 164.4

Advances in Management of Acute Respiratory Failure in Pregnancy based upon Clinical Trials

- Mechanical ventilation of a pregnant patient with ARDS should follow the guidelines of the ARDS Network Study [53]. B
- Unfractionated heparin remains the drug of choice for massive pulmonary embolism during pregnancy [60]. D
- Low molecular weight heparin is safe and effective in pregnancy, and may be used for anticoagulation for pulmonary embolism during pregnancy once the patient is stabilized [60]. D
- Pregnancy is a relative contraindication for thrombolytic therapy. Thrombolysis has been used safely in life-threatening pulmonary embolism during pregnancy with maternal mortality of 1% and fetal loss 6%. Recombinant tissue plasminogen activator and streptokinase are the recommended thrombolytics during pregnancy [63]. D

ARDS, acute respiratory distress syndrome; B, 1 RCT trial; D, nonrandomized, contemporaneous control group.

References

1. Creang AA, Berg CJ, Syverson C, et al: Pregnancy-related mortality in the United States, 2006–2010. *Obstet Gynecol* 125(1):5, 2015.
2. Lapinsky SE, Rojas-Suarez JA, Crozier TM, et al: Mechanical ventilation in critically-ill pregnant women: a case series. *Int J Obstet Anesth* 24(4):323, 2015.
3. Bobrowski RA: Pulmonary physiology in pregnancy. *Clin Obstet Gynecol* 53(2):285, 2010.
4. Mehta N, Chen K, Hardy E, et al: Respiratory disease in pregnancy. *Best Pract Res Clin Obstet Gynaecol* 29:598, 2015.
5. Carter AM: Placental gas exchange and oxygen supply to the fetus. *Compr Physiol* 5(3):1381, 2015.
6. Guntupalli KK, Karnad DR, Bandi V, et al: Critical illness in pregnancy, Part II: common medical conditions complicating pregnancy and pueperium. *Chest* 148(5):1333, 2015.
7. Chabada HL, Drobny J, Batorova A: Longitudinal evaluation of markers of hemostasis in pregnancy. *Bratisl Lek Listy* 115(3):140, 2014.
8. Guven S, Sonmez M, Caner Karahan S: The role of fibrinolytic and antifibrinolytic activities in the pathophysiology of HELLP syndrome. *Hypertens Pregnancy* 30:275, 2011.
9. Guimicheva B, Czuprynska J, Arya R: The prevention of pregnancy-related venous thromboembolism. *Brit J Haem* 168;163, 2015.
10. Reger B, Peterfalvi A, Litter I, et al: Challenges in the evaluation of D-dimer and fibrinogen levels in pregnant women. *Thromb Res* 131(4)e183, 2013.
11. Leung AN, Bull TM, Jaeschke R, et al: An official American Thoracic Society/Society of Thoracic Radiology clinical practice guideline-evaluation of suspected pulmonary embolism in pregnancy. *Radiology* 262:635, 2012.
12. Stein PD, Fowler SE, Goodman LR, et al: Multidetector computed tomography for acute pulmonary embolism. *N Engl J Med* 354:2317, 2006.
13. Nguyen CP, Goodman LH: Fetal risk in diagnostic radiology. *Sem Ultrasound CT MRI* 33:4, 2012.
14. Radiation and pregnancy: a fact sheet for clinicians. Centers for Disease Control and Prevention publication. Available at: https://emergency.cdc.gov/radiation/prenatalphysician.asp. Accessed July 7, 2017.
15. Revel MP, Cohen S, Sanchez O, et al: Pulmonary embolism during pregnancy: diagnosis with lung scintigraphy or CT angiography? *Radiology* 258(2):590, 2011.
16. Guntupalli KK, Hall N, Karnad DR, et al: Critical illness in pregnancy. Part I: an approach to a pregnant patient in the ICU and common obstetric disorders. *Chest* 148(4):1093, 2015.
17. Clark SL: Amniotic fluid embolism. *Obstet Gynecol* 123(2 Pt 1):337, 2014.
18. Rath WH, Hofer S, Sinicina I: Amniotic fluid embolism: an interdisciplinary challenge-epidemiology, diagnosis and treatment. *Dtsch Aztebl Int* 111(8):126, 2014.
19. Shaikh N, Ummunisa F: Acute management of vascular air embolism. *J Emerg Trauma Shock* 2(3):180, 2009.
20. Gordy S, Rowell S: Vascular air embolism. *Int J Crit Illn Inj Sci* 3:73,2013.
21. Mendelson CL: The aspiration of stomach contents into the lungs during obstetric anesthesia. *Am J Obstet Gynecol* 52:191, 1946.
22. Paranjothy S, Griffiths JD, Broughton HK, et al: Interventions at caesarean section for reducing the risk of aspiration pneumonitis. *Cochrane Database Syst Rev* 2:CD004943, 2014.
23. Raghavendran K, Nemzek J, Napolitano LM, et al: Aspiration-induced lung injury. *Crit Care Med* 39:818, 2011.
24. Graves CR. Pneumonia in pregnancy. *Clin Obstet Gyn* 53(2):329, 2010.
25. Mandell LA, Wunderlink RG, Anzueto A, et al: Infectious Diseases Society of America/American Thoracic Society Consensus Guidelines on the management of community-acquired pneumonia in adults. *Clin Inf Dis* 44 (S2):527–572, 2007.
26. Beigi RH: Influenza during pregnancy: a cause of serious infection in obstetrics. *Clin Obstet Gyn* 55(4):914, 2012.
27. Callaghan WM, Creanga AA, Jamieson DJ: Pregnancy-related mortality resulting from influenza in the United States during the 2009–2010 pandemic. *Obstet Gynecol* 126(3):486, 2015.
28. Zhang HJ, Patenaude V, Abenhaim HA: Maternal outcomes in pregnancies affected by varicella zoster infections:population-based study on 7.7 million pregnancy admissions. *J Obstet Gynaecol Res* 41(1):62, 2015.
29. WHO guidlelines for the global surveillance of severe acute respiratory syndrome. Updated recommendations, October 2004. Available at: World Health Organization Website, www.who.int/csr/resources/publications/WHO_CDS_CSR-ARO_2004_1/en/. Accessed November 24, 2015.
30. Bercovitch RS, Catanzaro A, Schwartz BS, et al: Coccidioidomycosis during pregnancy: a review and recommendations for management. *CID* 53(4):363, 2011.
31. Bates M, Ahmed Y, Kapata N, et al: Perspectives on tuberculosis in pregnancy. *Int J Infect Dis* 32:124, 2015.
32. Blumber HM, Burman WJ, Chaisson RE, et al: American Thoracic Society/Centers for Disease Control and Prevention/Infectious Diseases Society of America: treatment of tuberculosis. *Am J Respir Crit Care Med* 167(4):603, 2003.
33. Lazenby GB: Opportunistic infection in women with HIV AIDS. *Clin Obstet Gynecol* 55(4):927, 2012.

34. Mateus T, Silva J, Maia FL, et al: Listeriosis during pregnancy: a public health concern. *ISRN Obstet Gynecol* 2013:851712, 2013.
35. Centers for Disease Control and Prevention: Vital Signs: listeria illnesses, deaths, and outbreaks—United States, 2009–2011. *MMWR* 62:448–452, 2013.
36. Kelly W, Massoumi A, Lazarus A: Asthma in pregnancy: physiology, diagnosis, and management. *Postgrad Med* 127(4):349, 2015.
37. Murphy V, Namazy J, Powell H, et al: A meta-analysis of adverse perinatal outcomes in women with asthma. *BJOG* 118;1314, 2011.
38. Ali Z, Hansen AV, Ulrik CS: Exacerbations of asthma during pregnancy: impact on pregnancy complications and outcome. *J Obstet Gynaecol* 36:455–461, 2016. doi: 10.3109/01443615.2015.1065800.
39. Lim AS, Stewart K, Abramson MJ, et al: Multidisciplinary approach to management of maternal asthma (MAMMA): a randomized controlled trial. *Chest* 145(5):1046, 2014.
40. Maselli DJ, Adams SG, Peters JI, et al: Management of asthma during pregnancy. *Ther Adv Respir Dis* 7(2):87, 2013.
41. Kutuk MSA, Ozgun MT, Uludag S, et al: Acute pulmonary failure due to pulmonary edema during tocolytic therapy with nifedipine. *Arch Gynecol Obstet* 288:953, 2013.
42. Serena C, Begot E, Cros J, et al: Nicardipine-induced acute pulmonary edema: a rare but severe complication of tocolysis. *Case Rep Crit Care* 2014:242703, 2014. doi: 10.1155/2014/242703.
43. Dennis AT, Solnordal CB: Acute pulmonary oedema in pregnant women. *Anaesthesia* 67:646, 2012.
44. Kouki S, Fares AB: Postpartum spontaneous pneumomediastinum "Hamnnan's syndrome". *BMJ Case Rep* 2013. doi:10.1136/bcr-2013-010354.
45. MacDuff A, Arnold A, Harvey J: Management of spontaneous pneumothorax during pregnancy: British Thoracic Society pleural disease guideline. *Thorax* 65[Suppl 2]:II8–II31, 2010.
46. ARDS Definition Task Force; Ranieri VM, Rubenfeld GD, Thompson BT, et al: Acute respiratory distress syndrome: the Berlin Definition. *JAMA* 307(23):2526, 2012.
47. Duarte AG: ARDS in pregnancy. *Clin Obstet Gynecol* 57(4):862, 2014.
48. Expert Panel on MR Safety: ACR guidance document on MR safe practices: 2013. *J Magn Reson Imaging* 37:501, 2013.
49. Fujitani S, Baldisseri MR: Hemodynamic assessment in a pregnant and peripartum patient. *Crit Care Med* 33:S354, 2005.
50. Rajaram SS, Desai NK, Kalra A, et al: Pulmonary artery catheters for adult patients in intensive care. *Cochrane Database Syst Rev* 2:CD003408, 2013.
51. Dennis AT: Transthoracic echocardiography in obstetric anaesthesia and obsetric critical illness. *Int J Obstet Anesth* 20:160, 2011.
52. O'Neill E, Thorp J: Antepartum evaluation of the fetus and fetal well being. *Clin Obstet Gynecol* 55(3):722, 2012.
53. Acute Respiratory Distress Syndrome Network: Ventilation using low tidal volumes as compared with traditional tidal volumes in acute lung injury and the acute respiratory distress syndrome. *N Engl J Med* 342:1301, 2000.
54. Anselmi A, Ruggieri VG, Letheulle J, et al: Extracorporal membrane oxygenation in pregnancy. *J Card Surg* 30:781, 2015.
55. Pacheco LD, Saade GR, Hankins GD: Mechanical ventilation during pregnancy: sedation, analgesia, and paralysis. *Clin Obstet Gynecol* 57(4):844, 2014.
56. Mercier FJ, Riley ET, Frederickson WL, et al: Phenylephrine added to prophylactic ephedrine infusion during spinal anesthesia for elective cesarean section. *Anesthesiology* 95:668, 2001.
57. Dellinger RP, Levy MM, Rhodes A, et al: Surviving sepsis campaign: International guidelines for management of severe sepsis and septic shock: 2012. *Crit Care Med* 41:580, 2013.
58. Buchholz BM, Fuland A, Kiefer N, et al: Conception, pregnancy, and lactation despite chronic intestinal failure requiring home parenteral nutrition. *Nutr Clin Pract* 30:807, 2015.
59. Desai SV, McClave SA, Rice TW: Nutrition in the ICU, an evidence-based approach. *Chest* 145(5):1148, 2014.
60. Bates SM, Greer IA, Middeldorp S, et al: VTE, thrombophilia, antithrombotic therapy, and pregnancy: American College of Chest Physicians Evidence-Based Clinical Practice Guidelines (9th edition). *Chest* 141(2 Suppl):e691S–e736S, 2012.
61. Conti E, Zezza L, Ralli E, et al: Pulmonary embolism in pregnancy. *J Thromb Thrombolysis* 37:251, 2014.
62. Greer IA. Thrombosis in pregnancy: updates in diagnosis and management. *Hematology Am Soc Educ Program* 203, 2012.
63. Gartman EJ: The use of thrombolytic therapy in pregnancy. *Obstet Med* 6:105, 2013.
64. te Raa GD, Ribbert LS, Snijder RJ, et al: Treatment options in massive pulmonary embolism during pregnancy: a case report and review of literature. *Thromb Res* 124:1, 2009.
65. Goldhaber SZ: Contemporary pulmonary embolism thrombolysis. *Chest* 107:45S, 1995.
66. Horlocker TT, Wedel DJ, Rowlingson JC, et al: Regional anesthesia in the patient receiving antithrombotic or thrombolytic therapy. *Reg Anesth Pain Med* 35:64, 2010.
67. Sharma NS, Wille KM, Bellot SC, et al: Modern use of extracorporeal life support in pregnancy and postpartum. *ASAIO J* 61(1):110, 2015.
68. Nagarsheth NP, Pinney S, Bassiy-Marcu A, et al: Successful placement of a right ventricular assist device for treatment of a presumed amniotic fluid embolism. *Anesth Analg* 107:962, 2008.
69. Beiii RH, Venkataramanan R, Caritis SN: Oseltamivir for influenza in pregnancy. *Sem Perinat* 38:503, 2014.
70. Centers for Disease Control and Prevention (CDC): FDA approval of an extended period for adminstering VariAIG for postexposure prophylaxis of varicella. *MMWR Morb Mortal Wkly Rep* 61(12):212, 2012.
71. Gilroy SA, Bennett NJ: Pneumocystis pneumonia. *Sem Resp Crit Care Med* 32(6):775, 2011.
72. Committee on Obstetric Practice, American College of Obstetricians and Gynecologists, Committee Opinion No. 614: Management of pregnant women with presumptive exposure to *Listeria monocytogenes*. *Obstet Gynecol* 124(6):1241, 2014.
73. National Asthma Education and Prevention Program: Session 4. Expert panel report III: *Guidelines for the Diagnosis and Management of Asthma*. Bethesda, MD: National Heart, Lung, and Blood Institute, 2007; NIH publication no. 08-4051.
74. Namazy JA, Schatz M: Pharmacotherapy options to treat asthma during pregnancy. *Expert Opin Pharmacother* 16(12):1783, 2015.
75. Bain E, Pierides KL, Clifton VL, et al: Interventions for managing asthma in pregnancy. *Cochrane Database Syst Rev* 10:CD010660, 2014.
76. Lo JO Boltax J, Metz TD: Cesarean delivery for life-threatening status asthmaticus. *Obstet Gynecol* 121[2 Pt 2 Suppl 1]:422, 2013.
77. Nwaejike N, Aldam P, Pulimood T, et al: A case of recurrent spontaneous pneumothorax during pregnancy treated with video assisted thoracoscopic surgery. *BMJ Case Rep* 2012. doi:10.1136/bcr.05.2011.4282.
78. Gyte GML, Richens Y: Routine prophylactic drugs in normal labour for reducing gastric aspiration and its effects. *Cochrane Database Syst Rev* 3:CD005298, 2006.
79. Rasmussen SA, Watson AK, Kennedy ED, et al: Vaccines and pregnancy: past, present, and future. *Sem Fetal Neonatal Med* 19(3):161, 2014.

Chapter 165 ▪ Extrapulmonary Causes of Respiratory Failure

HELEN M. HOLLINGSWORTH • RICHARD S. IRWIN

The conditions that cause respiratory failure primarily by their effect on structures other than the lungs are discussed in this chapter. Severe impairment of the extrapulmonary compartment produces respiratory failure through the mechanism of hypoventilation, so the resultant respiratory failure is always hypercapnic. Extrapulmonary causes account for up to 17% of all cases of hypercapnic respiratory failure [1]. This chapter is organized to follow sequential sections of pathophysiology, diagnosis, differential diagnosis, and treatment.

PATHOPHYSIOLOGY

The extrapulmonary compartment includes the (a) central nervous system (CNS), (b) peripheral nervous system, (c) respiratory muscles, (d) chest wall, (e) pleura, and (f) upper airway [2]. Because many conditions can cause extrapulmonary respiratory failure, it is helpful to categorize them according to the specific component affected by the disease process (Fig. 165.1). We have limited the discussion that follows to descriptions of the individual diseases and conditions that are most important to the topic of respiratory failure. They are summarized in Tables 165.1 through 165.4.

Functionally, extrapulmonary disorders can lead to hypercapnic respiratory failure caused by a decrease in normal force generation (e.g., CNS dysfunction, peripheral nervous system abnormalities, or respiratory muscle dysfunction) or an increase in impedance to bulk flow ventilation (e.g., chest wall and pleural disorders or upper airway obstruction) [3].

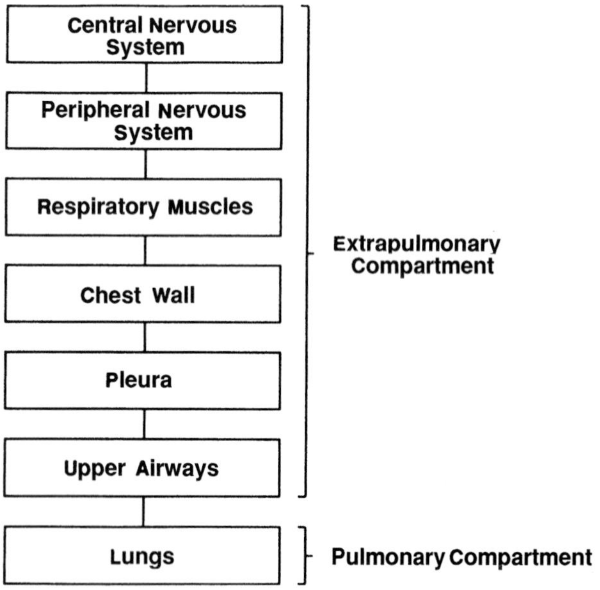

FIGURE 165.1 Schematic representation of the anatomy of the respiratory system.

DIAGNOSIS

General Considerations

Arterial hypercapnia in the presence of a normal alveolar–arterial oxygen tension [$P(A\text{–}a)O_2$] gradient on room air is the sine qua non of extrapulmonary respiratory failure [4]. The normal gradient reflects the fact that, in pure extrapulmonary failure, distal gas exchange is normal, and the decrease in the partial pressure of arterial oxygen (PaO_2) directly reflects the decrease in the partial pressure of alveolar oxygen (PAO_2). A $P(A\text{–}a)O_2$ gradient of less than 20 mm Hg in the presence of an elevated partial pressure of carbon dioxide ($PaCO_2$) is, with few exceptions, diagnostic of extrapulmonary respiratory failure [5–11]. The main exception occurs for patients with chronic obstructive pulmonary disease (COPD) who have increasing hypercapnia [12]. Their $P(A\text{–}a)O_2$ gradient can occasionally narrow to normal, probably related to substantial changes in the position of the alveolar and arterial points on the oxyhemoglobin dissociation curve related to ventilation–perfusion inequalities [12]. Thus, arterial hypercapnia with a normal $P(A\text{–}a)O_2$ gradient is consistent with pure extrapulmonary respiratory failure, but a normal $P(A\text{–}a)O_2$ cannot, by itself, rule out severe COPD.

Pulmonary parenchymal disease can also exist concomitantly with extrapulmonary dysfunction. For example, a patient with polymyositis can have respiratory muscle weakness in addition to interstitial lung disease. This coalescence of clinical processes may be suggested by the combination of hypercapnia and only mild-to-moderate widening of the $P(A\text{–}a)O_2$ gradient. A gradient between 20 and 30 mm Hg in the presence of arterial hypercapnia should raise the suspicion that a significant element of extrapulmonary dysfunction may be present. It is also important to realize that even when the $P(A\text{–}a)O_2$ gradient exceeds 30 mm Hg, some degree of extrapulmonary dysfunction can also be present in association with significant pulmonary impairment. For example, when hypercapnic respiratory failure results from an acute exacerbation of COPD, respiratory muscle fatigue often contributes to the development of carbon dioxide retention [13]. A less common example is the presence of a large abdominal ventral hernia in a patient with COPD. The resultant paradoxic breathing pattern can contribute significantly to abnormal gas exchange and increased dyspnea [14].

Decrease in Normal Force Generation

Because the inspiratory muscles generate the force that results in ventilation, any condition that directly or indirectly impairs respiratory muscle function can result in decreased force generation [3]. Dysfunction of the respiratory center, peripheral nervous system pathways, or the respiratory muscles themselves decreases the force available to produce ventilation. If this impairment is severe enough, the level of minute ventilation will be insufficient to clear the amount of carbon dioxide produced by ongoing metabolic processes and hypercapnic respiratory failure results.

An acute decrease in CNS output sufficient to result in hypercapnic respiratory failure (e.g., acute narcotic overdose) is usually accompanied by obvious evidence of generalized CNS depression. In contrast, a chronic (e.g., primary alveolar hypoventilation) or episodic (e.g., central sleep apnea) cause of decreased impulse formation may present a much more difficult diagnostic dilemma. Tests to evaluate respiratory center drive, such as voluntary hyperventilation, carbon dioxide stimulation, or polysomnography, may be necessary to define the problem.

Peripheral nervous system dysfunction or primary weakness of the respiratory muscles is often indicated by the presence of certain suggestive clinical findings that vary depending on the specific entity present (see the following discussion). Respiratory muscle fatigue or weakness may be suspected clinically and documented using a number of tests designed to evaluate respiratory muscle function.

Symptoms are usually nonspecific; patients may report dyspnea on exertion, either when supine (bilateral diaphragmatic paralysis) or when upright (C5 to C6 quadriplegia). Reports of weakness in other muscle groups, difficulty swallowing, and change in voice volume or tone may be other clues. Physical findings of changes in the rate, depth, and pattern of breathing suggest stressed, fatigued, or weakened respiratory muscles. For example, an increased respiratory rate, a decreased tidal volume, and paradoxic inward motion of the anterior abdominal wall during inspiration may be observed. The latter finding indicates a failure of the diaphragm to contract sufficiently to descend and move the abdominal contents downward and the abdominal wall outward during inspiration. A breathing pattern that cycles between predominantly chest wall and predominantly abdominal wall motion, called *respiratory alternans*, represents the alternating contraction of intercostal and accessory muscles, on the one hand, and the diaphragm, on the other. The assumption is that these two muscle groups alternate in their contribution to the work of breathing, allowing one another to rest during periods of muscle overload or fatigue.

Two readily available tests can be useful diagnostically to help assess respiratory muscle function. First, measurement of maximal inspiratory and expiratory pressures at the mouth is easy to perform, noninvasive, and can accurately predict the development of hypercapnic respiratory failure caused by decreased respiratory muscle force generation [15,16]. Arterial hypercapnia caused by respiratory muscle weakness is generally not seen until the maximal inspiratory pressure is reduced to 30% or less of normal [15,16]. Although normal predicted values vary (primarily on the basis of age and gender) [17,18], a maximal inspiratory pressure less negative than −30 cm H_2O is likely to be associated with arterial hypercapnia [16,19]. Maximal expiratory pressures are also reduced when there is respiratory muscle weakness, and, in some neuromuscular disorders, the decrease may be even greater than that of the corresponding inspiratory pressure [16]. A maximal expiratory pressure of less than 40 cm H_2O is generally associated with a poor cough and difficulty clearing secretions [19].

A second measurement that is valuable in predicting the development of arterial hypercapnia caused by neuromuscular weakness is the vital capacity. It can be performed either in the pulmonary function laboratory or at the bedside [15,19]. Although a vital capacity of less than 1 L, or less than 15 mL per kg of body weight is commonly associated with arterial hypercapnia [1,19], the vital capacity is a less sensitive predictor of arterial hypercapnia than is the maximal inspiratory pressure, particularly in patients with chest wall disorders such as kyphoscoliosis [16]. Significant arterial hypercapnia is unlikely to occur with an inspiratory pressure more negative than −30 cm H_2O; however, arterial hypercapnia may be present with a vital capacity as high as 55% or as low as 20% of the predicted value [15,16].

The measurement of transdiaphragmatic pressures (P_{di}) and diaphragmatic electromyograms (EMGs), although not commonly used clinically, may be helpful. An inspiratory effort associated with a P_{di} consistently more than 40% of maximum predictably results in diaphragmatic fatigue [20]. Therefore, it follows that patients with diaphragmatic weakness and a reduced maximum P_{di} are at risk for developing diaphragmatic fatigue and respiratory failure, even in the face of normal inspiratory pressure [20]. Similarly, a decrease of more than 20% from baseline in the high- to low-frequency ratio as measured by the diaphragmatic EMG indicates diaphragmatic fatigue and portends the development of hypercapnic failure [21,22].

For those readers interested in assessing diaphragm function with point of care ultrasonography, a section discussing this can be found in Chapter 168 on Discontinuation of Mechanical Ventilation.

Central Nervous System Dysfunction

The respiratory center, located in the brainstem, is composed of two main parts, the medullary center and the pneumotaxic center [23,24]. The medullary center is responsible for initiation and maintenance of spontaneous respiration, and the pneumotaxic center in the pons helps coordinate cyclic respiration. A decrease in central drive can occur owing to a direct central loss of sensitivity to changes in $PaCO_2$ and pH or a peripheral chemoreceptor loss of sensitivity to hypoxia as a result of CNS depressants, metabolic abnormalities, structural lesions, primary alveolar hypoventilation, and central sleep apnea (Table 165.1) [25–43].

Peripheral Nervous System Dysfunction

Disruption in impulse transmission from the respiratory center to the respiratory muscles can eventuate in respiratory failure. This disruption can be caused by spinal cord disease [44], anterior horn cell disease [45,46], peripheral neuropathy, or neuromuscular junction blockade [19] (Table 165.2) [5,25,44–88]. Denervation of the inspiratory muscles may occur as part of a generalized process (e.g., Guillain–Barré's syndrome, myasthenia gravis [19]) or as an isolated abnormality (e.g., phrenic nerve palsy secondary to hypothermic cardioplegia during cardiac surgery [67,89]).

Peripheral nervous system dysfunction severe enough to produce hypercapnic respiratory failure is always associated with pulmonary function test findings of a reduced vital capacity (usually less than 50% of the predicted value [15,19]) and markedly decreased maximal inspiratory and expiratory pressures (usually 30% of the predicted pressures [15,19,55]). This type of respiratory failure is characterized by an ineffective cough and a high incidence of aspiration, atelectasis, and pneumonia [5].

The effect on the respiratory system of interruption of CNS impulse transmission as a result of spinal cord abnormalities is highly dependent on the level of the injury [44,47]. A lesion at the C3 vertebral level or above abolishes both diaphragmatic and intercostal activities, leaving only some residual accessory muscle function [47]. The result is severe hypercapnic respiratory failure. Acute spinal cord lesions at the C5 and C6 levels produce an immediate fall in the vital capacity to 30% of the predicted value, owing to loss of intercostal and abdominal muscle function [44]. This is associated with a limitation of both inspiratory capacity and active expiration. Within approximately 3 months of injury, however, the denervated muscles become stiff, which enables improved diaphragmatic efficiency. This improvement usually leads to an increase in the vital capacity to 50% to 60% of normal. Mid-thoracic spinal cord lesions have relatively little impact on respiratory muscle function because they principally affect the abdominal muscles, resulting in only a limitation of active expiration and cough [5,47].

Most spinal cord diseases interrupt impulse transmission, resulting in respiratory muscle weakness, but two notable exceptions exist: tetanus and strychnine poisoning. In both conditions, inhibitory influences at the spinal cord and anterior horn cell

TABLE 165.1

Respiratory Failure Caused by Central Nervous System Dysfunction

Causes [References]	Salient clinical features	Diagnostic tests	Treatment
Central nervous system depressant drugs [25–27]	Pupillary changes Needle marks	Toxicology screen Electrocardiogram in tricyclic overdose	See "Pharmacology, Overdoses, and Poisonings" section
Hypothyroidism [28]	Myxedema	Thyroid function tests	Cautious thyroid replacement
Starvation [29]	Cachexia Diarrhea	↓ Albumin ↓ Cholesterol	Nutrition
Metabolic alkalosis [30]	Lethargy Confusion	Arterial blood gases Serum electrolytes	See Chapter 198
Structural brainstem damage [27,31,32]	Localizing neurologic findings		
Neoplasm	Headache	CT, MRI, cerebrospinal fluid cytology	Radiation, chemotherapy
Infection	Headache, fever	CT, MRI CT, MRI, cardiac echo	Antimicrobial therapy
Primary alveolar hypoventilation (Ondine's curse) [33–41]	Daytime hypersomnolence Headache Rarely dyspneic Polycythemia Cor pulmonale	Blunted or absent ventilator response to ↑ CO_2, ↓O_2 in inspired gas Normal pulmonary function tests	Nighttime ventilatory support Electrophrenic pacing Medroxyprogesterone acetate Supplemental oxygen
Central sleep apnea [31,41–43]	Same as primary alveolar hypoventilation	Polysomnography: apnea without respiratory effort Normal CO_2, O_2 response curves while awake	Nighttime ventilatory support Electrophrenic pacing Supplemental oxygen

↓, decreased; ↑ increased; CT, computed tomography; MRI, magnetic resonance imaging.

level decrease [51,52], causing a simultaneous increase in motor activity to groups of muscles that are normally antagonistic to one another. This results in intense muscle spasms, including involvement of the upper airway muscles, diaphragm, and intercostal muscles. The repetitive spasms and episodes of apnea result in severe arterial hypoxemia, hypercapnia, metabolic acidosis, and rhabdomyolysis [51,52].

Diseases that involve the anterior horn cells of the spinal cord interrupt efferent impulse transmission. Amyotrophic lateral sclerosis (ALS) is the most common anterior horn cell disease causing respiratory failure [5,45,47]. In most cases of ALS, the patient develops segmental muscular atrophy, weakness of the distal extremities, hyperreflexia, fasciculations, and bulbar paralysis [45]. Although respiratory failure usually develops late in the course of the disease, it may rarely be the presenting manifestation [45]. Repetitive episodes of aspiration secondary to bulbar dysfunction may contribute to respiratory impairment [5]. It has been speculated that antecedent poliomyelitis may be involved in some cases of ALS [53]. A post-polio syndrome, characterized by new, slowly progressive muscle weakness, may develop years after recovery from acute poliomyelitis [57].

Polyneuropathies with prominent motor neuron involvement, (e.g., Guillain–Barré's syndrome) can affect the respiratory nerves and lead to respiratory failure (see Chapter 152) [25]. Symmetric, predominantly distal muscle weakness with absent tendon reflexes is the typical presentation [25]. In one series of patients with Guillain–Barré's syndrome, 28% required mechanical ventilatory assistance. The average duration of mechanical ventilation was 9 weeks (range, 3 weeks to 7 months). Although the mortality rate is generally low, 21% of hospitalized patients died in one series [90]. Guillain–Barré's syndrome may be associated with autonomic dysfunction in approximately two-thirds of patients, including tachyarrhythmias and bradyarrhythmias, blood pressure fluctuations, abnormal hemodynamic responses to drugs, flushing and sweating, pupillary light unresponsiveness, and also bladder and bowel dysfunction (e.g., ileus) [90].

Dinoflagellate toxin poisoning, from red tide-contaminated shellfish and ciguatera-contaminated reef and other fish, is a dramatic but uncommon cause of peripheral neuropathy resulting that can produce respiratory failure [61–66]. The responsible agents are heat-stable neurotoxins that interfere with action potential propagation along peripheral nerves. During the warm summer months, the dinoflagellates that produce the toxins proliferate and are ingested by shellfish and fish. The clinical picture is virtually pathognomonic. Within 30 minutes of ingesting contaminated shellfish, tingling and numbness of the face, lips, and tongue develop. Paresthesias and muscle weakness follow, with rapid progression to limb and respiratory muscle paralysis [62,63]. Multiple-case presentations from one source of exposure are common.

Peripheral phrenic nerve palsies can contribute to or cause hypercapnic respiratory failure, particularly if they are bilateral [91]. Bilateral phrenic nerve palsies have been described as an uncommon complication of hypothermia used for cardioplegia during cardiac surgery (particularly when ice slush is used) [67], trauma [67,91], a variety of neurologic diseases (e.g., poliomyelitis and Guillain–Barré's syndrome) [67,68,91], Charcot–Marie–Tooth's disease [70], intrathoracic malignancies [92], and as a part of a paraneoplastic syndrome [93]. Bilateral diaphragmatic paralysis can also be idiopathic [94]. The characteristic clinical findings of bilateral diaphragmatic paralysis are severe orthopnea and marked abdominal paradoxic muscle movement in the supine position [69,89,91,95]. Fluoroscopy during a sniff test is more helpful in identifying unilateral than bilateral diaphragm paralysis, because upward motion of the ribs during inspiration when there is bilateral paralysis can make the diaphragm appear to descend. The diagnosis of diaphragmatic paralysis is usually confirmed by transdiaphragmatic pressure measurements that reveal a minimal or an absent P_{di} gradient [91]. Electromyography of the diaphragm and phrenic nerve conduction velocity studies may also be helpful.

TABLE 165.2

Respiratory Failure Caused by Peripheral Nervous System Dysfunction

Causes [References]	Salient features	Diagnostic tests	Supportive
Spinal cord disease [5,25,44,47–50]	Above C5, diaphragm, intercostal and abdominal activity abolished	Spinal X-ray film, CT, MRI	Supportive, vital capacity tends to improve more than 3 mo in traumatic lesions C5 and below
Traumatic	Below C5, diaphragm preserved, intercostal and abdominal activity abolished		Phrenic nerve pacing for high cervical cord lesions with intact phrenic nerve
Neoplasm	Below T5, abdominal activity diminished, impaired force expiration		
Hemorrhage			
Syrinx			
Infarct			
Transverse myelitis			
Tetanus [51]	Intense muscle spasms Trismus Apnea Metabolic acidosis History of penetrating wound	Clinical setting Gram's stain, anaerobic culture of wound History of inadequate immunization	Human antitetanus antiglobulin Wound debridement Penicillin, high dose Tetanus toxoid vaccination to prevent recurrence
Strychnine [52]	Intense muscle spasms Apnea Metabolic acidosis	Toxicology screen Clinical picture	Supportive Gastric lavage, charcoal
Anterior horn cell disease Amyotrophic lateral sclerosis [5,45,46,53,54]	Segmental muscle atrophy Hyperreflexia Fasciculations Distal extremity weakness	EMG	Supportive
Poliomyelitis [55,57]			
Polyneuropathy [25]	Viral illness, symmetric ascending distal muscle weakness	Elevated CSF protein without pleocytosis	Prevention with vaccine
Guillain–Barré's syndrome [25,58–60]	Ascending paralysis Areflexia Autonomic dysfunction	Demyelination by electrophysiology tests	See Chapter 152
Dinoflagellate poisoning	Paresthesias of face, progressive muscle weakness starting 30 min after ingestion of shellfish	History of contaminated shellfish ingestion	Supportive
Shellfish poisoning (red tide) [61–63]			
Ciguatera poisoning [64–66]	Gastrointestinal symptoms Paresthesias, abnormal temperature differentiation	Mouse bioassay, monoclonal antibody to ciguatoxin	Early gastric lavage, mannitol, avoid caffeine
Bilateral phrenic nerve palsy [67,69]	Severe orthopnea Abdominal paradoxic respiration	Fluoroscopy of diaphragm Surface EMG of diaphragm, transdiaphragmatic pressure	Diaphragmatic pacing
Charcot–Marie–Tooth's disease [70]	Peripheral muscle weakness and wasting, hereditary pes cavus, hammertoes	EMG	Supportive
Diphtheria [25]	Numbness of lips, paralysis of pharyngeal and laryngeal muscles	Throat culture	Diphtheria antitoxin Penicillin G or Erythromycin
Tick paralysis [25]	Tick exposure Age <10 y	Find tick Normal sensation	Remove tick
Acute intermittent porphyria [25]	Acute polyneuropathy-like Guillain–Barré's syndrome Mental disturbance Abdominal pain	Urine for porphobilinogen, δ-aminolevulinic acid	Hemin chloride, cimetidine Avoid exacerbating drugs such as phenytoin, barbiturates, ethosuximide
Myasthenia gravis (autoimmune and drug-induced) [25,71–76]	Muscle weakness Rapid fatigability Antecedent surgery, glucocorticoid, or aminoglycoside	EMG Tensilon test Antibodies to acetylcholine receptors	Anticholinesterase/calcium gluconate/thymectomy/glucocorticoids/immunosuppressants See Chapter 153 Plasmapheresis

TABLE 165.2

Respiratory Failure Caused by Peripheral Nervous System Dysfunction (*continued*)

Causes [References]	Salient features	Diagnostic tests	Supportive
Eaton–Lambert's syndrome [56,77]	Muscle wasting, hyporeflexia Associated cancer (e.g., small cell of lung)	Incremental pattern on EMG chest film	Treatment of associated cancer 3,4-diaminopyridine Anticholinesterase
Critical illness polyneuropathy [78–81]	Sepsis, multiorgan failure, generalized weakness, areflexia	Normal CSF, axonal degeneration by NCS	Supportive
Persistent drug-induced neuromuscular blockade [78,82,83]	Renal insufficiency Glucocorticoids	Creatinine phosphokinase, EMG, NCS, repetitive nerve stimulation	Limit use of neuromuscular blocking agents
Pseudocholinesterase deficiency [25]	Prolonged paralysis after succinylcholine Family history	Serum pseudocholinesterase EMG	Avoid succinylcholine
Botulism [85,86]	Wound infection, fever Ingestion of contaminate food: nausea and vomiting	Gram's stain and culture of stool, wound, or suspected food Demonstrate toxin in stool, serum, or food by mouse neutralization test	Trivalent antitoxin Wound debridement, penicillin G (or metronidazole if penicillin allergy) Nasogastric lavage
Organophosphates [87,88]	Dysphagia, diplopia, ptosis, dysarthria Use of insecticides Cholinergic toxicity (vomiting, diarrhea, weakness, cramps, sweating, ataxia, mental status changes)	History of exposure RBC acetyl cholinesterase level Atropine 1 mg challenge	Atropine Pralidoxime Benzodiazepine Cutaneous decontamination
Neuralgic amyotrophy [68]	Shoulder and neck pain, upper extremity weakness, breathlessness, orthopnea	Fluoroscopy of diaphragm, chest film, EMG	Analgesics, possible glucocorticoids

CSF, cerebrospinal fluid; CT, computed tomography; EMG, electromyogram; MRI, magnetic resonance imaging; NCS, nerve conduction study; RBC, red blood cell.

Several other causes of peripheral neuropathy can involve the efferent pathways to the respiratory muscles, including diphtheria, herpes zoster infection, tick paralysis, acute intermittent porphyria, beriberi, and a variety of metabolic disorders [25]. Respiratory failure associated with diphtheria is of delayed onset, usually occurring 4 to 6 weeks after the onset of illness [25]. Tick paralysis is seen mainly in children in whom the presence of the tick goes unnoticed for 5 to 6 days [25]. In acute intermittent porphyria, respiratory involvement may be a slowly progressive process or may cause an abrupt deterioration in respiratory function as a result of bilateral phrenic nerve paralysis [37]. Myasthenia gravis [19], botulism [84–86], organophosphate poisoning [25], and a variety of drugs can produce neuromuscular blockade that results in respiratory failure [76]. Although patients with myasthenia gravis typically show signs of obvious muscle weakness and rapid fatigability, particularly of the cranial muscles, before the development of respiratory failure, acute respiratory failure is occasionally a presenting manifestation [19,25,72]. More commonly, respiratory failure complicates myasthenia gravis after surgical procedures, following the institution of glucocorticoid therapy, or as a result of under- or overtreatment with anticholinesterase medications [19].

Although the diagnosis of myasthenia gravis is suspected on clinical grounds and a positive response to edrophonium chloride (Tensilon) is supportive, the diagnosis is confirmed by a typical EMG (decremental responses on repetitive nerve stimulation) and an elevated serum level of antibodies to acetylcholine receptors [19,71] (see Chapter 153). Part of the management of a patient with myasthenia gravis includes serial measurement of the maximum inspiratory pressure and vital capacity to assess the risk for respiratory failure [25]. A decrease in vital capacity to less than 20 mL per kg, in maximum inspiratory pressure to less negative than −30 cm H_2O, or in maximum expiratory pressure to less than 40 cm H_2O is a warning sign of impending respiratory failure [19].

Eaton–Lambert's syndrome, a form of neuromuscular blockade similar to myasthenia gravis, occurs in association with certain carcinomas, particularly small cell carcinoma of the lung [55,56]. The neuromuscular blockade in most cases precedes other evidence of the carcinoma, and the EMG shows an incremental pattern unlike that in true myasthenia.

Critical illness polyneuropathy occurs in the setting of sepsis and multiorgan failure in up to 30% of patients by clinical examination and up to 70% by electrophysiologic testing [78,81]. Profound generalized muscle weakness as a result of critical illness polyneuropathy is a major reason why these patients often require prolonged mechanical ventilatory support. Similar to patients with Guillain–Barré's Syndrome, patients with critical illness polyneuropathy also have areflexia, but in contrast, they may also have prominent sensory nerve deficits and a normal cerebrospinal fluid examination. Electrophysiologic testing helps to distinguish critical illness polyneuropathy from Guillain–Barré's syndrome; in critical illness, polyneuropathy nerve conduction studies show axon degeneration rather than demyelination. Although the etiology of critical illness polyneuropathy is not known, it is predominantly a disease of older patients who stay in the intensive care unit for more than 28 days and who have elevated serum glucose and decreased albumin levels at the time of diagnosis. Approximately half of patients with sepsis, multiorgan system failure, and critical illness polyneuropathy survive, and the prognosis of survivors for significant improvement from the neuropathy is good [79] (for additional details, see Chapter 154).

Prolonged administration (longer than 2 days) of neuromuscular blocking agents (NMBAs), such as pancuronium and vecuronium, has been associated with two distinct patterns of neuromuscular dysfunction [82]: (a) persistent neuromuscular junction blockade in patients with renal insufficiency who accumulate the parent drug and its active metabolites and (b) an acute noninflammatory myopathy that becomes apparent as neuromuscular transmission improves. The myopathy appears to be a consequence of an interaction between NMBAs and glucocorticoids and seems to be related to the total dose and duration of action of the NMBA [83]. This has been particularly dramatic in previously healthy asthmatic patients, approximately 15% of whom develop muscle weakness after short-term use of an NMBA and high-dose glucocorticoids [82]. In a systematic review of trials of cisatracurium administered by infusion for 48 hours to patients with acute respiratory distress syndrome (ARDS) (431 patients of which 190 received glucocorticoids), no increased risk of critical illness-acquired weakness was noted in the cisatracurium groups [83]. In general, it appears that NMBA given for short periods appear safe for patients with ARDS; further testing is needed in additional populations, particularly those receiving higher doses of systemic glucocorticoids.

Neuromuscular blockade may also occur as a result of administration of a variety of other drugs [76]. Certain cardiovascular drugs (e.g., lidocaine, quinidine, procainamide, and propranolol), anticonvulsants (e.g., phenytoin and trimethadione), D-penicillamine, and a number of antibiotics (most notably the aminoglycosides) can prolong postoperative respiratory depression, unmask underlying myasthenia gravis, or cause a drug-induced form of myasthenia gravis [76]. The definitive diagnosis of drug-induced neuromuscular blockade is usually made in retrospect if the abnormality reverses after elimination of the offending agent. In some cases, the administration of calcium gluconate has been reported to result in prompt improvement in neuromuscular transmission [76].

Prolonged neuromuscular blockade is occasionally seen after the administration of succinylcholine in individuals with pseudocholinesterase deficiency [25]. In contrast to the usual duration of paralysis of approximately 3 minutes, the effect in these individuals usually lasts 4 to 6 hours, during which time they require mechanical ventilatory support [25].

In botulism, neuromuscular blockade develops as a result of a neurotoxin produced by the bacteria *Clostridium botulinum*. Most cases are caused by neurotoxin-contaminated food [84–86], but, occasionally, botulism develops as a result of a wound infected with *C. botulinum* [51] (see Chapter 86). Certain findings help to predict whether respiratory failure requiring mechanical ventilation will develop. A vital capacity of 30% or less of the predicted value is generally associated with hypercapnic failure [50]. Other clues are the presence of nausea, vomiting, diarrhea, dyspnea, ptosis, or extremity weakness on initial examination.

Organophosphates, commonly used in insecticides, inhibit the enzyme cholinesterase, resulting in accumulation of acetylcholine at neurosynaptic junctions. The symptoms of organophosphate poisoning are those of cholinergic toxicity, including blurred vision, weakness, vomiting, diarrhea, cramps, sweating, increased secretions, incoordination, twitching, ataxia, mental status changes, and, if severe enough, respiratory failure and death [87,88]. Respiratory muscle paralysis combines with respiratory center depression, excessive secretions, and, possibly, bronchoconstriction to cause respiratory failure [87,88] (see Chapter 120). Neuralgic amyotrophy, a disorder of the peripheral nervous system affecting the brachial plexus, is associated with diaphragmatic dysfunction and dyspnea [68]. It usually presents with acute severe shoulder pain that may extend to the neck, back, and arm. Motor weakness of the ipsilateral shoulder and arm usually develops within 1 month of the onset of pain. A sensory defect may be present in one-fourth of patients. In one study [68], 12 of 16 patients had bilateral diaphragm paralysis, and 4 of 16 had unilateral diaphragm paralysis. Mild nocturnal desaturation, hypopneas, and obstructive sleep apneas (OSAs) were found in some patients, but alveolar hypoventilation was not found.

Respiratory Muscle Dysfunction

A number of systemic myopathies feature prominent respiratory muscle involvement, including the muscular dystrophies, myotonic disorders, inflammatory myopathies, periodic paralyses, metabolic storage diseases, endocrine myopathies, infectious myopathies, toxic myopathies, rhabdomyolysis, and electrolyte disturbances (Table 165.3) [16,25,82,83,96–126].

Generally, the clinical presentation is widespread skeletal muscle weakness. Muscle weakness is the inability of a muscle to generate the normal expected level of force and should be distinguished from muscle fatigue, which is the inability to generate the preexistent maximum force prior to putting the muscle under load or stress. Fatigue is reversible with rest; weakness may be reversible with reconditioning or the reversal or elimination of the causative factor (e.g., malnutrition, disuse atrophy). Respiratory muscle involvement and respiratory failure usually develop as the disease progresses. On occasion, however, respiratory failure may be the presenting manifestation of a generalized myopathy [97].

Myopathy-induced hypercapnic respiratory failure is almost invariably accompanied by a severely impaired cough mechanism and an inability to clear respiratory tract secretions [5]. Typical pulmonary function findings of respiratory muscle weakness are a decrease in maximum inspiratory and expiratory pressures and, as the disease progresses, a decrease in lung volumes [127].

The muscular dystrophies are inherited disorders that present with evidence of progressive proximal muscle weakness and atrophy [25,101]. Duchenne and Becker muscular dystrophies are caused by mutations in the dystrophin gene, located on the X chromosome [102]. Duchenne dystrophy usually presents at approximately 2 to 3 years of age and Becker dystrophy at approximately 15 to 20 years of age. The limb-girdle muscular dystrophies are a more heterogeneous group of disorders that show both autosomal recessive and autosomal dominant inheritance and include mutations in different members of the sarcoglycan complex, including motilin, dysferlin, caveolin, and sarcoglycan. Myofibrillar myopathy is also associated with mutations in the motilin gene, and both of these may eventuate in respiratory failure [103]. The limb-girdle muscular dystrophies frequently present later in adulthood than do the dystrophin-related muscular dystrophies [104]. The myotonic dystrophies are autosomal dominant disorders linked to two chromosome loci: 19q13, where a CTG repeat has been found in the intron of a serine threonine protein kinase gene, and 3q21, where a CCTG repeat has been found in the intron of zinc finger protein 9 [106,107]. The most prominent clinical features are myotonia (i.e., sustained contraction of muscles in response to direct stimulation), ptosis, prominent distal and facial muscle weakness, and atrophy [25,106,108].

The periodic paralyses are genetic disorders characterized by attacks of muscle weakness in response to a variety of precipitating factors such as exercise, emotional upset, exposure to cold, and, in some cases, exposure to alcohol [25]. Patients may exhibit hypokalemia, hyperkalemia, or normokalemia. In some patients, the disease is unmasked when they become hyperthyroid.

Glycogen storage diseases result from defects in muscle glycogenolysis or glycogen storage. Examples include α-glucosidase deficiency (also called acid maltase deficiency or glycogen

TABLE 165.3

Respiratory Failure Caused by Respiratory Muscle Dysfunction

Causes [References]	Salient features	Diagnostic tests	Specific treatment
Muscle dystrophies [101–105]	Proximal muscle weakness and atrophy Hereditary	Muscle biopsy Elevated CPK Genetic analysis	Supportive Duchenne: prednisone
Myotonic dystrophies [106–109]	Myotonia, ptosis Distal and facial muscle weakness and atrophy Hereditary	Muscle biopsy EMG genetic analysis	Supportive Possibly mexiletine and acetazolamide
Periodic paralyses [25,109,110]	Hypokalemic, hyperkalemic, or normokalemic Genetic Muscle weakness associated with exercise, emotional upset, cold, alcohol	Serum potassium Family history	Avoid precipitating factors Carbonic anhydrase inhibitor
Glycogen storage diseases [25,97,97,111] (Pompe and McArdle's diseases)	Exercise-related muscle cramping; slowly progressive muscle weakness and atrophy	CPK, muscle biopsy with assay for acid maltase, muscle phosphorylase levels	Supportive
Dermatomyositis/polymyositis [16,112–114]	Proximal muscle weakness Rash in dermatomyositis Difficulty swallowing	Elevated CPK, aldolase EMG Muscle biopsy	Glucocorticoids Immunosuppressants
Hyperthyroidism [115]	Thyrotoxicosis heat intolerance, tachycardia, hyperreflexia	TSH, TFTs	Propylthiouracil, methimazole See Chapter 141
Hypothyroidism [25]	Myxedema, cold intolerance Hyporeflexia, bradycardia	TSH, TFTs	Replace thyroid hormone See Chapter 142
Hyperadrenocorticalism [25,116]	Cushingoid appearance	Serum cortisol Dexamethasone suppression test, adrenal CT scan	Depends on cause
Rhabdomyolysis secondary to colchicine [117] or chloroquine toxicity [25]	Muscle pain, swelling, myoglobulinuria	↑ CPK	Supportive
Infectious myositis trichinosis [25,118] or viral [25]	Muscle tenderness, weakness, fever	Serology Muscle biopsy	Rest Glucocorticoids, thiabendazole or mebendazole
Hypophosphatemia [99,100,119,120]	Weakness Difficulty weaning	↓ Phosphate	Replete See Chapter 140
Hypermagnesemia or hypomagnesemia [100,121,122]	Weakness Difficulty weaning	↑ or ↓ Mg^{++}	
Hypokalemia [100]	Weakness	↓ K^{+}	Replete
Hypercalcemia [100,122]	Lethargy, confusion	↑ Ca^{++}	See Chapters 95 and 140
Eosinophilia-myalgia [123–125]	L-tryptophan ingestion Muscle tenderness and weakness, fasciitis Fasciitis	Eosinophilia Muscle biopsy	Discontinue L-tryptophan Supportive
Procainamide-induced myopathy [126]	Weakness Respiratory failure	Muscle biopsy, ↑ CPK	Discontinue procainamide
Acute myopathy secondary to neuromuscular blocking agents [82,83]	Neuromuscular blocking agents Glucocorticoids Rapid onset weakness	EMG Muscle biopsy	Supportive

↓, decreased; ↑, increased; CPK, creatinine phosphokinase; CT, computed tomography; EMG, electromyography; TFT, thyroid function test; TSH, thyroid-stimulating hormone.

storage disease type II) and muscle phosphorylase deficiency (also called McArdle's disease or glycogen storage disease type V). Patients exhibit exercise-induced muscle cramping and slowly progressive muscle weakness, with or without atrophy [25,97,98,111]. On occasion, respiratory failure may be the presenting manifestation [97,111]. The diagnosis is confirmed by muscle biopsy and chemical assay for muscle α-glucosidase or phosphorylase level [97,98].

Polymyositis and dermatomyositis are collagen vascular diseases that cause skeletal muscle inflammation. Proximal muscle weakness is prominent and usually develops over a period of weeks to months. Patients may have difficulty swallowing secondary to pharyngeal muscle involvement. Serum muscle enzyme levels are elevated. Typical EMG and muscle biopsy findings confirm the diagnosis [112]. Respiratory muscle failure is an uncommon, but not rare complication of inflammatory myositis [16,112]. Patients with polymyositis may also develop interstitial lung disease, organizing pneumonia, and alveolar hemorrhage [113,114].

Procainamide has been reported to cause a necrotizing myopathy with diaphragm involvement and respiratory failure [126]. Although anti–double-stranded DNA and antihistone antibodies were positive, antinuclear antibodies were absent, and the muscle biopsy did not reveal an inflammatory infiltrate. Neuromuscular junction transmission was normal, suggesting that this was not a drug-induced myasthenic syndrome. Slow improvement in muscle strength followed discontinuation of procainamide in this study.

Increased Impedance to Bulk Flow

In a number of pulmonary disorders, the development of hypercapnic respiratory failure is the result of a marked increase in impedance to ventilation (e.g., increased airflow resistance in COPD or asthma or increased elastic recoil in interstitial fibrosis) that even normal respiratory muscle force generation cannot overcome [3]. It may be less widely appreciated that increases in extrapulmonary impedance to ventilation can also result in hypercapnic respiratory failure. These disorders can be divided into those involving a decrease in chest wall or pleural compliance (e.g., kyphoscoliosis or pleural fibrosis) and those involving an increase in airflow resistance, resulting from upper airway obstruction (e.g., tracheal stenosis or laryngeal edema) (Table 165.4) [5,42,43,128–189].

Chest Wall and Pleural Disorders

Kyphoscoliosis is a common cause of extrapulmonary respiratory failure [5]. The severity of the scoliosis (i.e., lateral curvature of the spine) is usually the more important factor in the development of respiratory failure than is the kyphosis (i.e., dorsal curvature of the spine) [5]. In idiopathic kyphoscoliosis, chronic hypercapnic respiratory failure generally occurs when the angle of curvature is 120 degrees or greater [5]. In contrast, in paralytic kyphoscoliosis (e.g., as a result of poliomyelitis), the angle of curvature does not reliably predict either vital capacity or hypercapnic respiratory failure [128]. This appears to be owing to a greater element of muscle weakness in paralytic kyphoscoliosis [128]. Even in idiopathic kyphoscoliosis, however, the presence of markedly decreased chest wall compliance is further complicated by inspiratory muscle weakness [129] that contributes to the development of hypercapnic respiratory failure [94]. In addition, a modest element of pulmonary gas exchange abnormality is usually present [5].

Patients with kyphoscoliosis usually report progressive dyspnea on exertion and exercise limitation for a period of years before actual arterial hypercapnia develops [5]. In patients with moderately advanced kyphoscoliosis, acute hypercapnic respiratory failure may result from acute reversible complications such as pulmonary congestion, retained secretions, or pulmonary infection [130].

Massive chest wall obesity may be associated with significant hypoventilation and the development of hypercapnic respiratory failure [133]. This is termed the *obesity-hypoventilation syndrome*. The pathogenesis of respiratory failure appear to be multifactorial and include significant reduction in chest wall compliance, decreased respiratory muscle efficiency, reduced or blunted respiratory center drive, and impaired pulmonary gas exchange as a result of pulmonary congestion [133–135].

Upper Airway Obstruction

A variety of causes of upper airway obstruction involving the extrathoracic upper airway or intrathoracic trachea can result in the development of respiratory failure (Table 165.4).

Significant upper airway obstruction should be considered in the patient who reports dyspnea in association with inspiratory stridor (extrathoracic obstruction) or expiratory wheezing (intrathoracic obstruction), particularly if other symptoms suggest an upper airway process (e.g., dysphagia or dysphonia). Unless the patient is acutely ill, the diagnosis is usually evaluated by obtaining a flow–volume loop [190]. This technique not only demonstrates the presence of an upper airway obstruction but usually also helps determine whether it is extrathoracic or intrathoracic and variable or fixed [190]. Studies such as soft tissue neck radiographs, laryngoscopy, and bronchoscopy can identify the exact nature of the structural abnormality.

Upper airway obstruction from bilateral vocal cord paresis or paralysis may result from a variety of causes. The most common cause is trauma, particularly related to thyroid surgery [161] and, occasionally, after endotracheal intubation [162]. Other causes include tumors [142,166–170], cricoarytenoid arthritis [160], herpes simplex viral infection [163], and neurologic conditions, including Guillain–Barré's syndrome [160], extrapyramidal disorders such as Parkinson's disease [164], and myasthenia gravis [159]. Bilateral vocal cord paralysis should be considered when one of these conditions is present and the patient reports aspiration, dyspnea, or stridor [161]. Hoarseness is usually absent during normal speech in bilateral adductor paralysis. The results of flow–volume loop analysis can help confirm the presence of the typical extrathoracic variable obstruction associated with bilateral vocal cord paralysis [165].

OSA is increasingly recognized as a cause of intermittent functional upper airway obstruction [3,175,176]. Although obesity is a significant risk factor, OSA can occur in its absence [175,176]. Episodic loss of pharyngeal muscle tone caused by decreased respiratory center motor output, usually during rapid eye movement sleep, results in intermittent airway obstruction [175,177]. This disturbance in respiratory center control also accounts for the mixed apneas (i.e., combination obstructive and central apneas) frequently seen in these patients [175,177].

Approximately 10% to 20% of patients with OSA have chronic alveolar hypoventilation with elevation in $PaCO_2$ even while awake. These patients frequently have concomitant COPD or morbid obesity. Hypoxemia, whether just at night or all day, eventually causes cardiac arrhythmias, pulmonary hypertension, and cor pulmonale [3,175,178,179].

The diagnosis of OSA can be established by a sleep study (polysomnography) [174,175]. Other conditions that can cause or exacerbate OSA should be excluded, including adenotonsillar hypertrophy [180]; deviated nasal septum [176]; retrognathia or micrognathia [3]; macroglossia from acromegaly [183]; endocrine and metabolic abnormalities such as hypothyroidism [67,184,185]; CNS depression from ethanol, barbiturates, and benzodiazepines [175,186]; and exogenous androgen administration [187,188] (see Chapter 183).

DIFFERENTIAL DIAGNOSIS

The major differential diagnosis of extrapulmonary respiratory failure is hypercapnic respiratory failure from intrinsic lung diseases (e.g., COPD) (Fig. 165.1). These conditions, usually, can be readily distinguished because they are almost always associated with a markedly elevated $P(A–a)O_2$ gradient when calculated on room air, thus reflecting a severe derangement of distal gas exchange. Hypercapnic respiratory failure may also result from a combination of pulmonary and extrapulmonary abnormalities. This combined diagnosis is suggested by a P(A–a)

TABLE 165.4

Respiratory Failure Caused by Chest Wall, Plueral, and Upper Airway Diseases

Causes [Reference]	Salient features	Diagnostic tests	Specific treatment
Chest wall and pleural disorders			
Kyphoscoliosis [5,128–132]	Spinal curvature ≥120 degrees Progressive dyspnea on exertion over several years	Spinal X-ray films Restriction on PFTs	Nighttime ventilator support
Obesity-hypoventilation [133–135]	Massive chest wall obesity ± sleep apnea	Polysomnography ↓ CO_2 response curve ↓ Chest wall compliance	Weight loss Nasal CPAP or BPAP
Flail chest [136]	Multiple rib fractures, paradoxic respiration ± pleuritic chest pain	Chest film	Mechanical positive-pressure ventilation
Fibrothorax [5,137–139]	Asbestos exposure, pleural infection, pleural hemorrhage, uremia, collagen vascular disease	Observation of chest wall Restriction on PFTs Decreased maximum static elastic recoil pressure	Decortication
Thoracoplasty [5]	Chest wall deformity secondary to resection of ribs	Restriction on PFTs Chest film	Supportive
Ankylosing spondylitis [5]	Limited chest expansion Apical pulmonary fibrosis Limited lumbar mobility Chronic lower back pain	PFTs (↑ functional residual capacity, ↓ total lung capacity) HLA-B27 Spine and sacroiliac X-ray films	Anti-inflammatory agents Flexibility exercises
Upper airway obstruction			
Acute epiglottis [140–143]	Fever, sore throat, stridor, dysphagia	Soft tissue films of neck	See Chapter 180
Acute laryngeal edema			
Angioedema/anaphylaxis [142,144–148]	Stridor in setting of *Hymenoptera* sting, contrast media, or drug administration	Other evidence of angioedema/anaphylaxis; complement levels	Epinephrine parenterally Cricothyroidotomy
Traumatic [149,150]	Stridor after endotracheal extubation	History	Inhaled racemic epinephrine Reintubation Helium–oxygen mixture
Foreign body aspiration [151–156]	Unable to speak Stridor or apnea	X-ray film helpful when foreign body below cords	Heimlich maneuver Bronchoscopy Cricothyroidotomy
Retropharyngeal hemorrhage [157]	Associated with anticoagulation or head and neck surgery Sore throat	Soft tissue film of neck CT scan or tomography	Reverse anticoagulation
Bilateral vocal cord paralysis [158–165]	Stridor Aspiration	Flow–volume loop Laryngoscopy	See text
Laryngeal and tracheal tumors [142,166–170]	Dyspnea Hoarseness; dysphonia Stridor	Flow–volume loop Tomography Laryngotracheoscopy	Laser or surgical resection, radiation
Tracheal stenosis [150,162,171–173]	Progressive dyspnea History of endotracheal intubation	Flow–volume loop Tomography	Tracheostomy Stent, resection of stenosis
Tracheomalacia [171,172]		Laryngotracheoscopy	Stent
Idiopathic obstructive sleep apnea [42,43,174–188,132]	Snoring Daytime hypersomnolence Pulmonary hypertension Cor pulmonale	Polysomnography	Nasal CPAP, bilevel CPAP Protriptyline Uvulopalatopharyngoplasty Tracheostomy Nocturnal oxygen Weight loss
Adenotonsillar hypertrophy [180]	Daytime hypersomnolence Obstructive sleep apnea stridor	Direct visualization Lateral X-ray film	Resection
Obstructive goiter [189]	Enlarged thyroid	Tomography CT scan	Suppression with exogenous thyroid hormone Resection

↓, decreased; ↑, increased; CPAP, continuous positive airway pressure; CT, computed tomography; PFT, pulmonary function test.

O_2 gradient in the range of 25 to 30 mm Hg. If the extrapulmonary abnormality is predominant, the gradient, although abnormal, is generally less than 25 mm Hg [5]. When primary pulmonary disease is severe enough to cause hypercapnia, the gradient is generally above 30 mm Hg.

TREATMENT

The treatment of extrapulmonary respiratory failure can be divided into specific and supportive therapy. Supportive therapy involves the use of noninvasive or invasive mechanical ventilatory assistance (see Chapters 166 and 167), supplemental oxygen, and techniques of airway hygiene (see Chapter 169). In addition, regardless of the primary cause of respiratory muscle weakness, malnutrition exacerbates it and nutritional replacement can increase respiratory muscle strength and function [191,192]. In selected circumstances, inspiratory resistive training of the respiratory muscles and the use of theophylline as a positive respiratory muscle inotrope have been reported to improve respiratory muscle function and associated hypercapnic respiratory failure [193–196]. Only specific forms of therapy are discussed here and in Tables 165.1 through 165.4.

Central Nervous System Depression

A description of specific treatment modalities for CNS depression is given in Table 165.1.

Peripheral Nervous System Dysfunction

Treatment for peripheral nervous system disorders is outlined in Table 165.2. In general, there is little in the way of specific therapy for established spinal cord or anterior horn cell disease. The use of phrenic nerve pacemakers for high-level cervical cord transection may help treat the resultant respiratory failure when nerve conduction studies have determined that the phrenic nerves are intact and functioning [48–50,91]. If pacing brings on OSA, noninvasive positive airway pressure or tracheostomy may be necessary.

The availability and value of specific therapy for peripheral neuropathy depend on the cause. In the case of acute Guillain–Barré's syndrome, plasma exchange or intravenous infusion of pooled γ-globulin may be helpful when administered promptly for patients who reach or appear to be approaching the inability to walk without help or who have substantial decrease in ventilatory capacity or bulbar insufficiency (for more details on treating Guillain–Barré's syndrome, see Chapter 152).

Patients with severe respiratory muscle weakness because of Guillain–Barré's syndrome require supportive mechanical ventilatory assistance, usually for weeks to months [59]. If cranial nerve involvement is prominent and the patient is unable to swallow or clear oral secretions, intubation for airway protection should be considered, even in the absence of overt respiratory failure. Management is often complicated by autonomic nervous system dysfunction, which is a leading cause of death in this syndrome [90]. Characteristic abnormalities of increased or decreased sympathetic and parasympathetic nervous systems activity include hypertension, hypotension, bradyarrhythmias, tachyarrhythmias, flushing, diaphoresis, and ileus [90]. Because these events are often transient, minor fluctuations in heart rate or blood pressure should not be treated. When intervention is deemed necessary, short-acting and easily titratable drugs should be used [90]. Because patients are at increased risk for deep venous thrombosis and pulmonary embolism, prophylactic anticoagulation should be administered, according to guidelines for critically ill patients (for more details on anticoagulation in critically ill patients, see Chapter 93). Treatment of respiratory failure caused by myasthenia gravis is directed primarily at the myasthenia (see Chapter 153).

Drug-induced neuromuscular blockade often improves simply by discontinuing the offending agent [57]. Intravenous calcium gluconate may help to shorten the recovery time by reversing the presynaptic component of the neuromuscular blockade [76]. If this fails and the patient improves after an edrophonium chloride test, neostigmine bromide may be effective by reversing the postsynaptic component [52]. When myasthenia gravis is exacerbated or made manifest by a drug, therapy directed specifically at the myasthenic symptoms may be required [76].

Treatment of botulism is directed at minimizing further binding of toxin to nerve endings while supporting the patient until bound toxin dissipates [85] (see Chapter 86). Recovery of ventilatory and upper airway muscle strength in type A botulism occurs slowly; patients recover most of their strength in the first 12 weeks, but full recovery may take up to a year [86].

Respiratory Muscle Dysfunction

The treatment of myopathy depends on the cause (Table 165.3). Although the mechanism is not known, glucocorticoid therapy has resulted in some improvement in muscle strength in Duchenne muscular dystrophy, but adverse effects need to be monitored closely [102,105]. Mexiletine may be helpful in myotonic dystrophy, but is contraindicated in patients with heart block; other antiarrhythmic and anticonvulsive agents may also be of benefit [109]. These agents as well as sodium channel blockers can also worsen weakness while relieving myotonia.

Some patients with each of the different subtypes of periodic paralysis have responded well to acetazolamide, a carbonic anhydrase inhibitor that is kaliuretic [110]. Acetazolamide is often dramatically effective in preventing acute attacks of hypokalemic periodic paralysis, perhaps by causing a metabolic acidosis that, in turn, protects against the sudden decreases in potassium that provoke attacks. Certain patients benefit from low-carbohydrate or low-sodium diets in addition to acetazolamide. Inhalation of the β-adrenergic agonist albuterol alleviates acute attacks of weakness in some patients with hyperkalemic periodic paralysis [110].

Polymyositis-induced muscle weakness often responds to glucocorticoids or other immunosuppressants [112,114]. Muscle weakness from hypothyroidism, hypophosphatemia, hypomagnesemia, or hypokalemia responds to replacement therapy [25,115,116,119,121,122].

The specific treatment of trichinosis is less than satisfactory [118]. For patients with severe infection, albendazole or mebendazole together with systemic glucocorticoids may shorten the duration of myositis and muscle pain [118]. Albendazole is preferred over mebendazole owing to more consistent blood levels. The other mainstays of treatment are bed rest and anti-inflammatory analgesic agents.

Chest Wall and Pleural Disorders

Treatment for chest wall and pleural disorders is largely supportive (Table 165.4). If acute respiratory failure develops in kyphoscoliosis, reversible factors such as pulmonary congestion, infection, retained secretions, and other intercurrent illnesses should be sought and treated [130]. Episodes of acute respiratory failure in patients with kyphoscoliosis can often be managed with noninvasive positive-pressure ventilation (for details of noninvasive ventilation for acute respiratory failure, see Chapter 167).

When severe kyphoscoliosis is associated with significant chronic hypercapnic respiratory failure, nocturnal noninvasive positive-pressure ventilation often results in marked improvement in daytime function and gas exchange [131,197].

TABLE 165.5

Advances in the Treatment of Extrapulmonary Respiratory Failure

Disease	Treatment
Duchenne muscular dystrophy	Glucocorticoids improve pulmonary function and slow disease progression [105].
Guillain–Barré's syndrome	Both plasmapheresis and IVIG are effective when started within 4 wk of onset of symptoms [60].
Myasthenia gravis	Plasmapheresis is effective in short-term management of myasthenic crisis [74].
Trichinosis	Thiabendazole and mebendazole are effective in reducing muscle weakness in trichinosis [118].
Obstructive sleep apnea	Nasal continuous positive airway pressure is effective in the treatment of obstructive sleep apnea [200].

IVIG, intravenous immunoglobulin.

Upper Airway Obstruction

The first step in treating acute upper airway obstruction is to establish an adequate airway. Specific definitive therapy can then be used. In acute bacterial epiglottitis associated with significant respiratory distress, immediate steps are mandatory to prevent development of total obstruction [140]. Chapters 8, 9, 169, and 180 provide a complete discussion of this and other treatment issues.

Treatment of OSA is indicated when significant sleep-related apneas or hypopneas are noted in the setting of signs and symptoms such as morning headaches, daytime functional impairment, peripheral edema, cor pulmonale, and elevated hematocrit. In general, nasal continuous or bilevel positive-pressure devices (continuous positive airway pressure or bilevel continuous positive airway pressure) are effective [198–200] (see Chapters 169 and 183). In OSA complicated by life-threatening arrhythmias, severe arterial hypoxemia, or severe functional impairment [3,176], tracheostomy may rarely be necessary [3,42,176]. Other treatment modalities for OSA include weight loss [201], avoidance of alcohol and sedative drugs [175,186], mandibular and tongue repositioning appliances [202], and upper airway surgery other than tracheostomy (uvulopalatopharyngoplasty, tonsillectomy, adenoidectomy, and deviated septum repair), as appropriate [180,203]. When an identifiable cause of OSA is present (e.g., hypothyroidism), correction of the problem may be curative [184,185].

A summary of advances in the treatment of extrapulmonary respiratory failure is presented in Table 165.5.

References

1. Williams MH Jr, Shim CS: Ventilatory failure. *Am J Med* 48:477, 1970.
2. Pontoppidan H, Geffin B, Lowenstein E: Acute respiratory failure in the adult. *N Engl J Med* 287:690, 1972.
3. Pratter MR, Irwin RS: Extrapulmonary causes of respiratory failure. *J Intensive Care Med* 1:197, 1986.
4. Demers RR, Irwin RS: Management of hypercapnic respiratory failure: a systematic approach. *Respir Care* 24:328, 1979.
5. Bergofsky EH: Respiratory failure in disorders of the thoracic cage. *Am Rev Respir Dis* 119:643, 1979.
6. Aubier M, Murciano D, Fournier M, et al: Central respiratory drive in acute respiratory failure of patients with chronic obstructive pulmonary disease. *Am Rev Respir Dis* 122:191, 1980.
7. Bone RC, Pierce AK, Johnson RL Jr: Controlled oxygen administration in acute respiratory failure in chronic obstructive pulmonary disease. *Am J Med* 65:896, 1978.
8. Degaute JP, Domenighetti G, Naeije R, et al: Oxygen delivery in acute exacerbation of chronic obstructive pulmonary disease. *Am Rev Respir Dis* 124:26, 1981.
9. Weitzenblum E, Sautegeau A, Ehrhart M, et al: Long-term oxygen therapy can reverse the progression of pulmonary hypertension in patients with chronic obstructive pulmonary disease. *Am Rev Respir Dis* 131:493, 1985.
10. Marthan R, Castaing Y, Manier G, et al: Gas exchange alterations in patients with chronic obstructive lung disease. *Chest* 87:470, 1985.
11. Lejeune P, Mols P, Naeije R, et al: Acute hemodynamic effects of controlled oxygen therapy in decompensated chronic obstructive pulmonary disease. *Crit Care Med* 12:1032, 1984.
12. Gray BA, Blalock JM: Interpretation of the alveolar–arterial oxygen difference in patients with hypercapnia. *Am Rev Respir Dis* 143:4, 1991.
13. Braun NMT, Rochester DF: Respiratory muscle strength in obstructive lung disease. *Am Rev Respir Dis* 115:91, 1977.
14. Celli BR, Rassulo J, Berman JS, et al: Respiratory consequences of abdominal hernia in a patient with severe chronic obstructive pulmonary disease. *Am Rev Respir Dis* 131:178, 1985.
15. O'Donohue WJ Jr, Baker JP, Bell GM, et al: Respiratory failure in neuromuscular disease: management in a respiratory intensive care unit. *JAMA* 235:733, 1976.
16. Braun NMT, Arora NS, Rochester DF: Respiratory muscle and pulmonary function in polymyositis and other proximal myopathies. *Thorax* 38:616, 1983.
17. Smyth RJ, Chapman KR, Rebuck AS: Maximal inspiratory and expiratory pressures in adolescents: normal values. *Chest* 86:568, 1984.
18. Black LF, Hyatt RE: Maximal respiratory pressures: normal values and relationship to age and sex. *Am Rev Respir Dis* 99:696, 1969.
19. Chaudhuri A, Behan PO: Myasthenic crisis. *QJM* 102:97–107, 2009.
20. Roussos CS, Macklem PT: Diaphragmatic fatigue in man. *J Appl Physiol* 43:189, 1977.
21. Gross D, Grassino A, Ross WR, et al: Electromyogram pattern of diaphragmatic fatigue. *J Appl Physiol* 46:1, 1979.
22. Cohen CA, Zabelbaum G, Gross D, et al: Clinical manifestations of inspiratory muscle fatigue. *Am J Med* 73:308, 1982.
23. Mitchell RA, Berger AJ: Neural regulation of respiration. *Am Rev Respir Dis* 111:206, 1975.
24. Berger AJ, Mitchell RA, Severinghaus JW: Regulation of respiration. *N Engl J Med* 297:138, 1977.
25. Benditt JO, Boitano LJ: Pulmonary issues in patients with chronic neuromuscular disease. *Am J Respir Crit Care Med* 187:1046–1055, 2013.
26. Weil JV, McCullough RE, Kline JS, et al: Diminished ventilatory response to hypoxia and hypercapnia after morphine in normal man. *N Engl J Med* 292:1103, 1975.
27. Santiago TV, Pugliese AC, Edelman NH: Control of breathing during methadone addiction. *Am J Med* 62:347, 1977.
28. Skatrud J, Iber C, Ewart R, et al: Disordered breathing during sleep in hypothyroidism. *Am Rev Respir Dis* 124:325, 1981.
29. Doekel RC Jr, Zwillich CW, Scoggin CH, et al: Clinical semi-starvation depression of hypoxic ventilatory response. *N Engl J Med* 295:358, 1976.
30. Tuller MA, Mehdi F: Compensatory hypoventilation and hypercapnia in primary metabolic alkalosis. *Am J Med* 50:281, 1971.
31. Onders RP, Dimarco AF, Ignagni AR, et al: Mapping the phrenic nerve motor point: the key to a successful laparoscopic diaphragm pacing system in the first human series. *Surgery* 136:819, 2004.
32. Phillipson EA: Control of breathing during sleep. *Am Rev Respir Dis* 118:909, 1978.
33. Strohl KP, Hensley MJ, Saunders NA, et al: Progesterone administration and progressive sleep apneas. *JAMA* 245:1230, 1981.
34. Comroe JH Jr: Frankenstein, Pickwick and Ondine. *Am Rev Respir Dis* 111:689, 1975.
35. Hunt CE, Matalon SV, Thompson TR, et al: Central hypoventilation syndrome: experience with bilateral phrenic nerve pacing in 3 neonates. *Am Rev Respir Dis* 118:23, 1978.
36. Wolkove N, Altose MD, Kelsen SG, et al: Respiratory control abnormalities in alveolar hypoventilation. *Am Rev Respir Dis* 122:163, 1980.
37. Sugar O: In search of Ondine's curse. *JAMA* 240:236, 1978.
38. Butler J: Clinical problems of disordered respiratory control. *Am Rev Respir Dis* 110:695, 1974.
39. Skatrud JB, Dempsey JA, Kaiser DG: Ventilatory response to medroxyprogesterone acetate in normal subjects: time course and mechanism. *J Appl Physiol* 44:939, 1978.
40. Hyland RH, Jones NL, Powles AC, et al: Primary alveolar hypoventilation treated with nocturnal electrophrenic respiration. *Am Rev Respir Dis* 117:165, 1978.
41. Bubis MJ, Anthonisen NR: Primary alveolar hypoventilation treated by nocturnal administration of O_2. *Am Rev Respir Dis* 118:947, 1978.
42. Martin TJ, Sanders MH: Chronic alveolar hypoventilation: a review for the clinician. *Sleep* 18:617, 1995.
43. Shepard JWJ: Cardiorespiratory changes in obstructive sleep apnea, in Kryger MH, Roth T, Dement WC (eds): *Principles and Practice of Sleep Medicine*. 2nd ed. Philadelphia, PA, WB Saunders, 1994, p 657.
44. Ledsom JR, Sharp JM: Pulmonary function in acute cervical cord injury. *Am Rev Respir Dis* 124:41, 1981.
45. Fromm GB, Wisdom PJ, Block AJ: Amyotrophic lateral sclerosis presenting with respiratory failure. *Chest* 71:612, 1977.
46. Brooks BR: Natural history of ALS: symptoms, strength, pulmonary function and disability. *Neurology* 47:S71, 1996.

47. Mansel JK, Norman JR: Respiratory complications and management of spinal cord injuries. *Chest* 97:1446, 1990.
48. Glenn WW, Hogan JF, Loke JS, et al: Ventilatory support by pacing of the conditioned diaphragm in quadriplegia. *N Engl J Med* 310:1150, 1984.
49. McMichan JC, Piepgras DG, Gracey DR, et al: Electrophrenic respiration. *Mayo Clin Proc* 54:662, 1979.
50. Gibson G: Diaphragmatic paresis: pathophysiology, clinical features and investigation. *Thorax* 44:960, 1989.
51. Gibson K, Bonaventure Uwineza J, Kiviri W, et al: Tetanus in developing countries: a case series and review. *Can J Anaesth* 56:307–315, 2009.
52. Parker AJ, Lee JB, Redman J, et al: Strychnine poisoning: gone but not forgotten. *Emerg Med J* 28:84, 2011.
53. Mulder DW, Rosenbaum RA, Layton DD Jr: Late progression of poliomyelitis or forme fruste amyotrophic lateral sclerosis? *Mayo Clin Proc* 47:756, 1972.
54. Hopkins LC, Tatarian GT, Pianta TF: Management of ALS respiratory care. *Neurology* 47:S123, 1996.
55. Soliman MG, Higgins SE, El-Kabir DR, et al: Non-invasive assessment of respiratory muscle strength in patients with previous poliomyelitis. *Respir Med* 99:1217–1222, 2005.
56. Oh SJ, Claussen GG, Hatanaka Y, et al: 3,4-Diaminopyridine is more effective than placebo in a randomized, double-blind, cross-over drug study in LEMS. *Muscle Nerve* 40:795, 2009
57. Dalakas MC, Elder G, Hallett M, et al: A long-term follow-up study of patients with post-poliomyelitis neuromuscular symptoms. *N Engl J Med* 314:959, 1986.
58. Arcila-Londono X, Lewis RA: Guillain-Barré syndrome. *Semin Neurol* 32:179-186, 2012.
59. Koeppen S, Kraywinkel K, Wessendorf TE, et al: Long-term outcome of Guillain-Barré syndrome. *Neurocrit Care* 5:235–242, 2006.
60. Hughes RA, Wijdicks EF, Barohn R, et al: Quality Standards Subcommittee of the American Academy of Neurology. Practice parameter: immunotherapy for Guillain-Barre syndrome: report of the Quality Standards Subcommittee of the American Academy of Neurology. *Neurology* 61:736, 2003.
61. Massachusetts Department of Public Health: The red tide: a public health emergency. *N Engl J Med* 288:1126, 1973.
62. Ahles MD: Red tide: a recurrent health hazard. *Am J Public Health* 64:807, 1974.
63. Isbister GK, Kiernan MC: Neurotoxic marine poisoning. *Lancet Neurol* 4:219, 2005.
64. Eastaugh JA: Delayed use of mannitol in ciguatera (fish poisoning). *Ann Emerg Med* 28:105, 1996.
65. Dinubile MJ, Hokama Y: The ciguatera poisoning syndrome from farm-raised salmon. *Ann Intern Med* 122:113, 1995.
66. Defusco DJ, O'Dowd P, Hokama Y, et al: Coma due to ciguatera poisoning in Rhode Island. *Am J Med* 95:240, 1993.
67. Aguirre VJ, Sinha P, Zimmet A, et al: Phrenic nerve injury during cardiac surgery: mechanisms, management and prevention. *Heart Lung Circ* 22:895–902, 2013.
68. Mulvey DA, Aquilina RJ, Elliot MW, et al: Diaphragmatic dysfunction in neuralgic amyotrophy: an electrophysiologic evaluation of 16 patients presenting with dyspnea. *Am Rev Respir Dis* 147:66, 1993.
69. LaRoche C, Carroll N, Moxham J, et al: Clinical significance of severe diaphragm weakness. *Am Rev Respir Dis* 138:862, 1988.
70. Chan CK, Mohsenin V, Loke J, et al: Diaphragmatic dysfunction in siblings with hereditary motor and sensory neuropathy (Charcot-Marie-Tooth disease). *Chest* 91:567, 1987.
71. Drachman DB: Myasthenia gravis. *N Engl J Med* 298:186, 1978.
72. Dushay KM, Zibrak JD, Jensen WA: Myasthenia gravis presenting as isolated respiratory failure. *Chest* 97:232, 1990.
73. Zulueta J, Fanburg B: Respiratory dysfunction in myasthenia gravis. *Clin Chest Med* 15:683, 1994.
74. Sieb JP: Myasthenia gravis: an update for the clinician. *Clin Exp Immunol* 175:408, 2014.
75. Stricker RB, Kwiatkowska BJ, Habis JA, et al: Myasthenic crisis: response to plasma pheresis following failure of intravenous γ-globulin. *Arch Neurol* 50:837, 1993.
76. Barrons RW: Drug-induced neuromuscular blockade and myasthenia gravis. *Pharmacotherapy* 17:1220–1232, 1997.
77. McEvoy KM, Windebank AJ, Daube JR, et al: 3,4-Diaminopyridine in the treatment of Lambert-Eaton myasthenic syndrome. *N Engl J Med* 321:1567, 1989.
78. Raps EC, Bird SJ, Hansen-Flaschen J: Prolonged muscle weakness after neuromuscular blockade in the intensive care unit. *Crit Care Clin* 10:799, 1994.
79. Griffiths RD, Hall JB: Intensive care unit-acquired weakness. *Crit Care Med* 38:779–787, 2010.
80. Witt NJ, Zochodne DW, Bolton CR, et al: Peripheral nerve function in sepsis and multiple organ failure. *Chest* 99:176, 1991.
81. Gorson KC, Ropper AH: Acute respiratory failure neuropathy: a variant of critical illness polyneuropathy. *Crit Care Med* 21:267, 1993.
82. Peters JI, Stupka JE, Singh H, et al: Status asthmaticus in the medical intensive care unit: a 30-year experience. *Respir Med* 106:344–348, 2012.
83. Alhazzani W, Alshahrani M, Jaeschke R, et al: Neuromuscular blocking agents in acute respiratory distress syndrome: a systematic review and meta-analysis of randomized controlled trials. *Crit Care* 17:R43, 2013.
84. Schmidt-Nowara WW, Samet JM, Rosario PA: Early and late pulmonary complications of botulism. *Arch Intern Med* 143:451, 1983.
85. Gupta A, Sumner CJ, Castor M, et al: Adult botulism type F in the United States, 1981–2002. *Neurology* 65:1694, 2005.
86. Wilcox PC, Morrison NJ, Pardy RL: Recovery of the ventilatory and upper airway muscles and exercise performance after type A botulism. *Chest* 98:620, 1990.
87. Guven M, Sungur M, Eser B, et al: The effects of fresh frozen plasma on cholinesterase levels and outcomes in patients with organophosphate poisoning. *J Toxicol Clin Toxicol* 42(5):617, 2004.
88. Newmark J: Therapy for nerve agent poisoning. *Arch Neurol* 61:649, 2004.
89. Oliemy A, Singh S, Butler J: Role of topical application of iced slush in the development of phrenic nerve palsy after cardiac surgery. *J Cardiothorac Surg* 16:A8, 2015.
90. van Doorn PA, Ruts L, Jacobs BC: Clinical features, pathogenesis, and treatment of Guillain-Barré syndrome. *Lancet Neurol* 7:939–950, 2008.
91. Moorthy SS, Markand ON, Mahomed Y, et al: Electrophysiologic evaluation of phrenic nerves in severe respiratory insufficiency requiring mechanical ventilation. *Chest* 88:211, 1985.
92. Piehler JM, Pairolero PC, Gracey DR, et al: Unexplained diaphragmatic paralysis: a harbinger of malignant disease? *J Thorac Cardiovasc Surg* 84:861, 1982.
93. Thomas NE, Passamonte PM, Sunderrajan EV, et al: Bilateral diaphragmatic paralysis as a possible paraneoplastic syndrome from renal cell carcinoma. *Am Rev Respir Dis* 129:507, 1984.
94. Spitzer SA, Korczyn AD, Kalaci J: Transient bilateral diaphragmatic paralysis. *Chest* 64:355, 1973.
95. Kreitzer SM, Feldman NT, Saunders NA, et al: Bilateral diaphragmatic paralysis with hypercapnic respiratory failure. *Am J Med* 65:89, 1978.
96. Chausow AM, Kane T, Levinson D, et al: Reversible hypercapnic respiratory insufficiency in scleroderma caused by respiratory muscle weakness. *Am Rev Respir Dis* 130:142, 1984.
97. Rosenow RC III, Engel AG: Acid maltase deficiency in adults presenting as respiratory failure. *Am J Med* 64:485, 1978.
98. Wokke JH, Ausems MG, Van den Boogaard MJ, et al: Genotype–phenotype correlation in adult-onset acid maltase deficiency. *Ann Neurol* 38:450, 1995.
99. Newman JH, Neff TA, Ziporin P: Acute respiratory failure associated with hypophosphatemia. *N Engl J Med* 296:1101, 1977.
100. Knochel JP: Neuromuscular manifestations of electrolyte disorders. *Am J Med* 72:521, 1982.
101. Lynn D, Woda R, Mendell J: Respiratory dysfunction in muscular dystrophy and other myopathies. *Clin Chest Med* 15:661, 1994.
102. Hoffman EP, Fischbeck KH, Brown RH, et al: Characterization of dystrophin in muscle. *N Engl J Med* 318:1363, 1988.
103. Olive M, Goldfarb LG, Shatunov A, et al: Myotilinopathy: refining the clinical and myopathological phenotype. *Brain* 128[Pt 10]:2315, 2005.
104. ATS Consensus Statement: Respiratory care of the patient with Duchenne muscular dystrophy. *Am J Respir Crit Care Med* 170:456, 2004.
105. Moxley RT III, Ashwal S, Pandya S, et al: Quality Standards Subcommittee of the American Academy of Neurology. Practice Committee of the Child Neurology Society. Practice parameter: corticosteroid treatment of Duchenne dystrophy: report of the Quality Standards Subcommittee of the American Academy of Neurology and the Practice Committee of the Child Neurology Society. *Neurology* 64:13, 2005.
106. Thornton CA: Myotonic dystrophy. *Neurol Clin* 32:705–719, 2014.
107. Liquori CL, Ricker K, Moseley ML, et al: Myotonic dystrophy type 2 caused by a CCTG expansion in intron 1 of ZNF9. *Science* 293:864, 2001.
108. Begin R, Bureau MA, Lupien L, et al: Pathogenesis of respiratory insufficiency in myotonic dystrophy. *Am Rev Respir Dis* 125:312, 1982.
109. Suetterlin K, Männikkö R, Hanna MG: Muscle channelopathies: recent advances in genetics, pathophysiology and therapy. *Curr Opin Neurol* 27:583–590, 2014.
110. Statland J, Phillips L, Trivedi JR: Muscle channelopathies. *Neurol Clin* 32:801–815, 2014.
111. Boentert M, Karabul N, Wenninger S, et al: Sleep-related symptoms and sleep-disordered breathing in adult Pompe disease. *Eur J Neurol* 22:369–376, 2015.
112. Troyanov Y, Targoff IN, Tremblay JL, et al: Novel classification of idiopathic inflammatory myopathies based on overlap syndrome features and autoantibodies: analysis of 100 French Canadian patients. *Medicine (Baltimore)* 84:231, 2005.
113. Schwarz MI, Sutarik JM, Nick JA, et al: Pulmonary capillaritis and diffuse alveolar hemorrhage: a primary manifestation of polymyositis. *Am J Respir Crit Care Med* 151:2037, 1995.
114. NIH Conference: Myositis: immunologic contributions to understanding the cause, pathogenesis and therapy. *Ann Intern Med* 122:715, 1995.
115. Siafakas NM, Milona I, Salesiotou V, et al: Respiratory muscle strength in hyperthyroidism before and after treatment. *Am Rev Respir Dis* 146:1025, 1992.
116. Nieman LK, Ilias I: Evaluation and treatment of Cushing's syndrome. *Am J Med* 118:1340, 2005.
117. Kunci RW: Colchicine myopathy and neuropathy. *N Engl J Med* 316:1562, 1987.
118. Watt G, Saisorn S, Jongsakul K, et al: Blinded, placebo-controlled trial of antiparasitic drugs for trichinosis myositis. *J Infect Dis* 182:371, 2000.
119. Varsano S, Shapiro M, Taragan R, et al: Hypophosphatemia as a reversible cause of refractory ventilatory failure. *Crit Care Med* 11:908, 1983.
120. Aubier M, Murciano D, Lecocguic Y, et al: Effect of hypophosphatemia on diaphragmatic contractility in patients with acute respiratory failure. *N Engl J Med* 313:420, 1985.
121. Dhingra S, Solven F, Wilson A, et al: Hypomagnesemia and respiratory muscle power. *Am Rev Respir Dis* 129:497, 1984.
122. Agus ZS, Wasserstein A, Goldfarb S: Disorders of calcium and magnesium homeostasis. *Am J Med* 72:473, 1982.

123. Hertzman PA, Blevins WL, Mayer J, et al: Association of the eosinophilia-myalgia syndrome with the ingestion of tryptophan. *N Engl J Med* 322:869, 1990.
124. Silver RM, Heyes MP, Maize JC, et al: Scleroderma, fasciitis, and eosinophilia associated with the ingestion of tryptophan. *N Engl J Med* 322:874, 1990.
125. Medsger TA Jr: Tryptophan-induced eosinophilia-myalgia syndrome. *N Engl J Med* 322:926, 1990.
126. Ventayya RV, Poole RM, Pentz WH: Respiratory failure from procainamide-induced myopathy. *Ann Intern Med* 119:345, 1993.
127. Black LF, Hyatt RE: Maximal static respiratory pressures in generalized neuromuscular disease. *Am Rev Respir Dis* 103:641, 1971.
128. Kafer ER: Respiratory failure in paralytic scoliosis. *Am Rev Respir Dis* 110:450, 1974.
129. Lisboa C, Moreno R, Fava M, et al: Inspiratory muscle function in patients with severe kyphoscoliosis. *Am Rev Respir Dis* 132:48, 1985.
130. Libby DM, Briscoe WA, Boyce B, et al: Acute respiratory failure in scoliosis or kyphosis. *Am J Med* 73:532, 1982.
131. Garay SM, Turino GM, Goldring RM: Sustained reversal of chronic hypercapnia in patients with alveolar hypoventilation syndromes: long-term maintenance with noninvasive nocturnal mechanical ventilation. *Am J Med* 70:269, 1981.
132. Meyer TJ, Hill NS: Noninvasive positive pressure ventilation to treat respiratory failure. *Ann Intern Med* 120:760, 1994.
133. Rochester DF, Enson Y: Current concepts in the pathogenesis of the obesity-hypoventilation syndrome. *Am J Med* 57:402, 1974.
134. Sampson MG, Grassino A: Neuromechanical properties in obese patients during carbon dioxide rebreathing. *Am J Med* 75:81, 1983.
135. Mokhlesi B, Kryger MH, Grunstein RR: Assessment and management of patients with obesity hypoventilation syndrome. *Proc Am Thorac Soc* 5:218, 2008.
136. Trinkle JK, Richardson JD, Franz JL, et al: Management of flail chest without mechanical ventilation. *Ann Thorac Surg* 19:355, 1975.
137. Colp C, Reichel J, Park SS: Severe pleural restriction: the maximum static pulmonary recoil pressure as an aid in diagnosis. *Chest* 67:658, 1975.
138. Miller A, Teirstein AS, Selikoff IJ: Ventilatory failure due to asbestos pleurisy. *Am J Med* 75:911, 1983.
139. Gilbert L, Ribot S, Frankel H, et al: Fibrinous uremic pleuritis: a surgical entity. *Chest* 67:53, 1975.
140. Black MJ, Harbour J, Remsen KA, et al: Acute epiglottitis in adults. *J Otolaryngol* 10:23, 1981.
141. Lederman MM, Lowder J, Lerner PI: Bacteremic pneumococcal epiglottitis in adults with malignancy. *Am Rev Respir Dis* 125:117, 1982.
142. Schecter WP, Wilson RS: Management of upper airway obstruction in the intensive care unit. *Crit Care Med* 9:577, 1981.
143. Phelan DM, Love JB: Adult epiglottitis: is there a role for the fiberoptic bronchoscope? *Chest* 86:783, 1984.
144. Hunt KJ, Valentine MD, Sobotka AK, et al: A controlled trial of immunotherapy in insect hypersensitivity. *N Engl J Med* 299:157, 1978.
145. Valentine MD: Anaphylaxis and stinging insect hypersensitivity. *JAMA* 268:2830, 1992.
146. Greaves M, Lawlor F: Angioedema: manifestations and management. *J Am Acad Dermatol* 25:155, 1991.
147. Chevailler A, Arland G, Ponard D, et al: CI-inhibitor binding monoclonal immunoglobulins in three patients with acquired angioneurotic edema. *J Allergy Clin Immunol* 97:998, 1996.
148. Israiliz H, Hall WD: Cough and angioneurotic edema associated with angiotensin-converting enzyme inhibitor therapy. *Ann Intern Med* 117:234, 1992.
149. Stauffer JL, Olson DE, Petty TL: Complications and consequences of endotracheal intubation and tracheotomy: a prospective study of 150 critically ill adult patients. *Am J Med* 70:65, 1981.
150. Harley HR: Laryngotracheal obstruction complicating tracheostomy or endotracheal intubation with assisted respiration. *Thorax* 26:493, 1971.
151. Mittleman RE, Wetli CV: The fatal cafe coronary. *JAMA* 247:1285, 1982.
152. Irwin RS, Ashba JK, Braman SS, et al: Food asphyxiation in hospitalized patients. *JAMA* 237:2744, 1977.
153. Gelperin A: Sudden death in an elderly population from aspiration of food. *J Am Geriatr Soc* 22:135, 1974.
154. Haugen RK: The cafe coronary. *JAMA* 186:142, 1963.
155. Heimlich HJ: A life-saving maneuver to prevent food choking. *JAMA* 234:398, 1975.
156. Abdulmajid OA, Ebeid AM, Motaweh MM, et al: Aspirated foreign bodies in the tracheobronchial tree: report of 250 cases. *Thorax* 31:635, 1976.
157. Rosenbaum L, Thurman P, Krantz SB: Upper airway obstruction as a complication of oral anticoagulation therapy. *Arch Intern Med* 139:1151, 1979.
158. Rodrigues JF, York EL, Nair CP: Upper airway obstruction in Guillain-Barré syndrome. *Chest* 86:147, 1984.
159. Schmidt-Nowara WW, Marder EJ, Feil PA: Respiratory failure in myasthenia gravis due to vocal cord paresis. *Arch Neurol* 41:567, 1984.
160. Libby DM, Schley WS, Smith JP: Cricoarytenoid arthritis in ankylosing spondylitis. *Chest* 80:641, 1981.
161. Proctor DF: The upper airways. II. The larynx and trachea. *Am Rev Respir Dis* 115:315, 1977.
162. Kastanos N, Miro RE, Perez AM, et al: Laryngotracheal injury due to endotracheal intubation: incidence, evolution, and predisposing factors—a prospective long-term study. *Crit Care Med* 11:362, 1983.
163. Magnussen CR, Patanella HP: Herpes simplex virus and recurrent laryngeal nerve paralysis. *Arch Intern Med* 139:1423, 1979.
164. Vincken WG, Gauthier SG, Dollfuss RE, et al: Involvement of upper-airway muscles in extrapyramidal disorders: a cause of airflow limitation. *N Engl J Med* 311:438, 1984.
165. Cormier Y, Kashima H, Summer W, et al: Upper airway obstruction with bilateral vocal cord paralysis. *Chest* 75:423, 1979.
166. Fleetham JA, Lynn RB, Munt PW: Tracheal leiomyosarcoma: a unique cause of stridor. *Am Rev Respir Dis* 116:1109, 1977.
167. Olmedo G, Rosenberg M, Fonseca R: Primary tumors of the trachea. *Chest* 81:701, 1982.
168. Braman SS, Whitcomb ME: Endobronchial metastasis. *Arch Intern Med* 135:543, 175.
169. Weber AL, Grillo HC: Tracheal tumors: a radiological clinical and pathological evaluation of 84 cases. *Radiol Clin North Am* 16:227, 1976.
170. Kvale PA, Eichenhorn MS, Radke JR, et al: YAG laser photoresection of lesions obstructing the central airways. *Chest* 87:283, 1985.
171. Gamsu G, Borson DB, Webb WR, et al: Structure and function in tracheal stenosis. *Am Rev Respir Dis* 121:519, 1980.
172. Feist JH, Johnson TH, Wilson RJ: Acquired tracheomalacia: etiology and differential diagnosis. *Chest* 68:340, 1975.
173. Bergstrom B, Ollman B, Lindholm CE: Endotracheal excision of fibrous tracheal stenosis and subsequent prolonged stenting: an alternative method in selected cases. *Chest* 71:6, 1977.
174. Epstein LJ, Kristo D, Strollo PJ, et al: Clinical guideline for the evaluation, management, and long-term care of obstructive sleep apnea in adults. *J Clin Sleep Med* 5:263, 2009.
175. Flemons WW: Clinical practice. Obstructive sleep apnea. *N Engl J Med* 347:498, 2002.
176. Walsh RE, Michaelson ED, Harkleroad LE, et al: Upper airway obstruction in obese patients with sleep disturbance and somnolence. *Ann Intern Med* 76:185, 1972.
177. Onal E, Lopata M, O'Connor T: Pathogenesis of apneas in hypersomnia: sleep apnea syndrome. *Am Rev Respir Dis* 125:167, 1982.
178. Motta J, Guilleminault C, Schroeder JS, et al: Tracheostomy and hemodynamic changes in sleep-induced apnea. *Ann Intern Med* 89:454, 1978.
179. Shepard JW Jr, Garrison MW, Grither DA, et al: Relationship of ventricular ectopy to oxyhemoglobin desaturation in patients with obstructive sleep apnea. *Chest* 88:335, 1985.
180. Orr WC, Martin RJ: Obstructive sleep apnea associated with tonsillar hypertrophy in adults. *Arch Intern Med* 141:990, 1981.
181. Heimer D, Scharf SM, Lieberman A, et al: Sleep apnea syndrome treated by repair of deviated nasal septum. *Chest* 84:184, 1983.
182. Davies SF, Iber C: Obstructive sleep apnea associated with adult-acquired micrognathia from rheumatoid arthritis. *Am Rev Respir Dis* 127:245, 1983.
183. Mezon BJ, West P, Maclean JP, et al: Sleep apnea in acromegaly. *Am J Med* 69:615, 1980.
184. Rajagopal KR, Abbrecht PH, Derderian SS, et al: Obstructive sleep apnea in hypothyroidism. *Ann Intern Med* 101:491, 1984.
185. Orr WC, Males JL, Imes NK: Myxedema and obstructive sleep apnea. *Am J Med* 70:1061, 1981.
186. Remmers JE: Obstructive sleep apnea: a common disorder exacerbated by alcohol. *Am Rev Respir Dis* 130:153, 1984.
187. Sandblom RE, Matsumoto AM, Schoene RB, et al: Obstructive sleep apnea syndrome induced by testosterone administration. *N Engl J Med* 308:508, 1983.
188. Johnson MW, Anch AM, Remmers JE: Induction of the obstructive sleep apnea syndrome in a woman by exogenous androgen administration. *Am Rev Respir Dis* 129:1023, 1984.
189. Torres A, Arroyo J, Kastanos N, et al: Acute respiratory failure and tracheal obstruction in patients with intrathoracic goiter. *Crit Care Med* 11:265, 1983.
190. Acres JC, Kryger MH: Clinical significance of pulmonary function tests: upper airway obstruction. *Chest* 80:207, 1981.
191. Rochester DF, Esau SA: Malnutrition and the respiratory system. *Chest* 85:411, 1984.
192. Kelly SM, Rosa A, Field S, et al: Inspiratory muscle strength and body composition in patients receiving total parenteral nutrition therapy. *Am Rev Respir Dis* 130:33, 1984.
193. Aldrich TK, Karpel JP: Inspiratory muscle resistive training in respiratory failure. *Am Rev Respir Dis* 131:461, 1985.
194. Gross D, Ladd HW, Riley EJ, et al: The effect of training on strength and endurance of the diaphragm in quadriplegia. *Am J Med* 68:27, 1980.
195. Howell S, Fitzgerald RS, Roussos CH: Effects of aminophylline, isoproterenol, and neostigmine on hypercapnic depression of diaphragmatic contractility. *Am Rev Respir Dis* 132:241, 1985.
196. Vires N, Aubier M, Murciano D, et al: Effects of aminophylline on diaphragmatic fatigue during acute respiratory failure. *Am Rev Respir Dis* 129:396, 1984.
197. Gonzalez C, Ferris G, Diaz J, et al: Kyphoscoliotic ventilatory insufficiency: effects of long-term intermittent positive-pressure ventilation. *Chest* 124:857, 2003.
198. Remmers JE, Sterling JA, Thorarinsson B, et al: Nasal airway positive pressure in patients with occlusive sleep apnea. *Am Rev Respir Dis* 130:1152, 1984.
199. Sanders MH: Nasal CPAP effect on patterns of sleep apnea. *Chest* 86:839, 1984.
200. Kushida CA, Littner MR, Hirshkowitz M, et al: American Academy of Sleep Medicine. Practice parameters for the use of continuous and bilevel positive airway pressure devices to treat adult patients with sleep-related breathing disorders. *Sleep* 29:375, 2006.
201. Browman CP, Sampson MG, Yolles SF, et al: Obstructive sleep apnea and body weight. *Chest* 85:435, 1984.
202. American Sleep Disorders Association: Practice parameters for the treatment of snoring and obstructive sleep apnea with oral appliances. *Sleep* 18:511, 1995.
203. Conway W, Fugita S, Zorick F, et al: Uvulopalato-pharyngoplasty. *Chest* 88:385, 1985.

Chapter 166 ■ Invasive Mechanical Ventilation and Extracorporeal Life Support for Respiratory Failure

ROLANDO SANCHEZ SANCHEZ • GREGORY A. SCHMIDT

INTRODUCTION

Invasive mechanical ventilation (MV) describes controlled or assisted ventilation through an endotracheal tube, tracheostomy, or (rarely) esophageal obturator airway. Noninvasive ventilation is described in Chapter 167. This chapter describes ventilator modes, interpretation of respiratory system mechanical properties using pressure and flow waveforms, indications for MV and extracorporeal life support (ECLS), a patient-centered approach to ventilator settings, complications of MV, and the role for ECLS for patients with cardiopulmonary failure.

MV is used when the patient's spontaneous breathing is insufficient to sustain life, when it is useful to take control of respiration because of impending failure of other systems, or to support patients through deep sedation or therapeutic paralysis. Intensive care unit (ICU) ventilators operate by applying supra-atmospheric pressure to the invasive airway appliance, driving bulk gas flow along a pressure gradient into the alveoli (inspiration) and (usually) allowing passive expiration.

MODES OF MECHANICAL VENTILATION

Physiology of Positive Pressure Ventilation

Initial ventilator modes were designed to deliver breaths of air mixed with oxygen at a fixed volume (tidal volume, V_T) and frequency (*controlled modes*). These modes did not take into consideration the patient's effort, and consequently they were often associated with significant ventilator dyssynchrony, requiring deep levels of sedation and paralysis. Subsequently, new ventilator modes were developed that had the capacity to sense the patient's inspiratory effort, improving synchrony of breath onset and termination (*assisted modes*). Despite this progress, the general prevalence of ventilator dyssynchrony among mechanically ventilated patients (discussed in detail below) is still estimated at up to 25%, with higher values in specific populations like COPD and children. Lately, complex ventilator modes have been developed seeking to improve patient–ventilator synchrony; respond more readily to changing conditions; and adjust settings without clinician intervention.

In order to understand ventilator modes, it is essential to first describe the key components of individual breaths, characterized by (a) how the breath is initiated (trigger); (b) what governs gas flow during the breath (target); and (c) how the breath is terminated (cycle) (see Table 166.1). Ventilator modes are created based on which breath types are delivered and whether spontaneous breaths (SB) are allowed (Table 166.2).

Defining Characteristics of Breath Types

Trigger

MV breaths are triggered in one of four possible ways: (a) time, (b) pressure, (c) flow, or (d) neural sensing. Time is the trigger for controlled breaths, meaning that a breath will be delivered after a fixed time from the prior breath, defined by the set respiratory rate (time = 60 per frequency). In contrast, assisted breaths rely on the ventilator to detect patient effort. Most commonly, effort is sensed through a fall in pressure at the airway opening (pressure trigger) or by detecting a difference in the bias flow comparing the inspiratory and expiratory limbs of the ventilator circuit (flow triggering). In the majority of ventilated patients the means of effort detection has no significant impact on the efficiency of triggering or work of breathing, and is selected based on physician preference. However, in some clinical scenarios (such as in the presence of an air leak, for example when a bronchopleural fistula is present), choice of trigger can be important, because relying on flow can produce auto-triggering, a form of ventilator dyssynchrony. Neural sensing, in which the integrated

TABLE 166.1

Defining Characteristics of Breath Types

Breath Type	Trigger	Target	Cycle
Volume control (VC)	Time	Flow rate	Volume
Volume assist (VA)	Effort	Flow rate	Volume
Pressure control (PC)	Time	Pressure	Time
Pressure assist (PA)	Effort	Pressure	Time
Pressure support (PS)	Effort	Pressure	Flow rate

Effort describes triggering through pressure, flow, or the diaphragm electromyographic signal.

TABLE 166.2

Common Ventilator Modes are Composed of Breath Types

	VC	VA	PC	PA	PS	SB
Volume assist control (VACV)	x	x				
Volume SIMV (V-SIMV)	x	x			x	x
Pressure assist control (PACV)			x	x		
Pressure SIMV (P-SIMV)			x	x	x	x
Pressure support ventilation (PSV)					x	

SIMV, synchronized, intermittent, mandatory ventilation; SB, spontaneous breaths diaphragmatic electromyographic signal is used to initiate the breath, improves neuroventilatory coupling [1], especially for patients with severe airway obstruction and in children.

Target

Ventilator breaths are conventionally classified based on the targeted variable: pressure-targeted breaths versus flow-targeted breaths. For pressure-targeted breaths, the clinician sets and the ventilator produces a controlled pressure (P_I) throughout inspiration. Generally, P_I is constant although it can vary during proportional-assist breaths or those based on the diaphragm EMG. In contrast, during flow-targeted breaths, the clinician sets and the ventilator delivers a controlled inspiratory flow rate ($\dot{V}_I$). Generally, $\dot{V}_I$ is constant throughout the breath (constant flow or square wave), but can also decelerate or vary sinusoidally. Although clinicians tend to think of pressure- and flow-targeted breaths as differing fundamentally, in fact they are tightly coupled through the equation of motion for the respiratory system. This equation relates pressure at the airway opening (P_{ao}), volume above FRC (V), compliance of the respiratory system (C_{RS}), inspiratory flow ($\dot{V}_I$), respiratory system resistance (R), flow acceleration ($\ddot{V}_I$), inertance (I), and the pressure produced by the inspiratory muscles (P_{mus}) as follows:

$$P_{ao} = \frac{V}{C_{RS}} + \dot{V}_I R + \ddot{V} I - P_{mus}$$

According to this physiologic relationship, during pressure-targeted breaths (P_{ao} is generally constant and thus is the independent variable), volume and flow depend on P_{ao} along with C_{RS}, R, and P_{mus} (the inertance term is only relevant when there are rapid changes in flow, as during high frequency ventilation). Similarly, during flow-targeted breaths ($\dot{V}_I$ is generally constant and is the independent variable), P_{ao} becomes the dependent variable (Fig. 166.1). These points are crucial for two reasons: (1) the ventilatory impact of pressure- and flow-targeted breaths are linked by the mechanical properties of the respiratory system (in the passive patient these include only C_{RS} and R); and (2) this equation forms the basis for deriving clinically important information about the respiratory system from pressure and flow waveforms, as discussed further below.

Some unusual ventilator modes allow dual-control breaths, in which both pressure and flow can be targeted within a single breath. For example, "volume-assured pressure support" breaths begin as typical PS breaths but, if the projected tidal volume falls below the target, the breath switches to an AC, flow-targeted breath until completion. There are no apparent advantages to such dual-control breaths and modes.

Cycle

The cycle variable is the factor that terminates inspiration. There are four possible cycle variables: (a) time; (b) flow; (c) volume; (d) neural sensing. PC breaths are terminated by time (inspiratory time, T_I), often set between 0.5 and 1.0 seconds. At any given rate, inspiratory time determines expiratory time (because the number of seconds in each breath cycle = 60/frequency), so there are important consequences to the time chosen, especially in patients with airflow obstruction. Flow is the cycle variable for PS breaths, which terminate when flow falls to a specified fraction of the initial inspiratory flow or, on some ventilators, below an absolute threshold of flow. Because P_{ao} is (usually) constant during pressure-targeted breaths, $\dot{V}_I$ tends to decelerate throughout the breath as lung volume and lung recoil rise and effort falls, according to the equation of motion. Often, a value near 30% of initial flow is chosen to signal the ventilator to switch off because, in normal subjects, this tends to coincide with cessation of inspiratory effort (i.e., ventilator T_I approximates neural T_I, enhancing synchrony). The rate of fall of the flow depends on the mechanical properties of the respiratory system [2], however; for patients with severe airflow obstruction, this can lead to very long ventilator T_I (longer than neural T_I) and patient–ventilator dyssynchrony [3]. For these patients, synchrony can be improved by raising the cycle threshold to 50% or even higher.

The third means to cycle from inspiration to expiration is to rely on delivered volume, typical of flow-targeted breaths. When flow is constant, this is analogous to using time to cycle the breath, because $V = \dot{V}_I \times$ time. Finally, inspiration can be cycled off by using the declining signal from the diaphragm EMG. Regardless of the target, all ventilators have an additional maximal pressure limit as a safety feature to prevent lung overpressurization. This pressure is set by the clinician, often 10 cm H_2O above the peak pressure; whenever this pressure is exceeded,

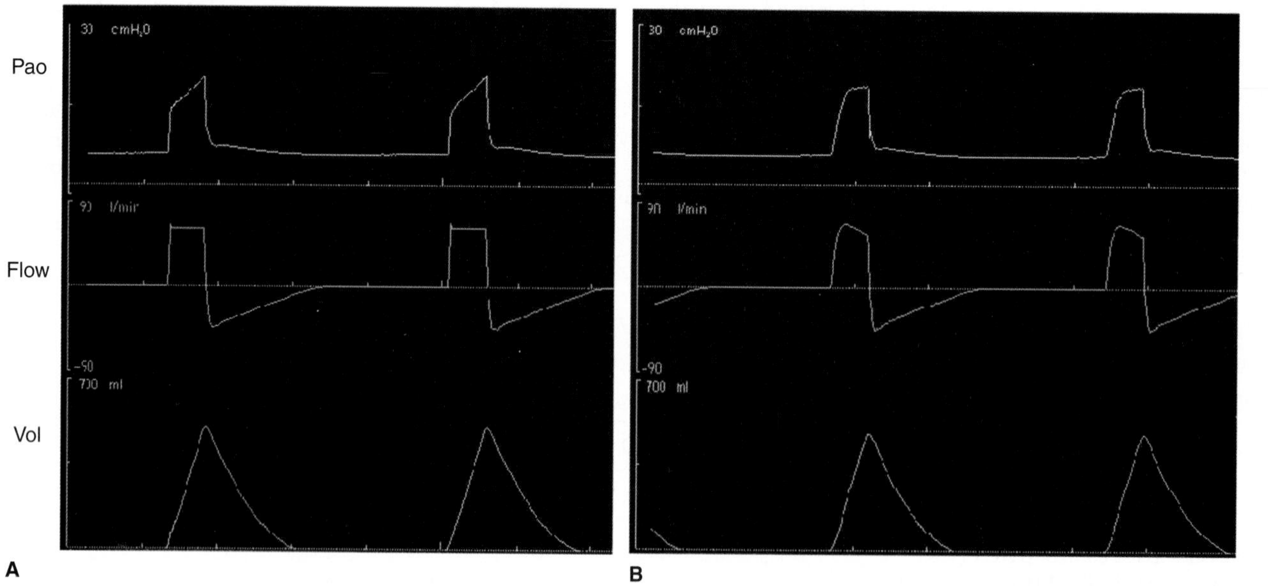

FIGURE 166.1 Passively ventilated patient on flow- (**A**) and pressure (**B**)-targeted mode. **A:** Flow remains constant and volume rises linearly throughout inspiration, while pressure is determined by the respiratory system mechanical properties. **B:** The pressure remains constant, being the independent variable, while the flow and volume are determined by the respiratory system mechanical properties. Note that expiratory flow, being mode independent, is identical during pressure-targeted and flow-targeted breaths.

the ventilator sets off an alarm and opens the expiratory valve to release the rest of the breath to the atmosphere.

Ventilator Modes

Ventilator modes are created based on which types of breaths are included, and whether spontaneous breathing is allowed. The profusion of modes can be confusing and is often driven by marketing imperatives and untested theories about what might confer benefits for critically ill patients. The evidence base supporting advantages for any particular mode is scant [4,5]. For each mode below, we describe the component breaths, settings the clinician must choose, and impact of patient effort. Positive end-expiratory pressure (PEEP) is discussed separately.

Volume Assist Control Ventilation

Volume assist control mode allows both VC and VA breaths, so is time- or effort-triggered, flow-targeted, and volume-cycled. In this mode the physician sets the tidal volume, inspiratory flow rate, and respiratory frequency. The I:E ratio, T_I, and the expiratory time (T_E) are determined by the combination of inspiratory flow rate, tidal volume, and frequency. At constant tidal volume, the higher the inspiratory flow rate, the shorter the T_I and the smaller the I:E ratio (Fig. 166.2).

In the passively ventilated patient a set tidal volume is delivered with each VC breath at a specified frequency. In the actively breathing patient, extra breaths can be triggered (VA), each at the same V_T and inspiratory flow rate as VC breaths: this will change the I:E ratio and T_E. When respiratory drive is high, or when neural T_I exceeds the ventilator T_I, patients may trigger a second breath (rarely a third) which is superimposed on the initial breath. This phenomenon, called double-triggering, is especially common during lung-protective ventilation of the acute respiratory distress syndrome (ARDS), and risks overdistention of lung or dynamic hyperinflation [6].

Volume-Synchronized Intermittent Mandatory Ventilation

Volume-synchronized intermittent mandatory ventilation (V-SIMV) entails VC, VA, PS, and SB, so is time- or effort triggered; flow- or pressure-targeted; and time- or flow-cycled. In the passive patient, it behaves the same way as volume assist control ventilation (VACV). In actively breathing patients, if the triggering effort occurs close to the next scheduled mandatory breath (defined interval or synchronization window), the ventilator delivers a VA breath and resets the interval until the next time-cycled breath. If the triggering effort occurs before the synchronization window, a PS or spontaneous breath follows (unsynchronized breath) (Fig. 166.3).

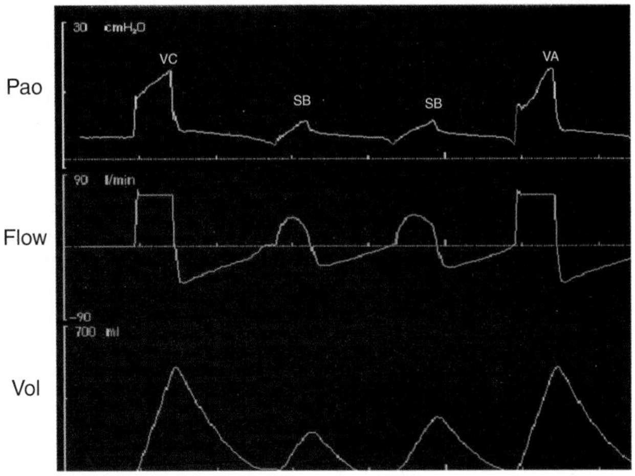

FIGURE 166.3 Volume-synchronized, intermittent, mandatory ventilation (V-SIMV). The different breath types delivered by V-SIMV mode in an actively breathing patient are shown: controlled breath (VC), followed by two unsynchronized spontaneous breaths (SB) and a synchronized-assisted breath (VA). Notice that the VA breath is composed of the same flow rate and volume as the VC breath but pressures are lower in accord with the patient's inspiratory effort. Here, the unsynchronized breaths are SBs, but these can also be pressure support breaths.

This ventilator mode has been used traditionally as a weaning strategy, although its use is decreasing, perhaps because it appears to prolong ventilator liberation.

Pressure Assist Control Ventilation

This mode consists of both pressure assist (PA) and PC breaths (time- or effort-triggered, pressure-targeted, and time-cycled). The respiratory rate (f), P_I, and T_I are set by the clinician, whereas the inspiratory to expiratory (I:E) ratio is determined indirectly based on f and T_I. With every breath, pressure rises quickly to the P_I, although a "rise time" can be set to slow the rate of rise. Most often the rise time is 0 during invasive ventilation, although a brief (0.1 to 0.2 second) rise time can aid synchrony in some patients (Fig. 166.4).

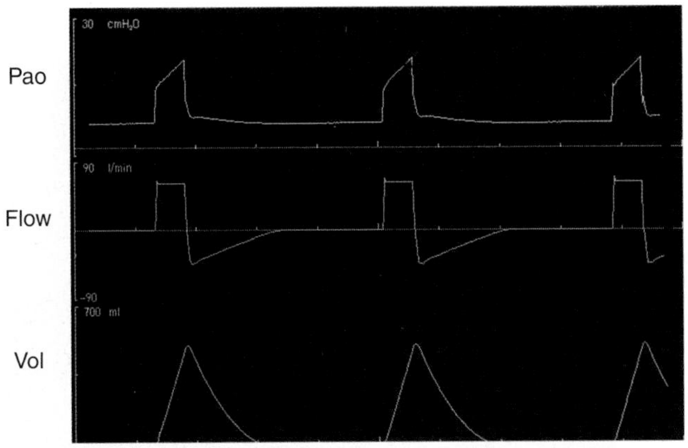

FIGURE 166.2 Volume assist-control ventilation. As in most flow-targeted modes, flow remains constant and volume rises linearly throughout inspiration, while pressure is determined by the respiratory system mechanical properties. The figure represents a passively ventilated patient; the V_T, T_I, and RR set by the clinician determine the I:E ratio and flow rate. If the patient triggers an extra breath, then the same tidal volume would be delivered at the same flow rate and T_I, but the I:E ratio would change.

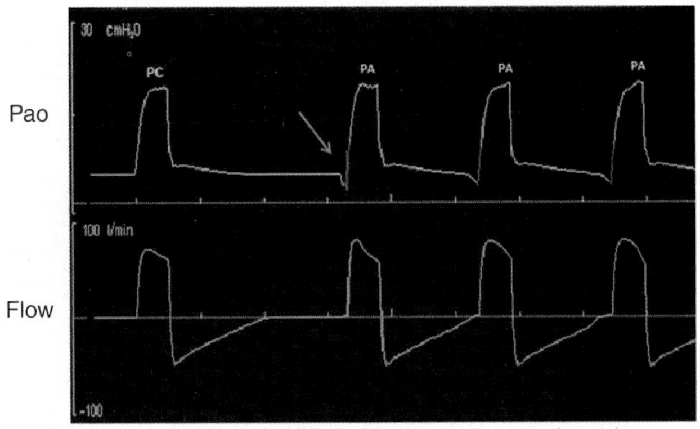

FIGURE 166.4 Pressure assist-control ventilation. Pressure is constant throughout inspiration, within the limits of the ventilator to control it. The inspiratory flow falls throughout the breath as the alveolar pressure rises. In this patient, the first breath is controlled (PC) while the next three are assisted (PA). The downward deflection of the pressure curve at the beginning of inspiration (PA breaths) represents the patient's inspiratory effort triggering the breath (arrow). Note the subtle differences in inspiratory flow during the PA breaths related to variable patient effort.

For the passive patient without airway obstruction and sufficiently long inspiratory time, P_I and alveolar pressure (P_{alv}) equilibrate at end inspiration (signaled by zero flow), and the tidal volume is predictable ($V_T = C_{RS} \times [P_I - PEEP]$). For patients with airflow obstruction or short T_I, there will not be equilibration between P_I and the alveolar pressure, flow does not fall to zero at end-inspiration, and V_T will be smaller than that predicted based on C_{RS} and P_I. For a patient who is actively breathing, V_T is often augmented by effort, and is usually larger than predicted by C_{RS} and P_I. In addition, active patients can trigger additional breaths increasing minute ventilation, reducing expiratory time (T_E), and increasing the I:E ratio.

Pressure Support Ventilation

Pressure support breaths (effort-triggered, pressure-targeted, and flow-cycled) comprise this mode. The patient must trigger the ventilator to deliver a breath, so this mode cannot be applied to passive patients. The clinician sets P_I and (optionally) the flow threshold for cycling the breath off: rate and minute ventilation depend on the patient's drive (Fig. 166.5). For patients with periodic breathing (relatively common in the critically ill), pressure support ventilation (PSV) can amplify the hyperpneic periods and extend the duration of apneas, especially when P_I is set to high levels. If this causes alarms to sound, reducing the level of P_I usually shortens or abolishes apneas.

Pressure SIMV

The combination of PC, PA, PS, and SB makes up pressure SIMV (Fig. 166.6). The clinician sets rate, P_I (PC and PA breath-related P_I is set independently of the P_I for PS breaths), and T_I. This mode is therefore effort- or time-triggered; pressure-targeted; and both time-cycled (PC and PA breaths) and flow-cycled (PS breaths). When the patient is passive, pressure SIMV becomes simply pressure control mode. When the patient triggers a breath in a brief window before a planned time-cycled PC breath, the breath becomes a PA breath. If patient effort precedes this window, the breath is instead PS or SB (depending on whether the clinician has enabled PS breaths). SIMV was created with the hope that it would ease the transition between full ventilatory support and spontaneous breathing, but instead IMV seems to impede weaning [7,8].

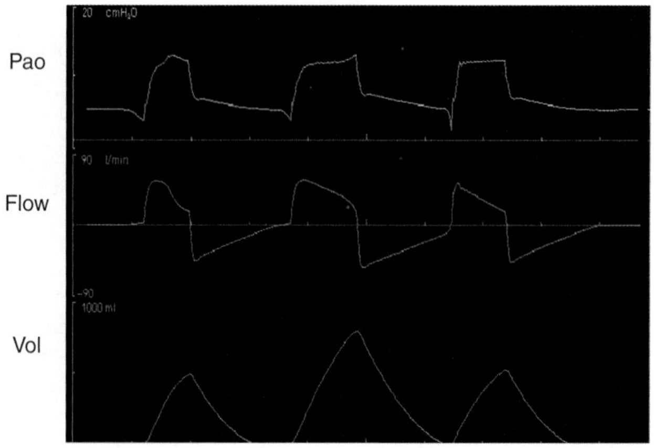

FIGURE 166.5 Pressure support. As is typical of most pressure-targeted modes, the inspiratory flow falls throughout the breath as the alveolar pressure rises (because of elastic recoil and falling inspiratory effort). Appreciate how tidal volume and inspiratory flow rate are determined, in part, by the patient's respiratory effort that can vary from breath to breath, while the P_{ao} is maintained constant (P_I + PEEP).

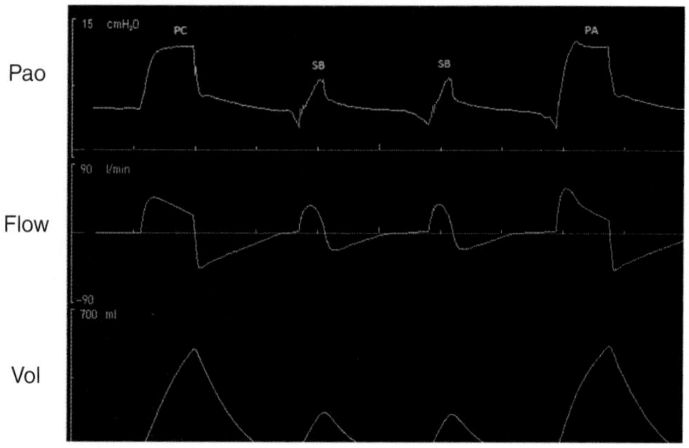

FIGURE 166.6 Pressure-synchronized, intermittent, mandatory ventilation (SIMV). Similar to volume-SIMV, several breath types can be delivered by this mode in an actively breathing patient: a controlled breath (PC) is followed by two unsynchronized spontaneous breaths (SB) and a synchronized assisted breath (PA). PA breaths have the same pressure profile and T_I as PC breaths. For unsynchronized breaths, pressure support is set at zero.

Pressure-Regulated Volume Control and Volume Support Ventilation

Although the name pressure-regulated volume control (PRVC) suggests that it targets flow (or volume), in fact PRVC is a pressure-targeted mode allowing only PC and PA breaths (Fig. 166.7). In this mode the clinician sets an initial P_I, T_I, frequency, and a tidal volume goal. The ventilator automatically and continually adjusts P_I to achieve the desired V_T. Therefore, if respiratory system mechanical properties or patient effort changes, so will P_I. This is one means of controlling tidal volume for patients with ARDS although, compared with VACV, it may increase the work of breathing [9]. No patient-centered benefits have been described [5]. A similar mode is volume support ventilation (VSV) which uses PS breaths also to achieve a target tidal volume. Because it uses PS rather than PC and PA breaths, VSV differs from PRVC in that T_I and frequency are not controlled by the clinician.

Airway Pressure Release Ventilation

PC, PS, and SB are combined during airway pressure release ventilation (APRV), making it time- and effort-triggered, pressure-targeted, and time- and flow-cycled, but this mode is

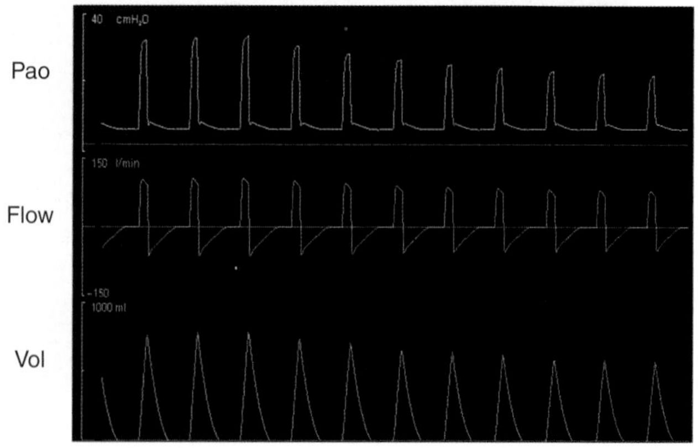

FIGURE 166.7 Pressure-regulated volume control. In this passively ventilated patient, the clinician switched the target V_T from 800 to 500 mL. Appreciate how the P_I is adjusted by the ventilator and decreases gradually to deliver the new target V_T. The time axis has been compressed for illustration purposes.

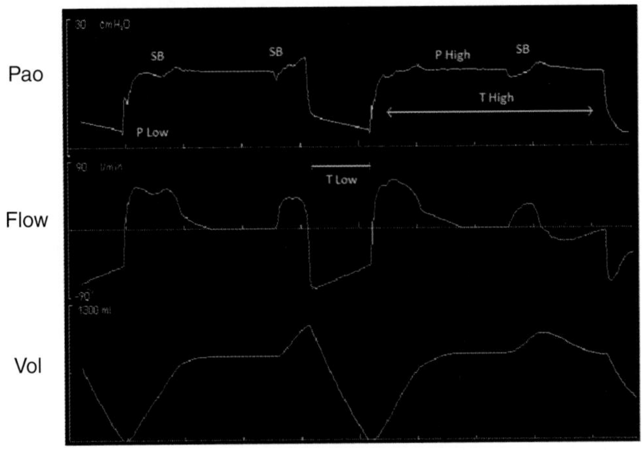

FIGURE 166.8 Airway pressure release ventilation in an actively breathing patient. The P_{HIGH} represents the P_I, and P_{LOW} the PEEP, while T_{LOW} represents the T_E, and T_{HIGH} the T_I. The patient can trigger spontaneous breaths (SB or pressure support) in combination with this mode during T_{HIGH} or T_{LOW}. T_{LOW} is typically quite short in order to produce autoPEEP (note that expiratory flow does not cease at the end of T_{LOW}).

characterized especially by a very long T_I (Fig. 166.8). This same mode is sometimes referred to as biphasic positive airway pressure, especially in Europe, and has also been termed "upside-down SIMV." The clinician enters frequency, T_{LOW} (which is simply T_E), P_{HIGH} (P_I), and P_{LOW} (PEEP). T_{LOW} is kept brief in order to produce auto-PEEP (autoPEEP), but there is no agreement as to how this should be done. Some users of APRV advocate setting T_{LOW} according to the expiratory flow curve; others base it on the expiratory time constant of the respiratory system. T_{HIGH} (T_I) is determined mathematically as a consequence of T_{LOW} and frequency (generally about 10 breaths/min). P_{HIGH} is often set below the upper inflection point of the pressure–volume (PV) curve or near the plateau airway pressure determined during VACV breaths. P_{LOW} can be set at zero, adjusted based on oxygenation, titrated to be just above the lower inflection point of the PV curve, or raised until V_T falls to 6 mL/kg predicted body weight.

In the absence of spontaneous respiratory efforts, APRV is identical to pressure assist-control ventilation (PACV) (albeit with inspiratory and expiratory times inverted—this is a form of inverse ratio ventilation). The point of APRV, however, is to facilitate spontaneous breathing. This mode allows unrestricted spontaneous ventilation throughout the respiratory cycle, both during T_{HIGH} and T_{LOW}, and these can be PS or SB. This mode was created as a more comfortable means for delivering inverse ratio ventilation and is often used in severe ARDS. There are three downsides to APRV: (a) tidal volume often exceeds values thought to be lung-protective; (b) derecruitment during T_{LOW} could produce atelectrauma; and (c) spontaneous breathing in early, severe ARDS may worsen outcomes [10]. Clinical trials have shown no patient-centered advantages to this mode [11–13].

High Frequency Oscillatory Ventilation

High frequency oscillatory ventilation (HFOV) is an alternative mode of ventilation in which the mean airway pressure (P_{aw}) is held constant while an oscillating pump delivers small tidal volumes at a rapid rate. HFOV has drawn interest in the management of ARDS for two reasons. First, it could be lung-protective by virtue of maintaining high P_{aw} (to keep the lungs open) while superimposing only very small tidal swings (to keep driving pressure and tidal volumes small). Second, the high P_{aw} characteristic of HFOV has the potential to recruit lung alveolar units when PEEP is ineffective, thereby treating refractory hypoxemia.

In HFOV, the clinician sets: P_{aw}, amplitude of the oscillatory pressure, frequency (Hz), bias flow, FiO_2, and inspiratory time. P_{aw} is the primary setting that regulates lung volume and alveolar recruitment so that, in conjunction with FiO_2, it exerts the most control over oxygenation. Amplitude determines the displacement of the piston in the ventilator; this displacement impacts the volume delivered to the patient (the "oscillatory volume"). Empirically, the $PaCO_2$ level correlates inversely with the product of the frequency and the square of the oscillatory volume. Because oscillatory volume (unlike tidal volume during conventional ventilation) is a complex function of amplitude, frequency, and duty cycle, the impact of ventilator changes on gas exchange is not self-evident. For example, reducing frequency tends to lower the $PaCO_2$ because oscillatory volume rises as a consequence, and this secondary effect has a greater impact on CO_2 exchange than the lower respiratory rate.

Two large, prospective, randomized trials compared HFOV to conventional lung-protective ventilation in adults [14,15]. In the first (OSCAR, Oscillation in ARDS) [14], 795 patients were randomized to HFOV (initial settings were P_{aw} 5 cm H_2O above the mean airway pressure at enrollment; frequency 10 Hz) or to conventional ventilation (local usual practice, although pressure-assist control ventilation and tidal volume 6 to 8 mL/kg predicted body weight (PBW) were encouraged). There was no difference in all-cause mortality 30 days after randomization (the primary outcome) or length of stay in the ICU or hospital. In the second trial, 548 subjects were randomized to HFOV (initial P_{aw} 30 cm H_2O, adjusted to oxygenation; frequency 3 to 12 Hz) or conventional ventilation (pressure-assist control, tidal volume 6 mL/kg PBW; high PEEP table) [15]. In-hospital mortality was significantly higher for the HFOV group (47% vs. 35%; $p = 0.005$) causing the study to be terminated early.

Based on these trials, HFOV should not be used routinely in adults. However, both of these studies address whether HFOV confers superior lung protection when used in moderate to severe ARDS, and not whether HFOV has a role as a rescue therapy. If HFOV is chosen as rescue therapy for adults with refractory hypoxemia, careful and serial assessment of fluid balance and right ventricular function is recommended.

Proportional Assist Ventilation

This mode is a form of PSV, but P_I varies throughout inspiration as a function of patient effort. Thus it is effort-triggered, pressure-targeted, and flow-cycled. Proportional assist ventilation (PAV) was created in response to a fundamental limitation of conventional flow- and pressure-targeted modes: ventilatory assistance is not proportional to patient effort. In contrast, PAV amplifies patient instantaneous effort throughout inspiration, leaving the patient in control of V_T, T_I, T_E, and $\dot{V}_I$. The theory behind PAV rests on the equation of motion for the respiratory system, as follows:

$$P_{mus} + P_{ao} = V \times E_{RS} + \dot{V}_I \times R_{RS}$$

where Pmus is the muscular pressure, P_{ao} is the airway opening pressure controlled by PAV, V is volume, E_{RS} is elastance, $\dot{V}_I$ is flow, and R_{RS} is resistance. The ventilator monitors instantaneous rate and volume of gas flow from the ventilator, then varies P_{ao} according to two functions: elastic assist and resistive assist. The clinician determines the degree of assistance, usually set at 40% to 80%. PAV matches the patient's respiratory neural activity very well; and several physiologic studies have suggested better ventilator synchrony with PAV compared to PSV [16–18].

Neurally Adjusted Ventilatory Assist

This novel mode provides a pressure targeted breath in proportion to the electrical activity of the diaphragm (EAdi), measured through microelectrodes built into a nasogastric tube and placed at the level of the diaphragmatic crura. Neurally adjusted ventilatory

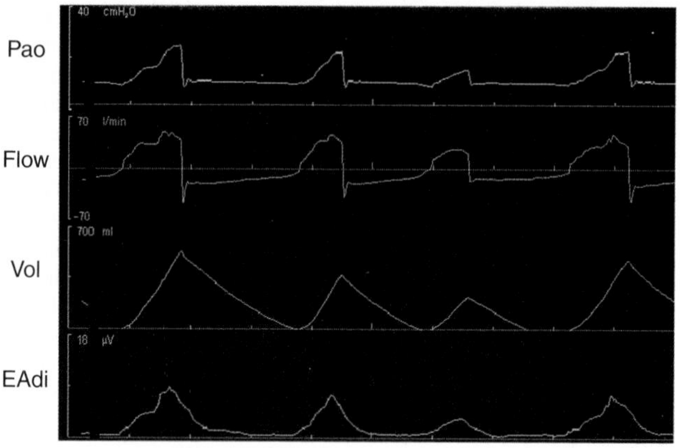

FIGURE 166.9 Neurally adjusted ventilator assist. In this mode, pressure-targeted breaths are delivered in proportion to the electrical activity of the diaphragm (EAdi). The lower part of the panel shows the timing and intensity of the diaphragmatic electrical activity, which determines the timing and intensity of ventilatory assist.

assist (NAVA) is electrically triggered; pressure-targeted; and electrically cycled. The timing and intensity of ventilatory assist is determined by the timing and intensity of the diaphragmatic electrical activity (Fig. 166.9).

$$P_{ao}\text{ (cm } H_2O) = \text{NAVA level (cm } H_2O/\mu v) \times \text{EAdi } (\mu v)$$

The NAVA level is set by the clinician through a titration process of stepwise changes in ventilatory assist. The end of inspiration and opening of the expiratory valve is determined by the EAdi signal reaching 40% to 70% of the peak EAdi. NAVA requires correct positioning of the electrode sensors, normal diaphragmatic anatomy, and intact ventilatory drive and breathing reflexes. The ventilator also has a safety mechanism: it switches to PACV or PSV if EAdi is not detected [19]. NAVA is thought to produce better neuroventilatory coupling than other conventional modes, decreasing the prevalence of ventilator asynchrony, especially for children [20], although the evidence in the adult population is limited [21,22]. A systematic review assessing the effectiveness and safety of NAVA in critically ill patients (adults and children) compared to conventional MV modes is currently underway [23].

Volume Assured Pressure Support

Rapid microprocessors allow ventilators to respond to changing conditions so rapidly that the level of ventilatory support can be changed within a single breath. With volume assured pressure support (VAPS), each breath begins as PS but, if the ventilator calculates that a target tidal volume will not be reached, switches (within that breath) to a VC breath. The clinician sets P_I and a target V_T.

Choosing a Ventilatory Mode

For the majority of ventilated patients, the choice of the ventilator mode is based on physician preference, and probably does not impact clinical outcomes. Indeed, a capable clinician can achieve similar degrees of ventilator support using almost any mode. It is likely more important to emphasize the principles of ventilator-induced lung injury (VILI), ventilator-induced diaphragm dysfunction (VIDD), and patient–ventilator dyssynchrony (PVD) than to focus on ventilator modes [4,5]. Nevertheless, there are some advantages and disadvantages of various available modes.

Advantages for Flow-Targeted Modes

One of the greatest benefits of using flow-targeted modes is that the mechanical properties of the respiratory system are readily apparent (as discussed further below). This is especially true when using constant-flow (square wave) ventilation. Another plus is that it is quite simple to limit tidal volume when one desires lung-protective ventilation, despite changing effort, sedation, and respiratory mechanics.

Advantages for Pressure-Targeted Modes

Pressure-targeted modes allow variable flow and some clinicians feel this enhances patient comfort. A second advantage is that when ventilating patients with severe airflow obstruction, pressure-targeted modes offer a built-in degree of protection against runaway dynamic hyperinflation: if autoPEEP rises while P_I remains constant, the driving pressure falls, lowering minute ventilation and tending to limit hyperinflation.

Positive End-Expiratory Pressure

During expiration, rather than opening the expiratory limb of the ventilator to the atmosphere, a valve is controlled in order to maintain positive pressure. This PEEP is used (a) to reduce the risk of atelectasis; (b) recruit alveoli and raise oxygenation in patients with pulmonary edema; (c) lower the inspiratory threshold load of autoPEEP in patients with airflow obstruction; and (d) reduce left ventricle (LV) afterload in patients with reduced systolic function. PEEP has important effects on the cardiovascular system, discussed below.

Reducing Atelectasis

The simple act of inserting an endotracheal tube lowers FRC, increasing the risk of atelectasis. This may be related to "laryngeal braking," an effect bypassed by the tube. When FRC falls, some lung regions (especially dependent zones) may fall below closing volume, producing resorptive atelectasis. For this reason, nearly all mechanically ventilated patients are given a minimum value of PEEP (usually 5 cm H_2O), sometimes referred to as "physiologic PEEP."

Use in Lung Edema

For patients with ARDS or cardiogenic pulmonary edema, PEEP is often effective for redistributing lung water from the alveolar space to the peribronchial, perivascular cuffs [24], raising FRC, recruiting alveoli, and raising PaO_2. Patients vary greatly in their response to PEEP, however, ranging from dramatic increments in oxygenation to little effect to "paradoxically" reduced PaO_2. The latter may be seen especially in focal consolidations. There is controversy regarding how to set PEEP in ARDS. Some advocate low levels, such as the least PEEP effective in maintaining adequate oxygenation or according to a low-PEEP table. Others argue that higher levels of PEEP are salutary by inhibiting atelectrauma. Clinical data have not resolved this question. Even if higher levels of PEEP are beneficial, there is no consensus regarding how to choose the level: analysis of PV curves, stress index, esophageal manometry, high-PEEP table, or other methodologies [25–30]. This topic is discussed in greater detail in Chapter 30.

In Obstructive Disease

During exacerbations of obstructive lung disease, the end-expiratory P_{alv} typically remains above atmospheric pressure (autoPEEP). This produces an inspiratory threshold load; that is, the patient has to expend significant effort to overcome autoPEEP even before inspiratory flow can be produced. Applying PEEP extrinsically reduces this load, lowering the work of breathing. Externally applied PEEP tends not to raise P_{alv} because the airways often behave like Starling resistors, rather than Ohmic resistors, analogous to waterfalls [31]. Externally applied PEEP set to roughly 75% of the autoPEEP lowers work of breathing usually without raising the degree of hyperinflation [32,33].

LV Dysfunction

PEEP raises mean and end-expiratory P_{pl}, reducing LV transmural pressure as described further below in "Heart–Lung Interaction." For patients with severe LV dysfunction, this effect is meaningful and can be effective when treating pulmonary edema, reducing mitral regurgitant fraction, and augmenting cardiac output. Withdrawal of PEEP can provoke clinical deterioration or weaning failure. This may be one of the reasons that extubation to noninvasive ventilation reduces the risk of extubation failure for patients with a cardiovascular basis for respiratory failure [34,35].

PHYSIOLOGY AND CLINICAL INTERPRETATION OF VENTILATOR WAVEFORMS

Flow and pressure waveforms provide valuable information about respiratory system mechanics and patient–ventilator interaction. Used properly, these signals allow the clinician to garner diagnostic information, customize ventilator settings for the individual patient, and follow the impacts of treatments and time on the underlying respiratory disease. The amount of information obtained depends upon which mode is used to ventilate the patient, as well as whether the patient is actively or passively ventilated [5]. It is easiest to discern the mechanical properties of the respiratory system when VACV is used and flow is constant. Although it is possible to calculate respiratory system resistance and compliance from the flow waveform during PACV, this cannot be done easily or in real time [2]. Expiratory flow is mode-independent, depending on elastic recoil, expiratory resistance, and (unless there is flow limitation) patient effort.

Evaluating Respiratory System Mechanics

When using flow-targeted modes with constant flow, P_{ao} during inspiration reflects the sum of three factors: (a) flow-related (resistive) pressure, P_{resist}; (b) elastic pressure due to lung volume and C_{RS}; and (c) total PEEP. With a few simple maneuvers, the total pressure can be partitioned into these three components, yielding insight into the underlying disease. In most mechanically ventilated patients, inspiratory P_{ao} is elevated above normal values in line with the derangement in the respiratory system. Completely normal ventilator waveforms suggest a mechanically normal respiratory system, such as seen with pure neuromuscular failure, or may reveal that the cause of respiratory failure has resolved or been bypassed (such as when the endotracheal tube relieves major airway obstruction). The following discussion assumes a passive patient, but patient–ventilator interaction is described below.

The peak inspiratory pressure (Ppk) represents the sum of P_{resist} and the elastic recoil pressure due to tidal distention of the respiratory system plus total PEEP. With an end-inspiratory pause, pressure falls from P_{pk} to a plateau (P_{plat}) by an amount equal to P_{resist} (Fig. 166.10). At normal inspiratory flows around 1 L per second, P_{resist} is between 4 and 10 cm H_2O/L/s. Elevated P_{resist} points to bronchospasm, airway edema, or other airway obstruction (tumor, secretion, mucus plugging, or partial endotracheal tube obstruction). It should be emphasized that a decelerating flow profile will lower P_{resist}, masking airflow obstruction.

With P_{resist} known, the remaining pressure (P_{plat}) is the sum of the elastic pressure (P_{el}) related to tidal inflation of the respiratory system and total PEEP. When there is no autoPEEP, total PEEP is simply the set PEEP. Many patients have autoPEEP, however, so this should be sought by examining the flow waveform at end expiration (normally, expiratory flow should taper exponentially toward zero before the subsequent breath). AutoPEEP is present when there is persistent expiratory flow

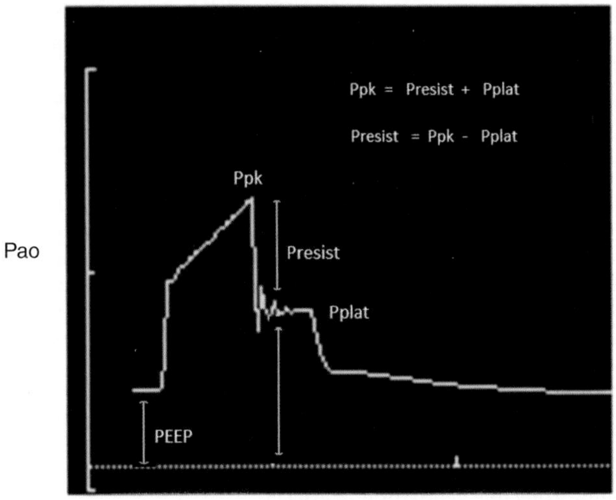

FIGURE 166.10 In passive patients ventilated with constant flow-targeted modes, the airway opening pressure is composed of resistive (Presist) and elastic (Pplat) elements, with the latter also including PEEP (or autoPEEP). An end-inspiratory pause allows the determination of each of these components in the pressure wave curve. Note that pressure rises in two distinct phases: an initial step rise related mostly to the inspiratory resistance (thus very similar to Presist), followed by a more gradual rise related to the respiratory system elastance.

at end expiration (Fig. 166.11). It should also be suspected in the presence of elevated P_{plat}, electromechanical dissociation following intubation, and whenever there is PVD. The most common method to quantify autoPEEP is the end-expiratory port occlusion technique, but this is successful only when patients are passive. Alternatively, one can measure the change in esophageal pressure at the start of inspiration, but this requires an esophageal balloon. The magnitude of autoPEEP is often rather small, only 1 to 3 cm H_2O, and so typically has only a modest impact on measurements of respiratory mechanics. Nevertheless, it can rise to very high values (10 to 20 cm H_2O or even higher) among patients with severe airflow obstruction, as discussed in Chapter 30. In such instances, it is critically important to detect and monitor autoPEEP and to adjust the ventilator accordingly (see below).

The final component of P_{ao} is that required to expand the alveoli against the elastic recoil forces of the lung and chest wall, an amount that depends upon V_T and the C_{RS} (or its inverse, elastance, Ers). This pressure is found by subtracting P_{resist} and total PEEP from Ppk. C_{RS} can be calculated by dividing V_T by

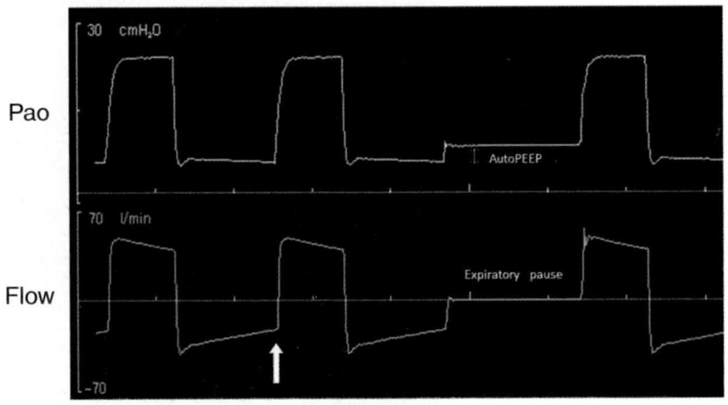

FIGURE 166.11 Pressure assist-control in a patient with airflow obstruction. Appreciate the persistent expiratory flow at end-expiration (arrow) revealing the presence of dynamic hyperinflation and autoPEEP. In passively ventilated patients, autoPEEP can be quantified by the end-expiratory port occlusion technique. At the time a breath is due, the ventilator closes the inspiratory and expiratory ports and withholds the expected breath, reflecting end-expiratory Palv, the autoPEEP pressure.

this pressure; normal values are around 70 mL/cm H_2O. When V_T is 400 mL, the compliance-related pressure should be about 6 cm H_2O (400 mL/70 mL/cm H_2O). Elevated pressures often signal high V_T, lung pathology (atelectasis, pulmonary edema, consolidation, etc.), or chest wall restriction (because of obesity, pleural disease, chest wall deformity, abdominal compartment syndrome, etc.).

A subtle but important feature of the inspiratory P_{ao} during constant-flow breaths is its normally linear rise, implying that C_{RS} is not changing during the breath. The degree of linearity is described by the "stress index" which is equal to 1 when P_{ao} rises in a straight line. If P_{ao} rises with a concave upward shape (stress index > 1), C_{RS} is falling during the breath, possibly revealing overdistention of lung. On the other hand, if P_{ao} rises with a convex upward shape (stress index < 1), C_{RS} is becoming greater during the breath—this may signal inspiratory recruitment (and implying expiratory derecruitment) (Fig. 166.12). This approach is one of many for setting the value of PEEP during lung-protective ventilation of ARDS.

Common disease patterns can be recognized by analyzing the pressure and flow waveforms (Fig. 166.13). The normal respiratory system (assuming a passive patient and typical ventilator settings) shows a P_{pk} of roughly 15 cm H_2O, P_{plat} 10 cm H_2O, P_{resist} 5 cm H_2O (calculated), and PEEP 5 cm H_2O. In addition, the early step-rise in pressure (in the first few milliseconds of the breath) is small (and similar to P_{resist}). Expiratory flow peaks at roughly 60% of the inspiratory flow and declines exponentially, falling to zero before the next breath. The patient with severe airflow obstruction, such as due to status asthmaticus, may have a P_{pk} of 65 cm H_2O, P_{plat} 20 cm H_2O, P_{resist} 45 cm H_2O, and total PEEP 14 cm H_2O. The early step rise in P_{ao} is abnormally large, related both to high P_{resist} and to the presence of autoPEEP. An end-expiratory occlusion will show a value higher than the set PEEP. Expiratory flow is usually very abnormal with low peak expiratory flow rates, a biphasic shape, and low flow rates persisting until end-expiration. Finally, the patient with a restrictive pulmonary process may exhibit P_{pk} of 40 cm H_2O, P_{plat} 33 cm H_2O, P_{resist} 7 cm H_2O, and PEEP 5 cm H_2O. The early step rise in P_{ao} is normal. Expiratory flow is normal to increased and often ceases before the next breath begins.

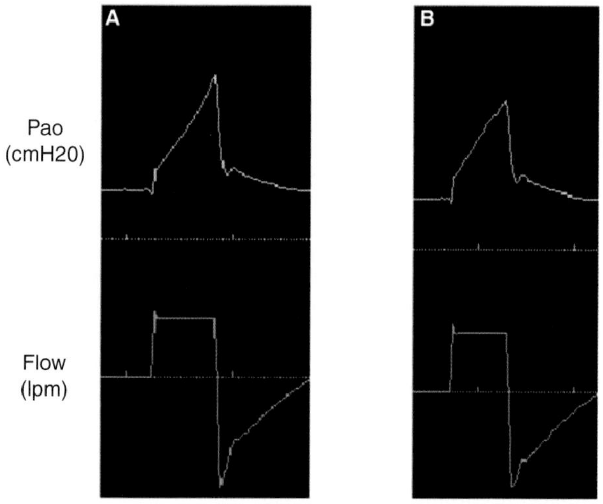

FIGURE 166.12 Volume assist-control ventilation with constant flow. **A:** A stress index > 1 (inspiratory P_{ao} rises with a concave upward shape). **B:** A stress index = 1 (inspiratory P_{ao} during constant-flow breaths rises linearly, signaling that compliance is not varying).

Although pressure-targeted modes are not recommended when seeking mechanical information about the respiratory system, some clues are available nevertheless. When P_{ao} is constant (PC breath), flow falls as alveolar pressure rises. Conditions characterized by a slow rise in P_{alv} because of reduced lung recoil and airflow obstruction (such as emphysema) will show only a very slowly diminishing inspiratory flow rate (Fig. 166.14). In contrast, something like pulmonary fibrosis, in which P_{alv} rises quickly during inspiration, is notable for a rapidly falling inspiratory flow rate. Finally, because expiration is mode independent, the same flow patterns seen during VACV will also be seen during pressure-targeted modes.

PATIENT VENTILATOR DYSSYNCHRONY

Definition

The degree of ventilatory support provided by MV extends from complete support to none. Both extremes of ventilatory support may be associated with structural injury of the respiratory muscles and subsequent muscle dysfunction and failure [36,37]. Thus, current strategies of MV aim to provide enough ventilatory support to achieve efficient gas exchange and match the patient's demand. The ventilator and patient share the ventilatory work, facilitating respiratory muscle recovery with less sedation or muscle paralysis. Ideally, the patient and ventilator should synchronize during the three phases of breath

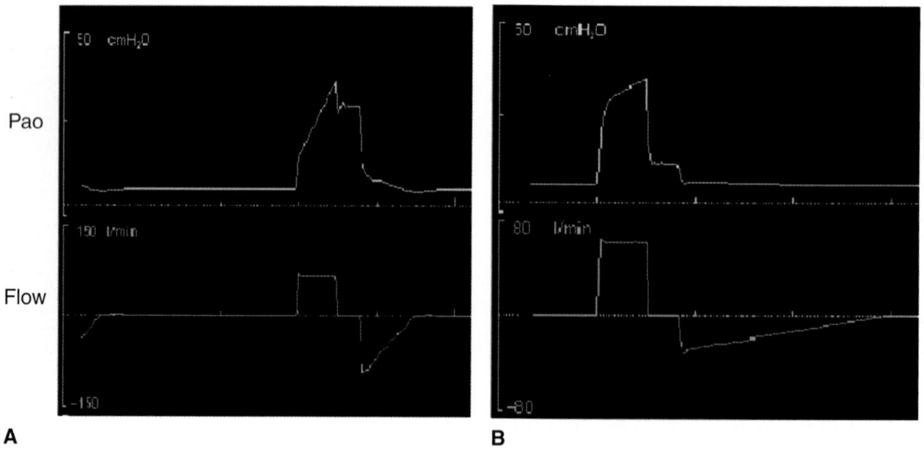

FIGURE 166.13 Volume assist-control ventilation. **A:** A patient with a restrictive pulmonary process: the pressure waveform shows an elevated Ppk and Pplat, while the Presist appears small. The flow waveform shows high expiratory flow that ceases before the next breath begins. **B:** A patient with severe airflow obstruction: the pressure waveform shows an elevated Ppk and Presist while the Pplat appears normal. The flow waveform shows low flow rates throughout expiration. Note also that the early step rise in pressure is much higher in **B**, in accord with the much higher Presist.

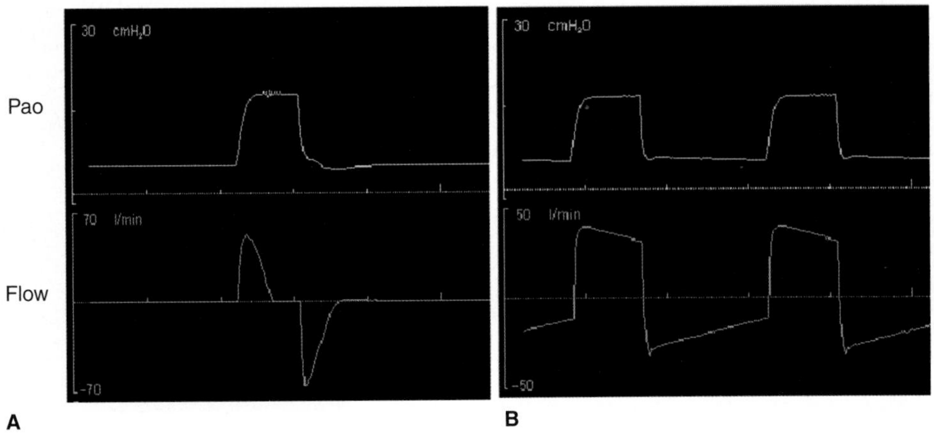

FIGURE 166.14 Restriction versus obstruction during pressure-targeted ventilation. **A:** A patient with a restrictive pulmonary process: the inspiratory portion of the flow waveform falls quickly, because of the rapid rise in Palv. The increased elastic recoil also drives rapid expiratory flow. **B:** A patient with severe airflow obstruction: the inspiratory portion of the flow waveform falls slowly, in line with the gradual rise in Palv. The expiratory flow is slow and prolonged.

delivery: triggering, flow delivery, and cycling off. The lack of optimal interaction is called PVD. This phenomenon results from inadequate or inappropriate ventilator settings (triggering, flow delivery, mode, and PEEP); excessive patient ventilatory drive; the presence of autoPEEP; and other poorly understand factors.

PVD is measured by three different methods: ventilator waveform analysis, esophageal pressure recordings, and electromyography of respiratory muscles, the last two being the most sensitive. Its prevalence can be as high as 80%, and is related to the type of dyssynchrony, ventilated population, method of detection used, the timing and duration of observation, the mode and settings of MV, and the presence of confounders like the degree of sedation [36,37].

Types

PVD can be classified by the phase of the breath in which it is seen but, for many patients, several types are present simultaneously. The origins of and responses to the different types of PVD are described below. Using NAVA greatly enhances synchrony during all breath phases, although any clinical benefits remain to be shown.

Triggering Phase

Ineffective Trigger. Also known as untriggered breath or trigger dyssynchrony. It is the most common form of PVD and refers to a patient's inspiratory effort (increase in transdiaphragmatic pressure or electrical activity of the diaphragm) after which there is no ventilator-delivered breath, or one that is delayed. Ventilator waveforms may show a subtle decrease in P_{ao} not followed by a triggered breath; a change in the slope of exponential decay of the expiratory flow waveform; or transient cessation of expiratory flow during the expiratory phase (Fig. 166.15). Trigger dyssynchrony may result from dynamic hyperinflation, reduced respiratory drive, high levels of PSV, respiratory muscle weakness, or insensitive trigger settings in the ventilator. Ineffective trigger is quite common, especially when autoPEEP is present. Raising the level of ventilator PEEP helps to counter the inspiratory threshold load of autoPEEP, enhancing synchrony. For many patients, however, ineffective trigger is probably not clinically important. It can be reduced by treating autoPEEP or by reducing the P_I during pressure-targeted breaths.

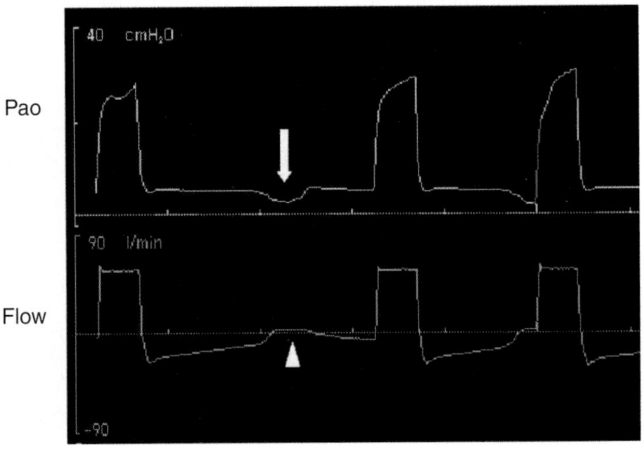

FIGURE 166.15 Ineffective trigger. Ineffective trigger is evidenced in this patient by a subtle decrease in P_{ao} not followed by a triggered breath (arrow) and a transient cessation of expiratory flow during the expiratory phase (arrowhead). Note also that expiratory flow ceases well before the third breath, marking a significant trigger delay (because the inspiratory threshold load of autoPEEP).

Extra-Triggering

a. *Auto-triggering* occurs when the ventilator delivers an unscheduled breath without a patient's effort. It may occur when the triggering threshold is too low, in the presence of circuit leaks or vigorous cardiac oscillations, and related to condensation in the exhalation limb of the ventilator tubing (Fig. 166.16). This form of PVD is readily solved once the source of auto-triggering is recognized. Nevertheless, it can be subtle and has been reported to obscure the diagnosis of brain death.
b. *Double-triggering or extra-triggering* consists of two consecutive inspirations with an interval of less than half of the mean inspiratory time (T_I) (Fig. 166.17). It usually accompanies high respiratory drive, low V_T settings, or when neural T_I exceeds machine T_I. Increasing the level of sedation appears largely ineffective in treating this type of PVD [38]. Raising minute ventilation or V_T can suppress drive, although this may run counter to other goals of MV, especially for patients with ARDS or severe airflow obstruction. Often inserting a brief (e.g., 0.2 second) end-inspiratory pause is effective.
c. *Reverse-triggering* (also called entrainment) [39], refers to the process whereby a machine breath elicits a spontaneous

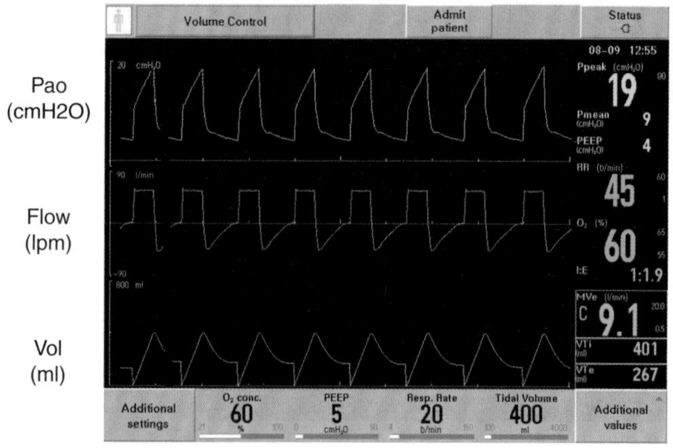

FIGURE 166.16 Auto-triggering. Auto-triggering was recognized in this therapeutically paralyzed patient by the discrepancy between the patient's respiratory rate (45/min) and the one set by the clinician (20). This patient had a circuit leak related to bronchopleural fistula: air lost through the chest tube mimicked the difference in flow between inspiratory and expiratory limbs of the ventilator that would be seen with inspiratory effort. (Note the discrepancy between inspiratory and expiratory tidal volumes). Auto-triggering resolved after switching flow- to pressure-triggering.

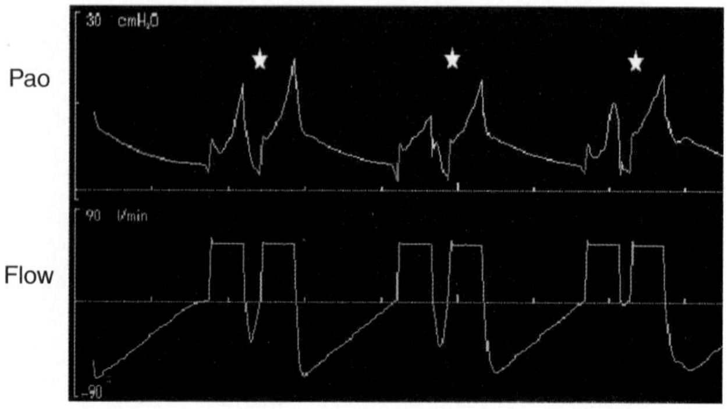

FIGURE 166.17 Double-triggering. Observe the presence of two consecutive inspirations (stars) with an inter-breath interval of less than half of the mean inspiratory time. Because little of each first breath is exhaled before the second breath is triggered, the effective tidal volume may be twice that set by the clinician.

effort, seemingly mediated by vasovagal pathways and mechanical stretch receptors.

Flow Delivery Phase

a. *Flow dyssynchrony* occurs when the delivered inspiratory flow is insufficient to meet the patient's ventilatory demand. This form of PVD is seen only during VA breaths. It can be detected by analyzing the pressure–time waveform, showing a concave appearance toward the Y axis (Fig. 166.18). If V_I is set too low, raising it to the range of 60 L per minute or higher may be effective. Flow dyssynchrony resolves when switching from flow-targeted to pressure-targeted breaths, although this may allow higher than desired tidal volumes.
b. *Excessive flow asynchrony* refers to the delivery of excessive flow, typically to patients with low inspiratory efforts. The rapid onset of flow can provoke discomfort and activate the expiratory muscles. Reducing V_I (flow-targeted breaths) or P_I (pressure-targeted breaths), or setting a rise-time of 0.1 to 0.2 seconds may ameliorate this form of PVD.

Cycling Phase

This type of asynchrony occurs when there is poor matching between machine T_I and the patient (neural) T_I. It can manifest as:

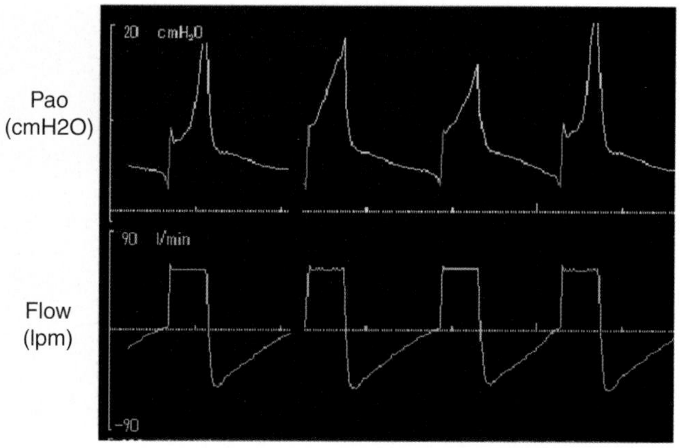

FIGURE 166.18 Volume-targeted mode in an active patient with flow dyssynchrony. Observe the concave appearance toward the Y-axis of the pressure waveform, most evident in the first and fourth breaths.

a. *Premature cycling* (machine T_I < neural T_I) manifested in very early expiration by a downward movement P_{ao} (pressure–time curve during flow-targeted modes) and slowed expiratory flow (flow–time curve). This is often associated with double-triggering (Fig. 166.19).
b. *Delayed cycling* (machine T_I > neural T_I) manifested by an elevation in P_{ao} at end inspiration as the patient recruits expiratory muscles to oppose the ventilator pressure (pressure–time curve and flow-targeted modes) (Fig. 166.20). Following PS breaths, delayed cycling is common (especially in obstructed patients) but difficult to recognize. It may be signaled by the shape of the flow-time waveform, with flow suddenly cycling off rather than gradually declining.

Consequences

Observational studies suggest that PVD is associated with poor outcomes, including longer MV duration, shorter ventilator-free survival, longer length of stay, higher rates of sleep pattern disruption, and lower likelihood of home discharge [18,40–42]. Although a causal relationship between PVD and poor outcomes has not been established, multiple mechanisms are postulated to explain these findings. PVD can compromise alveolar ventilation and gas exchange, worsen alveolar overdistention, and increase the work of breathing. Thus PVD could contribute to VILI, VIDD, intensive care unit acquired weakness (ICU-AW), or patient suffering. Furthermore, these consequences could worsen respiratory mechanics and potentiate further dyssynchrony, perpetuating this

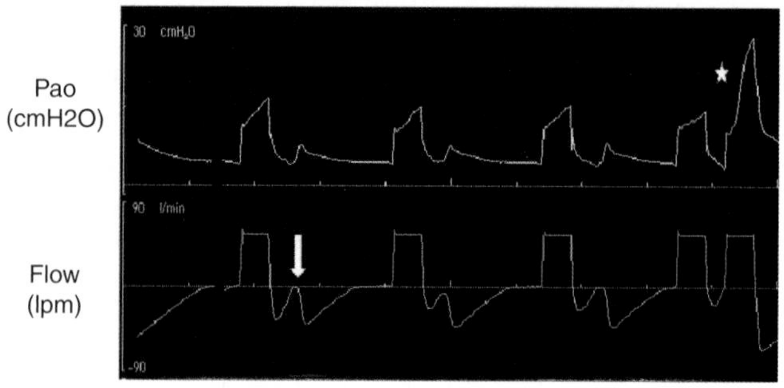

FIGURE 166.19 Premature cycling (machine T_I < neural T_I) in a patient ventilated on volume assist-control mode. Observe how inspiratory effort persists into machine T_E, slowing (and briefly stopping) expiratory flow (arrow). This is often associated with flow dyssynchrony (second breath) and double-triggering as evidenced in the last breath (star).

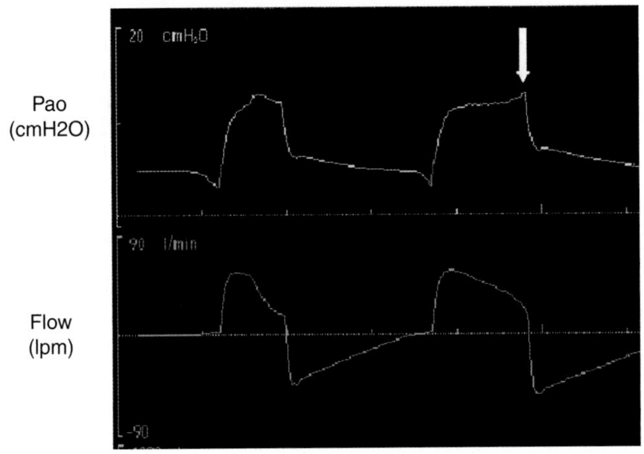

FIGURE 166.20 Patient ventilated on pressure support with delayed cycling (machine $T_I >$ neural T_I). Observe the sudden increase in the airway pressure at the end of inspiration (arrow), caused by expiratory effort from the patient. This can often be ameliorated by raising the flow threshold for breath termination, especially in patients with airflow obstruction.

pathologic process. Finally, PVD is a common indication for the use of higher levels of sedation by ICU physicians, which coupled with the factors mentioned before may increase the length of MV, ICU stay, and perhaps mortality [6,36,43,44].

VENTILATOR-INDUCED LUNG INJURY

Definition

The term VILI refers to the functional and structural alterations that occur in the lung as a direct consequence of MV. VILI usually perpetuates and worsens the damage in injured lungs, but it can also initiate injury in previously healthy lungs, and may lead to multiorgan dysfunction [5,45].

VILI is classified into macroscopic and microscopic injury. Macroscopic injury consists of the presence of extra-alveolar air, and it is commonly referred as barotrauma. It includes pneumothorax, pneumomediastinum, pneumoperitoneum, subcutaneous emphysema, and cystic lung spaces. Peak airway pressure, level of PEEP, tidal volume, minute ventilation, patient–ventilation interaction, lung blood flow, and airway damage have been associated with the development of barotrauma, although this association and the pathogenetic mechanisms behind it remain controversial. Microscopic injury refers to the constellation of histopathologic changes in the lung triggered by MV, including the disruption of the alveolar–capillary barrier, impaired surfactant production, distal airway injury, release of inflammatory mediators, and formation of hyaline membranes and pulmonary edema [5,45].

Pathophysiology

VILI occurs mainly because of the overdistention of lung units by the use of excessive tidal volumes (volutrauma); and the use of low distending pressures that allow repetitive opening and closing of airways and alveoli (atelectrauma). In addition, the release of intracellular mediators from injured cells in response to those forces may promote further damage to the lungs directly or indirectly by activating epithelial, vascular and inflammatory cells that release more injurious molecules (biotrauma). Other factors like body temperature, respiratory acidosis, and pulmonary vasculature pressures may also be relevant to the development of VILI, although their pathologic role appears to be secondary [5,45–49].

Prevention

The transpulmonary pressure, the pressure difference between the alveoli (P_{alv}) and the pleural space (P_{pl}), is the effective alveolar distending pressure and correlates closely with the development of VILI. In conditions where the pleural pressure is nonsignificant (chest wall elastance is normal and the patient is passively ventilated), the transpulmonary pressure relates mainly to the alveolar pressure at the end of inspiration when the airflow is zero (plateau pressure). Thus, restricting plateau pressure is a commonly used strategy to limit the transpulmonary pressure and avoid alveoli overdistention. An alternative (or complementary) hypothesis is that the difference between P_{plat} and PEEP (driving pressure) may be the key determinant of VILI [50].

Using low tidal volumes ($\approx$6 mL/kg of PBW) and limiting P_{plat} to less than 30 cm H_2O has been shown to reduce mortality by 22% in ventilated patients with ARDS, and is currently considered the standard of care in this patient population. A similar approach may also be beneficial in ventilated patients without ARDS [46,51,52]. Higher plateau pressures may be used in patients with poor chest wall compliance. Adequate levels of PEEP that minimize de-recruitment of alveoli and atelectasis may also be beneficial in preventing VILI. However, PEEP can also induce hyperinflation and alveolar overdistention in some patients. Thus, the appropriate level of PEEP has not been determined yet, and it may vary over time during the different stages of lung injury.

Measuring esophageal pressure allows for a more accurate calculation of the transpulmonary pressure to titrate PEEP and plateau pressure; this may improve outcomes in patients with ARDS [26]. Other suggested strategies for setting PEEP include the analysis of the PV curve and the shape of the pressure–time curve during constant flow inflation ("stress index") [53]. Unfortunately, there are insufficient data to support the application of these strategies in routine clinical practice. This topic is addressed more fully in Chapter 30.

Permissive hypercapnia may be a necessary consequence of lung protective ventilation, although it should probably be avoided in patients with intracranial hypertension and perhaps in pregnancy.

Heart–Lung Interaction

The respiratory and cardiovascular systems are closely interconnected. MV affects the circulatory system directly through cyclic changes in the pleural pressure and indirectly by reducing the work of breathing and altering pulmonary vascular resistance. Two important consequences of MV relate to cardiac loading conditions and interpretation of intravascular pressures.

Cardiac Loading

For the passively ventilated patient, both PEEP and tidal inspiration raise Ppl, and these effects are amplified when chest wall compliance is reduced. For the right ventricle (RV), the consequences include reduced preload and increased afterload. In severe ARDS, excessive V_T or PEEP impairs cardiac output, usually by impeding RV ejection (as opposed to dropping preload) [54–56]. Acute cor pulmonale in this population is probably less common than in the past because lung-protective tidal volumes have less impact on the RV. Prone positioning also reduces RV afterload and can boost cardiac output [57]. For the LV, raising the pleural pressure increases preload, reduces afterload, and lessens mitral regurgitation. When LV function is poor, withdrawal of PEEP or MV may be attended by circulatory decompensation.

MV and PEEP also affect the circulation indirectly by improving gas exchange, lowering the work of breathing, and (when PEEP recruits substantially) lowering pulmonary vascular resistance. One of the mechanisms of weaning failure appears to be an inability of the circulatory system to handle the increased demands of spontaneous ventilation [58].

Hemodynamic Interpretation

Because Ppl surrounds the heart, MV, PEEP, and spontaneous breathing alter the pressures measured in all cardiac chambers and the pulmonary circulation. These changes can be dramatic, especially when breathing effort is high or the chest wall compliance is greatly reduced. Because these effects are usually least at end expiration, all vascular pressures should be measured then. End expiration can be readily identified by ventilator waveform analysis. Patients with airflow obstruction often recruit expiratory muscles, artifactually raising end-expiratory Ppl. There is no value in altering the ventilator or reducing PEEP simply to record a "better" value for right atrial or wedge pressure.

Ventilator-Induced Diaphragmatic Dysfunction

VIDD refers to the constellation of histologic, biochemical, and physiologic modifications that occur in the diaphragm as a direct consequence of MV. VIDD may result from diaphragm inactivity, and contributes to weaning failure. VIDD correlates with the duration of MV and seems to be aggravated by sepsis and severity of illness. VIDD appears to be mediated by mitochondrial dysfunction with increase in oxidative stress, and activation of several catalytic pathways (ubiquitin–proteasome, caspases, calpains), which result in diaphragmatic muscle fiber injury and remodeling, decreased contractility, and atrophy. Lysosome-mediated autophagy is also upregulated in the diaphragm of ventilated patients, but this appears to be a beneficial adaptive response to remove the damaged mitochondria and alleviate VIDD [59–69].

Maintaining spontaneous respiratory efforts during MV is associated with decreased VIDD in animal models and in some observational human studies. Furthermore, the use of targeted therapies to block oxidative and catabolic pathways has also been shown to improve VIID in animal experiments. However, the lack of adequate data from human studies precludes the use of these strategies in current clinical practice [70–74].

Ventilator Settings According to Disease Type

Most ventilated patients can be classified into four phenotypes based on the mechanical properties of the respiratory system: (1) Normal gas exchange and respiratory mechanics; (2) ARDS; (3) Significant airflow obstruction; (4) Restriction of the chest wall. The principles underlying ventilator management differ between these groups so that initial settings should be individualized. Subsequently, the clinician should adjust these initial settings according to the patient–ventilator interaction and the respiratory system mechanical properties as revealed by pressure and flow waveform analysis. Thereafter, settings should be further altered as the underlying disease evolves. In addition, a "ventilator bundle," consisting of head-of-bed elevation; daily sedative interruption; readiness testing for spontaneous breathing; and other preventive steps should generally be provided to all ventilated patients.

Normal Gas Exchange and Mechanics

Patients with normal lungs may be ventilated in the perioperative setting; for drug overdose; in the setting of brain injury; or for other neuromuscular crises. These are the easiest patients to ventilate and, when they recover from the procedure or process, most are easily liberated from MV. Principles include achieving relatively normal arterial blood gas tensions and reducing the risk of complications, such as by using the ventilator bundle. Common ventilator settings include any of several modes (VACV, PACV, or, if drive and strength are adequate, PSV); PEEP 5 cm H_2O; FiO_2 0.3 to 0.4; tidal volume of 6 to 10 mL/kg PBW; and inspiratory flow rate 50 to 60 L per minute. Respiratory rate is often set at a value that encourages the patient to initiate breaths if this is clinically appropriate, because this may reduce the risk of VIDD. Periodic assessment of ventilator waveforms facilitates appropriate settings for rate. There is controversy about how much V_T should be limited. An association has been described between lower V_T (e.g., 6 mL/kg PBW) and reduced risk of developing ARDS and improved survival [75].

Acute Respiratory Distress Syndrome

Guiding principles involve providing adequate oxygenation and reducing the risk of VILI by limiting V_T or driving pressure. A large prospective trial showed a significant reduction in mortality simply by ventilating with 6, rather than 12 mL/kg PBW [46]. Whether to use higher or lower PEEP is controversial: any benefit may relate to whether an individual patient has a higher or lower potential for PEEP-induced lung recruitment. A retrospective analysis suggested that driving pressure (P_{plat} – PEEP) was more related to survival than the specific values of V_T and PEEP [50]. Patients ventilated with driving pressure ≤14 cm H_2O had better outcomes.

A consequence of limiting V_T or driving pressure is that some patients will experience hypercapnia. This appears to be well tolerated in adequately sedated patients, although it may be less safe in pregnancy, with intracranial hypertension, and during active myocardial ischemia. For most patients with ARDS, however, the benefits of lower V_T likely outweigh any potential harms from respiratory acidosis.

Typical ventilator settings in ARDS include: V_T 6 mL/kg PBW (best achieved using VACV or PRVC modes); rate 26 to 35 per minute; inspiratory flow rate 50 to 60 L per minute; and increased FiO_2. The preferred level of PEEP remains controversial [76].

Airflow Obstruction

The most important guideline for ventilating patients with severe airflow obstruction is to avoid dangerous degrees of hyperinflation. This is best achieved by limiting minute ventilation to less than 10 L per minute. This will be attended by hypercapnia far more often than in patients with ARDS, but appears safe. The degree of hyperinflation can be monitored by measuring autoPEEP or P_{plat}. PEEP should be used to ease the work of triggering; although 5 cm H_2O is often sufficient, some patients will benefit from values of 10 cm H_2O or higher. Some clinicians prefer pressure-targeted modes because these intrinsically limit the degree of hyperinflation (because hyperinflation tends to reduce V_T), but flow-targeted modes allow control over minute ventilation. Synchrony can be enhanced using NAVA, but no clinical benefit has yet been shown.

Chest Wall Restriction

Chest wall restriction is seen among patients with severe kyphoscoliosis, abdominal compartment syndrome, large ascites, circumferential burns, and massive obesity. The crucial challenge in these patients is that, during passive ventilation, the inspiratory rise in Ppl is proportional to chest wall elastance and V_T. Large tidal volumes risk hemodynamic compromise, so the principles of MV include limited V_T and minimum PEEP. In these patients it may be preferable to use higher fractions of oxygen than to raise PEEP. Although high values for P_{plat} may not signal lung overdistention, they are best avoided nevertheless to prevent cardiovascular effects.

EXTRACORPOREAL LIFE SUPPORT

Introduction

ECLS utilizes an extracorporeal circuit, membrane lung, and (usually) blood pump to support patients with severe respiratory or cardiac failure as a bridge to recovery or to definitive therapy (like organ transplantation). Although a highly complex therapy, recent refinements of circuit design and safety allow ECLS to be carried out in an ICU; sustained for days to months; and supervised by an intensivist and ICU nurse (assisted by an ECLS specialist—nurse or respiratory therapist—in many centers). Simpler, modular circuits facilitate interhospital transfer; transport for diagnostic testing or to the operating room; and mobilization for physical therapy and rehabilitation.

Currently, the most common indication for ECLS in adults is severe ARDS, where it has three major roles: (1) ECLS can be life-saving for catastrophic failure of gas exchange. This was the original concept, but is applicable to only a small proportion of ARDS patients. (2) For patients with ARDS, ECLS may limit VILI by relieving the native lung of the burden of gas exchange; (3) ECLS may facilitate early extubation and mobilization of patients, enhancing recovery and rehabilitation or improving the chances of surviving to transplantation [77]. ECLS plays a lesser role for patients with hypercapnic respiratory failure; postoperative circulatory failure; refractory cardiac arrest; and as a bridge to lung transplantation.

Key Circuit Components

Membrane Lung

The central feature of an ECLS circuit is the membrane lung, sometimes referred to as an oxygenator. This device has a semipermeable membrane separating blood and its cellular elements from the gas phase, while allowing diffusion of oxygen and carbon dioxide. Newer hollow-fiber, polymethylpentene membranes are highly efficient gas exchangers, have a large surface area for diffusion, and present low resistance to blood flow. These characteristics allow rapid blood flow rates using simple, centrifugal pumps, while being compact and reliable. The entire metabolic demand for oxygen can be met easily with a single device the size of a fist. Gas is supplied from wall oxygen or a gas cylinder, through a blender that regulates the fraction of oxygen, directed into the hollow fibers of the membrane, then out an exit port.

Vascular Cannulae

Blood exits and rejoins the circulation through vascular cannulae placed into large, central vessels. The size and location depend upon the mode of ECLS used, as described below. It is these cannulae that largely determine blood flow rates through the entire ECLS circuit, so it is critically important to use a size sufficient to achieve the aims of ELCS. Cannulae can be inserted by three different methods: (1) extrathoracic percutaneous approach by the Seldinger technique, (2) open surgical technique, usually used for cannulation of central arterial vessels, and (3) semiopen cutdown approach, which is a variation of the percutaneous technique, but with direct visualization of the vessel cannulation [30,59]. Dual-lumen cannulae allow both withdrawal and return of blood through a single access site, but fluoroscopic or echocardiographic guidance is recommended for insertion to reduce the risk of major vessel or right ventricular injury.

Blood Pump

Centrifugal pumps have largely replaced roller pumps, a major safety advantage afforded by the low blood resistance of modern membrane lungs. These pumps also are less traumatic to blood elements, producing less hemolysis. Some can be operated by hand in the event of power failure. By adjusting the speed of the pump, the operator controls blood flow rate.

Miscellaneous Components

ECLS circuits incorporate varying degrees of monitoring, often displaying pump speed; blood flow rates; hydrostatic pressures in the blood stream before and after the membrane; and temperature. Sensors may show blood gas tensions and other biochemical data and are used to detect bubbles within the circuit or signal other potential crises. Access points are provided for giving fluids and blood products; sampling blood for laboratory testing; removing air inadvertently introduced into the circuit; infusing heparin; or incorporating renal replacement therapies. A blood warmer is used to prevent hypothermia.

Extracorporeal Life Support Modes and Physiology

There are three conventional modes of ECLS, distinguished by the type of vascular access (venous or arterial) and the organ support provided (pulmonary and/or cardiovascular).

Venovenous (V-V) ECLS: This is the most common modality used for patients with severe respiratory failure. Blood is withdrawn from a large central vein, directed by the pump into the extracorporeal circuit, and returned to the venous circulation. Vascular access can be provided by a two-site approach in which a drainage cannula (23 to 29 Fr) is placed in a central vein, usually the femoral vein, extending to the vena cava. The return cannula (21 to 23 Fr) resides in another central vein (internal jugular or contralateral femoral vein) extending into the right atrium. Even though the cannulae are in separate locations, turbulence in the venous circulation may allow some oxygenated blood to be withdrawn again and sent to the extracorporeal circuit. This process, termed "recirculation" reduces the efficiency of gas exchange.

The single-site approach utilizes a dual-lumen cannula usually placed through the internal jugular vein and extended across the right atrium to the inferior vena cava. Blood is withdrawn through ports situated in both inferior and superior vena caval portions of the cannula, sent to the extracorporeal circuit, and returned through the second lumen into the right atrium where a jet is directed toward the tricuspid valve. When the dual-lumen cannula is well positioned, oxygenated blood passes through the tricuspid valve to the RV, reducing the degree of recirculation. Some degree of recirculation is seen nevertheless, especially if the cannula is positioned poorly or when blood flow rates are high. Other advantages of single-site cannulation are simplicity, fewer sites for vascular injury, and ease of getting the patient out of bed to sit, stand, or walk. On the other hand, these are very large catheters (often 31 Fr).

V-V ECLS is ideal for treating patients with ARDS as long as the native circulation is intact. Because this mode drains and returns equal volumes of blood, it does not directly support the circulation, although delivering highly oxygenated blood to the pulmonary artery may unload the RV when there is hypoxic pulmonary vasoconstriction. For ARDS patients with acute cor pulmonale or other causes of shock, venoarterial (V-A) ECLS is preferred. V-V ECLS readily bears the full oxygenation demand, as long as a sufficient fraction of the cardiac output (roughly 70%) can be captured and directed to the extracorporeal circuit. Thus good cannula positioning and adequate diameter are crucially important for treating ARDS. Arterial saturations are often in the mid-80s to low 90s, which is adequate for maintaining oxygen transport.

V-V ECLS can also emphasize carbon dioxide (CO_2) removal (extracorporeal CO_2 removal, $ECCO_2R$). In fact, the membrane lung is much more efficient at eliminating CO_2 than boosting oxygenation, so that less blood flow is required. For example, a circuit flow of roughly 1 L per minute is sufficient to eliminate the entire volume of CO_2 produced metabolically, meaning that smaller-bore catheters can be employed. V-V ECLS may be suitable for treating exacerbations of COPD or status asthmaticus if its complications (mostly bleeding) are outweighed by those of invasive ventilation. $ECCO_2R$ has also been used in ARDS in order to reduce V_T to 3 to 4 mL/kg PBW to further reduce the risk of VILI, so called "ultra-protective" ventilation.

Venoarterial (V-A) ECLS

This mode is used to provide circulatory support, in addition to oxygenation. Blood is withdrawn from the venous system, passed through the extracorporeal circuit for gas exchange, and returned to the patient's arterial system using the pump to produce sufficient pressure. The drainage cannula (23 to 29 Fr) is usually inserted into the femoral vein extending to the inferior vena cava. The cannula for blood return (17 to 19Fr) is inserted into the femoral artery (ipsilateral or contralateral) extending to the distal abdominal aorta. The returning blood will generate retrograde blood flow in the aorta which can increase the cardiac afterload with negative consequences for the failing heart. To prevent this phenomenon, the blood flow is usually maintained at somewhat lower rates than during V-V ECLS [78].

Unlike during V-V ECLS, blood captured by the withdrawal cannula bypasses the heart and the lungs completely, decreasing cardiac filling pressures and pulmonary blood flow, while maintaining adequate systemic perfusion. There are two peculiarities, however: (a) the systemic blood pressure lacks normal pulsatility unless there is residual native pump function; (b) oxygen saturation varies along the aorta (and its branches) as desaturated blood ejected from the dysfunctional heart mixes with highly oxygenated blood returned to the distal aorta. Thus the coronary vessels, right arm, and head may be supplied with blood much less oxygenated than that seen by the left arm or lower extremities. V-A ECLS is usually used in one of three clinical scenarios: (1) Failure to wean from cardiopulmonary bypass; (2) Biventricular or right heart failure combined with lung failure; or (3) Extracorporeal cardiopulmonary resuscitation (eCPR) [79].

Arteriovenous (A-V) Pumpless ECLS: This mode uses the same principle as venovenous $ECCO_2R$ removal but with a pumpless circuit, using the patient's own blood pressure as a driving force for circuit flow. This is made possible by the low blood flow resistance of polymethylpentene hollow-fiber membranes. The drainage cannula is inserted into the femoral artery extending to the distal abdominal aorta. The cannula for blood return is placed in the contralateral femoral vein. Even with relatively small cannulae, blood flow is sufficient for quite substantial CO_2 removal (although not for oxygenation), averaging about 150 mL per minute, about 75% of metabolic production [77,78].

Supportive Therapies during Extracorporeal Life Support

Mechanical Ventilation

Because ECLS supports gas exchange, the role of the mechanical ventilator is uncertain. Most often, ventilator settings similar to those thought to confer lung protection are chosen: low tidal volume (≤6 mL/kg PBW) or driving pressure (<14 cm H_2O); adequate PEEP (10 to 15 cm H_2O); low FiO_2 (0.3 to 0.4); and very low respiratory rate (6 to 10 breaths per minute) [78,80,81]. Low tidal volume ventilation with low end-inspiratory plateau pressures during ECLS was associated with lower levels of inflammatory biomarkers [82]. Some large observational studies in ECLS patients suggest that lower PEEP and high plateau pressures are associated with higher mortality, despite the use of low tidal volume [80,83].

Anticoagulation

Systemic anticoagulation is used during ECLS to avoid thrombus formation in the circuit, but brief periods off anticoagulation are often tolerated well. Heparin is traditionally employed, but argatroban has been used in patients with heparin-induced thrombocytopenia. Patients are at risk of both thrombosis and hemorrhage during ECLS, making the ideal anticoagulant drug, anticoagulation target, and means of monitoring controversial. Platelet number and function; coagulation proteins; endogenous anticoagulants such as antithrombin-III; and the fibrinolytic system are often abnormal relating to critical illness or ECLS itself. Some have proposed that monitoring with thromboelastography might provide additional insights into how best to reduce the risks of bleeding and clotting.

Mobilization

Critical illness and MV have been associated with ICU-AW and VIDD. Both processes involve complex inflammatory and catabolic muscle pathways that start early in the course of the critical illness, worsen progressively, and persist usually for years [77]. Early mobilization of ventilated patients inhibits catabolic pathways and is associated with improved ventilator-free days; reduced delirium; less risk of ICU-AW and VIDD; decreased length of hospitalization and ICU stay; and lower long-term disability [84]. Despite these benefits, historically most ECLS patients were managed with deep sedation or paralysis to avoid accidental decannulation, bleeding, or limb ischemia [77].

Safer ECLS circuits, increasing use of single-site, dual-lumen cannulae for VV-ECLS, and recognition that deep sedation is often not necessary has decreased the burden of mobilizing patients. Now it is common for patients to sit, stand, and walk while on ECLS [77]. This is especially true of the bridge-to-transplant population who often have single organ failure [77]. Nevertheless, this should only be attempted with a team experienced in mobilizing complex, critically ill patients.

Clinical Evidence and Indications

The first clinical trials comparing ECLS to ventilatory management in adults with ARDS failed to show benefit [85,86]. In retrospect, these trials were doomed by technologic limitations; use of the V-A mode with its attendant higher bleeding risk; and late initiation of ECLS (>9 days) after the ravages of VILI were probably irreversible [79]. The CESAR trial, published in 2009, is the largest randomized, multicenter, controlled trial performed using modern ECLS technology. In this study 180 adults age 18 to 65 with severe respiratory failure were randomized to conventional management at one of several designated hospitals in the UK, versus referral to a specialized center (Glenfield Hospital in Leicester, England) where they received a standardized management protocol (lung-protective ventilation, diuresis, prone positioning, and consideration for ECLS). This study produced new enthusiasm for ECLS when its positive findings were published: patients referred for ECLS had a lower rate of death or disability at 6 months compared to the conventional group (37% vs. 53%; RR: 0.69; 95 CI 0.05–0.97; $p = 0.03$). Despite the positive findings, this trial has important limitations. Of the subjects referred to Leicester, only 76% received ECLS. It is not possible to know whether outcomes were better because of ECLS or because of generally improved care at the referral center (which was more likely to provide lung-protective ventilation and other beneficial treatments) [87].

Subsequently, several observational studies of ECLS for patients with severe respiratory failure, dominated by populations with influenza A (H1N1), gave mixed results [88–90]. Thus, there is no consensus about the role for ECLS and little evidence base for guiding who might benefit from it. A better prediction tool for survival may improve the allocation of ECLS resources. The RESP score (http://www.respscore.com/) has been recently developed using the Extracorporeal Life Support Organization (ELSO) international registry, which includes 2,355 adult patients with severe acute respiratory failure treated by ECLS from 2000 to 2012. This score has been validated in large cohorts and is intended to help clinicians identify patients most likely to survive and benefit from ECLS. The RESP score uses 12 pre-ECLS clinical variables to classify patients into five different classes (I to V) of predicted hospital survival: 92% in class I, 76% in class II, 57% in class II, 33% in class IV, and 18% in class V. A limitation of this score is the lack of inclusion of prone positioning as one of the variables in the calculation of hospital survival probability [91].

Current indications for ECLS promulgated by the ELSO are listed in Table 166.3 [92]. Contraindications include significant comorbidities; advanced age; terminal illness; established VILI; or any condition precluding systemic anticoagulation. Many centers use the exclusion criteria from the CESAR trial: MV with FiO_2 greater than 0.80 and plateau airway pressure above 30 cm H_2O for more than 7 days [77,78].

An ongoing international, multicenter, randomized, and open trial (EOLIA; NCT01470703) will compare the 60-day all-cause mortality between patients treated with lung-protective MV in combination with early ECLS (within 3 to 6 hours after optimal medical management) versus those treated with lung protective ventilation alone. This trial is planning to enroll 331 participants with severe respiratory failure from October 2011 through February 2016.

The use of $ECCO_2R$ is based on limited clinical trial data. In one series of patients with ARDS and worsening hypercapnia, $ECCO_2R$ corrected CO_2 levels rapidly and modestly raised PO_2 [82,93,94]. In a prospective randomized trial, $ECCO_2R$ with ultraprotective ventilation (3 ml/kg) was compared to conventional low-tidal volume ventilation. Although there were no differences of ventilator-free days at 28 and 60 days, a post hoc analysis of patients with $PaO_2/FiO_2 \leq 150$ showed a significant improvement in the number of ventilator-free days at 60 days when treated with the ultra-protective strategy [95]. For patients with hypercapnic respiratory failure due to obstructive lung diseases, small case series show benefits such as early extubation and ambulation [96–98]. The lack of adequate clinical trials in this field precludes the generation of clear guidelines for the use of $ECCO_2R$.

The use of ECLS as a bridge to lung transplantation has been studied in small series with mixed results, and remains controversial [77,78,99,100]. MV preceding lung transplantation is associated with worse survival and higher rates of retransplantation, leading to interest in awake ECLS as a means to avoid MV [101–103]. A single-center, retrospective study using a historical control group suggested higher survival 6 months after lung transplantation among patients treated with awake ECLS versus those receiving MV (80% vs. 50%, $p = 0.02$) [102]. ECLS has been also studied in retrospective series as a rescue therapy for patients developing severe primary graft dysfunction following lung transplantation. These showed improved immediate survival, but mixed results in allograft function and long-term survival [78,104–106]. Early institution of ECLS for patients with lung transplant developing severe primary graft dysfunction may be associated with better outcomes [107].

The evidence supporting V-A ECLS for cardiac support is sparse [77,78]. Limited data suggest a role in refractory cardiac arrest, especially if this can be instituted rapidly [108–110].

Indications for Extracorporeal Life Support for Patients with Respiratory Failure

In the past, ECLS was considered just a rescue therapy for critically ill patients that failed to improve with conventional MV, prone positioning, and inhaled vasodilators. The advances of ECLS technology have decreased the complexity of the circuit and improved the oxygenation efficiency, making the respiratory support provided by MV less necessary. This may allow earlier extubation and liberation from MV, with a potential reduction of sedation use and delirium incidence, as well as an increase in early mobilization. Thus, ECLS may soon be seen as an early intervention that intensivist physicians can incorporate into their armamentarium to treat patients with respiratory failure, and avoid or potentiate adverse events like VILI, delirium, ICU-AW, VIDD, long-term disability, and perhaps even mortality [4]. ECLS should be performed at centers with physicians experienced in its use, and with established protocols. Centers with a higher volume of ECLS procedures have better outcomes. The ELSO recommends that ECLS centers should perform at least six cases per year, and

TABLE 166.3

Indications and contraindications of ECLS in adults with respiratory failure

Indications

1. Severe hypoxemia when the risk of mortality is 80% or greater ($PaO_2/FiO_2 < 150$ on $FiO_2 > 0.9$ and or Murray score 2–3)
2. CO_2 retention on mechanical ventilation despite high P_{plat} (>30 cm H_2O)
3. Severe air leak syndromes
4. Need for intubation in a patient on lung transplant list
5. Immediate cardiac or respiratory collapse (massive pulmonary embolism, airway obstruction, etc.)

Relative contraindications[a]

1. Mechanical ventilation at high settings ($FiO_2 > 0.9$; $P_{plat} > 30$ cm H_2O) for 7 days or more
2. Major pharmacologic immunosuppression (absolute neutrophil count < 400/mm^3)
3. CNS hemorrhage, recent or expanding
4. Nonrecoverable comorbidities, like terminal malignancy or major CNS damage
5. Age: No specific age is contraindicated, but consider increasing risk with increasing age

[a]There are no absolute contraindications to ECLS, and the risk-to-benefit ratio should be evaluated individually for each patient.
CNS, central nervous system; ECLS, extracorporeal life support

ideally 15 to 20 per year. Earlier initiation has also been associated with better outcomes in some observational studies [77,78].

Adverse Effects and Complications

The most common complications associated with the use of ECLS are infections, bleeding, thrombosis, and distal limb ischemia. The rates of complications are higher with V-A ECLS than with V-V ECLS.

References

1. Piquilloud L, Vignaux L, Bialais E, et al: Neurally adjusted ventilatory assist improves patient-ventilator interaction. *Intensive Care Med* 37(2):263–271, 2011.
2. Nassar BS, Collett ND, Schmidt GA: The flow-time waveform predicts respiratory system resistance and compliance. *J Crit Care* 27(4):418 e7–418e14, 2012.
3. Chiumello D, Polli F, Tallarini F, et al: Effect of different cycling-off criteria and positive end-expiratory pressure during pressure support ventilation in patients with chronic obstructive pulmonary disease. *Crit Care Med* 35(11):2547–2552, 2007.
4. Rittayamai N, Katsios CM, Beloncle F, et al: Pressure-controlled vs volume-controlled ventilation in acute respiratory failure: a physiology-based narrative and systematic review. *Chest* 148(2):340–355, 2015.
5. Hall S, Schmidt GA, Kress J: *Principles of Critical Care*. 4th ed. New York, McGraw Hill Education, 2015.
6. Pohlman MC, McCallister KE, Schweickert WD, et al: Excessive tidal volume from breath stacking during lung-protective ventilation for acute lung injury. *Crit Care Med* 36(11):3019–3023, 2008.
7. Brochard L, Rauss A, Benito S, et al: Comparison of three methods of gradual withdrawal from ventilatory support during weaning from mechanical ventilation. *Am J Respir Crit Care Med* 150(4):896–903, 1994.
8. Esteban A, Frutos F, Tobin MJ, et al: A comparison of four methods of weaning patients from mechanical ventilation. Spanish Lung Failure Collaborative Group. *N Engl J Med* 332(6):345–350, 1995.
9. Kallet RH, Campbell AR, Dicker RA, et al: Work of breathing during lung-protective ventilation in patients with acute lung injury and acute respiratory distress syndrome: a comparison between volume and pressure-regulated breathing modes. *Respir Care* 50(12):1623–1631, 2005.
10. Papazian L, Forel JM, Gacouin A, et al: Neuromuscular blockers in early acute respiratory distress syndrome. *N Engl J Med* 363(12):1107–1116, 2010.
11. Emr B, Gatto LA, Roy S, et al: Airway pressure release ventilation prevents ventilator-induced lung injury in normal lungs. *JAMA Surg* 148(11):1005–1012, 2013.
12. Roy S, Habashi N, Sadowitz B, et al: Early airway pressure release ventilation prevents ARDS-a novel preventive approach to lung injury. *Shock* 39(1):28–38, 2013.
13. Andrews PL, Shiber JR, Jaruga-Killeen E, et al: Early application of airway pressure release ventilation may reduce mortality in high-risk trauma patients: a systematic review of observational trauma ARDS literature. *J Trauma Acute Care Surg* 75(4):635–641, 2013.
14. Young D, Lamb SE, Shah S, et al: High-frequency oscillation for acute respiratory distress syndrome. *N Engl J Med* 368(9):806–813, 2013.
15. Ferguson ND, Cook DJ, Guyatt GH, et al: High-frequency oscillation in early acute respiratory distress syndrome. *N Engl J Med* 368(9):795–805, 2013.
16. Costa R, Spinazzola G, Cipriani F, et al: A physiologic comparison of proportional assist ventilation with load-adjustable gain factors (PAV+) versus pressure support ventilation (PSV). *Intensive Care Med* 37(9):1494–1500, 2011.
17. Ranieri VM, Giuliani R, Mascia L, et al: Patient-ventilator interaction during acute hypercapnia: pressure-support vs. proportional-assist ventilation. *J Appl Physiol (1985)* 81(1):426–436, 1996.
18. Bosma K, Ferreyra G, Ambrogio C, et al: Patient-ventilator interaction and sleep in mechanically ventilated patients: pressure support versus proportional assist ventilation. *Crit Care Med* 35(4):1048–1054, 2007.
19. Verbrugghe W, Jorens PG: Neurally adjusted ventilatory assist: a ventilation tool or a ventilation toy? *Respir Care* 56(3):327–335, 2011.
20. Beck J, Emeriaud G, Liu Y, et al: Neurally Adjusted Ventilatory Assist (NAVA) in children: a systematic review. *Minerva Anestesiol* 82(8):874–883, 2015.
21. Carteaux G, Cordoba-Izquierdo A, Lyazidi A, et al: Comparison between neurally adjusted ventilatory assist and pressure support ventilation levels in terms of respiratory effort. *Crit Care Med* 44(3):503–511, 2016.
22. Spahija J, de Marchie M, Albert M, et al: Patient-ventilator interaction during pressure support ventilation and neurally adjusted ventilatory assist. *Crit Care Med* 38(2):518–526, 2010.
23. Patthum A, Peters M, Lockwood C: Effectiveness and safety of Neurally Adjusted Ventilatory Assist (NAVA) mechanical ventilation compared to standard conventional mechanical ventilation in optimizing patient-ventilator synchrony in critically ill patients: a systematic review protocol. *JBI Database System Rev Implement Rep* 13(3):31–46, 2015.
24. Malo J, Ali J, Wood LD: How does positive end-expiratory pressure reduce intrapulmonary shunt in canine pulmonary edema? *J Appl Physiol Respir Environ Exerc Physiol* 57(4):1002–1010, 1984.
25. Brower RG, Lanken PN, MacIntyre N, et al: Higher versus lower positive end-expiratory pressures in patients with the acute respiratory distress syndrome. *N Engl J Med* 351(4):327–336, 2004.
26. Talmor D, Sarge T, Malhotra A, et al: Mechanical ventilation guided by esophageal pressure in acute lung injury. *N Engl J Med* 359(20):2095–2104, 2008.
27. Mercat A, Richard JC, Vielle B, et al: Positive end-expiratory pressure setting in adults with acute lung injury and acute respiratory distress syndrome: a randomized controlled trial. *JAMA* 299(6):646–655, 2008.
28. Meade MO, Cook DJ, Guyatt GH, et al: Ventilation strategy using low tidal volumes, recruitment maneuvers, and high positive end-expiratory pressure for acute lung injury and acute respiratory distress syndrome: a randomized controlled trial. *JAMA* 299(6):637–645, 2008.
29. Goligher EC, Kavanagh BP, Rubenfeld GD, et al: Oxygenation response to positive end-expiratory pressure predicts mortality in acute respiratory distress syndrome. A secondary analysis of the LOVS and ExPress trials. *Am J Respir Crit Care Med* 190(1):70–76, 2014.
30. Valentini R, Aquino-Esperanza J, Bonelli I, et al: Gas exchange and lung mechanics in patients with acute respiratory distress syndrome: comparison of three different strategies of positive end expiratory pressure selection. *J Crit Care* 30(2):334–340, 2015.
31. Tobin MJ, Lodato RF: PEEP, auto-PEEP, and waterfalls. *Chest* 96(3):449–451, 1989.
32. Georgopoulos D, Giannouli E, Patakas D. Effects of extrinsic positive end-expiratory pressure on mechanically ventilated patients with chronic obstructive pulmonary disease and dynamic hyperinflation. *Intensive Care Med* 1993;19(4):197–203.
33. Rossi A, Brandolese R, Milic-Emili J, et al: The role of PEEP in patients with chronic obstructive pulmonary disease during assisted ventilation. *Eur Respir J* 1990;3(7):818–822.
34. Ferrer M, Valencia M, Nicolas JM, et al: Early noninvasive ventilation averts extubation failure in patients at risk: a randomized trial. *Am J Respir Crit Care Med* 173(2):164–170, 2006.
35. Nava S, Gregoretti C, Fanfulla F, et al: Noninvasive ventilation to prevent respiratory failure after extubation in high-risk patients. *Crit Care Med* 33(11):2465–2470, 2005.
36. Epstein SK: How often does patient-ventilator asynchrony occur and what are the consequences? *Respir Care* 56(1):25–38, 2011.
37. Gilstrap D, MacIntyre N: Patient-ventilator interactions. Implications for clinical management. *Am J Respir Crit Care Med* 188(9):1058–1068, 2013.
38. Chanques G, Kress JP, Pohlman A, et al: Impact of ventilator adjustment and sedation-analgesia practices on severe asynchrony in patients ventilated in assist-control mode. *Crit Care Med* 41(9):2177–2187, 2013.
39. Akoumianaki E, Lyazidi A, Rey N, et al: Mechanical ventilation-induced reverse-triggered breaths: a frequently unrecognized form of neuromechanical coupling. *Chest* 143(4):927–938, 2013.
40. Thille AW, Rodriguez P, Cabello B, et al: Patient-ventilator asynchrony during assisted mechanical ventilation. *Intensive Care Med* 32(10):1515–1522, 2006.
41. de Wit M, Miller KB, Green DA, et al: Ineffective triggering predicts increased duration of mechanical ventilation. *Crit Care Med* 37(10):2740–2745, 2009.
42. Delisle S, Ouellet P, Bellemare P, et al: Sleep quality in mechanically ventilated patients: comparison between NAVA and PSV modes. *Ann Intensive Care* 1(1):42, 2011.
43. Leung P, Jubran A, Tobin MJ: Comparison of assisted ventilator modes on triggering, patient effort, and dyspnea. *Am J Respir Crit Care Med* 155(6):1940–1948, 1997.
44. Vitacca M, Bianchi L, Zanotti E, et al: Assessment of physiologic variables and subjective comfort under different levels of pressure support ventilation. *Chest* 126(3):851–859, 2004.
45. Slutsky AS, Ranieri VM: Ventilator-induced lung injury. *N Engl J Med* 369(22):2126–2136, 2013.
46. The Acute Respiratory Distress Syndrome Network. Ventilation with lower tidal volumes as compared with traditional tidal volumes for acute lung injury and the acute respiratory distress syndrome. *N Engl J Med* 342(18):1301–1308, 2000.
47. Bilek AM, Dee KC, Gaver DP 3rd: Mechanisms of surface-tension-induced epithelial cell damage in a model of pulmonary airway reopening. *J Appl Physiol (1985)* 94(2):770–783, 2003.
48. Dreyfuss D, Soler P, Basset G, et ak: High inflation pressure pulmonary edema. Respective effects of high airway pressure, high tidal volume, and positive end-expiratory pressure. *Am Rev Respir Dis* 137(5):1159–1164, 1988.
49. Webb HH, Tierney DF: Experimental pulmonary edema due to intermittent positive pressure ventilation with high inflation pressures. Protection by positive end-expiratory pressure. *Am Rev Respir Dis* 110(5):556–565, 1974.
50. Amato MB, Meade MO, Slutsky AS, et al: Driving pressure and survival in the acute respiratory distress syndrome. *N Engl J Med* 372(8):747–755, 2015.
51. Serpa Neto A, Cardoso SO, Manetta JA, et al: Association between use of lung-protective ventilation with lower tidal volumes and clinical outcomes among patients without acute respiratory distress syndrome: a meta-analysis. *JAMA* 308(16):1651–1659, 2012.
52. Guay J, Ochroch EA: Intraoperative use of low volume ventilation to decrease postoperative mortality, mechanical ventilation, lengths of stay and lung injury in patients without acute lung injury. *Cochrane Database Syst Rev* (12):CD011151, 2015.
53. Hata JS, Togashi K, Kumar AB, et al: The effect of the pressure-volume curve for positive end-expiratory pressure titration on clinical outcomes in acute respiratory distress syndrome: a systematic review. *J Intensive Care Med* 29(6):348–356, 2014.
54. Fougeres E, Teboul JL, Richard C, et al: Hemodynamic impact of a positive end-expiratory pressure setting in acute respiratory distress syndrome: importance of the volume status. *Crit Care Med* 38(3):802–807, 2010.

55. Schmitt JM, Vieillard-Baron A, Augarde R, et al: Positive end-expiratory pressure titration in acute respiratory distress syndrome patients: impact on right ventricular outflow impedance evaluated by pulmonary artery Doppler flow velocity measurements. *Crit Care Med* 29(6):1154–1158, 2001.
56. Gernoth C, Wagner G, Pelosi P, et al: Respiratory and haemodynamic changes during decremental open lung positive end-expiratory pressure titration in patients with acute respiratory distress syndrome. *Crit Care* 13(2):R59, 2009.
57. Jozwiak M, Teboul JL, Anguel N, et al: Beneficial hemodynamic effects of prone positioning in patients with acute respiratory distress syndrome. *Am J Respir Crit Care Med* 188(12):1428–1433, 2013.
58. Jubran A, Mathru M, Dries D, et ak: Continuous recordings of mixed venous oxygen saturation during weaning from mechanical ventilation and the ramifications thereof. *Am J Respir Crit Care Med* 1998;158(6):1763–1769.
59. Levine S, Nguyen T, Taylor N, et al: Rapid disuse atrophy of diaphragm fibers in mechanically ventilated humans. *N Engl J Med* 358(13):1327–1335, 2008.
60. Jaber S, Petrof BJ, Jung B, et al: Rapidly progressive diaphragmatic weakness and injury during mechanical ventilation in humans. *Am J Respir Crit Care Med* 183(3):364–371, 2011.
61. Vassilakopoulos T, Zakynthinos S, Roussos C: The tension-time index and the frequency/tidal volume ratio are the major pathophysiologic determinants of weaning failure and success. *Am J Respir Crit Care Med* 158(2):378–385, 1998.
62. Kim WY, Suh HJ, Hong SB, et al: Diaphragm dysfunction assessed by ultrasonography: influence on weaning from mechanical ventilation. *Crit Care Med* 39(12):2627–2630, 2011.
63. Hermans G, Agten A, Testelmans D, et al: Increased duration of mechanical ventilation is associated with decreased diaphragmatic force: a prospective observational study. *Crit Care* 14(4):R127, 2010.
64. Demoule A, Jung B, Prodanovic H, et al: Diaphragm dysfunction on admission to the intensive care unit. Prevalence, risk factors, and prognostic impact-a prospective study. *Am J Respir Crit Care Med* 188(2):213–219, 2013.
65. Jung B, Nougaret S, Conseil M, et al: Sepsis is associated with a preferential diaphragmatic atrophy: a critically ill patient study using tridimensional computed tomography. *Anesthesiology* 120(5):1182–1191, 2014.
66. Hooijman PE, Beishuizen A, Witt CC, et al: Diaphragm muscle fiber weakness and ubiquitin-proteasome activation in critically ill patients. *Am J Respir Crit Care Med* 191(10):1126–1138, 2015.
67. Picard M, Jung B, Liang F, et al: Mitochondrial dysfunction and lipid accumulation in the human diaphragm during mechanical ventilation. *Am J Respir Crit Care Med* 186(11):1140–1149, 2012.
68. Azuelos I, Jung B, Picard M, et al: Relationship between autophagy and ventilator-induced diaphragmatic dysfunction. *Anesthesiology* 122(6): 1349–1361, 2015.
69. Petrof BJ, Hussain SN: Ventilator-induced diaphragmatic dysfunction: what have we learned? *Curr Opin Crit Care* 22(1):67–72, 2016.
70. Ge H, Xu P, Zhu T, et al: High-level pressure support ventilation attenuates ventilator-induced diaphragm dysfunction in rabbits. *Am J Med Sci* 350(6): 471–478, 2015.
71. Hudson MB, Smuder AJ, Nelson WB, et al: Partial support ventilation and mitochondrial-targeted antioxidants protect against ventilator-induced decreases in diaphragm muscle protein synthesis. *PLoS One* 10(9):e0137693, 2015.
72. Goligher EC, Fan E, Herridge MS, et al: Evolution of diaphragm thickness during mechanical ventilation. impact of inspiratory effort. *Am J Respir Crit Care Med* 2015;192(9):1080–1088.
73. Kwon OS, Smuder AJ, Wiggs MP, et al: AT1 receptor blocker losartan protects against mechanical ventilation-induced diaphragmatic dysfunction. *J Appl Physiol (1985)* 2015;119(10):1033–10341, 2015.
74. Powers SK, Hudson MB, Nelson WB, et al: Mitochondria-targeted antioxidants protect against mechanical ventilation-induced diaphragm weakness. *Crit Care Med* 39(7):1749–1759, 2011.
75. Gajic O, Frutos-Vivar F, Esteban A, et al: Ventilator settings as a risk factor for acute respiratory distress syndrome in mechanically ventilated patients. *Intensive Care Med* 31(7):922–926, 2005.
76. Schmidt GA: Counterpoint: should positive end-expiratory pressure in patients with ARDS be set based on oxygenation? No. *Chest* 141(6):1382–1384; discussion 4–6, 2012.
77. al SGAe: *Extracoporeal Life Support for Adults*. Berlin: Springer; 2016.
78. Ventetuolo CE, Muratore CS: Extracorporeal life support in critically ill adults. *Am J Respir Crit Care Med* 190(5):497–508, 2014.
79. Blum JM, Lynch WR, Coopersmith CM: Clinical and billing review of extracorporeal membrane oxygenation. *Chest* 147(6):1697–1703, 2015.
80. Marhong JD, Munshi L, Detsky M, et al: Mechanical ventilation during extracorporeal life support (ECLS): a systematic review. *Intensive Care Med* 41(6):994–1003, 2015.
81. Marhong JD, Telesnicki T, Munshi L, et al: Mechanical ventilation during extracorporeal membrane oxygenation. An international survey. *Ann Am Thorac Soc* 11(6):956–961, 2014.
82. Terragni PP, Del Sorbo L, Mascia L, et al: Tidal volume lower than 6 ml/kg enhances lung protection: role of extracorporeal carbon dioxide removal. *Anesthesiology* 111(4):826–835, 2009.
83. Schmidt M, Stewart C, Bailey M, et al: Mechanical ventilation management during extracorporeal membrane oxygenation for acute respiratory distress syndrome: a retrospective international multicenter study. *Crit Care Med* 43(3):654–664, 2015.
84. Schweickert WD, Pohlman MC, Pohlman AS, et al: Early physical and occupational therapy in mechanically ventilated, critically ill patients: a randomised controlled trial. *Lancet* 373(9678):1874–1882, 2009.
85. Zapol WM, Snider MT, Hill JD, et al: Extracorporeal membrane oxygenation in severe acute respiratory failure. A randomized prospective study. *JAMA* 242(20):2193–2196, 1979.
86. Morris AH, Wallace CJ, Menlove RL, et al: Randomized clinical trial of pressure-controlled inverse ratio ventilation and extracorporeal CO_2 removal for adult respiratory distress syndrome. *Am J Respir Crit Care Med* 149 (2, pt 1):295–305, 1994.
87. Peek GJ, Mugford M, Tiruvoipati R, et al: Efficacy and economic assessment of conventional ventilatory support versus extracorporeal membrane oxygenation for severe adult respiratory failure (CESAR): a multicentre randomised controlled trial. *Lancet* 374(9698):1351–1363, 2009.
88. Noah MA, Peek GJ, Finney SJ, et al: Referral to an extracorporeal membrane oxygenation center and mortality among patients with severe 2009 influenza A(H1N1). *JAMA* 306(15):1659–1668, 2011.
89. Australia, New Zealand Extracorporeal Membrane Oxygenation Influenza I, Davies A, Jones D, Bailey M, Beca J, et al: Extracorporeal Membrane Oxygenation for 2009 Influenza A(H1N1) Acute Respiratory Distress Syndrome. *JAMA* 2009;302(17):1888–1895, 2011.
90. Pham T, Combes A, Roze H, et al: Extracorporeal membrane oxygenation for pandemic influenza A(H1N1)-induced acute respiratory distress syndrome: a cohort study and propensity-matched analysis. *Am J Respir Crit Care Med* 187(3):276–285, 2013.
91. Schmidt M, Bailey M, Sheldrake J, et al: Predicting survival after extracorporeal membrane oxygenation for severe acute respiratory failure. The Respiratory Extracorporeal Membrane Oxygenation Survival Prediction (RESP) score. *Am J Respir Crit Care Med* 189(11):1374–1382, 2014.
92. ELSO Guidelines for the Use of ECLS in Adult Respiratory Failure. 2013. Available at http://www.elso.org/Portals/0/IGD/Archive/FileManager/989d4d4d14cusersshyerdocumentselsoguidelinesforadultrespiratoryfailure1.3.pdf
93. Batchinsky AI, Jordan BS, Regn D, et al: Respiratory dialysis: reduction in dependence on mechanical ventilation by venovenous extracorporeal CO_2 removal. *Crit Care Med* 39(6):1382–1387, 2011.
94. Bein T, Weber F, Philipp A, et al: A new pumpless extracorporeal interventional lung assist in critical hypoxemia/hypercapnia. *Crit Care Med* 34(5):1372–1377, 2006.
95. Bein T, Weber-Carstens S, Goldmann A, et al: Lower tidal volume strategy (approximately 3 ml/kg) combined with extracorporeal CO_2 removal versus 'conventional' protective ventilation (6 ml/kg) in severe ARDS: the prospective randomized Xtravent-study. *Intensive Care Med* 39(5):847–856, 2013.
96. Burki NK, Mani RK, Herth FJ, et al: A novel extracorporeal CO(2) removal system: results of a pilot study of hypercapnic respiratory failure in patients with COPD. *Chest* 143(3):678–686, 2013.
97. Abrams DC, Brenner K, Burkart KM, et al: Pilot study of extracorporeal carbon dioxide removal to facilitate extubation and ambulation in exacerbations of chronic obstructive pulmonary disease. *Ann Am Thorac Soc* 10(4): 307–314, 2013.
98. Kluge S, Braune SA, Engel M, et al: Avoiding invasive mechanical ventilation by extracorporeal carbon dioxide removal in patients failing noninvasive ventilation. *Intensive Care Med* 38(10):1632–1639, 2012.
99. Del Sorbo L, Ranieri VM, Keshavjee S: Extracorporeal membrane oxygenation as "bridge" to lung transplantation: what remains in order to make it standard of care? *Am J Respir Crit Care Med* 185(7):699–701, 2012.
100. Dellgren G, Riise GC, Sward K, et al: Extracorporeal membrane oxygenation as a bridge to lung transplantation: a long-term study. *Eur J Cardiothorac Surg* 47(1):95–100; discussion, 2015.
101. Nosotti M, Rosso L, Tosi D, et al: Extracorporeal membrane oxygenation with spontaneous breathing as a bridge to lung transplantation. *Interact Cardiovasc Thorac Surg* 16(1):55–59, 2013.
102. Fuehner T, Kuehn C, Hadem J, et al: Extracorporeal membrane oxygenation in awake patients as bridge to lung transplantation. *Am J Respir Crit Care Med* 185(7):763–768, 2012.
103. Olsson KM, Simon A, Strueber M, et al: Extracorporeal membrane oxygenation in nonintubated patients as bridge to lung transplantation. *Am J Transplant* 10(9):2173–2178, 2010.
104. Hartwig MG, Walczak R, Lin SS, et al: Improved survival but marginal allograft function in patients treated with extracorporeal membrane oxygenation after lung transplantation. *Ann Thorac Surg* 93(2):366–371, 2012.
105. Fischer S, Bohn D, Rycus P, et al: Extracorporeal membrane oxygenation for primary graft dysfunction after lung transplantation: analysis of the Extracorporeal Life Support Organization (ELSO) registry. *J Heart Lung Transplant* 26(5):472–477, 2007.
106. Bermudez CA, Adusumilli PS, McCurry KR, et al: Extracorporeal membrane oxygenation for primary graft dysfunction after lung transplantation: long-term survival. *Ann Thorac Surg* 87(3):854–860, 2009.
107. Fiser SM, Kron IL, McLendon Long S, et al: Early intervention after severe oxygenation index elevation improves survival following lung transplantation. *J Heart Lung Transplant* 20(6):631–636, 2001.
108. Haneya A, Philipp A, Diez C, et al: A 5-year experience with cardiopulmonary resuscitation using extracorporeal life support in non-postcardiotomy patients with cardiac arrest. *Resuscitation* 83(11):1331–1337, 2012.
109. Wu MY, Lee MY, Lin CC, et al: Resuscitation of non-postcardiotomy cardiogenic shock or cardiac arrest with extracorporeal life support: the role of bridging to intervention. *Resuscitation* 83(8):976–981, 2012.
110. Chen YS, Lin JW, Yu HY, et al: Cardiopulmonary resuscitation with assisted extracorporeal life-support versus conventional cardiopulmonary resuscitation in adults with in-hospital cardiac arrest: an observational study and propensity analysis. *Lancet* 372(9638):554–561, 2008.

Chapter 167 ■ Mechanical Ventilation—Part II: Non-Invasive Mechanical Ventilation for the Adult Hospitalized Patient

NICHOLAS S. HILL

INTRODUCTION

Noninvasive ventilation (NIV) is the provision of mechanical ventilation without the need for an invasive artificial airway. NIV can be subdivided into a number of modalities with different mechanisms of action, including negative pressure ventilation that assists lung expansion by applying an intermittent negative pressure over the chest and abdomen, positive pressure ventilation that applies continuous or intermittent positive pressure to the upper airway, and abdominal displacement ventilators like pneumobelts and rocking beds that assist ventilation at least partly via the force of gravity on the abdominal contents [1–3]. Over the past two decades, noninvasive positive pressure ventilation (NPPV) [4] via the nose, mouth, or combination has become the predominant mode of NIV in both the outpatient and hospital settings, and henceforth will be referred to as "NIV" or "NPPV". In this chapter, we focus on acute applications, comparing and contrasting noninvasive and invasive approaches and describing epidemiologic trends of NIV. Next, we describe the equipment used for NIV and discuss indications and selection of patients for NIV in acute care settings. We then make recommendations regarding the practical and safe application of NIV, including selecting the proper location, appropriate monitoring, and avoiding complications. Finally, we consider the possible impact of newer approaches including high-flow nasal therapy (HFNT) and extracorporeal CO_2 removal ($ECCO_2R$) techniques.

TERMINOLOGY

As used in this chapter, NIV is a generic term for a number of different noninvasive approaches to assisting ventilation, whereas NPPV refers specifically to the form that facilitates ventilation by applying a positive pressure to the upper airway. This can be continuous positive airway pressure (CPAP) that can be used to successfully treat certain forms of respiratory failure or intermittent, combining a positive end-expiratory pressure (PEEP) with pressure support (PS) ventilation, the latter used to actively assist inspiration. Some ventilators are derived from portable positive pressure devices to treat sleep apnea and are commonly referred to as bilevel positive airway pressure (BPAP) devices. With these, the term expiratory positive airway pressure (EPAP) is used rather than PEEP and inspiratory positive airway pressure (IPAP) refers to the total inspiratory pressure. Thus, the difference between IPAP and EPAP equals the level of pressure support.

WHY NONINVASIVE MECHANICAL VENTILATION?

NIV has seen increasing popularity in acute care settings throughout Europe and the United States over the past two decades [5,6]. This trend is related to a number of advantages of NIV over invasive mechanical ventilation (IMV), but only for selected patients. By averting invasion of the upper airway, NIV avoids a number of well-known complications of intubation, including aspiration of gastric contents, dental trauma, trauma to the hypopharynx, larynx, and trachea including tracheal rupture [7], hypoglossal nerve paralysis, stimulation of the autonomic nervous system leading to arrhythmias, and hypotension [8]. Ongoing use of invasive ventilation increases the risk of ventilator-associated pneumonia (VAP) related to disruption of airway protective mechanisms, pooling of secretions above the tube cuff that leak into the lower airways, and formation of a bacterial biofilm within the tube that is distributed peripherally during suctioning. In addition, irritation from the tube stimulates mucus secretion and interferes with normal ciliary function. The need for repeated suctioning further traumatizes the airway and promotes bleeding and mucus secretion. Following extubation, immediate complications can include upper airway obstruction due to glottic swelling, negative pressure pulmonary edema, tracheal hemorrhage, and laryngospasm [9,10]. Complications of prolonged invasive ventilation (in association with tracheostomy) can include a spectrum of repeated airway and parenchymal infections, vocal cord dysfunction, tracheal stenosis, or malacia [4,11–13].

In addition, NIV is usually better tolerated than invasive ventilation, requiring less or no sedation. It usually permits short breaks that help to enhance tolerance. The avoidance of intubation-associated complications and sedation promotes more rapid weaning compared to invasive ventilation, shortening intensive care unit (ICU) stays and potentially reducing resource utilization and costs. On the other hand, NIV should not be considered as a replacement for IMV. When used appropriately, NIV serves as a way to avoid intubation and its attendant complications, but it must be used selectively, avoiding patients who have contraindications (see "Selection Guidelines for NIV in Acute Respiratory Failure" section). Appropriate candidates must be able to protect their airways and cooperate. Sometimes, NPPV is initiated for inappropriate or marginal candidates who fail to respond favorably. In this situation, it is important to intubate promptly, avoiding delays that can lead to cardiopulmonary arrest, necessitating emergency intubation and increased morbidity and mortality [14].

UTILIZATION AND EPIDEMIOLOGY

Rates of NIV utilization in acute care settings have increased in Europe and North America [15,16]. An observational study of NIV utilization for chronic obstructive pulmonary disease (COPD) and cardiogenic pulmonary edema (CPE) patients with acute respiratory failure (ARF) at a single 26-bed French ICU revealed an increase from 20% of ventilator starts in 1994 to nearly 90% in 2001 [15]. In association with this increase, the occurrence of health care–acquired pneumonias and ICU mortality fell from 20% and 21% to 8% and 7%, respectively. The authors speculated that increasing experience and skill with NPPV in their units contributed to the improved outcomes. In a US study examining utilization and outcomes of NPPV in 8 Massachusetts hospitals during 2004 to 2007, overall use of NIV as a percent of ventilator starts was 38.5% with a success rate of 73.9%. For ARF due to COPD exacerbation, use was 82.2% with a success rate of 75.7%, and for pneumonia, use and success rates were 41.4% and 47.2%, respectively [16]. This represents a substantial increase over prior surveys. Chandra et al. [6], using the US National Inpatient Sample of patient admissions, identified over 7.5 million COPD admissions during the years 1998 to 2008 and noted a 462% increase of the use of

NIV and a concomitant 42% decline for the use of IMV. These trends are apparent throughout the world. Esteban et al. have conducted worldwide prospective 1 month surveys from 40 countries that compared the trends of mechanical ventilation use and outcomes between 1998, 2004 and 2010, enrolling more than 18,000 patients. During this time period, the surveys showed a nearly threefold increase in percent NIV ventilator starts (5% to 14%) and a reduction of overall mortality of ventilated patients (31% to 28%) [17].

In the past, several studies reported variable use of NIV depending on the hospital. A 2003 national audit of COPD exacerbations in the United Kingdom revealed that NIV was unavailable 39% of ICUs and 36% of "high-dependency units" [18]. Similar results were seen by a North American survey of NIV use showing an estimated usage rate of 20% overall, but 30% of hospitals had estimated rates <15%. Reasons for low utilization were mostly attributed to lack of physician knowledge of NIV, inadequate equipment, and lack of staff training. Most disturbingly, estimated use of NIV for COPD exacerbations and CPE was only 29% and 39% of ventilator starts, respectively [19]. Even more disturbing, a Korean survey reported that NIV was used in just 2 of 24 university hospitals and comprised only 4% of ventilator starts. A majority of the physician staff (62%) and 42% of the nurses expressed a desire for additional educational programs on NIV [20].

Analyses of large databases have been helpful for highlighting these trends of increasing use of NIV. Using the Premier database consisting of 420 US hospitals, Lindenauer et al. [21] found that among 25,628 COPD patients, 70% were initially treated with NIV and 30% with IMV. Fifteen percent of patients who were initially treated with NIV later required IMV, indicative of NIV failure. Stefan et al. [22] using the same database for the years 2001 to 2011 observed a 15.1% annual increase in use of NIV for COPD patients and a 3.2% annual decrease of the use of IMV. NIV was used for a greater proportion of older patients (>85 years) than for those <65 years of age. Similar trends toward increased NIV use have been reported for patients with non-COPD diagnoses [22], raising the possibility of overzealous use of NIV for some of these patients. The observation by several investigators that mortality of NIV failures exceeds that of patients intubated in the first place also raises the possibility of overzealous use [6,22].

INDICATIONS FOR ACUTE APPLICATIONS OF NPPV

Indications for NIV depend on the etiology of ARF and specific settings in which ARF occurs (i.e., do-not-intubate [DNI] patients). As much as possible, our analysis is based on available evidence. We recommend application of NIV for those diagnoses that are those supported by multiple randomized trials. We consider NIV as an "option" when the application is supported by a single randomized trial, multiple historically controlled or cohort series, or evidence is not consistent. Successful application of NIV has been reported for all of these indications when applied for appropriately selected and monitored patients (Table 167.1).

TABLE 167.1

Indications for Noninvasive Positive Pressure Ventilation as Determined by Strength of Evidence

Recommended (supported by strong evidence[a])
COPD exacerbations
COPD—failure to wean from invasive mechanical ventilation
Acute cardiogenic pulmonary edema
Option (supported by weaker evidence[b])
Other obstructive airway diseases with acute respiratory failure
Asthma exacerbation
Cystic fibrosis
Immunosuppressed patients with acute respiratory failure
Hypoxemic respiratory failure[c]
ALI/ARDS (carefully selected patients)
Community-acquired pneumonia
Trauma
Extubation failure
Mainly patients with COPD or CHF
Postoperative respiratory failure
Prophylactic use of CPAP or "bilevel" after high-risk surgeries
Treatment of acute respiratory failure—mainly COPD or CHF
Do-not-intubate patients
To treat acute respiratory failure (COPD or CHF)
To palliate for relief of dyspnea or extend survival to settle affairs
Obesity hypoventilation
Neuromuscular disease
Partial upper airway obstruction (postextubation)
Not recommended
ALI/ARDS with multiorgan system dysfunction or hypotensive shock
End-stage pulmonary fibrosis with exacerbation
Total or near total upper airway obstruction

[a]Strong evidence refers to multiple randomized controlled trials and meta-analyses.
[b]Weaker evidence refers to mainly case series, case-matched series, single randomized trials, or some conflicting data.
[c]Must be monitored very carefully—not a routine indication.
ALI/ARDS, acute lung injury/acute respiratory distress syndrome; COPD, chronic obstructive pulmonary disease; CHF, congestive heart failure; CPAP, continuous positive airway pressure.

Recommended Indications

Chronic Obstructive Pulmonary Disease

COPD Exacerbations. The best established acute indication for NIV is to treat ARF due to COPD exacerbations. This is supported by a strong physiologic rationale. Studies demonstrate that the combination of extrinsic PEEP and PS reduce diaphragmatic work of breathing more than either modality alone, because the expiratory pressure counterbalances intrinsic PEEP and the higher inspiratory pressure (pressure support) actively assists the inspiratory muscles [23]. In the setting of COPD exacerbations, NIV thereby serves as a "crutch" to assist ventilation while medical therapies are given time to work.

Multiple randomized controlled trials (RCTs) and meta-analyses of COPD patients with ARF have established that NIV more rapidly reduces respiratory rate, improves dyspnea and gas exchange, reduces intubations from a rate of 50% to 20%, and lowers mortality compared to standard therapy [4,21,24–27]. This evidence has recently been bolstered by Lindenaur's study using the PREMIER database [21] which showed in a propensity adjusted analysis that NIV was associated with lower risks of mortality and hospital-acquired pneumonia, was associated with reduced costs and shorter hospital length of stay (LOS), but no significant difference of 30-day all-cause readmission rates. The above results justify the early use of NPPV for COPD exacerbations as a standard of care unless there are contraindications. COPD exacerbations also respond well to NPPV when complicated by pneumonia [28] or occurring in the setting of a DNI status [29–31] or postoperative or postextubation respiratory failure [32,33].

Facilitation of Weaning in COPD Patients. Some patients with COPD exacerbations require intubation because they are not candidates for NIV initially or fail a trial of NIV. Multiple controlled trials have demonstrated that NIV permits earlier extubation of these patients, even when they have failed multiple "T" piece weaning trials [34,35]. Early extubation to NIV increases eventual successful weaning rates, shortens the duration of ventilator use and hospital LOS, reduces the occurrence of nosocomial pneumonia, and reduces mortality. This approach should be considered whenever intubated COPD patients are failing spontaneous breathing trials, but it should be used with caution—only for patients who are otherwise appropriate candidates for NIV, can breathe without any assistance for long enough to permit initiation of NIV, can tolerate levels of pressure support deliverable by mask (i.e., inspiratory pressure <20 cm H_2O), and who are not a "difficult intubation."

Cardiogenic Pulmonary Edema

Positive airway pressure has well-known therapeutic effects for patients with acute pulmonary edema. The increased functional residual capacity opens collapsed alveoli and rapidly improves respiratory system compliance and oxygenation. The increased intrathoracic pressure reduces transmyocardial pressure and has preload and afterload reducing effects, thus enhancing cardiac function of patients with left ventricular dysfunction who are afterload-dependent.

Multiple RCTs have demonstrated that noninvasive CPAP (10 to 12.5 cm H_2O) alone dramatically improves dyspnea and oxygenation and lowers intubation rates among patients with acute pulmonary edema compared with standard O_2 therapy [16,36,37]. Subsequent studies evaluating the efficacy of NIV (i.e., pressure support plus PEEP or BPAP) either compared with O_2 therapy or CPAP alone [38–40] have shown benefits similar to those previously demonstrated for CPAP. In one large RCT [40], CPAP and NIV performed similarly, both improving dyspnea scores and pH more rapidly than oxygen alone, but neither lowered intubation nor mortality rate (the primary outcome variable) compared to controls. However, the intubation rate for this study was slightly below 3% in all of the groups, including controls, suggesting that the enrolled patients were too mildly ill for a study of this size to detect significant mortality benefits. Meta-analyses of the RCTs on CPAP or NIV compared with O_2 therapy alone have detected the benefits described above, even showing a significant reduction of mortality with CPAP [41,42]. Meta-analyses comparing the two modalities show equivalency of NPPV and CPAP with regard to rates of intubation, lengths of stay, and mortality, and with no increase of the myocardial infarction rate attributable to NIV use. However, some studies have found that NPPV reduces dyspnea and improves gas exchange more rapidly than CPAP alone [43,44]. Therefore, by virtue of its greater simplicity and potentially lower cost, CPAP alone is often regarded as the initial noninvasive modality of choice for cardiogenic edema patients, but NPPV is substituted when patients remain dyspneic or hypercapnic. The strong evidence favoring the use of CPAP or NIV to treat CPE establishes either one as standard therapy for initial ventilatory assistance of appropriately selected CPE patients.

The success of noninvasive positive pressure to treat CPE has encouraged its extension into the prehospital setting. An emerging trend is to provide CPAP devices on ambulances for initial therapy of CPE. The experience thus far with this practice has been favorable. In a RCT, Thompson et al. observed an absolute reduction of 30% of intubation rates (17 out of 34 patients, or 50% vs. 7/35 or 20%, unadjusted OR = 0.25 and CI = 0.09 to 0.73) and of 21% for mortality (OR 0.3; 95% CI 0.09 to 0.99) among CPE patients treated with CPAP compared to usual therapy with oxygen, including intubation and bag-valve-mask-ventilation when needed [45]. A subsequent pilot study reported an improved respiratory status for 12 DNI patients when managed with NPPV out-of-hospital by emergency medical services (EMS) professionals. Respiratory rate decreased from 34 to 27 per minute, $p = 0.009$, and pulse oximetry improved from 86% to 94%, $p < 0.01$, with only one intolerant patient [46]. A more recent RCT from Germany of 51 patients with CPE showed less frequent and shorter use of the ICU and a strong trend toward reduced rates of intubation among patients treated with NIV compared to standard O_2 therapy [47]. These studies suggest that outcomes of CPE patients can be improved by very early initiation of noninvasive positive pressure therapy in the field and adoption of this as a routine practice for EMS appears to be evolving.

Immunodeficient Patients with Acute Respiratory Failure

Based on studies showing that patients developing ARF with underlying immunodeficiency states such as human immunodeficiency virus and Pneumocystis pneumonia or post-transplantation have poor outcomes when treated with IMV [48] and RCTs demonstrating benefit of NIV over standard therapy for these patients [49], NIV has been suggested as a modality to be used early to avoid nosocomial infections, need for intubation and mortality. However, outcomes have improved among immunocompromised patients requiring IMV [50] and NIV was associated with worse outcomes than IMV for a RCT on patients with hematologic malignancies [51]. In addition, in a more recent RCT of 374 immunocompromised patients with "early" ARF ($PaO_2 < 60$ mm Hg on room air), most with hematologic malignancies, NIV failed to lower 28-day mortality, intubation rate, ICU-acquired infection rates or lengths of ICU or hospital stay [52]. In the latter study, 40% of the O_2 therapy group used nasal high-flow therapy (HFT), which may have improved outcomes for the O_2 therapy group. The latter view is supported by a recent RCT comparing use of HFT to standard oxygen (SO) therapy or NIV in 310 immunocompromised patients with ARF culled from a larger study [53]. This study showed a 44% reduction of intubation rate and a 2/3 reduction of 90-day mortality rate when HFT was compared to NIV. These more recent findings have tempered enthusiasm for NIV as a therapy for ARF of immunocompromised patients. Although we await more studies to better define its role for the management of ARF among immunocompromised patients, especially compared to HFT, NIV should still be considered for immunocompromised patients with early ARF and single organ system dysfunction. These patients should be closely monitored in an ICU and intubated without delay when the respiratory failure or underlying sepsis progresses in severity.

WEAKER INDICATIONS—NPPV IS AN OPTION

NIV can be used to treat ARF of other etiologies and in other settings, but the evidence to support these applications is weaker and use is optional but not necessarily recommended (Table 167.1).

Other Obstructive Diseases

Asthma Exacerbations

Retrospective cohort studies suggest that NPPV improves gas exchange and avoids intubation among patients with respiratory failure caused by asthma exacerbations [54,55]. However, there are only a few randomized trials supporting the use of NIV for this indication. In one, NIV improved the forced expired volume in 1 second (FEV_1) more rapidly and reduced the hospitalization rate compared with sham controls [56]. The second study [57] reported similar findings with "high" inflation pressures compared to lower pressures (IPAP and EPAP 8 and 6 cm H_2O and 6 and 4 cm H_2O, respectively—all lower than most other studies) or standard medical therapy. A third RCT from India enrolled patients with severe airway obstruction and respiratory distress (average FEV_1 21% predicted, respiratory rate 36 per minute) to receive NIV or standard therapy with oxygen supplementation [58]. NIV tended to improve FEV_1 more for the first hour, with less salbutamol use and a shorter hospital stay (38 vs. 54 hours). However, the clinical significance of these differences is in doubt because, in both NIV and control groups, intubation rates were similarly low and there was no mortality.

Pollack et al. demonstrated that NIV is an acceptable way to deliver bronchodilator aerosol, showing a greater improvement of peak expiratory flow 1 hour after administration via a "bilevel" device than a standard nebulizer [59]. This and the above studies suggest that when NIV is used as an early treatment for asthma exacerbations, it allows more effective beta-agonist bronchodilatation. However, for most clinical situations, NIV is reserved for patients with "status asthmaticus," that is, those with severe airway obstruction who are not responding adequately to initial bronchodilator therapy, an application that is not yet supported by RCTs.

Cystic Fibrosis

Ideally, NIV is initiated for patients with cystic fibrosis when they develop chronic respiratory failure before an acute crisis arises. For patients with acute exacerbations of cystic fibrosis, NIV has been used mainly as a bridge to transplantation [60]. These patients may remain severely hypercapnic and require aggressive management of secretion retention, but NPPV permits avoidance of intubation and can sustain them for months while they await availability of donor organs.

Hypoxemic Respiratory Failure

Hypoxemic respiratory failure consists of severe hypoxemia (PaO_2/FIO_2 <200), severe respiratory distress, tachypnea (>30 per minute), and a non-COPD cause of ARF such as ARDS, acute pneumonia, trauma, or acute pulmonary edema [61]. Some RCTs of hypoxemic respiratory failure patients have observed reductions in the need for intubation, shortened ICU lengths of stay, and even mortality in the NIV group as opposed to controls [62], but it is difficult to draw firm conclusions about individual diagnostic groups within this very broad category. A concern is that favorable responses in one subgroup, such as those with CPE, could obscure unfavorable responses in another, such as ARDS or pneumonia patients. Among studies examining subcategories specifically, Jolliet et al. found very high NPPV failure rates (>60%) in a cohort of patients with severe community-acquired pneumonia [63]. Confalonieri et al. [28] found that NIV was associated with lower rates of intubation, shorter ICU LOS, and lower 90-day mortality in a RCT of patients with severe community-acquired pneumonia. However, these benefits were seen only for the COPD subgroup—not for non-COPD patients. Thus, no convincing evidence supports the use of NIV over invasive ventilation for patients with severe community-acquired pneumonia lacking COPD, and although NIV remains an option for these patients, it should be used only for carefully selected and monitored patients, in a setting where prompt intubation is available to those who do not responding well within an hour of NIV initiation.

The situation with ARDS (which overlaps with severe community-acquired pneumonia) is quite similar, but few RCTs have been performed on the use of NIV for ARDS per se. One study used NPPV as a "first-line" therapy for ARDS, finding that the successful use of NIV was associated with much lower VAP and mortality rates than in NIV failures [64]. The authors suggested that an initial simplified acute physiology score (SAPS) II of 34 or less and an improvement of PaO_2/FIO_2 to greater than 175 during the first hour of NIV therapy could be used to identify patients likely to succeed. However, it is good to remember that this was not an RCT and that only 15% of the total patients with ARDS (two-thirds were intubated prior to ICU admission) actually succeeded with NIV. A pilot RCT of 40 patients with "early" ARDS (PaO_2/FIO_2 >200 and ≤300) found that NIV reduced the need for intubation, the number of organ failures and tended to reduce mortality [65]. More recently, the FLORALI trial demonstrated advantages of HFT over NIV for patients with ARDS mainly due to pneumonia [66]. In this trial, NIV administered via a full-face mask was compared to high-flow nasal oxygen (HFNO) and SO in a three-way RCT [6] of patients with ARDS (PaO_2/FIO_2 <300). Although the main outcome, intubation rate, was not different for the whole cohort, it was significantly lower with HFNO for the subgroup with PaO_2/FIO_2 <200. Even more recently, an analysis of patients in the Large Observational Study to Understand the Global Impact of Severe Acute Respiratory Failure (LUNG SAFE) study showed that patients with more severe ARDS (PaO_2/FIO_2 <150) treated with NIV had a higher mortality than those treated with IMV (36.2 vs. 24.7, $p < 0.05$) [67]. These latter results raise serious concerns about the advisability of using NIV for patients with severe ARDS. Furthermore, both ICU and 90-day mortality were lower for the HFT group than the NIV group. However, another recent RCT [68] showed that among ARDS patients treated with NIV via a helmet interface, intubation (18% vs. 62%) and mortality (34% vs. 56%) rates were much lower than with a full-face mask (both $p < 0.001$). The conflicting results of the various studies make it difficult to make firm recommendations on the use of NIV for ARDS. Certainly, if NIV is used, it should be used early and observed closely in an ICU, with prompt intubation if there is lack of improvement or signs of further deterioration. In the meantime, further studies are needed to determine whether HFT is preferable to face mask NIV and how NIV via the helmet compares with HFT for the treatment of ARDS.

Post-trauma Respiratory Failure

Flail chest or mild acute lung injury (ALI) are conditions that are posited to respond favorably to NPPV after traumatic chest wall injuries. Support for this view comes from retrospective studies such as that by Beltrame et al. [69], in which 46 trauma patients with respiratory insufficiency were treated with NIV and experienced rapid improvements of gas exchange and a 72% success rate, but burn patients responded poorly. More recently, a study that randomized thoracic trauma patients with PAO_2/FIO_2 <200 to NIV or high-flow oxygen was stopped early after enrollment of 50 patients because of significant reductions of intubation rate (12% vs. 40%) and hospital LOS (14 vs. 21 days) in the NIV group [70]. These results support the use of NIV for hypoxemic respiratory failure in post-thoracic trauma cases, but it is good to remember that these were carefully selected patients.

Extubation Failure

The recurrence of respiratory failure after extubation of patients initially intubated for about of ARF is referred to as *extubation failure* and is associated with a high risk of morbidity and mortality (rates exceeding 40% in some studies [71,72]). NIV has been proposed as a way to avoid extubation failure if begun early for patients at risk for extubation failure, reducing the need for reintubation and improving outcomes. However, some earlier randomized studies [73] comparing NIV to standard O_2 therapy found no reduction of reintubation attributable to NIV. In fact, Esteban et al. even found a significantly increased ICU mortality for the NIV group [14]. These studies were limited by low enrollment of COPD patients (only about 10% of patients), and the increased mortality was thought to be related to a 10-hour delay in reintubations for the NIV group compared with controls. Two subsequent randomized trials [74,75] of patients deemed to be at "high risk" for extubation failure found that NIV reduced the need for reintubation and ICU mortality. Forty to fifty percent of patients of these trials had COPD or CHF and one trial focusing on patients with postextubation hypercapnia showed a significant reduction in the occurrence of postextubation respiratory failure as well as 90-day mortality for the group randomized to NIV compared to oxygen-treated controls [76]. These studies support the use of NIV for patients at *high risk* of extubation failure, particularly if they have COPD, CHF, and/or hypercapnia. However, based on the Esteban study, NIV to prevent extubation failure should be used very cautiously in at-risk patients who do not have these favorable characteristics because of the higher risk of NIV failure and its attendant morbidity and mortality. More recently, HFT has garnered interest as a therapy for postextubation patients. Hernández et al. randomized more than 600 patients at high risk of extubation failure to NIV or HFT, finding that reintubation rates were similar (22.8% for the HFT and 19.1% in the NIV group) as were other secondary outcomes including hospital LOS and mortality [77]. The authors concluded that HFT was noninferior to NIV and may "offer advantages" for at-risk postextubation patients, especially considering that adverse effects leading to withdrawal of therapy occurred among 42.9% of the NIV patients and none receiving HFT.

Postoperative Respiratory Failure/Insufficiency

Noninvasive positive pressure techniques, both CPAP and NPPV, have been used for postoperative patients in either of two ways: to prevent complications after high-risk surgeries or to treat frank postoperative respiratory failure. When used prophylactically after major abdominal surgery [78–80] or thoracoabdominal aneurysm repair [81], CPAP (10 cm H_2O) reduces the incidence of hypoxemia, pneumonia, atelectasis, and intubations compared with standard treatment. For patients with ARF following extubation after surgery, an earlier randomized study of post–lung resection patients showed reduced intubation and mortality rates for the NIV group compared with standard management [81]. A more recent larger RCT (293 patients) of respiratory failure occurring after various types –of abdominal surgery showed significantly fewer reintubations with NIV (33.1%) than SO (45.5%) as well as fewer health care–associated infections [82].

As with postextubation failure, interest has been mounting for a possible role for HFT in the postoperative setting. Stephan et al. [83] randomized over 800 postcardiac surgery patients who were at risk for postsurgical respiratory failure to NIV or HFT [82]. They found no differences in treatment failures, re-intubations or mortality (about 22%, 14%, and 5% to 6% respectively) between the groups and concluded that HFT is not inferior to NIV in this setting and therefore is a reasonable alternative.

The above studies strongly support the idea that CPAP and NIV should be considered to prevent and treat postoperative respiratory complications and failure for at-risk patients, and that HFT is an option but needs more evaluation for this role.

Patients with a DNI Status

NIV to treat DNI and palliative care patients has been controversial. Some argue that when patients are dying of respiratory failure, there is little to lose by trying NIV. Contrariwise, others counter that this is apt to add to patient discomfort and prolong suffering during a patient's final hours. Prospective cohort series demonstrate that many DNI patients treated with NIV actually survive the hospitalization, depending on the diagnosis [31,84]. In one series, 43% of 114 such patients survived to hospital discharge, 75% of CHF patients, and 53% of COPD patients, whereas hospital survival for patients with pneumonia or an underlying malignancy had hospital survival in the range of 25% [31]. The presence of cough, awake mental status, and hypercapnia also imparted a favorable prognosis. Thus, it is possible to identify, on the basis of the diagnosis and some simple clinical observations, patients with a better than even chance of surviving the hospitalization, and NIV could be used for these patients as a form of life support with the hope of "bridging" them through their acute illness. NIV can also be used for palliation of patients with a poor prognosis for survival of the hospitalization, with the possible aims of alleviating dyspnea or to prolong survival slightly so that the patient has time to settle affairs or say goodbye to loved ones. In the only RCT examining palliative use of NIV, Nava et al. [85] randomized 200 dyspneic patients with end-stage malignancies to NIV or oxygen, observing that NIV reduced dyspnea more rapidly and reduced the need for morphine. As recommended by a consensus statement by a Society of Critical Care Medicine task force on NIV, it is necessary for the patient, family, and caregivers to agree on these goals and to cease promptly if NIV seems to be adding to suffering (via mask discomfort, for example) rather than alleviating it [86].

Other Acute Applications of NPPV

Endoscopic Procedures

In separate randomized trials, CPAP alone (up to 7.5 cm H_2O) or NIV both improved oxygenation and reduced postprocedure respiratory failure for patients with severe hypoxemia undergoing bronchoscopy compared with those receiving conventional O_2 supplementation [87,88]. The evidence supports the use of NIV to improve gas exchange and reduce potential complications during fiber-optic bronchoscopy, especially when the risk of intubation is deemed high such as among immunocompromised patients or among those with bleeding diatheses. However, patients must be monitored closely and the caregiver team must try to minimize the risk of aspiration and be prepared to provide emergent intubation. NIV is also being used for other endoscopic procedures, such as placement of percutaneous gastrostomy tubes for patients with respiratory compromise due to neuromuscular disease and performance of transesophageal echocardiography [89,90].

Preoxygenation before Intubation

A randomized trial of critically ill patients with hypoxemic respiratory failure showed that preoxygenation with NIV before intubation improved O_2 saturation during and after intubation and decreased the incidence of O_2 desaturations below 80% during intubation [91]. This approach is promising but needs further evaluation before its routine use can be recommended. This also begs the question whether, if NIV improves oxygenation substantially, intubation could be avoided for some of these patients.

SELECTION GUIDELINES FOR NPPV IN ACUTE RESPIRATORY FAILURE

Determinants of Success/Failure

Selection of appropriate patients for NIV is critical for optimizing success and providing benefit. Knowledge of factors that predict success or failure is helpful in selecting good candidates for NIV. Such factors, compiled from previous studies, are shown in Table 167.2. In effect, the predictors indicate that patients

TABLE 167.2

Predictors of NIV Failure

Inability to cooperate with therapy or Glasgow Coma Score (GCS) <12
Respiratory rate (RR) >30 and hypoxemia
Severe dyspnea
Excessive accessory muscle or paradoxical breathing
Paradoxical breathing
Hypercapnic respiratory failure with acidemia, pH <7.10
Acute hypoxemic respiratory failure with PaO_2/FIO_2 <100
SAPS II score ≥34 or APACHE II score >29
Age >40 but <70 y
Serum HCO_3 <22
Multiorgan dysfunction
ARDS, pneumonia, especially with high tidal volumes (>9.5 mL/kg ideal body weight)
Lack of improvement in respiratory rate within 1–2 h
Lack of increase in PaO_2/FIO_2 to >175 within 1 h

APACHE II, acute physiology and chronic health evaluation II; ARDS, acute respiratory distress syndrome; NIV, noninvasive ventilation; SAPS II, simplified acute physiology score II; RR, respiratory rate.

TABLE 167.3

Criteria to Select Patients to Receive NPPV for Acute Respiratory Failure

Hypercapnic respiratory failure	Hypoxemic respiratory failure
Subjective	
Moderate to severe dyspnea	Moderate to severe dyspnea
Physiologic	
Respiratory rate >24/min	Respiratory rate >30/min
Increased accessory muscle use	Increased accessory muscle use
Abdominal paradox	Abdominal paradox
Gas exchange	
pH <7.35, >7.10	pH >7.20
$PaCO_2$ >45 mm Hg, <98 mm Hg	PaO_2/FIO_2 >100, <300

From a composite of initiation criteria for randomized controlled trials. NPPV, noninvasive positive pressure ventilation.

who are most likely to succeed with NIV have incipient, milder respiratory failure than those who fail. This suggests that there is a "window of opportunity" for implementation of NIV when success is most likely. NIV should be started when patients have evidence of acute respiratory distress and increased acute physiology and chronic health evaluation II (APACHE II) scores, but not when patients are approaching respiratory arrest, have severe acidemia, high APACHE II scores, or are unable to cooperate.

Predictors of success differ slightly between patients with hypercapnic and hypoxemic forms of respiratory failure. A chart to predict NIV failure of COPD patients identified pH <7.25, respiratory rate ≥35, APACHE II score >29, and Glasgow Coma score ≤11 as independent predictors of NIV failure [92], whereas a recent prospective multicenter study of NIV to treat patients with ARDS identified a SAPS II score of ≥34 and a PaO_2/FIO_2 ratio <175 after the first hour as independent predictors of NIV failure [64]. In both analyses, the response to NIV after the first hour or two had more predictive value than baseline values.

For hypercapnic respiratory failure, a rise in pH and improving mental status within an hour or two of initiating NIV (presumably reflecting a drop in $PaCO_2$) predicts success, whereas, not surprisingly, a substantial early improvement of oxygenation bodes well for patients with hypoxemic respiratory failure. These observations highlight the importance of a "1- to 2-hour checkpoint" after which if the patient is not improving sufficiently, prompt intubation should be contemplated rather than risk further deterioration and the need for a riskier emergent intubation.

Selection Process

The selection of patients with ARF to receive NIV is based on criteria used in RCTs, and these are listed in Table 167.3. This is a simple three-step process, the first of which is to establish that the patient has a favorable diagnosis, ideally a condition like CPE or COPD, which is likely to respond to medical therapy fairly rapidly (a few days or less). Patients with weaker indications (i.e., acute asthma or pneumonia) can be tried on NIV but must be monitored very closely in an ICU, especially if they have risk factors for NIV failure. Patients at very high risk for

TABLE 167.4

Contraindications to NPPV in Acute Respiratory Failure

Cardiac/respiratory arrest
Medically unstable (hypotensive shock, uncontrolled cardiac ischemia, or arrhythmias)
Severe upper gastrointestinal bleeding
Unable to protect airway (impaired cough or swallowing)
Excessive secretions
Unable to apply mask due to facial surgery, trauma, burns, or facial deformity
Agitated or uncooperative
Undrained pneumothorax
Multiorgan system failure

NPPV, noninvasive positive pressure ventilation.

NIV failure, such as those with sepsis and evolving multiorgan dysfunction, are generally best managed invasively rather than to delay needed intubation.

Step two is to identify patients who need ventilatory assistance so that the modality is not wasted on patients who are too mildly ill to warrant ventilatory assistance. This is done on the basis of simple bedside observations of dyspnea, vital signs, and evidence of increased work of breathing (such as vigorous accessory muscle use). Arterial blood gas results showing acute-on-chronic CO_2 retention may be helpful, but needed ventilatory assistance should not be delayed pending availability of blood gas results. The third step is to exclude patients who have contraindications to NPPV and should be managed invasively (Table 167.4). Most of the contraindications are relative and judgment must be exercised when deciding whether patients have excessive secretions, medical instability, or uncooperativeness. Coma and severe obtundation are no longer considered absolute contraindications as long as they are related to hypercapnia. Patients with hypercapnic coma (Glasgow Coma Scale <8) have success and survival rates with NPPV that are equivalent to those of similar noncomatose patients [93].

TECHNIQUES AND EQUIPMENT FOR NPPV

Interfaces

Nasal Masks

Nasal masks are the most commonly used interfaces for outpatients with chronic respiratory failure because they are more comfortable than nasal prongs or oronasal masks, even if they are less efficient than oronasal masks at eliminating CO_2 [94]. In addition, they permit speech and expectoration and, with some practice, eating during use. Manufacturers offer numerous modifications of the nasal mask that fit into several basic categories.

Standard Nasal Masks

Standard nasal masks were first designed during the early 1980s to provide CPAP for obstructive sleep apnea (OSA) and consist of triangular clear plastic domes that fit over the nose (Fig. 167.1A). A soft, usually silicon cuff makes contact with the skin around the perimeter of the nose to form an air seal. These masks must be fit properly to minimize pressure over the bridge of the nose, which may induce redness, skin irritation, and occasionally ulceration. Forehead "spacers" are an adjustable joint often used to minimize pressure on the bridge of the nose. Various approaches have been used to enhance patient comfort, including an additional thin plastic flap or a baffle system to further reduce the strap tension necessary to maintain an air seal. Gel-containing seals, some that have heat-molding capabilities, may help to evenly distribute the pressure of the seal around the face.

Nasal Pillows

Nasal "pillows" consist of small rubber cones that are inserted directly into the nostrils. By removing the sealing surface from the eyes, these reduce claustrophobia and permit use of eyeglasses. They also eliminate contact with the nasal bridge and are helpful for patients with nasal bridge irritation or ulceration caused by standard nasal masks. However, they can cause irritation of the nostrils, and some patients alternate between different types of masks as a way of minimizing discomfort. Nasal pillows are less often used in the acute care setting.

Oronasal or Full-Face Masks

The main advantage of oronasal over nasal masks is that they reduce air leaking through the mouth because they cover both the nose and mouth. Mainly because of this advantage,

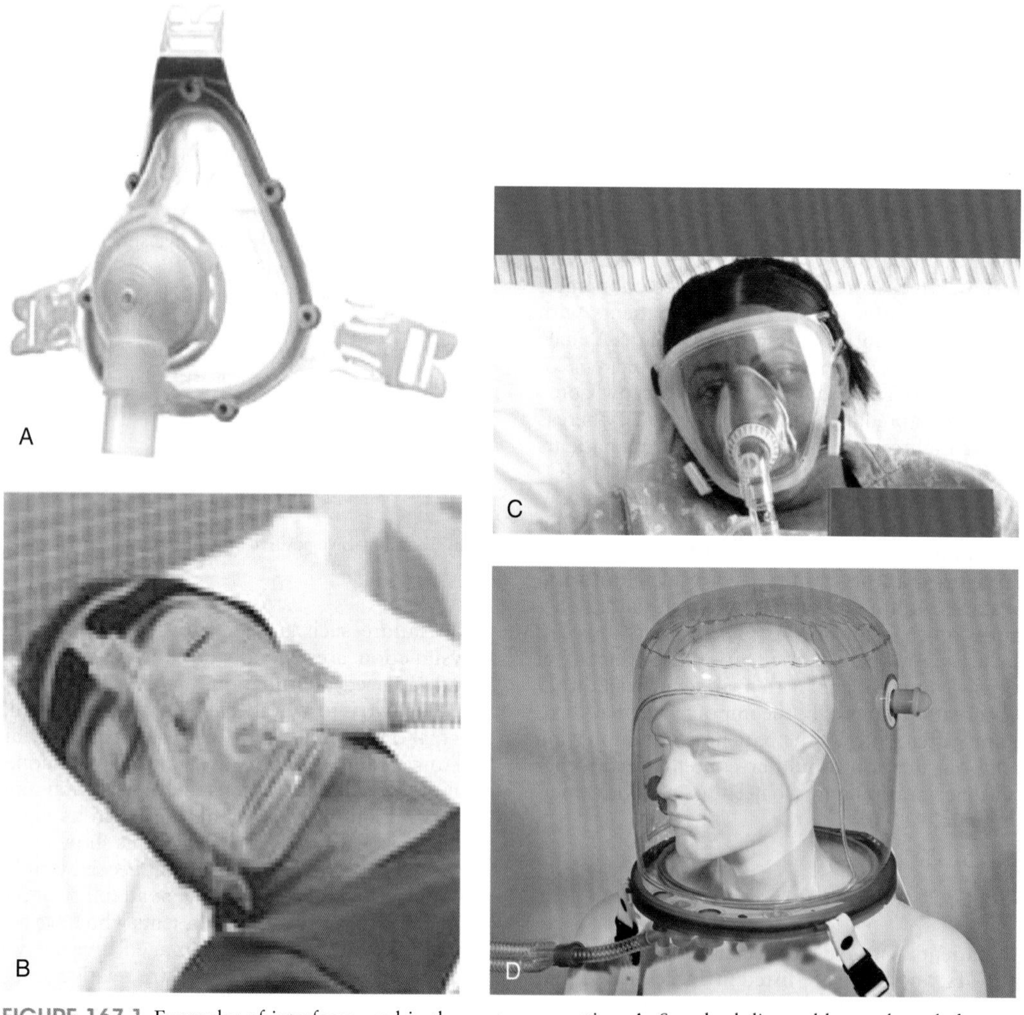

FIGURE 167.1 Examples of interfaces used in the acute care setting. **A:** Standard disposable nasal mask for use with "bilevel" ventilator. The single circuit of these ventilators necessitates an in-line exhaust valve shown by arrow (Mirage Quattro mask, ResMed, San Diego, CA). **B:** Disposable full-face mask with chin "shelf" to keep mandible in position and reduce air leaking under the seal (Model RT040, Fischer Paykel, Wellington, NZ). **C:** Total Face mask that resembles snorkel mask and situates mask seal farther from nose and mouth (Performax, Respironics, Inc., Murrysville, PA). **D:** "Helmet" interface that consists of clear plastic cylinder that fits over entire head and fits with strap under axillae.

Kwok et al. found that the oronasal was significantly better tolerated than the nasal mask in the acute setting [95]. Air seals of oronasal masks are similar to those of nasal masks, using a thin membrane of soft silicon to enhance comfort and minimize air leaks. Oronasal masks have built-in valves to prevent rebreathing or asphyxiation in the event of ventilator malfunction, especially for "bilevel"-type ventilators. Because of concerns that vomiting into an oronasal mask could cause aspiration, these masks have straps that allow rapid removal. Some oronasal masks incorporate a "shelf" that fits under the chin to stabilize it, aiming to minimize air leaking under the seal (Fig. 167.1B). Compared with nasal masks, oronasal masks interfere more with speech and eating, have more dead space, and are less comfortable. However, because of their better initial tolerability and more efficient CO_2 removal than nasal masks, they are usually preferred to treat ARF.

The Total Face Mask (Respironics, Inc.) is a larger version of an oronasal mask that seals around the perimeter of the face. It relocates the sealing surface from the nose and mouth to the perimeter of the face. It easily accommodates most facial shapes and sizes and can be rapidly applied by fastening just two Velcro straps behind the head. Although some patients find it frightening and refuse to try it, most find it comfortable and no more claustrophobic than standard oronasal masks (Fig. 167.1C). Two small RCTs comparing the Total Face Mask to a standard oronasal mask found no differences of outcomes between the masks, but one found that the Total face Mask was better tolerated and suggested that it could serve as an alternative for patients intolerant of standard full-face masks [96,97].

Helmet

The helmet (Fig. 167.1D) has been used primarily in Italy and has not yet been approved for use with NIV in the United States although a very similar device has been approved to avoid exposure of the lungs to hyperoxia in bariatric chambers. It consists of an inflatable plastic cylinder that fits over the head and seals around the neck and shoulders, sometimes secured by straps under the axillae. Some studies evaluating its use for COPD patients show that it is more comfortable and reduces facial ulcerations compared with an oronasal mask [98], but a recent RCT showed equivalent responses and tolerance between the helmet and full-face mask, except the mask lowered dyspnea scores more rapidly [99]. In another recent RCT [68] on patients with ARDS, the helmet avoided intubation and reduced mortality compared to a standard full-face mask. To prevent rebreathing, high airflow rates are necessary, which render the helmet much noisier than oronasal masks (100 vs. 70 dB, respectively) [100]. Although the helmet has some potential advantages over the full-face mask and may be more efficacious than the full-face mask for ARDS patients [68], it is also noisier, costlier, and unavailable in many countries. Nonetheless, it has the advantage of avoiding contact over the nose and mouth and may serve as a useful alternative when patients are having trouble tolerating other masks.

Oral Interfaces

Oral interfaces consisting of a mouthpiece inserted into a lip seal that is strapped tautly around the head to minimize air leakage have been used to treat patients with chronic neuromuscular conditions for many decades. A commercially available oral interface was introduced more recently for the treatment of occasional patients with sleep apnea. These interfaces are not often used in the acute care setting, although some studies have had patients hold interfaces in their mouths to enhance their sense of control when initiating NIV [101].

Headgear

The straps used to hold interfaces in place are important for interface comfort and stability as well as for control of air leaks. The number of strap connections varies from two to five, depending on the mask. In general, the more connections, the more stable the interface, but discomfort and claustrophobia become concerns. Most straps use soft, elastic material fastened with Velcro, but abrasions can occur if the edges are too rough. Minimizing strap tension just to the point of controlling air leaks is important to optimize comfort.

Ventilators for NPPV

The specific ventilator chosen is probably not as important to NIV success as the settings selected or the skill of the care team. Many ventilator options are available, including critical care ventilators (designed mainly for invasive ventilation in the acute setting), ventilators designed especially for applications of NIV in the acute care setting, "hybrid" ventilators that are designed mainly for use in the postacute setting or for sicker patients in the home, capable of providing pressure- or volume-limited ventilation invasively or noninvasively, and portable positive-pressure "bilevel" ventilators designed mainly for use in the home. The choice of ventilator depends mainly on availability, patient needs, and practitioner preferences. For example, patients with hypoxemic respiratory failure may be very difficult to manage noninvasively and the sophisticated monitoring and oxygen delivery capabilities of a critical care ventilator may be preferred, whereas a patient with an exacerbation of COPD who is oxygenating adequately might do just as well with a small, portable, inexpensive bilevel device.

Critical Care Ventilators

The microprocessor-controlled ventilators currently used mainly for IMV in critical care units can be adapted for NPPV. These offer an array of volume-limited or pressure-limited modes and sophisticated monitoring and alarm capabilities. Advantages over "bilevel" positive pressure devices include the universal presence of O_2 blenders, accurate tracking of tidal and minute volumes, and a dual-limb circuit with an active exhalation valve that minimizes rebreathing (Fig. 167.2A). Most practitioners use the pressure support mode for NPPV with these ventilators because of enhanced comfort, combining it with PEEP [102,103]. Shortcomings of these ventilators when used to deliver NPPV include intolerance of air leaks that inevitably occur with NPPV, causing difficulty with triggering and cycling which sets off annoying alarms.

Most critical care ventilators now incorporate NIV modes that automatically improve leak tolerance and compensating abilities, disable nuisance alarms, and permit multiple adjustments including those to limit inspiratory time, thus enabling improved expiratory synchrony. These modes have undergone little evaluation in clinical settings, but bench studies demonstrated that most NIV modes of critical care ventilators work well to deliver set pressures or volumes unless there are large air leaks, in which case most of them require additional adjustments to maintain delivery [104,105]. One of the studies also examined synchrony of ventilated patients in a crossover study and found that NIV-dedicated ventilators synchronized slightly better than critical care and transport ventilators using the NIV mode [105]. Masks and circuitry for the application of NIV via critical care ventilators should not have the built-in exhalation valves designed for use with single circuit bilevel devices because these will increase air leaking and interfere with proper function. Some mask manufacturers use blue coloration for plastic parts of masks meant for use with critical ventilators so that they can be easily identified.

Bilevel Pressure-Limited Ventilators

These devices were first conceived to enhance comfort for patients requiring high CPAP to treat sleep apnea [106], but it rapidly became apparent that they function as PS ventilators as well [107]. By virtue of their air leak tolerance and algorithms to enhance synchrony in the face of leaks, bilevel-type ventilators that deliver pressure assist or PS ventilation are the most commonly used ventilators today for delivery of NIV [15]. The prototype bilevel device was the "BiPAP S/T" (Respironics, Inc., Murrysville, PA), introduced during the late 1980s, but numerous versions are now available from many manufacturers (Fig. 167.2B).

Bilevel devices deliver two levels of positive pressure: preset inspiratory and expiratory positive airway pressures (IPAP and EPAP, respectively). The difference between the two is the level of inspiratory assistance, or pressure support. Pressure support modes provide sensitive inspiratory triggering and expiratory cycling mechanisms (usually by sensing changes in flow), permitting excellent patient–ventilator synchrony, reducing diaphragmatic work, and improving patient comfort [107,108]. Bilevel devices designed for home use are lighter (5 to 10 kg), more compact (<0.025 m^3), and have fewer alarms than critical care or "hybrid" ventilators. Most have limited IPAP (up to 20 to 35 cm H_2O, depending on the ventilator) and oxygenation capabilities and lack alarms or battery backup systems. O_2 supplementation is provided via a T-connector in the ventilator tubing or connector directly in the mask, the latter providing a slightly higher FIO_2. Even at flow rates of 15 L per minute, though, the maximum recommended by the manufacturer, the FIO_2 is still only 45% to 50% [109], insufficient for many patients with hypoxemic respiratory failure.

The BiPAP Vision and, more recently, its replacement the V60 (both Phillips Respironics, Inc.) (Fig. 167.2C) were designed for both invasive and noninvasive acute care applications, although they are used mainly for noninvasive. Equipped with an O_2 blender, they can provide high FIO_2s and have more sophisticated alarm and monitoring systems than the home-based bilevel devices (including graphic screens). They also feature adjustable rise times (the time taken to reach target inspiratory pressure) and inspiratory time limits that can help with comfort and synchrony. Because of these features, these devices have been well-received for the administration of NIV at acute care hospitals. The V60 (Fig. 167.2D) also incorporates battery backup, improved graphics with a touch screen, and some additional modes.

Because they have a single ventilator circuit, rebreathing can occur during use of bilevel ventilators and can interfere with the ability to enhance CO_2 elimination [110]. The rebreathing can be

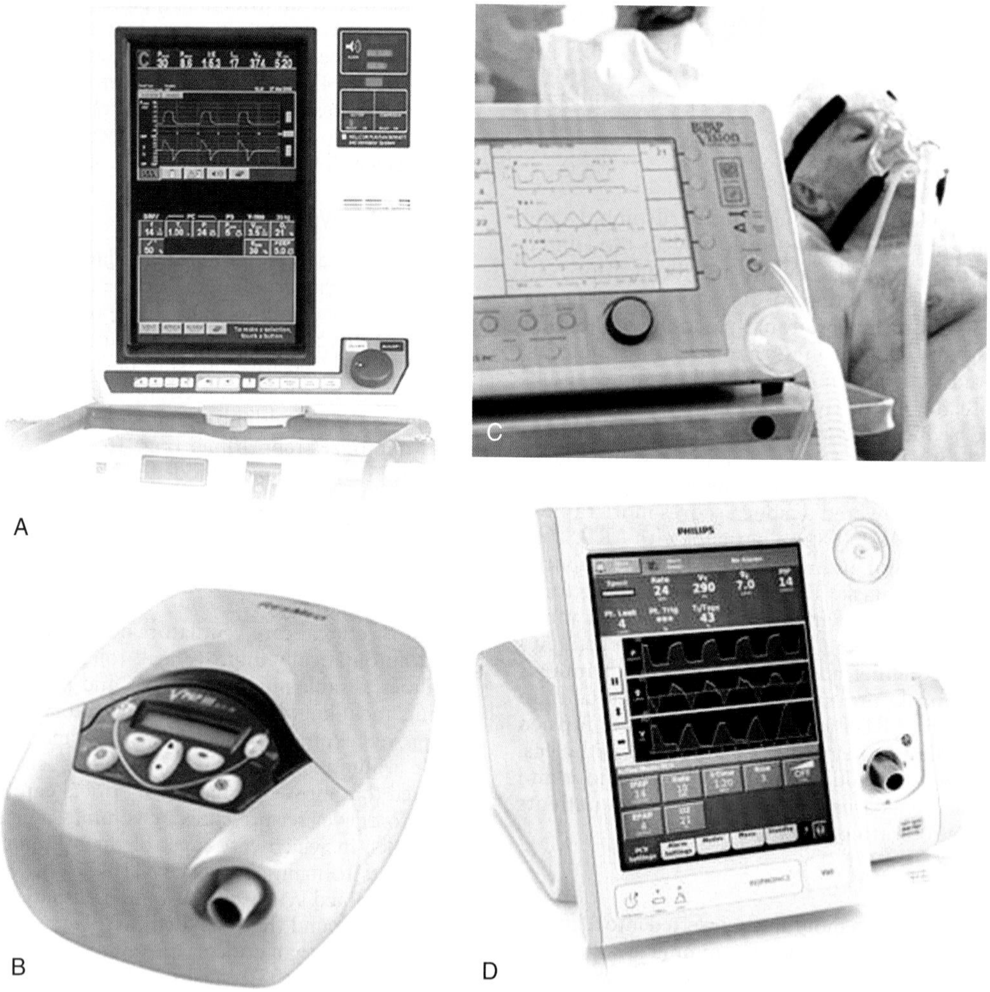

FIGURE 167.2 Examples of ventilators commonly used to deliver NPPV. **A:** "Critical care" ventilator that offers an "NIV" mode that permits multiple adjustments. May have trouble adapting to large leaks (Puritan Bennett 840, Covidien, Mansfield, MA). **B:** Typical "bilevel" ventilator designed mainly for home use but is capable of assisting ventilation in patients with acute respiratory failure as long as appropriate alarms are assured (S9 VPAP ST, ResMed, Inc.). **C:** Ventilator designed specifically for acute applications of NIV. Has oxygen blender and graphic monitoring screen (BiPAP Vision, Respironics, Inc.). **D:** Updated version of ventilator in (**C**). Offers internal battery for portability and improved graphic screen (V60, Philips Respironics, Inc., Andover, MA).

minimized by using masks with in-mask exhalation ports, which are associated with less rebreathing than in-circuit valves [111], use of nonrebreathing valves, and EPAP pressures of 4 cm H_2O or greater, which ensure higher bias flows during exhalation [109].

Adjuncts to NPPV

Humidification may enhance comfort during NIV and is advised when NIV is to be used for more than a few hours. For the acute care setting, a heated humidifier is preferred over a heat and moisture exchanger because the latter adds to work of breathing [112] and may interfere with triggering and cycling. Also, with excessive air leaking, a heated humidifier lowers nasal resistance [113]. Nasogastric tubes are not routinely recommended as adjuncts to NPPV, even when oronasal masks are used, but small bore flexible nasogastric tubes can be used for feeding when necessary and do not interfere much with mask sealing.

Ventilator Modes

Although pressure support (or bilevel) is the most commonly chosen mode to deliver NIV, others might be considered. Average volume-assured pressure support (AVAPS) is available on the V60 bilevel device (Phillips Respironics, Inc.). It tracks recent delivered tidal volumes and automatically adjusts inspiratory pressure to achieve a target minute volume. This can be advantageous for hypoventilating patients as has been shown in obesity-hypoventilation patients [114], but no efficacy advantages over standard BiPAP have been shown for acute care settings.

Proportional assist ventilation, a mode that uses the inspiratory flow signal and its integral, volume, to determine how much flow and volume assistance to provide to the patient, functions well as a NIV mode. It offers the potential advantages of enhanced comfort and synchrony [115]. Once again, studies have not been able to demonstrate improvements of efficacy over standard bilevel or pressure support modes in terms of reducing intubation or mortality rates. Neurally adjusted ventilator assistance (NAVA) uses the diaphragm electromyographic signal detected by an esophageal electrode to determine ventilatory assistance. Administered noninvasively, it improves synchrony compared to pressure support but without greater improvements in gas exchange or comfort [116].

Initiation of NIV

NIV is most often begun in the emergency department (ED) or ICU for acutely dyspneic patients who can become panicky when masks are strapped to their faces. Thus, unlike initiation of invasive ventilation with the patient heavily sedated or even paralyzed, initiation of NPPV requires skill on the part of the caregiver to rapidly gain the confidence of the patient and help them cooperate so that they can benefit from the technique. Explaining clearly what is happening and what to expect, using verbal cues like "try to let the ventilator breathe for you" and giving patients control by allowing them to hold the mask on their face can be quite helpful. Proper mask fit should be assured and the mask attached to the ventilator via tubing. Most practitioners start with PS ventilation using relatively low ventilator pressures (i.e., 8 to 10 cm H_2O for IPAP and 4 to 5 cm H_2O for EPAP) for at least several minutes to allow the patient to become familiar with the mask and airflow. It is then extremely important to increase the inspiratory pressure (and thereby the level of pressure support) to reduce respiratory distress and effort, targeting a respiratory rate in the low 20 s per minute and an increase in tidal volume to 6 to 7 mL per kg. Patients are often intolerant of higher pressures, especially initially, because of the sensation of burning in the sinuses or pressure in the ears, or because of the perceived effort of exhaling against an elevated pressure. Thus, the adjustment of inspiratory pressure becomes a titration, tailored for individual patients, balancing relief of respiratory distress and attainment of ventilatory targets against intolerance due to excessive pressures. Expiratory pressure is usually kept at 4 to 5 cm H_2O, but can be adjusted upward for patients who have difficulty triggering due to intrinsic PEEP, upper airway obstructions due to sleep apnea, or hypoxemia despite increases in FIO_2 to above 50% to 60%. L'Her et al. demonstrated that for patients with ALI that increases of PEEP during NPPV were quite effective for improving oxygenation and increases of pressure support are effective for relieving dyspnea [117]. However, it is well to recall that if EPAP is increased during NIV, IPAP must also be increased by the same amount to maintain the level of pressure support and tidal volume.

MONITORING

Location for NIV

Because of the importance of prompt initiation to avoid further patient deterioration that could necessitate intubation, NPPV should be started wherever the patient comes to medical attention, as long as appropriate equipment and personnel are available. Once initiated, transfer to an appropriately monitored location becomes important. This depends on the patient's need for monitoring as well as the unit's monitoring capabilities and skills of the staff for managing NPPV. Assessment of a patient's need for monitoring includes consideration of the severity of the respiratory failure as well as any comorbidities. When in doubt, a brief trial of NPPV withdrawal may be helpful. In one study of patients treated with NPPV in the ED for acute pulmonary edema or COPD, patients who remained stable during a 15-minute discontinuation trial were transferred to a regular ward and none subsequently required intubation [118]. NPPV is used on the regular wards of many hospitals because of the scarcity of ICU beds, but some guidelines have recommended that NPPV be applied only in the ICU because of concerns about patient safety [119]. Ozsancak Ugurlu et al. [120] reported that in eight Massachusetts, USA, hospitals, 42%, 37%, 18%, and 3% of patients were initiated on NIV in the ICU, ED, regular wards, and other wards, respectively. Of those on regular wards, 60% remained and 40% were transferred to the ICU. Those remaining on the wards succeeded with NIV in 82% of cases, exceeding success rates in the other units. These findings suggest that with proper training and availability of support personnel NPPV can be administered safely on regular floors for selected patients.

What to Monitor

Monitoring of NPPV shares similarities with that of IMV but also fundamental differences. Most importantly, subjective responses are critical to the success of NIV (Table 167.5). Alleviation of respiratory distress and good tolerance of the technique must be achieved without using large doses of analgesia and sedation as is commonly done with invasive ventilation. Thus, caregivers must observe patients closely for these responses and be prepared to make prompt adjustments as needed to maintain patient comfort and cooperation.

Physical signs of increased respiratory effort should also respond promptly when NIV is administered properly, including changed of accessory muscle use and respiratory rate. Air leaks should be sought and minimized. These are universal with NIV, and with bilevel devices, the continuous leak through the exhalation device is intentional, of course, to minimize rebreathing. But leaks under the seal of the mask can be large and interfere with synchronization and efficacy.

TABLE 167.5

What to Monitor During NPPV

Subjective responses
Comfort
Mask related
Air pressure and flow related
Dyspnea
Claustrophobia
Agitation
Delirium
Vital signs
Respiratory rate
Heart rate
Blood pressure
Breathing effort
Accessory muscle use
Paradoxical breathing
Gas exchange
Continuous oximetry
Baseline and 1–2 h arterial blood gases, then as indicated
Synchrony
Triggering
Expiratory asynchrony
Air leaks
Mask seal
Through mouth with nasal masks
Secretion clearance
Cough effectiveness
Quantity of secretions
Development of complications (see Table 167.6)

NPPV, noninvasive positive pressure ventilation.

Poor synchrony between the patient and ventilator, sometimes caused by excessive air leaking, patient agitation, ventilator maladjustment, or other factors, is common and contributes to NIV failure and must be identified and remediated [105]. Oximetry should be monitored continuously until the patient has stabilized and arterial blood gases should be drawn at baseline and after 1 to 2 hours of therapy to assure the desired gas exchange response. Tidal volumes of 6 to 8 mL per kg ideal body weight should be targeted. Tidal volume >9.5 mL per kg has been associated with NIV failure with 82% sensitivity and 87% specificity [121]. One important aspect of NIV monitoring is to determine early when patients are responding poorly to NIV so that the reasons can be reversed or failing that, the patient can be intubated promptly, avoiding undue delay and possible respiratory arrest with the emergent intubation and attendant risk of morbidity and mortality that entails.

Complications and Side Effects of NIV and Possible Remedies

NIV is successful for most patients and most adverse side effects are minor, but failure rates reported by studies representing "real-life" applications of NIV still approach 40% [15] and a knowledge of potential complications and ways of managing them can be helpful for minimizing NPPV failure rates. There are many possible adverse effects and complications, a variety of possible ways of categorizing them, and inevitable areas of overlap between the categories. For practical purposes, we distinguish between side effects related to the interface and those attributable to ventilator airflow and pressure, caregiver inexperience, or patient factors (Table 167.6).

Adverse Effects and Complications Associated with the Interface

Mask Discomfort

Mask discomfort is one of the most common reasons cited for NPPV failure. It may reflect a poorly fitted mask, a patient's difficulty accepting the interface chosen, excessively tight headstraps, a dyspneic patient's discomfort at having foreign material strapped to their face, or other factors. The clinician faced with a patient intolerant of NIV due to mask discomfort should quickly attempt to decipher the specific problem and correct it if possible. Often, inexperienced practitioners select masks that are too large and a trial with a smaller mask or a different mask type often helps. In the face of air leaks, reseating the mask and attempting to loosen the straps may help before resorting to tightening of the straps. As discussed earlier, an oronasal mask is usually the best initial mask choice, but some patients who are claustrophobic or expectorating frequently fare better with a nasal mask. Masks used in the acute setting are usually disposable after one use but some are reusable. They are relatively inexpensive compared to masks used for long-term applications of NIV, but it is still desirable to check that the mask selected is likely to fit (using a fitting gauge, for example) to minimize the need to dispose of multiple masks for each patient application. Noisiness can contribute to intolerance with some mask types such as the helmet [100].

Skin Irritation and Ulceration

Skin irritation and ulceration, mainly over the nasal bridge, is a less common complication of NIV as mask designs and skill at administering NIV has improved [15]. Contributors to NIV-related skin breakdown include excessive strap tension, mask type, poor mask fit, prolonged ventilation, high inspiratory pressures necessitating more strap tension to control leaks, hypersensitivity to mask material, and patient factors such as age and comorbidities such as congestive heart failure that can limit skin perfusion [122,123]. Facial structure and anatomical variation among patients also play a role. Prevention rather than treatment of skin breakdown is the best management strategy. This can be accomplished by optimizing mask fit while using the lowest effective positive pressures and strap tension and applying artificial skin to the affected area at the first sign of redness. Also, some newer mask types have softer, larger silicon sealing surfaces that minimize trauma to the facial skin. With these interventions, a significant nasal bridge ulcer should now be a rare event during NIV therapy.

Adverse Effects and Complications Associated with Airflow and Pressures

Nasal, Sinus and Ear Pain and Burning

Initiation of NIV is commonly associated with the sensation of nasal, sinus, and ear pain and burning. This is related to the patient's lack of familiarity with the sensation of air pressure and flow and usually subsides as the patient accommodates to the sensations. Using lower initial pressures and raising them gradually can help to minimize this problem as can making sure that any leak is minimized. Use of routine humidification can help with these side effects too.

Conjunctivitis

Conjunctivitis is another common adverse consequence of airflow during NIV. In this case, air leaks into the eyes due to a combination of high inspiratory pressure and incomplete mask sealing along the steep sides of the nose related to suboptimal mask fit and patient anatomic variations. This causes conjunctival

TABLE 167.6

Adverse Effects and Complications of NPPV and Possible Remedies

Adverse effect	Possible remedy
Interface related	
Mask discomfort	Check size and fit. Readjust headgear. Try different type.
Skin ulceration, irritation	Readjust mask. Loosen straps. Artificial skin prophylactically.
Air pressure and flow related	
Nasal, sinus pain, dryness	Lower pressure temporarily. Humidify gas. Nasal saline.
Conjunctivitis	Reseat mask. Check seal on nasal bridge. Artificial skin. Consider new mask type.
Gastric distension	Lower pressure if possible. Simethicone. Observe or distension, consider nasogastric drainage.
Patient–ventilator asynchrony	Eliminate leaks, treat agitation, assess for discomfort. Try lowering pressure support or limiting inspiratory time.
Rebreathing	Use mask with in-mask exhalation valve. Use adequate EPAP (≥4 cm H_2O). Use ventilator with active exhalation valve.
Air leaks	Reseat, readjust strap. Try different mask type. Chin strap if nasal mask. Lower pressure if possible.
Caregiver related	
Inadequate or excessive pressures	Monitor more carefully. Adjust upward as tolerated. Assure adequate training.
Inadequate equipment	Initiate NPPV program, with full selection of masks.
Patient related	
Agitation, anxiety	Assure proper mask fit, ventilator settings. Reassure, consider sedation.
Major complications	
NPPV failure	Optimal monitoring to detect and address problems before they lead to failure. If failure not responding to appropriate measures, intubate promptly to avoid delay.
Respiratory arrest	Monitor at-risk patients in ICU or closely in stepdown unit. Intubate before arrest occurs to avoid attendant morbidity and mortality.

EPAP, expiratory positive airway pressure; ICU, intensive care unit; NPPV, noninvasive positive pressure ventilation.

dryness, irritation, erythema, and discomfort after a period of hours and may respond to lowered inspiratory pressures (when possible), reseating the mask or tightening the straps, or trying a new type or size of mask.

Gastric Distension

Gastric distension among patients receiving NPPV is common but is usually well tolerated. However, extreme complications such as gastric perforation and abdominal compartment syndrome have been reported [124,125]. A study of obese patients found that those receiving NPPV with an inspiratory pressure of 16 cm H_2O had more gastric distension than those breathing spontaneously [126]. The authors cautioned that the increased gastric air might raise the risk of aspiration. As stated earlier, the amount of gastric distension during NPPV is usually clinically insignificant, but if it causes excessive abdominal distension, discomfort, nausea, bowel distension on a KUB exam, or a compartment syndrome, then drainage with a naso- or orogastric tube is the next logic step. Gas dispersing agents like simethicone can be tried but are usually ineffective. Lowering the inspiratory pressure as much as possible can also help. But if there is a high risk of vomiting and aspiration or if nasogastric suctioning is unsuccessful, then intubation and other methods to decompress the bowel should be considered.

Patient–Ventilator Asynchrony

Patient–ventilator asynchrony is the lack of coordination between a patient's own respiratory effort and the ventilator's output. The consequences of this phenomenon can include inefficient gas exchange, muscle fatigue, and ultimately, failure of NIV [127]. Asynchrony occurs frequently during NIV, mostly because of air leaks, rendering it difficult for the ventilator to sense the onset of patient inspiration and expiration, altered patient respiratory drive or agitation, ventilator mode, and inappropriately high inspiratory pressure for patients with COPD, contributing to ineffective triggering and cycling [128–130]. An observational study of three teaching hospital ICUs used an asynchrony index [the number of asynchrony events/(ventilator cycles + wasted respiratory effort) × 100] [127]. This study found that discomfort and air leaks were independent risk factors for asynchrony indices >10%. A follow-up study [131] found that an asynchrony index >10% occurred in 43% of patients and that double triggering and late cycling were the most common forms of asynchrony. Strategies to deal with asynchrony include minimizing air leaks, adjusting rise times and changing to timed modes (such as pressure control) to reduce the persistence of ventilator inspiration into patient expiration that occurs with bilevel modes [132], lowering pressure support when tidal volumes are large and breathing efforts fail to trigger the ventilator and giving sedation to control agitation or anxiety.

Rebreathing

Rebreathing has been a concern with bilevel ventilators in the past because of their single circuit design [133]. However, more recent studies have not demonstrated CO_2 rebreathing at levels deemed detrimental to patients, and rebreathing during NPPV has not been implicated in adverse patient outcomes [128,134] as long as the bias flow associated with expiratory pressures of 4 cm H_2O or greater are used flush CO_2 from the circuit to minimize rebreathing [129].

Air Leaks

Air leaks are universal during NIV because of its open circuit design. Some leaks are intentional as with bilevel ventilators, but air also leaks under the mask seal through the mouth and even into the gastrointestinal tract. Small leaks (<30 L per minute) are generally well tolerated as most ventilators compensate quite easily for them. However, large leaks (>60 L per minute) can have deleterious effects by interfering with ventilator assistance and synchrony, leading to increased work of breathing, fatigue, oxygen desaturations, and NIV failure. Leaks also contribute to patient discomfort, contributing to conjunctivitis, sleep disruption, and dry mouth [130]. Air leaks are associated with improperly sized or sealed masks, loose or excessively tightened headstraps, the presence of facial hair, unusual facial anatomy, high inspiratory pressure settings, and the presence of surgical dressings or catheters that disrupt the seal. Nasal masks are commonly associated with mouth leaks, reported to occur in as many as 94% of patients receiving NIV for hypercapnic ARF and contributing to the majority of mask failures [135]. In a comparison study of four different NIV interfaces among patients with ARF, the mouthpiece had the largest leak, while there was no significant difference between the Total Face Mask, oronasal mask, or nasal mask [136].

Measures that can be undertaken to minimize leaks include careful mask selection and fitting, proper strapping to the face, removal of facial hair, use of chin straps with nasal masks, and chin supports (built into certain mask types) for patients using oronasal masks. Leak-compensating ability of the ventilator is another consideration for patients having frequent or large leaks. Most bilevel ventilators compensate quite well, but newer critical care ventilators that have NIV modes may need additional adjustments when large leaks are present [104].

Caregiver-Related Factors

Complications of NIV are sometimes related to caregiver decisions that inadvertently predispose to NIV failure. Most commonly, these include selection of inappropriate candidates with excessively high risk of failure, such as ALI/ARDS patients who are septic and developing multiorgan failure or elderly pneumonia patients with poor cough and excessive secretions. Inadequate attention to detail during initiation predisposes to failure, including neglecting to spend time with the patient to instruct and win their confidence or to properly fit or attach the mask. Failure to increase the inspiratory pressure after initiation is a common cause of NIV failure because the patient never receives adequate ventilator assistance. Inadequate monitoring, either because an unstable patient is never sent from a regular ward to the ICU or because caregivers neglect the early signs of deterioration, permitting a respiratory crisis to occur, are other common reasons for NIV failures. Caregivers need to know when to intubate patients who are not responding adequately to NIV before an emergency or respiratory arrest occurs, avoiding delays of needed intubation. There is no substitute for having a skilled and experienced multidisciplinary team for optimizing NIV success rates. Evidence from studies indicates that as caregivers gain experience with NIV, patient outcomes improve, or they can sustain the same favorable outcomes for sicker patients [16].

Multidisciplinary Approach

NIV works best when it is administered as part of a team effort. Ideally, this is achieved in a specialized unit such as an ICU or step-down unit where members can gain experience by working together over time. Although team members may have different roles depending on the country they work in, all of the roles must be adopted by one team member or another in order for optimization of NIV delivery. In North America, physicians must be skilled at selecting appropriate patients for NPPV and writing proper orders for its initiation. The respiratory therapist then fits and applies the interface and makes initial ventilator adjustments. Nurses then monitor the patient, notifying the physician and therapist when problems arise. Physicians and therapists should also participate in monitoring so that they can intervene with timely adjustments to the mask or ventilator settings or with intubation, when needed. Pharmacologists assist in choosing the type and dose of sedation or analgesia if deemed indicated, and nutritionists assist in assuring that nutritional needs are met. Physical therapists may also become involved to help with secretion removal or early mobilization. In other countries such as in the United Kingdom, physiotherapists assume many of the roles of the respiratory therapist, and in many countries in the developing world, physicians are responsible for initiation and application of equipment in addition to their other duties. Regardless of how the responsibilities are distributed, most programs favor using protocols and having periodic training in-services that document NIV competencies for their team members.

Patient-Related Factors

Patients vary enormously in their ability to tolerate NIV, and this is reflected by success rates. Patients who are cognitively impaired due to congenital or acquired processes, such as strokes, dementia, or delirium, are unlikely to tolerate NIV because they cannot comprehend the purpose and become agitated. Other patients panic when a mask is strapped to their face, either because of claustrophobia or because of their already heightened anxiety and distress due to their respiratory condition. These factors must be kept in mind when selecting patients or when deciding that NIV has failed. Some anxious patients respond to reassurance and being given control of the mask and others require an anxiolytic. Patients with dementia or delirium can sometimes be managed successfully with antipsychotics like haloperidol, risperidone, or quetiapine.

Sedation and Analgesia during NPPV

Judicious use of sedation may help to calm patients having difficulty cooperating with NPPV, but most clinicians are very cautious, using smaller doses, mainly by intermittent bolus, than they use in invasively ventilated patients. Most respondents to a survey of critical care physicians from North America and Europe indicated that they used sedation or analgesia in less than 25% of patients [137]. They registered concerns about blunting the drive to breathe of spontaneously breathing patients. North Americans were more apt to use benzodiazepines alone and Europeans opioids alone as their preferred initial choice.

Dexmetetomidine, by virtue of its short duration of action, intravenous administration allowing rapid adjustment of effect, analgesic as well as sedative properties, and lack of respiratory depressant effects, has been considered an attractive agent for use with NIV. In a RCT, Devlin et al. [138] showed no benefit of dexmetetomidine compared to standard intermittent benzodiazepines and opioids when started routinely at initiation of NIV. However, in another RCT, Huang et al. [139] showed reduced intubation and shorter lengths of hospital stay in a study of patients with CPE failing NIV due to intolerance or agitation. In Europe, remifentanyl use was also associated with a reduced need for intubation for small cohorts of patients failing NPPV [140,141]. These observations suggest that these short-acting infusion medications may have advantages as rescue agents, but have no role as agents to be used routinely at the time of initiation of NIV. More information from clinical studies is needed before recommendations for specific medications and doses can be made, but use of sedation or analgesia should be considered for patients at risk of failing NPPV because of agitation, apprehension, or discomfort.

SUMMARY AND RECOMMENDATIONS

NIV has assumed an important role for the management of patients with ARF in critical care settings. Epidemiologic studies indicate that use of NIV has increased substantially over the past 15 years throughout the world. Current evidence indicates that NIV is well supported for therapy of ARF associated with COPD exacerbations and acute pulmonary edema. NIV is an option in a number of other settings, including immunocompromised patients with early ARF, facilitation of weaning of intubated COPD patients and for COPD or acute pulmonary edema patients in other settings, such as postoperative, postextubation, and patients with a DNI status. Less evidence supports use for acute asthma, obesity hypoventilation with an exacerbation, cystic fibrosis, or neuromuscular disease, but NPPV would be a consideration for these patients. Most patients with ARDS or severe community-acquired pneumonia should not be treated with NIV, but exceptions include those with minimal secretions, stable otherwise and with only one or at most two organ failures, when experienced personnel and a closely monitored setting is available. Initiation of NIV requires a properly fit and tolerable interface and a ventilator that is appropriately managed. Patients should be placed in a location that permits adequate monitoring of their state of physiologic stability, and monitoring should pay particular attention to subjective factors including mask tolerance and adaptation to mechanical ventilation. Administration should be by a skilled and experienced multidisciplinary team. Achievement of these goals should lead to appropriate and safe administration of NIV with better overall patient outcomes and more efficient utilization of scarce ICU resources. A recent development has been the increasing use of HFT to treat patients with acute hypoxemic respiratory failure and ARDS, or during the postextubation and postoperative periods. Recent high quality studies indicate that HFT is noninferior to NIV in these settings and may even exceed NIV efficacy for some situations. HFT is better tolerated than NIV, is an effective oxygenator, and can improve the efficiency of ventilation, but more studies are needed to better define its role relative to NIV.

Summary of Major Recommendations

- NIV should be considered the ventilator mode of first choice for ARF associated with COPD exacerbations [27] and acute CPE [42].
- NIV is an option for early ARF of immunocompromised patients, and facilitation of extubation in COPD patients.
- NIV can be considered to treat other patients with ARF such as those with asthma, exacerbations of cystic fibrosis, or obesity hypoventilation [15].
- For patients who decline invasive ventilation, NIV can be used as a form of life support or to palliate, but should be discontinued when goals are not being achieved [86].
- NIV should not be used routinely but very selectively and with close monitoring of patients with ARDS or pneumonia [64].
- NIV should be administered in an ICU, ED, or stepdown unit under close and continuous monitoring until stabilization has occurred [119].
- The full-face mask is the preferred initial interface for acute applications of NIV [95].
- Increases of expiratory pressure can be used to treat hypoxemia and increases in pressure support reduce work of breathing [117].
- Patient/ventilator asynchrony and air leaks can contribute to NIV failure and should be minimized [127].
- When NIV is failing, intubation should not be delayed [14].
- HFT may be considered as an alternative to NIV for selected patients with *de novo*, postoperative and postextubation hypoxemic respiratory failure, especially for patients intolerant of NIV [66,77,83].

References

1. Corrado A, Ginanni R, Villella G, et al: Iron lung versus conventional mechanical ventilation in acute exacerbation of COPD. *Eur Respir J* 23(3):419–424, 2004.
2. Hill NS: Use of negative pressure ventilation, rocking beds, and pneumobelts. *Respir Care* 39(5):532–545, 1994; discussion 545–539.
3. Tobin MJ: Mechanical ventilation. *N Engl J Med* 330(15):1056–1061, 1994.
4. Nava S, Hill N. Non-invasive ventilation in acute respiratory failure. *Lancet* 374(9685):250–259, 2009.
5. Demoule A, Girou E, Richard JC, et al: Increased use of noninvasive ventilation in French intensive care units. *Intensive Care Med* 32(11):1747–1755, 2006.
6. Chandra D, Stamm JA, Taylor B, et al: Outcomes of non-invasive ventilationfor acute exacerbations of COPD in the United States, 1998–2008. *Am J Respir Crit Care Med* 185(2):152–159, 2012.
7. Alagoz A, Ulus F, Sazak H, et al: Two cases of tracheal rupture after endotracheal intubation. *J Cardiothorac Vasc Anesth* 23(2):271–272, 2009.
8. Anzueto A, Frutos-Vivar F, Esteban A, et al: Incidence, risk factors and outcome of barotrauma in mechanically ventilated patients. *Intensive Care Med* 30(4):612–619, 2004.
9. Papaioannou V, Terzi I, Dragoumanis C, et al: Negative-pressure acute tracheobronchial hemorrhage and pulmonary edema. *J Anesth* 23(3):417–420, 2009.
10. Chuang YC, Wang CH, Lin YS: Negative pressure pulmonary edema: report of three cases and review of the literature. *Eur Arch Otorhinolaryngol* 264(9):1113–1116, 2007.
11. Elpern EH, Larson R, Douglass P, et al: Long-term outcomes for elderly survivors of prolonged ventilator assistance. *Chest* 96(5):1120–1124, 1989.
12. Rumbak MJ, Walsh FW, Anderson WM, et al: Significant tracheal obstruction causing failure to wean in patients requiring prolonged mechanical ventilation: a forgotten complication of long-term mechanical ventilation. *Chest* 115(4):1092–1095, 1999.
13. Griesdale DE, Bosma TL, Kurth T, et al: Complications of endotracheal intubation in the critically ill. *Intensive Care Med* 34(10):1835–1842, 2008.
14. Esteban A, Frutos-Vivar F, Ferguson ND, et al: Noninvasive positive-pressure ventilation for respiratory failure after extubation. *N Engl J Med* 350(24):2452–2460, 2004.
15. Ozsancak Ugurlu A, Sidhom SS, et al: Use and outcomes of noninvasive positive pressure ventilation in acute care hospitals in Massachusetts. *Chest* 145(5):964–971, 2014.
16. Girou E, Brun-Buisson C, Taille S, et al: Secular trends in nosocomial infections and mortality associated with noninvasive ventilation in patients with exacerbation of COPD and pulmonary edema. *JAMA* 290(22):2985–2991, 2003.
17. Esteban A, Frutos-Vivar F, Muriel A, et al. Evolution of mortality over time in patients receiving mechanical ventilation. *Am J Respir Crit Care Med* 188(2):220–230, 2013.
18. Kaul S, Pearson M, Coutts I, et al: Non-invasive ventilation (NIV) in the clinical management of acute COPD in 233 UK hospitals: results from the RCP/BTS 2003 National COPD Audit. *COPD* 6(3):171–176, 2009.
19. Maheshwari V, Paioli D, Rothaar R, et al: Utilization of noninvasive ventilation in acute care hospitals: a regional survey. *Chest* 129(5):1226–1233, 2006.
20. Hong SB, Oh BJ, Kim YS, et al: Characteristics of mechanical ventilation employed in intensive care units: a multicenter survey of hospitals. *J Korean Med Sci* 23(6):948–953, 2008.
21. Lindenauer PK, Stefan MS, Shieh MS et al: Outcomes associated with invasive and noninvasive ventilation among patients hospitalized with exacerbations of chronic obstructive pulmonary disease. *JAMA Intern Med.*174(12):1982–1993, 2014.
22. Stefan MS, Shieh MS, Pekow PS, et al: Trends in mechanical ventilation among patients hospitalized with acute exacerbation of COPD in the United States, 2001 to 2011.*Chest* 147:959–968, 2015.
23. Appendini L, Patessio A, Zanaboni S, et al; Physiologic effects of positive end-expiratory pressure and mask pressure support during exacerbations of chronic obstructive pulmonary disease. *Am J Respir Crit Care Med* 149(5):1069–1076, 1994.
24. Domenighetti G, Gayer R, Gentilini R: Noninvasive pressure support ventilation in non-COPD patients with acute cardiogenic pulmonary edema and severe community-acquired pneumonia: acute effects and outcome. *Intensive Care Med* 28(9):1226–1232, 2002.
25. Keenan SP, Mehta S: Noninvasive ventilation for patients presenting with acute respiratory failure: the randomized controlled trials. *Respir Care* 54(1):116–126, 2009.

26. Quon BS, Gan WQ, Sin DD: Contemporary management of acute exacerbations of COPD: a systematic review and metaanalysis. *Chest* 133(3):756–766, 2008.
27. Brochard L, Mancebo J, Wysocki M, et al: Noninvasive ventilation for acute exacerbations of chronic obstructive pulmonary disease. *N Engl J Med* 333(13):817–822, 1995.
28. Confalonieri M, Potena A, Carbone G, et al: Acute respiratory failure in patients with severe community-acquired pneumonia. A prospective randomized evaluation of noninvasive ventilation. *Am J Respir Crit Care Med* 160(5, Pt 1):1585–1591, 1999.
29. Bulow HH, Thorsager B: Non-invasive ventilation in do-not-intubate patients: five-year follow-up on a two-year prospective, consecutive cohort study. *Acta Anaesthesiol Scand* 53(9):1153–1157, 2009.
30. Fernandez R, Baigorri F, Artigas A: Noninvasive ventilation in patients with "do-not-intubate" orders: medium-term efficacy depends critically on patient selection. *Intensive Care Med* 33(2):350–354, 2007.
31. Levy M, Tanios MA, Nelson D, et al: Outcomes of patients with do-not-intubate orders treated with noninvasive ventilation. *Crit Care Med* 32(10):2002–2007, 2004.
32. Hilbert G, Gruson D, Portel L, et al: Noninvasive pressure support ventilation in COPD patients with postextubation hypercapnic respiratory insufficiency. *Eur Respir J* 11(6):1349–1353, 1998.
33. Ferrer M, Esquinas A, Arancibia F, et al: Noninvasive ventilation during persistent weaning failure: a randomized controlled trial. *Am J Respir Crit Care Med* 168(1):70–76, 2003.
34. Nava S, Ambrosino N, Clini E, et al: Noninvasive mechanical ventilation in the weaning of patients with respiratory failure due to chronic obstructive pulmonary disease. A randomized, controlled trial. *Ann Intern Med* 128(9):721–728, 1998.
35. Kilger E, Briegel J, Haller M, et al: Effects of noninvasive positive pressure ventilatory support in non-COPD patients with acute respiratory insufficiency after early extubation. *Intensive Care Med* 25(12):1374–1380, 1999.
36. Bersten AD, Holt AW, Vedig AE, et al: Treatment of severe cardiogenic pulmonary edema with continuous positive airway pressure delivered by face mask. *N Engl J Med* 325(26):1825–1830, 1991.
37. Ferrari G, Milan A, Groff P, et al: Continuous positive airway pressure vs. pressure support ventilation in acute cardiogenic pulmonary edema: a randomized trial. *J Emerg Med* 39:676–684, 2010.
38. Park M, Sangean MC, Volpe Mde S, et al: Randomized, prospective trial of oxygen, continuous positive airway pressure, and bilevel positive airway pressure by face mask in acute cardiogenic pulmonary edema. *Crit Care Med* 32(12):2407–2415, 2004.
39. Liesching T, Nelson DL, Cormier KL, et al. Randomized trial of bilevel versus continuous positive airway pressure for acute pulmonary edema. *J Emerg Med* 46(1):130–140, 2014
40. Gray A, Goodacre S, Newby DE, et al: Noninvasive ventilation in acute cardiogenic pulmonary edema. *N Engl J Med* 359(2):142–151, 2008.
41. Weng C-L, Zhao Y-T, Liu Q-H, et al: Meta-analysis: noninvasive ventilation in acute cardiogenic pulmonary edema. *Ann Intern Med* 152:590–600, 2010
42. Potts JM. Noninvasive positive pressure ventilation. Effect on mortality in acute cardiogenic pulmonary edema: a pragmatic meta-analysis. *Polskie Archiwum Medycyny Wewnętrznej* 119:349–352, 2009.
43. Mehta S, Jay GD, Woolard RH, et al: Randomized, prospective trial of bilevel versus continuous positive airway pressure in acute pulmonary edema. *Crit Care Med* 25(4):620–628, 1997.
44. Chadda K, Annane D, Hart N, et al: Cardiac and respiratory effects of continuous positive airway pressure and noninvasive ventilation in acute cardiac pulmonary edema. *Crit Care Med* 30(11):2457–2461, 2002.
45. Thompson J, Petrie DA, Ackroyd-Stolarz S, et al: Out-of-hospital continuous positive airway pressure ventilation versus usual care in acute respiratory failure: a randomized controlled trial. *Ann Emerg Med* 52(3):232–241, 241.e231, 2008.
46. Duchateau FX, Beaune S, Ricard-Hibon A, et al: Prehospital noninvasive ventilation can help in management of patients with limitations of life-sustaining treatments. *Eur J Emerg Med* 17(1):7–9, 2010.
47. Roessler MS, Schmid DS, Michels P, et al. Early out-of-hospital non-invasive ventilation is superior to standard medical treatment in patients with acute respiratory failure: a pilot study. *Emergency Medicine Journal* 29:409–414, 2012.
48. Ewig S, Torres A, Riquelme R, et al: Pulmonary complications in patients with haematological malignancies treated at a respiratory ICU. *Eur Respir J* 12(1):116–122, 1998.
49. Hilbert G, Gruson D, Vargas F, et al: Noninvasive ventilation in immunosuppressed patients with pulmonary infiltrates, fever, and acute respiratory failure. *N Engl J Med* 344(7):481–487, 2001.
50. Peigne V, Rusinova K, Karlin L, et al. Continued survival gains in recent years among critically ill myeloma patients. *Intensive Care Med* 35:512–518, 2009.
51. Molina R, Bernal T, Borges M, et al: Ventilatory support in critically ill hematology patients with respiratory failure. *Crit Care* 16:R133, 2012.
52. Lemiale V, Mokart D, Resche-Rigon M, et al: Effect of noninvasive ventilation vs oxygen therapy on mortality among immunocompromised patients with acute respiratory failure: a randomized clinical trial. *JAMA* 314:1711–1719, 2015.
53. Frat J-P, Ragot S, Girault C, et al:. Impact of non-invasive oxygenation strategies in immunocompromised patients with severe acute respiratory failure: post hoc analysis of a randomized trial. *Lancet Respir Med* 372(23):2185–2196, 2015.
54. Meduri GU, Cook TR, Turner RE, et al: Noninvasive positive pressure ventilation in status asthmaticus. *Chest* 110(3):767–774, 1996.
55. Fernandez MM, Villagra A, Blanch L, et al: Non-invasive mechanical ventilation in status asthmaticus. *Intensive Care Med* 27(3):486–492, 2001.
56. Soroksky A, Stav D, Shpirer I: A pilot prospective, randomized, placebo-controlled trial of bilevel positive airway pressure in acute asthmatic attack. *Chest* 123(4):1018–1025, 2003.
57. Soma T, Hino M, Kida K, et al: A prospective and randomized study for improvement of acute asthma by non-invasive positive pressure ventilation (NPPV). *Intern Med* 47(6):493–501, 2008.
58. Gupta D, Nath A, Agarwal R, et al:. A prospective randomized controlled trial on theefficacy of noninvasive ventilation in severe acute asthma. *Respir Care* 55:536–543, 2010.
59. Pollack CV Jr, Fleisch KB, Dowsey K: Treatment of acute bronchospasm with beta-adrenergic agonist aerosols delivered by a nasal bilevel positive airway pressure circuit. *Ann Emerg Med* 26(5):552–557, 1995.
60. Hill AT, Edenborough FP, Cayton RM, et al: Long-term nasal intermittent positive pressure ventilation in patients with cystic fibrosis and hypercapnic respiratory failure (1991–1996). *Respir Med* 92(3):523–526, 1998.
61. Ferrer M, Esquinas A, Leon M, et al: Noninvasive ventilation in severe hypoxemic respiratory failure: a randomized clinical trial. *Am J Respir Crit Care Med* 168(12):1438–1444, 2003.
62. Antonelli M, Conti G, Rocco M, et al: A comparison of noninvasive positive-pressure ventilation and conventional mechanical ventilation in patients with acute respiratory failure. *N Engl J Med* 339(7):429–435, 1998.
63. Jolliet P, Abajo B, Pasquina P, et al: Non-invasive pressure support ventilation in severe community-acquired pneumonia. *Intensive Care Med* 27(5):812–821, 2001.
64. Antonelli M, Conti G, Esquinas A, et al: A multiple-center survey on the use in clinical practice of noninvasive ventilation as a first-line intervention for acute respiratory distress syndrome. *Crit Care Med* 35(1):18–25, 2007.
65. Zhan Q, Sun B, Liang L, et al. Early use of noninvasive positive pressure ventilation for acute lung injury: a multicenter randomized controlled trial. *Crit Care Med* 40(2):455–460. 2012.
66. Frat JP, Thille AW, Mercat A, et al: High-flow oxygen through nasal cannula in acute hypoxemic respiratory failure. *N Engl J Med* 372(23):2185–2189, 2015.
67. Bellani G, Laffey JG, Pham T, et al: Noninvasive ventilation of patients with acute respiratory distress syndrome. Insights from the LUNG SAFE Study.*Am J Respir Crit Care Med* 195(1):67–77, 2017.
68. Patel BK, Wolfe KS, Pohlman AS,Hall JB, Kress JP. Effect of noninvasive ventilation delivered by helmet vs face mask on the rate of endotracheal intubation in patients with acute respiratory distress syndrome: a randomized clinical trial. *JAMA* 315:2435–2441, 2016.
69. Beltrame F, Lucangelo U, Gregori D, et al: Noninvasive positive pressure ventilation in trauma patients with acute respiratory failure. *Monaldi Arch Chest Dis* 54(2):109–114, 1999.
70. Hernandez G, Fernandez R, Lopez-Reina P, et al: Noninvasive ventilation reduces intubation in chest trauma-related hypoxemia: a randomized clinical trial. *Chest* 137(1):74–80, 2010.
71. Epstein SK: Etiology of extubation failure and the predictive value of the rapid shallow breathing index. *Am J Respir Crit Care Med* 152(2):545–549, 1995.
72. Boles JM, Bion J, Connors A, et al: Weaning from mechanical ventilation. *Eur Respir J* 29(5):1033–1056, 2007.
73. Keenan SP, Powers C, McCormack DG, et al: Noninvasive positive-pressure ventilation for postextubation respiratory distress: a randomized controlled trial. *JAMA* 287(24):3238–3244, 2002.
74. Nava S, Gregoretti C, Fanfulla F, et al: Noninvasive ventilation to prevent respiratory failure after extubation in high-risk patients. *Crit Care Med* 33(11):2465–2470, 2005.
75. Ferrer M, Valencia M, Nicolas JM, et al: Early noninvasive ventilation averts extubation failure in patients at risk: a randomized trial. *Am J Respir Crit Care Med* 173(2):164–170, 2006.
76. Ferrer M, Sellares J, Valencia M, et al: Non-invasive ventilation after extubation in hypercapnic patients with chronic respiratory disorders: randomised controlled trial. *Lancet* 374(9695):1082–1088, 2009.
77. Hernández G, Vaquero C, Colinas L, et al. Effect of postextubation high-flow nasal cannula vs noninvasive ventilation on reintubation and postextubation respiratory failure in high-risk patients: a randomized clinical trial. *JAMA* 316(15):1565–1574, 2016.
78. Ferreyra GP, Baussano I, Squadrone V, et al: Continuous positive airway pressure for treatment of respiratory complications after abdominal surgery: a systematic review and meta-analysis. *Ann Surg* 247(4):617–626, 2008.
79. Squadrone V, Coha M, Cerutti E, et al: Continuous positive airway pressure for treatment of postoperative hypoxemia: a randomized controlled trial. *JAMA* 293(5):589–595, 2005.
80. Kindgen-Milles D, Muller E, Buhl R, et al: Nasal-continuous positive airway pressure reduces pulmonary morbidity and length of hospital stay following thoracoabdominal aortic surgery. *Chest* 128(2):821–828, 2005.
81. Auriant I, Jallot A, Herve P, et al: Noninvasive ventilation reduces mortality in acute respiratory failure following lung resection. *Am J Respir Crit Care Med* 164(7):1231–1235, 2001.
82. Jaber S, Lescot T, Futier E, et al: Effect of noninvasive ventilation on tracheal reintubation amongpatients with hypoxemic respiratory failure following abdominalsurgery: a randomized clinical trial. *JAMA* 315(13):1345–1353, 2016.

83. Stephan F, Barrucand B, Petit P, et al. High-flow nasal oxygen vs noninvasive positive airway pressure in hypoxemic patients after cardiothoracic surgery. A randomized controlled trial. *JAMA* 313(23); 2331–2339, 2015.
84. Schettino G, Altobelli N, Kacmarek RM: Noninvasive positive pressure ventilation reverses acute respiratory failure in select "do-not-intubate" patients. *Crit Care Med* 33(9):1976–1982, 2005.
85. Nava S, Ferrer M, Esquinas A, et al. Palliative use of non-invasive ventilation in end-of-life patients with solid tumours: a randomised feasibility trial. *Lancet Oncol* 14(3):219–227, 2013.
86. Curtis JR, Cook DJ, Sinuff T, et al: Noninvasive positive pressure ventilation in critical and palliative care settings: understanding the goals of therapy. *Crit Care Med* 35(3):932–939, 2007.
87. Antonelli M, Conti G, Riccioni L, et al: Noninvasive positive-pressure ventilation via face mask during bronchoscopy with BAL in high-risk hypoxemic patients. *Chest* 110(3):724–728, 1996.
88. Antonelli M, Conti G, Rocco M, et al: Noninvasive positive-pressure ventilation vs. conventional oxygen supplementation in hypoxemic patients undergoing diagnostic bronchoscopy. *Chest* 121(4):1149–1154, 2002.
89. Pope JF, Birnkrant DJ, Martin JE, et al: Noninvasive ventilation during percutaneous gastrostomy placement in Duchenne muscular dystrophy. *Pediatr Pulmonol* 23(6):468–471, 1997.
90. Guarracino F, Cabrini L, Baldassarri R, et al: Non-invasive ventilation-aided transoesophageal echocardiography in high-risk patients: a pilot study. *Eur J Echocardiogr* 11:554–556, 2010.
91. Baillard C, Fosse JP, Sebbane M, et al: Noninvasive ventilation improves preoxygenation before intubation of hypoxic patients. *Am J Respir Crit Care Med* 174(2):171–177, 2006.
92. Confalonieri M, Garuti G, Cattaruzza MS, et al: A chart of failure risk for noninvasive ventilation in patients with COPD exacerbation. *Eur Respir J* 25(2):348–355, 2005.
93. Diaz GG, Alcaraz AC, Talavera JC, et al: Noninvasive positive-pressure ventilation to treat hypercapnic coma secondary to respiratory failure. *Chest* 127(3):952–960, 2005.
94. Navalesi P, Fanfulla F, Frigerio P, et al: Physiologic evaluation of noninvasive mechanical ventilation delivered with three types of masks in patients with chronic hypercapnic respiratory failure. *Crit Care Med* 28(6):1785–1790, 2000.
95. Kwok H, McCormack J, Cece R, et al: Controlled trial of oronasal versus nasal mask ventilation in the treatment of acute respiratory failure. *Crit Care Med* 31(2):468–473, 2003.
96. Chacur FH, Vilella Felipe LM, Fernandes CG, et al. The total face mask is more comfortable than the oronasal mask in noninvasive ventilation but is not associated with improved outcome. *Respiration* 82(5):426–430, 2011.
97. Ozsancak A, Sidhom SS, Liesching TN, et al. Evaluation of the total face mask for noninvasive ventilation to treat acute respiratory failure. *Chest* 139(5):1034–1041, 2011.
98. Antonelli M, Pennisi MA, Pelosi P, et al: Noninvasive positive pressure ventilation using a helmet in patients with acute exacerbation of chronic obstructive pulmonary disease: a feasibility study. *Anesthesiology* 100(1):16–24, 2004.
99. Pisani L, Mega C, Vaschetto R, et al: Oronasal mask versus helmet in acute hypercapnic respiratory failure. *Eur Respir J* 45(3):691–699, 2015.
100. Cavaliere F, Conti G, Costa R, et al: Noise exposure during noninvasive ventilation with a helmet, a nasal mask, and a facial mask. *Intensive Care Med* 30(9):1755–1760, 2004.
101. Patrick W, Webster K, Ludwig L, et al: Noninvasive positive-pressure ventilation in acute respiratory distress without prior chronic respiratory failure. *Am J Respir Crit Care Med* 153(3):1005–1011, 1996.
102. Fernandez R, Blanch L, Valles J, et al: Pressure support ventilation via face mask in acute respiratory failure in hypercapnic COPD patients. *Intensive Care Med* 19(8):456–461, 1993.
103. Ambrosino N, Nava S, Bertone P, et al: Physiologic evaluation of pressure support ventilation by nasal mask in patients with stable COPD. *Chest* 101(2):385–391, 1992.
104. Ferreira JC, Chipman DW, Hill NS, et al: Bilevel vs ICU ventilators providing noninvasive ventilation: effect of system leaks: a COPD lung model comparison. *Chest* 136(2):448–456, 2009.
105. Carteaux G, Lyazidi A, Cordoba-Izquierdo A, et al. Patient-ventilator asynchrony during noninvasive ventilation: a bench and clinical study. *Chest* 142(2):367–376, 2012.
106. Sanders MH, Moore SE, Eveslage J: CPAP via nasal mask: a treatment for occlusive sleep apnea. *Chest* 83(1):144–145, 1983.
107. Strumpf DC, Carlisle CC, Millman RP, et al: An evaluation of the Respironics BiPAP Bi-level CPAP device for delivery of assisted ventilation. *Respir Care* 35:415–422, 1990.
108. Fernandez-Vivas M, Caturla-Such J, Gonzalez de la Rosa J, et al: Noninvasive pressure support versus proportional assist ventilation in acute respiratory failure. *Intensive Care Med* 29(7):1126–1133, 2003.
109. Schwartz AR, Kacmarek RM, Hess DR: Factors affecting oxygen delivery with bi-level positive airway pressure. *Respir Care* 49(3):270–275, 2004.
110. Samolski D, Calaf N, Guell R, et al: Carbon dioxide rebreathing in non-invasive ventilation. Analysis of masks, expiratory ports and ventilatory modes. *Monaldi Arch Chest Dis* 69(3):114–118, 2008.
111. Schettino GP, Chatmongkolchart S, Hess DR, et al: Position of exhalation port and mask design affect CO_2 rebreathing during noninvasive positive pressure ventilation. *Crit Care Med* 31(8):2178–2182, 2003.
112. Lellouche F, Maggiore SM, Deye N, et al: Effect of the humidification device on the work of breathing during noninvasive ventilation. *Intensive Care Med* 28(11):1582–1589, 2002.
113. Richards GN, Cistulli PA, Ungar RG, et al: Mouth leak with nasal continuous positive airway pressure increases nasal airway resistance. *Am J Respir Crit Care Med* 154(1):182–186, 1996.
114. Storre JH, Seuthe B, Fiechter R, et al: Average volume-assured pressure support in obesity hypoventilation: a randomized crossover trial. *Chest* 130(3):815–821, 2006.
115. Gay PC, Hess DR, Hill NS: Noninvasive proportional assist ventilation for acute respiratory insufficiency. Comparison with pressure support ventilation. *Am J Respir Crit Care Med* 164(9):1606–1611, 2001.
116. Bertrand PM, Futier E, Coisel Y, et al: Neurally adjusted ventilatory assist vs pressure support ventilation for noninvasive ventilation during acute respiratory failure: a crossover physiologic study. *Chest* 143(1):30–36, 2013.
117. L'Her E, Deye N, Lellouche F, et al: Physiologic effects of noninvasive ventilation during acute lung injury. *Am J Respir Crit Care Med* 172(9):1112–1118, 2005.
118. Thys F, Roeseler J, Reynaert M, et al: Noninvasive ventilation for acute respiratory failure: a prospective randomised placebo-controlled trial. *Eur Respir J* 20(3):545–555, 2002.
119. Sinuff T, Cook DJ, Randall J, et al: Evaluation of a practice guideline for noninvasive positive-pressure ventilation for acute respiratory failure. *Chest* 123(6):2062–2073, 2003.
120. Ozsancak Ugurlu A, Sidhom SS, et al. Where is noninvasive ventilation actually delivered for acute respiratory failure? *Lung* 193(5):779–788, 2015.
121. Carteaux G, Millán-Guilarte T, De Prost N, et al. Failure of noninvasive ventilation for de novo acute hypoxemic respiratory failure: role of tidal volume. *Crit Care Med* 44(2):282–290, 2016.
122. Dellweg D, Hochrainer D, Klauke M, et al: Determinants of skin contact pressure formation during non-invasive ventilation. *J Biomech* 43(4):652–657, 2010.
123. Gregoretti C, Confalonieri M, Navalesi P, et al: Evaluation of patient skin breakdown and comfort with a new face mask for non-invasive ventilation: a multi-center study. *Intensive Care Med* 28(3):278–284, 2002.
124. De Keulenaer BL, De Backer A, Schepens DR, et al: Abdominal compartment syndrome related to noninvasive ventilation. *Intensive Care Med* 29(7):1177–1181, 2003.
125. Jean-Lavaleur M, Perrier V, Roze H, et al: Stomach rupture associated with noninvasive ventilation. *Ann Fr Anesth Reanim* 28(6):588–591, 2009.
126. Delay JM, Sebbane M, Jung B, et al: The effectiveness of noninvasive positive pressure ventilation to enhance preoxygenation in morbidly obese patients: a randomized controlled study. *Anesth Analg* 107(5):1707–1713, 2008.
127. Thille AW, Rodriguez P, Cabello B, et al: Patient-ventilator asynchrony during assisted mechanical ventilation. *Intensive Care Med* 32(10):1515–1522, 2006.
128. Lofaso F, Brochard L, Touchard D, et al: Evaluation of carbon dioxide rebreathing during pressure support ventilation with airway management system (BiPAP) devices. *Chest* 108(3):772–778, 1995.
129. Louis B, Leroux K, Isabey D, et al: Effect of manufacturer-inserted mask leaks on ventilator performance. *Eur Respir J* 35(3):627–636, 2010.
130. Storre JH, Bohm P, Dreher M, et al: Clinical impact of leak compensation during non-invasive ventilation. *Respir Med* 103(10):1477–1483, 2009.
131. Vignaux L, Vargas F, Roeseler J, et al: Patient-ventilator asynchrony during non-invasive ventilation for acute respiratory failure: a multicenter study. *Intensive Care Med* 35(5):840–846, 2009.
132. Calderini E, Confalonieri M, Puccio PG, et al: Patient-ventilator asynchrony during noninvasive ventilation: the role of expiratory trigger. *Intensive Care Med* 25(7):662–667, 1999.
133. Ferguson GT, Gilmartin M: CO_2 rebreathing during BiPAP ventilatory assistance. *Am J Respir Crit Care Med* 151(4):1126–1135, 1995.
134. Szkulmowski Z, Belkhouja K, Le QH, et al: Bilevel positive airway pressure ventilation: factors influencing carbon dioxide rebreathing. *Intensive Care Med* 36:688–691, 2010.
135. Girault C, Briel A, Benichou J, et al: Interface strategy during noninvasive positive pressure ventilation for hypercapnic acute respiratory failure. *Crit Care Med* 37(1):124–131, 2009.
136. Fraticelli AT, Lellouche F, L'Her E, et al: Physiological effects of different interfaces during noninvasive ventilation for acute respiratory failure. *Crit Care Med* 37(3):939–945, 2009.
137. Devlin JW, Nava S, Fong JJ, et al: Survey of sedation practices during noninvasive positive-pressure ventilation to treat acute respiratory failure. *Crit Care Med* 35(10):2298–2302, 2007.
138. Devlin JW, Al-Qadheeb NS, Chi A, et al. Efficacy and safety of early dexmedetomidine during noninvasive ventilation for patients with acute respiratory failure: a randomized, double-blind, placebo-controlled pilot study. *Chest* 145(6):1204–1212, 2014.
139. Huang Z, Chen YS, Yang ZL, et al: Dexmedetomidine versus midazolam for the sedation of patients with non-invasive ventilation failure. *Intern Med* 51:2299–2305, 2012.
140. Constantin JM, Schneider E, Cayot-Constantin S, et al. Remifentanil-based sedation to treat noninvasive ventilation failure: a preliminary study. *Intensive Care Med* 33:82–87, 2007.
141. Rocco M, Conti G, Alessandri E, et al. Rescue treatment for noninvasive ventilation failure due to interface intolerance with remifentanil analgosedation: a pilot study. *Intensive Care Med* 36: 2060–2065, 2010.

Chapter 168 ■ Discontinuation of Mechanical Ventilation

NICHOLAS A. SMYRNIOS • RICHARD S. IRWIN • ROLF D. HUBMAYR

A great deal of effort has been devoted to developing scientifically based strategies to achieve successful discontinuation of mechanical ventilation (MV), which is often referred to as "weaning." This chapter focuses on practical elements important for discontinuation. These include: (a) understanding the problem, (b) predicting successful discontinuation, and (c) managing discontinuation failure.

UNDERSTANDING THE PROBLEM

Who Are the Patients and What Are Their Outcomes?

Patients with respiratory failure are the individuals who require MV support. Although there is an overlap, respiratory failure can be generally categorized into lung failure and pump failure. *Lung failure* is pure gas-exchange failure and is manifested by hypoxemia. It is commonly caused by the acute respiratory distress syndrome or cardiogenic pulmonary edema. *Pump failure* is synonymous with ventilatory failure and is manifested by hypercapnia and hypoxemia. It is commonly caused by central nervous system depression (e.g., overdose and anesthesia) or respiratory muscle fatigue or weakness.

Early in a course of MV, patients require ventilation because of the original disease process that created their respiratory failure. For those who recover quickly from that original insult, most (80% to 90%) [1–4] can have MV easily discontinued and be extubated. For this group, MV can be discontinued in 77% of patients within 72 hours of the initiation of MV [4]. This group is composed predominantly of postoperative patients, patients with overdoses, and patients whose conditions cause pure lung failure that reverses rapidly. Later in their course of MV, the need for ventilation is usually less because of the original cause and more because of acquired barriers to weaning that have occurred during their hospitalization. Those patients, probably 10% to 20% of the total, are more difficult to wean from the ventilator and require additional attention. Data conflict regarding the impact of duration of MV on long-term survival. For example, 1-year survival for patients on MV for more than 21 days can be as high as 93% [5]. On the other hand, a recent study reported only a 56% 1-year survival and only 9% of those survivors were home without paid home care at 1 year [6]. Therefore, there is a great deal of improvement that can be realized for the treatment of this group of patients.

What Is Wrong with Patients on Prolonged Ventilator Support?

Acquired barriers to weaning generally affect the balance between the supply and demand for ventilation. These usually act in one of four ways [7].

1. *Inadequate respiratory drive* may be caused by nutritional deficiencies, sedatives, central nervous system abnormality, or sleep deprivation.
2. *Inability of the lungs to carry out gas exchange effectively* may continue if the underlying cause of respiratory failure has not sufficiently improved, or if the patient has preexisting lung disease. Causes of this include but are not limited to pneumonia, airway diseases such as asthma and chronic obstructive pulmonary disease (COPD), and pulmonary edema.
3. There may be profound *inspiratory respiratory muscle weakness* and possibly *fatigue*. Examples of causes include pulmonary and nonpulmonary infections, sedatives, neuromuscular blocking agents, and cardiovascular impairment.
4. *Psychologic dependency* may be an additional factor [8].

Of these, the literature suggests that pump failure caused by inspiratory respiratory muscle fatigue/weakness [9] is primarily responsible for failure of discontinuation of MV in the majority of these patients [3,10,11]. *Muscle fatigue* occurs when a muscle loses its ability to generate force because of being worked against a load. *Muscle weakness* is when a rested muscle is unable to generate force [12,13]. Although fatigue and weakness can be experimentally distinguished, this is not usually possible in the clinical setting. Therefore, the terms are often used interchangeably.

What Factors Lead to Respiratory Muscle Fatigue and Weakness?

The cause of inspiratory respiratory muscle fatigue is likely to be multifactorial. The major acquired barriers to weaning from MV are listed in Table 168.1. A few items deserve additional explanation.

Mechanical Ventilation

Although it is assumed that one of the benefits of MV is that it rests the respiratory muscles, this may not actually occur [14]. The responses of mechanical ventilators to rapid changes in patient effort are often inadequate. This is particularly true for older-generation ventilators. Positive pressure MV may increase minute volume without decreasing respiratory muscle work. In part, this is because ventilators used in either the assist control or synchronized intermittent mandatory ventilation (SIMV) modes do not synchronize their output with that of the patient's respiratory system. For extreme cases, the lack of synchronization causes patient effort to exceed that observed during unassisted breathing. Both SIMV and assist ventilation modes may cause problems in this regard. Also, SIMV systems expose patients to increases in airway resistance during spontaneous efforts that occur between machine breaths.

Continuous flow and demand valve systems have the potential for increasing the work of breathing. For instance, the continuous flow may not satisfy the patient's inspiratory flow demands. Demand valve SIMV systems may increase the work of breathing because they require substantial effort by the patient to breathe spontaneously. In assist control mode the patient's inspiratory muscles might work throughout the entire inspiratory cycle if tidal volume and inspiratory flow rate do not meet the patient's inspiratory demands. If auto–positive end-expiratory pressure (auto-PEEP) is present (see Chapters 30 and 166), the patient may not be able to trigger the ventilator or may be able to capture it only intermittently while performing a prohibitively large amount of work, because he or she must drop airway pressure below the amount of auto-PEEP before triggering the ventilator. If these events happen, the patient's diaphragm may develop an inflammatory injury that may not appear clinically for days

TABLE 168.1

Major Acquired Barriers to Weaning

1. Inadequate mechanical ventilation
2. Cardiac disease
    a. Coronary ischemia
    b. Left ventricular dysfunction
3. Volume overload
4. Infection
5. Nutritional deficiency
6. Neurologic dysfunction
    a. Neuromuscular abnormalities (including critical illness neuromyopathy)
    b. Altered mental status (including sedative effects)

afterward [15,16–18]. Paradoxically, although it is important to minimize the work of strenuous muscle activity while patients are receiving MV, it is also important to avoid prolonged muscle unloading because neuromuscular inactivity ("rest") can lead to ventilator-induced diaphragmatic dysfunction [18].

Cardiovascular Disease

Cardiac dysfunction affecting weaning may be categorized as ischemic disease or pump failure, or both. Failure of the cardiovascular system may prolong MV for a variety of reasons. Pulmonary edema may impair gas exchange, and this may contribute to an increased work of breathing during spontaneous breaths. Poor cardiac performance may contribute to an inadequate supply of oxygen to the respiratory muscles, whereas an increased work of breathing conversely may provoke myocardial ischemia [19]. Although MV may adversely affect cardiac output by increasing intrathoracic pressure, thereby decreasing venous return and cardiac output, it is also possible that some cardiovascular patients cannot have MV discontinued because the ventilator exerts a beneficial influence on cardiac function (i.e., unloading the left ventricle in left ventricular failure) [20]. Prematurely withdrawing MV from these patients may lead to deterioration of cardiac function.

Nutritional Factors

Nutritional deficiencies may prolong the discontinuation process by leading to myocardial and respiratory muscle dysfunction [21]. Older studies suggested that an appropriate amount of nutritional support may improve the success rate of discontinuation of MV [22], but these were not definitive. Randomized controlled trials comparing high-fat versus conventional feeds and growth hormone versus placebo showed no change in discontinuation success [23].

Other Factors

Important other factors that contribute to respiratory muscle fatigue and weakness are sedation and excess lung water. Further discussion of these factors may be found in the section on Managing Discontinuation Failure.

PREDICTING SUCCESSFUL DISCONTINUATION

When Is It Appropriate to Begin the Discontinuation Process?

There are no objective, rigorously generated data to determine the appropriate time to initiate weaning. Therefore, the authors recommend that clinicians consider a carefully monitored spontaneous breathing trial (SBT) when the following criteria, set forth in a national clinical practice guideline, have been met: (a) The underlying reason(s) for MV has been stabilized and the patient is improving, (b) the patient is hemodynamically stable on minimal-to-no pressors, (c) oxygenation is adequate (e.g., PaO_2/FiO_2 greater than 200, PEEP no more than 7.5 cm H_2O, FiO_2 less than 0.5), and (d) the patient is able to initiate spontaneous inspiratory efforts [24]. Because potentially harmful effects of suddenly having to take on the work of breathing occur early (albeit infrequently) during SBTs [25], patients should be closely monitored during the first 5 minutes. SBTs may be performed with a T-piece, with low-level pressure support ventilation (PSV), or with just a predetermined amount of continuous positive airway pressure (CPAP) using ventilators equipped with continuous flow internal circuits. There are no data that establish superiority of any of these approaches. There are also no data to show that attempts at starting the discontinuation of MV in this context lead to adverse consequences. On the contrary, screening patients daily to identify those who can breathe spontaneously can reduce the duration of MV and the cost of intensive care [26]. If the patient deteriorates or becomes distressed during this period of observation, MV should be restarted and a sufficient time given to allow the muscles to rest. That is generally done by performing the next trial the next day.

Predictive Indices for Total Discontinuation of Mechanical Ventilation (Weaning Indices)

A great deal of effort has gone into trying to find objective indices that will predict a patient's ability to be safely removed from the ventilator [27]. These studies yield conflicting data. A collective task force of clinician investigators cofacilitated by the American College of Chest Physicians, the American Association for Respiratory Care, and the American College of Critical Care Medicine developed evidence-based guidelines for weaning and discontinuing ventilatory support [24]. In their report, they evaluated the evidence for predicting success of weaning from MV [27]. A summary of their findings is as follows:

1. A large number of predictors have been found to be of no use in predicting the results of weaning.
2. A few predictors have been shown to be of some use, albeit inconsistent, for predicting discontinuation of the ventilator and successful extubation. Those include RR (RR) of less than 38 breaths per minute (sensitivity, 88%; specificity, 47%), a Rapid Shallow Breathing Index (RSBI) of less than 100 breaths/min/L (sensitivity, 65% to 96%; specificity, 0% to 73%), and an inspiratory pressure/maximal inspiratory pressure ratio less than 0.3. In addition, the combination of a RR of more than 38 breaths per minute and a RSBI more than 100 breaths/min/L appears to reduce the probability of successful extubation.
3. The ratio of airway pressure 0.1 second after the occlusion of the inspiratory port of unidirectional balloon occlusion valve ($P_{0.1}$) to maximal inspiratory pressure (PI_{max}) of 0.09 to 0.14 was highly predictive of successful extubation in two studies with a pooled Likelihood Ratio (LR) of 16.3 (>10 or <0.1 significant).
4. When LRs were calculated for RSBI, pooled results for a test predicting successful discontinuation showed a LR of 2.8; results for a test predicting failure of discontinuation showed a LR of 0.22. These results suggest mediocre accuracy [28].

Although clinical observation of the respiratory muscles during spontaneous breaths was initially thought to be reliable in predicting discontinuation failure, respiratory-inductive plethysmographic studies [29] cast this into question. Any time there is a substantial increase of load on the respiratory muscles, a change in the rate, depth, and pattern of breathing may be observed. Because these signs may also be manifestations of fatigue, it is useful to note them. If these signs never appear, successful discontinuation is likely. If they do appear, patients must be observed closely for further deterioration because discontinuation inevitably fails if these signs are owing to fatigue.

When Is It Appropriate to Extubate the Patient?

Patients will succeed following extubation if they are able to pump air in and out adequately, and if they are able to maintain the patency of their airway. Therefore, a patient must (1) successfully pass an SBT in one or another weaning mode, (2) meet expectations that they will not suffer from upper airway obstruction, and (3) have a reasonable expectation of secretion clearance.

Weaning Modes

A patient can be placed on an SBT abruptly or gradually. An abrupt approach is generally referred to as an SBT method. Gradual approaches are achieved by either progressively reducing the RR or reducing the pressure applied. Clinically, those approaches are generally known as either "intermittent mandatory ventilation (IMV)" and "PSV" approaches to ventilator liberation. In addition, some degree of support for ventilation can be applied even after removal from the ventilator. In common terms, that is usually referred to as the "noninvasive positive pressure ventilation (NIPPV)" approach (see Chapter 167).

Results of randomized controlled trials comparing methods for weaning subjects from MV show that both SBT and PSV trials are superior to SIMV trials [30–32]. Therefore, we strongly discourage the use of SIMV for weaning. There are no convincing data to support the superiority of SBT or PSV compared to each other, and no data to support the practice of changing modes in patients who are not weaning successfully. The use of NIPPV should be limited to use for patients with CO_2 retention [33]. In other situations, NIPPV has not been shown to avoid reintubation in comparison to standard modes and can be potentially dangerous by delaying reintubation time [34]. Because we do not recommend SIMV trials, we only provide examples of SBT, PSV, and NIPPV protocols.

Spontaneous Breathing Trials. SBTs consist of the sudden, complete withdrawal of machine support. Patients are closely observed as they breathe humidified gas mixtures delivered by the T-shaped tube that is connected to the endotracheal or tracheostomy tube; alternatively, they can remain connected to the ventilator and be allowed to breathe spontaneously in the CPAP mode. In contrast to techniques that involve the gradual withdrawal of machine support, during SBTs the patient's cardiorespiratory response patterns can be assessed without the confounding influence of machine settings. Although there is no generally agreed on standard of applying this method of discontinuation, most practitioners begin SBTs from assisted, not controlled, MV and assess the patient's tolerance.

Although CPAP is not universally used, the authors believe that it is physiologically sound to undertake SBTs in conjunction with CPAP irrespective of the underlying disease process. The addition of 5 cm H_2O of CPAP mitigates the fall in end-expired lung volume that results from having eliminated glottic regulation of upper-airway resistance and flow with an endotracheal tube [35]. Furthermore, for patients with airflow obstruction, CPAP can substantially lower the work of breathing by counterbalancing end-expiratory system recoil pressures (i.e., intrinsic PEEP) and by shifting loads from inspiratory to expiratory muscles [36–38]. It is not likely that the 5 cm H_2O of external PEEP will provoke hyperinflation by exceeding intrinsic PEEP.

An alternative mechanism by which CPAP can reduce inspiratory elastic work in airflow obstruction is by recruiting expiratory muscles during spontaneous breathing (SB). CPAP may result in exhalation below the new static equilibrium volume through the recruitment of expiratory muscles. Subsequent relaxation of the expiratory muscles inflates the lungs passively back to the new equilibrium volume. This may have the effect of unloading inspiratory muscles because the expiratory muscles do part of the inspiratory work. However, this mechanism is of limited value among patients with severe obstruction because low maximal flows prevent significant reductions of lung volume below static equilibrium volume.

In patients who continue to require MV only for oxygenation, CPAP may help maintain the benefits of improved oxygenation provided by PEEP without exposing the patient to the hazards of MV. It may also augment cardiac function during weaning.

Spontaneous Breathing Protocol. General guidelines are as follows:

1. When it has been decided that the patient is improving and stable, inform the patient that an attempt to remove MV will be made, why you believe he or she is ready, and what to expect. It is important to allow the patient to express fears whenever possible and to try to alleviate them [39].
2. Obtain baseline values and begin monitoring clinical parameters, such as pulse rate, RR, blood pressure, and subjective distress (e.g., have patients rate their dyspnea from 0 to 10), gas exchange (e.g., by pulse oximetry), and cardiac rhythm (e.g., by electrocardiographic monitoring). Record these values on a flow sheet that should be maintained and available. Arterial blood gases are generally not monitored during discontinuation trials.
3. Ensure a calm atmosphere by having the nurse, respiratory therapist, or physician remain at the bedside to offer encouragement and support.
4. Avoid sedation to ensure maximal patient effort. In most cases an interruption of continuous sedation is performed to coincide with the SBT.
5. Whenever possible, let the patient sit upright in bed or in a chair.
6. Fit the patient's endotracheal tube with a T-tube connected to a heated nebulizer with an inspired oxygen concentration 10% greater than that prevailing during the previous course of MV. Ensure that the T-tube flow exceeds the patient's peak inspiratory flow and that the inhaled gas is constantly humidified. If CPAP is being used, the T-tube setup becomes unnecessary and the ventilator system tubing is used.
7. Continue the trial to completion unless the following conditions develop:
    a. New onset diaphoresis
    b. New onset arrhythmias
    c. Systolic BP >180 mm Hg, or a change (increase or decrease) of ≥20% of the original systolic value or a new requirement for vasopressors.
    d. Heart rate >120, or a change (increase or decrease) of >30 beats per minute
    e. SaO_2 <90%, FiO_2 >0.6
    f. *If a blood gas is obtained*, pH <7.30; PaO_2 <60 mm Hg; SaO_2 <90%; rise in $PaCO_2$ of more than 10 mm Hg.
    g. Unstable pattern of ventilation
    h. RR <8 breaths per minute, >35 breaths per minute for >5 minutes, change of >50% of original RR, or a RSBI (f/V_T) >100
    i. New onset altered mental status
    j. Signs of respiratory muscle failure including new onset use of accessory muscles of breathing or thoracoabdominal paradox

k. Subjective discomfort of the patient with dyspnea or new pain rated as greater than 5/10
l. Failure as determined by the subjective assessment of the nurse, physician, or the respiratory therapist

If the trial is terminated, place the patient back on the previous MV settings. With few exceptions, such as patients recovering from general anesthesia or sedation with or without muscle paralysis, the authors usually do not have their patients undergo more than one (failed) discontinuation trial in any 24-hour period. This practice is supported by the work of Esteban et al. [40], who showed that twice-daily SBTs offered no advantage over once-daily trials. Moreover, the inspiratory effort associated with a failed weaning trial may be sufficient to induce muscle fatigue that may not recover [40], unless it is followed by an extended period of rest.

If a patient has no underlying lung disease, has been on MV for only a short time (e.g., less than 1 week), appears to be tolerating SB without dyspnea for 30 to 120 minutes, and maintains an adequate level of oxygenation, extubation may be performed after considering whether the patient is at risk of postextubation upper airway obstruction or not being able to clear secretions.

Pressure-Support Ventilation Trials. PSV discontinuation decreases MV gradually, making the patient responsible for a progressively increasing amount of ventilation. Although it is commonly assumed that PSV can be decreased to a low level (e.g., 5 to 7 cm H_2O) that compensates for endotracheal tube and circuit resistance, there is no simple way of predicting the level of PSV that compensates for this resistance.

PSV has become a popular mode of discontinuing MV for adults. In the PSV mode, a target pressure is applied to the endotracheal tube that augments the inflation pressure exerted by the inspiratory muscles on the respiratory system [41]. As the lungs inflate, inspiratory flow begins to decline because airway pressure and the inflation pressure exerted by the inspiratory muscles are opposed by rising elastic recoil forces. When inspiratory flow reaches a threshold value (that differs among vendors), the machine switches to expiration [42]. The popularity of PSV is based on the premise that discontinuation from MV should be a gradual process (meeting the definition of " weaning"). In addition, proponents of PSV over SBTs argue that the work of unassisted breathing through an endotracheal tube is unreasonably high and could lead to inspiratory muscle failure among susceptible patients [43]. For example, it has become popular to assume that PSV is an effective means to overcome the resistance of endotracheal tubes. However, this is conceptually incorrect because airway pressure during PSV does not vary with flow. Furthermore, a reduction of pulmonary resistance is not demonstrated after extubation [44], and the work of breathing may actually increase [45]. This suggests that, at least immediately after extubation, most patients manifest upper-airway resistance that is, in effect, equal to or greater than that of an 8-mm internal diameter endotracheal tube.

Enthusiasm for using PSV for all patients should be tempered by knowledge of its potential adverse patient–ventilator interactions. For example, elderly patients and even healthy individuals [46] are susceptible to PSV setting–induced central apneas. The mechanism appears to be intermittent hypocapnia, resulting from the uncoupling of tidal volume from inspiratory effort. Problems may arise when the physician feels compelled to rest susceptible subjects with PSV at night. Unless sufficiently high IMV backup rates are used in combination with PSV, the mechanical inhibition of inspiratory drive may result in apneas that trigger ventilator alarms and cause arousals and sleep fragmentation that can prolong the discontinuation process.

Pressure Support Protocol. General guidelines are as follows:

1. Repeat steps 1 through 5 of the SB protocol.
2. Switch the MV mode from volume-cycled breathing with assist or SIMV modes to PS, or, if the patient is already on PS as a ventilatory mode, decrease the amount of PS.
3. For patients who have received prolonged ventilator support (e.g., greater than 21 days), patients with neurologic diseases, or patients who have recently failed extubation, begin PS at a pressure of 25 cm H_2O if switching from another ventilatory mode, or less than the amount previously used during PS ventilation, and increase the fraction of inspired oxygen by 10%. Decrease airway inflation pressure slowly. If the patient fails to assume the increased work of breathing at a lower pressure, increase the pressure to the previously tolerated level and then higher, if necessary, until the patient is stable again. Then wait for 24 hours and begin the process again.
4. For patients who have no underlying lung disease and who have been on MV for only a short time (e.g., less than 1 week), PS can be set at 7 cm H_2O. If this pressure is well tolerated for 2 hours, the patient should be assessed for extubation [47].

Noninvasive Positive-Pressure Ventilation as a Mode of Discontinuing Mechanical Ventilation. A comprehensive description of NIPPV can be found in Chapter 167. Patients can receive this form of ventilation using either a ventilator specifically designed for noninvasive positive-pressure or an intensive care unit (ICU) ventilator, using PS mode plus PEEP. Ventilation can be delivered with a nose or face mask or, outside the USA, a helmet. Current literature indicates that the use of noninvasive ventilation as a "rescue" therapy for patients who are experiencing respiratory failure following extubation is ineffective for preventing reintubation [48]. Noninvasive ventilation may be an effective strategy for reducing reintubations and mortality among patients with chronic CO_2 retention when used routinely early after extubation [49].

Noninvasive Positive-Pressure Ventilation Protocol. General guidelines are as follows [50]:

1. Repeat steps 1 through 5 of the SB protocol.
2. Extubate the patient, apply a nose or face mask designed for NIPPV, and begin assisted breathing. Continuously adjust the ventilator settings (see Chapter 167) according to patient comfort, the presence of air leaks, and monitoring.
3. In between periods of 1 to 2 hours of SB with supplemental oxygen, intersperse intermittent periods of ventilation for 2 to 4 hours at a time. Then, gradually increase the duration of the SB periods as tolerated by the patient (e.g., monitor RR, gas exchange, and cardiorespiratory parameters and dyspnea).
4. When the period of SB spans the entire day and the patient is only receiving nocturnal ventilation, consideration should be given for discontinuing NIPPV.

Unconventional Modes of Discontinuing Mechanical Ventilation

A variety of unconventional techniques have been tried for discontinuing MV. These include inspiratory strength training [51], adaptive support ventilation [52], biofeedback [53,54], automatic tube compensation [55,56], and proportional assist ventilation. None of these techniques are supported by adequate evidence to justify recommendation as routine care.

Uncontrolled reports suggest that inspiratory muscle strength training [57] may be useful for preparing patients who are on prolonged ventilatory support for discontinuation. This method is thought to serve as a means of respiratory muscle endurance training; it is implemented by having patients perform low-repetition, high-resistance SB exercises.

During adaptive support ventilation [52], an automatic microprocessor-controlled mode of MV ensures the delivery of preset minute ventilation. It does this by continuously adapting to the patient's respiratory activity. Adaptive-support ventilation was developed in an attempt to automatically discontinue patients from MV by feedback from one or more ventilator-measured parameters.

Biofeedback, the detection and transmission back to the patient of some biologic functions that he or she cannot detect, may be helpful for selected patients [53,54]. For instance, by displaying respiratory volumes on bedside oscilloscopes and having patients make voluntary efforts to push volume tracings beyond limits taped on the screen, Corson et al. [53] allowed two patients with spinal cord lesions—one with a sensory level at C6 who lacked proprioceptive afferents from the chest wall—to gain control over their breathing. These authors assumed that the repeated practice of reaching the criteria of feedback increased the strength of the diaphragm and inspiratory muscles and may have had the net effect of enabling the medullary center to reinstate automatic breathing.

Automatic tube compensation (i.e., a means of resistive unloading during ventilator-assisted SB by compensating for the pressure drop across the endotracheal tube) has been best studied. Compared with SBT in a randomized controlled trial, there was no clear difference in clinically significant outcomes [57].

Proportional assist ventilation (PAV) is a mode of partial ventilatory support in which the ventilator applies pressure in proportion to the inspiratory effort [58]. This has potential value in liberating patients from MV. The theoretical advantage is that the support applied seems to coordinate well with the patient's own respiratory effort, thereby simulating SB but with less respiratory work. No studies have demonstrated a clinical advantage of this method over conventional methods.

How Long Should Discontinuation Trials Last?

The question regarding length of discontinuation trials has not been definitively answered. Therefore, the duration depends on the patient population, the weaning mode, and local practice. With respect to SBTs, a number of authors have set a maximum limit of 2 hours [25,30,47,59–62] and have extubated patients who were deemed stable by clinical, respiratory, and hemodynamic parameters. With respect to PSV trials, some have recommended that stable patients need only be on PSV at a setting of 5 to 7 cm H_2O for 2 hours before extubation. With these guidelines, reintubation rates range from 13% to 23% [30]. With respect to SBTs, other authors have found no difference in success of discontinuing MV when 30-minute and 2-hour trial intervals have been compared [61,62]. Nevertheless, because reintubation has been shown to be associated with a significantly greater risk of (a) in-hospital mortality, (b) ICU and hospital length of stay, and (c) transfer rate to a long-term care or rehabilitation facility [60], and because it is prudent to minimize the need for reintubation, we recommend the following:

- The authors prefer SBTs over other modes because they are the most direct way to assess the patient's performance without ventilatory support.
- Consider extubating patients who have well-tolerated SBTs of 30 to 120 minutes, with the following exceptions [63,64]: (a) patients with a tracheostomy who meet the definition of being on prolonged MV (i.e., at least 21 days for at least 6 hours per day), (b) neurologic patients who are predicted to have difficulty clearing their respiratory secretions, and (c) patients who have had to be reintubated after the recent discontinuation of MV. It is our practice to observe these patients breathing spontaneously for 2 to 24 hours before considering extubation. Factors discussed below related to upper airway obstruction and secretion clearance play a major role in determining the length of an SBT.
- Discontinuation should be performed using a clinical practice guideline that clearly defines responsibilities and empowers nurses and respiratory therapists to act within their scope of practice.

Upper Airway Obstruction

Patients at the highest risk of postextubation upper airway obstruction are those who have been on prolonged MV, are female, who have had repeated or traumatic intubations, or who have been intubated with a larger endotracheal tube size [65,66]. One method of assessing for the presence of upper airway obstruction during MV is the cuff-leak test. It is performed by comparing the exhaled volumes before and after the balloon of the endotracheal tube has been deflated. Although one study [67] showed that a cuff leak of less than 110 mL measured during assist-control ventilation within 24 hours of extubation identified patients at high risk of postextubation stridor, other studies have not [68]. Although the concept of measuring cuff leak is intuitively appealing, the benefits are not clearly identified, and the process and even the actual values for decision-making are not broadly agreed upon. Values of 110, 130, and 140 mL have all been published, and other studies used an approach of auscultation to detect leak. In addition, the appropriate course of action to take for an abnormal test is not defined. Some authors suggest treatment with steroids, some suggest delay of extubation, and some advocate having persons with advanced airway skills present for the extubation. Because we are unable to scientifically determine which patients should have a test, how we would conduct the test and what would constitute an abnormal result, and what we would do with an abnormal value if we had one, we do not advocate routinely performing or basing decisions on the results of a cuff-leak test. A provider may consider using a cuff-leak test for specific patients to gain a general appreciation of the airway status in a high-risk patient [69–71]. We also do not routinely administer systemic steroids to prevent postextubation stridor because of the inconsistent benefits reported by studies, and the uncertain timing of extubation encountered in clinical practice, which could potentially lead to extended courses of steroids with their associated side effects [72].

Secretion Clearance

Patients may also fail extubation because they are unable to clear their secretions. A prospective observational study [73] showed that the strongest predictors of extubation failure in patients who passed an SBT were (a) poor cough defined as a cough peak flow measurement of less than 60 L per minute, (b) secretion volume of 2.5 mL per hour or greater, and (c) poor mentation as determined by the inability to complete any of the four following tasks on command: open eyes, follow observer with eyes, grasp hand, and stick out tongue. In this series, reintubation took place in 12% of patients when one of these predictors was present and 80% when all were present.

Once extubation has taken place, the authors proceed cautiously before instituting feedings by mouth. Because there is no clinically reliable way of assessing the adequacy of swallowing at the bedside and picking up "silent aspiration," a formal swallowing evaluation (e.g., speech pathology consult and video fluoroscopic evaluation of swallow) should be considered for patients at increased risk of aspiration before resuming oral feedings. Although it is commonly appreciated that older age, debilitation, sedation, oral or nasal enteral feeding tubes, history of dysphagia, acute stroke, cervical spine surgery, muscle weakness, and/or tracheostomy are risk factors for aspiration, it is less commonly known that endotracheal intubation carries the same risk [74,75]. After extubation, swallowing difficulties exist among up to 50% of patients for 1 week, even when intubation has been of short duration, and the patient is awake and not seriously ill. In awake, postsurgical patients evaluated for aspiration following extubation, 50% of those who aspirated did so immediately when fed, whereas 25% and 5% aspirated when tested 4 and 8 hours later, respectively.

MANAGING DISCONTINUATION FAILURE

The authors' general approach to managing patients who have failed to have MV discontinued is based on three tenets: (a) protocol-based weaning yields superior outcomes when compared to nonprotocolized weaning; (b) SBT or PSV trials should be performed once daily; and (c) barriers to weaning are clinical conditions that promote muscle fatigue and weakness. Interventions that address and reverse these barriers are keys to successfully liberate patients from MV.

Protocol-Based Weaning

Multiple randomized controlled clinical trials [25,76] and nonrandomized controlled trials [77] have shown overwhelming advantages for clinically significant outcomes (e.g., decreased duration of MV, reintubation rates, ICU and hospital LOS) generated by the use of protocol-directed discontinuation implemented by nonphysician health care providers. These findings have been supported by a recent meta-analysis [78]. That report identified that reduced duration of MV, discontinuation duration, and ICU length of stay can be realized with use of standardized discontinuation protocols. These improvements are more consistent and of a larger magnitude than those generated by virtually any other intervention related to liberation from MV. Therefore, the authors strongly recommend that institutions employ protocols to guide interprofessional discontinuation efforts rather than wean by individual physician discretion.

Once-Daily Attempts at Liberation from Mechanical Ventilation

On the basis of multiple randomized controlled trials of methods for discontinuing patients from MV [32], the authors recommend that once-daily SBT or PSV trials be used as the discontinuation mode of choice. Because duration of MV is primarily determined by admitting diagnosis and degree of physiologic derangement [79], there does not appear to be anything to be gained by switching from one mode to another when the discontinuation process is prolonged. Switching to another mode and waiting to see the response directs the attention away from addressing factors that cause inspiratory muscle fatigue/weakness that we believe are the most important reason why patients are on prolonged MV.

Addressing Factors That Perpetuate Respiratory Muscle Fatigue

Respiratory muscle fatigue is almost always multifactorial in etiology (Table 168.2). Therefore, clinicians should systematically consider ways to increase muscle strength and decrease muscle demand.

The following measures should be considered to increase respiratory muscle strength:

1. Reverse malnutrition [22] and correct deficiencies of electrolytes.
2. Improve cardiovascular pump function and minimize cardiac ischemia [20]. Poor cardiac performance may contribute to an inadequate supply of oxygen to the respiratory muscles.

TABLE 168.2

Summary of Advances in Managing Discontinuation from Mechanical Ventilation Based on Randomized Controlled Clinical Trials

- Protocol-directed, ventilator management teams lead to favorable outcomes [25,76,77].
- SBTs or pressure support trials are superior to SIMV trials [32].
- 30- and 120-min trials are equally successful [61,74].
- Twice-daily spontaneous trials offer no advantage over once-daily trials [31,32].
- Daily interruption of sedation leads to better outcomes than continuous infusions [80].
- A combination of a daily sedation holiday with once-daily SBTs improves outcomes [83].
- Early physical and occupational therapy reduces ventilator time [89].
- Early tracheostomy leads to reduced ventilator time and ICU length of stay [98].

SIMV, synchronized intermittent mandatory ventilation; ICU, intensive care unit

3. Attempt to minimize the use of sedative drugs whenever possible. Whereas daily interruption of sedation compared to continuous infusions significantly decreases duration of MV and length of stay in a medical ICU [80], a more aggressive approach is to eliminate the use of continuous sedation and/or all sedation. One study of no sedation reported an increase of ventilator free days and a reduced ICU and hospital length of stay without any change in mortality [81]. Further study is needed to confirm these results. To assist in managing sedation, clinicians are encouraged to use validated and reliable monitoring scales such as the Richmond Agitation-Sedation Scale [82]. Pairing sedation and ventilator weaning protocols may yield a mortality benefit [83].
4. Efforts to reduce sedation overlap with attempts to reduce the incidence of delirium. A major component of these efforts is to reduce or eliminate the use of benzodiazepines by ventilated patients. Some authors have advocated for the use of dexmedetomidine for ventilated patients to reduce the incidence of delirium that leads to increased sedation. A randomized trial demonstrated reductions of the incidence of delirium and time on the ventilator seen with dexmedetomidine in comparison to midazolam [84]. Other components of delirium prevention include appropriate pain control, lighter levels of sedation, preservation of sleep-wake cycles, cognitive stimulation, and early mobilization among others.
5. Consider and evaluate for the possibilities of myopathy and polyneuropathy [85] and drug-induced neuromuscular dysfunction (e.g., neuromuscular blocking agents and antibiotics, especially aminoglycosides) [86,87]. Critical illness polyneuropathy and myopathy are major causes of persistent respiratory failure [88].
6. Mobilize patients to the maximum of their tolerance and initiate physical and occupational therapy early in their course. A protocol of early physical and occupational therapy combined with daily interruption of sedation demonstrated significant improvements in return to baseline functional status at hospital discharge and for the number of ventilator free days in the first 28 days of hospital stay [89].
7. Have the patient sit up to take advantage of gravity and maximize diaphragm function.
8. Reverse hypothyroidism.
9. Previously some authors have suggested improving respiratory muscle contractility with various interventions including

elimination of hypercapnia by increasing excretion of compensatory bicarbonate ions. However recently a randomized, placebo controlled trial controlled trial of acetazolamide failed to show any improvements in mortality, duration of MV or other clinically relevant end points [90]. Therefore, we do not recommend that approach.

10. Consider that progesterone may act as a respiratory center stimulant [91] in patients who take few or no spontaneous breaths despite a lack of sedative drugs. The effect of 20 mg of medroxyprogesterone acetate three times per day should begin within 2 days and be maximal within 7 days. This is a controversial therapy. Many believe the additional respiratory center stimulation may be inappropriate and precipitate worsening muscle fatigue.

The following measures should be considered to decrease respiratory muscle demand:

1. Maximize treatment of systemic disease (e.g., infection, acute and chronic uremia) to decrease metabolic requirements and mitigate production of chemical mediators with adverse effects on muscle.
2. Give bronchodilators for conditions associated with increased airway resistance (see Chapters 172 and 173); discontinue beta-blockers in asthmatic patients.
3. Use diuretics to reduce lung water in patients with pulmonary edema. Closely monitor renal function and serum sodium to avoid precipitating renal failure and hypernatremia.
4. Evaluate for compromised cardiac function. Echocardiography and assessments for myocardial ischemia such as 12 lead ECG or ST segment monitoring can diagnose underlying cardiac disorders. The increased work of breathing during discontinuation may steal oxygen from the heart as well as other organs and precipitate ischemia and heart failure among susceptible patients [20,92,93].
5. For average-size adults, endotracheal tubes less than 8 mm in internal diameter significantly increase airway resistance, although it is unlikely that tube size adversely affects the discontinuation process unless the tube is prohibitively small (i.e., <6 mm). If an effect on weaning success is suspected, replace the smaller tube with one with a larger internal diameter.
6. Consider CPAP for patients with marginal cardiac function. It may provide support for a failing heart by decreasing left ventricular preload [20,94].
7. Consider that the ventilator is increasing the work of breathing, and make adjustments [14]. Potential factors include (a) the appropriateness of the sensitivity/responsivity of the ventilator triggering system, (b) whether the ventilator flow pattern is synchronized with the patient's demand, (c) the appropriateness of the ventilator settings to avoid dynamic hyperinflation, (d) considering usage of extrinsic PEEP to overcome an increased triggering threshold load from $PEEP_i$, and (e) changing a heat and moisture exchanger to a heated humidifier to overcome the increased dead space and resistance of the exchanger [95].
8. Evaluate for overfeeding. Excess total caloric intake, but not disproportionate carbohydrate intake, may precipitate increased CO_2 production and respiratory acidosis for patients unable to increase their alveolar ventilation adequately when compensating for increased CO_2 production [96]. The treatment for this is to reduce caloric intake.
9. Consider performing tracheostomy when patients are predicted to require prolonged MV. Tracheostomy may improve patient comfort and mitigate the need for more sedation, decrease airway resistance, decrease ventilator-associated pneumonia, and decrease duration of MV. Although the best time to perform tracheostomy is not known, a recent meta-analysis of early versus late tracheostomy found improvements in ventilator-free days, length of ICU stay, shorter duration of sedation, and long-term mortality in the early tracheostomy cohort. However, the definition of early tracheostomy did vary in the studies analysed [97].
10. Consider draining large pleural effusions that may be compromising gas exchange and reducing lung compliance, thereby increasing demand on the respiratory muscles.
11. Before extubating weak patients, assess whether they are at increased risk of developing postextubation stridor and whether they are able to protect their airway and clear their respiratory secretions.

When managing patients with discontinuation failure, it is not likely that they fail for technologic reasons or the discontinuation mode but rather because of their diseases and causes of inspiratory muscle fatigue and how well these are managed. Advances for managing discontinuation from MV, based on randomized, controlled trials or meta-analyses of such trials, are summarized in Table 168.2. A number of studies have been published that show that the most favorable discontinuation outcomes are most likely achieved by protocol-directed weaning. Such programs can improve the quality of care of patients on MV and decrease their length of ICU stay and hospital costs, especially when the protocol includes a search for and correction of medical barriers that perpetuate inspiratory muscle fatigue. In our protocol, we focus on a daily basis on evaluating and managing altered mental status and neuromuscular disease, evaluating and managing cardiac pump failure or coronary ischemia, improving nutrition, treating infection, and reducing lung water without compromising renal function.

Utility of Ultrasonography for Assessment of Diaphragmatic Function for Discontinuation of Mechanical Ventilation

The diaphragm is the major inspiratory force generator, so assessment of its function is an important part of the evaluation of the patient with respiratory failure. Diaphragmatic dysfunction may contribute to difficulty of weaning the patient from mechanical ventilatory support as well being a factor in the development of respiratory failure. Ultrasonography is a convenient point-of-care technique for evaluation of diaphragmatic function [98,99].

Machine Requirements

For measurement of diaphragmatic excursion (DE), the ultrasonography examination is performed using a phased array cardiac probe (3.5 to 5.0 MHz) whose small footprint allows for examination between rib interspaces. A curvilinear abdominal probe may also be used. For measurement of diaphragmatic thickening (DT) during inspiration, the examination is performed using a linear vascular probe (7.5 MHz).

Patient Position and Ventilator Setting

In the ICU, the patient is examined in the supine or semirecumbent position appreciating that the weight of abdominal contents may have effect on DE, particularly if the patient is obese or has an elevation of intrabdominal pressure. The ventilator is set so as to provide minimal or no support during the measurement, because both PEEP and positive pressure ventilation may alter the degree of DE that results from patient effort [100]. The patient may be taken off pressure support or temporarily disconnected from the ventilator with provision of supplemental oxygen while performing the ultrasonography examination.

Scanning Technique

To measure DE on the right side, the phased array transducer is placed over the lower lateral chest wall in the mid-axillary line using a longitudinal scanning axis (coronal plane). Image depth is set deep in order to visualize the entire diaphragm. The hyperechoic curvilinear diaphragm is imaged by adjusting the scanning plane for maximal visualization (Video 168.1). If aerated lung blocks view of the diaphragm, the probe may be moved caudad and tilted upward to use the liver as a sonographic window to better visualize the diaphragm. Alternatively, using a transverse scanning plane, the probe is placed in the midclavicular line on the right side below the lower rib margin and angled cephalad. The liver serves as a sonographic window to image the curvilinear diaphragm.

To measure DE on the left side, the phased array transducer is placed over the lower lateral chest wall in the mid-axillary line using a longitudinal scanning axis (coronal plane). The hyperechoic curvilinear diaphragm is imaged by adjusting the scanning plane for maximal visualization. The left diaphragm is more difficult to image than the right, so it is often necessary to use the spleen as a sonographic window. The transverse plane mid-clavicular approach is not effective on the left side, because of the presence of bowel gas and absence of the liver forming a sonographic window.

Once the diaphragm is visualized, the examiner observes its movement during quiet breathing, during augmented effort, and with the patient performing a sharp inspiratory effort ("sniff test") (Video 168.2). The movement of the diaphragm is straightforward to assess on a qualitative basis: it either moves in a normal caudad direction with inspiration, or it moves in an inappropriate cephalad direction during inspiration (Video 168.2). Qualitative measurement of diaphragmatic function is made through simple visual assessment. Quantitative measurement of DE is performed with M mode ultrasonography where the interrogation line placed as perpendicular as possible to the major axis of movement of the dome of the diaphragm (Video 168.2). This may be difficult to achieve from the lateral position, but easier from the mid-clavicular upper quadrant approach on the right side. Some sophisticated cardiology type echocardiography machines have steerable M-mode that facilitates measurement along the correct axis [101]. Most machines used for point-of-care critical applications do not have this capability. As an alternative, a simple analogue measure with millimeter marks can be applied to the machine screen and adjusted to optimal measurement axis in order to measure the excursion directly.

To measure inspiratory diaphragmatic thickening, the linear vascular transducer is placed in the mid axillary line in longitudinal plane with the depth and gain adjusted in order to visualize the diaphragm. The image is frozen in inspiration and expiration and the thickness measured at the two points using the calipers function (Video 168.2). The degree of thickening is calculated using the following formula:

$$\text{Diaphragmatic Thickening (\%)} = \text{Diaphragmatic Thickness}_{\text{inspiratory}} - \text{Diaphragmatic Thickness}_{\text{expiratory}} / \text{Diaphragmatic Thickness}_{\text{inspiratory}}$$

Problems with Measurement

If the patient performs an active expiratory effort with abdominal muscle contraction that results in an end expiratory lung volume that is below FRC, the following inspiratory diaphragmatic movement will be in in caudad direction, but not due solely to diaphragmatic contraction. Rather, it results from inspiratory movement that derives from the elastic recoil of the chest wall. The operator watches for this breathing pattern, because it may mask a nonfunctioning diaphragm.

It may be difficult for the single operator to simultaneously time the inspiratory effort of the patient with diaphragmatic movement on the ultrasonography machine. It is useful to have a continuous tracing of the respiratory cycle running on the ultrasonography machine simultaneous with the ultrasonography image in order to correlate diaphragmatic movement with the respiratory cycle; however, most portable machines used for point-of-care ultrasonography do not have this capability. In this case, one operator is assigned to verbally identify inspiratory effort while the ultrasonographer watches for diaphragmatic movement on the screen, in order to correlate the movement with inspiration.

It may be difficult to make an accurate measurement of excursion unless the measurement axis is the same as the maximal movement axis of the diaphragm. In addition, the degree of excursion will vary according to the point of measurement because the apex of the curved structure moves more than its lateral aspects (Video 168.2).

Measurement of diaphragmatic thickening is in millimeter increments, so detail to correct caliper position is important. The operator averages several measurements and standardizes caliper position often by using an inner edge to inner edge technique (Video 168.2).

Clinical Applications of Ultrasonography Assessment of Diaphragmatic Function

Diaphragmatic dysfunction in patients receiving MV is most often secondary to neuromuscular disorders or non-myopathic diseases such as COPD, to ICU-acquired neuromyopathy, and/or to ventilator-induced diaphragmatic dysfunction, and is therefore symmetric [102–104]. Most studies performed in noncardiac surgery patients report on DE or DT on only one hemidiaphragm (usually on the right side) and use this as a proxy for the total diaphragmatic performance [105–108], although some studies take the lowest value or the mean value between left and right. Four studies describe the use of evaluating diaphragmatic function during weaning in noncardiac surgery patients. Jiang et al. measured the mean value of inspiratory excursions of the liver and the spleen (as a surrogate for DE) during a SBT [109] and demonstrated that patients who required reintubation within 72 hours had significantly lower mean values of liver and spleen displacements than those who did not require reintubation. With a cutoff value of 1.1 cm, the sensitivity and specificity to predict successful extubation were 84% and 83% respectively. Kim et al. reported that a DE value <10 mm for either hemidiaphragm was associated with longer weaning times and higher frequency of reintubation [110]. Both of these studies had unusually high rates of failed extubation thereby limiting their generalizability. Regarding the utility of DT, Di Nino et al. reported that a DT of greater than 30% was associated with positive predictive value of 91% and negative predictive value of 63% for extubation success [108]. Performance of DT was similar, if the measurements were performed during an SBT or a pressure support trial. Ferrari et al. observed in repeated weaning failure that a cutoff value of a DT >36% measured during an SBT on tracheostomy tube was associated with a positive predictive value of 92%, and a negative predictive value of 75% for success or failure from discontinuation of mechanical support at 48 hours [111]. When the performance of ultrasonographic measurements to predict extubation failure or success were compared with clinical parameters such as the rapid shallow breathing index the results were similar. Ultrasonography may be useful to monitor recovery of diaphragmatic recovery over time. Mariani et al. studied DE in patients with prolonged (>7 days) MV and followed DE with repeated measurements in patients with bilateral reduction of DE (E <11 mm) [112]. Some patients had a progressive improvement of DE over time. Grosu et al. observed progressive diaphragmatic thinning in patients receiving volume-controlled MV [113].

On occasion, the intensivist will manage the post-cardiac surgery patient who is difficult to wean from mechanical ventilatory support. Unilateral phrenic nerve injury may lead to asymmetric diaphragmatic dysfunction following cardiac surgery. Rarely, both hemidiaphragms are paralyzed, thereby precluding weaning form ventilatory support until there is return of function. In cardiac surgery patients, bilateral assessment of DE with identification of the best maximal DE is a useful functional parameter of diaphragmatic performance. Lerolle et al. reported that post-cardiac surgery patients with unilateral diaphragmatic paralysis could be weaned off the ventilator without difficulty, if the contralateral diaphragm had a maximal DE >25 mm [114].

Ultrasonography is useful in order to identify diaphragmatic dysfunction. However, it is an imperfect tool, like other indices that are used to predict the success or failure of extubation. It is possible that its utility will be improved when combined with other predictors, such as the lung aeration score or the rapid shallow breathing index. The causes of weaning failure are often multifactorial, only one of which may be diaphragmatic dysfunction.

References

1. Elpern EH, Larson R, Douglass P, et al: Long-term outcomes for elderly survivors of prolonged ventilator assistance. *Chest* 96:1120, 1989.
2. Frutos-Vivar F, Esteban A: Our paper 20 years later: how has withdrawal from mechanical ventilation changed? *Intensive Care Med* 40:1449, 2010.
3. Tobin MJ, Perez W, Guenther SM, et al: The pattern of breathing during successful and unsuccessful trials of weaning from mechanical ventilation. *Am Rev Respir Dis* 134:1111, 1986.
4. Morganroth ML, Grum CM: Weaning from mechanical ventilation. *J Intensive Care Med* 3:109, 1988.
5. Kurek CK, Cohen IL, Lamrinos J, et al: Clinical and economic outcome of patients undergoing tracheostomy for prolonged mechanical ventilation in New York State during 1993; analysis of 6,353 cases under diagnostic related group 483. *Crit Care Med* 25:983, 1997.
6. Unroe M, Kahn JM, Carson SS, et al: One-year trajectories of care and resource utilization for recipients of prolonged mechanical ventilation. A cohort study. *Ann Intern Med* 153:167, 2010.
7. Laghi F, Tobin MJ: Disorders of the respiratory muscles. *Am J Respir Crit Care Med* 168:10, 2003.
8. Arslanian-Engoren C, Scott LD: The lived experience of survivors of prolonged mechanical ventilation: a phenomenological study. *Heart Lung* 32:328, 2003.
9. Laghi F, Cattapan SE, Jubran A, et al: Is weaning failure caused by low-frequency fatigue of the diaphragm? *Am J Respir Crit Care Med* 167:120, 2003.
10. Polkey MI, Moxham J: Clinical aspects of respiratory muscle dysfunction in the critically ill. *Chest* 119:926, 2001.
11. Manthous CA, Schmidt GA, Hall JB: Liberation from mechanical ventilation: a decade of progress. *Chest* 114:886, 1998.
12. NHLBI Workshop Summary: Respiratory muscle fatigue: report of the Respiratory Muscle Fatigue Workshop Group. *Am Rev Respir Dis* 142:474, 1990.
13. Mador MJ: Respiratory muscle fatigue and breathing pattern. *Chest* 100:1430, 1991.
14. Tobin MJ, Jubran A, Laghi F: Patient-ventilator interaction. *Am J RespirCrit Care Med* 163:1059, 2001.
15. Vassilakopoulos T, Katsaounou P, Karatza M-H, et al: Strenuous resistive breathing induces plasma cytokines: role of antioxidants and monocytes. *Am J Respir Crit Care Med* 166:1572, 2002.
16. Jiang T-X, Reid WD, Belcastro A, et al: Load dependence of secondary diaphragm inflammation and injury after acute inspiratory loading. *Am J Respir Crit Care Med* 157:230, 1998.
17. van Gammeren D, Falk DJ, DeRuisseau KC, et al: Reloading the diaphragm following mechanical ventilation does not promote injury. *Chest* 127:2204, 2005.
18. Vassilakopoulos T, Petrof BJ: Ventilator-induced diaphragmatic dysfunction. *Am J Respir Crit Care Med* 169:336, 2004.
19. Lemaire F, Teboul J-L, Cinotti L, et al: Acute left ventricular dysfunction during unsuccessful weaning from mechanical ventilation. *Anesthesiology* 69:171, 1988.
20. Bradley TD, Holloway RM, McLaughlin PR, et al: Cardiac output response to continuous positive airway pressure in congestive heart failure. *Am Rev Respir Dis* 145:377, 1992.
21. Ulicny KS, Hiratzka LR: Nutrition and the cardiac surgical patient. *Chest* 101:836, 1992.
22. Larca L, Greenbaum DM: Effectiveness of intensive nutritional regimes in patients who fail to wean from mechanical ventilation. *Crit Care Med* 10:297, 1982.
23. Cook D, Mende M, Guyatt G, et al: Trials of miscellaneous interventions to wean from mechanical ventilation. *Chest* 120[Suppl]:438S, 2001.
24. MacIntyre NR, Cook DJ, Ely EW Jr, et al: Evidence-based guidelines for weaning and discontinuing ventilatory support. *Chest* 120[Suppl]:375S, 2001.
25. Ely EW, Baker AM, Dunagan DP, et al: Effect on the duration of mechanical ventilation of identifying patients capable of breathing spontaneously. *N Engl J Med* 335:1864, 1996.
26. Jubran A, Grant BJ, Laghi F, et al: Weaning prediction: esophageal pressure monitoring complements readiness testing. *Am J Respir Crit Care Med* 171:1252, 2005.
27. Meade M, Guyatt G, Cook D, et al: Predicting success in weaning from mechanical ventilation. *Chest* 120[Suppl]:400S, 2001.
28. Yang KL, Tobin MJ: A prospective study of indexes predicting the outcome of trials of weaning from mechanical ventilation. *N Engl J Med* 324:1445, 1991.
29. Tobin MJ, Guenther SM, Perez W, et al: Konno-Mead analysis of ribcage-abdominal motion during successful and unsuccessful trials of weaning from mechanical ventilation. *Am Rev Respir Dis* 135:1320, 1987.
30. Khemani RG, Randolph A, Markovitz B: Corticosteroids for the prevention and treatment of post-extubation stridor in neonates, children and adults. *Cochrane Database Syst Rev* (3):CD001000, 2009.
31. Girault C: Noninvasive ventilation for postextubation respiratory failure: perhaps not to treat but at least to prevent. *Crit Care Med* 33:2685, 2005.
32. Meade M, Guyatt G, Stinuff T, et al: Trials comparing alternative weaning modes and discontinuation assessments. *Chest* 120[Suppl]:425S, 2001.
33. Burns KE, Adhikari NK, Meade MO: Noninvasive positive pressure ventilation as a weaning strategy for intubated adults with respiratory failure. *Cochrane Database Syst Rev* CD004127, 2003.
34. Vallverdu I, Calaf N, Subirana M, et al: Clinical characteristics, respiratory functional parameters, and outcome of a two-hour T-piece trial in patients weaning from mechanical ventilation. *Am J Respir Crit Care Med* 158:1855, 1998
35. Quan SF, Falltrick RT, Schlobohm RM: Extubation from ambient or expiratory positive airway pressure in adults. *Anesthesiology* 55:53, 1981.
36. Martin JG, Shore S, Engel LA: Effect of continuous positive airway pressure on respiratory mechanics and pattern of breathing in induced asthma. *Am Rev Respir Dis* 126:812, 1982.
37. Reissmann HK, Ranieri VM, Goldberg P, et al: Continuous positive airway pressure facilitates spontaneous breathing in weaning chronic obstructive pulmonary disease patients by improving breathing pattern and gas exchange. *Intensive Care Med* 26:1764, 2000.
38. Petrof BJ, Legare M, Goldberg P, et al: Continuous positive airway pressure reduced work of breathing and dyspnea during weaning from mechanical ventilation in severe chronic obstructive pulmonary disease. *Am Rev Respir Dis* 141:281, 1990.
39. Bergbom-Engberg I, Haljamae J: Assessment of patients' experience of discomforts during respiratory therapy. *Crit Care Med* 17:1068, 1989.
40. Esteban A, Frutos F, Tobin MJ, et al: A comparison of four methods of weaning patients from mechanical ventilation. Spanish Lung Failure Collaborative Group. *N Engl J Med* 332:345, 1995.
41. MacIntyre NR: Respiratory function during pressure support ventilation. *Chest* 89:677, 1986.
42. MacIntyre NR, Ho L-I: Effects of initial flow rate and breath termination criteria on pressure support ventilation. *Chest* 99:134, 1991.
43. Fiastro JF, Habib MP, Quan SF: Pressure support compensation for inspiratory work due to endotracheal tubes and demand continuous positive airway pressure. *Chest* 93:499, 1988.
44. Brochard L, Rua F, Lorino H, et al: Inspiratory pressure support compensates for the additional work of breathing caused by the endotracheal tube. *Anesthesiology* 75:739, 1991.
45. Nathan SN, Ishaaya AM, Koerner, SK, et al: Prediction of pressure support during weaning from mechanical ventilation. *Chest* 103:1215, 1993.
46. Morrell MJ, Shea SA, Adams L, et al: Effects of inspiratory support upon breathing in humans during wakefulness and sleep. *Respir Physiol* 93:57, 1993.
47. Epstein SK, Ciubotaru RL, Wong JB: Effect of failed extubation on the outcome of mechanical ventilation. *Chest* 112:186, 1997.
48. Esteban A, Frutos-Vivar F, Ferguson N, et al: Noninvasive positive-pressure ventilation for respiratory failure after extubation. *N Engl J Med* 350: 2452–2460, 2004.
49. Ferrer M, Sellares J, Valencia M, et al: Non-invasive ventilation after extubation in hypercapnic patients with chronic respiratory disorders: randomized controlled trial. *Lancet* 374:1044–1045, 2009.
50. Girault C, Daudenthun I, Chevron V, et al: Noninvasive ventilation as a systematic extubation and weaning technique in acute-on-chronic respiratory failure: a prospective, randomized controlled study. *Am J Respir Crit Care Med* 160:86, 1999.
51. Sprague SS, Hopkins PD: Use of inspiratory strength training to wean six patients who were ventilator-dependent. *Phys Ther* 83:171, 2003.
52. Cassina T, Chiolero R, Mauri R, et al: Clinical experience with adaptive supportive ventilation for fast-tracking cardiac surgery. *J Cardiovasc Vasc Anesth* 17:571, 2003.
53. Corson JA, Grant JL, Moulton DP, et al: Use of biofeedback in weaning paralyzed patients from respirators. *Chest* 76:543, 1979.
54. Holliday JE, Hyers TM: The reduction of weaning time from mechanical ventilation using tidal volume and relaxation biofeedback. *Am Rev Respir Dis* 141:1214, 1990.
55. Haberthur C, Mols G, Elsasser S, et al: Extubation after breathing trials with automatic tube compensation, T-tube, or pressure support ventilation. *Acta Anaesthesiol Scand* 46:973, 2002.
56. Oczenski W, Kapka A, Krenn H, et al: Automatic tube compensation in patients after cardiac surgery. *Crit Care Med* 30:1467, 2002.
57. Cohen JD, Shapiro M, Grozovski E, et al: Extubation outcome following a spontaneous breathing trial with automatic tube compensation versus continuous positive airway pressure. *Crit Care Med* 34:682–686, 2006.

58. Bosma K, Ferreyra G, Ambrogio G, et al: Patient-ventilator interaction and sleep in mechanically ventilated patients: pressure support versus proportional assist ventilation. *Crit Care Med* 35:1048, 2007.
59. Hubmayr RD, Loosbrock LM, Gillespie DJ, et al: Oxygen uptake during weaning from mechanical ventilation. *Chest* 94:1148, 1988.
60. Brochard L, Rauss A, Benito S, et al: Comparison of three methods of gradual withdrawal from ventilatory support during weaning from mechanical ventilation. *Am J Respir Crit Care Med* 150:896, 1994.
61. Esteban A, Alia I, Gordo F, et al: Extubation outcome after spontaneous breathing trials with T-tube or pressure support ventilation. The Spanish Lung Failure Collaborative Group [published erratum appears in *Am J RespirCrit Care Med* 156:2028, 1997]. *Am J Respir Crit Care Med* 156:459, 1997.
62. Esteban A, Alia I, Tobin MJ, et al: Effect of spontaneous breathing trial duration on outcome of attempts to discontinue mechanical ventilation. Spanish Lung Failure Collaborative Group. *Am J Respir Crit Care Med* 159:512, 1999.
63. Perren A, Domenighetti G, Mauri S, et al: Protocol-directed weaning from mechanical ventilation: clinical outcome in patients randomized for a 30-min or 120-min trial with pressure support ventilation. *Intensive Care Med* 28:1058, 2002.
64. MacIntyre NR, Epstein SK, Carson S, et al: Management of patients requiring prolonged mechanical ventilation: report of a NAMDRC Consensus Conference. *Chest* 128:3937, 2005.
65. Epstein SK, Ciubotaru RL: Independent effects of etiology of failure and time to reintubation on outcome for patients failing extubation. *Am J Respir Crit Care Med* 158:489, 1998.
66. Pluijms WA, van Mook WNKA, Wittekamp BHJ, et al: Postextubation laryngeal edema and stridor resulting in respiratory failure in critically ill adult patients: updated review. *Crit Care.* 19:295, 2015.
67. Miller R, Cole R: Association between reduced cuff leak volume and postextubation stridor. *Chest* 110:1035, 1996.
68. Wang W, Zhou Y, Tong H, et al: Value of the cuff leak test is limited. *Crit Care* 19:446, 2015.
69. Chung YH, Chao TY, Chiu CT: The cuff leak test is a simple tool to verify severe laryngeal edema in patients undergoing long-term mechanical ventilation. *Crit Care Med* 34:409–414, 2006.
70. Jaber S, Chanques G, Matecki S, et al: Post extubation stridor in intensive care unit patients-risk factors evaluation and the importance of the cuff leak test. *Intensive Care Med* 29:69–74, 2003.
71. Wang CL, Tsai YH, Huang CC, et al: The role of the cuff leak test in predicting the effects of corticosteroid treatment on postextubation stridor. *Chang Gung Med J* 30:53–61, 2007.
72. Khemani RG, Randolph A, Markovitz B: Corticosteroids for the prevention and treatment of post-extubation stridor in neonates, children and adults. *Cochrane Database Syst Rev* (3):CD001000, 2009; doi:10.1002/14651858.CD001000.pub3.
73. Salam A, Tilluckdharry L, Amoateng-Adjepong Y, et al: Neurologic status, cough, secretions and extubation outcomes. *Intensive Care Med* 30:1334, 2004.
74. De Larminat V, Mongravers P, Dureuil B, et al: Alteration in swallowing reflex after extubation in intensive care patients. *Crit Care Med* 23:486, 1995.
75. Barquist E, Brown M, Cohn S, et al: Postextubationfiberoptic endoscopic evaluation of swallowing after prolonged endotracheal intubation: a randomized, prospective trial. *Crit Care Med* 29:1710, 2001.
76. Kollef MH, Shapiro SD, Silver P, et al: A randomized controlled trial of protocol-directed versus physician-directed weaning from mechanical ventilation. *Crit Care Med* 25:567, 1997.
77. Smyrnios NA, Connolly A, Wilson MM, et al: Effects of a multifaceted, multidisciplinary, hospital-wide quality improvement program on weaning from mechanical ventilation. *Crit Care Med* 30:1224, 2002.
78. Blackwood B, Burns KEA, Cardwell CR, et al: Protocolized versus non-protocolized weaning for reducing the duration of mechanical ventilation in critically ill adult patients. *Cochrane Database Syst Rev* (11):CD006904, 2014. DOI: 10.1002/14651858.CD006904.pub3.
79. Seneff MG, Zimmerman JE, Knaus WA, et al: Predicting the duration of mechanical ventilation: the importance of disease and patient characteristics. *Chest* 110:469, 1996.
80. Kress JP, Pohlman AS, O'Connor MF, et al: Daily interruption of sedative infusions in critically ill patients undergoing mechanical ventilation. *N Engl J Med* 342:1471, 2000.
81. Strom T, Martinussen T, Toft P: A protocol of no sedation for critically ill patients receiving mechanical ventilation: a randomized trial. *Lancet* 375:475, 2010.
82. Ely EW, Truman B, Shintani A, et al: Monitoring sedation status over time in ICU patients: reliability and validity of the Richmond Agitation-Sedation Scale (RASS). *JAMA* 289:2983, 2003.
83. Girard TD, Kress JP, Fuchs BD, et al: Efficacy and safety of a paired sedation and ventilator weaning protocol for mechanically ventilated patients in intensive care (awakening and breathing controlled trial): a randomised controlled trial. *Lancet* 371:126–134, 2008.
84. Riker RR, Shehabi Y, Bokessch PM, et al: Dexmedetomidine vs. midazolam for sedation of critically ill patients—a randomized trial. *JAMA* 301:489–499, 2009.
85. Bolton CF: Neuromuscular manifestations of critical illness. *Muscle Nerve* 32:140, 2005.
86. Arroliga A, Frutos-Vivar F, Hall J, et al: Use of sedatives and neuromuscular blockers in a cohort of patients receiving mechanical ventilation. *Chest* 128:496, 2005.
87. Argov Z, Mastaglia FL: Disorders of neuromuscular transmission caused by drugs. *N Engl J Med* 301:409, 1979.
88. Leitjen FSS, Harinck-de Ward JE, Poortvliet DCJ, et al: The role of polyneuropathy in Motor Convalescence after prolonged mechanical ventilation. *JAMA* 274:1221–1225, 1995.
89. Schweickert WD, Pohlman MC, Pohlman AS, et al: Early physical and occupational therapy in mechanically ventilated, critically ill patients: a randomized controlled trial. *Lancet* 373:1874–1882, 2009.
90. Faisy C, Meziani F, PLanquette B, et al: Effect of acetazolamide vs placebo on duration of invasive mechanical ventilation among patients with chronic obstructive pulmonary disease—a randomized trial. *JAMA* 315:480, 2016.
91. Skatrud JB, Dempsey JA, Kaiser DG: Ventilatory response to medroxyprogesterone acetate in normal subjects: time course and mechanism. *J Appl Physiol* 44:939, 1978.
92. Rasanen J, Vaisanen IT, Heikkila J, et al: Acute myocardial infarction complicated left ventricular dysfunction and respiratory failure: the effects of continuous positive airway pressure. *Chest* 87:158, 1985.
93. Rasanen J, Nikki P, Heikkila J: Acute myocardial infarction complicated by respiratory failure: the effects of mechanical ventilation. *Chest* 85:21, 1984.
94. Hess D, Branson RD: Ventilators and weaning modes. *Respir Clin North Am* 6:407, 2000.
95. Le Bourdelles G, Mier L, Fiquet B, et al: Comparison of the effects of heat and moisture exchangers and heated humidifiers on ventilation and gas exchange during weaning trials from mechanical ventilation. *Chest* 110:1294, 1996.
96. Talpers SS, Romberger DJ, Bunce SB, et al: Nutritionally associated increased carbon dioxide production: excess total calories vs. high proportion of carbohydrate calories. *Chest* 102:551, 1992.
97. Hosokawa K, Nishimura M, Egi M, et al: Timing of tracheotomy in ICU patients: asystematic review of randomized controlled trials. *Crit Care* 19:424, 2015.
98. Matamis D, Soilemezi E, Tsagourias M, et al: Sonographic evaluation of the diaphragm in critically ill patients. Technique and clinical applications. *Intensive Care Med* 39(5):801–810, 2013.
99. Summerhill EM. Monitoring recovery from diaphragm paralysis with ultrasound. *CHEST J* 1;133(3):737, 2008.
100. Pasero D, Koeltz A, Placido R, et al: Improving ultrasonic measurement of diaphragmatic excursion after cardiac surgery using the anatomical M-mode: a randomized crossover study. *Intensive Care Med* 41(4):650–656, 2015.
101. Beaumont M, Lejeune D, Marotte H, et al: Effects of chest wall counterpressures on lung mechanics under high levels of CPAP in humans. *J Appl Physiol.* 83(2):591–598, 1997.
102. Powers SK, Kavazis AN, Levine S. Prolonged mechanical ventilation alters diaphragmatic structure and function. Crit Care Med. 2009 Oct;37:S347–53.
103. Doorduin J, van Hees HWH, van der Hoeven JG, Heunks LMA. Monitoring of the respiratory muscles in the critically ill. Am J Respir Crit Care Med. 2013 Jan 1;187(1):20–7.
104. Demoule A, Jung B, Prodanovic H, Molinari N, Chanques G, Coirault C, et al. Diaphragm dysfunction on admission to the intensive care unit. Prevalence, risk factors, and prognostic impact-a prospective study. Am J Respir Crit Care Med. 2013 Jul 15;188(2):213–9.
105. Vivier E, Mekontso Dessap A, Dimassi S, Vargas F, Lyazidi A, Thille AW, et al. Diaphragm ultrasonography to estimate the work of breathing during non-invasive ventilation. Intensive Care Medicine. 2012 May;38(5):796–803.
106. Umbrello M, Formenti P, Longhi D, Galimberti A, Piva I, Pezzi A, et al. Diaphragm ultrasound as indicator of respiratory effort in critically ill patients undergoing assisted mechanical ventilation: a pilot clinical study. Critical Care [Internet]. 2015 Dec [cited 2015 Aug 29];19(1). Available from: http://ccforum.com/content/19/1/161
107. Ferrari G, De Filippi G, Elia F, Panero F, Volpicelli G, Aprà F. Diaphragm ultrasound as a new index of discontinuation from mechanical ventilation. Critical Ultrasound Journal. 2014;6(1):8.
108. DiNino E, Gartman EJ, Sethi JM, McCool FD. Diaphragm ultrasound as a predictor of successful extubation from mechanical ventilation. Thorax. 2014 May 1;69(5):431–5.
109. Jiang J-R, Tsai T-H, Jerng J-S, Yu C-J, Wu H-D, Yang P-C. Ultrasonographic evaluation of liver/spleen movements and extubation outcome. Chest. 2004;126(1):179–85.
110. Kim WY, Suh HJ, Hong S-B, Koh Y, Lim C-M. Diaphragm dysfunction assessed by ultrasonography: influence on weaning from mechanical ventilation. Crit Care Med. 2011 Dec;39(12):2627–30
111. Ferrari G, De Filippi G, Elia F, Panero F, Volpicelli G, Aprà F. Diaphragm ultrasound as a new index of discontinuation from mechanical ventilation. Critical Ultrasound Journal. 2014;6(1):8.
112. Mariani LF, Bedel J, Gros A, Lerolle N, Milojevic K, Laurent V, et al. Ultrasonography for Screening and Follow-Up of Diaphragmatic Dysfunction in the ICU: A Pilot Study. Journal of Intensive Care Medicine [Internet]. 2015 May 14 [cited 2015 Aug 29]; Available from: http://jic.sagepub.com/cgi/doi/10.1177/0885066615583639
113. Grosu HB. Diaphragm Muscle Thinning in Patients Who Are Mechanically Ventilated. CHEST Journal. 2012 Dec 1;142(6):1455.
114. Lerolle N, Guérot E, Zegdi R, Faisy C, Fagon J-Y, Diehl J-L. Ultrasonographic diagnostic criterion for severe diaphragmatic dysfunction after cardiac surgery. Chest. 2009 Feb;135(2):401–7.

Chapter 169 ■ Respiratory Adjunct Therapy

SCOTT E. KOPEC • RYAN G. SHIPE • RICHARD S. IRWIN

Various adjunct therapies are available to aid in the management of critically ill patients with existing or anticipated pulmonary dysfunction. In this chapter, we review several adjunct therapies, emphasizing any randomized trials determining efficacy and indications. We will specifically discuss the following: (a) aerosol therapy and humidification; (b) lung expansion techniques; (c) airway clearance techniques; (d) administration of medical gases; (e) nasal continuous positive airway pressure (CPAP) and bilevel positive airway pressure for sleep-related breathing disorders; and (f) communication alternatives for the patient with an artificial airway. A discussion of the use of bilevel positive airway pressure to provide noninvasive ventilatory support can be found in Chapter 167.

AEROSOL THERAPY

An *aerosol* is a stable suspension of solid or liquid particles dispersed in air as a fine mist. Bland aerosols are generally used to humidify inspired gases. Aerosol drug therapy represents the optimal modality for site-specific delivery of pharmacologic agents to the lungs in the treatment of a number of acute and chronic pulmonary diseases. Owing to the cost and potential hazards of aerosol therapy, use should be limited to aerosols whose clinical value has been objectively shown [1].

Bland Aerosols

Bland aerosols include sterile water or hypotonic, isotonic, and hypertonic saline delivered with or without oxygen. These are typically delivered via an ultrasonic nebulizer in an effort to decrease or aid in the clearance of pulmonary secretions. The routine use of bland aerosols in the treatment of some specific diseases has demonstrated mixed results. An evidence-based recommendation for the use of bland aerosols has been released by the British Thoracic Society (BTS) [2]. The use of bland aerosols for the treatment of chronic obstructive pulmonary disease (COPD) and croup appears not to be of any benefit [2,3]. For patients with cystic fibrosis (CF), the use of 7% (hypertonic) saline, administered twice daily, may result in a significantly higher forced vital capacity (FVC) and forced expiratory volume in 1 second (FEV_1), and a decrease in the number of acute exacerbations when compared to the use of normotonic saline [4]. The use of nebulized saline or sterile water may improve sputum clearance for patients with non-CF bronchiectasis [2]. Delivery of bland aerosols to the spontaneous breathing patient is ineffective for liquefying secretions because sufficient volumes of water fail to reach the lower airways. Furthermore, bland aerosols may provoke bronchospasm and place patients at risk for nosocomial pneumonia [3].

Mist therapy, the delivery of a continuous aerosol of sterile water or saline, is frequently used to treat upper-airway infections in children, but has not been shown to be more effective than air humidification [3].

Humidity Therapy

Theoretical reasons for using humidified inspired gas are to prevent drying of the upper and lower airways, hydrate dry mucosal surfaces in patients with inflamed upper airways (vocal cords and above), enhance expectoration of lower-airway secretions, and induce sputum expectoration for diagnostic purposes [3].

Humidity therapy is water vapor and, at times, heat added to inspired gas with the goal of achieving near-normal inspiratory conditions when the gas enters the airway [5]. Because adequate levels of humidity and heat are necessary to ensure proper function of the mucociliary transport system, humidification is imperative when the structures of the upper airway that normally warm and humidify inspired gases have been bypassed by an artificial airway. During mechanical ventilation, humidification is crucial to avoid hypothermia, atelectasis, inspissation of airway secretions, and destruction of airway epithelium because of heat loss, moisture loss, and altered pulmonary function [6]. Optimal humidification is the point at which normal conditions that prevail in the respiratory tract are simulated [7].

Several external devices are available to artificially deliver heat and moisture. Two such devices for mechanically ventilated patients are: (a) a heated waterbath humidifier, which is an external *active* source of heat and water, and (b) a heat and moisture exchanger filter (HMEF) that *passively* retains the heat and humidity leaving the trachea during expiration and recycles it during the next inspiration. HMEFs are also known as *hygroscopic condenser humidifiers* or *artificial noses*. The HMEF is designed to combine air-conditioning and bacterial filtration. In a randomized controlled trial, both devices were shown to be equally safe [8]. Potential advantages of HMEFs over heated waterbath humidifiers include reduced cost and avoidance of airway burns and overhydration. A potential disadvantage is that resistance of airflow through an HMEF may progressively rise, increasing the work of breathing and conceivably impeding weaning from the ventilator [8].

Cold-water devices such as bubble humidifiers are frequently used to add humidity to supplemental oxygen administered to spontaneously breathing patients. Owing to a lack of objective evidence to support the practice, the American College of Chest Physicians recommends elimination of the routine use of humidification of oxygen at flow rates of 1 to 4 L per minute when environmental humidity is sufficient [9], although the BTS does not recommend its use [2].

Patients requiring high-flow rates of oxygen (>10 L per minute) frequently develop discomfort due to upper-airway dryness. There are several devices available to deliver humidification via nasal cannulae at high-flow rates (high-flow oxygen delivery), including Vapotherm (Vapotherm, Annapolis, MD) and the Fisher & Paykel 850 (Fisher and Paykel Healthcare Corp., Auckland, New Zealand). These devices have been shown to improve patients' comfort [10], and may have some therapeutic benefit (see below).

Pharmacologically Active Aerosols

Inhaled therapy has several well-recognized advantages over other drug delivery routes. The drug is delivered directly to its targeted site of action; therefore, when compared to other routes of administration, a therapeutic response usually requires fewer drugs, there are fewer side effects, and the onset of action is generally faster [11]. A broad range of drugs is available as aerosols to treat obstructive lung diseases. These include β-adrenergic agonists, anticholinergics, anti-inflammatory agents, and anti-infectives. Additionally, the inhaled route is used to deliver drugs that are not effective when delivered by the oral route (e.g., pentamidine) [12].

Although a variety of drugs are currently available in aerosolized form, dosing to the lung remains inexact because deposition is affected by several patient-, environment-, and equipment-related factors. Potential hazards of aerosol drug therapy include (a) a reaction to the drug being administered, (b) the risk of infection, (c) bronchospasm, and (d) the potential for delivering too much or too little of the drug [12]. With respect to the use of aerosolized ribavirin, there are potential hazards to health care providers administering the medication (see later).

Bronchodilators

There are two classes of inhaled bronchodilators: (a) β_2-adrenergic receptor agonists (short-acting, long-acting, and ultra long-acting) and (b) anticholinergic agents.

Short-Acting β_2-Adrenergic Receptor Agonists. Although β_1- and β_2-adrenergic receptors are present in the lungs, β_2-adrenergic receptors appear to be entirely responsible for bronchodilation. Therefore, β_2-adrenergic receptor agonists (e.g., albuterol, pirbuterol, and terbutaline) are the agents commonly preferred for the relief of acute symptoms of bronchospasm. In addition to the bronchodilating properties of β_2-adrenergic receptor agonists, other actions include augmentation of mucociliary clearance; enhancement of vascular integrity; metabolic responses; and inhibition of mediator release from mast cells, basophils, and possibly other cells [3].

Inhalation of β_2-selective agonists is considered first-line therapy for the critically ill asthmatic [13] and COPD patient [3,14]. Although these agents can be administered orally, by inhalation, or parenterally, the inhaled route is generally preferred because fewer side effects occur for any degree of bronchodilation [3]. For most patients experiencing acute asthma attacks, inhalation is at least as effective as the parenteral route [3]. Inhaled β_2 agonists can be delivered as an aerosol from a jet or ultrasonic nebulizer or from a metered-dose inhaler (MDI). The relative efficacies of the nebulizer and MDI are dependent on the adequacy of technique. Although it was formerly a standard practice to deliver bronchodilators by nebulizer, several prospective, randomized controlled trials have challenged this practice. Delivering β_2 agonists by MDI with a spacer device (holding chamber) under the supervision of trained personnel is as effective in the emergency setting as delivery by nebulizer for adults and children [3]. For hospitalized patients, β_2 agonists delivered by MDI are as effective as therapy with a nebulizer and can result in considerable cost savings [3]. An analysis of 16 trials (686 children and 375 adults) to assess the effects of MDIs with holding chambers compared to nebulizers for the administration of β_2 agonists for acute asthma concluded that MDI with a holding chamber produced at least equivalent outcomes as nebulizer delivery [15].

Ideal frequency of administration and dosing of β_2 agonists has not been determined. For emergency department and hospital-based care of asthma, the National Institutes of Health Expert Panel Report 3 [13] recommends up to three treatments in the first hour, followed by 1 to 4 treatments every 1 to 4 hours as needed. These subsequent treatments should be titrated to the severity of symptoms and the occurrence of adverse side effects, ranging from hourly treatments for moderate severity to hourly or continuous treatments for severe exacerbations. Recommendations for initial treatment of severe acute exacerbations of COPD are for the administration of short-acting β_2 agonists every 2 to 4 hours if tolerated [3].

When given by jet nebulizer, the usual adult dose of albuterol is 0.5 mL of a 0.5% solution (2.5 mg) diluted in 2.5 mL of saline (or 3 mL of 0.083% unit-dose nebulizer solution). The frequency of dosing varies depending on the disease and the situation. It can range from every 4 to 6 hours for patients with COPD and stable asthma to every 20 to 30 minutes for six doses in patients with status asthmaticus [3]. For patients with acute asthma, albuterol solution has also been continuously nebulized for 2 hours [16]. In this randomized controlled trial of spontaneously breathing patients with FEV_1 less than 40% predicted, continuous delivery of high-dose (7.5 mg per hour) or standard-dose (2.5 mg per hour) albuterol were both superior to hourly intermittent treatments with 2.5 mg for increasing FEV_1. Although there was no difference in FEV_1 improvement between the two continuous doses, the standard dose had fewer side effects.

Although the usual dosage of bronchodilator by MDI is two puffs (90 μg per puff) every 4 to 6 hours in stable hospitalized and ambulatory adult patients, the dosage must be increased up to sixfold in acute severe asthma to achieve results equivalent to those achieved with small-volume nebulizers [3]. In an emergency department treatment study of severe asthma, four puffs of albuterol by MDI every 30 minutes for a total of six dosing intervals (24 puffs) was found to be safe and equivalent to 2.5 mg of albuterol diluted in 2 mL of saline given every 30 minutes for six doses [3]. Others have treated acute episodes of asthma in the emergency department in a dose-to-result fashion as follows: initially four puffs by MDI of bronchodilator of choice, followed by one additional puff every minute until the patient subjectively or objectively improved or side effects (e.g., tremor, tachycardia, and arrhythmia) occurred [3]. For mechanically ventilated patients, the bronchodilator effect obtained with four puffs (0.4 mg) of albuterol from an MDI with holding chamber is comparable to that obtained with 6 to 12 times the same dose given by a nebulizer and is likely to be more cost-effective [17].

Tremor is the principal side effect of β_2 agonists, due to the direct stimulation of β_2-adrenergic receptors in skeletal muscle. Tachycardia and palpitations are less frequent with the selective β_2 agonists (e.g., albuterol) than with nonselective β_1–β_2 agonists such as isoproterenol. Although vasodilation, reflex tachycardia, and direct stimulation of the heart can occur even with the use of selective β_2 agonists, cardiac adverse occurrences are uncommon when usual doses of inhaled β_2 agonists are administered. A transient decrease of arterial oxygen tension may occur among patients with acute, severe asthma. This response is likely due to the relaxation of the compensatory vasoconstriction in areas of decreased ventilation together with increased blood flow due to increased cardiac output [3].

β_2-Adrenergic agonists can cause acute metabolic responses including hyperglycemia, hypokalemia, and hypomagnesemia [3]. Although typically not seen in standard doses, if large and frequent doses of β agonists are given, electrocardiogram and serum potassium monitoring are indicated. After inhalation of 10- and 20-mg doses, the maximal decreases in potassium can be 0.62 ± 0.09 mmol per L and 0.98 ± 0.14 mmol per L, respectively [18].

Perinatal outcomes of 259 pregnant women with asthma who were treated with β_2-adrenergic agonists during pregnancy were compared to those of 101 women who were not treated with these agents, and 295 nonasthmatic women [3]. There were no differences in perinatal mortality rates, congenital abnormalities, preterm delivery, low birth weights, mean birth weights, or the number of small-for-gestational-age infants. In addition, there were no differences in Apgar scores, labor or delivery complications, or postpartum bleeding.

Levalbuterol (Xopenex, Sepracor Inc., Marlborough, MA) inhalation solution, the (R)-enantiomer of racemic albuterol, is a relatively selective, third-generation β_2-adrenergic receptor agonist approved for treatment of bronchospasm in adults and children aged 12 years or older. Levalbuterol appears to offer little benefit over albuterol for improving FEV_1 of patients with asthma, and is not associated with any fewer systemic side effects such as tachycardia and hypokalemia [19]. For further discussion of aerosolized β agonists in asthma and COPD, see Chapters 172 and 173.

Long-Acting and Ultra Long-acting Inhaled β_2 Agonists. Long-acting inhaled β_2 agonists (e.g., salmeterol and formoterol) and ultra long acting β_2 agonists (vilanterol and indacaterol) are currently not recommended for use in acute exacerbations of asthma (Expert Panel Report 2) [13] or COPD [3]. One prospective, double-blind, randomized, placebo-controlled trial demonstrated a possible role for salmeterol as an adjunct to conventional therapy for hospitalized asthmatic patients [20], but larger studies are needed to clarify whether there is a potential benefit in the setting of acute asthma. If patients are using these agents as controller medications for asthma or COPD and are hospitalized for other reasons, consider continuing them for asthma maintenance during the hospitalization. These agents should be administered at regular intervals; additional doses to relieve symptoms should not be prescribed.

Anticholinergics. Anticholinergics appear to have a role for acute asthma when combined with sympathomimetic drugs [3], for exacerbations of COPD when combined with albuterol [5], for intubated patients to prevent bradycardia induced by suctioning [21], and in selected patients with severe bronchorrhea [22]. Ipratropium bromide is dosed at 500 μg in 2.5 mL normal saline (1 unit 0.02% unit-dose vial) or 2 to 6 puffs by MDI (18 μg per puff) every 6 to 8 hours. For patients with a severe asthma exacerbation, 500 μg of ipratropium should be given every 20 minutes for three doses [13]. Ipratropium (18 μg per puff) and albuterol (103 μg per puff) are available as a combined MDI product (Combivent, Boehringer, Ingelheim; Ridgefield, CT). Ipratropium by MDI can be given to ventilated patients with the same spacer device used for β_2-agonist delivery. Tiotropium, a selective muscarinic antagonist, should be limited to the chronic management of patients with COPD. For further discussion of anticholinergic use in asthma and COPD, see Chapters 172 and 173.

Combined Bronchodilator Therapy. Although inhaled short-acting β_2-adrenergic receptor agonists remain first-line agents in the treatment of acute asthma, the addition of ipratropium bromide may result in an added benefit [23]. Anticholinergics may be of benefit as additive agents or as single agents in situations in which the patient cannot tolerate β_2-adrenergic side effects. Both agents appear effective in smoking-related chronic bronchitis.

Mucolytics

***N*-Acetylcysteine.** Theoretically, mucolytic agents facilitate expectoration of excessive lower-airway secretions and improve lung function [3]. Although *N*-acetylcysteine (Mucomyst, Apothecon, Princeton, NJ), the prototypic mucolytic agent, liquefies inspissated mucous plugs when administered by direct intratracheal instillation [24], it is of questionable clinical use when administered as an aerosol to nonintubated patients because very little of the drug is actually delivered to the lower respiratory tract. Inhaled *N*-acetylcysteine failed to prevent deterioration of lung function or exacerbations of patients with COPD [25], and nebulized *N*-acetylcysteine failed to demonstrate any benefit for patients with CF [26]. However, a small randomized trial suggested that nebulized *N*-acetylcysteine in combination with aerosolized heparin reduced the incidence of acute lung injury (ALI) and decreased mortality in patients with acute smoke inhalational injuries [27]. Because mucolytic instillations or aerosols can induce bronchospasm among patients with airway disease [28] (especially asthma), mucolytics should be administered to these patients in combination with a bronchodilator [3]. However, given the lack of evidence from randomized trials supporting its benefits, we do not recommend the routine use of aerosolized *N*-acetylcysteine.

Recombinant Human DNase. Recombinant human DNase (Pulmozyme, Genentech, South San Francisco, CA), when given as an aerosol in a dose of 2.5 mg once or twice a day to patients with CF, led to a moderate but significant decrease in dyspnea, a reduction of costs related to exacerbations of respiratory symptoms, and a modest improvement in FEV_1 after 3 months [2]. However, there may not be any statistically significant therapeutic benefit of rhDNase when added to antibiotics and chest physical therapy [29].

Two double-blind, placebo-controlled clinical trials evaluated the safety and efficacy of nebulized rhDNase in the treatment of non-CF–related bronchiectasis [30,31]. In these studies, rhDNase was consistently found ineffective (and possibly harmful [30]) to patients with non-CF–related bronchiectasis.

A randomized double-blind, placebo-controlled trial of patients with respiratory syncytial virus (RSV) bronchiolitis found significant improvement of chest radiographic findings that occurred with the use of nebulized rhDNase compared to significant worsening of those from a placebo group. Although further investigation is needed, results of this trial indicate a possible future role for this therapy in the treatment of RSV in infants and young children [32].

Other Mucolytics. Studies to determine the efficacy of other mucolytic agents, including water, have produced conflicting results. Current evidence does not appear to justify their use in clinical practice. Consensus guidelines for asthma [13] and COPD [3] do not recommend the use of mucolytic agents in the treatment of acute exacerbations of these diseases.

Anti-infectives

Aerosolization of antimicrobial solutions has been shown to be effective in CF patients with tracheobronchial infections and colonization [2]. In addition, inhaled antibiotics have also been used to treat tracheobronchial infections for patients with non-CF–related bronchiectasis, to treat and prevent ventilator-associated pneumonia, to treat chronic bronchitis for patients with COPD, to treat bronchiolitis of children, and to treat patients with multidrug-resistant tuberculosis (MDR-Tb) and mycobacterium avium complex (MAC) [11]. However, unlike their use in treating patients with CF, the benefits of using inhaled antibiotics for these other indications is less defined. Inhaled tobramycin has been demonstrated to decrease sputum bacterial counts, improve lung function, decrease the number of exacerbations, and improve quality of life for patients with pulmonary infections or colonization from CF [33]. For patients with non-CF–related bronchiectasis, inhaled antibiotics are not as well studied, but may decrease sputum bacterial counts and decrease the number of hospitalizations, but have no impact on lung function or survival [34]. Inhaled antibiotics have not been shown to provide any benefits for patients with chronic bronchitis or COPD [35]. Prophylactic use of inhaled antibiotics to decrease the risk of developing ventilator-associated pneumonia has not been shown to be of any benefit [35]. In addition, inhaled antibiotics appear to have no benefit over systemic antibiotics for treating ventilator-associated pneumonia [35]. A few small studies suggest that inhaled amikacin and rifampicin may be of some benefit for treating severe MDR-Tb and severe infections with MAC [36].

Currently only tobramycin, colistin, and aztreonam are FDA approved for inhalational use. Other antibiotics occasionally administered via an aerosol include amikacin, gentamicin, levofloxacin, azithromycin, vancomycin, ceftazidime, and imipenem. Inhaled colistin should be used with great caution as it decomposes into several toxic compounds that, if inhaled, can result in ALI and respiratory failure. Colistin suspension should be administered within 6 hours after it is prepared [37].

Inhaled tobramycin is approved for treatment of patients with CF who are (a) at least 6 years of age, (b) have FEV_1 greater than or equal to 25% and less than or equal to 75% predicted, (c) are colonized with *Pseudomonas aeruginosa*, and (d) are able to comply with the prescribed medical regimen [33]. When nebulizing tobramycin, it has been shown that different nebulizers and solutions and techniques may result in very different amounts of tobramycin being inhaled [38]. For example, the addition of albuterol lowered the surface tension of the solution in the nebulizer and resulted in a greater output of tobramycin. A prospective study [39] determined that antibiotics aerosolized by nebulizer could be effectively delivered to tracheostomized, mechanically ventilated patients. In this study, antibiotic concentrations similar to or greater than those achieved among spontaneously breathing individuals were "consistently demonstrated" in patients with a tracheostomy tube.

Aerosolized ribavirin has been used for patients with RSV infection and severe lower respiratory tract disease, or infants with chronic underlying conditions such as cardiac disease, pulmonary disease, or a history of prematurity [3]. However, proof of effectiveness in treating RSV infections is lacking. One study failed to establish the efficacy of inhaled ribavirin for immunocompromised adults with RSV infections [40]. Two prospective double-blind, randomized, placebo-controlled trials addressing the use of aerosolized ribavirin in treating children and adults with respiratory failure from RSV infections failed to show any improvement in the length of time requiring mechanical ventilation, length of stay in the intensive care unit, and oxygen requirements or alter immediate outcome [3]. Aerosolized ribavirin has been suggested to be beneficial for treating infections due to influenza A and B [41]. However, a randomized double-blind, placebo-controlled trial found that aerosolized ribavirin only resulted in accelerating normalization of temperature of children with influenza, but had no effect on respiratory rate, pulse rate, cough, or level of consciousness [42].

Ribavirin, in combination with systemic corticosteroids, was used empirically for the treatment of severe acute respiratory syndrome (SARS). However, a review of 14 clinical reports failed to demonstrate that ribavirin decreased the need for mechanical ventilation, or mortality, of patients with SARS [43].

There are several potential hazardous effects of aerosolized ribavirin. It can cause nausea, headaches, and bronchospasm [44]. In addition, it poses potential risks to health care workers who administer the medication. It has been shown to cause conjunctivitis as it can precipitate on contact lenses, and bronchospasm in health care workers administering the medication [44]. In addition, ribavirin is highly teratogenic. Although studies suggest that absorption of ribavirin by health care workers administering the medication is minimal [3], the short-term and long-term risks to women remain unknown. Therefore, conservative safety practices must be followed [3,44]. Given the lack of evidence supporting its efficacy, its known and potential side effects, and the availability of more efficacious treatment options, we do not recommend the use of aerosolized ribavirin for treating infections with RSV. Further studies are needed to determine its efficacy for treating influenza.

Although studies of patients with acquired immunodeficiency syndrome suggest that aerosolized pentamidine can be effective and well tolerated in mild *Pneumocystis jiroveci* pneumonia, it is not recommended for routine clinical practice [45]. Although aerosolized pentamidine has been used with success for primary and secondary *P. jiroveci* pneumonia prophylaxis [45], trimethoprim–sulfamethoxazole has been recommended as the drug of choice for prophylaxis in both situations. Aerosolized pentamidine (300 mg reconstituted with sterile water, administered every 4 weeks), delivered by a Respirgard II nebulizer (Marquest, Englewood, CO), has been approved for *P. jiroveci* pneumonia prophylaxis [45]. A retrospective study suggested that a standard ultrasonic nebulizer (Fisoneb, Fisons, NY) would yield similar effects to Respirgard II, a jet nebulizer, in providing primary and secondary prophylaxis with aerosolized pentamidine [46]. Because toxicity studies on the secondhand effects of aerosolized pentamidine exposure on health care personnel are limited [47], conservative safety practices are necessary.

Corticosteroids

At present, there is no indication for the use of inhaled corticosteroids for the treatment of the critically ill with acute exacerbations of obstructive lung disease. Systemic corticosteroids (oral or intravenous) are the recommended first-line agents for the treatment of acute asthma [13] and COPD [3]. Because inhaled corticosteroids are an integral component of asthma therapy, on discharge, they should be used for all patients receiving tapering doses of oral prednisone. They are considered the most effective anti-inflammatory therapy for control of persistent asthma [13]. Inhaled corticosteroids are available as MDIs, dry-powder inhalers, or inhalation suspension (budesonide) for aerosolized use.

When patients are hospitalized for reasons other than acute airway obstruction, inhaled corticosteroids may be continued if patients have been taking these agents for asthma or COPD maintenance therapy. To reduce the risk of oral candidiasis, mouth rinsing and use of a spacer device with MDI are recommended.

Racemic Epinephrine

Racemic epinephrine is effective for decreasing laryngeal edema by causing vasoconstriction [3]. The usual adult dose is 0.5 mL of a 2.25% solution diluted in 3 mL of normal saline every 4 to 6 hours. Because rebound edema frequently occurs, patients must be observed closely. Tachycardia is common during treatment and may precipitate angina among patients with coronary artery disease [3]. The role of racemic epinephrine aerosol for epiglottitis is not known. Similarly, inhaled racemic epinephrine is used to treat postextubation stridor, but this use has not been rigorously studied. Nebulized racemic epinephrine appears to have no benefit over nebulized albuterol for the management of bronchiolitis [48]. Because racemic epinephrine aerosol is associated with potentially serious side effects among patients with coronary artery disease, administration of inhaled mixtures of helium and oxygen should be considered first to decrease airway resistance and, therefore, the work of breathing associated with laryngeal edema or other upper-airway diseases (see 'Helium-Oxygen [Heliox]' section).

Aerosolized Vasodilators. Iloprost is an approved inhaled prostacyclin analog used for the chronic treatment of primary pulmonary hypertension and pulmonary hypertension due to use of appetite suppressants, portopulmonary syndrome, connective tissue disease, and chronic thromboembolic disease. It has also been used in patients with acute pulmonary hypertension after coronary bypass surgery, and may be more effective than inhaled nitric oxide (NO) [49]. It is currently FDA approved for patients with primary pulmonary hypertension and New York Heart Association (NYHA) class III (symptoms with minimal activity) and class IV (symptoms at rest) symptoms. Iloprost is administered as 2.5 to 5 μg doses, 6 to 9 times per day. It needs to be delivered via a specialized nebulizer system, the Prodose AAD system (Respironics, Murrysville, PA), to ensure proper dosing. A randomized double-blind, placebo-controlled trial demonstrated that iloprost produced improvements in 6-minute walk, hemodynamics, dyspnea, and quality of life after 12 weeks of therapy [50].

Inhaled prostocyclin has also been used to treat patients with severe acute respiratory distress syndrome (ARDS). Although aerosolized prostocyclin has been shown to improve oxygenation and reduce pulmonary arterial pressures, it does not improve overall outcomes and may be associated with adverse events including systemic hypotension [51]. Its routine use is not recommended, and it is typically reserved for patients with life-threatening hypoxemia refractory to other interventions.

Inhaled Cyclosporin. A randomized double-blind, placebo-controlled trial demonstrated improvement of survival and longer periods free of chronic rejection among lung transplant patients treated with inhaled cyclosporin [52]. The patients in the treatment group received 300 mg of aerosolized cyclosporin (Novartis, East Hanover, NJ) three times a week for the first 2 years after lung transplantation, in addition to usual systemic immunosuppression. There was no increased risk of side effects or opportunistic infections among the treated group.

Modes of Delivery

In the critical care setting, there are generally two types of aerosol delivery devices in use: those that create and deliver wet particles (air-jet nebulizers) and those that deliver preformed particles (pressurized MDIs) with or without MDI auxiliary delivery systems (spacers). Patients on mechanical ventilation or patients breathing through a tracheostomy cannot use dry-powder inhalers. Successful aerosol therapy is dependent on the percentage of the drug that is delivered to the lungs. Factors that influence aerosol deposition and effectiveness, such as flow rate, breathing pattern, and incoordination, have been largely overcome with newer and more advanced designs.

Nebulizers

Air-jet nebulizers are a nonpropellant-based option for inhaled drug delivery. Jet nebulizers rely on a high gas flow (provided by a portable compressor, compressed gas cylinder, or 50-psi wall outlet), Venturi orifices, and baffles to generate respirable particles, generally in the range of 1 to 5 μm in diameter [3]. Small-volume nebulizers, equipped with small fluid reservoirs, are used for drug delivery [3]. Factors that affect their performance include design, characteristics of the medication, and gas source. Large-volume nebulizers have reservoir volumes greater than 100 mL and can be used to deliver aerosolized solutions over an extended period. Large versions are used to deliver bland aerosols into mist tents.

Nebulizers are frequently used for pediatric and elderly populations as well as in the hospital setting. Nebulizer delivery of aerosolized drugs is indicated when a drug is not available in MDI form and when a patient cannot coordinate the use of an MDI. Disadvantages include the need for a gas flow source, lack of portability, cost, and the risk of bacterial contamination if not properly cleaned [53].

Metered-dose Inhalers

An MDI is a pressurized canister that contains drug suspended in a propellant and combined with a dispersing agent. The canister is inverted, placed in a plastic actuator, and, when pressed, delivers a metered dose of drug. The MDI is capable of delivering a more concentrated drug aerosol, as a bolus, than the solutions commonly available for nebulizers [3]. Delivery of a therapeutic dose is dependent on the quality of the patient's technique that requires a slow, deep inhalation followed by a breath hold (approximately 10 seconds). Because this maneuver can be difficult, especially if the patient is experiencing respiratory distress, it is essential that the technique be taught and supervised by trained personnel.

Older MDIs use chlorofluorocarbon propellants (CFCs). Their use has now been phased out after the United Nations passed the 1987 Montreal Protocol that called for the banning of substances that may adversely affect the ozone layer. Although medical devices were initially exempted, many pharmaceutical companies began to formulate alternative preparations and delivery systems. Hydrofluoroalkane-134a (HFA) has been found to be an effective alternative to CFCs. In addition, dry-powder inhalers for long- and short-acting β_2 agonists, corticosteroids, and tiotropium have been developed. Another advantage of the HFA-containing MDIs and the dry-powder inhalers is that lung deposition of the medication appears to be greater when compared to the CFC-containing MDIs.

Metered-dose Inhaler Auxiliary Devices. To overcome problems such as incorrect administration, oropharyngeal deposition, and inconsistent dosing associated with MDI aerosol delivery, several auxiliary devices (i.e., spacer, holding chamber) were developed [3]. When used properly, these devices have the following advantages: (a) a smaller, more therapeutic particle size is achieved; (b) oropharyngeal impaction is decreased; (c) fewer systemic side effects are experienced due to less oropharyngeal deposition compared to MDI alone; and (d) the risk of oral thrush associated with inhaled corticosteroids is decreased. It has been shown that among patients who have difficulty with coordination—particularly the elderly, handicapped, infants, and children younger than 5 years of age—spacer devices improve the efficacy of MDIs [54].

Choice of Delivery System

Since the development of the first MDI in the 1960s, there has been continuing debate about which aerosol delivery system, nebulizers, or MDI is superior. In 1997, Turner et al. [55] published a meta-analysis of 12 studies that compared bronchodilator delivery via nebulizer to delivery via MDI. Studies included in the review were all randomized clinical trials of adults with acute asthma or COPD who were treated in the emergency department or hospital and measured FEV_1 or peak expiratory flow rate. In all but two of the trials, spacers were used with MDIs. Based on the results of these studies, the authors concluded that there was no difference in effectiveness between the two delivery methods.

A Cochrane Library meta-analysis by Cates et al. [15] compared the clinical outcomes of adults and children with acute asthma who received β_2 agonists by nebulizer or MDI with spacer. In this review that included 16 randomized controlled trials, the authors concluded that the outcomes (hospital admission, length of stay in the emergency department, respiratory rate, heart rate, arterial blood gases, tremor and lung function) of both groups were equivalent.

In the United States, MDIs are underused in the acute care setting [3]. Barriers to selection of these devices include reimbursement issues and the misconception of clinicians regarding efficacy. Many third-party payors reimburse for the nebulizer/drug package but not for the MDI. In the critical care setting, selection of an aerosol delivery system for the spontaneously breathing patients should be based on several factors. In general, because the MDI with or without spacer is the most convenient and cost-effective method of delivery, it should be chosen whenever possible. Its use may be limited by factors such as the patient's ability to actuate and coordinate the device, either of which can affect aerosol deposition to the lungs; patient preference; practice situations; and economic evaluations. Additionally, parenchymal dosing with drugs such as pentamidine and ribavirin requires the use of a nebulizer [3]. Cost considerations may determine which delivery system is chosen in different settings. Studies show that use of MDIs with spacers likely produce considerable reductions in hospital costs [56]. The cost of a disposable nebulizer system in a hospital setting may be lower than the cost of a MDI and spacer device if patients are discharged with a second spacer device [15].

Aerosols can be delivered to intubated and mechanically ventilated patients with small-volume side-stream nebulizers connected to the inspiratory tubing or MDIs with an aerosol holding chamber. Although both delivery systems are effective for delivering aerosolized medications to the ventilated patient [3], drug delivery can be significantly reduced if proper technique in setting up and using both devices is not followed.

LUNG-EXPANSION TECHNIQUES

A *lung-expansion technique* is any technique that increases lung volume or assists the patient with increasing lung volume above that reached at his or her usual unassisted or uncoached inspiration. Rationales for the use of various strategies to promote lung inflation include (a) increasing pulmonary compliance, (b) increasing partial arterial pressure of oxygen (PaO_2), (c) decreasing work of breathing, and (d) increasing removal of secretions [57]. Lung-expansion techniques are meant to duplicate a normal sigh maneuver. Theoretically, sighs or periodic hyperinflations to near-total lung capacity reverse microatelectasis [3].

Lung-expansion techniques are indicated to prevent atelectasis and pneumonia among patients who cannot or will not take periodic hyperinflations [3], such as postoperative upper-abdominal and thoracic surgical patients and patients with respiratory disorders due to neuromuscular and chest wall diseases. Adequately performed, maximum inspirations 10 times each hour while awake significantly decrease the incidence of pulmonary complications after laparotomy [58]. Whatever technique is used postoperatively (e.g., coached sustained maximal inspiration with cough, incentive spirometry, volume-oriented intermittent positive-pressure breathing, intermittent CPAP, or positive expiratory pressure [PEP] mask therapy [59]), it should be taught and practiced preoperatively. When properly used, coached sustained maximal inspiration with cough and incentive spirometry—the least expensive and safest techniques—are as effective as any other method [60]. Of the several commercially available incentive spirometers, the one chosen should combine accuracy, low price, and maximum patient accessibility [61]. Because there are no definitive studies comparing the relative efficacy of volume- and flow-oriented incentive spirometers, the choice of equipment must be based on empiric assessment of patient acceptance, ease of use, and cost. When chest percussion with postural drainage is added to the previously mentioned expansion techniques for patients without prior lung disease, it has failed to affect the incidence of postoperative pulmonary complications [62].

AIRWAY CLEARANCE

Efficient mucociliary clearance and effective cough are the two basic processes necessary for normal clearance of the airways. In abnormal situations, this system may be dysfunctional and lead to mucus retention. Both the ACCP [63] and the BTS [2] have published evidence-based guidelines reviewing both pharmacologic and nonpharmacologic methods of augmenting pulmonary secretion clearance. Both guidelines are complete reviews on this topic. A summarized discussion of techniques aimed at enhancing airway clearance follows.

Augmentation of Mucociliary Clearance

Mucociliary clearance is one of the most important defense mechanisms of the respiratory system. Mucociliary dysfunction is any defect in the ciliary and secretory elements of mucociliary interaction that disturbs the normal defenses of the airway epithelium [64]. Ineffective mucociliary clearance leads to retention of tracheobronchial secretions. Mucociliary clearance may be ineffective because of depression of the clearance mechanisms or oversecretion in the face of normal mucous transport, or both. Mucus is ineffectively cleared and overproduced by smokers with or without chronic bronchitis and by asthmatic patients [3]. It is also ineffectively cleared in the following situations: (a) among patients with emphysema, bronchiectasis, and CF; (b) during and up to 4 to 6 weeks after viral upper respiratory tract infections; (c) during and for an unknown period after general anesthesia due to the inhalation of dry gas and cuffed endotracheal tubes used during surgery; and (d) during prolonged endotracheal intubation due to the presence of the cuffed tube, administration of elevated concentrations of inspired oxygen, and damage to the tracheobronchial tree from suctioning [3]. The most important consideration for improving mucociliary clearance is to remove the inciting cause(s) of ineffective clearance and overproduction of secretions.

Treatment

Mucociliary clearance can be enhanced pharmacologically and mechanically. Numerous drugs with potential mucociliary effect have been studied, but only a few are clinically useful. Pharmaceutical therapy is frequently used in conjunction with physical therapy.

Pharmacologic Augmentation. β agonists and aminophylline stimulate mucociliary clearance [3]. These drugs should be given in the same doses given for bronchodilatation. Mucolytics and expectorants (e.g., potassium iodide, glyceryl guaiacolate, guaifenesin, ammonium chloride, creosote, and cocillana) have not been shown to increase mucociliary clearance [3]. There is no evidence to support the use of mucokinetic agents for COPD exacerbations [3]. In a randomized controlled trail, healthy volunteers and patients with mild asthma showed no improvement of mucociliary clearance when given inhaled furosemide [65].

In vitro studies have demonstrated that corticosteroids reduce mucous secretion from human airway cells [66], and the use of inhaled corticosteroids has been recommended for the management of bronchorrhea (i.e., mucus secretions of more than 100 mL per day) [67]. However, we know of no randomized controlled trials demonstrating the benefit of inhaled corticosteroids in the management of bronchorrhea.

Mechanical Augmentation

Chest physiotherapy (CPT). Usually, CPT involves (a) gravity (therapeutic positioning), (b) percussion to the chest wall over the affected area, (c) vibration of the chest wall during expiration, and (d) coughing. Coughing appears to be the most important component of CPT (see 'Augmentation of Cough Effectiveness' section). It is felt to be beneficial for patients with CF and bronchiectasis, in the unusual COPD patient who expectorates more than 30 mL of sputum each day [63], and for patients with lobar atelectasis [2]. It is not indicated for asthmatic patients [63] or for those with uncomplicated pneumonias [2]. CPT does not improve FEV_1, provides only modest short-term effects, and long-term benefits are unproven [63]. For patients with COPD, alternative methods of airway clearance (see below) have not proven more effective than CPT, and the effects of CPT itself on patients with COPD may be minimal [68].

Complications of CPT are infrequent yet potentially severe [69]. They include massive pulmonary hemorrhage (perhaps caused by clots dislodged during percussion), decreased PaO_2 from positioning the "good" lung up in spontaneously breathing patients, rib fractures, increased intracranial pressure, decreased cardiac output, and decreased FEV_1.

Oscillatory devices. These devices include the flutter device (Varioraw SARL, Scandipharm Inc, Birmingham, AL), intrapulmonary percussive ventilation (Percussionator, IPV-1; Percussionaire, Sand Point, ID), and high-frequency chest wall oscillation. The flutter mucus clearance device is a small, handheld, pipe-like device used to facilitate the removal of mucus from the lungs. As patients exhale through the device, a steel ball rolls and bounces, producing vibrations that are transmitted throughout the airways. It is postulated that vibrations of the airways intermittently increase endobronchial pressure and accelerate expiratory airflow, thereby enhancing mucus clearance [70]. In a randomized controlled trial, the flutter device was compared to standard, manual chest therapy in hospitalized CF patients experiencing an acute exacerbation [71] and found to be a safe, efficacious, and cost-effective alternative to standard, manual chest percussion. Konstan et al. [70] compared periods of vigorous voluntary cough, postural drainage, and flutter-valve treatment. Among the therapies compared, the volume of sputum was three times greater with the flutter treatment. Although larger clinical trials are needed, it appears to be a useful device for self-administration of CPT and as an equal alternative to CPT [63].

Intrapulmonary percussive ventilation uses short bursts of air at 200 to 300 cycles per minute, along with entrained aerosols delivered via a mouthpiece [63]. In a study on patients with CF, this was found to be equal to CPT [72]. A small study suggested that high-frequency chest well oscillation decreased breathlessness and fatigue in patients with ALS [73]. High-frequency chest wall oscillation delivered through an inflatable vest appears to offer no benefit over standard CPT [3].

PEP mask. In PEP therapy, a mask is applied tightly over the mouth and nose, and a variable-flow resistor is adjusted to achieve PEP during exhalation between 5 and 20 cm H_2O. This, combined with "huff" coughing, allows mobilization of peripherally located secretions upward into larger airways. A Cochrane review of 20 studies in patients with CF failed to demonstrate that PEP had any short-term benefits over CPT [74].

Mechanical insufflation–exsufflation. Mechanical insufflation–exsufflation (cough in-exsufflator) increases the volume inhaled during the inspiratory phase of cough, thereby increasing cough effectiveness [63]. Cough efficiency can be further enhanced by applying negative airway pressure for 1 to 3 seconds after the initial inspiration. This method appears to be most beneficial for patients with impaired cough due to neuromuscular disease [75].

In summary, the data available, although not abundant, indicate that in patients with copious secretions, clearance of secretions can be enhanced with selected physical therapy procedures. Although these modalities appear to increase expectoration of mucus, it is not clear what clinical benefit this achieves. There is no information about the influence of physical therapy maneuvers on health care outcomes, including frequency of hospitalization, hospital length of stay, longevity, and quality of life. It is clear that these techniques are well entrenched in the management of patients with mucus hypersecretion, especially those with CF; it is time for us to prove that they lead to clinically important outcomes. Evidence-based guidelines for the use of these modalities can be found elsewhere [2,63].

Suctioning. Although mechanical aspiration or suctioning is routine in most hospitals, many are unaware of the numerous potential complications associated with suctioning, such as tissue trauma, laryngospasm, bronchospasm, hypoxemia, cardiac arrhythmias, respiratory arrest, cardiac arrest, atelectasis, pneumonia, misdirection of catheter, and death [3]. Complications are generally avoidable or reversible if proper technique and indications are adhered to strictly.

Endotracheal. Endotracheal suctioning is performed for patients with an artificial tracheal airway in place. It should be used only when there is definite evidence of excessive retained secretions. Routine suctioning according to a predetermined schedule may cause excessive mucosal tissue damage, excessive impairment of mucociliary clearance, unnecessary exposure to the potential risks of hypoxemia associated with the procedure, arrhythmias, atelectasis, and bronchoconstriction [3]. Endotracheal suctioning is indicated when there is a need to (a) remove accumulated secretions, (b) obtain a sputum specimen for microbiologic or cytologic examination, (c) maintain the patency and integrity of the artificial airway, and (d) stimulate cough in patients with ineffective cough [76].

Suction catheters are generally 22 inches long (adequate in length to reach the main stem bronchus) and sized in French units. Most have a side port to minimize mucosal damage. To avoid obstruction of the artificial airway, the outer diameter of the suction catheter should be less than half the size of the internal diameter of the endotracheal tube (rule of thumb: multiply the inner diameter of the endotracheal tube by 2 and use next smallest size [e.g., 8.0-mm endotracheal tube: $2 \times 8 = 16$, choose next smallest size $= 14$ French]) [77].

For patients receiving ventilatory support, closed, multiuse systems that are incorporated into the ventilator circuit are available. Because patients remain connected to the ventilator during suctioning, positive end-expiratory pressure (PEEP) and high fractional inspiration of oxygen (FiO_2) can be maintained, reducing the risk of hypoxemia. Preoxygenation with 100% O_2 is still necessary. The use of closed, multiuse systems may reduce costs and the risk of cross-contamination. However, these systems may increase tension on the tracheal tube and add resistance to the airway.

The practice of instilling normal saline into the airway before suctioning to aid secretion removal is common, but it is unclear whether it is effective and it may increase the risk of nosocomial pneumonia. The routine use of saline irrigation is not recommended [77].

Nasotracheal. Although nasotracheal suctioning may be considered for patients who do not have an artificial tracheal airway, it is not recommended because of the potential side effects, and there are other, safer alternatives. It is rarely indicated because CPT can be used in conscious patients, and semicomatose or comatose patients with retained secretions can be intubated. Nasotracheal suctioning has been associated with fatal cardiac arrest, life-threatening arrhythmias presumably due to hypoxemia, and bacteremia [3]. Because quantitative cultures acquired with plugged telescoping catheters at bronchoscopy can be obtained more safely and are definitely more reliable than nasotracheal suction (see Chapter 10) in obtaining uncontaminated lower respiratory tract secretions for culture, nasotracheal suction is not recommended for this purpose.

Nasopharyngeal. Nasopharyngeal suctioning is indicated to clear the upper airway. Because the catheter does not reach the vocal cords or enter the trachea, nasopharyngeal suctioning is associated with fewer complications than nasotracheal suctioning [3]. The catheter should not touch or go beyond the vocal cords. This requires insertion to a depth that corresponds to the distance between the middle of the patient's chin and the angle of the jaw, just below the earlobe.

Endotracheal extubation. Before removal of the endotracheal tube, perform nasopharyngeal and oropharyngeal suctioning to clear secretions that have pooled above the vocal cords for the inflated cuff. Replace the catheter and perform endotracheal suctioning. In preparation for deflating the cuff, place the endotracheal suction catheter tip just distal to the endotracheal tube to aspirate any secretions that gravitate downward when the cuff is deflated. Deflate the cuff and intermittently suction while removing the tube and catheter as a unit.

Augmentation of Cough Effectiveness

Although mucociliary transport is the major method of clearing the airway in healthy subjects, cough is an important reserve mechanism, especially in lung disease [3]. All studies suggest that cough is effective in clearing secretions only if secretions are excessive.

Pathophysiology of Ineffective Cough

The effectiveness of cough for clearing an airway theoretically depends on the presence of secretions of sufficient thickness to be affected by two-phase, gas–liquid flow and the linear velocity of air moving through its lumen [3]. The ineffectiveness of voluntary coughing in normal subjects to clear tagged aerosol particles in the lower airways is probably due to the inability of the moving airstream to interact appropriately with the normally thin mucus layer on which the particles were deposited [3]. Once there is sufficiently thick material in the airways, the effectiveness of cough depends on achieving a high expiratory flow rate of air and a small cross-sectional area of the airway during the expiratory phase of cough to achieve a high linear velocity (velocity equals flow/cross-sectional area); therefore, any condition associated with decreased expiratory flow rates or reduced ability to compress airways dynamically places affected patients at risk of having an ineffective cough.

All conditions that may lead to an ineffective cough interfere with the inspiratory or expiratory phases of cough; most conditions affect both. Cough effectiveness is likely to be most impaired in patients with respiratory muscle weakness because their ability to take in a deep breath in (flow rates are highest at high lung volumes) and to compress their airways dynamically during expiration are impaired, placing them at double liability. The muscles of expiration appear to be the most important determinant for producing elevated intrathoracic pressures, and they are capable of doing so even with an endotracheal tube in place [3]. Therefore, tracheostomy should not be performed in the intubated patient just to increase cough effectiveness.

Assessment of Cough Effectiveness

Ideally, clinicians would like to predict clinically or physiologically when a patient is at risk of developing atelectasis, pneumonia, or gas-exchange abnormalities because of an ineffective cough. There are no such studies, however. The existing data that relate to assessment of cough effectiveness were generated in patients with muscular dystrophy and myasthenia gravis [3,78]. These studies suggested that mouth maximum expiratory pressure (MEP) measurements may be useful for assessing cough strength, but they did not correlate these measurements with any clinical outcomes. Using the absence of peak flow transients (i.e., a spike of flow with a cough to the otherwise sustained maximal expiratory flow) during cough flow–volume curves as an indication that expiratory muscle strength during coughing was not adequate to compress the airways dynamically, investigators found that MEP was the most sensitive predictor of flow transient production during coughing [3]. All patients who could produce cough transients had MEP values greater than 60 cm H_2O; those who could not produce transients had MEP values of 45 cm H_2O or less. This latter value is consistent with the clinical observations of Gracey et al. [78], who found in patients with myasthenia gravis that MEP values less than 40 cm H_2O were frequently associated with difficulty in raising secretions without suctioning.

Bach and Saporito [79] prospectively evaluated measurement of peak cough flows (PCF) (assisted and unassisted) as a predictor of successful extubation and decannulation among 49 patients with primary neuromuscular ventilatory insufficiency. In this study, the ability to generate at least 160 L per minute of PCF (measured with Peak Flow Meter, HealthScan Inc, Cedar Grove, NJ) resulted in successful extubation or decannulation, whereas no patients with PCFs under 160 L per minute were successfully extubated or decannulated. The authors concluded that the assisted PCF could be used to predict the ability to safely extubate or decannulate patients with neuromuscular disease regardless of the extent of ventilatory insufficiency.

Protussive Therapy

When cough is useful yet inadequate, protussive therapy is indicated (e.g., bronchiectasis, CF, pneumonia, postoperative atelectasis) [3]. The goal of protussive therapy is to increase cough effectiveness with or without increasing cough frequency. It can be of a pharmaceutical or mechanical nature.

Only a small number of pharmacologic agents have been adequately evaluated as protussive agents [80]. Of these, aerosolized hypertonic saline in patients with chronic bronchitis and amiloride aerosol in patients with CF have been shown to improve cough clearance [3,81]. Although aerosolized ipratropium bromide diminished the effectiveness of cough for clearing radiolabeled particles from the airways in COPD, aerosolized terbutaline after CPT significantly increased cough clearance in patients with bronchiectasis [3]. The conflicting results with these two types of bronchodilators suggest that terbutaline achieved its favorable effect by increasing hydration of mucus or enhancing ciliary beating, and these overcame any negative effects that bronchodilation had on cough clearance. If bronchodilators result in too much smooth muscle relaxation of large airways, flow rates can actually decrease even in healthy individuals when more compliant large airways narrow too much because they cannot withstand dynamic compression during forced expirations [3]. Although hypertonic saline, amiloride, and terbutaline by aerosol after CPT have been shown to increase cough clearance, their clinical use remains to be determined in future studies that assess short-term and long-term effects of these agents on the patient's condition.

Expiratory Muscle Training

Because expiratory muscle weakness diminishes cough, strengthening the muscles may improve cough effectiveness. In quadriplegic subjects, there was a 46% increase in expiratory reserve volume after a 6-week period of isometric training to increase the clavicular portion of the pectoralis major [82]. This technique may improve cough by allowing patients with neuromuscular weakness to generate higher intrathoracic pressures [3].

Mechanical Measures

A variety of mechanical measures have been advocated as possible therapies to improve cough effectiveness [3], including (a) positive mechanical insufflation, followed by (b) manual compression of the lower thorax and abdomen in quadriparetic patients (an abdominal push maneuver that assists expiratory efforts in patients with spinal cord injuries), (c) mechanical insufflation–exsufflation, (d) abdominal binding and muscle training of the clavicular portion of the pectoralis major in tetraplegic patients, and (e) CPT in patients with chronic bronchitis. The usefulness of the first four measures for improving clinical outcomes has yet to be studied; and, among patients with CF, one technique does not appear to be superior to the others [3]. For patients with chronic bronchitis, the combination of short bouts of PEP breathing, forced expirations, and CPT resulted in reduced coughing, less mucus production, and fewer acute exacerbations compared with patients who received CPT alone. Except for patients with CF, there is no clear benefit of combining CPT with coughing over vigorous coughing alone [63].

The effects of deep lung insufflation on maximum insufflation capacities and PCF for patients with neuromuscular disease were investigated [83]. In this study, the authors concluded that with training, the capacity to stack air to deep insufflations can be enhanced despite neuromuscular weakness, and this can result in increased cough effectiveness.

ADMINISTRATION OF MEDICAL GASES

Oxygen Therapy

Indications for Oxygen Therapy

In the acute setting, administration of supplemental oxygen is indicated for (a) acute respiratory failure (hypoxemic and hypercapnic), (b) acute myocardial infarction (MI), (c) acute asthma, (d) normoxemic hypoxia (states characterized by the potential or actual documentation of tissue hypoxia despite a normal PaO_2 such as carbon monoxide [CO] poisoning), (e) the perioperative and postoperative states, and (f) cluster headaches [3,84,85]. Additionally, oxygen should be administered empirically in cases of cardiac or respiratory arrest, respiratory distress, hypotension, shock, and severe trauma [3].

A dosage sufficient to correct the hypoxemia should be prescribed. The goal of oxygen therapy is to correct hypoxemia to a PaO_2 greater than 60 mm Hg or arterial oxygen saturation (SaO_2) greater than 90%. Owing to the shape of the oxyhemoglobin dissociation curve, there is little benefit from increasing the PaO_2 to values much greater than 60 mm Hg, and in some cases, it may increase the risk, albeit small, of CO_2 retention [3].

Clinicians are cautioned regarding the haphazard use of oxygen, because there are potential complications associated with the administration of supplemental oxygen, particularly at high concentrations (e.g., $FiO_2 > 0.50$). Oxygen therapy should not be used in place of but in addition to mechanical ventilation when ventilatory support is indicated [84].

Respiratory Failure. Oxygen therapy is used in acute pulmonary conditions to prevent tissue hypoxia and the serious and often irreversible effects on vital organ function that can result from untreated hypoxemia. In the absence of hypercarbia, the risk of worsening alveolar hypoventilation with the administration of supplemental oxygen is essentially nonexistent. Even among patients with chronic hypercapnic respiratory failure, the administration of supplemental oxygen to achieve a PaO_2 of approximately 60 mm Hg is associated with only a small risk of worsening hypercapnia. The mechanism by which oxygen administration results in CO_2 elevation among patients with COPD is multifactorial. It cannot be explained solely by the effect of oxygen on ventilatory drives. It may also be due to an oxygen-induced increase in dead space resulting from relaxation of hypoxic vasoconstriction, and it also requires the presence of other respiratory abnormalities preventing compensatory hyperventilation [3]. Furthermore, in acute situations in which supplemental oxygen is necessary to maintain adequate tissue oxygenation, it should not be with held even if there is a risk that ventilatory support may be required. Care should be taken, however, to avoid the administration of excessively rich oxygen mixtures. See Chapter 173 for further discussion of oxygen therapy in COPD.

Acute Myocardial Infarction Without Respiratory Failure. Based on studies demonstrating that breathing enriched oxygen mixtures limited infarct size in animals, it has become common practice to administer oxygen to patients suspected of experiencing ischemic-type chest discomfort [84]. Because nitroglycerin dilates the pulmonary vascular bed and increases ventilation–perfusion abnormalities, supplemental oxygen has been recommended during nitroglycerine use and for the initial hours after an acute MI is first suspected. Experimental studies have shown that supplemental oxygen may limit ischemic myocardial injury [86,87] and reduce ST-segment elevation among patients experiencing a MI [88]. The routine use of supplemental oxygen, however, may be associated with an increased risk of death, questioning this practice [86,87]. In the setting of MI complicated by left ventricular failure, arrhythmias, or pneumonia, the appropriate oxygen concentration should be determined by monitoring of the PaO_2 or SaO_2 [84]. Supplemental oxygen should be administered to maintain an SaO_2 goal greater than 90% [84].

Acute Asthma. Supplemental oxygen protects against hypoxemia resulting from pulmonary vasodilation induced by β agonists and minimizes hypoxemia-induced vasoconstriction [89]. Normal levels of oxygen (normoxia) may protect against cardiac arrhythmias and may also help oxygen delivery to peripheral tissues [3].

Supplemental oxygen is recommended for patients with hypoxemia and for patients with FEV_1 or peak expiratory flow less than 50% of the predicted value during an acute attack when arterial oxygen monitoring is not available. The National Asthma Education and Prevention Program Expert Panel Report 3 recommends oxygen administered via nasal cannula or mask to maintain an SaO_2 greater than 90% (greater than 95% in pregnant women and in patients with a history of heart disease) [13]. SaO_2 monitoring should continue until a definite response to bronchodilatory therapy occurs.

Normoxemic Hypoxia. *Normoxemic hypoxia* encompasses conditions that are characterized by the potential or actual documentation of tissue hypoxia but with a normal PaO_2 [84]. Tissue hypoxia occurs as a result of abnormal hemoglobin function, deficient delivery, or inefficient use of oxygen by the tissues. Examples of such conditions include acute anemia, carboxyhemoglobinemia (perhaps the most lethal), and sickle-cell crisis.

Recommendations for the use of supplemental oxygen for normoxemic hypoxic conditions are outlined as follows:

1. *Acute anemia.* Although the definitive treatment is sufficient blood replacement, supplemental oxygen is a reasonable temporizing measure.
2. *Carboxyhemoglobinemia* (CO poisoning) [3]. Because a partial pressure of CO of less than 1 mm Hg can saturate 50% of hemoglobin and not interfere with lung function, measurements of oxygen tension are not useful for predicting the presence of CO poisoning or for directing oxygen therapy. Carboxyhemoglobin levels must be measured to detect CO poisoning. Administration of high concentrations of inspiratory oxygen is important when treating CO poisoning for two reasons: a higher amount of oxygen may be placed in the solution in the blood to supplement the oxygen already present, and a high PaO_2 accelerates the dissociation of CO from hemoglobin. In the absence of hyperbaric oxygen, a nonrebreathing mask driven by pure humidified oxygen is the treatment of choice. This should be given immediately and without interruption until it is verified that carboxyhemoglobinemia has fallen to less than 5%. Although hyperbaric oxygenation represents a potentially more effective alternative, it is not readily available for most patients. If it is available, patients with carboxyhemoglobin levels greater than 40% or with cardiac or neurologic symptoms should be considered for immediate transportation to a hyperbaric oxygen facility for treatment. (See Chapter 178 for further discussion of CO poisoning.)
3. *Sickle-cell crisis.* The role of oxygen therapy for sickle-cell crisis is unknown [90]. Because deoxygenation makes cells sickle, however, it seems reasonable to give supplemental oxygen in this setting. Because of the risk of oxygen toxicity, concentrations in excess of 50% should not be given for more than 48 hours.
4. *Cluster headache.* Several trials have shown that oxygen delivered at rates between 6 and 12 L per minute can reduce acute pain from cluster headaches [91]. Supplemental oxygen is a first-line therapy along with injectable triptans. The mechanism of action for oxygen therapy in this setting is unknown.

Prevention of Surgical Wound Infections. Routine perioperative administration of supplemental oxygen, regardless of the patient's SaO_2, may be advantageous in reducing the incidence of postoperative surgical site infections. The effect is more pronounced among patients undergoing colorectal surgery [92].

Postoperative State. An increase in the alveolar-arterial partial pressure of oxygen [$P(A\text{-}a)O_2$] gradient and a decrease of the functional residual capacity are common perioperatively and postoperatively. Ventilation–perfusion abnormalities and intrapulmonary shunting may occur, and while generally corrected within the first few hours after most types of surgery, it may be more significant among the elderly, the obese, for patients with pre-existing cardiopulmonary conditions, and after surgery of the upper abdomen and thorax. For these situations, PaO_2 may not normalize until postoperative Day 2. Because the PaO_2 usually increases with the administration of supplemental oxygen, low concentrations of supplemental oxygen should be administered to those at risk of postoperative hypoxemia [93]. In some cases, lung-expansion maneuvers may be necessary after oxygen fails to correct the PaO_2 [82].

Oxygen Delivery Systems

In the acute setting, bulk supply systems are used as a relatively inexpensive means of oxygen delivery. When transporting hospitalized patients, gas cylinders and liquid tanks are used.

Oxygen Delivery Devices

A variety of devices are available to deliver supplemental oxygen. Selection should be based on the amount of oxygen the system can deliver and its clinical performance. Factors capable of affecting performance include the type of device chosen, flow rates used by the device, the fit of the device, respiratory rate, inspiratory flows, and tidal volumes. Types of devices are as follows:

1. Standard dual-prong nasal cannulas are the most commonly used oxygen delivery devices for administering low-flow oxygen. Flow rates of 0.5 to 1.0 L per minute by nasal prongs approximate an inspired oxygen concentration of 0.24, and a rate of 2 L per minute approximates 0.28. Nasal cannulas are easy to use, relatively comfortable, fairly unobtrusive, do not interfere with eating or talking, and relatively inexpensive. Generally, it is unnecessary to humidify oxygen administered by nasal cannulae at flow rates of 4 L per minute or less [84].
2. Simple oxygen masks deliver FiO_2 of approximately 0.35 to 0.50 oxygen with flow rates of 5 L per minute or greater. Because nasal cannulas and simple oxygen masks deliver an overlapping range of FiO_2, the nasal cannulas should be used unless the nares are unavailable or prone to irritation from the cannula. Face masks must be removed when eating and drinking, and caution should always be exercised when using oxygen face masks for sedated, obtunded, or restrained patients. Because these masks have a reservoir of 100 to 200 mL, there is a risk of rebreathing CO_2. For this reason, flow rates of at least 5 L per minute are recommended. Because relatively high-flow rates are needed with simple masks, they are generally not appropriate for the delivery of a low FiO_2 (e.g., less than 0.30 to 0.35) [84].
3. Masks with reservoir bags, nonrebreathing and partial-rebreathing oxygen masks, can deliver a high FiO_2 (>0.50) with oxygen flowing into the reservoir at 8 to 10 L per minute to partially inflate the reservoir bag throughout inspiration. They are designed to deliver short-term high FiO_2 for situations when hypoxemia is suspected [94]. After the patient has been stabilized, if a high FiO_2 is required, a fixed performance device with a known FiO_2 should be substituted. Theoretically, the partial-rebreathing mask should deliver an FiO_2 of approximately 0.60, and the nonrebreathing mask should deliver 1.00. For the nonrebreathing mask to deliver an FiO_2 of 1.00, however, a tight-fitting mask is required.
4. A Venturi-type mask can be used if an accurate FiO_2 is required. Supplied by high oxygen flows, it maintains a fixed ratio of oxygen to room air so that the FiO_2 remains constant. These masks can deliver oxygen concentrations to the trachea of up to 0.50. Venturi-type masks have been designed to deliver FiO_2 settings of 0.24, 0.28, 0.31, 0.35, 0.40, and 0.50.
5. High-flow nasal cannula (HFNC) oxygen administers heated and humidified oxygen up to 60 L per minute. The physiologic consequences of HFNC include the application of a small amount of PEEP to the upper airway, an improvement of physiologic dead space, and improved work of breathing and oxygenation when compared to facemask oxygen for patients with hypoxemic respiratory failure. In a recent trial, while patients with nonhypercapneic respiratory failure treated with HFNC had equal rates of intubation as those treated with standard oxygen therapy and NIPPV, they had a better 90-day survival [95]. Clinical aspects of the use of HFNC such as who most benefits and when to escalate therapy remain undetermined.

Oxygen-Conserving Devices

Several devices have been developed to improve the efficacy of oxygen delivery. Three such methods are reservoir cannulas, demand-pulse oxygen delivery, and transtracheal catheters [3].

1. The reservoir nasal cannula stores 20 mL of oxygen during exhalation and delivers this oxygen as a bolus at the start of inspiration.
2. Electronic demand devices deliver a pulse of oxygen during early inspiration rather than continuously throughout the ventilatory cycle.
3. Transtracheal catheters bypass the anatomic dead space, and oxygen is delivered directly into the trachea using the central airways as a reservoir for oxygen during end-expiration [3]. When caring for patients with transtracheal catheters in place before admission to the hospital, it is important to secure them with tape or sutures to prevent accidental dislodging. There is no need to remove the catheter before or during endotracheal intubation. Although the patient is intubated, however, the transtracheal catheter should be capped.

Patients receiving transtracheal oxygen are at risk of developing inspissated secretions, mucus airway casts, and mucus balls, especially when the transtracheally delivered gas is not adequately humidified. Consequently, whenever a patient receiving transtracheal oxygen develops worsening hypoxemia or respiratory distress, mucus obstruction of the airway should be considered. In this setting, oxygen should be administered via nasal cannula and the transtracheal catheter removed. This maneuver can often shear off a mucus ball attached to the end of the catheter, allowing the patient to expectorate the accumulated mucus, and thereby improve the hypoxemia and eliminate the respiratory distress. The catheter can then be cleaned and reinserted with provision for adequate humidification of the transtracheally delivered gas.

Choice of Oxygen Delivery Device

For the hypercapnic, hypoxemic patient, therapy can begin with 0.5 to 2.0 L per minute by nasal cannula or 0.24 to 0.28 FiO_2 by Venturi-type mask. If the PaO_2 remains less than 55 mm Hg 30 minutes later, administration of progressive increments of inspired oxygen is undertaken. Assessment of gas exchange is measured at frequent intervals, usually every 30 minutes [3] for the first 1 to 2 hours or until it is certain that the PaO_2 is 55 mm Hg or greater and CO_2 narcosis is not developing. In the hypercapnic patient, titration of supplemental oxygen is best assessed by arterial blood gas analysis rather than oximetry because the arterial blood gas provides $PaCO_2$ and oxygenation data. An initial modest increase in $PaCO_2$ (5 to 10 mm Hg) is expected in most hypercapnic patients given supplemental oxygen [96].

If a well-fitted Venturi-type mask delivering FiO_2 of 0.50 fails to achieve an oxygen saturation of at least 90% or a PaO_2 of 60 mm Hg or greater, the patient usually has severe cardiogenic pulmonary edema, ARDS, overwhelming pneumonia, or a cardiac or pulmonary vascular shunt. In these settings, a nonrebreathing mask is recommended for two reasons. First, when properly worn, it has the potential to deliver the most predictable oxygen concentration (close to 100%) of all the high-concentration delivery mask devices (e.g., aerosol masks, partial rebreathing masks, or face tents). Second, it can reveal the presence of a right-to-left shunt. If the PaO_2 is 60 mm Hg or less in the face of a fractional concentration of inspired oxygen of close to 1.00, a right-to-left shunt of approximately 40% of the cardiac output is present. An alternative acceptable oxygen delivery method in this scenario is a high-flow nasal cannula. If the patient does not respond to these initial noninvasive modes of oxygen delivery, invasive mechanical ventilation should be considered.

Oxygen therapy should never be abruptly discontinued when hypercapnia has worsened and CO_2 narcosis is a possibility. This causes PaO_2 to fall to a level lower than it was before any oxygen was given [3] because the patient is breathing in a slower, shallower pattern.

Long-term Continuous Oxygen Therapy

Continuous (24-hour) oxygen therapy significantly prolongs and improves the quality of life in hypoxemic patients with COPD [3]. If used for 15 hours per day or more, it decreases mortality by 1.5- to 1.9-fold over the subsequent 3 years. Patients who should be given continuous oxygen during hospitalization and as outpatients include those with a PaO_2 of 55 mm Hg or less and those with a PaO_2 of 59 mm Hg or less plus peripheral edema, hematocrit of 55% or greater, or P pulmonale on electrocardiogram. Because many of these patients continue to improve as outpatients, the need for continuous oxygen therapy should be reassessed at 1 month [97].

Complications of Oxygen Therapy

Among adults, decreased mucociliary clearance, tracheobronchitis, and pulmonary oxygen toxicity are the major complications of oxygen therapy. Mucociliary clearance is decreased by 40% when 75% oxygen is breathed for 9 hours and by 50% when 50% oxygen is breathed for 30 hours [3]. Symptomatic tracheobronchitis is caused consistently by the inhalation of high concentrations of oxygen (0.90 or higher) for 12 hours or more; it is manifested by substernal pain, cough, and dyspnea [3].

To avoid clinically significant pulmonary oxygen toxicity, prolonged administration of concentrations greater than 0.50 should be restricted, whenever possible, to 48 hours [3]. The pathology of oxygen toxicity is that of ARDS; it can lead to death from refractory and progressive hypoxemia due to interstitial fibrosis. It is best avoided by restricting delivery of oxygen to the lowest concentration and shortest duration absolutely necessary to achieve a satisfactory PaO_2. Therefore, prophylaxis consists of using any and all measures that allow a decrease in the concentration of inspired oxygen to subtoxic levels. PEEP has been shown to be useful for achieving this goal.

For patients with previous bleomycin exposure, there appears to be a synergistic effect with subsequent exposure to high concentrations of inspired oxygen, resulting in the development of bleomycin associated pneumonitis [98]. Although it is unclear how long after bleomycin exposure that breathing high-inspired oxygen concentrations predisposes to pneumonitis, the risk appears highest within the first 6 months of bleomycin exposure.

A similar interaction can be seen among patients taking long-term amiodarone and exposure to high concentrations of inspired oxygen [99]. This risk appears higher for patients receiving high concentrations of inspired oxygen via mechanical ventilation. These patients can develop diffuse alveolar damage and ARDS, and mortality rates may be as high as 33% [100]. For patients with a history of either bleomycin or amiodarone exposure, we recommend using the lowest amounts of supplemental oxygen possible to maintain adequate oxygenation.

Although the complications of retrolental fibroplasia and bronchopulmonary dysplasia from oxygen toxicity have been limited in the past to pediatric patients, reports of adults with bronchopulmonary dysplasia, the eventual result of ARDS, have appeared [3]. Central nervous system dysfunction manifested by myoclonus, nausea, paresthesias, unconsciousness, and seizures is limited to hyperbaric oxygenation at pressures in excess of 2 atm [3].

Hyperbaric Oxygen Therapy

Hyperbaric therapy, 100% oxygen at 2 to 3 times the atmospheric pressure at sea level, is used as primary therapy in the treatment of patients with decompression sickness, arterial gas embolism, and severe CO poisoning [3]. In the case of CO poisoning, although hyperbaric therapy accelerates the resolution of symptoms, it does not appear to affect the rate of late sequelae or long-term mortality for non-life–threatening cases [3]. It is used as adjunctive therapy with supportive evidence in the treatment of crush injuries, clostridial myonecrosis/necrotizing fasciitis, compromised skin grafts, refractory osteomyelitis, and necrotizing skin infections [101]. Other conditions that may benefit from hyperbaric oxygen therapy include traumatic brain injury, acute ischemic stroke, acute coronary syndrome, and diabetic wounds. Data are inconclusive and further study is required [102–105].

Helium-Oxygen (Heliox)

Because helium is less dense and has a lower molecular weight than nitrogen, it often improves flow where airflow is turbulent (i.e., density and molecular weight dependent). However, this primarily occurs in large airways when there is tracheomalacia, laryngeal edema or an upper airway–obstructing lesion. Heliox has successfully decreased airway resistance for patients with postextubation upper-airway obstruction [3], for children with severe croup who were refractory to inhaled racemic epinephrine [106,107], and for upper-airway obstruction due to tracheal tumors or extrinsic compression [108]. Although there have been favorable physiologic effects shown by a number of randomized controlled trials of spontaneously breathing patients with acute severe asthma [3], one large meta-analysis of seven studies [109] and an extensive review by the Cochrane Database [110] failed to show any benefit of routinely using Heliox for the management of acute asthma patients. At this time, there is no definitive evidence to support the use of Heliox for the treatment of asthma exacerbations. Heliox has been used with nebulized albuterol for the treatment of asthma, but any benefit is unclear as there are conflicting results in the literature [111–113].

The effect of increasing concentrations of helium for decreasing airway resistance is linear, but most reduction has taken place when the concentration of helium approaches 40% [114]. Therefore, Heliox mixtures should contain a minimum of 40% helium, with the balance of the mixture being oxygen. For patients in respiratory distress with little hypoxemia due to laryngeal edema, a Heliox mixture of 80% helium and 20%

oxygen would suffice. For patients in respiratory distress with hypoxemia due to pulmonary edema associated with laryngeal edema, however, a Heliox mixture of 40% helium and 60% oxygen would be most advantageous.

In an uncontrolled trial, intubated patients with status asthmaticus on mechanical ventilation [115] were successfully ventilated with a mixture of 60% helium and 40% oxygen and experienced a decrease in airway pressures and $PaCO_2$ and resolution of acidosis. Others report improvements of airway mechanics among mechanically ventilated patients using an oxygen and helium mixture [116,117]. However, no definite improvement of outcomes were reported.

Because helium may affect how ventilators measure gas parameters, monitoring of ventilator outputs must be undertaken when helium is delivered through the ventilator.

Although Heliox may provide favorable short-term physiologic effects for patients with acute exacerbations of COPD [3], review of the literature has concluded that there is insufficient evidence to support the use of Heliox for the management of ventilated and nonventilated patients with acute exacerbations of COPD [118].

In summary, Heliox should only be considered a support modality that serves as a bridge, allowing specific therapies more time to work [3]. Only its use for the treatment of severe upper-airway obstruction and croup in children are supported by current studies. Current studies do not support its routine use in the management of acute exacerbations of COPD, asthma, or acute bronchiolitis among children. Nevertheless it is reasonable to consider the use of Heliox when conventional therapies have failed for patients with acute asthma or bronchiolitis.

Nitric Oxide

Inhaled NO is a potent, selective pulmonary vasodilator. Early studies reported the clinical application of inhaled NO in adult patients with primary pulmonary hypertension and since then, many trials have been conducted to identify additional applications [119]. Inhaled NO has been investigated for a variety of other areas, including (a) ALI and ARDS, (b) status asthmaticus, (c) intestinal ischemia and reperfusion, (d) thrombotic disorders, (e) sickle-cell crisis, and sepsis-related microcirulatory dysfunction [3,120]. An extensive review of the use of inhaled NO therapy for adults can be found elsewhere [121]. The effectiveness of using NO for these conditions is questionable. Inhaled NO appears to only transiently improve oxygenation, increases the concentrations of toxic oxides of nitrogen in the airways, and does not appear to decrease mortality among patients with severe lung injury [122]. High cost, exposure to toxic metabolites, safety concerns, and lack of efficacy of inhaled NO has led investigators to explore other inhaled vasodilator therapies such as prostacyclins and nitrosothiols for the treatment of patients with severe hypoxemia related to ARDS [123]. Studies to date have failed to detect significant mortality benefits, therefore, the effectiveness of inhaled prostacyclins remains unconfirmed [124].

CONTINUOUS POSITIVE AIRWAY PRESSURE FOR SLEEP-RELATED BREATHING DISORDERS

CPAP is an effective treatment for clinically significant obstructive sleep apnea/hypopnea syndrome, sleep-related oxyhemoglobin desaturation, and respiratory event-related sleep arousals. This therapy can be delivered by nasal, partial, or full-face mask and is associated with improved morbidity due to reductions of daytime somnolence and improved cardiopulmonary function. Although further study of the long-term effects of CPAP is necessary, data suggest a possible reduction of mortality [125]. Since 1981, its efficacy has been repeatedly demonstrated [126]. Multiple controlled studies have shown that CPAP can also be effective for patients with chronic left ventricular failure and Cheyne–Stokes respirations [3]. Among these patients, CPAP improved cardiac function and alleviated symptoms of heart failure and sleep-disordered breathing. CPAP has been shown to reverse central sleep apneas for some patients [127]. Simple snoring that is not associated with pauses in respiration or with clinical impairment is generally not treated with CPAP [127]. The use of CPAP and bilevel positive airways pressure (BiPAP) for the management of patients with acute respiratory failure is discussed in Chapter 167.

Application

CPAP acts as a pneumatic splint to prevent upper airway collapse. Patients usually respond rapidly to 3 to 15 cm H_2O. The minimal effective CPAP pressure is determined during a nocturnal polysomnogram during which pressure is titrated upward until sleep-related breathing events are eliminated [128]. Lack of response is often due to a poorly applied mask or patient intolerance [129]. Compliance rates can vary considerably (46% to 89%) [128].

Multiple delivery devices are available that may improve patient comfort, including a variety of nasal, partial, and full-face masks. Nasal pillows or the Helmet device can also be used to deliver CPAP. Rare serious complications [129] include bilateral bacterial conjunctivitis, massive epistaxis due to drying of the nasal mucosa of a patient with coagulopathy, and worsening obstruction among patients with large lax epiglotti.

Because CPAP is very effective, safe, and reasonably well tolerated, it has become the technique of choice for the treatment of idiopathic obstructive sleep apnea (i.e., no correctable anatomic abnormality identified). Relative contraindications include the presence of bullous lung disease or recurrent sinus or ear infections. There are no absolute contraindications [3]. It is important to realize that uvulopalatopharyngoplasty may compromise CPAP therapy by increasing mouth air leak and reducing the maximal level of pressure that can be tolerated, and it benefits only some patients [130].

Alternative Modalities

For patients with sleep apnea/hypopnea syndrome who cannot tolerate nasal or full-face mask CPAP because of the sensation of excessive pressure, nasal or full-face mask bilevel ventilation may be more tolerable. This permits independent adjustments of inspiratory positive airway pressure and expiratory positive airway pressure, setting a respiratory rate, and can eliminate sleep-disordered breathing at lower levels of expiratory airway pressure compared with conventional CPAP therapy for selected patients [3].

COMMUNICATION ALTERNATIVES FOR THE PATIENT WITH AN ARTIFICIAL AIRWAY

Anxiety and fear are common emotions experienced by patients during mechanical ventilation. These emotions have been associated with the experience of agony/panic and insecurity related to the inability to communicate [131]. Patients with endotracheal and tracheostomy tubes in place experience these feelings because the tubes interfere with normal verbal communication. Providing a means of communication for patients undergoing mechanical ventilation has been shown to significantly increase patient satisfaction [131].

Intubation with cuffed, inflated intratracheal tubes impairs verbal communication because they block the normal airflow through the vocal cords. Deflated cuffed or cuffless tubes, generally reserved for spontaneously breathing patients, allow verbal communication, provided there is no pathologic obstruction (e.g., edema and granulation tissue or excessive secretions) blocking the passage of air through or above the vocal cords.

Communication Aids and Devices

A variety of communication aids are available depending on the situation [132]. A speech therapist can be extremely valuable for helping to select which aid is best for your patient.

Partial cuff deflation methods can be used for nonventilator- and ventilator-dependent patients. They are most commonly used in the nonventilator situation. Their use in the ventilator situation requires extremely close monitoring of the patient along with ventilator adjustments.

In the nonventilator-dependent patient, one can use deflation of the tracheostomy cuff with intermittent gloved finger occlusion of the tube or a device with a one-way valve (e.g., Passy-Muir Valve [PMV], Passy-Muir, Inc., Irvine, CA). The PMV is a one-way, positive-closure, no-leak valve that attaches to the hub of tracheostomy tubes (including cuffless fenestrated and nonfenestrated tubes, metal tubes, and cuffed tubes with the cuff fully deflated) [133]. It is indicated for awake and alert tracheostomy patients who can generate sufficient air flow around the tracheostomy tube (or through a fenestrated tube) and through the vocal cords. When the patient inhales, the PMV opens, allowing air to enter the lungs through the tracheostomy tube. As exhalation begins, the PMV closes, and remains closed through exhalation so that air is redirected around the tracheostomy tube or through the tracheostomy tube fenestra (window), allowing for speech as the air passes through the vocal cords. Oxygen can be administered with the PMV in place at the tracheostomy tube site via oxygen mask, trach collar, or O_2 adapter. When using the PMV with tracheostomy tubes that have an inner cannula grasp ring that extends beyond the external end of the hub of the tracheostomy tube, the inner cannula should be removed when the PMV is in use to avoid obstruction of the valve's diaphragm movement.

For the ventilator-dependent patient, one can use partial deflation of the tracheostomy cuff alone or the one-way valve with *full* cuff deflation. During mechanical ventilation, both methods require close monitoring of the patient and the ventilator. Because use of the PMV with ventilator-dependent patients requires the cuff to be deflated, adjustments of the tidal volume may be necessary to offset the volume loss caused by the air leak. Contraindications to the use of the one-way valve include the presence of an inflated cuff, absolute necessity for the cuff to remain fully inflated, tracheal/laryngeal obstruction, or secretions preventing air from moving around or above the tube, laryngectomy, bilateral vocal cord paralysis, unconsciousness, and physiologic instability [3]. Use of the valve with an inflated cuff can result in breath stacking with resultant intrinsic PEEP and barotrauma [134]. Because less-exhaled volume is returned to the ventilator with the deflated cuff methods, ventilator-exhaled volume alarms have to be adjusted [135]. Lack of intact oral and laryngeal musculature for some patients with neuromuscular diseases may preclude effective use of the valve [135].

The electronic larynx is a handheld mechanical device that can be used by patients who have undergone laryngectomy. When pressed into the soft tissue of the neck, it generates a vibratory sound that escapes through the mouth and is articulated by the lips, tongue, and palate. Its disadvantage is the metallic-type sound that is produced [136]. The Blom–Singer tracheostoma valve (Forth Medical Ltd., Berkshire, UK) is available for prosthesis-assisted tracheoesophageal speech in postlaryngectomy voice rehabilitation [137]. Finally, a variety of computer-assisted communication devices and electric typewriters are available, but are usually considered for patients requiring long-term mechanical ventilation because of their complexity and expense [3].

Advances of respiratory adjunct therapy, based on randomized controlled trials or meta-analyses of such trials, are summarized in Table 169.1.

TABLE 169.1

Advances in Respiratory Adjunct Therapy

Topic	References	Findings
Aerosolized mist for croup	[2]	No benefit
Bland aerosols for CF	[2,4]	7% saline improved FVC and FEV_1 vs. 0.9% saline
Humidification for ventilated patients	[8]	No difference in safety between heated water baths and HMEFs
Delivery of inhaled β agonist	[3]	No difference between MDI and nebulizer
Salmeterol in acute asthma	[22]	Improvement in FEV_1 after 48 h with salmeterol vs. placebo
NAC for COPD	[27]	No improvement on lung function or exacerbations vs. placebo
DNase of CF	[2]	Decrease in dyspnea and exacerbations vs. placebo
DNase for bronchiectasis	[32,33]	No benefit over placebo
DNase for RSV bronchiolitis	[34]	Improvement in chest radiographic findings vs. placebo
Aerosolized ribavirin for RSV	[3,42]	No effect vs. placebo
Iloprost for PPH	[52]	Improved 6-min walk, dyspnea, and hemodynamics vs. placebo
Inhaled cyclosporin for lung transplant	[54]	Improved survival and less rejection vs. placebo
Furosemide for mucociliary clearance	[67]	No improvement vs. placebo
Flutter valve for CF	[72]	As efficacious as CPT
High-frequency oscillation for CF	[74]	As efficacious as CPT
High-flow oxygen for cluster headaches	[91]	Significantly decreases pain within 15 min
Inhaled NO	[121,122]	No improvement in survival in ARDS/ALI
Iloprost for acute pulmonary hypertension after cardiac surgery	[51]	More effective than inhaled NO
Perioperative supplemental O_2	[3]	Decreases wound infections with 80% FiO_2 vs. 30% FiO_2

ARDS/ALI, acute respiratory distress syndrome/acute lung injury; CF, cystic fibrosis; COPD, chronic obstructive pulmonary disease; CPT, chest physiotherapy; DNase, recombinant human deoxyribonuclease; FEV_1, forced expiratory volume in 1 second; FiO_2, fractional inspiration of oxygen; FVC, forced vital capacity; HMEF, hydroscopic condenser humidifier; MDI, metered-dose inhaler; NAC, *N*-acetylcysteine; PPH, primary pulmonary hypertension; RSV, respiratory syncytial virus; NO, nitric oxide.

References

1. Brain J: Aerosol and humidity therapy. *Am Rev Respir Dis* 122:12, 1990.
2. Bott J, Blumenthal S, Buxton M, et al: Guidelines for the physiotherapy management of the adult, medical, spontaneously breathing patient. *Thorax* 64[Suppl 1]:i1, 2009.
3. Kopec SE, Irwin RS: Respiratory adjunct therapy, in Irwin RS, Rippe JM (eds): *Intensive Care Medicine*. 7th ed. Philadelphia, PA, Lippincott Williams and Wilkins, 2007, p 684.
4. Elkins MR, Robinson M, Rose BR, et al: A controlled trial of long-term inhaled hypertonic saline in patients with cystic fibrosis. *N Engl J Med* 354:229, 2006.
5. Fink J: Humidity and bland aerosol therapy, in Wilkins RL, Stoller JK, Scanlan CL (eds): *Egan's Fundamentals of Respiratory Care*. 8th ed. St. Louis, Mosby, 2003, p 737.
6. AARC: Clinical practice guidelines. Humidification during mechanical ventilation. *Respir Care* 37:887, 1992.
7. Shelley MP, Lloyd GM, Park GR: A review of the mechanisms and the methods of humidification of inspired gas. *Intensive Care Med* 14:1, 1988.
8. Hurni J-M, Feihl F, Lazor R, et al: Safety of combined heat and moisture exchanger filters in long-term mechanical ventilation. *Chest* 111:686, 1997.
9. American College of Chest Physicians: NHLBI. National conference on oxygen therapy. *Respir Care* 29:922, 1984.
10. Chanques G, Constantin JM, Sauter M, et al: Discomfort associated with underhumidified high-flow oxygen therapy in critically ill patients. *Intensive Care Med* 35:996, 2009.
11. Robinson BR, Athota KP, Branson RD: Inhalational therapies for the ICU. *Current Opin in Crit Care* 15:1, 2009.
12. Fink J: Aerosol drug therapy, in Wilkins RL, Stoller JK, Scanlan CL (eds): *Egan's Fundamentals of Respiratory Care*. 8th ed. St. Louis, Mosby, 2003, p 761.
13. National Asthma Education and Prevention Program. Expert Panel Report 3: Guidelines for the diagnosis and management of asthma. Bethesda. 2007 update: National Institutes of Health, NHLBI, NIH Publication no. 08–4051. Available at www.nhlbi.nih.gov/guidelines/asthma/asthgdln.htm. Accessed July 13, 2017.
14. GOLD Scientific Committee: Global strategy for the diagnosis, management, and prevention of chronic obstructive pulmonary disease. Bethesda, MD, National Heart, Lung, and Blood Institute/World Health Organization, National Institute of Health, 2005 update. Available at http://www.goldcopd.com. Accessed July 13, 2017.
15. Cates CJ, Crilly JA, Rowe BH: Holding chambers versus nebulizers for beta-agonist treatment of acute asthma. *Cochrane Database Syst Rev* 6, 2010.
16. Shrestha M, Bidadi K, Gourlay S, et al: Continuous vs. intermittent albuterol, at high and low doses, in the treatment of severe acute asthma in adults. *Chest* 110:42, 1996.
17. Dhand R, Tobin MJ: Inhaled bronchodilator therapy in mechanically ventilated patients. *Am J Respir Crit Care Med* 156:3, 1997.
18. Allon M, Dunlay R, Copkney C: Nebulized albuterol for acute hyperkalemia in patients on hemodialysis. *Ann Intern Med* 110:426, 1989.
19. Lotvall J, Palmqvist M, Arvidsson P, et al: The therapeutic ratio of R-albuterol is comparable with that of RS-albuterol in asthmatic patients. *J Allergy Clin Immunol* 108:726, 2001.
20. Peters JI, Shelledy, DC, Jones AP, et al: A randomized, placebo-controlled study to evaluate the role of salmeterol in the in-hospital management of asthma. *Chest* 118:313, 2000.
21. Winston SJ, Gravelyn TR, Sitrin RG: Prevention of bradycardic responses to endotracheal suctioning by prior administration of nebulized atropine. *Crit Care Med* 15:1009, 1987.
22. Wick MM, Ingram RH: Bronchorrhea responsive to aerosolized atropine. *JAMA* 235:1356, 1976.
23. Rodrigo G, Rodrigo C, Burschtin O: A meta-analysis of the effects of ipratropium bromide in adults with acute asthma. *Am J Med* 107:363, 1999.
24. Irwin RS, Thomas HM III: Mucoid impaction of the bronchus: diagnosis and treatment. *Am Rev Respir Dis* 108:955, 1973.
25. Decramer M, Rutten-van Molken M, Dekhuijzen PN, et al: Effects of *N*-acetylcysteine on outcome in chronic obstructive pulmonary disease. *Lancet* 365:1552, 2005.
26. Duijvestijn YC, Brand PL: Systemic review of N-acetylcysteine in cystic fibrosis. *Acta Paediatr* 88:38, 1999.
27. Miller AC, Rivero A, Ziad S, et al: Influence of nebulized unfractionated heparin and N-acetylcysteine in acute lung injury after smoke inhalation injury. *J Burn Care Res* 30:249, 2009.
28. Rao S, Wilson DB, Brooks RC, et al: Acute effects of nebulization of N-acetylcysteine on pulmonary mechanics and gas exchange. *Am Rev Respir Dis* 102:17, 1970.
29. Wilmott RW, Amin RS, Colin AA, et al: Aerosolized recombinant human DNase in hospitalized cystic fibrosis patients with acute pulmonary exacerbations. *Am J Respir Crit Care Med* 153:1914, 1996.
30. O'Donnell AE, Barker AF, Ilowite JS, et al: Treatment of idiopathic bronchiectasis with aerosolised recombinant human DNase 1. *Chest* 113:1329, 1998.
31. Wills PJ, Wodehouse T, Corkery K, et al: Short-term recombinant human DNase in bronchiectasis. *Am J Respir Crit Care Med* 154:413, 1996.
32. Nasr SZ, Strouse PJ, Soskolone E, et al: Efficacy of recombinant human deoxyribonuclease I in the hospital management of respiratory syncytial virus bronchiolitis. *Chest* 120:203, 2001.
33. Fiel SB: Aerosolized antibiotics in cystic fibrosis: current and future trends. *Expert Rev Respir Med* 2:479, 2008.
34. LoBue PA: Inhaled tobramycin: not just for cystic fibrosis anymore. *Chest* 127:1098, 2005.
35. MacIntyre NR, Rubin BK: Should aerosolized antibiotics be administered to prevent or treat ventilator-associated pneumonia in patients who do not have cystic fibrosis. *Respir Care* 52:416, 2007.
36. Mutti P, Wang C, Hickey AJ. Inhaled drug delivery for tuberculosis therapy. *Pharm Res* 26:2401, 2009.
37. FDA MedWatch: www.fda.gov/medwatch/report.htm. Accessed June 28, 2007.
38. Coates AL, MacNeish CF, Meisner D, et al: The choice of jet nebulizer, nebulizing flow, and addition of albuterol affects the output of tobramycin aerosols. *Chest* 111:1206, 1997.
39. Palmer LB, Smaldone GC, Simon SR, et al: Aerosolized antibiotics in mechanically ventilated patients: delivery and response. *Crit Care Med* 26(1):31, 1998.
40. Ebbert JO, Limper AH: Respiratory syncytial virus pneumonitis in immunocompromised adults: clinical features and outcome. *Respiration* 72:263, 2005.
41. Knight V, Gilbert BE: Ribavirin aerosol treatment for influenza. *Infect Dis Clinic North Am* 1:441, 1987.
42. Rodriguez WJ, Hall CB, Welliver R, et al: Efficacy and safety of aerosolized ribavirin in young children hospitalized with influenza. *J Pediatr* 125:129, 1994.
43. Fujii T, Nakamura T, Iwamoto A: Current concepts in SARS treatment. *J Infect Chemo* 10:1, 2004.
44. Krilov L: Safety issues related to the administration of ribavirin. *Pediatr Infect Dis J* 21:479, 2002.
45. Masur H: Prevention and treatment of *Pneumocystis* pneumonia. *N Engl J Med* 327:1853, 1992.
46. McIvor RA, Berger P, Pack LL, et al: An effectiveness community-based clinical trial of Respirgard II and Fisoneb nebulizers for *Pneumocystis carinii* prophylaxis with aerosol pentamidine in HIV-infected individuals. *Chest* 110:141, 1996.
47. McDiarmid MA, Fujikawa J, Schaefer J, et al: Health effects and exposure assessment of aerosolized pentamidine handlers. *Chest* 104:382, 1993.
48. Walsh P, Caldwell J, McQuillan KK, et al: Comparison of nebulized epinephrine to albuterol in bronchiolitis. *Acad Emerg Med* 15:305, 2008.
49. Winterhalter M, Simon A, Fischer S, et al: Comparison of inhaled iloprost and nitric oxide in patients with pulmonary hypertension during weaning from cardiopulmonary bypass in cardiac surgery: a prospective study. *J Cardiovasc Vasc Anesth* 22:406, 2008.
50. Olschewski H, Simonneau G, Galie N, et al: Inhaled iloprost for severe pulmonary hypertension. *N Engl J Med* 347:322, 2002.
51. Fuller BM, Mohr NM, Skrupky L et al. The use of inhaled prostocyclin in patients with ARDS: a systematic review and meta-analysis. *Chest* 147:1510, 2015.
52. Iacono AT, Johnson BA, Grgurich WF, et al: A randomized trial of inhaled cyclosporin in lung-transplant recipients. *N Engl J Med* 354:141, 2006.
53. Grossman J: The evolution of inhaler technology. *J Asthma* 31(1):55, 1994.
54. Tinkelman DG, Berkowitz RB, Cole WQ III: Aerosols in the treatment of asthma. *J Asthma* 28:243, 1991.
55. Turner MO, Patel A, Ginsburg S, et al: Bronchodilator delivery in acute airflow obstruction: a meta-analysis. *Arch Intern Med* 157(15):1736, 1997.
56. Jasper AC, Mohsenifar Z, Kahan S, et al: Cost-benefit comparison of aerosol bronchodilator delivery methods in hospitalized patients. *Chest* 91(4):614, 1987.
57. Murray JF: Indications for mechanical aids to assist lung inflation in medical patients. *Am Rev Respir Dis* 122(1):121, 1980.
58. Bartlett RH: Postoperative pulmonary prophylaxis: breathe deeply and read carefully. *Chest* 81:1, 1982.
59. Mahlmeister MJ, Fink JB, Hoffman GL, et al: Positive-expiratory pressure mask therapy: theoretical and practical considerations and a review of the literature. *Respir Care* 36:1218, 1991.
60. Indihar FJ, Forsberg DP, Adams AB: A prospective comparison of three procedures used in attempts to prevent postoperative pulmonary complications. *Respir Care* 27:564, 1982.
61. Demers RR, Irwin RS, Braman SS, et al: Variable accuracy of five commercially available incentive spirometers. *Am Rev Respir Dis* 117[Suppl]:108, 1978.
62. Torrington KG, Sorenson DE, Sherwood LM: Postoperative chest percussion with postural drainage in obese patients following gastric stapling. *Chest* 86:891, 1984.
63. McCool FD, Rosen MJ: Nonpharmacologic airway clearance therapies. *Chest* 129[Suppl 1]:250S, 2006.
64. Salathe M, O'Riordan TG, Wanner A: Treatment of mucociliary dysfunction. *Chest* 110:1048, 1996.
65. Hasani A, Pavia D, Spitery MA, et al: Inhaled furosemide does not affect lung mucociliary clearance in healthy and asthmatic subjects. *Eur Respir J* 7:1497, 1994.
66. Marom Z, Shelhamer J, Alling D, et al: The effects of corticosteroids on mucous glycoprotein secretion from human airways in vitro. *Am Rev Respir Dis* 129:62, 1984.
67. Kaliner M, Maron Z, Patow C, et al: Human respiratory mucus. *J Allergy Clin Immunol* 73:318, 1986.
68. van der Schans CP: Conventional chest physical therapy for obstructive lung disease. *Respir Care* 52:1198, 2007.
69. Tyler ML: Complications of positioning and chest physiotherapy. *Respir Care* 27:458, 1982.
70. Konstan MW, Stern RC, Doershuk CF: Efficacy of the flutter device for airway mucous clearance in patients with cystic fibrosis. *J Pediatr* 124:689, 1994.

71. Homnick DN, Anderson K, Marks JH: Comparison of the flutter device to standard therapy in hospitalized patients with cystic fibrosis: a pilot study. *Chest* 114(4):993, 1998.
72. Homnick DN, White F, deCastro C: Comparison of effects of an intrapulmonary percussive ventilator to standard aerosol and chest physiotherapy in treatment of cystic fibrosis. *Pediatr Pulmonol* 20:50, 1995.
73. Lange DJ, Lechtzin N, Davey C, et al: High-frequency chest wall oscillation in ALS. *Neurology* 67:991, 2006.
74. Elkins MR, Jones A, vander Schans C: Positive expiratory pressure physiotherapy for airway clearance in people with cystic fibrosis. *Cochrane Database Syst Rev* 2, 2004.
75. Tzeng AC, Bach RJ: Prevention of pulmonary mortality for patients with neuromuscular disease. *Chest* 118:1390, 2000.
76. Endotracheal suctioning of mechanically ventilated adults and children with artificial airways. AARC clinical practice guideline. *Respir Care* 38:500, 1993.
77. Rau JL: Airway management, in Wilkins RL, Stoller JK, Scanlan CL (eds): *Egan's Fundamentals of Respiratory Care*. 8th ed. St. Louis, Mosby, 2003, p 627.
78. Gracey DR, Divertie MB, Howard FM Jr: Mechanical ventilation for respiratory failure in myasthenia gravis: two-year experience with 22 patients. *Mayo Clin Proc* 58:597, 1983.
79. Bach JR, Saporito LR: Criteria for extubation and tracheostomy tube removal for patients with ventilatory failure: a different approach to weaning. *Chest* 110:1566, 1996.
80. Irwin RS, Curley FJ, Bennett FM: Appropriate use of antitussives and protussives: a practical review. *Drugs* 46:80, 1993.
81. Donaldson SH, Bennett WD, Zeman KL, et al: Mucus clearance and lung function in cystic fibrosis with hypertonic saline. *N Engl J Med* 354:241, 2006.
82. Estenne M, Knoop C, Vanvaierenber J, et al: The effect of pectoralis muscle training in tetraplegic subjects. *Am Rev Respir Dis* 112:22, 1989.
83. Lang SW, Back JR: Maximum insufflation capacity. *Chest* 118:61, 2000.
84. American Association for Respiratory Care: Clinical practice guideline: oxygen therapy in the acute care hospital. *Respir Care* 36:1410, 1991.
85. Fulmer JD, Snider GL: ACCP-NHLBI National Conference on Oxygen Therapy. *Chest* 86:234, 1984.
86. Bateman NT, Leach RM: ABC of oxygen: acute oxygen therapy. *BMJ* 317:798, 1998.
87. O'Gara PT, Kushner FG, Ascheim DD, et al: 2013 ACCF/AHA guideline for themanagement of ST-elevation myocardial infarction: a report of the American College of Cardiology Foundation/American Heart Association Task Force on Practice Guidelines. *J Am Coll Cardiol* 61:e78–e140, 2013.
88. Maroko PR, Radvany P, Braunwald E, et al: Reduction of infarct size by oxygen inhalation following acute coronary occlusion. *Circulation* 52:360, 1975.
89. Ballester E, Reyes A, Roca J, et al: Ventilation-perfusion mismatching in acute severe asthma: effects of salbutamol and 100% oxygen. *Thorax* 44:258, 1989.
90. Embury SH, Garcia JF, Mohandas N, et al: Effects of oxygen inhalation on endogenous erythropoietin kinetics, erythropoiesis, and properties of blood cells in sickle-cell anemia. *N Engl J Med* 311:291, 1984.
91. Petersen AS, Barloese MC, Jensen RH: Oxygen treatment of Cluster Headache: a review. *Cephalalgia* 34(13):1079–1087, 2014.
92. Kao LS, Millas SG, Pedroza C, et al: Should perioperative supplemental oxygen be routinely recommended for surgery patients? A Bayesian meta-analysis. *Ann Surg* 256, 2012.
93. Fairley HB: Oxygen therapy for surgical patients. *Am Rev Respir Dis* 122:37, 1980.
94. Hunt G: Gas therapy, in Fink JB, Hunt GE (eds): *Clinical Practice in Respiratory Care*. Philadelphia, PA, Lippincott Williams & Wilkins, 1999, p 274.
95. Frat JP, Thille AW, Mercat A, et al: High-flow oxygen through nasal cannula in acute hypoxemic respiratory failure. *N Engl J Med* 372:2185, 2015.
96. Grant I, Heaton RK, McSweeney AJ, et al: Neuropsychologic findings in hypoxemic chronic obstructive pulmonary disease. *Arch Intern Med* 142:1470, 1982.
97. Sackner MA, Landa J, Hirsch J, et al: Pulmonary effects of oxygen breathing: a 6-hour study in normal man. *Ann Intern Med* 82:40, 1975.
98. Ingrassia TS, Ryu JH, Trastek VF, et al: Oxygen exacerbated bleomycin pulmonary toxicity. *Mayo Clin Proc* 66:173, 1991.
99. Kay GN, Epstein AE, Kirklin JK, et al: Fatal postoperative amiodarone pulmonary toxicity. *Am J Cardiol* 62:490, 1988.
100. Camus P, Martin WJ, Rosenow EC: Amiodarone pulmonary toxicity. *Clin Chest Med* 25:65, 2005.
101. Weaver L: Hyperbaric oxygen in the critically ill. *Crit Care Med* 39, 2011.
102. Bennett MH, Trytko B, Jonker B: Hyperbaric oxygen therapy for the adjunctive treatment of traumatic brain injury. *Cochrane Database Syst Rev* 12, 2012.
103. Bennett MH, Weibel S, Wasiak J, et al: Hyperbaric oxygen therapy for acute ischaemic stroke. *Cochrane Database Syst Rev* 11, 2014.
104. Bennett MH, Lehm J, Jepson N: Hyperbaric oxygen therapy for acute coronary syndrome. *Cochrane Database Syst Rev* 8, 2011.
105. Kranke P, Bennett MH, Martyn-St James M, et al. Hyperbaric oxygen therapy for chronic wounds. *Cochrane Database Syst Rev* 4, 2012.
106. Duncan PG: Efficacy of helium-oxygen mixtures in the management of severe viral and post-intubation croup. *Can Anesth Soc J* 26:206, 1979.
107. Moraa I, Sturman N, McGuire T, et al: Heliox for croup in children. *Cochrane Database Syst Rev* 12, 2013.
108. Lu T-S, Ohmura A, Wong KC, et al: Helium-oxygen in treatment of upper airway obstruction. *Anesthesiology* 45:678, 1976.
109. Rodrigo GJ, Rodrigo C, Pollack CV, et al: Use of helium-oxygen mixtures in the treatment of acute asthma: a systematic review. *Chest* 123:676, 2003.
110. Rodrigo GJ, Pollack CV, Rodrigo C, et al: Heliox for non-intubated acute asthma patients. *Cochrane Database Syst Rev* 4, 2003.
111. Kim IK, Phrampus E, Venkataraman S, et al: Helium/oxygen-driven albuterol nebulization in the treatment of children with moderate to severe asthma exacerbations: a randomized controlled trial. *Pediatrics* 116:1127, 2005.
112. Rivers ML, Kim TY, Stewart GM, et al: Albuterol nebulized in heliox in the initial ED treatment of pediatric asthma: a blinded, randomized trial. *Am J Emerg Med* 24:38, 2006.
113. Bighan MT, Jacobs BR, Monaco MA, et al: Helium/oxygen-driven albuterol nebulisation in the management of children with status asthmaticus: a randomized, placebo controlled trial. *Pediatr Crit Care* 11, 2010.
114. Pingleton SK, Bone RC, Ruth WC: Helium-oxygen mixtures during bronchoscopy. *Crit Care Med* 18:50, 1980.
115. Gluck EH, Onorato DJ, Castriotta R: Helium-oxygen mixtures in intubated patients with status asthmaticus and respiratory acidosis. *Chest* 98:693, 1990.
116. Lee DL, Lee H, Chang HW, et al: Heliox improves hemodynamics in mechanically ventilated patients with chronic obstructive pulmonary disease with systolic pressure variations. *Crit Care Med* 33:368, 2005.
117. Tassaux D, Gainnier M, Battisti A, et al: Helium-oxygen decreases inspiratory effort and work of breathing during pressure support in intubated patients with chronic obstructive pulmonary disease. *Intensive Care Med* 31:1501, 2005.
118. Rodrigo R, Pollack CV, Rodrigo GJ, et al: Heliox for treatment of exacerbations of chronic obstructive pulmonary disease. *Cochrane Database Syst Rev* 3, 2002.
119. Steudel W, Hurford WE, Zapol M: Inhaled nitric oxide: basic biology and clinical applications. *Anesthesiology* 91:1090, 1999.
120. Trzeciak S, Glaspey LJ, Dellinger RP, et al: Randomized controlled trial of inhaled nitric oxide for the treatment of microcirculatory dysfunction in patients with sepsis. *Crit Care Med* 42, 2014.
121. Griffiths MJ, Evans TW: Inhaled nitric oxide therapy in adults. *N Engl J Med* 353:2683, 2005.
122. Afshari A, Brok J, Moller AM: Inhaled nitric oxide for ARDS and acute lung injury in children and adults. *Cochrane Database Syst Rev* 7, 2010.
123. Puri N, Dellinger RP: Inhaled nitric oxide and inhaled prostacyclin in acute respiratory distress syndrome: what is the evidence? *Crit Care Clin* 27, 2011.
124. Afshar A, Brok J, Moller AM, et al: Aerosolized prostacyclin for acute lung injury (ALI) and acute respiratory distress syndrome (ARDS). *Cochrane Database Syst Rev* 8, 2010.
125. Indications and standards for use of nasal continuous positive airway pressure (CPAP) in sleep apnea syndromes. Official ATS Statement. *Am J Respir Crit Care Med* 150:1738, 1994.
126. Strohl KP, Cherniack NS, Gothe B: Physiologic basis of therapy for sleep apnea. *Am Rev Respir Dis* 134:791, 1986.
127. Issa FG, Sullivan CE: Reversal of central sleep apnea using nasal CPAP. *Chest* 90:165, 1986.
128. Piccirillo JF, Duntley S, Schotland H: Obstructive sleep apnea. *JAMA* 284(12):1492, 2000.
129. Hudgel DW: Treatment of obstructive sleep apnea: a review. *Chest* 109:1346, 1996.
130. Mortimore IL, Bradley PA, Murray JAM, et al: Uvulopalatopharyngoplasty may compromise nasal CPAP therapy in sleep apnea syndrome. *Am J Respir Crit Care Med* 154:1759, 1996.
131. Bergbom-Engberg I, Haljamae H: Assessment of patients' experience of discomfort during respirator therapy. *Crit Care Med* 17:1068, 1989.
132. Stovsky B, Rudy E, Dragonette P: Comparison of two types of communication methods used after cardiac surgery with patients with endotracheal tubes. *Heart Lung* 17:281, 1988.
133. Williams ML: An algorithm for selecting a communication technique with intubated patients. *Dimens Crit Care Nurs* 11:222, 1992.
134. Kaul K, Turcott JC, Lavery M: Passy-Muir speaking valve. *Dimens Crit Care Nurs* 15:298, 1996.
135. Manzano JL, Santiago L, Henriquez D, et al: Verbal communication of ventilator dependent patients. *Crit Care Med* 21:512, 1993.
136. Coltart L: Voice restoration after laryngectomy. *Nurs Standard* 13(12):36, 1998.
137. Vanden Hoogen FJ, Meevwic C, Oudes MJ, et al: The Blom-Singer tracheostoma valve as a valuable addition in the rehabilitation of the laryngectomized patient. *Eur Arch Otorhinolaryngol* 253:126, 1996.

Chapter 170 ■ Aspiration

KIMBERLY A. ROBINSON • RICHARD S. IRWIN

Aspiration is defined in *Webster's New Universal Unabridged Dictionary* as inhaling fluid or a foreign body into the bronchi and lungs [1]. The foreign material may be particulate matter, irritating fluids (e.g., HCl, mineral oil, animal fat), or oropharyngeal secretions containing infectious agents. Although infectious pneumonias can be caused by inhaling aerosolized infectious organisms, aspiration of oropharyngeal contents or regurgitated gastric material is the primary manner in which bacterial pathogens are introduced into the lower respiratory tract. In fact, studies indicate that 7% to 24% of cases of community-acquired pneumonia are aspiration pneumonia [2]. The term *aspiration pneumonia* strongly denotes infectious sequelae as a result of aspiration of oropharyngeal secretions colonized by pathogenic bacteria. However, there is a wide spectrum of conditions that result from aspirating foreign matter with varying clinical courses, not all of which are caused by infection [3–5]. It is difficult to predict exactly which course a patient will follow after an event. Although aspiration of a large volume of sterile gastric contents will likely lead to a chemical pneumonitis, aspiration of contaminated gastric contents will more likely result in an infectious pneumonia. Although the frequency of all clinically significant aspirations in the intensive care unit (ICU) setting is not known, a review of Table 170.1 suggests that aspiration syndromes are common causes of respiratory failure in the critically ill patient.

NORMAL DEFENSES AGAINST ASPIRATION AND THE MANNER IN WHICH THEY MAY FAIL

Pathogenesis

Syndromes caused by aspiration are determined by (a) the material aspirated, (b) the amount aspirated, and (c) the state of the patient's defenses at the time of the event. An understanding of the normal defenses and how and when they become impaired is also the cornerstone for an understanding of the pathogenesis of the various aspiration syndromes.

TABLE 170.1

Aspiration Syndromes

Mendelson's syndrome
Foreign body aspiration
Bacterial pneumonia and lung abscess
Chemical pneumonitis
Exogenous lipoid pneumonia
Recurrent pneumonias
Chronic interstitial fibrosis
Bronchiectasis
Mycobacterium fortuitum or *Mycobacterium chelonei* pneumonia
Diffuse aspiration bronchiolitis
Tracheobronchitis
Tracheoesophageal fistula
Chronic persistent cough
Bronchorrhea
Drowning

Because gastric acid prevents bacterial growth, the gastric contents are sterile under normal conditions. Nevertheless, it has long been thought that the pH of aspirated contents determined the clinical course, with lower pH aspirates portending a worse outcome. Elevation of gastric pH to protect the lung was cited as one reason to use prophylactic antacids for the critically ill patient. However, colonization of the stomach by pathogenic organisms may occur when the gastric pH is artificially elevated [6]. There is conflicting data as to whether or not proton pump inhibitors and H_2 blockers increase the risk of pneumonia [7–9]. Use of medications for stress ulcer prophylaxis in the ICU is entirely another issue and is discussed in Chapter 204.

Upper Gastrointestinal Defenses

Gastrointestinal mechanisms normally work in a coordinated, synchronized fashion. The teeth break up large food particles, and the tongue propels fluid and masticated food into the hypopharynx. Because the hypopharyngeal muscles prepare to move food into the esophagus, the epiglottis covers the laryngeal inlet and the vocal cords close and the upper esophageal sphincter (cricopharyngeus muscle) relaxes. Pharyngeal swallowing initiates primary peristaltic waves in the esophagus that carry fluid and food through a relaxed lower esophageal sphincter (LES) into the stomach. After the bolus enters the stomach, the LES then contracts and prevents, although not entirely, gastroesophageal reflux (GER).

Even in the absence of known trauma or a neurologic insult that could affect the swallowing cascade, some of the previously mentioned defenses may become impaired in a variety of situations, leading to silent aspiration. Aging can result in progressive loss of cough and swallowing reflexes resulting in aspiration pneumonia. The vocal cords close much more slowly after the age of 50 years and may not close at all during sleep or with sedation irrespective of age. Furthermore, the cough response to airway irritation is decreased during sleep compared to the waking state. It has been estimated that half of all healthy adults aspirate oropharyngeal secretions during sleep [3].

The risk of aspirating fluid and food is increased when the normal swallowing and upper gastrointestinal mechanisms fail to work in a coordinated, synchronized manner. Edentulous or neurologically impaired patients may not adequately masticate food resulting in higher aspiration risk. Aspiration also may occur when the bolus cannot readily be cleared from the pharynx owing to neuromuscular disorders of any cause [10]. Structural abnormalities such as Zenker's diverticulum place a patient at risk of aspiration because the diverticulum may empty "late" after the swallowing effort is completed, at the time when the vocal cords are abducted. Conditions in which vocal cord closure becomes excessively delayed (e.g., aging, debilitation, sedation, the presence of a tracheostomy, and after endotracheal extubation) place patients at high risk for aspiration.

Regurgitation and subsequent aspiration of stomach contents also occur among elderly, sedated, or sleeping patients, especially when their upper esophageal sphincter and LES have been rendered incompetent by an oral or a nasogastric tube [11]. The risk of aspiration is enhanced when such patient remains in the supine position, a scenario often encountered in the ICU setting.

Respiratory Defenses

For infectious agents to enter the lower respiratory tract, they must be small enough (<10 μm) to escape aerodynamic filtration in the nose, mouth, and larynx. Particles between 0.5 and 1.5 μm in diameter can reach the alveoli. This is particularly relevant because most bacteria are within this size range. Although mucociliary clearance removes the larger particles from the larger airways, additional defense mechanisms are needed to clear the smaller particles [12]. This is accomplished in respiratory bronchioles and alveoli primarily by the alveolar macrophages, aided by neutrophils [13]. Recent studies, utilizing newer, molecular biology, noncultural techniques, have revealed that the lungs have their own respiratory biome and may not be sterile as previously thought [14]. These results are consistent with chronic microaspiration during sleep, as mentioned earlier.

The first line of defense is mucociliary clearance. The respiratory filtration system and mucociliary clearance may become overwhelmed with large-volume fluid and food aspiration or with large amounts of inhaled infectious agents. Respiratory defenses may also become ineffective in the following settings: inhalational or systemic general anesthesia, endotracheal intubation, endotracheal suctioning, hypercapnia and hyperoxia, smoking, asthma, chronic bronchitis, cystic fibrosis and bronchiectasis, and respiratory infections with viruses and atypical organisms.

In the absence of mucociliary clearance, the airways can still be cleared of excessive secretions and foreign bodies if the patient has an effective cough. An effective cough generates a column of expired air moving quickly through the bronchi, thus dislodging mucus and debris from the bronchial mucosa and propelling it out of the lungs [14]. However, cough is not a primary defense mechanism and only provides clearance when mucociliary clearance is inefficient or overwhelmed. An effective cough is determined by both good expiratory flow rates and respiratory muscle strength. Thus, cough may be ineffective in patients with severe asthma, chronic obstructive pulmonary disease, respiratory neuromuscular disorders, painful incisions, or in those receiving excessive sedation and analgesia with antitussive effects [14].

When the mechanical airway defenses are overwhelmed, alveolar macrophages represent the initial phagocytic response. This response is followed by the influx of neutrophils into the alveolar spaces. Neutrophils are critical for the eradication of bacterial agents, and, therefore any impairment in their function would be detrimental [13]. Aspirated bacteria cause infectious pneumonia when the alveolar phagocytes become impaired, such as in alcoholism, pH less than 7.2, acute alveolar hypoxia, alveolar hyperoxia, corticosteroid therapy, respiratory viral infections, hypothermia, starvation, and exposures to nitrogen dioxide, sulfur dioxide, ozone, and cigarette smoking on a long-term basis [3].

Immunologic defenses such as complement, innate immunity proteins, and immunoglobulins augment the nonimmunologic mechanisms. Patients with hereditary and acquired immunologic abnormalities, such as immunoglobulin G and complement deficiencies, are susceptible to frequent and often severe bacterial pneumonias.

PREVALENCE OF ASPIRATION AMONG THE CRITICALLY ILL

Aspiration is the leading cause of pneumonia among the critically ill [15] and should be considered for all ICU patients with respiratory symptoms. This is especially true for the elderly, debilitated, or sedated patient. Oral or nasal enteral feeding tubes that compromise the LES, medications that decrease gastric motility, history of dysphagia, and poor dentition increase the probability. The presence of an endotracheal tube or a tracheostomy tube poses a high risk for aspiration and its consequences.

Translaryngeal Intubation

Clearly, no one would feed a patient with an oral or a nasal endotracheal tube in place, given the obvious mechanical barrier and distortion of the swallowing structures. What is often less intuitive is that dysphagia may persist for a variable time after the endotracheal tube has been removed. The reported prevalence of postextubation dysphagia ranges from 3% to 84% [16]. Factors that increase the likelihood of dysphagia after extubation include intubation >48 hours; laryngeal edema; and ulceration, erythema, and immobility of the vocal cords. Furthermore, neuromuscular weakness, loss of sensation, delirium, sedation, gastroesophageal reflux disease (GERD), and disorganized breathing all contribute to aspiration risk [16]. Should aspiration occur, ciliary clearance and other respiratory defenses might not respond appropriately because of the physical insult of the endotracheal tube. Flexible endoscopic evaluation of swallowing (FEES) aids in the identification of patients who are at high risk of aspiration after endotracheal intubation [17–19]. Studies have suggested that performing an FEES within 24 hours of extubation is safe and can potentially provide results that lead to avoidance of placing a nasogastric tube [16].

Aspiration Risk after Tracheostomy

Patients with a tracheostomy tube, with or without dependence on mechanical ventilation, are also at high risk for aspiration. The most commonly identified reasons for swallowing dysfunction for the patient with a tracheostomy tube are incomplete backward folding of the epiglottis, not allowing the glottis to rise and tilt forward with swallowing, pharyngeal retention, penetration, and aspiration [15]. The application of a speaking valve can restore subglottic air pressure and reduce aspiration and penetration [20].

Enteral Feeding Catheters

Many patients in an ICU have nasal or oral gastric tubes for nutritional support. The mere presence of an orogastric- or a nasogastric feeding tube increases the risk of reflux and aspiration by compromising the integrity and proper functioning of the LES by two mechanisms. First, the catheter prevents closure of the sphincter by direct mechanical interference. Second, the irritation of the pharynx by the tube promotes LES relaxation through vagally mediated pharyngeal mechanoreceptors [21]. In addition, the presence of a nasogastric feeding tube is associated with gram-negative bacterial contamination of the oropharynx, which, when aspirated, can result in infection of the lower airways [22].

Varying the size of the enteral feeding catheters and adjusting the location of the distal tip have been used in an attempt to minimize aspiration. However, decreasing the size of a nasal or an oral tube for enteral feeding does not reduce GER or microaspiration events [23]. Small-bore feeding tubes appear to provide no added benefit with respect to reflux events, even when advanced to the postpylorus position [24]. Patients with long-standing swallowing defects or on prolonged mechanical ventilation may be candidates for percutaneous gastrostomy or jejunostomy tubes; however, even percutaneous enteral feeding tubes alter lower esophageal tone and can allow reflux. This manner of enteral feeding is not completely protective against aspiration despite bypassing the LES. In fact, patients fed by gastrostomy tubes have the same incidence of pneumonia as those fed by nasogastric tubes [25,26]. Furthermore, although a percutaneous jejunostomy tube may minimize the large-volume aspiration events, it is a misconception that it prevents aspiration or decreases its incidence relative to a percutaneous gastrostomy tube [27].

There is little agreement over what constitutes excessive gastric residual volumes that place a patient on enteral feeds at increased risk of aspiration. In fact, one study showed that the absence of monitoring gastric residual volume was noninferior to residual gastric volume monitoring in terms of ventilator-associated pneumonia prevention. Additionally, there was less prokinetic drug use and improved nutrition in the nonmonitored group [28,29].

DIAGNOSIS OF AN ASPIRATION SYNDROME

Aspiration syndromes are underdiagnosed and challenging to diagnose. Although signs of wheezing, shortness of breath, cyanosis, and hypoxia may be present, aspiration may also be completely asymptomatic. There is also a misconception that aspiration must be witnessed before it can be assumed to have occurred because many aspiration events are silent [30]. There has been increasing research with regard to use of biomarkers (e.g., pepsin in bronchoalveolar lavage fluid, presence of lipid-laden pulmonary macrophages, and procalcitonin) to aid with diagnosis and prognosis of an aspiration syndrome. Although most biomarkers are easy to measure, they lack specificity and sensitivity [30].

Bedside Evaluation

Table 170.2 outlines all the studies that may be necessary to diagnose aspiration syndromes accurately (see "Differential Diagnosis and Treatment" section). In addition to taking a history, performing a physical examination and observing the patient drink 3 ounces of water when appropriate can uncover a swallowing problem. Although the bedside evaluation is not sensitive, a pharyngeal problem may be evident by watching the patient cough, sputter, and tilt his or her neck and head in an unnatural posture when drinking the water. An absent gag reflex is not a useful predictor of aspiration because many healthy individuals who do not have a gag reflex can swallow normally [31].

TABLE 170.2

Modalities for Diagnosing Aspiration Syndromes

History
Physical examination
Baseline examination
Observation of patient drinking water
Chest radiographs
Lower respiratory studies
Expectorated samples
Bronchoscopy
Protected specimen brush with quantitative cultures
Bronchoalveolar lavage
Lung biopsy
Upper gastrointestinal studies
Contrast films
Endoscopy
Esophageal manometry
GE scintiscan
24-Hour esophageal pH/impedance monitoring
Speech and swallow evaluation
FEES or modified barium swallow/video fluoroscopy

The order of when and in whom to order these tests depends on the patient populations and their presentations.
FEES, flexible endoscopic evaluation of swallowing; GE, gastroesophageal.

Modified Barium Swallow/Video Fluoroscopy

Although observing patients can be useful when there is obvious difficulty during swallowing, aspiration is often silent in the critically ill patient. The incidence of silent aspiration in stable patients receiving long-term mechanical ventilation via a tracheostomy is high, between 63% and 77%, as determined by modified barium swallow/video fluoroscopy (MBS/VF) [32,33]. Therefore, bedside evaluation alone, particularly for these high-risk populations, is insensitive. Because of this, a negative bedside examination should be confirmed by a more objective method to evaluate aspiration for high-risk patients.

The MBS incorporates the use of barium with VF and has been available since the 1950s. It defines the pharyngeal anatomy with swallowing of a radiopaque contrast material, and the swallowed bolus is followed in "real time" under fluoroscopy. This allows for the identification of abnormal anatomy and physiology and the response to modifications in dietary consistencies and postural changes [17]. Various consistencies of barium are used with the MBS/VF evaluation, such as thin liquids, paste consistency, and solid food. Findings indicative of swallowing dysfunction that can be assessed by MBS/VF examination include premature leakage of oral contents into the pharynx, penetration of swallowed material into the nasopharynx during a swallow, retention of material in the valleculae and pyriform recesses, and laryngeal penetration and aspiration. In addition, the elevation and tilting of the larynx that accompanies a normal swallow can be observed easily. Lower esophageal diseases, such as reflux or obstruction, can also be observed using the MBS/VF study.

The MBS/VF examination, however, has multiple limitations. MBS/VF is personnel intensive, requires transporting patients to the radiology department, and exposes patients to radiation. In addition, patients must adhere to a defined body position to accommodate the fixed fluoroscopy setup that may not be possible for all patients. The study is typically performed in the radiology department in the presence of a radiologist, radiology technician, and speech and language pathologist. Ideally, a speech pathologist should evaluate and accompany the patient to the examination so that specific recommendations can be made to prevent or minimize aspiration. Recommendations may consist of eliminating oral feeding or instituting various swallowing strategies such as the chin tuck, multiple swallows, turning of the head, or changing the consistency of solids and liquids.

Flexible Endoscopic Evaluation of Swallowing

Evaluation of swallowing under flexible endoscopic visualization has been shown to be sensitive in discerning a delay in swallowing initiation, penetration, aspiration, and pharyngeal residue [34–36]. The potential advantages include reduced cost and decreasing waiting time as compared with an MBS/VF evaluation. Patients avoid radiation exposure, and the examination can be performed at the bedside in varying body positions. FEES also allows visualization of pharyngeal secretions as well as identification of the source of the secretions that cannot be seen during MBS/VF. Potential risks associated with the procedure include gagging, laryngospasm, vasovagal syncope, topical anesthetic adverse reactions, and epistaxis. Furthermore, esophageal pathology and reflux cannot be concurrently evaluated as in MBS/VF.

FEES has now been extensively used in medical and surgical inpatients and, more specifically, in recently extubated ICU patients [16]. The decision to use MBS/VF versus FEES depends mainly on specific patient characteristics and available resources. Although there are some limitations of both approaches, both tests are comprehensive and show excellent agreement in diagnosing laryngeal penetration, aspiration, and pharyngeal residue, thus allowing for postural and dietary recommendations to decrease aspiration risk [17].

Culture Evaluation

Even when history or physical examination uncovers a swallowing defect, determining that an aspiration event has already occurred may also prove challenging. Furthermore, an infectious process is not always established with each aspiration event. It is often difficult to distinguish between an inflammatory or "chemical" pneumonitis and an infection because both may present with fever, cough, and an infiltrate on a chest radiograph. If an infection is suspected, identification of the responsible organism is oftentimes elusive because routine expectorated sputum smears and cultures can be inaccurate. Specimens obtained from quantitative bronchoalveolar lavage or telescoping plugged catheters at bronchoscopy can help identify the lower respiratory tract infectious agent more accurately and are used preferentially, although they require an invasive procedure and moderate sedation. When accurate lower respiratory sampling techniques are used and the culture and smear results are negative for a patient who has not recently received antibiotics, an exogenous lipoid pneumonia or chemical pneumonitis must be considered.

Detection of Aspirated Enteral Feeds

With respect to bedside methods for detecting aspiration in tube-fed patients, two methods have predominated; however, neither test is sufficiently sensitive to be recommended and both are problematic. In the first method, blue food coloring or methylene blue is added to enteral feeds and the tracheal secretions are assessed for blue discoloration. Potential problems with this method include tissue absorption of the dye as well as increased risk of infection if the dye is contaminated. The second method tests tracheal secretions with glucose oxidase reagent strips for aspirated carbohydrates. The glucose method is nonspecific because varying concentrations of glucose have been recovered from tracheal secretions in nonfed, parenterally fed, and enterally fed patients [37]. Therefore, the glucose test lacks specificity. Some FEES protocols involve mixing 1 mL of blue food coloring to both liquid and food to enhance visualization of the bolus, but studies have shown that this is not routinely required [17,19].

DIFFERENTIAL DIAGNOSIS AND TREATMENT

Treatment of the various aspiration syndromes should be prophylactic as well as specific. As previously mentioned, a formal speech and swallowing evaluation should be obtained whenever a swallowing condition is suspected or diagnosed. Specific recommendations can often be made to mitigate or eliminate aspiration from dysphagia. Precautionary rather than reactionary measures are likely to be far more effective, with less associated morbidity and mortality. However, the only preventive interventions that have been proven to be effective in the acute care setting are withholding oral feeding in sedated patients to prevent aspiration and elevating the head of the bed to at least 45 degrees to decrease GER and minimize subsequent aspiration [38,39].

A tracheoesophageal fistula is a rare complication resulting from injury to the posterior tracheal wall. This can occur from excessive endotracheal tube cuff pressure, direct injury during placement of a percutaneous tracheostomy, or erosion from the tip of a tracheostomy tube. For a mechanically ventilated patient, a tracheoesophageal fistula may present with increased secretions, evidence of aspiration of gastric contents, recurrent pneumonias, a persistent cuff leak, or severe gastric distention. Once a patient is extubated, the most frequent symptom is coughing after swallowing. The diagnosis can be made by bronchoscopy and esophagoscopy or by computed tomography scan of the mediastinum. Although definitive repair often requires surgical intervention, aspiration can be minimized by placing the cuff of the tracheostomy tube distal to the fistula [40].

Although a cuffed endotracheal tube does not offer complete protection against aspiration, all patients with severely altered consciousness with an enteral feeding tubes in place should be prophylactically intubated, whenever possible, for airway protection. Furthermore, once a patient is extubated, oral intake should not be resumed until an MBS/VF or FEES examination demonstrates swallowing competency [16]. Prophylactic antibiotics, corticosteroids, postpyloric feeding, gastric promotility agents, or gastric acid suppression cannot be routinely recommended at this time to prevent or minimize aspiration [3]. GERD with aspiration can be treated with a variety of measures, including head-of-the-bed elevation; a high-protein, low-fat antireflux diet; nothing to eat or drink for 2 to 3 hours before recumbency; no snacking between meals; acid suppression; and prokinetic drugs. If these measures fail, surgery with fundoplication can be effective. Oral hygiene should not be overlooked. Routine oral care has the potential to decrease colonization with pathogenic bacteria. Tongue cleaning should be considered for the edentulous patient [41]. Oral care with topical chlorhexidine has not shown any significant reductions in the frequency of ventilator-associated pneumonia for most patient populations, and routine use is not recommended [42,43].

Mendelson's Syndrome

Mendelson's syndrome is synonymous with the acute respiratory distress syndrome (ARDS) [3] owing to the parenchymal inflammatory reaction caused by a large volume of aspirated liquid gastric contents. After an aspiration event, clinical status and radiographic changes progress within the next 24 to 36 hours. Contrary to the general view that gastric aspirates with pH greater than 2.5 are benign, the same syndrome can occur at a pH of 5.9 [44]. Patients who develop this syndrome invariably have a marked disturbance of consciousness that can occur from sedative drug overdose or general anesthesia that interferes with vocal cord protection. The subsequent clinical course can include death in 30% to 62% of cases. Once liquid gastric content aspiration has occurred and the ARDS has supervened, ventilatory and medical strategies appropriate for treating the ARDS become the focus of care. Despite their frequent use, parenteral corticosteroids have not been shown to be helpful [3]. Antibiotics are indicated only when the syndrome is complicated by infection.

Foreign Body Aspiration

Aspiration of solid particles causes varying degrees of respiratory obstruction. Most cases occur in children. When foreign bodies are inhaled into the tracheobronchial tree, 38% of patients give a clear diagnostic history, 22% give a history of an acute choking and coughing episode, and 40% complain of cough, dyspnea, and wheezing. Although the chest radiograph may demonstrate the foreign object, atelectasis, or obstructive emphysema, it is normal in 80% of the cases.

Food asphyxiation is obstruction of the upper respiratory tract caused by food, usually at the level of the hypopharynx. It may occur whenever and wherever people eat, including hospitalized patients. In restaurants, it is called the *café coronary* because it is often mistaken for a heart attack. Food asphyxiation should be suspected in middle-aged or elderly patients with poor dentition or dentures that impair chewing adequately or in those sedated by alcohol or other drugs who attempt to swallow solid food. One key to a large foreign body aspiration that may obstruct the larynx or trachea is that the patient cannot speak. Particles that reach the lower respiratory tract and do not totally obstruct the trachea can be removed by coughing or bronchoscopically. Those that totally obstruct the trachea must be removed immediately by subdiaphragmatic abdominal thrusts sometimes followed by finger sweeps of the unconscious individual and chest thrusts in the markedly obese person and women in advanced stages of pregnancy [45].

Bacterial Pneumonia and Lung Abscess

Most bacterial pneumonias are a consequence of aspiration of oropharyngeal infectious material in association with impairment of lower respiratory tract defenses [41]. Preexisting gingival disease remains a prominent risk factor for anaerobic infections. The risk of aspiration pneumonia is lower among those with good oral hygiene. Initial studies from the 1960s to 1980s suggested anaerobes as the most common pathogens. However, we now find that aspiration pneumonia has a microbiologic spectrum that includes more *Staphylococcus aureus* and enteric gram-negative bacilli. Community-acquired pneumonia can occur when bacteria colonize the oropharynx prior to aspiration and are unable to be cleared by mucociliary clearance and detoxification by the alveolar phagocytes that have been rendered ineffective. Normal respiratory defenses and mucociliary clearance may be compromised by a preceding viral infection or underlying medical conditions that predispose to a bacterial "superinfection" [46]. Even the microbiology of abscesses has changed with the majority being due to aerobic (most commonly *Staphylococcus* species) organisms. Lung abscesses are now considered to be a result of more virulent community-acquired pneumonia pathogens and not because of aspiration of anaerobes alone [47]. The intubated patient is particularly susceptible to aspiration pneumonia because the endotracheal or tracheostomy tube bypasses the aerodynamic filtration protection of the upper respiratory tract and physically hinders mucociliary clearance. The intubated patient who requires a narcotic is at even greater risk because cough is also suppressed.

Once a bacterial pneumonia or lung abscess is suspected, the causative organism(s) should be identified and appropriate antibiotic therapy should be given (see Chapter 181).

Chemical Pneumonitis

Reminiscent of a chemical burn, airway and parenchymal injury may develop after an aspiration event that triggers a cascade of inflammatory mediators [5,41]. Fever, cough, rales, sputum production, hypoxemia, and infiltrates on chest radiograph may all be presenting signs and symptoms that are nonspecific. What distinguishes this syndrome from the other aspiration sequelae, however, is the rapid, self-limited course and clinical resolution over several days without the need for antimicrobial therapy. However, it should be noted that patients can progress to fulminant ARDS. Infectious aspiration pneumonia may not be a primary event but may develop as a superinfection of aspiration-induced pulmonary injury, depending on the contents of the aspirated material and the patient's underlying clinical condition.

Exogenous Lipoid Pneumonia

Exogenous lipoid pneumonia is the result of aspirating any kind of lipid or oil-based substance including mineral oil, animal oil (e.g., cod liver oil, milk products), vegetable oil, and formula feedings. Conditions more likely to be complicated by exogenous lipoid pneumonia include pharyngeal swallowing disorders, Zenker's diverticulum, cricopharyngeal achalasia, scleroderma involving the esophagus, epiphrenic diverticulum, esophageal carcinoma, esophageal achalasia, and GERD [3]. Although patients with exogenous lipoid pneumonia usually do not appear toxic, the clinical presentation occasionally cannot be distinguished from that of acute bacterial pneumonia.

The important clues to the diagnosis must come from the history, physical examination, and upper gastrointestinal studies. The presence of food particles in a bronchoscopy specimen is diagnostic. Although fat stains performed on unfixed expectorated sputum, bronchoalveolar lavage specimens, or lung biopsy may reveal numerous lipid-laden alveolar macrophages, this finding only supports the diagnosis of exogenous lipoid pneumonia. Lipid-laden macrophages can also arise from an endogenous source or represent a nonspecific response of the lung to injury [3] because the lung is capable of making its own lipid. Quantitative cultures obtained with telescoping plugged catheters at bronchoscopy may be needed to rule out a bacterial infection, and lung biopsy may be needed to rule out cancer and to make the appropriate diagnosis. After the diagnosis is made, however, the inciting agent is usually identified with pointed questioning of patient practices.

If not diagnosed promptly, recurrent aspirations of lipid or small amounts of liquid gastric contents, or both, can present as recurrent hemoptysis, recurrent pneumonias, chronic interstitial fibrosis, bronchiolitis, or bronchiectasis [4]. Rarely, exogenous lipoid pneumonias are complicated by organisms of the *Mycobacterium fortuitum* complex [48]. Although corticosteroids may be helpful for cases of acute lipid aspiration, acute exogenous lipoid pneumonias usually resolve on their own. The key to therapy is to prevent recurrences.

Tracheobronchitis

Tracheobronchitis must be considered not only for outpatients with GER and chronic, persistent cough [49] but also for hospitalized patients. Examples of conditions that predispose to an aspiration tracheobronchitis include a debilitated state, the postoperative period, endotracheal intubation, recent extubation, and neuromuscular diseases [3]. Aspiration tracheobronchitis should be suspected for patients with cough, wheezing, and bronchorrhea, defined as expectoration of more than 30 mL of phlegm in 24 hours. Treatment is the same as described previously in the "Exogenous Lipoid Pneumonia" section. In general, the bronchorrhea will disappear when oral intake is halted.

References

1. *Webster's New Universal Unabridged Dictionary*. New York, NY, Barnes & Noble Books, 1996, p 124.
2. Taylor JK, Fleming GB, Singanayagam A, et al: Risk factors for aspiration in community-acquired pneumonia: analysis of a hospitalized UK cohort. *Am J Med* 126:995, 2013.
3. Robinson KA, Markowitz DH, Irwin RS: Aspiration, in Irwin RS, Rippe JM (eds): *Intensive Care Medicine*. 6th ed. Philadelphia, PA, Lippincott Williams & Wilkins, 2008, pp 599–606.
4. Matsuse T, Oka T, Kida K, et al: Importance of diffuse aspiration bronchiolitis caused by chronic occult aspiration in the elderly. *Chest* 110:1289, 1996.
5. Nelson J, Lesser M: Aspiration-induced pulmonary injury. *J Int Care Med* 12:279, 1997.
6. Bonten MJ, Gaillard CA, van der Geest S, et al: The role of intragastric acidity and stress ulcer prophylaxis on colonization and infection in mechanically

ventilated ICU patients: a stratified, randomized, double-blind study of sucralfate versus antacids. *Am J Respir Crit Care Med* 152:1825, 1995.
7. Khorvash F, Abbasi S, Meidani M, et al: The comparison between proton pump inhibitors and sucralfate in the incidence of ventilator associated pneumonia in critically ill patients. *Adv Biomed Res* 3:52, 2014.
8. Cook D, Guyatt G, Marshall J, et al: A comparison of sucralfate and ranitidine for the prevention of upper gastrointestinal bleeding in patients requiring mechanical ventilation. Canadian Critical Care Trials Group. *N Engl J Med* 338:791–797, 1998.
9. Gulmez SE, Holm A, Frederiksen H, et al: Use of proton pump inhibitors and the risk of community-acquired pneumonia. *Arch Intern Med* 167:950–955, 2007.
10. Terzi N, Orlikowsi D, Aegerter P, et al: Breathing-swallowing interaction in neuromuscular patients. *Am J Respir Crit Care Med* 175:274–275, 2007.
11. Guilherme F, Gomes JC, Pisani ED, et al: The nasogastric feeding tube as a risk factor for aspiration and aspiration pneumonia. *Curr Opin Clin Nutr Metab Care* 6:327–333, 2003.
12. Lastbom L, Camner P: Deposition and clearance of particles in the human lung. *Scand J Work Environ Health* 26[Suppl 1]:23, 2000.
13. Zhang P, Summer WR, Bagby GJ, et al: Innate immunity and pulmonary host defense. *Immunol Rev* 175:39, 2000.
14. Bourke SJ: Mechanisms of cough, in Bourke SJ, Peel ET (eds): *Integrated Palliative Care of Respiratory Disease.* London, Springer-Verlag, 2013, p 48.
15. Macht M, Wimbish T, Clark BJ, et al: Postextubation dysphagia is persistent and associated with poor outcomes in survivors of critical illness. *Crit Care* 15:R231, 2011.
16. Varela JE, Varela K, Doherty J, et al: Incidence and predictors of aspiration after prolonged intubation in trauma patients. *J Am Coll Surg* 199:76, 2004.
17. Brady S, Donzelli J: The modified barium swallow and the functional endoscopic evaluation of swallowing. *Otolaryngol Clin North Am* 46:6, 2013.
18. Ajemian MS, Nirmul GB, Anderson MT, et al: Routine fiberoptic endoscopic evaluation of swallowing following prolonged intubation: implications for management. *Arch Surg* 136:434, 2001.
19. Barquist E, Brown M, Cohn S, et al: Postextubation fiberoptic endoscopic evaluation of swallowing after prolonged endotracheal intubation: a randomized, prospective trial. *Crit Care Med* 29:1710, 2001.
20. Prigent H, Lejalle M, Terzi N, et al: Effect of a trachesotomy speaking valve on breathing—swallowing interaction. *Intensive Care Med* 38:85–90, 2012.
21. Mittal R, Stewart W, Schirmer B: Effect of a catheter in the pharynx on the frequency of transient lower esophageal sphincter relaxation. *Gastroenterology* 103:1236, 1992.
22. Gomes GF, Pisani JC, Macedo ED, et al: The nasogastric feeding tube as a risk factor for aspiration and aspiration pneumonia. *Curr Opin Clin Nutr Metab Care* 6:327, 2003.
23. Ferrer M, Bauer T, Torres A, et al: Effect of nasogastric tube size on gastroesophageal reflux and microaspiration in intubated patients. *Ann Intern Med* 130:991, 1999.
24. Strong R, Condon S, Solinger M, et al: Equal aspiration rates from postpylorus and intragastric-placed small-bore nasoenteric feeding tubes: a randomized, prospective study. *JPEN J Parenter Enteral Nutr* 16:59, 1992.
25. Baeten C, Hoefnagels J: Feeding via nasogastric tube or percutaneous endoscopic gastrostomy: a comparison. *Scand J Gastroenterol Suppl* 194:95, 1992.
26. Kostadima E, Kaditis AG, Alexopoulos EI, et al: Early gastrostomy reduces the rate of ventilator-associated pneumonia in stroke or head injury patients. *Eur Res J* 26:106, 2005.
27. Montecalvo M, Steger K, Farber H, et al: Nutritional outcome and pneumonia in critical care patients randomized to gastric versus jejunal tube feedings. *Crit Care Med* 20:1377, 1992.
28. McClave SA, Lukan JK, Stefater JA, et al: Poor validity of residual volumes as a marker for risk of aspiration in critically ill patients. *Crit Care Med* 33(2):324–330, 2005.
29. Reignier J, Mercier E, Le Gouge A, et al: Effect of not monitoring residual gastric volume on risk of ventilator-associated pneumonia in adults receiving mechanical ventilation and early enteral feeding: a randomized controlled trial. *JAMA* 309:249, 2013.
30. Raghavendran K, Nemzek J, Napolitano LM, et al: Aspiration induced lung injury. *Crit Care Med* 39(4):818, 2011.
31. Bleach NR: The gag reflex and aspiration: a retrospective analysis of 120 patients assessed by videofluoroscopy. *Clin Otolaryngol Allied Sci* 18:303–307, 1993.
32. Tolep K, Getch C, Criner G: Swallowing dysfunction in patients receiving prolonged mechanical ventilation. *Chest* 109:167, 1996.
33. Elpern E, Scott M, Petro L, et al: Pulmonary aspiration in mechanically ventilated patients with tracheostomies. *Chest* 105:563, 1994.
34. Hiss SG, Postma GN: Fiberoptic endoscopic evaluation of swallowing. *Laryngoscope* 113:1386, 2003.
35. Wu CH, Hsiao TY, Chen JC, et al: Evaluation of swallowing safety with fiberoptic endoscope: comparison with videofluoroscopic technique. *Laryngoscope* 107:396, 1997.
36. Leder S, Sasaki C, Burrell M: Fiberoptic endoscopic evaluation of dysphagia to identify silent aspiration. *Dysphagia* 13:19, 1998.
37. Metheny N, Clouse R: Bedside methods for detecting aspiration in tube-fed patients. *Chest* 111:724, 1997.
38. Torres A, Serra-Batlles J, Ross E, et al: Pulmonary aspiration of gastric contents in patients receiving mechanical ventilation: the effect of body position. *Ann Intern Med* 116:540, 1992.
39. Orozco-Levi M, Torres A, Ferrer M, et al: Semirecumbent position protects from pulmonary aspiration but not completely from gastroesophageal reflux in mechanically ventilated patients. *Am J Respir Crit Care Med* 152:1387, 1995.
40. Reed MF, Mathisen DJ: Tracheoesophageal fistula. *Chest Surg Clin North Am* 13:271, 2003.
41. Marik PE: Pulmonary aspiration syndromes. *Curr Opin Pulm Med* 17:148–150, 2011.
42. Scannapieco FA, Binkley CJ: Modest reduction in risk for ventilator associated pneumonia in critically ill patients receiving mechanical ventilation following topical oral chlorhexidine. *J Evid Based Dent Pract* 12:103–106, 2012.
43. Klompas M, Speck K, Howell MD, et al: Reappraisal of routine oral care with chlorhexidine gluconate for patients receiving mechanical ventilation, systematic review and meta-analysis. *JAMA Intern Med* 174:751, 2014.
44. Schwartz D, Wynne J, Gibbs C, et al: The pulmonary consequences of aspiration of gastric contents at pH values greater than 2.5. *Am Rev Respir Dis* 121:119, 1980.
45. American Red Cross. *First Aid/CPR/AED Participants Manual.* 2nd ed. Dallas, TX, American Red Cross, 2014.
46. Rotta AT, Shiley KT, Davidson BA, et al: Gastric acid and particulate aspiration injury inhibits pulmonary bacterial clearance. *Crit Care Med* 32:747–754, 2004.
47. DiBardino DM, Wunderink RG: Aspiration pneumonia: a review of modern trends. *J Crit Care* 30:40–48, 2015.
48. Irwin R, Pratter M, Corwin R, et al: Pulmonary infection with *Mycobacterium chelonei*: successful treatment with one drug based on disk diffusion susceptibility data. *J Infect Dis* 145:772, 1982.
49. Irwin R, Corrao W, Pratter M: Chronic persistent cough in the adult: the spectrum and frequency of causes and successful outcome of specific therapy. *Am Rev Respir Dis* 123:413, 1981.

Chapter 171 ▪ Drowning

NICHOLAS A. SMYRNIOS • RICHARD S. IRWIN

OVERVIEW

Drowning is a process resulting in primary respiratory impairment from submersion/immersion in a liquid medium [1]. Implicit in this definition is that a liquid–air interface is present at the entrance of the victim's airway, preventing the victim from breathing air. A victim can be rescued at any time during the drowning process and may not require an intervention or may receive appropriate resuscitative measures. The victim may live or die after this process [1]. Older terms, such as near-drowning, submersion or immersion injury, and dry or wet drowning are discouraged to facilitate clearer communication.

Drowning is the fifth most common cause of unintentional injury death in the United States [2]. It is the third most common cause of accidental injury death worldwide, claiming approximately 372,000 lives annually [3]. For most countries, drowning statistics do not include additional water-related deaths from boating accidents which are categorized separately. Therefore, some large-scale tragedies may be missed with these statistics. Drowning is most common among men, children younger than 14 years, North American Native populations, and African-Americans [2]. The states with the highest drowning rates are Alaska and Mississippi [4]. Statistics on nonfatal drowning are less exact because many nonfatal drowning victims do not seek medical attention. Estimates for the incidence of nonfatal drowning vary widely enough that a definitive statement cannot be made at this time.

ETIOLOGY AND PATHOGENESIS

The following are considered risk factors for drowning.

Alcohol

Ethanol use is the major risk factor for submersion accidents. In all, 30% 70% of drownings are associated with alcohol consumption [5,6]. Alcohol use seems to be an issue for drowned men in particular [7]. Alcoholic beverages reduce the ability to deal with emergency situations by depressing coordination, increasing response time, and decreasing awareness of stimuli. Furthermore, alcohol consumption by a potential rescuer or by the adult responsible for supervising a child in the water can destroy that person's ability to function effectively, often resulting in a double tragedy. In addition, alcohol is frequently a factor in drownings that result from automobile accidents.

Inadequate Supervision

Children die in water because adults do not supervise them well enough. The backyard pool and family bathtub are common sites of pediatric drownings [5,8]. Lack of appropriate precautions and supervision play a major role in most of these cases. Studies have shown lower rates of drowning for areas where swimming pools are required by law to be surrounded by a fence [2,5]. The fence must completely isolate the pool from unsupervised access by children to be effective. Diving and sliding headfirst may produce serious head and neck injuries as a result of striking the bottom or side of a shallow body of water. Appropriate sign posting in hazardous areas, effective educational programs on the dangers of water recreation, and the presence of lifeguards minimize risk and improve survival [5,9].

Inattentive care givers also contribute to bathtub-related drownings. The use of infant bath seats, while providing some sense of security to parents, may actually predispose to submersion accidents because the child may slip and become trapped by the seat, making it impossible to escape the water [10]. The practice of leaving infants to bathe in the custody of a toddler is inappropriate and should be discouraged.

Child Abuse

Unfortunately, submersion injuries in children are sometimes inflicted intentionally. One study indicated that 29% of all nonfatal pediatric drownings in bathtubs were purposely caused to inflict harm on the child. Another 38% of all nonfatal pediatric drownings revealed evidence of severe neglect [11]. In general, these children are younger than average for submersion injuries, and many have signs of previous abuse on close examination.

Inadequate Swimming Skills

Both objective data and common sense support the idea that improved swimming skill can reduce the risk of drowning. Although the exact magnitude of this reduction is imprecise, some reports have estimated it as high as 88% for young children [12,13]. This factor may be more pronounced among males who may overestimate their swimming ability [7].

Seizures

Drowning is 15 to 19 times more common in people with epilepsy than in the general population [14]. Poor adherence to anticonvulsant regimens often plays a role. A large percentage of drowning deaths in epileptics occur in bathtubs [15]. Seizures that include a tonic component may be the most dangerous to victims. Tonic seizures include a forced exhalation component that increases body density and causes the victim to sink. When the tonic component relaxes, the negative intrathoracic pressure leads to an inhalation that will then be composed of water [16].

Boating Accidents

Of the 710 boating fatalities in the United States in 2006, 70% were caused by drowning [17]. A blood alcohol level of 0.10 g per 100 mL is estimated to increase the risk of death associated with boating by a factor of 10 [6]. Failure to use personal floatation devices may also contribute to these deaths [18]. In addition, injuries associated with the use of personal watercraft share many features with boating accidents and are associated with drowning [19].

Drugs

Centrally acting drugs cause disorientation, induce sleep, impair coordination, and reduce the ability to swim. Data implicate both therapeutic medications and illegal drugs [20].

PATHOPHYSIOLOGY

General Considerations

Two mechanisms produce the major pathologic changes responsible for morbidity in drowning: anoxia and hypothermia.

Anoxia

Most drownings are thought to follow a common pattern [21]. The drowning sequence begins with a period of breath holding. This voluntary breath holding may be followed by an intense laryngospasm that prevents breathing. This laryngospasm is usually owing to water present in the pharynx or larynx. This prolonged inability to breathe renders the patient hypoxemic and hypercapnic. In almost every case, there are eventually involuntary breaths with aspiration of varying amounts of water. In addition, water may be swallowed that is eventually regurgitated and aspirated. Eventually, the victim becomes unconscious and cardiac arrest occurs.

Hypothermia

The impact of hypothermia is complex. Survival after extremely long submersion is generally considered possible only when the victim has been submerged in icy water. Most authors believe that to achieve such spectacular survivals after long submersions, the core body temperature must be reduced quickly and the brain's metabolic activity slowed down in equally rapid fashion to prevent hypoxic damage to the brain. Factors that make this more likely for children include the increased relative body surface area, thin layer of subcutaneous fat, and smaller head size. In addition, children may aspirate water earlier after their submersion, and they may retain more water in the upper airway [22]. These factors may also play a role in rapid cooling. On the other hand, humans tolerate hypothermia poorly. In the most well-known example, the deaths after the sinking of the *Titanic* occurred not because of inability to float in most cases but because of hypothermia caused by exposure to extremely cold water. As if to highlight these contradictory effects of hypothermia on outcome, a recent study did not demonstrate any effect of water temperature on mortality [23].

Changes in human metabolism in response to hypothermia occur in two phases: the shivering phase and the nonshivering phase. Shivering occurs at a central temperature of 30°C to 35°C. The nonshivering phase occurs below 30°C, when muscle contractions nearly cease and oxygen consumption and metabolic rate decrease. Shivering and voluntary muscular movements, which in a cold dry environment work together to increase heat production with a minimal increase in heat loss, are ineffective in cold water. Both shivering and voluntary muscular movements increase blood flow to the extremities, thereby increasing conductive heat loss. Voluntary movements of the extremities also stir the surrounding water and can increase heat loss from convection. Body type may also play a major role. Water also nearly eliminates the insulative function of clothing by replacing the air between the fibers, thereby increasing heat conductance.

Submersion in very cold water can acutely lead to death. Hypothermia produces an increased tendency toward malignant arrhythmias. Cardiac arrest from ventricular fibrillation is common at core temperatures below 28°C, and asystole occurs at less than 20°C [24]. These arrhythmias may be refractory to resuscitative efforts until the body temperature has been increased. In addition, a decrease in core temperature can cause loss of consciousness and aspiration from the victim's inability to keep the head above water. This leads to aspiration of water and the sequence of events described previously.

Pulmonary Effects

The effects of aspiration of various water solutions on lung injury have been studied in animals [9]. Decreases in arterial oxygen saturation and dynamic compliance as well as increases in minute ventilation, mean pulmonary artery pressure, and shunt fraction are seen after bilateral aspiration of either freshwater or seawater.

On a microscopic level, freshwater and saline solutions may cause their adverse pulmonary effects by different mechanisms. Atelectasis as a result of increased surface tension, bronchoconstriction, and noncardiogenic pulmonary edema all play a role in the development of hypoxemia at different times after freshwater aspiration [9]. Freshwater acts in part by inactivating surfactant in the alveoli and in part by damaging type-II pneumocytes, thereby preventing the production of surfactant. The combination of these effects may damage the alveolar capillaries and interstitium and lead to the acute respiratory distress syndrome (ARDS). Hypertonic seawater may draw additional fluid from the plasma into the alveoli, thereby causing pulmonary edema despite a decreased intravascular volume [9]. The fluid-filled alveoli are then unavailable for efficient gas transfer, and a ventilation–perfusion mismatch occurs. Aspiration of gastric contents and particles in the water complicates both freshwater and saltwater drowning. Both saltwater and freshwater damage the alveolar–capillary interface and permit the influx of fluid into the alveolus. Therefore, in clinical practice, the difference between the injuries caused by freshwater and saltwater aspirations is small. In both cases, pulmonary edema causes decreased respiratory system compliance and hypoxemia.

Several other mechanisms of lung injury may occur with nonfatal drowning. Bacterial pneumonia, barotrauma, mechanical damage from cardiopulmonary resuscitation (CPR), chemical pneumonitis, centrally mediated apnea, and oxygen toxicity can cause respiratory deterioration in the postresuscitation period these must be considered along with ARDS in cases of respiratory distress occurring 1 to 48 hours after the event.

Neurologic Effects

The pathologic effects that most affect prognosis for drowning victims are related to the central nervous system. Cerebral injury is produced as a result of anoxia caused by gas exchange impairment and subsequent cardiopulmonary arrest.

Anoxic damage begins 4 to 10 minutes after cessation of cerebral blood flow in most situations [25]. The actual time course and clinical significance of anoxia in a specific drowning victim is notoriously uncertain because of the emotional condition of the witnesses and because the impact of hypothermia is difficult to judge. In addition, because drowning causes an asphyxial cardiac arrest, there will be persistence of perfusion for some time during the arrest that may provide some degree of protection from injury [25].

Many drowning victims suffer neurologic impairment. Victims display pathologic features similar to those of patients with anoxic encephalopathy from other causes, including diffuse cerebral edema, focal areas of necrosis, mitochondrial swelling, and other ischemic changes. These changes occur primarily in the cerebral cortex, hippocampus, and basal ganglia [25]. Severe anoxic encephalopathy with persistent coma, seizures, delayed language development, spastic quadriplegia, aphasia, and cortical blindness are seen as sequelae of submersion accidents. Unfortunately, despite a great deal of effort placed into trying to predict the ultimate neurologic outcome of drowning victims, it remains impossible to predict outcomes with accuracy for individual patients [26].

Musculoskeletal Effects

Children who develop anoxic encephalopathy because of drowning frequently develop musculoskeletal problems [27]. These problems result from spasticity, which appears to be more aggressive in these children than in those with other forms of spastic disorder. The most common of these are lower extremity contractures, hip subluxation or dislocation, and scoliosis [27].

Serum Electrolytes

Experimental studies with animals reveal significant differences in serum electrolytes between freshwater and saltwater drowning [28]. In the clinical setting, swallowing large amounts of seawater over an extended period of repeated submersions has been reported to cause significant changes in serum sodium, potassium, chloride, and magnesium levels [29]. This happens rarely, however, and the body corrects most of the alterations that do occur. Therefore, the actual clinical impact of electrolyte changes is minimal.

Hematologic Effects

Patients presenting with drowning episodes rarely require medical intervention for anemia. Studies have demonstrated near-normal hemoglobin values in both seawater and freshwater [28]. In the best study of the affect of drowning on coagulation, overt disseminated intravascular coagulation was 13 times more likely in victims of cardiac arrest from drowning as opposed to nondrowning cardiac arrest victims [30]. The authors speculated that ischemia-induced tissue plasminogen activator release plays a role in this phenomenon.

Renal Effects

Acute tubular necrosis, hemoglobinuria, and albuminuria have all been reported as consequences of submersion accidents [31]. Diuresis has traditionally been considered to be a result of changes in renal tubular function as a result of hypothermia [32]. However, diuresis is seen in experimental submersions at any temperature [32]. Drowning victims also frequently present with metabolic acidosis as a result of lactate accumulation [33].

Cardiac Effects

Submersion in water causes an increase in left atrial diameter and a decrease in heart rate [34]. Atrial fibrillation and sinus dysrhythmias are common but rarely require therapy. PR, QRS, and QT interval prolongations as well as J point elevation can be seen as in other causes of hypothermia [24]. The most common arrhythmias seen in cardiac arrests because of drowning are asystole followed by pulseless electrical activity [35].

The anoxia caused by drowning can also have an effect on hemodynamics. There may be transient increases in central venous and pulmonary artery occlusion pressures and a persistent decrease in cardiac output that may last more than 4 hours. These findings are independent of the tonicity of the solutions used and no different from those of anoxic controls.

Infectious Complications

Although a variety of infections are reported to be associated with drowning, pneumonia is the predominant infection described. Aspiration of mouth contents, gastric contents, and contaminated water all play a role in the development of pneumonia after drowning. A wide variety of organisms, including aerobic Gram-negative bacteria, aerobic Gram-positive bacteria, and fungi, have been described [36]. Combinations of infections, some with opportunistic organisms, have also been described [37]. Because organisms that can survive in very cold water usually cannot survive and proliferate at human body temperature, most pneumonia cases occur after warm-water drowning [37]. In addition to pneumonia, cases of brain abscess, meningoencephalitis, bacteremia, skin and soft tissue infections, and endophthalmitis are reported to occur.

DIAGNOSIS AND CLINICAL PRESENTATION

History

The minimum background historic information that must be obtained includes the patient's age; underlying cardiac, respiratory, or neurologic diseases; and medications used. It is also important to determine the activities precipitating the submersion, such as boating, diving, or ingestion of drugs or alcohol; the duration of submersion; and the temperature and type of water in which it occurred.

Physical Examination

The initial physical examination is often hurried, with more detailed assessment delayed until resuscitative efforts have been established. Tachypnea is the most frequent finding, and tachycardia is also common. Patients may also be apneic and pulseless. Hypothermia is common and depends on the temperature of the water and duration of submersion. It is important that an appropriate thermometer be used that can accurately measure hypothermic temperatures because the duration of resuscitation may depend on this value. Other findings include fever and signs of pulmonary edema. Any physical findings seen in cases of cerebral anoxia or severe hypothermia may also be seen in drowning. In addition to revealing the consequences of hypoxia/anoxia and hypothermia, the major importance of the physical examination is to uncover coexisting injuries that may have caused or resulted from the submersion.

Various classification systems have been proposed for use with drowning victims. None of them are uniformly applied, and their value has yet to be proven in the clinical arena.

Laboratory Studies

Hemoglobin, hematocrit, and serum electrolytes are usually normal on arrival in the emergency department whether the submersion occurred in freshwater or saltwater [9]. Arterial blood gas analysis frequently shows metabolic acidosis and hypoxemia. The blood alcohol level, prothrombin time, partial thromboplastin time, serum creatinine, urinalysis, and drug screen should also be obtained to help determine the cause of the accident and assess for complications of drowning. Cervical spine films should be performed whenever there is evidence of trauma. An electrocardiogram should be obtained and continuous monitoring performed whenever there is a significant chance of dysrhythmia. Chest radiographs frequently demonstrate some degree of pulmonary edema. Some films display confluent alveolar densities primarily in the perihilar regions, whereas others exhibit a diffuse, almost homogeneous nodular pattern bilaterally.

THERAPY

The treatment of nonfatal drowning should be approached in four phases.

Initial Resuscitation

Resuscitation of apneic or pulseless drowning victims should be initiated immediately and continue as needed throughout the prehospital phase into the emergency department. Mouth-to-mouth resuscitation may be begun in the water if the rescuer is a strong enough swimmer [39]. However, the rescuer must not put himself or herself in jeopardy. When performing rescue breathing, the rescuer should carefully support the victim's neck to prevent exacerbation of undiagnosed vertebral injuries. Full CPR with chest compressions should begin immediately on arrival on shore and proceed according to standard guidelines, advanced life support should begin as soon as appropriate providers arrive and all victims requiring resuscitation should ultimately be transported to a hospital [40]. The use of the Heimlich maneuver in the absence of a foreign body obstruction was strongly recommended against by an Institute of Medicine Report [41].

Resuscitation must be continued for victims of cold-water submersion at least until the patient has been rewarmed. Core temperature should be obtained immediately on arrival at the emergency department and monitored carefully during the first several hours. All drowning victims with cardiopulmonary arrest and hypothermia should be rewarmed rapidly only to a temperature between 32°C and 34°C and then maintained at that level (see following discussion) [42]. In the field, wet clothing should be removed and passive external rewarming plus inhalation of heated oxygen started. In the hospital, extracorporeal circulation should be used for cases of severe hypothermia from drowning, especially with circulatory collapse [43]. This method has the advantage of rapidly and directly rewarming the core. It can also correct the metabolic acidosis that commonly occurs. When this technique is not possible, rewarming with warmed peritoneal lavage, hemodialysis, or heated oxygen can be attempted (for an in-depth discussion of rewarming techniques, see Chapter 184).

A more difficult question is when and how long to resuscitate victims of warm-water submersion. As previously mentioned, there is no clearly established method of predicting ultimate neurologic recovery for individual patients. Therefore, until more information is available, the decision to terminate resuscitation must be based on a variety of factors particular to the individual case. On the other end of the clinical spectrum, victims who are asymptomatic and have normal oxygenation at 6 to 8 hours after presentation do not deteriorate during the subsequent 18 to 24 hours and do well in the long term [44,45].

Therapy of the Underlying Cause

If there is any question of possible head or neck trauma, the neck should be immobilized in a brace until cervical spine films are available. Hypoglycemia and severe electrolyte abnormalities can be detected on routine serum testing and corrected rapidly in the emergency department. Serum alcohol levels and a drug screen can detect potential intoxicants and prompt administration of necessary antidotes or other measures. Anticonvulsant levels can help tailor therapy for known epileptic patients.

Treatment of Respiratory and Other Organ Failure

The initial management of all pulmonary edema states involves monitoring PaO_2 and providing appropriate supplemental oxygen. Mechanical ventilation with positive end-expiratory pressure (PEEP) should be instituted if refractory hypoxic or hypercapnic respiratory failure develops. Excessive amounts of PEEP could adversely affect $PaCO_2$ and intracranial pressure and, therefore, have an adverse effect on cerebral perfusion. Moderate levels of PEEP used to enhance alveolar recruitment and enable adequate oxygenation are unlikely to have such an adverse impact. The standard of care for the management of ARDS from any cause is the use of low-tidal volume, low-pressure ventilation [46] (Table 171.1). Use of such a strategy has been shown to have a major effect on survival of ARDS patients. However, because of the potential impact of hypercapnia on cerebral blood volume, permissive hypercapnia should not be employed without intracranial pressure monitoring in comatose drowning victims [25].

Other therapies for the respiratory complications of drowning have been proposed, but none of those has demonstrated improvements of outcomes. Examples of these types of therapies include exogenous surfactant in respiratory failure and prophylactic antibiotics. We do not advocate the use of either of these therapies.

Treatment of other end-organ damage must be approached systematically. Serum electrolytes rarely require therapy. The treatment of renal failure focuses on optimizing fluid status and renal blood flow. Severe cases may require temporary dialysis. Lactic acidosis should be corrected by restoration of adequate ventilation and circulation. The only clinically significant hematologic effect is disseminated intravascular coagulation (DIC). The management of DIC is addressed in Chapter 88.

The cardiac dysrhythmogenic effects of hypothermia are corrected by rewarming. Sinus and atrial dysrhythmias as well as most interval prolongations rarely require additional therapy. For a discussion of the treatment of hypothermia-related malignant ventricular dysrhythmias, see Chapter 184.

Musculoskeletal complications of nonfatal drowning are treated in standard fashion. Contractures are treated with casts or splints; subluxated or dislocated hips can be approached with appropriate operative procedures; and scoliosis is treated with bracing or spinal instrumentation [27]. The relative success of these interventions for this population is unclear.

Neurologic Therapy

The quality of the evidence supporting any intervention is poor when addressing neurologic resuscitation of the drowning victim. Therefore, much of what is recommended is based on a consensus understanding of the available information supplemented by general principles of resuscitation. The following recommendations are based on the World Congress on Drowning and more recent publications.

- Restoration of spontaneous circulation is the highest priority goal. In-water rescue may be attempted by a trained lifeguard, but untrained individuals are likely to impair their own swimming by doing so and will probably be better served by bringing the victim to land. Because studies that established the efficacy of compression-alone CPR excluded drowning victims, and because the cause of drowning-related cardiac arrest is usually respiratory, conventional CPR with compressions and rescue breathing is recommended [25,47].
- Core temperature should be monitored continuously. It is not necessary to continue aggressively rewarming a drowning victim once spontaneous circulation has been recovered, unless the hypothermia is thought to be contributing to ongoing arrhythmias or other serious pathology. Hyperthermia should be prevented and normothermia maintained at all times in the acute recovery period. Therapeutic hypothermia to a core temperature of 32°C to 36°C is recommended for a period of 24 hours for comatose survivors [48,49,50].
- Seizures should be looked for and treated as necessary.
- The head of the bed should be elevated to 30 to 45 degrees while in the ICU.
- Blood glucose concentrations should be monitored and normoglycemia maintained.
- Hypoxemia and hypotension should be corrected.
- There is no pharmacologic therapy that has been shown to enhance brain recovery [25].

TABLE 171.1

Advances in the Management of Drowning Based on Randomized Clinical Trials

Intervention	Outcomes favorably affected	References
Small tidal volume ventilation for ARDS	Mortality, organ failure days, mechanical ventilation days	[46]
Therapeutic hypothermia for comatose survivors of cardiac arrest	Mortality	[49]
	Neurologic status	[48,49],50

ARDS, acute respiratory distress syndrome.

CONCLUSIONS

The course of nonfatal drowning is variable. Patients who receive prompt CPR, are rapidly restored to a perfusing rhythm, and regain neurologic function usually have dramatic and complete recoveries. On the other hand, patients with delayed resuscitation and those who do not rapidly recover neurologic function often have poor outcomes. Although freshwater and seawater drownings cause different clinical pictures in experimental animals, they are difficult to distinguish for human drowning victims. In general, patients who aspirate water present with hypoxemia and metabolic acidosis. They usually do not aspirate enough fluid to produce changes in blood volume, electrolytes, hemoglobin, and hematocrit of sufficient magnitude to be life-threatening.

The development of treatments specifically for drowning victims has been very slow. In general, most therapies are general treatments directed at cardiac arrest and ARDS. Treatment varies with the severity of the illness. For severely hypothermic patients, rewarming methods should be instituted immediately. These include removing wet clothing, covering with warm blankets, infusing warm fluids intravenously, and performing gastrointestinal irrigation with warm fluids. If the patient's temperature is less than 32°C, core rewarming may be most easily accomplished by cardiopulmonary bypass or peritoneal dialysis with a potassium-free dialysate warmed to 54°C. The desired core temperature for patients after cardiac arrest is 32°C to 36°C. Therapy for patients with severe hypoxemia includes institution of all the supportive modalities used for ARDS in Chapter 163. Abnormalities of multiple organ systems must be addressed systematically. The most important methods for reducing deaths from drowning currently reside in the area of drowning prevention.

References

1. Idris AH, Berg RA, Bierens J, et al: Recommended guidelines for uniform reporting of data from drowning—the "Utstein style." *Circulation* 108:2565, 2003.
2. Centers for Disease Control and Prevention, National Center for Injury Prevention and Control: Web-based injury statistics query and reporting system (WISQARS) (online). Accessed October 8, 2015.
3. Meddings D, Hyder AA, Ozanne-Smith J, et al (eds): Global report on drowning-preventing a leading killer. *WHO* 2014. ISBN 978-92-4-156478-6.
4. Centers for Disease Control and Prevention: National Center for injury prevention and control. *Drowning Prev* 2000.
5. Laosee OC, Gilchrist J, Rudd RA: Drowning—United States 2005–2009. *MMWR* 61:344, 2012.
6. Driscoll TR, Harrison JA, Steenkamp M: Review of the role of alcohol in drowning associated with recreational aquatic activity. *Inj Prev* 10:107, 2004.
7. Howland J, Hingson R, Mangione TW, et al. Why are most drowning victims men? Sex differences in aquatic skills and behaviours. *Am J Public Health* 86:93, 1996.
8. Saluja G, Brenner RA, Trumble AC: Swimming pool drownings among US residents aged 5–24 years: understanding racial/ethnic disparities. *Am J Public Health* 96:728, 2006.
9. Szpilman D, Bierens JJLM, Handley AJ, et al: Drowning. *N Engl J Med* 366:2102, 2012.
10. Byard RW, Donald T: Infant bath seats and near-drowning. *J Paediatr Child Health* 40:305, 2004.
11. Lavelle JM, Shaw KN, Seidl T, et al: Ten-year review of pediatric bathtub near drownings: evaluation for child abuse and neglect. *Ann Emerg Med* 25:344, 1995.
12. Brenner RA, Taneja GS, Haynie DL, et al: Association between swimming lessons and drowning in childhood—a case-control study. *Arch Pediatr Adolesc Med* 163:203, 2009.
13. Yang L, Nong Q, Li C, et al: Risk factors for childhood drowning in rural regions of a developing country: a case–control study. *Inj Prev* 13:178, 2007.
14. Bell GS, Gaitatzis A, Bell CL, et al: Drowning in people with epilepsy. *Neurology* 71:578, 2008.
15. Ryan CA, Doeling G: Drowning deaths in people with epilepsy. *Can Med Assoc J* 148:781, 1993.
16. Besag FMC: Tonic seizures are a particular risk factor for drowning in people with epilepsy. *BMJ* 321:975, 2000.
17. Centers for Disease Control and Prevention: Unintentional drowning: get the facts. (online). Accessed November 27, 2015.
18. Cummings P, Mueller BA, Quan L: Association between wearing a personal floatation device and death by drowning among recreational boaters: a matched cohort analysis of United States Coast Guard data. *Inj Prev* 17:156, 2011.
19. Branche CM, Conn JM, Annest JL: Personal watercraft related injuries: a growing public health concern. *JAMA* 278:663, 1997.
20. Gorniak JM, Jenkins AJ, Felo JA, et al: Drug prevalence in drowning deaths in Cuyahoga County, Ohio: a ten-year retrospective study. *Am J Foren Med Pathol* 26:240, 2005.
21. Layon AJ, Modell JH: Drowning update 2009. *Anesthesiology* 110:1211, 2009.
22. Xu X, Tikuisis P, Giesbrecht G: A mathematical model for human brain cooling during cold-water near-drowning. *J Appl Physiol* 86:265, 1999.
23. Quan L, Mack CD, Schiff MA: Association of water temperature and submersion duration and drowning outcome. *Resuscitation* 85:1304, 2014.
24. Steiner MK, Curley FJ, Irwin RS: Disorders of temperature control part I: hypothermia, in Irwin RS, Rippe JM (eds): *Irwin and Rippe's Intensive Care Medicine*. 7th ed. Philadelphia, PA, Lippincott Williams and Wilkins, 2012.
25. Topjian AA, Berg RA, Bierens JJLM, et al: Brain resuscitation in the drowning victim. *Neurocrit Care* 17:441, 2012.
26. Christensen DW, Jansen P, Perkin RM: Outcome and acute care hospital costs after warm water near drowning in children. *Pediatrics* 99:715, 1997.
27. Abrams RA, Mubarak S: Musculoskeletal consequences of near-drowning in children. *J Pediatr Orthop* 11:168, 1991.
28. Conn AW, Miyasaka K, Katayama M, et al: A canine study of cold water drowning in fresh versus salt water. *Crit Care Med* 23:2029, 1995.
29. Ellis RJ: Severe hypernatremia from sea water ingestion during near-drowning in a hurricane. *West J Med* 167:430, 1997.
30. Schwameis M, Schober A, Schorgenhofer C, et al: Asphyxia by drowning induces massive bleeding due to hyperfibrinolytic disseminated intravascular coagulation. *Crit Care Med* 43:2394, 2015.
31. Miki A, Takeda S, Yamamoto H, et al: A case of renal impairment after near-drowning: the universal nature of acute kidney injury. *Clin Exp Nephrol* 17:594, 2013.
32. Sramek P, Simeckova M, Jansky L, et al: Human physiological responses to immersion into water of different temperatures. *Eur J Appl Physiol* 81:436, 2000.
33. Opdahl H: Survival put to the acid test: extreme arterial blood acidosis (pH 6.33) after near drowning. *Crit Care Med* 25:1431, 1997.
34. Watenpaugh DE, Pump B, Bie P, et al: Does gender influence human cardiovascular and renal responses to water immersion? *J Appl Physiol* 89:621, 2000.
35. Dyson K, Morgans A, Bray J, et al: Drowning related out-of-hospital cardiac arrests. Characteristics and outcomes. *Resuscitation* 84:114, 2013.
36. Van Berkel M, Bierens JJLM, Lie RLK, et al: Pulmonary oedema, pneumonia, and mortality in submersion victims; a retrospective study in 125 patient. *Intensive Care Med* 22:101, 1996.
37. Chaney S, Gopalan R, Berggren RE: Pulmonary *Pseudoallescheria boydii* infection with cutaneous zygomycosis after near-drowning. *South Med J* 97:683, 2004.
38. Ender PT, Dolan MJ: Pneumonia associated with near-drowning. *Clin Infect Dis* 25:896, 1997.
39. Szpilman D, Soares M: In-water resuscitation—is it worthwhile? *Resuscitation* 63:25, 2004.
40. Vanden Hoek TL, Morrison LJ, Shuster M, et al: Cardiac arrest in special situations: 2010 American heart Association Guidelines for Cardiopulmonary Resuscitation and Emergency Cardiac Care. *Circulation* 122:S829, 2010.
41. Rosen P, Stoto M, Harley J: The use of the Heimlich maneuver in near drowning: Institute of Medicine Report. *J Emerg Med* 13:397, 1995.
42. van Dorp JC, Knape JTA, Bierens JJLM: *Final Recommendations of the World Congress on Drowning, Amsterdam 26–28 June 2002*. Amsterdam, the Netherlands, 2002.
43. Husby P, Anderson KS, Owen-Falkenberg A, et al: Accidental hypothermia with cardiac arrest: complete recovery after prolonged resuscitation and rewarming by extracorporeal circulation. *Intensive Care Med* 16:69, 1990.
44. Causey AL, Titelli JA, Swanson ME: Predicting discharge in uncomplicated near-drowning. *Am J Emerg Med* 18:9, 2000.
45. Noonan L, Howrey R, Ginsburg CM: Freshwater submersion injuries in children: a retrospective review of seventy-five hospitalized patients. *Pediatrics* 98:368, 1996.
46. The Acute Respiratory Distress Syndrome Network: Ventilation with lower tidal volumes as compared with traditional tidal volumes for acute lung injury and the acute respiratory distress syndrome. *N Engl J Med* 342:1301, 2000.
47. Bierens J: Recommendations of the World Congress on drowning—2002. Accessed October 22, 2015.
48. Bernard SA, Gray TW, Buist MD, et al: Treatment of comatose survivors of out-of-hospital cardiac arrest with induced hypothermia. *N Engl J Med* 346:612, 2002.
49. The Hypothermia After Cardiac Arrest Study Group: Mild therapeutic hypothermia to improve the neurologic outcome after cardiac arrest. *N Engl J Med* 346:549, 2002.
50. American Heart Association. Part 8: Post-Arrest Cardiac Care. In American Heart Association. Guidelines for Cardiopulmonary Resuscitation and Emergency Cardiovascular Care, 2015.

Chapter 172 ■ Acute Exacerbation of Asthma

J. MARK MADISON • RICHARD S. IRWIN

Asthma is a chronic inflammatory disease of the airways characterized by variable airway obstruction [1]. Inflammation of the airways causes airway obstruction by making airway smooth muscle more sensitive to contractile stimuli, by thickening the airway wall with edema and inflammatory cell infiltration, by stimulating glands to secrete mucus into the airway lumen, by damaging the airway epithelium, and by remodeling the architecture of the airways.

Acute exacerbations of asthma may punctuate the course of mild, moderate, or severe cases of chronic asthma. These exacerbations or flares of asthma can be life-threatening and are characterized by an acute, progressive worsening of respiratory symptoms and pulmonary function that is severe enough to warrant a change in treatment [1]. Typically, mild-to-severe exacerbations are triggered by poor adherence to asthma controller medications or by exposure to environmental factors such as inhaled allergens, irritants, or viral infections of the respiratory tract. Assessment, management, and prevention of exacerbations of asthma, especially those leading to respiratory failure, are the critical challenges of caring for adult patients with asthma [1–3]. Severe exacerbations of asthma leading to critical illness are the main focus of this chapter.

EPIDEMIOLOGY

According to the most recent data by the Center for Disease Control, the prevalence of asthma in the United States is 7.3% [4]. Worldwide, clinical asthma ranks among the most common chronic diseases, with a prevalence ranging from 1.04% in Vietnam to 21.5% in Australia [5]. In general, asthma prevalence increases with urbanization and westernization of societies.

Asthma exacerbation rates vary by season with peaks in emergency room visits and hospitalizations coinciding with respiratory viral infections, especially rhinoviral infections, in late summer and early autumn. In 2010 National Hospital Discharge Survey data, annual rates for inpatient hospital discharges for asthma in the United States were 18.3 per 10,000 population-age less than 18 years and 13 per 10,000 population-age 18 and over [4]. Although there remain important racial and gender differences in the rates of hospitalization, there was an overall decline in hospitalizations from 1995 to 2002, possibly due to better management and prevention [6].

In 2013, there were 3,630 deaths due to asthma in the United States indicating a death rate of 10.7 per million population of all ages [4]. Asthma mortality rates also have an annual cycle but do not strictly parallel the cycle for exacerbations. Among children, mortality peaks during the summer months, but, with increasing age, asthma mortality becomes more common during the winter months [7]. In 2013, the death rate for adults aged 18 years and older was 14.1 deaths per million population, but it is notable that there are large racial differences in the risk of death due to asthma. For all ages, non-Hispanic Blacks had a death rate of 25.9 per million population, while non-Hispanic Whites had a rate of only 8.4 per million population [4]. Deaths among patients hospitalized for asthma do account for one-third of asthma-related mortality, but potential differences of hospital care do not appear to account for racial disparities, and this suggests that prehospitalization factors are important [8].

PATHOPHYSIOLOGY

Pathology

Bronchial biopsy specimens from patients with asthma are pathologically abnormal [9–12], with collagen deposition beneath the epithelial basement membranes, mucosal infiltration by eosinophils and neutrophils, mast cell degranulation, and epithelial damage. These findings occur in both severe and mild asthma, suggesting that airway inflammation is of primary importance in the pathogenesis of asthma.

For exacerbations of asthma, the pathology of the airways is variable, reflecting at least two recognized clinical subtypes of exacerbation—slow onset and rapid onset. Slow onset exacerbations are the most common (approximately 80% of exacerbations) and the patient presents with more than 2 to 6 hours of symptoms—often days or weeks of symptoms [13–15]. This suggests that most such patients should have sufficient time to seek medical attention for worsening shortness of breath [16]. At autopsy, the lungs of patients who die of "slow-onset" asthma exacerbations are hyperinflated with thick tenacious mucus filling and obstructing the lumens of the airways. Microscopically, there is an eosinophilic bronchitis, with pronounced areas of mucosal edema and desquamation of the epithelium. Typically, hypertrophy and hyperplasia of smooth muscle are present and the muscle appears contracted [17].

The patient with the rapid-onset type of exacerbation presents with severe symptoms that have rapidly progressed over 2 to 6 hours [13–15]. These rapid-onset exacerbations may represent 8% to 14% of asthma exacerbations in general and can be fatal, leading to death in only a few hours after symptom onset [13,15]. Pathologically, airway obstruction by mucus is not prominent, and there is a neutrophilic, rather than eosinophilic, predominance of inflammatory cells in the airway submucosa [18]. There are no specific clinical characteristics that reliably predict which patients are prone to these rapid-onset asthma exacerbations. However, patients with rapid-onset asthma exacerbations may more commonly report sensitivity to nonsteroidal anti-inflammatory drugs [15].

Pathogenesis

Asthma is a disease or group of diseases with complex underlying genetics [19]. Why airway inflammation develops in the asthmatic patient is not understood entirely, but much evidence suggests an important role for Th2 cytokines [20]. Inhaled allergens, pollutants, smoke, and viral infections all may play a role in augmenting the baseline airway inflammation present in the asthmatic airway [1,2,21]. When these environmental triggers interact with the asthmatic airway, the inflammation is intensified and the released mediators have potent effects on smooth muscle cell function, epithelium and microvascular integrity, neural function, and mucus gland secretion [22]. All these factors contribute to increased narrowing of the asthmatic airway with smooth muscle contraction, mucus secretion, epithelial cell sloughing into the lumen, and edema and inflammatory cell infiltration of the airway wall. The resulting acute increase of airway obstruction is commonly referred to as an *acute exacerbation of asthma*.

Physiology

The major physiologic consequences of airway obstruction are hypoxemia and increased work of breathing. Understanding these physiologic disturbances is important for management of severe exacerbations of asthma.

Narrowing the caliber of airway lumens causes hypoxemia by two mechanisms. First, increases in the resistance to flow in the conducting airways result in uneven distribution of ventilation to the alveoli. Hypoxic vasoconstriction of vessels that supply underventilated alveoli partially compensates for this uneven ventilation, but overall ventilation–perfusion ($\dot{V}/\dot{Q}$) ratios remain abnormal and are the principal cause of hypoxemia during asthma exacerbations [23]. Consequently, even patients with severe exacerbations of asthma usually respond favorably to supplemental oxygen. A second, less common, cause of hypoxemia among asthmatics is right-to-left shunt due to atelectasis of lung distal to airways that are completely occluded by mucus or due to interatrial shunt precipitated by increased right atrial pressures from asthma-related increases of pulmonary vascular resistance [24,25].

The second physiologic consequence of severe airway obstruction is increased work of breathing. During acute exacerbations, respiratory muscles must expend increased energy, generating large changes of pleural pressure to overcome high airway resistance [26]. The resulting discordance between respiratory effort and the change in thoracic volume may play some role in the patient's sensation of dyspnea and central drive to increase minute ventilation. The ensuing rapid respirations further increase the work of breathing and worsen air trapping behind narrowed airways that prematurely close during expiration. The dynamic hyperinflation of the lung itself leads to increased respiratory muscle energy costs because it restricts vital capacity due to high thoracic volumes where alveolar dead space is increased, the respiratory muscles are at suboptimal mechanical advantage, and the lung is less compliant. All of these factors contribute to the significant increase of the work of breathing and the respiratory muscles must expend more energy to achieve the same alveolar ventilation. Initially, the respiratory muscles may be able to exert the force needed to maintain alveolar ventilation, but the muscles may fatigue if airway resistance increases rapidly, is sustained, or when there is inadequate oxygen delivery to theses muscles [27,28]. Dynamic hyperinflation due to severe airway obstruction also may impair cardiac performance by increasing right ventricular afterload, decreasing venous return to the left atrium, and by causing diastolic dysfunction [3,25].

TABLE 172.1

Differential Diagnosis of Wheezing

- Upper airway obstruction
  - Extrathoracic
    - Anaphylaxis
    - Arytenoid dysfunction
    - Bilateral vocal cord paralysis
    - Laryngeal edema
    - Laryngostenosis
    - Laryngocele
    - Mobile supraglottic soft tissue
    - Neoplasms
    - Postextubation granuloma
    - Postnasal drip syndrome
    - Relapsing polychondritis
    - Retropharyngeal abscess
    - Supraglottitis
    - Vocal cord dysfunction syndrome
    - Granulomatosis with polyangiitis (Wegener granulomatosis)
  - Intrathoracic
    - Acquired tracheomalacia
    - Airway neoplasms
    - Foreign body aspiration
    - Goiter
    - Herpetic tracheobronchitis
    - Right-side aortic arch
    - Tracheal stenosis due to intubation
    - Tracheobronchomegaly
- Lower airway obstruction
  - Aspiration
  - Asthma
  - Asthma-COPD overlap syndrome
  - Bronchiectasis
  - Bronchiolitis
  - Carcinoid syndrome
  - Chronic obstructive pulmonary disease
  - Cystic fibrosis
  - Lymphangitic carcinomatosis
  - Pulmonary edema
  - Parasitic infections
  - Pulmonary embolism

DIFFERENTIAL DIAGNOSIS

Not all wheezing is due to asthma (Table 172.1). Obstruction of the airway at any level can produce wheezing and dyspnea that can be confused with asthma. For example, vocal cord dysfunction syndrome [29] is an extrathoracic cause of episodic upper airway obstruction that can be confused with acute asthma. This diagnosis is suggested by the presence of stridor and wheeze in the absence of increased alveolar-arterial oxygen tension difference, extrathoracic variable obstruction on the flow-volume loop of pulmonary function tests, and by observing paradoxic closure of vocal cords during inspiration during laryngoscopy.

Furthermore, many disease processes other than asthma can obstruct the lower airways to produce wheezing and dyspnea (Table 172.1). Systemic anaphylaxis can cause wheezing and should be considered among the differential diagnoses especially when respiratory symptoms have been of rapid onset or progression [30]. A diagnosis of anaphylaxis is suggested by acute-onset wheezing, stridor, urticaria, nausea, diarrhea, and hypotension (especially after insect bites, drug administration, or intravenous contrast). Exacerbations of chronic obstructive pulmonary disease (COPD) present similarly to acute asthma, but chronic bronchitis or emphysema, or both, can usually be distinguished from asthma historically. However, consensus guidelines do recognize an asthma–COPD overlap syndrome that is characterized by chronic airflow obstruction and the presence of features that are associated with both asthma and COPD [1,31]. Pulmonary thromboembolism can masquerade as an exacerbation of asthma because the mediators released by platelets from thromboemboli sometimes cause bronchoconstriction and wheezing. However, hemoptysis, pleuritic pain, and pleural effusions rarely are seen in acute exacerbations of asthma.

Pulmonary edema, either cardiogenic or non-cardiogenic, can obstruct small airways with mucosal swelling to produce acute wheezing. However, in these cases the clinical history, physical examination, and chest radiographic changes that show vascular redistribution of blood flow and alveolar filling help exclude asthma as the primary diagnosis. Notably, however, acute, reversible left ventricular dysfunction (e.g., takotsubo cardiomyopathy) has been described as a possible complication of severe exacerbations of asthma; the underlying mechanism for this is unclear, but it may be due to the acute effects of intensive treatment with β-adrenergic agonists [32]. Aspiration can present with acute dyspnea and wheezing. In this case, a history of impaired consciousness or inability to protect the airway suggests the diagnosis and chest radiograph or ultrasound examination may show pulmonary infiltration.

ASSESSMENT

Failure of the physician to appreciate the severity of airway obstruction in acute asthma is not uncommon. The cornerstone of evaluation of patients with asthma exacerbations is the objective measurement of airflow. However, because some patients, especially those with severe exacerbations, may be unable to perform the necessary testing maneuvers, the physician also must be adept at recognizing certain historical features and physical findings that strongly suggest high risk for severe airway obstruction.

History

A history of baseline pulmonary function tests that show persistent decreases of the forced expired volume of air in 1 second (FEV_1), loss of lung elastic recoil, and hyperinflation at total lung capacity are associated with increased risk of near-fatal asthma [33]. A recent history of poorly controlled asthma (increases of dyspnea and wheezing, frequent nocturnal awakenings due to shortness of breath, increased use of β-adrenergic rescue medications, increased diurnal variability of peak expiratory flow, and recent hospitalizations or emergency department visits) and any history of a prior near-fatal asthma exacerbation (prior admission to an intensive care unit or intubation for asthma) are the most important predictors of a patient's propensity for severe life-threatening asthma exacerbations [1,2,34–37]. Current or recent use of oral corticosteroids, not currently using inhaled corticosteroids, a history of psychosocial problems, poor adherence with asthma medications, and a history of food allergies are other warnings that the patient is at risk of asthma-related death [1,2]. Patient complaints of severe breathlessness or chest tightness or difficulty walking more than 100 feet (30.48 m) also suggest severe airway obstruction. Cigarette smoking also has been associated with higher in-hospital and posthospitalization mortality [38]. In general, patients are somewhat better judges of the severity of their airway obstruction during an attack of asthma than are physicians who elicit their history at the bedside [39]. However, the patient's own assessment of airway obstruction should never be the exclusive means of assessing the severity of airway obstruction. Notably, patients with a history of severe asthma sometimes have a blunted perception of dyspnea [40,41]. When assessing risk for fatal asthma, other important historical details include identification of current medications and coexisting illnesses, such as psychiatric disease, that interfere with medical follow-up and cardiopulmonary disease. A history of known coronary artery disease is important because the patient may be more sensitive to the stimulatory effects of β_2-adrenergic agonists and to the cardiac complications of hypoxemia. These patients may also be receiving β_2-adrenergic antagonists that are making control of their asthma worse.

Physical Examination

Physical examination is important for excluding other causes of dyspnea (see Differential Diagnosis section) and assessing the degree of airway obstruction. Tachycardia (greater than 120 beats per minute), tachypnea (greater than 30 breaths per minute), diaphoresis, bolt-upright posture in bed, pulsus paradoxus greater than 10 mm Hg, and accessory respiratory muscle use all should be regarded as signs of severe airway obstruction [42]. However, because the absence of these signs does not rule out severe obstruction, physical examination cannot be relied on exclusively to estimate the severity of airway obstruction. The amount of wheezing heard on auscultation of the chest is a notoriously poor method of assessing the severity of airway obstruction [43]. Cyanosis is a late, insensitive finding of severe hypoxemia. Abnormal thoracoabdominal motion (e.g., respiratory muscle alternans, abdominal paradox) and depressed mental status due to hypoxemia and hypercapnia are ominous indicators and can herald the necessity for emergent mechanical ventilation [44].

Pulmonary Function Tests

To evaluate a patient who is having an acute exacerbation of asthma, an objective measure of maximal expiratory airflow should be performed [1,2]. An exception to this is the patient who is unable to perform a testing maneuver due to a severe, life-threatening exacerbation with obvious airway compromise and cyanosis. Peak expiratory airflow rate (PEFR) and FEV_1 are equally acceptable bedside measures to quantify the degree of airway obstruction. These tests are valuable for the initial assessment and for assessing responses to therapy, especially after 1 hour of treatment [1]. In general, a pretreatment PEFR or FEV_1 of less than 50% of baseline (either the predicted value or the patient's best-known value) indicates a severe exacerbation of asthma. Guidelines recommend reassessment of lung function one hour after initiation of treatment and then frequent reassessments thereafter (Table 172.2) [1,2,45].

Arterial Blood Gas Analysis

Analysis of arterial blood gases (ABGs) has a role in assessing and managing severe asthma exacerbations (see Chapter 27) and should be performed for suspected hypoventilation, severe respiratory distress, or when spirometric test results are less than 25% predicted [37]. Also, any patient who fails to respond to the first 30 to 60 minutes of intensive bronchodilator therapy should have an ABG analysis performed. Although ABG values are not predictive of overall patient outcomes, there is some correlation between hypoxemia and hypercapnia and the degree of airway obstruction measured by FEV_1. A partial pressure of arterial oxygen (PaO_2) less than 60 mm Hg or a pulse oximeter oxygen saturation value less than 90% on room air should be regarded as additional evidence that the patient's exacerbation is severe. Therefore, although ABG analysis is not recommended as routine during the initial evaluation of a patient with an acute exacerbation of asthma, it should be done for the evaluation

TABLE 172.2

Objective Assessment of Airway Obstruction after Initial One Hour of Intensive Therapy

Posttreatment PEFR or FEV_1	Response	Hospitalization?
>60% predicted	Good	No, unless risk factor
≥40% but ≤60% predicted	Incomplete	Consider risk factors
<40% predicted	Poor	Recommended

FEV_1, forced expired volume in 1 second; PEFR, peak expiratory flow rate.

of severe cases. One study did find that the frequency of ABG analysis in the initial evaluation of severe exacerbations decreased from 1997 to 2000 and that study suggested that ABG's may be underutilized in the evaluation of severe exacerbations [46].

Understanding the expected changes of the partial pressure of arterial carbon dioxide ($PaCO_2$) during an asthma exacerbation is important for recognition of a rapidly deteriorating course. With modest airway obstruction, the patient's mild dyspnea stimulates an increase in minute ventilation that meets or exceeds the level required to maintain normal alveolar ventilation. Thus, patients with modest obstruction have a normal or slightly below normal $PaCO_2$. As airway obstruction worsens, dyspnea becomes more severe and the central nervous system drive to increase minute ventilation becomes intense. Typically, the increase in minute ventilation exceeds the level required to maintain constant alveolar ventilation; consequently, patients with moderate-to-severe obstruction have lower than normal $PaCO_2$ and an acute respiratory alkalosis. As the airway obstruction becomes more severe and prolonged, high minute ventilation can no longer be maintained by the respiratory musculature and alveolar ventilation decreases. As a result, the $PaCO_2$ rises toward normal and then continues to climb, resulting in hypercapnia and respiratory acidosis. Thus, a normal or high $PaCO_2$ (greater than 40 mm Hg) during a severe exacerbation of asthma is a potentially ominous finding, often signifying the impending need for mechanical ventilation. Any coexisting conditions (malnutrition, advanced age) or medications (sedatives) that weaken respiratory muscle function or depress respiratory drive should be expected to accelerate the onset of hypercapnic ventilatory failure during acute exacerbations of asthma.

Other Laboratory Studies

For acute exacerbations of asthma, routine chest radiographs reveal few abnormalities other than hyperinflation [47]. However, although not recommended for routine assessment, for severe exacerbations chest radiography can be helpful when there is clinical suspicion of other causes of dyspnea and wheezing (see Differential Diagnosis section) or complications of severe airway obstruction [37]. Chest radiographs should be examined for evidence of enlarged cardiac silhouette, upper lung zone redistribution of blood flow, pleural effusions, and alveolar or interstitial infiltrates because any one of these findings suggests a diagnosis other than or in addition to acute asthma. In addition, chest radiography allows the early detection of common complications of severe airway obstruction, including pneumothorax, pneumomediastinum, and atelectasis. Also, lung infiltrates on chest radiographs can be compatible with a diagnosis of asthma complicated by mucoid impactions (e.g., V or Y or cluster of grapes-shaped densities) and/or complications associated with them (e.g., lobar collapse), allergic bronchopulmonary aspergillosis or eosinophilic granulomatosis with polyangiitis (Churg–Strauss syndrome).

Among the elderly, for patients with severe hypoxemia, and for individuals with suspected cardiac ischemia or arrhythmias, an electrocardiogram should be performed. Sinus tachycardia is common during acute exacerbations of asthma, but less common and transient findings include right-axis deviation, right ventricular hypertrophy and strain, P pulmonale, ST- and T-wave abnormalities, right bundle-branch block, and ventricular ectopic beats [48].

THERAPEUTIC AGENTS

Optimal management of an acute exacerbation of asthma begins with a careful assessment of the degree of airway obstruction. This initial assessment and repeated objective measures of airway obstruction guide treatment that combines supportive measures, bronchodilator therapy, and anti-inflammatory therapy (Table 172.3).

TABLE 172.3

Treatment of Severe Acute Exacerbations of Asthma

- Pharmacologic agents
  - Anti-inflammatory agents
    - Systemic corticosteroids (oral preferred unless impaired intestinal absorption)
  - Bronchodilators
    - Inhaled, short-acting β_2-adrenergic agonists
    - Inhaled, short-acting cholinergic antagonists
    - Intravenous $MgSO_4$ (not routine; consider in severe, refractory cases)
    - Oral or intravenous methylxanthines (not routine or recommended)
    - Systemic β_2-adrenergic agonists (not routine or recommended)
    - General anesthetics (not routine)
- Supportive measures
  - Frequent reassessment
  - Supplemental oxygen
  - Fluid management
  - Invasive mechanical ventilation if needed (controlled hypoventilation)
  - Helium–oxygen mixtures to drive nebulizer (not routine; consider in severe, refractory cases)
  - Lavage by bronchoscopy (not routine, intubated patients only)
- Education
  - Avoidance of asthma triggers
  - Medication use
  - Access to medical follow-up
  - Home monitoring of airway obstruction

Because the dominant causes of airway obstruction during an acute exacerbation of asthma are the result of airway inflammation, the cornerstone of treatment is anti-inflammatory therapy with systemic corticosteroids, administered within 1 hour of presentation [49]. Because corticosteroids take at least 4 to 6 hours to begin to have a beneficial effect and many of the inflammatory causes of airway obstruction may take days to resolve, the medical challenge is to support patients until the inflammatory processes have responded to corticosteroids.

β_2-Adrenergic agonists relieve airway obstruction due to airway smooth muscle contraction, and this is an important therapeutic maneuver during initial treatment. Although these bronchodilators relieve only one component of the airway obstruction during severe exacerbations of asthma, even small improvements of airflow can lead to important clinical benefits in the acute setting. Of the available bronchodilators, β_2-adrenergic agonists are the most effective and rapidly acting and, therefore, most useful during that critical time before the onset of corticosteroid action [50]. Other measures that support the patient until the inflammatory processes in the airways have resolved include supplemental oxygen, judicious fluid administration, and, when indicated, mechanical ventilation.

β_2-Adrenergic Agonists

β_2-Adrenergic agonists bind to β_2-adrenergic receptors on airway smooth muscle cells and cause relaxation of the muscle cell [51].

Although the primary cellular target of β_2-adrenergic agonists is airway smooth muscle, other cell types in the airways also express β_2-adrenergic receptors that may regulate mediator release by mast cells, epithelial cells, and nerves. There are three general classes of β_2-adrenergic agonists [52]. First, short-acting β_2-adrenergic agonists (SABA) have bronchodilatory effects that last for 3 to 5 hours. They include epinephrine, isoproterenol, terbutaline, metaproterenol, albuterol, and fenoterol. These short-acting agents are rapidly acting with an onset of action less than 5 minutes and are the mainstay of bronchodilator therapy for acute asthma, especially albuterol [1,2]. Second, there are the long-acting β_2-adrenergic agonists (LABA) that have either slowly or rapidly acting bronchodilatory effects lasting for at least 12 hours. Third, there are the ultra long-acting β_2-adrenergic agonists (ultra-LABA) that have half-lives suitable for once-daily dosing. Neither LABA nor ultra-LABA is currently recommended for the treatment of acute asthma exacerbations [1].

Among SABA medications, a single-isomer preparation (i.e., R-albuterol or levalbuterol) for inhalation is available. The potential advantage of this preparation is that the S-enantiomer present in racemic albuterol does not contribute to bronchodilation and might have deleterious effects on the airways. However, there have not been large, randomized, double-blind, and controlled trials in adults to show that this theoretical concern is clinically important. Moreover, a systematic review and meta-analysis of smaller studies concluded that levalbuterol was not superior to albuterol with respect to either efficacy or safety in the treatment of acute asthma exacerbations [53].

The major side effects of β_2-adrenergic agonists during the treatment of severe asthma exacerbations are tremor, cardiac stimulation, hypokalemia, and hyperlactatemia [52,54]. These side effects are potentially serious, especially in the elderly, who frequently have underlying cardiac disease. Cardiac toxicity can be minimized by using agonists with high β_2-adrenergic receptor selectivity, by avoiding systemic administration of β_2-adrenergic agonists, and by maintaining adequate oxygenation [55].

β_2-Adrenergic agonists can be administered to patients by inhalational, subcutaneous, or intravenous routes. Numerous studies have shown that the bronchodilator effects of inhaled β_2-adrenergic agonists are rapid in onset and equal to the effect achieved by systemic delivery [56]. Because the inhaled route allows administration of comparatively small doses directly to the airways with minimal systemic toxicity, this route is almost always preferable to systemic delivery [1,2].

Several options exist for the delivery of inhaled β_2-adrenergic agonists (see Chapter 169). A small-volume nebulizer is widely used. However, studies have shown that metered-dose inhalers (MDIs) equipped with spacer devices are as effective as small-volume nebulizers in the treatment of acute asthma, although some patients may have difficulty coordinating MDI use, especially during an acute exacerbation with severe respiratory distress [1,2,57,58]. Frequent, multiple inhalations of the medication may allow for progressively deeper penetration of the drug into peripheral airways. In fact, continuous administration by nebulizer may be more effective for severely obstructed patients [59,60]. For administration of inhaled albuterol in the treatment of severe exacerbations of asthma, National Institutes of Health guidelines recommend treatment with MDI (90 μg per puff; four to eight puffs every 20 minutes up to 4 hours, then every 1 to 4 hours as needed) or nebulizer treatments, either intermittent (2.5 to 5.0 mg every 20 minutes for three doses, then every 1 to 4 hours as needed) or continuous (10 to 15 mg per hour) [2] (see Management section).

Because of its lower density than oxygen, helium–oxygen (heliox)–powered nebulizer treatments have the potential to improve penetration of aerosols into the lungs. However, a systematic review with meta-analysis comparing heliox versus air–oxygen driven nebulization found no support for helium-powered nebulization in the routine care of acute exacerbations of asthma [61]. However, the method may be considered for patients not responding to standard therapies [1].

Theoretically, systemic administration of β-adrenergic agonists could deliver drugs via the bloodstream to obstructed airways that are poorly accessible to inhaled aerosols. However, this theoretical advantage has not been supported by most studies. Subcutaneous epinephrine (adults, 0.3 mL of a 1 to 1,000 solution every 20 minutes for three doses) was a traditional therapy for acute asthma in emergency departments, but it is not more effective than aerosol delivery of β_2-adrenergic agonists [1,2]. A major concern with the use of subcutaneous epinephrine to adults has been cardiac toxicity. More selective β_2-adrenergic agonists, such as terbutaline, are available for subcutaneous use, but cardiac toxicity among elderly individuals is still a significant concern even with these more selective agents. Formerly, intravenous isoproterenol (0.05 to 1.50 μg/kg/minute) was formerly used to treat severe exacerbations of asthma. However, intravenous delivery of β_2-adrenergic agonists is no longer recommended for the routine treatment of even severe exacerbations of asthma [1,2]. No convincing evidence has shown intravenous administration to be superior to inhaled delivery of β_2-adrenergic agonists [56,62]. Both the lack of enhanced efficacy and the potential cardiac toxicity of intravenous β_2-adrenergic agonists have led most authorities to reserve intravenous delivery for those rare adult patients, closely monitored, who continue to deteriorate on mechanical ventilation despite maximal routine therapy with inhaled β_2-adrenergic agonists. It is important to emphasize again that intravenous β_2-adrenergic agonists are not recommended in guidelines and are unlikely to be any more effective than inhaled β_2-adrenergic agonists such as albuterol [1,2].

Cholinergic Antagonists

For asthma, the muscarinic cholinergic antagonists (e.g., atropine, ipratropium, and tiotropium) are less effective and more slowly acting bronchodilators than β_2-adrenergic agonists [52,63,64]. In general, these agents should not be used as the sole bronchodilator therapy for acute asthma. Exceptions may be bronchospasm induced by acetylcholinesterase inhibitors or β_2-adrenergic antagonists and patients with severe cardiac disease who are unable to tolerate β_2-adrenergic agonists.

However, inhaled cholinergic antagonists have a low incidence of side effects and are a recommended adjunct to β_2-adrenergic agonists for the initial treatment of severe exacerbations of asthma [1,2,65,66]. Because even small improvements of airway caliber could prove clinically significant for the severely obstructed and deteriorating patient, it is recommended that ipratropium be routinely added to β_2-adrenergic agonist therapy during the initial treatment of severe asthma exacerbations in the emergency department [1] (see Management section). However, inhaled ipratropium bromide currently is not recommended for routine use once a patient is hospitalized with a severe exacerbation of asthma [1,2]. The long-acting anticholinergic, tiotropium, has a role in treating outpatients with difficult to control asthma, but it does not have any established role for treating hospitalized patients with acute exacerbations of asthma [1,2,67].

Methylxanthines

Because the literature does not demonstrate a benefit to adding methylxanthines to β_2-adrenergic agonists in the acute setting and because they increase toxicity, methylxanthines are no longer recommended for the treatment of asthma exacerbations [1,2,68–70].

For the rare, critically ill patient whose condition is acutely deteriorating despite maximal recommended therapy with bronchodilators, corticosteroids, and other adjuncts [1,2], the use of methylxanthines might be considered by some physicians, although data are not supportive [71]. For patients not already taking methylxanthines, a loading dose of aminophylline (6 mg/kg lean body weight) can be administered over 20 to 30 minutes, followed by an intravenous infusion at the rate of 0.6 mg/kg/h. This infusion rate should be decreased when conditions are present that decrease methylxanthine clearance, especially congestive heart failure, cirrhosis, and the use of drugs such as cimetidine, ranitidine, allopurinol, oral contraceptives, erythromycin, ciprofloxacin, or norfloxacin. Six hours after initiation of the infusion, the serum theophylline level should be checked and the infusion rate adjusted accordingly, with 10 to 15 μg/mL being therapeutic. Serum concentrations greater than 20 μg/mL are toxic.

Corticosteroids

Numerous studies have documented the safety and effectiveness of short courses of corticosteroids for the treatment of acute exacerbations of asthma [1,72–74]. Their beneficial effects are attributed to their many potent anti-inflammatory effects on multiple cell types [72,75].

Systemic corticosteroids are the principal therapy for acute exacerbations of asthma [1,2]. Prednisone, prednisolone, and methylprednisolone are the preferred agents. Compared with betamethasone and dexamethasone, neither prednisone nor methylprednisolone contain metabisulfites, and both have shorter half-lives. Although hydrocortisone has the shortest half-life, it has greater mineralocorticoid effect and may cause idiosyncratic bronchospasm in some aspirin-sensitive individuals [76].

The optimal route of corticosteroid administration (i.e., oral vs. intravenous) during the treatment of acute asthma is not well established by double-blind, placebo-controlled clinical studies. For initial treatment of an acute exacerbation of asthma, studies suggest that oral administration of corticosteroids is as effective as intravenous therapy [1,2,77,78]. Therefore, the oral route is preferred unless there is the possibility of impaired gastrointestinal tract transit time or absorption.

Inhaled corticosteroids do not have a well-established role for the treatment of acute exacerbations of asthma of hospitalized patients. However, in the Emergency Department setting inhaled, high-dose corticosteroids decrease hospitalization rates for patients not receiving systemic corticosteroids, but their benefit for patients receiving additional, systemic corticosteroids is not established [1,79].

The optimum dosages of corticosteroids for the treatment of acute asthma are also not well established by randomized controlled clinical trials [1,2,80]. One study compared 15, 40, and 125 mg methylprednisolone every 6 hours and suggested that patients improved most rapidly with the 125 mg dose [81]. However, most studies have failed to show a dose–response relationship for doses this high [80]. For example, one study showed no difference between 100 and 500 mg methylprednisolone for the emergency department treatment of asthma [82].

For adults, 2007 NIH guidelines recommend that prednisone, methylprednisolone, or prednisolone all be given at 40 to 80 mg per day in one or two divided doses until PEFR is 70% of predicted or personal best [2]. The Global Initiative for Asthma (GINA) guidelines updated in 2015 describe appropriate dosing as the equivalent of 50 mg of prednisone as a single daily dose or the equivalent of 200 mg of hydrocortisone in divided doses as being adequate in most cases [1]. According to NIH guidelines the duration of systemic corticosteroid treatment for a patient requiring an emergency department visit or a hospitalization is usually 3 to 10 days [2]. GINA guidelines recommend a 5- to 7-day course for adults [1,83,84]. For courses of treatment lasting less than 1 week and for courses lasting up to 10 days, there is no established benefit to slowly tapering the daily oral corticosteroid dose, especially when the patient is also using inhaled corticosteroids [1].

Oxygen

Supplemental oxygen therapy should be the initial intervention in the emergency department [1,2]. Because ventilation–perfusion mismatch is the dominant cause of hypoxemia with asthma, the PaO_2 usually increases readily in response to low levels (2 to 4 L per minute oxygen by nasal prongs) of supplemental oxygen therapy. Studies have shown that titrated, low-flow oxygen therapy to achieve oxygen saturations of 93% to 95% is associated with better outcomes than the routine use of untitrated, high flow, 100% oxygen therapy [85,86]. In addition to mitigating the cardiac and neurologic complications of severe hypoxemia, low-flow supplemental oxygen minimizes potential episodes of hypoxemia due to the acute administration of β_2-adrenergic agonists, decreases elevated pulmonary vascular pressures due to hypoxic vasoconstriction, decreases bronchospasm due to hypoxia, and improves oxygen delivery to respiratory muscles.

Fluids

No convincing evidence has shown that fluid administration in excess of euvolemia hastens mobilization of inspissated secretions from the airways. Fluid therapy should be used conservatively unless significant dehydration is present.

Other Agents

Intravenous magnesium sulfate (for adults, 2 g $MgSO_4$ in 50 mL saline during 20 minutes) has bronchodilator properties. Magnesium sulfate is not recommended for routine use of the treatment of asthma exacerbations, but it may be considered for the treatment of the most severe asthma exacerbations (FEV_1<25% to 30% or hypoxemia refractory to initial treatment) [1]. Additional study is needed, but some evidence suggests that its use may reduce hospitalization rates for the most severely obstructed patients who have an FEV_1 less than 25% of predicted [87]. Although the data are mixed, inhaled, rather than intravenous, magnesium sulfate may also have a role in the treatment of acute asthma. That is, for severe asthma exacerbations, albuterol nebulized diluted in magnesium sulfate solution may be a more effective bronchodilator than albuterol nebulized in normal saline [88,89].

Because of its lower gas density, some improvement in airway resistance may be achieved by delivering a mixture of helium and oxygen gases to patients with airway obstruction. However, guidelines do not recommend the routine use of heliox for the treatment of asthma and suggest that it be considered only for rare, severe cases unresponsive to standard therapies [1,2].

Some therapeutic agents that are used for the treatment of stable asthma have no established role in the treatment of severe exacerbations of asthma among hospitalized patients. These include aerosolized corticosteroids and sodium cromolyn as well as oral β_2-adrenergic agonists that may cause significant systemic toxicities. Although there is as yet no established role for the use of leukotriene antagonists for the treatment of acute asthma exacerbations, some evidence suggests a possible role and need for further study [90,91]. Mucus is an important cause of airway obstruction during acute exacerbations of asthma, but the routine use of mucolytics, such as acetylcysteine, potassium iodide, or human recombinant deoxyribonuclease (DNase), has not been shown to be effective for treating severe exacerbations of asthma, and at least one of these agents, acetylcysteine, may worsen cough and bronchospasm [92]. However, it is notable that acetylcysteine and DNase may be helpful during therapeutic bronchoscopy (see Additional and Unconventional Management Measures section).

Bacterial infections appear to play, at most, a minor role in the precipitation of severe asthma exacerbations [1,2]; for this reason, antibiotics are not routinely administered unless an active bacterial infectious process, particularly pneumonia or bacterial sinusitis, is suspected. However, intriguing evidence suggests that infections due to *Chlamydia pneumoniae* might play a role in the pathogenesis of asthma exacerbations for some patients [93].

Unless a patient is mechanically ventilated, sedation has no role in the treatment of severe exacerbations of asthma [1,2]. Opioids and other sedating medications may depress the respiratory central drive to breathe that is critical for adequate minute ventilation. Theoretically, some opioids also may cause mast cell degranulation and worsen bronchospasm.

TABLE 172.4

Factors Favoring Hospitalization after Initial Bronchodilator Therapy

Poor response to initial therapy
OR
Incomplete response to initial therapy and one or more of the following:
- History of endotracheal intubation or ICU admission for asthma
- Recent emergency department visit for asthma
- Recent hospitalization for asthma
- Multiple emergency department visits for asthma in last year
- Duration of current exacerbation >1 week
- Current use of oral corticosteroids
- Home situation inadequate for follow-up
- Psychiatric conditions that may interfere with medical compliance
- History of syncope or seizures during prior exacerbations

MANAGEMENT

Emergency Department

The National Asthma Education and Prevention Program and GINA have published and updated guidelines for the assessment and management of patients with asthma and these guidelines include the treatment of acute exacerbations [1,2]. These guidelines have been widely accepted, and we recommend them. Initial management of a patient with an acute exacerbation of asthma is based on the physician's assessment of the degree of airway obstruction and the patient's response to initial bronchodilator therapy using β_2-adrenergic agonists. If, during the initial assessment, the patient is in extreme distress and has evidence of fatigue, impaired consciousness, or hypercapnia such that respiratory arrest is judged imminent, endotracheal intubation and mechanical ventilation should be the first priorities and then systemic corticosteroids and nebulized β_2-adrenergic agonists and ipratropium should be started immediately. On the other hand, when respiratory arrest is not impending within minutes, 2 to 4 L per minute of supplemental oxygen should be initiated to keep oxygen saturation 93% to 95%; β_2-adrenergic agonists should be delivered by aerosol for three doses over 60 to 90 minutes (e.g., albuterol, 2.5 to 5.0 mg, every 20 minutes by small-volume nebulizer, then 2.5 to 10 mg every 1 to 4 hours as needed, or 10 to 15 mg per hour continuously or, alternatively, albuterol, 90 μg per puff, four to eight puffs by MDI with spacer every 20 minutes up to 4 hours, then every 1 to 4 hours as needed). When the PEFR is less than 50% of the predicted value, an oral (preferred) or intravenous systemic corticosteroid should be started immediately (e.g., prednisone 1 mg/kg/d up to 50 mg maximum or equivalent) and an inhaled anticholinergic as well (e.g., ipratropium bromide, 0.5 mg by nebulizer). After these treatments are initiated, a more detailed history and physical and laboratory examination can be completed. Close monitoring and repeated airflow measurements are critical for detecting further deterioration during this initial period of treatment.

After the initial treatment with a bronchodilator, patients are reassessed. Those who do not respond substantially (FEV_1 or PEFR greater than 60% of predicted) within 1 hour to initial treatment with β_2-adrenergic agonists should be given systemic corticosteroids (if not already given). Oral prednisone is generally recommended unless there is concern that gastrointestinal tract absorption will be less than optimal [1,2].

In addition to corticosteroids, treatment with β_2-adrenergic agonists and inhaled anticholinergics is continued for 1 to 3 hours with frequent reassessment. Patients who achieve an FEV_1 or PEFR of greater than 60% during this 1- to 3-hour period should be observed for at least 1 additional hour to ensure stability of the improvement. In one study, two-thirds of patients who presented to the emergency department responded to albuterol, with the FEV_1 increasing to at least 60% of predicted [94]. Many patients with such a good response do not require hospitalization. Exceptions are patients with a history that is suggestive of high risk for mortality from asthma (e.g., history of intubation and mechanical ventilation; Table 172.4). Patients discharged from the emergency department should be continued on systemic corticosteroids and β_2-adrenergic agonists, considered for initiation of inhaled corticosteroids, given instructions regarding medication use, given an action plan in case symptoms worsen, and given specific instructions for medical follow-up [1,2,67,95,96].

Patients who have an FEV_1 or PEFR that is greater than 40% but less than 60% after 4 hours of treatment have an incomplete response and require a careful triage decision. Some patients do well when discharged with detailed instructions, close medical follow-up, and continued systemic corticosteroids. However, other patients do poorly if discharged. It has been recommended that patients with incomplete responses be hospitalized when there is any clinical feature to suggest high risk for asthma mortality (Table 172.4). Patients with an FEV_1 or PEFR of less than 40% of predicted after 4 hours of intensive bronchodilator therapy (poor response) should be hospitalized, often in an intensive care unit (ICU) setting.

Treatment During Pregnancy

Pregnancy should not alter treatment of an acute exacerbation of asthma. Because severe asthma exacerbations have been associated with increased perinatal mortality, probably due to maternal hypoxia and respiratory alkalosis, the excellent control of asthma should be a main priority [97] (see Chapter 164). However, unfortunately, many pregnant women are suboptimally treated for asthma in the acute setting [98]. This is unfortunate because, in both the chronic and the acute setting, abundant evidence supports the safety of β_2-adrenergic agonist use during pregnancy [99]. Also, although chronic administration of systemic corticosteroids throughout pregnancy appears to carry some risk to the fetus, short courses of corticosteroids are considered safe for the fetus compared with the serious risks associated with poorly controlled asthma. Therefore, corticosteroids should not be withheld from pregnant women, who present with an acute asthma exacerbation. Treatment of chronic asthma during pregnancy should include inhaled corticosteroids [100], which is important for preventing development of acute asthma exacerbations [101].

Routine Inpatient Management

Most patients with severe exacerbations of asthma, who are admitted to the hospital, can be monitored and managed safely on a hospital ward that is well staffed by physicians, experienced nursing personnel, and respiratory therapists. However, patients with severe airway obstruction who are at high risk for mortality from asthma, especially those with an elevated $PaCO_2$ (greater than 42 mm Hg) or changes of mental status despite initial intensive bronchodilator therapy, need the close monitoring of an ICU setting for possible intubation and mechanical ventilation.

Pharmacotherapy for hospitalized patients includes a continuation of the inhaled β_2-adrenergic agonists and systemic corticosteroids begun in the emergency department [1,2]. Specifically, it is not recommended that ipratropium bromide be routinely continued once a patient is hospitalized [1]. For patients with severe airway obstruction and only transient relief from treatment, inhaled β_2-adrenergic agonists can be administered frequently as needed (e.g., every 20 minutes). For patients with less severe obstruction or those with intolerable side effects, frequency can be reduced accordingly. Most patients require β_2-adrenergic agonists a minimum of every 4 hours; however, a study has shown that ad libitum administration of albuterol every 4 hours is as effective as regularly timed administration of albuterol [102]. Evidence indicates that delivery of β_2-adrenergic agonists by small-volume nebulizer and delivery by MDI with spacer give equivalent results [1,2,71].

Most hospitalized patients begin to show improvement in expiratory airflow after 6 to 12 hours of systemic corticosteroid therapy, but improvement sufficient for hospital discharge frequently takes 2 to 7 days. In one series, mean length of hospital stay was 4 days, with a range of 0.5 to 17.0 days [103]. Expiratory airflow should be followed to assess the patient's progress. Patient exercise tolerance and PEFR usually improve incrementally during hospitalization, but it is common for patients recovering from exacerbations to have a hospital course punctuated by periods of worsening dyspnea, especially at night. These episodes of nocturnal worsening require patient assessment but generally respond well to inhaled β_2-adrenergic agonists. When the expiratory flow rate does not improve during the initial days of hospitalization, additional or alternative diagnoses, especially laryngeal dysfunction, congestive heart failure, and pulmonary thromboembolism, as well as gastroesophageal reflux disease and sinusitis, should be considered.

As the hospitalized patient recovers, the intensity of therapy is decreased gradually. When the patient has minimal or no wheezing, is no longer awakened by dyspnea at night, can tolerate activity without oxygen desaturation of hemoglobin, and has expiratory flow rates that have substantially improved, he or she is ready for hospital discharge. Patients generally should have a PEFR at least 70% of baseline at the time of discharge. Other patients with an incomplete response to therapy (50% to 70% of baseline) should be assessed individually.

Discharge planning is important for preventing future exacerbations (Table 172.5) [1,2]. Patients must be educated about asthma and the importance of seeking medical advice early in the course of exacerbations. Particularly important are detailed instructions on MDI use, routine measurement of PEFR, and keeping a symptom diary at home. On discharge, the patient is given medication instructions with particular attention to oral and inhaled corticosteroids (see Corticosteroids section). This is important because bronchial hyperresponsiveness remains high for at least 10 days after discharge from an ICU for severe asthma [104]. Patients who have recovered from an exacerbation of asthma should be instructed to use short-acting inhaled β_2-adrenergic agonists on an as-needed basis only.

TABLE 172.5

Discharge Planning

Medications
Inhaled β_2-adrenergic agonists
Inhaled corticosteroids
Oral corticosteroids (with plan for cessation)
Education
Avoidance of asthma triggers
Home monitoring of peak expiratory flow rates
Metered-dose inhaler techniques
Action plan if relapse starts
Appointment for medical follow-up
Asthma comanagement program

MANAGEMENT OF SEVERE RESPIRATORY FAILURE

Assessment

When acute hypoxemic or hypercapnic respiratory failure is severe, mechanical ventilation is potentially life-saving. Patients with severe obstruction can be supported with mechanical ventilation for the vital hours needed for corticosteroid action. However, mechanical ventilation for a severe asthma exacerbation can be complicated by morbidity and mortality, with associated mortality ranging from 0% to 38% in the literature [105–107].

The decision to initiate mechanical ventilation for a severe asthma exacerbation should be based on a number of considerations individualized for each patient [107]. For patients with severe distress for whom respiratory arrest has already occurred or is imminent, the need for intubation and mechanical ventilation is self-evident. The possibility of pneumothorax should be promptly addressed for these patients. Patients who are not *in extremis* should be monitored closely during initial bronchodilator therapy, and the physician should be prepared to perform intubation in case of substantial deterioration. The decision to intubate during a severe asthma exacerbation is a clinical judgment. For severely obstructed patients with decreasing objective measures of airflow, worsening mental status, or signs of respiratory muscle fatigue despite bronchodilator therapy, urgent intubation and mechanical ventilation should be strongly considered. In general, any patient who responds poorly to initial bronchodilator therapy and has an initial $PaCO_2$ of 40 mm Hg or more in association with moderately severe hypoxemia should have close serial clinical assessment and ABG monitoring. For patients with a $PaCO_2$ of greater than 55 to 70 mm Hg, increasing $PaCO_2$ (greater than 5 mm Hg per hour) in association with a PaO_2 of less than 60 mm Hg or the presence of metabolic acidosis, intubation, and mechanical ventilation should be very strongly considered. However, it is emphasized that when clinical signs indicate a need for intubation, the decision to intubate should be made immediately and never delayed, waiting for an ABG result. The role of noninvasive positive-pressure ventilation when managing patients with acute asthma is not established and guidelines do not make recommendations on its application, but they do emphasize close monitoring and avoidance of sedation if noninvasive mechanical ventilation is attempted [1,2,108] (see Chapter 167).

Endotracheal Intubation

Airway control should be established by the most experienced personnel available because even minor manipulation of the larynx and trachea can precipitate vagal reflexes that elicit laryngospasm and bronchospasm. Atropine can be given before intubation to attenuate these vagally mediated reflexes. Lidocaine can be used to achieve topical anesthesia of the hypopharynx and larynx, but even lidocaine has been associated with bronchospasm [109]. Administration of a short- and rapid-acting intravenous benzodiazepine often can facilitate patient relaxation and preoxygenation, allowing time for a controlled intubation that minimally irritates the larynx and trachea. Opiates are not used for intubation or sedation in asthmatic patients because some narcotics can provoke nausea and vomiting and theoretically can provoke histamine release that worsens bronchospasm.

Oral, rather than nasal, intubation is preferred for patients with a severe asthma exacerbation because nasal polyps and sinusitis are common in asthma and because the oral route allows placement of a larger endotracheal tube (internal diameter, 8 mm).

Invasive Mechanical Ventilation

The guiding principle for mechanical ventilation during a severe exacerbation of asthma is to provide adequate oxygenation while minimizing the risk of barotrauma (Table 172.6). Because the risk of barotrauma is related to dynamic hyperinflation of the lungs and high plateau airway pressures, a ventilatory strategy that minimizes lung volumes and airway pressures should be used [1,2,107]. (See Chapter 166 for a discussion of initiating mechanical ventilation.)

With outmoded mechanical ventilation strategies that aimed to normalize the $PaCO_2$, the required high tidal volumes and rapid frequencies of ventilation promoted increased air trapping and high airway pressures. Most authorities now believe that high airway pressures are to be avoided because they are a major cause of serious morbidity and mortality during mechanical ventilation of asthmatic patients [107,110–116].

The modern strategy for mechanical ventilation for a severe exacerbation of asthma is controlled hypoventilation with permissive hypercapnia [1,2,107,110–116] (see Chapter 166). This strategy seeks to mitigate gas trapping and dynamic hyperinflation and does not attempt to establish a normal $PaCO_2$ as long as the minute ventilation and fraction of inspired oxygen maintain adequate tissue oxygenation. Physician acceptance of hypercapnia in this setting is termed *permissive hypercapnia* [110–112]. Gas trapping and dynamic hyperinflation can be monitored, indirectly, by following plateau airway pressures, the level of intrinsic positive end expiratory pressure (PEEP) or auto-PEEP, and flow versus time graphics on the ventilator

TABLE 172.6

Goals of Mechanical Ventilation

Maintain oxygen saturation of hemoglobin (>90%; 95% during pregnancy)

Minimize dynamic hyperinflation
- Decrease minute ventilation
- Increase expiratory time
- Accept hypercarbia

Monitor closely for complications of mechanical ventilation

[115,116]. However, the most well-studied correlate of gas trapping and dynamic hyperinflation during mechanical ventilation for severe asthma is the volume of gas that remains in the lungs at end inspiration [114–116] (see Chapter 166). When the volume of air at end inspiration above functional residual capacity (VEI) exceeds 20 mL per kg, there is increased risk of hypotension and barotrauma. However, it should be noted that measurement of VEI requires the use of paralytics.

Although the use of sodium bicarbonate to treat acidosis is controversial, advocates for its use in severe acute respiratory acidosis have regarded a pH of 7.20 to be the minimum safe level [117]. This impression and the practice of infusing sodium bicarbonate to maintain a pH of more than 7.20 is based on two uncontrolled studies in which stuporous and comatose patients with acute respiratory acidosis markedly and quickly improved when infusion of sodium bicarbonate increased the pH to greater than 7.20 [118,119]. However, no controlled studies of respiratory acidosis support the use of sodium bicarbonate to maintain a specific pH value.

The physiologic responses to metabolic and respiratory acidosis include increases in cardiac output, pulmonary arterial pressure, and heart rate, whereas systemic vascular resistance decreases and mean systemic arterial pressure remains unchanged [120–122]. In diseased lungs, PaO_2 improves [120]. The hemodynamic changes are mediated directly by endogenous secretion of catecholamines, primarily norepinephrine, stimulated by decreases in pH. The effects of sodium bicarbonate infusions on these hemodynamic responses and gas exchange have been studied. As the acidosis lessens, cardiac output and PaO_2 worsen [121,122]. Moreover, sodium bicarbonate infusions have been shown neither to improve survival nor to enhance bronchodilation. Although studies from the 1950s and 1960s suggested that endogenous epinephrine release was depressed in acidosis, more recent studies have conclusively shown that it is either unchanged or augmented [122]. Because carbon dioxide is generated when infused sodium bicarbonate buffers hydrogen ions, infusion of sodium bicarbonate predictably raises carbon dioxide tensions in blood [123]. Because carbon dioxide readily diffuses across cell membranes, sodium bicarbonate therapy may cause paradoxic intracellular acidosis [124], and this may adversely affect survival. For these reasons, we suggest use of sodium bicarbonate only when the acidosis appears to be adversely affecting the patient's hemodynamic status.

In managing patients during mechanical controlled hypoventilation with permissive hypercapnia, the minimum safe pH is not known. In three uncontrolled studies, pH values were not maintained at greater than 7.2, and outcomes did not appear to be adversely affected. Sodium bicarbonate was not given in one study unless pH was less than 7.15 [114]; in the other two studies, it was not given to any patient even when pH was 7.02 and less than 7.00 [110,125].

Neuromuscular blocking agents, such as pancuronium, vecuronium, and atracurium, can be used to help maintain low airway pressures during delivery of mechanical ventilation (see Chapter 4). Paralyzing skeletal muscles prevents the development of high airway pressures due to the patient bucking or fighting the ventilator. Notably, a side effect of neuromuscular blocking agents can be severe bronchospasm. Vecuronium is often reported to be unlikely to cause bronchospasm, but case reports suggest that vecuronium too can rarely cause bronchospasm [126]. Another adverse effect of these agents is that patients who undergo even brief neuromuscular blockade in conjunction with corticosteroid administration have a risk of developing a prolonged and sometimes severe myopathy [127].

Because all patients with severe exacerbations of asthma are treated with corticosteroids, paralyzing agents should be avoided whenever possible. For patients who cannot be managed without neuromuscular blockade, continuous infusions of neuromuscular blocking agents should be avoided and muscle function should be allowed to recover partially between repetitive boluses.

Mechanical ventilation accomplishes the work of breathing, while the severely obstructed patient is treated intensively with inhaled bronchodilators and glucocorticoids. With this intensive pharmacologic therapy, mechanical ventilation usually can be discontinued in 1 to 3 days once discontinuation guidelines are met [107,128–130] (see Chapter 168). Some patients may require 2 to 4 weeks of mechanical ventilation, especially when pneumonia complicates an acute exacerbation of asthma.

Complications of Mechanical Ventilation

Serious complications have been reported as a result of mechanical ventilation for severe exacerbations of asthma [105–107,113,115,116]. Most of these are preventable or treatable if detected early. Problems with airway control, including traumatic and esophageal intubation, should always be anticipated. Intubation of the right mainstem bronchus is a serious problem of airway control because delivery of tidal volumes to one lung increases the risk of barotrauma. Once an airway is established and mechanical ventilation initiated, hypotension may occur because the high intrathoracic pressures that occur during mechanical ventilation during a severe asthma exacerbations impede venous return to the right ventricle of the heart. This is treated by administering intravenous fluids and adjusting tidal volumes, respiratory frequency, and inspiratory flow to decrease hyperinflation and intrinsic positive end-expiratory pressure.

Barotrauma is a major cause of morbidity and mortality among patients receiving mechanical ventilation for severe exacerbations of asthma [105–107,113,115,116]. High plateau airway pressures are associated with overdistended alveoli that rupture. Air may dissect along the bronchovascular interstitium and sometimes is evident on chest radiograph as parenchymal air cysts, linear air streaks emanating from the hila, and perivascular air halos [131,132]. As the air dissects centrally, mediastinal and subcutaneous emphysema develop. As an alternative, air from ruptured alveoli may dissect through the pleural surfaces into the pleural space to create a pneumothorax [133]. Ultrasound examination has high sensitivity for the rapid bedside detection of pneumothorax and should be considered for every ICU patient with deterioration of gas exchange or respiratory function. For patients on mechanical ventilation, pneumothorax progresses to tension pneumothorax rapidly and should always be treated immediately with tube thoracostomy. It must be presumed, emergently, that any pneumothorax during mechanical ventilation is under tension [134]. (See Chapter 166 for the discussion of minimizing barotrauma during mechanical ventilation.)

Mucous plugging commonly occurs during acute exacerbations of asthma. Large mucous plugs occluding the endotracheal tube should be considered when there is insurmountable difficulty ventilating a patient. Large mucous plugs also may cause lobar or lung atelectasis that impairs gas exchange and increases airway pressures. Cautiously, therapeutic bronchoscopy may be considered to relieve large mucous plugs if conservative measures, corticosteroids, and bronchodilators are not effective. Retained secretions and atelectasis also contribute to the significant risk of nosocomial pneumonia during mechanical ventilation [135].

Other complications are indirectly related to mechanical ventilation. Thromboembolism and gastric stress ulcers may occur with greater frequency in patients with severe exacerbations of asthma [136]. Arrhythmias and hypokalemia may occur during treatment for acute asthma because of therapy with sympathomimetic drugs. Hypophosphatemia may develop secondary to alkalosis [137].

TABLE 172.7

Special or Unconventional Therapeutic Measures

Intravenous β_2-adrenergic agonists
Methylxanthines
Helium–oxygen mixtures delivered through the ventilator
General anesthetics (e.g., ketamine, halothane)
Bronchoscopy with therapeutic lavage (intubated patients only)
Hypothermia
Extracorporeal life support

Additional and Unconventional Management Measures

Even after using bronchodilators, corticosteroids, sodium bicarbonate, and mechanical ventilation, airway obstruction sometimes is sufficiently severe to prevent maintenance of an acceptable arterial pH or adequate tissue oxygenation. In these rare cases, additional, sometimes unconventional, measures can be used to support the patient until corticosteroids have had time to suppress the underlying inflammatory process. Some of these measures are based only on anecdotal experience (Table 172.7).

If airway pressures remain high on mechanical ventilation despite the proper application of controlled hypoventilation with permissive hypercapnia, delivering heliox by mechanical ventilation has been suggested to allow adequate ventilation of the patient at reduced airway pressures [138]. Caution is necessary when using heliox in this setting because the low density of the gas mixture makes ventilator settings inaccurate (e.g., tidal volume) [139].

Bronchospasm usually is not the major factor limiting airflow of patients who are already being maximally treated for an acute exacerbation of asthma. However, for those who fail to respond to maximal conventional therapy, a variety of strategies have been advocated to maximize bronchodilation by relaxing airway smooth muscle. Some reports suggest that intravenous β_2-adrenergic agonists may significantly improve airway obstruction in select patients, but this treatment is not established and not recommended by current guidelines, in part because of danger of cardiac toxicity [1,2]. General anesthetics are excellent bronchodilators and an important option for patients whose conditions are refractory to maximal routine therapy. Anecdotally, halothane [140,141], thiopental [142], ketamine [143,144], and isoflurane [145] all have been used successfully to treat patients with severe asthma exacerbations. If general anesthetics are used, an anesthesiologist should be consulted.

Because a major cause of airway obstruction during an acute exacerbation of asthma is mucous plugging, therapeutic bronchoscopy with lavage has been used as an additional supportive measure for intubated patients who are extremely difficult to ventilate adequately [146–148]. While therapeutic bronchoscopy is not performed routinely because worsening bronchospasm is a recognized complication of bronchoscopy

TABLE 172.8

Treatment of Acute Asthma: Randomized Controlled Trials and Meta-analyses

- β-Adrenergic agonists are first-line therapy for acute asthma because they are rapidly acting and provide more bronchodilation than methylxanthines and cholinergic antagonists [56].
- Metered-dose inhalers with a holding chamber are at least as effective as wet nebulization for the delivery of β-adrenergic agonists in the treatment of acute asthma [71,72].
- Adding inhaled ipratropium bromide to treatment with β-adrenergic agonists provides benefit to adults with acute asthma in the emergency department [87].
- In hospitalized adult patients with acute asthma, systemic glucocorticoids speed improvement of symptoms and lung function [95].
- In addition to a short course of oral corticosteroids, initiate or continue daily inhaled corticosteroids on emergency room discharge of patients with persistent asthma [96].

among asthmatics, when necessary because standard therapy has failed, a flexible bronchoscope with a large suction channel should be used, and the mechanically ventilated patient should be sedated. *N*-acetylcysteine, a mucolytic agent, is associated with bronchospasm in asthmatic patients but, anecdotally, has been used successfully during therapeutic bronchoscopy by delivering a dilute solution (less than 1%) through the bronchoscope to dissolve mucous plugs [146]. DNase (2.5 mg in 10 mL of sterile normal saline) has been administered through a bronchoscope to relieve mucous plugging causing atelectasis in a child with asthma [149].

Case reports describe unconventional measures that might be considered for the management of rare, exceedingly difficult cases. For example, hypothermia and extracorporeal life support have been methods used to support critically ill patients whose conditions are refractory to conventional therapies [150,151].

Advances in asthma, based on randomized, controlled trials or meta-analyses of such trials, are summarized in Table 172.8.

References

1. Global Initiative for Asthma: Global Strategy for Asthma Management and Prevention, 2015. Available from: www.ginasthma.org.
2. National Asthma Education and Prevention Program: *Expert Panel Report 3: Guidelines for the Diagnosis and Management of Asthma. Publication No. 08-4051*. Bethesda, MD, National Institutes of Health, 2007.
3. Rodrigo GJ, Rodrigo C, Hall JB: Acute asthma in adults: a review. *Chest* 125:1081, 2004.
4. Centers for Diesase Control and Prevention: Most recent asthma data. http://www.cdc.gov/asthma/most_recent_data.htm. Last updated October 2, 2015.
5. To T, Stanojevic S, Moores G, et al: Global asthma prevalence in adults: findings from the cross-sectional world health survey. *BMC Public Health* 12:204, 2012.
6. Getahun D, Demissie K, Rhoads GG: Recent trends in asthma hospitalization and mortality in the United States. *J Asthma* 42:373, 2005.
7. Johnston NW, Sears MR: Asthma exacerbations 1: Epidemiology. *Thorax* 61:722, 2006.
8. Krishnan V, Diette GB, Rand CS, et al: Mortality in patients hospitalized for asthma exacerbations in the United States. *Am J Respir Crit Care Med* 174:633, 2006.
9. Bousquet J, Chanez P, Lacoste JY, et al: Eosinophilic inflammation in asthma. *N Engl J Med* 323:1033, 1990.
10. Kay AB: Pathology of mild, severe, and fatal asthma. *Am J Respir Crit Care Med* 154:566, 1996.
11. Wenzel S: Severe asthma in adults. *Am J Respir Crit Care Med* 172:149, 2005.
12. Kudo M, Ishigatsubo Y, Aoki I: Pathology of asthma. *Front Microbiol* 4:263, 2013.
13. Kolbe J, Fergusson W, Garrett J: Rapid onset asthma: a severe but uncommon manifestation. *Thorax* 53:241, 1998.
14. Rodrigo GJ, Rodrigo C: Rapid-onset asthma attack: a prospective cohort study about characteristics and response to emergency department treatment. *Chest* 118:1547, 2000.
15. Plaza V, Serrano J, Picado C, et al: Frequency and clinical characteristics of rapid-onset fatal and near-fatal asthma. *Eur Respir J* 19:846, 2002.
16. McFadden ER Jr, Warren EL: Observations on asthma mortality. *Ann Intern Med* 127:142, 1997.
17. Dunnill MS: The pathology of asthma, with special reference to changes in the bronchial mucosa. *J Clin Pathol* 13:27, 1960.
18. Sur S, Crotty TB, Kephart GM, et al: Sudden-onset fatal asthma: a distinct entity with few eosinophils and relatively more neutrophils in the airway submucosa? *Am Rev Respir Dis* 148:713, 1993.
19. Torgerson DG, Ampleford EJ, Chiu GY, et al: Meta-analysis of genome-wide association studies of asthma in ethnically diverse North American populations. *Nat Genet* 43:887, 2011.
20. Fahy JV: Type 2 inflammation in asthma—present in most, absent in many. *Nat Rev Immunol* 15:57, 2015.
21. Papadopoulos NG, Christodoulou I, Rohde G, et al: Viruses and bacteria in acute asthma exacerbations—a GA2LEN-DARE* systematic review. *Allergy* 66:458, 2011.
22. Jackson DJ, Makrinioti H, Rana BMJ, et al: IL-33-dependent type 2 inflammation during rhinovirus-induced asthma exacerbations in vivo. *Am J Respir Crit Care Med* 190:1373, 2014.
23. Rubinfield AR, Wagner PD, West JB: Gas exchange during acute experimental canine asthma. *Am Rev Respir Dis* 118:525, 1978.
24. Rodriguez-Roisin R, Ballester E, Roca J, et al: Mechanisms of hypoxemia in patients with status asthmaticus requiring mechanical ventilation. *Am Rev Respir Dis* 139:732, 1989.
25. Rossi A, Ganassini A, Brusasco V: Airflow obstruction and dynamic pulmonary hyperinflation, in Hall JB, Corbridge T, Rodrigo C, et al (eds): *Acute Asthma: Assessment and Management*. New York, NY, McGraw-Hill, 2000, p 57.
26. Freedman AR, Lavietes MH: Energy requirements of the respiratory musculature in asthma. *Am J Med* 80:215, 1986.
27. Martin JG, Powell E, Shore S, et al: The role of the respiratory muscles in the hyperinflation of bronchial asthma. *Am Rev Respir Dis* 121:441, 1980.
28. Bellemare F, Grassino A: Evaluation of human diaphragm fatigue. *J Appl Physiol* 53:1196, 1982.
29. Balkissoon R, Kenn K: Asthma: vocal cord dysfunction (VCD) and other dysfunctional breathing disorders. *Sem Respir Crit Care Med* 33:595, 2012.
30. Perskvist N, Edston E: Differential accumulation of pulmonary and cardiac mast cell-subsets and eosinophils between fatal anaphylaxis and asthma death: a postmortem comparative study. *Forensic Sci Int* 169:43, 2007.
31. Soler-Cataluna JJ, Cosio B, Izqierdo JL, et al: Consensus document on the overlap phenotype COPD-asthma in COPD. *Arch Bronconeumol* 48:331, 2012.
32. Marmoush FY, Barbour MF, Noonan TE, et al: Takotsubo cardiomyopathy: a new perspective in asthma. *Case Reports Cardiol*:640795, 2015.
33. Gelb AF, Schein A, Nussbaum E, et al: Risk factors for near-fatal asthma. *Chest* 126:1138, 2004.
34. Eisner MD, Lieu TA, Chi F, et al: Beta agonists, inhaled steroids, and the risk of intensive care unit admission for asthma. *Eur Respir J* 17:233, 2001.
35. Dhuper S, Maggiore D, Chung V, et al: Profile of near-fatal asthma in an inner-city hospital. *Chest* 124:1880, 2003.
36. Mitchell I, Tough SC, Semple LK, et al: Near-fatal asthma: a population-based study of risk factors. *Chest* 121:1407, 2002.
37. Camargo CA, Rachelefsky G, Schatz M: Managing asthma exacerbations in the emergency department. *Proc Am Throac Soc* 6:357, 2009.
38. Marquette CH, Saulnier F, Leroy O, et al: Long-term prognosis of near-fatal asthma: a 6-year follow-up study of 145 asthmatic patients who underwent mechanical ventilation for a near-fatal attack of asthma. *Am Rev Respir Dis* 146:76, 1992.
39. Shim CS, Williams MH: Evaluation of the severity of asthma: patients versus physicians. *Am J Med* 68:11, 1980.
40. Magadle R, Berar-Yanay N, Weiner P: The risk of hospitalization and near-fatal and fatal asthma in relation to the perception of dyspnea. *Chest* 121:329, 2002.
41. Eckert DJ, Catcheside PG, McEvoy RD: Blunted sensation of dyspnoea and near fatal asthma. *Eur Respir J* 24:197, 2004.
42. Sahn SA, Mountain RD: Clinical features and outcome in patients with acute asthma presenting with hypercapnia. *Am Rev Respir Dis* 138:535, 1988.
43. Shim CS, Williams MH: Relationship of wheezing to the severity of obstruction in asthma. *Arch Intern Med* 143:890, 1983.
44. Cohen CA, Zagelbaum G, Gross D, et al: Clinical manifestations of inspiratory muscle fatigue. *Am J Med* 73:308, 1982.
45. Grunfeld A, FitzGerald J: Discharge considerations for adult asthmatic patients treated in emergency departments. *Can Respir J* 3:322, 1996.
46. Lenhardt R, Malone A, Grant EN, et al: Trends in emergency department asthma care in metropolitan Chicago. *Chest* 124:1774, 2003.

47. Leong B, Vasu A, Cham Wai Ming G: Identifying adult asthmatic patients with an abnormal chest radiograph in the emergency department. *Eur J Emerg Med* 19:95, 2012.
48. Warnier MJ, Rutten FH, Kors JA, et al: Cardiac arrhythmias in adult patients with asthma. *J Asthma* 49:942, 2012.
49. Krishnan JA, Davis SQ, Naureckas ET, et al: An umbrella review: corticosteroid therapy for adults with acute asthma. *Am J Med* 122:977, 2009.
50. Rossing T, Fanta CH, Goldstein DH, et al: Emergency therapy of asthma: comparison of the acute effects of parenteral and inhaled sympathomimetics and infused aminophylline. *Am Rev Respir Dis* 122:365, 1980.
51. Cazzola M, Page CP, Rogliani P, et al: b2-Agonist therapy in lung disease. *Am J Respir Crit Care Med* 187:690, 2013.
52. Cazzola M, Page CP, Calzetta L, et al: Pharmacology and therapeutics of bronchodilators. *Pharmacol Rev* 64:450, 2012.
53. Jat KR, Krairwa A: Levalbuterol versus albuterol for acute asthma: a systematic review and meta-analysis. *Pulm Pharm Therap* 26:239, 2013.
54. Lewis LM, Ferguson I, House SL, et al: Albuterol administration is commonly associated with increases in serum lactate in patients with asthma treated for acute exacerbation of asthma. *Chest* 145:53, 2014.
55. Newhouse MT, Chapman KR, McCallum AL, et al: Cardiovascular safety of high doses of inhaled fenoterol and albuterol in acute severe asthma. *Chest* 110:595, 1996.
56. Williams SJ, Winner SJ, Clark TJH: Comparison of inhaled and intravenous terbutaline in acute severe asthma. *Thorax* 36:629, 1981.
57. Rodrigo C, Rodrigo G: Salbutamol treatment of acute severe asthma in the ED: MDI versus hand-held nebulizer. *Am J Emerg Med* 18:637, 1998.
58. Turner MO, Patel A, Ginsburg S, et al: Bronchodilator delivery in acute airflow obstruction. *Arch Intern Med* 157:1736, 1997.
59. Camargo CA, Spooner CH, Rowe BH: Continuous versus intermittent beta-agonists for acute asthma. *Cochrane Database Syst Rev* (4): CD001115, 2003. doi:10.1002/14651858.CD001115/.
60. Rodrigo GJ, Rodrigo C: Continuous vs intermittent β-agonists in the treatment of acute adult asthma: a systematic review with meta-analysis. *Chest* 122:160, 2002.
61. Rodrigo GJ, Castro-Rodriguez JA: Heliox-driven beta2-agonists nebulization for children and adults with acute asthma: a systematic review with meta-analysis. *Ann Allergy Asthma Immunol* 112:29, 2014.
62. Travers AH, Milan SJ, Jones AP, et al: Addition of intravenous beta(2)-agonists to inhaled beta(2)-agonists for acute asthma. *Cochrane Database Syst Rev* 12:CD010179, 2012.
63. Karpel JP, Appel D, Breidbart D, et al: A comparison of atropine sulfate and metaproterenol sulfate in the emergency treatment of asthma. *Am Rev Respir Dis* 133:727, 1986.
64. Storms WW, Bodman SF, Nathan RA, et al: Use of ipratropium bromide in asthma. *Am J Med* 81:61, 1986.
65. Rodrigo GJ, Castro-Rodriguez JA: Anticholinergics in the treatment of children and adults with acute asthma: a systematic review with meta-analysis. *Thorax* 60:740, 2005.
66. Griffiths B, Ducharme FM: Combined inhaled anticholinergics and short-acting beta2-agonists for initial treatment of acute asthma in children. *Cochrane Database Syst Rev* 8:CD000060, 2013.
67. Peters SP, Kunselman SJ, Icitovic N, et al: Tiotropium bromide step-up therapy for adults with uncontrolled asthma. *N Engl J Med* 363:1715, 2010. doi: 10.1056/NEJMoa1008770.
68. Fanta CH, Rossing TH, McFadden ER: Treatment of acute asthma: is combination therapy with sympathomimetics and methylxanthines indicated? *Am J Med* 80:5, 1986.
69. Siegal D, Sheppard D, Gelb A, et al: Aminophylline increases the toxicity but not the efficacy of an inhaled beta-adrenergic agonist in the treatment of acute exacerbations of asthma. *Am Rev Respir Dis* 132:283, 1985.
70. Rossing T, Fanta CH, McFadden ER, et al: A controlled trial of the use of single versus combined-drug therapy in the treatment of acute episodes of asthma. *Am Rev Respir Dis* 123:190, 1981.
71. Nair P, Milan SJ, Rowe BH: Addition of intravenous aminophyline to inhaled beta(2)-agonists in adults with acute asthma. *Cochrane Database Syst Rev* 12:CD002742, 2012.
72. McFadden ER: Acute severe asthma. *Am J Respir Crit Care Med* 168:740, 2003.
73. Manser R, Reid D, Abramson M: Corticosteroids for acute severe asthma in hospitalised patients. *Cochrane Database Syst Rev* (1):CD001740, 2001.
74. Rowe BH, Spooner CH, Ducharme FM, et al: Corticosteroids for preventing relapse following acute exacerbations of asthma. *Cochrane Database Syst Rev* CD00095, 2001.
75. Barnes PJ: Mechanisms of action of glucocorticoids in asthma. *Am J Respir Crit Care Med* 154:S21, 1996.
76. Partridge MR, Gibson GJ: Adverse bronchial reactions to intravenous hydrocortisone in two aspirin-sensitive asthmatic patients. *BMJ* 1:1521, 1978.
77. Ratto D, Alfaro C, Sipsey J, et al: Are intravenous corticosteroids required in status asthmaticus? *JAMA* 260:527, 1988.
78. Harrison BDW, Hart GJ, Ali NJ, et al: Need for intravenous hydrocortisone in addition to oral prednisolone in patients admitted to hospital with severe asthma without ventilatory failure. *Lancet* 1:181, 1986.
79. Edmonds ML, Milan SJ, Camargo CA Jr, et al: Early use of inhaled corticosteroids in the emergency department treatment of acute asthma. *Cochrane Database Syst Rev* (12):CD002308, 2012.
80. McFadden ER: Dosages of corticosteroids in asthma. *Am Rev Respir Dis* 147:1306, 1993.
81. Haskell RJ, Wang BM, Hansen JE: A double-blind, randomized trial of methylprednisolone in status asthmaticus. *Arch Intern Med* 143:1324, 1983.
82. Emerman CL, Cydulka RK: A randomized comparison of 100-mg vs 500-mg dose of methylprednisolone in the treatment of acute asthma. *Chest* 107: 1559, 1995.
83. Hasegawa T, Ishihara K, Takakura S, et al: Duration of systemic corticosteroids in the treatment of asthma exacerbation; a randomized study. *Intern Med* 39:794, 2000.
84. Jones AM, Munavvar M, Vail A, et al: Prospective, placebo-controlled trial of 5 vs 10 days of oral prednisolone in acute adult asthma. *Respir Med* 96:950, 2002.
85. Perrin K, Wijeskinghe M, Healy B, et al: Randomised controlled trial of high concentration versus titrated oxygen therapy in severe exacerbations of asthma. *Thorax* 66:937–941, 2011.
86. Chien JW, Ciufo R, Novak R, et al: Uncontrolled oxygen administration and respiratory failure in acute asthma. *Chest* 117:728, 2000.
87. Silverman RA, Osborn H, Runge J, et al: Acute Asthma/Magnesium Study Group. IV magnesium sulfate in the treatment of acute severe asthma: a multicenter randomized controlled trial. *Chest* 122:489, 2002.
88. Blitz M, Blitz S, Beasely R, et al: Aerosolized magnesium sulfate for acute asthma: a systematic review. *Chest* 128:337, 2005.
89. Powell C, Dwan K, Milan SJ, et al: Inhaled magnesium sulfate in the treatment of acute asthma. *Cochrane Database Syst Rev* (12):CD003898, 2012.
90. Silverman RA, Nowak RM, Korenblat PE, et al: Zafirlukast treatment for acute asthma: evaluation in a randomized, double-blind, multicenter trial. *Chest* 126:1480, 2004.
91. Ramsay CF, Pearson D, Mildenhall S, et al: Oral montelukast in acute asthma exacerbations: a randomised, double-blincd, placebo-controlled trial. *Thorax* 66:7, 2011.
92. Bernstein IL, Ausdenmoore RW: Iatrogenic bronchospasm occurring during clinical trials of a new mucolytic agent, acetylcysteine. *Dis Chest* 46:469, 1964.
93. Allegra L, Blasi F, Centanni S, et al: Acute exacerbations of asthma in adults: role of Chlamydia pneumoniae infection. *Eur Respir J* 7:2165, 1994.
94. Strauss L, Hejal R, McFadden ER Jr, et al: Observations on the effects of aerosolized albuterol in acute asthma. *Am J Respir Crit Care Med* 155:454, 1997.
95. Schatz M, Rachelefsky G, Krishnan JA: Follow-up after acute asthma episodes. *Proc Am Thorac Soc* 6:386, 2009.
96. Krishnan JA, Nowak R, Davis SQ, et al: Anti-inflammatory treatment after discharge home from the emergency department in adults with acute asthma. *Proc Am Thorac Soc* 6:380, 2009.
97. Schatz M, Dobrowski MP: Asthma in pregnancy. *N Engl J Med* 360:1862, 2009.
98. Cydulka RK, Emerman CL, Schreiber D, et al: Acute asthma among pregnant women presenting to the emergency department. *Am J Respir Crit Care Med* 160:887, 1999.
99. Schatz M, Zeiger RS, Harden KM, et al: The safety of inhaled beta-agonist bronchodilators during pregnancy. *J Allergy Clin Immunol* 82:686, 1988.
100. Joint Committee for American College of Obstetricians and Gynecologists and the American College of Allergy, Asthma and Immunology: The use of newer asthma and allergy medications during pregnancy. *Ann Allergy Asthma Immunol* 84:475, 2000.
101. Wendel PJ, Ramin SM, Barnett-Hamm C, et al: Asthma treatment in pregnancy: a randomized controlled study. *Int J Gynecol Obstet* 56:99, 1997.
102. Chandra A, Shim C, Cohen H, et al: Regular vs ad-lib albuterol for patients hospitalized with acute asthma. *Chest* 128:1115, 2005.
103. McFadden ER Jr, Elsanadi N, Dixon L, et al: Protocol therapy for acute asthma: therapeutic benefits and cost savings. *Am J Med* 99:651, 1995.
104. Rabbat A, Laaban JP, Orvoen-Frija E, et al: Bronchial hyperresponsiveness following acute severe asthma. *Intensive Care Med* 22:530, 1996.
105. Dales RE, Munt PW: Use of mechanical ventilation in adults with severe asthma. *Can Med Assoc J* 130:391, 1984.
106. Darioli R, Perret C: Mechanical controlled hypoventilation in status asthmaticus. *Am Rev Respir Dis* 129:385, 1984.
107. Brenner B, Corbridge T, Kazzi A: Intubation and mechanical ventilation of the asthmatic patient in respiratory failure. *Proc Am Thorac Soc* 6:371, 2009.
108. Ram FSF, Wellington SR, Rowe BH, et al: Non-invasive positive pressure ventilation for treatment of respiratory failure due to severe acute

exacerbations of asthma. *Cochrane Database Syst Rev* (3): CD004360, 2005. doi: 10.1002/14651858.CD004360.pub3.
109. Weiss EB, Patwardham AV: The response of lidocaine in bronchial asthma. *Chest* 72:429, 1977.
110. Bellomo R, McLaughlin P, Tai E, et al: Asthma requiring mechanical ventilation: a low morbidity approach. *Chest* 105:891, 1994.
111. Feihl F, Perret C: Permissive hypercapnia. *Am J Respir Crit Care Med* 150:1722, 1994.
112. Wilmoth DF, Carpenter RM: Preventing complications of mechanical ventilation: permissive hypercapnia. *AACN Clin Issues* 7:473, 1996.
113. Lazarus SC: Emergency treatment of asthma. *N Engl J Med* 363:755, 2010.
114. Williams TJ, Tuxen DV, Scheinkestel CD, et al: Risk factors for morbidity in mechanically ventilated patients with acute severe asthma. *Am Rev Respir Dis* 146:607, 1992.
115. Stather, DR, Stewart TE: Clinical review: mechanical ventilation in severe asthma. *Crit Care* 9:581, 2005.
116. Leatherman J: Mechanical ventilation for severe asthma. *Chest* 147:1671, 2015.
117. Menitove SM, Goldring RM: Combined ventilator and bicarbonate strategy in the management of status asthmaticus. *Am J Med* 74:898, 1983.
118. Westlake EK, Simpson T, Kaye M: Carbon dioxide narcosis in emphysema. *Q J Med* 24:155, 1955.
119. Addis GJ: Bicarbonate buffering in acute exacerbation of chronic respiratory failure. *Thorax* 20:337, 1965.
120. Brimioulle S, Vachiery J-L, Lejeune P, et al: Acid-base status affects gas exchange in canine oleic acid pulmonary edema. *Am J Physiol* 260:H1080, 1991.
121. Brofman JD, Leff AR, Munoz NM, et al: Sympathetic secretory response to hypercapnic acidosis in swine. *J Appl Physiol* 69:710, 1990.
122. Ebata T, Watanabe Y, Amaha K, et al: Haemodynamic changes during the apnoea test for diagnosis of brain death. *Can J Anaesth* 38:436, 1991.
123. Cooper DJ, Walley KR, Wiggs BR, et al: Bicarbonate does not improve hemodynamics in critically ill patients who have lactic acidosis. *Ann Intern Med* 112:492, 1990.
124. Shapiro JI, Whalen M, Kucera R, et al: Brain pH responses to sodium bicarbonate and carbicarb during systemic acidosis. *Am J Physiol* 69:710, 1990.
125. Hickling KG, Henderson SJ, Jackson R: Low mortality associated with low volume pressure limited ventilation with permissive hypercapnia in severe adult respiratory distress syndrome. *Intensive Care Med* 16:372, 1990.
126. Uratsuji Y, Konishi M, Ikegaki N, et al: Possible bronchospasm after administration of vecuronium. *Masui* 40:109, 1991.
127. Hansen-Flaschen J, Cowen J, Raps EC: Neuromuscular blockade in the intensive care unit. *Am Rev Respir Dis* 147:234, 1993.
128. Higgins B, Greening AP, Crompton GK: Assisted ventilation in severe asthma. *Thorax* 41:464, 1986.
129. Braman SS, Kaemmerlen JT: Intensive care of status asthmaticus: a 10-year experience. *JAMA* 264:366, 1990.
130. Mansel JK, Stogner SW, Petrini MF, et al: Mechanical ventilation in patients with acute severe asthma. *Am J Med* 89:42, 1986.
131. Johnson TH, Altman AR: Pulmonary interstitial gas: first sign of barotrauma due to PEEP therapy. *Crit Care Med* 7:532, 1979.
132. Jamadar DA, Kazerooni EA, Hirschl RB: Pneumomediastinum: elucidation of the anatomic pathway by liquid ventilation. *J Comput Assist Tomogr* 20:309, 1996.
133. Haake R, Schlichtig R, Ulstad DR, et al: Barotrauma. *Chest* 91:608, 1987.
134. Albelda SM, Giefter WB, Kelley MA, et al: Ventilator-induced subpleural air cysts: clinical, radiographic, and pathologic significance. *Am Rev Respir Dis* 127:360, 1983.
135. Zwillich CW: Complications of assisted ventilation: a prospective study of 354 consecutive episodes. *Am J Med* 57:161, 1974.
136. Pingleton SK, Bone RC, Pingleton WW, et al: The efficacy of low-dose heparin in prevention of pulmonary emboli in a respiratory intensive care unit. *Chest* 79:647, 1981.
137. Laaban J-P, Waked M, Laromiguiere M, et al: Hypophosphatemia complicating management of acute severe asthma. *Ann Intern Med* 112:68, 1990.
138. Gluck EH, Onorato DJ, Castriotta R: Helium-oxygen mixtures in intubated patients with status asthmaticus and respiratory acidosis. *Chest* 98:693, 1990.
139. Tassaux D, Jolliet P, Thouret JM, et al: Calibration of seven ICU ventilators for mechanical ventilation with helium-oxygen mixtures. *Am J Respir Crit Care Med* 160:22, 1999.
140. O Rourke PP, Crone RK: Halothane in status asthmaticus. *Crit Care Med* 10:341, 1982.
141. Schwartz SH: Treatment of status asthmaticus with halothane. *JAMA* 251:2688, 1984.
142. Grunberg G, Cohen JD, Keslin J, et al: Facilitation of mechanical ventilation in status asthmaticus with continuous intravenous thiopental. *Chest* 99:1216, 1991.
143. Sarma VJ: Use of ketamine in acute severe asthma. *Acta Anaesthesiol Scand* 36:106, 1992.
144. Hemming A, MacKenzie I, Finfer S: Response to ketamine in status asthmaticus resistant to maximal medical treatment. *Thorax* 49:90, 1994.
145. Maltais F, Sovilj M, Goldberg P, et al: Respiratory mechanics in status asthmaticus: effects of inhalational anesthesia. *Chest* 106:1401, 1994.
146. Millman M, Goldman AH, Goldstein IM: Status asthmaticus: use of acetylcysteine during bronchoscopy and lavage to remove mucus plugs. *Ann Allergy* 50:85, 1983.
147. Smith DL, Deshazo RD: Bronchoalveolar lavage in asthma. *Am Rev Respir Dis* 148:523, 1993.
148. Henke CA, Hertz M, Gustafson P: Combined bronchoscopy and mucolytic therapy for patients with severe refractory status asthmaticus on mechanical ventilation: a case report and review of the literature. *Crit Care Med* 22:1880, 1994.
149. Greally P: Human recombinant DNase for mucus plugging in status asthmaticus. *Lancet* 346:1423, 1995.
150. Browning D, Goodrum DT: Treatment of acute severe asthma assisted by hypothermia. *Anaesthesia* 47:223, 1992.
151. Shapiro MB, Kleaveland AC, Bartlett RH: Extracorporeal life support for status asthmaticus. *Chest* 103:1651, 1993.

Chapter 173 ■ Critical Care of Acute Exacerbations of COPD

MARK WEIR • GERARD CRINER

INTRODUCTION

An acute exacerbation of chronic obstructive pulmonary disease (AECOPD) is defined as "an event in the natural course of the disease characterized by a change in the patient's baseline dyspnea, cough, and/or sputum that is beyond normal day-to-day variations, is acute in onset, and may warrant a change in regular medication" (GOLD) [1]. AECOPDs contribute to morbidity, mortality, and reduced quality of life and also constitute the most important direct health care costs associated with COPD. The economic costs of COPD are considerable and have been increasing. In 1993, it was estimated to be >$15.5 billion in the United States, 6.1 billion of which corresponded to hospital stays [2]. In 2010, the cost to the United States for COPD was projected to be approximately $49.9 billion, including $29.5 billion in direct health care costs, $8.0 billion in indirect morbidity costs, and $12.4 billion in indirect mortality costs [3]. There is also a correlation between disease severity in terms of GOLD stage and health care cost [4]. The costs of inpatient care are estimated to represent 40% to 57% of the total direct costs generated by patients with COPD [2]. Exacerbations of COPD are important because they negatively affect quality of life, are associated with accelerated rates of decline of lung function for those with COPD, and are associated with significant morbidity and mortality. The goals of treatment for COPD exacerbations are to minimize their impact, recognize their significance, and try to prevent subsequent exacerbations.

RISK FACTORS FOR AECOPD

Exacerbations of COPD can be precipitated by several factors. The most common causes appear to be infection of the tracheobronchial tree with either bacteria or viruses; a minority are caused by eosinophilic inflammation similar to asthma and about 30% are of unknown cause. Environmental pollution has been linked with poorer respiratory symptoms, increased acute exacerbations, and COPD-associated mortality [5]. Because these phenotypes are clinically indistinguishable [6], methods for differentiating phenotypes are a current focus of research. For example, blood eosinophilia may be a method to identify a subgroup of COPD patients with steroid responsive exacerbations [7]. We know that exacerbations beget exacerbations, so factors associated with exacerbations are a history of previous exacerbation, increasing disease severity and comorbidities [8].

PATHOPHYSIOLOGY

The hallmark of COPD is airflow limitation measured by forced expiratory volume in 1 second to forced vital capacity (FEV_1/FVC) ratio <0.7 [9]. This is caused by increased resistance of the small conducting airways from peribronchial fibrosis and increased smooth muscle mass, mucous, and goblet cell hyperplasia. Emphysematous parenchymal destruction increases lung compliance and leads to early airway collapse. There are a variety of theories underlying these changes in the lung, but it is generally accepted that they are the result of "host factors" and exposures (i.e., chronic innate and adaptive inflammatory immune response of the host to a lifetime exposure to "environmental factors" such as inhaled toxic gases and particles) [10].

The natural history of COPD has a long preclinical stage of between 20 and 40 years during which time changes can be occurring in the lung. As the lung ages, FEV_1 deteriorates from about 35 years of age onward at a rate of about 25 to 30 mL per year in normal individuals and at an accelerated rate in susceptible smokers at about 60 mL per year [11]. People with normal rates of decline can develop COPD if they have achieved a low peak level of FEV_1 [11]. Symptoms are usually absent until 40% of FEV_1 has been lost. The airflow obstruction of COPD is caused by pathologic changes in the small conducting airways (<2 mm in diameter) that contribute about 25% to total airway resistance in healthy individuals. The changes include disruption of the epithelial barrier, mucus hyperplasia, and Goblet cell metaplasia that result in accumulation of mucous plugs in the small airway lumen, infiltration of the airway walls by inflammatory cells, smooth muscle hypertrophy, peribronchiolar fibrosis, and deposition of connective tissue in the airway wall [12]. These changes in the airway walls result in reduced cross-sectional area and impair the ability to increase caliber with lung inflation. These changes have been correlated with disease progression from GOLD stages 0 to 4 [13]. Emphysematous lung destruction is associated with a similar inflammatory infiltration of alveoli and airway walls. This causes abnormal dilation of the airways distal to the terminal bronchioles, perforations in alveolar walls, and obliteration of airway walls that coalesce to form bullae destroying large volumes of lung tissue [14]. This leads to both loss of lung elastic recoil and loss of anatomic tethering of small airways. Emphysema has been subtyped depending on its pattern of distribution in the lung. The centrilobular pattern of emphysematous destruction usually has an upper lobe predilection and is closely associated with cigarette smoking. The panacinar pattern of emphysema is usually more marked in the lower lobes and is characterized by a more uniform involvement of the acinus and is associated with α-1 antitrypsin deficiency [15].

Respiratory failure associated with COPD is usually a combination of lung failure and pump failure. Lung failure refers to the destruction of lung units, the alveoli and vascular beds, leading to reduced ventilation–perfusion ($\dot{V}/\dot{Q}$) matching and shunt [16]. Pump failure refers to mechanical disadvantage owing to increased workload, impaired chest wall and respiratory muscle performance, and impaired central or peripheral motor neuron function [17].

During AECOPD, inflammation within the lungs causes dynamic changes to occur. Increased bronchospasm and mucus hypersecretion results in further narrowing of the airway lumen and airflow limitation. Hypoxemia, anxiety, increased metabolic rate, and acidosis lead to an increased respiratory rate that shortens expiratory time and results in an increase of end-expiratory lung volume (EELV). This results in air trapping, which when extensive, leads to dynamic hyperinflation. The increase in EELV produces a positive alveolar pressure known as intrinsic positive end-expiratory pressure (PEEP). Intrinsic PEEP can occur with inappropriate ventilator settings (e.g., inappropriately high levels of minute ventilation or settings that result in insufficient expiratory time for exhalation relevant to the intrinsic ability of the lungs to passively exhale). Intrinsic PEEP can be associated with cardiac compromise, increased barotrauma, and alter the hemodynamic wave tracings during central venous pressure and pulmonary artery catheter monitoring. Dynamic hyperinflation leads to suboptimal muscle length to tension relationship and mechanical disadvantage for the muscles of respiration [18]. These changes induce severe dyspnea, increase dead space fraction, and aggravate $\dot{V}/\dot{Q}$ relationships resulting in hypoxemia and, when severe, hypercapnia. Resolution of exacerbation and improvement in symptoms correlate well with an improvement in FEV_1, inspiratory capacity, and reduced EELV [19].

SEVERITY SCORING

Knowledge about prognosis of AECOPD and factors that predict poor outcomes is important to enable intensive care unit (ICU) physicians to advise patients and families on the expected natural course of an illness, the likelihood of complications, and mortality [20]. Prognoses based on clinical judgment alone have been shown to be inherently uncertain and vulnerable to unconscious bias [21]. An accurate assessment tool like the numerous pneumonia scoring systems would be helpful. Currently, there is no assessment tool recommended by the major respiratory societies. Those available have not undergone external validation outside the population they were derived from, limiting there generalizability. Most of the scores have an area under the receiver operator curve of between 0.7 and 0.8, suggesting that they are only of moderate accuracy [22]. Singanayagam et al. [22] in a systematic review of the literature on **predictors of mortality** identified 12 factors with a consistent and statistically significant association with short-term mortality: age, male sex, low body mass index (BMI), cardiac failure, chronic renal failure, long-term oxygen therapy (LTOT), lower limb edema, GOLD stage 4, cor pulmonale, acidemia, confusion, and elevated plasma troponin level. In the subanalysis of patients managed in the ICU, three factors were associated with increased mortality: age, reduced Glasgow Coma Scale score, and acidemia. Messer et al. [23] reviewed the literature specific to management of AECOPD in the ICU for markers of **intermediate-term mortality**. They found that time spent in the hospital prior to ICU admission, low Glasgow Coma Scale on admission to the ICU, cardiorespiratory arrest prior to ICU admission, cardiac dysrhythmia prior to ICU admission, and higher values of acute physiology scoring systems were all prognostic of in-hospital mortality. Interestingly, they found a number of premorbid variables as not being associated with increased intermediate-term mortality, and these were age, functional capacity, oral steroid use, spirometry, previous ICU admission, BMI, smoking status, and LTOT.

ANTIBIOTICS AND BIOMARKERS

Overuse of antibiotics in the ICU is common and accelerates the development of drug resistance [24]. Quality ICU care involves the judicious use of antibiotics; the reduction of antibiotic prescription rates has been shown to reverse the occurrence of nosocomial infection and drug-resistant organisms [25]. However, the importance of antibiotics can be highlighted by the fact that mortality rates for patients in septic shock increase by 7% per hour within the first 6 hours of delayed antibiotic administration [26]. Patients with sepsis from ventilator-associated pneumonia who had a delay of more than 24 hours after diagnosis until initiation of antibiotics have a sevenfold higher mortality rate compared to those started on adequate therapy earlier [27]. Systematic reviews [28] of COPD exacerbations suggest that antibiotics have large and consistent beneficial effects across outcomes of patients admitted to ICU. They have not been shown to be as useful in mild-to-moderate exacerbations of COPD [28]. Recent strategies to reduce antibiotic overuse have included the development of biomarker-directed treatment algorithms wherein antibiotics are given or withheld depending on the level of biomarkers measured in the blood. Biomarkers that have been studied are highly sensitive C-reactive protein and procalcitonin. Procalcitonin is currently the most promising. Procalcitonin-guided therapy has been effective for reducing antibiotic use by approximately 40% to 50% in hospitalized patients presenting with acute lower respiratory tract infection symptoms [29–32]. In all of these randomized controlled studies, there was no increase in adverse events among patients who had antibiotics de-escalated.

MANAGEMENT

Oxygen

All patients with COPD exacerbations have the potential to develop hypoxemia and hypercapnia. We recommend an arterial blood gas to assess the degree of hypoxemia and hypercapnia. Supplemental oxygen therapy should be administered to patients suffering an exacerbation of COPD to maintain oxygen saturations between 88% and 92%, being careful to avoid hyperoxemia. Generally, the use of controlled oxygen therapy titrated to an acceptable goal of oxygen saturation (usually 88% to 92%) is considered appropriate [33].

Avoidance of hyperoxemia is important because of the well-described occurrence of worsening hypercapnia. There is evidence to show the indiscriminate use of oxygen therapy increases mortality and need for intubation [33]. The induction of hypercapnia through hyperoxemia is still poorly understood. It is thought to be a combination of mostly change in $\dot{V}/\dot{Q}$ mismatch, with a mild decrease in central respiratory drive and the Haldane effect [34]. The ability of the lungs to shunt blood away from areas of low alveolar oxygen tension is disrupted by the administration of high levels of oxygen; the resultant change in V/Q matching leads to increased dead space. The Haldane effect describes the binding ability of hemoglobin for CO_2 was increased oxygen shifts the hemoglobin CO_2 dissociation curve to the right and leads to an increase in $PaCO_2$. Patients who are already ventilating at their maximum are unable to increase minute ventilation further to counteract this.

High-flow nasal oxygen devices are increasingly used in critical care. There is a growing evidence base for their use in hypoxemic respiratory failure, but this form of oxygen therapy has been poorly studied in hypercapnic respiratory failure. One of the benefits of high-flow oxygen systems is the washout of CO_2 from anatomic dead space, effectively converting the oropharynx and conducting airways into a reservoir. The higher flow rates delivered match the patients inspiratory flow more effectively [35]. There is a small amount of PEEP delivered to the airway that can recruit lung units or potentially offset intrinsic PEEP. Probably, the greatest benefit is a reduced respiratory rate that leads to less air trapping. Evidence for the use of high-flow oxygen therapy in severe COPD or hypercapnic respiratory failure is limited mainly to case reports and a small study on exercise capacity [36,37]. A detailed discussion of oxygen therapy and delivery devices can be found in Chapter 169.

Bronchodilators

Patients in AECOPD have increased expiratory flow limitation. Nebulized short-acting bronchodilators are used to reduce bronchospasm. These medications have not been robustly studied in severe COPD exacerbations requiring critical care.

β-Agonists

Short-acting β-agonists include albuterol and levalbuterol. These drugs are selective β_2 receptor agonists that induce smooth muscle relaxation and relief of bronchospasm. They can be administered via inhaler or by nebulizer. They have been shown in randomized controlled trials and meta-analyses to improve symptoms and lung function [38,39]. Common side effects include tremor, tachycardia, and hypokalemia.

Anticholinergics

The short-acting anticholinergic ipratropium bromide blocks muscarinic acetylcholine receptors, thus promoting smooth muscle relaxation and inhibition of mucus secretion. These medications improve lung function and PaO_2 [38,40]. Common side effects include dry mouth, nausea, tachycardia, and sedation. There is a concern that nebulized anticholinergics may precipitate worsening glaucoma by coming into contact with the eyes in susceptible individuals.

In general, we use a combination of nebulized short-acting β-agonist and anticholinergic. A detailed discussion of inhaled bronchodilator therapy can be found in Chapter 169.

Antibiotics

Antibiotics are an intervention that is of proven benefit in AECOPD requiring ICU admission [28]. One must take into account potential pathogens, local resistance patterns, and antibiotic stewardship. The most common bacterial pathogens are *Haemophilus influenzae*, followed by *Streptococcus pneumoniae*, *Moraxella catarrhalis*, and *Pseudomonas aeruginosa*, and the common viral pathogens are *Rhinovirus*, *Parainfluenza*, *Influenza*, and *Respiratory Syncytial Virus* [41].

Prompt appropriate antibiotic therapy is the correct management of patients with severe COPD and symptomatic exacerbations that include at least two of the three cardinal symptoms (increased sputum purulence, volume or increased dyspnea; anthonisen type I or II exacerbations) [9].

Antivirals

Viral infections, in particular rhinovirus, account for approximately 30% of COPD exacerbations, and a variety of potential therapeutic agents have been investigated. Unfortunately, although the neuraminidase inhibitors such as oseltamivir and zanamivir are effective against influenza [42], antirhinoviral medications have failed to demonstrate a clinically significant benefit [43]. We do not routinely test for viral exacerbations outside the influenza season.

Steroids

Corticosteroids are routinely used for the treatment of COPD exacerbations. The evidence for the use of corticosteroids for COPD exacerbations admitted to the ICU is extrapolated from studies of individuals with milder disease [44]. To further confuse this picture, there is now evidence to support the use of systemic steroids in severe pneumonia [45], an often-coexisting diagnosis in exacerbations of COPD. We know that corticosteroids speed the recovery of FEV_1 and FVC in conjunction with bronchodilators [44]. Corticosteroids reduce the length of hospital stay and the risk of treatment failure in the first 3 months [46]. In two small studies performed in critically ill patients requiring ventilator support, there were conflicting results [47,48]. Clearly, some patients respond to steroid therapy and some do not, and this probably reflects the underlying inflammatory profile. Bafadhel et al. [49] showed peripheral blood eosinophil count as a promising biomarker to direct corticosteroid therapy during COPD exacerbations. The most appropriate dose is unclear and is generally at the discretion of the treating physician. The dosage should be cut down once a therapeutic response is evident and converted to oral once the patient is able to swallow. We acknowledge that there are adverse effects of corticosteroids with high dosage and extended treatment durations, but the current evidence base does not determine the most appropriate regimen. For patients admitted with very severe COPD exacerbations, we use methylprednisolone 40 mg every 6 hours consistent with the original study by Albert et al. [50].

Heliox

Helium is an inert gas that in combination with oxygen (heliox) has a lower density than oxygen and nitrogen. Heliox is a mixture of variable concentrations of helium and oxygen (60% to 80% helium and 40% to 20% oxygen). The benefit of using a lower density gas is its ability to improve flow in large airways where airflow is turbulent relative to laminar airflow. The increase in flow acts to decrease airway resistance and the work of breathing. In COPD, the addition of heliox to noninvasive ventilation (NIV) decreases respiratory effort and intrinsic PEEP, but does not improve outcomes such as requirement for intubation or mortality [51]. We do not routinely use heliox in the treatment of patients with AECOPD. A detailed discussion of heliox therapy can be found in Chapter 169.

Ventilatory Support

Indications for ventilator support in COPD patients include:

- Unsustainable increased work of breathing
- Severe hypoxemia
- Exacerbation leading to hypercapnia with reduced pH <7.35

Noninvasive Ventilation

The main benefits associated with noninvasive positive-pressure ventilation (NIPPV) in AECOPD are lower rates of intubation, shorter length of stay, and lower rates of the complications of invasive mechanical ventilation (MV). It has been shown to reduce the need for intubation, decrease length of stay, decrease mortality, and, in some areas, conserve the precious resource of ICU beds [52,53]. Patients with COPD who present with exacerbation and hypercapnic respiratory failure with acidosis (pH < 7.35) are the group most likely to benefit from NIPPV. Exacerbations increase the work of breathing often exceeding the patient's ability to compensate and result in hypoventilation. Increased intrinsic PEEP, dynamic hyperinflation, and weakened respiratory muscle force combine to produce ineffective tidal volume. NIV effectively unloads the respiratory muscles, increases tidal volume, reduces the respiratory rate, offsets intrinsic PEEP, and decreases the diaphragmatic work of breathing. These changes lead to more efficient ventilation with improved oxygenation and reduction in hypercapnia.

For effective treatment, NIV needs to be used for appropriate groups of patients, and combined with treatment of the underlying condition with bronchodilators, corticosteroids, and antibiotics. Exacerbations of COPD are ideally suited for treatment with NIV support, given the reversibility of exacerbations with treatment. However, failure rates of NIV of approximately 20% have been reported from controlled trials and may be much higher in some real-world settings [52]. We recommend prospectively establishing a management plan for NIPPV failure that takes the patient's wishes, comorbidities, and baseline functional status into consideration. If MV is felt to be inappropriate, goals of care should include symptom palliation and ongoing medical care [54]. A detailed discussion of NIPPV and how to institute it and deliver it can be found in Chapter 167.

Invasive Mechanical Ventilation

Indications for invasive mechanical ventilator support include:

- Reduced conscious level
- Inability to adequately control secretions
- Need for controlled ventilation with the use of sedation
- Persistent or worsening hypoxemia and/or worsening respiratory acidosis despite supplemental oxygen or NIPPV
- Hemodynamic instability and need for vasopressors

The goal of MV is to provide adequate respiratory muscle rest, improve gas exchange, and allow time for exacerbation resolution while not causing further harm.

Ventilator Settings

In general, initial ventilator settings are operator dependent and vary with local practices. We recommend the initial use of assist-control (AC) ventilation for invasive MV of AECOPD. AC ventilation is the most efficient at decreasing the work of breathing in COPD patients [55].

A major issue during ventilation for obstructive lung diseases (asthma and COPD) is the development of dynamic hyperinflation (interchangeable with auto-PEEP or intrinsic PEEP) [18]. This refers to increased EELV and the pressure it exerts. Dynamic hyperinflation can be minimized by reducing minute ventilation, prolonging expiration to allow deflation, and by reducing airflow resistance with targeted medication (Fig. 173.1).

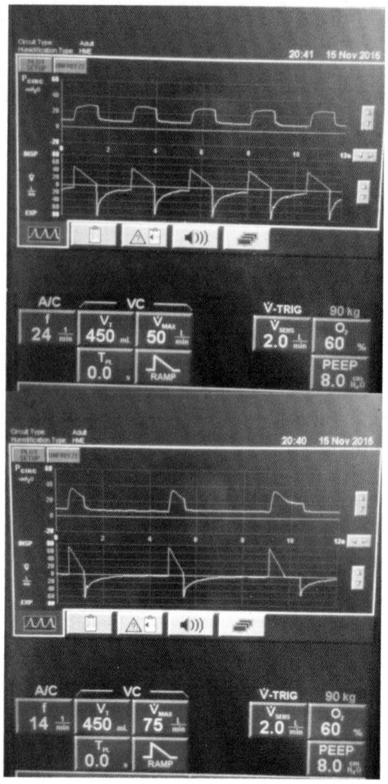

FIGURE 173.1 Inset of ventilator interface showing the effects that minute ventilation, respiratory rate, and inspiratory flow have on I:E ratio. Note that reducing the rate from 24 to 14 breaths per minute and increasing the inspiratory flow from 50 to 75 L per minute, the I:E ratio changes from 1:1.6 to 1:5.5. Also, note in A (**below left**) that the expired gas volume does not return to zero, leading to trapped air and intrinsic PEEP. I:E, inspiration:expiration; PEEP, positive end-expiratory pressure.

The aim of controlled ventilation should be to match minute ventilation to metabolic requirements while avoiding dynamic hyperinflation, lung injury, and extreme respiratory acidosis. It may be necessary to aggressively sedate the patient to achieve synchrony with the ventilator and reduce tachypnea. When selecting a tidal volume, it is important to provide sufficient volume to satisfy the patient and achieve synchrony with the ventilator. As guidance, tidal volumes of 5 to 8 mL per kg are often used [56].

When estimating the appropriate minute ventilation, it is important to be aware that, for many patients with severe COPD, the baseline state is a chronic compensated respiratory acidosis. For most individuals without chronic respiratory failure, we aim for a $PaCO_2$ 40 mm Hg, but, in this patient group, we aim to achieve their steady-state (baseline) $PaCO_2$ because this reflects the balance of their central respiratory drive and the ability of their lungs to ventilate. This can be estimated from stable blood gas records or serum bicarbonate ($PaCO_2 = 1.5 * [HCO_3] + 8 \pm 2$). Ventilator settings that produce a "normal" $PaCO_2$ in an individual with a chronic respiratory acidosis will lead to renal loss of bicarbonate. This can result to significant alkalosis (i.e., posthypercapnic metabolic alkalosis) with its potential central nervous system and cardiovascular complications, and difficulty when attempting to wean from the ventilator.

Optimization of the inspiration:expiration (I:E) ratio will reduce hyperinflation, and, in severely obstructed patients, >1:4 is often effective [56]. Adjustment of inspiratory flow to shorten the inspiratory phase of each breath can lead to better gas exchange by prolonging the expiratory phase and allowing more complete exhalation. In addition, reducing the respiratory rate will increase the I:E ratio. As guidance, flow rates between 70 and 100 L per minute are appropriate depending on peak airway pressures. Use of low tidal volumes and high-flow rates can lead to short insufflation time, with the risk of double triggering if the patient continues effort beyond ventilator insufflation time. Double triggering can lead to high tidal volumes and increased EELV. In this situation, use of a longer inspiratory time may resolve this; options include switching from constant flow to a decelerating flow waveform, or by reducing peak flow and/or adding an inspiratory pause [57].

The trigger for initiation of each breath depends on the mode of ventilation chosen. For controlled ventilation, the trigger is time. However, during AC, the patient initiates the breath, and this is thought to be more comfortable. The ventilator detects changes in the patient's effort and triggers a breath in response. Trigger types include pressure, volume, or flow. In pressure triggering, the patient must exert a predetermined amount of negative pressure to elicit a ventilator-assisted breath (-1 to -5 cm H_2O). In flow triggering, the patient's effort decreases the bias flow in the ventilator circuit by a predetermined value (1 to 3 L per minute), which then initiates a breath. We generally use flow triggering because it was thought to be more comfortable for the patient and can results in less work of breathing for some patients [17]. Patients with dynamic hyperinflation have greater difficulty triggering the ventilator. This is because they first must generate sufficient force to overcome the elastic recoil associated with the increased EELV (intrinsic PEEP) and then sufficient force to reach the trigger threshold [55].

The level of intrinsic PEEP can usually be estimated through the ventilator. Static intrinsic PEEP can be measured in patients without active respiratory effort. The ventilator executes an end-expiratory hold maneuver. This provides a measure of total PEEP by allowing lung units with different regional time constants to equalize with the ventilator. The intrinsic PEEP can then be calculated by subtracting the external PEEP from the total PEEP. For spontaneously breathing patients, the process is more complex and requires the use of esophageal pressure monitors and airflow tracings. Expiratory muscle activity and airway narrowing can all cause inaccurate measurements of intrinsic PEEP.

Elevated intrinsic PEEP can lead to nontriggered breaths that increase the work of breathing and sensation of dyspnea. In this situation, the addition of external PEEP set through the ventilator can decrease the inspiratory threshold load [18]. In general, setting external PEEP approximately 70% of the intrinsic PEEP is effective in patients with COPD. A reduction of nontriggered breaths is a good indication of more comfortable ventilator settings. The clinical assessment of the patient receiving MV is important in detecting the adequacy of patient ventilator interaction and respiratory distress. Analysis of ventilator waveforms can also provide vital information.

A detailed discussion of invasive ventilation and how to institute it and deliver it can be found in Chapter 166.

Weaning from Mechanical Ventilation

Patients with severe COPD can prove difficult when trying to liberate them from the ventilator. COPD patients can develop significant dynamic hyperinflation during weaning as a result of tachypnea and expiratory flow limitation. This will lead to respiratory distress and clinical signs of weaning failure [17]. All patients should be assessed for appropriateness of attempted weaning (Table 173.1) on a daily basis.

Rapid Shallow Breathing Index

Multiple studies have reported the development of rapid shallow breathing in patients who fail weaning from the ventilator. The development of rapid shallow breathing, asynchronous or paradoxic thoracoabdominal movements, and accessory muscle recruitment during a spontaneous breathing trial are physical examination findings of an unsuccessful weaning trial. The degree of rapid shallow breathing can be quantified by calculating the ratio of respiratory frequency to tidal volume (f/VT) in liters. An f/VT ratio of <105 breaths/min/L has been shown to be the best predictor of weaning outcome [17], and has become part of the routine assessment of suitability for weaning from MV. It is important to recognize that this test is most accurate in patients who have received MV for less than 7 days.

TABLE 173.1

Selection of COPD Patients for Weaning from Mechanical Ventilation

- Resolution of the underlying cause of respiratory failure
- Stable hemodynamics without need for significant vasopressors
- Stable metabolic state, that is, without sepsis or hyperthermia
- Cessation of neuromuscular blocking agents
- Patients should be alert, able to follow commands, and protect their airway
- Metabolic and electrolyte derangement should be corrected
- Adequate gas exchange, that is, PaO_2 to FiO_2 ratio greater than 200
- Require minimal assistance from the ventilator, that is, PEEP ≤ 5 cm H_2O and $FiO_2 \leq 50\%$
- Adequate respiratory muscle strength

Weaning Methods

There are three main types of weaning methods and these are daily spontaneous breathing trials, gradual reduction of pressure support (PS), and synchronized intermittent mandatory ventilation. Daily spontaneous breathing trials have been shown to be safe, effective, and faster at liberating patients from MV [58]. Comparing PS and spontaneous breathing trials, current evidence does not indicate which of these is superior [59]. We generally opt for a spontaneous breathing trial using the continuous positive airway pressure mode through the ventilator circuit to take advantage of ventilator alarms with or without PEEP for 30 minutes to 2 hours. At 30 to 120 minutes, if the patient looks favourable, we will extubate to humidified oxygen to maintain O_2 saturations 88% to 92%. Occasionally, we favour extubation to NIV in patients who are marginal as long as they can manage their own secretions, are mentally unimpaired, and don't have a difficult airway [60]. The development of rapid shallow breathing, asynchronous or paradoxic thoracoabdominal movements, and accessory muscle recruitment during a spontaneous breathing trial are physical examination findings indicating high risk for an unsuccessful trial of extubation [17]. When any of these findings are present, the patient should be placed back on ventilator support. Subsequently, there should be an assessment and correction of suspected causes of weaning failure.

A detailed discussion of weaning from MV can be found in Chapter 168.

Tracheostomy

Tracheostomy is commonly performed for mechanically ventilated patients with prolonged ventilator-dependent respiratory failure. Reasons to perform tracheostomy include the provision of a stable airway to facilitate rehabilitation, improved clearance of respiratory tract secretions and, in some cases, the reduction of sedation [61]. Sedation has been consistently associated with delirium and the length of ventilator-dependent respiratory failure [62]. Some patients appear to tolerate endotracheal intubation poorly and require sedation. In our experience, tracheostomy often reduces the need for sedation, because it can improve ability to communicate and reduce frustration. Complications of tracheostomy include bleeding, fistula formation, infection, and tracheal stenosis [63]. The use of a tracheostomy as an adjunct to the weaning process in COPD can be helpful for appropriate patients. COPD patients can occasionally require long periods of MV to allow time for their exacerbation to resolve sufficiently to allow weaning. Failure of weaning from the ventilator in COPD is complex to understand, because it results from an imbalance between respiratory muscle capacity and the applied resistive and elastic loads [64]. Endotracheal tubes can be small in diameter, and the development of biofilm (debris lining the endotracheal tube) can further decrease the internal diameter, leading to a greater resistive load [64]. Several groups have studied the effects that tracheotomies have on the ability to wean [64,65]. They found that tracheotomy significantly reduces work of breathing, the pressure time index, and measures of resistive and elastic workload.

A detailed discussion of endotracheal intubation and tracheotomy can be found in Chapters 8 and 9.

EXTRACORPOREAL LIFE SUPPORT, EXTRACORPOREAL CARBON DIOXIDE REMOVAL

Despite continued improvements in NIV, it is sometimes insufficient to overcome refractory hypercapnia and acidosis in AECOPD. In such cases, conversion to invasive MV is needed.

TABLE 173.2

Summary of the Main Randomized Controlled Trials of Noninvasive Ventilation in AECOPD Looking at Mortality

Author	Population	Design	NIPPV mode	Outcome	*p* value
Bott [74] 1993 The United Kingdom	N = 60 Adult AECOPD Mean pH NIPPV 7.35 vs. SMC 7.33	Multi center RCT NIPPV vs. SMC	Volume cycled NIPPV via nasal mask	Intention to treat: 30-d survival NIPPV 3/30 vs. SMC 9/30	0.106
Servillo 1994 Italy	N = 10 Adult AECOPD	Single-center parallel RCT NIPPV vs. SMC	Pressure support ventilation	Mortality: NIPPV 1/5 vs. SMC 1/5	NS
Brochard [75] 1995 France, Spain, and Italy	N = 85 Adult AECOPD Mean pH NIPPV 7.27 vs. SMC 7.28	Multicenter RCT NIPPV vs. SMC	Pressure support ventilation	In-hospital mortality: NIPPV 4/43 vs. 12/42	0.02
Barbe [76] 1996 Spain	N = 24 Adult AECOPD Mean pH NIPPV 7.34 vs. SMC 7.30	Single-center parallel RCT NIPPV vs. SMC	BiPAP via nasal mask	4/24 patients intolerant No mortality encountered	NS
Avdeev [77] 1998 Russia	N = 58 Adult AECOPD Mean pH NIPPV 7.28 vs. SMC 7.26	Single-center parallel RCT NIPPV vs. SMC	BiPAP via nasal/face mask	Mortality: NIPPV 2/29 vs. SMC 9/29	0.03
Celikel [78] 1998 Turkey	N = 30 Adult AECOPD Mean pH NIPPV 7.27 vs. SMC 7.28	Single-center parallel RCT NIPPV vs. SMC	Pressure support ventilation Initial settings CPAP 5 + PS 15 cm H_2O	Mortality: NIPPV 0/15 vs. SMC 1/15	NS
Plant [79] 2000 The United Kingdom	N = 236 Adult AECOPD Mean pH NIPPV 7.32 vs. SMC 7.31	Multicenter RCT NIPPV vs. SMC	BiPAP via nasal/face mask Initial settings EPAP 4 + PS 10 cm H_2O	In-hospital mortality: NIPPV 12/128 vs. 24/128	0.05
Khilnani [80] 2002 India	N = 40 Adult AECOPD Mean pH NIPPV 7.23 vs. SMC 7.23	Single-center parallel RCT NIPPV vs. SMC	BiPAP via nasal mask Initial settings IPAP 8 + EPAP 4 cm H_2O	In-hospital mortality: NIPPV 3/20 vs. 2/20	NS

N, number; NIPPV, noninvasive positive-pressure ventilation; SMC, standard medical care; RCT, randomized controlled trial; NS, nonsignificant; AECOPD, acute exacerbation of chronic obstructive pulmonary disease; BiPAP, bilevel positive airway pressure ventilation; CPAP, continuous positive airway pressure; EPAP, expiratory positive airway pressure; PS, pressure support; IPAP, inspiratory positive airway pressure.

This self-selecting group has a higher mortality up to 30% [66]. Mortality is increased because the patients are exposed to the associated risks of invasive ventilation, including ventilator-associated pneumonia [67], prolonged MV, and difficult weaning [68]. Advances in extracorporeal gas exchange technology have led to the evolution of systems designed for extracorporeal carbon dioxide removal ($ECCO_2R$). Currently, the evidence to support its use is based on case reports and small case series. Kluge et al. [69] studied 21 patients treated with $ECCO_2R$ at the point of failing support with NIV and compared them retrospectively to a historic cohort treated with invasive MV. Of the 21 patients, 14 who were treated had an AECOPD. Ninety percent of the patients treated with the $ECCO_2R$ did not require intubation and mechanical ventilatory support. There was no statistical difference in 28-day mortality or 6-month mortality. Burki et al. [70] also reported on a pilot study of $ECCO_2R$ in COPD patients with hypercapnic respiratory failure. There were three groups of patients: group 1 consisted of 7 patients who were receiving NIV and had a high likelihood of requiring intubation, group 2 consisted of 2 patients who had failed two weaning attempts from continuous NIV support, and group 3 consisted of 11 patients already on invasive MV that were placed on $ECCO_2R$ to assist with weaning. In the first group of patients, despite a mean arterial pH of 7.25 and PCO_2 of 83 mm Hg at baseline while on NIV, all seven avoided intubation and MV. Both patients in group 2 avoided invasive MV but remained on intermittent NIV support after weaning from $ECCO_2R$. In group 3, three patients were weaned off invasive MV, and, in three further patients, the level of invasive ventilatory support was reduced. Only one patient remained on the same level of ventilatory support. However, no patient in group 3 was able to be liberated from ventilator support altogether. The evidence from these studies would suggest that $ECCO_2R$ is an effective therapeutic modality for CO_2 removal but not without its associated risks, and it does not change the long-term survival. Complications related to the need for mobility limiting large-bore catheters, the need for anticoagulation, and the consequences of hemolysis and thrombocytopenia associated with ECMO all need to be considered. Patients who develop hypercapnic respiratory failure are at the severe end of the spectrum. The use of such lifesaving modalities should be seen as indication for consideration of lung transplantation or initiation of a palliative focused care plan.

Nutrition

Critical illness induces a highly catabolic state that can lead to loss of significant muscle mass. This catabolic state, prolonged immobility, and a series of other risk factors, including possible exposure to corticosteroids and paralytic agents, can contribute to critical care polyneuropathy [71]. Awareness of loss of respiratory muscle mass and diaphragm weakness is extremely important because it can lead to difficulty weaning from MV [72]. Nutrition should not be neglected for patients who are stable enough to feed. Nutrition should be balanced to meet the body's needs and avoid loss of muscle mass [73]. Unnecessary calories and excessive carbohydrate feeding can lead to carbon dioxide production which the patient's compromised respiratory system may be unable to clear.

A detailed discussion of nutritional support in critically ill patients can be found in Chapters 212–214.

References

1. Global strategy for the diagnosis, management, and prevention of chronic obstructive pulmonary disease (ATS journals). http://www.atsjournals.org.libproxy.temple.edu/doi/abs/10.1164/ajrccm.163.5.2101039?url_ver=Z39.88-2003&rfr_id=ori:rid:crossref.org&rfr_dat=cr_pub=pubmed#.VQXAnmZ-4jUU. 2015. Accessed March 15, 2015.
2. Chapman KR: Epidemiology and costs of chronic obstructive pulmonary disease. *Eur Respir J* 27(1):188–207, 2006. doi: 10.1183/09031936.06.00024505.
3. Confronting COPD in America: Executive summary. http://www.aarc.org/resources/confronting_copd/exesum.pdf. http://www.lung.org/assets/documents/EXESUM.pdf. 2015. Accessed Msrch 18, 2015.
4. Hilleman DE, Dewan N, Malesker M, et al: Pharmacoeconomic evaluation of copd. *Chest* 118(5):1278–1285, 2000.
5. MacIntyre N, Huang YC: Acute exacerbations and respiratory failure in chronic obstructive pulmonary disease. *Proc Am Thorac Soc* 5(4):530, 2008.
6. Bafadhel M, McKenna S, Terry S, et al: Acute exacerbations of chronic obstructive pulmonary disease: identification of biologic clusters and their biomarkers. *Am J Respir Crit Care Med* 184(6):662–671, 2011. doi: 10.1164/rccm.201104-0597OC.
7. Bafadhel M, Davies L, Calverley PMA, et al: Blood eosinophil guided prednisolone therapy for exacerbations of COPD: a further analysis. *Eur Respir J* 44(3):789–791, 2014. doi: 10.1183/09031936.00062614.
8. Mullerova H, Shukla A, Hawkins A, et al: Risk factors for acute exacerbations of COPD in a primary care population: a retrospective observational cohort study. *BMJ Open* 4(12):e006171, 2014. doi: 10.1136/bmjopen-2014-006171.
9. GOLD—the global initiative for chronic obstructive lung disease. http://www.goldcopd.com/guidelines-global-strategy-for-diagnosis-management.html. 2015. Accessed March 12, 2015.
10. Immunologic aspects of chronic obstructive pulmonary disease—NEJMra0804752. http://www.nejm.org.libproxy.temple.edu/doi/pdf/10.1056/NEJMra0804752. 2015. Accessed March 24, 2015.
11. Lange P, Celli B, Agusti A, et al: Lung-function trajectories leading to chronic obstructive pulmonary disease. *N Engl J Med* 373(2):111–122, 2015. doi: 10.1056/NEJMoa1411532.
12. Hirota N, Martin JG: Mechanisms of airway remodeling. *Chest* 144(3):1026–1032, 2013. doi: 10.1378/chest.12-3073.
13. McDonough JE, Yuan R, Suzuki M, et al: Small-airway obstruction and emphysema in chronic obstructive pulmonary disease. *N Engl J Med* 365(17):1567–1575, 2011. doi: 10.1056/NEJMoa1106955.
14. The definition of emphysema. Report of a national heart, lung, and blood institute, division of lung diseases workshop. *Am Rev Respir Dis* 132(1):182–185, 1985.
15. Parr DG, Stoel BC, Stolk J, et al: Pattern of emphysema distribution in alpha1-antitrypsin deficiency influences lung function impairment. *Am J Respir Crit Care Med* 170(11):1172–1178, 2004. doi: 10.1164/rccm.200406-761OC.
16. Roussos C, Koutsoukou A: Respiratory failure. *Eur Respir J Suppl* 47:3s–14s, 2003.
17. Tobin MJ, Laghi F, Jubran A: Ventilatory failure, ventilator support, and ventilator weaning. *Compr Physiol* 2(4):2871–2921, 2012. doi: 10.1002/cphy.c110030.
18. Reddy RM, Guntupalli KK: Review of ventilatory techniques to optimize mechanical ventilation in acute exacerbation of chronic obstructive pulmonary disease. *Int J Chron Obstruct Pulmon Dis* 2(4):441–452, 2007.
19. Parker CM, Voduc N, Aaron SD, et al: Physiological changes during symptom recovery from moderate exacerbations of COPD. *Eur Respir J* 26(3):420–428, 2005.
20. Connors AF Jr, Dawson NV, Thomas C, et al: Outcomes following acute exacerbation of severe chronic obstructive lung disease. The SUPPORT investigators (study to understand prognoses and preferences for outcomes and risks of treatments). *Am J Respir Crit Care Med* 154[4 Pt 1]:959–967, 1996. doi: 10.1164/ajrccm.154.4.8887592.
21. Wildman MJ, Sanderson C, Groves J, et al: Predicting mortality for patients with exacerbations of COPD and asthma in the COPD and asthma outcome study (CAOS). *QJM* 102(6):389–399, 2009. doi: 10.1093/qjmed/hcp036.
22. Singanayagam A, Schembri S, Chalmers JD: Predictors of mortality in hospitalized adults with acute exacerbation of chronic obstructive pulmonary disease. *Ann Am Thorac Soc* 10(2):81–89, 2013. doi: 10.1513/AnnalsATS.201208-043OC.
23. Messer B, Griffiths J, Baudouin SV: The prognostic variables predictive of mortality in patients with an exacerbation of COPD admitted to the ICU: an integrative review. *QJM* 105(2):115–126, 2012. doi: 10.1093/qjmed/hcr210.
24. Hawkey PM, Jones AM: The changing epidemiology of resistance. *J Antimicrob Chemother* 64 Suppl 1:i3–i10, 2009. doi: 10.1093/jac/dkp256.
25. Frank MO, Batteiger BE, Sorensen SJ, et al: Decrease in expenditures and selected nosocomial infections following implementation of an antimicrobial-prescribing improvement program. *Clin Perform Qual Health Care* 5(4):180–188, 1997.
26. Kumar A, Roberts D, Wood KE, et al: Duration of hypotension before initiation of effective antimicrobial therapy is the critical determinant of survival in human septic shock. *Crit Care Med* 34(6):1589–1596, 2006. doi: 10.1097/01.CCM.0000217961.75225.E9.
27. Iregui M, Ward S, Sherman G, et al: Clinical importance of delays in the initiation of appropriate antibiotic treatment for ventilator-associated pneumonia. *Chest* 122(1):262–268, 2002.
28. Vollenweider DJ, Jarrett H, Steurer-Stey CA, et al: Antibiotics for exacerbations of chronic obstructive pulmonary disease. *Cochrane Database Syst Rev* 12:CD010257, 2012. doi: 10.1002/14651858.CD010257.
29. Christ-Crain M, Stolz D, Bingisser R, et al: Procalcitonin guidance of antibiotic therapy in community-acquired pneumonia: a randomized trial. *Am J Respir Crit Care Med* 174(1):84–93, 2006. doi: 10.1164/rccm.200512-1922OC.
30. Schuetz P, Christ-Crain M, Thomann R, et al: Effect of procalcitonin-based guidelines vs standard guidelines on antibiotic use in lower respiratory tract infections: The ProHOSP randomized controlled trial. *JAMA* 302(10):1059–1066, 2009. doi: 10.1001/jama.2009.1297.
31. Stolz D, Smyrnios N, Eggimann P, et al: Procalcitonin for reduced antibiotic exposure in ventilator-associated pneumonia: a randomised study. *Eur Respir J* 34(6):1364–1375, 2009. doi: 10.1183/09031936.00053209.
32. Bouadma L, Luyt CE, Tubach F, et al: Use of procalcitonin to reduce patients' exposure to antibiotics in intensive care units (PRORATA trial): a multicentre randomised controlled trial. *Lancet* 375(9713):463–474, 2010. doi: 10.1016/S0140-6736(09)61879-1.
33. O'Driscoll BR, Howard LS, Davison AG; British Thoracic Society: BTS guideline for emergency oxygen use in adult patients. *Thorax* 63 Suppl 6:vi1–vi68, 2008. doi: 10.1136/thx.2008.102947.
34. Abdo WF, Heunks LM: Oxygen-induced hypercapnia in COPD: myths and facts. *Crit Care* 16(5):323, 2012. doi: 10.1186/cc11475.
35. Frat JP, Thille AW, Mercat A, et al: High-flow oxygen through nasal cannula in acute hypoxemic respiratory failure. *N Engl J Med* 372(23):2185–2196, 2015. doi: 10.1056/NEJMoa1503326.
36. Chatila W, Nugent T, Vance G, et al: The effects of high-flow vs low-flow oxygen on exercise in advanced obstructive airways disease. *Chest* 126(4):1108–1115, 2004.
37. Nishimura M: High-flow nasal cannula oxygen therapy in adults. *J Intensive Care* 3(1):15, 2015. doi: 10.1186/s40560-015-0084-5.
38. McCrory DC, Brown CD: Anti-cholinergic bronchodilators versus beta2-sympathomimetic agents for acute exacerbations of chronic obstructive pulmonary disease. *Cochrane Database Syst Rev* (4):CD003900, 2002. doi: 10.1002/14651858.CD003900.
39. Weber EJ, Levitt MA, Covington JK, et al: Effect of continuously nebulized ipratropium bromide plus albuterol on emergency department length of stay and hospital admission rates in patients with acute bronchospasm. A randomized, controlled trial. *Chest* 115:937–944, 1999. http://www-ncbi-nlm-nih-gov.libproxy.temple.edu/pubmed/10208189. Accessed November 21, 2015.
40. Karpel JP, Pesin J, Greenberg D, et al: A comparison of the effects of ipratropium bromide and metaproterenol sulfate in acute exacerbations of COPD. *Chest* 98(4):835–839, 1990.
41. Rangelov K, Sethi S: Role of infections. *Clin Chest Med* 35(1):87–100, 2014. doi: 10.1016/j.ccm.2013.09.012.
42. Jefferson T, Jones M, Doshi P, et al: Oseltamivir for influenza in adults and children: Systematic review of clinical study reports and summary of regulatory comments. *BMJ* 348:g2545, 2014. doi: 10.1136/bmj.g2545.
43. Martinez FJ: Pathogen-directed therapy in acute exacerbations of chronic obstructive pulmonary disease. *Proc Am Thorac Soc* 4(8):647–658, 2007.
44. Walters JA, Tan DJ, White CJ, et al: Systemic corticosteroids for acute exacerbations of chronic obstructive pulmonary disease. *Cochrane Database Syst Rev* 9:CD001288, 2014. doi: 10.1002/14651858.CD001288.pub4.
45. Torres A, Sibila O, Ferrer M, et al: Effect of corticosteroids on treatment failure among hospitalized patients with severe community-acquired pneumonia and high inflammatory response: a randomized clinical trial. *JAMA* 313(7):677–686, 2015. doi: 10.1001/jama.2015.88.
46. Woods JA, Wheeler JS, Finch CK, et al: Corticosteroids in the treatment of acute exacerbations of chronic obstructive pulmonary disease. *Int J Chron Obstruct Pulmon Dis* 9:421–430, 2014. doi: 10.2147/COPD.S51012.
47. Abroug F, Ouanes-Besbes L, Fkih-Hassen M, et al: Prednisone in COPD exacerbation requiring ventilatory support: an open-label randomised evaluation. *Eur Respir J* 43(3):717–724, 2014. doi: 10.1183/09031936.00002913.

48. Alia I, de la Cal MA, Esteban A, et al: Efficacy of corticosteroid therapy in patients with an acute exacerbation of chronic obstructive pulmonary disease receiving ventilatory support. *Arch Intern Med* 171(21):1939–1946, 2011. doi: 10.1001/archinternmed.2011.530.
49. Bafadhel M, McKenna S, Terry S, et al: Blood eosinophils to direct corticosteroid treatment of exacerbations of chronic obstructive pulmonary disease: a randomized placebo-controlled trial. *Am J Respir Crit Care Med* 186(1):48–55, 2012. doi: 10.1164/rccm.201108-1553OC.
50. Albert RK, Martin TR, Lewis SW: Controlled clinical trial of methylprednisolone in patients with chronic bronchitis and acute respiratory insufficiency. *Ann Intern Med* 92(6):753–758, 1980.
51. Maggiore SM, Richard JC, Abroug F, et al: A multicenter, randomized trial of noninvasive ventilation with helium-oxygen mixture in exacerbations of chronic obstructive lung disease. *Crit Care Med* 38(1):145–151, 2010. doi: 10.1097/CCM.0b013e3181b78abe.
52. Lightowler JV, Wedzicha JA, Elliott MW, et al: Non-invasive positive pressure ventilation to treat respiratory failure resulting from exacerbations of chronic obstructive pulmonary disease: cochrane systematic review and meta-analysis. *BMJ* 326(7382):185, 2003.
53. Lopez-Campos JL, Jara-Palomares L, Munoz X, Bustamante V, et al: Lights and shadows of non-invasive mechanical ventilation for chronic obstructive pulmonary disease (COPD) exacerbations. *Ann Thorac Med* 10(2):87–93, 2015. doi: 10.4103/1817-1737.151440.
54. Concise Guidance to Good Practice. https://www.brit-thoracic.org.uk/document-library/clinical-information/niv/niv-guidelines/the-use-of-non-invasive-ventilation-in-the-management-of-patients-with-copd-admitted-to-hospital-with-acute-type-ii-respiratory-failure/. https://www.brit-thoracic.org.uk/document-library/clinical-information/niv/niv-guidelines/the-use-of-non-invasive-ventilation-in-the-management-of-patients-with-copd-admitted-to-hospital-with-acute-type-ii-respiratory-failure/. 2015. Accessed November 12, 2015.
55. Leung P, Jubran A, Tobin MJ: Comparison of assisted ventilator modes on triggering, patient effort, and dyspnea. *Am J Respir Crit Care Med* 155(6):1940–1948, 1997. doi: 10.1164/ajrccm.155.6.9196100.
56. Garcia Vicente E, Sandoval Almengor JC, Diaz Caballero LA, et al: Invasive mechanical ventilation in COPD and asthma. *Med Intensiva* 35(5):288–298, 2011. doi: 10.1016/j.medin.2010.11.004.
57. Thille AW, Rodriguez P, Cabello B, et al: Patient-ventilator asynchrony during assisted mechanical ventilation. *Intensive Care Med* 32(10):1515–1522, 2006. doi: 10.1007/s00134-006-0301-8.
58. Blackwood B, Burns KE, Cardwell CR, et al: Protocolized versus non-protocolized weaning for reducing the duration of mechanical ventilation in critically ill adult patients. *Cochrane Database Syst Rev* 11:CD006904, 2014. doi: 10.1002/14651858.CD006904.pub3.
59. Ladeira MT, Vital FM, Andriolo RB, et al: Pressure support versus T-tube for weaning from mechanical ventilation in adults. *Cochrane Database Syst Rev* 5:CD006056, 2014. doi: 10.1002/14651858.CD006056.pub2.
60. Burns KE, Adhikari NK, Keenan SP, et al: Noninvasive positive pressure ventilation as a weaning strategy for intubated adults with respiratory failure. *Cochrane Database Syst Rev* (8):CD004127, 2010. doi: 10.1002/14651858.CD004127.pub2.
61. Astrachan DI, Kirchner JC, Goodwin WJ Jr: Prolonged intubation vs. tracheotomy: complications, practical and psychological considerations. *Laryngoscope* 98(11):1165–1169, 1988. doi: 10.1288/00005537-198811000-00003.
62. Shehabi Y, Bellomo R, Reade MC, et al: Early intensive care sedation predicts long-term mortality in ventilated critically ill patients. *Am J Respir Crit Care Med* 186(8):724–731, 2012. doi: 10.1164/rccm.201203-0522OC.
63. Stock MC, Woodward CG, Shapiro BA, et al: Perioperative complications of elective tracheostomy in critically ill patients. *Crit Care Med* 14(10):861–863, 1986.
64. Diehl JL, El Atrous S, Touchard D, et al: Changes in the work of breathing induced by tracheotomy in ventilator-dependent patients. *Am J Respir Crit Care Med* 159(2):383–388, 1999. doi: 10.1164/ajrccm.159.2.9707046.
65. Moscovici da Cruz V, Demarzo SE, Sobrinho JB, et al: Effects of tracheotomy on respiratory mechanics in spontaneously breathing patients. *Eur Respir J* 20(1):112–117, 2002.
66. Chandra D, Stamm JA, Taylor B, et al: Outcomes of noninvasive ventilation for acute exacerbations of chronic obstructive pulmonary disease in the United States, 1998–2008. *Am J Respir Crit Care Med* 185(2):152–159, 2012. doi: 10.1164/rccm.201106-1094OC.
67. Chastre J, Fagon JY: Ventilator-associated pneumonia. *Am J Respir Crit Care Med* 165(7):867–903, 2002. doi: 10.1164/ajrccm.165.7.2105078.
68. Mamary AJ, Kondapaneni S, Vance GB, et al: Survival in patients receiving prolonged ventilation: factors that influence outcome. *Clin Med Insights Circ Respir Pulm Med* 5:17–26, 2011. doi: 10.4137/CCRPM.S6649.
69. Kluge S, Braune SA, Engel M, et al: Avoiding invasive mechanical ventilation by extracorporeal carbon dioxide removal in patients failing noninvasive ventilation. *Intensive Care Med* 38(10):1632–1639, 2012. doi: 10.1007/s00134-012-2649-2.
70. Burki NK, Mani RK, Herth FJ, et al: A novel extracorporeal CO(2) removal system: results of a pilot study of hypercapnic respiratory failure in patients with COPD. *Chest* 143(3):678–686, 2013. doi: 10.1378/chest.12-0228.
71. Latronico N, Bolton CF: Critical illness polyneuropathy and myopathy: a major cause of muscle weakness and paralysis. *Lancet Neurol* 10(10):931–941, 2011. doi: 10.1016/S1474-4422(11)70178-8.
72. Laghi F, Tobin MJ: Disorders of the respiratory muscles. *Am J Respir Crit Care Med* 168(1):10–48, 2003. doi: 10.1164/rccm.2206020.
73. Alberda C, Gramlich L, Jones N, et al: The relationship between nutritional intake and clinical outcomes in critically ill patients: results of an international multicenter observational study. *Intensive Care Med* 35(10):1728–1737, 2009. doi: 10.1007/s00134-009-1567-4.
74. Bott J, Carroll MP, Conway JH, et al: Randomised controlled trial of nasal ventilation in acute ventilatory failure due to chronic obstructive airways disease. *Lancet* 341(8860):1555–1557, 1993.
75. Brochard L, Mancebo J, Wysocki M, et al: Noninvasive ventilation for acute exacerbations of chronic obstructive pulmonary disease. *N Engl J Med* 333(13):817–822, 1995. doi: 10.1056/NEJM199509283331301.
76. Barbe F, Togores B, Rubi M, et al: Noninvasive ventilatory support does not facilitate recovery from acute respiratory failure in chronic obstructive pulmonary disease. *Eur Respir J* 9(6):1240–1245, 1996.
77. Avdeev SN, Tret'iakov AV, Grigor'iants RA, et al: Study of the use of noninvasive ventilation of the lungs in acute respiratory insufficiency due exacerbation of chronic obstructive pulmonary disease. *Anesteziol Reanimatol* (3):45–51, 1998.
78. Celikel T, Sungur M, Ceyhan B, et al: Comparison of noninvasive positive pressure ventilation with standard medical therapy in hypercapnic acute respiratory failure. *Chest* 114(6):1636–1642, 1998.
79. Plant PK, Owen JL, Elliott MW: Early use of non-invasive ventilation for acute exacerbations of chronic obstructive pulmonary disease on general respiratory wards: a multicentre randomised controlled trial. *Lancet* 355(9219):1931–1935, 2000.
80. Khilnani GC, Saikia N, Banga A, et al: Non-invasive ventilation for acute exacerbation of COPD with very high PaCO(2): a randomized controlled trial. *Lung India* 27(3):125–130, 2010. doi: 10.4103/0970-2113.68308.

Chapter 174 ■ Pulmonary Hypertension in the Intensive Care Unit

KIMBERLY A. FISHER • HARRISON W. FARBER

INTRODUCTION

Pulmonary hypertension, defined as a mean pulmonary artery pressure (mPAP) greater than 25 mm Hg, is a common finding among critically ill patients. It can be related to the underlying critical illness (respiratory failure, pulmonary embolism, decompensated heart failure), pre-existing conditions (left-sided heart disease, chronic obstructive pulmonary disease [COPD], and interstitial lung disease), or may be the primary cause of critical illness, because in the case of decompensated right heart failure due to pulmonary arterial hypertension (PAH). Initiation of appropriate therapy requires differentiating among these possible etiologies.

CLASSIFICATION/ETIOLOGY

Pulmonary hypertension is classified into five groups based on similar pathology and response to treatment, according to the fifth World Symposium on Pulmonary Hypertension (Table 174.1) [1]. In this classification, groupings are based on whether the primary abnormality is in the precapillary arteries and arterioles (Group 1), postcapillary pulmonary veins and venules (Group 2), alveoli and capillary beds (Group 3), or due to chronic thromboemboli (Group 4). Group 5 comprises causes of pulmonary hypertension with multiple or unclear mechanisms.

PAH refers only to Group 1 and is distinct from other forms of pulmonary hypertension. PAH can be idiopathic (IPAH, formerly primary pulmonary hypertension or PPH), heritable (HPAH), or associated with underlying conditions such as collagen vascular disease, congenital heart disease, portal hypertension, HIV infection, and specific drugs (e.g., fenfluramine) or toxins (e.g., rapeseed oil). Pulmonary venous hypertension is the result of elevated pulmonary venous (e.g., sclerosing mediastinitis) or left-sided cardiac filling pressures that lead to passive elevation in pulmonary artery pressures (PAPs). This is typically caused by left ventricular (LV) systolic or diastolic heart failure, or valvular heart disease (mitral or aortic regurgitation or stenosis). Lung disease can cause pulmonary hypertension due to alveolar hypoxemia (hypoxic pulmonary vasoconstriction) and vascular destruction [2]. Chronic thromboembolic pulmonary hypertension (CTEPH) can be due to proximal and/or distal obstruction of the pulmonary vasculature by chronic thromboemboli.

Pulmonary hypertension related to critical illness can occur through multiple mechanisms, and therefore patients may fall into any of the above-described groups (Table 174.2). However, no matter the group, or the reason for admission to the intensive care unit (ICU), right heart failure in this setting is associated with a poor prognosis. Among patients with PAH or inoperable CTEPH admitted to the ICU with decompensated right heart failure, infection is the most commonly identified trigger (approximately 25%), with other causes including drug or dietary noncompliance, arrhythmia, pulmonary embolism, and pregnancy. For approximately 50% of cases of decompensated right heart failure, no precipitating etiology can be identified, suggesting it is due to underlying disease progression. Decompensated right heart failure requiring ICU admission is associated with a high mortality rate (32% to 41%) [3,4].

Decompensation of left heart disease can cause or worsen pulmonary venous hypertension. Exacerbations of chronic hypoxemic lung disease (chronic obstructive lung disease or interstitial lung disease) can be associated with pulmonary hypertension. Acute pulmonary embolism can cause pulmonary hypertension, depending on the degree of vascular obstruction. For a patient with normal pulmonary vasculature, greater than 50% obstruction of the pulmonary vasculature must occur before pulmonary hypertension occurs. Pulmonary hypertension may also occur following acute pulmonary embolism with a lesser degree of pulmonary vascular obstruction among patients with underlying cardiopulmonary disease [5].

Pulmonary hypertension complicates most cases of acute respiratory distress syndrome (ARDS), reported for 73% to 92%

TABLE 174.1

Updated Clinical Classification of Pulmonary Hypertension (Nice, 2013)

Group 1. Pulmonary arterial hypertension (PAH)
Idiopathic PAH
Heritable
Drug and toxin induced
Associated with connective tissues disease, HIV infection, portal hypertension, congenital heart diseases, and schistosomiasis
Pulmonary veno-occlusive disease and/or pulmonary capillary hemangiomatosis
Persistent pulmonary hypertension of the newborn
Group 2. Pulmonary hypertension owing to left heart disease
Systolic dysfunction
Diastolic dysfunction
Valvular disease
Congenital/acquired left heart inflow/outflow tract obstruction and congenital cardiomyopathies
Group 3. Pulmonary hypertension owing to lung disease and/or hypoxia
Chronic obstructive pulmonary disease
Interstitial lung disease
Other pulmonary diseases with mixed restrictive and obstructive pattern
Sleep-disordered breathing
Alveolar hypoventilation disorders
Chronic exposure to high altitude
Developmental abnormalities
Group 4. Chronic thromboembolic pulmonary hypertension
Group 5. Pulmonary hypertension with unclear multifactorial mechanisms
Hematologic disorders: chronic haemolytic anemia, myeloproliferative disorders, and splenectomy
Systemic disorders: sarcoidosis, pulmonary Langerhans cell histiocytosis, and lymphangioleiomyomatosis
Metabolic disorders: glycogen storage disease, Gaucher disease, and thyroid disorders
Others: tumoral obstruction, fibrosing mediastinitis, chronic renal failure, and segmental PH

Modified from Simonneau G, Gatzoulis M, Adatia I, et al: Updated clinical classification of pulmonary hypertension. *J Am CollCardiol* 52:D34–D41, 2013.

TABLE 174.2

Common Causes of Pulmonary Hypertension in the Intensive Care Unit

Hypoxemia/parenchymal lung disease
Acute respiratory distress syndrome
Pulmonary embolism
Interstitial lung disease
Obstructive sleep apnea
Chronic obstructive pulmonary disease
Left heart disease
Acute myocardial infarction
Valvular disease (mitral regurgitation/mitral stenosis)
Severe diastolic dysfunction
Cardiomyopathy
Postoperative states
Coronary artery bypass grafting
Cardiac transplantation
Lung/heart–lung transplantation
Pneumonectomy
Thromboembolic lung disease
Pulmonary embolism
Deterioration of chronic pulmonary arterial hypertension
Infection
Fluid overloaded state
Arrhythmias
Pulmonary embolism
Acute on chronic pulmonary hypertension
Medication withdrawal

Modified from Zamanian RT, Haddad F, Doyle RL, et al: Management strategies for patients with pulmonary hypertension in the intensive care unit. *Crit Care Med* 35:2037–2050, 2007.

of patients with ARDS [6,7]. However, it is almost always mild to moderate in severity; in one study, only 7% of patients with ARDS had severe pulmonary hypertension [7]. The magnitude of pulmonary hypertension in ARDS appears to be related to the severity of lung injury [8]. Approximately 25% of patients with ARDS have findings of right ventricular (RV) failure as detected by echocardiography [8–10]. It has been suggested that the incidence of RV failure in ARDS has decreased with widespread adoption of low tidal volume ventilation. The prognostic significance of pulmonary hypertension and RV failure for patients with ARDS is uncertain, with multiple studies yielding conflicting results [6,8,11,12].

PHYSIOLOGY OF THE PULMONARY CIRCULATION AND RIGHT VENTRICLE

The pulmonary circulation is the only vascular bed that accommodates the entire cardiac output while maintaining both low pressure and low vascular resistance. Normally, the pulmonary vasculature is able to accommodate increases in cardiac output without increases in pressure or resistance via dilation of pulmonary vessels and recruitment of previously closed vessels [13]. Pulmonary hypertension develops when abnormalities of the pulmonary vasculature lead to increases in pulmonary vascular resistance (PVR) and therefore increased RV afterload.

Because the RV normally ejects blood against a significantly lower afterload than the LV, it has a thinner wall and is therefore more compliant. This allows it to accommodate large increases in volume (preload). However, increases of afterload result in proportionate decreases of RV stroke volume [14]. Decreased RV stroke volume reduces blood return to the LV, thereby decreasing cardiac output. In addition, RV pressure overload causes "ventricular interdependence," in which elevated right ventricular end-diastolic pressure (RVEDP) causes bowing of the interventricular septum toward the LV during diastole, preventing LV diastolic filling and further reducing cardiac output [13]. RV pressure overload can also open the foramen ovale, allowing the shunting of blood from right to left, with resultant hypoxemia [14].

PATHOLOGY AND PATHOGENESIS

Patients with PAH share common pathologic findings including intimal fibrosis, increased medial thickness, pulmonary arteriolar occlusion, and plexiform lesions [15]. Multiple molecular pathways involved in the pathogenesis of IPAH have been identified. Patients with IPAH have an increase in mediators of vasoconstriction and vascular smooth muscle cell proliferation (thromboxane A2, Endothelin-1) and a decrease of substances that promote pulmonary vasodilation and inhibition of vascular smooth muscle cell proliferation (prostacyclin, nitric oxide, and vasoactive intestinal peptide) [16].

Pathologic findings of pulmonary hypertension associated with ARDS vary with the time course of illness. Micro- and macrothrombi have been demonstrated in most patients. Early in disease, there are findings of acute endothelial cell injury. During the intermediate phase, chronic capillary changes, fibrocellular obliteration of arteries, veins, and lymphatics can occur. Vascular remodeling with distorted, tortuous arteries and veins, arterial muscularization, and reduced capillary number are seen during the late stages [8].

DIAGNOSIS

Signs and Symptoms

Patients with PAH typically present with exertional dyspnea. Other presenting symptoms may include fatigue, syncope or near syncope, palpitations, and chest pain. Because the disease progresses, patients may develop symptoms referable to reduced cardiac output and RV failure including fatigue, abdominal bloating and distension, and lower extremity edema. The presence of orthopnea and paroxysmal nocturnal dyspnea is suggestive of pulmonary venous hypertension [17].

Signs of elevated PAP on physical examination include (a) prominent pulmonary component of the second heart sound or P2, (b) RV heave, (c) early systolic ejection click, (d) midsystolic ejection murmur, (e) RV S_4 gallop, and (f) prominent jugular "a" wave. With more advanced disease, patients may develop findings of tricuspid regurgitation, including a holosystolic murmur along the left lower sternal border, and elevated jugular venous pressure. Findings of RV failure include elevated jugular pressure, pulsatile hepatomegaly, peripheral edema, ascites, and hypotension [17,18]. Patients with non–Group 1 causes of pulmonary hypertension may also have findings related to the primary disease, such as wheezing, decreased breath sounds and prolonged expiratory phase in COPD, and crackles in interstitial lung disease. The presence of bruits over the lung fields is more specific for CTEPH, although present in only 30% of these patients [19].

Diagnostic Testing

Electrocardiography (ECG) findings suggestive of pulmonary hypertension include right axis deviation (RAD), right atrial enlargement (P-wave $\geq$ 2.5 mm), and right ventricular hypertrophy (RVH) [17]. However, ECG is not sufficiently sensitive or specific to screen patients suspected of PAH [20]. ECG findings in patients with IPAH have prognostic significance with findings of P-wave amplitude 2.5 mV or more in lead II, qR lead V1, and RVH by WHO criteria associated with significantly increased risk of death, even after controlling for hemodynamic parameters, functional class, and treatment [18,20,21].

Radiographic findings of pulmonary hypertension include enlarged main and hilar pulmonary arterial shadows (≥18 mm diameter in men, ≥16 mm diameter in women) with peripheral pulmonary vascular attenuation (pruning) and RV enlargement as evidenced by decreased size of the retrosternal clear space [20,22]. Other radiographic findings may suggest an underlying cause for pulmonary hypertension such as hyperinflation (COPD), prominent interstitial markings and fibrosis (interstitial lung disease), or cephalization and Kerley B lines (left-sided congestive heart failure).

Computerized tomography may be helpful in further delineating underlying parenchymal lung disease. Ventilation/perfusion (V/Q) scanning is the test of choice for identifying CTEPH; however, this cannot be performed on intubated patients and may be difficult to obtain in unstable patients, limiting its utility in critically ill patients. A normal or low probability V/Q scan virtually excludes the diagnosis of CTEPH [23]. Computerized tomographic angiography (CTA) can identify acute pulmonary emboli and often CTEPH as well. However, CTA has been found to be less sensitive than V/Q scanning at identifying CTEPH, and may underestimate the clot burden in this condition [23].

Laboratory evaluation may reveal underlying diseases associated with an increased risk of pulmonary hypertension, such as connective tissue disease positive antinuclear antibody (ANA), or HIV infection. Brain natriuretic peptide (BNP) may have prognostic value in patients with PAH [20]; however, BNP levels may be elevated in critically ill patients with shock, or cardiac dysfunction of any cause and is, therefore, a nonspecific finding of unclear clinical significance [14,24].

Pulmonary hypertension may be suggested among critically ill patients by echocardiography. Echocardiography can provide noninvasive estimates of pulmonary arterial pressures, assessment of right and LV function, and evaluation of valvular disease. Echocardiographic findings of pulmonary hypertension may include RV dilation and hypertrophy, D-shaped LV due to septal bowing in the LV during late systole, RV hypokinesis, tricuspid regurgitation, right atrial enlargement, and a dilated inferior vena cava (IVC) [13,20]. Echocardiography can provide prognostic information, with measures of RV dysfunction associated with worse outcomes, including increased RV diameter, a decreased tricuspid annular plane systolic excursion (TAPSE), an elevated RV myocardial performance index (Tei index), increased right atrial diameter, and the presence of a pericardial effusion [18]. Although echocardiographic estimates of PAP correlate well with invasively measured PAP for patients with left-sided heart disease [25], multiple studies have demonstrated that echocardiographic estimates of PAP for patients with suspected pulmonary hypertension or with underlying lung disease can be inaccurate; the false-positive rate is 30% to 40% under these circumstances [26–29].

Therefore, right heart catheterization remains the gold standard for diagnosis of pulmonary hypertension and must be performed to confirm the diagnosis, determine the appropriate etiology, and determine the treatment. As stated previously, pulmonary hypertension is defined as an mPAP of more than 25 mm Hg, measured by right heart catheterization. The finding of a pulmonary capillary wedge pressure (PCWP) greater than 15 mm Hg is indicative of pulmonary venous hypertension. Right heart catheter findings may include the following hemodynamic profiles: (a) elevated PAP, normal PCWP, elevated PVR, consistent with PAH or PH due to hypoxemic lung disease; (b) elevated PAP, elevated PCWP, normal pulmonary artery diastolic pressure (PAD)–PCWP gradient, consistent with pulmonary venous hypertension; and (c) elevated PAP, elevated PCWP, elevated PAD–PCWP gradient, consistent with pulmonary venous hypertension with an "active" component. Among patients with IPAH, findings at right heart catheterization of mPAP greater than or equal to 85 mm Hg, right atrial pressure (RAP) greater than or equal to 20 mm Hg, and cardiac index (CI) less than 2 L/min/m^2 an association with lower rates of survival has been reported [18].

Vasodilator testing may be performed at the time of right heart catheterization. This is done by measuring baseline hemodynamics, administering a short-acting pulmonary vasodilator (adenosine, inhaled nitric oxide [iNO], or prostacyclin), and then repeating the hemodynamic measurements. Vasodilator responsiveness is defined as a decrease of the mPAP by at least 10 mm Hg, to less than 40 mm Hg with no change or an increase of cardiac output [30]. Vasodilator responsiveness for patients with IPAH is predictive of response to treatment with high-dose calcium-channel blockers and suggests a better prognosis. Of note, patients with IPAH who are not acutely vasodilator responsive respond to long-term treatment with pulmonary vasodilators [31]; therefore, the finding of vasodilator responsiveness should only be used to decide which patients might be treated with calcium-channel blockers, not which patients should be treated in general. The clinical significance of vasodilator responsiveness for forms of pulmonary hypertension other than IPAH is unproven.

TREATMENT

Treatment of pulmonary hypertension is dictated by the underlying cause, according to the revised classification of pulmonary hypertension (Table 174.1). When treating pulmonary hypertension in the ICU, one must differentiate between patients with pulmonary hypertension associated with underlying critical illness and patients who are critically ill due to PAH with RV failure and hemodynamic compromise.

General Measures

Hypoxic pulmonary vasoconstriction may contribute to the pulmonary hypertension of critically ill patients. Supplemental oxygen results in a small, but statistically significant, decrease of PVR and an increase in cardiac output for patients with pulmonary hypertension of diverse etiologies [32]. Therefore, maintaining adequate oxygenation for critically ill patients with pulmonary hypertension is an important therapeutic goal.

Optimal fluid management in critically ill patients with decompensated RV failure can be extremely challenging. Because the RV is preload dependent, hypovolemia can result in decreased preload and therefore decreased cardiac output. However, hypervolemia can exacerbate RV pressure overload and ventricular interdependence, leading to decreased LV filling, also reducing cardiac output. Finding the optimal fluid balance for any given patient may require invasive hemodynamic monitoring.

Patients with RV dysfunction are poorly tolerant of loss of atrioventricular (AV) synchrony as occurs with atrial fibrillation and complete AV block. Therefore, maintenance of sinus rhythm may have salutary hemodynamic effects [33].

Retrospective and nonrandomized prospective studies of anticoagulation for patients with IPAH have demonstrated survival benefit with anticoagulation [34–36]. In the absence of contraindication, anticoagulation is therefore recommended for patients with PAH. However, there are no studies of anticoagulation for critically ill patients with pulmonary hypertension and thus no proven role for anticoagulation for this patient population.

Pulmonary Vasodilators

Significant advances in the outpatient treatment of PAH have been made since 1996 when the first pulmonary specific vasodilator was approved by the Food and Drug Administration (FDA). Patients with PAH (Group 1) benefit from treatment with prostacyclins (epoprostenol, treprostinil, and iloprost), endothelin-receptor antagonists (bosentan, ambrisentan, and macitentan), phosphodiesterase-5 inhibitors (sildenafil and tadalafil), and the soluble guanylate cyclase stimulator (riociguat). Table 174.3 summarizes the major randomized controlled trials that have demonstrated clinical benefits with each of these medications [37]. Choice of initial therapy for stable outpatients with PAH is dictated by patients' risk profile, as assessed by functional class, 6-minute walk distance, BNP level, hemodynamics, adverse events, and echocardiographic findings [38]. Oral pulmonary vasodilators are reserved for stable outpatients with low-risk profiles.

Patients with PAH and decompensated RV failure requiring admission to an ICU generally require treatment with intravenous prostanoids, although the initiation of pulmonary vasodilators as "rescue therapy" in the setting of decompensated right heart failure has not been well studied. In one small, retrospective study of patients with PAH and decompensated right heart failure, treatment with iloprost (inhaled) or treprostinil (intravenous or subcutaneous) was associated with decreased mortality [3]. However, in another study, treatment with intravenous epoprostenol or continuous iNO did not influence survival of patients with PAH or inoperable CTEPH and acute RV failure [4]. Of note, neither study was designed to study or compare the effects of pulmonary vasodilators on mortality from decompensated RV failure; therefore, no conclusions regarding which treatment may be most efficacious in this setting can be made.

Intravenous epoprostenol is the only medication with proven survival benefit in patients with IPAH [39] and is therefore the drug of choice for patients with severe PAH and a high-risk profile [40]. Epoprostenol therapy is typically initiated in the ICU with a right heart catheter in place. It is started at a dose of 1 to 2 ng/kg/min and uptitrated by 1 to 2 ng/kg/min at intervals of 15 to 30 minutes, with the hemodynamic goal of increased cardiac output and decreased PAP and PVR. Dose escalation is limited by side effects, such as headache, jaw pain, nausea, diarrhea, and systemic hypotension [39].

Treatment with epoprostenol can be complicated by the development of pulmonary edema, due to increased delivery of blood to the left side of the heart with resultant increased left-sided filling pressures. The development of pulmonary edema following the initiation of epoprostenol therapy should prompt consideration of pulmonary veno-occlusive disease or pulmonary capillary hemangiomatosis, but this can also be seen with more common conditions such as occult diastolic dysfunction [41,42]. Epoprostenol results in nonselective pulmonary vasodilation. This can worsen V/Q matching and cause clinically significant oxygen desaturation [43]. Among patients chronically treated with epoprostenol, this can cause severe hypoxemia if superimposed focal lung disease such as pneumonia occurs. Abrupt discontinuation of epoprostenol has been demonstrated to lead to severe rebound pulmonary hypertension and death.

Treatment of patients with non–Group 1 pulmonary hypertension is focused on treating the underlying disease. For patients with pulmonary venous hypertension, optimization of afterload reduction, and fluid management are the mainstays of therapy. Ensuring adequate oxygenation of patients with pulmonary hypertension due to parenchymal lung disease (Group 3) and treating the underlying disease are the main goals of therapy.

Given the frequent occurrence of pulmonary hypertension in patients with ARDS, much attention has been focused on treating this aspect of ARDS. Administration of intravenous and enteral pulmonary vasodilators to patients with ARDS and pulmonary hypertension increases intrapulmonary shunting with resultant deterioration in oxygenation without improving survival [8,44]. There is therefore no proven role for using these agents in patients with pulmonary hypertension related to ARDS.

Inhaled pulmonary vasodilators are only delivered to ventilated alveoli, and therefore improve V/Q matching and oxygenation for patients with ARDS, while reducing pulmonary pressures. Specifically, iNO improves oxygenation, reduces pulmonary shunting, and reduces PVR in patients with ARDS [45,46]. However, in two large, multicenter, randomized, controlled trials comparing treatment with iNO with conventional therapy for patients with ARDS, no mortality benefit was demonstrated [47,48]. Similarly, nebulized prostaglandin I_2 improves oxygenation and decreases PAPs in patients with ARDS, without improving survival [49,50].

TABLE 174.3

Results of Prospective, Randomized Trials of Pharmacologic Treatments for PAH [37]

Medication	No. of patients	WHO functional class	Results
Epoprostenol	81	III, IV	Improved survival, 6MWD, hemodynamics, and quality of life.
Treprostinil	470	II, III, IV	Improved 6MWD, signs and symptoms of PAH, hemodynamics; no difference in rates of death, transplantation, or clinical deterioration.
Iloprost	203	III, IV	Improved combined clinical endpoint of 10% increase in 6MWD, WHO functional class, and the absence of deterioration or death; improved individual endpoints of 6MWD, postinhalation hemodynamics, WHO functional class.
Bosentan	213	III, IV	Improved 6MWD, Borg dyspnea index, WHO functional class, delayed time to clinical worsening.
Ambrisentan	394	I, II, III, IV	Improved 6MWD, and delayed time to clinical worsening.
Macitentan	742	II, III, IV	Delayed time to clinical worsening, improved 6MWD.
Sildenafil	278	I, II, III, IV	Improved 6MWD, hemodynamics, WHO functional class; no delay in time to clinical worsening.
Tadalafil	405	I, II, III, IV	Improved 6MWD, delayed time to clinical worsening, decreased incidence of clinical worsening. No significant improvement in WHO functional class.
Riociguat	443	I, II, III, IV	Improved 6MWT, hemodynamics, WHO functional class, and delayed time to clinical worsening.

6MWD, 6-min walk distance; WHO, World Health Organization.

Vasopressors

Patients with pulmonary hypertension may develop hemodynamic instability requiring vasopressor support. This may be due to progression of pulmonary hypertension with the development of RV failure or due to the development of a superimposed process, such as sepsis. The main goals of vasopressor therapy for patients with pulmonary hypertension are to reduce PVR, preserve or improve cardiac output, and maintain systemic blood pressure. There are limited data to guide the choice of vasopressors in the setting of pulmonary hypertension and RV failure.

Dobutamine reduces PVR and increases cardiac output in animal models of pulmonary hypertension [14,51–53]. Among humans with mild-to-moderate pulmonary hypertension, dobutamine decreased PVR and increased CI; however, increased intrapulmonary shunting with resultant decrease in arterial oxygenation was also noted. Dobutamine administered in combination with iNO resulted in significant decreases of PVR with concomitant increases of CI and improved oxygenation [53,54]. Of note, these studies were performed in patients with stable cardiopulmonary hemodynamics. The physiologic effects of dobutamine for critically ill patients with pulmonary hypertension have not been well characterized. In a prospective, observational study of patients with PAH or inoperable CTEPH with acute RV failure requiring treatment with catecholamines, increasing dobutamine dose was associated with increased mortality [4]. However, this more likely reflects patients with more severe disease, rather than a deleterious effect of dobutamine on survival.

Norepinephrine administration for patients with pulmonary venous hypertension and systemic hypotension following induction of anaesthesia resulted in increased mPAP and PVR, but with decreased ratio of PAP to SBP (i.e., systolic blood pressure [SBP] increased more than PAP) and no change in CI. By contrast, phenylephrine administration resulted in decreased CI, without a concomitant decrease of the ratio of PAP to SBP [55]. Norepinephrine may be beneficial for restoring systemic blood pressure among patients with persistent hypotension despite treatment with pulmonary vasodilators and dobutamine, but should otherwise be avoided due to its pulmonary vasoconstrictive effects. Similarly, phenylephrine increases mPAP and PVR, with evidence of worsened RV function among patients with chronic pulmonary hypertension [56]. It should therefore be avoided for patients with hemodynamic compromise due to pulmonary hypertension.

Dopamine decreases PVR and increased cardiac output in an animal model of acute pulmonary embolism [57]. Similar effects were noted in patients with pulmonary hypertension due to chronic obstructive lung disease [58]. Among humans with pulmonary venous hypertension, dopamine infusions increased mPAP, but this effect was mediated through increased cardiac output, not by pulmonary vasoconstriction [59]. The effects of dopamine among patients with PAH have not been well studied. In a retrospective, single-center study of patients with PAH and decompensated RV failure, higher doses of dopamine were associated with increased mortality. However, patients requiring treatment with dopamine had significantly more severe disease, by both clinical and hemodynamic parameters [3].

Vasopressin has been found to have vasodilatory properties at low doses in animal studies. Among humans, administration of low dose vasopressin has resulted in greater increases in SVR than in PVR, as manifest by a reduced PVR/SVR ratio. There are case reports describing successful use of vasopressin as rescue therapy for patients with pulmonary hypertension and acute hemodynamic instability in a variety of clinical contexts, including following cardiac surgery, with spinal anesthesia, during caesarean section, and during sepsis [25].

In an animal model of pulmonary hypertension, isoproterenol reduces PVR and improves cardiac output [57]. However, these beneficial effects are largely offset by induction of tachyarrhythmias [60]. Although isoproterenol reduces PVR among patients with IPAH, the chronotropic effects limit its role for patients with PAH [14].

There are limited studies of the effects of epinephrine on pulmonary hemodynamics. In hypoxic piglets, epinephrine improved cardiac output without increasing PVR, and resulted in improved RV contractility in a case series of patients with septic shock and RV failure [13].

Mechanical Ventilation

Institution of mechanical ventilation has complex hemodynamic effects that can be of clinical significance, especially among patients with severe PAH and decompensated RV failure.

Mechanical ventilation increases RV afterload and decreases RV preload that can be of particular hemodynamic consequence for patients with pulmonary hypertension. The increased afterload effects appear to be mediated primarily through increased lung volume [18]. Many of the studies evaluating effects of mechanical ventilation on RV function were performed prior to the era of low tidal volume ventilation for ARDS; therefore, it is unknown whether these effects are as pronounced or clinically important at lower tidal volumes.

Permissive hypercapnia has become common with the widespread institution of low tidal volume ventilation. Hypercapnia increases pulmonary arterial pressures, although it is unclear whether this is due simply to increased cardiac output or by a direct pulmonary vasoconstrictive effect with one study demonstrating an increase in mPAP with no effect on PVR, while another has found an increase in mPAP, PVR, and decreased right ventricular ejection fraction (RVEF) [8]. Elevations of positive end-expiratory pressure (PEEP) also increase pulmonary arterial pressure and PVR [8]. In a recent study examining the hemodynamic effects of PEEP uptitration for patients with ARDS, mPAP increased from 25 to 28 mm Hg and PVR increased from 310 to 385 dynes s m^2 per cm^5 [61].

In addition to providing a mortality benefit for patients with severe ARDS, prone positioning has been found to result in reduction of $PaCO_2$ and the improvement of echocardiographic findings of RV pressure overload [18].

Although the net effect of mechanical ventilation is to increase pulmonary arterial pressure, this is typically well tolerated among patients with mild-to-moderate pulmonary hypertension. These effects, however, may be of particular hemodynamic consequence for patients with PAH and RV failure. Mechanical ventilation in these patients should ideally be with low tidal volume and low PEEP, while avoiding permissive hypercapnia.

Surgical Management

Atrial septostomy, or the creation of an atrial septal shunt via graded balloon dilation atrial septostomy, decompresses the RV by creating an alternative outflow tract for blood and increases left atrial filling. However, it is associated with very high morbidity and mortality among critically ill patients with RV failure. It is complicated by oxygen desaturation through the creation of a right-to-left shunt. It is contraindicated for patients with mean RAP greater than 20 mm Hg and significant hypoxemia (O_2 saturation $< 85\%$ on room air at rest) [37].

References

1. Simonneau G, Gatzoulis MA, Adatia I, et al: Updated clinical classification of pulmonary hypertension. *J Am Coll Cardiol* 62:D34–D41, 2013.
2. Seeger W, Adir Y, Barbera JA, et al: Pulmonary hypertension in chronic lung diseases. *J Am Coll Cardiol* 62:D109–D116, 2013.
3. Kurzyna M, Zylkowska J, Fijalkowska A, et al: Characteristics and prognosis of patients with decompensated right ventricular failure during the course

of pulmonary hypertension. *Kardiol Pol* 66:1033–1039, 2008; discussion 1040–1031.
4. Sztrymf B, Souza R, Bertoletti L, et al: Prognostic factors of acute heart failure in patients with pulmonary arterial hypertension. *Eur Respir J* 35:1286–1293, 2010.
5. Hargett CW, Tapson VF: Venous thromboembolism: pulmonary embolism and deep venous thrombosis, in Irwin RS, Rippe JM (eds): *Irwin and Rippe's Intensive Care Medicine*. 7th ed. Philadelphia, PA, Lippincott Williams & Wilkins, 2012, pp 566–567.
6. Bull TM, Clark B, McFann K, et al: Pulmonary vascular dysfunction is associated with poor outcomes in patients with acute lung injury. *Am J Respir Crit Care Med* 182:1123–1128, 2010.
7. Beiderlinden M, Kuehl H, Boes T, et al: Prevalence of pulmonary hypertension associated with severe acute respiratory distress syndrome: predictive value of computed tomography. *Intensive Care Med* 32:852–857, 2006.
8. Lai PS, Mita C, Thompson BT: What is the clinical significance of pulmonary hypertension in acute respiratory distress syndrome? A review. *Minerva Anestesiol* 80:574–585, 2014.
9. Vieillard-Baron A, Prin S, Chergui K, et al: Echo-doppler demonstration of acute cor pulmonale at the bedside in the medical intensive care unit. *Am J Respir Crit Care Med* 166:1310–1319, 2002.
10. Mekontso Dessap A, Boissier F, Charron C, et al: Acute cor pulmonale during protective ventilation for acute respiratory distress syndrome: prevalence, predictors, and clinical impact. *Intensive Care Med* 42:862–870, 2016.
11. Boissier F, Katsahian S, Razazi K, et al: Prevalence and prognosis of cor pulmonale during protective ventilation for acute respiratory distress syndrome. *Intensive Care Med* 39:1725–1733, 2013.
12. Osman D, Monnet X, Castelain V, et al: Incidence and prognostic value of right ventricular failure in acute respiratory distress syndrome. *Intensive Care Med* 35:69–76, 2009.
13. Ventetuolo CE, Klinger JR: Management of acute right ventricular failure in the intensive care unit. *Ann Am Thorac Soc* 11:811–822, 2014.
14. Zamanian RT, Haddad F, Doyle RL, et al: Management strategies for patients with pulmonary hypertension in the intensive care unit. *Crit Care Med* 35:2037–2050, 2007.
15. Humbert M: Pulmonary arterial hypertension and chronic thromboembolic pulmonary hypertension: pathophysiology. *Eur Respir Rev* 19:59–63, 2010.
16. Farber HW, Loscalzo J: Pulmonary arterial hypertension. *N Engl J Med* 351:1655–1665, 2004.
17. McGoon M, Gutterman D, Steen V, et al: Screening, early detection, and diagnosis of pulmonary arterial hypertension: ACCP evidence-based clinical practice guidelines. *Chest* 126:14S–34S, 2004.
18. Coz Yataco A, Aguinaga Meza M, Buch KP, et al: Hospital and intensive care unit management of decompensated pulmonary hypertension and right ventricular failure. *Heart Fail Rev* 21:323–346, 2016.
19. Fedullo PF, Auger WR, Kerr KM, et al: Chronic thromboembolic pulmonary hypertension. *N Engl J Med* 345:1465–1472, 2001.
20. Nef HM, Mollmann H, Hamm C, et al: Pulmonary hypertension: updated classification and management of pulmonary hypertension. *Heart* 96:552–559, 2010.
21. Bossone E, Paciocco G, Iarussi D, et al: The prognostic role of the ecg in primary pulmonary hypertension. *Chest* 121:513–518, 2002.
22. McGoon MD, Kane GC: Pulmonary hypertension: diagnosis and management. *Mayo Clin Proc* 84:191–207, 2009.
23. Jenkins D, Mayer E, Screaton N, et al: State-of-the-art chronic thromboembolic pulmonary hypertension diagnosis and management. *Eur Respir Rev* 21:32–39, 2012.
24. Maeder M, Fehr T, Rickli H, et al: Sepsis-associated myocardial dysfunction: diagnostic and prognostic impact of cardiac troponins and natriuretic peptides. *Chest* 129:1349–1366, 2006.
25. Price LC, Wort SJ, Finney SJ, et al: Pulmonary vascular and right ventricular dysfunction in adult critical care: current and emerging options for management: a systematic literature review. *Crit Care* 14:R169, 2010.
26. Colle IO, Moreau R, Godinho E, et al: Diagnosis of portopulmonary hypertension in candidates for liver transplantation: a prospective study. *Hepatology* 37:401–409, 2003.
27. Mukerjee D, St George D, Knight C, et al: Echocardiography and pulmonary function as screening tests for pulmonary arterial hypertension in systemic sclerosis. *Rheumatology (Oxford)* 43:461–466, 2004.
28. Hachulla E, Gressin V, Guillevin L, et al: Early detection of pulmonary arterial hypertension in systemic sclerosis: a french nationwide prospective multicenter study. *Arthritis Rheum* 52:3792–3800, 2005.
29. Fisher MR, Forfia PR, Chamera E, et al: Accuracy of doppler echocardiography in the hemodynamic assessment of pulmonary hypertension. *Am J Respir Crit Care Med* 179:615–621, 2009.
30. Sitbon O, Humbert M, Jais X, et al: Long-term response to calcium channel blockers in idiopathic pulmonary arterial hypertension. *Circulation* 111:3105–3111, 2005.
31. McLaughlin VV, Genthner DE, Panella MM, et al: Reduction in pulmonary vascular resistance with long-term epoprostenol (prostacyclin) therapy in primary pulmonary hypertension. *N Engl J Med* 338:273–277, 1998.
32. Roberts DH, Lepore JJ, Maroo A, et al: Oxygen therapy improves cardiac index and pulmonary vascular resistance in patients with pulmonary hypertension. *Chest* 120:1547–1555, 2001.
33. Goldstein JA, Harada A, Yagi Y, et al: Hemodynamic importance of systolic ventricular interaction, augmented right atrial contractility and atrioventricular synchrony in acute right ventricular dysfunction. *J Am Coll Cardiol* 16:181–189, 1990.
34. Fuster V, Steele PM, Edwards WD, et al: Primary pulmonary hypertension: natural history and the importance of thrombosis. *Circulation* 70:580–587, 1984.
35. Rich S, Kaufmann E, Levy PS: The effect of high doses of calcium-channel blockers on survival in primary pulmonary hypertension. *N Engl J Med* 327:76–81, 1992.
36. Kawut SM, Horn EM, Berekashvili KK, et al: New predictors of outcome in idiopathic pulmonary arterial hypertension. *Am J Cardiol* 95:199–203, 2005.
37. Galie N, Corris PA, Frost A, et al: Updated treatment algorithm of pulmonary arterial hypertension. *J Am Coll Cardiol* 62:D60–D72, 2013.
38. McLaughlin VV, Archer SL, Badesch DB, et al: ACCF/AHA 2009 expert consensus document on pulmonary hypertension a report of the American College of Cardiology Foundation Task Force on Expert Consensus Documents and the American Heart Association developed in collaboration with the American College of Chest Physicians; American Thoracic Society, Inc.; and the Pulmonary Hypertension Association. *J Am Coll Cardiol* 53:1573–1619, 2009.
39. Barst RJ, Rubin LJ, Long WA, et al: A comparison of continuous intravenous epoprostenol (prostacyclin) with conventional therapy for primary pulmonary hypertension. *N Engl J Med* 334:296–301, 1996.
40. Barst RJ, Gibbs JS, Ghofrani HA, et al: Updated evidence-based treatment algorithm in pulmonary arterial hypertension. *J Am Coll Cardiol* 54S78–S84, 2009.
41. Gugnani MK, Pierson C, Vanderheide R, et al: Pulmonary edema complicating prostacyclin therapy in pulmonary hypertension associated with scleroderma: a case of pulmonary capillary hemangiomatosis. *Arthritis Rheum* 43:699–703, 2000.
42. Montani D, Achouh L, Dorfmuller P, et al: Pulmonary veno-occlusive disease: clinical, functional, radiologic, and hemodynamic characteristics and outcome of 24 cases confirmed by histology. *Medicine (Baltimore)* 87:220–233, 2008.
43. Otulana B, Higenbottam T: The role of physiological deadspace and shunt in the gas exchange of patients with pulmonary hypertension: a study of exercise and prostacyclin infusion. *Eur Respir J* 1:732–737, 1988.
44. Cornet AD, Hofstra JJ, Swart EL, et al: Sildenafil attenuates pulmonary arterial pressure but does not improve oxygenation during ards. *Intensive Care Med* 36:758–764, 2010.
45. Melot C, Lejeune P, Leeman M, et al: Prostaglandin e1 in the adult respiratory distress syndrome. Benefit for pulmonary hypertension and cost for pulmonary gas exchange. *Am Rev Respir Dis* 139:106–110, 1989.
46. Zapol WM, Rimar S, Gillis N, et al: Nitric oxide and the lung. *Am J Respir Crit Care Med* 149:1375–1380, 1994.
47. Dellinger RP, Zimmerman JL, Taylor RW, et al: Effects of inhaled nitric oxide in patients with acute respiratory distress syndrome: results of a randomized phase ii trial. Inhaled nitric oxide in ards study group. *Crit Care Med* 26:15–23, 1998.
48. Lundin S, Mang H, Smithies M, et al: Inhalation of nitric oxide in acute lung injury: results of a european multicentre study. The european study group of inhaled nitric oxide. *Intensive Care Med* 25:911–919, 1999.
49. Walmrath D, Schneider T, Schermuly R, et al: Direct comparison of inhaled nitric oxide and aerosolized prostacyclin in acute respiratory distress syndrome. *Am J Respir Crit Care Med* 153:991–996, 1996.
50. Zwissler B, Kemming G, Habler O, et al: Inhaled prostacyclin (pgi2) versus inhaled nitric oxide in adult respiratory distress syndrome. *Am J Respir Crit Care Med* 154:1671–1677, 1996.
51. Bradford KK, Deb B, Pearl RG: Combination therapy with inhaled nitric oxide and intravenous dobutamine during pulmonary hypertension in the rabbit. *J Cardiovasc Pharmacol* 36:146–151, 2000.
52. Kerbaul F, Rondelet B, Motte S, et al: Effects of norepinephrine and dobutamine on pressure load-induced right ventricular failure. *Crit Care Med* 32:1035–1040, 2004.
53. Lahm T, McCaslin CA, Wozniak TC, et al: Medical and surgical treatment of acute right ventricular failure. *J Am Coll Cardiol* 56:1435–1446, 2010.
54. Vizza CD, Rocca GD, Roma AD, et al: Acute hemodynamic effects of inhaled nitric oxide, dobutamine and a combination of the two in patients with mild to moderate secondary pulmonary hypertension. *Crit Care* 5:355–361, 2001.
55. Kwak YL, Lee CS, Park YH, et al: The effect of phenylephrine and norepinephrine in patients with chronic pulmonary hypertension. *Anaesthesia* 57:9–14, 2002.
56. Rich S, Gubin S, Hart K: The effects of phenylephrine on right ventricular performance in patients with pulmonary hypertension. *Chest* 98:1102–1106, 1990.
57. Ducas J, Stitz M, Gu S, et al: Pulmonary vascular pressure-flow characteristics. Effects of dopamine before and after pulmonary embolism. *Am Rev Respir Dis* 146:307–312, 1992.
58. Philip-Joet F, Saadjian A, Vestri R, et al: Hemodynamic effects of a single dose of dopamine and l-dopa in pulmonary hypertension secondary to chronic obstructive lung disease. *Respiration* 53:146–152, 1988.
59. Holloway EL, Polumbo RA, Harrison DC: Acute circulatory effects of dopamine in patients with pulmonary hypertension. *Br Heart J* 37:482–485, 1975.
60. Prielipp RC, McLean R, Rosenthal MH, et al: Hemodynamic profiles of prostaglandin e1, isoproterenol, prostacyclin, and nifedipine in experimental porcine pulmonary hypertension. *Crit Care Med* 19:60–67, 1991.
61. Fougeres E, Teboul JL, Richard C, et al: Hemodynamic impact of a positive end-expiratory pressure setting in acute respiratory distress syndrome: importance of the volume status. *Crit Care Med* 38:802–807, 2010.

Chapter 175 ■ Managing Hemoptysis

PAULO J. OLIVEIRA • KIMBERLY A. ROBINSON • RICHARD S. IRWIN

OVERVIEW

Hemoptysis is defined in Stedman's Medical Dictionary as "the spitting of blood derived from the lungs or bronchial tubes." This common symptom may be the primary reason for seeking consultation in approximately 8% to 15% of an average chest clinic population. It elicits great apprehension in the patient and is likely to prompt early medical attention. The basis for this fear is the presumption that the hemoptysis is caused by a serious disease (e.g., cancer) and that it signals impending massive bleeding. The patient may describe an associated burning pain, vague discomfort, or bubbling sensation in the chest and shortness of breath. Hemoptysis may be scant, producing the appearance of streaks of bright red blood in the sputum, or profuse, with expectoration of a large volume of blood.

Massive hemoptysis warrants prompt medical attention and should always be considered life threatening. It is poorly defined in the literature with volumes of expectorated blood ranging from 100 mL per 24 hours to 1,000 mL per 24 hours; however, the expectoration of 600 mL per 24 hours is what is most reported in the literature [1]. Despite the wide range of definitions and lack of clear consensus, the volumetric rate of bleeding does appear to correlate with mortality with those who expectorated 600 mL within 4 hours having a mortality of 70% or greater. In comparison, many clinicians now cite and prefer the magnitude of clinical effect definition that implies that the consequences of expectorated blood are more important than the absolute volume. Mortality in the setting of massive hemoptysis is typically related primarily to asphyxiation and not exsanguination. Asphyxiating hemoptysis occurs with bleeding rates in excess of 150 mL per hour leading to potential immediate airway occlusion. This is supported by the knowledge that the average adult anatomical dead space of the tracheobronchial tree measures approximately 150 mL. Massive hemoptysis is estimated to occur in 5% to 15% of all patients with hemoptysis [2]. Nonmassive hemoptysis produces a quantity smaller than massive hemoptysis and greater than blood streaking. Dark red clots may also be expectorated when blood has been present in the lungs for days.

Pseudohemoptysis, on the other hand, is the expectoration of blood from a source other than the lower respiratory tract (below the larynx). It may cause diagnostic confusion when patients cannot clearly describe the source of their bleeding, which is not unusual. Pseudohemoptysis may occur when blood from the oral cavity, nares, pharynx, or tongue drains to the back of the throat and initiates the cough reflex; when blood emanating from the gastrointestinal tract is aspirated into the lower respiratory tract among patients who have hematemesis; and when the oropharynx is colonized with a red, pigment-producing, aerobic, gram-negative rod, *Serratia marcescens* [3]. Other rare causes of pseudohemoptysis are self-inflicted injuries, other bizarre tactics in the malingering patient seeking hospitalization (factitious hemoptysis), and rifampin overdose (red man syndrome) imbuing a reddish hue to secretions. The causes and distinguishing features of pseudohemoptysis are listed in Table 175.1.

This chapter deals with managing hemoptysis in the intensive care unit (ICU) in the context of a general discussion of hemoptysis. The management of tracheoarterial fistula, traumatic rupture of the pulmonary artery caused by balloon flotation catheters, and diffuse intrapulmonary hemorrhage or diffuse alveolar hemorrhage (DAH) are highlighted.

TABLE 175.1

Differential Features of Pseudohemoptysis

Cause	History	Physical examination	Laboratory tests
Upper respiratory tract	Little or no cough; epistaxis, bleeding from gums when brushing teeth	Gingivitis, telangiectasias, ulcerations, lacerations, or varices of the tongue, nose, or nasopharynx, oropharynx, or hypopharynx	Observing actively bleeding lesion
Upper gastrointestinal tract	Coffee-ground appearance of blood because of mixture with HCl; usually lacks the bubbly, frothy appearance of bloody sputum; nausea, vomiting, or history of gastrointestinal disease	Epigastric tenderness; signs of chronic liver disease	Acid pH of blood; blood in nasogastric aspirate; barium swallow, esophagoscopy, and gastroscopy
Serratia marcescens	Previous hospitalization, broad-spectrum antibiotics, mechanical ventilation	Normal	No red blood cells in red sputum; culture of organism
Malingering	Psychiatric illness; unconfirmed history of massive hemoptysis	Normal unless self-induced lesions seen; patients unable to cough up blood on command (most patients with true hemoptysis will)	True hemoptysis usually must be ruled out (see Table 175.4)

TABLE 175.2

Categories of Causes of Hemoptysis

- Tracheobronchial disorders
  - Acute tracheobronchitis
  - Amyloidosis
  - Aspiration of gastric contents
  - Bronchial adenoma
  - Bronchial endometriosis
  - Bronchial telangiectasia
  - Bronchiectasis
  - Bronchogenic carcinoma
  - Broncholithiasis
  - Chronic bronchitis
  - Cystic fibrosis
  - Endobronchial hamartoma
  - Endobronchial metastases
  - Endobronchial tuberculosis
  - Foreign body aspiration
  - Mucoid impaction of the bronchus
  - Thyroid cancer
  - Tracheobronchial trauma
  - Tracheoesophageal fistula
  - Tracheoarterial fistula
- Cardiovascular disorders
  - Aortic aneurysm
  - Bronchial artery rupture
  - Congenital heart disease
  - Congestive heart failure
  - Coronary artery bypass graft
  - Fat embolization
  - Hughes–Stovin syndrome
  - Mitral stenosis
  - Neonatal intrapulmonary hemorrhage
  - Postmyocardial infarction syndrome
  - Pulmonary arteriovenous fistula
  - Pulmonary artery aneurysm
  - Pulmonary embolism
  - Pulmonary venous varix
  - Schistosomiasis
  - Subclavian artery aneurysm
  - Superior vena cava syndrome
  - Thoracic endometriosis (catamenial)
  - Tumor embolization
- Hematologic disorders
  - Antithrombotic therapy
  - Disseminated intravascular coagulation
  - Leukemia
  - Thrombocytopenia
  - Hemophilia
- Localized parenchymal diseases
  - Acute and chronic nontuberculous pneumonia
  - Actinomycosis
  - Amebiasis
  - Ascariasis
  - Aspergilloma
  - Bronchopulmonary sequestration
  - Coccidioidomycosis
  - Congenital and acquired cyst
  - Cryptococcosis
  - Exogenous lipoid pneumonia
  - Histoplasmosis
  - Hydatid mole
  - Lung abscess
  - Lung contusion
  - Metastatic cancer
  - Mucormycosis
  - Nocardiosis
  - Paragonimiasis
  - Pulmonary endometriosis
  - Pulmonary tuberculosis
  - Sporotrichosis
  - Thoracic splenosis
- Diffuse parenchymal disease
  - Disseminated angiosarcoma
  - Drugs[a] (Alemtuzumab, abciximab, gemtuzumab, anti-CD 33 monoclonal antibody)
  - Farmer's lung
  - Goodpasture's syndrome (anti-glomerular basement disease)
  - Idiopathic pulmonary hemosiderosis
  - Immunoglobulin A nephropathy
  - Inhaled isocyanates
  - Charcoal lighter fluid injection
  - Legionnaires' disease
  - Mixed connective tissue disease
  - Mixed cryoglobulinemia
  - Polyarteritis nodosa
  - Scleroderma
  - Systemic lupus erythematosus
  - Trimellitic anhydride toxicity
  - Viral pneumonitis
  - ANCA-Associated Vasculitides:
  - GPA
  - MPA
  - Isolated pulmonary pauci-immune capillaritis
  - Pulmonary capillaritis associated with systemic vasculitides
  - Bone marrow transplantation
  - Lysinuric protein intolerance
- Other
  - Idiopathic/Cryptogenic
  - Iatrogenic
  - Bronchoscopy
  - Cardiac catheterization
  - Needle biopsy of lung

Common causes; For a complete list of references, see Robinson KA, Irwin RS: Managing Hemoptysis, in Irwin RS, Rippe JM (eds): *Intensive Care Medicine*. 7th ed. Philadelphia, Lippincott Williams & Wilkins, 2012, pp 578–587.
[a]Sachdeva A, Matuschak M: Diffuse alveolar hemorrhage following alemtuzumab. *Chest* 133:133, 2008.
ANCA, anti-neutrophilic cytoplasmic antibody; GPA, granulomatosis with polyangiitis; MPA, microscopic polyangiitis

TABLE 175.3

Common Causes of Massive Hemoptysis

Infectious	
	Bronchitis
	Bronchiectasis
	Tuberculosis
	Cystic fibrosis
	Aspergilloma
	Sporotrichosis
	Lung abscess
	Pneumonia in human immunodeficiency virus–infected patients
Malignant	
	Bronchogenic cancer
	Metastatic cancer
	Leukemia
Cardiovascular	
	Arteriobronchial fistula
	Congestive heart failure
	Pulmonary arteriovenous fistula
Diffuse parenchymal disease	
	Diffuse alveolar hemorrhage
Trauma	
	Iatrogenic
	Pulmonary artery rupture
	Malposition of chest tube
	Tracheoarterial fistula

ETIOLOGY

Hemoptysis can be caused by a wide variety of disorders (Table 175.2) [4]. The etiology of hemoptysis is considered here in three general categories: nonmassive, massive, and idiopathic/cryptogenic. Patients in the ICU frequently have nonmassive hemoptysis, and the spectrum of the causes of hemoptysis for these patients probably differs little from that reported by major series. Commonly, the causes include trauma (secondary to suctioning), overzealous anticoagulation, and infection. Unlike the general ICU patient, patients with massive hemoptysis are frequently in the ICU because of their hemoptysis and thereby constitute a different subgroup of patients.

Nonmassive Hemoptysis

Although bronchiectasis, pneumonia, lung carcinoma, and tuberculosis have always been among the most common causes of hemoptysis, their incidence has varied depending on the study population, geographic location, and era. For example, among immunocompromised patients, *Pneumocystis jiroveci*, fungal diseases, *Mycobacterium tuberculosis*, and *Mycobacterium avium intracellulare* may be at the top of the differential diagnosis, and tuberculosis may be a more common cause of hemoptysis in China than in the USA [5,6].

Although bleeding from tracheoarterial fistula complicating tracheostomy; rupture of pulmonary artery from a balloon flotation catheter; and DAH may be submassive, they are discussed in the following section.

Massive Hemoptysis

The more frequent causes of massive hemoptysis likely to be seen in the ICU are listed in Table 175.3. Virtually, all causes of hemoptysis may result in massive hemoptysis, but it is most frequently caused by tuberculosis, bronchiectasis, infection, and lung cancer [2]. Infection is also a cause of bleeding from aspergilloma [7] or cystic fibrosis [8]. Hemoptysis due to cystic fibrosis has become more common because of the longer survival of affected patients [8]. Idiopathic or cryptogenic hemoptysis has been reported in 11% to 19% of patients despite extensive diagnostic evaluation [2].

Rupture of a pulmonary artery complicates balloon flotation catheterizations in less than 0.2% of cases [9]. It is fortunate that it is uncommon because it carries a mortality rate of 40% to 70% [9–11]. With the less frequent use of this procedure, this complication has become uncommon and is now rarely seen. Tracheoarterial fistula is also an unusual but devastating condition, complicating approximately 0.7% of tracheostomies with a mortality rate exceeding 80% [12]. DAH, usually caused by an immunologically mediated disease, should also be considered in the differential diagnosis of massive hemoptysis in the ICU; however, 30% to 40% of patients may initially not present with hemoptysis and only diffuse pulmonary infiltrates on radiologic imaging.

Idiopathic Hemoptysis

Using the systematic diagnostic approach outlined later and in Tables 175.4 and 175.5, the cause of hemoptysis can be found in most instances. In 11% to 19% of patients [2], the cause cannot be determined. This condition, called idiopathic, cryptogenic or essential hemoptysis, is seen most commonly among men between the ages of 30 and 50 years. Prolonged follow-up studies with rare exceptions usually fail to reveal the source of bleeding, even though 10% of patients continue to have occasional episodes of hemoptysis [13]. In a subset of patients, Dieulafoy disease of the bronchus (i.e., an abnormal ectatic bronchial arterial superficial vessel contiguous to the epithelium of the bronchial mucosa) has been demonstrated at pathologic examination when surgery has been performed for massive bleeding and may be related to conditions associated with chronic airway inflammation [14].

PATHOGENESIS

To appreciate fully the pathogenesis of hemoptysis, it is necessary to review briefly the normal anatomy of the nutrient blood supply to the lungs. The bronchial arteries are the chief source of blood of the airways (from mainstem bronchi to terminal bronchioles); the supporting framework of the lung that includes the pleura, intrapulmonary lymphoid tissue; and large branches of the pulmonary vessels and nerves in the hilar regions. The pulmonary arteries supply the pulmonary parenchymal tissue, including the respiratory bronchioles. Communications between these two blood supplies, bronchopulmonary arterial and venous anastomoses, occur near the junction of the terminal and respiratory bronchioles. These anastomoses allow the two blood supplies to complement each other. Arteriographic studies of patients with active hemoptysis have shown that the systemic circulation (bronchial arteries) is primarily responsible for the bleeding in approximately 92% of cases [15]. When performing an exhaustive angiographic search for the cause of hemoptysis, one must always be suspicious for pulmonary arterial and nonbronchial systemic arterial collaterals as sources of hemoptysis when no clear bronchial arterial source is found.

The pathogenesis of hemoptysis depends on the type and location of the disease. In general, if the lesion is endobronchial, the bleeding is from the bronchial circulation, and if the lesion is parenchymal, the bleeding is from the pulmonary circulation. Moreover, for chronic diseases, repetitive episodes are most likely caused by increased vascularity at the involved area [4].

For bronchogenic carcinoma, hemoptysis results from necrosis of the tumor, with its increased blood supply from bronchial arteries, or from local invasion of a large blood vessel. For bronchial adenomas, bleeding is usually from rupture of the prominent surface vessels. For bronchiectasis, granulation tissue often replaces the normal bronchial wall and, with infection, this area can become irritated and bleed. In acute bronchitis, bleeding results from irritation of the unusually friable and vascular mucosa [4].

The mechanism of hemoptysis with mitral stenosis is controversial, but the most likely explanation is rupture of the dilated varices of the bronchial veins in the submucosa of large bronchi because of pulmonary venous hypertension [16]. Pulmonary venous hypertension may also be responsible for the bleeding with congestive heart failure because it is associated with widening of the capillary anastomoses between bronchial and pulmonary arteries [17].

Hemoptysis from pulmonary embolism may be caused by infarction, with necrosis of parenchymal tissue, or caused by hemorrhagic consolidation secondary to increased bronchial artery blood flow that forms collaterals with the pulmonary circulation to bypass the obstructing clot [18].

With tuberculosis, bleeding can occur for a variety of reasons. In the acute parenchymal exudative lesion, scant hemoptysis may result from necrosis of a small branch of a pulmonary artery or vein. In the chronic parenchymal fibroulcerative lesion, massive hemoptysis may result from rupture of a pulmonary artery aneurysm bulging into the lumen of a cavity (Rasmussen's aneurysm) [19,20]. The aneurysm occurs from tuberculous involvement of the adventitia and media of the vessel within or adjacent to a tuberculous cavity. When a healed and calcified tuberculous lymph node erodes the wall of a bronchus because of pressure necrosis, the patient may cough up blood as well as the calcified node (broncholith). With endobronchial tuberculosis, hemoptysis may result from acute tuberculous ulceration of the bronchial mucosa. With healed and fibrotic parenchymal areas of tuberculosis, bleeding may arise from irritation of granulation tissue in the walls of bronchiectatic airways in the same areas.

In traumatic rupture of the pulmonary artery by a balloon flotation catheter, risk factors include pulmonary hypertension, distal location of the catheter tip, excessive catheter manipulation in an attempt to obtain a pulmonary artery-occluded pressure measurement, a large catheter loop in the right ventricle, and advanced age [9–11].

In tracheoarterial fistula complicating tracheostomy, bleeding is caused by trauma from the tracheostomy cannula or balloon [12]. Bleeding usually is caused by the rupture of the innominate artery. The fistula can form at three tracheal locations: the stoma, the intratracheal cannula tip, and the balloon. Trauma at the stoma is caused by pressure necrosis, usually because the tracheostomy was created too low (below the fourth tracheal ring); at the cannula tip because of excessive angulation of the cannula; or at the balloon site because of pressure necrosis caused by use of excessive inflation pressures. Other risk factors include high cuff pressures, tubes that are malpositioned (too short and angulated) and stomal wound infections. These bleeds are devastating with mortality rates nearing 100% and typically occur 3 days to 6 weeks post-tracheostomy. They can reportedly be heralded by a sentinel bleed among 50% of cases in association occasionally with a pulsating tracheostomy tube. Because of this most-feared potential complication, it is recommended that any post-tracheotomy bleeding occurring 3 days to 6 weeks after insertion should be considered a tracheoarterial fistula until proven otherwise, requiring multimodality, vigilant approach with direct inspection, angiography, etc.

DAH associated with immunologic diseases is caused by an inflammatory lesion, usually of the capillaries [4].

DIAGNOSIS

General Considerations

The success rate for determining the cause of hemoptysis is excellent but variable. If one accepts the diagnosis of idiopathic (essential) hemoptysis as a distinct entity [14], the cause of hemoptysis can be determined in nearly 100% of cases [13]. The diagnostic work-up of hemoptysis involves routine (Table 175.4) as well as special evaluations (Table 175.5). Routine evaluations are initially performed for every patient, whereas special studies are ordered only when the clinical setting suggests that they are indicated. In general, each category of disease (Table 175.2) has its special studies (Table 175.5).

Routine Evaluation

As in any diagnostic problem, a detailed history and physical examination must be performed. These should be performed in a systematic fashion to rule in not only the common causes of hemoptysis but also the category of the cause (Table 175.2).

Although the amount of bleeding usually is not indicative of the seriousness of the underlying disease process, a history of the frequency, timing, and duration of hemoptysis may be helpful. For example, repeated episodes of hemoptysis occurring during months to years suggest a more chronic etiology such as bronchiectasis. Hemoptysis is typically a late finding in bronchogenic carcinoma although history may reveal small amounts of hemoptysis occurring every day for weeks. Hemoptysis that coincides with the menses (catamenial) suggests the rare diagnostic possibility of pulmonary endometriosis [21], whereas bleeding associated with sexual intercourse or other forms of exertion suggests passive congestion of the lungs [22].

Although hemoptysis may be a symptom at any age, it is distinctly uncommon in the young. When hemoptysis is present before the third decade of life, it suggests an acute tracheobronchitis, a congenital cardiac or lung defect, an unusual tumor, cystic fibrosis, a blood dyscrasia, trauma, or infectious pneumonia. No matter what the age, if a patient with pneumonia who is undergoing appropriate therapy has hemoptysis that persists for more than the usual 24 hours, an endobronchial lesion or coagulopathy should be suspected.

A travel history can often be helpful for bringing certain endemic diseases to mind. This is true of coccidioidomycosis and histoplasmosis in the USA; paragonimiasis and ascariasis in East Asia; and schistosomiasis in South America, Africa, and East Asia.

TABLE 175.4

Routine Evaluation of Hemoptysis

History
Physical examination
Complete blood cell count
Urinalysis
Coagulation studies
Electrocardiogram
Chest radiographs
±Flexible bronchoscopy[a]

[a]Although flexible bronchoscopy should not be performed in patients with some conditions (e.g., pulmonary embolism, aortopulmonary fistula), it should be routinely considered (see text).

TABLE 175.5

Special Evaluation of Hemoptysis

Tracheobronchial disorders
- Expectorated sputa for tubercle bacilli, parasites, fungi, and routine cytologic testing
- Bronchoscopy
- High-resolution chest CT scan
- Cardiovascular disorders
- Echocardiogram
- Arterial blood gases on 21% and 100% oxygen
- Ventilation and perfusion lung scans, venous duplex scanning
- Pulmonary angiogram, MRI, spiral chest CT scan with contrast
- Multidetector CT angiography of chest, aortogram
- Cardiac catheterization

Hematologic disorders
- Coagulation studies
- Bone marrow

Localized parenchymal diseases
- Expectorated sputa for parasites, tubercle bacilli, fungi, and routine cytologic testing
- Chest CT scan and MRI
- *Aspergillus* precipitins in serum
- Lung biopsy with special stains

Diffuse parenchymal diseases[a]
- Expectorated sputa for cytologic testing
- Blood urea nitrogen, creatinine, antinuclear antibody, rheumatoid factor, complement, cryoglobulins, lupus erythematosus preparation
- Serum for circulating antiglomerular basement membrane antibody and antineutrophilic cytoplasmic antibody
- Serum for precipitins for hypersensitivity pneumonitis screen
- Acute and convalescent serum antibody studies for Legionnaires' disease and respiratory viruses
- Lung or kidney biopsy with special stains, including immunofluorescence

[a]Diffuse implies involvement of all lobes.
CT, computed tomography; MRI, magnetic resonance imaging.

Chronic sputum production before hemoptysis suggests a diagnosis of chronic bronchitis, bronchiectasis, and cystic fibrosis. The presence of orthopnea and paroxysmal nocturnal dyspnea suggests the diagnoses of passive congestion of the lungs. A history of antithrombotic therapy suggests an intrapulmonary bleed due to supratherapeutic anticoagulation or possibly recurrent thrombotic disease if the anticoagulant is subtherapeutic or the patient is no longer anticoagulated. The possibility of pulmonary embolism should always be considered when a patient who presents with hemoptysis has been at an increased risk for deep venous thrombosis (e.g., meets Virchow's triad).

The possibility of traumatic rupture of a pulmonary artery caused by balloon flotation catheterization should always be considered when these catheters are used [9–11].

Although tracheoarterial fistula must be considered in the differential diagnosis of hemoptysis in every patient with a tracheostomy, it is an infrequent cause in this setting. When it occurs, the onset is almost always at least 48 to 72 hours after the procedure [13]. Although the peak incidence is between the first and third week and 72% of fistulas bleed during the first 21 days after tracheostomy, hemorrhage from this complication can also occur as late as 18 months after the procedure [13]. There is a sentinel bleed in 34% to 50% of cases [12]. Before 48 hours, bleeding from the stoma is usually caused by capillary bleeding from inadequate hemostasis. Whenever hemoptysis occurs in a patient with an endotracheal tube or tracheostomy in place, trauma from suctioning should be considered, especially when coagulation is abnormal.

Although patients with DAH typically have hemoptysis, they occasionally do not expectorate at all but just complain of dyspnea, fever, cough, and malaise. Therefore, lack of hemoptysis does not rule out a substantial intrapulmonary hemorrhage because the alveoli can accommodate large volumes of blood [2].

The diagnosis of trimellitic anhydride–induced pulmonary hemorrhage should be suspected in workers exposed to high-dose trimellitic anhydride fumes. Exposure occurs when heated metal surfaces are sprayed with corrosion-resistant epoxy resin coatings. The syndrome requires a latent period of exposure and appears to be antibody mediated [23]. Respiratory failure with pulmonary infiltrates and hemoptysis has also been reported in a patient with a documented exposure and antibodies to isocyanates [24].

For a patient with the triad of known upper airway disease, lower airway disease, and renal disease, antineutrophil cytoplasmic autoantibody (ANCA)–associated vasculitides, namely granulomatosis with polyangiitis (GPA)—formerly referred to as Wegener's granulomatosis—should be suspected. Pulmonary hemorrhage can occur at any point during the course of the illness in the patient with systemic lupus erythematosus (SLE) and can also be the initial manifestation of the disease. Goodpasture's syndrome (anti-glomerular basement membrane antibody mediated disease) typically occurs in young men and it has been reported to be associated with influenza infection, inhalation of hydrocarbons, and penicillamine ingestion. Therefore, it should be considered in these historical contexts [4].

DAH should be suspected for patients who have undergone recent hematopoietic stem cell transplantation when they present with cough, dyspnea, hypoxemia, and diffuse pulmonary infiltrates. This typically occurs with marrow recovery. It has been reported to occur in approximately 20% of patients during autologous bone marrow transplantation, and it has been associated with mortality rates of 64% to 100% [25–27]. Lung tissue injury, inflammation, and cytokine release are implicated in the pathogenesis of DAH of hematopoietic stem cell transplant patients.

Physical examination may be helpful in several ways. Inspection of the skin and mucous membranes may show telangiectasias, suggesting hereditary hemorrhagic telangiectasia, or ecchymoses and petechiae, suggesting a hematologic abnormality. Pulsations transmitted to a tracheostomy cannula should heighten suspicion, or risk, of a tracheoartery fistula. Inspection of the thorax may show evidence of recent or old chest trauma, and unilateral wheeze or rales may herald localized disease such as bronchial adenoma or carcinoma. Although pulmonary embolism is not definitively diagnosed on physical examination, tachypnea, phlebitis, and pleural friction rub suggest this disorder. If crackles are heard diffusely on chest examination, passive congestion as well as other diseases causing DAH should be considered (Table 175.2). Careful cardiovascular examination and echocardiography may identify mitral stenosis, pulmonary artery stenosis, or pulmonary hypertension.

The routine laboratory studies listed in Table 175.4 are useful for the following reasons.

The complete blood cell count results may suggest the presence of an infection, hematologic disorder, or chronic blood loss. Sputum should be sent for Gram stain and culture, including studies for acid-fast organisms. In addition, sputum should be sent for cytologic evaluation if the patient is a smoker and older than 40 years. Idiopathic hemosiderosis or other causes of DAH (Table 175.2) may present only with diffuse pulmonary infiltrates and iron deficiency anemia from chronic bleeding into the lungs. Urinalysis may reveal hematuria and suggest the presence of a systemic disease associated with diffuse parenchymal disease (e.g., pulmonary renal hemorrhage syndrome due to SLE, Goodpasture's syndrome, (ANCA)-associated vasculitides such as GPA and microscopic polyangiitis (MPA, and other systemic vasculitides; Table 175.2). Although there is simultaneous evidence of clinical involvement of the lungs and kidneys in 33% of cases of Goodpasture's syndrome, there can be clinical lung involvement without renal disease and clinical renal involvement without lung disease.

Coagulation studies may uncover a hematologic disorder that is primarily responsible for the hemoptysis or that contributes to excessive bleeding from another disease. The electrocardiogram may help suggest the presence of a cardiovascular disorder. Although as many as 30% of patients with hemoptysis have negative chest radiographs [4], routine posteroanterior and lateral films may be diagnostically valuable. If unrevealing, one should strongly consider obtaining computed tomography (CT) of the chest not only for diagnosis, but when combined with intravenous contrast, modern multidetector CT angiography (MDCTA) of the chest can more accurately localize potential intrathoracic sources of the bleeding and provide a potential roadmap for subsequent interventions (e.g., bronchial arterial embolization [BAE]) [28,29].

When pulmonary tumor or infection is not readily apparent, there are other radiographic signs that may help to elucidate the cause and source of bleeding. Radiopaque foreign bodies may give rise to hemoptysis even years after entry into the lungs. One may note the disappearance of a calcified mediastinal lymph node after it has eroded the bronchial wall and is expectorated as a broncholith. Aortic or pulmonary aneurysms may erode into the bronchial tree. Single or multiple pulmonary cavities may suggest pulmonary tuberculosis, fungal disease, parasitic disease, acute or chronic lung abscess, neoplasm, septic pulmonary emboli, or GPA. The finding of a mass within a cavitary lesion raises the possibility of a fungus ball (aspergilloma), whereas localized honeycombing may be indicative of bronchiectasis. The presence of a new infiltrate localized to the area subtending a balloon flotation catheter suggests a rupture of the pulmonary artery [9–11]. The appearance of a new air-fluid level in a preexisting cavity or cyst suggests the location of the source of bleeding, as does a nonsegmental alveolar pattern that clears within a few days. A solitary pulmonary nodule with vessels going toward it suggests an arteriovenous fistula. Among patients with hemoptysis due to pulmonary embolism, a parenchymal density abutting a pleural surface with evidence of pleural reaction or effusion is usually present. The cardiac silhouette, vascular or parenchymal patterns, and the presence of Kerley B lines may be useful in documenting cardiovascular disease.

When chest radiography shows diffuse pulmonary infiltrates, hemorrhage from bleeding disorders (e.g., thrombocytopenia in the compromised host), lung contusion from blunt chest trauma, freebase cocaine use, and passive congestion of the lungs should be considered, in addition to the diseases listed under "Diffuse Parenchymal Disease" in Table 175.2. In the earliest stages of DAH, chest radiographs may appear normal, but usually the hemorrhage first appears in a diffuse alveolar pattern. This progresses to a mixed alveolar–interstitial pattern and then, when bleeding ceases entirely, to an interstitial pattern, as hemosiderin deposition accumulates [25–27].

Bronchoscopy and Computed Tomography

Even if the history, physical examination, and chest radiograph are normal, or there is an "obvious" cause of hemoptysis on the chest radiograph, bronchoscopy is invaluable not only for accurate diagnosis but also for precise localization of the pulmonary hemorrhage. It is not uncommon for bronchoscopy to establish sites of bleeding different from those suggested by chest radiography. But not all patients with hemoptysis require bronchoscopy. Bronchoscopy may not be needed in patients with stable chronic bronchitis with one episode of blood streaking (especially those who are younger than 40 years of age with short-lived hemoptysis of less than 1 week duration where the likelihood of occult malignancy is low), particularly if associated with an exacerbation of acute tracheobronchitis, or in patients in whom the site of bleeding was recently documented by bronchoscopic examination. In addition, patients with acute lower respiratory tract infections, and patients with obvious cardiovascular causes of hemoptysis, such as congestive heart failure and pulmonary embolism, may not require bronchoscopic examination.

For localizing the bleeding site, the best results are obtained when bronchoscopy is performed during or within 24 hours of active bleeding. The bleeding site can be localized in up to 93% of patients with a flexible bronchoscope and in up to 86% with the rigid instrument [30,31]. When the procedure is done within 48 hours, localization of bleeding can drop to 51% [30,31]. When bronchoscopy is done after bleeding has ceased, accurate localization is likely to be reduced even further [30–32]. Although the flexible bronchoscope is usually the instrument of choice for diagnosing lower respiratory tract problems, rigid bronchoscopy is preferred in cases of massive, uncontrolled hemorrhage because patency of the airway is maintained more effectively during the procedure (see Interventional Pulmonary Chapter 182). There are data that show that obtaining high-resolution chest CT scanning before bronchoscopy may enhance the yield of bronchoscopy [30–32]. With the exception of tracheoarterial fistula, the tracheobronchial disorders that can be diagnosed by a bronchoscopic examination are listed in Table 175.2.

Bedside bronchoscopy should not be performed to rule in the diagnosis of tracheoarterial fistula. In tracheostomized patients with hemoptysis, bronchoscopy should be performed to rule out other causes, such as bleeding from suction ulcers, tracheitis, or lower respiratory tract disorders. If no other cause for hemoptysis can be found and bleeding has stopped, or anterior and downward pressure on the cannula on the stomal site or overinflation of the tracheostomy balloon slows down or stops the bleeding, a surgical consultation (cardiothoracic and vascular) should be sought immediately and the patient brought to the operating room for examination in a more controlled environment. As long as tracheoarterial fistula remains a diagnostic possibility, the tracheostomy balloon should not be deflated, and the tracheostomy tube should not be removed without protecting the airway below the tracheostomy tube [12,33].

When there is no active bleeding, bronchoscopy with bronchoalveolar lavage can be helpful for diagnosing DAH. Return of bright red or progressively bloodier lavage fluid from multiple lobes (at least two segments) on serial lavage aliquots usually from both lungs suggests an active, DAH; lavage fluid containing more than 20% hemosiderin-laden macrophages (i.e., siderophages) on cytologic analysis from these same specimens suggest bleeding that has been ongoing and is also suggestive of DAH [34]. Because carbon monoxide–diffusing capacity is increased because of binding of carbon monoxide by intra-alveolar red blood cells for 24 to 48 hours after bleeding stops, this test may be helpful for suggesting intra-alveolar hemorrhage of the stable patient without hemoptysis but is rarely utilized currently.

In general, CT scanning plays an important role in the evaluation of hemoptysis and it has been shown by some studies to be as good as bronchoscopy for localizing the bleeding and superior to bronchoscopy at diagnosing the cause of bleeding [32]. Chest CT is superior to plain films and bronchoscopy in diagnosing bronchiectasis, tuberculous-related lesions, aspergillomas, and tumors, the most common causes of massive hemoptysis. CT, however, also has its limitations because it cannot provide direct visualization of the mucosa and associated abnormalities such as bronchitis, vascular anomalies including telangiectasias, early mucosal based carcinomas, benign papillomas and Kaposi's sarcomas. Clearly for these cases, flexible bronchoscopy will be superior and bronchoscopy also provides the ability to additionally provide stabilizing, temporizing therapeutic interventions in some cases. Ultimately, CT scan of the chest and flexible bronchoscopy should be essentially viewed as complementary to each other, and most clinicians would consider performing a CT scan without contrast on all cases of moderate to massive hemoptysis when feasible. As previously stated, the addition of IV contrast with performance of MDCTA can further enhance the ability of CT to further localize the source of bleeding particularly when one is planning on moving ahead with an interventional angiographic treatment modality to more precisely localize the anatomical circulatory source of the bleeding [35].

Angiography

Angiography can determine the site of bleeding in 90% to 93% of cases. When performed routinely, diagnostic angiography establishes a diagnosis not identified by bronchoscopy in only 4% of patients [15]. Although angiography may not be initially helpful in confirming the rupture of the pulmonary artery caused by balloon flotation catheterization if the rent has sealed, it can be extremely helpful for detecting a pseudoaneurysm that has formed during the healing process [10,11]. Identification of an unstable lesion is important because it should be obliterated to prevent future rupture and death [10,11]. Angiography has not been shown to be routinely useful for diagnosing tracheoarterial fistula and if the suspicion is high, one should proceed to direct inspection in the operating room with surgical consultant backup and involvement available [12,33]. Again, in recent years, MDCTA has gained popularity and become a key modality for the algorithmic approach to the diagnosis and management of massive hemoptysis at many institutions given its improved ability to localize the source of bleeding (bronchial arterial, pulmonary arterial, or nonbronchial systemic collaterals) with lower doses of contrast and provide valuable preplanning information to the interventional radiologist prior to embolization efforts [36].

Special Evaluation

Depending on the results of the initial evaluation and the possible categories of cause of hemoptysis (Table 175.2), additional diagnostic evaluations should be systematically performed (Table 175.5).

The diagnosis of Goodpasture's syndrome, for example, is made by demonstrating linear deposition of immunoglobulin (Ig) G along the basement membrane of the lung or kidney and the presence of high titers of circulating anti–glomerular basement membrane antibody in the blood. Antibodies from patients with traditional Goodpasture's syndrome react with the α_3 (IV) chain of type IV collagen.

Definitive diagnosis of the pulmonary vasculitides depends on histologic examination, including special stains and cultures that rule out tuberculosis and fungal diseases. Pulmonary capillaritis with hemorrhage has been reported in an ever-increasing number of conditions [4,25–27]. The diagnosis can on rare occasion be made on transbronchial biopsy, thus avoiding the need for open or video-assisted thoracoscopic wedge lung biopsy [37], but care must be taken to exclude infectious etiologies by using special stains. Antineutrophil cytoplasmic autoantibodies are helpful for diagnosing GPA (formerly Wegener's) and MPA and for potentially following disease activity [4,25–27]. The complete evaluation of GPA, MPA, SLE, and mixed cryoglobulinemia is reviewed in Chapters 66 and 67. The diagnostic features of polyarteritis nodosa, the hypersensitivity vasculitides, giant cell and Takayasu's arteritis, and Behçet's disease are also presented in detail in Chapter 67. For all of these, pulmonary involvement is rare. Several cases of Henoch–Schönlein syndrome, one of the hypersensitivity vasculitides, have been reported with severe alveolar hemorrhage, including one in which immunofluorescent stains of the lung revealed granular deposits of IgA consistent with an immune complex mediation. Giant cell arteritis involvement of the lung is suggested by upper respiratory tract symptoms of sore throat, cough, and hoarseness [4].

Although high levels of IgG, IgA, and IgM antibody to trimellitic-coupled protein and trimellitic-conjugated erythrocytes have been found among patients with trimellitic anhydride-induced pulmonary disease [23], the diagnosis can be made clinically by obtaining a history of the exposure and ruling out other diseases (Table 175.2).

It is important to be aware that diseases may be considered and therefore evaluated in more than one category. For instance, a patient with hemoptysis due to overzealous antithrombotic therapy may be evaluated in three categories: (a) a hematologic disorder that may cause, (b) localized, and (c) diffuse parenchymal disease. A patient with chronic bleeding from the tracheobronchial disorder of diffuse bronchial telangiectasis could present with diffuse as well as localized parenchymal disease (aspiration hemosiderosis). A patient with long-standing passive congestion of the lungs, a cardiovascular disorder, might present with diffuse pulmonary hemosiderosis, whereas a patient with acute pulmonary edema usually presents with diffuse pulmonary infiltrates.

DIFFERENTIAL DIAGNOSIS

When evaluating patients with hemoptysis, it is necessary to rule out the causes of pseudohemoptysis. Features that can help to differentiate the causes of pseudohemoptysis from one another and pseudohemoptysis from true hemoptysis are found in Table 175.1. In addition to history and routine physical examination, it is important to perform a meticulous examination of the nose and entire pharynx, preferably with a nasopharyngoscope. Unless the cause of pseudohemoptysis is definitively determined, the spitting up of blood must be assumed to be true hemoptysis until proven otherwise. An upper-airway lesion must not be assumed to be the cause of the bleeding unless it is seen bleeding actively at the time of examination. Not infrequently, the evaluation may require a team approach with the interprofessional involvement and input from a gastroenterologist and an otolaryngologist, as well as the primary evaluating pulmonary and/or critical care specialist.

TREATMENT

The treatment of hemoptysis can be divided into supportive and definitive categories. When prescribing definitive therapy, it is important to consider the cause, the amount and rate of bleeding, and the patient's underlying lung function. The assessment and management of the patient is frequently occurring concurrently based on the pace and urgency of the overall presentation. The basic tenets of management include the following: (1) stabilization, (2) localization/lateralization, and (3) isolation and containment with potential definitive therapy.

Supportive Care

Supportive care usually includes bed rest and mild sedation. Drugs with antitussive effects (e.g., all narcotics) should not be used. An effective cough may be necessary to clear blood from the airways and avoid asphyxiation. Drugs with antiplatelet effects also should not be used and any underlying bleeding diathesis should be reversed when possible. Depending on the results of pulse oximetry or arterial blood gas analysis, supplemental oxygen should be given. If bleeding continues and gas exchange becomes further compromised, endotracheal intubation and mechanical ventilation may become necessary. To facilitate flexible bronchoscopy with a sufficiently large suction port, an endotracheal tube with an internal diameter of 8 mm or greater should be used, when possible. When the expertise is available at your facility, a strong consideration for moving directly to the operating room for rigid bronchoscopy should be strongly considered when the patient is actively bleeding, compromised, or at high risk for progressive decline. Other traumatic respiratory adjunctive therapies, such as chest physiotherapy and postural drainage, should be avoided. Fluid and blood product resuscitation as well as reversal agents for antithrombotic agents should be given when indicated.

The amount and rate of hemoptysis should be continuously monitored until bleeding stops. These parameters in addition to the patient's clinical/functional status help determine the patient's subsequent care. Current evolving management of massive hemoptysis focuses on an integrated, multipronged, and multidisciplinary approach to streamline efficient care and optimize outcomes [5].

Definitive Care

Nonmassive Hemoptysis

For patients with scant or frank (submassive) hemoptysis, treatment is directed at the specific cause. For instance, suppurative bronchiectasis is treated with antibiotics plus a mucociliary escalator drug (e.g., β-adrenergic agonists). Chronic bronchitis associated with cigarette smoking is treated with a mucociliary escalator and cessation of cigarette smoking. Broad-spectrum antibiotic therapy should be considered if hemoptysis occurs in the context of an acute exacerbation of chronic bronchitis. In severe exacerbations of ICU patients, gram-negative enteric rods, *Pseudomonas aeruginosa*, *Stenotrophomonas maltophilia*, and penicillin-resistant *Streptococcus pneumoniae* may be playing a role approximately 30% of the time [38]. Cystic fibrosis is treated with appropriate antibiotics to cover the likely pathogens [39], plus a mucociliary escalator. Bronchial adenoma and bronchogenic carcinoma should be resected whenever possible based on the patients underlying lung function and pulmonary reserves, when available. Recently, radiofrequency and microwave ablation has been used in stages III and IV non–small cell lung cancer for palliation of hemoptysis, cough, and pain, because reduction in tumor volume can lead to symptomatic improvement. However, hemoptysis has been reported as a complication of radiofrequency ablation in up to 12% of cases [40]. Congestive heart failure is treated with combinations of drugs for preload and afterload reductions, mitral stenosis with diuretics, and pulmonary embolism with anticoagulation. There are no data showing that patients with hemoptysis due to pulmonary embolism bleed more with anticoagulation; therefore, do not initially withhold treatment or undertreat these patients with nonmassive hemoptysis. The effects of overzealous anticoagulation are treated with cessation of blood thinning and perhaps fresh-frozen plasma and/or prothombin complex concentrate and vitamin K. Tuberculosis is treated with antituberculous drugs (see Chapter 82). Appropriate antibiotic therapy is prescribed for acute infectious pneumonias (see Chapters 73 and 181).

Massive Hemoptysis

For patients with massive hemoptysis, treatment is directed not only at the specific cause but also at abrupt cessation of bleeding. Death from massive hemoptysis is predominantly because of asphyxiation, and the likelihood of death appears directly related to the rate of bleeding. Urgent management of all cases of massive hemoptysis must emphasize protecting the uninvolved lung from aspiration of blood and tamponading the bleeding site.

When tracheoarterial fistula may be present, the following steps should be considered. If bleeding is immediate and profuse, there may be time only to overinflate the balloon, tamponading the potential bleeding site at the balloon, and apply downward and forward pressure on the top of the tracheostomy tube, tamponading the potential bleeding site at the stoma. When the arterial rupture is at the cannula tip, these efforts are not helpful. If bleeding stops or slows down either by these efforts or spontaneously, an endotracheal tube should be placed distal to the tip of the tracheostomy tube and a surgical consultation requested immediately. Ideally, a surgeon should be present when the tracheostomy tube is removed; should crisp bleeding start again, the surgeon can attempt to finger-tamponade/compress the bleeding artery (usually the innominate) by bluntly dissecting down the anterior tracheal wall and behind the sternum to the vessel. The vessel, once reached, can be compressed against the back of the sternum [12,33]. When the situation has been stabilized, clots can be gently suctioned from the distal trachea and the patient taken to the operating room for definitive repair. A review of the definitive surgical options can be found elsewhere [12,33]. There have also been reports recently of using the skills of interventional radiologists to place endovascular grafts in these acute settings to halt the bleeding from tracheoarterial fistulas but care must occur expeditiously to have any reasonable chance of survival [41].

When bleeding originates from below the primary carina, the bleeding lung should be kept dependent to minimize aspiration of expectorated blood ("bleeding side down"). Numerous techniques have been advocated to help minimize aspiration by isolating the involved lung or lung segments and have proved helpful. Simple, selective intubation of the uninvolved lung when possible and tolerable can be performed and augmented with bronchoscopic guidance. A bronchoscopically positioned endobronchial balloon or blocker may provide effective tamponade. Hemoptysis due to bleeding from all lobes except the right upper lobe, because of the acute angle takeoff, has been managed with balloon occlusion [2,42]. This technique involves positioning a balloon to completely occlude a bronchus, thus allowing the lung to collapse distally. Small-caliber catheters with balloons can be inserted in segmental airways with bronchoscopy. Placement of a double-lumen endotracheal tube that intubates each mainstem bronchus separately is helpful, but the tubes can be difficult to place and have a tendency to dislodge, and once in position, their small diameter may prevent subsequent diagnostic flexible bronchoscopy. In cases of persistent massive hemoptysis, diagnostic considerations may need to be delayed because placement of a double-lumen endotracheal tube may be necessary to ensure patient survival.

Urgent treatment to stop massive hemoptysis may involve laser bronchoscopy, argon plasma coagulation (APC)/electrocautery, installation of antifibrinolytic tranexamic acid, fibrinogen–thrombin complex solution installation, topically instilled epinephrine/vasoconstrictor solutions, iced saline lavage, angiographic embolization, supportive treatment only, or surgical resection. Use of laser or APC/electrocautery to stop hemoptysis can be successful for patients with cancer, but is only temporizing and recurrence of bleeding within a few weeks is typical. No large studies of patients with massive hemoptysis have been reported. Because "hot" therapies, such as laser, APC and electrocautery, are useful only for patients with proximal, central airway lesions and are difficult to use during massive hemoptysis, they have not evolved into a common primary therapeutic tools for these patients but do have a place in a multimodality approach in the face of an actively bleeding and decompensating patient.

Bronchoscopically directed iced-saline lavage of the bronchi leading to the site of hemorrhage has been reported to be successful for stopping hemorrhage in an uncontrolled series [2,42]. In addition, in a small number of patients, bronchoscopy-guided topical hemostatic therapy using oxidized regenerated cellulose has been successful in controlling life-threatening hemoptysis [43]. An excellent review of the overall contemporary bronchoscopic treatment strategies for massive hemoptysis can be found in the aforementioned references.

Angiography can identify the bleeding site in more than 90% of cases [15,44], and, when combined with an embolization procedure, has been successful in initially stopping bleeding in massive hemoptysis in 77% to 95% of cases [44]. Several angiographic sessions may be required, and systemic and pulmonary vessels may need to be studied. Approximately 16% of patients bleed again within 1 to 4 days, and multiple procedures are frequently necessary [15,44]. Once active bleeding ceases, 20% of patients bleed again during the next 6 months [44] and 22% of patients by 3 to 5 years [15]. More recent studies have shown similar results [44]. Angiographic embolization has been achieved with the use of polyurethane particles, polyvinyl alcohol particles, and steel coils. Sclerosing agents have led to subsequent massive lung necrosis and should be avoided [15,44]. Although early studies included several cases complicated by accidental embolization of the spinal artery, the prevalence is less than 1% and occurs when the spinal artery arises from the bronchial artery, an uncommon anatomical variant [44]. Other complications, such as pleurisy or hematoma formation, are infrequent and usually minor [15].

For patients with hemoptysis due to trauma, urgent thoracotomy has been advocated, with the recommendation that it is performed with the patient in the lateral decubitus position to minimize aspiration, and that the bronchovascular trunk of the involved lung is clamped while the patient is stabilized to minimize the chance of air embolism while on positive-pressure ventilation [45].

Survival from iatrogenic rupture of the pulmonary artery has been reported. Several urgent maneuvers may prove helpful, and balloon tamponade and selective intubation should always be attempted. Balloon tamponade of the ruptured vessel with the Swan–Ganz balloon has been helpful [46]. With the balloon deflated, the catheter should be withdrawn 5 cm and the balloon inflated with 2 mL of air and allowed to float back into the hemorrhaging vessel to occlude it. Ideally, patients should immediately be intubated in the mainstem bronchus opposite the involved lung to minimize aspiration. In most patients, death from pulmonary artery rupture occurs before the bleeding lung can be identified. Because the catheter usually floats to the right pulmonary artery, when it is not known which pulmonary artery has been ruptured, selective intubation of the left mainstem bronchus or placement of a double-lumen endotracheal tube should be attempted. Selective intubation of the left mainstem bronchus can be facilitated by using a bronchoscope or suction catheter designed specifically to enter the left lung. All patients who stop bleeding require angiographic evaluation to help localize the arterial tear and check for the formation of a pseudoaneurysm [11]. At the time of angiography, embolization of the affected vessel should be performed if a pseudoaneurysm or a tear is found. Hemoptysis from a pseudoaneurysm usually occurs in the first day after formation but may occur weeks later [10,11].

The role of emergency surgery for hemoptysis has changed during the past 20 years since the first report of bronchial artery embolization. Bronchial artery embolization has increasingly become first-line treatment for control of massive hemoptysis [5,44]. Nonetheless, surgery remains the procedure of choice when massive hemoptysis is caused by arteriovenous malformations, leaky aortic aneurysm, hydatid cyst, iatrogenic pulmonary rupture, chest trauma, bronchial adenoma, and fungal balls resistant to medical therapy [1].

In patients with cystic fibrosis, even with normal lung function, resection should be avoided because repeated episodes in other areas are likely to occur. A patient with a 1-second forced expiratory volume of less than 2 L or a maximum voluntary ventilation of less than 50% of predicted should not undergo surgery unless split-lung function studies reveal that the patient is not likely to be left a respiratory cripple because of disabling dyspnea.

With respect to surgery, it is clear that no treatment preference can be recommended for all patients on the basis of reported studies. The trials of therapy span different decades of practice, have widely differing causes of hemoptysis in their populations, and use several different definitions for massive hemoptysis. A review of the literature suggests the following strategy: (a) patients who are not candidates for surgery because of their pulmonary function, general medical condition, or diffuse nature of their lesions should be treated with selective embolization; (b) resectional surgery should be performed in operable patients when surgery is the definitive treatment for the underlying disease; and (c) all potentially operable patients who continue to bleed at rates of more than 1 L per day despite supportive, conservative care and subsequent embolization should undergo surgical resection. The correct therapy in a given patient depends on the cause of the bleeding, lung function, availability of resources, and local expertise.

For patients with DAH, selective arterial embolization and surgery are not options. Recombinant factor VIIa has been used successfully for treatment of DAH due to disseminated aspergillosis, bone marrow transplantation, small-vessel vasculitis, and cystic fibrosis [47,48]. For immunologically mediated diseases, corticosteroids, cytotoxic agents, and other interventions (e.g., plasmapheresis in Goodpasture's syndrome) are available (see Chapters 67 and 68).

When corticosteroid therapy is given alone for critically ill patients with immunologic lung diseases, the dose is 1 mg/kg/d of intravenous methylprednisolone or the equivalent dose of another corticosteroid. Larger doses, on the order of 7 to 15 mg/kg/d for 1 to 3 days, have been recommended to control progressive pulmonary hemorrhage and hypoxemia of Goodpasture's syndrome, SLE, and the vasculitides (see Chapters 66 and 67). In general, corticosteroids should be administered initially in round-the-clock divided doses until substantial improvement has occurred. They can then be given once per day and tapered as the patient's condition dictates.

When combined corticosteroid and cytotoxic drug therapy is given, it is usually prescribed for immunologic lung diseases caused by vasculitides (e.g., GPA, MPA, and rheumatoid vasculitis) and anti-GBM disease (Goodpasture's syndrome). For details regarding specific therapy for these conditions, see Chapters 66 and 67.

References

1. Jean-Baptiste E: Clinical assessment and management of massive hemoptysis. *Crit Care Med* 28:1642–1647, 2000.
2. Sakr L, Dutau H: Massive hemoptysis: An update on the role of bronchoscopy in diagnosis and management. *Respiration* 80:39–41, 2010.
3. Gale D: Overgrowth of *Serratia marcescens* in respiratory tract, simulating hemoptysis. *JAMA* 164:1328, 1957.
4. Robinson KA, Irwin RS: Managing Hemoptysis, in Irwin RS, Rippe JM (eds): *Intensive Care Medicine*. 7th ed. Philadelphia, Lippincott Williams & Wilkins, 2012, pp 578–587.
5. Shigemura N, Wan IY, Yu SCH: Multidisciplinary management of life-threatening massive hemoptysis: a 10 year experience. *Ann Thorac Surg* 87:849–853, 2009.
6. Hsiao, EI, Kirsch CM, Kagawa FT, et al: Utility of fiberoptic bronchoscopy before bronchial artery embolization for massive hemoptysis. *Am J Roentgenol* 177:861–867, 2001.
7. Kravitz JN, Berry MW, Schabel SI, et al: A modern series of percutaneous intracavitary instillation of amphotericin B for the treatment of severe hemoptysis from pulmonary aspergilloma. *Chest* 143:1414–1421, 2013.

8. Flume PA, Yankaskas JR, Ebeling M, et al: Massive hemoptysis in cystic fibrosis. *Chest* 128:729–738, 2005
9. Kearney TJ, Shabot MM: Pulmonary artery rupture associated with the Swan-Ganz catheter. *Chest* 108:1349–1352, 1995
10. Abreu AR, Campo MA, Krieger BP: Pulmonary artery rupture induced by a pulmonary artery catheter: A case report and review of the literature. *J Intens Care Med* 19:291–296, 2004.
11. Bartter T, Irwin RS, Phillips DA, et al: Pulmonary artery pseudoaneurysm: a potential complication of pulmonary artery catheterization. *Arch Intern Med* 148:471, 1988.
12. Schaefer OP, Irwin RS: Tracheo-artery fistula. *J Int Care Med* 10:64, 1995.
13. Adelman M, Haponik EF, Bleeker ER, et al: Cryptogenic hemoptysis: clinical features, bronchoscopic findings, and natural history in 67 patients. *Ann Intern Med* 102:829, 1985.
14. Savale L, Parrot A, Khalil A, et al: Cryptogenic hemoptysis: from a benign to a life-threatening pathologic vascular condition. *Am J Respir Crit Care Med* 175:1181, 2007.
15. Remy J, Remy-Jardin M, Voisin C: Endovascular management of bronchial bleeding; in Butler J (ed): The *Bronchial Circulation*. New York, Dekker, 1992, pp 667–723.
16. Ferguson FC, Kobilak RE, Deitrick JE: Varices of bronchial veins as source of hemoptysis in mitral stenosis. *Am Heart J* 28:445, 1944.
17. Wood DA, Miller M: Role of dual pulmonary circulation in various pathologic conditions of lungs. *J Thorac Surg* 7:649, 1938.
18. Dalen JE, Haffajee CI, Alpert JS, et al: Pulmonary embolism, pulmonary hemorrhage, and pulmonary infarction. *N Engl J Med* 296:1431, 1977.
19. Kneeling AN, Costello R, Lee MJ: Rasmussen's aneurysm: a forgotten entity? *Cardiovasc Intervent Radiol* 31:196, 2008.
20. Rasmussen V: On hemoptysis, especially when fatal, in its anatomical and clinical aspects. *Edinburgh Med J* 14:385, 1968.
21. Rodman MH, Jones CW: Catamenial hemoptysis due to bronchial endometriosis. *N Engl J Med* 266:805, 1962.
22. Fagin ID: Hemoptysis with intercourse. *JAMA* 240:22, 1978.
23. Patterson R, Zeiss CR, Pruzansky JJ: Immunology and immunopathology of trimellitic anhydride pulmonary reactions. *J Allergy Clin Immunol* 70:19, 1982.
24. Patterson R, Nugent KM, Harris KE, et al: Immunologic hemorrhagic pneumonia caused by isocyanates. *Am Rev Respir Dis* 141:226, 1990.
25. Sisson JH, Thompson AB, Anderson JR, et al: Airway inflammation predicts diffuse alveolar hemorrhage during bone marrow transplantation in patients with Hodgkin disease. *Am Rev Respir Dis* 146:439, 1992.
26. Lara AR, Schwarz MI: Diffuse alveolar hemorrhage. *Chest* 137(5): 1164–1171, 2010.
27. Green RJ, Ruoss SJ, Kraft SA, et al: Pulmonary capillaritis and alveolar hemorrhage: update on diagnosis and management. *Chest* 110:1305, 1996.
28. Khalil A, Fartouk, M, Parrot A, et al: Impact of MDCT Angiography on the management of patients with hemoptysis. *Am J Roentgenol* 195: 772–778, 2010.
29. Larici AR, Franchi P, Occhipinti M, et al: Diagnosis and management of hemoptysis. *Diag Interv Radiol* 20: 229–309, 2014.
30. Saumench J, Escarrabill J, Padro L, et al: Value of fiberoptic bronchoscopy and angiography for diagnosis of the bleeding site in hemoptysis. *Ann Thorac Surg* 48:272, 1989.
31. McGuinness G, Beacher JR, Harkin TJ, et al: Hemoptysis: prospective high-resolution CT/bronchoscopic correlation. *Chest* 105:1155, 1994.
32. Revel MP, Fournier LS, Hennebicque AS, et al: Can CT replace bronchoscopy in the detetction of the site and cause of bleeding in patients with large or massive hemoptysis? *Am J Roentgenol* 179 (5):1217–1224, 2002.
33. Grant CA, Dempsey G, Harrison J, et al: Tracheo-innominate artery fistula after percutaneous trachesostomy: three case reports and a clinical review. *Br J Anaesth* 96(1):127–131, 2006.
34. De Lassence A, Fleury-Feith J, Escudier E, et al: Alveolar hemorrhage: diagnostic criteria and results in 194 immunocompromised hosts. *Am J Respir Crit Care Med* 151:157, 1995.
35. Noe GD, Jaffe SM, Molam MP: CT and CT angiography in massive hemoptysis with emphasis on pre-embolization assessment. *Clin Radiol* 66: 869–875, 2011.
36. Lin Y, Ziqian C, Xizhang Y, et al: Bronchial and non-bronchial systemic arteries: value of multidetector CT angiography in diagnosis and angiographic embolization feasibility analysis. *J Med Imag Radiat Oncol* 57: 644–651, 2013.
37. Kopec SE, Irwin RS: Lung Biopsy, in Irwin RS, Rippe JM (eds): *Intensive Care Medicine*. 7th ed. Philadelphia, Lippincott Williams & Wilkins, 2012, pp 815-822.
38. Ewig S, Soler N, Gonzalez J, et al: Evaluation of antimicrobial treatment in mechanically ventilated patients with severe chronic obstructive pulmonary disease exacerbations. *Crit Care Med* 28:692, 2000.
39. Sood N, Paradowski LJ, Yankaskas JR: Outcomes of intensive care unit care in adults with cystic fibrosis. *Am J Respir Crit Care Med* 163:335, 2001.
40. Rose SC, Thistlewaite PA, Sewell PE, et al: Lung cancer and radiofrequency ablation. *J Vasc Interv Radiol* 17:927, 2006.
41. Hamaguchi S, Nakajima Y: Two cases of tracheoinnominate artery fistula following tracheostomy treated successfully by endovascular embolization of the innominate artery. *J Vasc Surg* 55 (2): 545–547, 2011.
42. Subramanian A, Kate AH, Chhajed PN: Role of bronchoscopy in massive hemoptysis, in Mehta A, Jain P (eds): *Interventional Bronchoscopy—A Clinical Guide*. New York, Humana Press, 2013, pp 245-257.
43. Valipour A, Kreuzer A, Koller H, et al: Bronchoscopy-guided topical hemostatic tamponade therapy for the management of life-threatening hemoptysis. *Chest* 127:2113, 2005.
44. Chun JY, Morgan R, Belli AM: Radiological management of hemoptysis: a comprehensive review of diagnostic imaging and bronchial arterial embolization. *Cardiovasc Intervent Radiol* 33:240–250, 2010.
45. Wilson RF, Soullier GW, Wiencek RG: Hemoptysis in trauma. *J Trauma* 27:1123, 1987.
46. Remy T, Siproudhis L, Laurent JF, et al: Massive hemoptysis from iatrogenic balloon catheter rupture of pulmonary artery: successful early management by balloon tamponade. *Crit Care Med* 15:272, 1987.
47. Macdonald JA, Fraser JF, Foot CL, et al: Successful use of recombinant factor VII in massive hemoptysis due to community-acquired pneumonia. *Chest* 130:577, 2006.
48. Lau EMT, Yozghatlian V, Kosky C, et al: Recombinant activated Factor VII for massive hemoptysis in patients with cystic fibrosis. *Chest* 136:277–281, 2009.

Chapter 176 ■ Pleural Diseases of the Critically Ill Patient

PETER DOELKEN • JOHN TERRILL HUGGINS

Pleural disease is an unusual cause for admission to the intensive care unit (ICU). Exceptions are a large hemothorax for monitoring bleeding rate and hemodynamic status and an unstable secondary spontaneous pneumothorax or large unilateral or bilateral pleural effusions that have caused acute respiratory failure.

Pleural disease can be overlooked among critically ill patients because it may be overshadowed by the presenting illness that has resulted in ICU admission. Furthermore, it is often a subtle finding on the clinical examination and supine chest radiograph. A pleural effusion may not be seen on the supine chest radiograph because a diffuse alveolar filling process can mask the posterior layering of fluid or because bilateral effusions without parenchymal infiltrates are misinterpreted as an underexposed film or objects outside the chest. Pneumothorax may remain undetected in the supine patient because pleural air tends to be situated anteriorly and does not produce the diagnostic visceral pleural line seen on an upright radiograph. However, it is clear that pleural ultrasound is a superior modality for the detection of pleural fluid and pneumothorax when compared to standard chest radiographs and is comparable to chest computed tomography (CT).

When the patient on mechanical ventilation is at increased risk for barotrauma because airway pressures are high, the index of suspicion for pneumothorax should be heightened; if there is evidence of pulmonary interstitial gas (see the following discussion) or subcutaneous emphysema, appropriate radiologic studies should be obtained.

RADIOLOGIC SIGNS OF PLEURAL DISEASE

Because the distribution of fluid and air in the normal pleural space tends to follow gravitational influences, and because the lung has a tendency to maintain its normal shape as it becomes smaller, fluid initially accumulates between the bottom of the lung and the diaphragm, and air accumulates between the top of the lung and the apex of the thorax in the upright position. When chest radiographs are obtained in other than the erect position, free pleural fluid and air change position and result in a different radiographic appearance.

PLEURAL FLUID

Standard Chest Radiograph

In healthy humans in the supine position, the radiolucency of the lung base is equal to or greater than that in the lung apex [1]. Furthermore, when in the supine position, breast and pectoral tissue tend to fall laterally away from the lung base. Thus, an effusion should be suspected if there is increased homogeneous density over the lower lung fields compared to the upper lung fields. As the pleural effusion increases, the increased radiodensity involves the upper hemithorax as well. However, failure of chest wall tissue to move laterally, cardiomegaly, prominent epicardial fat pad, and lung collapse or consolidation may obscure a pleural effusion on a supine radiograph. Patient rotation or an off-center X-ray beam can mimic a unilateral homogeneous density. An absent pectoral muscle, prior mastectomy, unilateral hyperlucent lung, scoliosis, previous lobectomy, hypoplastic pulmonary artery, or pleural or chest wall mass may lead to unilateral homogeneous increased density and mimic an effusion.

Approximately 175 to 525 mL of pleural fluid results in blunting of the costophrenic angle on an erect radiograph. This quantity of effusion can be detected on a supine radiograph as an increased density over the lower lung zone. Failure to visualize the hemidiaphragm, absence of the costophrenic angle meniscus, and apical capping are less likely to be seen with effusions of less than 500 mL [1]. The major radiographic finding of a pleural effusion in a supine position is increased homogeneous density over the lower lung field that does not obliterate normal bronchovascular markings, does not show air bronchograms, and does not show hilar or mediastinal displacement until the effusion is massive. If a pleural effusion is suspected in the supine patient, ultrasonography (US) should be performed.

Other Radiographic Imaging

Ultrasonography

US provides rapid identification and characterization of pleural effusions for critically ill patients. US is well suited for the identification and evaluation of fluid, because fluid is less echogenic than soft tissue. Many studies have demonstrated the usefulness of ultrasound for this indication. Pleural effusions as small as 3 to 5 mL can be detected by ultrasound [1]. Pleural US is superior to standard chest radiography for detecting the presence of pleural effusions and in distinguishing pleural effusions from atelectasis or pleural thickening [2,3].

Compared to chest CT scan, pleural ultrasound has 93% sensitivity and specificity for pleural effusions [4]. More importantly, the complexity of the pleural effusion is better appreciated on ultrasound when compared to chest CT [5].) (Fig. 176.1A–D).

US takes less time and is less expensive than CT, can be done at the bedside, and can be repeated serially. Disadvantages include hindrance of the ultrasonic wave by air, in either the lung or the pleural space, a restricted field of view, inferior evaluation of the lung parenchyma compared with CT, and operator dependence. US was helpful for diagnosis among 27 (66%) of 41 patients and treatment of 37 (90%) of 41 patients, and had an important influence on treatment planning for 17 (41%) of 41 critically ill patients [4].

US has also been demonstrated to be a useful modality to guide bedside thoracentesis in the mechanically ventilated patient, resulting in high success rate and excellent safety of the procedure [6].

Free-flowing pleural effusions will layer posteriorly in the thorax of the supine patient. Patients with multiple lines or compromised hemodynamic and oxygenation status will be difficult to position sitting upright in bed. If the patient is supine, the bed may prevent the easy visualization of small pleural effusions. One option is for the examiner to place the transducer in the posterior axillary line while angling the probe up toward the center of the body to visualize smaller effusions. For unstable patients who have effusions that are difficult to visualize, positioning the patient in a lateral decubitus position may be helpful. The examiner should always use a systematic approach to identify the following three findings to confirm the presence of a pleural effusion (see Video 1-25 in Chapter 12 Cases).

1. Anatomic boundaries: An identification of the diaphragm and subdiaphragmatic organs (the liver or the spleen, depending on the side), the chest wall, and the lung, which should be clearly differentiated from the pleural effusion.
2. Echo-free space: The relatively echo-free space surrounded by typical anatomic boundaries is the pleural effusion.
3. Dynamic changes: Characteristic changes of the echo-free space should be identified.

These dynamic changes would be respirophasic change and lung flap. Another characteristic sign of pleural effusions is the plankton sign, which is caused by swirling debris agitated by cardiac or respiratory motion in a pleural effusion. Fibrin strands may be seen moving in synchronization with cardiac pulsations or respiratory motion. The hematocrit sign may be observed in cases of hemothorax or empyema. By gravitational effect, the effusion is layered into two phases of different echogenicity.

Debris, strands, or septations may be visible. In the case of parapneumonic effusions, these findings typically indicate the presence of a complicated parapneumonic effusion or an empyema [7].

Patients with septated effusions visible on US require longer hospital stays, longer chest tube drainage, and more often require fibrinolytic therapy or surgery for adequate drainage [8]. Pleural ultrasound is superior to CT scan for visualizing septations within a pleural effusion [9]. The identification and characterization of pleural fluid is discussed in detail in Chapter 12. In addition, the reader is referred to the video image library that is associated with this textbook that contains a comprehensive collection of US findings of pleural effusion.

Computed Tomography

CT is recognized as providing increased resolution compared with conventional imaging. Although moving a critically ill patient for CT has potential risks, the diagnostic advantage is justified for the stable patient when the clinical course is not congruent with the proposed diagnosis suggested by the portable chest radiograph or US. Among selected patients with multisystem trauma, chest CT often provides additional diagnostic information and positively affects patient management and outcomes.

PNEUMOTHORAX

When supine, pneumothorax gas migrates along the anterior surface of the lung, making detection on the anteroposterior radiograph problematic. The base, lateral chest wall, and juxtacardiac area should be carefully visualized for evidence of pneumothorax. Accumulation of air along the mediastinal parietal pleura may simulate pneumomediastinum. An erect or

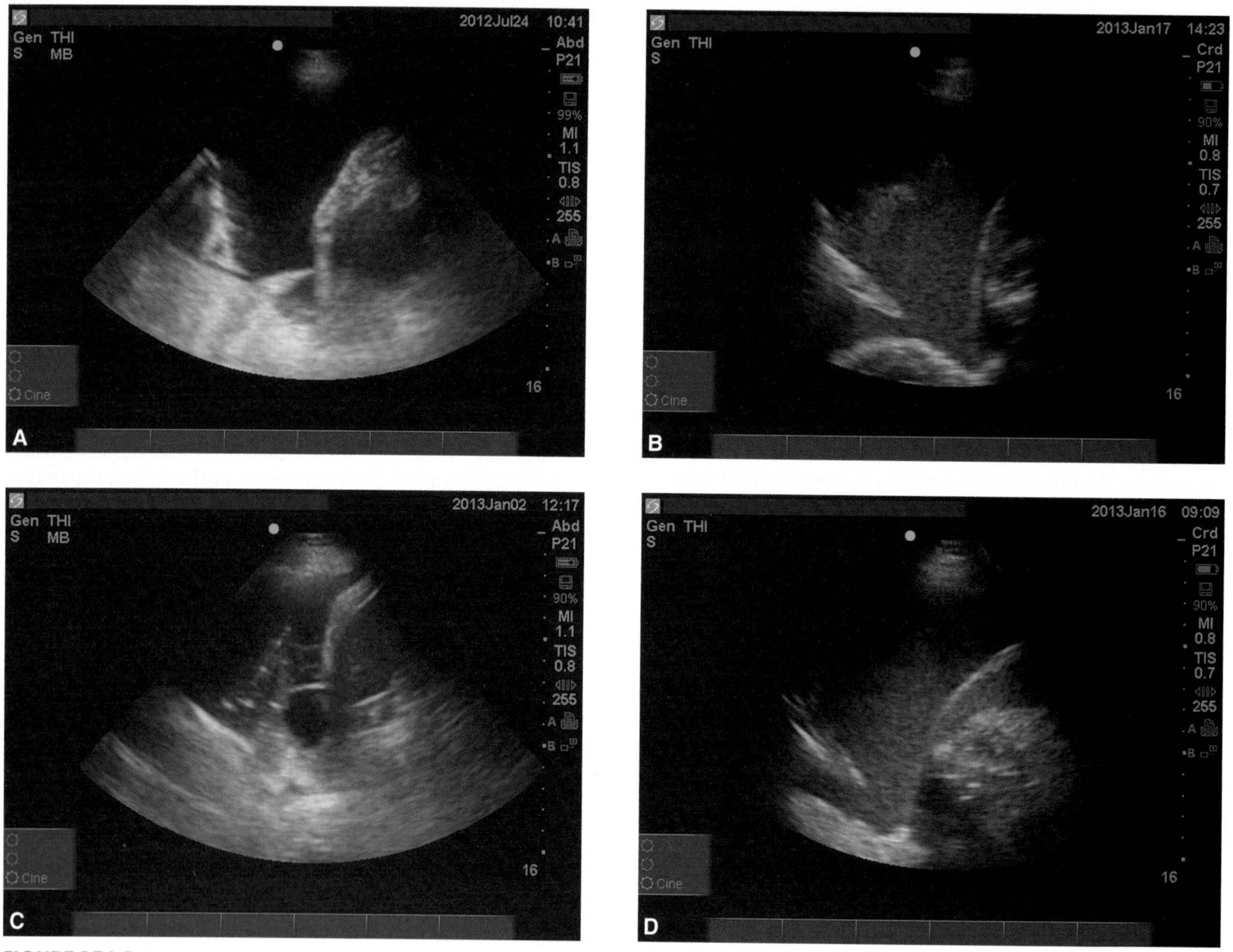

FIGURE 176.1 **A:** An anechoic pleural effusion in a patient with decompensated congestive heart failure. **B:** A complex, nonseptate pleural effusion seen in a patient with malignant pleural effusion. **C:** A complex, septae pleural effusion seen in a patient with severe sepsis owing to the presence of an empyema. **D:** A complex pleural effusion with an anechoic area assoicated with an increased echogenic density in the dependent area of the fluid collection. This is called the "hematocrit sign" and occurred in a patient who developed a hemothorax as a result of extravascular migration of a central line into the pleural space.

a decubitus (suspected hemithorax up) radiograph should be obtained to assess for the presence of a pneumothorax. US is sensitive for the detection of pneumothorax by determining the presence or absence of "lung sliding" [10]. Among individuals without pneumothorax, the lung–chest wall interface, which represents a to-and-fro movement synchronized with respiration, can be identified. US visualization of lung sliding is correlated with the absence of pneumothorax, and from this sign alone, at least anterior pneumothorax can be excluded rapidly at the bedside of a mechanically ventilated patient. However, the absence of lung sliding may be caused by the presence of large bullae or pleural symphysis caused by previous pleurodesis or pleural adhesions as a result of previous pleural disease. Hence, the absence of lung sliding is not specific for pneumothorax, but detection of lung sliding reliably excludes the presence of pleural air in the examined area. We recommend that preprocedural scanning be performed to determine the presence of lung sliding prior to the placement of a central venous line. The presence of lung sliding before and after the placement of a central venous catheter is reassuring for excluding an iatrogenic pneumothorax.

The most common radiographic signs of tension pneumothorax are contralateral mediastinal shift, ipsilateral diaphragmatic depression, and ipsilateral chest wall expansion. Underlying lung disease may prevent total lung collapse, even if tension is present; for patients on mechanical ventilation, little or no midline mediastinal shift may result from the tension. Among the latter, a depressed ipsilateral diaphragm is a more reliable sign of tension than mediastinal shift.

For patients with acute respiratory distress syndrome (ARDS), barotrauma can result in a localized tension pneumothorax with a subtle contralateral mediastinal shift, flattening of the cardiac contour, and depression of the ipsilateral hemidiaphragm [11]. Pleural adhesions and relative compressibility and mobility of surrounding structures, in addition to the supine position, probably account for these loculated tension pneumothoraces.

A study of 88 critically ill patients with 112 pneumothoraces found that the anteromedial and subpulmonic recesses were involved for 64% of patients in the supine and semierect positions [12]. Furthermore, in 30% of the pneumothoraces of this study that were not initially detected by the clinician or radiologist, half of the patients progressed to tension pneumothorax. Therefore, a high index of suspicion is necessary to avoid catastrophic situations.

Factors that may contribute to an improved ability to diagnose this potentially lethal problem include (a) familiarity with atypical locations of pneumothoraces in critically ill patients, usually caused by the supine or semierect position; (b) the consequence of underlying cardiopulmonary disease; and (c) knowledge of other risk factors contributing to misdiagnosis (e.g., mechanical ventilation, altered mental status, prolonged ICU stay, and development of pneumothorax after peak physician staffing hours) [13].

EVALUATION OF THE PATIENT WITH A PLEURAL EFFUSION

Diagnostic Thoracentesis

Indications

Patients with a pleural effusion provide the opportunity to diagnose, at least presumptively, the underlying process responsible for pleural fluid accumulation. Pleural effusions are most commonly caused by primary lung disease but may also result from disease in the gastrointestinal tract, liver, kidney, heart, or reticuloendothelial system.

Although disease of any organ system can cause a pleural effusion in critically ill patients, the diagnoses listed in Table 176.1 represent the majority of the causes seen in ICUs. The types of pleural effusions seen in medical and surgical ICUs are similar, but some causes related to surgical (coronary artery bypass grafting, chylothorax, and abdominal surgery) and nonsurgical trauma (hemothorax) represent a substantial percentage of surgical ICU effusions.

When a pleural effusion is suspected on physical examination and confirmed radiologically, a diagnostic thoracentesis under ultrasonographic guidance should be performed in an attempt to establish the cause. Exceptions are patients with a secure clinical diagnosis and a small amount of pleural fluid, as in atelectasis, or patients with uncomplicated congestive heart failure (CHF) [14]. Observation may be warranted in these situations, but thoracentesis should be performed if there are adverse changes [15].

The indications for diagnostic thoracentesis do not change simply because the patient is in the ICU or on mechanical ventilation. In fact, establishing the diagnosis quickly for these critically ill patients may be more important and life-saving than in noncritically ill patients. It has been well documented that even among patients on mechanical ventilation, diagnostic thoracentesis is safe if there is strict adherence to the general principles of the procedure and US is used (see Chapter 12) [16]. Pneumothorax, the most clinically important complication of thoracentesis [11], is no more likely to occur during mechanical ventilation; however, when a pneumothorax does develop, the patient on mechanical ventilation is likely to develop a tension pneumothorax.

TABLE 176.1

Causes of Pleural Effusions

In the medical ICU	In the surgical ICU
Atelectasis	Atelectasis
Congestive heart failure	Congestive heart failure
Pneumonia	Pneumonia
Hypoalbuminemia	Pancreatitis
Pancreatitis	Hypoalbuminemia
ARDS	Coronary artery bypass surgery
Pulmonary embolism	ARDS
Hepatic hydrothorax	Pulmonary embolism
Esophageal sclerotherapy	Esophageal rupture
Postmyocardial infarction	Hemothorax
Iatrogenic	Chylothorax
	Abdominal surgery
	Iatrogenic

ARDS, acute respiratory distress syndrome; ICU, intensive care unit.

Contraindications

There are no absolute contraindications to diagnostic thoracentesis. If clinical judgment dictates that the information gained from the pleural fluid analysis may help in diagnosis and therapy, thoracentesis should be performed (see Chapter 12). Diagnostic thoracentesis with a small-bore needle can be performed safely in virtually any patient if meticulous technique is used. The major relative contraindications to thoracentesis are a bleeding diathesis or an anticoagulation. A patient with a small amount of pleural fluid and a low benefit to risk ratio also represents a relative contraindication. Thoracentesis should not be attempted through an area of active skin infection.

Complications

Complications of diagnostic thoracentesis include pain at the needle insertion site, bleeding (local, intrapleural, or intra-abdominal), pneumothorax, empyema, and spleen or liver puncture (see Chapter 12). Pneumothorax has been reported in prospective studies to occur in 4% to 30% of patients [17,18]. However, when ultrasound-guided thoracentesis is performed by experienced physician sonographers, pneumothorax or other injuries caused by organ puncture appear to be rare events. Liver or spleen puncture tends to occur when the patient is not sitting absolutely upright because movement toward recumbency causes cephalad migration of the abdominal viscera. The upward displacement of abdominal organs is readily detected by US. However, even if the liver or the spleen is punctured with a small-bore needle, generally the outcome is favorable if the patient is not receiving anticoagulants and does not have a bleeding diathesis.

Therapeutic Thoracentesis

Indications and Contraindications

The primary indication for therapeutic thoracentesis is relief of dyspnea. Contraindications to therapeutic thoracentesis are similar to those for diagnostic thoracentesis. However, there appears to be an increased risk of pneumothorax, thus making a therapeutic thoracentesis in patients on mechanical ventilation potentially hazardous.

The technique for therapeutic thoracentesis is essentially the same as for diagnostic thoracentesis, except that a blunt-tip needle or plastic catheter, rather than a sharp-tip needle, should be used (see Chapter 12). This reduces the risk of pneumothorax, which may occur because fluid is removed and the lung expands toward the chest wall. Again, the use of sonographic guidance is recommended.

The amount of fluid that can be removed safely from the pleural space at one session is controversial. Ideally, monitoring pleural pressure should dictate the amount of fluid that can be removed. As long as intrapleural pressure does not fall to less than -20 cm H_2O, fluid removal can continue [19]. However, intrapleural pressure monitoring is not done routinely. In the patient with contralateral mediastinal shift on chest radiograph who tolerates thoracentesis without chest tightness, cough, or light-headedness, probably several liters of pleural fluid can be removed safely. However, neither the patient nor the operator may be aware of a precipitous drop in pleural pressure. In patients without a contralateral mediastinal shift or with ipsilateral shift (suggesting an endobronchial obstruction), the likelihood of a precipitous drop in intrapleural pressure is increased, and pleural pressure should be monitored during thoracentesis. Alternatively, a small-bore catheter connected to a standard thoracostomy pleural drainage system may be temporarily inserted, thus avoiding excessively negative pleural pressure development during drainage. Simple gravity drainage or drainage using any system incorporating a nonreturn valve does not reliably guard against the development of excessively negative pressure.

Physiological Effects and Complications

Improvement in lung volumes up to 24 hours after therapeutic thoracentesis does not correlate with the amount of fluid removed, despite relief of dyspnea in those patients [20]. In some patients, however, maximum spirometric improvement may not occur for several days. Patients with initial negative pleural pressures and those with more precipitous falls in pleural pressure with thoracentesis tend to have the least improvement in pulmonary function after therapeutic thoracentesis because many have a trapped lung or an endobronchial obstruction [18]. The mechanism of dyspnea from a large pleural effusion probably is related to the increase in chest wall resting volume resulting in shortening of the respiratory muscles resting length and consequent decrease in contractile efficiency [21]. Drainage of moderately sized pleural effusions (1,495 mL) does not appear to result in predictable changes of respiratory system compliance or resistances although a systematic decrease of work performed by the ventilator as a consequence of thoracentesis has been reported [22].

Complications of therapeutic thoracentesis are the same as those seen with diagnostic thoracentesis (see Chapter 12). Three complications that are unique to therapeutic thoracentesis are hypoxemia, unilateral pulmonary edema, and hypovolemia. After therapeutic thoracentesis, hypoxemia may occur despite relief of dyspnea [23,24] from worsening ventilation–perfusion relationships in the ipsilateral lung or clinically occult unilateral pulmonary edema.

Some investigators have concluded that the change in partial pressure of arterial oxygen (PaO_2) after therapeutic thoracentesis is unpredictable [24]; some have observed a characteristic increase in PaO_2 within minutes to hours [19], whereas others suggest a systematic decrease in PaO_2 that returns to prethoracentesis values by 24 hours [23]. In the largest study, including 33 patients with various causes of unilateral pleural effusions, a significant increase of PaO_2 was found 20 minutes, 2 hours, and 24 hours after therapeutic thoracentesis [25]. This was in conjunction with a decrease in the alveolar–arterial oxygen gradient [$P(A\text{–}a)O_2$] and was accompanied by a small but significant decrease in shunt, without a change in V_D/V_T. Data suggest an improved ventilation–perfusion relationship after therapeutic thoracentesis, with an increase in ventilation of parts of the lung that were previously poorly ventilated but well perfused. The relief of dyspnea among these patients cannot be explained by improved arterial oxygen tension. The increases have been modest, and, in some cases, there has been a fall in PaO_2. Improvement in lung volumes is a constant finding after therapeutic thoracentesis but may take days or even weeks to maximize; immediate changes are usually modest and highly variable. Therefore, the relief of dyspnea cannot be adequately explained by changes in lung volume or in the mechanics of breathing but may be the result of decreased stimulation of lung or chest wall receptors, or both [20].

PLEURAL EFFUSIONS OF THE CRITICALLY ILL

The types of pleural effusions in critically ill patients are listed in Table 176.2.

Atelectasis

Atelectasis is a common cause of small pleural effusions among comatose, immobile, pain-ridden patients in ICUs [26] and after upper abdominal surgery [27]. Other causes include major bronchial obstruction from lung cancer or a mucous plug. Atelectasis causes pleural fluid because of decreased pleural pressure. With alveolar collapse, the lung and chest wall separate further, creating local areas of increased negative pressure. This decrease of pleural pressure favors the movement of fluid into the pleural space, presumably from the parietal pleural surface. The fluid accumulates until the pleural or parietal-pleural interstitial pressure gradient reaches a steady state.

Pleural fluid from atelectasis is a serous transudate with a low number of mononuclear cells, a glucose concentration equivalent to serum, and pH in the range of 7.45 to 7.55. When atelectasis resolves, pleural fluid dissipates during several days.

Congestive Heart Failure

CHF is the most common cause of transudative pleural effusions and a common cause of pleural effusions among the critically ill. Pleural effusions as aresult of CHF are associated with increases of pulmonary venous pressure [28]. Most patients with subacute or chronic elevation of pulmonary venous pressure (pulmonary capillary wedge pressure of at least 24 mm Hg) have evidence of pleural effusion on US or lateral decubitus radiograph. Isolated increases in systemic venous pressure tend not to produce pleural effusions. Thus, patients with chronic obstructive pulmonary disease (COPD) and cor pulmonale rarely have pleural effusions, and the presence of pleural fluid implies another cause.

Most patients with pleural effusions secondary to CHF have the classic signs and symptoms. The chest radiograph shows cardiomegaly and bilateral small-to-moderate pleural effusions of similar size (right slightly greater than left). There is usually radiographic evidence of pulmonary congestion, with the severity of pulmonary edema correlating with the presence of pleural effusion.

The effusion is a transudate, with mesothelial cells and lymphocytes accounting for the majority of the less than 1,000 cells per μL. Acute diuresis can raise the pleural fluid protein and lactate dehydrogenase into the range of an exudate [29,30]. In the patient with secure clinical diagnosis of CHF, observation is appropriate. Thoracentesis should be performed if the patient is febrile, has pleural effusions of disparate size, has a unilateral pleural effusion, does not have cardiomegaly, has pleuritic chest pain, or has a PaO_2 inappropriate for the degree of pulmonary edema.

Treatment consists of decreasing pulmonary venous hypertension and improving cardiac output with diuretics, ionoropes, or afterload reduction. In successfully managed heart failure, the effusions resolve during days to weeks after the pulmonary edema has cleared.

Hepatic Hydrothorax

Pleural effusions occur in approximately 6% of patients with cirrhosis of the liver and clinical ascites. The effusions result from movement of ascitic fluid through congenital or acquired diaphragmatic defects [31].

TABLE 176.2

Differential Diagnosis of Pleural Effusions in Critically Ill Patients

	Clinical presentation	Chest radiograph	Pleural fluid analysis	Diagnosis	Comments
Transudates					
Congestive heart failure	Usual signs and symptoms plus I >O, weight gain, worsening $P(A–a)O_2$, ↓ C_{ST}	Bilateral effusions, right >left, cardiomegaly, extravascular lung water	Serous, nucleated cells <1,000/μL, lymphocytes, mesothelial cells, pH 7.45–7.55	Presumptive	Associated with ↑ pulmonary capillary wedge pressure, acute diuresis may result in ↑ protein and LDH
Atelectasis	Asymptomatic or dyspnea, worsening $P(A–a)O_2$	Small unilateral or bilateral effusions, volume loss	Serous, nucleated cells <1,000/μL, lymphocytes, mesothelial cells, pH 7.45–7.55	Presumptive	Common after upper abdominal surgery, also with pulmonary embolism, mucous plug
Hepatic hydrothorax	Stigmata of liver disease, clinical ascites, asymptomatic or dyspnea, worsening $P(A–a)O_2$, poor response to low-flow O_2	Unilateral right or bilateral effusions, small to massive, normal heart size, no other CXR abnormalities	Serous-serosanguineous nucleated cells <1,000/μL, lymphocytes, mesothelial cells, pH 7.40–7.55	Presumptive, PF protein and LDH similar to ascitic fluid	6% of patients with clinical ascites, fluid movement from abdomen to chest via diaphragm defect
Hypoalbuminemia	Asymptomatic or dyspnea, anasarca	Small-to-moderate bilateral effusions, normal heart size, no other CXR abnormalities	Serous, nucleated cells <1,000/μL, lymphocytes, mesothelial cells, pH 7.45–7.55	Presumptive	Serum albumin <1.5 g/dL, never have isolated pleural effusion
Iatrogenic: extravascular migration of central venous catheter	Chest pain, dyspnea	Abnormal position of catheter, widening of mediastinum, small-to-large unilateral effusion	Serous-hemorrhagic or white, may contain PMNs, chemistries similar to infusate, PF/S glucose >1.0	Presumptive	Highest incidence with left external jugular vein placement, aspiration or retrograde flow of blood confirms intravascular placement
Exudates					
Parapneumonic effusions: uncomplicated	Fever, chest pain, ↑ WBC, purulent sputum	New alveolar infiltrate, minimal-to-moderate ipsilateral free-flowing effusion	Turbid, PMNs, glucose >60 mg/dL, LDH <700 IU/L, pH ≥7.30	Presumptive	Effusion resolves without sequelae on antibiotics only
Parapneumonic effusions: complicated	Fever, chest pain, ↑ WBC, purulent sputum	New alveolar infiltrate, moderate-to-large ipsilateral effusion with or without loculation	Pus, positive bacteriology, pH <7.10, glucose <40 mg/dL, LDH >1,000 IU/L	Based on PF acidosis, positive bacteriology, aspiration of pus, loculation	Putrid odor defines anaerobic empyema, requires pleural space drainage for resolution
Pancreatitis	Acute abdominal pain, nausea, vomiting, fever	Small, unilateral, left effusion (60%), atelectasis	Turbid, nucleated cells 10,000–50,000/μL, PMNs, pH 7.30–7.35, PF/S amylase >1.0	PF/S amylase >1.0 or >upper limits of normal for serum	Effusion resolves as pancreatitis resolves without need for pleural space drainage

(continued)

TABLE 176.2

Differential Diagnosis of Pleural Effusions in Critically Ill Patients (*continued*)

	Clinical presentation	Chest radiograph	Pleural fluid analysis	Diagnosis	Comments
Pulmonary embolism	Acute dyspnea, tachypnea, chest pain, ↑ $P(A–a)O_2$	Unilateral, small-to-moderate effusion, peripheral infiltrate, atelectasis	Serous-bloody nucleated cells 100–50,000/μL, PMNs or lymphocytes	Presumptive	20% transudates, effusion present on admission, $^1/_3$ of hemithorax, reaches maximum volume by 72 h
Postcardiac injury syndrome	Chest pain, pericardial rub, fever, dyspnea 3 d to 3 wk after cardiac injury, ↑ WBC, ↑ erythrocyte sedimentation rate	Left or bilateral small-to-moderate effusion, left lower lobe infiltrates	Serosanguineous-bloody, nucleated cells 500–39,000/μL, PMNs or lymphocytes, pH >7.30	Presumptive	Effusion resolves in 1–3 wk, may require steroids
Esophageal sclerotherapy	Chest pain following sclerotherapy with large sclerosant volume, effusion appears by 48–72 h	Small, unilateral, or bilateral effusion	Serosanguineous, nucleated cells 100–38,000/μL, PMNs or mononuclear, pH >7.30	Presumptive	Requires no specific therapy, resolves in days to weeks
ARDS	Depends on cause	Bilateral alveolar infiltrates tend to mask small bilateral effusions	Serous-serosanguineous, PMNs	Presumptive	Requires no specific therapy, effusions resolve as ARDS resolves
Spontaneous esophageal rupture	Severe retching or vomiting followed by thoracoabdominal pain, fever, subcutaneous air	Subcutaneous/mediastinal air; left pneumothorax, followed by left effusion	Early: serous, pH >7.30; later: turbid-purulent effusion, PMNs, pH approaches 6.00, ↑ amylase	Pleural fluid pH <7.00, with ↑ salivary amylase and positive bacteriology	With early diagnosis prognosis good with primary closure and drainage
Hemothorax	Following blunt and penetrating chest trauma, invasive procedures, malignancy, anticoagulation	Small-to-massive unilateral effusion, other abnormalities depending on cause of hemothorax	Gross blood, PF/blood Hct >50%	PF/blood Hct >50%	Often not appreciated on initial radiograph in setting of trauma; should be drained with chest tube
Coronary artery bypass graft	Asymptomatic, dyspnea	Small-to-moderate left effusion without parenchymal infiltrates, left lower lobe atelectasis, elevation of left hemidiaphragm	Hemorrhagic PF/blood Hct <5%, nucleated cells <10,000/μL, lymph predominant, pH >7.40	Presumptive	May require weeks for resolution, rarely results in trapped lung
Abdominal surgery	Asymptomatic 48–72 h after upper abdominal surgery	Small bilateral effusions, atelectasis	Serous nucleated cells <10,000/μL (75%), pH usually >7.40	Presumptive	Larger left effusions following splenectomy, most commonly found with atelectasis and diaphragmatic irritation, resolves spontaneously
Chylothorax (traumatic)	Asymptomatic or dyspnea following intrathoracic surgery, especially coarctation repair and esophagectomy	Small-to-massive left, right, or bilateral effusion	Milky fluid, nucleated cells <7,000/μL almost all lymphocytes, pH 7.40–7.80, ↑ triglycerides	Triglycerides >110 mg/dL, chylomicrons on lipoprotein electrophoresis	Defect in thoracic duct frequently closes spontaneously with tube drainage and minimizing chyle formation

ARDS, acute respiratory distress syndrome; CXR, chest radiograph; ↓, decreased; Hct, hematocrit; ↑, increased; I, input; LDH, lactate dehydrogenase; O, output; PF, pleural fluid; PF/S, pleural fluid/serum; PMN, polymorphonuclear leukocyte; WBC, white blood cell.

The patient usually has the classic stigmata of cirrhosis and clinically apparent ascites. The usual chest radiograph shows a normal cardiac silhouette and a right-sided pleural effusion, which can vary from small to massive; effusions are less likely isolated to the left pleural space or are bilateral [31]. Rarely, a massive pleural effusion may be found without clinical ascites (demonstrated only by US), implying the presence of a large diaphragmatic defect. The pleural fluid is a serous transudate with a low nucleated cell count and a predominance of mononuclear cells, pH greater than 7.40, and a glucose level similar to that of serum. The fluid can be hemorrhagic owing to an underlying coagulopathy or rupture of a diaphragmatic bleb. Demonstrating that pleural and ascitic fluids have similar protein and lactate dehydrogenase concentrations, substantiates the diagnosis. If diagnosis is problematic, injection of a radionuclide into the ascitic fluid with detection on chest imaging within 1 to 2 hours supports a pleuroperitoneal communication through a diaphragmatic defect [32]; delayed demonstration of the tracer suggests that the pathogenesis of the effusion is via convection through the mesothelium.

Hepatic hydrothorax may be complicated by spontaneous bacterial empyema (SBE), which is analogous to spontaneous bacterial peritonitis. The criteria for diagnosis of SBE are similar to those for the diagnosis of spontaneous bacterial peritonitis. SBE must be considered in the differential diagnosis of the infected cirrhotic patient, even in the absence of clinical ascites [33,34]. The pleural fluid culture and analysis may reveal positive culture, a total neutrophil count of more than 500 cells per μL, and a serum to pleural fluid albumin gradient greater than 1.1. The chest radiograph should not show a pneumonic process. Treatment of SBE is conservative with antibiotics unless purulence is present, in which case tube thoracostomy must be considered.

Treatment of hepatic hydrothorax is directed at resolution of the ascites, using sodium restriction and diuresis. The effusion frequently persists unchanged until all ascites is mobilized. If the patient is acutely dyspneic or in respiratory failure, therapeutic thoracentesis should be done as a temporizing measure. Care should be exercised with paracentesis or thoracentesis because hypovolemia can occur with rapid evacuation of fluid. Chest tube insertion should be avoided because it can cause infection of the fluid, and prolonged drainage can lead to protein and lymphocyte depletion and renal failure. Chemical pleurodesis via a chest tube is often unsuccessful owing to rapid movement of ascitic fluid into the pleural space. Treatment options in hepatic hydrothorax refractory to medical management include transjugular intrahepatic portal systemic shunt and video-assisted thoracoscopy to patch the diaphragmatic defect, followed by pleural abrasion or talc poudrage for the properly selected patient [35,36].

Hypoalbuminemia

Many patients admitted to a medical ICU have a chronic illness and associated hypoalbuminemia. When the serum albumin level falls below 1.8 g per dL, pleural effusions may be observed [37]. Because the normal pleural space has an effective lymphatic drainage system, pleural fluid tends to be the last collection of extravascular fluid that occurs in patients with low oncotic pressure. Therefore, it is unusual to find a pleural effusion solely because of hypoalbuminemia in the absence of anasarca. Patients with hypoalbuminemic pleural effusions tend not to have pulmonary symptoms unless there is underlying lung disease, because the effusions are rarely large. Chest radiograph shows small-to-moderate bilateral effusions and a normal heart size. The pleural fluid is a serous transudate with less than 1,000 nucleated cells per μL, predominantly lymphocytes and mesothelial cells. The pleural fluid glucose level is similar to that of serum, and the pH is in the range of 7.45 to 7.55. Diagnosis is presumptive if other causes of transudative effusions can be excluded. The effusions resolve when hypoalbuminemia is corrected.

Iatrogenic

Extravascular migration of a central venous catheter can cause pneumothorax, hemothorax, chylothorax, or a transudative pleural effusion [38,39]. Its incidence is estimated at less than 1% but may be considerably higher. Malposition of the catheter on placement should be suspected if there is absence of blood return or questionable central venous pressure measurements. The immediate postprocedure chest radiograph should be assessed for proper catheter placement; a catheter placed from the right side should not cross the midline. If the catheter is not in the appropriate vessel, phlebitis, perforation of a vein or the heart, or instillation of fluid into the mediastinum or pleural space can occur. In the alert patient, acute infusion of intravenous fluid into the mediastinum usually results in new-onset chest discomfort and dyspnea. Depending on the volume and the rate at which it is introduced into the mediastinum, tachypnea, worsening respiratory status, and cardiac tamponade may ensue. The chest radiograph shows the catheter tip in an abnormal position [40,41], a widened mediastinum, and evidence of unilateral or bilateral pleural effusions. The effusion can have characteristics similar to those of the infusate (milky if lipid is being given) and may be hemorrhagic and neutrophil predominant as a result of trauma and inflammation. The pleural fluid to serum glucose ratio is greater than 1.0 if glucose is being infused [39]. The pleural fluid glucose concentration can fall rapidly after glucose infusion into the pleural space, probably explaining the relatively low glucose concentrations of pleural fluid compared to the infusate. Extravascular migration of a central venous catheter appears to be more common with placement in the external jugular vein, particularly on the left side. Left-sided catheters appear to put the patient at increased risk of perforation because of the horizontal orientation of the left brachiocephalic vein compared to the right brachiocephalic vein. When catheters are introduced from the left side, they should be of adequate length for the tip to rest in the superior vena cava.

Free flow of fluid and proper fluctuation of central venous pressure during the respiratory cycle may not be reliable indicators of intravascular placement. This is probably because intrathoracic pressure changes are transmitted to the mediastinum and, thus, the venous pressure catheter. Aspiration of blood or retrograde flow of blood when the catheter is lowered below the patient's heart level should confirm intravascular catheter placement. If blood cannot be aspirated and the effusate is aspirated instead, extravascular migration is assured. The central venous catheter should be removed immediately. If there is a small effusion, observation is warranted. If the effusion is large, causing respiratory distress, or a hemothorax is discovered, thoracentesis or tube thoracostomy should be performed.

Parapneumonic Effusions

Community-acquired or nosocomial pneumonia is common among critically ill patients. The classic presentation is fever, chest pain, leukocytosis, purulent sputum, and a new alveolar infiltrate on chest radiograph. For the elderly, debilitated patient, however, many of these findings may not be present. The chest radiograph commonly shows a small-to-large ipsilateral pleural effusion [42]. When the effusion is free flowing and anechoic on ultrasound, and thoracentesis shows a nonpurulent, polymorphonuclear (PMN) predominant exudate with a pH of 7.30 or greater, it is highly likely that the effusion will resolve during 7 to 14 days without sequelae with antibiotics alone (uncomplicated effusion). If the chest radiograph or CT demonstrates loculation and pus is aspirated, the diagnosis of empyema is established, and immediate drainage is needed. In the free-flowing nonpurulent fluid, if Gram's stain or culture is positive or pH is less than 7.30, the likelihood of a poor outcome increases, and the pleural space should be drained.

Although a meta-analysis found that low-risk patients with fluid pH between 7.20 and 7.30 may be managed without tube drainage, the patient admitted to the ICU typically cannot be considered low risk, and pH values of less than 7.30 should prompt drainage in most cases [43–45]. Drainage can be accomplished by standard chest tube or small-bore catheter. When loculations occur, pleural space drainage should be accomplished by placement of image-guided tubes or catheters with fibrinolytics plus DNAse or empyectomy and decortication [46–48]. Most thoracic surgeons routinely begin with thoracoscopy and, if not successful, proceed directly to a standard thoracotomy for empyectomy and decortication [49–52].

Pancreatitis

Pleuropulmonary abnormalities are commonly associated with pancreatitis, largely because of the close proximity of the pancreas to the diaphragm. Approximately half of patients with pancreatitis have an abnormal chest radiograph, with pleural effusions in 3% to 17% [53,54]. Mechanisms that may be involved in the pathogenesis of pancreatic pleural effusion include (a) direct contact of pancreatic enzymes with the diaphragm (sympathetic effusion), (b) transfer of ascitic fluid via diaphragmatic defects, (c) communication of a fistulous tract between a pseudocyst and the pleural space, and (d) retroperitoneal movement of fluid into the mediastinum with mediastinitis or rupture into the pleural space [53,54]. Ascitic amylase moves into the pleural space via the previously mentioned mechanisms. The pleural fluid to serum amylase ratio is greater than unity in pancreatitis because of slower lymphatic clearance from the pleural space compared with more rapid renal clearance.

The effusion associated with acute pancreatitis is usually small and left sided (60%), but may be isolated to the right side (30%) or be bilateral (10%). The patient usually presents with abdominal symptoms of acute pancreatitis. The diagnosis is confirmed by an elevated pleural fluid amylase concentration that is greater than that of serum. A normal pleural fluid amylase may be found early in acute pancreatitis, but increases on serial measurements. The fluid is a PMN-predominant exudate with glucose values approximating those of serum. Leukocyte counts may reach 50,000 cells per μL. The pleural fluid pH is usually 7.30 to 7.35 [54].

No specific treatment is necessary for the pleural effusion of acute pancreatitis; the effusion resolves as the pancreatic inflammation subsides. Drainage of the pleural space does not appear to affect residual pleural damage. If the pleural effusion does not resolve in 2 to 3 weeks, pancreatic abscess or pseudocyst should be excluded.

Pulmonary Embolism

The presence of a unilateral pleural effusion may suggest pulmonary embolism or obscure the diagnosis by directing attention to a primary lung or cardiac process. Pleural effusions occur in approximately 40% of patients with pulmonary embolism [54,55]. These effusions result from several different mechanisms, including increased pleural capillary permeability, imbalance in microvascular and pleural space hydrostatic pressures, and pleuropulmonary hemorrhage ischemia from pulmonary vascular obstruction, in addition to release of inflammatory mediators from platelet-rich thrombi, can cause capillary leak into the lung and, subsequently, the pleural space, explaining the usual finding of an exudative effusion. Transudates, described in approximately 20% of patients with pulmonary embolism, result from atelectasis [54].

With pulmonary infarction, necrosis and hemorrhage into the lung and pleural space may result. More than 80% of patients with infarction have bloody pleural effusions, but more than 35% of patients with pulmonary embolism without radiographic infarction also have hemorrhagic fluid [55]. The presence of a pleural effusion does not materialy alter the signs or symptoms for patients with pulmonary embolism. Chest pain, usually pleuritic, occurs amomg most patients with pleural effusions complicating pulmonary embolism, and is invariably ipsilateral [56]. The chest radiograph virtually always shows a unilateral effusion that occupies less than one-third of the hemithorax. An associated pulmonary infiltrate (infarction) is seen in approximately half of patients with pulmonary embolism and effusion.

Pleural fluid analysis is variable and nondiagnostic [54]. The pleural fluid is hemorrhagic in two-thirds of patients, but the number of red blood cells exceeds 100,000 per μL in less than 20% [57]. The nucleated cell count ranges from less than 100 (atelectatic transudates) to greater than 50,000 per μL (pulmonary infarction) [54]. There is a predominance of PMNs when a thoracentesis is performed near the time of the acute injury and of lymphocytes with later thoracentesis. The effusion as a result of pulmonary embolism is usually (92%) apparent on the initial chest radiograph and reaches a maximum volume during the first 72 hours. Patients with pleural effusions that progress with therapy should be evaluated for recurrent embolism, hemothorax secondary to anticoagulation, an infected infarction, or an alternate diagnosis. When consolidation is absent on chest radiograph, effusions usually resolve in 7 to 10 days; with consolidation, the resolution time is 2 to 3 weeks [54].

The association of pleural effusion with pulmonary embolism does not alter therapy. Furthermore, the presence of a bloody effusion is not a contraindication to full-dose anticoagulation because hemothorax is a rare complication of heparin therapy. An enlarging pleural effusion on therapy necessitates thoracentesis to exclude hemothorax, empyema, or another cause. Active pleural space hemorrhage necessitates discontinuation of anticoagulation, tube thoracostomy, and placement of a vena cava filter.

Postcardiac Injury Syndrome

Postcardiac injury syndrome (PCIS) is characterized by fever, pleuropericarditis, and parenchymal infiltrates 3 weeks (2 to 86 days) after injury to the myocardium or pericardium [58–61]. PCIS has been described after myocardial infarction, cardiac surgery, blunt chest trauma, percutaneous left ventricular puncture, and pacemaker implantation. The incidence after myocardial infarction has been estimated at up to 4% of cases [58], but with more extensive myocardial and pericardial involvement, it may be higher. It occurs with greater frequency (up to 30%) after cardiac surgery [60]. The pathogenesis of PCIS remains obscure but is probably on an autoimmune basis in patients with myocardial or pericardial injury and, possibly, concomitant viral illness [61].

The diagnosis of PCIS remains one of exclusion, for no specific criteria exist. It is important to diagnose or exclude PCIS presumptively. Failure to diagnose accurately could lead to iatrogenic complications from inappropriate therapy, such as cardiac tamponade from anticoagulation for presumed pulmonary embolism and adverse effects related to antimicrobial therapy for presumed pneumonia.

Pleuropulmonary manifestations are the hallmark of PCIS. The most common presenting symptoms are pleuritic chest pain, found in virtually all patients, and fever, pericardial rub, dyspnea, and rales, which occur in half of patients [59]. Rarely, hemoptysis occurs, an important differential point when pulmonary embolism with infarction is in the differential diagnosis.

Fifty percent of patients have leukocytosis, and almost all have an elevated erythrocyte sedimentation rate (average, 62 mm per hour) [59].

The chest radiograph is abnormal among virtually all patients, with the most common abnormality being left-sided and bilateral pleural effusions; a unilateral right effusion is unusual [59]. Pulmonary infiltrates are present in 75% of patients and are most commonly seen in the left lower lobe [58]. The pleural fluid is a serosanguineous or bloody exudate with a glucose level greater than 60 mg per dL and pleural fluid pH greater than 7.30. Nucleated cell counts range from 500 to 39,000 per μL, with a predominance of PMNs early in the course [59]. Pericardial fluid on echocardiogram is an important finding suggesting PCIS. The pleural fluid characteristics should help differentiate PCIS from a parapneumonic effusion and CHF, but do not exclude pulmonary embolism.

PCIS is usually self-limited and may not require therapy if symptoms are trivial. It usually responds to aspirin or nonsteroidal anti-inflammatory agents, but some patients require corticosteroid therapy for resolution. In those who respond, the pleural effusion resolves within 1 to 3 weeks.

Esophageal Sclerotherapy

Pleural effusions are found in approximately 50% of patients 48 to 72 hours after esophageal sclerotherapy with sodium morrhuate and in 19% of patients after absolute alcohol sclerotherapy [62–64]. Effusions may be unilateral or bilateral, with no predilection for side. Effusion appears more likely with larger total volumes of sclerosant injected and larger volume injected per site [62,63]. The effusions tend to be small, serous exudates with variable nucleated (90 to 38,000 per μL) and red cell counts (126 to 160,000 per μL) and glucose concentration similar to that of serum [62]. These effusions probably result from an intensive inflammatory reaction after extravasation of the sclerosant into the esophageal mucosa, resulting in mediastinal and pleural inflammation. The effusion is not associated with fever, chest pain, or evidence of perforation is of little consequence, requires no specific therapy, and resolves during several days to weeks [62,63]. However, late perforation may evolve among patients with apparent innocuous effusions. For patients with symptomatic effusions for 24 to 48 hours, diagnostic thoracentesis should be done and an esophagram considered.

Acute Respiratory Distress Syndrome

The presence of pleural effusions in ARDS has not been well appreciated. In a retrospective study of 25 patients with ARDS, a 36% incidence of pleural effusions was found, a percentage similar to that found with hydrostatic pulmonary edema [56]. All patients had extensive alveolar pulmonary edema and endotracheal tube fluid that was compatible with increased permeability edema. Several experimental models of increased permeability pulmonary edema, including α-naphthyl thiourea, oleic acid, and ethchlorvynol, have been shown to produce pleural effusions. In the oleic acid and ethchlorvynol models, the development of pleural effusions lagged behind interstitial and alveolar edema by several hours. In the oleic acid model, 35% of the excess lung water is collected in the pleural spaces. It appears that the pleura act as a reservoir for excess lung water in increased permeability and hydrostatic pulmonary edema. These effusions tend to be underdiagnosed clinically because the patient has bilateral alveolar infiltrates, and the radiograph is taken with the patient in a supine position. Experimentally, the effusion is serous to serosanguineous, with a predominance of PMNs. These effusions usually require no specific therapy and resolve as ARDS resolves. However, in a series of positive end-expiratory pressure (PEEP) unresponsive patients with ARDS, drainage of pleural effusion via tube thoracostomy has been shown to result in improved oxygenation [57]. The decision to proceed to pleural space drainage in ARDS should be approached on a case-by-case basis and is not generally recommended.

Spontaneous Esophageal Rupture

Esophageal rupture, a potentially life-threatening event, requires immediate diagnosis and therapy. The history in spontaneous esophageal rupture is usually severe retching or vomiting or a conscious effort to resist vomiting. In some patients, the perforation may be silent. Early recognition of spontaneous rupture depends on interpretation of the chest radiograph. Several factors influence chest radiograph findings: the time between perforation and chest radiograph examination, site of perforation, and mediastinal pleural integrity. A chest radiograph taken within minutes of the acute injury is usually unremarkable. Mediastinal emphysema probably requires at least 1 to 2 hours to be demonstrated radiographically and is present in less than half of patients; mediastinal widening may take several hours. Pneumothorax, present in 75% of patients with spontaneous rupture, indicates violation of the mediastinal pleura; 70% of pneumothoraces are on the left, 20% are on the right, and 10% are bilateral [65]. Mediastinal air is seen early if pleural integrity is maintained, whereas pleural effusion secondary to mediastinitis tends to occur later. Pleural fluid, with or without associated pneumothorax, occurs in 75% of patients. A presumptive diagnosis should immediately be confirmed radiographically. Esophagrams are positive in approximately 90% of patients [65]. In the upright patient, rapid passage of the contrast material may not demonstrate a small rent; therefore, the study should be done with the patient in the appropriate lateral decubitus position [66].

Pleural fluid findings depend on the degree of perforation and the timing of thoracentesis from injury. Early thoracentesis without mediastinal perforation shows a sterile, serous exudate with a predominance of PMNs, a pleural fluid amylase less than serum, and pH greater than 7.30 [67]. Once the mediastinal pleura tears, amylase of salivary origin appears in the fluid in high concentration [68]. Because the pleural space is seeded with anaerobic organisms from the mouth, the pH falls rapidly and progressively to approach 6.00 [67]. Other pleural fluid findings suggestive of esophageal rupture include the presence of squamous epithelial cells and food particles. The diagnosis of spontaneous esophageal rupture dictates immediate operative intervention. If diagnosed and treated appropriately within the first 24 hours with primary closure and drainage, survival is greater than 90%. Delay from the time of initial symptoms to diagnosis results in a reduced survival with any form of therapy.

Hemothorax

Hemothorax (blood in the pleural space) should be differentiated from a hemorrhagic pleural effusion, because the latter can be the result of only a few drops of blood in pleural fluid. An arbitrary, but practical, definition of a hemothorax with regard to therapy is a pleural fluid to blood hematocrit ratio greater than 30%. The majority of hemothoraces results from penetrating or blunt chest trauma. Hemothorax can also result from invasive procedures, such as placement of central venous catheters, thoracentesis, and pleural biopsy, and pulmonary infarction, malignancy, or ruptured aortic aneurysm. Bleeding can occur from vessels of the chest wall, lung, diaphragm, or mediastinum. Blood that enters the pleural space clots, rapidly undergoes fibrinolysis, and becomes defibrinogenated; thus, it rarely causes significant pleural fibrosis.

Hemothorax should be suspected for any patient with blunt or penetrating chest trauma. If a pleural effusion is found on the admitting chest radiograph, thoracentesis should be performed immediately and the hematocrit measured on the fluid. The hemothorax may not be apparent on the initial chest radiograph, which may be because of the supine position of the patient. Because bleeding may be slow and not appear for several hours, it is imperative that serial radiographs be obtained for these patients. The incidence of concomitant pneumothorax is high (approximately 60%). Patients with traumatic hemothorax should be treated with immediate tube thoracostomy [69]. Large diameter chest tube drainage evacuates the pleural space, may tamponade the bleeding (especially if the origin is from a pleural laceration), allows monitoring of the bleeding, and decreases the likelihood of subsequent fibrothorax [69]. If bleeding continues without signs of slowing, thoracotomy should be performed, depending on the individual circumstance [69]. Pleural effusions occasionally occur after removal of the chest tube from traumatic hemothoraces [70]. A diagnostic thoracentesis is indicated to exclude empyema. If empyema is excluded, the pleural effusion usually resolves without specific treatment and without residual pleural fibrosis.

Hemothorax is a rare complication of anticoagulation that has been reported among patients receiving heparin and warfarin. Coagulation studies are usually within the therapeutic range. The hemothorax tends to occur on the side of the pulmonary embolism. Anticoagulation should be discontinued immediately, a chest tube inserted to evacuate the blood, and a vena cava filter considered.

Coronary Artery Bypass Surgery

A small, left pleural effusion is virtually always present after coronary artery bypass surgery. This is associated with left lower lobe atelectasis and elevation of the left hemidiaphragm on chest radiograph. Left diaphragm dysfunction is secondary to intraoperative phrenic nerve injury from cold cardioplegia, stretch injury, or surgical trauma [71,72]. The larger and grossly bloody effusions tend to be associated with internal mammary artery grafting, which causes marked exudation from the bed where the internal mammary artery was harvested [73].

The pleural fluid is a hemorrhagic exudate with a low nucleated cell count, a glucose level similar to that of serum, and a pH greater than 7.40. Rarely, a loculated hemothorax may develop with trapped lung, resulting in clinically significant restriction [74]. If there is a large effusion that qualifies as a hemothorax (see previous section), the fluid should be drained by tube thoracostomy. It is also prudent to drain moderately large, bloody effusions to avoid later necessity for decortication.

Abdominal Surgery

Approximately half of the patients who undergo abdominal surgery develop small unilateral or bilateral pleural effusions within 48 to 72 hours of surgery [27]. The incidence is higher after upper abdominal surgery, in patients with postoperative atelectasis, and in patients who have free ascitic fluid at the time of surgery. Larger left-sided pleural effusions are common after splenectomy [27]. The effusion is usually an exudate with less than 10,000 nucleated cells per μL. The glucose level is similar to that of serum, and pH is usually greater than 7.40. The effusion usually is related to diaphragmatic irritation or atelectasis. Small effusions generally do not require diagnostic thoracentesis, are of no clinical significance, and resolve spontaneously. Pleural effusion from subphrenic abscess or pulmonary embolism is unlikely to occur within 2 to 3 days of surgery. The only indication for diagnostic thoracentesis would be to exclude infection if the effusion is relatively large or loculated.

Chylothorax

Trauma from surgery accounts for approximately 25% of cases of chylothorax, second only to lymphoma. Most series estimate an incidence of chylothorax of less than 1% after thoracic surgery [75], but a 3% incidence has been reported after esophagectomy [76,77]. Virtually all intrathoracic procedures, including lobectomy, pneumonectomy, and coronary artery bypass grafting, have been reported to cause chylothorax. Other iatrogenic chylothoraces can be caused by complications of prolonged central vein catheterization. Nonsurgical trauma, such as penetrating and nonpenetrating neck, thoracic, and upper abdominal injuries, has also been associated with chylothorax.

When the thoracic duct is torn by stretching during surgery, chyle leaks into the mediastinum and subsequently ruptures through the mediastinal pleura. In the nonsurgical setting, penetrating injuries and fractures may directly tear the thoracic duct. Chylothorax from a central venous catheter usually involves venous thrombosis. Other rare causes of chylothorax include sclerotherapy of esophageal varices and translumbar aortography [78,79].

The patient may be asymptomatic if the effusion is small and unilateral, or may present with dyspnea with a large unilateral effusion or bilateral effusions. The pleural fluid is usually milky, but 12% can be serous or serosanguineous [80], with less than 7,000 nucleated cells per μL, virtually all lymphocytes. The pleural fluid pH is alkaline (7.40 to 7.80), and triglyceride levels are greater than plasma levels. Finding a pleural fluid triglyceride concentration of greater than 110 mg per dL makes the diagnosis of chylothorax highly likely. If the triglyceride level is less than 50 mg per dL, chylothorax is highly unlikely. Triglyceride levels of 50 to 110 mg per dL indicate the need for lipoprotein electrophoresis [80]; the presence of chylomicrons confirms a chylothorax. The thoracic duct defect after trauma usually closes spontaneously within 10 to 14 days, with chest tube drainage as well as bed rest and total parenteral nutrition to minimize chyle formation. A pleuroperitoneal shunt relieves dyspnea, recirculates chyle, and prevents malnutrition and immunocompromise.

Duropleural Fistula

Disruption of the dura and parietal pleura by surgical and nonsurgical trauma may result in a duropleural fistula with subsequent development of a pleural effusion [81–84]. The pleural fluid characteristics depend on the severity of the trauma and the delay between the trauma and the pleural fluid analysis. Pleural fluid because of a chronic duropleural fistula is usually a colorless transudate with low mononuclear cell count; a duropleural fistula associated with recent trauma may be a transudate or an exudate [83,84]. The diagnosis may even be delayed because of a coexisting process such as hemothorax. The diagnosis of duropleural fistula is established by the detection of β_2-transferrin in the pleural fluid [85]. Confirmation of the fistula by conventional or radionuclide myelography is recommended if surgical management is contemplated.

PNEUMOTHORAX

Definition and Classification

Pneumothorax refers to air in the pleural space. Free air may also be found in the adventitial planes of the lung or the mediastinum (pneumomediastinum).

Spontaneous pneumothorax occurs without an obvious cause as a consequence of the natural course of a disease process.

Primary spontaneous pneumothorax occurs without clinical findings of lung disease. Secondary spontaneous pneumothorax occurs as a consequence of clinically manifest lung disease, the most common being COPD. Traumatic pneumothorax results from penetrating or blunt chest injury. Iatrogenic pneumothorax occurs as an inadvertent consequence of diagnostic or therapeutic procedures.

Pathophysiology

Pressure in the pleural space is subatmospheric throughout the normal respiratory cycle, averaging approximately −9 mm Hg during inspiration and −5 mm Hg during expiration. Because of airways resistance, pressure in the airways is positive during expiration (+3 mm Hg) and negative (−2 mm Hg) during inspiration. Thus, in normal breathing, airway pressure is greater than pleural pressure throughout the respiratory cycle. Airway pressure may be increased markedly with coughing or strenuous exercise; however, pleural pressure rises concomitantly so that the transpulmonary pressure gradient is usually not substantially changed. When there are rapid fluctuations in intrathoracic pressure, however, a large transpulmonary pressure gradient occurs transiently. Bronchial and bronchiolar obstruction, resulting in air trapping, can significantly increase the transpulmonary pressure gradient. The alveolar walls and visceral pleura maintain the pressure gradient between the airways and pleural space. When the pressure gradient is transiently increased, alveolar rupture may occur; air enters the interstitial tissues of the lung and may enter the pleural space, resulting in a pneumothorax. If the visceral pleura remains intact, the interstitial air moves toward the hilum, resulting in pneumomediastinum. Because mean pressure within the mediastinum is always less than in the periphery of the lung, air moves proximally along the bronchovascular sheaths to the hilum and mediastinal soft tissues. The development of pneumomediastinum after alveolar rupture requires continual cyclic respiratory efforts, which result in slow movement of air from the ruptured alveolus along a pressure gradient to the mediastinum. Mediastinal air may decompress into the cervical and subcutaneous tissues or the retroperitoneum. With abrupt rise in mediastinal pressure or insufficient decompression to subcutaneous tissue, the mediastinal pleura may rupture, causing pneumothorax. Inadequate decompression of the mediastinum, rather than direct rupture of subpleural blebs into the pleural space, may be the major cause of pneumothorax.

When pneumothorax occurs, the elasticity of the lung causes it to collapse. Lung collapse continues until the pleural defect seals or pleural and alveolar pressures equalize. When a ball valve effect occurs at the site of communication between the pleural space and the alveolus, permitting only egress of air from the lung, there is a progressive accumulation of air within the pleural space, which can result in markedly increased positive pleural pressure, resulting in tension pneumothorax. Tension pneumothorax compresses mediastinal structures, resulting in impaired venous return to the heart, decreased cardiac output, and, at times, fatal cardiovascular collapse [86,87]. Rarely, tension along the bronchovascular sheaths and in the mediastinum can cause collapse of the pulmonary arteries and veins, resulting in cardiovascular collapse.

Patients with primary spontaneous pneumothorax have a decrease in vital capacity and an increase in the $P(A–a)O_2$ gradient, and usually present with hypoxemia owing to predominantly development of an intrapulmonary shunt and areas of low ventilation–perfusion in the atelectatic lung [88]. Hypercapnia does not occur because there is adequate function in the uninvolved lung to maintain necessary alveolar ventilation. Patients with secondary spontaneous pneumothorax, in contrast, commonly develop hypercapnia because the gas exchange abnormality caused by the pneumothorax is superimposed on lungs with preexisting abnormal pulmonary gas exchange.

Pneumothorax of the Critically Ill

Patients with secondary spontaneous pneumothorax may be admitted to an ICU because they develop severe hypoxemic and, at times, hypercapnic respiratory failure. Patients with primary spontaneous pneumothorax rarely require ICU admission because the contralateral lung can maintain necessary alveolar ventilation, and the hypoxemia can be managed with supplemental oxygen. The most common causes of pneumothoraces among ICU patients are invasive procedures and barotrauma.

Iatrogenic Pneumothorax

Central Venous Catheters. Central venous catheters are used routinely for critically ill patients for volume resuscitation, parenteral nutrition, and drug administration. Approximately 3 million central venous catheters are placed annually in the United States, and this procedure continues to be associated with clinically relevant morbidity and some mortality. The morbidity and mortality associated with central venous catheter use are most commonly physician related. Pleural complications of acquisition of venous access and the indwelling phase of central venous catheters include pneumothorax, hydrothorax, hemothorax, and chylothorax. In a recent study of mechanical complications of central venous catheters, 1.1% of 534 patients had pneumothorax [89]. This translates into approximately 33,000 pneumothoraces per year from central venous catheter insertions in critically ill patients in the United States. In the same study, none of the 405 patients developed pneumothorax when the central venous catheter was replaced over a guidewire.

The subclavian and internal jugular routes have been associated with pneumothorax, hemothorax, chylothorax, and catheter placement into the pleural space. Cannulation of the subclavian vein is associated with a higher risk of pneumothorax (less than 5%) [90] than cannulation of the internal jugular vein (less than 0.2%) [91]; with the external jugular venous approach, pneumothorax is avoided. There is a greater risk of pneumothorax with the infraclavicular compared to the supraclavicular approach to the subclavian vein. All complications of insertion, regardless of approach, can be reduced by appropriate physician training and experience. Operator inexperience appears to increase the number of complications with the internal jugular approach. It probably does not have as much impact on the incidence of pneumothorax with the subclavian vein approach, which accounts for 25% to 50% of all complications [92].

Most pneumothoraces occur at the time of the procedure from direct lung puncture, but delayed pneumothoraces have been noted; therefore, it is prudent to perform an ultrasonographic examnation or view a chest radiograph 12 to 24 hours after the procedure. Up to half of the patients with needle puncture pneumothorax may be managed expectantly without the need for tube drainage. Bilateral pneumothoraces have been reported to occur from unilateral attempts [92], and death can occur when there is a delay in the diagnosis of pneumothorax. As stated previously, a pneumothorax may be more difficult to detect while the patient is supine. Additional views should be taken, especially if the venous cannulation does not proceed as anticipated. With any newly placed central venous catheter, a postprocedure chest radiograph should be obtained, regardless of the site cannulated, to assure that the catheter tip is properly positioned. If a small pneumothorax is diagnosed by chest radiograph and the patient is asymptomatic and not on mechanical ventilation, the patient can be followed expectantly with repeat chest radiographs to assure that the leak has ceased. If the patient is on mechanical ventilation or the pneumothorax is large or has caused significant symptoms or gas exchange abnormalities, then tube thoracostomy should be performed as soon as possible.

Barotrauma. Pulmonary barotrauma is an important clinical problem because of the widespread use of mechanical ventilation. Barotrauma occurs in approximately 3% to 10% of mechanically ventilated patients and includes parenchymal interstitial gas, pneumomediastinum, subcutaneous emphysema, pneumoperitoneum, and pneumothorax [75,93–95]. The most clinically important form is pneumothorax, occurring in 1% to 15% of all mechanically ventilated patients. For patients with ARDS, rates of 6.5% to 87% have been reported [94,95]. The number of ventilator days, underlying disease (ARDS, COPD, or necrotizing pneumonia), and use of PEEP have an impact on the incidence of pneumothorax. When a pneumothorax develops during mechanical ventilation, 30% to 97% of patients develop tension. The reported incidence of barotrauma varies widely between the studies with the lowest incidences reported among the most large series [95]. This may be partly explained by the adoption of less aggressive ventilation strategies over time.

The initial radiographic sign of barotrauma is often pulmonary interstitial gas or emphysema [96]. In the early stages, however, interstitial gas may be difficult to detect radiographically. This harbinger of pneumothorax may be detected as distinct subpleural air cysts, linear air streaks emanating from the hilum, and perivascular air halos. Subpleural air cysts, most commonly seen among patients with ARDS, tend to appear abruptly on the chest radiograph as single or multiple thin-walled, round lucencies, and are most often visualized at the lung bases, medially or diaphragmatically [97]. The cysts, which may expand rapidly, are usually 3 to 5 cm in diameter. Differentiating between peripheral subpleural air cysts and a localized basilar pneumothorax may be problematic. Pleural air cysts appear to be more common among younger patients, possibly because connective tissue planes of the lung are looser in younger patients than in older patients. The risk of tension pneumothorax is substantial among patients who have developed subpleural lung cysts with continued mechanical ventilation. When mechanical ventilation is discontinued, the cyst may resolve spontaneously or become secondarily infected.

Ultrasound has emerged as a bedside modality for the detection of pneumothorax. The absence of lung sliding is the finding associated with pneumothorax [5]. False-positive results may occur and are because of bullous lung disease or preexisting pleural symphysis [5,98,99]. The disappearance of lung sliding that was present previously may be more specific for the development of pneumothorax; for example, after line placement. However, this subject awaits further study.

When evidence of barotrauma without pneumothorax is observed in any patient requiring continued mechanical ventilation, immediate attempts should be made to lower the plateau airway pressure. Among those with ARDS, tidal volumes [100] and inspiratory flow rates should be lowered, an attempt should be made to reduce or remove PEEP, and neuromuscular blockers and sedation should be considered [101]. Among those with status asthmaticus, in addition to the aforementioned maneuvers, controlled hypoventilation should be accomplished [102,103]. There is no evidence supporting the use of prophylactic chest tubes. However, the patient should be monitored closely for tension pneumothorax and provisions made for emergency bedside tube thoracostomy.

Tension Pneumothorax

Pneumothorax among the mechanically ventilated patient usually presents as an acute cardiopulmonary emergency, beginning with respiratory distress and, if unrecognized and untreated, progressing to cardiovascular collapse. In one report of 74 patients, the diagnosis of pneumothorax was made clinically for 45 patients (61%) based on hypotension, hyperresonance, diminished breath sounds, and tachycardia. The mortality rate was 7% among these patients diagnosed clinically. In the remaining 29 patients, diagnosis was delayed between 30 minutes and 8 hours, and 31% of these patients died of pneumothorax. Other series of barotrauma in the setting of mechanical ventilation have reported mortality rates from 58% to 77% [75].

Tension pneumothorax can be lethal when diagnosis and treatment are delayed. The diagnosis should be made clinically at the bedside for the patient on mechanical ventilation who develops a sudden deterioration characterized by apprehension, tachypnea, cyanosis, decreased ipsilateral breath sounds, subcutaneous emphysema, tachycardia, and hypotension. The diagnosis may be problematic among the unconscious, the elderly, and the patient with bilateral tension, which may be more protective of the mediastinal structures and lessen the impact on cardiac output.

For the unconscious or critically ill patient, hypoxemia may be one of the earlier signs of tension pneumothorax. For the patient on mechanical ventilation, increasing peak and plateau airway pressure, decreasing compliance, and auto-PEEP should raise the possibility of tension pneumothorax. Difficulty with bag valve mask ventilation, the patient with greater than expected force required to delver adequate tidal volumes should prompt consideration of tension pneumothorax.

When the clinical signs and symptoms are noted among mechanically ventilated patients, treatment should not be delayed to obtain radiographic confirmation. If a chest tube is not immediately available, placement of a large-bore needle into the anterior second intercostal space on the suspected side is life-saving and confirms the diagnosis, because a rush of air is noted on entering the pleural space. An appropriately large chest tube can then be placed and connected to an adequate drainage system that can accommodate the large air leak that may develop among mechanically ventilated patients [103].

On relief of the tension, there is a rapid improvement in oxygenation, increase of blood pressure, decrease of heart rate, and fall in airway pressures. In experimental tension pneumothorax, it has been observed that the inability to raise cardiac output in response to hypoxemia leads to a reduction in systemic oxygen transport and a decrease in mixed venous partial pressure of oxygen (PO_2), partially explaining the cardiovascular collapse seen in these patients [87]. For mechanically ventilated patients, a decrease in cardiac output is an inevitable consequence of tension pneumothorax.

BRONCHOPLEURAL FISTULA

Definition and Causes

Communication between the bronchial tree and the pleural space is a dreaded complication of mechanical ventilation. There are three presentations of bronchopleural fistula (BPF): (a) failure to reinflate the lung despite chest tube drainage or continued air leak after evacuation of the pneumothorax in the setting of chest trauma; (b) complication of a diagnostic or therapeutic procedure, such as thoracic surgery; and (c) complication of mechanical ventilation, usually for those with ARDS [86]. Among those with ARDS, a pneumothorax often occurs under tension and is later associated with empyema, multiple sites of leakage, and a poor prognosis. A large air leak through a BPF can result in failure of lung reexpansion, loss of a significant amount of each delivered tidal volume, loss of the ability to apply PEEP, inappropriate cycling of the ventilator, and inability to maintain alveolar ventilation (Table 176.3).

If there is a continued air leak for longer than 24 hours after the development of pneumothorax, then a BPF exists. The main factors that perpetuate BPF are high airway pressures that increase the leak during inspiration, increased mean intrathoracic pressures throughout the respiratory cycle (PEEP, inflation hold, high inspiratory to expiratory ratio) that increase the leak throughout the breath, and high negative suction. Among those with severe ARDS, all of these factors are present because they usually are necessary to support gas exchange.

Management

Given the frequency of barotrauma in BPF among mechanically ventilated patients, intensivists are called to give advice on the management of these difficult patients. Definitive therapy of BPF frequently involves invasive surgical approaches that include thoracoplasty, mobilization of the pectoralis or intercostal muscles, bronchial stump stapling, and decortication [104,105]. Although some of these techniques are still used today, there is a trend toward more conservative management of acute and chronic BPF, using innovations of standard techniques and new modalities that include chest tube management, drainage systems, ventilatory support, and definitive nonoperative therapy (Table 176.4). Insertion of an endobronchial valve designed for the treatment of emphysema may be considered in selected patients [106]. Nonoperative therapy provides an alternative to the surgical approaches in patients who are poor operative candidates. Each patient with a BPF is unique and requires individual management based on the specific clinical setting. Attention to the basics of medical care of patients with BPF should not be neglected in the face of the potentially dramatic events related to the BPF. Nutritional status must be maintained, appropriate antibiotics used for the infected pleural space, and the space adequately drained.

Chest Tubes

The initial therapy for pneumothorax for a patient on mechanical ventilation is placement of a chest tube in an attempt to reexpand the lung (see Chapter 13). The chest tube is initially necessary, can be detrimental later, and may play a role more important than that of a passive conduit. Air leaks in the setting of BPF range from less than 1 to 16 L per minute [107]; therefore, a chest tube that permits prompt and efficient drainage of this level of airflow is required. The smallest internal diameter that allows a maximum flow of 15.1 L per minute at −10 cm H_2O suction is 6 mm (a 32-Fr chest tube has an internal diameter of 9 mm). A chest tube with a diameter adequate to convey the potentially large airflow of the BPF must be considered. A chest tube with too small diameter can lead to lung collapse and tension pneumothorax in the setting of a mobile mediastinum.

Not only can the chest tube be used to drain pleural air, it can also be used to limit the air leak in certain situations. One modality is the application of intrapleural pressure equivalent to the level of PEEP during the expiratory phase of ventilation [108,109]. With positive intrapleural pressure applied through the chest tube, the air leak persists during the inspiratory phase of ventilation but decreases during expiration, allowing maintenance of PEEP in patients in whom it is necessary for adequate oxygenation. Synchronized closure of the chest tube during the inspiratory phase has also been used to limit air leak [110,111]. A combination of these techniques has been suggested for patients with significant BPF air leaks during both the inspiratory and expiratory phases of mechanical ventilation [111,112]. These techniques pose potential hazards, including increased pneumothorax and tension pneumothorax [110,112], necessitating extremely close patient monitoring when such manipulations are used.

Instillation of chemical agents through the chest tube may potentially help close the BPF if the anatomic defect is small and single, but it is unlikely to be successful if the fistula is large or if there are multiple fistulas. Various agents have been successful in preventing recurrent pneumothoraces in patients who are not on mechanical ventilation [113–115], but BPF in the setting of mechanical ventilation is a different situation. One study compared the recurrence of pneumothorax in 39 patients with BPF randomized to intrapleural tetracycline or placebo groups [116]. There was no evidence that intrapleural tetracycline facilitated closure of the BPF. No adverse effects were encountered from the instillation of tetracycline in patients with persistent air leaks.

The chest tube may be associated with adverse effects among patients with BPF. The gas escaping through the chest tube represents part of the minute ventilation delivered to the patient and makes maintenance of an effective tidal volume problematic. Maintenance of a specific level of ventilation is not only affected by the amount of gas escaping through the fistula. The escaping gas does not passively flow from the airways into the BPF but is involved in physiologic gas exchange [117,118]. Approximately 25% of the minute ventilation has been found to escape via the BPF among patients with ARDS, with more than 20% of CO_2 excretion occurring by this route for half of the patients [118]. The role of the BPF in active CO_2 exchange is complex: Proposed mechanisms include drainage of gas from alveoli in the area of the BPF and removal of gas from remote alveolar areas by pressure gradients created by the BPF [119].

Carbon dioxide excretion and a reduction of minute ventilation occur to a lesser extent in BPF trauma victims [117]. In these patients, variable CO_2 excretion and loss of minute ventilation were dynamic and depend on the level of chest tube suction. The difference between trauma and ARDS patients may have been because of the variability of lung compliance and the use of different ventilators [118]. Also, BPF may affect oxygen use,

TABLE 176.3

Consequences of a Large Bronchopleural Fistula

- Failure of lung reexpansion
- Loss of delivered tidal volume
- Inability to apply positive end-expiratory pressure
- Inappropriate cycling of ventilator
- Inability to maintain alveolar ventilation

TABLE 176.4

Management of Bronchopleural Fistula in Patients Requiring Mechanical Ventilation

- Conservative
  - Adequate-size chest tube
  - Use of drainage system with adequate capabilities
  - Mechanical ventilation
    - Conventional (controlled, assist-control, intermittent mandatory ventilation)
    - High frequency
    - Independent lung
    - Flexible bronchoscopy
    - Direct application of sealant
- Invasive
  - Mobilization of intercostal or pectoralis muscles
  - Thoracoplasty
  - Bronchial stump stapling
  - Pleural abrasion and decortication

which generally decreases the use of inspired oxygen before it escapes through the fistula [117]. This relationship is variable but requires consideration for patients with impaired oxygenation.

Negative pressure applied to the chest tube may be transmitted beyond the pleural space and into the airways, creating inappropriate cycling of the ventilator [119]. The increased flow through a BPF can occur with increased negative pleural pressure and may interfere with closure and healing of the fistulous site [112]. Therefore, the least amount of chest tube suction that keeps the lung inflated should be maintained in patients with BPF. The chest tube is a potential source of infection, both at the insertion site and within the pleural space.

Drainage Systems

As with the chest tube, the resistance of flow of gases is a consideration for the choice of the drainage system for the patient with a BPF [107]. The size of the air leak and the flow that the drainage system can accommodate are necessary considerations. In an experimental model of BPF that simulated the type of air leak seen clinically (mean maximal flow, 5 L per minute), four pleural drainage units (PDUs) (Emerson Post-Operative Pump, Emerson; Pleur-Evac, Teleflex Medical; Sentinel Seal, Tyco; and Thora-Klex, Avilor) were tested at water seal, −20 cm H_2O, and −40 cm H_2O suction [107]. Compared with the water seal, −20 cm H_2O suction significantly increased the ability of all four PDUs to evacuate air via the chest tube, but an increase in suction to −40 cm H_2O did not significantly alter flow. When the air leak reached 4 to 5 L per minute, use of the Thora-Klex or Sentinel Seal became clinically impractical. The Pleur-Evac can handle flow rates up to 34 L per minute, but its use with rates greater than 28 L per minute is impractical owing to intense bubbling in the suction control chamber. Air leaks of this magnitude are infrequent clinically in BPF and are likely to be seen only with major airway disruption or diffuse parenchymal leak secondary to ARDS with severe barotraumas [119]. In the latter situations, the low-pressure, high-volume Emerson suction pump remains the only PDU capable of handling the air leak [107]. The choice of PDU should be influenced by its physiologic capabilities and the type of BPF air leak that is encountered.

Mechanical Ventilation

Conventional Ventilation. The dilemma with a BPF in a mechanically ventilated patient is achieving adequate ventilation and oxygenation while allowing repair of the BPF to occur. Because air flow escaping through a BPF theoretically delays healing of the fistulous site, reducing flow through the fistula has been a major goal in promoting repair. The BPF provides an area of low resistance to flow and acts as a conduit for the escape of a variable percentage of delivered tidal volume during conventional positive-pressure mechanical ventilation. Thus, the goal of management is to maintain adequate ventilation and oxygenation while reducing the fistula flow [112]. Using the lowest possible tidal volume, fewest mechanical breaths per minute, lowest level of PEEP, and shortest inspiratory time (see Chapter 166) can do this. Avoidance of expiratory retard also reduces airway pressures. Using the greatest number of spontaneous breaths per minute, thereby reducing use of positive pressure, may also be advantageous. Intermittent mandatory ventilation or pressure modes of ventilation may have advantages over assist-control ventilation for managing the air leak of BPF.

In a retrospective study of 39 patients with BPF who were maintained on conventional ventilation, only two patients developed a pH less than 7.30 despite air leaks of up to 900 mL per breath [119]. Overall, mortality was higher when the BPF developed late in the illness and was higher with larger leaks (more than 500 mL per breath).

High-Frequency Ventilation. Despite anecdotal reports, experimental data, and clinical studies involving high-frequency ventilation (HFV) in the setting of BPF, controversy exists. However, there appear to be subgroups of patients with BPF in whom HFV may be beneficial. Both animal [120] and human [121] studies suggest that HFV is superior to conventional ventilation in controlling PO_2 and partial pressure of carbon dioxide (PCO_2) when there is a proximal (tracheal or bronchial) unilateral or bilateral fistula in the presence of normal lung parenchyma.

The use of HFV in BPF in patients with parenchymal lung disease, such as ARDS, is more controversial. Although some studies have shown that HFV improves or stabilizes gas exchange for patients with extensive parenchymal lung disease, others have not shown a beneficial effect on gas exchange or a reduction in fistula outflow [122,123]. A trial of HFV appears reasonable for the patient with a proximal BPF and normal lung parenchyma; however, it is unclear whether HFV should be considered the primary mode of ventilation in this setting. Despite discrepancies of clinical results, a trial of HFV for selected critically ill patients with a BPF and diffuse parenchymal disease who appear to be failing conventional ventilation may be justified. Caution must be exercised, however, with close monitoring of gas exchange parameters and fistula flow whenever HFV is used.

Other Modes of Ventilation. Other maneuvers during both conventional ventilation and HFV can be potentially helpful in patients with BPF. Selective intubation and conventional ventilation of the unaffected lung in patients with unilateral BPF may be useful but predisposes to the collapse of the nonintubated lung [124,125]. The use of differential lung ventilation with conventional ventilation may be of benefit for some patients [122]. Positioning of the patient such that the BPF is dependent has been shown to decrease fistula flow [125].

Case reports and animal studies suggest other potential applications of HFV for BPF, including the use of independent lung ventilation with HFV applied to the BPF lung and conventional ventilation to the normal lung [126]. Another mode of HFV, ultra–high-frequency jet ventilation, is being explored and has been used with some success for reducing BPF in humans [127] and animal models [128]. Independent lung ventilation with ultra–high-frequency lung ventilation applied to the BPF lung and conventional ventilation to the normal lung led to rapid BPF closure in two of three patients [127].

Flexible Bronchoscopy

The flexible bronchoscope can be valuable in the diagnosis of BPF. Bronchoscopic therapy of BPF has several potential advantages, including low cost, shortened hospital stay, and relative noninvasiveness, particularly in poor operative candidates [129–133] (see Chapter 10). Proximal fistulas, such as those associated with lobectomy or pneumonectomy or stump breakdown, can be directly visualized through the bronchoscope. Distal fistulas cannot be visualized directly and require bronchoscopic passage of an occluding balloon to localize the bronchial segment leading to the fistula [132,133]. A balloon is systematically passed through the working channel of the bronchoscope and into each bronchial segment in question and then inflated; a reduction in air leak indicates localization of a bronchial segment communicating with the BPF. Once the fistula has been localized, various materials can be passed through a catheter in the working channel of the bronchoscope and into the area of the fistula [129–137]. Direct application of a sealant through the working-channel catheter onto the fistula site is the method generally used for directly visualized proximal fistulas. For distal fistulas, a multiple-lumen Swan–Ganz's catheter has been used to localize the BPF and pass the occluding material of choice [132].

Several agents have been used through the bronchoscope in an attempt to occlude BPF. These include fibrin agents cyanoacrylate-based agents, absorbable gelatin sponge (Gelfoam,

Pfizer), blood tetracycline, and lead shot [131–133]. The reports on all of these agents are limited to only a few patients. The cyanoacrylate-based and fibrin agents have received the most attention but still have had less than 20 total cases reported. These patients have had at least a 50% reduction of fistula flow, and most had closure of the fistula subsequent to sealant application, although multiple applications were necessary in some patients. These agents appear to work in two phases, with the agent initially sealing the leak by acting as a plug and subsequently inducing an inflammatory process with fibrosis and mucosal proliferation permanently sealing the area [129]. They are not useful with large proximal tracheal or bronchial ruptures or multiple distal parenchymal defects [132].

References

1. Woodring JH: Recognition of pleural effusion on supine radiographs: how much fluid is required? *AJR Am J Roentgenol* 142:59, 1984.
2. Diacon AH, Brutsche MH, Soler M: Accuracy of pleural puncture site: a prospective comparison of clinical examination with ultrasound. *Chest* 2003;123:436–441.
3. Kelbel C, Borner N, Schadmand S, et al: Diagnosis of pleural effusions and atelectasis: sonography and radiology compared. *Rofo* 154:159–163, 1991.
4. Lichtenstein D, Goldstein I, Mourgeon E, et al: Comparative diagnostic performances of auscultation, chest radiography, and lung ultrasonography in acute respiratory distress syndrome. *Anesthesiology* 100:9–15, 2004.
5. Yu C-J, Yang P-C, Chang D-B, et al: Diagnostic and therapeutic use of chest sonography: value in critically ill patients. *AJR Am J Roentgenol* 159:695, 1992.
6. Mayo PH, Goltz HR, Tafreshi M, et al: Safety of ultrasound-guided thoracentesis in patients receiving mechanical ventilation. *Chest* 125:1059, 2004.
7. Chian CF, Su WL, Soh LH, et al: Echogenic swirling pattern as a predictor of malignant pleural effusions in patients with malignancies. *Chest* 126:129–134, 2004.
8. Tu CY, Hsu WH, Hsia TC, et al: Pleural effusions in febrile medical ICU patients chest ultrasound study. *Chest* 126:1274–1280, 2004.
9. Qureshi NR, Rahman NM, Gleeson FV: Thoracic ultrasound in the diagnosis of malignant pleural effusion. *Thorax* 64:139–143, 2009.
10. Lichtenstein DA, Menu Y: A bedside ultrasound sign ruling out pneumothorax in the critically ill. Lung sliding. *Chest* 108:1345, 1995.
11. Gobien RP, Reines HD, Schabel SI: Localized tension pneumothorax: unrecognized form of barotrauma in adult respiratory distress syndrome. *Radiology* 142:15, 1982.
12. Tocino IM, Miller MH, Fairfax WR: Distribution of pneumothorax in the supine and semirecumbent critically ill adult. *AJR Am J Roentgenol* 144:901, 1985.
13. Kollef MH: Risk factors for the misdiagnosis of pneumothorax in the intensive care unit. *Crit Care Med* 19:906, 1991.
14. Collins TR, Sahn SA: Thoracentesis: clinical value, complications, technical problems, and patient experience. *Chest* 91:817, 1987.
15. Godwin JE, Sahn SA: Thoracentesis: a safe procedure in mechanically ventilated patients. *Ann Intern Med* 113:800, 1990.
16. Bartter T, Mayo PD, Pratter MR, et al: Lower risk and higher yield for thoracentesis when performed by experienced operators. *Chest* 103:1873, 1993.
17. Seneff MG, Corwin W, Gold LH, et al: Complications associated with thoracentesis. *Chest* 89:97, 1986.
18. Grogan DR, Irwin RS, Channick R, et al: Complications associated with thoracentesis. *Arch Intern Med* 150:873, 1990.
19. Heidecker J, Huggins JT, Sahn SA, et al: Pathophysiology of pneumothorax following ultrasound-guided thoracentesis. *Chest* 130:1173, 2006.
20. Light RW, Jenkinson SG, Minh V, et al: Observations on pleural pressures as fluid is withdrawn during thoracentesis. *Am Rev Respir Dis* 121:799, 1980.
21. Estenne M, Yernault J-C, Detroyer A: Mechanism of relief of dyspnea after thoracentesis in patients with large effusions. *Am J Med* 74:813, 1983.
22. Doelken P, Abreu R, Sahn SA: Effect of thoracentesis on respiratory mechanics and gas exchange in the patient receiving mechanical ventilation. *Chest* 130:1354, 2006.
23. Brandstetter RD, Cohen RP: Hypoxemia after thoracentesis: a predictable and treatable condition. *JAMA* 242:1060, 1979.
24. Karetzky M, Kothari GA, Fourre JA, et al: The effect of thoracentesis on arterial oxygen tension. *Respiration* 36:96, 1978.
25. Perpina M, Benlloch E, Marco V, et al: The effect of thoracentesis on pulmonary gas exchange. *Thorax* 38:747, 1983.
26. Mattison L, Coppage L, Alderman D, et al: Pleural effusions in the medical intensive care unit: prevalence, causes and clinical implications. *Chest* 111:1018, 1997.
27. Nielsen PH, Jepsan SB, Olsen AD: Postoperative pleural effusion following upper abdominal surgery. *Chest* 96:1133, 1989.
28. Wiener-Kronish JP, Matthay MA, Callen PW, et al: Relationship of pleural effusions to pulmonary hemodynamics in patients with congestive heart failure. *Am Rev Respir Dis* 132:1253, 1987.
29. Shinto RA, Light RW: Effects of diuresis on the characteristics of pleural fluid in patients with congestive heart failure. *Am J Med* 88:230, 1990.
30. Chakko SC, Caldwell SH, Sforza PP: Treatment of congestive heart failure: its effect on pleural fluid chemistry. *Chest* 95:798, 1989.
31. Strauss RM, Boyer TD: Hepatic hydrothorax. *Semin Liver Dis* 17:227, 1997.
32. Frazer IH, Lichtenstein M, Andrews JT: Pleuroperitoneal effusion without ascites. *Med J Aust* 2:520, 1983.
33. Xiol X, Castellvi JM, Guardiola J, et al: Spontaneous bacterial empyema in cirrhotic patients: a prospective study. *Hepatology* 23:719, 1996.
34. Abba AA, Laajam MA, Zargar SA: Spontaneous neutrocytic hepatic hydrothorax without ascites. *Respir Med* 90:631, 1996.
35. Strauss RM, Martin LG, Kaufman SL, et al: Transjugular intrahepatic portal systemic shunt for the management of symptomatic cirrhotic hydrothorax. *Am J Gastroenterol* 89:1520, 1994.
36. Mouroux J, Perrin C, Venissac N, et al: Management of pleural effusion of cirrhotic origin. *Chest* 109:1093, 1996.
37. Eid AA, Keddissi JI, Kinasewitz GT: Hypoalbuminemia as a cause of pleural effusions. *Chest* 115:1066, 1999.
38. Scott WL: Complications associated with central venous catheters: a survey. *Chest* 94:1221, 1988.
39. Duntley P, Siever J, Korwes ML, et al: Vascular erosion by central venous catheters: clinical features and outcome. *Chest* 101:1633, 1992.
40. Aslamy Z, Dewald LL, Heffner JE: MRI of central venous anatomy: implications for central venous catheter insertion. *Chest* 114:820, 1998.
41. Wechsler RJ, Byrne KJ, Steiner RM: The misplaced thoracic venous catheter: detailed anatomical consideration. *Crit Rev Diagn Imaging* 21:289, 1982.
42. Heffner JE, McDonald J, Bareberi C, et al: Management of parapneumonic effusions: an analysis of physician practice patterns. *Arch Surg* 130:433, 1995.
43. Heffner JE: Indications for draining a parapneumonic effusion: an evidence-based approach. *Semin Respir Infect* 14:48, 1999.
44. Heffner JE, Brown LK, Barberi C, et al: Pleural fluid chemical analysis in parapneumonic effusions: a meta-analysis. *Am J Respir Crit Care Med* 151:1700, 1995.
45. Lesho EP, Roth BJ: Is pH paper an acceptable, low-cost alternate to the blood gas analyzer for determining pleural fluid pH? *Chest* 112:1291, 1997.
46. Ashbaugh DG: Empyema thoracis: factors influencing morbidity and mortality. *Chest* 99:1162, 1991.
47. Sahn SA: Use of fibrinolytic agents in the management of complicated parapneumonic effusions. *Thorax* 53[Suppl]:S65, 1998.
48. Rahman NM, Maskell NA, West A, et al: Intrapleural use of tissue plasminogen activator and DNase in pleural infection. *N Engl J Med* 356(6):518–526, 2011.
49. Ridley PD, Brainbridge MV: Thoracoscopic débridement and pleural irrigation in the management of empyema thoracis. *Ann Thorac Surg* 51:461, 1991.
50. Landreneau RJ, Keenan RJ, Hazelrigg SR, et al: Thoracoscopy for empyema and hemothorax. *Chest* 109:18, 1995.
51. Podbielski FJ, Maniar HS, Rodriguez HE, et al: Surgical strategy of complex empyema thoracis. *JSLS* 4:287, 2000.
52. Cunniffe MG, Maguire D, McAnena OJ, et al: Video-assisted thoracoscopic surgery in the management of loculated empyema. *Surg Endosc* 14:175, 2000.
53. Maringhini A, Ciambra M, Patti R, et al: Ascites, pleural, and pericardial effusions in acute pancreatitis: a prospective study of the incidence, natural history, and prognostic role. *Dig Dis Sci* 41:848, 1996.
54. Sahn SA: Getting the most of pleural fluid analysis. *Respirology* 17(2): 270–277, 2012.
55. Bynum LJ, Wilson JE 3rd: Characteristics of pleural effusions associated with pulmonary embolism. *Arch Intern Med* 136:159, 1976.
56. Aberle DR, Wiener-Kronish JP, Webb WR, et al: Hydrostatic versus increased permeability pulmonary edema: diagnosis based on radiographic criteria in critically ill patients. *Radiology* 168:73, 1988.
57. Talmor M, Hydo L, Gershenwald JG, et al: Beneficial effects of chest tube drainage of pleural effusion in acute respiratory failure refractory to positive end-expiratory pressure ventilation. *Surgery* 123:137, 1998.
58. Dressler W: The post-myocardial infarction syndrome: a report of 44 cases. *Arch Intern Med* 103:28, 1959.
59. Stelzner TJ, King TE Jr, Antony VB, et al: The pleuro-pulmonary manifestations of the postcardiac injury syndrome. *Chest* 84:383, 1983.
60. Kaminsky ME, Rodan BA, Osborne DR, et al: Post-pericardiotomy syndrome. *AJR Am J Roentgenol* 138:503, 1982.
61. Kim S, Sahn SA: Postcardiac injury syndrome: an immunologic pleural fluid analysis. *Chest* 109:570, 1996.
62. Bacon BR, Bailey-Newton RS, Connors AF Jr: Pleural effusions after endoscopic variceal sclerotherapy. *Gastroenterology* 88:1910, 1985.
63. Saks BJ, Kilby AE, Dietrich PA: Pleural and mediastinal changes following endoscopic injection sclerotherapy of esophageal varices. *Radiology* 149:639, 1983.
64. Parikh SS, Amarapurkar DN, Dhawan PS, et al: Development of pleural effusion after sclerotherapy with absolute alcohol. *Gastrointest Endosc* 39:404, 1993.
65. Bladergroen MR, Lowe JE, Postlethwait RW: Diagnosis and recommended management of esophageal perforation and rupture. *Ann Thorac Surg* 42:235, 1986.
66. DeMeester TR: Perforation of the esophagus. *Ann Thorac Surg* 42:231, 1986.
67. Maulitz RM, Good JT Jr, Kaplan RL, et al: The pleuropulmonary consequences of esophageal rupture: an experimental model. *Am Rev Respir Dis* 120:363, 1979.
68. Sherr HP, Light RW, Merson MH, et al: Origin of pleural fluid amylase in esophageal rupture. *Ann Intern Med* 76:985, 1972.

69. Weil PH, Margolis IB: Systematic approach to traumatic hemothorax. *Am J Surg* 142:692, 1981.
70. Wilson JM, Boren CH, Peterson SR, et al: Traumatic hemothorax: is decortication necessary? *J Thorac Cardiovasc Surg* 77:489, 1979.
71. Iverson L, Mittal A, Dugan D, et al: Injuries to the phrenic nerve resulting in diaphragmatic paralysis with special reference to stretch trauma. *Am J Surg* 132:263, 1976.
72. Wheeler W, Rubis L, Jones C, et al: Etiology and prevention of topical cardiac hypothermia-induced phrenic nerve injury and left lower lobe atelectasis during cardiac surgery. *Chest* 88:680, 1985.
73. Landymore RW, Howell F: Pulmonary complications following myocardial revascularization with the internal mammary artery graft. *Eur J Cardiothorac Surg* 4:156, 1990.
74. Kollef MH: Trapped-lung syndrome after cardiac surgery: a potentially preventable complication of pleural injury. *Heart Lung* 19:671, 1990.
75. Cullen DJ, Caldera DL: The incidence of ventilator-induced pulmonary barotrauma in critically ill patients. *Anesthesiology* 50:185, 1979.
76. Ferguson MK, Little AG, Skinner DB: Current concepts in the management of postoperative chylothorax. *Ann Thorac Surg* 45:542, 1985.
77. Orringer MB, Bluett M, Deeb GM: Aggressive treatment of chylothorax complicating transhiatal esophagectomy without thoracotomy. *Surgery* 104:720, 1988.
78. Hillerdal G: Chylothorax and pseudochylothorax. *Eur Respir J* 10:1157, 1997.
79. Nygaard SD, Berger HA, Fick RB: Chylothorax as a complication of oesophageal sclerotherapy. *Thorax* 47:134, 1992.
80. Staats BA, Ellefson RD, Budhan LL, et al: The lipoprotein profile of chylous and nonchylous pleural effusions. *Mayo Clin Proc* 55:700, 1980.
81. Monla-Hassan J, Eichenhorn M, Spickler E, et al: Duro-pleural fistula manifested as a large pleural transudate. *Chest* 114:1786, 1998.
82. D'Souza R, Doshi A, Bhojraj S, et al: Massive pleural effusion as the presenting feature of a subarachnoid-pleural fistula. *Respiration* 69:96, 2002.
83. Pollack II, Pang D, Hall W: Subarachnoid-pleural and subarachnoid mediastinal fistulae. *Neurosurgery* 26:519, 1990.
84. Assietti R, Kibble MB, Bakay R: Iatrogenic cerebrospinal fluid fistula to the pleural cavity: case report and literature review. *Neurosurgery* 33:1004, 1993.
85. Skedros DG, Cass SP, Hirsch BE, et al: Beta-2 transferrin assay in clinical management of cerebral spinal fluid and perilymphatic fluid leaks. *J Otolaryngol* 22:341, 1993.
86. Gustman P, Yerger L, Wanner A: Immediate cardiovascular effects of tension pneumothorax. *Am Rev Respir Dis* 127:171, 1983.
87. Hurewitz AN, Sidhu U, Bergofsky B, et al: Cardiovascular and respiratory consequence of tension pneumothorax. *Bull Eur Physiopathol Respir* 22:545, 1986.
88. Moran JF, Jones RH, Wolfe WG: Regional pulmonary function during experimental unilateral pneumothorax in the awake state. *J Thorac Cardiovasc Surg* 74:394, 1977.
89. Hagley MT, Martin B, Gast P, et al: Infectious and mechanical complications of central venous catheters placed by percutaneous venipuncture and over guide wires. *Crit Care Med* 20:1426, 1992.
90. Eerola R, Kaukinen L, Kaukinen S: Analysis of 13,800 subclavian catheterizations. *Acta Anesthesiol Scand* 29:193, 1985.
91. Tyden H: Cannulation of the internal jugular vein: 500 cases. *Acta Anesthesiol Scand* 26:485, 1982.
92. Weiner P, Sznajder I, Plavnick L, et al: Unusual complications of subclavian vein catheterization. *Crit Care Med* 12:538, 1984.
93. Kumar A, Pontoppidan H, Falke KJ, et al: Pulmonary barotrauma during mechanical ventilation. *Crit Care Med* 1:1, 1973.
94. Tocino I, Westcott JL: Barotrauma. *Radiol Clin North Am* 34:59, 1996.
95. Anzueto A, Frutos-Vivar F, Esteban A: Incidence, risk factors and outcome of barotrauma in mechanically ventilated patients. *Intensive Care Med* 30:612, 2004.
96. Johnson TH, Altman AR: Pulmonary interstitial gas: first sign of barotrauma due to PEEP therapy. *Crit Care Med* 7:532, 1979.
97. Albelda SM, Gefter WB, Kelley MA, et al: Ventilator-induced subpleural air cysts: clinical, radiographic, and pathologic significance. *Am Rev Respir Dis* 127:360, 1983.
98. Kirkpatrick AW, Ng AK, Dulchavsky SA, et al: Sonographic diagnosis of pneumothorax inapparent on plain radiography: confirmation by computed tomography. *J Trauma* 50:750, 2001.
99. Dulchavsky SA, Hamilton DR, Diebel LN, et al: Thoracic ultrasound diagnosis of pneumothorax. *J Trauma* 47:970, 1999.
100. Snyder J, Carrol G, Schuster DP, et al: Mechanical ventilation: physiology and application. *Curr Probl Surg* 21:1, 1984.
101. Willetts SM: Paralysis of ventilated patients: yes or no? *Intensive Care Med* 11:2, 1985.
102. Darioli E, Perret C: Mechanical controlled hypoventilation in status asthmaticus. *Am Rev Respir Dis* 129:385, 1984.
103. Baumann MH, Sahn SA: Tension pneumothorax: diagnostic and therapeutic pitfalls. *Crit Care Med* 21:177, 1993.
104. Steiger Z, Wilson RF: Management of bronchopleural fistulas. *Surgery* 158:267, 1984.
105. Beltrami V: Surgical transsternal treatment of bronchopleural fistula post-pneumonectomy. *Chest* 95:379, 1989.
106. Ferguson JS, Sprenger K, VanNatta T: Closure of a bronchopleural fistula using bronchoscopic placement of an endobronchial valve designed for the treatment of emphysema. *Chest* 129:479, 2006.
107. Rusch VW, Capps JS, Tyler ML, et al: The performance of four pleural drainage systems in an animal model of bronchopleural fistula. *Chest* 4:859, 1988.
108. Phillips YY, Lonigan RM, Joyner LR: A simple technique for managing a bronchopleural fistula while maintaining positive pressure ventilation. *Crit Care Med* 7:351, 1979.
109. Weksler N, Ovadia L: The challenge of bilateral bronchopleural fistula. *Chest* 95:938, 1989.
110. Gallagher TJ, Smith RA, Kirby RR, et al: Intermittent inspiratory chest tube occlusion to limit bronchopleural cutaneous air leaks. *Crit Care Med* 4:328, 1976.
111. Bevelaqua FA, Kay S: A modified technique for the management of bronchopleural fistula in ventilator-dependent patients: a report of 2 cases. *Respir Care* 31:904, 1986.
112. Powner DJ, Grenvik A: Ventilatory management of life-threatening bronchopleural fistulae: a summary. *Crit Care Med* 9:54, 1981.
113. Goldszer RC, Bennett J, VanCampen J, et al: Intrapleural tetracycline for spontaneous pneumothorax. *JAMA* 241:724, 1979.
114. Macoviak JA, Stephenson LW, Ochs R, et al: Tetracycline pleurodesis during active pulmonary-pleural air leak for prevention of recurrent pneumothorax. *Chest* 81:78, 1982.
115. Verschoof AC, Vende T, Greve LH, et al: Thoracoscopic pleurodesis in the management of spontaneous pneumothorax. *Respiration* 53:197, 1988.
116. Light RW, O'Hara VS, Moritz TE, et al: Intrapleural tetracycline for the prevention of recurrent spontaneous pneumothorax. *JAMA* 264:2224, 1990.
117. Powner DJ, Cline CD, Rodman GH: Effect of chest-tube suction on gas flow through a bronchopleural fistula. *Crit Care Med* 13:99, 1985.
118. Bishop MJ, Benson MS, Pierson DJ: Carbon dioxide excretion via bronchopleural fistulas in adult respiratory distress syndrome. *Chest* 91:400, 1987.
119. Pierson DJ, Horton CA, Bates PW: Persistent bronchopleural air leak during mechanical ventilation: a review of 39 cases. *Chest* 90:321, 1986.
120. Kuwik RJ, Glass D, Coombs DW: Evaluation of high-frequency positive pressure ventilation for experimental bronchopleural fistula. *Crit Care Med* 9:164, 1981.
121. Turnbull AD, Carlon GC, Howland WS, et al: High-frequency jet ventilation in major airway or pulmonary disruption. *Ann Thorac Surg* 32:468, 1981.
122. Albeda SM, Hansen-Flaschen JH, Taylor E, et al: Evaluation of high-frequency jet ventilation in patients with bronchopleural fistulas by quantitation of the airleak. *Anesthesiology* 63:551, 1985.
123. Bishop MJ, Benson MS, Sato P, et al: Comparison of high-frequency jet ventilation with conventional mechanical ventilation for bronchopleural fistula. *Anesth Analg* 66:833, 1987.
124. Rafferty TD, Palma J, Motoyama EK, et al: Management of a bronchopleural fistula with differential lung ventilation and positive end-expiratory pressure. *Respir Care* 25:654, 1980.
125. Lau K: Postural management of bronchopleural fistula. *Chest* 94:1122, 1988.
126. Feeley TW, Keating D, Nishimura T: Independent lung ventilation using high-frequency ventilation in the management of a bronchopleural fistula. *Anesthesiology* 69:420, 1988.
127. Crimi G, Candiani A, Conti G, et al: Clinical applications of independent lung ventilation with unilateral high-frequency jet ventilation (ILV-UHFJV). *Intensive Care Med* 12:90, 1986.
128. Orlando R, Gluck EH, Cohen M, et al: Ultra-high-frequency jet ventilation in a bronchopleural fistula model. *Arch Surg* 123:591, 1988.
129. Torre M, Chiesa G, Ravine M, et al: Endoscopic gluing of bronchopleural fistula. *Ann Thorac Surg* 43:295, 1987.
130. Hoier-Madsen K, Schulze S, Pedersen VM, et al: Management of bronchopleural fistula following pneumonectomy. *Scand J Thorac Cardiovasc Surg* 18:263, 1984.
131. Glover W, Chavis TV, Daniel TM, et al: Fibrin glue application through the flexible fiberoptic bronchoscope: closure of bronchopleural fistula. *J Thorac Cardiovasc Surg* 93:470, 1987.
132. Regel G, Sturm JA, Neumann C, et al: Occlusion of bronchopleural fistula after lung injury: a new treatment by bronchoscopy. *J Trauma* 29:223, 1989.
133. Lan R, Lee C, Tsai Y, et al: Fiberoptic bronchial blockade in a small bronchopleural fistula. *Chest* 92:944, 1987.
134. Ellis JH, Sequeira FW, Weber TR, et al: Balloon catheter occlusion of bronchopleural fistulae. *AJR Am J Roentgenol* 138:157, 1982.
135. Roksvaag H, Skalleberg L, Nordberg C, et al: Endoscopic closure of bronchial fistula. *Thorax* 38:696, 1983.
136. Menard JW, Prejean CA, Tucker YW: Endoscopic closure of bronchopleural fistulas using a tissue adhesive. *Am J Surg* 155:415, 1980.
137. Jones DP, David I: Gelfoam occlusion of peripheral bronchopleural fistulas. *Ann Thorac Surg* 42:334, 1986.

Chapter 177 ■ Gas Embolism Syndromes

MARK M. WILSON

The gas embolism syndromes occur in many different settings and may result in life-threatening emergencies. The clinical manifestations of these disorders are varied, and the final pathophysiologic consequences depend on where the gas bubbles obstruct the circulation and how they impact the function of the surrounding tissue. The nervous system, heart, lungs, and skin are the organ systems most frequently involved. The diagnosis of a gas embolism syndrome can be very difficult to establish. Clinicians must depend on a high level of suspicion in the appropriate settings to rapidly identify the problem, prevent further gas entry into the circulation, and begin effective treatment. Each of these entities is discussed in more detail based on the predominant location of the gas collections, although they are not always separate and distinct.

VENOUS GAS EMBOLISM

Although the actual incidence of venous gas embolism (VGE) in the United States is unknown, it has been estimated conservatively that at least 20,000 cases of "air" embolism occur annually [1]. The consequences of VGE range from clinically undetectable to being rapidly fatal.

Etiology

Clinical reports emphasize the high incidence of VGE in association with traumatic injuries and invasive procedures involving the head, neck, and chest (Table 177.1) [1]. Only the most common causes are discussed in detail in this chapter.

Surgical

Virtually, any surgical procedure that transiently exposes an open vein to a relative negative pressure may be associated with VGE. The best-studied surgical procedure known to be commonly associated with VGE is craniotomy performed in the Fowler's (sitting) position. When monitors for VGE are prospectively used [1], VGE has been documented in 21% to 32% of all craniotomies and up to 58% of occipital craniotomies. Air may also enter the venous system via the occipital emissary veins, the dural sinuses, the diploic veins, the veins of tumors, or through burr holes.

Childbirth, hysterectomy, and abortion have been associated with an increased incidence of VGE [1]. It has been estimated that VGE causes 1% of maternal deaths. The incidence of VGE during cesarean section has been reported to be on the order of 39% to 71% overall, and the majority of episodes occur during uterine repair and placenta removal. During pregnancy, the veins of the uterus are exposed and fixed; when traumatized; they remain open and may serve as a portal of entry for gaseous emboli.

Prospective Doppler monitoring studies have documented a 31% to 83% incidence of VGE during total hip replacement [1]. The presumptive mechanism of embolization involves the forcible entry of air into the venous circulation through vascular openings of the bony medulla of the femur as a result of the high pressures generated in the distal shaft when the prosthesis is inserted.

Sinus lavage and dental surgical procedures have resulted in fatal cases of VGE [1]. Emboli are the result of intraosseous irrigation with water or air under pressure (at least 80 cm water). The cause of VGE during these procedures is not well understood.

TABLE 177.1

Causes of Venous Gas Embolism

Surgical
Any head/neck/cardiothoracic surgery
Orthopedic surgery (arthroscopy, endoprosthesis placement)
Hysterectomy, cesarean section
Transurethral resection of the prostate
Abortion, uterine curettage
Normal childbirth, childbirth with placenta previa or extraction procedure
Liver transplantation/resection
Traumatic
Open/penetrating wounds
Vena cava lacerations
Positive-pressure mechanical ventilation
Self-contained underwater breathing apparatus diving
Decompression sickness
Pneumothorax/pneumoperitoneum
Cunnilingus/intercourse during pregnancy
Self-induced
Diagnostic and therapeutic procedures
Central venous catheter insertion/removal
Pulmonary artery catheterization
Thoracoscopy, thoracentesis
Pleurodesis, percutaneous lung biopsy
Gravity infusion of blood/intravenous products
Pressurized injections/infusions (including contrast media)
Any involving gas insufflation
Hemodialysis
Pericardiocentesis
Pacemaker/defibrillator placement
Radiofrequency cardiac ablation
Endoscopic retrograde cholangiopancreatography
Epidural catheter insertion
Neodymium:yttrium-aluminum-garnet laser therapy
Liquid nitrogen cryosurgery
Hydrogen peroxide irrigation/ingestion
Blood donation

Trauma

Open or penetrating wounds—especially of the chest, neck, head, heart, spine, abdomen, and pelvis—may result in VGE owing to the exposure of an open vein to a relative positive pressure gradient (i.e., atmospheric pressure as compared with central venous pressure) [1]. Pneumothorax or pneumoperitoneum may result in VGE by the inadvertent puncture of intrathoracic or intraabdominal blood vessels during the mechanism of injury.

Some of the more unusual cases of traumatic embolization include reports of self-induced VGE caused by urethral insufflation with an atomizer bulb, scrotal injection of air with a bicycle pump, and attempted in hospital suicide by forcible breathing into an intravenous line [1].

Diagnostic and Therapeutic Procedures

Air embolism in the setting of central venous catheterization has an unknown overall incidence, probably because the diagnosis is made only with large emboli. This fact also impacts the reported mortality rate in the literature of 29% to 50% [1]. Morbidity is also significant because 42% of all survivors of recognized VGE experienced residual neurologic deficits. Air can enter the central venous system in several different ways: (a) during needle/wire/catheter insertion; (b) with fracture of the catheter, malfunction of a self-sealing diaphragm, or detachment of external connections; (c) after removal of a catheter that has been in place for several days, such that air is "sucked" into an open subcutaneous tissue tunnel that has formed a skin tract; and (d) as a result of a piggyback infusion running dry [1].

Thoracoscopy may produce VGE presumably as a result of the associated pneumothorax. Lung biopsy by percutaneous or bronchoscopic techniques creates a direct traumatic opening at the blood–air interface. Significant embolization might result whenever a medium-sized vein is exposed [1].

Gas insufflation procedures have been associated with gaseous embolization [1]. Diagnostic procedures involving the female genital tract, urethra, urinary bladder, kidney, retroperitoneal and perirenal spaces, peritoneal and pleural cavities, joints, cerebral ventricles, epidural space, and paranasal sinuses all carry a risk for VGE. To minimize this risk, the volume of gas introduced, the pressure resulting within the cavity, and the rate of injection should always be as low as possible. It has been suggested that carbon dioxide (CO_2) should be used as the insufflating agent whenever possible because of its high blood solubility and rapid clearance. This last recommendation begs a word of caution, however, because VGE-associated deaths have been reported even with the use of CO_2 [1].

Placement of epidural catheters for anesthesia has been noted prospectively to be associated with Doppler-detectable VGE [1]. Among pregnant women placed in the left lateral decubitus position, VGE was noted to occur in 43%, almost half of whom were at least briefly symptomatic. The underlying mechanism relates to the rich plexus of veins of the epidural space, mostly anterior and lateral to the spinal cord. These veins are susceptible to trauma from a needle if the puncture is not directly in the midline or if the needle is rotated once in the epidural space. Because there are no valves in this plexus of veins, the intravascular pressure likely closely follows the central venous pressure. In the left lateral decubitus position, the site of puncture is above the level of the right atrium (RA), and, for pregnant women, uterine compression of the inferior vena cava is relieved, both of which serve to create a subatmospheric pressure in the epidural venous plexus.

Thermal tissue-ablation procedures using application of heat or cold have been associated with VGE [1]. Laser ablation/coagulation of tissues requires a continuous method for cooling of the laser tip. In general, these methods have involved using liquid (saline) or gas (air, nitrogen [N_2], CO_2). Reports exist in the literature of the entry of these compressed gases into the venous circulation owing to opening of vascular channels during the ablative procedure [1]. At the other temperature extreme, cryosurgery with instillation of liquid N_2 is used to extend the surgical margin of excision during cancer operations. Direct contact between the tissues and the liquid N_2 may lead to entry of N_2 into the circulation in the gaseous state [1]. N_2 gas expands because it is warmed to a volume of greater than 500 times that it occupied in the liquid state. Gas emboli of this magnitude could be rapidly fatal.

Ingestion or use of hydrogen peroxide (H_2O_2) in closed spaces or body cavities has been shown to result in fatal VGE [1]. Animal and human studies have shown that H_2O_2 is readily absorbed from the intestines and the peritoneum. Oxygen (O_2) emboli arise from the systemic absorption of H_2O_2 because catalase-induced decomposition causes release of water and molecular O_2. One milliliter of a 3% H_2O_2 solution releases an estimated 10 mL of O_2 in reaction with catalase [1], which is abundant in human blood.

Case reports of VGE during blood donation and insertion of peripheral intravenous catheters illustrate that whenever a vein is exposed to atmospheric pressure, there is a hazard of embolization [1].

Pathophysiology

Entry of Gas into the Circulation

VGE has been shown to occur among patients in essentially any position [1]. The critical factor common to all VGE lies in the pressure gradient produced between the right side of the heart and the level of the open vessel. Any increase in the distance of the open vessel above the level of the heart or any decrease in intrathoracic pressure would increase the likelihood of air entering the venous circulation and traveling to the heart. For each 5 in. in vertical height above the level of the RA, there is an approximately 9.3 mm Hg decrease in local blood pressure. Any decrease of mean intrathoracic pressure or mechanisms resulting in a contracted blood volume or low central venous pressure will tend to enhance any existing venous pressure gradient.

Large amounts of gas can rapidly pass into the venous system under the proper conditions. Calculations indicate that approximately 100 mL of air per second would enter a vessel via a No. 14G needle with only a 5 cm H_2O pressure gradient across it.

Travel of Gas to the Heart

Once the gas has entered the venous circulation, it travels toward the point of lower pressure until it becomes lodged at an area of obstruction or its passage is impeded or prevented by electrostatic forces between the interface of the bubble with the vascular endothelium overcoming the laminar flow in that vessel. Animal studies have found that passage of air emboli through the superior vena cava (SVC) can be retarded or the air even retained at sites proximal to the SVC for an indefinite period [1].

Large venous gas emboli are capable of lodging and then obstructing blood flow in the heart and the pulmonary vasculature [1]. Grossly, these events have been observed to cause immediate dilation of the RA, the right ventricle (RV), and the pulmonary outflow tract. A rapidly expanding zone of RV ischemia follows soon thereafter. Functional obstruction of the RV outflow tract may result owing to an "air lock" phenomenon. A blood–froth mixture results from systolic compression of the compressible gas phase with the noncompressible whole-blood phase. This concoction is then able to expand during diastole, the net result being an inadequate pumping action of the RV. It has been postulated that turbulent blood flow results from this "whipping" type of action or from vortex flow around partially obstructing collections of air bubbles. This whipping subsequently enhances fibrin formation, platelet aggregation, and coalescence of intravascular fat.

Smaller collections of air may not impair the heart, and they may pass directly to the pulmonary arteries. Larger collections enter the pulmonary arteries with associated collections of fat and fibrin emboli.

Fate of Gas Emboli

Bubbles with the smallest initial radii have the shortest life span and are occasionally seen to pass directly through a capillary bed after attaining a radius of approximately 5 μm [1]. The bulk of excretion of gaseous emboli is accounted for by molecular diffusion across the capillary wall into the alveolar spaces. The rate of washout is related to RV performance and mean pulmonary artery (PA) pressure [1].

Surface–tension relationships, vascular pressures, and the size range of the bubbles are additional factors that influence passage of emboli across the lungs. In addition, the composition of the gas influences the size of the bubbles and the rate of dissolution in the blood. Bubbles of air or N_2 would be expected to remain in the blood for longer periods of time than O_2 or CO_2, especially if the ventilatory gases resemble room air composition. This relationship is because of the similarity of the partial pressures of the gases inside the bubbles with those of the surrounding blood, as well as to the different solubilities of the gases. Tonic factors affecting the diameter of pulmonary vessels (e.g., anesthetic agents, neurogenic or hypoxic pulmonary vasoconstriction, arterial tension of CO_2, endogenous mediators) also influence the passage of bubbles across the lungs.

Cardiopulmonary Consequences of Embolization

Pulmonary vascular obstruction is a major consequence of VGE and can lead to death. Obstruction to blood flow through the RV and through the pulmonary vascular system results from pulmonary vasoconstriction and from the mechanical impediment to flow imposed by the gas bubbles [1]. The change in PA pressures depends on whether the gas emboli are the result of a slow continuous infusion or a rapid bolus injection. In the first instance, a brisk increase in PA pressure to a level of up to 300% of baseline is seen [1]. This rapid increase phase is believed to be as a result of pulmonary vascular vasoconstriction and is followed by a plateau phase. The plateau response likely represents the opening of anatomic intrapulmonary shunts or a balance between the rate of gas infusion and rate of elimination. In contrast, when approximately 100 mL of air is injected as a bolus, PA pressure declines by as much as 20%, because the right heart is acutely stressed beyond its capabilities. Larger bolus injections (125 to 200 mL) are consistently fatal.

Pulmonary edema from VGE has been described anecdotally among humans [1]. Increased hydrostatic pulmonary vascular pressures (from mechanical occlusion of the PA and from induced vasoconstriction) and increased capillary permeability have been suggested as mechanisms for edema formation [1]. Regardless, the edema proves to be transient and reverses because the gas emboli are rapidly absorbed.

Maldistribution of ventilation–perfusion ($\dot{V}/\dot{Q}$) matching is the major factor leading to hypoxemia and changes in CO_2 concentrations. With small amounts of continuous gas bubble infusion (0.2 mL/min/kg) into the venous circulation, there is an increase in high $\dot{V}/\dot{Q}$ areas in the lung. With larger volume gas emboli (0.75 to 2 mL per kg), however, shunting and an increase in the physiologic dead space have been shown to occur and to increase proportionally as the volume of embolic gas increases. This effect can involve as much as 35% of the total cardiac output, and it may be severe enough to cause CO_2 retention in addition to hypoxemia.

The end-tidal CO_2 concentration ($ETCO_2$) decreases during VGE as a result of the increase in dead space caused by vascular obstruction. More simply, $ETCO_2$ decreases as CO_2 is "washed out" of alveoli that are ventilated but not perfused adequately. Inadequate matching may further worsen in the setting of a reduced cardiac output, resulting directly from VGE or indirectly as a consequence of non–embolic-related events (e.g., blood loss, myocardial ischemia, vasoactive medications). Any reduction in pulmonary blood flow decreases the delivery of CO_2 in the venous blood to the alveoli, thereby further decreasing the $ETCO_2$.

Paradoxic Embolism

A paradoxic embolism may occur in the presence of intrapulmonary arteriovenous anastomoses (IPAVA; owing to their larger diameter as compared with the general pulmonary microcirculation) or via an anatomic intracardiac shunt. A gas embolism may elevate right-sided heart pressures, thus facilitating right-to-left shunting through a patent foramen ovale (PFO). Autopsy studies of patients with no history of cardiac disease document the presence of a probe-patent PFO in 25% to 35% of the general population [1].

Considered an anatomic variant, a probe-patent PFO is generally 1 to 10 mm in diameter and remains functionally closed as long as left atrial (LA) pressure exceeds RA pressure. A reversal of the normal interatrial pressure gradient might be expected to increase the risk of paradoxic embolization. RA pressure has been demonstrated to be higher than LA pressure in the seated position in up to 54% of adult humans monitored during neurosurgical procedures [1]. The critical pressure necessary for gas bubbles to be forced through a PFO is not known, but it is likely to be small. After cardiac surgery, it has been shown that as little as a 4 mm Hg gradient can produce a 50% right-to-left intracardiac shunt [1].

Clinically, it may be important to distinguish between an anatomic PFO and a functional PFO because it is only the latter that has an impact on any morbidity and mortality experienced. It has been reported that paradoxic embolization occurs in only 15% to 25% of patients with a PFO [1]. Contrast echocardiography using agitated sterile saline given as a rapid intravenous bolus has documented a lower prevalence of functional PFO (i.e., 10% to 20%) [1], as compared to the known prevalence of 25% to 35% for anatomic PFO. The amount of contrast material crossing from the right heart to the left heart does not correlate with the magnitude of shunt flow, nor does the Valsalva maneuver provoke shunting in all patients with PFO [1]. The question remains as to whether this finding represents a low sensitivity of this method for detecting PFO or whether there are some anatomic PFOs that have no functional role. Consensus opinion is that all PFOs should be considered to have the potential for allowing paradoxic embolization. Multiple reports have documented that the absence of any agitated saline or color flow through the interatrial septum by echocardiography does not exclude the presence of a PFO; it only excludes the presence of a right-to-left interatrial shunt at that moment in time [1].

Bubble passage through the pulmonary circulation has been shown to occur in the absence of intracardiac communications when the rate of venous air infusion exceeds the rate of pulmonary filtration and excretion [1]. Paradoxic air embolization during cardiopulmonary bypass has been reported to occur in the absence of an intracardiac defect when the mean PA pressure exceeds approximately 30 mm Hg [1]. Animal research suggests the existence of this same "critical value" of PA pressure that, once exceeded, dramatically increases the tendency for paradoxic embolization [1]. This increase occurs presumably on the basis of IPAVA (which may be as large as 500 μm in diameter), bronchopulmonary anastomoses (i.e., flow is from the PA to the bronchial veins and then to the pulmonary veins), or by routine transpulmonary passage of the gas across the capillary beds.

Factors Affecting Mortality

The size of the embolus, its rate of delivery, and the final destinations of the gaseous emboli are the most important factors influencing the severity of injury produced by VGE. Among humans, accidental bolus injections of 100 and 300 mL of air have been reported to be fatal [1]. In critically ill patients with minimal cardiopulmonary reserve, smaller emboli could be expected to have a greater morbidity.

In the context of equal volumes, mortality is decreased if the embolism is of CO_2 rather than air or O_2. Animal work indicates that CO_2 may be injected to five times the volume of O_2 before symptoms of embolism appear, presumably because of its greater solubility in blood [1]. Although tolerated to a larger extent, it must be remembered that CO_2 emboli are not entirely benign and may lead to similar clinical consequences as air embolization.

When nitrous oxide (N_2O) is used for anesthesia, mortality is increased in the setting of VGE [1]. N_2O attains a high blood concentration because of its high solubility (approximately 20-fold that of O_2 and 34-fold that of N_2). Because a large concentration gradient would exist between this blood and any air embolus, N_2O would be expected to diffuse from the blood into the embolus. As a result, the embolus increases geometrically in size in direct relation to the partial pressure of N_2O because the N_2O molecules can diffuse from the blood into the air embolus much more rapidly than the N_2 can be removed. The end result is a potential worsening of any generated physiologic abnormalities or delay of the ultimate resolution of the embolus. The presence of N_2O in the anesthetic mixture has been shown to reduce the median lethal dose of a given volume of air by a factor of 3.4 [1].

Diagnosis

Clinical Manifestations

The symptoms of VGE are generally nonspecific. Patients may report feeling faint or dizzy, express a fear of impending doom, or even complain of dyspnea or substernal chest pain. This presentation, with or without paradoxic embolism, may mimic an acute cardiopulmonary or central nervous system (CNS) event. Severe VGE may present dramatically with elevated neck veins, "clear lungs," and hypotension, and it may be rapidly followed by altered mental status and death. Because signs and symptoms are nonspecific, the importance of a detailed history, familiarity with the clinical situations in which VGE occurs, and a high degree of clinical suspicion cannot be overemphasized if one is to make an accurate diagnosis.

Physical Examination

Physical examination is usually not helpful for making the diagnosis. The only "specific" sign attributed to VGE is the classic mill-wheel murmur, otherwise reported only to occur in the rare syndrome of hydropneumopericardium. This murmur has been described as the rhythmic splashing or churning sound generated by the agitation of gas trapped with fluid in a closed space. Most often, it is only audible transiently and is heard infrequently at best, even with severe VGE. With large emboli and resultant cardiovascular collapse, a sound resembling the "squeezing of a wet sponge" has been described over the precordium [1].

VGE may occur without any change of vital signs. Wheezing as a result of acute bronchospasm may occasionally be heard. In a prospective study of seated neurosurgical patients, marked hypotension was noted in 78%, respiratory changes in 61%, and ventricular ectopy in 50% [1].

Laboratory Data

Abnormal results may include electrocardiogram (ECG) changes consistent with myocardial ischemia or acute cor pulmonale, premature ventricular contractions, and/or arterial blood gas findings of hypoxemia and hypercapnia.

Radiographic Findings

Chest radiography may verify the presence of VGE, but it should not be relied on for the diagnosis, especially in emergent situations. Air in the main PA is pathognomonic of pulmonary VGE, and it is recognized as a characteristic bell-shaped lucency in the distal main PA. This sign is seen very infrequently, especially in supine patients. Other patterns seen are focal upper lung zone oligemia, central PA dilation, and air in the systemic veins or the arterial circulation [1]. Pulmonary edema ranging from hilar haziness to generalized vascular redistribution may occur soon after VGE, and it usually persists for at least 16 to 24 hours [1]. Noncardiogenic pulmonary edema has been reported [1], is usually self-limited, and resolves over several days. Progression of noncardiogenic pulmonary edema to full-blown acute respiratory distress syndrome has also been described [1].

Ventilation–Perfusion Lung Scans

On $\dot{V}/\dot{Q}$ imaging, VGE may produce patterns consistent with "high probability" for pulmonary venous thromboembolism. Prompt and complete resolution of these scintigraphic perfusion defects within 24 hours has been documented [1], and it is probably characteristic for VGE. In contrast, perfusion defects produced by venous thromboembolism resolve more slowly over a period of weeks to months and may not ever resolve completely. Areas of $V/\dot{Q}$ matching (i.e., "indeterminate probability") may coexist with $V/\dot{Q}$ mismatches, and they are believed to represent reflex bronchoconstriction in conjunction with occlusion of the PA or its branches. The decreased ventilation is apparently because of the release of bronchoconstricting agents, such as serotonin, from the occluded segments of the PA. This phenomenon is readily reversible within several hours if the PA occlusion is transient, and it is related to rapid resolution of the gaseous emboli.

Detection and Monitoring Method

Precordial Doppler monitoring is generally considered one of the more sensitive techniques for detecting emboli. Because a gas–blood interface is an excellent acoustic reflector, when an ultrasonographic beam strikes a moving gas bubble, a distinctive and characteristic artifact above the background flow signal is produced.

VGE may be missed by this technique owing to the position of the probe or completeness of the examination. False-positive reports of VGE may arise as a result of arrhythmia. The sound pattern induced by a junctional rhythm may easily mimic changes produced by VGE. With a junctional rhythm, cannon A waves may be present because of contraction of the RA against a closed tricuspid valve. The resultant turbulence in the RA is detected and confused for VGE.

Serial measurements of PA pressure can be a useful monitoring technique because even small emboli may produce significant increases in PA pressures. Major increases of PA pressure do not occur unless at least 10% of the vasculature is obstructed and the rise in PA pressure is roughly proportional to the size of the embolus. Finally, the likelihood of a paradoxic embolism increases above a mean PA pressure of 30 mm Hg, and serial monitoring would potentially allow the clinician a chance to prevent or minimize this complication [1].

$ETCO_2$ and N_2 levels fluctuate with VGE. Because these changes probably result primarily from significant mismatch of ventilation and perfusion, it would be anticipated that they would detect emboli later than Doppler techniques or changes in PA pressure and that they would be more likely to miss small emboli. Like PA pressure changes, however, variations in $ETCO_2$ stay abnormal longer, and they are more closely related to the volume of gas embolized [1]. Potential confounding factors exist that may also cause a reduction in $ETCO_2$ in the absence of a VGE-related event, and they include any set of circumstances that result in an acute decrease of cardiac output, increases of alveolar ventilation, or increases of physiologic dead space.

Consideration of the advantages and disadvantages of the available VGE detection technology suggests that a combination of transesophageal echocardiography or precordial Doppler ultrasonography with PA pressure, $ETCO_2$, or transcutaneous O_2 devices would provide the highest sensitivity, the quantitative determination, and the best available physiologic response monitoring. Across the United States, use of $ETCO_2$ monitoring in combination with precordial Doppler ultrasonography has become the primary, if not the standard, approach for VGE detection perioperatively.

Treatment

Because a fatal outcome may occur long before any confirming diagnostic tests can be performed, treatment must be initiated promptly at the earliest suspicion of gas embolization. In combined retrospective and prospective analyses of seated neurosurgical procedures, a significant beneficial role was found for the use of routine precordial Doppler monitoring [1]. Before the advent of routine Doppler monitoring, VGE was clinically detected less often (5.7% before vs. 32% after), but the episodes noted had more severe sequelae. Once precordial Doppler monitoring became standard, the morbidity and mortality directly related to venous or arterial emboli was documented to be 0.5%. This improvement of event detection and reduction in the severity of VGE was ascribed to earlier recognition, allowing for earlier institution of therapy and prevention of further occurrences.

Routine Treatment Measures

Immediate measures should include identification of the site of gas entry and prevention of further gas entry, cessation or correction of exacerbating factors, administration of 100% O_2, and changing position to the left lateral decubitus position. For most patients, the site of gas entry is readily apparent. Failure to stop gas entry in a timely fashion may be fatal. If there is suspicion of a low central blood volume, volume should be rapidly repleted. Immediate cessation of delivery of N_2O and ventilating with 100% O_2 facilitates resolution of any gas emboli experienced during anesthesia with this agent.

Because air emboli are composed of approximately 79% N_2 and 21% O_2, any maneuver that rapidly increases the elimination of dissolved N_2 should decrease the size of the embolus. Administration of 100% O_2 achieves this goal by washing N_2 out of the alveoli and by creating a favorable gradient for N_2 to cross into the alveolus from the blood.

Placing patients in the left lateral decubitus position may facilitate movement of any air obstructing the pulmonary outflow tract toward the apex of the RV, thereby relieving the obstruction and improving survival.

Aspiration and Dislodgement

For patients with witnessed gas embolism or in whom monitoring techniques suggest that the gas is still trapped in the heart, attempts can be made to aspirate or dislodge the gas. Gas may be aspirated from the heart by placing a central venous catheter into the RA or the RV or by pulling back a PA catheter and then aspirating serially from each successive heart chamber [1]. In unwitnessed gas embolism, this early phase has usually passed before the embolism is detected, and these interventions may result in more harm than benefit. Closed-chest compression may dislodge the embolus from the RV.

Hyperbaric Oxygen

When available, use of hyperbaric oxygen (HBO) may be helpful. HBO is the only therapy demonstrated to have any benefit well after VGE has been clinically established [1]. Even after emboli of 150 to 500 mL, HBO produced rapid improvement of all cardiopulmonary and neurologic abnormalities despite delays in initiating therapy of up to 20 hours. The most common HBO treatment protocols in use today are the US Navy Treatment Tables 5, 6, and 6A [2]. Use of these Tables is briefly discussed later in "Treatment" section of Decompression Sickness. Although it is accepted that HBO should be instituted as early as possible, the literature supports that special consideration be given to this modality at late stages, even in a seemingly irrecoverable situation [1,3].

Managing Unwitnessed Venous Gas Embolism

Given that VGE may mimic or cause a clinical presentation that is difficult to distinguish from venous pulmonary thromboembolism (PE), RV infarct, myocardial infarction (MI), or stroke, clinicians may frequently feel reluctant to consider the difficult to establish diagnosis of VGE and to begin treatment until other causes are ruled out. The simple measures indicated for the immediate management of VGE outlined herein are not contraindicated for the management of any of the other conditions typically in the differential diagnosis.

Little has been published on the clinical management of cardiovascular consequences of VGE. Because MI and RV infarct may frequently accompany large VGE, urgent, routine evaluation with ECG and echocardiography would be indicated for most cases. Because myocardial ischemia and subsequent MI of VGE probably result from hypoxemia, the effects of massive overdistention of the ventricle, and perhaps direct embolization of coronary vessels, the value of traditional management techniques for MI is not clearly established. There are no theoretical contraindications to the use of nitrates, aspirin, β-blockers, calcium channel blockers, or vasodilators in patients with ECG changes. The role of anticoagulation or thrombolytic therapy in VGE is unclear.

Discrimination between PE and VGE in patients with unwitnessed, unmonitored events can be difficult. Patients at risk for VGE are frequently at risk for PE as well. Once the gas has left the RV, changes in PA pressures and $ETCO_2$ values may be similar in both conditions. As noted earlier, the radiologic findings may be similar, but they may resolve within 24 hours with VGE. If the clinical suspicion of PE is high, there is no known contraindication to initiating appropriate anticoagulation for patients with suspected VGE.

Prevention

Preventive measures are likely the most valuable management strategy for VGE. All patients undergoing the procedures listed in Table 177.1 [1] should be considered at high risk. In addition, hyperventilation, obstructive lung disease, and hypovolemia are common clinical conditions that increase the natural pressure gradient between atmospheric air and the central venous compartment; they may, therefore, also increase the chances of VGE during predisposing manipulations. Patients with a known PFO, pulmonary hypertension, previous MI with markedly reduced RV function, known right-to-left shunts, or congenital heart disease with any of the mentioned abnormalities should also be considered at high risk, not for experiencing an embolism per se but for being susceptible for increased morbidity and mortality of a paradoxic embolism. A high false-negative rate (sensitivity, 64%) limits the usefulness of preoperative transthoracic echocardiography with Valsalva maneuver in predicting the presence of PFO and the risk of paradoxic emboli [1].

In general, patients should have procedures performed in a supine rather than upright position, and the point of potential air entry should be kept lower than the RA. Placement, manipulation, and removal of subclavian and internal jugular venous catheters are probably the most common clinical procedures during which specific measures can be performed to prevent substantial air embolization [1]. All patients should be placed in the Trendelenburg position, and they should be asked to perform the Valsalva maneuver or to hold their breath during needle/wire/catheter insertion. The operator should completely occlude the hub of the needle during manipulations to prevent open communication with atmospheric pressure. During removal of central catheters, patients should also be placed in the Trendelenburg position, the entry site should be compressed, and an occlusive dressing applied.

ARTERIAL GAS EMBOLISM

Arterial gas embolism (AGE) probably occurs daily in most hospitals owing to the prevalence of the situations known to be associated with AGE (Table 177.2) [1]. Although the prevalence of AGE is likely not as high as VGE, the clinical significance is potentially much greater than VGE (Fig. 177.1). In the clinical setting, most causes of AGE are preventable, and prompt treatment is frequently effective.

TABLE 177.2

Risk Factors and Causes of Arterial Gas Embolism

All causes listed for venous gas embolism in Table 177.1, via paradoxic embolization
Cardiopulmonary bypass/coronary artery bypass graft/ open-heart procedures
Coronary angiography/angioplasty/stenting
Cardioplegic solution infusion
Misuse/malfunction of pump oxygenator
Intraaortic balloon pump
Penetrating lung injury/resection
Bronchovenous fistula (as a result of trauma, mechanical ventilation, biopsy, thoracentesis)
Arterial line, arteriography
Self-contained underwater breathing apparatus diving
Decompression sickness
Carotid endarterectomy

Etiology

Cardiac Surgery and Bypass

AGE during cardiopulmonary bypass has an estimated incidence that ranges from 0.1% to 11.0% [1]. There is evidence that the use of in line filters and preferential use of membrane oxygenators over bubble oxygenators may decrease this risk significantly.

The importance of trapped air in the left heart as a potential source of AGE after an open cardiotomy has been appreciated for years. Air may remain adherent to the endocardium, sutures, and prosthetic valves, and in cul-de-sacs in the atria, ventricles, or aorta even after the heart is closed and beating spontaneously again. Complete air evacuation, even after specific and meticulous venting techniques, is nearly impossible to achieve [1]. Residual air has been shown to be present in the heart after discontinuation of bypass in approximately two-thirds of patients undergoing open cardiotomies and in approximately 12% of patients undergoing coronary artery bypass grafting (CABG) only, for an overall incidence of approximately 45%. The source of intracardiac air resulting from CABG operations is thought to be because of the ascending aorta being cross-clamped and suction then being applied to the left heart or the aortic root for the purpose of venting. The resultant pressure decrease is transmitted to the coronary arterial circulation, thus allowing air entry via the coronary arteriotomy site, with subsequent passage into the aortic root or the left ventricle. Any gases trapped in a proximal coronary artery or in a distally attached vein graft may also pass into the aortic root in the absence of venting if the graft is injected under pressure, as occurs commonly during the administration of cardioplegic hypothermia.

Transcranial Doppler monitoring of the middle cerebral artery during open-heart operations has confirmed the occurrence of cerebral gas embolization [1]. With refined surgical techniques, over time there has been a considerable reduction in the incidence of major neurologic injury after cardiac surgery and CABG, with a currently reported incidence of approximately 5% to 10% [1]. Detailed neuropsychiatric function testing, however, has shown persistent impairment of cerebral function in up to 70% of patients after CABG [1].

Lung Trauma

Systemic AGE is a frequent and unrecognized cause of death among patients with blunt or penetrating lung trauma [1]. The mode of air entry after percutaneous lung puncture, penetrating or blunt lung trauma, or with positive-pressure mechanical ventilation is via production of a bronchovenous fistula. Risk factors enhancing the chance of AGE include underlying emphysema, uncooperative patients, sneezing or coughing bouts, use of large diameter needles, hypotension, hypovolemia, Valsalva maneuver, and a site of involvement that is in close proximity to the hila. For patients with preexisting pulmonary fibrosis, one should expect an increased frequency and severity of systemic embolism because of the inability of the injured veins to retract and constrict. What has been referred to in the past as "pleural shock" (i.e., fainting, seizures, or even sudden death during a thoracentesis or therapeutic pneumothorax for treatment of tuberculosis) has since become recognized as a manifestation of AGE. Percutaneous procedures with needle calibers less than 20G (0.9 mm) have generally been considered safe, despite a case report describing a cerebral AGE after transthoracic aspiration with a 23G (0.6-mm) needle. The reported incidence for this

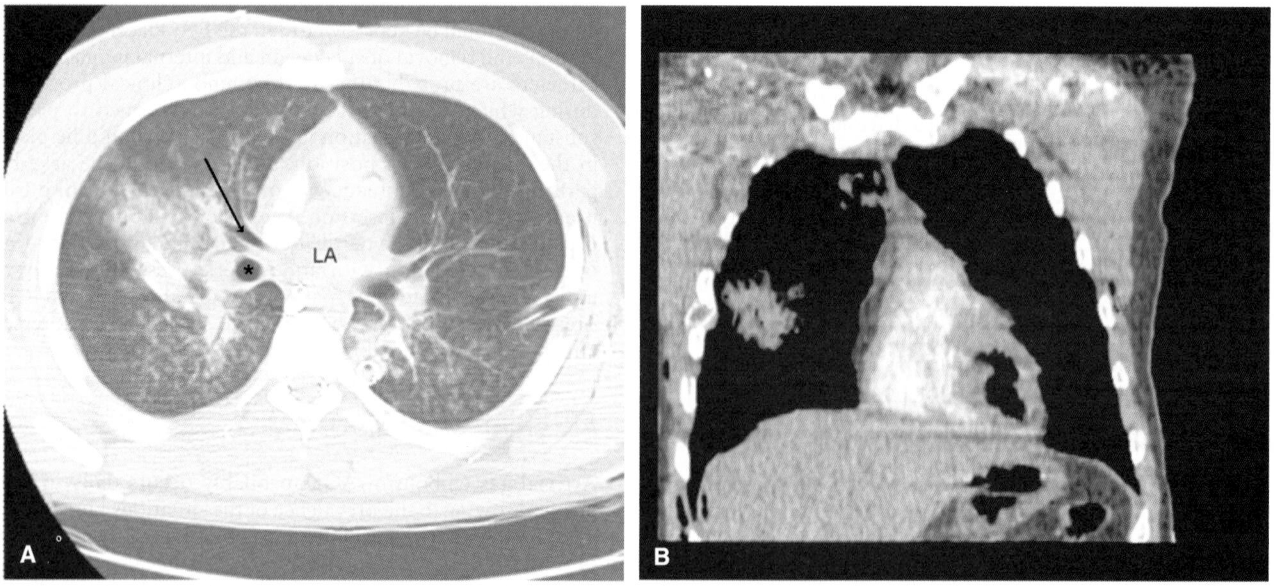

FIGURE 177.1 Fatal air embolism after massive facial trauma and prolonged extrication in an unbelted, backseat passenger in a car accident. A: Cross section of the chest showing air outlining the right superior pulmonary vein (*black arrow*) emptying into the LA. *Black** indicates the bronchus intermedius. B: Coronal reconstruction showing a massive air collection in the LA. LA, left atrium.

complication for needles of 16G to 20G (0.9 to 1.6 mm) has been variably estimated at 0.5 to 0.8 in 1,000 cases [1].

Arterial Lines

Cerebral AGE via retrograde flow from an indwelling radial arterial line has been reported as a case study and then followed up with a laboratory investigation [1]. Radioactive xenon mixed with 2 to 5 mL of air and injected at a rate of 0.6 to 2.5 mL per second into the radial artery resulted in demonstrable retrograde passage into the cerebral circulation. This low-flow rate is approximately 5- to 25-fold less than the reported "safe range" of previous work [1]. Because the true "safe" amount of air that can remain in an arterial flush catheter without the risk of retrograde embolization remains unknown, medical personnel need to be vigilant and meticulous in ensuring removal of any entrapped air in arterial flush lines.

Percutaneous Transluminal Coronary Angioplasty/Coronary Artery Stents

Most coronary artery gas emboli resulting from percutaneous transluminal coronary angioplasty or stenting of a coronary artery are reportedly extremely small, and they do not result in symptoms or hemodynamic consequences [1]. Of the symptomatic episodes, most cause rapid onset of chest pain with ECG evidence of ischemia or infarction. The systemic blood pressure may be unaffected, or it may be mildly decreased. For almost all patients, these effects resolve spontaneously within 5 to 10 minutes, similar to findings from experimental models. Only rarely does percutaneous transluminal coronary angioplasty–related AGE result in bradycardia, hypotension, ventricular fibrillation, MI, or asystole [1].

Pathophysiology

In AGE, the gas enters the arterial system by the direct rupture of a blood–air interface, by direct passage from the PA to pulmonary venous system, or through a functional right-to-left cardiac shunt. Gas bubbles distribute themselves throughout the body primarily directed by the relative blood flow at the time. Bubble buoyancy is actually a minor factor unless there is a significant depression of forward systemic flow [1]. Because the heart, lung, and brain receive the greatest amount of blood flow, the consequences of embolization are most frequently reported for these organs. Pulmonary manifestations of AGE are uncommon, perhaps because the redundancy of the pulmonary vascular supply limits the consequences of bubble occlusion.

Systemic Mechanical and Biophysical Effects

Bubble formation results in two broad categories of effects: mechanical—physical obstruction to blood flow with distortion or tearing of tissues as the bubble forms and expands, and biophysical—where the blood–gas, blood–tissue, or gas–endothelial interfaces stimulate a cascade of leukocyte, platelet, coagulation, fibrinolytic, and complement-mediated activations [1]. Research over the last few decades now recognizes the importance of oxidative stressors causing impairment of endothelium-dependent vasorelaxation (i.e., the endothelial dysfunction hypothesis). This is primarily caused by loss of nitric oxide activity in the vessel wall [1,3,4].

Similar to VGE, the trapped bubbles may pass through the circulation and exit via the lungs, or they may be slowly metabolized by body tissues. Unlike the situation when bubbles are trapped in a vein, an arterial occlusion may have an immediate clinical impact. Uptake and release of inert gas by a particular tissue depends on the rate of blood flow to that tissue, as well as the rate of gas diffusion out of the blood into the tissue.

When bubbles do form, the inert gas becomes isolated from the circulation, and it cannot be removed by blood flow until it diffuses back into tissues. The speed of diffusion is the result of the difference between the N_2 partial pressure in the air bubble and the N_2 partial pressure in the tissue. The partial pressure of the inert gas in the bubble also varies directly with the bubble's loss of O_2 through metabolic conversion into CO_2, which is 21 times more soluble than O_2.

Cardiovascular Effects

The heart is extremely intolerant of even minute amounts of arterial gas. AGE may produce MI, loss of left ventricular function, dysrhythmias, hypotension, or hypertension. As little as 0.025 to 0.05 mL of air directly entering a coronary artery may result in transient impairment of ventricular function, focal MI, ventricular fibrillation, or death [1].

Central Nervous System Effects

Cerebral embolism produces stroke-like symptoms and cerebral edema. Injury is probably more a result of damage from endothelial mediators, oxidant stress, and neuronal hypoxia rather than being directly a result of vascular obstruction or edema. After 5 to 30 seconds of arrested cerebral blood flow, most gas bubbles easily pass through the pial arteries. Significant volumes of gas may subsequently be collected in "air traps" in the jugular veins [1]. Larger emboli (e.g., large enough to obstruct several generations of arteriolar branching) are also generally only temporarily obstructing, and they relocate to the cerebral and the jugular veins during the period of reactive hyperemia that follows periods of arrested cerebral blood flow. Cerebral air emboli have been shown to persist in the circulation for 40 hours after initial insult [5]. It has been proposed, therefore, that the CNS dysfunction that follows cerebral AGE is not the result of bubble entrapment alone; it is instead, in large part, caused by effects on vascular endothelium or blood components.

Diagnosis

AGE, whether traumatic, iatrogenic, or dysbaric (i.e., solely as a result of changes in ambient pressures) in origin, presents immediately after the insult occurs, typically within 10 minutes. A myriad array of dramatic manifestations is possible, typically with symptoms suggestive of coronary or CNS involvement. If pain is the only symptom, however, AGE is unlikely. Two general clinical patterns have been recognized: fulminant collapse and isolated CNS injury. In the former, the initial presentation is apnea, coma, and cardiac arrest. This pattern is known to occur in 4% to 5% of patients with dysbaric air embolism but has an unknown incidence for other types of AGE. The responsible mechanism is believed to be direct coronary artery embolization with resultant MI or gaseous embolization of the cerebral circulation, resulting in hypertension and marked dysrhythmias. This subgroup is generally unresponsive to resuscitative efforts (Fig. 177.1).

In the latter group, the initial presentation is that of stable respiratory and heart rates, but with a wide spectrum of neurologic signs and symptoms. Usually, the symptoms are abrupt in onset, and they progress rapidly to overt signs. Patients may feel faint or dizzy or have an apprehensive fear of death. There may be loss of consciousness, convulsions, visual disturbances (including blindness), headache, confusion or other mental status changes, coma, vertigo, nystagmus, aphasia, sensory disturbances, weakness or hemiparesis, or even focal or more widespread paralysis. The pupils are usually dilated, and, occasionally, air may be seen in the retinal vessels. Liebermeister's sign may be present and is recognized as sharply defined areas of tongue pallor. Marbling of the skin of the uppermost portions of the body is another pathognomonic sign of AGE (along with retinal gas and

Liebermeister's sign) [1]. With prompt recompression therapy, the majority of these cases have the potential for full recovery.

Other clinical manifestations of extra-alveolar gas are related to the traumatic entry of air into the interstitium after alveoli rupture. The air may dissect along the perivascular sheaths into the mediastinum, causing pneumomediastinum, usually associated with a substernal aching or tightness that may have a pleuritic nature and may radiate to the neck, back, or shoulders. There may be coexistent subcutaneous emphysema and a notable "crunching" sound with each heartbeat (Hamman's sign) caused by air in the pericardium. Air may dissect further to cause a pneumothorax in up to 10% of cases [1]. Tension pneumothorax may occur in patients on positive-pressure mechanical ventilation or during decompression. Pneumopericardium and air in the retroperitoneum and subcutaneous tissues of the neck, trunk, or limbs may also occur. This extra-alveolar gas also has access to torn pulmonary blood vessels when the intrathoracic pressure decreases during normal inspiration after barotrauma has occurred. Once egress into the pulmonary venous circulation has occurred, migration to the left side of the heart and then to the arterial circulation may follow. Hemoptysis has often been mentioned as a cardinal sign of dysbaric air embolism, but it actually occurs in a minority (approximately 5%) of patients [1].

Treatment

Management of AGE and decompression sickness (DCS) is similar. Appropriate therapy involves prompt recognition, initial stabilization (with emphasis on preventing further damage), and definitive specific therapy (Table 177.3). All patients undergoing cardiopulmonary procedures or with recent lung trauma must be considered at high risk for AGE. Therefore, it cannot be emphasized strongly enough that a high index of suspicion for these diagnoses is one of the most important elements of care. Like many other true medical emergencies, therapeutic interventions should not be delayed to implement diagnostic testing. Details of therapy are found in the next section.

TABLE 177.3

Treatment Summary of Arterial Gas Embolism and Decompression Sickness

- Of time-tested benefit
  - Prevent further bubble formation and extension of other injuries
  - Cardiopulmonary life support as needed
  - 100% concentration of inspired oxygen
  - Maintain intravascular volume with isotonic fluids
  - Treat coexisting problems
  - Transport as soon as possible to recompression facility
  - Hyperbaric therapy
- Unproven benefit (but generally believed to be helpful)
  - Supine position (avoid head-down position)
  - Avoid glucose-containing infusions
  - Avoid hypertension, anxiety, hyperthermia
  - Lidocaine for the treatment of AGE
  - Diazepam for seizures, severe agitation, intractable vomiting (not used prophylactically)
  - DVT prophylaxis for patients with lower extremity weakness/paralysis.
- Experimental or of questionable benefit
  - Antiplatelet agents
  - Corticosteroids (possible central nervous system toxicity)
  - Calcium channel blockers
  - Lidocaine in the treatment of DCS
  - Combination nonsteroidal anti-inflammatory drug, heparin, and prostaglandin I2
  - Perfluorochemicals and/or other surface-active agents
  - Induced hypothermia
  - Cerebral venoarterial perfusion
- Proven detrimental
  - Recompression while submerged (used only as a last resort)
  - Alcohol/analgesics
  - Volume overload in AGE or with cardiopulmonary symptoms
  - Delayed transport to hyperbaric oxygen facility
  - Additional hypobaric exposures

AGE, arterial gas embolism; DVT, deep venous thrombosis; DCS, decompression sickness.

DECOMPRESSION SICKNESS

DCS occurs only when a transition is made to an environment with a relatively lower ambient pressure. Any rapid lowering of ambient pressure, regardless of the initial pressure level or saturation of inert gas, results in the release of bubbles of inert gas into the blood and tissues. This is equally true for too quick a return to a normobaric state after a hyperbaric exposure (as in diving or compressed air mining), or for rapid progression from a normobaric state into a hypobaric exposure (as in aviators, astronauts, or mountain climbers). It is estimated that around 10 million divers are currently active worldwide, performing more than 250 million dives annually and that at least 1 in 20 divers will experience DCS in their diving careers [6]. Statistics compiled by the Divers Alert Network (www.diversalertnetwork.org) indicate that there are more than 1,000 diving-related injuries annually in the United States alone, of which nearly 10% to 15% are fatal. DCS is the most frequent serious complication of self-contained underwater breathing apparatus (scuba) diving with an overall incidence of 1 to 35 cases per 10,000 dives [1,6,7] depending on the region of the world and the type of diving involved. DCS ranks third, after drowning and barotrauma/AGE (estimated incidence of 7 cases per 100,000 dives), as a cause of death among divers [1,6]. Strict enforcement of work regulations for tunnel workers and pilots has greatly decreased the incidence of DCS in these two groups. Interestingly and for unknown reasons, in hypobaric-related DCS, symptoms of spinal cord involvement are less common, whereas symptoms of brain involvement are more frequent as compared with hyperbaric-related DCS.

Etiology

Diving

The turn of the 20th century saw the origin of decompression tables, which define set depths and time limits of hyperbaric exposure to be used by divers to minimize the risk of DCS. Although derived empirically by J. S. Haldane, all common schedules since have been based on his original methods. Haldane's work demonstrated that the human body could tolerate a twofold reduction in ambient pressure without symptoms of DCS. Haldane also formulated the concept that the tissues of the body absorb nitrogen at varying rates, depending on the type of tissue and its vascularity. It is important to remember that dive tables are not infallible, and DCS may still occur despite following a "no decompression" profile. Experience has shown that modern scuba divers and aviators can have a significant net accumulation of inert gas (VGE) and yet remain without symptoms [1,8]. There is an important inter- and intraindividual variation in the degree of "bubbling" after a dive, indicating a significant, but as yet poorly characterized, influence of personal factors affecting gas saturation and desaturation [1,8].

Flying

DCS because of rapid hypobaric exposures is a syndrome indistinguishable from that produced in divers, and it is usually the result of accidental loss of cabin pressure in a pressurized aircraft. The altitude threshold for DCS is generally reported to be approximately 18,000 ft., but unless a person has had a hyperbaric exposure within the past 24 hours, there are rarely any difficulties with exposure to altitudes of up to 25,000 ft. [1]. Exposures above this level up to approximately 48,000 ft. for durations of 30 minutes to 3 hours have resulted in a DCS incidence of 1.5% [1]. More prolonged exposures and even greater altitudes increase the severity of an episode of DCS. Modern airline transportation has minimized these risks by pressurizing aircraft to maintain cabin pressures equivalent to 8,000 ft. while flying at actual altitudes of greater than 40,000 ft. DCS may also occur while flying after a diving trip, and it may be produced by exposure to altitudes of as little as 4,000 ft., even when "no-decompression" type of diving took place. Current recommendations are to avoid all flying for at least 12 hours after any dive. For flights exceeding a cabin pressure equivalent of approximately 8,000 ft., or for the case of divers requiring decompression stops, at least a 24-hour delay is recommended before flying.

At the extreme of human hypobaric exposures is the astronaut. Astronauts performing activities outside their space vehicles are decompressed from a cabin pressure equivalent to sea level, down to a suit pressure equivalent of approximately 30,000 ft. [1]. To minimize the risk of DCS, astronauts breathe 100% O_2 before decompression ("prebreathing") to reduce the partial pressure of N_2 before entering the space-suit environment. Only time and further space exploration will elucidate the risks of DCS from these types of exposures [9].

Pathophysiology

Bubble Formation

During DCS, the gas previously dissolved in body tissues and blood is released as gas bubbles into the tissues and the bloodstream. Boyle's law states that the volume of a gas varies inversely with its surrounding absolute pressure. At sea level, the weight of air that we breathe is equal to 14.7 lb per square in, 760 mm Hg, or 1 atmosphere absolute (ATA), depending on the choice of units. Table 177.4 indicates that for every 33 ft. of seawater a diver descends, the ambient pressure increases by 1 ATA and that the volume occupied by that same gas decreases proportionally. This table also demonstrates the reduction of pressure and volume expansion that accompanies increases of altitude.

The gear divers use to allow them to breathe underwater is designed to deliver air at the ambient pressure of the surrounding water, allowing the diver's lungs to remain fully expanded. As a scuba diver ascends slowly from depth, pressure in the lungs equalizes with ambient pressure as long as proper exhalation is achieved. If, for some reason, these expanding gases are not allowed to escape from the lungs (e.g., breath holding, localized gas trapping), overdistention of the alveoli may occur, which can result in pulmonary barotrauma. The fragility of alveoli is not generally appreciated, but it is highlighted by the fact that with the lungs fully expanded on compressed air, a pressure differential of only 95 to 110 cm H_2O (equivalent to an ascent from a depth of only 4 to 6 ft.) may be sufficient to rupture alveolar architecture [1]. With very few exceptions, all scuba diving is done at pressures less than 7 ATA, and most is done in the 2 to 4 ATA range [1,6].

Dalton's law of partial pressures states that the total pressure exerted by a mixture of gases is equal to the sum of the partial pressures of its constituent gases. The composition of gases that make up our atmosphere remains essentially constant up through an altitude of approximately 70,000 ft.: 78.08% N_2, 20.95% O_2, and the remaining fraction of CO_2, hydrogen, helium, argon, and neon [1]. In most settings, N_2 is the predominant constituent of any inhaled gas mixture. N_2 is inert (i.e., it is unused/unchanged by passage through the body). This fact is in contrast to CO_2 and O_2, which are actively transported and, therefore, do not depend entirely on purely physical laws for removal. N_2 is more soluble in fat than in water, which suggests that during decompression, bubbles more likely form in lipophilic tissues such as bone marrow, fat, and spinal cord.

Henry's law of gas solubility states that the amount of gas that dissolves in a fluid is directly proportional to the pressure of that gas on that fluid. The deeper one descends underground or in the ocean, the greater the driving pressure for the gas on the blood and the bodily fluids. The total accumulation of dissolved N_2 into the tissues of the body, therefore, depends on the depth achieved and the time spent at that depth. As ambient pressure decreases on ascent, solubility decreases and gas is released from body fluids.

TABLE 177.4

Pressure–Volume Relationships

	Pressure equivalents			
Distance from sea level (ft)	**lb/in^2**	**mm Hg**	**Atmosphere absolute**	**Bubble volume (%)**
+48,000	1.85	96	0.126	794
+40,000	2.72	141	0.185	541
+32,000	3.98	206	0.271	369
+24,000	5.70	295	0.388	258
+16,000	7.97	412	0.542	185
+8,000	10.92	565	0.743	135
Sea level	14.70	760	1	100
–33	29.40	1,520	2	50
–66	44.10	2,280	3	33
–99	58.80	3,040	4	25
–132	73.50	3,800	5	20
–165	88.20	4,560	6	17

Studies of bubble formation suggest that of the total absorption of inert gas that occurs during a dive, only 5% to 10% is released as bubbles after a rapid decompression [1]. The site of origin of intravascular bubbles is controversial, but overwhelming human and animal experimental evidence shows that gas bubbles are first detected in the venous circulation during decompression. Whereas the inability to detect venous bubbles is a good predictor of safety from developing DCS (NPV 99%), the occurrence of venous bubbles (even high grade) is a poor predictor of DCS (PPV 4%) [4]. It is most probable that AGE in DCS arises from the venous circulation or from pulmonary barotrauma with entry of gas bubbles into the pulmonary veins (i.e., dysbaric air embolism).

Biophysical effects result from the blood–gas, blood–tissue, and gas–endothelial interfaces, where an enormous chemical and physical discontinuity activates and amplifies reactive systems that are usually quiescent during normal blood flow. Electrochemical forces also exist at any blood-damaged endothelial interfaces, and they activate coagulation, complement, kinin, and fibrinolytic systems and allow for the denaturation of proteins. During DCS, and presumably with AGE, a localized hypercoagulable state develops, with a coexistent reduction in platelet count because of aggregation at the blood–bubble interface with leukocytes, red blood cells, and formed fibrin strands. The end result of this diffuse activation is to amplify any existing mechanical obstruction to blood flow with progressive sludging and clotting [1]. Further tissue injury then results from a decrease of local blood flow, edema formation, leukocyte chemotaxis, and oxidant stress. Newer studies also suggest impaired endothelial function owing to altered nitric oxide (NO) production or availability may play a significant role in the formation of vascular bubbles [4]. These effects are likely to be most important among cases of CNS involvement, for which small areas of reduced blood flow can produce severe disability or death. A disturbance of barrier function would best account for the well-established features of AGE and DCS which are otherwise difficult to reconcile with simple vascular occlusion as the sole explanatory mechanism.

It is important to emphasize that divers perform safe decompressions millions of times each year. For most, this process involves only a slow ascent after a short-duration dive. Others may require staged ascents, with one or more stops at intermediate depths to give more time for N_2 elimination. Still others require planned periods of chamber recompression after diving to prevent DCS. The overall safety of decompression exposures has withstood the test of time, and it has improved with experience and use of preventive measures. Safe decompression is by far the rule, rather than the exception.

Diagnosis

The clinical manifestations of DCS are protean, reflecting the effects of bubbles distorting tissues, obstructing blood flow, and perhaps, most importantly, by endothelial activation and initiation of oxidant stress and a pro-inflammatory response. Symptoms will generally occur within 1 hour of a decompression event among approximately 42%, and within 8 hours for over 80% of afflicted individuals [2]. A gross classification system is in common use based on the perceived severity of the clinical situation and the anticipated response to therapy. Type I DCS encompasses 75% to 90% of patients and includes those with musculoskeletal pain; skin or lymphatic manifestations; or nonspecific symptoms of anorexia, malaise, and fatigue. Generally, these patients require only a brief period of repressurization. Caution is still in order because up to 20% to 30% of this group may progress to a type II illness. Type II DCS is characterized by those cases with CNS or peripheral nerve involvement or any cardiorespiratory dysfunction. Overall, 10% to 25% of patients have type II DCS, and it generally represents a more severe illness with the potential for greater difficulties during treatment. The presence of a PFO is associated with a four- to sixfold increase in the odds ratio of developing a type II DCS [1,10–13].

Type I Decompression Sickness

Type I DCS includes the most common and classic manifestations usually associated with DCS. The majority of patients report a deep, dull "aching" pain in a limb during decompression or within the first 36 hours after surfacing (98% of patients experience onset within 24 hours of surfacing). Initially, there may be a vague feeling that "something is wrong," and the limb discomfort is dull and poorly localized. With time, this may progress to an intense throbbing pain within a more circumscribed and specific location. The affected area is generally nontender to palpation, and movement of any affected joints does not exacerbate the pain, except among severe cases.

The limbs are the most common sites of symptoms of DCS (in approximately 92% of cases of DCS overall and as the initial clinical manifestations of DCS in approximately 77%) [1,6]. Shoulders, elbows, and knees are the most commonly affected joints. More than one site may be involved, but rarely is the distribution bilaterally symmetric. Any pain occurring in the abdominal or thoracic areas, including the hips, should be considered a symptom arising from spinal cord involvement and treated instead as type II DCS. Heat, ice, immobilization, and potent analgesics do not relieve the pain, which is caused by the collections of gas in the periarticular and perivascular tissues. The most striking characteristic of this pain is its rapid relief with recompression. This rapid relief of discomfort with the application of pressure, and especially the tendency for this pain to return to the same site if recompression is inadequate, distinguishes the pain of "the bends" from any coexistent musculoskeletal strain or from the ischemic pain resulting from AGE.

Usually, there are no objective physical signs associated with limb DCS, except for a potential "peau d'orange" appearance of the skin from local lymphatic obstruction. The skin exhibits two distinct types of manifestations of DCS: (a) a transient pruritus involving ears, trunk, wrists, and hands (more common after exposure in hyperbaric chambers) and (b) a more intense itching, usually limited to the trunk, that begins as erythema (from dermal vasodilation) and progresses to a characteristic mottling with confluent rings of pallor surrounding areas of cyanosis. This lesion blanches to the touch and is known as *cutis marmorate*. These changes are thought to result from bubble obstruction of the skin's venous drainage or bubble-induced vasospasm [1]. These abnormalities generally resolve spontaneously over a few days. Importantly, *cutis marmorate* is considered a manifestation of type II DCS and treated as such.

Type II Decompression Sickness

Type II DCS may occur separately or in combination with the musculoskeletal pain of type I DCS in up to 30% of patients [1,2,6]. The primary organ systems affected in this category are pulmonary, nervous, and vestibular.

Pulmonary DCS, known as "the chokes," occurs rarely in diving (approximately 2% of the overall cases [1]), and it is generally the result of very rapid or emergency-type ascents. Aviators, astronauts, and submarine trainees are also in situations in which sudden dramatic decompression may occur, and pulmonary DCS has been noted in nearly 6% in these groups [1]. Clinically, this condition usually begins with a substernal discomfort that starts within minutes of reaching the surface. As it progresses, the discomfort may take on a respirophasic nature. The respiratory pattern becomes more rapid and shallow, with occasional paroxysms of a nonproductive cough. Evidence of right heart strain or failure may develop and may progress to full-blown cardiovascular collapse. The underlying mechanism involves both direct and indirect effects of massive pulmonary gas embolization from VGE.

Neurologic DCS has a varied incidence among different populations [1]. A wide range of possible presenting signs and symptoms may be produced by neurologic DCS, and all must be taken seriously even when there are no objective findings on neurologic examination. The spectrum of neurologic dysfunction ranges from pruritus with skin rash or "pins and needles" sensation (15% of cases) to full paralysis (6%) or convulsions (1%) and death. Personality changes and agitation occur in 3%, but they are very rarely the presenting symptoms. Visual disturbances (7%) and difficulties with cerebellar function (18%) are also frequently seen. The pathogenesis underlying CNS injury from DCS is the subject of much debate and controversy. Most researchers would agree that the notion of CNS tissue ischemia arising from obstructing arterial gas bubbles is too simplistic. As mentioned previously, the endothelial dysfunction hypothesis is currently under investigation as a better candidate mechanism to explain the varied manifestations of DCS.

Vestibular DCS, "the staggers," occurs relatively commonly as the initial manifestation of DCS, and it comprises a syndrome of nausea, vomiting, dizziness, and nystagmus. Frequently, tinnitus or hearing loss may also be present. Typical onset is immediately after decompression, and it occurs in 13% to 72% of patients with type II DCS. The underlying pathology has been demonstrated in animals to be the result of rupture of the fragile membranes in the cochlea and semicircular canals.

Treatment

Prompt Recognition and Diagnosis

The most common problem in DCS and AGE is making the initial diagnosis. Particularly in the case of DCS, there is an early tendency by patients for denial of the existence of any problems. Any neurologic or cardiorespiratory symptoms after diving must be assumed to relate to AGE or DCS until proven otherwise.

Stabilization

Nonspecific therapy may help to stabilize the patient and prevent an extension of injury. Immediate institution of cardiopulmonary resuscitation may be needed, and it takes precedence over all other measures. Endotracheal intubation is sometimes necessary to ensure patency and protection of the airway. All balloon cuffs (endotracheal and Foley) should be inflated with sterile water rather than air to minimize the volume changes of these compartments during recompression therapy.

When AGE is suspected, most authorities recommend the flat, supine position initially. If the patient is unconscious or vomiting, the left lateral decubitus (Durant) position is also recommended. The Trendelenburg position is no longer advocated with the concern that maintaining this body position for extended periods may worsen any associated cerebral edema, and the knowledge that keeping the head lower than the heart does not prevent migration of bubbles into the cerebral circulation unless the patient is in total circulatory arrest or an extremely low-output state [1].

Once any life-threatening concerns have been addressed, administration of 100% O_2 and the maintenance of intravascular volume become the next most important features of treatment while arranging transport to a hyperbaric facility. The 100% O_2 can be delivered intermittently or continuously for extended periods (generally up to 12 hours) without serious concern for any resulting significant pulmonary toxicity. The high fraction of inspired O_2 is used to alleviate any tissue hypoxia and to provide a strong concentration gradient that will wash out as much inert gas as rapidly as possible. Note that if the symptoms of AGE or DCS resolve or are improved after breathing 100% O_2, the patient will still require recompression therapy.

As a result of capillary endothelial injury, the more severe the DCS syndrome, the greater the magnitude of plasma leakage from the vascular space, the reduction in blood volume, and the resultant hemoconcentration [1]. Increased blood viscosity resulting from hemoconcentration may further impair any compromised microcirculation; therefore, normovolemia should be the goal of infusion therapy. Fluids should be administered to all individuals suffering from DCS except for cardiopulmonary DCS ("the chokes") owing to concerns for exacerbating any pulmonary edema injury. In addition, because patients who suffer AGE are typically less dehydrated than those with DCS and because CNS injury in AGE may be complicated by cerebral edema, care should be taken not to overload the patient with AGE. Intravascular volume maintenance can be achieved with isotonic fluids given at a rate sufficient to keep the urine output at 0.5 to 1 mL/kg/h or more, and is recommended for patients who are vomiting, unconscious, or having any symptoms more severe than isolated limb bends. Glucose-containing solutions are probably best avoided in the first 12 hours after suspected cerebral embolization because an increased serum glucose level is one of the major determinants of the brain's lactate production, which has been associated with increased neuronal damage in the ischemic state [1]. Conscious patients may be given judicious amounts of oral liquids, such as nonacidic fruit juices or balanced electrolyte solutions. Alcohol-containing beverages should be strictly avoided.

When the diagnosis of cerebral air embolism is evident on clinical grounds, comprehensive diagnostic testing is not necessary. Diagnostic testing should never delay transport to a facility equipped to provide HBO therapy or initiation of this specific therapy. If HBO is not immediately available, a noncontrast head computed tomography scan, chest radiography, and an ECG should be obtained while awaiting transport. For coma as a result of AGE or DCS, the head computed tomography will typically reveal multiple, small, well-defined, low-density areas in the brain. Head computed tomography scanning is also useful in ruling out possible correctable causes of intracerebral bleeding. Magnetic resonance imaging and single-photon emission tomography techniques, where available, are likewise potentially useful to document the presence of cerebral gas collections. Because these tests are highly insensitive, negative studies alone should never deny patients' access to HBO therapy in the appropriate clinical situation.

Patient Transport

When air evacuation is necessary to transfer a patient to a recompression facility, it is of utmost importance that the patient not be exposed to any further decreases in barometric pressure, as occurs with travel at increasing altitudes. In general, unless the aircraft is capable of maintaining a cabin pressure equivalent to sea-level pressure, flight altitude should not exceed 500 to 1,000 ft. above the departure point because deaths have resulted from exposure to altitudes of only 4,000 to 5,000 ft. [1,14]. It is believed to be preferable to await the arrival of a pressurized transport than to risk exposing a patient with DCS or AGE to further hypobaric insult.

To obtain a listing of the nearest recompression facility as well as advice on treatment options from a medical diving specialist on a 24-hour emergency basis, contact the Divers Alert Network Emergency Hotline at Duke University at (919) 684-9111. For nonemergency questions during regular business hours, contact the DAN Medical Information Line at (919) 684-2948.

Adjunctive Therapy

To date, other than supplemental O_2, there are no drugs of proven benefit for treating DCS or AGE. There is an unfortunate paucity of randomized controlled trials to guide treatment options. Several agents are used frequently, but this therapy is primarily based on expert opinion and limited trials involving small numbers of animal and human subjects [1,15]. For a discussion of the use of oxygen and fluids, see "Stabilization" section. As noted previously, there are some small but important differences in the recommendations for adjunctive therapies between AGE and DCS, and these will be briefly addressed below.

Steroids. Steroids are no longer recommended for the treatment of AGE or DCS.

Lidocaine. Lidocaine is not currently recommended for the treatment of any type of DCS. Clinical evidence does support its use for the treatment of AGE (reduces cerebral metabolism and stabilizes neural membranes by decreasing the flux of sodium and potassium) [2]. Lidocaine may be given as a 0.5 to 1 mg per kg intravenous bolus at a rate of 25 to 50 mg per minute, followed by 0.5 mg per kg intravenously every 5 to 10 minutes as needed, to a maximum total of 225 mg or 3 mg per kg, whichever is lower. Patients with hypotension, cardiac arrest, or biventricular heart failure should receive only a single loading dose of 100 mg. After the loading doses, a continuous intravenous infusion at 2 to 4 mg per minute may be used to achieve and maintain a blood level of 2 to 4 µg per mL. If an intravenous infusion cannot be established, intramuscular administration of 4 to 5 mg per kg will typically produce therapeutic plasma concentrations within 15 minutes and lasting for approximately 90 minutes. Supratherapeutic doses may be associated with paresthesias, ataxia, and seizures.

Diazepam. Intravenous diazepam is effective in the control of seizures, severe agitation, and the intractable vomiting resulting from "the staggers." The typical regimen is a 5-mg intravenous bolus given over 3 minutes and then repeated every 5 minutes as needed (maximum dose, 20 to 30 mg) to control seizures. If intravenous access is not available, the intravenous preparation may be given rectally to adults in a dose of 7.5 to 10 mg every 5 minutes as needed. Diazepam is not recommended for use prophylactically in AGE or DCS because of its sedative properties and its propensity to mask the onset of CNS toxicity, thus affecting the ability to assess response to hyperbaric treatment. Generalized seizures unresponsive to benzodiazepine therapy may be suppressed with barbiturates [1,15].

Anticoagulants. Anticoagulants should not be used routinely in the treatment of AGE or DCS. The exception to this is the patient suffering from lower extremity weakness or paralysis. In these cases, low molecular weight heparin should be initiated as soon as possible after injury to reduce the risk of deep venous thrombosis (DVT) and pulmonary embolism. Enoxaparin 30 mg, or its equivalent, is given subcutaneously every 12 hours. Intermittent pneumatic compression is an alternative although less effective for preventing DVT [2].

Aspirin and other Nonsteroidal Anti-inflammatories. Routine use of agents with antiplatelet effects is not recommended in AGE or DCS owing to concerns for worsening any neurologic hemorrhage.

Antipyretic Therapies. Any AGE or DCS with evidence of brain or spinal cord injury should receive aggressive treatment for elevated body temperature to prevent further neurologic insult [2].

Until further studies are performed, discretionary therapy with these adjunctive agents should be considered the realm of "clinical judgment" and "expert opinion." Evidence-based recommendations await results from further controlled trials.

Hyperbaric Therapy

Hyperbaric therapy involves exposing the entire body to prolonged periods of higher than atmospheric pressure; it specifically treats AGE and DCS [1,2,16]. Anecdotal reports of success in isobarically occurring AGE lends credence to the recommendation for early consideration of HBO therapy for any suspected cerebral gas embolism [1]. Many treatment protocols have been proposed [17,18], and none would be expected to be fully efficacious and life sustaining for all cases. As of 2015, no randomized controlled human studies exist that compare these different treatment options. A review of the pertinent literature on humans since the 1960s reveals a decrease in cerebral air embolism mortality from 93% for those not receiving therapy to 28% to 33% with closed-chest massage and "conventional therapy," and then to 7% with addition of HBO [1], and would seem to argue strongly for this modality for AGE.

Fully 80% to 90% of all patients with DCS or AGE effectively respond to recompression therapy [1,6,18]. Although there is generally an inverse relationship between any delay to treatment and complete symptom resolution, evidence supports the use of HBO for AGE and DCS even after delays of more than 24 hours. Delays of initiating recompression therapy for up to 10 days have been anecdotally reported in the literature to be successful in up to 90% of these patients [1]. Recompression treatments may be repeated as needed until symptoms resolve entirely or until improvement reaches a plateau and there is no further improvement [2,6]. Approximately 40% of injured divers show complete resolution after the first treatment, and only 20% require more than three rounds of recompression therapy [2,6].

The mechanism of action of HBO therapy involves a decrease in volume of any gas-filled spaces and resorption of bubbles back into body fluids. This process presumably results in a diminution of tissue distortion, resolution of vascular compromise, and reduced bubble–endothelial surface contact. HBO therapy should be undertaken for at least 4 hours because elimination of bubbles may be reduced in areas of poor flow where sludging and edema exist [1]. It must be remembered that recompression acts only on the primary cause of these syndromes and not necessarily on any of the secondary effects that may result (e.g., endothelial dysfunction, activation of the inflammatory cascade).

Hyperoxygenation results from a markedly enhanced arterial O_2 content, primarily from O_2 dissolving more readily into the plasma. Although the oxyhemoglobin dissociation curve remains unchanged, the arterial partial pressure of O_2 may reach 2,000 mm Hg on a fractional inspired oxygen concentration of 100% and an ambient pressure of 3 ATA [1,19]. In the clinical setting, however, these high plasma O_2 concentrations are never transmitted fully to the tissue level as a result of progressive arteriolar vasoconstriction from the disease process itself, as well as a direct effect from the increasing O_2 concentration. Local tissue perfusion, although reduced further by HBO, is still sufficient to cause supranormal tissue partial pressure of O_2 levels of approximately 500 mm Hg. HBO allows the delivery of nearly 60 mL of oxygen per L of blood (vs. 3 mL per L at atmospheric pressure), a rate sufficient to support resting tissues just on the basis of the O_2 dissolved in solution alone. In practice, the physiologic effects of high concentrations of O_2 to induce generation of O_2 free radicals and pulmonary O_2 toxicity necessitates that periods of hyperoxygenation be alternated with periods of lower fraction of inspired O_2 breathing to avoid potentially severe complications [1,2,17,19].

Opinions regarding the optimal hyperbaric regimen for AGE and DCS have varied in terms of the simulated depth (i.e., pressure) required, recompression time necessary, and inspired gas concentrations used. Common recompression guidelines in use today include US Navy Treatment Tables 5, 6 and 6A. Tables 6 and 6A are illustrated in Figure 177.2 and Table 177.5 [1,2,17]. Other popular recompression tables in use worldwide include COMEX Table 30 and Royal Navy Tables 71 and 72 [6].

Hyperbaric treatment recommendations for DCS are loosely based on the general category of illness patterns described previously [1,2,17]. In general, those patients with type I "pain-only" DCS (except for *cutis marmorate*) are generally in

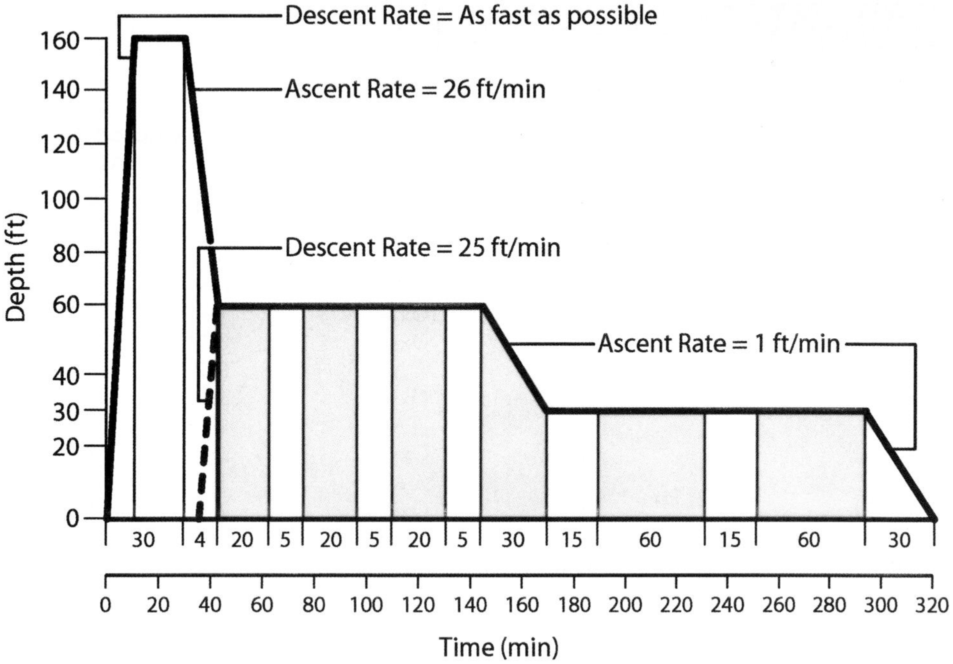

FIGURE 177.2 US Navy Treatment Tables 6 and 6A. Treatment Table 6A is shown in its entirety and is used when symptoms are suspected to be as a result of arterial gas embolism or severe decompression sickness. Treatment Table 6 is superimposed (starting at *dotted line*) and is seen to begin with a simulated pressure descent on 100% fractional concentration of oxygen to 60 ft. at a rate of 25 ft. per minute. Thereafter, the tables are the same. Treatment Table 6 is recommended for treatment of type II or type I decompression sickness when symptoms are not relieved within 10 minutes at 60 ft. Nonshaded areas are periods of breathing room air. Shaded areas are periods of breathing 100% fractional concentration of oxygen. Individual time periods are shown first, with total elapsed time indicated underneath. [Adapted from U.S. Navy Diving Manual, Washington, DC, Department of the Navy, 2008, NAVSEA Technical Manual, Volume 5, Chapter 20. Revision 6; and Wilson MM, Curley FJ: Gas embolism: part II. Arterial gas embolism and decompression sickness. *J Intensive Care Med* 11:261, 1996, with permission.]

a more stable medical condition on arrival to a recompression facility; therefore, more time is available to perform a thorough and detailed physical examination before chamber treatment. Particular emphasis should be placed on the neurologic examination so that serial examinations can document the presence of any subtle findings that can be used to monitor the response to therapy. If type I DCS subjects have complete relief of symptoms within the first 10 minutes of recompression at a pressure of 2.8 ATA (equivalent to 60 ft seawater), US Navy Treatment Table 5 (basically a shortened version of US Navy Table 6) is appropriate [2].

Subjects with type I DCS with an inadequate response to initial recompression at 2.8 ATA, the presence of *cutis marmorate* or with any neurologic abnormality, no matter how subtle (i.e., type II DCS or AGE), requires initial treatment according to at least US Navy Treatment Table 6 [2]. This would allow for more optimal therapy of any developing neurologic deficits, and it would, therefore, be expected to decrease the overall occurrence of progression to type II DCS.

Extensive clinical experience has found no objective benefits to starting recompression at levels greater than 2.8 ATA [1,17]. Consensus opinion now recommends that subjects experiencing type II DCS or AGE who have an improvement of symptoms within the first O_2 breathing period (20 minutes) should continue recompression therapy using Treatment Table 6 [2]. If instead, these same subjects have symptoms that are unchanged or worsen within 20 minutes of recompression on air at 2.8 ATA, additional recompression on air to a depth equivalent to cause symptom relief or significant improvement (not to exceed 6 ATA or 165-feet seawater pressure) is performed. These subjects then follow Treatment Table 6A [2]. For patients who do not respond adequately to standard protocols, extension periods or change to other established protocols might be indicated and are decided on an individual basis [1,2,17].

Prevention

There are a limited number of time-tested recommendations that can be made in an effort to minimize the occurrence of DCS. These would include (a) following prescribed "no-decompression" limit diving profiles that factor in the duration of time spent at specific depths and duration of surface intervals between repetitive dives; (b) limiting ascent rates from depth to speeds slower than the ascent rate of the diver's exhaled air bubbles; and (c) avoiding any hypobaric insults in the postdive period with no flying for at least 12 hours in all divers, delay in flying for 24 hours or more if a dive profile included any mandatory decompression stops, and finally, flying should be prohibited for at least 72 hours after recompression therapy has been administered for DCS or AGE. As alluded to earlier, hypobaric stresses in these instances may result in new onset of one of these syndromes or for the recurrence of one of these previously treated disorders.

Extensive ongoing research is underway to evaluate the potential preventative roles of predive aerobic exercise [20,21], during-dive exercise [22,23], exogenous nitric oxide [21,24], predive normobaric O_2 [25], and predive hyperbaric O_2 [26,27]. These preconditioning agents are hypothesized to upregulate endogenous antioxidants, moderate inflammatory injury, and/or inhibit reperfusion injury. All studies have noted the existence of substantial variability among individuals in the degree of bubble formation detected and the resultant incidence of DCS.

The higher-than-expected incidence of PFO among divers with severe or unexplained DCS suggests an increased risk for DCS in the presence of a PFO and raises the question that PFO closure procedures may represent another possible avenue of prevention of AGE and DCS. While it has been shown by small studies that PFO closure can decrease or eliminate the arterialization of VGE [28], available data does not confirm that PFO closure

TABLE 177.5

Depth and Time Profiles for US Navy Treatment Tables 6 and 6A

Simulated depth (ft)	Time (min)	Breathing medium	Total elapsed time (h:min) 6A	6
165	30	Air	0:30	—
165–60	4	Air	0:34	—
(0–60)[a]	(2.4)	(Oxygen)	(—)	0:02
60	20	Oxygen	0:54	0:22
60	5	Air	0:59	0:27
60	20	Oxygen	1:19	0:47
60	5	Air	1:24	0:52
60	20	Oxygen	1:44	1:12
60	5	Air	1:49	1:17
60–30	30	Oxygen	2:19	1:47
30	15	Air	2:34	2:02
30	60	Oxygen	3:34	3:02
30	15	Air	3:49	3:17
30	60	Oxygen	4:49	4:17
30–0	30	Oxygen	5:19	4:47

[a]Parentheses indicate profile when following the dotted line in Figure 177.2. This applies *only* to Table 6 profile and is not used when following Table 6A profile.

procedures reduce the incidence of DCS [13,28,29]. Further, the risk–benefit assessment for surgical or catheter-delivered PFO closure procedures is still debated. The reported risk for serious complications from PFO closure procedures is estimated at 1% or higher, which is an order of magnitude greater than the risk of DCS or AGE for recreational divers. Current consensus is that routine screening for PFO is not warranted for the general diving population. Screening (following a strict protocol) can be considered for certain high-risk subgroups for DCS or AGE (e.g., those with prior DCS or AGE events; family history of PFO or atrial septal defect; divers who perform heavy exertions at deeper depths or repetitive dives). PFO closure can be offered on an individual basis for those who desire to continue higher risk dive profiles. Avoidance of risk is generally a better option than attempts at risk mitigation or cure after the fact.

References

1. Wilson MM: Gas embolism syndromes: venous gas emboli, arterial gas emboli and decompression sickness, in: Irwin RS, Rippe JM (eds): *Intensive Care Medicine*, 7th ed, Philadelphia, Wolters Kluwer/Lippincott Williams & Wilkins, 2012, pp 669–683.
2. US Navy Department: *U.S. Navy Diving Manual. Rev. 6, Vol. 5. Diagnosis and Treatment of Decompression Sickness and Arterial Gas Embolism. Publication no. NAVSEA 0910-LP-106-0957*. Washington, DC, US Navy Department, 2008. Available at: www.usu.edu/scuba/navy_manual6.pdf
3. Madden LA, Laden G: Gas bubbles may not be the underlying cause of decompression illness—the at-depth endothelial dysfunction hypothesis. *Med Hypotheses* 72:389–392, 2009.
4. Mollerlokken A, Gaustad SE, Havnes MB, et al: Venous gas embolism as a predictive tool for improving CNS decompression safety. *Eur J Appl Physiol* 112:401–409, 2012.
5. Bessereau J, Genotelle N, Chabbaut C, et al: Long-term outcome of iatrogenic gas embolism. *Intensive Care Med* 36:1180–1187, 2010.
6. Divers Alert Network: DAN Annual Diving Report 2012–2015 Edition. A report on 2010–2013 data on diving fatalities, injuries, and incidents. Durham, NC, Divers Alert Network, 2015. Available at www.diversalertnetwork.org
7. Hall J: The risks of scuba diving: a focus on decompression illness. *Hawai'i J Med Public Health* 73(11):13–16, 2014.
8. Bove AA: Diving medicine. *Am J Resp and Crit Care Med* 189:1479–1486, 2014.
9. Foster PP, Butler BD: Decompression to altitude: assumptions, experimental evidence, and future directions. *J Appl Physiol* 106:678–690, 2009.
10. Lairez O, Cournot M, Minville V, et al: Risk of neurological decompression sickness in the diver with right-to-left shunt: literature review and meta-analysis. *Clin J Sport Med* 19:231–235, 2009.
11. Liou K, Wolfers D, Turner R, et al: Patent foramen ovale influences the presentation of decompression illness in SCUBA divers. *Heart Lung Circ* 24:26–31, 2015.
12. Billinger M, Zbinden R, Mordasini R, et al: Patent foramen ovale closure in recreational divers: effect on decompression illness and ischaemic brain lesions during long-term follow-up. *Heart* 97:1932–1937, 2011.
13. Bove AA: The PFO gets blamed again...perhaps this time it is real. *JACC: Cardiovasc Interv* 7:409–410, 2014.
14. MacDonald RD, O'Donnell C, Allan GM: Interfacility transport of patients with decompression illness: literature review and consensus statement. *Prehosp Emerg Care* 10:482–487, 2006.
15. Bennett MH, Lehm JP, Mitchell SJ, et al: Recompression and adjunctive therapy for decompression illness: A systematic review of randomized controlled trials. *Anesth Analg* 111:757–762, 2010.
16. Vann RD, Butler FK, Mitchell SJ, et al: Decompression illness. *Lancet* 377:153–164, 2010.
17. Antonelli C, Franchi E, Della Marta ME, et al: Guiding principles in choosing a therapeutic table for DCI hyperbaric therapy. *Minerva Anesthesiol* 75:151–161, 2009.
18. Cianci P, Slade JB Jr: Delayed treatment of decompression sickness with shunt, no-air-break tables: review of 140 cases. *Aviat Space Environ Med* 77:1003–1008, 2006.
19. Thom SR: Hyperbaric oxygen: its mechanisms and efficacy. *Plast Reconstr Surg* 127:S131–S141, 2011.
20. Dujic Z, Duplancic D, Marinovic-Terzic I, et al: Aerobic exercise before diving reduces venous gas bubble formation in humans. *J Physiol* 555:637–642, 2004.
21. Wisloff U, Richardson RS, Brubakk AO: Exercise and nitric oxide prevent bubble formation: a novel approach to the prevention of decompression sickness? *J Physiol* 555:825–829, 2004.
22. Jankowski LW, Tikuisis P, Nishi RY: Exercise effects during diving and decompression on postdive venous gas emboli. *Aviat Space Environ Med* 75:489–495, 2004.
23. Dujic D, Palada I, Obad A, et al: Exercise during a 3-min decompression stop reduces postdive venous gas bubbles. *Med Sci Sports Exerc* 37:1319–1323, 2005.
24. Dujic D, Palada I, Zoran V, et al: Exogenous nitric oxide and bubble formation in divers. *Med Sci Sports Exerc* 38:1432–1435, 2006.
25. Castagna O, Gempp E, Blatteau J-E: Pre-dive normobaric oxygen reduces bubble formation in scuba divers. *Eur J Appl Physiol* 106:167–172, 2009.
26. Butler BD, Little T, Cogan V, et al: Hyperbaric oxygen pre-breathe modifies the outcome of decompression sickness. *Undersea Hyperb Med* 33:407–417, 2006.
27. Katsenelson K, Arieli Y, Abramovich A, et al: Hyperbaric oxygen pretreatment reduces the incidence of decompression sickness in rats. *Eur J Appl Physiol* 101:571–576, 2007.
28. Honek J, Sramek M, Sefc L, et al: Effect of catheter-based patent foramen ovale closure on the occurrence of arterial bubbles in scuba divers. *JACC: Cardiovasc Interv* 7:403–408, 2014.
29. Madden D, Ljubkovic M, Dujic Z: Intrapulmonary shunt and SCUBA diving: another risk factor? *Echocardiography* 32:S205–S210, 2015.

Chapter 178 ■ Acute Inhalation Injury

ANNA NOLAN • MICHAEL D. WEIDEN • LAWRENCE C. MOHR, JR • DAVID J. PREZANT

OVERVIEW

Chemicals are a main component of most industrial processes. These industries generate many trillion dollars of economic activity in the United States and Europe and are integral to many local economies. Owing to the close proximity of these industries, communities must be equipped to medically manage acute exposures. If inhaled, many have the potential to cause asphyxiation or life-threatening acute lung injury. Although recent events have increased concern that toxic gases may be used as weapons of mass destruction, accidental exposures remain the greatest health threat [1]. Individuals may be exposed to the accidental release of toxic gases in the workplace [2] or in the general environment, including the home [1].

Smoke inhalation is another major cause of acute inhalation injury [3]. Thousands of individuals are smoke inhalation victims each year, having been exposed to toxic gases and airborne particulate matter from the burning of a variety of materials [4]. Smoke inhalation most commonly occurs as a result of industrial or residential fires, where large amounts of carbon monoxide (CO), hydrogen cyanide (HCN), hydrogen chloride, acrolein, sulfur dioxide, phosgene, and other toxic, irritant gases are produced and released into the environment in various respirable forms (Table 178.1).

Toxic agents can be inhaled in several different forms or physical states. A gas at standard temperature and pressure has the ability for its molecules to diffuse freely and be distributed uniformly throughout any container. The density of a gas is expressed relative to air. The denser the gas, the heavier it is. Gases that are denser than air will typically gravitate to low areas. Cold gases are denser than the same gas at higher temperatures. A vapor is a substance in the gaseous state that normally exists as a liquid or solid and is formed when a substance is heated above its critical temperature, which is the temperature at which it cannot be liquefied regardless of the amount of pressure. A fog is a liquid aerosol formed by condensation of a substance from a gaseous to a liquid state. Dusts are fine particles of a solid organic or an inorganic material that are small enough to be airborne, typically ranging from 0.1 to 25.0 μm in diameter. Fumes are extremely fine solid particles that are dispersed into the air by the combustion or melting of solid materials, particularly metals. Fumes usually consist of particles that range from 0.001 to 1.0 μm in diameter. Smoke consists of airborne particles resulting from the incomplete combustion of organic materials. These particles either contain or are coated with multiple chemical substances resulting from combustion and range in size from less than 0.3 μm to greater than 10 μm in diameter.

The nature of the acute injury will depend on the chemical and physical properties of the inhaled toxicant, the pathophysiologic mechanism by which the toxicant causes injury, the dose received, and whether prior pulmonary disease exists. This chapter focuses on the diagnosis and treatment of acute inhalation injury resulting from asphyxiant gases, toxic irritant gases, and smoke.

ASPHYXIANT GASES

Background

Asphyxiants cause tissue hypoxia. They are classified as either *simple* or *chemical asphyxiants* based on their mechanism of toxicity. Simple asphyxiants displace or dilute oxygen in the ambient atmospheric air, causing a decrease in the fraction of oxygen in inspired air (FiO_2). Chemical asphyxiants, on the other hand, interfere with physiologic processes associated with the uptake, transport, or utilization of oxygen. Simple asphyxiants include common gases such as carbon dioxide, natural gas, propane, methane, nitrogen, and acetylene. They may be lighter or heavier than air (Table 178.2). Simple asphyxiants that are lighter than air accumulate and displace oxygen in higher areas first, whereas those that are heavier than air accumulate and displace oxygen in low-lying areas first. Chemical asphyxiants can be further characterized as those that decrease oxygen-carrying capacity, such as carbon monoxide, and those that inhibit oxygen utilization by cells, such as HCN (Table 178.3). Medical problems related to the inhalation of the most common asphyxiants are discussed in the subsequent sections.

Carbon Dioxide

Pathophysiology

Carbon dioxide (CO_2) is the most common simple asphyxiant. It is produced by aerobic metabolism and is exhaled into the atmosphere by humans and other animals. It is also a by-product of carbohydrate fermentation, the combustion of carbonaceous material, and the oxidation of coal contaminants. It has many uses such as for cooling, fire extinguishing, hydrofracking, and when used for cooling in the solid form is known as dry ice [5].

TABLE 178.1

Toxic Products of Combustion in Residential Fires

Acetaldehyde	Hydrogen fluoride
Acrolein	Hydrogen sulfide
Ammonia	Isocyanates
Carbon monoxide	Metals (Pb, Zn, Mn, Cd, Co)
Chlorine	Oxides of nitrogen
Hydrogen chloride	Phosgene
Hydrogen cyanide	Sulfur dioxide

TABLE 178.2

Simple Asphyxiants

Heavier than air	Lighter than air
Argon	Acetylene
Butane	Ethylene
Carbon dioxide	Methane
Ethane	Neon
Natural gas	Nitrogen
Propane	

TABLE 178.3

Chemical Asphyxiants

Agents that decrease oxygen-carrying capacity
Carbon monoxide
Hydrogen sulfide
Oxides of nitrogen
Agents that inhibit cellular oxygen utilization
Acrylonitrile
Hydrogen cyanide
Hydrogen sulfide

CO_2 is heavier than air and reduces FiO_2 simply by diluting and displacing oxygen in ambient air. The National Institute of Occupational Safety and Health occupational standards for CO_2 are 5,000 ppm for an 8-hour time weighted average, and 30,000 ppm for a 15 minute short-term exposure limit [5]. However, studies investigating the effect of CO_2 at lower concentrations show that even at 1,000 ppm, a level often exceeded in classrooms in California and Texas, cognition and mentation can be significantly affected [6]. Most deaths from CO_2 asphyxiation result from the confinement of an individual in a poorly ventilated space. Such closed-space confinement prevents air with a normal FiO_2 from entering while exhaled CO_2 is accumulating and displacing oxygen inside. Simple asphyxiation from CO_2 has also been reported from environmental exposures. In 1986, for example, simple asphyxiation caused approximately 1,700 deaths from a cloudy mist of CO_2 and water droplets that rose suddenly from a lake in Cameroon [7]. Asphyxiation from CO_2 has also been reported by off-gassing from dry ice in a confined space [8,9].

In general, once the ambient CO_2 increases to the point where the FiO_2 has decreased to 0.15, acute signs and symptoms of hypoxia begin to appear within minutes. These include dyspnea, tachypnea, tachycardia, confusion, incoordination, and dizziness. As the FiO_2 decreases below 0.10, lethargy or coma may develop as a result of cerebral edema, and cardiopulmonary arrest may occur. Brain damage sustained as a result of extensive cerebral edema or prolonged hypoxia may be permanent in individuals with these conditions who are resuscitated and survive. It is unlikely that life can be sustained for more than several minutes with a FiO_2 less than 0.06 [10].

Diagnosis and Management

CO_2 asphyxiation should be considered for any patient who presents with clinical signs of hypoxia, is unconscious, or is found to be in cardiopulmonary arrest after removal from an enclosed space or another source of potential CO_2 exposure. Clinical signs are nonspecific and related to the magnitude of hypoxia, as indicated earlier. Arterial blood gases, serum electrolytes, and measurement of the anion gap should be obtained. During and shortly after CO_2 asphyxiation, arterial blood gas analysis would be expected to show decreased arterial oxygen tension (PaO_2) and elevated carbon dioxide tension ($PaCO_2$). However, both PaO_2 and $PaCO_2$ typically return to normal shortly after the patient is removed from the source of CO_2 exposure. Once the patient breathes oxygenated air, CO_2 is rapidly excreted by hyperventilation. Most patients will be acidotic at the time of presentation as a result of respiratory acidosis from CO_2 retention and concurrent lactic acidosis from hypoxia. Lactic acidosis will cause an elevated anion gap. The respiratory acidosis typically resolves shortly after removal from the source of CO_2 exposure. The lactic acidosis will resolve once tissue oxygenation returns to normal but usually takes longer to resolve than the respiratory acidosis. The hypoxia caused by CO_2 asphyxiation can cause cardiac dysrhythmias and myocardial infarction, especially for individuals with underlying heart disease. Canine models of acute exposure to lethal levels of CO_2 show hypoxia, acidosis, and severe hypokalemia [5]. Possible electrocardiographic changes include inverted T-waves, depressed ST segments, and prominent U-waves. Therefore, it is recommended that an electrocardiogram and serial cardiac biomarkers be obtained for all patients.

Removal from the source of exposure and administration of oxygen are the only specific therapies for CO_2 asphyxiation. If the patient is alert, has spontaneous respirations, and has a patent airway, it is recommended that high-flow oxygen be administered by a nonrebreather mask. Endotracheal intubation will be required if adequate oxygenation cannot be achieved by the use of a face mask or the patient has suffered mental status changes or cardiopulmonary arrest. Additional supportive care, such as cardiopulmonary resuscitation, hemodynamic support, and mechanical ventilation should be used as required by the patient's overall condition. Cardiac dysrhythmias and myocardial infarction should be aggressively treated. Most victims of CO_2 asphyxiation will recover completely if removed from the source of CO_2 exposure prior to cardiopulmonary arrest and given medical treatment as soon as possible. Individuals who have experienced a prolonged period of hypoxia, however, may have irreversible brain damage and chronic neurologic sequelae even after they are successfully resuscitated.

Carbon Monoxide

Pathophysiology

Carbon monoxide (CO) is a colorless, odorless, tasteless, nonirritating gas. It is the most common chemical asphyxiant and the second most common atmospheric pollutant after CO_2. CO is produced in a variety of ways, including incomplete combustion from fires, faulty heating systems, internal combustion engines (including gas-powered generators placed in poorly ventilated areas during electrical failures), wood stoves, charcoal grills, volcanic eruptions, and a variety of industrial processes. Hepatic production of CO occurs with poisoning from methylene chloride that is commonly found in paint thinners and is easily absorbed through the skin.

More than 5,000 deaths are attributed to CO poisoning in the United States each year [11]. Most are intentional from exposures to motor vehicle exhaust. The minority are accidental and caused by fires or the use of poorly ventilated generators following storms, blackouts, or other disasters [12,13]. CO poisoning is responsible for 80% of fatalities related to smoke inhalation [14]. Twenty-five percent of fatalities from CO poisoning occur in persons with underlying cardiopulmonary disease [15].

CO easily diffuses across alveolar-capillary membranes in the lung and is rapidly taken up by erythrocytes in the pulmonary capillary blood. It binds to the iron moiety of hemoglobin with an affinity that is approximately 240 times greater than the affinity of hemoglobin for oxygen. Thus, CO competes with oxygen for hemoglobin binding sites and, as a result of its greater affinity, displaces oxygen from hemoglobin. The binding of CO to the iron moiety also creates an allosteric change in the hemoglobin molecule that inhibits the off-loading of oxygen in the peripheral tissues and causes a shift of the oxyhemoglobin dissociation curve to the left. CO also interferes with intracellular oxygen utilization by inactivating intracellular respiratory enzymes, such as cytochrome oxidase [16]. Thus, the cumulative effect on peripheral oxygen delivery and utilization is greater than that expected from decreased oxygen transport alone. Reoxygenation injury of the brain has also been described [17]. One mechanism for reoxygenation injury appears to be lipid peroxidation of the brain by xanthine oxidase that is generated by peroxidases and reactive oxygen species produced by activated neutrophils that become sequestered in the microvasculature of the brain following, but not during, CO poisoning [18]. In summary, CO toxicity involves four pathophysiologic mechanisms: (a) a decrease in the oxygen-carrying capacity of blood; (b) decreased oxygen delivery to peripheral tissues as a result of the left shift in the oxyhemoglobin dissociation curve; (c) mitochondrial dysfunction and impairment of cellular respiration by inhibition of cytochrome oxidase activity; and (d) lipid peroxidation of the brain during reoxygenation. Lipid peroxidation leads to reversible demyelination in areas of the central nervous system, including corpus callosum, the internal/external capsule, optic tracts, and periventricular parenchyma [12].

The presentation of individuals with CO poisoning is highly variable with nonspecific symptoms and signs that are loosely correlated to carboxyhemoglobin levels (Table 178.4). Early symptoms of CO poisoning include headache, dizziness, sore throat, nausea, shortness of breath, and fatigue. These symptoms can mimic those of a nonspecific viral syndrome, especially when an entire family is affected from CO exposure related to a faulty home heating system during the winter months. Impaired ability to concentrate occurs in more than half of affected individuals, and 6% have been reported to experience loss of consciousness. The severity of symptoms appears to correlate better with duration of exposure than with carboxyhemoglobin levels [19]. The brain and heart are very sensitive to CO intoxication, and both neurologic and cardiovascular impairment predominate with prolonged exposures. Mental status changes, and seizures, sudden loss of consciousness, tachypnea, tachycardia, cardiac dysrhythmias, hypotension, and myocardial ischemia are likely to occur when the carboxyhemoglobin concentration exceeds 20%. Cardiovascular disorders may occur at lower concentrations among subjects with preexisting cardiopulmonary diseases. Evidence of myocardial ischemia has been observed in one-third of individuals with moderate to severe CO intoxication, and it has recently been reported that myocardial injury, as determined by elevation of serial cardiac biomarkers, is an independent predictor of mortality from CO poisoning [15,20,21]. Metabolic acidosis, owing to increased lactate production from anaerobic metabolism, is a common consequence of tissue hypoxia. Rhabdomyolysis can occur as a consequence of impaired aerobic metabolism in skeletal muscle cells. Renal failure can develop as a consequence of rhabdomyolysis, but this occurs infrequently [22]. Carbon monoxide poisoning is almost always fatal when the carboxyhemoglobin concentration exceeds 60% [14,23].

Fetal hemoglobin has a much greater affinity for CO than adult hemoglobin. Therefore, during pregnancy, the fetus may be more susceptible to CO poisoning than the mother. Once the mother is removed from the source of CO, clearance of carboxyhemoglobin may take four to five times longer in the fetus than it did in the mother [24]. Thus, the effective duration of CO exposure is considerably longer for the fetus than it is for the mother. It has been reported that severe CO toxicity in pregnant women can produce ischemic brain damage to the fetus and increase the risk of stillbirth [25,26].

CO poisoning can result in a delayed neuropsychiatric syndrome that may present at any time between 3 days and 4 months after apparent recovery from acute effects [14,27]. The syndrome has been reported to occur in 10% to 30% of individuals who survive CO poisoning. Symptoms include cognitive impairment, personality changes, Parkinsonism, incontinence, focal neurologic deficits, dementia, and psychosis. There is poor correlation between the development of the delayed neuropsychiatric syndrome and carboxyhemoglobin levels. Loss of consciousness during the acute illness phase, carboxyhemoglobin 25% or more, duration of exposure, and age appear to be significant risk factors [19]. Brain imaging studies have shown that the areas most affected are the globus pallidus and deep white matter [14]. The exact mechanism for the development of this syndrome is unclear, but it is thought to be associated with reoxygenation brain injury, as discussed earlier. Most affected individuals recover within 1 year, although some may have chronic, long-term neurologic or psychiatric impairment [14]. A more comprehensive discussion of the neurologic aspects of carbon monoxide poisoning is presented in chapter (Chapter 156).

TABLE 178.4

Carbon Monoxide Toxicity

HbCO level (%)	Clinical manifestations of carbon monoxide intoxication
0–5	Normal nonsmoker
5–10	Mild headache, shortness of breath with exertion, decreased exercise tolerance, decreased angina threshold
10–20	Moderate headache, fatigue, dizziness, blurred vision, nausea, decreasing threshold for exertional shortness of breath with possibly shortness of breath at rest
20–30	Severe headache, confusion and impaired judgment, vomiting, shortness of breath at rest, decreased cardiac arrhythmia threshold
30–40	Muscle weakness, incapacitation, cardiac arrhythmias, decreased seizure threshold
40–50	Seizures, syncope, cardiac arrest
50–60	Fatal

HbCO, carboxyhemoglobin.

Diagnosis and Management

Because CO poisoning can present with a variety of nonspecific signs and symptoms, a high index of suspicion is needed to make the diagnosis. History of potential exposure to a source of CO and elevation of arterial or venous blood carboxyhemoglobin level can point to the diagnosis [12]. Cherry-red lips, cyanosis, and retinal hemorrhages have been reported in some cases of high-dose CO poisoning, but these signs occur infrequently, and diagnosis depends on clinical history substantiated by increased levels of carboxyhemoglobin in arterial or venous blood [14]. Carboxyhemoglobin is most accurately measured by CO-oximetry because routine pulse oximetry cannot distinguish between carboxyhemoglobin and oxyhemoglobin, which both read at 660 nm [28]. PaO_2 is also of little value, because in the absence of coexistent lung injury, it is normal. This is owing to the fact that a CO partial pressure of only 1 mm Hg in arterial blood can saturate more than 50% of hemoglobin without affecting gas exchange or the amount of dissolved oxygen. Exposure to CO generally causes elevation of carboxyhemoglobin to greater than 3% to 4% in nonsmokers and higher than 10% in smokers [28]. Recently, noninvasive CO-oximetry has become commercially available. Studies show that it has a high degree of specificity but poor sensitivity [29,30]. Using a cutoff of 15% carboxyhemoglobin, noninvasive CO-oximetry had a poor sensitivity of 48% (correctly identified only 11 of 23 patients with elevated levels) but an excellent specificity of 99% (correctly identify 96 of 97 patients with levels below 15%) [30]. Until further studies are done, this would suggest that its primary value is for ruling out the diagnosis when there are no symptoms. It is probably most useful in environments where it is difficult or not possible to obtain blood measurement such as by emergency medical service (EMS) units in the prehospital environment, but should be used cautiously [31].

Patients with CO poisoning resulting from smoke inhalation should also be examined for evidence of thermal injury to the skin or airways. If CO poisoning is the result of a suicide attempt, a drug screen and serum ethanol, salicylate, and acetaminophen levels should be obtained. Another advantage of measuring the arterial carboxyhemoglobin level is that it also allows for simultaneous measurement of arterial pH. The pH can be used in conjunction with the anion gap and the serum lactate level to assess the degree of metabolic acidosis which when elevated is an independent predictor of poor prognosis [14]. $PaCO_2$ is only helpful in assessing the ventilatory response to hypoxia and ventilatory compensation for lactic acidosis and should be obtained when mental status is abnormal or there is a prior history of chronic pulmonary disease. The serum creatine kinase level will be elevated if rhabdomyolysis has occurred. An electrocardiogram and serial cardiac biomarkers should be obtained in all patients to evaluate the possibility of myocardial ischemia or infarction. Single-photon emission computed tomography (CT) perfusion scintigraphy (Table 178.5) has been cited as a technique of choice to diagnose cardiac involvement after CO exposure [32]. Because CO lowers the threshold for the development of ventricular dysrhythmias, patients should be carefully monitored until they are discharged from the emergency department or hospital [33]. The chest radiograph is usually normal, but signs of noncardiogenic pulmonary edema can rarely be seen in cases of severe CO poisoning [23], especially if there is coexistent smoke inhalation. CT of the head is useful if there is a need to rule out other causes of neurologic impairment in this acute setting.

The initial treatment of CO poisoning is prompt removal from the source of exposure and administration of 100% oxygen via a nonrebreather mask to reduce the half-life of carboxyhemoglobin from 4 to 6 hours and 40 to 80 minutes [14,34]. Patients who are unconscious or have cardiopulmonary compromise should be intubated and receive 100% oxygen by mechanical ventilation and hyperbaric oxygen therapy (HBOT) may be considered (see later). Oxygen should be administered until the carboxyhemoglobin level returns to normal. Pregnant women typically require oxygen for a longer period of time, because it takes longer for CO to be excreted from the fetus as a result of the greater affinity of fetal hemoglobin for CO [24].

TABLE 178.5

New Advances and Observations in Acute Inhalation Injury

Intervention	Year	Study	*N*	Findings	Ref.
SPECT for diagnosing cardiac involvement in CO poisoning	2012	Review	88	99mTc-MIBI SPECT changes were observed in the majority of acutely CO-poisoned patients with ECG evidence of ischemia	[32]
Inhaled anticoagulation in smoke inhalation–induced lung injury.	2009	Single-center, retrospective study with historical control	30	Inhaled anticoagulation regimens improve survival and decrease morbidity in smoke inhalation–induced lung injury	[124]
Extracorporeal life support in zinc chloride inhalation with ARDS.	2010	Case report	1	Extracorporeal life support improves the outcome in zinc Chloride inhalation victims suffering from ARDS.	[89]
Sulfur dioxide pollution and increased incidence of cardiovascular mortalities.	2015	Case crossover	849,127	Based on data about deaths from cardiovascular diseases in areas with increased concentration of sulfur dioxide daily exposure results showed increased incidence of mortality by 0.70	[88]
Significant morbidity and mortality with accidental chlorine exposure following train derailment	2007	Prospective study	605	Majority developed symptoms and needed medical care, 25 developed pulmonary edema, 9 deaths from asphyxia and pulmonary edema and its complications.	[79]
Lung function in fire Department Rescue Workers followed for 7 years after exposure to World Trade Center Dust.	2010	Prospective Study	12,781	Exposure to World Trade Center dust led to large declines in FEV_1 during the first year. Overall, these declines were persistent, without recovery over the next 6 y, leaving a substantial proportion with abnormal lung function.	[132]

SPECT, single-photon emission computed tomography; ECG, electrocardiogram; ARDS, acute respiratory distress syndrome; FEV_1, forced expiratory volume in 1 second.

Most patients with mild to moderate CO poisoning can be treated in the emergency department and discharged after the carboxyhemoglobin level has returned to normal and all abnormal signs and symptoms have resolved. Patients with severe CO poisoning, coexistent smoke inhalation, serious underlying diseases, neurologic or cardiopulmonary instability, or whose poisoning was an intentional suicide attempt should be admitted to the hospital for treatment and close observation.

HBOT has been used to treat patients with either extreme levels of CO poisoning (≥25% carboxyhemoglobin) or end-organ sensitivity to CO at elevated but lower levels. Examples of this might include neurologic abnormalities or hemodynamic instability that are felt to be caused by CO poisoning. Although as many as 18 possible different HBOT protocols exist, there is no general consensus and it is considered the mainstay of treatment for severe CO poisoning [35]. HBOT is performed by placing the patient in a chamber that is highly pressurized with 100% oxygen. HBOT produces a large increase in the amount of dissolved oxygen in blood that in turn greatly increases the partial pressure of oxygen in the blood. The half-life of carboxyhemoglobin decreases as the partial pressure of oxygen in the blood increases. HBOT with 100% oxygen at a pressure of 2.5 to 3.0 atmosphere will reduce the half-life of carboxyhemoglobin from 4 to 6 hours to approximately 20 minutes [14,23,36].

Several animal studies suggest that HBOT may attenuate the development of delayed neuropsychiatric symptoms following CO exposure [37]. Although the efficacy of HBOT for preventing the development of the delayed neuropsychiatric syndrome in humans following CO poisoning has not been conclusively established [38], many experts argue for its use when the levels exceed 20% to 25% [38,39]. HBOT will, however, hasten the resolution of symptoms and when available is currently recommended for patients with CO poisoning meeting any of the following criteria: any period of unconsciousness, coma, or persistent neurologic abnormalities; carboxyhemoglobin level of 25% or more; metabolic lactic acidosis; or cardiac dysrhythmias [14,15,19,27,40–42]. If myocardial ischemia is present, most experts believe cardiac catheterization with stenting of the blocked vessel to be the urgently required procedure. In a pregnant patient, fetal distress even at lower percentage of carboxyhemoglobin elevations would prompt consideration for HBOT if available.

The clearance of CO can also be accelerated by use of normocapnic, hyperoxic, and hyperpnea. In this technique, the patient breathes a hyperoxic gas mixture that contains an FiO_2 of 95.2% to 95.5% and a small amount of CO_2, in the range of 4.5% to 4.8%, through a nonrebreathing circuit. The resulting increase in minute ventilation increases the partial pressure gradient for oxygen and CO between pulmonary capillary blood and alveolar gas but does not increase the partial pressure gradient for CO_2. In a clinical study, normocapnic hyperoxic hyperpnea reduced the half-life of carboxyhemoglobin to 31 minutes compared with 78 minutes for individuals treated with 100% oxygen at normal minute ventilation [43]. CO-poisoned patients in hospitals without access to hyperbaric chambers might benefit from this technique.

The potential benefit of HBOT must be weighed against its inherent risks. HBOT can cause barotrauma, tympanic membrane rupture, increased anxiety, pulmonary edema, hemorrhage, tension pneumothorax, decompression sickness, nitrogen emboli, seizures, and brain damage because of superoxide production [12]. Moreover, there is insufficient evidence that HBOT reduces neurologic damage from CO intoxication. In addition to controversy concerning which patients with CO intoxication might benefit most from HBOT, there is controversy surrounding the need to treat for HCN toxicity (see later) for patients suffering severe CO poisoning from smoke inhalation. The likelihood for cyanide toxicity in smoke inhalation victims increases with increasing carboxyhemoglobin levels and increasing acidosis [44].

Hydrogen Cyanide

Pathophysiology

HCN is a chemical asphyxiant produced by the combustion of nitrogen-containing polymers during fires [44–46]. It is also part of jewelry making and various manufacturing processes (metal plating) and in the reclamation of silver from photographic and radiographic film. It has the potential to be used as a chemical agent during terrorist attacks [47]. It is a colorless, volatile liquid at room temperature, but readily vaporizes into a gas. The gaseous form of HCN easily diffuses across the alveolar membrane after inhalation. Inhaled HCN is lethal in high doses, and its inhalation during a fire may contribute to the mortality of smoke inhalation victims [44–46]. The inhalation of lethal doses of HCN may also occur following accidental releases at industrial facilities or from its use in a terrorist attack.

After inhalation, HCN is rapidly distributed to tissues throughout the body. At the cellular level, HCN molecules bind to iron-containing sites on cytochrome a_3 in mitochondria that inhibits the enzyme's activity toxicity and decreases the cellular utilization of oxygen [44,48]. Cytochrome a_3 is a key enzyme in the cytochrome oxidase system that is important for carrying out and sustaining aerobic metabolism within cells. Inhibition of cytochrome a_3 by HCN blocks cellular respiration and oxidative phosphorylation, forcing affected cells into anaerobic metabolism.

The binding of HCN to cytochrome a_3, and the resulting inhibition of cellular respiration, occurs very rapidly after HCN inhalation, with clinical signs and symptoms occurring within 15 seconds. The clinical effects of HCN intoxication are directly related to its ability to stop cellular respiration. They are nonspecific and identical to the signs and symptoms typically seen during hypoxia. Hyperpnea, dyspnea, tachycardia, agitation, anxiety, dizziness, headache, confusion, nausea, muscle weakness, and trembling are common. Lactic acidosis occurs as a result of anaerobic metabolism and may be severe. Hypotension, flushing, seizures, and Parkinson-like symptoms may occur among cases of severe intoxication. Coma, apnea, and cardiac dysrhythmias are poor prognostic signs unless prompt treatment is given [49,50].

Diagnosis and Management

The diagnosis of HCN poisoning requires a high index of suspicion. It should be suspected in every individual with any of the above signs or symptoms for which there is no other obvious cause and a pertinent history such as smoke inhalation victims, victims of industrial accidents in which cyanide could have been released, and victims of terrorist attacks. Blood and urine cyanide concentrations can be obtained, but because these tests are not routinely performed in most laboratories, results take days to return and, therefore, are only be used to confirm the diagnosis. Treatment for this potentially life-threatening poisoning must be initiated immediately based on diagnostic suspicion alone.

There are several important clues that can be helpful for making a clinical diagnosis of HCN intoxication. In smoke inhalation victims, HCN toxicity should be suspected whenever CO intoxication occurs, and in fact, the likelihood increases with increasing carboxyhemoglobin levels [44]. Regardless of the etiology of HCN exposure, metabolic acidosis with an increased anion gap and an elevated serum lactate concentration should typically be present. Arterial and venous blood gases can provide potentially useful information, with a high index of suspicion when the arteriovenous O_2 difference is far less than normal. Because of poor cellular extraction and utilization of oxygen, the arterial oxygen tension is usually above 90 mm Hg, whereas venous oxygen tension may be significantly elevated above the normal range of 35 to 45 mm Hg. Similarly, arterial oxygen saturation is typically in the normal range of 95% to 100%, whereas the oxygen saturation of mixed venous blood may be in the vicinity of 85% or greater, significantly higher than the normal range of 60% to 80%. This so-called arteriolarization of venous blood can be a useful clue in considering the diagnosis of HCN intoxication [51].

Because HCN poisoning can rapidly progress, treatment must begin as soon as possible in patient presenting with seizures, coma, hypotension, or cardiac arrest in whom HCN toxicity is suspected [52,53]. The US Food and Drug Administration approved two forms of therapy for cyanide toxicity. The Cyanokit antidote consisting of hydroxocobalamin—a precursor to vitamin B_{12}. It is a relatively benign substance (see below for adverse reactions) with rapid onset of action. For these reasons, it may be a superior antidote to the older more commonly available cyanide antidote kit (CAK) consisting of sodium nitrite and sodium thiosulfate [54,55]. Hydroxocobalamin has no adverse effect on the oxygen-carrying capacity of the red blood cells and no negative impact on the patient's blood pressure—significant benefits when treating victims of smoke inhalation. The mechanism of action is surprisingly simple: hydroxocobalamin binds to cyanide forming vitamin B_{12} (cyanocobalamin), a nontoxic compound excreted in the urine.

Victims presenting with seizures, hypotension, or a coma in a setting consistent with cyanide toxicity should be considered candidates for empiric administration of hydroxocobalamin 5 g intravenously over 15 minutes through two intravenous or intraosseous lines. Consideration should be given to obtaining a blood sample for subsequent analysis for HCN and for baseline laboratory tests that could be interfered with by the presence of hydroxocobalamin.

The most common adverse reactions (>5%) include transient chromaturia, erythema, rash (predominantly acneiform), hypertension, nausea, headache, decreased lymphocyte percentage, and injection site reactions. Less common allergic reactions include anaphylaxis, chest tightness, angioneurotic edema, and dyspnea. Because of its deep red color, hydroxocobalamin may cause hemodialysis machines to shut down because of an erroneous detection of a "blood leak." Reddish color of the blood and urine may interfere with some colorimetric laboratory tests (i.e., blood glucose, iron levels, creatinine, total hemoglobin concentration, carboxyhemoglobin, oxyhemoglobin, and methemoglobin) [56,57].

Sodium nitrite and sodium thiosulfate can also be used for the treatment of HCN poisoning. These antidotes are found in the CAK, along with ampules of amyl nitrite inhalant. Sodium nitrite generates methemoglobin by changing the normal ferrous state of iron in the heme molecule of hemoglobin (Fe^{+2}) to the ferric state (Fe^{+3}). The ferric heme molecules in methemoglobin have a high affinity for HCN. Thus, HCN molecules preferentially bind to the methemoglobin generated by sodium nitrate, which in turn prevents HCN from entering cells and inhibiting cellular respiration. The adult dose of sodium nitrite is 300 mg in 10 mL of diluent (30 mg per mL) administered intravenously over 2 to 4 minutes, and the pediatric dose is 0.33 mL per kg of a 3% solution, intravenously over 2 to 4 minutes, not to exceed 10 mL [49,58]. Following the administration of sodium nitrite, sodium thiosulfate should be administered intravenously. Sodium thiosulfate acts as a substrate for rhodanese, a detoxifying enzyme found in the liver. In the presence of sodium thiosulfate, rhodanese catalyses the conversion of HCN cyanide to thiocyanate that is then excreted in the urine. The adult dose is 12.5 g of sodium thiosulfate in 50 mL of diluent (25% solution), administered intravenously at a rate of 3 to 5 mL per minute. The pediatric dose of sodium thiosulfate is 412.5 mg per kg (1.65 mL per kg) of a 25% solution, given intravenously at a rate of 3 to 5 mL per minute [51,58].

The inhalation of amyl nitrite from ampules can be used as a temporizing measure until venous access for the administration of sodium nitrite and sodium thiosulfate is obtained. The inhalation of amyl nitrite should never be considered a substitute for the administration of intravenous sodium nitrite and sodium thiosulfate. In fact, amyl nitrite can itself be associated with serious reactions such as hypotension, syncope, methemoglobinemia, and hemolysis in G6PD-deficient patients. These effects are more pronounced in children, the elderly, and in patients with cardiopulmonary diseases. Dose regimen is difficult to control and could even result in exposure of the health care provider to amyl nitrite's adverse effects. For these reasons, administration of amyl nitrite may be unwarranted, especially because hydroxocobalamin is now available [59].

One hundred percent oxygen should be administered to all patients with HCN poisoning to maximize the oxygen-carrying capacity of blood. Ventilatory support should be provided as needed. The administration of sodium bicarbonate should be considered for the treatment of severe lactic acidosis in patients who are unconscious or hemodynamically unstable. Arterial blood gas analysis should be used to guide the need for repeat doses of sodium bicarbonate to ensure that metabolic alkalosis does not develop.

Hydrogen Sulfide

Pathophysiology

Hydrogen sulfide (H_2S) is a colorless, highly flammable gas that has the characteristic odor of "rotten eggs." It is produced in a variety of settings, most commonly sewer systems, manure pits on farms, oil fields, and petroleum refining plants [60–62]. It's noxious, "rotten eggs" odor is detectable by smell at low concentrations but may not be detectable at high concentrations or after prolonged exposure because of olfactory fatigue. Inhaled H_2S is both a chemical asphyxiant and a respiratory tract irritant. As such, it can produce a variety of clinical effects, including central nervous system dysfunction [63], cardiac dysrhythmias, and pulmonary edema as a result of acute lung injury. The severity of symptoms and prognosis are dependent on the dose of H_2S inhaled.

H_2S blocks the cellular utilization of oxygen by inhibiting the activity of cytochrome a_3, a mitochondrial enzyme of the cytochrome oxidase system that is involved in aerobic metabolism. The pathophysiologic mechanism of H_2S asphyxiation is identical to that of HCN. As with HCN intoxication, disruption of aerobic metabolism leads to arteriolarization of venous blood and causes a shift to anaerobic metabolism within affected cells that, in turn, leads to metabolic acidosis and an elevated anion gap because of increased lactate production. H_2S is lipid soluble and readily crosses the alveolar membrane after inhalation. Inhalation is the primary route of H_2S toxicity. After absorption through the lungs, H_2S easily dissolves in the blood and is rapidly distributed to tissues throughout the body. The respiratory system and organs with high oxygen demand, such as the brain and heart, are particularly vulnerable.

The severity of clinical signs and symptoms associated with H_2S toxicity depends on the exposure dose. Signs and symptoms of asphyxiation and mucosal irritation typically exist simultaneously. Local irritant effects dominate at low exposure doses, whereas pulmonary edema and life-threatening chemical asphyxiation dominate at higher exposure doses. Clinically detectable eye, mucous membrane, and respiratory tract irritation begin to occur at low exposure doses in the vicinity of 50 parts per million (ppm). Low-dose exposures in the range of 50 to 200 ppm are typically characterized by burning of the eyes, increased lacrimation, sore throat, nausea, cough, and occasional wheezing. Because olfactory function is lost at around 100 to 200 ppm, if exposed individuals can still smell the "rotten eggs" odor of H_2S, the concentration is usually not high enough to cause severe asphyxiation or irritant injury. At exposure concentrations of

200 to 250 ppm, H_2S produces intense irritation of mucous membranes, corneal ulceration, blepharospasm, and dyspnea. Pulmonary edema may occur at these concentrations as a result of irritant-induced acute lung injury [64]. At concentrations greater than 500 ppm, chemical asphyxiation of the brain may produce headache, seizures, delirium, confusion, and lethargy. The central nervous system effects of H_2S toxicity may be exacerbated by hypoxemia secondary to severe pulmonary edema. In survivors, long-term neurologic sequelae, such as ataxia, intention tremor, sensorineural hearing loss, muscle spasticity, and memory impairment, have been reported [61].

Concentrations in the range of 750 to 1,000 ppm will cause severe inhibition of aerobic metabolism within the central nervous system and heart. Myocardial ischemia, arrhythmias, and dilated cardiomyopathy have all been reported after significant exposures [65,66]. As doses increase, loss of consciousness, cessation of brainstem function, and cardiopulmonary arrest will occur.

Diagnosis and Management

A high index of suspicion is the key to making the diagnosis of H_2S intoxication. Although blood levels of thiosulfate are helpful in confirming the diagnosis of H_2S poisoning [67], these tests are not readily available in most clinical laboratories. When available, atmospheric measures of H_2S concentration can be used to increase diagnostic suspicion and in classifying the expected the severity of exposure and intoxication. In the absence of specific exposure information, signs of ocular irritation, inflammation of mucosal membranes, and the smell of "rotten eggs" on the clothing or breath of a patient should suggest the diagnosis of H_2S intoxication.

The inhibition of cytochrome a_3 by H_2S toxicity causes a decrease in the extraction and utilization of oxygen by affected cells. As a result, blood gas analyses typically show a PaO_2 in the normal range and an elevated mixed venous oxygen tension (PvO_2), typically in the range of 35 to 45 mm Hg. There may also be a "saturation gap" between the saturation of oxygen (SaO_2 or SvO_2) calculated from blood gas data and the SaO_2 measured by CO-oximetry as a result of sulfide ions binding to some oxygen binding sites on hemoglobin molecules, forming molecules of sulfhemoglobin. In addition, both methemoglobin and sulfhemoglobin are produced during the treatment of H_2S poisoning with sodium nitrite and amyl nitrite, as discussed later. Therefore, if H_2S poisoning is known or suspected, SaO_2 should be measured by CO-oximetry. A rapid decline in either PaO_2 or SaO_2 could indicate the development or progression of pulmonary edema. Serum lactate concentration is typically elevated as a result of the inhibition of aerobic metabolism. The elevated lactate concentration causes a metabolic acidosis and elevation of the anion gap.

The treatment for H_2S intoxication is similar to that for HCN intoxication—100% oxygen, antidote, and, possibly, HBOT. One hundred percent oxygen should be given to all patients. Assisted ventilation should be provided as necessary. Sodium nitrite can be used as an antidote to generate methemoglobin by changing the normal ferrous state of iron in the heme molecule of hemoglobin (Fe^{+2}) to the ferric state (Fe^{+3}). The ferric heme molecules in methemoglobin have a high affinity for H_2S [68]. The preferential binding of H_2S molecules to methemoglobin results in the formation of sulfhemoglobin that prevents circulating H_2S from entering cells and inhibiting cellular respiration. Sodium nitrite should be administered as soon as possible after exposure. Inhalation of amyl nitrite from ampules contained in CAKs can be administered as a temporizing measure until venous access is obtained for the administration of sodium nitrite. The detoxifying enzyme rhodanese is not involved in H_2S metabolism, because it is in HCN metabolism. Therefore, sodium thiosulfate or hydroxocobalamin should not be given for the treatment of H_2S intoxication. Several case reports argue for a beneficial effect of HBOT in H_2S intoxication [69,70]. Basic supportive measures should not be forgotten and include irrigation of the eyes with sterile saline and the treatment of irritant-induced bronchospasm with inhaled β_2-agonists. Consideration should be given to the administration of sodium bicarbonate for the treatment of severe metabolic acidosis in unconscious or hemodynamically unstable patients. A benzodiazepine, such as diazepam, or a barbiturate can be used to control seizures if present. If a benzodiazepine or barbiturate is given, patients should be carefully monitored for signs of respiratory insufficiency.

TABLE 178.6

Determinants of Severity of Lung Injury

- Duration of exposure
- Minute ventilation
- Age of victim
- Proximity to source
- Density of gas and height of victim
- Temperature of gas
- Toxicity of gas
- Water solubility of gas
- Particle size of mist, fog, or vapor
- Breathing pattern oronasal vs. mouth breathing
- Host factors such as preexisting asthma, coronary disease, chronic obstructive pulmonary disease
- Orthopedic problems that affect the ability to evacuate quickly

IRRITANT GASES

Irritant gases are those that cause chemical injury to the airways and lung tissue upon inhalation. The nature, location, and severity of respiratory tract injuries associated with the inhalation of an irritant gas depend on the physical and chemical properties of the gas, exposure dose, and host factors of exposed individuals. The most important physical and chemical properties are the water solubility and density of the gas. Exposure dose is determined by the concentration of the gas in the environment and the duration of exposure. Minute ventilation, age, and the presence of preexisting respiratory disease are the most important host factors (Table 178.6).

The sites of injury following inhalation of an irritant gas depend on the water solubility of the gas that determines where most of the gas will be deposited in the respiratory tract (Table 178.7). Highly soluble gases, such as ammonia and sulfur dioxide, generally cause irritant damage to exposed mucous membranes, such as the eyes and upper airway (nose, lips, pharynx, and larynx), while sparing the lower airways. At high concentrations, however, a highly soluble irritant gas can overwhelm the upper

TABLE 178.7

Solubility of Irritant Gases

High	Intermediate	Low
Ammonia	Chlorine	Hydrogen sulfide
Methyl isocyanate		Oxides of nitrogen
Sulfur dioxide		Phosgene
Hydrogen Chloride		Ozone

respiratory tract, and significant amounts may reach the upper and lower airways, thereby producing both mucous membrane and airway injury. Irritant gases of intermediate solubility, such as chlorine, may produce significant upper airway injury, especially in the pharynx and larynx, but the mucous membrane irritation is usually not as intense as that caused by highly soluble gases. Because of its intermediate solubility, the irritant effects of chlorine will extend more distally at higher concentrations. Thus, high concentrations of inhaled chlorine can produce both upper and lower airway injuries, as well as pulmonary edema as a result of alveolar damage. The inhalation of low-solubility irritant gases, such as phosgene and oxides of nitrogen, typically produces minimal upper airway irritation but can cause intense lower airways and alveolar damage. As a result of lung tissue injury, the development of noncardiogenic pulmonary edema is more likely following inhalation of a low-solubility irritant gas or at high concentrations of gases with intermediate solubility. Irritant gases that are associated with the development of pulmonary edema are listed in Table 178.8. The inhalation of gases that are lipid soluble, but not water soluble, such as chloroform, ether, or other halogenated hydrocarbons, will produce central nervous system effects and little, if any, respiratory injury. Methylene chloride, found in paint remover and other solvents, is an exception to this rule in that high doses may cause pulmonary edema [71].

Irritant gases cause damage to airways and lung tissues by direct cellular injury, cellular injury secondary to the production of free radicals, and production of an inflammatory response. Direct cellular injury is commonly produced by irritant gases that possess either a highly acidic or a highly alkaline pH. Chlorine and phosgene, for example, produce hydrochloric acid when they come in contact with water in mucous membranes. Ammonia forms a strong alkali, ammonium hydroxide, when it comes in contact with water in mucous membranes and airways.

TABLE 178.8

Toxic Gases and Fumes that can Produce Pulmonary Edema

Acetaldehyde	Methylene chloride
Acrolein	Nickel carbonyl
Ammonia	Nitrogen dioxide
Antimony tri- or pentachloride	Osmium tetroxide
Beryllium	Ozone
Bismuth pentachloride	Paraquat
Boranes	Perchloroethylene
Cadmium and cadmium salts	Phosgene
Chloramine	Phosphine
Chlorine	Polytetrafluoroethylene
Cobalt metal	Selenium dioxide
Dichlorosilane	Silanes
Dimethyl sulfate	Silicone tetrachloride
Dioxane dimethyl sulfate	Silicone tetrafluoride
Fire smoke	Sulfur dioxide
Glyphosate herbicides	TDI in high concentrations
Hydrogen chloride	Titanium tetrachloride
Hydrogen fluoride	Trimellitic anhydride
Hydrogen selenide	Vanadium
Hydrogen sulfide	War gases
Lithium hydride	Zinc oxide and chloride
Mercury	Zirconium chloride
Methyl bromide	

TDI, toluene diisocyanate.

Ammonium hydroxide causes liquefaction damage to cells and tissues on contact, with the severity of damage directly related to the hydroxyl ion concentration. Damage to respiratory tract cells and tissues can also be caused by irritant gases that generate the production of free radicals. Oxides of nitrogen, for example, cause the production of free radicals that cause cellular damage by lipid peroxidation. Both direct cell damage and cell damage secondary to free-radical formation result in the release of a variety of inflammatory mediators that elicit an inflammatory response, thereby causing further oxidant damage to respiratory tract cells. In the airways, the damage caused by irritant gases is manifested by mucosal edema, mucus production, increased smooth muscle contraction, and airway obstruction. At the alveolar level, damage of type 1 pneumocytes occurs followed by capillary leakage caused by epithelial cell damage, disruption of epithelial cell tight junctions, endothelial damage, and increased vascular permeability.

Specific Irritant Toxic Gases

Ammonia

Ammonia (NH_3) is a colorless, pungent, alkaline gas that is less dense than air and highly soluble in water where it forms ammonium hydroxide (NH_4OH). Most inhalational injuries from NH_3 occur as a result of exposures during fertilizer production, chemical manufacturing, oil refining, or the use of cleaning solutions [72]. NH_3 exposures may also occur during the illicit production of methamphetamine [73]. The strong, pungent smell associated with NH_3 is readily detected at a concentration as low as 50 ppm. Few individuals can tolerate a concentration greater than 100 ppm without experiencing nasal stuffiness and irritating cough.

As a highly soluble gas, NH_3 primarily causes irritation to the eyes, mucous membranes of the nasal–oral pharynx, and mucosa of the upper respiratory airways. The reaction of NH_3 with water in the conjunctivae, mucous membranes, and upper airway mucosa results in the formation of NH_4OH that causes liquefaction necrosis and intense pain in the eyes, mouth, nose, and throat. The voice is lost shortly after exposure, and patients typically experience sensations of choking and suffocation. The eyes are erythematous, swollen, and may show signs of corneal opacification or ulceration. Edema, ulceration, necrosis, and sloughing of the mucous membranes are typically seen. Airway obstruction as a result of laryngeal edema, bronchial inflammation, bronchoconstriction, and plugs of sloughed epithelium may cause dyspnea, wheezing, and hypoxemia [74]. Death from laryngospasm can occur within minutes after exposure to high concentrations ($\geq$1,500 ppm). With exposure to high concentrations, alveolar damage and pulmonary edema can occur within 24 hours [74]. Secondary bacterial bronchopneumonia may occur within days. Long-term sequelae of NH_3 inhalation at moderate to severe concentrations include persistent airway obstruction from reactive airways dysfunction syndrome (RADS), asthma, bronchitis, bronchiectasis, and bronchiolitis obliterans [74,75].

Chlorine

Chlorine (Cl_2) is a dense, greenish-yellow gas under ambient conditions. It is highly reactive, has intermediate solubility, and has the characteristic pungent odor of bleach. Industrial uses of Cl_2 include the production of chemicals and bleaches, paper manufacturing, textile processing, and the production of polyvinyl chloride. Most Cl_2 exposures result from accidental releases at industrial sites, from ruptured tanks during its transportation, or at swimming pools [76–78]. The relatively high density of Cl_2 causes it to accumulate in low-lying areas, which should be avoided following its accidental release.

Chlorine is detectable by smell at levels of 1 ppm. On contact with mucous membranes, chlorine reacts with water to produce hydrochloric acid (HCl), hypochlorous acid (HClO), and free oxygen radicals. Individuals exposed to low concentrations of Cl_2 typically experience burning of the eyes and mucous membranes, as well as choking and coughing as a result of inflammation of the nasal–oral pharynx and upper airway. At higher concentrations, laryngeal edema, lower airway inflammation, bronchoconstriction, and pulmonary edema can develop. In 2005, a train derailment in Graniteville, South Carolina (Table 178.5) released about 60 tons of chlorine gas [79]. Although the majority presented with wheezing or rales, 17% and 11%, respectively, developed these symptoms later over the next 24 hours [2]. Of the 9 victims of the acute chlorine poisoning, 8 showed cardiomegaly on autopsy, but it is unclear whether it was from a preexisting condition that contributed to their mortality, versus a result of severe lung injury or hypoxemia and subsequent release of vasoactive mediators [2]. The potentially delayed onset of symptoms from acute inhalation of chlorine suggests that exposed individuals with an initial paucity of significant signs and symptoms may not reflect the true severity of the inhalational injury, and exposed individuals may be sent home from the emergency department prematurely. For example, an exposure concentration of 50 ppm may produce relatively mild signs and symptoms initially but can cause death from laryngospasm or massive pulmonary edema within 1 to 2 hours after exposure. The onset of pulmonary edema may also be delayed up to 24 hours after exposure. At any time within 2 days after Cl_2 exposure, airway inflammation and mucosal desquamation may cause plugging of medium and small bronchi, leading to airflow obstruction and atelectasis. Individuals with a history of asthma or airway hyperactivity may have, particularly, severe bronchospasm.

Secondary bacterial bronchopneumonia may develop as a consequence of ulceration and desquamation of airway mucosa and/or alveolar damage. Fortunately, most exposed individuals will recover completely if they receive prompt medical treatment and survive the acute effects of Cl_2 exposure. However, chronic pulmonary problems may develop in some individuals, including RADS, asthma, bronchiectasis, and bronchiolitis obliterans [78,80,81].

Phosgene

Phosgene ($COCl_2$) is a heavy, poorly soluble, colorless gas that has the smell of freshly mown hay. Upon contact with water, it hydrolyzes to form CO_2 and HCl. $COCl_2$ has been used as a chemical warfare agent and was responsible for most gas fatalities during World War I [47]. It is currently use as a chlorinating agent in a variety of industrial processes, including the production of isocyanates, pesticides, dyes, and pharmaceutic agents. Firefighters, welders, and paint strippers may be exposed to $COCl_2$ as a result of its release from heated chlorinated hydrocarbons, such as polyvinyl chloride [82]. Phosgene is approximately four times as dense as air and tends to accumulate close to the ground and in low-lying areas. Therefore, individuals should avoid low-lying areas following an accidental release.

As a gas with low solubility, $COCl_2$ is less irritating to the eyes and mucous membranes than NH_3 or Cl_2 and causes mostly irritant damage in the lower airways and cellular damage at the alveolar level. Immediate symptoms include burning of the eyes, increased lacrimation, sore throat, rhinorrhea, cough, choking, dyspnea, and chest tightness, are often mild and resolve within several minutes after cessation of $COCl_2$ exposure. With high-concentration exposures, laryngeal edema can occur, with stridor and the potential for sudden death. As a result of its low solubility, the mucous membranes and upper airways are typically spared, and there may be few, if any, additional symptoms for 2 to 24 hours following the acute inhalation of $COCl_2$. However, inhaled $COCl_2$ will eventually hydrolyze to form HCl in the lower airways and alveoli, causing oxidative and inflammatory injury. As a result, bronchospasm and pulmonary edema typically develop between 2 and 6 hours following exposure, but pulmonary edema may be delayed for up to 24 hours. The pulmonary edema can progress to the acute respiratory distress syndrome (ARDS) and respiratory failure. Most victims survive without long-term sequelae if they receive prompt medical care. Those with ARDS have the worst prognosis and will require assisted ventilation and circulatory support as needed. Chronic problems may develop in some individuals with RADS, asthma, bronchiectasis, and bronchiolitis obliterans [83].

Nitrogen Oxides

The four stable oxides of nitrogen are nitrous oxide (N_2O), nitric oxide (NO), nitrogen dioxide (NO_2), and nitrogen tetroxide (N_2O_4). Oxides of nitrogen are used in the production of dyes, lacquer, and fertilizer. They are also generated in a variety of processes, including arc welding [82], chemical engraving, explosives, and the storage of fresh silage [84]. All oxides of nitrogen can produce serious acute respiratory tract injury upon inhalation. However, NO_2 is the most common and clinically important toxicant in this group. NO_2 is an irritating, low-solubility, dense orange-brown gas. It forms nitric acid (HNO_3) and nitrous acid (HNO_2) upon contact with water.

NO_2 causes silo filler's disease, one of the best-characterized syndromes of toxic gas exposure. Silo filler's disease develops following exposure to NO_2 gas that accumulates just above the silage in recently filled, top-loading silos. During the first 2 weeks in the silo, carbohydrates in the silage ferment and produce organic acids. The organic acids then oxidize nitrates in the silage into NO_2. Within hours after it starts to be produced, NO_2 rapidly accumulates to toxic levels of 200 to 2,000 ppm. High concentrations of NO_2 typically persist for 1 to 2 weeks, then decrease. Entry into a silo without proper respiratory protection, especially within the first 2 weeks of the silo being filled with fresh silage, can cause a rapid loss of consciousness and sudden death. The incidence of this disorder is estimated to be 5 cases per 100,000 silo-associated farm workers per year [84].

The lower airways and lung are the primary sites of injury following acute inhalation of NO_2. The low water solubility of NO_2 results in a paucity of eye, mucous membrane, and upper airway irritant symptoms. The most significant effects occur in the lower airways and lungs as a result of the conversion of NO_2 to HNO_3 upon contact with water in bronchial mucosa and alveoli. The clinical response to inhaled NO_2 occurs in three phases [84,85]. The first phase is the *acute illness phase* that typically occurs within the first hour after exposure. The severity of symptoms in this first phase is dose related. At doses up to 100 ppm, cough, wheezing, dyspnea, and chest pain develop as a result of lower airway irritation and bronchospasm. Hypotension may occur in severe cases. At doses greater than 100 ppm, pulmonary edema may develop within 1 to 2 hours after exposure. The hypoxemia resulting from pulmonary edema is further exacerbated by NO_2-induced methemoglobinemia.

Without further NO_2 exposure, symptoms of the *acute illness phase* usually resolve over a period of 2 to 8 weeks. During this *latent phase*, the patient may have mild cough and wheezing, or may be totally asymptomatic. The patient may then develop a *delayed illness phase* that is characterized by the sudden onset of fever, chills, cough, dyspnea, and generalized lung crackles on exam [84,85]. The *delayed illness phase* is characterized by bronchiolitis obliterans. Lung biopsies show this bronchiolitis to be proximal and without organizing pneumonia [64,84,85]. The bronchioles are packed with inflammatory exudate and fibrin that may obliterate the entire lumen. The bronchiolitis obliterans of the *delayed illness phase* may be extensive and cause severe, life-threatening hypoxemia. Symptom severity in the *acute illness phase* does not always correlate with the severity of bronchiolitis obliterans in the *delayed illness phase*. Therefore, patients with relatively mild symptoms in the days following acute NO_2 exposure may experience severe, life-threatening bronchiolitis obliterans and pulmonary edema in the *delayed illness phase*.

Sulfur Dioxide

Sulfur dioxide (SO_2) is a colorless, dense, irritating gas that is highly soluble in water. It has a readily identifiable, strong, pungent, odor. SO_2 is a common atmospheric pollutant from the combustion of coal and gasoline. It is used in a variety of industrial process, such as bleaching, refrigeration, and paper manufacturing [64,86]. SO_2 forms sulfuric acid (H_2SO_4) upon contact with water in human tissues. As a highly soluble gas, the predominant effects of SO_2 exposure are irritation of the eyes, nose, mucous membranes, pharynx, and upper respiratory tract. Exposure doses greater than 10 ppm typically cause bronchospasm with symptoms of cough, wheezing, dyspnea, and chest pain. Symptom severity increases with increasing exposure doses. Individuals with preexisting asthma or chronic obstructive lung disease are more likely to develop severe exacerbations [87]. These include RADS, asthma, bronchiolitis obliterans, and restrictive lung disease. Sulfur dioxide in air pollution was also associated with increased cardiovascular mortality (Table 178.5) [88].

Zinc Chloride

Zinc chloride exposure occurs most commonly with the use of smoke bombs when synthetic smoke is created (police operations, military drills, and firefighter training) [89]. After inhalation, the zinc oxide reacts with hexachloroethane. Zinc chloride is an ultrafine particle that can penetrate into the lower respiratory tract. Exposure to the smoke for as little as 1 to 5 minutes can progress to ARDS and death. Initial symptoms can include dry cough, sore throat, shortness of breath, and chest tightness, and often the onset of severe respiratory distress is delayed [89]. Positive findings on auscultation or chest X-ray may not appear until 48 hours later in at least one case report of zinc chloride inhalation [89]. The inhalation of zinc chloride causes tracheobronchitis and pneumonitis. High-resolution CT (HRCT) taken 1 to 3 days after exposure may show ground-glass opacities bilaterally with consolidation in the posterior region of the lungs [90]. Pulmonary function tests on these patients showed mostly restrictive lung disease, and follow-up HRCTs showed varying degrees of pulmonary fibrosis.

Literature on the treatment of zinc chloride-lung injury is sparse, and supportive care is primarily what is used. There is some evidence that the use of N-acetyl cysteine may facilitate zinc clearance. At least one group reported success with the use of extracorporeal oxygen life support in an exposed patient with ARDS [89]. The use of corticosteroids in these patients with lung injury remains controversial.

Heavy Metals

Two common sources of inhalational exposure to heavy metals occur in the occupational setting: cadmium and mercury. Although the most common environmental source for cadmium is smoking, and thus associated with chronic exposure, exposure can occur in the occupational setting in battery factories, zinc smelters, pigment plants, and welding fumes. Symptoms may manifest up to 2 days after exposure, and include respiratory distress, cough, shivering, and fever [91]. Mortality is frequently because of cadmium's interference with pulmonary cellular function such as repair of DNA and integrity of membrane structure [92]. This direct toxicity leads to pulmonary edema, chemical pneumonitis, bronchitis, and emphysema [91,92]. Cadmium exposure also causes renal toxicity. A 15-year follow-up study on residents of the polluted Kakehashi river basin in Japan showed that those with cadmium-induced renal damage had higher risk of mortality [93]. Although cadmium exposure has been shown to be a carcinogen in animal studies, human studies are less conclusive and demonstrate varying levels of association with lung and prostate cancer [93].

Although there is no gold standard for treatment of cadmium toxicity, ethylenediaminetetraacetic acid (EDTA) is the most widely accepted chelator [94]. Concomitant administration of glutathione also shows protection against nephrotoxicity. Dosage of EDTA should not exceed 1 g per h, and no more than 3 g per session.

SMOKE

Smoke is a toxic, mixture of gases, vapors, fumes, liquid droplets, and carbonaceous particles generated by the incomplete combustion or pyrolysis of multiple substances at very high temperatures. Approximately 80% of all fire-associated deaths are attributed to inhalational injury [95]. Smoke inhalation is the most common cause of death among fire victims without surface burns. Inhalation injury exerts a greater influence than burn size or age in determining burn mortality [96]. Patients being treated in burn centers have a mortality rate of 29% in the presence of inhalation injury, in comparison with a mortality rate of 2% in its absence [97].

Combustion occurs when oxygen reacts with molecules under intense heat and they become oxidized to smaller compounds. Pyrolysis occurs as a result of heat alone, does not require oxygen, and consists of the melting or boiling of heated material. The toxic products of incomplete combustion or pyrolysis generated in a given setting are determined by multiple factors, including the type of fuel consumed, temperature, rate of heating, and distance from the source [95]. Black smoke results from particles of carbon or soot generated during the combustion or pyrolysis of carbon-containing materials. Common combustible materials in a fire include wood, paper, plastics, polyurethane, paints, and other polymers present in carpeting and upholstery.

Toxic gases are released during combustion and pyrolysis. These gases include both asphyxiants and irritants. CO and HCN are common asphyxiants found in smoke. Aldehydes, acrolein, NO_2, SO_2, and HCl are common irritants found in smoke. These irritant gases are more likely to be released during pyrolysis than combustion [98]. Particulates present in smoke adsorb these irritant chemicals to their surface, which can concentrate the chemicals and increase irritant damage to the respiratory tract upon inhalation [99].

Victims of smoke inhalation are exposed to multiple irritant gases [95,100], but several are particularly notable. *Acrolein* is an aldehyde released in fires involving polyethylene, polypropylene, vinyl materials, wood, and other organic fuels. At low concentrations, acrolein is intensely irritating to the upper respiratory tract and can cause significant upper airway edema. At high concentrations (>10 ppm), acrolein inhalation can cause life-threatening pulmonary edema [101]. *Isocyanate*, a known cause of asthma, is also among the toxic products produced in fires. The inhalation of isocyanate contained in smoke can precipitate severe bronchospasm in individuals with or without a history of airway disease.

Smoke particles cause airway damage as a result of direct injury from heat and steam, irritation of the airway mucosa by the particles themselves, and from inflammation as a result of the irritant effects of toxic chemicals absorbed to their surface. Heat injury from hot gases and steam is usually limited to the upper respiratory tract because heat rapidly dissipates across the upper airways [101]. Smoke particles greater than 10 μm in diameter also contribute to upper airway injury (rhinosinusitis, pharyngitis, laryngitis, and upper airway edematous obstruction), because they do not penetrate into the lower airways unless present at high concentrations. Subglottic or supraglottic edema following smoke inhalation can lead to significant upper airway obstruction. Upper airway obstruction occurs for up to 30% of burn patients and may occur as early as 4 hours or as late as 24 hours after exposure [102]. The production of upper airway edema is because of a variety of factors, including direct mucosal damage and ulceration from heat and superheated steam, the release of inflammatory mediators from the damaged mucosa, and the production of oxygen free radicals from toxic chemicals on the surface of smoke particles. Acute upper airway edema following smoke inhalation usually resolves within 3 to 4 days. Rarely, thermal injury can produce circumferential, constricting eschars, or scarring of the upper airway after the acute edema resolves. Such eschars can produce chronic upper airway obstruction.

In the large- to medium-sized airways of the chest, tracheobronchitis can develop as a result of smoke inhalation. Severe cough and chest tightness without bronchoconstriction are common presenting symptoms. Tracheobronchitis is as a result of irritant chemical and/or particulate injury. Heat injury is rare and occurs only after the inhalation of superheated steam [101].

Particles less than 3 μm in diameter travel to the distal portions of the respiratory tract and can cause small airways and alveolar injury. Lower airway penetration by small smoke particulates can cause irritation, inflammation, and bronchoconstriction. Individuals with preexisting asthma or chronic obstructive pulmonary disease may experience exacerbations, but bronchoconstriction can also occur in individuals with no prior history of airway disease. Small smoke particles can also cause alveolar-capillary injury in the lung parenchyma by direct oxidative damage from adsorbed irritants and by oxygen free radicals and inflammatory mediators released by neutrophils that migrate to areas of irritant damage. Rarely, pulmonary edema can occur as a consequence of alveolar-capillary injury and may occur hours to days after smoke inhalation. Although pulmonary edema occurs among far less than 10% of smoke inhalation victims, it has a high mortality rate [103].

Airway injury, whether it is tracheobronchitis or small airway bronchoconstriction, can cause sloughing of necrotic tissue into the lower airways that can lead to mucous plugging, bronchial obstruction, atelectasis, hyperinflation, and altered mucociliary clearance. Secondary bacterial pneumonia can develop in obstructed lung segments or as a result of alveolar damage adversely affecting local immunodefenses.

Most smoke inhalation deaths are caused by asphyxiation as a result of CO or HCN in the inhaled smoke [44–46,104]. CO intoxication is responsible for 80% of smoke inhalation fatalities, and approximately one-fourth of these occur in victims with underlying cardiac or pulmonary disease [14]. NO_2 may also be a component of inhaled smoke. In addition to being a potent irritant, NO_2 can cause the development of methemoglobinemia, which further decreases the already impaired oxygen-carrying capacity resulting from carboxyhemoglobinemia. Coexisting HCN intoxication should be considered in all smoke inhalation victims with CO intoxication, especially those with clinical evidence of altered neurologic or cardiac status. In a study from Paris, a clear association was found between blood HCN levels and percent carboxyhemoglobin levels [44]. This association was strongest in patients with metabolic acidosis and elevated lactate levels [44]. In a study from the Dallas County Fire Department, an HCN blood level above 1.0 mg per L was a strong predictor of death, but the association between CO and HCN levels was not strong [105]. In this study, of the 144 patients who reached the emergency room alive, 12 had blood cyanide concentrations exceeding 1.0 mg per L and 8 of the 12 subsequently died. Among these 12 patients, the relationship between percent carboxyhemoglobin levels and HCN blood levels was poor. For example, the highest percent carboxyhemoglobin level found was 40.0%, in a patient with a blood HCN level of 1.20 mg per L. The highest HCN level found was 11.50 mg per L in a patient with a percent carboxyhemoglobin level of 22.4%.

Diagnosis and Management of Irritant Toxic Gases, Including Smoke Inhalation

The most important factors for the diagnosis of toxic inhalational injury are a history of circumstances that caused the exposure, identification of the specific toxic gas to which an individual has been exposed, and an estimate of the exposure concentration. Exposure duration is based not only on exposure time but also on the patient's minute ventilation during that time. Chemical analyses of material at the site of exposure, if available, can be particularly helpful in identifying the offending toxicant and estimating its exposure concentration. The relative solubility of a toxic gas can be helpful in determining the areas of the respiratory tract where irritant injuries are most likely to occur, and obviously patients with preexisting pulmonary disease are most at risk. When the irritant toxic gases are in the setting of smoke inhalation, the exposure will be to multiple gases and particulates. Facial burns, singed eyebrows, soot in the upper airway, and carbonaceous sputum make smoke inhalation highly likely.

The management of acute inhalational injury from toxic irritants is at first supportive. All contaminated clothing should be removed to prevent further inhalation and percutaneous absorption of the toxic substance. Superficial burns should be treated conservatively with a topical antibiotic such as silver sulfadiazine. The eyes should be thoroughly flushed with sterile normal saline as soon as possible. Careful attention to the eyes is important because cataracts can occur following heavy exposures. Humidified oxygen should be given by face mask. Not everyone exposed to fire smoke warrants hospital admission. Victims with mild inhalation exposures may be treated and released if they are (i) asymptomatic with normal mental status and absent of confusion; (ii) no burns, carbon material, or edema in the upper airway; (iii) normal pulmonary examination without signs of respiratory distress, stridor, or wheeze; and (iv) if available a pulse oximeter and noninvasive carboxyhemoglobin reading that are normal or at baseline. Upon release, patients should be advised to seek medical attention if symptoms occur or reoccur, because the clinical manifestations of inhalation injury may take 4 to 24 hours to develop [103]. It is for this reason that borderline patients or patients with significant comorbidity should be observed rather than released whenever possible.

The medical evaluation after any exposure to potentially toxic irritant gases should focus on assessing the nature and extent of upper and lower respiratory tract injury, the adequacy of oxygenation, cardiac function, and the hemodynamic stability of the patient. Inhalation victims may be unconscious or have altered mental status at the time of presentation. Typical patient complaints include eye irritation, headaches, confusion, sore throat, cough, chest tightness, and difficulty breathing. Common physical findings include irritation of the eyes, skin and other exposed mucosal surfaces, tachypnea, cough, stridor, wheezing, and rhonchi. Rales on presentation are unusual, because pulmonary edema is a later complication [103].

Arterial blood gases, oxygen saturation, should be obtained on all patients. The methemoglobin level should be measured in patients with suspected NO_2 exposure or after treatment with amyl or sodium nitrites for suspected HCN toxicity. Serum lactate concentration should be measured, and the magnitude of metabolic acidosis should be assessed. Although chest radiographs may be normal shortly after acute exposure, serial radiographs are useful for detecting the development of pulmonary edema and secondary bacterial pneumonia in hypoxemic individuals. An electrocardiogram should be obtained to detect the presence of myocardial ischemia and cardiac dysrhythmias. Hemodynamic monitoring may be necessary in complex, critically ill patients with pulmonary edema.

The carboxyhemoglobin level, a measure of CO intoxication, should be obtained in all patients with suspected exposure to smoke, fires, or other sources of combustion. If high levels of carboxyhemoglobin, methemoglobin, or HCN exist, the arterial oxygen tension (PaO_2) is not useful in assessing the adequacy of oxygen transport or tissue oxygenation. Arterial oxygen saturation should be measured by CO-oximetry because pulse oximetry and the calculation of SaO_2 from the PaO_2 will overestimate the actual oxygen saturation of hemoglobin.

All individuals with known or suspected inhalational injury should be given 100% humidified oxygen as soon as possible. This will help improve the oxygen-carrying capacity of hemoglobin when high levels of carboxyhemoglobin or methemoglobin are present. High levels of methemoglobin are unusual but, if present, can be treated with intravenous methylene blue. The fraction of inspired oxygen can be titrated down to maintain a PaO_2 greater than 60 mm Hg once carboxyhemoglobin and methemoglobin levels have returned to normal. When available, HBOT should be considered for the treatment of CO intoxication according to the criteria for previously delineated in the section in this chapter. HBOT has been used to treat patients with extreme levels of CO poisoning (≥25% carboxyhemoglobin) or end-organ sensitivity to CO at elevated but lower levels. Examples of this might include neurologic abnormalities or hemodynamic instability that was felt to be caused by CO poisoning.

Severely ill smoke inhalation patients presenting with seizures, coma, hemodynamic instability, and/or severe lactic acidosis should be suspected of having both CO and HCN intoxication [44–46,105]. Blood HCN levels can be measured, but results cannot be obtained in time to make therapeutic decisions, and, therefore, the decision to treat for HCN toxicity should be based on the exposure characteristics and clinical presentation. The NYC Fire Department's protocol is to intubate such patients; provide hemodynamic support as needed; empirically treat for HCN poisoning with hydroxocobalamin; and, if noninvasive carboxyhemoglobin levels are elevated, to transport to an HBOT center. In addition, all smoke inhalation victims found in cardiac arrest receive hydroxocobalamin during cardiac resuscitation.

For smoke inhalation patients, with suspected HCN poisoning, hydroxocobalamin is preferable to sodium thiosulfate because of its rapid onset of action. Inhaled amyl nitrite and intravenous sodium nitrite should be avoided because they generate methemoglobin that can further impair the oxygen-carrying capacity of blood hemoglobin if high levels of carboxyhemoglobin or methemoglobin are already present. The Paris Fire Brigade routinely administers hydroxocobalamin to smoke inhalation patients and published their experience in 2006 [53]. Of the 29 patients in cardiac arrest, 18 (62%) recovered with cardiac resuscitation and hydroxocobalamin treatment. The average time between hydroxocobalamin administration and recovery of spontaneous cardiac activity was 19 minutes. In 15 hemodynamically unstable patients not in cardiac arrest, 12 (80%) showed hemodynamic improvement (blood pressure >90 mm Hg) after hydroxocobalamin. The average time for hemodynamic improvement was 49 minutes from the start of and 29 minutes from the end of hydroxocobalamin infusion. In a second study, 28 of 42 patients (67%) admitted to the ICU with smoke inhalation and confirmed a posteriori HCN poisoning survived after hydroxocobalamin administration [54].

Respiratory symptoms and distress are not only related to oxygen delivery/utilization problems. Irritant, toxic gases can also cause tachypnea, stridor, and hoarseness as a result of upper and lower airway disease. Patients are at risk for developing progressive laryngeal edema with complete obstruction of the upper airway. Smoke inhalation further adds to this risk owing to heat and particulate matter exposure. Patients with laryngeal edema can be difficult to intubate and, if intubation is delayed, may require an emergency tracheostomy. However, not all patients require intubation [106]. Prompt inspection of the larynx with a laryngoscope is imperative [102]. Immediate intubation should be considered if there is evidence of significant upper airway edema or blisters. All patients with upper airway edema should be treated with nebulized racemic epinephrine and systemic corticosteroids. If edema is minimal and early intubation is not required, airflow can usually be maintained with positive pressure breathing administered by the use of continuous positive-airway pressure (CPAP) or bilevel positive-airway pressure (BiPAP). An inhaled mixture of helium and oxygen can also improve upper airway airflow by reducing turbulence as a result of its low density. If the clinical decision is not for immediate or early intubation [106], then patients with upper airway edema should be admitted to the hospital and closely monitored for signs of edema progression and the need for emergent intubation at a later time.

Lower airway involvement from irritant gas or smoke inhalation is typically diagnosed by history and physical examination. However, additional diagnostic evidence can be provided by laryngoscopic or bronchoscopic demonstration of edema, hemorrhage, or carbonaceous material distal to the vocal cords. Inhalation injury to the smaller airways and lung parenchyma can be confirmed by Xenon 133 ventilation scanning [107] or noncontrast chest CT scans [90,108]. Inhalation injury on chest CT should be suspected with findings of ground-glass infiltrates (more central than peripheral). Sensitivity for both types of scans is high, but there are false positives, especially in patients with obstructive airway disease, and their value in determining the need for intubation, treatment, and prognosis has not been determined [90,107,108].

Lower airway involvement should be suspected on physical examination when wheezing is present or when spirometry or challenge testing demonstrates acute reductions in lung function, bronchodilator responsiveness, or airway hyperreactivity [109–112]. Acute bronchospasm should be treated with β_2-agonists. Ipratropium can be added if significant improvement is not obtained with a β_2-agonist alone. In the presence of significant burn injuries, treatment with systemic corticosteroids is usually contraindicated, because their use is associated with increased mortality from sepsis [113]. Systemic corticosteroids should be reserved for severe upper airway obstruction, severe bronchospasm resistant to bronchodilator therapy, and failed extubation as a result of stridor or bronchospasm [113]. Low-dose inhaled corticosteroids have not been studied in large case series, but it is unlikely that they would negatively impact on mortality in burn patients. A placebo-controlled, double-blind, randomized control trial conducted in France showed that low-dose hydrocortisone reduced the need for vasopressors in severe burn patients [114]. Animal studies have shown that inhaled corticosteroids improve oxygenation and attenuate the development of acute lung injury following chlorine exposure [115,116]. Although inhaled corticosteroids are often given following chlorine and phosgene inhalation, there are no controlled clinical trials regarding their efficacy. Chest physiotherapy and frequent suctioning may be helpful in those patients with mucus plugs and thick secretions. Intubation may be necessary if bronchial secretions are excessive and frequent bronchoscopic suctioning needed.

Noncardiogenic pulmonary edema from acute lung injury (ARDS) is far less common than airway injury but should be suspected in patients with worsening oxygenation and increasing dyspnea. A chest radiograph should be obtained if signs of respiratory distress, abnormal breath sounds, or worsening hypoxemia are noted. Pulmonary edema or ARDS from inhalation injury typically presents as scattered, nodular alveolar infiltrates on chest radiographs, although large, diffuse, confluent infiltrates may occur as the illness progresses. Careful attention to fluid and electrolyte balance is essential, especially if surface burns are present. If gas exchange abnormalities are severe, positive-pressure ventilation with CPAP or BiPAP may help to support adequate oxygenation. If there is no response or secretions are burdensome, then intubation and assisted ventilation are required. Nasotracheal intubation should be avoided because of the severe nasal inflammation that typically occurs following the inhalation of chemical irritants and because the smaller endotracheal tube diameters needed for nasotracheal intubation do not allow for the repeated bronchoscopic suctioning that may be needed if secretions become a problem. Positive end-expiratory pressure in the range of 5 to 10 cm H_2O may help to improve oxygenation in mechanically ventilated patients [117–119]. The use of systemic corticosteroids for the treatment of pulmonary edema or ARDS following toxic irritant inhalation remains controversial [120]. Again, there are no controlled clinical trials evaluating the efficacy of corticosteroid treatment. Most experts believe that corticosteroids are not useful as pulmonary edema, or ARDS typically resolves 48 to 72 hours after inhalation exposure, with most patients surviving if appropriate supportive treatment is given. However, whether corticosteroids might be useful for preventing the few that develop pulmonary bronchiolitis obliterans or pulmonary fibrosis remain to be determined. Experimental studies suggest that treatment to block inflammatory mediators and free radicals may be effective for smoke inhalation victims [121–123]. Recent examples include retrospective analyses of mechanically ventilated smoke inhalation patients, adult [124], and pediatric [125], demonstrating successful treatment with nebulized unfractionated heparin and *N*-acetylcysteine (Table 178.5). Other anticoagulants, including tissue plasminogen activator, antithrombin, and thromboxane have been studied to decrease inflammation and have shown promise in treating smoke inhalation [126]. However, prospective controlled clinical trials have not been conducted for any of the above experimental agents.

Secondary bacterial pneumonia can occur as a complication of irritant-induced airway or lung injury [127]. There is no evidence that the administration of prophylactic antibiotics reduces the incidence of secondary bacterial pneumonia. Antibiotics should be given only if pneumonia occurs, and the specific antibiotics chosen should be based on standard practice according to known community organisms and sensitivities until culture results return.

LONG-TERM COMPLICATIONS OF ACUTE INHALATION INJURY

Although most patients exposed to irritant gases or smoke will recover completely, others may develop long-term sequelae. The most common long-term complications are listed in Table 178.9. Some of these disorders may become evident in the days or weeks following acute exposure, whereas others may take months, or rarely even years, before clinical symptoms and signs become evident. Therefore, all patients with acute inhalational injury require medical follow-up for the potential development of these disorders, even if they are initially asymptomatic after resolution of acute signs and symptoms.

TABLE 178.9

Agents that can Produce Bronchiolitis Obliterans

Ammonia	Methyl isocyanate
Chlorine	Mustard gas
Cocaine free-base	Oxides of nitrogen
Fire smoke	Phosgene
Hydrogen selenide	Sulfur dioxide

Some may develop a chronic cough syndrome, dyspnea, and/or wheezing following recovery from acute inhalation injury. Pulmonary function tests, chest radiographs, and high-resolution CT scans of the chest can be helpful for determining the etiology of chronic cough among such patients. When chest radiographs and chest CT scans are normal, the chronic cough is usually as a result of to asthma, RADS, bronchitis, rhinosinusitis, and/or gastroesophageal reflux [128,129]. Pulmonary function tests may be normal. Such patients could have rhinosinusitis, gastroesophageal reflux disease, and could also have RADS/irritant asthma. The diagnostic evaluation of such patients should be guided by a careful history and physical examination. RADS is characterized by immediate and persistent, nonspecific airway hyperreactivity following inhalation of a toxic substance in individuals with no prior history of cigarette smoking, allergen, or airway disease [130]. Irritant asthma is the more proper terminology if symptoms were not immediate or if there is a history of prior allergies, pulmonary disease, or smoking. When pulmonary function tests are normal, bronchial challenge testing (methacholine, histamine, mannitol, cold air, or exercise) may be performed to evaluate airway hyperreactivity in patients suspected of having RADS or irritant asthma. Transient, self-limited bronchial hyperreactivity may occur in the weeks following irritant gas or smoke exposures, so the detection of early bronchial hyperreactivity may not always be predictive of RADS [109–112]. The evaluation of firefighters with heavy exposure to dust and irritant gases during the first days after the World Trade Center (WTC) collapse showed that bronchial hyperreactivity demonstrated by methacholine challenge testing after 1 month or 3 months after exposure was predictive of persistent airway hyperreactivity and RADS [112]. It can take months or years for the symptoms of RADS to resolve, and some patients may never have complete resolution. Treatment with an inhaled bronchodilator should be considered if a significant bronchodilator response is found. Even in the absence of a documented bronchodilator response, a trial should be considered if there is a history of symptoms with exercise, irritants, or change in temperature/humidity. Inhaled corticosteroids should be considered not only for symptom control but also for the possibility, albeit unproven concept, that early treatment may prevent progression or lead to resolution [131].

If symptoms persist, serial measurements of spirometry, lung volumes, and diffusion capacity should be assessed to determine whether there is accelerated decline in lung function, hyperinflation, bronchiolitis obliterans, emphysema, or pulmonary fibrosis. A study of more than 12,000 firefighters and EMS workers exposed to dust and gases from the September 11, 2001, attack on the WTC found that the decline in lung function during the first 6 to 12 months after the attack was 12 times the expected annual decline and even more important for the majority of those exposed to this decline persisted for the next 6 years [132]. Another study of firefighters exposed to WTC dust and gases demonstrated that interstitial pulmonary fibrosis was exceedingly rare and that airway obstruction was probable cause of the persistent lung injury [133].

Bronchiolitis obliterans is a rare but particularly ominous complication following the inhalation of certain toxic gases, particularly NO_2, other oxides of nitrogen, SO_2, mustard gas, and/or smoke [134–138]. Inhaled toxicants that can produce bronchiolitis obliterans are listed in Table 178.10. Bronchiolitis obliterans can take two forms following acute inhalation injury. The first form is manifested by the acute onset of fever, chills, cough, dyspnea, and generalized lung crackles that develop 2 to 8 weeks after acute exposure to an offending gas, as discussed in "Nitrogen Oxides" section. Chest radiographs or high-resolution CT scans typically show a diffuse "miliary" pattern of small nodules and/or areas of ground-glass inflammation. Although lung biopsies are usually not necessary to make the diagnosis with a history of acute inhalation injury, they show a proximal

TABLE 178.10

Long-Term Effects of Acute Inhalation Injury

Complete resolution of symptoms
Sinusitis/rhinitis
Gastroesophageal reflux
Asthma
RADS
Chronic bronchitis or chronic obstructive pulmonary disease
Bronchiectasis
Bronchiolitis obliterans
Bronchostenosis
Restrictive interstitial fibrosis
Vocal cord dysfunction syndrome or RUDS

RADS, reactive airways dysfunction syndrome; RUDS, reactive upper airways disorders.

bronchiolitis with occlusion of the bronchioles by inflammatory exudates and fibrin, but without organizing pneumonia [139]. Bronchiolitis obliterans can be life threatening if untreated, but, for many, may improve or resolve with systemic corticosteroid therapy [139]. It is recommended that patients with this form of bronchiolitis obliterans be treated with 40 to 60 mg of prednisone daily for at least 2 months, with the dose tapered after all symptoms and radiographic findings resolve. The second type of bronchiolitis obliterans occurs in patients who have persistent cough and dyspnea with an obstructive ventilatory impairment on pulmonary function tests that does not respond to inhaled corticosteroids or bronchodilators [139,140]. Chest radiographs may appear normal, but high-resolution CT scans of the chest often show hyperinflation and air trapping. Lung biopsy may be necessary to make a definitive diagnosis and typically shows a pure constrictive bronchiolitis. This form of bronchiolitis obliterans is usually not responsive to systemic corticosteroid therapy, and the prognosis for improvement is poor. Patients affected with this form of bronchiolitis obliterans may get progressively worse and suffer life-long disability. The administration of prophylactic corticosteroids to prevent bronchiolitis obliterans following inhalation injury is controversial with treatment effects in either direction [141,142].

References

1. Bronstein AC, Spyker DA, Cantilena Jr LR, et al: 2006 Annual Report of the American Association of Poison Control Centers' National Poison Data System (NPDS). *Clin Toxicol (Phila)* 45(8):815–917, 2007.
2. White CW, Martin JG: Chlorine gas inhalation: human clinical evidence of toxicity and experience in animal models. *Proc Am Thorac Soc* 7(4):257–263, 2010.
3. Pruitt BA Jr., Cioffi WG: Diagnosis and treatment of smoke inhalation. *J Intensive Care Med* 10(3):117–127, 1995.
4. Stefanidou M, Athanaselis S, Spiliopoulou C: Health impacts of fire smoke inhalation. *Inhal Toxicol* 20(8):761–766, 2008.
5. Langford NJ: Carbon dioxide poisoning. *Toxicol Rev* 24(4):229–235, 2005.
6. Satish U, Mendell MJ, Shekhar K, et al: Is CO_2 an indoor pollutant? Direct effects of low-to-moderate CO_2 concentrations on human decision-making performance. *Environ Health Perspect* 120(12):1671–1677, 2012.
7. Baxter PJ, Kapila M, Mfonfu D: Lake Nyos disaster, Cameroon, 1986: the medical effects of large scale emission of carbon dioxide? *BMJ* 298(6685):1437–1441, 2012.
8. Rupp WR, Thierauf A, Nadjem H, et al: Suicide by carbon dioxide. *Forensic Sci Int* 231(1–3):e30–e32, 2013.
9. La Harpe R, Shiferaw K, Mangin P, et al: Fatality in a wine vat. *Am J Forensic Med Pathol* 34(2):119–121, 2013.
10. DeBehnke DJ, Hilander SJ, Dobler DW, et al: The hemodynamic and arterial blood gas response to asphyxiation: a canine model of pulseless electrical activity. *Resuscitation* 30(2):169–175, 1995.
11. Centers for Disease Control and Prevention: Nonfatal, unintentional, non—fire-related carbon monoxide exposures—United States, 2004–2006. *Morb Mortal Wkly Rep* 57(33):896–899, 2008.
12. Huzar TF, George T, Cross JM: Carbon monoxide and cyanide toxicity: etiology, pathophysiology and treatment in inhalation injury. *Expert Rev Respir Med* 7(2):159–170, 2013.
13. Chen BC, Shawn LK, Connors NJ, et al: Carbon monoxide exposures in New York City following Hurricane Sandy in 2012. *Clin Toxicol (Phila)* 51(9):879–885, 2013.
14. Weaver LK: Clinical practice. Carbon monoxide poisoning. *N Engl J Med* 360(12):1217–1225, 2009.
15. Henry CR, Satran D, Lindgren B, et al: Myocardial injury and long-term mortality following moderate to severe carbon monoxide poisoning. *JAMA* 295(4):398–402, 2006.
16. Jaffe FA: Pathogenicity of carbon monoxide. *Am J Forensic Med Pathol* 18(4):406–410, 1997.
17. Zhang J, Piantadosi CA: Mitochondrial Oxidative Stress after Carbon-Monoxide Hypoxia in the Rat-Brain. *J Clin Invest* 90(4):1193–1199, 1992.
18. Thom SR: Leukocytes in carbon monoxide-mediated brain oxidative injury. *Toxicol Appl Pharmacol* 123(2):234–247, 1993.
19. Weaver LK, Valentine KJ, Hopkins RO: Carbon monoxide poisoning: risk factors for cognitive sequelae and the role of hyperbaric oxygen. *Am J Respir Crit Care Med* 176(5):491–497, 2007.
20. Kao HK, Lien TC, Kou YR, et al: Assessment of myocardial injury in the emergency department independently predicts the short-term poor outcome in patients with severe carbon monoxide poisoning receiving mechanical ventilation and hyperbaric oxygen therapy. *Pulm Pharmacol Ther* 22(6):473–477, 2009.
21. Satran D, Henry CR, Adkinson C, et al: Cardiovascular manifestations of moderate to severe carbon monoxide poisoning. *J Am Coll Cardiol* 45(9):1513–1516, 2005.
22. Wolff E: Carbon monoxide poisoning with severe myonecrosis and acute renal failure. *Am J Emerg Med* 12(3):347–349, 1994.
23. Kao LW, Nanagas KA: Carbon monoxide poisoning. *Med Clin North Am* 89(6):1161–1194, 2005.
24. Hill EP, Hill JR, Power GG, et al: Carbon monoxide exchanges between the human fetus and mother: a mathematical model. *Am J Physiol* 232(3):H311–H323, 1977.
25. Koren G, Sharav T, Pastuszak A, et al: A multicenter, prospective study of fetal outcome following accidental carbon monoxide poisoning in pregnancy. *Reprod Toxicol* 5(5):397–403, 1991.
26. Yildiz H, Aldemir E, Altuncu E, et al: A rare cause of perinatal asphyxia: maternal carbon monoxide poisoning. *Arch Gynecol Obstet* 281(2):251–254, 2010.
27. Thom SR, Taber RL, Mendiguren II, et al: Delayed neuropsychologic sequelae after carbon monoxide poisoning: prevention by treatment with hyperbaric oxygen. *Ann Emerg Med* 25(4):474–480, 1995.
28. Hampson NB, Piantadosi CA, Thom SR, et al: Practice recommendations in the diagnosis, management, and prevention of carbon monoxide poisoning. *Am J Respir Crit Care Med* 186(11):1095–1101, 2012.
29. Suner S, Partridge R, Sucov A, et al: Non-invasive pulse CO-oximetry screening in the emergency department identifies occult carbon monoxide toxicity. *J Emerg Med* 34(4):441–450, 2008.
30. Touger M, Birnbaum A, Wang J, et al: Performance of the RAD-57 pulse CO-oximeter compared with standard laboratory carboxyhemoglobin measurement. *Ann Emerg Med* 56(4):382–388, 2010.
31. Ben-Eli D, Peruggia J, McFarland J, et al: Detecting CO. FDNY studies prehospital assessment of COHb. *J Emerg Med Serv* 32(10):S36–S37, 2007.
32. Lippi G, Rastelli G, Meschi T, et al: Pathophysiology, clinics, diagnosis and treatment of heart involvement in carbon monoxide poisoning. *Clin Biochem* 45(16/17):1278–1285, 2012.
33. DeBias DA, Banerjee CM, Birkhead NC, et al: Effects of carbon monoxide inhalation on ventricular fibrillation. *Arch Environ Health* 31(1):42–46, 1976.
34. Kasten KR, Makley AT, Kagan RJ: Update on the critical care management of severe burns. *J Intensive Care Med* 26(4):223–236, 2011.
35. Chiew AL, Buckley NA: Carbon monoxide poisoning in the 21st century. *Crit Care* 18(2):221, 2014.
36. Pace N, Strajman E, Walker EL: Acceleration of carbon monoxide elimination in man by high pressure oxygen. *Science* 111(2894):652–654, 1950.
37. Thom SR: Functional inhibition of leukocyte B2 integrins by hyperbaric oxygen in carbon monoxide-mediated brain injury in rats. *Toxicol Appl Pharmacol* 123(2):248–256, 1993.
38. Juurlink DN, Buckley N, Stanbrook MB, et al: Hyperbaric oxygen for carbon monoxide poisoning. *Cochrane Database Syst Rev* (1):CD002041, 2005.
39. Weaver LK, Hopkins RO, Chan KJ, et al: Hyperbaric oxygen for acute carbon monoxide poisoning. *N Engl J Med* 347(14):1057–1067, 2002.
40. Scheinkestel CD, Bailey M, Myles PS, et al: Hyperbaric or normobaric oxygen for acute carbon monoxide poisoning: a randomised controlled clinical trial. *Med J Aust* 170(5):203–210, 1999.
41. Piantadosi CA: Perspective—Carbon monoxide poisoning. *N Engl J Med* 347(14):1054–1055, 2002.
42. Isbister GK, McGettigan P, Harris I: Hyperbaric oxygen for acute carbon monoxide poisoning. *N Engl J Med* 348(6):558–558, 2003.
43. Takeuchi A, Vesely A, Rucker J, et al: A simple "new" method to accelerate clearance of carbon monoxide. *Am J Respir Crit Care Med* 161(6):1816–1819, 2000.
44. Baud FJ, Barriot P, Toffis V, et al: Elevated blood cyanide concentrations in victims of smoke inhalation. *N Engl J Med* 325(25):1761–1766, 1991.
45. Wetherell HR: The occurrence of cyanide in the blood of fire victims. *J Forensic Sci* 11(2):167–173, 1966.
46. Eckstein M, Maniscalco PM: Focus on smoke inhalation—the most common cause of acute cyanide poisoning. *Prehosp Disaster Med* 21(2):s49–s55, 2006.

47. Ganesan K, Raza SK, Vijayaraghavan R: Chemical warfare agents. *J Pharm Bioallied Sci* 2(3):166–178, 2010.
48. Marziaz ML, Frazier K, Guidry PB, et al: Comparison of brain mitochondrial cytochrome c oxidase activity with cyanide LD(50) yields insight into the efficacy of prophylactics. *J Appl Toxicol* 33(1):50–55, 2013.
49. Lazarus AA, Devereaux A: Potential agents of chemical warfare. Worst-case scenario protection and decontamination methods. *Postgrad Med* 112(5):133–140, 2002.
50. Busl KM, Bleck TP: Treatment of neuroterrorism. *Neurotherapeutics* 9(1):139–157, 2012.
51. Johnson RP, Mellors JW: Arteriolization of venous blood gases: a clue to the diagnosis of cyanide poisoning. *J Emerg Med* 6(5):401–404, 1988.
52. Barillo DJ: Diagnosis and treatment of cyanide toxicity. *J Burn Care Res* 30(1):148–152, 2009.
53. Fortin JL, Giocanti JP, Ruttimann M, et al: Prehospital administration of hydroxocobalamin for smoke inhalation-associated cyanide poisoning: 8 years of experience in the Paris Fire Brigade. *Clin Toxicol (Phila)* 44 Suppl 1:37–44, 2006.
54. Borron SW, Baud FJ, Barriot P, et al: Prospective study of hydroxocobalamin for acute cyanide poisoning in smoke inhalation. *Ann Emerg Med* 49(6):794–801, 801 e1–e2, 2007.
55. Hall AH, Dart R, Bogdan G: Sodium thiosulfate or hydroxocobalamin for the empiric treatment of cyanide poisoning? *Ann Emerg Med* 49(6):806–813, 2007.
56. Beckerman N, Leikin SM, Aitchinson R, et al: Laboratory interferences with the newer cyanide antidote: hydroxocobalamin. *Semin Diagn Pathol* 26(1):49–52, 2009.
57. Lee J, Mukai D, Kreuter K, et al: Potential interference by hydroxocobalamin on cooximetry hemoglobin measurements during cyanide and smoke inhalation treatments. *Ann Emerg Med* 49(6):802–805, 2007.
58. Reade MC, Davies SR, Morley PT, et al: Review article: management of cyanide poisoning. *Emerg Med Australas* 24(3):225–238, 2012.
59. Lavon O, Bentur Y: Does amyl nitrite have a role in the management of pre-hospital mass casualty cyanide poisoning? *Clin Toxicol* 48(6):477–484, 2010.
60. Ballerino-Regan D, Longmire AW: Hydrogen sulfide exposure as a cause of sudden occupational death. *Arch Pathol Lab Med* 134(8):1105, 2010.
61. Poli D, Solarino B, Di Vella G, et al: Occupational asphyxiation by unknown compound(s): environmental and toxicological approach. *Forensic Sci Int* 197(1–3):e19–e26, 2010.
62. Yalamanchili C, Smith MD: Acute hydrogen sulfide toxicity due to sewer gas exposure. *Am J Emerg Med* 26(4):518 e5–e7, 2008.
63. Byungkuk NA, Hyokyung KI, Hun LE, et al: Neurologic sequela of hydrogen sulfide poisoning. *Ind Health* 42(1):83–87, 2004.
64. Gorguner M, Akgun M: Acute inhalation injury. *Eurasian J Med* 42(1):28–35, 2010.
65. Amino M, Yoshioka K, Suzuki Y, et al: Improvement in a patient suffering from cardiac injury due to severe hydrogen sulfide poisoning: a long-term examination of the process of recovery of heart failure by performing nuclear medicine study. *Intern Med* 48(19):1745–1748, 2009.
66. Lee EC, Kwan J, Leem JH, et al: Hydrogen sulfide intoxication with dilated cardiomyopathy. *J Occup Health* 51(6):522–525, 2009.
67. Ago M, Ago K, Ogata M: Two fatalities by hydrogen sulfide poisoning: variation of pathological and toxicological findings. *Leg Med (Tokyo)* 10(3):148–152, 2008.
68. Ravizza AG, Carugo D, Cerchiari EL, et al: The treatment of hydrogen sulfide intoxication: oxygen versus nitrites. *Vet Hum Toxicol* 24(4):241–242, 1982.
69. Stine RJ, Slosberg B, Beacham BE: Hydrogen sulfide intoxication. A case report and discussion of treatment. *Ann Intern Med* 85(6):756–758, 1976.
70. Gunn B, Wong R: Noxious gas exposure in the outback: two cases of hydrogen sulfide toxicity. *Emerg Med (Fremantle)* 13(2):240–246, 2001.
71. Buie SE, Pratt DS, May JJ: Diffuse pulmonary injury following paint remover exposure. *Am J Med* 81(4):702–704, 1986.
72. Fedoruk MJ, Bronstein R, Kerger BD: Ammonia exposure and hazard assessment for selected household cleaning product uses. *J Expo Anal Environ Epidemiol* 15(6):534–544, 2005.
73. Bloom GR, Suhail F, Hopkins-Price P, et al: Acute anhydrous ammonia injury from accidents during illicit methamphetamine production. *Burns* 34(5):713–718, 2008.
74. Leduc D, Gris P, Lheureux P, et al: Acute and long term respiratory damage following inhalation of ammonia. *Thorax* 47(9):755–757, 1992.
75. Tonelli AR, Pham A: Bronchiectasis, a long-term sequela of ammonia inhalation: A case report and review of the literature. *Burns* 35(3):451–453, 2009.
76. Becker M, Forrester M: Pattern of chlorine gas exposures reported to Texas poison control centers, 2000 through 2005. *Tex Med* 104(3):52–57, 51, 2008.
77. LoVecchio F, Blackwell S, Stevens D: Outcomes of chlorine exposure: a 5-year poison center experience in 598 patients. *Eur J Emerg Med* 12(3):109–110, 2005.
78. Babu RV, Cardenas V, Sharma G: Acute respiratory distress syndrome from chlorine inhalation during a swimming pool accident: a case report and review of the literature. *J Intensive Care Med* 23(4):275–280, 2008.
79. Wenck MA, Van Sickle D, Drociuk D, et al: Rapid assessment of exposure to chlorine released from a train derailment and resulting health impact. *Public Health Rep* 122(6):784–792, 2007.
80. Schwartz DA, Smith DD, Lakshminarayan S: The pulmonary sequelae associated with accidental inhalation of chlorine gas. *Chest* 97(4):820–825, 1990.
81. Parimon T, Kanne JP, Pierson DJ: Acute inhalation injury with evidence of diffuse bronchiolitis following chlorine gas exposure at a swimming pool. *Respir Care* 49(3):291–294, 2004.
82. Antonini JM, Lewis AB, Roberts JR, et al: Pulmonary effects of welding fumes: review of worker and experimental animal studies. *Am J Ind Med* 43(4):350–360, 2003.
83. Sciuto AM, Hurt HH: Therapeutic treatments of phosgene-induced lung injury. *Inhal Toxicol* 16(8):565–580, 2004.
84. Douglas WW, Hepper NG, Colby TV: Silo-filler's disease. *Mayo Clin Proc* 64(3):291–304, 1989.
85. Weinberger B, Laskin DL, Heck DE, et al: The toxicology of inhaled nitric oxide. *Toxicol Sci* 59(1):5–16, 2001.
86. Andersson E, Murgia N, Nilsson T, et al: Incidence of chronic bronchitis in a cohort of pulp mill workers with repeated gassings to sulphur dioxide and other irritant gases. *Environ Health* 12:113, 2013.
87. Johns DO, Linn WS: A review of controlled human SO(2) exposure studies contributing to the US EPA integrated science assessment for sulfur oxides. *Inhal Toxicol* 23(1):33–43, 2011.
88. Bravo MA, Son J, de Freitas CU, et al: Air pollution and mortality in Sao Paulo, Brazil: Effects of multiple pollutants and analysis of susceptible populations. *J Expo Sci Environ Epidemiol*, 2016;26(2):150–161.
89. Chian CF, Wu CP, Chen CW, et al: Acute respiratory distress syndrome after zinc chloride inhalation: survival after extracorporeal life support and corticosteroid treatment. *Am J Crit Care* 19(1):86–90, 2010.
90. Hsu HH, Tzao C, Chang WC, et al: Zinc chloride (smoke bomb) inhalation lung injury: clinical presentations, high-resolution CT findings, and pulmonary function test results. *Chest* 127(6):2064–2071, 2005.
91. Seidal K, Jörgensen N, Elinder CG, et al: Fatal cadmium-induced pneumonitis. Scand J *Work Environ Health* 19(6):429–431, 1993.
92. Mannino DM, Holguin F, Greves HM, et al: Urinary cadmium levels predict lower lung function in current and former smokers: data from the Third National Health and Nutrition Examination Survey. *Thorax* 59(3):194–198, 2004.
93. Jarup L: Cadmium overload and toxicity. *Nephrol Dial Transplant* 17[Suppl 2]:35–39, 2002.
94. Bernhoft RA: Cadmium toxicity and treatment. *Sci World J* 2013:394652, 2013.
95. Haponik EF, Crapo RO, Herndon DN, et al: Smoke inhalation. *Am Rev Respir Dis* 138(4):1060–1063, 1988.
96. Thompson PB, Herndon DN, Traber DL, et al: Effect on mortality of inhalation injury. *J Trauma* 26(2):163–165, 1986.
97. Saffle JR, Davis B, Williams P: Recent outcomes in the treatment of burn injury in the United States: a report from the American Burn Association Patient Registry. *J Burn Care Rehabil* 16(3, pt 1):219–232; discussion 288–289, 1995.
98. Levin BC, Paabo M, Fultz ML, et al: Generation of hydrogen-cyanide from flexible polyurethane foam decomposed under different combustion conditions. *Fire Mater* 9(3):125–134, 1985.
99. Zikria BA, Floch HF, Ferrer JM: Chemical factors contributing to pulmonary damage in smoke poisoning. *Surgery* 71(5):704, 1972.
100. Treitman RD, Burgess WA, Gold A: Air contaminants encountered by firefighters. *Am Ind Hyg Assoc J* 41(11):796–802, 1980.
101. Haponik EF, Summer WR: Respiratory complications in burned patients—diagnosis and management of inhalation injury. *J Crit Care* 2(2):121–143, 1987.
102. Haponik EF, Munster AM, Wise RA, et al: Upper airway function in burn patients. Correlation of flow-volume curves and nasopharyngoscopy. *Am Rev Respir Dis* 129(2):251–257, 1984.
103. Cancio LC: Airway management and smoke inhalation injury in the burn patient. *Clin Plast Surg* 36(4):555–567, 2009.
104. Douglas CG, Haldane JS, Haldane JBS: The laws of combination of hemoglobin with carbon monoxide and oxygen. *J Physiol Lond* 44(4):275–304, 1912.
105. Silverman SH, Purdue GF, Hunt JL, et al: Cyanide toxicity in burned patients. *J Trauma* 28(2):171–176, 1988.
106. Cochran A: Inhalation injury and endotracheal intubation. *J Burn Care Res* 30(1):190–191, 2009.
107. Agee RN, Long III JM, Hunt JL, et al: Use of 133xenon in early diagnosis of inhalation injury. *J Trauma* 16(3):218–224, 1976.
108. Masaki Y, Sugiyama K, Tanaka H, et al: Effectiveness of CT for clinical stratification of occupational lung edema. *Ind Health* 45(1):78–84, 2007.
109. Sherman CB, Barnhart S, Miller MF, et al: Firefighting acutely increases airway responsiveness. *Am Rev Respir Dis* 140(1):185–190, 1989.
110. Chia KS, Jeyaratnam J, Chan TB, et al: Airway responsiveness of firefighters after smoke exposure. *Br J Ind Med* 47(8):524–527, 1990.
111. Kinsella J, Campbell D, Carter R, et al: Increased airways reactivity after smoke inhalation. *Lancet* 337(8741):595–597, 1991.
112. Banauch GI, Alleyne D, Sanchez R, et al: Persistent hyperreactivity and reactive airway dysfunction in firefighters at the World Trade Center. *Am J Respir Crit Care Med* 168(1):54–62, 2003.
113. Mlcak RP, Suman OE, Herndon DN: Respiratory management of inhalation injury. *Burns* 33(1):2–13, 2007.
114. Venet F, Plassais J, Textoris J, et al: Low-dose hydrocortisone reduces norepinephrine duration in severe burn patients: a randomized clinical trial. *Crit Care* 19:21, 2015.
115. Gunnarsson M, Walther SM, Seidal T, et al: Effects of inhalation of corticosteroids immediately after experimental chlorine gas lung injury. *J Trauma* 48(1):101–107, 2015.
116. Wang J, Winskog C, Edston E, et al: Inhaled and intravenous corticosteroids both attenuate chlorine gas-induced lung injury in pigs. *Acta Anaesthesiol Scand* 49(2):183–190, 2015.
117. Peck MD, Harrington D, Mlcak RP, et al: Potential studies of mode of ventilation in inhalation injury. *J Burn Care Res* 30(1):181–183, 2015.

118. Dries DJ: Key questions in ventilator management of the burn-injured patient (first of two parts). *J Burn Care Res* 30(1):128–138, 2015.
119. Dries DJ: Key questions in ventilator management of the burn-injured patient (second of two parts). *J Burn Care Res* 30(2):211–220, 2009.
120. Greenhalgh DG: Steroids in the treatment of smoke inhalation injury. *J Burn Care Res* 30(1):165–169, 2009.
121. Sterner JB, Zanders TB, Morris MJ, et al: Inflammatory mediators in smoke inhalation injury. *Inflamm Allergy Drug Targets* 8(1):63–69, 2009.
122. Dries DJ, Endorf FW: Inhalation injury: epidemiology, pathology, treatment strategies. *Scand J Trauma Resusc Emerg Med* 21:31, 2013.
123. Toon MH, Maybauer MO, Greenwood JE, et al: Management of acute smoke inhalation injury. *Crit Care Resusc* 12(1):53–61, 2010.
124. Miller AC, Rivero A, Ziad S, et al: Influence of nebulized unfractionated heparin and N-acetylcysteine in acute lung injury after smoke inhalation injury. *J Burn Care Res* 30(2):249–256, 2009.
125. Desai MH, Mlcak R, Richardson J, et al: Reduction in mortality in pediatric patients with inhalation injury with aerosolized heparin/N-acetylcystine [correction of acetylcystine] therapy. *J Burn Care Rehabil* 19(3):210–212, 1998.
126. Miller AC, Elamin EM, Suffredini AF: Inhaled anticoagulation regimens for the treatment of smoke inhalation-associated acute lung injury: a systematic review. *Crit Care Med* 42(2):413–419, 2014.
127. Edelman DA, Khan N, Kempf K, et al: Pneumonia after inhalation injury. *J Burn Care Res* 28(2):241–246, 2007.
128. Prezant DJ, Weiden M, Banauch GI, et al: Cough and bronchial responsiveness in firefighters at the World Trade Center site. *N Engl J Med* 347(11):806–815, 2002.
129. Rafael E, Shohet MR, Chasan R, et al: Occupational toxicant inhalation injury: the World Trade Center (WTC) experience. *Int Arch Occup Environ Health* 81(4):479–485, 2008.
130. Brooks SM, Weiss MA, Bernstein IL: Reactive airways dysfunction syndrome (RADS). Persistent asthma syndrome after high level irritant exposures. *Chest* 88(3):376–384, 1985.
131. Banauch GI, Izbicki G, Christodoulou V, et al: Trial of prophylactic inhaled steroids to prevent or reduce pulmonary function decline, pulmonary symptoms, and airway hyperreactivity in firefighters at the world trade center site. *Disaster Med Public Health Prep* 2(1):33–39, 2008.
132. Aldrich TK, Gustave J, Hall CB, et al: Lung function in rescue workers at the world trade center after 7 years. *N Engl J Med* 362(14):1263–1272, 2010.
133. Weiden MD, Ferrier N, Nolan A, et al: Obstructive airways disease with air trapping among firefighters exposed to World Trade Center dust. *Chest* 137(3):566–574, 2010.
134. King MS, Eisenberg R, Newman JH, et al: Constrictive bronchiolitis in soldiers returning from Iraq and Afghanistan. *N Engl J Med* 365(3):222–230, 2011.
135. Saber H, Saburi A, Ghanei M: Clinical and paraclinical guidelines for management of sulfur mustard induced bronchiolitis obliterans; from bench to bedside. *Inhal Toxicol* 24(13):900–906, 2012.
136. Pirjavec A, Kovic I, Lulic I, et al: Massive anhydrous ammonia injury leading to lung transplantation. *J Trauma* 67(4):E93–E97, 2009.
137. Ainslie G: Inhalational injuries produced by smoke and nitrogen dioxide. *Respir Med* 87(3):169–174, 2009.
138. Beheshti J, Mark EJ, Akbaei HM, et al: Mustard lung secrets: long term clinicopathological study following mustard gas exposure. *Pathol Res Pract* 202(10):739–744, 2006.
139. Barker AF, Bergeron A, Rom WN, et al: Obliterative bronchiolitis. *N Engl J Med* 370(19):1820–1828, 2014.
140. Lynch JP, Weigt SS, DerHovanessian A, et al: Obliterative (constrictive) bronchiolitis. *Semin Respir Crit Care Med* 33(5):509–532, 2012.
141. Moylan JA: Supportive therapy in burn care. Smoke inhalation. Diagnostic techniques and steroids. *J Trauma* 19(11 Suppl):917, 1979.
142. Moulick ND, Banavali S, Abhyankar AD, et al: Acute accidental exposure to chlorine fumes—a study of 82 cases. *Indian J Chest Dis Allied Sci* 34(2):85–89, 1992.

Chapter 179 ■ Chest Radiographic Examination

CAROLE A. RIDGE • BENEDIKT H. HEIDINGER • JERRY P. BALIKIAN • DIANA E. LITMANOVICH

INTRODUCTION

Radiographic examination of the critically ill patient in the intensive care unit (ICU) or coronary care unit (CCU) is often necessary to follow the patient's progress or changes in status after admission or after surgery. Radiographic examinations are requested to evaluate the course of the primary disease and to diagnose complications that may ensue. The bedside chest radiograph has been shown to alter management 85% of 258 consecutive radiographs analyzed by Palazzetti and colleagues [1]. A similar retrospective study analyzing 1,354 radiographs from a respiratory ICU found a 34.5% incidence of new or increased abnormalities or tube or catheter malpositions [2]. These studies suggest that routine daily radiographic examinations frequently demonstrate unexpected or changing abnormalities, many of which prompt changes in clinical management. In 2013, American College of Radiology published appropriateness criteria for the need of ICU studies advising that a portable chest radiograph is appropriate after placement of an endotracheal tube, central venous line, Swan–Ganz catheter, nasogastric tube, feeding tube, or chest tube or if a clinical indication mandates chest radiography in a stable or ventilated patient [3].

Critically ill patients in the ICU or CCU often cannot take advantage of radiologic investigations that are readily available to mobile patients. Because some of these patients cannot be transported while their circulatory functions are labile and they are connected to electrocardiogram monitors, ventilators, catheters, and surgical appliances, usually the only examination that is readily available to them is the portable bedside radiographic examination. The chest radiograph is especially important because physical examination to determine the presence of complications such as atelectasis, pneumothorax, pneumonia, or pulmonary edema is limited in the intubated and ventilated patient.

The main advances in portable screen-film radiographic examinations include the advent of computed radiography and flat panel detectors [4]. Computed radiography technology uses a photostimulable barium halide phosphor cassette similar to that used in screen-film radiography. After exposure, the cassette is transported to a computed radiography reader device, which is scanned by a laser; the image is then available in digital soft copy format. The main advantages include the reduced need for cassette handling leading to improved workflow and the ability to manipulate the image after acquisition to improve visualization of subtle structures (e.g., a central venous catheter tip). Flat panel technology is based on thin layers of amorphous silicon thin-film transistors (TFTs) deposited on a piece of glass. The TFT layer is coupled with an X-ray absorptive layer. Because the silicon film transistors are thin, the X-ray absorptive layer can be thick, leading to increased X-ray detection efficiency. This development has addressed the limitation of long exposure times inherent to prior iterations of radiographic systems and has thus enabled a reduction in radiation dose while continuing to possess the described advantages of computed radiography. Both flat panel and computed radiography imaging systems can now be used for portable chest radiographic examination.

Interpretation of portable examinations is fraught with pitfalls. Magnification of the cardiac silhouette cannot be eliminated because of the short tube–detector distance and the often supine position of the patient. Signs used to evaluate pulmonary venous hypertension are not valid on the supine

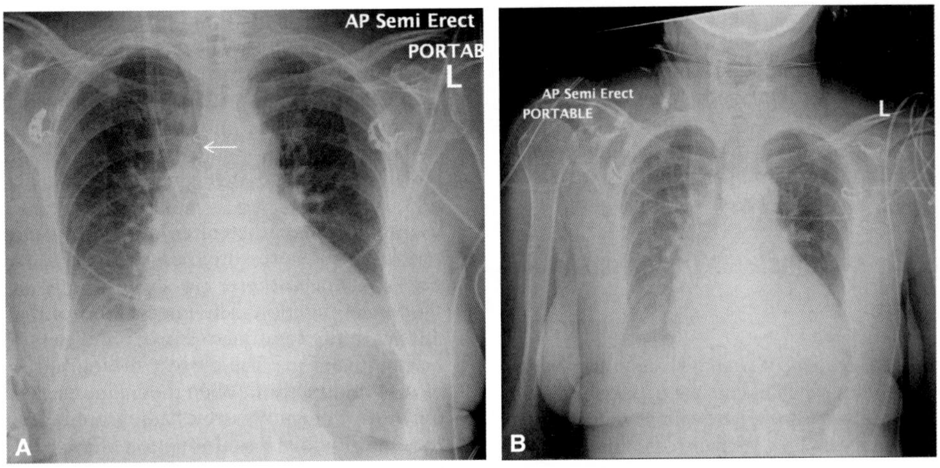

FIGURE 179.1 The degree of inflation of the lung may cause pulmonary opacities to appear more or less dense indicating an apparent disimprovement which is in fact secondary to decreased aeration (e.g., the removal of an endotracheal tube). This is demonstrated on this anteroposterior portable chest radiograph of a 70-year-old male who is day 2 after uncomplicated mitral valve repair. The first radiograph (**A**) demonstrates a low lying endotracheal tube tip in the lower trachea (*arrow*), two satisfactorily positioned right internal jugular venous catheters, intact sternotomy wires, two mediastinal drains, and moderate cardiomegaly. Five hours later (**B**), the endotracheal tube has been removed because of clinical stability and as a result, lung density increases due to the absence of mechanical ventilation.

radiograph. Furthermore, the meniscus of a pleural effusion is often not visible using supine or semi-erect radiographic positioning. Radiographs are often acquired after a poor inspiratory effort because of the patient's inability to follow breath-hold instructions. As a result, the appearance of parenchymal abnormalities is difficult to evaluate. Increased inflation of the lung may cause the opacities to appear less dense, but the apparent improvement secondary to increased aeration does not correspond to a true improvement. The reverse situation can occur as well, particularly after a patient has been extubated (Fig. 179.1).

EVALUATION OF TUBES AND CATHETERS

Endotracheal Tubes

The location of endotracheal tubes should be checked as soon as possible after insertion (see Chapter 1). To evaluate the position of the tube properly, Goodman et al. [5] showed that one must evaluate the head and neck position simultaneously because tube position can change with flexion and extension of the neck [6] by as much as 4 cm [5,7]. If the radiograph includes the mandible, the following guidelines may be of use:

1. When the inferior border of the mandible is at or above C4, the tip should be 7 ± 2 cm from the carina.
2. When the inferior border of the mandible is at the C5 to C6 levels, the tip of the tube should be 5 ± 2 cm from the carina.
3. When the inferior border of the mandible is at T1 or below, the tip of the tube should be 3 ± 2 cm from the carina.

If, however, the mandible is not visible, and the technologist has ensured that the head is in a neutral position, an endotracheal tube position 5 ± 2 cm from the carina is acceptable (Fig. 179.2). When the tube is too high, it may slip into the pharynx. If it is just below the vocal cords, its inflated cuff can cause glottic or subglottic edema, ulceration, and, ultimately, scarring. If it is too low, it can enter a bronchus and cause atelectasis of the lung supplied by the obstructed bronchus (Fig. 179.3).

Ideally, the tube should be one-half to two-thirds the width of the trachea, and the inflated cuff should fill the trachea without causing the lateral walls to bulge. Repeated overdistension of the

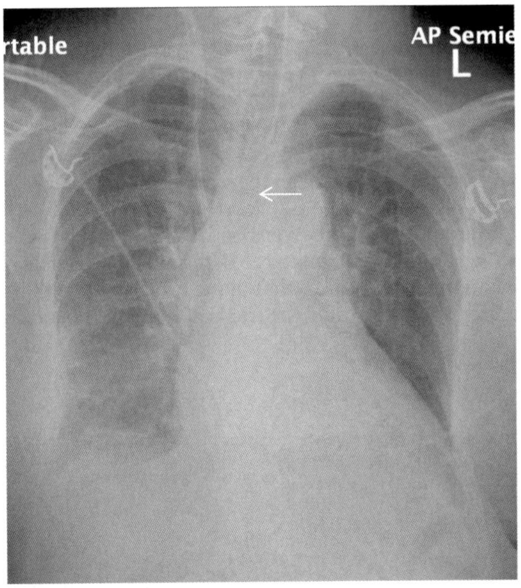

FIGURE 179.2 Correct endotracheal tube position. Anteroposterior portable chest radiograph of a 70-year-old male who is day 1 after mitral valve repair. The radiograph demonstrates appropriate endotracheal tube position in the lower trachea 3 cm from the carina (*arrow*), two satisfactorily positioned right internal jugular venous catheters, intact sternotomy wires, two mediastinal drains, acute perihilar "batwing" opacities indicating pulmonary edema which resolved after diuresis (Fig. 179.1) and moderate cardiomegaly.

cuff on chest film, despite careful cuff inflation to the minimal leak level may predispose to tracheomalacia (Fig. 179.4) [6].

Immediately after intubation, and especially after difficult intubation, an image should be obtained to define the position of the endotracheal tube. The radiologist should also look for signs of perforation of the pharynx, such as new subcutaneous emphysema, pneumomediastinum, and pneumothorax. Dislodging of teeth, dental caps, and portions of dentures into the tracheobronchial tree has been reported after intubation. If this is suspected, a foreign body in the tracheobronchial tree should be carefully sought.

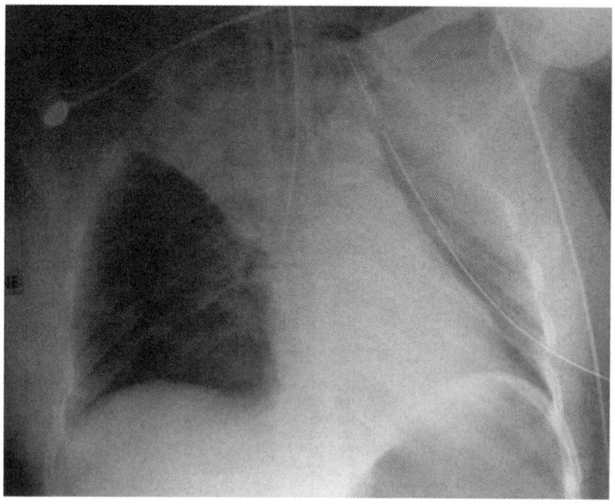

FIGURE 179.3 Endotracheal tube malposition. Anteroposterior chest radiograph of a 25-year-old male admitted to the ICU after a motor vehicle accident. The radiograph demonstrates the tip of the endotracheal tube in the right main bronchus (*arrow*), causing right upper lobe atelectasis; in addition, there is complete collapse of the left lung owing to a large pneumothorax which has been treated with emergent left chest tube placement, the tip of which is in satisfactory position. ICU, intensive care unit.

Tracheostomy Tubes

The tip of the tracheostomy tube should be located one-half to two-thirds of the way between the stoma and the carina. Unlike the endotracheal tube, the tracheostomy tube does not change position with flexion and extension of the neck. The tracheostomy tube should be evaluated to determine its inner diameter (which should be two-thirds that of the tracheal lumen); its long axis (which should parallel the tracheal lumen); the location of its distal end (Fig. 179.2) (which should not about the tracheal wall laterally, anteriorly, or posteriorly); and for development of new pneumothorax, pneumomediastinum, or subcutaneous emphysema, which may indicate tracheal rupture.

Central Venous Catheters

Central venous catheters should be evaluated to ensure accurate central venous pressure measurement and central venous drug delivery. The catheter tip should be located at the superior cavoatrial junction. The intersection of the bronchus intermedius with the right heart border and the inflection of the right heart border are the closest radiographic landmarks to the cavoatrial junction. When these landmarks are not identifiable, the most uniformly visible radiographic landmark is the carina; the superior cavoatrial junction is approximately 4 cm above this structure (Fig. 179.5) [8]. Complications of central venous catheter placement include infection, vascular perforation or dissection, inadvertent arterial cannulation (Fig. 179.6A), and cardiac perforation, leading to cardiac tamponade (Fig. 179.6B) and catheter fragment embolization.

Swan-Ganz Catheters

Swan-Ganz catheters are used to perform right heart catheterizations [9]. Ideally, the tip of the Swan-Ganz catheter should be located in the right or left branch of the pulmonary artery (Fig. 179.7). Occasionally, the tip may be malpositioned (Fig. 179.6); a radiograph should be routinely taken to check its position. If the catheter tip is more than 3 cm from the midline, the catheter could potentially produce pulmonary infarction (Fig. 179.8A–C) by blocking the artery directly or from a clot in or around the tip. Other rare complications include perforation of the pulmonary artery, the resulting focal hemorrhage leading to the formation of “traumatic pseudoaneurysm” (Fig. 179.8D), balloon rupture, and

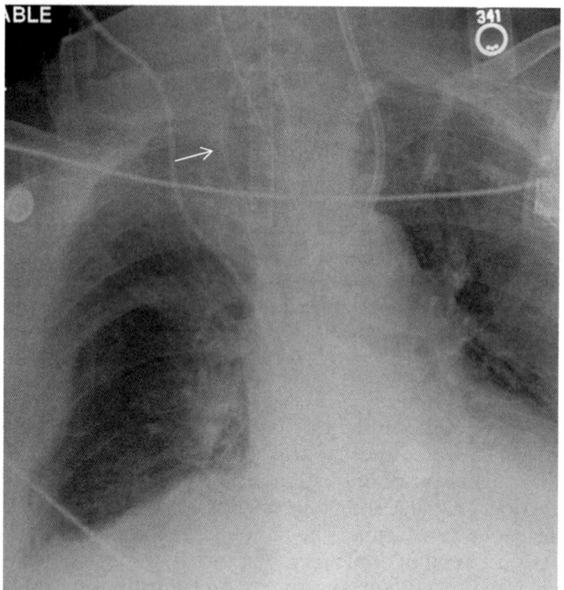

FIGURE 179.4 Endotracheal cuff overinflation. Anteroposterior portable chest radiograph of a 64-year-old male who is day 1 after colectomy. The balloon of the endotracheal tube (*arrow*) is wider than the transverse diameter of the trachea indicating overdistension.

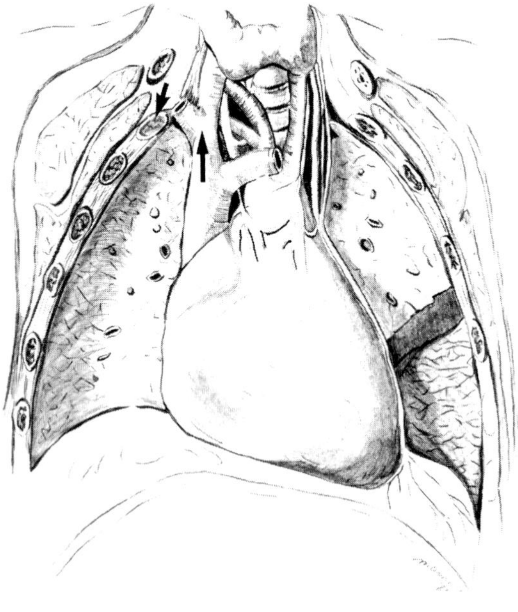

FIGURE 179.5 Junction of internal jugular vein and right subclavian vein. Veins shown in relation to the first rib. The junction of the internal jugular and right subclavian veins (*long arrow*) occurs at approximately the level of the first rib (*short arrow*). The central venous pressure line should be at or beyond this point to measure true venous pressure. (Drawing by Mary Cunnion).

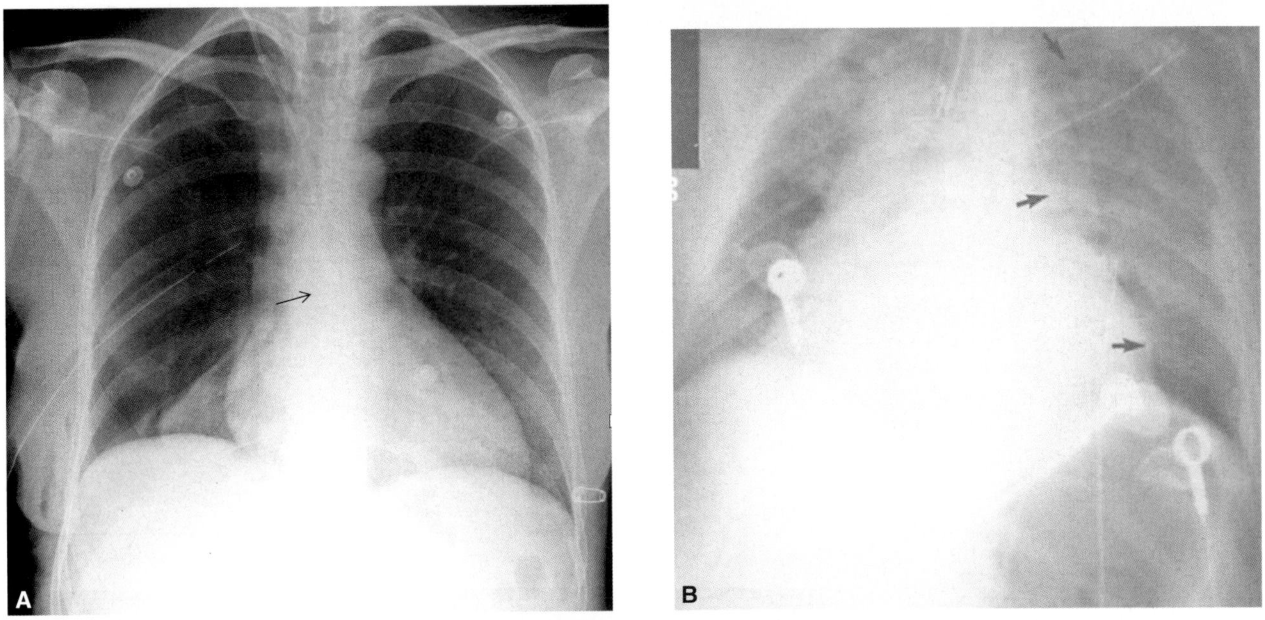

FIGURE 179.6 **A:** Central line complications. Inadvertent arterial cannulation. Anteroposterior chest radiograph in a 50-year-old female day 1 after hysterectomy and central line insertion who complained of dizziness. The central venous catheter crosses the midline consistent with an intra-arterial course (*arrow*), an iatrogenic right pneumothorax has been treated with chest tube placement. A subsequent CT confirmed catheter position in the right subclavian artery and a posterior circulation cerebral infarct owing to occlusion of the right vertebral artery. **B:** Central line complications. Portable anteroposterior view of a different patient with pulmonary edema in whom a central venous pressure line extends from the left subclavian vein. The line entered the pericardium (*arrows*) and caused tamponade from the bleeding resulting from the vascular perforation. CT, computed tomography.

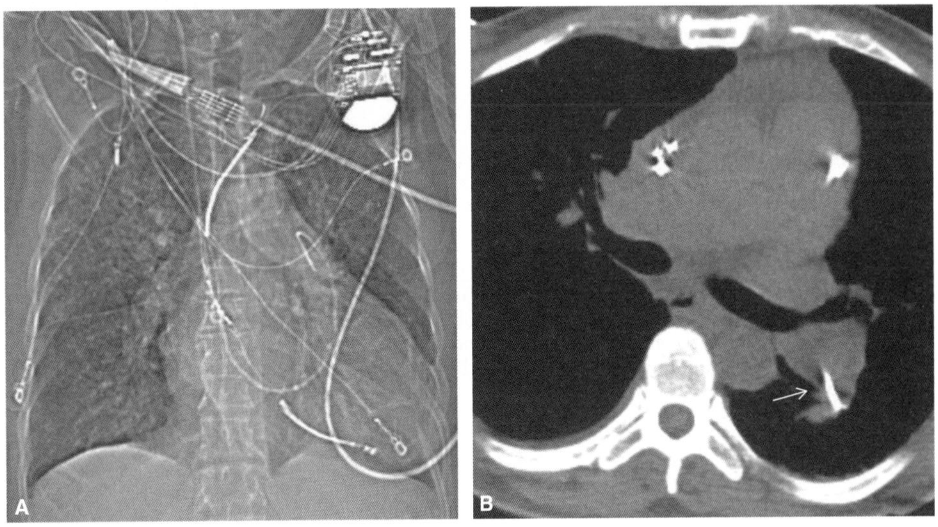

FIGURE 179.7 Thoracic CT scout (A) and axial images (B) in a 52-year-old female with dilated cardiomyopathy shows a right internal jugular approach Swan–Ganz catheter with its tip in the left lower lobar pulmonary artery (*arrow*). CT, computed tomography.

pulmonary artery–bronchial tree fistula. Once correct position is confirmed radiographically, clinical criteria can be used to confirm ongoing correct position which include >1.25 mL volume of air required to insufflate the catheter tip balloon and obtain a pulmonary capillary wedge pressure tracing and the absence of >1 cm migration from initial catheter position according to the centimeter markings from the catheter hub [10].

Intra-aortic Balloon Pump

The intra-aortic balloon pump (IABP) was designed to improve cardiac function and coronary perfusion in a setting of cardiogenic shock, and this remains the major indication for its use [11]. Ideally, the tip of the IABP should be positioned at the level of the aortic arch below the origin of the left subclavian artery to augment coronary artery perfusion during diastole maximally without occluding the subclavian and cerebral vessels (Fig. 179.9). A position too low in the thoracic aorta may limit its effectiveness and can give rise to occlusion of the abdominal aortic branches. On the chest radiograph, the ideal IABP position was defined as below the aortic arch, between T2 and T5 vertebrae [12]. Complications related to IABP placement include major vessel obstruction (Fig. 179.10), embolization from a clot formed in or around the catheter, and aortic dissection with balloon rupture.

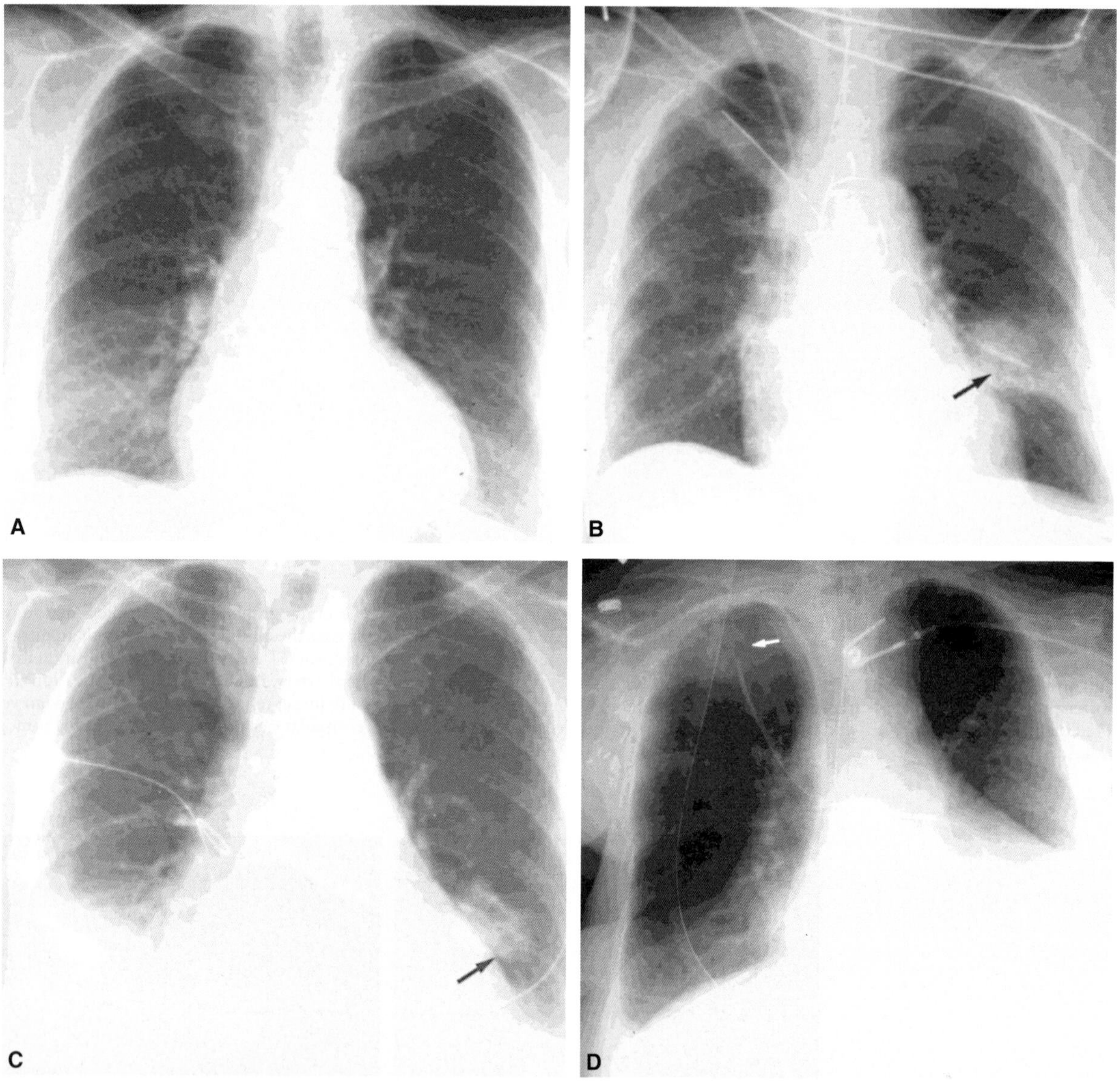

FIGURE 179.8 A–D: Infarction caused by Swan-Ganz catheter. **A:** Preoperative posteroanterior view of the chest shows bilaterally clear lung parenchyma. **B:** Postoperative posteroanterior view of the chest shows overly distal position of the Swan-Ganz catheter. An area of density (*arrow*) surrounds the tip of the catheter, representing a pulmonary infarct in the area supplied by the occluded artery. **C:** Posteroanterior film after 5 days shows a persistent left lower lobe density (*arrow*)—the resolving infarct. Right pleural effusion is also present. **D:** Note tip of Swan-Ganz catheter line at periphery of right upper lobe pulmonary artery and showing a round opacity representing "traumatic pseudoaneurysm" (*arrow*).

Chest Tubes

Chest tubes (thoracostomy or pleural drainage tubes) are used to drain either fluid or air from the pleural space (see Chapter 8). If placed for a pneumothorax, the tube tip should be projected over the lung apex where pleural air typically collects on the chest radiograph; if placed to drain a pleural effusion, the tube should be projected over the posterior lower pleural space (Fig. 179.11A, B). If a wide bore chest tube is used, the side hole of the tube (where there is an interruption in the opaque marker) should be seen within the pleural space. If a locking pigtail catheter is used, the catheter should form a round loop in the pleural space, thus ensuring sidehole position within the pleura because sideholes are typically located only in the region of the pigtail; if present, a radio-opaque marker indicates the position of the most distal sidehole.

Nasogastric Tubes

The tip of the nasogastric tube should be visible below the diaphragm projected over the expected location of the stomach. Malposition in the esophagus or bronchi should be excluded radiographically prior to nasogastric tube use (Fig. 179.12A, B). Malposition in the lungs can rarely lead to bronchopleural fistula formation (Fig. 179.12C).

Transvenous Pacemakers

Pacemaker leads are passed under fluoroscopic guidance into the right atrium, apex of the right ventricle, and/or through the coronary sinus into the left ventricular cardiac vein; the latter is used for biventricular pacing in severe heart failure

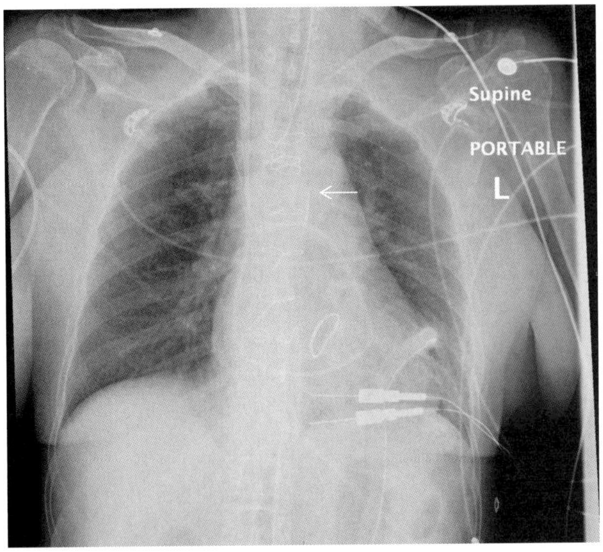

FIGURE 179.9 Correct IABP position. The tip of the IABP should be positioned at the level of the aortic arch below the origin of the left subclavian artery (*arrow*) to augment coronary artery perfusion during diastole maximally without occluding the subclavian and cerebral vessels. IABP, intra-aortic balloon pump.

[13] (see Heading V). Films should be checked for breaks or fractures in the wire (Fig. 179.13). A lateral view should be obtained to ascertain that the right ventricular pacemaker tip is directed anteriorly 3 to 4 mm beneath the pericardial fat [14]. A posteriorly directed tip on the lateral view, coupled with a cephalad direction in the anteroposterior (AP) view, suggests that the pacer is in the coronary sinus or a tributary [15]. Projection of the pacemaker tip anterior to the pericardial fat stripe suggests myocardial perforation [14]. Subcutaneous emphysema may signify air entrapment in the pulse generator pocket. This can produce a system malfunction with unipolar pulse generators [16].

Assessment of the position of the tubes and lines with computed tomography (CT) is precise and usually achieved with a combination of axial, coronal, and sagittal reformatted images.

EVALUATION OF THE LUNG PARENCHYMA

Densities of the Lung Parenchyma

Pulmonary parenchymal densities in the critically ill patient may be caused by either infectious or noninfectious conditions, such as atelectasis, cardiogenic pulmonary edema, acute respiratory

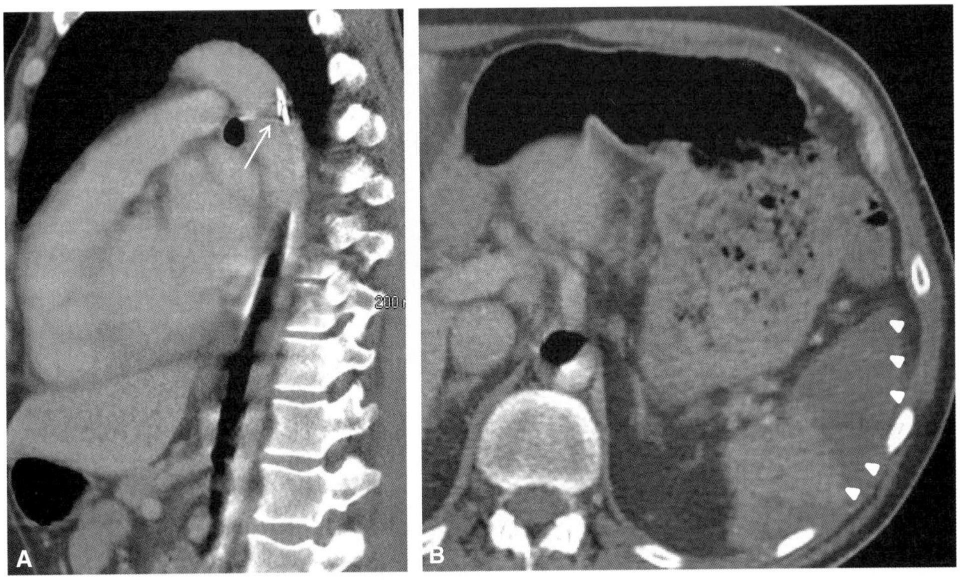

FIGURE 179.10 Sagittal (A) and axial (B) CT images of a 41-year-old male with a myocardial infarct requiring intra-aortic balloon pump placement demonstrates appropriate distal tip position distal to the left subclavian artery origin of the aortic arch (*arrows*). The balloon is inflated during image acquisition, and is shown to be too long, descending below the coeliac artery origin resulting in splenic infarction. CT, computed tomography.

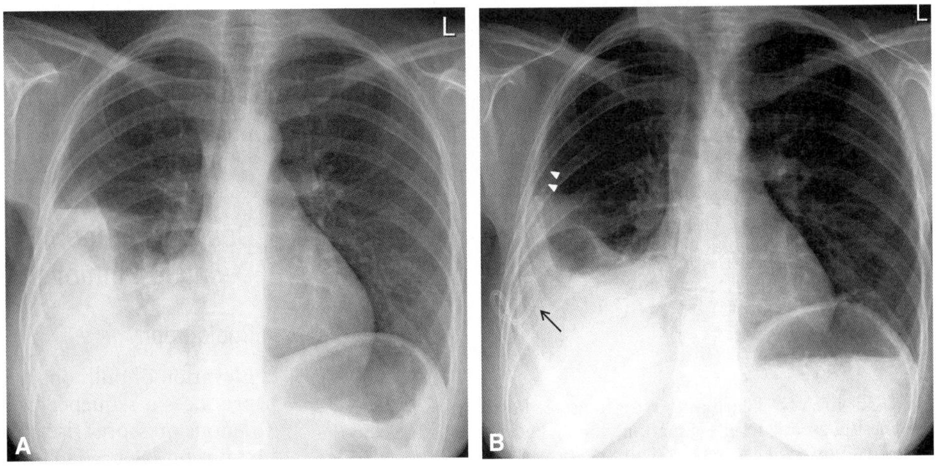

FIGURE 179.11 **A, B:** Satisfactory pleural drainage catheter position. Chest radiographs of a 33-year-old female with dyspnea secondary to stage 4 ALK mutant lung carcinoma with a malignant right pleural effusion. A right pleural catheter was placed with symptomatic improvement; the pigtail and its sideholes are shown within the right lateral pleural space (*arrow*). A small right lateral pneumothorax is likely owing to ex vacuo phenomenon in a chronically atelectatic lung because of the large right effusion. ALK, anaplastic lymphoma kinase.

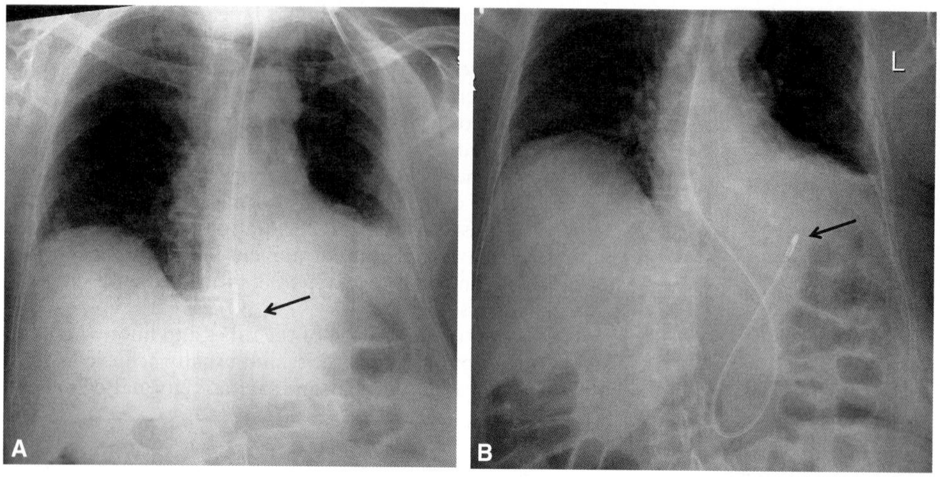

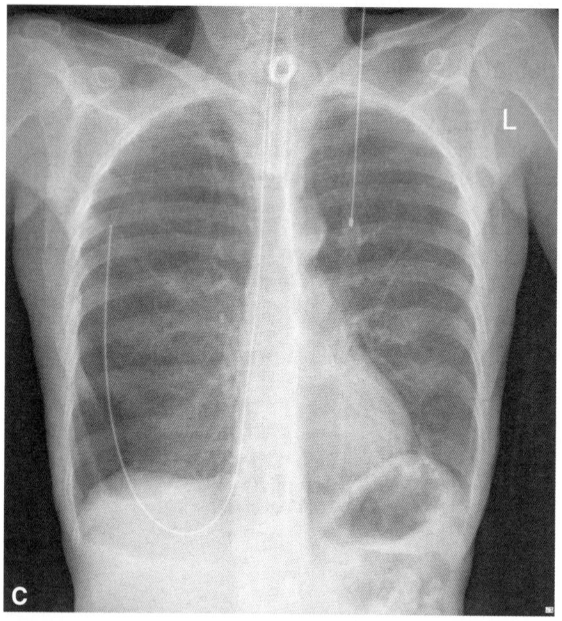

FIGURE 179.12 Nasogastric tube malposition. **A:** Anteroposterior chest radiograph in a patient requiring nasoenteric feeding. The initial radiograph demonstrated too proximal a tube tip position in the lower esophagus (*arrow*). **B:** A repeat anteroposterior radiograph after nasogastric tube repositioning confirms satisfactory position in the stomach with the distal tip coiled in the gastric fundus (*arrow*). **C:** Posteroanterior chest radiograph in a 57-year-old female with supraglottic squamous cell carcinoma and recurrent aspiration pneumonia requiring nasoenteric feeding. A nasogastric tube was placed at the bedside, and a radiograph demonstrates malposition with the distal tip of the nasogastric tube projected over a large right pneumothorax indicating perforation of the lung owing to endobronchial placement of the tube.

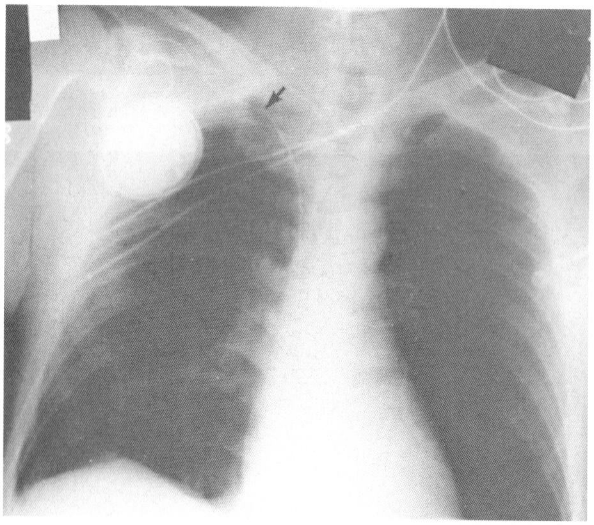

FIGURE 179.13 Pacemaker wire fracture. Posteroanterior view of the chest in a patient with a malfunctioning pacemaker. A break in the pacer wire (*arrow*) caused the malfunction.

distress syndrome (ARDS), pulmonary infarction, or contusion. Radiologic evaluation to determine whether parenchymal densities are secondary to pulmonary edema, or other causes, or a combination is often necessary so that appropriate therapy can be started.

Evaluation of densities in the retrocardiac area was traditionally performed using an overpenetrated radiograph before the introduction of computed radiography. Computed radiography and flat panel detector technology have helped overcome these challenges owing to the ability of the radiologist to manipulate image from computed radiographic images digitally and the improved X-ray detection efficiency of silicon film transistors [4].

Congestive Heart Failure and Pulmonary Edema Owing to Pulmonary Venous Hypertension

Radiography

Elevation of pulmonary venous pressure, irrespective of cause, produces a sequence of radiologic findings. When pulmonary venous pressures rise above normal, pulmonary vascular redistribution occurs [17], producing distention of the upper lobe vessels with a concomitant decrease in caliber of those in the lower lobe in the upright patient. For patients in the supine position, the equivalent of the upper lobe vessels is the anterior or ventral pulmonary vessels and the equivalent of the lower lobe vessels is the posterior or dorsal vessels. The change in caliber of the vessels in the supine position may be discernible on a cross-table lateral film of the chest.

At pulmonary capillary wedge pressures of 20 to 25 mm Hg, lymphatic drainage is exceeded and the alveolar interstitium, bronchovascular interstitium, interlobular septa, and subpleural tissues fill with fluid. The visible radiologic changes include:

1. Thickening of the interlobular septa (Kerley A and B lines) (Fig. 179.14A, B).
2. Peribronchial cuffing: The bronchial walls (which normally manifest as thin well-defined radiodense rings when imaged en face) become ill-defined and more radiodense (Fig. 179.2).
3. Blurring or haziness of the perivascular outlines (Fig. 179.14C)
4. Widening of the pleural layer over the convexity of the lungs secondary to the presence of fluid in the subpleural space
5. Pulmonary vascular redistribution (Fig. 179.14C)

At pulmonary capillary wedge pressures of 25 to 40 mm Hg, fluid fills the alveolar spaces and alveolar edema is seen. The air space consolidation may extend to the subpleural zone, or the more characteristic butterfly or bat-wing edema pattern may be seen (Fig. 179.2).

Unilateral pulmonary edema in the ICU may relate to patient positioning; however, acute unilateral pulmonary edema is a typical manifestation of acute mitral regurgitation (Fig.179.14D) [18]. Unilateral diminution in pulmonary blood flow, as seen in Swyer–James syndrome, right or left pulmonary artery thromboembolism, and surgical corrections of congenital heart disease (e.g., shunts for tetralogy of Fallot), are other causes of unilateral edema.

Atypical patterns of congestive failure and pulmonary edema have been described in patients with chronic pulmonary disease [19]. It is postulated that the thick-walled spaces in which thickened fibrous septa replace normal alveolar walls impair collateral ventilation and prevent dispersion of edema fluid throughout the lungs [19]. Fluid is then trapped in relatively larger spaces that have replaced normal alveoli. Shadows produced do not coalesce, and the images are seen on radiographs as miliary nodular patterns. The other two patterns, interstitial and reticular, are also seen without chronic lung disease.

Pulmonary edema can be owing to cardiac or noncardiac causes. Different radiologic indices distinguish between hydrostatic (cardiac) edema, overhydration pulmonary edema, and edema secondary to increased capillary permeability (see "Acute Respiratory Distress Syndrome" section) [20]. In overhydration edema (e.g., edema secondary to renal failure), the cardiac output is large, and, consequently, pulmonary blood flow is large. All vessels are recruited, and no redistribution

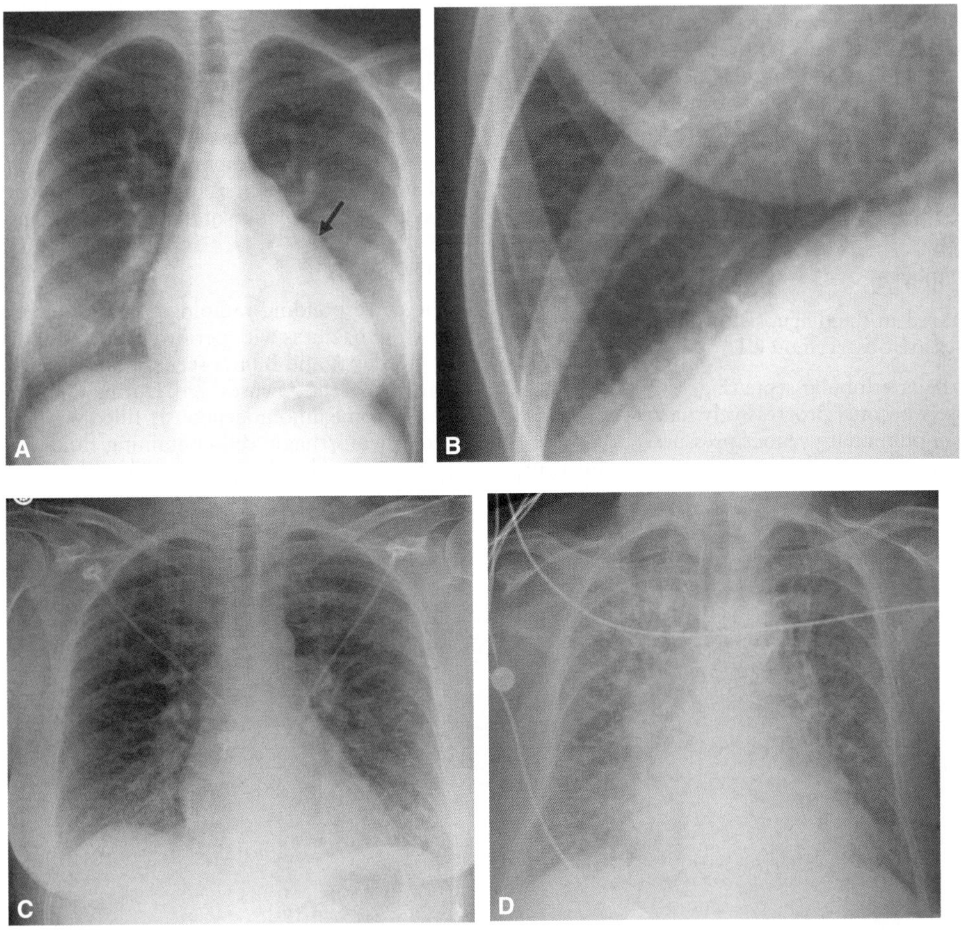

FIGURE 179.14 Pulmonary edema. **A:** Frontal chest radiograph in a 54-year-old male with mitral valve regurgitation demonstrates enlargement of the left atrium (*arrow*). **B:** Magnified view of the same patient's chest radiograph confirms thickening of the interlobular septa, likely indicating chronic pulmonary edema. **C:** Frontal chest radiograph of a 63-year-old demonstrates blurring of the perivascular outlines, diffuse ground glass opacity, and enlargement of the upper lobe pulmonary vein redistribution consistent with pulmonary edema. **D:** Frontal chest radiograph of an 85-year-old female with mitral regurgitation and dyspnea demonstrates asymmetric ground glass opacity in the right lung likely secondary to a flail posterior mitral leaflet.

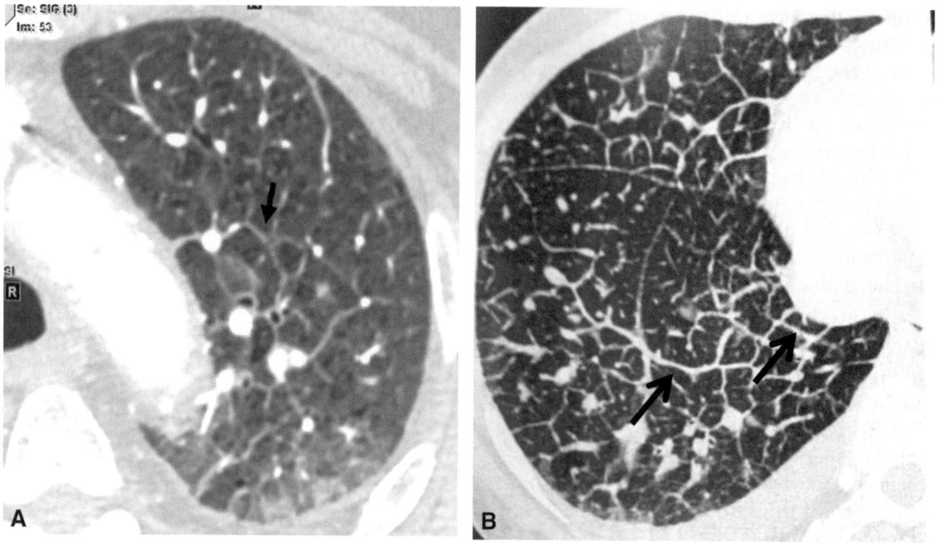

FIGURE 179.15 Interlobular septal thickening. Axial CT images of two patients, one with acute pulmonary edema owing to fluid overload (A) and another with chronic pulmonary edema because of mitral valve regurgitation (B). The secondary pulmonary lobules that are outlined by a thin septum containing lymphatic channels and veins are not normally visible on CT, but the edematous septa become thickened in the setting of pulmonary edema and therefore become perceptible on CT (*arrows*). CT, computed tomography.

of flow occurs. Because blood volume is also increased, the vascular pedicle, azygos vein, and hilar vessels are large. In pure capillary permeability edema, there is no increase in blood volume, and therefore the vascular pedicle and azygos vein remain normal in size; no signs of pulmonary venous hypertension are present, and heart size is also normal. When different types of edema coexist, edema may occur at lower left atrial pressures, and wedge pressure readings may be low or only slightly elevated [21].

Computed Tomography

Although not required in the diagnosis of pulmonary edema, specific CT features are observed on CT:

1. Thickening of the interlobular septa (Fig. 179.15)
2. The dorsal vessels become progressively narrower because of the increase in pulmonary venous pressure.
3. Diffuse ground glass opacity throughout the lung parenchyma
4. Pleural effusions.

Acute Respiratory Distress Syndrome

ARDS is a progressive hypoxic condition with radiographic bilateral lung infiltration, which is not derived from hydrostatic edema. Numerous diseases cause ARDS, but the common denominator is diffuse alveolar damage [22]. The pathologic alterations with corresponding radiologic changes occur 12 to 24 hours after the first appearance of respiratory symptoms. Insidious accumulation of fluid in the extravascular space occurs.

Radiography

The corresponding radiologic picture includes perihilar, perivascular haziness with peribronchial cuffing. Only occasionally are Kerley A and B lines seen; in one series, they were noted in only five of the 75 cases [23]. During the acute stage, the alveoli also become inhomogeneously filled with a proteinaceous and often hemorrhagic cell-containing fluid. Hyaline membranes form in the alveoli and sometimes in the alveolar ducts. The radiologic picture is one of heterogeneous or confluent ground glass opacity that is not rapidly reversible (Fig. 179.16A). The

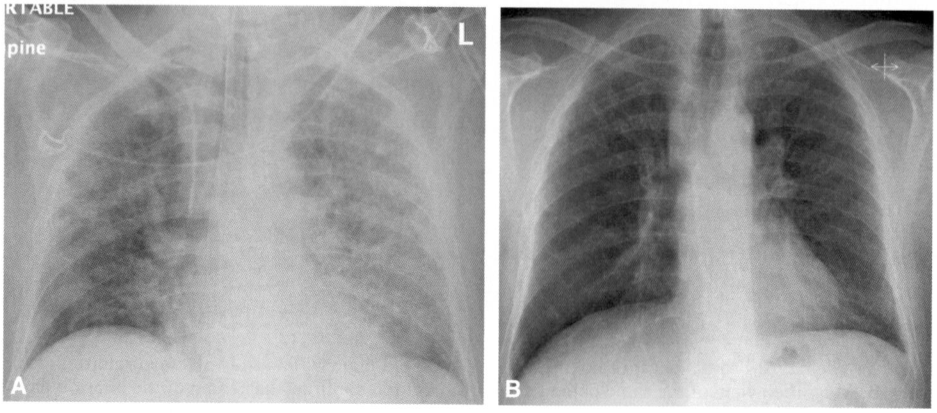

FIGURE 179.16 Acute respiratory distress syndrome: Sequential chest radiographs of a 54-year-old male admitted to the ICU with hypoxia after femorofemoral bypass surgery. Initial chest radiography demonstrated diffuse ground glass opacity which persisted for 2 months (A), 1-year follow-up chest radiograph (B) performed to assess the cause of an ongoing oxygen requirement confirmed apical predominant pulmonary fibrosis consistent with the long-term sequelae of acute respiratory distress syndrome. ICU, intensive care unit.

course of ARDS is highly variable. In some patients, reabsorption of the exudates is complete within a few days, thereby producing radiologic clearing of the densities. In some, there is a delayed clearing of the exudates, with a corresponding delay in clearing of the radiologic picture. In a third group, progressive fibrosis occurs, predominantly in the nondependent lung, where barotrauma from mechanical ventilation is worst.

After the first week, the radiologist's main concern is the recognition of superimposed complications, such as pulmonary infections, oxygen toxicity, barotrauma, and pulmonary embolism with infarction. When clinical signs and symptoms of infection are present and the radiographic picture deteriorates, pneumonia should be suspected. Development of cavities and a change in the character of the densities should lead to suspicion of superimposed abscess, infarction, or cardiac failure. Only direct hemodynamic measurements of the pulmonary capillary wedge pressure provide a dependable means of detecting superimposed failure in cases of ARDS [24]. Radiographic findings in the chronic phase of ARDS serve as independent predictors of mortality and include cyst formation, ground glass opacity, and bronchiectasis (Fig. 179.16B) [25].

Computed Tomography

The following specific features are observed on CT [26]:

1. Acute phase
   a. Dense consolidation in the dependent portions of the lung (Fig. 179.17A)
   b. Diffuse ground glass opacity throughout the lung parenchyma (Fig. 179.17B)
   c. Bronchiectasis is occasionally observed
2. If parenchymal abnormalities persist after the acute phase, findings include:
   a. Pulmonary cysts in the nondependent lung (Fig. 179.17C)
   b. Reticulation and ground glass opacity in the nondependent lung (Fig. 179.17D)

Atelectasis and Pneumonia

Radiography

Atelectasis is easily diagnosed when a characteristic linear or triangular density is accompanied by volume loss (shift of fissures or mediastinum or diaphragmatic elevation, or both). Densities that fall between these categories, however, such as scattered opacities, are often indistinguishable from pneumonia on a single study.

In the presence of opacities that are not readily diagnosed as atelectasis, pneumonia should be strongly considered. Bronchial aspirates for culture should be obtained from the lung periphery, with care to bypass the upper airway because the central airways become readily colonized after placement of a tracheostomy or endotracheal tube [27].

Computed Tomography

Evidence of volume loss, such as hyperexpansion of adjacent lung or migration of mediastinal structures toward the atelectatic lung,

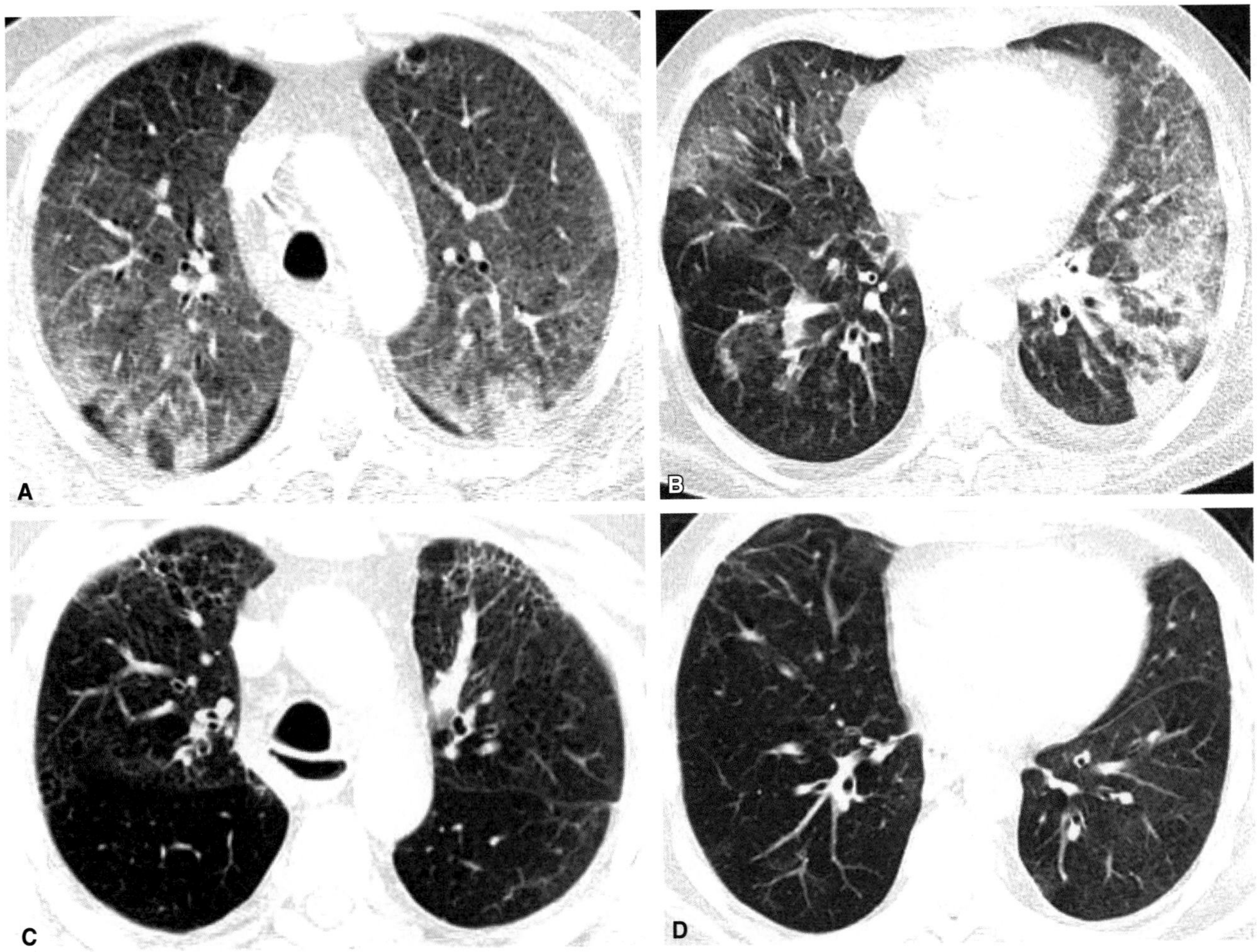

FIGURE 179.17 Acute respiratory distress syndrome: Axial CT images of a 54-year-old male admitted to the ICU with hypoxia after femorofemoral bypass surgery. Initial chest radiography and CT demonstrated diffuse ground glass opacity (A) which persisted for 2 months (B), 1-year follow-up chest CT performed to assess the cause of an ongoing oxygen requirement confirmed nondependent apical predominant pulmonary fibrosis (C,D) consistent with the long-term sequelae of acute respiratory distress syndrome. CT, computed tomography; ICU, intensive care unit.

favors atelectasis on both contrast-enhanced and noncontrast-enhanced thoracic CT. Contrast-enhanced CT helps to differentiate between the normal enhancement pattern of atelectatic lung and the expected hypoenhancing appearance of pneumonia.

Aspiration

The extent and severity of pulmonary injury after aspiration of gastric contents depend on the volume and character of the aspirated material (see Chapter 170). Aspiration pneumonitis (Mendelson syndrome) is a chemical injury caused by the inhalation of sterile gastric contents [28]. Pathologically, the lungs show areas of atelectasis within minutes; up to 1 hour after aspiration, however, only mild microscopic abnormalities are present (interstitial edema with capillary congestion). These progress to complete desquamation of the bronchial epithelium and polymorphonuclear leukocyte infiltration of the airways (bronchiolitis). Alveolar spaces fill with fluid, red blood cells, and polymorphonuclear leukocytes, progressing to consolidation in 24 to 48 hours. Formation of hyaline membranes occurs by 48 hours and organization or resolution within 72 hours [29,30].

Radiography

Findings of aspiration pneumonitis are often concurrent with those of aspiration bronchiolitis and include airway thickening with ground-glass opacities in centrilobular and peribronchovascular distribution. Aspiration pneumonia is an infectious process caused by the inhalation of oropharyngeal secretions that are colonized by pathogenic bacteria [28], which manifests as segmental or lobar consolidation. In supine patients, typically, the posterior segments of the upper lobes and superior segments of the lower lobes are involved; and in upright patients, the posterior segments of the lower lobes are involved (Fig. 179.18) [31,32].

Computed Tomography

CT findings usually consist of multiple patchy and ill-defined consolidations of relatively low-density with posterobasal predisposition (Fig. 179.18). Occasionally, consolidation contains areas of fluid density or cavities as a sign of necrotizing pneumonia or abscess.

Diffuse aspiration bronchiolitis is characterized by chronic inflammatory reaction to repeatedly aspirated foreign particles in the bronchioles. Patients with esophageal conditions such as achalasia, Zenker's diverticulum, or esophageal carcinoma are at risk for aspiration bronchiolitis. These patients often develop moderate to marked dilatation of the esophagus, with associated signs and symptoms such as dysphagia, regurgitation, and aspiration. At thin-section CT, aspiration bronchiolitis manifests as unilateral or bilateral foci of branching areas of increased attenuation with a tree-in-bud appearance or as mottled, poorly defined acinar areas of increased attenuation (Fig. 179.18). Consolidation is not a major radiologic finding of aspiration bronchiolitis. Esophageal dilatation with an air-fluid level may also be present.

Fat Embolism

Fat embolism usually follows trauma associated with fracture, but conditions such as severe burns, diabetes mellitus, fatty liver, pancreatitis, steroid therapy, sickle cell anemia, surgery for prosthetic hip placement, and acute osteomyelitis can also result in fat embolism. Most of the fat is believed to originate from the bone marrow, entering the circulation via torn veins in the injured area and, to a lesser extent, through the lymphatic system. Fats are then transported to the lungs in the form of neutral triglycerides. The fat globules also appear to induce platelet and erythrocyte aggregation and stimulation of intravascular coagulation.

Continuous fat embolization, conversion of triglycerides to fatty acids, and intravascular coagulation occur as an ongoing process over 1 to 3 days. Emboli pass from the pulmonary circulation into the systemic circulation and lodge in different organs, notably the brain, kidney, and skin.

The chest radiographic manifestation of fat embolism is that of acute pulmonary edema which develops within 72 hours of trauma [33,34]. The pulmonary opacities clear in 7 to 10 days but may take 4 weeks to resolve completely [34]. Acute cor pulmonale with cardiac failure may also be seen.

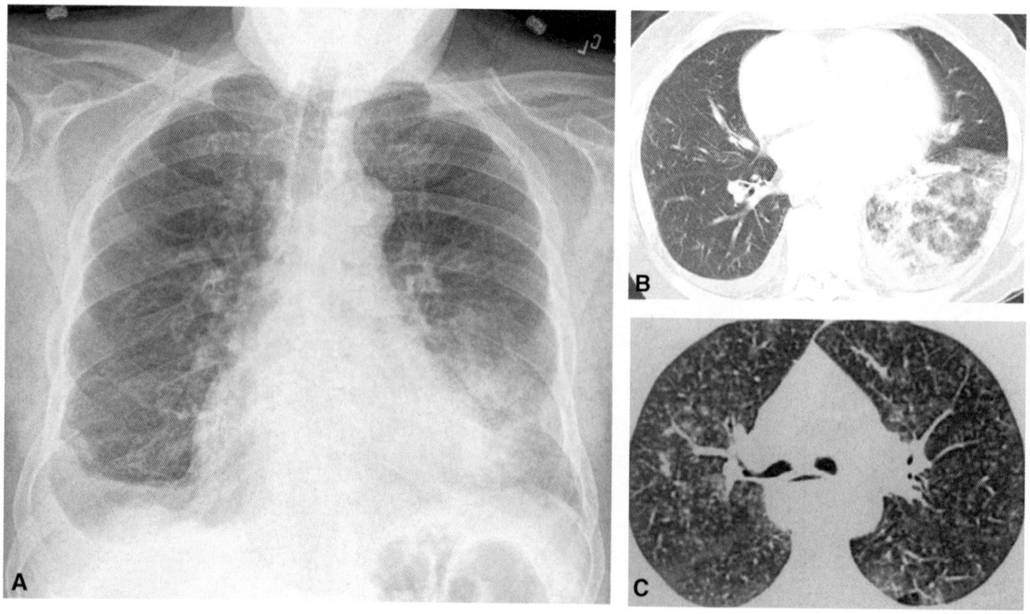

FIGURE 179.18 A: Chest radiograph of a 53-year-old male who experienced an aspiration event in the early postoperative period after colectomy. Left lower lobe ground glass opacities represent aspiration pneumonitis and are better delineated on CT (B). C: aspiration bronchiolitis in a 63-year-old female with recurrent episodes of silent aspiration. Aspiration bronchiolitis manifests as unilateral bilateral tree-in-bud nodules.

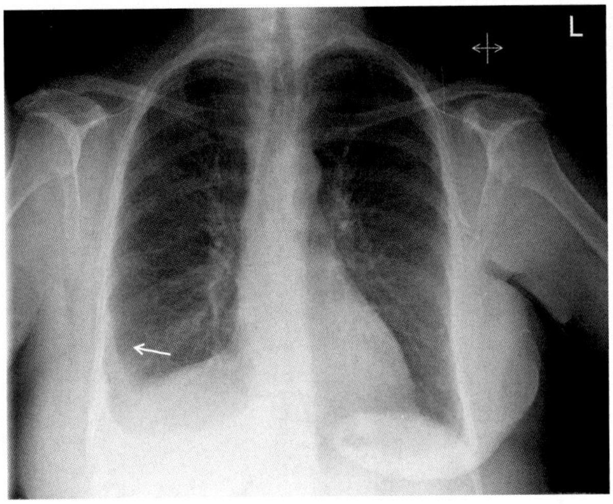

FIGURE 179.19 Pleural effusion in a 35-year-old female after cholecystectomy demonstrates a homogenous right basal opacity with a curvilinear upper meniscus (*arrow*) consistent with right pleural effusion.

Computed Tomography

Although CT is not typically used to diagnose fat embolism, reported CT findings include scattered ground-glass opacities, consolidation, and centrilobular nodules in the order of frequency [35].

ABNORMALITIES OF THE PLEURA, MEDIASTINUM, AND DIAPHRAGM

Pleural Effusion

Radiography

The radiographic appearance of fluid in the pleural space is the same whether the fluid is serous, chylous, purulent, or sanguinous. The degree of opacity of the effusion depends on the amount of fluid and presence or absence of underlying pulmonary disease. It is easily identifiable when tangential to the X-ray beam as a homogenous opacity that is free from lung markings, displaces the lung, and is most often located in the dependent portion of the thorax, with a meniscus along its superior margin. However, when the X-ray beam is parallel to the meniscus of the effusion, it appears as a homogeneous area of increased density in the thorax through which vascular markings may be seen.

Free pleural fluid is not confined to any portion of the thoracic cavity, and the distribution changes with patient position. Distribution is influenced by gravity, capillary action, and resistance of the underlying lung to expansion. In the upright position, the fluid collects first in the posterior costophrenic sulcus and subsequently in the lateral costophrenic sulcus. The typical meniscal configuration of pleural fluid (Fig. 179.19) is attributed to several factors, including capillary attraction drawing the fluid superiorly between the visceral and parietal pleural surfaces, the relation of the fluid surface to the radiograph beam, the greater retractility of the lung periphery, and the tendency of the lung to preserve its shape while recoiling from the chest.

Subpulmonic pleural fluid is the typical pattern of free fluid collection in the upright position if no pleural adhesions are present [36]. Radiologically, the fluid presents as an opaque density, parallel to the diaphragm and simulating an elevated hemidiaphragm (Fig. 179.20). Subpulmonic effusion is recognized in the posteroanterior (PA) film when the apex of the pseudodiaphragmatic shadow peaks more laterally than usual. The pulmonary vessels in the lung posterior to the subpulmonic collection cannot be seen through the pseudodiaphragmatic contour because of the greater density of the fluid collection. On the left side, there is increased distance between the gastric bubble and the base of the lung. Often, the costophrenic sulcus is blunted.

The appearance of interlobar fluid depends on the shape and orientation of the fissure, location of fluid within the fissure, and direction of the radiograph beam. Often, an elliptic or rounded, sharply marginated density is identified on PA or lateral films and has been described as a "pseudotumor" (Fig. 179.21).

A lateral decubitus view can be obtained to confirm the presence of pleural effusion, rule out a parenchymal process coexisting with an effusion, or quantify the amount of fluid in the pleural cavity. In the lateral decubitus view, fluid forms an opacity parallel to the thoracic wall (Fig. 179.22). When a decubitus view cannot be obtained for a completely immobile patient, an ultrasonographic evaluation can be performed. Sonographically guided thoracentesis enhances the likelihood of a successful tap in these cases and when the fluid is loculated.

Pleural effusion occurs quite frequently in the first week after thoracic or abdominal surgery (Fig. 179.19). After pneumonectomy, increasing amounts of fluid are noted to accumulate in the thorax. This accumulation occurs over a period of 1.5 to 2

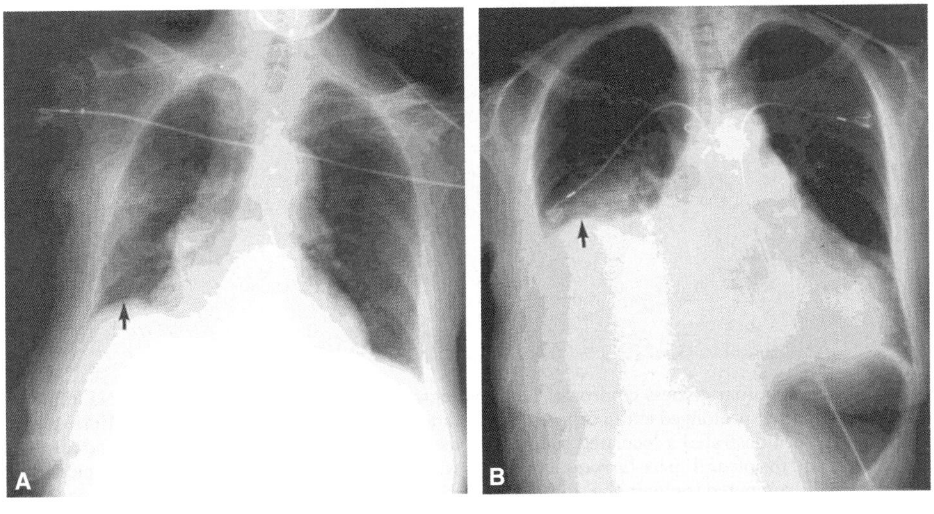

FIGURE 179.20 Subpulmonic effusion. Anteroposterior views of two different patients (**A, B**) with the subpulmonic effusion simulating elevated hemidiaphragms, with a more lateral than usual peak (*arrows*).

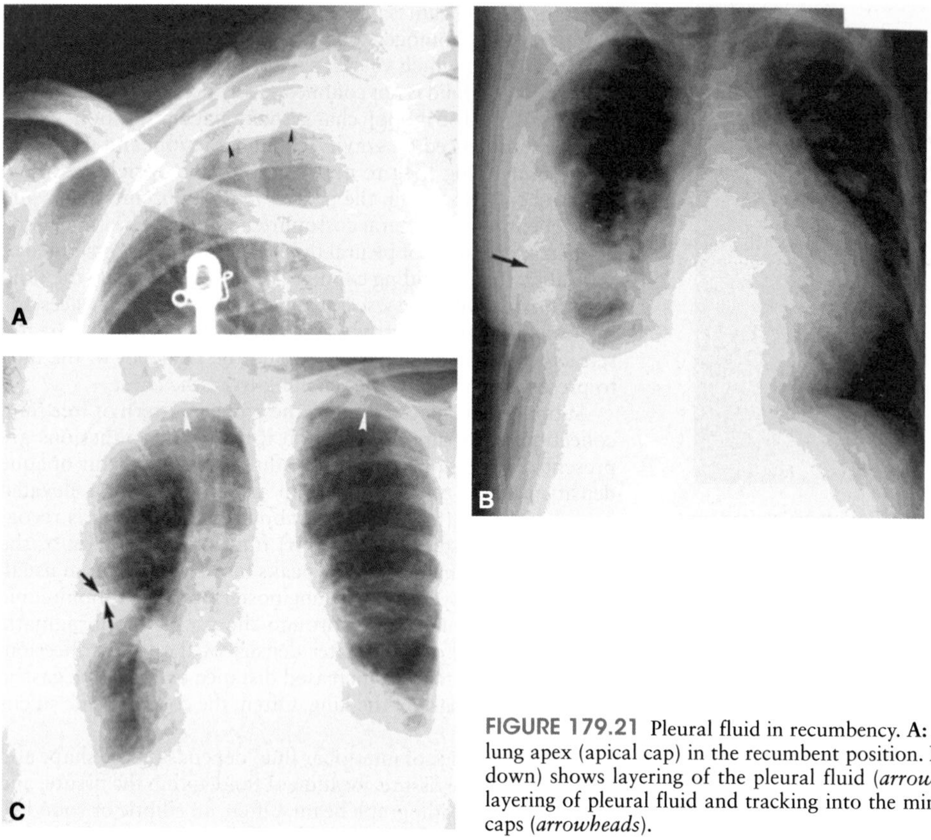

FIGURE 179.21 Pleural fluid in recumbency. **A:** Arrowheads show fluid tracking over the lung apex (apical cap) in the recumbent position. **B:** Right lateral decubitus view (right side down) shows layering of the pleural fluid (*arrow*). **C:** Right lateral decubitus view shows layering of pleural fluid and tracking into the minor fissure (*arrows*). Note bilateral apical caps (*arrowheads*).

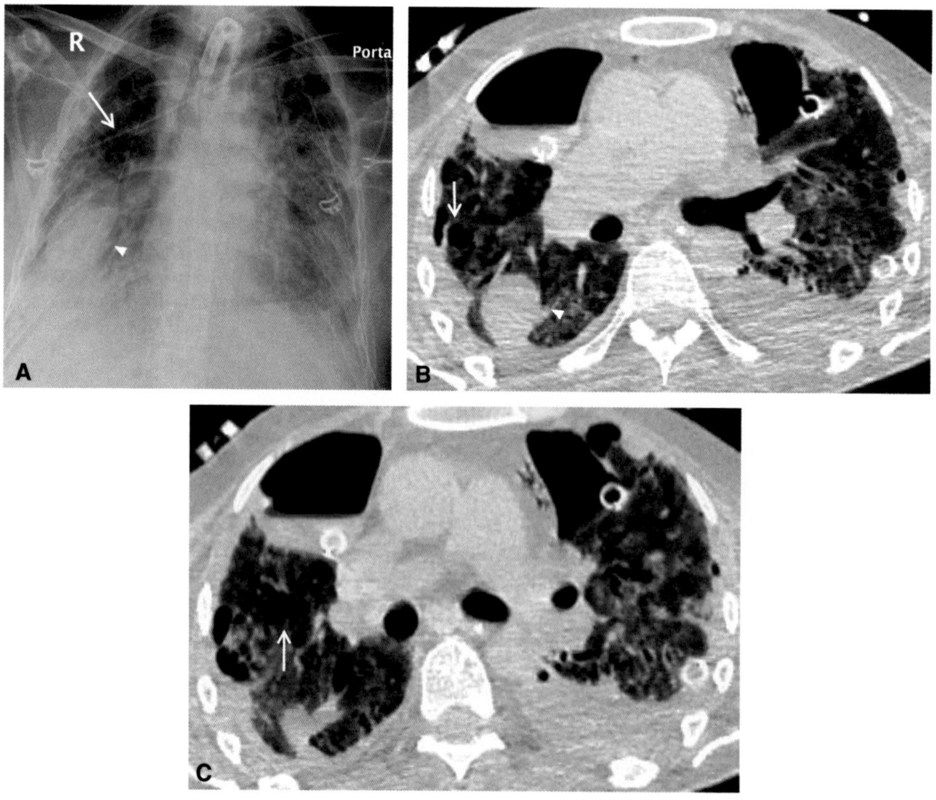

FIGURE 179.22 Loculated pleural effusion and acute respiratory distress syndrome. Chest radiograph in a 42-year-old male with H1N1 influenza pneumonia and acute respiratory distress syndrome requiring prolonged extracorporeal membrane oxygenation resulting in pleural effusions, PIE and pneumothoraces. **A–C:** Chest radiography and CT demonstrated a loculated right major fissural pleural effusion (*arrowheads*) and air-filled perivascular spaces that are separate from the airways and the pleural space (*arrows*) consistent with PIE. In addition, there are bilateral apical chest drains and a correctly positioned tracheostomy tube. CT, computed tomography; PIE, pulmonary interstitial emphysema.

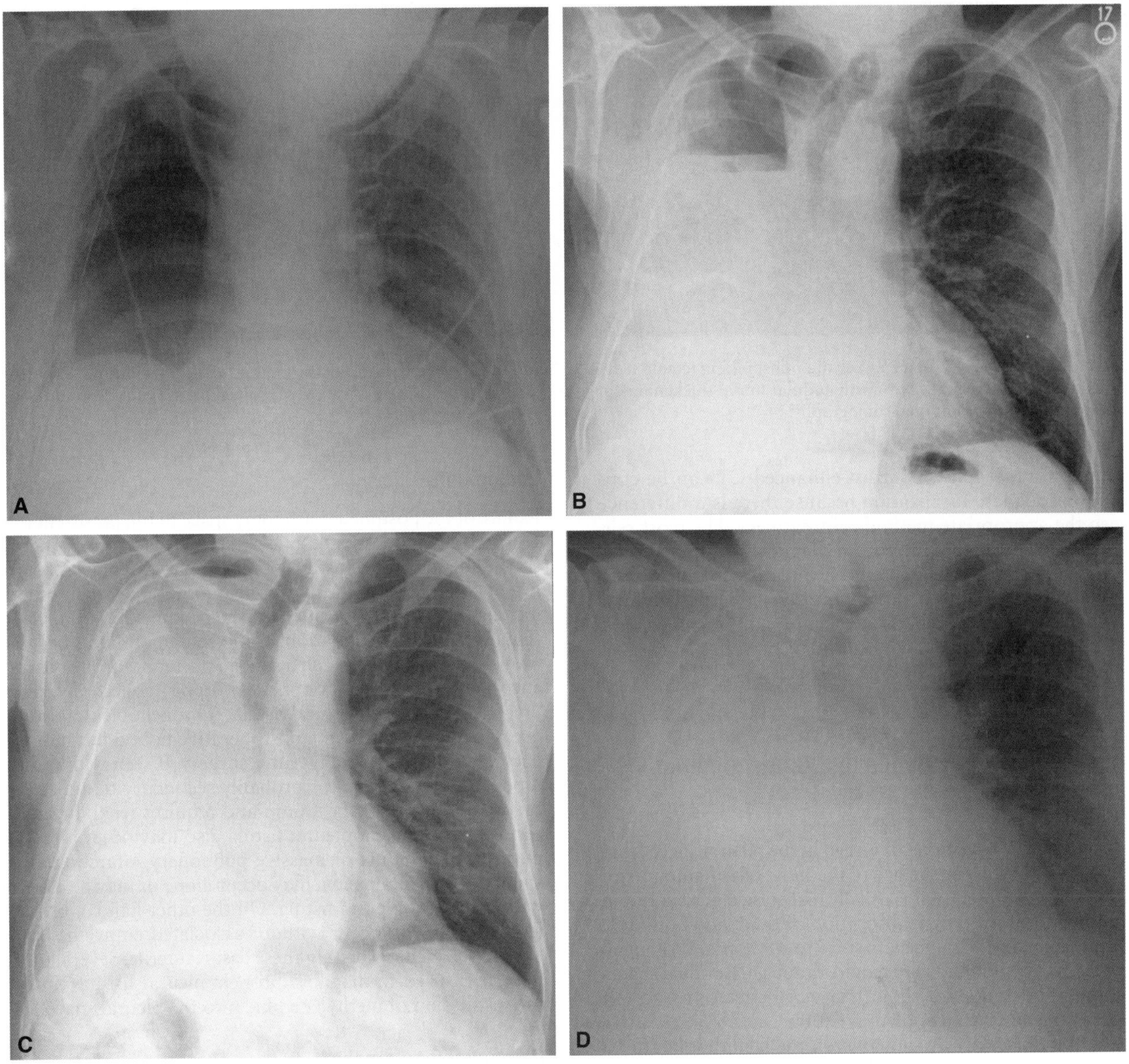

FIGURE 179.23 Expected radiographic changes post-pneumonectomy: Serial chest radiographs (A–D) immediately, 2 weeks, 2 months, and 1 year after pneumonectomy demonstrate gradual opacification of the pneumonectomy space with progressive resolution of pleural air.

months after surgery, ultimately leading to complete hemithoracic opacification by 2 months (Fig. 179.23) [37].

Computed Tomography

Although it is rarely necessary to perform CT to diagnose pleural effusion, it may be used as a tool to differentiate between a simple pleural effusion, hemothorax, or an empyema. A simple pleural effusion is typically located in the dependent portion of the pleural space, is homogenously low in attenuation, and does not enhance. A hemothorax is higher in attenuation, may exhibit internal layering, and may not lie in the dependent portion of the lung. The CT features of empyema are discussed in the next section.

Empyema and Peripheral Lung Abscess

An intrathoracic fluid-containing cavitary lesion adjacent to the chest wall may represent either a lung abscess or an empyema.

Lung Abscess

Radiography. Conventional radiography may show a thick-walled cavity and an air fluid level within the cavity. There may be associated consolidation or atelectasis.

Computed Tomography. Typically, CT is performed to differentiate between lung abscess and empyema. The lung abscess cavity will typically create an acute angle with the adjacent pleura whereas an empyema will form an obtuse angle with the pleura (Fig. 179.24). Additional similar cavitating lesions on CT would raise the differential diagnosis of septic emboli rather than lung abscess.

Empyema

Radiography. By conventional radiography, visualization of the three-dimensional shape of the pleural lesion as oblong, flattened, and conforming to the shape of the thorax with an obtuse angle with the pleura helps differentiate between the two lesions. Abscesses are more rounded than empyemas and exhibit an acute angle with the pleural surface.

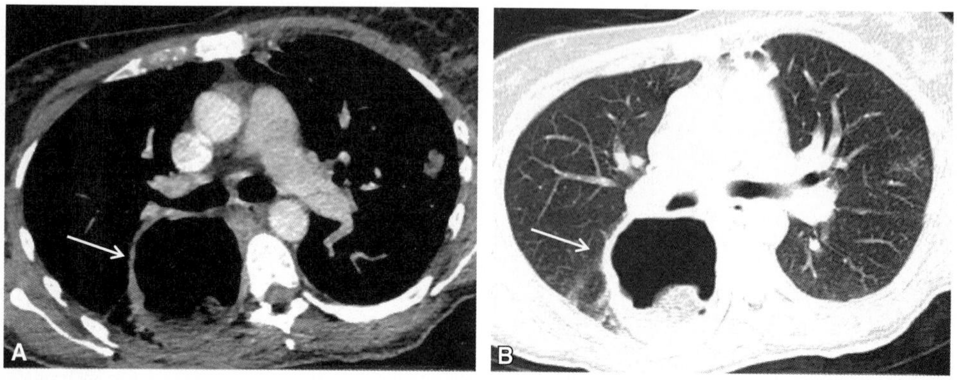

FIGURE 179.24 Axial CT of a 39-year-old nonsmoking female with cough and fever viewed on soft tissue (A) and lung (B) windows demonstrates a rounded intraparenchymal cavity with nodular mural thickening consistent with a lung abscess. The cavity resolved after 2 months of intravenous antibiotic therapy. CT, computed tomography.

Computed Tomography. Contrast-enhanced CT can be considered for adequate localization because there is a difference between the appropriate methods of treatment. The most reliable CT features for the differential diagnosis of lung abscess and empyema are wall characteristics, pleural separation, and lung compression. A lung abscess typically has a thick nodular wall and does not compress the adjacent lung. An empyema is surrounded by two enhancing pleural layers (split pleura sign) and compresses the adjacent lung (Fig. 179.25) [38].

Postpneumonectomy Space and Bronchopleural Fistula

After a pulmonary resection, air is seen in the pleural space from small air leaks in the cut surface of the lung. Small amounts of fluid also may be present. Air is usually reabsorbed gradually and continuously, followed by reabsorption of fluid, and both may be completely gone within the first 24 to 48 hours. Prolonged persistence of air and fluid may require drainage. Residual spaces may remain indefinitely without untoward effects and do not necessarily suggest bronchopleural fistula.

Air and fluid are always apparent in the hemithorax after a pneumonectomy and may be loculated in some cases. The normal evolution is that of resorption of air and replacement by fluid. The rate of air resorption is variable, but the space left by a pneumonectomy is usually completely obliterated with fluid within 2 months [37]. If the quantity of air increases rather than decreases, one must consider the presence of a bronchopleural fistula.

Radiography

Failure of the postpneumonectomy space to fill; persistent or progressive pneumothorax despite chest tube placement; progressive subcutaneous or mediastinal emphysema; a 2-cm increase in the lucent component of the hydropneumothorax, with a shift of the mediastinum to the side opposite the postpneumonectomy space (Fig. 179.23); consolidation in the remaining lung because of transbronchial spillage; and a sudden pneumothorax or reappearance of air in a previously opaque postpneumonectomy space are predictive of bronchopleural fistula. A bronchopleural fistula can occur any time during the postoperative period but more often occurs within 8 to 12 days after surgery. If seen within the first 4 postoperative days, it is probably secondary to a mechanical failure of closure of the stump and requires reexploration and reclosure. A bronchopleural fistula also may occur after a suppurative pneumonia or massive pulmonary infarction, or even spontaneously. Empyema may occur alone or may be associated with a bronchopleural fistula. On the other hand, a bronchopleural fistula can occur without associated empyema, and the fluid in the pleural space in these cases is sterile. Several methods have been used to diagnose bronchopleural fistulas, including the instillation of methylene blue into the pleural space [39].

Computed Tomography

If bronchopleural fistula is suspected, increasing pneumothorax, hydropneumothorax, or mediastinal shift may be evident. CT is more sensitive than bronchoscopy for the direct imaging of bronchopleural fistula. Bronchopleural fistula can be confirmed if an airway is shown to communicate with gas in the pleural space [40].

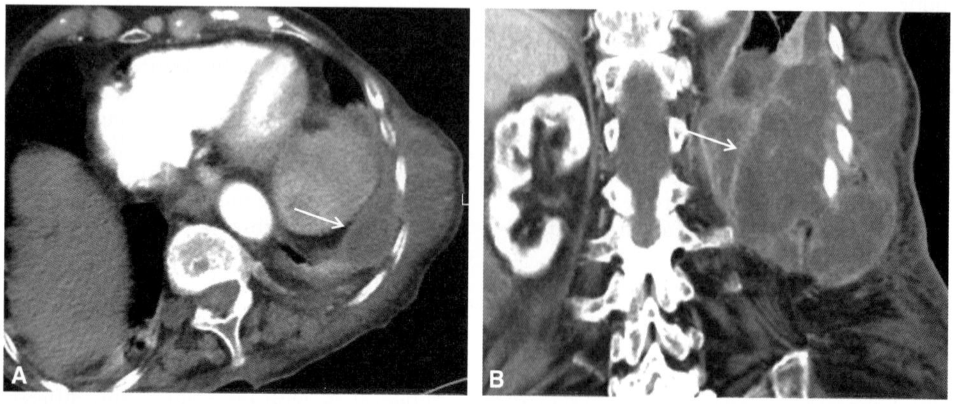

FIGURE 179.25 Empyema. Axial (**A**) and coronal (**B**) CT images of a 73-year-old female with a left staghorn calculus complicated by pyonephrosis and left empyema. The axial CT images exhibit enhancement of both layers of pleura (split pleura sign). The pleural collection has decompressed onto the chest wall (empyema necessitans). The empyema was successfully managed with intravenous antibiotics and pleural drainage. CT, computed tomography.

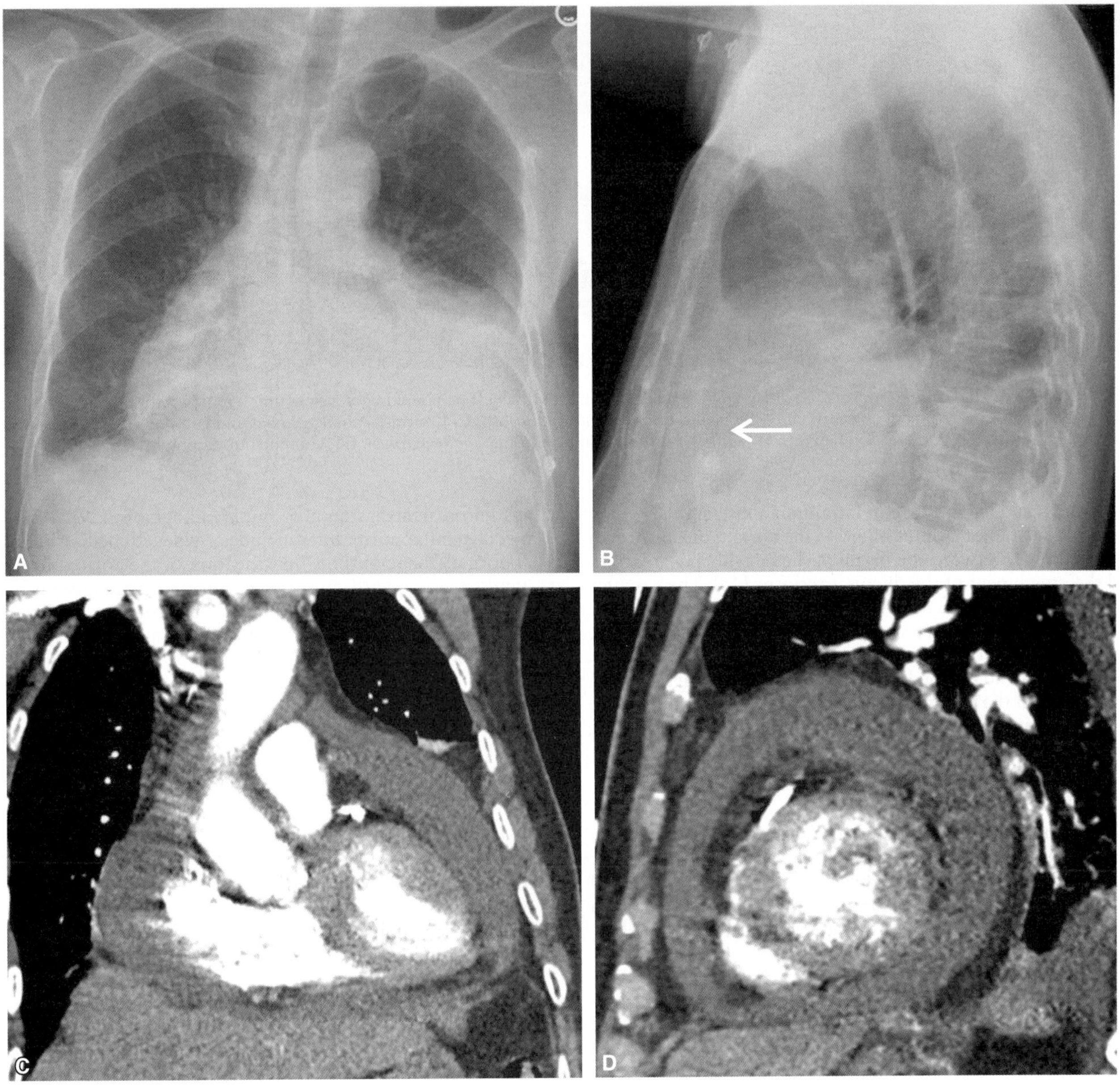

FIGURE 179.26 Pericardial effusion. Chest radiographs and coronal and sagittal CT images of a 51-year-old patient with tuberculous pericarditis and dyspnea. Anteroposterior and lateral radiographs (A,B) demonstrate enlargement of the cardiac silhouette and a 2-cm rim of increased density surrounding the epicardial fat on the lateral radiograph (*arrow*, the epicardial fat sign). Coronal (C) and true short axis (D) contrast-enhanced CT reconstructions confirm the presence of a large circumferential pericardial effusion. CT, computed tomography.

CARDIAC ABNORMALITIES

Pericardial Effusion, Hemopericardium, and Tamponade

Radiography

Fluid or blood in the pericardial cavity is suspected when there is enlargement of the cardiac silhouette. The two layers of the normal pericardium are often seen as a pencil-thin line on the lateral chest radiograph. The normal pericardium is often seen anterior to the heart, separated from it by abundant epicardial fat. A line wider than 2 mm is diagnostic of pericardial fluid or thickening (Fig. 179.26). The epicardial fat sign on the lateral radiograph is thought to be the most sensitive radiographic sign of pericardial effusion [41,42]. Other described radiographic signs of pericardial effusion include a symmetrically enlarged "water bottle" cardiac silhouette and widening of the tracheal bifurcation angle [43]. CT and ultrasound remain the definitive tools for the diagnosis of pericardial effusion; ultrasound possesses the advantages of avoiding ionizing radiation and can be performed at the bedside.

TRAUMA

Vascular Trauma

The initial diagnosis of injury to the thoracic aorta and the brachiocephalic arteries may be suspected on the basis of clinical signs. Laceration of the aorta and brachiocephalic vessels most frequently follows rapid deceleration with vehicular accidents or falls. The differences in the degree of fixation of the different segments of the aorta may cause sufficient stresses between segments in forceful deceleration to cause closed rupture. Flexion

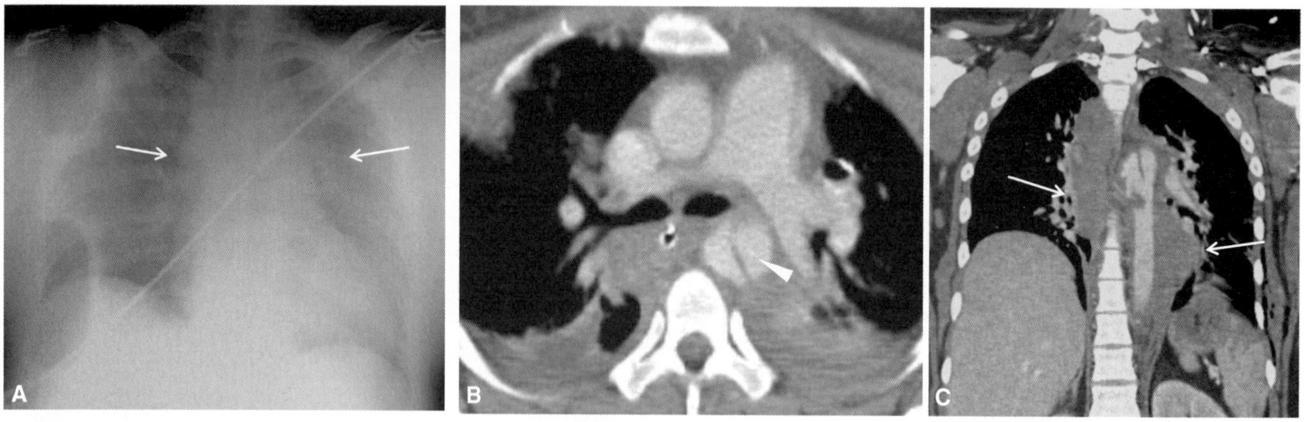

FIGURE 179.27 Chest radiograph and CT images of a 25-year-old male with chest pain and hypotension after a motor vehicle accident. **A:** Chest radiograph demonstrates biconvex widening of the mediastinum (*white arrows*). **B, C:** Contrast-enhanced axial and coronal CT images confirm a descending thoracic aortic dissection flap (*arrowhead*) and mediastinal hematoma (*white arrows*). CT, computed tomography.

stress and a sudden increase in intraluminal pressure also may be the cause of injury. Blunt injury to the aorta typically occurs at the isthmus, between the origin of the left subclavian artery and the attachment of the ductus arteriosus [44]. The vascular injury is almost always transverse and may involve only one or all layers. When all layers are involved, exsanguination occurs; if the tear is only through the intima or the intima and media, the adventitia and the mediastinal pleura can contain the blood temporarily. If the diagnosis is missed, up to 90% of those who survive the initial impact will die within 4 months [45]. Therefore, the diagnosis must be very aggressively pursued.

Radiography

The presence of fractures of the first and second ribs suggests the possibility of associated vascular injuries. Confirmation by cross-sectional imaging is recommended, regardless of a normal radiologic appearance on plain radiographs, if the mechanism of injury could potentially affect the thoracic aorta and brachiocephalic vessels.

In an adequately penetrated radiograph of the chest, mediastinal widening appears to be the most useful sign suggesting a mediastinal hematoma (Fig. 179.27). A normal aortic outline without mediastinal widening makes the diagnosis of aortic or brachiocephalic vessel injury unlikely. A large meta-analysis reports that 92.7% of patients with traumatic aortic rupture have an abnormal mediastinum on initial radiography [39]. Described mediastinal abnormalities include a widened mediastinum, an abnormal aortic outline, opacification of the aortopulmonary window, downward displacement of the left mainstem bronchus, deviation of trachea to the right of midline, deviation of nasogastric tube to the right of midline, and a widened right paratracheal stripe [39,46].

Computed Tomography

Aortic and brachiocephalic injuries should be confirmed with cross-sectional imaging. Magnetic resonance imaging (MRI), transesophageal color-flow Doppler echocardiography, contrast-enhanced CT, and aortography all have high sensitivities (see Chapter 36 for a complete discussion of the circumstances under which each method is preferred). Direct signs of aortic injury on CT include an intramural hematoma (Fig. 179.28) or an aortic dissection (Fig. 179.27). Intramural hematoma is radiologically defined as crescentic thickening of the vessel wall in the absence of an intimal flap or entry tear, resulting from a hemorrhage within the aortic wall [47], it is often of higher CT density relative to unopacified blood on a noncontrast CT. Aortic dissection is defined as disruption of the media layer of the aorta with bleeding within and along the wall of the aorta caused by a tear in the intima of the aortic wall leading to the radiologic appearance of an intimal flap and false lumen

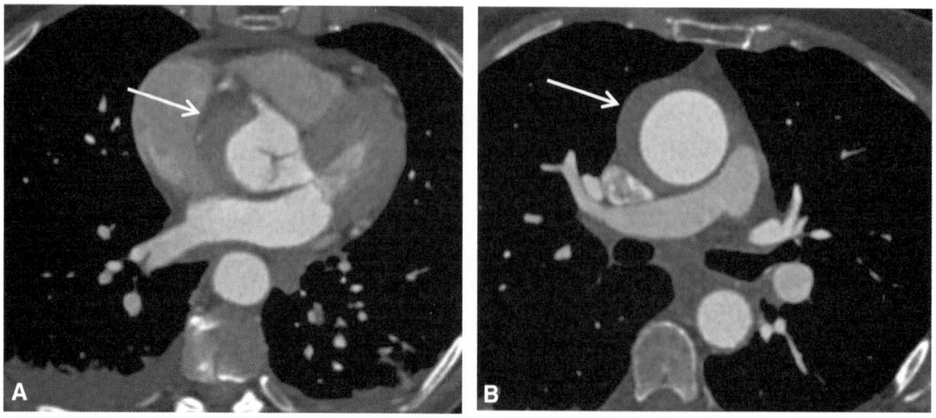

FIGURE 179.28 **A, B:** CT of intramural hematoma. Axial CT of a 79-year-old female who presented with acute chest pain. Crescentic thickening of the aortic wall from the origin of the right coronary artery to the aortic arch (*arrows*) in the absence of an intimal flap or a tear characterizes a type I intramural hematoma. CT, computed tomography.

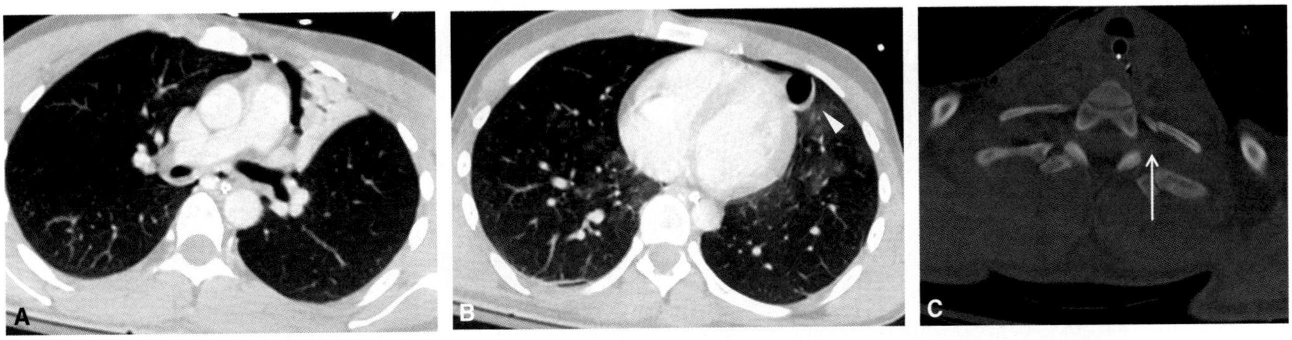

FIGURE 179.29 A: Axial CT images of a 24-year-old male after a motor vehicle accident demonstrated a left upper lobe pulmonary contusion manifesting as consolidation; pneumomediastinum is also present. B: CT, 2 months later, confirms resolution of consolidation but formation of a single spheric cystic space in a subpleural location in the left upper lobe (*arrowhead*) consistent with a traumatic lung cyst. C: Axial CT with bone windows confirms a left first rib injury indicating the severity of trauma (*arrow*). CT, computed tomography.

(Fig. 179.27B). Indirect radiologic signs include periaortic hematoma, hemothorax, an increase in aortic caliber, and an irregular aortic luminal contour [48]. Associated rib fractures are common, seen in 75% of patients in one autopsy series [49].

Pulmonary Contusion, Hematoma, and Traumatic Lung Cyst

Radiography

Pulmonary contusion is a frequent cause of posttraumatic pulmonary opacification (Fig. 179.29). Radiologically, it manifests as increased density and/or consolidation with poorly defined margins that do not conform to the shape of the lobes or lung segments. The lack of sharp demarcation of consolidation is because of intra-alveolar blood or fluid. Increased density and consolidation usually manifest within the first 6 hours. Improvement of the lesion is rapid, occurring within 24 to 48 hours. Complete clearing is usually seen in 3 to 10 days. When laceration of a lung occurs as a result of a penetrating injury or surgical resection, a pulmonary hematoma form. The cavity formed by retraction of the torn elastic tissues may be completely dense or partially air filled if bronchial communication occurs. The lesion may progressively increase in size in the next few days because of edema or hemorrhage which both manifest as ground glass opacity. This is in contrast to a contusion, which typically decreases in size. The lesion may take weeks or months to clear. Resolution may be incomplete, resulting in a pulmonary nodule.

Computed Tomography

These findings and their complications are better characterized by CT. Pulmonary contusion manifests as ground glass opacity and consolidation when severe (Fig. 179.29). The abnormalities do not respect bronchopulmonary segmental anatomy. Subpleural sparing may be seen [50]. Pulmonary laceration manifests as rounded opacity rather than a linear opacity as is seen in other organs [50]. The laceration can also become air filled, giving rise to an air-fluid level. Secondary infection leads to liquefaction of dead tissues and bronchial communication, producing an air-filled cavity with or without an associated fluid level.

Lung cysts also may occur after trauma. They may appear immediately after blunt trauma or may form after several hours or days. Single, multiple, or multilocular thin-walled, oval to spheric cystic spaces may be seen in the lung periphery or subpleurally. Bleeding into the cyst from ruptured capillaries may occur. The lung cysts persist for long periods, often more than 4 months, but progressively decrease in size during this period (Fig. 179.29).

Traumatic Diaphragmatic Hernia

Severe diaphragmatic injury after blunt or penetrating trauma to the thoracoabdominal area may allow escape of abdominal contents into the thorax. The presence of a gas-containing viscus within the thoracic cavity is the hallmark of traumatic diaphragmatic rupture with an associated hernia. Most hernias occur on the left side, because the liver acts as a buffer on the right. Very often, the condition may be initially overlooked. Coexistent radiographic abnormalities such as atelectasis and pleural effusion may obscure the radiographic signs of herniation, and positive pressure ventilatory support may delay herniation of abdominal contents through a ruptured diaphragm [51]. Symptomatic patients may experience intermittent incarceration of the herniated viscus.

Radiography

Findings suggestive of diaphragmatic rupture include a distorted elevated diaphragmatic outline, mediastinal shift, intrathoracic herniation of a hollow viscus (stomach, colon, small bowel), and visualization of a nasogastric tube above the diaphragm on the left side (Fig. 179.30) [52].

Computed Tomography

The CT features include discontinuity of the diaphragm (Fig. 179.30A), intrathoracic herniation of abdominal contents, a constriction of the herniating hollow viscus at the site of the diaphragmatic tear (known as the collar sign, Fig. 179.30B), and posterior displacement of the herniated viscera in the thorax (dependent viscera sign) confirming the absence of diaphragmatic support [52].

Extra-alveolar Air and Signs of Barotrauma

Pneumothorax

Radiography. The diagnosis of pneumothorax is made when air is seen superior, inferior, lateral, or anterior to the lung, and the visceral pleural line is identified. The air creates a zone of radiolucency devoid of lung markings between the lung and the thoracic wall. The lung partially (Fig. 179.31A) or more completely (Fig. 179.31B) collapses and drops to the most dependent position, slung by its fixed attachment at the pulmonary ligament.

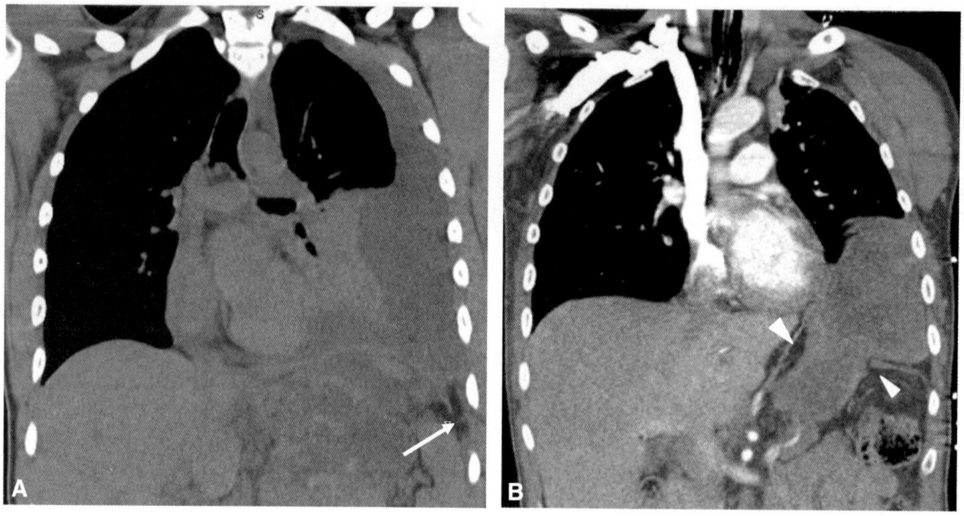

FIGURE 179.30 Coronal CT images of two patients with traumatic diaphragmatic injury; features include discontinuity of the diaphragm (**A**, *arrow*), intrathoracic herniation of abdominal contents, and constriction of the herniating hollow viscus at the site of the diaphragmatic tear known as the collar sign (**B**, *arrowheads*). CT, computed tomography.

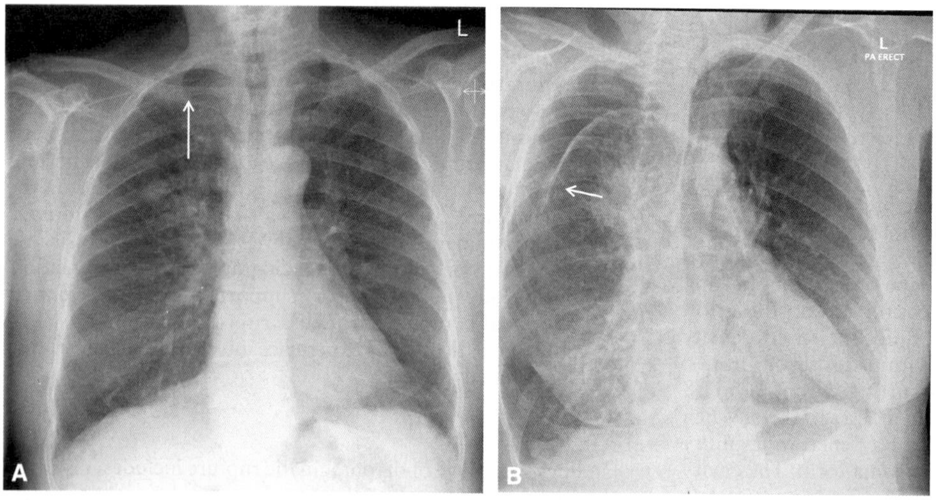

FIGURE 179.31 Frontal chest radiographs demonstrate small (**A**) and large (**B**) pneumothoraces after lung biopsy as evidenced by vertical pleural lines in the right hemithoraces (*arrows*).

As air accumulates in the pleura, the mediastinum tends to shift to the opposite side. This is best seen in a film taken during the expiratory phase of respiration. For the mediastinum to shift, the intrapleural pressure need only become less negative, not necessarily positive, on the side of the pneumothorax. Diminished negative pressure on the side of the pneumothorax creates sufficient imbalance between the pleural pressures of the two sides to cause mediastinal displacement during the expiratory phase of respiration. Tension pneumothorax causes a shift of the mediastinum to the opposite side during inspiratory and expiratory phases of respiration. In addition, diaphragmatic flattening, with progression to reversal of its normal curve, occurs in tension pneumothorax. The percentage of pneumothorax present in upright PA and lateral radiograph can be calculated by means of an average interpleural distance, using the total lung volume of the partially collapsed lung and the total hemithoracic volume as parameters [53]. Pneumothorax size can be predicted using a nomogram based on average interpleural distance.

The distribution of air in the pleural cavity is affected by pleural adhesions and by disease of the underlying lung. Adhesions prevent lung retraction; therefore, extensive adhesions may lead to a loculated pneumothorax. A diseased lung, especially one with scarring or atelectasis secondary to bronchial obstruction, tends to retract to a greater degree than the adjacent lung. Obstructive emphysema, consolidation, and interstitial emphysema make the lung rigid and interfere with retraction, keeping the lung or the involved segment expanded. The distribution of air is also influenced by patient position because air rises to the nondependent portion of the thorax.

Early recognition of a pneumothorax is mandatory for ICU patients because of the risk of barotrauma or rapid progression to tension pneumothorax in an intubated patient. For the supine patient, air collects in the anterior portion of the thorax, between the medial portion of the lung and the anterior mediastinum, or in the subpulmonic area.

Subpulmonic pneumothorax is seen as a lucent area outlining the anterior costophrenic sulcus projected over the right or left upper quadrant or only as a deep lateral costophrenic sulcus on the involved side (Fig. 179.32) [54,55]. Flattening of the cardiac border or a lateral depression of the hemidiaphragm are additional signs of tension pneumothorax that should be sought in a supine patient with suspected pneumothorax if a pleural gas collection is not immediately apparent.

Computed Tomography. CT is not typically required to identify a pneumothorax, unless percutaneous drainage is intended, and CT is used for pre- and intraprocedural guidance.

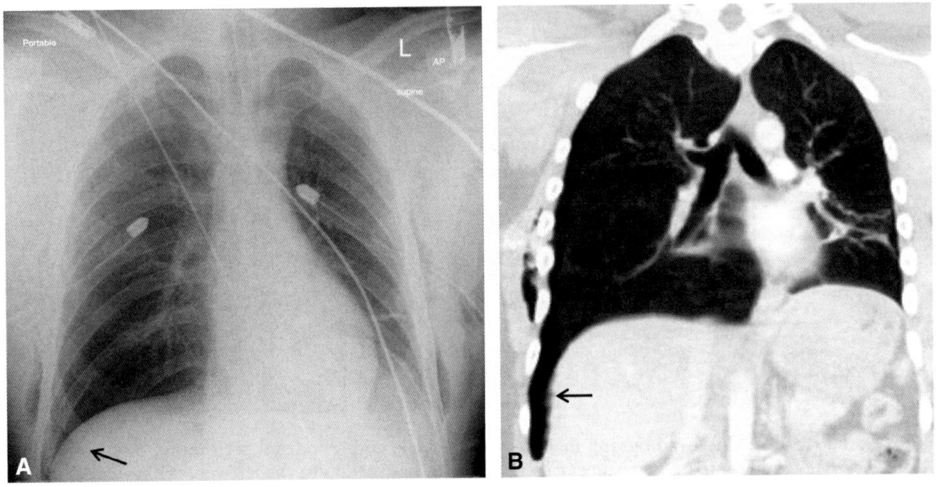

FIGURE 179.32 Deep sulcus sign. Frontal supine chest radiograph in a 25-year-old male involved in a motor vehicle accident. The radiograph (A) and CT (B) demonstrate lucency outlining the anterior and lateral costophrenic sulcus projected indicating accumulation of air in the nondependent portion of the thorax. CT, computed tomography.

Pulmonary Interstitial Emphysema

Pulmonary interstitial emphysema (PIE) occurs when air dissects through alveolar walls into the adjacent interstitial tissues where it forms cystic spaces and in adults and is typically associated with a medical intervention such as ventilation or biopsy. As a result, air dissects along the interstitium of the lungs, into the perivascular connective tissues, the interlobular septa, and the subpleural connective tissue, most extensively around the pulmonary veins [56].

Radiography. Radiologically, these spaces are seen as irregular radiolucent mottling in the medial one-half to two-thirds of the lungs or as discrete areas of radiolucency (Fig. 179.22). Radiolucencies are 2 cm or more in diameter and are best seen at the lung bases. PIE also may appear as radiolucent streaks radiating toward the hila or as a lucent halo around vessels on end. Subpleural blebs may be present most frequently around the hilar areas.

Interstitial emphysema changes rapidly, decreasing in size and disappearing completely in a matter of days. Differentiation of interstitial emphysema from necrotizing bronchopneumonia is sometimes difficult or impossible. Extensive PIE makes the lung appear better aerated than it actually is. PIE may progress to pneumothorax; infradiaphragmatic dissection; or mediastinal, cervical, or subcutaneous emphysema [57].

Computed Tomography. CT is not part of the routine investigation of PIE. When seen on CT, it manifests as cystic air spaces in the lung parenchyma, typically in a perivascular location and is typically accompanied by pneumothorax and pneumomediastinum (Fig. 179.22).

Subcutaneous Emphysema

Radiography. Air in the subcutaneous tissues is seen as linear streaks of lucency outlining tissue planes or as bubbles of lucency within the soft tissues (Fig. 179.33). Localized subcutaneous emphysema usually follows thoracostomy tube insertion, tracheostomy placement, and is usually of no significance. It may also be the earliest sign of pulmonary barotrauma. Extensive air in the subcutaneous tissues may occur in patients on ventilators, those with malfunctioning chest tubes, or those with bronchopleural fistulas. CT is not necessary to confirm subcutaneous emphysema but is usually incidentally noted when air has collected in other spaces such as the pleura or mediastinum (Fig. 179.33).

Pneumomediastinum

Radiography. Pneumomediastinum is manifested radiologically as vertical streaks of lucency just lateral to the borders of the heart, with the parietal and visceral pleura reflected by the lucent stripe (Fig. 179.33). When air extends into the soft tissues of the

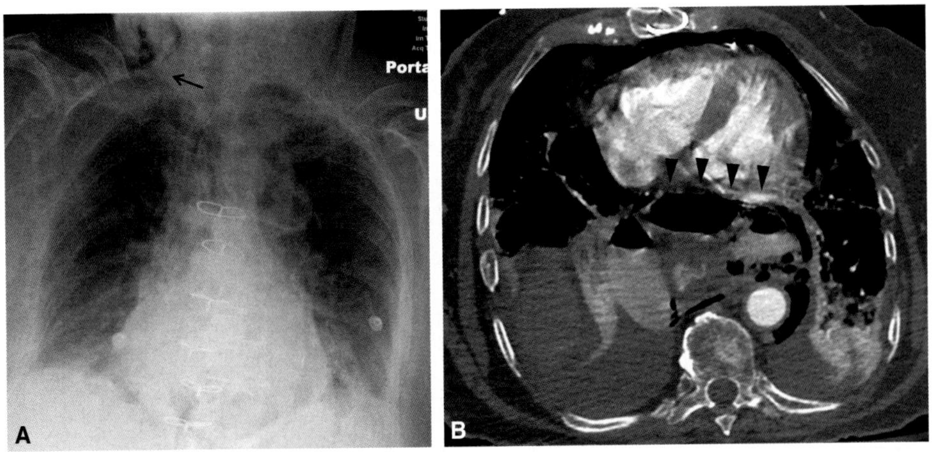

FIGURE 179.33 A: Chest radiograph in a 51-year-old male with esophageal rupture owing to Boerhaave syndrome. Air in the subcutaneous tissues is represented by linear streaks of lucency outlining tissue (*arrow*). B: Axial CT confirms the cause of subcutaneous emphysema: esophageal perforation which has resulted in extensive pneumomediastinum (*arrowheads*), pleural effusions, and atelectasis. CT, computed tomography.

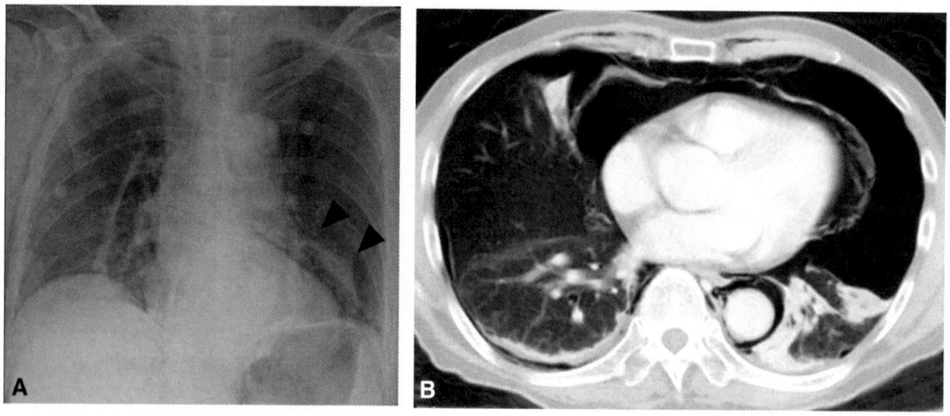

FIGURE 179.34 A: Chest radiograph in a 56-year-old male with duodenal perforation after esophagoduodenoscopy. Air in the pericardial space (*arrowheads*) is represented by curvilinear lucency which lies medial to the left ventricular free wall pericardium. B: Axial CT confirms extensive pneumopericardium, pneumomediastinum, and bilateral pneumothoraces which have tracked superiorly from the retroperitoneum. CT, computed tomography.

neck or into the retroperitoneum, it is most likely secondary to a pneumomediastinum.

Computed Tomography. Air can enter the mediastinum from a ruptured bronchus, trachea, or esophagus; from the neck (especially during the course of tracheostomy or line placement, when the negative pressure of the thorax draws air in through the incision). The site of rupture may be better characterized with CT.

Pneumopericardium

Radiography. Radiologic diagnosis of a pneumopericardium is made when a lucent stripe is seen around the heart extending to, but not beyond, the proximal pulmonary artery and outlining a thickened pericardium (Fig. 179.34). It may be difficult to differentiate from a pneumothorax or pneumomediastinum. Pneumopericardium is almost always the result of surgery but also may follow trauma or infection.

Computed Tomography. CT is more sensitive than radiography at detecting small quantities of pericardial air and may also be used to differentiate pneumopericardium from pneumomediastinum.

PULMONARY THROMBOEMBOLISM AND INFARCTION

Episodes of pulmonary thromboembolism usually show some changes on plain chest radiographs, such as linear atelectasis, elevation of a hemidiaphragm, or pleural effusion [58]. Most embolic occlusions occur in the lower lobes, the right more often than the left, probably as a result of hemodynamic flow patterns (see Chapter 92).

Radiography

Although pulmonary embolism is not typically perceptible on chest radiography, pulmonary oligemia, pulmonary infarction, and cor pulmonale can have radiographic manifestations. An area of increased radiolucency (local oligemia) of the lung within the distribution of the occluded artery is referred to as Westermark's sign [59]. Pulmonary infarction manifests as parenchymal consolidation owing to tissue necrosis or hemorrhage and edema. The consolidation is almost always subpleural with a rounded medial edge (Hampton's hump) (Fig. 179.35A). Infarcts vary in size, but most are 3 to 5 cm in diameter. Air bronchograms are rarely present; cavitation is unusual and, if present, suggests septic embolization. If infarction leads to necrosis, resolution averages 20 days and may take as long as 5 weeks. Cor pulmonale manifests as right ventricular cardiac enlargement, main pulmonary artery enlargement, increased size of the major hilar vessels with sudden tapering of the vessels, and dilatation of the azygos vein and superior vena cava are seen. These changes occur with massive or submassive pulmonary embolism. Pleural effusion is at least as common as parenchymal consolidation; the amount of fluid is frequently small, and the fluid is often unilateral.

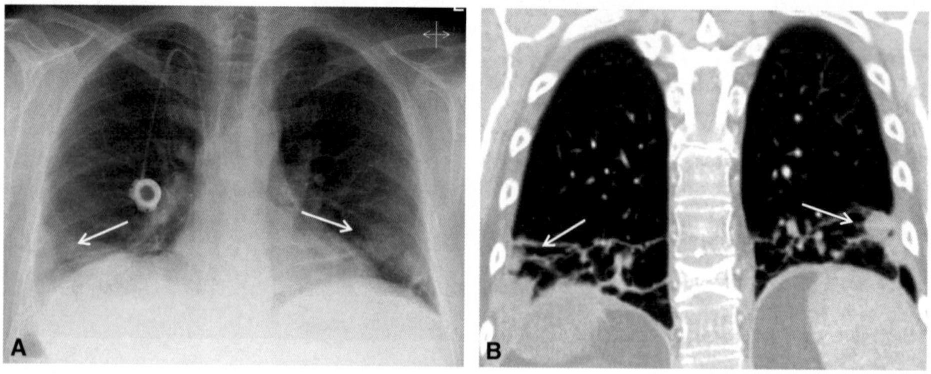

FIGURE 179.35 Chest radiograph and CT pulmonary angiogram in a 41-year-old male with colorectal carcinoma, dyspnea, and CT confirmation of bilateral pulmonary emboli. The chest radiograph (A) and CT (B) demonstrate peripheral subpleural rounded opacities consistent with pulmonary infarcts (*arrows*). CT, computed tomography.

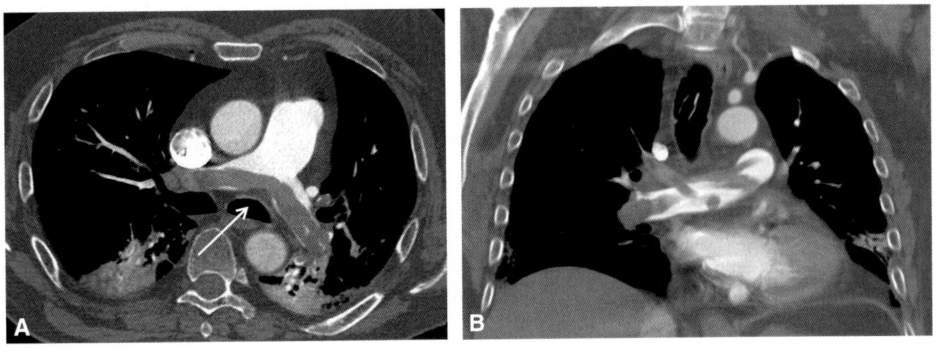

FIGURE 179.36 CT pulmonary angiogram in a 41-year-old male with colorectal carcinoma and dyspnea. Axial (A) and coronal (B) CT images confirm bilateral intravascular filling defects which complete or partially occlude the pulmonary arteries (*arrows*). CT, computed tomography.

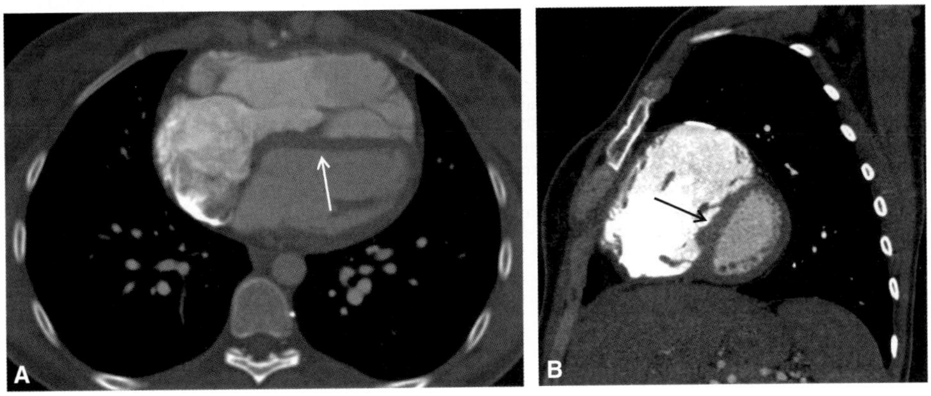

FIGURE 179.37 Axial (A) and true cardiac short axis (B) images of a gated CT pulmonary angiogram in a patient with long-standing pulmonary hypertension. The right ventricle is moderately dilated, and the interventricular septum is straightened toward the left ventricle (*arrows*) (rather than the normal configuration of bowing toward the right ventricle) consistent with raised right ventricular pressures. CT, computed tomography.

Computed Tomography

The frequent presence of underlying chest disorders, such as ARDS, pulmonary edema, associated pneumonia, or chronic obstructive lung changes, often makes the radiologic diagnosis of pulmonary embolism virtually impossible on plain chest radiographs in the ICU patient. Radioisotopic scanning and CT provide superior sensitivity for pulmonary embolism. CT scanning is typically preferred in the acutely ill patient because it is more reliable in the setting of chronic obstructive pulmonary disease, requires a shorter imaging time, and can indicate alternative diagnoses, if negative for pulmonary embolism. The direct CT signs of pulmonary embolism include:

1. An intravascular filling defect(s) that either partially or completely occludes the vessel. Acute pulmonary emboli are typically centrally located in the vessel and may produce dilatation of the affected vessel (Fig. 179.36). In the case of chronic pulmonary embolism, the filling defect may either be curvilinear or weblike and lies within peripheral pulmonary arteries, often at arterial branch points. Pulmonary arterial occlusion is typically absent owing to recanalization.
2. Indirect CT signs of pulmonary embolism include peripheral wedge-shaped or rounded areas of hyperattenuation (pulmonary infarction) (Fig. 179.35) or linear parenchymal bands in the subpleural lung. In the case of large pulmonary emboli or chronic pulmonary embolism, features of right heart strain should be sought, including right ventricular dilatation, contrast material reflux into the hepatic veins, and deviation or straightening of the interventricular septum toward the left ventricle (Fig. 179.37) [60].

EXTRAPULMONARY STRUCTURES

Evaluation of the chest radiograph is never complete unless the extrapulmonary, extrapleural, and extracardiac structures (extrathoracic soft tissues and bones of the thorax) are carefully assessed for possible pathology. It is not the purpose of this chapter to deal with these pathologic processes in depth; suffice it to say that one should look for masses, calcifications, and abnormal air collections such as abscesses in the cervical and thoracic soft tissues and subphrenic areas. The osseous structures also may provide clues to disease of a systemic nature (e.g., H-shaped vertebrae and bone infarcts in sickle cell anemia) or to metastases in the form of lytic or blastic bone lesions. Fractures after trauma, and occasionally rib fractures from resuscitation procedures after cardiac arrest, may be seen on the chest radiograph.

References

1. Palazzetti V, Gasparri E, Gambini C, et al: Chest radiography in intensive care: an irreplaceable survey? *Radiol Med* 118(5):744–751, 2013.
2. Bekemeyer WB, Crapo RO, Calhoon S, et al: Efficacy of chest radiography in a respiratory intensive care unit. A prospective study. *Chest* 88(5):691–696, 1985.
3. Amorosa JK, Bramwit MP, Mohammed TL, et al: ACR appropriateness criteria routine chest radiographs in intensive care unit patients. *J Am Coll Radiol* 10(3):170–174, 2013.
4. McAdams HP, Samei E, Dobbins J 3rd, et al: Recent advances in chest radiography. *Radiology* 241(3):663–683, 2006.
5. Conrardy PA, Goodman LR, Lainge F, et al: Alteration of endotracheal tube position. Flexion and extension of the neck. *Crit Care Med* 4(1):8–12, 1976.
6. Ravin CE, Handel DB, Kariman K: Persistent endotracheal tube cuff overdistension: a sign of tracheomalacia. *AJR Am J Roentgenol* 137(2):408–409, 1981.

7. Goodman LR, Conrardy PA, Laing F, et al: Radiographic evaluation of endotracheal tube position. *AJR Am J Roentgenol* 127(3):433–434, 1976.
8. Ridge CA, Litmanovich D, Molinari F, et al: Radiographic evaluation of central venous catheter position: anatomic correlation using gated coronary computed tomographic angiography. *J Thorac Imaging* 28(2):129–133, 2013.
9. Swan HJ, Ganz W, Forrester J, et al: Catheterization of the heart in man with use of a flow-directed balloon-tipped catheter. *N Engl J Med* 283(9):447–451, 1970.
10. Houghton D, Cohn S, Schell V, et al: Routine daily chest radiography in patients with pulmonary artery catheters. *Am J Crit Care* 11(3):261–265, 2002.
11. Westaby S, Anastasiadis K, Wieselthaler GM: Cardiogenic shock in ACS. Part 2: role of mechanical circulatory support. *Nat Rev Cardiol* 9(4):195–208, 2012.
12. Siriwardena M, Pilbrow A, Frampton C, et al: Complications of intra-aortic balloon pump use: does the final position of the IABP tip matter? *Anaesth Intensive Care* 43(1):66–73, 2015.
13. Godoy MC, Leitman BS, de Groot PM, et al: Chest radiography in the ICU: Part 2, Evaluation of cardiovascular lines and other devices. *AJR Am J Roentgenol* 198(3):572–581, 2012.
14. Ormond RS, Rubenfire M, Anbe DT, et al: Radiographic demonstration of myocardial penetration by permanent endocardial pacemakers. *Radiology* 98(1):35–37, 1971.
15. Hall WM, Rosenbaum HD: The radiology of cardiac pacemakers. *Radiol Clin North Am* 9(2):343–353, 1971.
16. Hearne SF, Maloney JD: Pacemaker system failure secondary to air entrapment within the pulse generator pocket. A complication of subclavian venipuncture for lead placement. *Chest* 82(5):651–654, 1982.
17. Savoca CJ, Gamsu G, Brito AC: The effect of acute pulmonary edema on pulmonary vascular resistance: significance for the interpretation of dilated upper lobe vessels on chest radiographs. *Invest Radiol* 12(6):488–495, 1977.
18. Attias D, Mansencal N, Auvert B, et al: Prevalence, characteristics, and outcomes of patients presenting with cardiogenic unilateral pulmonary edema. *Circulation* 122(11):1109–1115, 2010.
19. Hublitz UF, Shapiro JH: Atypical pulmonary patterns of congestive failure in chronic lung disease. The influence of pre-existing disease on the appearance and distribution of pulmonary edema. *Radiology* 93(5):995–1006, 1969.
20. Meria P, Corbel L, Mendelsberg M, et al: Peritonitis after spontaneous rupture of a pyonephrosis into the peritoneal cavity. Apropos of a case. *J Chir (Paris)* 129(11):477–478, 1992.
21. Milne EN: Chest radiology in the surgical patient. *Surg Clin North Am* 60(6):1503–1518, 1980.
22. Fujishima S: Pathophysiology and biomarkers of acute respiratory distress syndrome. *J Intensive Care* 2(1):32, 2014.
23. Jacobson JT, Johnson D, Horvath G, et al: Effect of underlying heart disease on the frequency content of ventricular fibrillation in the dog heart. *Pacing Clin Electrophysiol* 23(2):243–252, 2000.
24. Unger KM, Shibel EM, Moser KM: Detection of left ventricular failure in patients with adult respiratory distress syndrome. *Chest* 67(1):8–13, 1975.
25. Ichikado K, Suga M, Muranaka H, et al: Prediction of prognosis for acute respiratory distress syndrome with thin-section CT: validation in 44 cases. *Radiology* 238(1):321–329, 2006.
26. Ichikado K: High-resolution computed tomography findings of acute respiratory distress syndrome, acute interstitial pneumonia, and acute exacerbation of idiopathic pulmonary fibrosis. *Semin Ultrasound CT MR* 35(1):39–46, 2014.
27. Matthew EB, Holstrom FM, Kaspar RL: A simple method for diagnosing pneumonia in intubated or tracheostomized patients. *Crit Care Med* 5(2):76–81, 1977.
28. Marik PE: Aspiration pneumonitis and aspiration pneumonia. *N Engl J Med* 344(9):665–671, 2001.
29. Greenfield LJ, Singleton RP, McCaffree DR, et al: Pulmonary effects of experimental graded aspiration of hydrochloric acid. *Ann Surg* 170(1):74–86, 1969.
30. Landay MJ, Christensen EE, Bynum LJ: Pulmonary manifestations of acute aspiration of gastric contents. *AJR Am J Roentgenol* 131(4):587–592, 1978.
31. Yousem SA, Faber C: Histopathology of aspiration pneumonia not associated with food or other particulate matter: a clinicopathologic study of 10 cases diagnosed on biopsy. *Am J Surg Pathol* 35(3):426–431, 2011.
32. Prather AD, Smith TR, Poletto DM, et al: Aspiration-related lung diseases. *J Thorac Imaging* 29(5):304–309, 2014.
33. Muangman N, Stern EJ, Bulger EM, et al: Chest radiographic evolution in fat embolism syndrome. *J Med Assoc Thai* 88(12):1854–1860, 2005.
34. Glas WW, Grekin TD, Musselman MM: Fat embolism. *Am J Surg* 85(3):363–369, 1953.
35. Newbigin K, Souza CA, Torres C, et al: Fat embolism syndrome: state-of-the-art review focused on pulmonary imaging findings. *Respir Med* 113:93–100, 2016.
36. Hessen I: Roentgen examination of pleural fluid; a study of the localization of free effusions, the potentialities of diagnosing minimal quantities of fluid and its existence under physiological conditions. *Acta Radiol Suppl* 86:1–80, 1951.
37. Munden RF, O'Sullivan PJ, Liu P, et al: Radiographic evaluation of the pleural fluid accumulation rate after pneumonectomy. *Clin Imaging* 39(2):247–250, 2015.
38. Stark DD, Federle MP, Goodman PC, et al: Differentiating lung abscess and empyema: radiography and computed tomography. *AJR Am J Roentgenol* 141(1):163–167, 1983.
39. Woodring JH: The normal mediastinum in blunt traumatic rupture of the thoracic aorta and brachiocephalic arteries. *J Emerg Med* 8(4):467–476, 1990.
40. Stern EJ, Sun H, Haramati LB: Peripheral bronchopleural fistulas: CT imaging features. *AJR Am J Roentgenol* 167(1):117–120, 1996.
41. Carsky EW, Mauceri RA, Azimi F: The epicardial fat pad sign: analysis of frontal and lateral chest radiographs in patients with pericardial effusion. *Radiology* 137(2):303–308, 1980.
42. Carrafiello G, Mangini M, Fontana F, et al: Radiofrequency ablation for single lung tumours not suitable for surgery: seven years' experience. *Radiol Med* 117(8):1320–1332, 2012.
43. Chen JT, Putman CE, Hedlund LW, et al: Widening of the subcarinal angle by pericardial effusion. *AJR Am J Roentgenol* 139(5):883–887, 1982.
44. Carter Y, Meissner M, Bulger E, et al: Anatomical considerations in the surgical management of blunt thoracic aortic injury. *J Vasc Surg* 34(4):628–633, 2001.
45. Parmley LF, Mattingly TW, Manion WC, et al: Nonpenetrating traumatic injury of the aorta. *Circulation* 17(6):1086–1101, 1958.
46. O'Conor CE: Diagnosing traumatic rupture of the thoracic aorta in the emergency department. *Emerg Med J* 21(4):414–419, 2004.
47. Ridge CA, Litmanovich DE: Acute aortic syndromes: current status. *J Thorac Imaging* 30(3):193–201, 2015.
48. Cullen EL, Lantz EJ, Johnson CM, et al: Traumatic aortic injury: CT findings, mimics, and therapeutic options. *Cardiovasc Diagn Ther* 4(3):238–244, 2014.
49. Williams JS, Graff JA, Uku JM, et al: Aortic injury in vehicular trauma. *Ann Thorac Surg* 57(3):726–730, 1994.
50. Kaewlai R, Avery LL, Asrani AV, et al: Multidetector CT of blunt thoracic trauma. *Radiographics* 28(6):1555–1570, 2008.
51. Killeen KL, Mirvis SE, Shanmuganathan K: Helical CT of diaphragmatic rupture caused by blunt trauma. *AJR Am J Roentgenol* 173(6):1611–1616, 1999.
52. Iochum S, Ludig T, Walter F, et al: Imaging of diaphragmatic injury: a diagnostic challenge? *Radiographics* 22 Spec No:S103–S116, 2002; discussion S16-8.
53. Rhea JT, DeLuca SA, Greene RE: Determining the size of pneumothorax in the upright patient. *Radiology* 144(4):733–736, 1982.
54. Rhea JT, vanSonnenberg E, McLoud TC: Basilar pneumothorax in the supine adult. *Radiology* 133[3 Pt 1]:593–595, 1979.
55. Gordon R: The deep sulcus sign. *Radiology* 136(1):25–27, 1980.
56. Barcia SM, Kukreja J, Jones KD: Pulmonary interstitial emphysema in adults: a clinicopathologic study of 53 lung explants. *Am J Surg Pathol* 38(3):339–345, 2014.
57. Johnson TH, Altman AR: Pulmonary interstitial gas: first sign of barotrauma due to PEEP therapy. *Crit Care Med* 7(12):532–535, 1979.
58. Bynum LJ, Wilson JE 3rd: Radiographic features of pleural effusions in pulmonary embolism. *Am Rev Respir Dis* 117(5):829–834, 1978.
59. Westermark N: Studies of the circulation by roentgen cinematography. *Radiology* 50(6):791–802, 1948.
60. Wittram C, Maher MM, Yoo AJ, et al: CT angiography of pulmonary embolism: diagnostic criteria and causes of misdiagnosis. *Radiographics* 24(5):1219–1238, 2004.

Chapter 180 ■ Severe Upper Airway Infections

SUMERA R. AHMAD • STEPHEN J. KRINZMAN • SUNIL RAJAN • RICHARD S. IRWIN

The components of the upper airway include the nose, mouth, nasopharynx, oropharynx, and hypopharynx. It communicates with the paranasal sinuses and tympanic cavities. Although minor infections of these areas are commonly observed in the outpatient setting, occasionally, they may become severe and life threatening. This class of disease requires intense observation and aggressive management and is the focus of this chapter.

SINUSITIS

For patients on mechanical ventilatory support, sinusitis is one of four common causes of fever, along with pneumonia, catheter-related infection, and urinary tract infection [1–4]. Sinusitis is encountered in the intensive care unit (ICU) in two situations: as an uncommon, potentially fatal complication of a community-acquired sinus infection such as meningitis, osteomyelitis, orbital infection, or brain abscess and as a hospital-acquired sinus infection that may be a frequent cause of occult fever for a critically ill patient.

Incidence

The frequency of radiographically documented sinusitis among mechanically ventilated patients varies greatly from 18% to 88%, with a mean of 56% in one recent meta-analysis [5]. Of note, 67% of the patients reviewed were nasally intubated. Using criteria to identify patients with clinical evidence of sinus infection—fever; leukocytosis or leukopenia; and purulent sinus secretions—clinical sinus infection was present in one half of patients with radiographically demonstrated sinusitis [5]. In one series, 95% of nasotracheally intubated patients developed radiographic evidence of pansinusitis [6], as did 25% of patients who were orotracheally intubated.

Pathogenesis

Critically ill patients are predisposed to develop nosocomial sinusitis for several reasons. The diameter of the ostia, normally as small as 1 or 2 mm, has been shown to decrease with recumbency as much as 23% because of venous hydrostatic pressures [7]. In addition, the maxillary sinus ostia are poorly located for gravitational drainage [7]. Nasotracheal and nasogastric tubes strongly predispose patients to develop radiographic changes of sinusitis (OR 4.66 for nasally vs. orally intubated patients), and in one series, 73% of mechanically ventilated patients developed culture-proven sinusitis within 7 days of placement of nasogastric or nasotracheal tubes [6]. Larger intranasal tubes (tracheal) induce radiographic sinus changes more quickly than smaller tubes (gastric) [4]. Using multiple logistic regression analysis, risk factors for nosocomial sinusitis, of strongest association, are sedative use; nasogastric feeding tubes; Glasgow coma scale less than 8; and nasal colonization with enteric gram-negative bacteria [8].

Etiology

The microbiology of nosocomial sinusitis is quite distinct from that of community-acquired sinusitis, and is similar to that of other nosocomial respiratory infections. Nosocomial sinusitis is polymicrobial in 54% of cases, with gram-negative aerobic organisms being the most common causative agents (49%), followed by gram-positive aerobic organisms (37%), fungi (7.5%) and anaerobes (7.5%). The most commonly isolated pathogens are *Streptococcus* spp. including *Streptococcus pneumonia* (13%); *Pseudomonas* spp. (13%); *Staphylococcus aureus* (11%); *E. coli* (9%); coagulase negative staphylococci (6%); *Acinetobacter* spp. (5%); and *Klebsiella* spp. (5%) [5]. The organisms isolated in nosocomial sinusitis are the ones frequently identical to those cultured from the lower respiratory tract [3,9]. Such findings support the concept of general colonization of the airway mucosa of critically ill patients.

Specific situations warrant consideration of infection with more unusual pathogens. Acute invasive fungal rhinosinusitis (AIFR) is a rare condition, but has a mortality rate of 40% to 50% [10]. Affected patients are usually immunocompromised, with the most common comorbidities being hematologic malignancy, diabetes, medical immunosuppression, renal failure, and HIV. Aspergillus and species of Zygomycetes such as Mucor are identified in the majority of cases, with Mucor spp. being more commonly found in diabetic patients, and Aspergillus spp. being found in patients with severe HIV-associated immunosuppression or hematologic malignancies. The most common presenting symptoms are fever, purulent nasal drainage, facial pain, facial swelling, nasal crusting, and visual symptoms [10]. Common nasal endoscopic findings include necrotic mucosa and hyaline or thick mucus secretion. Radiographically, sinus opacity and bony erosion are seen in all cases, and these findings are usually unilateral [11]. Treatment consists of surgical debridement and systemic antifungal therapy. *Cryptococcus neoformans* can cause sinusitis with a high relapse rate and significant mortality in immunocompetent and immunocompromised patients [12]. *Candida* spp. [13]; *Pseudoallescheria boydii* and *Cytomegalovirus* spp.; and other unusual organisms have been isolated in patients with acquired immunodeficiency syndrome with sinusitis [14].

Complications

Complications of acute sinusitis are rare but can be rapidly fatal and are best managed in an ICU. Orbital complications include edema, predominantly of the eyelids, orbital cellulitis, orbital abscess, subperiosteal abscess, and cavernous sinus thrombosis [15,16]. The last one is the most severe, with a mortality of greater than 20% [17–19]. Intracranial complications have an overall mortality of 40% and include osteomyelitis, meningitis, epidural abscess, subdural empyema, and brain abscesses [17–19]. For these cases, sinus drainage is imperative and antibiotics are started early and redirected by culture results.

Several investigators have examined the relationship between nosocomial sinusitis and ventilator-associated pneumonia. In adult, intubated patients with clinically evident sinusitis, ventilator-associated pneumonia (VAP) is also present in 41%, and the incidence of VAP is higher among patients with sinusitis than for those without. The same organism can be isolated from both the lung and sinuses among 59% of such patients. In addition, clinically evident sinusitis increases the risk of bloodstream infections, and in patients with sinusitis and bloodstream infections, the same organism is identified among 20% of cases [5]. A prospective, randomized study of a strategy to systematically detect and treat nosocomial sinusitis, both radiographic evidence and bacteriologic evidence of sinusitis were reported for 55% of febrile, mechanically ventilated patients [20]. All patients in the study were nasotracheally intubated. Seventy percent of patients with positive radiographs had positive quantitative cultures. VAP occurred for significantly fewer patients (34% vs. 47%, $p = 0.02$) of the group for which there was systematic screening for and treatment of sinusitis. Taken together, these findings suggest a causal relationship between nosocomial sinusitis and VAP.

Nosocomial sinusitis may also cause fever of unknown origin (FUO) in mechanically ventilated patients. van Zanten and colleagues prospectively studied 351 orotracheally intubated patients with fever for more than 48 hours despite treatment with broad-spectrum antibiotics [3]. In 198 patients, the cause of the fever remained unknown despite initial investigations that included chest radiographs. Based on the results of sinus radiographs and subsequent sinus cultures, infectious sinusitis was confirmed for 30% of patients with FUO and was found to be the sole cause of fever for 16% of cases.

Diagnosis

Computed Tomography Scans and Radiographs

Computed tomography (CT) scanning has become the imaging modality of choice for the diagnosis of nosocomial sinusitis. Compared with plan sinus radiographs, sinus CT scans can more accurately visualize the ethmoid and sphenoid sinuses and are also superior in differentiating mucosal thickening from air–fluid levels [21]. Portable sinus radiographs performed in the supine position have been recommended to identify sinus infections among critically ill patients who cannot travel for standard sinus films or a CT scan [22]. As discussed earlier, patients may have sterile cultures despite radiographic evidence of sinusitis.

Ultrasonography

With the increasing use of ultrasound in the ICU, there has been a renewed interest in this modality to diagnose nosocomial sinusitis. Although bone often presents obstacles to ultrasound imaging, the anterior walls of the maxillary sinuses are flat bones composed of compact tissue, allowing adequate ultrasound penetration. Prior investigations had demonstrated that ultrasound was 67% sensitive and 87% specific for maxillary sinusitis visualized on CT scans [23]. Accuracy is improved when the patient is in the semi-recumbent position, rather than supine [24].

More recent investigations have shown further improvements of diagnostic accuracy. Vargas and coworkers used B-mode ultrasound in the semi-recumbent position in 120 patients with suspected sinusitis [24]. They found that among 36 patients with negative sinus ultrasounds, none had evidence of maxillary sinusitis on CT scan. Extensive maxillary sinus disease is indicated by hyperechogenic visualization of the posterior wall and extension to the internal and external walls was, in one investigation, found to be 100% specific for total opacification of the sinus on CT scan [25]. On transnasal puncture, fluid could be aspirated from all such patients, and the cultures were positive for 67% of patients [24]. In patients where only the posterior wall of the maxillary sinus is hyperechogenic, 80% of transnasal punctures yield fluid, and cultures are positive in half of those where fluid is obtained.

Rhinoscopy and Antral Aspiration

As reviewed earlier, opacification of the paranasal sinuses among the critically ill patient does not necessarily indicate infectious sinusitis; in some series, half or more of such patients have sterile cultures. Rhinoscopy can add significantly to the diagnostic yield for patients with suspected sinusitis. In patients with both purulent secretions in the middle meatus by rhinoscopy and radiographic evidence of sinusitis, 92% have positive cultures by antral lavage. Although cultures obtained from the maxillary sinus by antral puncture had previously been considered the gold standard for diagnosis of nosocomial sinusitis, endoscopically guided middle meatal cultures accurately reflect cultures obtained from direct maxillary sinus aspiration in 85% to 100% of patients [26]. Bilateral cultures should be obtained, as in one series, two-thirds of the positive cultures were negative on the contralateral side [26].

Treatment

Nosocomial sinusitis is most often related to the presence of nasopharyngeal and oropharyngeal catheters and tubes [4,27,28]. Therefore, in addition to antibiotics and decongestants, treatment includes removal of all nasal tubes to eliminate the source of obstruction and irritation in addition to decongestants and antibiotics. Because the spectrum of bacteria causing nosocomial sinusitis is similar to that causing other nosocomial respiratory infections [4,29,30], broad-spectrum gram-positive and gram-negative coverage is indicated. With removal of nasal tubes and antibiotic therapy, 67% of patients become afebrile within 48 hours [31]. The optimal treatment for nosocomial sinusitis remains uncertain and antibiotic selection should take local antibiograms into account. In a prospective randomized trial demonstrating clinic improvement when sinusitis was systematically investigated and treated, the treatment consisted of endoscopic transnasal puncture for culture, broad spectrum antibiotics, and serial catheter directed sinus lavage [20]. To our knowledge, no study has randomized patients to medical versus surgical treatment.

SPHENOID SINUSITIS

Sphenoid sinusitis deserves separate mention because of its potentially fulminant nature and difficulty of diagnosis. Delay in its diagnosis has been associated with serious morbidity and mortality [32,33]. The typical presentation of acute infection is severe headache that interferes with sleep, often accompanied by fever and nasal discharge [32,33]. Neurologic deficits can be prominent features; trigeminal hyperesthesia or hypoesthesia occurs in one third of cases [33]. Gram-positive organisms have been isolated from the cultures of most patients with acute sinusitis, whereas equal numbers of gram-positive and facultative gram-negative pathogens have been cultured from those with chronic sphenoid sinusitis [32,33]. Serious sequelae including permanent neurologic deficits and death can result from the spread to nearby structures (e.g., cavernous sinus, pituitary gland, optic chiasm). When findings suggest extension of the infection, early CT scan of the sinuses is essential. Surgical drainage may be necessary if symptoms persist or neurologic signs develop while the patient is receiving appropriate antibiotic therapy.

OTOGENIC INFECTIONS

Serious complications of otologic infection occur rarely [34,35]. Anatomically, the external auditory canal is one-half cartilaginous, and the medial half tunnels through the temporal bone. The auditory tubes (pharyngotympanic tube) pass into the nasopharynx along the superior border of the lateral pharyngeal spaces (LPS). Other structures that are accessible to pathogens include the mastoid air cells, the jugular foramen, cranial nerves (especially the facial nerve), the internal carotid artery, and the dura mater of the posterior cranial fossa.

Mastoiditis

Acute mastoiditis is an uncommon complication of otitis media, seen primarily in children and young adults. Inflammation spreads from the middle ear to the modified respiratory mucosa lining of the mastoid air cells, by direct invasion of the bone or through the mastoid emissary veins. The closed space infection leads to accumulation of purulent exudate, increased pressure, and bony necrosis. Pain, typically postauricular, fever, and abnormal tympanic membranes are the most common findings on presentation, and a fluctulent mass may be noted, causing anterior displacement of the auricle [36]. The duration of symptoms averages 10 days [36]. In a review of 202 hospitalized children, the most frequent culture result was "no growth" (30%), followed by *Streptococcus pneumoniae* (21%), *skin flora* (14%), *Pseudomonas aeruginosa* (7%), *Streptococcus pyogenes* (7%), and *Staphylococcus aureus (4%)* [37]. Radiographic abnormalities may be evident on CT or MRI imaging that can reveal opacification or cloudiness of the mastoid air cells and, less frequently, evidence of bone destruction [38]. Although uncommon (1.9%), complications can include conductive hearing loss, facial palsy, sinus thrombosis, subdural and epidural abscess, and meningitis [36,38]. Treatment includes broad-spectrum antibiotics that can adequately penetrate cerebrospinal fluid and surgical intervention for those who fail to improve within 24 to 72 hours.

Chronic mastoiditis and chronic otitis media result from a progressive inflammatory process that usually leads to obstruction of the communication between the middle ear and mastoid (aditus) or the middle ear and nasopharynx (eustachian tube) [39]. Often a cholesteatoma or epidermal inclusion cyst within the tympanomastoid compartment may be involved and may become secondarily infected [39]. Presenting symptoms include hearing loss, painless otorrhea, and tympanic membrane perforation [39]. Other symptoms (e.g., facial nerve paresis, headache, ear pain, fever) may be present if complications have occurred. Uncomplicated chronic otitis media and mastoiditis are treated medically with local hygiene, topical antibiotics often including a corticosteroid, and oral, or infrequently parenteral, antibiotics [39]. Broad-spectrum antibiotics are required to cover a wide range of aerobic and anaerobic organisms. Surgery is usually reserved for recurrent disease, often associated with a cholesteatoma, which can be identified by CT scan of the temporal bone [39].

Malignant External Otitis

Malignant, or necrotizing, external otitis (MEO) most often affects elderly diabetic patients. Diabetic microangiopathy, impaired chemotaxis and phagocytosis, combined with the ability of *Pseudomonas aeruginosa* to invade vessel walls, causes vasculitis with thrombosis, leading to the characteristic pathophysiology of this of this disorder [40]. The majority of patients (65% to 100%) have diabetes mellitus, but MEO may also develop in patients with other forms of immunosuppression, including HIV/AIDS, hematologic malignancies, after chemotherapy and with solid organ transplantation [40,41]. MEO most commonly presents with otalgia, granulation tissue in the external auditory canal, most prominently at the osteocartilaginous junction, and often purulent and fetid otorrhea [42]. Spread of infection is anteriorly toward the parotid compartment or downward into the temporal bone; spread to the mastoid is less common [34]. Extension leads to pain and tenderness of the tissues around the ear. *P. aeruginosa* is the most commonly implicated pathogen (85%) [42]. Patients with acquired immunodeficiency syndrome may develop infection from a wider variety of organisms and may accumulate less granulation tissue in the external auditory canal [43]. *Aspergillus* spp. have been identified, primarily in immunocompromised patients [44,45]. Osteomyelitis [46], cranial nerve paralysis [47], and central nervous system (meningitis) and vascular (thrombophlebitis) spread [48] are potential severe and fatal complications of MEO.

CT and magnetic resonance imaging scanning, along with technetium-99 bone scans, are valuable components of the diagnostic evaluation of MEO [48]. CT scans may show erosion of the tympanic bone (80%), and clouding of the mastoid cells in 19.5% [41]. CT scans may be normal among 11% of cases [41]. Thus, if there is a high clinical suspicion, technetium-99 bone scans should be obtained, and are positive in close to 100% of cases [40]. Surgical interventions may not be required, but management does require biopsy and culture, and may require debridement and drainage of associated abscess [40]. Therapy for MEO includes prolonged antibiotics directed against *P. aeruginosa* unless the culture data suggest another pathogen. This may include a semisynthetic penicillin, ceftazidime, or oral fluoroquinolones [48]. The duration of treatment is not clearly defined and complete response is defined by resolution of signs and symptoms.

SUPRAGLOTTITIS (EPIGLOTTITIS)

Acute supraglottitis is an uncommon infection of the structures located above the glottis. These structures include the epiglottis, aryepiglottic folds, arytenoids, pharynx, uvula, and tongue base. The true vocal cords are rarely involved. The infection may progress to abrupt and fatal airway obstruction. This entity is well described in children, in whom the presentation and course are usually fulminant. In the pediatric population, increased awareness and prophylactic airway control have reduced overall mortality to less than 1% [49,50]. Although this disease at one time affected primarily children, with the introduction of the conjugate vaccine for *Hemophilus influenza* type b (Hib), there has been a dramatic decline in pediatric infections, and supraglottitis is becoming a disease of adults. In children, *H. influenzae* type B is still the most commonly identified causative organism.

Incidence

In the post–*H. influenzae* type B vaccine era, the annual incidence of acute supraglottitis is estimated between 0.6 and 0.78 cases per 100,000 immunized children [51]. Among adults, the incidence of acute supraglottitis has increased from 0.79 cases per 100,000 adults in 1986 to 2.1 cases per 100,000 adults in 2005 [52]. Adults with acute supraglottitis usually present in their 40s and 50s, with a male preponderance, and children usually present between the ages of 2 and 5 years [52].

Pathogenesis and Pathophysiology

Among children, the inflammation is mainly restricted to the epiglottis because of loose mucosa on its lingual aspect. This provides a readily available space for edema to collect within. Swelling reduces the airway aperture by curling the epiglottis posteriorly and inferiorly, accentuating the juvenile omega shape. When edema spreads to involve the aryepiglottic folds, respiratory distress can occur as inspiration draws these structures downward, further exacerbating the obstruction and resulting in stridor. The adult airway is relatively protected because the larynx is larger and the epiglottis is shaped more like a spatula.

Etiology

H. influenzae type B is the most common cause identified among pediatric cases, even in the post-vaccine era [51,53]. In adults, numerous bacterial, viral, and fungal organisms have been implicated, including *Hemophilus influenza* type B, *Streptococcus pneumonia*, *Staphylococcus aureus*, *Streptococcus* spp., *Moraxella catarrhalis*, *Pseudomonas* spp., *methicillin-resistant Staphylococcus aureus* (MRSA), and *Neisseria* spp. Non-bacterial agents include *Candida albicans*, and viruses such as Herpes simplex, Parainfluenza, Varicella zoster, and Epstein-Barr. Among adults, blood cultures are positive in less than 20% of cases, and *H. influenzae* is the isolate for one-third of these cases [53,54].

Noninfectious causes of acute supraglottitis have been described and include thermal injuries related to inhalation drug use, ingestion of hot food, apparent caustic injury from aspiration, and posttransplant lymphoproliferative disorder [55,56]. McKinney and Grigg [57] described a case of epiglottitis after general anesthesia administered via a laryngeal mask.

Diagnosis

History and Physical Examination

For children, the classic presentation is of a 3-year-old child who initially complains of a sore throat followed by dysphagia and/or odynophagia, which then progresses within hours to stridor. The child prefers to sit, leaning forward, and usually appears pale and frightened. Breathing is slow and quiet with characteristic drooling noted. These symptoms may lead to sudden respiratory depression and arrest. The progression of symptoms can be remembered as the four "Ds": dysphagia, dysphonia, drooling, and distress. Children with acute supraglottitis rarely present with coughing that may help to distinguish them from those with laryngotracheobronchitis or croup [51].

Among adults, the classic presentation is more the exception than the rule, and as such, the frequency of misdiagnosis has been reported as high as 60% to 75% [49,52]. More than 90% of adults seek medical attention complaining of sore throat with or without dysphagia [56,59]. Many patients report antecedent upper respiratory tract infections [59,60], and between 60 and 90% will have an elevated temperature [51]. Other less common signs and symptoms are respiratory distress, muffled voice, drooling, and stridor [49,50,53,55,58]. Hoarseness or true dysphonia is not observed because the process usually spares the true vocal cords. Children and adults often prefer an upright posture with the neck extended and mouth slightly open [59].

The duration of symptoms varies, ranging from hours to several days [61]. Patients who present early in their disease course have more severe symptoms, fever, and leukocytosis, and those presenting within 8 hours of the onset of symptoms are more likely to have signs of upper airway obstruction [62]. They are also more likely to be infected with *H. influenzae* [61]. These patients are at increased risk of needing artificial airways and of dying [63].

Evaluation of patients with suspected supraglottitis depends, in part, on their age and the severity of their symptoms. For young children with a classical presentation, pharyngeal examination should not be attempted. An artificial airway should be established in the controlled setting of an operating room, where an examination can be performed with less risk of airway obstruction.

For older children and adults, supraglottitis should be considered when sore throat and dysphagia seem to be out of proportion to visible signs of pharyngitis. In this situation, if the patient has no respiratory distress, examination of the larynx and supralaryngeal structures is recommended. The epiglottis may appear cherry red in color but more commonly is pale and edematous. Other supraglottic structures may be edematous as well, resulting in the inability to visualize the vocal cords [51].

Diagnostic Tests

Although considered the classic radiographic finding, the "thumb sign," indicating a swollen epiglottis (Fig. 180.1), may be negative in up to 56% of cases [51], so its absence should never be used to exclude the diagnosis. When there is significant clinical suspicion, direct visualization of the structures should be performed [64]. The radiograph should be taken in the upright position to avoid pooling of secretions posteriorly and potentially increasing the obstruction, and the patient must be observed at all times by someone skilled in airway management.

Few laboratory tests are helpful at the time of initial evaluation. An elevated white blood cell count and C-reactive protein level may identify a patient at higher risk. Throat cultures are positive in less than 33% of the cases, and blood cultures detect a causative agent in less than 20% of the cases [52,55]. Swab culture of the epiglottis obtained under direct visualization may better reflect the causative agent, and has been positive in up to 75% of the cases [55,58].

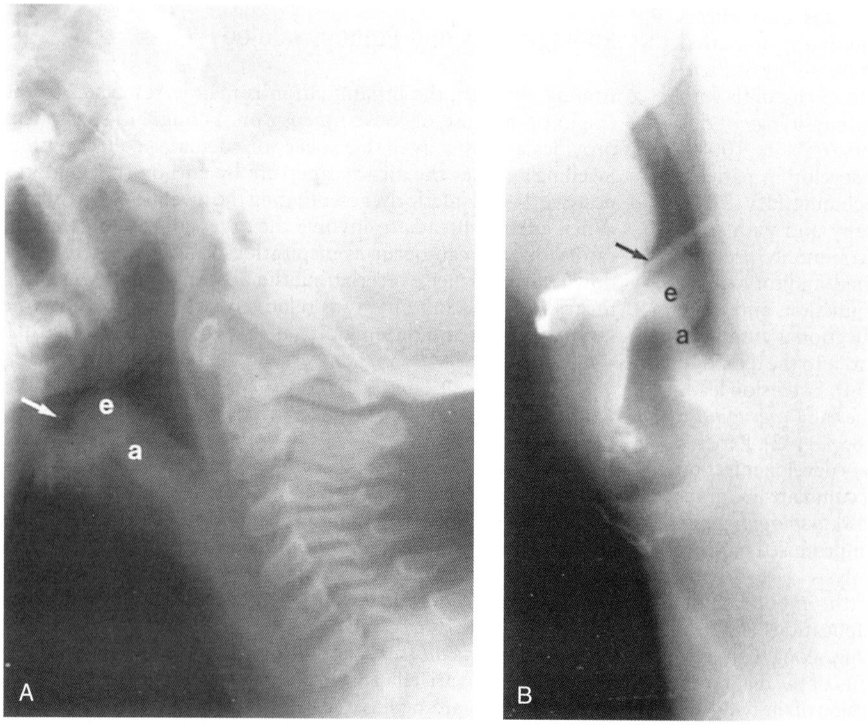

FIGURE 180.1 Acute supraglottitis. Lateral radiographs of the neck obtained with soft tissue technique in a 2-year-old child (**A**) and a 42-year-old adult (**B**). There is epiglottic (*e*) swelling (thumb sign), thickening of the aryepiglottic folds (*a*), and narrowing of the vallecula (*arrow*) in both patients. Compare with normal epiglottis in Figure 180.11(*a*).

Differential Diagnosis

Supraglottitis of children is a clinical diagnosis. Because immediate airway control is a priority, recognizing other pediatric illnesses presenting with a sore throat and not requiring this intervention is important [65,66]. The most common infection is croup, a predominantly viral laryngotracheobronchitis that occurs up to 40 times more frequently than epiglottitis [66]. Typically, the child is younger than 3 years and has had an upper respiratory tract infection of at least 48 hours' duration. Hoarseness develops initially and is followed by a distinctive barking cough. Although respiratory distress with stridor is common, intubation is rarely needed [65,66]. Anteroposterior and lateral views of the neck may show the classic, "steeple sign" (Fig. 180.2), a gradual narrowing of the proximal tracheal air column secondary to subglottic edema. Other less common infectious considerations for children include pseudomembranous croup (bacterial laryngotracheobronchitis), retropharyngeal abscess, lingual tonsillitis, and diphtheria [65,66].

Among adults, infectious mononucleosis, often with massive tonsillar hypertrophy leading to stridor, and a unilateral pharyngeal mass should be considered when patients complain of sore throat and dysphagia. Pharyngitis may present a picture indistinguishable from that of mild or early supraglottitis [63].

Bacterial tracheitis is a potentially life-threatening illness with features similar to those of supraglottitis and viral croup. Although more often seen among the pediatric population, adults can also be affected [67]. These patients present with a brief, progressive upper respiratory tract prodrome including a brassy cough, stridor, high fever, and toxicity but do not exhibit dysphagia or drooling [65,66]. Airway obstruction is caused by subglottic mucosal edema and thick, inspissated, mucopurulent tracheal secretions [67]. Bacterial superinfection of a preceding viral tracheitis occurs most commonly with *S. aureus* and *H. influenzae* [66]. Rare cases of membranous tracheobronchitis due to a fungal agent have been described among immunocompromised hosts [60], but these infections have involved primarily the lower respiratory tract. Lateral neck radiographs demonstrate subglottic narrowing and may show mucosal irregularities or membranes in the tracheal air column [68]. Chest radiographs may show signs of atelectasis due to central bronchial obstruction by mucus or necrotic debris [69]. Management is similar to that for supraglottitis, and bronchoscopy should be performed for diagnosis [70]. Intubation or tracheostomy is usually necessary to relieve obstruction and provide adequate tracheal suctioning [67,70]. Antibiotic therapy should be directed against *S. aureus* and other common causative respiratory pathogens.

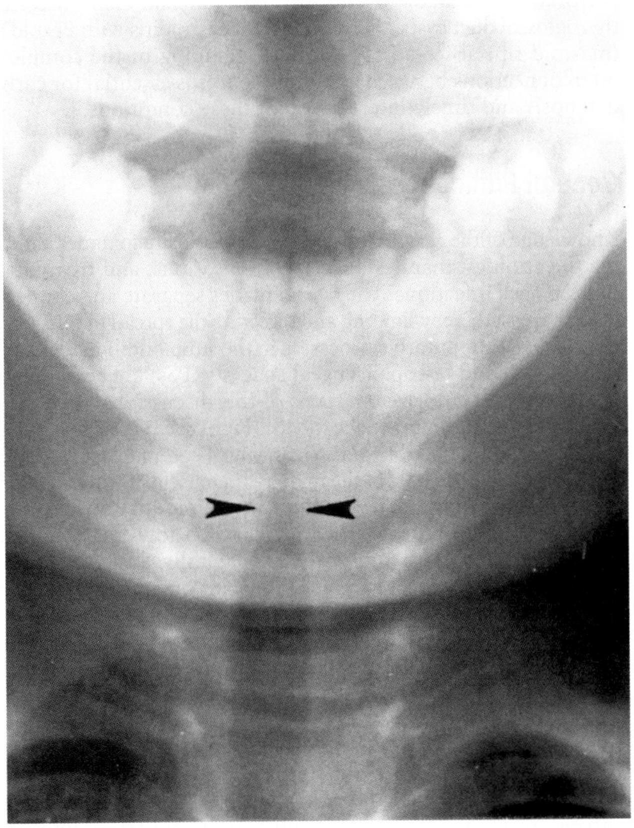

FIGURE 180.2 Croup. Anteroposterior radiograph of the neck in a 19-month-old child. Subglottic edema produces smooth tapering (*arrowheads*) of the tracheal air column (the steeple sign).

Rhinoscleroma should also be considered in the differential diagnosis. *Klebsiella rhinoscleromatis* is the etiologic agent of this chronic granulomatous disorder [71,72]. Although nasal and oral mucous membranes are the most common sites of infection, patients have presented acutely with upper airway obstruction due to indolent spread to the larynx and tracheobronchial tree. This condition may be seen in immigrants to the USA from endemic areas such as Central America, Central Europe, Africa, and Asia. The nodular and indurated endoscopic appearance is nondiagnostic, so multiple biopsy specimens for culture and histologic examination are required. Treatment is with a prolonged course of oral antibiotics. Repeated cultures of biopsy specimens may be needed to ascertain whether bacteriologic cure has been achieved [72].

Noninfectious causes of acute upper airway obstruction are usually suggested by the history obtained and by the patient's nontoxic appearance. These include foreign body aspiration; allergic edema; chemical laryngitis from gastroesophageal reflux; and necrotizing tracheobronchitis as a complication of mechanical ventilation [73]. Paraquat poisoning can cause a pharyngeal membrane similar to diphtheria that is accompanied by signs of shock and sepsis [74].

Treatment

The treatment of supraglottitis has two major components: airway management and medical therapy. The early placement of an artificial airway for children has significantly reduced mortality. Moreover, because airway obstruction is the most common cause of death among adults for whom airways are not secured when the diagnosis of supraglottitis is made, some authors favor establishing an artificial airway prophylactically, as is performed in children [50,52,61]. In one series [75], adult patients who presented with stridor within 24 hours of onset of symptoms had a rapidly progressive course, requiring airway interventions, whereas those presenting with similar symptoms but with a longer interval since symptom onset responded to medical therapy. For these reasons, we favor reserving intubation for adult patients with early signs of airway obstruction [56,61,76], or those with recent onset and rapid progression of symptoms. All patients should be observed in an ICU with the immediate availability of equipment and personnel for emergent intubation.

Both tracheostomy and translaryngeal endotracheal intubation have been performed. No difference in mortality has been reported when comparing these two modalities [77,78]. Significant reductions for duration of airway control, incidence of upper airway complications, and length of hospital stay have been observed in patients with endotracheal intubation when compared with tracheostomy [78,79]. The acute complications of tracheostomy, including pneumothorax, hemorrhage, and subcutaneous or mediastinal emphysema, occur with increased frequency among patients younger than 12 years [77]. Accidental extubation, particularly for children, is the greatest risk of endotracheal intubation [77,78]. Much of the morbidity of the artificial airway is associated with its prolonged maintenance, which is unlikely to occur with supraglottitis. In one large series, 90% of children were extubated in less than 24 hours [80]. The choice of an artificial airway should be determined by the skill of available personnel in placing and maintaining the airway. Endotracheal intubation is preferred, with surgical backup, should the attempt fail.

The appropriate time for extubation in a patient recovering from acute supraglottitis varies. Some physicians remove the artificial airway when the patient's general toxic appearance and fever have subsided [80]. Others wait until repeat laryngoscopy or lateral neck radiographs show decreased edema of the involved structures [81]. One can deflate the cuff of the endotracheal tube to test for an air leak around the tube or the patient's ability to breathe with the tube plugged for a brief moment [82]. It is important to remember that if the tube fills the trachea, the patient may not be able to breathe even if supraglottitis has completely resolved.

Medical therapy is crucial for rapid recovery from supraglottitis. All patients require close observation, humidification, and, often, mild sedation [53]. Many antibiotics are effective, and the regimens must cover *H. influenzae* infection. With the high frequency of β-lactamase–producing strains of *H. influenzae*, ampicillin is no longer adequate as an initial single agent. The initial drug of choice is a second- or third-generation cephalosporin that covers ampicillin-resistant *H. influenzae* as well as the other possible pathogens in adults: *S. aureus*, *S. pneumoniae*, and other streptococcal species [64]. Cefotaxime has been considered the antibiotic of choice; ceftriaxone and ampicillin/sulbactam have also been found to be effective [53]. Trimethoprim–sulfamethoxazole can be used as an alternative agent for penicillin-allergic patients. With the rising frequency of penicillin-resistance and multidrug-resistant *S. pneumoniae*, the initial antibiotic regimen may require modification based upon culture data. The antibiotics should be initially administered intravenously for several days, depending on the response, and then continued by mouth for 7 to 10 days [82].

Corticosteroid therapy is controversial for patients with infectious supraglottitis. Many authors, finding no contraindications, use steroids empirically [53,77]. There have been no randomized, controlled trials assessing the effectiveness of corticosteroids for patients with acute epiglottitis (Table 180.1). Steroids have been noted to be effective in a large, randomized, controlled trial of children with moderate-to-severe croup, lending some support to the hypothesis that steroids may be beneficial in infectious upper airway disease [83]. The use of a helium–oxygen mixture (Heliox) could be considered to diminish the work of breathing and provide a bridge to avoid intubation while antibiotics take effect.

Complications of the disease differ between the pediatric and adult populations. The former has a higher incidence of pneumonia and accidental extubation [84]. Pulmonary edema immediately after intubation for severe stridor has been described among children [85]. For adults, an epiglottic abscess may be suggested by a persistent or deteriorating clinical condition [86,76]. CT scan of the neck may be helpful for making this diagnosis, particularly if direct visualization is not adequate [86,87]. Both groups face risks and complications associated with intubation and tracheostomy [79]. Treatment recommendations are outlined in Figure 180.3.

TABLE 180.1

Organisms Implicated in Acute Epiglottitis

Organism	References
Hemophilus influenzae	[3,30]
Streptococcus pneumoniae	[12]
β-Hemolytic streptococci	[13,14]
Staphylococcus aureus	[14,16,17]
Klebsiella pneumoniae	[17,18]
Neisseria meningitides	[27]
Bacteroides spp.	[19]
Haemophilus parainfluenzae	[21,30]
Candida albicans[a]	[22,25]
Pasteurella multocida	[28]
Herpes simplex virus type 1[b]	[31,32]

[a]Cultured from epiglottic swab or seen on autopsy; all others recovered from blood.
[b]Epiglottis biopsy specimen histology and viral culture.

INFECTIONS OF THE DEEP SPACES OF THE NECK

Deep neck infections can be fatal extensions of upper airway infections. These potentially catastrophic infections are infrequently encountered today because of the prompt treatment of pharyngitis, tonsillitis, odontogenic, and otologic infections with antibiotics [88]. Deep neck infections are more common in males, smokers, alcoholics, and intravenous drug users [88]. They can be fatal for patients who are immunocompromised such those with HIV, diabetes mellitus, chronic steroid use and those undergoing chemotherapy [89]. In a retrospective analysis of 365 patients, the presence of diabetes mellitus and multiple deep neck space infections were the strongest predictors of complications [90]. Airway obstruction and mediastinitis were the most troublesome of complications [90], but patients may also develop jugular vein thrombosis, pneumonia, pericarditis, and arterial erosion [91]. Tonsillitis remains the most common cause of this disease in children, whereas poor dental hygiene and injection drug abuse are the most common causes in adults [91]. Other causes include trauma, surgical trauma, esophageal perforation, laryngopyocele, infected branchial cleft, infected thyroglossal duct cysts, thyroiditis, and mastoiditis with Bezold's (mastoid tip) abscess [91]. An understanding of the complex interconnections between anatomic spaces is essential for early diagnosis and timely intervention of these conditions.

General Pathogenesis and Anatomy

Knowledge of the cervical fasciae is a prerequisite to understanding the etiology, manifestations, complications, and treatment of deep neck infections. The fascial planes separate and connect distant areas, thereby limiting and directing the spread of infection (Fig. 180.4). Suppurative processes in the submandibular, lateral pharyngeal, and retropharyngeal spaces (RPSs) are considered life threatening and are the focus of this discussion.

The submandibular space (SMS) (Fig. 180.5) consists of the sublingual and submylohyoid spaces, which communicate around the free posterior border of the mylohyoid muscle. It extends from the mucous membrane of the floor of the mouth above to the superficial layer of the deep cervical fascia below. It is bounded by the mandible both anteriorly and laterally. Superolaterally is the buccopharyngeal gap, an important opening behind the styloglossus muscle, which connects the SMS to the LPS.

The LPS (Fig. 180.6), also called the pharyngomaxillary or parapharyngeal space, is shaped like an inverted cone with its apex at the hyoid bone and its base at the base of the skull. The styloid process penetrates the space and divides it into two functional units: anterior (muscular) and posterior (neurovascular) compartments. The former lies lateral to the tonsillar fossa and connects inferomedially to the SMS. The latter contains the carotid sheath and its contents (internal carotid artery, internal jugular vein, vagus nerve, and lymph nodes), cranial nerves IX through XII, and the cervical sympathetic trunks. Both compartments abut the RPS.

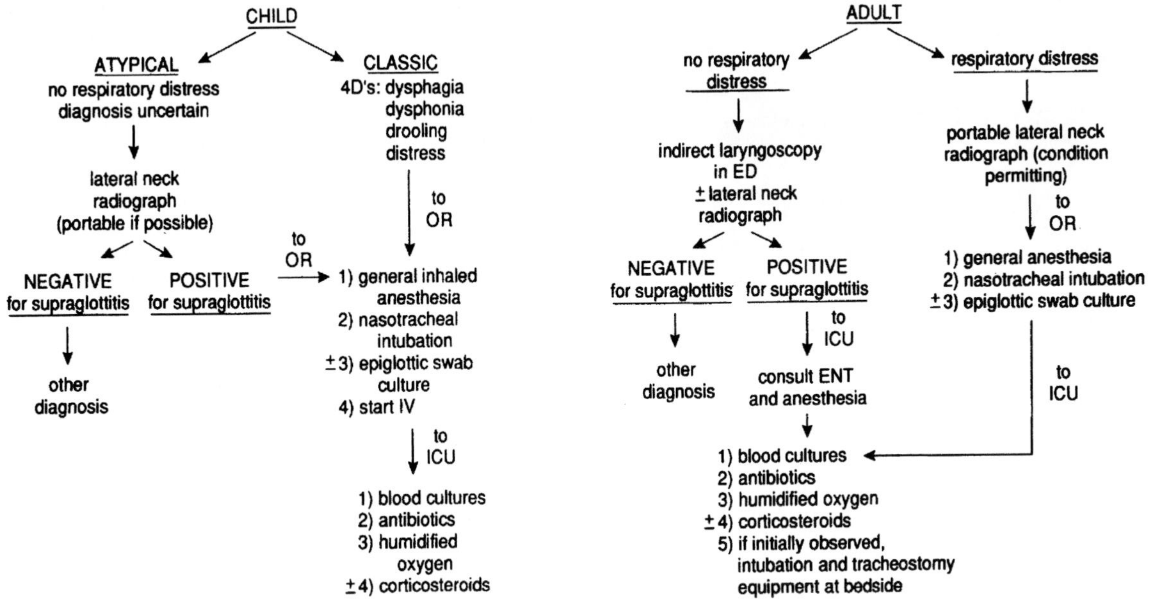

FIGURE 180.3 Management algorithm for acute supraglottitis; ± for epiglottic swab relates to questionable use; for corticosteroids reflects inconclusive study data. ED, emergency department; ENT, ear, nose, and throat specialist; ICU, intensive care unit; OR, operating room.

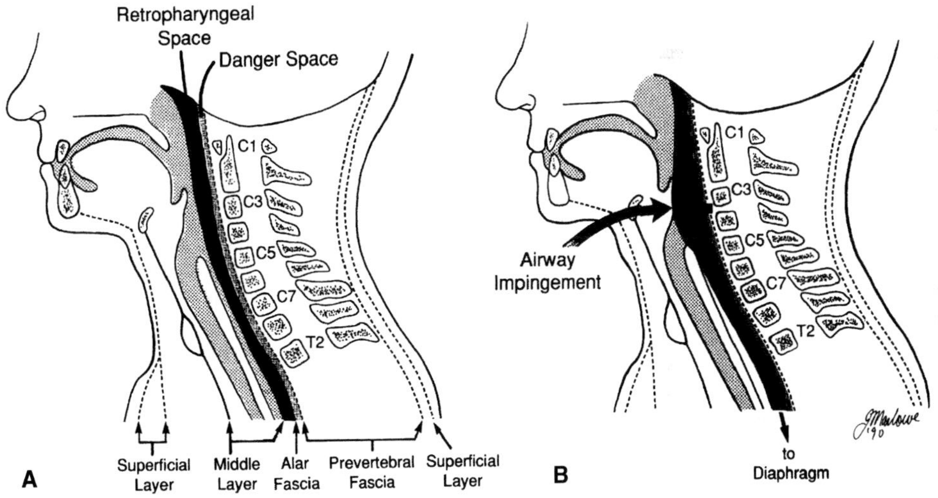

FIGURE 180.4 Schematic representation of cervical fascial planes and spaces. **A:** Normal. **B:** Retropharyngeal space abscess. (Adapted from Netter FH: *Atlas of Human Anatomy*. Summit, NJ, Ciba-Geigy, 1989.)

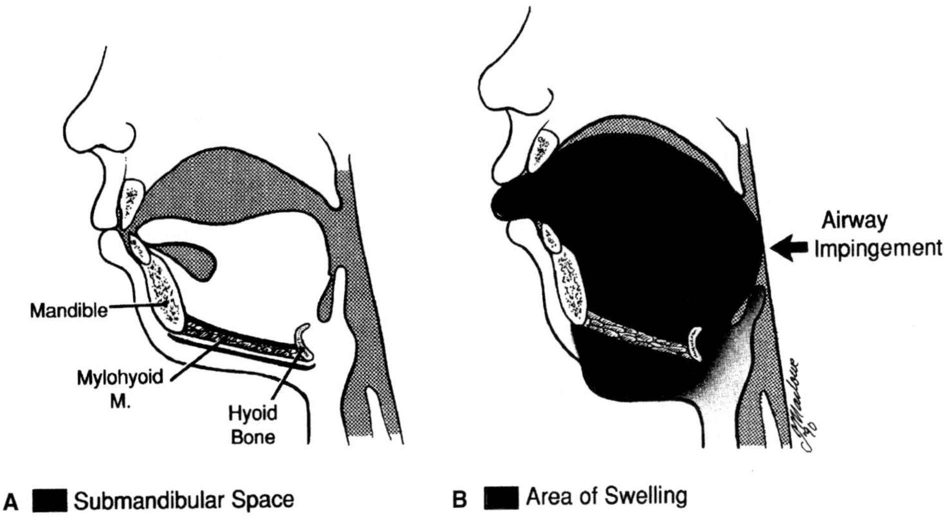

FIGURE 180.5 Schematic representation of submandibular space. **A:** Normal. **B:** Ludwig's angina. The submandibular space consists of sublingual and submylohyoid spaces. Area of swelling in **B** fills the submandibular space.

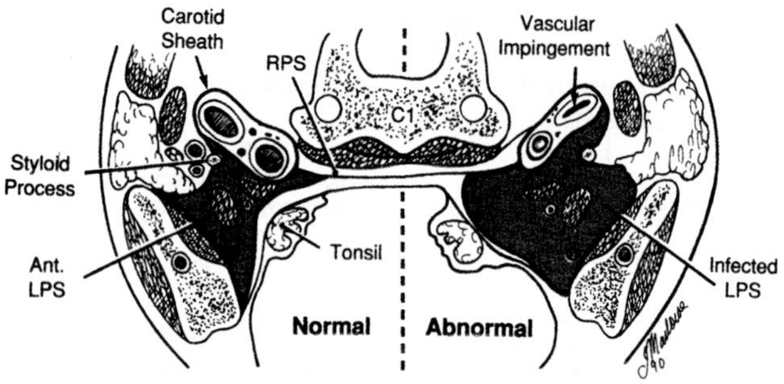

FIGURE 180.6 Cross-sectional view of LPS, showing normal anatomic landmarks and effects of space infection on them. RPS, retropharyngeal space; LPS, lateral pharyngeal space.

The RPS, also called the posterior visceral space (see Fig. 180.4), lies between the middle layer of the deep cervical fascia, which surrounds the pharynx and esophagus anteriorly, and the alar layer of the deep cervical fascia posteriorly. It extends from the base of the skull to the level of T1 or T2 in the superior mediastinum. Laterally, it abuts the LPS. Two chains of lymph nodes that drain many structures of the head are located on either side of the midline.

Immediately posterior to the RPS is the danger space (see Fig. 180.4), so named because it is the pathway into the chest for all neck infections. It extends from the base of the skull to the diaphragms and is bounded posteriorly by the prevertebral layer of the deep cervical fascia. Involvement of this space by infection is a result of extension from the RPS or prevertebral space and can result in life-threatening complications.

The prevertebral space (see Fig. 180.4) lies between the vertebral bodies and the prevertebral layer of the deep cervical fascia. Infections at this location most often represent chronic processes arising from cervical spine injuries or infections.

Etiology

Bacteria found in normal oral flora are primarily responsible for deep cervical infections. When mucosal barriers are interrupted, bacteria can penetrate into the deeper spaces. Infections are typically polymicrobial with anaerobes predominating over aerobes. Fungi and mycobacteria are uncommon etiologic agents in these infections. The role of biofilms in deep neck infections has been observed with electron microscopy, resulting in failure of antimicrobial therapy, particularly in larger abscesses [92]. Numerous bacteria naturally form biofilms, such as *staphylococcus epidermidis*, *Pseudomonas aeruginosa*, *E. coli*, *Streptococci*, *Candida*, and other gram-positive and gram-negative species [92].

Correct identification of the causal pathogen requires careful culture techniques. Several factors contribute to the difficulty of obtaining meaningful bacteriologic data. Most patients receive antibiotics before hospitalization, many deep infections resolve with empiric antibiotic therapy without the need for aspiration procedures, and cultures obtained perorally are often contaminated by nonpathogenic organisms colonizing the oropharynx [91,93,94]. With proper anaerobic collection and transport techniques, three anaerobic isolates are most commonly identified: *Peptostreptococcus*, *Fusobacterium* (mostly *F. nucleatum*), and *Bacteroides* (mostly *B. melaninogenicus*) [93,94]. Although obligate anaerobes as a class are recovered most often, aerobic streptococci (mostly *Streptococcus viridans*) and staphylococci are the most frequent individual isolates [93]. Among 148 adults, *Klebsiella pneumoniae* was found to be the most prevalent bacterial isolate [95].

Among other facultative gram-negative organisms *Escherichia coli*, *P. aeruginosa*, *K. pneumoniae*, *H. influenzae*, *Enterobacter*, *Proteus mirabilis*, *Citrobacter freundii*, and *Actinomyces* spp. have been isolated from deep cervical infections [91]. *Eikenella corrodens*, a facultative anaerobic gram-negative rod, is an emerging pathogen in head and neck infections that is uniformly resistant to clindamycin [94]. Staphylococci should be considered in deep neck infections, particularly with cases of penetrating trauma, including cervical intravenous (IV) drug use [94]. *Staphylococcus aureus*, including resistant forms (MRSA), have been found to be more prevalent among the pediatric population in younger age group with subsequent higher rate of complications, such as mediastinitis [96]. Among patients with diabetes, *K. pneumoniae* is most commonly isolated, followed by Streptococcus spp. [97].

When microbiologic confirmation is lacking, clinical clues may help suggest the presence of anaerobes. A foul-smelling discharge, gas production, tissue necrosis, and abscess formation can be suggestive, but the sensitivity of these findings is low. Gram's stain may reveal anaerobic organisms with specific morphologic characteristics (e.g., *Clostridia*, *Fusobacterium*). Because anaerobes are more fastidious, failure of the more rapidly available aerobic cultures to reveal a causative organism may suggest an anaerobic pathogen.

Diagnosis

It is important to distinguish the space or spaces involved by deep neck infections to allow for early recognition and prevention of potentially devastating complications. The clinical picture may be confusing because of involvement of multiple spaces and interference with the physical examination by trismus. Fever and systemic toxicity are common early symptoms. Other signs and symptoms may be helpful to localize the primary site of infection (Table 180.2) [98]. Serologic testing contributes little to the diagnostic evaluation. Although initial assessment often includes a lateral neck radiograph to screen for widening of the retropharyngeal tissues, the sensitivity of this test is lower than contrast-enhanced computed tomomography (CECT). CECT has a sensitivity of 80% to 90% [99] and a positive predicted value 76.9% for the diagnosis of deep neck infections [100]. Plain chest x-ray can be used to screen for complications such as pleural effusions, mediastinitis and pneumonia [99]. False positive CT scans may be caused by cellulitis or by metastatic cervical lymph nodes with necrosis, and thus biopsy of necrotic lymph nodes is recommended to assure these changes are caused by infection and not malignancy. The ability of CT scans to diagnose a deep neck abscess is much better when multiple spaces are involved (PPV 91.3%) than when the infection is confined to a single pocket (PPV 50%) [100]. Ultrasound is useful for superficial abscesses, which would have the added advantage of drainage and limited radiation exposure, though it is less helpful for deeper locations [99]. MRI can be more precise than CECT in multiple space involvement, though has greater acquisition time and requires more patient cooperation [100].

Submandibular Space Infections

Infection in the SMS is exemplified by Ludwig's angina. This is a potentially life-threatening, bilateral cellulitis originating in the SMS. It spreads rapidly by direct extension, rather than via lymphatics, and can involve the submental and sublingual spaces [101]. Glandular structures are spared, and gangrene occurs without abscess formation (see Fig. 180.5) [102]. Dental infections are the most common source, specifically those involving the roots of the second and third molar area lying immediately superior to this region [99,103]. The next most common cause is extension from an upper airway infection such as peritonsillary abscess [103]. Symptoms range from fever, malaise, submandibular swelling, erythema, to dyphagia, dyspnea, and endangerment of airway from tongue swelling, trismus, and neck swelling [101,103]. Among early cases, conservative

TABLE 180.2

Comparative Features of Infections of the Deep Cervical Spaces

		Clinical features				
Space infections	Usual site of origin	Pain	Trismus	Swelling	Dysphagia	Dyspnea
Submandibular	Second and third mandibular molars	Present	Minimal	Submandibular	Absent	Absent
Sublingual	Mandibular incisors	Present	Minimal	Floor of mouth (tender)	Present if involvement is bilateral	Present if involvement is bilateral
Lateral pharyngeal						
Anterior	Masticator spaces	Intense	Prominent	Angle of jaw	Present	Occasional
Posterior	Masticator spaces	Minimal	Minimal	Posterior pharynx (unilateral)	Present	Severe
Retropharyngeal	Lateral pharyngeal space; distant via lymphatics	Present	Minimal	Posterior pharynx (often unilateral)	Present	Present
Prevertebral	Cervical vertebrae	Present	None	Posterior pharynx (usually midline)	Occasional	Occasional

Modified from Megran DW, Scheifele DW, Chow AW: Odontogenic infections. *Pediatr Infect Dis* 3:257, 1984.

management with antibiotics and critical care observation can be considered because endoscopically assisted nasotracheal intubation or bedside tracheostomy tube may be needed with for airway management [103].

Ludwig's angina is essentially a clinical diagnosis. Physical examination (Fig. 180.7) reveals bilateral, firm submandibular swelling [102]; most patients with SMS involvement demonstrate soft tissue swelling, prompting further radiographic examination (Fig. 180.8). With aggressive airway management, antibiotics and surgical decompression of indurated submandibular glands, mortality from Ludwig's angina has decreased to less than 10% [94] Mortality rates have decreased significantly because of a more effective antibiotic therapy and early airway control [7,54].

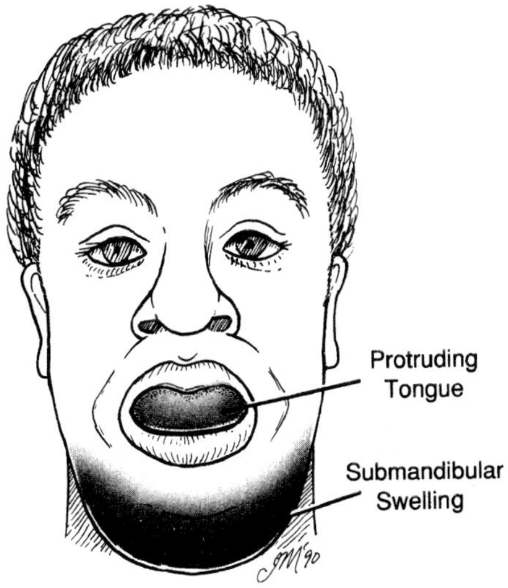

FIGURE 180.7 Schematic representation of salient clinical findings of Ludwig's angina.

Lateral Pharyngeal Space Infections

The signs and symptoms of LPS infections are determined by which of the two compartments is affected (see Fig. 180.6). The four major clinical signs of anterior compartment involvement include systemic toxicity with high fever and rigors; unilateral trismus due to irritation of the internal pterygoid muscle; induration and swelling along the angle of the jaw; and medial bulging of the lateral pharyngeal wall with the palatine tonsil protruding into the airway [104] (Fig. 180.9). Other symptoms may include dysphagia and pain involving the jaw or side of the neck. Pain may be referred to the ipsilateral ear and may worsen with turning the head to the unaffected side, which compresses the inflamed space by contraction of the sternocleidomastoid muscle. Common sources of involvement arise from pharyngitis, tonsillitis, otitis, matoiditis, parotitis, and cervical lymphadenitis [94,104]. Peritonsillar abscess are a particularly common cause of this infection [104]. Extension from the SMS and RPS has also been observed.

For infection of the posterior compartment, trismus and tonsillar prolapse are notably absent. Edema may involve the larynx and epiglottis, resulting in marked dyspnea [104]. External swelling may be visible when it spreads to the parotid space (see Fig. 180.9), but most patients have no localizing signs.

Many symptoms and signs in LPS infections are caused by the involvement of the neurovascular structures. Suppurative jugular venous thrombosis, or Lemierre's syndrome, is the most common complication. Bacteremia and septic emboli, the most frequent consequences of this entity, occur in one half of the cases [105–107]. Suppurative subclavian thrombosis, lateral sinus thrombosis, cavernous sinus thrombosis, and metastatic infections have also been reported [104,105,107].

Signs suggestive of carotid sheath involvement include persistent tonsillar swelling after resolution of a peritonsillar abscess, ipsilateral Horner's syndrome, and cranial nerve IX to XII palsies [104]. Carotid artery aneurysm or rupture can present as a pulsatile mass, resulting in sentinel bleeding from the ear or pharynx after a protracted course of illness of 7 to 14 days, as hematoma of the neck or hemodynamic collapse [94] It can be result of direct inoculation of infection after intravenous drug use [94]. CT scan has been used to define neck masses, particularly in the LPS, with excellent results (Fig. 180.10) [108]. Because the complications of deep neck abscesses are potentially fatal, CT scan of the neck is indicated for all cases, especially when surgical intervention is contemplated. The scan can be extended inferiorly to include the chest and mediastinum. Ultrasound

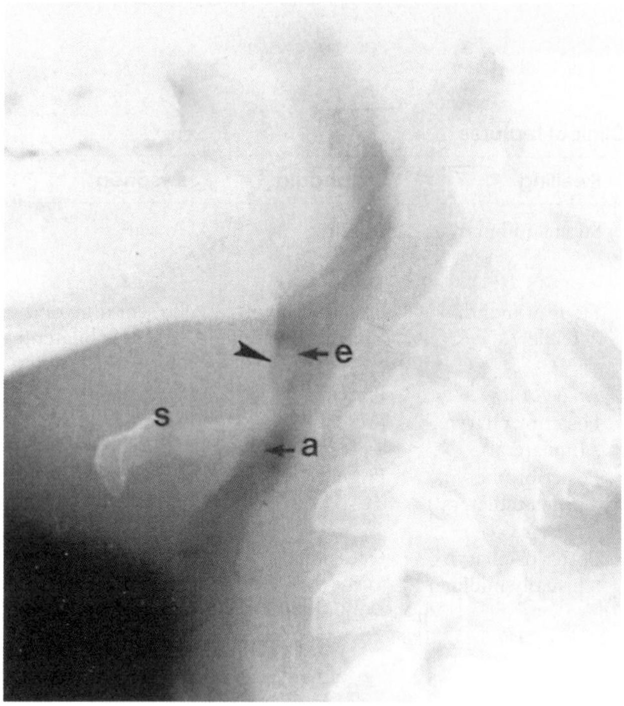

FIGURE 180.8 Ludwig's angina. Lateral radiographs of the neck obtained with soft tissue technique in a 7-year-old child. There is soft tissue swelling of the submandibular space (*s*), producing a smooth impression on the airway anteriorly, compressing and practically ablating the vallecula (*arrowhead*): the epiglottis (*e*) and aryepiglottic folds (*a*) are normal.

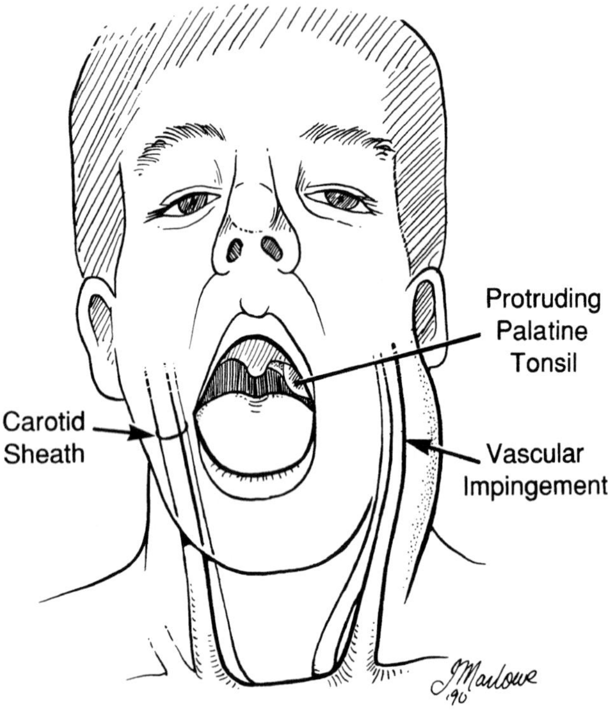

FIGURE 180.9 Schematic representation of salient clinical findings of lateral pharyngeal space abscess.

may quickly and accurately identify thrombus and perivenous changes due to suppurative adenitis [99], although pain from the probe can limit accuracy. CT findings include inflammatory changes in the perivascular space, enhancement of venous walls and the presence of thrombus within the lumen [99].

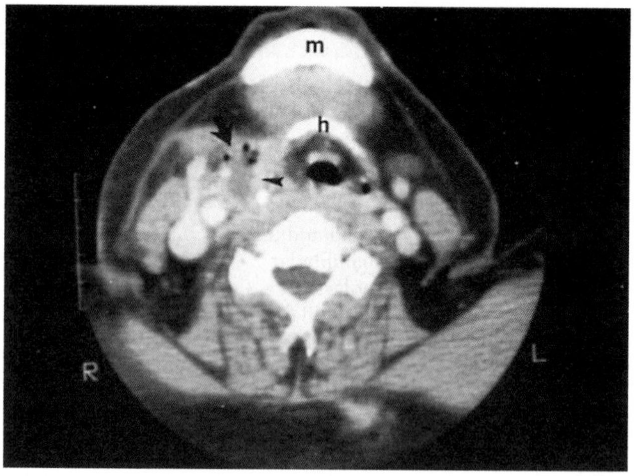

FIGURE 180.10 Abscess in the lateral pharyngeal space. Computed tomography at the level of the hyoid bone (*h*), at the apex of the inverted lateral pharyngeal space cone. There is a cystic mass (*arrow*) with floating air bubbles and enhancing rim (*arrowhead*), findings virtually pathognomonic of abscess caused by gas-forming organisms. *m*, base of mandible.

Retropharyngeal Space Infections

RPS abscesses are uncommon but potentially fatal infections, most often seen in children younger than 6 years old because the lymph nodes regress with age [94,109]. The two chains of lymph nodes in this space drain adjacent muscles, nose, nasopharynx, pharynx, middle ear, eustachian tubes, and paranasal sinuses and are the source of most RPS abscesses. Among children, it is typically secondary to acute pharyngitis, whereas for adults, it can occur from penetrating injury from fish bone ingestion, nasogastric tube placement or intubation [99]. Among children, the initial symptoms include fever, irritability, and refusal to eat [94]. The neck is often stiff and sometimes tilted away from the involved side [109]. Dyspnea and dysphagia occur as the swelling increases. Adults can present with neck pain, fever, dyspnea, snoring, and nasal obstruction [94]. Respiratory distress can occur as the abscess protrudes anteriorly (see Fig. 180.4).

Among children, spontaneous rupture of a retropharyngeal abscess may result in aspiration and asphyxiation or upper airway obstruction from a combination of a child's high larynx and anterior displacement of the pharyngeal wall [94]. Severe respiratory distress, particularly if accompanied by chest pain or pleurisy, suggests mediastinal extension.

The lateral neck radiograph can aid in making the diagnosis by its ability to detect prevertebral soft tissue swelling (Fig. 180.11) The radiograph should be a true lateral view, with the neck in full extension, and should be made during inspiration. Exhalation, crying, and swallowing, especially in children, may cause thickening of the upper cervical soft tissues. Normal dimensions have been defined as less than 7 mm in all age groups at the C2 (retropharyngeal) level and less than 14 mm in children or 22 mm in adults at the C6 (retrotracheal) level [110]. Loss or reversal of the normal cervical lordosis secondary to inflammation-induced muscle spasm also suggests an RPS infection. CT scans can be valuable as well for the diagnosis of retropharyngeal abscess. It is of paramount importance to extend the CT to include the upper mediastinum. Large paramedian nodes will be seen with central low density and an enhancing ring, whereas in cellulitis, there is symmetric low attenuation of the RPS [99].

The most feared complications are airway obstruction and rupture of abscess. Hence, patients with impending airway obstruction should be examined in the operating room, intubated in Trendelenberg's position along the opposite side of the pharyngeal swelling. Needle aspiration should precede intra-oral incision and drainage [94].

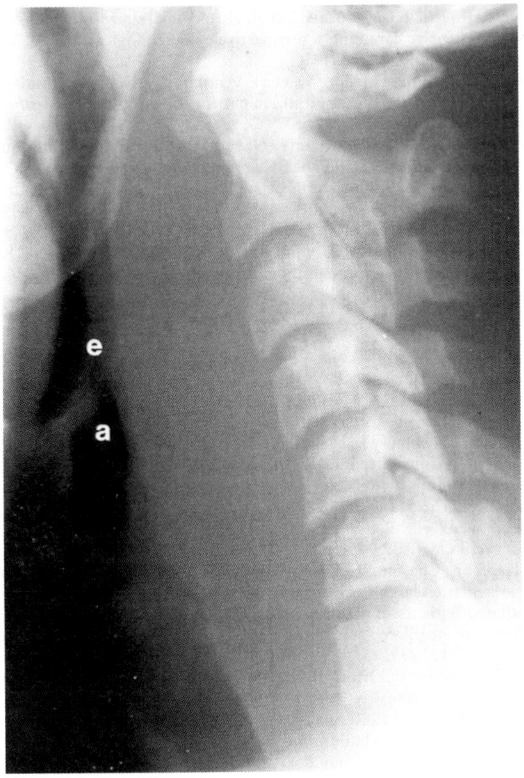

FIGURE 180.11 Retropharyngeal abscess. Lateral neck radiograph. There is marked swelling of the prevertebral soft tissues extending from the base of the skull to the base of the neck, with bulging and anterior displacement of the airway. There is mild reversal of the normal lordosis of the neck secondary to muscle spasm. The epiglottis (*e*) and aryepiglottic folds (*a*) are normal.

Descending Infections

Any deep neck infection can have access to the posterior mediastinum and diaphragm by the common pathways of the RPS and danger space [111,112]. Descending necrotizing mediastinitis can carry a mortality of greater than 36% [112]. The process can develop within 12 hours to as long as 2 weeks from the onset of the primary infection. The diagnosis may be difficult to make early in the course of the illness. Severe dyspnea and pleuritic or retrosternal chest pain concomitant with or subsequent to the onset of symptoms of an oropharyngeal infection suggest this process. The infection may progress, producing a widespread necrotizing process extending to the diaphragms and occasionally into the retroperitoneal space; a mediastinal abscess that may rupture into the pleural cavity; or purulent pleural and pericardial effusions [112]. Suggestive physical findings include diffuse, bulky induration of the neck and upper chest associated with pitting edema or crepitation [94].

Cervical necrotizing fasciitis, a fascial infection with muscle necrosis, often without pus or abscess formation, can progress superficially along the fascial planes of the neck and chest wall [113]. Early in the course of this disease, the physical appearance may be deceptively benign. Skin erythema occurs initially and progresses to dusky skin discoloration, blisters, or bullae and eventually to visible skin necrosis [114]. Crepitation may be absent, but gas in the tissues can readily be seen using CT. Surgical exploration with wide excision is essential to determine the full extent of necrosis and to improve prognosis [113].

Infections of the prevertebral space comprises of spinal epidural collection that can result in spinal cord compression and irreversible paralysis in 4% to 22% of patients [104]. Psoas muscle collections may also be seen because of the open communication with the PVS [104].

Differential Diagnosis

Few clinical entities must be distinguished from deep cervical infections. Common causes of submandibular swelling include cervical adenitis and submandibular sialoadenitis. In the proper settings, the differential diagnosis includes anticoagulant overdose with sublingual hematoma, tumor of the floor of the mouth, superior vena cava syndrome, and angioedema. None of these presents with the classical physical findings or respiratory symptoms of SMS infection due to Ludwig's angina.

The major entities from which LPS infection must be differentiated are peritonsillar abscess, anaerobic tonsillitis, and masticator space infections. Peritonsillar abscess becomes evident with fever and tonsillar prolapse but without extreme toxicity, trismus, or parotid swelling [115]. Vincent's angina is an anaerobic tonsillitis caused by *Fusobacterium necrophorum*, which produces a foul smelling discharge that forms a pseudomembrane and can be associated with bacteremia and metastatic abscesses [106].

Acute suppurative parotitis can occur as a complication of pharmacologic therapy (e.g., diuretics and anticholinergics) [115]. Reduced salivary flow allows normal oral flora to spread to Stensen's duct and into the gland. The most common pathogen is *S. aureus*, but infection is also seen with hemolytic streptococcus, gram-negative bacilli, and anaerobes]. The mainstays of therapy are hydration, sialagogues, and often a broad-spectrum antibiotic with anti–β-lactamase activity. Despite appropriate treatment, complications may include spread to the mastoid, entrapment of the facial nerve, severe swelling of the pharynx and neck resulting in airway obstruction, and problems typical of involvement of the LPS. Mortality may approach 25% [115].

Retropharyngeal swelling can be seen secondary to tumors such as leiomyoma, hemangioma, ectopic parathyroid adenoma, or hyperplasia. It can also be as a result of prevertebral tendinitis, tortuous carotid artery, lymphatic malformations, congenital lesions such as branchial cleft cyst and fluid accumulation after radiation therapy for head and neck tumors [116]. For children presenting with fever, sore throat, nuchal rigidity, drooling, or respiratory distress, RPS abscess, severe croup, epiglottitis, and meningitis must also be considered.

Treatment

All patients with deep neck infections require hospitalization. Therapy has three components: airway management, IV antibiotics, and timely surgical exploration.

Airway Management

Establishment of an artificial airway is not universally required, but it should be done when evidence of airway obstruction exists, such as dyspnea and stridor or inability to handle secretions. The method of airway protection in patients with deep cervical infections must be individualized for the patient and to the expertise of the available personnel [117]. Upper airway obstruction is most often a complication of infections involving the SMS, for which one approach to control the airway has been tracheostomy [118,119]. Because the surgical risks of tracheotomy may be increased by the distortion of the neck with edema, cricothyroidotomy has been recommended as an alternative, particularly in emergent situations [120], given that it can be performed rapidly, and has low complication rates. Distortion of neck landmarks may equally complicate this procedure, but fewer critical structures are in proximity, which may reduce some procedure-related risks.

Endotracheal intubation can be difficult to achieve because of trismus and intraoral swelling. Trismus may be a more significant problem when infection has spread to the LPS. Blind intubation is unsafe because of the risk of trauma to the posterior pharyngeal wall, rupture of abscesses in the LPS or RPS, and possibly laryngospasm precipitating lower airway obstruction [118,119]. Intubation utilizing a flexible laryngoscope may be useful but requires a cooperative, stable patient and may therefore be useful only for selected cases [117]. Inhaled anesthesia to relieve trismus, along with an antisialagogue, may allow for intubation under direct vision [118,119]. If this is attempted, skilled personnel should be available to establish an emergent surgical airway if needed.

Antimicrobial Therapy

Antibiotic therapy should be given intravenously for all neck infections. Optimum empiric coverage is recommended with either penicillin in combination with a β-lactamase inhibitor (such as amoxicillin; ticarcillin with clavulanic acid; or piperacillin/tazobactam) or a β-lactamase–resistant antibiotic (such as cefoxitin, cefuroxime, imipenem, or meropenem) in combination with a drug that is highly effective against most anaerobes (such as clindamycin or metronidazole) [90,94]. Vancomycin should be considered for patients with immune dysfunction, neutropenia, and in IV drug abusers at risk for infection with MRSA [94]. If needed, other agents including linezolid, daptomycin, and quinupristin/dalfopristin can be substituted in place of vancomycin. The addition of gentamicin for effective Gram-negative coverage against *K. pneumoniae*, which is resistant to clindamycin, is highly recommended for diabetic patients with intact renal function [94]; Parenteral antibiotic therapy should be continued until the patient has been afebrile for at least 48 hours, followed by oral therapy using amoxicillin with clavulanic acid, clindamycin, ciprofloxacin, trimethoprim–sulfamethoxazole, or metronidazole [94]. The antibiotic regimen can be de-escalated based on culture data.

Resection of a thrombosed vein is not widely recommended but may be unavoidable in a patient who deteriorates despite drainage of the LPS, or in one whose vein is frankly suppurative [104].

Surgery

Conservative therapy using antibiotics and selective needle aspirations can be successful [93,94,121]. In general, if signs of clinical improvement are not observed after treatment with IV antibiotics for 24 to 48 hours, then reimaging and surgical intervention are likely warranted. Surgical drainage is the cornerstone of treatment for anterior LPS, RPS, and PVS infections [104]. For SMS infections, an initial trial of antibiotics can be considered. Selected patients, such as those with cellulitis, abscess size less than 3 cm, and without involvement of more than one danger space and general stability may not require surgical intervention [93]. Once surgical intervention is indicated, dental extraction is included as well [93,104]. Recommendations for surgical treatments are individualized and can include cervical drainage; thoracotomy with radical surgical debridement of the mediastinum; and excision of necrotic tissue, decortication, and irrigation [122]. A less invasive thoracoscopic approach has also been described [123].

References

1. Meduri GU, Mauldin GL, Wunderink RG, et al: Causes of fever and pulmonary densities in patients with clinical manifestations of ventilator-associated pneumonia. *Chest* 106:221–235, 1994.
2. Marik PE: Fever in the ICU. *Chest* 117:855–869, 2000.
3. van Zanten ARH, Dixon JM, Nipshagen MD, et al: Hospital-acquired sinusitis is a common cause of fever of unknown origin in orotracheally intubated critically ill patients. *Crit Care* 9:R583–R590, 2005.
4. Westergren V, Lunblad L, Hellquist HB: Ventilator-associated sinusitis: a review. *Clin Infect Dis* 27:851–864, 1998.
5. Agrafiotis M, Vardakas KZ, Gkegkes ID, et al: Ventilator-associated sinusitis in adults: systematic review and meta-analysis. *Respir Med* 106(8):1082–1095, 2012.
6. Rouby JJ, Laurent P, Gosnach M, et al: Risk factors and clinical relevance of nosocomial maxillary sinusitis in the critically ill. *Am J Respir Crit Care Med* 150:776–783, 1994.
7. Rohr AS, Spector SL: Paranasal sinus anatomy and pathophysiology. *Clin Rev Allergy* 2:387–395, 1984.
8. George DL, Falk PS, Meduri UG, et al: Nosocomial sinusitis in patients in the medical intensive care unit: a prospective epidemiological study. *Clin Infect Dis* 27:463–470, 1998.
9. Souweine B, Mom T, Traore O, et al: Ventilator-associated sinusitis: microbiological results of sinus aspirates in patients on antibiotics. *Anesthesiology* 93:1255–1260, 2000.
10. Monroe MM, McLean M, Sautter N, et al: Invasive fungal rhinosinusitis: a 15-year experience with 29 patients. *Laryngoscope* 123(7):1583–1587, 2013.
11. Valera FC, do Lago T, Tamashiro E, et al: Prognosis of acute invasive fungal rhinosinusitis related to underlying disease. *Int J Infect Dis* 15(12):e841–e844, 2011.
12. Choi SS, Lawson W, Bottone EJ, et al: Cryptococcal sinusitis: a case report and review of the literature. *Otolaryngol Head Neck Surg* 99:414–418, 1988.
13. Dooley DP, McAllister CK: Candidal sinusitis and diabetic ketoacidosis: a brief report. *Arch Intern Med* 149:962–964, 1989.
14. Marks SC, Upadhyay S, Crane L: Cytomegalovirus sinusitis: a new manifestation of AIDS. *Arch Otolaryngol Head Neck Surg* 122:789–791, 1996.
15. Shahin J, Gullane PJ, Dayal VS: Orbital complications of acute sinusitis. *J Otolaryngol* 16:23–27, 1987.
16. Gallagher RM, Gross CW, Phillips CD: Suppurative intracranial complications of sinusitis. *Laryngoscope* 108:1635–1642, 1998.
17. Dolan RW, Chowdhury K: Diagnosis and treatment of intracranial complications of paranasal sinus infections. *J Oral Maxillofac Surg* 53:1080–1087, 1995.
18. Parker GS, Tami TA, Wilson JF, et al: Intracranial complications of sinusitis. *South Med J* 82:563–569, 1989.
19. Singh B, Van Dellen J, Ramjettan S, et al: Sinogenic intracranial complications. *J Laryngol Otol* 109:945–950, 1995.
20. Holzapfel L, Chastang C, Demigeon G, et al: A randomized study assessing the systematic search for maxillary sinusitis in nasotracheally mechanically ventilated patients. Influence of nosocomial maxillary sinusitis on the occurrence of ventilator-associated pneumonia. *Am J Respir Crit Care Med* 159:695–701, 1999.
21. Witte RJ, Heurter JV, Orton DF, et al: Limited axial CT of the paranasal sinuses in screening for sinusitis. *Am J Radiol* 167:1313–1315, 1996.
22. Aebert H, Hunefeld G, Regel G: Paranasal sinusitis and sepsis in ICU patients with nasotracheal intubation. *Intensive Care Med* 15:27–30, 1988.
23. Hilbert G, Vargas F, Valentino R, et al: Comparison of B-mode ultrasound and computed tomography in the diagnosis of maxillary sinusitis in mechanically ventilated patients. *Crit Care Med* 29:1337–1342, 2001.
24. Vargas F, Bui HN, Boyer A: Transnasal puncture based on echographic sinusitis evidence in mechanically ventilated patients with suspicion of nosocomial maxillary sinusitis. *Intensive Care Med* 32:858–866, 2006.
25. Lichtenstein D, Biderman P, Meziere G, et al: The "sinusogram", a real-time ultrasound sign of maxillary sinusitis. *Intensive Care Med* 24:1057–1061, 1998.
26. Elwany S, Helmy SA, El-Reweny EM, et al: Endoscopically directed middle meatal cultures vs computed tomographic scans in the diagnosis of bacterial sinusitis in intensive care units. *J Crit Care*. 2012;27(3):315.e1–315.e5.
27. Bert F, Lambert-Zechovsky N: Sinusitis in mechanically ventilated patients and its role in the pathogenesis of nosocomial pneumonia. *Eur J Clin Microb Infect Dis* 15:533–544, 1996.
28. Salord F, Gaussorgues P, Marti-Flich J, et al: Nosocomial maxillary sinusitis during mechanical ventilation: a prospective comparison of orotracheal versus the nasotracheal route for intubation. *Intensive Care Med* 16:390–393, 1990.
29. Stein M, Caplan ES: Nosocomial sinusitis: a unique subset of sinusitis. *Curr Opin Infect Dis* 18:147–150, 2005.
30. Bert F, Lambert-Zechhovsky N: Microbiology of nosocomial sinusitis in intensive care unit patients. *J Infect* 31:5–8, 1995.
31. Deutschman CS, Wilton P, Sinow J, et al: Paranasal sinusitis associated with nasotracheal intubation: a frequently unrecognized and treatable source of sepsis. *Crit Care Med* 14:111–114, 1986.
32. Grillone GA, Kasznica P: Isolated sphenoid sinus disease. *Otolaryngol Clin North Am* 37:435–451, 2004.
33. Wang ZM, Kanoh N, Dai CF, et al: Isolated sphenoid sinus disease: an analysis of 122 cases. *Ann Otol Rhinol Laryngol* 111:323–327, 2002.
34. Leskinen K, Jero J: Acute complications of otitis media in adults. *Clin Otolaryngol* 30:511–516, 2005.
35. Agrawal S, Husein M, MacRae D: Complications of otitis media: an evolving state. *J Otolaryngol* 34[Suppl 1]:S33–S39, 2005.
36. Bunik M. Mastoiditis. *Pediatr Rev*. 2014;35(2):94–95; discussion 94–95.
37. Anthonsen K, Hostmark K, Hansen S, et al: Acute mastoiditis in children: a 10-year retrospective and validated multicenter study. *Pediatr Infect Dis J* 32(5):436–440, 2013.
38. Minks DP, Porte M, Jenkins N. Acute mastoiditis—the role of radiology. *Clin Radiol* 68(4):397–405, 2013.
39. Nadol JB Jr, Eavey RD: Acute and chronic mastoiditis: clinical presentation, diagnosis, and management. *Curr Clin Top Infect Dis* 15:204–229, 1995.
40. Carfrae MJ, Kesser BW: Malignant otitis externa. *Otolaryngol Clin North Am* 41(3):537–549, viii–ix, 2008.
41. Franco-Vidal V, Blanchet H, Bebear C, et al: Necrotizing external otitis: a report of 46 cases. *Otol Neurotol* 2007;28(6):771–773.
42. Rubin Grandis J, Branstetter BF, Yu VL: The changing face of malignant (necrotising) external otitis: clinical, radiological, and anatomic correlations. *Lancet Infect Dis* 4:34–39, 2004.
43. Ress BD, Luntz M, Telischi FF, et al: Necrotizing external otitis in patients with AIDS. *Laryngoscope* 107:456–460, 1997.
44. Gordon G, Giddings NA: Invasive otitis externa due to *Aspergillus* species: case report and review. *Clin Infect Dis* 19:866–870, 1994.

45. Harley WB, Dummer JS, Anderson TL, et al: Malignant external otitis due to *Aspergillus flavus* with fulminant dissemination to the lungs. *Clin Infect Dis* 20:1052–1054, 1995.
46. Murray ME, Britton J: Osteomyelitis of the skull base: the role of high resolution CT in diagnosis. *Clin Radiol* 49:408–411, 1994.
47. Boringa JB, Hoekstra OS, Roos JW, et al: Multiple cranial nerve palsy after otitis externa: a case report. *Clin Neurol Neurosurg* 97:332–335, 1995.
48. Amorosa L, Modugno GC, Pirodda A: Malignant external otitis: review and personal experience. *Acta Ololaryngol Suppl (Stockh)* 521:3–16, 1996.
49. Guldfred LA, Lyhne D, Becker BC: Acute epiglottitis: epidemiology, clinical presentation, management and outcome: *J Laryngol Otol* 122, 818–823, 2008.
50. Nakamura H, Tanaka H, Matsuda A, et al: Acute epiglottitis: a review of 80 patients. *J Laryngol Otol* 115:31–34, 2001.
51. Glynn F, Fenton JE: Diagnosis and management of supraglottitis (epiglottitis). *Curr Infect Dis Rep* 10:200–204, 2008.
52. Ames WA, Ward VM, Tranter RM, et al: Adult epiglottitis: an under-recognized, life-threatening condition. *Br J Anaesth* 85:795–797, 2000.
53. Anderson B: Airway management in Ludwig's anginaShah RK, Roberson DW, Jones DT: Epiglottitis in the *Haemophilus influenzae* type B vaccine era: changing trends; Laryngoscope 114:557–560, 2004.
54. Trollfors B, Nylen O, Carenfelt C, et al: Aetiology of acute epiglottis in adults. *Scand J Infect Dis* 30:49–51, 1998.
55. Mayo-Smith MF, Spinale JW, Donskey CJ, et al: Acute epiglottitis: an 18-year experience in Rhode Island. *Chest* 108:1640–1647, 1995.
56. Kornak JM, Freije JE, Campbell BH: Caustic and thermal epiglottitis in the adult. *Otolaryngol Head Neck Surg* 114:310–312, 1996.
57. McKinney B, Grigg R: Epiglottitis after anaesthesia with a laryngeal mask. *Anaesth Intensive Care* 23:618–619, 1995.
58. Frantz TD, Rasgon BM, Quesenberry CP Jr: Acute epiglottitis in adults: analysis of 129 cases. *JAMA* 272:1358–1360, 1994.
59. Park KW, Darvish A, Lowenstein E: Airway management for adult patients with acute epiglottitis: a 12-year experience at an academic medical center (1984–1995). *Anesthesiology* 88:254–261, 1998
60. Edmonds LC, Prakash UB: Lymphoma, neutropenia, and wheezing in a 70-year-old man. *Chest* 103:585–587, 1993.
61. Mustoe T, Strome M: Adult epiglottitis. *Am J Otolaryngol* 4:393–399, 1983.
62. Deeb ZE, Yenson YC, DeFries HO: Acute epiglottitis in the adult. *Laryngoscope* 95:289–291, 1985.
63. MayoSmith MF, Hirsch PJ, Wodzinski SF, et al: Acute epiglottitis in adults: an eight-year experience in the state of Rhode Island. *N Engl J Med* 314:1133–1139, 1986.
64. Schamp S, Pokiesser P, Danzer M, et al: Radiologic findings in acute epiglottitis. *Eur Radiol* 9:1629–1631, 1999.
65. Schroeder LL, Knapp JF: Recognition and emergency management of infectious causes of upper airway obstruction in children. *Semin Respir Infect* 10:21–30, 1995.
66. Stroud RH, Friedman NR: An update on inflammatory disorders of the pediatric airway: epiglottitis, croup, and tracheitis. *Am J Otolaryngol* 22:268–275, 2001.
67. Valor RR, Polnitsky CA, Tanis DJ, et al: Bacterial tracheitis with upper airway obstruction in a patient with the acquired immunodeficiency syndrome. *Am Rev Respir Dis* 146:1598–1599, 1992.
68. Nemzek WR, Katzenberg RW, Van Slyke MA, et al: A reappraisal of the radiologic findings of acute inflammation of the epiglottis and supraglottic structures in adults. *Am J Neuroradiol* 16:495–502, 1995.
69. Seigler RS: Bacterial tracheitis: an unusual radiographic presentation. *Clin Pediatr (Phila)* 33:374–377, 1994.
70. Donnelly BW, McMillan JA, Weiner LB: Bacterial tracheitis: report of eight new cases and review. *Rev Infect Dis* 12:729–735, 1990.
71. Yigla M, Ben-Izhak O, Oren I, et al: Laryngotracheobronchial involvement in a patient with nonendemic rhinoscleroma. *Chest* 117:1795–1798, 2000.
72. Amoils CP, Shindo ML: Laryngotracheal manifestations of rhinoscleroma. *Ann Otol Rhinol Laryngol* 105:336–340, 1996.
73. Chechani V, Vasudevan VP, Kamholz SL: Necrotizing tracheobronchitis: complication of mechanical ventilation in an adult. *South Med J* 84:271–273, 1991.
74. Bismuth C, Garnier R, Baud FJ, et al: Paraquat poisoning. An overview of the current status. *Drug Saf* 5:243–251, 1990.
75. Madhotra D, Fenton JE, Makura ZG, et al: Airway intervention in adult supraglottitis. *Ir J Med Sci* 173(4):197–199, 2004.
76. Deeb ZE: Acute supraglottitis in adults: early indicators of airway obstruction. *Am J Otolaryngol* 18:112–115, 1997.
77. Cantrell RW, Bell RA, Morioka WT: Acute epiglottitis: intubation versus tracheostomy. *Laryngoscope* 88:994–1005, 1978.
78. Oh TH, Motoyama EK: Comparison of nasotracheal intubation and tracheostomy in management of acute epiglottitis. *Anesthesiology* 46:214–216, 1977.
79. Wood DE: Tracheostomy. *Chest Surg Clin North Am* 6:749–764, 1996.
80. Butt W, Shann F, Walker C, et al: Acute epiglottitis: a different approach to management. *Crit Care Med* 16:43–47, 1988.
81. Sheikh KH, Mostow SR: Epiglottitis—an increasing problem for adults. *West J Med* 151:520–524, 1989.
82. Cummings CW: Supraglottitis (Epiglottitis), in Cummings CW, Haughey BH, Regan Thomas J (eds): *Cummings Otolaryngology: Head & Neck Surgery*. 4th ed. St. Louis, Mosby Elsevier, 2005.
83. Tibballs J, Shann FA, Landau LI: Placebo-controlled trial of prednisolone in children intubated for croup: *Lancet* 340(8822):745–748, 1992.
84. Crockett DM, McGill TJ, Healy GB, et al: Airway management of acute supraglottitis at the Children's Hospital, Boston: 1980–1985. *Ann Otol Rhinol Laryngol* 97:114–119, 1988.
85. Bonadio WA, Losek JD: The characteristics of children with epiglottitis who develop the complication of pulmonary edema. *Arch Otolaryngol Head Neck Surg* 117:205–207, 1991.
86. Berger G, Landau T, Berger S, et al: The rising incidence of adult acute epiglottitis and epiglottic abscess. *Am J Otolaryngol* 24:374–383, 2003.
87. Smith MM, Mukherji SK, Thompson JE, et al: CT in adult supraglottitis. *Am J Neuroradiol* 17:1355–1358, 1996.
88. Hasegawa J, Hidaka H, Tateda M et al. An analysis of clinical risk factors of deep neck infection. *Auris Nasus Larynx*. 2011;38(1):101-107.
89. Hedge A, Mohan S, Lim WE. Infections of the deep neck spaces. *Singapore Med J* 53(5):305–311; quiz 312, 2012.
90. Boscolo-Rizzo P, Stellin M, Muzzi E, et al: Deep neck infections: a study of 365 cases highlighting recommendations for management and treatment. *Eur Arch Otorhinolaryngol* 269(4):1241–1249, 2012.
91. Eftekharian A, Roozbahany NA, Vaezeafshar R, et al: Deep neck infections: a retrospective review of 112 cases. *Eur Arch Otorhinolaryngol* 266:273–277, 2009.
92. May JG, Shah P, Sachdeva L et al: Potential role of biofilms in deep cervical abscess. *Int J Pediatr Otorhinolaryngol* 78(1):10–13, 2014.
93. Boscolo-Rizzo P, Marchiori C, Montolli F, et al: Deep neck infections: a constant challenge. *J Otorhinolaryngol Relat Spec* 68(5):259–265, 2006.
94. Vieira F, Allen SM, Stocks RMS, et al: Deep neck infection. *Otolaryngol Clin North Am* 41:459–483, 2008.
95. Chi TH, Tsao YH, Yuan CH: Influences of patient age on deep neck infection: clinical etiology and treatment outcome. *Otolaryngol Head Neck Surg* 151(4):586–590, 2014.
96. Baldassari CM, Howell R, Amorn M, et al: Complications in pediatric deep neck space abscesses. *Otolaryngol Head Neck Surg* 144(4):592–595, 2011.
97. Lin RH, Huang CC, Tsou YA et al. Correlation between imaging characteristics and microbiology in patients with deep neck infections: a retrospective review of one hundred sixty-one cases. *Surg Infect (Larchmt)* 15(6):794–799, 2014.
98. Tovi F, Fliss DM, Zirkin HJ: Necrotizing soft-tissue infections in the head and neck: a clinicopathological study. *Laryngoscope* 101:619–625, 1991.
99. Maroldi R, Farina D, Ravanelli M, et al: Emergency imaging assessment of deep neck space infections. *Semin Ultrasound CT MR* 33(5):432–442, 2012.
100. Chuang SY, Lin HT, Wen YS, et al: Pitfalls of CT for deep neck abscess imaging assessment: a retrospective review of 162 cases. *B-ENT* 9(1):45–52, 2013.
101. Chou YK, Lee CY, Chao HH, et al: An upper airway obstruction emergency: Ludwig angina. *Pediatr Emerg Care* 23(12):892–896, 2007.
102. Britt JC, Josephson GD, Gross CW: Ludwig's angina in the pediatric population: report of a case and review of the literature. *Int J Pediatr Otorhinolaryngol* 52:79–87, 2000.
103. Hodgdon A: Dental and related infections. *Emerg Med Clin North Am* 31(2):465–480, 2013.
104. Reynolds SC, Chow AW: Life-threatening infections of the peripharyngeal and deep fascial spaces of the head and neck. *Infect Dis Clin North Am* 21(2):557–576, 2007.
105. Chirinos JA, Lichtstein DM, Garcia J, et al: The evolution of Lemierre syndrome: report of 2 cases and review of the literature. *Medicine* 81:458–465, 2002.
106. Brook I: Current management of upper respiratory tract and head and neck infections. *Eur Arch Otorhinolaryngol* 266(3):315–323, 2009.
107. Bentham JR, Pollard AJ, Milford CA, et al: Cerebral infarct and meningitis secondary to Lemierre's syndrome. *Pediatr Neurol* 30:281–283, 2004.
108. Wang LF, Kuo WR, Tsai SM, et al: Characterizations of life-threatening deep cervical space infections: a review of one hundred ninety-six cases. *Am J Otolaryngol* 24:111–117, 2003.
109. Lalakea M, Messner AH: Retropharyngeal abscess management in children: current practices. *Otolaryngol Head Neck Surg* 121:398–405, 1999.
110. Furst I, Ellis D, Winton T. Unusual complication of endotracheal intubation: retropharyngeal space abscess, mediastinitis, and empyema. *J Otolaryngol*. 2000;29(5):309–311.
111. Sancho LM, Minamoto H, Fernandez A, et al: Descending necrotizing mediastinitis: a retrospective surgical experience. *Eur J Cardiothorac Surg* 16:200–205, 1999.
112. Kiernan PD, Hernandez A, Byrne WD, et al: Descending cervical mediastinitis. *Ann Thorac Surg* 65:1483–1488, 1998.
113. Mohammedi I, Ceruse P, Duperret S, et al: Cervical necrotizing fasciitis: 10 years' experience at a single institution. *Intensive Care Med* 25:829–834, 1999.
114. Stoykewych AA, Beecroft WA, Cogan AG: Fatal necrotizing fasciitis of dental origin. *J Can Dent Assoc* 58:59–62, 1992.
115. Herzon FS, Nicklaus P: Pediatric peritonsillar abscess: management guidelines. *Curr Probl Pediatr* 26:270–278, 1996.
116. Debnam JM, Guha-Thakurta N: Retropharyngeal and prevertebral spaces: anatomic imaging and diagnosis. *Otolaryngol Clin North Am* 45(6):1293–1310, 2012.
117. Ovassapian A, Tuncbilek M, Weitzel EK, et al: Airway management in adult patients with deep neck infections: a case series and review of the literature. *Anesth Analg* 100:585–589, 2005.
118. Neff SP, Merry AF, Anderson B: Airway management in Ludwig's angina. *Anaesth Int Care* 27:659–661, 1999.
119. Marple BF: Ludwig angina: a review of current airway management. *Arch Otolaryngol Head Neck Surg* 125:596–599, 1999.
120. Isaacs JH Jr, Pedersen AD: Emergency cricothyroidotomy. *Am Surg* 63:346–349, 1997.
121. Plaza Mayor G, Martinez-San Millan J, Martinez-Vidal A: Is conservative treatment of deep neck space infections appropriate? *Head Neck* 23:126–133, 2001.
122. Iwata T, Sekine Y, Shibuya K, et al: Early open thoracotomy and mediastinopleural irrigation for severe descending necrotizing mediastinitis. *Eur J Cardiothorac Surg* 28:384–388, 2005.
123. Isowa N, Yamada T, Kijima T, et al: Successful thoracoscopic debridement of descending necrotizing mediastinitis. *Ann Thorac Surg* 77:1834–1837, 2004.

Chapter 181 ■ Acute Infectious Pneumonia

GIRISH B. NAIR • MICHAEL S. NIEDERMAN

Pneumonia is a common community- and hospital-acquired infection that is managed in the intensive care unit (ICU) when it leads to acute respiratory failure or septic shock, or when it complicates the course of an otherwise serious illness. Modern medical technology has not been able to eliminate this infection. Rather, it has promoted its emergence by the application of novel, life-sustaining therapies in specific at-risk populations who have impairments in respiratory tract host defenses. This chapter reviews the scope of the problem among seriously ill patients.

Sir William Osler described pneumonia as "the captain of the men of death." The Centers for Disease Control and Prevention (CDC) surveillance data from 2010 reported 1.1 million pneumonia-related discharges with an average of 5.2 days of hospital stay [1]. There is a significant economic impact associated with pneumonia and the greatest burden of care, which is linked with inpatient management. One recent study estimated the direct and indirect costs of caring for pneumococcal pneumonia per year in patients over 50 years of age to be $3.7 billion and $1.8 billion, respectively [2]. Since the discovery of penicillin in 1928, antibiotics have remained the mainstay of disease management, but the indiscriminate use of broad-spectrum antibiotics has resulted in the emergence of drug-resistant pathogens, even among common organisms such as *Streptococcus pneumoniae*. The U.S. Government has recently announced the "National Action Plan for combating Antibiotic-resistant Bacteria" in 2015 [3].

Community-acquired pneumonia (CAP) refers to pneumonia developing in the outpatient setting or within 48 hours after hospitalization, whereas nosocomial pneumonia (NP) by definition occurs at least 48 hours after admission [4,5]. NP, or hospital-acquired pneumonia (HAP), includes ventilator-associated pneumonia (VAP) which develops at least 48 hours after endotracheal intubation. Health care–associated pneumonia (HCAP) is pneumonia developing in patients with previous exposure to the health care environment, such as nursing homes, dialysis centers, or previous hospitalization for more than 2 days in the preceding 3-month period. These individuals can become infected with hospital-associated drug-resistant pathogens and the latest treatment guidelines recommended initial, empirical, broad-spectrum antibiotics targeting resistant pathogens [4]. However, it is now clear that this population represent a heterogeneous group, and that some patients can be treated with antimicrobials targeted at community acquired pathogens, so the classification of HCAP is in flux [6].

The incidence of pneumonia among hospitalized patients is directly related to the degree of underlying systemic illness, being more common in medical than in surgical patients, and in those requiring prolonged mechanical ventilation [4]. Certain patient populations are at increased risk for pneumonia, primarily as a result of disease-associated impairments in lung host defenses. These include the elderly and those with cardiac disease, alcoholism, chronic obstructive pulmonary disease (COPD), congestive heart failure (CHF), malnutrition, head injury, cystic fibrosis, bronchiectasis, malignancy, splenic dysfunction, renal failure, liver failure, diabetes mellitus, and other immunosuppressive illnesses or therapies [4,6]. In addition, hospitalized patients often receive therapeutic interventions that predispose them to pneumonia, including antibiotic therapy, enteral feeding, endotracheal intubation, tracheostomy, and the use of certain medications (such as corticosteroids, aspirin, digitalis, morphine, and pentobarbital) [6].

The mortality implications of pneumonia (along with influenza) rank it as the eighth leading cause of death in the United States, the sixth leading cause of death in those older than 65 years, and the number one cause of death from infectious diseases [5]. Although CAP can vary from a mild to a severe illness, those who enter the ICU with this infection have a mortality rate that can vary from 20% to greater than 50% [7]. The indications for ICU admission and the definitions for severe CAP are changing, and with good reason, since the later in the hospital course that the ICU is used, the higher the mortality [8]. Among patients with severe CAP, delayed admission to the ICU or delayed intubation (after 3 days), are associated with increased mortality and longer length of ICU stay [9,10]. Although sepsis increases CAP mortality, bacteremia by itself is not a mortality risk [11].

Poor prognostic factors associated with CAP mortality include the presence of multilobar pneumonia (bilateral may be worse than unilateral multilobar), respiratory rate greater than 30 breaths per minute on admission, severe hypoxemia, abnormal liver function, low serum albumin, signs of clinical sepsis, and delayed or inappropriate antibiotic therapy [5,12]. There is also a biphasic relation with platelet count, with increased mortality outside the range of 100,000 to 400,000 per μL [13,14]. Arterial partial pressure of carbon dioxide ($PaCO_2$ <35 or >45 mm Hg) on admission is also related to increased mortality in hospitalized CAP patients, independent of the presence of COPD [13,14]. Hospitalized pneumonia patients are also at increased risk of cardiac ischemia and arrhythmias, and the event may be abrupt and without warning potentially causing cardiorespiratory arrest [15]. In a recent study evaluating factors predicting in-hospital versus postdischarge mortality of hospitalized pneumonia patients aged 65 or older, mortality was 12.1% within 30 days of admission (52.4% of the deaths occurred during the hospital stay) [16]. In that study, the timing of death was unrelated to baseline patient demographic factors or comorbidities, but in-hospital mortality was related to the severity of illness [16].

The adverse prognostic factors discussed above are particularly applicable to the elderly, and those with nursing home–acquired pneumonia often have a higher mortality rate than those with simple CAP [7]. One factor that may explain this finding is that older patients often have atypical clinical presentations of pneumonia, which may lead to their being diagnosed at a later, more advanced stage of illness, resulting in an increased risk of death. In general, the mortality associated with severe CAP is a reflection of how accurately the ICU is used, what organisms are causing the infection, what complications develop in the hospital, and how effective is the initial empiric therapy [17] (Table 181.1).

NP is associated with a high mortality rate (ranging from 20% to 50%) and a significant economic impact with additional hospital costs of ≥10,019 to 40,000 USD [18,19]. HAP has been the second most common nosocomial infection in the United States accounting for up to 25% of all ICU infections and for more than 50% of the antibiotics prescribed [4]. However, in recent years, with the application of effective prevention strategies, the frequency of VAP has been declining. The presence of HAP increases hospital stay by an average of 7 to 9 days per patient [6]. Available data suggest critically ill patients who develop VAP appear to be twice as likely to die compared with

TABLE 181.1

Risk Factors for Pneumonia Mortality in Patients with CAP

Physical findings	
	Abnormal vital signs
	Respiratory rate >30/min
	Hemodynamic compromise: systolic or diastolic hypotension
	Tachycardia (>120/min)
	Afebrile or high fever (>38°C)
	Altered mental status or coma
Laboratory findings	
	Respiratory failure: hypoxemic or hypercarbic
	Multilobar infiltrates
	Rapidly progressive infiltrates
	Positive blood culture
	Multiple organ failure
	Hypoalbuminemia
	Renal insufficiency
	Thrombocytopenia
	Thrombocytosis
	Hypercapnia
	Hypocapnia
	Polymicrobial infection
Historical information	
	Serious comorbidity or advanced age
	Poor functional status at presentation
	Recent hospitalization
	Immunosuppression (including systemic corticosteroids)
	Nonrespiratory clinical presentation
	Delayed or inappropriate therapy
	Prolonged mechanical ventilation

CAP, community-acquired pneumonia.

similar patients without VAP (pooled odds ratio [OR], 2.03; 95% confidence interval, 1.16 to 3.56) [18].

Factors associated with NP mortality include severity of illness, poor functional status before the onset of mechanical ventilation, development of shock, acute renal failure, worsening of hypoxemia during the period of mechanical ventilation, inappropriate therapy, delay in the initiation of therapy, failure to de-escalate therapies, prolonged mechanical ventilation, coma on admission, chronic liver disease, nonsurgical primary diagnosis, bilateral infiltrates, septic shock, multiple system organ failure, and use of prior antibiotic therapy [6]. Patients usually develop HAP because of an underlying chronic illness, and thus the question arises, if they die, whether their death was due to the pneumonia itself or a result of the underlying, predisposing illness. This issue of "attributable mortality" has been studied, and in older studies, as many as 60% of those who die did so as a direct result of their pneumonia [18]. However, more recent data suggest a much lower attributable mortality, and lower death rates from pneumonia among patients with ARDS than previously reported. In a study including 4,479 ventilated patients, mortality related with VAP (24.1%) was not substantially different from mortality in non-VAP patients (23.1%) [20]. However, these studies were performed on patients already on antibiotics; and thus, it is difficult to differentially evaluate the impact of pneumonia on mortality, as inappropriate or no therapy would increase mortality. Bacteriology is another important factor adding to mortality in HAP, with Kollef et al. reporting a high attributable mortality for late-onset VAP caused by potentially drug-resistant organisms such as *Pseudomonas aeruginosa*, *Acinetobacter* spp, and *Stenotrophomonas maltophilia* [21]. Thus, similar to the data with severe CAP, mortality in NP is also affected by patient characteristics, bacteriology, and the efficacy of therapy.

TYPES OF PNEUMONIA ENCOUNTERED IN THE INTENSIVE CARE UNIT

Serious pneumonia occurs when a potential pathogen overwhelms a patient's host defenses, and then, because of either overwhelming infectious challenge or an excessive inflammatory response to infection, the patient develops respiratory failure or septic shock. Certain pathogens are so virulent that they can even overcome an intact, and normal, host defense system, as is the case with epidemic viral illness. Normal host defenses can also be overcome if the inoculum of the pathogen is large (as with massive aspiration), but smaller inocula can be pathogenic if disease-associated factors interfere with immune function. Certain patients seem to become ill because of an excessive inflammatory response to a localized infection, and genetic differences of the immune system are one increasingly implicated explanation.

Community-Acquired Pneumonias Leading to Intensive Care Unit Admission

Although less than 20% of all patients with CAP require hospitalization, those patients ill enough to enter the hospital may have a substantial mortality rate, and mortality is even greater for those admitted to the ICU. For a general ICU population, the mortality rate of CAP, reported in a meta-analysis of 788 patients, was just more than 35%, but other series have reported lower rates [12].

Pathogens that have been described as causing severe CAP include *S. pneumoniae* (pneumococcus), *Legionella pneumophila*, *Haemophilus influenzae*, enteric Gram-negative bacteria, *Staphylococcus aureus* (including community-acquired methicillin-resistant strains), *Mycoplasma pneumoniae*, *Pneumocystis jiroveci*, *Mycobacterium tuberculosis*, *Chlamydophila pneumoniae*, endemic fungi (blastomycosis and histoplasmosis), influenza virus, respiratory syncytial virus, varicella, severe acute respiratory syndrome virus (SARS, caused by a coronavirus), and the bacteria associated with aspiration pneumonia [5].

Definition of Severe CAP and Prognostic Factors/Scoring Systems

Although "severe" CAP does not have a uniform definition, the term has been used to refer to patients with CAP who require ICU care. Some investigators have focused on defining patients with CAP who need intensive respiratory or vasopressor support (IRVS), independent of the site of admission [5,7]. Torres et al. [22] estimated that CAP accounted for 10% of all admissions to an ICU over a 4-year period, and that these patients were admitted directly to the ICU 42% of the time, after admission to a hospital ward 37% of the time, and after transfer from another hospital 21% of the time.

Over the past decade, a number of studies have examined prognostic scoring systems for patients with CAP. In general, there are two widely used approaches, the Pneumonia Severity Index (PSI) and the British Thoracic Society approach (CURB-65). Each uses a point scoring system to predict a patient's mortality risk, with the CURB-65 being simpler and more focused on acute illness parameters, whereas the PSI is a more complex system that incorporates measurements of both chronic and acute disease factors [7]. Although both tools predict mortality risk, neither is a direct measure of severity of illness. For example, as many as 37% of those admitted to the ICU in one study were in PSI classes I–III, pointing out that even those with a low risk for death (which PSI can measure) may benefit from aggressive intensive care support [23]. Conversely, patients in higher PSI classes do not always need ICU care if they fall into these high mortality risk groups because of advanced age and comorbid illness in the absence of physiologic findings of severe pneumonia.

In another study, both tools were applied to the same patients, and each was similarly accurate for identifying low-risk patients [24]. However, the CURB-65 was more discriminating for predicting mortality risk of patients with more severe illnesses. This approach gives one point for each of five abnormalities: confusion, elevated blood urea nitrogen (BUN) (>19.6 mg per dL), respiratory rate 30 per minute or more, low blood pressure (BP) (either systolic <90 mm Hg or diastolic ≤60 mm Hg), and whether the patient is at least 65 years old. If three of these five criteria are present the predicted mortality rate is greater than 20%, and these patients are generally considered for ICU admission [25]. A similar approach has been developed by the Japanese Respiratory Society, using the A-DROP scoring system, that assesses **A**ge (male ≥70 years, female ≥75 years); **D**ehydration (BUN ≥210 mg per L); **R**espiratory failure (SaO(2) ≤90% or PaO(2) ≤60 mm Hg); **O**rientation disturbance (confusion); and low blood **P**ressure (systolic BP ≤90 mm Hg) [26].

España et al. developed a severe pneumonia scoring system (CURXO-80), based on data from 1,057 patients in Spain, suggested that the need for ICU admission could be defined by the presence of one of two major criteria (arterial pH <7.39 or a systolic BP <90 mm Hg), or the presence of two of six minor criteria, which included confusion, BUN greater than 30 mg per dL, respiratory rate greater than 30 per minute, PaO_2/FiO_2 ratio less than 250, multilobar infiltrates, and age 80 years or older. This approach gave different point values to each abnormality, and when severity criteria were met, the tool was 92% sensitive for identifying those with severe CAP and was more accurate than the PSI or the CURB-65 [27]. Another tool, SMART-COP, was developed to predict the need for IRVS using eight clinical features, in which the acronym referred to systolic BP less than 90 mm Hg, multilobar infiltrates, albumin less than 3.5, respiratory rate elevation (>25 for those younger than 50 years, and >30 for those older than 50 years), tachycardia (>125 per minute), confusion, low oxygen (<70 mm Hg if younger than 50 years or <60 mm Hg if older than 50 years), and arterial pH less than 7.35 [28]. Using specific cutoffs, the sensitivity for the need for IRVS was 92.3% and the specificity of 62.3%, with a positive and negative predictive value of 22% and 98.6%, respectively. Both PSI and CURB-65 did not perform as well overall.

Recently, the accuracy of prognostic scoring systems has been enhanced by biomarker measurements. Most data have focused on procalcitonin (PCT), a "hormokine" that has increased plasma concentrations in the presence of severe bacterial infections, but not in viral illness. Masiá et al. reported PCT levels to correlate well with the PSI score and the development of complications such as empyema, mechanical ventilation, and septic shock in a study of 185 patients [29]. Krüger and associates found that PCT identified low-risk patients in all severity classes, and that the finding of a low PCT value had a 98.9% negative predictive value for mortality, regardless of the results of prognostic scoring tools [30]. Similarly in a study of 1,651 patients admitted with CAP, there were 546 in high PSI classes (IV and V), but in the 126 of these who had low PCT levels, only two died, suggesting the advantage of combining serum markers with the commonly used prognostic indices [31].

Although there are no absolute criteria for severe pneumonia, or need for ICU admission, in the 2007 American Thoracic Society/Infectious Society Diseases of America (ATS/IDSA) guidelines, severe CAP was defined as the presence of one of two major criteria (need for mechanical ventilation, or septic shock requiring pressors) or the presence of three of nine minor criteria [5]. These minor criteria were a PaO_2/FiO_2 ratio of 250 or less, respiratory rate 30 per minute or more, confusion, multilobar infiltrates, systolic BP less than 90 mm Hg despite aggressive fluid resuscitation, BUN greater than 20 mg per dL, leukopenia (<4,000 cells per μL), thrombocytopenia (<100,000 cells per μL), and hypothermia (<36°C) [5]. In a study of 2,102 CAP episodes over 7-year period, the ATS/IDSA predictive rule had a sensitivity of 71% and a specificity of 88% for determining the need for ICU admission [32]. Phua and colleagues showed that the ATS minor criteria had greater discriminatory power in the prediction of severity, ICU admission, and mortality than the PSI and CURB [33]. Brown and associates noted that both the positive and negative predictive value of minor criteria exceeded 80% if four criteria were used to define the need for ICU admission rather than just three criteria [34]. In a recent study, investigators simplified the ATS/IDSA criteria by excluding variables that occurred in <5% of cases—leukopenia, thrombocytopenia, and hypothermia, and noted similar predictive value for mortality and intensive care admission as compared to the original ATS/IDSA criteria [35]. In the same study, addition of another variable—acidosis (pH <7.35) improved the prediction for mortality and for ICU admission.

Another score, the "CAP—PIRO score" is calculated within 24 hours of ICU admission and assigns 1 point for each variable: comorbidities (COPD, immunocompromise), age greater than 70 years, multilobar opacities on chest radiograph, shock, severe hypoxemia, acute renal failure, bacteremia, and acute respiratory distress syndrome [36]. Patients are stratified into four levels of risk, and the score performed well as a 28-day mortality prediction tool in patients with CAP requiring ICU admission, with a better performance than APACHE II and the IDSA/ATS criteria. The Risk of Early Admission to ICU (REA-ICU) index was derived from a data set of nearly 5,000 patients and is helpful as a tool on admission to identify patients who had no obvious indication for ICU management, but subsequently required ICU care. It categorizes individuals into four risk groups based on 11 criteria independently associated with ICU admission: male gender, age younger than 80 years, comorbid conditions, respiratory rate of 30 breaths per minute or higher, heart rate of 125 beats per minute or higher, multilobar infiltrate or pleural effusion, white blood cell count less than 3 or 20,000 per μL or above, hypoxemia (oxygen saturation <90% or arterial partial pressure of oxygen (PaO_2) <60 mmHg), blood urea nitrogen of 11 mmol/L or higher, pH less than 7.35 and sodium less than 130 mEq/L [37]. The mortality and likelihood of needing ICU care increased with each risk group with the highest in class IV with a score ≥9. In a recent validation study including 850 CAP patients, who had no obvious need for ICU care on admission, the REA-ICU index performed better than PSI but was similar to other tools (like SMART-COP, CURXO-80, the 2007 IDSA/ATS minor severity criteria, and CURB-65) at defining the need for early ICU admission [38].

CAP Prognostic Factors Defined After Initial Management

The above discussion has focused on data available on admission to guide the site of care decision, but after admission, as the results of cultures become available, and therapy (accurate or not) is given, these events can impact prognosis. Garau et al. found that late and overall CAP mortality are reduced when patients have negative blood cultures, and when antibiotic therapy is given according to guidelines [39]. Among patients with severe CAP, the most important prognostic finding during therapy is radiographic progression [22]. Ineffective initial empirical therapy has also been identified as a potent predictor of death, being associated with a 60% mortality rate, compared with an 11% mortality rate when patients received initial effective therapy [40]. Similarly, among other studies of CAP, the use of a combination of a β-lactam and a macrolide antibiotic was associated with a lower mortality than when other therapies were given, and the use of guideline compliant therapy was associated with a reduced duration of mechanical ventilation [5,41]. In the setting of severe pneumococcal bacteremia, the use of combination therapy is associated with reduced mortality, compared with monotherapy, particularly among patients treated in the ICU [5]. Not only must initial therapy be accurate, it must be timely, and in patients with septic shock (from all sources, including pneumonia), mortality increases by 7% for each hour of delay in initiating therapy [42]. Retrospective data have also shown a reduced mortality for admitted CAP patients who were treated within 4 hours of arrival to the hospital compared with those who were treated later [5].

The interaction between prognostic factors related to therapy and bacteriology is most evident when patients with CAP are infected with drug-resistant organisms, particularly drug-resistant pneumococcus. Studies have defined the clinical features of patients at risk for drug-resistant pneumococcus (drug-resistant *S. pneumoniae* [DRSP]) and these include older than 65 years, *β*-lactam therapy in the past 3 months, multiple medical comorbidities, alcoholism, nosocomial acquisition, and contact with a child in day care [5]. Most investigators have found no difference of mortality for patients infected with resistant or sensitive organisms, after controlling for comorbid illness [43], although patients with resistant organisms may have a more prolonged hospital stay, and suppurative complications such as empyema [44], and the presence of high-level penicillin resistance has been associated with increased mortality among those infected with HIV [45].

Recently, the definitions of resistance have been changed for nonmeningeal infection, with sensitive being defined by a penicillin minimum inhibitory concentration (MIC) ≤2 mg/L, intermediate as an MIC of 4 mg/L, and resistant as an MIC ≥8 mg/L [46]. Although the clinical impact of resistance on outcomes such as mortality was hard to show using older definitions, with the new definitions of resistance, very few pathogens will be defined as resistant, but those that are, may affect outcomes.

Nosocomial Pneumonia in the Intensive Care Unit

Risk Factors for HAP and VAP

As mentioned, pneumonia is the nosocomial infection most likely to contribute causally to the death of patients, particularly those treated with mechanical ventilation (VAP). Risk factors for this infection fall into four categories: the underlying primary critical illnesses leading to ICU admission; coexisting medical illness; factors associated with therapies that are frequently used in the ICU; and malnutrition. Thus, some of the common conditions associated with NP include risk factors present on admission such as immune-suppressive illness, risk of aspiration (coma and impaired consciousness), serious comorbid illnesses (chronic heart or lung disease, renal failure, malignancy, and diabetes mellitus), ARDS, malnutrition (serum albumin <2.2 mg per dL), obesity, age greater than 60 years, smoking and drug abuse, need for major surgery, and recent major trauma or burns. Other nonmodifiable risk factors that increase the risk of NP are treatment related such as prior antibiotic therapy, immune-suppressive therapy (including corticosteroids), need for multiple transfusions, transport out of the ICU, mechanical ventilation with positive end-expiratory pressure (PEEP), tracheostomy, nasogastric tube use, supine position in the first 24 hours after admission, and intestinal bleeding prophylaxis [4,47].

Among ICU patients, nearly 90% of episodes of HAP occur during mechanical ventilation. Further, intubation increases the risk of acquiring pneumonia by as much as 6- to 20-fold [4]. Older studies estimated that the risk of NP was 1% per day of mechanical ventilation, but other data show a risk of 3% per day for the first 5 days, 2% per day for days 6 to 10, and 1% per day for days 11 to 15[48]. Although VAP occurs in 9% to 27% of all intubated patients, since many patients are intubated for only a short time, up to half of all VAP episodes begin within the first 4 days of mechanical ventilation (early-onset pneumonia) [4].

The relation between pneumonia and ARDS is particularly interesting. In older studies, as many as one-third of all cases of ARDS were the result of pneumonia, but secondary pneumonia was the most common nosocomial infection acquired by patients with established ARDS [4]. When patients with ARDS develop pneumonia, it is generally a late event, occurring after at least 7 days of mechanical ventilation, and when it occurs, it can be the start of a progressive downhill course characterized by multiple organ failure [4]. Using quantitative diagnostic methods, Chastre et al. found an incidence of 55% of VAP among patients with ARDS; however, there were no significant differences of survival between ARDS patients with and without VAP [49]. Thus, NP among patients without ARDS is clearly associated with a higher mortality; there is insufficient data to substantiate an increased mortality due to pulmonary infection for patients with ARDS, partly due to a high intrinsic mortality related with ARDS.

Health Care–Associated Pneumonia

HCAP refers to patients who develop infection while having contact with the health care environment, such as those residing in nursing homes, those treated in dialysis units, patients who have been in the hospital in the past 90 days, and those getting home infusion therapy or home wound care (Table 181.2), and some of these patients are at risk for infection with multidrug-resistant (MDR) organisms. This has also been addressed in the 2005 ATS/IDSA guidelines as a form of HAP, but some investigators prefer to consider it a form of CAP in complex hosts [4]. HCAP patients with severe illness or poor functional status as defined by activities of daily living score, or who are taking immunosuppressive medications, are at increased risk of developing MDR infections, and need broad-spectrum empiric antimicrobial therapy. However, recent studies have shown that patients who qualify as having HCAP are a heterogeneous population, and that when HCAP patients are managed in the ICU, the frequency of MDR pathogens is much greater than when they are not as ill and do not need ICU care [50].

TABLE 181.2

Hospital-Acquired Pneumonia and Healthcare-Associated Pneumonia: Risk Factors for Multidrug Resistant Organisms

Current hospitalization of ≥5 d
Antibiotic treatment in prior 90 d
High frequency of antibiotic resistance in the community/specific hospital unit
Immunosuppressive disease/therapy
Presence of multiple risk factors for healthcare-associated pneumonia
Hospitalization for 2 d or more in the preceding 90 d
Residence in a nursing home or extended care facility
Home infusion therapy (including antibiotics)
Chronic dialysis within 30 d
Home wound care
Family member with multidrug-resistant pathogen

Adapted from Niederman MS, Craven DE, Bonten MJ, et al: Guidelines for the management of adults with hospital-acquired, ventilator-associated, and healthcare-associated pneumonia. *Am J RespirCrit Care Med* 171:388–416, 2005, with permission.

PATHOGENESIS OF PNEUMONIA

Normal Host Defenses

When an organism enters the respiratory tract, it encounters a host defense system designed to repel and remove it from every anatomic site in the airway. Pneumonia develops when the size of the organism inoculum overcomes the host defense system, when the organism is so virulent that it cannot be repelled, or when the patient is so impaired that he/she is unable to resist an organism type or inoculum size that could ordinarily be handled by a fully functioning host defense system. With a variety of acute illnesses, such as malnutrition, uremia, and general surgery, Gram-negative bacteria can bind more avidly to the oral epithelium, and colonization can occur, the first step toward lower respiratory tract infection [51].

The lower respiratory tract (starting beneath the vocal cords) has a complex host defense system that keeps this site sterile for normal people, although recent studies of the respiratory microbiome have questioned whether this site is ever free of bacteria. For the lower respiratory tract to become infected, organisms must overcome the physical barrier of the vocal cords and the tracheobronchial protective mechanisms of cough, bronchoconstriction, airway angulation, and the upward transport of the mucociliary blanket. Protective substances in respiratory secretions include IgA, the predominant immunoglobulin of the upper airway; IgG, which dominates in the lower respiratory tract; complement; lysozymes; surfactant; and fibronectin [52]. The resident phagocytic cell of the lower respiratory tract is the alveolar macrophage, but its function can be augmented by the production of inflammatory cytokines which can promote the recruitment of blood neutrophils and the development of cell-mediated and humoral immunity.

In the setting of focal lung infection, the cytokine inflammatory response is normally localized to the site of initial infection [53]. Severe pneumonia occurs when the inflammatory response is not localized (due to overwhelming infection or inappropriate bilateral inflammation) and the inflammatory response extends to the systemic circulation (sepsis syndrome). The innate immune response is organized to recognize pathogens and initiate an immune response. Pathogen recognition is mediated by toll-like receptors for Gram-negative bacteria and their activation contributes to pathogen-stimulated production of interleukin 1 (IL-1) or tumor necrosis factor (TNF). When pathogens are recognized through these mechanisms, nuclear factor κB is produced by inflammatory cells, which in turn leads to cytokine production that can recruit more inflammatory cells. In addition, the lower airway handles individual pathogens in specific ways. For example, *S. aureus* is removed by resident alveolar macrophages, whereas certain enteric Gram-negative bacteria and the pneumococcus require the recruitment of neutrophils (presumably in response to interleukin-8) to be cleared [53]. Cell-mediated immunity is required to resist infection with *L. pneumophila* and *M. tuberculosis*. Viruses are handled somewhat differently from bacteria, and important factors in defense against these agents include the alveolar macrophage, neutralizing antibodies (IgG, IgA, and IgM), cytotoxic T lymphocytes, and cytokines such as the interferons. Specific genetic immune impairments or acquired immune dysfunction can cause specific aspects of the inflammatory response to malfunction and lead to infection with specific, predictable pathogens.

How Microorganisms Reach the Lung

Bacteria and other infectious agents can reach the lung by inhalation from ambient air, hematogenously from distal sites of infection, by direct extension or exogenous penetration, and by aspiration from a colonized oropharynx and nasopharynx. Inhalation is an uncommon route of organism entry except for pathogens such as *L. pneumophila*, viruses, and *M. tuberculosis*. Hematogenous spread can occur with septic emboli from such sites as the valves of the right cardiac chambers. Exogenous penetration is an unlikely route of bacterial entry but can occur, for example, with extension of an abdominal infection into the pleural space and then the lung parenchyma. Most pneumonias result when microorganisms are aspirated from a previously colonized oropharynx. The source of bacteria that colonize the upper airway is most likely the patient's own lower intestinal flora, but the nasal sinuses and stomach can also harbor bacteria that can subsequently reach the lung. The coexistence of nosocomial sinusitis and pneumonia has been documented, often with the same organisms, and both infections can be promoted by the presence of a nasogastric or nasotracheal tubes [4].

In addition to promoting sinusitis, the endotracheal tube and the nasogastric tube can also serve as additional pathways for bacterial entry to the lung. Insertion of an endotracheal tube allows micro-organism direct access to the lung from the hands of the ICU staff, thereby avoiding the defense mechanisms present above the vocal cords. Any organisms that reach the inside of the endotracheal tube can proliferate to large numbers because this site is free from host defenses, and a biofilm commonly lines the interior of the endotracheal tube and can contain as many as 10^6 organisms per cm of the tube surface [54]. These organisms can reach the lung every time an intubated patient is suctioned. A silver-coated endotracheal tube with antibacterial properties was shown to reduce the incidence of VAP, but had no impact on mortality [55]. In a recent prospective study, investigators found endotracheal tubes to be coated with biofilm, as early as after 24 hours of intubation, and the biofilm was not associated with the duration of intubation, the administration of selective digestive decontamination (SDD), systemic antibiotics, or immunosuppression. In that study, the persistence of biofilm was commonly associated with treatment failure for VAP [56]. Another factor in VAP pathogenesis is the ventilator circuit tubing, which can easily be contaminated by large numbers of bacteria [4]. Interestingly, the ventilator circuits are usually contaminated by the patient, as the circuit becomes colonized in large numbers, as bacteria proliferate in the water condensate in the tubing. If handled carefully, the circuits are not a major source of pneumonia pathogens, and the incidence of pneumonia is not increased even when ventilator circuit tubing is never changed during the course of therapy [4].

The gastrointestinal tract, particularly the stomach, can serve as a reservoir for bacteria, and several investigators have shown that Gram-negative bacilli can move retrograde from the stomach to the oropharynx and then antegrade into the lung [57]. The stomach can be the source of 20% to 40% of the enteric Gram-negative bacteria that colonize the trachea of intubated patients, but it is difficult to determine if these colonizing gastric bacteria also lead to pneumonia. One of the ways that the stomach can be an important source of pneumonic organisms is through the mechanism of reflux and aspiration. When a nasogastric tube is used for feeding, it can promote aspiration, especially when a large-bore tube is used with a bolus feeding method rather than with a continuous infusion of enteral nutrients, and when the patient is kept in a supine position [58]. When a nasogastric tube is present, it may promote pneumonia if the gastric contents have a pH above 4 to 6, as can occur with the use of antacids, H_2 blockers, and enteral feeding. An elevated pH can increase the number of Gram-negative bacteria in the stomach, increasing to as many as 1 to 100 million per mL of gastric juice, and elevation of gastric pH has been reported as a risk factor for NP, although not in all studies [59]. The Canadian Critical Care Trials Group reported that acidified enteral feeds preserve gastric acidity and substantially reduce gastric colonization among critically ill patients; however, in one study, there was no impact on the incidence of pneumonia with this intervention [59]. Increases of gastric volume can be detrimental and promote aspiration, thus accounting for the observation that when continuous enteral feeding leads to an elevation of gastric pH (and presumably an elevation of gastric volume), the incidence of pneumonia is higher than when continuous feeding is used but does not raise pH [60]. Another way to minimize the impact of the stomach and to avoid aspiration is to keep patients in a semierect position whenever possible, particularly because the supine position can favor aspiration when a nasogastric tube is in place [58]. However, this position may not favor secretion clearance from the lung, and the lateral Trendelenburg position may be better for this purpose.

Airway Colonization and Nosocomial Pneumonia

Colonization (the persistence of organisms in the absence of a host response and without an adverse effect to the host) of the respiratory tract by enteric Gram-negative bacilli is the first step toward the development of NP. Risk factors for Gram-negative colonization of the upper and lower respiratory tract are similar and include antibiotic therapy, endotracheal intubation, smoking, malnutrition, general surgery, and therapies that raise gastric pH [52]. Additional risk factors for oropharyngeal colonization include azotemia, diabetes, coma, hypotension, advanced age, and underlying lung disease. Additional risk factors for tracheobronchial colonization include chronic bronchitis, cystic fibrosis, ciliary dysfunction, tracheostomy, bronchiectasis, acute lung injury, and viral infection [51]. The distinction between colonization and infection among mechanically ventilated patients is less clear than in the past, with recognition and focus on ventilator-associated tracheobronchitis (VAT) [61]. Some patients who are mechanically ventilated can have high concentrations of pathogenic organisms in the tracheobronchial tree, in the absence of pneumonia, yet may become clinically ill with purulent sputum due to VAT, and therapy could potentially prevent some from progressing to VAP.

One pathogenetic mechanism that links many of the clinical risk factors for upper and lower airway colonization is a cell–cell interaction termed bacterial mucosal adherence. Many clinical disease states can alter the oropharyngeal or tracheal epithelium, making the cell surface more receptive for binding by such bacteria as *P. aeruginosa* [51]. Diseases that result in an increased number of oropharyngeal and tracheal cell bacterial receptors are many of the same processes that promote colonization of these sites [51]. One study of intubated patients demonstrated the rapidity with which the endotracheal tube itself became colonized with enteric Gram-negatives and found that colonization took place despite the use of bacterial filters in the ventilator circuit [62]. Colonization is a common finding among intubated patients, and the presence of potential pathogens in the respiratory secretions of intubated patients is to be expected, and does not require therapy unless there are clinical signs of infection.

Host Defense Impairments in Acute and Chronic Illness that Predispose to Pneumonia

Many systemic diseases increase the risk of pneumonia as a result of disease-associated malfunctions in the respiratory host defense system, including ARDS, sepsis, CHF, malnutrition, renal failure, diabetes mellitus, chronic liver disease, alcoholism, cancer, and collagen vascular diseases [63]. In addition, many illnesses can be complicated by pneumonia because they require therapy with medications that interfere with immune function. Several studies have shown that acute and chronic malnutrition (Table 181.3) can increase the risk of bacterial and viral infections both in and out of the hospital. Genetic variation may explain why patients, who have certain inherited patterns of immune responses, are more prone to severe forms of pneumonia, and even mortality, than others. CAP severity is increased with genetic changes in the IL-10-1082 locus that are often present along with changes in the TNF-α-308 locus. Another genetic change associated with an increased risk of septic shock from CAP is a modification of heat shock protein 70-2 [64]. Currently, there are a large number of genes that are associated with the severity and outcome of CAP, but the clinical application of this information is not yet well defined. One recent observation about gender differences in the immune response was that men have a higher degree of systemic inflammation on admission for CAP (higher levels of TNF, IL-6, and IL-10), and that higher levels of these mediators increased pneumonia mortality risk [65]. Recently, Rautanen and colleagues reported the first Genome-wide association studies (GWAS) on survival from sepsis due to pneumonia in three independent cohorts of patients admitted to ICU [66]. Of more than 6 million single nucleotide polymorphisms (SNPs) examined, the authors noted common variants in the FER gene (one C/T SNP in chromosome 5) to be strongly associated with survival [66].

TABLE 181.3

Lung Host Defense Impairments with Malnutrition

Increased tracheal and buccal cell adherence
Altered macrophage function and migration
Reduced recruitment of neutrophils
Impaired cell-mediated immunity and T-cell depletion
Diminished secretory immunoglobulin A
Complement deficiency

ETIOLOGY OF PNEUMONIA

Community-Acquired Pneumonia

Even with extensive diagnostic testing, a specific etiologic agent can be identified in only approximately 50% of pneumonias that develop outside of the hospital, although the rate of pathogen recovery may be higher among intubated and mechanically ventilated patients [67]. Although the exact incidence of viral pneumonias is unknown, these agents may account for up to one third of all community-acquired cases. The most common pathogen identified in pneumonias arising out of the hospital is the pneumococcus, and among the elderly, although pneumococci are still the most common pathogens, enteric Gram-negative organisms may be responsible for 20% to 40% of all cases of pneumonia, and anaerobes and *H. influenzae* are other common agents [68]. However, age alone has little impact on the bacterial etiology of CAP, but rather, the comorbid illnesses that become more common in the elderly affect bacteriology [69]. The most common CAP pathogens leading to ICU admission (severe pneumonia) are pneumococcus, *L. pneumophila*, epidemic viruses (influenza), *S. aureus* (including methicillin-resistant *S. aureus* [MRSA]), and enteric Gram-negative bacilli, including, for some patients, *P. aeruginosa* [17]. The incidence of CAP caused by the USA 300 clone of *S. aureus*—community-acquired MRSA (CA-MRSA) is on the rise, but the exact frequency and the impact on mortality and other outcomes remain to be defined [70]. Although Gram-negatives are more common in VAP and HCAP than in CAP, risk factors for Gram-negative pneumonia (in addition to nursing home residence, an HCAP risk factor) are cardiac disease, smoking history, and clinical features of

TABLE 181.4

Likely Pathogens for Pneumonia in the Critically Ill

Database	Suspected pathogen
Alcoholism—acute or chronic	*Streptococcus pneumoniae* (including DRSP), anaerobes, Gram-negative bacilli, *Mycobacterium* sp.
Chronic obstructive pulmonary disease	*S. pneumoniae, Haemophilus influenzae, Moraxella catarrhalis*
Recent viral infection and postinfluenza	*S. pneumoniae, Staphylococcus aureus* (including MRSA), *H. influenzae*, Gram-negative bacilli
Nursing home (age >75 y)	Gram-negative bacilli (including resistant ones such as *Pseudomonas aeruginosa, Acinetobacter* spp.), *S. pneumoniae, H. influenzae*, aspiration (anaerobes), *S. aureus, Chlamydophila, Mycobacterium tuberculosis*
AIDS (risk groups: intravenous drug abuser, hemophilia, homosexual)	*S. pneumoniae, Salmonella*, cytomegalovirus, *H. influenzae, Cryptococcus, P. jiroveci*, anaerobes, *M. tuberculosis*
Hospital acquired	Gram-negative bacilli (including *P. aeruginosa*), *S. aureus* (including MRSA)
High-risk aspiration	Anaerobes (if aspirate while not intubated), Gram-negative bacilli, chemical pneumonitis
Cardiac disease	*S. pneumoniae*, Gram-negative bacilli
Neutropenia	*P. aeruginosa, Aspergillus* sp., Gram-negative bacilli
Recent antibiotic therapy	DRSP, *P. aeruginosa*, MRSA (especially in HAP)
Endobronchial obstruction	Anaerobes, Gram-negative bacilli
Structural lung disease (cystic fibrosis, bronchiectasis)	*P. aeruginosa, P. cepacia, S. aureus*

AIDS, acquired immunodeficiency syndrome; DRSP, drug-resistant *S. pneumoniae*; HAP, hospital-acquired pneumonia; MRSA, methicillin-resistant *S. aureus*

severe illness including hyponatremia, septic shock, and severe tachypnea [71].

Other pathogens that can lead to respiratory failure include *H. influenzae*, pathogens associated with aspiration (such as anaerobes), *P. jiroveci, tuberculosis*, varicella, and respiratory syncytial virus. Mixed infection occurs in more than 10% of patients with CAP requiring hospitalization, and in one study, in patients with mixed CAP, *S. pneumoniae* was the most prevalent microorganism (44 out of 82; 54%) [72]. In that study, the most frequent combination was *S. pneumoniae* with *H. influenzae* (17 out of 82; 21%), and influenza A occurred with *S. pneumoniae* in 5 out of 28 (18%). Of note, patients with mixed pyogenic pneumonia more frequently developed shock when compared with patients with single pyogenic pneumonia (18% vs. 4%) [72].

Polymicrobial infection with viruses and bacteria is not uncommon in patients with severe pneumonia. In a recent study, investigators reported the role of viruses in 198 patients with severe pneumonia (64 with CAP and 134 with HCAP) and noted 35.9% (n = 71) had positive bacterial culture, 36.4% (n = 72) had viral infections, and 9.1% (n = 18) had bacterial–viral co-infections with no difference in mortality between the three groups [73]. Bacterial co-infection was more common with parainfluenza and influenza viruses and less common with respiratory syncytial virus and rhinoviruses.

When evaluating a patient with pneumonia, it is important to understand the status of each individual's respiratory host defense system to predict which possible pathogen is most likely (Table 181.4). Thus, CAP in a previously healthy person is most likely due to a pathogen of such intrinsic virulence that it can overcome even an intact host defense system. These pathogens include *S. pneumoniae, Legionella* sp., *S. aureus*, viruses, and *M. pneumoniae*. If the patient has a serious underlying illness, then organisms of less intrinsic virulence that would ordinarily be eliminated by a normal host can be responsible. When an alcoholic has pneumonia, anaerobes and *Klebsiella pneumoniae* become more likely; those with chronic bronchitis may be infected with nontypeable *H. influenzae* and *Moraxella catarrhalis*; cardiac patients commonly have pneumococcal infection; those with cystic fibrosis are commonly infected by *S. aureus* and *P. aeruginosa*; and those with risk factors for aspiration can have enteric Gram-negative bacterial or anaerobic lung infection. Other associations are listed in Table 181.4. Certain historical information can be valuable, such as an appropriate travel or exposure history that suggests specific etiologic pathogens (Table 181.5).

TABLE 181.5

Historical and Physical Features Useful in Pneumonia Diagnosis

Clinical setting	Organisms
Environmental contact	
Birds, bats	*Chlamydophila psittaci, Cryptococcus neoformans, Histoplasma capsulatum*
Bird droppings	*C. psittaci, H. capsulatum* (histoplasmosis)
Ungulates	*Coxiellaburnetii* (Q fever)
Hunting (animal and insect bites)	*Yersinia pestis* (plague), *Francisella tularensis* (tularemia)
Infected hides	Anthrax
Travel or location	
Southeast Asia	*Pseudomonas pseudomallei*, SARS (coronavirus)
Southwestern United States	*Coccidioides immitis* (coccidioidomycosis)
Midwestern United States	*H. capsulatum* (histoplasmosis)
Prison environment	*Mycobacterium* sp. (tuberculosis)
Poor dental hygiene	Anaerobes

SARS, severe acute respiratory syndrome.

Nosocomial Pneumonia

Both VAP and HCAP may be caused by a variety of Gram-positive and Gram-negative bacteria, many of which are MDR. These infections may be polymicrobial and are seen more often among patients with ARDS than among other ventilated patients [74]. Viral or fungal pathogens are rarely causative for immunocompetent hosts [75]. Among patients who have a prolonged hospital stay, therapy with corticosteroids or antibiotics, need for long-term mechanical ventilation, and in those with ARDS, the pathogen most likely to cause pneumonia is *P. aeruginosa*, but at many hospitals, *Acinetobacter* is becoming an increasing concern. Contamination with *Legionella* sp. in the water system can lead to infection, especially among patients treated with corticosteroids. Another pathogen that should be considered when NP arises in the setting of corticosteroid therapy for COPD is *Aspergillus* sp. [76].

In the National Nosocomial Infections Surveillance (NNIS) system data examining changes in the organisms from 1986 to 2003, Gram-negative aerobes persisted as being the most frequent organisms in HAP (65.9%), with little change in their distribution over this period, except for a rise in the proportion of *Acinetobacter* from 1.5% in 1975 to 6.9% in 2003 [77]. The most common Gram-negative organism reported was *Pseudomonas aeruginosa* (18.1%), and others included *Klebsiella* spp. (7.2%), *Acinetobacter* spp. (6.9%), and *Escherichia coli* (5%). The Gram-positive organisms included *S. aureus* (27.8%), *Enterobacter* spp. (10%), coagulase-negative *Staphylococcus* (1.8%), and *Enterococci* (1.3%) [77]. This pattern was similar to a recent antimicrobial surveillance program from 1997 to 2008 of hospitalized patients with pneumonia from North America, Europe, and Latin America -the SENTRY surveillance data [78]. In that study, *P. aeruginosa* (26.6%) and *Acinetobacter* species were more common among VAP than HAP patients. The EPIC study was a point prevalence evaluation of infection and the etiologic pathogens, in ICUs throughout the world, on a given day in 2007 and among 13,796 patients, 64% had respiratory tract infections and among all infections, Gram-negatives were more common than Gram-positives (62.2% vs. 46.8%) [79]. The most common organisms were *P. aeruginosa* and *S. aureus* (half of which was methicillin-resistant). Some studies have compared the bacteriology of pneumonia among ventilated and nonventilated patients. In one study, investigators evaluated NP over a 3-year period in ventilated (n = 164) and nonventilated patients (n = 151), finding no significant difference in the relative proportion of etiologic pathogens isolated from both the groups, except for *S. pneumoniae*, which was more common in nonventilated ICU patients than VAP patients [80]. However, another prospective surveillance study comparing 327 episodes of VAP in 309 patients with 261 episodes of HAP among 247 patients, the patients with VAP had more episodes of Gram-negative bacilli, compared to patients with HAP (59% vs. 39.6%, $p < 0.001$) and HAP patients had a higher incidence of *S. pneumoniae* and viruses [81].

HAP involving anaerobic organisms may follow aspiration among nonintubated patients but is rare among patients with VAP [4]. Gram-negative organisms are more common with aspiration, especially in the health care environment, including the nursing home [68]. Oropharyngeal commensals such as viridans group streptococci, coagulase-negative staphylococci, *Neisseria* species, and *Corynebacterium* species can produce infection of immunocompromised hosts and some immunocompetent patients. The identity of specific MDR pathogens causing HAP varies from one ICU to another, and depends on the patient population treated and the degree of prior antibiotic exposure, but the dominant organisms change over time [4,77]. Risk factors for infection with MDR pathogens are summarized in Table 181.2.

The bacteriology of HCAP is widely variable depending on the types of patients evaluated. Current data show that HCAP is a heterogeneous disease, including a wide range of patients, some severely ill and others not. In the severely ill population, often treated in the ICU, MDR Gram-negatives, and MRSA are common and must be considered when designing empiric therapy. Elderly residents of long-term care facilities have been found to have a spectrum of pathogens similar to late-onset HAP and VAP [4,82]. In patients aged 75 years and older with severe pneumonia, El-Solh et al. found *S. aureus* (29%), enteric Gram-negative rods (15%), *S. pneumoniae* (9%), and *Pseudomonas* species (4%) as the most frequent causes of nursing home–acquired pneumonia [75]. These resistant organisms are a particular concern for severely ill patients with other risk factors, including poor functional status, prior antibiotic therapy, immune-suppressive therapy, and a history of recent hospitalization.

CLINICAL FEATURES OF PNEUMONIA

General Features of Community-Acquired Pneumonia

The signs and symptoms of pneumonia depend on both host and bacterial factors, and in the past, the presentation was classified as being either "typical" or "atypical," but studies have shown that this approach is not clinically useful [5]. The common clinical features of CAP include fever, cough, sputum production, dyspnea, and occasionally pleuritic chest pain. Gastrointestinal symptoms that may be seen include nausea, vomiting, and diarrhea. Because many of the symptoms of pneumonia result from the host inflammatory response, patients who have altered immune function have less dramatic symptoms. Thus, those with advanced age, chronic lung disease, cardiac disease, renal failure, diabetes, immunosuppressive therapy, and other chronic illnesses have not only an increased incidence of pneumonia but also a less distinct and subtler clinical presentation. In the elderly patient, pneumonia can have a nonrespiratory presentation with symptoms of confusion, falling, failure to thrive, altered functional capacity, or deterioration in a preexisting medical illness, such as CHF.

General Features of Nosocomial Pneumonia

A major controversy is how to determine when hospital-acquired (particularly ventilator-associated) pneumonia is present. On clinical grounds alone, the diagnosis is imprecise and in the presence of diseases such as ARDS, atelectasis, pulmonary embolism, lung contusion, and CHF, all of which may be associated with lung infiltrates, pneumonia may be overlooked, or these processes may be incorrectly diagnosed as lung infection. In addition, the elderly and immunosuppressed may have few clinical findings when pneumonia develops in the hospital. Limited sputum production due to impaired immunologic status and mobilization of leukocytes compound the difficulties of diagnosis. Conversely, those on a mechanical ventilator with VAT may have purulent sputum, fever, and pathogens colonizing the sputum but not have invasive parenchymal lung infection.

Fagon et al. using quantitative cultures collected with a protected specimen brush (PSB) to define this infection for mechanically ventilated patients, have reported that up to two-thirds of cases that are diagnosed based on clinical criteria alone are not truly pneumonia [83]. Most clinical definitions of NP require the patient to be hospitalized 48 to 72 hours before the onset of purulent sputum, leukocytosis, fever, and a new and persistent infiltrate. If these features exist along with isolation of a potential pathogen from the sputum, then this organism is deemed to be responsible for the infection. The findings of a positive blood culture or radiographic cavitation add to the likelihood of pneumonia being present. Positive blood cultures when NP is suspected can support the diagnosis, but if the organism present in the blood culture is different from the one in the respiratory tract, the bacteremia may be secondary to an extra-pulmonary infection [4]. One approach to the clinical definition of VAP, developed by Pugin et al. [84], has been to use a scoring system that weigh six clinical variables: fever, white blood cell count and differential, the presence of pathogens in the sputum, sputum purulence, radiographic patterns, and oxygenation changes. When this Clinical Pulmonary Infection Score (CPIS) has been used, the clinical and quantitative bacteriologic definitions of pneumonia have correlated very well.

The CDC definition of VAP is subject to significant interobserver variability. Klompas and associates developed a simplified streamlined surveillance definition of VAP excluding the criteria of delirium and rales, and defined worsening oxygenation as at least 2 days of stable or decreasing daily minimum PEEP, followed by an increase of at least 2.5 cm H_2O of PEEP for more than 2 days; or at least 2 days of stable or decreasing fraction of inspired oxygen (FiO_2), followed by a sustained increase of at least 0.15 in FiO_2 over 2 days [85]. Compared to the conventional definition, the streamlined definition identified patients with VAP faster (3.5 vs. 39 minute per patient) and more objectively, with no major difference in hospital mortality, ICU length of stay, and ventilator days between the two definitions. More recently, hospitals have begun to look at a new condition, ventilator-associated complications (VAC), which relies heavily on changes in oxygenation, and is related to pneumonia, but includes a number of other illnesses, as discussed below.

The use of biomarkers, both in the serum and in the respiratory secretions, may help in making this difficult diagnosis. For patients with VAP, studies have used PCT, C-reactive protein, soluble triggering receptors expressed on myeloid 1 (STREM), and IL-6, among others [86–88]. Ramirez and colleagues found that a combination of CPIS of at least 6 points and serum PCT levels of at least 2.99 ng per mL had 100% specificity and negative predictive value of 92% (AUC = 0.961) for the diagnosis of VAP [89]. In another prospective study, serial PCT measurements on days 1, 3, and 7 were significantly higher among microbiologically proven VAP patients who had an unfavorable outcome than those with a favorable outcome, while serial CPIS values were less discriminatory [90]. The difficulty to accurately diagnose NP, especially VAP in the absence of a gold standard test, is a concern, and clinicians often start broad-spectrum antibiotics based on clinical judgment.

DIAGNOSTIC APPROACH TO THE PATIENT WITH SEVERE PNEUMONIA

Once the presence of severe pneumonia has been defined, the patient should be categorized by place of origin of infection, defining the illness as CAP, HCAP, or HAP (including VAP). Then the immune competence of the patient, the types of comorbid diseases present, and the existence of risk factors for specific pathogens should be defined to identify the most likely etiologic pathogens. Historical data, physical examination, and laboratory findings pertinent to diagnoses will also be helpful for determining which etiologic agent is responsible and what specific therapy should be instituted (see Tables 181.4 and 181.5). For example, contact with animals, especially birds, rats, and rabbits, can suggest the diagnosis of psittacosis, plague, and tularemia, respectively.

Historical Information

The history can be used to determine if the patient has pneumonia as the cause of his or her acute illness, recognizing that certain populations, such as the elderly, may have an altered, nonclassical presentation. Among elderly and compromised hosts, the infection may be heralded only by lethargy and confusion [69]. Among compromised hosts with malignancy or immunosuppressive therapy, the presentation may be so stunted that pneumonia may only be discovered only at autopsy.

Hemoptysis is an important historical feature, since it implies tissue necrosis and is most common with pyogenic streptococcal pneumonia (groups A to D), anaerobic lung abscess, *S. aureus*, necrotizing Gram-negative organisms, and invasive aspergillosis. Microaspiration of anaerobic organisms leading to pneumonia is more likely with a history of preexisting severe periodontal disease or with a history of seizure disorder, altered consciousness, or esophageal obstructive disease. Extrapulmonary symptoms may give clues to specific etiologic agents, with diarrhea and abdominal discomfort being seen in patients with *Legionella* sp. and otitis media and pharyngitis with *M. pneumoniae* (Table 181.6).

For the patient with NP, the history should focus on whether the patient has recently received antibiotics and how long the patient has been in the hospital prior to the onset of infection. Both are risk factors for infection with MDR Gram-positive and Gram-negative bacteria. In addition, the specific antibiotics used in the past 2 weeks should be recorded, since the pathogens causing the current infection are likely to be resistant to those agents. Other risk factors for MDR pathogens that can be present in those with HAP and HCAP include hospitalization in the past 90 days, poor functional status, and immunosuppressive therapy (including corticosteroid use).

Physical Examination

The physical examination is valuable for suggesting the presence of pneumonia and for grading its severity. Tachypnea (>20 breaths per minute) may be the earliest sign of pneumonia among the elderly, and findings of consolidation are more specific for

TABLE 181.6

Extrapulmonary Findings in Pneumonia

Findings	Organisms
Dermatologic findings	
Herpes labialis	*Streptococcus pneumoniae*
Erythema multiforme	*Mycoplasma* sp., *Chlamydophila psittaci*
Erythema nodosum	*Mycobacterium tuberculosis*, *Coccidioides immitus*
	Histoplasma capsulatum
Skin nodules	*Nocardia* sp.
	Aspergillus sp.
	Coccidioides immitus
	Blastomyces sp.
Pharyngitis, bullous myringitis	*Mycoplasma* sp.
Splenomegaly	*Francisella tularensis*
	C. psittaci
	Coxiella burnetii (Q fever)
Pleural effusion	*Haemophilus influenzae*
	S. pneumonia
	Pyogenic streptococci
	Aspergillus sp.
	F. tularensis

pneumonia than crackles, especially in the ICU [91]. In patients with CAP, an admission respiratory rate greater than 30 breaths per minute is an important negative prognostic feature, and in some studies mortality increases dramatically when respiratory rate exceeds this level [92]. Signs of pleural effusion are particularly common with *H. influenzae*, pneumococcal, streptococcal, and aspergillus pneumonia, where pleural friction rubs may be detected. Pleural involvement can be seen, although less often, in *Legionella* and *M. pneumonia*. Relative bradycardia is a frequent finding in many pneumonias caused by *Mycoplasma*, *Legionella*, and *Chlamydophila* organisms [93].

Dermatologic manifestations (erythema nodosum, erythema multiforme, and skin nodules) may be observed with *Mycoplasma*, fungal, *Nocardia*, and tuberculous infections. Horder spots (pale macular rash), long considered part of the presentation of psittacosis, should lead the clinician to look for other evidence of this infection. Ecthyma gangrenosum, an indurated, round skin lesion with a central dark area surrounded by erythema, is characteristic of Gram-negative septicemia, especially with *P. aeruginosa*. Central nervous system abnormalities can be found in infections with pneumococcus, *M. tuberculosis*, *H. influenzae*, Gram-negative organisms, cryptococci, *Aspergillus* sp., *Legionella* sp., *Toxoplasma gondii*, varicella zoster, and cytomegalovirus (CMV). Other physical findings that narrow the differential diagnosis include splenomegaly in the case of psittacosis and tularemia, herpes labialis in pneumococcal infection, bullous myringitis with *M. pneumoniae* infection, and lymphadenopathy with tularemia. The predictive value of many of these observations has not been evaluated rigorously (Table 181.6).

Routine Diagnostic Testing

The IDSA/ATS guidelines for CAP recommend a relatively streamlined evaluation, including chest radiograph, routine blood chemistries and blood counts, blood cultures (for the critically ill), assessment of oxygenation (oximetry or blood gas), and a clinical evaluation of severity of illness. Although the routine use of sputum culture or Gram stain of sputum is not recommended, these tests should be done for critically ill patients to identify unusual or drug-resistant organisms. If a sputum sample is obtained, it should be prior to therapy, rapidly transported to the lab, and of good quality with little evidence of oral contamination. The critically ill, intubated patient should have an endotracheal aspirate sent for culture, and *Legionella* and pneumococcal urinary antigen testing should be considered. The routine use of serologic testing is not encouraged [5]. The impact of diagnostic testing for patients with severe CAP remains uncertain, and several studies have shown that even when the etiologic diagnosis is known, outcome may not be affected, whereas the use of early and effective empirical therapy has been associated with improved outcomes [5,40]. However, Rello et al. have shown that knowing the etiologic pathogen can help to focus and simplify treatment in nearly one-third of cases of severe CAP [93].

Most routine laboratory results are not specific for individual pathogens, and the focus of diagnostic testing is to assess disease severity. Extremes of white blood cell count (<4,000 or >30,000 per μL) may indicate overwhelming sepsis and may be a poor prognostic finding [5]. Elevated liver function tests are not a specific finding but can be seen in a variety of viral and bacterial pneumonias, including those associated with *Legionella* sp., *M. tuberculosis*, *Mycoplasma* sp., Q fever, tularemia, and psittacosis, as well as in pneumococcal infection. Similarly, electrolyte disturbances, including hypophosphatemia and hyponatremia, are not predictive of a specific pathogen for the individual patient with pneumonia, but hyponatremia (<130 mEq per L) on admission may predict a poor outcome [94].

Serology, Urinary Antigen, and PCR Testing

As mentioned, routine serologic testing is not recommended because results are rarely positive at the time of presentation (i.e., convalescent serologic testing is usually needed), and even if positive, results are usually not available during the first 24 to 48 hours of critical illness [5]. Serologic responses are useful for retrospective epidemiologic purposes to document viral and so-called atypical pathogen infection and may be useful if the patient is not responding to appropriate empiric therapy (discussed later). Many patients with CAP have serologic evidence for recent atypical pathogen infection, but in the setting of an illness like *Legionella* pneumonia, convalescent titers are essential and less than 10% of those with acute illness have a positive serologic result. To make the diagnosis of *Legionella* pneumonia acutely, urinary antigen testing has the highest yield (approximately 50%), but is specific for serogroup I infection [5]. The direct immunofluorescent stain of sputum for *L. pneumophila* has a sensitivity of between 25% and 50% and a specificity of more than 90% for this organism. The urinary antigen for the detection of pneumococcal pneumonia has also been described for patients with severe disease, asplenia, liver disease, alcoholism, or leukopenia. Genetic probes for specific viral DNA and RNA are available for CMV, varicella zoster, herpes simplex, influenza virus, and adenovirus.

Chest Radiographic Interpretation

The chest radiograph is essential for the diagnosis of pneumonia for the critically ill patient (Table 181.7), and the use of pattern reading can help to narrow the differential diagnosis of CAP and HAP, particularly when used in concert with other available information. For example, the rapid development of a diffuse alveolar pattern frequently implies a hematogenously disseminated infection such as varicella or CMV, or the development of ARDS as a pneumonic complication. Hyperinflation is characteristic of respiratory syncytial virus pneumonia. A more subacute presentation of diffuse alveolar infiltrates may represent hematogenous dissemination of tuberculosis. *P. jiroveci* must be considered in the setting of a diffuse alveolar or reticulonodular pattern for groups at risk for HIV infection. Noninfectious causes of pulmonary infiltrates such as heart failure, bronchiolitis obliterans and organizing pneumonia (BOOP), drug toxicity, and lymphangitic carcinomatosis can also have this presentation. Focal infiltrates (i.e., confined to single segments or lobes) are most likely to represent bacterial pneumonia related to microaspiration into a particular area of the lung.

Acute bacterial pneumonias generally progress more rapidly (hours to days) than fungal or mycobacterial infections (days to weeks). Pleural effusions occur commonly in *H. influenzae* pneumonia (>50%) and pneumococcal infection (25%) but can also be seen in patients with group A streptococcal pneumonia. Cavitation can occur in both infectious and noninfectious lung disease, but the finding of multiple cavitary nodules suggests septic embolization from right-sided endocarditis. Rapid cavitation is also common among Gram-negative pneumonias, whereas a subacute course with cavitation suggests anaerobic or mycobacterial infection. Cavitation and necrotizing pneumonia also are present in CA-MRSA pneumonia, and its presence is often used to guide initial empirical antibiotic treatment. Occasionally, ventilator-associated bacterial pneumonia can progress rapidly and fatally, emphasizing the need for timely recognition and therapy. Chronic cavitation (weeks to months) is more likely due to a noninfectious problem, such as carcinoma, lymphoma, or granulomatosis with polyangiitis (Wegener granulomatosis), especially in the absence of the systemic signs of acute infection.

The limitations of the chest radiograph for critically ill patients are considerable, especially for the detection of VAP, when the clinician must rely on a portable film, which may not

TABLE 181.7

Radiographic Patterns in Diagnosis of Pneumonia

Diffuse infiltrates		
Acute	**Chronic**	
Pneumocystis jiroveci pneumonia Viral Cardiogenic edema Drug reaction Alveolar hemorrhage	Tuberculosis (typical or atypical) Fungi Radiation injury Drug reaction Lymphangitic cancer	
Focal infiltrates		
Acute	**Chronic**	**Cavitation**
Streptococcus pneumoniae *Staphylococcus aureus* *Legionella* sp. Gram-negative bacilli Lung infarction Bronchiolitis obliterans and organizing pneumonia	Fungi Tuberculosis Malignancy	Fungi/*Nocardia* sp. Anaerobes Gram-negative bacilli *S. aureus* Tuberculosis Malignancy Wegener granulomatosis

show findings very clearly. Also, among ICU patients, coexisting and preexisting lung disease may obscure the findings of pneumonia. Chest radiographs are of limited value for predicting the causative pathogen of CAP, but are useful for determining the extent of pneumonia and detecting complications such as parapneumonic effusions [95]. CT scans of the chest generally have a higher sensitivity for diagnosing occult pneumonia, with an initially negative chest radiograph [96].

Sputum Examination and Evaluation of Other Respiratory Secretions

Although Gram stain of the sputum has been the traditional first step for the evaluation of patients with suspected pneumonia, this is problematic for the critically ill patient who is not intubated and may be unable to expectorate. When a specimen is obtained from a nonintubated patient, the sample should have more than 25 polymorphonuclear cells and less than 10 epithelial cells per low-power field. When such criteria are met and intracellular organisms are identified, a bacterial density above 10^5 colony-forming units per mL of secretions is usually present [5]. In addition to not always being able to distinguish airway colonization from pneumonia, the sputum Gram stain may be falsely negative up to 50% of the time compared with blood cultures. Some findings from the sputum may suggest specific etiologies. For example, an inflammatory Gram stain (polymorphonuclear cells) without organisms in a patient with pneumonia is presumptive evidence of an atypical (*Legionella* or *Mycoplasma*) or viral cause. Gram stain may be best used to broaden initial empirical therapy, rather than to narrow it, especially if an unusual pathogen that is not routinely treated is thought to be present. For example, the finding of Gram-positive cocci in clusters in a patient with influenza would lead to empiric therapy for *S. aureus*. The use of special stains for tuberculosis and silver or staining for *P. jiroveci* may provide definitive evidence for these organisms. With the use of rapid point-of-care diagnostic tests for influenza virus, treatment and chemoprevention can be offered. Rapid influenza testing can sometimes differentiate influenza A from influenza B and this can guide treatment decision. Other diseases caused by agents of bioterrorism and endemic diseases can be identified by examination of respiratory secretions.

Cultures

A definitive etiologic diagnosis of pneumonia can be made when cultures of blood, pleural fluid, or spinal fluid are positive in the presence of a lung infiltrate and a compatible clinical picture. Bacteremia is uncommon for most pneumonias, occurring among less than 15% of patients with CAP, in 20% of pneumococcal infections, and in only 8% to 15% of NPs [97]. For CAP initial PCT levels on admission may predict risk for bacteremia with levels of <0.25 mg per L identifying patients at very low risk for bacteremic episodes [98]. In a study including 3,786 patients from two large prospective studies, predictors of bacteremia with CAP were found to be younger age, high C-reactive protein, leukocytosis or leukopenia, low platelet count, low sodium level, elevated urea, and elevated arterial pH [99]. Among those with NP, the presence of bacteremia may imply an extrapulmonary infection, especially when the organism presents in the blood culture is different from the one in the respiratory tract. Blood cultures are indicated for all patients admitted to the ICU with a diagnosis of pneumonia but are most valuable if collected prior to antibiotic therapy [100].

Sputum cultures can be difficult to interpret because of the problem of separating infection from colonization among the critically ill. In a study of bacteremic NP, sputum culture yielded both false-positive and false-negative findings compared with blood cultures, with only 49% of the cases having the same organism recovered from both blood and sputum [97]. Among intubated patients, colonization is present after several days, so the culture should be interpreted in the clinical context of the patient, and a sample should not be cultured in the absence of clinical signs of infection. Viruses may be cultured from respiratory secretions, but this procedure may take up to 20 days, depending on the virus. Thus, cytologic evidence of viral infection that can be recognized sooner may provide helpful information. For example, inclusion bodies and multinucleated giant cells are suggestive of CMV or herpesvirus infection.

Invasive Diagnostic Sampling and Quantitative Cultures

Because of the inherent problems distinguishing colonizing from infecting pathogens in samples of lower respiratory tract secretions, investigators have advocated for the collection of deep respiratory secretions through invasive (bronchoscopic) or semi-invasive (catheter-lavage) means, combined with analysis of the results using quantitative cultures. Bronchoscopic sampling has been used for the critically ill, particularly among those who are immunosuppressed or who already have an endotracheal tube in place, such as patients with VAP and severe CAP. Cultures are obtained by using the bronchoscopically directed PSB, or bronchoalveolar lavage (BAL), and the samples cultured quantitatively. When PSB samples are cultured quantitatively, patients with NP will have greater than 10^3 organisms per mL of respiratory secretions. When BAL is used, a threshold concentration of 10^4 to 10^5 organisms per mL is used to define pneumonia [4]. In some studies, lower airway cells recovered by lavage have been examined for the presence of intracellular organisms, and the finding of more than 5% to 25% of cells with intracellular bacteria may predict the diagnosis of pneumonia, confirmed by PSB. Quantitative endotracheal aspirates have also been used, particularly for patients with severe nursing home pneumonia, and this technique has a very good correlation with results of BAL when a threshold of 10^4 colony-forming organisms per mL is used [4,101]. Although the role of bronchoscopy for patients with suspected VAP is still controversial, most investigators agree that BAL is valuable for establishing a nonbacterial cause of infection, especially for the immunocompromised host or the patient with HIV infection, where it can reliably diagnose *P. jiroveci* pneumonia and CMV infection [102].

Quantitative cultures have been proposed as the most accurate way to establish the presence of VAP and to define the etiologic pathogen. Although the clinical diagnosis of VAP has been much maligned, it may be very accurate, particularly when it is objectively defined by calculating the CPIS and if the score incorporates a Gram stain of a lower respiratory tract sample [103]. Once the clinical diagnosis of VAP is made, a culture is needed to identify the etiologic pathogen, but this culture could be quantitative or semiquantitative (light, moderate, or heavy growth), and collected as an endotracheal aspirate or via bronchoscopy or catheter lavage. Studies of the impact of quantitative culture methods on VAP outcome have been mixed, but a meta-analysis showed no effect on mortality [104]. Singh et al. used clinical diagnosis and management with the CPIS and showed that patients with suspected VAP and a low score could be safely managed with a short course of antibiotics [105]. In a large multicenter trial, Heyland et al. compared management of VAP using cultures obtained via endotracheal aspirates with those obtained by BAL [106]. They found no difference of mortality between the two groups, and similar rates of adjusting antibiotic therapy after initial empiric management. Unlike an earlier study, in this investigation, all patients initially received antibiotic therapy, so cultures were used to adjust antibiotics but never to withhold them. One of the limitations of these data is that less than 15% had MDR pathogen pneumonia. A recent systematic review using Cochrane Database including five randomized controlled trials with 1367 VAP patients, comparing quantitative microbiologic sample to qualitative sampling found no differences of mortality, ICU length of stay, or higher rates of antibiotic change between the two groups [107]. Fewer studies have been done to investigate the impact of quantitative lower respiratory secretion cultures for patients with severe CAP. Rello et al. have shown that information from bronchoscopic sampling can help to narrow and focus antibiotic therapy for patients with severe CAP [93]. However, among patients with severe CAP, PSB and BAL only give an etiologic diagnosis in one-quarter to one-third of all patients (which is less than with sputum or endotracheal aspirate cultures), but among this group, antibiotics were changed in nearly 75%.

Guidelines for NP have recommended that all patients have a lower respiratory tract sample collected prior to starting therapy, and that the technique and culture method should be one that the clinician is expert at performing and interpreting. Lower respiratory tract cultures can be obtained bronchoscopically or nonbronchoscopically and can be cultured quantitatively or semiquantitatively. Quantitative cultures increase specificity of the diagnosis of HAP but may potentially delay the initiation of therapy for patients with early pneumonia. Nonquantitative cultures are sensitive but may lead to some colonizing organisms being treated. Regardless of which method is used, it should only be initiated once the clinician has made a clinical diagnosis of pneumonia and is ready to initiate therapy. Therapy should be prompt and not delayed for the purpose of collecting a diagnostic sample, especially for patients who are clinically unstable or septic from pneumonia [4].

Percutaneous needle aspiration of the lung in an area of infiltrate has also been studied, but it is limited by a high incidence of false-negative results and an unacceptable complication rates, including pneumothorax in up to 30% of patients and a 10% rate of hemoptysis. Although open lung biopsy is the unequivocal standard for the diagnosis of infection, it has been applied primarily for the immunocompromised host with rapidly advancing, life-threatening infection. *Aspergillus*, CMV, herpes simplex, and *T. gondii* infections are more readily diagnosed by open lung biopsy than by other described techniques. For patients with CAP, open lung biopsy is rarely needed, and its potential for demonstrating a treatable infection that will alter outcome is low, and similar findings have been reported when it is used in patients with HAP [108] (Table 181.8).

Lung Ultrasound (LUS)

Bedside, noninvasive, real time echography of the lung is increasingly being adopted by intensivists for diagnosing pleural and pulmonary diseases. Various patterns with B and M mode ultrasound techniques including—"tissue sign" and "dynamic airbronchograms" are seen with pulmonary consolidation. (The utility of lung ultrasound for diagnosis of pneumonia is reviewed in Chapter 11.) Multiple studies have compared LUS to CT chest and the sensitivity and specificity ranges from 90% to 100% [109]. Reissig and associates in a prospective, multicenter study, including 362 patients with suspected CAP found LUS to have a sensitivity of 93.4% and specificity of 97.7% compared to chest X-ray and CT chest [110]. In another study, investigators proposed a new score for diagnosing VAP using PCT level and chest echography: the Chest Echography and Procalcitonin Pulmonary Infection Score (CEPPIS) [111]. In that study, a CEPPIS >5 performed better than CPIS >6 for diagnosing VAP (OR, 23.78; sensitivity, 80.5%; specificity, 85.2%) [111]. Although LUS is operator dependent, a recent meta-analysis of 10 studies with 1,172 patients supports the use of LUS by skilled practitioners [112].

Ventilator Associated Events

A CDC working group has proposed monitoring for a new entity, ventilator associated events (VAE), in order to "objectively" measure the complications related to mechanical ventilation, as an alternative to looking for VAP, which as discussed, is difficult to define. VAE is recognized by assessing for worsening oxygenation (defined by ventilator settings and not by physiologic measurements) and systemic signs of infection [113]. VAE includes VAC, infectious ventilator-associated complications (IVAC), and probable, as well as possible VAP (Table 181.9). Muscedere et al. studied the clinical impact and preventability of VAC and IVAC, and the relationship to VAP, using prospectively collected data from 1,320 patients [114]. They found VAC developed in 10.5% and patients who had VAC were more likely to develop VAP than those who

TABLE 181.8

Diagnostic Techniques in Pneumonia

Test	Advantages	Disadvantages
Expectorated sputum Gram stain	Easy to perform; rapidly available; inexpensive	High false-positive and false-negative rates
Expectorated sputum culture	Easy to obtain	High false-positive and false-negative rates
Blood culture	High specificity	Low sensitivity, not always a lung source
Transtracheal aspiration	Less contamination than expectorated sputum	High false-positive rates in colonized patients; bleeding; impractical to do
Needle aspiration (percutaneous)	High specificity; useful for children and malignancy	High risk of pneumothorax especially in patients with chronic obstructive pulmonary disease and in ventilated patients; not widely done
Bronchoscopy (protected brush, bronchoalveolar lavage [BAL])	Low morbidity and mortality; useful in ventilated patients and for nonbacteriologic diagnosis and in compromised host	"Invasive"; requires special training; less useful if patient already on antibiotics; wide range of sensitivity; may bias against the treatment of early infection
Nonbronchoscopic BAL	May give quantitative culture data in ventilated patients; can be done any time of the day by respiratory therapists or physicians	Variable accuracy, assumes that random sampling is reflective of bacteriology throughout the lung; same benefits/disadvantages of relying on other quantitative methods
Open lung biopsy	Excellent for nonbacterial diagnosis and in compromised host	Most invasive; critically ill may not be able to undergo procedure; may not change prognosis

TABLE 181.9

New CDC definition for Ventilator associated Events

Ventilator-associated complication	At least *one of the* following indicators of *worsening oxygenation*: 1. Minimum daily FiO_2 values increase ≥0.20 (20 points) over baseline and remains at or above that increased level for ≥2 calendar days. 2. Minimum daily PEEP values increase ≥3 cm H_2O over baseline and remains at or above that increased level for ≥2 calendar days.
Infection-related ventilator-associated complication	Patient has VAC and also fits *both* of the two following criteria: 1. Temperature greater than 38°C or WBC greater than 12,000 or less than 4,000/μL. 2. A new antimicrobial agent is started and is continued for 4 or more calendar days.
Possible VAP	On or after calendar day 3 of mechanical ventilation and within 2 calendar days before or after the onset of worsening oxygenation, *one* of the following criteria is met: 1. Purulent respiratory secretions (defined as secretions from the lungs, bronchi, or trachea that contain >25 neutrophils and <10 squamous epithelial cells per low power field [lpf, ×100]; If the laboratory reports semiquantitative results, those results must be equivalent to the above quantitative thresholds). 2. Positive culture (qualitative, semiquantitative or quantitative) of sputum, endotracheal aspirate, bronchoalveolar lavage, lung tissue, or protected specimen brushing.
Probable VAP	On or after calendar day 3 of mechanical ventilation and within 2 calendar days before or after the onset of worsening oxygenation, ONE of the following criteria is met: 1. Purulent respiratory secretions (from one or more specimen collections—and defined as for possible VAP) AND one of the following: Positive culture of endotracheal aspirate, ≥10^5 CFU/mL or equivalent semiquantitative result, or positive culture of bronchoalveolar lavage, ≥10^4 CFU/mL or equivalent semiquantitative result, or positive culture of lung tissue, ≥10^4 CFU/mL or equivalent semiquantitative result, or positive culture of protected specimen brush, ≥10^3 CFU/mL or equivalent semiquantitative result. 2. One of the following (without requirement for purulent respiratory secretions): positive pleural fluid culture (where specimen was obtained during thoracentesis or initial placement of chest tube and NOT from an indwelling chest tube), or positive lung histopathology, or positive diagnostic test for *Legionella* spp., or positive diagnostic test on respiratory secretions for influenza virus, respiratory syncytial virus, adenovirus, and parainfluenza virus.

CDC, Centers for Disease Control and Prevention; PEEP, positive end-expiratory pressure; VAP, ventilator-associated pneumonia.

did not (28.1% vs. 9.2%, $p < 0.001$). However, only 39 of 139 with VAC had VAP, and most patients with VAP did not have VAC or IVAC. When prevention efforts were undertaken, they were able to reduce the incidence of VAC and VAP, but not IVAC. In another study, patients with VAC had a higher ICU length of stay (22 vs. 11 days), duration of mechanical ventilation (20 vs. 5 days), and use of antibiotics than non-VAC patients, but no difference of overall ICU mortality

[115]. VAC definitions were not specific for VAP and included atelectasis in 16.3%, acute pulmonary edema in 11.8%, and acute respiratory distress syndrome in 6.5%. Thus the VAC definition identified sick patients, but not all VAC patients had pneumonia. In a recent study only 32% of patients with VAP identified by prospective surveillance were detected using the VAE algorithm [116]. Bouadma and associates analyzed a large prospective cohort of ventilated patients, and found a significant correlation between VAP and IVAC episodes [117]. Although the VAE definitions track episodes of sustained respiratory deterioration among mechanically ventilated patients after a period of stability or improvement, VAC and IVAC are not always VAP, and the prevention efforts for VAP do not always affect VAC and IVAC rates, raising doubt about the utility of these new definitions as a measure of the quality of care for ventilated patients [118].

Differential Diagnosis

In the evaluation of a patient with lung infiltrates, it is necessary to determine (a) if it is pneumonia, or another infiltrative or inflammatory process, that is responsible for the constellation of symptoms and signs being evaluated and (b) if it is pneumonia, what is the etiologic pathogen. Since the features of pneumonia are nonspecific, it is necessary to consider such alternative noninfectious processes such as aspiration with chemical pneumonitis, acute pulmonary embolism, pulmonary infarction, pulmonary hemorrhage, ARDS, CHF, BOOP, radiation pneumonitis, bronchoalveolar carcinoma, and atelectasis. An increasingly common problem is the differentiation of acute infectious pneumonia from drug-induced pneumonitis caused by agents such as amiodarone, bleomycin, busulfan, methotrexate, and newer cancer treatments, such as immune checkpoint inhibitors.

Among immunocompromised patients, a new lung infiltrate may represent infection, progression of the underlying primary disease, or drug-induced lung disease. As for all patients, the nature of the immune impairment determines which pathogens are most likely. Although *P. jiroveci* pneumonia is a cause of rapidly progressive hypoxemic respiratory failure in the patient with HIV infection, a similar picture may be seen with tuberculosis, and pneumococcus is also a common respiratory pathogen among these patients [119]. Many have suggested that tuberculosis is poorly recognized in the intensive care setting and should be considered for patients with a history of inadequately treated tuberculosis or radiographic evidence of previous infection. The use of corticosteroid therapy in doses more than 20 mg per day increases the risk of opportunistic fungi, with reports stressing the occurrence of invasive aspergillosis among patients receiving high-dose steroid therapy for exacerbations of COPD. Patients with impaired B-cell function such as multiple myeloma are particularly prone to pneumonia with encapsulated organisms, including pneumococcus and *H. influenzae*. A similar organism profile can be seen among splenectomized patients and among those with complement defects. Even in the setting of established pneumonia, patients may have a second infectious process such as extrapulmonary infection (catheter-associated bacteremia) or complications of antibiotic therapy, such as antibiotic-induced colitis.

THERAPY

Supportive Therapies

Supportive therapies for pneumonia in the critically ill are crucial, because the use of antibiotics may not impact the course of disease during the first 24 to 72 hours of treatment. Many of the commonly applied measures are based on traditional practice, with little documentation of efficacy.

Nutritional Support

Evidence implicating malnutrition as a cofactor for pneumonia is substantial, but the evidence that nutritional intervention alters the outcome of severe pneumonia is lacking [69]. Enteral nutrition is preferred, if this can be practically accomplished, because data suggest better preservation of immune function using this route compared with total parenteral nutrition [120]. When enteral feedings are given, a small-bore tube, preferably placed in the small bowel, should be used along with a continuous infusion method to prevent aspiration and to optimize the delivery of calories [121]. All patients should be kept semierect (greater than 30 degrees upright) and not supine as much as possible, to reduce the risk of reflux and aspiration [58]. The optimal time for initiating enteral feeding has not been determined.

Chest Physiotherapy

There is little support for the routine application of chest physiotherapy in patients who have an effective cough and scant amounts of respiratory secretions. Because of the labor-intensive nature of this intervention, techniques such as percussion, vibration, and postural drainage should be specifically targeted to patients with large volumes of purulent secretions (>30 mL per day) and an ineffective clearance by coughing. For patients at bed rest in the ICU, the use of positioning and rotation may be helpful for clearing secretions. In several studies, particularly of surgical trauma patients, the preventive use of beds that rotate patients from side to side, and presumably accelerate mucus clearance, has led to a reduced incidence of NP [122].

Aerosols and Humidification

Humidification has been a traditional practice of respiratory therapy aimed at reducing sputum viscosity and promoting mucociliary clearance. Because the deposition of water vapor depends on particle size and the degree of airway obstruction, it is likely that most aerosols are deposited above the glottis and act only to stimulate cough. Although mucolytic agents such as acetylcysteine offer the theoretic benefit of reducing the viscosity of purulent secretions, they may act as irritants that can provoke bronchospasm, and thus must be used selectively. Bronchodilator therapy with β_2 agents can enhance mucociliary clearance and ciliary beat frequency, but there have been no controlled trials that have demonstrated improved outcomes with their use for pneumonia, in the absence of underlying bronchospasm. The greatest benefit of bronchodilator therapy may be expected in the patient with COPD in whom pneumonia develops.

Antibiotic and Other Pharmacologic Therapies

Among the critically ill, timely initiation of appropriate antimicrobial therapy has been shown to improve survival for patients with both severe CAP and VAP [4,5,42]. Because it is often impossible to identify a specific etiologic agent at the time that therapy is started, initial therapy is necessarily empirical but can be modified and focused (de-escalated) once the results of diagnostic testing become available. The ATS and IDSA have developed algorithms for initial empiric therapies of severe pneumonia arising in both the community and the hospital.

Community-Acquired Pneumonia

Because the use of clinical syndromes or sputum Gram stain to guide therapy is often inaccurate and not recommended, initial therapy is empirical, based on the likely etiologic pathogens. For patients treated in the ICU, monotherapy is not recommended, regardless of agent, all patients require initial therapy directed at pneumococcus (including DRSP), atypical pathogens (especially *Legionella*), *H. influenzae*, and enteric Gram-negatives (including *P. aeruginosa* for some patients). For selected patients, particularly following influenza or other viral infections, empirical therapy for *S. aureus*, including MRSA, may be necessary. Aspiration pneumonia, including anaerobic pathogens, can occasionally present as severe illness, needing ICU care. Endemic viruses can also cause severe CAP, and the use of antiviral agents depends on local epidemiology and whether influenza or another viral agent is suggested by rapid testing or is prevalent at the time that the patient is being evaluated. Among the critically ill, initial therapy is determined by whether the patient has risks for *P. aeruginosa*, which include structural lung disease (bronchiectasis), therapy with broad-spectrum antibiotics for more than 7 days in the last month, use of corticosteroids (>10 mg of prednisone daily), malnutrition, or HIV infection [5].

For the patient with severe CAP, mixed infection, involving a bacterial pathogen and an atypical pathogen, is also common and should be covered by the initial empiric regimen. Every patient should receive therapy directed at these organisms, which can be either as a primary pathogen or copathogen, but studies have shown that the use of a macrolide may be of specific value. In patients with bacteremic pneumococcal pneumonia, particularly in those with severe illness, dual therapy including a macrolide has been associated with improved outcomes [123,124]. A quinolone can also be used to treat atypical pathogen infection and may have an advantage for the patient with suspected *Legionella* infection, where the outcomes using quinolones have been exceptionally good [125].

When the patient has no risk factors for *Pseudomonas*, therapy should be with an intravenous β-lactam (ceftriaxone or cefotaxime) with activity against DRSP plus either intravenous azithromycin or an intravenous quinolone (levofloxacin 750 mg or moxifloxacin 400 mg). When the patient has risk factors for *Pseudomonas*, therapy should involve two antipseudomonal agents, in addition to providing coverage for DRSP and *Legionella* [5]. For these patients, therapy can be a two-drug regimen, using a selected antipseudomonal β-lactam (cefepime, piperacillin/tazobactam, imipenem, and meropenem), in combination with an antipseudomonal quinolone (ciprofloxacin, high-dose levofloxacin 750 mg daily). Alternatively, the above-mentioned β-lactams can be combined with an aminoglycoside and either azithromycin or an antipneumococcal quinolone (levofloxacin 750 mg or moxifloxacin 400 mg). For the penicillin-allergic patient, aztreonam can be combined with an aminoglycoside and an antipneumococcal fluoroquinolone [5]. Occasionally, these broad-empiric approaches should be modified, particularly when clinical or culture data suggest an organism that is not included in the initial regimen (e.g., *S. aureus* or MRSA). In addition, certain comorbidities predispose to specific pathogens, and these should be covered by the chosen empiric regimen (see Table 181.4).

In a recent cluster-randomized crossover study, Postma and colleagues compared β-lactam monotherapy (BL, $n = 656$), β-lactam–macrolide combination therapy (BLM, $n = 739$), and fluoroquinolone monotherapy (FQ, $n = 889$) for hospitalized non-ICU CAP patients [126]. The investigators found no difference in 90 day mortality between the three groups (BL = 9%, BLM = 11% and FQ = 8.8%), but 38.7% of patients in β-lactam monotherapy group received an additional agent during their hospital stay for atypical coverage, which was not considered a deviation from the protocol. Adrie et al. compared the impact of dual (β-lactam plus macrolide or fluoroquinolone [$n = 394$]) versus monotherapy (β-lactam alone [$n = 471$]) forimmunocompetent severe CAP, and there was no difference of 60-day mortality between the two groups [127]. However, there was survival advantage for patients, who had initial adequate antibiotic therapy and those who received dual therapy had a higher frequency of initial adequate antibiotics. In another report, Garin et al. found patients treated with β-lactam monotherapy were less likely to reach clinical stability compared to β-lactam–macrolide combination, if they were infected with atypical pathogens or if they had severe pneumonia with PSI category IV [128]. Sligl and colleagues conducted a meta-analysis of macrolide use for severe CAP, including 28 studies and nearly 10,000 patients [129]. They found a significant reduction of mortality from 24% to 21% ($p < 0.05$) when a macrolide was used in this patient population.

As mentioned earlier, no patient with severe CAP should receive monotherapy, even with a quinolone, since studies have not proven the efficacy of this approach [130]. Although quinolones are acceptable as monotherapy for patients who are not critically ill, it is currently uncertain if the outcome is different when a quinolone is used in place of macrolide, as part of a combination regimen for patients in the ICU. Moxifloxacin is safe and efficacious for CAP, even for the elderly, but few patients with severe CAP have been studied with monotherapy. In the Community-Acquired Pneumonia Recovery in the Elderly (CAPRIE) study, comparing moxifloxacin with levofloxacin for CAP among the elderly who were hospitalized outside of the ICU, although the cure rate for moxifloxacin (94.7%) was greater than levofloxacin (84.6%) in the severe CAP subgroup, the difference was not statistically significant [131]. One study of nearly 400 patients with severe CAP compared monotherapy with high-dose levofloxacin (500 mg twice daily) with the combination of ceftriaxone/ofloxacin, and although an equivalent clinical response was observed in both treatment groups (79.1% with levofloxacin compared with 79.5% with combination therapy), patients with shock were excluded from the study, and among patients with mechanical ventilation, treatment with levofloxacin resulted in a lower clinical cure rate (63% compared with 72% with combination therapy) [130]. Therefore, quinolone monotherapy is not recommended for patients with severe CAP, especially in the setting of septic shock and respiratory failure.

In one report, the use of initial empiric therapy with a β-lactam plus a fluoroquinolone for severe CAP was associated with increased short-term mortality (OR, 2.71; 95% confidence interval, 1.2 to 6.1), compared to other guideline-recommended antimicrobial regimes [132]. On the other hand, a meta-analysis of 23 randomized trials of CAP therapy outside the ICU compared the use of fluoroquinolones with other antibiotics, including β-lactams, macrolides, or both. Although there was no mortality difference in favor of the fluoroquinolones, for patients with more severe pneumonia, those who required hospitalization and those requiring intravenous therapy, the quinolones were more effective [133].

If DRSP is present, any of the recommended regimens will be effective. Although pneumococcal resistance to multiple agents is present at rates up to 40%, using older definitions of resistance, the outcome in CAP is generally not worsened by the presence of penicillin-resistant organisms, compared with penicillin-sensitive organisms, and that these resistant organisms can still be effectively treated by high doses of penicillin, amoxicillin, amoxicillin/clavulanate, the third-generation cephalosporins (ceftriaxone or cefotaxime), or the antipneumococcal fluoroquinolones [5]. If highly resistant pneumococcus (but not cephalosporin resistant) is documented and meningitis is present, therapy should be initiated with vancomycin, cefotaxime, or ceftriaxone. Discordant therapy of DRSP usually has no impact on outcomes, but even for studies when it was independently associated with death (OR, 27.3), it was very unlikely that discordant therapy would be given with ceftriaxone or cefotaxime [134]. Ceftriaxone is usually used at doses of 1 to 2 mg per day, but if DRSP and severe infection are present, the dose can be increased to 2 g every 12 hours. A notable exception to using cephalosporins for severe CAP is cefuroxime. Yu et al. [135] studied patients with bacteremic pneumococcal pneumonia, and found that discordant therapy with cefuroxime did increase mortality in the presence of in vitro resistance. *H. influenzae* is also becoming increasingly resistant to common antimicrobials because of the production of β-lactamases, and these organisms can be treated with second- or third-generation cephalosporins, quinolones, macrolides, or ampicillin/sulbactam. Other new antibiotics may become available for the therapy of CAP. Tigecycline is a novel glycylcycline antibacterial agent, with an expanded broad spectrum of activity including proven utility against Gram-positive, Gram-negative, anaerobic, and atypical pathogens. It is effective in vitro against clinically important community- and hospital-acquired resistant organisms—*Acinetobacter*, MRSA, DRSP, vancomycin-resistant *Enterococcus* spp., *E. coli*, and *K. pneumoniae* expressing extended-spectrum β-lactamases (ESBLs). Currently, it is approved for CAP, but not as monotherapy for NP [136]. New anti-Staphylococcal agents are also being developed, and may have utility for severe CAP, including telavancin and ceftaroline [137]. Ceftaroline fosamil is a cephalosporin approved by FDA for use in the treatment of acute bacterial skin infections and CAP [138]. Nemonoxacin is a newly developed quinolone with broad-spectrum activity against Gram-positive, Gram-negative and atypical pathogens, including drug-resistant *S. pneumoniae* and methicillin-resistant Staphylococcus aureus, and is being investigated in pneumonia [139].

Duration of Treatment

Currently there are insufficient data on the appropriate duration of treatment for critically ill CAP patients. Generally, *S. pneumoniae* can be treated for 5 to 7 days if the patient is responding rapidly and has received the correct dose of an accurate therapy. Longer duration of treatment is necessitated by the presence of extrapulmonary infection (e.g., meningitis), and the identification of certain pathogens (such as bacteremic *S. aureus* and *P. aeruginosa*). *L. pneumophila* pneumonia may require at least 14 days of therapy, although shorter duration therapy has been effective using quinolones. Antibiotics can be switched from intravenous to oral once the patient is afebrile for at least two occasions 8 hours apart, is able to take food by mouth, and there are clinical signs of improvement [140]. Initial PCT level may accurately predict positive blood cultures among pneumonia patients and serial measurements help with antibiotic de-escalation and withdrawal in CAP patients [98,141]. In a randomized trial of antibiotic therapy in the ICU, PCT-guidance led to a reduction in duration of therapy compared to standard care for all patients, including those with severe CAP [142]. A recent meta-analysis of 14 randomized trials favored a PCT based treatment algorithm for antibiotic de-escalation without an increase in either mortality or treatment failures [143].

Treatment of Community-Acquired Methicillin-resistant S. aureus

Patients with recent influenza should be treated for *S. aureus*, including community-acquired methicillin-resistant *S. aureus* (CA-MRSA), in addition to the other usual severe CAP pathogens. CA-MRSA is different from nosocomial MRSA, as it occurs in previously healthy people, can carry the Panton–Valentine leukocidin gene (a virulence factor which is associated with tissue necrosis), and causes a necrotizing, often bilateral severe pneumonia [70]. The best therapy for CA-MRSA is unclear, but the options include vancomycin, linezolid, or the combination of vancomycin and clindamycin. The latter two regimens have the ability to inhibit bacterial toxin synthesis (by linezolid or clindamycin), which may be part of the pathogenesis of severe CA-MRSA infection, but current recommendations are not definitive about whether antitoxin therapy is needed [5]. In a recent study of 133 patients with PVL positive CAP, treatment with antibiotics having antitoxin effects (clindamycin, rifampin, and linezolid) was associated with a reduced mortality compared to those who did not get antitoxin therapy (6.1% vs. 52.3%, $p < 0.001$), although only about one-third of patients received this therapy [144].

Role of Steroids for CAP

The role of low-dose (replacement) steroids in septic shock has been the topic of numerous studies, and relative adrenal insufficiency occurs in a high proportion of patients with severe CAP [145]. Salluh et al. [146] have shown that in patients with severe CAP, median cortisol levels were 15.5 μg per dL, and 65% of patients met the criteria for adrenal insufficiency (cortisol levels <20 μg per dL). When patients with septic shock were evaluated, 63% had adrenal insufficiency. A recent meta-analysis of nine trials involving 1,001 patients did not support routine use of corticosteroids for CAP patients, but may improve mortality in a subset with severe CAP [147]. Torres and associates in a randomized, prospective study found that in patients with severe CAP and high levels of inflammation (elevated CRP >15 mg per L) at admission, administration of intravenous methylprednisolone (bolus of 0.5 mg/kg/12 h) led to less treatment failure compared to placebo, but there was no significant difference in hospital mortality between the two groups [148]. In another recent meta-analysis of 13 randomized controlled trials, adjunctive systemic corticosteroid therapy reduced mortality by approximately 3%, need for mechanical ventilation by approximately 5%, and hospital stay by approximately 1 day among patients with CAP and PSI score IV or higher, and CURB-65 score of two or higher [149]. These results suggest that steroid use in the setting of severe CAP does not appear to be harmful, but routine use in severe CAP is not recommended, but may have value for selected patients with high levels of systemic inflammation. Another setting in which corticosteroids may have benefit is in pneumococcal pneumonia that is complicated by meningitis, where pre-treatment with corticosteroids, prior to antibiotic therapy, may lead to more favorable neurologic outcomes [150]. In addition, corticosteroids have benefit in the therapy of *P. jiroveci* pneumonia with hypoxemia (PaO_2 <70 mm Hg on room air).

Hospital-Acquired Pneumonia, Including VAP and HCAP

To select the optimal therapy for these infections, it is important to have knowledge of patterns of bacterial infection and antibiotic resistance in a given ICU, understanding that the bacteriology varies from one ICU to another. As with CAP, for most patients, initial therapy is empirical, and if that therapy is "inappropriate" (i.e., not active against the etiologic pathogen), then mortality is higher than if the therapy was appropriate [4]. The key decision point in initial empiric therapy is to determine whether the patient has risk factors for MDR pathogens, as outlined in Table 181.2. Early onset of HAP, within the first 4 days of hospitalization, is only one factor to consider when defining whether the patient is at risk for MDR pathogen infection [4]. To be considered not at risk for MDR pathogens, the patient must have both early onset of infection, and no risks for HCAP such as recent hospitalization, treatment in a health care–associated facility (nursing home, dialysis center, among others), and the patient should not have received antibiotic therapy in the past month. However, we may not know all the risk factors for MDR pathogens, and some recent data have shown that even among patients with early-onset infection, and no known MDR risks, up to half of these patients may still have MDR pathogen infection. This may relate to a high frequency of MDR pathogens, even without other risk factors, in patients with severe sepsis and in those treated in an ICU with more than 25% of the pathogens being MDR [151]. On the other hand, patients with either late-onset infection, or the presence of any of the other MDR risk factors, regardless of time of onset of infection, are at risk for infection with MDR Gram-negative and Gram-positive pathogens (Table 181.2). It is essential that initial empirical therapy be appropriate, and that it be given as soon as possible, since changing antimicrobial therapy once culture results are available may not reduce the excess mortality associated with initial inappropriate treatment. The need to get initial therapy correct has led to many patients receiving a broader spectrum regimen than may be needed, and thus it is necessary to obtain cultures prior to therapy, and to use the results to de-escalate to fewer drugs, and narrower spectrum therapy, after 2 to 3 days.

Guidelines make a distinction between appropriate therapy and adequate therapy, with both requiring the use of an agent to which the etiologic pathogen is sensitive. However, adequate therapy also requires that the drug penetrates to the site of infection, and that it is administered in the correct dose and with multiple agents if required. The regimens listed in Table 181.10 are directed at providing appropriate therapy that is targeted to the most likely pathogens. Therapy for those who are not at risk for MDR pathogen infection can be with a second- or third-generation cephalosporin, a β-lactam/β-lactamase inhibitor combination, ertapenem, a quinolone (moxifloxacin or levofloxacin), or, for penicillin-allergic patients, quinolone monotherapy, or the combination of clindamycin and aztreonam. Therapy for those at risk for MDR pathogens is directed at *P. aeruginosa*, *Acinetobacter* spp., ESBL-producing *K. pneumonia* and *Enterobacter* spp., and MRSA [4]. Patients at risk for infection with these organisms should initially receive a combination of an antipseudomonal β-lactam plus either an antipseudomonal quinolone (ciprofloxacin or levofloxacin) or an aminoglycoside (amikacin, gentamicin, or tobramycin). The antipseudomonal β-lactams include cefepime, imipenem, meropenem, and piperacillin/tazobactam. Aztreonam can be used for penicillin-allergic patients. This combination regimen is often supplemented with therapy for MRSA with either vancomycin or linezolid.

To ensure adequate therapy, the right doses have to be used—typically, for critically ill patients with normal renal function, the correct doses of common antibiotics include cefepime 1 to 2 g every 8 to 12 hours; imipenem 500 mg every 6 hours or 1 g every 8 hours; meropenem 1 g every 8 hours; piperacillin–tazobactam 4.5 g every 6 hours; levofloxacin 750 mg daily or ciprofloxacin 400 mg every 8 hours; vancomycin 15 mg per kg every 12 hours leading to a trough level of 15 to 20 mg per L; linezolid 600 mg every 12 hours; and aminoglycosides of 7 mg/kg/d of gentamicin

TABLE 181.10

Initial Empiric Antibiotic Therapy for Nosocomial Pneumonia

Hospital-acquired pneumonia and ventilator-associated pneumonia: early onset, no known risk factors for multidrug resistant (MDR) pathogens, any disease severity

Potential pathogen	Recommended antibiotic for patient type; drugs listed are meant as a group to treat all listed pathogens
Streptococcus pneumonia	Ceftriaxone
	or
Haemophilus influenza	Levofloxacin, moxifloxacin, or ciprofloxacin
or	*or*
Methicillin-sensitive *Staphylococcus aureus*	
Antibiotic-sensitive enteric Gram-negative bacilli	Ampicillin/sulbactam
	or
Escherichia coli	Ertapenem
Klebsiella pneumonia	
Proteus spp.	
Serratia marcescens	
Enterobacter spp.	

Hospital-acquired pneumonia, ventilator-associated pneumonia, and healthcare-associated pneumonia: late onset, or with risk factors for MDR pathogens, any disease severity

Potential pathogens	Combination antibiotic therapy (for patient type; drugs listed are meant as a group to treat all listed pathogens)
Pathogens listed above	Antipseudomonal cephalosporin (cefepime, ceftazidime) or
Plus	
MDR pathogens	
Pseudomonas aeruginosa	Antipseudomonal carbapenem (imipenem or meropenem)
	or
K. pneumonia	β-Lactam/β-lactamase inhibitor (piperacillin–tazobactam)
Acinetobacter spp.	
Plus	*Plus*
Consider[a]	Antipseudomonal fluoroquinolone (ciprofloxacin or levofloxacin)
	or
Legionella pneumophila	Aminoglycoside (amikacin/gentamicin/tobramycin)
	Plus
Methicillin-resistant *S. aureus*	Linezolid or vancomycin

[a]If an environmental source of Legionella is present, with a known nosocomial outbreak, use fluoroquinolone in the regimen.
Adapted from Niederman MS, Craven DE, Bonten MJ, et al: Guidelines for the management of adults with hospital-acquired, ventilator-associated, and healthcare-associated pneumonia. *Am J RespirCrit Care Med* 171:388–416, 2005, with permission.

or tobramycin and 20 mg per kg of amikacin [4]. There is interest in optimizing dosing of antibiotics, and this means using continuous or prolonged infusions of β-lactams which are bactericidal in a time-dependent fashion, or giving once-daily high doses of aminoglycosides or quinolones, which are bactericidal in a concentration-dependent fashion. Doripenem has similar efficacy to other antipseudomonal β-lactams for treatment of HAP/VAP and can be given as a 4-hour infusion to ICU patients, with some enhanced efficacy against *P. aeruginosa* when this dosing approach is used, but at least 10 days of therapy are required to treat *P. aeruginosa* [152].

For patients at risk for infection with MDR pathogens, initial empirical therapy should involve a combination of agents, but the role of continued combination therapy is uncertain. One advantage of combination therapy is to provide synergy for the therapy of *P. aeruginosa*, which is accomplished when an aminoglycoside is combined with a β-lactam. Synergy has only been proven to be of value for patients with neutropenia and pseudomonal bacteremia, both uncommon in the therapy of VAP [153]. Although combination therapy could theoretically prevent the emergence of resistance that is common with monotherapy, this has not been proven to be a benefit [154]. The major utility of combination therapy is to provide broader spectrum coverage than is possible with one agent alone, since most hospitals do not have a single agent that is able to cover all the likely pathogens with a high enough frequency. Adding a second agent increases the likelihood that initial empirical therapy will be appropriate, if MDR pathogens are present. In the Canadian Clinical Trials Group study of VAP, the use of combination therapy increased the likelihood of appropriate therapy for patients who had MDR pathogens from 11% to 84%, with an associated improvement in microbiologic eradication [155].

Combination therapy should include agents from different antibiotic classes to avoid antagonism of therapeutic mechanisms. For Gram-negatives, regimens usually involve the combination of a β-lactam with either a quinolone or an aminoglycoside. Although quinolones can penetrate into the lung better than aminoglycosides and have less potential for nephrotoxicity, a trend toward improved survival has been seen with aminoglycoside-containing, but not with quinolone-containing, combinations [156]. In some studies, combination therapy has been continued for less than the full course of therapy, with discontinuation of the aminoglycoside after 5 days if the patient is improving [157]. Monotherapy should be used when possible because combination therapy is often expensive and exposes patients to unnecessary antibiotics, thereby increasing the risk of drug toxicity and the selection of antibiotic-resistant organisms. Once cultures are available, if the etiologic pathogen is susceptible, it is possible to change to monotherapy, using one of the agents that has proven to be effective in critically ill ventilated patients with pneumonia due to susceptible pathogens: ciprofloxacin, levofloxacin, imipenem, meropenem, cefepime, and piperacillin/tazobactam [4].

The choice of initial therapy should be based on local patterns of antimicrobial susceptibility and anticipated side effects, and should also take into account which therapies patients have recently received (within the past 2 weeks), striving not to repeat the same antimicrobial class, if possible. In addition, some studies have shown that recent therapy with quinolones promotes not only Gram-negative resistance to quinolones but also to β-lactams, and they can lead to the emergence of MRSA and MDR Gram-negatives [158]. Therefore, it may be better not to use quinolones for a first episode of hospital infection, because it may make both β-lactams and quinolones less effective when therapy is needed for a subsequent infection [159]. In addition, at many hospitals, Gram-negative susceptibility to quinolones has declined and empiric coverage is improved only if an aminoglycoside is added to a β-lactam, but not if a quinolone is added [160].

For the initial antimicrobial therapy regimen to account for local bacteriologic patterns, each ICU should ideally have its own antibiogram that is updated as often as possible in order to increase the likelihood of appropriate initial antibiotic treatment. Each ICU should establish its own "go to" empiric antibiotic regimen, tailored to the antibiotic susceptibility patterns of the local flora. If patients develop HAP during or shortly after antibiotic treatment for a different infection, the empiric therapy should involve an agent from a different antibiotic class. Recent exposure to a class of antibiotics can predict subsequent resistance to a variety of agents, usually to the same class but occasionally to other classes of agents as well [161].

For the treatment of NP, the guidelines emphasize the need for a "de-escalation" strategy of usage [4]. After 2 to 3 days, the clinical course can be assessed and the culture data reviewed, and in responding patients, efforts can be made to change the initial broad-spectrum therapy. This de-escalation can involve focusing to a more narrow spectrum agent, reducing the number of antibiotics, stopping therapy altogether in patients not likely to have infection, and making efforts to reduce duration of therapy [162]. When this strategy has been used, outcomes such as the frequency of secondary infection, antimicrobial resistance, and mortality have improved. De-escalation can best be accomplished when lower respiratory tract cultures are obtained prior to initiating therapy, although rates can be high with either a nonquantitative endotracheal aspirate or a quantitatively cultured bronchoscopic sample [106]. Negative lower respiratory tract cultures can be used to stop antibiotic therapy for a patient who has had cultures obtained in the absence of an antibiotic change in the past 72 hours and who is clinically doing well. In retrospect, such a patient may not have pneumonia but rather another diagnosis such as CHF or atelectasis. Combination therapy can be de-escalated to monotherapy once culture data are available, and aminoglycosides may be used for a short duration (5 days), when used in combination with a β-lactam to treat *P. aeruginosa* pneumonia. In clinical practice, physicians do not de-escalate often enough, even though data do not show adverse outcomes when this approach is applied to patients who are responding to initial empirical therapy [163].

The recommended duration of therapy for VAP has been the subject of recent studies. Luna et al. [164] observed that patients who survived VAP after receiving appropriate therapy tended to have clinical improvement by days 3 to 5, especially reflected by improved PaO_2/FiO_2 ratio, whereas nonresponding patients did not have such a response during the same time period. On the other hand, prolonged antibiotic therapy simply leads to colonization with resistant bacteria, which may be a risk factor for recurrent VAP. A multicenter, randomized, controlled trial demonstrated that patients who received appropriate, initial empiric therapy of VAP for 8 days had outcomes similar to those patients who received therapy for 14 days [165]. A trend to greater rates of relapse for short-duration therapy was seen if the etiologic agent was *P. aeruginosa* or *Acinetobacter* spp. In another study, investigators prospectively randomized VAP patients to receive 15 days ($n = 109$) versus 8 days ($n = 116$) of therapy [166], finding no difference in mortality, ICU length of stay and mechanical ventilation days between both the groups, but more secondary infection in the shorter course cohort than the longer treatment cohort (35.3% vs. 19.3%, $p = 0.01$). Thus, for patients who receive initially appropriate antibiotics and have a good clinical response to therapy, the duration of therapy should be as short as 7 days, provided that the etiologic pathogen is not *P. aeruginosa*. The optimal duration of therapy for VAP due to MDR organisms such as *P. aeruginosa* or *Acinetobacter*spp is not known. Serial measurement of PCT can help guide therapy discontinuation for VAP and help decrease number of days on antibiotic, without having an adverse effect on mortality [86]. Bouadma et al. [142] compared 307 patients with ICU infection who had therapy guided by PCT, compared to 314 controls.

The number of antibiotic-free days was approximately 2.7 days less for the PCT group, with no differences in 28- or 60-day mortality between the two groups.

Although aminoglycosides are used in VAP, there is concern about nephrotoxicity (especially among the elderly) and these drugs are less active in areas of the lung that have a low pH level, as may occur with pneumonia. Also, these antibiotics achieve only 40% of the serum concentration in respiratory secretions, when given intravenously. Although once-daily dosing has been proposed to take advantage of the postantibiotic effects of aminoglycosides to enhance efficacy, while reducing the need for monitoring serum levels and reducing the toxicity, a meta-analysis has shown neither enhanced efficacy nor reduced toxicity with once-daily dosing [4]. Another approach used by some investigators is the direct delivery of aminoglycosides into the airway in an effort to achieve high levels of antibiotic at the site of infection, with little risk of systemic absorption and toxicity [167]. One side effect of aerosolized antibiotics has been bronchospasm, which can be induced by the antibiotic or the associated diluents present in certain preparations. Pending further investigation, this therapy should be used as an adjunct to systemic antibiotics, for patients with severe Gram-negative pneumonias who are not responding to intravenous therapy, or for patients infected by a relatively resistant organism that might be eliminated only with high local drug concentrations.

HCAP Treatment

Some patients with health care–associated infections are bacteriologically similar to hospital-acquired infections and also at risk for infection with MDR pathogens [82], but some studies have shown that not all HCAP patients are at the same risk [168]. In the 2005 ATS/IDSA guidelines patients with HCAP were thought to be at risk for infection with MDR pathogens, needing empiric broad-spectrum therapy [4]. However, some studies have shown efficacy for antibiotic regimens for HCAP that are often monotherapy, and similar to CAP therapy [169–172]. Falcone and colleagues found that HCAP patients receiving a guideline concordant regimen had a significantly shorter duration of antibiotic therapy (median 15 vs. 12 days), a shorter duration of hospitalization (median 18 vs. 14 days), and a lower mortality rate (17.8% vs. 7.1%) than those receiving other therapies [170].

Shindo and associates in a prospective study including 1,413 patients (887 CAP and 526 HCAP) determined the risk factors for drug-resistant pathogens (DRPs) to macrolides, β-lactam and respiratory fluoroquinolones (CAP-DRPs) [173]. They found HCAP patients had a higher frequency of CAP- DRPs than patients with CAP (26.6% vs. 8.6%) and higher 30-day mortality (20.3% vs. 7.0%). Independent risk factors for CAP-DRPs in this population included - prior hospitalization, immunosuppression, previous antibiotic use, gastric acid-suppressive agents, tube feeding, and nonambulatory status. In a prospective study, Maruyama and colleagues evaluated 425 patients (CAP = 124, HCAP = 321), and applied a therapeutic algorithm based on the presence of MDR risk factors (immunosuppression, hospitalization within the last 90 days, poor functional status—Barthel Index score <50, and antibiotic therapy within the past 6 months) and severity of illness (need for ICU admission or requiring mechanical ventilation) to determine outcomes [174]. HCAP patients admitted to the ICU, with at least one MDR risk factor were treated with a HAP regimen based on the ATS/IDSA 2005 guidelines. This represented only two-third of the ICU admitted patients, so that one-third were treated with a narrower spectrum, CAP-type regimen, and the outcomes for all were good. In the entire study group, using the algorithm, 92.9% received appropriate therapy for the identified pathogens. Thus not all HCAP patients need MDR coverage, and some can be effectively treated with a narrower spectrum regimen.

Other Issues

For the therapy of NP, in addition to *P. aeruginosa*, the other challenging Gram-negative organisms are *Acinetobacter* spp. and ESBL-producing *Enterobacteriaceae*. For both groups of pathogens, a carbapenem is the most effective therapy, if the organisms are sensitive, but if not, then novel therapies may be needed. *Acinetobacter* can be treated with tigecycline but generally not as monotherapy, since it has not shown efficacy in clinical trials when utilized this way. In a large double-blind, randomized, multicenter trial comparing imipenem/cilastatin to tigecycline in 945 HAP patients, those patients with VAP who were treated with tigecycline had a significantly lower cure rate and more deaths compared to patients with imipenem [175]. Colistin, a polymyxin, may be necessary in this setting, with some risk of nephrotoxicity. For multidrug-resistant *Acinetobacter* infection, a combination regimen is usually recommended and can include colistin, sulbactam, tigecycline and/or an inhaled antimicrobial [176].

The treatment options for suspected MRSA pneumonia have been expanded with the availability of agents such as the oxazolidinones (linezolid), telavancin, teicoplanin and streptogramins. Linezolid achieves higher lung epithelial lining fluid concentrations compared to glycopeptides and could therefore have an advantage for MRSA lung infections. However, results from two older meta-analyses demonstrated comparable clinical and microbiologic success with using linezolid and glycopeptides and a significant twofold increase in the risk of thrombocytopenia and gastrointestinal events with linezolid [177,178]. In a subset analysis of two prospective, randomized trials, linezolid had a clinical and microbiologic advantage over vancomycin for patients with documented MRSA VAP [179]. This advantage may be due to the higher penetration of linezolid into the epithelial lining fluid than with vancomycin [180]. Since those analyses, a multicenter prospective randomized trial of linezolid versus vancomycin for patients with documented MRSA pneumonia was completed, and linezolid led to a significantly higher rate of clinical response than optimally dosed vancomycin [181]. However, there was no difference in mortality between the two groups, but this could potentially be explained by the fact that patients, who failed vancomycin, were able to be salvaged with linezolid, and any survival in this setting was attributed to vancomycin. Linezolid may also be preferred if patients have renal insufficiency or are receiving other nephrotoxic agents such as aminoglycosides, because of concerns of synergistic nephrotoxicity with vancomycin, but this is not conclusively proven. Linezolid is generally well tolerated, but patients must be monitored for drug-induced thrombocytopenia, especially after prolonged use (>14 days). Another recent meta-analysis that also included the new randomized controlled trial of linezolid versus vancomycin did find a higher microbiologic eradication rate for linezolid and more nephrotoxicity when glycopeptides (vancomycin or teicoplanin) were used [182]. Quinupristin/dalfopristin is an option but was less efficacious compared with vancomycin in treatment of NP caused by MRSA [183].

STRATEGIES FOR PREVENTION OF PNEUMONIA

Community-Acquired Pneumonia

Preventive strategies can be applied in the outpatient (prehospital) setting or in the hospital and ICU. Outpatient measures proven to reduce the incidence of severe lower respiratory tract infection are immunization against pneumococcal and influenza infection in susceptible populations. The pneumococcal polysaccharide vaccine (PPV) is directed at 23 strains of pneumococcus (accounting for 85% to 90% of all infections), and it is both cost-effective and potentially cost saving among individuals older than 65 years for the prevention of bacteremia. In a study of US hospitals, prior vaccination against pneumococcus was associated with improved survival (adjusted OR, 0.50; 95% confidence interval, 0.43 to 0.59), decreased chance of respiratory failure or other complications, and decreased length of stay among hospitalized patients with CAP [184]. With documented effectiveness of 75% in this age group, the recommendation is that all immune-competent patients aged 65 years or older should be immunized [5]. If prior history of vaccination is not available, revaccination is also safe, as there was no difference in the risk of adverse events following more than three doses of PPV, compared with one or two doses [185]. This may be relevant following vaccination with 23-valent PPV, because pneumococcal antibody levels decline to prevaccination levels within 6 to 10 years. Two protein-conjugated pneumococcal vaccines have been licensed and are more immunogenic than the older vaccine, but contain only 7 and 13 serotypes [5]. The 13-valent pneumococcal conjugate vaccine (PCV13) was approved by the Food and Drug Administration (FDA) in late 2011 for use among adults aged ≥50 years [186]. Based on a randomized, placebo-controlled trial evaluating the efficacy of PCV13 for preventing CAP among adults aged ≥65 years (CAPITA—Community Acquired Pneumonia Immunization Trial in Adults), the Advisory Committee on Immunization Practices recommended routine use of PCV13 among adults aged ≥65 years since Aug 2014 [186]. PCV13 should be administered in series with the 23-valent PPV, giving PCV 13 first, if possible. PCV 13 and PPV 23-valent vaccination are also recommended for patients with chronic pulmonary diseases, receiving steroids or immunomodulating therapy, or who have concurrent sickle cell disease or other hemoglobinopathies, primary immunodeficiency disorders, human immunodeficiency virus infection/acquired immunodeficiency syndrome, nephrotic syndrome, and hematologic or solid malignancies [187].

Annual influenza vaccination has reduced the frequency and severity of influenza among the elderly and chronically ill patients, and vaccination of medical personnel may reduce nosocomial transmission of influenza from staff to patients. For those above 65 years of age an higher dose influenza vaccine (60 μg of hemagglutinin per strain) has been shown to provide better protection [188,189]. In one study, patients ≥65 years, who had received high-dose inactivated influenza vaccine during the 2012 to 2013 influenza seasons were less likely to have influenza-related medical encounters and hospitalization than standard-dose vaccine [190]. Antiviral chemoprophylaxis (with oseltamivir, zanamivir, amantadine, or rimantadine) may be adjunctive to immunization and is 70% to 90% effective in avoiding infections with influenza A, if it is started at the earliest recognition of an outbreak, and if the circulating strain is sensitive to these agents (which has not always been the case in recent epidemics). The neuraminidase inhibitors, zanamivir and oseltamivir, are active against both influenza A and B, for prophylaxis and if treatment is started within 36 hours of the onset of symptoms [191].

Nosocomial Pneumonia

In the ICU, several general strategies may be used to reduce the incidence of pneumonia (Table 181.11). In general, it is possible to reduce the incidence of VAP, but this requires the use of multiple interventions together, which are often administered in the form of a "Ventilator bundle." The use of these bundles has been effective at reducing the incidence of VAP, particularly if the implementation of the bundle is closely monitored [192].

TABLE 181.11

Preventive Strategies Available in Intensive Care Unit Pneumonia

To be used in all patients based on strong data

- "Ventilator bundles": individualize to each ICU
- Oral care, possibly with chlorhexidine
- 24 h of prophylactic systemic antibiotics following emergent intubation
- Change ventilator circuits only when soiled
- Noninvasive ventilation when possible
- Reduce use of nasogastric tubes (place orally, and if possible postpyloric)
- Daily interruption of sedation
- Infection control: hand washing, isolate patients with resistant organisms

To be considered in most patients

- Prophylactic PEEP of 5–8 cm
- Closed suction catheter systems
- Maintain endotracheal tube cuff pressure to avoid aspiration
- Avoid immunosuppressants
- Restricted blood transfusion policy
- Glycemic control
- Influenza and pneumococcal vaccine: consider hospital-based programs

Require further data prior to being adopted for routine use

- Ideal head position: elevated vs. lateral Trendelenburg
- Endotracheal tube biofilm removal or avoidance: silver-coated endotracheal tube, other devices when available
- Subglottic secretion drainage endotracheal tubes
- "Selective digestive decontamination"—oropharynx and GI tract
- Probiotics into the GI tract
- Early tracheostomy
- Silver-coated endotracheal tube
- Polyurethane and conical endotracheal tube cuffs

GI, gastrointestinal; ICU, intensive care unit; PEEP, positive end-expiratory pressure.

Typically a bundle includes: hand washing, daily interruption of sedation, daily weaning trial, head of bed elevation, oral care (possibly with chlorhexidine), deep venous thrombosis prophylaxis, and stress ulcer prophylaxis. Bundles have been effective for reducing VAP rates but it is controversial whether it is possible to achieve a "zero VAP" goal [193].

Infection Control and Ventilator Equipment Handling

Handwashing, although simple and effective in reducing the spread of resistant organisms, is frequently neglected in the ICU. Proper disinfection of nebulization equipment should be done after each use. Heat moisture exchangers in the ventilator circuit can eliminate the need for cascade humidification but have not been shown to reduce the incidence of NP. Ventilator circuit changes should be made no more often than every 48 hours, and more frequent changes and manipulations may add to the risk of infection [4]. In fact, there is no increased infection risk if tubing is never changed [194]. Micro-aspiration of gastric contents is facilitated by the underinflation of the tracheal cuff pressure and can be effectively prevented by maintaining the tracheal cuff pressure by use of an automated pneumatic device, or by close monitoring of the cuff pressure [195]. In addition, maintenance of PEEP at 5 to 8 cm may also keep the endotracheal tube cuff sealed, and minimize secretion leakage around the cuff. Biofilm formation on the inner surface of the endotracheal tube can be inhibited by using an endotracheal tube coated with silver. In a multicenter trial involving intubated patients, those who had silver-coated endotracheal tubes had lower rates of microbiologically confirmed VAP compared to the control group with uncoated tube (4.8% vs. 7.5%; $p = 0.03$), but there were no differences in the duration of intubation, or mortality among the two groups [55]. There are also a variety of devices under development that can remove the biofilm once it has formed.

Prophylactic Antibiotics

Intense interest has been focused on "SDD" as a means of preventing both NP and sepsis. This approach attempts to sterilize the intestine and oral cavity of all Gram-negative organisms, assuming that the gastrointestinal tract is the source of the organisms that cause pneumonia. Several large meta-analyses and four recent prospective trials have shown a benefit for SDD in preventing VAP and in reducing mortality [196]. The full regimen is usually a combination of topical (polymyxin, tobramycin, and amphotericin or related compounds) and systemic antibiotics (nonpseudomonal third-generation cephalosporin), but the use of only topical oral antibiotics (selective oral decontamination [SOD]) or oral antiseptics (such as chlorhexidine) has also reduced the incidence of infection. In a large randomized trial, both SDD and SOD reduced ICU mortality rates [197]. In spite of these possible benefits, widespread use of SDD in all ICU patients has not been adopted outside of certain European centers and in many studies, the benefits have applied only to selected populations such as surgical and trauma patients, with less benefit to medical patients. In addition, those at the extremes of disease severity (mild or severely ill) may not benefit, and the incremental benefit of these approaches when added to an effective ventilator bundle, has not been evaluated. To be fully effective, SDD needs to be used in all patients in a given ICU, and this widespread use has been shown in some studies to promote the emergence of resistant bacteria, particularly Gram-positives such as MRSA. This is likely to be an even greater problem for ICUs with a high baseline rate of resistance. SDD may also lead to an increased rate of hospital-acquired infections in patients after they leave the ICU [198]. In a prospective, randomized, double-blind study of 350 patients undergoing cardiac surgery, use of chlorhexidine gluconate 0.12% oral rinse reduced the incidence of pneumonia by 69% in comparison with controls (5/173 vs. 17/180; $p < 0.05$). There was no difference in antibiotic resistance patterns in either group [199]. Recently, there is some question about whether oral chlorhexidine can be harmful, possibly related to toxicity if aspirated, and a limited efficacy and higher mortality among noncardiac surgery patients [200]. Another recent meta-analysis of 28 randomized controlled trials supported the use of SOD in the prevention of VAP. In fact, the entire regimen of SDD may not be any more effective than the use of oral antiseptics [201].

The concept of antibiotic rotation or cycling has also been investigated as a resistance control strategy [145,157,182,202], and although there was initial enthusiasm for this approach, recent studies have been less supportive, and most ICUs focus on antimicrobial stewardship, focusing on monitoring local patterns of resistance and introducing heterogeneity into the choice of antibiotics [157,203].

Control of Respiratory Secretions

Stagnation of respiratory secretions can lead to both pneumonia and atelectasis, and efforts to remove these secretions could reduce the incidence of pneumonia. One way to achieve this objective is through the use of continuous lateral rotation delivered by a rotating bed that is used in place of a traditional hospital bed to improve mucociliary clearance and help mobilize secretions. Another way to control respiratory secretions is to remove oropharyngeal contents before they can be aspirated into the lung. Continuous aspiration of subglottic secretions, through the use of a specially designed endotracheal tube, has significantly reduced the incidence of early-onset VAP in several studies [4]. Subglottic drainage aspiration (SSD) can be achieved by a specially adapted endotracheal tube that will allow suctioning of secretions that pool above the endotracheal tube cuff, thereby interrupting the aspiration of secretions into the tracheobronchial tree. A recent randomized control trial showed a significant reduction of microbiologically confirmed VAP with the use of SSD, compared to the control population (14.8% vs. 25.6%; $p = 0.02$) but no difference in duration of mechanical ventilation or mortality [204]. In another randomized study enrolling over 700 patients comparing continuous aspiration of subglottic secretions (CASS) versus controls after cardiac surgery, the CASS group had lower VAP rate (26.7% vs. 47.5%; $p = 0.04$), and fewer days in the ICU (7 vs. 16.5 days; $p = 0.01$) [205].

Stress Ulcer Prophylaxis

Several clinical studies have documented that neutralization of gastric pH with antacids or H_2 blockers can add to the risk of NP (especially late-onset infection) among mechanically ventilated patients [4]. Although not all studies have shown that the gastric reservoir is an important source of infection, prevention strategies should take into account its potential influence by minimizing gastric volume and preventing aspiration of gastric contents; however, ventilator bundles have been able to reduce VAP rates, even when H_2 blockers are used. This is likely because gastric acid neutralization is combined with elevation of the head of the bed, which may prevent aspiration of gastric contents. Although some studies have suggested a benefit of performing stress ulcer prophylaxis with sucralfate, at least one large, double-blind, randomized trial comparing ranitidine with sucralfate, demonstrated a trend toward lower rates of VAP with sucralfate, but reported that clinically significant gastrointestinal bleeding was 4% higher in the sucralfate group [206].

Ventilator Bundles

The incidence of VAP can be reduced substantially if there is a high rate of compliance with all the interventions in a ventilator bundle. Bundle use has been reported to lead to almost 45% reduction in the incidence of VAP and the benefit was greatest when adherence to the protocol was high [192]. In the last several years, this approach has become so popular and apparently effective that many believe that it can lead to a "zero VAP" rate. However, there is concern that the benefits of ventilator bundles have been overstated, and that it is impossible to eliminate VAP in certain high-risk patients [207]. Thus, it is unclear if VAP is really being prevented, or if the disease is being diagnosed less often, especially given the subjective nature of the VAP definition, and the possibility of treating patients for another diagnosis. In addition, although studies have shown a reduction of VAP rates, secondary benefits such as reduction in mortality and antibiotic use have not generally been reported.

Advances for managing acute infectious pneumonia, based on randomized, controlled trials or meta-analyses of such trials, are summarized in Table 181.12.

TABLE 181.12

Recent Advances in Pneumonia Management Based on Randomized Trials, Large Database Analyses, and Meta-analysis

- Antibiotic duration in VAP should be as short as possible. In patients with a low clinical suspicion, based on serial clinical observations and improvement, therapy can be stopped after 3 d, while those with microbiologically confirmed VAP can be safely treated for 8 d, provided that initial therapy is appropriate and that a nonfermenting Gram-negative is not responsible [61,150].
- Linezolid is associated with a lower mortality and higher bacteriologic eradication rate than vancomycin in patients with VAP that is proven to be caused by MRSA, but quinupristin/dalfopristin is not superior to vancomycin [122,137,139].
- Quinolone monotherapy should not be used for patients with severe CAP, since it has not been proven to be safe and effective for all of the types of patients admitted to the ICU [4,118].
- Patients with severe CAP should receive combination therapy, generally with a beta-lactam and a macrolide. Meta-analysis has shown reduced mortality for severe CAP patients treated with a macrolide [129].
- Mortality in CAP can be reduced by administering the first dose of antibiotics as soon as possible after a patient's arrival to the hospital [4].
- In patients with VAP, an etiologic diagnosis can be made with either endotracheal aspirate culture or bronchoscopic culture, with no difference in mortality, comparing the 2 methods [2].
- Combination antimicrobial therapy in VAP increases the likelihood of initially effective empiric therapy for patients who are likely to have multidrug-resistant pathogen infection, but the use of combination therapy has not been definitively proven to reduce mortality [2].
- When cephalosporins are used for empiric therapy of severe CAP, and drug-resistant *S. pneumoniae* is suspected, ceftriaxone and cefotaxime are reliable choices, while cefuroxime is not [4].
- In the presence of CAP with pneumococcal bacteremia, use of dual antibiotic therapy is associated with reduced mortality, compared with monotherapy, especially for patients with severe pneumonia [115,116].

CAP, community-acquired pneumonia; ICU, intensive care unit; MRSA, methicillin-resistant *Staphylococcus aureus*; VAP, ventilator-associated pneumonia.

References

1. Centers for Disease Control and Prevention: Pneumonia Facts. Available at: http://www.cdc.gov/nchs/fastats/pneumonia.htm. Accessed November 22, 2015.
2. Weycker D, Strutton D, Edelsberg J, et al: Clinical and economic burden of pneumococcal disease in older US adults. *Vaccine* 28:4955–4960, 2010.
3. *National Action Plan for Combating Antibiotic-Resistant Bacteria*. 2015; Available from: https://www.whitehouse.gov/sites/default/files/docs/national_action_plan_for_combating_antibotic-resistant_bacteria.pdf. Accessed December 12, 2015.
4. Niederman MS, Craven DE, Bonten MJ, et al: Guidelines for the management of adults with hospital-acquired, ventilator-associated, and healthcare-associated pneumonia. *Am J Respir Crit Care Med* 171:388–416, 2005.
5. Mandell LA, Wunderink RG, Anzueto A, et al: Infectious Diseases Society of America/American Thoracic Society consensus guidelines on the management of community-acquired pneumonia in adults. *Clin Infect Dis* 44:S27–S72, 2007.
6. Nair GB, Niederman MS: Nosocomial pneumonia: lessons learned. *Crit Care Clin* 29: 521–546, 2013.
7. Niederman MS: Making sense of scoring systems in community acquired pneumonia. *Respirology* 14:327–335, 2009.
8. Woodhead M, Welch CA, Harrison DA, et al: Community-acquired pneumonia on the intensive care unit: secondary analysis of 17,869 cases in the ICNARC Case Mix Programme Database. *Crit Care* 10[Suppl 2]:S1, 2006.
9. Renaud B, Santin A, Coma E, et al., Association between timing of intensive care unit admission and outcomes for emergency department patients with community-acquired pneumonia *Crit Care Med* 37:2867–2874, 2009.
10. Hraiech S, Alingrin J, Dizier S, et al: Time to intubation is associated with outcome in patients with community-acquired pneumonia. *PLoS One* 8:e74937, 2013.
11. Bordón J, Peyrani P, Brock GN, et al: The presence of pneumococcal bacteremia does not influence clinical outcomes in patients with community-acquired pneumonia: results from the Community-Acquired Pneumonia Organization (CAPO) International Cohort study. *Chest* 133:618–624, 2008.
12. Fine MJ, Smith MA, Carson CA, et al: Prognosis and outcomes of patients with community-acquired pneumonia: a meta-analysis. *JAMA* 275:134–141, 1996.
13. Prina E, Ferrer M, Ranzani OT, et al: Thrombocytosis is a marker of poor outcome in community-acquired pneumonia *Chest* 143:767–775, 2013.
14. Laserna E, Sibila O, Aguilar PR, et al: Hypocapnia and hypercapnia are predictors for ICU admission and mortality in hospitalized patients with community-acquired pneumonia. *Chest* 142:1193–1199, 2012.
15. Carr GE, Yuen TC, McConville JF, et al: Early cardiac arrest in patients hospitalized with pneumonia: a report from the American Heart Association's Get With The Guidelines-Resuscitation Program. *Chest* 141:1528–1536, 2012.
16. Metersky ML, Waterer G, Nsa W, et al: Predictors of in-hospital vs postdischarge mortality in pneumonia *Chest* 142: 476-81, 2012.
17. Ruiz M, Ewig S, Torres A, et al: Severe community-acquired pneumonia: risk factors and follow-up epidemiology. *Am J RespirCrit Care Med* 160:923–929, 1999.
18. Safdar N, Dezfulian C, Collard HR, et al: Clinical and economic consequences of ventilator-associated pneumonia: a systematic review. *Crit Care Med* 33:2184–2193, 2005.
19. Rello J, Ollendorf DA, Oster G, et al: Epidemiology and outcomes of ventilator-associated pneumonia in a large US database. *Chest* 122: 2115–2121, 2002.
20. Bekaert M, Timsit JF, Vansteelandt S, et al: Attributable mortality of ventilator-associated pneumonia: a reappraisal using causal analysis. *Am J Respir Crit Care Med* 184:1133–1139, 2011.
21. Kollef MH, Silver P, Murphy DM, et al: The effect of late-onset ventilator associated pneumonia in determining patient mortality. *Chest* 108:1655–1662, 1995.
22. Torres A, Serra-Batlles J, Ferrer A, et al: Severe community-acquired pneumonia. Epidemiology and prognostic factors. *Am Rev Respir Dis* 144:312–318, 1991.
23. Restrepo M, Motersen E, Velez J, et al: A comparative study of community-acquired pneumonia patients admitted to the ward and the ICU. *Chest* 133:610–617, 2008.
24. Aujesky D, Auble TE, Yealy DM, et al: Prospective comparison of three validated prediction rules for prognosis in community-acquired pneumonia. *Am J Med* 118:384–392, 2005.
25. Lim WS, van der Eerden MM, Laing R, et al: Defining community acquired pneumonia severity of presentation to hospital: an international derivation and validation study. *Thorax* 58:377–382, 2003.
26. Shindo Y, Sato S, Maruyama E, et al: Comparison of severity scoring systems A-DROP and CURB-65 for community-acquired pneumonia. *Respirology* 13:731–735, 2008.
27. España PP, Capelastegui A, Gorordo I, et al: Development and validation of a clinical prediction rule for severe community-acquired pneumonia. *Am J Respir Crit Care Med* 174:1249–1256, 2006.
28. Charles PG, Wolfe R, Whitby M, et al: SMART-COP: a tool for predicting the need for intensive respiratory or vasopressor support in community-acquired pneumonia. *Clin Infect Dis* 47:375–384, 2008.
29. Masiá M, Gutiérrez F, Shum C, et al: Usefulness of procalcitonin levels in community-acquired pneumonia according to the patients outcome research team pneumonia severity index. *Chest* 128:2223–2229, 2005.
30. Krüger S, Ewig S, Marre R, et al: Procalcitonin predicts patients at low risk of death from community-acquired pneumonia across all CRB-65 classes. *Eur Respir J* 31:349–355, 2008.
31. Huang DT, Weissfeld LA, Kellum JA, et al: Risk prediction with procalcitonin and clinical rules in community-acquired pneumonia. *Ann Emerg Med* 52:48–58, 2008..
32. Liapikou A, Ferrer M, Polverino E, et al: Severe community-acquired pneumonia: validation of the Infectious Diseases Society of America/American Thoracic Society guidelines to predict an intensive care unit admission. *Clin Infect Dis* 48:377–385, 2009.
33. Phua J, See KC, Chan YH, et al: Validation and clinical implications of the IDSA/ATS minor criteria for severe community-acquired pneumonia. *Thorax* 64:598–603, 2009.
34. Brown SM, Jones BE, Jephson AR, et al: Validation of the Infectious Disease Society of America/American Thoracic Society 2007 guidelines for severe community-acquired pneumonia. *Crit Care Med* 37:3010–3016, 2009.
35. Salih W, Schembri S, Chalmers JD: Simplification of the IDSA/ATS criteria for severe CAP using meta-analysis and observational data. *Eur Respir J* 43:842–851, 2014.
36. Rello J, Rodriguez A, Lisboa T, et al: PIRO score for community-acquired pneumonia: a new prediction rule for assessment of severity in intensive care unit patients with community-acquired pneumonia. *Crit Care Med* 37:456–462, 2009.
37. Renaud B, Labarère J, Coma E, et al: Risk stratification of early admission to the intensive care unit of patients with no major criteria of severe community-acquired pneumonia: development of an international prediction rule. *Crit Care* 13:R54, 2009.

38. Labarere J, Schuetz P, Renaud B, et al: Validation of a clinical prediction model for early admission to the intensive care unit of patients with pneumonia. *Acad Emerg Med* 19:993–1003, 2012.
39. Garau J, Baquero F, Pérez-Trallero E, et al: Factors impacting on length of stay and mortality of community-acquired pneumonia. *Clin Microbiol Infect* 14:322–329, 2008.
40. Leroy O, Santré C, Beuscart C, et al: A five-year study of severe community-acquired pneumonia with emphasis on prognosis in patients admitted to an intensive care unit. *Intensive Care Med* 21:24–31, 1995.
41. Shorr AF, Bodi M, Rodriguez A, et al: Impact of antibiotic guideline compliance on duration of mechanical ventilation in critically ill patients with community-acquired pneumonia. *Chest* 130:93–100, 2006.
42. Kumar A, Roberts D, Wood K, et al: Duration of hypotension before initiation of effective antimicrobial therapy is the critical determinant of survival in human septic shock. *Crit Care Med* 34:1589–1596, 2006.
43. Moroney JF, Fiore AE, Harrison LH, et al: Clinical outcomes of bacteremic pneumococcal pneumonia in the era of antibiotic resistance. *Clin Infect Dis* 33:797–805, 2001.
44. Metlay JP, Hofmann J, Cetron MS, et al: Impact of penicillin susceptibility on medical outcomes for adult patients with bacteremic pneumococcal pneumonia. *Clin Infect Dis* 30:520–528, 2000.
45. Turett GS, Blum S, Fazal BA, et al: Penicillin resistance and other predictors of mortality in pneumococcal bacteremia in a population with high human immunodeficiency virus seroprevalence. *Clin Infect Dis* 29:321–327, 1999.
46. Patel JB, Cockerill FR, Alder J, et al: Performance Standards for Antimicrobial Susceptibility Testing; Twenty-Fourth Informational Supplement. CLSI document M100-S24; 2014. Available at: http://ncipd.org/control/images/NCIPD_docs/CLSI_M100-S24.pdf.
47. Uçkay I, Ahmed QA, Sax H, et al: Ventilator-associated pneumonia as a quality indicator for patient safety? *Clin Infect Dis* 16:557–563, 2008.
48. Cook DJ, Walter SD, Cook RJ: Incidence of and risk factors for ventilator-associated pneumonia in critically ill patients. *Ann Intern Med* 129:433–440, 1998.
49. Chastre J, Trouillet JL, Vuagnat A, et al: Nosocomial pneumonia in patients with acute respiratory distress syndrome. *Am J Respir Crit Care Med* 157:1165–1172, 1998.
50. Brito V, Niederman MS: Healthcare-associated pneumonia is a heterogenous disease, and all patients do not need the same broad-spectrum antibiotic therapy as complex nosocomial pneumonia. *Curr Opin Infect Dis* 22:316–325, 2009.
51. Niederman MS: The pathogenesis of airway colonization: lessons learned from the study of bacterial adherence. *Eur Respir J* 7:1737–1740, 1994.
52. Ahmed QA, Niederman MS: Respiratory infection in the chronically critically ill patient. Ventilator-associated pneumonia and tracheobronchitis. *Clin Chest Med* 22:71–85, 2001.
53. Boutten A, Dehoux MS, Seta N, et al: Compartmentalized IL-8 and elastase release within the human lung in unilateral pneumonia. *Am J Respir Crit Care Med* 153:336–342, 1996.
54. Inglis TJ, Millar MR, Jones G, et al: Tracheal tube biofilm as a source of bacterial colonization of the lung. *J Clin Microbiol* 27:2014–2018, 1989.
55. Kollef MH, Afessa B, Anzueto A, et al: Silver-coated endotracheal tubes and incidence of ventilator-associated pneumonia: the NASCENT randomized trial. *JAMA* 300:805–813, 2008.
56. Gil-Perotin S, Ramirez P, Marti V, et al: Implications of endotracheal tube biofilm in ventilator-associated pneumonia response: a state of concept. *Crit Care*, 16:R93, 2012.
57. Niederman MS, Craven DE: Devising strategies for preventing nosocomial pneumonia—should we ignore the stomach? *Clin Infect Dis* 24:320–323, 1997.
58. Torres A, Serra-Batlles J, Ros E, et al: Pulmonary aspiration of gastric contents in patients receiving mechanical ventilation: the effect of body position. *Ann Intern Med* 116:540–543, 1992.
59. Heyland DK, Cook DJ, Schoenfeld PS, et al: The effect of acidified enteral feeds on gastric colonization in critically ill patients: results of a multicenter randomized trial. Canadian Critical Care Trials Group. *Crit Care Med* 27:2399–2406, 1999.
60. Jacobs S, Chang RW, Lee B, et al: Continuous enteral feeding: a major cause of pneumonia among ventilated intensive care unit patients. *J Parenter Enteral Nutr* 14:353–356, 1990.
61. Craven DE, Chroneou A, Zias N, et al: Ventilator-associated tracheobronchitis: the impact of targeted antibiotic therapy on patient outcomes. *Chest* 135:521–528, 2009.
62. Feldman C, Kassel M, Cantrell J, et al: The presence and sequence of endotracheal tube colonization in patients undergoing mechanical ventilation. *Eur Respir J* 13:546–551, 1999.
63. Mason CM, Nelson S: Pulmonary host defenses and factors predisposing to lung infection. *Clin Chest Med* 26:11–17, 2005.
64. Waterer GW, Quasney MW, Cantor RM, et al: Septic shock and respiratory failure in community-acquired pneumonia have different TNF polymorphism associations. *Am J Respir Crit Care Med* 163:1599–1604, 2001.
65. Reade MC, Yende S, D'Angelo G, et al: Differences in immune response may explain lower survival among older men with pneumonia. *Crit Care Med* 37:1655–1662, 2009.
66. Rautanen A, Mills TC, Gordon AC, et al: Genome-wide association study of survival from sepsis due to pneumonia: an observational cohort study. *Lancet Respir Med* 3:53–60, 2015.
67. Ruiz M, Ewig S, Marcos MA, et al: Etiology of community-acquired pneumonia: impact of age, comorbidity, and severity. *Am J Respir Crit Care Med* 160:397–405, 1999.
68. Arancibia F, Bauer TT, Ewig S, et al: Community-acquired pneumonia due to gram-negative bacteria and Pseudomonas aeruginosa: incidence, risk, and prognosis. *Arch Intern Med* 162:1849–1858, 2002.
69. Riquelme R, Torres A, el-Ebiary M, et al: Community-acquired pneumonia in the elderly: clinical and nutritional aspects. *Am J Respir Crit Care Med* 156:1908–1914, 1997.
70. Francis JS, Doherty MC, Lopatin U, et al: Severe community-onset pneumonia in healthy adults caused by methicillin-resistant Staphylococcus aureus carrying the Panton-Valentine leukocidin genes. *Clin Infect Dis* 40:100–107, 2005.
71. Kang CI, Song JH, Oh WS, et al: Clinical outcomes and risk factors of community-acquired pneumonia caused by gram-negative bacilli. *Eur J Clin Microbiol Infect Dis* 27:657–661, 2008.
72. de Roux A, Ewig S, Garcia E, et al: Mixed community-acquired pneumonia in hospitalised patients. *Eur Respir J* 27:795–800, 2006.
73. Choi SH, Hong SB, Ko GB, et al: Viral infection in patients with severe pneumonia requiring intensive care unit admission. *Am J Respir Crit Care Med* 186:325–332, 2012.
74. Markowicz P, Wolff M, Djedaïni K, et al: Multicenter prospective study of ventilator-associated pneumonia during acute respiratory distress syndrome. Incidence, prognosis, and risk factors. ARDS Study Group. *Am J Respir Crit Care Med* 161:1942–1948, 2000.
75. El-Solh AA, Pietrantoni C, Bhat A, et al: Microbiology of severe aspiration pneumonia in institutionalized elderly. *Am J Respir Crit Care Med* 167:1650–1654, 2003.
76. Rodrigues JM, Niederman MS, Fein AM, et al: Nonresolving pneumonia in steroid-treated patients with obstructive lung disease. *Am J Med* 93:29–34, 1992.
77. Gaynes R, Edwards JR: Overview of nosocomial infections caused by gram-negative bacilli. *Clin Infect Dis* 41:848–854, 2005.
78. Jones RN: Microbial etiologies of hospital-acquired bacterial pneumonia and ventilator-associated bacterial pneumonia. *Clin Infect Dis* 51[Suppl 1]: S81–S87, 2010.
79. Vincent JL, Rello J, Marshall J, et al: International study of the prevalence and outcomes of infection in intensive care units. *JAMA* 302:2323–2329, 2009.
80. Esperatti M, Ferrer M, Theessen A, et al: Nosocomial pneumonia in the intensive care unit acquired by mechanically ventilated versus nonventilated patients. *Am J Respir Crit Care Med* 182:1533–1539, 2010.
81. Weber DJ, Rutala WA, Sickbert-Bennett EE, et al: Microbiology of ventilator-associated pneumonia compared with that of hospital-acquired pneumonia. *Infect Control Hosp Epidemiol* 28:825–831, 2007.
82. Kollef MH, Shorr A, Tabak YP, et al: Epidemiology and outcomes of health-care-associated pneumonia: results from a large US database of culture positive patients. *Chest* 128:3854–3862, 2005.
83. Fagon JY, Chastre J, Domart Y, et al: Nosocomial pneumonia in patients receiving continuous mechanical ventilation. Prospective analysis of 52 episodes with use of a protected specimen brush and quantitative culture techniques. *Am Rev Respir Dis* 139:877–884, 1989.
84. Pugin J, Auckenthaler R, Mili N, et al: Diagnosis of ventilator-associated pneumonia by bacteriologic analysis of bronchoscopic and nonbronchoscopic "blind' bronchoalveolar lavage fluid. *Am Rev Respir Dis* 143:1121–1129, 1991.
85. Klompas M, Kleinman K, Khan Y, et al: Rapid and reproducible surveillance for ventilator-associated pneumonia.*Clin Infect Dis* 54: 370–377, 2012.
86. Stolz D, Smyrnios N, Eggimann P, et al: Procalcitonin for reduced antibiotic exposure in ventilator-associated pneumonia: a randomised study. *Eur Respir J* 34:1364–1375, 2009.
87. Gibot S, Cravoisy A, Levy B, et al: Soluble triggering receptor expressed on myeloid cells and the diagnosis of pneumonia *N Engl J Med* 350:451–458, 2004.
88. Ramirez P, Ferrer M, Gimeno R, et al: Systemic inflammatory response and increased risk for ventilator-associated pneumonia: a preliminary study.*Crit Care Med* 37:1691–1695, 2009.
89. Ramirez P, Garcia MA, Ferrer M, et al: Sequential measurements of procalcitonin levels in diagnosing ventilator-associated pneumonia. *Eur Respir J* 31:356–362, 2008.
90. Luyt CE, Guérin V, Combes A, et al: Procalcitonin kinetics as a prognostic marker of ventilator-associated pneumonia. *Am J Respir Crit Care Med* 171:48–53, 2005.
91. McFadden JP, Price RC, Eastwood HD, et al: Raised respiratory rate in elderly patients: a valuable physical sign. *Br Med J (Clin Res Ed)* 284:626–627, 1982.
92. Farr BM, Sloman AJ, Fisch MJ: Predicting death in patients hospitalized for community-acquired pneumonia. *Ann Intern Med* 115:428–436,1991.
93. Rello J, Bodi M, Mariscal D, et al: Microbiological testing and outcome of patients with severe community-acquired pneumonia. *Chest* 123:174–180, 2003.
94. Nair V, Niederman MS, Masani N, et al: Hyponatremia in community-acquired pneumonia. *Am J Nephrol* 27:184–190, 2007.
95. Boersma WG, Daniels JM, Löwenberg A, et al: Reliability of radiographic findings and the relation to etiologic agents in community-acquired pneumonia. *Respir Med* 100:926–932, 2006.
96. Syrjala H, Broas M, Suramo I, et al: High-resolution computed tomography for the diagnosis of community-acquired pneumonia. *Clin Infect Dis* 27:358–363, 1998.
97. Bryan CS, Reynolds KL: Bacteremic nosocomial pneumonia. Analysis of 172 episodes from a single metropolitan area. *Am Rev Respir Dis* 129:668–671, 1991.
98. Muller F, Christ-Crain M, Bregenzer T, et al: Procalcitonin levels predict bacteremia in patients with community-acquired pneumonia: a prospective cohort trial. *Chest* 138:121–129, 2010.

99. van Werkhoven CH, Huijts SM, Postma DF, et al: Predictors of bacteraemia in patients with suspected community-acquired pneumonia. *PLoS One* 10:e0143817, 2015.
100. Metersky ML, Ma A, Bratzler DW, et al: Predicting bacteremia in patients with community-acquired pneumonia. *Am J Respir Crit Care Med* 169:342–347, 2004.
101. El Solh AA, Akinnusi ME, Pineda LA, et al: Diagnostic yield of quantitative endotracheal aspirates in patients with severe nursing home-acquired pneumonia. *Crit Care* 11:R57, 2007.
102. Feller-Kopman D, Ernst A: The role of bronchoalveolar lavage in the immunocompromised host. *Semin Respir Infect* 18:87–94, 2003.
103. Fartoukh M, Maitre B, Honoré S, et al: Diagnosing pneumonia during mechanical ventilation: the clinical pulmonary infection score revisited. *Am J Respir Crit Care Med* 168:173–179, 2003.
104. Berton DC, Kalil AC, Teixeira PJ: Quantitative versus qualitative cultures of respiratory secretions for clinical outcomes in patients with ventilator-associated pneumonia. *Cochrane Database Syst Rev* (1):CD006482, 2012.
105. Singh N, Rogers P, Atwood CW, et al: Short-course empiric antibiotic therapy for patients with pulmonary infiltrates in the intensive care unit. A proposed solution for indiscriminate antibiotic prescription. *Am J Respir Crit Care Med* 162:505–511, 2000.
106. Heyland DK, Dodek P, Muscedere J, et al: Randomized trial of combination versus monotherapy for the empiric treatment of suspected ventilator-associated pneumonia. *Crit Care Med* 36:737–744, 2008.
107. Berton DC, Kalil AC, Teixeira PJ: Quantitative versus qualitative cultures of respiratory secretions for clinical outcomes in patients with ventilator-associated pneumonia. *Cochrane Database Syst Rev* (10):CD006482, 2014.
108. Dunn IJ, Marrie TJ, Mackeen AD, et al: The value of open lung biopsy in immunocompetent patients with community-acquired pneumonia requiring hospitalization. *Chest* 106:23–27, 1994.
109. Lichtenstein DA: Lung ultrasound in the critically ill. *Ann Intensive Care* 4:1, 2014.
110. Reissig A, Copetti R, Mathis G, et al: Lung ultrasound in the diagnosis and follow-up of community-acquired pneumonia: a prospective, multicenter, diagnostic accuracy study. *Chest* 142: 965–972, 2012.
111. Zagli G, Cozzolino M, Terreni A, et al: Diagnosis of ventilator-associated pneumonia: a pilot, exploratory analysis of a new score based on procalcitonin and chest echography. *Chest* 146:1578–1585, 2014.
112. Chavez MA, Shams N, Ellington LE, et al: Lung ultrasound for the diagnosis of pneumonia in adults: a systematic review and meta-analysis. *Respir Res* 15:50, 2014.
113. Magill SS, Klompas M, Balk R, et al: Executive summary: Developing a new, national approach to surveillance for ventilator-associated events. *Ann Am Thorac Soc* 10:S220–S223, 2013.
114. Muscedere J, Sinuff T, Heyland DK, et al: The clinical impact and preventability of ventilator-associated conditions in critically ill patients who are mechanically ventilated. *Chest* 144:1453–1460, 2013.
115. Hayashi Y, Morisawa K, Klompas M, et al: Toward improved surveillance: the impact of ventilator-associated complications on length of stay and antibiotic use in patients in intensive care units. *Clin Infect Dis* 56:471–477, 2013.
116. Klein Klouwenberg PM, van Mourik MS, Ong DS, et al: Electronic implementation of a novel surveillance paradigm for ventilator-associated events: feasibility and validation. *Am J Respir Crit Care Med* 189:947–955, 2014.
117. Bouadma L, Sonneville R, Garrouste-Orgeas M, et al: Ventilator-associated events: prevalence, outcome, and relationship with ventilator-associated pneumonia. *Crit Care Med* 43:1798–1806, 2015.
118. Niederman MS, Nair GB: Managing ventilator complications in a "VACuum" of data. *Chest* 147:5–6, 2015.
119. Noskin GA, Glassroth J: Bacterial pneumonia associated with HIV-1 infection. *Clin Chest Med* 17:713–723, 1996.
120. Moore FA, Moore EE, Jones TN, et al: TEN versus TPN following major abdominal trauma: reduced septic mortality. *J Trauma* 29:916–922, 1989.
121. Heyland DK, Drover JW, MacDonald S, et al: Effect of postpyloric feeding on gastroesophageal regurgitation and pulmonary microaspiration: results of a randomized controlled trial. *Crit Care Med* 29:1495–1501, 2001.
122. Sahn SA: Continuous lateral rotational therapy and nosocomial pneumonia. *Chest* 99:1263–1267, 1991.
123. Waterer GW, Somes GW, Wunderink RG: Monotherapy may be suboptimal for severe bacteremic pneumococcal pneumonia. *Arch Intern Med* 161:1837–1842, 2001.
124. Baddour LM, Yu VL, Klygkan KP, et al: Combination antibiotic therapy lowers mortality among severely ill patients with pneumococcal bacteremia. *Am J RespirCrit Care Med* 170:440–444, 2004.
125. Yu VL, Greenberg RN, Zadeikis N, et al: Levofloxacin efficacy in the treatment of community-acquired legionellosis. *Chest* 125:2135–2136, 2004.
126. Postma DF, van Werkhoven CH, van Elden LJ, et al: Antibiotic treatment strategies for community-acquired pneumonia in adults. *N Engl J Med* 372:1312–1323, 2015.
127. Adrie C, Schwebel C, Garrouste-Orgeas M, et al: Initial use of one or two antibiotics for critically ill patients with community-acquired pneumonia: impact on survival and bacterial resistance. *Crit Care* 17:R265, 2013.
128. Garin N, Genné D, Carballo S, et al: β-Lactam monotherapy vs β-lactam-macrolide combination treatment in moderately severe community-acquired pneumonia: a randomized noninferiority trial. *JAMA Intern Med* 174:1894–1901, 2014.
129. Sligl WI, Asadi L, Eurich DT, et al: Macrolides and mortality in critically ill patients with community-acquired pneumonia: a systematic review and meta-analysis. *Crit Care Med* 42:420–432, 2014.
130. Leroy O, Saux P, Bédos JP, et al: Comparison of levofloxacin and cefotaxime combined with ofloxacin for ICU patients with community-acquired pneumonia who do not require vasopressors. *Chest* 128:172–183, 2005.
131. Anzueto A, Niederman MS, Pearle J, et al: Community-acquired pneumonia recovery in the elderly (CAPRIE): efficacy and safety of moxifloxacin therapy versus that of levofloxacin therapy. *Clin Infect Dis* 41:73–81, 2006.
132. Mortensen EM, Restropo MI, Anzueto A, et al: The impact of empiric antimicrobial therapy with a beta-lactam and fluoroquinolone on mortality for patients hospitalized with severe pneumonia. *Crit Care* 10:R8, 2005.
133. Vardakas KZ, Siempos II, Grammatikos A, et al: Respiratory fluoroquinolones for the treatment of community-acquired pneumonia: a meta-analysis of randomized controlled trials. *Can Med Assoc J* 179:1269–1277, 2008.
134. Lujan M, Gallego M, Fontanals D, et al: Prospective observational study of bacteremic pneumococcal pneumonia: effect of discordant therapy on mortality. *Crit Care Med* 32:625–631, 2004.
135. Yu VL, Chiou CC, Feldman C, et al: An international prospective study of pneumococcal bacteremia: correlation with in vitro resistance, antibiotics administered, and clinical outcome. *Clin Infect Dis* 37:230–237, 2003.
136. Falagas ME, Metaxas EI: Tigecycline for the treatment of patients with community-acquired pneumonia requiring hospitalization. *Expert Rev Anti Infect Ther* 7:913-23, 2008.
137. Boucher HW, Talbot GH, Bradley JS, et al: Bad bugs, no drugs: no ESKAPE! An update from the Infectious Diseases Society of America. *Clin Infect Dis* 48:1–12, 2009.
138. Lodise TP, Low DE: Ceftaroline fosamil in the treatment of community-acquired bacterial pneumonia and acute bacterial skin and skin structure infections. *Drugs* 72:1473–1493, 2012.
139. Lai CC, Lee KY, Lin SW, et al: Nemonoxacin (TG-873870) for treatment of community-acquired pneumonia. *Expert Rev Anti Infect Ther* 12:401–417, 2014.
140. Nair GB, Niederman MS: Community-acquired pneumonia: an unfinished battle. *Med Clin North Am* 95:1143–1161, 2011.
141. Schuetz P, Briel M, Christ-Crain M, et al: Procalcitonin to guide initiation and duration of antibiotic treatment in acute respiratory infections: an individual patient data meta-analysis. *Clin Infect Dis* 55:651–662, 2012.
142. Bouadma L, Luyt CE, Tubach F, et al: Use of procalcitonin to reduce patients' exposure to antibiotics in intensive care units (PRORATA trial): a multicentre randomised controlled trial. *Lancet* 375:463–474, 2010.
143. Schuetz P, Müller B, Christ-Crain M, et al: Procalcitonin to initiate or discontinue antibiotics in acute respiratory tract infections. *Cochrane Database Syst* Rev (9):CD007498, 2012.
144. Sicot N, Khanafer N, Meyssonnier V, et al: Methicillin resistance is not a predictor of severity in community-acquired Staphylococcus aureus necrotizing pneumonia-results of a prospective observational study. *Clin Microbiol Infect* 19:E142–E148, 2013.
145. Salluh JI, Póvoa P, Soares M, et al: The role of corticosteroids in severe community-acquired pneumonia: a systematic review. *Crit Care* 12:R76, 2008.
146. Salluh JI, Bozza FA, Soares M, et al:Adrenal response in severe community-acquired pneumonia: impact on outcomes and disease severity. *Chest* 134:947–954, 2008.
147. Nie W, Zhang Y, Cheng J, et al: Corticosteroids in the treatment of community-acquired pneumonia in adults: a meta-analysis. *PLoS One* 7:e47926, 2012.
148. Torres A, Sibila O, Ferrer M, et al: Effect of corticosteroids on treatment failure among hospitalized patients with severe community-acquired pneumonia and high inflammatory response: a randomized clinical trial. *JAMA* 313:677–686, 2015.
149. Siemieniuk RA, Meade MO, Alonso-Coello P, et al: Corticosteroid therapy for patients hospitalized with community-acquired pneumonia: a systematic review and meta-analysis. *Ann Intern Med* 163:519–528, 2015.
150. de Gans J, van de Beek D: Dexamethasone in adults with bacterial meningitis. *N Engl J Med* 347:1549–1556, 2002.
151. Martin-Loeches I, Deja M, Koulenti D, et al: Potentially resistant microorganisms in intubated patients with hospital-acquired pneumonia: the interaction of ecology, shock and risk factors. *Intensive Care Med* 39: 672–681, 2013.
152. Kollef MH, Chastre J, Clavel M, et al: A randomized trial of 7-day doripenem versus 10-day imipenem-cilastatin for ventilator-associated pneumonia. *Crit Care* 16:R218, 2012.
153. Safdar N, Handelsman J, Maki DG: Does combination antimicrobial therapy reduce mortality in Gram-negative bacteraemia? A meta-analysis. *Lancet Infect Dis* 4:519–527, 2004.
154. Cometta A, Baumgartner JD, Lew D, et al: Prospective randomized comparison of imipenem monotherapy with imipenem plus netilmicin for treatment of severe infections in nonneutropenic patients. *Antimicrob Agents Chemother* 38:1309–1313, 1994.
155. Aarts MA, Hancock JN, Heyland D, et al: Empiric antibiotic therapy for suspected ventilator-associated pneumonia: a systematic review and meta-analysis of randomized trials. *Crit Care Med* 36:108–117, 2008.
156. Fowler RA, Flavin KE, Barr J, et al: Variability in antibiotic prescribing patterns and outcomes in patients with clinically suspected ventilator-associated pneumonia. *Chest* 123:835–844, 2003.
157. Gruson G, Gilles H, Vargas F, et al: Rotation and restricted use of antibiotics in a medical intensive care unit. Impact on the incidence of ventilator-associated pneumonia caused by antibiotic-resistant gram-negative bacteria. *Am J Respir Crit Care Med* 162:837–842, 2000.

158. Nseir S, Di Pompeo C, Soubrier S, et al: First-generation fluoroquinolone use and subsequent emergence of multiple drug-resistant bacteria in the intensive care unit. *Crit Care Med* 33:283–289, 2005.
159. Niederman MS: Reexamining quinolone use in the intensive care unit: use them right or lose the fight against resistant bacteria. *Crit Care Med* 33:443–444, 2005.
160. Beardsley JR, Williamson JC, Johnson JW, et al: Using local microbiologic data to develop institution-specific guidelines for the treatment of hospital-acquired pneumonia. *Chest* 130:787–793, 2006.
161. Trouillet JL, Vuagnat A, Combes A, et al: *Pseudomonas aeruginosa* ventilator-associated pneumonia: comparison of episodes due to piperacillin-resistant versus piperacillin-susceptible organisms. *Clin Infect Dis* 34:1047–1054, 2002.
162. Niederman MS: De-escalation therapy in ventilator-associated pneumonia. *Curr Opin Crit Care* 12:452–457, 2006.
163. Kollef MH, Morrow LE, Niederman MS, et al: Clinical characteristics and treatment patterns among patients with ventilator-associated pneumonia. *Chest* 129:1210–1218, 2006.
164. Luna CM, Blanzaco D, Niederman MS, et al: Resolution of ventilator-associated pneumonia: prospective evaluation of the clinical pulmonary infection score as an early clinical predictor of outcome. *Crit Care Med* 31:676–682, 2003.
165. Chastre J, Wolff M, Fagon JY, et al: Comparison of 8 vs 15 days of antibiotic therapy for ventilator-associated pneumonia in adults: a randomized trial. *JAMA* 290:2588–2598, 2003.
166. Capellier G, Mockly H, Charpentier C, et al: Early-onset ventilator-associated pneumonia in adults randomized clinical trial: comparison of 8 versus 15 days of antibiotic treatment.*PLoS One* 7:e41290, 2012.
167. Palmer L, Smaldone G, Simon S, et al: Aerosolized antibiotics in mechanically ventilated patients: delivery and response. *Crit Care Med* 26:31–39, 1998.
168. Carratalá J, Mykietiuk A, Fernández-Sabé N, et al: Health care-associated pneumonia requiring hospital admission: epidemiology, antibiotic therapy, and clinical outcomes. *Arch Intern Med* 167:1393–1399, 2007.
169. Grenier C, Pépin J, Nault V, et al: Impact of guideline-consistent therapy on outcome of patients with healthcare-associated and community-acquired pneumonia. *J Antimicrob Chemother* 66:1617–1624, 2011.
170. Falcone M, Corrao S, Licata G, et al: Clinical impact of broad-spectrum empirical antibiotic therapy in patients with healthcare-associated pneumonia: a multicenter interventional study. *Intern Emerg Med* 7:523–531, 2012.
171. Chalmers JD, Taylor JK, Singanayagam A, et al: Epidemiology, antibiotic therapy, and clinical outcomes in health care-associated pneumonia: a UK cohort study. *Clin Infect Dis* 53:107–113, 2011.
172. Attridge RT, Frei CR, Restrepo MI, et al: Guideline-concordant therapy and outcomes in healthcare-associated pneumonia. *Eur Respir J* 38:878–887, 2011.
173. Shindo Y, Ito R, Kobayashi D, et al: Risk factors for drug-resistant pathogens in community-acquired and healthcare-associated pneumonia. *Am J Respir Crit Care Med* 188:985–995, 2013.
174. Maruyama T, Fujisawa T, Okuno M, et al: A new strategy for healthcare-associated pneumonia: a 2-year prospective multicenter cohort study using risk factors for multidrug-resistant pathogens to select initial empiric therapy. *Clin Infect Dis* 57:1373–1383, 2013.
175. Freire AT, Melnyk V, Kim MJ, et al: Comparison of tigecycline with imipenem/cilastatin for the treatment of hospital-acquired pneumonia. *Diagn Microbiol Infect Dis* 68:140–151, 2010.
176. Garnacho-Montero J, Dimopoulos G, Poulakou G, et al: Task force on management and prevention of Acinetobacter baumannii infections in the ICU. *Intensive Care Med* 41:2057–2075, 2015.
177. Walkey AJ, O'Donnell MR, Wiener RS: Linezolid vs glycopeptide antibiotics for the treatment of suspected methicillin-resistant *Staphylococcus aureus* nosocomial pneumonia: a meta-analysis of randomized controlled trials. *Chest* 139:1148–1155, 2011.
178. Kalil AC, Murthy MH, Hermsen ED, et al: Linezolid versus vancomycin or teicoplanin for nosocomial pneumonia: a systematic review and meta-analysis. *Crit Care Med* 38:1802–1808, 2010.
179. Wunderink RG, Rello J, Cammarata SK, et al: Linezolid vs vancomycin: analysis of two double-blind studies of patients with methicillin-resistant *Staphylococcus aureus* nosocomial pneumonia. *Chest* 124:1789–1797, 2003.
180. Conte JE Jr, Golden JA, Kipps J, et al: Intrapulmonary pharmacokinetics of linezolid. *Antimicrob Agents Chemother* 46:1475–1480, 2002.
181. Wunderink RG, Niederman MS, Kollef MH, et al: Linezolid in methicillin-resistant Staphylococcus aureus nosocomial pneumonia: a randomized, controlled study. *Clin Infect Dis* 54:621–629, 2012.
182. Jiang H, Tang RN, Wang J: Linezolid versus vancomycin or teicoplanin for nosocomial pneumonia: meta-analysis of randomised controlled trials. *Eur J Clin Microbiol Infect Dis* 32:1121–1128, 2013.
183. Fagon JY, Patrick H, Haas DW, et al: Treatment of Gram-positive nosocomial pneumonia. Prospective randomized comparison of quinupristin/dalfopristin versus vancomycin. *Am J Respir Crit Care Med* 161: 753–762, 2000.
184. Fisman DN, Abrutyn E, Spaude KA, et al: Prior pneumococcal vaccination is associated with reduced death, complications, and length of stay among hospitalized adults with community-acquired pneumonia. *Clin Infect Dis* 42:1093–1101, 2006.
185. Walker FJ, Singleton RJ, Bulkow LR, et al: Reactions after 3 or more doses of pneumococcal polysaccharide vaccine in adults in Alaska. *Clin Infect Dis* 40:1730–1735, 2005.
186. Tomczyk S, Bennett NM, Stoecker C, et al: Use of 13-valent pneumococcal conjugate vaccine and 23-valent pneumococcal polysaccharide vaccine among adults aged >/=65 years: recommendations of the Advisory Committee on Immunization Practices (ACIP). *MMWR Morb Mortal Wkly Rep* 63: 822–825, 2014.
187. Mirsaeidi M, Ebrahimi G, Allen MB, et al: Pneumococcal vaccine and patients with pulmonary diseases. *Am J Med* 127: 886 e1–e8, 2014.
188. DiazGranados CA, Dunning AJ, Kimmel M, et al: Efficacy of high-dose versus standard-dose influenza vaccine in older adults. *N Engl J Med* 371:635–645, 2014.
189. Nace DA, Lin CJ, Ross TM, et al: Randomized, controlled trial of high-dose influenza vaccine among frail residents of long-term care facilities. *J Infect Dis* 211:1915–1924, 2015.
190. Izurieta HS, Thadani N, Shay DK et al: Comparative effectiveness of high-dose versus standard-dose influenza vaccines in US residents aged 65 years and older from 2012 to 2013 using Medicare data: a retrospective cohort analysis. *Lancet Infect Dis* 15:293–300, 2015.
191. Jefferson T, Jones M, Doshi P, et al: Neuraminidase inhibitors for preventing and treating influenza in healthy adults: systematic review and meta-analysis. *BMJ* 339:b5106, 2009.
192. Resar R, Pronovost P, Haraden C, et al: Using a bundle approach to improve ventilator care processes and reduce ventilator-associated pneumonia. *Jt Comm J Qual Patient Saf* 31:243, 2005.
193. Niederman MS: New strategies to prevent ventilator-associated pneumonia: what to do for your patients. *Curr Treat Options Infect Dis* 8:1–15, 2016.
194. Dreyfuss D, Djedaini K, Weber P, et al: Prospective study of nosocomial pneumonia and of patient and circuit colonization during mechanical ventilation with circuit changes every 48 hours versus no change. *Am Rev Respir Dis* 143:738–743, 1991.
195. Nseir S, Zerimech F, Fournier C, et al: Continuous control of tracheal cuff pressure and microaspiration of gastric contents in critically ill patients. *Am J Respir Crit Care Med* 184:1041–1047, 2011.
196. Roquilly A, Marret E, Abraham E, et al: Pneumonia prevention to decrease mortality in intensive care unit: a systematic review and meta-analysis. *Clin Infect Dis* 60:64–75, 2015.
197. de Smet AM, Kluytmans JA, Cooper BS, et al: Decontamination of the digestive tract and oropharynx in ICU patients. *N Engl J Med* 360:20–31, 2009.
198. de Smet AM, Hopmans TE, Minderhoud AL, et al: Decontamination of the digestive tract and oropharynx: hospital acquired infections after discharge from the intensive care unit. *Intensive Care Med* 35:1609–1613, 2009.
199. DeRiso AJ 2nd, Ladowski JS, Dillon TA, et al: Chlorhexidine gluconate 0.12% oral rinse reduces the incidence of total nosocomial respiratory infection and nonprophylactic systemic antibiotic use in patients undergoing heart surgery.*Chest* 109:1556–1561, 1996.
200. Klompas M, Speck K, Howell MD, et al: Reappraisal of routine oral care with chlorhexidine gluconate for patients receiving mechanical ventilation: systematic review and meta-analysis. *JAMA Intern Med* 174:751–761, 2014.
201. Pileggi C, Bianco A, Flotta D, et al: Prevention of ventilator-associated pneumonia, mortality and all intensive care unit acquired infections by topically applied antimicrobial or antiseptic agents: a meta-analysis of randomized controlled trials in intensive care units. *Crit Care* 15:R155, 2011.
202. Niederman MS: Is "crop rotation" of antibiotics the solution to a "resistant" problem in the ICU? *Am J Respir Crit Care Med* 156:1029–1031, 1997.
203. Dellit TH, Owens RC, McGowan JE Jr, et al: Infectious Diseases Society of America and the Society for Healthcare Epidemiology of America guidelines for developing an institutional program to enhance antimicrobial stewardship. *Clin Infect Dis* 44:159–177, 2007.
204. Lacherade JC, De Jonghe B, Guezennec P, et al: Intermittent subglottic secretion drainage and ventilator-associated pneumonia: a multicenter trial. *Am J Respir Crit Care Med* 182:910–927, 2010.
205. Bouza E, Pérez MJ, Muñoz P, et al: Continuous aspiration of subglottic secretions in the prevention of ventilator-associated pneumonia in the postoperative period of major heart surgery. *Chest* 134:938–946, 2008.
206. Cook D, Guyatt G, Marshall J, et al: Canadian Critical Care Trials Group. A comparison of sucralfate and ranitidine for the prevention of upper gastrointestinal bleeding in patients requiring mechanical ventilation. *N Engl J Med* 338:791, 1998.
207. Klompas M, Platt R: Ventilator-associated pneumonia—the wrong quality measure for benchmarking. *Ann Intern Med* 147:803–805, 2007.

Chapter 182 ▪ Interventional Pulmonary in the Intensive Care Unit

ANDRES F. SOSA • PAULO J. OLIVEIRA

Interventional pulmonology (IP) is a relatively new field in pulmonary and critical care medicine that involves the use of advanced procedures for the diagnosis and treatment of tracheobronchial and pleural disorders. Since the introduction of endobronchial laser therapy and the "dedicated tracheobronchial silicone stent" by Dumon in 1990 [1] mainly in response to the rising prevalence of lung cancer in the 1980s [2], the specialty has evolved to target a wide spectrum of benign and malignant respiratory pathologies.

The treatment of complex airway diseases needs specialized training that is beyond the scope of a general pulmonary and critical care fellowship [3]. Guidelines that attempt to ensure basic skill and competency for all procedures encompassed within the specialty have been published by major societies, including the American College of Chest Physicians (ACCP), the American Thoracic Society (ATS), and the European Respiratory Society (ERS) [3,4]. Starting in 2013, the American Association of Bronchology and Interventional Pulmonolgy (AABIP) has started board examinations and certification to ensure competency within the field (Table 182.1). Interventional Pulmonary Fellowships now participate in the National Residency Matching Program (NRMP).

As a main feature, the uses of the rigid bronchoscope, and its many applications for treatment and palliation, require expertise not only in the procedures themselves, but, as importantly, in selecting those patients who might benefit from an intervention. Given the nature of the disease processes the field encounters, an important proportion of patients will have significant comorbidities and limited functional status that need to be considered prior to any procedure.

There are multiple applications for the field of IP in the intensive care unit (ICU). Because, the subspecialty frequently serves patients requiring ICU level of care, the interventional pulmonologist is a valuable member of the ICU team. In the current chapter, we address some of the techniques at the disposal of the interventional pulmonologist and how these may be applied to the ICU setting (Table 182.2); it is not the intention of this chapter to describe in detail the entire range of procedures performed by the subspecialty of IP.

AIRWAY PROCEDURES

Rigid Bronchoscopy

The first successful removal of an aspirated foreign body by a translaryngeal approach was done with a rigid bronchoscope by Gustav Killian in 1897 [5]. Until that time, foreign body aspiration could be severely incapacitating and resulted in chronic illness from recurrent infections, atelectasis, hemorrhage, or death [5]. The rigid bronchoscope was later used for other diagnostic and

TABLE 182.1

Current Requirements for Interventional Pulmonary Board Certification by the AABIP

Core procedural groups	Minimum number of procedures (3 years total)
Complex Airway Diseases Rigid or Flexible Bronchoscopy Airway interventions—benign and malignant Any combination of mechanical debulking, laser, APC, electrocautery, cryotherapy, stents (hybrid/silicone), or other endoscopic modality, brachytherapy, PDT, or emerging technologies Other flexible or rigid interventions not easily classified elsewhere: endobronchial valves, blockers, bronchial thermoplasty, etc.	90
Advanced Diagnostic Bronchoscopy Peripheral lung lesions and mediastinal assessment Any combination of navigation; radial probe EBUS or virtual bronchoscopy guided transbronchial sampling; Convex Probe EBUS; and other emerging technologies	90
Pleural disease management (Medical thoracoscopy/pleuroscopy optional) Any combination of minimally invasive diagnostic and therapeutic procedures including thoracic ultrasound-guided thoracentesis, tube thoracostomy, indwelling pleural catheter, closed pleural biopsies, and thoracoscopy.	90
Percutaneous tracheostomy and percutaneous endoscopic gastrostomy	Optional for IP fellowship training and board eligibility
Multidisciplinary patient management conferences or other didactic conferences Any combination of tumor board, multidisciplinary clinics, transplant selection committee meetings, etc.	Yes

AABIP, American Association for Bronchology and Interventional Pulmonology; APC, argon-plasma coagulation; PDT, percutaneous dilatational tracheostomy; EBUS, Endobronchial ultrasound; IP, interventional pulmonology.
Adapted from the AABIP. Available at http://aabronchology.org/education/board-certification/board-eligibility-criteria. Accessed May 13, 2017.

TABLE 182.2

Procedures that May Be Performed by Interventional Pulmonologists in the ICU

Airway procedures	Pleural procedures	Other procedures
Flexible and rigid bronchoscopy	• Chest ultrasonography	• *Percutaneous endoscopic gastrostomy*
Diagnostic:	• Thoracentesis	
Transbronchial lung biopsy	• Tube thoracostomy	
Transbronchial needle aspiration	• Placement of pleural catheters	
Endobronchial ultrasound		
Therapeutic:	• Transthoracic needle aspiration/biopsy	
Airway stent placement		
APC		
Nd:YAG Laser		
Electrocautery		
Cryotherapy		
Balloon dilatation		
Endobronchial valves		
Percutaneous Tracheostomy		

ICU, intensive care unit; APC, argon plasma coagulation; Nd:YAG, neodymium-doped yttrium aluminum garnet.

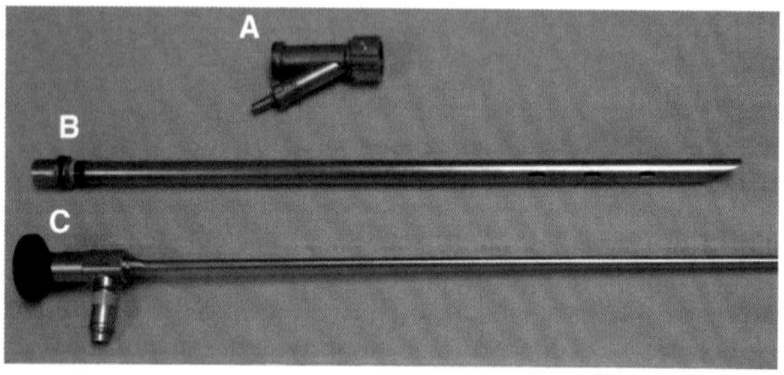

FIGURE 182.1 **A:** Universal Instrumentation Barrel and Anesthesia Connector. **B:** Rigid Bronchoscope Tube. **C:** Rigid Telescope.

therapeutic procedures. Since the invention of the flexible bronchoscope by Shigeto Ikeda in 1968 [6], the rigid bronchoscope has served a role mainly for therapeutic interventions, removal of foreign bodies, and the management of massive hemoptysis. After the spike of lung cancer prevalence during the 1980s that spurred the use of endobronchial laser therapy and the silicone stent, the rigid bronchoscope has recovered a more prominent role for the management of both benign and malignant airway disease [1,7].

The rigid bronchoscope is a stiff metallic tube that is introduced by a trans-laryngeal approach and allows for ventilation and passage of different instruments. There is a longer bronchial barrel with side fenestrations to allow for collateral ventilation while intubating the right or left bronchus, and a shorter tracheal barrel that has no side fenestrations and is used for intubation of the trachea. At its proximal end, the rigid bronchoscope provides the connections for mechanical ventilation and passage of the light source. The distal end has a beveled tip that can be used for coring out endoluminal lesions. The airway lumen may be projected to a screen using a telescope with a camera attachment or may be visualized directly through an eye piece (Fig. 182.1).

Massive Hemoptysis

The anatomical dead space of the central airways is approximately 100 to 200 mL; a rapid bleed close to this volume may be enough to cause central airway obstruction (CAO), asphyxiation, and death. The exact quantity of blood that defines massive hemoptysis has been estimated to be from >200 to 1,000 mL in a 24-hour-period, but it seems more practical to keep in mind that any bleed that could be life-threatening should be considered massive [8]. Causes of massive hemoptysis include malignancies; tuberculosis; fistulas from major vessels; and bronchiectasis.

When confronted with massive hemoptysis, one should start by ensuring stability of the patient by providing appropriate means for oxygenation and ventilation. It is important to keep in mind that the patient with hemoptysis may already have a very limited functional status and that respiratory failure may happen very rapidly. For the unstable patient, endotracheal intubation should not be delayed and—in addition to general measures that include placing the patient with the bleeding side down, establishing appropriate intravenous access, and sending appropriate laboratory testing—no time should be wasted in identifying and controlling the source of bleeding. Oftentimes, the source of bleeding may be identified by radiologic studies and controlled by angiographic embolization, but in cases when chest imaging is unrevealing or the bleeding source is thought to be within the airways, one should proceed with diagnostic and therapeutic bronchoscopy [9].

Massive hemoptysis has a high mortality rate, and it is paramount to secure airway patency, identify the bleeding source and apply therapeutic interventions to stop the bleeding. The rigid bronchoscope is superior to the flexible bronchoscope for all these functions because it allows for ventilation and more vigorous suctioning that may help secure the airway and visualize more thoroughly the source of bleeding. Also, if the cause of hemorrhage is endobronchial, rigid bronchoscopy provides a way to control the bleeding with cauterizing modalities such as electrocautery, argon plasma coagulation (APC), or laser therapy. The use of other hemostatic therapies such as iced saline, epinephrine, fibrin glue, oxidized regenerated cellulose, or the placement of occlusive balloons, may all be applied successfully through the rigid barrel while maintaining airway patency [8–13]. For these reasons, the rigid bronchoscope remains the instrument of choice for the endoscopic assessment and treatment of massive hemoptysis.

Central Airway Obstruction

CAO is a problem that may be encountered in the ICU. It may be because of either benign or malignant etiologies. Patients often experience progressive dyspnea on exertion when the narrowing involves 50% of the airway lumen, then developing dyspnea at rest when the stenosis reaches 70% of the airway lumen [14]. When the stenosis is severe, a seemingly stable patient may rapidly develop an acute, critical occlusion of the central airway because, for one example, an otherwise mild respiratory tract infection has caused an increase of secretions that are poorly cleared by ineffective cough, occluding the already severely narrowed airway at or near the site of the stenosis.

Nonmalignant Central Airway Obstruction

Nonmalignant CAO may result from inflammatory conditions such as sarcoidosis, amyloidosis, antineutrophil cytoplasmic autoantibodies (ANCA)-associated vasculitis, or relapsing polychondritis. Benign disease processes also may occlude the central airway by extrinsic compression and this may be seen in large goiters, post-pneumonectomy and post-lung transplantation stenosis and vascular malformations. Finally, tracheobronchomalacia also may result in CAO because the abnormally collapsible airway can occlude the central airway lumen during expiration. However, the most common cause of nonmalignant CAO is stenosis caused by artificial airways, either postintubation or posttracheostomy tracheal stenosis (Table 182.3) [15,16].

Postintubation and Posttracheostomy Tracheal Stenosis. This is the most common cause of benign tracheal stenosis and results from granulation and fibrotic responses to artificial airways at anatomic loci from the supraglottic space to the lower trachea. The endotracheal tube may cause pressure ulceration and necrosis at any point where the tube contacts the airway wall; this may be the posterior commissure of the glottic space, the balloon site or at the tip of the tube. The same applies for a tracheostomy tube where pressure ulcerations and granulation tissues may form immediately above the stoma within the trachea, at the balloon site or at the tip of a tube that rubs against the airway mucosa. Inflammation, ulceration, and necrosis may in turn result in constriction of the airway wall caused by a loss of support from damaged cartilage, obstruction from granulation tissue, fibrosis, and formation of synechiae. Damage from the balloon has been reduced by the development of high-volume, low-pressure cuffs; however, it remains important not to exceed the normal mucosal capillary perfusion pressure of 20 to 30 mm Hg or tracheal injury may occur because of tissue ischemia. If after achieving a cuff pressure of 25 mm Hg there is still an air leak present, it is advisable to use a larger tracheostomy tube rather than to overinflate the balloon [17].

Tracheal stenosis may become apparent soon after what should have been a successful wean from mechanical ventilation when the patient fails extubation because of stridor and respiratory distress requiring immediate reintubation. However, severe airway narrowing also may present as an airway emergency weeks or months after extubation or tracheostomy decannulation. Not uncommonly, these late deteriorations are preceded by ongoing complaints of worsening stridor or dyspnea on exertion that progress to dyspnea at rest. Frequently, these patients may have been misdiagnosed as having asthma or COPD and gone through treatment with different bronchodilators and systemic steroids without improvement before recognition.

It is important to understand that airway patency is the priority for patients with tracheal stenosis. When the presentation is one of acute respiratory failure, the patient must be intubated with an endotracheal tube immediately. If an endotracheal tube cannot be advanced, then the patient must be taken to rigid bronchoscopy immediately. More importantly, when confronted with tracheal stenosis the specialist must keep in mind that there needs to be a multidisciplinary approach. Ideally, the intensivist; emergency department physician; thoracic surgeon or otorhinolaryngologist; anesthesiologist; and the interventional pulmonologist collaborate to develop a coherent plan of action that considers different alternatives for a safe and successful approach. When the patient is symptomatic but stable, there may be sufficient time to plan for a procedure that will both assess the stenotic segment and potentially relieve the obstruction. However, if the patient is unstable with acute respiratory failure, restoration of airway patency must occur immediately. If it is not possible to pass an endotracheal tube and the stenosis is felt to be proximal, emergent bedside tracheotomy may become the best option because there may not be enough time to transport the patient to the operating room. However, the latter presentation is unusual when patients first arrive at the emergency department and, often, subsequent deterioration may be averted by carefully planning and by quickly treating the stenosis before overt decompensation occurs.

The rigid bronchoscope is an invaluable tool because it provides the means to successfully maintain the patency of the airway while the patient is being treated endoscopically, either definitively when the stenosis is simple, or temporarily as a bridge to a planned tracheal resection and reconstruction when the stenosis is complex [16–19]. The interventionalist has multiple, different therapeutic modalities that may be applied through the rigid bronchoscope to restore airway patency. One method is to use sequentially larger diameter rigid barrels to dilate the airway in a secure and gentle manner. For this method, the patient is intubated with a larger diameter tracheal barrel immediately proximal to the stenosed area and then a smaller diameter bronchial barrel is advanced through the stenosis, allowing for the subsequent advancement of larger caliber bronchial barrels until enough of the lumen is restored for spontaneous breathing. Alternatively, after intubation with a tracheal barrel immediately proximal to the stenotic area, Jackson–Pratt dilators can be advanced sequentially under direct visualization with the rigid telescope. Balloon dilatation may also be done, keeping in mind that the airway is completely occluded while the balloon is inflated. With a very tight stenosis one must use gentle maneuvers because dilating against a fixed stenosis can

TABLE 182.3

Causes of Central Airway Obstruction

Malignant	Nonmalignant

Primarily intrinsic obstruction
• Primary lung carcinoma
• Adenoid cystic
• Mucoepidermoid
• Carcinoid
• Metastatic head and neck cancer
• Breast
• Renal cell
• Colon
• Melanoma
Extrinsic
• Esophageal
• Thymus
• Thyroid
• Germ cell
• Lymphadenopathy:
  • Lymphoma
  • Metastatic cancer
Mixed
• Any of the above
	• Postintubation and posttracheostomy tracheal stenosis
	• Lymphadenopathy
	• Vascular malformation
	• Inflammatory:
	  • Relapsing polychondritis
	  • ANCA-associated granulomatous vasculitis
	• Post-lung transplant stenosis
	• Post-pneumonectomy syndrome
	• Goiter
	• Pseudotumor
	  • Hamartomas
	  • Amyloid
	  • Papillomatosis
	• Tracheobronchomalacia

This table is not all-inclusive.
ANCA, antineutrophil cytoplasmic autoantibodies.

result in tracheal tears, especially where the anterior wall meets the posterior membrane of the trachea. Such tracheal tears can result in more scarring and further restenosis, possibly involving an even longer segment of the trachea.

Simple airway stenosis typically involves short (<1 cm long) segments of the airway without malacia or loss of cartilaginous support and may have thin web scarring or acute granulation tissue [18,19]. This type of stenosis may be treated definitively with endoscopic treatment [18,19]. The interventional pulmonologist has different therapeutic modalities at his or her disposal and these include coagulation modalities (i.e., electrocautery, laser therapy, and APC) that relieve obstructions by coagulation necrosis and vaporization of scar tissue. A commonly referenced technique involves the use of neodymium-doped yttrium aluminum garnet (Nd:YAG) laser vaporization of scar tissue followed by gentle dilatation [15].

Complex airway stenoses show more extensive scarring (>1 cm long), sometimes featuring a circumferential hourglass-like constriction or malacia. Complex stenoses may also be "A" shaped because of bilateral collapse of the walls of a fractured cartilage (Figs. 182.2 and 182.3) [16]. For complex airway stenoses, tracheal resection and reconstruction is the standard of care and, in experienced hands, this is a highly effective surgical procedure with low morbidity and mortality [17]. For the patient with poor reserve, a temporizing endoscopic procedure, as already described, may be attempted and this is often followed with airway stenting. When airway stenting is done, one approach is to leave the stent in place until the patient is able to undergo definitive surgery or, alternatively, to remove the stent after approximately 6 months to 1 year to assess for resolution of the stenosis, an outcome that is possible but uncommon [19].

Malignant Central Airway Obstruction

Lung cancer is the leading cause of death from cancer in the USA. It is responsible for one-third of deaths from cancer of both men and women. It outnumbers prostate, breast, and colon cancers combined [2]. There may be airway complications associated with lung cancer up to 30% of the time. When there is airway involvement, patients often present to the ICU with lobar or complete lung collapse, sepsis from post-obstructive pneumonia, or severe dyspnea [20]. It is well established that the relief of malignant CAO may lead to symptomatic and quality of life improvements, reduce work of breathing, and decreased health care utilization [21–23]. Moreover, survival appears to be the same after successful endoscopic treatment of malignant CAO when compared to cancer patients without CAO [24,25].

Malignant CAO may be caused by endobronchial tumor growth, extrinsic compression, or mixed causes (Table 182.3). The rigid bronchoscope may be used for immediate relief of malignant CAO by gently advancing the instrument and, while carefully remaining parallel to the airway wall, rotating the beveled tip around the base of a polypoid lesion to core it out and restore patency of the airway lumen [26]. The rigid bronchoscope also ensures a means to ventilate the patient during the procedure. The flexible videobronchoscope can be advanced through the lumen of the rigid barrel to reach into segmental airways not approachable by rigid bronchoscopy. This technique increases the maneuverability that is needed to apply therapies (e.g., laser, electrocautery, or APC) aiming to eradicate tumor and achieve hemostasis [27].

Since the introduction of the tracheobronchial silicone stent by Dumon in 1990, stents have become an integral part of the relief of both benign and malignant CAO (mostly silicone for the former, and both metallic and silicone for the latter) and are a main feature of the interventional pulmonologists' skill set [28]. In some instances, airway stents can be a valuable tool for maintaining airway patency once it has been restored. With both benign and malignant disease causing extrinsic compression

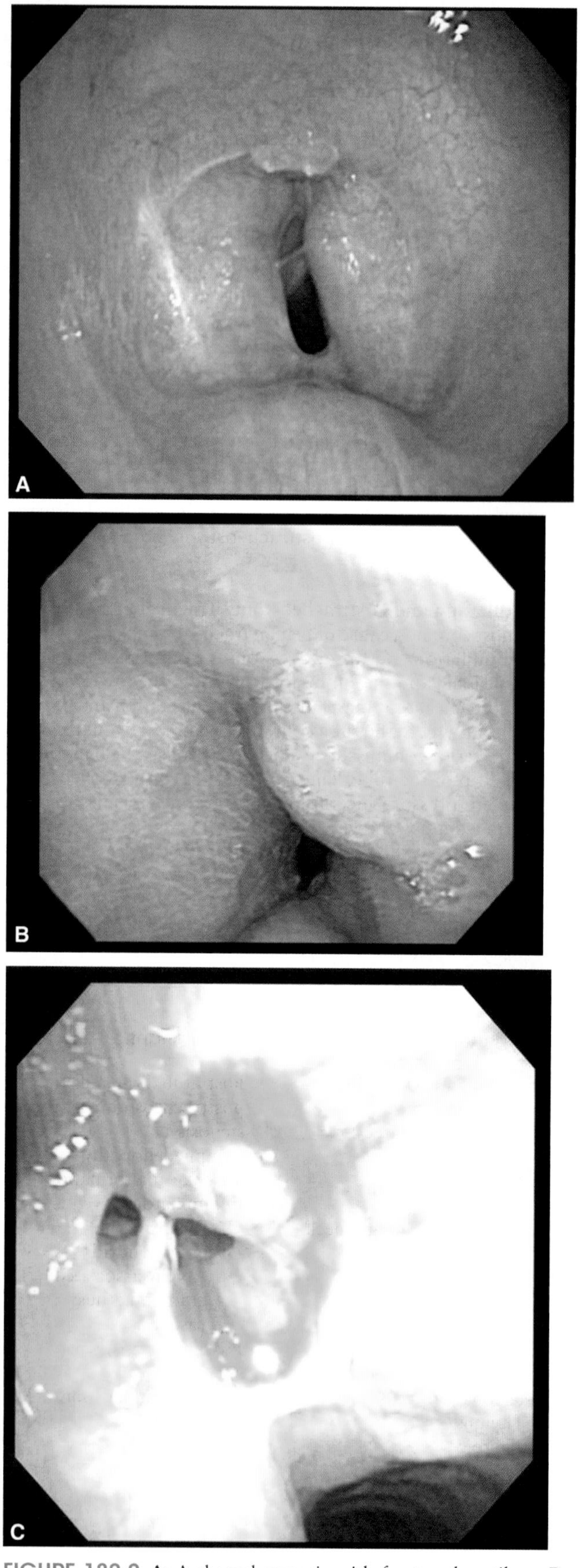

FIGURE 182.2 A: A-shaped stenosis with fractured cartilage. B: Complex stenosis with chronic granulation above stoma site. C: Simple stenosis cause by a thin web in ANCA-associated vasculitis, easily broken with the flexible bronchoscope; ANCA, antineutrophil cytoplasmic autoantibodies.

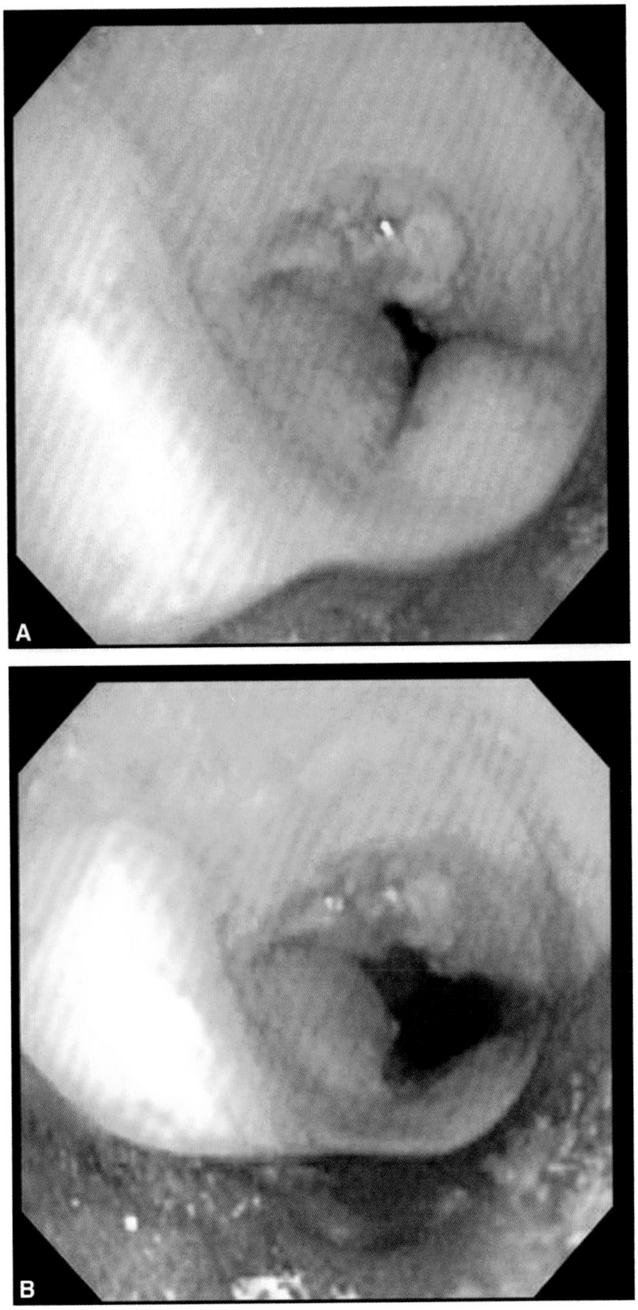

FIGURE 182.3 Complex post-tracheostomy tracheal stenosis with malacia. A: Very narrow trachea lumen with passive expiration. B: notice dilatation of the tracheal lumen under positive pressure ventilation.

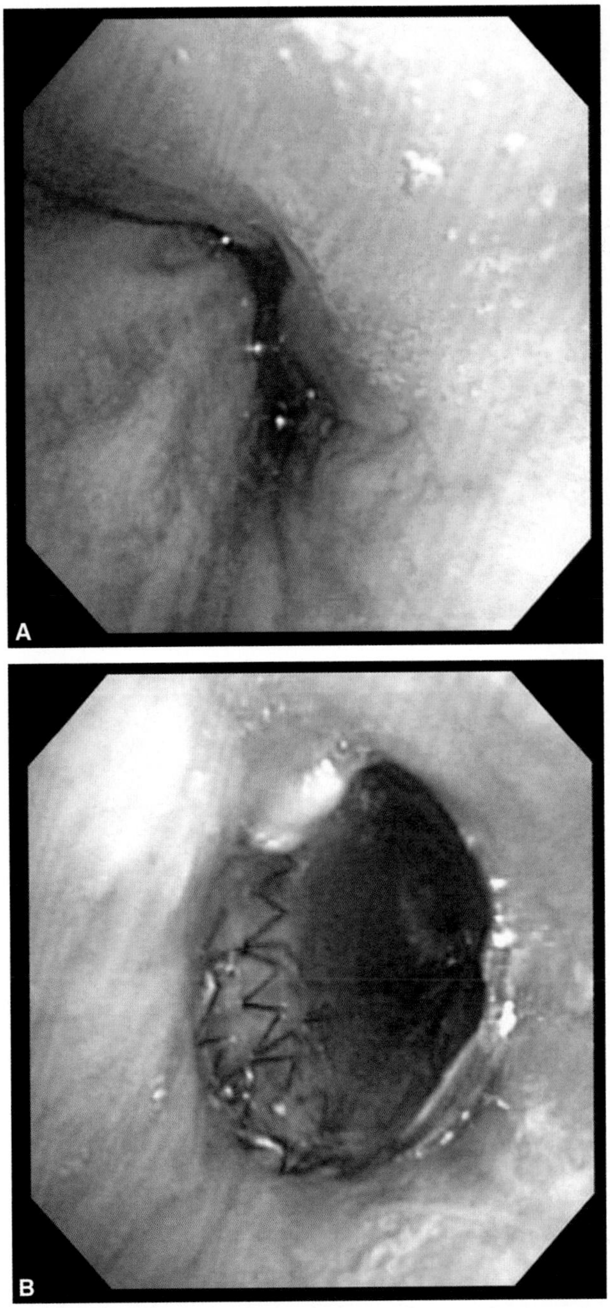

FIGURE 182.4 A: Malignant extrinsic compression left mainstem bronchus. B: Relief of obstruction after stent placement.

and sometimes with intrinsic and mixed obstruction as well, it may be necessary to leave an airway stent in place to ensure the stability and patency of the airway lumen (Figs. 182.4 and 182.5). There are two main types of stent, silicone and metallic, and it is generally accepted that, except for very carefully selected situations, metallic stents should be used primarily for malignant disease-related CAO [28]. The rigid bronchoscope provides the only means for deployment of a silicone stent and, it is arguably the best means for the deployment of any type of stent because it ensures control of the airway throughout the entire procedure (Fig. 182.6). It is up to the interventionalist to decide when a stent may benefit a patient; what type and size to place; how to care for it; and how to follow up the patient after insertion.

Recent data from the American College of Chest Physicians Quality Improvement Registry, Evaluation, and Education (AQuIRE) program have shown the benefits of therapeutic bronchoscopy for malignant CAO. The data from fifteen centers performing 1,115 procedures showed successful restoration of airway patency in 93% of all cases. Endobronchial obstruction and stent placement were associated with success, whereas failure was more likely in patients with American Society of Anesthesiology (ASA) score >3, renal failure, primary lung cancer, left mainstem disease, and tracheoesophageal fistula. Symptomatic improvement as assessed by Borg score for dyspnea occurred in 48% of patients, and it seemed to be more significant among patients with greater baseline dyspnea. Health-related quality of life (HRQOL) as measured by the SF-6D was improved for 42% of patients, and again greater improvements were found in patients with greater baseline dyspnea. The overall complication

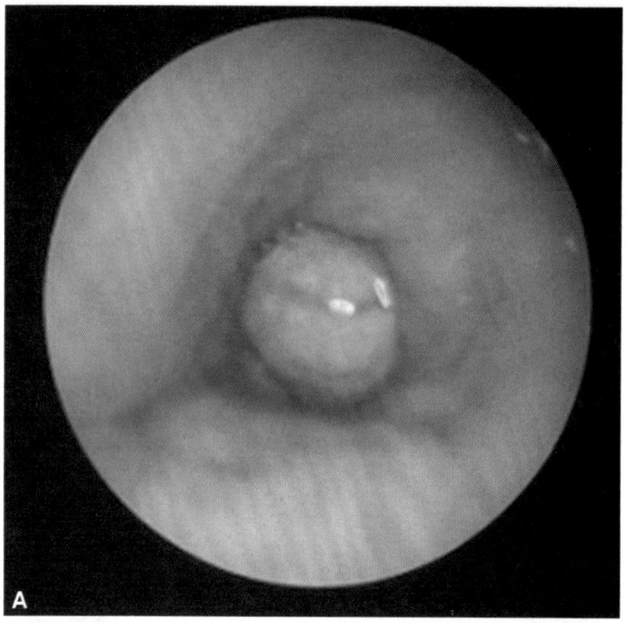

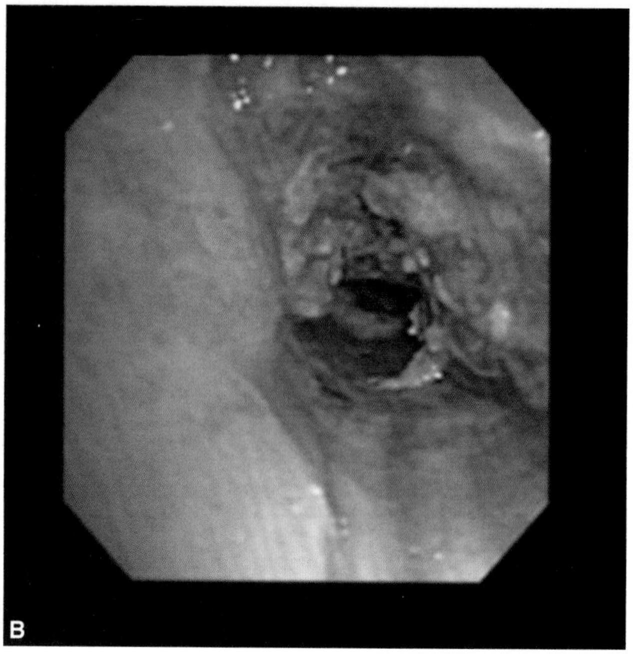

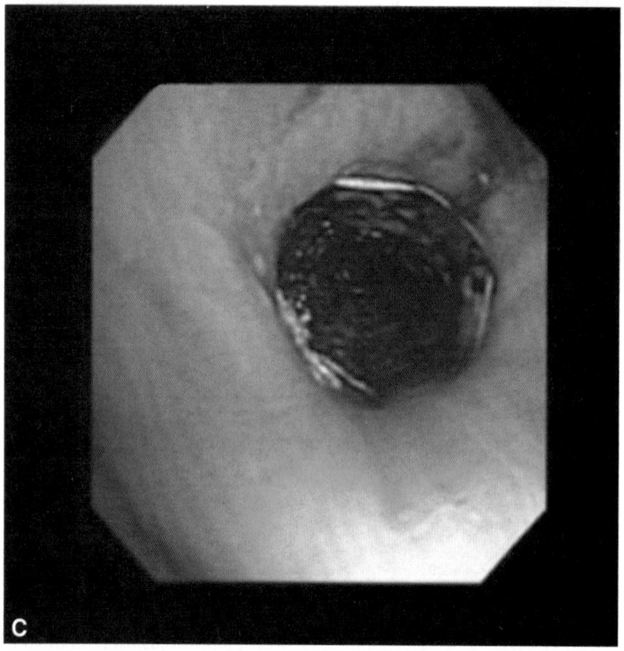

FIGURE 182.5 **A:** Malignant intrinsic obstruction right middle lobe. **B:** Post-debridement with argon plasma coagulation. **C:** Stent placed because of residual tumor obstruction in bronchus intermedius.

rate was 3.9%, but there was a significant variation among centers (0.9% to 11.7%; $p = 0.002$) and ASA score >3, redo therapeutic bronchoscopy, and moderate sedation were all found to be risk factors for complications. The 30-day mortality rate was 14.8%, and this again varied among different centers (7.7% to 20.2%; $p = 0.02$). The findings of the ACQuIRE program reinforce the concept that malignant airway obstruction can often be treated to achieve significant palliation of symptoms and improved quality of life [20].

Airway Obstruction Caused by Aspiration of Foreign Bodies

A more common occurrence among children, non-asphyxiating foreign body aspiration may also be seen in adults. Failure to have an effective swallowing mechanism or lack of a strong cough may be a problem encountered by patients with certain predisposing conditions such as alcohol intoxication, narcotic abuse, neuromuscular diseases, and advanced dementia.

The rigid bronchoscope, initially conceived for the removal of aspirated foreign bodies, has lost its central role for this application since the advent of the flexible bronchoscope. There are many accessories that may be employed with a flexible bronchoscope for retrieval of foreign bodies. Some of these include forceps, balloons, baskets, and cryotherapy, the latter being particularly useful for soft, water-rich material. However, for certain instances, it may be more advisable to use the rigid bronchoscope, instead. Through the rigid bronchoscope, one can ensure ventilation even during sometimes laborious and lengthy procedures, especially, for example, when larger instruments are required or when there is granulation tissue covering the foreign body.

Bronchopleural Fistula

A bronchopleural fistula (BPF) is a communication between the airway and the pleural space. BPFs occur 1.5% to 28.5% of the time after lung resection with the highest incidence following

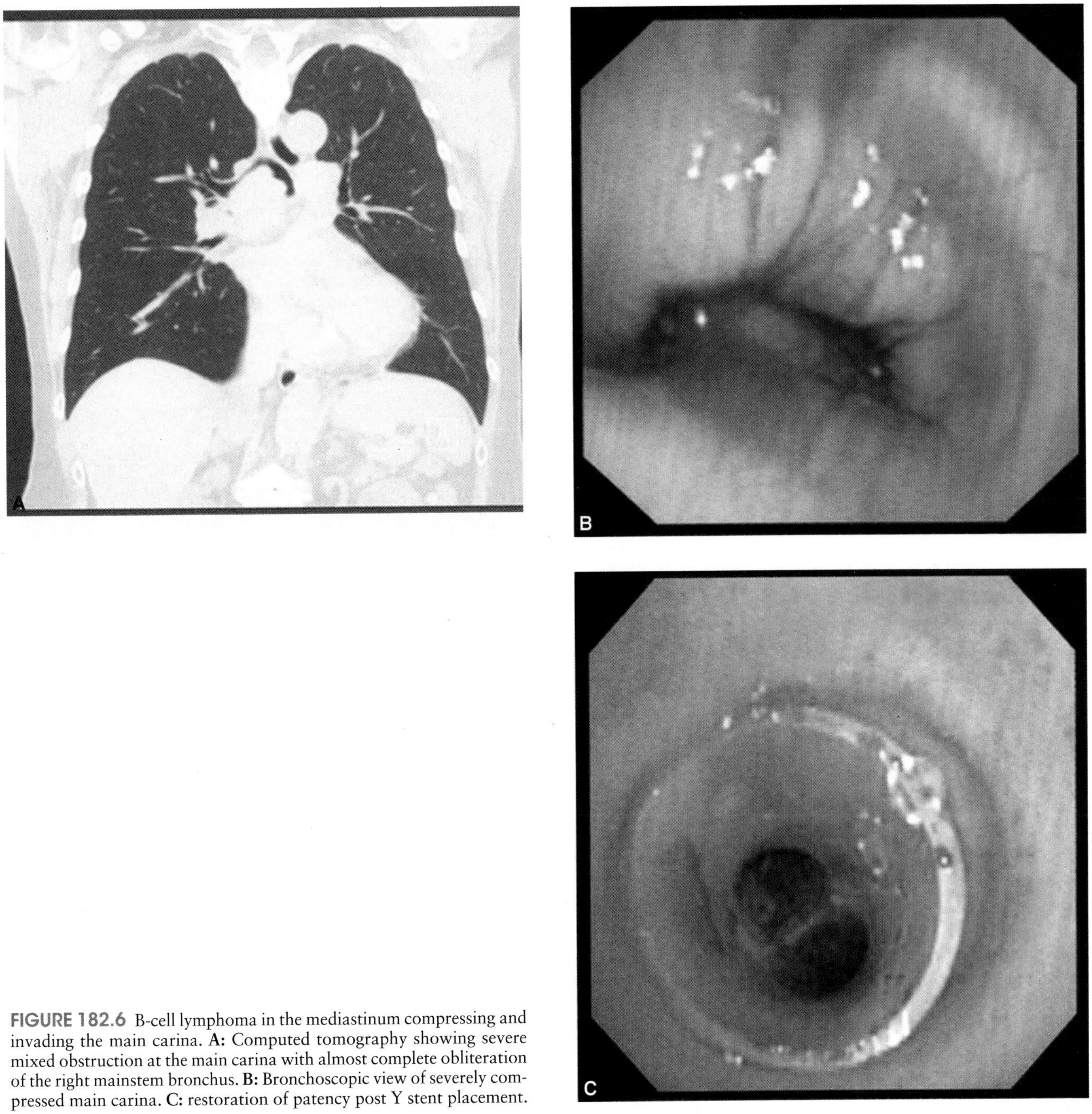

FIGURE 182.6 B-cell lymphoma in the mediastinum compressing and invading the main carina. A: Computed tomography showing severe mixed obstruction at the main carina with almost complete obliteration of the right mainstem bronchus. B: Bronchoscopic view of severely compressed main carina. C: restoration of patency post Y stent placement.

right pneumonectomy and right lower lobectomy. An air leak through the chest tube postoperatively indicates a communication between lung parenchyma and the pleural space, and these leaks are considered prolonged air leaks (PAL) when they persist more than 7 days. These PAL are commonly seen after lung resection and seem to be particularly frequent and of longer duration among patients with underlying emphysema or bullous disease. In a review of the National Emphysema Trial (NETT), 90% of patients developed some form of an air leak. Patients with BPF and air leaks have significantly higher morbidity and mortality rate [27,28].

The patient with a BPF may present acutely with severe dyspnea, respiratory distress, or hypotension due to tension pneumothorax. Alternatively, the presentation may be subacute or chronic, when an infected pleural space causes fatigue, wasting, fever, and cough, sometimes with expectoration of purulent material and sepsis. The chest radiograph will reveal an air fluid level. Because the pleural space becomes infected with airway secretions, a drainage procedure is always warranted. The ultimate treatment of a BPF is surgical and usually involves placing a muscle flap over the affected airway. Other risk factors for the development of an air leak include the acute respiratory distress syndrome (ARDS), chest trauma, necrotizing infection, and pulmonary fibrosis [29].

The management of a BPF or an air leak involves general and specific measures [29]. At all times, the pressure gradient between the airway and the pleural space should be minimized, positive pressure ventilation should be avoided when feasible and chest tubes should have the minimal amount of suction required to maintain gas exchange, the goal should not always be to achieve complete lung reexpansion but rather to maintain ventilation and oxygenation [30]. For more detailed management of the patient on the ventilator, please refer to the section on the topic of BPF of Chapter 176 on Pleural Diseases.

For endoscopic management of BPF, there are several options when the defect is small and either parenchymal or an airway defect less than 3 mm in diameter. Endoscopic treatment is very

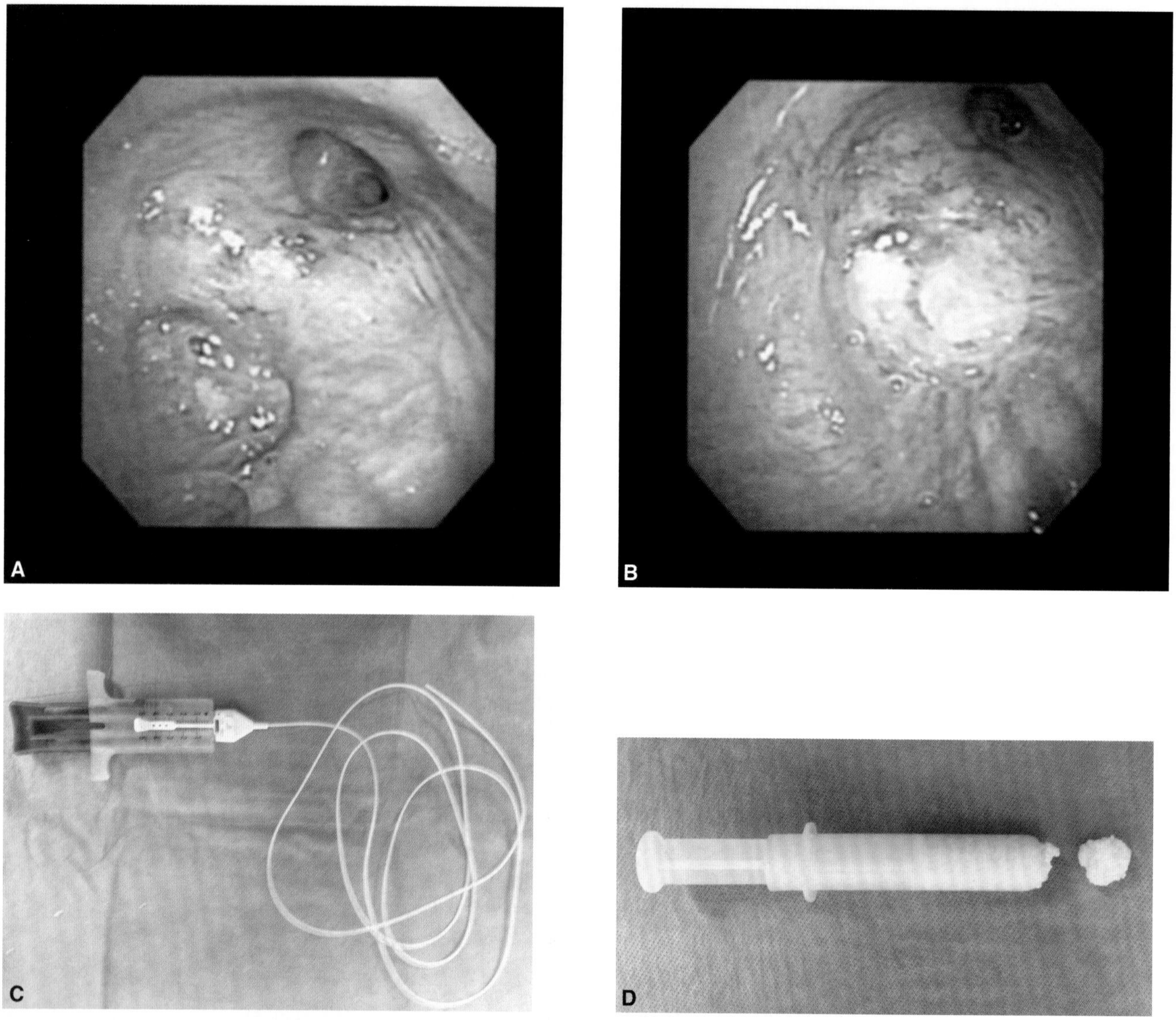

FIGURE 182.7 A: Bronchopleural fistula at right lower lobe stump. B: Fistula closed with fibrin derivative over a bone graft substitute previously introduced into the fistula opening. C: Catheter and double syringe used to inject the thrombin and fibrinogen combination. D: synthetic bone graft used to fill the defect in the stump.

unlikely to work when the airway defect is >8 mm [31,32]. First, if the defect is not immediately visible by bronchoscopy, one option is to advance a Fogarty balloon and selectively occlude different lung segments, starting proximally, until the leak is observed to decrease or disappear. When the site of the leak is localized, several sealants may be applied, such as fibrinogen–fibrin compound; tetracycline and blood clot; ethanol; cyanoacrylate glue; gel foam; coils; silver nitrate; calf bone; amplatzer occlusion devices; spigots; or stents [30–33] (Fig. 182.7). In a study involving 60 patients with an air leak, spigots were placed with reduction in the air leak in 38% and resolution in 40% [34]. In 2008, the FDA approved Spiration IBV endobronchial valves for the treatment of PAL after lung resection. These one-way valves are placed bronchoscopically into the affected lung segments. Typically, several valves may be needed to effectively stop or reduce the leak [35].

The standard treatment of a BPF should be surgical if at all possible. When the patient is too frail to undergo a major surgical procedure, endoscopic options may be contemplated. However, the approach to these often challenging cases should be multidisciplinary, involving the intensivist, the thoracic surgeon, and the interventional pulmonologist [36].

Percutaneous Dilatational Tracheostomy

Since its description by Ciaglia in 1985, percutaneous dilatational tracheostomy (PDT) has become a very commonly performed procedure in the ICU [37]. Indications are typically the same as those for surgical tracheostomy (ST), including a requirement for long-term ventilatory support; inability to clear secretions; and airway obstruction.

There are several potential advantages of PDT over ST. In a meta-analysis including 17 randomized clinical trials and 1,212 patients, there was a lower risk of infection among patients of the PDT group, possibly related to less manipulation and trauma of pre-tracheal tissues during PDT. There also was a decreased incidence of bleeding and death when patients with PDT were compared to those who had undergone ST performed in the operating room [38]. Another meta-analysis of critically ill patients also compared PDT to ST, and this study showed that although technical difficulties were more common, PDT was associated with less procedural time and less stoma inflammation [39].

Percutaneous tracheostomy has become a part of the skills set of many intensivists. However, given the steep learning curve and the need for a minimal volume to maintain competency, it seems reasonable to have a few designated physicians performing this procedure at a given institution. The interventional pulmonologists are well suited to be the designated specialists for this technique given their familiarity with airway interventions, especially when considering that short and long-term complications such as bleeding at the stoma site and posttracheostomy tracheal stenosis are often treated by the subspecialty. When performed by an IP team, PDT is safe and has a complication rate that is similar to that of ST performed by a surgical team [40].

Complications of PDT mimic those of ST, and may be short and long term. The short-term complications most often encountered include bleeding and infection; other more rare ones include posterior tracheal injury, subcutaneous emphysema, pneumomediastinum, and pneumothorax. Bleeding is usually venous and non-life threatening, being external or from the endotracheal mucosa at the level of the stoma. Locally, a mixture of lidocaine and epinephrine can be injected to control bleeding. We also have successfully used oxidized regenerated cellulose strips (Surgicel) applied within the bleeding area in the stoma. Movement of the tracheostomy tube or forceful coughing may also cause bleeding within the endotracheal mucosa at the level of the stoma and this may present as frank blood being suctioned by the bedside nurse or respiratory therapist. For this type of bleeding, the interventional pulmonologist can use electrocoagulation techniques such as electrocautery or APC to control severe hemorrhage. A trachea–innominate artery fistula may present as a massive bleeding a few weeks after tracheostomy placement and should be prevented by placing the tracheostomy between the first and second or second and third tracheal rings. Tracheal stenosis and trachea–esophageal fistula may also present as long-term complications and may be occurring more commonly as the number of ICU survivors increases. It remains to be determined whether PDT or ST is superior for avoiding these serious complications.

To minimize the potential complications of PDT, some authorities have proposed the use of bedside ultrasonography to detect large vessels that may pose a significant bleeding risk, as well as for the identification of anatomical landmarks when they are difficult to visualize or palpate, such as in morbidly obese patients [41,42]. Videobronchoscopy also is widely employed to ensure proper placement of the initial needle in the space between either the first and second or second and third tracheal rings. Again, both techniques are within the typical skills set of the interventional pulmonologist.

Percutaneous Gastrostomy Tube Placement

Since its first inception by Gauderer and colleagues in 1980 [43], the placement of percutaneous gastrostomy (PEG) tubes has gained widespread acceptance for long-term enteral nutrition of patients unable to swallow effectively. The procedure is now routinely performed by surgeons, gastroenterologists, or interventional radiologists. Given their advanced endoscopic and procedural training, interventional pulmonologists may also safely perform placement of PEG tubes in the ICU setting at the patient bedside. When indicated, the PDT and PEG tubes can often both be placed together, at a single procedural session [44].

PEG is usually performed by inserting an endoscope into the stomach and then transilluminating the puncture site through the gastric and abdominal walls. Finger indentation can be seen within the insufflated gastric lumen at the site of transillumination. A skin incision then is made under local anesthetic and an angiocath is advanced through the abdominal wall and into the stomach. A loop is inserted through the angiocath and then grabbed and brought out through the mouth attaching it to the gastrostomy tube. The loop is then attached to the gastrostomy tube such that the tube can be pulled down the esophagus, into the stomach, and through the gastric and abdominal walls for securement at the skin surface. An alternate method uses a pull-away sheath and introduces the tube through the abdominal wall.

The safety and efficacy of PEG placement by an IP team has been demonstrated. In one review of 72 patients undergoing the procedure, PEG tube insertion was successful in 97.2%, with no major complications [44].

Ultrasound Guided Thoracentesis and Placement of Pleural Catheters

Pleural effusions may be seen in up to 62% of ICU patients. Although these are often small effusions not contributing to the patient's condition, many times they may need to be sampled or drained for diagnostic or therapeutic reasons [45]. The characterization of a pleural effusion as a transudate or exudate, either uncomplicated or complicated, may be very helpful in the management of the ICU patient.

Over the last decade, the use of ultrasonography in the ICU setting has become widespread. Bedside ultrasound allows for the characterization of the lung and pleural space in a quick, safe and noninvasive way that spares the patient the radiation of chest radiography or computed tomography (CT) [46].

For the assessment and drainage of pleural fluid in patients with or without mechanical ventilation, chest ultrasonography is more sensitive and specific than chest radiographs and is more reliable than physical examination for selecting an appropriate puncture site [47,48]. Chest ultrasonography is also helpful for characterizing pleural effusions because transudates are usually anechoic. Exudates may sometimes be anechoic, but when the fluid is complex (septated, loculated, etc.) or hypoechoic an exudate is more likely [49].

Interventional pulmonologists are thoroughly trained in thoracentesis and placement of pleural catheters under ultrasound guidance, a procedure that may often be indicated for ICU patients with empyema or other effusions requiring complete drainage. The interventionalist considers the entire medical picture to decide whether a thoracentesis or a pleural catheter is best indicated. Pleural catheters also facilitate instillation of fibrinolytics for complicated effusions and chemical pleurodesis for malignant effusions. Additionally, pleural catheters and chest tubes may also be placed by an IP specialist for evacuation of a pneumothorax.

Workup of Solid Lung and Pleural Lesions

Chest ultrasound also may be useful for safely sampling solid lung or pleural lesions. With a large enough acoustic window, a 22G to 25G needle may be advanced, under local anesthetic, into the lesion to aspirate material for cytologic analysis. In addition, a core needle biopsy may be performed. These biopsy samples may be obtained safely by marking the entry site and then using ultrasound to define the safe range, direction and depth of the puncture. Sonographic evaluation for a potential pneumothorax may be done immediately after the aspiration with relative ease. The IP specialist, thoroughly trained in chest ultrasonography and pleural procedures, is often able to safely and effectively obtain valuable histopathologic sampling using these techniques for carefully selected cases.

Related Considerations

Although not exclusive to the realm of interventional pulmonologists, we briefly discuss the role of lung biopsy in the management of critically ill patients with respiratory failure and parenchymal infiltrates. The available approaches include not only surgical lung biopsy but also the use of nonsurgical, bronchoscopic diagnostic modalities such as transbronchial lung biopsies (TBBx), and the burgeoning utilization of transbronchial cryobiopsies, a newer biopsy technique that may obviate the need for surgical biopsy. For a comprehensive discussion of lung biopsy in the ICU setting the reader is referred to prior editions of this textbook [50].

Lung Biopsy procedures can be grouped into two main categories: invasive, open surgical procedures (e.g., open thoracotomy lung biopsy and video-assisted thoracoscopic (VATS) lung biopsy) and semi-invasive, closed nonsurgical procedures (e.g., percutaneous transthoracic needle biopsy under fluoroscopic, ultrasound, or more commonly computed tomography (CT) guidance; transbronchial lung biopsy; and the more recently described, transbronchial cryobiopsy). In the setting of localized or diffuse parenchymal pulmonary disease, many factors are considered when developing a diagnostic plan, including the history of a probable inciting event (e.g., ARDS), the patient's immune status, the severity of disease, the pace of the presentation, the timing of the diagnostic intervention, the diagnostic yield, the likelihood that the results obtained will alter management (the concept of a "contributive result") [51], the risks of bleeding or other complications, and the availability of local expertise for performing the various types of procedures. Prior to proceeding with lung biopsy one should strongly consider the utilization and contribution of BAL (bronchoalveolar lavage) when specimens are sent for culture, viral PCR (polymerase chain reaction), cell counts, and cytology. In many situations, BAL, without tissue biopsy, is the least invasive and safest sampling method (even in a patient with a bleeding diathesis) and, when combined with the probable clinical diagnosis, is completely adequate and sufficient for directing appropriate therapy. Of course, when considering various lung biopsy approaches, contraindications must be taken into account (see Table 182.4) and also the likelihood that a particular method of biopsy can establish or rule out a given diagnosis based on pretest probability (see Table 182.5).

Open lung biopsy (OLB) has the advantage of providing a large tissue sample for pathology and is sometimes performed for critically ill patients, especially those with ARDS featuring extensive lung infiltration of uncertain etiology. Two recent systematic reviews on the role of OLB of critically ill patients have shed light on its performance characteristics and utility. Libby and colleagues found that OLB in ARDS provided a specific diagnosis in 84% of patients and led to a change in management in 73% of cases. Moreover, there was acceptable mortality (43%, rarely because of the OLB itself) and morbidity (complication rate of 22% with PAL being the most common complication) [52]. Wong and colleagues combined the Libby study with other case series and found that OLB had a more modest diagnostic yield of only 54%. They additionally reported that the most common diagnoses made by OLB were fibrosis/pneumonitis and infection [53]. Therapeutic changes did occur for most (78%) of the patients and complication rates were similar to the Libby study. VATS may also be utilized as a biopsy technique for ARDS and has been reported to have yields and complications similar to OLB. However, severely critically ill patients and moribund patients may not tolerate VATS, a surgical procedure that requires single lung ventilation during general anesthesia.

Transbronchial lung biopsy via a flexible bronchoscope is an important biopsy technique because it may obviate the need for OLB in certain circumstances (e.g., immunocompromised patients or lung transplant patients when graft rejection and infection are considered). As stated above, a decision to proceed with TBBx (and OLB) should only be taken after careful risk-benefit analysis of inherent limitations and potential complications (TBBx bleeding risk of 1% to 4% and risk of pneumothorax up to 25% of mechanically ventilated patients) [54]. Fluoroscopy can increase yield and possibly safety and is generally recommended, especially when targeting focal parenchymal disease which is difficult in the ICU, resource-limited settings, and is associated with radiation exposure. The diagnostic yield of TBBx is limited by the size of the specimens obtained (1 to 3 mm), crush artifact, and sampling error. TBBx results are frequently nonspecific and, therefore, the technique has a limited role for the assessment of most idiopathic interstitial pneumonias and vasculitides. However, it does have significant yield for diseases such as sarcoidosis, eosinophilic pneumonia, various infections, and lymphangitic carcinomatosis.

Small sample size and tissue artifacts associated with TBBx create considerable problems in interpreting pathologic specimens and thus limit its diagnostic accuracy in many settings. In order to obtain larger tissue samples and avoid artifact, proceduralists and investigators have recently explored flexible bronchoscopic transbronchial cryobiopsy to obtain lung specimens. The technique of transbronchial cryobiopsy has been thoroughly described elsewhere [55]. Results from various case series have demonstrated that large tissue specimens can be obtained (median size three to five times greater than TBBx) and these have preserved histologic characteristics, often free of artifacts. When correlated with clinical and radiologic findings, this technique has allowed the diagnosis of interstitial pneumonias such as NSIP (nonspecific interstitial pneumonia) and UIP (usual interstitial pneumonia), producing diagnostic yields as high as 70% to 80%. Complications include pneumothorax in up to 23% of cases and minor bleeding that is readily controlled. More severe bleeding sometimes requires

TABLE 182.4

Contraindications and Relative Contraindications to Lung Biopsy [1–5]

Open thoracotomy biopsy
Contraindication
Too ill to undergo general anesthesia
Thorascopic lung biopsy
Contraindications
Too ill to undergo general anesthesia
Extensive pleural adhesions
Uncorrectable coagulopathy
Postpneumonectomy patient
Severe pulmonary hypertension
Relative contraindications
Inability to place a double-lumen endotracheal tube
Inability to tolerate single lung ventilation
Closed biopsy
Contraindications
Uncorrectable coagulopathy (including uremia)[a]
Unstable cardiovascular status
Severe hypoxia likely to worsen during bronchoscopy
Inadequately trained bronchoscopist
Poor patient cooperation
Relative Contraindications
Recent myocardial infarction or unstable angina
Adjacent vascular abnormalities
Positive-pressure ventilation
Cavitating lesions (especially with air-fluid levels, or >10 cm diameter)
Severe pulmonary hypertension
Adjacent emphysematous lung disease
Suspected echinococcal disease
Uncontrollable cough

[a]Bronchoalveolar lavage can be performed with relative safety in patients with thrombocytopenia.

TABLE 182.5

Potentially High Yielding Biopsy Procedures for a Variety of Underlying Disease Processes

Bronchoalveolar lavage
- Infections (PCP, mycobacteria, and endemic fungal)
- Alveolar proteinosis
- Alveolar hemorrhage
- Acute eosinophilic pneumonia
- Lung cancer
- Lymphoma
- Exogenous lipoid pneumonia

Transbronchial needle aspiration
- Lung cancer
- Lymphoma
- Infections (endemic fungi, mycobacteria, and nocardia)

Bronchial brush biopsy
- Lung cancer
- Metastatic cancers

Transbronchial lung biopsy
- Sarcoidosis
- Lymphangitic carcinomatosis
- Alveolar proteinosis
- Lung cancer
- Chronic eosinophilic pneumonia
- Amyloidosis
- Lymphocytic interstitial pneumonia
- Cryptogenic organizing pneumonitis
- Hypersensitivity pneumonitis
- Invasive aspergillosis

Open lung biopsy or video-assisted thoracoscopic biopsy
- Pulmonary capillaritis (vasculitides)
- Diffuse alveolar damage
- Idiopathic pulmonary fibrosis
- Nonspecific interstitial pneumonitis
- Inorganic pneumoconiosis

PCP, Pneumocystis pneumonia.

placement of an endobronchial blocker. The future is promising for this newer technique and we await further studies that are specific to the critical care setting.

CONCLUSIONS

The still growing specialty of IP deals with many complex airway and pleural diagnoses and features a variety of diagnostic and therapeutic bronchoscopic and pleural procedures that are helpful in the ICU setting. Given the complexities of the critically ill patient population, a multidisciplinary approach to clinical management is ideal. One key to success is a close collaboration among intensivists; IP physicians; thoracic surgeons; ENT specialists; radiation and medical oncologists; and interventional radiologists.

References

1. Dumon JF: A dedicated tracheobronchial stent. *Chest* 97:328–332, 1990.
2. Siegel R, Naishadham D, Jemal A: Cancer statistics, 2012. *CA Cancer J Clin* 62:10–29, 2012.
3. Bolliger CT, Mathur PN: ERS/ATS Statement on Interventional Pulmonology. *Eur Respir J* 19:356–373, 2002.
4. Ernst A, Silvestri GA, Johnstone D: Interventional pulmonary procedures: guidelines from the American College of Chest Physicians. *Chest* 123:1693–1717, 2003.
5. Becker HD: History of the rigid bronchoscope, in Ernst A, Herth FJF (eds): *Principles and Practice of Interventional Pulmonology*. 1st ed. Berlin, Springer, 2013, pp 3-13.
6. Ikeda S, Yanai N: Flexible Bronchofiberscope. *Kejo J Med* 17:1–16, 1968.
7. Laforet EG, Berger RL, Vaughan CW: Carcinoma Obstructing the Trachea: treatment by laser resection. *N Eng J Med* 294:941, 1976.
8. Sakr L, Dutau H: Massive hemoptysis: an update on the role of bronchoscopy in diagnosis and management. *Respiration* 80:38–58, 2010.
9. Sosa A, Madison JM, Oliveira P: Hemoptysis, in SK Jindal (ed): *Textbook of Pulmonary and Critical Care Medicine*. 1st ed. New Delhi, Jaypee Brothers Medical Publishers, 2011, pp 204–221.
10. Chowla M, Getzen T, Simoff MJ: Medical pneumonectomy. Interventional bronchoscopic and endovascular management of massive hemoptysis due to Pulmonary Pseudoaneurysm, a consequence of endobronchial brachytherapy. *Chest* 135:1355–1358, 2009.
11. Shigemura N, Wan IY, CH Yu S, et al: Multidisciplinary Management of Massive Hemoptysis: a 10-year experience. *Ann Thorac Surg* 87:849–853, 2009.
12. Worrell SG, DeMeester SA. Thoracic emergencies. *Surg Clin N Am* 94:183–191, 2014.
13. Valipows A, Kreuzer A, Koller H, et al: Bronchoscopic guided hemostatic therapy for the management of life-threatening hemoptysis. *Chest* 127:2113–2118, 2005.
14. Brouns M, Jayaraju ST, Lacor C, et al: Tracheal Stenosis: a flow dynamics study. *J Appl Physiol* 102:1178–1184, 2007.
15. Ernst A, Feller-Kopman D, Becker HD, et al: Central airway obstruction. *Am J Respir Crit Care Med* 169:1278–1297, 2004.
16. Murgu SD, Egressy K, Laxmanan B, et al: Central Airway Obstruction: benign strictures, tracheobronchomalacia and malignancy related obstruction. *Chest* 150:426–441, 2016.
17. Grillo HC: Postintubation stenosis, in Grillo (ed): *Surgery of the Trachea and Bronchi*. 1st ed. Hamilton, ON, BC Decker, 2004, pp 301–340.
18. Brichet A, Verkindre C, Dupont J, et al: Multidisciplinary approach to management of postintubation tracheal stenosis. *Eur Respir J* 13:888–893, 1999.
19. Galluccio G, Lucantoni G, Battistoni P, et al: Interventional bronchoscopy in the management of benign tracheal stenosis. *Eur J Cardiothorac Surg* 35:429–434, 2009.
20. Simoff MJ, Lally B, Slade M, et al: Symptoms management in lung cancer. Diagnosis and management of lung cancer, 3rd edition: American College of Chest Physicians evidence-based clinical practice guidelines. *Chest* 143:e455s–e497s, 2013.
21. Colt H, Harrell JH: Therapeutic rigid bronchoscopy allows level of care changes in patients with acute respiratory failure from central airway obstruction. *Chest* 112:202–206, 1997.
22. Oviatt PL, Stather DR, Michaud G, et al: Exercise capacity, lung function, and quality of life after interventional bronchoscopy. *J Thorac Oncol.* 6:38–42, 2011.
23. Ost DE, Ernst A, Grosu H, et al: Therapeutic bronchoscopy for malignant central airway obstruction, success rates and impact on dyspnea and quality of life. *Chest* 147:1282–1298, 2015.
24. Saji H, Furukawa K, Tsutsui H, et al. Outcomes of airway stenting for advanced lung cancer with central airway obstruction. *Interact Cardiovasc Thorac Surg* 11:425–428, 2010.
25. Razi SS, Lebovics RS, Schwartz G, et al. Timely airway stenting improves survival in patients with malignant central airway obstruction. *Ann Thorac Surg* 90:1088–1093, 2010.
26. Alraiyes AH, Machuzak MS. Rigid bronchoscopy. *Semin Respir Crit Care Med* 35:671–680, 2014.
27. Mahmood K, Wahidi MM: Ablative therapies for central airway obstruction. *Semin Respir Crit care Med* 35:681–692, 2014.
28. Defranchi HA, Defranchi S: Interventional pulmonology in the intensive care unit, in Díaz-Jiménez JP, Rodriguez AN (eds): *Interventions in Pulmonary Medicine*. 1st ed. Berlin, Springer, 2013, pp 451–468.
29. Shekar K, Foot C, Fraser J, et al: Bronchopleural fistula: an update for intensivists. *J Crit Care* 25:47–55, 2010.
30. Baumann MH, Sahn SA. Medical management and therapy of bronchopleural fistulas in the mechanically ventilated patient. *Chest* 97:721–728, 1990.
31. Noppen LM. Bronchopleural fistulas. An overview of the problem with special focus on endoscopic management. *Chest* 128:3955–3965, 2005.
32. Kollaus PH, Lax F, Janikier D: Endoscopic treatment of postoperative bronchopleural fistula: Experience with 45 cases. *Ann Thorac Surg* 66:923–927, 1998.
33. Fruchter O, Kramer MR, Dagan T, et al: Endobronchial closure of bronchopleural fistula using Amplatzer devices. Our experience and literature review. *Chest* 139:682–687, 2011.
34. Watanabe Y, Keisuke M, Akihiko T, et al. Bronchial occlusion with endobronchial Watanabe Spigot. *J Bronchol* 10:264–267, 2003.
35. U.S. Department of Health and Human Services: Press announcements. Available at http://www.fda.gov/NewsEvents/Newsroom/PressAnnouncement/2008/ucm116970.htm. Accessed May 13, 2017.
36. Slade M. Management of pneumothorax and prolonged air leak. *Semin Respir Crit care Med* 35:706–714, 2014.
37. Dennis BM, Eckert MJ, Guter O, et al. Safety of bedside percutaneous tracheostomy in the critically ill: Evaluation of more than 3,000 procedures. *J Am Coll Surg* 216:858–867, 2013.
38. Delaney A, Bagshaw SM, Nalos M. Percutaneous dilatational tracheostomy versus surgical tracheostomy in critically ill patients: a systematic review and meta-analysis. *Crit Care* 10: R55, 2006.
39. Putensen C, Theuerkauf N, Guenther U, et al. Percutaneous and surgical tracheostomy in critically ill adult patients: a meta-analysis. *Crit Care* 18:544, 2014.

40. Yarmus L, Pandian V, Gilbert C, et al: Safety and efficiency of interventional pulmonologists performing percutaneous tracheostomy. *Respiration* 84:123–127, 2012.
41. Alansari M, Alotais H, Al Aseri Z, et al: Use of ultrasound guidance to improve safety of percutaneous dilatational tracheostomy: a literature review. *Crit Care* 19:229, 2015.
42. Guinot P-G, Zogheib E, Petiot S, et al: Ultrasound-guided percutaneous tracheostomy in critically ill obese patients. *Crit Care*16:R40, 2012.
43. Belanger A, Akulian J: Interventional pulmonology in the intensive care unit: Percutaneous tracheostomy and gastrostomy. *Semin Respir Crit Care Med* 35:744–775, 2014.
44. Yarmus L, Gilbert C, Lechtzi N, et al: Safety and feasibility of interventional pulmonologists performing bedside percutaneous endoscopic gastrostomy tube placement. *Chest* 144:436–440, 2013.
45. Mattison LE, Coppagge L, Alderman DF, et al: Pleural effusions in the medical ICU. Prevalence, causes and clinical implications. *Chest* 111:1018–1023, 1997.
46. Lichtenstein DA: Lung ultrasound in the critically ill. *Ann Intensive Care* 4:1, 2014.
47. Lichtenstein D, Hulot J-S, Rabiller A, et al: Feasibility and safety of ultrasound-aided thoracentesis in mechanically ventilated patients. *Intensive Care Med* 25:955–958, 1999.
48. Diacon AH, Butsche MH, Soler M: Accuracy of pleural puncture sites. A prospective comparison of clinical examination with ultrasound. *Chest* 123:436–441, 2003.
49. Yan P-C, Lu K-T, Chang D-B, et al. Value of sonography in determining the nature of pleural effusions: Analysis of 320 cases. *Am J Roentgenol* 159:29–33, 1992.
50. Kopec SE, Irwin RS. Lung biopsy, in Irwin RS, Rippe JM (eds): *Intensive Care Medicine*. 7th ed. Philadelphia, PA, Lippincott Williams & Wilkins, 2012, pp 815–822.
51. Palakshappa JA, Meyer NJ: Which patients with ARDS benefit from lung biopsy? *Chest* 148(4): 1073–1082, 2015.
52. Libby LJ, Glebman BD, Altorki NK: Surgical lung biopsy in adult respiratory distress syndrome: a meta-analysis. *Ann Thorac Surg* 98:1254–1260, 2014.
53. Wong AK, Walkey AJ: Open lung biopsy among critically ill, mechanically ventilated patients: a metaanalysis. *Annals ATS* 12(8):1226–1230, 2015.
54. Jain P, Hadique S, Mehta AC. Transbronchial lung biopsy, in Jain P, Mehta AC (eds): Interventional Bronchoscopy: A Clinical Guide. New York, NY, Springer Science & Business Media, 2013, pp 15–44.
55. Poletti V, Casoni GL, Gurioli C, et al: Lung cryobiopsies: a paradigm shift in diagnostic bronchoscopy? *Respirology* 19: 645-654, 2014.

Chapter 183 ■ Sleep Issues in the Intensive Care Unit Setting

BIREN B. KAMDAR • NANCY A. COLLOP

INTRODUCTION

Although its precise function is complex and incompletely understood, sleep is considered a vital process necessary for physical, emotional, and psychologic well-being and survival. In the intensive care unit (ICU) setting, critically ill patients often experience poor sleep quality owing to underlying baseline comorbidities, severe illness, loud noises, bright lights, care-related disturbances, and noxious medications. Although the contribution of poor sleep to the ICU recovery process remains largely unknown, interventions to improve sleep have garnered significant attention as part of recent efforts to improve outcomes during and following critical illness. This chapter provides a summary of current knowledge surrounding sleep in the ICU, including an overview of normal sleep, causes and potential consequences of sleep disruption in the ICU, and strategies to improve sleep for critically ill patients.

OVERVIEW OF NORMAL ADULT SLEEP

Sleep Architecture

A basic knowledge of normal adult sleep physiology is necessary to appropriately understand and improve sleep in the ICU setting. Adults are recommended to obtain 7 to 9 hours of consolidated sleep during each 24-hour cycle [1]. Sleep is divided into non-rapid eye movement (NREM) and rapid eye movement (REM) stages, which alternate over four to six 90- to 100-minute cycles across the sleep period (**Fig. 183.1**). NREM is comprised of N1, N2, and N3 stages, which account for 2% to 5%, 45% to 55%, and 13% to 24% of the sleep period, respectively, whereas REM comprises 20% to 25%. In general, stages N1 and N2 are "lighter" than stage N3, which is also known as "slow wave" or "deep" sleep and is believed to play a key role in the body's restorative processes. REM, on the other hand, is characterized by muscle atonia but involves autonomic variability and substantial brain activity, including dreaming. Although NREM predominates in the first third of the sleep period and tends to occur soon after sleep onset, most REM occurs in the latter half of the sleep period.

Circadian Rhythms

Achieving a normal duration and pattern of sleep relies on individual factors such as age, comorbid conditions, intrinsic sleep–wake cycle, volitional control of sleep duration, and drugs, along with environmental factors such as ambient temperature, noise, and light [2]. The sleep–wake cycle is regulated through

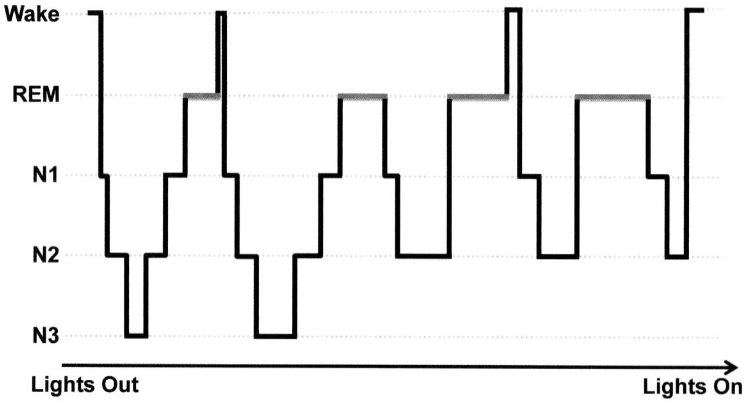

FIGURE 183.1 One night hypnogram of normal adult sleep, demonstrating typical sleep stage transitions. (From Kamdar BB: Sleep deprivation in critical illness: its role in physical and psychological recovery. *J Intensive Care Med* 27(2):97–111, 2012, with permission).

two complementary processes, the sleep homeostat and circadian pacemaker. The sleep homeostat, or process S, dictates sleepiness and is influenced by buildup of melatonin and the neurotransmitter adenosine, the end product of ATP metabolism. Process S is similar to thirst: the longer you are without sleep, the sleepier you become. As an opposing process, the circadian pacemaker, or process C, dictates wakefulness and is largely synchronized to environmental light–associated suppression of melatonin release from the pineal gland. In nocturnal sleepers, melatonin secretion occurs in the absence of light, between 9 p.m. and 3 a.m., with lowest values between 7 a.m. and 9 a.m. [3].

Physiologic Processes during Sleep

During sleep, a complex interplay of physiologic processes occur, which are believed to play a fundamental role in growth and homeostasis. The physiologic processes most relevant for critically ill patients are discussed here.

Thermoregulation

Sleep and circadian rhythms play an integral role in body temperature and thermoregulation. In healthy adults, body temperature peaks late in the day, falls during sleep, nadirs late in sleep, and rises before awakening. During NREM, temperature sensitivity decreases, whereas poikilothermia (body temperature variation based on surroundings) and a loss of compensatory responses (i.e., sweating and shivering) occur during REM.

Respiratory Processes

N1 sleep is characterized by decreased respiratory drive and muscle activity, irregular breathing, and increased upper airway collapsibility. During N2 and N3, respiratory rate and tidal volume stabilize whereas minute ventilation falls, resulting in a rise in arterial $PaCO_2$ of 4 to 6 mm Hg and concomitant drop in pH of 0.03 to 0.05 units. This hypoventilation is believed to occur in the setting of decreased central ventilatory drive, upper airway muscle relaxation, and increased airway resistance [1].

Cardiovascular Processes

Alterations of blood flow and electrical activity that occur during sleep can increase one's risk of life-threatening cardiovascular events, especially in those with diminished cardiorespiratory reserve [4]. During NREM, increased parasympathetic tone leads to a drop in blood pressure, heart rate, and systemic vascular resistance. Alternatively, during REM, a relative increase in sympathetic tone leads to increased (up to 35%) blood pressure and heart rate [4]. Bursts of vagal activity during REM can also potentiate sinus pauses and bradycardia.

Endocrine Processes

Growth hormone (GH), prolactin, cortisol, and thyroid-stimulating hormone (TSH) undergo fluctuations during the sleep–wake cycle [1] (**Fig. 183.2**). GH and prolactin, cell differentiation and proliferation hormones possibly involved in preservation of muscle mass and immune function during critical illness, peak during early and late sleep, respectively, and remain at low levels during wakefulness. More specifically, GH secretion has been shown to correlate with depth of sleep and is therefore highest during N3 [5]. Alternatively, cortisol, a key hormone involved in glucose metabolism, stress, and wound healing, follows a diurnal cycle, rising in the morning and falling toward bedtime. TSH secretion follows a similar circadian pattern, peaking before sleep onset and falling during sleep.

SLEEP IN THE INTENSIVE CARE UNIT

A typical night in an ICU is characterized by a busy whirlwind of beeping alarms, loud voices, bright lights, and visits from providers to administer medications, gather vital signs, draw blood, perform X-rays, and perform routing assessments. As a consequence, sleep suffers, leading patients to list poor sleep quality as an important cause of anxiety and stress in the ICU and among the worst memories of their ICU experience [4].

Sleep Architecture of the Critically Ill

Studies of medical and surgical ICU populations have demonstrated that mechanically and nonmechanically ventilated critically ill patients generally experience exceptionally poor sleep quality as compared to healthy adults. Regardless of sedation or mechanical ventilation status, critically ill patients experience marked variability in sleep duration, with reported ranges of 3.6 to 6.2 hours per day [6–9] in some studies and 7.0 to 10.4 hours in others [10–12]. Whether patients experience short- or long duration of sleep, numerous investigations involving polysomnography (PSG) have demonstrated that sleep in the ICU is characterized by a predominance of N1 and N2, reduced or near absent N3 and REM, and marked fragmentation, with over 50% of sleep occurring during daytime hours [1] (**Fig. 183.3**). In a notable study involving polysomnographic recordings from 22 critically ill patients, of whom 20 were mechanically ventilated, patients averaged 41 ± 28 episodes of sleep per 24-hour period, each averaging 15 ± 9 minutes, highlighting the profound level of sleep fragmentation in this population [12].

Sleep Measurement in the ICU

Measuring sleep in the ICU is exceedingly challenging. Whether limited by logistical, environmental, or patient-related factors, instrument reliability, or cost, existing challenges in measuring sleep accurately and on a large-scale remain a key barrier hindering efforts to understand and improve sleep in the ICU setting [13].

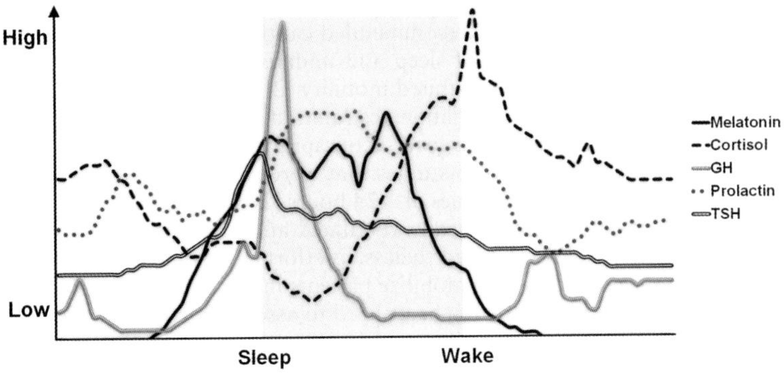

FIGURE 183.2 Hormone levels in healthy adults maintaining standard sleep–wake cycles, activities, and meal times. Lines represent levels of melatonin, cortisol, growth hormone, prolactin, and thyroid-stimulating hormone across the sleep–wake cycle. A typical sleep period is represented by the shaded rectangular box. (From Knauert M: Sleep and sleep disordered breathing in hospitalized patients. *Semin Respir Crit Care Med* 35:582, 2014, with permission).

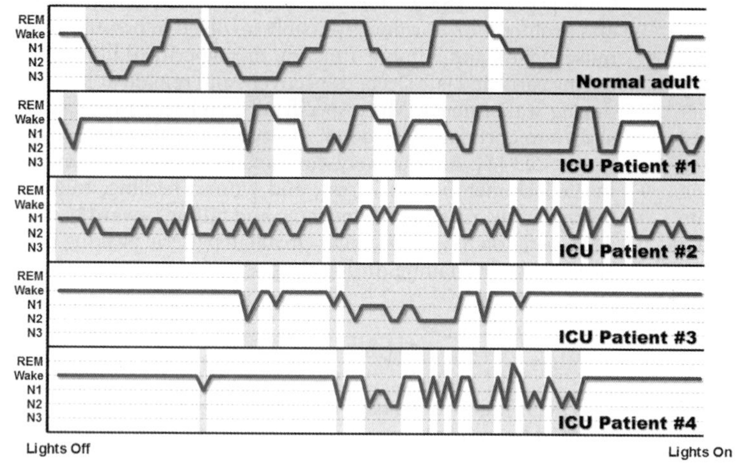

FIGURE 183.3 Sleep patterns of typical patients in an ICU. The tracings summarize polysomnography recordings of overnight sleep in one normal adult and four different ICU patients. Shaded areas represent sleep, and unshaded areas represent wake. Notable in the ICU patients is the lack of REM and absence of restorative N3 sleep. ICU, intensive care unit; REM, rapid eye movement. (From Knauert M: Sleep and sleep disordered breathing in hospitalized patients. *Semin Respir Crit Care Med* 35:582, 2014, with permission).

Polysomnography

PSG, the most widely used mode of sleep measurement, involves simultaneous electroencephalogram (EEG), electromyogram (EMG), and electrooculogram (EOG) recordings. Although PSG is the gold standard for sleep measurement, its large-scale use in the ICU is challenging because it is costly, laborious, and requires bulky equipment, skilled technicians, and interpretation by a sleep expert. Moreover, interpretation of PSG is especially challenging in the presence of common ICU medications and illnesses such as sepsis, shock, hepatic encephalopathy, and renal failure [1,4,14]. More recently, a multisite investigation involving continuous PSG recordings in 37 mechanically ventilated patients revealed EEG recordings suggestive of sleep despite patients being interactive and awake, and others suggesting wakefulness despite patients being comatose [15]. Moreover, 36 of 37 patients, and 85% of recorded EEG data, demonstrated monotonous, atypical tracings uncharacteristic of conventional sleep stages or sleep/wake transitions, highlighting the challenges of interpreting PSG recordings and applying existing PSG scoring systems to the ICU population. Additionally, unattended PSG, which is likely required for large-scale ICU-based studies, was recently shown in a medical ICU population to be infeasible, because 26 of 28 (93%) patients were unable to tolerate PSG for 24 hours owing to reasons such as discomfort, mobility limitation, and, ironically, the PSG devices themselves causing inability to sleep [9]. Hence, PSG is impractical for large-scale ICU sleep investigations and is therefore discouraged [13].

Actigraphy

Actigraphy, which involves accelerometer-based sleep estimation using a wristwatch-like interface, is a well-established research instrument. As compared to PSG, actigraphy is affordable, involves a comfortable interface, is practical for prolonged and large-scale use, and allows for assessments of physical activity unavailable with other sleep measurement modalities [16–19]. Although actigraphy seems ideal for sleep estimation, its use for the critically ill is recommended cautiously out of concern for overestimation of sleep and underestimation of wakefulness in the setting of limited mobility [20] because of common ICU factors such as sedation, restraints, neuromuscular weakness, or severe illness. Moreover, actigraphy measurement in the ICU has been limited to studies that were small in size [20–30], involved recording times of <24 hours [16,20,21,31], or enrolled primarily mechanically ventilated and/or sedated patients [17,20,21,32,33]. Nevertheless, as efforts to promote sleep, minimize sedation, and mobilize patients in the ICU setting grow [34], actigraphy may be utilized to assess the effect of ICU-based interventions.

Bispectral Index

Bispectral index (BIS) involves a single forehead sensor containing multiple EEG electrodes, whose signals are processed to provide a 0 to 100 integer value corresponding to level of consciousness. Often used to assess depth of anesthesia during surgery, BIS can evaluate sleep depth, similar to PSG, and provide continuous, unsupervised recordings using a simple interface, similar to actigraphy. Although BIS poses a potentially attractive option for sleep evaluation in the ICU, its interpretation is complicated by variability and overlap of cutoffs for sleep stages and sedated states [4,35]. Moreover, similar to PSG [9], BIS in the ICU is susceptible to electrode detachment and artifact with subject movement [35], thus complicating its potential use for continuous, unattended recordings on a large scale.

Subjective Measures of Sleep

Subjective sleep measurement, whether by patients or their proxies, represents the most practical option for evaluating patient sleep in the ICU. The most commonly used instruments in the ICU are the Richards-Campbell Sleep Questionnaire (RCSQ) [36,37] and Verran/Snyder-Halpern Sleep Scale [38,39], which both involve 5- and 14-item visual analogue scales, respectively, assessing various characteristics of sleep. Although both instruments are reliable, only the RCSQ has been validated against PSG for a critically ill population [37,39]. Nevertheless, both instruments have been utilized extensively as an endpoint of ICU-based interventions to improve sleep [40–45]. Despite their low cost and ease of use, these instruments are potentially limited by recall bias, rater fatigue across repeated daily assessments, noncompliance, impaired patient cognition or consciousness, and lack of daytime sleep ratings. Although bedside nurses may complete these instruments on their patients' behalf [41,46,47], a recent interrater reliability study of the RCSQ demonstrated that nurses tend to overestimate patient sleep quality [48]. Hence, the use of nurse proxies to subjectively assess sleep in the ICU, whether by observation or validated instruments, must be performed with caution.

Causes of ICU Sleep Disruption

Noise

Whether attributed to staff conversations, alarms, ventilators, or nightly floor waxing, most ICUs are loud at all hours of the day (Fig. 183.4). Studies of both medical and surgical ICUs have demonstrated that noise levels frequently approach and exceed 80 decibels (dB) [8,12,49–56], the threshold necessary to maintain

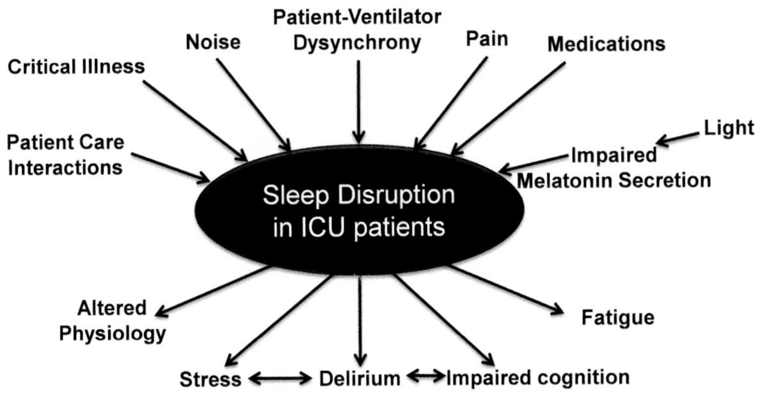

FIGURE 183.4 Risk factors and potential outcomes of poor sleep in the intensive care unit (ICU). (Adapted from Kamdar BB: Sleep deprivation in critical illness: its role in physical and psychological recovery. *J Intensive Care Med* 27:97, 2012, with permission).

sleep, and far surpassing the 35 dB and 45 dB nighttime and daytime ICU limits outlined by the Environmental Protection Agency [1,4,14,18]. When correlated with PSG recordings, these loud noises have been attributed to 11% to 18% of sleep arousals and 17% to 24% of awakenings in critically ill patients [8,12,51,57].

Subjectively, patients in the ICU consistently report staff conversations and alarms as the most disruptive noises affecting sleep [8,58]. When measured, these factors comprised 26% and 31%, respectively, of ICU noises ≥75 dB in an observational study [59], and 57% and 30% in a detailed soundscape analysis [54]. Interestingly, a recent investigation commented that the traditional ICU design, with closely spaced beds facing a central nurse station, strongly contributes to noise pollution [60]. This study also noted that although staff conversations were loudest in the rooms of the sickest patients, they were often unrelated to patient care and held directly over patients under the assumption that sedation rendered patients unaware of their surroundings. These findings highlight potentially important and underrecognized design and behavioral issues worth considering during ICU-based sleep improvement efforts.

Light and Melatonin

In addition to promoting well-being, improving mood, and possibly preventing ICU delirium [61], light plays a key role in synchronizing circadian rhythms, and therefore in regulating sleep and wake. When light levels falls below 100 lux (normal indoor light ~180 lux), melatonin is secreted from the pineal gland, promoting sleep. Conversely, in the presence of light, melatonin secretion is suppressed, promoting wakefulness. Moreover, light levels above 1,500 lux are considered sufficient to disrupt sleep. Although ICU-based studies are lacking on this topic, one study involving continuous light measurement of four ICUs demonstrated mean maximum nocturnal light levels of 128 to 1,445 lux, high enough to suppress melatonin release but below the threshold to disrupt sleep [53].

Melatonin, and melatonin supplementation in particular, has received recent attention [62]. Independent of light levels, impaired melatonin secretion has been described in patients with sepsis [63] and delirium [64,65], suggesting that factors other than light influence circadian rhythms in the critically ill. As small trials involving melatonin have demonstrated both positive [24,32] and negative [66] findings regarding improvements in ICU sleep quality, further research is needed in this area.

Patient Care Interactions

Although difficult to measure accurately, critically ill patients experience approximately 7.8 patient care interactions per hour during sleep [67] and 43 to 51 per night shift [68,69]. These interactions include care-related activities such as vital sign checks, blood draws, medication administration, radiographs, baths, wound care, respiratory care (e.g., suctioning and ventilator adjustments), and general assessments, along with care-unrelated activities such as family visitation. When correlated with PSG in one study, 20% of these activities precipitated a sleep arousal or awakening, accounting for 7% of all observed sleep disruptions [8]. These data are supported by patient reports that blood draws, vital sign checks, and nurse visits are the most disruptive ICU factors affecting sleep [41,58].

Efforts to minimize patient care interactions should involve engagement of staff to evaluate the timing and necessity of interactions during patient sleep. Although minimizing interactions with unstable patients is not feasible, a recent interventional study demonstrated that for more stable patients, engaged ICU staff were able to bundle closely scheduled orders and conduct baths earlier, resulting in less nighttime interactions [41,70].

Mechanical Ventilation

Mechanical ventilation, which is administered to roughly 40% of ICU patients [71], improves gas exchange during respiratory failure but can also affect sleep quality. In general, ICU patients receiving mechanical ventilation report worse sleep quality than their nonventilated counterparts [58], experiencing greater sleep fragmentation, lower sleep efficiency, and more sleep during daytime hours [10,72]. When quantified, patients receiving mechanical ventilation average 20 to 63 sleep arousals per hour [8–12], which can be precipitated by issues related to patient-ventilator synchrony, or by noxious factors associated with mechanical ventilation, such as suctioning, repositioning, ventilator alarms, physical restraints, provider assessments, and discomfort from endotracheal, nasogastric, or orogastric tubes.

The effect of ventilator mode on sleep quality has been studied extensively. In a study of 11 mechanically ventilated ICU patients receiving pressure support (PSV) and assist control (ACV) ventilator modes, PSV precipitated more central apneas and subsequent sleep arousals and awakenings per hour than ACV (79 ± 7 vs. 54 ± 7), in particular when PCO_2 levels dropped below the sleep-induced apnea threshold [73]. By adding dead space to the ventilator circuitry during PSV, the investigators observed a significant rise in PCO_2 and a concomitant decline in central apneas and sleep disruptions. Adding to these findings, a study of 20 patients alternating between ASV and lower pressure PSV (6 cm H_2O) during sleep noted markedly increased wakefulness during PSV, but no central apneas [74]. Although this study suggested that mode and not level of support had a greater effect on sleep, a subsequent study of 15 patients alternating between ACV, clinician-adjusted PSV, and PSV that automatically adjusted to patient effort, compliance and end-tidal CO_2 demonstrated equally fragmented sleep with all three modes [51]. Moreover, 13 patients receiving PSV and proportional assist ventilation (PAV), which promotes patient-ventilator synchrony by delivering pressure support proportional to patient inspiratory effort, suggested improved sleep quality during PAV as compared to PSV [56]. However,

TABLE 183.1

Effect of Commonly Used ICU Medications on Sleep

Drug class/Medication	Mechanism of action	Effect on sleep
Sedatives		
Benzodiazepines	GABA receptor agonist	↓W, ↑TST, ↓N3, ↓REM
Dexmedetomidine	α_2-Agonist	↑N3, ↓SL, ↓REM
Propofol	GABA receptor agonist	↑TST, ↓SL, ↓W
Analgesics		
Opioids	μ-Receptor agonist	↓N3, ↓REM
Cardiovascular		
Norepinephrine/epinephrine	α- and β-receptor agonist	↓N3, ↓REM, Insomnia
Dopamine	D_2-, β_1-, α_1-receptor agonist	↓N3, ↓REM, Insomnia
Phenylephrine	α_1-Receptor agonist	↓N3, ↓REM
β-Blockers	CNS β-receptor antagonist	↑W, ↓REM, Nightmares, Insomnia
Amiodarone	Various pathways	Nightmares
Clonidine	α_2-Agonist	↓REM
Immunosuppressants		
Corticosteroids	Decreased melatonin secretion	↑W, ↓N3, ↓REM, Insomnia
Tacrolimus	Calcineurin inhibitor	Insomnia
Cyclosporine	Inhibits production and release of IL-2	Insomnia
Antipsychotics		
Haloperidol	Dopamine-receptor antagonist	↑TST, ↑N3, ↑SE, ↓SL, ↓W
Olanzapine	$5HT_2$-, D_2-receptor antagonist	↑TST, ↑N3, ↑SE, ↓SL, ↓W
Antimicrobial		
Fluoroquinolones	GABA type A receptor inhibition	Insomnia

GABA, gamma-aminobutyric acid; W, wake; TST, total sleep time; N3, slow-wave sleep; REM, rapid eye movement sleep; SL, sleep latency; CNS, central nervous system.

as confirmed in another study of 17 patients [75], the authors noted that patients who were synchronous with PSV experienced similar sleep quality as during PAV. Finally, a study of 14 awake, nonsedated patients alternating between neutrally adjusted ventilator assist (NAVA) and PSV demonstrated reduced apneas, increased REM, and improved sleep quality during NAVA, as neuromechanical coupling during NAVA presumably improved patient-ventilator synchrony [57].

Synthesizing this literature, a recent meta-analysis of randomized controlled trials of interventions to improve sleep in the ICU revealed significantly improved sleep efficiency, but not sleep fragmentation, when comparing timed with spontaneous modes of ventilation [76]. As important limitations, the authors acknowledged the small sample size and single-site design of the included studies. Hence, until larger multisite trials are performed, practitioners should adopt an individualized approach to ventilator management during sleep, and consider use of less conventional ventilator modes to optimize patient-ventilator synchrony.

Although noninvasive ventilation (NIV) is administered frequently in the ICU and in the outpatient setting for sleep-disordered breathing (SDB), little is known regarding sleep during NIV in the ICU. Two investigations conducted by a single research group on 27 and 24 patients receiving NIV for hypercapnic respiratory failure demonstrated that, overall, whereas total sleep time and efficiency were low during NIV, the majority of sleep occurred at night, was of normal architecture, and was of higher duration and quality when compared to spontaneous breathing periods without NIV [77,78]. Interestingly, in the first study, patients exhibiting worse sleep architecture were more likely to fail NIV, defined as requiring intubation or dying. These findings demonstrated that, in select patients, NIV was well tolerated during sleep and may aid in promoting sleep. Further research is needed to corroborate these findings.

Medications

Several common ICU medications can affect sleep architecture (**Table 183.1**). Sedative medication is frequently prescribed in the ICU, particularly for mechanically ventilated patients, to alleviate pain and anxiety and presumably to reduce agitation. Despite these properties, these agents can also affect sleep. For example, opioids such as fentanyl and morphine profoundly inhibit N3 and REM in addition to precipitating arousals and central apneas [4,79]. Additionally, benzodiazepines such as lorazepam and midazolam, which are often co-administered with opioids, may lower sleep latency and increase N2 and total sleep time, but profoundly reduce N3 and REM sleep [4,79]. Additionally, agents such as dexmedetomidine and propofol, which have gained popularity as less deliriogenic non-benzodiazepine sedative options [34,80–82], may also contribute to fragmented sleep [83] but are considered less disruptive to sleep than benzodiazepines and opioids [80,81,84,85]. Until research expands in this area, practitioners should aim to administer minimal or no sedation and perform daily interruptions of sedation, consistent with current guidelines [34], as a strategy to minimize sedation-related disruptions to sleep architecture.

A number of other common ICU medications can also affect sleep (**Table 183.1**). Vasopressor medications such as norepinephrine, dopamine, and phenylephrine may diminish N3 and REM sleep via sympathomimetic pathways. However, in critically ill patients with various types and degrees of shock, it is unclear to what extent these drugs penetrate the blood–brain barrier [79]. Additionally, patients receiving β-blockers can experience REM suppression and, subsequently, nightmares and insomnia; however, this effect is likely dependent on lipid solubility of the drug administered [79]. Immunosuppressive drugs such as corticosteroids, which are prescribed often including during asthma and chronic obstructive pulmonary disease (COPD) exacerbations, and tacrolimus and cyclosporine, which are common among transplantation patients, are also known to disrupt sleep and cause insomnia [86,87]. Finally, haloperidol and olanzapine, antipsychotics receiving attention for their possible role in ICU delirium prevention [88], may promote restorative sleep stages and, in one study, were recommended as part of a pharmacologic guideline to promote sleep [41].

Withdrawal from medications may also affect sleep in the ICU. Abrupt discontinuation of prolonged, high-dose opioid and benzodiazepine infusions may precipitate sleep disruptions and insomnia, lending further support to strategies for sedation minimization, daily sedation interruption, and gradual tapering of prolonged sedation [79]. Additionally, because antidepressant medications such as tricyclic antidepressants, selective serotonin reuptake inhibitors, and monoamine oxidase inhibitors are often held in the setting of critical illness, patients should be monitored closely for associated withdrawal reactions including insomnia, nightmares, and REM rebound [79]. Finally, withdrawal from alcohol, nicotine, and illicit drugs such as cannabis and amphetamines can lead to profound insomnia and sleep disruption, and, in extreme cases, delirium [79].

Finally, medications prescribed specifically for sleep in the ICU can both promote and impair sleep. "Z-drugs," which include zolpidem, zopiclone, eszopiclone, and zaleplon are non-benzodiazepine γ-aminobutyric acid ($GABA_A$)-receptor agonists commonly used for insomnia. These drugs possess hypnotic properties similar to benzodiazepines, but, unlike benzodiazepines, bind different $GABA_A$ receptor subunits and have a shorter half-life, therefore disturbing sleep architecture minimally [89]. Although these drugs can promote restorative sleep, their use in sick, frail, or elderly ICU patients is recommended cautiously owing to risk of oversedation, delirium, and drug–drug interactions.

Additionally, various medications are prescribed off-label for sleep in the ICU setting. Trazodone, while being the most commonly prescribed medication for sleep in the US, is a sedating antidepressant studied little for insomnia and carrying adverse side effects including hypotension and anticholinergic syndrome. Additionally, antihistamines such as diphenhydramine and doxylamine, commonly found in over-the-counter sleep preparations, can be oversedating and deliriogenic, particularly among the elderly. Therefore, trazodone and antihistamines were not recommended for sleep by an expert NIH panel on chronic insomnia [90].

In summary, developing a pharmacologic strategy to optimize sleep in the ICU requires a detailed review of potential benefits, side effects, and drug–drug interactions of existing medications, and consideration of underlying withdrawal states. Given a lack of evidence supporting pharmacologic strategies to promote sleep in the ICU, nonpharmacologic interventions and medication minimization (i.e., lowering sedation) should be considered as first-line therapies to promote sleep, before prescription of new medications.

Illness

A variety of factors related to existing and preexisting illness can affect ICU sleep quality. Although the sickest patients likely deserve and theoretically should experience the most restorative sleep, studies on the association of severity of illness and sleep architecture are limited. Additionally, for sepsis, acute respiratory distress syndrome, shock, renal failure, encephalopathy, and coma, EEG recordings are often markedly atypical, making sleep interpretation difficult [4,15]. Nevertheless, critically ill patients with sepsis have demonstrated perturbed melatonin levels, suggesting poorer sleep quality in this population [63].

A number of preexisting comorbidities can predispose patients to worse sleep quality in the ICU setting. For example, COPD, a common cause of respiratory failure in the ICU, is associated with insomnia, sleep arousals, and reduced total sleep time, N3 and REM [91]. Additionally, SDB, which includes obstructive sleep apnea (OSA) and central sleep apnea, Cheyne-Stokes respiration, and obesity hypoventilation syndrome, can markedly disrupt sleep. More specifically, OSA and Cheyne-Stokes respiration are often seen with congestive heart failure and stroke, comorbidities common in the critically ill [1].

Finally, critically ill patients often experience pain, which has been shown to contribute to arousals, sleep fragmentation, and reduced total sleep time [7,8]. Additionally, anxiety and stress regarding one's illness or the ICU environment have been reported by patients to impair sleep [92].

CONSEQUENCES OF DISRUPTED SLEEP IN THE ICU

A large body of research, primarily from healthy and noncritically ill patient populations, has described a constellation of physical and neuropsychologic disruptions that occur in the sleep-deprived state. Theoretically, sick and often frail individuals with organ dysfunction and diminished reserve, similar to those in the ICU, would be most susceptible to dramatic physiologic changes following even the smallest amounts of sleep loss. However, research has yet to corroborate this hypothesis. Nevertheless, an understanding of potential short- and long-term consequences of sleep loss may be helpful to better deal with complex clinical problems and target interventions to improve sleep in the ICU.

Cardiorespiratory Consequences

Among noncritically ill adults, sleep deprivation of 24 hours or more has been shown to result in diminished respiratory muscle strength (Forced expiratory volume in 1 second [1], Forced vital capacity [FVC], and maximal inspiratory pressure), especially for those with COPD, along with increased respiratory muscle fatigability, a blunted hypercapnic ventilatory response, and increased upper airway collapsibility [4]. How these findings apply to critically ill patients has not been investigated, but suggest that poor sleep may impair the respiratory aspects of the ICU recovery process, especially for those receiving mechanical ventilation or with altered baseline respiratory dynamics.

From a cardiovascular standpoint, during sleep deprivation, a surge in sympathetic tone and catecholamine release can lead to blood pressure, heart rate lability, and an elevated risk of myocardial ischemia [4]. As another potential fascinating consequence during the recovery from illness and illness-associated sleep deprivation, "REM rebound" occurs because individuals repay sleep debt and specifically REM sleep, and is characterized by an increased amount of REM with its associated autonomic variability leading to irregular breathing, labile heart rate, and hypoxemia [11]. REM rebound may therefore increase the risk of hemodynamic instability, especially for those with compromised cardiorespiratory physiology. Whether these phenomena occur in critically ill patients is unknown.

Immunologic Consequences

It is a popular belief that proper sleep is necessary to prevent and fight infection. At an extreme level, animal studies have

TABLE 183.2

Studies of Multicomponent Interventions to Promote Sleep in the Intensive Care Unit

			Intervention							
Author	**Study design**	**Setting**	**Quiet Time Protocol**	**Eye masks**	**Ear-plugs**	**Back massage**	**Relaxation / Music**	**Guided imagery**	**Pharmaco-logic Aids**	**Delirium Prevention**
Patel et al. [42] (UK, n = 338)	P	S	√	√	√					√
Foster and Kelly [131] (USA, n = 32)	P	M	√				√			√
Kamdar et al. [41] (USA, n = 300)	P	M	√	√	√		√		√	
Maidl et al. [130] (USA, n = 129)	Q	G	√							
Faraklas et al. [129] (USA, n = 130)	P	B	√							
Jones and Dawson [134] (UK, n = 100)	P	G		√	√					
Li et al. [43] (Asia, n = 55)	P	S	√							
Hu et al. [133] (Asia, n = 14)	R	L		√	√					
Dennis et al. [128] (USA, n = 50)	P	N	√							
Richardson [133] (UK, n = 64)	Q	C		√	√					
Monsén and Edéll-Gustafsson [128] (Europe, n = 23)	P	N	√							
Richardson [136] (USA, n = 36)	R	G					√	√		
Olson et al. [127] (USA, n = 239)	P	N	√							
Walder et al. [125] (Europe, n = 17)	P	S	√							
Richards et al. [40] (USA, n = 69)	R	C				√	√	√		

ICU, intensive care unit; RCSQ, Richards-Campbell Sleep Questionnaire; PSG, polysomnography; SICUQ, Sleep in the ICU Questionnaire; REM, Rapid eye movement; TST, total sleep time; P, Pre–post observational; Q, quasi-experimental; R, randomized; B, Burn ICU; C, Cardiac ICU; G, General/Multiple ICUs; L, Laboratory/simulated ICU; M, Medical ICU; N, Neurologic ICU; S, Surgical ICU.

From Kamdar BB: Bundling sleep promotion with delirium prevention: ready for prime time? *Anaesthesia* 69:527–531, 2014, with permission [141].

Outcomes							Primary outcomes	
Sleep								Main limitations
Polysomnography	RCSQ	SICUQ	Observation / Other	Noise levels	Lights levels	Delirium		
	√	√		√	√	√	↓ delirium, noise, light; improved perceived sleep	Unadjusted analyses; one-time sleep measurement
			√	√		√	No improvement in delirium, sleep, or noise	Small sample size, missing data
	√	√				√	↓ adjusted odds of daily and incident delirium/coma; improved noise	RCSQ instead of PSG, no noise/light measurement
	√						No improvement in sleep ratings	No pre-intervention group, nurses not blinded
	√						↓ sleep latency and complaints of disruptions and noise	Intervention stopped early (loss of study coordinator)
			√				↑ perceived sleep quantity but not quality	Small sample size, frequent intervention refusal
	√	√		√			Improved perceived sleep quality, ↓ interruptions and noise	Small sample size, one-time sleep assessment
√							↑ REM sleep, ↓ arousals, improved perceived sleep quality	Use of laboratory setting and healthy subjects
			√	√	√		↓ light and noise, ↑ odds of observed sleep	Small sample size, same-day pre-post assessment
			√				Increased perceived sleep quantity	Small sample size, unvalidated measure of sleep
			√	√			↓ minimum noise level (8 of 14 nights) and patient care interactions	Bias in reporting of patient care interactions
			√				No pre-post improvement in sleep; MICU sleep worse than SICU/CCU	Varied gender response to intimate intervention, short duration, small sample size
			√	√	√		↑ observed sleep; ↓ noise and light; noise/light and sleep association	Unblinded and non-continuous sleep assessments
			√	√	√		↓ noise and light; no improvement in sleep	Subjective measure of sleep
√							↑ Sleep efficiency, TST, REM and ↓ sleep latency with back-massage	Inclusion of only males aged 55–79

demonstrated that profound sleep deprivation leads to an immunocompromised state, with decreased lymphocytes, leukocytes, and spleen weight, followed by septicemia and death [4]. Although studies in humans have fortunately not produced similar results, they have instead yielded some more complex ones. For example, although multiple studies have demonstrated that sleep-deprived individuals have an attenuated response to vaccination and alterations in markers and modulators of immunity, these data are inconsistent and are not supported by microbiologic studies [4]. Additionally, sleep deprivation can suppress proliferation of T-helper cells and the release of interleukin 2 (IL-2), whereas triggering the proliferation of leukocytes, monocytes, and natural killer cells, and the release of tumor necrosis factor-α, interleukin 1 (IL-1), interleukin-6 (IL-6), intercellular adhesion molecule 1, E-selectin, and C-reactive protein [4]. Although notable, the mechanisms and implications surrounding these alterations are poorly understood and have not been studied in the critically ill.

Metabolic and Endocrine Consequences

For the body, sleep deprivation is a state of catabolism and stress, characterized by a rise in oxygen consumption ($\dot{V}O_2$) and carbon dioxide production ($\dot{V}CO_2$), and the release of cortisol and catecholamines [4]. Although similar responses have been seen in critically ill patients with sepsis [93,94], it is unknown to what degree ICU-related sleep disruption plays a role in these processes, or whether improved sleep may alleviate this vigorous response.

The thyroid axis, GH, and prolactin are also affected by sleep deprivation. During sleep deprivation, TSH, T_3, and T_4 rise and GH and prolactin fall; however, interestingly, the opposite trends tend to occur during critical illness [4]. How these opposing processes interact in the setting of ICU-related sleep disruption is unknown, but poses an interesting avenue for research.

Finally, sleep restriction has been shown among healthy subjects to blunt insulin secretion, decrease sensitivity to insulin, and impair glucose regulation [4]. How these alterations impact the critically ill, who often develop hyperglycemia and suffer adverse consequences from it [95], is unclear, and represents another important area of investigation.

Mobility-Related Consequences

Prolonged immobilization is common during critical illness and contributes to short- and long-term physical, functional, and cognitive impairments, along with early death [96,97]. Hence, early mobilization of ICU patients is now widely recommended and has been shown to reduce delirium, length of stay, and mortality, while improving physical and functional outcomes [96,98,99]. Poor sleep quality in the ICU has been identified as a key modifiable barrier preventing these mobilization efforts [100], based on studies in noncritically ill populations demonstrating reduced energy, diminished activity levels, weakness, and physical disabilities following sleep deprivation [101–103]. As interest in ICU early mobilization continues to grow, it is likely that sleep will also gain attention and further motivate efforts to improve sleep.

Delirium and Other Consequences

Delirium affects up to 80% of critically ill patients and has been shown in numerous studies to be associated with devastating short- and long-term outcomes including prolonged mechanical ventilation and length of stay, cognitive and physical disability, and early death [104]. Because delirium and sleep deprivation share similar characteristics, such as inattention and mood disturbances, their association and potential overlap have received particular attention during efforts to understand and prevent delirium in the ICU [46,105]. Nevertheless, the true association of delirium and sleep remains unknown. Observational studies in this area have described greater mental status changes among medical–surgical patients experiencing the most nurse-observed sleep interruptions [106] and increased delirium incidence in patients reporting sleep deprivation after thoracic surgery [107]. Additionally, a study involving single-night PSG in 29 mechanically ventilated surgical ICU patients demonstrated higher incidence of delirium among patients experiencing <6% REM [108]. Although these studies established an important foundation, additional larger, multisite studies involving validated instruments for sleep and delirium are necessary to clearly evaluate the delirium–sleep association.

Additionally, a large and expanding body of literature has revealed that survivors of critical illness often experience disabling psychiatric, neurocognitive, and psychologic complications after intensive care, including depression [109], posttraumatic stress [110,111], anxiety [111,112], cognitive impairments [113,114], and impaired health-related quality of life (HRQOL) [115–118]. Similarly, the sleep-deprived state has been demonstrated in many studies to be associated with depressed mood, anxiety, and stress [119,120]; cognitive deficits [121,122]; and reduced HRQOL [123]. Given that most of the sleep deprivation studies involved healthy subjects who overcame their deficits with recovery sleep, it is unclear what impact the acute and often prolonged sleep loss experienced by sick ICU patients would have on long-term outcomes. Because studies on this topic would be complicated by confounding factors related to critical illness and the challenges of measuring sleep in the ICU, investigations in this area should focus on whether interventions to improve sleep in the ICU can attenuate adverse psychiatric, neurocognitive, and psychologic outcomes following critical illness.

METHODS TO IMPROVE SLEEP IN THE INTENSIVE CARE UNIT

In its 2013 Clinical Practice Guidelines for Management of Pain, Agitation, and Delirium (PAD) in the ICU, the Society of Critical Care Medicine (SCCM) introduced "promoting sleep in adult ICU patients by optimizing patients' environments, using strategies to control light and noise, clustering patient care activities, and decreasing stimuli at night to protect patients' sleep cycles" as new guideline with a level 1C recommendation [34]. This recommendation was motivated by the hypothesized association of poor sleep with delirium in the ICU and, subsequently, by the association of delirium with adverse short- and long-term outcomes (see "Delirium and Other Consequences" section). Hence, in addition to sedation minimization and early mobilization, sleep promotion has established itself as a cornerstone of ICU delirium prevention efforts.

Efforts to promote sleep in the ICU should address patient- and ICU-level disruptors of sleep, such as noise, light, patient care interactions, patient-ventilator dyssynchrony, and discomfort from uncontrolled pain [124] or anxiety, while maintaining circadian rhythmicity during waking hours via provision of zeitgebers (circadian cues), such as ambient light and physical activity. Studies in a number of ICU settings have supported the feasibility of simple interventions such as environmental noise, light, and/or disturbance reduction [43,125–131], earplugs and/or eye masks [132–135], and relaxation techniques [40,131,136,137], and some have even demonstrated modest improvements of measures of sleep quality [40,43,126,128,137].

More recently, multidisciplinary, multi-intervention "bundled" approaches have been applied for sleep promotion in the ICU (**Table 183.2**), given the ease of performing multiple similar interventions simultaneously (i.e., turning off hallway and room lights, televisions, and alarms at the same time), low incremental costs of added interventions, and success of prior bundled interventions [138]. In particular, two larger studies demonstrated feasibility and efficacy of bundled ICU sleep promotion interventions, which resulted in improvements of normal mental status (i.e., less delirium and coma) [41,42]. Notably, one study also involved a pharmacologic guideline recommending medications to promote restorative sleep (i.e., zolpidem and haloperidol), while discouraging commonly prescribed medications (i.e., benzodiazepines, opioids, and antihistamines) known to impair sleep [41].

Regarding mechanical ventilation, although a recent small meta-analysis suggested that timed modes of ventilation may promote sleep better than spontaneous modes [76], the PAD guidelines deemed insufficient evidence to support particular modes of mechanical ventilation to promote sleep (see "Mechanical Ventilation" section). Finally, a few small studies ($n \leq 32$ ICU patients) evaluating melatonin and melatonin receptor agonists (e.g., ramelteon) for sleep promotion suggested that these medications are safe to administer, but the studies were underpowered or not designed to demonstrate clinically meaningful improvements in sleep quality or other important ICU outcomes [24,32,66,139].

It should be emphasized that despite recent SCCM PAD guidelines highlighting the previously underrecognized issue of sleep in the ICU, no guidelines currently exist to specifically guide ICU sleep promotion strategies. Hence, as with most ICU-wide intervention efforts, to achieve buy-in and sustain a sleep promotion protocol, practitioners should consider an established implementation approach involving engagement of a multidisciplinary stakeholder team, identification of dedicated champions, evaluation of local implementation barriers, and development and evaluation of interventions unique to their ICU environment and patient population [70,140]. Continued research is needed to identify and address common barriers to ICU-based sleep improvement efforts and standardize a sleep improvement protocol for use across multiple ICU settings.

References

1. Knauert MP, Malik V, Kamdar BB: Sleep and sleep disordered breathing in hospitalized patients. *Semin Respir Crit Care Med* 35:582–592, 2014.
2. Kryger M, Roth T, Dement WC (eds): *Principles and Practice of Sleep Medicine*. 4th ed. Philadelphia, PA, Elsevier/Saunders, 2005, p xxxiii, 1517.
3. Brzezinski A: Melatonin in humans. *N Engl J Med* 336:186–195, 1997.
4. Kamdar BB, Needham DM, Collop NA: Sleep deprivation in critical illness: its role in physical and psychological recovery. *J Intensive Care Med* 27:97–111, 2012.
5. Gronfier C, Luthringer R, Follenius M, et al: A quantitative evaluation of the relationships between growth hormone secretion and delta wave electroencephalographic activity during normal sleep and after enrichment in delta waves. *Sleep* 19:817–824, 1996.
6. Hilton BA: Quantity and quality of patients' sleep and sleep-disturbing factors in a respiratory intensive care unit. *J Adv Nurs* 1:453, 1976.
7. Aurell J, Elmqvist D: Sleep in the surgical intensive care unit: continuous polygraphic recording of sleep in nine patients receiving postoperative care. *BMJ* 290:1029, 1985.
8. Gabor JY, Cooper AB, Crombach SA, et al: Contribution of the intensive care unit environment to sleep disruption in mechanically ventilated patients and healthy subjects. *Am J Respir Crit Care Med* 167:708, 2003.
9. Knauert MP, Yaggi HK, Redeker NS, et al: Feasibility study of unattended polysomnography in medical intensive care unit patients. *Heart Lung* 43:445–452, 2014.
10. Cooper AB, Thornley KS, Young GB, et al: Sleep in critically ill patients requiring mechanical ventilation. *Chest* 117:809–818, 2000.
11. Gottschlich MM, Jenkins ME, Mayes T, et al: The 1994 Clinical Research Award. A prospective clinical study of the polysomnographic stages of sleep after burn injury. *J Burn Care Rehabil* 15:486–492, 1994.
12. Freedman NS, Gazendam J, Levan L, et al: Abnormal sleep/wake cycles and the effect of environmental noise on sleep disruption in the intensive care unit. *Am J Respir Crit Care Med* 163:451–457, 2001.
13. Watson PL: Measuring sleep in critically ill patients: beware the pitfalls. *Crit Care* 11:159, 2007.
14. King LM, Bailey KB, Kamdar BB: Promoting sleep in critically ill patients. *Nurs Crit Care* 10:37–43, 2015.
15. Watson PL, Pandharipande P, Gehlbach BK, et al: Atypical sleep in ventilated patients: empirical electroencephalography findings and the path toward revised ICU sleep scoring criteria. *Crit Care Med* 41:1958–1967, 2013.
16. Raj R, Ussavarungsi K, Nugent K: Accelerometer-based devices can be used to monitor sedation/agitation in the intensive care unit. *J Crit Care* 29:748–752, 2014.
17. Verceles AC, Hager ER: Use of accelerometry to monitor physical activity in critically ill subjects: a systematic review. *Respir Care* 60:1330–1336, 2015.
18. Pisani MA, Friese RS, Gehlbach BK, et al: Sleep in the intensive care unit. *Am J Respir Crit Care Med* 191:731–738, 2015.
19. Martin JL, Hakim AD: Wrist actigraphy. *Chest* 139:1514–1527, 2011.
20. Beecroft JM, Ward M, Younes M, et al: Sleep monitoring in the intensive care unit: comparison of nurse assessment, actigraphy and polysomnography. *Intensive Care Med* 34:2076–2083, 2008.
21. Grap MJ, Borchers CT, Munro CL, et al: Actigraphy in the critically ill: correlation with activity, agitation, and sedation. *Am J Crit Care* 14:52–60, 2005.
22. Mistraletti G, Taverna M, Sabbatini G, et al: Actigraphic monitoring in critically ill patients: preliminary results toward an "observation-guided sedation". *J Crit Care* 24:563–567, 2009.
23. Shilo L, Dagan Y, Smorjik Y, et al: Patients in the intensive care unit suffer from severe lack of sleep associated with loss of normal melatonin secretion pattern. *Am J Med Sci* 317:278–281, 1999.
24. Shilo L, Dagan Y, Smorjik Y, et al: Effect of melatonin on sleep quality of COPD intensive care patients: a pilot study. *Chronobiol Int* 17:71–76, 2000.
25. Kroon K, West S: 'Appears to have slept well': assessing sleep in an acute care setting. *Contemp Nurse* 9:284–294, 2000.
26. Winkelman C: Investigating activity in hospitalized patients with chronic obstructive pulmonary disease: a pilot study. *Heart Lung* 39:319–330, 2010.
27. Winkelman C, Higgins PA, Chen YJ: Activity in the chronically critically ill. *Dimens Crit Care Nurs* 24:281–290, 2005.
28. Winkelman C, Higgins PA, Chen YJ, et al: Cytokines in chronically critically ill patients after activity and rest. *Biol Res Nurs* 8:261–271, 2007.
29. Koldobskiy D, Diaz-Abad M, Scharf SM, et al: Long-term acute care patients weaning from prolonged mechanical ventilation maintain circadian rhythm. *Respir Care* 59:518–524, 2014.
30. van der Kooi AW, Tulen JH, van Eijk MM, et al: Sleep monitoring by actigraphy in short-stay ICU patients. *Crit Care Nurs Q* 36:169–173, 2013.
31. Grap MJ, Munro CL, Wetzel PA, et al: Responses to noxious stimuli in sedated mechanically ventilated adults. *Heart Lung* 43:6–12, 2014.
32. Bourne RS, Mills GH, Minelli C: Melatonin therapy to improve nocturnal sleep in critically ill patients: encouraging results from a small randomised controlled trial. *Crit Care* 12:R52, 2008.
33. Grap MJ, Munro CL, Wetzel PA, et al: Sedation in adults receiving mechanical ventilation: physiological and comfort outcomes. *Am J Crit Care* 21:e53–e63, 2012.
34. Barr J, Fraser GL, Puntillo K, et al: Clinical practice guidelines for the management of pain, agitation, and delirium in adult patients in the intensive care unit. *Crit Care Med* 41:263, 2013.
35. Bourne RS, Minelli C, Mills GH, et al: Clinical review: sleep measurement in critical care patients: research and clinical implications. *Crit Care* 11:226, 2007.
36. Richards KC, O'Sullivan PS, Phillips RL: Measurement of sleep in critically ill patients. *J Nurs Meas* 8:131, 2000.
37. Shahid A, Wilkinson K, Marcu S, et al: Richards–Campbell Sleep Questionnaire (RCSQ), in Shahid A, Wilkinson K, Marcu S, et al (eds): *STOP, THAT and One Hundred Other Sleep Scales*. New York, NY, Springer, 2012, pp 299–302.
38. Snyder-Halpern R, Verran JA: Instrumentation to describe subjective sleep characteristics in healthy subjects. *Res Nurs Health* 10:155–163, 1987.
39. Shahid A, Wilkinson K, Marcu S, et al: Verran and Snyder-Halpern sleep scale (VSH), in Shahid A, Wilkinson K, Marcu S, et al (eds): *STOP, THAT and One Hundred Other Sleep Scales*. New York, NY, Springer, 2012, pp 397–398.
40. Richards KC: Effect of a back massage and relaxation intervention on sleep in critically ill patients. *Am J Crit Care* 7:288, 1998.
41. Kamdar BB, King LM, Collop NA, et al: The effect of a quality improvement intervention on perceived sleep quality and cognition in a medical ICU. *Crit Care Med* 41:800–809, 2013.
42. Patel J, Baldwin J, Bunting P, et al: The effect of a multicomponent multidisciplinary bundle of interventions on sleep and delirium in medical and surgical intensive care patients. *Anaesthesia* 69:540–549, 2014.
43. Li SY, Wang TJ, Vivienne Wu SF, et al: Efficacy of controlling night-time noise and activities to improve patients' sleep quality in a surgical intensive care unit. *J Clin Nurs* 20:396–407, 2011.
44. Scotto CJ, McClusky C, Spillan S, et al: Earplugs improve patients' subjective experience of sleep in critical care. *Nurs Crit Care* 14:180–184, 2009.
45. Yazdannik AR, Zareie A, Hasanpour M, et al: The effect of earplugs and eye mask on patients' perceived sleep quality in intensive care unit. *Iran J Nurs Midwifery Res* 19:673–678, 2014.
46. Figueroa-Ramos MI, Arroyo-Novoa CM, Lee KA, et al: Sleep and delirium in ICU patients: a review of mechanisms and manifestations. *Intensive Care Med* 35:781, 2009.
47. Nicolas A, Aizpitarte E, Iruarrizaga A, et al: Perception of night-time sleep by surgical patients in an intensive care unit. *Nurs Crit Care* 13:25, 2008.
48. Kamdar BB, Shah PA, King LM, et al: Patient-nurse interrater reliability and agreement of the Richards-Campbell sleep questionnaire. *Am J Crit Care* 21:261–269, 2012.

49. Aaron JN, Carlisle CC, Carskadon MA, et al: Environmental noise as a cause of sleep disruption in an intermediate respiratory care unit. *Sleep* 19:707, 1996.
50. Topf M, Davis JE: Critical care unit noise and rapid eye movement (REM) sleep. *Heart Lung* 22:252, 1993.
51. Cabello B, Thille AW, Drouot X, et al: Sleep quality in mechanically ventilated patients: comparison of three ventilatory modes. *Crit Care Med* 36:1749, 2008.
52. Elliott RM, McKinley SM, Eager D: A pilot study of sound levels in an Australian adult general intensive care unit. *Noise Health* 12:26, 2010.
53. Meyer TJ, Eveloff SE, Bauer MS, et al: Adverse environmental conditions in the respiratory and medical ICU settings. *Chest* 105:1211–1216, 1994.
54. Park M, Kohlrausch A, de Bruijn W, et al: Analysis of the soundscape in an intensive care unit based on the annotation of an audio recording. *J Acoust Soc Am* 135:1875–1886, 2014.
55. Tainter CR, Levine AR, Quraishi SA, et al: Noise levels in surgical ICUs are consistently above recommended standards. *Crit Care Med* 44:147–152, 2015.
56. Bosma K, Ferreyra G, Ambrogio C, et al: Patient-ventilator interaction and sleep in mechanically ventilated patients: pressure support versus proportional assist ventilation. *Crit Care Med* 35:1048, 2007.
57. Delisle S, Ouellet P, Bellemare P, et al: Sleep quality in mechanically ventilated patients: comparison between NAVA and PSV modes. *Ann Intensive Care* 1:42, 2011.
58. Freedman NS, Kotzer N, Schwab RJ: Patient perception of sleep quality and etiology of sleep disruption in the intensive care unit. *Am J Respir Crit Care Med* 159:1155–1162, 1999.
59. Kahn DM, Cook TE, Carlisle CC, et al: Identification and modification of environmental noise in an ICU setting. *Chest* 114:535, 1998.
60. Christensen M: Noise levels in a general intensive care unit: a descriptive study. *Nurs Crit Care* 12:188–197, 2007.
61. Van Rompaey B, Elseviers MM, Schuurmans MJ, et al: Risk factors for delirium in intensive care patients: a prospective cohort study. *Crit Care* 13:R77, 2009.
62. Mo Y, Scheer CE, Abdallah GT: Emerging role of melatonin and melatonin receptor agonists in sleep and delirium in intensive care unit patients. *J Intensive Care Med* 31:451–455, 2016.
63. Mundigler G, Delle-Karth G, Koreny M, et al: Impaired circadian rhythm of melatonin secretion in sedated critically ill patients with severe sepsis. *Crit Care Med* 30:536, 2002.
64. Yoshitaka S, Egi M, Morimatsu H, et al: Perioperative plasma melatonin concentration in postoperative critically ill patients: its association with delirium. *J Crit Care* 28:236–242, 2013.
65. Miyazaki T, Kuwano H, Kato H, et al: Correlation between serum melatonin circadian rhythm and intensive care unit psychosis after thoracic esophagectomy. *Surgery* 133:662, 2003.
66. Ibrahim MG, Bellomo R, Hart GK, et al: A double-blind placebo-controlled randomised pilot study of nocturnal melatonin in tracheostomised patients. *Crit Care Resusc* 8:187–191, 2006.
67. Malik V, Parthasarathy S: Sleep in intensive care units. *Curr Resp Care Rep* 3:35–41, 2014.
68. Tamburri LM, DiBrienza R, Zozula R, et al: Nocturnal care interactions with patients in critical care units. *Am J Crit Care* 13:102, 2004.
69. Celik S, Oztekin D, Akyolcu N, et al: Sleep disturbance: the patient care activities applied at the night shift in the intensive care unit. *J Clin Nurs* 14:102, 2005.
70. Kamdar BB, Yang J, King LM, et al: Developing, implementing, and evaluating a multifaceted quality improvement intervention to promote sleep in an ICU. *Am J Med Qual* 29:546–554, 2014.
71. Esteban A, Anzueto A, Alia I, et al: How is mechanical ventilation employed in the intensive care unit? An international utilization review. *Am J Respir Crit Care Med* 161:1450–1458, 2000.
72. Hardin KA, Seyal M, Stewart T, et al: Sleep in critically ill chemically paralyzed patients requiring mechanical ventilation. *Chest* 129:1468, 2006.
73. Parthasarathy S, Tobin MJ: Effect of ventilator mode on sleep quality in critically ill patients. *Am J Resp Crit Care Med* 166:1423, 2002.
74. Toublanc B, Rose D, Glerant JC, et al: Assist-control ventilation vs. low levels of pressure support ventilation on sleep quality in intubated ICU patients. *Intensive Care Med* 33:1148, 2007.
75. Alexopoulou C, Kondili E, Vakouti E, et al: Sleep during proportional-assist ventilation with load-adjustable gain factors in critically ill patients. *Intensive Care Med* 33:1139, 2007.
76. Poongkunran C, John SG, Kannan AS, et al: A meta-analysis of sleep-promoting interventions during critical illness. *Am J Med* 128:1126–1137, 2015.
77. Roche Campo F, Drouot X, Thille AW, et al: Poor sleep quality is associated with late noninvasive ventilation failure in patients with acute hypercapnic respiratory failure. *Crit Care Med* 38:477–485, 2010.
78. Cordoba-Izquierdo A, Drouot X, Thille AW, et al: Sleep in hypercapnic critical care patients under noninvasive ventilation: conventional versus dedicated ventilators. *Crit Care Med* 41:60–68, 2013.
79. Bourne RS, Mills GH: Sleep disruption in critically ill patients—pharmacological considerations. *Anaesthesia* 59:374, 2004.
80. Riker RR, Shehabi Y, Bokesch PM, et al: Dexmedetomidine vs midazolam for sedation of critically ill patients: a randomized trial. *JAMA* 301:489, 2009.
81. Pandharipande PP, Pun BT, Herr DL, et al: Effect of sedation with dexmedetomidine vs lorazepam on acute brain dysfunction in mechanically ventilated patients: the MENDS randomized controlled trial. *JAMA* 298:2644, 2007.
82. Lonardo NW, Mone MC, Nirula R, et al: Propofol is associated with favorable outcomes compared with benzodiazepines in ventilated intensive care unit patients. *Am J Respir Crit Care Med* 189:1383–1394, 2014.
83. Kondili E, Alexopoulou C, Xirouchaki N, et al: Effects of propofol on sleep quality in mechanically ventilated critically ill patients: a physiological study. *Intensive Care Med* 38:1640–1646, 2012.
84. Tung A, Bergmann BM, Herrera S, et al: Recovery from sleep deprivation occurs during propofol anesthesia. *Anesthesiology* 100:1419, 2004.
85. Tung A, Lynch JP, Mendelson WB: Prolonged sedation with propofol in the rat does not result in sleep deprivation. *Anesth Analg* 92:1232, 2001.
86. Zhao J, Dai YH, Xi QS, et al: A clinical study on insomnia in patients with cancer during chemotherapy containing high-dose glucocorticoids. *Pharmazie* 68:421–427, 2013.
87. Neuhaus P, McMaster P, Calne R, et al: Neurological complications in the European multicentre study of FK 506 and cyclosporin in primary liver transplantation. *Transpl Int* 7:S27–S31, 1994.
88. Rea RS, Battistone S, Fong JJ, et al: Atypical antipsychotics versus haloperidol for treatment of delirium in acutely ill patients. *Pharmacotherapy* 27:588–594, 2007.
89. Gunja N: The clinical and forensic toxicology of Z-drugs. *J Med Toxicol* 9:155–162, 2013.
90. NIH State-of-the-Science Conference Statement on manifestations and management of chronic insomnia in adults. *NIH Consens State Sci Statements* 22:1–30, 2005.
91. Stege G, Vos PJ, van den Elshout FJ, et al: Sleep, hypnotics and chronic obstructive pulmonary disease. *Respir Med* 102:801, 2008.
92. Wong FY, Arthur DG: Hong Kong patients' experiences of intensive care after surgery: nurses' and patients' views. *Intensive Crit Care Nurs* 16:290, 2000.
93. Hamrahian AH, Oseni TS, Arafah BM: Measurements of serum free cortisol in critically ill patients. *N Engl J Med* 350:1629, 2004.
94. Moriyama S, Okamoto K, Tabira Y, et al: Evaluation of oxygen consumption and resting energy expenditure in critically ill patients with systemic inflammatory response syndrome. *Crit Care Med* 27:2133, 1999.
95. Schiffner L: Glucose management in critically ill medical and surgical patients. *Dimens Crit Care Nurs* 33:70–77, 2014.
96. Kress JP, Hall JB: ICU-acquired weakness and recovery from critical illness. *N Engl J Med* 370:1626–1635, 2014.
97. Fan E, Cheek F, Chlan L, et al: An official American Thoracic Society Clinical Practice guideline: the diagnosis of intensive care unit-acquired weakness in adults. *Am J Respir Crit Care Med* 190:1437–1446, 2014.
98. Needham DM, Korupolu R, Zanni JM, et al: Early physical medicine and rehabilitation for patients with acute respiratory failure: a quality improvement project. *Arch Phys Med Rehabil* 91:536–542, 2010.
99. Schweickert WD, Pohlman MC, Pohlman AS, et al: Early physical and occupational therapy in mechanically ventilated, critically ill patients: a randomised controlled trial. *Lancet* 373:1874, 2009.
100. Hopkins RO, Spuhler VJ: Strategies for promoting early activity in critically ill mechanically ventilated patients. *AACN Adv Crit Care* 20:277–289, 2009.
101. Reyes S, Algarin C, Bunout D, et al: Sleep/wake patterns and physical performance in older adults. *Aging Clin Exp Res* 25:175–181, 2013.
102. Martin JL, Fiorentino L, Jouldjian S, et al: Sleep quality in residents of assisted living facilities: effect on quality of life, functional status, and depression. *J Am Geriatr Soc* 58:829–836, 2010.
103. Zarrabian MM, Johnson M, Kriellaars D: Relationship between sleep, pain, and disability in patients with spinal pathology. *Arch Phys Med Rehabil* 95:1504–1509, 2014.
104. Reade MC, Finfer S: Sedation and delirium in the intensive care unit. *N Engl J Med* 370:444–454, 2014.
105. Kamdar BB, Niessen T, Colantuoni E, et al: Delirium transitions in the medical ICU: exploring the role of sleep quality and other factors. *Crit Care Med* 43:135–141, 2015.
106. Helton MC, Gordon SH, Nunnery SL: The correlation between sleep deprivation and the intensive care unit syndrome. *Heart Lung* 9:464, 1980.
107. Yildizeli B, Ozyurtkan MO, Batirel HF, et al: Factors associated with postoperative delirium after thoracic surgery. *Ann Thorac Surg* 79:1004, 2005.
108. Trompeo AC, Vidi Y, Locane MD, et al: Sleep disturbances in the critically ill patients: role of delirium and sedative agents. *Minerva Anestesiol* 77:604–612, 2011.
109. Davydow DS, Gifford JM, Desai SV, et al: Depression in general intensive care unit survivors: a systematic review. *Intensive Care Med* 35:796–809, 2009.
110. Parker AM, Sricharoenchai T, Raparla S, et al: Posttraumatic stress disorder in critical illness survivors: a metaanalysis. *Crit Care Med* 43:1121–1129, 2015.
111. Bienvenu OJ, Colantuoni E, Mendez-Tellez PA, et al: Cooccurrence of and remission from general anxiety, depression, and posttraumatic stress disorder symptoms after acute lung injury: a 2-year longitudinal study. *Crit Care Med* 43:642–653, 2015.
112. Stevenson JE, Colantuoni E, Bienvenu OJ, et al: General anxiety symptoms after acute lung injury: predictors and correlates. *J Psychosom Res* 75:287–293, 2013.
113. Pandharipande PP, Girard TD, Jackson JC, et al: Long-term cognitive impairment after critical illness. *N Engl J Med* 369:1306–1316, 2013.
114. Needham DM, Dinglas VD, Bienvenu OJ, et al: One year outcomes in patients with acute lung injury randomised to initial trophic or full enteral feeding: prospective follow-up of EDEN randomised trial. *BMJ* 346:f1532, 2013.
115. Parsons EC, Hough CL, Vitiello MV, et al: Insomnia is associated with quality of life impairment in medical-surgical intensive care unit survivors. *Heart Lung* 44:89–94, 2015.
116. Needham DM, Davidson J, Cohen H, et al: Improving long-term outcomes after discharge from intensive care unit: report from a stakeholders' conference. *Crit Care Med* 40:502–509, 2012.

117. Cuthbertson BH, Roughton S, Jenkinson D, et al: Quality of life in the five years after intensive care: a cohort study. *Crit Care* 14:R6, 2010.
118. Dowdy DW, Eid MP, Dennison CR, et al: Quality of life after acute respiratory distress syndrome: a meta-analysis. *Intensive Care Med* 32:1115, 2006.
119. Salas RE, Gamaldo CE: Adverse effects of sleep deprivation in the ICU. *Crit Care Clin* 24:461, 2008.
120. Dinges DF, Pack F, Williams K, et al: Cumulative sleepiness, mood disturbance, and psychomotor vigilance performance decrements during a week of sleep restricted to 4–5 hours per night. *Sleep* 20:267, 1997.
121. Banks S, Dinges DF: Behavioral and physiological consequences of sleep restriction. *J Clin Sleep Med* 3:519, 2007.
122. Tucker AM, Whitney P, Belenky G, et al: Effects of sleep deprivation on dissociated components of executive functioning. *Sleep* 33:47, 2010.
123. Faubel R, Lopez-Garcia E, Guallar-Castillon P, et al: Sleep duration and health-related quality of life among older adults: a population-based cohort in Spain. *Sleep* 32:1059, 2009.
124. Jones J, Hoggart B, Withey J, et al: What the patients say: a study of reactions to an intensive care unit. *Intensive Care Med* 5:89–92, 1979.
125. Walder B, Francioli D, Meyer JJ, et al: Effects of guidelines implementation in a surgical intensive care unit to control nighttime light and noise levels. *Crit Care Med* 28:2242–2247, 2000.
126. Olson DM, Borel CO, Laskowitz DT, et al: Quiet time: a nursing intervention to promote sleep in neurocritical care units. *Am J Crit Care* 10:74, 2001.
127. Monsen MG, Edell-Gustafsson UM: Noise and sleep disturbance factors before and after implementation of a behavioural modification programme. *Intensive Crit Care Nurs* 21:208–219, 2005.
128. Dennis CM, Lee R, Woodard EK, et al: Benefits of quiet time for neuro-intensive care patients. *J Neurosci Nurs* 42:217–224, 2010.
129. Faraklas I, Holt B, Tran S, et al: Impact of a nursing-driven sleep hygiene protocol on sleep quality. *J Burn Care Res* 34:249–254, 2013.
130. Maidl CA, Leske JS, Garcia AE: The influence of "quiet time" for patients in critical care. *Clin Nurs Res* 23:544–559, 2014.
131. Foster J, Kelly M: A pilot study to test the feasibility of a nonpharmacologic intervention for the prevention of delirium in the medical intensive care unit. *Clin Nurse Spec* 27:231–238, 2013.
132. Richardson A, Allsop M, Coghill E, et al: Earplugs and eye masks: do they improve critical care patients' sleep? *Nurs Crit Care* 12:278–286, 2007.
133. Hu RF, Jiang XY, Zeng YM, et al: Effects of earplugs and eye masks on nocturnal sleep, melatonin and cortisol in a simulated intensive care unit environment. *Crit Care* 14:R66, 2010.
134. Jones C, Dawson D: Eye masks and earplugs improve patient's perception of sleep. *Nurs Crit Care* 17:247–254, 2012.
135. Van Rompaey B, Elseviers MM, Van Drom W, et al: The effect of earplugs during the night on the onset of delirium and sleep perception: a randomized controlled trial in intensive care patients. *Crit Care* 16:R73, 2012.
136. Richardson S: Effects of relaxation and imagery on the sleep of critically ill adults. *Dimens Crit Care Nurs* 22:182–190, 2003.
137. Su CP, Lai HL, Chang ET, et al: A randomized controlled trial of the effects of listening to non-commercial music on quality of nocturnal sleep and relaxation indices in patients in medical intensive care unit. *J Adv Nurs* 69:1377–1389, 2013.
138. Pronovost P, Needham D, Berenholtz S, et al: An intervention to decrease catheter-related bloodstream infections in the ICU. *N Engl J Med* 355:2725, 2006.
139. Hatta K, Kishi Y, Wada K, et al: Preventive effects of ramelteon on delirium: a randomized placebo-controlled trial. *JAMA Psychiatry* 71:397–403, 2014.
140. Pronovost PJ, Berenholtz SM, Needham DM: Translating evidence into practice: a model for large scale knowledge translation. *BMJ* 337:a1714, 2008.
141. Kamdar BB, Kamdar BB, Needham DM: Bundling sleep promotion with delirium prevention: ready for prime time? *Anaesthesia* 69:527–531, 2014.

Chapter 184 ■ Disorders of Temperature Control, Part I: Hypothermia

MARY KATHRYN STEINER • RICHARD S. IRWIN

This chapter reviews the normal physiology of temperature regulation and the major hypothermic syndromes. Iatrogenic and intentional hypothermia are also reviewed. Three hyperthermic syndromes—heat stroke, malignant hyperthermia, and neuroleptic malignant syndrome—are reviewed in Chapter 185.

NORMAL PHYSIOLOGY OF TEMPERATURE REGULATION

The equilibrium between heat production and heat loss determines the body temperature. For healthy, resting individuals, this equilibrium is tightly regulated, producing an average oral temperature of 36.60°C ± 0.38°C [1]. Table 184.1 is a conversion chart of temperatures in Celsius to Fahrenheit. Small shifts of this temperature set point occur, with a normal diurnal variation producing a peak temperature usually near 6:00 p.m. Minute-to-minute changes in body temperature are quickly sensed, and appropriate changes are made in body heat production and loss to restore a normal balance.

Heat Production

In a neutral environment (28°C for humans), humans generate all net body heat from the energy released in the dissociation of high-energy bonds during the metabolism of dietary fats, proteins, and carbohydrates. At rest, the trunk and viscera supply 56% of the body heat, but, during exercise, up to 90% may be generated by the muscles. Although shivering or an increase in muscle tone may produce a fourfold rise in net heat production [2], vigorous exercise may cause a sixfold increase.

Heat Loss

Under usual environmental conditions, heat exchange with the environment takes the form of heat loss. Heat may be exchanged by radiation, conduction, convection, or evaporation [3–6]. Radiation exchange—the transfer of thermal energy between objects with no direct contact—accounts for 50% to 70% of heat lost by humans at rest in a neutral environment. Conduction (10% to 15% of heat loss) involves the direct exchange of heat with

TABLE 184.1

Fahrenheit to Celsius Temperature Conversions

°C	°F	°C	°F
45	113.0	32	89.6
44	111.2	31	87.8
43	109.4	30	86.0
42	107.6	29	84.2
41	105.8	28	82.4
40	104.0	27	80.6
39	102.2	26	78.8
38	100.4	25	77.0
37	98.6	24	75.2
36	96.8	23	73.4
35	95.0	22	71.6
34	93.2	21	69.8
33	91.4	20	68.0

objects in direct contact with the body. Larger quantities of heat may be rapidly exchanged when the body is submerged in water; this is caused by the much greater thermal conductivity of water as compared with air. Convection involves the exchange of heat with the warmer or cooler molecules of air that pass by the skin. Heat exchange by this mechanism increases rapidly with greater temperature differences between the skin and the air and with rapid airflow (e.g., wind). Evaporative heat loss of humans occurs primarily through perspiration. Evaporation of sweat from the skin requires that energy be supplied by the skin, resulting in a net loss of heat from the body of 0.6 kcal per g of sweat absorbed. Unlike the other methods of heat exchange, evaporation can exchange heat loss even when a warmer environment surrounds the skin. Therefore, evaporation is the major means by which the body prevents hyperthermia in a warm environment.

Temperature Control Systems

The anatomy and regulation of the system that controls the body temperature has been reviewed in-depth by several investigators [2–6], as outlined in the previous edition and are only briefly described here. Neurons that are directly responsive to temperature ascend from the skin, the deep viscera, and the spinal cord through the lateral spinothalamic tract to the preoptic anterior hypothalamus. When the hypothalamus perceives a temperature increase, it modulates autonomic tone to produce (a) an increase in evaporative heat loss through increased sweat output by the body's 2.5 million sweat glands, (b) cutaneous vasodilation that allows direct flow of heat to the skin to increase convective and conductive heat losses, and (c) decreased muscle tone and activity to prevent any unnecessary heat production. When the hypothalamus perceives a temperature decrease, it modulates autonomic tone to cause (a) sweat production to cease or decrease, (b) cutaneous vasculature to constrict, and (c) muscle tone to increase involuntarily and shivering to begin. The immediate defense of thermoregulation is via the autonomic nervous system, whereas delayed control is mediated by the endocrine system. Prolonged exposure to cold stimulates the thyroid axis, leading to an increased metabolic rate.

The monoamines, baroreceptor data, hypothalamic calcium and sodium concentrations, and inflammatory cytokines (interleukin-1, interleukin-6, and tumor necrosis factor-α) are believed to be modulators of the anterior hypothalamic thermostat. They produce effects slowly, and they have little to do with the regulation of acute temperature changes.

Voluntary responses play an important role in thermoregulation. Humans may respond to thermal stress by (a) adding or removing clothes (affecting evaporative, conductive, and radiant heat exchange), (b) moving to a warmer or cooler climate, (c) changing the level of activity, and (d) changing posture. Impairment of voluntary control places an unnecessary stress on autonomic control mechanisms, thereby predisposing to an imbalance in heat exchange and a change in body temperature.

The ability to regulate temperature effectively declines with age [7,8], probably as a result of deterioration in sensory afferents. Although younger individuals usually notice temperature changes as low as 0.8°C, older persons may not notice changes of up to 2.3°C. Moreover, because the sweat threshold increases and sweat volume decreases with age, an older individual may be more susceptible to hyperthermia than a younger person [9]. Old age may also be a liability for hypothermia because of (a) a lower basal metabolic rate, (b) a higher heat conductance owing to a decline in body mass, (c) a decrease in the heat generated by shivering owing to a smaller muscle mass, and (d) an inability to vasoconstrict cutaneous vessels in response to cold. In the elderly, restricted mobility or deterioration of cortical function can lead to a greater impact on the voluntary responses to temperature changes compared with the young.

UNINTENTIONAL HYPOTHERMIA

Hypothermia, defined as a core temperature less than 35°C, may occur at all ambient temperatures and in patients of all ages but more commonly among the elderly. The stage of hypothermia, defined by core temperature, has a large impact on both recognition and treatment. The most commonly used definitions are as follows [227,228]. Mild hypothermia is a core temperature of 32°C to 35°C, moderate hypothermia is a core temperature of 28°C to 32°C, and severe hypothermia is a core temperature below 28°C. In addition, some experts regard a temperature of <24°C or <20°C as profound hypothermia [229,230]. Because the clinical features of hypothermia differ among patients, and because core temperature measurement is imprecise, the recognition of each stage is more important than its exact boundaries. Prehospital personnel, while carefully measuring core temperatures, may also refer to the clinical staging scheme described by the International Commission for Mountain Emergency Medicine, or the "Swiss System" [229].

Mild hypothermia I—normal mental status with shivering-estimated core temperature of 32°C to 35°C
Moderate hypothermia II—altered mental status without shivering-core temperature of 28°C to 32°C
Severe hypothermia III—unconscious-estimated core temperature of 24°C to 28°C
Severe hypothermia IV—apparent death-estimated core temperature of 13.7°C to 24°C
Death V—death as a result of irreversible hypothermia-estimated core temperature of <9°C to 13.7°C

Hypothermia often occurs within 24 hours of admission in more than 3% of intensive care unit admissions [10]. Hypothermia is a diagnosis that is frequently missed and underreported. When all data are reviewed, the overall mortality from hypothermia in the United States has been conservatively estimated at 30 deaths per 1 million population per year [11]. The mortality for treated hypothermia ranges from 12% [12] to 73% [13].

Causes and Pathogenesis

The most frequent causes of hypothermia appear to be exposure, use of depressant drugs, and hypoglycemia. Understanding the causes of hypothermia (Table 184.2) and their pathogenesis enables one to develop a rational approach to treatment.

Exposure to Cold

Wet, wind, and exhaustion contribute to increased loss of body heat. Wet clothing loses 90% of its insulating value [14], rendering soaked individuals effectively nude. Exposure to rain or snow contributed greatly to the development of hypothermia in 15 of 23 incidents among hikers discussed in one review [14]. Convective

TABLE 184.2

Causes of Unintentional Hypothermia

Normal aging
Exposure to cold
Drugs (e.g., alcohol)
Endocrine dysfunction (e.g., hypoglycemia)
Central nervous system disorders
Spinal cord transection
Skin disorders
Debility
Trauma

heat loss because of wind may increase to more than five times baseline values, increasing with wind velocity [15]. Hikers with poor selection of clothing, campers who fail to seek appropriate shelter, or skiing in unfavorable weather can result in fatal hypothermia [15]. Victims of hypothermia display inappropriate behavior that worsens hypothermia. Up to 25% may remove their clothing and burrow, hiding under a bed or on a shelf [16]. Many quickly experience loss of coordination and then stupor or collapse. Death may occur within an hour of the onset of symptoms [15]. Immersion in water at a temperature colder than 24°C leads to extremely rapid heat loss. Core temperature drops at a rate proportional to the temperature of the water [17]. Although survival periods of 1 to 2 hours have been reported for individuals immersed in water at 0°C to 10°C, death may occur within minutes.

Drugs

Alcohol, phenothiazines, barbiturates, and paralytic agents frequently produce hypothermia by depressing sensory afferents, the hypothalamus, or effector responses reducing centrally mediated vasoconstriction. Alcohol impairs the perception of cold, clouds the sensorium, and acts as a direct vasodilator [18,19]. Alcoholics are also thought to be more susceptible to exposure because of a state of relative starvation, increased conductive losses from decreased subcutaneous fat, and high levels of blood alcohol that potentially impair the metabolic response to hypothermia by decreasing blood sugar and increasing acidosis. Most sedative–hypnotic drugs cause hypothermia by inhibiting shivering and impairing voluntary control. Phenothiazines increase the threshold necessary to produce shivering and lead to hypothalamic depression [10]; barbiturates decrease effective shivering [20]. Paralytic agents used to suppress ventilation prevent shivering and eliminate all voluntary control mechanisms [21,22]. Unexplained hypothermia has resulted from the administration of common antibiotics, such as penicillin [23] and erythromycin [24]. Bromocriptine may cause hypothermia by altering central dopaminergic tone [25].

Endocrine Dysfunction

Diabetic ketoacidosis, hyperosmolar coma, and hypoglycemia are frequently reported causes of hypothermia [18]. In one survey, 20% of patients with blood glucose levels less than 60 mg per dL had temperatures of less than 35°C. Hypoglycemia lowers cerebral intracellular glucose concentrations and impairs hypothalamic function [26]. In acute hypoglycemia (e.g., insulin administration), hypothermia occurs as a result of peripheral vasodilation and sweating. At glucose concentrations of less than 45 mg per dL, subjects fail to perceive cold environments and fail to shiver [27]. This impairment appears transient because normal regulatory mechanisms and euthermia may be restored when normal serum glucose levels are restored.

The prevalence of hypothyroidism in hypothermic patients ranges from 0% to 10%. Several patients with mild hypothyroidism have been safely rewarmed to euthermia without administration of exogenous thyroid hormone. In contrast, myxedema coma, a rare presentation of hypothyroidism, is associated with subnormal temperatures in 82% of cases [28]. It has a high mortality if not treated with exogenous thyroxine. Myxedema coma occurs most frequently among middle-aged to older women, and more than 90% of cases occur in winter [28]. Severe hypothermia with temperatures less than 30°C occurs in 15% of patients [28]. Coma arises because of a cerebral thyroxine deficiency. Hypothermia then results from a combination of loss of voluntary control mechanisms, from stupor or coma, decreased calorigenesis from thyroid deficiency, and decreased shivering, presumably from impaired hypothalamic regulation [28,29].

Panhypopituitarism and adrenal insufficiency are also rare causes of hypothermia. Unless profound insufficiency exists, these conditions rarely produce significant hypothermia in the absence of some other insults to the thermoregulatory system.

Central Nervous System Disorders

Diseases such as stroke, primary and metastatic brain tumors, luetic gliosis, and sarcoidosis may produce hypothermia by direct anatomic impingement on the hypothalamus [30,31]. Metabolic derangements from carbon monoxide poisoning or thiamine deficiency (Wernicke–Korsakoff syndrome) can also produce hypothermia by affecting the hypothalamus [32–37]. Patients with anorexia nervosa have been shown to have multiple hypothalamic abnormalities, resulting in the lack of shivering and vasoconstriction and a rapid drop in core temperature when they are exposed to cold [38]. Shapiro syndrome has been reported to cause spontaneous periodic hypothermia by an unclear mechanism [20,39]. Several patients with multiple sclerosis have experienced transient hypothermia with flares of their neuropathy, suggesting the presence of hypothalamic plaques [40].

Spinal Cord Transection

Acute spinal cord injury disrupts autonomic pathways, such as skin and core temperature afferents. In addition, they develop a reduced body muscle mass, resulting in the inability to shiver effectively, loss of cold-induced reflex vasoconstriction responses, and immobility [41–43].

Skin Disorders

Skin disorders characterized by vasodilatation or increased transepithelial water loss may lead to hypothermia. Inappropriate conductive and convective heat losses in psoriasis, ichthyosis, and erythroderma have been shown to be associated with increased evaporative losses of up to 3 L per day [44,49]. Patients with extensive third-degree burns have been reported to have an even larger evaporative heat loss, losing up to 6 L fluid. When an additional cause of hypothermia is present, these patients may be in danger of severe drops in temperature. Heat loss and caloric requirements can be decreased dramatically by covering the skin with impermeable membranes to decrease evaporative losses [50–52].

Debility

Case reports suggest that hypothermia may occur in patients with debilitating illnesses, such as Hodgkin disease [49]; systemic lupus erythematosus [50,51]; and severe cardiac, renal, hepatic, or septic failure. Most debilitated patients are also compromised by some degree of immobility or decreased voluntary control.

Trauma

Trauma patients often are hypothermic [52,53] because of multiple insults to the thermoregulatory system [53]. In patients with moderately elevated injury severity scores, during the first day of hospitalization, 42% experience hypothermia, with 13% having temperatures less than 32°C [52]. The presence of shock [52] and massive transfusion [53] significantly contributed to the development of hypothermia in these patients.

Pathophysiology

Profound metabolic alterations occur in every organ system in response to a core temperature less than 35°C. Metabolic changes that appear to be temperature dependent occur in two phases: shivering (35°C to 30°C) and nonshivering (less than 30°C).

Shivering is characterized by intense energy production from the breakdown of stored body fuels. It involves an increase in muscle tone and rhythmic contraction of small and large muscle groups. In different patient populations with different measurement

TABLE 184.3

Common Effects of Hypothermia

Metabolic depletion	Anemia, hemoconcentration
Cardiac arrhythmia	Thrombocytopenia
Hypotension	Ileus
Hypopnea	Pancreatitis
Dehydration	Hyperglycemia
Coma	Pneumonia
Granulocytopenia	Sepsis
Altered drug clearance	

techniques, heat production has been shown to increase by four times the normal amount [54], oxygen consumption by two to five times, and metabolic rate by six times [55]. Central pooling of blood resulting from peripheral vasoconstriction may raise central venous pressure and slightly elevate cardiac output. Because cardiac output remains relatively close to normal and oxygen demand increases dramatically, mixed venous oxygen saturation decreases [56]. Hepatic and muscular glycogenolysis may cause blood sugar levels to rise, which is not seen in starved or exhausted patients or those with prolonged hypothermia [57,58]. The catabolism of fat increases the serum levels of glycerol, nonesterified fatty acids, and ketones. Anaerobic metabolism causes a rise in lactate levels, and levels as high as 25.2 mmol per L have been reported [59]. The metabolic acidosis induced by this intense catabolism is compensated for the most part by the increased metabolism of lactate in the liver and increased minute ventilation [58]. Cortisol levels rise [13]. Most of these metabolic changes peak near 34°C or 35°C and become much less pronounced near the temperature of 30°C.

As core temperature falls toward 30°C, shivering nearly ceases and metabolism slows down dramatically. Near 30°C, metabolic rate approaches basal levels [60], and it may be half basal value by 28°C [55]. As shivering and metabolism slow down, oxygen consumption declines. At 30°C, oxygen consumption decreases to approximately 75% of basal value [60]; at 26°C to 35% to 53%; and at 20°C to only 25% of basal value. This profound decrease in metabolism is reflected by changes in every organ system (Table 184.3).

Cardiovascular Function

Increasing degrees of hypothermia are associated with malignant arrhythmias, depressed cardiac function, and hypotension. A decrease in cardiac conductivity and automaticity [61–63] and an increase in the refractory period [64,65] begin during the shivering phase and progress as core temperature decreases. The electrocardiogram (ECG) of mild hypothermia may show bradycardia with prolongation of the PR, QRS, and QT intervals. Below 30°C, first-degree block is usual, and, at 20°C, third-degree block may be seen [57,66]. Below 33°C, the ECG commonly shows the characteristic J-point elevation (Fig. 184.1). As temperature drops below 25°C, the likelihood of appearance of J waves increases [67,68], most prominent in the mid-precordial and lateral precordial leads [69]. J waves may persist 12 to 24 hours after restoration of normal temperature [70,71].

Atrial fibrillation is common at temperatures of 34°C to 25°C, and ventricular fibrillation frequently occurs at temperatures less than 28°C. The incidence of ventricular fibrillation increases with physical stimulation of the heart and is associated with intracardiac temperature gradients of greater than 2°C [72]. Purkinje cells show marked decreases in excitability in the range of 14°C to 15°C [63], and asystole is common when core temperatures drop below 20°C.

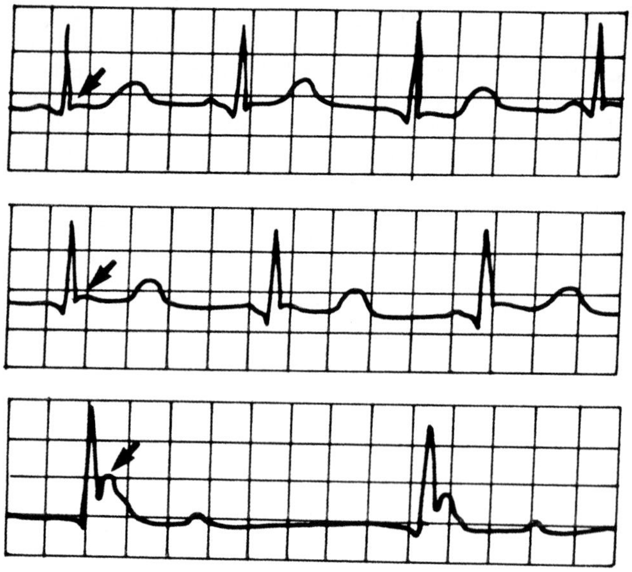

FIGURE 184.1 The electrocardiographic changes of hypothermia. As temperature decreases (*top to bottom*), the rate slows down and the PR and QT intervals become prolonged. J waves (*arrows*) appear at a temperature less than 35°C and become prominent by a temperature near 25°C. The J wave initially is seen (*top*) as a widened QRS interval with a slight ST elevation at the J point.

Consequently, there is a gradual decrease in cardiac output. Systole may become extremely prolonged [73], greatly decreasing ejection fraction and aortic pressures. Ventricular compliance is severely reduced [74]. Output decreases to approximately 90% of normal at 30°C and may decrease rapidly at lower temperatures, with increasing bradycardia or arrhythmia. Regional blood flow is altered to preserve myocardial and cerebral perfusion [75]. Although blood pressure appears to be initially maintained by an increase in systemic vascular resistance (SVR) [76], systemic resistance decreases and hypotension is common [57] at temperatures less than 25°C. Oxygen demand usually decreases more rapidly than does cardiac output, causing mixed venous oxygen content to increase as the nonshivering phase begins.

Pulmonary Function

Pulmonary mechanics and gas exchange appear to change little with hypothermia [57,77–79]. Although the ventilatory response to an elevation in carbon dioxide tension (PCO_2) may be blunted [77], there is no clear decrease in hypoxic drive [57]. As the increased oxygen demand and acidosis of the shivering phase decline, minute ventilation decreases. Tidal volume and respiratory rate decline at lower temperatures. At 25°C, respirations may be only 3 or 4 per minute [19]; at temperatures less than 24°C, respiration may cease [55]. Apnea is presumed to be secondary to failure of respiratory drive at a brainstem level.

Renal Function

As blood pressure decreases during the nonshivering phase, glomerular filtration rate (GFR) may decrease by 85% [57] and renal blood flow by 75%, without a significant change in urine production. Maintenance of a good urine output, despite decreases in blood pressure and GFR in hypothermia, has been termed *cold diuresis*. This results from a defect in tubular reabsorption. The urine may be extremely dilute, with an osmolarity of as low as 60 mOsm per L and a specific gravity of 1.002 [80]. The stimulus for this dilute diuresis may be the triggering of volume receptors as central volume increases with peripheral vasoconstriction [73], a relative insensitivity to antidiuretic hormone [71], or a direct suppression of antidiuretic hormone release [19]. Although kaliuresis and glycosuria may accompany the dilute diuresis, the net result for the patient is dehydration and a relatively hyperosmolar serum.

Neurologic Function

Hypothermic patients present with coma. Complete neurologic recovery has been described in hypothermic adults after 20 minutes of complete cardiac arrest [18] and up to 3.5 hours of cardiopulmonary resuscitation (CPR) [80]. The mechanism by which hypothermia produces a seemingly protective effect is not well understood, because it probably relates to a significant decrease in cerebral metabolism and a smaller injury by the no-reflow phenomenon [81], a mechanism whereby the brain is protected from injury until reperfusion.

Cerebral oxygen consumption decreases by approximately 55% for each 10°C decrease in temperature [82]. Cerebral blood flow decreases from 75% of normal at 30°C to only 20% of normal at 20°C [57]. The supply of nutrients and removal of wastes are adequate at these extremes given patient recovery and experimental evidence that the intracellular pH of brain tissue cooled to 20°C is unchanged even after 20 minutes of anoxia [83].

Visual [84,85] and auditory [86,87] evoked potentials demonstrate delayed latencies; latency increases as temperature decreases. The spectrum of electroencephalographic frequencies also changes with hypothermia. In healthy men cooled to 33°C by immersion, θ and β activities increased by 17% and α activity decreased by 34% compared with control values [85]. Electromyography during hypothermia has been reported to be normal [88].

Hematologic Function

Hypothermia affects white blood cells (WBCs), red blood cells, platelets, and perhaps coagulation mechanisms. The WBC count in mild hypothermia remains normal to slightly elevated and drops severely at temperatures lower than 28°C [89,90]. The hematocrit usually rises in hypothermic patients at a temperature of 30°C, in part, because of hemoconcentration from dehydration caused by cold diuresis and in part as a result of to splenic contraction [91]. The increase in blood viscosity in hypothermic patients appears to be because of decreased deformability of the red cell membrane [92]. After intravascular volume and euthermia have been restored, a mild anemia may last up to 6 weeks. Bone marrow aspirates obtained from these patients show erythroid hypoplasia and increased ringed sideroblasts, suggesting a maturation arrest [93]. Platelet counts drop as temperature decreases, and prolongation of the bleeding time has been noted at 20°C [89]. The decrease in platelet count is thought to be secondary to hepatic or splenic sequestration.

No clear evidence indicates that a coagulopathy is associated with hypothermia. Deep venous thrombosis and disseminated intravascular coagulopathy (DIC) have been reported in hypothermic patients [33,94].

Gastrointestinal Tract Function

Ileus, pancreatitis, and hepatic dysfunction accompany hypothermia. Ileus is present at temperatures 30°C and lower. Subclinical pancreatitis appears to be common. Although patients usually lack symptoms of acute pancreatitis, more than half have amylase elevations greater than 550 S units and up to 80% of patients who die of hypothermia have evidence of pancreatitis at autopsy [95]. The relationship between alcohol use and pancreatitis in these patients is unclear. Hepatic dysfunction occurs commonly and involves synthetic and detoxification abilities. Postmortem studies of patients who died from exposure-induced hypothermia commonly have gastric submucosal hemorrhage [96] and, to a lesser extent, duodenal ulceration and perforation [97].

Endocrine Function

Hypothermia directly suppresses the release of insulin from the pancreas and increases resistance to insulin's action in the periphery [98,99]. The blood glucose level rises in early hypothermia because of glycogenolysis and increased corticosteroid levels, and remains elevated because of a decreased concentration and the action of insulin. Elevations in blood glucose, however, are usually mild; only 9% of patients in one series had blood glucose levels higher than 200 mg per dL. The responses to thyroid-stimulating hormone (TSH) and adrenocorticotrophic hormone appear blunted [57]. In hypothyroid patients, TSH increases in response to cold [100]. Corticosteroid levels vary, but rarely appear to be severely depressed [58,101,102]. Urinary catecholamine levels are increased threefold to sevenfold on average in hypothermic deaths compared with death owing to other causes [96].

Immune Function

Infection is a major cause of death in hypothermic patients. Hypoperfusion increases the risk of bacterial invasion in ischemic regions of the skin and intestine. Pneumonia risk is increased as a result of central nervous system depression reducing the cough reflex, an increase in atelectasis because of decrease in tidal volume and minute ventilation, impaired killing of bacteria by pulmonary alveolar macrophages, and the severity of cold-induced granulocytopenia [90,103]. Evidence from hypothermic animals with induced sepsis indicates an impaired release of PMNs from the marrow [90], impaired phagocytosis, migration [105], and a decrease in the half-life for circulating PMNs during hypothermia [103], leading to delayed clearance of staphylococcal [104] and Gram-negative organisms from the blood. Ineffective clearance of organisms may permit a continued low-grade bacteremia [104]. The role of changes in antigen–antibody interactions, complement activation, and innate immune pathways that are known to be impaired by cold in vitro, has not been clearly defined in hypothermic patients. Wound healing is delayed in patients with mild perioperative hypothermia [106]. Cytokine production, for example, interleukin-6 may be delayed and prolonged [107]. Thus, the hypothermic host with temperature dependant compromised barrier functions is more susceptible to invasion by pathogens and less equipped to defend itself when invasion occurs.

Drug Clearance

Little is known about the clearance of drugs in hypothermic adults. Complex interactions of reduced cardiac output, dehydration, slowed hepatic metabolism, decreased GFR, abnormal renal tubular filtration and reabsorption, and altered protein–drug dissociation constant alter the volume of distribution and total body clearance of many drugs [108].

Diagnosis

The diagnosis of hypothermia may be suggested by a history of exposure or immersion, clinical examination, and laboratory abnormalities. Elderly, alcoholic, diabetic, quadriparetic, or severely debilitated patients are at high risk of hypothermia. Signs of hypothermia vary with the patient's temperature. Cool skin, muscle rigidity, shivering, and acrocyanosis are present for most noncomatose patients. In obtunded patients, myxedema-type facies have been reported [95,109]. Although mental status changes vary widely among patients, they follow a typical pattern: between 35°C and 32°C, the patient may be stuporous or confused; between 32°C and 27°C, the patient may be verbally responsive but incoherent; and, at temperatures less than 27°C,

83% of patients are comatose but able to respond purposefully to noxious stimuli [110]. Muscle tone remains increased after shivering stops. Reflexes remain normal until body temperature is lower than 27°C, when they become depressed and/or absent. Plantar reflexes may be upgoing. The pupillary reflex may be sluggish below 30°C and may become fixed at temperatures less than 27°C. ECG changes are almost always present.

In the absence of an accurate temperature reading, the ECG can be used to gauge the degree of hypothermia [67,69]. J waves become prominent as temperature decreases and, in the absence of a cerebrovascular accident, appear to be pathognomonic for hypothermia. Prolonged PR or QT intervals in the presence of muscle tremor artifact and bradycardia strongly suggest the diagnosis. Because of the increased solubility of carbon dioxide and oxygen, arterial blood gases reported at 37°C may show a value of partial pressure of oxygen (PaO_2) + $PaCO_2$ greater than 150 mm Hg on room air, a biochemical impossibility at euthermia. An elevated hematocrit, a good output of dilute urine with hypotension, ileus, and an elevated amylase are helpful but nonspecific indicators of hypothermia.

Because the symptoms of hypothermia frequently mimic those of other disorders, the diagnosis may be missed unless there is a clear history of exposure or an accurate temperature reading is taken. Proper diagnosis depends on the use of a low-reading thermometer to determine core temperature. Electronic temperature probes that are accurate at low temperatures, can be used in several body sites, have a rapid response time, and can be left indwelling to provide online temperature readings during treatment.

The site for recording the temperature is important (see Chapter 27). Oral or nasopharyngeal temperatures may not reflect core temperature because of the influence of surrounding airflow. Bladder temperatures are commonly used and are accurate in mild-to-moderate hypothermia [111,112]. In patients with severe hypothermia, especially those requiring endotracheal intubation, an esophageal probe inserted into the lower one-third of the esophagus (about 24 cm below the larynx) provides a near approximation of cardiac temperature. Esophageal temperature is the most accurate method to track the progress of rewarming. Rectal probe readings may rise with peritoneal lavage or fall if adjacent to cold feces; esophageal probes not inserted into the lower third of the esophagus may read falsely high if heated humidified oxygen is used. Infrared tympanic thermometers and the so-called temporal artery thermometers are not accurate.

Bladder and rectal temperatures should not be used for critical patients during rewarming. Changes in rectal and bladder temperatures significantly lag behind core temperature changes during rewarming. Great vessel temperature can be measured using the thermistor on a Swan-Ganz catheter, but is highly affected by the infusion of heated fluids. During extracorporeal rewarming, bladder and pulmonary artery temperatures may increase faster than esophageal and rectal temperatures [112]. It may be helpful to monitor at least two core sites.

Differential Diagnosis

Clinical changes produced by hypothermia can mask and mimic other diseases. For example, rigidity of the cervical musculature, a rigid abdomen and absent bowel sounds, or shock and coma may be because of other diagnoses, and clinical judgment is required.

Deviation from the temperature–symptom relationship should suggest that the cause of a symptom may be other than hypothermia. For example, ventricular fibrillation or coma with a temperature higher than 30°C or shock with a low hematocrit or heme-positive stools, or hypoglycemia for relative tachycardia should alert the physician to suspect another diagnosis and pursue further diagnostic evaluations. Relative hyperventilation implies an underlying organic acidosis (e.g., diabetic ketoacidosis or aspirin overdose), because CO_2 production should be decreased in moderate-to-severe hypothermia.

Certain medications directly or indirectly cause hypothermia, either by impairing thermoregulatory mechanisms, decreasing awareness of cold, or by clouding judgment.

Establishing a diagnosis of myocardial infarction, after vigorous resuscitation attempts, can be difficult. Creatine kinase, lactate dehydrogenase, and serum glutamic oxaloacetic acid transaminase values may be elevated because of hepatic hypoperfusion and presumed skeletal muscle damage. Elevations in creatinine kinase MB and BB fractions have been reported in hypothermic patients with no evidence of cerebral infarct [60]. ECG changes in hypothermia do not mimic those seen in myocardial infarction, and are thus more reliable.

The neurologic manifestations of hypothermia vary widely, but the level of consciousness should be consistent with the core temperature. If the level of the consciousness is not proportional to the degree of hypothermia, suspect a head injury, central nervous system infection, or overdose.

Treatment

With immediate appropriate treatment, mortality should be low. Accumulated statistics suggest that mortality varies with the severity of the underlying disease and the temperature at initial examination. The overall mortality in a series of city-dwelling hypothermic patients was 12%, but this increased to nearly 50% if a serious underlying disease was present [13]. In the same series of patients, mortality increased to 1.8% for each 1°C decrease in temperature on admission. Mortality was higher when hypothermia occurred indoors [113]. In healthy young mountain climbers, mortality was also found to vary with body core temperature on admission: mortality was 25% for temperatures higher than 32°C versus 66% for temperatures lower than 27°C [55]. Multivariate analyses indicated that the strongest predictors of mortality were prehospital cardiac arrest, low or absent blood pressure, elevated blood urea nitrogen, and the need for tracheal intubation or nasogastric tube placement in the emergency department [114]. The Mount Hood tragedy suggests that serum potassium levels greater than 10 mEq per L, fibrinogen less than 50 mg per dL, and ammonia greater than 350 μg per dL at the time of diagnosis predict very low survival probability [111]. Asphyxia caused by submersion resulting in severe hypothermia may be associated with up to a 95% mortality rate [115]. The higher survival rates in city-dwelling patients are believed to represent the benefits of immediately accessible care. Many experts believe that without treatment, mortality for profound hypothermia may approach 100%.

Treatment should be aggressive. Functional survival in adults has been reported even after 6.5 hours of CPR [116]. Treatment includes initial field care and transport, stabilizing cardiopulmonary status, treating the cause of hypothermia, preventing the common complications of hypothermia, and rewarming.

Initial Field Care and Transport

Field management of hypothermia from exposure or immersion includes removal of wet clothes replacing with dry ones, and insulate from cold and wind with blankets. Sharing the body heat of another person in the same sleeping bag appears to offer no significant advantage [117]. Drinking hot drinks is not encouraged because it may increase hypothermia by producing peripheral vasodilation through a pharyngeal reflex [118]. Glucose drinks have been advocated, but recent work has shown that glycogen depletion does not impair shivering or rewarming [119].

The following precautions should be taken to transport the victim: transport in the supine position to prevent seizures from orthostatic hypotension [16], avoid rough handling owing to risk of ventricular fibrillation [74,118,119], cut clothing off, and carry the victim gently by a team of rescuers. A patient without a blood pressure or palpable pulse may already be in fibrillation and should be resuscitated until adequate ECG and pressure monitoring are available (see Chapters 27 and 28) [120].

Stabilizing Cardiopulmonary Status

Because early death from hypothermia is as a result of hypotension and arrhythmia, the goal of initial in-hospital management of hypothermic patients should be to achieve a safe, stable cardiopulmonary status. Shock among those with mild hypothermia is usually caused by the dehydration that results from cold diuresis; in more profound hypothermia, it may be cardiogenic. Fluid resuscitation should be attempted in all patients with hypothermic shock. Delivery of fluids through a central rather than a peripheral catheter is preferable for several reasons: vasoconstriction makes insertion of peripheral intravenous (IV) catheters difficult, vasoconstriction may impair delivery of peripherally injected medications, peripheral IV catheters may cause unnecessary damage to frostbitten extremities, and central catheter placement permits monitoring of central venous pressure. Because most patients are hemoconcentrated and hyperosmolar, slightly hypotonic crystalloid fluids should be given. Whenever possible, all IV fluids should be warmed to at least room temperature before infusion. If fluid resuscitation fails, pressor agents should be administered. Although pressor agents increase the risk of ventricular fibrillation, they have been used safely in patients with hypothermia [120,121]. The use of arterial and central venous pressure monitors may help guide treatment. The increased risk of hemorrhage from hypothermia-induced thrombocytopenia and prolongation of bleeding times must, however, be considered when undertaking invasive procedures, such as central venous catheter placement or intubation.

The management of arrhythmias must be approached in a nontraditional manner because many pharmacologic agents, pacing efforts, and defibrillation attempts do not work in the hypothermic patient [122–124]. Because supraventricular arrhythmias and heart block generally resolve spontaneously on rewarming [68,79], therapy is usually unnecessary. Digitalis should be avoided because the efficacy of the drug is unclear in hypothermia, and toxicity increases as the patient is warmed [64]. Little is known regarding the efficacy of calcium channel blockers in treating supraventricular tachyarrhythmias in hypothermic patients.

For hypothermic patients experiencing ventricular fibrillation, procainamide has been of little help and lidocaine has been of only modest benefit [119]. Bretylium or amiodarone appears to be the drug of choice [118,125–127]. Electrical defibrillation should probably be attempted at least once, but it is unlikely to succeed until core temperature surpasses 30°C [18, 72,128]. The role of pacing in patients with fibrillation and asystole is unclear [64,129]. If other avenues of support are unavailable, however, pacing should be tried [130].

Acid–base status and oxygenation should be assessed immediately. Accurate assessment of acid–base status for hypothermic patients is complicated by several issues. First, arterial blood gases measured at 37°C produce different values of pHa and $PaCO_2$ than those exist in a patient at a lower temperature. Second, normal values for pHa and $PaCO_2$ also change with temperature. Third, body buffer systems respond differently at colder temperatures. When blood is drawn from a hypothermic patient and then rewarmed to and measured at 37°C, the solubility of carbon dioxide decreases, resulting in higher $PaCO_2$ and lower pHa values than actually exist [131].

Normal values for pHa and $PaCO_2$ also change with temperature. At a temperature of 20°C, a pHa of approximately 7.65 permits continued cellular function, and this value, not a pHa of 7.40, should be regarded as normal. Normal values for $PaCO_2$ are altered because of the higher content of carbon dioxide in cooled blood, decreased rate of production of carbon dioxide, and slower rate of carbon dioxide elimination from relative alveolar hypoventilation. Respiratory exchange ratio values as low as 0.32 have been reported. On balance, these changes result in lower $PaCO_2$ values at colder temperatures.

Temperature changes the protein–drug dissociation constant of chemical reactions and reduces the ionization level of buffer proteins [131]. This produces a smaller effective protein buffer pool and places a greater reliance for buffering on the less efficient carbonic acid system. Because of this less effective buffering, acid–base disturbances that would be well tolerated at 37°C might be poorly tolerated at lower temperatures.

Because of a decrease in the solubility of oxygen on warming the blood to 37°C, arterial oxygen tension values reported at 37°C may be substantially higher than the actual value in colder patients. Therefore, PaO_2 values must be corrected for temperature, or the presence of significant hypoxemia may be overlooked. Several nomograms to permit correction exist [132,138–140]. For clinical purposes, the following formula can be used to correct PaO_2 for temperature: decrease the PaO_2 measured at 37°C by 7.2% for each degree that the patient's temperature is less than 37°C.

Because acute respiratory distress syndrome may, and pneumonia [97] frequently does, accompany hypothermia, a chest radiograph should be obtained. In all, 90% to 100% oxygen should be administered until adequate oxygenation has been demonstrated. Oxygen saturation, after correction for temperature, should be maintained at greater than 90% to help prevent hypoxic damage. Stuporous or comatose patients should have prophylactic intubation to decrease the risk of aspiration pneumonia. Blind nasotracheal intubation may be required; orotracheal intubation may be difficult because of the rigidity of upper airway muscles [122]. If respiratory failure is evident on blood gas analysis, the trachea should be intubated and the lungs mechanically ventilated. Experiences during hypothermic surgery and in the treatment of unintentional hypothermia indicate that the initial ventilator settings should be similar to those normally used at temperatures of 37°C [132,133] (see Chapter 166).

Treating the Cause of Hypothermia

Hypoglycemia is rapidly detected by a glucose test strip and confirmed by blood glucose value. As a result of the ineffective action of insulin at low temperatures and the relatively high serum osmolarity from water diuresis, serious and difficult-to-treat hyperosmolarity may result from boluses of high concentrations of glucose [58,79]. Therefore, treatment with highly concentrated glucose solutions should be delayed until measure of the blood glucose has been obtained. Once hypoglycemia has been documented, 25 to 50 g glucose as a 50% dextrose solution is given to the patient. Some patients have been reported to shiver on correction of hypoglycemia and to correct their hypothermia rapidly.

Alcohol or sedative drug use or overdose is usually indicated by history and confirmed by toxicologic screening. No reports indicate adverse effects of naloxone in hypothermia; it should routinely be given if coma is present.

A thorough neurologic examination may suggest central nervous system or peripheral nervous system disease. If the patient has a history of trauma, the neck should be stabilized until a cervical spine radiograph has been obtained. Flaccid extremities suggest a cord or peripheral nerve injury. Cerebral edema secondary to tumor may be seen on funduscopic examination. Treatment with thiamine is benign and is given routinely for stuporous hypothermic patients until Wernicke–Korsakoff syndrome is ruled out. Thiamine is given with glucose, if hyperglycemia is absent, to decrease the chance of cerebral dysfunction. If the patient has Wernicke–Korsakoff encephalopathy, response to thiamine treatment may be seen within hours; if thiamine is not given, efforts to increase temperature may be futile [35,39]. Cyclic hypothermia is rarely fatal and responds to cyproheptadine, ephedrine, and naloxone [141,142].

Thyroid hormone is not given routinely to every patient with hypothermia because it is potentially harmful and hypothyroid coma is rare. In all cases of suspected myxedema, treatment with thyroid hormone is mandatory because it may be lifesaving. Conventional treatment of myxedema hypothermic coma begins with immediate IV administration of 0.2 to 0.5 mg thyroxine. If the patient has not clearly responded in 24 hours, this dose is repeated, and the patient is maintained on 0.05 to 0.10 mg thyroxine IV daily until clinically stable (see Chapter 142).

Debilitating diseases such as congestive heart failure, sepsis, hepatic, or renal failure should be treated in a conventional manner. For diabetic patients, insulin resistance increases rapidly below 30°C; insulin administration should be delayed when possible until the patient's temperature is more than 30°C. If insulin is given during hypothermia, it must be administered IV because subcutaneous absorption is impaired by hypoperfusion. In addition, insulin should be given in small doses because its degradation may be delayed at low temperature and cumulative doses may produce hypoglycemia and rebound hypothermia as the patient is warmed.

Preventing Common Complications

Early attention to the prevention, diagnosis, and treatment of diseases that are commonly associated with hypothermia may significantly reduce morbidity and mortality [143]. Diabetic patients who have hypothermia and infection have a particularly grave prognosis. In patients with diabetic ketoacidosis, the prevalence of hypothermia was four times higher in those with underlying infection and mortality was three times higher [144]. The possibility of infection should be carefully evaluated in diabetic patients with hypothermia, and early intervention with antibiotics should be considered.

Pneumonia is a common complication in hypothermic patients who survive the rewarming period. The incidence of pneumonia can probably be reduced by early intubation in stuporous or comatose patients to protect the airway, thereby minimizing aspiration. In addition, periodic hyperinflation [78], elevation of the head of the bed, and attention to periodic clearance of respiratory tract secretions may decrease the incidence of pneumonia in hypothermic patients. Antibiotics should only be given when infection is already likely to be present [143,145]. A study demonstrated that a low SVR in patients with mild-to-moderate hypothermia strongly indicates the presence of infection [76]. When SVR is low or diabetic ketoacidosis is present, we believe it is reasonable to give broad-spectrum antibiotic coverage for 24 to 48 hours pending results of respiratory tract cultures.

Because pancreatitis and ileus are both commonly associated with hypothermia, a nasogastric tube should be passed, a baseline amylase level should be obtained, and the patient should not be allowed to eat or drink until hypothermia has resolved, and pharyngeal swallowing function testing indicates minimal aspiration risk.

Prophylaxis of deep vein thrombosis (DVT) in patients with hypothermia is a difficult task. Subcutaneous heparin should not be used because it may be poorly absorbed for several days until skin function returns to normal. Pneumatic boots should not be placed on frostbitten extremities. Because of these concerns and because it is not clear that the risk of DVT from hypothermia outweighs that of systemic anticoagulation, we do not routinely recommend immediate prophylaxis for DVT. Because DIC has been reported, baseline clotting studies may be of value. DIC has occurred even in heparinized patients [146].

Acute tubular necrosis has been reported with hypothermia [66], but it is infrequent and probably results from shock and hypoxia, not as a direct action of hypothermia itself. Renal damage may be minimized by careful cardiovascular support. Hypermagnesemia reduces temperatures in hypothermic patients with renal failure and should be avoided [147]. Hypophosphatemia may result from treatment [148]. Electrolyte levels may vary greatly during treatment.

In cases of exposure, frostbite frequently occurs on the ears, nose, face, penis, scrotum, and extremities. It may be painless and go unrecognized by the victim until he or she is rewarmed. Frostbite is detectable on physical examination because recently frozen tissue usually appears gray, white, or waxy. Soon after warming, the skin may become edematous, blister, or turn red or black because of hemorrhage or necrosis. The extent of damage and eschar formation is usually demarcated within 10 days. Limbs should be handled gently. Thawing frostbitten areas is best postponed until core temperatures have risen to normal and the patient's condition is stable. It is best accomplished by immersion for 30 to 60 minutes in water heated to 38°C to 43°C. After thawing, whirlpool debridement, intra-arterial reserpine, and anticoagulation with heparin or dextran may be helpful. Amputation may be necessary but should always be delayed as long as possible to allow a clear demarcation of viable tissue [118].

Because of the risk of relapse, hypothermic patients require prolonged monitoring. Elderly patients who have had one episode of hypothermia may experience relapse and, in addition, may be at greater risk for future hypothermic episodes [149]. Any patient who has sustained severe hypothermia under conditions other than extreme exposure should be monitored closely for recurrent episodes.

Rewarming

Rewarming methods can be divided into three categories: passive external rewarming, active external rewarming, and active central rewarming.

Passive External Rewarming. Passive external rewarming is the least invasive and slowest rewarming technique. The patient is kept dry, sheltered from wind, and covered with blankets to decrease heat loss, thereby allowing thermogenesis to restore normal temperature. Temperature increase varies inversely with patient age; the average rate of temperature increase with this method is only 0.38°C per hour [60]. Passive rewarming is appropriate only when the patient's core temperature is >30°C.

Active External Rewarming. Active external rewarming is the most controversial method. It involves raising the core temperature by heating the skin with hot blankets, electric heating pads, and hot water bottles; circulating warmed air immediately adjacent to the skin [150,151]; or immersion in a tub of warm water. This method works [18,55,118,149,152] and has been successful in patients with temperatures as low as 17°C [153]. Initial reports [150,151] suggest that rewarming by covering the patient with a plastic blanket that contains tubes of circulating heated air is helpful for the mild hypothermia seen in the perioperative setting. Several studies have now documented that rewarming by the heated air method is safe and effective for moderate hypothermia of numerous etiologies. Mortality with active external rewarming appears to be higher than with passive or central rewarming methods [13]. This possible increase in mortality may be because of a (a) less accurate control over the rate of temperature increase, (b) increased risk of shock from warming the skin before the core, and (c) increased incidence of acidosis resulting from abrupt return of blood to the core from relatively hypoperfused areas. Treatment by immersion is impossible for patients who require continuous ECG and temperature monitoring, central venous access, and artificial ventilation and who are in imminent danger of shock or arrest. Experience with patients undergoing external rewarming suggests that aggressive hydration and central catheter monitoring are helpful [124].

Active Central Rewarming. The fastest and most invasive warming methods are those designed to permit active central rewarming. Although commercial Food and Drug Administration–approved warmers limit fluid warming to 40°C, heated IV crystalloid to temperatures as high as 65°C has been shown to be safe in animal trials [154]. Oxygen that has been humidified and heated to 40°C to 46°C is a safe [13,155] and effective [153] rewarming technique; it can be delivered by face mask or an endotracheal tube. Temperature must be monitored orally to ensure that inspired air does not exceed 46°C, or mucosal damage or burns might occur. Temperature increase with heated oxygen is usually less than 1°C per hour.

Lavage by gastric or esophageal balloons also produces a slow temperature increase and has been shown to be effective [156]; however, this method involves risk of aspiration and ventricular fibrillation during balloon insertion. Peritoneal lavage safely raises temperatures at a rate of up to 4°C per hour [80,94,157–159]. Average warming rates, however, are closer to 2°C per hour. Saline or dialysate fluid is heated to 38°C to 43°C and exchanged every 15 to 20 minutes. Alternatively, two peritoneal trocars can be placed and a continuous infusion and drainage circuit can be established. Pleural lavage with two chest tubes also appears to be effective [160,161].

Insertion of femoral artery and vein catheters allows blood to be removed, heated, and returned to the body. This is usually performed with a hemodialysis machine [144] or pump oxygenator that used during cardiopulmonary bypass. Rewarming at a rate of 1°C to 2°C per hour has been reported by passing the blood from a surgically created arteriovenous fistula through a countercurrent fluid warmer with [162] or without [163,164] a roller pump. For patients with severe cardiopulmonary collapse, a pump oxygenator offers the advantage of hemodynamic support, rapid elevation of temperature, and nearly complete regulation of acid–base and oxygen disorders [66,74,111,119,142,165,166]. In one review of 68 patients presenting with a mean core temperature of 21°C and being treated with cardiopulmonary bypass primarily by the femoral route, there was a 60% survival, and 80% of survivors returned to their previous level of function [166]. No survival is reported in patients presenting with temperatures of less than 15°C. In cases of profound hypothermia, a median sternotomy approach may be preferable because of the possibilities of direct cardiac massage, improved blood flow, and easy access [111].

The desired rate of rewarming varies according to the patient's cardiopulmonary status and underlying disease. Results of experiments performed on hypothermic dogs suggest that if intramyocardial temperature gradients can be maintained at less than 2°C, the risk of fibrillation decreases [72]. This research argues that safe warming should be either slow enough to allow uniformity in tissue temperatures or fast enough to minimize the period of risk. Slower warming techniques allow a prolonged period of hypothermia and presumably should produce a higher risk of infection because of prolonged immune suppression and a higher incidence of acid–base and intravascular volume problems. A diagnosis of diabetes or myxedema may also influence the desired rate of rewarming. For diabetic ketoacidosis, for example, insulin resistance and the severity of the acidosis could be substantially improved by rapid rewarming [95].

The rewarming method selected must be appropriate for the individual patient being rewarmed. In one study of 55 patients with accidental hypothermia, extracorporeal membrane oxygenation was used for those in cardiopulmonary arrest; peritoneal dialysis for those with unstable hemodynamics; and airway rewarming, insulation, and warmed fluids for those with stable hemodynamics. Survival was 100% [167].

IATROGENIC HYPOTHERMIA

Iatrogenic hypothermia occurs frequently in surgical recovery rooms and intensive care units [168–171], is associated with increased morbidity, and can be minimized with a systematic team approach. Although subnormal temperatures occur frequently during the postoperative period, frank hypothermia (temperature <35°C) is uncommon. In a series of 195 patients who underwent noncardiothoracic surgery, 60% had temperatures less than 36°C, 29% had less than 35.5°C, and 13% had less than 35°C [172]. Iatrogenic hypothermia results from the infusion of blood products or fluids at lower than body core temperatures [168,172], from continuous ultrafiltration at high flow rates in the intensive care unit [173], and from anesthesia and surgery performed in cool (<23°C) operating rooms [21,22,69,174,175]. In another series of 101 patients undergoing elective surgery under general anesthesia, 78% had temperatures less than 36°C. The average temperature decrease was 0.77°C, and maximal decrease was 2.5°C [175].

Causes and Pathogenesis

Perioperative hypothermia results from increased heat loss, decreased heat production, and compromised thermoregulation [176]. Heat loss may be increased by loss of behavioral control mechanisms, decreased insulation because of exposure of larger skin surfaces, cutaneous vasodilation resulting from anesthetics, increased evaporative losses from serosal surfaces and volatile antiseptics applied to skin, and exposure to air-conditioned environments. Decreased heat production results from muscular paralysis. Impaired thermoregulation results from slowed or compromised afferent and efferent nerve impulses and hypothermic reflexes because of sedative anesthetics. Redistribution of heat from the core to the periphery is felt to be a primary factor for perioperative hypothermia. Temperature change may be abrupt with a 1°C core heat loss within 30 minutes of induction because of redistribution of heat from the core to the periphery [177].

The frequency and severity of heat loss increases with patient age [168,170,171], open chest or abdominal surgery [168,170,178], low-operating room temperature [21,22], length of surgery [169], infusion of cool IV solutions, and certain types of anesthetics. Elderly patients experience a decrease in temperature, shiver less frequently, and take longer to rewarm than do younger patients [168,171]. Temperature decrease during surgery involving open body cavities may result in almost twice the decrease in temperature seen in extremity surgery [170]. Lightly anesthetized, paralyzed, draped patients who are not provided with active warming experience a temperature decrease of 0.3°C per hour at ambient temperatures less than 21°C [22]. Surgery involving muscle paralysis with curare-type agents produces twice the temperature decrease in nonparalyzing procedures [170]. Although halothane and epidural anesthesia may increase heat loss because of vasodilation, no major differences have been detected in the heat loss from most inhalational agents [170,171]. Laparoscopic procedures produce hypothermia that may be more severe than open laparotomy. Massive infusion of chilled solutions can induce hypothermia, as heat loss from infusion of room temperature solutions approximates 16 kcal per L [171]. Blood infused at its stored temperature of 4°C produces a heat loss of 32 kcal per L [172]. In an average human, infusion of 1 L of 4°C blood produces a 0.5°C decrease in temperature [168]. The mean temperature of patients given more than 20 units of blood in 24 hours has been reported to be 32.9°C ± 1.7°C [53]. The rapid transfusion of blood not warmed to body temperature must be considered a risk factor for the development of mild hypothermia. There was no difference in mean temperature of survivors and nonsurvivors after massive transfusion.

Pathophysiology

Perioperative complications from mild hypothermia arise directly from the hypothermia and from the hypermetabolism triggered by the patient's efforts to restore body temperature. An otherwise healthy individual with a temperature ranging from 34°C to 36°C will have (a) a slightly increased cardiac output, (b) an oxygen consumption up to five times basal levels, (c) an elevated SVR because of peripheral vasoconstriction, (d) a decrease in mixed venous oxygen saturation because of increased oxygen extraction, (e) shivering or muscle rigidity, and (f) a slightly depressed mental status. The alveolar–arterial oxygen gradient and even the arteriovenous oxygen difference [76] may be in the normal range [124]. Therefore, deviations from this pattern during the perioperative period and subsequent morbidity must reflect the additive effects of surgery and anesthesia on metabolism.

For critically ill postoperative patients with cardiac depression, one must be concerned about the potential effects of mild hypothermia because an increase in oxygen consumption could lead to acidosis and hypoxemia. Although acidosis results from an increase in anaerobic metabolism as metabolic demand outstrips oxygen delivery, minute ventilation is usually maintained to the degree necessary to preserve acid–base balance [179]. Hypoxemia may result from the combination of increased pulmonary parenchymal shunt (venous admixture) after surgery and lower mixed venous PO_2. In one study, shivering appeared to be accompanied by a drop in PaO_2; arterial oxygen saturation fell below 90% in 53% of shivering patients and remained above 90% in all nonshivering patients [179]. Decreased temperature and shivering can elevate oxygen consumption and, in some patients, lower PaO_2 [171,180]. Increased perioperative cardiac ischemia, ventricular tachycardia [181], delayed wound healing [106], perioperative bleeding requiring transfusion [107,182,183], increased length of stay in recovery, and increased length of stay in hospital [106] may occur with perioperative hypothermia. Patients with prolonged postoperative hypothermia have a higher mortality than those who return to normal temperatures in the first postoperative hour [184].

Prevention and Treatment

Numerous interventions have been attempted to minimize perioperative temperature decrease and shivering. The use of postoperative warming blankets alone does not prevent significant temperature loss because the body surface area exposed to heat is small [18,174,185]. The use of warming blankets along with heating of all infused liquids can maintain average temperature on arrival in the recovery room above 36°C [185]. Heating and humidifying the carbon dioxide used for laparoscopic insufflation to 30.0°C to 30.5°C decrease the heat loss associated with laparoscopic procedures [186]. Crystalloids can be easily warmed in a microwave oven to 39°C in 2 minutes [187]. The inhalation of heated, humidified air can be safely applied to most intubated patients and is effective for preventing temperature loss [180,188,189] and shivering [180]. Most publications clearly favor the use of preoperative, intraoperative, and postoperative forced air warmers [190–192]. One hour of prewarming with an air warmer set to 43°C may minimize redistribution loss and decrease hypothermia for brief procedures. Vasodilators such as nitroprusside or nifedipine may be started hours preoperatively, resulting in peripheral vasodilation and minimizing redistribution loss by prewarming the peripheral tissues. Cutaneous rewarming minimizes shivering. Meperidine may lower the shivering threshold and control pain in postoperative patients. Prewarming is felt to be the most effective strategy for high-risk patients [177].

Prevention of the development of hypothermia in summary includes minimizing preoperative and postoperative time in chilled rooms, covering the patient with drapes or blankets whenever possible, and infusing all solutions at least at room temperature. High-risk patients including those undergoing major abdominal or cardiothoracic surgery, surgery involving intentional hypothermia, or surgery with anesthesia times in excess of 4 hours; patients older than 60 years undergoing surgery; or those with known or expected cardiac depression should receive preventive measures, including preoperative [193–195] and intraoperative [191,196] forced warm air, heating of infused solutions to 37.5°C, and inhalation of heated humidified oxygen. In any patient undergoing extracorporeal bypass, a heat exchanger to the bypass circuit should be used [197]. Blood and colloid solutions should be heated to 37.5°C [198].

INTENTIONAL HYPOTHERMIA

Intentional hypothermia has been induced by partial immersion or surface or central cooling techniques to treat cancer, limit the toxicity of sepsis, help prevent the alopecia of chemotherapy, reduce carbon dioxide production in refractory status asthmaticus, assist in the amputation of limbs, and minimize the hypoperfusion injury associated with cardiothoracic surgery. Currently, mild-to-moderate hypothermia (32°C to 36°C) is the first treatment with proven efficacy for postischemic neurologic injury, and employing intentional hypothermia to retard postcardiac arrest brain injury is now recommended by the American Heart Association [226,220].

Therapeutic Hypothermia after Cardiac Arrest

Therapeutic hypothermia improves survival and neurologic outcomes after sudden cardiac arrest, and has been summarized in a systematic review and meta-analysis of six randomized trials including 1,413 patients [199–201,225]. According to this review, patients treated with therapeutic hypothermia were more likely to survive than patients whose temperature was not managed similarly (relative risk: 1.41; 95% confidence interval [CI]: 1.09 to 1.82); however, no difference for outcomes was found based on the target temperature of 33°C versus 36°C. Conclusion about the absence of any difference of outcomes based on the target temperature is based primarily on the findings of a large, well-performed, multinational randomized trial of 939 unconscious survivors of out-of-hospital cardiac arrest that reported no differences of mortality or neurologic function between patient's treated with a target temperature of 33°C (n = 473) compared to patients with a targeted temperature of 36°C (n = 466) [220].

Cardiac arrest results in immediate termination of blood flow and loss of oxygen, leading to neurologic ischemic injury after only several minutes and permanent loss after 5 to 10 minutes. If resuscitation results in restoration of circulation, then an additional reperfusion injury occurs. Several animal models, including dogs, showed that cooling after prolonged cardiac arrest provided considerable neurologic benefits [203]. Subsequently, two pivotal, randomized, controlled trials were conducted and confirmed efficacy [200,201]. The first of these was a large, multicenter, randomized controlled trial that enrolled 275 patients in 9 European hospitals who had sustained a cardiac arrest with an initial rhythm of ventricular fibrillation. The second randomized controlled trial enrolled 77 patients from 4 hospitals in Victoria, Australia, with similar inclusion criteria, however, did not exclude older patients or those who were hypoxic. The American Heart Association recommended, in review of these two studies, therapeutic hypothermia for 12 to 24 hours following resuscitation from out-of-hospital cardiac arrest for the treatment of neurologic injury when the initial rhythm is ventricular fibrillation [204].

Therapeutic hypothermia is of potential benefit for minimizing brain injury in all postcardiac arrest patients, regardless of their arrhythmia or the location of their arrest according to the 2010 Guidelines for Advanced Cardiac Life Support [226]. Nonetheless, evidentiary support for therapeutic hypothermia in nonshockable rhythms is primarily limited to nonrandomized studies using historic or concurrent controls [205]. One subgroup analysis of 186 patients with a nonshockable rhythm reported no difference in mortality between those treated with temperature management using a target of 33°C versus a target of 36°C [220].

In addition, the trials used therapeutic hypothermia several hours after resuscitation; therefore, the role for earlier cooling or prolonged cooling was not evaluated. In a Cochrane database systematic review, when combined with standard postcardiac arrest care, lowering the body temperature to the range of 32°C to 34°C during the first hours after cardiac arrest improves neurologic outcomes compared to not controlling body temperature [219]. A large randomized trial reports similar improvements in outcome whether the temperature is maintained at 33°C or 36°C [220]. Given that the induction of hypothermia has become more feasible, the side effects are generally easily managed in the critical care setting, and there is a benefit for anoxic brain injury; consideration may be given to treat comatose postcardiac arrest nonventricular fibrillation patients with therapeutic hypothermia [205].

Hyperthermia must be avoided following cardiac arrest. Failure to control a patient's core temperature is associated with the development of fever and worse neurologic outcomes [221,222]. According to an observational study of 151 patients, the risk of death increases for each degree over 37°C during the first 48 hours after cardiac arrest (odds ratio: 2.26; 95% CI: 1.24 to 4.12) [221]. Earlier onset of fever is associated with worse outcomes, whereas delayed fever onset has not shown the same deleterious effects [222]. Overall, these data suggest that active control of the postcardiac arrest patient's core temperature, with a target between 32°C and 36°C, followed by active avoidance of fever, is the optimal strategy to promote patient's survival.

For Acute Myocardial Infarction

Timely myocardial reperfusion using thrombolytic therapy or angioplasty is the most effective therapy for patients with ST elevation myocardial infarction. Although mild hypothermia appears feasible and safe, its ability to limit infarct size or reduce rates of adverse cardiac events has not been proven [206].

For Spinal Cord Injury

Hypothermia strategies date back to the 1960s for the treatment of acute spinal cord injury, but no randomized phase III trials have been conducted to confirm efficacy and safety, let alone the appropriate therapeutic window. Hypothermia remains an experimental treatment with unknown clinical relevance for patients with acute spinal cord injury [207].

For Ischemic and Hemorrhagic Stroke

Hypothermia reduces brain edema and intracranial pressure (ICP) in patients with traumatic brain injury; however, only very few small pilot studies have investigated the role hypothermia may have in the treatment of acute ischemic stroke. There are no controlled trials performed for hypothermia in hemorrhagic stroke [208]. The use of normothermia protocols is being actively studied.

For Acute Liver Toxicity

Patients with rapidly progressive acute liver failure, such as with acetaminophen overdose, are at high risk for developing cerebral edema, intracranial hypertension, brainstem herniation, brain death or anoxic brain injury, and permanent brain impairment. Techniques such as manipulating the body position, increasing sedation, and increasing osmolarity through medications can temporarily control this phenomenon. However, these steps often postpone but do not stop the development of brain herniation unless liver transplantation or spontaneous liver regeneration follows immediately. Using therapeutic hypothermia has been shown to effectively bridge patients to transplant by reducing cerebral edema and intracranial hypertension by decreasing splanchnic ammonia production, lowering oxidative metabolism within the brain, and restoring normal regulation of cerebral hemodynamics [209]. However, hypothermia has not been adequately studied for its safety, and concerns of increasing the risk of infection, cardiac arrhythmias, and bleeding may be accentuated. Multicenter, randomized control trials are needed to determine whether hypothermia protects the brain and improves survival without causing harm.

In Multisystem Trauma

Hypothermia may be helpful in attenuating the damage to tissues before adequate blood volume resuscitation can be restored in traumatic blood loss. Clinical trials to determine its efficacy are needed [210].

Advances in hypothermia, based on randomized controlled trials or meta-analyses of such trials, are summarized in Table 184.4.

Methods of Cooling

Induction and maintenance of hypothermia requires blocking the body's normal thermoregulation mechanism as well as active heat exchange. Therapeutic hypothermia can be achieved through four mechanisms individually or in combination, which include conduction, convection, radiation, and evaporation as previously described. There are four phases of temperature modulation during therapeutic hypothermia: induction, maintenance, rewarming, and normothermia [211]. Induction is

TABLE 184.4

Advances in Management of Hypothermia Based on Randomized Controlled Trials

Induced hypothermia benefits survivors of cardiac arrest:

Unconscious adult patients with recovery of spontaneous circulation after out-of-hospital cardiac arrest should be cooled with a target between 32°C and 36°C for 12–24 h when the initial rhythm was VF, followed by active avoidance of fever for at least 48 h following cardiac arrest.

Similar therapy may be beneficial for patients with non-VF arrest out-of-hospital or for in-hospital arrest

VF, ventricular fibrillation.

typically initiated prehospital, especially in out-of-hospital cardiac arrests, but can occur in hospital for patients awaiting a liver transplantation, with cerebral edema from acute liver failure and for control of refractory elevated ICP. In cardiac arrest survivors, contraindications to perform therapeutic hypothermia would include if the patient can follow verbal commands, more than 8 hours have elapsed since return of spontaneous circulation, life-threatening bleeding or infection, cardiopulmonary collapse is imminent despite vasopressor or mechanical hemodynamic support, or an underlying terminal condition exists.

Induction is commonly achieved by rapid bolus administration of 30 to 40 mL per kg cold (4°C) isotonic resuscitation fluid [211] targeting a goal temperature of 32°C to 36°C. Serum potassium will drop, and empirically repleting potassium for a goal of more than 3.8 mEq per dL is needed. Close monitoring and treatment for seizures are necessary. Simultaneous sedation, paralysis (for shivering), and use of commercial surface or intravascular cooling devices are concomitant therapeutic strategies [211].

Maintenance phase occurs in the intensive care unit and is a phase where both metabolic and hemodynamic homeostasis are maintained. The core temperature is kept at 33°C for 18 to 24 hours. Maintenance of brain perfusion by keeping mean arterial perfusion pressure at 65 mm Hg or more (cerebral perfusion pressure [CPP] may need to be monitored given cerebral autoregulatory failure [212]), normocarbia with volume-cycled mechanical ventilation to maintain a normal pH as hypercarbia is to be avoided; maintain a perfusing rhythm, antibiotic prophylaxis if pulmonary infiltrates present [211,213], maintenance of a blood glucose of 120 to 160 mg per dL [212], maintenance of normal electrolyte levels and appropriate medication dosing given the reduction in drug metabolism and duration of action, skin care, and aggressive treatment of shivering with neuromuscular blockade [211].

After 24 hours of therapeutic hypothermia, the gradual rewarming phase starts and is associated with hemodynamic instability often referred to as the postresuscitation syndrome. It is characterized by an increase in inflammatory cytokine levels, vasodilatation, and hypotension. The patient is also at increased risk for an elevation in the ICP and a decrease in the CPP. Gradual rewarming at a goal rate of 0.2°C to 0.33°C per hour until the patient is at 36.5°C or 37°C is preferred to avoid large hemodynamic fluctuations. Supportive fluid boluses, inotropes, and vasopressors may be necessary to maintain CPP, especially if there are signs of elevated ICP. The use of neuromuscular blockade until the temperature reaches 35°C to avoid shivering and sedation is weaned once the body temperature reaches 36°C is recommended [211].

For patients who have undergone therapeutic hypothermia postcardiac arrest, a rebound fever can occur and is harmful [214,221,222]. Brain injury may be attenuated by fever control [215]. Maintaining normothermia for at least 72 hours from return of circulation is thus common practice [211]. This is easily achieved by employing commercial cooling devices and resetting target temperature to 36.5°C to 37.5°C. Nursing attention to onset of fever spikes and frequent adjustments to the cooling device set points need to be closely observed.

A number of issues occur with induction, maintenance, and withdrawal of therapeutic hypothermia and require close attention. (i) Serum potassium needs to be aggressively replaced if levels are less than 3.8 mEq per dL as soon as therapeutic hypothermia is employed and the levels should be followed every 3 to 4 hours during the induction phase. (ii) Accurately measure the core temperature continuously, preferably achieved by esophageal measurements. (iii) With neuromuscular blockade, a thorough neurologic examination and adequate sedation a priori are important. (iv) There is no evidence demonstrating the superiority of any cooling method, and, in clinical practice, a combination of intravascular and surface cooling is commonly employed. (v) The incidence of pneumonia in postcardiac arrest patients treated with hypothermia is 30% to 50% [201]. The etiology may be related to aspiration at the time of cardiac arrest or from the immunosuppressive effects from hypothermia. Preliminary data support therapeutic antibiotics for presumed pneumonia with de-escalation based on culture results [213]. (vi) Seizures can occur 19% to 34% of the time and go undetected with neuromuscular blockade [216]. Thus, continuous electroencephalography monitoring of the paralyzed patient may be necessary. If continuous monitoring is not available, then empirically using antiepileptic drugs with sedative effects to sedate the patient may be warranted [211]. (vii) Hemodynamic instability is common during the rewarming phase because of cutaneous vasodilatation and the inflammatory state [211]. Close attention to monitoring adequate cardiac output, global tissue perfusion, and brain perfusion using IV isotonic fluids, inotropes, and/or vasopressor agents may be necessary. Hemodynamic monitoring may be achieved using invasive or noninvasive cardiac output devices, urinary output if kidney function is normal, and central venous oxyhemoglobin saturation for tissue perfusion or direct invasive monitoring of brain metabolism [211]. (viii) To reduce shivering, focal counter rewarming [211] can be employed in which the face, neck, and extremities are actively warmed, whereas the torso and central venous system are cooled. This paradoxically increases the cooling process by enhancing the cutaneous vasodilatation.

COOLING TECHNIQUES

The conventional method involves the infusion of cold saline or ringer's lactate solution at 4°C administered at 30 to 40 mL per kg through a peripheral vein and has been shown to decrease core temperature by 2°C to 4°C without left ventricular systolic dysfunction and a reduction in cardiac output [217]. This method is supported by multiple safety and efficacy trials [211] and should be the preferred method for induction in conventional cooling. Thereafter, cooling can be maintained with ice packs applied to the neck, groin, and axilla and rubber cooling mats or blankets as used in the operating room. Ongoing infusion of cold fluid has not been shown to be an effective method to maintain hypothermia [218]. A number of issues associated with this method include the lack of an internal feedback loop making accurate temperature maintenance difficult, a high incidence of overcooling, and the need for a high level of nursing care. Nonetheless, it is widely available and cost-effective.

Patients with a history of heart failure or severely compromised renal function, or signs of acute pulmonary edema, should not receive rapid cooled infusions to induce therapeutic hypothermia. Surface cooling measures or an IV cooling device should be used instead. There is no evidence demonstrating the superiority of any cooling method, and, in clinical practice, a combination of intravascular and surface cooling is commonly employed. The lone observation study comparing intravascular and surface cooling methods found that neither the time needed to reach the goal temperature nor neurologic outcomes were significantly different between the two groups [223]. The effect of mild temperature fluctuations and excessive hypothermia on patient outcomes is unknown, and thermostatically controlled devices provide the most precise minute-to-minute temperature regulation and can avoid fever [224].

ACKNOWLEDGMENTS

The authors wish to thank Dr. Frederick J. Curley for his efforts in co-authoring earlier editions of this chapter upon which much of the newer information has been added.

References

1. Dinarello CA, Wolff SM: Pathogenesis of fever in man. *N Engl J Med* 298:607, 1978.
2. Iampietro PF, Vaughn JA, Goldman RF, et al: Heat production from shivering. *J Appl Physiol* 15:632, 1960.
3. Cabanac M: Regulation and modulation in biology. A re-examination of temperature regulation. *Ann N Y Acad Sci* 15:813, 1997.
4. Cabanac M: Temperature regulation. *Annu Rev Physiol* 37:415, 1975.
5. Kenney WL, Munce TA: Invited review: aging and human temperature regulation. *J Appl Physiol* 95(6):2598, 2003.
6. Nomoto S, Shibata M, Iriki M, et al: Role of afferent pathways of heat and cold in body temperature regulation. *Int J Biometeorol* 49(2):67, 2004.
7. Wagner JA, Robinson S, Marino RP: Age and temperature regulation of humans in neutral and cold environments. *J Appl Physiol* 37:562, 1974.
8. Collins KJ, Dore C, Exton-Smith AN, et al: Accidental hypothermia and impaired temperature homeostasis in the elderly. *BMJ* 1:353, 1977.
9. Ellis FP, Exton-Smith AN, Foster KG, et al: Eccrine sweating and mortality during heat waves in very young and very old persons. *Isr J Med Sci* 12:815, 1976.
10. Whittle JL, Bates JH: Thermoregulatory failure secondary to acute illness: complications and treatment. *Arch Intern Med* 139:418, 1979.
11. Centers for Disease Control and Prevention: Hypothermia-related deaths, Georgia—January 1996–December 1997, and United States, 1979–1995. *Morb Mortal Wkly Rep* 47:1037, 1998.
12. Miller JW, Danzl DF, Thomas DM: Urban accidental hypothermia: 135 cases. *Ann Emerg Med* 9:456, 1980.
13. Mathews JA: Accidental hypothermia. *Postgrad Med* 43:662, 1967.
14. Pugh LG: Accidental hypothermia in walkers, climbers and campers: reports to the medical commission on accident prevention. *BMJ* 1:123, 1966.
15. Rothschield MA, Schneider V: Terminal burrowing behaviour: a phenomenon of lethal hypothermia. *Int J Legal Med* 108:116, 1995.
16. Milner JE: Hypothermia. *Ann Intern Med* 89:565, 1978.
17. Hayward JS, Eckerson JD, Collis ML: Thermal balance and survival time prediction of man in cold water. *Can J Physiol Pharmacol* 53:21, 1974.
18. Jessen K, Hagelsten JO: Search and rescue service in Denmark with special reference to accidental hypothermia. *Aerosp Med* 43:787, 1972.
19. Raheja R, Puri BK, Schaeffer RC: Shock due to profound hypothermia and alcohol ingestion. *Crit Care Med* 9:644, 1984.
20. Duff RS, Farrant PC, Leveaux VM, et al: Spontaneous periodic hypothermia. *Q J Med* 30:329, 1961.
21. Morris RH: Operating room temperature and the anesthetized, paralyzed patient. *Arch Surg* 102:95, 1971.
22. Morris RH, Wilkey BR: The effects of ambient temperature on patient temperature during surgery not involving body cavities. *Anesthesiology* 32:102, 1972.
23. Hassel B: Acute hypothermia due to penicillin. *BMJ* 304:882, 1992.
24. Hassel B: Hypothermia from erythromycin. *Ann Intern Med* 115:69, 1991.
25. Pfeiffer RF: Bromocriptine-induced hypothermia. *Neurology* 40:383, 1990.
26. Freinkel N, Metzger BE, Harris E, et al: The hypothermia of hypoglycemia: studies with 2-deoxy-D-glucose in normal human subjects and mice. *N Engl J Med* 287:841, 1972.
27. Gale EA, Bennett T, Green JH, et al: Hypoglycemia, hypothermia and shivering in man. *Clin Sci* 61:463, 1981.
28. Forrester CF: Coma in myxedema. *Arch Intern Med* 111:100, 1963.
29. Hamburger S, Collier RE: Myxedema coma. *Ann Emerg Med* 11:156, 1982.
30. Fitzgerald FT: Hypoglycemia and accidental hypothermia in an alcoholic population. *West J Med* 133:105, 1980.
31. Branch EF, Burger PC, Brewer DL: Hypothermia in a case of hypothalamic infarction and sarcoidosis. *Arch Neurol* 25:245, 1971.
32. Kearsley JH, Musso AF: Hypothermia and coma in the Wernicke–Korsakoff syndrome. *Med J Aust* 2:504, 1980.
33. Koeppen AH, Daniels JC, Baroron KD: Subnormal body temperatures in Wernicke's encephalopathy. *Arch Neurol* 21:493, 1969.
34. Hansen B, Larsson C, Wiren J, et al: Hypothermia and infection in Wernicke's encephalopathy. *Acta Med Scand* 215:185, 1984.
35. Ackerman WJ: Stupor, bradycardia, hypotension and hypothermia: a presentation of Wernicke's encephalopathy with rapid response to thiamine. *West J Med* 121:428, 1974.
36. Philip G, Smith JF: Hypothermia and Wernicke's encephalopathy. *Lancet* 2:122, 1973.
37. Donnan GA, Seeman E: Coma and hypothermia in Wernicke's encephalopathy. *Aust N Z J Med* 10:438, 1980.
38. Mechlenburg RS, Loriaux DL, Thompson RH, et al: Hypothalamic dysfunction in patients with anorexia nervosa. *Medicine* 53:147, 1974.
39. Shapir WR, Williams GH, Plum F: Spontaneous recurrent hypothermia accompany agenesis of the corpus callosum. *Brain* 92:423, 1969.
40. Lammens M, Lissoir F, Carton H: Hypothermia in three patients with multiple sclerosis. *Clin Neurol Neurosurg* 91:117, 1989.
41. Randall WC, Wurster RD, Lewin RJ: Responses of patients with high spinal transection to high ambient temperatures. *J Appl Physiol* 21:985, 1966.
42. Pledger HG: Disorders of temperature regulation in acute traumatic tetraplegia. *J Bone Joint Surg* 44B:110, 1962.
43. Altus P, Hickman JW, Nord J: Accidental hypothermia in a healthy quadriplegic patient. *Neurology* 35:427, 1985.
44. Krook G: Hypothermia in patients with exfoliative dermatitis. *Acta Derm Venereol* 40:142, 1960.
45. Grice KA, Bettley FR: Skin water loss and accidental hypothermia in psoriasis, ichthyosis, and erythroderma. *BMJ* 2:195, 1967.
46. Moncrief JA: Burns. *N Engl J Med* 288:444, 1973.
47. Roe CF, Kinney JM, Blair C: Water and heat exchange in third-degree burns. *Surgery* 56:212, 1964.
48. Stoner HB: Mechanism of body temperature changes after burns and other injuries. *Ann N Y Acad Sci* 150:722, 1968.
49. Buggini RV: Hypothermia in Hodgkin's disease. *N Engl J Med* 312:244, 1985.
50. Csuka ME, McCarty DJ: Transient hypothermia after corticosteroid treatment of subacute cutaneous lupus erythematosus. *J Rheumatol* 11:112, 1984.
51. Kugler SL, Costakos DT, Aron AM, et al: Hypothermia and systemic lupus erythematosus. *J Rheumatol* 17:680, 1990.
52. Jurkovich GJ, Greiser WB, Luterman A: Hypothermia in trauma victims: an ominous predictor of survival. *J Trauma* 27:1019, 1987.
53. Wilson RF, Dulchavsky SA, Soullier G, et al: Problems with 20 or more blood transfusions in 24 hours. *Am Surg* 53:410, 1987.
54. Iampietro PF, Faughn JA, Goldman RF, et al: Heat production from shivering. *J Appl Physiol* 15:632, 1960.
55. Martyn JW: Diagnosing and treating hypothermia. *Can Med Assoc J* 125:1089, 1981.
56. Michenfelder JD, Uihlein A, Daw EF, et al: Moderate hypothermia in man: hemodynamic and metabolic effects. *Br J Anaesth* 37:738, 1965.
57. Hardy JD, Bard P: *Body Temperature Regulation in Medical Physiology.* St. Louis, MO, Mosby, 1974.
58. Stoner HB, Frayn KN, Little RA, et al: Metabolic aspects of hypothermia in the elderly. *Clin Sci* 59:19, 1980.
59. Cohen DJ, Cline JR, Lepinski SM, et al: Resuscitation of the hypothermic patient. *Am J Emerg Med* 6:475, 1988.
60. MacLean D, Griffiths PD, Browning MC, et al: Metabolic aspects of spontaneous rewarming in accidental hypothermia and hypothermic myxoedema. *Q J Med* 43:371, 1974.
61. Cooper KE: The circulation in hypothermia. *Br Med Bull* 17:48, 1961.
62. Trevino A, Rasi B, Beller BM: The characteristic electrocardiogram of accidental hypothermia. *Arch Intern Med* 127:470, 1971.
63. Southwick FS, Dalglish PH: Recovery after prolonged asystolic cardiac arrest in profound hypothermia. *JAMA* 243:1250, 1980.
64. Angelakos ET, Torres J, Driscoll R: Ouabain on the hypothermic dog heart. *Am Heart J* 56:458, 1958.
65. Bjornstad H, Tande PM, Refsum H: Cardiac electrophysiology during hypothermia and implications for medical treatment. *Arctic Med Res* 50[Suppl]:71, 1991.
66. Kugelberg J, Schuller H, Berg B, et al: Treatment of accidental hypothermia. *Scand J Thorac Cardiovasc Surg* 1:142, 1967.
67. Thompson R, Rich J, Chmelik F, et al: Evolutionary changes in the electrocardiogram of severe progressive hypothermia. *J Electrocardiol* 10:67, 1977.
68. Rankin AC, Rae AP: Cardiac arrhythmias during rewarming of patients with accidental hypothermia. *BMJ* 289:874, 1984.
69. Clements SD, Hurst JW: Diagnostic value of electrocardiographic abnormalities observed in subjects accidentally exposed to cold. *Am J Cardiol* 29:729, 1972.
70. Yan GX, Antxzelevitch C: Cellular basis of the electrocardiographic J wave. *Circulation* 93:372, 1996.
71. Van Mieghem C, Sabbe M, Knockaert D: The clinical value of the ECG in non cardiac conditions. *Chest* 125(4):1561, 2004.
72. Mouritzen CV, Andersen MN: Myocardial temperature gradients and ventricular fibrillation during hypothermia. *J Thorac Cardiovasc Surg* 49:937, 1965.
73. Hervey GR: Hypothermia. *Proc R Soc Med* 66:1055, 1973.
74. Althaus U, Aeberhard T, Schupbach P, et al: Management of profound accidental hypothermia with cardiorespiratory arrest. *Ann Surg* 195:492, 1982.
75. Zarins CK, Skinner DB: Circulation in profound hypothermia. *J Surg Res* 14:97, 1973.
76. Morris DL, Chambers HF, Morris MG, et al: Hemodynamic characteristics of patients with hypothermia due to occult infection and other causes. *Ann Intern Med* 102:153, 1985.
77. Blair E, Esmond WG, Attar S, et al: The effect of hypothermia on lung function. *Ann Surg* 160:814, 1964.
78. Hedley-Whyte J, Pontoppidan H, Laver MB, et al: Arterial oxygenation during hypothermia. *Anesthesiology* 26:595, 1965.
79. Rosenfeld JB: Acid–base and electrolyte disturbances in hypothermia. *Am J Cardiol* 12:678, 1963.
80. Pickering BG, Bristow GK, Craig DB: Core rewarming by peritoneal irrigation in accidental hypothermia with cardiac arrest. *Anesth Analg* 56:574, 1977.
81. Norwood WI, Norwood CR: Influence of hypothermia on intracellular pH during anoxia. *Am J Physiol* 243:C62, 1982.
82. Michenfelder JD, Theye RA: Hypothermia: effect on canine brain and whole-body metabolism. *Anesthesiology* 29:1107, 1965.
83. Norwood WI, Norwood CR, Castaneda AR: Cerebral anoxia: effect of deep hypothermia and pH. *Surgery* 86:203, 1979.
84. Russ W, Kling D, Lofsevitz A, et al: Effect of hypothermia on visual evoked potentials (VEP) in humans. *Anesthesiology* 61:207, 1984.
85. FitzGibbon T, Hayward JS, Walker D: EEG and visual evoked potentials of conscious man during moderate hypothermia. *Electroencephalogr Clin Neurophysiol* 58:48, 1984.

86. Stockard JJ, Sharbrough FW, Tinker JA: Effects of hypothermia on the human brainstem auditory response. *Ann Neurol* 3:368, 1978.
87. Marshall NK, Donchin E: Circadian variation in the latency of brainstem responses and its relation to body temperature. *Science* 212:356, 1981.
88. Maclean D, Griffiths PD, Emslie-Smith D: Serum-enzymes in relation to electrocardiographic changes in accidental hypothermia. *Lancet* 2:1266, 1968.
89. Blair E: A physiologic classification of clinical hypothermia. *Surgery* 58:607, 1965.
90. Doherty P, Bohn D, Bigger D: Hyperthermia and neutrophil dysfunction: clinical and experimental observations. *Crit Care Med* 12:233, 1984.
91. Kanter GS: Hypothermic hemoconcentration. *Am J Physiol* 214:856, 1968.
92. Poulos ND, Mollitt DL: The nature and reversibility of hypothermia-induced alterations in blood viscosity. *J Trauma* 31:996, 1991.
93. O'Brien H, Ames JA, Mollin LD: Recurrent thrombocytopenia, erythroid hypoplasia and sideroblastic anaemia associated with hypothermia. *Br J Haematol* 51:451, 1982.
94. Schissler P, Parker MA, Scott SJ: Profound hypothermia: value of prolonged cardiopulmonary resuscitation. *South Med J* 74:474, 1981.
95. Maclean D, Murison J, Griffiths PD: Acute pancreatitis and diabetic ketowacidosis in accidental hypothermia and hypothermic myxoedema. *BMJ* 4:757, 1973.
96. Hirvonen J, Huttunen P: Increased urinary concentration of catecholamines in hypothermia deaths. *J Forensic Sci* 27:264, 1982.
97. Mant AK: Autopsy diagnosis of accidental hypothermia. *J Forensic Med* 16:126, 1969.
98. Baum D, Dillard DH, Porte D: Inhibition of insulin release in infants undergoing deep hypothermic cardiovascular surgery. *N Engl J Med* 279:1309, 1968.
99. Curry DL, Curry KP: Hypothermia and insulin secretion. *Endocrinology* 87:750, 1970.
100. O'Malley BP, Davies TJ, Rosenthal FD: TSH responses to temperature in primary hypothyroidism. *Clin Endocrinol* 13:87, 1980.
101. Maclean D, Browning MC: Plasma 11-hydroxycorticosteroid concentrations and prognosis in accidental hypothermia. *Resuscitation* 52:249, 1974.
102. Woolff PD, Hollander CS, Mitsuma T, et al: Accidental hypothermia: endocrine function during recovery. *J Clin Endocrinol Metab* 34:460, 1972.
103. Bohn D, Baker C, Kent G, et al: Accidental and induced hypothermia: effects on neutrophil migration in vivo. *Crit Care Med* 129:A112, 1984.
104. DeGuzman VC, Webb WR, Grogan JB: The effect of hypothermia on clearance of staphylococcal bacteremia. *Clin Res* 10:58, 1962.
105. Biggar WD, Bohn DJ, Kent G, et al: Neutrophil migration in vitro and in vivo during hypothermia. *Infect Immun* 46:857, 1984.
106. Kurz A, Sessler DI, Lenhardt R: Perioperative normothermia to reduce the incidence of surgical wound infection and shorten hospitalization. Study of wound infection and temperature group. *N Engl J Med* 334:1209, 1996.
107. Fairchild KD, Viscardi RM, Hester L, et al: Effects of hypothermia on cytokine production by cultured mononuclear phagocytes from adults and newborns. *J Interferon Cytokine Res* 20(12):1049, 2000.
108. Koren G, Barker C, Bohn D, et al: Influence of hypothermia on the pharmacokinetics of gentamicin and theophylline in piglets. *Crit Care Med* 13:844, 1985.
109. Rosin AJ, Exton-Smith AN: Clinical features of accidental hypothermia, with some observations on thyroid function. *BMJ* 1:16, 1964.
110. Fischbeck KH, Simon RP: Neurological manifestations of accidental hypothermia. *Ann Neurol* 10:384, 1981.
111. Hauty MG, Esrig BC, Hill JG, et al: Prognostic factors in severe accidental hypothermia: experience from the Mt. Hood tragedy. *J Trauma* 27:1107, 1987.
112. Lilly JK, Boland JP, Zekan S: Urinary bladder temperature monitoring: a new index of body core temperature. *Crit Care Med* 8:742, 1980.
113. Megarbane B, Axler O, Chary I, et al: Hypothermia with indoor occurrence is associated with a worse outcome. *Intensive Care Med* 26(12):1843, 2000.
114. Danzl DF, Hedges JR, Pozos RS: Hypothermia outcome score: development and implications. *Crit Care Med* 17:227, 1989.
115. Farstad M, Anderson KS, Koller ME, et al: Rewarming from accidental hypothermia by extracorporeal circulation—a retrospective study. *Eur J Cardiothorac Surg* 20:58, 2001.
116. Lexow K: Severe accidental hypothermia: survival after 6 hours 30 minutes of cardiopulmonary resuscitation. *Arctic Med Res* 50[Suppl]:112, 1991.
117. Giesbrecht GG, Sessler DI, Mekjavic IB, et al: Treatment of mild immersion hypothermia with direct body to body contact. *J Appl Physiol* 76:2373, 1994.
118. Bangs C, Hamelt M: Out in the cold: management of hypothermia, immersion and frostbite. *Top Emerg Med* 2:19, 1980.
119. Neufer PD, Young AJ, Sawka MN, et al: Influence of skeletal muscle glycogen on passive rewarming after hypothermia. *J Appl Physiol* 65:805, 1988.
120. 2005 American Heart Association Guidelines for emergency resuscitation and emergency cardiovascular care. *Circulation* 112:24[Suppl]:136–138, 2005.
121. Towne WD, Geiss WP, Yanes HO, et al: Intractable ventricular fibrillation associated with profound accidental hypothermia: successful treatment with partial cardiopulmonary bypass. *N Engl J Med* 287:1135, 1972.
122. DaVee TS, Reineberg EJ: Extreme hypothermia and ventricular fibrillation. *Ann Emerg Med* 9:100, 1980.
123. Nicodemus HF, Chaney RD, Herold R: Hemodynamic effects of inotropes during hypothermia and rapid rewarming. *Crit Care Med* 9:325, 1981.
124. Harari A, Regnier B, Rapin M, et al: Haemodynamic study of prolonged deep accidental hypothermia. *Eur J Intensive Care Med* 1:65, 1975.
125. Danzl DF, Sowers MB, Vicario SJ, et al: Chemical ventricular defibrillation in severe accidental hypothermia. *Ann Emerg Med* 11:698, 1982.
126. Dronen S, Nowak RM, Tomlanovich MC: Bretylium tosylate and hypothermic ventricular fibrillation. *Ann Emerg Med* 9:335, 1980.
127. Buckley JJ, Bosch OK, Bacaner MB: Prevention of ventricular fibrillation during hypothermia with bretylium tosylate. *Anesth Analg* 50:587, 1971.
128. Alexander L: *The Treatment of Shock from Prolonged Exposure to Cold, Especially in Water*. London, Combined Intelligence Objectives Subcommittee, APO 413, CIOS Item 24, HMSO, 1945.
129. Truscott DG, Frior WB, Clein LJ: Accidental profound hypothermia: successful resuscitation by core rewarming and assisted circulation. *Arch Surg* 106:216, 1973.
130. Dixon RG, Dougherty JM, White LJ, et al: Transcutaneous pacing in a hypothermic dog model. *Ann Emerg Med* 29:602, 1997.
131. Reeves RB: Temperature-induced changes in blood acid-base status: pH and PCO_2 in a binary buffer. *J Appl Physiol* 40:752, 1976.
132. Severinghaus JW: Respiration and hypothermia. *Ann N Y Acad Sci* 80:384, 1959.
133. Rhan H, Reeves RB, Howell BJ: Hydrogen ion regulation, temperature, and evolution. *Am Rev Respir Dis* 112:165, 1975.
134. Blayo MC, Lecompte Y, Pocidalo JJ: Control of acid-base status during hypothermia in man. *Respir Physiol* 42:287, 1980.
135. Ream AK, Reitz BA, Silverberg G: Temperature correction of PCO_2 and pH in estimating acid-base status: an example of the emperor's new clothes? *Anesthesiology* 56:41, 1982.
136. Kroncke GM, Nichols RD, Mendenhall JT, et al: Ectothermic philosophy of acid-base balance to prevent fibrillation during hypothermia. *Arch Surg* 121:303, 1986.
137. Swain JA: Hypothermia and blood pH. *Arch Intern Med* 148:1643, 1988.
138. Malan A: Blood acid-base state at a variable temperature: a graphical representation. *Respir Physiol* 31:259, 1977.
139. Kelman GR, Nunn JF: Nomograms for correction of blood PO_2, PCO_2, pH, and base excess for time and temperature. *J Appl Physiol* 21:1484, 1966.
140. Brooks DK: The meaning of pH at low temperatures during extra-corporeal circulation. *Anaesthesia* 19:337, 1964.
141. Flynn MD, Mawson DM, Tooke JE, et al: Cyclical hypothermia: successful treatment with ephedrine. *J R Soc Med* 84:753, 1991.
142. Kloos RT: Spontaneous periodic hypothermia. *Medicine* 74:268, 1995.
143. Hudson LD, Conn RD: Accidental hypothermia: associated diagnoses and prognosis in a common problem. *JAMA* 227:37, 1974.
144. Guerin JM, Meyer P, Segrestaa JM: Hypothermia in diabetic ketoacidosis. *Diabetes Care* 10:801, 1987.
145. Lewis S, Brettman LR, Holzman RS: Infections in hypothermic patients. *Arch Intern Med* 141:920, 1981.
146. Carr ME Jr, Wolfert AI: Rewarming by hemodialysis for hypothermia: failure of heparin to prevent DIC. *J Emerg Med* 6:277, 1988.
147. Freeman RM: The role of magnesium in the pathogenesis of azotemic hypothermia. *Proc Soc Exp Biol Med* 137:1069, 1971.
148. Levy LA: Severe hypophosphatemia as a complication of the treatment of hypothermia. *Arch Intern Med* 140:128, 1980.
149. Ledingham IM, Mone JG: Treatment of accidental hypothermia: a prospective clinical study. *BMJ* 280:1102, 1980.
150. Sessler DI, Moayeri A: Skin surface warming: heat flux and central temperature. *Anesthesiology* 73:218, 1990.
151. Grange C, Clery G, Purcell G, et al: Evaluation of the Bair Hugger warming device. *Anaesth Intensive Care* 20:122, 1992.
152. Myers RA, Britten JS, Cowley RA: Quantitative aspects of therapy. *JACEP* 8:523, 1979.
153. Anderson S, Herbring BG, Widman B: Accidental profound hypothermia. *Br J Anaesth* 42:653, 1970.
154. Sheaff CM, Fildes JJ, Keogh P, et al: Safety of 65°C intravenous fluid for the treatment of hypothermia. *Am J Surg* 172:52, 1996.
155. Hayward JS, Steinman AM: Accidental hypothermia: an experimental study of inhalation rewarming. *Aviat Space Environ Med* 46:1236, 1975.
156. Ledingham IM, Douglas IH, Rauth GS, et al: Central rewarming system for treatment of hypothermia. *Lancet* 1:1168, 1980.
157. Edwards HA, Benstead JG, Brown K, et al: Apparent death with accidental hypothermia. *Br J Anaesth* 42:906, 1970.
158. Johnson LA: Accidental hypothermia: peritoneal dialysis. *JACEP* 6:556, 1977.
159. Troelsen S, Rybro L, Knudsen F: Profound accidental hypothermia treated with peritoneal dialysis. *Scand J Urol Nephrol* 20:221, 1986.
160. Brunette DD, Sterner S, Robinson EP, et al: Comparison of gastric lavage and thoracic cavity lavage in the treatment of severe hypothermia in dogs. *Ann Emerg Med* 16:1222, 1987.
161. Winegard C: Successful treatment of severe hypothermia and prolonged cardiac arrest with closed thoracic cavity lavage. *J Emerg Med* 15(5):629, 1997.
162. Gregory JS, Bergstein JM, Aprahamian C, et al: Comparison of three methods of rewarming from hypothermia: advantages of extracorporeal blood warming. *J Trauma* 31:1247, 1991.
163. Gentilello LM, Cobean RA, Offner PJ, et al: Continuous arteriovenous rewarming: rapid reversal of hypothermia in critically ill patients. *J Trauma* 32:316, 1992.
164. Gentillello LM, Rifley WJ: Continuous arteriovenous rewarming: report of a new technique for treating hypothermia. *J Trauma* 31:1151, 1991.
165. Maresda L, Vasko JS: Treatment of hypothermia by extracorporeal circulation and internal rewarming. *J Trauma* 27:89, 1987.
166. Vretenar DF, Urschel JD, Parrot JC, et al: Cardiopulmonary bypass resuscitation for accidental hypothermia. *Ann Thorac Surg* 58:895, 1994.
167. Kornberger E, Mair P: Important aspects in the treatment of severe accidental hypothermia: the Innsbruck experience. *J Neurosurg Anesth* 8:83, 1996.
168. Roe CF, Goldberg MJ, Blair CS, et al: The influence of body temperature on early postoperative oxygen consumption. *Surgery* 60:85, 1966.

169. Jones HD, McLaren CA: Postoperative shivering and hypoxaemia after halothane, nitrous oxide and oxygen anesthesia. *Br J Anaesth* 37:35, 1965.
170. Goldberg MJ, Roe CF: Temperature changes during anesthesia and operations. *Arch Surg* 93:365, 1966.
171. Vaughn MS, Vaughn RW, Cork RC: Postoperative hypothermia in adults: relationship of age, anesthesia, and shivering to rewarming. *Anesth Analg* 60:746, 1981.
172. Flacke JW, Flacke WE: Inadvertent hypothermia: frequent, insidious, and often serious. *Anesthesia* 3:183, 1983.
173. Matamis D, Tsagourias M, Koletsos K, et al: Influence of continuous haemofiltration-related hypothermia on haemodynamic variables and gas exchange in septic patients. *Intensive Care Med* 20:43, 1994.
174. Morris RH, Kumar A: The effect of warming blankets on maintenance of body temperature of the anesthetized, paralyzed adult patient. *Anesthesiology* 36:408, 1972.
175. Kean M: A patient temperature audit within a theatre recovery unit. *Br J Nurs* 9(23):150, 2000.
176. Sessler DI: Mild perioperative hypothermia. *N Engl J Med* 336(24):1730, 1997.
177. Leslie K, Sessler DI: Perioperative hypothermia in the high risk surgical patient. *Best Pract Res Clin Anaesthesiol* 17(4):485, 2003.
178. Roe CF: Effect of bowel exposure on body temperature during surgical operations. *Am J Surg* 122:13, 1971.
179. Bay J, Nunn JF, Prys-Roberts C: Factors influencing arterial PO_2 during recovery from anesthesia. *Br J Anaesth* 40:398, 1968.
180. Pflug AE, Aasheim GM, Foster C, et al: Prevention of post-anaesthesia shivering. *Can Anaesth Soc J* 25:43, 1978.
181. Frank SM, Fleisher LA, Breslow MJ, et al: Perioperative maintenance of normothermia reduces the incidence of morbid cardiac events: a randomized clinical trial. *JAMA* 277:1127, 1997.
182. Schmied H, Kurz A, Sessler D, et al: Mild intraoperative hypothermia increases blood loss and allogeneic transfusion requirements following total hip arthroplasty. *Lancet* 347:289, 1996.
183. Kahn HA, Faust GR, Richard R, et al: Hypothermia and bleeding during abdominal aortic aneurysm repair. *Ann Vasc Surg* 8:6, 1994.
184. Slotman GJ, Jed EH, Burchard KW: Adverse effects of hypothermia in postoperative patients. *Am J Surg* 149:495, 1985.
185. Roizen MF, Sohn YJ, L'Hommedieu CS, et al: Operating room temperature prior to surgical draping: effect on patient temperature in recovery room. *Anesth Analg* 59:852, 1980.
186. Ott DE: Correction of laparoscopic insufflation hypothermia. *J Laparoendosc Surg* 1:183, 1991.
187. Leaman PL, Martyak GG: Microwave warming of resuscitation fluids. *Ann Emerg Med* 14:876, 1985.
188. Newton DE: The effect of anaesthetic gas humidification on body temperature. *Br J Anaesth* 47:1026, 1975.
189. Caldwell C, Crawford R, Sinclair I: Hypothermia after cardiopulmonary bypass in man. *Anesthesiology* 55:86, 1981.
190. Ciufo D, Dice S, Coles C: Rewarming hypothermic postanesthesia patients: a comparison between a water coil warming blanket and a forced-air warming blanket. *J Post Anesth Nurs* 10:309, 1995.
191. MacKenzie MA, Herman AR, Wollersheim HC, et al: Thermoregulation and afterdrop during hypothermia in patients with poikilothermia. *Q J Med* 86:205, 1993.
192. Taguchi A, Arkilic CF, Ahluwalia A, et al: Negative pressure rewarming vs. forced hot air warming in hypothermic postanaesthetic volunteers. *Anesth Analg* 92(1):261, 2001.
193. Glosten B, Hynson J, Sessler DI, et al: Preanesthetic skin-surface warming reduces redistribution hypothermia caused by epidural block. *Anesth Analg* 77:488, 1993.
194. Camus Y, Delva E, Sessler DI, et al: Pre-induction skin-surface warming minimizes intraoperative core hypothermia. *J Clin Anesth* 7:384, 1995.
195. Just B, Trevien V, Delva E, et al: Prevention of intraoperative hypothermia by preoperative skin-surface warming. *Anesthesiology* 79:214, 1993.
196. Russell SH, Freeman JW: Prevention of hypothermia during orthotopic liver transplantation: comparison of three different intraoperative warming methods. *Br J Anaesth* 74:415, 1995.
197. Ireland KW, Follette DM, Iguidbashian J, et al: Use of a heat exchanger to prevent hypothermia during thoracic and thoracoabdominal aneurysm repairs. *Ann Thorac Surg* 55:534, 1993.
198. Dalili H, Andriani J: Effects of various blood warmers on the components of bank blood. *Anesth Analg* 53:125, 1974.
199. Hachimi-Idrissi S, Corne L, Ebinger G, et al: Mild hypothermia induced by a helmet device: a clinical feasibility study. *Resuscitation* 51:275–281, 2001.
200. Bernard SA, Gray TW, Buist MD, et al: Treatment of comatose survivors of out of hospital cardiac arrest with induced hypothermia. *N Engl J Med* 346:557–563, 2002.
201. HACA Investigators: Mild therapeutic hypothermia to improve neurologic outcome after cardiac arrest. *N Engl J Med* 346:549–556, 2002.
202. Sagalyn E, Band RA, Gaieski DF, et al: Therapeutic hypothermia after cardiac arrest in clinical practice: review and compilation of recent experiences. *Crit Care Med* 37(7):S223–S226, 2009.
203. Stertz F, Safar P, Tisherman SA, et al: Mild hypothermic cardiopulmonary resuscitation improves outcome after cardiac arrest in dogs. *Crit Care Med* 19:379–389, 1991.
204. American Heart Association: 2005 Guidelines for cardiopulmonary resuscitation and emergency cardiovascular care. *Circulation* 112:IV1–IV203, 2005.
205. Bernard S: Hypothermia after cardiac arrest: expanding the therapeutic scope. *Crit Care Med* 37(7):S227–S233, 2009.
206. Parham W, Edelstein K, Unger B, et al: Therapeutic hypothermia for acute myocardial infarction: past, present, and future. *Crit Care Med* 37(7): S234–S237, 2009.
207. Dietrich WD: Therapeutic hypothermia for spinal cord injury. *Crit Care Med* 37(7):S238–S242, 2009.
208. Linares G, Mayer AS: Hypothermia for the treatment of ischemic and hemorrhagic stroke. *Crit Care Med* 37(7):S243–S249, 2009.
209. Stravitz RT, Larsen FS: Therapeutic hypothermia for acute liver failure. *Crit Care Med* 37(7):S258–S264, 2009.
210. Fukodome EY, Alam HB: Hypothermia in multisystem trauma. *Crit Care Med* 37(7):S265–S272, 2009.
211. Seder DB, Van der Kloot TE: Methods of cooling: practical aspects of therapeutic temperature management. *Crit Care Med* 37(7):S211–S222, 2009.
212. Sundgreen C, Larsen FS, Herzog TM, et al: Autoregulation of cerebral blood flow in patients resuscitated from cardiac arrest. *Stroke* 32:128–132, 2001.
213. Sirvent JM, Torres A, El-Ebiary M, et al: Protective effect of intravenously administered cefuroxime against nosocomial pneumonia in patients with structural coma. *Am J Respir Crit Care Med* 155:1729–1734, 1997.
214. Bergman R, Tjan DH, Adriaanse MW, et al: Unexpected fatal neurological deterioration after successful cardiopulmonary resuscitation and therapeutic hypothermia. *Resuscitation* 76:142–145, 2008.
215. Oddo M, Frangos S, Milby A, et al: Induced normothermia attenuates cerebral metabolic distress in patients with aneurysmal subarachnoid hemorrhage and refractory fever. *Stroke* 40:1913–1916, 2009.
216. Jordan K: Nonconvulsive status epilepticus in acute brain injury. *J Clin Neurophysiol* 16:332–340, 1999.
217. Polderman KH, Rijnsburger ER, Peerdeman SM, et al: Induction of hypothermia in patients with various types of neurological injury with use of large volumes of ice cold intravenous fluid. *Crit Care Med* 33:2744–2751, 2005.
218. Kliegel A, Janata A, Wandaller C, et al: Cold infusions alone are effective for induction of therapeutic hypothermia but do not keep patients cool after cardiac arrest. *Resuscitation* 73:46–53, 2007.
219. Arrich J, Holzer M, Havel C, et al: Hpothermia for neuroprotection in adults after cardiopulmonary resuscitation. *Cochrane Database Syst Rev* (9):CD004128, 2012.
220. Nielson N, Wetterslev J, Cronberg T, et al: Targeted temperature managementat 33 °C versus 36 °C after cardiac arrest. *N Eng J Med* 369:2197, 2013.
221. Zeiner A, Holzer M, Sterz F, et al: Hyperthermia after cardiac arrest is associated with an unfavourable neurologic outcome. *Arch Intern Med* 161:2007, 2001.
222. Gebhart K, Guette FX, Doshi AA, et al: Prevalence and effect of fever on outcome following resuscitation from cardiac arrest. *Resuscitation* 84:1062, 2013.
223. Tomte O, Draegni T, Mangschau A, et al: A comparison of intravascular and surface cooling techniques in comatose cardiac arrest survivors. *Crit Care Med* 39:443, 2011.
224. Merchant RM, Abella BS, Peberdy MA, et al: Therapeutic hypothermia after cardiac arrest: unintentional overcooling is common using ice packs and conventional cooling blankets. *Crit Care Med* 34:S490, 2006.
225. Vargas M, Servillo G, Sutherasan Y, et al. Effects of in-hospital low targeted temperature after out of hospital cardiac arrest: a systematic review with meta-analysis of randomized controlled trials. *Resuscitation* 91:8, 2015.
226. Peberdy MA, Callaway CW, Neumar RW, et al: Part 9: Post cardiac arrest care: 2010 American Heart Association Guidelines for Cardiopulmonary Resuscitaion and Emergency Cardiovascular Care. *Circulation* 122:S768, 2010.
227. Giesbrecht GG. Cold stress, near drowning and accidental hypothermia: a review. *Aviat Space Environ Med* 71:733, 2000.
228. Soar J, Perkins GD, Abbas G, et al: European Resuscitation Council Guidelines for Resuscitation 2010 Section 8. Cardiac arrest in special circumstances: electrolye abnormalities, poisoning, drowning, accidental hpothermia, hyperthermia, asthma, anaphylaxis, cardiac sugery, trauma, pregnancy, electrocution. *Resuscitation* 81:1400, 2010.
229. Durrer B, Brugger H, Syme D, et al: The medical on site treatment of hypothermia: ICAR-MEDCOM recommendation. *High Alte Med Biol* 4:99, 2003.
230. Danzl D: Accidental hypothermia, in: Auerbach PS (Ed): *Wilderness Medicine*, 6th ed, Elsevier, Philadelphia, 2012, p 115.

Chapter 185 ■ Disorders of Temperature Control, Part II: Hyperthermia

MARY KATHRYN STEINER • RICHARD S. IRWIN

This chapter reviews the pathobiology, pathophysiology, diagnosis, differential diagnosis, and treatment of four major hyperthermic syndromes—heat stroke, malignant hyperthermia (MH), neuroleptic malignant syndrome, and drug-induced hyperthermia (DIH).

HEAT STROKE

Heat stroke is defined as a core body temperature usually in excess of 40°C (104°F) characterized by central nervous system (CNS) dysfunction in the setting of a large environmental heat load that cannot be dissipated.

Causes and Pathogenesis

There are two types of heat stroke: exertional and nonexertional (classic, heat stroke). Exertional heat stroke is seen in younger individuals, otherwise healthy, exercising at higher than normal ambient temperatures and humidity. Typical patients are athletes and military recruits in basic training. The thermoregulatory mechanisms are intact, but overwhelmed by the thermal challenge of the environment and the increase in endogenous heat production. Nonexertional heat stroke occurs in individuals >70 years with underlying chronic medical conditions during a heat wave. Patients frequently have some impairment of thermoregulatory control, and temperatures rise easily with increased thermal challenge.

The causes of heat stroke fall into two categories (Table 185.1): increased heat production and impaired heat loss.

Increased Heat Production

Endogenous heat production during exertion ranges from 300 to 900 kcal per hour. Even in conditions favoring the maximal evaporation of sweat, only 500 to 600 kcal per hour of heat may be lost. Endogenous heat production may also be increased by fever, thyrotoxicosis, or the hyperactivity associated with amphetamine and hallucinogen use. In these conditions of increased thermogenesis, especially during maximal exercise, a healthy individual with intact regulatory mechanisms may develop hyperthermia.

Impaired Heat Loss

Schizophrenic, comatose, senile, or mentally deficient patients are at increased risk of heat stroke when ambient temperatures are high, owing to impaired voluntary control [5,6]. These patients may fail to perceive a temperature rise and to take appropriate action. Impermeable clothing in hot environments prevents evaporative heat loss, and individuals may suffer heat stroke [7,8].

Acclimatization increases heat tolerance by increasing cardiac output, decreasing peak heart rate, and increasing stroke volume. This lowers the threshold necessary to induce sweating, increases the volume of sweating, and, via an increase in aldosterone, expands extracellular volume and minimizes sodium loss in sweat [9,10]. However, unacclimatized individuals who do not mount an adaptive response are at increased risk of suffering exertional heat stroke [11].

Dehydration and impaired cardiovascular performance increases the risk of heat stroke owing to a decrease in skin or muscle blood flow, thus decreasing the movement of heat from the core to the environment [10,12]. Hypokalemia increases the risk of heat stroke by decreasing muscle blood flow, impairing cardiovascular performance, and decreasing sweat gland function [9,10]. Adequate fluid intake and maintenance of a normal vascular volume prevents heat stroke.

Many drugs are known to predispose to heat stroke. Anticholinergic drugs such as phenothiazines, butyrophenones, thiothixenes, and anti-Parkinson's medications reduce sweat activity [14]. Barbiturate overdose may produce sweat gland necrosis [10]. Diuretics promote dehydration and hypokalemia. β-Blockers may increase the risk of heat stroke by cardiac depression. Alcohol consumption may increase the risk of heat stroke 15-fold because of dehydration secondary to antidiuretic hormone inhibition and inappropriate vasodilation [6].

Skin disorders that impair sweat gland function, such as cystic fibrosis and chronic idiopathic anhydrosis, predispose to heat stroke [15].

Hypothalamic lesions impair thermoregulation. During the early stages of heat stroke, the hypothalamus regulates autonomic responses to limit hyperthermia. In the later stages, once thermal toxicity occurred, hypothalamic regulation is impaired [16]. Anhydrosis has been reported in up to 100% of heat stroke victims in some series [17]. The hypothalamic set point may be elevated. The exact cause of hypohidrosis remains unclear and may reflect hypothalamic dysfunction or the secondary effects of dehydration and cardiovascular collapse. Electron microscopic studies of eccrine sweat glands in a patient with fatal exertional heat stroke show changes suggestive of sweat gland fatigue [18]. Heat stroke can, however, occur among individuals who perspire profusely, indicating that sweat gland malfunction is not the only factor contributing to the pathogenesis of the syndrome.

The increased risk of heat stroke among the elderly is predominantly owing to a decreased ability to sweat and a compromised cardiovascular response to heat exposure when compared with younger individuals [8,19]. In one report, 84% of elderly patients showed no evidence of sweating at the time heat stroke was diagnosed [20]. Elderly patients are more likely to have deficient voluntary control, poor acclimatization, and they take drugs that adversely affect thermoregulation.

Pathophysiology

The primary injury of heat stroke is caused by direct cellular toxicity of temperatures above 42°C, the *critical thermal maximum* [21]. Cell function deteriorates owing to cessation of mitochondrial activity, alterations in chemical bonds involved in enzymatic reactions, and cell membrane instability. This toxic effect may account for the widespread organ damage seen in all three of the major hyperthermic syndromes [22].

Heat stress activates numerous cytokines that modulate the body's response to increased temperature [23]. For most cases, the inflammatory response of heat stroke parallels that seen for heat stress from exertion. Tumor necrosis factor α, interleukin (IL)-1β, IL-2, IL-6, IL-8, IL-10, IL-12, and interferon γ are typically increased with heat stroke. IL-6 is activated in the

TABLE 185.1

Causes of Heat Stroke

Increased heat production
Exercise
Fever
Thyrotoxicosis
Amphetamines
Hallucinogens
Impaired heat loss
High ambient temperature or humidity
Ineffective voluntary control
Lack of acclimatization
Dehydration
Cardiovascular disease
Hypokalemia
Drugs
Anticholinergics
Phenothiazines
Butyrophenones
Thiothixenes
Barbiturates
Anti-Parkinson's agents
Diuretics
β-Blockers
Alcohol
Debilitating conditions
Skin diseases
Cystic fibrosis
Central nervous system lesions
Older age

muscles and modulates inflammatory response by controlling cytokine levels and hepatic production of acute phase proteins. Endotoxemia from bacterial translocation of an ischemic gut further exacerbates the inflammatory response. Endothelial injury activates the coagulation cascade, promoting a prothrombotic state. Heat shock proteins are transcribed in response to heat stress and act on the brain to induce tolerance to heat stress [24].

Dehydration, metabolic acidosis, and local hypoxia alter the pathophysiologic consequences and clinical presentation of each of the hyperthermic syndromes. For example, classic heat stroke may occur with relatively little metabolic acidosis because no exertion was involved in its onset; however, it may be associated with more pronounced dehydration caused by the gradual rise in temperature and prolonged sweating. Exertional heat stroke, alternatively, may be accompanied by a severe metabolic acidosis and hypoxia caused by muscular exercise. It is typically associated with a more normal volume status because the onset of temperature elevation is abrupt.

Muscle Effects

Muscle degeneration and necrosis occur as a direct result of high temperatures. Muscle damage is more severe with exertional heat stroke owing to local increases of heat, hypoxia, and metabolic acidosis associated with exertion. Significant muscle enzyme elevation and severe rhabdomyolysis are extremely common among exertional heat stroke victims [12,25,26] but rare with classic heat stroke [27].

Cardiac Effects

Cardiac output is increased [28] owing to increased demands and low peripheral vascular resistance secondary to vasodilation and dehydration. Dehydration frequently results from sweat rates that may easily reach 1.5 to 2.0 L per hour during episodes of heat stroke [29]. Central venous pressure is initially elevated [30]. Hypotension occurs commonly as a result of high-output failure or temperature-induced myocardial hemorrhage and necrosis with subsequent cardiac depression and failure [9,12,31]. Tachyarrhythmias are frequent. Postmortem specimens show focal myocytolysis, myocyte necrosis, and hemorrhage in subepicardial, intramuscular, subendocardial, or intravalvular tissues [32].

Central Nervous System Effects

Direct thermal toxicity to brain and spinal cord rapidly produces cell death, cerebral edema, and local hemorrhage. These may lead to profound stupor or coma, almost universal features of all the hyperthermic syndromes. Seizures secondary to edema and hemorrhage are not uncommon. Because Purkinje cells of the cerebellum are particularly sensitive to the toxic effects of high temperatures, ataxia, dysmetria, and dysarthria may be seen acutely and in survivors of hyperthermia [10,33]. Progressive cerebellar atrophy has been documented by computed tomography (CT) and magnetic resonance imaging (MRI) [34]. Lumbar puncture from those with classic and exertional heat stroke may reveal increased protein levels, xanthochromia, and a slight lymphocytic pleocytosis [12,20]. Survivors of severe heat stroke may show premature cataract formation, considered to be secondary to dehydration [35]. Up to 33% of survivors of heat stroke have at least moderate neurologic impairment after discharge from the hospital [36].

Renal Effects

Renal damage occurs in nearly all hyperthermia patients; it is potentiated by dehydration, cardiovascular collapse, and rhabdomyolysis. In classic heat stroke, acute renal failure occurs on average in 5% of patients as a result of dehydration [9]. In exertional heat stroke, acute renal failure occurs in up to 35% of cases [9,31]. Dehydration, pigment load, hypoperfusion, and urate nephropathy are thought to contribute to a clinical picture of acute tubular necrosis [31]. Other features include low serum osmolarity, moderate proteinuria, active sediment, and characteristic machine-oil appearance of the urine. In one series, the incidence of acute tubular necrosis increased with survival time [32]. Hypocalcemia and creatinine phosphokinase values above 10,000 U per L increase the risk of acute renal failure [37]. Respiratory alkalosis is common for mild hyperthermia, with metabolic acidosis predominating at temperatures greater than 41°C [24].

Gastrointestinal Tract Effects

The combination of direct thermotoxicity and relative hypoperfusion of the intestines during hyperthermia leads to ischemic intestinal ulcerations that may result in frank bleeding [9]. Hepatic necrosis and cholestasis occurs 2 to 3 days after hyperthermic insult, and 5% to 10% of the cases result in death [10].

Hematologic Effects

White blood cell counts are elevated owing to catecholamine release and hemoconcentration. Anemia and a bleeding diathesis [29] are present owing to (a) direct compromise of platelets and bleeding factor functions by heat, (b) a decrease in coagulation factor synthesis from liver failure, (c) a decrease in platelet and megakaryocyte counts, (d) platelet aggregation [38], and (e) disseminated intravascular coagulation (DIC). Megakaryocyte counts are reduced in up to 50% of specimens, and surviving megakaryocytes are morphologically abnormal [32]. DIC is present among most cases of fatal hyperthermia [32,39], most frequently appearing on days 2 and 3 after hyperthermic insult. It is considered to be caused by activation of the clotting cascade by vascular endothelial damage and generalized cell necrosis [40]. Among cases of DIC, cardiac, CNS, pulmonary, gastrointestinal (GI) tract, and renal complications are more frequent and severe. An increase in blood viscosity up to 24% has been postulated to facilitate thromboses [41].

Endocrine Effects

Hypoglycemia may occur among severe exertional heat stroke victims caused by metabolic exhaustion [26]. Among milder heat stroke patients, hyperglycemia and elevations of serum cortisol have been reported [42]. Although at autopsies the adrenal glands frequently show pericortical hemorrhages, survivors show little evidence of adrenal dysfunction [22,31]. Growth hormone and aldosterone levels actually increase abruptly during severe, acute heat exposure and are thought to act to preserve volume.

Electrolyte Effects

Hyperthermia produces frequent imbalances in potassium, sodium, phosphate, and calcium levels [29,43]. Among heat stroke victims, sweating involves the active excretion of potassium from the body, producing normal to low serum potassium levels and decreased total body potassium concentrations. Among cases of exertional heat stroke with severe cell injury, potassium levels may be extremely elevated because of cell lysis. Although mild hypophosphatemia occurs frequently as a result of intracellular trapping and parathyroid hormone resistance, phosphate levels may decrease to less than 1 mg per 100 mL in cases of hyperthermia with severe rhabdomyolysis [43]. Calcium values may fall 2 to 3 days after cellular injury owing to intracellular precipitation. Among patients with severe tissue injury, rebound hypercalcemia may occur 2 to 3 weeks after hyperthermia as a result of parathyroid hormone activation [43].

Pulmonary Effects

Direct thermal injury to the pulmonary vascular endothelium may lead to cor pulmonale or acute respiratory distress syndrome. This and the tendency toward myocardial dysfunction make pulmonary edema common. Increased oxygen demands and acidosis frequently produce a respiratory alkalosis. Metabolic acidosis is, however, the most common acid–base disorder [44].

Diagnosis

The diagnosis of classic heat stroke is made clinically based on an elevated rectal temperature above 40°C (>104°F), CNS dysfunction, and exposure to severe environmental heat.

Heat stroke should be expected for any patient exercising in hot weather or in susceptible individuals during heat waves (see Table 185.1). Coma or profound stupor is nearly always present, but other traditional criteria of anhidrosis and core temperature above 41°C may be absent. Although anhidrosis occurs in 84% of elderly patients with classic heat stroke [20], profuse sweating is typically present in exertional heat stroke [10]. Thus, the presence of anhidrosis is helpful, but its absence is not. Likewise, by the time the patient receives medical care, the temperature may have fallen significantly owing to cessation of exertion, removal from a hot environment, or cooling measures undertaken during transport. Most patients do have a temperature above 40°C, however. Other examination findings include vital sign abnormalities (e.g., tachycardia, tachypnea, and hypotension), flushing, pulmonary crackles, and oliguria.

Risk Factors for Increased Mortality

Patients who present to the hospital with heat stoke have high mortality, with rates ranging from 21% to 63% [241]. Mortality correlates with the degree of temperature elevation, time to initiation of cooling measures, and the number of organ systems affected [242]. According to one prospective cohort study, the risk of death increases for patients who present with anuria, coma, or cardiovascular failure [243]. Patients who take antihypertensives, lack air conditioning, are socially isolated, or are unable to take care of themselves are also at high risk [17, 20–22].

Diagnostic Evaluation

Serial rectal temperatures (accurate at high temperatures) should be obtained for all patients with heat stroke to assess and monitor. A chest radiograph may show pulmonary edema. The electrocardiogram may show dysrhythmias, conduction disturbances, nonspecific ST-T changes, or heat-related myocardial ischemia or infarction [244,245]. Laboratory studies may reveal coagulopathy, acute kidney injury, acute hepatic necrosis, and a leucocytosis as high as 40,000 per mm^3 [246]. Arterial blood gas may reveal metabolic acidosis and respiratory alkalosis. Serum creatinine kinase and urine myoglobin help detect rhabdomyolysis and its complications (e.g., hypocalcemia, hyperphosphatemia, elevated BUN and creatinine). Toxicology screening, a head CT, and analysis of the cerebrospinal fluid (CSF) may be helpful when altered mental status is present.

Differential Diagnosis

The differential diagnosis of severe hyperthermia includes infectious, endocrine, CNS, toxic, and oncologic causes [54]. Table 185.2 lists the common causes of hyperthermia. Classic heat stroke is often distinguished from other conditions by history and examination. However, the clinical picture can be unclear. No single diagnostic test definitively confirms or excludes heat stroke, and laboratory abnormalities may overlap in patients with heat stroke and with hyperthermia owing to other causes. For example, patients with heat stroke will meet the criteria for systemic inflammatory response syndrome. In such circumstances, it is prudent to initiate cooling measures while other diagnoses are evaluated. Rapid improvement with active cooling suggests that heat stroke is the main diagnosis but not always. The most important causes of severe hyperthermia owing to failure of thermoregulation are heat stroke, neuroleptic malignant syndrome, and MH.

Treatment

The management of classic heat stroke requires adequate airway protection, breathing and circulation, rapid cooling, and treatment of complications.

Cooling Measures to Decrease Thermogenesis

Evaporative cooling is the method used most often because it is effective, noninvasive, easily done, and allows for other medical care to occur. It is associated with decreased morbidity and mortality in the elderly [247]. Some cooling may be achieved in the field by moving the victim to a shaded cooler area, removing the clothes, constantly wetting the skin, and fanning or transporting in an open vehicle to create a breeze. Once the victim reaches the hospital, cooling and subsequent supportive care are best provided in an intensive care setting.

With evaporative cooling, the naked patient is placed in a cool room and sprayed with a mist of lukewarm water while fans are used to blow air over the moist skin. In one specially designed evaporative cooling unit, patients were sprayed with

TABLE 185.2

Differential Diagnosis of Hyperthermia

- Hyperthermic syndromes
  - Exertional heat stroke
  - Nonexertional heat stroke
  - Malignant hyperthermia
  - Neuroleptic malignant syndrome
  - Drug-induced hyperthermia/serotonin syndrome
- Infection
  - Meningitis
  - Encephalitis
  - Sepsis
  - Brain abscess
  - Tetanus
  - Typhoid fever
  - Malaria
- Endocrinopathy
  - Thyroid storm
  - Pheochromocytoma
  - Diabetic ketoacidosis
- Central nervous system
  - Hypothalamic stroke
  - Cerebral hemorrhage
  - Status epilepticus
  - Acute hydrocephalus
- Oncologic
  - Lymphoma
  - Leukemia

15°C water and their skin was fanned at 30 times per minute with air heated to 45°C to 48°C. Temperature reduction was rapid and mortality was 11% [57]. There was no mortality in 25 patients with nonexertional heat stroke treated with cooling by covering with a cool, wet, 20°C sheet and fanning with two 35-cm electric fans. Fanning was adjusted to maintain skin temperature at 30°C to 32°C; skin temperature fell 1°C every 11 minutes [58]. Among 14 patients with nonexertional heat stroke, there was one death when evaporative/convective cooling was used. The median time to return to temperature less than 39.4°C was 60 minutes.

Direct external cooling (DEC) involves immersing the patient in ice water or packing the patient in ice. Ice water immersion with massage has been effective with few reported complications [59], but it complicates monitoring and intravenous (IV) access. Colder water cools more rapidly (up to 0.35°C per minute), with one study demonstrating that 2°C water cooled volunteers twice as rapidly as 8°C water [60]. Because cold skin temperatures produce vasoconstriction, however, constant massage may be necessary to allow circulation to carry heat from the core. DEC is highly effective but makes patient monitoring and management extremely inconvenient. Therefore, some authors advocate evaporative cooling as a safer cooling method in patients at high risk of cardiovascular collapse [52]. Because comparative studies of cooling techniques use different water temperatures for immersion and different evaporative cooling protocols, there is no consensus on which lowering technique is superior. In most cases, treatment will be determined by what resources are immediately available. The Israeli Defense Forces protocol involves moving the collapsed patient to the shade, removing clothing, splashing the skin with water while fanning, and transporting to the hospital in an open vehicle. These measures yielded a cooling rate of 0.11°C per minute [61]. The US Marine Corps protocol calls for covering the patient with sheets covered with ice and then fanning the patient. This has had no mortalities in 200 cases and has reduced temperatures to below 39°C in 10 to 40 minutes [62].

In rare instances in which evaporative and DEC methods fail to reduce the temperature, peritoneal lavage with iced saline cooled to 20°C or 9°C, gastric lavage, hemodialysis, or cardiopulmonary bypass with external cooling of the blood may be necessary to reduce the temperature. Temperature should be continuously monitored and cooling stopped as it approaches 39°C. Although IV chlorpromazine of 10 to 25 mg has been advocated to prevent shivering during cooling, it is usually unnecessary. Cooling blankets, commonly used, are ineffective and are not recommended [63].

Pharmacologic Therapy

It is not required in heat stroke. There is no role for antipyretic agents such as acetaminophen or aspirin because the underlying mechanism does not involve a change in the hypothalamic set—point and they may worsen hepatic injury or DIC. Dantrolene is ineffective in patients with hyperthermia not because of MH [248].

Complications

Arrhythmias, metabolic acidosis, and cardiogenic failure complicate the early management of hyperthermic crises. Supraventricular tachyarrhythmias usually require no treatment because they respond to restoration of normal temperature and metabolism. Digitalis should be avoided owing to the likelihood of hyperkalemia.

Hypotension should be treated initially with normal saline and, if necessary, isoproterenol. Dopaminergic and α-agonists should be avoided because they produce peripheral vasoconstriction. Volume expansion with dextran is contraindicated owing to its anticoagulating effect. Pulmonary artery and arterial catheter monitoring may be helpful in the management of hypotension because patients frequently have low peripheral resistance, dehydration, and impaired cardiac function and are at a high risk of congestive heart and renal failure. Because 64% of patients may have a normal central venous pressure before resuscitation, volume expansion in most cases should be guided by intravascular pressure monitoring where available [66]. Seizures, quite common in heat stroke, usually respond to diazepam.

Blood gas status should be determined early in treatment. Blood gases drawn at temperatures above 39°C should be corrected for temperature, although to our knowledge no studies have demonstrated that this is clinically necessary. The solubility of oxygen and carbon dioxide increases as blood drawn from the patient is cooled to 37°C for analysis. This lowers the carbon dioxide and oxygen tensions and elevates the pH when compared with values present in the patient. Therefore, the patient is more acidotic and less hypoxemic than the uncorrected values indicate. Normal values of intracellular pH and changes on the body's buffering system in hyperthermia have been poorly described. Because normal values for blood gases in hyperthermic patients are unavailable, by convention the blood gas values are corrected for temperature, using any reliable nomogram, and clinical decisions are made as if the patient were euthermic [67–69]. The following approximate corrections have been used: for each 1°C that the patient's temperature is above 37°C, the oxygen tension is increased by 7.2%, carbon dioxide (CO_2) tension increased by 4.4%, and pH is lowered by 0.015 units. More research is needed before definite conclusions can be made. Nevertheless, 100% oxygen should be delivered until adequate oxygenation is ensured. Bicarbonate should be administered, guided by frequently obtained arterial blood gas values. The base deficit is frequently large, and up to 30 g of bicarbonate has been required for correction. Comatose patients should have prophylactic intubation to protect their airways from aspiration.

Urine output should be closely monitored with an indwelling bladder catheter. Patients should be routinely given 1 to 2 mg per kg of mannitol over 15 to 20 minutes to promote continued urine flow and to possibly decrease cerebral edema. Continuous urine output should then be maintained with intermittent doses of furosemide. In all cases of hyperthermia, serum potassium levels should be closely followed. In cases of oliguria or potential renal failure, polystyrene sulfonate should be given early for hyperkalemia.

Moderate-to-severe liver failure is common, may prolong illness, and, in combination with renal failure, may make administration of several drugs difficult. Histamine receptor type 2 (H_2)–blocking drugs or proton pump inhibitors given prophylactically may decrease the incidence of GI tract bleeding.

Most patients who die of heat stroke have evidence of DIC [70]. Coagulation parameters such as prothrombin time, partial thromboplastin time, platelet count, and fibrinogen should be carefully followed. Should DIC occur, traditional recommendations for treatment should be followed (see Chapter 88).

Steroids are of no known benefit in heat stroke. Infection has not been reported as a major cause of morbidity and mortality in hyperthermia, and antibiotics are associated with superinfections [20,26].

Prognosis

Morbidity and mortality are directly related to the peak temperature reached and time spent at elevated temperatures. A delay in treatment of only 2 hours may result in increased mortality up to 70% [11,52]. When heat stroke is swiftly recognized and aggressively treated, mortality should be minimal. For example, in one series of 15 patients with exertional heat stroke, all were successfully treated with no mortality and little morbidity [11]. Another study predicts mortality of only 5% when heat stroke patients are managed properly [10]. A recent review of 34 elderly patients with classic heat stroke revealed 18% mortality. Seventy-three percent recovered without sequelae, and 9% had some residual neurologic deficit.

Although patients with temperatures as high as 46.5°C have survived without sequelae [71], mortality is increased with premorbid debility and higher maximal temperatures [44]. When ventricular fibrillation, DIC, or coma last more than 6 to 8 hours, or high lactate levels complicate hyperthermia, mortality is predictably increased. A continued rise in growth hormone levels despite therapy has been reported to be associated with a worse prognosis [72].

With respect to morbidity, neurologic function usually rapidly returns to normal after restoration of euthermia; however, some patients may be left with a mild cerebellar disorder [73]. Hepatic and renal failure in mild and moderate cases completely resolves. Moderate muscle weakness may persist for several months among patients with severe muscle damage.

Although it has not been proven, patients who have experienced hyperthermic crises are at increased risk of recurrence upon exposure to similar heat stresses.

MALIGNANT HYPERTHERMIA

MH is a drug- or stress-induced hypermetabolic syndrome characterized by vigorous muscle contractions, an abrupt increase in temperature, and subsequent cardiovascular collapse. MH occurs, on average, in 1 in every 50,000 to 150,000 adult patients given anesthesia [71,74]. This may be an underestimation because of unrecognized, mild, or atypical reactions owing to variable penetrance of the inherited trait. MH occurs in all ethnic groups, more frequently in males than females (2:1), children under the age of 19 accounts for about 52% of reported events, 21% have had previous uneventful anesthesia, and 76% have no family history of MH [94,95].

Cause and Pathogenesis

The cause of the temperature increase in MH is because of sustained muscle contraction over time, generating more heat than one can dissipate. When exposed to various drugs, muscles may develop sustained or repeated contractions (Table 185.3). Current evidence indicates that patients with MH have a defect in calcium metabolism in skeletal muscle cell membranes [76–79]. In most cases, a defect in the ryanodine receptor (RYR1) results in release of calcium from the sarcoplasmic reticulum, resulting in muscle contraction and heat generation [80]. This leads to hydrolysis of adenosine triphosphate and the activation of catabolic pathways, hepatic and muscular glycogenolysis, and catecholamine-induced accelerated turnover of substrates and the production of lactate.

Although halothane and succinylcholine are involved in more than 80% of cases, MH has developed after the use of many other agents as well (see Table 185.3). Heat stress, vigorous exercise, excitement, anoxia, viral infections, and lymphoma have also been reported to trigger MH [81,82]. Some data suggest that conditions of ischemia or hypoxia are the common triggers to hyperthermia in susceptible individuals.

The hyperthermic reaction to anesthetics is not allergic in nature; patients may have received the same anesthetic previously or may be exposed later without developing a reaction. There is little evidence that impaired heat dissipation or altered hypothalamic regulation is instrumental in producing acute hyperthermia in these patients. However, sympathetic activity and heat dissipation may be abnormal during vigorous exercise [83].

Pathophysiology

MH-susceptible patients have genetic skeletal receptor abnormalities, allowing excessive calcium accumulation in the presence of certain anesthetic triggering agents. During an episode of MH, downstream effects from unregulated passage of calcium from the sarcoplasmic reticulum into the intracellular space lead to sustained muscle contraction and production of more heat than the body can dissipate. Temperature levels above 42°C lead to similar physiologic and pathologic changes described for patients with exertional heat stroke [84]. DIC, hepatic failure, seizures, ventricular dysrhythmias, and electrolyte abnormalities are more common and severe than in heat stroke.

Vigorous muscle contracture at the onset of MH almost immediately precipitates a severe metabolic acidosis, with increased CO_2 production and compensatory hyperventilation. High elevations of creatinine kinase, lactate dehydrogenase, and aldolase are present [65] and reflect ongoing rhabdomyolysis. Hyperkalemia follows within minutes to hours [76]. Renal failure frequently occurs in MH, most likely secondary to myoglobinuria. Dehydration and low cardiac output do not contribute until later. The degree of hypocalcemia, hypophosphatemia, and hyperkalemia varies with the duration and peak of hyperthermia and degree of secondary myonecrosis. All three are more severe in MH than in heat stroke. Direct thermal injury producing cerebral edema and cerebral hemorrhage can result in coma. Seizures occur among most uncontrolled cases. DIC is a nearly universal finding [85]. Initially, volume status is normal because little volume has been lost in sweat. Cardiac output increases to meet metabolic demands and in response to the vasodilation of muscle beds. Sinus tachycardia, supraventricular tachyarrhythmias, and ventricular fibrillation occur soon after temperature exceeds 40°C. Tissue hypoxia, acidosis, and hyperkalemia make ventricular arrhythmias common. Because

TABLE 185.3

Drugs and Malignant Hyperthermia

Drugs known to trigger malignant hyperthermia
Halothane
Methoxyflurane
Enflurane
Succinylcholine
Decamethonium
Gallamine
Diethyl ether
Ethylene
Ethyl chloride
Trichloroethylene
Ketamine
Phencyclidine
Cyclopropane
Drugs generally considered safe for patients with malignant hyperthermia
Nitrous oxide
Barbiturates
Diazepam
Tubocurarine
Pancuronium, vecuronium
Opiates

higher maximal temperatures are usually seen in MH, hepatic failure and GI tract bleeding are more frequent than in heat stroke [85]. Among survivors, hepatic necrosis and cholestasis peak in 2 to 3 days and may be severe.

Diagnosis

The metabolic predisposition to MH appears to be inherited in an autosomal dominant fashion, with variable penetrance and expressivity. Although multiple screening strategies have been attempted [76,86–89], tests using caffeine or halothane stimulation of excised muscle are the standard screening tests recommended by the MH Association of the United States [90]. Their false-positive rate is near 10% and false-negative rate is near zero [91]. Because there is no noninvasive test suitable for screening the general population, screening of family members of proven cases remains the best method of identifying susceptible individuals before hyperthermic crisis occurs. RYR1 gene mutation analysis of cells from buccal samples may help identify high-risk individuals. Only 25% of those susceptible have an identified mutation. Although an identified mutation would suggest susceptibility, the absence of a mutation does not rule it out [92,93].

Clinical Signs

Early signs of hyperthermic crisis vary with the anesthetic agent administered but include masseter muscle contracture after the administration of succinylcholine, muscle rigidity, sinus tachycardia, supraventricular tachyarrhythmias, mottling or cyanosis of the skin, increased CO_2 production resistant to increasing minute ventilation, and hypertension. Hyperthermia is typically a late sign during an acute crisis, but it may be rapidly followed by hypotension, acidosis, peaked T-waves on the electrocardiogram owing to hyperkalemia, and malignant ventricular arrhythmias [85], as well as myoglobinuria and excessive bleeding. In one case report, desaturation measured by oximetry preceded temperature elevation by 40 minutes [96].

Two signs may be helpful in making a prehyperthermic diagnosis: increased end-tidal CO_2 and masseter spasm [97–103]. Monitoring of end-tidal CO_2 is recommended for all anesthetic procedures and is mandatory for patients at risk of MH [91,94,95]. Severe masseter spasm after succinylcholine has been recognized as an early warning sign of MH; however, the decision to discontinue anesthesia for patients with succinylcholine-induced spasm remains controversial [100–104]. If surgery must be continued, dangerous triggering anesthetics should be avoided, dantrolene should be given or at least be immediately accessible, and temperature and end-tidal CO_2 should be monitored.

Differential Diagnosis

Because MH occurs almost exclusively in the perioperative setting, the differential diagnosis is more limited than that for heat stroke (see Table 185.2) [104]. Endocrinopathies and drug reactions, not infection, are the most frequent diseases in the differential diagnosis. Thyroid storm and pheochromocytoma may be very difficult to distinguish from MH in the anesthetized patient [105]. Thyroid storm is now infrequent, owing to preoperative thyroid function test screening and prophylaxis of patients at risk. Dantrolene in doses used for MH has been shown to decrease temperature in perioperative thyroid storm [106]. The temperature rise in pheochromocytoma is typically much slower than that in MH [107]. Hyperthermia, owing to narcotic administration in patients taking monoamine oxidase inhibitors, also must be considered.

Treatment

Dantrolene, a hydantoin derivative, acts by uncoupling the excitation–contraction mechanism in skeletal muscle and lowering myoplasmic calcium. This action takes place directly at the RYR1 receptor [108]. Dantrolene used for less than 3 weeks rarely causes toxicity [109]. In an acute crisis, 1.0 to 2.5 mg per kg of fresh dantrolene should be administered intravenously every 5 to 10 minutes. Effects may be seen 2 to 3 minutes after injection. Although cases that required 42 mg per kg have been reported [110], most authorities advise not to exceed 10 mg per kg [75,76,110,111]. The half-life of action is approximately 5 hours [76], and because relapse may occur, oral or IV dosages of 1 mg per kg IV or 2 mg per kg by mouth every 6 hours should continue for at least 24 to 48 hours [76]. Oral dantrolene may be substituted once the patient is alert [112], given its bioavailability. With dantrolene, temperatures often rapidly decrease; without it, they may increase 1°C to 2°C every 15 minutes [95,97,110].

In the United States, there are two types of dantrolene preparations. The older form is a lyophilized powder in a 20-mg vial containing 3 g of mannitol and sodium hydroxide, and each 20 mg vial requires mixing with 60 mL of sterile water requiring additional personnel to assist in drug preparation given that for an initial bolus in a 70-kg patient, nine vials are needed. It is however the least expensive. The new dantrolene formulation (Ryanodex) is rapidly dissolved, supplied in 250-mg vials, reconstituted with only 5 mL of sterile water, and warming is not needed. It is double the price but because it is hyperconcentrated, blood concentrations are achieved faster, it requires less time, and fewer staff to prepare the vial, making it clinically more efficient to deliver.

Because even minute quantities of the triggering agent may continue to produce the syndrome, anesthesia should be immediately stopped, and the anesthesia apparatus, tubing, and ventilation equipment should be immediately changed.

As with heat stroke, iced saline, gastric or peritoneal lavage, evaporative cooling, and infusion of chilled electrolyte solutions may be helpful. Aggressive management with cardiopulmonary bypass with external cooling of the blood may be necessary when dantrolene fails to slow down thermogenesis promptly [113]. When patients respond to therapy quickly, before severe temperature elevation occurs, only minimal supportive measures may be necessary. Once temperature exceeds 41°C, complications are widespread and patients frequently require long-term intensive care unit (ICU) support.

Ventricular fibrillation with subsequent cardiac collapse is the most common cause of death for the early stages of the syndrome. Procainamide should be given to all patients prophylactically as soon as MH is diagnosed [76]. Procainamide acts to increase the uptake of calcium from the myoplasm directly and in early stages may help reduce hyperthermia. Administration of digitalis should be avoided because of the increased likelihood of hyperkalemia. Hypotension should be treated with saline infusion and isoproterenol. Avoid dopaminergic and α-agonists because they reduce heat dissipation owing to peripheral vasoconstriction. Seizures often occur among MH patients. Prophylactic treatment with phenobarbital is strongly recommended because seizures may increase heat production, metabolic acidosis, and hypoxia. Arterial blood gas values should be adjusted for temperature. Mannitol and furosemide may be needed to promote continued urine output and may reduce the likelihood of cerebral edema and acute tubular necrosis. The serum potassium level increases over several hours and is treated with polystyrene sulfonates. Hepatic failure and DIC require supportive treatment. With prolonged supportive care, hepatic, renal, and neurologic functions typically normalize. Muscle weakness, however, may last for months.

Prognosis

With current management techniques, mortality resulting from MH should be less than 30% [75]. In one review, prompt dantrolene therapy in cases of confirmed MH resulted in a 100% survival rate [25].

NEUROLEPTIC MALIGNANT SYNDROME

Neuroleptic malignant syndrome (NMS) is a life-threatening neurologic emergency associated with the use of neuroleptic agents and is characterized by hyperthermia, muscular rigidity, dysautonomia, and altered mental status. Most current knowledge is derived from case reports rather than systematic study. Since the NMS was first described in 1968 [114], fewer than 3,000 cases have been reported in the world's literature, and most are from the 1980s and 1990s.

Incidence rates for NMS vary from 0.02% to 3% among patients taking neuroleptic agents [115–120]. The variation reflects differences among the populations sampled, surveillance methods, and definitions of the disease. NMS has been described for all age groups, and it is more common in men by twofold [115,162,163]. The larger muscle mass in men may predispose to the development of hyperthermia. There is, however, no difference in mean maximal temperature between men and women. A case control study has shown that environmental temperature does not affect the incidence of the NMS but several factors do: total neuroleptic dose; mental retardation; intramuscular administration of a neuroleptic, psychomotor agitation, or increasing dose; or recent introduction of a neuroleptic drug [164]. Early estimates of mortality were as high as 30% [121]. Incidence also appears to be declining [122]. Mortality rates since 1986 has fallen to less than 12% [123]. Two prospective series reported 24 and 68 cases, with mortality rates of 0% [124] and 5% [125], respectively.

Cause and Pathogenesis

The cause of NMS is unknown. An animal model for NMS has been developed, but it does not correspond with the human syndrome [115]. Because the syndrome is found among patients on dopamine receptor blockade agents or inpatients after withdrawal of dopaminergic agents (Table 185.4), dopamine receptor blockade is considered to be central to most theories of its pathogenesis. Butyrophenones [126–140], phenothiazines [126,128,131,134,141,142], thioxanthenes [143–145], and dibenzoxazepines [146] are believed to act as dopamine receptor–blocking agents. Atypical antipsychotics, such as risperidone [147], molindone [148], clozapine [149], and fluoxetine [150], and dopamine blockers used to treat GI tract disease, such as metoclopramide and domperidone [151], have also caused the syndrome. The incidence of the syndrome with the newer atypical antipsychotics has not changed [152]. Drugs acting at the D_2 dopamine–binding sites appear to have the greatest potential for causing the syndrome. Most cases occur among patients taking butyrophenones or piperazines, agents with a high incidence of extrapyramidal reactions. The rate of increase in dose appears more important than the maximal dose achieved [123]. Dopamine-depleting agents such as tetrabenazine and α-methyltyrosine produced NMS in a patient with Huntington's disease [121]. Abrupt withdrawal of levodopa (L-dopa), dopa-carbidopa, or amantadine produced the syndrome in patients suspected of having Parkinson's disease [153–155]. Initiation of metoclopramide therapy has produced the syndrome, presumably owing to alteration in central dopaminergic tone [156–158].

An alternative theory is that rigidity and muscle damage represent a primary effect on the peripheral muscle system, possibly from direct changes in muscle mitochondrial function. This is because of either a primary muscle defect or a direct toxic effect by neuroleptics. A peripheral muscle abnormality is possible because the sarcoplasmic calcium concentration

TABLE 185.4

Drugs Associated with the Onset of Neuroleptic Malignant Syndrome

Butyrophenones
Haloperidol
Bromperidol
Phenothiazines
Chlorpromazine
Levomepromazine
Trifluoperazine
Fluphenazine
Thioxanthenes
Thiothixene
Dibenzoxazepines
Loxapine
Dihydroindolones
Molindone
Flurooxypropylamines
Fluoxetine
Tricyclic-dibenzodiazepines
Clozapine
Dopamine-depleting agents
Tetrabenazine
α-Methyltyrosine
Withdrawal of levodopa, carbidopa, amantadine
Domperidone
Metoclopramide

is higher among patients who have had the syndrome [125], resolves with nifedipine use [159], and has been reported to be triggered by hypoparathyroidism [160]. However, the muscular effects are typical of the parkinsonian type of extrapyramidal reactions, frequently seen at low therapeutic doses soon after treatment begins, and the muscle spasm resolves with the use of centrally acting dopaminergic agents such as bromocriptine, amantadine, and L-dopa.

Hyperthermia results from an increase in endogenous heat production, impaired heat dissipation, loss of voluntary temperature regulation, and possibly an elevation of the hypothalamic set point. This suggests that there may also be a disrupted modulation of the sympathetic nervous system. The fact that the degree of temperature increase varies directly with the severity of rigidity evident on examination strongly suggests that muscle contracture is responsible for increased thermogenesis [126]. A decrease in muscle rigidity by uncoupling contraction with dantrolene or by paralysis with succinylcholine results in a decrease in temperature [161]. Impaired heat dissipation from the anticholinergic-induced hypohidrosis of neuroleptics may also occur. The most likely hypothesis is that regulatory reflexes remain intact, but muscle rigidity from the hypothalamus and subsequent increased thermogenesis exceed dissipative capacity.

Familial clusters of NMS suggest a genetic predisposition. Genetic studies have shown that the presence of a specific allele of the dopamine D_2 receptor gene is overrepresented in NMS patients. This allele is associated with reduced density and function of dopamine receptors as well as decreased dopaminergic activity and metabolism [239].

Clinical Presentation

Onset of symptoms may occur within hours after the initial neuroleptic treatment or up to 4 weeks later [162]. Among the majority of cases, onset occurs within 1 week from initial neuroleptic drug use, and 88% occur within 2 weeks of a dosage increase of an already prescribed neuroleptic agent [162]. Most reported cases have occurred among patients with underlying neuropsychiatric disorders. Most cases have a slow progression of symptoms over at least 24 to 48 hours and last 2 weeks after stopping the inciting drug [171].

Early symptoms include dysphagia or dysarthria, pseudo-Parkinsonism, dystonia, or catatonic behavior. In one series, 96% of patients demonstrated rigidity, 92% of patients demonstrated tremor, and 96% of patients demonstrated muteness or hypophonia in the 48 hours before diagnosis [124]. Rigidity precedes hyperthermia in 59% of patients, is concurrent in 23%, and is subsequent in only 8%. Changes of mental status or rigidity are the presenting symptoms in 82% of patients [172]. Autonomic signs of hypermetabolism such as diaphoresis, tachycardia, changes in blood pressure, and tachypnea, reflect efforts to dissipate the thermogenesis of muscle contracture and to expel CO_2 effectively. Peak temperatures are reached within 48 hours after the onset of symptoms in 88% of patients [124]. Temperatures may reach as high as 42.2°C [132] but are typically lower: 53% are more than 40°C and 13% are higher than 41°C [124]. Rectal or core, rather than oral, temperatures are needed to ensure accuracy (see Chapter 26). Elevations in creatinine kinase and transaminase levels and leucocytosis parallel the body temperature.

Complications

Because of the relatively low maximal temperatures—39.9°C, on average [163]—among patients with NMS compared with those of patients with heat stroke and MH, it is not surprising that direct thermal injury occurs less often. Only 40% of patients have temperatures above 40°C [165]. The complications of NMS are summarized in Table 185.5. Cardiovascular collapse, renal failure, and electrolyte abnormalities are less common and less severe than in classic heat stroke.

Rhabdomyolysis, most probably secondary to hyperthermia and muscle rigidity, is frequently seen, with typical creatinine kinase elevations in the range of 1,000 to 5,000 IU. Although rhabdomyolysis is usually mild, creatinine kinase elevations of greater than 100,000 IU have been reported [145,166,167] and may occur in up to one-third of patients [124]. Prolonged muscle weakness or dysfunction in survivors has not been described.

Renal failure occurs in 9% to 30% of patients [124,162]. Proteinuria occurs in up to 91% of patients [124]. Renal failure is owing to myoglobin-induced acute tubular necrosis and the dehydration that results from diaphoresis. Renal dysfunction of most patients is transient and mild and, even among cases with acute tubular necrosis, and may return to premorbid values after brief periods of dialysis support [129]. Mortality among renal failure patients, however, may be as high as 56% [123].

NMS has been associated with worsening of underlying psychiatric conditions, amnesia, cognitive impairments, and peripheral neuropathy [168,169]. Coma is not uncommon among severe cases. Grand mal seizures have rarely been reported [129,144]. The electroencephalogram (EEG) typically is normal or shows nonspecific diffuse slowing [124]. CT scans of the brain are normal in 95% of patients. CSF analysis after lumbar puncture is normal in 97% of patients, showing an elevated protein level in the other 3% [162,170]. In one case, an MRI scan revealed hyperintensity of the occipitoparietal white matter [171]. Pathologic examinations of patients at autopsy have revealed no specific lesions [154].

Although death from cardiovascular collapse has been reported [126], specific cardiac abnormalities have been poorly described. There is no evidence that severe atrophy, heart block, or congestive heart failure occurs frequently in NMS.

Hematologic alterations are mild. The white blood cell count is elevated among 78% of cases [124,162], usually less than 20,000 cells per mm^3, and rarely exceeding 25,000 cells per mm^3. Elevation may be caused by hemoconcentration and catecholamine release. Platelet count is elevated in 56% of patients [124]. A hemolytic coagulopathy, possibly DIC, has been infrequently reported [132]. Deep venous thrombosis or antemortem embolic phenomena are not reported in the English literature. Thrombotic events, when they do occur, may be a result of the patient's immobility owing to coma and muscle rigidity rather than to any temperature-mediated change.

Mild elevations of lactate dehydrogenase, serum glutamic oxaloacetic acid transaminase, serum glutamic pyruvic transaminase, and alkaline phosphatase are common.

Pulmonary complications occur because of the extrapyramidal actions of the neuroleptics. Dysphagia [126] and sialorrhea can lead to aspiration pneumonias and necessitate intubation in 13%

TABLE 185.5

Complications of Neuroleptic Malignant Syndrome

Rhabdomyolysis
Renal failure
Seizure
Cardiovascular collapse
Disseminated intravascular coagulation
Hepatic failure
Aspiration pneumonia
Respiratory failure
Death

to 21% of patients [124,131,132,134,140,145,153,161–163,166] and are probably the most serious frequent sequelae of NMS.

Diagnosis

There is no diagnostic test for NMS, the laboratory abnormalities help confirm and rule out other conditions or help trend the patients for complications. MRI and CT imaging of the brain are typically normal but can show diffuse cerebral edema with severe metabolic derangements. CSF is typically normal but may have nonspecific protein elevation in 3% of the cases [162,170]. EEG is helpful to rule out nonconvulsive status epilepticus. NMS patients have generalized slow-wave activity. An international multispecialty consensus group published diagnostic criteria for NMS in 2011 [240]. This criterion requires independent validation before its use can be recommended in clinical practice.

Differential Diagnosis

A thorough examination and diagnostic evaluation for other causes of hyperthermia should be conducted (see Table 185.2). In one series, all patients referred to an ICU with a suspicion of NMS had another diagnosis that would explain fever [119]. Because many patients taking neuroleptic agents develop extrapyramidal side effects and few cases of hyperthermia are a result of NMS, other more common causes of hyperthermia (e.g., meningitis or streptococcal pharyngitis) are more likely. Appropriate cultures, chest radiograph, lumbar puncture, and physical examination are mandatory. Patients without classic symptoms are more likely to have another cause of hyperthermia [173].

Catatonia, heat stroke, MH, and hyperthermic reactions to other drugs may occasionally be confused with the NMS. Acute lethal catatonia presents with psychotic excitement and automatisms a few weeks before motor deficit [174]. Laboratory values are typically normal. The treatment and prognosis for these patients remain unclear [163,175,176]. If rigidity and hyperthermia subsequently develop in a catatonic patient, however, the development of NMS should be presumed and all neuroleptic agents should be stopped. If catatonia has been induced or exacerbated by neuroleptics, withdrawal of the neuroleptic drug should aid in clarifying the diagnosis.

Heat stroke must be considered when temperature elevation develops in a patient taking neuroleptics during periods of high ambient temperature or after vigorous exercise. Unlike NMS, however, heat stroke is usually accompanied by flaccid obtundation, and muscle rigidity is rare.

MH resembles NMS in that both conditions have increased thermogenesis secondary to muscular rigidity as well as similar laboratory findings, and both respond to dantrolene. In most cases, an adequate history should clearly separate the two syndromes; MH results from the use of different agents (compare Tables 185.3 and 185.4). Moreover, the symptoms of MH are much more rapid in onset and more severe. Extrapyramidal symptoms are also very unusual in MH. In the rare circumstance in which the two syndromes cannot be distinguished, attempts at paralysis with curare or pancuronium may aid diagnosis. These agents produce a flaccid paralysis in NMS but should have no effect on the postsynaptically mediated muscle contracture of MH.

Serotonin syndrome (SS) is the most commonly diagnosed related disorder and is caused by the use of selective serotonin reuptake inhibitors. It has a similar presentation and is difficult to distinguish from NMS. Typical features in these patients that are not often seen in NMS are shivering, hyperreflexia, myoclonus, and ataxia. Nausea, vomiting, and diarrhea are also a common part of the prodrome in SS and are rarely seen in NMS.

Idiosyncratic drug reactions and anaphylaxis accompanying severe hyperthermia may usually be diagnosed by their distinct clinical presentations. Monoamine oxidase inhibitors may produce hyperthermia, especially when administered with meperidine, linezolid, or dextromethorphan [177–180]. In patients with neuropsychiatric disorders who are receiving neuroleptic agents and monoamine oxidase inhibitors, MH may result from either agent. In these cases, both agents should be stopped. Therapies for NMS, such as bromocriptine or L-dopa, however, are contraindicated in these patients because of their recent use of monoamine oxidase inhibitors.

Treatment

Stopping the causative agent is the most important treatment followed by supportive care. The goal of treatment for NMS is to reduce the temperature, reverse extrapyramidal side effects, and prevent sequelae.

Supportive care is essential in the ICU [181] and includes maintaining cardiorespiratory stability, and euvolemic state with crystalloid IV therapy (and possibly urine alkalinization to reduce renal failure from rhabdomyolysis) [126], lowering fever using cooling blankets (or more aggressive measures including ice water gastric lavage) and possibly acetaminophen or aspirin, lower the blood pressure if markedly elevated (clonidine is effective and possibly nitroprusside), prophylactic intubation if sialorrhea is present, prevention of deep vein thrombosis, and the use of benzodiazepines to control agitation [191].

Specific agents used to decrease thermogenesis by reducing muscle contracture include dantrolene, curare, pancuronium, amantadine, bromocriptine, and L-dopa (Table 185.6). The use of these agents is based upon case reports and clinical experience, not from clinical trials. The efficacy is unclear and disputed [124,162,181–182,192–197].

Dantrolene reduces thermogenesis by uncoupling muscle contracture at the membrane level and in doses as small as 1 mg per kg may result in a temperature decrease of 1°C to 2°C within hours [135,136,140,183]. Dantrolene may also favorably alter CNS dopaminergic metabolism [184]. Although doses of up to 10 mg per kg have been used, current practice would recommend doses of 1.0 to 2.5 mg per kg IV every 6 hours until a dose of 100 to 300 mg per day by mouth can be given [185,186]. Dantrolene therapy does carry a risk of hepatotoxicity, but in patients with temperatures greater than 40°C, its use is specific and should be beneficial. Paralysis with curare or pancuronium should produce a similar prompt decrease in temperature, but this treatment necessitates mechanical ventilation and extensive support [161]. Bromocriptine, amantadine, and carbidopa/L-dopa increase central dopaminergic tone; this decreases the central drive, reducing muscular rigidity and thermogenesis. These agents also are beneficial in that they act directly to reduce extrapyramidal side effects. Prompt decreases in temperature have been reported after the use of 2.5 mg of bromocriptine three times per day [134,138,167,187], 100 or 200 mg of amantadine twice per day [139,188], or 10 to 100 mg of carbidopa/L-dopa three times per day [127,155].

TABLE 185.6

Treatments for Neuroleptic Malignant Syndrome

Dantrolene
Paralysis (curare, pancuronium)
Bromocriptine
Amantadine
Levodopa
Electroconvulsive therapy

Failures of these therapies, however, have also been published [141,143,153,187]. The appropriate dosing remains an important question. Some authorities have advocated bromocriptine doses as high as 60 mg per day [185]. Use of a centrally acting dopamine agonist is warranted when NMS occurs because of withdrawal of anti-Parkinson's agents. The use of dantrolene, bromocriptine, and amantadine has yet to be shown to reduce mortality significantly [123]. Electroconvulsive therapy has been successful for several patients [131,132,189,190] and is the only therapeutic modality that may be used successfully to treat simultaneously hyperthermia, the extrapyramidal side effects, and the underlying neuropsychiatric disorder for which the neuroleptic drug was prescribed. Because of several reports of cardiovascular collapse among patients undergoing electroconvulsive therapy, this therapy should be given only to patients at low risk of cardiovascular disease who have failed other therapy.

Less-specific agents, such as diphenhydramine, benztropine, diazepam, and trihexyphenidyl, have been used successfully [127,130,134,137,139,146] but more typically have not been helpful [121,134,140,141,161,187,188].

Prognosis

Most episodes resolve within 2 weeks. The average time to recovery with supportive care is 9.6 days [165]. Typically, ICU stay is prolonged owing to the frequency of complications and slow response to therapy. Although dopaminergic therapy lowers the mean time to response from 6.8 to 1.1 days [199], the mean time to recovery is long—13 days when the syndrome results from nondepot neuroleptics and 26 days for depot neuroleptics [162]. One patient receiving haloperidol decanoate was symptomatic for months [200]. Rechallenge with neuroleptics may cause the syndrome to recur, but this occurs much more frequently during the first 2 weeks [201,202], concomitant use of lithium, high potency drugs, and parenteral neuroleptics.

Although mortality rates as high as 20% to 30% have been reported [115], this rate can probably be reduced to less than 10% with appropriate support and treatment. Age and sex do not appear to influence mortality. Mortality rate does appear to be influenced by peak temperature, inciting neuroleptic drug, and renal failure. No death among patients with maximal temperatures lower than 40°C has been reported. Haloperidol is statistically less likely to result in death than other neuroleptics [123]. Death has been reported as a result of cardiovascular collapse [126], pneumonia [131,161], renal failure [129,145], and hepatic failure [145]. More than 57 cases of acute renal failure caused by NMS have been reported [198]. The development of renal failure is particularly ominous; in some series, 46% of patients with myoglobinuria and 56% of those with renal failure died [123].

DRUG-INDUCED HYPERTHERMIA

Most of our knowledge about DIH is derived from case reports. Numerous drugs have been suggested to cause hyperthermia. Drugs that blunt cardiovascular performance, such as β-blockers, or alter heat dissipation, such as chlorpromazine, are widely used and can contribute to temperature elevation. These drugs rarely result in clinically significant hyperthermia without some other precipitant. Patients on regimens of such agents typically present with heat stroke. This section focuses on drugs that independently produce significant elevations of temperature (Table 185.7).

Commonly abused street drugs may result in severe hyperthermia without other pharmacologic or environmental stimuli. Temperature elevation accompanies phencyclidine use in 2.6% of cases [204]. Temperatures as high as 41.9°C have been reported [205]. Amphetamine use may result in temperatures higher than 43°C [205,206]. Although ecstasy (3, 4-methylenedioxymethamphetamine [MDMA]) has resulted in fatal hyperthermia, use is usually associated with a more mild temperature elevation [207]. Hyperthermia (temperatures greater than 37.5°C) was more prevalent (36%) in patients admitted to emergency departments because of overdose of paramethoxyamphetamine than MDMA [208]. Although all these drugs have a low incidence of producing severe hyperthermia, owing to the prevalence of their use, they may account for a large percentage of cases of hyperthermia presenting to an emergency department.

TABLE 185.7

Drugs that may Cause Hyperthermia and/or Serotonin Syndrome

Monoamine oxidase inhibitors	
	Phenelzine = Nardil
	Tranylcypromine = Parnate
	Linezolid
Serotonin releasers	
	Amphetamines
	Ecstasy (MDMA)
	LSD
SRI	
Citalopram = Celexa	
	Fluoxetine = Prozac
	Fluvoxamine = Luvox
	Paroxetine = Paxil
	Sertraline = Zoloft
Tricyclics:	
	Clomipramine = Anafranil
	Imipramine = Tofranil
	Venlafaxine = Effexor
Analgesics:	
	Tramadol
	Methadone
	Dextromethorphan
	Dextropropoxyphene
	Chlorpheniramine
Antihistamines:	
	Brompheniramine
Other	
	Withdrawal of baclofen

MDMA, 3,4-methylenedioxymethamphetamine; LSD, Lysergic acid diethylamide; SRI, Serotonin reuptake inhibitors.

Common prescription drugs that alter central serotonin levels and lysergic acid diethylamine, a serotonin analog, may result in hyperthermia greater than 41°C [209]. These drugs may produce a characteristic constellation of symptoms now known as the *serotonin syndrome* (SS) [209–214]. Monoamine oxidase inhibitors and selective serotonin reuptake inhibitors may produce hyperthermia, especially when administered with meperidine or dextromethorphan [177–179], tricyclic antidepressant [177,215], or each other. Severe hyperthermia is rare. Increasingly, combinations of drugs that independently would not cause serotonin toxicity act in concert to result in hyperthermia and the SS [216]. For example, a postoperative patient who receives linezolid, a weak monoamine oxidase inhibitor, and tramadol, a weak serotonin reuptake inhibitor, may present with fever, confusion, and clonus. Tramadol, meperidine, fentanyl, dextromethorphan, dextropropoxyphene, pentazocine, brompheniramine, chlorpheniramine, and linezolid in combination with other drugs may cause fever and the SS [180]. In addition, abrupt withdrawal of baclofen, especially after intrathecal administration, has resulted in severe sequelae including hyperpyrexia and potential multiorgan failure and death [180].

Aspirin receives mention as a cause of hyperthermia secondary to increased metabolism, but few hard data are available on this association [217].

Pathogenesis

These drugs are thought to cause hyperthermia as a result of muscular contracture or hypermetabolism. Virtually, all case reports of DIH mention increased muscle tone, rigidity, or tremor. Cocaine, amphetamine, phencyclidine, and hallucinogens appear to produce hyperthermia by centrally and peripherally inducing vigorous muscle contractions [218,219]. Repeated cocaine use may elevate temperature by depletion of postsynaptic dopamine [218].

Many drugs such as tricyclics, amphetamines (paramethoxyamphetamine, MDMA), monoamine oxidase inhibitors, and the serotonin reuptake inhibitors may elevate CNS serotonin, resulting in hyperthermia [177,179,219–221]. Buspirone, serotonin agonists, lithium, and carbamazepine stimulate postsynaptic serotonin receptors. Monoamine oxidase inhibitors increase serotonin release and inhibit serotonin metabolism [222]. Selective serotonin reuptake inhibitors, dextromethorphan, and meperidine inhibit serotonin reuptake and, in susceptible patients, increase already high serotonin levels and trigger a hyperthermic crisis [200]. In many patients, combination drug therapy contributes to triggering the syndrome. In general, a 2-week, drug-free period after stopping a monoamine oxidase inhibitor before starting a selective serotonin reuptake inhibitor is indicated. Any opiate may trigger the syndrome when another drug already predisposes the patient.

Some patients may exhibit exertional heat stroke, in that they are frequently found running in an agitated or confused manner. Almost all suffer from loss of voluntary control of temperature.

Status epilepticus frequently accompanies DIH but is unlikely to contribute to hyperthermia, in that status epilepticus is rarely associated with significant temperature elevation in the absence of drug use [223].

DIH reactions are idiosyncratic and infrequent in comparison with the total number of persons using the drug. It can occur by IV, enteral, or nasal insufflation usage, and after low-dose use and massive overdose [224].

Pathophysiology

The pathophysiology of DIH is most similar to that of exertional heat stroke or MH. In the SS, direct stimulation of the 5-HT_{1A} and 5-HT_2 receptors in the raphe nuclei may directly result in hyperthermia. Rise in temperature is frequently rapid, and multiple organ failure rapidly ensues with prolonged elevation of temperature. Patients, however, may also be affected by the direct toxic action of the drug, and it may be difficult to separate the sequelae of hyperthermia from those of direct drug toxicity. Amphetamine overdose, for example, may result in severe rhabdomyolysis, DIC, and renal failure at temperatures less than 40°C. Hyperthermia can be assumed to have the same physiologic sequelae in these patients as others, but prompt correction of temperature may not be adequate to ensure survival.

Diagnosis

In most case reports, patients are described as agitated, hyperexcited, and diaphoretic and have increased muscle tone. Because nonexertional heat stroke is uncommon in youth, hyperthermia at a young age always suggests possible drug intoxication. The diagnosis of DIH should be considered mostly when the patient is young, is an outpatient, has not engaged in recent heavy exertion, has a history of drug abuse, or is on a drug or combination of drugs that may result in the SS.

Patients with the SS typically display tremor, hyperreflexia, myoclonus, tachycardia, diarrhea, confusion, and diaphoresis [210–214]. SS should be suspected and treated whenever patients have spontaneous clonus and are on a serotonergic agent. Nausea and diarrhea are atypical in NMS and may help suggest the SS in complicated cases [225]. The onset of symptoms is within 2 hours of medication ingestion in 50% of cases and within 24 hours in 75% of cases [222]. Myoclonus or rigidity is present in 50% of cases, and mental status changes in 40% of cases. Severe hyperthermia occurs in approximately one-third of cases [211]. Diagnosis may be confirmed by toxicologic screen or history.

Treatment

For all cases, treatment should be directed at minimizing the toxicity of the causative drug. Suspected offending drugs should be discontinued. Treatment of hyperthermia should be symptomatic and directed at the underlying physiology. Treatment in general parallels that for exertional heat stroke and is extensively outlined in that section. Evaporative cooling and external cooling with ice are the preferred methods of cooling and should be instituted in any patient with a temperature above 39°C. Many patients may be dehydrated from diaphoresis and require volume replacement. As for MH and exertional heat stroke, hyperkalemia, acidosis, and myoglobinuria demand careful attention. Because the temperature appears to be generated from muscular contraction, paralysis or use of dantrolene would appear to be useful therapy. Paralysis has been effective in several cases. Paralysis and support with mechanical ventilation should be considered in any patient with a temperature above 40°C not responding promptly to symptomatic cooling. If therapeutic drug levels persist, rebound hyperthermia may occur when paralysis resolves.

When SS is suspected, therapy with benzodiazepines, propranolol, chlorpromazine, cyproheptadine, or postsynaptic serotonin blockers such as methysergide has been advocated, but clinical experience is minimal [218–220,226]. No study to date reports a systematic trial of therapy. Because hyperthermia may be mediated by central serotonin receptors, doses of cyproheptadine high enough to block central receptors, 20 to 50 mg, should be considered [227]. One regimen advises 12 mg by mouth or nasogastric tube then 4 to 8 mg every 4 to 6 hours [216].

Prognosis

Hyperthermia owing to amphetamine overdose appears to be well tolerated, with 10 of 11 patients reported in the literature surviving [205,206,228,229]. Hyperthermia in cocaine overdose is frequently accompanied by renal failure [224,230,231], DIC [231,232], and seizures [231,232] and several fatalities [224,231–233] have been reported. Survival despite high temperature has been recorded as well [224,230,234]. Phencyclidine with hyperthermia has resulted in renal failure [235], respiratory and liver failure with coma, and subsequent death [236].

Death and serious morbidity caused by SS appear to be rare [208]. No large series involving significant hyperthermia have been reported, and death and cure with appropriate treatment have been reported [179]. Because severe hyperthermia would likely signify a much more severe case than usual, the physician should always consider the patient at risk of death and ICU level care would always be warranted.

TABLE 185.8

Distinguishing Characteristics of the Hyperthermic Syndromes

	Heat stroke	Malignant hyperthermia	Neuroleptic malignant syndrome	Acute lethal catatonia	Serotonin syndrome
Inciting factor	Ambient temperature: max >32°C, min >27°C	Triggering anesthetic	Triggering neuroleptic or withdrawal of dopaminergic agent	Excitement and automatisms prior to neuroleptic use	Serotonin active drug(s)
Time to fever	Hours to days	Minutes	Hours to days	Weeks	Minutes to hours
Mental status	Obtunded	Anesthetized	Mute, stuporous	Excited transitioning to catatonia	Confused, agitated
Muscle tone	Flaccid	Rigid, spasm	Extrapyramidal rigid	Variable	Clonus, hyperreflexia, tremor, pyramidal rigidity

TABLE 185.9

Advances in Management of Hyperthermia Based on Randomized Controlled Trials

- No randomized clinical trials have been conducted comparing the effectiveness of different cooling methods for any hyperthermic syndrome [237].
- Dantrolene sodium is ineffective in heat stroke [64]. Dantrolene did not alter survival in heat stroke [65].
- There are no other randomized studies involving the treatment of heat stroke or malignant hyperthermia or drug-induced hyperthermia.
- In neuroleptic malignant syndrome, treatment with dantrolene and bromocriptine may offer no advantage over supportive care [176].
- Solu-Medrol may benefit patients with neuroleptic malignant syndrome owing to withdrawal from Parkinson's medications [182].

Table 185.8 compares the distinguishing characteristics of the hyperthermic syndromes. Advances in hyperthermia based on randomized, controlled trials or meta-analyses of such trials are given in Table 185.9.

HYPERTHERMIA AND FEVER CONTROL AFTER BRAIN INJURY

Fever among neurocritical care patients is frequent and often results in an adverse neurologic outcomes. Morbidity and mortality are increased among patients who have ischemic brain injury, intracerebral hemorrhage, and cardiac arrest. Fever appears to have a longer impact after subarachnoid hemorrhage and traumatic brain injury. New techniques (see hypothermia Chapter 67) have made treatment of fever and maintaining normothermia possible.

ACKNOWLEDGMENT

The authors wish to thank Dr. Frederick J. Curley for his efforts in coauthoring earlier editions of this chapter upon which much of the newer information has been added.

References

1. Gauss H, Meyer KA: Heat stroke: a report of 158 cases from Cook County Hospital, Chicago. *Am J Med Sci* 154:554, 1917.
2. Clowes GHA, O'Donnell TF: Heat stroke. *N Engl J Med* 291:564, 1974.
3. Ellis EP: Mortality from heat illness and heat-aggravated illness in the United States. *Environ Res* 5:1, 1972.
4. Heat stroke: United States, 1980. *MMWR Morb Mortal Wkly Rep* 30:277, 1981.
5. Wise TN: Heat stroke in three chronic schizophrenics: case reports and clinical considerations. *Compr Psychiatry* 14:263, 1973.
6. Kilbourne EM, Choi K, Jones S, et al: Risk factors for heat stroke: a case control study. *JAMA* 247:3332, 1982.
7. Cole RD: Heat stroke during training with nuclear, biological, and chemical protective clothing. Case report. *Mil Med* 148:624, 1983.
8. Centers for Disease Control (CDC): Fatalities from occupational heat exposure. *MMWR Morb Mortal Wkly Rep* 33:410, 1984.
9. Stine FJ: Heat illness. *JACEP* 8:154, 1979.
10. Knochel JP: Environmental heat illness: an eclectic review. *Arch Intern Med* 133:841, 1974.
11. O'Donnell TF: Acute heat stroke: epidemiologic, biochemical, renal, and coagulation studies. *JAMA* 234:824, 1975.
12. Shibolet S, Coll R, Gilat T, et al: Heat stroke: its clinical picture and mechanism in 36 cases. *Q J Med* 36:525, 1967.
13. Ansari A, Burch GE: Influence of hot environments on the cardiovascular system. *Arch Intern Med* 123:371, 1969.
14. Adams BE, Manoguerra AS, Lilja GP, et al: Heat stroke: associated with medications having anticholinergic effects. *Minn Med* 60:103, 1977.
15. Dann EJ, Berkman N: Chronic idiopathic anhydrosis: a rare cause of heat stroke. *Postgrad Med J* 68:750, 1992.
16. Chun-Jen S, Mao-Tsun L, Shih-Han T: Experimental study on the pathogenesis of heat stroke. *J Neurosurg* 60:1246, 1984.
17. Attia M, Khogali M, El-Khatib G: Heat stroke: an upward shift of temperature regulation set point at an elevated body temperature. *Int Arch Occup Environ Health* 53:9, 1983.
18. Baba N, Ruppert RD: Alteration of eccrine sweat gland in fatal heat stroke. *Arch Pathol* 85:669, 1968.
19. Sprung CL: Hemodynamic alterations of heat stroke in the elderly. *Chest* 75:361, 1979.
20. Levine JA: Heat stroke in the aged. *Am J Med* 47:251, 1969.
21. McElroy CR: Update on heat illness. *Top Emerg Med* 2:1, 1980.
22. Fajardo LF: Pathologic effects of hyperthermia in normal tissues. *Cancer Res* 44[Suppl]:4826S, 1984.

23. Bouchama A, Knockel J: Heat stroke. *N Engl J Med* 346:1978, 2002.
24. Bouchama A, De Vol EB: Acid base alterations in heat stroke. *Intensive Care Med* 27:680, 2001.
25. Vertel RM, Knochel JP: Acute renal failure due to heat injury: an analysis of 10 cases associated with the high incidence of myoglobinuria. *Am J Med* 43:435, 1967.
26. Costrini AM, Pitt HA, Gustafson AB, et al: Cardiovascular and metabolic manifestations of heat stroke and severe heat exhaustion. *Am J Med* 66:296, 1979.
27. Hart GR, Anderson RJ, Crumpler CP, et al: Epidemic classical heat stroke: clinical characteristics and course of 28 patients. *Medicine (Baltimore)* 61:189, 1982.
28. Dahmash NS, Al Harthi SS, Akhtar J: Invasive evaluation of patients with heat stroke. *Chest* 103:1210, 1993.
29. Knochel JP: Heat stroke and related heat disorders. *Dis Mon* 35:306, 1989.
30. Atar S, Rozner E, Rosenfeld T: Transient cardiac dysfunction and pulmonary edema in exertional heat stroke. *Mil Med* 168:671, 2003.
31. Kew MC, Abrahams C, Levin NW, et al: The effects of heat stroke on the function and structure of the kidney. *Q J Med* 36:277, 1967.
32. Malamud N, Haymaker W, Custer RP: Heat stroke: a clinicopathologic study of 125 fatal cases. *Mil Surg* 97:397, 1946.
33. Manto MU: Isolated cerebellar dysarthria associated with a heat stroke. *Clin Neurol Neurosurg* 98:55, 1996.
34. Grohan H, Hopkins PM: Heat stroke: implications for clinical care. *Br J Anaesth* 88:700, 2002.
35. Minassian DC, Mehra V, Jones BR: Dehydrational crises from severe diarrhea or heat stroke and risk of cataract. *Lancet* 1:751, 1984.
36. Dematte JE, O'Mara K, Buescher J, et al: Near-fatal heat stroke during the 1995 heat wave in Chicago. *Ann Intern Med* 129:173, 1998.
37. Shieh SD, Lin YF, Lu KC, et al: Role of creatine phosphokinase in predicting acute renal failure in hypocalcemic exertional heat stroke. *Am J Nephrol* 12:252, 1992.
38. Gader AM, Al-Mashhadani SA, Al-Harthy SS: Direct activation of platelets by heat is the possible trigger of coagulopathy of heat stroke. *Br J Haematol* 74:86, 1990.
39. Jones TS, Liang AP, Kilbourne EM, et al: Morbidity and mortality associated with the July 1980 heat wave in St. Louis and Kansas City, MO. *JAMA* 247:3328, 1982.
40. Bouchamma A, Hammami MM, Haq A, et al: Evidence for endothelial cell activation/injury in heat stroke. *Crit Care Med* 24:1173, 1996.
41. Keatinge WR, Coleshaw SR, Easton JC, et al: Increased platelet and red cell counts, blood viscosity, and plasma cholesterol levels during heat stress, and mortality from coronary and cerebral thrombosis. *Am J Med* 81:795, 1986.
42. Al-Harthi SS, Karrar O, Al-Mashhadani SA: Metabolite and hormonal profiles in heat stroke patients at Mecca pilgrimage. *J Intern Med* 228:343, 1990.
43. Knochel JP, Caskey JH: The mechanism of hypophosphatemia in acute heat stroke. *JAMA* 238:425, 1977.
44. Tucker CE, Stanford J, Graves B, et al: Classic heat stroke: clinical and laboratory assessment. *South Med J* 78:20, 1985.
45. Buck CW, Carscallen HB, Hobbs GE: Temperature regulation in schizophrenia. *Arch Neurol Psych* 64:828, 1950.
46. Litman RE: Heat stroke in Parkinsonism. *Arch Intern Med* 89:562, 1952.
47. Randall WC, Wurster RD, Lewin RJ: Responses of patients with high spinal transection to high ambient temperatures. *J Appl Physiol* 21:985, 1966.
48. McLeod RN: Heat illness in early season football practice. *J Ky Med Assoc* 70:613, 1972.
49. Hanson PG, Zimmerman SW: Exertional heat stroke in novice runners. *JAMA* 242:154, 1979.
50. Rose RC, Hughes RD, Yarbrough DR, et al: Heat injuries among recreational runners. *South Med J* 73:1038, 1980.
51. Whitworth JAG, Wolfman MJ: Fatal heat stroke in a long distance runner. *Lancet* 1:545, 1984.
52. Wyndham CH: Heat stroke and hyperthermia in marathon runners. *Ann N Y Acad Sci* 301:128, 1977.
53. O'Donnell J, Axelrod P, Fischer C, et al: Use and effectiveness of hypothermia blankets for febrile patients in the intensive care unit. *Clin Infect Dis* 24(6):1214, 1997.
54. Marik PE: Fever in the ICU. *Chest* 117(3):855, 2000.
55. Talman WT, Florek G, Bullard DE: A hyperthermic syndrome in two subjects with acute hydrocephalus. *Arch Neurol* 45:1037, 1988.
56. Chesanow RL: A 65-year-old woman with heat stroke. *Am J Med* 41:415, 1961.
57. Khogali M, Weiner JS: Heat stroke: report on 18 cases. *Lancet* 2:276, 1980.
58. Al-Aska AK, Abu-Aisha H, Yaqub B, et al: Simplified cooling bed for heat-stroke. *Lancet* 1:381, 1987.
59. Costrini A: Emergency treatment of exertional heatstroke and comparison of whole body cooling techniques. *Med Sci Sports Exerc* 22(1):15, 1990.
60. Proulx CL, Ducharme MB, Kenny GP: Effect of water temperature on cooling efficiency during hypothermia in humans. *J Appl Physiol* 94(4):1317, 2003.
61. Haddad E, Moran DS, Epstein Y: Cooling heat stroke patients by available field measures. *Intensive Care Med* 30(2):338, 2004.
62. Gaffin SL, Garner JW, Flinn SD: Cooling methods for heatstroke victims. *Ann Intern Med* 132(8):678, 2000.
63. O'Grady NP, Barie PS, Bartlett J, et al: Practice parameters for evaluating new fever in critically ill adult patients. *Crit Care Med* 26:392, 1998.
64. Bouchama A, Cafege A, Devol EB, et al: Ineffectiveness of dantrolene sodium in the treatment of heat stroke. *Crit Care Med* 19:176, 1991.
65. Channa AB, Seraj MA, Saddique AA, et al: Is dantrolene effective in heat stroke patients? *Crit Care Med* 18(3):290, 1990.
66. Seraj MA, Channa AB, Al Harthi SS, et al: Are heat stroke patients volume depleted? Importance of monitoring central venous pressure as a simple guideline to therapy. *Resuscitation* 21:33, 1991.
67. Severinghaus JW: Respiration and hypothermia. *Ann N Y Acad Sci* 80:384, 1959.
68. Malan A: Blood acid base state at variable temperature, a graphical representation. *Respir Physiol* 31:259, 1977.
69. Kelman GR, Nunn JF: Nomograms for correction of blood Po_2, PCO_2, pH, and base excess for time and temperature. *J Appl Physiol* 21:1484, 1966.
70. Chao TC, Simniah R, Pakiam JE: Acute heat stroke deaths. *Pathology* 13:145, 1981.
71. Slovis CM, Anderson GF, Casolaro A: Survival in a heat stroke victim with a core temperature in excess of 46.5°C. *Ann Emerg Med* 11:269, 1982.
72. Alzeer A, Arifi A, el-Hazmi M, et al: Thermal regulatory dysfunction of growth hormone in classic heat stroke. *Eur J Endocrinol* 134:727, 1996.
73. Lee S, Merriam A, Skim TS, et al: Cerebellar degeneration in neuroleptic malignant syndrome: neuropathologic findings and review of the literature concerning heat-related nervous system injury. *J Neurol Neurosurg Psychiatry* 52:387, 1989.
74. Ali SZ, Taguchi A, Rosenberg H: Malignant hyperthermia. *Best Pract Res Clin Anaesthesiol* 17(4):519, 2003.
75. Aldrete JA: Advances in the diagnosis and treatment of malignant hyperthermia. *Acta Anaesthesiol Scand* 25:477, 1981.
76. Gronert GA: Malignant hyperthermia. *Anesthesiology* 53:395, 1980.
77. Michelson JR, Gallant EM, Litterer LA, et al: Abnormal sarcoplasmic reticulum ryanodine receptor in malignant hyperthermia. *J Biol Chem* 263:9310, 1988.
78. Wallace AJ, Woolridge W, Kingston HM, et al: Malignant hyperthermia: a large kindred linked to the RYR1 gene. *Anaesthesia* 51:16, 1996.
79. McCarthy TV, Healy JM, Heffron JJ, et al: Localization of the malignant hyperthermia susceptibility locus to human chromosome 19q12–13.2. *Nature* 343:562, 1990.
80. Denborough M: Malignant hyperthermia. *Lancet* 352:1131, 1998.
81. Schiller HH: Chronic viral myopathy and malignant hyperthermia. *N Engl J Med* 292:1409, 1975.
82. Tsueda K, Dubick MN, Wright BD, et al: Intraoperative hyperthermic crisis in two children with undifferentiated lymphoma. *Anesth Analg* 57:511, 1978.
83. Campbell IT, Ellis FR, Evans RT, et al: Studies of body temperatures, blood lactate, cortisol and free fatty acid levels during exercise in human subjects susceptible to malignant hyperpyrexia. *Acta Anaesthesiol Scand* 27:349, 1983.
84. Denborough MA: Etiology and pathophysiology of malignant hyperthermia. *Int Anesthesiol Clin* 7:11, 1979.
85. Steward DJ: Malignant hyperthermia: the acute crisis. *Int Anesthesiol Clin* 17:1, 1979.
86. Kalow W, Britt BA, Chan F-Y: Epidemiology and inheritance of malignant hyperthermia. *Int Anesthesiol Clin* 17:119, 1979.
87. Lutsky I, Witkowski J, Henschel EO: HLA typing in a family prone to malignant hyperthermia. *Anesthesiology* 56:224, 1982.
88. Harriman DGF: Preanesthetic investigations of malignant hypothermia: microscopy. *Int Anesthesiol Clin* 17:97, 1979.
89. Payen JF, Bosson JL, Bourdon L, et al: Improved noninvasive diagnostic testing for malignant hyperthermia: susceptibility from a combination of metabolites determined in vivo with 31P-magnetic resonance spectroscopy. *Anesthesiology* 78:848, 1993.
90. Britt BA: Preanesthetic diagnosis of malignant hyperthermia. *Int Anesthesiol Clin* 17:63, 1979.
91. Glisson SN: Malignant hyperthermia. *Compr Ther* 14:33, 1988.
92. Litman RS, Rosenberg H: Malignant hyperthermia: update on susceptibility screening. *JAMA* 293(23):2918, 2005.
93. Sei Y, Sambuughin NN, Davis E, et al: Malignant hyperthermia in North America: genetic screening of the three hot spots in the type 1 ryanodine receptor gene. *Anesthesiology* 101(4):824, 2004.
94. Strazis KP, Fox AW: Malignant hyperthermia: a review of published cases. *Anesth Analg* 72:297, 1993.
95. Felice-Johnson J, Sudds T, Bennett G: Malignant hyperthermia: current perspectives. *Am J Hosp Pharm* 38:646, 1981.
96. Bacon AK: Pulse oximetry in malignant hyperthermia. *Anaesth Intensive Care* 17:208, 1989.
97. Baudendistel L, Goudsouzian N, Cote C, et al: End tidal CO_2 monitoring: its use in the diagnosis and management of malignant hyperthermia. *Anesthesia* 39:1000, 1984.
98. Liebenschutz F, Mai C, Pickerodt VW: Increased carbon dioxide production in two patients with malignant hyperpyrexia and its control by dantrolene. *Br J Anaesth* 51:899, 1979.
99. Triner L, Sherman J: Potential value of expiratory carbon dioxide measurement in patients considered to be susceptible to malignant hyperthermia. *Anesthesiology* 55:482, 1981.
100. Badgwell JM, Heaver JE: Masseter spasm heralds malignant hyperthermia or merely academia gone mad? *Anesthesiology* 61:230, 1984.
101. Schwartz L, Rockoff MA, Koka BV: Masseter spasm with anesthesia: incidence and implications. *Anesthesiology* 61:772, 1984.
102. Flewellen E, Nelson TE: Halothane-succinylcholine induced masseter spasm: indicative of malignant hyperthermia susceptibility? *Anesth Analg* 63:693, 1984.
103. Ellis FR, Halsall PJ: Suxamethonium spasm: a differential diagnostic conundrum. *Br J Anaesth* 56:381, 1984.
104. Larach MG, Rosenberg H, Larach DR, et al: Prediction of malignant hyperthermia susceptibility by clinical signs. *Anesthesiology* 66:547, 1987.
105. Peters KR, Nance P, Wingard DW: Malignant hyperthyroidism or malignant hyperthermia? *Anesth Analg* 60:613, 1981.

106. Bennett MH, Wainwright AP: Acute thyroid crisis on induction of anaesthesia. *Anaesthesia* 44:28, 1989.
107. Crowley KG, Cunningham AJ, Conroy B, et al: Phaeochromocytoma: a presentation mimicking malignant hyperthermia. *Anaesthesia* 43:1031, 1988.
108. Nelson TE, Lin M, Zapata-Sudo G, et al: Dantrolene sodium can increase or attenuate activity of skeletal muscle ryanodine receptor calcium release channel. Clinical implications. *Anesthesiology* 84:1368, 1996.
109. Gallant EM, Ahern CP: Malignant hyperthermia: responses of skeletal muscles to general anesthetics. *Mayo Clin Proc* 58:758, 1983.
110. Blank JW, Boggs SD: Successful treatment of an episode of malignant hyperthermia using a large dose of dantrolene. *J Clin Anesth* 5:69, 1993.
111. Kolb ME, Horne ML, Martz R: Dantrolene in human malignant hyperthermia: a multicenter study. *Anesthesiology* 56:254, 1982.
112. Allen GC, Cattran CB, Peterson RG, et al: Plasma levels of dantrolene following oral administration in malignant hyperthermia-susceptible patients. *Anesthesiology* 69:900, 1988.
113. Ryan JF, Donlon JV, Malt RA, et al: Cardiopulmonary bypass in the treatment of malignant hyperthermia. *N Engl J Med* 290:1121, 1974.
114. Delay J, Deniker P: Drug-induced extrapyramidal syndromes, in Vinken PJ, Bruyn GW (eds): *Diseases of the Basal Ganglia*. Amsterdam, the Netherlands, North Holland Publishing Company, 1968, p 248.
115. Caroff SN: The neuroleptic malignant syndrome. *J Clin Psychiatry* 41:79, 1980.
116. Modestin J, Toffler G, Drescher JP: Neuroleptic malignant syndrome: results of a prospective study. *Psychiatry Res* 44:251, 1992.
117. Gelenberg AJ, Bellinghausen B, Wojcik JD, et al: A prospective survey of neuroleptic malignant syndrome in a short-term psychiatric hospital. *Am J Psychiatry* 145:517, 1988.
118. Friedman JH, Davis R, Wagner RL: Neuroleptic malignant syndrome: the results of a 6-month prospective study of incidence in a state psychiatric hospital. *Clin Neuropharmacol* 11:373, 1988.
119. Keck PE Jr, Pope HG Jr, McElroy SL: Frequency and presentation of neuroleptic malignant syndrome: a prospective study. *Am J Psychiatry* 144:1344, 1987.
120. Hermesh H, Aizenber D, Weizman A, et al: Risk for definite neuroleptic malignant syndrome: a prospective study of 223 consecutive inpatients. *Br J Psychiatry* 161:254, 1992.
121. Burke RE, Fahn S, Mayeaux R, et al: Neuroleptic malignant syndrome caused by dopamine-depleting drugs in a patient with Huntington's disease. *Neurology (NY)* 31:1022, 1981.
122. Keck PE, Pope HG, McElroy SL: Declining frequency of neuroleptic malignant syndrome in a hospital population. *Am J Psychiatry* 148:880, 1991.
123. Shalev A, Hermesh H, Munitz H: Mortality from neuroleptic malignant syndrome. *J Clin Psychiatry* 50:18, 1989.
124. Rosebush PI, Stewart TD: A prospective analysis of 24 episodes of neuroleptic malignant syndrome. *Am J Psychiatry* 146:717, 1989.
125. Lopez JR, Sanchez V, Lopez MJ: Sarcoplasmic ionic calcium concentration in neuroleptic malignant syndrome. *Cell Calcium* 10:223, 1989.
126. Itoh H, Ohtsuka N, Ogita K, et al: Malignant neuroleptic syndrome: its present status in Japan and clinical problems. *Folia Psychiatr Neurol Jpn* 31:565, 1977.
127. Stoudemire A, Luther JS: Neuroleptic malignant syndrome and neuroleptic induced catatonia: differential diagnosis and treatment. *Int J Psychiatry Med* 14:57, 1984.
128. Oppenheim G: Mutism and hyperthermia in a patient treated with neuroleptics. *Med J Aust* 2:228, 1973.
129. Eiser AR, Neff MS, Slifkin RF: Acute myoglobinuric renal failure: a consequence of the neuroleptic malignant syndrome. *Arch Intern Med* 142:601, 1982.
130. Geller B, Greydanus DE: Haloperidol induced comatose state with hyperthermia and rigidity in adolescence: two case reports with a literature review. *J Clin Psychiatry* 40:102, 1979.
131. Jesse SS, Anderson GF: ECT in the neuroleptic malignant syndrome: case report. *J Clin Psychiatry* 44:186, 1983.
132. Eles GR, Songer JE, DiPette DJ: Neuroleptic malignant syndrome complicated by disseminated intravascular coagulation. *Arch Intern Med* 144:1296, 1984.
133. Liskow BI: Relationship between neuroleptic malignant syndrome and malignant hyperthermia. *Am J Psychiatry* 142:390, 1985.
134. Mueller PS, Vester JW, Fermaglich J: Neuroleptic malignant syndrome: successful treatment with bromocriptine. *JAMA* 249:386, 1983.
135. May DC, Morns SW, Stewart RM, et al: Neuroleptic malignant syndrome: response to dantrolene sodium. *Ann Intern Med* 98:183, 1983.
136. Coons DJ, Hillman FJ, Marshall RW: Treatment of neuroleptic malignant syndrome with dantrolene sodium: a case report. *Am J Psychiatry* 139:944, 1982.
137. Feibel JM, Schiffer RB: Sympathoadrenal medullary hyperactivity in the neuroleptic malignant syndrome: a case report. *Am J Psychiatry* 138:1115, 1981.
138. Dhib-Jalbut S, Messelbrock R, Brott T, et al: Treatment of the neuroleptic malignant syndrome with bromocriptine. *JAMA* 250:484, 1983.
139. Amdurski S, Radwan M, Levi A, et al: A therapeutic trial of amantadine in haloperidol-induced malignant neuroleptic syndrome. *Curr Ther Res* 33:225, 1983.
140. Goulon M, de Rohan-Chabot P, Elkharrat D, et al: Beneficial effects of dantrolene in the treatment of neuroleptic malignant syndrome: a report of two cases. *Neurology* 33:516, 1983.
141. Tollefson GD, Garvey MJ: The neuroleptic syndrome and central dopamine metabolites. *J Clin Psychopharmacol* 4:150, 1984.
142. Lew T, Tollefson G: Chlorpromazine-induced neuroleptic malignant syndrome and its response to diazepam. *Biol Psychiatry* 18:1441, 1983.
143. Downey GP, Rosenberg M, Carroff S, et al: Neuroleptic malignant syndrome patient with unique clinical and physiologic features. *Am J Med* 77:338, 1984.
144. McAllister RG: Fever, tachycardia and hypertension with acute catatonic schizophrenia. *Arch Intern Med* 138:1154, 1978.
145. Weinberg S, Twersky RS: Neuroleptic malignant syndrome. *Anesth Analg* 62:848, 1983.
146. Tollefson G: A case of neuroleptic malignant syndrome: in vitro muscle comparison with malignant hyperthermia. *J Clin Psychopharmacol* 2:266, 1982.
147. Bonwick RJ, Hopwood MJ, Morris PL: Neuroleptic malignant syndrome and risperidone: a case report. *Aust N Z J Psychiatry* 30:419, 1996.
148. Gradon JD: Neuroleptic malignant syndrome possibly caused by molindone hydrochloride. *Ann Pharmacother* 25:1071, 1991.
149. Anderson ES, Powers PS: Neuroleptic malignant syndrome associated with clozapine use. *J Clin Psychiatry* 52:102, 1991.
150. Halman M, Goldbloom DS: Fluoxetine and neuroleptic malignant syndrome. *Biol Psychiatry* 28:518, 1990.
151. Spirt MJ, Chan W, Thieberg M, et al: Neuroleptic malignant syndrome induced by domperidone. *Dig Dis Sci* 37:946, 1992.
152. Anath J, Parameswaran S, Gunatilake S, et al: Neuroleptic malignant syndrome and atypical antipsychotic drugs. *J Clin Psychiatry* 65:464, 2004.
153. Henderson VW, Wooten GF: Neuroleptic malignant syndrome: a pathogenetic role for dopamine receptor blockade? *Neurology (NY)* 31:132, 1981.
154. Sechi GP, Tanda F, Mutani R: Fatal hyperpyrexia after withdrawal of levodopa. *Neurology* 34:249, 1984.
155. Toru M, Matsuda O, Makiguchi K, et al: Neuroleptic malignant syndrome-like state following withdrawal of anti-parkinsonian drugs. *J Nerv Ment Dis* 1969:324, 1981.
156. Patterson JF: Neuroleptic malignant syndrome associated with metoclopramide. *South Med J* 81:674, 1988.
157. Samie MR: Neuroleptic malignant-like syndrome induced by metoclopramide. *Mov Disord* 2:57, 1987.
158. Friedman LS, Weinrauch LA, D'Elia JA: Metoclopramide-induced neuroleptic malignant syndrome. *Arch Intern Med* 147:1495, 1987.
159. Hermesh H, Molcho A, Aizenberg D, et al: The calcium antagonist nifedipine in recurrent neuroleptic malignant syndrome. *Clin Neuropharmacol* 11:552, 1988.
160. Lim R: Idiopathic hypoparathyroidism presenting as the neuroleptic malignant syndrome. *Br J Hosp Med* 41:182, 1989.
161. Morris HH, McCormick WF, Reinarz JA: Neuroleptic malignant syndrome. *Arch Neurol* 37:462, 1980.
162. Keck PE, Caroff SN, McElroy SL: Neuroleptic malignant syndrome and malignant hyperthermia: end of a controversy? *J Neuropsychiatry Clin Neurosci* 7:135, 1995.
163. Curley FJ, Irwin RS: Disorders of temperature control, Part I. Hyperthermia, Part 2. *J Intensive Care Med* 1:591, 1986.
164. Viejo LF, Morales V, Punal P, et al: Risk factors in neuroleptic malignant syndrome. A case-control study. *Acta Psychiatr Scand* 107:45, 2003.
165. Caroff SN, Mann SC: Neuroleptic malignant syndrome. *Med Clin North Am* 77:185, 1993.
166. Denborough MA, Collins SP, Hopkinson KC: Rhabdomyolysis and malignant hyperpyrexia. *BMJ* 288:1878, 1984.
167. Granato JE, Stern BJ, Ringel A, et al: Neuroleptic malignant syndrome: successful treatment with dantrolene and bromocriptine. *Ann Neurol* 4:89, 1983.
168. Adityanjee, Sajatovic M, Munshi K: Neuropsychiatric sequelae of the neuroleptic malignant syndrome. *Clin Neuropharmacol* 28(4):197, 2005.
169. Becker T, Kornhuber J, Hofmann E, et al: MRI white matter hyperintensity in neuroleptic malignant syndrome (NMS): a clue to pathogenesis? *J Neural Transm* 90:151, 1992.
170. Caroff SN, Mann SC: Neuroleptic malignant syndrome. *Psychopharmacol Bull* 24:25, 1988.
171. Susman VL: Clinical management of the neuroleptic malignant syndrome. *Psychiatr Q* 72(4):325, 2001.
172. Velamoor VR, Norman RM, Caroff SN, et al: Progression of symptoms in the neuroleptic malignant syndrome. *J Nerv Ment Dis* 182:168, 1994.
173. Sewell DD, Jeste DV: Distinguishing neuroleptic malignant syndrome (NMS) from NMS-like acute medical illnesses: a study of 34 cases. *J Neuropsychiatry Clin Neurosci* 4:265, 1992.
174. Banushali MJ, Tuite PJ: The evaluation and management of patients with the neuroleptic malignant syndrome. *Neurol Clin North Am* 23:389, 2004.
175. Anderson WH: Lethal catatonia and the neuroleptic malignant syndrome. *Crit Care Med* 19:1333, 1991.
176. Chiang WK, Herschman Z: Lethal catatonia and the neuroleptic malignant syndrome. *Crit Care Med* 20:1622, 1992.
177. Gong SNC, Rogers KJ: Role of brain monoamines in the fatal hyperthermia induced by pethidine or imipramine in rabbits pretreated with a monoamine oxidase inhibitor. *Br J Pharmacol* 48:12, 1978.
178. Browne B, Linter S: Monoamine oxidase inhibitors and narcotic analgesics: a critical review of the implications for treatment. *Br J Psychiatry* 151:210, 1987.
179. Meyer D, Halfin V: Toxicity secondary to meperidine in patients on monoamine oxidase inhibitors: a case report and critical review. *J Clin Psychopharmacol* 1:319, 1981.
180. McAllen, KJ, Schwartz DR: Adverse drug reactions resulting in hyperthermia in the intensive care unit. *Crit Care Med* 38[Suppl]:S244–S252, 2010.

181. Rosebush PI, Stewart T, Mazurek MF: The treatment of neuroleptic malignant syndrome: are dantrolene and bromocriptine useful adjuncts to supportive care? *Br J Psychiatry* 159:709, 1991.
182. Sato Y, Asoh T, Metoki N, et al: Efficacy of methylprednisolone pulse therapy on neuroleptic malignant syndrome in Parkinson's disease. *J Neurol Neurosurg Psychiatry* 74:574, 2003.
183. Goekoop JG, Carboat PA: Treatment of neuroleptic malignant syndrome with dantrolene. *Lancet* 2:49, 1982.
184. Nisijima K, Ishiguro T: Does dantrolene influence central dopamine and serotonin metabolism in the neuroleptic malignant syndrome? A retrospective study. *Biol Psychiatry* 33:45, 1993.
185. Olmsted TR: Neuroleptic malignant syndrome: guidelines for treatment and reinstitution of neuroleptics. *South Med J* 81:888, 1988.
186. Harpe C, Stondemire A: Aetiology and treatment of neuroleptic malignant syndrome. *Med Toxicol* 2:166, 1987.
187. Zubenko G, Pope MG: Management of a case of neuroleptic malignant syndrome with bromocriptine. *Am J Psychiatry* 40:1619, 1983.
188. McCarron MM, Boettger ML, Peck JJ: A case of neuroleptic malignant syndrome successfully treated with amantadine. *J Clin Psychiatry* 43:381, 1982.
189. Hermesh H, Aizenberg D, Weizman A: A successful electroconvulsive treatment of neuroleptic malignant syndrome. *Acta Psychiatr Scand* 75:237, 1987.
190. Addonizio G, Susman VL: ECT as a treatment alternative for patients with symptoms of neuroleptic malignant syndrome. *J Clin Psychiatry* 48:102, 1987.
191. Lotstra F, Linkowski P, Mendlewicz J: General anesthesia after neuroleptic malignant syndrome. *Biol Psychiatry* 18:243, 1983.
192. Maling TJB, MacDonald AD, Davis M, et al: Neuroleptic malignant syndrome: a review of the Wellington experience. *N Z Med J* 101:193, 1988.
193. Smego RA, Durack DT: The neuroleptic malignant syndrome. *Arch Intern Med* 142:1183, 1982.
194. Birkhimer LJ, DeVane CL: The neuroleptic malignant syndrome: presentation and treatment. *Drug Intell Clin Pharm* 18:462, 1984.
195. Conner CS: Therapy of syndrome malin. *Drug Intell Clin Pharm* 17:639, 1983.
196. Neuroleptic malignant syndrome. *Lancet* 1:545, 1984.
197. Dallman JH: Neuroleptic malignant syndrome: a review. *Mil Med* 149:471, 1984.
198. Nishioka Y, Miyazaki M, Kubo S, et al: Acute renal failure in neuroleptic malignant syndrome. *Ren Fail* 24(4):539, 2002.
199. Rosenberg MR, Green M: Neuroleptic malignant syndrome. *Arch Intern Med* 149:1927, 1989.
200. Legras A, Hurel D, Dabrowski G, et al: Protracted neuroleptic malignant syndrome complicating long-acting neuroleptic administration. *Am J Med* 85:875, 1988.
201. Wells AJ, Sommi RW, Crismon ML: Neuroleptic rechallenge after neuroleptic malignant syndrome: case report and literature review. *Drug Intell Clin Pharm* 22:475, 1988.
202. Rosebush PI, Stewart TD, Gelenberg AJ: Twenty neuroleptic rechallenges after neuroleptic malignant syndrome in 15 patients. *J Clin Psychiatry* 50:295, 1989.
203. Koponen H, Repo E, Lepola U: Long-term outcome after neuroleptic malignant syndrome. *Acta Psychiatr Scand* 84:550, 1991.
204. McCarron MM, Schulze BW, Thompson GA, et al: Acute phencyclidine intoxication: incidence of clinical findings in 1,000 cases. *Ann Emerg Med* 10:237, 1981.
205. Ginsberg MD, Hertzman M, Schmidt-Nowara WW: Amphetamine intoxication with coagulopathy, hyperthermia, and reversible renal failure: a syndrome resembling heatstroke. *Ann Intern Med* 73:81, 1970.
206. Krisko I, Lewis E, Johnson JE: Severe hyperpyrexia due to tranylcypromine-amphetamine toxicity. *Ann Intern Med* 70:559, 1969.
207. Ling LH, Marchant C, Buckley NA, et al: Poisoning with the recreational drug paramethoxyamphetamine (death). *Med J Aust* 174(9):453, 2001.
208. Dar KJ, McBrien ME: MDMA-induced hyperthermia: report of a fatality and review of current therapy. *Intensive Care Med* 22(9):995, 1996.
209. Friedman SA, Hirsch SE: Extreme hyperthermia after LSD ingestion. *JAMA* 217:1549, 1971.
210. Mills KC: Serotonin syndrome. *Crit Care Clin* 13(4):763, 1997.
211. Mason PJ, Morris VA, Balcezak TJ: Serotonin syndrome: presentation of 2 cases and review of the literature. *Medicine (Baltimore)* 79(4):201, 2000.
212. Sporer KA: The serotonin syndrome: implicated drugs, pathophysiology, and management. *Drug Saf* 13(2):94, 1995.
213. Brown TM, Skop BP, Mareth TR: Pathophysiology and management of the serotonin syndrome. *Ann Pharmacother* 30(5):527, 1996.
214. Martin TG: Serotonin syndrome. *Ann Emerg Med* 28(5):520, 1996.
215. Schuckit M, Robins E, Feighner J: Tricyclic antidepressants and monoamine oxidase inhibitors. *Arch Gen Psychiatry* 24:509, 1971.
216. Gillman PK: Monoamine oxidase inhibitors, opioid analgesics and serotonin toxicity. *Br J Anaesth* 95(4):431–441, 2005.
217. Leatherman JW, Schmitz PG: Fever, hyperdynamic shock, and multiple-system organ failure: a pseudo sepsis syndrome associated with chronic salicylate intoxication. *Chest* 100:1391, 1991.
218. Kosten TR, Kleber HD: Rapid death during cocaine abuse: a variant of the neuroleptic malignant syndrome? *Am J Drug Alcohol Abuse* 14:335, 1988.
219. Kline SS, Mauro LS, Scala-Barnett DM, et al: Serotonin syndrome versus neuroleptic malignant syndrome as a cause of death. *Clin Pharm* 8:510, 1989.
220. Nijhawan PK, Katz G, Winter S: Psychiatric illness and the serotonin syndrome: an emerging adverse drug effect leading to intensive care unit admission. *Crit Care Med* 24:1086, 1996.
221. Mueller PD, Korey WS: Death by ecstasy: the serotonin syndrome? *Ann Emerg Med* 32(3):377, 1998.
222. Ener RA, Meglathery SB, Van Decker WA, et al: Serotonin syndrome and other serotonergic disorders. *Pain Med* 4(1):63, 2003.
223. Rosenberg J, Pentel P, Pond S, et al: Hyperthermia associated with drug intoxication. *Crit Care Med* 14:964, 1986.
224. Merigian KS, Roberts JR: Cocaine intoxication: hyperpyrexia, rhabdomyolysis and acute renal failure. *Clin Toxicol* 25:135, 1987.
225. Carbone JR: The neuroleptic malignant and serotonin syndromes. *Emerg Med Clin North Am* 18(2):317, 2000.
226. Graudis A, Stearman A, Chan B: Treatment of the serotonin syndrome with cyproheptadine. *J Emerg Med* 16(4):615, 1998.
227. Gillman PK: The serotonin syndrome and its treatment. *J Psychopharmacol* 13(1):100, 1999.
228. Kendrick WC, Hull AR, Knochel JP: Rhabdomyolysis and shock after intravenous amphetamine administration. *Ann Intern Med* 86:381, 1977.
229. Zalis E, Parmley L Jr: Fatal amphetamine poisoning. *Arch Intern Med* 112:822, 1963.
230. Menashe PI, Gottlieb JE: Hyperthermia, rhabdomyolysis, and myoglobinuric renal failure after recreational use of cocaine. *South Med J* 81:379, 1988.
231. Campbell BG: Cocaine abuse with hyperthermia, seizures and fatal complications. *Med J Aust* 149:387, 1988.
232. Bauwens JE, Boggs JM, Hartwell PS: Fatal hyperthermia associated with cocaine use. *West J Med* 150:210, 1989.
233. Loghmanee F, Tobak M: Fatal malignant hyperthermia associated with recreational cocaine and ethanol abuse. *Am J Forensic Med Pathol* 7:246, 1986.
234. Bettinger J: Cocaine intoxication: massive oral overdose. *Ann Emerg Med* 9:429, 1980.
235. Patel R, Das M, Palazzolo M, et al: Myoglobinuric acute renal failure in phencyclidine overdose: report of observations in eight cases. *Ann Emerg Med* 9:549, 1980.
236. Armen R, Kanel G, Reynolds T: Phencyclidine-induced malignant hyperthermia causing submassive liver necrosis. *Am J Med* 77:167, 1984.
237. Yeo TP: Heat Stroke: a comprehensive review. *AACN Clin Issues* 15(2):280, 2004.
238. Badjatia N: Hyperthermia and fever control in brain injury. *Crit Care Med* 37(7):S250–S257, 2009.
239. Mihara K, Kondo T, Suzuki A, et al: Relationship between functional dopamine D2 and D3 receptors gene polymorphisms and neurologic malignant syndrome. *Am J Med Genet B Neuropsychiatr Genet* 117B:57, 2003.
240. Guerera RJ, Caroff SN, Cohen A, et al: An international consensus study of neuroleptic malignant syndrome diagnostic criteria using the Delphi method. *J Clin Psychiatry* 72:1222, 2011.
241. Misset B, De Jonghe B, Bastuji-Garin S, et al: Mortality of patients with heatstroke admitted to intensive care units during the 2003 heat wave in France: a national multiple-center risk factor study. *Crit Care Med* 34:1087, 2006.
242. Pease S, Bouadma L, Kermarrec N, et al: Early organ dysfunction course, cooling time and outcome in classic heatstroke. *Intensive Care Med* 35:144, 2009.
243. Argaud L, Ferry T, Le QH, et al: Short and long term outcomes of heatstroke following the 2003 heat wave in Lyon, France. *Arch Intern Med* 167:2177, 2007.
244. Akthar MJ, al-Nozha M, al-Harthi S, et al: Electrocardiographic abnormalities in patients with heat stroke. *Chest* 104:411, 1993.
245. Garcia-Rubira JC, Aquilar J, Romero D: Acute myocardial infarction in a young man after heat exhaustion. *Int J Cardiol* 47:297, 1995.
246. Bouchama A, Knochel JP. Heat Stroke. *N Engl J Med* 346:1978, 2002.
247. Bouchama A, Dehbi M, Chaves-Carballo E: Cooling and hemodynamic management in heatstroke: practical recommendations. *Crit Care* 11:R54, 2007.
248. Bouchama A, Cafege A, Devol EB, et al: Ineffectiveness of dantrolene sodium in the treatment of heatstroke. *Crit Care Med* 19:176, 1991.

Section 17

CARDIOVASCULAR PROBLEMS AND CORONARY CARE

AKSHAY S. DESAI • PATRICK T. O'GARA • DAVID A. MORROW

Chapter 186 ■ The Evolution of the Modern Cardiovascular Intensive Care Unit

HANNAH BENSIMHON • JASON N. KATZ

INTRODUCTION

There has been a striking evolution in the management of patients with cardiovascular diseases. Novel technologies and therapeutics have empowered clinicians to tackle conditions once considered untreatable. Created initially to support life-saving interventions following acute myocardial infarction (MI), Coronary Care Units (CCUs) began to rapidly proliferate in the 1960s, and were subsequently lauded for their ability to improve patient survival. Now heavily embedded in contemporary health care systems, the CCU has evolved into a Cardiovascular Intensive Care Unit (CICU)—home to patients with complex cardiac and noncardiac critical illnesses. This chapter highlights the historical underpinnings of the CCU and describes the evolving patient characteristics, disease severity, and care processes that have helped to shape the modern CICU.

FROM CORONARY TO INTENSIVE CARE

Historical Advances in the Management of Acute Myocardial Infarction

In a 1923 study entitled, "Thrombosis of the Coronary Arteries with Infarction of the Heart," Dr. Joseph Wearn, a physician at the Peter Bent Brigham Hospital, described the course of 19 patients who survived an acute MI [1]. At that time, the condition was described as "one of the great rarities of medicine." Given that it was "impossible to diagnose," it was believed to be of little clinical import, and hence little effort had gone into improving either its evaluation or management. In fact, most afflicted individuals received little more than prolonged convalescence, and every effort was made to "spare the patient from bodily exertion."

In the 40 years following the publication of Dr. Wearn manuscript, the incidence of death from coronary disease and acute MI steadily increased, becoming the most common cause of mortality in the United States (US) by the 1930s, and reaching a peak in the mid-1960s [2]. This epidemiologic shift was attributed largely to a decrease in death from other causes (i.e., infection) and a simultaneous increase in coronary atherosclerosis. Lifestyle changes, dominated by increasing tobacco use and an evolving diet, were implicated in this emerging epidemic, and the development of novel ways to diagnose and treat acute MI became a national priority.

The invention of the electrocardiogram (ECG) in 1902 by Dutch physiologist Willem Einthoven was a major step in that process [3]. Initially the ECG was celebrated for its ability to characterize electrical rhythm disturbances of the heart, but slowly gained prominence for its capacity to demonstrate particular waveform distortions in the setting of acute myocardial ischemia and infarction. Several decades later, William Kouwenhoven, an electrical engineer with no formal medical training, published data on the earliest form of cardiac defibrillation [4]. Since most of his seminal work was performed on animal models, it would take another decade for the first successful open cardiac defibrillation to be performed by Dr. Claude Beck on cardiac surgical patients at Case Western Reserve University. For patients suffering sudden death, this open defibrillation and cardiac massage became standard of care. The evolution of contemporary cardiopulmonary resuscitation and closed chest defibrillation soon followed from additional work by Guy Knickerbocker, Paul Zoll, and others [4].

With these advancements of resuscitation techniques, along with developments in cardiac monitoring (i.e., telemetry), clinicians were finally equipped with tools to identify and rapidly treat the life-threatening sequelae of acute MI. As Desmond Julian, a senior registrar of the royal infirmary of Edinburgh, would later articulate, "many cases of cardiac arrest associated with myocardial ischemia could be treated successfully if all medical, nursing, and auxiliary staff were trained in closed chest massage, and if the cardiac rhythm of patients were continuously monitored by an ECG" [5]. This vision became the foundation for the development and subsequent rapid proliferation of CCUs throughout the world (Fig. 186.1) [6,7].

One of the earliest CCUs, founded by Dr. Lawrence Meltzer in Philadelphia, was no more than a pair of adjacent rooms between which an early model defibrillator could be passed. Another, in Toronto, Ontario, emphasized arrhythmia surveillance with archetypal telemetry monitoring [8]. In general, nurses were empowered to act immediately and autonomously to resuscitate unstable patients. Despite their relatively narrow scope, early CCUs nonetheless were suggested to have had an enormous impact on survival. As an example, Killip and Kimball reported a decrease in mortality from 27% to 6% for acute MI patients cared for in the New York Hospital/Cornell Medical Center CCU [9]. Similar results were reported by others and led to a rapid proliferation of CCUs embedded within most large hospitals.

Shifting Care in the CCU—Addressing Complications of MI

In 1967, Lown and colleagues were credited with a paradigm shift in CCU care. These clinicians publicly bemoaned many of the challenges with MI management, noting in particular that there was little available with which to "alter the inexorable course of overwhelming shock or unyielding pulmonary edema," so often contributing to postinfarction death. Although acknowledging that their CCU was "equipped, organized, and oriented to treat (fatal) rhythm disturbances," they were one of the earliest to emphasize the staggering impact of cardiogenic shock and heart failure on mortality following MI. They called for a shift

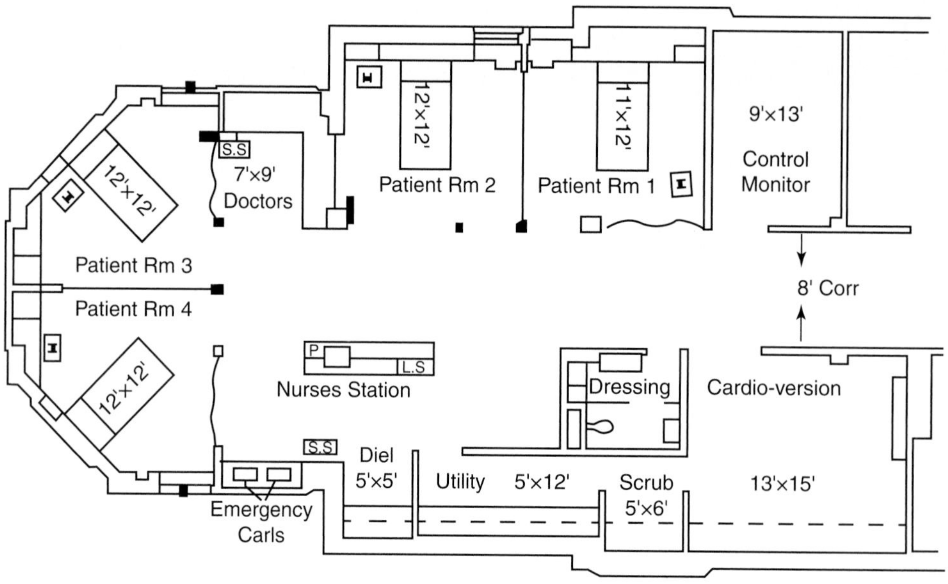

FIGURE 186.1 Prototypical design of the earliest Coronary Care Unit. A design of the Samuel A. Levine Cardiac Unit at Brigham and Women's Hospital, Boston, MA [10]. Monitoring was carried out from the bedside units (M) and from two four-channel oscilloscopes visible from the central nursing station. A central monitoring room was employed for continuous tape recording.

the focus of management in the CCU from resuscitation to the prevention of adverse events [10].

Lown's appeal was addressed by several major advances in the 1960s and 1970s. The intra-aortic balloon pump (IABP), for instance, utilized counter-pulsation technology to support the failing heart, and could be employed as a means for treating cardiogenic shock. First used clinically in 1968 by Adrian Kantrowitz, the IABP enhanced coronary perfusion while decreasing left ventricular work [11]. In 1970, Swan and Ganz introduced their pulmonary arterial catheter which would have a major impact on the way critically ill cardiac patients were managed [12]. Though their device was not the first of its kind, it advanced CCU care because it could be inserted quickly at the bedside. Use of the Swan–Ganz catheter led to important new insights into cardiac hemodynamics, and altered our understanding of the complications of and treatments for acute MI.

This technology gradient continued to evolve with the introduction of echocardiography. First used in the 1950s in Europe, echocardiography was subsequently promoted in the US in the late 1960s by many practitioners, including Dr. Harvey Feigenbaum [13], who embraced this tool in the face of growing frustrations with the "tediousness and inaccuracies of catheterization techniques for the measurement of cardiac output, volumes, and pressures." Echocardiography became increasingly more commonplace in the CCU and was championed for its ability to provide portable, rapid, and comprehensive information about a critically ill cardiac patient.

Additional Maturation of the CCU

A powerful endorsement of the CCU came from Goldman and Cook who attributed much of the declining morality seen from ischemic heart disease between 1968 and 1976 to the development of specific medical interventions, including the CCU [14]. Julian [15] and Reader [16] separately surmised that the steady decline of mortality among individuals 35 to 64 years of age within the US, Australia, and New Zealand may have been a direct effect of specialized CCU care. Similar support for the CCU could be found even after the introduction and validation of fibrinolytic therapy for acute MI, as treatment received in a CCU was still considered a major predictor of contemporary survival [17].

Although cardiologists became better equipped to treat MI, a condition once considered terminal, the population of patients admitted to the modern CCU concurrently changed substantially with the proportion of patients admitted to the CCU with MI declining. The population is more diverse, with greater representation of older, female, and minority patients. Patients admitted to CCUs are more likely to suffer from additional comorbid conditions, including chronic lung, liver, and kidney disease. Illness severity has worsened in parallel. Many CCUs have now evolved into intensive care units (ICUs) for patients with cardiovascular diseases. In a longitudinal study of nearly 30,000 patients admitted to a single-center CCU over a two-decade period, presenting disease severity increasingly worsened and the impact of noncardiovascular critical illness had intensified [18]. In response to these changes, many institutions have since accepted a new moniker for contemporary CCU care, and have begun to use the term "Cardiovascular Intensive Care Unit (CICU)" to reflect their broadened approach to the management of all critically ill cardiac patients. Figure 186.2 illustrates many of the key historical events that have been essential to the maturation of the CICU.

UNDERSTANDING THE NEEDS OF TODAY'S CICU

Clinical research initiatives have been paramount in the field of cardiology, and have led to substantial improvements of outcomes for patients with cardiovascular diseases. Critically ill cardiac patients have also benefited from many of these advances. Examples include revascularization for cardiogenic shock [19], targeted temperature management for cardiac arrest [20], and the use of left ventricular assist devices (LVADs) for end-stage heart failure [21]. Although disease-specific investigative efforts have influenced the care of today's CICU patients, research into optimal care pathways and platforms for critical care delivery in the CICU have unfortunately lagged behind.

Recognizing an increasing overlap between the contemporary CICU and other medical and surgical ICUs has helped clinicians and investigators better evaluate technologies and practices

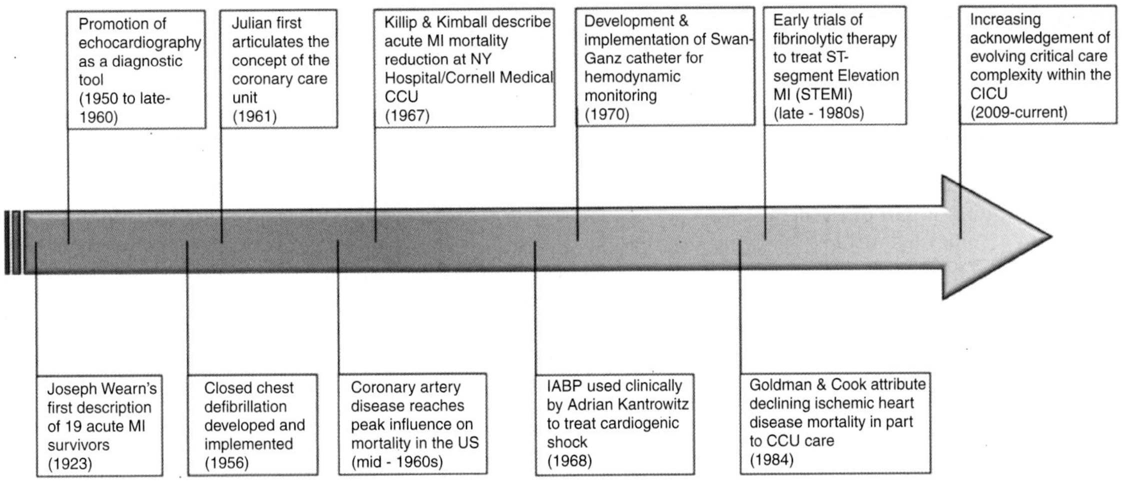

FIGURE 186.2 Historical events key to the maturation of the contemporary Cardiovascular Intensive Care Unit (CICU).

available for critically ill patients with cardiac conditions. Several studies have demonstrated that prognostic markers once reserved for general critical care populations may also have value within the CICU [22,23]. Recognizing key differences of these units has likewise been important. The increasing influence of nonsurgical cardiac interventions, including percutaneous valve replacement platforms and mechanical circulatory support (MCS) devices will undoubtedly lead to additional divergence.

As the utilization of the CICU increases and costs associated with it escalate, a more comprehensive understanding of the highest impact practices will be imperative. Halpern and Pastores reported a 200% increase in ICU costs between 1985 and 2000 [24], and went on to identify an additional 44% increase in costs between 2000 and 2005. They noted that while the total number of hospital beds had decreased in the US by over 4%, the number of critical care beds had increased by 6.5% [24]. The increasing representation of critical care in the modern medical landscape has appropriately directed research efforts towards the identification of technologies, practices, and system structures which deliver the highest value care to the sickest patients. Large databases which exist for medical ICUs have not been replicated specifically for the CICU. Therefore, much of our understanding of practice in the CICU comes from smaller, and commonly retrospective or descriptive studies.

Organizational Structure in the Contemporary CICU

Many of today's ICUs are considered "closed" units, in which responsibility of care for patients admitted to the intensive care setting falls to a dedicated critical care team. This structure stands in direct contrast to historical "open" units, wherein any physician may admit patients to the ICU and continue to maintain the primary role in managing them throughout their hospital course, including their intensive care. Importantly, a "closed" unit structure does not exclude involvement of a patient's long-term providers but rather creates an environment of team-based care in which moment-to-moment care is directed by the dedicated critical care team in collaboration with the patient's primary outpatient providers, involved specialists, and a broad group of multidisciplinary staff.

Studies of these two models within medical ICUs have generally showed better outcomes with the "closed ICU approach" [25,26]; although a more recent multicenter analysis failed to corroborate this association [27]. No studies evaluating optimal organizational structure have yet been conducted specifically in dedicated CICUs. Nonetheless, a recent survey of largely academic CICUs showed that 55% operated in a "closed" model of care. More research will be valuable to understand the impact of staffing patterns on CICU outcomes.

Who is in Charge of the CICU?

Defining the optimal staffing and training for today's CICU is an important issue facing the field. Research conducted in general critical care units has demonstrated superior outcomes for patients managed by intensivists with dedicated training in the care of critically ill populations. In a systematic review, a 29% mortality reduction along with significant improvements of resource consumption was attributed to intensivist care [28]. The specialized pharmacopeia necessary for care of critically ill patients, along with the routine use of critical care procedures such as mechanical ventilation, central venous catheterization, and flexible bronchoscopy within the modern ICU create a need for clinicians with advanced critical care experience or training. Direction of care by intensivists is also believed to improve patient triage, minimize the risk for iatrogenic complications, and to reduce ICU lengths-of-stay and direct costs. Although it would seem reasonable to extrapolate these findings to CICU populations—a group of patients who have previously been shown to suffer from high rates of noncardiovascular critical illness and to require the frequent use of critical care interventions—the impact of intensivist care on outcomes in the CICU has not been directly established. At present, the prevalence of intensivist-staffing models in CICUs remains low. In a 2013 survey conducted by members of an American Heart Association Scientific Statement Writing Group, a mere 8.1% of CICU medical directors reported that intensivists served as primary physicians for patients admitted to their units [29]. The lack of evidence directly examining an intensivist model in the CICU, combined with an acknowledgement from the general critical care community indicating a lack of complete comfort managing cardiovascular disease [30], points to a need for studies aimed at understanding optimal staffing for the CICU [31].

Critical care consultation allows for the contribution of both intensivists and cardiologists to participate in the care of CICU patients. This comanagement strategy depends upon the availability of critical care-trained physicians—specialists who are already at a significant shortage due to increasing demand and stagnating supply [32]. Telemedical consultation has also been proposed as an alternative strategy for achieving this "high-intensity staffing," and has been successfully employed in general or mixed ICUs [33,34]. Major considerations related to costs-of-care and the lack of direct patient–physician

TABLE 186.1

Potential Levels of Certification to Distinguish the Critical Care Cardiologist

Level of training	Mechanism	Specifics of training	Competency
Level 1	Inclusion of critical care rounding as part of a general cardiology fellowship	Typically ≥8 wk of cardiology critical care exposure designed to allow the trainee to acquire the knowledge, skills, and experience necessary to achieve basic competencies in this area.	Allows for competency to provide cardiovascular consultation in an intensive care setting
Level 2	Advanced critical care exposure and/or additional ICU electives as part of a general cardiology fellowship	Involves more advanced knowledge and skills than Level I training, with greater experience with bedside procedures and the skills needed for leading interdisciplinary teams managing critically ill patients. An additional 3–6 mo of clinical training within the 3-y CV medicine fellowship may support these skills.	Allows for competency to lead or comanage an interdisciplinary team in the CICU
Level 3	Additional training to prepare for specialization in critical care cardiology, and may lead to dual board-certification in cardiology and critical care medicine	Experience beyond the standard 3-y CV fellowship for the trainee to acquire specialized knowledge and competencies in performing, interpreting, and training others to perform specific critical care functions and procedures or provide advanced, specialized critical care at a high level of skill. Trainees should obtain additional critical care medicine training within the department of medicine, a portion of which may be spent in cardiac surgical intensive care units.	Allows for competency to lead a CICU team, to manage critically ill patients in other ICU settings, to spearhead ICU research initiatives, and to direct health care system efforts aimed at quality improvement for critical care delivery

ICU, intensive care unit; CICU, Cardiovascular Intensive Care Unit.

contact, among others, require additional study before tele-ICU platforms can be widely entertained or implemented in the CICU setting.

An additional approach towards appropriate staffing of the CICU is to avail critical care training opportunities to cardiologists. Several proposed training frameworks exist by which this goal may be accomplished [31,35]. Most commonly, multiple tiers of proficiency are proposed, wherein fellows of general cardiology training programs can obtain proficiency in cardiovascular critical care delivery. A summary of one possible framework is included in Table 186.1. The optimal design and implementation such training pathways remain in evolution [31,35].

Key Members of the CICU Team

Nurses have been pivotal members of the CICU team since its inception in the 1960s. Equipped with defibrillators and empowered to act autonomously to resuscitate post-MI patients, nurse-led CICU care has been associated with pronounced reductions of mortality. More recent data also suggests that nurse-to-patient ratios are significant predictors of survival [36].

In addition to nurses, the inclusion of critical care pharmacists as part of the multidisciplinary team has been associated with improved patient outcomes, reduced adverse drug events, and medication cost savings [37,38]. Respiratory therapists reduce the number of ventilator-patient days and can likewise decrease critical care costs [39,40]. Early mobility in the ICU, led by physical therapists, can also contribute to improved outcomes in several clinical domains [41]. Though all vetted in general ICU environments, there is no reason to believe that these team members should not have similar favorable impacts in the modern CICU. Additionally, palliative care expertise will likely take on increasing importance given the evolving population of today's CICU. These specially trained clinicians can help facilitate goals-of-care discussions, address end-of-life care, and are already being called upon to support patient selection for durable MCS [42]. Potential members of the CICU team are further highlighted in Figure 186.3.

Processes and Protocols for Cardiac Critical Care Delivery

A key mechanism through which multidisciplinary teams likely affect care is through the early implementation of proven critical care interventions. The need for data on such processes and protocols in the CICU is great. Some interventions with a strong base of evidence from research in general ICUs have already been applied in CICUs. Among these are the use of bundled care to reduce ventilator-associated pneumonia, management techniques for decreasing catheter-associated urinary tract infections, and protocols for unfractionated heparin adjustment and electrolyte replacement. There may be benefit for bundled CICU care practices in more cardiac-specific disease processes such as cardiac arrest and cardiogenic shock, but more research is needed to validate and systematize these approaches. ICU care has been compared to air traffic control, where algorithms and mechanisms for checks-and-balances are necessary to avoid serious errors. The development and validation of consistent

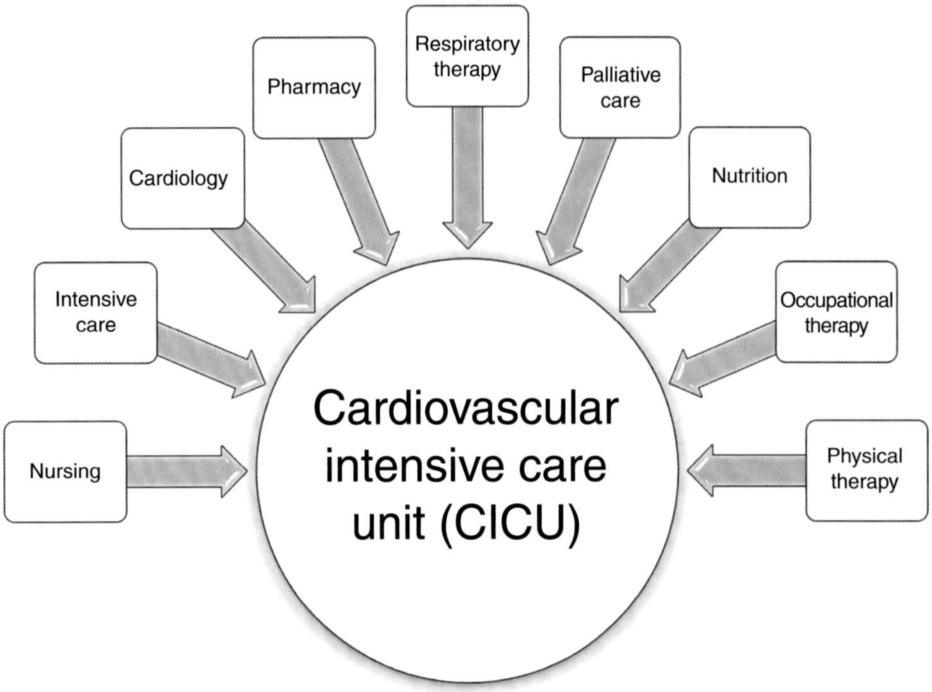

FIGURE 186.3 Important members of the modern CICU team.

care protocols and processes unique to the CICU must be part of the evolution of these specialized units, and comprehensive quality measures should likewise be created.

CONCLUSIONS

The modern CICU has evolved quickly and substantially from its origins as a monitoring unit specific to patients with acute MI. Now home to an increasingly diverse and complex population of patients with cardiovascular critical illness, the CICU must continue to grow responsibly. Many challenges face this maturing critical care setting. Included among these challenges are the need to determine the appropriate staffing, training, and organizational models necessary to deliver the highest quality of evidence-based care. Well-constructed responses to these challenges will only come through collaborative investigative efforts and dialogue among key stakeholders.

References

1. Wearn JT: Thrombosis of the coronary arteries, with infarction of the heart. *Am J Med Sci* 165(2):250–276, 1923.
2. Dalen J, Alpert J, Goldberg RJ, et al: The epidemic of the 20(th) century: coronary heart disease. *Am J Med* 127(9):807–812, 2014.
3. Fye WB: A history of the origin, evolution, and impact of electrocardiography. *Am J Cardiol* 73(13):937–949, 1994.
4. Acosta P, Varon J, Sternbach GL, et al: Resuscitation great. Kouwenhoven, Jude and Knickerbocker: The introduction of defibrillation and external chest compressions into modern resuscitation. *Resuscitation* 64(2):139–143, 2005.
5. Julian D: Treatment of cardiac arrest in acute myocardial ischaemia and infarction. *Lancet* 2:840–844, 1961.
6. Meltzer LE: Coronary units can help decrease deaths. *Mod Hosp* 104:102–104, 1965.
7. Brown KW, MacMillan RL, Forbath N, et al: Coronary unit: an intensive-care centre for acute myocardial infarction. *Lancet* 2:349–352, 1963.
8. Day HW: History of coronary care units. *Am J Cardiol* 30(4):405–407, 1972.
9. Killip T, Kimball J: Treatment of myocardial infarction in a coronary care unit. Two year experience with 250 patients. *Am J Cardiol* 20:457–464, 1967.
10. Lown B, Fakhro A, Hood W, et al: The coronary care unit: new perspectives and directions. *J Am Med Assoc* 199:188–198, 1967.
11. Kantrowitz A, Tjonneland S, Feed PS, et al: Initial clinical experience with intraaortic balloon pumping in cardiogenic shock. *J Am Med Assoc* 203:113–118, 1968.
12. Swan HJC, Ganz W, Forrester JS, et al: Cardiac catheterization with a flow-directed balloon-tipped catheter. *N Engl J Med* 283:447–451, 1970.
13. Feigenbaum H: Clinical applications of echocardiography. *Prog Cardiovasc Dis* 14(6):531–558, 1972.
14. Goldman L, Cook EF: The decline in ischemic heart disease mortality rates: an analysis of the comparative effects of medical interventions and changes in lifestyle. *Ann Intern Med* 101:825–836, 1984.
15. Julian DG: The history of coronary care units. *Br Heart J* 57:497–502, 1987.
16. Reader R: Why the decreasing mortality from coronary heart disease in Australia? *Circulation* 58[Suppl II]:32, 1978.
17. Rotstein Z, Mandelzweig L, Lavi B, et al: Does the coronary care unit improve prognosis of patients with acute myocardial infarction? A thrombolytic era study. *Eur Heart J* 20:813–818, 1999.
18. Katz JN, Shah BR, Volz EM, et al: Evolution of the coronary care unit: clinical characteristics and temporal trends in healthcare delivery and outcomes. *Crit Care Med* 38:375–381, 2010.
19. Hochman J, Sleeper J, Webb J, et al for the Should We Emergently Revascularize Occluded Coronaries for Cardiogenic Shock (SHOCK) investigators: Early revascularization in acute myocardial infarction complicated by cardiogenic shock. *N Engl J Med* 341:625–634, 1999.
20. Nolan J, Morley P, Vandenhoek T, et al: Therapeutic hypothermia after cardiac arrest. An advisory statement by the advanced life support task force of the International Liaison Committee on Resuscitation. *Circulation* 108:118–121, 2003.
21. Rose E, Geligns A, Moskowitz A, et al for the Randomized evaluation of mechanical assistance for the treatment of congestive heart failure (REMATCH) study group: Long-term use of a left ventricular assist device for end-stage heart failure. *N Engl J Med* 345:1435–1443, 2001.
22. Pauley E, LishmanovA, Schumann S, et al: Delirium is a robust predictor of morbidity and mortality among critically ill patients treated in the cardiac intensive care unit. *Am Heart J* 170:79–86, 2015.
23. Teskey J, Calvin R, McPhail I: Disease severity in the coronary care unit. *Chest* 100:1637–1642, 1991.
24. Halpern N, Pastores S, Greenstein R: Critical care medicine in the United States 1985–2000. An analysis of bed numbers, use, and costs. *Crit Care Med* 32:1254–1259, 2004.
25. Carson S, Stocking C, Podscadecki T, et al: Effects of organizational change in the medical intensive care unit of a teaching hospital: a comparison of open and closed formats. *J Am Med Assoc* 276:322–328, 1996.
26. Multz A, Chalfin D, Samson I, et al: A closed medical intensive care unit improves resource utilization when compared with an open MICU. *Am J Respir Crit Care Med* 157:1468–1473, 1998.
27. Checkley W, Martin G, Brown S, et al for the United States Critical Illness and Injury Trials Group Critical Illness Outcomes Study Investigators: Structure, process, and annual ICU mortality across 69 centers. *Crit Care Med* 42:344–356, 2014.
28. Pronovost P, Angus D, Dorman T, et al: Physician staffing patterns and clinical outcomes in critically ill patients. *J Am Med Assoc* 288:2151–2162, 2002.
29. O'Malley RG, Olenchock B, Bohula-May E, et al: Organization and staffing practices in US cardiac intensive care units: a survey on behalf of the American

Heart Association Writing Group on Evolution of Critical Care Cardiology. *Eur Heart J Acute Cardiovasc Care* 2(1):3–8, 2013.
30. Hill T, Means G, van Diepen S, et al: Cardiovascular critical care: a perceived deficiency among US trainees. *Crit Care Med* 43(9):1853–1858, 2015.
31. Morrow D, Fang J, Fintel D, et al: Evolution of critical care cardiology. Transformation of the cardiovascular intensive care unit and the emerging need for new medical staffing and training models. *Circulation* 126:1408–1428, 2012.
32. Angus D, Kelley M, Schmitz R, et al, for the Committee on Manpower for Pulmonary and Critical Care Societies (COMPACCS). Care for the critically ill patient: Current and projected workforce requirements for care of the critically ill patients with pulmonary disease: can we meet the requirements of an aging population? *J Am Med Assoc* 284(21):2762–2770, 2000.
33. Young L, Chan P, Lu X, et al: Impact of telemedicine intensive care unit coverage on patient outcomes: a systematic review. *Arch Intern Med* 171(6):498–506, 2011.
34. Wilcox M, Adhikari N: The effect of telemedicine in critically ill patients: systematic review and meta-analysis. *Crit Care* 16(4):R127, 2012.
35. Sinha S, Julien H, Krim SR, et al: Securing the future of cardiovascular medicine. *J Am Coll Cardiol* 65:1907–1914, 2015.
36. Neuraz A, Guerin C, Payet C, et al: Patient mortality is associated with staff resources and workload in the ICU: a multicenter observational study. *Crit Care Med* 43(8):1587–1594, 2015.
37. Horn E, Jacobi J: The critical care clinical pharmacist: evolution of an essential team member. *Crit Care Med* 34:S46–S51, 2006.
38. Leape L, Cullen D, Clapp M, et al: Pharmacist participation on physician rounds and adverse drug events in the intensive care unit. *J Am Med Assoc* 282:267–270, 1999.
39. Burns S, Marshall M, Burns J, et al: Design, testing, and results of an outcomes-managed approach to patients requiring prolonged mechanical ventilation. *Am J Crit Care* 7:45–57, 1998.
40. Wood G, MacLeod B, Moffatt S: Weaning from mechanical ventilation: physician-directed vs a respiratory-therapist-directed protocol. *Respir Care* 40:219–221, 1995.
41. Cameron S, Ball I, Cepinskas G, et al: Early mobilization in the critical care unit: a review of adult and pediatric literature. *J Crit Care* 30(4):664–672, 2015.
42. Decision memo for ventricular assist devices for bridge-to-transplant and destination therapy. Available at: https://www.cms.gov/medicare-coverage-database/details/nca-decision-memo.aspx?NCAId=268&NcaName=Ventricular+Assist+Devices+for+Bridge-to-Transplant+and+Destination+Therapy&MEDCACId=65&IsPopup=y&bc=AAAAAAAACAAAAA%3d%3d&. Accessed May 3, 2016.

Chapter 187 ■ ST-Segment Elevation Myocardial Infarction

HURST M. HALL • DAVID A. MORROW • JAMES A. DE LEMOS

Advances in the prevention, diagnosis, and management of patients with acute ST-segment elevation myocardial infarction (STEMI) have led to reductions both in the incidence and in case fatality from this condition [1]. Rapid delivery of reperfusion therapy is the cornerstone of STEMI management. The development of integrated systems of STEMI care has resulted in delivery of timely reperfusion therapy to larger numbers of eligible individuals, improving patient outcomes. This chapter describes the pathophysiology of STEMI, its diagnosis, risk stratification, and management. Mechanical complications of myocardial infarction (MI) are discussed in Chapter 191. The management of cardiogenic shock, including mechanical circulatory support, is addressed in Chapters 190, 196, and 197.

PATHOPHYSIOLOGY

The initial pathophysiologic event leading to STEMI is usually rupture or erosion of a lipid-rich atherosclerotic plaque. The atherosclerotic plaque "vulnerable" to rupture tends to have a dense lipid-rich core and a thin protective fibrous cap and is often not associated with critical narrowing of the arterial lumen. Molecular factors that regulate synthesis and dissolution of the extracellular matrix appear to modulate integrity of the protective fibrous cap. In unstable atherosclerotic lesions, inflammatory cells accumulate at the "shoulder" region of the plaque and release proteinases that degrade extracellular matrix and weaken the fibrous cap at this critical site [2].

Following plaque rupture, platelets adhere to subendothelial collagen, von Willebrand factor, or fibrinogen, and become activated by various local mediators such as adenosine diphosphate (ADP), collagen, and thrombin. Activated platelets undergo a conformational change and secrete the contents of their α-granules, promoting vasoconstriction and clot retraction. Activated platelets also express glycoprotein (GP) IIb/IIIa receptors in increased number and with greater binding affinity; fibrinogen-mediated cross-linking at this critical receptor leads to platelet aggregation. On the phospholipid surface of the platelet membrane, prothrombin is converted to thrombin, catalyzing the conversion of fibrinogen to fibrin [3].

The distinguishing feature of the platelet–fibrin clot in STEMI is that it completely occludes the epicardial coronary artery, leading to transmural myocardial injury, manifested by ST-segment elevation on the electrocardiogram (ECG). Despite similar initial pathophysiological features, unstable angina and non-STEMI (NSTEMI) are infrequently associated with complete occlusion of the culprit coronary artery and do not benefit from fibrinolytic therapy. Without reperfusion therapy, most patients with STEMI suffer transmural infarction and evolve Q-waves over the first few days after MI. Successful reperfusion therapy, however, may limit necrosis to the subendocardial regions and prevent development of Q-waves. The distinction between Q-wave and non-Q-wave MI can only be made retrospectively, and thus is not useful for early patient management.

DIAGNOSIS AND RISK ASSESSMENT

History and Physical Examination

The pain of acute MI is qualitatively similar to angina and is classically described as a severe pressure-type pain in the midsternum, often radiating to the left arm, neck, or jaw. Associated symptoms include dyspnea, diaphoresis, nausea, vomiting, and weakness. In the elderly and those with diabetes, pain is often atypical and may not be present at all [4]. Commonly, inferior STEMI presents with nausea and vagal symptoms rather than chest pain. Characterization of the quality of the pain may help to distinguish MI from other conditions that cause chest discomfort, such as aortic dissection, pulmonary embolism, pericarditis, and gastrointestinal (GI) disorders such as cholecystitis and peptic ulcer (Table 187.1).

Patients with acute MI often appear pale and clammy; in many cases, they are in obvious distress. Elderly patients, in particular, may be agitated and incoherent. In contrast, patients with cardiogenic shock may be listless and confused. The objective of the initial examination should be to rapidly narrow the differential diagnosis and assess the clinical stability of the patient. A focused examination can help to differentiate ischemia from

TABLE 187.1

Differential Diagnosis of Acute MI

Condition	Characterization of pain	Physical findings	ECG findings	Helpful diagnostic tests
Acute coronary syndrome	Pressure-type pain at rest, often radiating to neck or left arm	Examination often normal; check for signs of cardiogenic shock or HF	ST-segment elevation, ST-segment depression, T-wave abnormalities, LBBB	Measurement of cardiac enzymes
Tako-Tsubo cardiomyopathy	Similar to AMI, but commonly precipitated by emotional stress	Examination often normal; may have signs of HF	Anteroapical ST-segment elevation commonly with T-wave inversion	Cardiac enzymes only minimally elevated; anteroapical akinesis; normal coronary arteries
Aortic dissection	"Tearing" pain radiating to back	Diminished pulse or blood pressure in left arm	Nonspecific changes, LVH; ST-segment elevation if dissection involves coronary ostia	Chest X-ray, CT scan, or MRI; transesophageal echocardiography
Pulmonary embolism	Pleuritic chest pain with dyspnea and cough	Tachypnea; tachycardia; pleural rub; right ventricular heave	Sinus tachycardia with nonspecific ST and T-wave changes; $S_1Q_3T_3$ pattern classic, but rarely seen	CT angiogram; ventilation-perfusion lung scan; pulmonary angiogram
Pericarditis	Positional pain (worse lying flat)	Pericardial friction rub	Diffuse, concave ST-segment elevation with PR-segment depression	Echocardiogram

CT, computed tomography; CHF, congestive heart failure; ECG, electrocardiogram; LBBB, left bundle branch block; LVH, left ventricular hypertrophy MRI, magnetic resonance imaging.

conditions such as pneumothorax, pericarditis, aortic dissection, and cholecystitis (Table 187.1). Concomitant conditions, such as valvular heart disease, peripheral vascular disease, and cerebrovascular disease, may complicate patient management and can be rapidly detected by physical examination. A brief survey for signs of congestive heart failure (HF) should be performed. Cool extremities or impaired mental status suggests decreased tissue perfusion, whereas elevated jugular venous pressure and rales suggest elevated cardiac filling pressures. Finally, the hemodynamic and mechanical complications of acute MI can often be detected by careful attention to physical findings.

An important condition that may mimic acute MI is Tako-Tsubo cardiomyopathy (also called apical ballooning syndrome or stress cardiomyopathy). This syndrome, more common among elderly women, is typically precipitated by acute emotional distress or noncardiac medical illness. The chest pain associated with anteroapical ST-segment elevation and T-wave inversions is usually indistinguishable from an evolving anterior infarct. The diagnosis is typically made when normal coronary arteries and the distinctive anteroapical wall motion abnormality (Fig. 187.1) are seen at the time of emergent cardiac catheterization. In contrast to acute MI, cardiac enzymes usually elevate only modestly

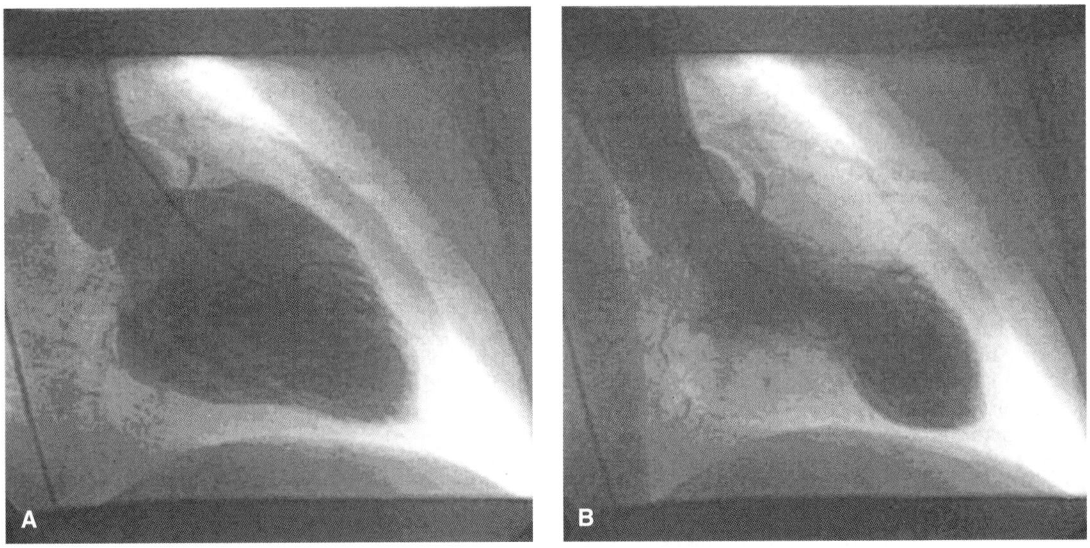

FIGURE 187.1 Representative contrast ventriculogram from a patient with Tako-Tsubo cardiomyopathy, demonstrating an anteroapical wall motion abnormality. The ventriculogram in Panel A was obtained at end diastole and in Panel B at end systole. (From the *Libyan J Med*, AOP: 070707, published July 19, 2007.)

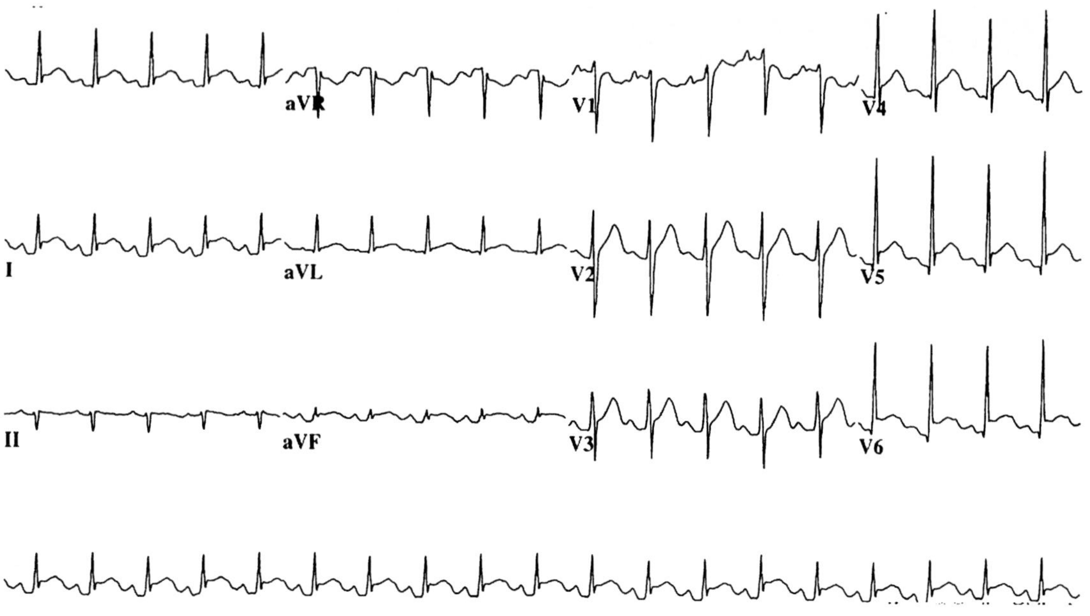

FIGURE 187.2 Electrocardiogram changes characteristic of pericarditis. Concave (upsloping) ST-segment elevation is seen diffusely, together with PR-segment depression. Importantly, T-waves are essentially normal, another distinguishing feature from ST elevation MI.

and the left ventricular (LV) functional abnormalities tend to be transient. The pathophysiology of this syndrome is considered to be caused by catecholamine-mediated myocardial stunning.

Electrocardiogram

Performance of the 12-lead ECG in the prehospital setting allows activation of a STEMI team prior to hospital arrival, significantly reducing time to reperfusion and leading to improved mortality [5]. The ST-segment elevation of acute MI must be distinguished from that caused by pericarditis or even the normal early repolarization variant. Ischemic ST-segment elevation typically has a convex configuration, is limited to selected ECG leads, and is often associated with reciprocal ST-segment depression (Table 187.1). Diagnostic criteria in the absence of left bundle branch block (LBBB) are based on ST-segment elevation at the J point in two contiguous leads $\geq$0.1 mV in all leads other than V_2–V_3. In V_2–V_3, $\geq$0.2 mV is required in men $\geq$40 years and $\geq$0.25 mV in men <40 years, or $\geq$0.15 mV in women. Reversible ischemic ST-segment elevation is also seen with coronary vasospasm (Prinzmetal's variant angina). Pericarditis, on the other hand, is typically associated with diffuse ST-segment elevation and depression of the PR segment (Fig. 187.2). The contour of the elevated ST segment in pericarditis and early repolarization variant is typically concave (upward sloping).

LBBB masks ischemic ST-segment elevation. A *new* (or presumed new) LBBB in a patient with ischemic chest discomfort suggests a large anterior infarction and is an indication for reperfusion therapy. It should be emphasized that an acute STEMI leading to LBBB requires a very large ischemic territory and would not be expected to be a subtle clinical event. Old LBBB and LBBB of unknown age present a diagnostic dilemma because most of these patients do not have ongoing transmural myocardial ischemia. The Sgarbossa ECG criteria are specific but very insensitive for masked STEMI [6,7]. Among patients not meeting Sgarbossa criteria, emergent echocardiography (to look for an anterior wall motion abnormality), rapid testing of cardiac biomarkers, and even emergent cardiac catheterization should be considered (Fig. 187.3) [7].

Cardiac Biomarkers and Other Tools for Risk Assessment

Cardiac biomarkers are much more important for the initial diagnosis of NSTEMI than for STEMI. For patients with STEMI, cardiac marker measurements are used to confirm the diagnosis in patients with equivocal electrocardiographic changes and may help to gauge prognosis. Patients with an elevated cardiac troponin or B-type natriuretic peptide level *prior* to initiation of reperfusion therapy are at higher risk for death and HF, even after accounting for baseline variables such as infarct location and time to treatment [8,9]. The peak levels of troponin, creatine kinase (CK), or creatine kinase myocardial band (CKMB) provide a crude estimation of infarct size. It should be noted that with successful reperfusion, although the total amount of biomarker released is reduced, the peak value may actually increase, with an earlier peak and more rapid fall in biomarker levels.

Information from the patient's clinical presentation and physical examination are also very valuable for assessing the patient's prognosis. Evidence for HF or hemodynamic stress (Killip Classification) at the time of presentation is weighted heavily in this assessment. For example, it is possible to use the patient's age and vital signs at presentation to rapidly and accurately obtain a preliminary estimate of short-term survival [10]. Anterior infarct location, delays to therapy, and information regarding medical comorbidity offer additional prognostic information [11]. As such, tools such as the Thrombolysis in Myocardial Infarction (TIMI) risk score and the Global Registry of Acute Coronary Events (GRACE) model that integrate age, the physical examination, the ECG, and other clinical parameters such as serum creatinine provide very strong discrimination of short- and long-term mortality risk, and should be implemented using simple bedside calculation [11,12], handheld devices, or web-based tools [13,14] (Fig. 187.4).

REPERFUSION THERAPY

Rapid provision of reperfusion therapy is the primary treatment objective in patients presenting with STEMI. Both primary percutaneous coronary intervention (PCI) and pharmacologic reperfusion are accepted reperfusion strategies, with primary

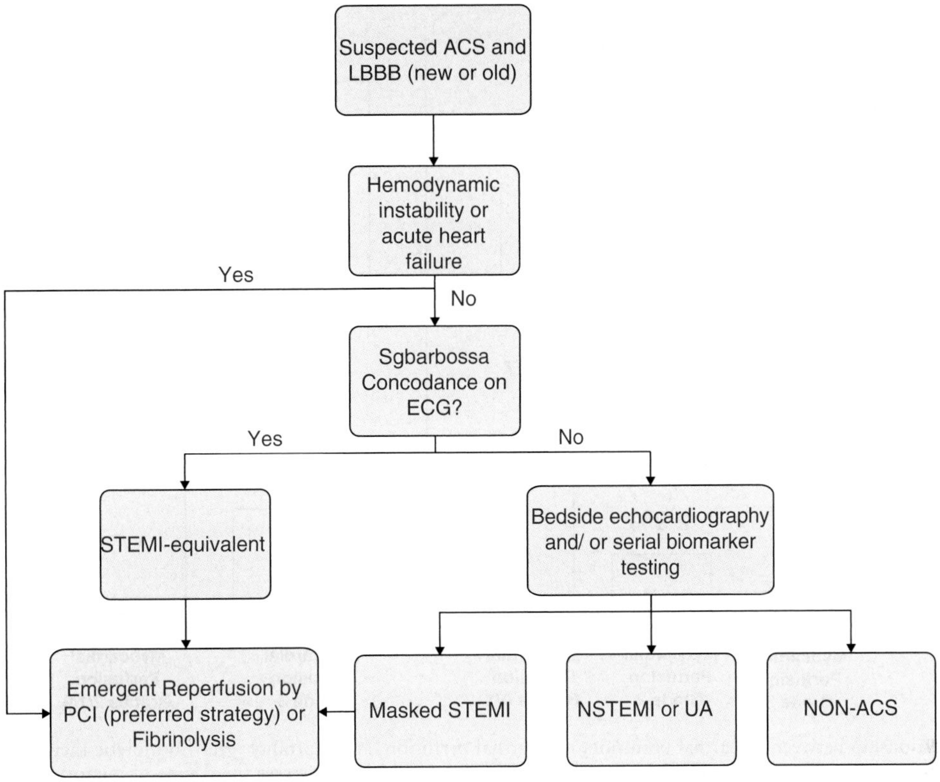

FIGURE 187.3 Proposed diagnostic algorithm for suspected myocardial infarction and LBBB. (Adapted from Neeland IJ, Kontos MC, de Lemos JA: Evolving considerations in the management of patients with left bundle branch block and suspected myocardial infarction. *J Am Coll Cardiol* 60(2):96–105, 2012).

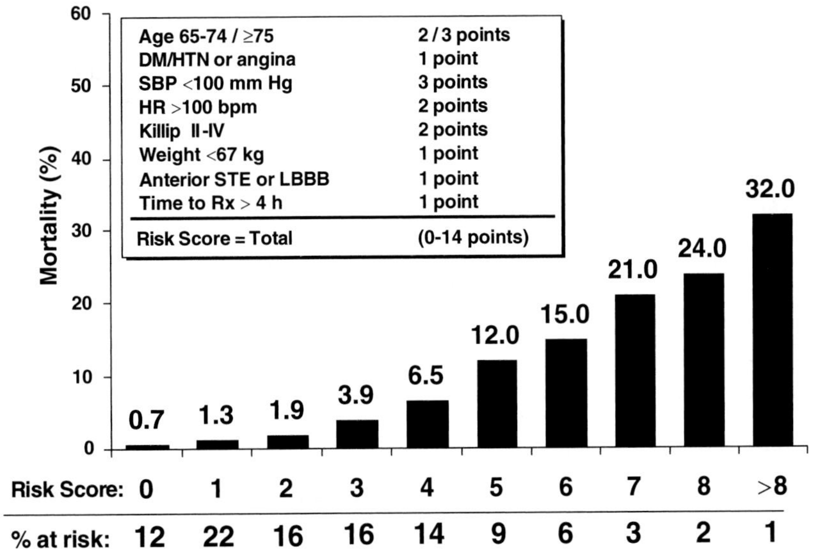

FIGURE 187.4 TIMI risk score for STEMI: a simple, bedside, clinical tool for predicting 30-day mortality. At the high end, a score of more than 5 identified 12% of patients with a mortality risk at least twofold higher than the mean for the population. In contrast, the 12% of patients with a risk score of zero had a mortality rate of less than 1%. Discriminating among the lower risk groups, nearly two-thirds of the population had risk scores of 0 to 3 with a 5.3-fold gradient in mortality over this range where smaller differences in absolute risk may have clinical impact. h/o, history of; HTN, hypertension; LBBB, left bundle branch block; STEMI, ST-segment elevation myocardial infarction; TIMI, thrombosis in myocardial infarction. (Adapted from Morrow DA, Antman EM, Charlesworth A, et al: TIMI risk score for ST-elevation myocardial infarction: a convenient, bedside, clinical score for risk assessment at presentation: an intravenous nPA for treatment of infarcting myocardium early II trial substudy. *Circulation* 102(17):2031–2037, 2000.)

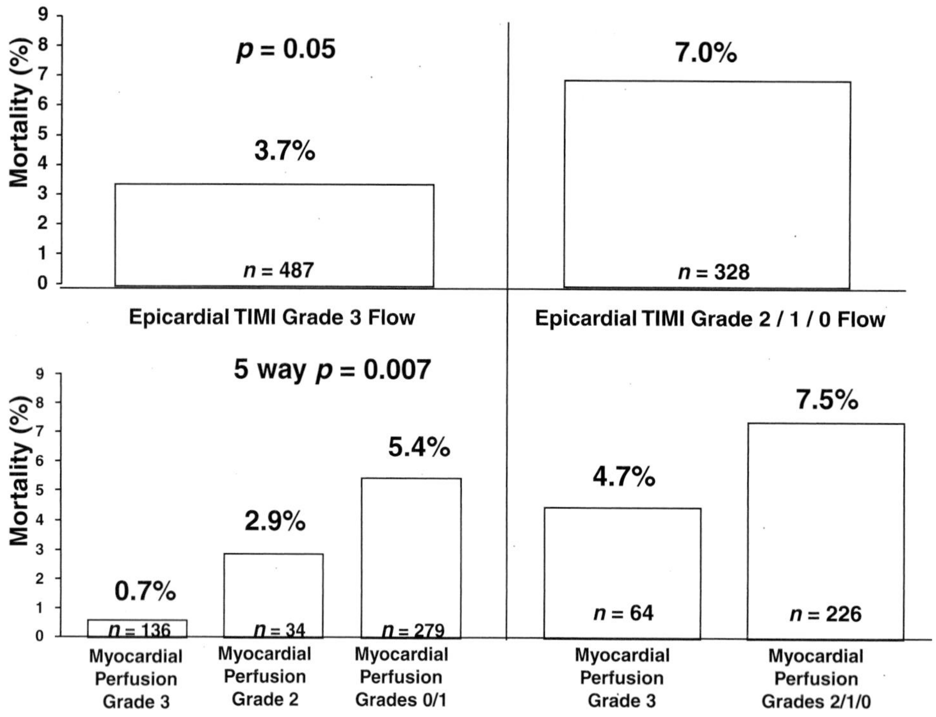

FIGURE 187.5 Relationship between epicardial perfusion, myocardial perfusion, and mortality after fibrinolytic therapy in the TIMI 10B trial. Myocardial perfusion was assessed using the TIMI Myocardial Perfusion Grade, which assesses the degree of microvascular "blush" seen on the routine coronary angiogram. This study found that myocardial perfusion was significantly associated with mortality independent of epicardial blood flow; using these two measures together provided incremental risk prediction. TIMI, thrombosis in myocardial infarction. (Adapted from Gibson CM, Cannon CP, Murphy SA, et al; for the TIMI Study Group: The relationship of the TIMI Myocardial Perfusion Grade to mortality after thrombolytic administration. *Circulation* 101:125–130, 2000.)

PCI being the preferred method of reperfusion when it can be performed in a timely manner by experienced operators.

What Constitutes "Optimal" Reperfusion?

Early successful coronary reperfusion limits infarct size and improves LV dysfunction and survival. These benefits are at least in part owing to the early restoration of antegrade flow in the infarct-related artery (IRA). In a retrospective analysis of six angiographic trials of different fibrinolytic regimens, patients who achieved normal (TIMI grade 3) antegrade flow in the IRA had a 30-day mortality rate of 3.6% versus 6.6% in patients with slow (TIMI grade 2) antegrade flow and 9.5% in patients with an occluded artery (TIMI grade 0 or 1 flow) [15].

With primary PCI, normal (TIMI grade 3) epicardial blood flow is achieved in >90% of STEMI patients, in contrast to ~50% with fibrinolytic therapy. However, even among patients who achieve TIMI grade 3 flow in the IRA after reperfusion therapy, tissue-level perfusion may be inadequate. Using a number of different diagnostic tools, investigators have demonstrated that measures of tissue and microvascular perfusion provide prognostic information that is independent of TIMI flow grade [16] (Fig. 187.5). For example, Ito and colleagues, using myocardial contrast echocardiography, found impaired tissue and microvascular perfusion in approximately one-third of patients with TIMI grade 3 blood flow after primary PCI: these patients were at increased risk for the development of HF and death [17]. Microvascular dysfunction is thought to occur in the setting of MI as a result of distal embolization of microthrombi, tissue inflammation from myocyte necrosis, and arteriolar spasm caused by tissue injury.

Perhaps the most clinically relevant measure of tissue perfusion is a simple bedside assessment of the degree of resolution of ST-segment elevation on the 12-lead ECG. Greater degrees of ST-segment resolution are associated with improved IRA epicardial blood flow [18]. Furthermore, patients who have normal epicardial blood flow, but persistence of ST-segment elevation on the 12-lead ECG after reperfusion, have abnormal tissue and microvascular perfusion [19,20], which leads to poor recovery of infarct zone wall motion and higher rates of death and HF [21]. As a result, ST-segment resolution appears to integrate epicardial and myocardial (microvascular) reperfusion, and as such may actually provide a more clinically useful assessment of reperfusion than coronary angiography [22].

Time to Reperfusion

Regardless of the choice of reperfusion strategy, several common themes are evident. First, the benefits of reperfusion therapy are time dependent. Patients who receive fibrinolytic therapy within 1 hour from the onset of chest pain have an approximately 50% reduction in mortality, whereas those presenting more than 12 hours after onset of symptoms derive little, if any, benefit. For each hour earlier that a patient is treated with a fibrinolytic, there is an absolute 1% decrease in mortality [23]. Similarly, for primary PCI, the "door-to-balloon" time has been shown to be directly correlated with clinical benefits [24].

Although performance metrics like door-to-balloon time have catalyzed important quality improvement efforts at the institutional level after initial presentation, broader initiatives at the systemic level aimed at reducing the *total ischemic time* (time from initial symptom onset to perfusion) have been equally important because total ischemic time is the principal determinant of outcome. To this end, both the American College of Cardiology (ACC) and American Heart Association (AHA) have established system-wide initiatives aimed at reducing

TABLE 187.2

Contemporary Components of Early STEMI Care

- Prehospital Care
  - EMS personnel perform 12-lead ECG at time of FMC
  - Activation of the catheterization laboratory prior to patient arrival
  - Transport directly to a PCI-capable hospital for primary PCI (if available) in <90 min
- ED
  - Emergency medicine physician activates the catheterization laboratory (if patient initially presents to ED at PCI-capable hospital)
  - A single call to a central page operator activates the PCI team
  - Immediate transfer to PCI-capable hospital for primary PCI if FMC-to-device time <120 min if patient arrives at non-PCI-capable hospital
  - Administer fibrinolytic therapy in <30 min at non-PCI-capable hospitals when anticipated FMC-to-device time at PCI capable hospital >120 min
- Cardiac catheterization laboratory
  - Expectation that staff will arrive in the catheterization laboratory within 20–30 min after being paged
- Real-time data feedback is provided to emergency department and the catheterization laboratory staff

ED, Emergency Department; EMS, emergency medical services FMC, first medical contact; PCI, percutaneous coronary intervention.

both in-hospital and prehospital system efficiency in order to reduce total ischemic time. For example, the ACC initiated the Door-to-balloon (D2B) Alliance as a quality initiative that utilizes strategies that discriminate between hospitals with short and long door-to-balloon times [25] to successfully reduce the majority of participating hospitals' door-to-balloon times to <90 minutes [26]. In a similar manner, the AHA established the "Mission:Lifeline" program to improve health system readiness and response to STEMI, with an emphasis on Emergency Medical System activation for primary PCI. These system-wide initiatives are paramount in reducing total ischemic time and subsequently improving outcomes in patients with STEMI (Table 187.2).

Fibrinolytic Therapy

The use of fibrinolytic therapy worldwide has decreased substantially. Nevertheless, fibrinolytic therapy remains the primary approach to reperfusion therapy for some countries and in a few regions in the United States where there is no access to timely primary PCI.

Placebo-controlled trials using streptokinase, anistreplase (APSAC), and recombinant tissue plasminogen activator (tPA [Alteplase]) established a clear benefit of fibrinolytic therapy for patients with STEMI. The Fibrinolytic Therapy Trialists' overview of all the large placebo-controlled studies reported a 2.6% absolute reduction in mortality for patients with STEMI treated within the first 12 hours after the onset of symptoms [23]. This benefit has been shown to persist through 10 years of follow-up. Highlights of differences in dosing, pharmacokinetics, recanalization rates, and cost between agents are shown in Table 187.3.

Several genetic alterations of tPA have led to prolonged half-life (to allow bolus administration), as well as increased fibrin specificity and resistance to endogenous inhibitors of plasminogen, such as PAI-1. Reteplase is a double-bolus agent whereas

TABLE 187.3

Fibrinolytic Agents

	Alteplase	Reteplase	Tenecteplase	Streptokinase
Fibrin selective	+++	++	++++	–
Half-life	5 min	14 min	17 min	20 min
Dose	15 mg bolus; then 0.75 mg/kg over 30 min; then 0.5 mg/kg over 60 min (max 100 mg total dose)	Two 10 unit bolus doses given 30 min apart	0.53 mg/kg as a single bolus	1.5 million units over 30–60 min
Weight adjusted	Partial	No	Yes	No
Adjunctive heparin	Yes	Yes	Yes	Probably
Possible allergy	No	No	No	Yes
TIMI grade 2 or 3 flow (90 min)	80%	80%	80%	60%
TIMI grade 3 flow (90 min)	55%–60%	60%	55% to 65%	32%
Efficacy vs. tPA	NA	Similar	Equivalent	1% ↑ mortality
Safety	NA	Similar	Similar ICH ↓ Non-ICH bleeding	↓ ICH ↓ Overall bleeding
Cost	+++	+++	+++	+

ICH, intracranial hemorrhage; tPA, Alteplase.

TABLE 187.4

Contraindications to Fibrinolytic Therapy

Absolute contraindications	Relative contraindications
Any prior intracranial hemorrhage	Blood pressure > 180/110[a]
Ischemic stroke within 3 mo	History of prior ischemic stroke >3 mo
Recent head trauma	Known bleeding diathesis
Known brain tumor	Proliferative diabetic retinopathy
Active internal bleeding	Prolonged CPR (>10 min
Suspected aortic dissection	Pregnancy
Intracranial or intraspinal surgery within 2 mo	Dementia
Significant closed head or facial trauma within 3 mo	Major surgery <3 wk
Severe uncontrolled hypertension (unresponsive to emergency therapy)	Chronic oral anticoagulation therapy
	Active peptic ulcer or recent internal bleeding

[a]Prior recommendations have considered only a *sustained* blood pressure >180/110 a relative contraindication; however, even a single blood pressure greater than this threshold is associated with an increased risk for intracranial hemorrhage.
CPR, cardiopulmonary resuscitation; TIA, transient ischemic attack.

tenecteplase is administered in a single weight-adjusted bolus. Bolus administration may minimize the risk for dosing errors, decrease "door-to-needle" time, and allow for prehospital administration.

Although the bolus fibrinolytic agents have not been demonstrated in placebo-controlled trials to reduce mortality or intracranial hemorrhage (ICH), they are easier to use and have largely replaced Alteplase for this reason in the United States. Tenecteplase appears to offer a modest advantage in safety over other agents and has emerged as a preferred fibrinolytic agent for patients not able to receive primary PCI.

Current Guidelines for Fibrinolysis

Fibrinolytic therapy is indicated as an option for reperfusion therapy in patients presenting within 12 hours of symptom onset if they have ST-segment elevation or new LBBB and no contraindications to lytic therapy (Table 187.4), and are unable to be transferred to a PCI-capable hospital for primary PCI within 120 minutes [27]. Patients who are older than 75 years of age, those who present more than 12 to 24 hours after the onset of acute MI, and those who are hypertensive but present with high-risk MI have a less favorable balance of risk and potential benefit, but may be considered for treatment with a fibrinolytic therapy when primary PCI is not available. Dose reduction has been suggested for elderly patients being treated with tenecteplase.

Limitations of Fibrinolytic Therapy

Current fibrinolytic regimens achieve patency (TIMI grade 2 or 3 flow) in approximately 80% of patients, but complete reperfusion (TIMI grade 3 flow) in only 50% to 60% of cases. In addition, as noted previously in this chapter, approximately one-third of patients with successful epicardial reperfusion have inadequate myocardial and microvascular reperfusion [17]. Finally, even after successful fibrinolysis, a 10% to 20% risk of reocclusion is present. Reocclusion and reinfarction are associated with a two- to threefold increase in mortality [28].

Bleeding is the most common complication of fibrinolytic therapy. Major hemorrhage occurs in 5% to 15% of patients. ICH is the most devastating of the bleeding complications, causing death in the majority of patients affected and almost universal disability in survivors. In major clinical trials, ICH has occurred in 0.5% to 0.9% of patients, but in clinical practice, where patient selection is less rigorous, rates are higher. Patients particularly at high risk of ICH include the elderly (particularly elderly females), patients with low body weight, and those who receive excessive doses of heparin.

Rescue Percutaneous Coronary Intervention

Because failure of fibrinolytic therapy is associated with high rates of morbidity and mortality, "rescue" PCI is frequently performed for such patients. Because tools to diagnose failed reperfusion are only modestly effective, and clinical trials evaluating rescue PCI have enrolled very slowly, data to support rescue PCI in patients with an occluded infarct artery are limited. In the MERLIN trial, 307 patients with ECG evidence of failed reperfusion (ST-segment resolution <50% measured 60 minutes after fibrinolytic therapy) were randomized to rescue PCI or conservative therapy. Rescue PCI was performed an average of approximately 90 minutes after the qualifying ECG and was associated with a 26% reduction in the composite endpoint of death, reinfarction, stroke, HF, and revascularization at 30 days. However, mortality was not significantly reduced. The most recent study performed was the REACT trial, in which 427 patients with ECG evidence of failed fibrinolysis at 90 minutes were randomized to repeat fibrinolysis, conservative treatment, or rescue PCI. Repeat fibrinolysis did not confer a benefit in this trial, but rescue PCI reduced the primary endpoint of death, reinfarction, stroke, or severe HF at 6 months by 53%. Mortality was also reduced from 12.8% for the conservative therapy arm to 6.2% in the rescue PCI arm. We recommend urgent catheterization and PCI for all patients with persistent ST-segment elevation and ongoing chest pain 90 minutes after the administration of reperfusion therapy, unless they are at particularly low risk for complications (i.e., a young patient with an uncomplicated inferior MI). For patients who are pain free, but in whom the ST segments remain elevated, urgent catheterization should also be strongly considered, particularly if the patient has high-risk features, such as older age, anterior location of infarction, diabetes, or prior CAD. Performance of routine PCI after fibrinolytic therapy will be discussed under "Pharmacoinvasive strategies."

Primary Percutaneous Coronary Intervention

Immediate or "primary" PCI has emerged as the clearly preferred reperfusion method for patients with STEMI. Randomized trials

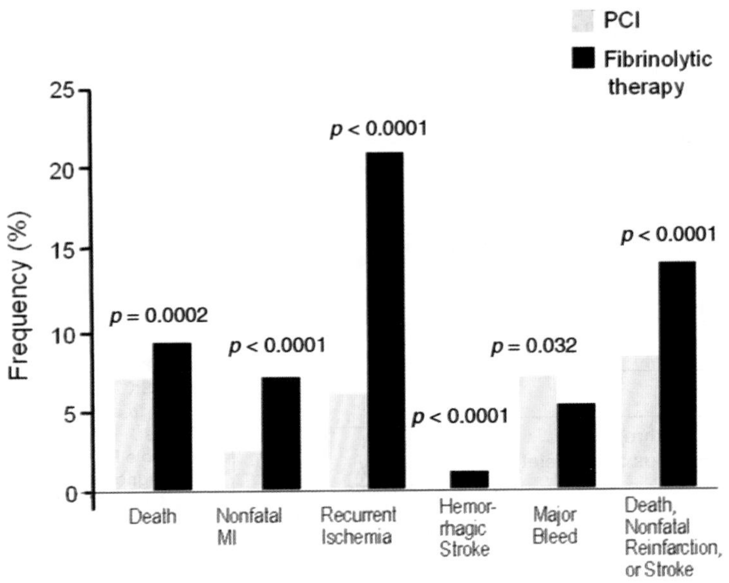

FIGURE 187.6 Short-term (4- to 6-week) outcomes from a meta-analysis of 23 randomized controlled trials comparing fibrinolytic therapy with primary percutaneous coronary intervention. (Adapted from Keeley EC, Boura JA, Grines CL: Primary angioplasty versus intravenous thrombolytic therapy for acute myocardial infarction: a quantitative review of 23 randomised trials. *Lancet* 361(9351):13–20, 2003.)

performed at both referral centers and experienced community hospitals have shown that primary PCI reduces the likelihood of death or MI when compared to fibrinolytic therapy [29]. Moreover, rates of major bleeding and stroke are also significantly lower with primary PCI than with fibrinolytic therapy (Fig. 187.6). The relative benefits of primary PCI are greatest in patients at highest risk, including those with cardiogenic shock, right ventricular infarction, large anterior MI, and increased age (partly owing to an increased ICH rate with fibrinolytic therapy). However, as with fibrinolytic therapy, rapid time to treatment is paramount to success [24]. In addition, although operator and institutional experience are critical to realize the full benefit of primary PCI, excellent results with primary PCI have been demonstrated in well-trained community hospitals without on-site cardiac surgery [30]. Current ACC/AHA guidelines recommend primary PCI of the infarct artery over fibrinolytic therapy when time-to-treatment delays are short and the patient presents to a high-volume, well-equipped center with experienced interventional cardiologists (ideal first medical contact (FMC)-to-device time <90 minutes at PCI-capable hospitals). When the FMC-to-device time is expected to be longer than 120 minutes, fibrinolysis is generally preferred for patients presenting within 12 hours of symptom onset unless contraindications are present (Fig. 187.7) [27].

Advances in PCI technology have been rapidly translated from elective to emergent PCI. Compared with primary percutaneous transluminal coronary angioplasty PTCA, primary stenting is associated with similar rates of death and reinfarction but lower subsequent target vessel revascularization rates [31,32]. Initial fears about stent thrombosis when drug-eluting stents (DES) were placed in the setting of STEMI have not been realized, and the advantages of DES over bare metal stents (BMS) with regard to in-stent restenosis and target vessel revascularization extend to patients with STEMI [33,34].

Nonetheless, current ACC/AHA guidelines recommend that BMS be used for patients in whom there is uncertainty regarding their ability to comply with prolonged dual-antiplatelet therapy (DAPT), whether related to bleeding risk or adherence concerns. However, recent data comparing BMS and newer generation everolimus-eluting stents (EES) show that EES have lower rates of stent thrombosis [35]. In addition, there is a growing body of evidence suggesting that shorter duration DAPT (<12 months) following DES placement is associated with fewer bleeding complications and acceptable rates of stent thrombosis [36]. Therefore, newer generation EES utilizing everolimus are generally preferred over BMS, even if prolonged DAPT use is uncertain. BMS may still be an acceptable option when these stents are not available, or if treatment with DAPT for at least 3 months is not possible.

Arterial Access

Vascular access bleeding is the most common complication after primary PCI for STEMI. One strategy that appears to decrease bleeding complications is the use of radial artery access. Among the 1,958 patients with STEMI in the Radial Versus Femoral Access for Coronary Angiography and Intervention in Patients with Acute Coronary Syndromes (RIVAL) trial [37], randomization to radial access was associated with a 40% reduction in the composite primary outcome of death, MI, stroke and non-coronary artery bypass graft (CABG)-related bleeding when compared with femoral access (heart rate [HR] 0.60, 95% confidence interval [CI] 0.38 to 0.94, $p = 0.026$). In a post hoc analysis of STEMI patients included in the RIVAL trial, there also appeared to be reduction in all-cause mortality with radial compared to femoral artery access (1.3% vs. 3.2%; HR 0.39; $p = 0.006$), a benefit not observed among the NSTEMI subgroup [38]. The Minimizing Adverse Hemorrhagic Events by TRansradial Access Site and Systemic Implementation of angioX (MATRIX) trial [39] was a randomized superiority trial comparing radial versus femoral access in 8,404 patients with acute coronary syndrome (48% with STEMI). Compared with femoral artery access, radial access was associated with less death, MI, and stroke (8.8% vs. 10.3%, relative risk (RR) 0.85; 95% CI 0.74 to 0.99; $p = 0.03$). All-cause mortality was also reduced (1.6% vs. 2.2%; RR 0.72; 95% CI 0.53 to 0.99; $p = 0.045$), consistent with results from the RIVAL trial. Based on these data, radial artery access is becoming the preferred route of vascular access for patients with STEMI in many parts of the world, with increasing use in the United States. Data from 593,094 procedures in the National Cardiovascular Data Registry (NCDR) showed that when compared to femoral artery access, radial artery access was associated with similar

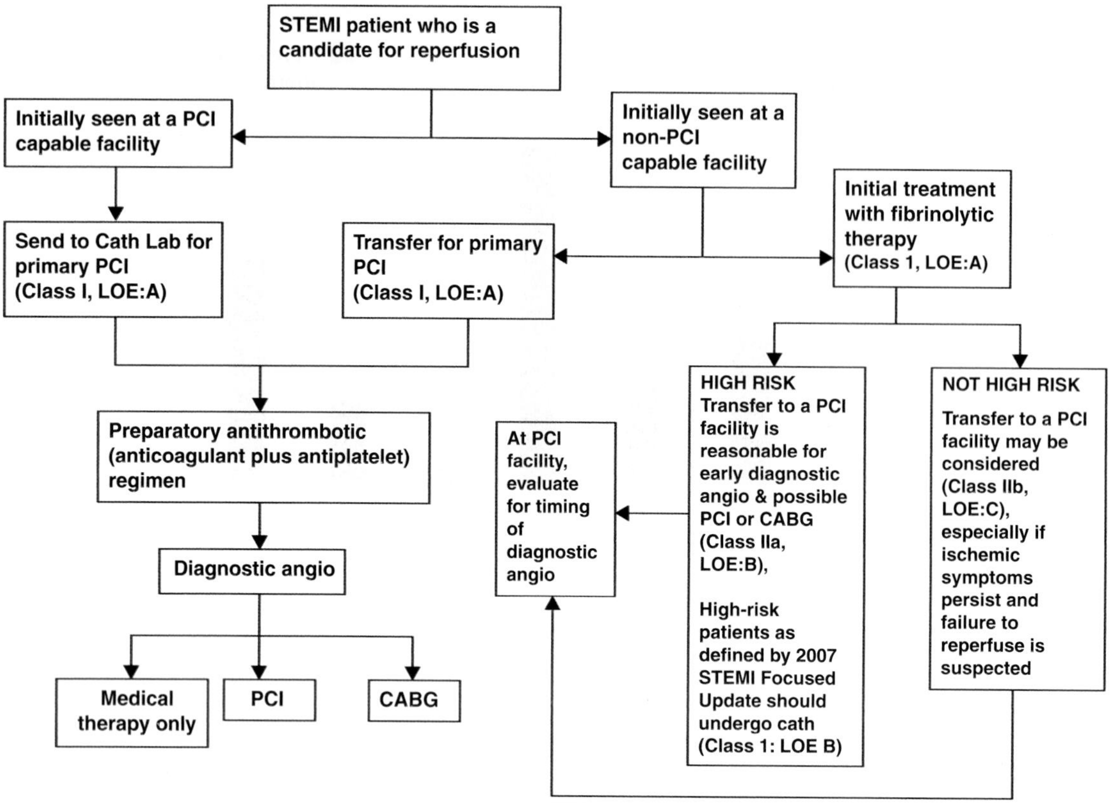

FIGURE 187.7 An algorithm for triage and transfer for primary percutaneous coronary intervention among patients with ST elevation myocardial infarction. (Adapted from O'Gara PT, Kushner FG, Ascheim DD, et al: 2013 ACCF/AHA guideline for the management of st-elevation myocardial infarction: a report of the American College of Cardiology Foundation/American Heart Association Task Force on Practice Guidelines. *Circulation* 127(4):e362–e425, 2013.)

procedural success (odds ratio [OR] 1.02, 95% CI 0.93 to 1.12) but significantly lower bleeding complications (OR 0.42, 95% CI 0.31 to 0.56) [40].

Multivessel CAD

Approximately 50% of patients presenting with STEMI have multivessel disease [41,42]. Percutaneous treatment options for patients with STEMI and multivessel CAD include culprit-vessel-only PCI, multivessel PCI performed at the time as primary PCI, or immediate culprit PCI with "staged" PCI of nonculprit vessels at a later time during the index hospitalization. Previous clinical practice guidelines recommended *against* PCI of a noninfarct artery at the time of primary PCI in hemodynamically stable patients (class III), based exclusively on observational data. However, recent small randomized controlled trials have led to a shift in practice recommendations. In the Preventative Angioplasty in Acute Myocardial Infarction trial that included 465 patients with STEMI and multivessel CAD, multivessel primary PCI was associated with a significant decrease in the composite primary outcome of cardiac death, nonfatal MI, or refractory angina when compared with culprit-artery-only PCI (9% vs. 22%, HR 0.35, 95% CI 0.21 to 0.58; $p < 0.001$), with directionally concordant changes in each element of the primary endpoint [43]. In the Complete Versus Culprit-Lesion Only Primary PCI trial, 296 patients with STEMI were randomized to culprit-only versus multivessel PCI, performed either during the index procedure or during the index hospitalization (72% performed during the index procedure). A significant reduction in the composite primary outcome of death, reinfarction, HF, and ischemic-driven revascularization was seen among patients randomized to multivessel PCI versus culprit-only PCI (10% vs. 21%, HR 0.49, 95% CI 0.24 to 0.84, $p = 0.009$) [44]. Based on these trials and data from other similar studies [45,46], the prior Class III (harm) recommendation was upgraded to a Class IIb recommendation with regard to the consideration of multivessel PCI in patients presenting with STEMI, either at the time of primary PCI or as a planned, staged procedure [47].

Thrombus Aspiration

Because of the large thrombus burden in STEMI, distal embolization at the time of PCI is common and may cause additional tissue and microvascular injury. Strategies to prevent distal embolization using embolic protection devices, which are commonly used when PCI is performed in saphenous vein grafts, cause delays in reperfusion and do not appear to improve outcomes when STEMI is caused by native vessel obstruction [48]. An alternative approach to decrease distal embolization is manual aspiration thrombectomy, which was previously supported by a class IIa recommendation [27], based on favorable results from a small trial [49]. However, several large and recent multicenter trials have prompted a shift in guideline recommendations. In the Thrombus Aspiration During ST-Segment Elevation Myocardial Infarction trial of 7,244 patients with STEMI, aspiration thrombectomy prior to primary PCI was not associated with improved short-term differences in death (2.8% vs. 3.0%, $p = 0.63$), reinfarction (0.5% vs. 0.9%, $p = 0.09$), stent thrombosis (0.2% vs. 0.5%, $p = 0.06$), or target vessel revascularization (1.8% vs. 2.2%, $p = 0.27$), when compared with primary PCI only [50]; these results were similar at 1 year follow-up [51]. In the Trial of Routine Aspiration Thrombectomy With PCI Versus PCI Alone in Patients with STEMI (TOTAL) trial, 10,732 patients with STEMI were randomized to either aspiration thrombectomy prior to primary PCI or primary PCI only. There were no significant differences between the two groups at 6 months with regard to the composite of cardiovascular death, recurrent MI, cardiogenic shock, or New York Heart Association Class IV HF (6.9% vs. 7.0%, $p = 0.86$) [52]. Collectively, these data have led to routine aspiration thrombectomy before primary PCI being downgraded from a class IIa recommendation to a class III recommendation [47]. It is unclear whether selective use or "bailout" thrombectomy in patients with large thrombus burden is beneficial (class IIb).

Transfer to Primary Percutaneous Coronary Intervention

Although primary PCI is the preferred reperfusion option for most patients who present to dedicated centers that can perform interventional procedures quickly and expertly, many patients with STEMI present to centers without primary PCI readily available. In such cases, a decision must be made as to whether immediate pharmacologic reperfusion therapy or transfer for primary PCI (if possible) is the best alternative. For patients transported to a non-PCI-capable hospital in whom a rapid transfer is possible (time from FMC-to-device system time <120 minutes or less), transfer for primary PCI is preferable (Fig. 187.7) [28]. Unfortunately, data from the AHA Mission:Lifeline Program between 2008 and 2012 showed 35% of STEMI patients transferred for primary PCI failed to achieve FMC-to-device time of <120 minutes [53]. Independent predictors of delay in this population included patient comorbidities (cardiogenic shock, cardiac arrest), process variables (prolonged door-in door-out time, rural hospital locations), and lower PCI hospital annual STEMI volumes. These data reemphasize the importance of ongoing efforts to improve access to rapid care in patients with STEMI. For patients with contraindications to fibrinolytic therapy, evidence of failed fibrinolytic therapy, cardiogenic shock, presentation more than 12 hours after symptom onset, or transfer to a center that can perform emergent PCI is indicated, even if delay times are longer [27].

Several studies have compared various strategies of routine transfer for primary PCI of patients eligible for fibrinolytic therapy versus immediate fibrinolysis with or without transfer. Although these studies have reported a lower incidence of adverse cardiac events among those randomized to transfer for primary PCI [54,55], generalizability of the results has been questioned because the very rapid transfer times in these studies are significantly shorter than those typically occur in the United States [56] and the rates of referral for rescue PCI were unusually low in these trials.

Subsequent analyses have helped to define the influence of symptom duration and transfer-related time delay on the benefits of transfer for primary PCI. For example, among the 850 patients enrolled in the PRAGUE-2 study, there was a significant and quantitatively large reduction in mortality (6.0% vs. 15.3%; $p < 0.02$) among those who were randomized more than 3 hours after symptom onset. In contrast, there was no reduction in mortality among patients presenting within 3 hours [57]. Similar findings were observed in the Comparison of Angioplasty and Prehospital Thrombolysis in Acute Myocardial Infarction (CAPTIM) trial in which the control arm received prehospital fibrinolytic [58]. A meta-analysis of randomized studies has suggested that if the delay between immediate administration of a fibrinolytic and initiation of PCI is more than 1 hour, the pharmacological therapy becomes favored with respect to survival [59]. These data form the basis of the recommendation in the AHA/ACC guidelines that fibrinolysis, in the absence of contraindications, should be used in patients with STEMI and ischemic symptom onset <12 hours when it is anticipated that primary PCI cannot be performed within 120 minutes of FMC [27].

Pharmacoinvasive Strategies

In light of the deleterious impact of delays to primary PCI on myocardial salvage, an approach in which reperfusion is initiated with a pharmacological regimen and followed by angiography and PCI is potentially attractive, particularly for patients being transferred for primary PCI who are anticipated to have longer FMC device times. In the modern era, it is clear that PCI can be performed effectively and safely early after fibrinolytic therapy [60]. In addition, it is well known that patients who arrive in the catheterization laboratory with a patent IRA prior to "primary" PCI, owing to either spontaneous lysis or pharmacologic reperfusion, have an extraordinarily low risk of mortality [61].

The term "facilitated" PCI has been coined to signify the administration of a pharmacological reperfusion regimen en route to the cardiac catheterization laboratory for a planned "primary" PCI. A number of different pharmacological pretreatment regimens have been proposed, including fibrinolytic agents alone (at full or reduced dose), combinations of GP IIb/IIIa inhibitors and reduced-dose fibrinolytics, or GP IIb/IIIa inhibitors alone. Clinical trial results regarding facilitated PCI using regimens that contain a fibrinolytic have been disappointing: although surrogate measures of early reperfusion are enhanced, no favorable efficacy outcomes have been observed and bleeding rates are clearly increased [62,63]. Moreover, the usefulness of administration of a GP IIb/IIIa inhibitor alone prior to the arrival in the catheterization laboratory is uncertain [27,63].

An alternative pharmacoinvasive strategy that may be logistically attractive for patients presenting to non-PCI centers is to perform initial pharmacologic reperfusion therapy followed by transfer for routine *nonemergent* coronary angiography and revascularization if needed. This pathway has shown favorable results in several relatively small studies [64–66] and the larger Trial of Routine Angioplasty and Stenting after Fibrinolysis to Enhance Reperfusion in Acute Myocardial Infarction (TRANSFER-AMI) trial [67]. In TRANSFER-AMI, 1,059 high-risk patients with STEMI presenting to hospitals without PCI capability received pharmacological reperfusion with a regimen that contained tenecteplase and were randomized to standard treatment on site or to immediate transfer and PCI within 6 hours after fibrinolysis. Interestingly, most patients in the standard treatment arm underwent coronary angiography, but this was performed approximately 1 day later than in the transfer arm. The primary endpoint of death, MI, recurrent ischemia, HF, or cardiogenic shock within 30 days was reduced from 17.2% in the standard treatment arm to 11.0% in the early PCI arm (HR 0.64; $p = 0.004$). For patients who present to hospitals without PCI capability and in whom the door-to-balloon time is expected to be longer than 90 minutes, these data support a strategy of "drip and ship," in which standard pharmacological reperfusion therapy is administered and the patient transferred for subsequent catheterization and PCI. The timing of the catheterization and PCI remains controversial. Data from studies of facilitated PCI suggest that very early PCI (i.e., within 2 hours) is not helpful and may be harmful. However, the accumulated data described previously suggest favorable outcomes if the PCI is performed between 3 and 24 hours after successful fibrinolytic therapy. Current ACC/AHA guidelines provide a class IIa recommendation for coronary angiography in STEMI patients treated with fibrinolytic therapy, either as soon as logistically possible (in the case of suspected failed reperfusion) or between 3 and 24 hours after successful reperfusion with fibrinolytic therapy [27].

STEMI and Out-of-hospital Cardiac Arrest

Sudden cardiac death caused by cardiac arrest accounts for the majority of coronary heart disease deaths annually in the United States [68]. Although only 23% of out-of-hospital cardiac arrest cases have a shockable initial rhythm, the majority of neurologically intact survivors arise from this subgroup [28]. Two randomized controlled trials showed improved rates of neurologically intact survival of comatose patients presenting with out-of-hospital ventricular fibrillation (VF) or pulseless ventricular tachycardia (VT), who are cooled to between 32°C and 34°C for 12 and 24 hours on presentation. However, the ideal temperature target to best improve clinical outcomes remains unclear. A randomized control trial comparing targeted temperature management to 33°C versus 36°C for patients surviving out-of-hospital cardiac arrest observed no significant differences in death or poor neurologic function at 6 months (54% vs. 52%, $p = 0.78$) [69], suggesting that perhaps preventing hyperthermia may be a more important treatment goal than achieving hypothermia. Current professional society recommendations advise that patients with STEMI and out-of-hospital cardiac arrest should receive targeted temperature management before or at the time of cardiac catheterization [28]. Observational studies indicate that reasonable clinical outcomes can be expected for comatose patients after cardiac arrest who have diagnostic ST-elevation and undergo primary PCI. Neither the presenting cardiac arrest nor initiation of targeted temperature management should delay or deter primary PCI in patients with STEMI.

ADJUNCTIVE ANTIPLATELET AND ANTITHROMBOTIC THERAPY

Aspirin and $P2Y_{12}$ Inhibitors

For patients with STEMI, aspirin decreases reocclusion and reinfarction rates by nearly 50% and mortality by approximately 25% [70]. The benefits of aspirin are comparable to those of fibrinolytic therapy, and when used together, aspirin and fibrinolytic therapy provide additive benefits [71]. Aspirin should be initiated at an oral dose of 162 to 325 mg (preferably chewed) at the time the patient is first encountered by medical personnel in the field or emergency department. Following MI, lifelong therapy with aspirin is indicated to prevent recurrent cardiac events. Efficacy appears to be similar at all doses greater than 75 mg, whereas bleeding risk clearly increases with higher aspirin dose. However, despite increased bleeding risk, evidence from the NCDR from 2007 to 2011 shows the majority of acute coronary syndrome patients in the United States are discharged on high-dose aspirin [72]. Following the initial higher dose (162 to 325 mg) administered acutely in STEMI, the authors strongly favor an 81-mg dose of aspirin over higher dosages for long-term secondary prevention for all patients with STEMI [27,73].

In addition to aspirin, a second antiplatelet agent should be added for the acute management and secondary prevention in patients with STEMI. In particular, a series of trials established the benefits of inhibiting the binding of ADP to the $P2Y_{12}$ receptor on the platelet surface, thereby decreasing platelet activation and aggregation. Clopidogrel is a thienopyridine derivative that is a $P2Y_{12}$ antagonist. The Clopidogrel as Adjunctive Reperfusion Therapy-Thrombolysis in Myocardial Infarction 28 (CLARITY-TIMI 28) trial compared clopidogrel (300-mg loading dose followed by 75 mg per day) with placebo in 3,491 patients with STEMI who were treated with standard pharmacological reperfusion including fibrinolytic therapy, aspirin, and heparin. The primary composite endpoint of death, MI, or an occluded IRA assessed at the time of protocol-mandated angiography (average 3 to 4 days) was reduced from 21.7% in the placebo arm to 15.0% in the clopidogrel arm ($p < 0.001$). At 30 days, the clinical composite of death, MI, or urgent revascularization was reduced by 20% ($p = 0.03$) [74]. The much larger Clopidogrel and Metoprolol in Myocardial Infarction Trial (COMMIT) trial was performed in more than 45,000 patients in China and was designed to evaluate the impact of adjunctive clopidogrel (administered at 75 mg per day without a loading dose) on death and major clinical events. Clopidogrel reduced death, reinfarction, or stroke by 9% and death alone by 7%, both of which were statistically significant [75]. Based on the results of these two trials, clopidogrel should now routinely be added to standard fibrinolytic regimens in patients younger than 75 years [27].

For patients undergoing primary PCI, similarly, an oral $P2Y_{12}$ receptor antagonist should be administered in addition to aspirin: a loading dose followed by a *minimum* of 12 months of maintenance therapy is recommended for patients with STEMI receiving a stent (BMS or DES) [27]. Presently available alternatives include clopidogrel, prasugrel, and ticagrelor.

If clopidogrel is used, a loading dose of 600 mg is preferred and should be given as early as possible before or at the time of PCI [27]. In the CURRENT/OASIS 7 trial, which compared high-dose (600-mg loading dose, 150 mg per day for 7 days, and then 75 mg per day) with standard-dose (300-mg loading dose and then 75 mg per day) clopidogrel, the higher dose clopidogrel strategy was associated with a lower rate of cardiovascular death, MI, or stroke at 30 days and a lower rate of stent thrombosis (4.0% vs. 2.8%) among the subgroup with STEMI ($n = 6{,}346$). The higher dose clopidogrel regimen was also associated with a higher rate of major bleeding (1.1% vs. 1.6%; $p = 0.006$) [76].

Prasugrel is a second-generation thienopyridine that is more rapidly acting, more potent, and associated with less response variability than clopidogrel. The Trial to Assess Improvement in Therapeutic Outcomes by Optimizing Platelet Inhibition with Prasugrel-Thrombolysis in Myocardial Infarction (TRITON-TIMI) 38 trial [77] enrolled 13,608 patients with acute coronary syndrome who were scheduled to undergo PCI. Patients were randomized to prasugrel (60-mg loading dose and then 10 mg per day) or clopidogrel (300-mg loading dose and then 75 mg per day): both the drugs were initiated at the time of PCI with no pretreatment given. In the subgroup of patients with STEMI ($n = 3{,}534$), the primary efficacy endpoint of CV death, MI, and stroke at a median of 14.5 months was reduced from 12.4% in the clopidogrel arm to 10.0% in the prasugrel arm (HR 0.79; $p = 0.02$; Table 187.5). Stent thrombosis occurred in 2.8% STEMI patients randomized to clopidogrel versus 1.6% randomized to prasugrel ($p = 0.008$). Importantly, in the STEMI subgroup, no significant differences were noted in non-CABG bleeding between treatment arms. Prasugrel was associated with net harm among patients with prior stroke or transient ischemic attack (largely caused by an excess in ICH) and is contraindicated in such patients. In addition, there were two important subgroups in whom prasugrel was associated with excess bleeding that nullified clinical benefit, including patients >75 years of age and those <60 kg [77].

Ticagrelor is a direct acting and *reversible* non-thienopyridine oral $P2Y_{12}$ antagonist. This agent provides more rapid onset (and offset) of action and a more potent and predictable antiplatelet response than clopidogrel. It does not require activation by the cytochrome p450 system. In the Study of Platelet Inhibition and Patient Outcomes (PLATO) trial [78], ticagrelor (180-mg loading dose, 90 mg twice daily) was compared with clopidogrel (300- to 600-mg loading dose, 75 mg daily) in 18,624 patients with ACS, 38% of whom had STEMI. At the end of the 12-month follow-up period, the primary endpoint of CV death, MI, and stroke occurred in 11.7% of subjects in the clopidogrel arm versus 9.8% in the ticagrelor arm (HR 0.84; 95% CI 0.77 to 0.92; $p < 0.001$). The risk reduction was similar in the STEMI subgroup (HR 0.84; 95% CI 0.72 to 0.98; Table 187.5). Similar to the findings in the CURRENT/OASIS 7 and TRITON-TIMI 38 trials, stent thrombosis was reduced significantly with the more potent oral antiplatelet regimen. Also consistent with prior studies, ticagrelor increased non-CABG major bleeding (4.5% vs. 3.8%, $p = 0.03$) [78]. Notably, in the PLATO trial,

TABLE 187.5

Comparison of Novel P2Y12 Inhibitors with Clopidogrel: Results from Subgroups with STEMI

	TRITON-TIMI 38			PLATO		
	N = 3,534			N = 7,026		
Endpoint	Prasugrel (%)	Clopidogrel (%)	HR (95% CI)	Ticagrelor (%)	Clopidogrel (%)	HR (95% CI)
CV death, MI, stroke	10.0	12.4	0.79 (0.65–0.97)	8.5	10.1	0.84 (0.72–0.98)
Stent thrombosis[a]	1.6	2.8	0.58 (0.36–0.93)	2.2	2.9	0.75 (0.59–0.95)
Non-CABG TIMI major bleeding[a,b]	2.4	2.1	1.11 (0.70–1.77)	4.5	3.8	1.19 (1.02–1.38)

Note that endpoint assessment was at 15 months in TRITON-TIMI 38 and 12 months in PLATO.
[a]The stent thrombosis and bleeding results from PLATO are from the entire study because the specific data for STEMI have not yet been reported.
[b]TIMI major bleeding (non-CABG) was the primary bleeding endpoint in TRITON-TIMI 38 and was an additional bleeding endpoint in PLATO.
STEMI, ST-segment elevation myocardial infarction; MI, myocardial infarction.

treatment with ticagrelor resulted in a significant 21% relative risk reduction in vascular mortality and a 22% reduction in total mortality (5.9% vs. 4.5%; $p < 0.001$). This mortality reduction was unique to PLATO among the trials of $P2Y_{12}$ antagonists.

Ticagrelor has side effects that are likely mediated by increases in circulating adenosine. Dyspnea occurs in 10% to 15% of patients early after treatment initiation, is not associated with HF, and is usually transient. Ventricular pauses may also be triggered by ticagrelor early after treatment initiation, but these pauses also decrease in frequency over time, are rarely symptomatic, and have not required an excess of clinical intervention. Because of these side effects, the clinician should be aware of a history of reactive airway disease or significant ECG conduction abnormalities when considering ticagrelor.

The onset of action of oral $P2Y_{12}$ inhibitors may be delayed among patients with STEMI; possibly owing to reduced gut perfusion that is common early after presentation. Morphine administration also appears to reduce absorption of $P2Y_{12}$ inhibitors and contribute to delayed onset of action [79–81]. Cangrelor is a novel intravenous, fast-acting, and reversible $P2Y_{12}$ inhibitor that may offer an alternative strategy for patients to achieve rapid $P2Y_{12}$ inhibition. However, the available data are limited to comparisons with clopidogrel and do not provide strong support for a favorable risk/benefit profile of this drug in STEMI [82]. Given the high cost, at the present time, we generally limit cangrelor use to patients unable to take oral $P2Y_{12}$ inhibitors.

GP IIb/IIIa Inhibitors

Although use of GP IIb/IIIa inhibitors in elective PCI has been decreasing, these agents remain useful adjuncts to primary PCI for patients with STEMI when heparin is the anticoagulant used. In a meta-analysis involving 3,266 patients enrolled in four randomized trials comparing abciximab with placebo, patients receiving abciximab had a 46% reduction in 30-day death, reinfarction, and urgent target vessel revascularization compared to those who received placebo [83]. Fewer data are available for the other GP IIb/IIIa inhibitors (tirofiban and eptifibatide) in the primary PCI setting. Moreover, data are very limited in the current era of more potent and rapidly acting $P2Y_{12}$ inhibitors. Current ACC/AHA guidelines recommend selective use of GP IIb/IIIa inhibitors at the time of primary PCI (class IIa recommendation) for selected patients who are receiving unfractionated heparin [27].

Antithrombin Therapies in Patients Receiving Fibrinolytic Therapy

The AHA/ACC guidelines recommend administration of an anticoagulant (unfractionated heparin (UFH), enoxaparin, or fondaparinux) as adjunctive therapy in all patients receiving pharmacologic reperfusion therapy with the fibrin-specific agents alteplase, reteplase, or tenecteplase. For UFH, recommended dosing is a 60 U per kg bolus (maximum bolus of 4,000 U) plus an initial infusion of 12 U/kg/h (with a maximum initial infusion rate of 1,000 U per hour) for up to 48 hours. Low molecular weight heparins (LMWHs) represent an attractive alternative to UFH for patients receiving fibrinolytic therapy. In the Enoxaparin and Thrombolysis Reperfusion for Acute Myocardial Infarction Treatment - Thrombolysis in Myocardial Infarction (ExTRACT-TIMI) 25 trial [84], which randomized 20,506 patients treated with fibrinolytic therapy to intravenous UFH for 48 hours or enoxaparin through hospital discharge, the primary endpoint of death or reinfarction was reduced from 12.0% in the UFH arm to 9.9% in the enoxaparin arm (RR 0.83; $p < 0.001$). Major bleeding occurred in 1.4% of UFH-treated patients versus 2.1% of those treated with enoxaparin ($p < 0.001$), but there was no significant difference in ICH, and the net clinical benefit (death/MI/major bleeding) favored enoxaparin. The direct antithrombin agents have also been extensively studied as adjuncts to fibrinolytic therapy but appear to offer no significant advantage over UFH when given with any of the currently available fibrinolytic agents [85–87]. Thus, of the currently available antithrombin agents, LMWH administered for the duration of the hospitalization (up to 8 days, or until PCI) has been shown to be superior to short-term use of UFH and represents the most attractive strategy for patients managed with a fibrinolytic.

Antithrombin Therapy as an Adjunct to Primary PCI

Intravenous UFH, with or without a GP IIb/IIIa receptor antagonist, and titrated to an appropriate activated clotting time, has been a cornerstone adjunctive therapy for patients with STEMI undergoing primary PCI. Multiple studies have compared bivalirudin, a direct-acting antithrombin, as alternative to UFH in this setting. In the Harmonizing Outcomes with Revascularization and Stents in Acute Myocardial Infarction (HORIZONS-AMI) trial [88], 3,602 patients undergoing primary PCI for STEMI were randomized to standard care with heparin plus a GP IIb/IIIa inhibitor or to bivalirudin alone. The primary outcome, which was a composite of efficacy and safety endpoints at 30 days, was significantly lower in the bivalirudin versus heparin/GP IIb/IIIa inhibitor arm (9.2% vs. 12.1%; RR 0.76; $p = 0.005$). This was mediated by lower rate of major bleeding with bivalirudin (4.9% vs. 8.3%; RR 0.60; $p < 0.001$) and similar rates of the ischemic outcomes. Total mortality (2.1% vs. 3.1%; $p = 0.05$) and cardiac mortality (1.8% vs. 2.9%; $p = 0.03$) trended lower in the bivalirudin arm. An issue of concern was an increased risk of stent thrombosis within the first 24 hours in the bivalirudin group. Subsequent studies confirmed lower rates of bleeding but higher rates of stent thrombosis with bivalirudin compared with UFH plus GP IIb/IIIa inhibitor therapy and did not substantiate the reduction in all-cause mortality [89].

An important limitation of these trials is that they all compared bivalirudin versus UFH *plus* a GP IIb/IIIa inhibitor, which may have contributed to the higher risk of bleeding with UFH rather than to UFH alone. This limitation is of particular relevance, given the declining use of GP IIb/IIIa inhibitors in contemporary STEMI treatment. The Unfractionated heparin versus bivalirudin in primary percutaneous coronary intervention (HEAT-PPCI) trial randomized 1,829 patients undergoing primary PCI for STEMI to either heparin or bivalirudin [90]. Importantly, the use of GP IIb/IIIa inhibitor use was similar in each arm (13% and 15%, respectively), and over 90% of patients were treated with either prasugrel or ticagrelor. Patients randomized to bivalirudin were more likely to have stent thrombosis (3.4% vs. 0.9%, RR 3.91, 95% CI 1.61 to 9.52), as well as a numerically greater (but not statistically significant) trend in the composite primary outcome of all-cause mortality, stroke, reinfarction, or revascularization (8.7% vs. 5.7%, RR 1.52, 95% CI 0.9 to 2.13; Fig.187.8). Interestingly, there was no significant difference in bleeding between the two treatment groups, likely related to lower dosages of heparin used compared with prior studies, balanced and low rates of GP IIb/IIIa inhibitor use in both arms, as well as significant utilization of radial artery access (~80%).

These findings highlight the conflicting data regarding the optimal antithrombin regimen for patients with STEMI. A meta-analysis including 16 randomized control trials comparing bivalirudin with heparin found that bivalirudin use was associated with increased risk of MI and stent thrombosis, but a decreased risk of bleeding, with the magnitude of the bleeding reduction dependent on concomitant GP IIb/IIIa use [91]. However, comparisons of trials are difficult owing to varying dosages of heparin and GP II/IIIa inhibitor use, as well as radial versus femoral access use. In our opinion, given its markedly lower cost, UFH should be the anticoagulant of choice for primary PCI for STEMI, with bivalirudin restricted to patients at high risk for bleeding in whom radial access is not utilized.

Warfarin/Oral Anticoagulation

In the era of DAPT, the use of warfarin, either alone or in combination with DAPT, must be weighed carefully. The availability of $P2Y_{12}$ inhibitors has virtually eliminated the past reliance on warfarin for aspirin-allergic patients. However, because warfarin is superior to aspirin in preventing systemic emboli in patient with atrial fibrillation, and reduces systemic emboli in patients with documented LV dysfunction following MI, there are some circumstances warranting consideration of warfarin use, particularly when the risk of thromboembolism exceeds the risk of bleeding. Current ACC/AHA guidelines support warfarin use in addition to DAPT for patients who have mechanical heart valves, recent venous thromboembolism, hypercoagulable disorders, or atrial fibrillation with an elevated stroke risk (class I). Warfarin use is also reasonable for STEMI patients with asymptomatic LV mural thrombi (class IIa), and perhaps for some STEMI patients with anterior apical akinesis (class IIb) [27]. For patients with or at risk for LV thrombus, the duration of warfarin use can be limited to 3 months. It should be noted that the newer direct oral anticoagulants have not been evaluated in this clinical context, so their use cannot be recommended.

An increasingly challenging scenario relates to the combination of aspirin, a $P2Y_{12}$ inhibitor, and warfarin. "Triple therapy" is associated with substantially increased risks for bleeding. In a registry analysis of 480 patients, triple therapy was associated with a 50% increase in bleeding compared to DAPT alone [92]. It may be expected that risks will be even higher with combinations that include the newer and more potent antiplatelet agents such as prasugrel and ticagrelor. As such, we recommend attempting to avoid altogether or to minimize the duration of triple therapy. Consideration should be given to using BMS instead of DES, which would allow the duration of clopidogrel to be reduced to 1 month. For patients who require triple therapy, the international normalized ratio (INR) should be maintained at the lowest end of the therapeutic range (2.0 to 2.5), aspirin dose should be 81 mg, and GI prophylaxis with a proton pump inhibitor (other than omeprazole if possible) should be considered. For patients with atrial fibrillation, a reevaluation of the risks of bleeding and stroke (using a tool such as the $CHADS_2$-VASCscore) should be performed and the threshold to initiate or continue warfarin may be higher among patients on aspirin and $P2Y_{12}$ inhibitor [93].

Another strategy being evaluated is withdrawal of the aspirin component of triple therapy. In the What is the Optimal antiplatElet and Anticoagulant Therapy in Patients With Oral Anticoagulation and Coronary StenTing (WOEST) trial [94], 573 patients on oral anticoagulation and undergoing PCI were randomized to warfarin + clopidogrel alone versus warfarin + clopidogrel plus aspirin (triple therapy). Patients treated with warfarin + clopidogrel had significantly fewer bleeding episodes when compared with those patients treated with triple therapy (HR 0.36, 95% CI 0.26 to 0.50; $p < 0.0001$). Surprisingly, the group randomized to withhold aspirin also had markedly lower rates of all-cause mortality than the triple therapy group (2.5% vs. 6.3%, $p = 0.03$). However, owing to the small size of the study, and because most patients enrolled did not have ACS, it is difficult to extrapolate these results to patients with STEMI. Ongoing research efforts continue to search for the optimal risk/benefit profile in this complex patient population.

ANTI-ISCHEMIC THERAPY

β-Blockers

β-blockers were among the first therapeutic interventions used to limit the size of acute MI. Previous trials that excluded patients with HF, hypotension, or bradycardia demonstrated that very early administration of a β-blocker decreases infarct size and prevents recurrent MI and death [95]. The fact that β-blockers were particularly effective in reducing sudden death and reducing mortality among patients with complex ventricular ectopy at baseline suggests that β-blockers exert much of their beneficial effect by reducing the frequency and severity of arrhythmias [96]. In addition, they appear to significantly decrease the risk of cardiac rupture. Data from the COMMIT trial in more than 45,000 patients, however, failed to demonstrate benefit from a strategy of immediate intravenous metoprolol followed by 200 mg metoprolol daily on in-hospital outcomes, including death and MI. Although early β blockade reduced the risks of reinfarction and VF compared to placebo, this was counterbalanced by an increased risk of cardiogenic shock during the first few days after admission [97]. Post hoc analyses indicate that this increased risk was predominantly among patients with indicators of or risk factors for hemodynamic compromise. In addition, the outcome may have been influenced by the high dose of metoprolol used in this study. ACC/AHA guidelines now recommended that β-blockers be initiated orally, within the first 24 hours, once it has been determined that the hemodynamic status is stable and there is

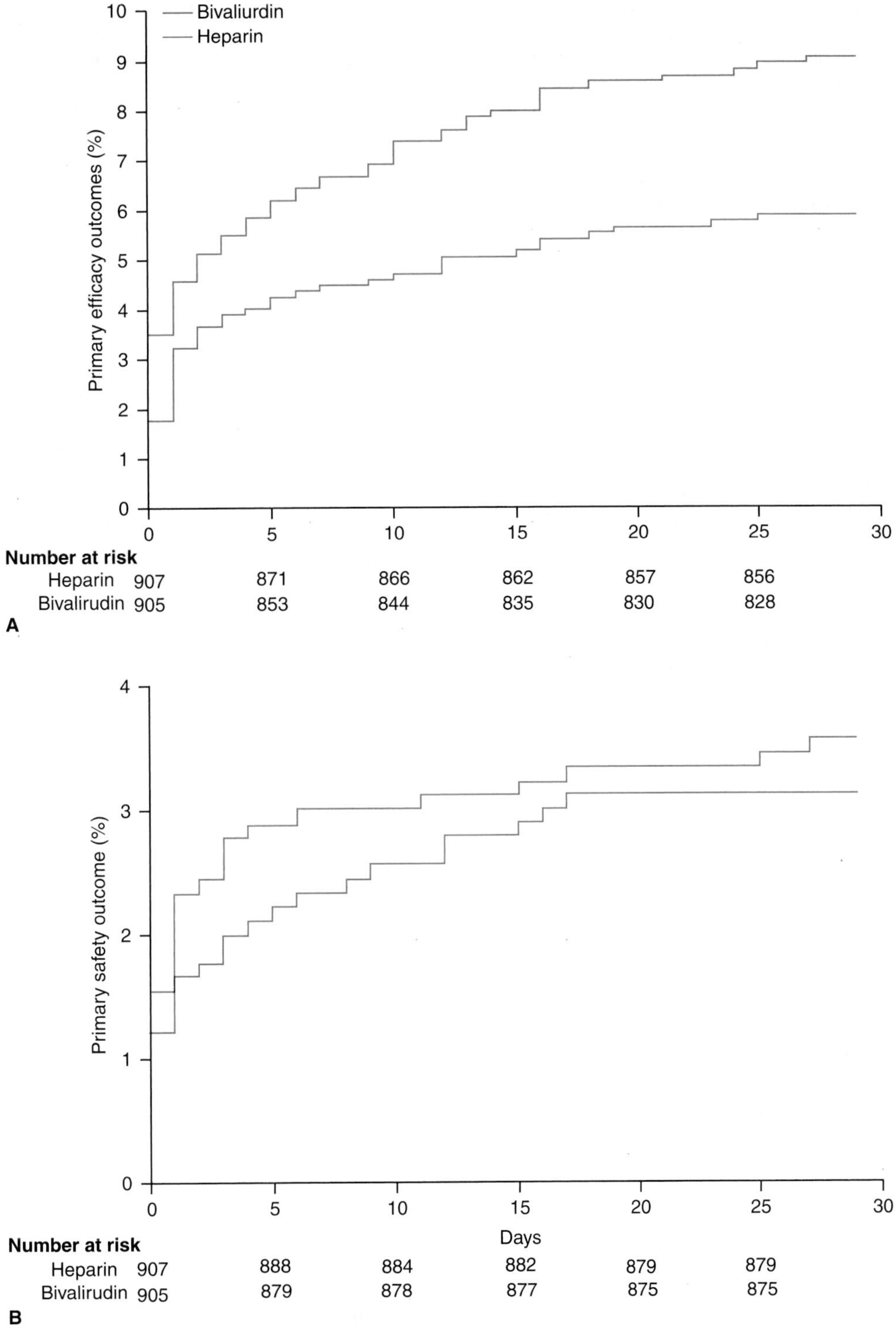

FIGURE 187.8 Results from the HEAT-PPCI Trial. Compared with bivalirudin, heparin reduced the incidence of major adverse ischemic events in the setting of primary percutaneous coronary intervention, with no increase in bleeding complications. (Adapted from Shahzad A, Kemp I, Mars C, et al: Unfractionated heparin versus bivalirudin in primary percutaneous coronary intervention (HEAT-PPCI): an open-label, single centre, randomised controlled trial. *Lancet* 384(9957):1849–1858, 2014.]

no evidence of HF. Parenteral β-blockers should be used only if there is a clear indication such as ongoing chest pain or an atrial tachyarrhythmia with normal or elevated blood pressure [27].

When given long-term following MI, β-blockers significantly reduce the incidence of nonfatal reinfarction and mortality, an effect that extends to most members of this class of agents [96]. The Carvedilol Post-Infarct Survival Control in LV Dysfunction (CAPRICORN) trial examined the incremental effects of β blockade to angiotensin-converting enzyme (ACE) inhibition in post-MI in patients with LV dysfunction but no clinical HF. Over a mean follow-up of 1.3 years, the composite of death and MI was reduced from 20% in the placebo arm to 14% in the carvedilol arm, a 29% relative reduction. On the basis of robust clinical data and a very favorable cost-to-benefit ratio, long-term oral β blockade should be continued for at least 3 years in patients without HF following MI [98].

Renin-Angiotensin-Aldosterone System Inhibitors

ACE inhibitors are routinely used following STEMI to prevent adverse LV chamber remodeling, a gradual process by which the left ventricle assumes a more globular shape and dilates; remodeling is associated with an increased risk for HF and death. A large overview of almost 100,000 patients found a 7% reduction of 30-day mortality when ACE inhibitors were given to all patients with acute MI, with most of the benefit observed in the first week. The benefit was greatest in high-risk groups, such as those in Killip class II or III, those with LV dysfunction, and those with an anterior MI [99]. In addition to preventing remodeling and HF, ACE inhibitors prevent recurrent ischemic events after MI [100]. As opposed to aspirin and reperfusion therapy, it is not crucial to introduce the ACE inhibitor in the hyperacute phase of acute MI.

Angiotensin receptor blockers (ARBs) are effective alternatives to ACE inhibitors for patients with LV dysfunction or HF following acute MI and provide similar long-term benefits [101]. However, combination therapy with ACE inhibitors and ARBs is not more effective [101]. Because of the larger evidence base and lower cost of ACE inhibitors, they are preferred over ARBs unless side effects to ACE inhibitors develop.

Aldosterone antagonists should also be considered for use in appropriate high-risk patients following STEMI, who are receiving adequate doses of ACE inhibitors. In the Eplerenone Post-Acute Myocardial Infarction Heart Failure Efficacy and Survival (EPHESUS) trial, which included patients with an LV ejection fraction <40% following an MI and either HF symptoms or diabetes, eplerenone treatment (compared to placebo) was associated with a 15% reduction of the risk of mortality [102]. Because of its much lower cost, spironolactone may be considered as an alternative to eplerenone. Aldosterone antagonists should be avoided in patients with hyperkalemia or significant renal dysfunction (Table 187.7). Despite strong evidence and a class I recommendation, and in contrast to other post-MI recommendations, aldosterone antagonists remain dramatically underutilized in contemporary practice [103].

Nitrates

Nitrates dilate large coronary arteries and arterioles, peripheral veins, and to a lesser extent, peripheral arterioles. Venodilation decreases preload, thus reducing both myocardial oxygen demand and symptoms of pulmonary congestion that may complicate MI. The Gruppo Italiano per lo Studio della Sopravvivenza nell'Infarto (GISSI) 3 May favor leaving as GISSI 3 [104] and the Fourth International Study of Infarct Survival (ISIS-4) [105] trials collectively enrolled almost 80,000 patients and evaluated the role of long-term (4- to 6-week) nitrate therapy post-MI. Neither study found a significant reduction in mortality with nitrates, although the ability to detect such a difference may have been reduced because more than 50% of patients received off-protocol nitrates. Although evidence from randomized clinical trials does not support routine long-term nitrate therapy for patients with uncomplicated MI, it is reasonable to give intravenous nitroglycerin for the first 24 to 48 hours in patients with acute MI who have HF, recurrent ischemia, or hypertension. Intravenous therapy is preferred in the early phases of MI because of its immediate onset of action and ease of titration. Nitrates should be avoided in patients with right ventricular infarction.

Calcium Channel Blockers

Calcium channel blockers block the entry of calcium into cells via voltage-sensitive calcium channels. In vascular smooth muscle cells, this causes coronary and peripheral vasodilation, whereas in cardiac tissue, it leads to depression of myocardial contractility, sinus rate, and atrioventricular (AV) nodal conduction. The dihydropyridine calcium channel antagonists, of which nifedipine is the prototype, cause coronary and peripheral artery dilation without blocking sinus or AV nodal function. As a result, the potential benefit of these agents is counterbalanced by reflex tachycardia. The short-acting preparations of nifedipine, in particular, appear to be dangerous in the setting of acute MI because they may cause rapid hemodynamic fluctuations. Sustained-release preparations of nifedipine, on the other hand, can be used safely in combination with a β-blocker. Amlodipine is a third-generation agent that causes less reflex tachycardia than other dihydropyridines, but with other calcium channel blockers, there is no documented benefit of this agent following MI; as such, it should only be used in patients who remain hypertensive after full-dose β blockade and ACE inhibition.

Diltiazem and verapamil slow HR and modestly reduce myocardial contractility, thereby decreasing myocardial oxygen demand. Of the two agents, verapamil has greater negative inotropic and chronotropic effects. A pooled analysis indicated that verapamil and diltiazem had no effect on mortality following acute MI, but that they did significantly reduce the rate of reinfarction (6.0% vs. 7.5%; $p < 0.01$) [106]. Despite an overall neutral effect of these agents on mortality, among patients with depressed LV function or evidence of HF, mortality is increased in patients treated with diltiazem or verapamil.

It should be emphasized that there have not been studies comparing the efficacy of verapamil or diltiazem to a β-blocker. β-blockers consistently reduce both mortality and reinfarction and should be recommended for all patients who can tolerate them. Verapamil or diltiazem may be a reasonable alternative for patients who cannot tolerate a β-blocker, provided LV function is normal, but they should not be given routinely following MI.

ARRHYTHMIAS COMPLICATING ST ELEVATION MYOCARDIAL INFARCTION

Ventricular Arrhythmias

Ventricular arrhythmias are common following the onset of STEMI, but the impact on outcomes depends on the timing of onset (Table 187.6. Previously, it had been thought that VT occurring early after presentation (within the first 48 hours) did not influence long-term survival if it was rapidly terminated, whereas VT occurring beyond 48 hours had ominous implications. However, in a more recent analysis of 5,745 patients with STEMI from the Assessment of Pexelizumab in Acute Myocardial Infarction (APEX-AMI) trial [107], 5.7% developed VT or VF, which was associated with worse overall 90-day mortality (adjusted HR 3.63, 95% CI 2.59 to 5.09). Of those who developed ventricular arrhythmia, 64% occurred before the end of the index cardiac catheterization, and 90% occurred within the first 48 hours of STEMI presentation.

TABLE 187.6

Electrical Complications of Acute MI

Complication	Prognosis	Treatment
Ventricular tachycardia/fibrillation		
In the catheterization lab	Good	Usually none
Within first 48 h	Fair	Immediate cardioversion; amiodarone or lidocaine; β-blockers
After 48 h	Poor	Immediate cardioversion; electrophysiology study/implantable defibrillator; amiodarone
Sinus bradycardia	Excellent	Atropine for hypotension or symptoms
Second-degree heart block		
Mobitz type I (Wenckebach)	Excellent	Atropine for hypotension or symptoms
Mobitz type II	Guarded	Temporary pacemaker
Complete heart block		
Inferior MI	Good	Temporary pacemaker
Anterior MI	Poor	Temporary pacemaker followed by permanent pacemaker

MI, myocardial infarction.

Those patients whose ventricular arrhythmia occurred after index catheterization but less than 48 hours after presentation had an increased incidence of mortality at 90 days (adjusted HR 5.59, 95% CI 3.71 to 8.43).

VF is the primary mechanism of arrhythmic sudden death. In patients with acute MI, most episodes of VF occur early (<4 to 12 hours) after infarction. As with sustained VT, *late* VF occurs more frequently in patients with severe LV dysfunction or HF and is a poor prognostic marker. Patients with VF or sustained VT associated with symptoms or hemodynamic compromise should be cardioverted emergently. Underlying metabolic and electrolyte abnormalities must be corrected, and ongoing ischemia should be addressed. We aim to maintain the serum potassium level between 3.5 and 4.5 mEq per L [108] and serum magnesium level of 2 mEq per L or more. Intravenous amiodarone is a particularly effective antiarrhythmic agent in patients with acute MI because it lowers HR and does not have pro-arrhythmic properties. Lidocaine remains an effective alternative if amiodarone is not tolerated or is unsuccessful in controlling the arrhythmia. Prophylactic use of antiarrhythmic agents, other than β-blockers, is not indicated.

Bradyarrhythmias

The usual cause of bradycardia is increased vagal tone or ischemia/infarction of conduction tissue. Sinus bradycardia is typically caused by irritation of cardiac vagal receptors, which are located most prominently on the inferior surface of the left ventricle (Table 187.6. Thus, this arrhythmia is usually seen with inferior MI. If the HR is extremely low (<40 to 50) and is associated with hypotension, intravenous atropine should be given.

Mobitz type I (Wenckebach) second-degree AV block is also very common among patients with inferior wall MI and may be caused by ischemia or infarction of the AV node or to increased vagal tone. The level of conduction block is usually located within the AV node, and therefore the QRS complex is narrow and the risk for progression to complete heart block is low. Atropine should be reserved for patients with hypotension or symptoms, and temporary pacing is rarely required. Mobitz type II block is observed much less often than Mobitz type I block in acute MI. As opposed to Mobitz type I block, Mobitz type II block is more frequently associated with anterior MI, an infranodal lesion, and a wide QRS complex. Because Mobitz type II block can progress suddenly to complete heart block, a temporary pacemaker is indicated.

Although compete heart block may occur with either inferior or anterior MI, the implications differ markedly depending on the location of the infarct. With inferior MI, heart block often progresses from first-(or Wenckebach) to third-degree AV block. The level of block is usually within or above the level of the AV node, the escape rhythm is often stable, and the effect is transient. Although temporary pacing is often indicated, a permanent pacemaker is rarely required. With anterior MI, complete heart block is usually a result of extensive infarction involving the bundle branches. The escape rhythm is usually unstable and the AV block permanent. Mortality is extremely high, and permanent pacing is almost always required for survivors.

Supraventricular Arrhythmias

Atrial fibrillation may occur in up to 15% of patients early after MI, but atrial flutter and paroxysmal supraventricular tachycardia are not commonly seen (Table 187.). Although atrial fibrillation is usually transient, it is a marker for increased morbidity and mortality, probably because it is associated with other adverse risk predictors such as LV dysfunction and congestive heart failure. Management of supraventricular arrhythmias in the setting of acute MI is similar to management in other settings; however, there should be a lower threshold for cardioversion, and the ventricular rate should be more aggressively controlled. Because of their beneficial effects for acute MI, β-blockers are the agents of choice for control rate. Diltiazem or verapamil may serve as alternatives for patients without significant HF or LV dysfunction, whereas digoxin should be reserved for patients with concomitant LV dysfunction. Of the antiarrhythmic agents available, amiodarone is safest for patients with recent MI because it has a low risk for causing arrhythmias.

TRANSITION TO DISCHARGE

Risk assessment is a continuous process that should be consistently reevaluated throughout the hospital stay. Continuing care must be individualized using lifestyle interventions, disease-modifying pharmacological therapies, and additional coronary revascularization when indicated. All patients with STEMI are considered at high

TABLE 187.7

Summary of Advances in Managing STEMI Based on Randomized Controlled Clinical Trials

• Performance of a prehospital ECG reduces reperfusion times in STEMI [5]
• Fibrinolytic therapy reduces mortality vs. placebo if administered within 12 h of symptom onset but is associated with a small risk of intracranial hemorrhage [24]
• Aspirin reduces mortality to a similar extent as fibrinolytics [70]
• Primary PCI is superior to fibrinolytic therapy for patients who can be treated within 90 min of presentation in a high-volume center [38]
• Transfer to another facility for early nonemergent PCI should be considered following successful fibrinolytic therapy [68]
• The addition of clopidogrel to aspirin, antithrombins, and fibrinolytic therapy reduces recurrent MI and mortality [72,73]
• Prasugrel and ticagrelor represent alternatives to clopidogrel that reduce stent thrombosis and recurrent ischemic events, but at an increased risk for bleeding [75,76]
• Enoxaparin is superior to unfractionated heparin as an adjunct to fibrinolytic therapy but is associated with slightly more bleeding [79]
• Radial artery access (as opposed to femoral artery) may decrease bleeding complications and should be considered when feasible [40]
• β-Blockers improve long-term outcomes following STEMI but may increase risk when given early to unstable patients [93,94]
• ACE inhibitors prevent adverse remodeling after STEMI and reduce death and heart failure events [95]
• Aldosterone antagonists reduce mortality in patients with LV dysfunction or heart failure following MI but should be used in caution in individuals with renal dysfunction [98]

ACE, angiotensin-converting enzyme; ECG, electrocardiogram; STEMI, ST-segment elevation myocardial infarction; LV, left ventricular; MI, myocardial infarction; PCI, percutaneous coronary intervention.

risk and therefore warrant aggressive intervention for secondary prevention. All patients should undergo a transthoracic echocardiogram prior to hospital discharge to assess ventricular systolic function and to ensure that appropriate medications are initiated prior to discharge (i.e., ACE inhibitor, aldosterone antagonists) [27]. In addition, all patients without contraindications should be initiated on high-intensity statin therapy, and considered for ezetimibe, prior to discharge. Referral to cardiac rehabilitation is also indicated for all patients admitted with STEMI. The objectives of exercise-based cardiac rehabilitation are to increase functional capacity, decrease or alleviate anginal symptoms, reduce disability, improve quality of life, and reduce morbidity and mortality rates [109]. Finally, perhaps the most powerful secondary prevention strategy is smoking cessation. A meta-analysis of cohort studies in patients with ACS showed that smoking cessation reduces the subsequent cardiovascular mortality rate by almost 50% [110]. All of these interventions, together with appropriate patient and family education regarding medication adherence and timely follow-up, will serve to reduce rates of rehospitalization and improve patient outcomes (Table 187.7) [111,112].

References

1. Gibson CM, Pride YB, Frederick PD, et al: Trends in reperfusion strategies, door-to-needle and door-to-balloon times, and in-hospital mortality among patients with ST-segment elevation myocardial infarction enrolled in the National Registry of Myocardial Infarction from 1990 to 2006. *Am Heart J* 156(6):1035–1044, 2008.
2. Libby P: Molecular bases of the acute coronary syndromes. *Circulation* 91(11):2844–2850, 1995.
3. Theroux P, Fuster V: Acute coronary syndromes: unstable angina and non-Q-wave myocardial infarction. *Circulation* 97(12):1195–1206, 1998.
4. Canto JG, Shilpak MG, Rogers WJ, et al: Prevalence, clinical characteristics, and mortality among patients with myocardial infarction presenting without chest pain. *JAMA* 283(24):3223–3229, 2000.
5. Diercks DB, Kontos MC, Chen AY, et al: Utilization and impact of pre-hospital electrocardiograms for patients with acute ST-segment elevation myocardial infarction: data from the NCDR (National Cardiovascular Data Registry) ACTION (Acute Coronary Treatment and Intervention Outcomes Network) Registry. *J Am Coll Cardiol* 53(2):161–166, 2009.
6. Shlipak MG, Lyons WL, Go AS, et al: Should the electrocardiogram be used to guide therapy for patients with left bundle-branch block and suspected myocardial infarction? *JAMA* 281(8):714–719, 1999.
7. Neeland IJ, Kontos MC, de Lemos JA: Evolving considerations in the management of patients with left bundle branch block and suspected myocardial infarction. *J Am Coll Cardiol* 60(2):96–105, 2012.
8. Ohman EM, Armstrong PW, White HD, et al: Risk stratification with a point-of-care cardiac troponin T test in acute myocardial infarction. GUSTOIII Investigators. Global Use of Strategies To Open Occluded Coronary Arteries. *Am J Cardiol* 84(11):1281–1286, 1999.
9. Mega JL, Morrow DA, De Lemos JA, et al: B-type natriuretic peptide at presentation and prognosis in patients with ST-segment elevation myocardial infarction: an ENTIRE-TIMI-23 substudy. *J Am Coll Cardiol* 44(2):335–339, 2004.
10. Morrow DA, Antman EM, Giugliano RP, et al: A simple risk index for rapid initial triage of patients with ST-elevation myocardial infarction: an InTIME II substudy. *Lancet* 358(9293):1571–1575, 2001.
11. Morrow DA, Antman EM, Charlesworth A, et al: TIMI risk score for ST-elevation myocardial infarction: a convenient, bedside, clinical score for risk assessment at presentation: an intravenous nPA for treatment of infarcting myocardium early II trial substudy. *Circulation* 102(17):2031–2037, 2000.
12. Morrow DA, Antman EM, Parsons L, et al: Application of the TIMI risk score for ST-elevation MI in the National Registry of Myocardial Infarction 3. *JAMA* 286(11):1356–1359, 2001.
13. Eagle KA, Lim MJ, Dabbous OH, et al: A validated prediction model for all forms of acute coronary syndrome: estimating the risk of 6-month postdischarge death in an international registry. *JAMA* 291(22):2727–2733, 2004.
14. Jacobs DR Jr, Kroenke C, Crow R, et al: PREDICT: A simple risk score for clinical severity and long-term prognosis after hospitalization for acute myocardial infarction or unstable angina: the Minnesota heart survey. *Circulation* 100(6):599–607, 1999.
15. Cannon CP, Braunwald E: GUSTO, TIMI and the case for rapid reperfusion. *Acta Cardiol* 49(1):1–8, 1994.
16. Gibson CM, Cannon CP, Murphy SA, et al: Relationship of TIMI myocardial perfusion grade to mortality after administration of thrombolytic drugs. *Circulation* 101(2):125–130, 2000.
17. Ito H, Tomooka T, Sakai N, et al: Lack of myocardial perfusion immediately after successful thrombolysis. A predictor of poor recovery of left ventricular function in anterior myocardial infarction. *Circulation* 85(5):1699–1705, 1992.
18. de Lemos JA, Antman EM, Giugliano RP, et al: ST-segment resolution and infarct-related artery patency and flow after thrombolytic therapy. Thrombolysis in Myocardial Infarction (TIMI) 14 investigators. *Am J Cardiol* 85(3):299–304, 2000.
19. Santoro GM, Valenti R, Buonamici P, et al: Relation between ST-segment changes and myocardial perfusion evaluated by myocardial contrast echocardiography in patients with acute myocardial infarction treated with direct angioplasty. *Am J Cardiol* 82(8):932–937, 1998.
20. Angeja BG, Gunda M, Murphy SA, et al: TIMI myocardial perfusion grade and ST segment resolution: association with infarct size as assessed by single photon emission computed tomography imaging. *Circulation* 105(3):282–285, 2002.
21. Schroder R, Dissmann R, Brüggemann T, et al: Extent of early ST segment elevation resolution: a simple but strong predictor of outcome in patients with acute myocardial infarction. *J Am Coll Cardiol* 24(2):384–391, 1994.
22. de Lemos JA, Braunwald E: ST segment resolution as a tool for assessing the efficacy of reperfusion therapy. *J Am Coll Cardiol* 38(5):1283–1294, 2001.

23. Indications for fibrinolytic therapy in suspected acute myocardial infarction: collaborative overview of early mortality and major morbidity results from all randomised trials of more than 1000 patients. Fibrinolytic Therapy Trialists' (FTT) Collaborative Group. *Lancet* 343(8893):311–322, 1994.
24. Cannon CP, Gibson CM, Lambrew CT, et al: Relationship of symptom-onset-to-balloon time and door-to-balloon time with mortality in patients undergoing angioplasty for acute myocardial infarction. *JAMA* 283(22):2941–2947, 2000.
25. Bradley EH, Herrin J, Wang Y, et al: Strategies for reducing the door-to-balloon time in acute myocardial infarction. *N Engl J Med* 355(22):2308–2320, 2006.
26. Nallamothu BK, Krumholz HM, Peterson ED, et al: Door-to-balloon times in hospitals within the get-with-the-guidelines registry after initiation of the door-to-balloon (D2B) Alliance. *Am J Cardiol* 103(8):1051–1055, 2009.
27. O'Gara PT, Kushner FG, Ascheim DD, et al: 2013 ACCF/AHA guideline for the management of ST-elevation myocardial infarction: a report of the American College of Cardiology Foundation/American Heart Association Task Force on Practice Guidelines. *Circulation* 127(4):e362–e425, 2013.
28. Gibson CM, Karha J, Murphy SA, et al: Early and long-term clinical outcomes associated with reinfarction following fibrinolytic administration in the Thrombolysis in Myocardial Infarction trials. *J Am Coll Cardiol* 42(1):7–16, 2003.
29. Keeley EC, Boura JA, Grines CL: Primary angioplasty versus intravenous thrombolytic therapy for acute myocardial infarction: a quantitative review of 23 randomised trials. *Lancet* 361(9351):13–20, 2003.
30. Aversano T, Lemmon CC, Liu L; Atlantic CPORT Investigators: Outcomes of PCI at hospitals with or without on-site cardiac surgery. *N Engl J Med* 366(19):1792–1802, 2012.
31. Zhu MM, Feit A, Chadow H, et al: Primary stent implantation compared with primary balloon angioplasty for acute myocardial infarction: a meta-analysis of randomized clinical trials. *Am J Cardiol* 88(3):297–301, 2001.
32. Stone GW, Grines CL, Cox DA, et al: Comparison of angioplasty with stenting, with or without abciximab, in acute myocardial infarction. *N Engl J Med* 346(13):957–966, 2002.
33. Kastrati A, Dibra A, Spaulding C, et al: Meta-analysis of randomized trials on drug-eluting stents vs. bare-metal stents in patients with acute myocardial infarction. *Eur Heart J* 28(22):2706–2713, 2007.
34. Stone GW, Lansky AJ, Pocock SJ, et al: Paclitaxel-eluting stents versus bare-metal stents in acute myocardial infarction. *N Engl J Med* 360(19):1946–1959, 2009.
35. Palmerini T, Biondi-Zoccai G, Della Riva D, et al: Stent thrombosis with drug-eluting and bare-metal stents: evidence from a comprehensive network meta-analysis. *Lancet* 379(9824):1393–1402, 2012.
36. Navarese EP, Andreotti F, Schulze V, et al: Optimal duration of dual antiplatelet therapy after percutaneous coronary intervention with drug eluting stents: meta-analysis of randomised controlled trials. *BMJ* 350:h1618, 2015.
37. Jolly SS, Yusuf S, Cairns J, et al: Radial versus femoral access for coronary angiography and intervention in patients with acute coronary syndromes (RIVAL): a randomised, parallel group, multicentre trial. *Lancet* 377(9775):1409–1420, 2011.
38. Mehta SR, Jolly SS, Cairns J, et al: Effects of radial versus femoral artery access in patients with acute coronary syndromes with or without ST-segment elevation. *J Am Coll Cardiol* 60(24):2490–2499, 2012.
39. Valgimigli M, Gagnor A, Calabró P, et al: Radial versus femoral access in patients with acute coronary syndromes undergoing invasive management: a randomised multicentre trial. *Lancet* 385(9986):2465–2476, 2015.
40. Rao SV, Ou FS, Wang TY, et al: Trends in the prevalence and outcomes of radial and femoral approaches to percutaneous coronary intervention: a report from the National Cardiovascular Data Registry. *JACC Cardiovasc Interv* 1(4):379–386, 2008.
41. Sorajja P, Gersh BJ, Cox DA, et al: Impact of multivessel disease on reperfusion success and clinical outcomes in patients undergoing primary percutaneous coronary intervention for acute myocardial infarction. *Eur Heart J* 28(14):1709–1716, 2007.
42. Park DW, Clare RM, Schulte PJ, et al: Extent, location, and clinical significance of non-infarct-related coronary artery disease among patients with ST-elevation myocardial infarction. *JAMA* 312(19):2019–2027, 2014.
43. Wald DS, Morris JK, Wald NJ, et al: Randomized trial of preventive angioplasty in myocardial infarction. *N Engl J Med* 369(12):1115–1123, 2013.
44. Gershlick AH, Khan JN, Kelly DJ, et al: Randomized trial of complete versus lesion-only revascularization in patients undergoing primary percutaneous coronary intervention for STEMI and multivessel disease: the CvLPRIT trial. *J Am Coll Cardiol* 65(10):963–972, 2015.
45. Hofsten DE, Kelbµk H, Helqvist S, et al: The Third DANish Study of Optimal Acute Treatment of Patients with ST-segment Elevation Myocardial Infarction: ischemic postconditioning or deferred stent implantation versus conventional primary angioplasty and complete revascularization versus treatment of culprit lesion only: rationale and design of the DANAMI 3 trial program. *Am Heart J* 169(5):613–621, 2015.
46. Hlinomaz O, Groch L, PolokovβK: Multivessel coronary disease diagnosed at the time of primary PCI for STEMI: complete revascularization versus conservative strategy. PRAGUE 13 trial. Available at http://sbhci.org.br/wpcontent/uploads/2015/05/PRAGUE-13-Trial.pdf. Accessed September 10, 2015.
47. Levine GN, Bates ER, Blankenship JC, et al: 2015 ACC/AHA/SCAI Focused Update on Primary Percutaneous Coronary Intervention for Patients With ST-Elevation Myocardial Infarction: An Update of the 2011 ACCF/AHA/SCAI Guideline for Percutaneous Coronary Intervention and the 2013 ACCF/AHA Guideline for the Management of ST-Elevation Myocardial Infarction: A Report of the American College of Cardiology/American Heart Association Task Force on Clinical Practice Guidelines and the Society for Cardiovascular Angiography and Interventions. *Circulation* 133:1135–1147, 2016.
48. Stone GW, Webb J, Cox DA, et al: Distal microcirculatory protection during percutaneous coronary intervention in acute ST-segment elevation myocardial infarction: a randomized controlled trial. *JAMA* 293(9):1063–1072, 2005.
49. Vlaar PJ, Svilaas T, van der Horst IC, et al: Cardiac death and reinfarction after 1 year in the Thrombus Aspiration during Percutaneous coronary intervention in Acute myocardial infarction Study (TAPAS): a 1-year follow-up study. *Lancet* 371(9628):1915–1920, 2008.
50. Frobert O, Lagerqvist B, Olivecrona GK, et al: Thrombus aspiration during ST-segment elevation myocardial infarction. *N Engl J Med* 369(17):1587–1597, 2013.
51. Lagerqvist B, Fröbert O, Olivercrona GK, et al: Outcomes 1 year after thrombus aspiration for myocardial infarction. *N Engl J Med* 371(12):1111–1120, 2014.
52. Jolly SS, Cairns JA, Yusuf S, et al: Randomized trial of primary PCI with or without routine manual thrombectomy. *N Engl J Med* 372(15):1389–1398, 2015.
53. Dauerman HL, Bates ER, Kontos MC, et al: Nationwide analysis of patients with st-segment-elevation myocardial infarction transferred for primary percutaneous intervention: findings from the American Heart Association Mission: lifeline program. *Circ Cardiovasc Interv* 8(5), 2015.
54. Widimsky P, Groch L, Zelízko M, et al: Multicentre randomized trial comparing transport to primary angioplasty vs immediate thrombolysis vs combined strategy for patients with acute myocardial infarction presenting to a community hospital without a catheterization laboratory. The PRAGUE study. *Eur Heart J* 21(10):823–831, 2000.
55. Andersen HR, Nielsen TT, Rasmussen K, et al: A comparison of coronary angioplasty with fibrinolytic therapy in acute myocardial infarction. *N Engl J Med* 349(8):733–742, 2003.
56. Nallamothu BK, Bates ER, Herrin J, et al: Times to treatment in transfer patients undergoing primary percutaneous coronary intervention in the United States: National Registry of Myocardial Infarction (NRMI)-3/4 analysis. *Circulation* 111(6):761–767, 2005.
57. Widimsky P, Budesínský T, Vorβc D, et al: Long distance transport for primary angioplasty vs immediate thrombolysis in acute myocardial infarction. Final results of the randomized national multicentre trial—PRAGUE-2. *Eur Heart J* 24(1):94–104, 2003.
58. Steg PG, Bonnefoy E, Chabaud S, et al: Impact of time to treatment on mortality after prehospital fibrinolysis or primary angioplasty: data from the CAPTIM randomized clinical trial. *Circulation* 108(23):2851–2856, 2003.
59. Nallamothu BK, Bates ER: Percutaneous coronary intervention versus fibrinolytic therapy in acute myocardial infarction: is timing (almost) everything? *Am J Cardiol* 92(7):824–826, 2003.
60. Ross AM, Coyne KS, Reiner JS, et al: A randomized trial comparing primary angioplasty with a strategy of short-acting thrombolysis and immediate planned rescue angioplasty in acute myocardial infarction: the PACT trial. PACT investigators. Plasminogen-activator Angioplasty Compatibility Trial. *J Am Coll Cardiol* 34(7):1954–1962, 1999.
61. Brodie BR, Stuckey TD, Hansen C, et al: Benefit of coronary reperfusion before intervention on outcomes after primary angioplasty for acute myocardial infarction. *Am J Cardiol* 85(1):13–18, 2000.
62. Keeley EC, Boura JA, Grines CL: Comparison of primary and facilitated percutaneous coronary interventions for ST-elevation myocardial infarction: quantitative review of randomised trials. *Lancet* 367(9510):579–588, 2006.
63. Ellis SG, Tendera M, de Belder MA, et al: Facilitated PCI in patients with ST-elevation myocardial infarction. *N Engl J Med* 358(21):2205–2217, 2008.
64. Fernandez-Aviles F, Alonso JJ, Castro-Beiras A, et al: Routine invasive strategy within 24 hours of thrombolysis versus ischaemia-guided conservative approach for acute myocardial infarction with ST-segment elevation (GRACIA-1): a randomised controlled trial. *Lancet* 364(9439):1045–1053, 2004.
65. Zeymer U, Uebis R, Vogt A, et al: Randomized comparison of percutaneous transluminal coronary angioplasty and medical therapy in stable survivors of acute myocardial infarction with single vessel disease: a study of the Arbeitsgemeinschaft Leitende Kardiologische Krankenhausarzte. *Circulation* 108(11):1324–1328, 2003.
66. Armstrong PW; WEST Steering Committee: A comparison of pharmacologic therapy with/without timely coronary intervention vs. primary percutaneous intervention early after ST-elevation myocardial infarction: the WEST (Which Early ST-elevation myocardial infarction Therapy) study. *Eur Heart J* 27(13):1530–1538, 2006.
67. Cantor WJ, Fitchett D, Borgundvaag B, et al: Routine early angioplasty after fibrinolysis for acute myocardial infarction. *N Engl J Med* 360(26):2705–2718, 2009.
68. Lloyd-Jones D, Adams RJ, Brown TM, et al: Executive summary: heart disease and stroke statistics—2010 update: a report from the American Heart Association. *Circulation* 121(7):948–954, 2010.
69. Nielsen N, Wetterslev J, Cronberg T, et al: Targeted temperature management at 33 degrees C versus 36 degrees C after cardiac arrest. *N Engl J Med* 369(23):2197–2206, 2013.
70. Roux S, Christeller S, Ludin E: Effects of aspirin on coronary reocclusion and recurrent ischemia after thrombolysis: a meta-analysis. *J Am Coll Cardiol* 19(3):671–677, 1992.
71. Randomised trial of intravenous streptokinase, oral aspirin, both, or neither among 17,187 cases of suspected acute myocardial infarction: ISIS-2. ISIS-2 (Second International Study of Infarct Survival) Collaborative Group. *Lancet* 2(8607):349–360, 1988.

72. Hall HM, de Lemos JA, Enriquez JR, et al: Contemporary patterns of discharge aspirin dosing after acute myocardial infarction in the United States: results from the National Cardiovascular Data Registry (NCDR). *Circ Cardiovasc Qual Outcomes* 7(5):701–707, 2014.
73. Antithrombotic Trialists Collaboration: Collaborative meta-analysis of randomised trials of antiplatelet therapy for prevention of death, myocardial infarction, and stroke in high risk patients. *BMJ* 324(7329):71–86, 2002.
74. Sabatine MS, Cannon CP, Gibson CM, et al: Addition of clopidogrel to aspirin and fibrinolytic therapy for myocardial infarction with ST-segment elevation. *N Engl J Med* 352(12):1179–1189, 2005.
75. Chen ZM, Jiang LX, Chen YP, et al: Addition of clopidogrel to aspirin in 45,852 patients with acute myocardial infarction: randomised placebo-controlled trial. *Lancet* 366(9497):1607–1621, 2005.
76. Mehta SR, Tanguay JF, Eikelboom JW, et al: Double-dose versus standard-dose clopidogrel and high-dose versus low-dose aspirin in individuals undergoing percutaneous coronary intervention for acute coronary syndromes (CURRENT-OASIS 7): a randomised factorial trial. *Lancet* 376(9748):1233–1243, 2010.
77. Montalescot G, Wiviott SD, Braunwald E, et al: Prasugrel compared with clopidogrel in patients undergoing percutaneous coronary intervention for ST-elevation myocardial infarction (TRITON-TIMI 38): double-blind, randomised controlled trial. *Lancet* 373(9665):723–731, 2009.
78. Wallentin L, Becker RC, Budaj A, et al: Ticagrelor versus clopidogrel in patients with acute coronary syndromes. *N Engl J Med* 361(11):1045–1057, 2009.
79. Hobl EL, Stimpfl T, Ebner J, et al: Morphine decreases clopidogrel concentrations and effects: a randomized, double-blind, placebo-controlled trial. *J Am Coll Cardiol* 63(7):630–635, 2014.
80. Parodi G, Valenti R, Bellandi B, et al: Comparison of prasugrel and ticagrelor loading doses in ST-segment elevation myocardial infarction patients: RAPID (Rapid Activity of Platelet Inhibitor Drugs) primary PCI study. *J Am Coll Cardiol* 61(15):1601–1606, 2013.
81. Montalescot G, van't Hof AW: Prehospital ticagrelor in ST-segment elevation myocardial infarction. *N Engl J Med* 371(11):1016–1027, 2014.
82. White HD, Bhatt DL, Gibson CM, et al: Outcomes with cangrelor versus clopidogrel on a background of bivalirudin: insights from the CHAMPION PHOENIX (A Clinical Trial Comparing Cangrelor to Clopidogrel Standard Therapy in Subjects Who Require Percutaneous Coronary Intervention [PCI]). *JACC Cardiovasc Interv* 8(3):424–433, 2015.
83. Kandzari DE, Hasselblad V, Tcheng JE, et al: Improved clinical outcomes with abciximab therapy in acute myocardial infarction: a systematic overview of randomized clinical trials. *Am Heart J* 147(3):457–462, 2004.
84. Antman EM, Morrow DA, McCabe CH, et al: Enoxaparin versus unfractionated heparin with fibrinolysis for ST-elevation myocardial infarction. *N Engl J Med* 354(14):1477–1488, 2006.
85. Global Use of Strategies to Open Occluded Coronary Arteries (GUSTO) IIb investigators. A comparison of recombinant hirudin with heparin for the treatment of acute coronary syndromes. *N Engl J Med* 335(11):775–782, 1996.
86. Antman EM: Hirudin in acute myocardial infarction. Thrombolysis and Thrombin Inhibition in Myocardial Infarction (TIMI) 9B trial. *Circulation* 94(5):911–921, 1996.
87. White H; Hirulog and Early Reperfusion or Occlusion (HERO)-2 Trial Investigators: Thrombin-specific anticoagulation with bivalirudin versus heparin in patients receiving fibrinolytic therapy for acute myocardial infarction: the HERO-2 randomised trial. *Lancet* 358(9296):1855–1863, 2001.
88. Stone GW, Witzenbichler B, Guagliumi G, et al: Bivalirudin during primary PCI in acute myocardial infarction. *N Engl J Med* 358(21):2218–2230, 2008.
89. Steg PG, van't Hof A, Hamm CW, et al: Bivalirudin started during emergency transport for primary PCI. *N Engl J Med* 369(23):2207–2217, 2013.
90. Shahzad A, Kemp I, Mars C, et al: Unfractionated heparin versus bivalirudin in primary percutaneous coronary intervention (HEAT-PPCI): an open-label, single centre, randomised controlled trial. *Lancet* 384(9957):1849–1858, 2014.
91. Cavender MA, Sabatine MS: Bivalirudin versus heparin in patients planned for percutaneous coronary intervention: a meta-analysis of randomised controlled trials. *Lancet* 384(9943):599–606, 2014.
92. Lamberts M, Olesen JB, Ruwald MH, et al: Bleeding after initiation of multiple antithrombotic drugs, including triple therapy, in atrial fibrillation patients following myocardial infarction and coronary intervention: a nationwide cohort study. *Circulation* 126(10):1185–1193, 2012.
93. Holmes DR Jr, Kereiakes DJ, Kleiman NS, et al: Combining antiplatelet and anticoagulant therapies. *J Am Coll Cardiol* 54(2):95–109, 2009.
94. Dewilde WJ, Oirbans T, Verheugt FW, et al: Use of clopidogrel with or without aspirin in patients taking oral anticoagulant therapy and undergoing percutaneous coronary intervention: an open-label, randomised, controlled trial. *Lancet* 381(9872):1107–1115, 2013.
95. TIMI Study Group: Comparison of invasive and conservative strategies after treatment with intravenous tissue plasminogen activator in acute myocardial infarction. Results of the thrombolysis in myocardial infarction (TIMI) phase II trial. *N Engl J Med* 320(10):618–627, 1989.
96. Yusuf S, Peto R, Lewis J, et al: Beta blockade during and after myocardial infarction: an overview of the randomized trials. *Prog Cardiovasc Dis* 27(5):335–371, 1985.
97. Chen ZM, Pan HC, Chen YP, et al: Early intravenous then oral metoprolol in 45,852 patients with acute myocardial infarction: randomised placebo-controlled trial. *Lancet* 366(9497):1622–1632, 2005.
98. Smith SC Jr, Benjamin EJ, Bonow RO, et al: AHA/ACCF Secondary Prevention and Risk Reduction Therapy for Patients with Coronary and other Atherosclerotic Vascular Disease: 2011 update: a guideline from the American Heart Association and American College of Cardiology Foundation. *Circulation* 124(22):2458–2473, 2011.
99. Indications for ACE inhibitors in the early treatment of acute myocardial infarction: systematic overview of individual data from 100,000 patients in randomized trials. ACE Inhibitor Myocardial Infarction Collaborative Group. *Circulation* 97(22):2202–2212, 1998.
100. Rutherford JD, Pfeffer MA, Moyé LA, et al: Effects of captopril on ischemic events after myocardial infarction. Results of the Survival and Ventricular Enlargement trial. SAVE Investigators. *Circulation* 90(4):1731–1738, 1994.
101. Pfeffer MA, McMurray JJ, Velazquez EJ, et al: Valsartan, captopril, or both in myocardial infarction complicated by heart failure, left ventricular dysfunction, or both. *N Engl J Med* 349(20):1893–1906, 2003.
102. Pitt B, Remme W, Zannad F, et al: Eplerenone, a selective aldosterone blocker, in patients with left ventricular dysfunction after myocardial infarction. *N Engl J Med* 348(14):1309–1321, 2003.
103. Rao KK, Enriquez JR, de Lemos JA, et al: Use of aldosterone antagonists at discharge after myocardial infarction: results from the National Cardiovascular Data Registry Acute Coronary Treatment and Intervention Outcomes Network (ACTION) Registry-Get with the Guidelines (GWTG). *Am Heart J* 166(4):709–715, 2013.
104. GISSI-3: effects of lisinopril and transdermal glyceryl trinitrate singly and together on 6-week mortality and ventricular function after acute myocardial infarction. Gruppo Italiano per lo Studio della Sopravvivenza nell'infarto Miocardico. *Lancet* 343(8906):1115–1122, 1994.
105. ISIS-4: a randomised factorial trial assessing early oral captopril, oral mononitrate, and intravenous magnesium sulphate in 58,050 patients with suspected acute myocardial infarction. ISIS-4 (Fourth International Study of Infarct Survival) Collaborative Group. *Lancet* 345(8951):669–685, 1995.
106. Yusuf S, Held P, Furberg C: Update of effects of calcium antagonists in myocardial infarction or angina in light of the second Danish Verapamil Infarction Trial (DAVIT-II) and other recent studies. *Am J Cardiol* 67(15):1295–1297, 1991.
107. Mehta RH, Starr AZ, Lopes RD, et al: Incidence of and outcomes associated with ventricular tachycardia or fibrillation in patients undergoing primary percutaneous coronary intervention. *JAMA* 301(17):1779–1789, 2009.
108. Goyal A, Spertus JA, Gosch K, et al: Serum potassium levels and mortality in acute myocardial infarction. *JAMA* 307(2):157–1564, 2012.
109. Leon AS, Franklin BA, Costa F, et al: Cardiac rehabilitation and secondary prevention of coronary heart disease: an American Heart Association scientific statement from the Council on Clinical Cardiology (Subcommittee on Exercise, Cardiac Rehabilitation, and Prevention) and the Council on Nutrition, Physical Activity, and Metabolism (Subcommittee on Physical Activity), in collaboration with the American association of Cardiovascular and Pulmonary Rehabilitation. *Circulation* 111(3):369–376, 2005.
110. Wilson K, Gibson N, Willan A, et al: Effect of smoking cessation on mortality after myocardial infarction: meta-analysis of cohort studies. *Arch Intern Med* 160(7):939–944, 2000.
111. Bernheim SM, Grady JN, Lin Z, et al: National patterns of risk-standardized mortality and readmission for acute myocardial infarction and heart failure. Update on publicly reported outcomes measures based on the 2010 release. *Circ Cardiovasc Qual Outcomes* 3(5):459–467, 2010.
112. Krumholz HM, Merrill AR, Schone EM, et al: Patterns of hospital performance in acute myocardial infarction and heart failure 30-day mortality and readmission. *Circ Cardiovasc Qual Outcomes* 2(5):407–413, 2009.

Chapter 188 ■ Unstable Angina/Non–ST-Segment Elevation Myocardial Infarction, the Non–ST-Elevation Acute Coronary Syndromes

MICHAEL G. SILVERMAN • MARC S. SABATINE

The spectrum of acute coronary syndromes (ACS) ranges from unstable angina (UA) to non–ST-segment elevation myocardial infarction (NSTEMI) to ST-segment elevation myocardial infarction (STEMI) [1]. The latter condition is usually caused by acute total obstruction of a coronary artery [2,3], and urgent reperfusion is the mainstay of therapy. In contrast, the non–ST-segment elevation acute coronary syndromes (NSTE-ACS)—UA and NSTEMI—are usually associated with a severe, nonocclusive lesion in the culprit coronary artery [4].

Every year in the USA, approximately 1.1 million patients are hospitalized with ACS; about 800,000 of these patients suffer from MI, with approximately 25% of patients with MI presenting with STEMI [5]. Worldwide, these numbers are each several times the respective total in the USA. In recent years, numerous advances have advanced our understanding of the pathophysiology, diagnosis, risk stratification, and management of NSTE-ACS.

DEFINITION

ACS traditionally present with specific clinical features that can help distinguish ACS from stable angina: (a) occurring at rest (or with minimal exertion), usually lasting more than 20 minutes; (b) being severe and of new onset (i.e., within 1 month); or (c) occurring with a crescendo pattern (i.e., more severe, prolonged, or frequent) [6]. In the absence of ST-segment elevations on electrocardiogram (ECG), these patients are characterized as having NSTE-ACS. Among patients with NSTE-ACS, those with evidence of myocardial necrosis on the basis of serum biomarkers have a diagnosis of NSTEMI, whereas those without evidence of myocardial necrosis are diagnosed with UA. With increasingly sensitive biomarkers for myocardial necrosis, among patients with NSTE-ACS the diagnosis of NSTEMI is increasing whereas that of UA is decreasing [7,8].

PATHOPHYSIOLOGY

The development of NSTE-ACS is caused by either a reduction in the supply of blood flow and oxygen, or an increase in myocardial oxygen demand, or both. The five broad etiologies are (a) plaque rupture or erosion with superimposed nonocclusive thrombus; (b) dynamic obstruction (i.e., coronary spasm); (c) progressive mechanical obstruction (i.e., restenosis); (d) inflammation and arteritis; and (e) conditions leading to increased myocardial oxygen demand, such as anemia, sepsis, or hypoxia [9]. Individual patients may have several of these processes contribute to the onset of their NSTE-ACS.

Plaque Rupture and Erosion

Atherosclerosis is a silent process that usually begins 20 to 30 years prior to a patient's clinical presentation [10,11]. Plaque rupture and erosion can be precipitated by multiple factors, including endothelial dysfunction [12], plaque lipid content [13], local inflammation [14], coronary artery tone at the site of irregular plaques and local shear stress forces, platelet function [15,16], and the status of the coagulation system (i.e., a potentially prothrombotic state) [17,18]. These processes culminate in formation of platelet-rich thrombi at the site of the plaque rupture or erosion and the resultant ACS [19–21].

Thrombosis

Coronary artery thrombosis plays a central role during the pathogenesis of NSTE-ACS [4,19,20,22–26], as demonstrated in the Thrombolysis in Myocardial Infarction (TIMI) IIIA trial, in which 35% of patients had definite thrombus and an additional 40% had possible thrombus [4]. Thrombosis occurs in two interrelated stages: (a) primary hemostasis and (b) secondary hemostasis [27,28]. The first stage of hemostasis is initiated by platelets as they adhere to damaged vessels and form a platelet plug. With rupture or ulceration of an atherosclerotic plaque, the subendothelial matrix (e.g., collagen and tissue factor) is exposed to the circulating blood. Platelets then adhere to the subendothelial matrix via the glycoprotein (GP) Ib receptor and von Willebrand's factor (platelet adhesion). After adhering to the subendothelial matrix, the platelet undergoes a conformational change from a smooth discoid shape to a spiculated form, which increases the surface area on which thrombin generation can occur. This leads to degranulation of the α- and dense granules and the subsequent release of thromboxane A2, adenosine diphosphate (ADP), serotonin, and other platelet aggregatory and chemoattractant factors, as well as the expression and activation of GP IIb/IIIa receptors on the platelet surface such that it can bind fibrinogen. This process is called platelet activation. The final step is platelet aggregation, that is, the formation of the platelet plug. Fibrinogen (or von Willebrand's factor) binds to the activated GP IIb/IIIa receptors of two platelets, thereby creating a growing platelet aggregate. Antiplatelet therapy has been directed at decreasing the formation of thromboxane A2 (aspirin), inhibiting the ADP pathway of platelet activation (thienopyridines), and directly inhibiting platelet aggregation.

Secondary Hemostasis

Simultaneous with the formation of the platelet plug, the plasma coagulation system is activated (Fig. 188.1). Following plaque rupture or ulceration, the injured endothelial cells on the vessel wall become activated and release protein disulfide isomerase, which acts to cause a conformational change in circulating tissue factor [29–32]. Tissue factor can then bind to factor VIIa and form a protein complex, leading to the activation of factor X. With the activation of factor X (to factor Xa), thrombin is generated and acts to cleave fibrinogen to form fibrin. Thrombin plays a central role during arterial thrombosis: (a) it converts fibrinogen to fibrin in the final common pathway for clot formation; (b) it is a powerful stimulus for platelet aggregation; and (c) it activates factor XIII, which leads to cross-linking and stabilization of the fibrin clot [27].

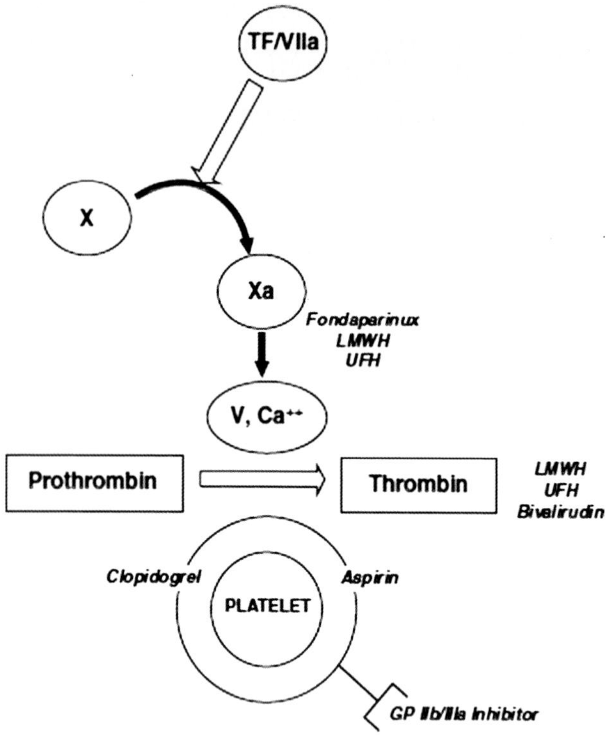

FIGURE 188.1 Diagram of the major components of the clotting cascade and the areas targeted by antithrombotic agents.

Coronary Vasoconstriction

Another etiologic factor of NSTE-ACS is dynamic obstruction, that is, coronary vasoconstriction. The process is identified in three settings: (a) vasospasm in the absence of obstructive plaque, (b) vasoconstriction in the setting of atherosclerotic plaque, and (c) microcirculatory angina. Vasospasm can occur among patients without coronary atherosclerosis or among those with a nonobstructive atheromatous plaque. Vasospastic angina appears to be caused by hypercontractility of vascular smooth muscle and endothelial dysfunction occurring in the region of spasm. Prinzmetal's variant angina, with intense focal spasm of a segment of an epicardial coronary artery, is the prototypical example [33]. Such patients have rest pain accompanied by transient ST-segment elevation. Vasoconstriction more commonly occurs in the setting of significant coronary atherosclerotic plaque, especially those with superimposed thrombus. Vasoconstriction can occur as the result of local vasoconstrictors released from platelets, such as serotonin and thromboxane A2 [34–36]. Vasoconstriction can also result from a dysfunctional coronary endothelium, which has reduced the production of nitric oxide and increased the release of endothelin. Adrenergic stimuli, cold immersion [37], cocaine [38,39], or mental stress [40] can also cause coronary vasoconstriction among susceptible vessels. A third setting in which vasoconstriction is identified is microcirculatory angina ("syndrome X"). In this condition, ischemia results from constriction of the small intramural coronary resistance vessels [41]. Although no epicardial coronary artery stenoses are present, coronary flow is usually slowed and does not increase appropriately in response to a variety of signals.

Progressive Mechanical Obstruction

Another etiology of NSTE-ACS results from progressive luminal narrowing. This is most commonly seen in the setting of restenosis following percutaneous coronary intervention (PCI). However, angiographic [42] and atherectomy studies [43,44] have demonstrated that many patients without previous PCI show progressive luminal narrowing of the culprit vessel, likely related to rapid cellular proliferation, in the period preceding the onset of NSTE-ACS.

Secondary Myocardial Infarction

Secondary MI is defined as MI precipitated by conditions extrinsic to the coronary arteries, typically among patients with prior coronary stenosis and chronic stable angina. This change could occur either as a result of an increase of myocardial oxygen demand or as a decrease of coronary blood flow. Conditions that increase myocardial demand include tachycardia (e.g., a supraventricular tachycardia or new-onset atrial fibrillation with rapid ventricular response), fever, thyrotoxicosis, hyperadrenergic states, and elevations of left ventricular (LV) afterload, such as hypertension or aortic stenosis. Secondary MI can also occur as a result of impaired oxygen delivery, as in anemia, hypoxemia (e.g., caused by pneumonia or congestive heart failure), hyperviscosity states, or hypotension.

CLINICAL PRESENTATION AND DIAGNOSIS

History and Physical Examination

A description of "ischemic pain" is the hallmark of ACS. Ischemic chest pain is usually described as a discomfort or pressure (rarely as a pain) that is brought on by exertion and relieved by rest. It is generally located in the retrosternal region but sometimes in the epigastrium and frequently radiates to the anterior neck, left shoulder, and left arm. The physical examination may be unremarkable or may support the diagnosis of cardiac ischemia [45]. Signs that suggest ischemia are sweatiness, pale cool skin, sinus tachycardia, and a fourth heart sound. Elevated jugular venous pressure, a third heart sound, or rales on lung examination suggest the presence of heart failure complicating ACS.

Electrocardiogram

The ECG is the most widely used tool for the evaluation of ischemic heart disease and should be performed within minutes for patients presenting with suspected ACS. In NSTE-ACS, ST-segment depression (or transient ST-segment elevation) and T-wave changes occur in up to 50% of patients [46–48]. A normal ECG does not exclude ACS, and should be repeated at regular intervals among individuals with suspected ACS [7]. Additionally, a normal ECG may occur when the left circumflex coronary artery is occluded. Among patients with signs and symptoms of persistent myocardial ischemia, and the standard 12 lead ECG is nondiagnostic, then additional leads such as V_7 to V_9 to look for a posterior MI can be helpful. Among patients presenting with an inferior MI, checking right-sided leads (e.g., V_{3R} and V_{4R}) is helpful to screen for a concomitant right ventricular MI [7,8].

Cardiac Biomarkers

UA is not associated with any detectable damage to the myocyte. The diagnosis of NSTEMI is made if there is biochemical evidence of myocardial necrosis, preferably cardiac troponin T or I, in the appropriate clinical setting. The biomarker criteria include at least one value greater than the 99th percentile of the upper reference range. If the initial value is positive, a subsequent value must demonstrate an increase or decrease of

≥20% [7,49]. Although false-positive troponin elevations do occur [50], elevations of cardiac biomarkers in the absence of other clinical data consistent with an ACS usually do represent true myocardial damage. In these cases, myocyte damage is because of etiologies besides atherosclerotic coronary artery disease, such as myocarditis; LV strain from congestive heart failure; hypertensive crisis; or right ventricular strain from pulmonary embolus [51].

A limitation of standard troponin assays is that they tend to have a low sensitivity in the first few hours of symptom onset. Thus, the current recommendation is to check troponin levels on presentation and then 3 to 6 hours after symptom onset (and repeat 6 hours later if the patient has any intermediate- or high-risk clinical features or any ECG changes). More sensitive assays show better diagnostic performance for patients presenting early after symptom onset [52,53]. High-sensitivity troponin assays, which have a coefficient of variation <10% at the 99th percentile of the upper limit of normal and can quantify troponin levels in >50% of a healthy cohort, can further improve the early diagnosis of MI. Using a high-sensitivty assay, values below the 99th percentile at presentation and 1 hour later have a negative predictive value >99.5%. Moreover, values below the limit of detection at presentation (seen in ~25% of patients) have a negative predictive value of >99.5% [54,55].

Cardiac Imaging

Cardiac imaging continues to assume increasing importance for the early diagnosis of patients presenting with suspected NSTE-ACS, especially when the ECG is normal, nonspecific, or obscured by a left bundle branch block or paced rhythm. Myocardial perfusion imaging using technetium sestamibi has been useful for patients presenting with chest pain in the emergency department without a diagnostic ECG or positive biomarkers to discriminate patients with coronary artery disease from those with noncardiac chest pain [56,57]. Similarly, echocardiography is useful to screen for regional or global LV dysfunction, which may help in establishing (or excluding) the diagnosis of ischemic heart disease for patients who present to the emergency department with chest pain [58]. Coronary computed tomography angiogram (CTA) has also been shown to be effective for excluding coronary artery disease among patients presenting to the emergency department with a low-risk story of chest pain, nondiagnostic ECG, and negative biomarkers [59]. All of these modalities can also assess LV function, a powerful determinant of subsequent prognosis after MI (and presumably after UA) [60–62]. Coronary angiography is also used to establish the diagnosis of ACS and is considered the gold-standard modality to define the extent of coronary disease, and as a prelude to percutaneous revascularization (see section on treatment strategies and interventions) [4,47,63,64].

RISK STRATIFICATION

The process of risk stratification for patients with NSTE-ACS refers to two simultaneous processes (frequently carried out at the time of hospital presentation): (a) risk assessment (i.e., prediction of mortality/morbidity risk), and (b) selection of a management strategy (i.e., an early invasive vs. early conservative approach).

Risk assessment using clinical, electrocardiographic, and laboratory markers identifies which patients are at highest risk for adverse outcomes. Moreover, data from several trials have demonstrated that early risk assessment (especially using troponin) has also been useful for predicting which patients will derive the greatest benefit from more potent antithrombotic therapies, such as low-molecular-weight heparin (LMWH) and GP IIb/IIIa inhibitors. Risk assessment can similarly be used to determine the most appropriate level of care and monitoring (i.e., between the coronary intensive care unit and the step-down/telemetry unit). The "management strategy" refers to whether early angiography is performed (with revascularization as appropriate) directly following the index event or whether a conservative or ischemia-driven strategy is carried out, first with noninvasive assessment of residual ischemia, followed by angiography and revascularization only if recurrent ischemia is demonstrated (see section on, "Early Routine Invasive" vs. "Ischemia-Guided" Strategy of Coronary Angiography and Revascularization).

Risk Assessment Using Clinical Predictors

The initial clinical evaluation can be used to risk-stratify patients quickly and to assist with triage and early management strategy [7,8,65]. In addition to age, gender, and significant comorbidities, certain aspects of the clinical presentation can yield valuable information. High-risk patients can be identified by the presence of pain at rest and increasing frequency of symptoms leading up to the index event. Furthermore, tachycardia, hypotension, and signs of heart failure portend a poor prognosis. In particular, the Killip classification of heart failure severity has been shown to predict both short and long-term mortality for patients with NSTE-ACS [7,8,66,67].

Risk Assessment by Electrocardiography

The admission ECG can be quite useful for predicting early and long-term adverse outcomes [47,68]. In the Global Use of Strategies to Open Occluded Coronary Arteries (GUSTO) IIb study, The presence of ST segment depressions of more than 0.5 mm was associated with a higher risk of 30-day and 6-month death or reinfarction compared with T-wave changes alone [68]. In the TIMI III registry of patients with NSTE-ACS, multivariable predictors of 1-year death or MI included left bundle branch block and ST-segment deviation of 0.5 mm or greater [46]. In contrast, the presence of isolated T-wave changes was not associated with a significantly increased risk of death or MI compared with no ECG changes [46].

The presence of ECG changes has also been associated with greater treatment benefit from more aggressive therapies. The presence of ST-segment deviation identified patients in both the Efficacy and Safety of Subcutaneous Enoxaparin in Non-Q-Wave Coronary Events (ESSENCE) and TIMI 11B trials who benefit the most from antithrombotic therapy with enoxaparin vs. unfractionated heparin (UFH) for NSTE-ACS [69,70]. Similarly, in both the Fragmin and Fast Revascularization during Instability in Coronary Artery Disease (FRISC) II, and Treat Angina with Aggrastat and Determine Cost of Therapy with an Invasive or Conservative Strategy (TACTICS)-TIMI 18 trials, an invasive strategy had a particular benefit for patients with ST-segment depression at presentation [71,72]. Thus, ST-segment deviation not only is a marker of increased risk for adverse outcomes but also identifies those patients who may derive greater benefit from aggressive antithrombotic and invasive therapy.

Risk Assessment by Cardiac Markers

Troponin

Patients with NSTEMI have a worse long-term prognosis than those with UA [73,74]. Patients with an elevated troponin, even with a normal CK-MB, have a significantly worse prognosis [75–77]. Beyond a binary positive vs. negative test result, there is a linear relationship between the level of troponin T or I in the

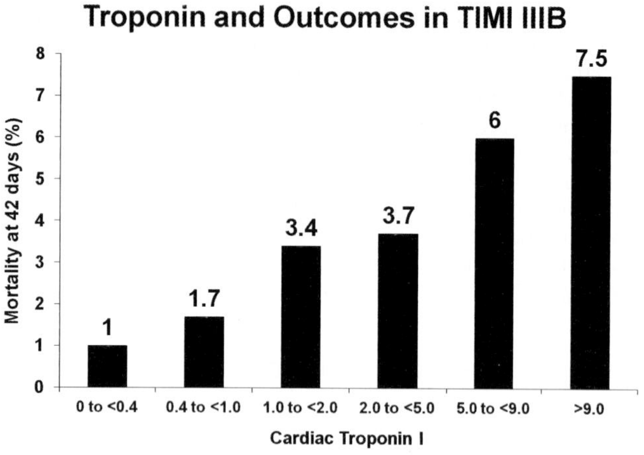

FIGURE 188.2 TIMI IIIB: a direct relationship was observed between increasing levels of troponin I and a higher 42-day mortality. cTnI, cardiac specific troponin I; Ng, negative (Adapted from Antman EM, Tanasijevic MJ, Thompson B, et al: Cardiac-specific troponin I levels to predict the risk of mortality in patients with acute coronary syndromes. *N Engl J Med* 335:1342–1349, 1996.).

blood and the subsequent risk of death: the higher the troponin, the higher the mortality risk (Fig. 188.2). Thus, troponin is useful not only for diagnosing infarction [78] but also for assessing risk among patients who present with NSTE-ACS. Given the enhanced sensitivity and specificity, troponin is the preferred marker of myocardial necrosis for both diagnosis and prognosis [7,8].

The presence of elevated troponin levels also correlates with the utility of particular therapies. In a trial examining the benefit of abciximab among patients with NSTEMI, the reduction of death or MI at 6 months was 70% for those who were troponin T positive, whereas there was no significant benefit for those who were troponin T negative ($p < 0.001$) [79]. In the TIMI 11B trial, even when looking at patients who were CK-MB negative, those who were troponin I positive derived a significantly greater benefit from enoxaparin vs. UFH, compared with those who had both markers negative [80]. Research has also demonstrated that troponin levels are useful when choosing an invasive vs. conservative strategy for patients with NSTE-ACS. In both the FRISC II and TACTICS-TIMI 18 trials, patients who had a positive troponin T or I (including those who had very low levels of troponin) had a dramatic reduction of cardiac events after allocation to an invasive strategy [76,81]. Thus, there is evidence from multiple trials that the use of troponins can assist in both assessing the risk and determining which patients will accrue the most benefit from more potent antithrombotic agents and an invasive management strategy.

Other Biomarkers

NSTE-ACS patients with an elevated C-reactive protein (CRP) have an increased risk of death and adverse cardiovascular events [82,83]. Even among patients with negative troponin I at baseline, CRP is able to discriminate high- and low-risk groups [84]. B-type natriuretic peptide (BNP) as well as N-terminal pro B-type natriuretic peptide (NT-proBNP), both biomarkers of LV wall stress, has also been shown to be a powerful predictor of mortality and heart failure among patients with NSTE-ACS [85–88]. Growth-differentiation factor 15 (GDF-15), a member of the transforming growth factor-β family induced by inflammation and cellular injury, has been shown to be a similarly powerful predictor of adverse cardiovascular outcomes after NSTE-ACS [89]. Researchers have even suggested that GDF-15 may be able to identify which NSTE-ACS patients will benefit most from an invasive treatment strategy. A retrospective analysis from the FRISC-II trial looked at GDF-15 levels among patients with NSTE-ACS and found that patients with markedly elevated GDF-15 levels had lower mortality when an invasive treatment strategy was used as opposed to conservative management. In contrast, among patients with ST-segment depression or an elevated troponin T level, those with a low GDF-15 level did not benefit from an invasive treatment strategy [90]. Larger prospective studies are needed to see if GDF-15 will be a useful tool when deciding on the management of patients with NSTE-ACS. Multimarker strategies have also been employed to improve risk stratification. The combination of troponin, CRP, and BNP can predict up to a 13-fold gradient of mortality post-ACS [91]. However, it should be noted that although CRP and BNP can be used as prognostic indicators, only troponin and potentially GDF-15 can identify patients who may derive greater benefit from specific interventions.

Combined Risk Assessment Scores

The current AHA/ACC and ESC guidelines for the management of NSTE-ACS recommend the use of risk scores to facilitate decisions regarding triage and management strategy [7,8]. The TIMI risk score uses readily available clinical factors, ECG changes, and cardiac markers. It consists of the following seven risk factors: age 65 years or older, more than three risk factors for coronary artery disease, documented coronary artery disease at catheterization, ST-segment deviation of 0.5 mm or greater, more than two episodes of angina in the past 24 hours, aspirin use within the prior week, or elevated serum cardiac markers. Use of this scoring system was able to risk-stratify patients across a 10-fold gradient of risk, from 4.7% to 40.9% ($p < 0.001$) [92]. Most importantly, this risk score identified patients who derived the greatest benefit from enoxaparin vs. UFH [92], from use of a GP IIb/IIIa inhibitor [93], and from an early invasive management strategy [72].

The GRACE (Global Registry of Acute Coronary Events) risk score incorporates multiple characteristics on admission to identify patients at greatest risk of in-hospital and 6-month mortality following an ACS. The model includes age; heart rate; systolic blood pressure; serum creatinine; presence and severity of heart failure according to Killip class, whether or not there was a cardiac arrest at admission; ST-segment deviation; and elevated cardiac markers at presentation [94,95]. When applied to patients with NSTE-ACS, the GRACE risk score is also able to identify those patients most likely to benefit from an early invasive strategy. In the Timing of Intervention in Patients with Acute Coronary Syndromes (TIMACS) trial, NSTE-ACS patients with a GRACE risk score of greater than 140 (the highest risk tertile) had a 35% reduction in the primary end point (composite of death, MI, or stroke) with early coronary angiography (median time, 14 hours) when compared to delayed intervention (median time, 50 hours): 13.9% vs. 21%; $p = 0.006$. In patients with a GRACE risk score of less than 140, there was no difference between the two groups: 7.6% vs. 6.7%; $p = 0.48$ [96]. Therefore, combined risk assessment scores can not only identify those patients at the highest risk for an adverse cardiovascular event, but can also assist the clinician with management decisions regarding antithrombotic therapy and coronary angiography.

MEDICAL THERAPIES

Treatment Goals

The treatment objectives for patients with NSTE-ACS are focused on stabilizing and "passivating" the acute coronary lesion, treatment of residual ischemia, and long-term secondary prevention. Antithrombotic therapy (e.g., aspirin, P_2Y_{12} ADP receptor blockers such as ticagrelor, prasugrel and clopidogrel, anticoagulants, and GP IIb/IIIa inhibitors) is used to prevent further clotting in the coronary artery and allow endogenous fibrinolysis to dissolve the thrombus and reduce the degree of coronary stenosis. Antithrombotic therapy is continued long term so that if future events occur, the degree of thrombosis is reduced. Anti-ischemic therapies (e.g., β-blockers, nitrates, and sometimes calcium channel blockers) are used to reduce myocardial oxygen demand. Coronary revascularization is frequently needed to treat recurrent or residual ischemia. After stabilization of the acute event, the many factors that led up to the event need to be addressed. Treatment of atherosclerotic risk factors such as hypercholesterolemia, hypertension, and smoking, which contributes to stabilization of the cholesterol-laden plaque and healing of the endothelium, is critical.

Antiplatelet Therapy

Aspirin

Aspirin is a cornerstone of therapy for patients who present with NSTE-ACS. Through irreversible inhibition of cyclooxygenase (thus limiting the production of thromboxane A_2), aspirin decreases platelet activation and has demonstrated clear beneficial effects for patients who present with NSTE-ACS [74,97–99]. The randomized Clopidogrel and Aspirin Optimal Dose Usage to Reduce Recurrent Events - Seventh Organization to Assess Strategies in Ischemic Syndromes (CURRENT-OASIS 7) trial evaluated 25,086 ACS patients (who were referred for an invasive strategy) and demonstrated no differences of outcomes between the low-dose (75 to 100 mg) and high-dose (300 to 325 mg) aspirin groups. Importantly, each arm received an initial loading dose of aspirin of at least 300 mg on day 1 [100]. These results were similar for the prespecified subset of individuals who underwent PCI [101]. A subsequent meta-analysis demonstrated comparable benefit between low-dose (less than 160 mg) and high-dose (greater than or equal to 160 mg) aspirin with an increased risk of bleeding in the high-dose group [102]. Additionally, patients treated with ticagrelor in the Platelet Inhibition and Patient Outcomes (PLATO) trial had better outcomes when they were concomitantly treated with low vs. high maintenance dose of aspirin [103]. Thus, for patients presenting with NSTE-ACS, an initial loading dose of non-enteric coated aspirin of 325 mg followed by maintenance dose of 75 to 81 mg daily is a reasonable approach [7,8]. For patients with an allergy to aspirin, a loading dose of clopidogrel followed by daily maintenance dosing is a reasonable alternative [7].

P_2Y_{12} ADP Receptor Blockers

Clopidogrel is a thienopyridine derivative that inhibits platelet activation and aggregation by irreversibly inhibiting the binding of ADP to the P_2Y_{12} receptor on the surface of the platelet. In the Clopidogrel in Unstable Angina to Prevent Recurrent Events (CURE) trial the addition of clopidogrel plus aspirin led to a 20% reduction of recurrent cardiovascular events when compared with aspirin alone for 12,562 randomized NSTE-ACS patients [104]. For patients who underwent PCI, those treated with clopidogrel experienced a 30% reduction of ischemic events [105]. The combination of clopidogrel plus aspirin was however associated with a relative 35% increase of major bleeding (using the CURE trial definition), but the absolute increase was only 1% (from 2.7% to 3.7%). Furthermore, using the standard TIMI definition of bleeding, there was no significant increase of major bleeding risk and no increase of intracranial hemorrhage.

Clopidogrel is an inactive prodrug that requires hepatic metabolism via the cytochrome P450 (CYP) system to produce the active metabolite (Table 188.1). Roughly, 85% of the prodrug is hydrolysed to an inactive metabolite by circulating esterases [8,106]. There are several notable pharmacogenetic and drug–drug interactions for clopidogrel that can affect patient outcomes. Approximately 25% to 30% of the population has a reduced-function genetic variant of *CYP2C19*, a member of the CYP450 enzyme family. When treated with clopidogrel, these individuals have lower circulating levels of the clopidogrel active metabolite, thereby leading to less platelet inhibition, and a higher rate of ischemic events including stent thrombosis [107–109].

Metabolism of clopidogrel may also be affected by certain drugs. Several pharmacodynamic studies had shown that proton pump inhibitors (PPIs) that inhibit *CYP2C19* could decrease clopidogrel activity. However, the safety of combination therapy with clopidogrel and omeprazole was demonstrated in the Clopidogrel and the Optimization of Gastrointestinal Events Trial (COGENT), which randomized patients to clopidogrel alone or a combination pill of clopidogrel plus omeprazole following PCI. There was no difference of cardiovascular outcomes over 6 months, although they did note a significant reduction in GI events among patients taking the PPI [110]. Given the dependence of clopidogrel metabolism on the CYP450 system and the large number of PPIs available, including some that do not inhibit CYP2C19, extra vigilance should be taken when prescribing other drugs with clopidogrel.

Prasugrel is a third-generation P_2Y_{12} ADP receptor blocker. Although also a prodrug and an irreversible P_2Y_{12} inhibitor, prasugrel has a quicker onset of action when compared to clopidogrel (30 to 90 minutes for prasugrel vs. 2 to 6 hours for clopidogrel). Prasugrel has more predictable and more potent platelet inhibition than clopidogrel [106]. The Trial to Assess Improvement in Therapeutic Outcomes by Optimizing Platelet Inhibition with Prasugrel - Thrombolysis in Myocardial Infarction (TRITON-TIMI) 38 compared prasugrel to clopidogrel in 13,608

TABLE 188.1

Comparison of P_2Y_{12} Receptor Blockers

	Clopidogrel	Prasugrel	Ticagrelor	Cangrelor
Inhibitor reversibility	Irreversible	Irreversible	Reversible	Reversible
Administration	Oral	Oral	Oral	Intravenous
Loading dose	300–600 mg	60 mg	180 mg	30 μg/kg bolus
Maintenance dose	75 mg daily	10 mg daily	90 mg twice daily	4 μg/kg/min
Prodrug vs. Active drug	Prodrug	Prodrug	Active drug	Active drug
Loading dose Onset of action	2–6 h	30 min	30 min	2 min
Effect Duration	7–10 d	7–10 d	3–5 d	30–120 min
Cessation before surgery	5 d	7 d	5 d	60 min

Adapted from Franchi F, Angiolillo DJ: Novel antiplatelet agents in acute coronary syndrome. *Nat Rev Cardiol* 12(1):30–47, 2015; and Roffi M, Patrono C, Collet JP, et al. 2015 ESC Guidelines for the management of acute coronary syndromes in patients presenting without persistent ST-segment elevation: Task Force for the Management of Acute Coronary Syndromes in Patients Presenting without Persistent ST-Segment Elevation of the European Society of Cardiology (ESC). *Eur Heart J* 37(3):267–315, 2016.

ACS patients who were scheduled to undergo PCI. Notably, study medication was administered after coronary anatomy was known, either during or after PCI. Patients receiving prasugrel had a 19% reduction of the rate of cardiovascular death, MI, and stroke (9.9% vs. 12.1%; $p < 0.001$) as well as a 52% reduction in stent thrombosis (1.1% vs. 2.4%; $p < 0.001$) [111,112]. These positive effects come at the price of significantly increased rates of major bleeding with prasugrel after PCI (2.4% vs. 1.8%; $p < 0.001$) [111]. Comparable effects to the overall trial results were seen among the 10,074 patients with NSTE-ACS. Prasugrel is contraindicated for patients with a history of cerebrovascular events due to net harm in this subgroup, whereas there was no clinical benefit for patients older than 75 years of age or for patients who weighed less than 60 kg [111]. The Targeted Platelet Inhibition to Clarify the Optimal Strategy to Medically Manage Acute Coronary Syndromes (TRILOGY ACS) trial evaluated aspirin plus either clopidogrel or prasugrel in NSTE-ACS patients managed medically without revascularization. There was no difference in ischemic or bleeding events [113]. As a result of these findings, for patients treated with PCI who are not at high risk for bleeding, prasugrel is preferred over clopidogrel [7].

Ticagrelor is another oral P_2Y_{12} ADP inhibitor; however, unlike clopidogrel or prasugrel, it has reversible binding and is administered twice daily. Similar to prasugrel, ticareglor has a faster and more predictable onset of action than clopidogrel (Table 188.1). The PLATO trial compared clopidogrel and ticagrelor in 18,624 patients presenting with ACS [114]. Similar to the overall trial, for the subset of 11,080 NSTE-ACS patients, ticagrelor reduced the primary end point of CV death, MI, or stroke (10.0% vs. 12.3%, $p = 0.0013$) when compared with clopidogrel. There was also a reduction in the rates of CV death (3.7% vs. 4.9% $p = 0.007$), and all-cause mortality (4.3% vs. 5.8% $p = 0.002$) [115]. Bleeding outcomes were also similar to the overall trial for the subset of patients with NSTE-ACS: No overall difference of major bleeding, but the ticagrelor group did have a higher rate of non-CABG related major bleeding (4.8% vs. 3.8% $p = 0.0139$). The lower event rates with ticagrelor vs. clopidogrel were independent of revascularization status within the first 10 days following randomization [115]. Two additional notable side effects observed from the PLATO trial were dyspnea (occurred in 15% and led to drug discontinuation in <1% of patients) and asymptomatic ventricular pauses which were not associated with increased rates of syncope or pacemaker implantation [114]. Ticagrelor is preferred over clopidogrel for patients treated with medical therapy or with PCI [7].

Cangrelor is an intravenous P_2Y_{12} ADP inhibitor with a short half-life (less than 10 minutes) that has a fast and predictable onset and offset of action. Within minutes of an initial bolus the desired antiplatelet effect is achieved, and within 60 minutes of stopping the infusion platelet function is restored. In the CHAMPION-PHOENIX trial, there was a significant reduction of the composite of death from any cause, myocardial infarction, ischemia-driven revascularization, or stent thrombosis at 48 hours with cangrelor compared to clopidogrel (4.7% vs. 5.9% $p = 0.005$), with the results mainly driven by periprocedural stent thrombosis and MI. There was no increase in the rate of primary safety end point, GUSTO-defined severe bleeding (0.16% for the cangrelor group vs. 0.11% for the clopidogrel group $p = 0.44$) [116].

Cangrelor's short half-life with quick onset and offset make it an appealing option for use as a bridge for patients planned for surgery. The phase II pharmacodynamic BRIDGE study evaluated the use of cangrelor as a bridge to CABG for 210 patients (More than 1/3 with NSTE-ACS) who had an indication for thienopyridine treatment [117]. Continuous infusion at a dose of 0.75 μg/kg/min provided comparable platelet inhibition to daily thienopyridine therapy. There was no increase of major bleeding complications; however, the study was not powered for clinical end points. The use of cangrelor as a bridge for noncardiac surgery or for other clinical scenarios appears to be an attractive strategy, although it has not yet been evaluated in these additional settings [106].

Although the use of P_2Y_{12} inhibition in NSTE-ACS has become standard of care, the optimal timing of P_2Y_{12} inhibitor administration (before or after coronary angiography) remains quite uncertain [118,119]. Previous guidelines recommended that P_2Y_{12} inhibitor therapy be initiated as soon as possible after the diagnosis of NSTE-ACS [120,121]. However, these recommendations were based on data from studies of clopidogrel, which is a prodrug and for which the clinical data suggested a benefit to pretreatment [105,122]. Subsequent to the previous guidelines, the only randomized controlled trial to evaluate the effect of pretreatment with P_2Y_{12} inhibition (the ACCOAST trial) demonstrated no ischemic benefit with the administration of prasugrel prior to angiography, whereas pretreatment was associated with increased bleeding [123]. As a result, prasugrel is not recommended prior to coronary angiography for patients with NSTE-ACS. In contrast, there are no randomized controlled data to support or refute pretreatment with either clopidogrel or ticagrelor. As a result, the current guidelines provide no substantive recommendations regarding when to initiate clopidogrel or ticagrelor for patients with NSTE-ACS undergoing an invasive strategy, whereas for patients undergoing a noninvasive strategy, P_2Y_{12} inhibition with clopidogrel or ticagrelor is recommended as soon as the diagnosis of NSTE-ACS is made [7,8].

Duration of Dual Antiplatelet Therapy

For patients who have tolerated dual antiplatelet therapy well for 12 months, it may be reasonable to continue dual antiplatelet therapy for longer than 12 months [124]. For patients who had been on dual antiplatelet therapy for 12 months following PCI, the Dual Antiplatelet Therapy (DAPT) study demonstrated a significant reduction in major adverse cardiovascular and cerebrovascular events with prolonged dual antiplatelet therapy (for an additional 18 months) compared to aspirin alone [125]. This benefit was consistent for the subgroup of patients with a prior MI. This concept was reaffirmed in the Prevention of Cardiovascular Events in Patients with Prior Heart Attack Using Ticagrelor Compared to Placebo on a Background of Aspirin—Thrombolysis in Myocardial Infarction 54 (PEGASUS-TIMI 54) [126]. The combination of aspirin plus 2 different doses of ticagrelor (60 or 90 mg twice daily) reduced the composite outcome of cardiovascular death, MI, or stroke when compared with aspirin plus placebo among patients with a prior MI more than 1 year before study entry (Fig. 188.3). A meta-analysis of DAPT for patients with prior MI also showed similar benefit

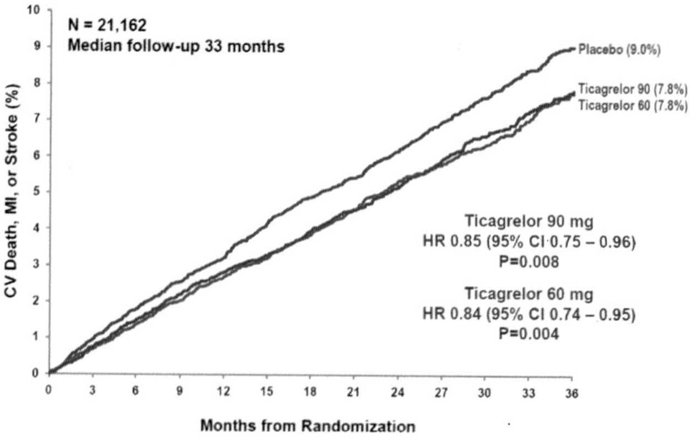

FIGURE 188.3 Kaplan–Meier curves demonstrating the benefit of ticagrelor (60 mg or 90 mg) vs. placebo in reducing rates of major adverse cardiovascular events (Adapted from Bonaca MP, Bhatt DL, Cohen M, et al. Long-term use of ticagrelor in patients with prior myocardial infarction. *N Engl J Med* 372:1791–800, 2015.).

with prolonged DAPT vs. aspirin alone [127]. This benefit was seen across several high-risk subgroups including patients with diabetes, multivessel coronary artery disease, renal impairment, and peripheral arterial disease [128]. Importantly, prolonged DAPT did increase the overall risk of bleeding (although there was no increase in the risk of intracranial hemorrhage or of fatal bleeding). [125–127]. Thus, the increased risk of bleeding must be weighed against the ischemic benefit, with treatment decisions tailored to the individual patient, potentially targeting individuals with risk factors associated with increased recurrent events [128].

Glycoprotein IIb/IIIa Inhibitors

Glycoprotein (GP) IIb/IIIa inhibitors prevent the final common pathway of platelet aggregation, that is, fibrinogen-mediated cross-linkage of platelets via the GP IIb/IIIa receptor (Fig. 188.1). Currently available GP IIb/IIIa inhibitors are all administered intravenously and include abciximab, eptifibatide, and tirofiban. Abciximab is a monoclonal antibody Fab fragment directed at the GP IIb/IIIa receptor, whereas eptifibatide, a synthetic heptapeptide, and tirofiban, a nonpeptide molecule, are antagonists of the GP IIb/IIIa receptor whose structure mimics the arginine–glycine–aspartic acid amino acid sequence by which fibrinogen binds to the GP IIb/IIIa receptor.

The efficacy of the GP IIb/IIIa inhibitors for the treatment of NSTEMIs has been evaluated by several studies. A meta-analysis of six randomized controlled trials (with nearly 30,000 NSTE-ACS patients) demonstrated a modest 9% relative reduction of rates of 30 day death or MI (10.7% vs. 11.5% $p = 0.02$) with the use of GP IIb/IIIa inhibitors. Notably, this benefit was predominantly seen among individuals who underwent PCI [129]. These trials, however, were largely performed before the era of routine P_2Y_{12} inhibition. The ISAR-REACT 2 trial addressed whether GP IIb/IIIa inhibition with abciximab provided additional benefit for 2,022 NSTE-ACS patients who were scheduled to undergo PCI after pretreatment with clopidogrel. The use of abciximab was associated with a 25% reduction of adverse cardiovascular events (8.9% vs. 11.9%, $p = 0.03$). The benefits afforded by the addition of abciximab to clopidogrel were limited to patients with an elevated troponin [130].

Although these earlier trials demonstrated the benefit of GP IIb/IIIa inhibition for the management of patients with NSTEMIs undergoing PCI, the optimal timing for drug initiation was unclear. Subsequent randomized controlled trials compared upstream GP IIb/IIIa inhibitor initiation prior to angiography vs. deferred initiation at the time of PCI. The Acute Catheterization and Urgent Intervention Triage Strategy (ACUITY) Timing trial demonstrated that a deferred treatment strategy was noninferior to the upstream treatment strategy for ischemic events (7.9% vs. 7.1%, relative risk 1.12, 95% CI 0.97 to 1.29, $p = 0.044$ for noninferiority, $p = 0.13$ for superiority), whereas the deferred treatment strategy was associated with lower bleeding rates (4.9% vs. 6.1%, $p < 0.001$ for noninferiority, $p = 0.009$ for superiority) [131]. Similar findings were observed from the more recent Early Glycoprotein IIb/IIIa Inhibition in Non–ST-Segment Elevation Acute Coronary Syndrome (EARLY ACS) trial which evaluated the use of routine use of upstream GP IIb/IIIa inhibitor eptifibatide vs. delayed provisional use of the medication at the time of PCI [132]. There was no significant difference of the composite rate of death, MI, urgent revascularization, or thrombotic complication during PCI between the two groups, whereas the patients randomized to upstream eptifibatide had higher rates of non–life-threatening bleeding and more blood transfusions.

Based on these data demonstrating no benefits but increased bleeding with upstream initiation of GPIIb/IIIa inhibitors, their role prior to PCI is limited. The current AHA/ACC guidelines provide a class IIb recommendation that for high-risk patients (e.g., those with positive troponin) treated with an early invasive strategy and dual antiplatelet therapy, a GP IIb/IIIa inhibitor may be considered as part of initial antiplatelet therapy [7]. Alternatively, the current ESC guidelines recommend against the use of GP IIb/IIIa inhibitors for patients in whom the coronary anatomy is not known, and provide a class IIa recommendation for their use during PCI in bailout situations or for thrombotic complications [8].

Vorapaxar

Vorapaxar is an oral selective platelet thrombin receptor PAR-1 inhibitor that prevents thrombin mediated platelet activation. The Thrombin Receptor Antagonist for Clinical Event Reduction in Acute Coronary Syndrome (TRACER) trial randomized 12,944 patients with NSTE-ACS to either vorapaxar (40 mg loading dose followed by 2.5 mg daily) or placebo [133]. Most patients were treated with aspirin (97%) and clopidogrel (92%). There was no significant difference in ischemic events between the two treatment groups (18.5% vorapaxar vs. 19.9% placebo; $p = 0.07$); however, there were significantly increased rates of moderate or severe bleeding for the vorapaxar group (7.2% vs. 5.2%; HR 1.35; 95% CI, 1.16 to 1.58; $p < 0.001$). Rates of intracranial hemorrhage were also significantly higher with vorapaxar compared to placebo (1.1% vs. 0.2%; HR 3.39; 95% CI, 1.78 to 6.45; $p < 0.001$).

In a non-acute setting, the Thrombin Receptor Antagonist in Secondary Prevention of Atherothrombotic Ischemic Events (TRA 2P—TIMI 50) trial evaluated the effect of vorapaxar (2.5 mg once daily) for the secondary prevention of ischemic events among patients with a history of MI, stroke, or peripheral arterial disease [134]. There was a reduction of ischemic events with vorapaxar compared with placebo (9.3% vs. 10.5%; $p < 0.001$) at the expense of excess moderate or severe bleeding (4.2% vs. 2.5%; $p < 0.001$) and increased intracranial bleeding (1% vs. 0.5%; $p < 0.001$). Among the 17,779 patients with a history of MI, the vorapaxar group had a lower rate or ischemic events (8.1% vs. 9.7%; $p < 0.001$), but also had higher rates of moderate or severe bleeding (3.4% vs. 2.1%; $p < 0.001$).

Anticoagulation

Heparin

Among patients with NSTE-ACS, anticoagulation on top of antiplatelet therapy reduces the risk of events [135]. Unfractionated heparin (UFH) is a widely used anticoagulant that works by blocking both thrombin and factor Xa. UFH is administered as a continuous infusion in patients with ACS owing to its short half-life. A meta-analysis showed a 33% reduction in death or MI when comparing UFH plus aspirin vs. aspirin alone [136].

The optimal regimen appears to be weight-adjusted dosing (60 units/kg bolus with a maximum of 4,000 units and 12 units/kg/h infusion with a maximum of 1,000 units per hour), with frequent monitoring of the activated partial thromboplastin time (aPTT) (every 6 hours until in the target range and every 12 to 24 hours thereafter), and titration using a standardized normogram, with a target range of aPTT between 1.5 and 2.5 times control or approximately 50 to 70 seconds. UFH should be continued for 48 hours or until PCI is performed [7].

Low-Molecular-Weight Heparin

Compared with UFH, LMWH has a higher ratio of anti-Xa to antithrombin activity, and thus has more effective inhibition of thrombin generation [137]. LMWH has additional potential advantages over standard UFH. LMWH has less binding with platelet factor 4 (PF4), a heparin-neutralizing protein, which may explain the lower rates of heparin induced thrombocytopenia (HIT) with LMWH vs. UFH [137]. Additionally, higher bioavailability and a more predictable dose response allow for weight-based subcutaneous dosing without frequent monitoring. The recommended enoxaparin dose is 1 mg/kg every 12 hours. Importantly, because enoxaparin is affected by renal dysfunction, dose adjustment is necessary for patients with reduced renal function (creatinine clearance 15 to 30 mL per min: dose 1 mg/kg once daily), and for patients with severe renal dysfunction (creatinine clearance < 15 mL per minute) LMWH should not be used.

Several trials have compared UFH with enoxaparin in patients with NSTE-ACS. The earlier studies, Efficacy and Safety of Subcutaneous Enoxaparin in Non-Q-Wave Coronary Events (ESSENCE) and TIMI 11b, demonstrated a reduction of ischemic events among patients treated with enoxaparin vs. UFH [70,138]. Importantly, these trials were conducted on a background of predominantly noninvasive management strategies. In contrast, the subsequent Superior Yield of the New Strategy of Enoxaparin, Revascularization and Glycoprotein IIb/IIIa Inhibitors (SYNERGY) trial, conducted among high-risk NSTE-ACS patients who were planned for an early invasive strategy, demonstrated no reduction in ischemic events with enoxaparin vs. UFH, but that enoxaparin was associated with increased bleeding (9.1% vs. 7.6%; $p = 0.008$) [139]. Given the differing results, a meta-analysis was performed including 49,088 ACS patients that demonstrated a significant reduction of ischemic events with enoxaparin vs. UFH and no differences of bleeding [140]. Similar results were noted for the subset of NSTE-ACS patients; enoxaparin reduced ischemic events (odds ratio 0.90; 95% CI 0.81 to 0.996, $p = 0.043$), without a significant increase of major bleeding (odds ratio 1.13, 95% CI 0.84 to 1.54, $p = 0.419$).

Fondaparinux

Fondaparinux is a synthetic pentasaccharide and a specific factor Xa inhibitor. In the Organization to Assess Strategies in Ischemic Syndromes (OASIS)-5 study, fondaparinux was found to be noninferior to enoxaparin in terms of ischemic events and nearly halved the rate of major bleeding over the first 9 days in patients with NSTE-ACS [141]. By 30 days, mortality was significantly lower in the fondaparinux arm (hazard ratio 0.83; 95% CI 0.71 to 0.97; $p = 0.02$). Notably, in the subset of patients undergoing PCI, fondaparinux was associated with an increased risk of catheter-related thrombi. Standard-dose UFH during PCI appeared to minimize this risk [142], and consequently, the AHA/ACC and ESC recommend that standard-dose UFH be used during PCI for patients treated with fondaparinux beforehand [7,8].

Bivalirudin

Bivalirudin is another antithrombotic drug used in the treatment of NSTE-ACS, which acts by directly inhibiting thrombin and thus inhibiting clot formation. Bivalirudin was evaluated in the Acute Catheterization and Urgent Intervention Triage Strategy (ACUITY) trial, which randomized 13,819 patients with NSTE-ACS, who were to be managed with an early invasive strategy, to one of three treatments: UFH or enoxaparin plus a GP IIb/IIIa inhibitor, bivalirudin plus a GP IIb/IIIa inhibitor, or bivalirudin alone. The study found no differences of the primary end point of death, MI, unplanned revascularization for ischemia, and major bleeding at 30 days between bivalirudin plus GP IIb/IIIa inhibitor and UFH/enoxaparin plus a GP IIb/IIIa inhibitor [143]. For the bivalirudin-alone group, when compared with the group receiving UFH/enoxaparin plus a GP IIb/IIIa inhibitor, there was no difference of the composite ischemic end point, but there was a lower rate of bleeding (3.0% vs. 5.7%; $p < 0.001$). Similar results were noted for the Intracoronary Stenting and Antithrombotic Regimen: Rapid Early Action for Coronary Treatment 4 (ISAR-REACT 4) trial [144]. A meta-analysis including 16 trials comparing bivalrudin-based regimens with heparin-based regimens demonstrated that bivalrudin was associated with a reduction of bleeding events, but with an increased risk of MI and stent thrombosis [145]. The Minimizing Adverse Hemorrhagic Events by Transradial Access Site and Systemic Implementation of Angiox (MATRIX) study demonstrated no benefit with bivalrudin for either major adverse cardiovascular events or for net clinical adverse events (a composite of major bleeding and major adverse cardiovascular events) [146]. The AHA/ACC guidelines recommend that bivalirudin only be used for patients managed with an early invasive strategy whereas the ESC guidelines recommend bivalirudin as an alternative to UFH-GP IIb/IIIa inhibitors during PCI [7,8].

Oral Anticoagulation

Oral anticoagulation with warfarin following ACS has been examined by several trials, because prolonged treatment might extend the benefits of early anticoagulation. The Warfarin Reinfarction Study II randomized 3,630 patients with acute MI to three arms: aspirin 160 mg daily; warfarin alone (target INR 2.8 to 4.2; mean 2.8); and warfarin (target INR 2.0 to 2.5; mean 2.2) plus 75 mg aspirin [147]. When compared with aspirin alone, the combination of warfarin plus aspirin lowered the rate of ischemic events, but at the expense of increased bleeding.

Two more recent trials have evaluated the addition of non-vitamin K antagonist oral anticoagulants (NOACs) to dual antiplatelet therapy following ACS. The Apixaban for Prevention of Acute Ischemic Events (APPRAISE) 2 trial compared the addition of apixaban 5mg twice daily to placebo in addition to standard antiplatelet therapy following ACS. The trial was stopped early to a significant increase of bleeding without a reduction of ischemic events [148].

The Anti-Xa Therapy to Lower Cardiovascular Events in Addition to Aspirin with or without Thienopyridine Therapy in Subjects with Acute Coronary Syndrome (ATLAS ACS 2)—TIMI 51 evaluated the effect of adding rivaroxaban (2.5 or 5 mg twice daily) vs. placebo in 15,526 patients with a recent ACS. Roughly 50% of the population had NSTE-ACS and 93% were on clopidogrel in addition to aspirin, and it included patients with a history of intracranial bleeding, ischemic stroke, or TIA [149]. At mean follow-up of 13 months, the addition of rivaroxaban led to a 16% lower rate of death, MI, or stroke at the expense of increased bleeding. The 2.5 mg dose led to a significant 32% reduction in all-cause mortality whereas the 5 mg dose did not. Although both doses led to a significant increase of bleeding (including intracranial bleeding), the 2.5 mg dose had less of an increased bleeding risk than the 5 mg dose. As a result, the 2.5 mg twice daily dose is currently available in Europe with a class IIb recommendation from the ESC for patients with a recent NSTE-ACS, to be used in combination with aspirin and clopidogrel. It is not recommended to be used in combination with ticagrelor or prasugrel and is contraindicated in patients with a history of ischemic stroke or TIA [8]. Rivaroxaban has not been approved for this indication in the USA and is not included in the current AHA/ACC guidelines. However, supporting the benefit of this approach, the results of the COMPASS trial have recently been announced in which very low-dose rivaroxaban added to aspirin was superior to low-dose aspirin monotherapy in patients with a history of vascular disease.

Thrombolytic Therapy for NSTE-ACS

Because thrombolytic therapy is beneficial for the treatment of patients with acute MI presenting with ST-segment elevation, it was hoped that it might play a role in other ACS. In TIMI IIIB, 1,473 patients with UA and non–Q-wave MI were treated with aspirin and heparin and were randomized to receive either tissue-type plasminogen activator (t-PA) or placebo. No difference was found for the primary end point comparing t-PA with placebo: the incidence of death, postrandomization infarction, or recurrent, objectively documented ischemia through 6 weeks (54.2% for t-PA and 55.5% for placebo; p = not significant [NS]) [47].

The TIMI IIIB results are corroborated by the Fibrinolytic Therapy Trialists' Collaborative Group overview, in which patients with suspected MI and ST-segment depression on the ECG had a higher mortality when treated with a fibrinolytic [150,151]. Accordingly, fibrinolytic therapy is not indicated in NSTE-ACS [7].

Anti-ischemic Therapy

Oxygen

Patients who are in respiratory distress and/or have an arterial oxygen saturation <90% should receive supplemental oxygen [7,8]. Previous guidelines recommended for the routine use of supplemental oxygen in all patients with NSTE-ACS during the first 6 hours after presentation, even in the absence of low arterial oxygen saturation [120]. In normoxic NSTE-ACS patients, there is no evidence that routine supplemental oxygen is beneficial; however, there is evidence of potential harm with routine supplemental oxygen among normoxic STEMI patients [152].

Nitrates

Nitrates can be helpful for the management of ischemic symptoms of patients with NSTE-ACS. Importantly, they are provided for symptom relief and do not impart a mortality benefit. Both the Gruppo Italiano per lo Studio della Sopravvivenza nell'Infarto miocardico (GISSI) 3 and International Study of Infarct Survival (ISIS) four trials failed to demonstrate a survival benefit with nitrates for patients with confirmed or suspected ACS [153,154]. If there is persistent pain or hypertension after three sublingual tablets and initiation of β-blockade, intravenous nitroglycerin is recommended [7]. Nitrates should not be given to patients who have recently taken a phosphodiesterase inhibitor because of an increased risk of hypotension.

β-Blockers

β-Blockers lower heart rate, blood pressure, and contractility, leading to decreased myocardial oxygen consumption. A recent meta-analysis demonstrated that early initiation of β-blockade was associated with a reduction of ischemic events and a modest reduction in near term all-cause mortality [155]. The Clopidogrel and Metoprolol in Myocardial Infarction Trial (COMMIT) demonstrated the importance of selecting the right population for early initiation of β-blockade in ACS [156]. In the overall population of 45,852 patients, the beneficial effects of metoprolol on reinfarction and ventricular fibrillation were balanced by an increased risk of cardiogenic shock. When the population was stratified according to risk of cardiogenic shock, those considered low risk demonstrated a significant benefit associated with early initiation of β-blockade. The clinical features identified as high risk for cardiogenic shock included age >70 years, systolic blood pressure <120 mmHg, heart rate >110 beats per minute, and overt heart failure on initial examination (Killip class III). The current guidelines recommend for initiation of oral β-blockade within the first 24 hours for patients who are not in heart failure, in a state of low cardiac output, have a high risk of cardiogenic shock, or have significant AV block [7]. For patients with initial contraindications to early β-blocker therapy, once patients have hemodynamically stabilized, initiation of β-blockade should be considered. Additionally, a history of chronic obstructive lung disease or asthma is not a contraindication to the initiation of β-blockade in the absence of active airway disease [7].

Calcium Channel Blockers

Nondihydropyridine calcium channel blockers (i.e., diltiazem and verapamil) slow heart rate, lower blood pressure, decrease myocardial contractility, and provide mild coronary vasodilation. The Diltiazem Reinfarction Study, which involved 576 patients with non–Q-wave MI, showed that diltiazem reduced the rate of recurrent MI from 9.3% with placebo to 5.2% with diltiazem [157]. Similarly, the Danish Verapamil Infarction Trial (DAVIT) II demonstrated a reduction of events, especially among patients without heart failure [158]. Not all trials, however, have shown a benefit with calcium channel blockade [159,160]. In fact, in patients with acute MI with significant LV dysfunction or heart failure, a harmful effect has been observed with the administration of diltiazem [161]. Short acting nifedipine (a dihydropyridine calcium channel blocker) has been shown to have harmful effects for patients with acute MI and is not recommended for patients with NSTE-ACS [162]. Thus, the current guidelines recommend that nondihydropyridine calcium channel blockers be used only for patients with preserved LV function and without heart failure, and then only if needed for recurrent ischemia despite the use of nitrates and β-blockade or for patients in whom β-blockade is contraindicated [7]. Calcium channel blockers should not be administered to patients at increased risk for cardiogenic shock or with significant AV block.

Ranolazine

Although the exact mechanism of its antianginal effects is unknown, ranolazine has been shown to partially inhibit fatty acid oxidation and may improve the efficiency of oxygen utilization in cardiac myocytes. In the Combination Assessment of Ranolazine in Stable Angina (CARISA) trial, researchers found that patients with stable angina who were treated with ranolazine in addition to β-blockers or calcium channel blockers had fewer episodes of angina (one episode less per week than placebo; $p < 0.02$) and showed increased exercise capacity (115.6 vs. 91.7 seconds; $p = 0.01$) [163]. Similar results reflecting the antianginal effects of ranolazine for patients with chronic stable angina were demonstrated by the MARISA (Monotherapy Assessment of Ranolazine in Stable Angina) trial [164]. The Metabolic Efficiency with Ranolazine for Less Ischemia in Non-ST Elevation Acute Coronary Syndrome (MERLIN)-TIMI 36 trial expanded the use of ranolazine to the NSTE-ACS population by evaluating 6,560 patients with NSTE-ACS, 3,279 of whom were randomized to receive ranolazine and 3,281 of whom received placebo. Although there was no difference of the primary end point (a composite of cardiovascular death, MI, or recurrent ischemia) between the two groups (21.8% vs. 23.5%; $p = 0.11$), there was a significant reduction of the rates of recurrent ischemia with ranolazine (13.9% vs. 16.1%; $p = 0.03$) [165]. Follow-up analyses of the MERLIN-TIMI 36 trial confirmed the results of the CARISA and MARISA trials and demonstrated that anginal symptoms were improved with ranolazine (HR 0.77; 95% CI 0.59 to 1.00; $p = 0.048$) [166]. Hence, ranolazine remains an attractive addition to β-blockers and nitrates for treatment of chronic, severe angina.

Angiotensin-Converting Enzyme Inhibitors

Angiotensin-converting enzyme (ACE) inhibitors have been shown to reduce mortality for patients after MI, who have either LV systolic dysfunction (ejection fraction <40%) or heart failure [167,168]. A meta-analysis of nearly 100,000 patients demonstrated a statistically significant albeit small 0.48% absolute decrease (7% relative risk reduction) in 30-day mortality with the early initiation of ACE inhibitors following MI [169]. Benefit was seen as early as 24 hours; however, there was also an increase of hypotension and renal dysfunction seen with early initiation of ACE inhibition. These results suggest that ACE inhibitors may be safely initiated early following MI, but the benefits must be weighed against the risk for hypotension and renal dysfunction.

The long-term use of ACE inhibition has also been evaluated in a less acute setting for patients with a history of MI, peripheral arterial disease, or diabetes in the Heart Outcomes Prevention Evaluation trial [170]. Patients at increased risk of cardiovascular events without a history of heart failure or reduced LV systolic function randomized to ACE inhibition had a 22% reduction in ischemic events compared to placebo. Similar results were also seen in the European Trial on Reduction of Cardiac Events with Perindopril in Stable Coronary Artery Disease (EUROPA) trial [171]. A third trial, however, the Prevention of Events with Angiotensin Converting Enzyme inhibition (PEACE) trial, did not show any benefit with the routine use of trandolapril for patients with stable coronary heart disease and preserved LV systolic function, possibly because this was a lower risk population treated with more aggressive baseline therapy [172]. The current guidelines recommend the use of ACE inhibitors for patients with NSTE-ACS with systolic dysfunction (LVEF < 40%), heart failure, hypertension, diabetes, or stable CKD [7].

Angiotensin Receptor Blockers

Angiotensin receptor blockers (ARBs) provide an alternative to ACE inhibitors, and may block the renin–angiotensin system more completely than ACE inhibitors, because angiotensin II can be generated via pathways that are independent of ACE [173]. The Valsartan in Acute Myocardial Infarction Trial (VALIANT) randomized nearly 15,000 patients with a recent MI complicated by heart failure to receive an ARB (valsartan), an ACE inhibitor (captopril), or a combination of the two drugs [174]. Valsartan was found to be noninferior to captopril at 2 years with regard to mortality ($p = 0.004$) and recurrent cardiovascular events ($p < 0.001$). VALIANT was subsequently followed by the On-going Telmisartan Alone and In Combination with Ramipril Global Endpoint Trial (ON-TARGET), which randomized patients with known vascular disease or diabetes to receive either telmisartan (an ARB), ramipril (an ACE inhibitor) or both drugs together [175]. Again, the ARB was shown to be noninferior to the ACE inhibitor with similar rates of death, MI, stroke, or hospitalization for heart failure at 56 months (16.5% vs. 16.7%; RR 1.01; 95% CI 0.94 to 1.09). Furthermore, patients who received telmisartan had less complaints of cough (1.1% vs. 4.2%; $p < 0.001$) when compared to those receiving the ACE inhibitor. Hence, ARBs are effective alternatives for patients who are intolerant of ACE inhibitors.

Mineralocorticoid Receptor Antagonism

Aldosterone blockade in addition to ACE inhibition lowers the rate of all-cause mortality of patients with severe heart failure and reduced systolic function [176]. The main adverse effect with aldosterone blockade is hyperkalemia. The Eplerenone Post–Acute Myocardial Infarction Heart Failure Efficacy and Survival Study (EPHESUS) randomized 6,642 patients stabilized from a recent MI with LV dysfunction (LVEF <40%), plus heart failure or diabetes, to receive eplerenone (selective aldosterone blocker) vs. placebo in addition to optimal medical therapy [177]. At 24 months, eplerenone led to a 30% reduction in all-cause mortality. Aldosterone blockade is recommended for patients post-MI who are receiving ACE inhibition, β-blockade, have an LVEF of ≤ 40%, and either heart failure or diabetes. It is not recommended for patients with renal dysfunction (men with creatinine >2.5 mg/dL or for woman with creatinine >2.0 mg/dL) or hyperkalemia ($K^+ > 5.0$ meq/L) [7].

Lipid-Lowering Therapy

Long-term treatment with lipid-lowering therapy with statins has been shown to be beneficial in patients with a prior history of NSTE-ACS [178–180]. Furthermore, the Pravastatin or Atorvastatin Evaluation and Infection Therapy (PROVE-IT) TIMI 22 trial demonstrated the benefit of intensive lipid-lowering therapy with atorvastatin 80 mg compared to moderate lipid lowering therapy with pravastatin 40 mg in patients with a recent ACS [181]. Intensive lipid-lowering therapy resulted in a 16% reduction of the risk of recurrent ischemic events when compared with moderate lipid-lowering therapy. The benefits emerged after only 30 days post-ACS [182], highlighting the importance of early initiation of intensive statin therapy post-ACS. The average LDL-C achieved was 62 mg/dL for the atorvastatin 80 mg group and 95 mg/dL for the pravastatin 40 mg group. Based in part on these results, the adult treatment panel III of the National Cholesterol Education Program issued an update in which they recommended a new optional very low LDL-C goal of less than 70 mg/dL for patients with high-risk coronary heart disease [183]. More recently, the Improved Reduction of Outcomes: Vytorin Efficacy International Trial (IMPROVE-IT) evaluated the effects of ezetimibe plus simvastatin vs. simvastatin alone for stable patients with a recent ACS [184]. The addition of ezetimibe reduced LDL-C (54 mg/dL in the ezetimibe/simvastatin group vs. 70 mg/dL in the simvastatin monotherapy group). Over 7-year follow-up, there was a 6.4% relative risk reduction of recurrent ischemic events for the combination therapy group vs. the monotherapy group (Fig. 188.4). The relative risk reduction was consistent with what was expected based on the degree of LDL-C lowering [184,185]. The most recent AHA/ACC NSTE-ACS guidelines were published prior to completion of IMPROVE-IT; however, the current ESC NSTE-ACS guidelines recommend considering ezetimibe as adjunctive lipid-lowering therapy for patients with LDL ≥70 mg/dL despite a maximally tolerated statin [8]. A consensus statement from the ACC suggests a possible role for ezetimibe in addition to maximally tolerated statin for patients with a history of cardiovascular disease who are unable to achieve adequate LDL-C levels with a statin alone [186]. Similarly, the proprotein convertase subtilisin/kexin type 9 (PCSK9) inhibitor evolocumab was shown in the FOURIER trial to reduce major cardiovascular events when added to statin therapy in patients with a history of MI [201]. These recommendations are

Cardiovascular death, MI, documented unstable angina requiring rehospitalization, coronary revascularization (≥30 days), or stroke

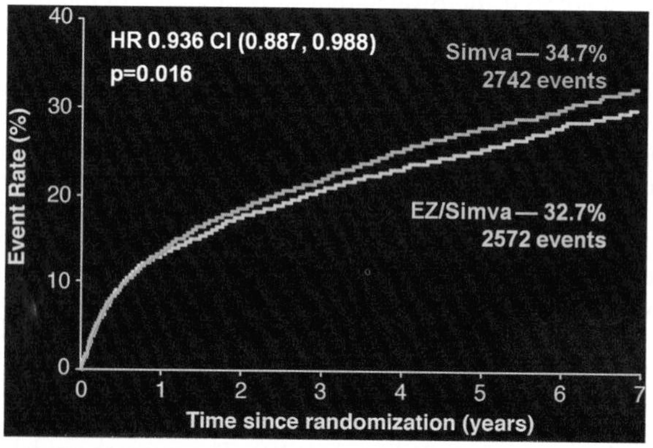

FIGURE 188.4 Kaplan–Meier curves demonstrating the benefit of ezetimibe added simvastatin vs. simvastatin alone in reducing the 7-year event rates of the primary composite end point [death from cardiovascular disease, a major coronary event (nonfatal myocardial infarction, documented unstable angina requiring hospital admission, or coronary revascularization occurring at least 30 days after randomization), or nonfatal stroke] in patients with acute coronary syndrome (Adapted from The IMPROVE-IT Investigators: Ezetimibe Added to Statin Therapy after Acute Coronary Syndromes. *N Engl J Med* 372:21887–2397, 2015.).

supported by a meta-regression analysis demonstrating similar reductions of cardiovascular risk per degree of LDL-C lowering for therapies that lower LDL-C through modulation of the LDL receptor (i.e., statins, ezetimibe, bile acid sequestrants, and PCSK9 inhibitors) [185].

TREATMENT STRATEGIES AND INTERVENTIONS

"Routine Invasive" vs. "Ischemia-Guided" Strategy of Coronary Angiography and Revascularization

Two general approaches to the use of coronary angiography and revascularization in NSTE-ACS exist. The first is a "routine invasive" strategy, involving routine coronary angiography within the first 72 hours and revascularization with PCI or bypass surgery as appropriate [7,8]. The other is a more conservative approach with initial medical management with coronary angiography and revascularization only for recurrent ischemia, which could be termed an "ischemia-guided" strategy. Several trials have compared these two treatment strategies; overall a routine invasive strategy lowers the risk of ischemic events compared with an ischemia-guided approach.

A seven trial meta-analysis demonstrated 25% lower rates of death and 17% lower rates of MI over 2-year follow-up with a routine invasive approach [187]. A subsequent meta-analysis including eight trials demonstrated similar findings with a 22% lower rate in the composite of death, MI, or rehospitalization for ACS over 1-year follow-up (Fig. 188.5) [188]. The second meta-analysis demonstrated that whereas men overall seemed to benefit from a routine invasive approach, only high-risk women (identified by a positive cardiac biomarker) benefit from a routine invasive approach, and low-risk women (those without positive cardiac biomarkers) had a nonsignificant trend toward harm with a routine invasive approach. The current guidelines reflect these findings and recommend for a routine invasive approach for most patients except those who are low risk, notably low-risk women without an elevated troponin [7,8].

Timing of Invasive Strategy

Urgent Invasive

An urgent invasive strategy (ideally within 2 hours) is recommended for NSTE-ACS patients considered "very high risk" identified by one of the following clinical features: Angina refractory to medical therapy, hemodynamic instability, recurrent malignant arrhythmias, acute heart failure, or evidence of mechanical complications (Table 188.2) [7,8]. These recommendations are largely based on expert consensus, because patients with the above characteristics are traditionally excluded from randomized controlled trials [8].

"Early" Invasive vs. "Delayed" Invasive

Routine invasive strategies have generally been defined as coronary angiography within 72 hours; however, a key question is whether patients benefit from an early invasive strategy (within the first 24 hours) vs. a delayed invasive strategy (24 to 72 hours). Two meta-analyses attempted to address this question and demonstrated no benefit for death or MI; however, both demonstrated lower rates of recurrent ischemia [189,190].

There is data suggesting improved outcomes with an early invasive strategy for high-risk NSTE-ACS patients. The TIMACS trial randomized 3031 patients with NSTE-ACS to undergo an early invasive strategy (coronary angiography within 24 hours of randomization, median 14 hours) vs. a delayed invasive strategy (coronary angiography more than 36 hours after randomization, median 50 hours). Although the primary end point (composite of death, MI, or stroke) at 6 months was no different between the two groups, the prespecified analysis according to GRACE risk score demonstrated a significant 35% reduction of the primary end point for high-risk patients with a GRACE risk score >140 [96]. Accordingly the guidelines recommend that NSTE-ACS patients at high risk (i.e., GRACE score >140, or an elevated troponin compatible with MI) should undergo an early invasive strategy within the first 24 hours of presentation [7,8], whereas the remaining individuals should undergo coronary angiography within 72 hours of presentation.

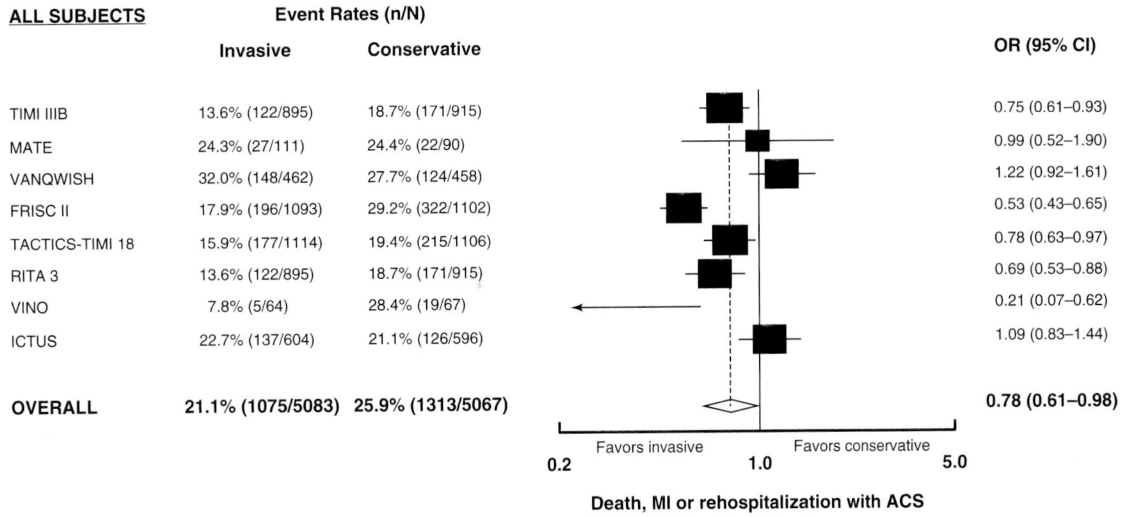

ALL SUBJECTS
Event Rates (n/N)
Invasive
Conservative
OR (95% CI)
TIMI IIIB 13.6% (122/895) 18.7% (171/915) 0.75 (0.61–0.93)
MATE 24.3% (27/111) 24.4% (22/90) 0.99 (0.52–1.90)
VANQWISH 32.0% (148/462) 27.7% (124/458) 1.22 (0.92–1.61)
FRISC II 17.9% (196/1093) 29.2% (322/1102) 0.53 (0.43–0.65)
TACTICS-TIMI 18 15.9% (177/1114) 19.4% (215/1106) 0.78 (0.63–0.97)
RITA 3 13.6% (122/895) 18.7% (171/915) 0.69 (0.53–0.88)
VINO 7.8% (5/64) 28.4% (19/67) 0.21 (0.07–0.62)
ICTUS 22.7% (137/604) 21.1% (126/596) 1.09 (0.83–1.44)
OVERALL 21.1% (1075/5083) 25.9% (1313/5067) 0.78 (0.61–0.98)
Favors invasive
Favors conservative
0.2
1.0
5.0
Death, MI or rehospitalization with ACS

FIGURE 188.5 Meta-analysis of the benefit of a routine invasive vs. "selective" invasive (i.e., conservative) strategy for patients with unstable angina or NSTEMI. ACS, acute coronary syndrome. Rate of death or MI or rehospitalization with ACS through follow-up [Adapted from O'Donoghue M, Boden WE, Braunwald E, et al: Early invasive vs conservative treatment strategies in women and men with unstable angina and non-ST-segment elevation myocardial infarction: a meta-analysis. *JAMA* 300(1):71–80, 2008.].

TABLE 188.2

Matching Clinical Risk Criteria with Invasive vs. Ischemia-Guided Management Strategies in NSTE-ACS Patients

Urgent Invasive (within 2 hours)	Very High Risk • Hemodynamic instability • Sustained VT or VF • Refractory ischemia • Acute Heart Failure or mechanical complications
Early Invasive (within 24 hours)	High Risk • GRACE risk score >140 • Elevated troponin consistent with MI
Delayed Invasive (24–72 hours)	Intermediate Risk • Diabetes • Renal insufficiency (eGFR <60 mL/min/1.73 m^2) • Reduced LV systolic function (EF <40%) • Prior PCI or CABG • GRACE risk score 109–140; TIMI risk score ≥2
Ishcemia-guided	Low Risk • Grace risk score <109, TIMI risk score <2 • Low-risk troponin-negative female patients

CABG, coronary artery bypass graft; EF, ejection fraction; eGFR, estimated glomerular filtration rate; GRACE, Global Registry of Acute Coronary Events; LV, left ventricular; MI, myocardial infarction; NSTE-ACS, non–ST-elevation acute coronary syndrome; PCI, percutaneous coronary intervention; TIMI, thrombolysis in myocardial infarction; VF, ventricular fibrillation; VT, ventricular tachycardia.

Adapted from Amsterdam EA, Wenger NK, Brindis RG, et al: 2014 AHA/ACC guideline for the management of patients with non-ST-elevation acute coronary syndromes: a report of the American College of Cardiology/American Heart Association Task Force on Practice Guidelines. *Circulation* 130(25):e344–426, 2014, and from Roffi M, Patrono C, Collet JP, et al: 2015 ESC Guidelines for the management of acute coronary syndromes in patients presenting without persistent ST-segment elevation: Task Force for the Management of Acute Coronary Syndromes in Patients Presenting without Persistent ST-Segment Elevation of the European Society of Cardiology (ESC). *Eur Heart J* 37(3):267–315, 2016.

High-Risk Subgroups

Elderly Patients

Age is a significant predictor of adverse outcomes among patients with NSTE-ACS [191]. Despite the increased risk, elderly NSTE-ACS patients are less likely to receive recommended evidenced based medical therapy or undergo an early invasive strategy [192]. Although some elderly patients may have contraindications to medications, registry data have shown lower mortality rates for patients on evidenced based medical therapy [193]. Similarly, an early invasive strategy for elderly NSTE-ACS patients has been associated with a lower risk of recurrent ischemic events from both registry and randomized controlled trial data [192,194]. The reduction in ischemic events, however, comes at the price of an increased risk of bleeding [194]. Therefore, in elderly patients with NSTE-ACS, the treatment strategy and use of evidence based medical therapy should be based on an individualized assessment, with careful consideration to weight and renal function when determining the optimal dose of medication.

Patients with Diabetes

In the setting of NSTE-ACS, patients with diabetes have worse outcomes compared to patients without diabetes. In a pooled analysis involving 15,459 NSTE-ACS patients, those with diabetes had an increased 30-day and 1-year mortality rate (2.1% and 7.2%, respectively) compared to those without diabetes (1.1% and 3.1%, respectively) [195]. Given the increased risk of adverse events, NSTE-ACS patients with diabetes should undergo a routine invasive strategy with coronary angiography within the first 72 hours [7,8].

In regard to antithrombotic therapy, patients with diabetes should be treated similarly to patients without diabetes. Both prasugrel and ticagrelor were associated with decreased ischemic events compared to clopidogrel in NSTE-ACS patients with diabetes [196,197]. Although outcomes in PLATO were similar regardless of diabetes status [195], in TRITON-TIMI 38, compared to patients without diabetes, patients with diabetes had a significantly greater net clinical benefit with prasugrel over clopidogrel [196].

Patients with Chronic Kidney Disease

NSTE-ACS patients with chronic kidney disease (CKD) have more comorbidities and a worse prognosis than those without CKD, yet they are less likely to receive evidence based medical therapy or undergo routine coronary angiography [198,199]. Although there is limited data comparing a routine invasive vs. an ischemia-guided approach for patients with CKD, there is some evidence that a routine invasive approach may be preferred. A meta-analysis of 1,453 CKD patients from five randomized controlled trials comparing a routine invasive vs. an ischemia-guided strategy demonstrated a significant reduction of rehospitalization and trends toward decreased mortality and MI with a routine invasive approach [200].

These findings were supported by results from the Swedish Web-System for Enhancement and Development of Evidence-Based Care in Heart Disease Evaluated According to Recommended Therapies (SWEDEHEART) registry. Among 23,262 NSTEMI patients, the frequency of an invasive strategy decreased with worsening renal function. After adjustment for propensity score and discharge medications, an invasive strategy was associated with an overall 36% decrease of 1-year mortality throughout all patients with CKD. When the population was stratified according to CKD stage, the benefits seen with an invasive strategy were noted among patients with stage I though III CKD. For patients with stage IV CKD there was a trend toward benefit, but there was no benefit in stage V CKD [199]. In NSTE-ACS patients with stage I through III CKD, a routine invasive strategy is reasonable.

Evidence based pharmacotherapy for patients with CKD should be the same as for patients with normal renal function, although with dose modification or alternative therapies when appropriate based on degree of renal impairment.

CONCLUSIONS

Using the medical history, physical exam, ECG, and cardiac markers, clinicians can diagnose and risk-stratify patients with NSTE-ACS. These patients are treated with aspirin, a P_2Y_{12} ADP receptor blocker (ticagrelor or prasugrel, or if cannot use either of those, then clopidogrel), an anticoagulant (UFH, LMWH, fondaparinux, or bivalirudin), and anti-ischemic therapy with nitrates and β-blockers. Risk stratification is used to properly match treatment strategy to patient risk (Fig. 188.6). For patients at intermediate to high risk, a routine invasive strategy is warranted. For patients at low risk, medical therapy is appropriate, and a more conservative ischemia-guided approach is reasonable.

Advances in NSTE-ACS, based on randomized controlled trials or meta-analyses of such trials, are summarized in Table 188.3.

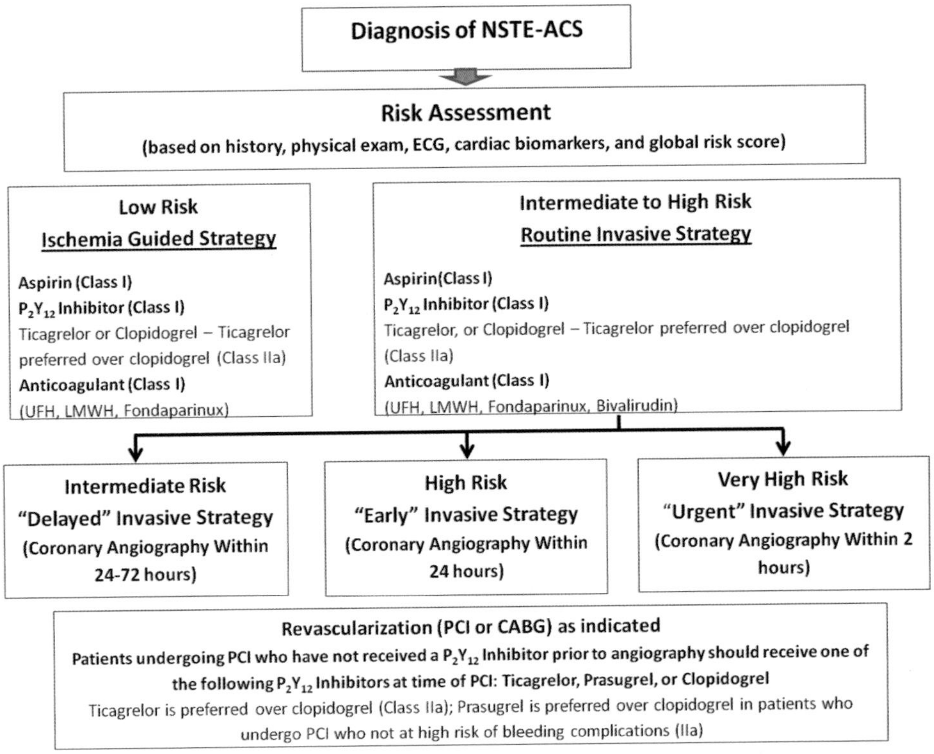

FIGURE 188.6 Algorithm for risk stratification and treatment of patients with NSTE-ACS. ECG, electrocardiogram; LMWH, low-molecular-weight heparin; UFH, unfractionated heparin.

TABLE 188.3

Advances in Managing NSTE-ACS

- Identification of high-risk patients is key to management of NSTE-ACS [7,8]
- Aspirin leads to a significant reduction in the risk of death or MI [74,97–99]
- The addition of clopidogrel to aspirin further reduces risk by 20% [104]. Prasugrel and ticagrelor are alternative oral P_2Y_{12} ADP receptor blockers that have been shown to be superior to clopidogrel for the reduction of ischemic events, at the expense of an increased risk of bleeding [111,114]. Cangrelor is a recently approved intravenous P_2Y_{12} receptor blocker with a short onset and offset of action [8,106].
- Glycoprotein IIb/IIIa inhibitors can be considered in high-risk troponin-positive patients [130]; however, the benefit of upstream administration in patients undergoing urgent coronary angiography and percutaneous coronary intervention is questionable [131,132].
- Anticoagulation has been shown to be beneficial in treating patients with NSTE-ACS: Options include unfractionated heparin [136], low-molecular-weight heparin [138,139], fondaparinux [141], and bivalirudin [143].
- Early, intensive statin therapy is beneficial [181–183]
- The addition of ezetimibe and/or a PCSK9 inhibitor to statin therapy is beneficial [8,184,201]
- An early invasive strategy is beneficial in intermediate- and high-risk patients [187]

MI, Myocardial Infarction; NSTE-ACS, non–ST-elevation acute coronary syndrome.

References

1. Cannon CP, Braunwald E: The spectrum of myocardial ischemia. The paradigm of acute coronary syndromes, in Cannon CP (ed): *Contemporary Cardiology: Management of Acute Coronary Syndromes*. 2nd ed. Totowa, NJ, Humana Press, 2003, pp 3–18.
2. DeWood MA, Spores J, Notske R, et al: Prevalence of total coronary occlusion during the early hours of transmural myocardial infarction. *N Engl J Med* 303:897–902, 1980.
3. TIMI Study Group: The thrombolysis in myocardial infarction (TIMI) trial; phase I findings. *N Engl J Med* 312:932–936, 1985.
4. The TIMI IIIA Investigators: Early effects of tissue-type plasminogen activator added to conventional therapy on the culprit lesion in patients presenting with ischemic cardiac pain at rest. Results of the thrombolysis in myocardial ischemia (TIMI IIIA) trial. *Circulation* 87:38–52, 1993.
5. Mozaffarian D, Benjamin EJ, Go AS, et al: Heart disease and stroke statistics 2016 update. A report from the American Heart Association. *Circulation* 133(4):e38–w360, 2015.
6. Braunwald E, Antman EM, Beasley JW, et al: ACC/AHA guideline update for the management of patients with unstable angina and non-ST-segment elevation myocardial infarction-2002: summary article: a report of the American College of Cardiology/American Heart Association Task Force on Practice Guidelines (Committee on the Management of Patients With Unstable Angina). *Circulation* 106(14):1893–1900, 2002.
7. Amsterdam EA, Wenger NK, Brindis RG, et al: 2014 AHA/ACC guideline for the management of patients with non-ST-elevation acute coronary syndromes: a report of the American College of Cardiology/American Heart Association Task Force on Practice Guidelines. *Circulation* 130(25):e344–e426, 2014.
8. Roffi M, Patrono C, Collet JP, et al: 2015 ESC Guidelines for the management of acute coronary syndromes in patients presenting without persistent ST-segment elevation: Task Force for the Management of Acute Coronary Syndromes in Patients Presenting without Persistent ST-Segment Elevation of the European Society of Cardiology (ESC). *Eur Heart J* 37(3):267–315, 2016.
9. Braunwald E: Unstable angina: an etiologic approach to management. *Circulation* 98(21):2219–2222, 1998.
10. Fuster V, Badimon L, Cohen M, et al: Insights into the pathogenesis of acute ischemic syndromes. *Circulation* 77:1213–1220, 1988.
11. Fuster V, Badimon L, Badimon JJ, et al: The pathophysiology of coronary artery disease and the acute coronary syndromes. *N Engl J Med* 326:242–250, 310–218, 1992.
12. Ludmer PL, Selwyn AP, Shook TL, et al: Paradoxical vasoconstriction induced by acetylcholine in atherosclerotic coronary arteries. *N Engl J Med* 315(17):1046–1051, 1986.

13. Lee RT, Libby P: The unstable atheroma. *Arterioscler Thromb Vasc Biol* 17(10):1859–1867, 1997.
14. Moreno PR, Bernardi VH, Lopez-Cuellar J, et al: Macrophages, smooth muscle cells, and tissue factor in unstable angina. Implications for cell-mediated thrombogenicity in acute coronary syndromes. *Circulation* 94:3090–3097, 1996.
15. Weiss EJ, Bray PF, Tayback M, et al: A polymorphism of a platelet glycoprotein receptor as an inherited risk factor for coronary thrombosis. *N Engl J Med* 334:1090–1094, 1996.
16. Ault K, Cannon CP, Mitchell J, et al: Platelet activation in patients after an acute coronary: results from the TIMI 12 trial. *J Am Coll Cardiol* 33:634–639, 1999.
17. Merlini PA, Bauer KA, Oltrona L, et al: Persistent activation of coagulation mechanism in unstable angina and myocardial infarction. *Circulation* 90:61–68, 1994.
18. Becker RC, Tracy RP, Bovill EG, et al: Surface 12-lead electrocardiogram findings and plasma markers of thrombin activity and generation in patients with myocardial ischemia at rest. *J Thromb Thrombolysis* 1:101–107, 1994.
19. Falk E: Unstable angina with fatal outcome: dynamic coronary thrombosis leading to infarction and/or sudden death. *Circulation* 71:699–708, 1985.
20. Davies MJ, Thomas A: Plaque fissuring—the cause of acute myocardial infarction, sudden ischemic death, and crescendo angina. *Br Heart J* 53:363–373, 1985.
21. Libby P. Mechanisms of acute coronary syndromes and their implications for therapy. *N Engl J Med* 2013 368; 2004–2013, 2013.
22. Sherman CT, Litvack F, Grundfest W, et al: Coronary angioscopy in patients with unstable angina pectoris. *N Engl J Med* 315:913–919, 1986.
23. Brunelli C, Spallarossa P, Ghigliotta G, et al: Thrombosis in refractory unstable angina. *Am J Cardiol* 68:110B–118B, 1991.
24. Mizuno K, Satumo K, Miyamoto A, et al: Angioscopic evaluation of coronary artery thrombi in acute coronary syndromes. *N Engl J Med* 326:287–291, 1992.
25. Sullivan E, Kearney M, Isner JM, et al: Pathology of unstable angina: analysis of biopsies obtained by directional coronary atherectomy. *J Thromb Thrombolysis* I:63–71, 1994.
26. Harrington RA, Califf RM, Holmes DR Jr, et al: Is all unstable angina the same? Insights from the coronary angioplasty versus excisional atherectomy trial (CAVEAT-I). *Am Heart J* 137(2):227–233, 1999.
27. Colman RW, Marder VJ, Salzman EW, et al: Overview of hemostasis, in Colman RW, Hirsh J, Marder VJ, et al (eds): *Hemostasis and Thrombosis: Basic Principles and Clinical Practice*. 3rd ed. Philadelphia, JB Lippincott Company, 1994, pp 3–18.
28. Handin RI, Loscalzo J: Hemostasis, thrombosis, fibrinolysis, and cardiovascular disease, in Braunwald E (ed): *Heart Disease*. 4th ed. Philadelphia, WB Saunders, 1992, pp 1767–1789.
29. Broze GJ Jr: The role of tissue factor pathway inhibitor in a revised coagulation cascade. *Semin Hematol* 29:159–169, 1992.
30. Furie B, Furie BC: Molecular and cellular biology of blood coagulation. *N Engl J Med* 326:800–806, 1992.
31. Badimon JJ, Lettino M, Toschi V, et al: Local inhibition of tissue factor reduces the thrombogenicity of disrupted human atherosclerotic plaques: effects of tissue factor pathway inhibitor on plaque thrombogenicity under flow conditions. *Circulation* 99(14):1780–1787, 1999.
32. Furie B, Furie BC: Mechanisms of thrombus formation. *N Engl J Med* 359(9):938–949, 2008.
33. Prinzmetal M, Kennamer R, Merliss R, et al: A variant form of angina pectoris. *Am J Med* 27:375–388, 1959.
34. Hirsch PD, Hillis LD, Campbell WB, et al: Release of prostaglandins and thromboxane into the coronary circulation in patients with ischemic heart disease. *N Engl J Med* 304:685–691, 1981.
35. Willerson JT, Golino P, Eidt J, et al: Specific platelet mediators and unstable coronary artery lesions. Experimental evidence and potential clinical implications. *Circulation* 80:198–205, 1989.
36. Eisenberg PR, Kenzora JL, Sobel BE, et al: Relation between ST segment shifts during ischemia and thrombin activity in patients with unstable angina. *J Am Coll Cardiol* 18(4):898–903, 1991.
37. Nabel EG, Ganz P, Gordon JB, et al: Dilation of normal and constriction of atherosclerotic coronary arteries caused by the cold pressor test. *Circulation* 77(1):43–52, 1988.
38. Daniel WC, Lange RA, Landau C, et al: Effects of the intracoronary infusion of cocaine on coronary arterial dimensions and blood flow in humans. *Am J Cardiol* 78(3):288–291, 1996.
39. Pitts WR, Lange RA, Cigarroa JE, et al: Cocaine-induced myocardial ischemia and infarction: pathophysiology, recognition, and management. *Prog Cardiovasc Dis* 40(1):65–76, 1997.
40. Yeung AC, Vekshtein VI, Krantz DS, et al: The effect of atherosclerosis on the vasomotor response of coronary arteries to mental stress. *N Engl J Med* 325(22):1551–1556, 1991.
41. Epstein SE, Cannon RO: Site of increased resistance to coronary flow in patients with angina pectoris and normal epicardial coronary arteries. *J Am Coll Cardiol* 8(2):459–461, 1986.
42. Kaski JC, Chester MR, Chen L, et al: Rapid angiographic progression of coronary artery disease in patients with angina pectoris. The role of complex stenosis morphology. *Circulation* 92(8):2058–2065, 1995.
43. Arbustini E, De Servi S, Bramucci E, et al: Comparison of coronary lesions obtained by directional coronary atherectomy in unstable angina, stable angina, and restenosis after either atherectomy or angioplasty. *Am J Cardiol* 75(10):675–682, 1995.
44. Flugelman MY, Virmani R, Correa R, et al: Smooth muscle cell abundance and fibroblast growth factors in coronary lesions of patients with nonfatal unstable angina. A clue to the mechanism of transformation from the stable to the unstable clinical state. *Circulation* 88(6):2493–2500, 1993.
45. Giugliano RP, Cannon CP, Braunwald E: Non-ST elevation acute coronary syndromes, in Mann DL, Zipes DP, Libby P, Bonow RO (eds): *Braundwald's Heart Disease*. 10th ed. Philadelphia, Saunders, 2015, pp 1155–1181.
46. Cannon CP, McCabe CH, Stone PH, et al: The electrocardiogram predicts one-year outcome of patients with unstable angina and non-Q wave myocardial infarction: results of the TIMI III registry ECG ancillary study. *J Am Coll Cardiol* 30:133–140, 1997.
47. The TIMI IIIB Investigators: Effects of tissue plasminogen activator and a comparison of early invasive and conservative strategies in unstable angina and non-Q-wave myocardial infarction: results of the TIMI IIIB trial. *Circulation* 89:1545–1556, 1994.
48. The platelet receptor inhibition for ischemic syndrome management in patients limited by unstable signs and symptoms (PRISM-PLUS) trial investigators: Inhibition of the platelet glycoprotein IIb/IIIa receptor with tirofiban in unstable angina and non-Q-wave myocardial infarction. *N Engl J Med* 338:1488–1497, 1998.
49. Thygesen K, Alpert JS, Jaffe AS, et al: Third universal definition of myocardial infarction. *J Am Coll Cardiol* 60:1581–1598, 2012.
50. Wright SA, Sawyer DB, Sacks DB, et al: Elevation of troponin I levels in patients without evidence of myocardial injury. *JAMA* 278(24):2144, 1997.
51. Jeremias A, Gibson CM: Narrative review: alternative causes for elevated cardiac troponin levels when acute coronary syndromes are excluded. *Ann Intern Med* 142(9):786–791, 2005.
52. Reichlin T, Hochholzer W, Bassetti S, et al: Early diagnosis of myocardial infarction with sensitive cardiac troponin assays. *N Engl J Med* 361(9):858–867, 2009.
53. Keller T, Zeller T, Peetz D, et al: Sensitive troponin I assay in early diagnosis of acute myocardial infarction. *N Engl J Med* 361(9):868–877, 2009.
54. Shah AS, Anand A, Sandoval Y, et al. High-sensitivity cardiac troponin I at presentation in patients with suspected acute coronary syndrome: a cohort study. *Lancet* 386:2481–2488, 2015
55. Morrow DA. Evidence-based algorithms using high-sensitivity cardiac troponin in the emergency department. *JAMA Cardiol.* 1:379–381, 2016.
56. Veretto T, Cantalupi D, Altieri A, et al: Emergency room technetium-99 m sestamibi imaging to rule out acute myocardial ischemic events in patients with nondiagnostic electrocardiograms. *J Am Coll Cardiol* 22:1804–1808, 1993.
57. Tatum JL, Jesse RL, Kontos MC, et al: Comprehensive strategy for the evaluation and triage of the chest pain patient. *Ann Emerg Med* 29:116–125, 1997.
58. Berning J, Launbjerg J, Appleyard M: Echocardiographic algorithms for admission and predischarge prediction of mortality in acute myocardial infarction. *Am J Cardiol* 69:1538–1544, 1992.
59. Hoffmann U, Truong QA, Schoenfeld DA, et al. Coronary CT angiography versus standard evaluation in acute chest pain. *N Engl J Med* 367:299–308, 2012.
60. Multicenter Postinfarction Research Group: Risk stratification and survival after myocardial infarction. *N Engl J Med* 309:331–336, 1983.
61. Zaret BL, Wackers FJT, Terrin ML, et al: Value of radionuclide rest and exercise left ventricular ejection fraction is assessing survival of patients after thrombolytic therapy for acute myocardial infarction: results of the thrombolysis in myocardial infarction (TIMI) phase II study. *J Am Coll Cardiol* 26:73–79, 1995.
62. Nicod P, Gilpin E, Dittrich H, et al: Influence on prognosis and morbidity of left ventricular ejection fraction with and without signs of left ventricular failure after acute myocardial infarction. *Am J Cardiol* 61:1165–1171, 1988.
63. Diver DJ, Bier JD, Ferreira PE, et al: Clinical and arteriographic characterization of patients with unstable angina without critical coronary arterial narrowing (from the TIMI-IIIA trial). *Am J Cardiol* 74:531–537, 1994.
64. McCullough PA, O'Neill WW, Graham M, et al: A prospective randomized trial of triage angiography in acute coronary syndromes ineligible for thrombolytic therapy. Results of the medicine versus angiography in thrombolytic exclusion (MATE) trial. *J Am Coll Cardiol* 32(3):596–605, 1998.
65. Cannon CP, Thompson B, McCabe CH, et al: Predictors of non-Q-wave acute myocardial infarction in patients with acute ischemic syndromes: an analysis from the thrombolysis in myocardial ischemia (TIMI) III trials. *Am J Cardiol* 75:977–981, 1995.
66. Khot UN, Jia G, Moliterno DJ, et al. Prognostic importance of physical examination for heart failure in non-ST-elevation acute coronary syndromes: the enduring value of Killip classification. *JAMA*. 290(16):2174–2181, 2003.
67. Mello BH, Oliveira GB, Ramos RF, et al. Validation of the Killip-Kimball classification and late mortality after acute myocardial infarction. *Arq Bras Cardiol* 103(2):107–117, 2014.
68. Savonitto S, Ardissino D, Granger CB, et al. Prognostic value of the admission electrocardiogram in acute coronary syndromes. *JAMA* 281(8):707–713, 1999.
69. Cohen M, Stinnett SS, Weatherley BD, et al: Predictors of recurrent ischemic events and death in unstable coronary artery disease after treatment with combination antithrombotic therapy. *Am Heart J* 139(6):962–970, 2000.
70. Antman EM, McCabe CH, Gurfinkel EP, et al: Enoxaparin prevents death and cardiac ischemic events in unstable angina/non-Q-wave myocardial infarction: results of the thrombolysis in myocardial infarction (TIMI) 11B trial. *Circulation* 100(15):1593–1601, 1999.
71. Diderholm E, Andren B, Frostfeldt G, et al: ST depression in ECG at entry identifies patients who benefit most from early revascularization in unstable coronary artery disease: a FRISC II substudy. *Circulation* 100[Suppl I]:I-497–I-498, 1999.
72. Cannon CP, Weintraub WS, Demopoulos LA, et al: Comparison of early invasive and conservative strategies in patients with unstable coronary syndromes treated with the glycoprotein IIb/IIIa inhibitor tirofiban. *N Engl J Med* 344(25):1879–1887, 2001.

73. Anderson HV, Cannon CP, Stone PH, et al: One-year results of the thrombolysis in myocardial infarction (TIMI) IIIB clinical trial. A randomized comparison of tissue-type plasminogen activator versus placebo and early invasive versus early conservative strategies in unstable angina and non-Q-wave myocardial infarction. *J Am Coll Cardiol* 26:1643–1650, 1995.
74. Theroux P, Ouimet H, McCans J, et al: Aspirin, heparin or both to treat unstable angina. *N Engl J Med* 319:1105–1111, 1988.
75. Antman EM, Tanasijevic MJ, Thompson B, et al: Cardiac-specific troponin I levels to predict the risk of mortality in patients with acute coronary syndromes. *N Engl J Med* 335:1342–1349, 1996.
76. Morrow DA, Cannon CP, Rifai N, et al: Ability of minor elevations of troponin I and T to predict benefit from an early invasive strategy in patients with unstable angina and non-ST elevation myocardial infarction: results from a randomized trial. *JAMA* 286:2405–2412, 2001.
77. Heidenreich PA, Alloggiamento T, Melsop K, et al: The prognostic value of troponin in patients with non-ST elevation acute coronary syndromes: a meta-analysis. *J Am Coll Cardiol* 38(2):478–485, 2001.
78. Antman EM, Grudzien C, Mitchell RN, et al: Detection of unsuspected myocardial necrosis by rapid bedside assay for cardiac troponin T. *Am Heart J* 133(5):596–598, 1997.
79. Hamm CW, Heeschen C, Goldmann B, et al: Benefit of abciximab in patients with refractory unstable angina in relation to serum troponin T levels. *N Engl J Med* 340(21):1623–1629, 1999.
80. Morrow DA, Antman EM, Tanasijevic M, et al: Cardiac troponin I for stratification of early outcomes and the efficacy of enoxaparin in unstable angina: a TIMI 11B substudy. *J Am Coll Cardiol* 36:1812–1817, 2000.
81. Laqerqvist B, Diderholm E, Lindahl B, et al: An early invasive treatment strategy reduces cardiac events regardless of troponin levels in unstable coronary artery (UCAD) with and without troponin-elevation: a FRISC II substudy. *Circulation* 100[Suppl I]:I-497, 1999.
82. Haverkate F, Thompson SG, Pyke SDM, et al: Production of C-reactive protein and risk of coronary events in stable and unstable angina. *Lancet* 349:462–466, 1997.
83. Toss H, Lindahl B, Siegbahn A, et al: Prognostic influence of increased fibrinogen and C-reactive protein levels in unstable coronary artery disease. *Circulation* 96(12):4204–4210, 1997.
84. Morrow DA, Rifai N, Antman EM, et al: C-reactive protein is a potent predictor of mortality independently and in combination with troponin T in acute coronary syndromes: a TIMI 11 A substudy. *J Am Coll Cardiol* 31:1460–1465, 1998.
85. De Lemos JA, Morrow DA, Bentley JH, et al: The prognostic value of B-type natriuretic peptide in patients with acute coronary syndromes. *N Engl J Med* 345:1014–1021, 2001.
86. James SK, Lindahl B, Siegbahn A, et al: N-terminal pro-brain natriuretic peptide and other risk markers for the separate prediction of mortality and subsequent myocardial infarction in patients with unstable coronary artery disease: a global utilization of strategies to open occluded arteries (GUSTO)-IV substudy. *Circulation* 108(3):275–281, 2003.
87. Morrow DA, de Lemos JA, Blazing MA, et al: Prognostic value of serial B-type natriuretic peptide testing during follow-up of patients with unstable coronary artery disease. *JAMA* 294(22):2866–2871, 2005.
88. Eggers KM, Lagerqvist B, Venge P, et al: Prognostic value of biomarkers during and after non-ST-segment elevation acute coronary syndrome. *J Am Coll Cardiol* 54(4):357–364, 2009.
89. Wollert KC, Kempf T, Timo P, et al: Prognostic value of growth-differentiation factor-15 in patients with non-ST-elevation acute coronary syndrome. *Circulation* 115(8):962–971, 2007.
90. Wollert KC, Kemph T, Lagerqvist B, et al: Growth differentiation factor 15 for risk stratification and selection of an invasive treatment strategy in non-ST-elevation acute coronary syndrome. *Circulation* 116:1540–1548, 2007.
91. Sabatine MS, Morrow DA, de Lemos JA, et al: Multimarker approach to risk stratification in non-ST-elevation acute coronary syndromes: simultaneous assessment of troponin I, C-reactive protein, and B-type natriuretic peptide. *Circulation* 105(15):1760–1763, 2002.
92. Antman EM, Cohen M, Bernink PJ, et al: The TIMI risk score for unstable angina/non-ST elevation MI: a method for prognostication and therapeutic decision making. *JAMA* 284:835–842, 2000.
93. Morrow DA, Antman EM, Snapinn SM, et al: An integrated clinical approach to predicting the benefit of tirofiban in non-ST elevation acute coronary syndromes. Application of the TIMI risk score for UA/NSTEMI in PRISM-PLUS. *Eur Heart J* 23(3):223–229, 2002.
94. Granger CB, Goldberg RJ, Dabbous O, et al. Predictors of hospital mortality in the Global Registry of Acute Coronary Events. *Arch Intern Med* 163:2345–2353, 2003.
95. Eagle KA, Lim MJ, Dabbous OH, et al: A validated prediction model for all forms of acute coronary syndrome. Estimating the risk of 6-month postdischarge death in an international registry. *JAMA* 291(22):2727–2733, 2004.
96. Mehta S, Granger CB, Boden WE, et al: Early versus delayed invasive intervention in acute coronary syndromes. *N Engl J Med* 360(21):2165–2175, 2009.
97. Lewis HD, Davis JW, Archibald DG, et al: Protective effects of aspirin against acute myocardial infarction and death in men with unstable angina. *N Engl J Med* 309:396–403, 1983.
98. Cairns JA, Gent M, Singer J, et al: Aspirin, sulfinpyrazone, or both in unstable angina. *N Engl J Med* 313:1369–1375, 1985.
99. The RISC Group: Risk of myocardial infarction and death during treatment with low dose aspirin and intravenous heparin in men with unstable coronary artery disease. *Lancet* 336:827–830, 1990.
100. CURRENT-OASIS 7 Investigators: Dose comparisons of clopidogrel and aspirin in acute coronary syndromes. *N Engl J Med* 363(10):930–942, 2010.
101. Mehta SR, Tanguay JF, Eikelboom JW, et al: Double-dose versus standard-dose clopidogrel and high-dose versus low-dose aspirin in individuals undergoing percutaneous coronary intervention for acute coronary syndromes (CURRENT-OASIS 7): a randomised factorial trial. *Lancet* 376(9748):1233–1243, 2010.
102. Berger JS, Sallum RH, Katona B, et al. Is there an association between aspirin dosing and cardiac and bleeding events after treatment of acute coronary syndrome? A systematic review of the literature. *Am Heart J* 164:153–162, 2012.
103. Mahaffey KW, Wojdyla DM, Carroll K, et al: Ticagrelor compared with clopidogrel by geographic region in the Platelet Inhibition and Patient Outcomes (PLATO) trial. *Circulation* 124:544–554, 2011.
104. CURE Study Investigators: The clopidogrel in unstable angina to prevent recurrent events (CURE) trial programme; rationale, design and baseline characteristics including a meta-analysis of the effects of thienopyridines in vascular disease. *Eur Heart J* 21(24):2033–2041, 2000.
105. Mehta SR, Yusuf S, Peters RJ, et al: Effects of pretreatment with clopidogrel and aspirin followed by long-term therapy in patients undergoing percutaneous coronary intervention: the PCI-CURE study. *Lancet* 358(9281):527–533, 2001.
106. Franchi F, Angiolillo DJ. Novel antiplatelet agents in acute coronary syndrome. *Nat Rev Cardiol* 12(1):30–47, 2015.
107. Mega JL, Close SL, Wiviott SD, et al: Cytochrome P-450 polymorphisms and response to clopidogrel. *N Engl J Med* 360(4):354–362, 2009.
108. Simon T, Verstuyft C, Mary-Krause M, et al: Genetic determinants of response to clopidogrel and cardiovascular events. *N Engl J Med* 360(4):363–375, 2009.
109. Collet JP, Hulot JS, Pena A, et al: Cytochrome P450 2C19 polymorphism in young patients treated with clopidogrel after myocardial infarction: a cohort study. *Lancet* 373(9660):309–317, 2009.
110. Bhatt DL, Cryer BL, Contant CF, et al for the COGENT Investigators. Clopidogrel with or without omeprazole in coronary artery disease. *N Engl J Med* 363(20): 1909–1917, 2010.
111. Wiviott SD, Braunwald E, McCabe CH, et al: Prasugrel versus clopidogrel in patients with acute coronary syndromes. *N Engl J Med* 357(20):2001–2015, 2007.
112. Wiviott SD, Braunwald E, McCabe CH, et al: Intensive oral antiplatelet therapy for reduction of ischaemic events including stent thrombosis in patients with acute coronary syndromes treated with percutaneous coronary intervention and stenting in the TRITON-TIMI 38 trial: a subanalysis of a randomized trial. *Lancet* 371(9621):1353–1363, 2008.
113. Roe MT, Armstrong PW, Fox KA et al for the TRILOGY ACS Investigators. Prasugrel versus clopidogrel for acute coronary syndromes without revascularization. *N Engl J Med* 367(14):1297–1309, 2012.
114. Wallentin L, Becer RC, Budaj A, et al for the PLATO Investigators: Ticagrelor versus clopidogrel in patients with acute coronary syndrome. *N Engl J Med* 361(11):1045–1057, 2009.
115. Lindholm D, Varenhorst C, Cannon CP, et al: Ticagrelor vs. clopidogrel in patients with non-ST-elevation acute coronary syndrome with or without revascularization: results from the PLATO trial. *Eur Heart J* 35(31):2083–2093, 2014.
116. Bhatt DL, Stone GW, Mahaffey KW, et al for the CHAMPION PHOENIX Investigators: Effect of platelet inhibition with cangrelor during PCI on ischemic events. *N Engl J Med* 368(14):1303–1313, 2013.
117. Angiolillo DJ, Firstenberg MS, Price MJ, et al for the BRIDGE investigators: Bridging antiplatelet therapy with cangrelor in patients undergoing cardiac surgery: a randomized controlled trial. *JAMA* 307(3):265–2674, 2012.
118. Valgimigli M. Pretreatment with P2Y12 inhibitors in non-ST-segment-elevation acute coronary syndrome is clinically justified. *Circulation* 130:1891–1903, 2014.
119. Collet JP, Silvain J, Bellemain-Appaix A, Montalescot G. Pretreatment with P2Y12 inhibitors in non-ST-segment-elevation acute coronary syndrome: an outdated and harmful strategy. *Circulation* 130:1904–1914, 2014.
120. Anderson JL, Adams CD, Antman EM, et al: 2012 ACCF/AHA focused update incorporated into the ACCF/AHA 2007 guidelines for the management of patients with unstable angina/non-ST-elevation myocardial infarction: a report of the American College of Cardiology Foundation/American Heart Association Task Force on Practice Guidelines. *J Am Coll Cardiol* 61(23):e179–e347, 2013.
121. Hamm CW, Bassand JP, Agewall S, et al: ESC guidelines for the management of acute coronary syndromes in patients presenting without persistent ST-segment elevation: the Task Force for the management of acute coronary syndromes (ACS) in patients presenting without persistent ST-segment elevation of the European Society of Cardiology (ESC). *Eur Heart J* 32:2999–3054, 2011
122. Bellemain-Appaix A, O'Connor SA, Silvain J, et al. Association of clopidogrel pretreatment with mortality, cardiovascular events, and major bleeding among patients undergoing percutaneous coronary intervention: a systematic review and meta-analysis. JAMA 308; 2507–2516, 2012.
123. Montalescot G, Bolognese L, Dudek D, et al for the ACCOAST Investigators. Pretreatment with prasugrel in non-ST-segment elevation acute coronary syndromes. *N Engl J Med* 369(11):999–1010, 2013.
124. Levine GN, Bates ER, Bittl JA, et al. 2016 ACC/AHA Guideline Focused Update on Duration of Dual Antiplatelet Therapy in Patients With Coronary Artery Disease: A Report of the American College of Cardiology/American Heart Association Task Force on Clinical Practice Guidelines. *J Am Coll Cardiol* 68:1082–1115, 2016.
125. Mauri L, Kereiakes DJ, Yeh RW, et al. Twelve or 30 months of dual antiplatelet therapy after drug-eluting stents. *N Engl J Med* 371:2155–2166, 2014.
126. Bonaca MP, Bhatt DL, Cohen M, et al. Long-term use of ticagrelor in patients with prior myocardial infarction. *N Engl J Med* 372:1791–1800, 2015.

127. Udell JA, Bonaca MP, Collet JP, et al. Long-term dual antiplatelet therapy for secondary prevention of cardiovascular events in the subgroup of patients with previous myocardial infarction: a collaborative meta-analysis of randomized trials. *Eur Heart J* 37:390–399, 2016.
128. Bonaca MP, Sabatine MS. Antiplatelet Therapy for Long-term Secondary Prevention After Myocardial Infarction. *JAMA Cardiol* 1:627–628, 2016.
129. Roffi M, Chew DP, Mukherjee D, et al: Platelet glycoprotein IIb/IIIa inhibition in acute coronary syndromes. Gradient of benefit related to the revascularization strategy. *Eur Heart J* 23:1441–1448, 2002.
130. Kastrati A, Mehilli J, Neumann FJ, et al: Abciximab in patients with acute coronary syndromes undergoing percutaneous coronary intervention after clopidogrel pretreatment: the ISAR-REACT 2 randomized trial. *JAMA* 295(13):1531–1538, 2006.
131. Stone GW, Bertrand ME, Moses JW, et al: Routine upstream initiation vs deferred selective use of glycoprotein IIb/IIIa inhibitors in acute coronary syndromes. The ACUITY timing trial. *JAMA* 297:591–602, 2007.
132. Giugliano RP, White JA, Bode C, et al: Early versus delayed provisional eptifibatide in acute coronary syndromes. *N Engl J Med* 360(21):2176–2190, 2009.
133. Tricoci P, Huang Z, Held C, et al: Thrombin-receptor antagonist vorapaxar in acute coronary syndromes. *N Engl J Med* 366:20–33, 2012.
134. Morrow DA, Braunwald E, Bonaca MP, et al for the TRA 2P–TIMI 50 Steering Committee and Investigators: Vorapaxar in the secondary prevention of atherothrombotic events. *N Engl J Med* 366:1404–1413, 2012.
135. Eikelboom JW, Anand SS, Malmberg K, et al: Unfractionated heparin and low-molecular-weight heparin in acute coronary syndrome without ST elevation: a meta-analysis. *Lancet* 355:1936–1942, 2000.
136. Oler A, Whooley MA, Oler J, et al: Adding heparin to aspirin reduces the incidence of myocardial infarction and death in patients with unstable angina. A meta-analysis. *JAMA* 276:811–815, 1996.
137. Hirsh J, Anand SS, Halperin JL, et al: Guide to anticoagulant therapy: Heparin: a statement for healthcare professionals from the American Heart Association. *Circulation* 103(24):2994–3018, 2001.
138. Cohen M, Demers C, Gurfinkel EP, et al: A comparison of low-molecular-weight heparin with unfractionated heparin for unstable coronary artery disease. *N Engl J Med* 337:447–452, 1997.
139. The SYNERGY Trial Investigators. Enoxaparin vs unfractionated heparin in high-risk patients with non–ST-segment elevation acute coronary syndromes managed with an intended early invasive strategy: primary results of the SYNERGY randomized trial. *JAMA* 292:45–54, 2004.
140. Murphy SA, Gibson CM, Morrow DA, et al: Efficacy and safety of the low-molecular weight heparin enoxaparin compared with unfractionated heparin across the acute coronary syndrome spectrum: a meta-analysis. *Eur Heart J* (28):2077–2086, 2007.
141. Yusuf S, Mehta SR, Chrolavicius S, et al for the Fifth Organization to Assess Strategies in Acute Ischemic Syndromes Investigators: Comparison of fondaparinux and enoxaparin in acute coronary syndromes. *N Engl J Med* 354(14):1464–1476, 2006.
142. Steg PG, Jolly SS, Mehta SR et al for the FUTURA/OASIS-8 Trial Group: Low-dose vs standard-dose unfractionated heparin for percutaneous coronary intervention in acute coronary syndromes treated with fondaparinux: the FUTURA/OASIS-8 randomized trial. *JAMA* 304(12):1339–1349, 2010.
143. Stone GW, McLaurin BT, Cox DA, et al: Bivalirudin for patients with acute coronary syndromes. *N Engl J Med* 355:2203–2216, 2006.
144. Kastrati A, Neumann FJ, Schulz S, et al: Abciximab and heparin versus bivalirudin for non-ST-elevation myocardial infarction. *N Engl J Med* 365:1980–1989, 2011.
145. Cavender MA, Sabatine MS. Bivalirudin versus heparin in patients planned for percutaneous coronary intervention: a meta-analysis of randomised controlled trials. *Lancet* 384; 599–606, 2014.
146. Valgimigli M, Frigoli E, Leonardi S, et al. Bivalirudin or unfractionated heparin in acute coronary syndromes. *N Engl J Med* 373; 997–1009, 2015.
147. Hurlen M, Abdelnoor M, Smith P, et al: Warfarin, aspirin, or both after myocardial infarction. *N Engl J Med* 347(13):969–974, 2002.
148. Alexander JH, Lopes RD, James S, et al: Apixaban with antiplatelet therapy after acute coronary syndrome. *N Engl J Med* 365(8):699–708, 2011.
149. Mega JL, Braunwald E, Wiviott SD, et al: Rivaroxaban in patients with a recent acute coronary syndrome. *N Engl J Med* 366(1):9–19, 2012.
150. Fibrinolytic Therapy Trialists' (FTT) Collaborative Group: Indications for fibrinolytic therapy in suspected acute myocardial infarction: collaborative overview of early mortality and major morbidity results from all randomised trials of more than 1000 patients. *Lancet* 343:311–322, 1994.
151. ISIS-2 (Second International Study of Infarct Survival) Collaborative Group: Randomised trial of intravenous streptokinase, oral aspirin, both, or neither among 17,187 cases of suspected acute myocardial infarction: ISIS-2. *Lancet* 2:349–360, 1988.
152. Stub D, Smith K, Bernard S, et al: Air versus oxygen in ST-segment-elevation myocardial infarction. *Circulation* 131:2143–2150, 2015.
153. Gruppo Italiano per lo Studio della Sopravvivenza nell'Infarto Miocardico: GISSI-3: effect of lisinopril and transdermal glyceryl trinitrate singly and together on 6-week mortality and ventricular function after acute myocardial infarction. *Lancet* 343:1115–1122, 1994.
154. ISIS-4 Collaborative Group: ISIS-4: randomized factorial trial assessing early oral captopril, oral mononitrate, and intravenous magnesium sulphate in 58,050 patients with suspected acute myocardial infarction. *Lancet* 345:669–685, 1995.
155. Chatterjee S, Chaudhuri D, Vedanthan R, et al: Early intravenous beta-blockers in patients with acute coronary syndrome—a meta-analysis of randomized trials. *Int J Cardiol* 168:915–921, 2013.
156. Chen ZM, Pan HC, Chen YP, et al: Early intravenous then oral metoprolol in 45,852 patients with acute myocardial infarction: randomised placebo controlled trial. *Lancet* 366:1622–1632, 2005.
157. Gibson RS, Boden WE, Theroux P, et al: Diltiazem and reinfarction in patients with non-Q wave myocardial infarction. Results of a double-blind, randomized, multicenter trial. *N Engl J Med* 315:423–429, 1986.
158. The Danish Study Group: Effect of verapamil on mortality and major events after acute myocardial infarction (the Danish Verapamil Infarction Trial II–DAVIT II). *Am J Cardiol* 66:779–785, 1990.
159. Smith NL, Reiber GE, Psaty BM, et al: Health outcomes associated with beta-blocker and diltiazem treatment of unstable angina. *J Am Coll Cardiol* 32:1305–1311, 1998.
160. Rengo F, Carbonin P, Pahor M, et al: A controlled trial of verapamil in patients after acute myocardial infarction: results of the calcium antagonist reinfarction Italian study (CRIS). *Am J Cardiol* 77:365–369, 1996.
161. The Multicenter Diltiazem Postinfarction Trial Research Group: The effect of diltiazem on mortality and reinfarction after myocardial infarction. *N Engl J Med* 319:385–392, 1988.
162. Furberg CD, Psaty BM, Meyer JV: Nifedipine.Dose-related increase in mortality in patients with coronary heart disease. *Circulation* 92:1326–1331, 1995.
163. Chaitman BR, Pepine CJ, Parker JO: Effects of ranolazine with atenolol, amlodipine, or diltiazem on exercise tolerance and angina frequency in patients with severe chronic angina: a randomized controlled trial. *JAMA* 291(3):309–316, 2004.
164. Chaitman BR, Skettino SL, Parker JO: Anti-ischemic effects and long-term survival during ranolazine monotherapy in patients with chronic severe angina. *J Am Coll Cardiol* 43(8):1375–1382, 2004.
165. Morrow DA, Scirica BM, Karwatowska-Prokopszuk E, et al: Effects of ranolazine on recurrent cardiovascular events in patients with non-ST-elevation acute coronary syndromes: the MERLIN-TIMI 36 randomized trial. *JAMA* 297(160):1775–1783, 2007.
166. Wilson SR, Scirica BM, Braunwald E, et al: Efficacy of ranolazine in patients with chronic angina observations from the randomized, double-blind, placebo-controlled MERLIN-TIMI (Metabolic Efficiency with Ranolazine for Less Ischemia in Non-ST-Segment Elevation Acute Coronary Syndromes) 36 trial. *J Am Coll Cardiol* 53(17):1510–1516, 2009.
167. Pfeffer MA, Braunwald E, Moye LA, et al: Effect of captopril on mortality and morbidity in patients with left ventricular dysfunction after myocardial infarction. *N Engl J Med* 327:669–677, 1992.
168. The Acute Infarction Ramipril Efficacy (AIRE) Study Investigators: Effect of ramipril on mortality and morbidity of survivors of acute myocardial infarction with clinical evidence of heart failure. *Lancet* 342:821–828, 1993.
169. ACE Inhibitor Myocardial Infarction Collaborative Group: Indications for ACE inhibitors in the early treatment of acute myocardial infarction: systematic overview of individual data from 100,000 patients in randomized trials. *Circulation* 97:2202–2212, 1998.
170. Yusuf S, Sleight P, Pogue J, et al: Effects of an angiotensin-converting-enzyme inhibitor, ramipril, on cardiovascular events in high-risk patients. *N Engl J Med* 342:145–153, 2000. [Published erratum appears in *N Engl J Med* 342(10):748, 2000.]
171. Fox KM: Efficacy of perindopril in reduction of cardiovascular events among patients with stable coronary artery disease: randomised, double-blind, placebo-controlled, multicentre trial (the EUROPA study). *Lancet* 362(9386):782–788, 2003.
172. Braunwald E, Domanski MJ, Fowler SE, et al: Angiotensin-converting-enzyme inhibition in stable coronary artery disease. *N Engl J Med* 351(20): 2058–2068, 2004.
173. Petrie MC, Padmanabhan N, McDonald JE, et al: Angiotensin converting enzyme (ACE) and non-ACE dependent angiotensin II generation in resistance arteries from patients with heart failure and coronary artery disease. *J Am Coll Cardiol* 37:1056–1061, 2001.
174. Pfeffer MA, McMurray JV, Velazquez EJ, et al: Valsartan, captopril, or both in myocardial infarction complicated by heart failure, left ventricular dysfunction or both. *N Engl J Med* 349(20):1893–1906, 2003.
175. The ONTARGET Investigators: Telmisartan, ramipril, or both in patients at high risk for vascular events. *N Engl J Med* 358:1547–1559, 2008.
176. The Randomized Aldactone Evaluation Study Investigators: The Effect of Spironolactone on Morbidity and Mortality in Patients with Severe Heart Failure. *N Engl J Med* 341:709–717, 1999.
177. Pitt B, Remme W, Zannad F, et al. Eplerenone, a selective aldosterone blocker, in patients with left ventricular dysfunction after myocardial infarction. *N Engl J Med* 348:1309–1321, 2003.
178. Scandinavian Simvastatin Survival Study Group: Randomised trial of cholesterol lowering in 4444 patients with coronary heart disease: the Scandinavian simvastatin survival study (4S). *Lancet* 344:1383–1389, 1994.
179. Sacks RM, Pfeffer MA, Moye LA, et al: The effect of pravastatin on coronary events after myocardial infarction in patients with average cholesterol levels. *N Engl J Med* 335:1001–1009, 1996.
180. The Long-Term Intervention with Pravastatin in Ischaemic Disease (LIPID) Study Group: Prevention of cardiovascular events and death with pravastatin in patients with coronary heart disease and a broad range of initial cholesterol levels. *N Engl J Med* 339(19):1349–1357, 1998.

181. Cannon CP, Braunwald E, McCabe CH, et al: Intensive versus moderate lipid lowering with statins after acute coronary syndromes. *N Engl J Med* 350(15):1495–1504, 2004.
182. Ray KK, Cannon CP, McCabe C, et al: Early late benefits of high-dose Atorvastatin in patients with acute coronary syndromes: results from the PROVE-IT TIMI 22 trial. *J Am Coll Cardiol* 46:1405–1410, 2005.
183. Grundy SM, Cleeman JI, Merz CN, et al: Implications of recent clinical trials for the National Cholesterol Education Program Adult Treatment Panel III guidelines. *Arterioscler Thromb Vasc Biol Aug* 24(8):e149–e161, 2004.
184. The IMPROVE-IT Investigators: Ezetimibe Added to Statin Therapy after Acute Coronary Syndromes. *N Engl J Med* 372:2387–2397, 2015.
185. Silverman MG, Ference BA, Im K, et al. Association between lowering LDL-C and cardiovascular risk reduction among different therapeutic interventions: a systematic review and meta-analysis. *JAMA* 316:1289–1297, 2016.
186. Lloyd-Jones DM, Morris PB, Ballantyne CM, et al. 2016 ACC Expert Consensus Decision Pathway on the Role of Non-Statin Therapies for LDL-Cholesterol Lowering in the Management of Atherosclerotic Cardiovascular Disease Risk: A Report of the American College of Cardiology Task Force on Clinical Expert Consensus Documents. *J Am Coll Cardiol* 68:92–125, 2016.
187. Bavry AA, Kumbhani DJ, Rassi AN, et al: Benefit of early invasive therapy in acute coronary syndromes: a meta-analysis of contemporary randomized clinical trials. *J Am Coll Cardiol* 48(7):1319–1325, 2006.
188. O'Donoghue M, Boden WE, Braunwald E, et al: Early invasive vs conservative treatment strategies in women and men with unstable angina and non-ST-segment elevation myocardial infarction: a meta-analysis. *JAMA* 300(1):71–80, 2008.
189. Katritsis DG, Siontis GC, Kastrati A, et al: Optimal timing of coronary angiography and potential intervention in non-ST-elevation acute coronary syndromes. *Eur Heart J* 32:32–340, 2011.
190. Navarese EP, Gurbel PA, Andreotti F, et al: Optimal timing of coronary invasive strategy in non-ST-segment elevation acute coronary syndromes: a systematic review and meta-analysis. *Ann Intern Med* 158:261–270, 2013.
191. Rosengren A,Wallentin L, Simoons M, et al: Age, clinical presentation, and outcome of acute coronary syndromes in the Euroheart acute coronary syndrome survey. *Eur Heart J* 27:789–795, 2006.
192. Devlin G, Gore JM, Elliott J, et al: Management and 6-month outcomes in elderly and very elderly patients with high-risk non-ST-elevation acute coronary syndromes: The Global Registry of Acute Coronary Events. *Eur Heart J* 29:1275–1282, 2008
193. Skolnick AH, Alexander KP, Chen AY, et al: Characteristics, management, and outcomes of 5,557 patients age ≥90 years with acute coronary syndromes: results from the CRUSADE initiative. *J Am Coll Cardiol* 49:1790–1797, 2007.
194. Bach RG, Cannon CP, Weintraub WS, et al: The effect of routine, early invasive management on outcome for elderly patients with non-ST-segment elevation acute coronary syndromes. *Ann Intern Med* 141(3):186–195, 2004.
195. Donahoe SM, Stewart GC, McCabe CH, et al: Diabetes and mortality following acute coronary syndromes. *JAMA* 298(7):765–775, 2007.
196. Wiviott SD, Braunwald E, Angiolilo DJ, et al: Greater clinical benefit of more intensive oral antiplatelet therapy with prasugrel in patients with diabetes mellitus in the trial to assess improvement in therapeutic outcomes by optimizing platelet inhibition with prasugrel thrombolysis in myocardial infarction 38. *Circulation* 118(16):1626–1636, 2008.
197. James S, Angiolillo DJ, Cornel JH, et al: Ticagrelor vs. clopidogrel in patients with acute coronary syndromes and diabetes: a substudy from the PLATelet inhibition and patient Outcomes (PLATO) trial. *Eur Heart J* 31: 3006–3016, 2010.
198. Szummer K, Lundman P, Jacobson SH, et al: Relation between renal function, presentation, use of therapies and in-hospital complications in acute coronary syndrome: data from the SWEDEHEART register. *J Intern Med* 268:40–49, 2010.
199. Szummer K, Lundman P, Jacobson SH, et al: Influence of renal function on the effects of early revascularization in non-ST-elevation myocardial infarction: data from the Swedish Web-system for Enhancement and Development of Evidence-based care in Heart disease Evaluated According to Recommended Therapies (SWEDEHEART). *Circulation* 120:851–858 2009.
200. Charytan DM, Wallentin L, Lagerqvist B, et al: Early angiography in patients with chronic kidney disease: a collaborative systematic review. *Clin J Am Soc Nephrol* 4:1032–1043, 2009.
201. Sabatine MS, Giugliano RP, Keech AC, et al. Evolocumab and Clinical Outcomes in Patients with Cardiovascular Disease. *NEJM* 376:1713–1722, 2017.

Chapter 189 ■ Management of Common Arrhythmias in Intensive Care Unit

NIYADA NAKSUK • VAIBHAV R. VAIDYA • OMAR Z. YASIN • SAMUEL J. ASIRVATHAM

Patients admitted to the intensive care unit (ICU) are vulnerable to arrhythmias [1], which can cause hemodynamic compromise. The first priority is, therefore, to determine whether the patient has poor perfusion related to the dysrhythmia and whether emergent management is required [2]. In this situation, advanced cardiac life support (ACLS) should be promptly applied. Providers should always seek to reverse underlying processes (Table 189.1). The use of a pragmatic algorithm based on the electrocardiogram (ECG) can aid the diagnosis of arrhythmia; tachyarrhythmias and bradyarrhythmias are simply distinguished by a ventricular rate of >100 beats per minute (bpm) and <60 bpm, respectively. Tachyarrhythmias are broadly divided into wide complex tachycardias (WCTs) that have a QRS width >120 ms and narrow complex tachycardias, most of which are supraventricular tachycardias (SVTs). If the patient is sufficiently stable, providers may have time to perform a detailed assessment focusing on a relevant history, including ongoing symptoms, underlying cardiovascular disease, and medications, as well as pertinent laboratory tests. Continuous ECG monitoring should be implemented, and serial assessments are warranted because the patient can rapidly deteriorate at any time.

This chapter reviews commonly encountered arrhythmias among critically ill patients, including (I) ventricular arrhythmias (VAs), (II) supraventricular arrhythmias, and (III) bradyarrhythmias. A summary of an approach to common arrhythmias and their management is provided in Figures 189.1 through 189.5 and Table 189.2. Treatment of arrhythmias in patients with an existing implantable cardioverter defibrillator (ICD) or pacemaker is discussed in Chapters 15 and 18.

SECTION I: VENTRICULAR ARRHYTHMIAS

Ventricular arrhythmias (VAs) are abnormal electrical signals arising below the level of the His bundle. VAs have a characteristic QRS width >120 ms and have clinical consequences that fall along a spectrum ranging from asymptomatic to cardiac arrest. VAs include ventricular fibrillation, polymorphic ventricular tachycardia, torsade de pointes, monomorphic-sustained ventricular tachycardia, premature ventricular complexes, nonsustained ventricular tachycardia, and accelerated idioventricular rhythm. Figure 189.1 summarizes the approach and common mechanisms of these arrhythmias.

Ventricular Fibrillation (VF)

VF is a disorganized rhythm that always causes inadequate cardiac output. VF or pulseless ventricular tachycardia (VT) accounts for 21% of in-hospital cardiac arrest. Approximately 40% of patients with in-hospital VF or pulseless VT survive hospitalization if prompt and effective ACLS is delivered [3].

The 2015 ACLS guidelines emphasize an integrated strategy of early defibrillation and effective chest compressions [4].

TABLE 189.1

Extrinsic and Intrinsic Factors Associated with an Increase in Risk of Arrhythmias

Common factors for arrhythmias	Risk factors for prolonged QT interval
Cerebrovascular event	Advanced age
Drugs (especially inotropes)	Female
Electrolyte abnormalities and acidosis	Bradycardia, heart block, pauses
Hypoxia	Electrolyte abnormalities (hypokalemia, hypomagnesemia, hypocalcemia)
Structural heart disease	Structural heart disease
Pulmonary disease (pulmonary embolism, tension pneumothorax)	Impaired hepatic drug metabolism
Inflammatory process of multiorgan systems	Impaired renal function
Vascular cannulation	Neurologic disease
	Occult congenital long QT syndrome
	Premature complexes
	Use of QT-prolonging drugs[a]

[a]An updated list can be found at www.qtdrugs.org.

Witnessed cardiac arrest because of VF, pulseless VT, or TDP, should be treated with immediate defibrillation and effective cardiopulmonary resuscitation (CPR). Provision of uninterrupted pre- and postshock CPR is emphasized because it may take up to 200 seconds after a shock attempt until an organized rhythm returns [5]; uninterrupted CPR increases the likelihood of return of spontaneous circulation (ROSC) [6]. After two unsuccessful attempts of defibrillation, epinephrine can be used as a first-line vasopressor agent [4]. When VF or pulseless VT persists after three shocks, the administration of amiodarone is recommended [7]. Effort should be made to identify and correct the primary or precipitating causes. The management of cardiac arrest in special situations is summarized in Table 189.3 [8,9].

Two small randomized controlled trials that enrolled patients with in-hospital cardiac arrest, including shockable VF/VT, suggested that combination of vasopressin-epinephrine and methylprednisone during early CPR cycles and subsequent stress-dose hydrocortisone for those who remained in shock were associated with an increase in ROSC and hospital survival [10,11]. Therefore, the 2015 guidelines recommend that this combined therapy may be considered (class IIb) for such cases [4]. After ROSC is achieved, lidocaine may be considered to reduce the risk of recurrence [4]. The guidelines recommend (class I) controlled temperature management between 32°C and 36°C for a patient with in-hospital arrest, irrespective of initial rhythms (shockable vs. nonshockable rhythms), who

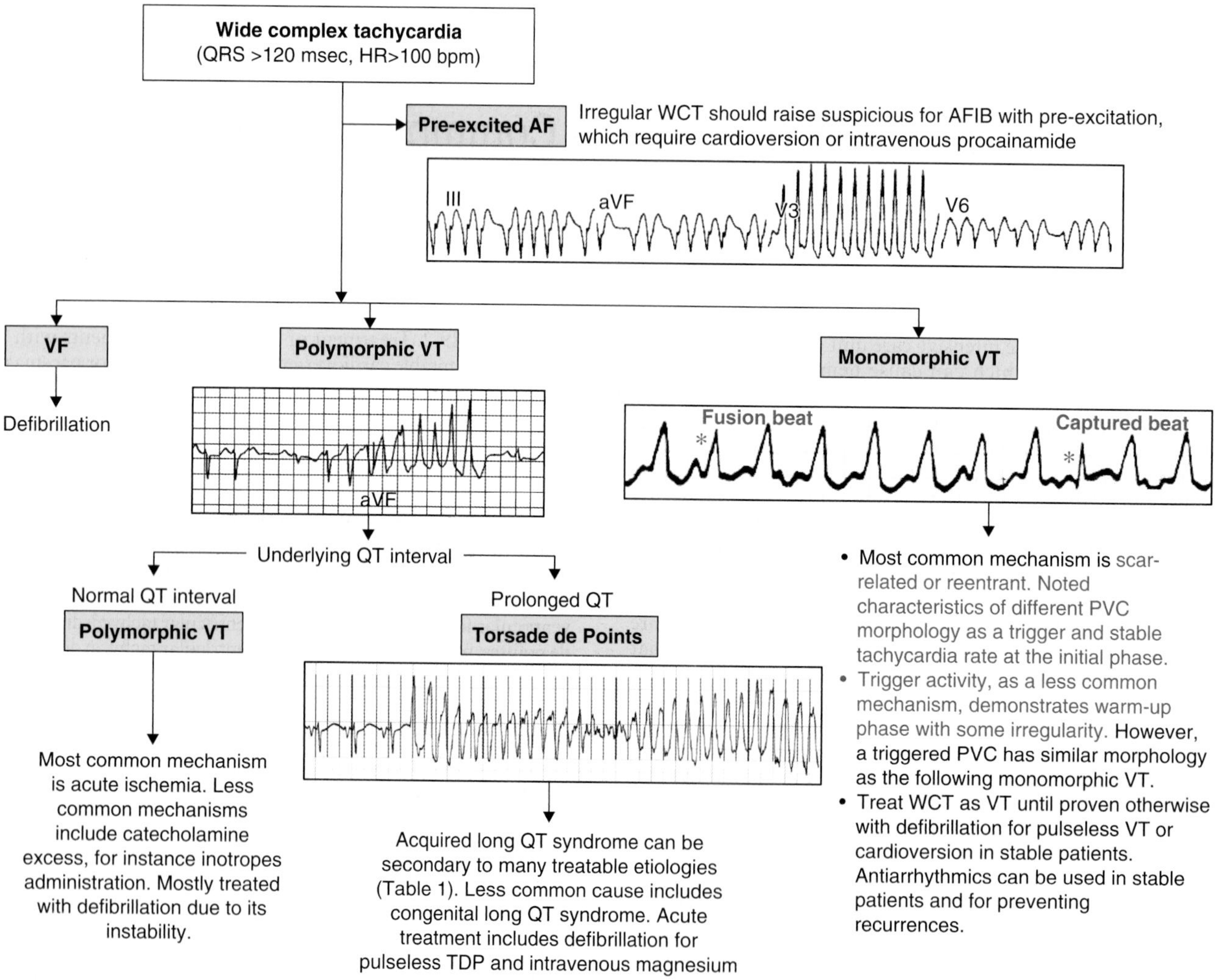

FIGURE 189.1 Approach to wide complex tachycardia (WCT). Courtesy of Stephen C. Hammill, MD.

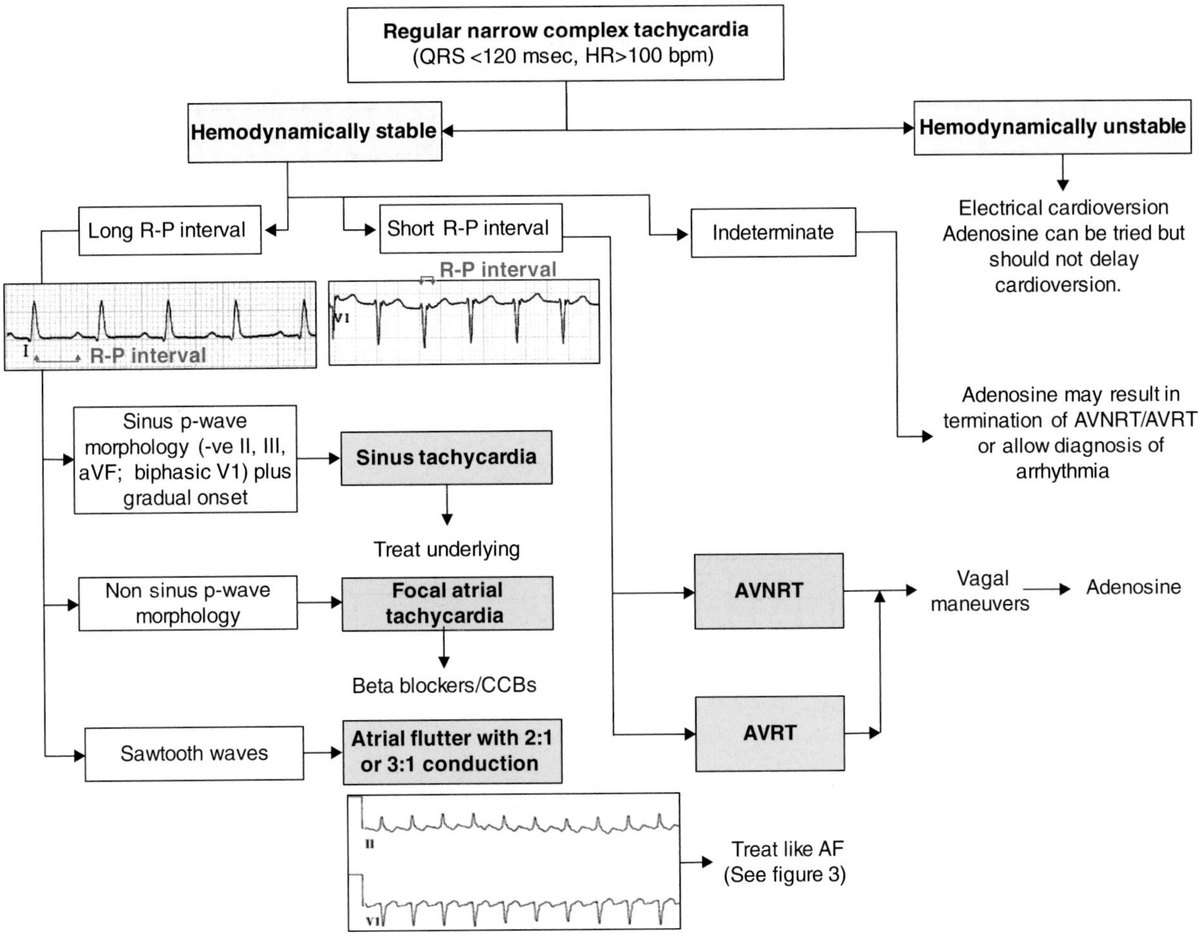

FIGURE 189.2 Approach to regular narrow complex tachycardia.

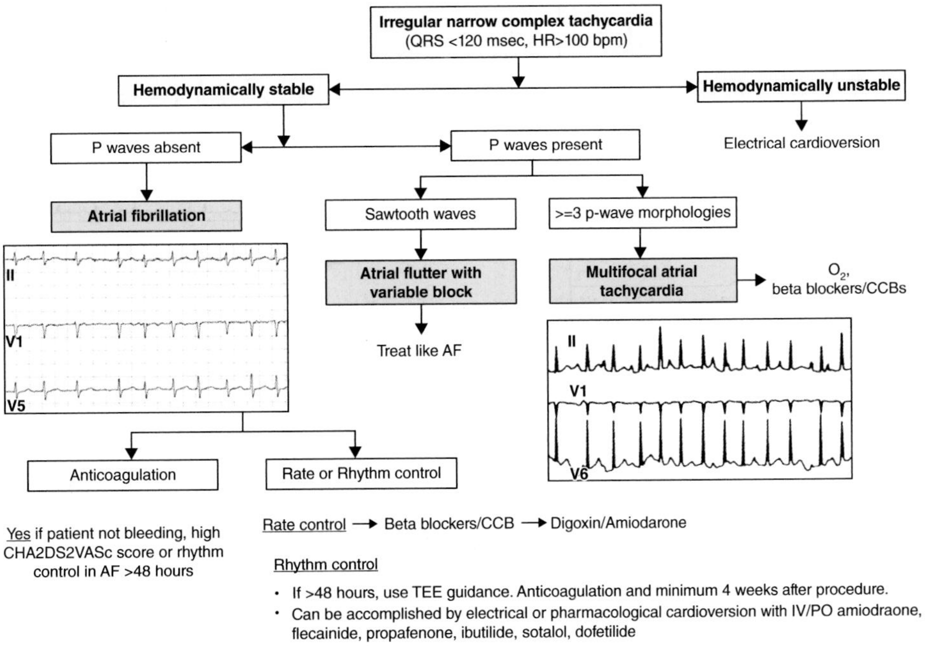

FIGURE 189.3 Approach to irregular narrow complex tachycardia.

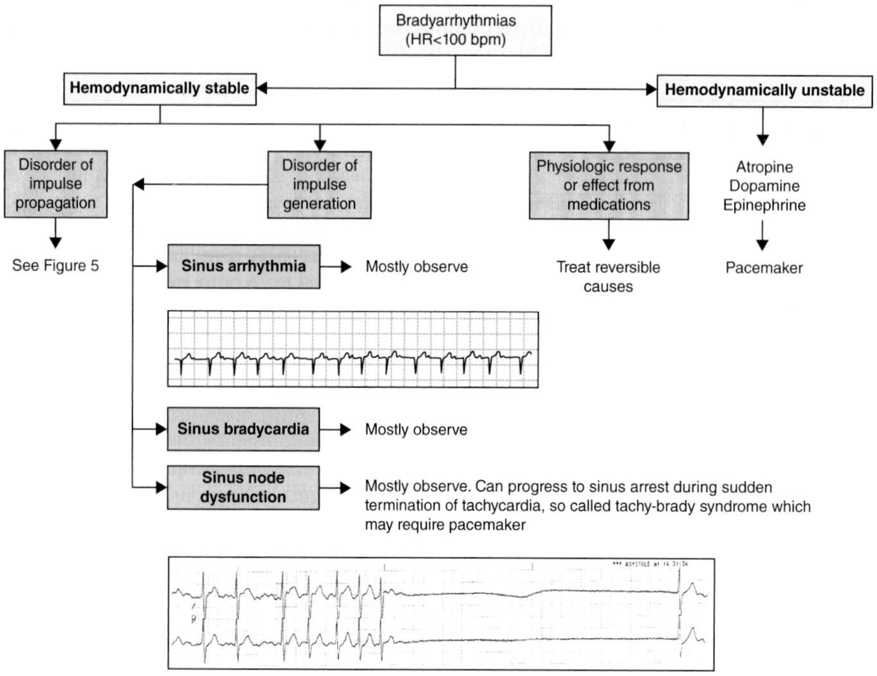

FIGURE 189.4 Approach to bradyarrhythmias.

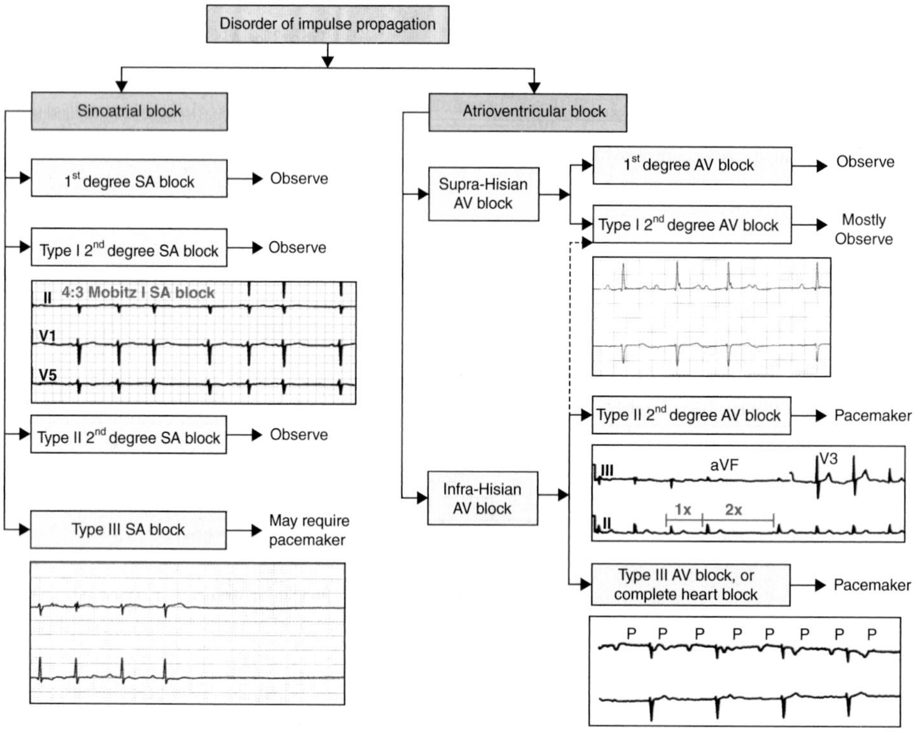

FIGURE 189.5 Approach to bradyarrhythmias (continue). Note that type I second-degree sinoatrial (SA) block with group beating and progressing shortening P-P interval before missing P and QRS complex. Figure presents 4:3 Mobitz I SA block. For AV block, type I second-egree AV block or Mobtiz type I or Wenckebach-type block with progressive prolongation of the PR interval before failure of conduction of a P wave. Type II second-degree AV block or Mobtiz type II with characteristics of constant P-P interval and pause duration of two times P-P intervals. This feature is distinguished from a premature atrial complex with physiologic block. Third-degree atrioventricular block or complete heart block with atrioventricular dissociation and ventricular escape rhythm.

TABLE 189.2

Summary of Evidence-based Recommendations for Acute Management of Arrhythmias

Arrhythmias	Management
Ventricular arrhythmias	
VF and pulseless VT	Defibrillation Epinephrine Amiodarone
Monomorphic VT	Amiodarone, lidocaine, procainamide Electrical cardioversion
Torsade de pointes	Magnesium Pacing
In-hospital cardiac arrest	Combined vasopressin, steroids, and epinephrine
Supraventricular tachycardia	
AVNRT/AVRT	Valsalva maneuver Adenosine Calcium channel blocker (diltiazem or verapamil) β-Blocker (metoprolol or esmolol) Electrical cardioversion
Preexcited atrial fibrillation	Urgent cardioversion Procainamide
Atrial tachycardia	β-Blocker (metoprolol or esmolol) Calcium channel blocker (diltiazem or verapamil)
Atrial fibrillation/atrial flutter	**Rate control:** β-Blocker (metoprolol or esmolol) Calcium channel blockers (diltiazem or verapamil) Digoxin **Rhythm control:** Electrical cardioversion Pharmacologic cardioversion: Propafenone, flecainide, dofetilide, ibutilide and sotalol, amiodarone,
Bradyarrhythmias	
First-degree AVB	Observe
Second-degree AVB, Mobitz type I	Mostly observe
Second-degree AVB, Mobitz type II	Pacemaker implant in the absence of reversible cause
Third-degree AVB	Pacemaker implant in the absence of reversible cause

VT, ventricular tachycardia; AVNRT, atrioventricular nodal reentrant tachycardia; AVRT, atrioventricular reentrant tachycardia; AVB, atrioventricular block.

remains comatose after ROSC [4,12]. It is noteworthy that a prospective study of targeted temperature for patients with in-hospital cardiac arrest is not available.

Polymorphic Ventricular Tachycardia (PMVT)

PMVT is an unstable rhythm with a varying QRS morphology and axis from beat to beat. PMVT can look like VF and tends to degenerate into VF. Similar to VF, PMVT is commonly caused by acute myocardial ischemia, and, therefore, exclusion of an acute coronary syndrome is warranted [13]. Other less common causes include digoxin toxicity and catecholamine excess, for example, from inotropes commonly used in the ICU. The differential diagnosis of PMVT includes artifact (marked by normal QRS complexes visibly marching at the sinus rate through the artifact), atrial fibrillation (AF) with aberrancy, and preexcited AF (see "Section II: Supraventricular tachycardia" section). PMVT with an underlying prolonged QTc is called torsade de pointes (TDP).

Emergent defibrillation is warranted for all unstable patients with PMVT. In hemodynamically stable patients, cardioversion, administration of intravenous magnesium, and lidocaine are initial steps. Antiarrhythmic drugs that can prolong QT interval (e.g., class IA and III agents, Table 189.4) should be avoided. For PMVT for which the baseline QTc interval is absolutely known to be normal, amiodarone can be administered. Use of atrioventricular nodal blockers for wide complex, irregular tachycardia of unclear etiology may precipitate VF and is contraindicated.

Torsade de Pointes (TDP)

TDP is a subtype of PMVT with an underlying prolonged QT interval during sinus rhythm and twisting of QRS complex around the isoelectric baseline during tachycardia (Fig. 189.1). TDP differs from PMVT in both underlying mechanism and treatment. TDP often has a characteristic onset with a slowing

TABLE 189.3

Modification of Management of Cardiac Arrest in Special Situations Based on the 2010 and 2015 BLS and ACLS Guidelines and the 2015 Updated Guidelines for Cardiac Arrest in Pregnancy

Diagnosis	Clinical relevance and management
Asthma	Severe asthma may result in severe auto-PEEP. Strategy to reduce this PEEP includes low respiratory rate and tidal volume and a brief disconnection from the bag mask or ventilator.
Anaphylaxis	Early and advanced airway management is critical. Patients require aggressive fluid resuscitation with isotonic crystalloid. Epinephrine intravenous route may not be effective after 15 min of resuscitation, and vasopressin may be successfully used.
Pregnancy	ACLS consists of multidisciplinary care team. Continuous manual left uterine displacement is recommended during cardiac arrest. Providers should anticipate the difficult airway management, and no more than two attempts should be made for intubation. Perimortem cesarean delivery at the site of the arrest for patients with >20 wk of gestation is advisable if ROSC is not achieved with usual resuscitation.
Pulmonary embolism	In patients with confirmed PE, the guidelines provide a class IIa recommendation for considering thrombolysis, surgical embolectomy, and mechanical embolectomy during resuscitation.
Hyperkalemia	Severe hyperkalemia (>6.5 mmol/L) can cause a variety of abnormal rhythms, including VT, slow ventricular rate response, and sinus arrest. Stabilizing the myocardium with calcium chloride is the first-line treatment. Other treatment to shift potassium intracellularly (e.g., sodium bicarbonate) and promote potassium excretion should be followed in order of urgency.
Hypokalemia	No evidence to support intravenous bolus of potassium supplement during CPR. Replacement is generally achieved by infusion.
Hypomagnesemia	Especially in the setting of TDP, 1 to 2 g of $MgSO_4$ bolus is recommended. Administration of large, repeated doses of magnesium should be avoided in the presence of severe renal insufficiency because of its potential toxicity.
Drug toxicity	
Opioid	Naloxone may be reasonable to use.
Benzodiazepines	The use of flumazenil, as an antidote, in patients with undifferentiated coma is not recommended because it may be associated with seizures, arrhythmias, and hypotension.
β-Blockers	Therapeutic antidotes include glucagon, insulin, and calcium.
Calcium channel blockers	Antidotes with high-dose insulin and calcium have been described.
Cyclic antidepressants	Cyclic antidepressants inhibit cardiac Na channel and cause widened QRS complex and VT. Many of these drugs also have a characteristic known as use-dependency, such that the administration of *β*-blockers can decrease their electrophysiologic effect. Administration of sodium bicarb during cardiac arrest may be considered.
Digoxin	Antidigoxin Fab antibody should be administered to patients with severe life-threatening cardiac glycoside toxicity after resuscitation. Hyperkalemia is a marker of severity in acute cardiac glycoside poisoning and is associated with poor prognosis. Antidigoxin Fab may be administered empirically to patients with acute poisoning from digoxin whose serum potassium level >5.0 mEq/L.
Local anesthetic toxicity	Guidelines recommend considering intravenous long-chain fatty acid emulsion as an initial bolus during cardiac arrest, particularly in bupivacian toxicity.

PEEP, positive end-expiratory pressure; ACLS, advanced cardiac life support; ROSC, return of spontaneous circulation; PE, pulmonary embolism; VT, ventricular tachycardia; CPR, cardiopulmonary resuscitation; TDP, torsade de pointes.

heart rate followed by a premature ventricular complex which interrupts the T wave, known as pause-dependent or a long–short ventricular cycle length. It is strongly related with QT-prolonging drugs, electrolyte abnormalities, or a congenital ion channel disorder. Hence, a meticulous search for these predisposing factors is critical (Table 189.1) [14]. Unlike VF or PMVT, TDP is generally not caused by acute myocardial ischemia.

Acute management for pulseless TDP includes emergent defibrillation. For unstable patients, synchronized cardioversion can be applied. As for hemodynamically stable patients, intravenous magnesium can be given for the purpose of treatment and prevention, irrespective of serum magnesium level. If baseline rhythm is bradycardia, atrial pacing at a rate of at least 90 bpm or isoproterenol administration may suppress the TDP [15].

Monomorphic Ventricular Tachycardias (VT)

VT is defined as three or more consecutive ventricular beats at a rate greater than 100 bpm. Sustained VT is defined as VT causing hemodynamic compromise or VT that lasts more than 30 seconds. Different from PMVT, monomorphic VT has uniform QRS morphology. VT is the most common cause of wide complex tachycardia (WCT) encountered in clinical practice [16]. Therefore, WCT should be managed as VT until proven otherwise [17]. Lack of significant symptoms should not exclude the diagnosis of VT; minimal symptoms may occur for a patient without underlying cardiopulmonary disease and relatively slow VT.

Differential diagnosis of WCT includes SVT with rate-related aberrant interventricular conduction, SVT with abnormal baseline QRS configuration or ventricular pacing rhythms, and SVT with nonspecific wide QRS complexes because of medications

TABLE 189.4

Drug Therapy Commonly Used in Acute Management of Arrhythmias

	Clinical use	Contraindications	Common side effects during acute administration	Comments
Adenosine	• AVNRT • AVRT (but not preexcited AF)	• Preexcited AF • Second- or third-degree heart block	• Heart block • Chest discomfort • Dyspnea	• Adenosine has rapid half-life; adverse effect is brief and generally well tolerate
Amiodarone	• AF/AFL • VT • VF	• Severe hepatic disease • Second- or third-degree heart block • Hypersensitivity to iodine	• Hypotension, deteriorating heart failure owing to *β*-blocker mechanism • Prolonged QTc, rarely proarrhythmic • Bradycardia, heart block	
β-Blocker	• AVNRT • AVRT (but not preexcited AF) • AF/AFL with rapid ventricular response • MAT • VT storm	• Preexcited AF • Severe pulmonary disease • Reduced dose in CHF with acute exacerbation • Caution in ACS	• Hypotension • Bradycardia, heart block • Bronchospasm • Deteriorating heart failure, cardiogenic shock in patients with depressed ventricular function or ACS	• Esmolol has short half-life; preferred agent in relatively unstable patients • Metoprolol metabolized by liver ∩ *β*-Blockers have less evidence supporting its use in SVT, in comparison to calcium blocker. However, its safety profile has made *β*-blocker as one of common choices
Calcium channel blocker	• AVNRT • AVRT (but not preexcited AF) • AF/AFL with rapid ventricular response • MAT	• Preexcited AF • Second- or third-degree heart block • ACS • CHF	• Bradycardia, heart block • Negative inotropic effect, resulting deteriorating heart failure or cardiogenic shock	• Including diltiazem and verapamil which have similar profile • Calcium channel blocker has more data supporting its use in SVT, compared to *β*-blocker
Digoxin	• AF/AFL with rapid ventricular response	• Adjusted dose in severe renal failure	• Various forms of arrhythmias • Digoxin toxicity; central nervous and gastrointestinal systemic manifestation • Interacts with several medications	• Use is not considered the first-line therapy for SVT. However, digoxin is reasonable in hear failure. • Long-term use may be associated with an increase in mortality • Check digoxin level
Flecainide	• Rhythm control for AF/AFL	• Second- or third-degree heart block • CHF	• Proarrhythmic in structural heart disease • Worsens CHF	
Isoproterenol	• Heart block		• Hypotension	
Lidocaine	• Ventricular tachycardia	• Seizure disorders • Severe hepatic dysfunction	• Neurotoxicity • May increase defibrillator threshold	• Check lidocaine level
Magnesium	• TDP	• Severe renal failure	• Neurotoxicity at high level	• Serum magnesium may not reflect intracellular level
Procainamide	• Preexcited atrial fibrillation	• Hypotension • Second- or third-degree heart block • CHF • Reduce dosage in renal failure • Prolonged QT, previous TDP • Systemic lupus erythematosus	• Proarrhythmia • Hypotension • Positive ANA, lupus like syndrome	

AVNRT, atrioventricular nodal reentrant tachycardia; AVRT, atrioventricular reentrant tachycardia; AF, atrial fibrillation; AFL, atrial flutter; VT, ventricular tachycardia; VF, ventricular fibrillation; MAT, multifocal atrial tachycardia; ACS, acute coronary syndrome; SVT, supraventricular tachycardia; CHF, congestive heart failure; TDP, torsade de pointes; ANA, antinuclear antibody.

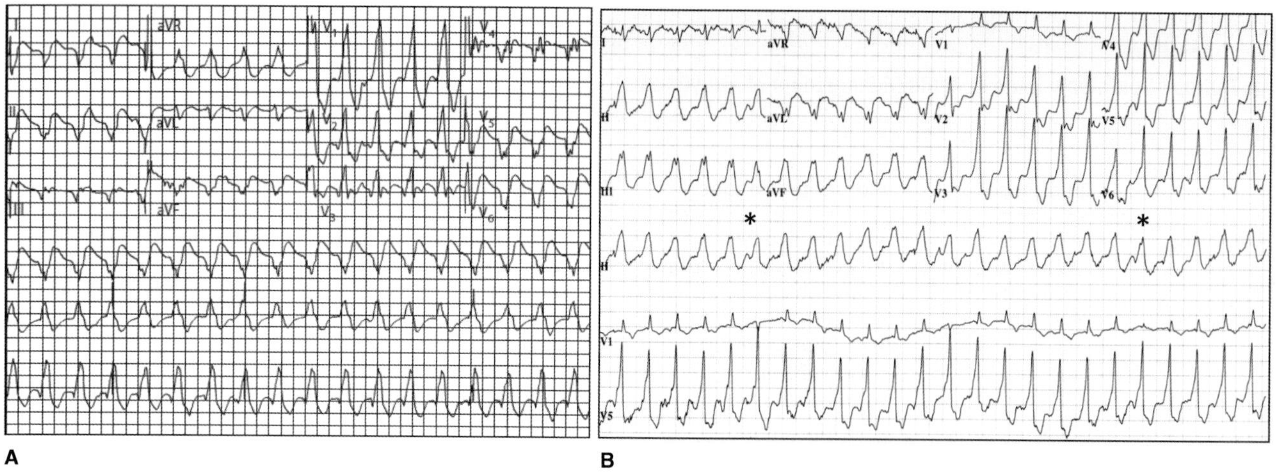

FIGURE 189.6 Monomorphic ventricular tachycardia (VT). Figure A demonstrates regular wide complex tachycardia with northwest axis and atypical RBBB pattern (single R wave in V1, and prominent S wave in V6). Atrioventricular dissociation, fusion beat (*, Fig. B), and positive concordance of QRS complexes. Courtesy of Thomas M. Munger, MD and Stephen C. Hammill, MD.

TABLE 189.5

Atypical Bundle Branch Pattern and QRS Criteria Indicative of the Diagnosis of Ventricular Tachycardia

	Typical RBBB pattern	RBBB pattern suggestive of VT	Typical LBBB pattern	LBBB pattern suggestive of VT
V1	rSR′, rSr′, rR′	Rsr′, Rr′, qR, monophasic R	QS or rS with QRS onset to the S wave nadir ≤60 ms and the duration of R wave ≤30 ms	Other patterns with QRS onset to the S wave nadir >60 ms and the duration of R wave >30 ms
V6	Small S (rS)	Large S (rS, QS)	No Q wave	Presence of Q wave
QRS		>140 ms		>160 ms

RBBB, right bundle branch block; LBBB, left bundle branch block.

or electrolyte abnormalities [2]. SVT with antegrade conduction over an accessory pathway or preexcitation syndrome is a less common cause of WCT and is discussed in "Section II: Supraventricular tachycardia" section.

Characteristic ECG for the Diagnosis of Ventricular Tachycardia

Careful evaluation of 12-lead ECGs often provides the distinction between VT and SVT (Fig. 189.6). It is necessary to integrate several ECG features for the diagnosis of VT because there is no perfect single criterion. In unstable patients, relatively simple criteria using the QRS axis, the presence of AV dissociation and concordance on the precordial leads can be used to differentiate VT. It is important to note that among patients with known structural heart disease, VT is the most likely cause of WCT.

- Regularity—VT is generally regular; irregular WCT is most commonly as a result of AF (Fig. 189.1).
- AV relationship—AV dissociation or ventricular rhythm faster than an independent atrial rhythm is the hallmark of VT. AV dissociation can be suggested by the presence of fusion (QRS morphology with mixed features between a normal beat and a ventricular beat Fig. 189.6) and captured complexes (QRS complex identical to one seen in sinus rhythm but that occurs in the midst of WCT). Related to AV dissociation, examination may reveal irregular cannon A waves in the jugular venous pulses resulting from periodic atrial contraction dissociated with tricuspid valve closure.
- QRS axis—WCT with axis of -60° to -120°, particular that WCT falling in to the northwest axis (-90° to -180°) and the axis that shifts from the baseline >40° are suggestive of VT [8].
- Precordial leads—If QRS polarities of the precordial leads are all negative or positive from V1 through V6 (i.e., concordance), WCT is likely VT.
- Right bundle branch block (RBBB) and left bundle branch block (RBBB) patterns—Generally, any patterns of atypical RBBB or atypical LBBB are considered VT (Table 189.5).
- Brugada criteria—Including four stepwise approaches, these criteria are the most widely known algorithm for identifying VT (Fig. 189.7) [18]. Its diagnostic performance varies among clinicians with the sensitivity >79% and specificity ~60% [17,19].

Pathophysiology and Etiology

Different from VF, PMVT and TDP, the most common mechanism of monomorphic VT is underlying myocardial scarring, as a substrate for reentry, in patients with a prior infarction or cardiomyopathy [15]. Precipitating factors should be considered and excluded (Table 189.1); such triggers commonly encountered in the ICU include a hyperdynamic state and intracardiac catheters. All antiarrhythmic drugs can be proarrhythmic, and the decision whether to continue or discontinue

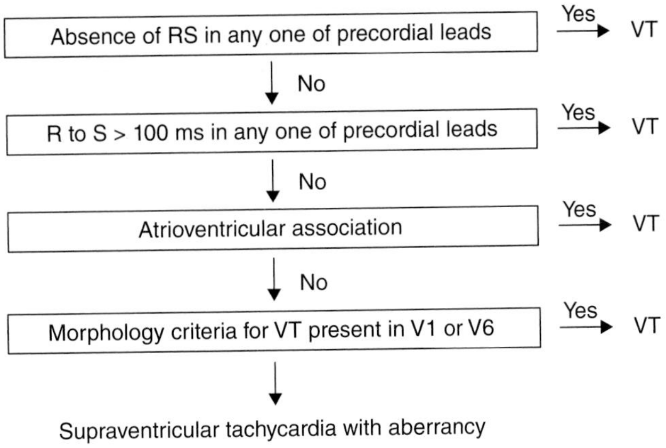

FIGURE 189.7 Brugada criteria for the diagnosis of ventricular tachycardia (VT).

therapy should be discussed with a cardiologist. If available, a serum drug level (e.g., amiodarone, digoxin, quinidine, procainamide) may be obtained. Digoxin toxicity can cause a variety of arrhythmias, including AV block, tachyarrhythmias, and bidirectional VT which is characteristic but rare. Tricyclic antidepressants and other sodium channel blocking drugs (e.g., flecainide, propafenone, quinidine, procainamide, disopyramide, phenothiazines) can slow ventricular conduction (reflected by a widened QRS complex), and cause very rapid VT known as ventricular flutter [20,21].

Initiation of the ACLS algorithm and defibrillation is warranted for pulseless VT [4]. Unstable patients with palpable pulses require immediate cardioversion with appropriate sedation and analgesia. Medical therapy can be administrated in hemodynamically stable patients. Antiarrhythmic drugs in a patient with unknown etiology of VT include class I (procainamide or lidocaine) or class III antiarrhythmic drugs (amiodarone or sotalol). Amiodarone has superior efficacy for terminating most VA and rarely has an absolute contraindication in the acute setting [15]. Preference of each drug's profile and possible side effects are summarized in Table 189.4. Synchronized cardioversion can be used for persistent VT. Maintenance antiarrhythmic therapy may be required to prevent acute recurrence, and a cardiology consult is recommended for all patients with VT. Vagal maneuvers or adenosine administration may be attempted in the rare circumstance of very high suspicion for SVT in hemodynamically stable patients with a regular WCT. These maneuvers inhibit the AV node and often terminate SVT but have little effect on VT. Vagal maneuvers or adenosine administration are contraindicated for PMVT suspicious for AF with preexcitation.

Ventricular Tachycardia Storm

VT storm is defined as an occurrence of ≥3 episodes of sustained VT/VF within 24 hours. VT storm is a true emergency and requires a multidisciplinary approach. VT storm is commonly associated with a hyperadrenergic state, and treatment with β-blockers has been shown to improve mortality [22]. Choices include intravenous metoprolol or esmolol which has a shorter half-life and is attractive for patients with severe hemodynamic compromise. In addition, amiodarone should be administered during the acute phase even if the patient is already receiving an oral formulation [15,23]. Amiodarone is recommended over lidocaine owing to its superior effectiveness for treatment of most VAs. Treatment of reversible causes is always critical. Additionally, medical optimization of heart failure is necessary because electrical instability can be a manifestation of pump failure [24].

If medical therapy is not successful, sedation and intubation may significantly suppress electrical storm. Neuraxial modulation for suppression of hyperdynamic state may also be warranted [25]. Mechanical circulatory support may facilitate suppression of VT storm in patients for whom ischemia or hemodynamic stress are driving triggers. Thoracic epidural anesthesia with intrathecal clonidine or bupivacaine at bedside can reduce the arrhythmic burden [24,25]. Further, sympathetic denervation and stellate ganglionectomy by a video-assisted thoracoscopic approach may be considered for refractory cases [24].

Non-Sustained Ventricular Tachycardia

NSVT is relatively common and generally not associated with symptoms. Little is known about the prognostic implications of NSVT in a structurally normal heart or nonischemic cardiomyopathy. NSVT, however, is associated with a higher risk of sudden cardiac death among patients with a history of myocardial infarction. Polymorphic NSVT should prompt a thorough evaluation for acute ischemia. General management focuses on correction of triggers and identifying underlying structural heart disease, which will dictate subacute and long-term management. A primary prevention ICD may be considered for postinfarct patients with left ventricular ejection fraction <40% and a positive electrophysiology study [26].

Premature Ventricular Contraction

Premature ventricular contractions (PVCs) are ectopic ventricular contractions with wide QRS complex occurring for <3 consecutive beats. PVCs are very common and can be found in a healthy population [15]. In rare circumstances, PVCs may be associated with poor outcomes; for example, in patients with severely depressed ventricular function or dyssynchronization, PVCs can precipitate heart failure. Very frequent PVCs >10,000 to 20,000 beats per 24 hours, or >20% of all beats, may cause PVC induced cardiomyopathy. Management focuses on identifying any underlying structural heart disease and correctable triggers. In patients without structural heart disease, specific medical therapy for PVCs is rarely warranted.

Accelerated Idiopathic Ventricular Rhythm

Accelerated idiopathic ventricular rhythm (AIVR) is a wide complex ventricular rhythm at a lower rate of VT (i.e., 40 to 100 bpm). This rhythm often occurs during the first 12 hours

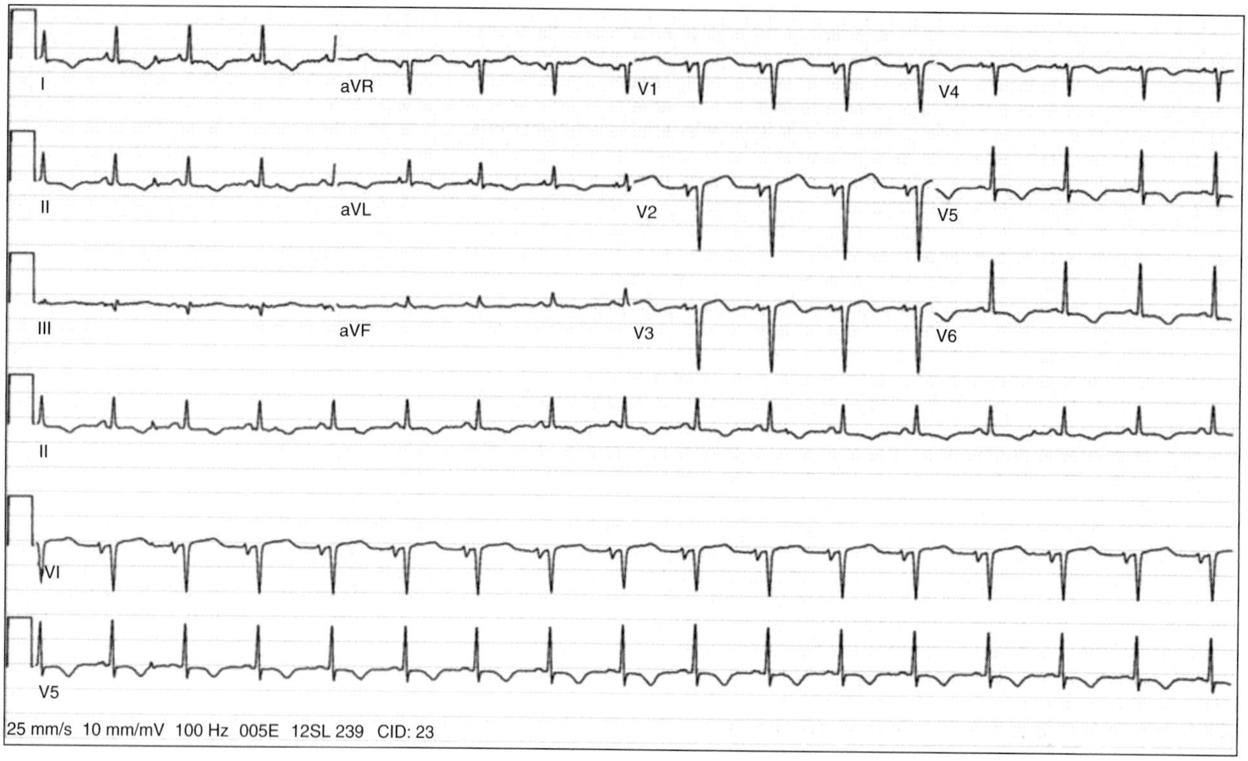

FIGURE 189.8 An electrocardiogram of a patient hospitalized for sepsis and complicated stress-induced cardiomyopathy. Noted ST-T changes in V1 to V3 and T wave inversion in V4 to V6 and I and II with prolongation of the QT interval. Courtesy of Faisal F. Syed, MD.

following reperfusion of an acute myocardial infarction during periods of elevated sympathetic tone. AIVR usually resolves without specific therapy. Electrolyte abnormalities (e.g., hyperkalemia) and ventricular pacing rhythm can mimic AIVR.

Subacute and Long-Term Management

Subacute and long-term management of VAs requires an assessment for the underlying structural cardiac disease [15]. After cardiac arrest, ventricular function may initially be depressed because of myocardial stunning, and, therefore, repeat imaging is required during follow-up. VF and PMVT are most commonly caused by acute coronary ischemia, and prompt revascularization can significantly improve prognosis even in cases without ST elevation myocardial infarction [13]. While TDP and monomorphic VT are not generally related to ischemia, other treatable triggers commonly observed in the ICU should be evaluated (Table 189.1).

The choice and duration to maintain antiarrhythmic drugs should be directed by a multispecialty team. Reassessment of ventricular function 40 days after myocardial infarction or 90 days after revascularization will determine the need for ICD implantation. However, in patients with persistent VAs, ICD implantation is indicated prior to dismissal. Postmyocardial infarction patients with impaired left ventricular ejection fraction are at a higher risk of sudden cardiac death in the first 3 months. Although not yet adequately studied by adequately powered randomized trials, such patients may benefit from a wearable defibrillator upon hospital discharge.

Long-term management following an episode of VAs is largely dictated by the residual risk and the underlying structural heart disease. Among patients with cardiomyopathy, β-blockers and an angiotensin-converting enzyme inhibitor are associated with a significant reduction in risk of sudden cardiac death [27–29].

Arrhythmias in Stress-Induced Cardiomyopathy

Reversible cardiomyopathy as a result of acute severe illness known as stress-induced cardiomyopathy or apical ballooning syndrome or takotsubo cardiomyopathy, can be found in approximately 28% of critically ill patients [18]. It is associated with remarkable ECG changes that are relatively similar to acute myocardial ischemia. Therefore, stress-induced cardiomyopathy is a diagnosis of exclusion. Gigantic T wave inversion and prominent QT prolongation are frequently evident with peak prolongation occurring 2 to 3 days postadmission (Fig. 189.8). Arrhythmias are common in this setting, with reported frequencies of 4.7% for AF, 2.2% sustained VT, and 1.2% VF. Risk of VAs appears to be highest at the peak of longest QT interval and maximal T wave inversion [30]. Therefore, patients should be monitored during this critical period.

Given that catecholamine surge during critical illness is likely a culprit of stress-induced cardiomyopathy, early administration of a β-blocker is a mainstay of treatment. However, β-blockers for patients with bradycardia or severe QTc prolongation should be prescribed cautiously because TDP could be related to pause or bradycardia. Noteworthy, an increase in the awareness of genetic syndromes predisposing patients with stress-induced cardiomyopathy to have markedly prolonged QT interval has been recognized. Thus, a careful personal and family history should be collected, and referral to an electrophysiologist should be considered [30].

SECTION II: SUPRAVENTRICULAR TACHYCARDIA

SVTs are among the most commonly encountered arrhythmias in the ICU setting, and can cause considerable morbidity and mortality for critically ill patients. A structured approach to facilitate prompt diagnosis and management of these rhythms is displayed in Figures 189.2 and 189.3.

The 2015 American College of Cardiology/American Heart Association and the Heart Rhythm Society (ACC/AHA/HRS) guidelines for the management of the adult patients with SVT define SVT as a tachycardia originating above the level of the His bundle [31]. A ventricular rate that exceeds 100 bpm and a narrow QRS complex (QRS width < 120 ms) are the hallmarks of SVT. Less commonly, a WCT can be owing to SVT with bundle branch block or aberrant conduction. Differentiation of SVT from VT using the 12-lead ECG is discussed in Section I.

SVTs are classified as regular narrow complex tachycardias, characterized by regular intervals between successive R waves or as irregular narrow complex tachycardias, with irregular R-R intervals. The differential diagnosis of regular narrow complex tachycardia includes sinus tachycardia, atrioventricular nodal reentrant tachycardia (AVNRT), atrioventricular reentrant tachycardia (AVRT), and focal atrial tachycardia. Irregular narrow complex tachycardias include AF and multifocal atrial tachycardia (MAT). Atrial flutter (AFL) can present as a regular narrow complex tachycardia, but can be irregular owing to variable AV conduction block. Furthermore, the management approach to AF and AFL is very similar, and, hence, AFL is discussed in "Irregular Narrow Complex Tachycardia" section.

Regular Narrow Complex Tachycardia

Ventricular response greater than 100 bpm, QRS width <120 ms, and regular R-R intervals define regular narrow complex tachycardia. Sinus tachycardia, AVNRT, AVRT, focal atrial tachycardia, and AFL are the most important considerations for the differential diagnosis of these rhythms (Fig. 189.9). Particular attention to three key electrocardiographic features will allow differentiation of regular narrow complex tachycardias. First, the onset and termination of tachycardia can be sudden (AVNRT and AVRT) or gradual (sinus tachycardia). Atrial tachycardia can present in either fashion (Figs. 189.2 and 189.3). Second, the ECG should be scrutinized for the presence and timing of P waves. If the P wave occurs closer to the preceding QRS complex (short R-P tachycardia), AVNRT and AVRT are more likely, although important exceptions exist (Fig. 189.2) [32]. If the P wave occurs closer to the succeeding QRS complex (long R-P tachycardia), sinus tachycardia and atrial tachycardia are more likely. Finally, the morphology of the P wave can differentiate sinus tachycardia from atrial tachycardia. Sinus P waves are upright in leads II, III, and aVF and biphasic in lead V1. An abrupt change in P wave morphology should alert the clinician to an atrial tachycardia [32–34].

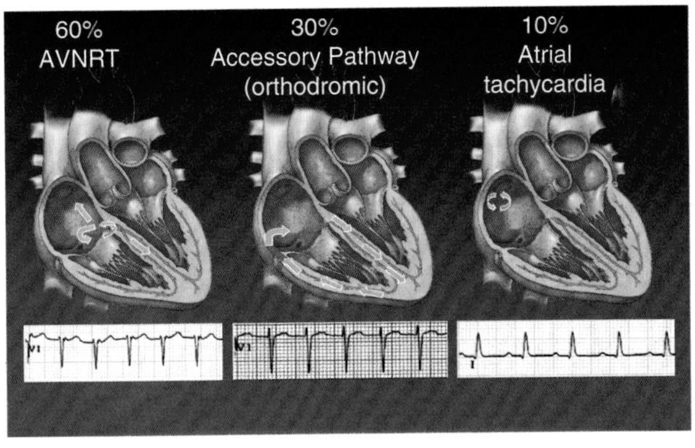

FIGURE 189.9 Genesis of commonly encountered regular narrow complex tachycardia.

Sinus Tachycardia

Sinus tachycardia is a commonly encountered rhythm in the ICU setting. It is usually a normal physiologic response to a hyperadrenergic state caused by shock, pain, systemic inflammation, adrenergic medications, or rarely endocrine disturbances such as hyperthyroidism. It is characterized by a ventricular rate greater than 100 bpm, sinus P wave morphology, long R-P interval, and gradual onset and offset. Sinus tachycardia will resolve with treatment of the underlying cause.

Occasionally, sinus tachycardia can result in cardiac ischemia in patients with severe coronary artery disease. Other conditions where maximizing the diastolic interval is important are severe mitral stenosis and restrictive cardiac physiology as seen in heart failure with preserved ejection fraction. In these situations, temporary use of short-acting β-blockers or calcium channel blockers to reduce the sinus rate is warranted.

Focal Atrial Tachycardia

Focal atrial tachycardias are regular narrow complex, long R-P interval SVTs that arise from regions other than the sinus node. The mechanism can be automatic, triggered activity, or reentry. The morphology of the P waves can help differentiate focal atrial tachycardias from sinus tachycardia. Atrial tachycardias can have sudden onset, especially if a reentrant mechanism is involved.

In contrast to sinus tachycardia, the fast heart rates with focal atrial tachycardia are usually inappropriate, and treatment with β-blockers or calcium channel blockers is reasonable in acute situations if the increased heart rate is poorly tolerated [31]. Vagal maneuvers and adenosine can slow the ventricular response and allow for diagnosis of the atrial rhythm, and can terminate atrial tachycardia owing to triggered activity [35]. Second-line options for termination include intravenous class IC agents such as flecainide [36] and intravenous class III agents such as ibutilide and amiodarone (Table 189.4) [37,38]. Overdrive pacing through an existing atrial lead can terminate the tachycardia, and should only be performed under expert guidance [31].

Atrioventricular Nodal Reentrant Tachycardia

AVNRT is often categorized as a paroxysmal SVT, because of abrupt onset and offset. It is the most common regular SVT, and is more common in women than in men [39]. There is usually a history of previous episodes beginning in second or third decade of life. The ventricular rate is often between 150 and 250 bpm, but can occasionally exceed 250 bpm [40].

Impulses from the sinus node are conducted to the AV node via the "fast" pathway and the "slow" pathway. The fast pathway is typically anatomically located anteriorly in the right atrium and conducts impulses rapidly to the AV node. The slow pathway is anatomically located posteriorly along the ostium of the coronary sinus. During normal conduction, impulses travel down the fast pathway to the Atrioventricular node (AV node), resulting in ventricular conduction. There is retrograde activation of the slow pathway, and, as a result, the antegrade activation of the slow pathway does not reach the AV node. Differences in the refractory periods of the two pathways can result in initiation and maintenance of AVNRT [41,42]. When a premature atrial contraction (PAC) occurs, the fast pathway can be refractory from the previous sinus beat, and the wavefront travels down the slow pathway. If the PAC is timed critically, the fast pathway may have recovered by the time the wavefront reaches the AV node, resulting in retrograde conduction up the fast pathway, establishing a reentrant circuit.

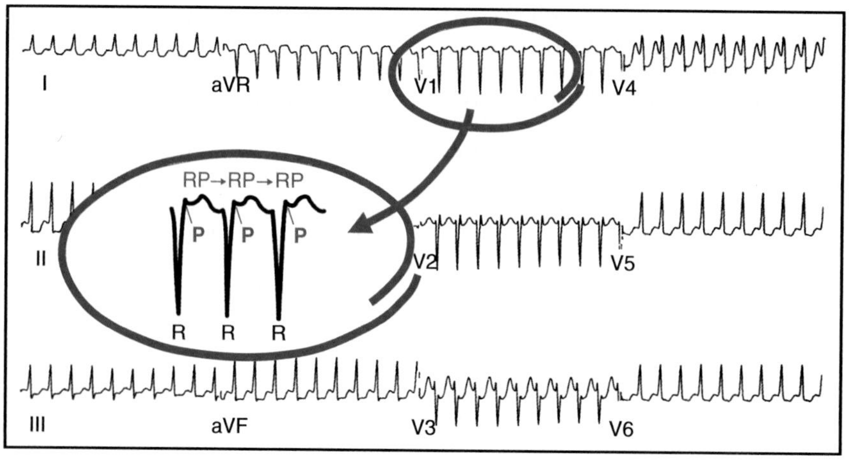

FIGURE 189.10 Example of short RP interval tachycardia. Note typical atrioventricular nodal reentrant tachycardia (AVNRT) with pseudo-R′ in V1.

This is the underlying pathophysiology of "typical" AVNRT, which occurs in about 80% cases.

The surface ECG shows a PAC with prolonged PR interval (owing to conduction down the slow pathway), followed by a sudden onset regular narrow complex tachycardia. Retrograde P waves can be seen after each QRS complex, and, hence, this tachycardia has a short R-P interval (Fig. 189.10). Although this tachycardia is usually well tolerated, older patients and critically ill young patients may not tolerate it well.

AVNRT usually responds well to vagal maneuvers which is the first-line therapy in acute management (Fig. 189.2) [43,44]. The Valsalva maneuver can be performed easily at the bedside and can terminate AVNRT. Other maneuvers, such as carotid massage (after exclusion of a bruit), applying an ice cold towel to the face, can also be effective. Eyeball pressure is no longer recommended as a vagal maneuver owing to the potential for harm [31]. If these fail, intravenous adenosine is almost always successful in terminating AVNRT [45,46]. It can also help unmask a cause for SVT other than AVNRT by slowing the ventricular response and allowing the diagnosis of unrecognized atrial tachycardia or flutter. Intravenous β-blockers and calcium channel blockers are rarely required for treatment [47]. If patients have recurrent AVNRT in the ICU, oral therapy with calcium channel blockers or β-blockers can be effective in preventing recurrences [48]. Catheter ablation is widely utilized in the outpatient setting for definite management of AVNRT, but very rarely performed during an acute illness [49].

Atrioventricular Reentrant Tachycardia

Accessory pathways are myocardial fibers that connect atrial myocardium directly to ventricular myocardium [31]. The presence of an accessory pathway can permit conduction of impulses directly from the atrium to the ventricle (anterograde conduction or antidromic AVRT) or conduction of impulses from the ventricle to the atrium (retrograde conduction or orthodromic AVRT). In sinus rhythm, the surface ECG may reveal short PR interval, a "delta wave" and some degree of fusion between impulses conducted down the accessory pathway and the AV node (Fig. 189.11).

Presence of an accessory pathway can result in three clinical presentations relevant to intensive care physicians. First, a PAC can conduct down the AV node and up the accessory pathway, resulting in a reentrant tachycardia (orthodromic AVRT).The ECG will show a regular narrow complex tachycardia with a short R-P interval, similar to AVNRT. This is the most common tachycardia in patients with accessory pathways. Second, there can be a reentrant tachycardia with conduction down the accessory pathway and up AV node (antidromic AVRT: Fig. 189.12).

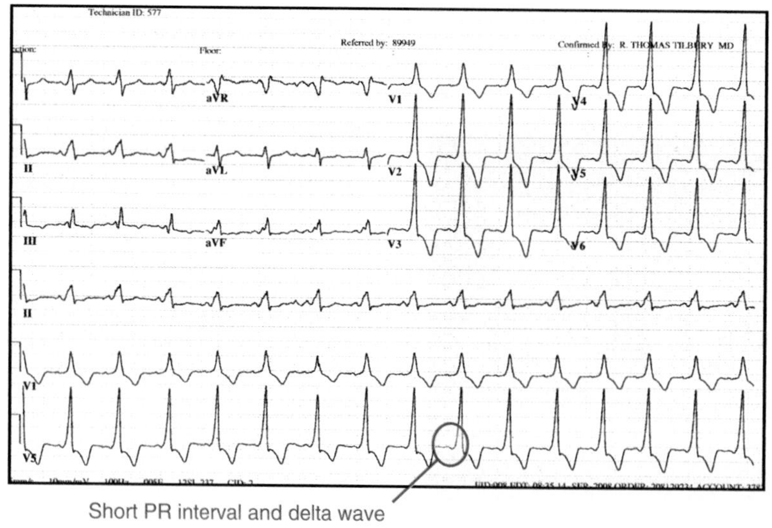

FIGURE 189.11 An electrocardiogram demonstrates short PR interval and "delta wave" in sinus rhythm.

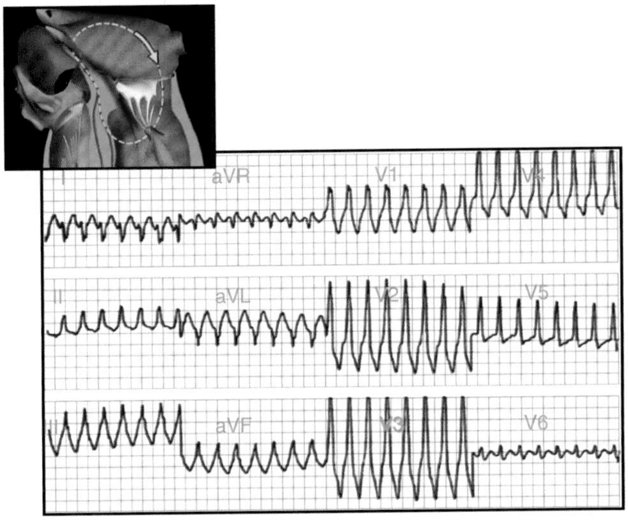

FIGURE 189.12 Antidromic atrioventricular reentrant tachycardia (AVRT). The anterograde impulses travel through the accessory pathway resulting in widen QRS complex.

Antidromic AVRT is a regular tachycardia with a wide complex QRS on the surface ECG, because conduction is directly to the ventricular tissue and not through the usual conduction system.

Finally, an atrial arrhythmia such as AF or AFL can conduct down the accessory pathway, resulting in extremely rapid heart rate (preexcited AF/AFL: Fig. 189.13). The difference between preexcited AF and antidromic AVRT is that the AV node is not involved in the tachycardia circuit. Presence of preexcitation on the surface ECG and an associated SVT is diagnostic for Wolff–Parkinson–White (WPW) syndrome. Preexcited AF is commonly associated hemodynamic instability and is best treated with cardioversion in unstable patients [31]. VF can occur among patients with preexcited AF. If patients are hemodynamically stable, intravenous procainamide [50] or ibutilide [51] can be administered (Table 189.4). The use of any AV nodal blocking agents is contraindicated in preexcited AF, because these agents increase conduction down the accessory pathway and can precipitate VF.

It is uncommon for orthodromic or antidromic AVRT to cause hemodynamic instability, because the circuit involves the AV node, which has decremental conduction properties. Nevertheless, hemodynamically unstable patients with either of these rhythms should undergo cardioversion. In hemodynamically stable patients, the management is similar to AVNRT. Vagal maneuvers should be attempted first [52] followed by intravenous adenosine [53]. Intravenous β-blockers or calcium channel blockers can also terminate the tachycardia. Catheter ablation of the accessory pathway is the definitive treatment and is usually performed in the outpatient setting.

Irregular Narrow Complex Tachycardia

When evaluating an irregular narrow complex tachycardia, AF, AFL with variable block, and MAT should be considered. Among these, AF is the most common, and is actually the most common arrhythmia worldwide [54].

Atrial Fibrillation (AF)

AF is present in about 1% of the general population and in 9% of adults older than 80 years [55]. AF occurs as the result of chaotic and uncoordinated atrial activation and is characterized by the absence of P waves and irregular R-R intervals on the surface ECG (Fig. 189.3). Morbidity from AF is a consequence of rapid ventricular rates, lack of atrial contraction, and the propensity for clot formation in the left atrium with consequent risk of systemic embolization. AF is classified as valvular or nonvalvular according to the presence or the absence of significant mitral stenosis or prosthetic valve. It is also classified based on duration of AF as paroxysmal (terminates spontaneously or within 7 days of onset), persistent (AF for >7 days), long-standing persistent (AF > 12 months), or permanent (persistent AF with no further attempts at restoration of sinus rhythm) [56].

Among ICU patients, AF can result in hemodynamic instability because of rapid ventricular rates. This is especially true for cases with restrictive left ventricular filling, such as diastolic dysfunction, hypertrophic cardiomyopathy, or restrictive cardiomyopathy. AF can cause instability for any patient in whom a longer diastolic filling period is desirable, such as patients with severe mitral stenosis, constrictive pericarditis, or severe coronary artery disease. As discussed previously, patients with WPW syndrome can experience severe hemodynamic instability and even VF if they develop AF and antegrade conduction down the accessory pathway.

Etiology and Pathophysiology

AF can be considered a final common manifestation of several processes that favor increased ectopy and reentry in the left atrial

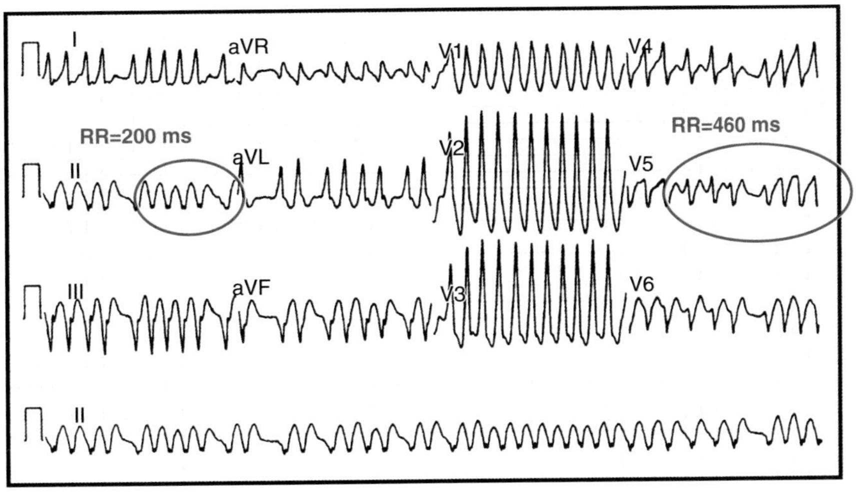

FIGURE 189.13 Preexcited AF with characteristics of irregularly regular tachycardia and variable QRS complex morphology and RR intervals. AF, atrial fibrillation.

myocardium. The interplay of rapidly discharging foci, usually of the pulmonary veins, atrial substrate abnormalities that favor reentry, and autonomic disturbances that trigger atrial activation results in initiation and maintenance of AF [57].

There are several well-recognized risk factors that contribute to these aforementioned processes. Apart from increasing age, hypertension is the most prevalent risk factor for AF. Congestive heart failure arising from ischemic heart disease, dilated cardiomyopathy, myocarditis, valvular heart disease, or congenital heart disease is a common and important risk factors for AF. Ischemia itself can precipitate AF, without an accompanying cardiomyopathy. In addition to the classic risk factors, obesity and metabolic syndrome, obstructive sleep apnea, hyperthyroidism, chronic kidney disease, and any process resulting in systemic inflammation can contribute to AF [58–60]. It is important to recognize pulmonary embolism as a trigger for AF. Excessive alcohol consumption (holiday heart syndrome), toxicities from drugs of abuse such as cocaine, and medications such as inotropes can result in AF [61,62].

A special mention must be made of AF in the postoperative period. Increased sympathetic tone in postoperative states as a result of inflammation, fluid shifts, and pain contribute to increased incidence of AF. Cardiac surgery patients are particularly at risk of developing AF, and up to 40% of postcardiac surgery patients can develop AF [63]. Postoperative amiodarone and β-blockers can decrease the incidence of AF in this group of patients [64,65]. The genesis of AF among cardiac surgery patients is multifactorial, and atrial incisions, pericardial inflammation, and atrial ischemia are all thought to contribute.

The electrophysiologic basis for AF requires a trigger for initiation and substrate for maintenance. Triggers for AF include rapid discharges from the myocardial sleeves that surround pulmonary veins, electrolyte abnormalities causing increased atrial ectopy, and abnormal intracellular calcium handling, resulting in triggered after depolarization [66]. Conditions favoring reentry form the substrate for maintenance of AF. The haphazard orientation of pulmonary venous myocytes, atrial fibrosis from atrial dilation, and scar tissue formation from ischemia or previous surgery are all foci of reentry and favor maintenance of AF. In addition, AF itself results in structural and electrical remodeling, and, hence, the tenet "AF begets AF [67]."

Management

The ultimate clinical goals of AF treatment include amelioration of symptoms, including palpitations, fatigue, dyspnea, lightheadedness, prevention and treatment of heart failure including tachycardia-induced cardiomyopathy, and prevention of stroke. These goals are usually achieved through either adequate control of the ventricular rate or restoration of sinus rhythm.

AF is associated with increased mortality after adjustment of confounders. However, in the outpatient setting, it is unclear whether long-term treatment of AF improves outcomes [68]. Among ICU patients, AF can result in hemodynamic instability or ischemia or both. For the hemodynamically unstable patient, synchronized direct cardioversion is indicated. A careful search must be made for precipitating factors for all patients once stabilized. Any condition causing sympathetic activation can precipitate AF. Common ICU-associated causes include sepsis, myocardial ischemia, pulmonary embolism, systemic inflammation, pericarditis, and stroke (Table 189.1). Addressing and treating these conditions can result in spontaneous resolution of new-onset AF. Administration of sympathomimetic agents is common in ICU settings and can cause AF. Electrolytes must be checked, and hypokalemia and hypomagnesemia in particular must be corrected.

Apart from controlling these precipitants of AF, a rate control or rhythm control approach may be pursued for management [56]. Rate control refers to a strategy of using drugs that increase the refractoriness of the AV node to impulse propagation, resulting in a controlled ventricular rate. Oral or intravenous β-blockers, calcium channel blockers, digoxin, and even amiodarone can be used for rate control. Rhythm control is a strategy of converting AF into sinus rhythm and can be achieved by electrical synchronized cardioversion or pharmacologic cardioversion with medications. From a standpoint of long-term management, a large multicenter randomized controlled trial found no difference in endpoints when rhythm control was compared with rate control [69]. In the ICU setting, because of high rates of recurrent AF, rate control is the most commonly adopted management strategy for AF; rhythm control is reserved for AF that is difficult to rate control.

Prevention of Thromboembolic Complications

The association of stroke and AF is well described. Stasis of blood in the left atrial appendage, a hypercoagulable state induced by AF itself result in left atrial thrombosis and systemic embolization. Risk factors for stroke among patients with AF are easily recalled by the CHA2DS2VASc scoring system recommended be the ACC/AHA/HRS 2014 AF guidelines [56]. Increasing scores are indicative of increasing annual incidence of stroke, 6.7% per year in patients with a score of 9 [70]. Anticoagulation can be avoided for patients with a score of 0, and anticoagulants are indicated for patients with a score of ≥2. A score of 1 represents a gray area, and no therapy, aspirin alone, or anticoagulation can be considered for management based on patient preference and the clinical scenario. Stroke prevention with anticoagulation is counterbalanced by the risk of intracranial and extracranial bleeding with anticoagulation [56]. While warfarin was the mainstay of anticoagulation for AF in the past, novel oral anticoagulants, including dabigatran, rivaroxaban, apixaban, and edoxaban, are now commonly utilized for thromboprophylaxis.

There are no clear guidelines for anticoagulation and bridging for patients with AF in the ICU setting [56]. For patients already on anticoagulation for AF, in the absence of bleeding or significant risk factors for bleeding, anticoagulation should be continued in the ICU. Bridging anticoagulation for AF patients needing a procedure remains a controversial topic. A recent randomized controlled trial found that forgoing bridging anticoagulation was noninferior to perioperative bridging and offered less risk of bleeding [71]. It is noteworthy that the BRIDGE study excluded patients at high risk for thromboembolic events (mean CHADS2 score of the study patients was 2.3 and only 8% had previous history of stroke). Bridging therapy may offer adequate thromboprophylaxis for patients with a higher risk of stroke with the option to rapidly cease anticoagulation if bleeding occurs. Anticoagulation must, of course, be discontinued for patients with AF with active bleeding in the ICU. A discussion of reversal of warfarin and novel oral agents in the actively bleeding patient for actively bleeding patients can be found in Chapters 88 and 93 is, and is the subject of authoritative reviews [72].

The role of anticoagulation for new-onset AF in the ICU setting is also uncertain. AF that terminates spontaneously within 48 hours of onset is rarely associated with stroke, and anticoagulation can be withheld in these patients. If AF persists for >48 hours, or it is suspected that AF has been ongoing for >48 hours at the time of admission, anticoagulation can be considered for patients with a high CHA2DS2VASc score or for those in whom cardioversion is to be considered. Intravenous heparin can achieve therapeutic anticoagulation rapidly, and its anticoagulant effect should dissipate in about an hour when stopped.

Regardless of the CHA2DS2VASc score, anticoagulation should be administered, unless contraindicated, for 4 weeks after cardioversion for AF. Atrial stunning and reduction in atrial contractility result in a thrombogenic environment and a high risk for embolic complications in the absence of anticoagulation in patients undergoing cardioversion.

Rate Control Strategy

The rate control strategy can ameliorate symptoms of AF and improve hemodynamic stability. In the outpatient setting, a heart rate <80 bpm at rest and <110 bpm with exertion were criteria for adequate rate control in the AFFIRM trial [69]. A single randomized controlled study, the RACE-II trial, demonstrated similar outcomes with a "lenient" rate control strategy with heart rate <110 bpm at rest [73]. This study had few patients with left ventricular systolic dysfunction, and most patients had heart rates <100 bpm and, hence, must be interpreted in this context.

Intravenous administration of AV nodal blocking agents can achieve timely rate control of AF with rapid ventricular response within minutes. β-Blockers such as metoprolol and esmolol and calcium channel blockers such as diltiazem and verapamil are widely used for acute rate control in the ICU [74]. The choice between these classes of agents is usually decided by individual provider preferences and the side effect profile of these medications (Table 189.1). Although rare, even cardioselective β-blockers can worsen bronchospasm, especially among ICU patients who are actively wheezing as a result of obstructive airway disease. Calcium channel blockers should be avoided for patients with poor ventricular function and heart failure. A special note must be made of preexcited AF in WPW syndrome. AV nodal blocking agents must not be used in this setting, because it can precipitate VF by increasing conduction down the accessory pathway.

Digoxin is a second-line agent for rate control of AF, and can be administered intravenously. Compared with β-blockers and calcium channel blockers, intravenous digoxin takes longer to achieve its effects (>1 hour for onset and >6 hours for maximal effect) [74]. In addition to slower onset of action, dose adjustment for elderly and renally impaired patients, potential for lethal toxicity, including AV block and VAs, association with mortality in long-term studies all make digoxin a less favorable agent. However, it remains the only rate control medication that does not have negative inotropic effects, and can be a useful medication in the right clinical setting, for acute decompensated heart failure in particular.

Intravenous amiodarone is another option for cases of difficult rate control [75]. Clinicians with adequate experience in the use of amiodarone should guide therapy because hypotension, decompensation of heart failure, and VAs can result with its use (Table 189.1). Pharmacologic conversion to sinus rhythm can also occur, and anticoagulation must be considered based on the clinical setting as discussed previously. Dronedarone is rarely used for rate or rhythm control in ICUs and is contraindicated in patients with permanent AF and patients with acute decompensated heart failure [76].

Rhythm Control Strategy

The rhythm control strategy aims to restore sinus rhythm which can be achieved by electrical cardioversion, antiarrhythmic drug therapy, or a combination of the two. Intravenous conscious sedation is used for patients undergoing electrical cardioversion.

In the ICU setting, rhythm control is often reserved for patients who have persistently rapid ventricular rates or adverse hemodynamic consequences of AF despite an adequate trial of pharmacotherapy. As mentioned previously, hemodynamically unstable patients should be managed with cardioversion. For hemodynamically stable patients, electrical cardioversion can be performed within 48 hours of onset, and should be followed by 4 weeks of anticoagulation [77]. For patients with >48 hours or unknown duration of AF, left atrial appendage thrombus may have formed, and there are two options for management. One option is to perform transesophageal echocardiography, which can exclude a left atrial thrombus before performing cardioversion and continuing anticoagulation. If an atrial thrombus is detected, anticoagulation should be initiated and continued for 3 weeks prior to attempting cardioversion.

It is important to determine and document whether a cardioversion attempt is followed by at least temporary conversion to sinus rhythm or immediate resumption of AF [56]. If sinus rhythm is not present after cardioversion, even temporarily, approaches to improve energy delivery such as increasing the electric output, using biphasic waveforms, adjusting location of the electrodes, or even applying pressure to optimize electrode-skin contact can be useful. Ibutilide decreases the defibrillation threshold and can be useful in this situation. If sinus rhythm is temporarily present, use of antiarrhythmics may increase the likelihood of maintenance of sinus rhythm.

For patients with long-standing AF undergoing cardioversion, there can be significant underlying sinus node dysfunction, resulting in long pauses and even sinus arrest with a ventricular escape rhythm. Providers must be ready to institute temporary transcutaneous pacing and placement of temporary transvenous pacemaker in such cases.

Pharmacologic agents can be used primarily for rhythm control or as an adjunct to electrical cardioversion. Amiodarone is perhaps the most widely used medication for this purpose. Amiodarone has a very long half-life, and there are several loading regimens available for initiation. It can be loaded intravenously and can have rate control effects in addition to enabling cardioversion. Oral amiodarone loading takes much longer to exert its antiarrhythmic effects.

Other drugs used for rhythm control include class IC agents, including propafenone and flecainide, which should be avoided in patients with structural heart disease owing to proarrhythmic effects. Class III antiarrhythmics, including dofetilide, ibutilide, and sotalol, can be used with caution in patients with structural heart disease, but can result in pro-arrhythmia because of QT prolongation (Table 189.4) [56]. These drugs should be used under expert guidance.

Atrial Flutter (AFL)

AFL is another commonly encountered arrhythmia in the ICU setting, and frequently coexists in patients with AF. "Typical" AFL is the most common type of flutter and occurs because of a reentrant circuit involving the cavotricuspid isthmus in the right atrium. The surface ECG shows sawtooth-like flutter waves, which are negative in leads II, III, and aVF and positive in lead V1. The flutter rate is typically around 300 bpm, and the refractoriness of the AV node results in 2:1, 3:1, or even 4:1 block, resulting in ventricular rates around 150, 100, and 75 bpm, respectively. Variable AV block is also common among patients receiving AV blocking agents, and can result in irregular R-R intervals. "Atypical" AFL involves reentrant circuits around atrial scars from previous surgery or ablation and can manifest with different morphology and rates on the surface ECG.

Regardless of the type of AFL, the clinical effects are similar to AF, and the management approach is similar to AF as well [56]. Rate control in AFL can actually be more challenging than AF, and rhythm control may need to be used more often for problematic cases. Unlike AF, pharmacologic rhythm control may result in acute hemodynamic instability owing to 1:1 ventricular conduction, and immediate cardioversion may be required.

Prevention of AF for Surgical Patients

The postcardiothoracic surgery patient is particularly prone to development of AF, and an incidence as high has 25% to 50% has been reported in this group of patients. Perioperative amiodarone and β-blockade are both reasonable options to prevent AF in patients at particularly high risk of AF [64,65]. Sotalol and colchicine have both demonstrated efficacy for preventing the AF of cardiac surgery patients [78,79].

Multifocal Atrial Tachycardia

MAT is an irregular narrow complex tachycardia, characterized by at least three distinct morphologies of P waves. There is variability of both the P-R and R-R intervals [80]. MAT is most commonly associated with chronic medical conditions causing hypoxemia such as chronic obstructive pulmonary disease. Intravenous β-blockers or calcium channel blockers can be used for treatment of acute episodes. Correcting hypoxemia through oxygen supplemental therapies is also a key component of treatment. If more than three distinct P wave morphologies are present, but the heart rate is less than 100 bpm, then the rhythm is referred to as a wandering atrial pacemaker.

Approach to the Hemodynamically Unstable SVT

Shock is commonly encountered in the ICU setting and may be because of hypovolemic, cardiogenic, distributive, or obstructive etiologies. A variety of SVTs, including sinus tachycardia, AVNRT, AVRT, AF/AFL, and preexcited AF, can occur in patients with shock. Sinus tachycardia usually represents the physiologic compensation to hypotension. The other SVTs can be innocent bystanders or can contribute to hypotension caused by rapid ventricular rates, poor ventricular filling, and reduction in stroke volume and cardiac output. Hemodynamic instability owing to these rhythms usually occurs when the ventricular rates are very poorly controlled (>150 bpm).

All ICU providers must be familiar with the ACLS protocols for tachycardia [81]. If there is hypotension, altered mental status or ischemic chest pain as a result of the SVT, immediate synchronized cardioversion must be performed. Vagal maneuvers can be attempted if the patient is cooperative and the rhythm has a narrow complex. If the arrhythmia is definitely narrow complex, adenosine can terminate AVNRT and AVRT, and can allow diagnosis of other atrial arrhythmias.

Preexcited AF presents with a bizarre wide complex rhythm owing to rapid conduction of impulses down the accessory pathway (Fig. 189.12). Patients are frequently hemodynamically unstable, and VF can result if nodal blocking agents are used. Procainamide, a class 1a anti-arrhythmic, is the drug of choice for preexcited AF.

SECTION III: BRADYARRHYTHMIAS

Bradyarrhythmias are generally defined as heart rate below 60 bpm in symptomatic patients. Bradyarrhythmias can be largely classified into two types, (1) disorders of impulse generation, which refers to failure of the sinoatrial (SA) node to generate an initial electrical impulse and (2) disorders of impulse conduction which refers to failure in propagation electrical impulse to the myocardium (Figs. 189.4 and 189.5). Bradycardias are not always pathologic. Examples include sinus bradycardia or bradyarrhythmias in the setting of vagal response as seen in athletes or during sleeping, or a result of increased vagal tone from various factors such as carotid sinus hypersensitivity, pain, gastrointestinal distress (i.e., bowel obstruction, nausea, and vomiting), genitourinary dysfunction (i.e., urinary retention), increased intracranial pressure, hypoxia, and hypothermia [82].

Disorders of Impulse Generation

Sinus Arrhythmia

Sinus arrhythmia is the change in beat-to-beat P-P interval with unchanged morphology of the P waves (sinus rhythm) (Fig. 189.4). It is usually a normal physiologic response to alteration of vagal tone during respiration or external irritation. Certain pathology such as digitalis toxicity, ischemic heart disease, or intracranial hemorrhage can mimic the benign form of this sinus arrhythmia [83]. However, sinus arrhythmia usually does not cause hemodynamic instability, and treatment is not required.

Sinus Bradycardia

Sinus bradycardia, or sinus rhythm, with heart rate below 60 bpm, is secondary to reduced automaticity of the SA node. This happens as a result of alteration of vagal tone or pharmacologic agents such as parasympathomimetics, β-Blockers, calcium antagonists, and digitalis. Sinus bradycardia is not always indicative of pathology.

Sinus Node Dysfunction

Also referred as sick sinus syndrome, sinus node dysfunction is an intrinsic dysfunction of the SA node that leads to inappropriate automaticity and other pacemaker foci (or junctional escape) take over control of the heart rate. Sinus node dysfunction can manifest as a combination of bradycardia and atrial tachycardia, known as "tachy-brady syndrome," which occurs in approximately half of the patients with sinus node dysfunction [84]. Sinus node dysfunction is commonly related to age and can occur as a result of hypothyroidism, infiltrative disease, collagen vascular disease, trauma, ischemia, infection, or ion channel dysfunction [4]. Sinus node dysfunction often coexists with AV nodal disease [85].

The ability of the SA node to respond to stress decreases with age which manifests as delayed recovery after an episode of tachycardia [86]. These can be dangerous in the ICU setting, in which preexisting SA and AV nodal diseases are often exacerbated through the use of cardioinhibitory medications as well as an increase in vagal tone as a result of pain. Patients can develop sinus arrest especially immediately after sudden termination of a tachyarrhythmia which may require immediate intervention (Fig. 189.4). Further, there can be an abrupt increase in repolarization time (QT interval) during bradycardia, and the patient may be predisposed to TDP.

Disorders of Impulse Propagation

Sinoatrial Block

SA block, or SA exit block, is a failure of propagation of impulse generated by the SA node to the atrial myocardium. There are three degrees of SA block. First-degree SA block is a delayed conduction within the SA node and is undetectable on ECG. Second-degree SA block presents as intermittent conduction of SA impulse and can be divided into two types. Type I second-degree SA block is a result of progressive lengthening of the interval between impulse generation and transmission, causing successive P waves closer together with a characteristic of group beating and progressive shortening of the P-P interval until a pause is detected on ECG (Fig. 189.5). Type II second-degree SA block is a result of intermediate block where there is no progressive shortening of the P-P interval, but a sinus pause occurs. The ECG, hence, presents a missing P wave, making the duration of a P-P interval an exact multiple of the preceding P-P interval (Fig. 189.5). Finally, third-degree SA block manifests as sinus arrest (Fig. 189.5), which may require temporary pacing especially when subsidiary pacemakers (i.e., junctional rhythm) do not provide sufficient cardiac output.

Atrioventricular Block

AV block is a failure of impulse propagation at the level of the AV node that is composed of the supra- and infrahisian conduction system. The etiologies behind AV nodal disease are similar to those causing SA dysfunction. Just like SA block, there are three degrees of AV block. In first-degree AV block, there is a prolongation of the PR interval to greater than 200 ms [86,87]. There are two types of second-degree AV block. Type I second-degree AV block, also called Mobitz type I or Wenckebach-type block, is characterized by regular and progressive prolongation of the PR interval before conduction of a P wave fails to propagate to the ventricles (Fig. 189.5) [86,87]. It also involves a regular and progressive shortening of the R-R interval until an R wave is dropped. The dysfunction in impulse propagation in first- and second-degree type I AV blocks is thought to occur at the suprahisian level and generally result in a stable rhythm with narrow QRS complex and may present a physiologic response of decremental conduction in the AV node because of increasing heart rate and, therefore, rarely require intervention. Type I second-degree AV block can be a result of infrahisian disease that has a poorer prognosis. One way in a clinical setting to distinguish the level of AV block is to observe the heart rate response to physiologic need (e.g., exercise in outpatient setting) or atropine.

Type II second-degree AV block or Mobitz type II block manifests as sudden failure in the propagation of an atrial impulse (dropped R wave) without a change in the preceding PR interval (Fig. 189.5) [87]. Third-degree AV block is a complete failure of propagation of the atrial impulse to the ventricles with a hallmark of AV dissociation (Fig. 189.5). In this setting, latent pacemaker foci below the level of conduction may assume control of the ventricular rhythm such as junctional or ventricular escape rhythm. Second-degree type II and third-degree AV blocks are often called high-grade AV block, which indicates the abnormal propagation at the infrahisian level. Hence, it is often unstable and requires temporary or permanent pacemaker depending on their reversibility [87].

Treatment

Providers need to evaluate hemodynamic stability of the patients and distinguish reversible causes from permanent etiologies (Fig. 189.4). In the ICU setting, common causes include electrolyte disturbance, adverse effects from medications particularly β-blockers, nondihydropyridine calcium channel blockers, digoxin, antiarrhythmics, inferior or anteroseptal myocardial infarction, myocarditis, or endocarditis (particularly involving the aortic valve), any peri-AV inflammation as in Lyme's disease, systemic lupus erythematous, and trauma from cardiac surgery, catheter, or radiation.

Pharmacotherapy

Atropine may be administered in patients with bradyarrhythmias. However, atropine does not have much effect on high-grade AV blocks (i.e., infrahisian disease). It also has a short half-life, thus implementing the next treatment plan should be prepared. According to the 2015 ACLS guidelines, β-adrenergic agonists such as epinephrine and dopamine as well as cardiac pacing are the first or next step after trial of atropine [4]. In addition, isoproterenol infusion may be used to stimulate heart rate via the β-1 agonist (Table 189.4). One should be careful when using chronotropic infusions because they can exacerbate ischemia in the setting of cardiogenic shock by reducing coronary perfusion. Other treatments can be tailored toward the factors that precipitated the bradyarrhythmia. For instance, glucagon can be used in the setting of β-blocker overdose; sodium bicarbonate and hemodialysis can be used for acidosis; calcium, insulin, and hemodialysis can be used in the setting of hyperkalemia (Table 189.3).

Pacemaker Therapy

Pacemakers are used to improve circulatory hemodynamics by improving cardiac output by controlling the heart rate and/or rhythm. Pacemakers can be used as a permanent treatment or can be instituted as a temporizing measure [88]. There are several modalities of temporary cardiac pacing. Transcutaneous cardiac pacing is usually used in an emergent setting for patients not responsive to intravenous medications. However, owing to its instability and painful pacing, this modality should only be used as a temporizing measure for a short period of time. The pacing system is consisted of a pulse generator attached to high-impedance external patch electrode pads that are applied to the anteroposterior or anterolateral positions of the patient's bare chest. With the application of extra electrodes, these systems can sense native QRS discharge that allows them to have antibradycardia, antitachycardia, and defibrillation capacity. The need for continued pacing can be evaluated by gradually decreasing pacing output, resulting in returning of stable rhythm.

Transvenous endocardial pacing is predominantly used for patients with unstable bradyarrhythmias that will last for a period of time while waiting for permanent pacemaker implantation or resolving of underlying etiology. In transvenous pacing, the heart is directly paced using catheters placed in the apex of the right ventricle. Central venous access is achieved using an introducer sheath through the jugular, subclavian, femoral, or brachial veins [89]. Pacing catheters are then advanced under fluoroscopic guidance. A chest X-ray is then used to confirm placement of the catheter, and the pacing and sensing thresholds are tested. The catheters are then connected to an external pacing generator. Transvenous pacing is more easily tolerated and more reliable than transcutaneous pacing but is associated with a greater risk of complications, including hematoma, induction of VA, myocardial puncture, pneumothorax, bleeding, lead dislodgment, and infection leading to sepsis [89–91].

References

1. Yoshida T, Fujii T, Uchino S, et al: Epidemiology, prevention, and treatment of new-onset atrial fibrillation in critically ill: a systematic review. *J Intensive Care* 3(1):19, 2015.
2. Das MK, Zipes DP: *Assessment of the Patient with a Cardiac Arhythmia*. Elsevier, 2013, pp 567–573.
3. Girotra S, Nallamothu BK, Spertus JA, et al: Trends in survival after in-hospital cardiac arrest. *N Engl J Med* 367(20):1912–1920, 2012.
4. Neumar RW, Shuster M, Callaway CW, et al: Part 1: Executive Summary: 2015 American Heart Association guidelines update for cardiopulmonary resuscitation and emergency cardiovascular care. *Circulation* 132[18 Suppl 2]:S315–S367, 2015.
5. Pierce AE, Roppolo LP, Owens PC, et al: The need to resume chest compressions immediately after defibrillation attempts: An analysis of post-shock rhythms and duration of pulselessness following out-of-hospital cardiac arrest. *Resuscitation* 89:162–168, 2015.
6. Sell RE, Sarno R, Lawrence B, et al: Minimizing pre- and post-defibrillation pauses increases the likelihood of return of spontaneous circulation (ROSC). *Resuscitation* 81(7):822–825, 2010.
7. Kudenchuk PJ, Cobb LA, Copass MK, et al: Amiodarone for resuscitation after out-of-hospital cardiac arrest due to ventricular fibrillation. *N Engl J Med* 341(12):871–878, 1999.
8. Griffith MJ, de Belder MA, Linker NJ, et al: Multivariate analysis to simplify the differential diagnosis of broad complex tachycardia. *Br Heart J* 66(2):166–174, 1991.
9. Lavonas EJ, Drennan IR, Gabrielli A, et al: Part 10: special circumstances of resuscitation: 2015 American Heart Association guidelines update for cardiopulmonary resuscitation and emergency cardiovascular care. *Circulation* 132[18 Suppl 2]:S501–S518, 2015.
10. Mentzelopoulos SD, Zakynthinos SG, Tzoufi M, et al: Vasopressin, epinephrine, and corticosteroids for in-hospital cardiac arrest. *Arch Intern Med* 169(1):15–24, 2009.
11. Mentzelopoulos SD, Malachias S, Chamos C, et al: Vasopressin, steroids, and epinephrine and neurologically favorable survival after in-hospital cardiac arrest: a randomized clinical trial. *JAMA* 310(3):270–279, 2013.
12. Donnino MW, Andersen LW, Berg KM, et al: Temperature management after cardiac arrest: an advisory statement by the advanced life support task force of the International Liaison Committee on Resuscitation and the American Heart Association Emergency Cardiovascular Care Committee and the Council on cardiopulmonary, critical care, perioperative and resuscitation. *Circulation* 132:2448–24456, 2015.

13. Hollenbeck RD, McPherson JA, Mooney MR, et al: Early cardiac catheterization is associated with improved survival in comatose survivors of cardiac arrest without STEMI. *Resuscitation* 85(1):88–95, 2014.
14. Drew BJ, Ackerman MJ, Funk M, et al: Prevention of torsade de pointes in hospital settings: a scientific statement from the American Heart Association and the American College of Cardiology Foundation. *J Am Coll Cardiol* 55(9):934–947, 2010.
15. Pedersen CT, Kay GN, Kalman J, et al: EHRA/HRS/APHRS expert consensus on ventricular arrhythmias. *Heart Rhythm* 11(10):e166–e196, 2014.
16. Akhtar M, Shenasa M, Jazayeri M, et al: Wide QRS complex tachycardia. Reappraisal of a common clinical problem. *Ann Intern Med* 109(11):905–912, 1988.
17. Tchou P, Young P, Mahmud R, et al: Useful clinical criteria for the diagnosis of ventricular tachycardia. *Am J Med* 84(1):53–56, 1988.
18. Brugada P, Brugada J, Mont L, et al: A new approach to the differential diagnosis of a regular tachycardia with a wide QRS complex. *Circulation* 83(5):1649–1659, 1991.
19. Neumar RW: Part 8: adult advanced cardiovascular life support: 2010 American Heart Association Guidelines for cardiopulmonary resuscitation and emergency cardiovascular care (vol 122, pg S729, 2010). *Circulation.* 128(25):E480–E480, 2013.
20. Bou-Abboud E, Nattel S: Relative role of alkalosis and sodium ions in reversal of class I antiarrhythmic drug-induced sodium channel blockade by sodium bicarbonate. *Circulation* 94(8):1954–1961, 1996.
21. Goldman MJ, Mowry JB, Kirk MA: Sodium bicarbonate to correct widened QRS in a case of flecainide overdose. *J Emerg Med* 15(2):183–186, 1997.
22. Nademanee K, Taylor R, Bailey WE, et al: Treating electrical storm: sympathetic blockade versus advanced cardiac life support-guided therapy. *Circulation* 102(7):742–747, 2000.
23. Tarditi DJ, Hollenberg SM: Cardiac arrhythmias in the intensive care unit. *Semin Respir Crit Care Med* 27(3):221–229, 2006.
24. Tung R, Shivkumar K: Neuraxial modulation for treatment of VT storm. *J Biomed Res* 29(1):56–60, 2015.
25. Douglas P, Zipes JJ: Cardiac electrophysiology: from cell to bedside. *Chapter 41: Sympathetic Innervation, Denervation, and Cardiac Arrhythmias.* 6th ed. Elsevier, 2014, pp 409–417.
26. Buxton AE, Lee KL, Fisher JD, et al: A randomized study of the prevention of sudden death in patients with coronary artery disease. Multicenter Unsustained Tachycardia Trial Investigators. *N Engl J Med* 341(25):1882–1890, 1999.
27. Cohn JN, Johnson G, Ziesche S, et al: A comparison of enalapril with hydralazine–isosorbide dinitrate in the treatment of chronic congestive heart failure. *N Engl J Med* 325(5):303–310, 1991.
28. Pitt B, Segal R, Martinez FA, et al: Randomised trial of losartan versus captopril in patients over 65 with heart failure (Evaluation of Losartan in the Elderly Study, ELITE). *Lancet* 349(9054):747–752, 1997.
29. Effect of metoprolol CR/XL in chronic heart failure: Metoprolol CR/XL Randomised Intervention Trial in Congestive Heart Failure (MERIT-HF). *Lancet* 353(9169):2001–2007, 1999.
30. Zipes DP, Camm AJ, Borggrefe M, et al: ACC/AHA/ESC 2006 guidelines for management of patients with ventricular arrhythmias and the prevention of sudden cardiac death: a report of the American College of Cardiology/American Heart Association Task Force and the European Society of Cardiology Committee for Practice Guidelines (Writing Committee to Develop Guidelines for Management of Patients With Ventricular Arrhythmias and the Prevention of Sudden Cardiac Death). *J Am Coll Cardiol* 48(5):e247–e346, 2006.
31. Page RL, Joglar JA, Caldwell MA, et al: 2015 ACC/AHA/HRS guideline for the management of adult patients with supraventricular tachycardia: a report of the American College of Cardiology/American Heart Association Task Force on Clinical Practice Guidelines and the Heart Rhythm Society. *Circulation* 2015.
32. Delacrétaz E: Supraventricular tachycardia. *N Engl J Med* 354(10):1039–1051, 2006.
33. Olgin J, Zipes DP: *Specific Arrhythmias. Braunwald's Heart Disease: A Textbook of Cardiovascular Medicine*: Elsevier BV, 2012, pp 771–824.
34. Asirvatham S: *Supraventricular Tachycardia. Concise Textbook*. Informa UK Limited, 2006, pp 379–387.
35. Markowitz SM, Stein KM, Mittal S, et al: Differential effects of adenosine on focal and macroreentrant atrial tachycardia. *J Cardiovasc Electrophysiol* 10(4):489–502, 1999.
36. Creamer JE, Nathan AW, Camm AJ: Successful treatment of atrial tachycardias with flecainide acetate. *Heart* 53(2):164–166, 1985.
37. Eidher U, Freihoff F, Kaltenbrunner W, et al: Efficacy and safety of ibutilide for the conversion of monomorphic atrial tachycardia. *Pacing Clin Electrophysiol* 29(4):358–362, 2006.
38. Mehta AV, Sanchez GR, Sacks EJ, et al: Ectopic automatic atrial tachycardia in children: clinical characteristics, management and follow-up. *J Am Coll Cardiol* 11(2):379–385, 1988.
39. Porter MJ, Morton JB, Denman R, et al: Influence of age and gender on the mechanism of supraventricular tachycardia. *Heart Rhythm* 1(4):393–396, 2004.
40. Gonzalez-Torrecilla E, Almendral J, Arenal A, et al: Combined evaluation of bedside clinical variables and the electrocardiogram for the differential diagnosis of paroxysmal atrioventricular reciprocating tachycardias in patients without pre-excitation. *J Am Coll Cardiol* 53(25):2353–2358, 2009.
41. Srivathsan K, Gami AS, Barrett R, et al: Differentiating atrioventricular nodal reentrant tachycardia from junctional tachycardia: novel application of the delta H-A interval. *J Cardiovasc Electrophysiol* 19(1):1–6, 2008.
42. Jackman WM, Beckman KJ, McClelland JH, et al: Treatment of supraventricular tachycardia due to atrioventricular nodal reentry by radiofrequency catheter ablation of slow-pathway conduction. *N Engl J Med* 327(5):313–318, 1992.
43. Wen ZC, Chen SA, Tai CT, et al:Electrophysiological mechanisms and determinants of vagal maneuvers for termination of paroxysmal supraventricular tachycardia. *Circulation* 98(24):2716–2723, 1998.
44. Luber S, Brady WJ, Joyce T, et al: Paroxysmal supraventricular tachycardia: outcome after ED care. *Am J Emerg Med* 19(1):40–42, 2001.
45. DiMarco JP, Miles W, Akhtar M, et al: Adenosine for paroxysmal supraventricular tachycardia: dose ranging and comparison with verapamil. Assessment in placebo-controlled, multicenter trials. The Adenosine for PSVT Study Group. *Ann Intern Med* 113(2):104–110, 1990.
46. Rankin AC, Oldroyd KG, Chong E, et al: Value and limitations of adenosine in the diagnosis and treatment of narrow and broad complex tachycardias. *Br Heart J* 62(3):195–203, 1989.
47. Gupta A, Naik A, Vora A, et al: Comparison of efficacy of intravenous diltiazem and esmolol in terminating supraventricular tachycardia. *J Assoc Physicians India* 47(10):969–972, 1999.
48. D'Este D, Zoppo F, Bertaglia E, et al: Long-term outcome of patients with atrioventricular node reentrant tachycardia. *Int J Cardiol* 115(3):350–353, 2007.
49. O'Hara GE, Philippon F, Champagne J, et al: Catheter ablation for cardiac arrhythmias: a 14-year experience with 5330 consecutive patients at the Quebec Heart Institute, Laval Hospital. *Can J Cardiol* 23 Suppl B:67B–70B, 2007.
50. Sellers TD Jr, Campbell RW, Bashore TM, et al: Effects of procainamide and quinidine sulfate in the Wolff-Parkinson-White syndrome. *Circulation* 55(1):15–22, 1977.
51. Glatter KA, Dorostkar PC, Yang Y, et al: Electrophysiological effects of ibutilide in patients with accessory pathways. *Circulation* 104(16):1933–1939, 2001.
52. Smith GD, Dyson K, Taylor D, et al: Effectiveness of the Valsalva Manoeuvre for reversion of supraventricular tachycardia. *Cochrane Database Syst Rev* 3:CD009502, 2013.
53. Delaney B, Loy J, Kelly AM: The relative efficacy of adenosine versus verapamil for the treatment of stable paroxysmal supraventricular tachycardia in adults: a meta-analysis. *Eur J Emerg Med* 18(3):148–152, 2011.
54. Chugh SS, Blackshear JL, Shen WK, et al: Epidemiology and natural history of atrial fibrillation: clinical implications. *J Am Coll Cardiol* 37(2):371–378, 2001.
55. McManus DD, Rienstra M, Benjamin EJ: An update on the prognosis of patients with atrial fibrillation. *Circulation* 126(10):e143–e146, 2012.
56. January CT, Wann LS, Alpert JS, et al: 2014 AHA/ACC/HRS guideline for the management of patients with atrial fibrillation: executive summary: a report of the American College of Cardiology/American Heart Association Task Force on practice guidelines and the Heart Rhythm Society. *Circulation* 130(23):2071–2104, 2014.
57. Calkins H, Kuck KH, Cappato R, et al: 2012 HRS/EHRA/ECAS expert consensus statement on catheter and surgical ablation of atrial fibrillation: recommendations for patient selection, procedural techniques, patient management and follow-up, definitions, endpoints, and research trial design: a report of the Heart Rhythm Society (HRS) Task Force on Catheter and Surgical Ablation of Atrial Fibrillation. Developed in partnership with the European Heart Rhythm Association (EHRA), a registered branch of the European Society of Cardiology (ESC) and the European Cardiac Arrhythmia Society (ECAS); and in collaboration with the American College of Cardiology (ACC), American Heart Association (AHA), the Asia Pacific Heart Rhythm Society (APHRS), and the Society of Thoracic Surgeons (STS). Endorsed by the governing bodies of the American College of Cardiology Foundation, the American Heart Association, the European Cardiac Arrhythmia Society, the European Heart Rhythm Association, the Society of Thoracic Surgeons, the Asia Pacific Heart Rhythm Society, and the Heart Rhythm Society. *Heart Rhythm* 9(4):632.e621–696.e621, 2012.
58. Gami AS, Hodge DO, Herges RM, et al: Obstructive sleep apnea, obesity, and the risk of incident atrial fibrillation. *J Am Coll Cardiol* 49(5):565–571, 2007.
59. Pathak RK, Middeldorp ME, Meredith M, et al: Long-term effect of goal-directed weight management in an atrial fibrillation cohort: A Long-Term Follow-Up Study (LEGACY). *J Am Coll Cardiol* 65(20):2159–2169, 2015.
60. Cappola AR, Fried LP, Arnold AM, et al: Thyroid status, cardiovascular risk, and mortality in older adults. *JAMA* 295(9):1033–1041, 2006.
61. Kodama S, Saito K, Tanaka S, et al: Alcohol consumption and risk of atrial fibrillation: a meta-analysis. *J Am Coll Cardiol* 57(4):427–436, 2011.
62. Stankowski RV, Kloner RA, Rezkalla SH: Cardiovascular consequences of cocaine use. *Trends Cardiovasc Med* 25(6):517–526, 2015.
63. Mathew JP. A multicenter risk index for atrial fibrillation after cardiac surgery. *JAMA* 291(14):1720, 2004.
64. Crystal E, Garfinkle MS, Connolly SS, et al: Interventions for preventing post-operative atrial fibrillation in patients undergoing heart surgery. *Cochrane Database Syst Rev.* (4):CD003611, 2004.
65. Koniari I, Apostolakis E, Rogkakou C, et al: Pharmacologic prophylaxis for atrial fibrillation following cardiac surgery: a systematic review. *J Cardiothorac Surg* 5:121, 2010.
66. Haïssaguerre M, Jaïs P, Shah DC, et al: Spontaneous initiation of atrial fibrillation by ectopic beats originating in the pulmonary veins. *N Engl J Med.* 339(10):659–666, 1998.
67. Nattel S, Burstein B, Dobrev D: Atrial remodeling and atrial fibrillation: mechanisms and implications. *Circ Arrhythm Electrophysiol* 1(1):62–73, 2008.
68. Benjamin EJ, Wolf PA, D'Agostino RB, et al: Impact of atrial fibrillation on the risk of death: The Framingham Heart Study. *Circulation* 98(10):946–952, 1998.

69. Wyse DG, Waldo AL, DiMarco JP, et al: A comparison of rate control and rhythm control in patients with atrial fibrillation. *N Engl J Med* 347(23):1825–1833, 2002.
70. Lip GY, Nieuwlaat R, Pisters R, et al: Refining clinical risk stratification for predicting stroke and thromboembolism in atrial fibrillation using a novel risk factor-based approach: the euro heart survey on atrial fibrillation. *Chest* 137(2):263–272, 2010.
71. Douketis JD, Spyropoulos AC, Kaatz S, et al: Perioperative bridging anticoagulation in patients with atrial fibrillation. *N Engl J Med* 373(9):823–833, 2015.
72. Daniels PR: Peri-procedural management of patients taking oral anticoagulants. *BMJ* 351:h2391, 2015.
73. Van Gelder IC, Groenveld HF, Crijns HJ, et al: Lenient versus strict rate control in patients with atrial fibrillation. *N Engl J Med* 362(15):1363–1373, 2010.
74. Siu CW, Lau CP, Lee WL, et al: Intravenous diltiazem is superior to intravenous amiodarone or digoxin for achieving ventricular rate control in patients with acute uncomplicated atrial fibrillation. *Crit Care Med* 37(7):2174–2179, 2009; quiz 2180.
75. Delle Karth G, Geppert A, Neunteufl T, et al: Amiodarone versus diltiazem for rate control in critically ill patients with atrial tachyarrhythmias. *Crit Care Med* 29(6):1149–1153, 2001.
76. Connolly SJ, Camm AJ, Halperin JL, et al: Dronedarone in high-risk permanent atrial fibrillation. *N Engl J Med* 365(24):2268–2276, 2011.
77. Gallagher MM, Hennessy BJ, Edvardsson N, et al: Embolic complications of direct current cardioversion of atrial arrhythmias: association with low intensity of anticoagulation at the time of cardioversion. *J Am Coll Cardiol* 40(5):926–933, 2002.
78. Imazio M, Brucato A, Ferrazzi P, et al: Colchicine reduces postoperative atrial fibrillation: results of the Colchicine for the Prevention of the Postpericardiotomy Syndrome (COPPS) atrial fibrillation substudy. *Circulation* 124(21):2290–2295, 2011.
79. Shepherd J, Jones J, Frampton GK, et al: Intravenous magnesium sulphate and sotalol for prevention of atrial fibrillation after coronary artery bypass surgery: a systematic review and economic evaluation. *Health Technol Assess* 12(28):iii–iv, ix–95, 2008.
80. Kastor JA: Multifocal atrial tachycardia. *N Engl J Med* 322(24):1713–1717, 1990.
81. Neumar RW, Otto CW, Link MS, et al: Part 8: adult advanced cardiovascular life support: 2010 American Heart Association Guidelines for Cardiopulmonary Resuscitation and Emergency Cardiovascular Care. *Circulation* 122[18 Suppl 3]:S729–S767, 2010.
82. Kiss O, Sydo N, Vargha P, et al: Prevalence of physiological and pathological electrocardiographic findings in Hungarian athletes. *Acta Physiol Hung* 102(2):228–237, 2015.
83. Deboor SS, Pelter MM, Adams MG: Nonrespiratory sinus arrhythmia. *Am J Crit Care* 14(2):161–162, 2005.
84. Semelka M, Gera J, Usman S: Sick sinus syndrome: a review. *Am Fam Physician* 87(10):691–696, 2013.
85. Stockburger M, Trautmann F, Nitardy A, et al: Pacemaker-based analysis of atrioventricular conduction and atrial tachyarrhythmias in patients with primary sinus node dysfunction. *Pacing Clin Electrophysiol* 32(5):604–613, 2009.
86. Kumar P, Kusumoto FM, Goldschlager N: Bradyarrhythmias in the elderly. *Clin Geriatr Med* 28(4):703–715, 2012.
87. Chow GV, Marine JE, Fleg JL: Epidemiology of arrhythmias and conduction disorders in older adults. *Clin Geriatr Med* 28(4):539–553, 2012.
88. Epstein AE, DiMarco JP, Ellenbogen KA, et al: 2012 ACCF/AHA/HRS focused update incorporated into the ACCF/AHA/HRS 2008 guidelines for device-based therapy of cardiac rhythm abnormalities: a report of the American College of Cardiology Foundation/American Heart Association Task Force on Practice Guidelines and the Heart Rhythm Society. *Circulation* 127(3):e283–e352, 2013.
89. Sullivan BL, Bartels K, Hamilton N: Insertion and management of temporary pacemakers. *Semin Cardiothorac Vasc Anesth* 20:52–62, 2016.
90. Kornberger A, Schmid E, Kalender G, et al: Bridge to recovery or permanent system implantation: an eight-year single-center experience in transvenous semipermanent pacing. *Pacing Clin Electrophysiol* 36(9):1096–1103, 2013.
91. Munoz Bono J, Prieto Palomino MA, Macias Guarasa I, et al: Efficacy and safety of non-permanent transvenous pacemaker implantation in an intensive care unit. *Med Intensiva* 35(7):410–416, 2011.

Chapter 190 ■ Pharmacologic Management of Cardiogenic Shock and Hypotension

MICHAEL M. GIVERTZ • JAMES C. FANG

Hypotension and hemodynamic instability are frequently encountered clinical problems in the intensive care setting. When the mean arterial blood pressure falls below approximately 60 mmHg, end-organ perfusion becomes compromised and is manifested clinically as cool skin, decreased urine output, and altered mental status. Cornerstones of management include volume resuscitation and therapy directed toward the underlying cause of hypotension (e.g., cardiac pacing for bradycardia; cardioversion or defibrillation for tachyarrhythmias; blood transfusion for gastrointestinal bleeding; and corticosteroids for adrenal insufficiency). When these measures fail to restore blood pressure and vital organ perfusion or while awaiting their availability, administration of intravenous vasoactive agents may be necessary. This chapter reviews the general management of the hypotensive patient with an emphasis on coronary care and the pharmacologic properties of commonly used vasopressor and positive inotropic agents. An overview of shock (see Chapter 37); volume resuscitation (see Chapter 37); sepsis (see Chapter 39); and the use of intra-aortic balloon counterpulsation and mechanical circulatory support devices (see Chapter 196) is given elsewhere.

GENERAL APPROACH TO THE HYPOTENSIVE PATIENT IN THE CORONARY CARE UNIT

The assessment of the hypotensive patient begins with accurate measurement of the blood pressure and rapid correlation with clinical signs of hypoperfusion. Blood pressure should be measured in both arms and confirmed by another examiner. This practice is especially important when automated devices are used to make these measurements in the setting of tachyarrhythmias or respiratory distress. For patients with peripheral arterial disease, upper extremity blood pressure should also be compared to measurements in the legs in the supine position. In rare circumstances, true central aortic pressure may differ significantly from peripherally obtained blood pressures and can only be confirmed by invasive measurement during diagnostic catheterization. This situation should be suspected when clinical features of hypoperfusion do not accompany low blood pressure.

Hypotension is generally defined as a mean arterial pressure of less than 60 mmHg and/or a systolic blood pressure less than 100 mmHg. However, higher values may be consistent with clinically relevant hypotension if there are concomitant clinical signs of hypoperfusion such as mental status changes, oliguria, pallor, and cool extremities. If clinically relevant hypotension cannot be rapidly corrected, invasive monitoring with an arterial line should be considered, especially when vasoactive medications are employed. Central venous catheterization should also be considered to monitor intravascular volume, because volume status is often dynamic in the hypotensive patient and multiple mechanisms of hypotension may be simultaneously present. A central venous catheter can also be used for rapid administration of drugs and intravenous fluids. Indwelling urinary catheterization should also be employed to assess hourly urine output as an index of end-organ perfusion.

The history and physical examination should be directed toward establishing the primary mechanism and etiology of hypotension. Primary mechanisms include hypovolemia, low cardiac output, and vasodilation. Assessing volume status is critical; if not discernible from the bedside evaluation (jugular venous pressure, skin turgor, urine output, and orthostasis), echocardiography or invasive measurement of the central venous pressure should be obtained. If there are clinical reasons to suggest a dissociation of right and left ventricular hemodynamics (i.e., right ventricular infarction), pulmonary artery catheterization may be required to measure the left ventricular filling pressure. Warm well-perfused skin and extremities despite hypotension may suggest low systemic vascular resistance and a vasodilatory state, whereas cool clammy skin and extremities suggest vasoconstriction as a compensatory response to a low output syndrome. A narrow pulse pressure may also suggest reduced cardiac output. If a putative mechanism of hypotension cannot be ascertained from bedside assessment, pulmonary artery catheterization can be used to characterize the hemodynamic profile. This strategy is especially useful when more than one mechanism is present (for example, a large myocardial infarction complicated by pneumonia, leading to cardiogenic shock along with vasodilatory shock).

Initial management strategies are directed at the primary cause of hypotension and addressed later in this chapter. In general, therapy is guided by the primary pathophysiologic mechanism underlying the hypotension (e.g., volume resuscitation for hypovolemia; positive inotropes for low cardiac output; and vasopressors for vasoplegia). The pace and aggressiveness of therapeutic intervention are guided by the presence or absence of clinical signs of hypoperfusion. For example, holding vasodilators may be sufficient for the hypotensive patient without changes in mental status or urine output. In contrast, the acutely hypotensive patient with clinical shock needs rapid resuscitation with intravascular volume expansion and usually vasoactive therapy.

ADRENERGIC RECEPTOR PHYSIOLOGY

Most vasopressor and positive inotropic agents currently available for use are sympathomimetic amines that exert their action by binding to and stimulating adrenergic receptors. To better understand the similarities and differences among these agents, a basic knowledge of adrenergic receptor distribution and function is helpful [1].

The adrenergic receptors that are most relevant to the management of hypotension are the α_1, β_1, and β_2 receptors. α_1-Adrenergic receptors are present in smooth muscle cells of many vascular beds, including the arterioles supplying the skin, mucosa, skeletal muscle, and kidneys, as well as the peripheral veins. α_1-Adrenergic stimulation causes vasoconstriction and is the most common mechanism of vasopressor action. The presence of α_1 receptors has also been demonstrated in the myocardium, where stimulation appears to result in a positive inotropic effect with little change in heart rate. β_1-Adrenergic receptors are the predominant adrenergic receptor type in the heart and they mediate positive inotropic, chronotropic, and lusitropic responses. Stimulation of β_2-adrenergic receptors causes relaxation of smooth muscle cells in bronchial, gastrointestinal, and uterine muscle, as well as vasodilation of skeletal muscle. β_3-adrenergic receptors, which are located mainly in adipose tissue, are involved in the regulation of lipolysis and thermogenesis and do not play a role in hemodynamic stability. Other relevant receptors are the dopaminergic receptors (DA_1 and DA_2), which mediate renal, coronary, cerebral, and mesenteric vasodilation, and cause a natriuretic response.

The receptor selectivity of sympathomimetic amines can be drug and dose dependent. For example, β_2 receptors are more sensitive to epinephrine than are α_1 receptors. Thus, at low doses of epinephrine, the vasodilatory effect of β_2 receptors predominates, whereas at high doses, α_1-mediated vasoconstriction overcomes the β_2 effect and increases systemic vascular resistance. The dose-dependent actions of dopamine have also been well established.

The overall clinical effects of vasoactive agents depend not only on the outcome of direct adrenergic receptor stimulation, but also on the reflex response of homeostatic forces. For example, stimulation of β_1-adrenergic receptors by norepinephrine would be expected to cause an increase of heart rate; however, norepinephrine-mediated α_1-adrenergic stimulation induces a reflex increase of vagal tone that cancels out its positive chronotropic effects. The action of some drugs (e.g., dopamine and ephedrine) is further complicated by their ability to stimulate release of stored endogenous catecholamines.

COMMONLY USED VASOPRESSORS AND POSITIVE INOTROPES

The armamentarium of vasoactive agents has changed little since the 1980s [2]. Commonly used drugs with vasopressor activity are dopamine, epinephrine, norepinephrine, phenylephrine, and ephedrine. Vasopressin is a newer alternative to adrenergic vasopressors. Agents with positive inotropic activity that are useful for the treatment of hypotension include dobutamine, dopamine, epinephrine, and isoproterenol. Table 190.1 summarizes the receptor activity and hemodynamic effects of these drugs.

TABLE 190.1

Dose Range, Receptor Activity, and Predominant Hemodynamic Effects of Vasoactive Drugs Commonly Used to Treat Hypotension

Drug	Dose range	Dopaminergic	α_1	β_1	β_2	Heart rate	Cardiac output	Systemic vascular resistance
Dobutamine	2.5–20 μg/kg/min	–	+	+++	++	↔↑	↑↑	↓
Dopamine	1–5 μg/kg/min	+++	–	–	–	↔	↔	↔
	5–10 μg/kg/min	++	+	++	–	↑	↑↑	↔↑
	10–20 μg/kg/min	++	+++	++	–	↑↑	↔↑	↑↑
Epinephrine	1–10 μg/min	–	+++	++	++	↑↑	↑	↑↑
Isoproterenol	2–10 μg/min	–	–	+++	+++	↑↑	↑↑	↓
Norepinephrine	0.5–30 μg/min	–	+++	++	–	↔	↔	↑↑
Phenylephrine	40–180 μg/min	–	+++	–	–	↔↓	↔	↑↑
Ephedrine	10–25 mg IV q5–10 min	–	++	++	++	↑	↔	↑↑
Vasopressin	0.01–0.07 units/min	–	–	–	–	↔	↔↓	↑↑

Dopamine

Dopamine is an endogenous catecholamine that functions as a central neurotransmitter and a synthetic precursor of norepinephrine and epinephrine. When administered intravenously, the effects of dopamine are mediated by dose-dependent stimulation of dopaminergic and adrenergic receptors, and by stimulation of norepinephrine release from nerve terminals.

At low doses (less than 5 μg/kg/min), dopamine predominantly stimulates dopaminergic receptors in renal, mesenteric, and coronary vessels with minimal adrenergic effects. In normal subjects, the so-called renal-dose dopamine augments renal blood flow, glomerular filtration rate, and natriuresis, with little effect on blood pressure. Low-dose dopamine has frequently been used by itself or in combination with other drugs as a renoprotective agent. However, the efficacy and safety of this strategy remain controversial [3]. Although mechanistic studies have demonstrated renal vasodilatory effects of dopamine among patients with heart failure [4], a randomized placebo-controlled trial in 360 patients with acute heart failure and renal dysfunction demonstrated no effect of low-dose dopamine on renal function or decongestion, and no difference in symptoms or clinical outcomes compared to placebo [5]. Similar neutral effects of low-dose dopamine on renal function, and intensive care unit (ICU) and hospital length of stay have been observed in critically ill patients with early renal dysfunction [6]. Moderate doses of dopamine (5 to 10 μg/kg/min) stimulate β_1-adrenergic receptors in the myocardium, augmenting cardiac output by increasing contractility and, to a lesser extent, heart rate (Fig. 190.1). In addition, venoconstriction mediated by serotonin and dopaminergic receptors may occur [7]. At higher doses (greater than 10 μg/kg/min), α_1-adrenergic receptor stimulation predominates, resulting in systemic arteriolar vasoconstriction. The overall effects of dopamine at the highest doses resemble those of norepinephrine (see later). However, it should be remembered that there is a great deal of overlap in the dose-dependent effects of dopamine in critically ill patients [1,3].

Moderate- to high-dose dopamine is a mainstay in the treatment of hypotension. In studies of fluid-resuscitated patients with septic shock, dopamine produced a mean increase in mean arterial pressure of approximately 25%, primarily owing to an increase of cardiac index and, to a lesser extent, systemic vascular resistance [3]. In the setting of hyperdynamic septic shock when excessive vasodilation is the primary source of hypotension, addition or substitution of a more potent α-adrenergic agonist such as norepinephrine may be more effective. Moreover, evidence of worsening splanchnic oxygen utilization with the use of high-dose dopamine has made it a less attractive agent.

By itself or in combination with other agents, dopamine may be used at moderate doses for the management of patients with acute heart failure and hypotension. Venodilating agents (e.g., nitroprusside and nitroglycerin) may be added to moderate the tendency of dopamine to increase cardiac-filling pressures [8]. Dopamine may also be combined with dobutamine for added inotropic effects or used at low doses to augment diuresis [9], although the benefits of "renal-dose" dopamine remain unproven and other agents may be more effective for preserving renal function of critically ill patients [10]. For patients with symptomatic bradycardia unresponsive to atropine, particularly when associated with hypotension, dopamine can be effective while preparing for emergent transvenous temporary pacing [11].

The use of dopamine is associated with several adverse effects, including tachycardia, tachyarrhythmias, and excessive vasoconstriction. Although these effects are generally dose dependent, in individual patients there may be substantial overlap of receptor affinity such that even at low doses dopamine may result in toxicity [5]. For patients with ischemic heart disease, increased myocardial oxygen consumption coupled with some degree of coronary vasoconstriction with high-dose dopamine can result in myocardial ischemia. As with other positive inotropes, dopamine can increase flow to poorly oxygenated regions of the lung and cause shunting and hypoxemia. In addition, dopamine has been shown to depress minute ventilation of normoxic

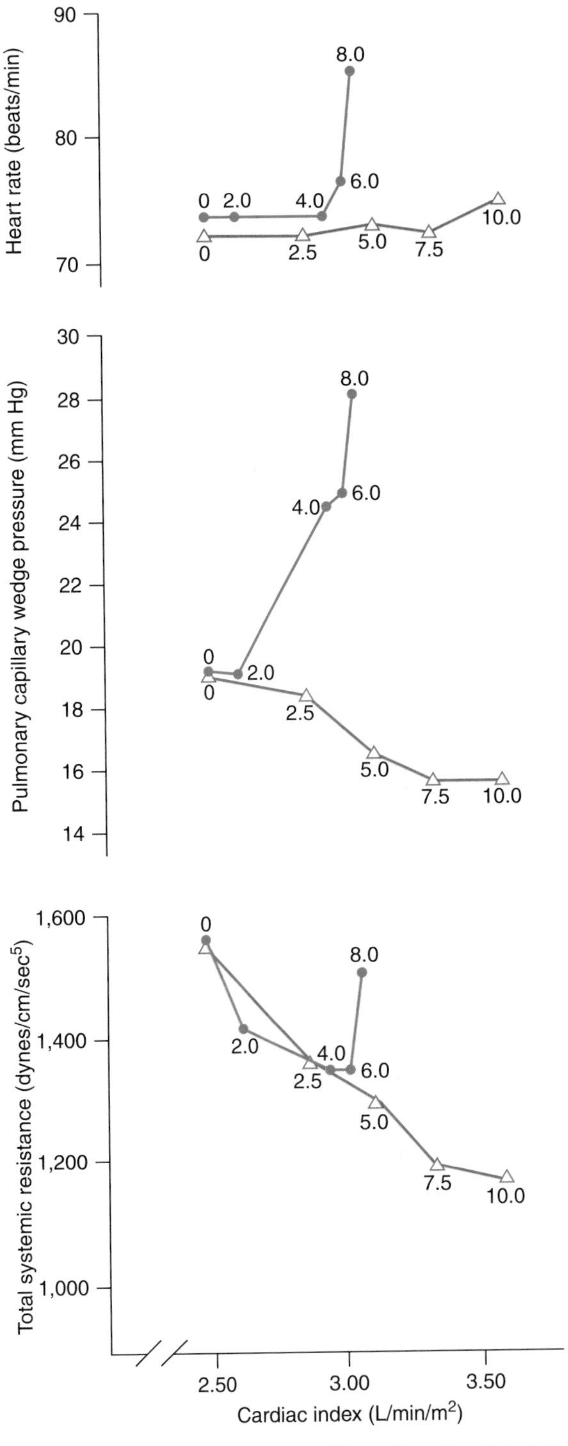

FIGURE 190.1 Comparative effects of dopamine (*closed circles*) and dobutamine (*open triangles*) on heart rate, pulmonary capillary wedge pressure, and total systemic resistance in patients with advanced heart failure. The numbers shown on the figures are infusion rates in μg/kg/min. These data demonstrate that dopamine at doses greater than 2 to 4 μg/kg/min exerts a vasoconstrictor effect and increases heart rate and left ventricular filling pressure (Adapted from Leier CV, Heban PT, Huss P, et al: Comparative systemic and regional hemodynamic effects of dopamine and dobutamine in patients with cardiomyopathic heart failure. *Circulation* 58:466–475, 1978, with permission.).

patients with heart failure [12]. When dopamine is used for patients with acute heart failure, increased venous tone and pulmonary arterial pressure may exacerbate pulmonary edema in the setting of already high cardiac filling pressures. Despite these caveats, oxygen saturation generally remains constant owing to improved hemodynamics.

There is mounting evidence that dopamine adversely effects splanchnic perfusion at doses usually required to treat septic shock. A small, randomized study of patients with sepsis using selective splanchnic and hepatic cannulation showed that infusion of dopamine was associated with a disproportionate increase of splanchnic oxygen delivery compared with oxygen extraction (65% vs. 16%). In contrast, norepinephrine produced better-matched increases in oxygen delivery and extraction (33% vs. 28%) [13]. Another study showed that among patients with septic shock randomly assigned to treatment with norepinephrine or dopamine, gastric intramucosal pH worsened significantly among patients treated with dopamine despite similar improvements in mean arterial pressure [14]. Thus, the use of dopamine for septic shock may be associated with splanchnic shunting, impairment of gastric mucosal oxygenation, and increased risk of gastrointestinal bleeding [3].

Epinephrine

Epinephrine is an endogenous catecholamine that is a potent nonselective agonist of α- and β-adrenergic receptors. Stimulation of myocardial β_1 and β_2 receptors increases contractility and heart rate, resulting in a rise in cardiac output (Fig. 190.2). Cardiac output is further augmented by an increase in venous return as a result of α_1-mediated venoconstriction. Blood flow to skeletal muscles is increased owing to β_2-mediated vasodilation. With very low-dose infusions of epinephrine (0.01 to 0.05 μg/kg/min), β-adrenergic–mediated positive chronotropic and inotropic effects predominate. Diastolic blood pressure and overall peripheral vascular resistance may actually decrease owing to vasodilation of skeletal muscle. With higher doses of epinephrine, stimulation of α-adrenergic receptors in precapillary resistance vessels of the skin, mucosa, and kidneys outweighs β_2-mediated vasodilation in skeletal muscle, causing increased mean and systolic blood pressure [1].

Epinephrine plays a central role in cardiovascular resuscitation (see Chapter 14) and the management of anaphylaxis (see Chapter 69). Epinephrine is also used to reverse hypotension with or without bradycardia after cardiopulmonary bypass or cardiac transplantation [15]. Because of its adverse effects on splanchnic [16] and renal blood flow and potential for inducing myocardial ischemia and tachyarrhythmias, epinephrine has generally been regarded as a second-line agent in the management of septic shock [3,17]. However, a randomized trial showed no difference in efficacy or safety between epinephrine alone versus norepinephrine plus dobutamine for patients with septic shock [18]. For patients with symptomatic bradycardia and hypotension who have failed atropine or external pacing, epinephrine may be used to stabilize the patient while awaiting more definitive therapy (e.g., transvenous placement of a temporary or permanent pacemaker) [19]. When used to treat hypotension, epinephrine is given as a continuous infusion starting at a low dose (0.5 to 1.0 μg per minute) and titrating up to 10 μg per minute as needed. Continuous infusions of epinephrine may cause restlessness, tremor, headache, and palpitations. Epinephrine should be avoided for patients taking β-adrenergic antagonists, because unopposed α-adrenergic vasoconstriction may cause severe hypertension and cerebral hemorrhage.

Norepinephrine

Norepinephrine is an endogenous catecholamine that is a potent β_1- and α_1-adrenergic agonist, with little β_2 activity. The main cardiovascular effect of norepinephrine is dose-dependent arterial and venous vasoconstriction owing to α-adrenergic stimulation (Fig. 190.2). The positive inotropic and chronotropic effects of β_1 stimulation are generally counterbalanced by the increased afterload and reflex vagal activity induced by the elevated systemic vascular resistance. Thus, heart rate and cardiac output usually do not change significantly, although cardiac output may increase or decrease depending on vascular resistance, left ventricular function, and reflex responses [7].

Norepinephrine, when infused at doses ranging from 0.5 to 30.0 μg per minute, is a potent vasopressor. Although traditionally reserved as a second-line agent or used in addition to other vasopressors in cases of severe distributive shock, norepinephrine has emerged as the agent of choice for the management of hypotension in hyperdynamic septic shock [18,20]. In a small, prospective double-blind trial, Martin et al. [21] randomized patients with hyperdynamic septic shock to dopamine or

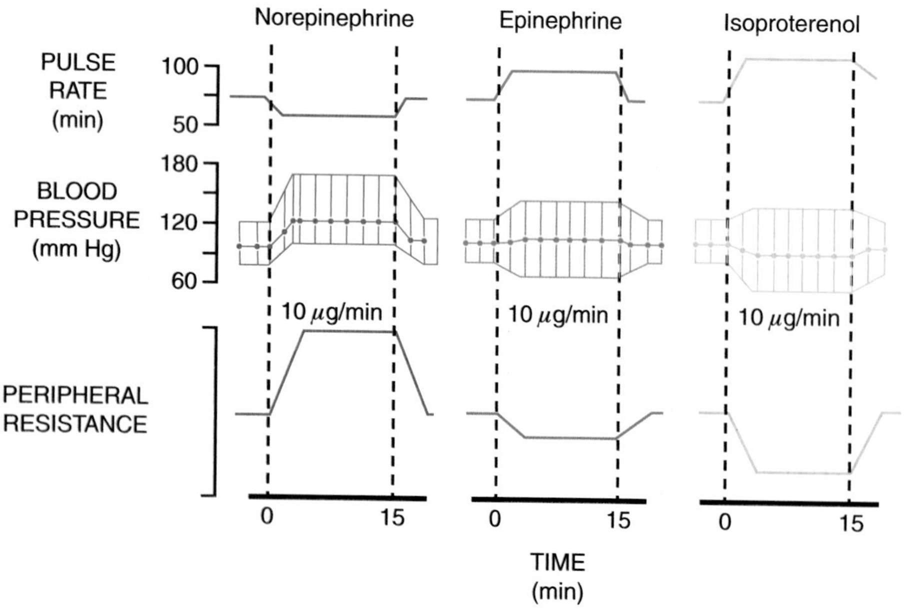

FIGURE 190.2 Cardiovascular effects of intravenous infusions of norepinephrine, epinephrine, and isoproterenol in normal human subjects (Modified from Westfall TC, Westfall DP: Adrenergic agonists and antagonists, in Brunton LL (ed): *Goodman & Gilman's The Pharmacological Basis of Therapeutics*. 11th ed. New York, McGraw-Hill, 2005, pp 237–295, with permission.).

norepinephrine titrated to a mean arterial pressure greater than or equal to 80 mmHg or systemic vascular resistance greater than 1,100 dynes/s/cm^{-5}, or both. Although only 5 of 16 patients randomized to dopamine were able to achieve these endpoints, 15 of 16 patients randomized to norepinephrine were successfully treated with a mean dose of 1.5 μg/kg/min. Moreover, 10 of the 11 patients who remained hypotensive on high-dose dopamine improved with the addition of norepinephrine. A subsequent prospective, nonrandomized, observational study suggested that in adults with septic shock treated initially with high-dose dopamine or norepinephrine, the use of norepinephrine was associated with improved survival [22]. More recently, the Sepsis Occurrence in Acutely Ill Patients (SOAP) II trial group randomized 1,679 patients with shock to receive either dopamine or norepinephrine as first-line vasopressor therapy to restore and maintain blood pressure [23]. There was no significant difference between the groups in rate of death at 28 days (52.5% vs. 48.5%, respectively; OR with dopamine, 1.17; 95% confidence interval, 0.97 to 1.42; $p = 0.10$) (Fig. 190.3A); however, there were more arrhythmic events with dopamine (24.1% vs. 12.4%, $p < 0.0001$). In a subgroup analysis of patients with cardiogenic shock ($n = 280$), dopamine was associated with an increased risk of death ($p = 0.03$) (Fig. 190.3B). Meta-analyses of norepinephrine versus dopamine in the treatment of septic shock have also suggested that norepinephrine is associated with reduced mortality and less arrhythmic events [24]. In the setting of sepsis, norepinephrine improves renal blood flow and urine output [25], although large doses may be required to achieve these effects because of α-receptor downregulation [3].

Adverse effects of norepinephrine include increased myocardial oxygen consumption causing ischemia and renal and mesenteric vasoconstriction. Renal ischemia may be of particular concern for patients with hemorrhagic shock. Norepinephrine can also cause necrosis and sloughing at the site of intravenous injection owing to drug extravasation. Norepinephrine is relatively contraindicated for patients with hypovolemia. As previously discussed, the overall effect of norepinephrine on gut mucosal oxygenation of septic patients compares favorably with that of high-dose dopamine.

Phenylephrine

Phenylephrine is a synthetic sympathomimetic amine that selectively stimulates α_1-adrenergic receptors. When administered intravenously, phenylephrine causes dose-dependent arterial vasoconstriction and increases peripheral vascular resistance. As blood pressure rises, activation of vagal reflexes causes slowing of the heart rate.

Phenylephrine, infused at 40 to 180 μg per minute, is commonly used for the management of anesthesia-induced hypotension [26,27] and hyperdynamic septic shock. Its rapid

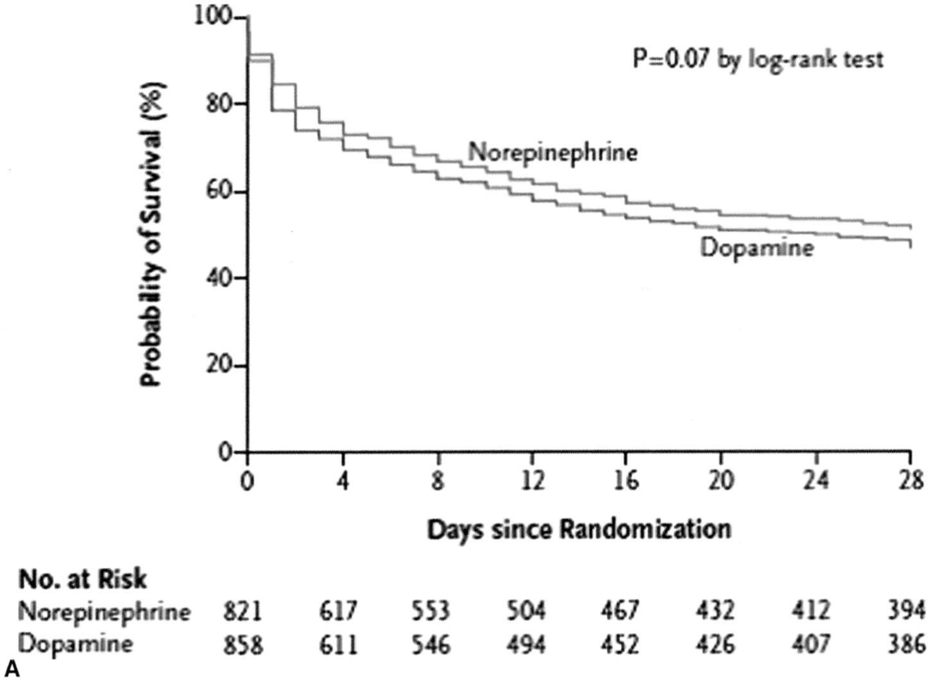

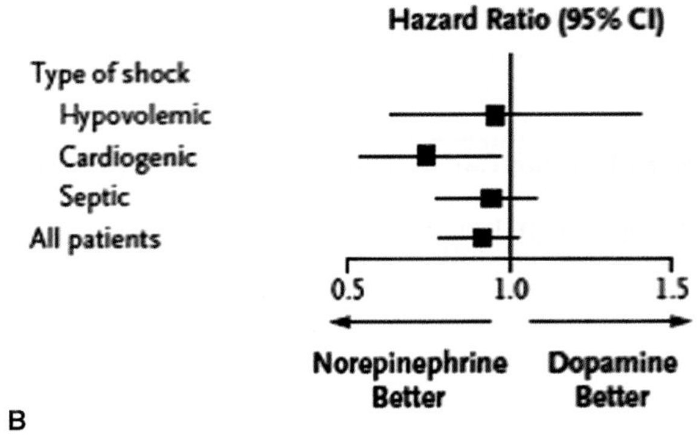

FIGURE 190.3 *Panel A*, Kaplan–Meier curves for 28-day survival in patients with shock randomized to norepinephrine (*blue line*) or dopamine (*red line*). *Panel B*, Forest plot for predefined subgroup analysis according to type of shock. A total of 1,044 patients were in septic shock, 280 were in cardiogenic shock, and 263 were in hypovolemic shock (From De Backer D, Biston P, Devriendt J, et al: Comparison of dopamine and norepinephrine in the treatment of shock. *N Engl J Med* 362:779–789, 2010, with permission.).

onset of action, short duration, and primary vascular effects make it an ideal agent for treating hemodynamically unstable patients in the intensive care setting. However, there are few data regarding its relative efficacy compared with older vasopressors such as norepinephrine and dopamine. In one small study of fluid-resuscitated patients with septic shock, the addition of phenylephrine to dobutamine or dopamine increased mean arterial pressure and systemic vascular resistance without a change in heart rate [28]. In addition, urine output improved, whereas serum creatinine remained stable. In another study, patients with septic shock were randomized to initial hemodynamic support with phenylephrine or norepinephrine [29]. There were no differences in systemic or regional hemodynamics between the groups. The absence of β-adrenergic agonist activity at usual doses (phenylephrine activates β receptors only at much higher doses) makes phenylephrine an attractive agent for the management of hypotension in clinical situations where tachycardia or tachyarrhythmias, or both, limit the use of other agents [3]. As with other vasopressors, high-dose phenylephrine may cause excessive vasoconstriction. In addition, patients with poor ventricular function may not tolerate the increased afterload induced by α_1-stimulation [28]. Compared to epinephrine and norepinephrine, phenylephrine is less likely to decrease microcirculatory blood flow in the gastrointestinal tract [30]. When used to treat hypotension during spinal anesthesia for cesarean delivery, phenylephrine dose requirements may be affected by β_2-adrenoceptor genotype [31].

Ephedrine

Ephedrine is a naturally occurring sympathomimetic amine derived from plants. Its pharmacologic action results from direct nonselective activation of adrenergic receptors, as well as stimulation of norepinephrine release from storage sites. Although ephedrine is less potent and longer acting (half-life, 3 to 6 hours) than epinephrine, its hemodynamic profile is similar and includes cardiac stimulation and peripheral vasoconstriction.

Ephedrine is rarely used in the critical care setting except in the temporary treatment of hypotension induced by spinal anesthesia [26]. Ephedrine does not appear to compromise uterine blood flow and is considered an alternative to phenylephrine in the treatment of anesthesia-induced hypotension of the obstetric patient [32]. However, prophylactic use for pregnant woman undergoing Caesarean section is not recommended because it may cause hypertension and tachycardia [33]. Ephedrine can be administered at doses of 10 to 25 mg, given as an intravenous bolus every 5 to 10 minutes, with the total dose not to exceed 150 mg in 24 hours. For healthy women undergoing elective cesarean delivery that develop hypotension, pharmacogenomic data suggests that β_2-adrenoceptor genotype may affect dose requirements [34]. Adverse effects of ephedrine include myocardial ischemia and excessive vasoconstriction; in the setting of delivery, ephedrine can cause fetal acidosis.

Isoproterenol

Isoproterenol is a synthetic sympathomimetic amine with potent nonselective β-adrenergic activity and little effect on α-adrenergic receptors. Its major cardiovascular effect is increased cardiac output owing to direct positive inotropic and chronotropic effects (Fig. 190.2). Isoproterenol also increases heart rate by increasing atrioventricular nodal conduction. Systemic and pulmonary vascular resistances decrease owing to β_2-mediated vasodilation of skeletal muscle and pulmonary vasculature, respectively. Reduced peripheral resistance typically causes a fall of mean arterial and diastolic blood pressure, whereas systolic blood pressure is unchanged or rises modestly owing to increased cardiac output. Coronary blood flow remains unchanged, which in the face of increased myocardial oxygen demand can produce ischemia among patients with ischemic heart disease. In addition, stimulation of myocardial β_2-receptors can cause arrhythmias via increased dispersion of repolarization [35].

Stimulation of β-adrenergic receptors in the heart by isoproterenol increases the risk of excessive tachycardia, tachyarrhythmias, and myocardial ischemia. Given the likelihood of toxicity and the availability of alternative drugs, isoproterenol is no longer used as an inotropic agent; rather, its use is limited to the temporary treatment of hemodynamically significant bradycardia unresponsive to atropine while awaiting more definitive treatment with an external or transvenous pacemaker. The starting infusion rate for isoproterenol is 1 μg per minute, and this can be titrated up to 10 μg per minute to achieve the desired response (e.g., for bradycardia, titrated to a heart rate of 60 beats per minute or higher, depending on the blood pressure response). Other uses for isoproterenol include "chemical" overdrive pacing for torsades de pointes refractory to magnesium [36], and temporary inotropic and chronotropic support after cardiac transplantation [37]. Side effects of isoproterenol include palpitations, headache, flushing, and rarely paradoxical bradycardia [38].

Dobutamine

Dobutamine is a synthetic sympathomimetic amine that was derived from isoproterenol in an attempt to create a less arrhythmogenic positive inotrope with minimal vascular effects. Although initially thought to be a selective β_1-adrenergic agonist, its mechanism of action appears to be more complex. Dobutamine is available for clinical use as a mixture of two enantiomeric forms with different pharmacologic properties. Ruffolo et al. [39] showed that although both stereoisomers are nonselective β-agonists, the positive isomer is several times more potent. In addition, the two isomers have opposing effects on α-adrenergic receptors: the positive isomer is an α-antagonist and the negative isomer is a potent α_1-agonist. The overall effect of the racemic mixture is potent nonselective β- and mild α-adrenergic stimulation [39].

Cardiac contractile force is enhanced by β_1- and α-adrenergic stimulation. Heart rate may also increase, but to a lesser extent than occurs with isoproterenol or dopamine (Fig. 190.1). In contrast to dopamine, dobutamine decreases cardiac filling pressures, making it a preferred agent for the treatment of patients with acute heart failure [40]. Systemic vascular resistance is modestly reduced or may remain unchanged, because α_1-mediated vasoconstriction is counterbalanced by β_2-mediated vasodilation and reflex withdrawal of sympathetic tone that typically occurs in response to increased cardiac output. Dobutamine has no effect on dopaminergic receptors; however, renal blood flow often increases in proportion to the increase of cardiac output [41] because of reduced renal sympathetic activity [42].

Dobutamine, by itself or in combination with other vasoactive drugs, is useful in the temporary support of myocardial function of patients with hypotension and poor end-organ perfusion, including those with acute heart failure as well as patients with concomitant septic shock and depressed cardiac function. Among patients with cardiogenic shock, the effect of dobutamine on systemic vascular resistance and blood pressure is difficult to predict. Therefore, when used in this setting, it is often administered in combination with dopamine [9,40].

Dobutamine is generally initiated at an infusion rate of 2 μg/kg/min and can be titrated up to 15 μg/kg/min or higher to achieve the desired hemodynamic or clinical effects, or both. Side effects that may limit dose titration include increased heart rate and exacerbation of supraventricular and ventricular arrhythmias. As with other positive inotropic agents, increased myocardial oxygen consumption can worsen cardiac ischemia,

TABLE 190.2

Summary of Advances in the Management of Hypotension

- Norepinephrine is recommended as a first-line agent to treat hypotension in the setting of septic shock [3,23].
- Vasopressin improves blood pressure in patients with sepsis [48] or vasodilatory shock after cardiopulmonary bypass [49]. Newer analogs of vasopressin, terlipressin and selepressin, are under development [58,59].
- Stress-dose steroids improve hemodynamics and may reduce mortality in septic shock if adrenocortical insufficiency is present [83,85]. Doses of hydrocortisone should not exceed 200–300 mg/d [3].
- Methylene blue is effective for refractory hypotension following cardiopulmonary bypass [69,70] and may be useful in preventing vasoplegia in high-risk surgical patients [71].

and short-term dobutamine therapy has been associated with excess mortality [43,44]. Although systolic and mean arterial blood pressures typically increase, hypotension may occur when dobutamine is administered to a volume-depleted patient. Some patients with advanced heart failure may be resistant to dobutamine owing to β-receptor hyporesponsiveness or may develop tolerance after several days of a continuous infusion [45]. Chronic dobutamine therapy may also cause an eosinophilic or hypersensitivity myocarditis [46], leading to further hemodynamic deterioration, as well as late acute cellular rejection following heart transplantation [47].

Vasopressin

Arginine vasopressin, an antidiuretic hormone, has emerged as a safe alternative to adrenergic vasopressors for the treatment of refractory vasodilatory shock. The mechanism of action of vasopressin has not been fully elucidated, but likely involves binding to V_1 receptors on vascular smooth muscle cells. Although it has minimal pressor activity among normal subjects, vasopressin has been shown to improve blood pressure for patients with sepsis [48] and in patients with vasodilatory shock after cardiopulmonary bypass [49] (Table 190.2). In these initial studies, vasopressin was initiated at a dose of 0.1 units per minute; for subjects maintaining a mean arterial pressure greater than 70 mmHg, vasopressin was tapered to 0.01 units per minute and then discontinued. Notably, many patients in these studies were poorly responsive to intravenous catecholamine support and had inappropriately low vasopressin levels before treatment consistent with a defect in baroreflex-mediated vasopressin secretion. It remains unclear, however, whether the benefits of vasopressin are confined to patients with relative vasopressin deficiency, hypersensitivity, or both.

Russell et al. [50] randomized 778 patients with septic shock who were receiving a minimum of 5 μg per minute of norepinephrine to receive either low-dose vasopressin (0.01 to 0.03 units per minute) or norepinephrine (5 to 15 μg per minute) in addition to open-label vasopressors. After 28 days, there was no significant difference in mortality rates between the vasopressin and norepinephrine groups (35.4% and 39.3%, respectively; $p = 0.26$) (Fig. 190.4). However, for patients with less severe septic shock (prospectively defined as those receiving treatment with less than 15 μg per minute of norepinephrine), mortality was lower for the vasopressin group (26.5% vs. 35.7%, $p = 0.05$). In a meta-analysis of 9 trials covering 998 participants, vasopressin use for vasodilatory shock was associated with a 13% reduced risk of mortality compared to norepinephrine [51].

Vasopressin may also be effective for the treatment of cardiac arrest unresponsive to epinephrine and defibrillation [52]. In 2010, revised guidelines for advanced cardiovascular life support (ACLS) recommended vasopressin as an alternative to epinephrine for the treatment of adult shock-refractory ventricular fibrillation, as well as an adjunctive agent in the treatment of patients with vasodilatory shock, such as septic shock or sepsis syndrome, refractory to standard therapy [53]. However, vasopressin was removed from the 2015 ACLS Cardiac Arrest Algorithm [7] in recognition of equivalence of effect with other available interventions (e.g., epinephrine). A meta-analysis of cardiac arrest trials demonstrated no significant differences between vasopressin and epinephrine groups in failure of return of spontaneous circulation, death within 24 hours, or death before hospital discharge [54]. In a randomized clinical trial of 2,894 patients with out-of-hospital cardiac arrest receiving advanced cardiac life support, the combination of vasopressin (40 International Units) and epinephrine (1 mg) did not improve outcomes compared to epinephrine alone: return of spontaneous circulation, 28.6% versus 29.5%; survival to hospital admission, 20.7% versus 21.3%; and survival to hospital discharge, 1.7% versus 2.3%; respectively [55]. In the setting of vasodilatory shock, vasopressin can be administered as a continuous infusion

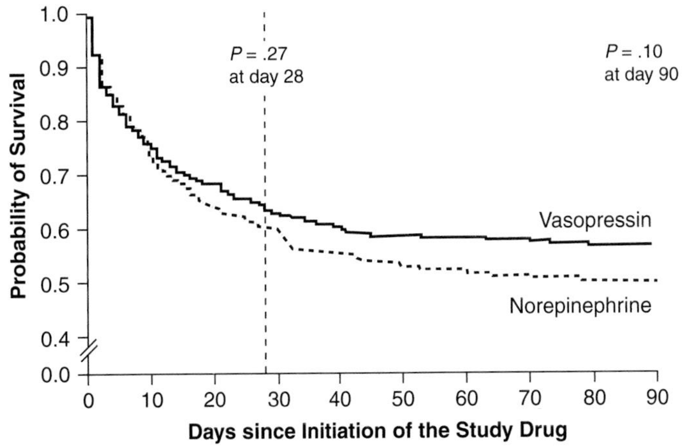

No. at Risk										
Vasopressin	397	301	272	249	240	234	232	230	226	220
Norepinephrine	382	289	247	230	212	205	200	194	193	191

FIGURE 190.4 Kaplan–Meier survival curves for patients with septic shock randomized to vasopressin (*solid line*) or norepinephrine (*dashed line*). The *dashed vertical line* marks day 28. *P* values are calculated with use of the log rank test (From Russell JA, Walley KR, Singer J, et al: Vasopressin versus norepinephrine infusion in patients with septic shock. *N Engl J Med* 358:877–887, 2008, with permission.).

at 0.01 to 0.07 units per minute. Potential adverse effects of vasopressin include excess vasoconstriction causing end-organ ischemia including myocardial ischemia and mesenteric ischemia, and hyponatremia. Cardiac output may also worsen owing to increased afterload. Rebound hypotension is common following withdrawal of vasopressin and can be avoided by slowly tapering the dose.

Newer vasopressin receptor agonists, including terlipressin and selepressin, are undergoing clinical investigation [51,56]. Terlipressin is a synthetic, long-acting analog of vasopressin that is approved in Europe for the treatment of esophageal variceal bleeding and hepatorenal syndrome. In a pilot study of patients with septic shock despite adequate volume resuscitation, a continuous infusion of low-dose terlipressin (1.3 μg/kg/h) was effective for reversing arterial hypotension and reducing catecholamine requirements [57]. Compared with vasopressin or norepinephrine, terlipressin was associated with less rebound hypotension upon discontinuation. Adverse effects associated with terlipressin include hypertension, bradycardia, skin pallor, and reduction of platelet count. In preclinical studies, selepressin, a selective, short-acting vasopressin V_{1a} agonist, has been shown to limit myocardial ischemia, reduce pulmonary edema and improve short-term outcomes compared to vasopressin and norepinephrine [58,59].

Adjunctive and Investigational Agents

In addition to the agents discussed previously, the phosphodiesterase inhibitor milrinone is commonly used for the management of acute heart failure. Milrinone increases cardiac contractility by directly inhibiting the breakdown of cyclic adenosine monophosphate, resulting in an increase of intracellular calcium [60]. In addition, phosphodiesterase inhibition of vascular smooth muscle causes systemic and pulmonary vasodilation [61]. Because milrinone does not require binding to adrenergic receptors to exert its effects, it is particularly useful for the treatment of patients taking β-adrenergic antagonists [62] or those with advanced heart failure that may be resistant to β-agonist stimulation with dobutamine [45]. Milrinone is generally administered as an intravenous loading dose (50 μg per kg), followed by a continuous infusion at doses ranging from 0.25 to 0.75 μg/kg/min. As it is renally excreted, milrinone should be dose-adjusted when renal failure is present; and for all patients, milrinone should be titrated cautiously, using invasive hemodynamic monitoring. Because it is a potent vasodilator, however, milrinone should be avoided in the treatment of patients with frank hypotension, and is contraindicated in patients with severe aortic stenosis. Similarly, the use of levosimendan [63], a calcium sensitizer with phosphodiesterase and potassium channel inhibitor properties, may be limited by hypotension [64]. In a randomized, double-blind study of 1,327 patients with acute heart failure, intravenous levosimendan showed no benefit compared to dobutamine for reducing all-cause mortality at 180 days (26% vs. 28%, respectively; hazard ratio, 0.91; 95% confidence interval, 0.74 to 1.13; $p = 0.40$), and increased the incidence of atrial fibrillation [65]. Although approved for use in Europe, levosimendan remains an investigational agent in the USA.

With the exception of vasopressin, all currently available vasopressors exert their action through stimulation of α-adrenergic receptors. This approach is often associated with worsening splanchnic perfusion, and in some patients may prove ineffective for restoring mean arterial pressure. Evidence of the central role of endothelium-derived nitric oxide (NO) for mediating vasodilation [66] led to the development of substances that interfere with NO production or activity. Several investigators have shown that analogs of L-arginine, the synthetic precursor of NO, can competitively inhibit NO synthetic enzymes, thereby decreasing NO production and increasing mean arterial pressure of patients with septic shock [67]. Others have shown that inhibition of guanylate cyclase, the target enzyme of NO, with methylene blue is effective in increasing mean arterial pressure, reducing the need for vasopressors and maintaining oxygen transport during septic shock [68]. Methylene blue has also been used successfully to treat refractory hypotension for patients with vasoplegia following cardiopulmonary bypass (Table 190.2) [69,70], and may be used to prevent vasoplegia of high-risk cardiac surgical patients [71]. However, the overall safety and efficacy of NO inhibition remains unproven. A large, randomized, placebo-controlled trial of the NO synthase inhibitor 546C88 for sepsis was stopped prematurely owing to excess mortality at 28 days (59% vs. 49%, $p < 0.001$) in the active treatment arm [67]. As with adrenergic agents, lack of selectivity may have contributed to undesirable effects. In addition, the FDA warns that the coadministration of methylene blue with certain selective serotonin reuptake inhibitors may trigger the serotonin syndrome, a potentially lethal condition with cognitive, autonomic, and somatic manifestations [72,73]. More selective NO inhibitors are currently under investigation.

Another novel agent that was approved for the treatment of patients with severe sepsis, but then withdrawn from the market, is recombinant human activated protein C (drotrecogin alfa activated) [74]. In the Recombinant Human Activated Protein C Worldwide Evaluation in Severe Sepsis study, 1,690 patients with systemic inflammation and organ failure owing to acute infection (71% of whom presented with shock) were randomized to receive drotrecogin alfa activated or placebo as a continuous infusion for 4 days [75]. Drotrecogin alfa activated reduced all-cause mortality by 19%, but tended to increase the risk of serious bleeding. Based on this study, drotrecogin alfa activated was recommended for the treatment of patients with severe sepsis and high risk of death (Apache II score greater than 25). In a subsequent study of patients with severe sepsis and low risk of death (Apache II score less than or equal to 25), there was no beneficial effect of drotrecogin alfa activated on either in-hospital or 28-day mortality [76]. The risk of serious bleeding was higher (2.4% vs. 1.2%, $p = 0.02$) in the drotrecogin alfa activated group. Finally, in a randomized, controlled trial (PROWESS-SHOCK) of 1,697 patients with septic shock and clinical hypoperfusion despite fluids and vasopressors, the addition of drotrecogin alfa activated did not significantly reduce mortality at 28 or 90 days [77]. A randomized controlled study of drotrecogin alfa activated in children with severe sepsis also showed no benefit [78]. The 28-day mortality rates were 17.2% and 17.5% in the drotrecogin alfa activated and placebo groups, respectively ($p = 0.93$).

Several hormones including cortisol and thyroxine are known to play important roles in the maintenance of vascular tone, and their absolute or relative deficiency may contribute to hypotension in the critically ill patient. The adverse effects of hypothyroidism (see Chapter 142) and adrenal insufficiency (see Chapter 139) on central and peripheral hemodynamics have been well described. Although the routine use of high-dose corticosteroids has not been shown to be beneficial in the treatment of sepsis, the administration of stress-dose steroids to patients suspected of having relative impairment of adrenocortical response may be helpful for restoring normal hemodynamics and improving outcomes.

In the 1990s, three small trials of patients with septic shock demonstrated decreased duration of shock with steroid treatment [79–81]. Subsequently, Annane et al. [82] randomized 300 patients with septic shock to receive hydrocortisone (50 mg intravenous bolus every 6 hours) and fludrocortisone (50 μg by mouth once daily) or matching placebos for 7 days. Patients were enrolled after undergoing a short corticotropin stimulation test. In the 229 nonresponders to corticotropin (i.e., with relative adrenal insufficiency), treatment with corticosteroids increased vasopressor withdrawal (57% vs. 40%, $p = 0.001$) and decreased mortality (53% vs. 63%, $p = 0.02$) at 28 days. There were no differences of outcomes between steroid and placebo groups in the corticotropin responders. Although this trial was criticized

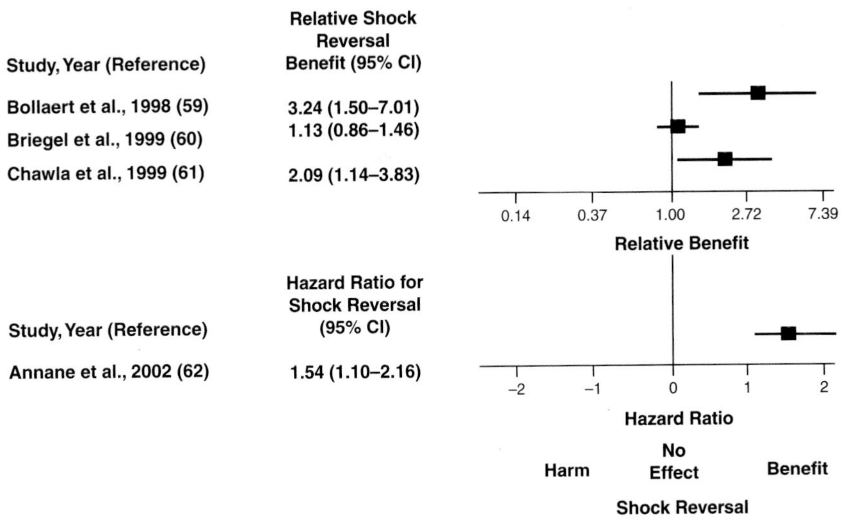

FIGURE 190.5 The relative benefit and hazard ratio (with 95% CI) of shock reversal for sepsis trials published after 1997. In three of the four trials, the discontinuation of vasopressor therapy was significantly improved with steroid treatment (From Minneci PC, Deans KJ, Banks SM, et al: Meta-analysis: the effect of steroids on survival and shock during sepsis depends on the dose. *Ann Intern Med* 141:47–56, 2004, with permission.).

on both methodological and clinical grounds, a subsequent meta-analysis (Fig. 190.5) showed that a 5- to 7-day course of physiologic hydrocortisone doses increased survival for patients with vasopressor-dependent septic shock [83].

In a follow-up study (CORTICUS), 499 patients with septic shock who remained hypotensive after fluid and vasopressor resuscitation were randomized to receive 50 mg of intravenous hydrocortisone or placebo every 6 hours for 5 days [84]. At 28 days, there was no significant difference in mortality between patients of the two study groups whose plasma cortisol levels did not rise appropriately after administration of corticotropin (39.2% vs. 36.1% in the hydrocortisone and placebo groups, respectively; $p = 0.69$) or between those who had a response to corticotropin (28.8% vs. 28.7%, respectively; $p = 1.00$) (Fig. 190.6). In a meta-analysis of 12 trials investigating prolonged low-dose corticosteroid treatment, 28-day mortality was lower for treated vs. control patients (38% vs. 44%; RR 0.84, 95% CI 0.72 to 0.97, $p = 0.02$) [85]. However, in an observational registry of 17,847 patients who required vasopressor therapy despite fluid resuscitation, the use of low-dose systemic corticosteroids was associated with higher in-hospital mortality (41% vs. 35%; OR 1.18, 95% CI 1.09 to 1.23, $p < 0.001$) [86]. As discussed previously, correction of relative vasopressin deficiency is an alternative or adjunctive therapeutic strategy in refractory shock.

Calcium

The routine use of intravenous calcium has been shown to have no benefit in the setting of cardiac arrest and may be detrimental by causing cellular injury [19]. Indications for acute calcium administration in the hypotensive patient include correction of clinically significant hyperkalemia (e.g., with acute kidney injury) or hypocalcemia (e.g., following multiple blood transfusions) and as an antidote to calcium channel blocker or β-blocker overdose [87,88]. Calcium chloride (100 mg per mL in a 10-mL vial) is usually given as a slow intravenous push of 5 to 10 mL, and may be repeated as needed. Rapid intravenous administration of calcium may cause bradycardia or asystole particularly in patients receiving digoxin. In critically ill patients, ionized calcium rather than total calcium concentration should be followed.

CHOOSING AN AGENT

There are few large, randomized, well-controlled studies to guide the pharmacologic management of hypotension. The use of vasopressors and positive inotropes is generally based on data from animal studies and small, often poorly controlled clinical trials. Useful consensus recommendations can be found in the recently revised Advanced Cardiovascular Life Support guidelines [7] and the International Guidelines for Management of Severe Sepsis and Septic Shock updated in 2013 [3].

The selection of the appropriate vasoactive agent can be individualized with attention to the known or suspected underlying cause of hypotension (Table 190.3). However, the clinician is commonly faced with a patient who presents with life-threatening hypotension of unknown etiology. In this setting, it may be necessary to initiate a vasopressor as a temporizing measure even before the adequacy of intravascular volume repletion can be ensured. Consensus guidelines for management of septic shock recommend norepinephrine as a first-line vasopressor agent, with dopamine as an alternative for patients with low risk of tachyarrhythmias or who have bradycardia [3]. Although dopamine in moderate to high doses can provide both positive inotropic and vasopressor effects, atrial or ventricular arrhythmias may be provoked. For severe hypotension in the coronary care unit (systolic blood pressure less than 70 mmHg), a more potent α_1-adrenergic agonist such as norepinephrine should be considered. If greater control of heart rate is required, the addition of esmolol may be considered. In an open-label study of 154 patients with septic shock and a heart rate greater than or equal to 90 beats per minute, the addition of esmolol titrated to maintain heart rate between 80 and 94 beats per minute improved stroke volume index and renal function, decreased serum lactate and fluid requirements, and reduced 28-day mortality (49% vs. 81%, adjusted HR 0.39, 95% CI 0.26 to 0.59, $p < 0.001$) (Fig. 190.7) [89].

For the hypotensive patient with significant cardiac pump dysfunction (cardiac index less than 2.2 L/min/m^2 associated with end-organ dysfunction), dobutamine should be considered. Milrinone is often not tolerated in this situation owing to its vasodilating properties. With frank cardiogenic shock and concomitant vasoplegia, a drug with pressor action is usually needed. In this setting, vasopressin and norepinephrine can be used in combination with dobutamine. Rarely, epinephrine may be required. In patients with septic shock and related myocardial dysfunction, dobutamine up to 15 μg/kg/min or higher can be added for additional inotropic support [3]. Although dopamine is also often considered for this clinical situation owing to its combined inotropic and pressor properties, there has been concern that mortality may be increased when compared to norepinephrine based on a subgroup of patients with cardiogenic shock in the SOAP II trial (Fig. 190.3B) [23].

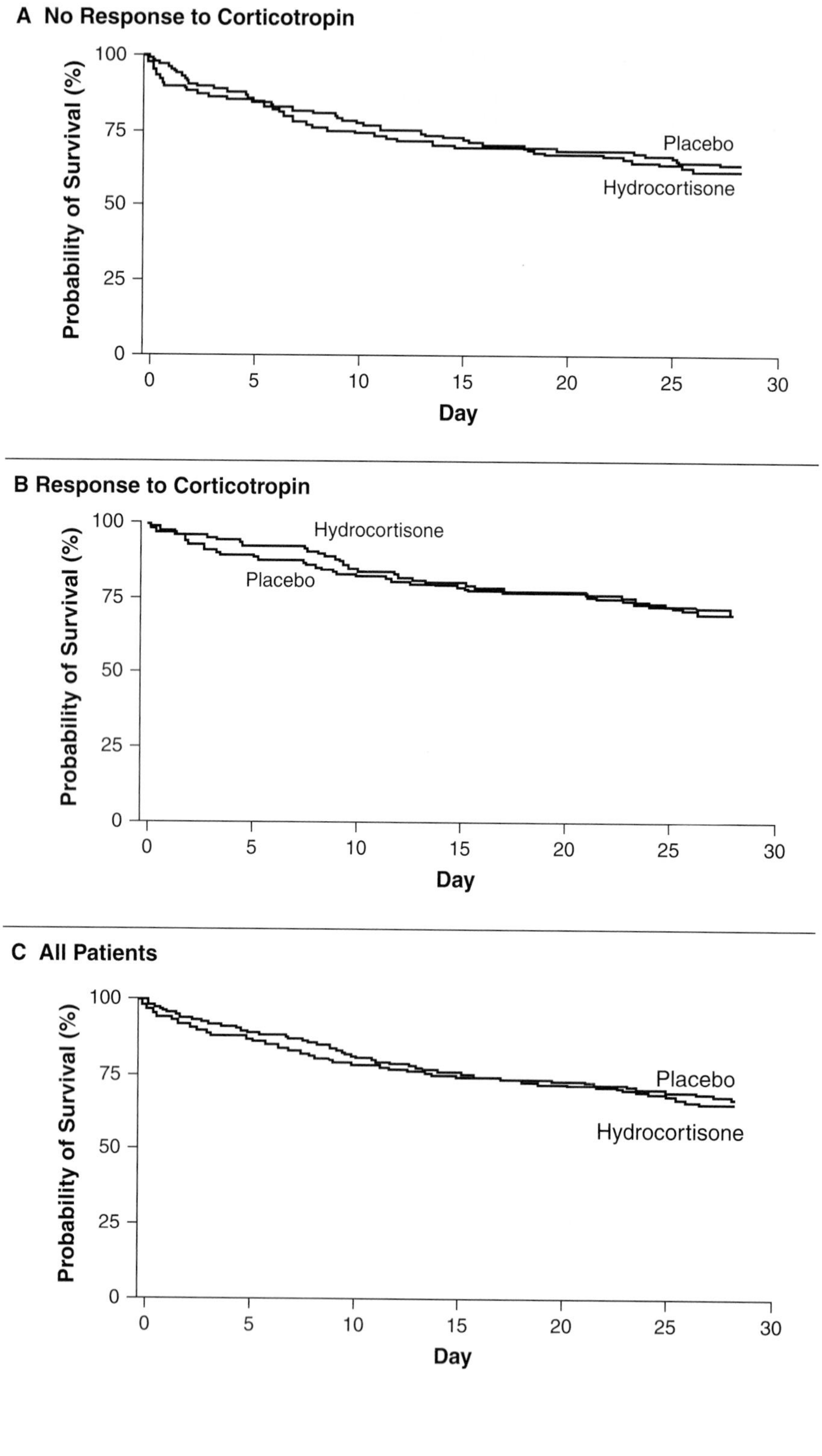

FIGURE 190.6 Shown are Kaplan–Meier curves for survival at 28 days comparing patients with septic shock who received hydrocortisone versus placebo. There was no difference among patients who did not have a response to a corticotropin test (*Panel A*), those who had a response to corticotropin (*Panel B*) and all patients randomized (*Panel C*) (From Sprung CL, Annane D, Keh D, et al: Hydrocortisone therapy for patients with septic shock. *N Engl J Med* 358: 111–124, 2008, with permission.).

Current experience with phenylephrine is insufficient to assess its efficacy relative to older agents, although its peripheral selectivity and lack of positive chronotropic effects make it a theoretically useful agent for cases in which tachycardia, tachyarrhythmias, or both limit the use of other drugs. Epinephrine is the least selective of the catecholamines and is occasionally added for refractory septic shock. Vasopressin is emerging as an alternative to adrenergic agents, but its use for hypotension may be limited to patients with hemodynamic collapse that is resistant to adequate fluid resuscitation and high-dose conventional vasopressors. For patients with vasoplegic shock refractory to multiple pressors, including those status post cardiopulmonary bypass, a trial of methylene blue should be considered [68–70].

CLINICAL USE OF VASOACTIVE DRUGS

For the volume-resuscitated patient with persistent hypotension, vasoactive medications are administered with the goal of improving arterial pressure while avoiding myocardial ischemia, arrhythmias, and excess vasoconstriction. Although a mean arterial blood pressure of greater than 60 mmHg is usually

TABLE 190.3

Hemodynamic Profiles of Selected Causes of Hypotension and Commonly Used First-Line Agents

Cause of hypotension	Pulmonary capillary wedge pressure	Cardiac output	Systemic vascular resistance	Preferred agent(s)
Unknown	?	?	?	Dopamine, norepinephrine
Hypovolemia	↓	↓	↑	None[a]
Acute decompensated heart failure	↑	↓	↑	Dopamine, dobutamine
Cardiogenic shock	↑ ↔	↓	↑	Norepinephrine
Hyperdynamic sepsis	↓ ↔	↑	↓	Norepinephrine
Sepsis with depressed cardiac function	?	↓	↓	Dopamine, norepinephrine plus dobutamine
Anaphylaxis	?	?	↓	Epinephrine
Anesthesia-induced hypotension	?	?	↓	Phenylephrine, ephedrine[b]

[a]Volume resuscitation with intravenous fluids and/or blood products recommended.
[b]For obstetric patients.

adequate to maintain autoregulatory blood flow to vital organs [90], some patients may require considerably higher pressures [91]. Therefore, it is essential to use other indicators of global and regional perfusion in addition to the mean arterial pressure to guide therapy. Altered mental status, oliguria, and cool skin are important clinical signs of poor perfusion, but are somewhat nonspecific. The clinical use of mixed venous oxygen saturation and serum lactate level, as well as intramucosal pH monitoring by gastric tonometry remains unproven [3]. Although some clinicians have advocated achieving "supranormal" levels of oxygen delivery in the treatment of critically ill patients, this approach is controversial [92], and adverse effects of hyperoxia have been demonstrated on coronary blood flow and myocardial function among patients with coronary artery disease [93] and heart failure [94], respectively. A meta-analysis in critically ill patients found that various approaches to hemodynamic optimization reduced mortality when patients were treated early to achieve hemodynamic goals before the development of organ failure and when therapy produced differences of oxygen delivery [95].

Vasopressors and positive inotropes are powerful drugs with considerable potential for toxicity. Diligent monitoring and careful adjustment of medications based on changes in clinical status are essential. Patients should be treated in an intensive care setting with continuous monitoring of cardiac rhythm, urine output, and arterial oxygenation. Fluid resuscitation and careful attention to intravascular volume are paramount, because up to 50% of patients with hypotension related to sepsis may stabilize with fluids alone [3]. Moreover, the administration of vasopressors to intravascularly depleted patients can worsen end-organ perfusion. The routine use of pulmonary artery catheters in this setting remains unproven, because overaggressive treatment may increase the risk of adverse events [96]. For patients who do not respond adequately to initial fluid boluses and brief infusion of vasopressors, bedside echocardiography or invasive hemodynamic monitoring may help to optimize cardiac filling pressures and performance [97-99]. Intra-arterial cannulation and direct monitoring of blood pressure is suggested during prolonged vasopressor use. Drugs should be administered through central venous catheters via volumetric infusion pumps that deliver precise flow rates. In the event of vasopressor extravasation, an α_1-adrenergic antagonist (e.g., phentolamine, 5 to 10 mg, diluted in 10 to 15 mL of saline) can be infiltrated into the area to limit local vasoconstriction and tissue necrosis.

With few exceptions, the drugs discussed in this chapter are short-acting agents with rapid onset and offset of action. They are generally initiated without a bolus and can be titrated frequently. Abrupt lowering or discontinuation of vasoactive drugs should be avoided to prevent rebound hypotension. Common dose ranges are provided in Table 190.1, but there may be a considerable variation of the dose required to restore adequate hemodynamics. Furthermore, an individual patient's response to an agent may diminish with time owing to several mechanisms, including adrenergic receptor desensitization [100,101].

Critically ill patients in the ICU are generally treated with multiple drugs in addition to vasoactive agents (e.g., other cardiovascular medications and antibiotics). Careful attention

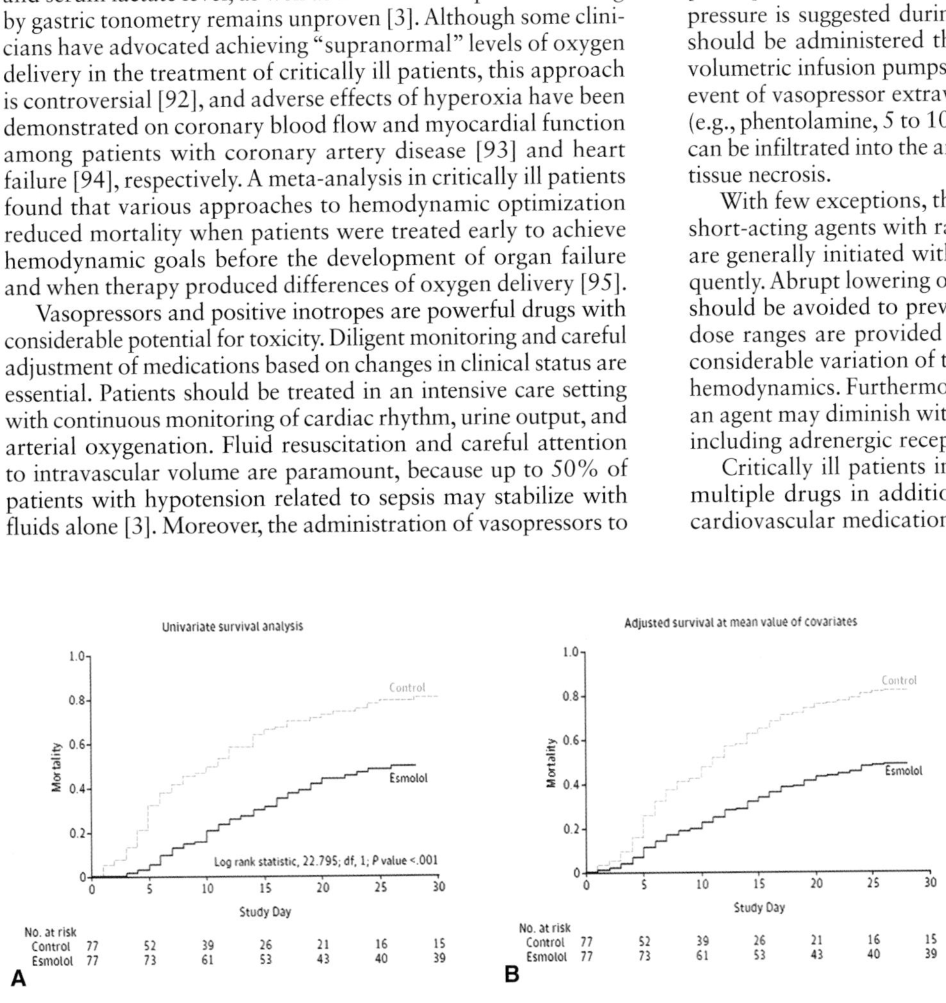

FIGURE 190.7 *Panel A*, Unadjusted Kaplan–Meier survival plots of patients with septic shock and tachycardia randomized to receive esmolol or standard care. *Panel B*, Multivariable Cox-adjusted survival at mean values of Simplified Acute Physiology Score II (From Morelli A, Ertmer C, Westphal M, et al: Effect of heart rate control with esmolol on hemodynamic and clinical outcomes in patients with septic shock: a randomized clinical trial. *JAMA* 310:1683–1691, 2013, with permission.).

should be paid to potential drug–drug interactions, because they can significantly alter the response to a given sympathomimetic amine. For example, prior or current treatment with a β-adrenergic antagonist can cause resistance to the action of dobutamine or other β-adrenergic agonists. The administration of less-selective drugs (e.g., norepinephrine) to a patient receiving chronic β-blockade can result in unopposed α-adrenergic stimulation. Another well-described interaction is the exaggerated response to some catecholamines among individuals taking monoamine oxidase inhibitors. The starting dose for these patients should be less than 10% of the usual dose [1]. ICU rounding with a dedicated ICU pharmacist is recommended.

References

1. Westfall TC, Westfall DP: Chapter 12. Adrenergic agonists and antagonists, in Brunton LL, Chabner BA, Knollmann BC (eds): *Goodman & Gilman's The Pharmacological Basis of Therapeutics*. 12 ed. New York, NY, McGraw-Hill, 2011.
2. Overgaard CB, Dzavík V: Inotropes and vasopressors: review of physiology and clinical use in cardiovascular disease. *Circulation* 118:1047–1056, 2008.
3. Rhodes A, Evans LE, Alhazzani W, et al: Surviving sepsis campaign: International guidelines for management of sepsis and septic shock. *Crit Care Med*. 45:486–552, 2017.
4. Elkayam U, Ng TM, Hatamizadeh P, et al: Renal vasodilatory action of dopamine in patients with heart failure: magnitude of effect and site of action. *Circulation* 117:200–205, 2008.
5. Chen HH, Anstrom KJ, Givertz MM, et al: Low-dose dopamine or low-dose nesiritide in acute heart failure with renal dysfunction: the ROSE acute heart failure randomized trial. *JAMA* 310:2533–2543, 2013.
6. Bellomo R, Chapman M, Finfer S, et al: Low-dose dopamine in patients with early renal dysfunction: a placebo-controlled randomised trial. Australian and New Zealand Intensive Care Society (ANZICS) Clinical Trials Group. *Lancet* 356:2139–2143, 2000.
7. Neumar RW, Shuster M, Callaway CW, et al. Part 1: executive summary: 2015 American Heart Association Guidelines Update for Cardiopulmonary Resuscitation and Emergency Cardiovascular Care. *Circulation* 132:S315–S367, 2015.
8. Loeb HS, Ostrenga JP, Gaul W, et al: Beneficial effects of dopamine combined with intravenous nitroglycerin on hemodynamics in patients with severe left ventricular failure. *Circulation* 68:813–820, 1983.
9. Leier CV, Heban PT, Huss P, et al: Comparative systemic and regional hemodynamic effects of dopamine and dobutamine in patients with cardiomyopathic heart failure. *Circulation* 58:466–475, 1978.
10. Givertz MM, Teerlink JR, Albert NM, et al. Acute decompensated heart failure: update on new and emerging evidence and directions for future research. *J Card Fail* 19:371–389, 2013.
11. Neumar RW, Otto CW, Link MS, et al: Part 8: adult advanced cardiovascular life support: 2010 American Heart Association Guidelines for Cardiopulmonary Resuscitation and Emergency Cardiovascular Care. *Circulation* 122:S729–S767, 2010.
12. Van de Borne P, Oren R, Somers VK: Dopamine depresses minute ventilation in patients with heart failure. *Circulation* 98:126–131, 1998.
13. Ruokonen E, Takala J, Kari A, et al: Regional blood flow and oxygen transport in septic shock. *Crit Care Med* 21:1296–1303, 1993.
14. Marik PE, Mohedin M: The contrasting effects of dopamine and norepinephrine on systemic and splanchnic oxygen utilization in hyperdynamic sepsis. *JAMA* 272:1354–1357, 1994.
15. Ahmed I, House CM, Nelson WB. Predictors of inotrope use in patients undergoing concomitant coronary artery bypass graft (CABG) and aortic valve replacement (AVR) surgeries at separation from cardiopulmonary bypass (CPB). *J Cardiothorac Surg* 12;4:24, 2009.
16. Piton G, Cypriani B, Regnard J, et al. Catecholamine use is associated with enterocyte damage in critically ill patients. *Shock* 43:437-442, 2015.
17. De Backer D, Creteur J, Silva E, et al: Effects of dopamine, norepinephrine, and epinephrine on the splanchnic circulation in septic shock: which is best? *Crit Care Med* 31:1659–1667, 2003.
18. Annane D, Vignon P, Renault A, et al: Norepinephrine plus dobutamine versus epinephrine alone for management of septic shock. *Lancet* 370:676–684, 2007.
19. Link MS, Berkow LC, Kudenchuk PJ, et al. Part 7: adult advanced cardiovascular life support: 2015 American Heart Association Guidelines Update for Cardiopulmonary Resuscitation and Emergency Cardiovascular Care. *Circulation* 132:S444–S464, 2015.
20. Nasraway SA: Norepinephrine: no more "leave 'em dead"? *Crit Care Med* 28:3096–3098, 2000.
21. Martin C, Papazian L, Perrin G, et al: Norepinephrine or dopamine for the treatment of hyperdynamic septic shock? *Chest* 103:1826–1831, 1993.
22. Martin C, Viviand X, Leone M, et al: Effect of norepinephrine on the outcome of septic shock. *Crit Care Med* 28:2758–2765, 2000.
23. De Backer D, Biston P, Devriendt J, et al. Comparison of dopamine and norepinephrine in the treatment of shock. *N Engl J Med* 362:779–789, 2010.
24. De Backer D, Aldecoa C, Njimi H, et al. Dopamine versus norepinephrine in the treatment of septic shock: a meta-analysis*. *Crit Care Med* 40:725–730, 2012.
25. Bellomo R, Giantomasso DD: Noradrenaline and the kidney: friends or foes? *Crit Care* 5:294–298, 2001.
26. Ngan Kee WD, Lee A, Khaw KS, et al: A randomized double-blinded comparison of phenylephrine and ephedrine infusion combinations to maintain blood pressure during spinal anesthesia for cesarean delivery: the effects on fetal acid-base status and hemodynamic control. *Anesth Analg* 107:1295–1302, 2008.
27. Heesen M, Kölhr S, Rossaint R, et al. Prophylactic phenylephrine for caesarean section under spinal anaesthesia: systematic review and meta-analysis. *Anaesthesia* 69:143–165, 2014.
28. Gregory JS, Bonfiglio MF, Dasta JF, et al: Experience with phenylephrine as a component of the pharmacologic support of septic shock. *Crit Care Med* 19:1395–1400, 1991.
29. Morelli A, Ertmer C, Rehberg S, et al. Phenylephrine versus norepinephrine for initial hemodynamic support of patients with septic shock: a randomized, controlled trial. *Crit Care* 12:R143, 2008.
30. Krejci V, Hiltebrand LB, Sigurdsson GH: Effects of epinephrine, norepinephrine, and phenylephrine on microcirculatory blood flow in the gastrointestinal tract in sepsis. *Crit Care Med* 34:1456–1463, 2006.
31. Odekon L, Landau R, Blouin JL, et al. The effect of β2-adrenoceptor genotype on phenylephrine dose administered during spinala nesthesia for cesarean delivery. *Anesth Analg* 120:1309–1316, 2015.
32. Mitra JK, Roy J, Bhattacharyya P, et al. Changing trends in the management of hypotension following spinal anesthesia in cesarean section. *J Postgrad Med* 59:121–126, 2013.
33. Lee A, Ngan Kee WD, Gin T: A dose-response meta-analysis of prophylactic intravenous ephedrine for the prevention of hypotension during spinal anesthesia for elective cesarean delivery. *Anesth Analg* 98:483–490, 2004.
34. Smiley RM, Blouin J, Negron M, et al: Beta2-adrenoceptor genotype affects vasopressor requirements during spinal anesthesia for cesarean delivery. *Anesthesiology* 104:644–650, 2006.
35. Lowe MD, Rowland E, Brown MJ, et al: Beta(2) adrenergic receptors mediate important electrophysiological effects in human ventricular myocardium. *Heart* 86:45–51, 2001.
36. Roden DM: Drug-induced prolongation of the QT interval. *N Engl J Med* 350:1013–1022, 2004.
37. De Broux E, Lagace G, Chartrand C: Efficacy of isoproterenol on the failing transplanted heart during early acute rejection. *Ann Thorac Surg* 53:1062–1067, 1992.
38. Brembilla-Perrot B, Muhanna I, Nippert M, et al: Paradoxical effect of isoprenaline infusion. *Europace* 7:621–627, 2005.
39. Ruffolo RR Jr: The pharmacology of dobutamine. *Am J Med Sci* 294:244–248, 1987.
40. Givertz MM, Colucci WS: Strategies for management of acute decompensated heart failure, in Antman E, Sabatine M (eds): *Cardiovascular Therapeutics: A Companion to Braunwald's Heart Disease*, 4th ed. Philadelphia, PA, Elsevier Saunders, 2013, pp 281-306.
41. Wimmer A, Stanek B, Kubecova L, et al: Effects of prostaglandin E1, dobutamine and placebo on hemodynamic, renal and neurohumoral variables in patients with advanced heart failure. *Jpn Heart J* 40:321–334, 1999.
42. Al-Hesayen A, Parker JD. The effects of dobutamine on renal sympathetic activity in human heart failure. *J Cardiovasc Pharmacol* 51:434–436, 2008.
43. Abraham WT, Adams KF, Fonarow GC, et al: In-hospital mortality in patients with acute decompensated heart failure requiring intravenous vasoactive medications: an analysis from the Acute Decompensated Heart Failure National Registry (ADHERE). *J Am Coll Cardiol* 46:57–64, 2005.
44. Mebazaa A, Parissis J, Porcher R, Gayat et al. Short-term survival by treatment among patients hospitalized with acute heart failure: the global ALARM-HF registry using propensity scoring methods. *Intensive Care Med* 37:290–301, 2011.
45. Hare JM, Givertz MM, Creager MA, et al: Increased sensitivity to nitric oxide synthase inhibition in patients with heart failure: potentiation of beta-adrenergic inotropic responsiveness. *Circulation* 97:161–166, 1998.
46. Takkenberg JJ, Czer LS, Fishbein MC, et al: Eosinophilic myocarditis in patients awaiting heart transplantation. *Crit Care Med* 32:714–721, 2004.
47. Kanai-Yoshizawa S, Sugiyama Kato T, Mancini D, et al: Hypersensitivity myocarditis and outcome after heart transplantation. *J Heart Lung Transplant* 32:553–559, 2013.
48. Landry DW, Levin HR, Gallant EM, et al: Vasopressin pressor hypersensitivity in vasodilatory septic shock. *Crit Care Med* 25:1279–1282, 1997.
49. Argenziano M, Chen JM, Choudhri AF, et al: Management of vasodilatory shock after cardiac surgery: identification of predisposing factors and use of a novel pressor agent. *J Thorac Cardiovasc Surg* 116:973–980, 1998.
50. Russell JA, Walley KR, Singer J, et al: Vasopressin versus norepinephrine infusion in patients with septic shock. *N Engl J Med* 358:877–887, 2008.
51. Serpa Neto A, Nassar AP, Cardoso SO, et al. Vasopressin and terlipressin in adult vasodilatory shock: a systematic review and meta-analysis of nine randomized controlled trials. *Crit Care* 14;16:R154, 2012.
52. Lindner KH, Prengel AW, Brinkmann A, et al: Vasopressin administration in refractory cardiac arrest. *Ann Intern Med* 124:1061–1064, 1996.
53. Field JM, Hazinski MF, Sayre MR, et al: Part 1: executive summary: 2010 American Heart Association Guidelines for Cardiopulmonary Resuscitation and Emergency Cardiovascular Care. *Circulation* 122:S640–S656, 2010.

54. Aung K, Htay T: Vasopressin for cardiac arrest: a systematic review and meta-analysis. *Arch Intern Med* 165:17–24, 2005.
55. Gueugniaud PY, David JS, Chanzy E, et al: Vasopressin and epinephrine vs. Epinephrine alone in cardiopulmonary resuscitation. *N Engl J Med* 359:21–30, 2008.
56. Delmas A, Leone M, Rousseau S, et al: Clinical review: vasopressin and terlipressin in septic shock patients. *Crit Care* 9:212–222, 2005.
57. Morelli A, Ertmer C, Rehberg S, et al: Continuous terlipressin versus vasopressin infusion in septic shock (TERLIVAP): a randomized, controlled pilot study. *Crit Care* 13:R30, 2009.
58. Boucheix OB, Milano SP, Henriksson M, et al. Selepressin, a new V1A receptor agonist: hemodynamic comparison to vasopressin in dogs. *Shock* 39:533–538, 2013.
59. He X, Su F, Taccone FS, et al. A selective V1A receptor agonist, selepressin, is superior to arginine vasopressin and to norepinephrine in ovine septic shock. *Crit Care Med* 44:23–31, 2016.
60. DiBianco R: Acute positive inotropic intervention: the phosphodiesterase inhibitors. *Am Heart J* 121:1871–1875, 1991.
61. Givertz MM, Hare JM, Loh E, et al: Effect of bolus milrinone on hemodynamic variables and pulmonary vascular resistance in patients with severe left ventricular dysfunction: a rapid test for reversibility of pulmonary hypertension. *J Am Coll Cardiol* 28:1775–1780, 1996.
62. Kobayashi S, Susa T, Tanaka T, et al. Low-dose β-blocker in combination with milrinone safely improves cardiac function and eliminates pulsus alternans in patients with acute decompensated heart failure. *Circ J* 76:1646–1653, 2012.
63. Slawsky MT, Colucci WS, Gottlieb SS, et al: Acute hemodynamic and clinical effects of levosimendan in patients with severe heart failure. *Circulation* 102:2222–2227, 2000.
64. Kivikko M, Lehtonen L, Colucci WS: Sustained hemodynamic effects of intravenous levosimendan. *Circulation* 107:81–86, 2003.
65. Mebazaa A, Nieminen MS, Packer M, et al: Levosimendan vs dobutamine for patients with acute decompensated heart failure: the SURVIVE Randomized Trial. *JAMA* 297:1883–1891, 2007.
66. Kelly RA, Balligand JL, Smith TW: Nitric oxide and cardiac function. *Circ Res* 79:363–380, 1996.
67. Lopez A, Lorente JA, Steingrub J, et al: Multiple-center, randomized, placebo-controlled, double-blind study of the nitric oxide synthase inhibitor 546C88: effect on survival in patients with septic shock. *Crit Care Med* 32:21–30, 2004.
68. Kirov MY, Evgenov OV, Evgenov NV, et al: Infusion of methylene blue in human septic shock: a pilot, randomized, controlled study. *Crit Care Med* 29:1860–1867, 2001.
69. Levin RL, Degrange MA, Bruno GF, et al: Methylene blue reduces mortality and morbidity in vasoplegic patients after cardiac surgery. *Ann Thorac Surg* 77:496–499, 2004.
70. Omar S, Zedan A, Nugent K. Cardiac vasoplegia syndrome: pathophysiology, risk factors and treatment. *Am J Med Sci* 349:80-88, 2015.
71. Ozal E, Kuralay E, Yildirim V, et al: Preoperative methylene blue administration in patients at high risk for vasoplegic syndrome during cardiac surgery. *Ann Thorac Surg* 79:1615–1619, 2005.
72. Ng BK, Cameron AJ. The role of methylene blue in serotonin syndrome: a systematic review. *Psychosomatics* 51:194–200, 2010.
73. Boyer EW, Shannon M. The serotonin syndrome. *N Engl J Med* 352:1112–1120, 2005.
74. Toussaint S, Gerlach H: Activated protein C for sepsis. *N Engl J Med* 361:2646–2652, 2009.
75. Bernard GR, Vincent JL, Laterre PF, et al: Efficacy and safety of recombinant human activated protein C for severe sepsis. *N Engl J Med* 344:699–709, 2001.
76. Abraham E, Laterre PF, Garg R, et al: Drotrecogin alfa (activated) for adults with severe sepsis and a low risk of death. *N Engl J Med* 353:1332–1341, 2005.
77. Ranieri VM, Thompson BT, Barie PS, et al. Drotrecogin alfa (activated) in adults with septic shock. *N Engl J Med* 366:2055–2064, 2012.
78. Nadel S, Goldstein B, Williams MD, et al: Drotrecogin alfa (activated) in children with severe sepsis: a multicentre phase III randomised controlled trial. *Lancet* 369:836–843, 2007.
79. Bollaert PE, Charpentier C, Levy B, et al: Reversal of late septic shock with supraphysiologic doses of hydrocortisone. *Crit Care Med* 26:645–650, 1998.
80. Briegel J, Forst H, Haller M, et al: Stress doses of hydrocortisone reverse hyperdynamic septic shock: a prospective randomized, double-blind, single-center study. *Crit Care Med* 27:723–732, 1999.
81. Chawla K, Kupfer Y, Goldma I: Hydrocortisone reverses refractory septic shock [Abstract], *Crit Care Med* 27:A23, 1997.
82. Annane D, Sebille V, Charpentier C, et al: Effect of treatment with low doses of hydrocortisone and fludrocortisone on mortality in patients with septic shock. *JAMA* 288:862–871, 2002.
83. Minneci PC, Deans KJ, Banks SM, et al: Meta-analysis: the effect of steroids on survival and shock during sepsis depends on the dose. *Ann Intern Med* 141:47–56, 2004.
84. Sprung CL, Annane D, Keh D, et al: Hydrocortisone therapy for patients with septic shock. *N Engl J Med* 358:111–124, 2008.
85. Annane D, Bellissant E, Bollaert PE, et al. Corticosteroids for treating sepsis. *Cochrane Database Syst Rev* (12):CD002243, 2015.
86. Casserly B, Gerlach H, Phillips GS, et al. Low-dose steroids in adult septic shock: results of the Surviving Sepsis Campaign. *Intensive Care Med* 38:1946–1954, 2012.
87. DeWitt CR, Waksman JC: Pharmacology, pathophysiology and management of calcium channel blocker and beta-blocker toxicity. *Toxicol Rev* 23:223–238, 2004.
88. Palatnick W, Jelic T. Emergency department management of calcium-channel blocker, beta blocker, and digoxin toxicity. *Emerg Med Pract* 16:1–19, 2014.
89. Morelli A, Ertmer C, Westphal M, et al. Effect of heart rate control with esmolol on hemodynamic and clinical outcomes in patients with septic shock: a randomized clinical trial. *JAMA* 310:1683–1691, 2013.
90. LeDoux D, Astiz ME, Carpati CM, et al: Effects of perfusion pressure on tissue perfusion in septic shock. *Crit Care Med* 28:2729–2732, 2000.
91. Leone M, Asfar P, Radermacher P, et al. Optimizing mean arterial pressure in septic shock: a critical reappraisal of the literature. *Crit Care* 10;19:101, 2015.
92. Huang YC: Monitoring oxygen delivery in the critically ill. *Chest* 128:554S–560S, 2005.
93. McNulty PH, King N, Scott S, et al: Effects of supplemental oxygen administration on coronary blood flow in patients undergoing cardiac catheterization. *Am J Physiol Heart Circ Physiol* 288:H1057–H1062, 2005.
94. Mak S, Azevedo ER, Liu PP, et al: Effect of hyperoxia on left ventricular function and filling pressures in patients with and without congestive heart failure. *Chest* 120:467–473, 2001.
95. Kern JW, Shoemaker WC: Meta-analysis of hemodynamic optimization in high-risk patients. *Crit Care Med* 31:1598–1599, 2003.
96. Shah MR, Hasselbland V, Stevenson LW, et al: Impact of the pulmonary artery catheter in critically ill patients: meta-analysis of randomized critical trials. *JAMA* 294:1664–1670, 2005.
97. Rivers E, Nguyen B, Havstad S, et al: Early goal-directed therapy in the treatment of severe sepsis and septic shock. *N Engl J Med* 345:1368–1377, 2001.
98. Berger RE, Rivers E, Levy MM: Management of septic shock. N Engl J Med 376:2282-2285, 2017.
99. PRISM Investigators, Rowan KM, Angus DC, et al: Early, goal-directed therapy for septic shock: A patient-level meta-analysis. N Eng J Med 376:2223-2234, 2017.
100. Geloen A, Chapelier K, Cividjian A, et al: Clonidine and dexmedetomidine increase the pressor response to norepinephrine in experimental sepsis: a pilot study. *Crit Care Med* 41:e431–e438, 2013.
101. Alcántara Hernández R, García-Sáinz JA: Roles of phosphoinositide-dependent kinase-1 in α1B-adrenoceptor phosphorylation and desensitization. *Eur J Pharmacol* 674:179–187, 2012.

Chapter 191 ■ Mechanical Complications of Myocardial Infarction

CHRISTOS GALATAS • ANNABEL A. CHEN-TOURNOUX

CONSEQUENCES OF ISCHEMIA

Within 8 to 10 seconds after occlusion of an epicardial coronary artery, myocardial oxygen supply is exhausted, resulting in a shift from aerobic to anaerobic metabolism [1]. With continued ischemia, high-energy phosphates become depleted, while hydrogen ions, lactate, and other metabolic byproducts accumulate. Disruption of the cell membrane allows protein leakage out of the cell, producing serologic evidence of myocyte injury. The onset and extent of irreversible tissue injury depend on many factors, such as myocardial oxygen consumption, ischemic preconditioning, and collateral blood flow. In the absence of collateral vessels, irreversible injury begins after 20 minutes of coronary occlusion. The benefits of reperfusion diminish with time, with salvage of only 10% of potentially viable myocardium at 180 minutes of ischemia [2].

Patency of the epicardial vessel does not necessarily indicate adequate perfusion at the microvascular level. The "no-reflow" phenomenon, indicating microvascular obstruction, has an incidence between 5% and 50% after primary percutaneous coronary intervention (PCI) for ST-segment elevation myocardial infarction (STEMI) depending on the imaging technique employed. Several mechanisms appear to be responsible for microvascular obstruction, including distal embolization, endothelial dysfunction, and external compression of vessels from interstitial and myocyte edema [3,4]. To date, a wide range of mechanical and pharmacologic strategies have been studied to reduce microvascular obstruction, with variable effects. Although early restoration of flow is necessary for myocardial survival, reperfusion also leads to injury through oxidative stress and impaired calcium homeostasis [5]. In addition, an intense inflammatory response is activated to clear the infarcted area of debris and prepare for later phases of healing [6].

Ischemia and reperfusion may be followed by a prolonged period of contractile dysfunction known as myocardial stunning. Importantly, the dysfunction associated with stunning is completely reversible. By definition, myocardial perfusion must be restored to normal or near normal to distinguish stunning from myocardial dysfunction due to continued ischemia (hibernation). In general, the myocardium is stunned for a period longer than that of the ischemic insult, often requiring hours to days to regain function [5]. Stunning is observed in clinical scenarios of ischemia–reperfusion, whether global, as with cardioplegia during cardiac surgery or transplant harvest, or regional, as with acute coronary syndromes. Stunning from repeated episodes of demand ischemia may lead to chronic left ventricular (LV) dysfunction. Stunning is clinically important to recognize: since dysfunction may be fully reversible, continued hemodynamic and/or mechanical support may be indicated until ventricular function has recovered. In addition, stunning has implications for the timing of evaluation of LV function to guide therapeutic decisions after myocardial infarction (MI). For example, LV ejection fraction assessment for implantable cardiac defibrillator implantation is generally deferred for at least 1 month following MI.

DIAGNOSIS, TREATMENT, AND OUTCOME OF SHOCK DUE TO LEFT VENTRICULAR PUMP FAILURE

Approximately 5% to 8% of patients with STEMI and 2.5% of those with NSTEMI (non-ST–segment elevation myocardial infarction) develop cardiogenic shock (CS), the leading cause of death among patients hospitalized with MI. CS is a clinical condition of inadequate end-organ perfusion due to cardiac dysfunction. Hemodynamic parameters of CS include persistent hypotension (systolic blood pressure [SBP] 80 to 90 mm Hg or mean arterial pressure [MAP] 30 mm Hg lower than baseline) with severe reduction in cardiac index (1.8 L/min/m^2 without support or 2.0 to 2.2 L/min/m^2 with support) and adequate or elevated filling pressure (LV end-diastolic pressure > 18 mm Hg or right ventricular [RV] end-diastolic pressure > 10 to 15 mm Hg). Clinical evidence of systemic hypoperfusion includes altered mental status, cold and clammy skin, and oliguria.

LV dysfunction due to extensive infarction or ischemia is the most common cause of CS after MI. Mechanical complications of MI such as ventricular septal rupture (VSR), papillary muscle rupture (PMR), and free wall rupture (FWR) can also result in CS, albeit less often; the combined incidence of VSR, PMR, and FWR is <1% in contemporary series [7].

The observation of normal to low systemic vascular resistance among many patients with CS suggests an important role for inappropriate vasodilation in CS. Indeed, neurohormonal and cytokine abnormalities consistent with the systemic inflammatory response syndrome (SIRS) have been observed [8]. Despite the growing recognition of SIRS associated with CS, therapies targeting it remain unproven at this time.

The cornerstone of CS treatment is percutaneous or surgical revascularization of the infarct-related artery. In the prospective, multicenter SHOCK trial, over 300 patients were randomized to early (within 6 hours) percutaneous or surgical revascularization or initial medical stabilization with subsequent revascularization (54 hours after randomization) [9,10]. Despite an excess of death in the early revascularization group, likely related to procedural complications, early revascularization improved the secondary outcome in the trial of survival at 6 months and 1 year (46.7% vs. 33.6%; $p < 0.03$). This benefit persisted at 3 and 6 years [11]. The benefit of revascularization appears similar to different patient subgroups (patients with diabetes, women, prior MI, and early vs. late shock) and whether revascularization is achieved with PCI or CABG. Consequently, early revascularization with either PCI or CABG is a class I recommendation for CS complicating STEMI or NSTEMI in American and European guidelines [12–15]. In STEMI patients with CS who are not suitable candidates for PCI or CABG, fibrinolytic therapy should be administered in the absence of contraindications [12].

Supportive measures for patients in CS include inotropes, vasopressors, and mechanical circulatory support (MCS). Diuretics or intravenous fluids may be required depending on the intravascular volume status. Commonly used inotropes and vasopressors in CS include dobutamine, dopamine, and norepinephrine. In a randomized trial comparing dopamine and norepinephrine for multiple etiologies of shock, dopamine was associated with increased arrhythmic events (24.1% vs. 12.4%, $p < 0.05$) and increased 28-day mortality in the predefined subgroup of patients with CS [16]. Routine use of a pulmonary artery catheter (PAC) to guide hemodynamic management of CS has not been specifically studied in adequately sized randomized trials in the post-MI setting and has not been shown to decrease mortality in any randomized trials in other settings [17].

For several decades, the principal mechanical therapy for CS has been the intra-aortic balloon pump (IABP) and it remains the most commonly used form of MCS in CS. More recently, the routine use of IABP for CS has been questioned. The IABP-SHOCK II trial, a prospective multicenter, open-label trial, randomized 600 patients with CS complicating acute MI to IABP versus no IABP [18]. All patients were planned for early revascularization by either PCI or CABG and received guideline-directed medical therapy. There was no difference in the primary efficacy endpoint of 30-day mortality (HR 0.96, 95% CI 0.79 to 1.17, $p = 0.69$) or in the safety endpoints (major bleeding, stroke, or peripheral ischemic complications). Other parameters of CS, such as serum creatinine or lactate, were not significantly different between the groups. A Cochrane Collaboration meta-analysis of seven studies including IABP-SHOCK II found that IABP may have a beneficial effect on some hemodynamic parameters, but this does not result in a survival benefit [19]. The authors concluded that there is no convincing randomized data to support the use of IABP in MI-related CS. In the 2013 American College of Cardiology Foundation and American Heart Association Guidelines for the management of STEMI, IABP received a class IIa recommendation (changed from a previous class I recommendation) in patients with CS after MI who do not quickly stabilize with pharmacologic therapy [12].

Newer forms of MCS in adult patients with CS include left ventricular assist devices (LVADs) such as the Impella and TandemHeart. To date, there is a paucity of data comparing LVADs to IABP, and the former is currently given a class IIb recommendation for treatment of refractory CS [12]. A meta-analysis of 100 patients from three randomized trials (two comparing TandemHeart with IABP and one comparing Impella 2.5 with IABP) showed that while LVADs resulted in higher cardiac index (mean difference 0.35 L/min/m^2, 95% CI 0.09 to 0.61); higher MAP (mean difference 12.8 mm Hg, 95% CI 3.6 to 22.0); and lower PCWP (mean difference 25.3 mm Hg, 95% CI 29.4 to 21.2), there was no improvement in 30-day mortality (RR 1.06, 95% CI 0.68 to 1.66) [20]. In addition, there are no randomized data demonstrating that use of LVADs in CS is associated with decreased mortality compared to standard therapy. Observational data from the Impella-EUROSHOCK Registry demonstrated that Impella insertion is feasible and results in decreased serum lactate [21]. However, 30-day mortality remains high. Decreased lactate as well as faster weaning of inotropes was also reported in a 40-patient, retrospective, single-center study [22]. Data from the American USPella Registry of patients in CS undergoing PCI demonstrated a potential benefit of Impella insertion prior to PCI (survival to discharge 65.1% vs. 40.7% in pre-PCI and post-PCI Impella groups, respectively; OR of in-hospital mortality 0.37, 95% CI 0.19 to 0.72) [23]. The ideal patient selection strategy, MCS device type, and timing of insertion have yet to be determined [24].

Extracorporeal membrane oxygenation (ECMO) is another option for mechanical support in CS; data are limited to retrospective, nonrandomized studies and no mortality benefit has been demonstrated [25,26]. The ideal use of this technology in this setting will require further study.

Despite advances in revascularization, pharmacotherapy and mechanical support, mortality in CS remains high. Registry data from the United States and Europe demonstrate an in-hospital mortality rate of close to 50% [27,28]. Independent predictors of mortality in CS include older age; history of hypertension, MI, or heart failure; lower blood pressure and worse renal function on presentation; failed reperfusion; and low LV ejection fraction [11,27,29,30].

RIGHT VENTRICULAR INFARCTION

Right ventricular infarction (RVI) has long been recognized for its distinct clinical and hemodynamic features. Most cases of RVI are caused by proximal occlusion of a dominant right coronary artery (RCA) and RVI may complicate 50% of inferior MI (IMI). Very rarely, the left anterior descending (LAD) artery may be the culprit vessel. RVI causes RV hypokinesis which leads to decreased LV preload and decreased cardiac output (CO). In addition, acute RV dilation in the face of the restraining effects of the pericardium leads to elevated intrapericardial pressure and leftward shifting of the interventricular septum, further compromising LV filling and CO [31].

RV anatomy and physiology are distinct from those of the LV and provide a more favorable oxygen supply to demand profile. In many instances, the RV myocardium may actually be stunned or hibernating and not infarcted. In one cardiac magnetic resonance (CMR) study, RV edema and late gadolinium enhancement (LGE) were relatively common early after MI (51% and 31%, respectively) [32]. At 4-month follow-up, the frequency and extent of LGE were markedly reduced, suggesting limited permanent myocardial damage. In fact, some authors would even consider the term RVI a misnomer and that chronic right heart failure secondary to MI is rare [31].

Early recognition of RVI is crucial because of its implications for management and prognosis. Clinical manifestations of RVI include hypotension in the setting of clear lungs and elevated jugular venous pressure, although the latter may not be evident if the patient is relatively hypovolemic. Conversely, a volume-depleted patient may exhibit sensitivity to preload reduction, such as with the use of nitrates or diuretics. Evidence of interventricular dependence, such as Kussmaul sign (distension of jugular veins during inspiration), may also be present. However, the physical examination is not sensitive for the diagnosis of RVI.

Electrocardiogram (ECG) indicators of RVI include ST-segment elevation in lead III greater than II, ST-segment elevation in lead V1, and >1 mm ST-segment elevation in right-sided precordial lead V_{4R}, the latter being most predictive. These ECG abnormalities may resolve quickly (50% within 10 hours), underscoring the importance of obtaining a right-sided ECG on presentation for all patients with IMI. RVI is also associated with bradyarrhythmias (sinoatrial or atrioventricular [AV] block) and tachyarrhythmias (atrial fibrillation and ventricular tachyarrhythmias). Echocardiography may reveal RV dilation, RV and inferior LV hypokinesis, and paradoxical septal motion. It may also demonstrate complications of RVI such as RV mural thrombus and pulmonary embolism; right-to-left shunting across a patent foramen ovale; and severe tricuspid regurgitation from acute RV and tricuspid annular dilation or from primary papillary muscle ischemia or rupture. Two small studies have demonstrated that CMR has superior sensitivity to detect RVI compared to physical examination, ECG, and echocardiography [33,34]. Finally, right heart catheterization demonstrating a right atrial pressure >10 mm Hg or >80% of the PCWP supports the diagnosis of RVI.

Treatment of RVI should emphasize urgent reperfusion. Successful reperfusion is associated with significantly improved RV function and clinical outcomes [35]. Intravenous fluid should be judiciously administered to maintain optimal RV preload; 1 to 2 L of isotonic fluid is a reasonable start. Conversely, preload reducing medications should be avoided. Central venous pressure (CVP) monitoring may be helpful for avoiding RV volume overload (CVP > 10 to 14 mm Hg), which may compromise LV preload via ventricular interdependence. As right atrial contraction is an important contributor to right-sided output, AV sequential pacing for complete heart block or direct-current cardioversion for atrial fibrillation should be considered. Inotropic support may be required but pure α-adrenergic agonists should be avoided because they may increase pulmonary vascular resistance, further compromising RV function.

Mechanical support may be necessary until RV function has recovered. IABP may be useful independent of LV systolic function, with increases in MAP, SBP, and diastolic blood pressure [36]. Percutaneous right ventricular assist devices (RVADs) may also be considered. A retrospective cohort of patients treated with the Tandem-Heart RVAD demonstrated improved MAP, CO, and right atrial pressure [37]. Similarly, the prospective, open-label, nonrandomized RECOVER RIGHT study utilizing the Impella RP demonstrated improved hemodynamics with use of this RVAD [38]. Of note, both studies included multiple etiologies of RV dysfunction. Finally, ECMO has also been used in a limited number of patients with RVI [39].

Hemodynamic instability associated with RVI represents only 5% of cases of CS complicating MI but portends high in-hospital mortality, ranging from 23% to 53% [40,41]. A meta-analysis showed that the presence of RVI more than doubles the relative risk of mortality among patients with acute MI (RR 2.59, 95% CI 2.02 to 3.31) [42]. Despite this high mortality, patients surviving the acute insult generally have a good prognosis with recovery of RV function [43].

MYOCARDIAL RUPTURE

Myocardial rupture is a rare, but immediately life-threatening complication of MI, occurring 1 to 7 days after MI and accounting for 10% to 15% of deaths. The pathogenesis of rupture depends on timing and whether reperfusion has occurred, with intramural hemorrhage causing rupture in the first 48 hours following fibrinolysis, and coagulation necrosis, inflammation, and myocardial disintegration occurring over 3 to 5 days in the absence of reperfusion. In the National Registry of Myocardial Infarction, older age, female gender, and fibrinolysis were independent predictors of myocardial rupture [44].

Myocardial rupture may occur despite a limited infarct area and relatively preserved systolic function because of increased shear stress in the necrotic zone and its borders. Rupture is possible at three sites: a PMR, the VSR, or the ventricular FWR. The specific presentations and sequelae depend on the location of the defect(s) (Table 191.1), but in all cases, prompt diagnosis and management, with expertise from critical care, imaging, interventional and surgical specialities, are critical to prevent irreversible end-organ malperfusion.

Papillary Muscle Rupture

PMR complicates 0.25% of AMI patients treated with PCI and is the etiology of CS for 7% of cases [7]. The posteromedial papillary muscle is affected three times more often than the anterolateral papillary muscle as the former has a single vascular supply (RCA or left circumflex artery [LCx], depending on dominance) while the latter has a dual vascular supply (LAD and LCx). Complete or partial rupture of the papillary muscle can lead to varying degrees of mitral regurgitation (MR). PMR can occur despite a limited territory of infarction and it is not uncommon to observe PMR with relatively preserved LV function.

Patients with PMR present with acute dyspnea secondary to pulmonary congestion. Physical examination may reveal a systolic murmur best heard at the apex, diminished air entry and

TABLE 191.1

Characteristics of Myocardial Rupture

Characteristic	Ventricular septal rupture	Free wall rupture	Papillary muscle rupture
Incidence	1%–3% without reperfusion therapy; 0.2%–0.34% with fibrinolysis; 3.9% in patients with cardiogenic shock	0.8%–6.2%; primary angioplasty, but not fibrinolysis, appears to reduce risk	1%; posteromedial more frequent than anterolateral papillary muscle
Time course	Bimodal peak: <24 h and 3–5 d; range 1–14 d	Bimodal peak: <24 h and 3–5 d; range 1–14 d	Bimodal peak: <24 h and 3–5 d; range 1–14 d
Clinical manifestations	Chest pain, dyspnea, hypotension	Anginal, pleuritic, or pericardial chest pain; syncope, hypotension, arrhythmia, nausea, restlessness, hypotension, sudden death	Abrupt onset of dyspnea due to pulmonary edema; hypotension
Physical findings	Harsh holosystolic murmur, thrill, accentuated S_2, S_3, pulmonary edema, RV, and LV failure, cardiogenic shock	Jugular venous distention, pulsus paradoxus, electromechanical dissociation, and cardiogenic shock	Soft murmur in some cases, no thrill, variable signs of RV overload, severe pulmonary edema (may be asymmetric), cardiogenic shock
Echocardiographic findings	VSR, color Doppler left-to-right shunt across septum, RV dilation, and hypokinesis	Myocardial tear >5 mm pericardial effusion not always visualized; clot within pericardial space, tamponade	Hypercontractile LV, torn papillary muscle or chordae tendineae, flail leaflet, severe MR by color Doppler
Cardiac catheterization	Oxygen saturation step-up from RA to RV, large V-waves	Ventriculography insensitive; equalization of diastolic pressures	No oxygen saturation step-up from RA to RV (may occur from RV to PA); large V-waves, high PCWP

LV, left ventricle; MR, mitral regurgitation; PA, pulmonary artery; PCWP, pulmonary capillary wedge pressure; RA, right atrial; RV, right ventricle; VSR, ventricular septal rupture.

Adapted from Antman EM, Anbe DT, Armstrong PW, et al: ACC/AHA guidelines for the management of patients with ST-elevation myocardial infarction: a report of the American College of Cardiology/American Heart Association Task Force on Practice Guidelines (Committee to Revise the 1999 Guidelines for the Management of Patients With Acute Myocardial Infarction). *Circulation* 110:e82–e292, 2004.

crackles. The murmur may be absent due to equalization of the left atrial and LV pressures. The diagnosis is suggested by the presence of large V-waves in the PCWP tracing, however this finding may also be seen with severe LV dysfunction, VSR, or other etiologies of MR. Indeed, a much more common mechanism of MR following MI is tethering of the mitral leaflet(s) due to ischemia and dysfunction of the papillary muscle and/or underlying LV segments. The diagnosis of PMR is made by echocardiography with visualization of a flail portion of the mitral leaflet or a ruptured papillary muscle head prolapsing into the left atrium, along with color Doppler evidence of MR (Video 191.1), which has a distinct appearance from ischemic MR (Video 191.1). Transesophageal echocardiography (TEE) should be performed if there is inadequate visualization by the transthoracic approach.

Initial stabilization may be accomplished with inotropic agents, afterload reduction as tolerated, and placement of an IABP. However, in-hospital mortality is as high as 80% when medical therapy is used alone and surgical intervention is indicated for patients who are suitable surgical candidates. The use of ECMO or LVAD prior to surgery has been described in a limited number of patients [45,46]. Surgical repair may consist of chordal-sparing mitral valve replacement or, if necrosis is limited, papillary muscle re-implantation with or without ring annuloplasty. Coronary angiography should be performed prior to surgery so that CABG can be performed concomitantly if necessary. Thirty-day mortality ranges from 22.5% to 39.3% with surgery. Mortality is reduced with concomitant CABG whereas low CO, renal failure, complete PMR, and the need for ECMO or intraoperative IABP portend a worse prognosis [47–49]. Percutaneous repair with the MitraClip device has been successfully employed in this setting but data is limited to case reports [50,51]. Long-term survival after surgery ranges from 60% to 80% and is similar to that of matched patients with MI but no PMR [49].

Ventricular Septal Rupture

VSR is a rare but devastating complication of transmural MI, typically associated with total occlusion of the infarct-related artery and poor collateral flow. Infarctions from the LAD, dominant RCA, or dominant LCx may all involve branch arteries to the septum. Anterior infarctions are more likely to cause apical defects and inferior or lateral infarctions are more likely to cause basal defects. Complex VSRs, serpiginous lesions with an exit site remote from the entry site, are more frequently noted with IMI. Five to 10% of patients have multiple defects.

Prior to the advent of fibrinolytics and percutaneous reperfusion therapies, VSR occurred in 1% to 2% of patients with acute MI, an average of 3 to 5 days after MI. More contemporary series report an incidence between 0.17% and 0.31% [52]. Despite this decline, mortality remains high (41% to 80%) and essentially unchanged. Risk factors for developing a VSR include advanced age, female sex, chronic kidney disease, and cerebrovascular disease [53]. Positive biomarkers, CS, higher Killip class, and longer time to reperfusion are additional risk factors [7].

VSR causes an abrupt shunting of flow from the LV to the lower pressure RV. Consequently, there is acute volume overload of the right heart and impaired forward CO. The degree of shunting and hemodynamic compromise, which may vary from complete stability to acute shock, depends on the rupture size, the relative resistance of the pulmonary and systemic circulations, and the relative function of the ventricles. Symptoms include chest pain, dyspnea, and altered mental status. Physical examination reveals hypotension with a harsh, pansystolic murmur best heard at the left sternal border, as opposed to at the apex, which would be more suggestive of PMR. A parasternal thrill is present in half of patients. Signs of RV failure including jugular venous distension, a loud pulmonic component of the second heart sound, and lower extremity edema may also be present; a third heart sound may result from LV or RV volume overload. ECG findings include persistent ST-segment elevation and AV nodal or infranodal conduction abnormalities. As the LV fails and systolic pressure decreases, left-to-right shunting decreases. If RV pressures exceed those on the left, right to left shunting occurs, resulting in hypoxemia.

The diagnosis of VSR is most commonly made using echocardiography, which can demonstrate a dropout of the interventricular septum on 2D imaging and flow across the septum on Doppler imaging (Video 191.2). Moreover, echocardiography provides information about LV and RV function. Right heart catheterization demonstrates a step-up in oxygen saturation (>8%) in the RV; increased pulmonary-to-systemic flow ratios ($Q_p/Q_s > 1.4$); and increased right-sided pressures, but is generally not required if echocardiography is readily available. Left ventriculography can also identify a VSR.

Nonsurgical therapies, such as afterload reduction, diuretics, inotropes, and IABP are purely temporizing and when used alone result in mortality greater than 90%. Surgical repair of a VSR, first performed in 1957, is the definitive treatment. Operative management should also take into account the presence of concomitant CAD and potential revascularization targets, the degree of MR, and the severity of LV and RV dysfunction. Despite surgical repair, mortality remains high: a large cohort from the Society of Thoracic Surgeons database showed a mortality of 54.1% if repair was required within 7 days of MI [54]. Mortality may be significantly reduced if the patient's clinical status allows surgery to be delayed until myocardial scar tissue has formed [55].

Evidence for use of LVADs, such as the Impella or TandemHeart, and ECMO to stabilize patients until surgery is limited to small case series [56–58], and their role in VSR management is yet to be defined. Percutaneous closure of VSR has been reported with a procedural success rate of 73.6% to 91% [59–61]. In parallel with the surgical experience, the presence of CS and VSR closure in the acute phase are risk factors for mortality. VSR with acute CS is associated with extremely high mortality no matter what the approach. Optimal patient selection and timing of various strategies such as mechanical support and surgical or percutaneous repair remain to be defined.

Free Wall Rupture

LV FWR is the most common type of cardiac rupture with an incidence of 0.52% in patients treated with primary PCI [7]. The temporal pattern of rupture has two peaks: the first within 24 hours and the second between 3 and 5 days after acute MI [62]. As with VSR, FWR can be classified as simple or complex. In addition, risk factors for FWR are similar to those for VSR with successful, early reperfusion and the presence of flow from collateral vessels being protective. The culprit vessel is the LAD or LCx for >80% of cases. Rupture occurs most commonly in the posterolateral free wall close to the papillary muscle insertion.

FWR results in blood rapidly entering the pericardial space and commonly presents as pericardial tamponade, electromechanical dissociation, or sudden cardiac death (Video 191.3). Physical examination is consistent with tamponade and can demonstrate hypotension, a pulsus paradoxus (decrease in SBP >10 mm Hg with inspiration) and elevated JVP. An LV pseudoaneurysm occurs when FWR is contained by adherent pericardium or pericardial adhesions, thus preventing immediate pericardial tamponade and death. Symptoms of contained rupture include recurrent chest pain or pleurisy, emesis without preceding nausea, unexplained restlessness, and syncope. Hypotension may be accompanied by "inappropriate" bradycardia. New ST-segment elevation or

T-wave abnormalities may be evident. Pseudoaneurysms can be diagnosed by echocardiography, contrast or radionuclide ventriculography, or CMR. Diagnostic pericardiocentesis may yield blood; therapeutic pericardiocentesis may destabilize a contained effusion and result in death. Surgical repair is usually necessary, although survival with pericardiocentesis and supportive medical therapy has been reported for selected patients [63].

LEFT VENTRICULAR REMODELING

Acute MI triggers a cascade of molecular and cellular events that leads to changes in LV shape, dimension, and function. This process of remodeling is initially compensatory but becomes maladaptive as increased ventricular wall stress leads to progressive hypertrophy, dilation, spherical distortion, and impairment of contractile function. MR [64] and mechanical dyssynchrony [65,66], if present, further exacerbate ventricular wall stress and adverse remodeling. Because LV remodeling is concordant with clinical outcomes over the natural history of heart failure, its prevention is accepted as a reasonable therapeutic target.

Among patients with MI, infarct size is a major determinant of negative LV remodeling. Thus, timely and effective reperfusion of the occluded artery is central to reduction of infarct size, preservation of ventricular function and long-term prognosis. Various adjunctive cardioprotective strategies for use in the acute setting are under investigation but their clinical impact is uncertain [67].

The renin–angiotensin–aldosterone (RAAS) and sympathetic nervous systems are central mediators of remodeling. Myocyte stretch from increased wall stress stimulates the local production of angiotensin II, which in turn promotes myocyte hypertrophy, fibroblast proliferation, and collagen production. Adrenergic stimulation, in response to myocardial injury and/or hemodynamic compromise, leads to myocardial production of cytokines, such as tumor necrosis factor-α (TNF-α), interleukin-1β (IL-1β), and interleukin-6 (IL-6), that mediate myocyte hypertrophy, apoptosis, and changes in the extracellular matrix. Furthermore, adrenergic stimulation enhances the activity of the RAAS.

Blockade of the RAAS and sympathetic nervous system is the cornerstone of pharmacologic therapy directed at interrupting remodeling and improving long-term outcome. Angiotensin-converting enzyme (ACE) inhibitors have not only beneficial effects on hemodynamics and loading conditions but also direct effects on remodeling, and confer a survival benefit in patients with MI [68–71]. ACE inhibitors thus carry a class I recommendation for patients with STEMI with an anterior location, heart failure or LV ejection fraction <40%, and a class IIa indication for all patients with STEMI, who have no contraindications [12]. Patients who are intolerant of ACE inhibitors appear to derive similar benefit from angiotensin-receptor blockers (ARBs) [72]. Aldosterone blockade for patients without contraindication has also been shown to improve survival in patients with LV dysfunction after MI [73].

β-Blockers reduce myocyte apoptosis, collagen deposition, and hypertrophy; they reduce myocardial oxygen demand by reducing heart rate and blood pressure; and they directly oppose catecholamine stimulation of myocytes. β-Blockers reduce not only infarct size when administered early after MI [74], but also future remodeling [75,76], and carry a class I recommendation for patients with STEMI in the absence of contraindications [12].

Finally, novel strategies to prevent LV remodeling after MI are under investigation, including regenerative therapies utilizing stem cell and paracrine factors and pharmacologic interventions targeting oxidant stress, inflammatory and matrix-metalloproteinase pathways.

Recommendations for the management of the mechanical complications of MI based on randomized controlled trials are summarized in Table 191.2.

TABLE 191.2

Summary of Recommendations Based on Randomized Controlled Clinical Trials

- Cardiogenic shock: Early revascularization by PCI or CABG in suitable patients reduces mortality [10,11].
- Remodeling: ACE inhibition, angiotensin-receptor blockade and aldosterone blockade in patients with evidence of LV dysfunction after MI attenuates LV remodeling and improves survival [68–73].
- Remodeling: β-blockade in patients after MI attenuates LV remodeling and improves survival [74–76].

ACE, angiotensin-converting enzyme; CABG, coronary artery bypass graft; LV, left ventricular; MI, myocardial infarction; PCI, percutaneous coronary intervention.

VIDEO 191.1 Papillary muscle rupture complicating inferior MI as seen by trans-esophageal echocardiography. **A.** The ruptured papillary muscle is seen prolapsing into the left atrium during systole, associated with flail motion of the anterior mitral leaflet. **B.** Color Doppler imaging demonstrates severe, eccentric mitral regurgitation. **C.** A short-axis view of the left ventricle showing only the anterolateral papillary muscle.

VIDEO 191.2 Ventricular septal rupture complicating a late-presentation anterior MI as seen by trans-thoracic echocardiography. **A.** The rupture is clearly seen in the mid-septum in this apical 4-chamber view. The right ventricle is noted to be dilated and akinetic due to acute volume overload. **B.** Color Doppler imaging demonstrates bi-directional flow across the interventricular septum.

VIDEO 191.3 Trans-esophageal echocardiography in a patient with late-presentation of inferolateral MI. **A.** In this long-axis view, the inferolateral wall is akinetic, resulting in severe tethering of the posterior mitral leaflet. **B.** Color Doppler imaging demonstrates severe ischemic mitral regurgitation. **C.** A new small pericardial effusion is noted during the echocardiogram. **D.** The effusion increases quickly over the next few minutes leading to compression of the right ventricle and pericardial tamponade. Note the spontaneous echo contrast in the left heart reflecting stasis from low cardiac output. A free wall rupture was suspected and the patient immediately underwent surgical exploration and repair of a lateral wall rupture, as well as coronary artery bypass and mitral valve replacement.

References

1. Kloner RA, Jennings RB: Consequences of brief ischemia: stunning, preconditioning, and their clinical implications: part 1. *Circulation* 104:2981–2989, 2001.
2. Westaby S, Kharbanda R, Banning AP: Cardiogenic shock in ACS. Part 1: prediction, presentation and medical therapy. *Nat Rev Cardiol* 9(3):158–171, 2011.
3. Durante A, Camici PG: Novel insights into an "old" phenomenon: the no reflow. *Int J Cardiol* 187:273–280, 2015.
4. Bekkers SC, Yazdani SK, Virmani R, et al: Microvascular obstruction: underlying pathophysiology and clinical diagnosis. *J Am CollCardiol* 55(16):1649-60, 2010.
5. Kloner RA, Jennings RB: Consequences of brief ischemia: stunning, preconditioning, and their clinical implications: part 2. *Circulation* 104:3158–3167, 2001.
6. Frangogiannis NG: The inflammatory response in myocardial injury, repair, and remodeling. *Nat Rev Cardiol* 11(5):255–265, 2014.
7. French JK, Hellkamp AS, Armstrong PW, et al: Mechanical complications after percutaneous coronary intervention in ST-elevation myocardial infarction (from APEX-AMI). *Am J Cardiol* 105(1):59–63, 2010.
8. Reynolds HR, Hochman JS: Cardiogenic shock: current concepts and improving outcomes. *Circulation* 117(5):686–697, 2008.
9. Hochman JS, Sleeper LA, Webb JG, et al: Early revascularization in acute myocardial infarction complicated by cardiogenic shock. SHOCK Investigators. Should we emergently revascularize occluded coronaries for cardiogenic shock. *N Engl J Med* 341:625–634, 1999.
10. Hochman JS, Sleeper LA, White HD, et al: One-year survival following early revascularization for cardiogenic shock. *JAMA* 285:190–192, 2001.
11. Hochman JS, Sleeper LA, Webb JG, et al: Early revascularization and long-term survival in cardiogenic shock complicating acute myocardial infarction. *JAMA* 295(21):2511–2515, 2006.
12. O'Gara PT, Kushner FG, Ascheim DD, et al: 2013 ACCF/AHA guideline for the management of ST-elevation myocardial infarction: a report of the American College of Cardiology Foundation/American Heart Association Task Force on Practice Guidelines. *Circulation* 127:529–555, 2013.

13. Amsterdam EA, Wenger NK, Brindis RG, et al: 2014 AHA/ACC Guideline for the management of patients with non-ST-elevation acute coronary syndromes: a report of the American College of Cardiology/American Heart Association Task Force on Practice Guidelines. *J Am CollCardiol* 64(24):e139–e228, 2014.
14. Steg G, James SK, Dan Atar, et al: ESC Guidelines for the management of acute myocardial infarction in patients presenting with ST-segment elevation. *Eur Heart J* 33:2569–2619, 2012.
15. Roffi M, Patrono C, Collet JP, et al: 2015 ESC Guidelines for the management of acute coronary syndromes in patients presenting without persistent ST-segment elevation. *Eur Heart J* 37:267–315, 2016.
16. De Backer D, Biston P, Devriendt J, et al: Comparison of dopamine and norepinephrine in the treatment of shock. *N Engl J Med* 362:779–789, 2010.
17. Gidwani UK, Goel S: The pulmonary artery catheter in 2015: the swan and the phoenix. *Cardiol Rev* 24(1):1–13, 2016.
18. Thiele H, Zeymer U, Neumann FJ, et al: Intraaortic balloon support for myocardial infarction with cardiogenic shock. *N Engl J Med* 367:1287–1296, 2012.
19. Unverzagt S, Buerke M, de Waha A, et al: Intra-aortic balloon pump counterpulsation (IABP) for myocardial infarction complicated by cardiogenic shock. *Cochrane Database Syst Rev* 3:CD007398, 2015.
20. Cheng JM, Uil CA, Hoeks SE, et al: Percutaneous left ventricular assist devices vs. intra-aortic balloon pump counterpulsation for treatment of cardiogenic shock: a meta-analysis of controlled trials. *Eur Heart J* 30:2102–2108, 2009.
21. Lauten A, Engström AE, Jung C, et al: Percutaneous left-ventricular support with the Impella-2.5–assist device in acute cardiogenic shock: results of the Impella–EUROSHOCK-Registry. *Circulation: Heart Fail* 6:23–30, 2013.
22. Gaudard P, Mourad M, Eliet J, et al: Management and outcome of patients supported with Impella 5.0 for refractory cardiogenic shock. *Crit Care* 19:363, 2015.
23. O'Neill WW, Schreiber T, Wohns W, et al: The current use of Impella 2.5 in acute myocardial infarction complicated by cardiogenic shock: results from the USpella registry. *J Interv Cardiol* 27(1):1–11, 2014.
24. Rihal CS, Naidu SS, Givertz MM, et al: 2015 SCAI/ACC/HFSA/STS clinical expert consensus statement on the use of percutaneous mechanical circulatory support devices in cardiovascular care. *J Am Coll Cardiol* 65(19):e7–e26, 2015.
25. Kim H, Lim SH, Hong J, et al: Efficacy of veno-arterial extracorporeal membrane oxygenation in acute myocardial infarction with cardiogenic shock. *Resuscitation* 83(8):971–975, 2012.
26. Tang GHL, Malekan R, Kai M, et al: Peripheral venoarterial extracorporeal membrane oxygenation improves survival in myocardial infarction with cardiogenic shock. *J Thorac Cardiovasc Surg* 145(3):e32–e33, 2013.
27. Goldberg RJ, Spencer FA, Gore JM, et al: Thirty-year trends (1975–2005) in the magnitude of, management of, and hospital death rates associated with cardiogenic shock in patients with acute myocardial infarction: a population-based perspective. *Circulation* 119(9):1211–1219, 2009.
28. Jeger RV, Radovanovic D, Hunziker PR, et al: Ten-year trends in the incidence and treatment of cardiogenic shock. *Ann Intern Med* 149(9):618–626, 2008.
29. Sutton AG, Finn P, Hall JA, et al: Predictors of outcome after percutaneous treatment for cardiogenic shock. *Heart* 91:339–344, 2005.
30. Picard MH, Davidoff R, Sleeper LA, et al: Echocardiographic predictors of survival and response to early revascularization in cardiogenic shock. *Circulation* 107:279–284, 2003.
31. Goldstein JA: Acute right ventricular infarction: insights for the interventional era. *Curr Probl Cardiol* 37(12):533–557, 2012.
32. Masci PG, Francone M, Desmet W, et al: Right ventricular ischemic injury in patients with acute ST-segment elevation myocardial infarction: characterization with cardiovascular magnetic resonance. *Circulation* 22(14):1405–1412, 2010.
33. Galea N, Francone M, Carbone I, et al: Utility of cardiac magnetic resonance (CMR) in the evaluation of right ventricular (RV) involvement in patients with myocardial infarction (MI). *Radiol Med* 119:309–317, 2014.
34. Kumar A, Abdel-Aty H, Kriedemann I, et al: Contrast-enhanced cardiovascular magnetic resonance imaging of right ventricular infarction. *J Am Coll Cardiol* 48(10):1969–1976, 2006.
35. Bowers TR, O'Neill WW, Grines C, et al: Effect of reperfusion on biventricular function and survival after right ventricular infarction. *N Engl J Med* 338:933–940, 1998.
36. McNamara MW, Dixon SR, Goldstein JA: Impact of intra-aortic balloon pumping on hypotension and outcomes in acute right ventricular infarction. *Coronary Artery Dis* 25:602–607, 2014.
37. Kapur NK, Paruchuri V, Korabathina R, et al: Effects of a percutaneous mechanical circulatory support device for medically refractory right ventricular failure. *J Heart Lung Transplant* 30:1360–1367, 2011.
38. Anderson MB, Goldstein J, Milano C, et al: Benefits of a novel percutaneous ventricular assist device for right heart failure: The prospective RECOVER RIGHT study of the Impella RP device. *J Heart Lung Transplant* 34(12):1549–1560, 2015.
39. Hisata Y, Hashizume K, Tanigawa K, et al: Right infarction response to coronary artery bypass and the Abiomed BVS 5000. *Asian Cardiovasc Thorac Ann* 22(3):329–331, 2014.
40. Brodie BR, Stuckey TD, Hansen C, et al: Comparison of late survival in patients with cardiogenic shock due to right ventricular infarction versus left ventricular pump failure following primary percutaneous coronary intervention for ST-elevation acute myocardial infarction. *Am J Cardiol* 99(4):431–435, 2007.
41. Jacobs AK, Leopold JA, Bates E, et al: Cardiogenic shock caused by right ventricular infarction: a report from the SHOCK registry. *J Am Coll Cardiol* 41:1273–1279, 2003.
42. Hamon M, Agostini D, Le Page O, et al: Prognostic impact of right ventricular involvement in patients with acute myocardial infarction: meta-analysis. *Crit Care Med* 36(7):2023–2033, 2008.
43. Gumina RJ, Murphy JG, Rihal CS, et al: Long-term survival after right ventricular infarction. *Am J Cardiol* 98(12):1571–1573, 2006.
44. Becker RC, Gore JM, Lambrew C, et al: A composite view of cardiac rupture in the United States National Registry of Myocardial Infarction. *J Am Coll Cardiol* 27:1321–1326, 1996.
45. Harmon L, Boccalandro F: Cardiogenic shock secondary to severe acute ischemic mitral regurgitation managed with an Impella 2.5 percutaneous left ventricular assist device. *Catheter Cardiovasc Interv* 79:1129–1134, 2012.
46. Obadia B, Theron A, Gariboldi V: Extracorporeal membrane oxygenation as a bridge to surgery for ischemic papillary muscle rupture. *J Thorac Cardiovasc Surg* 147:e82–e84, 2014.
47. Schroeter T, Lehmann S, Misfeld M, et al: Clinical outcome after mitral valve surgery due to ischemic papillary muscle rupture. *Ann Thorac Surg* 95:820–824, 2013.
48. Bouma W, Wijdh-den Hamer IJ, Koene BM, et al: Predictors of in-hospital mortality after mitral valve surgery for post-myocardial infarction papillary muscle rupture. *J Cardiothorac Surg* 18(9):171, 2014.
49. Russo A, Suri RM, Grigioni F, et al: Clinical outcome after surgical correction of mitral regurgitation due to papillary muscle rupture. *Circulation* 118(15):1528–1534, 2008.
50. Wolff R, Cohen G, Peterson C et al: MitraClip for papillary muscle rupture in patient with cardiogenic shock. *Can J Cardiol* 30(11):1461, 2014.
51. Bahlmann E, Frerker C, Kreidel F, et al: MitraClip implantation after acute ischemic papillary muscle rupture in a patient with prolonged cardiogenic shock. *Ann Thorac Surg* 99:e41–e42, 2015.
52. Jones BM, Kapadia SR, Smedira NG, et al: Ventricular septal rupture complicating acute myocardial infarction: a contemporary review. *Eur Heart J* 35:2060–2068, 2014.
53. Crenshaw BS, Granger CB, Birnbaum Y, et al: Risk factors angiographic patterns, and outcomes in patients with ventricular septal defect complicating acute myocardial infarction. *Circulation* 100(1):27–32, 2000.
54. Arnaoutakis GJ, Zhao Y, George TJ, et al: Surgical repair of ventricular septal defect after myocardial infarction: outcomes from the Society of Thoracic Surgeons National Database. *Ann Thorac Surg* 94:436–444, 2012.
55. Papalexopoulou N, Young CP, Attia RQ: What is the best timing of surgery in patients with post-infarct ventricular septal rupture? *Interact Cardiovasc Thoracic Surg* 16(2):193–196, 2013.
56. Gregoric ID, Bieniarz MC, Arora H, et al: Percutaneous ventricular assist device support in a patient with a postinfarction ventricular septal defect. *Tex Heart Inst J* 35(1):46–48, 2008.
57. La Torre MW, Centofanti P, Attisani M, et al: Posterior ventricular septal defect in presence of cardiogenic shock: early implantation of the Impella recover LP 5.0 as a bridge to surgery. *Tex Heart Inst J* 38(1):42–49, 2011.
58. Rohn V, Spacek M, Belohlavek J, et al: Cardiogenic shock in patient with posterior postinfarctionseptal rupture—successful treatment with extracorporeal membrane oxygenation (ECMO) as a ventricular assist device. *J Card Surg* 24(4):435–436, 2009.
59. Attia R, Blauth C: Which patients might be suitable for a septal occlude device closure of postinfarction ventricular septal rupture rather than immediate surgery? *Interact Cardiovasc Thorac Surg* 11(5):626–629, 2010.
60. Assenza GE, McElhinney DB, Valente AM, et al: Transcatheter closure of post-myocardial infarction ventricular septal rupture. *Circ Cardiovasc Interv* 6(1):59–67, 2013.
61. Risseeuw F, Diebels I, Vandendriessche T, et al: Percutaneous occlusion of post-myocardial infarction ventricular septum rupture. *Neth Heart J* 22(2):47–51, 2014.
62. Oliva PB, Hammill SC, Edwards WD: Cardiac rupture, a clinically predictable complication of acute myocardial infarction: report of 70 cases with clinicopathologic correlations. *J Am Coll Cardiol* 22:720–726, 1993.
63. Figueras J, Cortadellas J, Evangelista A, et al: Medical management of selected patients with left ventricular free wall rupture during acute myocardial infarction. *J Am Coll Cardiol* 29:512–518, 1997.
64. Amigoni M, Meris A, Thune JJ, et al: Mitral regurgitation in myocardial infarction complicated by heart failure, left ventricular dysfunction, or both: prognostic significance and relation to ventricular size and function. *Eur Heart J* 28(3):326–333, 2007.
65. Mollema SA, Liem SS, Suffoletto MS, et al: Left ventricular dyssynchrony acutely after myocardial infarction predicts left ventricular remodeling. *J Am Coll Cardiol* 50(16):1532–1540, 2007.
66. Shin SH, Hung CL, Uno H, et al: Mechanical dyssynchrony after myocardial infarction in patients with left ventricular dysfunction, heart failure, or both. *Circulation* 121(9):1096–1103, 2010.
67. Lønborg JT: Targeting reperfusion injury in the era of primary percutaneous coronary intervention: hope or hype? *Heart* 101(20):1612–1618, 2015.
68. Pfeffer MA, Lamas GA, Vaughan DE, et al: Effect of captopril on progressive ventricular dilatation after anterior myocardial infarction. *N Engl J Med* 319:80–86, 1988.

69. Pfeffer MA, Braunwald E, Moye LA, et al: Effect of captopril on mortality and morbidity in patients with left ventricular dysfunction after myocardial infarction. Results of the survival and ventricular enlargement trial. The SAVE Investigators. *N Engl J Med* 327:669–677, 1992.
70. Effect of ramipril on mortality and morbidity of survivors of acute myocardial infarction with clinical evidence of heart failure. The Acute Infarction Ramipril Efficacy (AIRE) Study Investigators. *Lancet* 342:821–828, 1993.
71. Køber L, Torp-Pedersen C, Carlsen JE, et al: A clinical trial of the angiotensin-converting enzyme inhibitor trandolapril in patients with left ventricular dysfunction after myocardial infarction. Trandolapril Cardiac Evaluation (TRACE) Study Group. *N Engl J Med* 333(25):1670–1676, 1995.
72. Pfeffer MA, McMurray JJ, Velazquez EJ, et al: Valsartan, captopril, or both in myocardial infarction complicated by heart failure, left ventricular dysfunction, or both. *N Engl J Med* 349:1893–1906, 2003.
73. Pitt B, Remme W, Zannad F, et al: Eplerenone, a selective aldosterone blocker, in patients with left ventricular dysfunction after myocardial infarction. *N Engl J Med* 348:1309–1321, 2003. Erratum in *N Engl J Med* 348:2271, 2003.
74. Ibanez B, Macaya C, Sánchez-Brunete V, et al: Effect of early metoprolol on infarct size in ST-segment elevation myocardial infarction patients undergoing primary percutaneous coronary intervention. *Circulation* 128(14):1495–1503; 2013.
75. Dargie HJ: Effect of carvedilol on outcome after myocardial infarction in patients with left-ventricular dysfunction: the CAPRICORN randomised trial. *Lancet* 357:1385–1390, 2001.
76. Doughty RN, Whalley GA, Walsh HA, et al: Effects of carvedilol on left ventricular remodeling after acute myocardial infarction: the CAPRICORN echo substudy. *Circulation* 109:201–206, 2004.

Chapter 192 ■ Valvular Heart Disease

GARRICK C. STEWART • PATRICK T. O'GARA

The incidence of valvular heart disease continues to rise owing to the increasing longevity of the population and, thus, remains a source of significant morbidity and mortality [1]. More than 5 million Americans are living with valvular heart disease, and nearly 100,000 undergo valve surgery each year [2]. Patients with native or prosthetic valvular heart disease constitute a significant proportion of intensive care unit (ICU) admissions. Many patients will come to medical attention during an acute illness that triggers an abrupt change of cardiac physiology. Although stabilization with medical management is possible for patients with mild-to-moderate disease, surgery may be urgently required when severe valvular heart disease is present. A prompt diagnosis requires a high index of suspicion as defined by the clinical history and a careful physical examination [3]. Timely cardiac imaging with transthoracic echocardiography (TTE) can define valve anatomy and lesion severity. Transesophageal echocardiography (TEE) may be required in selected circumstances for better visualization of valve structures and characterization of the hemodynamics. The need for an invasive hemodynamic assessment may follow. An early collaboration among intensivists, cardiologists, and cardiac surgeons is critical for optimizing patient outcomes. This chapter highlights an integrated approach to the diagnosis and treatment of the native and prosthetic valve disease most commonly encountered in an ICU setting.

AORTIC STENOSIS

Aortic stenosis (AS) is a progressive disease for which there is no medical treatment. The ICU management of patients with AS may be quite challenging, particularly in the setting of concomitant medical illness. Characterizing the severity of stenosis is critical for determining the timing of surgical intervention and requires a careful history, physical examination, and initial imaging with TTE (Fig. 192.1)

Etiology

AS accounts for one-quarter of all chronic valvular heart disease, with approximately 80% of symptomatic cases occurring in adult males. Common etiologies of valvular AS include age-related calcific degeneration, stenosis of a congenitally bicuspid valve, and rheumatic heart disease. Age-related degenerative calcific AS is the most common cause of AS among adults in the USA, but

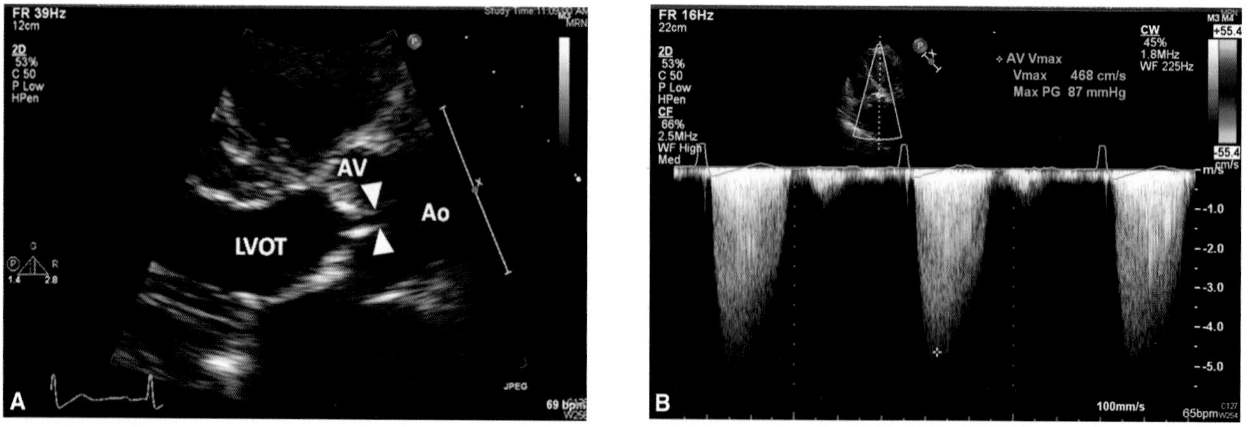

FIGURE 192.1 Transthoracic echocardiogram of severe valvular aortic stenosis. **A:** Transthoracic echocardiogram parasternal long axis view of the aortic valve during systole. Aortic valve leaflets are thickened with severely restricted motion consistent with severe aortic stenosis. *Solid arrowheads* point out minimal leaflet excursion consistent with stenosis. Ao, aortic root; AV, aortic valve, LVOT, left ventricular outflow track. **B:** Transaortic continuous wave Doppler jet from the apical five chamber view. Peak transaortic velocity is 4.68 m per second, producing an estimated peak transaortic gradient of 87 mm Hg.

bicuspid disease has become the most common etiology noted at time of isolated aortic valve replacement (AVR) surgery for AS [4]. Over 30% of adults >65 years of age exhibit aortic valve sclerosis, whereas 2% have more severe valvular stenosis. The valve cusps are focally thickened or calcified in aortic sclerosis, with production of a systolic ejection murmur, but without significant outflow obstruction (peak jet velocity <2.5 m per second). Recent studies suggest that calcific AS is the end result of an active disease process rather than the inevitable consequence of aging [5,6]. There may also be a genetic predisposition to calcific degeneration of trileaflet valves [7]. The histologic appearance of a sclerotic valve is similar to atherosclerosis, with inflammation, calcification, and thickening, though the pathologic processes of valve fibrosis/calcification and atherosclerosis are not identical [8]. Both calcific AS and aortic sclerosis appear to be a marker for coronary heart disease events [9]. Older age, male sex, smoking, diabetes mellitus, hypertension, chronic kidney disease, and hypercholesterolemia are all risk factors for calcific AS. High-dose lipid-lowering therapy has not been shown to retard the progression of AS in randomized trials [10,11].

Congenitally bicuspid aortic valves are present in 1% to 2% of the population, with a 4 to 1 male predominance, and seldom result in serious narrowing of the aortic orifice in childhood [12]. Abnormal valve architecture makes the two cusps susceptible to hemodynamic stresses, ultimately leading to thickening, calcification, and fusion of leaflets; and narrowing of the orifice [13] AS develops earlier in bicuspid valves, usually in the fifth or sixth decades, compared with trileaflet aortic valves, which usually do not develop calcific AS until the sixth or seventh decade of life [14]. Bicuspid aortic valves are also associated with aortic regurgitation, aortic root dilatation, and aortic coarctation (Fig. 192.2). Up to 25% to 40% of patients with bicuspid aortic valve will have a root or ascending aortic aneurysm unrelated to the severity of the valve lesion. Patients with bicuspid aortic valves are susceptible to aortic dissection [15]. Cystic medial degeneration similar to that seen in Marfan syndrome is responsible for aneurysm development with a bicuspid aortic valve [16]

Rheumatic disease may affect the aortic leaflets, leading to commissural fusion, fibrosis, and calcification, with narrowing of the valve orifice. Rheumatic AS is almost always accompanied by involvement of the mitral valve and concomitant aortic regurgitation. Radiation-induced AS as a sequela of cancer radiotherapy often occurs in conjunction with proximal coronary artery disease. Rare causes of valvular AS include Paget's disease of the bone; rheumatoid arthritis; and ochronosis. By the time AS becomes severe, dense calcification and thickening may make it difficult to determine the underlying valve architecture and the precise etiology of AS.

In addition to valvular AS, other causes of left ventricular (LV) outflow obstruction include hypertrophic obstructive cardiomyopathy (HOCM); discrete congenital subvalvular AS resulting from a fibromuscular membrane; and supravalvular AS. The various causes of LV outflow obstruction can be differentiated by careful physical examination and TTE.

Pathophysiology

Obstruction to LV outflow produces a pressure gradient between the LV and the aorta (Fig. 192.3). The ventricle responds to this pressure overload by slowly developing concentric hypertrophy, which is initially adaptive because it reduces wall stress. The law of Laplace states that wall stress is directly proportional to the product of LV pressure and radius, and inversely proportional to LV wall thickness. Compensatory hypertrophy may accommodate a large pressure gradient for years before it becomes maladaptive and LV function declines, with chamber dilatation and reduced cardiac output [17]. In the setting of AS with preserved ejection fraction, cardiac output may be normal at rest but fail to rise appropriately with exercise. Coronary flow reserve may be reduced because of the increased oxygen demand of the hypertrophied LV;

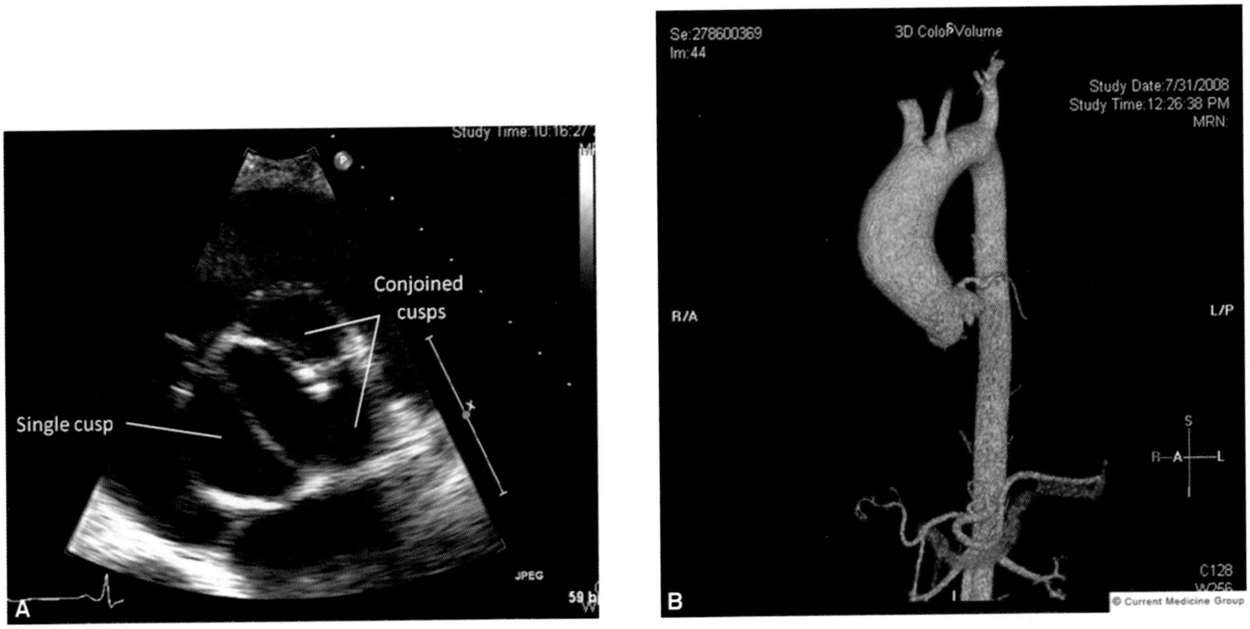

FIGURE 192.2 Bicuspid aortic valve and aortic root aneurysm. A: Transthoracic echocardiogram with parasternal short axis view at the level of the aortic valve reveals a bicuspid aortic valve with fusion of the right and left coronary cusps. B: A 5.1-cm ascending aortic aneurysm in a 37-year-old man with bicuspid aortic valve disease and only moderate aortic stenosis (valve area, 1.2 cm^2). Patients with bicuspid disease frequently develop aneurysms of the ascending aorta independent of the severity of hemodynamic valvular impairment, and are at risk for aortic dissection. Resection is indicated for maximal aneurysm size larger than 5.0 cm, an increase in aneurysm size of more than 0.5 cm per year, or at the time of aortic valve replacement if the aneurysm size exceeds 4.5 cm (From Libby P (ed.): *Essential Atlas of Cardiovascular Disease*. Berlin, Springer, 2009, p 216, Figure 9-6, with permission.).

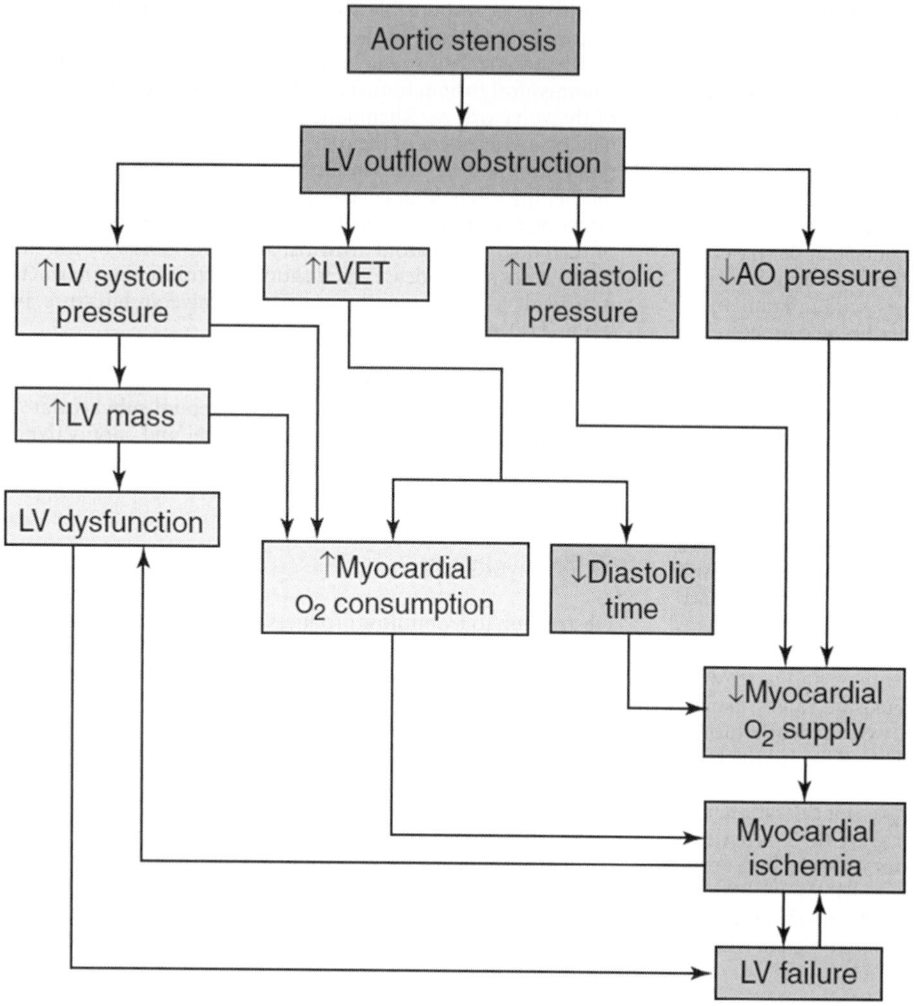

FIGURE 192.3 Pathophysiology of AS. LV outflow obstruction results in a gradual increase in LV systolic pressure, an increase in LVET, an increase in LV diastolic pressure, and a decrease in mean Ao pressure. Increased LV systolic pressure results in compensatory LVH, which may lead to LV dysfunction and failure. Increased LV systolic pressure, LVH, and LVET increase myocardial oxygen (O_2). consumption. Increased LVET results in a decrease in LV diastolic time (myocardial perfusion time), and increased LV diastolic pressure and decreased Ao diastolic pressure decrease coronary perfusion pressure, thereby decreasing myocardial supply. Increased myocardial O_2 consumption and decreased myocardial O_2 supply produce myocardial ischemia, which further compromises LV function. AS, aortic stenosis; LV, left ventricular; LVET, left ventricular ejection time; Ao, aortic root; LVH, left ventricular hypertrophy. (Adapted from Bonow R, Braunwald E: Valvular heart disease, in Zipes D, et al. (ed): *Braunwald's Heart Disease*. Philadelphia, Elsevier, 2005, p 1585, with permission.).

the increased transmural pressure gradient; the decreased capillary density, and the increased distance across the hypertrophied LV that blood must travel to reach the subendocardium [18]. Taken together, these factors can contribute to subendocardial ischemia even in the absence of epicardial coronary artery disease [19]. The loss of appropriately timed atrial contraction, such as that occurs with atrial fibrillation (AF), may cause rapid progression of symptoms because of the reliance on atrial systole to fill the stiff, hypertrophied LV.

No single parameter of valve structure or function is sufficient to define the severity of AS. Integration of the clinical history, physical examination, and TTE is required to place the lesion in context [20]. The physical examination of AS in the ICU may be particularly challenging, contributing to the greater importance of timely TTE. Echocardiographic criteria for severe AS among patients with normal underlying LV function include calcified leaflets with reduced excursion, maximal transaortic jet velocity of >4 m per second, mean gradient transaortic gradient of >40 mm Hg or an effective aortic valve orifice of <1 cm^2 (Table 192.1). When there is underlying LV systolic dysfunction, severe AS may be present despite low transaortic velocities, reduced flow, and low mean gradient (low-flow, low-gradient severe AS with low ejection fraction). Such patients are at particularly high risk for complications and require further evaluation (usually with dobutamine stress echocardiography) to determine if true valvular AS is present, or whether the reduced valve area relates to an underlying cardiomyopathy (pseudo-severe AS) [21]. Elderly, hypertensive patients might exhibit severe AS (valve area index <0.6/cm^2/m^2) with reduced flow (stroke volume index < 35 mL/m^2) despite a normal ejection fraction. Such "paradoxical" low-flow, low-gradient severe AS requires aggressive treatment of systemic hypertension and reevaluation with TTE [22].

Clinical Presentation

History

The cardinal symptoms of AS are dyspnea, angina, and syncope [23]. Exertional dyspnea is typically the first reported symptom

TABLE 192.1

Severity of Aortic Stenosis (normal LV systolic function, normal cardiac output [flow])

Severity of stenosis	Valve area (cm^2)	Mean gradient (mm Hg)	Jet velocity (m/s)
Mild	>1.5	<25	<3.0
Moderate	1.0–1.5	25–40	3.0–4.0
Severe	<1.0	>40	>4.0

LV, left atrial.

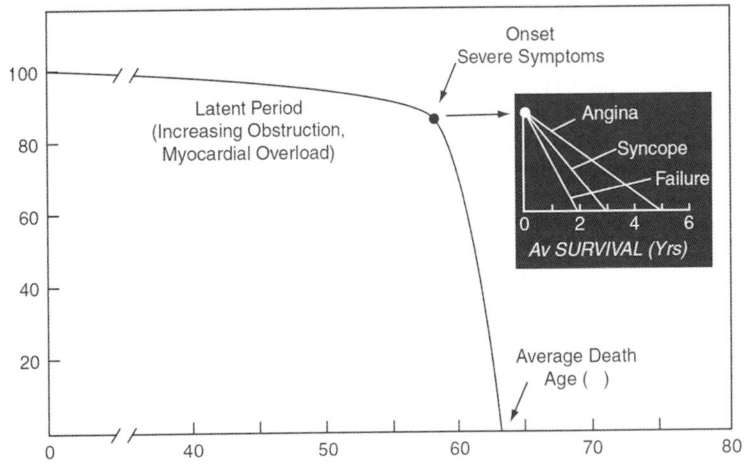

FIGURE 192.4 The onset of symptoms in patients with AS initiates a rapid rise in the risk of mortality. Patients with angina have a better prognosis than those with syncope. (From Ross J Jr, Braunwald E: Aortic stenosis. *Circulation* 38(1S5):61–67, 1968, with permission.)

and reflects an elevation in LV end-diastolic pressure transmitted to the pulmonary venous circulation. Some patients, particularly the elderly, may report generalized fatigue and weakness rather than dyspnea. Angina occurs in two-thirds of patients with AS and is similar to that reported by patients with flow-limiting coronary atherosclerosis [24]. Syncope is effort related and caused by cerebral hypoperfusion from a drop of mean arterial pressure produced by the combination of peripheral vasodilatation in the presence of a fixed cardiac output or an inappropriate baroreceptor reflex. Severe AS is also rarely associated with acquired von Willebrand's disease related to sheering of von Willebrand multimers passing through the stenotic orifice [25]. As a result, gastrointestinal bleeding, epistaxis, or ecchymoses may be present among patients with severe AS [25].

Most patients with AS have gradually increasing LV obstruction over many years, producing a long latent phase. During this clinically silent period, there is a very low risk of sudden death (<1% per year) [26]. The rate of AS progression is variable, with an average increase in mean gradient of 7 mm Hg and reduction of valve area of 0.1 cm^2 per year [27]. Symptoms from valvular AS are rare until the valve orifice has narrowed to approximately <1 cm^2. The onset of symptoms is a critical turning point in the natural history of the disease, usually indicates severe AS, and heralds the need for surgical evaluation and treatment because of the markedly reduced survival with symptomatic severe AS [23] (Fig. 192.4). An abrupt change in the natural history of AS may occur with AF, endocarditis, or myocardial infarction, each of which may trigger acute decompensation [28].

Physical Examination

The hallmark of AS is a carotid arterial pulse that rises slowly to a delayed peak, known as *pulsus parvus et tardus*. Among the elderly, stiffened carotid arterial walls may mask this finding. Similarly, patients with AS and concomitant aortic regurgitation may have preservation of the arterial pulsation caused by an elevated stroke volume. The LV apical impulse may be displaced laterally with a sustained contour caused by LV hypertrophy and prolonged systolic ejection in the face of valve obstruction.

The murmur of AS is a systolic ejection murmur commencing shortly after S1; rising in intensity with a peak in mid ejection; and then ending just before aortic valve closure. It is characteristically low-pitched; harsh or rasping in character; and best heard at the base of the heart in the second right intercostal space. The AS murmur is transmitted upward along the carotid arteries, though may sometimes be transmitted to the apex where it may be confused with the murmur of mitral regurgitation (Gallavardin phenomenon). The murmur of AS is diminished with the Valsalva maneuver and standing, in contrast to the murmur of LV outflow tract obstruction in hypertrophic cardiomyopathy, which gets louder with these maneuvers. Often, S2 becomes paradoxically split in severe AS because of prolonged LV ejection. An S4 is audible at the apex and reflects LV hypertrophy with an elevated LV end-diastolic pressure. An S3 generally occurs late in the course of AS when LV dilatation is present. Murmur intensity does not necessarily correspond to AS severity. The best predictors of AS severity on physical exam are a late peak to the systolic murmur, a single S2 (absent aortic valve closure sound) and *pulsus parvus et tardus*. Among patients with heart failure and a low cardiac output, the clinical examination may be misleadingly unimpressive.

Investigations

Electrocardiography

Most patients with severe AS will have electrocardiography (ECG) evidence of LVH. Left atrial (LA) enlargement is common. Nonspecific ST and T wave abnormalities may be seen or evidence of LV strain may be apparent. Rarely, atrioventricular conduction defects may develop because of extension of perivalvular calcium into the adjacent conduction system. This finding is more common after AVR. There is poor correlation between ECG findings and AS severity. The presence of left bundle branch block may equate with a higher risk of advanced AV block after valve replacement (either surgical or transcatheter).

Chest Radiography

The chest radiograph may be normal with severe AS. There may be "post-stenotic" dilation of the ascending aorta, or a widened mediastinum if aortic aneurysmal dilatation is present in patients with a bicuspid aortic valve. LV chamber size is usually normal, though aortic valve calcification may be seen, especially on the lateral film. Valvular calcium deposits can be visualized using fluoroscopy during cardiac catheterization, chest CT, or TTE. A normal chest X-ray does not exclude severe AS. In the later stages of AS, the LV dilates, leading to a widened cardiac silhouette, often accompanied by pulmonary congestion.

Echocardiography

TTE with Doppler is indicated for assessing the severity of AS. TTE visualized aortic valve structure, including the number of cusps; the degree of calcification; leaflet excursion; annular size; and supravalvular anatomy. Eccentric valve cusps are characteristic of congenitally bicuspid aortic valves and are often accompanied by aneurysmal enlargement of the root or ascending aorta. TTE is also useful for identifying coexisting valvular disease; differentiating valvular AS from other forms of LV outflow tract obstruction; checking for secondary pulmonary hypertension; and evaluating underlying biventricular function. The peak transvalvular jet velocity on continuous wave Doppler is critical for assessing AS severity. Peak and mean transvalvular gradients are derived from the jet velocity using the modified Bernoulli equation, and the aortic valve area is estimated from the continuity equation. The dimensionless index, which is the ratio of the LV outflow tract velocity time integral (VTI) to aortic VTI, can also be used to estimate AS severity when measurement of LV outflow tract diameter is difficult because of extensive calcification. A dimensionless index <0.25 is consistent with severe AS [20]. Advanced TTE techniques may be required to evaluate patients with suspected low-flow, low-gradient severe AS. Transesophageal echocardiography can be used when TTE images are inadequate to assess the severity of AS.

Cardiac Catheterization

Noninvasive assessment with TTE is now standard, but catheterization may be helpful when there is a discrepancy between the clinical and echocardiographic findings. Calculation of aortic valve area by invasive hemodynamic assessment requires accurate assessment of the transvalvular flow and mean transvalvular pressure gradient to calculate effective orifice area using the Gorlin formula [29]. Concerns have been raised about the risk of cerebral embolization during attempts to cross the aortic valve and directly measure the transaortic gradient. Angiography is indicated to detect coronary artery disease for patients >45 years old who are being considered for operative treatment of severe AS [30]. Coronary CT angiography is now performed more often for this indication.

Special Case: Low-flow/Low-gradient Aortic Stenosis

The appropriate diagnosis and management of patients with AS and a depressed ejection fraction (EF) can be vexing. Patients with anatomically severe AS and reduced EF (<40%) often have a relatively low pressure gradient (<30 mm Hg) because of a weakened ventricle. The true severity of AS can be difficult to determine when the cardiac output and transaortic gradient are low. If the ventricle itself is diseased and unable to generate sufficient systolic force to open the leaflets adequately, a reduced aortic valve area may be present at rest, overestimating AS severity. This condition is known as pseudo-severe AS [31]. In such cases, LV dysfunction is the predominant pathology and may be caused by prior MI or a primary cardiomyopathy. Patients with either true severe AS with reduced EF or pseudo-severe AS have a low-flow state with low trans-aortic gradients contributing to calculated aortic valve areas <1 cm^2. Pseudo-severe AS patients must be distinguished from those with true severe AS and poor LV function, since patients with true severe AS and flow reserve will usually benefit from valve surgery, whereas patients with pseudo-severe AS are not operative candidates [32–34].

Dobutamine stress echocardiography has a well-defined diagnostic role in this setting [35] (Fig. 192.5). The inotropic effects of low-dose dobutamine will increase transvalvular flow in patients with flow reserve [36]. Flow reserve is defined as

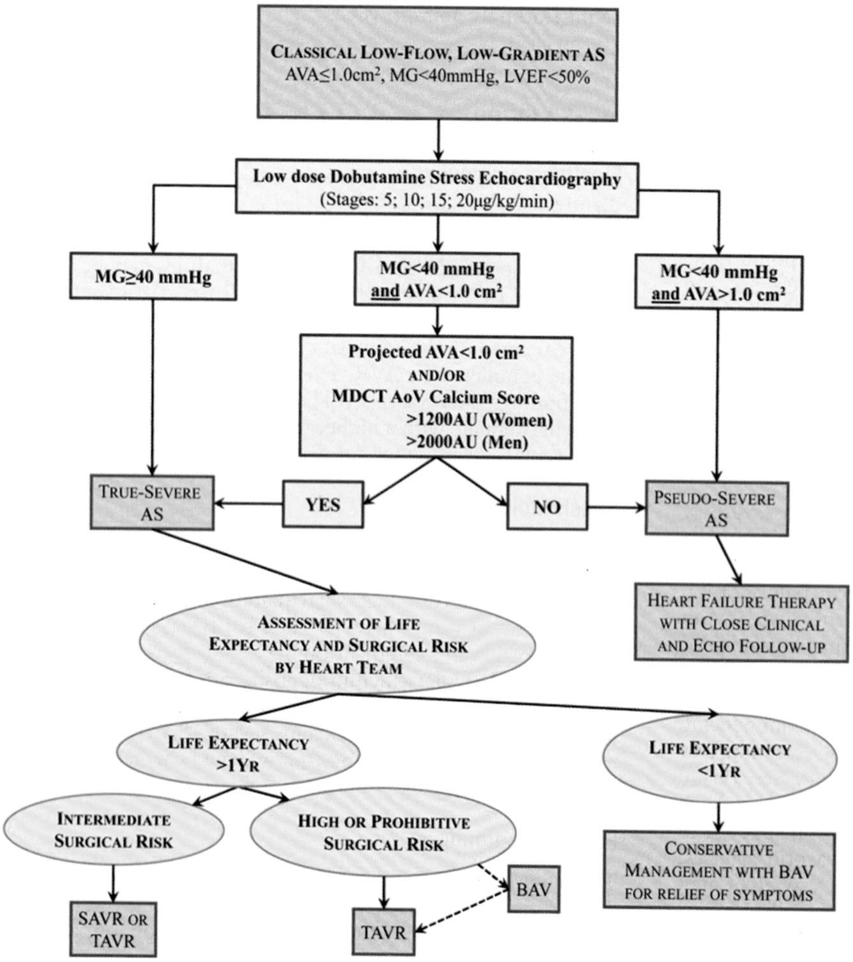

FIGURE 192.5. Algorithm for the management of classical (reduced left ventricular ejection fraction) low-flow, low-gradient AS. AS, aortic stenosis; AoV, aortic valve; AVA, aortic valve area; BAV, bicuspid aortic valve; LVEF, left ventricular ejection fraction; MDCT, multidetector computed tomography; MG, mean gradient; SAVR, surgical aortic valve replacement; TAVR, transcatheter aortic valve replacement (From Clavel MA, Magne J, Pibarot P. Low-gradient aortic stenosis. *Eur Heart J* 2016;37:2645–2657, used with permission.).

an increase in stroke volume with inotropic infusion of >20%. Dobutamine infusion, particularly at doses <20 μg/kg/min, is generally well tolerated, but should only be performed at experienced centers with a cardiologist in attendance. In patients with genuine severe AS and LV dysfunction, dobutamine will increase cardiac output and mean transvalvular gradient but calculated aortic valve area will remain low (<1 cm^2). Patients with pseudo-severe AS will have an increase in aortic valve area into a range no longer considered severe (>1.2 cm^2) with little change in transvalvular gradient. Some patients will not have any flow response to dobutamine, signaling a poor prognosis [37]. Surgery is indicated in true severe AS with flow reserve after dobutamine challenge, and generally contraindicated for patients with pseudo-severe AS or those without contractile reserve [30]. Patients with low-flow, low-gradient AS with reduced EF undergoing AVR have a significantly higher perioperative and long-term mortality if multivessel coronary artery disease is also present [33,38]. The evaluation of patients with low-flow, low-gradient severe AS and preserved EF can also be challenging and requires input from an imaging and valve disease expert.

Intensive Care Unit Management

AVR is the preferred treatment strategy for patients with symptomatic severe AS and for asymptomatic patients with severe AS who have a reduced ejection fraction (<50%). In contrast, surgery may be postponed for patients with severe, asymptomatic AS and normal LV function, as these patients may do well for years [39]. AVR is also indicated for patients with moderate AS who require other cardiac surgery, such as coronary artery bypass grafting (CABG) or aortic aneurysm repair. Patients with severe AS and cardiogenic shock may have percutaneous aortic balloon valvuloplasty (PABV) as a bridge to AVR.

The choice between surgical and transcatheter AVR (SAVR, TAVR) is determined by a multidisciplinary heart valve team that includes cardiologists, interventionalists, imaging specialists, and cardiac surgeons. TAVR is now considered for patients deemed to be a prohibitive, high, or intermediate surgical risk as assessed by the Society for Thoracic Surgeons (STS) Predicted Risk of Mortality (PROM) Score in combination with an assessment for frailty, procedure-specific risk (e.g., a highly calcified ascending aorta), and the presence of vital organ system dysfunction [40]. Many ICU patients have advanced comorbidities that make TAVR an attractive means for treatment of AS.

Medical Management

Medical interventions for severe AS are largely supportive until surgery is feasible. In patients with severe AS with heart failure or cardiogenic shock, management should be guided by invasive hemodynamic monitoring with a pulmonary artery catheter. Diuresis may relieve pulmonary congestion, but caution is advised. For patients in cardiogenic shock, arterial pressure should be supported with inotropes and/or vasopressors until valve surgery can be performed. Vasodilators are generally contraindicated, except for selected patients with depressed ejection fraction [41]. In these select patients with EF <35%; severe AS; and cardiogenic shock accompanied by high systemic vascular resistance, sodium nitroprusside infusion has been shown to modestly improve hemodynamics, and can serve as a bridge to the operating room [42].

Aortic Valve Replacement

AVR is the preferred treatment for severe symptomatic AS [30,43]. Choice of surgical valve prosthesis depends on patient age, anticipated lifespan, and preference for and tolerance of anticoagulation [44]. The perioperative mortality for isolated SAVR ranges from <1% in healthy, younger patients with normal LV systolic function, to 10% or more in elderly patients with coexisting CAD and reduced EF who require concomitant CABG. Age alone is not a contraindication to SAVR. Other factors associated with reduced survival after SAVR include chronic kidney disease, obstructive lung disease, coronary artery disease, reoperation, emergency operation, and age >65 years. The overall 10-year survival for patients with SAVR is approximately 60%.

Balloon aortic valvuloplasty (BAV) is often used instead of an operation for children and young adults with congenital, noncalcific AS. During the procedure in adults, a balloon in placed across the stenotic aortic valve and inflated to high pressure to fracture adherent calcium and increase effective orifice area [45]. A technically successful procedure can reduce the transaortic valve gradient to a mild degree, but rarely increase valve area to >1 cm^2. Valvuloplasty is not widely used among adults with severe calcific AS because of high restenosis rates, high frequency of embolic complications (particularly stroke), and the development of aortic regurgitation [46] among adults with acutely decompensated AS, BAV is particularly high risk and has no proven long-term benefits [47]. BAV is almost entirely restricted to its performance during TAVR.

TAVR has an established and growing role in the management of patients with symptomatic severe AS (Fig. 192.6) [40]. The transfemoral access route is strongly preferred whenever

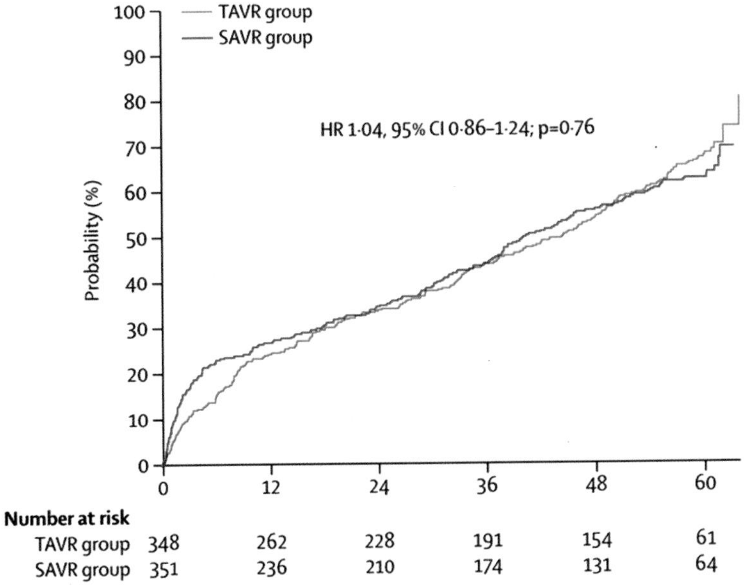

FIGURE 192.6 Five-year outcomes of transcatheter (TAVR, *blue*) or surgical aortic valve replacement (SAVR, *red*) in high surgical risks patients with aortic stenosis. Kaplan–Meier analysis of all-cause death in the intention-to-treat analysis of the PARTNER 1 randomized trial (From Mack MJ, Leon MB, et al. 5-year outcomes of transcatheter aortic valve replacement or surgical aortic valve replacement for high surgical risk patients with aortic stenosis (PARTNER 1). *Lancet* 2015;385:2477–2484, used with permission.).

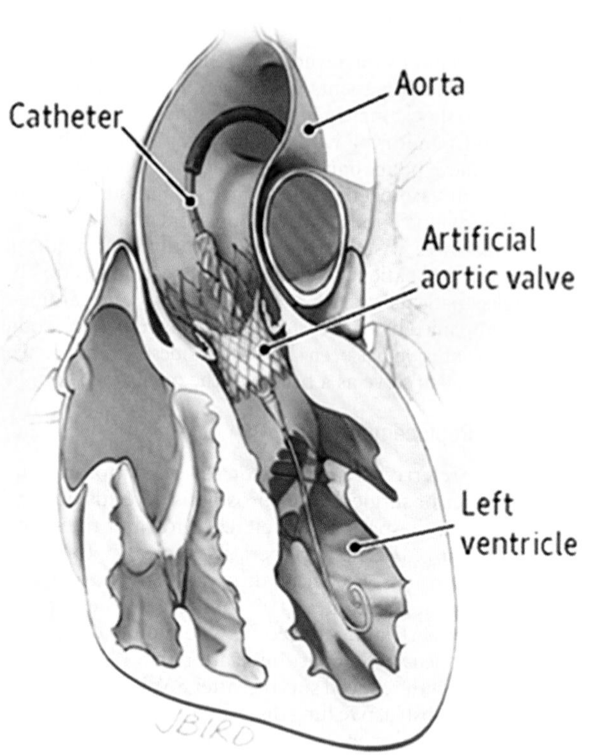

FIGURE 192.7 Placement of a transcatheter aortic valve via the femoral approach (Adapted from Jin J. Transcatheter aortic valve replacement. *JAMA* 312:2059, 2014, used with permission.).

possible and is largely dictated by the iliofemoral and aortic anatomy, although other access sites are available (subclavian, transaortic, transapical) (Fig. 192.7). Early and late results have been excellent, but concerns remain about vascular injury, stroke, paravalvular leak, the need for permanent pacing and long-term durability of the prosthesis [48,49]. Transcatheter valve-in-valve implantation is available in many centers for treatment of high-risk patients with structural deterioration of a previously implanted bioprosthesis [50].

AORTIC REGURGITATION

Acute severe aortic regurgitation (AR) may occur in previously normal or only mildly diseased valves and often results in abrupt hemodynamic decompensation and respiratory compromise requiring ICU admission. Acute valvular regurgitation is a surgical emergency, but accurate diagnosis may be a challenge since exam findings may be subtle and the clinical presentation nonspecific [51]. Patients with acute AR appear gravely ill and have tachycardia, significant dyspnea, and often hypotension. The presentation of acute AR may even be mistaken for other acute conditions like sepsis, pneumonia, or nonvalvular heart failure. In marked contrast, chronic severe AR may be asymptomatic or minimally symptomatic and is rarely encountered in the ICU setting. In cases of acute valvular regurgitation, a high index of suspicion is required, along with timely TTE, and prompt surgical consultation.

Etiology

Most cases of acute severe AR are caused by infective endocarditis (IE), but other causes include aortic dissection and blunt chest trauma. Staphylococci have emerged as the most important causative agents of native valve endocarditis [52,53]. Patients with antecedent aortic valve disease or a congenital bicuspid valve are at increased risk for IE, though organisms like *S. aureus* can infect a normal trileaflet valve [54]. IE is a particular problem among injection drug users, patients with indwelling catheters, and those on hemodialysis. Acute severe AR from IE is the consequence of tissue destruction, leaflet perforation, or bulky vegetations impairing leaflet coaptation [55].

AR is present in up to 65% of patients with Stanford Type A aortic dissection [56]. Ascending aortic dissection may be seen in the setting of Marfan syndrome, bicuspid aortic valve, or in patients following previous CABG or AVR surgery. Retrograde extension of the dissection flap into the annulus may cause prolapse or eversion of the aortic valve leaflets. Type A aortic dissection with AR is a surgical emergency requiring prompt diagnosis and intervention [57]. Aneurysmal enlargement of the aortic root without dissection may also lead to AR. Though AR is usually chronic when produced by aortic root dilatation, an acute-on-chronic decompensation may occur if there is superimposed dissection or abrupt aneurysm enlargement [58]. Important causes of aortic root pathology producing AR include connective tissue disorders (Marfan syndrome and Ehlers–Danlos syndrome) and vasculitis (syphilitic aortitis, giant cell arteritis, or Takayasu's arteritis). Aortic leaflet tears, perforation, or detachment producing AR may also follow blunt chest trauma or occur as a complication of BAV for AS [59].

Pathophysiology

Unlike in chronic AR, the LV in acute AR has not had time to develop compensatory eccentric hypertrophy in response to elevated afterload and preload (Fig. 192.8). The nondilated, noncompliant LV receives a significant diastolic volume load from the regurgitant flow, resulting in an abrupt rise in LV end-diastolic pressure. This pressure may in turn be transmitted to the pulmonary bed, resulting in pulmonary edema. Since the LV cannot dilate acutely in response to the volume load, forward stroke volume is decreased, and tachycardia develops to maintain cardiac output. Impaired forward stroke volume leads to decreased systolic pressure and a narrower than anticipated pulse pressure. Patients may present with signs of impending cardiogenic shock. LV diastolic pressure may equilibrate with aortic pressure during the latter half of diastole (diastasis), resulting in attenuation of the AR murmur in the acute setting. The elevation of end-diastolic pressure and tachycardia can increase myocardial oxygen demand and, when coupled with decreased diastolic coronary blood flow owing to lower aortic diastolic pressure, can reduce myocardial perfusion and result in coronary ischemia. Ischemia from AR can be compounded by impaired coronary flow from preexisting atherosclerosis or an aortic dissection flap. In acute severe AR, LV failure and cardiogenic shock develop if surgery is not promptly performed.

Clinical Presentation

History

Acute AR may present with little or no warning. Symptoms like weakness, profound dyspnea, angina, and presyncope are common. Antecedent valve disease, fever, and skin findings may suggest IE. Severe, ripping chest or back pain with hypertension may indicate aortic dissection. Signs of blunt chest trauma may be disarmingly subtle. The natural history of acute severe AR is one of LV failure and death in the absence of rapid intervention. Patients with chronic AR may present acutely with a sudden worsening of their underlying pathology.

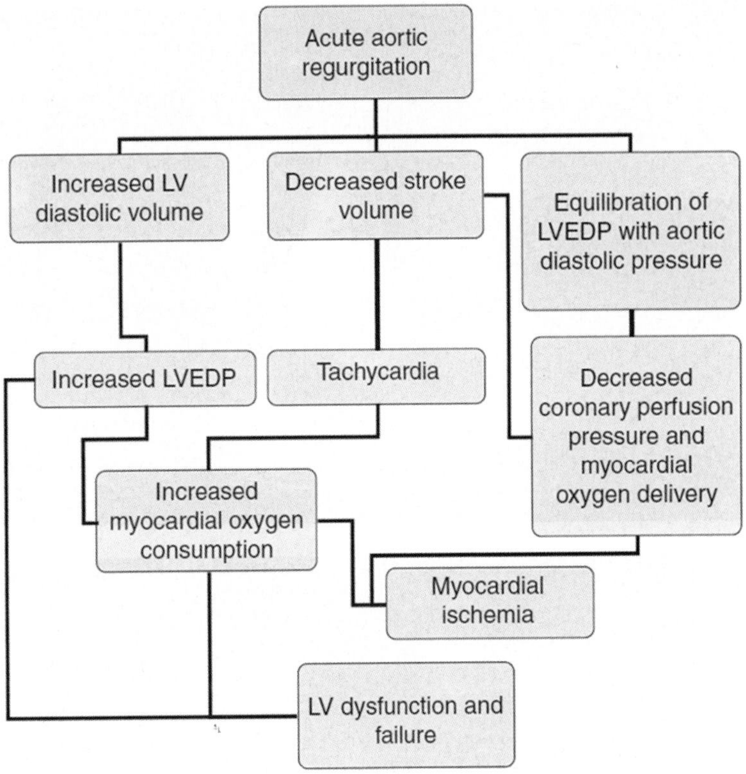

FIGURE 192.8 Pathophysiology of acute aortic regurgitation. LV, left ventricle; LVEDP, left ventricular end diastolic pressure (Adapted from Bonow R, Braunwald E: Valvular heart disease, in Zipes D, et al. (ed): *Braunwald's Heart Disease*. Philadelphia, Elsevier, 2005, with permission.).

Physical Examination

The classic eponymous signs observed in chronic AR are attenuated or absent in acute AR so the degree of AR may be greatly underestimated. Patients are often tachycardic with low or low–normal blood pressure. Pulse pressure may underestimate AR severity in the acute setting. Tachypnea, accessory muscle use, and hypoxemia are worrisome findings, and pulmonary rales are common. LV apical impulse is not displaced unless prior LV dysfunction was present. The first heart sound (S1) is often soft owing to premature closure of the mitral valve from the rapid LV diastolic pressure rise. There is often a low-pitched systolic ejection murmur from increased flow across the aortic valve, whereas the diastolic murmur is of grade 1 or 2 intensity and is of short duration. A pulse deficit or relative decrease may be appreciated in the setting of AR from aortic dissection.

Investigations

Electrocardiography

Sinus tachycardia is often present, though the ECG may be entirely normal in acute severe AR. In contrast, LV hypertrophy is a feature of chronic AR. Nonspecific ST-segment and T-wave abnormalities or signs of LV strain are common. With IE, if there is paravalvular extension of the infection in the region of the atrioventricular node, a heart block of varying degree may be present. In the setting of acute heart failure, supraventricular and ventricular tachycardias may occur.

Chest radiography

The cardiac silhouette may be normal, unless AR is chronic or there was a preexisting heart disease. Pulmonary edema is common and characterized by cephalization of pulmonary vein flow and Kerley B lines. A widened mediastinum may signify aortic dissection or thoracic aortic aneurysm.

Echocardiography

Urgent TTE is mandated whenever acute AR is suspected. Echocardiography can determine the etiology and hemodynamic severity of AR while providing information about the underlying LV function, aortic size, and coexisting valvular heart disease (Fig. 192.9). Severe AR is characterized by a wide regurgitant jet (vena contracta >7 mm) and holodiastolic flow reversal in the descending thoracic aorta [60,61]. The rapid rise in LV diastolic pressure with acute severe AR produces a short pressure half time (<250 ms) and premature mitral valve closure [62]. CT angiography has become the preferred imaging test to assess for acute dissection, but TEE may be indicated if the study is nondiagnostic and is crucial for intraoperative planning [63–65].

Cardiac catheterization

Establishing the hemodynamic severity of AR seldom requires catheterization, which can delay surgery [66]. Younger patients without coronary risk factors may proceed directly to emergency valve replacement without angiography. Patients with Type A dissection should proceed directly to surgical repair.

Intensive Care Unit Management

Medical management

Acute severe AR has a high mortality rate. Medical management should not delay urgent or emergent surgery. Congestive heart failure and cardiogenic shock are the principal targets of acute medical therapies. Use of vasodilators, particularly sodium

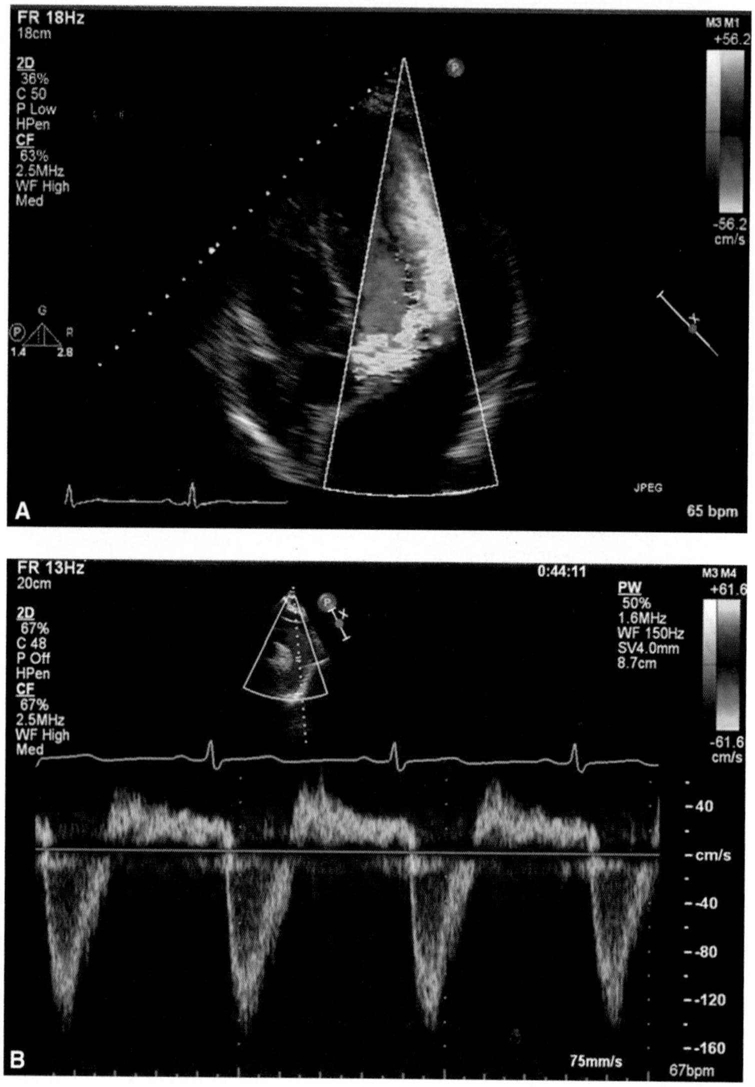

FIGURE 192.9 Echocardiographic appearance of severe aortic regurgitation. **A:** Transthoracic echocardiogram apical four chamber view with severe aortic regurgitation from infective endocarditis. Color Doppler shows ventricular filling from the aorta during diastole. **B:** Pulse wave Doppler of the descending thoracic aortic reveals holodiastolic flow reversal consistent with severe aortic regurgitation.

nitroprusside, and diuretics is the mainstay of medical therapy, as the systemic blood pressure allows [67,68]. Inotropes such as dopamine or dobutamine may be used to augment forward cardiac output. Pulmonary edema from acute AR frequently requires intubation and mechanical ventilation. Intra-aortic balloon counterpulsation (IABP) is strictly contraindicated. β-Blockers should only be considered for cases of acute aortic dissection. Antibiotics are indicated for IE, but surgery must not be delayed once heart failure intervenes [30].

Surgical treatment

Surgery is indicated for acute severe AR, unless overwhelming patient comorbidities dictate otherwise. AVR is often performed, but valve repair may be possible for many cases of dissection. Many surgeons favor the use of homograft material for management of aortic valve/root IE, given the low reinfection rates with cadaveric tissue. A composite valve–graft conduit may be used when disease dictates replacement of both the aortic root and the valve [69]. Perioperative risk depends largely on age; preoperative LV function; etiology; and urgency of surgery. Debridement of periaortic abscess or aortic root replacement compounds operative risk.

MITRAL STENOSIS

Widespread use of programs to detect and treat of Group A streptococcal pharyngitis has reduced the incidence of rheumatic fever in the developed world, the leading cause of MS [70]. The burden of rheumatic valve disease in the developing world remains considerable and is a significant cause of premature death. Most cases of rheumatic MS in the USA are seen in patients who have recently emigrated from endemic areas [1]. MS often presents as acute heart failure and, when symptomatic, requires mechanical relief of LV inflow obstruction. ICU management goals include treatment of heart failure, rate control of AF, and preparation for valvotomy or valve replacement surgery.

Etiology

Rheumatic fever produces valvular inflammation and scarring, though nearly half of patients may not recall as history of acute rheumatic fever or chorea. Two-thirds of patients with rheumatic MS are female and 40% of patients with rheumatic valvular disease will have isolated MS [71]. Screening TTE in endemic areas may detect up to 10 times as many cases of rheumatic valve disease compared to clinical screening alone [72]. By contrast, in developed countries, MS is more commonly produced by calcific degeneration of the annulus and mitral leaflets, congenital abnormalities of mitral inflow, or collagen vascular diseases such as lupus or rheumatoid arthritis [73]. Atrial myxoma may mimic MS by causing obstruction to LV inflow. The natural history of MS is often dependent on the patient's socioeconomic status. In developing countries patients tend to be younger with a more pliable valve, whereas in developed countries patients are older with comorbid conditions [74]. Patients in low- or middle-income countries also have relatively less access to programs for screening; detection; medical and surgical treatment; and anticoagulation management.

Pathophysiology

Rheumatic fever leads to inflammation and scarring of the mitral valve, with fusion of the valve commissures and subvalvular apparatus [70]. Although the initial insult is rheumatic, altered flow patterns may lead to calcification and further valve deformity, leading to a narrow funnel-shaped valve. Calcific degeneration of acquired mitral valve thickening may also produce MS. The mitral orifice is normally 4 to 6 cm^2. MS develops when the area is reduced to <2 cm^2 so that an elevated left atrioventricular pressure gradient is required to propel blood across the mitral valve. Severe MS is present when the valve area is <1.5 cm^2; the mean gradient is usually >10 mm Hg. An elevated LA pressure leads to pulmonary hypertension (PA pressure >30 mm Hg), exercise intolerance and eventually right-sided heart failure. Adequate transit time is required to allow blood to flow across the stenotic mitral valve during diastole.

Clinical Manifestations

History

MS is a slowly progressive disease with a latent period of up to two decades between the episode of rheumatic carditis and symptom onset. Progression of MS in developing countries is more rapid and may be associated with recurrent episodes of rheumatic fever. The typical patient will have an asymptomatic period with an abnormal physical exam. As MS progresses, lesser stresses precipitate the symptoms, making the patient limited in daily activities; orthopnea and paroxysmal nocturnal dyspnea develop. Pulmonary edema in previously asymptomatic individuals may be triggered by tachyarrhythmias (AF), volume overload, fever, anemia, hyperthyroidism, or pregnancy [75]. Each of these circumstances shortens the diastolic filling period and elevates the LA to LV transvalvular gradient. Development of persistent AF marks a turning point in the patient's course, with an accelerated rate of symptom progression. Systemic embolization may be the first clue to the presence of MS, irrespective of underlying rhythm [76]. Patients may also suffer from hemoptysis because of shunting between the pulmonary and bronchial veins, leading to rupture. Underappreciated calcific MS may also be identified after failure to wean from mechanical ventilation.

The overall 10-year survival with untreated MS is 50% to 60% [77]. Asymptomatic patients have a survival of >80% at 10 years, whereas symptomatic MS led to death within 2 to 5 years in the era before the development of mitral valvotomy [78]. Once pulmonary hypertension develops (>50 mm Hg PA systolic pressure), mean survival is less than 3 years. The common causes of death associated with MS are heart failure, systemic embolism, and infections, including endocarditis.

Physical Examination

MS produces signs of heart failure, including pulmonary rales, peripheral edema, ascites, an elevated jugular venous pressure, and congestive hepatomegaly. Patients with severe MS may also have a malar flush with pinched and blue facies. The first heart sound (S1) is usually accentuated in the early phases of the disease. The opening snap (OS) of MS is best appreciated in early diastole during expiration near the cardiac apex. The time interval between aortic valve closure (A2) and OS varies inversely with the severity of MS, and the height of the LA pressures. The OS is followed by a low-pitched rumbling diastolic murmur best heard at the apex with the patient in the left lateral decubitus position. Presystolic accentuation of the murmur may be present in sinus rhythm. In general, the duration of the murmur corresponds to the severity of stenosis. If the valve is heavily calcified and immobile, with low cardiac output or AF, it may be relatively "silent" with a soft S1, absent presystolic accentuation, and an inaudible diastolic rumble. Associated valvular lesions, including the murmurs of AR, pulmonic regurgitation (PR), and tricuspid regurgitation (TR), may be present, along with a loud P2 from pulmonary hypertension or a parasternal lift from right ventricle (RV) pressure or volume overload.

Investigations

Electrocardiogram

The ECG in sinus rhythm may reveal LA enlargement, but AF can be present at any stage in the natural history. A vertical QRS axis may be present along with nonspecific ST-segment and T-wave abnormalities. Signs of RV hypertrophy signify advanced disease.

Chest Radiograph

Radiographic changes with MS include LA enlargement; dilation of the main PA and its central branches; RV enlargement; and signs of pulmonary vascular congestion. Interstitial or alveolar edema signifies a marked and often acute elevation of pulmonary capillary wedge pressure.

Echocardiography

Rheumatic MS is characterized by thickened mitral leaflet tips, immobility of the posterior leaflet, and restricted anterior leaflet motion. Calcific MS is marked by dense echogenic deposits throughout the mitral apparatus and turbulent LV diastolic inflow. Direct planimetry to measure valve area may be difficult in heavily calcified valves [79]. Continuous wave Doppler can be used to estimate the LA–LV pressure gradient. Estimates of mitral valve area can be made by the pressure half-time technique or the continuity equation [80]. Careful assessment of the degree and location of valvular calcification; thickening of the leaflet and subvalvular apparatus; and leaflet mobility can determine suitability for percutaneous mitral balloon valvuloplasty (PMBV) [81]. Routine assessment of chamber dimension and ventricular function should be performed. TEE is required to exclude LA thrombus in patients being considered for PMBV.

Cardiac catheterization

Catheterization may be necessary to determine the severity of stenosis when noninvasive and clinical data are discordant or as a prelude to PMBV (Fig. 192.10). Cardiac output and mean transvalvular gradient measurements are used to calculate mitral valve area using the Gorlin formula [29].

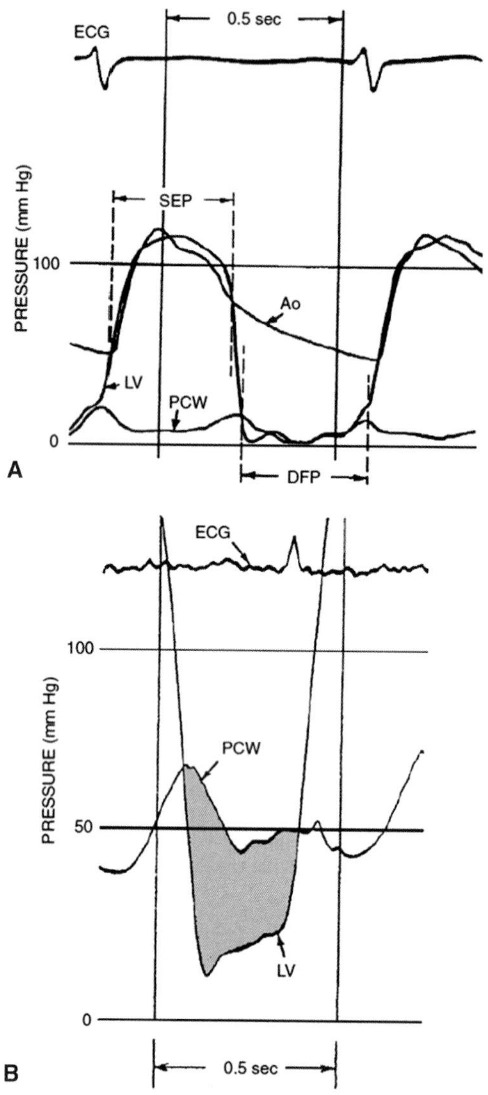

FIGURE 192.10 Hemodynamic measurements in mitral stenosis. **A:** Depicts normal LV, LA, and Ao pressure tracings. **B:** depicts the pressure gradient between PCW and LV in a patient with MS (*shaded area*). LV, left ventricle; LA, left atrial; Ao, aortic; PCW, pulmonary capillary wedge pressure; DFP, diastolic filling period; SEP, systolic ejection period (Adapted from Carabello BA: Modern management of mitral stenosis. *Circulation* 112(3):432–437, 2005, with permission.).

Intensive Care Unit Management

Medical Therapy

Acute MS typically manifests as pulmonary edema. Reversible precipitants must be identified, such as rapid AF, anemia, sepsis, volume overload, or thyrotoxicosis. Medical therapy is directed at rate control of AF, and alleviation of pulmonary and systemic congestion by loop diuretics. Nodal blocking agents such as β-blockers or non-dihydropyridine calcium-channel blockers are the preferred rate controlling agents and may be administered intravenously [82]. Cardioversion may be required in the acute setting to restore hemodynamic stability, though most patients respond to rate control. Anticoagulation should be initiated promptly. For patients with only mild-to-moderate MS, addressing one or more underlying precipitants will suffice without the need for mechanical intervention. Patients with severe MS have a poor prognosis without intervention, which may consist of PMBV, surgical commissurotomy, or mitral valve replacement (MVR) (Fig. 192.11).

Percutaneous Mitral Balloon Valvuloplasty

PMBV is the preferred treatment for symptomatic (NYHA Class II–IV) patients with isolated severe MS and favorable valve morphology. Unlike BAV, PMBV has achieved durable results. Ideal patients for PMBV are younger (<45 years old), have lower NYHA functional class, and have pliable mitral leaflets [83,84]. PMBV is performed by transseptal puncture, passing a guidewire across the mitral valve, and inflating a balloon (Inoue balloon) across the mitral orifice to split the commissures and widen the stenotic valve [46,85].

Successful PMBV doubles the mitral valve area, reduces mean transmitral gradient by half, and improves symptoms without development of significant mitral regurgitation (MR) [86]. Acute complications of PMBV include severe MR, residual atrial septal defect after transseptal puncture, and, less commonly, LV perforation, cardiac tamponade, and systemic emboli [30]. Overall procedural morality is between 0.4% and 3.0% [87]. Patients have excellent event-free survival after PMBV with rates of 80% to 90% over 3 to 7 years when performed by a skilled operator at a high-volume center [88]. Short and intermediate-term outcomes from PMBV are commensurate with open surgical commissurotomy, but with reduced morbidity and at lower cost [89]. There is a significant rate of restenosis after both percutaneous and surgical commissurotomy with most patients requiring a repeat procedure within 10 to 15 years.

Surgical Treatment

If the anatomy is unfavorable for PMBV or the procedure is unsuccessful, open surgical valvotomy may be performed, which requires cardiopulmonary bypass [90]. MVR is necessary in patients with MS and significant MR, and those in whom valve anatomy is too distorted to respond to commissurotomy repair alone. MVR is often performed with preservation of the chordal attachments to facilitate LV recovery. A surgical maze procedure of the LA or isolation of the pulmonary veins may also be performed to treat concomitant AF, though success rates are relatively lower for rheumatic MS patients. The average operative risk for MVR is 5%, with an overall 10-year survival in surgical survivors of 70%. Long-term prognosis is influenced by patient age, comorbid conditions, and the presence of concomitant pulmonary hypertension and RV dysfunction [91,92].

MITRAL REGURGITATION

Acute, severe mitral regurgitation (MR) presents with pulmonary edema and hemodynamic compromise because of the lack of time for the cardiopulmonary circuit to adapt to the additional volume load. Examination findings may be subtle and presentation may be mistaken for other acute conditions like pneumonia or nonvalvular decompensated heart failure. A high clinical index of suspicion; timely evaluation by TTE; and prompt referral for surgical consultation are of critical value in the management of this condition [51]. Many patients in the ICU will have MR accompanied by reduced LV systolic function, from either myocardial infarction (MI) or chronic cardiomyopathy. The surgical management of patients with MR and advanced systolic heart failure remains controversial.

Etiology

MR may be caused by abnormalities of any component of the mitral apparatus: annulus, valve leaflets, chordae tendineae, papillary muscles, and adjacent LV free wall [93] (Table 192.2). Common causes of acute MR include chordal rupture from mxyomatous degeneration, blunt trauma, or endocarditis; leaflet perforation from endocarditis or leaflet avulsion from trauma;

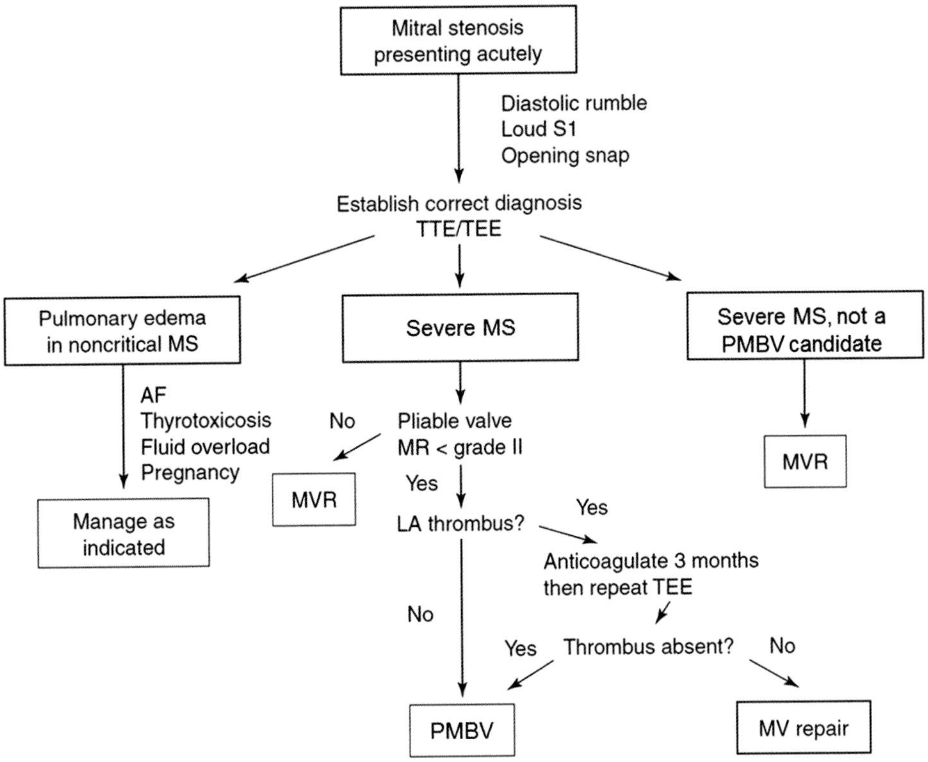

FIGURE 192.11 Management of the acute presentation of mitral stenosis. AF, atrial fibrillation; LA, left atrial; MR, mitral regurgitation; MS, mitral stenosis; MV, mitral valve; MVR, mitral valve replacement; PMBV, percutaneous mitral balloon valvuloplasty; S1, first heart sound; TEE, transesophageal echocardiography; TTE, transthoracic echocardiography (Adapted from Bellamy MF, Enriquez-Sarano M: Valvular heart disease, in Irwin RS, Rippe JM (eds): *Intensive Care Medicine* Philadelphia, Lippincott Williams & Wilkins, 2003, pp 313–328, with permission.).

TABLE 192.2

Causes of Chronic Mitral Regurgitation

- Mitral Annulus Disorders
  - Infective endocarditis (abscess formation)
  - Trauma (valvular heart surgery)
  - Paravalvular leak due to suture interruption (surgical technical problems or infective endocarditis)
- Mitral Leaflet Disorders
  - Infective endocarditis (perforation or interfering with valve closure by vegetation)
  - Trauma (tear during percutaneous balloon mitral valvuloplasty or penetrating chest injury)
  - Tumors (atrial myxoma)
  - Myxomatous degeneration
  - Systemic lupus erythematosus (Libman–Sacks lesion)
- Chordae Tendineae
  - Idiopathic (spontaneous)
  - Myxomatous degeneration (mitral valve prolapse, Marfan syndrome, and Ehlers–Danlos syndrome)
  - Infective endocarditis
  - Acute rheumatic fever
  - Trauma (percutaneous balloon valvuloplasty, blunt chest trauma)
- Papillary Muscle Disorders
  - Coronary artery disease (causing dysfunction and rarely rupture)
  - Acute global left ventricular dysfunction
  - Infiltrative diseases (amyloidosis, sarcoidosis)
  - Trauma

Bonow R, Braunwald E: Valvular heart disease, in Zipes D, et al. (eds): *Braunwald's Heart Disease*. Philadelphia, Elsevier Saunders, 2005, pp 1553–1621.

papillary muscle infarction with rupture; displacement of the papillary muscles from adverse LV remodeling due to ischemic or nonischemic cardiomyopathy; acute rheumatic carditis or other acute condition like stress cardiomyopathy; and mitral prosthetic paravalvular leak [94–97]. Often, the causes of MR are divided into primary disorders involving the mitral valve leaflets or chordae, or "functional" disorders in which the leaflets are relatively normal, but the MR is secondary and is caused by tethering of the mitral apparatus from ventricular remodeling; LV and annular dilatation; and increased sphericity. This classification emphasizes on when attention should be directed toward mitral valve surgery and/or to address an underlying cardiomyopathy.

Ischemic MR refers to MR that develops in the wake of an MI. The most important mechanism of ischemic MR is mitral valve leaflet tethering due to chronic post-infarction remodeling, resulting in apical and lateral displacement of the papillary muscles [98]. This shape change occurs after an inferior or posterior transmural MI leads to displacement of the posteromedial papillary muscle [99]. After MI, the presence of MR can augment post-infarction remodeling, further exacerbating the degree of functional MR [100]. Papillary rupture is a rare complication of acute MI (1% to 3%) with a bimodal peak at 1 day, then 3 to 5 days post-MI. The posteromedial papillary muscle has a single blood supply from the right coronary or left circumflex artery and, thus, is 6 to 10 times more likely to rupture than the anterolateral papillary, which has a dual blood supply. Dynamic MR can occur during episodes of transient ischemia involving the papillary muscles, but is not usually severe [101]. Dynamic MR is also a feature of HOCM and has been observed in some patients with stress cardiomyopathy.

Pathophysiology

In acute MR, the LV ejects blood into a small, noncompliant LA, leading to a rapid rise in LA pressure during systole. The difference of LA compliance explains why chronic MR (increased compliance) can be well tolerated, and why acute MR (reduced compliance) is not. The rise of LA pressure is transmitted to the pulmonary venous bed and leads to pulmonary edema, which may be asymmetric if there is an eccentric jet of MR directed to a particular pulmonary vein. The severity of pulmonary edema may be relatively less for patients whose LA has been conditioned by some degree of chronic MR. Large V waves are typically inscribed in the LA and PCW tracings during ventricular systole in acute MR [102]. Such V waves may also be seen with other conditions as well, including LV failure and acute ventricular septal rupture. During acute MR, LV systolic function may be normal, hyperdynamic, or low, depending on the etiology of MR. Tachycardia may temporarily preserve forward cardiac output, but hypotension, organ failure, and cardiogenic shock may evolve.

Clinical Manifestations

History

With acute severe MR, symptoms of left heart failure predominate, including dyspnea, orthopnea, and cough. Patients with post-MI papillary muscle rupture may have concurrent angina, dyspnea, and abrupt hemodynamic compromise. Spontaneous chordal rupture from myxomatous degeneration may be accompanied by chest pain in nearly half of patients. Symptoms like fevers, chills, malaise, and anorexia may be present in patients with endocarditis (Table 192.3).

Physical Examination

Patients with acute severe MR are tachycardic and tachypnic. Blood pressure is variable, though pulse pressure is often narrow owing to reduced forward stroke volume. Jugular venous pressure may be normal or elevated. Rales or wheezes may be audible over the lung fields, and may be asymmetric. The precordium is often hyperdynamic with a palpable apical thrill. S1 is normal or decreased in intensity, whereas S2 may be widely split because of early closure of the aortic valve. A diastolic filling complex may be appreciated and consists of a third heart sound (S3). and a short mid-diastolic rumble from increased transmitral diastolic flow. The systolic murmur of acute MR may be highly variable, and even absent in up to half of cases of post-MI papillary muscle rupture. The murmur of acute MR is usually not holosystolic, but rather early to mid-systolic in timing, with a crescendo–decrescendo configuration, and is coarse rather than high pitched. These features reflect the rapid LA pressure rise and diminution of the LV–LA pressure gradient throughout systole. The murmur of chronic MR, in contrast, is holosystolic (plateau) owing to the persistent LV–LA gradient during systole. The murmur of acute MR is usually loudest at the left sternal border or apex and the location of radiation may provide a clue as to etiology. Anterior leaflet prolapse or flail produces a posteriorly directed jet, so the murmur typically radiates to the axilla and back. With posterior leaflet involvement, the jet is directed anteriorly and is transmitted to the base, where it may be confused with AS.

Investigations

Electrocardiogram

ECG may show sinus tachycardia or an atrial arrhythmia, such as AF. LA abnormality may be discernible if P waves are present, though signs of LV chamber enlargement are rare in the acute

TABLE 192.3

Clinical Findings in Acute Severe Mitral Regurgitation

	Acute primary MR	Papillary muscle rupture	Functional MR with CHF
Etiology	Ruptured chordae, endocarditis, trauma	1 or 3–5 d post-MI	Ischemic heart disease, dilated cardiomyopathy
Presentation	Acute pulmonary edema	Sudden onset pulmonary edema and cardiogenic shock	CHF and pulmonary edema
Clinical Examination			
Point of maximum impulse/ apex beat	Normal or displaced thrill	Usually normal if no prior LV dysfunction	Displaced
Murmur	Holosystolic, Loud	May be very soft or absent	Early systolic, rarely holosystolic Soft
Sounds	Third heart sound, second heart sound split	Decreased sounds	Third heart sound
Investigations			
Electrocardiogram	Normal	Acute MI	Left bundle branch block
Chest radiograph	Normal heart size	Usually normal	Cardiomegaly
Echocardiogram			
Two-dimensional	LV and LA size normal Ruptured chord	Normal LV Ruptured head of papillary muscle	LV and LA dilated Annular dilatation Tenting of mitral valve leaflets
Doppler	Pulmonary venous flow reversal	Unimpressive color	Restrictive filling
Quantitation	Large regurgitation volume Large effective regurgitation orifice	Free-flow MR	Variable regurgitation volume Dynamic effective regurgitation orifice

CHF, congestive heart failure; LA, left atrial; LV, left ventricular; MI, myocardial infarction; MR, mitral regurgitation.
From Parikh S, O'Gara PT: Valvular heart disease, in Rippe JM, Irwin RS (eds): *Intensive Care Medicine*, Philadelphia, Lippincott Williams & Wilkins, 2006.

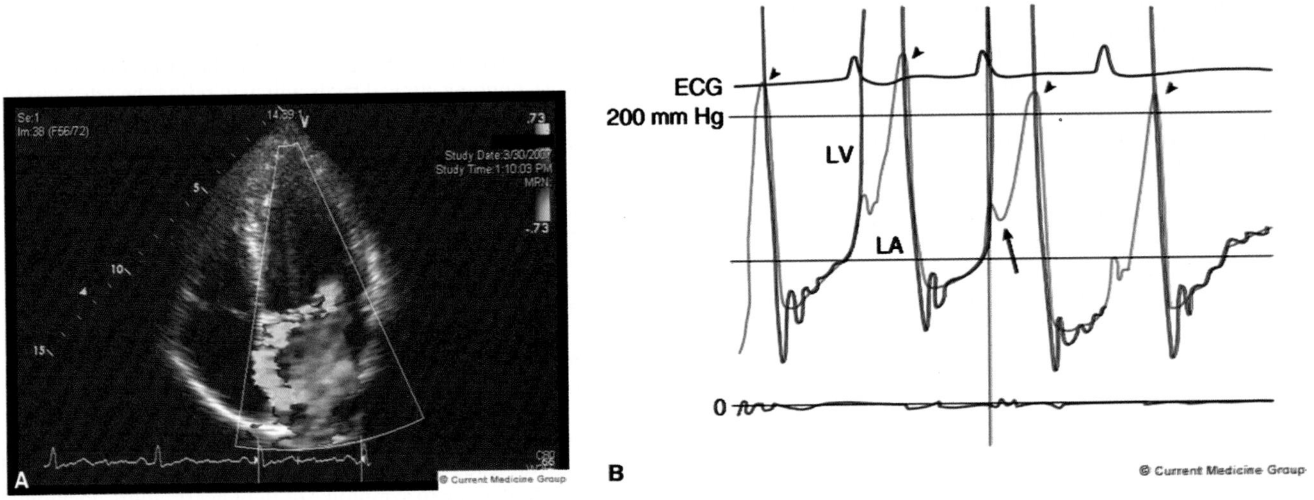

FIGURE 192.12 Mitral regurgitation. A: Color-flow Doppler image from the apical four chamber view of a patient with myxomatous degeneration of the mitral valve with posterior leaflet prolapse producing an anteromedially directed jet of severe mitral regurgitation against the inter-atrial septum. Eccentric jets are common in prolapse and/or flail leaflet and are directed opposite the involved leaflet. B: The "V" wave of mitral regurgitation. This hemodynamic tracing shows a large LA "V" wave (arrowheads) occurring during ventricular systole in a patient with atrial fibrillation ("A" wave absent). Following the "V" wave there is a rapid fall in LA pressure, along the course of the declining LV pressure. In diastole, LA and LV pressures are equalized. The arrow indicated the "C" wave deflection. Giant "V" waves are defined by an increase in >10 mm Hg from mean pressure and are consistent with mitral regurgitation, but may be blunted in patients with large and compliant left atria. LV, left atrial; LV, left ventricular; ECG, electrocardiogram (From O'Gara PT: Valvular Heart Disease, in Libby P (ed.): *Essential Atlas of Cardiovascular Disease*. Berlin, Springer, 2009; p 216, Figures 9-20 and 9-22.).

phase. With post-MI papillary muscle rupture evidence of an evolving inferior-posterior or lateral MI may be seen.

Chest Radiograph

In acute MR, the cardiac silhouette is normal in size despite the present of alveolar pulmonary edema. Asymmetric edema may be present in patients with a flail leaflet producing an eccentric MR jet, particularly in the right upper lobe [103]. Decompensated chronic MR may have associated cardiomegaly, LA enlargement, and prominent pulmonary arteries.

Echocardiography

Prompt TTE is the most important study for patients with suspected acute MR (Fig. 192.12). TTE can delineate mitral anatomy, characterize severity, and document underlying LV function and coexisting valvular pathology. Flail leaflet may be diagnosed by rapid movement of a portion of leaflet/chordal tissue posteriorly into the LA during systole. Chordal rupture, leaflet vegetations, and periannular abscess may be identified in endocarditis. Among patients with functional MR, LV remodeling may be evident along with annular dilatation, papillary muscle displacement and leaflet tethering. Semiquantitative assessment of MR severity can be performed with color flow and continuous wave Doppler interrogation. MR severity correlates with vena contracta width; LA jet width area; pulmonary vein systolic flow reversal; effective regurgitant orifice area; and regurgitant fraction and volume [104,105]. An integrated approach is necessary (Table 192.4). TEE can further characterize mitral valve anatomy and MR severity if TTE images are suboptimal or when complicated IE is suspected. TEE is routinely performed at the time of MV surgery.

Cardiac Catheterization

Catheterization is rarely required to define MR etiology or severity. If there is a discrepancy between clinical findings and noninvasive imaging or when estimated pulmonary artery pressures are out of proportion to the degree of MR, then invasive hemodynamic assessment is indicated. MR severity may be qualitatively assessed by contrast ventriculography. Coronary angiography typically precedes surgery for patients with coronary risk factors and in those with suspected post-MI papillary rupture or dynamic, ischemic MR. Right heart catheterization with oximetry can be done to distinguish acute post-infarction MR from VSD when the TTE is not diagnostic.

Intensive Care Unit Management

Medical Therapy

The goal of medical therapy for acute severe MR is to stabilize the patient in anticipation of surgery. Afterload reduction with intravenous vasodilators is the mainstay of therapy. Sodium nitroprusside is preferred, though its extended use requires monitoring of thiocyanate levels [67]. Inotropes such as dobutamine

TABLE 192.4

Echocardiographic Findings Consistent with Severe Mitral Regurgitation

Qualitative
Vena contracta width >0.7 cm with large central MR jet (area >40% left atrial area) or with a wall-impinging jet of any size, swirling in left atrium (Echo, Doppler)
Pulmonary vein systolic flow reversal (Doppler)
Dense contrast in left atrium (Angiography)
Quantitative
Regurgitant volume ≥60 mL/beat
Regurgitant fraction ≥50%
Effective regurgitant orifice ≥0.40 cm^2

From Zoghbi WA, Enriquez-Sarano M, Foster E, et al: Recommendations for evaluation of the severity of native valvular regurgitation with two-dimensional and Doppler echocardiography. *J Am Soc Echocardiogr* 16:777–802, 2003, with permission.

or dopamine may occasionally be required to support cardiac output and arterial pressure. IABP for mechanical afterload reduction may be particularly helpful for reducing regurgitant volume and decreasing LV end-diastolic pressure. If end-organ hypoperfusion or hypotension indicates that cardiogenic shock is present, IABP should be promptly initiated as a bridge to surgery. Loop diuretics may help ameliorate pulmonary edema.

Adjunctive medical therapy is driven in part by suspected etiology. For example, antibiotics are indicated for IE and anti-ischemic therapy is required for post-MI papillary muscle rupture [106]. With medical therapy alone, the mortality after papillary rupture is 80% [107]. Although percutaneous coronary intervention (PCI) may help relieve MR in the setting of acute MI, severe MR even without papillary muscle rupture will most often require surgical correction, despite successful coronary reperfusion. Despite recent advances of percutaneous valve repair techniques, none has yet been tested in the setting of acute MR [108,109]. Percutaneous mitral leaflet edge-to-edge repair has been approved in the USA for the treatment of patients with chronic, primary MR, severe heart failure and high surgical risk. It is not yet approved in the USA for the treatment of functional MR. There are numerous trans-catheter devices under investigation for use in the treatment of chronic, functional MR. Cardiac resynchronization therapy, when indicated by heart failure symptoms and a wide left bundle branch QRS complex, may help reduce chronic, functional MR related to contractile dyssynchrony, but has no role in the acute setting [110].

Surgical Therapy

Surgery is indicated for the treatment of acute severe MR [30]. In contrast to acute severe AR, many patients with acute severe MR may be stabilized over the course of a few days with IABP or inodilators to allow operation under less urgent circumstances. Also, unlike acute AR, acute severe MR may be treated with either repair or replacement, depending on the anatomic findings. Valve repair is the preferred surgical therapy when possible for patients with primary MR. Replacement is necessary, however, with papillary muscle rupture [111]. Mitral repair involves valve reconstruction using a variety of valvuloplasty techniques and insertion of an annuloplasty ring. In addition to reducing the need for anticoagulation and the risk of late prosthetic valve failure, valve repair preserves the integrity of the subvalvular apparatus, which maintains LV function to a greater degree. Valve replacement with chordal sparing is needed when there is destruction, distortion or infection of the native tissue that makes repair impossible. The decision between repair and replacement for severe ischemic MR can be challenging and is usually left to the discretion of the surgeon [112,113]. There is a high rate of recurrent MR after annuloplasty repair of ischemic MR [40]. Surgical strategy can be guided by intraoperative TEE and direct visual inspection after the patient is placed on cardiopulmonary bypass.

Surgical outcomes depend on age; underlying LV function; presence of concomitant coronary disease; patient comorbidities; and the etiology of MR [114]. IE has a high mortality rate even with medical and surgical therapy, though mortality has decreased with improvements of operative technique and more widespread use of mitral repair [115,116].

The surgical approaches for patients with MR accompanied by advanced systolic heart failure continue to evolve and remain controversial [117]. There is a broad consensus that patients with chronic functional MR and heart failure should be optimized with medical therapy; evaluated for revascularization when coronary disease is present; and considered for cardiac resynchronization therapy (CRT) when indicated [118]. After these steps, reconfirmation of MR severity is required before considering MV surgery. When severe MR is present, a careful integrated assessment of viability, mitral anatomy, and patient comorbidities must be made in consultation with the heart valve team [117]. As percutaneous and alternative approaches to mitral valve disease for patients with heart failure continue to evolve, ongoing clinical trials will help refine the selection of candidates for mitral surgery and determine outcomes of mitral repair versus replacement.

TRICUSPID REGURGITATION

Most ICU patients with TR have functional TR rather than a primary valvular abnormality. Functional TR is produced when the tricuspid annulus is dilated owing to RV enlargement for any reason, including left heart disease or pulmonary hypertension. The most important cause of primary TR encountered in the ICU is IE, particularly among injection drug users [52]. TR can also be produced by leaflet trauma from pacemaker or defibrillator leads or after endomyocardial biopsy. When severe, TR may contribute to symptoms of right heart failure, including fatigue, edema, and ascites. The murmur of TR usually increases in intensity with inspiration (Carvallo's sign). Examination of the neck veins reveals CV waves. A pulsatile liver edge may also be felt in the right upper quadrant.

Treatment of TR depends on its cause and severity. The vast majority of patients with acute TR due to IE are managed medically. TV surgery during the acute phase of the disease and prior to completion of a course of antibiotics is rarely indicated. Surgery for other causes of primary TR, such as carcinoid, is not a scenario that is encountered in an ICU setting. TV surgery at the time of left-sided surgery (usually MV surgery) is routinely performed when TR is severe or when TR is only mild–moderate, but the TV annulus is dilated beyond 40 mm. Late reoperation for isolated severe TR many years after MV surgery is associated with high morbidity and mortality [40].

PROSTHETIC VALVE DYSFUNCTION

The choice of valve prosthesis (Fig. 192.13) is informed by consideration of patient age; the need for anticoagulation; hemodynamic profile; expected durability; and patient preferences and values [119]. Mechanical valves have excellent durability and hemodynamic performance, but require life-long anticoagulation to prevent thromboembolic complications [120]. In contrast, the principal advantage of bioprosthetic valves is the reduced risk of thromboembolic complications after 3 months, except when there are other risk factors such as a hypercoagulable state or chronic AF [121]. Bioprosthetic valves are usually xenografts (porcine or cryopreserved, mounted bovine pericardium); homografts from human cadavers are often used to treat aortic valve and root endocarditis [122]. The Ross procedure for treatment of bicuspid aortic valve disease involves using the patient's native pulmonary valve to replace the aortic valve (pulmonary autograft) and a homograft to replace the native RV outflow tract. Bioprostheses may develop structural valve deterioration (SVD), which is mostly a function of patient age at implant. SVD occurs more rapidly among patients less than 40 years of age, compared with patients over 65 years of age. Rates of SVD may not differ between homograft and xenograft valves. Over the past 10 years, there has been a clear and significant trend toward the use of bioprosthetic valves in relatively younger patients (ages 50–65), despite the inherent risk of SVD and need for reoperation, given the increased durability of the current generation xenograft valves; decreased risk at reoperation; availability of transcatheter valve-in-valve implantation; aggregate risks of long-term anticoagulation; and patient values and preferences [50,123].

All prosthetic valves are subject to dysfunction that can lead to significant hemodynamic compromise. Common prosthetic

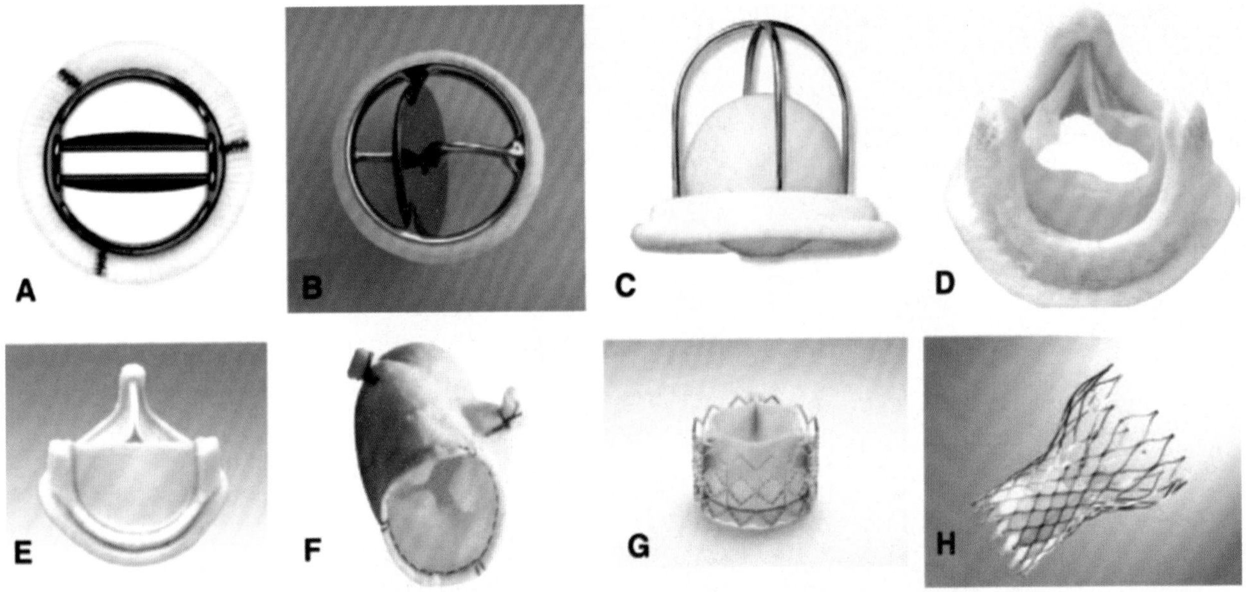

FIGURE 192.13. Different types of prosthetic heart valves. **A:** Bileaflet mechanical valve (St. Jude's). **B:** Monoleaflet, tilting disk mechanical valve (Medtronic Hall). **C:** Caged ball valve (Starr-Edwards). **D:** stented porcine bioprosthesis (Medtronic Mosaic). **E:** Stented pericardial bioprosthesis (Carpentier-Edwards Magna). **F:** Stentless porcine bioprosthesis (Medtronic Freestyle). **G:** percutaneous bioprosthesis expanded over a balloon (Edwards Sapien). **H:** Self-expandable percutaneous bioprosthesis (CoreValve) (From Pibarot P, Dumesnil JG: Prosthetic heart valves: selection of the optimal prosthesis and long-term management. *Circulation* 119:1034–1048, 2009, with permission.).

valve abnormalities include mechanical valve thrombosis; prosthetic valve endocarditis; structural deterioration and failure; and paravalvular regurgitation with or without hemolysis.

Prosthetic Valve Thrombosis

Prosthetic valve thrombosis (PVT) is any valve thrombus attached to or near an operated valve that occludes part of the blood flow path or interferes with the function of the valve [30]. PVT is a rare but life-threatening condition (Fig. 192.14). It is more common with older generation mechanical valves, particularly in the setting of inadequate anticoagulation. The incidence is estimated to be between 0.3% and 1.3% per year in patients with mechanical valves [122, 124, 125].

Clinical Presentation and Investigations

PVT follows a rapid clinical course, unlike the in-growth of pannus tissue within a prosthetic valve ring, which slowly gives rise to valve dysfunction and stenosis [126]. PVT manifests as abrupt onset of systemic embolization; congestive heart failure; or cardiogenic shock. The degree of hemodynamic compromise is determined by valve position and degree of resulting dysfunction. The physical examination may be unrevealing, though soft mechanical valve closure sounds or a pathologic murmur may be present. Mitral PVT is more common than aortic PVT.

A subtherapeutic international normalized ratio (INR) of a patient with a mechanical valve is a red flag for PVT [127]. Rapid diagnosis depends on prompt TTE or fluoroscopy, though both modalities may be complementary [128]. TTE can diagnose the presence of valve thrombus, its composition, and associated functional stenosis or regurgitation. TEE usually provides further risk stratification, particularly for cases of suspected mitral PVT and when TTE windows are inadequate [129]. Fluoroscopy can be useful to characterize tilting-disc or bileaflet mobility. Excursion of tilting-disc mechanical valves is much better appreciated with fluoroscopy than with TTE. There is increasing use of cardiac CT for characterization of prosthetic valve function when thrombosis is suspected [130]. A multimodality imaging approach is usually employed in rapid succession, beginning with TTE, followed by TEE, and then the other modalities as needed. Measurement of thrombus burden by TEE may be important for therapeutic decision-making.

Intensive Care Unit Management

Initial management should focus on systemic anticoagulation with intravenous heparin to prevent thrombus extension. Small thrombi without hemodynamic compromise are often treated with anticoagulation alone, whereas larger thrombi require either systemic fibrinolytic therapy or surgery [131,132]. Fibrinolytic therapy is associated with risks of life-threatening hemorrhage and systemic embolization and thus is often delivered in the ICU for purposes of monitoring. The risk is low with right-sided PVT and higher with left-sided PVT, with a risk of cerebral embolism of 12% to 15% [133–135]. Fibrinolysis is considered the first-line therapy for patients with right-sided PVT, and for those with left-sided PVT, small thrombus burden, and NYHA Class I–II symptoms [30]. Fibrinolysis is less useful and potentially more harmful if LA thrombus is present, if the valve thrombus is >2 weeks old, or if PVT is accompanied by shock. TTE after fibrinolysis can monitor for thrombus resolution and dictate additional fibrinolysis for residual thrombus [136]. Alteplase is the most commonly used fibrinolytic for PVT, though urokinase and streptokinase have been used. The typical dose is 10 mg bolus followed by an infusion of 90 mg over 2 hours. An alternative protocol utilizing a slow infusion of low-dose alteplase (e.g., 25 mg over 5 hours without a bolus) has been shown to be effective and safer for pregnant women with mitral PVT [137]. After successful fibrinolysis, unfractionated heparin should be initiated along with warfarin until an INR of 3.0 to 4.0 is achieved for patients with a prosthetic aortic valve or INR 3.5 to 4.5 for a prosthesis in the mitral position [30].

Emergency operation is recommended for patients with hemodynamic instability, NYHA Class 3 to 4 symptoms, or a large clot burden ($> 0.8\ cm^2$) [30,43]. Perioperative mortality

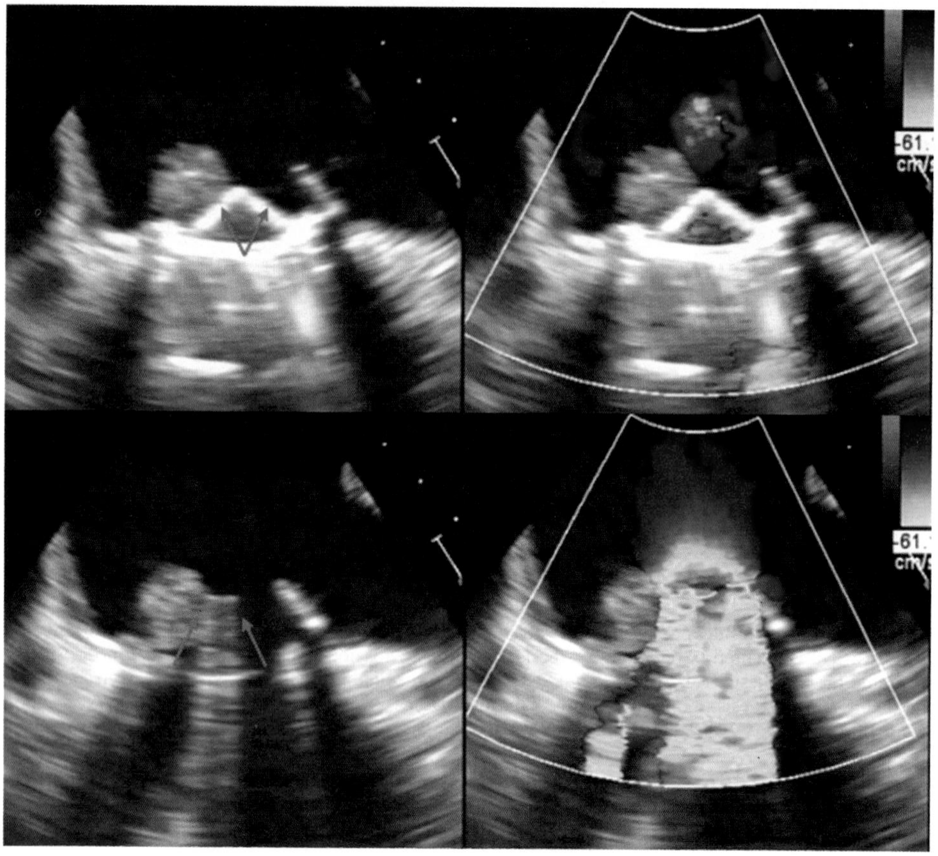

FIGURE 192.14 Prosthetic valve thrombosis transesophageal echocardiography reveals a large obstructive prosthetic thrombus with normal mobility of both leaflets (*arrows*) but unilateral transprosthetic flow (From Messika-Zeitoun D, Cimadevilla C. Mechanical valve thrombosis, http://www.escardio.org/Education/E-Learning/Clinical-cases/Valvular-heart-disease/Mechanical-Valve-Thrombosis#, with permission.).

rates approach 15% and are highest for PVT in the mitral position. A bioprosthesis is recommended after surgery for PVT to reduce future risk of valve thrombosis.

Prosthetic Valve Endocarditis

The incidence of prosthetic valve endocarditis (PVE) is 0.5% per year even with appropriate antibiotic prophylaxis and accounts for 7% to 25% of all cases of endocarditis in the developed world [53]. Endocarditis of a prosthetic valve is a devastating disease that carries a mortality rate of 30% to 50% over 6 months. This high mortality reflects not only a more serious infection but also the difficulty in eradicating the infection with antibiotics alone [138,139]. Infection may involve any part of the valve prosthesis, but the sewing ring may be particularly vulnerable. Sewing ring infection may result in abscess formation, paravalvular regurgitation, and further penetration into adjacent cardiac structures. The risk of PVE may be higher with mechanical valves during the first few months after implantation, but long-term risk is comparable for mechanical and bioprosthetic valves [52]. Infection with coagulase-negative staphylococci is common within the first postoperative year; *S. aureus* and streptococci species dominate in later years [140–142].

Fever is the most common symptom and may be associated with other signs of prosthetic valve dysfunction including congestive heart failure, a new murmur, or embolic phenomena. Blood cultures should be drawn prior to antibiotic therapy in any patient with a fever and a prosthetic valve. TEE is essential because of its greater sensitivity and specificity in detecting signs of PVE including vegetations, paraprosthetic abscess, or new paravalvular regurgitation [143,144]. There is increasing experience with PET-CT to visualize the extent of infection and screen for extracardiac foci of infection when clinically appropriate.

Eradication of the infecting pathogen with antimicrobial therapy alone is often impossible and depends on the virulence of the organism and extent of infection. Medical therapy is more likely to be successful for late PVE or with non-staphylococcal bacterial infections [145]. Surgical consultation should be sought early in the course of PVE. Indications for surgical therapy include failure of medical treatment marked by persistent bacteremia; hemodynamically significant prosthesis regurgitation with LV dysfunction; large vegetations; paravalvular extension with abscess or conduction defects; or development of intracardiac fistulas [30]. Surgery is almost always required for cases of *S. aureus* PVE. Infection with *S. aureus* is a marker for hospital mortality.

Structural Valve Deterioration

Failure of mechanical valves in the absence of infection is rare. Mechanical failure from strut fracture often presents with dyspnea; acute heart failure; and hemodynamic collapse with a physical examination marked by absent valve clicks. Death from mechanical valve strut fracture ensues rapidly if the valve is in the aortic position; patients with mitral valve failure can often be stabilized prior to surgery.

With conventional stented bioprostheses, freedom from SVD is 70% to 90% at 10 years, and 50% to 80% at 15 years [139,146]. SVD of bioprostheses is often related to tearing or rupture of one prosthetic valve cusp or progressive calcification and immobility [147]. Risk factors for SVD include younger age at implant; mitral valve position; renal insufficiency; and hyperparathyroidism [148]. Evaluation for SVD requires TTE and often TEE with care to exclude endocarditis as a complicating feature. SVD is the most common cause of reoperative valve replacement in patients with a bioprosthesis. Indications for reoperation are similar for those with native valve disease and are dominated by the development of heart failure. Transcatheter

TABLE 192.5

Advances in Valvular Heart Disease

- TAVR for calcific AS is now considered for prohibitive-, high-, and intermediate-risk patients as assessed by the STS Risk Score in conjunction with frailty assessment and patient preference. Challenging decision-making around transcatheter valve therapies has led to establishment of multidisciplinary heart valve teams that include interventional cardiologists, cardiac surgeons, imaging specialists, anesthesiologists, and intensivists.
- Bioprostheses are now in more widespread use than mechanical valves to treat aortic stenosis owing to improved bioprosthetic durability and the absence of obligate anticoagulation. Bioprosthesis are nevertheless prone to degeneration and restenosis. Valve-in-valve TAVR can now be considered for use to treat aortic stenosis due to prosthetic valve degeneration [50]
- Low-flow, low-gradient aortic stenosis, though traditionally recognized in patients with reduced EF, has also been appreciated in patients with normal EF (≥50%) [153]. Referred to as "paradoxical" low-flow, low-gradient AS, patients often have concentric LV hypertrophy and carry worse prognosis than patients with high-gradient severe AS.
- For patients with a congenital bicuspid aortic valve, the aortic root or ascending aorta should be repaired or replaced in asymptomatic patients if the diameter of the aortic root or ascending aorta is ≥5.5 cm. However, if the patient has an additional risk factor such as a family history of aortic dissection or an aortic growth rate ≥0.5 cm/y, surgery should be considered when the aorta measures ≥5 cm. Aortic surgery in patients with bicuspid valve should also be performed in patients undergoing aortic valve replacement for stenosis of regurgitation if the aortic root or ascending aorta is ≥4.5 cm [154]
- Mitral regurgitation has been reclassified according to primary and secondary etiologies. Primary MR results from mitral leaflet prolapse, restricted leaflet motion from rheumatic or radiation heart disease, or infective endocarditis. Secondary causes include coronary artery disease and cardiomyopathy resulting in displacement of the mitral apparatus. There is a Class I recommendation for surgery only for primary MR when both symptoms and LVEF >30% are present, or in asymptomatic patients with severe primary MR who demonstrate progressive LV remodeling manifested as LVEF 30%–60% or LV end-systolic dimension ≥40 mm [30]
- Endovascular edge-to-edge mitral valve clipping can reduce mitral regurgitation and stimulate reverse remodeling, offering an alternative to surgical repair for primary degenerative mitral valve regurgitation [155]. Clinical trials are ongoing for the use of percutaneous edge-to-edge repair in high surgical risk patients with symptomatic severe functional (secondary) mitral regurgitation.
- Direct oral anticoagulants are not recommended for use in patients with mechanical heart valves owing to concerns about increased risk of thromboembolic and bleeding events [156]

TAVR, transcatheter aortic valve replacement; AS, aortic stenosis; STS, Society for Thoracic Surgeons; EF, ejection fraction; LV, left ventricular; MR, mitral regurgitation; LVEF, left ventricular ejection fraction.

valve-in-valve implantation offers an alternative to reoperation for selected patients [50].

Paravalvular Regurgitation

Paravalvular regurgitation is most often caused by infection; suture dehiscence; or fibrosis and calcification of the native annulus, leading to inadequate contact between the sewing ring and annulus. Mild paravalvular regurgitation on perioperative echocardiography has a benign course with reoperation required in <1% of patients at 2 years [149]. For patients with more severe paravalvular leak, a close follow-up is required, and surgical intervention is warranted for those who develop symptoms, progressive LV dysfunction, or hemolysis. A large proportion (>50%). of mechanical valve patients have some degree of mild intravascular hemolysis marked by anemia and an elevated lactate dehydrogenase (LDH). Paravalvular leaks, particularly small leaks, can lead to more severe anemia caused by shearing of red blood cells. Severe, refractory anemia that is not responsive to iron, folate, and erythropoietin is an indication for repeat valve operation or closure of the paravalvular leak with transcatheter techniques [150]. For high-risk patients not suitable for reoperation, transcatheter closure of the paravalvular leak may be achieved in selected cases with the use of a septal or ductal occluder device [151,152].

PREVENTING INFECTIVE ENDOCARDITIS

Emerging data on the lifetime risk of IE, as well as trends of antibiotic resistance and antibiotic-associated adverse events, have led to changes in guideline recommendations for antibiotic prophylaxis [54]. Infective endocarditis is much more likely to occur from frequent exposure to random bacteremia associated with daily activities than from medical or dental procedures. Antibiotic prophylaxis for IE should only be provided to patients at greatest risk for complications from endocarditis, including patients with prosthetic valves, previous endocarditis, complex congenital heart disease, or cardiac transplantation. Routine antibiotic prophylaxis for mitral valve prolapse is no longer recommended [30,145].

Advances for valvular heart disease are summarized in Table 192.5.

References

1. Nkomo VT, Gardin JM, Skelton TN, et al: Burden of valvular heart diseases: a population-based study. *Lancet* 368:1005–1011, 2006.
2. Mozaffarian D, Benjamin EJ, Go AS et al: Heart disease and stroke statistics—2015 update: a report from the American Heart Association. *Circulation* 131:e29–e322, 2015.
3. O'Gara PT, Braunwald E: Approach to the patient with a heart murmur, in Braunwald E, Fauci AS, Kasper DL, et al, ed. *Harrison's Principles of Internal Medicine*. 15th ed. New York, NY, McGraw-Hill, 2001, pp 207–211.
4. Roberts WC, Ko JM: Frequency by decades of unicuspid, bicuspid, and tricuspid aortic valves in adults having isolated aortic valve replacement for aortic stenosis, with or without associated aortic regurgitation. *Circulation* 111:920–925, 2005.
5. Freeman RV, Otto CM: Spectrum of calcific aortic valve disease: pathogenesis, disease progression, and treatment strategies. *Circulation* 111:3316–3326, 2005.
6. Goldbarg SH, Elmariah S, Miller MA, et al: Insights into degenerative aortic valve disease. *J Am Coll Cardiol* 50:1205–1213, 2007.
7. Probst V, Le Scouarnec S, Legendre A et al: Familial aggregation of calcific aortic valve stenosis in the western part of France. *Circulation* 113:856–860, 2006.
8. Rajamannan NM, Evans FJ, Aikawa E et al: Calcific aortic valve disease: not simply a degenerative process: A review and agenda for research from the National Heart and Lung and Blood Institute Aortic Stenosis Working Group. Executive summary: Calcific aortic valve disease-2011 update. *Circulation* 124:1783–1791, 2011.
9. Otto CM, Lind BK, Kitzman DW, et al: Association of aortic-valve sclerosis with cardiovascular mortality and morbidity in the elderly. *N Engl J Med* 341:142–147, 1999.
10. Cowell SJ, Newby DE, Prescott RJ, et al: A randomized trial of intensive lipid-lowering therapy in calcific aortic stenosis. *N Engl J Med* 352:2389–2397, 2005.

11. Rossebo AB, Pedersen TR, Boman K, et al: Intensive lipid lowering with simvastatin and ezetimibe in aortic stenosis. *N Engl J Med* 359:1343–1356, 2008.
12. Hoffman JI, Kaplan S: The incidence of congenital heart disease. *J Am Coll Cardiol* 39:1890–1900, 2002.
13. Fedak PW, Verma S, David TE, et al: Clinical and pathophysiological implications of a bicuspid aortic valve. *Circulation* 106:900–904, 2002.
14. Michelena HI, Desjardins VA, Avierinos JF et al: Natural history of asymptomatic patients with normally functioning or minimally dysfunctional bicuspid aortic valve in the community. *Circulation* 117:2776–2784, 2008.
15. Tzemos N, Therrien J, Yip J et al: Outcomes in adults with bicuspid aortic valves. *JAMA* 300:1317–1325, 2008.
16. Tadros TM, Klein MD, Shapira OM: Ascending aortic dilatation associated with bicuspid aortic valve: pathophysiology, molecular biology, and clinical implications. *Circulation* 119:880–890, 2009.
17. Spann JF, Bove AA, Natarajan G, et al: Ventricular performance, pump function and compensatory mechanisms in patients with aortic stenosis. *Circulation* 62:576–582, 1980.
18. Gaasch WH, Zile MR, Hoshino PK, et al: Tolerance of the hypertrophic heart to ischemia. Studies in compensated and failing dog hearts with pressure overload hypertrophy. *Circulation* 81:1644–1653, 1990.
19. Marcus ML, Doty DB, Hiratzka LF, et al: Decreased coronary reserve: a mechanism for angina pectoris in patients with aortic stenosis and normal coronary arteries. *N Engl J Med* 307:1362–1366, 1982.
20. Otto CM: Valvular aortic stenosis: disease severity and timing of intervention. *J Am Coll Cardiol* 47:2141–2151, 2006.
21. Carabello BA, Paulus WJ: Aortic stenosis. *Lancet* 373:956–966, 2009.
22. Tribouilloy C, Rusinaru D, Marechaux S, et al: Low-gradient, low-flow severe aortic stenosis with preserved left ventricular ejection fraction: characteristics, outcome, and implications for surgery. *J Am Coll Cardiol* 65:55–66, 2015.
23. Ross J Jr, Braunwald E: Aortic stenosis. *Circulation* 38:61–67, 1968.
24. Hakki AH, Kimbiris D, Iskandrian AS, et al: Angina pectoris and coronary artery disease in patients with severe aortic valvular disease. *Am Heart J* 100:441–449, 1980.
25. Vincentelli A, Susen S, Le Tourneau T et al: Acquired von Willebrand syndrome in aortic stenosis. *N Engl J Med* 349:343–349, 2003.
26. Rosenhek R, Binder T, Porenta G, et al: Predictors of outcome in severe, asymptomatic aortic stenosis. *N Engl J Med* 343:611–617, 2000.
27. Nassimiha D, Aronow WS, Ahn C, et al: Rate of progression of valvular aortic stenosis in patients > or = 60 years of age. *Am J Cardiol* 87:807–809, A9, 2001.
28. Ware LB, Matthay MA: Clinical practice. Acute pulmonary edema. *N Engl J Med* 353:2788–2796, 2005.
29. Gorlin R, Gorlin SG: Hydraulic formula for calculation of the area of the stenotic mitral valve, other cardiac valves, and central circulatory shunts. I. *Am Heart J* 41:1–29, 1951.
30. Nishimura RA, Otto CM, Bonow RO, et al: 2014 AHA/ACC guideline for the management of patients with valvular heart disease: executive summary: a report of the American College of Cardiology/American Heart Association Task Force on Practice Guidelines. *J Am Coll Cardiol* 63:2438–2488, 2014.
31. Carabello BA: Clinical practice. Aortic stenosis. *N Engl J Med* 346:677–682, 2002.
32. Tribouilloy C, Levy F, Rusinaru D, et al: Outcome after aortic valve replacement for low-flow/low-gradient aortic stenosis without contractile reserve on dobutamine stress echocardiography. *J Am Coll Cardiol* 53:1865–1873, 2009.
33. Clavel MA, Fuchs C, Burwash IG, et al: Predictors of outcomes in low-flow, low-gradient aortic stenosis: results of the multicenter TOPAS Study. *Circulation* 118:S234–S242, 2008.
34. Quere JP, Monin JL, Levy F, et al: Influence of preoperative left ventricular contractile reserve on postoperative ejection fraction in low-gradient aortic stenosis. *Circulation* 113:1738–1744, 2006.
35. Picano E, Pibarot P, Lancellotti P, et al: The emerging role of exercise testing and stress echocardiography in valvular heart disease. *J Am Coll Cardiol* 54:2251–2260, 2009.
36. Grayburn PA: Assessment of low-gradient aortic stenosis with dobutamine. *Circulation* 113:604–606, 2006.
37. Carabello BA: Is it ever too late to operate on the patient with valvular heart disease? *J Am Coll Cardiol* 44:376–383, 2004.
38. Levy F, Laurent M, Monin JL, et al: Aortic valve replacement for low-flow/low-gradient aortic stenosis operative risk stratification and long-term outcome: a European multicenter study. *J Am Coll Cardiol* 51:1466–1472, 2008.
39. Pellikka PA, Sarano ME, Nishimura RA, et al: Outcome of 622 adults with asymptomatic, hemodynamically significant aortic stenosis during prolonged follow-up. *Circulation* 111:3290–3295, 2005.
40. Nishimura RA, Otto CM, Bonow RO, et al: 2014 AHA/ACC guideline for the management of patients with valvular heart disease: a report of the American College of Cardiology/American Heart Association Task Force on Practice Guidelines. *J Am Coll Cardiol* 63:e57–e185, 2014.
41. Khot UN, Novaro GM, Popovic ZB, et al: Nitroprusside in critically ill patients with left ventricular dysfunction and aortic stenosis. *N Engl J Med* 348:1756–1763, 2003.
42. Popovic ZB, Khot UN, Novaro GM, et al: Effects of sodium nitroprusside in aortic stenosis associated with severe heart failure: pressure-volume loop analysis using a numerical model. *Am J Physiol Heart Circ Physiol* 288:H416–H423, 2005.
43. Vahanian A, Alfieri O, Andreotti F, et al: Guidelines on the management of valvular heart disease (version 2012): the Joint Task Force on the Management of Valvular Heart Disease of the European Society of Cardiology (ESC) and the European Association for Cardio-Thoracic Surgery (EACTS). *Eur J Cardiothorac Surg* 42:S1–S44, 2012.
44. Rahimtoola SH: Choice of prosthetic heart valve for adult patients. *J Am Coll Cardiol* 41:893–904, 2003.
45. Safian RD, Berman AD, Diver DJ, et al: Balloon aortic valvuloplasty in 170 consecutive patients. *N Engl J Med* 319:125–130, 1988.
46. Vahanian A, Palacios IF: Percutaneous approaches to valvular disease. *Circulation* 109:1572–1579, 2004.
47. Kuntz RE, Tosteson AN, Berman AD, et al: Predictors of event-free survival after balloon aortic valvuloplasty. *N Engl J Med* 325:17–23, 1991.
48. Holmes DR Jr, Nishimura RA, Grover FL, et al: Annual outcomes with transcatheter valve therapy: from the STS/ACC TVT registry. *J Am Coll Cardiol* 66:2813–2823, 2015.
49. Mack MJ, Leon MB, Smith CR et al: 5-year outcomes of transcatheter aortic valve replacement or surgical aortic valve replacement for high surgical risk patients with aortic stenosis (PARTNER 1): a randomised controlled trial. *Lancet* 385:2477–2484, 2015.
50. Dvir D, Webb JG, Bleiziffer S, et al: Transcatheter aortic valve implantation in failed bioprosthetic surgical valves. *JAMA* 312:162–170, 2014.
51. Stout KK, Verrier ED. Acute valvular regurgitation. *Circulation* 119:3232–3241, 2009.
52. Baddour LM, Wilson WR, Bayer AS, et al: Infective endocarditis: diagnosis, antimicrobial therapy, and management of complications: a statement for healthcare professionals from the Committee on Rheumatic Fever, Endocarditis, and Kawasaki Disease, Council on Cardiovascular Disease in the Young, and the Councils on Clinical Cardiology, Stroke, and Cardiovascular Surgery and Anesthesia, American Heart Association: endorsed by the Infectious Diseases Society of America. *Circulation* 111:e394–e434, 2005.
53. Mylonakis E, Calderwood SB. Infective endocarditis in adults. *N Engl J Med* 345:1318–1330, 2001.
54. Wilson W, Taubert KA, Gewitz M et al: Prevention of infective endocarditis: guidelines from the American Heart Association: a guideline from the American Heart Association Rheumatic Fever, Endocarditis, and Kawasaki Disease Committee, Council on Cardiovascular Disease in the Young, and the Council on Clinical Cardiology, Council on Cardiovascular Surgery and Anesthesia, and the Quality of Care and Outcomes Research Interdisciplinary Working Group. *Circulation* 116:1736–1754, 2007.
55. Haldar SM, O'Gara PT: Infective endocarditis: diagnosis and management. *Nat Clin Pract Cardiovasc Med* 3:310–317, 2006.
56. Mehta RH, Suzuki T, Hagan PG, et al: Predicting death in patients with acute type a aortic dissection. *Circulation* 105:200–206, 2002.
57. Januzzi JL, Eagle KA, Cooper JV, et al: Acute aortic dissection presenting with congestive heart failure: results from the International Registry of Acute Aortic Dissection. *J Am Coll Cardiol* 46:733–735, 2005.
58. Isselbacher EM: Thoracic and abdominal aortic aneurysms. *Circulation* 111:816–828, 2005.
59. Obadia JF, Tatou E, David M: Aortic valve regurgitation caused by blunt chest injury. *Br Heart J* 74:545–547, 1995.
60. Tribouilloy CM, Enriquez-Sarano M, Fett SL, et al: Application of the proximal flow convergence method to calculate the effective regurgitant orifice area in aortic regurgitation. *J Am Coll Cardiol* 32:1032–1039, 1998.
61. Tribouilloy CM, Enriquez-Sarano M, Bailey KR, et al: Assessment of severity of aortic regurgitation using the width of the vena contracta: a clinical color Doppler imaging study. *Circulation* 102:558–564, 2000.
62. Bekeredjian R, Grayburn PA: Valvular heart disease: aortic regurgitation. *Circulation* 112:125–134, 2005.
63. Nienaber CA, Eagle KA: Aortic dissection: new frontiers in diagnosis and management. Part I: from etiology to diagnostic strategies. *Circulation* 108:628–635, 2003.
64. Cigarroa JE, Isselbacher EM, DeSanctis RW, et al: Diagnostic imaging in the evaluation of suspected aortic dissection. Old standards and new directions. *N Engl J Med* 328:35–43, 1993.
65. Hagan PG, Nienaber CA, Isselbacher EM et al: The International Registry of Acute Aortic Dissection (IRAD): new insights into an old disease. *JAMA* 283:897–903, 2000.
66. Penn MS, Smedira N, Lytle B, et al: Does coronary angiography before emergency aortic surgery affect in-hospital mortality? *J Am Coll Cardiol* 35:889–894, 2000.
67. Evangelista A, Tornos P, Sambola A, et al: Role of vasodilators in regurgitant valve disease. *Curr Treat Options Cardiovasc Med* 8:428–434, 2006.
68. Miller RR, Vismara LA, DeMaria AN, et al: Afterload reduction therapy with nitroprusside in severe aortic regurgitation: improved cardiac performance and reduced regurgitant volume. *Am J Cardiol* 38:564–567, 1976.
69. Stevens LM, Madsen JC, Isselbacher EM, et al: Surgical management and long-term outcomes for acute ascending aortic dissection. *J Thorac Cardiovasc Surg* 138:1349–1357.e1, 2009.
70. Chandrashekhar Y, Westaby S, Narula J. Mitral stenosis. *Lancet* 374:1271–1283, 2009.
71. Waller BF, Howard J, Fess S. Pathology of mitral valve stenosis and pure mitral regurgitation—Part I. *Clin Cardiol* 17:330–336, 1994.
72. Marijon E, Ou P, Celermajer DS, et al: Prevalence of rheumatic heart disease detected by echocardiographic screening. *N Engl J Med* 357:470–476, 2007.
73. Carabello BA. Modern management of mitral stenosis. *Circulation* 112:432–437, 2005.
74. Iung B, Baron G, Butchart EG, et al: A prospective survey of patients with valvular heart disease in Europe: The Euro Heart Survey on Valvular Heart Disease. *Eur Heart J* 24:1231–1243, 2003.

75. Elkayam U, Bitar F: Valvular heart disease and pregnancy part I: native valves. *J Am Coll Cardiol* 46:223–230, 2005.
76. Chiang CW, Lo SK, Ko YS, et al: Predictors of systemic embolism in patients with mitral stenosis. A prospective study. *Ann Intern Med* 128:885–889, 1998.
77. Rowe JC, Bland EF, Sprague HB, et al: The course of mitral stenosis without surgery: ten- and twenty-year perspectives. *Ann Intern Med* 52:741–749, 1960.
78. Horstkotte D, Niehues R, Strauer BE: Pathomorphological aspects, aetiology and natural history of acquired mitral valve stenosis. *Eur Heart J* 12[Suppl B]:55–60, 1991.
79. Martin RP, Rakowski H, Kleiman JH, et al: Reliability and reproducibility of two dimensional echocardiograph measurement of the stenotic mitral valve orifice area. *Am J Cardiol* 43:560–568, 1979.
80. Hatle L, Brubakk A, Tromsdal A, et al: Noninvasive assessment of pressure drop in mitral stenosis by Doppler ultrasound. *Br Heart J* 40:131–140, 1978.
81. Wilkins GT, Weyman AE, Abascal VM, et al: Percutaneous balloon dilatation of the mitral valve: an analysis of echocardiographic variables related to outcome and the mechanism of dilatation. *Br Heart J* 60:299–308, 1988.
82. Alan S, Ulgen MS, Ozdemir K, et al: Reliability and efficacy of metoprolol and diltiazem in patients having mild to moderate mitral stenosis with sinus rhythm. *Angiology* 53:575–581, 2002.
83. Iung B, Garbarz E, Michaud P, et al: Late results of percutaneous mitral commissurotomy in a series of 1024 patients. Analysis of late clinical deterioration: frequency, anatomic findings, and predictive factors. *Circulation* 99:3272–3278, 1999.
84. Palacios IF, Sanchez PL, Harrell LC, et al: Which patients benefit from percutaneous mitral balloon valvuloplasty? Prevalvuloplasty and postvalvuloplasty variables that predict long-term outcome. *Circulation* 105:1465–1471, 2002.
85. Inoue K, Owaki T, Nakamura T, et al: Clinical application of transvenous mitral commissurotomy by a new balloon catheter. *J Thorac Cardiovasc Surg* 87:394–402, 1984.
86. Iung B, Cormier B, Ducimetiere P, et al: Immediate results of percutaneous mitral commissurotomy. A predictive model on a series of 1514 patients. *Circulation* 94:2124–2130, 1996.
87. Orrange SE, Kawanishi DT, Lopez BM, et al. Actuarial outcome after catheter balloon commissurotomy in patients with mitral stenosis. *Circulation* 95:382–389, 1997.
88. Palacios IF, Tuzcu ME, Weyman AE, et al. Clinical follow-up of patients undergoing percutaneous mitral balloon valvotomy. *Circulation* 91:671–676, 1995.
89. Reyes VP, Raju BS, Wynne J, et al: Percutaneous balloon valvuloplasty compared with open surgical commissurotomy for mitral stenosis. *N Engl J Med* 331:961–967, 1994.
90. Ben Farhat M, Ayari M, Maatouk F, et al: Percutaneous balloon versus surgical closed and open mitral commissurotomy: seven-year follow-up results of a randomized trial. *Circulation* 97:245–250, 1998.
91. Edwards FH, Peterson ED, Coombs LP, et al: Prediction of operative mortality after valve replacement surgery. *J Am Coll Cardiol* 37:885–892, 2001.
92. STS Adult Cardiovascular National Surgery Database—STS national database risk calculator. Available at http://www.sts.org/sections/stsnationaldatabase/riskcalculator/.
93. Carabello BA: The current therapy for mitral regurgitation. *J Am Coll Cardiol* 52:319–326, 2008.
94. Levine RA, Hung J: Ischemic mitral regurgitation, the dynamic lesion: clues to the cure. *J Am Coll Cardiol* 42:1929–1932, 2003.
95. Chaput M, Handschumacher MD, Guerrero JL, et al: Mitral leaflet adaptation to ventricular remodeling: prospective changes in a model of ischemic mitral regurgitation. *Circulation* 120:S99–S103, 2009.
96. Simmers TA, Meijburg HW, de la Riviere AB: Traumatic papillary muscle rupture. *Ann Thorac Surg* 72:257–259, 2001.
97. Freed LA, Levy D, Levine RA, et al: Prevalence and clinical outcome of mitral-valve prolapse. *N Engl J Med* 341:1–7, 1999.
98. Otsuji Y, Levine RA, Takeuchi M, et al: Mechanism of ischemic mitral regurgitation. *J Cardiol* 51:145–156, 2008.
99. Levine RA, Schwammenthal E: Ischemic mitral regurgitation on the threshold of a solution: from paradoxes to unifying concepts. *Circulation* 112:745–758, 2005.
100. Beeri R, Yosefy C, Guerrero JL, et al: Mitral regurgitation augments post-myocardial infarction remodeling failure of hypertrophic compensation. *J Am Coll Cardiol* 51:476–486, 2008.
101. Kaul S, Spotnitz WD, Glasheen WP, et al: Mechanism of ischemic mitral regurgitation. An experimental evaluation. *Circulation* 84:2167–2180, 1991.
102. Grose R, Strain J, Cohen MV: Pulmonary arterial V waves in mitral regurgitation: clinical and experimental observations. *Circulation* 69:214–222, 1984.
103. Schnyder PA, Sarraj AM, Duvoisin BE, et al: Pulmonary edema associated with mitral regurgitation: prevalence of predominant involvement of the right upper lobe. *Am J Roentgenol* 161:33–36, 1993.
104. Enriquez-Sarano M, Dujardin KS, Tribouilloy CM, et al: Determinants of pulmonary venous flow reversal in mitral regurgitation and its usefulness in determining the severity of regurgitation. *Am J Cardiol* 83:535–541, 1999.
105. Enriquez-Sarano M, Sinak LJ, Tajik AJ, et al: Changes in effective regurgitant orifice throughout systole in patients with mitral valve prolapse. A clinical study using the proximal isovelocity surface area method. *Circulation* 92:2951–2958, 1995.
106. Picard MH, Davidoff R, Sleeper LA, et al: Echocardiographic predictors of survival and response to early revascularization in cardiogenic shock. *Circulation* 107:279–284, 2003.
107. Kishon Y, Oh JK, Schaff HV, et al: Mitral valve operation in postinfarction rupture of a papillary muscle: immediate results and long-term follow-up of 22 patients. *Mayo Clin Proc* 67:1023–1030, 1992.
108. Feldman T, Wasserman HS, Herrmann HC, et al: Percutaneous mitral valve repair using the edge-to-edge technique: six-month results of the EVEREST Phase I Clinical Trial. *J Am Coll Cardiol* 46:2134–2140, 2005.
109. Babaliaros V, Cribier A, Agatiello C. Surgery insight: Current advances in percutaneous heart valve replacement and repair. *Nat Clin Pract Cardiovasc Med* 3:256–264, 2006.
110. Solis J, McCarty D, Levine RA, et al: Mechanism of decrease in mitral regurgitation after cardiac resynchronization therapy: optimization of the force-balance relationship. *Circ Cardiovasc Imaging* 2:444–450, 2009.
111. Verma S, Mesana TG. Mitral-valve repair for mitral-valve prolapse. *N Engl J Med* 361:2261–2269, 2009.
112. Goldstein D, Moskowitz AJ, Gelijns AC, et al: Two-Year Outcomes of Surgical Treatment of Severe Ischemic Mitral Regurgitation. *N Engl J Med* 374:344–353, 2016.
113. Smith PK, Puskas JD, Ascheim DD, et al: Surgical treatment of moderate ischemic mitral regurgitation. *N Engl J Med* 371:2178–2188, 2014.
114. Roques F, Nashef SA, Michel P. Risk factors for early mortality after valve surgery in Europe in the 1990s: lessons from the EuroSCORE pilot program. *J Heart Valve Dis* 10:572–577; discussion 577–578, 2001.
115. Iung B, Rousseau-Paziaud J, Cormier B, et al: Contemporary results of mitral valve repair for infective endocarditis. *J Am Coll Cardiol* 43:386–392, 2004.
116. Murdoch DR, Corey GR, Hoen B, et al: Clinical presentation, etiology, and outcome of infective endocarditis in the 21st century: the International Collaboration on Endocarditis-Prospective Cohort Study. *Arch Intern Med* 169:463–473, 2009.
117. Di Salvo TG, Acker MA, Dec GW, et al: Mitral valve surgery in advanced heart failure. *J Am Coll Cardiol* 55:271–282.
118. Tracy CM, Epstein AE, Darbar D, et al: 2012 ACCF/AHA/HRS focused update of the 2008 guidelines for device-based therapy of cardiac rhythm abnormalities: a report of the American College of Cardiology Foundation/American Heart Association Task Force on Practice Guidelines. *J Am Coll Cardiol* 60:1297–1313, 2012.
119. Vongpatanasin W, Hillis LD, Lange RA: Prosthetic heart valves. *N Engl J Med* 335:407–416, 1996.
120. Goldsmith I, Turpie AG, Lip GY: Valvar heart disease and prosthetic heart valves. *BMJ* 325:1228–1231, 2002.
121. Cannegieter SC, Rosendaal FR, Wintzen AR, et al: Optimal oral anticoagulant therapy in patients with mechanical heart valves. *N Engl J Med* 333:11–17, 1995.
122. Durrleman N, Pellerin M, Bouchard D, et al: Prosthetic valve thrombosis: twenty-year experience at the Montreal Heart Institute. *J Thorac Cardiovasc Surg* 127:1388–1392, 2004.
123. Chiang YP, Chikwe J, Moskowitz AJ, et al: Survival and long-term outcomes following bioprosthetic vs mechanical aortic valve replacement in patients aged 50 to 69 years. *JAMA* 312:1323–1329, 2014.
124. Grunkemeier GL, Li HH, Naftel DC, et al: Long-term performance of heart valve prostheses. *Curr Probl Cardiol* 25:73–154, 2000.
125. Roudaut R, Serri K, Lafitte S: Thrombosis of prosthetic heart valves: diagnosis and therapeutic considerations. *Heart* 93:137–142, 2007.
126. Barbetseas J, Nagueh SF, Pitsavos C, et al: Differentiating thrombus from pannus formation in obstructed mechanical prosthetic valves: an evaluation of clinical, transthoracic and transesophageal echocardiographic parameters. *J Am Coll Cardiol* 32:1410–1417, 1998.
127. Hering D, Piper C, Horstkotte D: Drug insight: an overview of current anticoagulation therapy after heart valve replacement. *Nat Clin Pract Cardiovasc Med* 2:415–422, 2005.
128. Shapira Y, Herz I, Sagie A: Fluoroscopy of prosthetic heart valves: does it have a place in the echocardiography era? *J Heart Valve Dis* 9:594–599, 2000.
129. Tong AT, Roudaut R, Ozkan M, et al: Transesophageal echocardiography improves risk assessment of thrombolysis of prosthetic valve thrombosis: results of the international PRO-TEE registry. *J Am Coll Cardiol* 43:77–84, 2004.
130. Makkar RR, Fontana G, Jilaihawi H, et al: Possible Subclinical Leaflet Thrombosis in Bioprosthetic Aortic Valves. *N Engl J Med* 373:2015–2024, 2015.
131. Vahanian A, Baumgartner H, Bax J, et al: Guidelines on the management of valvular heart disease: The Task Force on the Management of Valvular Heart Disease of the European Society of Cardiology. *Eur Heart J* 28:230–268, 2007.
132. Nishimura RA, Carabello BA, Faxon DP, et al: ACC/AHA 2008 Guideline update on valvular heart disease: focused update on infective endocarditis: a report of the American College of Cardiology/American Heart Association Task Force on Practice Guidelines endorsed by the Society of Cardiovascular Anesthesiologists, Society for Cardiovascular Angiography and Interventions, and Society of Thoracic Surgeons. *J Am Coll Cardiol* 52:676–685, 2008.
133. Roudaut R, Lafitte S, Roudaut MF, et al: Fibrinolysis of mechanical prosthetic valve thrombosis: a single-center study of 127 cases. *J Am Coll Cardiol* 41:653–658, 2003.
134. Alpert JS. The thrombosed prosthetic valve: current recommendations based on evidence from the literature. *J Am Coll Cardiol* 41:659–660, 2003.
135. Piper C, Hering D, Langer C, et al. Etiology of stroke after mechanical heart valve replacement--results from a ten-year prospective study. *J Heart Valve Dis* 17:413–417, 2008.
136. Shapira Y, Herz I, Vaturi M, et al: Thrombolysis is an effective and safe therapy in stuck bileaflet mitral valves in the absence of high-risk thrombi. *J Am Coll Cardiol* 35:1874–1880, 2000.

137. Ozkan M, Cakal B, Karakoyun S, et al: Thrombolytic therapy for the treatment of prosthetic heart valve thrombosis in pregnancy with low-dose, slow infusion of tissue-type plasminogen activator. *Circulation* 128:532–540, 2013.
138. Akowuah EF, Davies W, Oliver S, et al: Prosthetic valve endocarditis: early and late outcome following medical or surgical treatment. *Heart* 89:269–272, 2003.
139. Vesey JM, Otto CM: Complications of prosthetic heart valves. *Curr Cardiol Rep* 6:106–111, 2004.
140. Moreillon P, Que YA: Infective endocarditis. *Lancet* 363:139–149, 2004.
141. Hill EE, Herregods MC, Vanderschueren S, et al: Management of prosthetic valve infective endocarditis. *Am J Cardiol* 101:1174–1178, 2008.
142. Chu VH, Miro JM, Hoen B, et al: Coagulase-negative staphylococcal prosthetic valve endocarditis—a contemporary update based on the International Collaboration on Endocarditis: prospective cohort study. *Heart* 95:570–576, 2009.
143. Bach DS: Transesophageal echocardiographic (TEE) evaluation of prosthetic valves. *Cardiol Clin* 18:751–771, 2000.
144. Tornos P: Management of prosthetic valve endocarditis: a clinical challenge. *Heart* 89:245–246, 2003.
145. Habib G, Hoen B, Tornos P, et al: Guidelines on the prevention, diagnosis, and treatment of infective endocarditis (new version 2009): the Task Force on the Prevention, Diagnosis, and Treatment of Infective Endocarditis of the European Society of Cardiology (ESC). *Eur Heart J* 30:2369–2413, 2009.
146. Pibarot P, Dumesnil JG: Prosthetic heart valves: selection of the optimal prosthesis and long-term management. *Circulation* 119:1034–1048, 2009.
147. Schoen FJ, Levy RJ: Calcification of tissue heart valve substitutes: progress toward understanding and prevention. *Ann Thorac Surg* 79:1072–1080, 2005.
148. Ruel M, Kulik A, Rubens FD, et al: Late incidence and determinants of reoperation in patients with prosthetic heart valves. *Eur J Cardiothorac Surg* 25:364–370, 2004.
149. Davila-Roman VG, Waggoner AD, Kennard ED, et al: Prevalence and severity of paravalvular regurgitation in the Artificial Valve Endocarditis Reduction Trial (AVERT) echocardiography study. *J Am Coll Cardiol* 44:1467–1472, 2004.
150. Shapira Y, Vaturi M, Sagie A: Hemolysis associated with prosthetic heart valves: a review. *Cardiol Rev* 17:121–124, 2009.
151. Hourihan M, Perry SB, Mandell VS, et al: Transcatheter umbrella closure of valvular and paravalvular leaks. *J Am Coll Cardiol* 20:1371–1377, 1992.
152. Kim MS, Casserly IP, Garcia JA, et al: Percutaneous transcatheter closure of prosthetic mitral paravalvular leaks: are we there yet? *JACC Cardiovasc Interv* 2:81–90, 2009.
153. Hachicha Z, Dumesnil JG, Bogaty P, et al: Paradoxical low-flow, low-gradient severe aortic stenosis despite preserved ejection fraction is associated with higher afterload and reduced survival. *Circulation* 115:2856–2864, 2007.
154. Hiratzka LF, Creager MA, Isselbacher EM et al: Surgery for Aortic Dilatation in Patients With Bicuspid Aortic Valves: A Statement of Clarification From the American College of Cardiology/American Heart Association Task Force on Clinical Practice Guidelines. *J Am Coll Cardiol* 67:724–731, 2016.
155. Feldman T, Kar S, Rinaldi M, et al: Percutaneous mitral repair with the MitraClip system: safety and midterm durability in the initial EVEREST (Endovascular Valve Edge-to-Edge REpair Study) cohort. *J Am Coll Cardiol* 54:686–694, 2009.
156. Eikelboom JW, Connolly SJ, Brueckmann M, et al: Dabigatran versus warfarin in patients with mechanical heart valves. *N Engl J Med* 369:1206–1214, 2013.

Chapter 193 ■ Acute Aortic Syndromes

MARC P. BONACA[1]

INTRODUCTION

Acute aortic syndromes represent a spectrum of entities characterized by disruption of the integrity of the aorta wall threatening central pressure, vital organ perfusion and survival. They include acute aortic dissection, intramural hematoma (IMH), penetrating aortic ulcer (PAU), expanding aortic aneurysm, and aortic trauma [1,2]. Although the classical presentation of "aortic agony" is characterized by severe, sudden-onset pain in the chest or back, this presentation, although recognizable, occurs only among a minority of cases [3]. As the initial manifestations of acute aortic syndromes are highly variable and establishing the diagnosis requires specific testing, arriving at the appropriate diagnosis in a timely manner is often challenging. Owing to the early mortality risk [4], prompt recognition of the acute aortic syndromes enables early treatment decision-making potentially improving outcomes. Frequently, the clinician must depend on subtle findings gleaned from history, detailed physical examination, and imaging in order to decide on an appropriate treatment plan [5]. This chapter reviews the spectrum of acute aortic syndromes, including acute aortic dissection, acute aortic IMH, PAU, and rupture of aortic aneurysm. Because patients with suspected acute aortic syndromes are frequently critically ill and require rapid disposition to treatment, evaluation, and treatment algorithms are described, with each individual section serves as a guide to a syndrome-specific evaluation. Key features of a focused history and physical examination are emphasized. In addition, critical laboratory and imaging tests are reviewed.

[1]With acknowledgement to Leon M. Ptaszek, Eric M. Isselbacher and Amy E. Spooner

AORTIC DISSECTION

Definition and Classification

Dissection of the aortic wall involves longitudinal cleavage of the muscular media, leading to the formation of a second (or false) vessel lumen. The inciting event for a typical aortic dissection is thought to be a tear in the intima that leads to exposure of the underlying media, generally weakened by medial degeneration. Once created, this cleavage front advances due to wall strain that can be created at physiologic levels of blood pressure. The cleavage front typically advances in the direction of blood flow, but dissection against the direction of flow is also observed.

There are multiple consequences of dissection. The false lumen may have little or now outflow leading to increased pressure relative to the native (or true) lumen, leading to compression and potentially compromised downstream blood flow. The resulting intimal flap may also involve or obstruct branch vessels leading to end-organ malperfusion that can result in stroke, limb ischemia, or visceral malperfusion. Owing to the resulting weakening of the aortic wall, the damaged aorta may therefore be more prone to rupture.

Aortic dissections are generally classified by location and extent. There are two commonly used classification systems (Fig.193.1). The DeBakey system includes three types of aortic dissection [6]. Type I involves dissection of both the ascending and descending aorta, and/or the arch. Type II dissection involves only the ascending aorta proximal to the brachiocephalic artery, and type III involves only the descending aorta distal to the left subclavian artery [6]. The Stanford system includes two dissection types. All dissections involving the ascending aorta are included in Type A: this includes Types I and II in the DeBakey system. Stanford Type B includes all dissections

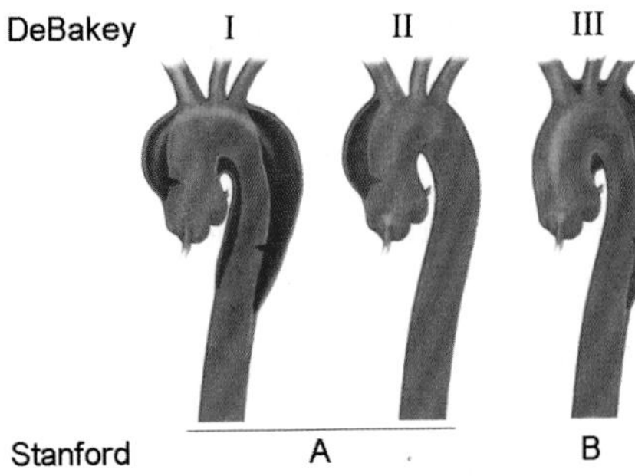

FIGURE 193.1 Dissection classification (DeBakey/Stanford). [© Massachusetts General Hospital Thoracic Aortic Center. Used with permission.]

that do not involve the ascending aorta [7]. Classification of the location of a dissection carries prognostic and treatment importance. Surgery is indicated for dissection of the ascending aorta, whereas medical management is frequently the treatment of choice for descending dissection without associated end-organ malperfusion or impending rupture. The optimal treatment for isolated arch dissection (also called non-A and non-B dissection) is debated [8].

Chronicity of the dissection is defined as the time interval between onset of symptoms and evaluation. Dissections that are present for less than 2 weeks are defined as acute, whereas those that are present longer are defined as chronic [1]. This has been further divided into hyperacute (<24 hours), acute (2 to 7 days), subacute (8 to 30 days), and chronic (>30 days) with these time categories associated with survival [9]. It is noteworthy that the mortality associated with untreated ascending aortic dissection reaches up to 75% at 2 weeks [10].

CLASSIC AORTIC DISSECTION

Epidemiology

Estimates of the incidence of aortic dissection range from 3 to 16 cases per 100,000 per year [1,4,11]. The highest incidence occurs in the sixth and seventh decades of life among patients with hypertension [1,4,11]. Although a male predominance is traditionally described, at age 75 or above the incidence is similar in men and women [4,5]. Younger patients without a history of hypertension may present with acute aortic syndromes generally in the setting of a family history, connective tissue disease, vascular inflammatory disease, or trauma; therefore, this diagnosis should not be discounted for the young. Age may also influence presentation with complicated Type B dissection [12]. The aorta may be disrupted in the setting of trauma or during procedures (iatrogenic) with the latter described occurring at approximately 0.15% [13]. A proportion of patients suffering iatrogenic dissection may infact have medial degeneration and therefore an underlying susceptibility [13]. Acute aortic syndromes have been described in the setting of cocaine use, possibly related to abrupt changes in heart rate in blood pressure, and are most often Type B in young, urban, male smokers.

Mortality rates associated with dissection are very high, and many patients do not survive to hospital admission. Overall 30-day mortality for aortic dissection of any type is greater than 50% [3,4]. In one community-based cohort study, nearly 50% of patients with dissection died before hospitalization. Thirty-day survival for those admitted alive was only ~50% [3,4].

Outcomes of patients presenting with acute aortic syndromes vary by type and the presence of anatomic complications. Recent studies describe the mortality for medically managed Type A dissection at 0.77% per hour with historical data sets quoting even higher rates [3,14]. Early mortality may be due to complications including cardiac tamponade, aortic regurgitation, stroke, or compromised myocardial perfusion [15,16]. For iatrogenic dissection, mortality may be as high as 30% to 40% [17].

Overall, Type B dissection is associated with a lower mortality than Type A with early rates of 13% and 5-year rates of 33% [4,18]. In reality, however, the morbidity and mortality of Type B dissection are variable and depend on the anatomic exent as well as the presence of complications. It is estimated that as many as one in five patients with Type B dissection develop malperfusion and approximately 25% require an intervention during the index hospitalization [1,2,19]. When also including other complications such as periaortic hematoma, refractory pain, or refractory hypertension, the proportion of patients with complications during the index hospitalization for Type B dissection approaches 50% [18]. For patients who present with or develop complications, in-hospital mortality is ~20% while it is 6% for uncomplicated Type B dissection [18]. Age has been shown to have an important impact for patients with complicated Type B dissection with mortality among patients less than 70 years old of 10% versus 30% among patients older than 70 with a ~2.4-fold risk of mortality after adjustment for baseline differences [20]. For patients who present without complications and are medically managed, there is long-term risk of complication including aneurysm and expansion necessitating close follow-up [21].

Etiology and Pathophysiology

Any process that causes damage to the aortic tunica media, leading to medial degeneration, increases the risk for aneurysm or dissection. Although this medial disruption is a defining feature of acute aortic syndromes, cases of isolated intimal tears without hematoma formation have been described [1]. In the case of typical aortic dissection, the precipitating event is thought to be the creation of a tear in the intimal layer overlying a damaged area of the media. In the elderly patient with dissection, the presence of medial degeneration is correlated with the effects of aging, hypertension, and atherosclerotic disease [1]. Indeed, hypertension is found among 70% to 80% of patients with aortic dissection [1,4]. A number of underlying biological processes have been considered as contributing to the etiology of dissection including inflammation, endothelial reactive oxidative stress, and disturbed P53-MDM2 signaling [22,23].

For the younger patient with aortic dissection, medial degeneration is still the culprit, but the constellation of correlated risk factors tends to differ [1,4]. Typically, young patients are more likely to have hereditary connective tissue disorders that compromise the integrity of the extracellular matrix in the tunica media, most notably Marfan syndrome, Loeys–Dietz syndrome, Ehlers–Danlos syndrome, bicuspid aortic valve, or familial thoracic aortic aneurysm syndrome (FTAAS) [24–27]. Among patients presenting with recurrent aortic dissection, approximately 5% of all dissections, Marfan syndrome is often present [28]. Patients, 40 years of age or younger, are also less likely to be hypertensive, and may have a larger aortic diameter on presentation. Paradoxically, mortality of this younger cohort does not appear to be lower than that of older patients. All of these syndromes have been associated with breakdown of the fibrillin and collagen components of the extracellular matrix in the media, leading to medial degeneration. Aortic dissection risk is also increased in patients with Turner and Noonan syndromes [25]. Increased risk for dissection is found in a number of other conditions, including aortitis, especially in the context of giant cell arteritis and Takayasu arteritis [1,2,29]. Cocaine use has also been associated with dissection, ostensibly on the basis of increases in cardiac output, blood pressure, or as a consequence of direct vascular injury from cocaine itself (i.e., cocaine-induced vasculitis/endarteritis). In particular, crack cocaine has been identified as a potential precipitant of dissection.

Notably, pregnancy is an independent risk factor for aortic dissection [30]. The highest incidence of dissection is observed during the third trimester or early postpartum period [30]. This risk is high particularly among pregnant women with a bicuspid aortic valve, Marfan, Ehlers–Danlos, or Turner syndrome [25,30,31]. Among pregnant women with Turner syndrome, the risk of dissection or rupture exceeds 2%, and the risk of death is increased 100-fold [25,30]. Sporadic aortic dissections may occur among women without these predisposing conditions, possibly due to the elevated expression of relaxin and inhibin associated with pregnancy.

Iatrogenic injury to the aortic wall, sustained in the context of cardiac catheterization, intra-aortic balloon pump placement, or cardiac surgery, increases the risk of future aortic dissection [13,32,33]. Cardiac surgery involving the aortic valve appears to pose the greatest risk [17]. Iatrogenic dissection of the ascending aorta at the time of cardiac surgery is also associated with increased mortality risk with the highest rates for those that occur during the early (42%) or late (32%) postoperative periods compared to those that are discovered intraoperatively (17% mortality) and presumably addressed as part of the index procedure [13,17,34,35]. Aortic dissection after prior aortic valve replacement for bicuspid aortic valve has also been described [36].

Damage sustained by the aorta may take up to several years to develop into aneurysm and/or dissection. Blunt trauma or rapid deceleration injury is frequently associated with injury to the aortic isthmus.

Clinical Manifestations

There is no single physical examination finding or lab test that allows for positive identification of dissection: only imaging of the aorta verifies the diagnosis with a high degree of sensitivity and specificity. Consequently, the initial evaluation and examination must incorporate a high index of suspicion and careful assessment.

The classic initial symptom of acute aortic dissection is classically described as the abrupt onset of severe chest or back pain. The severity of this pain is characteristically at its maximum at the point of inception. This is in sharp contrast with the typical crescendo onset of myocardial infarction pain [1,4]. The quality of the pain is often described as being “tearing” or “stabbing” and the pain may radiate or be migratory [1,37]. Although severe pain is described by the majority of patients presenting with acute aortic syndromes, symptoms can be variable depending on the location and extent of the disruption as well as patient factors including gender. A minority of patients present with syncope which is associated with poor outcomes as it may occur in the setting of complications such as stroke or tamponade [38,39]. Focal neurologic symptoms may also be the primary manifestation and may be transient in nature potentially complicating diagnosis [14,37]. The initial location of the pain is correlated to the location of the dissection: of the patients from reported clinical series who presented with anterior chest or neck pain, 65% to 90% were found to have dissection of the ascending aorta. Interscapular or back may also represent dissection of the descending aorta [1]. This variability of presenting symptom presents a challenge for clinicians and may delay diagnosis particularly for those with atypical symptoms [37].

The physical examination of patients with acute aortic syndromes may also be variable. The most common finding at the time of presentation is hypertension; however, the frequency depends on the anatomic classification [1]. Of the patients of the IRAD series, 36% of patients with Type A dissection had elevated blood pressure, whereas 70% of patients with Type B dissection had hypertension. Hypotension may also be a presenting feature of aortic dissection and portends developing shock more frequently for Type A compared to Type B dissections. It is also noteworthy that patients with dissections who present with a “deadly triad” of hypotension/shock, an absence of pain, and evidence of branch vessel involvement exhibit a markedly higher mortality [1,38,40,41]. Pericardial tamponade in the context of Type A aortic dissection is a surgical emergency, as it represents a tenuously compensated rupture of the aorta [39]. Unless the patient is in extremis, pericardiocentesis should not be performed, as the release of pressure from the pericardial space may precipitate a rise in blood pressure, recurrent hemorrhage into the pericardium, and cardiovascular collapse [16,38,39]. Dissection into the pleural space may also lead to hypotension and syncope, and similarly requires immediate surgical intervention. These findings are sometimes attributed to alternative diagnoses such as pleural effusion (either reactive or from hemorrhage) and may occur in as many as 16% of patients [1,3]. On occasion, Type A dissection may extend proximally to the ostia of the coronary arteries, leading to myocardial infarction or involve the aortic valve leading to severe aortic regurgitation [42].

A number of other vascular complications of aortic dissection may be apparent on initial evaluation. A pulse deficit is described in approximately 30% of patients with Type A dissection and is associated with increased mortality [41]. Focal neurologic deficits are described among 17% of patients. These occlusion events are typically the result of the extension of the dissection into a branch vessel (“static” occlusion), occlusion of the ostium of the vessel due to migration of the intimal flap (“dynamic” occlusion), or impaired flow in the true lumen due to distention of the false lumen. The spectrum of clinical findings associated with aortic side-branch involvement ranges from no signs and symptoms, to subtle findings, to florid manifestations, including severe ischemia of the affected territories. The mass effects of the dissection may lead to focal neurologic defects for rare cases. Involvement of a subclavian artery may lead to a difference in measured blood pressure between the two arms or pulse deficit. Impaired flow in the mesenteric arteries leads to signs and symptoms consistent with mesenteric ischemia. Dissections may also lead to occlusion of the renal arteries, leading to acute renal failure, or renal infarction. A pulse deficit is described in approximately 30% of patients with Type A dissection and is associated with increased mortality [41]. Focal neurologic deficits are described in 17% of patients. Rarely, dissection leads to spinal artery occlusion with resultant paraparesis or paraplegia. Lower limb ischemia may also occur in Type B dissection.

Diagnosis

A focused history and examination should be performed to assess the pretest likelihood of acute aortic syndrome [1]. Evaluation should include known genetic, connective tissue, or familial conditions associated with aortic disease, history of recent aortic manipulation, typical pain, or high-risk signs such as pulse deficit, blood pressure differential, focal neurologic signs or symptoms, and new murmur of aortic regurgitation [1,29]. Risk scores based on the AHA/ACC consensus guidelines for the diagnosis of acute coronary syndrome have been evaluated and shown to be highly sensitive [43].

The electrocardiogram (ECG) is often (69%) abnormal, but is generally nonspecific [3]. Chest X-ray (CXR) is likewise generally performed and is abnormal for most cases (80%), but findings are rarely specific for acute aortic syndrome [3]. The presence of ST-segment elevation in lead aVR in patients with Type A dissection has been shown to be of prognostic value [44]. Widening of the mediastinum and displacement of aortic calcification are also more common among cases than controls. CXR and ECG may provide value but neither are sensitive for acute aortic syndromes and normal findings should not delay definitive imaging for patients in whom there is clinical suspicion [1].

There is not yet a specific biomarker in common clinical use that allows the clinician to confirm the diagnosis. D-Dimer, a fibrin degradation product indicative of intravascular coagulation, is widely available and well established for the diagnostic algorithm for pulmonary embolism. A D-dimer >500 ng per mL has been shown to be highly sensitive for acute dissection (~97%, negative predictive value 96%) but relatively nonspecific (56%, positive predictive value 60%) [45–49]. Based on this high sensitivity, D-dimer may be a potential screening tool to "rule out" acute aortic dissection [45]. The kinetics of D-dimer after dissection are not well described posing one possible limitation. One study reported that almost 1 in 5 patients with aortic dissection had D-dimer levels <400 ng per mL illustrating variability of performance [50,51]. In addition, the sensitivity in the setting of isolated IMH or not established. Other biomarkers under investigation include smooth muscle myosin heavy chain protein; however, diagnostic performance still does not exceed that of computed tomographic (CT) or magnetic resonance (MR) angiography [52,53]. Soluble elastin fragment (sELAF) levels have also evaluated, but the performance of assays for this biomarker has not been widely validated [54]. Other available biomarkers such as cardiac troponin and natriuretic peptides are important prognostic markers in most clinical settings but are nonspecific for aortic disruption.

Imaging

Prompt imaging is critical during the evaluation of suspected aortic dissection. Multiple modalities are at the disposal of the clinician; however, the patient is best served by the modality that offers high sensitivity and specificity without delay or transport time. The specific technique of choice may differ among hospitals, as not all facilities have the same capabilities. Following is a discussion of the relative strengths and weaknesses of the commonly available imaging techniques used for the diagnosis of aortic dissection. The decision regarding the optimal technique to be used in a specific context is left to the individual clinician. Frequently, multiple imaging modalities must be used for a single patient. In addition, a single patient may require serial studies if his/her signs or symptoms evolve [1].

In most hospital settings, a CXR is performed as a matter of course in the evaluation of chest pain. The CXR may offer much useful information. In the patient with an aortic dissection, the CXR may reveal an abnormal aortic silhouette, widening of the mediastinum, separation of intimal calcium, pleural effusions, and blunting of the heart boarders representing extravasation of blood into the pericardial space. Although useful, CXR rarely establishes the diagnosis of acute aortic syndrome and is unable to define the total extent or the presence of complications. Therefore, other modalities must be used.

Transthoracic echocardiography (TTE) is a readily available, noninvasive, and portable imaging modality that may be considered. Sensitivity is highest for disruption of the ascending aorta particularly if it involves the root or aortic valve. In addition, complications such as aortic regurgitation and pericardial effusion can be visualized. It should be noted that sensitivity for Type A dissection varies between 70% and 90%, and sensitivity for Type B dissection is approximately 40%. Given this suboptimal sensitivity, performing a TTE should not delay a more sensitive imaging study [1].

In terms of definitive imaging, computed tomographic angiography (CTA), magnetic resonance angiography (MRA) and transesophageal echocardiography (TEE) have enabled diagnosis of acute aortic syndromes with high sensitivity (>95%) and specificity (>95%) (Table 193.1) [1,55–59].

By virtue of the close proximity of the aorta to the ultrasound probe in the esophagus, TEE offers clear views of most portions of the thoracic aorta and affords excellent information regarding aortic valve function. TEE may be useful to guide surgical intervention for Type A aortic dissection. TEE, like TTE, is portable and can be performed easily at the bedside, which makes it the procedure of choice for evaluation of critically ill or physiologically unstable patients who may be at higher risk during transportation for radiographic examinations. In addition, TEE does not require the use of nephrotoxic contrast agents. For aortic dissection, TEE has a sensitivity between 90% and 100%, and specificity is approximately 90%. Color Doppler imaging may identify the blood flow between the true and false lumens. Perhaps the most important procedural drawback regarding TEE is the need for conscious sedation, which may be difficult to administer to a patient who is hemodynamically unstable.

CT scanning allows for a full view of the entire aorta. Consequently, the sensitivity (90% to 100%) and specificity (90%) for visualization of the intimal flap in aortic dissection are comparable to TEE [57]. Specific CT techniques, such as spiral CT, also allow for facile three-dimensional reconstruction. The "double barrel" produced by dissection can be distinct. In classic aortic dissection, an intimal flap can be seen, separating a true and false lumen. Pericardial and pleural effusions are often easily visualized, but blood flow and tamponade physiology cannot be assessed directly. Dedicated aortic CT scans should compensate for cardiac motion through tools such as ECG gating [57]. In addition, noncontrast images should also be obtained for greater sensitivity for isolated IMH. When obtaining aortic imaging, the full aorta from chest to pelvis should be visualized to determine the full extent of aortic and branch vessel involvement. Imaging only the chest, for example, may result in incomplete characterization and require follow-up testing. The intravenous (IV) contrast required is associated with risks of allergic reactions and contrast nephropathy. Many patients presenting with the acute aortic syndromes may also have renal insufficiency or failure; however, for the critically ill patient in whom aneurysmal rupture is suspected, definitive diagnosis and treatment of the aortic process should take priority.

CT scanning and magnetic resonance imaging (MRI) share several of the same advantages, such as high image resolution and the ability to scan the entire aorta. Overall, the sensitivity and specificity of intimal flap detection by MRI are nearly 100%. MRI does not require the use of IV contrast, which represents an advantage over CT scanning; however, MRI is more expensive and not as readily available or as rapidly performed as CT scanning. The primary limitation of MRI is lack of availability: not all hospitals have MR scanners available for emergent use. Even when available, issues of transporting a potentially unstable patient are still present. MRI is also contraindicated for patients in who have vascular clips, implantable cardioverter-defibrillators (ICDs) or pacemakers.

In the past, retrograde aortography was considered the gold-standard technique for aortic imaging. Because aortography is an invasive test that requires the assembly of a catheterization laboratory team and the use of IV contrast and ionizing radiation, it is typically reserved for those cases where diagnostic uncertainty remains after one or more other imaging studies have been obtained. The ability of aortography to detect aortic dissection depends on the presence of blood flow between the true and false lumens; therefore, for cases where blood flow between these chambers is limited, the aortogram may be nondiagnostic. Overall, among patients with classic aortic dissection, the sensitivity and specificity for intimal flap visualization are 80% to 90% and 90% to 95%, respectively [49]. Aortography is still the study of choice for visualization of aortic branch vessels, which may not be visualized by other imaging modalities as well. In addition, aortography is particularly useful when endovascular treatment is contemplated.

TABLE 193.1

Imaging Modalities for Patients with Suspected Acute Aortic Syndromes

	Key findings	Advantages	Disadvantages
TTE	Intimal flap in ascending aorta Dilatation of aortic root Aortic valve regurgitation Pericardial effusion Color Doppler differentiation of flow in dissection-related "true" and "false" lumens	Readily available Noninvasive Quickly performed at bedside No ionizing radiation Intravenous contrast not required Aortic valve function can be directly assessed	Only aortic root and ascending aorta can be reliably assessed Image quality may be affected by body habitus Branch vessels and intramural hematomas are not reliably visualized
TEE	Intimal flap in aorta Dilatation of aorta Aortic valve regurgitation Pericardial effusion Color Doppler differentiation of flow in dissection-related "true" and "false" lumens	Readily available Noninvasive Quickly performed at bedside No ionizing radiation Intravenous contrast not required Image quality not affected by body habitus Ascending aorta, arch, and proximal descending aorta may be visualized Aortic valve function can be assessed directly	Distal thoracic and abdominal aorta cannot be visualized May only be performed by trained personnel Sedation required Branch vessels are not reliably visualized
CT	Intimal flap in aorta Dilatation of aorta in any segment Pericardial effusion Dissection-related "true" and "false" lumens or intramural hematoma accentuated with contrast	Readily available Noninvasive Quickly performed Image quality not affected by body habitus Full aorta may be assessed in single scan Most widely used first imaging test in suspected dissection	Requires use of ionizing radiation and intravenous contrast Transportation to scanner may be required in some centers Patient monitoring during scan may be difficult Aortic valve function cannot be assessed directly
MRI	Intimal flap in aorta Dilatation of aorta in any segment Pericardial effusion Dissection-related "true" and "false" lumens or intramural hematoma may be differentiated	Noninvasive No ionizing radiation Image quality not affected by body habitus Full aorta may be assessed in single scan Branch vessel visualization is excellent Contrast not required to visualize intramural hematoma or to differentiate between true and false lumen Aortic valve function can be directly assessed	Not readily available at many hospitals Transportation to scanner may be required in some centers Patient monitoring during scan may be difficult Scan time longer than other modalities
Aortogram	Intimal flap in aorta Dilatation of aorta in any segment True and false lumens may be differentiated with contrast	Best modality for branch vessel visualization Allows for assessment of full aorta	Invasive Study not as readily available due to required assembly of trained personnel Ionizing radiation and intravenous contrast required Intramural hematoma cannot be reliably assessed

Consultation with an imaging specialist may be useful particularly for determining the optimal diagnostic protocol. At some centers scans protocoled to exclude several acute diagnosis such as pulmonary embolism, dissection, and myocardial infarction, called "Triple Rule-Out" may be obtained; however, they are associated with higher doses of radiation and the clinical utility is debated [55]. In addition, the sensitivity and specificity of CT or MR may be altered if they are optimized to detect other diagnosis such as pulmonary embolism.

Management

The primary goal of treatment for a patient with aortic dissection is to minimize the effects of the dissection while rapidly evaluating the necessity of urgent intervention, if indicated (Fig. 193.5) [60]. Diagnosis, management, and interventional decision-making are complex and time sensitive and acute multidisciplinary response teams may allow for optimized management [61]. Clinical stability should first be assessed to evaluate for acute complications such as

TABLE 193.2

Commonly Used Medications with Routes/Doses

Class	Medication	Dosing[a]
β-Blockers	Metoprolol	2.5–5.0 mg IV q 5 min, up to three doses followed by 5–10 mg IV q 4–6 h
	Labetalol	20 mg IV administered over 2 min followed by 40–80 mg IV q 10 min with maximum initial dose 300 mg, to be followed by 2 mg/min IV infusion with 10 mg/min maximum rate
	Esmolol	500 μg/kg IV bolus dose, followed by 50 μg/kg/min IV infusion with 300 μg/kg/min maximum rate
Calcium-channel blockers	Diltiazem	Bolus 5–10 mg IV, maximum dose 25 mg IV infusion 5–15 mg/h for up to 24 h 30–90 mg PO qid, maximum 360 mg/d
	Verapamil	80–120 mg PO tid–qid maximum 480 mg/d
	Nifedipine	10–20 mg PO tid, start with 10 mg dose, maximum 180 mg/d
	Nicardipine	20–40 mg PO tid, start with 20 mg dose, maximum 120 mg/d
	Nisoldipine	20–40 mg PO qd, start with 10 mg dose, maximum 60 mg/d
Vasodilators	Nitroprusside	0.3–10 μg/kg/min IV infusion up to 3 d

[a]Therapeutic goals include maintenance of systolic blood pressure 100–110 mm Hg, heart rate approximately 60 beats per minute.

tamponade or aortic regurgitation, where traditional pharmacologic interventions may be harmful and urgent surgery is needed. Initial medical management of stable patient while waiting for possible intervention should focus on management of pain, decrease of blood pressure to a minimum acceptable level, and decrease in the force of left ventricular contraction (d*P*/d*t*). In general, short acting parenteral therapies are favored in the acute setting to allow titration. Early observation should occur in an intensive care setting, with continuous arterial pressure monitoring. For patients presenting with evidence of heart failure, pulmonary artery catheter placement may be considered, but is usually not necessary.

Pain management is titrated aggressively for patients with dissection. The goals of pain treatment are patient comfort and decrease of adrenergic tone. Narcotic analgesics are effective for the rapid reduction of symptom severity, especially when administered in IV form. Long-acting oral formulations of narcotics are not recommended.

Blood pressure and d*P*/d*t* can be decreased with a β-blocker. Noncardioselective agents such as propranolol, labetalol, and esmolol have been used extensively in this context [62]. β-Blockers should be considered even for patients who are not hypertensive at presentation, as the reduction in d*P*/d*t* is thought to be beneficial for reducing the advancement of the dissection front. The goal heart rate is 60 beats per minute, and the goal systolic blood pressure is no higher than 120 mm Hg. For patients with hypertension, agents with both α- and β-antagonism such as labetalol may be useful. In the event that a patient's blood pressure is still elevated even after a goal heart rate has been reached with β-blockade, a vasodilator such as nitroprusside or an IV angiotensin converting enzyme inhibitor, such as enalaprilat may also be administered; however, vasodilator therapy should not be used without concomitant β-blockade, given the possibility of an increase in heart rate and d*P*/d*t* accompanying its potent vasodilatory effects [62].

In the rare event that a β-blocker cannot be used, due to contraindications such as bronchospasm, the nondihydropyridine calcium-channel blockers are the second-line agents. Verapamil and diltiazem, both of which have vasodilator and negative inotropic/chronotropic effects, may be used.

Close monitoring, including pulse and perfusion monitoring, is required for all patients as complications such as limb or visceral malperfusion may develop after the initial assessment. Hypotension may be seen in conjunction with dissection. It should be noted that the mode of blood pressure measurement should be scrutinized before changing a treatment plan; "pseudo-hypotension" may occur when dissection propagates into the limb in which blood pressure is being measured. In such cases, it is recommended that hypotension be verified by measurement of blood pressure in other limbs prior to discontinuation of β-blockers or calcium-channel blockers (Table 193.2).

Intervention

The primary concept that relates to the optimal choice of therapy has not changed for nearly 30 years. In most cases, the location of the dissection determines whether the patient should undergo immediate surgery. Patients who present with acute dissection in the context of pregnancy require additional consideration and multidisciplinary evaluation [63]. Type A dissection is treated with surgery in virtually all cases, as the outcomes associated with surgical repair are superior to outcomes with medical management: ~25% versus ~50% to 70% mortality at 30 days [3,4,64]. In general, preoperative coronary angiography has not been shown to be beneficial and is not recommended [65]. The one potential contraindication to urgent surgical repair of Type A dissection is stroke in evolution depending on severity, due to high risk of hemorrhagic transformation during surgery [15,16]. In aggregate, survival of patients with acute Type A dissection who are treated with surgical repair has improved over the last 25 years [10]. Aortic dissection repair is complex surgery, and each patient's medical comorbidities need to be addressed in detail before surgery as time allows. In the past, patients older than 80 were thought to have an operative survival rate too low to justify attempted repair. A multicenter study reported acceptable outcomes for aortic dissection repair performed in selected octogenarians. Although this study raises the possibility of aortic dissection repair in this age group, this approach remains controversial and each patient must be approached individually [66]. There is an evolving role of endovascular Type A dissection repair, however, surgical management remains the current standard [67–69].

Patients with Type B dissections are generally managed conservatively. Urgent intervention is warranted in the setting of complications including visceral or limb malperfusion, aortic expansion or impending rupture, progression of dissection, refractory pain, or refractory hypertension [70]. Risk stratification for Type B aortic dissection may be complex and benefit from specialty and multidisciplinary evaluation [71]. Interventional options include open surgery or endovascular techniques including fenestration and stent grafting.

Although there are no randomized assessments in the acute setting, observational studies suggest that outcomes may be better with endovascular therapy when feasible. Although percutaneous fenestration of the "false" lumen had previously been the therapeutic option of choice in this setting, this technique has been largely supplanted by the more definitive endovascular stent repair. The theory that closure of the primary entry tear may reduce the risk of propagation and further complications, as well as increase the likelihood of false lumen thrombosis, has led to the development and investigation of the use of covered stent grafts for selected patients with aortic dissection. It is thought that the minimally invasive nature of this technique may decrease perioperative mortality and thus improve outcomes [72,73]. Initial results and short-term outcomes with endovascular therapy of acute Type B dissections are promising [74,75]. Case series have described this strategy for pregnant women with Type B dissection [76]. Newer technologies using conformable aortic grafts in the aortic arch and thoracic aorta show promising early outcomes [77].

The increasing use of endovascular repair for Type B dissection prompted an expert consensus statement from an interdisciplinary group [72]. Data from 63 studies published between 2006 and 2012, and including 6,729 patients were reviewed [72]. The authors recommended medical treatment for uncomplicated acute Type B dissection but felt that complicated acute Type B dissection should be treated with TEVAR rather than surgery, when feasible and combined with other endovascular interventions such as fenestration, noting a survival benefit with the less invasive approach [72]. Intervention for subacute and chronic Type B dissection was recommended only when complications developed; in these settings as well, TEVAR was favored over surgery when feasible [72]. Nonrandomized observations from IRAD also found that TEVAR was associated with lower 5-year mortality when compared to medical therapy, suggesting that improved techniques may be associated with better outcomes, and prompting a call for further randomized trials [73].

There has been a growing utilization of endovascular stent grafting for uncomplicated Type B dissection in the subacute or chronic phase, particularly when there are markers suggesting an increased risk of adverse remodeling. Prognostic factors described include false lumen size, entry tear size and location, maximum aortic diameter of 40 mm or greater, number of vessels originating from the false lumen, and the patency of the false lumen [78–83]. The INSTEAD trial randomized patients with uncomplicated Type B dissection to medical management or stent grafting [84]. Patients were randomized to treatment between 2 and 52 weeks after dissection (mean time intervals from dissection to randomization 45 days for optimal medical therapy (OMT) vs. 39 days for TEVAR + OMT group). The primary endpoint was all-cause death at 2 years. Secondary endpoints included aortic-related deaths, progression, and aortic remodeling. No differences between groups in either the primary or secondary endpoint were seen at 2 years [84]. A subsequent exploratory analysis at 5 years suggested remodeling benefit as well as aortic-related mortality and all-cause mortality [85]. A subsequent trial called ADSORB also suggested benefits in terms of aortic modeling parameters [86]. Other nonrandomized assessments of TEVAR for acute uncomplicated Type B dissection in selected patients have also shown lower rates of aortic adverse events and mortality with TEVAR versus medical therapy alone [87]. Although these outcomes have not driven broad utilization of this strategy, there is growing interest in those patients believed to be at risk for complications such as aneurysm formation. Trials exploring composite devices are ongoing [88]. In the chronic phase traditional criteria for intervention are driven by aortic size (≥5.5 cm ascending aorta and ≥5.5 to 6.0 cm descending aorta), its rate of growth over time, and the presence of associated complications such as aortic regurgitation and left ventricular dysfunction of some patients with Type A disease.

Observational series of patients presenting with traumatic aortic disruption have suggested alternative classification systems which may clarify imaging characteristics and their impact on interventional decision-making.

Outpatient Follow-up and Medical Therapy

Outpatient medications for patients generally should generally be oral long-acting therapies of similar classes to those used in the acute setting [1]. There may be specific benefits to certain classes of agents for patients with connective tissue disease [89]. Patients should be advised to avoid heavy lifting, Valsalva, or other activities that put undue stress on the aorta; however, moderate cardiovascular activity should be encouraged [90–92]. Close follow-up is required for all patients as adverse remodeling may occur in as many as a third of patients, however, achieving high rates of long-term follow-up can be challenging [93].

INTRAMURAL HEMATOMA

Not all cases of apparent aortic dissection involve communication between the true and false lumens via a tear in the intima. In 1988, the first cases of an "atypical" form of dissection without intimal rupture were described [94]. IMH is defined as a spontaneous collection of blood within the aortic media that does not apparently communicate with the lumen. The natural history of IMH is not fully understood. It is thought that it may represent a predecessor of aortic dissection with eventual intimal rupture.

Both classic aortic dissection and IMH are generally associated with the same set of risk factors and may be indistinguishable clinically. Diagnostic imaging studies, notably TEE, CT angiography, or MRI, are required to distinguish them (Fig.193.2). Characteristic features include a crescentic or circumferential thickening of the aortic wall indicating the presence of fresh thrombus. CT imaging with and without contrast facilitates diagnosis as the hematoma has a higher tissue density than unenhanced blood on noncontrast CT but is without enhancement after contrast administration [1]. Consequences of untreated IMH have traditionally suggest a similar risk for adverse outcomes as with typical aortic dissection; however, more recent data sets suggest variable outcomes.

Epidemiology

IMH occurs among a minority of the patients presenting with an apparent aortic dissection. Acute dissection events included in the IRAD registry were found to be due to IMH 10% of the time. Serial imaging of IRAD patients with IMH revealed that 16% evolved to dissection with intimal tear [5,95]. There was no statistically significant difference of mortality rates for typical dissection and IMH in this series [96]. Other reports suggest that patients with IMH may have better survival and may more often be managed more conservatively than patients with dissection [95,97]. An IRAD report of 178 patients with IMH noted an incidence between 0% and 25% of patients presenting with acute aortic syndromes [94]. The descending thoracic aorta was involved more often (58% Type B, 42% Type A, $p < 0.001$) [94]. Overall outcomes for Type A and Type B IMH were similar to those for dissection in the same anatomic distributions. IMH was associated with a higher rate of pericardial effusions and periaortic hematomas, but a lower incidence of pulse deficits and aortic regurgitation [94]. In-hospital mortality was high for Type A IMH (26.6%) and higher for those treated medically (40%) compared to those treated surgically (24.1%) although treatment was not randomized [94]. One observational review

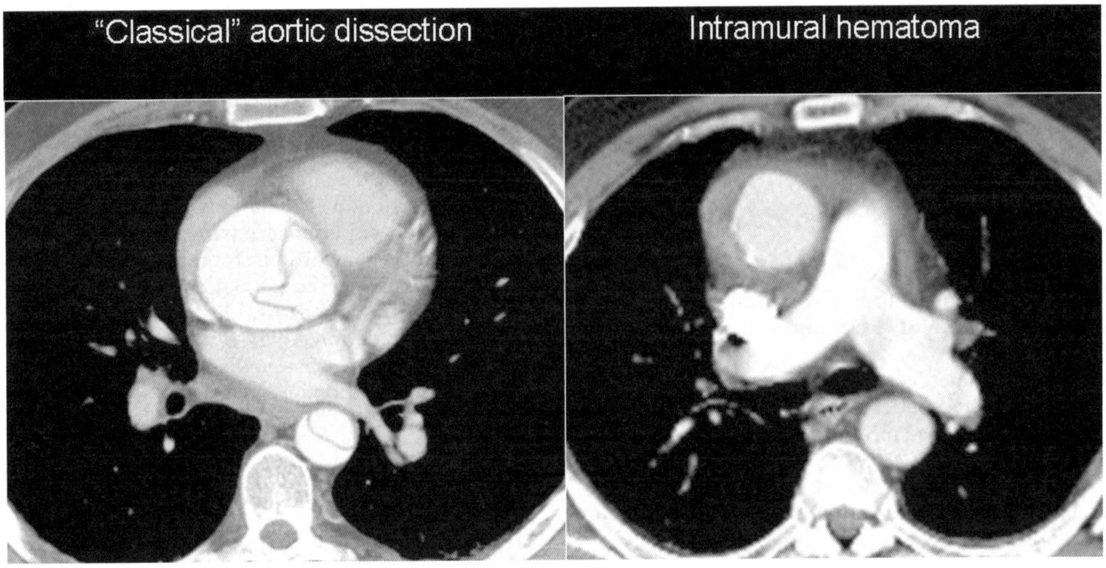

FIGURE 193.2 CT angiograms demonstrating the typical appearance of a "classical" aortic dissection versus that of an aortic intramural hematoma. Note the smooth crescentic thickening of the wall of the ascending aorta in the patient with intramural hematoma and the obvious intimal flap seen in the patient with the acute dissection. [© Massachusetts General Hospital Thoracic Aortic Center. Used with permission.]

of 65 patients with IMH found that those with an associated PAU progressed more frequently than IMH without PAU (48% vs. 8% $p = 0.002$) [98].

Although the risk factors and clinical presentations of classic aortic dissection and IMH are indistinguishable, certain important differences are recognized. Compared to those with typical aortic dissection, patients with IMH tend to be older, tend to have more atherosclerotic disease, and are more likely to have a distal acute aortic syndrome; two-thirds of IMH cases are Type B, in contrast with typical dissections, 65% of which are Type A.

Long-term follow-up of patients with IMH reveals that the hematoma evolves most commonly into a true or false aortic aneurysm or especially when associated with penetrating atherosclerotic ulcer (PAU). Up to 45% of such aneurysms that are located in the ascending aorta lead to rupture. Spontaneous regression occurs in up to one-third of cases. Regression is most likely with IMH not associated with increased aortic diameter at the time of presentation. Some observational data suggest that Type B IMH may have a more benign course than Type B dissection [99]. Clinical and radiographic progression of IMH is more likely when PAU is present (Fig.193.3). IMH in the absence of PAU appears to follow a more stable course, especially when located in the descending thoracic aorta [63].

Etiology and Pathophysiology

There are two proposed mechanisms by which an IMH may form. The first is the rupture of the vasa vasorum in the aortic wall, which may be the result of medial degeneration. The other leading mechanism is the invasion of a PAU beyond the internal elastic lamina of the vessel, compromising the integrity of the media. Once in the media, this ulceration can lead to hematoma formation. Both of these events could ostensibly be at work simultaneously.

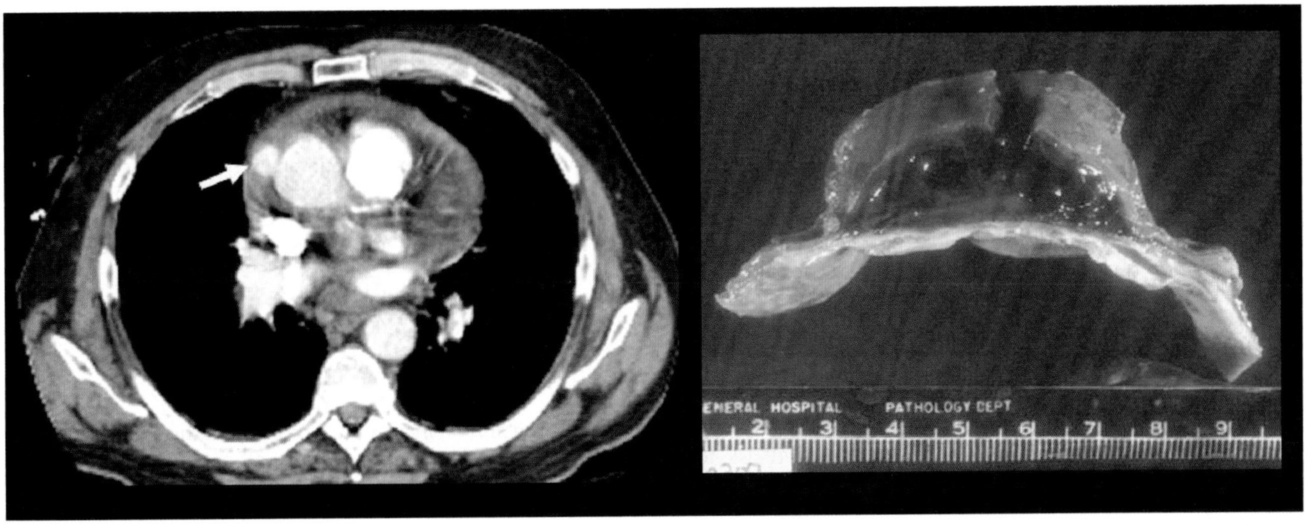

FIGURE 193.3 CT angiogram of an acute penetrating atherosclerotic ulcer, with corresponding pathologic specimen from the patient after ascending aortic repair.

Clinical Manifestations

The clinical presentation of IMH mirrors that of typical aortic dissection, and the two cannot be reliably distinguished on the basis of clinical criteria alone.

Imaging

Because the clinical presentation of IMH can overlap with that of classic dissection, prompt imaging is critical. The same set of imaging modalities used for classic aortic dissection is to be used to image IMH.

CXR findings associated with IMH mirror those for classic aortic dissection. Affected patients may exhibit an abnormal aortic silhouette or a widened mediastinum, but this finding is not as well validated as in classic dissection. Separation of intimal calcium from the aortic border may also be visible. These are simply associated findings; differentiation of IMH from classic dissection requires other imaging modalities.

TTE does not allow for definitive, reliable diagnosis of IMH. With TEE, IMH may appear as an echogenic, crescent-shaped segment of aortic wall. This is not a definitive modality, as in some cases, the thickened wall segment can be difficult to distinguish from atherosclerotic thickening.

With CT scanning, IMH appears as a crescent-shaped thickening of the aortic wall, but with a normal-appearing aortic lumen. CT imaging with and without contrast facilitates diagnosis as the hematoma has a higher tissue density than unenhanced blood on noncontrast CT but is without enhancement after contrast administration [1]. A contrast study is required for a definitive diagnosis. The most important feature that distinguishes an IMH from a classic dissection is the absence of contrast within the aortic wall. MRI allows for diagnosis of IMH without the use of contrast. The intensity of the hematoma can be determined by the signal sequence. Aortography is not a useful method for evaluating IMH, as the sensitivity for identification of IMH is less than 20%.

Management

As is the case for management of typical dissection, early imaging and surgical consultation are the central components of the management of a patient with an IMH, which can be a rapidly progressive disease. Frequent re-evaluation of the diseased aortic segment may also be warranted, especially if the patient presents with new hypotension or progressive symptoms. The most dangerous consequence of IMH is continued expansion and progression to typical dissection and/or aortic rupture. Given the high-risk nature of IMH in the ascending aorta, management is similar to typical aortic dissection: surgery for Type A syndromes and medical management for Type B syndromes [1,2]. The recent literature contains some controversy regarding the optimal management of acute Type A IMH [97,100].

For Type B IMH, medical management appears to be the consistently validated early treatment approach, unless a surgical indication is present. In-hospital mortality for patients in the IRAD series is less than 10% for patients receiving medical management.

There may be a role for prophylactic endovascular stent placement for patients with IMH who are thought to be in imminent danger of hematoma expansion and aortic rupture [101]. Type B IMH should be frequently reassessed and reimaged as indicated, as these patients are at increased risk for evolution into classical dissection or rupture. Several studies have suggested that a small proportion of IMH will resorb in short-term follow-up, and this appears to be correlated with smaller aneurysm size at presentation. However, a significant proportion of patients will go on to develop enlarging aortic aneurysm and/or pseudoaneurysm, classic aortic dissection, or rupture. The role of endovascular stents is evolving similar to that for Type B dissection [101]. The use of endovascular stent grafting to manage a complication of a Type B IMH with subsequent dissection is demonstrated in Figure 193.4. A summary of recommended management strategies for patients with acute aortic dissection or IMH is shown in Figure 193.5.

Although experience has varied, management of IMH should proceed according to the principles outlined for classic dissection. Specifically, patients with Type A IMH should receive surgery. The natural history of Type B IMH has been well delineated. Some may resorb spontaneously, while others go on to evolve classic dissection, false aneurysm, or true aneurysm formation.

EXPANDING AORTIC ANEURYSM AND RUPTURE

Definition and Classification

An aortic aneurysm is broadly defined as a segment of the aortic lumen whose diameter exceeds 1.5 times the normal diameter for that segment [1]. The risk of aneurysm rupture increases as a function of diameter. In addition, rupture risk is thought to be higher for rapidly expanding aneurysms. Aneurysms are also classified according to location (e.g., thoracic vs. abdominal), morphology, and etiology. All segments of the aorta can be affected and multiple aneurysms may be found in a single patient. Up to 13% of patients with an identified aortic aneurysm are found to have multiple aneurysm; as such, for patients in whom a single aneurysm has been detected, consideration should be given to scanning the entire aorta for additional aneurysms. In the general population, abdominal aneurysms are more common than thoracic aneurysms. Overall, aortic aneurysm is the eighth leading cause of cardiovascular mortality and was estimated to have caused more than 150,000 deaths globally in 2013.

The most commonly encountered aortic aneurysm morphology is fusiform—specifically, a symmetrical dilatation of an aortic segment, involving the entire circumference of the vessel wall (Fig.193.6). Aneurysms may also be saccular, or may involve only a portion of the vessel, leading to an asymmetric dilatation. It is also important to distinguish between true and false aneurysms: a true aneurysm involves all three layers of the vessel wall, whereas a false aneurysm is typically a collection of blood underneath the adventitia or outside the vessel altogether. This collection is frequently the result of a defect in the aortic wall. The presence of a suspected saccular aneurysm deserves special note, as it may actually represent a false aneurysm caused by a partially contained rupture of the aortic wall.

Aortic aneurysms are frequently asymptomatic at the time of diagnosis, and tend to be detected with tests ordered for other reasons. Indeed, an aortic aneurysm may not be associated with any symptoms until the time of rupture. As the clinical presentations of ruptured thoracic and abdominal aortic aneurysms (AAAs) frequently differ, they are discussed separately.

ANEURYSMS OF THE THORACIC AORTA

Epidemiology

The overall annual incidence of thoracic aortic aneurysm (TAA) is 6 per 100,000, and up to 40% of all patients are asymptomatic at the time of diagnosis. The risk of aneurysm rupture or dissection increases as a function of size. An abrupt increase in risk has been noted at a diameter of 6 cm: for aneurysms greater than 6 cm, the rupture rate has been observed to be 3.7% per

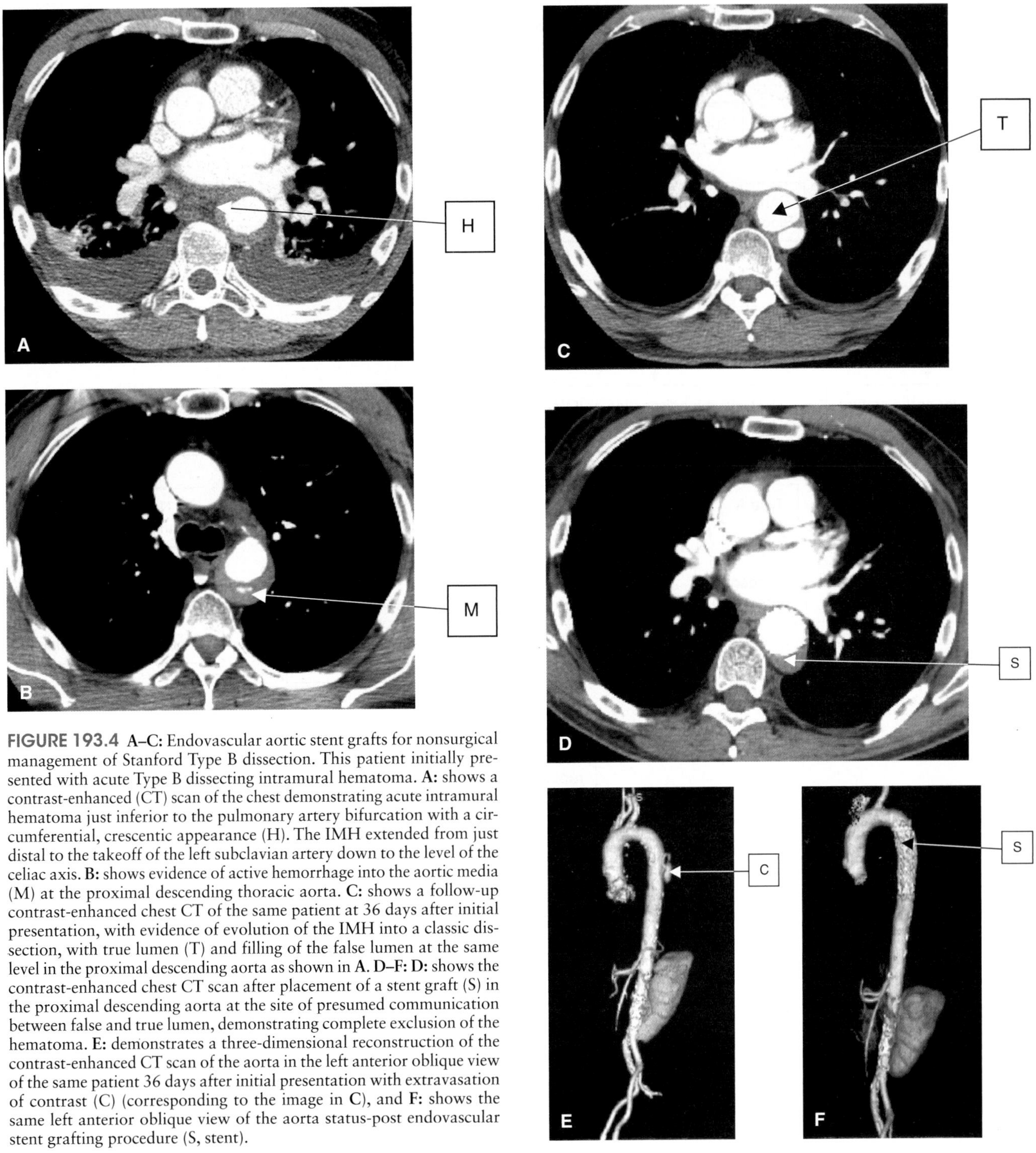

FIGURE 193.4 A–C: Endovascular aortic stent grafts for nonsurgical management of Stanford Type B dissection. This patient initially presented with acute Type B dissecting intramural hematoma. **A:** shows a contrast-enhanced (CT) scan of the chest demonstrating acute intramural hematoma just inferior to the pulmonary artery bifurcation with a circumferential, crescentic appearance (H). The IMH extended from just distal to the takeoff of the left subclavian artery down to the level of the celiac axis. **B:** shows evidence of active hemorrhage into the aortic media (M) at the proximal descending thoracic aorta. **C:** shows a follow-up contrast-enhanced chest CT of the same patient at 36 days after initial presentation, with evidence of evolution of the IMH into a classic dissection, with true lumen (T) and filling of the false lumen at the same level in the proximal descending aorta as shown in **A. D–F: D:** shows the contrast-enhanced chest CT scan after placement of a stent graft (S) in the proximal descending aorta at the site of presumed communication between false and true lumen, demonstrating complete exclusion of the hematoma. **E:** demonstrates a three-dimensional reconstruction of the contrast-enhanced CT scan of the aorta in the left anterior oblique view of the same patient 36 days after initial presentation with extravasation of contrast (C) (corresponding to the image in **C**), and **F:** shows the same left anterior oblique view of the aorta status-post endovascular stent grafting procedure (S, stent).

year [1]. The most commonly affected segments are the aortic root and ascending aorta; 60% of observed cases involve these segments. Aneurysms of the descending aorta account for 40% of cases, and the aortic arch accounts for 10%.

The surgical treatment strategy for asymptomatic aortic aneurysms differs on the basis of location, size, and etiology: for an aneurysm of the aortic root or the ascending aorta, surgical repair is indicated for a diameter of 5.5 cm or more or for aneurysms expanding at a rate >0.5 cm per year [1]. Patients who by nature of their underlying disease state are at increased risk of rupture, such as patients with Marfan syndrome, 5 cm (or less in certain cases, such as in patients with strong family histories for premature aortic dissection or rupture) is the recommended operative threshold [102]. For patients with aneurysm in the setting of bicuspid aortic valve the rate of dissection or rupture at diameters below 5.0 cm is low and a recent consensus statement suggested that using 5.5 cm was reasonable although treatment at lower dimensions should be considered if expanding rapidly or if valve surgery was warranted [103]. Endovascular aortic repair with aortic arch vessel revascularization has been described and may be an option in the future for patients at heightened surgical risk [104]. In the descending thoracic aorta, size remains the principal predictor of adverse outcomes with low rates of complications at sizes below 5.0 to 5.5 cm [105].

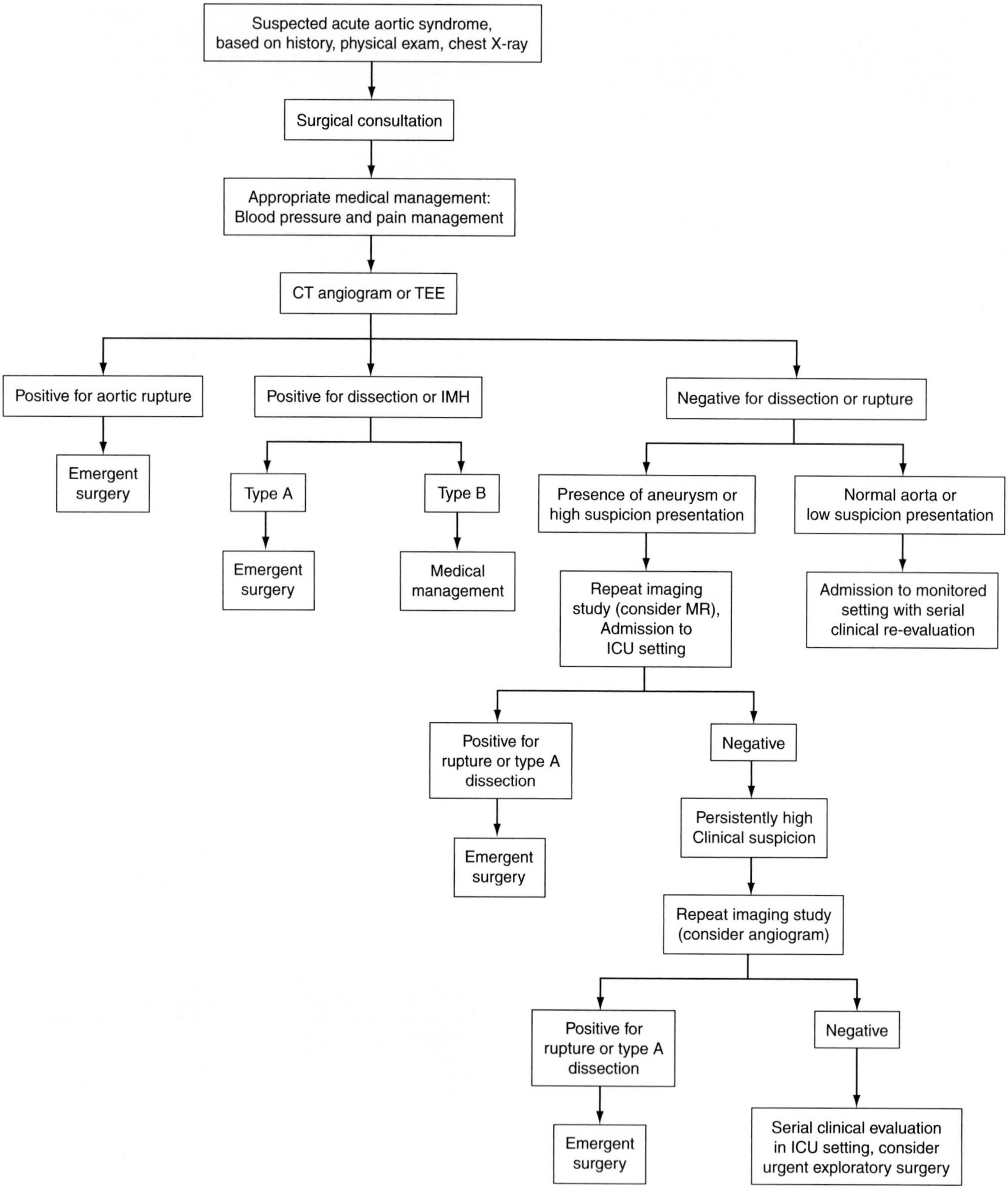

FIGURE 193.5 A suggested management strategy for patients with suspected acute aortic syndrome.

For patients with large TAAs, survival without surgical repair is poor, with 5-year survival after initial identification at 20%. Rupture occurs in 32% to 68% of patients whose TAAs are not repaired surgically [1]. Of those patients whose rupture occurs outside a hospital setting, it is thought that less than half will arrive to a hospital alive. For those patients who survive until hospital admission, mortality at 6 hours is 54%. At 24 hours, mortality without surgery is 76%.

Etiology and Pathophysiology

Multiple factors have been implicated for the formation of TAAs, including atherosclerotic disease, specific gene defects, and infectious processes. In many cases, a central pathophysiologic process is medial degeneration, which leads to the loss of elastic fibers and smooth muscle cells. This process, which is frequently correlated with aging, causes progressive stiffening and weakening of the vessel wall, leading to progressive dilatation. Hypertension accelerates dilatation due to the increase of wall strain.

The inciting factors that lead to aneurysm formation influences which portion of the aorta is affected and the age at which the abnormality tends to be diagnosed. Aneurysms of the aortic root and ascending aorta are frequently associated with inherited defects of structural genes or with inflammation caused either by infection or by vasculitis. In general, aneurysms associated with structural genetic mutations tend to occur at a younger age, in some cases during the second and third decades of life [25]. Identified connective tissue disorders, such as Marfan and Ehlers–Danlos syndromes, have been established as causes for aneurysms of this portion of the aorta [25]. These syndromes are caused by deficits in fibrillin-1 and type III collagen, respectively [25]. In addition, mutations of transforming growth factor beta (TGF-β) signaling have been associated with aneurysm and dissection [24]. Mutations in LRP1, LOX, FBN1, ULK4, ACTA2, SMAD1, the X-linked biglycan gene, and other genes have all been described in the setting of dissection [26,27,106–108]. The specific protein deficits lead to weakening of the vessel wall due to medial necrosis with resultant ectasia. A growing body of evidence reveals a hereditary syndrome (FTAAS) that does not lead to overt manifestations of connective tissue disease but is associated with aneurysm of the ascending aorta. Multiple loci have been identified, but routine genetic testing for this spectrum of disorders is not yet available. A bicuspid aortic valve is also associated with aneurysm of the aortic root/ascending aorta [109–111]. Dilation of this segment of the aorta has been shown to be due to medial degeneration that is independent of the potential hemodynamic effects of the abnormal valve. An acquired defect of the integrity of fibrillin-1 may also occur in some of these patients. A growing body of evidence suggests that the enzymatic activity of several matrix metalloproteinases (MMPs) may play a central role in the loss of connective tissue integrity for patients with bicuspid aortic valve [112]. Turner syndrome is associated with an increased incidence of bicuspid aortic valve, as well as with aortic coarctation and aneurysm of the ascending aorta [25].

Ascending aortic aneurysm may also be caused by infectious processes, such as bacterial endaortitis or chronic spirochetal infection. Syphilis, once a common cause of aneurysm in the ascending aorta but less frequently dissection, is now rarely seen in the developed world. The aortitis caused by bacterial infection leads to both fusiform and saccular aneurysms. Inflammation-related aneurysm in this area may also be caused by vasculitic processes, most notably Takayasu or giant cell arteritis. Although typically associated with stenotic lesions of the aorta or great vessels, Takayasu arteritis may present acutely, with the development of aortic aneurysms that are associated with signs of systemic and focal aortic inflammation; in rare cases, patients with acute aortic dilatation associated with Takayasu arteritis have suffered acute aortic rupture. Patients with Takayasu arteritis are typically younger Asian females, who may show involvement of the pulmonary arteries as well. In contrast, aneurysms associated with giant cell arteritis are more frequently diagnosed in older Caucasian females with prior polymyalgia rheumatica and/or symptomatic temporal arteritis.

Aneurysms of the descending aorta are generally caused by atherosclerosis. As such, these aneurysms are more commonly found in men and are not frequently seen before the sixth decade

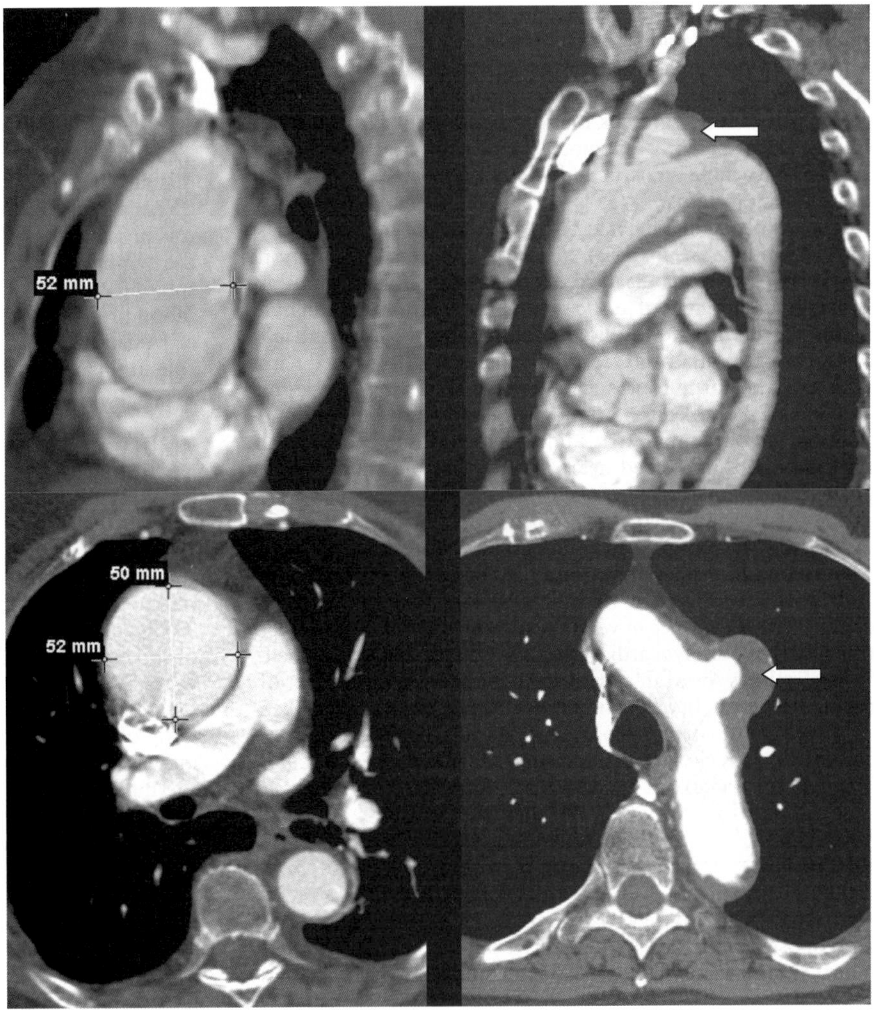

FIGURE 193.6 CT angiograms of a fusiform aneurysm (left-hand panels, with dimensions) and a saccular aneurysm (right-hand panels, *white arrows*).

of life. These aneurysms are found beyond the branch point of the left subclavian artery and are typically fusiform. Saccular aneurysms may be found at the aortic isthmus, and are frequently the result of rapid deceleration trauma.

Clinical Manifestations

Expanding aneurysms of the ascending and descending thoracic aorta produce symptoms due to compression of neighboring thoracic structures and compromise of aortic valve function (see later in the chapter). Compression leads to chest and back pain in as many as 37% and 21% of cases, respectively. Specific thoracic structures, when compressed by the aorta, lead to distinct signs and symptoms, including superior vena cava syndrome, pulmonary symptoms due to tracheal compression, or dysphagia due to esophageal compression. In addition, stretching of the recurrent laryngeal nerve may lead to unilateral vocal cord paralysis, with hoarseness (Ortner syndrome).

Symptoms from rupture of a TAA are largely related to mechanical effects of blood extending into adjoining thoracic spaces. The sudden onset of acute chest or back pain is a common feature of aneurysm rupture for all segments of the thoracic aorta. Perhaps the most salient feature of this pain is the fact that its maximal intensity occurs at onset. In patients whose aneurysms have produced prior symptoms, the pain at the time of rupture may be a more intense form of the same sensation, often at the same location. The pain does not necessarily have a tearing quality, as is often the case with dissection.

The most common area of blood flow from a rupture of the ascending aorta is the left pleural space, followed by the intrapericardial space. Blood flow into these areas lead to hemothorax and hemopericardium. Tamponade physiology may be present. Rupture of the descending aorta can lead to erosion into the esophagus: over time, an aortoesophageal fistula may form, leading to severe hematemesis. No matter where the point of blood egress is found, rapid loss of intravascular volume leads promptly to hypotension and shock if unrepaired. Ancillary warning signs include decreased urine output and altered mental status.

The heart examination may also exhibit distinct abnormalities with expanding aneurysm and rupture. Progressive dilatation of the aortic root may lead to dilatation of the valve annulus with consequent signs of aortic regurgitation. This phenomenon is associated with a diastolic murmur heard best over the left sternal border with the exception of aneurysms associated with ectasia of the aortic root, such as syphilitic aortitis, where the murmur of aortic regurgitation may be more noticeable along the right sternal border. Critical levels of regurgitation may be associated with left-sided heart failure. This murmur may be present in the absence of rupture. When rupture of one of the sinuses of Valsalva occurs, the murmur may be continuous; in this setting, the ruptured area may communicate with a cardiac chamber, such as the right atrium or ventricle.

In the context of acute rupture, the electrocardiography frequently shows evidence of ventricular "strain" or ischemia. Over time, markers of myocardial necrosis may be elevated as well. Several studies show an elevation of D-dimer in the context of aortic dissection, but elevation of this marker has not yet been validated for aneurysm progression or rupture [104]. There is currently no widely available biomarker in use to detect vascular injury in the context of aneurysm or rupture.

Imaging

Aortic aneurysm may be visualized as a widened mediastinum on anteroposterior views. Although this technique offers invaluable information, it cannot be considered a definitive study. TTE allows for the evaluation of the aortic root and ascending aorta. TEE is well suited to the evaluation of potentially aneurysmal segments in the aortic arch and descending aorta. As noted previously, perhaps the most important procedural drawback regarding TEE is the need for conscious sedation, which may be difficult to administer to a patient who is hemodynamically unstable.

CT scanning allows for evaluation of potentially aneurysmal segments in the entire aorta. Contrast CT imaging may also be helpful in identification of areas of blood extravasation in ruptured aortic aneurysms. MRI may be used for aortic measurement and identification of aneurysmal segments without contrast. Evaluation of blood extravasation with MRI is possible, but thought to be less sensitive than CT with contrast, especially for slow or low-volume extravasation. Aortography is a highly sensitive technique for assessing extravasation. The use of this technique in the acute setting is ordinarily reserved for those cases where neither CT scanning nor MRI is available.

Rupture of a Thoracic Aortic Aneurysm: Management

Rupture of a TAA is a surgical emergency. Open repair of the vessel is the most established repair technique. Typically, the procedure is performed with deep hypothermic circulatory arrest. The type of repair is determined by the location of the rupture and the presence or absence of aortic valve involvement. Dacron grafts are generally placed to replace the diseased vessel segment, with various strategies for aortic valve repair or replacement when necessary. Recent work indicates that a less invasive form of repair, retrograde endovascular stent placement, may be useful for the repair of aneurysms of the descending aorta.

Patients with aneurysm of both ascending and descending segments present an additional challenge. Standard methods entail surgical replacement of diseased segments in a "staged" fashion; however, newer methods involving a hybrid approach of surgical replacement of the ascending aorta, with subsequent endovascular therapy of the distal segments, appear promising.

It may be that a particular patient presents with complaints raising concern for a ruptured aortic aneurysm. In the event that no rupture is found and the patient is hemodynamically stable, it is possible that expansion of the aneurysm is responsible for the symptoms. In such a case, the focus of immediate clinical treatment should be to decrease aortic wall strain and systemic blood pressure through the use of β-blockers in the context of a critical care setting. Prompt surgical consultation plays a vital role in the continuing care of these patients.

ANEURYSMS OF THE ABDOMINAL AORTA

Epidemiology

AAAs are far more common than TAAs. The estimated prevalence of AAAs ranges between 1.3% and 8.9% in men and between 1.0% and 2.2% in women older than 60 years. Most cases are observed in men older than 55 years and women older than 70 years. AAAs have been found to be correlated with smoking. Overall prevalence of abdominal aneurysms has risen substantially over the past 30 years. This trend has been linked to the increased prevalence of atherosclerosis, which is thought to be the major etiology responsible for abdominal aneurysms. In addition, improvements in imaging technology have increased the rate of detection.

Rupture of AAAs is estimated to cause approximately 15,000 deaths per year in the United States. The total mortality rate for patients with rupture ranges from 65% to 85%. One prospective study revealed that 25% of patients with AAA rupture die before arriving at a hospital. Of those who arrived at the hospital alive, 51% died before surgery. Patients who did have surgery sustained a 46% operative mortality rate. Total 30-day survival rate for this population was 11%. Given the poor prognosis associated with rupture, elective repair is recommended when possible. As is the case with TAAs, the risk of rupture increases as a function of aortic diameter.

Etiology and Pathophysiology

Incidence of AAA is closely correlated with the presence of atherosclerotic disease in the aorta. In general, the infrarenal segment of the aorta is most heavily affected by atherosclerosis, and this is also the segment where most abdominal aneurysms are observed. These aneurysms are typically fusiform, but saccular aneurysms may also be found.

The risk factor most closely associated with abdominal aneurysms is smoking, followed by age, hypertension, and hyperlipidemia. There is also a strong association between gender and abdominal aneurysm formation. Family history of AAA is associated with a 30% increase of risk for AAA formation, but there are not yet any specific genes linked with this finding.

Damage to the vessel wall, caused by atherosclerotic plaque, has been shown to cause local inflammation. This inflammatory process is thought to cause degradation of extracellular matrix proteins, notably elastin and collagen. In addition, it is thought that the proinflammatory cytokine milieu leads to cell death within the vessel wall. Weakening of the vessel wall follows, potentially accelerated by the action of multiple proteases, including MMP and cathepsin L [112]. There is some speculation that MMP polymorphisms may lead to a change in susceptibility to abdominal aneurysms, but there are no screening tests currently available to the clinician [112]. Hypertension increases the wall strain on the weakened vessel wall, leading to accelerated expansion. The full effects of smoking on aneurysm formation and expansion are not known, but increased atherosclerosis and hypertension are thought to be contributors.

Aneurysms of the descending thoracic aorta tend to be caused by atherosclerosis. These aneurysms often extend into the abdominal cavity, superior to the renal arteries. Such aneurysms are referred to as thoracoabdominal, and their management mirrors the management of aneurysms in the abdominal cavity.

Aneurysms of the descending thoracic or abdominal aorta may also be caused by acute bacterial infections. This is not a common finding, but tends to be found more often in patients who are IV drug users or who have traveled recently from a country where exposure to typical organisms (*Salmonella* and *Brucella*) is more likely to occur. Chronic tuberculosis is rarely associated with abdominal aneurysms. Syphilis may also be associated with abdominal aneurysms, but it is more commonly associated with the ascending aorta. Connective tissue disorders, such as Marfan and Ehlers–Danlos syndromes, do not typically affect the abdominal aorta; however, some systemic inflammatory disorders, notably Takayasu arteritis or Behcet disease, may be associated with abdominal aneurysms.

Clinical Manifestations

As is the case with thoracic aneurysms, most abdominal aneurysms are asymptomatic and tend to be discovered with testing performed for other reasons. Those patients who do have aneurysm-related complaints tend to report pain in the hypogastric area and/or pain in the lower back. This pain is caused by the expansion of the aneurysm and tends to last for hours or days at a time, and is usually dull and steady. In the abdomen, fewer structures tend to be affected by the expanding aorta. The most common consequence of aortic expansion is compression of the ureter or kidney, leading to hydronephrosis.

An episode of rupture tends to be announced by a sudden onset or increase in abdominal and/or back pain. The most notable feature of this pain is that it is at its maximum at the time of onset. Rupture most frequently leads to blood leakage into the left retroperitoneal space. These patients may present with an initial episode of pain associated with the first rupture, followed by temporary tamponade of the retroperitoneal space. A larger, life-threatening bleed inevitably follows. Less frequently, the aneurysm may erode into surrounding structures, most notably the duodenum, leading to either formation of an aortoduodenal fistula or potentially massive gastrointestinal (GI) bleeding.

Physical examination of a patient with an AAA may reveal a palpable, pulsatile mass in the midline. This mass is easiest to palpate in the hypogastric or paraumbilical region. The sensitivity of the manual examination is suboptimal: 82% for aneurysms 5 cm or greater. Furthermore, a mass may be difficult to appreciate. Consequently, the absence of a pulsatile mass on physical examination should not be interpreted as an absence of aneurysm. On rupture of an abdominal aneurysm, most patients become hypotensive, tachycardic, and diaphoretic. Patients may also exhibit signs of peritoneal irritation on examination. As noted, the patient may also present with evidence of GI bleeding. Laboratory analysis may reveal evidence of elevation in D-dimer or an elevation in cardiac biomarkers, due to demand-related myocardial ischemia. The incidence of popliteal aneurysm is higher among patients with AAA so a careful popliteal pulse examination should be performed with ultrasound imaging where abnormal.

Imaging

Transcutaneous ultrasound is a noninvasive and readily available technique for the evaluation of the abdominal aorta. This method is frequently used to track the size of abdominal aneurysms, though it is not the imaging modality of choice for the acute aortic syndromes. Like TTE, abdominal ultrasound is often limited by body habitus. As with thoracic aneurysms, the most definitive evaluations are provided by CT scanning and MRI. Aortography may provide useful information regarding aortic aneurysm, but it is not the modality of choice in the acute setting unless CT scanning and MRI are not available.

Rupture of an Abdominal Aortic Aneurysm: Management

Rupture of an AAA is a surgical emergency. Open repair, with replacement of the diseased segment with a Dacron graft, is the most established technique. Intraoperative mortality after rupture is very high, as noted previously. Retrograde endovascular stent placement is a promising technique [113–115], but it is not yet in common use in the acute setting [116,117]. Timely, but elective, surgical or endovascular intervention on the basis of size criteria, as assessed with longitudinal imaging, is the most effective means to prevent progression to rupture.

References

1. Hiratzka LF, Bakris GL, Beckman JA, et al: 2010 ACCF/AHA/AATS/ACR/ASA/SCA/SCAI/SIR/STS/SVM guidelines for the diagnosis and management of patients with thoracic aortic disease: a report of the American College of Cardiology Foundation/American Heart Association Task Force on Practice Guidelines, American Association for Thoracic Surgery, American College of Radiology, American Stroke Association, Society of Cardiovascular Anesthesiologists, Society for Cardiovascular Angiography and Interventions, Society of Interventional Radiology, Society of Thoracic Surgeons, and Society for Vascular Medicine. *Circulation* 121:e266–e369, 2010.
2. Erbel R, Aboyans V, Boileau C, et al: 2014 ESC guidelines on the diagnosis and treatment of aortic diseases: document covering acute and chronic aortic

diseases of the thoracic and abdominal aorta of the adult. The task force for the diagnosis and treatment of aortic diseases of the European Society of Cardiology (ESC). *Eur Heart J* 35:2873–2926, 2014.
3. Hagan PG, Nienaber CA, Isselbacher EM, et al: The international registry of acute aortic dissection (IRAD): new insights into an old disease. *JAMA* 283:897–903, 2000.
4. Howard DP, Banerjee A, Fairhead JF, et al: Population-based study of incidence and outcome of acute aortic dissection and premorbid risk factor control: 10-year results from the oxford vascular study. *Circulation* 127:2031–2037, 2013.
5. Mussa FF, Horton JD, Moridzadeh R, et al: Acute aortic dissection and intramural hematoma: a systematic review. *JAMA* 316:754–763, 2016.
6. DeBakey M, Beall AJ, Cooley D, et al: Dissecting aneurysms of the aorta. *Surg Clin North Am* 46:1045–1055, 1966.
7. Daily P, Trueblood HW, Stinson EB, et al: Management of acute aortic dissections. *Ann Thorac Surg* 10:237–247, 1970.
8. Nienaber CA, Clough RE: Management of acute aortic dissection. *Lancet* 385:800–811, 2015.
9. Booher AM, Isselbacher EM, Nienaber CA, et al: The IRAD classification system for characterizing survival after aortic dissection. *Am J Med* 126:730.e19–730.e24, 2013.
10. 2010 ACCF/AHA/AATS/ACR/ASA/SCA/SCAI/SIR/STS/SVM Guidelines for the Diagnosis and Management of Patients with Thoracic Aortic Disease Representative Members, Hiratzka LF, Creager MA, et al: Surgery for aortic dilatation in patients with bicuspid aortic valves: A statement of clarification from the American College of Cardiology/American Heart Association Task Force on Clinical Practice Guidelines. *J Thorac Cardiovasc Surg* 151:959–966, 2016.
11. Pape LA, Awais M, Woznicki EM, et al: Presentation, diagnosis, and outcomes of acute aortic dissection: 17-year trends from the international registry of acute aortic dissection. *J Am Coll Cardiol* 66:350–358, 2015.
12. Jonker FH1, Trimarchi S, Muhs BE, et al: The role of age in complicated acute type B aortic dissection. *Ann Thorac Surg*. 96(6):2129–34, 2013.
13. Stanger O, Schachner T, Gahl B, et al: Type-A aortic dissection after non-aortic cardiac surgery. *Circulation*. 2013.
14. Strauss C, Harris K, Hutchison S, et al: "Time is Life": early mortality in type A acute aortic dissection: insights form the IRAD Registry. *J Am Coll Cardiol* 61:1159–1107, 2013.
15. Bossone E, Corteville DC, Harris KM, et al: Stroke and outcomes in patients with acute type A aortic dissection. *Circulation* 128:S175–S179, 2013.
16. Conzelmann LO, Hoffmann I, Blettner M, et al: Analysis of risk factors for neurological dysfunction in patients with acute aortic dissection type A: Data from the german registry for acute aortic dissection type A (GERAADA). *Eur J Cardiothorac Surg* 42:557–565, 2012.
17. Cleveland JC Jr: A perfect storm: type A aortic dissection and prior cardiac surgery. *Circulation* 128:1593–1594, 2013.
18. Trimarchi S, TolenaarJL, Tsai TT, et al: Influence of clinical presentation on the outcome of acute B aortic dissection: evidences from IRAD. *J Cardiovasc Surg (Torino)* 53:161–168, 2012.
19. Jonker FH, Patel HJ, Upchurch GR, et al: Acute type B aortic dissection complicated by visceral ischemia. *J Thorac Cardiovasc Surg* 149:1081.e1–1086.e1, 2015.
20. Jonker FH, Trimarchi S, MuhsBE, et al: The role of age in complicated acute type B aortic dissection. *Ann Thorac Surg* 96:2129–2134, 2013.
21. Jonker FH, Trimarchi S, Rampoldi V, et al: Aortic expansion after acute type B aortic dissection. *Ann Thorac Surg* 94:1223–1229, 2012.
22. Fan LM, Douglas G, Bendall JK, et al: Endothelial cell-specific reactive oxygen species production increases susceptibility to aortic dissection. *Circulation* 129:2661–2672, 2014.
23. Gong B, Wang Z, Zhang M, et al: Disturbed P53-MDM2 feedback loop contributes to thoracic aortic dissection formation and may be a result of TRIM-25 overexpression. *Ann Vasc Surg* 40:243–251, 2017.
24. Bertoli-Avella AM, Gillis E, Morisaki H, et al: Mutations in a TGF-beta ligand, TGFB3, cause syndromic aortic aneurysms and dissections. *J Am Coll Cardiol* 65:1324–1336, 2015.
25. Isselbacher EM, Lino Cardenas CL, Lindsay ME: Hereditary influence in thoracic aortic aneurysm and dissection. *Circulation* 133:2516–2528, 2016.
26. Lee VS, Halabi CM, Hoffman EP, et al: Loss of function mutation in LOX causes thoracic aortic aneurysm and dissection in humans. *Proc Natl Acad Sci USA* 113:8759–8764, 2016.
27. Lemaire SA, McDonald ML, Guo DC, et al: Genome-wide association study identifies a susceptibility locus for thoracic aortic aneurysms and aortic dissections spanning FBN1 at 15q21.1. *Nat Genet* 43:996–1000, 2011.
28. Isselbacher EM, Bonaca MP, Di Eusanio M, et al: Recurrent aortic dissection: observations from the international registry of aortic dissection. *Circulation* 134:1013–1024, 2016.
29. Bonaca MP, O'Gara PT: Diagnosis and management of acute aortic syndromes: dissection, intramural hematoma, and penetrating aortic ulcer. *Curr Cardiol Rep* 16:536, 2014.
30. Kamel H, Roman MJ, Pitcher A, et al: Pregnancy and the risk of aortic dissection or rupture: a cohort-crossover analysis. *Circulation* 134:527–533, 2016.
31. Kuperstein R, Cahan T, Yoeli-Ullman R, et al: Risk of aortic dissection in pregnant patients with the marfan syndrome. *Am J Cardiol* 119:132–137, 2017.
32. Moza A, Al-Hudaif A, Sheikh M: Isolated aortic dissection during coronary intervention: rare but challenging. *Cardiovasc Interv Ther* 31:300–303, 2016.
33. Nunez-Gil IJ, Bautista D, Cerrato E, et al: Incidence, management, and immediate- and long-term outcomes after iatrogenic aortic dissection during diagnostic or interventional coronary procedures. *Circulation* 131:2114–2119, 2015.
34. Collins JS, Evangelista A, Nienaber CA, et al: Differences in clinical presentation, management, and outcomes of acute type a aortic dissection in patients with and without previous cardiac surgery. *Circulation* 110:II237–II242, 2004.
35. Teman NR, Peterson MD, Russo MJ, et al: Outcomes of patients presenting with acute type A aortic dissection in the setting of prior cardiac surgery: an analysis from the international registry of acute aortic dissection. *Circulation* 128:S180–S185, 2013.
36. Girdauskas E, Rouman M, Disha K, et al: Aortic dissection after previous aortic valve replacement for bicuspid aortic valve disease. *J Am Coll Cardiol* 66:1409–1411, 2015.
37. Harris KM, Strauss CE, Eagle KA, et al: Correlates of delayed recognition and treatment of acute type A aortic dissection: the international registry of acute aortic dissection (IRAD). *Circulation* 124:1911–1918, 2011.
38. Conzelmann LO, Weigang E, Mehlhorn U, et al: Mortality in patients with acute aortic dissection type A: analysis of pre- and intraoperative risk factors from the german registry for acute aortic dissection type A (GERAADA). *Eur J Cardiothorac Surg* 49:e44–e52, 2016.
39. Gilon D, Mehta RH, Oh JK, et al: Characteristics and in-hospital outcomes of patients with cardiac tamponade complicating type A acute aortic dissection. *Am J Cardiol* 103:1029–1031, 2009.
40. Czerny M, Schoenhoff F, Etz C, et al: The impact of pre-operative malperfusion on outcome in acute type A aortic dissection: results from the GERAADA registry. *J Am Coll Cardiol* 65:2628–2635, 2015.
41. Di Eusanio M, Trimarchi S, Patel HJ, et al: Clinical presentation, management, and short-term outcome of patients with type A acute dissection complicated by mesenteric malperfusion: observations from the international registry of acute aortic dissection. *J Thorac Cardiovasc Surg* 145:385.e1–390.e1, 2013.
42. Ho MY, Yeh JK, Wang CY, et al: Aortic dissection with severe aortic regurgitation. *Circulation* 133:e398–e399, 2016.
43. Rogers AM, Hermann LK, Booher AM, et al: Sensitivity of the aortic dissection detection risk score, a novel guideline-based tool for identification of acute aortic dissection at initial presentation: results from the international registry of acute aortic dissection. *Circulation* 123:2213–2218, 2011.
44. Kosuge M, Uchida K, Imoto K, et al: Prognostic value of ST-segment elevation in lead aVR in patients with type A acute aortic dissection. *J Am Coll Cardiol* 65:2570–2571, 2015.
45. Suzuki T, Distante A, Zizza A, et al: Diagnosis of acute aortic dissection by D-dimer: the international registry of acute aortic dissection substudy on biomarkers (IRAD-bio) experience. *Circulation* 119:2702–2707, 2009.
46. Marill KA: Serum D-dimer is a sensitive test for the detection of acute aortic dissection: a pooled meta-analysis. *J Emerg Med* 34:367–376, 2008.
47. Salvagno GL, Targher G, Franchini M, et al: Plasma D-dimer in the diagnosis of acute aortic dissection. *Eur Heart J* 29:1207, 2008; author reply 1207-8.
48. Martin T, Shariq S: D-dimer is elevated in acute aortic dissection. *BMJ Case Rep* 2010:2943, 2010.
49. Shimony A, Filion KB, Mottillo S, et al: Meta-analysis of usefulness of d-dimer to diagnose acute aortic dissection. *Am J Cardiol* 107:1227–1234, 2011.
50. Ohlmann P, Morel O, Radulescu B, et al: D-dimer in ruling out acute aortic dissection: sensitivity is not 100%. *Eur Heart J* 29:828–829, 2008; author reply 829.
51. Paparella D, Malvindi PG, Scrascia G, et al: D-dimers are not always elevated in patients with acute aortic dissection. *J Cardiovasc Med (Hagerstown)* 10:212–214, 2009.
52. Suzuki T, Katoh H, Tsuchio Y, et al: Diagnostic implications of elevated levels of smooth-muscle myosin heavy-chain protein in acute aortic dissection. the Smooth Muscle Myosin Heavy Chain Study. *Ann Intern Med* 133:537–541, 2000.
53. Suzuki T, Katoh H, Watanabe M, et al: Novel biochemical diagnostic method for aortic dissection. Results of a prospective study using an immunoassay of smooth muscle myosin heavy chain. *Circulation* 93:1244–1249, 1996.
54. Shinohara T, Suzuki K, Okada M, et al: Soluble elastin fragments in serum are elevated in acute aortic dissection. *Arterioscler Thromb Vasc Biol* 23:1839–1844, 2003.
55. Ayaram D, Bellolio MF, Murad MH, et al: Triple rule-out computed tomographic angiography for chest pain: a diagnostic systematic review and meta-analysis. *Acad Emerg Med* 20:861–871, 2013.
56. Bossone E, Evangelista A, Isselbacher E, et al: Prognostic role of transesophageal echocardiography in acute type A aortic dissection. *Am Heart J* 153:1013–1020, 2007.
57. Chiu KW, Lakshminarayan R, Ettles DF: Acute aortic syndrome: CT findings. *Clin Radiol* 68:741–748, 2013.
58. Valente T, Rossi G, Lassandro F, et al: MDCT in diagnosing acute aortic syndromes: reviewing common and less common CT findings. *Radiol Med* 117:393–409, 2012.
59. Shiga T, Wajima Z, Apfel CC, et al: Diagnostic accuracy of transesophageal echocardiography, helical computed tomography, and magnetic resonance imaging for suspected thoracic aortic dissection: systematic review and meta-analysis. *Arch Intern Med* 166:1350–1356, 2006.
60. Aggarwal B, Raymond CE: Therapeutic goals in patients with acute aortic dissection: management before surgery. *J Am Coll Cardiol* 65:1599–1600, 2015.

61. Harris KM, Strauss CE, Duval S, et al: Multidisciplinary standardized care for acute aortic dissection: design and initial outcomes of a regional care model. *Circ Cardiovasc Qual Outcomes* 3:424–430, 2010.
62. Suzuki T, Isselbacher EM, Nienaber CA, et al: Type-selective benefits of medications in treatment of acute aortic dissection (from the International Registry of Acute Aortic Dissection [IRAD]). *Am J Cardiol* 109:122–127, 2012.
63. Sawlani N, Shroff A, Vidovich MI: Aortic dissection and mortality associated with pregnancy in the United States. *J Am Coll Cardiol* 65:1600–1601, 2015.
64. Evangelista A, Rabasa JM, Mosquera VX, et al: Diagnosis, management and mortality in acute aortic syndrome: results of the spanish registry of acute aortic syndrome (RESA-II). *Eur Heart J Acute Cardiovasc Care* 2048872616682343, 2016.
65. Ramanath VS, Eagle KA, Nienaber CA, et al: The role of preoperative coronary angiography in the setting of type A acute aortic dissection: insights from the international registry of acute aortic dissection. *Am Heart J* 161:790.e1–796.e1, 2011.
66. Piccardo A, Regesta T, Zannis K, et al: Outcomes after surgical treatment for type A acute aortic dissection in octogenarians: a multicenter study. *Ann Thorac Surg* 88:491–497, 2009.
67. Horton JD, Kolbel T, Haulon S, et al: Endovascular repair of type A aortic dissection: current experience and technical considerations. *Semin Thorac Cardiovasc Surg* 28:312–317, 2016.
68. Li Z, Lu Q, Feng R, et al: Outcomes of endovascular repair of ascending aortic dissection in patients unsuitable for direct surgical repair. *J Am Coll Cardiol* 68:1944–1954, 2016.
69. Preventza O, Cervera R, Cooley DA, et al: Acute type I aortic dissection: traditional versus hybrid repair with antegrade stent delivery to the descending thoracic aorta. *J Thorac Cardiovasc Surg* 148:119–125, 2014.
70. Trimarchi S, Eagle KA, Nienaber CA, et al: Importance of refractory pain and hypertension in acute type B aortic dissection: insights from the international registry of acute aortic dissection (IRAD). *Circulation* 122:1283–1289, 2010.
71. Nienaber CA: The art of stratifying patients with type B aortic dissection. *J Am Coll Cardiol* 67:2843–2845, 2016.
72. Fattori R, Cao P, De Rango P, et al: Interdisciplinary expert consensus document on management of type B aortic dissection. *J Am Coll Cardiol* 61:1661–1678, 2013.
73. Fattori R, Montgomery D, Lovato L, et al: Survival after endovascular therapy in patients with type B aortic dissection: a report from the international registry of acute aortic dissection (IRAD). *JACC Cardiovasc Interv* 6:876–882, 2013.
74. Hanna JM, Andersen ND, Ganapathi AM, et al: Five-year results for endovascular repair of acute complicated type B aortic dissection. *J Vasc Surg* 59:96–106, 2014.
75. Midulla M, Renaud A, Martinelli T, et al: Endovascular fenestration in aortic dissection with acute malperfusion syndrome: immediate and late follow-up. *J Thorac Cardiovasc Surg* 142:66–72, 2011.
76. Brener MI, Keramati AR: Type B dissection in a pregnant woman managed with peripartum thoracic endovascular aortic repair. *Circulation* 133:e369–e373, 2016.
77. Bockler D, Brunkwall J, Taylor PR, et al: Thoracic endovascular aortic repair of aortic arch pathologies with the conformable thoracic aortic graft: early and 2 year results from aeuropeanmulticentre registry. *Eur J Vasc Endovasc Surg* 51:791–800, 2016.
78. Gasparetto A, Park KB, Sabri SS, et al: Factors related to late false lumen enlargement after thoracic stent-graft placement for type B aortic dissection. *J Vasc Interv Radiol* 28:44–49, 2017.
79. Girish A, Padala M, Kalra K, et al: The impact of intimal tear location and partial false lumen thrombosis in acute type B aortic dissection. *Ann Thorac Surg* 102:1925–1932, 2016.
80. Kamman AV, Brunkwall J, Verhoeven EL, et al; ADSORB trialists: Predictors of aortic growth in uncomplicated type B aortic dissection from the acute dissection stent grafting or best medical treatment (ADSORB) database. *J Vasc Surg* 65:964–971, 2017.
81. Kudo T, Mikamo A, Kurazumi H, et al: Predictors of late aortic events after stanford type B acute aortic dissection. *J Thorac Cardiovasc Surg* 148:98–104, 2014.
82. Li DL, Zhang HK, Chen XD, et al: Thoracic endovascular aortic repair for type B aortic dissection: analysis among acute, subacute, and chronic patients. *J Am Coll Cardiol* 67:1255–1257, 2016.
83. Teraa M, van Herwaarden JA, Trimarchi S, et al: Morphologic characteristics for treatment guidance in uncomplicated acute type B aortic dissection. *Circulation* 130:1723–1725, 2014.
84. Nienaber CA, Rousseau H, Eggebrecht H, et al: Randomized comparison of strategies for type B aortic dissection: the INvestigation of STEnt grafts in aortic dissection (INSTEAD) trial. *Circulation* 120:2519–2528, 2009.
85. Nienaber CA, Kische S, Rousseau H, et al: Endovascular repair of type B aortic dissection: long-term results of the randomized investigation of stent grafts in aortic dissection trial. *Circ Cardiovasc Interv* 6:407–416, 2013.
86. Brunkwall J, Kasprzak P, Verhoeven E, et al: Endovascular repair of acute uncomplicated aortic type B dissection promotes aortic remodelling: 1 year results of the ADSORB trial. *Eur J Vasc Endovasc Surg* 48:285–291, 2014.
87. Qin YL, Wang F, Li TX, et al: Endovascular repair compared with medical management of patients with uncomplicated type B acute aortic dissection. *J Am Coll Cardiol* 67:2835–2842, 2016.
88. Lombardi JV, Cambria RP, Nienaber CA, et al: Prospective multicenter clinical trial (STABLE) on the endovascular treatment of complicated type B aortic dissection using a composite device design. *J Vasc Surg* 55:629.e2–640.e2, 2012.
89. Lacro RV, Dietz HC, Sleeper LA, et al: Atenolol versus losartan in children and young adults with marfan's syndrome. *N Engl J Med* 371:2061–2071, 2014.
90. Chaddha A, Kline-Rogers E, Woznicki EM, et al: Cardiology patient page. activity recommendations for postaortic dissection patients. *Circulation* 130:e140–e142, 2014.
91. Delsart P, Maldonado-Kauffmann P, Bic M, et al: Post aortic dissection: gap between activity recommendation and real life patients aerobic capacities. *Int J Cardiol* 219:271–276, 2016.
92. Fuglsang S, Heiberg J, Hjortdal VE, et al: Exercise-based cardiac rehabilitation in surgically treated type-A aortic dissection patients. *Scand Cardiovasc J* 1–7, 2016.
93. Kret MR, Azarbal AF, Mitchell EL, et al: Compliance with long-term surveillance recommendations following endovascular aneurysm repair or type B aortic dissection. *J Vasc Surg* 58:25–31, 2013.
94. Harris KM, Braverman AC, Eagle KA, et al: Acute aortic intramural hematoma: an analysis from the international registry of acute aortic dissection. *Circulation* 126:S91–S96, 2012.
95. Song JK, Yim JH, Ahn JM, et al: Outcomes of patients with acute type A aortic intramural hematoma. *Circulation* 120:2046–2052, 2009.
96. Evangelista A, Mukherjee D, Mehta RH, et al: Acute intramural hematoma of the aorta: a mystery in evolution. *Circulation* 111:1063–1070, 2005.
97. Kitai T, Kaji S, Yamamuro A, et al: Clinical outcomes of medical therapy and timely operation in initially diagnosed type A aortic intramural hematoma: a 20-year experience. *Circulation* 120:S292–S298, 2009.
98. Ganaha F, Miller DC, Sugimoto K, et al: Prognosis of aortic intramural hematoma with and without penetrating atherosclerotic ulcer: a clinical and radiological analysis. *Circulation* 106:342–348, 2002.
99. Tolenaar JL, Harris KM, Upchurch GR Jr, et al: The differences and similarities between intramural hematoma of the descending aorta and acute type B dissection. *J Vasc Surg* 58:1498–1504, 2013.
100. Evangelista A, Eagle KA: Is the optimal management of acute type a aortic intramural hematoma evolving? *Circulation* 120:2029–2032, 2009.
101. Bischoff MS, Meisenbacher K, Wehrmeister M, et al: Treatment indications for and outcome of endovascular repair of type B intramural aortic hematoma. *J Vasc Surg* 64:1569.e2–1579.e2, 2016.
102. Cameron D: Surgery for congenital diseases of the aorta. *J Thorac Cardiovasc Surg* 149:S14–S17, 2015.
103. Kim JB, Spotnitz M, Lindsay ME, et al: Risk of aortic dissection in the moderately dilated ascending aorta. *J Am Coll Cardiol* 68:1209–1219, 2016.
104. Iida Y, Kawaguchi S, Koizumi N, et al: Thoracic endovascular aortic repair with aortic arch vessel revascularization. *Ann Vasc Surg* 25:748–751, 2011.
105. Kim JB, Kim K, Lindsay ME, et al: Risk of rupture or dissection in descending thoracic aortic aneurysm. *Circulation* 132:1620–1629, 2015.
106. Guo DC, Grove ML, Prakash SK, et al: Genetic variants in LRP1 and ULK4 are associated with acute aortic dissections. *Am J Hum Genet* 99:762–769, 2016.
107. Meester JA, Vandeweyer G, Pintelon I, et al: Loss-of-function mutations in the X-linked biglycan gene cause a severe syndromic form of thoracic aortic aneurysms and dissections. *Genet Med* 19:386–395, 2017.
108. Murana G, PantaleoA, Parolari A, et al: Genetically triggered thoracic aortic aneurysms and cardiovascular conditions (GenTAC) registry predicting predictors for aortic dissection: a new thought around the corner? *J Thorac Dis* 8:E1093–E1095, 2016.
109. Itagaki S, Chikwe JP, Chiang YP, et al: Long-term risk for aortic complications after aortic valve replacement in patients with bicuspid aortic valve versus marfan syndrome. *J Am Coll Cardiol* 65:2363–2369, 2015.
110. Sherrah AG, Andvik S, van der Linde D, et al: Nonsyndromic thoracic aortic aneurysm and dissection: outcomes with marfan syndrome versus bicuspid aortic valve aneurysm. *J Am Coll Cardiol* 67:618–626, 2016.
111. Weinsaft JW, Devereux RB, Preiss LR, et al: Aortic dissection in patients with genetically mediated aneurysms: incidence and predictors in the GenTAC registry. *J Am Coll Cardiol* 67:2744–2754, 2016.
112. Liu O, Xie W, Qin Y, et al: MMP-2 gene polymorphisms are associated with type A aortic dissection and aortic diameters in patients. *Medicine (Baltimore)* 95:e5175, 2016.
113. Carrel T, Do DD, Triller J, et al: A less invasive approach to completely repair the aortic arch. *Ann Thorac Surg* 80:1475–1478, 2005.
114. Garzon G, Fernandez-Velilla M, Marti M, et al: Endovascular stent-graft treatment of thoracic aortic disease. *Radiographics* 25[Suppl 1]:S229–S244, 2005.
115. Larzon T, Lindgren R, Norgren L: Endovascular treatment of ruptured abdominal aortic aneurysms: a shift of the paradigm? *J Endovasc Ther* 12:548–555, 2005.
116. Criado F, Abul-Khoudoud OR, Domer GS, et al: Endovascular repair of the thoracic aorta: lessons learned. *Ann Thorac Surg* 80:857–863, 2005.
117. Katzen B, Dake MD, MacLean AA, et al: Endovascular repair of abdominal and thoracic aortic aneurysms. *Circulation* 112:1663–1675, 2005.

Chapter 194 ■ Management of Acute Decompensated Heart Failure

G. WILLIAM DEC

DEFINITION/EPIDEMIOLOGY

Acute decompensated heart failure (ADHF) is the most common indication for hospitalization in the USA and results in nearly 1 million hospitalizations annually [1]. In-hospital mortality for all patients in the Acute Decompensated Heart Failure National Registry (ADHERE) averaged 4% but was substantially higher in the cohort of patients over 75 years of age [2]. Potential explanations for the higher prevalence of heart failure in the elderly include the high rate of hypertension; ventricular remodeling from prior myocardial infarction; age-related loss of functional myocytes; and increased extracellular matrix that contributes to alterations in left ventricular compliance. Several of these features combine to create a ventricular phenotype of "heart failure with preserved ejection fraction." Thus, 40% to 50% of heart failure admissions in the elderly occur in the setting of preserved systolic function; however, these episodes carry the same in-hospital mortality rate. Indications for hospitalization for patients with ADHF have been summarized by the Heart Failure Society of America in their Practice Guidelines (Table 194.1) [3].

Most (>70%) acute heart failure admissions occur among patients with chronic heart failure. The differentiation of new-onset decompensated heart failure from subacute or acute worsening of chronic heart failure is important, because their pathophysiologies differ. Patients with new-onset heart failure have intense sympathetic activation and enhanced microvascular permeability [4]. Consequently, jugular venous distention may be more difficult to assess in these patients because of venous vasoconstriction and redistribution of fluids. Over 60% of patients hospitalized with ADHF have a history of coronary artery disease, hypertension, atrial fibrillation, diabetes mellitus, or renal dysfunction. Although dramatic, only 5% to 10% of patients with acute decompensation present with "sudden-onset" pulmonary edema.

TABLE 194.1

Indication for Hospitalization in Acute Decompensated Heart Failure

Definite	Evidence for severe decompensation with:
	Hypotension
	Worsening renal function or oliguria
	Mental obtundation
	Dyspnea at rest (resting tachypnea; oxygen saturation <90%)
	Significant atrial or ventricular arrhythmias
	Acute coronary syndrome
Possible	Evidence for moderate decompensation with:
	Signs of pulmonary or systemic congestion
	Major electrolyte abnormalities (hyponatremia, hypokalemia or hyperkalemia)
	Associated comorbid conditions (pneumonia, pulmonary embolism, uncontrolled diabetes mellitus)
	Symptoms of stroke or transient ischemic attack
	Repeated ICD firings
	New-onset heart failure

Adapted from Lindenfeld J, Albert NM, Boehmer JP, et al: Executive summary: HFSA2010 comprehensive heart failure practice guidelines. *J Card Fail* 16:498, 2010 (Table 12.1) (with permission).

Pathophysiologic Considerations

A variety of pathophysiologic mechanisms may be responsible for an ADHF episode. The key feature is volume overload with pulmonary and/or venous congestion. Hemodynamic measurements typically reveal increased right- and left-sided ventricular filling pressures; cardiac index is often, but not always, depressed. Congestion may be related to poor adherence to diet or medications or progression of left ventricular dysfunction with concomitant activation of vasoconstrictor neurohormones and/or worsening renal function. Other comorbidities, particularly poorly controlled hypertension, new onset atrial fibrillation, or active myocardial ischemia may also contribute to acute decompensation.

Deterioration of renal function may result from diminished cardiac output and a corresponding reduction of glomerular filtration rate, high venous filling pressures, intra-renal vasoregulation, alterations of circulatory volume, more intense neurohormonal activation, and/or the nephrotoxic effects of medications administered during hospitalization. Angiotensin II actively induces secretion of endothelin-1 and vasopressin. Further elevation of these neurohormones leads to sodium and water retention, increased myocardial wall stress, and decreased renal perfusion. A deleterious positive feedback loop is often established resulting in chronic elevation of vasoconstrictor neurohormones and worsening heart failure [1].

Myocardial injury is now recognized as an important element of the ADHF syndrome [5–7]. Myocyte loss is triggered by subendocardial myocardial ischemia, myocardial strain (consequent to elevated filling pressures), neurohormonal activation (via angiotensin II, endothelin, and aldosterone), systemic inflammation, and oxidative stresses [1]. Strategies aimed at preventing or limiting acute myocardial injury should be considered a treatment goal during management of any acute episode.

Predictors of Prognosis

Patients hospitalized for ADHF have a 2.5-fold higher 4 year mortality than that observed for stable chronic heart failure patients (60% versus 15%) [2]. Findings on physical examination also predict prognosis and should influence treatment during hospitalization. The presence of a chronic third heart sound or elevation in jugular venous pressure establish more advanced disease and predict increased long-term mortality. Moderate-to-severe mitral or tricuspid regurgitation are also both associated with increased symptoms, morbidity and mortality.

Table 194.2 lists independent parameters that have been correlated with clinical outcomes of hospitalized heart failure patients. These parameters include older age, male sex, heart failure etiology, history of previous heart failure hospitalization, respiratory rate, anemia, comorbid conditions, and biomarker levels. The utility of biomarkers, particularly B-type natriuretic

TABLE 194.2

Predictors of Adverse Outcome during Hospitalization for Acute Decompensated Heart Failure

Hypotension
Renal dysfunction
Older age
Male sex
Ischemic heart failure etiology
Prior heart failure hospitalizations
Respiratory rate on admission >30/min
Anemia
Hyponatremia or hypochloremia
Elevated serum troponin T or I
Elevated serum B-type natriuretic peptide or ST2 at discharge
Left ventricular ejection fraction <35%
Major medical comorbid conditions:
Chronic obstructive pulmonary disease
Dementia
Cerebrovascular or peripheral vascular disease
End stage kidney disease or hepatic cirrhosis
Malignancy
Fragility

Adapted from Dec GW: *Curr Probl Cardiol* 32:331, 2007 (Table 3) (With permission).

peptide (BNP), NT-pro BNP and ST2, have been shown useful in identifying patients at increased risk for readmission or deaths [8]. Serial assessment of BNP during hospitalization is useful for predicting post-discharge prognosis and suggests that this approach may soon help guide heart failure inpatient management. However, it should be recognized that a variety of etiologies including pulmonary embolism, acute coronary syndromes, and sepsis may also lead to markedly elevated BNP. Troponin I or T release occurs in 30% to 70% of ADHF patients; its elevation is associated with a twofold increase in post-discharge mortality and a threefold increase of rehospitalization rates [6,7]. Further, the combination of elevated BNP and troponin has been associated with a 12-fold increased risk of mortality. Several studies have demonstrated lower systolic blood pressure, higher blood urea nitrogen, and severity of hyponatremia as independent predictors of in-hospital mortality [9]. Renal dysfunction is also recognized as an extremely powerful predictor of heart failure outcome. The presence of chronic renal insufficiency, defined as a serum creatinine >1.4 mg per dL for women and >1.5 mg per dL for men, predicts an increased risk of death (risk ratio = 1.43). Unfortunately, approximately 25% of hospitalized patients with decompensated heart failure will exhibit a deterioration of renal function despite appropriate medical therapy. In these hospitalized patients, a modest rise in serum creatinine (i.e., 0.30 to 0.5 mg per dL) has been associated with a longer length of hospital stay and increased in-hospital mortality in some but not all series. This constellation of poorly understood physiologic mechanisms has been termed the "cardiorenal syndrome" and its optimal management remains to be defined [10].

Fonarow et al, using ADHERE data on over 33,000 patients, performed an extensive risk stratification of in-hospital mortality during ADHF [2]. Recursive partitioning of 32 key variables indicated that the best single predictor of in-hospital mortality was a high admission level of blood urea nitrogen (>43 mg per dL), followed by admission systolic blood pressure <115 mm Hg and a serum creatinine >2.75 mL per dL. On the basis of these three simple variables, patients can be readily stratified into groups at low, medium, and high risk for in-hospital mortality

TABLE 194.3

Potential Reversible Causes of Acute Decompensated Heart Failure

Dietary or medication noncompliance
Systemic infection
Active myocardial ischemia
Acute or worsening valvular insufficiency
Supraventricular tachycardias
Uncontrolled hypertension
Alcohol consumption
Cocaine, amphetamines, or excessive bronchodilator use
Sleep disordered breathing (central or obstructive apneas)
Hyperthryoidism or hypothyroidism
Anemia
Pulmonary embolism
Peripartum cardiomyopathy

From Dec GW: *Curr Probl Cardiol* 32:325, 2007 (Table 1) (with permission).

with rates ranging from 2.1% to 21.9%. Additional predictive variables from other studies include troponin release, markedly elevated natriuretic peptide levels, hyponatremia, and pulmonary hypertension [8,11]. Early identification of high-risk patients may ultimately lead to better strategies designed to improve their in-hospital outcomes.

PHARMACOLOGIC MANAGEMENT OF ADVANCED HEART FAILURE

Congestion is the most common cause for admission for ADHF and should be aggressive treated with diuretics. Renal function will often worsen transiently during aggressive in-hospital diuresis. Although earlier studies suggested increased mortality for modest increases of serum creatinine (e.g., >0.3 mg per dL), recent findings by Metra et al. and Testani et al. have shown that persistent congestion due to inadequate diuresis rather than transient changes of renal function greatly increases the risk of adverse outcomes following hospital discharge [12,13]. The importance of this finding is that diuresis should not be curtailed during ADHF treatment because of a modest decline of baseline renal function.

Almost 50% will have heart failure with preserved ejection fraction rather than systolic dysfunction. The acute treatment for volume overload should not differ by etiology. The treatment of HF-pEF is largely empirical as clinical trials have failed to find effective therapies to improve prognosis. The goals of medical therapy in HF-pEF should include adequate control of hypertension, rate control or restoration of normal sinus rhythm for new onset atrial fibrillation, and evaluation and management of myocardial ischemia or valvular heart disease. The remaining sections discuss treatment of heart failure with reduced ejection fraction (HF-rEF).

Systolic heart failure that persists after correction of potentially reversible causes (Table 194.3) should be treated with dietary sodium restriction, diuretics for volume overload, vasodilator therapy (particularly ACE inhibitors or angiotensin receptor antagonists), and a β-adrenergic blocker [14]. Sodium restriction (<4 g per day) is generally indicated for patients with advanced symptoms. Likewise, many ADHF patients require a 1.5 to 2 L per day fluid restriction.

Diuretics

Diuretics remain the mainstay for "congestive symptoms" but have not been shown to improve survival during hospitalization

TABLE 194.4

Intravenous Diuretic Regimens for Treating Decompensated Heart Failure

Drug	Initial dose	Maximal single dose
Loop diuretics		
Furosemide	40 mg	200 mg
Bumetanide	1 mg	4 to 8 mg
Torsemide	10 mg	100 to 200 mg
Thiazide diuretics		
Chlorothiazide	500 mg	1,000 mg
Synergistic nephron blockade		
Chorothiazide		500 to 1,000 mg + loop diuretics 1–4 X per day
Metolazone	2.5 to 10 mg PO + loop diuretic 1–2 X per day	
Intravenous infusions		
Furosemide	40 mg IV loading dose; then 5–40 mg/h infusion	
Bumetanide	1–2 mg IV loading dose; then 0.5 to 2 mg/h infusion	
Torsemide	20 mg IV loading dose; then 5 to 20 mg/h infusion	

mg, milligrams; IV, intravenous.

or long-term treatment. Neurohormonal activation (as measured by circulating renin, angiotensin II, endothelin-1, and BNP) has been shown to acutely decrease during short-term diuretic therapy administered to lower markedly elevated filling pressures. Two pharmacologic classes of agents are relevant to acute heart failure management: loop diuretics and distal tubular agents (Table 194.4). Loop diuretics (e.g., furosemide, torsemide, bumetanide, and ethacrynic acid) are the most potent. Some data suggest that oral torsemide and bumetanide may be more effective than furosemide for advanced heart failure, perhaps because of superior absorption from the gastrointestinal tract in the setting of elevated right-sided filling pressures. Although once daily dosing of loop diuretic is usually effective for outpatient therapy, patients with persistent symptoms or those with marked hemodynamic instability during hospitalization often require dosing two or three times a day to adequately manage volume overload.

Thiazide diuretics such as hydrochlorothiazide and metolazone act mainly by inhibiting reabsorption of sodium and chloride in the distal convoluted tubules of the kidneys. Thiazides produce a fairly modest diuresis; however, these agents are ineffective when glomerular filtration rate (GFR) falls below 40 mL per minute.

Diuretic tolerance is often encountered in ADHF patients. Lack of response to diuretic therapy may be caused by excessive sodium intake; use of agents that antagonize their effects (particularly nonsteroidal anti-inflammatory drugs); worsening renal dysfunction; addition of potentially nephrotoxic agents during hospitalization; or compromised renal blood flow due to worsening cardiac function. Combined intravenous loop diuretic plus thiazide creates a synergistic response and should be considered for patients who fail to diurese despite optimal doses of an intravenous loop diuretic alone [15]. Metolazone is particularly effective when administered with a loop diuretic.

Two recent randomized controlled trials have evaluated various diuretic dosing strategies in ADHF. The DOSE-HF trial demonstrated that there were no significant differences in patient global assessment of symptoms,or in renal function when loop diuretics were administered by intermittent boluses compared to continuous infusion [16]. Similarly, high-dose loop diuretics did not improve dyspnea more quickly than low-dose intravenous diuretics [16]. In a second study, neither low-dose ("renal") dopamine nor low-dose nesiritide increased urine output at 72 hours compared to loop diuretics alone [17]. Finally, high-dose diuretics, when needed, have not been shown to produce greater activation of the renin–angiotensin–aldosterone system (RAAS) than low-dose diuretics [18].

Elevated vasopressin levels play an important role for mediating fluid retention and contributing to hyponatremia. Short-term treatment with the V2-receptor antagonist, tolvaptan, has been shown to lower filling pressures, enhance diuresis, correct hyponatremia, and improve renal function. Ongoing trials are evaluating the role of vaptan therapy in ADHF management.

Ultrafiltration (UF) using a venovenous access approach is now feasible and potentially useful for acutely lowering markedly elevated ventricular filling pressures when conventional high-dose combination diuretic therapy fails to produce adequate diuresis. Contrary to initial suggestions, UF has not been shown to produce less activation of the RAAS than loop diuretic therapy [18]. Small, short-term observational studies suggested increased weight loss during hospitalization but have not demonstrated decreased length of stay or better preservation of renal function. The UNLOAD trial randomized 200 patients with ADHF to standard intravenous diuretics versus UF and demonstrated greater weight loss at 48 hours in the UF cohort [19]. Readmissions for heart failure were also lower at 90 days (32% versus 18%) for the UF group. However, no comment was made on overall rehospitalization rates and renal function was not improved. A recent randomized controlled trial for ADHF with worsening renal function demonstrated that UF resulted in an identical degree of weight loss, but worse renal function and more adverse events than standard loop diuretic therapy [20]. Despite early hopes, UF does not improve renal function; in fact,

TABLE 194.5

Inhibitors of the Renin–Angiotensin–Aldosterone System and β-Blockers Used for Advanced Heart Failure due to Systolic Dysfunction

Drug	Initial dose	Maximal dose
ACE inhibitors		
Captopril	6.25 mg three times daily	50 mg three times daily
Enalapril	2.5 mg twice daily	20 mg twice daily
Lisinopril	2.5 mg daily	40 mg daily
Fosinopril	5 mg daily	40 mg daily
Ramapril	1.25 mg daily	10 mg daily
Quinapril	5 mg twice daily	20 mg twice daily
Trandolapril	1 mg daily	4 mg daily
Angiotensin receptor blockers		
Losartan	25 mg daily	100 mg daily
Valsartan	20 mg twice daily	160 mg twice daily
Candesartan	4 mg daily	32 mg daily
Aldosterone antagonists		
Spironolactone	12.5 mg every other day	25 mg twice daily
Eplerenone	25 mg daily	50 mg daily
β-adrenergic blockers		
Metoprolol XL/CR[a]	12.5 mg daily	200 mg daily
Carvedilol	3.125 mg twice daily	50 mg twice daily
Bisoprolol	1.25 mg daily	10 mg daily

[a]Metoprolol succinate, extended release.
mg, milligrams.

worsening renal function occurs quite frequently during UF and is associated with an extraordinarily high 1-year mortality [21]. Importantly, hemodynamic instability has been an exclusion criterion in all published studies. The latest ACC/AHA practice guidelines recommend ultrafiltration as a class IIA therapeutic option for heart failure that remains refractory to conventional diuretic therapy [14]. Several ongoing controlled trials should better define the therapeutic niche for this treatment modality.

Vasodilator Therapy

Vasodilators remain a cornerstone of acute and chronic heart failure management (Table 194.5) [22,23]. Mechanisms of action vary and include direct effects on venous capacitance vessels (e.g., nitrates), arterioles (e.g., hydralazine), or balanced effects (sodium nitroprusside, angiotensin-converting enzyme (ACE) inhibitors, and angiotensin II receptor blockers). Drugs that produce balanced venous and arteriolar dilatation should generally be chosen as a first-line therapy because both preload and afterload are elevated during ADHF. However, in the ICU setting, it may sometimes be useful to use nitrates to reduce markedly elevated preload or hydralazine to treat elevated afterload for short periods of time. ACE inhibitors play a crucial role by altering the vicious cycle of hemodynamic abnormalities and neurohormonal activation that characterize advanced heart failure [23]. Randomized, controlled clinical trials have demonstrated the beneficial effects of ACE inhibitors on functional capacity; neurohormonal activation; quality of life; and long-term survival for patients with chronic heart failure due to left ventricular systolic dysfunction [23]. There is compelling evidence that ACE inhibitor therapy should be continued whenever feasible for all ADHF patients [14,23]. It is especially important to recognize that for patients with advanced heart failure that even low doses of vasodilator treatment confer benefits. Low-dose treatment should be considered for patients with marginal blood pressure (i.e., systolic pressure >85 to 90 mm Hg) in order to permit the subsequent introduction of β-blockers. An ACE inhibitor should be initiated for any patient who experiences a transmural myocardial infarction during hospitalization, because post-infarction trials have shown 10% to 27% reductions in all-cause mortality and 20% to 50% reductions in the risk of developing overt heart failure.

Alternative therapy with combination hydralazine and nitrates should be considered for patients with marginal renal function (creatinine >2.5 mg per dL) and those with previously documented intolerance to ACE inhibitors or angiotensin receptor blockers [14]. Similar hemodynamic goals can be achieved with these agents among patients with advanced NYHA Class III or IV heart failure. Women appear somewhat less responsive to ACE inhibitor therapy than do men. Important racial differences may also exist in pharmacologic responsiveness to different vasodilator regimens. Two retrospective analyses from large trials confirmed ACE inhibitor therapy to be less effective in blacks than whites with heart failure of comparable severity. The African-American Heart Failure trial (A-HeFT) confirmed the benefit of hydralazine and isosorbide dinitrate for this population; this combination should be considered when initiating therapy for hospitalized black patients [14,23].

Angiotensin receptor blockers (ARBs) are now also considered a suitable first-line therapy for heart failure patients [14]. These drugs should be selected for ACE inhibitor–intolerant, non–African-American patients who experience rash or cough with an ACE inhibitor. They cannot be used for patients who experience ACE inhibitor-related deterioration in renal function, hypotension or hypokalemia. Symptomatic and mortality benefits appear comparable between ACE inhibitors and ARBs. Combination therapy with and ACE inhibitor and ARB has largely been replaced by the use of an aldosterone antagonist as third agent to go along with an ACE inhibitor and β-adrenergic blocker [14]. A novel drug that combines neprilysin inhibitior with an ARB (sacubitril-valsatan) has recently been shown superior to standard ACE inhibitor therapy for outpatient management [24]. It has not been studied in ADHF and should not be initiated during hospitalization.

Digitalis

Digoxin continues to have a role for the management of patients with advanced NYHA class III to IV symptoms [14]. The drug has mild positive inotropic effect on cardiac muscle, reduces activation of the sympathetic and renin angiotensin systems, and partially restores the favorable inhibitory effects of cardiac baroreceptor function [25]. Short- and long-term controlled trials have provided unequivocal evidence that chronic digoxin administration increases left ventricular ejection fraction, improves exercise capacity, decreases advanced heart failure symptoms, and reduces heart failure associated hospitalizations [25]. Post hoc analysis has shown that patients most likely to demonstrate a favorable response had severe symptoms, greater degrees of left ventricular dysfunction, lower ejection fractions, and the presence of a third heart sound. A prespecified subgroup analysis of patients enrolled in the Digitalis Investigation Group (DIG) trial provided confirmatory evidence that patients with severe heart failure (LVEF <25% or CT ratio >0.55) showed the greatest benefit [26]. Because renal function may fluctuate considerably during hospitalization, measurement of serum digoxin levels is important. Retrospective subgroup analysis has suggested an increased risk of all-cause mortality among both women and men who have digoxin levels >1.0 ng per dL [26]. Poor renal function, small lean body mass, and elderly patients are at greatest risk for developing digoxin toxicity during standard maintenance dosing. In addition, a number of commonly utilized drugs including verapamil, flecainide, spironolactone, and amiodarone will significantly increase serum digoxin levels. Recent data from the TREAT-AF study have suggested increased mortality rates of patients without heart failure who are treated with digoxin for rate control in new-onset atrial fibrillation [27]. In general, digoxin should be not be used as a first-line therapy for rate control. For adult patients with advanced heart failure, sinus rhythm, and normal renal function, a dosage of 0.25 mg per day is appropriate. For patients at increased risk of toxicity, the initial starting dose should be 0.125 mg daily and uptitrated as necessary to achieve a trough level of 0.5 to 0.9 ng per dL.

β-Adrenergic Blockers

β-adrenergic blockers have been shown to lower all-cause mortality and decrease heart failure hospitalizations in a variety of randomized controlled trials in patients with NYHA class II to IV symptoms (Table 194.5) [14]. The mortality benefits of β-blocker therapy for patients with advanced (NYHA class IV) heart failure symptoms is clearly established [14]. The Carvedilol Perspective Randomized Cumulative Survival (COPERNICUS) trial evaluated patients with severe symptoms and LVEF < 25% [28]. Carvedilol reduced all-cause mortality by 35%, the combined risk of death or cardiovascular hospitalization by 27%, and the risk of death or heart failure hospitalization by 31% [28]. Importantly, carvedilol-treated patients spent 40% fewer days in the hospital for acute heart failure decompensation [28]. It appears that not all β-blockers have equivalent benefits for heart failure. For example, bucindolol, a third generation non-selective β-blocker with intrinsic sympathomimetic activity, was not associated with statistically significant reductions of overall mortality. Unlike ACE inhibitors or ARBs, the specific β-blockers (e.g., bisoprolol, carvedilol, or metoprolol succinate) that have been validated as effective by clinical trials should be prescribed. The effectiveness of these agents appears to be equal among men and women [14]. Clinicians should consider initiating carvedilol as a first-line therapy, given its broader antiadrenergic effects whenever possible. However, for patients with marginal blood pressure for whom partial α-blockade may be deleterious, metoprolol succinate or bisoprolol may be suitable first-line agents.

A β-blocker should be initiated for all β-blocker–tolerant ADHF patients for whom it has not been previously prescribed. In the intensive care unit setting, treatment should be initiated at very low doses and gradually uptitrated every few days or within 1 week. The usual starting doses are carvedilol 3.125 mg twice daily or metroprolol succinate 6.25 mg twice daily. Importantly, β-blockers should not be initiated until optimal volume status and hemodynamic stability have been achieved. The majority of ADHF patients will already be receiving β-blocker treatment. In general, β-blockers should not be withdrawn unless marked bradycardia or hemodynamic instability develops, owing to the risk of rebound hypertension and tachycardia. When necessary to achieve active diuresis for ADHF with hemodynamic instability, a 50% reduction in the ambulatory dose is often preferable to drug cessation. In a retrospective observational study of over 2,300 patients eligible to receive β-blocker during hospitalization, Fonarow and colleagues demonstrated that continuation of β blocker was associated with a significantly lower risk of propensity-adjusted post-discharge death and rehospitalization rates compared to those who had β-blockers withdrawn [29].

Aldosterone Antagonists

Circulating aldosterone levels are elevated in relationship to heart failure severity, adversely affect prognosis, and contribute to deterioration of function and left ventricular remodeling following acute myocardial infarction. Potential deleterious effects include endothelial dysfunction, increased oxidative stress, enhanced platelet aggregation, activation of matrix metalloproteinases, and increased activation of the sympathetic nervous system. The mineralocorticoid receptor antagonist (MRA) spironolactone has been shown to reduce mortality of patients with severe heart failure by 30% [30]. Results of the EPHESUS trial confirm that eplerenone, a more selective MRA, can also reduce morbidity and mortality amongst patients with evidence of systolic dysfunction and heart failure following acute myocardial infarction [30]. The beneficial effects of MRA's appear to be independent of their diuretic actions, and likely relate to interruption of the downstream adverse effects of aldosterone activation.

Spironolactone or eplerenone should generally not be initiated in the ICU setting. Both can be associated with serious hyperkalemia, particularly in the presence of impaired renal function or other medications which impair potassium excretion. An MRA (Table 194.5) should be added to the patient's medical regimen prior to discharge following optimization of other heart failure therapies, provided that significant renal dysfunction (creatinine >2.5 mg per dL) or hyperkalemia (K^+ >5.0 mEq per L) is not present. Patients who have been receiving these agents should continue taking them during hospitalization, unless marked hemodynamic instability, electrolyte disturbances, or worsening renal function are present.

INTENSIVE CARE MANAGEMENT OF ACUTE DECOMPENSATED HEART FAILURE

Congestive symptoms (pulmonary and/or systemic) are the most frequent reason for hospitalization in ADHF. Establishing the patient's prior euvolemic weight and achieving it through diuretic dosing adjustments is critical for treating acute decompensation. Diuretics should be switched to intravenous administration whenever questionable oral absorption (i.e., postoperative state) is expected. Once daily ACE inhibitor or ARB therapy is ideal for outpatient management to enhance compliance; however, if hemodynamic instability is anticipated during hospitalization, a temporary switch to a short-acting agent (e.g., captopril in place of lisinopril) should be considered. Among patients with deteriorating renal function, it may be necessary to withhold the ACE-inhibitor or ARB and transiently substitute hydralazine and nitrates, particularly when serum creatinine exceeds 3.0 mg per dL. β-blocker dosing should remain unchanged and may require a modest increase if atrial tachyarrhythmias are encountered in the postoperative state (see below). Serum electrolytes should be followed frequently, given the potential for electrolyte imbalance (e.g., hypokalemia or hypomagnesemia) to potentiate atrial and ventricular arrhythmias among vulnerable patients.

Stevenson has popularized a 2-minute clinical assessment to ascertain the hemodynamic profiles for heart failure patients (Fig. 194.1) [31]. Patients are characterized in a 2×2 fashion according to the presence or absence of congestion and low or adequate perfusion on physical examination [31]. The clinical profiles thus defined have been shown to correlate reasonably well with direct hemodynamic measurements of filling pressure and cardiac output and are correlated with prognosis following hospital discharge [32]. "Warm and dry" patients have normal resting hemodynamics and are well compensated. For these patients, other potential etiologies for dyspnea or fatigue should be considered. The majority (70% to 80%) of patients admitted with worsening symptoms fit the "warm and wet" profile. These individuals are volume overloaded but have adequate end-organ perfusion. The primary treatment goal is thus relief of "congestive" symptoms using intravenous loop diuretics alone or in combination with a thiazide. Those who fail to respond to escalating doses of intravenous loop diuretics may benefit from a continuous intravenous loop diuretic infusion. A small minority of patients with refractory volume overload may benefit from continuous venovenous hemofiltration (CVVH) or ultrafiltration [14]. Although neurohormonal antagonists including ACE-inhibitors, ARBs, and β-blockers should ideally be maintained during hospitalization, downward dose adjustment or temporary suspension (particularly of β-blockers) should be considered for patients who are difficult to diurese or who are hypotensive. A very small minority of patients (<5%) fall into the "cold and dry" profile. These individuals have impaired cardiac output but do not adequately utilize the Starling mechanism to increase preload. Judicious hydration should be attempted with assessment for obstructive cardiomyopathy by echocardiography. Patients who fail to demonstrate improvement of end-organ perfusion and impaired ventricular function may require a short-term infusion of a positive inotropic agent such as dobutamine or milrinone.

Echocardiography during ICU Management

Transthoracic echocardiography is an essential tool for the evaluation and management of the ADHF patient [33]. An echocardiogram should be performed for all patients with a new diagnosis of heart failure to determine its etiology (i.e., systolic dysfunction, diastolic dysfunction, or unsuspected valvular disease). It is also useful for assessing right ventricular function, estimating pulmonary artery pressures and whether regional or global wall motion abnormalities are present. For patients with chronic heart failure, it can be useful for assessing potential causes for acute decompensation such as worsening left or right ventricular function, or the development of more severe valvular disease.

In addition to providing clinical essential information about cardiac structure and function, echo-Doppler can now provide estimates of right and left ventricular filling pressures and cardiac output measures that correlate well with catheter-based hemodynamics [33]. Central venous pressure can be estimated via measurement of the inferior vena caval diameter and respiratory variation; systolic pulmonary artery pressure is calculated as CVP + peak pressure gradient between the right atrium and right ventricle during systole. Left atrial pressure (LAP) is typically assessed using mitral valve inflow velocity; tissue Doppler of the septal and lateral mitral annulus; and pulmonary venous flow patterns. Echocardiography is most useful for differentiating high from low LAPs; however, there may be a considerable overlap in the intermediate range of pressures. These parameters can be measured serially to assess responses to therapy [33].

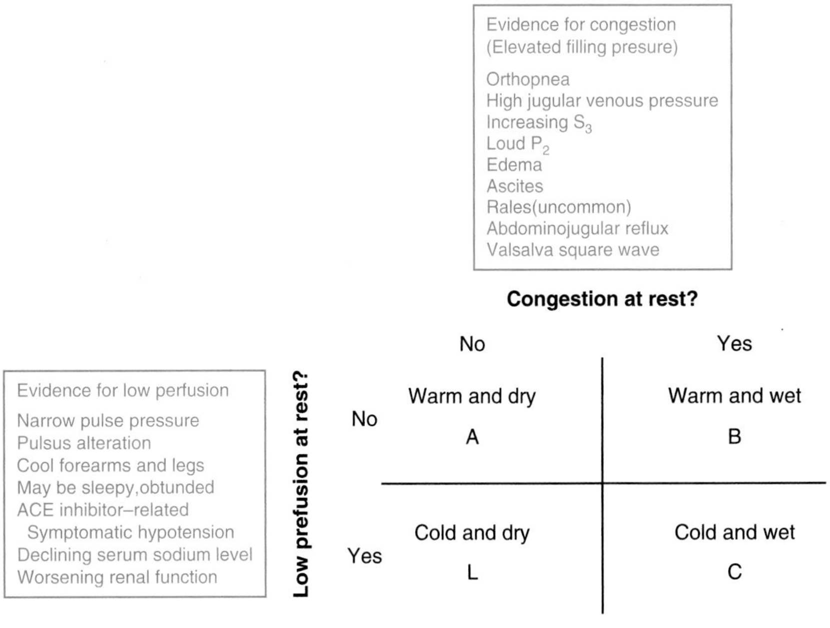

FIGURE 194.1 Hemodynamic profiles of patients presenting with acute decompensated heart failure. Most patients can be classified in a 2-minute bedside assessment according to their physical signs and symptoms. This classification is useful in guiding therapy and predicting prognosis. (From Nohria A, Lewis E, Stevenson LW: Medical management of advanced heart failure. *JAMA* 287:628–640, 2002 [Figure 4], used with permission).

TABLE 194.6

Indications for Hemodynamic Monitoring in Decompensated Heart Failure

- Ongoing Congestive Symptoms and Suspected End-Organ Hypoperfusion
  - Narrow pulse pressure: Cool extremities
  - Declining renal function: Hypotension on ACE or ARB treatment
  - Mental confusion: Progressive hyponatremia
- Heart failure and other Medical Comorbidities
  - Cardiac: unstable angina pectoris; stenotic valvular lesions, and hypertrophic cardiomyopathy
  - Noncardiac: severe obstructive or restrictive pulmonary disease, advanced renal disease, and sepsis
- Other Situations
  - Perioperative monitoring to optimize status for a high-risk procedure
  - Symptoms disproportionate to clinical assessment of degree of compensation
  - Uncertain volume status
  - Inability to wean inotropic support

ACE, angiotensin-converting enzyme; ARB, angiotensin receptor blocker.

TABLE 194.7

Principles of Hemodynamic Tailored Heart Failure Therapy

Measure baseline resting hemodynamics (CVP, PAP, PCW, CI, and SVR)
Administer intravenous diuretics, vasodilator (nitroprusside, nitroglycerin, or nesiritide) or inotropic agent (milrinone or dobutamine) dosed to achieve specific hemodynamic goals:
  Pulmonary capillary wedge pressure <16 mm Hg
  Right atrial pressure <8 mm Hg
  Cardiac index >2.2 L/min/m^2
  Systemic vascular resistance <1,000–1,200 dynes-sec-cm^{-5}
  Systolic blood pressure >80 mm Hg
Maintain optimal hemodynamics for 24–48 hours
Uptitration of oral vasodilators as intravenous vasodilators are weaned
Adjust oral diuretics to keep optimal volume status

CVP, central venous pressure; PAP, pulmonary artery pressure; PCW, pulmonary capillary wedge pressure; CI, Cardiac index; SVR, systemic vascular resistance. Adapted from Stevenson LW: *Eur J Heart Failure* 1:251–257, 1999 (Table 2, page 254); Used with permission.

Hemodynamically Guided Therapy

Approximately 10% to 15% of patients with advanced heart failure will demonstrate marked hemodynamic deterioration on admission ("cold and wet" profile). These patients have impending cardiogenic shock [31,32]. Potential causes for acute decompensation such as recent myocardial infarction, rhythm change, worsening valvular disease, or medical/dietary noncompliance should be sought. The ESCAPE trial randomized patients with acute decompensation without hemodynamic compromise to conventional medical management based on physical findings and symptoms versus tailored hemodynamic monitoring following insertion of a pulmonary artery catheter. Somewhat surprisingly, outcomes did not differ between the two management strategies [34]. Certain high-risk subgroups may, nonetheless, benefit from short-term hemodynamic monitoring for management of ADHF. Principal indications for hemodynamic monitoring with a pulmonary artery catheter include evidence of worsening end-organ dysfunction, need for withholding vasoactive medications because of hypotension, heart failure associated with other comorbidities (i.e., unstable angina or valvular heart disease) or inability to wean positive inotropic support (Table 194.6). "Tailored" hemodynamic treatment for refractory heart failure is outlined in Table 194.7 [32]. Following initial assessment of baseline hemodynamics, intravenous diuretics, vasodilators, or positive inotropes are administered to achieve desired hemodynamic goals which generally include a pulmonary capillary wedge pressure below 15 mm Hg and a cardiac index above 2.2 L/min/m^2. This intravenous program is maintained for 48 to 72 hours to affect desired diuresis and improve end-organ perfusion. Following this stage, oral vasodilators are uptitrated as intravenous agents are weaned. Further adjustment of diuretic dose and ambulation should be completed during the final 24 to 48 hours of hospitalization. This "tailored approach" produces sustained improvement of filling pressures, forward cardiac output, decreased mitral regurgitation, and decreased neurohormonal activation [32]. Oral vasodilator therapy and β-blockers should be withheld during treatment with intravenous vasoactive agents.

Considerable controversy continues to exist regarding the relative roles of intravenous vasodilator drugs (i.e., nitroglycerin, nitroprusside, or nesiritide) versus positive inotropic agents (dobutamine, dopamine, or milrinone) in this population (Table 194.8). Previously, inotropic infusions have been used for patients with moderate heart failure in order to promote brisk diuresis. These agents, however, are associated with an increased risk of ischemic events and tachyarrhythmias [35]. A second major limitation of short-term inotropic support is the additional complexity needed to readjust oral regimens as the infusions are weaned [36]. Although positive inotropes should not be routinely used for "warm and wet" patients, these agents can be life saving for patients with progressive hemodynamic collapse [14,36]. Patients who present or develop obtundation, anuria, persistent hypotension, or lactic acidosis may only respond to inotropic support, which should be continued until the cause of cardiac deterioration is determined and definitive therapy implemented. A brief inotropic treatment may also be appropriate for patients who develop the cardiorenal syndrome [36]. It should be emphasized, however, that many patients with

TABLE 194.8

Intravenous Vasoactive Agents for Decompensated Heart Failure

Drug	Initial dose	Maximal dose
Vasodilator		
Nitroprusside	0.20 μg/kg/min	10 μg/kg/min
Nitroglycerin	10 μg/kg/min	1,000 μg/kg/min
Nesiritide	Loading dose: 2 μg/kg/min Maintenance dose: 0.01 μg/kg/min	0.030 μg/kg/min
Positive inotropic agents		
Dobutamine	2.5 μg/kg/min	20 μg/kg/min
Milrinone	Loading dose: 50 μg/kg Maintenance dose: 0.375 μg/kg/min	0.75 μg/kg/min
Dopamine	2.5 μg/kg/min	20 μg/kg/min

low cardiac output have high systemic vascular resistance that predictably improves with vasodilator therapy alone, obviating the need for inotropic support [37]. In-hospital mortality has also been shown to be lower for nonhemodynamically compromised patients treated with intravenous vasodilators compared to positive inotropes [37]. Intravenous nitroprusside, a direct nitrosodilator, rapidly lowers filling pressures and improves cardiac output, which in turn, improves diuretic responsiveness. Hemodynamically monitored nitroprusside infusions rarely cause systematic hypotension but may be complicated by thiocyanate toxicity, particularly when high doses are required for prolonged periods of time for patients with preexisting hepatic or renal dysfunction. Intravenous nitroglycerin also produces arterial and venous dilatation but is less effective than nitroprusside. Nesiritide, a human recombinant form of endogenous BNP, rapidly improves symptoms. It has largely been utilized for patients demonstrating the "warm and wet" hemodynamic profile rather than those with more advanced "cool and wet" profiles. A small study suggested that short-term in-hospital nesiritide administration resulted in fewer heart failure rehospitalizations and lower 6-month mortality following discharge compared to dobutamine [38]. Further, perioperative nesiritde has been reported to improve renal function and enhance urine output following coronary bypass surgery [39]. However, the safety of nesiritide has been questioned, and the hope that this agent would attenuate renal dysfunction during heart failure treatment has not been realized. Neither the ASCEND-HF trial nor the DOSE-HF trial demonstrated any benefit of short-term nesiritide therapy for the treatment of ADHF [16,40]. Table 194.9 summarizes randomized clinical trials of ADHF therapies.

Biomarker-Guided Therapy

Serial BNP or NT-pro-BNP measurements to guide therapies for ambulatory patients are increasingly utilized. Small, controlled trials of chronic heart failure patients demonstrated fewer heart failure rehospitalizations using BNP levels to adjust pharmacologic therapy. However, this approach recently failed to improve survival free of repeat hospitalizations or quality of life in a large cohort of patients. A reasonable approach for inpatients with ADHF should include the measurement of BNP or NT-pro-BNP on admission and prior to discharge when the patient is euvolemic, both for prognostic purposes as well as to aid in tailoring post-discharge treatment [41]. Daily biomarker measurement does not add significant prognostic value. A fall of 30% or greater in BNP or NT-pro-BNP at discharge identifies patients at low risk for readmission [42]. Conversely, a rise in either biomarker suggests worsening disease or inadequate therapy and should prompt a review of the patient's heart failure regimen.

PERIOPERATIVE MANAGEMENT OF ADVANCED HEART FAILURE PATIENTS

Hernandez et al. have reported that patients with heart failure undergoing major noncardiac surgical procedures experience substantially increased morbidity and mortality compared to patients with ischemic heart disease or an age-matched population [43]. After adjusting for demographics, type of surgery, and co-morbidities, the risk-adjusted operative mortality (death before discharge or within 30 days of surgery) was 11.7% for heart failure patients,

TABLE 194.9

Results of Randomized Trials of Pharmacologic Treatment and Ultrafiltration in Acute Decompensated Heart Failure

Intervention	Trial	Year	Study	No. of patients	Findings	References
Milrinone	OPTIME-CHF	2002	RCT	951	No reduction in hospitalizations for cardiac causes within 60 days of treatment with milrinone for ADHF	[35]
Ultrafiltration	UNLOAD	2007	RCT	200	UF resulted in greater weight loss and fewer rehospitalizations for heart failure	[19]
PAC placement	ESCAPE	2005	RCT	433	PAC for tailoring of therapy did not lower mortality or rehospitalizations	[34]
Nesiritide versus dobutamine	—	2002	Open label randomized	261	Nesiritide resulted in fewer readmissions and lower 6-month mortality than dobutamine	[38]
Nesiritide	NAPA	2007	RCT	279	Nesiritide improved renal function after CABG	[39]
Diuretic Dosing	DOSE-HF	2011	RCT	308	No significant differences high-versus low-dose loop diuretic or bolus versus continuous infusion on weight loss or renal function	[16]
Dopamine Nesiritide	ROSE-HF	2013	RCT	360	Neither dopamine nor nesiritide enhanced diuresis or improved renal function when added to a diuretic	[17]
Ultrafiltration	CARESS	2012	RCT	188	UF was not superior to loop diuretics and was associated with more adverse events	[20]

ADHF, acute decompensated heart failure; CABG, coronary artery bypass grafting; PAC, pulmonary artery catheter; RCT, randomized controlled trial; UF, ultrafiltration; OPTIME-CHF, outcomes of a prospective trial of intravenous milrinone for exacerbation of chronic heart failure trial; ESCAPE, evaluation study of congestive heart failure and pulmonary artery catheterization effectiveness trial; NAPA, nesiritide administered peri-anesthesia in patients undergoing cardiac surgery trial; DOSE-HF, diuretic optimization strategies evaluation trial; ROSE-HF, renal optimization strategies evaluation trial; CARESS-HF, CARdioRenal ReScue Study in acute decompensated heart failure trial.

6.6% for ischemic heart disease patients, and 6.2% for controls. Further, the risk-adjusted 30-day readmission rates were 20% for the heart failure cohort compared with 14% for the ischemic population and 11% for age-match controls. The presence of a third heart sound or signs of overt heart failure signs clearly identifies patients at increased risk for adverse outcome during noncardiac surgical procedures [43]. Every effort must be made to detect unsuspected heart failure by careful evaluation and to optimize therapy before embarking on nonemergent procedures.

Nonemergent surgical procedures should be delayed for ADHF patients. Volume overload should be corrected and adequate oxygenation insured. Maintenance pharmacologic therapy including vasodilators, β-blockers, and digitalis should be continued. A trough digoxin level should be checked and maintained < 1 ng per dL to minimize potential toxicity. Spironolactone should be withheld until stable hemodynamics and renal function have been achieved. Patients with refractory symptoms or deteriorating end-organ function should have a pulmonary catheter inserted in order to optimize their hemodynamics. Current evidence does not support the routine use of a pulmonary artery catheter for perioperative monitoring [44]. A single large scale randomized clinical trial of pulmonary artery catheterization in high-risk surgical patients demonstrated no improvement of survival [45]. However, only 16% of patients enrolled in this trial had symptomatic heart failure. Ejection fraction alone is insufficient to recommend the use of continuous hemodynamic monitoring. The majority of patients with markedly impaired ventricular function (LVEF < 20%) may be well compensated on optimized pharmacologic therapies and undergo surgery without invasive monitoring. Conversely, some patients with only moderate impairment of LVEF may benefit from pulmonary artery monitoring when hemodynamic instability is anticipated. Practice guidelines for intraoperative hemodynamic monitoring published by the American Society of Anesthesiologists consider the severity of the patient's underlying cardiovascular disease, the type of surgical procedure, and the likelihood of major hemodynamic lability [46]. The extent of anticipated intraoperative and perioperative fluid shifts is another key factor. Current ACC/AHA guidelines recommend intraoperative pulmonary artery monitoring as a Class 2B indication, as indicated for patients at risk for major hemodynamic disturbances that are easily detected by pulmonary artery catheter who are scheduled to undergo a procedure that is likely to cause these hemodynamic changes [44].

MECHANICAL CIRCULATORY SUPPORT

A small minority (1% to 2%) of patients admitted with ADHF will progress to cardiogenic shock that fails to respond to intropic or vasodilator support. If a potentially reversible cause is identified (e.g., acute myocarditis) or if the patient qualifies to be a candidate for heart transplantation, short-term mechanical circulatory support should be considered [47]. An intra-aortic balloon pump can increase cardiac output and improve diastolic coronary artery filling. However, it has not been shown to improve survival when shock complicates acute myocardial infarction and its role for refractory ADHF has not been established [48]. Newer percutaneous support devices (i.e., Tandem Heart, Impella 5.0) provide greater hemodynamic benefits than IABP but have not yet been demonstrated to improve outcomes [47,49]. Extracorporeal membrane oxygenation (ECMO) may be lifesaving for patients with advanced biventricular dysfunction or those with shock and inadequate oxygenation. Short-term support is well tolerated with the newer devices, but in-hospital mortality remains high [49].

MANAGEMENT OF ARRHYTHMIAS

Atrial and ventricular arrhythmias are nearly ubiquitous among advanced heart failure patients and often contribute to clinical decompensation. Atrial fibrillation and flutter are the most commonly encountered supraventricular arrhythmias. The likelihood of atrial fibrillation increases with heart failure severity and approaches 40% for NYHA class III and IV patients [50]. The potential adverse effects of atrial fibrillation include loss of atrioventricular synchrony, rapid or inappropriately slow ventricular response rates, variable diastolic filling times, and thromboembolic complications. Patients with a known history of chronic atrial fibrillation should have adequate heart rate control and anticoagulation whenever feasible (see below). Uncontrolled, sustained, rapid (>120 beats per minute) atrial fibrillation can result in a reversible dilated cardiomyopathy or, more typically, can worsen preexisting left ventricular systolic dysfunction [50]. A heart rate below 100 beats per minute during modest ambulation is a reasonable goal. β-adrenergic blockers remain the most effective rate-control treatment option [51]. Addition of digoxin may be considered when necessary for adequate rate control. A large recent registry analysis found no increase of mortality risk by treating new-onset atrial fibrillation of heart failure patients [50]. Calcium channel blockers (e.g., diltiazem and verapamil) should generally be avoided during ADHF owing to their negative inotropic effects. Amiodarone is a highly effective drug for rate control, and is frequently useful for controlling persistent atrial arrhythmias for ICU patients [51].

Atrial fibrillation commonly occurs during hospitalization owing to enhanced sympathetic stimulation. For all patients, thyroid function should be assessed to exclude hyperthyroidism as a contributing factor. For ADHF patients who are hemodynamically stable, initial therapy should focus on adequate rate control (HR < 100 per minute). For patients who experience active angina pectoris or hemodynamic instability during rapid atrial fibrillation, urgent synchronized cardioversion should be performed followed by initiation of an atrial stabilizing agent to prevent recurrence. For ADHF, restoration or maintenance of sinus rhythm is often desirable; amiodarone or dofetilide remain the most useful antiarrhythmic drugs [50,51]. Amiodarone is particularly well tolerated from a hemodynamic standpoint; the loading dose of amiodarone should be kept below 1,000 mg per day to prevent further exacerbation of heart failure symptoms. Dronedarone, a non-iodinated derivative of amiodarone, has also been shown to be effective for maintenance of sinus rhythm and rate control for rapid atrial fibrillation. However, increased mortality due to worsening heart failure has been reported among patients with depressed LV function; this agent should not be utilized for heart failure patients [52].

Dofetilide is a class III anti-arrhythmic drug that blocks the repolarizing potassium current. It is highly effective for restoring sinus rhythm but has been associated with torsades de pointes in up to 3% of patients [51]. Continuous ECG monitoring for the first 48 hours after initiation in the hospitalized patient is essential. Sotalol, an additional class III antiarrhythmic drug, may occasionally be substituted for other β-blockers, following improvement in ADHF, but it carries with it a similar risk of torsades, and is generally less effective than amiodarone.

Asymptomatic nonsustained ventricular tachycardia (NSVT) occurs among over 50% of patients with NYHA class III/IV heart failure [53]. Pharmacologic suppression of NSVT does not lower the risk of sudden death. Asymptomatic ventricular ectopy should be viewed as a marker of disease severity rather than a specific marker for sudden cardiac death risk [53]. Heart failure patients often develop frequent ventricular premature beats or short runs of NSVT during their ICU stay. Precipitating causes such as electrolyte disturbances (e.g., hypokalemia or hypomagnesemia), enhanced sympathetic tone, a decrease of β-blocker dose, or withholding of prior anti-arrhythmic therapy should be considered. The majority of patients have no symptoms and do not require pharmacologic suppression. Frequent runs of ventricular tachycardia or sustained monomorphic VT require anti-arrhythmic treatment. Amiodarone (intravenous 0.50 to 1.0

mg per minute) or lidocaine (0.5 to 2 mg per minute) are generally most effective for acute management [54]. β-blockers, sotalol, and amiodarone are effective long-term oral treatment options [54].

A growing percentage of advanced heart failure patients have implantable cardioverter defibrillators (ICDs) to treat symptomatic ventricular tachyarrhythmias or for primary prevention of sudden cardiac death. The ICD should be interrogated for any recent atrial or ventricular arrhythmias prior to admission, and the device temporarily inactivated prior to surgical procedures that involve electrocautery. It should be reactivated and its function checked by an electrophysiologist in the early perioperative period.

Anticoagulation

Systemic anticoagulation is often a part of a heart failure patient's outpatient management. Studies have suggested that the risk of thromboembolic complications is lower than previously expected, averaging 1.5 to 3 episodes/100 patient years when normal sinus rhythm is present. Current indications for systemic anticoagulation include paroxysmal or chronic atrial fibrillation, a history of thromboembolism, or echocardiographically documented left ventricular thrombus [55,56]. Relative indications include a markedly dilated left ventricle (>75 mm) with severe systolic dysfunction and spontaneous echocardiographic contrast ("smoke"), indicating sluggish intracavitary blood flow. The presence of a low ejection fraction alone is *insufficient* to warrant systemic anticoagulation. A non–vitamin K antagonist agent or Warfarin should be continued with an INR goal of 2.0 to 3.0 when invasive procedures are not planned. If surgery or central venous catheter placement are required, warfarin can be reversed with vitamin K or fresh frozen plasma, agent specific reversal of selected non–vitamin K antagonist can be accomplished, and transiently substituted with intravenous heparin or subcutaneous low-molecular weight heparin as feasible. For those patients who require anticoagulation but are unable to receive heparin (e.g., owing to heparin-induced thrombocytopenia), alternative anticoagulants including the direct thrombin inhibitors argatroban and hirudin, or the pentasaccharide fondaparinux can be considered. Non–vitamin K antagonist anticoagulants (i.e., dabigatran, rivaroxaban, and apixaban) are increasingly replacing warfarin for outpatient management of nonvalvular atrial fibrillation [57]. These agents should be continued unless invasive procedures are anticipated.

CONCLUSIONS

The patient with advanced heart failure or ADHF requires special considerations. Meticulous attention to volume status and maintenance of appropriate vasodilator therapy and β-adrenergic blockade form the cornerstones of acute management. Negative inotropic drugs and agents that might further impair renal function should be avoided. Patients with refractory symptoms or recent decompensation may require hemodynamic monitoring via a pulmonary artery catheter, and initiation of short-term vasoactive therapy including nitroprusside, nitroglycerin, milrinone, or dobutamine. Maintenance of sinus rhythm should be considered, and pharmacological suppression of recurrent ventricular tachyarrhythmias is often necessary. With careful management, hospital morbidity and mortality can be minimized despite the presence of advanced symptomatic heart failure.

References

1. Gheorghiade M, Pang PS: Acute heart failure syndromes. *J Am Coll Cardiol* 53:557–573, 2009.
2. Fonarow GC, Adams KF, Abraham WT, et al; for the ADHERE Scientific Advisory Committee: Risk stratification for in-hospital mortality in acutely decompensated heart failure: classification and regression tree analysis. *JAMA* 293:572–580, 2005.
3. Lindenfeld J, Albert N, Boehmer JP, et al: Executive summary: HFSA2010 comprehensive heart failure practice guidelines. *J Card Fail* 16:475–539, 2010.
4. Nieminen MS, Harjola VP: Definition and epidemiology of acute heart failure syndromes. *Am J Cardiol* 96 (Suppl):5G–10G, 2005.
5. Tarvasmaki T, Harjola VP, Nieminen MS, et al: Acute heart failure with and without concomitant acute coronary syndromes: patient characteristics, management, and survival. *J Cardiac Fail* 20:723–730, 2014.
6. Braga JR, Tu JV, Austin PC, et al: Outcomes and care of patients with acute heart failure syndromes and cardiac troponin elevation. *Circ Heart Fail* 6:193–202, 2013.
7. Kociol RB, Pang PS, Gheorghiade M, et al: Troponin elevation in heart failure. Prevalence, mechanism and clinical implications. *J Am Coll Cardiol* 56:1071–1078, 2010.
8. Fonarow G, Peacock WP, Phillips CO, et al: Admission B-type natriuretic peptide levels and in-hospital mortality in acute decompensated heart failure. *J Am Coll Cardiol* 49:1943–1950, 2007.
9. Abraham WT, Fonarow GC, Albert NM, et al: Predictors of in-hospital mortality in patients hospitalized for heart failure. Insights from the Organized Program to Initiate Lifesaving Treatment in Hospitalized Patients with Heart Failure (OPTIMIZE-HF). *J Am Coll Cardiol* 52:347–356, 2008.
10. Kazury A, Elkayam U: Cardiorenal interactions in acute decompensated heart failure: contemporary concepts facing emerging controversies. *J Cardiac Fail* 20:1004–1011, 2014.
11. Aronson D, Darawsha W, Atamna A, et al: Pulmonary hypertension, right ventricular function, and clinical outcome in acute decompensated heart failure. *J Cardiac Fail* 19:665–671, 2013.
12. Metra M, Davison B, Bettari L, et al: Is worsening renal function an ominous prognostic sign in patient with acute heart failure? The role of congestion and its interaction with renal function. *Circ Heart Fail* 5:54–62, 2012.
13. Testani JM, Chen J, McCauley BD, et al: Potential effects of aggressive decongestion during the treatment of decompensated heart failure on renal function and survival. *Circulation* 122:265–272, 2010.
14. Jessup M, Silver MA, Stevenson LW, et al: 2009 Focused update: ACCF/AHA guidelines for the diagnosis and management of heart failure in adults. A report of the American College of Cardiology Foundation/American Heart Association Task Force on Practice Guidelines. *J Am Coll Cardiol* 53:1343–1382, 2009.
15. Jentzer JC, DeWald TA, Hernandez AF: Combination of loop diuretics with thiazide-like diuretic in heart failure. *J Am Coll Cardiol* 56:1527–1534, 2010.
16. Felker GM, Lee KL, Bull DA, et al: Diuretic strategies in patients with acute decompensated heart failure. *N Engl J Med* 364:797–805, 2011.
17. Chen HH, Anstrom KJ, Givertz MM, et al: Low-dose dopamine or low-dose nesiritide in acute heart failure with renal dysfunction. The ROSE acute heart failure randomized trial. *JAMA* 310:2533–2543, 2013.
18. Metz RJ, Stevens SR, DeVore AD, et al: Decongestion strategies and renin-angiotensin-aldoseterone system activation in acute heart failure. *J Am Coll Cardiol HF* 3:97–107, 2015.
19. Costanzo MR, Guglin ME, Saltzberg MT, et al: Ultrafiltration versus intravenous diuretics for patients hospitalized for acute decompensated heart failure. *J Am Coll Cardiol* 49:675–668, 2007.
20. Bart BA, Goldsmith SR, Lee KL, et al: Ultrafiltration in decompensated heart failure with cardiorenal syndrome. *N Engl J Med* 367:2296–2304, 2012.
21. Raichlin E, Haglund NA, Mumitru I, et al: Worsening renal function in patients with acute decompensated heart failure treated with ultrafiltration: predictors and outcomes. *J Cardiac Fail* 19:787–794, 2013.
22. Felker GM, Pang PS, Adams KF, et al: Clinical trials of pharmacological therapies in acute heart failure syndromes. Lessons learned and directions forward. *Circ Heart Fail* 3:314–325, 2010.
23. Carlson MD, Eckman PM: Review of vasodilators in acute decompensated heart failure: the old and the new. *J Cardiac Fail* 7:478–493, 2013.
24. McMurray JJ, Packer M, Desai AS, et al: Angiotensin-neprilysin inhibiton versus enalapril in heart failure. *N Engl J Med* 371:993–1004, 2014.
25. Gheorghiade M, van Veldhuisen DJ, Colucci WS: Contemporary use of digoxin in the management of cardiovascular disorders. *Circulation* 113:2556–2564, 2006.
26. Adams KR, Patterson JH, Gattis WA, et al: Relationship of serum digoxin concentration to mortality and morbidity in women in the Digitalis Investigation Group trial. A retrospective analysis. *J Am Coll Cardiol* 46:497–504, 2005.
27. Turakhia MP, Santageli P, Winkelmayer WC, et al: Increased mortality associated with digoxin in contemporary patients with atrial fibrillation. Findings from the TREAT-AF study. *J Am Coll Cardiol* 64:660–668, 2014.
28. Packer M, Fowler MB, Roecker EB, et al: Effect of carvedilol on morbidity of patients with severe chronic heart failure. Results of the Carvedilol Prospective Randomized Cumulative Survival (COPERNICUS) trial. *Circulation* 106:2194–2199, 2002.
29. Fonarow GC, Abraham WT, Albert NM, et al: Influence of beta-blocker continuation or withdrawal on outcomes in patients hospitalized with heart failure. Findings from the OPTIMIZE-HF Program. *J Am Coll Cardiol* 52:190–199, 2008.
30. Butler J, Ezekowitz JA, Colins SP, et al: Update on aldosterone antagonists use in heart failure with reduced ejection fraction Hear Failure Society of America Guidelines Committee. *J Card Fail* 18:265–281, 2012.
31. Nohria A, Tsang SW, Fang JC, et al: Clinical assessment identifies hemodynamic profiles that predict outcomes in patients with advanced heart failure. *J Am Coll Cardiol* 41:1797–1804, 2003.

32. Stevenson LW: Are hemodynamic goals viable in tailoring heart failure therapy? *Circulation* 113:1020–1033, 2006.
33. Biegel R, Cereck B, Siegel RJ, et al: Echo-Doppler hemodynamics. An important management tool for today's heart failure care. *Circulation* 131:1031–1034, 2015.
34. The ESCAPE Investigators and Study Coordinators: Evaluation study of congestive heart failure and pulmonary artery catheterization effectiveness. The ESCAPE trial. *JAMA* 294:1625–1633, 2005.
35. Francis GS, Bartos JA, Adatya S: Intotropes. *J Am Coll Cardiol* 63:2069–2078, 2014.
36. Goldhaber UI, Hamilton MA: Role of inotropic agents in the treatment of heart failure. *Circulation* 121:1655–1660, 2010.
37. Abraham WT, Adams KF, Fonarow GC, et al: In-hospital mortality in patients with acute decompensated heart failure requiring intravenous vasoactive medications. An analysis for the Acute Decompensated Heart Failure National Registry (ADHERE). *J Am Coll Cardiol* 46:57–64, 2005.
38. Silver MA, Horton DP, Ghali JK, et al: Effect of nesiritide versus dobutamine on short-term outcomes in the treatment of patients with acutely decompensated heart failure. *J Am Coll Cardiol* 39:798–803, 2002.
39. Mentzer RM, Oz MC, Sladen RN, et al: Effects of perioperative nesiritide in patients with left ventricular dysfunction undergoing cardiac surgery. The NAPA trial. *J Am Coll Cardiol* 49:716–722, 2007.
40. O'Connor CM, Starling RC, Hernandez AF, et al: Effect of nesiritide in patients with acute deompensated heart failure. *N Engl J Med* 365:32–43, 2011.
41. Daniels LB, Maisel AS: Natriuretic peptides. *J Am Coll Cardiol* 50:2357–2368, 2007.
42. Logeart D, Thabut G, Jourdain P, et al: Predischarge B-type natriuretic peptide assay for identifying patients at high risk of re-admission after decompensated heart failure. *J Am Coll Cardiol* 43:635–641, 2004.
43. Hernandez AF, Whellan DF, Htroud S, et al: Outcomes in heart failure patients after major non-cardiac surgery. *J Am Coll Cardiol* 44:1446–1453, 2004.
44. Fleisher LA, Fleischmann KE, Ting HH, et al: 2014 ACC/AHA guidelines on perioperative cardiovascular evaluation and management of patients undergoing non-cardiac surgery: executive summary. A report of the American College of Cardiology/American Heart Association Task Force on Practice Guidelines. *J Am Coll Cardiol* 64:2372–2405, 2014.
45. Sandham JD, Hull RD, Brant RE, et al; for the Canadian Critical Care Clinical Trials Group: A randomized, controlled trial of the use of pulmonary-artery catheters in high risk surgical candidates. *N Engl J Med* 348:5–14, 2003.
46. Practice Guidelines for Pulmonary Artery Catheterization: An updated report of the American Society of Anesthesiologists Task Force on Pulmonary Artery Catheterization. *Anesthesiology* 99:988–1014, 2003.
47. Rahil CS, Naidu SS, Givertz MM, et al: 2015 ACAI/ACC/HFSA/STS clinical expert consensus statement on the use of percutaneous mechanical circulatory support devices in cardiovascular care. *J Am Coll Cardiol* 65:2140–2141, 2015.
48. Seyfarth M, Sibbing D, Bauer I, et al: A randomized clinical trial to evaluate the safety and efficacy of a percutaneous left ventricular assist device versus intra-aortic balloon pumping for treatment of cardiogenic shock caused by myocardial infarction. *J Am Coll Cardiol* 52:1584–1588, 2008.
49. Kar B, Gregoric ID, Basra SS, et al: The percutaneous ventricular assist device in severe refractory cardiogenic shock. *J Am Coll Cardiol* 57:686096, 2011.
50. Anter E, Jessup M, Callans DJ: Atrial fibrillation and heart failure. Treatment considerations for a dual epidemic. *Circulation* 119:2516–2525, 2009.
51. Zimetbaum P: Antiarrhythmic drug therapy for atrial fibrillation. *Circulation* 125:381–389, 2012.
52. Allen LA, Fonarow GC, Simon DN, et al: Digoxin use and subsequent outcomes among patients in a contemporary atrial fibrillation cohort. *J Am Coll Cardiol* 65:2691–2698, 2015.
53. Kober L, Torp-Pedersen C, McMurray JJ, et al: Increased mortality after dronedarone therapy for severe heart failure. *N Engl J Med* 358:2678–2687, 2008.
54. Chen T, Koene R, Benditt DG, et al: Ventricular ectopy in patients with left ventricular dysfunction: should it be treated? *J Card Fail* 19:40–49, 2013.
55. Zipes DP, Camm JA, Borggrefe M, et al: ACC/AHA/ESC 2006 guidelines for management of patients with ventricular arrhythmias and the prevention of sudden death-executive summary. *J Am Coll Cardiol* 48:1064–1108, 2006.
56. Wann SL, Curtis AB, Ellenbogen KA, et al: 2011 ACCF/AHA/HRS focused update on the management of patients with atrial fibrillation. *Circulation* 123:1144–1150, 2011.
57. Spinler SA, Shafir V: New oral anticoagulants for atrial fibrillation. *Circulation* 126:133–137, 2012.

Chapter 195 ■ Management of the Cardiac Arrest Survivor

MICHAEL G. SILVERMAN • BENJAMIN M. SCIRICA

More than 500,000 people suffer a cardiac arrest (CA) each year in the USA. Out-of-hospital (OH) CA affects almost 350,000 people annually, and only 10% to 12% survive to hospital discharge [1]. Although survival has improved over the last several years, the mortality associated with CA remains extremely high [2]. Among those with an OHCA who survive to hospital presentation, the mortality rate is almost 60%. For the nearly 210,000 people who suffer an in-hospital (IH) CA each year, the mortality rate approaches 75% [1].

Although there are multiple causes of CA, hypoxemia–ischemia–reperfusion that arises during a CA and resuscitation can lead to a common pathophysiology that often results in multisystem organ dysfunction and neurologic injury, irrespective of the precipitating event [3]. In this chapter, we discuss the general approach to managing patients post-return of spontaneous circulation (ROSC) following a CA.

THE ROLE OF CORONARY ANGIOGRAPHY

Acute coronary syndrome (ACS) is a common cause of CA, and guidelines recommend performing a 12-lead electrocardiogram (ECG) as soon as possible following ROSC [3]. An observational analysis of post-CA patients taken for coronary angiography demonstrated that almost all patients (96%) with ST elevation on ECG had a significant coronary artery lesion [4]. Several observational studies have reported improved outcomes associated with coronary angiography among patients with ST elevation following OHCA [5–19]. In fact, the current guidelines recommend emergent coronary angiography for patients with OHCA with ST elevation on ECG (Class I recommendation) [3].

For patients without ST elevation on ECG, the role of emergent coronary angiography is less clear. An analysis from the PROCAT registry demonstrated that among individuals without ST segment elevation following OHCA, percutaneous intervention (PCI) was associated with improved outcomes [20]. It is important to recognize, however, that there are no randomized controlled trials evaluating the role of coronary angiography and PCI for comatose individuals following OHCA. The current guidelines provide a class IIa recommendation that the decision to proceed with coronary angiography should be made regardless of neurologic status and that coronary angiography is reasonable for comatose individuals following OHCA of suspected cardiac etiology but without ST-segment elevation in the setting of hemodynamic or electrical instability [3].

HEMODYNAMIC TARGETS

Hypotension is common following CA and is associated with worse outcomes [21,22]; however, there is limited randomized clinical trial data to support specific targets and the observational data is mixed. The current guidelines consider it reasonable (class IIb) to avoid and treat hypotension (systolic blood pressure [SBP] less than 90 mm Hg or mean arterial pressure [MAP] less than 65 mm Hg), but do not provide specific blood pressure targets. Similarly, owing to a lack of data, the guidelines

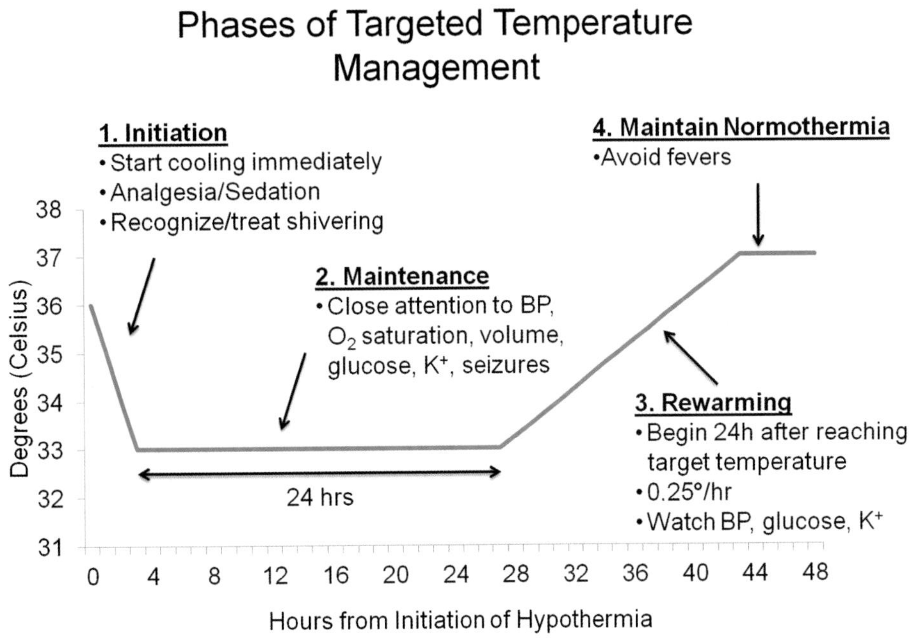
Phases of Targeted Temperature Management
1. Initiation
• Start cooling immediately
• Analgesia/Sedation
• Recognize/treat shivering
2. Maintenance
• Close attention to BP, O2 saturation, volume, glucose, K+, seizures
3. Rewarming
• Begin 24h after reaching target temperature
• 0.25°/hr
• Watch BP, glucose, K+
4. Maintain Normothermia
•Avoid fevers
24 hrs
Degrees (Celsius)
38
37
36
35
34
33
32
31
0
4
8
12
16
20
24
28
32
36
40
44
48
Hours from Initiation of Hypothermia

FIGURE 195.1 Phases of targeted temperature management. Adapted from Scirica BM. Therapeutic hypothermia after cardiac arrest. Circulation 127:244–250, 2013.

do not provide definitive recommendations regarding other hemodynamic measures.

Observational studies have targeted MAP goals of greater than 65 mm Hg up to greater than 90 mm Hg [23–25], with no difference seen in cerebral tissue oxygenation among individuals with a MAP of 70 mm Hg compared to a MAP of 90 mm Hg [25]. Therefore, a MAP goal of 70 to 75 may be reasonable [26]. Given the potential vasodilation from the post-CA inflammatory state, targeting a central venous pressure greater than 10 to 12 mm Hg is reasonable to help prevent hypotension and decrease vasopressor requirements [27].

TARGETED TEMPERATURE MANAGEMENT

Among individuals with ROSC following CA, neurologic mortality and morbidity is substantial. Roughly 80% of patients with ROSC remain comatose [28] and many of the deaths are attributed to neurologic injury [29]. Targeted temperature management (TTM) for comatose individuals post-CA has the potential to improve survival and neurologic outcomes. Figure 195.1 demonstrates the phases of targeted temperature management.

Indications for TTM

Two randomized clinical trials published in 2002 led to the initial adoption of therapeutic hypothermia (TH) following OHCA [30,31]. Both studies included comatose patients with ROSC following a ventricular fibrillation (VF) OHCA. Patients were randomized to either cooling to a temperature between 32°C and 34°C over 12 to 24 hours, or no temperature management at all. Both trials demonstrated significantly improved outcomes, with very low numbers needed to treat (roughly 6) for both improved survival and neurologic outcomes [32].

The TTM trial [33], the largest randomized clinical trial of temperature management following OHCA, randomized all individuals to 1 of 2 actively managed temperatures: 33°C versus 36°C for 28 hours, at which time gradual rewarming (0.5°C per hour) was initiated. At 6 month follow-up, there was no difference in mortality (50% for the 33°C group versus 48% for the 36°C group, $p = 0.51$) or in rates of poor neurologic outcome (52% for each group, $p = 0.87$). Importantly, nearly 20% of individuals in the TTM trial had an initial nonshockable rhythm. The similar outcomes between treatment strategies were observed for all important subgroups of patients (e.g., shockable versus nonshockable rhythms; time to return of normal circulation; and age).

The current American Heart Association and International Consensus on Cardiopulmonary Resuscitation guidelines now provide strong recommendations for the use of TTM for all comatose patients with ROSC following CA (Table 195.1). This includes OHCA with shockable and nonshockable rhythms, as well as all individuals with an in-hospital CA (IHCA) regardless of rhythm [3,34]. It is worth noting that the American Heart Association increased the strength of the recommendation for TTM for patients with nonshockable rhythms from class IIb to I, despite the absence of any appropriately powered randomized studies in this population.

TABLE 195.1

Recommendations for the Use of Targeted Temperature Management in Patients Following Cardiac Arrest

Indications	Comatose adult patients with ROSC after: • VF/pVT OHCA (Class I, level of evidence B) • non – VF/pVT OHCA (Class I, level of evidence C) • any IHCA (class I, level of evidence C)
Target temperature	Select and maintain a constant temperature between 32°C and 36°C (class I, level of evidence B)
Duration	Reasonable for TTM to be maintained for at least 24 hours after achieving target temperature (Class IIa, level of evidence C)

ROSC, return of spontaneous circulation; VF, ventricular fibrillation; pVT, pulse-less ventricular tachycardia; OHCA, out-of-hospital cardiac arrest; IHCA, in-hospital cardiac arrest; TTM, targeted temperature management.

Initiation of TTM

The optimal timing for TTM initiation and time to target temperature remain uncertain; however, observational patient data and animal data suggest worse outcomes with delayed initiation of TTM. Given these findings, there has been interest in the potential for prehospital initiation of TTM. However, Kim et al. demonstrated that prehospital cooling with cold saline did not lead to better survival or neurologic outcomes, and in fact was associated with higher rates of pulmonary edema and rearrest [35]. The detrimental effects of iced saline infusions were confirmed by the RINSE Trial, which found that early infusion of up to 2 L of iced saline was associated with a lower rate of successful ROSC [36]. As a result, the current guidelines recommend against the routine initiation of prehospital cooling with cold fluids. Therefore, it seems reasonable to initiate TTM as soon as possible on hospital arrival for comatose patients with ROSC following OHCA using ice packs, standard cooling blankets, or intravenous or surface cooling devices. The need for invasive coronary angiography should not delay initiation of TTM, because the use of TTM during invasive coronary angiography and PCI is both safe and feasible [4,17,37].

Target Temperature

The initial TH trials from 2002 targeted a goal temperature of 32°C to 34°C and 33°C [30,31]. A subsequent smaller pilot study demonstrated improved outcomes associated with 32°C versus 34°C [38], suggesting that lower temperatures might be better. In contrast, the more recent and larger TTM trial demonstrated similar outcomes between individuals randomized to 33°C versus 36°C [33]. Although there was no difference in outcomes between these two treatment groups, it is crucial to remember that this was a trial of two active temperature management interventions (33°C versus 36°C). The current guidelines recommend for a target temperature of 32°C to 36°C for at least 24 hours. The temperature range in the guideline recognizes uncertainty regarding the hypothesis that some individuals may benefit from greater degrees of hypothermia, whereas others may be at an increased risk of complications at lower temperatures (such as bradycardia), and thus can be effectively treated at a more moderate target temperature.

Methods of Cooling

Several methods for cooling have been used in the setting of TTM. Traditional methods have included cold intravenous fluid and ice packs. Alternative methods have included surface cooling methods such as blankets and gel pads with circulating cold water. Intravascular methods also exist that function via heat exchange [39]. An intranasal approach has also been used in the intra-arrest setting [40]. Although there is data demonstrating different rates of achieving and maintaining target temperature, no particular method has been associated with better outcomes than the others. As mentioned above, intravenous iced saline should not be used to initiate TTM.

Routine Care during Targeted Temperature Management

Sedation, Analgesia, and Shivering

Sedation and analgesia are an integral part of TTM until the patient has returned to normothermia [26]. All patients undergoing TTM should receive appropriate sedation and analgesia, typically a low dose, continuous infusion. Between 35°C and 37°C, shivering occurs frequently as a physiologic reaction. Shivering slows the time to target temperature and increases metabolic activity, so it should be treated aggressively. Blankets and a hot air warmer are nonpharmacologic methods to prevent and treat shivering. A bolus of intravenous magnesium can also help raise the shivering threshold. Increasing analgesia and sedation can also reduce shivering. If, however, shivering persists after these measures, then neuromuscular blockade can be effective. There are varying approaches to the use of neuromuscular blockade (selective versus continuous), which are currently being evaluated in ongoing clinical trials. If a patient is not cooling at a rate of 1°C per hour, then an empiric bolus of a neuromuscular blockade may help reduce subclinical shivering and achieve the target temperature more quickly.

Seizure Surveillance

The evaluation and management of seizures is another key component of neurologic care post-CA, because up to 12% to 22% of patients following CA will have seizure activity [3]. Nonconvulsive status epilepticus is a potential reason for patients not to regain consciousness and can be associated with secondary brain injury. In addition to potentially further injuring the brain, seizure activity also carries a poor prognosis. Therefore, it is important to recognize and manage nonconvulsive status epilepticus appropriately. Frequent or continuous EEGs are recommended for all comatose patients with ROSC following CA.

Ventilation and Oxygenation

Management of mechanical ventilation is an important component of post-arrest care. Ventilation should be targeted to maintain a $PaCO_2$ in the normal range (35 to 45 mm Hg). Hypocapnia has been associated with decreased cerebral perfusion [25] and worse outcomes in observational studies [41,42]. Similarly, oxygenation should be targeted within a range to avoid episodes of hypoxia (PaO_2 less than 60 mm Hg) as well as hyperoxia (PaO_2 greater than 300 mm Hg), with current recommendations to titrate FiO_2 to maintain oxygen saturation greater than 94% [3].

Hypergylcemia

Hypothermia decreases pancreatic insulin secretion and increases insulin resistance, leading to hyperglycemia [26]. Blood glucose should be monitored hourly. The optimal glucose target remains debated. No difference in 30-day survival was seen in one randomized clinical trial comparing tight control (72 to 108 mg per dL) versus moderate control (108 to 144 mg per dL) in the post-CA setting. There is currently no data to support that glycemic control for post-CA patients should differ from any other critical care setting [3], though avoidance of hypoglycemia is key because it could exacerbate neurologic damage.

Potassium

Hypokalemia is also a common occurrence during the cooling process because of both the inward cellular shift of potassium, and the modest diuresis and kaliuresis in the setting of hypothermia. Electrolytes should therefore be monitored frequently (every 4 to 6 hours) and repleted appropriately. Potassium repletion should then be held starting 4 hours prior to the rewarming phase because of the reversal of cellular shift as potassium returns to the serum.

Infection

Infection can occur frequently among post-CA patients undergoing TTM. This can be from a combination of exposure from possible aspiration, emergent intubation, mechanical ventilation, and possible catheter related infections in the setting of potential immune suppression from TTM.

Electrocardiography

The most common arrhythmia of TTM is sinus bradycardia. At cooler temperatures, the PR interval will prolong and patients can experience a junctional escape rhythm. Rewarming by 1°C to 2°C will resolve conduction abnormalities. Cooling can also prolong the QT interval, again in a "dose-dependent" fashion, though there is no evidence to suggest it precipitates torsade-de-pointes. Osborn, or J waves, may be present in up to 20% of patients, depending on the target temperature [43]. No specific therapy is required for any non–life-threatening arrhythmia, but rewarming by 1°C to 2°C will resolve most conduction abnormalities.

Hemodynamics

A substudy from the Targeted Temperature Management trial [44] demonstrated the effect of hypothermia on hemodynamics (Fig. 195.2). A target temperature of 33°C was associated with an increase of systemic and pulmonary vascular resistance when compared with a target temperature of 36°C. Although the lower temperature was associated with decreased cardiac index, this was thought to be largely mediated by a reduction in heart rate, and there was no difference in left ventricular ejection fraction between the groups.

Return to Normothermia

Gradual rewarming (0.25°C to 0.5°C per hour) should be initiated at least 24 hours after TTM initiation [3]. Rewarming faster than this raises the risk of hypoglycemia, hyperkalemia, and hypotension (from vasodilation). Once the TTM protocol has been completed and the patient has achieved normothermia, actively avoiding fever among patients who remain comatose is reasonable, because hyperthermia has been associated with worse neurologic outcomes in other critical care settings [45,46]. This can often be achieved by leaving the temperature management system in place [3] and by the use of antipyretics.

NEUROLOGIC PROGNOSTICATION

Providing a neurologic prognosis following CA is a complicated task that often requires multimodality tools including physical examination, EEG, neuroimaging, somatosensory evoked potentials (SSEPs), and serologic biomarkers. Despite advances in post-resuscitation care, neuroprognostication remains the most challenging aspect of care, because no test has acceptable levels of certainty. Few patients meet formal criteria for brain death after resuscitation and most patients have intact brainstem function, such that the patient has spontaneous ventilation. Ideally, a test would identify patients at an early stage with the potential for a good neurologic outcome while also indicating which patients have no chance of meaningful neurologic recovery.

Timing

The ideal timing for neurologic prognostication for comatose patients following CA remains uncertain. The ultimate goal is

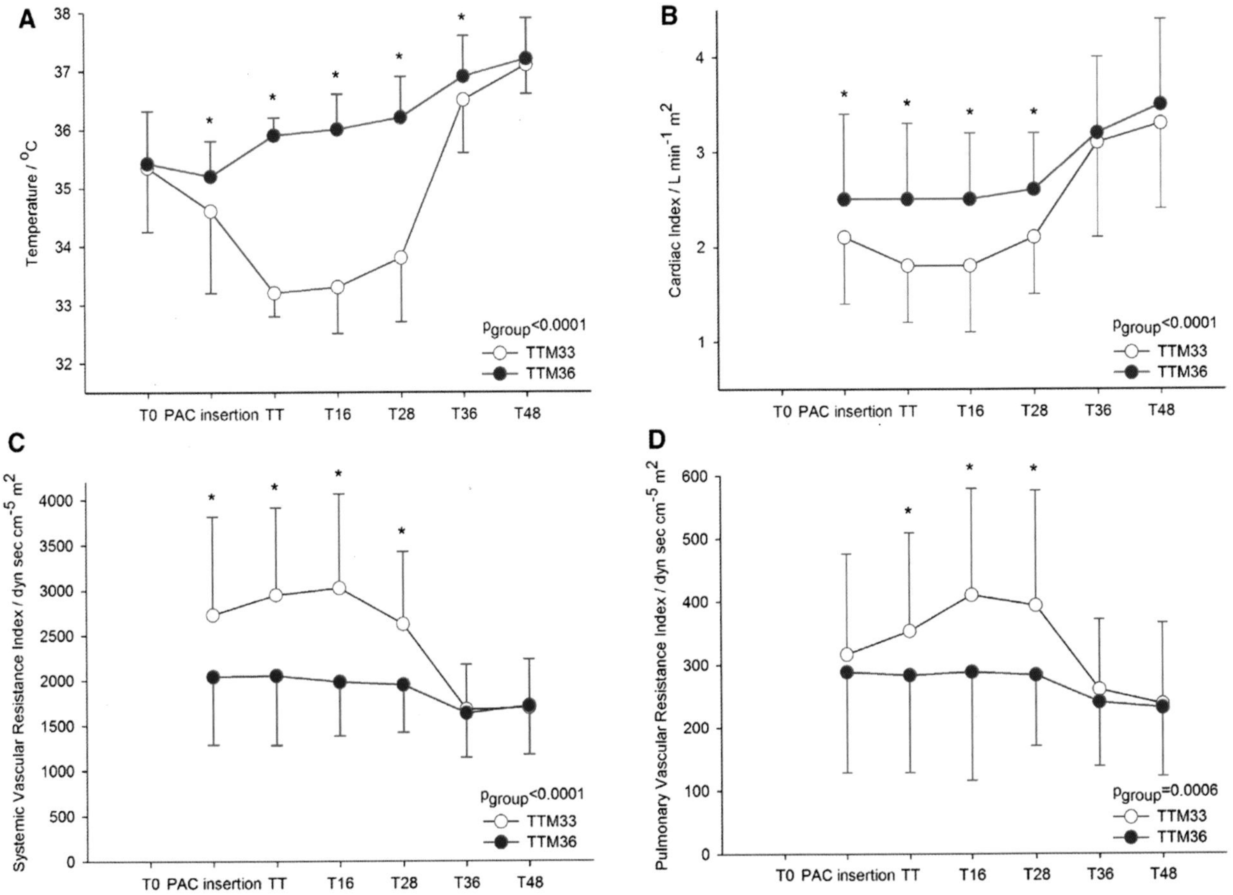

FIGURE 195.2 Hemodynamic effects of targeted temperature management. **A:** The change in temperature. **B:** The change in cardiac index. **C:** The change in systemic vascular resistance. **D:** The change in pulmonary vascular resistance. From Bro-Jeppesen J, Hassager C, Wanscher M, et al: Targeted temperature management at 33°C versus 36°C and impact on systemic vascular resistance and myocardial function after out-of-hospital cardiac arrest: a sub-study of the Target Temperature Management Trial. *Circ Cardiovasc Interv* 7(5):663–672, 2014.

TABLE 195.2

Acceptable Neurologic Criteria for Discontinuation of Care in the Targeted Temperature Management Trial

- Brain death due to cerebral herniation[a]
- Severe myoclonus status in the first 24 hours after admission and a bilateral absence of N20-peak on median nerve SSEP[a]
- Minimum 72 hours after intervention period: Glasgow motor score 1–2 and bilateral absence of N20-peak on median nerve SSEP
- Minimum 72 hours after intervention period: Glasgow motor score 1–2 and treatment refractory status epilepticus

[a]This finding was permitted for poor neurologic prognostication prior to 72 hours after targeted temperature management.

TABLE 195.3

Principles of Management for the Post-Cardiac Arrest Patient

- Identify and treat the underlying cause of cardiac arrest
- Acute Cardiovascular Care
  - Obtain EKG
  - STEMI → Coronary Angiography
  - NSTEMI with hemodynamic or electrical instability → coronary angiography
- Hemodynamics
  - Avoid and treat hypotension (SBP < 90 mm Hg, MAP < 65 mm Hg)
  - Consider goal MAP ~70–75
- Mechanical Ventilation
  - Maintain normocarbia: $PaCO_2$ 35–45 mm Hg
  - Maintain oxygen saturation > 94%
- Targeted Temperature Management (TTM) for comatose patients (regardless of rhythm)
  - Initiate TTM as soon as possible on hospital arrival
    - TTM can be started prior to and continued during coronary angiography
  - Target temperature: 32°C–36°C
  - Initiate gradual rewarming ≥ 24 h after starting TTM protocol
  - Check blood glucose every hour
  - Check electrolytes every 4–6 h
- Neurologic monitoring for comatose patients
  - Continuous EEG as soon as possible following cardiac arrest
  - Consider somatosensory evoked potentials (SSEPs) 24–72 h post-arrest
- Neurologic prognostication should be delayed until:
  - at least 72 h post-return to normothermia for patients treated with TTM
  - at least 72 h post-arrest for patients not treated with TTM

to identify a time point that minimizes (or eliminates) the risk of inaccurately predicting a poor neurologic outcome, thus avoiding a "false positive." For patients who have not been treated with TTM, a minimum of 72 hours following ROSC is suggested [3,47]. Patients undergoing TTM experience delayed neurologic recovery; therefore it is important to wait a minimum of 72 hours post-return to normothermia when the patient is off of all potentially sedating medications and free of other confounding illnesses, before assessing for neurologic prognosis [3,48].

There are few clinical criteria that clearly identify patients with a poor neurologic prognosis. The TTM trial specified the clinical scenarios listed in Table 195.2 as acceptable criteria for poor prognosis that would justify the transition to comfort care. Many patients will not fulfil these criteria, thus leaving the clinician to use the diagnostic tests discussed below to help guide therapy and prognosis.

Diagnostic Testing

The absence of pupillary light reflexes at 72 hours following CA is considered a reasonable predictor of poor neurologic outcome for TTM and non–TTM-treated patients [3]. The absence of motor movements, extensor posturing, and myoclonus have fairly high false-positive rates (up to nearly 10%), and therefore should not be used to predict poor neurologic outcome [3].

A lack of EEG reactivity at 72 hours post-CA, and persistent burst suppression after rewarming are considered reasonable

TABLE 195.4

Advances in Post-cardiac Arrest Care Based on Randomized Controlled Trials

Intervention	Year	Study	No. of patients	Findings	References
Therapeutic hypothermia 32–34°C versus "normothermia"	2002	Multicenter	275	Lower mortality, improved neurologic outcomes	[30]
Therapeutic hypothermia 33°C versus "normothermia"	2002	Multicenter	77	Improved survival with good neurologic outcome	[31]
Targeted temperature management 33°C versus 36°C (both active temperature management interventions)	2013	Multicenter	939	No difference between groups	[33]
Pre-hospital intravenous cold saline	2014	Multicenter	1359	No benefit, increased risk of pulmonary edema and rearrest	[34]
Pre-hospital intra-arrest intravenous cold saline	2016	Multicenter	1198	No benefit in survival at hospital discharge. Decrease in the rate of ROSC for patients with a shockable rhythm	[35]

predictors of poor neurologic outcomes for TTM-treated patients [49]. Status epilepticus for more than 72 hours is also a reasonable marker of poor neurologic outcome. In non–TTM-treated patients, burst suppression at 72 hours post-CA is a reasonable marker of poor neurologic prognosis when combined with other predictors [3]. Research into earlier EEG patterns post-arrest is ongoing to identify both good and poor prognostic patterns.

SSEPs test the cortical response to peripheral median nerve stimulation. Independent of whether patients undergo TTM, an SSEP 24 to 72 hours post-CA demonstrating the bilateral absence of the N20 waveform is a reasonable predictor of poor neurologic outcome [3].

Computed tomography (CT) or magnetic resonance imaging (MRI) of the brain to evaluate for edema can provide useful measures in support of poor neurologic outcome. Imaging immediately post-arrest it is less likely to help with prognosis, unless there is evidence of hemorrhage, trauma, or herniation. Many patients without long-term neurologic recovery will have normal CT imaging within the first 24 hours. The optimal timing for MRI is after re-warming.

Neuron-specific enolase (NSE) and S-100B, two of the more commonly evaluated serologic tests for predicting poor neurologic outcomes, have been shown to have high false-positive rates. As a result, they are not recommended for use in isolation and should only be used as supportive information in combination with other tests and clinical findings [3].

In general, a combination of certain diagnostic testing can help to increase the specificity for a poor neurologic prognosis [50]. Rarely will one test be the deciding factor in prognosis; rather, the integration of all testing, combined with the patient's age and co morbidities, will allow a multidisciplinary team to provide the most appropriate prognosis for patients.

CONCLUSIONS

Caring for post-CA patients involves a multifaceted and multisystem approach to evaluate and treat the underlying cause of arrest and to minimize and prevent further progression of end organ damage (Table 195.3). For patients who remain comatose following ROSC, TTM can improve survival and neurologic outcomes, and is now recommended as standard of care regardless of the presenting rhythm. Despite the advances of post-arrest care that have led to improved outcomes (Table 195.4), many questions regarding the routine care and prognostication of these patients remain. Care for the post-CA patients requires a multidisciplinary team of intensivists, cardiologists, neurologists, social workers, and nurses. Only through team-based care at centers with resources and experience can the most contemporary treatments be delivered.

References

1. Mozaffarian D, Benjamin EJ, Go AS, et al; on behalf of the American Heart Association Statistics Committee and Stroke Statistics subcommittee: heart disease and stroke statistics 2016 update. A report from the American Heart Association. *Circulation* 133:447–454, 2016.
2. Fugate JE, Brinjikji W, Mandrekar JN, et al: Post-cardiac arrest mortality is declining: a study of the US National Inpatient Sample 2001 to 2009. *Circulation* 126: 546–550, 2012.
3. Callaway CW, Donnino MW, Fink EL, et al: Part8: Post-cardiac arrest care: 2015 American Heart Association Guidelines update for cardio-pulmonary resuscitation and emergency cardiovascular care. *Circulation* 132(Suppl 2):S465–S482, 2015.
4. Dumas F, Cariou A, Manzo-Silberman S, et al: Immediate percutaneous coronary intervention is associated with better survival after out-of-hospital cardiac arrest: insights from the PROCAT (Parisian Region Out of hospital Cardiac ArresT) registry. *Circ Cardiovasc Interv* 3:200–207, 2010.
5. Hollenbeck RD, McPherson JA, Mooney MR, et al: Early cardiac catheterization is associated with improved survival in comatose survivors of cardiac arrest without STEMI. *Resuscitation* 85:88–95, 2014.
6. Mooney MR, Unger BT, Boland LL, et al: Therapeutic hypothermia after out-of-hospital cardiac arrest: evaluation of a regional system to increase access to cooling. *Circulation* 124:206–214, 2011.
7. Gräsner JT, Meybohm P, Lefering R, et al; German Resuscitation Registry Study Group: ROSC after cardiac arrest–the RACA score to predict outcome after out-of-hospital cardiac arrest. *Eur Heart J* 32:1649–1656, 2011.
8. Cronier P, Vignon P, Bouferrache K, et al: Impact of routine percutaneous coronary intervention after out-of-hospital cardiac arrest due to ventricular fibrillation. *Crit Care* 15:R122, 2011.
9. Bulut S, Aengevaeren WR, Luijten HJ, et al: Successful out-of hospital cardiopulmonary resuscitation: what is the optimal in-hospital treatment strategy? *Resuscitation* 47:155–161, 2000.
10. Bro-Jeppesen J, Kjaergaard J, Wanscher M, et al: Emergency coronary angiography in comatose cardiac arrest patients: do real-life experiences support the guidelines? *Eur Heart J Acute Cardiovasc Care* 1:291–301, 2012.
11. Aurore A, Jabre P, Liot P, et al: Predictive factors for positive coronary angiography in out-of-hospital cardiac arrest patients. *Eur J Emerg Med* 18:73–76, 2011.
12. Nanjayya VB, Nayyar V: Immediate coronary angiogram in comatose survivors of out-of-hospital cardiac arrest–an Australian study. *Resuscitation* 83:699–704, 2012.
13. Reynolds JC, Callaway CW, El Khoudary SR, et al: Coronary angiography predicts improved outcome following cardiac arrest: propensity-adjusted analysis. *J Intensive Care Med* 24:179–186, 2009.
14. Strote JA, Maynard C, Olsufka M, et al: Comparison of role of early (less than six hours) to later (more than six hours) or no cardiac catheterization after resuscitation from out-of hospital cardiac arrest. *Am J Cardiol* 109:451–454, 2012.
15. Tømte O, Andersen GØ, Jacobsen D, et al: Strong and weak aspects of an established post-resuscitation treatment protocol-A five-year observational study. *Resuscitation* 82:1186–1193, 2011.
16. Waldo SW, Armstrong EJ, Kulkarni A, et al: Comparison of clinical characteristics and outcomes of cardiac arrest survivors having versus not having coronary angiography. *Am J Cardiol* 111:1253–1258, 2013.
17. Nielsen N, Hovdenes J, Nilsson F, et al; Hypothermia Network. Outcome, timing and adverse events in therapeutic hypothermia after out-of-hospital cardiac arrest. *Acta Anaesthesiol Scand* 53:926–934, 2009.
18. Werling M, Thorén AB, Axelsson C, et al: Treatment and outcome in post-resuscitation care after out-of-hospital cardiac arrest when a modern therapeutic approach was introduced. *Resuscitation* 73:40–45, 2007.
19. Zanuttini D, Armellini I, Nucifora G, et al: Impact of emergency coronary angiography on in-hospital outcome of unconscious survivors after out-of-hospital cardiac arrest. *Am J Cardiol* 110:1723–1728, 2012.
20. Dumas F, Bougouin W, Geri G, et al: Emergency percutaneous coronary intervention in post-cardiac arrest patients without ST-segment elevation pattern: insights from the PROCAT II registry. *J Am Coll Cardiol Interv* 9:1011–1018, 2016.
21. Trzeciak S, Jones AE, Kilgannon JH, et al: Significance of arterial hypotension after resuscitation from cardiac arrest. *Crit Care Med* 37:2895–2903, 2009.
22. Bray JE, Bernard S, Cantwell K, et al; VACAR Steering Committee: The association between systolic blood pressure on arrival at hospital and outcome in adults surviving from out-of-hospital cardiac arrests of presumed cardiac aetiology. *Resuscitation* 85:509–515, 2014.
23. Sunde K, Pytte M, Jacobsen D, et al: Implementation of a standardised treatment protocol for post resuscitation care after out-of-hospital cardiac arrest. *Resuscitation* 73:29–39, 2007.
24. Gaieski DF, Band RA, Abella BS, et al: Early goal-directed hemodynamic optimization combinedwith therapeutic hypothermia in comatose survivors of out-of-hospital cardiac arrest. *Resuscitation* 2009;80:418–424.
25. Bouzat P, Suys T, Sala N, et al: Effect of moderate hyperventilation and induced hypertension on cerebral tissue oxygenation after cardiac arrest and therapeutic hypothermia. *Resuscitation* 84:1540–1545, 2013.
26. Silverman MG, Scirica BM: Cardiac arrest and therapeutic hypothermia. *Trends Cardiovasc Med* 26:337–344, 2016.
27. Scirica BM: Therapeutic hypothermia after cardiac arrest. *Circulation* 127:244–250, 2013.
28. Booth CM, Boone RH, Tomlinson G, et al: Is this patient dead, vegetative, or severely neurologically impaired? Assessing outcome for comatose survivors of cardiac arrest. *J Am Med Assoc* 291:870–879, 2004.
29. Laver S, Farrow C, Turner D, et al: Mode of death after admission to an intensive care unit following cardiac arrest. *Intensive Care Med* 30:2126–2128, 2004.
30. Hypothermia after Cardiac Arrest Study Group: Mild therapeutic hypothermia to improve the neurologic outcome after cardiac arrest. *N Engl J Med* 346:549–556, 2002.
31. Bernard SA, Gray TW, Buist MD, et al: Treatment of comatose survivors of out-of-hospital cardiac arrest with induced hypothermia. *N Engl J Med* 346:557–563, 2002.
32. Walters JH, Morley PT, Nolan JP: The role of hypothermia in post-cardiac arrest patients with return of spontaneous circulation: a systematic review. *Resuscitation* 82:508–516, 2011.
33. Nielsen N, Wetterslev J, Cronberg T, et al: Targeted temperature management at 33°C versus 36°C after cardiac arrest. *N Engl J Med* 369:2197–2206, 2013.
34. Callaway CW, Soar J, Aibiki M, et al; Advanced Life Support Chapter Collaborators: Part 4: Advanced Life Support: 2015 International Consensus on cardiopulmonary resuscitation and emergency cardiovascular care science with treatment recommendations. *Circulation* 132(Suppl 1):S84–S145, 2015.

35. Kim F, Nichol G, Maynard C, et al: Effect of prehospital induction of mild hypothermia on survival and neurological status among adults with cardiac arrest: a randomized clinical trial. *JAMA* 31:45–52, 2014.
36. Bernard SA, Smith K, Finn J, et al: Induction of therapeutic hypothermia during out-of-hospital cardiac arrest using a rapid infusion of cold saline the RINSE trial (Rapid Infusion of Cold Normal Saline). *Circulation* 134:797–805, 2016.
37. Hovdenes J, Laake JH, Aaberge L, et al: Therapeutic hypothermia after out-of-hospital cardiac arrest: experiences with patients treated with percutaneous coronary intervention and cardiogenic shock. *Acta Anaesthesiol Scand* 51;137–142, 2007.
38. Lopez-de-Sa E, Rey JR, Armada E, et al: Hypothermia in comatose survivors from out-of-hospital cardiac arrest: pilot trial comparing 2 levels of target temperature. *Circulation* 126:2826–2833, 2012.
39. Alkadri ME, Peters MN, Katz MJ, et al: State-of-the-art paper: therapeutic hypothermia in out of hospital cardiac arrest survivors. *Catheter Cardiovasc Interv* 82:E482–E490, 2013.
40. Castrén M, Nordberg P, Svensson L, et al: Intra-arrest transnasal evaporative cooling: a randomized, prehospital, multicenter study (PRINCE: Pre-ROSC IntraNasal Cooling Effectiveness). *Circulation* 122:729–736, 2010.
41. Roberts BW, Kilgannon JH, Chansky ME, et al: Association between postresuscitation partial pressure of arterial carbon dioxide and neurological outcome in patients with post-cardiac arrest syndrome. *Circulation* 127:2107–2113, 2013.
42. Lee BK, Jeung KW, Lee HY, et al: Association between mean arterial blood gas tension and outcome in cardiac arrest patients treated with therapeutic hypothermia. *Am J Emerg Med* 32:55–60, 2014.
43. Salinas P, Lopez-de-Sa E, Pena-Conde L, et al: Electrocardiographic changes during induced therapeutic hypothermia in comatose survivors after cardiac arrest. *World J Cardiol* 7(7):423–430, 2015.
44. Bro-Jeppesen J, Hassager C, Wanscher M, et al: Targeted temperature management at 33°C versus 36°C and impact on systemic vascular resistance and myocardial function after out-of-hospital cardiac arrest: a sub-study of the Target Temperature Management Trial. *Circ Cardiovasc Interv* 7(5):663–672, 2014.
45. Bohman LE, Levine JM: Fever and therapeutic normothermia in severe brain injury: an update. *Curr Opin Crit Care* 20:182–188, 2014.
46. Badjatia N: Hyperthermia and fever control in brain injury. *Crit Care Med* 37(7 Suppl):S250–S257, 2009.
47. Sandroni C, Cavallaro F, Callaway CW, et al: Predictors of poor neurological outcome in adult comatose survivors of cardiac arrest: a systematic review and meta-analysis. Part 1: patients not treated with therapeutic hypothermia. *Resuscitation* 84:1310–1323, 2013.
48. Sandroni C, Cavallaro F, Callaway CW, et al: Predictors of poor neurological outcome in adult comatose survivors of cardiac arrest: a systematic review and meta-analysis. Part 2: Patients treated with therapeutic hypothermia. *Resuscitation* 84:1324–1338, 2013.
49. Westhall E, Rossetti AO, van Rootselaar AF, et al: Standardized EEG interpretation accurately predicts prognosis after cardiac arrest. *Neurology* 86(16):1482–1490, 2016.
50. Rossetti AO, Rabinstein AA, Oddo M: Neurological prognostication of outcome in patients in coma after cardiac arrest. *Lancet Neurol* 15(6):597–609, 2016.

Chapter 196 ■ Management of Cardiac Devices in the ICU

MELANIE MAYTIN

INTRODUCTION

Cardiac device technology has made great advancements since the introduction of the first implantable pacemaker in 1958. Since then, the number of cardiac device implants continues to increase annually. The driver of this increase includes a larger burden of cardiac dysfunction related to the aging of the general population, expanding indications for device therapy, and ongoing innovation of the technology for cardiac pacing and defibrillation. As a result, many patients presenting to the intensive care unit (ICU) with noncardiac illnesses may have implanted cardiac devices. This chapter aims to briefly review basic cardiac device function and programming with emphasis on device malfunction and troubleshooting. A discussion of the indications for permanent pacing, defibrillator, or resynchronization therapy is beyond the scope of this text; for additional information regarding these topics, the reader is referred to the American College of Cardiology/American Heart Association/Heart Rhythm Society 2012 Focused Update of the 2008 Guidelines for Device-Based Therapy of Cardiac Rhythm Abnormalities [1].

GENERAL DEVICE MANAGEMENT

Normal Device Function and Special Considerations

Identification of the type of device is critical for interpretation of its function. Although patients would ideally be able to provide information regarding the type of device that has been implanted (pacemaker, implantable cardioverter defibrillator [ICD], cardiac resynchronization device, among others) or carry a device identification card with them at all times, this is frequently not the case for hospitalized patients. Substantial device information can be gleaned from a chest radiograph, including the lead configuration, the type of device, abnormalities of lead position or integrity, and even the device manufacturer (Fig. 196.1A to E). Identification of the device manufacturer is essential when formal device interrogation or reprogramming is planned as each device company uses different software and programs to communicate with their respective devices (Fig. 196.2). The overwhelming majority of devices implanted are manufactured by 1 of 3 companies, and patient device information and technical support are available 24 hours a day (Table 196.1).

Conventional device systems consist of a pulse generator or battery, logic circuits, pacing lead(s), and/or defibrillator lead(s). Cardiac implantable electronic device (CIED) therapy is rapidly evolving with novel technologies aimed at limiting vascular access or avoiding the vasculature entirely. The first subcutaneous ICD (S-ICD) was approved for use in the United States by the Food and Drug Administration in 2012 while, to date, no leadless pacemakers are approved by the FDA although postmarket studies are currently enrolling subjects. All implantable cardiac devices have programmable pacemaker functions with the exception of the current S-ICD device. Although the S-ICD can deliver transient backup pacing following defibrillator therapy, pacing is delivered transcutaneously and is not currently a viable long-term pacing option. Apart from the S-ICD, CIED both sense intrinsic electrical depolarization and excite myocardial tissue through an artificial electrical stimulus delivered near the lead/device tip. Electrical stimuli can be delivered in many ways depending upon how the device is programmed. Pacing nomenclature is standardized to easily communicate information regarding the device and the pacing mode (Table 196.2). Pacing algorithms are best understood as a function of timing cycles. A pacemaker operates like a timer with programmable intervals to coordinate all sensed and paced events. Nontracking modes of pacing (AAI, VVI, and DDI) deliver electrical impulses at set intervals (*lower rate limit*) unless a sensed electrophysiologic cardiac event occurs in the appropriate chamber before the end of the programmed interval (in which case the timer resets, Fig. 196.3). Dual chamber devices programmed to a tracking mode can provide pacing at the programmed lower rate or track sensed intrinsic conduction up to a programmed *upper rate limit*. There is no sensing in asynchronous pacing modes (AOO, VOO, and DOO) and electrical stimuli are produced at programmed intervals unaffected by intrinsic conduction.

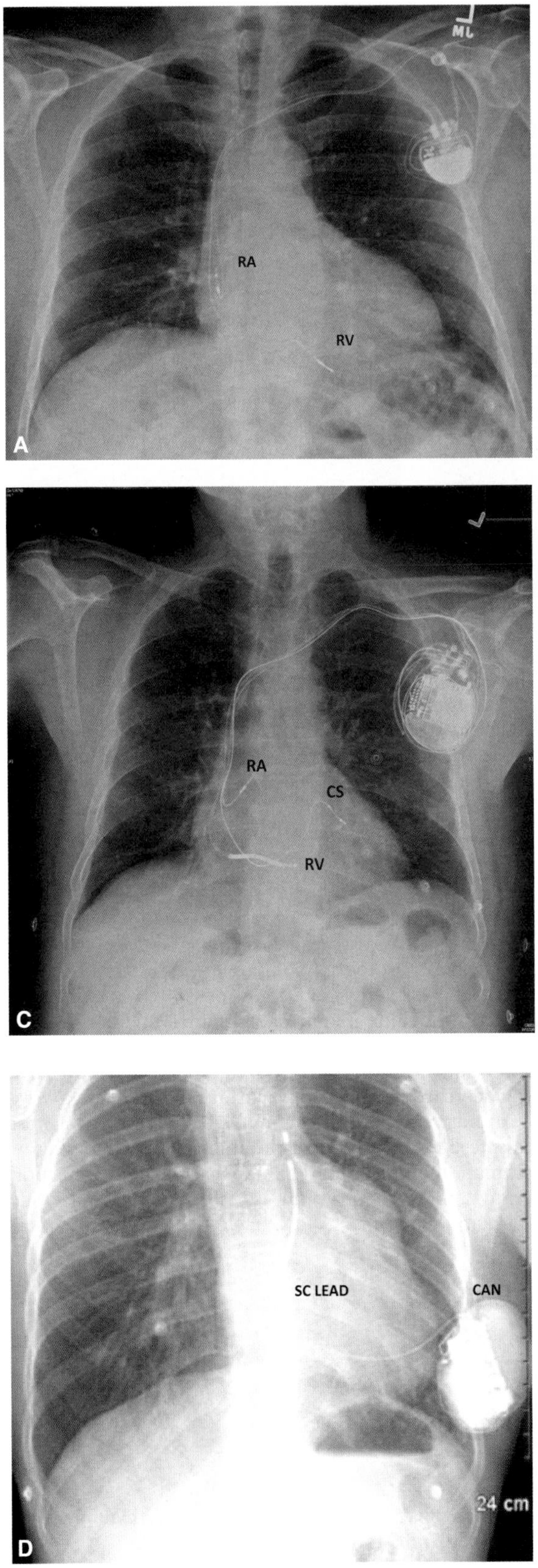

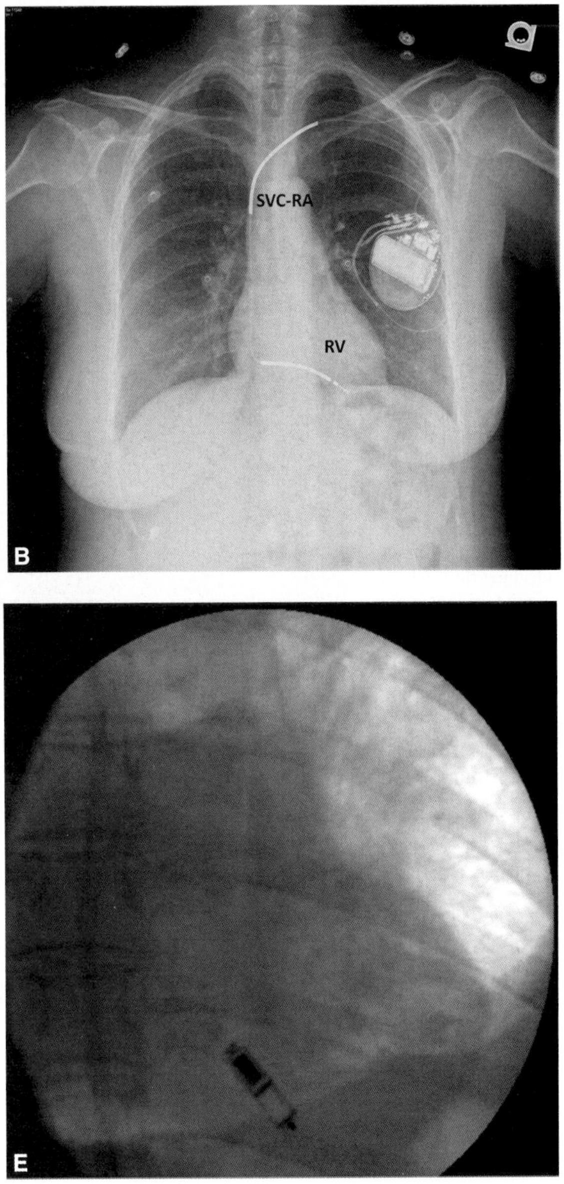

FIGURE 196.1 Information regarding implantable cardiac devices can be gained from chest radiograph. **A:** Dual chamber pacemaker with leads in the RA and RV. **B:** Single chamber, dual coil defibrillator with high voltage conductors in the RV and SVC–RA junction. **C:** Cardiac resynchronization device with leads in the RA, RV, and CS. These devices may or may not have defibrillator function. **D:** Subcutaneous implantable cardioverter defibrillator (S-ICD) with generator in the left anterior-to-mid axillary line and defibrillator lead tunneled subcutaneously to the left parasternal region with the coil between the xyphoid process and suprasternal notch. **E:** Leadless pacemaker implanted in the RV. RA, right atrium; RV, right ventricle; SVC, superior vena cava; CS, coronary sinus; CAN, generator; SQ LEAD, subcutaneous lead.

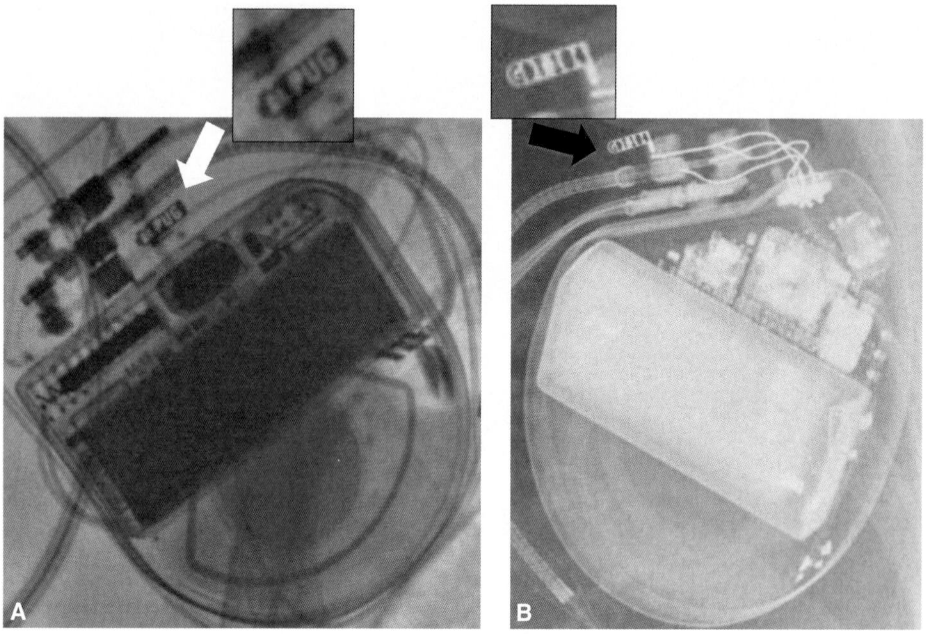

FIGURE 196.2 Many cardiac devices are marked with a radiopaque code that specifically identifies the manufacturer and model of the device. **A:** Chest radiograph in patient with implanted CRT-D. Arrow points to radiopaque marker. Inset shows enlarged image of code. Symbol at beginning of code represents Medtronic. **B:** Chest radiograph in patient with implanted CRT-D. Arrow points to radiopaque marker. Inset shows enlarged image of code. First three letters of code "GDT" represent Guidant (now Boston Scientific).

TABLE 196.1

Device Manufacturers' Contact Information

Medtronic	1.800.MEDTRONIC
Boston Scientific	1.800.CARDIAC
St. Jude Medical	1.800.PACEICD
Biotronik	1.800.547.0394
Sorin Group	1.800.352.6466

Magnets

The placement of a magnet over a device affects pacemakers and defibrillators differently. Application of a magnet to a pacemaker will cause the reed switch to close and result in asynchronous pacing. The pacing rate is company-specific with a different rate once battery depletion has occurred. Thus, placement of a magnet over the device can assist with the determination of battery status and device identification. If exposure to electromagnetic interference (EMI) is anticipated, positioning a magnet over the device can prevent inappropriate pacing inhibition. Upon removal of the magnet, the pacing mode will revert to the originally programmed settings, and, in general, formal device interrogation is not required. In contrast, application of a magnet to a defibrillator will disable all antitachycardia therapies but will *not* affect the pacing mode. Therefore, magnets can be used to prevent inappropriate therapies due to supraventricular tachycardia (SVT), lead fracture, or EMI. Upon removal of the magnet, defibrillator therapies will be restored, and, in general, formal device interrogation is not required.

Electromagnetic Interference

CIEDs are susceptible to strong electromagnetic fields [2]. In the hospital, many potential sources of EMI exist. Sources of electromagnetic energy that could possibly interfere with device function include magnetic resonance imaging (MRI), electrocautery, defibrillation, radiation therapy, neurostimulators, TENS units, radiofrequency ablation, electroconvulsive therapy, video capsule endoscopy, extracorporeal shock-wave lithotripsy, and therapeutic diathermy [3,4]. EMI exposure most commonly results in inappropriate inhibition or triggering of pacing stimuli, inappropriate ICD tachyarrhythmia detection and therapy and reversion to an asynchronous pacing mode (*noise-reversion mode*).

TABLE 196.2

Pacing Designation

	NASPE/BPEG Generic (NBG) Code				
Position	**I**	**II**	**III**	**IV**	**V**
Category	Chamber(s) pace	Chamber(s) sensed	Response to sensing	Programmability, rate modulation	Antitachyarrhythmia function(s)
Letters used	O-None A-Atrium V-Ventricle D-Dual (A+V)	O-None A-Atrium V-Ventricle D-Dual (A+V)	O-None T-Triggered I-Inhibited D-Dual (T+I)	O-None P-Simple programmable M-Multi-programmable C-Communicating R-Rate modulation	O-None P-Pacing (antitachy-arrhythmia) S-Shock D-Dual (P+S)
Manufacturer's designation only	S-Single (A or V)	S-Single (A or V)			

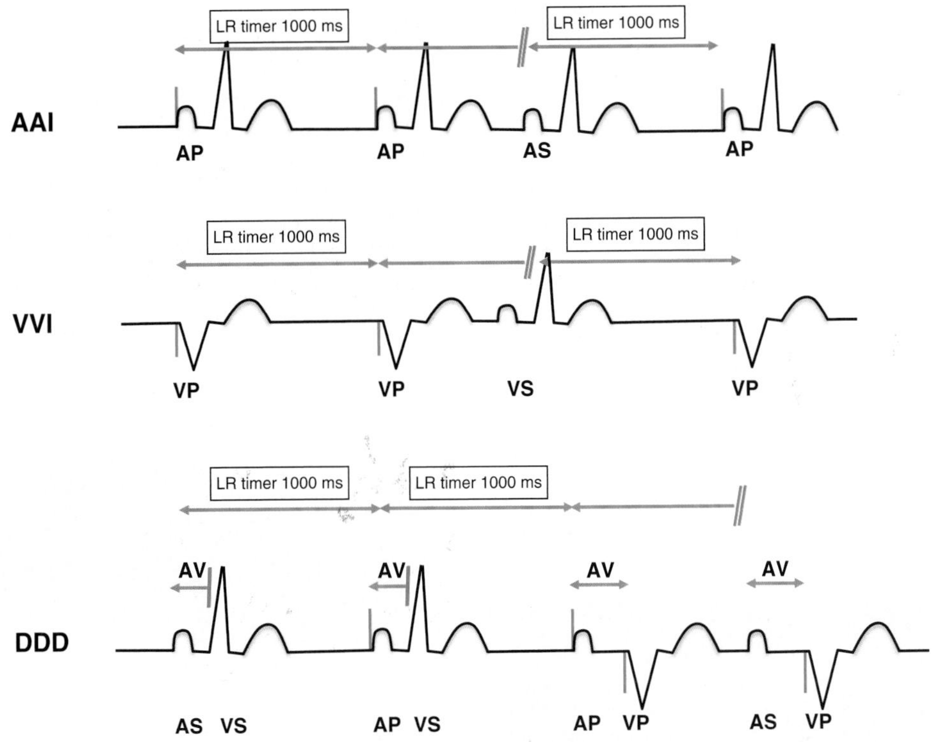

FIGURE 196.3 Timing of events in various pacing modes. AAI is an atrial nontracking mode of pacing that provides backup atrial pacing at the programmed lower rate limit. Similarly, VVI is a ventricular nontracking mode of pacing that provides backup ventricular pacing at the programmed lower rate limit. DDD is a dual chamber mode of pacing that can both inhibit and trigger events in both the atrium and the ventricle. AS, atrial sensed event; AP, atrial paced event; VS, ventricular sensed event; VP, ventricular paced event; LR, lower rate limit.

Inappropriate inhibition of ventricular pacing can be catastrophic for the pacemaker-dependent patient; similarly atrial oversensing with inappropriate ventricular tracking could result in a myriad of symptoms and induce heart failure, hypotension, or angina. Improper ICD tachyarrhythmia detection due to EMI could potentially be arrhythmia-inducing as a result of unsynchronized inappropriate shock delivery during the vulnerable period of repolarization. Noise-reversion mode is an algorithm that reverts transiently to asynchronous pacing in response to rapid frequency signals. The algorithm is designed to protect against inappropriate inhibition of pacing when high frequency signals are sensed. Although this algorithm is present in all pacemakers regardless of manufacturer, this is not the case for ICDs. Less frequently, EMI can result in reprogramming of the device parameters or permanently damage circuitry or a lead. When EMI exposure is unavoidable, certain measures can be taken to minimize the potential risks. For example, pacemaker or defibrillator patients requiring surgery with electrocautery should have a magnet placed over the device during the operation. Other forms of EMI (e.g. MRI, radiation therapy, among others) carry substantial risk and may prompt the revision or removal of the entire cardiac device system prior to the magnetic exposure. Care should be taken to avoid sources of EMI for device patients or, if exposure to EMI cannot be avoided, at a minimum, measures should be taken to minimize potential harm with consideration of device interrogation following exposure.

Mode Switch

Mode switch is a programmable pacing algorithm that automatically changes the pacing mode to a nontracking mode in response to a sensed atrial arrhythmia. The purpose of this algorithm is to prevent inappropriately fast ventricular tracking at the upper rate limit in response to a rapid atrial tachyarrhythmia. Once the device has mode switched, it will remain in a nontracking mode until the atrial rate has fallen below the mode switch threshold for a specific number of intervals. This algorithm is very useful for patients with paroxysmal atrial arrhythmias (e.g. SVT, atrial fibrillation, or atrial flutter). The atrial rate at which mode switch occurs is programmable in most devices and the feature can even be programmed "off."

Line Management

The placement of central venous catheters in cardiac device patients warrants special consideration. Depending upon the location and age of the device and the planned location of central venous access, a number of potential complications can occur. Reported complications associated with central venous catheters in cardiac device patients include lead damage from needle puncture [5], lead dislodgement and inappropriate ICD therapies [6]. Additionally, central venous stenosis as a consequence of prior cardiac device implantation may present a challenge to central venous catheter placement ipsilateral to the device [7]. Cardiac device infections and device-related endocarditis represent a particularly serious hazard of indwelling central venous catheters necessitating removal of the entire device system [8]. Central venous access should be performed contralateral to the device whenever possible.

MRI

The likelihood that patients with cardiac devices will require an MRI is high but this imaging modality is not without potential risks for these patients. To minimize these risks, MRI-conditional pacemakers, ICDs and CRT-Ds have been developed and have received FDA approval for use in the United States. The potential hazards of MRI for cardiac device patients include movement of the device, programming changes, asynchronous pacing, activation of tachyarrhythmia therapies, inhibition of pacing output, and induced lead currents that could lead to heating and cardiac

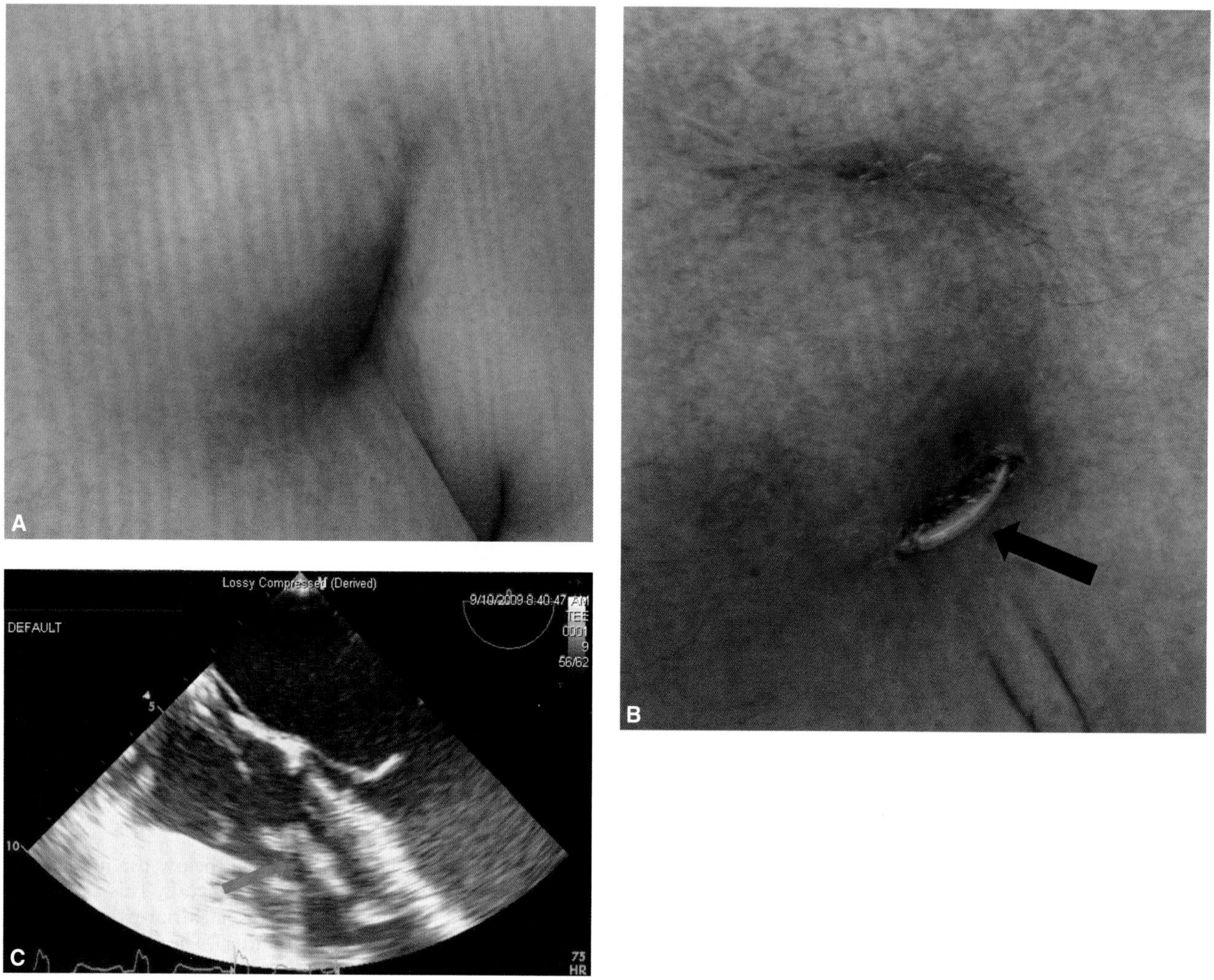

FIGURE 196.4 Different manifestations of device-related infections. **A:** Swelling and erythema suggest pocket infection although local signs of inflammation may be absent. **B:** Erosion of either the lead(s) or device by definition is a manifestation of infection. In this example, the pocket appears swollen with areas of erythema and a pacing electrode (*arrow*) is seen eroding through the skin at the inferior margin of the pocket. **C:** Device-related infection could result in bactermia, vegetations, and sepsis. Here, transesophageal echocardiography demonstrated a large vegetation (*arrow*) adherent to the atrial pacing lead and seen to prolapse across the tricuspid valve.

stimulation [9], resulting in altered pacing and defibrillation thresholds (DFT), device damage, asystole, arrhythmias, or even death [10]. Although an implantable cardiac device remains a strong relative contraindication to MRI, certain centers have developed protocols for performing MRIs for cardiac device patients [11] without MRI-conditional devices. If an MRI is the only diagnostic imaging option in such a patient, imaging at 1.5 Tesla with appropriate programming and monitoring can often be undertaken safely with careful assessment of the risk–benefit ratio on a case-by-case basis [11–14].

External Defibrillation

In the event of a cardiac arrest or hemodynamically unstable arrhythmia of a patient with an implantable cardiac device, resuscitative efforts should proceed as per guidelines without deviation. Defibrillation or cardioversion can result in permanent damage to the cardiac device; to minimize these risks, the defibrillation pads should be placed at least 10 cm from the pulse generator [15]. Other potential risks of external defibrillation include device reprogramming [16] and myocardial damage at the interface with the lead resulting in an acute rise in threshold [17]. Following defibrillation or cardioversion, cardiac devices should be interrogated formally to insure proper function and programming. Again, the low potential risk of damage to the device should *not* impede usual and necessary resuscitative efforts for the patient.

Infections

Cardiac device-related infection encompasses a disease spectrum from pocket infection to device-related endocarditis. The clinical manifestations of cardiac device-related infection are protean and can range from pain at the implant site without cutaneous manifestations to minor erythema or swelling of the device pocket (Fig. 196.4A) to overt erosion of the system (Fig. 196.4B) to device-related endocarditis (Fig. 196.4C, Video 196.1) [18,19]. In the absence of bacteremia, systemic manifestations and leukocytosis are rare. Cultures of the device leads yield the highest results and, *Staphylococci* are the pathogens most frequently identified [20]. A high index of suspicion is warranted for a patient with implanted pacemaker or ICD and signs and symptoms of infection or documented bacteremia. Cardiac device-related infection requires prompt removal of the entire device system for complete treatment unless significant comorbidities preclude extraction [8,18]. Although no specific vegetation size has been established as a contraindication to transvenous extraction, most experts agree

TABLE 196.3

Troubleshooting Pacemaker Malfunction

Problem	Etiology	Causes	Management
Failure to pace, no PPM stimuli	Oversensing	Physiological events P, R, or T waves Myopotentials Nonphysiological events EMI Lead fracture Loose set-screw	Reprogram. Avoid EMI sources. Device revision.
Failure to pace with PPM stimuli	Noncapture	Elevated threshold Exit block MI, fibrosis Medications Electrolytes Hardware failure Lead dislodgement Lead fracture Lead perforation Battery depletion	Reprogram, if possible. Correct reversible causes. May require device revision. Device revision.
Inappropriate pacing	Undersensing	Low EGM amplitude Low at implant MI, fibrosis Medications Electrolytes Lead dislodgement Lead fracture ERI Noise reversion	Reprogram, if possible. Correct reversible causes. May require device revision. Lead revision Lead revision Replace PPM Reprogram

that vegetations greater than 3 cm in size are better treated surgically [8]. Patients with device-related endocarditis require a minimum of 6 weeks of intravenous antibiotics and pose a particular challenge with respect to the timing of re-implant in pacemaker-dependent patients.

Pacemaker Malfunction

Oversensing

Sensing problems are one of the most common causes of pacemaker malfunction (Table 196.3). Oversensing is defined as the sensing of physiologic or nonphysiologic events that should not be sensed. Consequently, oversensing can lead to inappropriate inhibition of pacemaker output (Fig. 196.5). Physiologic events that can be the cause of oversensing include far-field P waves, wide QRS complexes, T waves, and myopotentials, either pectoral or diaphragmatic. Typically, oversensing due to physiologic events can be overcome by decreasing the programmed sensitivity. Nonphysiologic oversensing may be the result of EMI or hardware problems such as loose set-screw or lead dislodgement or fracture and will likely require device revision to correct. Oversensing and failure to pace for a pacemaker-dependent patient can be catastrophic. Application of a magnet over the device will change the device to an asynchronous pacing mode and insure more reliable delivery of pacing until a formal evaluation can be performed.

Undersensing

In contrast, undersensing occurs when the device fails to sense intrinsic events. This results the generation of unnecessary pacemaker impulses and "over-pacing." Undersensing may be a result of alterations in electrogram amplitude of physiologic events or may represent hardware failure. Antiarrhythmic drug therapy, myocardial infarction and metabolic derangements can alter electrogram amplitude transiently or permanently. Undersensing may be potentially corrected by changing the programmed sensitivity. Other etiologies of undersensing are similar to those of noncapture (lead dislodgement, perforation or fracture). Asynchronous pacing modes, due to EMI or battery depletion, can mimic undersensing on surface electrocardiogram.

Noncapture

Noncapture occurs when electrical impulses emitted from the device fail to capture the myocardium. The surface electrocardiogram will demonstrate pacing stimuli without evidence of capture (Fig. 196.6). Loss of capture can be intermittent or permanent, but often necessitates device revision. Causes of noncapture can be divided into changes in capture threshold and hardware malfunction. The capture threshold can rise in the first 4 to 6 weeks following lead implantation due to inflammatory changes at the lead-myocardial border although this has become less relevant clinically with the advent and widespread use of steroid-eluting leads. A rise of capture threshold myocardial fibrosis or infarction near the exit of the pacing stimulus, metabolic derangements (specifically, hyperkalemia, acidemia, or hyperglycemia) and certain medications. Class Ia, Ic, and III antiarrhythmic drugs [21–24] can increase capture thresholds as can mineralocorticoids and hypertonic saline [25]. When the capture threshold exceeds the maximal programmable output, this is termed *exit block*. Primary hardware problems such as lead dislodgement, perforation or fracture and battery depletion can all result in noncapture. A chest radiograph can help diagnose specific lead issues (Fig. 196.7A to C), as can transthoracic echocardiography (Video 196.2) or other imaging modalities.

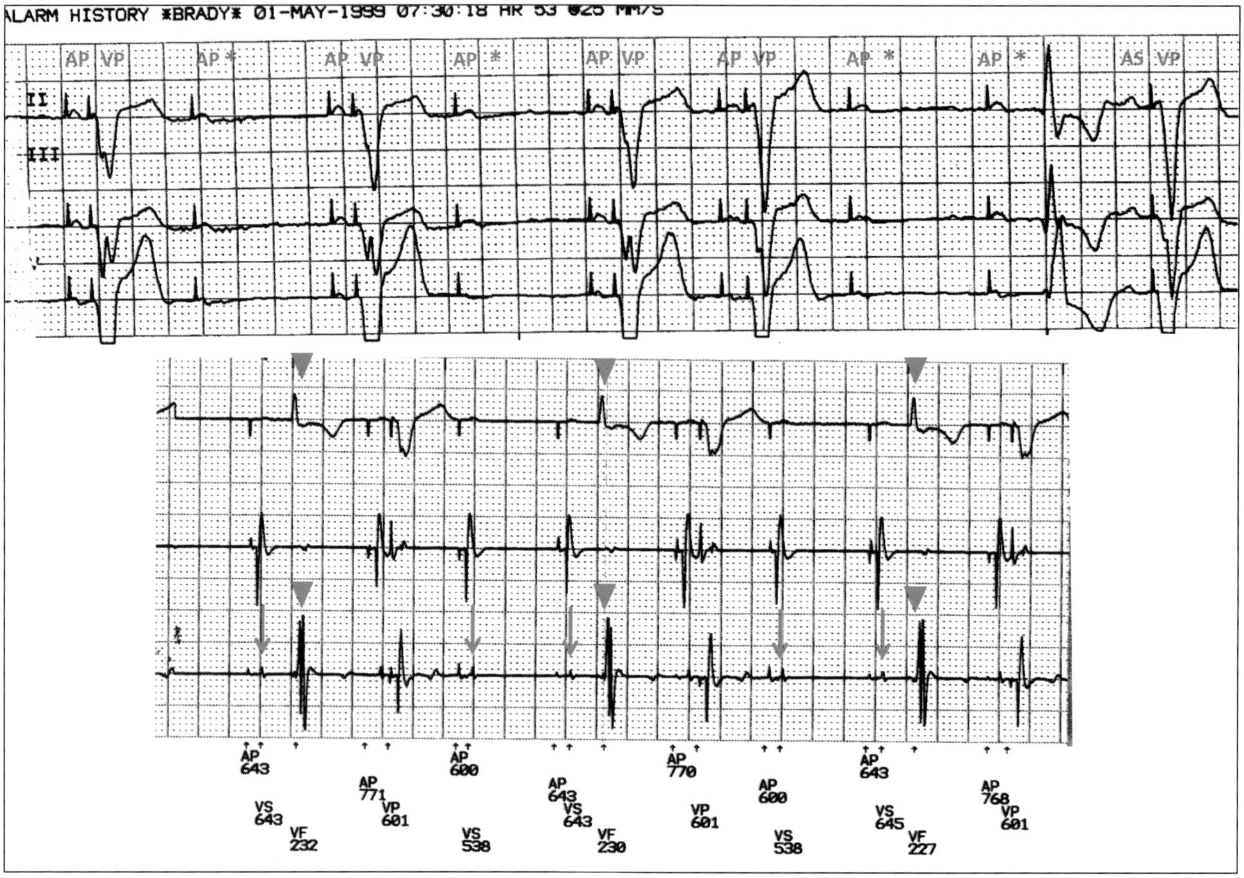

FIGURE 196.5 Dual chamber defibrillator with evidence of ventricular oversensing. The top panel demonstrates atrial (AP) and ventricular (VP) sequential pacing with the intermittent absence of ventricular pacing stimuli (*asterisks*) following atrial paced events. The bottom panel represents the intracardiac electrograms from the same device with ventricular oversensing of atrial events (*arrows*). When intrinsic ventricular conduction does occur (*arrowheads*), the device incorrectly labels the event as "VF" (*arrowheads*) or a ventricular event that because of timing falls into the programmed ventricular fibrillation detection zone.

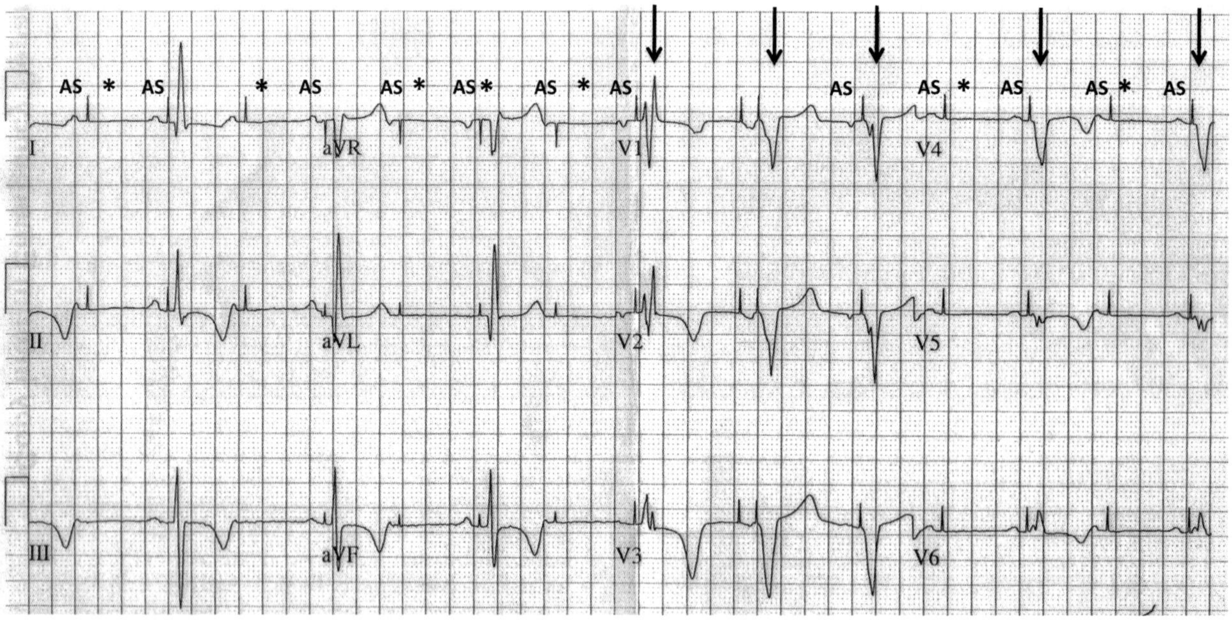

FIGURE 196.6 Surface electrocardiogram with intermittent loss of ventricular capture. There is appropriate atrial sensing (AS) and tracking as evidence by pacing stimuli at a fixed interval following the P wave but intermittent failure of ventricular output to capture the myocardium (*asterisks*). Evidence of varying degrees of fusion between intrinsic conduction and ventricular pacing is also observed (*arrows*).

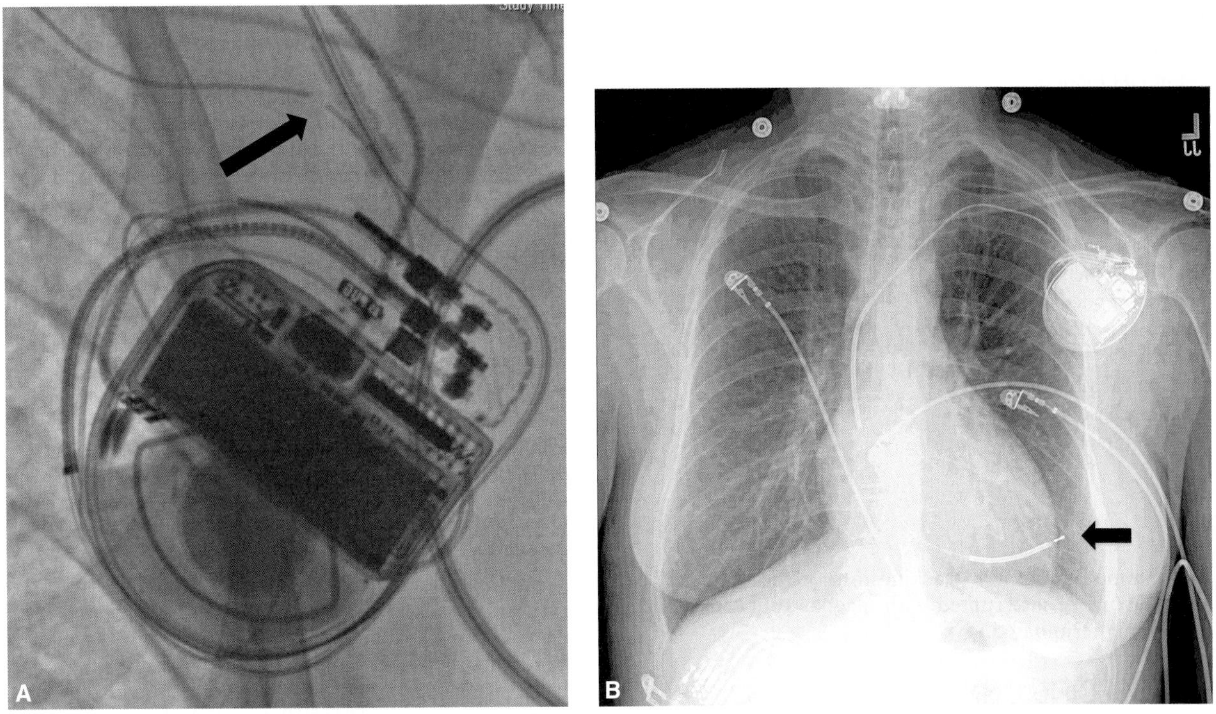

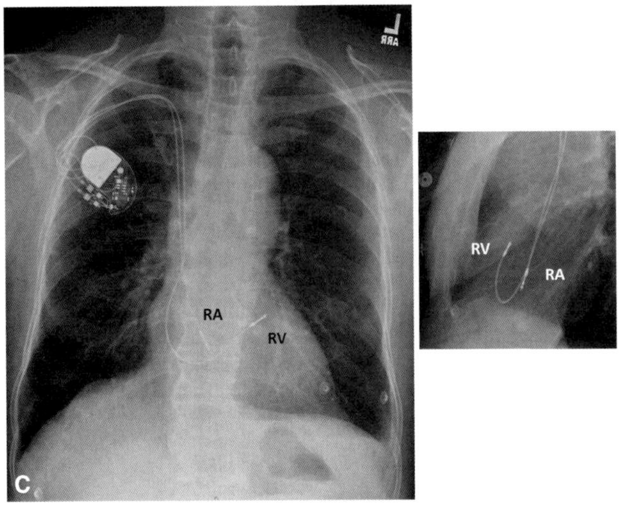

FIGURE 196.7 Chest radiography can identify device hardware problems. **A:** Lead fractures (*arrow*) can sometimes been seen on X-ray and detailed attention should be paid to the leads along their entire length when a hardware problem is suspected. **B:** Overt lead perforation can be diagnosed by X-ray. In this example, the entire distal electrode of the defibrillator lead extends beyond the cardiac silhouette (*arrow*). **C:** Chest radiography can also confirm lead dislodgement. PA and lateral films of a dual chamber pacing system with the ventricular lead in the right ventricular outflow tract demonstrate dislodgement of the atrial lead. There is evidence of atrial lead dislodgement in the PA view with the distal electrode pointing inferiorly and no visible slack on the lead with absence of the typical "J"-shaped appearance. Atrial lead dislodgement is confirmed by the lateral view that demonstrates the distal electrode of the lead residing below the tricuspid valve annulus.

Formal pacemaker interrogation or magnet application can identify battery depletion.

No Output

The complete absence of pacemaker stimuli despite magnet application suggests complete battery depletion or generator damage. Damage to the generator can occur rarely as a result of direct trauma [26] or external defibrillation [15].

Pacemaker-Mediated Tachycardia (PMT)

PMT refers to any sustained tachyarrhythmia that is dependent upon continued pacemaker participation in the circuit. Classically, the term PMT is used to describe an endless loop tachycardia of dual chamber devices consisting of ventricular pacing, retrograde atrial activation, appropriate sensing and triggered ventricular pacing perpetuating the tachycardia (Fig. 196.8). PMT should be suspected when ventricular pacing occurs at

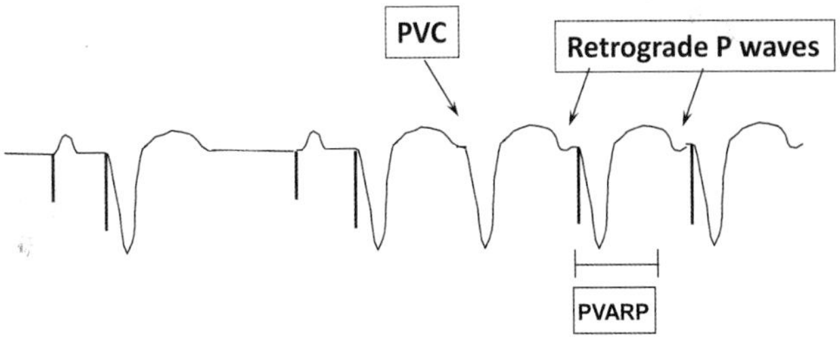

FIGURE 196.8 Pacemaker-Mediated Tachycardia (PMT). A premature ventricular complex (PVC) occurs in a patient with a dual chamber pacemaker. The PVC results in retrograde conduction back to the atrium that is subsequently tracked by the ventricular lead and incessant tachycardia ensues. Retrograde atrial activation is sensed by the pacemaker because it falls outside the postventricular atrial refractory period (PVARP). One means of eliminating PMT is to extend the PVARP.

TABLE 196.4

Causes of Electrical Storm

Acquired long QT
Decompensated heart failure
Electrolyte disturbances
Fever/sepsis
Hyperthyroidism
Lead dislodgement/position
Medication noncompliance
Myocardial ischemia
Myocarditis
Psychological stressors
Substance abuse
Sympathomimetics

the programmed maximum tracking rate of the device. The PMT circuit can be interrupted with magnet application and the arrhythmia terminated.

DEVICE-SPECIFIC CONSIDERATIONS

Implantable Cardioverter Defibrillator

Electrical Storm

Electrical or ventricular tachycardia (VT) storm is defined as three or more episodes of VT or ventricular fibrillation within a 24-hour period. When a patient presents with electrical storm, suppression of the arrhythmias are of paramount importance. Identifying the trigger can be difficult [27] but attempts should be made to identify and correct potentially treatable causes (Table 196.4). Repeated defibrillator therapy is painful and highly stressful, can cause heightened sympathetic tone and result in early battery depletion, myocardial ischemia/stunning and recurrent ventricular arrhythmias [28]. Thus, initial treatment should consist primarily of sympathetic blockade with β-blockers and anxiolysis with benzodiazepines. Amiodarone is often the antiarrhythmic agent of choice [29]. Refractory cases may require intubation and deep anesthesia [30]; stellate ganglion blockade can be considered for extreme cases [31]. Catheter ablation can be effective for the treatment of electrical storm and should be considered for electrical storm refractory to antiarrhythmic therapies [32].

Ineffective Defibrillation

Successful defibrillation occurs when a critical mass of myocardium is successfully depolarized and depends upon shock vector, lead position, and the electrical milleu (Fig. 196.9). The optimal three-dimensional orientation of the ICD shock vector should deliver energy uniformly throughout the left ventricle. The vector is dependent on the position of the high-voltage coils in the right ventricle (RV) and superior vena cava (SVC)–right atrial (RA) junction and their anatomic relations to the left ventricle. Typically, the RV coil is the cathode and the SVC-RA coil and ICD can form the anode with current traveling from cathode to anode.

Implantable defibrillators can fail to deliver effective defibrillation therapy in certain situations. Elevated DFT can occur as a result of metabolic derangements, myocardial ischemia, pneumothorax, hypoxia, multiple defibrillations, drug therapy, delays in arrhythmia detection, and device hardware malfunction (Table 196.5). Immediate management should consist of external defibrillation and treatment of potential reversible causes. Long-term management may require device revision or cessation/addition of specific anti-arrhythmic medications.

Inappropriate Activations

Inappropriate activations are common among patients with implantable defibrillators regardless of indication [33] and are associated with significant morbidity and mortality [34,35]. Common causes of inappropriate activations include SVT, ventricular sensing problems, lead failure, and EMI. The detection algorithms of ICDs are based primarily on heart rate and any ventricular sensed event that exceeds the programmed detection rate will trigger ICD activation. Supraventricular discriminators

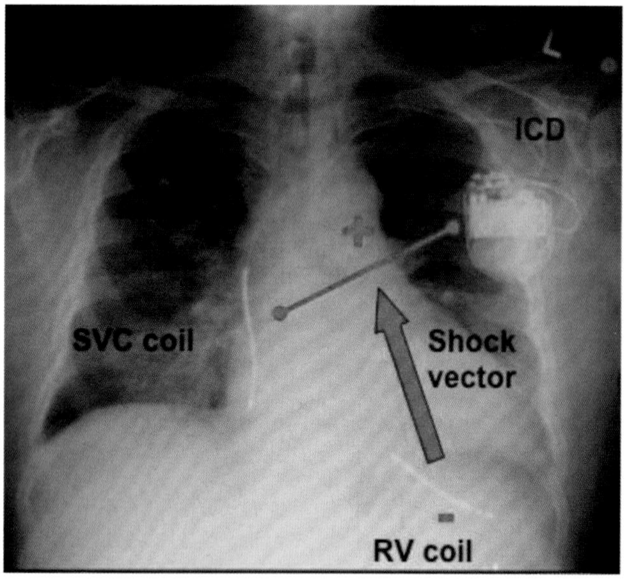

FIGURE 196.9 Defibrillator vector. With a dual coil ICD lead implanted in the RV apex and active ICD can, the shock vector is from the RV coil to the summation of the superior vena caval (SVC) coil and ICD generator (ICD). The SVC coil directs some of the current towards the posterior base of the heart. ICD, implantable cardioverter defibrillator.

TABLE 196.5

Effects of Common Drugs on Defibrillation Thresholds

Drug	Effect on DFT
Anti-arrhythmics	
Amiodarone	↑
Disopyramide	↔
Dofetilide	↓
Ibutilide	↓
Flecainide	↑↔
Lidocaine	↑
Mexilitine	↑
Quinidine	↑↔
Procainamide	↑↔
Propafenone	↔
Sotalol	↓
β-Blockers	
Atenolol	↔↓
Carvedilol	↑
Propanolol	↑
Calcium-channel blockers	
Diltiazem	↑
Verapamil	↑
Others	
Digoxin	↔
Fentanyl	↑
Ranolazine	↔
Sildenafil	↑

related to arrhythmia onset, cycle length stability, and electrogram morphology are also programmable but reduce inappropriate activations only slightly [36,37]. Repeated inappropriate ICD activations for hemodynamically stable patients should prompt magnet application or device deactivation with backup external defibrillation available and definitive treatment directed at the underlying rhythm or problem.

The most common cause of inappropriate defibrillator activations is atrial fibrillation although sinus tachycardia and other SVTs can result in inappropriate activations. Surface electrocardiogram and clinical status may aid with the diagnosis when formal interrogation is not immediately available. The device should be inactivated and treatment directed at the underlying atrial arrhythmia. Ventricular sensing problems also result in inappropriate activations when other electrical events (P waves, T waves, and wide QRS) are misinterpreted as a ventricular event. This "double counting" is erroneously interpreted as a tachyarrhythmia and prompts inappropriate ICD activation. Ventricular oversensing may be transient as a result of metabolic derangements (e.g. peaked T waves with hyperkalemia) or may sometimes be successfully eradicated with reprogramming of the device although some sensing problems may require device revision. The S-ICD is particularly susceptible to inappropriate therapies as a result of both ventricular oversensing and undersensing (with a resultant autogain algorithm) as sensing is based upon surface QRS vectors that can change with position and activity. Hardware problems such as lead fracture, insulation break, lead dislodgement or a loose set-screw may result in noise and short ventricular cycle lengths that can be mistakenly detected as VT. The surface electrocardiogram is extremely useful and will demonstrate sinus rhythm or tachycardia at the time of defibrillation. Device hardware problems cannot be overcome with reprogramming. The ICD should be deactivated until the system can be revised. Similarly, EMI can produce noise and result in inappropriate activation.

Device Management at the End of Life

Patients with ICDs and end-stage heart failure or other fatal illness warrant special considerations. Successful defibrillation may prolong life but it cannot prevent death. In addition, repeated ICD shocks to a patient with end-stage disease may cause unnecessary pain and anxiety. Defibrillation can be deactivated for ICDs without deactivating pacemaking functions. Discussions regarding ICD deactivation occur rarely even for patients with do-not-resuscitate orders [38]. It is important that patients and their families understand that deactivation of defibrillator therapies is always an option [39].

Cardiac Resynchronization Therapy (Bi-Ventricular Pacing)

Cardiac resynchronization therapy (CRT) improves symptoms, decreases hospitalizations, assists with reversing remodeling of the left ventricle and reduces mortality among patients with symptomatic heart failure, severe left ventricular dysfunction or mechanical dyssynchrony (QRS > 120 ms) [1,40–43]. Ventricular resynchronization aims to achieve myocardial coordination through left ventricular pre-excitation ideally at the site of latest activation. This can be achieved through an endovascular approach with left ventricular lead placement via coronary sinus cannulation or epicardially with a direct surgical approach (typically via left lateral thoracotomy). Approximately 70% of CRT patients demonstrate clinical improvements including reduction of symptoms [44,45]; fewer show improvement of left ventricular function [46].

Loss of Resynchronization

Achieving resynchronization appears dependent upon not only stimulating the ventricle at the site of latest activation but also providing reliable biventricular pacing. There appears to be a threshold effect of CRT related to the frequency of biventricular pacing. A recent retrospective analysis demonstrated a significant decrease of hospitalizations and mortality at biventricular pacing above 92% [47]. Among CRT responders, loss of resynchronization can result in recurrent symptoms, diminished functional capacity, repeat hospitalization, and significant hemodynamic alterations. Although formal device interrogation is necessary to assess the degree of biventricular pacing over the long-term, careful observation of the telemetry monitor often can provide significant insights. Similarly, the 12-lead electrocardiogram can identify the site of ventricular stimulation and can be used to detect loss of biventricular pacing (Fig. 196.10A,B). Atrial arrhythmias with intact ventricular conduction exceeding the programmed lower rate of the CRT device are the most common reason for failure to achieve sufficient resynchronization. Other potential reasons for suboptimal biventricular pacing include elevated pacing threshold, lead fracture, or lead migration to an unfavorable location. Common reasons for a lack of response to CRT are lead location, suboptimal programming and underlying narrow QRS [48]. If the left ventricular pacing lead is not stimulating a late activation site in the basal posterolateral left ventricle, the degree of biventricular pacing is irrelevant. The electrocardiogram and chest radiograph are useful for identifying issues with left ventricular lead placement.

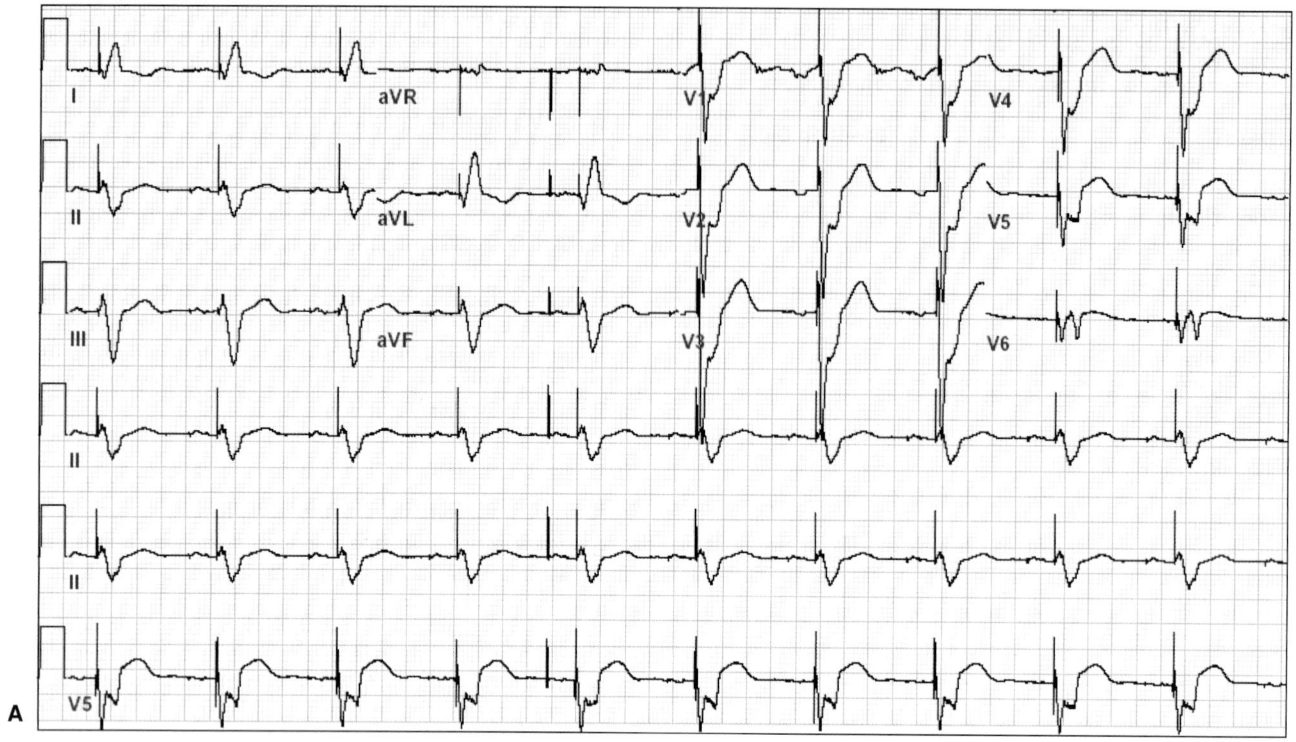

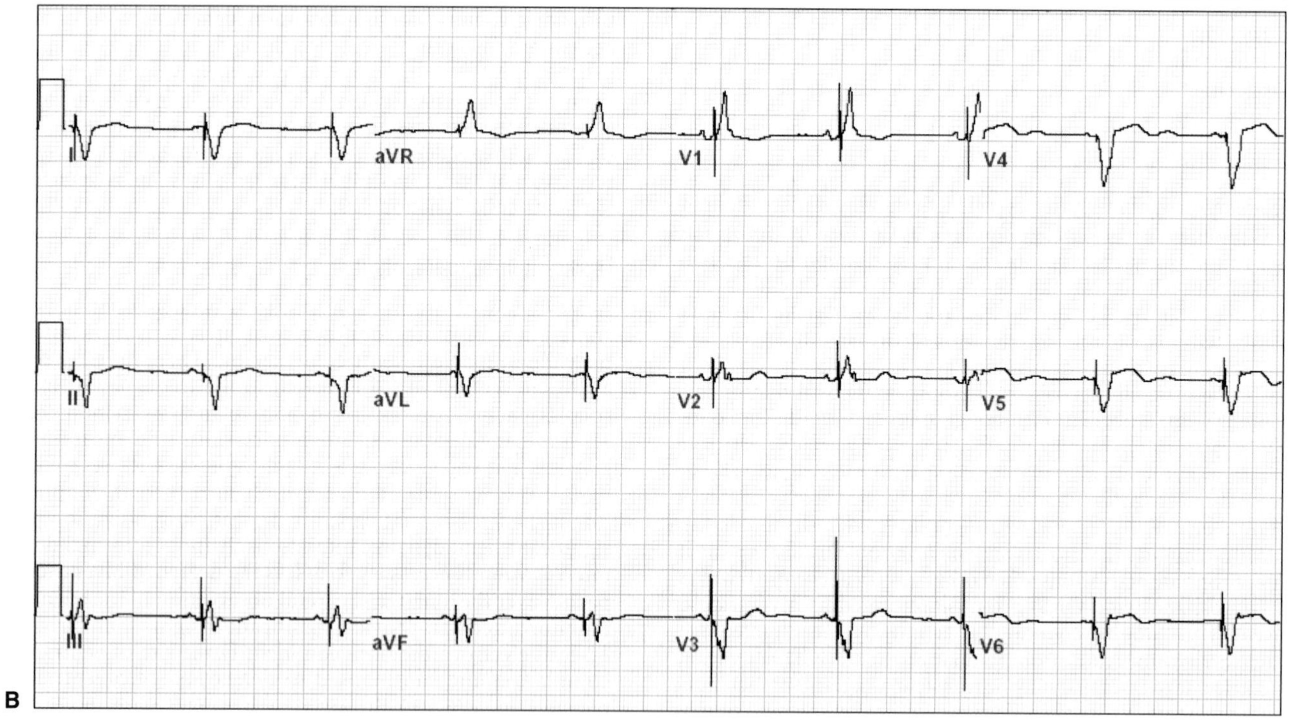

FIGURE 196.10 Electrocardiographic assessment of pacing site. **A:** Right ventricular apical pacing with left bundle branch morphology and superior frontal plane axis. **B:** In contrast, biventricular stimulation with right bundle morphology in V1 and QS waves in leads I and aVL.

Summary

In the modern era, patients with implantable pacemakers, defibrillators, and cardiac resynchronization devices are increasingly commonly admitted to the care of an intensivist. Attention to and understanding of the implanted device as a critical portion of the patient's acute care is warranted. Early involvement of electrophysiologist colleagues for the care of critically ill patients especially with device malfunction or infection is prudent.

References

1. Tracy CM, Epstein AE, Darbar D, et al: 2012 ACCF/AHA/HRS Focused Update of the 2008 Guidelines for Device-Based Therapy of Cardiac Rhythm Abnormalities: a report of the American College of Cardiology Foundation/American Heart Association Task Force on Practice Guidelines. *Heart Rhythm* 9:1737–1753, 2012.
2. Napp A, Stunder D, Maytin M, et al: Are patients with cardiac implants protected against electromagnetic interference in daily life and occupational environment? *Eur Heart J* 36:1798–1804, 2015.
3. Dyrda K, Khairy P: Implantable rhythm devices and electromagnetic interference: myth or reality? *Expert Rev Cardiovasc Ther* 6:823–832, 2008.
4. Ellenbogen K, Kay GN, Lau C-P, et al (eds): *Clinical Cardiac Pacing, Defibrillation, and Resynchronization Therapy*. 3rd ed. Philadelphia, PA, Saunders Elsevier, 2007.
5. Stokes K, Staffeson D, Lessar J, et al: A possible new complication of subclavian stick: conductor fracture. *Pacing Clin Electrophysiol* 10:748, 1987.
6. Varma N, Cunningham D, Falk R: Central venous access resulting in selective failure of ICD defibrillation capacity. *Pacing Clin Electrophysiol* 24:394–395, 2001.
7. Gurjar M, Baronia AK, Azim A, et al: Should blind internal jugular venous catheterization be avoided in a patient with ipsilateral permanent pacemaker implant? *Am J Emerg Med* 24:501–502, 2006.
8. Wilkoff BL, Love CJ, Byrd CL, et al: Transvenous lead extraction: Heart Rhythm Society Expert consensus on facilities, training, indications, and patient management: this document was endorsed by the American Heart Association (AHA). *Heart Rhythm* 6:1085–1104, 2009.
9. Levine GN, Gomes AS, Arai AE, et al: Safety of magnetic resonance imaging in patients with cardiovascular devices: an American Heart Association scientific statement from the Committee on Diagnostic and Interventional Cardiac Catheterization, Council on Clinical Cardiology, and the Council on Cardiovascular Radiology and Intervention: endorsed by the American College of Cardiology Foundation, the North American Society for Cardiac Imaging, and the Society for Cardiovascular Magnetic Resonance. *Circulation* 116:2878–2891, 2007.
10. Gimbel JR: Unexpected asystole during 3T magnetic resonance imaging of a pacemaker-dependent patient with a 'modern' pacemaker. *Europace* 11:1241–1242, 2009.
11. Nazarian S, Halperin HR: How to perform magnetic resonance imaging on patients with implantable cardiac arrhythmia devices. *Heart Rhythm* 6:138–143, 2009.
12. Naehle CP, Zeijlemaker V, Thomas D, et al: Evaluation of cumulative effects of MR imaging on pacemaker systems at 1.5 tesla. *Pacing Clin Electrophysiol* 32:1526–1535, 2009.
13. Naehle CP, Strach K, Thomas D, et al: Magnetic resonance imaging at 1.5-T in patients with implantable cardioverter-defibrillators. *J Am Coll Cardiol* 54:549–555, 2009.
14. Faris OP, Shein M: Food and Drug Administration perspective: magnetic resonance imaging of pacemaker and implantable cardioverter-defibrillator patients. *Circulation* 114:1232–1233, 2006.
15. Gould L, Patel S, Gomes GI, et al: Pacemaker failure following external defibrillation. *Pacing Clin Electrophysiol* 4:575–577, 1981.
16. Barold SS, Ong LS, Scovil J, et al: Reprogramming of implanted pacemaker following external defibrillation. *Pacing Clin Electrophysiol* 1:514–520, 1978.
17. Aylward P, Blood R, Tonkin A: Complications of defibrillation with permanent pacemaker in situ. *Pacing Clin Electrophysiol* 2:462–464, 1979.
18. Klug D, Wallet F, Lacroix D, et al: Local symptoms at the site of pacemaker implantation indicate latent systemic infection. *Heart* 90:882–886, 2004.
19. Wilkoff BL: How to treat and identify device infections. *Heart Rhythm* 4:1467–1470, 2007.
20. Anselmino M, Vinci M, Comoglio C, et al: Bacteriology of infected extracted pacemaker and ICD leads. *J Cardiovasc Med (Hagerstown)* 10:693–698, 2009.
21. Hellestrand KJ, Burnett PJ, Milne JR, et al: Effect of the antiarrhythmic agent flecainide acetate on acute and chronic pacing thresholds. *Pacing Clin Electrophysiol* 6:892–899, 1983.
22. Soriano J, Almendral J, Arenal A, et al: Rate-dependent failure of ventricular capture in patients treated with oral propafenone. *Eur Heart J* 13:269–274, 1992.
23. Reiffel JA, Coromilas J, Zimmerman JM, et al: Drug-device interactions: clinical considerations. *Pacing Clin Electrophysiol* 8:369–373, 1985.
24. Jung W, Manz M, Luderitz B: Effects of antiarrhythmic drugs on defibrillation threshold in patients with the implantable cardioverter defibrillator. *Pacing Clin Electrophysiol* 15:645–648, 1992.
25. Preston TA, Judge RD: Alteration of pacemaker threshold by drug and physiological factors. *Ann N Y Acad Sci* 167:686–692, 1969.
26. Hai AA, Kalinchak DM, Schoenfeld MH: Increased defibrillator charge time following direct trauma to an ICD generator: blunt consequences. *Pacing Clin Electrophysiol* 32:1587–1590, 2009.
27. Brigadeau F, Kouakam C, Klug D, et al: Clinical predictors and prognostic significance of electrical storm in patients with implantable cardioverter defibrillators. *Eur Heart J* 27:700–707, 2006.
28. Huang DT, Traub D: Recurrent ventricular arrhythmia storms in the age of implantable cardioverter defibrillator therapy: a comprehensive review. *Prog Cardiovasc Dis* 51:229–236, 2008.
29. Kowey PR: An overview of antiarrhythmic drug management of electrical storm. *Can J Cardiol* 12 Suppl B:3B–8B, 1996; discussion 27B-8B.
30. Burjorjee JE, Milne B: Propofol for electrical storm; a case report of cardioversion and suppression of ventricular tachycardia by propofol. *Can J Anaesth* 49:973–977, 2002.
31. Nademanee K, Taylor R, Bailey WE, et al: Treating electrical storm: sympathetic blockade versus advanced cardiac life support-guided therapy. *Circulation* 102:742–747, 2000.
32. Carbucicchio C, Santamaria M, Trevisi N, et al: Catheter ablation for the treatment of electrical storm in patients with implantable cardioverter-defibrillators: short- and long-term outcomes in a prospective single-center study. *Circulation* 117:462–469, 2008.
33. Wilkoff BL, Hess M, Young J, et al: Differences in tachyarrhythmia detection and implantable cardioverter defibrillator therapy by primary or secondary prevention indication in cardiac resynchronization therapy patients. *J Cardiovasc Electrophysiol* 15:1002–1009, 2004.
34. Gehi AK, Mehta D, Gomes JA: Evaluation and management of patients after implantable cardioverter-defibrillator shock. *JAMA* 296:2839–2847, 2006.
35. Messali A, Thomas O, Chauvin M, et al: Death due to an implantable cardioverter defibrillator. *J Cardiovasc Electrophysiol* 15:953–956, 2004.
36. Boriani G, Occhetta E, Pistis G, et al: Combined use of morphology discrimination, sudden onset, and stability as discriminating algorithms in single chamber cardioverter defibrillators. *Pacing Clin Electrophysiol* 25:1357–1366, 2002.
37. Srivatsa UN, Hoppe BL, Narayan S, et al: Ventricular arrhythmia discriminator programming and the impact on the incidence of inappropriate therapy in patients with implantable cardiac defibrillators. *Indian Pacing Electrophysiol J* 7:77–84, 2007.
38. Goldstein NE, Lampert R, Bradley E, et al: Management of implantable cardioverter defibrillators in end-of-life care. *Ann Intern Med* 141:835–838, 2004.
39. Sears SF, Matchett M, Conti JB: Effective management of ICD patient psychosocial issues and patient critical events. *J Cardiovasc Electrophysiol* 20:1297–1304, 2009.
40. Bristow MR, Saxon LA, Boehmer J, et al: Cardiac-resynchronization therapy with or without an implantable defibrillator in advanced chronic heart failure. *N Engl J Med* 350:2140–2150, 2004.
41. Abraham WT, Fisher WG, Smith AL, et al: Cardiac resynchronization in chronic heart failure. *N Engl J Med* 346:1845–1853, 2002.
42. St John Sutton MG, Plappert T, Abraham WT, et al: Effect of cardiac resynchronization therapy on left ventricular size and function in chronic heart failure. *Circulation* 107:1985–1990, 2003.
43. Cleland JG, Daubert JC, Erdmann E, et al: Longer-term effects of cardiac resynchronization therapy on mortality in heart failure [the CArdiac REsynchronization-Heart Failure (CARE-HF) trial extension phase]. *Eur Heart J* 27:1928–1932, 2006.
44. Lecoq G, Leclercq C, Leray E, et al: Clinical and electrocardiographic predictors of a positive response to cardiac resynchronization therapy in advanced heart failure. *Eur Heart J* 26:1094–1100, 2005.
45. Molhoek SG, VAN Erven L, Bootsma M, et al: QRS duration and shortening to predict clinical response to cardiac resynchronization therapy in patients with end-stage heart failure. *Pacing Clin Electrophysiol* 27:308–313, 2004.
46. Nelson GS, Curry CW, Wyman BT, et al: Predictors of systolic augmentation from left ventricular preexcitation in patients with dilated cardiomyopathy and intraventricular conduction delay. *Circulation* 101:2703–2709, 2000.
47. Koplan BA, Kaplan AJ, Weiner S, et al: Heart failure decompensation and all-cause mortality in relation to percent biventricular pacing in patients with heart failure: is a goal of 100% biventricular pacing necessary? *J Am Coll Cardiol* 53:355–360, 2009.
48. Mullens W, Grimm RA, Verga T, et al: Insights from a cardiac resynchronization optimization clinic as part of a heart failure disease management program. *J Am Coll Cardiol* 53:765–773, 2009.

Chapter 197 ■ Long-Term Mechanical Support for Advanced Heart Failure

JONATHAN E. HOLTZ • JEFFREY J. TEUTEBERG

In 2015, the American Heart Association estimated that there were 5.7 million American adults with heart failure (HF). Projections estimate that number will grow to >8 million adults by the year 2030. Each year, there are an estimated 650,000 new cases of HF, 1 million annual hospital admissions, and 300,000 deaths as a result of HF [1,2]. In 2012, the total cost for HF was estimated to be almost $31 billion with an expected rise to $70 billion by 2030—$244 for every US adult [3]. The subset of patients with systolic HF is estimated to be 3 to 3.5 million, and of those, about 10% or 200,000 to 300,000 will have advanced HF [1–3]. The mortality from HF remains very high, approximately 50% at 5 years. Those who are inotrope dependent have a mortality of 78% at 6 months and nearly 90% at 1 year. In comparison, the 1-year mortality for pancreatic cancer is 80% [4,5].

Cardiac transplantation still represents the most definitive therapy for advanced HF with estimated survival of 85% at 1 year and 70% at 5 years. The current generation of continuous flow left ventricular asssist devcies (LVADs) have an estimated survival of 80% at 1 year and 70% at 2 years (Fig. 197.1) [6]. The use of an LVAD pretransplant has traditionally conferred an increased risk posttransplant, but with modern continuous flow devices, that is no longer the case [7]. Given that there are approximately 2,200 donor hearts available each year targeted to eligible candidates, the role of long-term mechanical circulatory support (MCS) has become a fundamental tenet of advanced HF treatment. The proper application of MCS requires knowledge of the underlying mechanism of HF, understanding of the potential benefits and limitations of both medical and device therapy, familiarity with the full range of devices available for support, and, perhaps most critically, careful selection of the appropriate timing for intervention.

MECHANICAL CIRCULATORY SUPPORT

Over the past five decades, MCS technology has evolved substantially from partial temporary support with intra-aortic balloon counterpulsation to a broad array of ventricular assist devices (VADs) capable of providing long-term complete support for one or both ventricles. The first successful implantation of a paracorporeal LVAD was performed by Dr. DeBakey in 1966 and supported a 37-year-old woman for 10 days. Initial Food and Drug Administration (FDA) approval was granted to the first VAD system in 1995 [8]. Through the 1990s, extensive experience with bridging patients to transplantation spurred the evolution from bulky extracorporeal devices to smaller, implantable designs, which allowed patients to be discharged from the hospital with substantial improvements of functional status and quality of life. In 2008, the first modern-generation continuous flow LVAD, the HeartMate II (HM II; Thoratec Corp., Pleasanton, CA, USA) was approved by the FDA as a bridge to transplantation (BTT) and then received approval for a destination therapy (DT) indication in 2010 [9]. More recently, a series of landmark trials have demonstrated the superiority of continuous flow LVADs with increased survival, enhanced quality of life, and fewer adverse events, compared to the prior generations of larger pulsatile pumps [10–13]. As of November 2015, the longest continuous support that a patient has recieved from an LVAD was 11.5 years, requiring three HM II pumps becauseof driveline infections. The longest continuous support on a single pump (HM II) is 10.3 years (Thoratec Corp., personal communication, 11/25/2015).

BENEFITS OF MECHANICAL CIRCULATORY SUPPORT

Continuous Flow LVAD Technology

Continuous flow LVADs have become the dominant technology, primarily because of their smaller size and greater durability. Continuous flow pumps consist of an inflow cannula, outflow cannula, and a single impeller that spins continuously. Current generation devices are valveless pumps that use a magnetic field to spin a single impeller that is supported by mechanical, hydrodynamic, or magnetic bearings (Fig. 197.2) [14]. Axial

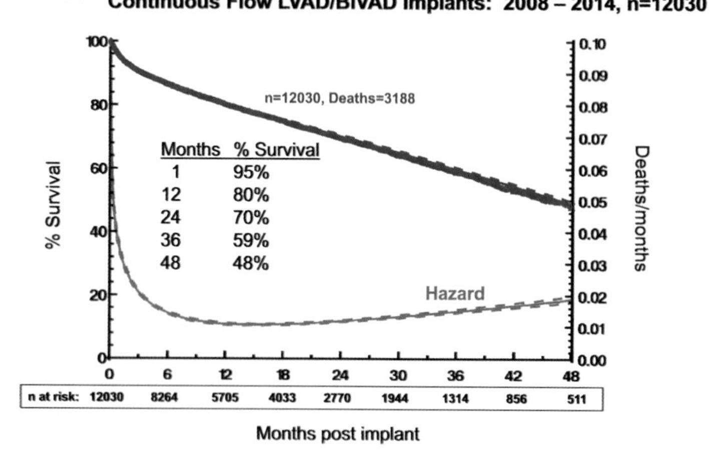

FIGURE 197.1 Parametric survival curve and associated hazard function with the 70% confidence limit for survival after implnatation of a continuous flow LVAD or BiVAD. The number of patients at risk during each time interval is indicated below. LVAD, left ventricular assist device; BiVAD, biventricular assist device. (From Kirklin JK, Naftel DC, Pagani FD, et al: Seventh INTERMACS annual report: 15,000 patients and counting. *J Heart Lung Transplant* 34(12):1495–1504, 2015. © Elsevier, Inc., with permission.)

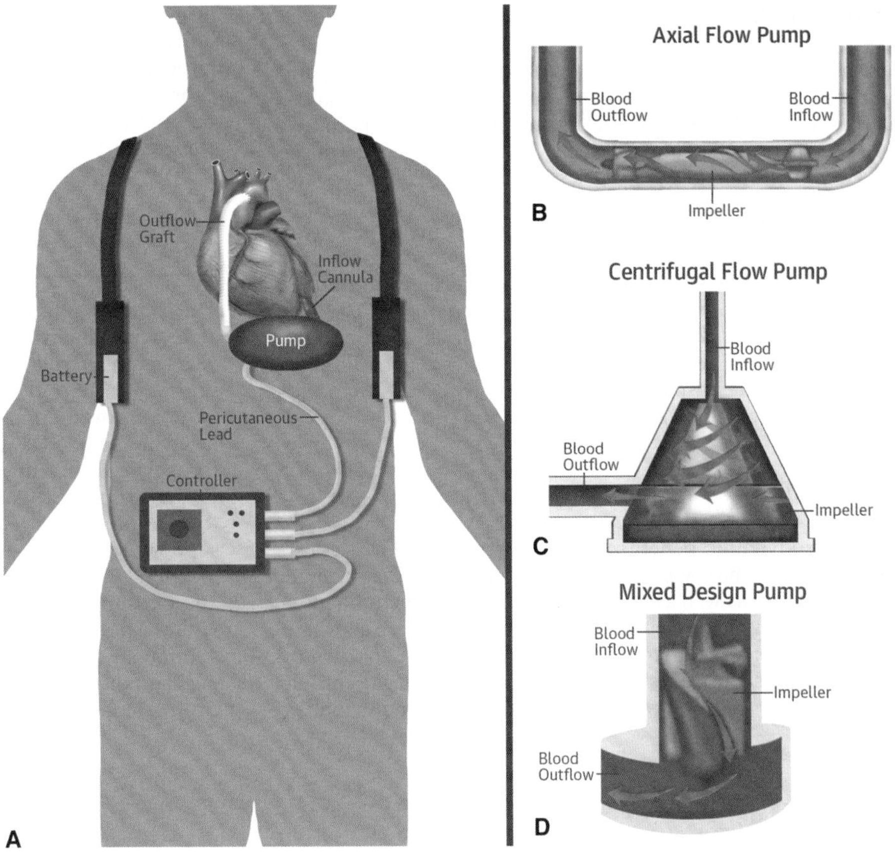

FIGURE 197.2 Schematic of an LVAD system. Components include a surgically implanted pump that works in parallel with the native heart via an inflow cannula to the left ventricle and an outflow graft to the ascending aorta, a percutaneous driveline, a system controller, and electrically powered batteries with a life span up to 12 hours (**A**). Features of continuous flow axial (**B**), centrifugal (**C**), and mixed design pumps, where the pump is axial but blood exits perpendicular to the inflow like in centrifugal pumps (**D**), are also shown. LVAD, left ventricular asssist devcie. (From Mancini D, Colombo PC: Left ventricular assist devices: a rapidly evolving alternative to transplant. *J Am Coll Cardiol* 65(23):2542–2555, 2015. © Elsevier, Inc., with permission.)

flow pumps direct blood flow parallel to the axis of rotation, whereas centrifugal flow pumps have the impeller direct flow perpendicular to the axis of rotation [15]. The impeller's position may be maintained by mechanical bearings (St. Jude, HeartMate II), hydrodynamic thrust bearings (Heartware, HVAD), or full magnetic levitation (St. Jude, HeartMate 3).

One important concept regarding axial and centrifugal flow devices is that of hydrodynamic performance, which is demonstrated by pump head curves (Fig. 197.3). A pump head curve illustrates the relationship between pump flow and pressure difference across the inflow (left ventricular pressure) and outflow (aortic pressure) of a pump at a set speed. When the pressure differential across the pump is lower, such as during ventricular systole, pump flow is greater. Axial flow pumps have a steeper relationship between flow and head pressure than centrifugal flow pumps; thus, the same change in pressure across the pump will result in smaller changes in flow across the cardiac cycle and hence less pulsatilty.

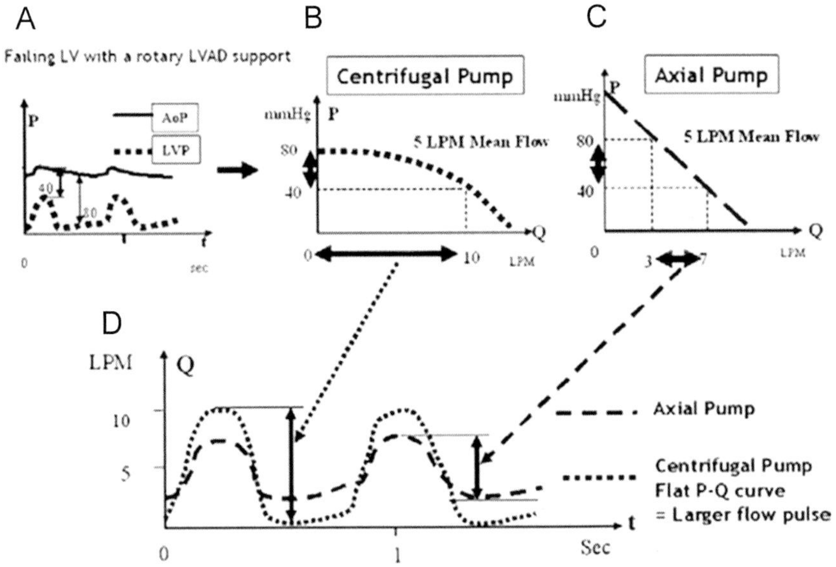

FIGURE 197.3 (**A**) Representation of the systemic AoP and LVP relationship is shown during rotary LVAD support in a failing ventricle. Comparison of (**B**) centrifugal flow and (**C**) axial rotary pump performance characteristics are shown as pressure differential across pump inlet and outlet in mm Hg and pump flow in L/min. (**D**) Representative centrifugal and axial rotary pump flow waveforms during rotary LVAD support in a failing ventricle are compared. AoP, arterial pressure; LVP, left ventricular pressure; LVAD, left ventricular asssist devcie. (From Pagani FD: Continuous-flow rotary left ventricular assist devices with "3rd generation" design. *Semin Thorax Cardiovasc Surg* 2008;20:255–263. © 2008 Elsevier, Inc., with permission.)

Hemodynamics

As the left ventricle (LV) begins to fail, cardiac output falls and intracardiac filling pressures rise. The main goals of MCS are to decompress the failing ventricle and augment systemic perfusion [6]. Mechanical unloading of the LV leads to a decrease of the severity of mitral regurgitation, less pulmonary congestion, and a reduction of pulmonary hypertension, all of which, in turn, can result in improved right ventricular (RV) function. Partial support pumps provide several liters of flow to augment the reduced native ventricular contribution to the total output, whereas full support pumps provide upward of 7 to 10 L per minute of flow with the native heart contributing little to the total output. Restoration of forward flow and the normalization of filling pressures also reduces neurohormonal activation, with attendant benefits on cardiorenal function [16].

Biological

The hemodynamic benefits of MCS with an LVAD are also associated with biologic changes such as improved β-adrenergic responsiveness as well as favorable myocardial structural, functional, and contractile changes. LVAD support has been shown to alter gene expression that is linked to improving the β-receptor density and responsiveness that is downregulated during chronic HF. Likewise, studies have shown improved calcium handling properties, as well as a reduction of maladaptive neurohormonal upregulation. In vivo, mechanical unloading with an LVAD is known to be associated with alteration of gene and protein expression within the cardiac myocyte, a reduction of nuclear size and DNA content, and reductions of fibrosis and collagen content within the cardiac extracellular matrix [17].

SELECTION OF APPROPRIATE MECHANICAL SUPPORT

The clinical application of MCS grew from early experience as temporary support in the operating room to providing support for years as an alternative to transplant. A broad array of different ventricular support devices is now available, and all currently FDA–approved durable devices included in INTERMACS are listed in Table 197.1. In general, the devices may be configured for isolated left ventricular (LVAD), right ventricular (RVAD), or biventricular (BiVAD) support and for short-term (bridge to decision [BTD], recovery, or transplant), or long-term (DT) support. Some devices are extracorporeal or paracorporeal in location, with cannulae traversing the skin allowing for inflow and outflow of blood, whereas others are totally implantable with the pump and the cannulae housed in the thoracic and/or abdominal cavity with only a single percutaneous line supplying the power and providing the connections to the external control systems.

TABLE 197.1

FDA–approved Durable Mechanical Circulatory Support Devices

	Description	Approved devices	Advantages	Disadvantages
Permanent—LV Support				
Pulsatile extracorporeal	Inflow cannula from LV and outflow cannula to ascending aorta	• Thoratec PVAD	• Ease of implantation	• Total of two large cannula traversing skin • External pumps
Pulsatile intracorporeal	Pump implanted in the abdomen or preperitoneally, allowing increased mobility and ability to discharge	• HeartMate XVE • HeartMate VE • HeartMate IP • Thoratec IVAD • NovaCor PC • NovaCor PCq	• Requires only an aspirin, no Coumadin • Approved as DT • Durable	• Less durable if duration of support >9–12 mo • BSA ≥ 1.5 m^2 • INR 2.5–3.5 • Less portable peripherals
Continuous flow	Pump implanted in the thoracic cavity with only one moving part	• Thoratec HeartMate II • HeartWare HVAD • MicroMed DeBakey Child VAD	• Reduced size and noise • Much greater durability than pulsatile devices • Better adverse event profile than pulsatile pumps	• Difficult to assess BP and pulse owing to lack of pulsatility • "Suck-down" caused by over unloading ventricle
Permanent—Biventricular support				
Extracorporeal	Two pumps—one supporting the RV and one supporting the LV, but native heart remains in place	• Thoratec PVAD	• Easy to insert for unstable patients	• Two pumps with a total of four cannula transversing the skin • External pumps
Intracorporeal	Native heart removed	• AbioCor and SynCardia CarioWest	• Removes cardiac tissues which may contribute to inflammation and be susceptible to clots, arrhythmias or interference with pump	• Available only in select centers • Not applicable to most patients

FDA, Food and Drug Administration; DT, destination therapy; BSA, body surface area; INR, international normalized ratio; BP, blood pressure; RV, right ventricle; LV, left ventricle.

Cannulation of Ventricular Assist Devices

VADs are typically implanted in parallel with the native right- or left-sided circulation. For long-term LVADs, the pump inflow is from a cannula placed directly into the LV apex, and the pump outflow is a cannula that is anastomosed to the ascending aorta just distal to the aortic valve (AV). Pulsatile systems typically have valves in the inflow and outflow cannulae, whereas continuous flow devices do not. RVADs typically have inflow from the right atrium, or alternatively from the cavae or femoral veins, rather than the RV apex, because RV apical cannulation typically provides less reliable flow. Outflow is directed to the main pulmonary artery just distal to the pulmonic valve through either direct or transvenous cannulation.

The LV is continuously and actively unloaded; therefore, the LV less frequently fills to the point where it can eject blood during systole. As a result, patients often have minimal contribution from their native ventricles leading to a greatly reduced pulse pressure. Historically, the blood pressure has been referred to as a mean blood pressure; however, this terminology is currently under scrutiny because research is demonstrating that there is significant heterogeneity in the pulse pressure that patients are able to produce, often under dynamic circumstances of preload and afterload [18]. Based on clinical experience, the pulse pressure may vary from 0 to greater than 25 mm Hg. Patients supported with continuous flow LVADs often require Doppler ultrasound to assess their blood pressure owing to the lack of pulsatility. As previously mentioned, continuous flow pumps are generally one of two major types: axial or centrifugal flow. The HM II is an axial flow LVAD with typical operating speeds ranging from 9,000 to 10,000 × *g* and is approved for both BTT and DT. The Heartware HVAD is a centrifigual flow LVAD with hydrodynamic bearings and is approved for BTT and is currently undergoing study for a desination therapy clinical trial. Continuous flow pumps are the preferred technology, compared to pulsatile pumps, because of demonstrated superior survival rates and lower rates of adverse events.

LONG-TERM INDICATIONS FOR MECHANICAL CIRCULATORY SUPPORT

VAD support can be divided into four device strategies at the time of implant: (1) BTT, (2) DT, (3) BTD, and (4) bridge to recovery (BTR). As the field has evolved, DT has become the most common indication for durable MCS with nearly 46% of implants assigned as DT in 2014, whereas 30% were listed as BTT candidates. BTR remains uncommon at 1% to 2%. Approximately 20% to 25% are assigned as BTD [6].

The survival following cardiac transplantation has been excellent with a median survival of almost 11 years [7]. With increased numbers of patients waiting for a cardiac transplantation and little to no growth in organ availability, bridging patients with an LVAD has become increasingly common with 37% of patients having an LVAD at some point before transplantation [7]. DT specifically refers to the long-term use of an LVAD as an alternative therapy to transplantation for patients who are ineligible because of contraindications. This is the largest growing VAD indication having increased to almost half of all indications as of 2014 [6]. As of 2014, almost one in four patients were designated as BTD for an LVAD. The rationale for this designation is often owing to a temporary contraindication to transplantation listing such as end-organ function that is expected to improve after mechanical correction of the maladaptive mechanisms of HF (e.g., pulmonary hypertension, cardiorenal syndrome, etc.). BTR is a hotly contested topic with incidences ranging as low as <1% to as high as 20%, in highly selected cohorts. In the HM II trials, 1% to 2% of patients were explanted owing to LV recovery. LV recovery is most likely to occur among young patients with nonischemic cardiomyopathies of <1-year duration [19,20].

UNIVENTRICULAR VERSUS BIVENTRICULAR SUPPORT

Selection of the appropriate device for MCS depends initially on the type of support that is required. Most patients presenting with acute HF or shock predominantly have LV failure and may be candidates for isolated LV support with an LVAD. Successful LVAD implantation relies heavily on confirmation of adequate native RV function, because RV function is required for LVAD filling. For patients with concomitant, severe RV dysfunction, biventricular support may be necessary. Although recent experience suggests that selected BiVAD patients can be successfully discharged to home, 1-year survival with a BiVAD is 50%, which remains markedly less than the 80% 1-year survival with an LVAD alone. This discrepancy is partially owing to greater severity of illness and end-organ dysfunction among patients presenting initially with biventricular failure [6,21]. Because there is no approved BiVAD device for DT, this therapy is only available for patients who are potentially candidates for cardiac transplantation. Those patients with prolonged shock, giant cell myocarditis, refractory ventricular tachyarrhythmias, or a high likelihood of postoperative right ventricular failure (RVF) may be considered for BiVADs. Even with the current generation of continuous flow LVADs, RVF complicates 10% to 40% of LVAD implants, underscoring the need for careful assessment of RV function prior to VAD implantation [22]. At select centers, explant of the native heart and implantation of a total artificial heart may provide an alternative to the use of BiVADs [23].

CANDIDATE SELECTION FOR LONG-TERM MCS THERAPY

Patient selection and timing of implantation are critical features of successful mechanical support [6]. Guidelines for the clinical management of the HM II was published in 2010. In 2013, The International Society for Heart and Lung Transplantation (ISHLT) published guidelines for the selection, implantation, and device management for MCS patients [24,25]. The most salient recommendations are summarized below.

Illness Assessment

The criteria for use of MCS as BTT are based on several factors that include being a cardiac transplantation candidate with impaired systemic perfusion and end-organ function. In general, a patient must have a cardiac index less than 2.0 L per minute with evidence of elevated filling pressures after optimal medical management. Other reasons to use MCS as BTT include an expected long wait list time owing to uncommon blood type and/or larger body size. Additional factors include a worsening clinical status with evidence of new or worsening end-organ dysfunction such as renal or hepatic dysfunction, prolonged coagulation levels, and progressive HF.

In contrast to BTT, the Centers for Medicare and Medicaid Services adopted the entry criteria for the REMATCH trial as reimbursement requirements for DT:

1. New York Heart Association (NYHA) functional class IV or stage D HF symptoms, despite use of maximally tolerated optimal medical therapy for at least 45 of the last 60 days, or have been intra-aortic balloon pump (IABP) dependent

for 7 or more days, or intravenous (IV) inotrope dependent for 14 or more days;
2. Left ventricular ejection fraction less than 25%; and
3. Functional limitation with a peak oxygen consumption ≤14 mL/kg/min, unless on inotropic therapy, IABP support, or physically unable to perform the test. In general, any patient who is inotrope dependent and expected to have a sufficient 1- to 2-year survival with a reasonable quality of life should be referred for consideration of VAD therapy.

Several predictive models, such as the Heart Failure Survival Score and the Seattle Heart Failure Model, exist to help clinicians estimate survival [26,27]. However, these models were derived from a less critically ill population and have not been validated for patients who are being considered for MCS [28]. Older models also, exist but are limited by describing risk attributable to an antiquated device [29,30] or were derived from a previous era of MCS support [31]. The HM II Risk Score was derived and validated within 1,122 patients who received continuous flow HM II devices and identified the following factors as being associated with higher mortality: increasing age, hypoalbumnemia, renal dysfunction, coagulopathy, and LVAD implantation at less experienced centers [32].

INTERMACS has provided a means by which to assess risk for patients undergoing MCS by their preimplant acuity of illness. INTERMACS established seven different profiles for patients being implanted with MCS from advanced NYHA class III patients, through inotrope dependence, to critical cardiogenic shock despite maximal medical management (Table 197.2) [33]. Data from INTERMACS have shown that risk stratification based solely upon the preimplant profiles does indeed predict outcomes when applied to both pulsatile and continuous flow devices [6,34–36]. There is a significant survival difference at 1 year between those who were INTERMACS Level 1 (76%) versus 2 to 3 (80%) or 4 to 7 (82%). Notably, INTERMACS Level 1 primarily confers an early hazard for mortality with a sharp drop of survival occurring within the first 3-months postimplantation.

Unfortunately, all predictive models have had limited use in clinical practice because of their inability to accurately predict outcomes across a heterogeneous HF population. Recently, a Bayesian model was developed to predict survival with some of the important predictor variables for mortality, including intervention within the last 48 hours (such as extracorporeal membrane oxygenation, dialysis, and ventilators), events during the hospitalization, prior cardiac operations, INTERMACS profile, renal dysfunction, and implant year [37]. A recent study of DT patients from the INTERMACS cohort developed a predictive model to determine a composite outcome of mortality and quality of life. Notably, one in three patients had a poor outcome at 1 year, which was mostly driven by death. The most significant predictors of a poor outcome at 1 year were older age, lower baseline quality of life scores, larger body mass indices (BMIs), INTERMACS profiles 1 and 2, and a history of solid organ cancer. Still, the model was not able to broadly separate patient risk [38]. In summary, LVAD prediction risk models can help guide clincians' decision-making and help to calibrate patients' expectations; however, they can not be solely relied upon for these complex decisions. Comorbidities that may be life-threatening at the time of implantation or postoperatively should be carefully excluded prior to MCS candidacy. In general, the most common contraindications to transplant in DT patients are advanced age, renal dysfunction, high BMI, pulmonary hypertension, and other significant comorbidities [34].

TABLE 197.2

Intermacs Profiles and Time to MCS

Profile	Description	Time to MCS
1	Acutely decompensating	Hours
2	Failing inotropes	Days
3	Inotrope dependent, stable	Weeks
4	Recurrent, but not refractory advanced HF	Weeks to months
5	Exertion intolerant, but no dyspnea at rest	Variable
6	Exertion limited, dyspnea with only mild activity	Variable
7	Advanced NYHA class III	Not a candidate for MCS

MCS, mechanical circulatory support; HF, hear failure; NYHA, New York Heart Association.

Right Ventricular Function

RVF remains a common complication and important cause of morbidity and mortality after LVAD implantation [22]. Most LVAD candidates have some degree of RV dysfunction prior to implant, rendering the assessment of RV function and prediction of RVF paramount to achieving good outcomes.

RVF is defined by INTERMACS as documented elevations of central venous pressure (CVP) and its manifestations, such as edema, ascites, or worsening hepatic or renal dysfunction. Severe RVF is defined as the need for prolonged postimplant inotropes, inhaled nitric oxide or IV vasodilators continued beyond postoperative day 14, or a requirement for RV mechanical support. Patients must meet the criteria for RVF mentioned above as well as any of the following: (1) need for inotropes at any time since last evaluation, (2) two or more readmissions requiring treatment for RVF, (3) RVAD support, or (4) death as a result of RVF [39].

LV mechanical support is generally beneficial for RV function, with chronic unloading of the LV resulting in a reduction of pulmonary pressures and RV afterload with resulting improved RV function. However, there may be deleterious effects of an LVAD on RV function, particularly when RV function is marginal. Profound unloading of the LV, particularly with continuous flow devices, can result in shifting of the septum away from the RV and, thus, decrease the septal contribution to RV output [40]. LV contraction contributes 20% to 40% of RV output [41]. The RV may also struggle to accommodate the increased venous return as a result of the improved cardiac output from the LVAD [40,42]. In addition, tricuspid regurgitation can intensify in the setting of a known regurgitant valve that may be further tethered by the septal shift with increased RV volume from venous return. Lastly, perioperative volume resusitation can exacerbate RV dilation and TR [43]. The same processes that lead to LV dysfunction can also cause RVF [42]. Lastly, other processes that may exacerbate pulmonary hypertension, such as blood product-induced lung injury, hypoxic lung disease, sleep apnea, chronic thromboembolic disease, or pulmonary vasculopathy, can also contribute to RV dysfunction.

Similar to the overall patient selection process, investigators have developed risk scores to attempt to predict RVF among LVAD candidates [44–51]. Identified clinical and biochemical risk factors for RVF include female gender, nonischemic etiology, prior cardiac surgery, need for an IABP, inotrope dependency, vasopressor use, need for mechanical ventilation, and elevated renal/liver biomarkers. Echocardiographic assessment of RV function has been aggressively studied with various predictors identified: tricuspid annular motion <7.5 mm [52], spherical RV geometry [53], severe TR [53], increased RV to LV end-diastolic diameter ratio [54,55], RV fractional area contraction, and left atrial volume index [56], as well as some LV parameters [57].

Assessment of RV function is problematic owing to its complex three-dimensional geometry [58]. The current imaging gold standard to assess the RV is cardiac MRI, but data are lacking, often owing to ferromagnetic contraindications of advanced HF patients, such as mechanical valves, pacemaker, and defibrillators. Multiple hemodynamic alternations have been associated with RVF but lack consistency. An elevated CVP or CVP to pulmonary capillary wedge pressure ratio has been reported as risk factors in multiple studies [44,47,49,59]. Despite the aforementioned risk factors, few exist across multiple studies, and the risk scores also lack consistent validation.

The treatment goals for RVF are similar to LV failure—decrease excess preload and afterload, while increasing contractility. RV preload should be reduced with aggressive diuresis and, if needed, mechanical volume removal if there is a renal limitation to diuresis. The dysfunctional RV may need slightly more preload to maintain output, but a goal should be to reduce the RA pressure to at least less than 15 mm Hg, and preferably as low as tolerated [20]. If inotropes are needed, milrinone, an ionodilator, offers theoretical benefits for RV support in the setting of concomitant pulmonary hypertension owing to its vasodilatory properties [60]. Afterload is addressed through strategies to reduce elevated pulmonary pressures. Reducing the left-sided filling pressures is the first and most important therapeutic targets and can be accomplished through a combination of diuresis, inotropy, IABP, and even a temporary LVAD. Patients must have adequate oxygenation to avoid hypoxic pulmonary vasoconstriction and, if intubated, positive end-expiratory pressure should be minimized [61]. Nitric oxide may be considered for the intubated patient, but such patients may be too ill to consider LV support alone. There is little evidence for the use of other vasodilators such as prostaglandins, preoperatively, and some evidence that such therapies may be deleterious in the setting of LV failure [62]. Consideration may be given to surgical repair of moderate to severe tricuspid regurgitation, but this remains controversial [24,63]. The management of RV function is outlined in Table 197.3.

Arrhythmias

Ventricular tachyarrhythmias are common in the setting of acutely decompensated HF. Many patients with chronic HF will have a history of ventricular tachycardia or have an implantable cardioverter defibrillator (ICD) with or without resynchronization therapy [58]. Aside from their impact on the patient's stability in the acute phase of their presentation, the persistence of ventricular tachyarrhythmias has implications for outcomes after mechanical support. The presence of sustained ventricular tachycardia or ventricular fibrillation during LVAD support can substantially affect RV function, particularly when it is borderline. Although ventricular tachyarrhythmias are not typically lethal in the setting of LVAD support alone, they may result in lower pump output, hypotension, and recurrent symptoms. For patients with an ICD, they may also result in frequent ICD discharges. Preoperative ventricular tachyarrhythmias in the setting of substantially elevated filling pressures or acute ischemia often resolve after MCS as the HF state resolves. However, patients with treatment-refractory and recurrent ventricular arrhythmias in the presence of an untreatable substrate are at higher risk of recurrence or persistence of these arrhythmias post-MCS and should be considered for biventricular support or a total artificial heart [24]. Patients with medically refractory atrial tachyarrhythmias may benefit from ablative procedures prior to long-term MCS [24].

Valvular Disease

In the presence of an LVAD, aortic insufficiency (AI) leads to a circulatory loop with a portion of LVAD output regurgitating through the AV into the LV and back again through the device, limiting effective forward flow and ultimately leading to organ malperfusion and increased LV diastolic pressures. The prognosis of moderate to severe AI of LVAD patients is generally poor and leads to a higher rate of AV replacement and potentially reduced survival. Current, evidence-based guidelines for valvular repair all have a level of evidence C classification [24]. Preoperatively, assessment of the degree of AI should be performed with echocardiography. If more than mild AI is present, consideration should be given to surgical intervention during device implantation such as a central aortic suture (commonly referred to as the "Park stitch"), bioprosthetic replacement, or oversewing the AV [24]. With adequate decompression by the LVAD, the LV generates very little effective forward flow, which often results in minimal AV opening. Among patients with mechanical aortic prostheses, this lack of flow across the valve may result in the formation of thrombosis and subsequent embolism [64]. Consequently, guidelines recommend that mechanical AVs be replaced with tissue valves at the time of surgery or oversewn [24]. Mitral regurgitation essentially resolves post-MCS with adequate LV decompression, but significant mitral stenosis can impede LVAD filling and should be addressed at the time of implantation [65]. A summary of other valvular recommendations can be seen in Table 197.3.

Other Cardiac Abnormalities

Per the ISHLT guidelines, atrial septal defects and patent formaen ovales should be closed at the time of MCS implantation. In the setting of a ventricular septal defect, an LVAD alone is not recommended without concomitant repair of the VSD, if otherwise indicated by guidelines. LV thrombus can form in the setting of acute ischemia or with chronic LV dysfunction. Such thrombi are usually located in the LV apex, which is the site of cannulation for the LVAD. Echocardiography or computed tomography (CT), with contrast when needed, should be used to screen preoperatively. Although the ventricle is routinely inspected before insertion of the cannula, knowledge of the presence of thrombus preoperatively is important because retained thrombus may systemically embolize or, worse, be suctioned into the impeller of a continuous flow pump, possibly resulting in pump failure. For patients with congenital heart disease, it is important to establish the anatomic position of the systemic ventricle and aorta as well as the type and location of any previous corrective surgeries. Complex congenital heart disease may necessitate placement of the pump or inflow/outflow cannulae in atypical positions. The presence of aortic root disease should be screened for with a CT scan prior to implantation, particularly when there is a history of vascular and/or coronary artery disease [24,25].

Noncardiac Preoperative Assessment

Other chronic medical conditions, many of which are exacerbated by acute HF, should be optimized if possible prior to implantation of long-term MCS. Patients must be assessed for signs of infection, and when daignosed, treated aggressively prior to implant. Active infection at the time of implantation can be catastrophic because bacteremia can result in device infection which may be chronically suppressed but rarely cured with antibiotic therapy. If the pump or the pump pocket becomes infected, the most definitive recourse is urgent cardiac transplantation, when indicated, because device exchanges in these situations often result in recurrent infection [66]. ISHLT guidelines recommend documented clearance of bacteremia for at least 5 days with at least a prior 7 day course of appropriate antimicrobial therapy prior to LVAD implantation [24]. Preimplant renal dysfunction is very common, with almost 90% of patients having at least mild kidney dysfunction. The presence of renal dysfunction often

TABLE 197.3

Organ System Review of Candidates for Mechanical Circulatory Support

Organ system	Review	Organ system	Review
LV dysfunction			
Preload	• Diuresis • Mechanical volume removal	**Pulmonary disease**	• Avoid hypoxia • Attempt to quantify extent/ severity of lung disease
Cardiac output	• Support with inotropy • IABP or temporary support as needed	**Liver disease**	• Occult liver disease in the presence of persistently high right atrial pressures • Ultrasound/CT scan to assess for cirrhosis
After load	• Treat hypertension, if present • IABP		
RV dysfunction	• Assess with invasive hemodynamics	**Coagulation**	• Stop any unneeded anticoagulants/antiplatelets • Review for history of hypercoagulable state
Preload	• Diurese to CVP <15 mm Hg • Mechanical volume removal		
Inotropy	• Milrinone if concomitant pulmonary hypertension • Maintain pump speed to keep septum midline • Consider low-dose digoxin • Mechanical RV support	**Vascular disease**	• Review history • Confirmatory ultrasound/CT scanning
Afterload	• Decreasing left-sided filling pressures • Milrinone • Pulmonary vasodilators • Wean from cardiopulmonary bypass with pharmacologic RV support • Avoid hypoxia	**Nutrition**	• Screen with prealbumin • Nutritional support
Arrhythmias	• Rate control • Antiarrhythmics • Cardioversion if hemodynamically tenuous. • Persistent ventricular tachyarrhythmia despite adequate treatment of left HF may need consideration for BiVADs	**Surgical Identify**	• ASD/VSD • Number of prior sternotomies • Location and number of prior bypass grafts • Congenital abnormalities • Prior cardiac surgeries • Intracardiac thrombus • Mitral stenosis
Valvular disease	• Consider surgical repair for: • ≥ mild AI, severe AS, ≥ moderate MS, ≥ moderate TR. • Consider replacement of a preexisting mechanical AV.	**Other limitations**	
		Emotional	• Careful assessment and support
Noncardiac infection	• Aggressive assessment and treatment	**Physical**	• Ability to care for and utilize device
Renal dysfunction	• Decrease high right atrial pressures • Inotropy or IABP • Avoid nephrotoxic agents, contrast	**Cognitive** **Social** **Financial**	• Understanding device • Support system available • Adequate resources as both inpatient and outpatient

LV, left ventricle; IABP, intra-aortic balloon pump; CT, computed tomography; RV, right ventricle; CVP, central venous pressure; ASD, atrial septal defect; VSD, ventricular septal defect; HF, heart failure; BiVADs; AI, aortic insufficiency; AV, aortic valve.

negatively impacts patients' advanced therapies options [67]. Many of the causes of the renal dysfunction are often related to the hemodynamic perturbations of HF (poor renal perfusion, renal venous congestion, high doses of diuretics, the adverse neurohormonal milieu of HF, etc.); fortunately, substantial early improvement of renal function often occurs post-MCS implant [67–71]. Still, there is a population of patients with worsening renal function post-MCS implantation associated with morbid outcomes, and there is no effective clinical algorithm to risk stratify those patients. Preoperatively, it is recommended to optimize HF management with inotropy, IABP, or even temporary mechanical support when necessary to help promote renal recovery. The need for renal replacement therapy post-MCS remains a highly morbid event, likely reflecting the level of illness entering the surgery [72].

Intrinsic pulmonary disease also has a number of implications for long-term MCS. Advanced lung disease impacts mortality and morbidity from the implantation surgery itself as well as the ability to rehabilitate and attain a good postoperative functional status. Hypoxic pulmonary vasoconstriction from intrinsic lung disease may also exacerbate preexisting pulmonary hypertension. Patients with severe obstructive or restrictive pulmonary disease are not candidates for long-term MCS [65]. Though there are no strict pulmonary function testing exclusion criteria, outcomes are often unfavorable when the forced expiratory volume at 1 second, forced vital capacity, and carbon monoxide diffusing capacity are all less than 50% of predicted values and LVAD eligibility should be scrutinized [25]. Intubation and mechanical ventilation prior to implantation are also strong risk factors for mortality and RVF [6,47].

Preoperative hepatic dysfunction, most notably elevated bilirbuin levels and low albumin levels, have been associated with poor outcomes [6,73]. Hepatic dysfunction is occasionally a result of shock from acute decompensation, but chronic occult hepatic dysfunction is not uncommon with chronic HF, especially in the setting of poor RV function with persistently high right atrial pressures or those with Fontan circulation. These patients may have significant hepatic dysfunction without substantial baseline abnormalities of transaminases or total bilirubin. There should be a low threshold to screen such patients with hepatic Doppler ultrasonography, CT, or even biopsy to assess hepatic architecture for signs of cirrhosis. If there is evidence of cirrhosis, then early involvement of a hepatologist and liver biopsy is suggested. The distinction between hepatic dysfunction secondary to chronic hepatic congestion as a result of RVF and cirrhosis is paramount, because the former will likely improve with MCS support (LVAD or BiVAD) and the latter will not. Patients with cirrhotic physiology do very poorly and, in general, are not eligible for LVAD therapy. The Model for End Stage Liver Disease (MELD) score has been used as a risk stratification score, and it has been shown to predict mortality, perioperative bleeding, RVF, renal failure, and postoperative infections [74]. The utility of the MELD score for the MCS population lies in its incorporation of multisystem dysfunction and coagulopathy. Specific interventions to optimize hepatic function preoperatively include preload and afterload reduction to decrease right atrial pressure and pulmonary vascular resistance and treatment of viral infections. Temporary MCS may be considered when medical therapy is insufficient. Vitamin K supplementation and nutritional optimization should be considered when significant coagulopathy exists to help mitigate perioperative bleeding. Bleeding, especially from the gastrointesintal tract, is recognized as one of the most common adverse events of continuous flow devices and is associated with a high morbidity [75–77]. There is a high rate of gastrointesintal arteriovenous malformations (AVMs) and acquired von Willebrand deficiency among patients supported with continuous flow devices, which may be secondary to a combination of low flow pulsatility as well as shear stress on blood components [76,78–81]. Given the need for systemic anticoagulation with LVADs, patients with recurrent gastrointesintal bleeding should be evaluated by gastroenterology for treatable sources of the bleeding. If there is no remediable source of bleeding, then the patient's eligibility for MCS should be questioned.

Minimizing perioperative bleeding surrounding MCS implantation can also be achieved through careful management of antiplatelet and anticoagulant therapy. Ideally, antiplatelet agents should be stopped at least 5 days prior to implantation [25]. On the contrary, patients with a history of thrombophilia should undergo a hypercoagulable workup, given the elevated risk of pump thrombosis.

Extensive carotid or peripheral vascular disease may increase the risk of extracardiac vascular events such as mesenteric ischemia, lower extremity ischemia, and neurologic events, and must be evaluated appropriately with preoperative noninvasive testing. Notably, patients with peripheral vascular disease have been excluded from many of the MCS trials. Screening should consist of carotid dopplers, ankle-brachial index testing, and abdominal ultrasound or CT abdominopelvic testing for those with risk factors. Among patients who present acutely, nutrition is not often a pressing issue, but nutritional impairment among patients with chronic HF can be quite profound, and low BMI is a risk factor for poor outcomes [66]. Poor nutrition impacts T-cell function and is another risk factor for infection and poor postoperative wound healing. For patients at nutritional risk, supplemental feeding may be of some use, but should not delay implantation when MCS is indicated. Obesity is also common among patients with HF but is not a contraindication to MCS. In the HM II trials, a BMI >40 kg per m^2 was an exclusion criteria. Observational studies have mixed results regarding an association of obesity with poor outcomes [6,38,82–84]. Based on data from INTERMACS, the largest registry available, obesity incrementally portends a risk for mortality and poor quality of life [38]. Based on the authors' clinical experience, obesity increases the risk of driveline complications owing to mechanical stress. Though there are small case series reporting on simultaneous sleeve gastrectomies and LVAD implantation for patients with class III obesity (BMI $\geq$ 40 kg per m^2) with both promising weight loss results and medium-term outcomes, these are preliminary experiences in need of more observational and clinical trial data [85,86]. Clinical prudence should be used when evaluating MCS eligibility for those with class II or higher obesity (BMI $\geq$ 35 kg per m^2) [24].

In general, the estimated life expectancy of patients with a history of malignancy will guide their candidacy for MCS. If they have an active or recently treated cancer with a reasonable life expectancy (e.g., >2 years), then DT MCS is an option. If their cancer is in long-term remission, they may be candidates for MCS as BTT or DT. However, if their life expectancy is <2 years, then long-term MCS is not recommended [24].

COMPLICATIONS OF MECHANICAL CIRCULATORY SUPPORT

Though VAD technology and increased clinical experience have led to improved outcomes over time, adverse events still occur and account for considerable morbidity and mortality [6]. The overall 1-year adverse event rate is lower in the most recent era (2012 to 2014) of MCS devices. Nevertheless, certain events such as hemolysis, renal dysfunction, stroke, and respiratory failure have increased in the current era [6]. Based on the INTERMACS registry, the most common adverse event rates (events/100 patients months) in the first year postimplant are bleeding (7.8), infection (7.3), arrhythmia (4.1), respiratory failure (2.7), and stroke (1.6) [6]. (These are based on standard definitions of adverse events, which can be found on the INTERMACS website) [39]. In addition, acquired AI occurs frequently with an incidence of >30% at 3 years [87].

EARLY POSTOPERATIVE HEMODYNAMIC MANAGEMENT

Per the 2013 ISHLT guidelines, early postoperative hemodynamic management recommendations are listed in Table 197.4. An algorithm for low pump output treatment is presented in Figure 197.4. A systematic approach to treating hypotension has been proposed (Fig. 197.5) [24].

Bleeding

Bleeding is the most common adverse event after VAD implantation with transfusions, leading to a higher risk of infection, allosensitization, and acute lung injury [88,89]. Though major bleeding episodes can often be managed successfully with transfusions and/or procedures, the 1-year mortality rate is significantly higher than for those without bleeding episodes. The degree of perioperative bleeding can be affected by preexisting coagulopathy, liver congestion, and prior sternotomies or other concomitant corrective surgeries at the time of MCS. Most

TABLE 197.4

Treatment Recommendations for Early Postoperative Hemodynamic Management

Cardiac index (L/min/m²)	MAP (mm Hg)	LV ejection	Primary recommendation	Alternative
<2.2	<65	No	Epinephrine Vasopressin Norepinephrine	Dopamine
		Yes	Increase pump speed	Volume for low CVP
	>65	No	Dobutamine	Milrinone
		Yes	Increase pump speed	
	>90	No	Milrinone	Sodium nitroprusside
		Yes	Sodium nitroprusside Nitroglycerin Hydralazine	Milrinone Nicardipine
>2.2	<65	No	Norepinephrine	Vasopressin
		Yes	Norepinephrine	Vasopressin
	>65 and <90	No	No intervention	
		Yes	No intervention	
	>90	No	Sodium nitroprusside Nitroglycerin Hydralazine	Milrinone Nicardipine
		Yes	Sodium nitroprusside	Nicardipine

MAP, mean arterial pressure; LV, left ventricle; CVP, central venous pressure.
From Feldman D, Pamboukian SV, Teuteberg JJ, et al: The 2013 International Society for Heart and Lung Transplantation Guidelines for mechanical circulatory support: executive summary. *J Heart Lung Transplant* 32(2):157–187, 2013. © Elsevier, Inc., with permission.

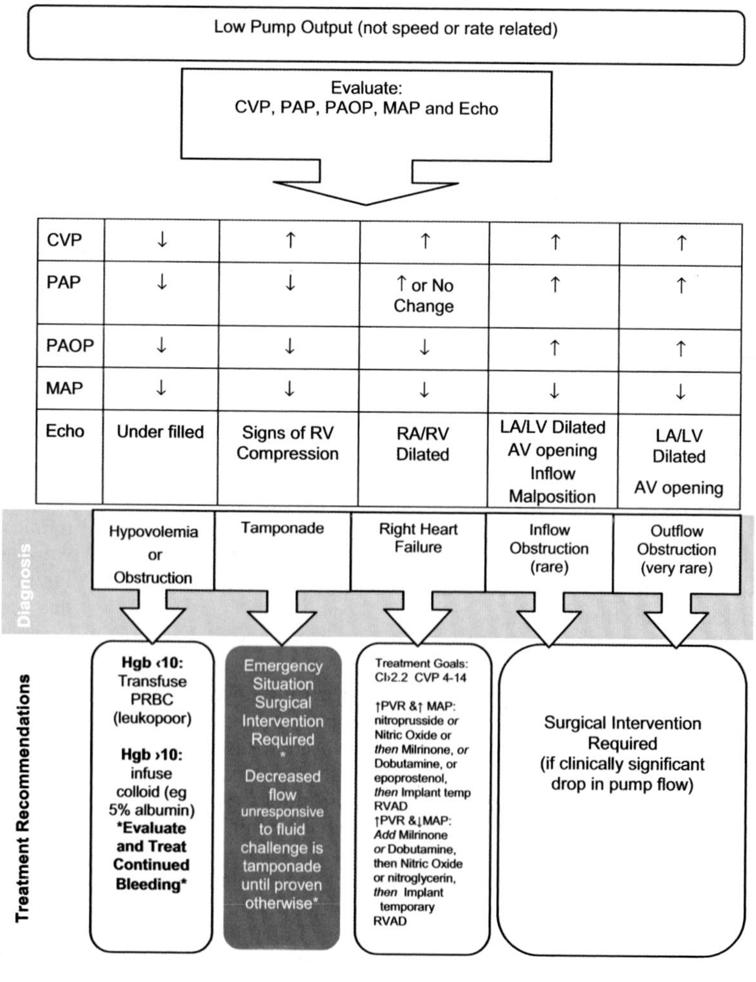

FIGURE 197.4 Treatment algorithm for low pump output. AV, arteriovenous; CI, cardiac index; CVP, central venous pressure; Hgb, hemoglobin; LA, left atrium; LV, left ventricle; MAP, mean arterial pressure; PAOP, pulmonary artery occlusion pressure; PAP, pulmonary artery pressure; PRBC, packed red blood cells; PVR, peripheral vascular resistance; RA, right atrium; RV, right ventricular; RVAD, right ventricular assist device. (From Feldman D, Pamboukian SV, Teuteberg JJ, et al: The 2013 International Society for Heart and Lung Transplantation Guidelines for mechanical circulatory support: executive summary. *J Heart Lung Transplant* 32(2):157–187, 2013. © Elsevier, Inc., with permission.)

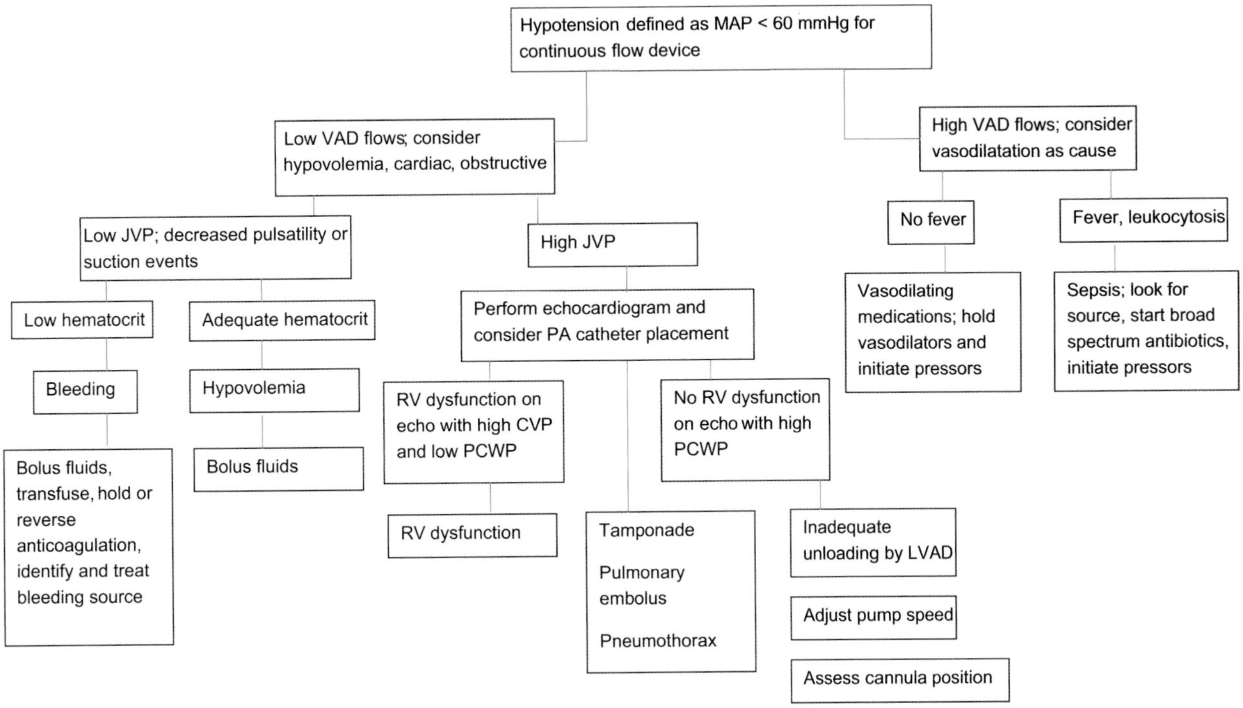

FIGURE 197.5 Algorithm for assessment of hypotension after implant. CVP, central venous pressure; JVP, jugular venous pressure; LVAD, left ventricular assist device; MAP, mean arterial pressure; PA, pulmonary artery; PCWP, pulmonary capillary wedge pressure; RV, right ventricular; VAD, left ventricular assist device. (From Feldman D, Pamboukian SV, Teuteberg JJ, et al: The 2013 International Society for Heart and Lung Transplantation Guidelines for mechanical circulatory support: executive summary. *J Heart Lung Transplant* 32(2):157–187, 2013. © Elsevier, Inc., with permission.)

current generation devices require anticoagulation with heparin after postoperative bleeding subsides and then chronically with oral anticoagulation and, depending on the center and device, an antiplatelet agent(s).

Continuous flow pumps present a unique risk for gastrointestinal bleeding. The high shear stress from the impeller on blood can cause destruction of large multimers of von Willebrand factor (vWF), which results in a picture of acquired von Willebrand's disease [79,90,91]. Although bleeding risk is mostly manifest from gastrointestinal AVM, it is unknown if the loss of vWF multimers results in bleeding from preexisting AVMs or the lack of pulsatile flow predisposes to the development of AVMs [76,79]. Although most patients have a demonstrable loss of vWF multimers, only a minority of patients develop bleeding. For those who are awaiting cardiac transplantation, bleeding requiring transfusion carries the additional risk of sensitization to human leukocyte antigens that may limit the pool of suitable donor hearts [92].

Anticoagulation and antiplatelet therapy should be initiated postoperatively in the intensive care unit setting and targeted to device-specific goals. Though there is some institutional variation, the recommended international normalized ratio (INR) goal for the two most common continuous flow devices (HM II and HVAD) is 2.0 to 3.0. Chronic antiplatelet therapy with aspirin (81 to 325 mg daily) should be considered in addition to warfarin [24].

If bleeding occurs, it should be immediately evaluated and anticoagulation should be lowered, discontinued and/or reversed as needed [24]. In the setting of clinically significant bleeding with an elevated INR, the ISHLT MCS guidelines recommend reversing anticoagulation [24]. During a sentinel gastrointestinal bleed, gastroenterology consultation should assist with management, and patients should at least undergo endoscopy and colonoscopy. If the evaluation does not reveal a source, subsequent diagnostic testing may include small bowel evaluation (capsule endoscopy or push enteroscopy), tagged red blood scan, or angiography [24]. Sometimes despite extensive evaluation, no source of bleeding can be identified or is not amenable to therapy. In those cases, reevaluation of the goals and necessity of anticoagulation and antiplatelet agents should be considered.

Infection

The most common time for blood-borne infections related to VADs occurs within the first 30 days after implantation, although infections also arise later, just at a lower risk [93]. Risk factors associated with VAD infections consist of the severity of preoperative illness, biventricular support, age, and higher blood urea nitrogen levels [94]. Aside from the infection risks associated with surgery and indwelling lines postoperatively, there are additional chronic risks associated with the presence of the VAD itself and the associated driveline or cannulae. However, sepsis from any source can result in seeding of interior of the VAD or its components, which may necessitate more urgent and higher risk cardiac transplantation or even device replacement [95]. Vegetations on LVAD prosthetic valves may also be a source of thromboembolism [96]. The education of patients and their caregivers about percutaneous lead and exit-site care with aseptic technique for dressing changes is crucial.

Several recommendations can be made for the evaluation of MCS patients with a suspected infection. Aside from routine infectious workup, at least three sets of blood cultures should be drawn within 24 hours with at least one culture from any indwelling central venous catheter. Any suspected source of infection should be swabbed or aspirated when clinically indicated (e.g., purulence from driveline infection, etc.). Inflammatory markers (such as erythrocyte sedimentation rate or serial C-reactive protein) should be considered. The ISHLT guidelines define the criteria for MCSD-specific infections and pocket infections [24].

Thrombosis, Thromboembolism, and Stroke

Based on clinical trials and postmarketing surveillance of the HM II, thrombosis rates of 2% to 4% have been reported [10,13,97]; however, a multicenter study noted an increased rate of pump thrombosis events of 8.4% at 3 months after implantation [98]. The risk of pump thrombosis was heralded by elevated lactate dehydrogenase levels, confirming its usefulness as a clinical biomarker. Pump thrombosis rates peaked at 1 month after implantation and began to decrease by 6 months. Treatment of pump thrombosis included heart transplantation, device replacement, medical therapy with anticoagulation augmentation, and/or thrombolytics. The morbidity and mortality of pump thrombosis was striking with a mortality of 48% among patients with device thrombosis who did not receive a heart transplantation or device replacement [98]. Based on multiple studies, the estimates of 1-year pump thrombosis incidence ranges between 6% to 12% for the HM II device and 5% to 13% for the HVAD [99]. Overall, one can conclude that the risk of thrombosis in the HM II has increased from levels seen during the 2008 to 2010 period, with the highest rates seen in 2013, and some evidence suggests that thrombosis risk may have declined in 2014 [100–102]. The exact cause of the increased rates of device thrombosis is currently unknown and is under active investigation.

Embolism may result from the pump as a result of inadequate anticoagulation, the cardiac chambers as a result of arrhythmias such as atrial fibrillation, or may arise from the native vasculature as a result of the patients' preexisting vascular atherosclerosis. The overall incidence of ischemic stroke varies greatly by type of device; however, with the current generation devices, the rate is 0.09 per patient-year overall and 0.05 per patient-year after 30 days [103]. The overall prevalence of ischemic cerebrovascular accidents (ICVA) and hemorrhagic cerebrovascular accidents (HCVA) in HVAD patients has been cited at 7% and 8%, respectively. Predictors of suffering an ICVA were the use of aspirin ≤81 mg and atrial fibrillation, whereas predictors of an HCVA were mean arterial pressure >90 mm Hg, aspirin ≤81 mg, and an INR >3.0. Likewise, sites that had established improved blood pressure management protocols demonstrated markedly lower rates of HCVA (1.8% vs. 10.8%) [104]. The strongest predictor of HCVA was an elevated mean arterial pressure, underscoring the importance of tight blood pressure management.

For patients who present with a new neurocognitive deficit, neurology consultation in conjunction with CT and angiography of the head and neck is recommended. An interrogation of device parameters to evaluate for signs of pump thrombosis or malfunction is warranted. A review of INR and lactate dehydrogenase trends should be done to look for patterns that would increase the risk of bleeding or thrombosis. In the setting of an HCVA, anticoagulation should be stopped and/or reversed.

Blood pressure management is critical to mitigate the risk of HCVA in this population, and guidelines advise a target mean arterial pressure of ≤80 mm Hg in all nonpulsatile VAD patients [24]. This is a level of evidence C recommendation and needs to be individualized to each patient based on their degree of pulsatility. Blood pressure measurement can be challenging because of the markedly low pulse pressure that is often encountered. Doppler probes are the current clinical standard to measure blood pressure, and the opening Doppler pressure has been shown to correlate with the systolic blood pressure of patients with significant pulsatility to allow discrimination between a systolic and mean blood pressure. In other words, the Doppler opening pressure closely approximates the mean arterial pressure for patients with low pulsatility.

PSYCHOSOCIAL CONSIDERATIONS

Aside from the plethora of medical and surgical considerations, there are emotional, physical, and social considerations that require equal consideration. The acute nature of many patients' illness often precludes a detailed assessment of such issues, but devoted addressal of these issues in nonemergent situations is vital to achieving both optimal outcomes, clinically and programatically. Physical limitations that may impact the patient's ability to care for the device such as the manual dexterity to change batteries or auditory acuity to hear alarms are important and practical considerations. Adequate cognitive ability is needed to understand the importance of the device and its components, the ability to troubleshoot problems, and recognize when to ask for assistance. The emotional ability to adapt to the device, its implications, potential limitations, and adverse events is also important for maximizing long-term outcomes and quality of life. Finally, patients must have an adequate social support network; although having an implanted VAD does not typically involve constant supervision, there must be a background of reliable support for assistance in an emergency and for long-term emotional support.

In support of the above considerations, all patients should have a screen for psychosocial risk factors, cognitive dysfunction, and support structures prior to MCS. Routine cognitive testing may use a screening metric such as the Montreal Cognitive Assessment test [105,106]. If a history of psychiatric illness is present, a thorough evaluation by the psychiatry service should be performed to identify risk factors as well as initiate and/or optimize therapy. Medical compliance and coping capacity must also be assessed, given that poor compliance and coping are associated with adverse outcomes. If noncompliance has been demonstrated on repeated occassions, then, in most cases, MCS should not be offered [24].

Tobacco use is not an absolute contraindication for MCS; however, ongoing efforts should be made to counsel the importance of cessation. A timetable for tobacco cessation may be set a prior by individual programs. At least 6 months of tobacco cessation is required prior to cardiac transplantation. On the other hand, alcohol and substance abuse are strict contraindications to MCS. The timeline for abstinence can be determined by individual programs [40].

TIMING

When patients present to the intensive care unit with shock and are subsequently stabilized with aggressive medical therapy, the decision to transition to MCS rests on the expectation of improvement in the patient's condition. Since 2008, the proportion of patients implanted in critical cardiogenic shock, INTERMACS Level 1, has remained stable at 15% [6]. The majority (65%) of patients are INTERMACS Level 2 (failing inotropes) or 3 (stable on inotropes), whereas 20% of patients have ambulatory, noninotrope-dependent HF (Levels 4 to 7) [6]. For those who received an intervention, such as revascularization, waiting to see the impact of this intervention on the patient's clinical status is reasonable in the absence of further clinical deterioration. Many patients, however, will not have a readily identifiable or treatable proximate cause of their deterioration. For those who are eligible or are already listed for transplantation, the risk of continued medical therapy awaiting transplantation must be weighed against the risk of proceeding with MCS [107]. The advantages of waiting for transplantation in the setting of stable, yet critical illness are an increased likelihood of receiving an organ owing to a higher status, avoiding a second surgery, and bypassing the potential morbidity and mortality of MCS itself. Disadvantages to delaying MCS include the high-risk nature of transplantation during acute illness, further decompensation prior to transplantation that may require higher risk emergent univentricular or biventricular support, becoming too ill for either transplantation or mechanical support, or death. Proceeding with MCS early allows for surgery to be performed when the patient is less ill followed by a lower risk transplant once the patient is rehabilitated. Certain patients may be expected to have a short wait for transplantation based on their size, blood type, and level of sensitization, and the disadvantages of waiting for transplantation may be minimized. Others may have clear indications for early MCS such as persistent pulmonary hypertension not responsive to medical therapy [108]. Unfortunately, most patients do not have a clear delineation of risk, and determining the optimal timing of MCS can be quite difficult. There is an emerging consensus that earlier institution of mechanical support is preferable to waiting, because further decompensation will yield worse outcomes with both MCS and transplantation. For patients with multiorgan failure or on mechanical ventilation, strong consideration should be given to temporary MCS in order to optimize clinical status and assess long-term goals prior to placement of long-term MCS [24]. The ROADMAP (Risk Assessment and Comparative effectiveness of Left Ventricular Assist Device and Medical Management in Ambulatory Heart Failure Patients) study examined the question of earlier implantation of DT LVAD in a less sick population of HF patients. The cohort was DT LVAD versus optimal medical therapy in NYHA functional class IIIB to IV chronic HF patients, not on inotropic therapy. Both showed a similar 20% mortality at 1 year. While the LVAD group had better functional capacity and quality of life, the group also experienced significantly more adverse events [109]. The optimal timing of device implantation remains controversial, but implanting patients who are INTERMACS profiles 6 and 7 likely results in no mortality benefit and a higher rate of adverse events.

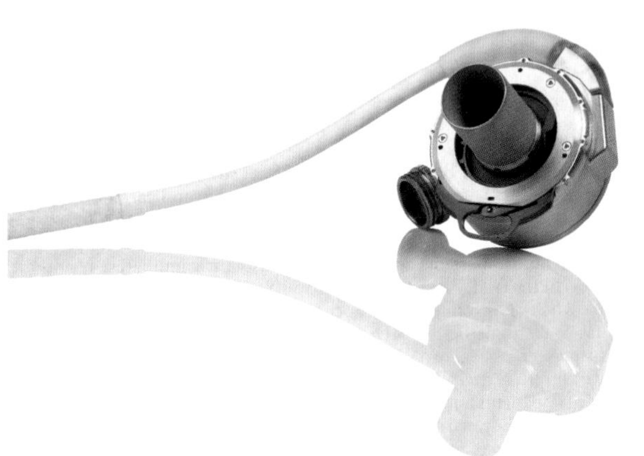

A

B

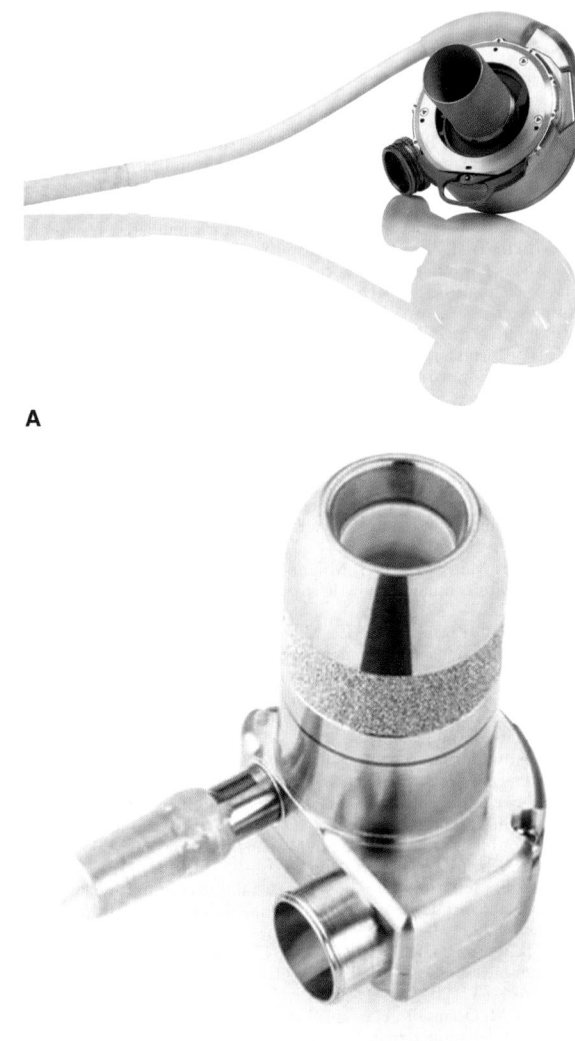

FIGURE 197.6 Future devices currently under investigation, neither available for clinical use. **A:** HeartMate III LVAD; **B:** HeartWare MVAD. Images reprinted with permission from HeartWare International, Inc., and Thoratec Corp.

FUTURE DIRECTIONS

MCS has evolved over the past 25 years from an investigational strategy reserved only for the moribund to a standard therapy supporting patients with stable advanced HF. Today, a wide variety of devices are available for short-, medium-, and long-term support at numerous centers worldwide.

A number of newer MCS devices are now in clinical use or clinical trials. The HeartWare Miniaturized Ventricular Asssist Device (MVAD) and the HeartMate 3 (Thoratec Corporation, Pleasanton, CA, USA) are both enrolling patients for multicenter, prospective trials titled the MVAD Advantage CE trial and The MOMENTUM 3 U.S. IDE Clinical trial, respectively (Fig. 197.6) [110,111]. The unique characteristics of the HeartWare MVAD include a magnetically suspended rotor that is housed within the inflow cannula as well as a wide-bladed design to minimize cellular trauma, while providing up to 10 L per minute of axial blood flow [112]. The HeartMate 3 LVAS provides magnetically levitated centrifugal flow with an artificial pulse mode allowing for enhanced pulsatility and an intended life span of at least 10 years [113]. Advances of pump technology are moving toward smaller pumps that still allow for full support, pumps that can be either implanted percutaneously or through minimally invasive surgeries, increased durability, totally implantable systems with transcutaneous energy transfer, and an improved device–patient interface. Research is also focused on improving biocompatibility, lowering risk of thrombosis, and better responsiveness to physiologic demands.

Medical Arm of Mechanically Assisted Circulatory Support (MedaMACS) is a medical arm of the INTERMACS database that was started in December 2012 with 154 patients enrolled, as of the Seventh INTERMACS report. It has enrolled INTERMACS Level 4 to 7 patients, and 1-year VAD/transplant-free survival has approached 75% [6]. MedaMACS will provide information about the risk of events among "stable" patients with advanced HF and offer guidance on the optimal timing of MCS therapy.

CONCLUSIONS

Einstein once quipped, "I never think of the future – it comes soon enough." Though MCS was once considered to be science fiction, the reality of its place as an increasingly common HF therapy has arrived, and the future of its success depends on a continued commitment to further advances [114]. Though the field is still hindered by adverse events and technological limitations, those too are improving. Devices technology continues to evolve rapidly. Further desirable advances include freedom from an external drive line, as well as alternative energy sources, such as transcutaneous energy. As the number of patients with advanced HF increases, one can anticipate that the demand for and role of MCS, particularly DT, will expand significantly. Ideally, it is hoped MCS will be available to a greater proportion of patients with advanced HF, while resulting in continued improvement of outcomes and reduction of costs.

References

1. Roger VL: Epidemiology of heart failure. *Circ Res* 113(6):646–659, 2013.
2. Braunwald E: The war against heart failure: the Lancet lecture. *Lancet* 385(9970):812–824, 2015.
3. Mozaffarian D, Benjamin EJ, Go AS, et al: Heart disease and stroke statistics-2015 update: a report from the american heart association. *Circulation* 131(4):e29, 2015.
4. Rogers JG, et al: Chronic mechanical circulatory support for inotrope-dependent heart failure patients who are not transplant candidates: results of the INTrEPID Trial. *J Am Coll Cardiol* 50(8):741–747, 2007.
5. Howlader N, Noone AM, Krapcho M, et al: *SEER Cancer Statistics Review 1975–2010*. Bethesda, MD: National Cancer Institute, 2007. Available at: http://seer.cancer.gov/csr.
6. Kirklin JK, Naftel DC, Pagani FD, et al: Seventh INTERMACS annual report: 15,000 patients and counting. *J Heart Lung Transplant* 34:1495–1504, 2015.
7. Lund LH, Edwards LB, Kucheryavaya AY, et al: The registry of the International Society for Heart and Lung Transplantation: thirty-second official adult heart transplantation report-2015; focus theme: early graft failure. *J Heart Lung Transplant* 34(10):1244, 2015.
8. Cowell JL: Thoratec corporation, in Pederson JP (ed): *International Directory of Company Histories*. Vol. 122. St. James Press, 2011.
9. Thoratec HeartMate II LVAS. September 5, 2013 [cited 2015. December 15, 2015]; Available from: http://www.thoratec.com/downloads/HeartMate-II-Fact-Sheet-03312011.pdf.
10. Slaughter MS, Rogers JG, Milano CA, et al: Advanced heart failure treated with continuous-flow left ventricular assist device. *N Engl J Med* 361(23):2241–2251, 2009.
11. Slaughter MS, Pagani FD, McGee EC, et al: HeartWare ventricular assist system for bridge to transplant: combined results of the bridge to transplant and continued access protocol trial. *J Heart Lung Transplant* 32(7):675–683, 2013.
12. Rose EA, Gelijns AC, Moskowitz AJ, et al: Long-term use of a left ventricular assist device for end-stage heart failure. *N Engl J Med* 345(20):1435–1443, 2001.
13. Miller LW, Pagani FD, Russell SD, et al: Use of a continuous-flow device in patients awaiting heart transplantation. *N Engl J Med* 357(9):885–896, 2007.
14. Mancini D, Colombo PC: Left ventricular assist devices: a rapidly evolving alternative to transplant. *J Am Coll Cardiol* 65(23):2542–2555, 2015.
15. Moazami N, Fukamachi K, Kobayashi M, et al: Axial and centrifugal continuous-flow rotary pumps: a translation from pump mechanics to clinical practice. *J Heart Lung Transplant* 32(1):1–11, 2013.
16. James KB, McCarthy PM, Thomas JD, et al: Effect of the implantable left ventricular assist device on neuroendocrine activation in heart failure. *Circulation* 92(9):191–195, 1995.
17. Hall JL, Fermin DR, Birks EJ, et al: Clinical, molecular, and genomic changes in response to a left ventricular assist device. *J Am Coll Cardiol* 57(6):641–652, 2011.
18. Lanier GM, Orlanse K, Hayashi Y, et al: Validity and reliability of a novel slow cuff-deflation system for noninvasive blood pressure monitoring in patients with continuous-flow left ventricular assist device. *Circ Heart Fail* 6(5):1005–1012, 2013.
19. Goldstein DJ, Maybaum S, MacGillivray TE, et al: Young patients with nonischemic cardiomyopathy have higher likelihood of left ventricular recovery during left ventricular assist device support. *J Card Fail* 18(5):392–395, 2012.
20. Kormos RL, Miller LW: *Mechanical Circulatory Support: A Companion to Braunwald's Heart Disease*. Elsevier Health Sciences, 2011.
21. Farrar DJ, Hill JD, Pennington DG, et al: Preoperative and postoperative comparison of patients with univentricular and biventricular support with the Thoratec ventricular assist device as a bridge to cardiac transplantation. *J Thorac Cardiovasc Surg* 113(1):202–209, 1997.
22. Lampert BC, Teuteberg JJ: Right ventricular failure after left ventricular assist devices. *J Heart Lung Transplant* 34(9):1123–1130, 2015.
23. Morris RJ: *Total Artificial Heart—Concepts and Clinical Use. Seminars in Thoracic and Cardiovascular Surgery*. Elsevier, 2008.
24. Feldman D, Pamboukian SV, Teuteberg JJ, et al: The 2013 International Society for Heart and Lung Transplantation Guidelines for mechanical circulatory support: executive summary. *J Heart Lung Transplant* 32(2):157–187, 2013.
25. Slaughter MS, Pagani FD, Rogers JG, et al: Clinical management of continuous-flow left ventricular assist devices in advanced heart failure. *J Heart Lung Transplant* 29(4):S1–S39, 2010.
26. Aaronson KD, Schwartz JS, Chen TM, et al: Development and prospective validation of a clinical index to predict survival in ambulatory patients referred for cardiac transplant evaluation. *Circulation* 95(12):2660–2667, 1997.
27. Levy WC, Mozaffarian D, Linker DT, et al: The seattle heart failure model prediction of survival in heart failure. *Circulation* 113(11):1424–1433, 2006.
28. Levy WC, Mozaffarian D, Linker DT, et al: Can the Seattle heart failure model be used to risk-stratify heart failure patients for potential left ventricular assist device therapy? *J Heart Lung Transplant* 28(3):231–236, 2009.
29. Deng MC, Loebe M, El-Banayosy A, et al: Mechanical circulatory support for advanced heart failure effect of patient selection on outcome. *Circulation* 103(2):231–237, 2001.
30. Lietz K, Long JW, Kfoury AG, et al: Outcomes of left ventricular assist device implantation as destination therapy in the post-rematch era implications for patient selection. *Circulation* 116(5):497–505, 2007.
31. Oz MC, Goldstein DJ, Pepino P, et al: Screening scale predicts patients successfully receiving long-term implantable left ventricular assist devices. *Circulation* 92(9):169–173, 1995.
32. Cowger J, et al: Predicting survival in patients receiving continuous flow left ventricular assist devices: the HeartMate II risk score. *J Am Coll Cardiol* 61(3):313–321, 2013.
33. Stevenson LW, Pagani FD, Young JB, et al: INTERMACS profiles of advanced heart failure: the current picture. *J Heart Lung Transplant* 28(6):535–541, 2009.
34. Kirklin JK, Naftel DC, Pagani FD, et al: Sixth INTERMACS annual report: a 10,000-patient database. *J Heart Lung Transplant* 33(6):555–564, 2014.
35. Kirklin JK, Naftel DC, Stevenson LW, et al: INTERMACS database for durable devices for circulatory support: first annual report. *J Heart Lung Transplant* 27(10):1065–1072, 2008.
36. Boyle AJ, Ascheim DD, Russo MJ, et al: Clinical outcomes for continuous-flow left ventricular assist device patients stratified by pre-operative INTERMACS classification. *J Heart Lung Transplant* 30(4):402–407, 2011.
37. Loghmanpour NA, Kanwar MK, Druzdzel MJ, et al: A new Bayesian network-based risk stratification model for prediction of short-term and long-term LVAD mortality. *ASAIO J* 61(3):313–323, 2015.
38. Arnold SV, Jones PG, Allen LA, et al: Abstract 11601: identifying patients at high risk for poor global outcome after left ventricular assist device for destination therapy: results from the INTERMACS Registry. *Circulation* 132[Suppl 3]:A11601, 2015.
39. Interagency Registry for Mechanically Assisted Circulatory Support (INTERMACS). Appendix A: Adverse event definitions: adult and pediatric patients. 2013 [cited 2015 December 1]. Available from: https://www.uab.edu/medicine/intermacs/intermacs-documents.
40. Farrar D: *Ventricular Interactions During Mechanical Circulatory Support. Seminars in Thoracic and Cardiovascular Surgery*. 1994.
41. Santamore WP, Dell'Italia LJ: Ventricular interdependence: significant left ventricular contributions to right ventricular systolic function. *Prog Cardiovasc Dis* 40(4):289–308, 1998.
42. Haddad F, Doyle R, Murphy DJ, et al: Right ventricular function in cardiovascular disease, part II pathophysiology, clinical importance, and management of right ventricular failure. *Circulation* 117(13):1717–1731, 2008.
43. Krishan K, Nair A, Pinney S, et al: Liberal use of tricuspid-valve annuloplasty during left-ventricular assist device implantation. *Eur J Cardiothorac Surg* 41(1):213–217, 2012.
44. Dang NC, Topkara VK, Mercando M, et al: Right heart failure after left ventricular assist device implantation in patients with chronic congestive heart failure. *J Heart Lung Transplant* 25(1):1–6, 2006.
45. Patel ND, Weiss ES, Schaffer J, et al: Right heart dysfunction after left ventricular assist device implantation: a comparison of the pulsatile HeartMate I and axial-flow HeartMate II devices. *Ann Thorac Surg* 86(3):832–840, 2008.
46. Matthews JC, Koelling TM, Pagani FD, et al: The right ventricular failure risk score: a pre-operative tool for assessing the risk of right ventricular failure in left ventricular assist device candidates. *J Am Coll Cardiol* 51(22):2163–2172, 2008.
47. Kormos RL, Teuteberg JJ, Pagani FD, et al: Right ventricular failure in patients with the HeartMate II continuous-flow left ventricular assist device: incidence, risk factors, and effect on outcomes. *J Thorac Cardiovasc Surg* 139(5):1316–1324, 2010.
48. Ochiai Y, McCarthy PM, Smedira NG, et al: Predictors of severe right ventricular failure after implantable left ventricular assist device insertion: analysis of 245 patients. *Circulation* 106[12 Suppl 1]:1198–1202, 2002.
49. Atluri P, Goldstone AB, Fairman AS, et al: Predicting right ventricular failure in the modern, continuous flow left ventricular assist device era. *Ann Thorac Surg* 96(3):857–864, 2013.
50. Drakos SG, et al: Risk factors predictive of right ventricular failure after left ventricular assist device implantation. *Am J Cardiol* 105(7):1030–1035, 2010.
51. Fitzpatrick JR, Frederick JR, Hsu VM, et al: Risk score derived from pre-operative data analysis predicts the need for biventricular mechanical circulatory support. *J Heart Lung Transplant* 27(12):1286–1292, 2008.
52. Puwanant S, Hamilton KK, Klodell CT, et al: Tricuspid annular motion as a predictor of severe right ventricular failure after left ventricular assist device implantation. *J Heart Lung Transplant* 27(10):1102–1107, 2008.
53. Potapov EV, Stepanenko A, Dandel M, et al: Tricuspid incompetence and geometry of the right ventricle as predictors of right ventricular function after implantation of a left ventricular assist device. *J Heart Lung Transplant* 27(12):1275–1281, 2008.
54. Kukucka M, Stepanenko A, Potapov E, et al: Right-to-left ventricular end-diastolic diameter ratio and prediction of right ventricular failure with continuous-flow left ventricular assist devices. *J Heart Lung Transplant* 30(1):64–69, 2011.
55. Vivo RP, Cordero-Reyes AM, Qamar U, et al: Increased right-to-left ventricle diameter ratio is a strong predictor of right ventricular failure after left ventricular assist device. *J Heart Lung Transplant* 32(8):792–799, 2013.
56. Raina A, Seetha Rammohan HR, Gertz ZM, et al: Postoperative right ventricular failure after left ventricular assist device placement is predicted by preoperative echocardiographic structural, hemodynamic, and functional parameters. *J Card Fail* 19(1):16–24, 2013.
57. Kato TS, Farr M, Schulze PC, et al: Usefulness of two-dimensional echocardiographic parameters of the left side of the heart to predict right ventricular failure after left ventricular assist device implantation. *Am J Cardiol* 109(2):246–251, 2012.
58. Simon MA: Assessment and treatment of right ventricular failure. *Nat Rev Cardiol* 10(4):204–218, 2013.
59. Dandel M, Potapov E, Krabatsch T, et al: Load dependency of right ventricular performance is a major factor to be considered in decision making before ventricular assist device implantation. *Circulation* 128[11 Suppl 1]:S14–S23, 2013.

60. Overgaard CB, Džavík V: Inotropes and vasopressors review of physiology and clinical use in cardiovascular disease. *Circulation* 118(10):1047–1056, 2008.
61. Vieillard-Baron A, Jardin F: Why protect the right ventricle in patients with acute respiratory distress syndrome? *Curr Opin Crit Care* 9(1):15–21, 2003.
62. McLaughlin VV, McGoon MD: Pulmonary arterial hypertension. *Circulation* 114(13):1417–1431, 2006.
63. Robertson JO, Grau-Sepulveda MV, Okada S, et al: Concomitant tricuspid valve surgery during implantation of continuous-flow left ventricular assist devices: a Society of Thoracic Surgeons database analysis. *J Heart Lung Transplant* 33(6):609–617, 2014.
64. John R, Mantz K, Eckman P, et al: Aortic valve pathophysiology during left ventricular assist device support. *J Heart Lung Transplant* 29(12):1321–1329, 2010.
65. Holman WL, Kormos RL, Naftel DC, et al: Predictors of death and transplant in patients with a mechanical circulatory support device: a multi-institutional study. *J Heart Lung Transplant* 28(1):44–50, 2009.
66. Schulman AR, Martens TP, Russo MJ, et al: Effect of left ventricular assist device infection on post-transplant outcomes. *J Heart Lung Transplant* 28(3):237–242, 2009.
67. Brisco MA, Kimmel SE, Coca SG, et al: Prevalence and prognostic importance of changes in renal function after mechanical circulatory support. *Circ Heart Fail* 7(1):68–75, 2014.
68. Hasin T, Topilsky Y, Schriger JA, et al: Changes in renal function after implantation of continuous-flow left ventricular assist devices. *J Am Coll Cardiol* 59(1):26–36, 2012.
69. Sandner SE, Zimpfer D, Zrunek P, et al: Renal function and outcome after continuous flow left ventricular assist device implantation. *Ann Thorac Surg* 87(4):1072–1078, 2009.
70. Singh M, Shullo M, Kormos RL, et al: Impact of renal function before mechanical circulatory support on posttransplant renal outcomes. *Ann Thorac Surg* 91(5):1348–1354, 2011.
71. Butler J, Geisberg C, Howser R, et al: Relationship between renal function and left ventricular assist device use. *Ann Thorac Surg* 81(5):1745–1751, 2006.
72. Topkara VK, Dang NC, Barili F, et al: Predictors and outcomes of continuous veno-venous hemodialysis use after implantation of a left ventricular assist device. *J Heart Lung Transplant* 25(4):404–408, 2006.
73. Reinhartz O, Farrar DJ, Hershon JH, et al: Importance of preoperative liver function as a predictor of survival in patients supported with Thoratec ventricular assist devices as a bridge to transplantation. *J Thorac Cardiovasc Surg* 116(4):633–640, 1998.
74. Matthews JC, Pagani FD, Haft JW, et al: Model for end-stage liver disease score predicts left ventricular assist device operative transfusion requirements, morbidity, and mortality. *Circulation* 121(2):214–220, 2010.
75. Crow S, John R, Boyle A, et al: Gastrointestinal bleeding rates in recipients of nonpulsatile and pulsatile left ventricular assist devices. *J Thorac Cardiovasc Surg* 137(1):208–215, 2009.
76. Geisen U, Heilmann C, Beyersdorf F, et al: Non-surgical bleeding in patients with ventricular assist devices could be explained by acquired von Willebrand disease. *Eur J Cardiothorac Surg* 33(4):679–684, 2008.
77. Stern DR, Kazam J, Edwards P, et al: Increased incidence of gastrointestinal bleeding following implantation of the HeartMate II LVAD. *J Card Surg* 25(3):352–356, 2010.
78. Uriel N, Pak SW, Jorde UP, et al: Acquired von Willebrand syndrome after continuous-flow mechanical device support contributes to a high prevalence of bleeding during long-term support and at the time of transplantation. *J Am Coll Cardiol* 56(15):1207–1213, 2010.
79. Crow S, Chen D, Milano C, et al: Acquired von Willebrand syndrome in continuous-flow ventricular assist device recipients. *Ann Thorac Surg* 90(4):1263–1269, 2010.
80. Letsou GV, Shah N, Gregoric ID, et al: Gastrointestinal bleeding from arteriovenous malformations in patients supported by the Jarvik 2000 axial-flow left ventricular assist device. *J Heart Lung Transplant* 24(1):105–109, 2005.
81. Demirozu ZT, Radovancevic R, Hochman LF, et al: Arteriovenous malformation and gastrointestinal bleeding in patients with the HeartMate II left ventricular assist device. *J Heart Lung Transplant* 30(8):849–853, 2011.
82. Butler J, Howser R, Portner PM, et al: Body mass index and outcomes after left ventricular assist device placement. *Ann Thorac Surg* 79(1):66–73, 2005.
83. Mano A, Fujita K, Uenomachi K, et al: Body mass index is a useful predictor of prognosis after left ventricular assist system implantation. *J Heart Lung Transplant* 28(5):428–433, 2009.
84. Musci M, Loforte A, Potapov EV, et al: Body mass index and outcome after ventricular assist device placement. *Ann Thorac Surg* 86(4):1236–1242, 2008.
85. Shah SK, Gregoric ID, Nathan SS, et al: Simultaneous left ventricular assist device placement and laparoscopic sleeve gastrectomy as a bridge to transplant for morbidly obese patients with severe heart failure. *J Heart Lung Transplant* 34(11):1489, 2015.
86. Chaudhry UI, Kanji A, Sai-Sudhakar CB, et al: Laparoscopic sleeve gastrectomy in morbidly obese patients with end-stage heart failure and left ventricular assist device: medium-term results. *Surg Obes Relat Dis* 11(1):88–93, 2015.
87. Holtz J, Teuteberg J: Management of aortic insufficiency in the continuous flow left ventricular assist device population. *Curr Heart Fail Rep* 11(1):103–110, 2014.
88. McKenna DH, Eastlund T, Segall M, et al: HLA alloimmunization in patients requiring ventricular assist device support. *J Heart Lung Transplant* 21(11):1218–1224, 2002.
89. Sihler KC, Napolitano LM: Complications of massive transfusion. *Chest* 137(1):209–220, 2010.
90. Klovaite J, Gustafsson F, Mortensen SA, et al: Severely impaired von Willebrand factor-dependent platelet aggregation in patients with a continuous-flow left ventricular assist device (HeartMate II). *J Am Coll Cardiol* 53(23):2162–2167, 2009.
91. Meyer AL, Malehsa D, Budde U, et al: Acquired von Willebrand syndrome in patients with an axial flow left ventricular assist device. *Circ Heart Fail* 3(6):675–681, 2010.
92. Mehra MR, Uber PA, Uber WE, et al: Allosensitization in heart transplantation: implications and management strategies. *Curr Opin Cardiol* 18(2):153–158, 2003.
93. Gordon SM, Schmitt SK, Jacobs M, et al: Nosocomial bloodstream infections in patients with implantable left ventricular assist devices. *Ann Thorac Surg* 72(3):725–730, 2001.
94. Holman WL, Kirklin JK, Naftel DC, et al: Infection after implantation of pulsatile mechanical circulatory support devices. *J Thorac Cardiovasc Surg* 139(6):1632.e2–1636.e2.
95. Holman WL, Park SJ, Long JW, et al: Infection in permanent circulatory support: experience from the REMATCH trial. *J Heart Lung Transplant* 23(12):1359–1365, 2004.
96. Fischer SA, Trenholme GM, Costanzo MR, et al: Infectious complications in left ventricular assist device recipients. *Clin Infect Dis* 24(1):18–23, 1997.
97. Starling RC, Naka Y, Boyle AJ, et al: Results of the post-US Food and Drug Administration-approval study with a continuous flow left ventricular assist device as a bridge to heart transplantation: a prospective study using the INTERMACS (Interagency Registry for Mechanically Assisted Circulatory Support). *J Am Coll Cardiol* 57(19):1890–1898, 2011.
98. Starling RC, Moazami N, Silvestry SC, et al: Unexpected abrupt increase in left ventricular assist device thrombosis. *N Engl J Med* 370(1):33–40, 2014.
99. Stewart GC, Givertz MM, Mehra MR: Pump thrombosis redux. *J Heart Lung Transplant* 34(12):1512, 2015.
100. Kirklin JK, Naftel DC, Pagani FD, et al: Pump thrombosis in the Thoratec HeartMate II device: an update analysis of the INTERMACS Registry. *J Heart Lung Transplant* 34:1515–1526, 2015.
101. Smedira NG, Blackstone EH, Ehrlinger J, et al: Current risks of HeartMate II pump thrombosis: non-parametric analysis of Interagency Registry for Mechanically Assisted Circulatory Support data. *J Heart Lung Transplant* 34(12):1527–1534, 2015.
102. Jeffries N, Miller MA, Taddei-Peters WC, et al: What is the truth behind pump thrombosis in the HeartMate II device? A National Heart, Lung, and Blood Institute perspective based on data from the Interagency Registry for Mechanically Assisted Circulatory Support. *J Heart Lung Transplant* 34(12):1506, 2015.
103. Pagani FD, Miller LW, Russell SD, et al: Extended mechanical circulatory support with a continuous-flow rotary left ventricular assist device. *J Am Coll Cardiol* 54(4):312–321, 2009.
104. Teuteberg JJ, Slaughter MS, Rogers JG, et al: The HVAD left ventricular assist device: risk factors for neurological events and risk mitigation strategies. *JACC Heart Fail* 3(10):818–828, 2015.
105. Cordell CB, Borson S, Boustani M, et al: Alzheimer's Association recommendations for operationalizing the detection of cognitive impairment during the Medicare Annual Wellness Visit in a primary care setting. *Alzheimers Dement* 9(2):141–150, 2013.
106. Chow WB, Rosenthal RA, Merkow RP, et al: Optimal preoperative assessment of the geriatric surgical patient: a best practices guideline from the American College of Surgeons National Surgical Quality Improvement Program and the American Geriatrics Society. *J Am Coll Surg* 215(4):453–466, 2012.
107. Taylor DO, Edwards LB, Aurora P, et al: Registry of the International Society for Heart and Lung Transplantation: twenty-fifth official adult heart transplant report—2008. *J Heart Lung Transplant* 27(9):943–956, 2008.
108. Torre-Amione G, Southard RE, Loebe MM, et al: Reversal of secondary pulmonary hypertension by axial and pulsatile mechanical circulatory support. *J Heart Lung Transplant* 29(2):195–200, 2010.
109. Rogers JG, Boyle AJ, O'Connell JB, et al: Risk assessment and comparative effectiveness of left ventricular assist device and medical management in ambulatory heart failure patients: Design and rationale of the ROADMAP clinical trial. *Am Heart J* 169(2):205.e20-210.e20, 2015.
110. Schmitto JD, Hanke JS, Rojas SV, et al: First implantation in man of a new magnetically levitated left ventricular assist device (HeartMate III). *J Heart Lung Transplant* 34:858–860, 2015.
111. McGee E, Chorpenning K, Brown MC, et al: In vivo evaluation of the HeartWare MVAD pump. *J Heart Lung Transplant* 33(4):366–371, 2014.
112. LaRose JA, Tamez D, Ashenuga et al: Design concepts and principle of operation of the HeartWare ventricular assist system. *ASAIO J* 56(4):285–289, 2010.
113. Farrar DJ, Kevin B, Charles DP, et al: Design features, developmental status, and experimental results with the Heartmate III centrifugal left ventricular assist system with a magnetically levitated rotor. *ASAIO J* 53(3):310–315, 2007.
114. Fang JC: Rise of the machines—left ventricular assist devices as permanent therapy for advanced heart failure. *N Engl J Med* 361(23):2282–2285, 2009.

Section 18

RENAL PROBLEMS IN THE INTENSIVE CARE UNIT

PANG-YEN FAN

Chapter 198 ■ Metabolic Acidosis and Metabolic Alkalosis

ROBERT M. BLACK • JASON M. KURLAND

NORMAL ACID–BASE PHYSIOLOGY

Acidemia and alkalemia denote, respectively, blood pH below or above the normal value of 7.40. A simple (single) acid–base disturbance always causes the blood pH to change. In comparison, the coexistence of two opposing primary acid–base disturbances, such as a metabolic acidosis as a result of diarrhea with metabolic alkalosis as a result of vomiting, may result in little or no deviation of the blood pH from normal. Maintenance of blood pH at approximately 7.40 is necessary to stabilize intracellular pH at 7.20, a crucial chemical condition for optimal cell physiology.

Renal Regulation of H^+ Secretion

Maintenance of a normal plasma bicarbonate (HCO_3^-) concentration depends on reclamation of the 4,500 mEq of HCO_3^- filtered by the kidneys each day. Reabsorption of filtered HCO_3^- takes place almost entirely in the proximal tubule (Fig. 198.1). In this process, luminal HCO_3^- combines with H^+ secreted into the tubular lumen by a Na–H antiporter. The formation and subsequent dissociation of carbonic acid (H_2CO_3) to carbon dioxide (CO_2) and water (H_2O), catalyzed by carbonic anhydrase, permits CO_2 to enter the luminal membrane of the proximal tubular cell. Once inside the cell, CO_2 combines with OH^- to form HCO_3^-. A Na-3HCO_3 cotransporter then carries HCO_3^- across the peritubular membrane into the blood. As a result, filtered HCO_3^- is returned to the circulation without any net loss of H^+.

A fall in proximal tubular bicarbonate reabsorption causes urinary HCO_3^- losses and may lead to a fall in plasma HCO_3^- concentration and to metabolic acidosis. The carbonic anhydrase inhibitor acetazolamide, for example, reduces the activity of luminal carbonic anhydrase, thereby decreasing the entry of H_2O and CO_2 across the luminal membrane, which decreases HCO_3^- reabsorption by the tubular cell (Fig. 198.1).

The process of reclamation for all filtered HCO_3^- by itself is not sufficient to maintain a normal blood pH. The kidney must also excrete the 50 to 100 mEq per kg of H^+ generated each day from the metabolism of dietary proteins, particularly

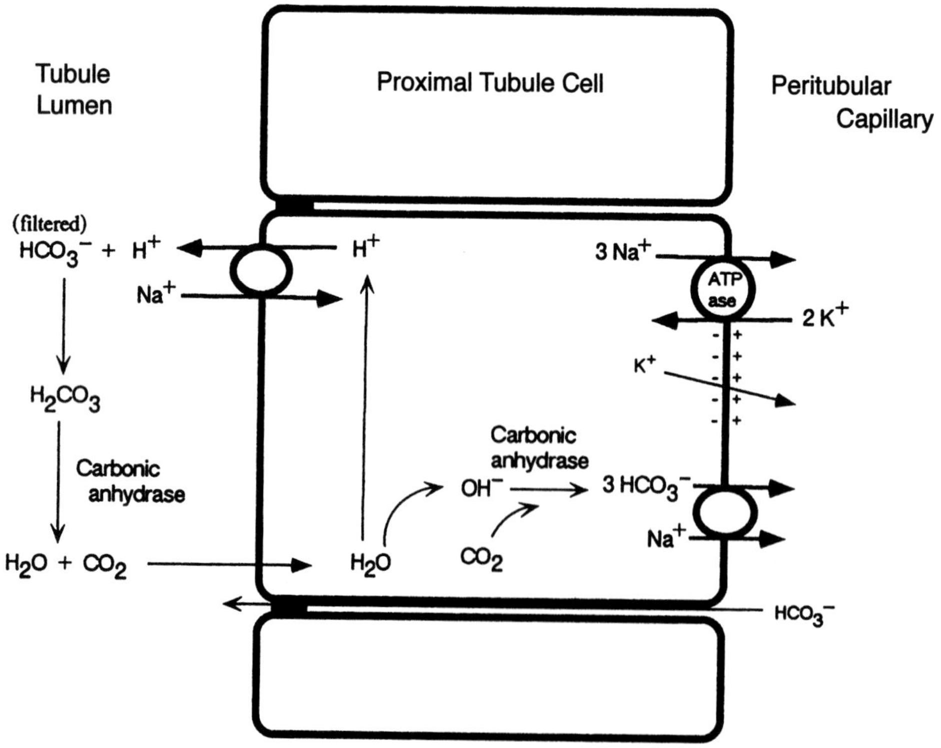

FIGURE 198.1 Proximal tubular reclamation of filtered bicarbonate (HCO_3). The first step in maintaining normal acid–base balance is the reabsorption of all filtered HCO_3. Inability to accomplish this results in metabolic acidosis (proximal, type 2, renal tubular acidosis) (see text for details). ATPase, adenosine triphosphatase.

sulfur-containing amino acids (i.e., methionine, cysteine), which are converted to sulfuric acid. This acid load is initially buffered in the body to minimize changes in blood pH, causing a clinically undetectable decrease in the plasma HCO_3^- concentration. The kidney must eventually excrete this daily acid increment to replete the HCO_3^- used in this process or more severe acidemia will develop over time.

Energy requirements limit the ability of the kidney to excrete acid (H^+ ions) when the urine pH falls below 4.5. To offset this limitation, urinary buffers present in the urine maintain the urine pH above this critical value, permitting ongoing excretion of the daily acid load.

Two distinct urinary buffering systems enable continued H^+ secretion: titratable acids and ammonia. Titratable acids (primarily HPO_4) are freely filtered through the glomerulus and can combine with H^+:

$$HPO_4^- + H^+ \rightarrow H_2PO_4$$

Titratable acidity is determined by adding alkali to the daily urine volume and equals the number of milliequivalents of base required to return the urine pH to 7.4. Approximately one-half of the daily acid load is excreted in this way.

By comparison, the most important urinary buffer is ammonia, because the abundance of this buffer can be varied according to physiologic needs. Ammonia synthesis occurs in the proximal tubule, derived principally from the breakdown of glutamine to α-ketoglutarate (Fig. 198.2). This process is stimulated by intracellular acidosis and by hypokalemia, both of which act by decreasing the intracellular pH (see the following discussion). Ammonia thus generated can combine with intracellular H^+, forming ammonium (NH_4^+). NH_4^+ is then secreted into the proximal tubule lumen by substituting for H^+ on the Na–H antiporter. Ammonia

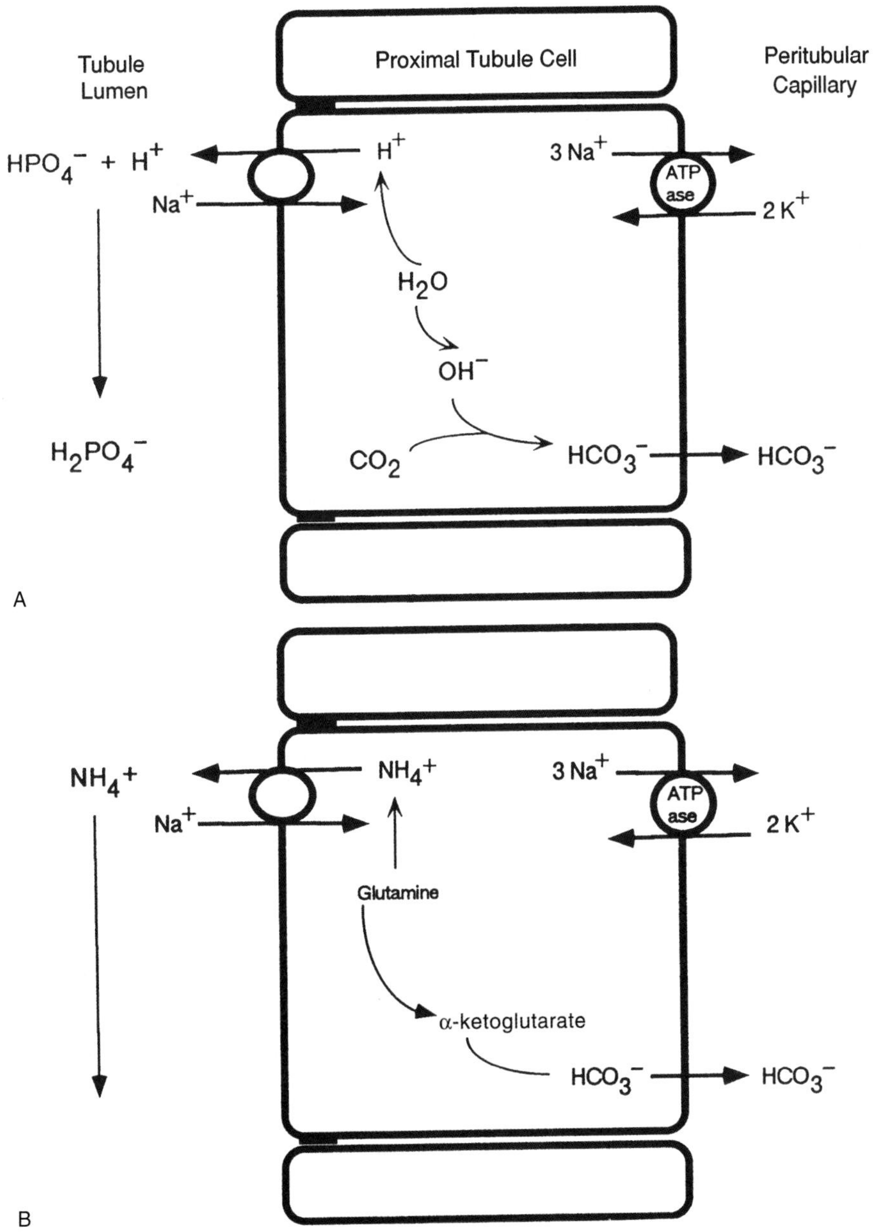

FIGURE 198.2 Excretion of the daily acid load permits the regeneration of bicarbonate (HCO_3) that was used as a buffer. Two processes are involved: the excretion of titratable acid (**A**) and the excretion of ammonium (NH_4^+) (**B**). The latter is particularly important because acidosis stimulates the breakdown of glutamine to ammonia. By comparison, hyperkalemia impairs the capacity of the proximal tubule to make ammonia, thus contributing to the metabolic acidosis observed in hyperkalemic disorders. ATPase, adenosine triphosphatase.

(NH_3) that forms by the dissociation of H^+ from NH_4^+ is largely reabsorbed, recycled, and then secreted into the collecting tubule. There, it is trapped in the tubular lumen as NH_4^+ by combining with secreted H^+ and excreted as ammonium chloride (NH_4Cl). For each molecule of buffered H^+ excreted in the urine, an HCO_3^- is regenerated (Fig. 198.2), thus replenishing the HCO_3^- used initially by the body to buffer daily metabolic acid load.

METABOLIC ACIDOSIS

Metabolic acidosis can be categorized by the presence or absence of an increased anion gap (AG). The *anion gap* (AG) refers to the difference between measured cations (Na^+) and measured anions (chloride [Cl^-] and HCO_3^-):

$$AG = Na^+ - (Cl^- + HCO_3^-)$$

Potassium (K^+) is usually not included in the calculation of the AG because changes large enough to alter the gap significantly are uncommon or incompatible with life.

The normal AG varies between 3 and 11 mEq per L and averages approximately 7 to 8 mEq per L. These unmeasured anions consist of proteins (primarily albumin), sulfates, phosphates, and circulating organic acids. Uric acid is a large molecule and, therefore, does not contribute significantly to the AG even when hyperuricemia is present.

A reduction in the plasma albumin concentration can lower the baseline AG (approximately 2.5 mEq per L for every 1 g per dL fall in the albumin concentration) [1]. Thus, the hypoalbuminemic patient may not have a high AG even in the presence of a disorder that typically causes an elevation (e.g., lactic acidosis; see later).

Metabolic Acidosis with an Increased Anion Gap

The causes of metabolic acidosis associated with an increased AG are listed in Table 198.1. Lactic acidosis is the most frequent form in hospitalized patients, whereas chronic renal failure is the principal cause of an increased AG for ambulatory persons.

Chronic Kidney Disease

Renal disease represents an interesting example of the potential overlap between normal and elevated AG acidosis. The high AG in patients with advanced chronic kidney disease is usually a late finding and reflects a severe reduction in glomerular filtration rate (GFR). As the GFR falls below 20 to 30 mL per minute (plasma creatinine >3 to 4 mg per dL), anions, such as sulfate and phosphate, that would normally be excreted by filtration are retained. With lesser degrees of renal dysfunction, however, metabolic acidosis appears primarily because H^+ (HCl) secretion is reduced, with little or no effect on the AG.

The metabolically generated daily acid load on a typical American diet approximates 50 to 100 mEq. This acid, mainly sulfuric, is immediately buffered by $NaHCO_3$:

$$H_2SO_4 + 2NaHCO_3 \rightarrow Na_2SO_4 + 2CO_2 + 2H_2O$$

The excess sulfate is excreted in the urine. If glomerular and tubular function decline in parallel, then the H^+ and the SO_4^{2-} are retained, producing metabolic acidosis with a high AG. If, however, there is differential tubular dysfunction, the excretion of acid is diminished, but excretion of sulfate may be maintained owing to reduced reabsorption. In the latter setting, the AG may not rise as the serum HCO_3^- concentration decreases.

Therefore, the decrease in plasma HCO_3^- (severity of acidemia) need not correlate with extent of the rise in AG in renal dysfunction. Typically, the plasma bicarbonate concentration is greater than 12 mEq per L in patients with uncomplicated chronic kidney disease. A search for a second acid–base disorder is indicated when a lower HCO_3^- concentration is identified.

TABLE 198.1

Causes of Metabolic Acidosis with an Increased Anion Gap

Chronic kidney diseasea
Lactic acidosis
Ketoacidosis[a]
Rhabdomyolysis
Ingestions
Salicylates
Methanol
Ethylene glycol
Pyroglutamic acid (also known as 5-oxoproline)[b]
Toluene[c]

[a]May be associated with normal anion gap early in course or during therapy (ketoacidosis) (see text for details).
[b]Usually as a result of acetaminophen.
[c]Toluene may also cause a non–anion gap acidosis (see Table 198.3).

Lactic Acidosis

Lactic acidosis is the most common cause of severe metabolic acidosis encountered in the intensive care unit. The AG is always increased above baseline (normal lactate level is <1.0 mmol per L) because lactate does not appear in the urine until a higher plasma concentration (at least 6 to 8 mmol per L) is achieved. Lactate levels greater than 5 mmol per L are considered diagnostic of lactic acidosis, although levels between 2 and 5 mmol per L may be significant in the appropriate clinical circumstances. Metformin, a biguanide commonly used in the treatment of type II diabetes mellitus, can cause lactic acidosis, particularly in patients who present with acute or chronic renal insufficiency. Hemodialysis has been used in the treatment of metformin-induced acidosis [2].

Most cases of lactic acidosis involve the L-isomer. By comparison, D-lactic acidosis, a disorder observed most commonly in patients with short bowel syndrome, results in a rise in the AG, but the lactate level is normal [3]. D-Lactate, generated by intestinal bacteria, is not detected by the usual lactate assay, and a specific enzymatic assay must be requested to diagnose this disorder.

Ketoacidosis

Ketoacidosis occurs when acetoacetic acid and β-hydroxybutyric acid are overproduced by the liver (for a complete discussion, see Chapter 137). Acetone, a breakdown product of acetoacetic acid, is not an acid and does not contribute to the acidemia or to the increased AG observed in this disorder.

Although ketoacidosis is generally associated with an elevated AG, loss of ketoanions in the urine, particularly during intravenous fluid therapy, may attenuate the expansion of the AG. Once formed, ketones may be excreted in the urine before, under the influence of insulin, they can be metabolized back to HCO_3^-. Because ketoacids titrate the plasma HCO_3^- concentration downward, the loss of urinary ketoanions (as sodium or potassium salts) is tantamount to the renal loss of HCO_3^-. Thus, a high AG metabolic acidosis is often present before therapy in individuals with ketoacidosis, but may convert to a normal AG metabolic acidosis with saline repletion and cessation of ketogenesis. Sodium-glucose cotransporter-2 inhibitors, used in the treatment of type 2 diabetes, may increase the risk of ketoacidosis.

Rhabdomyolysis

Massive muscle breakdown is an important cause of metabolic acidosis with an increased AG. Acute kidney injury as a result of myoglobinuria can cause retention of anions (e.g., phosphate) that have been released from damaged myocytes.

Ingestions

The most common acid–base abnormality observed with salicylate intoxication is a respiratory alkalosis caused by direct stimulation of the medullary respiratory center. With moderate-to-severe salicylate intoxication, the AG increases as salicylic acid promotes formation of lactic acid, rather than accumulation of salicylate in the blood. The consequence is a mixed respiratory alkalosis with a high AG metabolic acidosis.

Methanol and ethylene glycol ingestions require early diagnosis because prompt treatment may be lifesaving. Inhibitors of alcohol dehydrogenase such as ethanol and fomepizole can limit the conversion of the alcohols to their more toxic metabolic products, with fomepizole being the preferred agent. The clinical features of these ingestions are discussed in detail in Chapter 119.

Detection of an osmolal gap suggests methanol or ethylene glycol poisoning and may avoid delayed treatment while awaiting lab measurement of these toxins. The *osmolal gap* refers to the difference between the plasma osmolality (P_{Osm}) measured by the laboratory and that calculated using the following formula:

$$\text{Calculated } P_{Osm} \text{ (mOsm/kg)} = (2 \times Na^+) + (\text{glucose}/18) + (\text{BUN}/2.8) + (\text{ethanol}/3.7) \quad [4]$$

Normally, the measured P_{Osm} is higher than the calculated value by 10 mOsm per kg. A larger osmolal gap indicates the presence of osmotically active substances not normally present. The most frequent causes of an increased osmolal gap are ethyl alcohol, isopropyl alcohol, ketones, lactate, mannitol, ethylene glycol, and methanol. If ethanol, lactate, or ketones cannot be identified in a patient with an AG metabolic acidosis with an osmolal gap, the diagnosis of ethylene glycol or methanol intoxication should be strongly suspected. In the intensive care unit setting, a high osmolal gap acidosis has also been associated with the use of continuous high-dose intravenous infusions of lorazepam for more than 48 hours. Propylene glycol, which is used as a solvent for intravenous medications including lorazepam, has been implicated as the cause of the hyperosmolar metabolic acidosis in this scenario [5]. It is important to understand that the presence of an osmolal gap that results from an ingested alcohol may only be detected when P_{Osm} is measured in the laboratory by freezing-point depression [6]. In addition, after the alcohol is metabolized, the osmolal gap may disappear.

Toluene (present in glue and metabolized to hippuric acid) is a rare cause of metabolic acidosis. The AG rises early and then returns toward normal, because hippurate is excreted by the kidneys, a process that is similar to the renal handling of ketones (see previous discussion).

Rarely, acetaminophen administration in therapeutic doses can lead to an elevated AG metabolic acidosis in metabolically stressed individuals, including pregnant women. In this setting, reduced glutathione stores permit the generation of pyroglutamic acid (5-oxoproline) [7].

Metabolic Acidosis with a Normal Anion Gap

Metabolic acidosis with a normal AG, which may also be called a *hyperchloremic acidosis*, is associated with the conditions listed in Table 198.2. The decrement in the plasma HCO_3^- concentration is matched by a rise in the plasma Cl^- level, maintaining electroneutrality.

Acid and Chloride Administration

The infusion of amino acid solutions during hyperalimentation is an abundant source of hydrochloric acid (HCl). The development of a metabolic acidosis is more common in patients with renal insufficiency.

Oral administration of cholestyramine chloride reportedly occasionally also causes acidemia. This resin, which is sometimes used in the management of hypercholesterolemia, is nonresorbable and can act as an anion-exchange resin, exchanging its Cl^- for endogenous HCO_3^- and producing a metabolic acidosis. Sevelamer hydrochloride, a compound used as a phosphorous binder in chronic kidney disease, has been associated with lower bicarbonate levels than in those patients treated with calcium-based binders. The mechanism of the metabolic acidosis is believed to be similar to cholestyramine [8].

TABLE 198.2

Causes of Metabolic Acidosis with a Normal Anion Gap

- Acid administration
  - Hyperalimentation with HCl-containing amino acid solutions
- Bicarbonate losses
  - Gastrointestinal
    - Diarrhea
    - Pancreatic or biliary drainage
    - Cholestyramine and sevelamer hydrochloride
    - Urinary diversions (ureterosigmoidostomy)
  - Renal
    - Proximal (type 2) renal tubular acidosis
    - Ketoacidosis (particularly during therapy)
    - Postchronic hypocapnia
- Impaired renal acid excretion
  - With hypokalemia
    - Classic distal (type 1) renal tubular acidosis
  - With hyperkalemia
    - Hyperkalemic distal renal tubular acidosis
    - Hypoaldosteronism (type 4 renal tubular acidosis)
- Reduced renal perfusion

Bicarbonate Losses

Loss of HCO_3^- from the gastrointestinal tract or kidneys can lead to a reduction in the plasma HCO_3^- level. Bowel contents are alkaline compared to blood because HCO_3^- is added by pancreatic and biliary secretions. Most of the secreted alkali is reclaimed by as HCO_3^- is exchanged for Cl^- in the ileum and colon. Gastrointestinal losses of HCO_3^- are most commonly observed in patients with diarrhea so severe that colonic transit time is too rapid for alkali reabsorption. At times, the resulting HCO_3^- losses can approach 40 mEq per L of stool. Less frequently, metabolic acidosis from HCO_3^- depletion is a result of pancreatic fistulae, biliary drainage, or a ureterosigmoidostomy. In the last circumstance, the excretion of acid (as NH_4Cl) urine directly into the colon permits the exchange of HCl for HCO_3^- because the colon is permeable to H^+ and Cl^-, unlike the urinary bladder. This problem does not usually occur with an ileal bladder.

Pancreatic HCO_3^- losses are also observed in essentially all patients with a pancreatic allograft anastomosed directly to the urinary bladder. Bicarbonate secreted into the bladder cannot be reabsorbed.

Renal tubular acidosis (RTA) can be classified as type 1 (distal), type 2 (proximal), and type 4 (hypoaldosteronism). Type 3 refers to what is now considered to be an infantile variant of type 1; therefore, type 3 RTA is a term not generally applied to adults. Renal bicarbonate losses can cause or contribute to acidemia in type 2 (proximal) RTA (Table 198.2), during recovery from ketoacidosis (see previous discussion), and for patients who are posthypocapnia. For patients with proximal RTA (Table 198.3),

TABLE 198.3

Some Causes of Types 1 and 2 RTA

Distal (type 1) RTA	Proximal (type 2) RTA
Idiopathic	Hereditary disorders
Genetic	Cystinosis
Familial	Wilson's disease[c]
Marfan's syndrome	Glycogen storage disease, type 1
Ehlers–Danlos syndrome	Acquired disorders
Disorders of calcium metabolism	Multiple myeloma[c]
Idiopathic hypercalciuria	Primary hyperparathyroidism
Hypergammaglobulinemic states	Toxins and drugs
Amyloidosis[a]	Lead
Cryoglobulinemia	Cadmium
Drugs and toxins	Mercury
Amphotericin B	Copper (Wilson's disease)[c]
Lithium carbonate	Carbonic anhydrase inhibitors
Toluene[b]	Topiramate
Autoimmune diseases	
Sjögren's syndrome[a]	
Thyroiditis	
Chronic active hepatitis	
Primary biliary cirrhosis	
Miscellaneous	
Cirrhosis	
Medullary sponge kidney	
Associated with hyperkalemia	
Urinary tract obstruction	
Sickle cell anemia	
Systemic lupus erythematosus	
Renal transplant rejection[a]	

[a]Also may cause proximal RTA.
[b]Metabolism to hippuric acid may cause the anion gap to increase.
[c]Also may cause distal RTA.
RTA, renal tubular acidosis.

the normal reabsorptive threshold for HCO_3^- is reduced. As a result, HCO_3^- can no longer be reabsorbed at a rate adequate to maintain the normal plasma level of approximately 25 mEq per L. As a consequence, the urine pH is initially alkaline (>5.3), and the fractional excretion of HCO_3^- is elevated (>15% of the filtered load, with normal <3%). However, HCO_3^- wasting ceases, and the urine becomes acidic (pH <5.3) once the plasma HCO_3^- concentration drops below the new (lower) HCO_3^- reabsorptive threshold. This process explains why the urine pH may be high or low in proximal RTA.

Renal HCO_3^- losses also occur as compensation for chronic respiratory alkalosis (chronic hypocapnia). During chronic hyperventilation, the blood pH increases as the PCO_2 decreases. As can be seen in Figure 198.1, an increase in intracellular pH diminishes H^+ excretion, thereby leading to a concomitant decrease in HCO_3^- reabsorption. These changes cause the plasma HCO_3^- concentration to fall, partially compensating for the alkalemia. If the stimulus for hyperventilation (e.g., hypoxemia) is suddenly eliminated, the PCO_2 rapidly returns to normal. Renal compensation, by comparison, continues for 1 to 2 more days, causing a persistent reduction in the plasma HCO_3^- concentration. The resulting posthypocapnic metabolic acidosis normally resolves spontaneously.

Reduced Renal H^+ Excretion

Reduced renal acid excretion can be observed in four conditions: chronic kidney disease, type 1 (distal) RTA (Table 198.3), type 4 RTA (hypoaldosteronism), and states of reduced renal perfusion. The acidosis of chronic kidney disease is primarily caused by a reduction in ammonia production. Patients with chronic renal insufficiency have a substantial decline in the number of functioning nephrons. Nephrons that continue to filter, however, characteristically have filtration rates and acid excretion rates per nephron that are above normal. Impaired acid excretion in these patients occurs because the number of hyperfiltering nephrons is inadequate to compensate for those that are nonfunctioning. The AG is frequently normal in mild-to-moderate kidney disease (plasma creatinine < 3 mg per dL) because Cl^- replaces the HCO_3^- used to buffer the retained acid. At this time, the GFR is still high enough to permit the excretion of anions like phosphate, which contribute to the rise in AG as renal function declines further.

The classic form of type 1 (distal) RTA (Table 198.3) occurs when H^+ cannot be pumped into the tubule lumen by the intercalated cells of the collecting tubules. The result is that urine cannot be maximally acidified (urine pH is always ≥5.5). In addition to metabolic acidosis, hypokalemia is typically present. The K^+ deficit is caused, in part, by enhanced distal nephron Na–K exchange, a process that is necessary to maintain Na^+ balance because H^+ cannot be secreted in response to Na^+ reabsorption. Distal RTA may also result from a translocation of the bicarbonate–chloride exchanger from the peritubular to the luminal membrane, leading to secretion of bicarbonate into the collecting tubule lumen.

The most important clinical complication of distal RTA is the formation and deposition of calcium throughout the kidney (nephrocalcinosis). This process begins in the collecting tubules, where the urine is most concentrated, and is commonly accompanied by the formation of calcium phosphate calculi. The factors that may contribute to the renal stone disease in this disorder include hypercalciuria, because metabolic acidosis causes a release of bone calcium that can then be filtered and excreted; the alkaline urine pH, which predisposes to the precipitation of calcium phosphate crystals; and, most importantly, hypocitraturia. The reduction in urinary citrate is a direct result of the metabolic acidosis, which increases proximal tubular citrate reabsorption. Because calcium citrate is significantly more soluble than calcium phosphate, hypocitraturia facilitates the precipitation of calcium phosphate crystals in the tubular lumen. In comparison with distal RTA, stone formation is less common and less severe in patients with proximal RTA, possibly because a proportion of these patients may have the full Fanconi's syndrome, in which proximal tubular reabsorption of HCO_3^- and many other substances, including citrate, is impaired [9].

In addition to the classic form of type 1 (distal) RTA, in which hypokalemia is characteristic, a hyperkalemic variety has also been described. This disorder, as well as type 4 (hypoaldosteronism) RTA, is discussed in Chapter 199.

Clinical Signs and Symptoms of Metabolic Acidosis

Kussmaul's respirations on physical examination suggest the presence of metabolic acidosis. This unusual respiratory pattern reflects an increase in tidal volume rather than a rise in respiratory rate and is caused by stimulation of the respiratory center in the brainstem by the low blood pH. As acidemia becomes more severe, nausea and vomiting or mental status changes, including coma, may occur.

Secondary hypotension also may be observed in severely acidemic patients, the hypotension resulting from depressed myocardial contractility and arterial vasodilation. Although circulating catecholamines may initially counteract the adverse cardiovascular effects of acidemia, such compensation becomes insufficient as the blood pH falls below 7.20.

The plasma K^+ concentration may be altered by the degree of metabolic acidosis. Infusion of a mineral acid such as arginine HCl, for example, causes a prompt rise in the plasma K^+ concentration as K^+ moves out of cells in exchange for H^+. By comparison, a shift of K^+ is less likely to occur in those patients with metabolic acidosis caused by organic acids, such as lactic and ketoacidosis. The reason for this apparent difference is uncertain, but it may relate to the release of insulin by organic substrates (e.g., lactate), which would drive K^+ into cells.

Diagnosis

Metabolic acidosis is easily diagnosed by the presence of a low blood pH and plasma bicarbonate concentration. The detection of a widened AG can then be used to identify a specific cause for the disorder. The likelihood of identifying a specific acid(s) in a patient with a high AG acidosis increases as the width of the AG increases.

While patients may have a simple metabolic acidosis, many individuals have a concomitant respiratory or second metabolic acid–base disorder. To distinguish mixed from simple acid–base disorders, knowledge of the appropriate respiratory compensation as well as an understanding of the ratio of the increment in AG to decrement in plasma HCO_3^- concentration is useful.

Respiratory Compensation

Stimulation of the brainstem respiratory center by acidemia causes a fall in the PCO_2. In uncomplicated metabolic acidosis, the PCO_2 is expected to fall by 1.2 mm Hg for each 1 mEq per L decrease in the HCO_3^-. Alternatively, the PCO_2 can be estimated from the following equation:

$$\text{Expected } PCO_2 \text{ (mm Hg)} = [(1.5 \times HCO_3^-) + 8] \pm 2$$

A PCO_2 that is substantially different from the expected value indicates a superimposed respiratory acidosis or alkalosis. For example, if the plasma bicarbonate concentration was 10 mEq per L, the expected PCO_2 would be approximately 23 mm Hg $[(1.5 \times 10) + 8 = 23]$. A lower PCO_2 would indicate the presence of a concomitant respiratory alkalosis (as might be seen with a salicylate overdose), whereas a higher PCO_2 would signify a simultaneous respiratory acidosis. *This calculation is useful only in the evaluation of the respiratory response to metabolic acidosis and it is inaccurate when the plasma bicarbonate concentration is more than 20 mEq per L.*

By a quirk of mathematics, the last two digits of the pH equal the PCO_2 in moderate metabolic acidosis if respiratory compensation is appropriate. For example, the PCO_2 in a patient with a pH of 7.27 should be 27 mm Hg. A lower PCO_2 indicates a superimposed respiratory alkalosis, whereas a higher value signifies a primary respiratory acidosis. This approach is invalid for severe acidosis with pH approaching or below 7.00, given the limitations of respiratory compensation.

Change in Anion Gap to Change in Bicarbonate Concentration Ratio

In patients with a high AG metabolic acidosis, the identification of a second metabolic acid–base disorder (normal AG acidosis) can be made by comparing the change in the AG to the change in the plasma HCO_3^- concentration.

The elevation in AG is because of the increase in the unmeasured anions. However, there is not always a one-to-one relationship between the increase in AG (ΔAG) and the fall in plasma bicarbonate (ΔHCO_3^-) because some of the excess hydrogen ions are buffered by nonbicarbonate buffers (including intracellular proteins and bone) and the ΔAG, therefore, generally exceeds ΔHCO_3^-. In lactic acidosis, the $\Delta AG/\Delta HCO_3^-$ ratio averages approximately 1.4 to 1.6:1. In contrast, the $\Delta AG/\Delta HCO_3^-$ ratio averages approximately 1:1 in ketoacidosis caused by the loss of ketoacid anions in the urine which lowers the elevated AG without affecting the plasma HCO_3^- concentration. Patients with relatively normal renal function can lose large quantities of ketoacids in the urine and may have a $\Delta AG/\Delta HCO_3^-$ ratio below 1. In fact, the loss of ketoacid anions in the urine causes the frequent development of a hyperchloremic (normal AG) metabolic acidosis during the treatment (recovery phase) of diabetic ketoacidosis. In contrast, urinary anion loss is minimal in lactic acidosis because shock is typically associated with reduced urinary flow rate, and most of the lactate that is filtered can be reabsorbed by a specific sodium-L-lactate cotransporter in the luminal membrane of the proximal tubular cells. Thus, when the ΔAG is more than double the ΔHCO_3^-, a coexisting metabolic alkalosis and metabolic acidosis is likely. An example of this situation would be severe vomiting in a patient with ketoacidosis. A ΔAG less than the ΔHCO_3^- suggests concomitant high AG and normal AG metabolic acidosis as could occur in a patient with bicarbonate losses from diarrhea combined with lactic acidosis from hypotension.

Changes in the concentration of other unmeasured cations or anions in the plasma can also lead to miscalculation of the AG. As an example, hypoalbuminemia (decreased unmeasured anions) and severe hypercalcemia (increased unmeasured cations) can lower the AG. Thus, a patient with one or both of these disorders may have a baseline AG of 4 rather than 8 or 9 mEq per L. As a result, calculation of the $\Delta AG/\Delta HCO_3^-$ ratio is most accurate when the preacidosis AG is known.

Urinary Anion Gap

Another useful tool in the evaluation of a metabolic acidosis is the urinary AG (UAG). UAG is the difference between the sum of the urinary Na^+ and K^+ and the urinary Cl^-:

$$UAG = (Na^+ + K^+) - Cl^-$$

The most frequent use of the UAG is to identify the etiology of a normal AG metabolic acidosis with hypokalemia. The most common nonrenal cause is diarrhea, which provokes an appropriate increase in renal H^+ secretion. These additional H^+ ions are buffered in the urine by ammonia and excreted primarily as NH_4Cl. Because NH_4^+ is not measured in the calculation of the UAG, but Cl^- is, an increased rate of renal H^+ secretion causes the UAG to become a negative number. Conversely, the presence of a positive UAG in an individual with a non-AG metabolic acidosis suggests that the disorder is caused by impaired renal H^+ excretion (e.g., distal RTA). In this setting, impaired H^+ secretion leads to a fall in urinary Cl^- (which would be excreted as NH_4Cl) and a positive calculated UAG. It is important to note, however, that underlying renal insufficiency may also be associated with impaired NH_4Cl excretion owing to a limitation in ammonia synthesis; in these individuals, the UAG may remain positive even in the presence of diarrhea.

Treatment of Metabolic Acidosis

Treatment of metabolic acidosis must be directed at correction of acidemia as well as the cause of the acid–base disturbance. The likelihood that alkali administration is necessary and that it will be effective depends on the blood pH, compensatory mechanisms, and the underlying cause.

The degree of acidemia and hypobicarbonatemia should be evaluated before administering alkali. As a general rule, alkali therapy generally is not needed until the arterial blood pH drops below 7.15 to 7.20. An exception may occur when the plasma HCO_3^- concentration falls to less than 10 to 12 mEq per L, despite a blood pH of more than 7.15. Alkali administration is usually unnecessary if the acidosis is likely to resolve spontaneously (e.g., lactic acidosis after a grand mal seizure).

Alkali Administration

HCO_3^- therapy should be considered in patients with moderate-to-severe metabolic acidosis. However, depending on the etiology, the use of exogenous bicarbonate remains controversial. The initial goal of alkali therapy is to raise the arterial blood pH to 7.20, a typically safe level at which the patient is at less risk of cardiovascular compromise. The pH does not need to be corrected back to normal because the potential risks of HCO_3^- therapy (e.g., hypernatremia, hypercapnia, fluid overload, cerebrospinal fluid acidosis, and "overshoot" alkalosis) are likely to outweigh the benefits, as long as renal function (and therefore acid-excretory ability) is relatively intact.

The quantity of exogenous bicarbonate required to produce a change in pH is determined by estimating the total body HCO_3^- deficit. The apparent HCO_3^- space is about 50% of lean body weight in healthy subjects. In patients with more severe metabolic acidosis (plasma HCO_3^- concentration <10 mEq per L), cellular and bone buffering become more prominent owing to the marked reduction in the quantity of available extracellular buffer (primarily HCO_3^-). This preferential entry of H^+ into cells causes the HCO_3^- space to expand to approximately 70% of the lean body weight. The volume of distribution for bicarbonate (bicarbonate space) can be estimated by the following equation:

$$\text{Bicarbonate space} = (0.4 + [2.6/\{HCO_3^-\}]) \times \text{lean body weight (in kg)}$$

These are only rough guidelines and cannot replace ongoing monitoring of serum bicarbonate level and arterial pH during the correction phase. Furthermore, if there is continuing alkali loss from diarrhea, then the HCO_3^- requirements are substantially increased because the apparent volume of distribution of HCO_3^- is much greater than 70% of body weight in this setting.

Treatment of Specific Causes of Metabolic Acidosis

Renal Disease. Treatment of the metabolic acidosis of renal dysfunction depends on the clinical manifestations and the severity of the acidosis. Most individuals with acute kidney injury can be managed with dialysis or using the guidelines for alkali administration listed previously. There is some recent data suggesting that alkali therapy can slow down the rate of decline in chronic kidney disease and reduce mortality in this setting [10].

Ketoacidosis. While correction of volume depletion is an essential part of initial management of patients with diabetic ketoacidosis, the utility of intensive fluid administration may be limited after the intravascular volume has been restored because volume expansion then leads to the excretion of ketone anions in the urine. Moreover, excessive expansion of the plasma volume reduces proximal tubular HCO_3^- reabsorption, in part, by reducing Na–H exchange. The net effect is normalization of the AG without a significant increase in the plasma HCO_3^- concentration. In this setting, spontaneous correction of the metabolic acidosis requires regeneration of new bicarbonate by the kidney (a process that may take several days), in contrast to the rapid increase in HCO_3^- that occurs when ketone anions are metabolized back to HCO_3^- in the liver as insulin is given. Consequently, fluid administration should be tempered after intravascular volume compromise has been corrected.

Alkali administration is not usually necessary for patients with ketoacidosis. There appears to be no difference in mortality between patients treated with $NaHCO_3$ and controls [11]. Insulin therapy should raise the plasma HCO_3^- concentration because ketone anions are metabolized. Patients who may benefit from cautious alkali therapy include those with severe acidemia and cardiovascular compromise and those with a normal AG acidosis. As already discussed, the latter condition pertains to those who have sustained major urinary losses of ketones, rendering them depleted of potential bicarbonate substrate.

Lactic Acidosis. Correction of any predisposing disorder is the primary therapy for lactic acidosis. Reversal of circulatory failure, hypoxemia, or sepsis reduces the rate of lactate production and enhances its removal.

The benefit of $NaHCO_3$ in the treatment of lactic acidosis remains unproven [11]. The potential benefits of alkali administration principally involve the maintenance of normal cardiovascular homeostasis through correction of acidosis. This potential advantage must be weighed against possible deleterious effects, such as volume overload, hypernatremia, and overshoot alkalosis, after restoration of tissue perfusion. As a result of these potential problems, no concrete recommendations can be made regarding alkali therapy in lactic acidosis. One approach might be to administer HCO_3^- to maintain the arterial blood pH above 7.15 to 7.20 and the plasma HCO_3^- concentration above 10 to 12 mEq per L, as suggested previously (see "Alkali Administration" section). However, if the lactate level increases without a significant improvement in clinical status or blood pH, the benefit of continuing alkali administration should be questioned. It appears that correction of the underlying cause of lactic acidosis is the most important goal, because measures to raise the bicarbonate level without a fall in lactate have not been associated with a reduction in mortality. These findings are consistent with the hypothesis that the high mortality in lactic acidosis results from the underlying disorder causing the acidosis, but not from the acidemia per se.

Drug and Toxin Ingestions. The treatment of toxins and ingestions is discussed in Section on Pharmacology, Overdoses, and Poisonings.

Renal Tubular Acidosis. The acidemia of type 1 (distal) RTA can be corrected with HCO_3^- or a precursor such as citrate. The usual requirement is 1 to 3 mEq/kg/d, which should be sufficient to buffer that fraction of the daily acid load (50 to 100 mEq per day) that is not being excreted. In general, a potassium salt is administered (e.g., potassium citrate) because this repairs the K^+ deficit as well. Large doses of oral $NaHCO_3$ can cause gastrointestinal symptoms by generating CO_2 in the stomach. This problem can be minimized by the use of citrate, most of which is ultimately metabolized in the body to HCO_3^-. Solutions are available that contain 1 to 2 mEq per mL of sodium, potassium, or sodium and potassium citrate.

The initial step in the management of type 2 (proximal) RTA is to determine the presence of a treatable underlying disorder, such as vitamin D deficiency, multiple myeloma, or the use of a carbonic anhydrase inhibitor. Even if no specific therapy is available, correction of the acidemia may not be required in adults if the patient is asymptomatic and if there is only mild-to-moderate reduction in the plasma HCO_3^- concentration. In comparison, treatment is always indicated in young children because restoring acid–base balance can permit normal growth to resume.

The evaluation and treatment of the hyperkalemic form of distal RTA and of type 4 RTA (hypoaldosteronism), in which hyperkalemia is also present, can be found in Chapter 199.

METABOLIC ALKALOSIS

Primary metabolic alkalosis is characterized by an elevated plasma HCO_3^- concentration in the presence of an arterial pH above 7.40. Hyperbicarbonatemia may represent an appropriate response to chronic respiratory acidosis, which can be easily diagnosed by measurement of the arterial blood pH.

Pathophysiology and Etiology

There are two steps involved in the development of metabolic alkalosis. The factors that generate alkalosis may differ from those that maintain it. A primary rise in the plasma HCO_3^- concentration can be induced by several mechanisms: (a) loss of acid from the gastrointestinal tract or in the urine, (b) administration of HCO_3^- or a precursor such as citrate, or (c) loss of fluid with a Cl^- to HCO_3^- ratio that is higher than that of plasma. The third condition is sometimes referred to as *contraction alkalosis* because the total HCO_3^- content remains relatively unchanged while the extracellular fluid volume "contracts around it," thereby elevating the HCO_3^- concentration. In contrast to the first two mechanisms, contraction alkalosis is rarely responsible for more than a mild increase in the plasma HCO_3^- concentration. Loss of fluid with an electrolyte composition similar to that of plasma, as might occur with hemorrhage, does not result in a contraction alkalosis because HCO_3^- is lost proportionately to the other molecular components of plasma.

The excess in HCO_3^- generated by any of these processes should be rapidly excreted in the urine. The maintenance of a metabolic alkalosis, therefore, indicates an impairment of renal HCO_3^- excretion. The most common hindrances to renal disposal of bicarbonate are volume and potassium depletion.

Under ordinary conditions, HCO_3^- appears in the urine when the plasma level rises above the normal value of approximately 25 mEq per L. In the presence of volume depletion, however, the capacity of the proximal tubule to reabsorb HCO_3^- increases, allowing the plasma HCO_3^- level to rise without triggering bicarbonaturia. Several mechanisms account for these changes, including stimulation of luminal Na–H countertransport (Fig. 198.1) by angiotensin II, generated in response to volume contraction. Most hypovolemic states are associated with Cl^- depletion. Because tubular luminal Cl^- appears to be important in distal nephron Cl^-–HCO_3^- exchange, it is not surprising that correction of the metabolic alkalosis usually requires Cl^- repletion as well. In comparison, giving Cl^- may be ineffective when primary or secondary hyperaldosteronism, severe hypokalemia, or renal insufficiency is responsible for the defect in HCO_3^- excretion. The cause of a metabolic alkalosis can usually be identified by how readily it responds to administration of Cl^- (see "Diagnosis" section). The effect of hypokalemia in the maintenance of metabolic alkalosis is discussed later in this chapter.

Alkali Administration

Because administered HCO_3^- is normally excreted rapidly in the urine, alkali administration must be massive, or renal impairment must limit the excretion of HCO_3^- if metabolic alkalosis is to develop. Milk-alkali syndrome is an uncommon disorder characterized by hypercalcemia and metabolic alkalosis. The chronic ingestion of milk and calcium carbonate–containing antacids can lead to the development of metabolic alkalosis when the increased HCO_3^- load cannot be excreted as a result of renal impairment from chronic hypercalcemia. This condition is now rarely seen, probably because nonabsorbable antacids, proton-pump inhibitors, and H_2-blockers have largely supplanted the use of large quantities of baking soda and milk as treatment of gastritis and peptic ulcer disease.

Chloride-Responsive Metabolic Alkalosis

Generation of Chloride-Responsive Metabolic Alkalosis. The two most common causes of metabolic alkalosis are diuretic therapy and loss of gastric secretions (resulting from nasogastric suction or vomiting) (Table 198.4). Thiazide and loop diuretics can induce H^+ loss from increased distal Na^+ presentation in the presence of elevated aldosterone levels, which causes enhanced distal nephron Na–H exchange. Hydrogen secretion in this nephron segment is associated with increased HCO_3^- generation. The proximal tubule may also play an important role because stimulation of the renin–angiotensin system by volume depletion enhances the activity of the Na–H antiporter, thereby increasing H^+ secretion and HCO_3^- reabsorption. To the degree that the urinary anion losses represent primarily Cl^-, a component of contraction alkalosis may also occur.

Although volume contraction may contribute to the metabolic alkalosis caused by vomiting and nasogastric suction, and occasionally with intestinal Cl^- wasting, gastric H^+ losses are primarily responsible for the generation of metabolic alkalosis in this setting. Secretion of gastric acid results in the retention of 1 mEq of HCO_3^- for each milliequivalent of H^+ that is secreted because both of the ions are derived from the intracellular dissociation of carbonic acid:

$$H_2CO_3 \rightarrow HCO_3^- + H^+$$

This process does not normally lead to metabolic alkalosis because the 80 to 200 mEq of HCl secreted by the stomach each day enters the duodenum, where it stimulates an equivalent amount of HCO_3^- secretion from the pancreas. By comparison, when vomiting or nasogastric suctioning occurs, the H^+ secreted by the stomach never reaches the duodenum and, therefore,

TABLE 198.4

Major Causes of Metabolic Alkalosis

Hydrogen loss		
	Gastrointestinal	
		Loss of gastric secretions (vomiting or nasogastric suction)[a]
		Chloride-losing diarrheal states
	Renal	
		Loop or thiazide-type diuretic[a]
		Mineralocorticoid excess[a]
		Postchronic hypercapnia
		Hypercalcemia[b]
		High-dose intravenous penicillins
		Bartter's and Gitelman's syndromes
Bicarbonate retention		
	Massive blood transfusion	
	Administration of large amounts of $NaHCO_3$	
	Milk-alkali syndrome	
Contraction alkalosis		
	Diuretics[a]	
		Loss of high chloride/low bicarbonate gastrointestinal secretions[a] (vomiting and some diarrheal states)
Hydrogen movement into cells		
	Hypokalemia	
	Refeeding	

[a]Most common causes.
[b]Primary hyperparathyroidism is frequently associated with a mild metabolic acidosis (see text for details).

cannot induce pancreatic HCO_3^- secretion. Hence, there is a net retention of HCO_3^-. As in diuretic use, distal nephron Na–H exchange also contributes to the development of this disorder because aldosterone levels are stimulated by the loss of extracellular volume.

Metabolic alkalosis may also be observed after the rapid correction of chronic respiratory acidosis. This *posthypercapnic metabolic alkalosis* occurs because chronic respiratory acidosis activates compensatory renal mechanisms that induce HCl loss in the urine; the ensuing rise in the plasma HCO_3^- concentration is appropriate in that it returns the arterial pH toward normal. The plasma HCO_3^- generally increases by approximately 3.5 mEq per L for every 10 mm Hg rise in the arterial PCO_2. If hypercapnia is rapidly reversed, however (most frequently by artificial ventilation), the excess HCO_3^- that has been generated may persist, and alkalemia ensues.

Maintenance of Chloride-Responsive Metabolic Alkalosis. As reviewed previously, renal excretion of HCO_3^- normally begins when the plasma level exceeds 25 mEq per L. The normal kidney can excrete large quantities (>1,000 mEq per L) without a substantial increase in the plasma HCO_3^- concentration. As a result, maintenance of a Cl^--responsive alkalosis implies a reduction in renal HCO_3^- excretion. Reduced GFR and, more importantly, enhanced proximal tubular $NaHCO_3$ reabsorption limit HCO_3^- excretion, allowing the increase in plasma HCO_3^- to persist. Normally, Cl^- is the major anion reabsorbed with Na^+. In states of Cl^- depletion, as occurs in Cl^--responsive metabolic alkalosis, however, Na^+ must be reabsorbed with the next most abundant anion, HCO_3^-. Consequently, the need to preserve volume prevents correction of the alkalosis.

Hypokalemia also promotes renal HCO_3^- reabsorption and contributes to the maintenance of metabolic alkalosis. K^+ losses frequently occur with diuretic administration or gastric acid losses. If the plasma HCO_3^- concentration exceeds the reabsorptive capacity of the proximal renal tubule, the resultant bicarbonaturia obligates excretion of a cation (e.g., Na^+). Some of the Na^+ leaving the proximal tubule with HCO_3^- is then reabsorbed distally in exchange for K^+. These urinary K^+ losses are primarily responsible for the hypokalemia seen with vomiting; gastric K^+ losses are usually less important because these secretions have a K^+ concentration of less than 10 mEq per L. As a result of K^+ depletion, relative intracellular acidosis occurs as H^+ shifts into cells to maintain electroneutrality as K^+ moves extracellularly in response to hypokalemia. Ultimately, this intracellular acidosis stimulates proximal tubular Na–H exchange, which further reduces renal HCO_3^- excretion (Fig. 198.1).

Chloride-Resistant Metabolic Alkalosis

Metabolic alkalosis in some individuals is not responsive to the administration of Cl^--containing solutions. In these disorders, a primary increase in mineralocorticoid activity, potassium depletion, or disorders of renal tubular Cl^- wasting (Bartter's and Gitelman's syndromes) are usually responsible for the generation and maintenance of the alkalosis. In all of these circumstances, there is enhanced renal H^+ excretion and HCO_3^- reabsorption. Either there is no Cl^- depletion or there is an inability to reabsorb Cl^- explaining why NaCl and KCl do not correct the metabolic alkalosis in these individuals. Edematous states, such as congestive heart failure and cirrhosis, are also generally unresponsive to volume (and Cl^-) replacement, despite the reduction in effective arterial blood volume.

Mineralocorticoid Excess. Mineralocorticoids, such as aldosterone, act in the cortical collecting tubule (see Chapter 72), where they enhance Na–K exchange as well as H^+ secretion. As a result, overproduction of an endogenous mineralocorticoid (as occurs in primary aldosteronism) or with the ingestion of a substance that can increase the mineralocorticoid activity of cortisol (e.g., glycyrrhizic acid in licorice) leads to hypokalemia and metabolic alkalosis. Hypertension is characteristically present in these disorders. In contrast to patients with secondary increases in mineralocorticoid activity (e.g., as in congestive heart failure), edema does not occur. This phenomenon, called *aldosterone escape*, results at least in part from the high renal interstitial pressures generated by the hypertension that limits further NaCl reabsorption; it is also possible that atrial natriuretic peptide, released in response to volume expansion, contributes to this phenomenon.

In addition to the direct effect of aldosterone on H^+ secretion, hypokalemia also appears to be necessary for the maintenance of a significant metabolic alkalosis in patients with primary mineralocorticoid excess. The mechanism of this effect involves the development of intracellular acidosis with increased H^+ secretion and HCO_3^- reabsorption by the proximal tubule and enhanced distal nephron Na–H exchange.

Severe Hypokalemia. The effect of mild-to-moderate hypokalemia on the generation and maintenance of metabolic alkalosis has been discussed. Severe hypokalemia (plasma $K^+ < 2$ mEq per L) can additionally impair distal Cl^- reabsorption by an unknown mechanism. In this setting, some of the Na^+ that is normally reabsorbed with Cl^- must be reabsorbed in exchange for H^+.

Bartter's and Gitelman's Syndromes. Bartter's syndrome is a rare cause of metabolic alkalosis typically seen in children and young adults. The loop of Henle appears to be the site responsible for this disorder. Metabolic alkalosis is also present in patients with Gitelman's syndrome, in which the defect occurs in the thiazide-sensitive site of the distal tubule. In contrast to patients with primary aldosteronism, patients with Bartter's and Gitelman's syndromes are normotensive or slightly hypotensive.

The associated volume depletion causes chronic activation of the renin–angiotensin–aldosterone system, increasing distal nephron K^+ and H^+ secretion, as in patients receiving to a loop or thiazide diuretic.

Clinical Manifestations

Most patients with metabolic alkalosis do not suffer clinically from the effects of alkalemia [12]. When symptoms are present, they are typically those associated with volume depletion (e.g., weakness, muscle cramps, postural dizziness) or hypokalemia (e.g., muscle weakness, polyuria, polydipsia). The usual symptoms of alkalemia are because of increased neuromuscular excitability and are exhibited as paresthesias, carpopedal spasm, or lightheadedness, although these findings are relatively more common in patients with acute respiratory alkalosis.

Diagnosis

The cause of metabolic alkalosis can usually be elicited from the history and physical examination. One of the most important aspects of the physical examination in identifying a cause is the determination of blood pressure. Except for the hypertensive individual taking a diuretic, hypokalemia in the presence of metabolic alkalosis and hypertension should suggest the presence of a primary mineralocorticoid-induced disease, such as hyperaldosteronism. Normotensive individuals with no obvious cause most often have surreptitious vomiting or diuretic ingestion (*pseudo-Bartter's syndrome*) as the precipitating event; Bartter's and Gitelman's syndromes are much rarer.

The urinary Cl^- concentration is important because urinary Na^+ wasting may occur in the presence of a high plasma HCO_3^- concentration even if volume depletion is present. $NaHCO_3^-$ losses develop when the plasma HCO_3^- level exceeds the renal reabsorptive threshold, a condition that obligates the excretion of HCO_3^- with a cation to maintain electroneutrality. The most abundant cation in the filtrate is Na^+, even in low perfusion states. As a result, the urine Na^+ concentration should not be used to infer the volume status of an individual with an increased plasma HCO_3^- concentration, unless it is less than 20 mEq per L. By comparison, the urinary Cl^- concentration characteristically is low in hypoperfusion states because Cl^- is not affected by bicarbonaturia.

Measurement of the urinary Cl^- concentration is useful in differentiating these disorders (Table 198.5). The urinary Cl^- concentration is typically less than 15 mEq per L, with hypovolemia caused by vomiting or diuretic therapy (if the effect of the diuretic has worn off). Higher values are found if the diuretic is still in effect, if Bartter's or Gitelman's syndromes or severe hypokalemia are present, or if there is primary mineralocorticoid excess (e.g., primary aldosteronism). Diuretic abuse may be distinguished from Bartter's or Gitelman's syndromes in some cases by screening the urine for diuretics.

TABLE 198.5

Urine Chloride Concentration in Metabolic Alkalosis

Less than 15 mEq/L	Greater than 20 mEq/L
Vomiting	Mineralocorticoid excess
Nasogastric suction	Alkali loading
Postdiuretic administration	During diuretic administration
Posthypercapnia	Severe hypokalemia
High-dose penicillin therapy	Bartter's and Gitelman's syndromes
Alkali loading[a]	

[a]Because the maintenance of metabolic alkalosis requires impairment of renal bicarbonate excretion, the pathophysiology of the renal limitation determines the urinary chloride concentration. If, for example, there is underlying hypovolemia, the urinary chloride concentration is low (<15 mEq/L); in comparison, the urinary chloride concentration is >20 mEq/L when the cause of renal bicarbonate retention is a reduction in glomerular filtration rate, as in the milk-alkali syndrome, or in patients with acute tubular necrosis who received large alkali loads.

Mixed Acid–Base Disturbances with Metabolic Alkalosis

Respiratory Compensation. The increased arterial pH in metabolic alkalosis leads to a compensatory rise in the PCO_2. This decrease in respiration is owing to direct suppression of the medullary respiratory center by alkalemia. In general, the PCO_2 rises approximately 0.7 mm Hg for every 1 mEq per L elevation in the plasma HCO_3^- concentration [14], a relationship that pertains until PCO_2 rises to approximately 60 mm Hg (corresponding to a plasma HCO_3^- concentration = 53 mEq per L); values above this level are unusual because further hypoventilation is limited by the development of hypoxemia. The identification of a PCO_2 greater or less than predicted suggests the presence of a second primary acid–base disturbance, respiratory acidosis or respiratory alkalosis, respectively.

Metabolic Alkalosis with Metabolic Acidosis. As previously discussed, the ratio of the increment in AG to decrement in the plasma HCO_3^- concentration ($\Delta AG/\Delta HCO_3^-$) can be used to identify the presence of a metabolic alkalosis in a patient with metabolic acidosis. In such cases, the increment in the serum AG is more than twofold greater in magnitude than the apparent fall in the bicarbonate level.

Treatment of Metabolic Alkalosis

Rapid correction of metabolic alkalosis is usually not necessary because of the general rarity of adverse effects directly related to the rise in pH. As a result, there is ordinarily time to identify the cause of the disorder and to institute specific therapy. Any exogenous sources of alkali (e.g., preparations containing HCO_3^-, acetate, lactate, or citrate) should be discontinued.

Because hypomagnesemia may be present in some patients with metabolic alkalosis, a serum magnesium level should be checked, particularly in patients with refractory hypokalemia, because hypomagnesemia predisposes to renal potassium wasting.

Chloride-Responsive Metabolic Alkalosis

Chloride replacement (as NaCl or KCl or both) is appropriate for management of most individuals with a low urinary Cl^- concentration. Administration of Cl^--containing fluid with K^+ ameliorates the alkalosis by permitting renal excretion of the excess HCO_3^-. It allows more Na^+ to be reabsorbed with Cl^-, rather than in exchange for H^+; it reduces the volume stimulus for Na^+ retention, permitting HCO_3^- excretion in the urine; and it increases the plasma K^+ concentration, which raises the tubular cell pH and reduces renal H^+ secretion. Replacement of the volume deficit with non–Cl^--containing solutions of Na^+ or K^+ does not correct the alkalosis or hypokalemia because non-Cl^- anions obligate further K^+ and H^+ excretion. Patients with vomiting or nasogastric suction may also benefit from H_2-blockers or other medications that reduce gastric acid secretion. They are not, however, substitutes for Cl^- replacement, which is still necessary to correct the already present chloride deficit.

The therapy of metabolic alkalosis in edematous patients (e.g., those with congestive heart failure and advanced liver disease) is more difficult. Although renal perfusion is characteristically reduced, leading to a low urinary Cl^- concentration, Cl^- administration (e.g., as 0.9% saline) does not enhance HCO_3^- excretion because the reduced effective arterial blood volume is not corrected by this therapy. In this setting, the carbonic anhydrase inhibitor acetazolamide (at a dose of 250 to 500 mg once- or twice-daily orally or intravenously) may be useful because it permits fluid mobilization while decreasing HCO_3^- reabsorption in the proximal tubule. An adverse consequence of acetazolamide administration is the tendency for more K^+ wasting. Careful monitoring of the plasma K^+ concentration is necessary. When the plasma K^+ level is low, the use of a distally acting K^+-sparing diuretic (e.g., amiloride or spironolactone) can be considered.

In extremely rare instances, these maneuvers may be insufficient, or the metabolic alkalosis may be so severe that adverse neurologic symptoms of alkalemia are present. In such instances, HCl can be given intravenously to lower the plasma HCO_3^- concentration. HCl is usually given as a solution isotonic to plasma (150 mEq H^+ and 150 mEq Cl^- in each liter of distilled H_2O). The volume needed to reduce the plasma HCO_3^- concentration can be estimated from calculation of the HCO_3^- excess. Because the volume of distribution of HCO_3^- is approximately 50% of the lean body weight, the amount of HCl needed to lower the plasma HCO_3^- concentration from 45 to 35 mEq per L in a 70-kg man can be calculated as follows (assuming there are no ongoing HCO_3^- losses):

$$HCO_3^- \text{ excess} = 0.5 \times 70 \text{ L} \times (45 - 35 \text{ mEq/L}) = 350 \text{ mEq}$$

This would require administration of slightly more than 2 L of an isotonic HCl solution. Because the very low pH of this solution can injure small veins and tissues, particularly if extravasation occurs, administration should generally occur over at least 24 hours using a large (central) vein. As a result, the administration of HCl may outweigh the potential benefits.

Dialytic therapy may be helpful in the unusual patient presenting with metabolic alkalosis, volume overload, and renal failure. Peritoneal dialysis typically contains lactate as the HCO_3^- precursor at a concentration of approximately 40 mEq per L, an amount that may worsen the alkalosis. By comparison, the alkali level can be adjusted with most current hemodialysis machines. It is important to note that citrate used for anticoagulation in some continuous dialytic therapies can lead to metabolic alkalosis as well [13].

Chloride-Resistant Metabolic Alkalosis

Individuals with a urinary chloride concentration greater than 15 mEq per L are unlikely to respond to Cl^--containing solutions such as physiologic saline, with correction of the metabolic alkalosis. Because the effective renal blood flow is already normal or Cl^- reabsorption must be impaired, the administered Cl^- is rapidly excreted in the urine. Moreover, enhanced distal Na^+ presentation increases Na–K exchange, leading to a rise in urinary K^+ excretion with more severe hypokalemia in states of primary mineralocorticoid excess.

In a hypertensive patient, primary aldosteronism should be considered. Removing the source of aldosterone (by adrenalectomy when an aldosterone-secreting adenoma is present) or blocking its action (with a K^+-sparing diuretic, such as spironolactone) is usually sufficient to correct the hypokalemia and metabolic alkalosis and to control hypertension in this disorder.

The abnormality in Bartter's and Gitelman's syndromes, impaired Cl^- reabsorption, cannot be corrected with treatment. Therapy is, therefore, directed at improving the laboratory abnormalities, particularly hypokalemia and metabolic alkalosis. Nonsteroidal anti-inflammatory drugs (including cyclooxygenase-2 inhibitors) reduce renin secretion (a prostaglandin-dependent process) and may be effective in correcting the plasma HCO_3^- and K^+ levels to or near normal, although K^+ supplementation may also be required. Angiotensin-converting enzyme inhibitors or K^+-sparing diuretics may be useful alone or in combination, but they have the potential risk of causing the already slightly low blood pressure to fall. It is important to exclude surreptitious diuretic use or forced vomiting in these individuals before assigning a diagnostic or therapeutic regimen used for Bartter's syndrome or Gitelman's syndrome because the former are far more common disorders.

References

1. Kraut JA, Madias NE: Serum anion gap: its uses and limitations in clinical medicine. *Clin J Am Soc Nephrol* 2:162, 2007.
2. Nyirenda MJ, Sandeep T, Grant I, et al: Severe acidosis in patients taking metformin-rapid reversal and survival despite high APACHE score. *Diabet Med* 23:432, 2006.
3. Uribarri J, Oh MS, Carroll, HJ: D-Lactic acidosis. A review of clinical presentation, biochemical features, and pathophysiologic mechanisms. *Medicine* 77:73, 1998.
4. Purssell RA, Pudek M, Brubacher J, et al: Derivation and validation of a formula to calculate the contribution of ethanol to the osmolal gap. *Ann Emerg Med.* 38(6):653, 2001.
5. Arroliga AC, Shehab N, McCarthy K, et al: Relationship of continuous infusion lorazepam to serum propylene glycol concentration in critically ill adults. *Crit Care Med* 32:1709, 2004.
6. Sweeney TE, Beuchat CA: Limitations of methods of osmometry: measuring the osmolality of body fluids. *Am J Physiol* 264:R469, 1993.
7. Fenves AZ, Kirkpatrick HM, Patel VV, et al: Increased anion gap metabolic acidosis as a result of 5-oxoproline (pyroglutamic acid): a role for acetaminophen. *Clin J Am Soc Nephrol* 1:441, 2006.
8. Brezina B, Qunibi W, Nolan CR: Acid loading during treatment with sevelamer hydrochloride: mechanisms and clinical implications. *Kidney Int* 66:S-39, 2004.
9. Messiaen T, Deret S, Mougenot B, et al: Adult Fanconi syndrome secondary to light chain gammopathy. *Medicine* 79:135, 2000.
10. de Brito-Ashurst I, Varagunam M, Raftery MJ, et al: Bicarbonate supplementation slows progression of CKD and improves nutritional status. *J Am Soc Nephrol* 20(9):2075, 2009.
11. Kraut JA, Kurtz I: Use of base in the treatment of severe acidemic states. *Am J Kidney Dis* 38:703, 2001.
12. Galla JH: Metabolic alkalosis. *J Am Soc Nephrol* 11:369, 2000.
13. Gupta M, Wadhwa NK, Bukovsky R, et al: Regional citrate for continuous venovenous hemodiafiltration using calcium-containing dialysate. *Am J Kidney Dis* 43:67, 2004.
14. Adrogue HJ, Madias NE: Secondary responses to altered acid-base status: the rules of engagement. *J Am Soc Nephrol* 21(6):920-923, 2010.

Chapter 199 ■ Disorders of Plasma Sodium and Plasma Potassium

ROBERT M. BLACK • GARY O. NOROIAN

DISORDERS OF PLASMA SODIUM

Hyponatremia and hypernatremia are conditions commonly observed in the intensive care unit. They are defined as plasma Na^+ concentration below 135 mEq per L and above 145 mEq per L, respectively. The correct management of patients with these disorders depends on an understanding of normal salt (NaCl) and water (H_2O) physiology.

It is important to appreciate that hyponatremia represents a disorder of water balance; the plasma sodium concentration reflects the ratio of water to sodium in the body. However, the presence of hyponatremia or hypernatremia cannot be used to assess the volume status of a patient. Furthermore, the plasma sodium concentration has little relationship to the urinary sodium concentration.

Hypothalamic osmoreceptors influence thirst and the release of antidiuretic hormone (ADH). The latter increases U_{Osm}, causing water retention by enhancing the permeability of the collecting tubules to water. ADH is also released in response to effective volume depletion (hypovolemia). Although water retention causes extracellular volume expansion, this is slight, as approximately two-thirds of the water enters the cells. As a result, volume-mediated ADH release can occur even in states of hyponatremia.

Relationship between Plasma Na^+ and Plasma Osmolality

The osmolality of plasma (P_{Osm}) is determined by the sum of the osmolar contributions of the individual osmotically active substances. In plasma, Na^+ salts, glucose, and urea (blood urea nitrogen [BUN]) are the major determinants of osmolality. Therefore, the P_{Osm} can be estimated by the following formula:

$$P_{Osm} \approx 2 \times \text{plasma } Na^+ + \text{glucose}/18.0 + \text{BUN}/2.8$$

Using this equation,[1] it is evident that the major determinant of the P_{Osm} in healthy individuals is the plasma Na^+ concentration.

The ability of a solute (such as sodium) to promote shifts of water between the intracellular and the extracellular compartments depends not only on its capacity to increase the P_{Osm} but also on its exclusion from one of these compartments. Because urea can cross almost all cell membranes readily, it cannot promote the movement of water between the intracellular and extracellular spaces. As such, urea is referred to as an *ineffective osmole*. A rise in the BUN is detected as an increase in the measured (by the laboratory) and calculated P_{Osm}, but there is no change in the plasma Na^+ concentration because urea does not obligate water movement from the intracellular to the extracellular space. Because urea is an ineffective osmole and because glucose normally contributes less than 8 mOsm per kg, the effective P_{Osm} correlates best with the plasma Na^+. Thus, effective P_{Osm} can be described as follows:

$$P_{Osm} \text{ (effective)} \approx 2 \times \text{plasma } Na^+ \text{ concentration}$$

Sodium is confined primarily to the extracellular fluid by the Na-K antiporter present in most cells. This pump also maintains a high (approximately 130 mEq per L) intracellular K^+ concentration; thus, potassium is the principal effective osmole inside cells. The ability of water to cross almost all cell membranes indicates that the P_{Osm} must be in equilibrium with the intracellular osmolality. In fact, osmolality is equal throughout all body compartments, explaining the need for only one osmoreceptor.

Because osmotic equilibrium exists throughout body water, calculation of water deficits or excesses, when dealing with a hyponatremic or hypernatremic individual, respectively, must be based on total body water (TBW) and not merely on the extracellular fluid volume. Moreover, loss of potassium from the body, as might occur with diuretic administration, affects the plasma Na^+ concentration.

Two processes participate in the reduction in plasma Na^+ concentration induced by potassium losses. Sodium movement into cells to maintain electroneutrality lowers the plasma Na^+, and loss of potassium from the gastrointestinal tract or kidneys causes a fall in the plasma potassium with a larger fall in the intracellular potassium. The result is a reduction in the intracellular osmolality that leads to water movement from cells to the extracellular compartment.

Finally, although plasma hypoosmolality is always associated with hyponatremia, a high P_{Osm} can occur in the absence of hypernatremia. Other ineffective osmoles (in addition to urea) have the ability to raise the measured P_{Osm} without affecting water shifts. The most important of these are the alcohols: ethanol, ethylene glycol, and methanol. By contrast, severe hyperglycemia can induce hyponatremia by pulling water out of cells, but the P_{Osm} will be elevated. This phenomenon, seen most often in diabetics, is referred to as *hyperosmolar hyponatremia*.

Regulation of Plasma Osmolality

Maintenance of the plasma Na^+ concentration within narrow limits (285 to 292 mOsm per kg) depends on the ability of the kidneys to excrete water and on a normal thirst mechanism with access to water. Under normal conditions, the quantity of water that can be excreted in the urine far exceeds the amount ingested.

Renal water excretion is determined by two factors: urinary solute excretion and the ability to generate maximally dilute urine (U_{Osm} <100 mOsm per kg). The typical American diet affords a solute intake between 600 and 1,200 mOsm—average 900 mOsm—per day. Assuming an output that approximates intake, the daily urinary solute excretion of a typical adult would also average 900 mOsm. Dietary NaCl, KCl, and protein, which is broken down to urea, make up most of this solute load. The individual who excretes 900 mOsm of solute per day and who can dilute urine maximally (down to 50 mOsm per kg) has the capacity to excrete up to 18 L of water in a 24-hour period:

$$900 \text{ mOsm}/50 \text{ mOsm/kg} = 18 \text{ L}$$

[1]The molecular weights of glucose and nitrogen are 180 and 14, respectively. As a result, the osmotic effect of glucose is determined by dividing by 18 (because the concentration is in 100 mL of plasma and not 1 L), whereas that of BUN is obtained by dividing by 2.8 (there are two nitrogens on each molecule of urea).

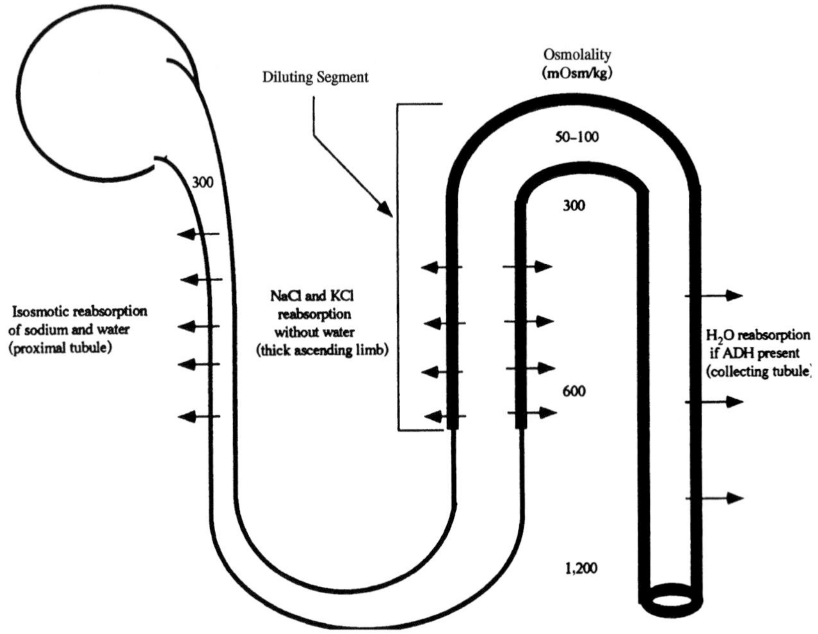

FIGURE 199.1 Excretion of a dilute urine. Solute entering the early proximal tubule has an osmolality identical to that of plasma; fluid is isotonically reabsorbed in this nephron segment. Separation of solute from water (H_2O) within the tubule begins in the thick ascending limb of Henle, which is impermeable to H_2O. Excretion of urine with a minimum osmolality of 50 to 100 mOsm per L requires intact function of this nephron segment as well as suppression of antidiuretic hormone (ADH) release. (Adapted from Iwasaki Y, Oiso Y, Yamauchi K, et al: Osmoregulation of plasma vasopressin in myxedema. *J Clin Endocrinol Metab* 70:534, 1990.)

The capacity to dilute urine begins in the loop of Henle and continues to the collecting tubule. This portion of the nephron, which is impermeable to water, is often referred to as the *diluting segment* (Fig. 199.1). As filtrate passes through the loop of Henle, solute is removed by the Na/K/2Cl transporter located in the cells of thick ascending limb and by the NaCl carrier in the distal tubule. Filtrate leaving the diluting segment and entering the early collecting tubule characteristically is very dilute, with a urinary osmolality (U_{Osm}) of less than 100 mOsm per kg.

A maximally dilute urine cannot be excreted if the removal of salt by the pumps and carriers in the diluting segment is impaired or if the collecting tubule is rendered permeable to water by the presence of ADH. Inability to dilute the urine may have serious consequences. For example, for a patient unable to achieve urinary dilution below an osmolality of 300 mOsm per kg, the amount of water that can be excreted on a normal diet is reduced to 3 L:

$$900 \text{ mOsm}/300 \text{ mOsm/kg} = 3 \text{ L}$$

As discussed earlier, solute excretion is normally determined by dietary intake. A reduction in dietary sodium and protein intake, as is seen in the patient on a "tea-and-toast" diet, limits the capacity to excrete water. If solute intake falls to 150 mOsm per day, for instance, water excretion is limited to approximately 3 L even when urinary dilution is normal:

$$150 \text{ mOsm}/50 \text{ mOsm/kg} = 3 \text{ L}$$

It is easy to see that the combination of impaired diluting ability with a concomitant reduction in solute intake is more likely to impair water excretion and result in hyponatremia than either disturbance alone.

Regulation of Antidiuretic Hormone

Healthy adults are able to excrete very large or very small volumes of urine, the concentration of which varies according to the P_{Osm}. The primary hormone regulating water excretion in health is ADH. ADH (called *arginine vasopressin* in humans) is synthesized in the supraoptic and paraventricular nuclei of the hypothalamus. Hypothalamic osmoreceptors for ADH release are stimulated by hyperosmolality and inhibited by hypoosmolality. A change in osmoreceptor cell volume is probably the factor that modifies ADH secretion in response to changes in the P_{Osm}. The concentration of urea, an ineffective osmole incapable of altering cell volume, does not affect ADH release.

A 1% to 2% reduction in P_{Osm} (P_{Osm} <280 mOsm per kg) maximally inhibits ADH release, leading to a U_{Osm} that is less than 100 mOsm per kg [1]. By contrast, a 1% to 2% increase in P_{Osm} above normal, or a 7% to 10% decrease in blood pressure or volume (even in the presence of plasma hypoosmolality), stimulates ADH release. In the presence of ADH, the luminal membranes of the cortical and medullary collecting tubules become permeable because water channels (aquaporins) are inserted into the luminal membrane. Water can then pass into the surrounding medullary interstitium because of the osmotic gradient.

Hyponatremia

In most settings, the development of hyponatremia with hypoosmolality represents the retention of ingested or administered water. Thus, the causes of hyponatremia can be divided into those in which water excretion is abnormal and those in which water excretion is normal, but water ingestion is considerably increased.

Hypoosmolar Disorders with Impaired Water Excretion

The U_{Osm} is typically greater than 100 mOsm per kg in patients with reduced water excretion (Table 199.1). An exception to this rule occurs when solute intake is markedly reduced, as in the patient subsisting on a solute-poor diet.

Renal Hypoperfusion-Induced Hyponatremia. A fall in effective perfusion pressure stimulates release of ADH [2]. Hypovolemic

TABLE 199.1

Causes of Hyponatremia

- Impaired water excretion (U_{Osm} >100 mOsm/kg and usually >300 mOsm/kg)
  - Hypovolemic states
    - True volume depletion (by gastrointestinal, skin, or renal losses)
    - Edematous states with reduced effective arterial blood volume (advanced liver and heart disease)
  - Diuretics (particularly thiazides)
  - Advanced chronic kidney disease
  - Endocrine deficiencies (hypothyroidism and hypoadrenalism)
  - Syndrome of inappropriate antidiuretic hormone secretion
  - Cerebral salt wasting
  - Reduced solute intake (tea-and-toast diet, beer drinkers' hyponatremia)[a]
- Normal water excretion (U_{Osm} <100 mOsm/kg)
  - Primary polydipsia
    - Psychiatric disorders (particularly with phenothiazines)
    - Hypothalamic disorders
- Hyponatremia without hypoosmolality
  - Normal P_{Osm}
    - Pseudohyponatremia (hypertriglyceridemia, hyperproteinemia, genitourinary tract irrigation)
  - Increased P_{Osm}
    - Hyperosmolar hyponatremia (hyperglycemia, mannitol infusion in renal failure)
    - Azotemia (effective osmolality is reduced)

[a]U_{Osm} <100 mOsm/kg, but normal water excretion is impaired by the reduced solute load (see text for details).
P_{Osm}, osmolality of plasma; U_{Osm}, osmolality of urine.
Adapted from Iwasaki Y, Oiso Y, Yamauchi K, et al: Osmoregulation of plasma vasopressin in myxedema. *J Clin Endocrinol Metab* 70:534, 1990; and Stasior D, Kikeri D, Duel B, et al: Nephrogenic diabetes insipidus responsive to indomethacin plus dDAVP [letter]. *N Engl J Med* 324:850, 1991.

hyponatremia can occur in states of volume depletion or in edematous individuals with congestive heart failure (CHF) or advanced liver disease because each of these conditions is associated with a reduced effective arterial blood volume. As discussed previously, the resulting increase in the U_{Osm} (e.g., to 600 mOsm per kg) would limit renal water excretion on a 900 mOsm per day diet to 1.5 L, assuming all of the ingested solute were excreted (900/600 mOsm per kg). Solute excretion tends to be reduced in these settings, which are characterized by enhanced tubular salt reabsorption. In addition, most stimuli that activate angiotensin II release stimulate thirst and lead to increased water ingestion, despite concurrent hypoosmolality.

Diuretic-Induced Hyponatremia. The ability to excrete dilute urine is impaired by diuretics, whether they act in the thick ascending limb of Henle (loop diuretics) or in the distal tubule (thiazide diuretics) (Fig. 199.2). Each class reduces salt transport out of the diluting segment, thus raising the minimum achievable U_{Osm}. Raising the minimum U_{Osm}, however, does not usually lead to hyponatremia because a large volume of urine can still be excreted by most patients.

Almost all cases of diuretic-induced hyponatremia in otherwise healthy individuals have been caused by thiazide, rather than loop, diuretics. This observation is attributable, in part, to different sites of the action within the renal tubule (Fig. 199.2). Loop diuretics, which act in the outer medulla, reduce the solute concentration in the renal medullary interstitium. Although

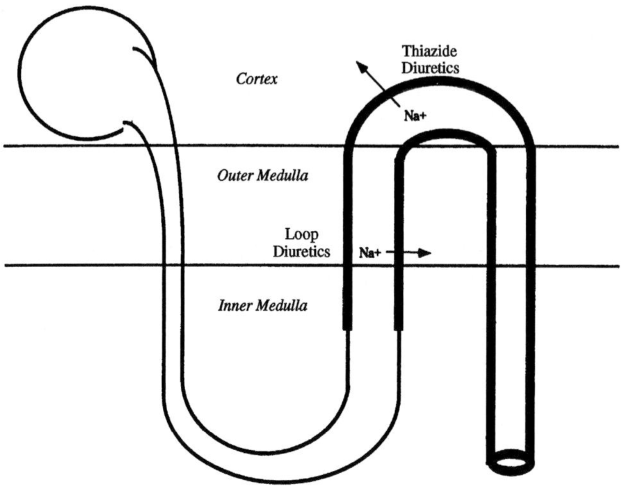

FIGURE 199.2 Site of action of loop and thiazide diuretics. Loop diuretics inhibit the Na-K-2Cl cotransporter in the medullary portion of the thick ascending limb of Henle, whereas thiazides block a simple NaCl carrier in the cortical portion of the distal tubule. These differences explain, in part, the susceptibility of individuals treated with thiazide-type diuretics to the development of hyponatremia (see text for details). (Adapted from Iwasaki Y, Oiso Y, Yamauchi K, et al: Osmoregulation of plasma vasopressin in myxedema. *J Clin Endocrinol Metab* 70:534, 1990.)

ADH *permits* water reabsorption from the collecting tubule, medullary osmolality *drives* the process. A fall in the interstitial osmolality from 1,200 to 300 mOsm per kg, for instance, would limit the maximum U_{Osm} that can be generated from 1,200 to 300 mOsm per kg. By comparison, thiazide diuretics, which act in the cortex, impair diluting capacity but have a lesser effect on concentrating ability. Thus, the U_{Osm} may be 600 mOsm per kg in the thiazide-treated individual; if the urinary osmoles are primarily NaCl and KCl, urinary electrolyte losses can exceed those contained in an equal volume of plasma. In these patients, therefore, the plasma Na^+ may actually fall in the absence of ongoing water intake. For reasons that are not well understood, however, most individuals with thiazide-induced hyponatremia gain weight, indicating that the hyponatremia is at least in part a result of increased water intake. This disorder occurs more frequently in women, typically occurs early in therapy (within 1 to 4 weeks), and is more likely to be observed in elderly individuals [3]. As discussed previously, accompanying hypokalemia may also contribute to the fall in P_{Osm}.

Advanced Chronic Kidney Disease. The normal glomerular filtration rate (GFR) is approximately 180 L per day. As renal function decreases, the ability to excrete water also decreases. The limitation in water excretion occurs for two reasons: tubular dysfunction leads to an inability to dilute the urine maximally, even in the absence of ADH, and the drop in GFR, particularly when severe, reduces daily solute excretion.

Endocrine Deficiency. Hypothyroidism and hypocortisolism can impair water excretion. Both may reduce cardiac output or stroke volume, leading to increased ADH release. The resulting fall in GFR adversely affects free water excretion by diminishing delivery of filtrate to the diluting segments. Decreased delivery may be particularly important in patients with myxedema in whom hyponatremia may develop despite appropriate suppression of ADH release [4].

Another factor contributing to the hyponatremia of hypocortisolism is that corticotropin-releasing factor promotes the co-release of adrenocorticotropic hormone (ACTH) and ADH [5].

It is important to note that adrenocortical dysfunction (as in Addison's disease) leads to reduced cortisol and aldosterone levels, the latter predisposing to hyperkalemia. The presence of a low cortisol level alone, because of either pituitary or hypothalamic disease, or the abrupt withdrawal from prolonged exogenous corticosteroid administration may cause hyponatremia but should not alter potassium homeostasis, because aldosterone release is normal.

Syndrome of Inappropriate Antidiuretic Hormone Secretion. The syndrome of inappropriate ADH secretion (SIADH) is characterized by the following: plasma hypoosmolality, U_{Osm} more than 100 to 150 mOsm per kg (because ADH should be absent in the hypoosmolar state), urinary Na^+ concentration of more than 20 mEq per L (reflecting normal renal perfusion); normal adrenal, renal, and thyroid function; and normal potassium and acid–base balance. *The* U_{Osm} *does not need to exceed the* P_{Osm} *to make this diagnosis.* SIADH may be caused by enhanced hypothalamic ADH secretion, ectopic hormone production (usually by cancer), or administration of medications with ADH activity (Table 199.2).

In approximately one-third of patients, SIADH is associated with resetting of the hypothalamic osmostat. This disorder has been described in patients with hypovolemia, psychosis, and chronic malnutrition, as well as in normal pregnancy (in which the plasma Na^+ concentration decreases by the second trimester from 140 to 135 mEq per L). ADH release is not suppressed until the P_{Osm} falls well below normal in this disorder. As a result, the P_{Osm} may vary between 240 and 250 mOsm per kg (plasma Na^+ approximately 120 to 125 mEq per L), compared with the normal value of approximately 285 to 292 mOsm per kg. In contrast to the classic form of the SIADH, in which nonsuppressible ADH release is seen, ADH secretion ceases when the P_{Osm} falls below this new, reset level. Because suppression of ADH prevents a further fall in the plasma Na^+ concentration, the severity of hyponatremia is limited in this condition.

The presence of a reset osmostat should be suspected in any patient with apparent SIADH who has mild hyponatremia (usually between 125 and 135 mEq per L) that is stable over many days despite variations in sodium and water intake. The diagnosis can be confirmed clinically by observing the response to a water load (10 to 15 mL per kg given orally or intravenously during 30 minutes). Healthy subjects and those with a reset osmostat should excrete more than 80% within 4 hours, whereas excretion is impaired in classic SIADH.

Elevated ADH levels have been reported with the use of medications and various recreational drugs. Hyponatremia associated with ingestion of 3,4-methylenedioxy-methamphetamine (Ecstasy) is reportedly caused by increased water drinking and inappropriate ADH and has led to fatalities [1]. Similar effects may be seen with the commonly prescribed selective serotonin reuptake inhibitors (SSRIs) used for the treatment of depression [6].

Cerebral Salt Wasting. Cerebral salt wasting is a rare disorder characterized by a low P_{Osm}, a U_{Osm} above 100 to 150 mOsm per kg, and a urine Na^+ concentration greater than 20 mEq per L. Unlike SIADH, however, evidence of volume depletion (including low central filling pressures) is present. In affected individuals, therefore, the high urinary Na^+ represents inappropriate salt wasting rather than a response to normal tissue perfusion (as in SIADH patients). The cause of this putative syndrome is unclear. Mineralocorticoid replacement therapy with fludrocortisone acetate has been effective in some patients.

Reduced Solute Intake. As discussed previously, a reduction in salt and protein intake can lead to hypoosmolality if water intake exceeds output. Severely reduced solute intake, as occurs with a "tea-and-toast diet," can cause hyponatremia even with normal degrees of water intake. "Beer drinkers' hyponatremia" occurs for a similar reason; the limited amount of solute in beer relative to its water content may be inadequate to permit excretion of the ingested water. In both conditions, the U_{Osm} should be maximally dilute (U_{Osm} <100 mOsm per kg). The absence of polyuria and the development of hyponatremia with normal or slightly above normal fluid intake distinguish these individuals from those with primary polydipsia.

Hypoosmolar Disorders with Normal Water Excretion. Psychiatric patients, particularly those with schizophrenia, often have abnormalities in water balance. Evaluation of psychotic patients has revealed that a variety of defects in water handling can occur that affect thirst, the release of ADH, and the renal response to ADH. Depending on the abnormality that is

TABLE 199.2

Major Causes of the Syndrome of Inappropriate ADH Secretion

Disorders	Comments
Pulmonary diseases	Acute asthma, atelectasis, empyema, pneumothorax, acute respiratory failure, tuberculosis, carcinoma, pneumonia
Neurologic disorders	Meningitis, tumors, psychiatric disorders, subarachnoid hemorrhage, herpes zoster, Wernicke's encephalopathy
Ectopic production	Cancer (particularly oat-cell carcinoma of lung)
Drugs	Intravenous cyclophosphamide, SSRIs, carbamazepine, chlorpropamide, nonsteroidal anti-inflammatory drugs (because prostaglandins block ADH effect), cisplatin[a]
After major surgery	Pain stimulates hypothalamic ADH release
Administration of exogenous ADH or oxytocin	Oxytocin can reduce plasma Na^+ concentration in mother and fetus
Symptomatic human immunodeficiency virus infection	Likely multifactorial
Idiopathic	Important to continue periodic monitoring for an underlying disorder, particularly carcinoma; vasculitis (such as temporal arteritis) should be considered in elderly patients when no other cause is apparent
Cerebral salt wasting	See text for details

[a]Hyponatremia induced by cisplatin may be because of renal salt wasting.
ADH, antidiuretic hormone; SSRIs, selective serotonin reuptake inhibitors.

present, the patient may present with polydipsia and polyuria or hyponatremia.

Hyponatremia has been reported in as many as 13% of marathon runners and may occasionally be fatal. Although the exact mechanism has not been elucidated, risk factors for developing low serum sodium levels include weight gain during the race, female sex, racing time, and lower body mass index [7]. Exercise-induced hyponatremia has been described after intense physical activity during marathons, triathlons, and high-intensity competitions. Again, the pathophysiology involves a combination of excessive fluid intake as well as a defect in renal water excretion. Athletes have been encouraged to drink more fluids c/w recommendations 30 years ago [8]. There may be a variety of pathways that stimulate ADH secretion, including muscle injury and release of cytokines with vigorous activity.

Primary Polydipsia. This disorder is most often seen in anxious, middle-aged women and in patients with psychiatric illnesses, including those taking medications that can lead to the sensation of dry mouth. These individuals drink large volumes of water for social, dietary, or health reasons. This may be manifested clinically by exaggerated weight gain during the day associated with a transient reduction in the plasma sodium concentration. Primary polydipsia can also be induced by hypothalamic lesions that directly affect the thirst center, as may occur with an infiltrative disease such as sarcoidosis. For example, the osmotic threshold for thirst may be reduced below the threshold for the release of ADH. These patients continue to drink until the P_{Osm} is less than the threshold level. This implies truly prodigious water intake, because ADH secretion is suppressed by the fall in P_{Osm}, resulting in rapid excretion of the excess water. The mechanism responsible for abnormal thirst regulation in this setting is unclear. Drug therapy may contribute to the increase in water intake if the medication induces the sensation of a dry mouth.

Because people with normally functioning kidneys and regulation of ADH secretion are capable of excreting more than 10 to 15 L of urine per day, hyponatremia as a result of polydipsia is unusual. Despite this, there are rare patients in whom severe, and potentially fatal, hyponatremia has developed even though the U_{Osm} was appropriately dilute. More commonly, however, polydipsic patients manifesting hyponatremia have a concurrent abnormality in ADH release or response. Concurrent thiazide diuretic therapy for systemic hypertension can lead to a marked and symptomatic reduction in the plasma sodium concentration in these patients.

Hyponatremia without Hypoosmolality

Hyponatremia may occur without plasma hypoosmolality. An increase in the plasma concentration of proteins (as immunoglobulins in multiple myeloma) or lipids (primarily triglycerides in lipemic plasma) can reduce the plasma Na^+ concentration. Lipids and proteins displace water from a given volume of plasma but do not affect the Na^+ concentration in the water phase of plasma. As a result, the measured P_{Osm} is normal in this condition, which is called *pseudohyponatremia*. Because the sodium concentration in the aqueous component of plasma is normal, this form of hyponatremia is not of pathophysiologic consequence. The methods of electrolyte determination currently used in many laboratories (ion-selective electrodes) are not affected by plasma lipids or proteins.

An unusual form of hyponatremia, sometimes associated with a normal P_{Osm} but occasionally with hypoosmolality, can occur after transurethral prostatectomy, uterine irrigation after endometrial ablation, or with lithotripsy [9–11], which often requires the use of as much as 20 to 30 L of nonconductive flushing solutions containing glycine, sorbitol, or mannitol. Some patients absorb 3 L or more of fluid through the exposed mucosal vascular plexus, leading to a dilutional reduction in the plasma sodium concentration that may fall below 100 mEq per L. Even when P_{Osm} is not notably reduced, confusion, disorientation, twitching, seizures, and hypotension may occur. Several methods have been devised to attempt to monitor the amount of fluid absorbed so that patients at risk for severe hyponatremia can be detected. Frequent determinations of the plasma sodium concentration are important.

There are instances in which patients with plasma hyperosmolality may develop hyponatremia (*hyperosmolar hyponatremia*). This most commonly occurs with severe hyperglycemia or when mannitol is given to patients with renal failure, resulting in an osmotic shift of water from cells into the extracellular fluid, diluting the plasma Na^+ concentration. In contrast to hypoosmolar hyponatremia, treatment is directed at correcting the high glucose concentration with insulin and free water repletion because cellular dehydration is present. For every 100 mg per dL rise in the blood sugar, the plasma Na^+ concentration falls by approximately 1.6 mEq per L, although this estimate varies with body size, falling more in a smaller individual.

Symptoms of Hypoosmolality

The neurologic manifestations of hyponatremia appear to be entirely because of the consequences of plasma hypoosmolality. A fall in P_{Osm} causes water movement from the extracellular space into cells. The resulting increase in cell water, which is of particular importance in the central nervous system, can lead to brain swelling. A variety of symptoms may be found, including lethargy, confusion, nausea, vomiting, and, in severe cases, seizures and coma. Focal neurologic symptoms are uncommon. Hyponatremic encephalopathy is generally reversible, although permanent neurologic damage or death has been reported, chiefly in premenopausal women [12]. Hyponatremic women may progress rapidly from minimal symptoms (such as headache and nausea) to respiratory arrest. Cerebral edema and herniation have been found in those women who died, suggesting a possible hormonally mediated decrease in the efficiency of the osmotic adaptation. The reason for the higher morbidity in this patient population is not well understood.

The likelihood that symptoms will develop is related to the level of hyponatremia and the rapidity with which it develops. For example, a rapid decline in the plasma Na^+ concentration during several hours or days (e.g., from 140 to 115 mEq per L) may be associated with severe neurologic findings. In comparison, a similar fall in plasma sodium occurring during 1 week or more may not cause any symptoms. In the latter circumstance, the degree of cerebral edema is much less. This protective response, which begins on the first day and is complete within several days, occurs in two major steps:

1. The initial cerebral edema elevates the interstitial hydraulic pressure, creating a gradient for extracellular fluid movement out of the brain into the cerebrospinal fluid.
2. The brain cells lose solutes, leading to the osmotic movement of water out of the cells and less brain swelling [13]. The volume regulatory response begins with the movement of potassium and sodium salts out of the cells, followed by organic solutes, particularly the amino acids glutamine, glutamate, and taurine, and, to a lesser degree, the carbohydrate inositol. Electrolyte movement occurs quickly because it is mediated by the activation of quiescent cation channels in the cell membrane; organic solute loss occurs later because it requires synthesis of new transporters.

The organic solutes (called *osmolytes*) account for approximately one-third of the cellular solute loss in chronic hyponatremia. Changes in the concentration of these solutes offer the advantage of restoring cell volume without interfering with protein function; in comparison, a potentially deleterious effect on protein function would occur if the volume adaptation was mediated *entirely* by changes in the cell cation (potassium plus sodium) concentration.

This adaptation is so efficient that it is not uncommon to see patients with heart failure or SIADH who are asymptomatic despite a plasma sodium concentration of 115 to 120 mEq per L. The occurrence of symptoms in patients with chronic hyponatremia usually signifies a profoundly low serum sodium concentration of less than 110 to 115 mEq per L.

Diagnosis of Hyponatremia

Three laboratory findings provide important information in the differential diagnosis of hyponatremia: P_{Osm}, U_{Osm}, and urinary sodium concentration.

Plasma Osmolality

Because P_{Osm} is mainly determined by the plasma sodium concentration, it is reduced in most hyponatremic patients. In some cases, however, the P_{Osm} is either normal (as in pseudohyponatremia) or elevated (as in hyperosmolar hyponatremia).

Urine Osmolality

In patients with hypoosmolar hyponatremia, the U_{Osm} can be used to distinguish between patients with impaired water excretion, accounting for most cases, and primary polydipsia, in which water excretion is normal but intake is so high that it exceeds excretory capacity. Hyponatremia caused by primary polydipsia should completely suppress ADH secretion, resulting in the excretion of maximally dilute urine with an osmolality less than 100 mOsm per kg and a specific gravity less than 1.003. A higher U_{Osm} indicates an inability to excrete free water normally, which suggests continued secretion of ADH.

Urinary Sodium Concentration

The two major causes of hyponatremia are hypovolemia and SIADH. These disorders can usually be distinguished by measuring the urinary sodium concentration. The urinary sodium concentration of patients with hypovolemia is typically less than 20 mEq per L, assuming the patient is not receiving diuretics. Because patients with SIADH have normal renal perfusion, unless they are on a very low sodium intake, the urinary sodium concentration is greater than 40 mEq per L. Patients with the SIADH can conserve urinary sodium normally and raise the urine osmolality further if intravascular volume depletion occurs.

The fractional excretion of sodium (FENa) is typically used as an assessment of volume status in acute kidney injury; in this setting, a level less than 1% suggests volume depletion. However, with normal kidney function, the expected value of FENa in euvolemia is less than 1%. As a result, random urinary sodium concentration is more accurate. FENa should not be used in the workup of hyponatremia.

Evaluation of acid–base and potassium balance may aid in the diagnosis in some hyponatremic patients. As examples, metabolic alkalosis and hypokalemia suggest diuretic use or vomiting; metabolic acidosis and hypokalemia suggest diarrhea or laxative abuse; and metabolic acidosis and hyperkalemia suggest adrenal insufficiency. On the contrary, plasma bicarbonate and potassium concentrations are typically normal in patients with SIADH. Although water retention tends to lower these values by dilution, as it does the plasma sodium and chloride concentrations, normal levels are restored by the factors that normally regulate acid–base and potassium balance.

The initial water retention and volume expansion in patients with SIADH are typically associated with hypouricemia (plasma uric acid concentration of ≤3 mg per dL) because of increased uric acid excretion in urine. In addition, urinary urea losses may cause a fall in the BUN to less than 5 mg per dL. These findings are the opposite of what is typically seen in volume depletion and thiazide-induced hyponatremia.

All of the findings seen in SIADH have also been described in the controversial syndrome of *cerebral salt wasting*, a disorder in which the high urinary sodium concentration occurs as a result of defective tubular reabsorption, and the elevation in ADH and subsequent development of hyponatremia are because of the associated volume depletion. Hypouricemia may also be present, which presumably is another manifestation of impaired renal tubular function.

Treatment of Hyponatremia

Saline or Water Restriction

In general, the plasma sodium concentration can be raised by giving patients salt (either as saline or salt tablets) or by restricting their water intake to below the level of excretion. The choice of therapy is primarily governed by the cause of the hyponatremia. The more recent additions of antagonists to the ADH receptor in the collecting tubule (vaptans) are also discussed.

Salt administration, usually as isotonic saline, is appropriate in those with true volume depletion or adrenal insufficiency, in which cortisol replacement is also indicated. Water restriction is used in patients without neurologic symptoms who have edematous states such as heart failure and hepatic cirrhosis and in those with SIADH, primary polydipsia, or advanced chronic kidney disease.

With volume depletion, isotonic saline corrects the hyponatremia by two mechanisms. Each liter of saline infused raises the plasma sodium by 1 to 2 mEq per L because saline has a higher sodium concentration (154 mEq per L) than plasma. In addition, volume repletion removes the stimulus to ADH release, thereby allowing the water surfeit to be excreted. At this time, the plasma sodium concentration will return rapidly toward normal.

In primary polydipsia, the initiation of water restriction may result in a dramatic rise in the plasma sodium concentration. These patients may be less predisposed to osmotic demyelination because their hyponatremia often is of rapid onset, with less brain cell adaptation apt to occur.

The optimal rate of correction of hyponatremia varies with the clinical state of the patient. In asymptomatic patients, who are more likely to have chronic hyponatremia, the plasma sodium concentration should be raised at a maximum rate of approximately 0.5 mEq/L/h and less than 8 mEq/L/d [2]. A more rapid rise can increase the risk of osmotic demyelination.

More rapid initial correction is indicated for patients with symptomatic hyponatremia, particularly those presenting with seizures or other severe neurologic manifestations, which primarily result from cerebral edema induced by acute (developing during 2 to 3 days) hyponatremia. Here, the plasma sodium concentration can be raised at an initial rate of 1.5 to 2.0 mEq/L/h for the first 3 to 4 hours (or longer, if the patient remains symptomatic) because the risk of persistent severe hyponatremia outweighs that of overly rapid correction. This appears to be particularly important in premenopausal women, who may progress from minimal symptoms (headache and nausea) to coma and respiratory arrest; furthermore, irreversible neurologic damage or death is relatively common in younger women with symptomatic hyponatremia, even if the hyponatremia is corrected at an appropriate rate. In comparison, men are at much less risk of symptomatic hyponatremia and of permanent neurologic injury. After the initial 3 to 4 hours of rapid correction, the rate should be slowed down so that the total rise in plasma sodium does not exceed approximately 8 mEq during the initial 24 hours.

The quantity of sodium required to achieve the desired elevation in the plasma sodium concentration *in patients with true volume depletion* can be estimated from the product of the plasma sodium deficit per liter and the TBW, which represents the osmotic space of distribution of the plasma sodium concentration. Normal values for the TBW are 0.5 and 0.6 times the lean body weight in women and men, respectively. If the initial aim in an asymptomatic hyponatremic 60-kg woman is to raise the plasma sodium concentration from 110 to 120 mEq per L, then

$$\text{Sodium deficit for initial therapy} = 0.5 \times 60 \times (120 - 110) = 300 \text{ mEq}$$

Thus, 600 mL of 3% hypertonic saline (which contains roughly 1 mEq of sodium per 2 mL, 500 mEq Na, and 500 mEq Cl per L) should be given during 20 hours at a rate of 30 mL per hour. This regimen should raise the plasma sodium concentration at the desired rate of 0.5 mEq/L/h, and serial monitoring of the plasma sodium concentration (beginning at 2 to 3 hours) is still required.

The preceding formula may be less accurate in patients with SIADH [3]. In this setting, the administered salt in the hypertonic 3% saline is excreted because plasma volume expansion is present. Therefore, the rise in plasma sodium is not because of sodium retention. Because there are approximately 1,000 mEq of solute (Na and Cl) in a liter of 3% saline, the fluid in the renal collecting tubule is relatively hyperosmotic. This causes water to be retained in the urine and excreted simultaneously with the salt load. If, for example, the U_{Osm} were 500 mOsm per kg, the 1,000 mEq of salt excreted would obligate the elimination of 2 L of urine (a net loss of 1 L of free water, because 1 L of water was administered with the hypertonic saline). The result would be no change in total body sodium and that the plasma sodium concentration would increase because of the loss of 1 L of water. Administration of the same hypertonic saline solution to an individual with SIADH and a U_{Osm} of 250 mOsm per kg would result in the loss of 4 L of urine (a net water loss of 3 L). The serum sodium would increase by a greater amount than it did in the person with the higher U_{Osm}. As a consequence of the excretion of the salt load and varying levels of U_{Osm} in patients with SIADH, the sodium replacement formula is frequently misleading in this setting.

Effects of Potassium

Potassium is as osmotically active as sodium, and giving potassium can raise the plasma sodium concentration and osmolality in a hyponatremic subject. Because most of the excess potassium goes into the cells, electroneutrality is maintained in one of three ways, each of which raises the plasma sodium concentration: (a) intracellular sodium moves into the extracellular fluid; (b) extracellular chloride moves into the cells with potassium; the increase in cell osmolality promotes free water entry into the cells; and (c) intracellular hydrogen moves into the extracellular fluid. These hydrogen ions are buffered by extracellular bicarbonate and, to a much lesser degree, by plasma proteins. This buffering renders the hydrogen ions osmotically inactive; the ensuing fall in extracellular osmolality leads to water movement into the cells.

Thus, any administration of potassium must be taken into account when calculating the sodium deficit. This relationship becomes clinically important in the patient with severe diuretic or vomiting-induced hyponatremia who is also hypokalemic.

Risk of Osmotic Demyelination

Severe hyponatremia, especially if acute in onset, can lead to cerebral edema, potentially irreversible neurologic damage, and death. This most often occurs when large volumes of hypotonic fluids are given to postoperative patients who have pain-induced ADH release that impairs the ability of the kidneys to excrete water or to patients with acute thiazide-induced hyponatremia. Within 24 hours, however, the brain begins to lose extracellular water into the cerebrospinal fluid and loses intracellular water by extruding sodium and potassium salts and osmolytes, thereby lowering the brain volume toward normal.

Hyponatremia that develops slowly (i.e., during >2 to 3 days) is associated with a lesser likelihood of neurologic symptoms. In this setting, in which brain volume has fallen toward normal, rapid correction of severe hyponatremia may lead within 1 to several days to the development of a neurologic disorder called *osmotic demyelination* or *central pontine myelinolysis*. These lesions are detectable by cerebral computed tomography or magnetic resonance imaging. Results of these diagnostic tests may not become positive for as long as 4 weeks, however [14].

The mechanisms responsible for osmotic demyelination are not completely understood. Rapid elevation in the plasma sodium concentration leads to water movement out of the brain, which can lower the brain volume below normal. Such osmotically induced shrinkage in axons could sever their connections with surrounding myelin sheaths. Alternatively, the initial brain cell response to brain shrinkage may be the uptake of potassium and sodium from the extracellular fluid; this elevation in cell cation concentration could be toxic to the cells.

The manifestations of osmotic demyelination, which may be irreversible, include mental status changes, dysarthria, dysphagia, paraparesis or quadriparesis, and coma; seizures may occur but are less common. Patients in whom the plasma sodium concentration is raised to more than 20 mEq per L in the first 24 hours or is overcorrected to greater than 140 mEq per L are at greatest risk. Other putative risk factors for osmotic demyelination include chronic alcoholism, malnutrition, prolonged diuretic use, liver failure and transplantation, and burns [15]. On the contrary, late neurologic deterioration is rare if the hyponatremia is corrected at an average rate equal to or less than 0.5 mEq/L/h [2].

Studies in experimental animals indicate that the total rate of correction during the first 24 hours is more important than the maximum rate in any given hour [16]. Demyelinating lesions are most common when the plasma sodium concentration in severe hyponatremia is raised by more than 20 mEq/L/d and are rare at a rate less than 10 to 12 mEq/L/d. This is similar to the safe average rate of correction of 0.5 mEq/L/h observed in humans.

Recommendations

The preferred rate at which the plasma sodium concentration should be increased varies with the clinical presentation. Owing to the cerebral adaptation previously described, patients with chronic asymptomatic hyponatremia are generally at little risk for neurologic symptoms. In this setting, rapid correction is not indicated and may be harmful. Although the optimal rate of correction is not clearly proven, the current recommendation in asymptomatic patients is that the plasma sodium concentration be raised at a maximum rate of 4 to 8 mEq/L/d (which represents an average correction of 0.5 mEq/L/h). Although it may be safe to increase the plasma sodium concentration at a rate of more than 8 mEq per day, there is no reason to correct it more rapidly *in the absence of symptoms*.

It is not known whether there is a potential benefit to administering water to previously hypoosmolar patients whose hyponatremia has been corrected much too rapidly. In rodents, a marked reduction in the incidence and severity of brain lesions was demonstrated if overly rapid correction (30 mEq per L or more during several hours) was partially reversed so that the net daily elevation in the plasma sodium concentration was less than 20 mEq per L [17]. This improvement was seen if therapy was begun before the onset of neurologic symptoms; benefit was much less likely in animals with symptomatic demyelination. The applicability of these findings to humans is uncertain.

More aggressive initial correction, at a rate of 1.5 to 2.0 mEq/L/h, is indicated for the first 3 to 4 hours (or until the symptoms resolve) in patients who present with seizures or other severe neurologic abnormalities as a result of untreated and usually acute hyponatremia. The primary problem in these patients is cerebral edema, and the risk of delayed therapy is greater than the potential risk of too rapid correction. Even in this setting, however, the plasma sodium concentration should probably not be raised by more than 8 mEq per L in the first 24 hours because partial cerebral adaptation has already occurred. It is usually not necessary to continue hypertonic saline once the plasma sodium concentration is greater than 120 mEq per L.

Treatment of Hyponatremia for the Syndrome of Inappropriate Antidiuretic Hormone Secretion. Hyponatremia for the SIADH results primarily from ADH-induced retention of ingested water. Appropriate therapy for this disorder depends on the severity of the hyponatremia and, on the fact that, although water excretion is impaired, sodium handling is intact because there is no abnormality in volume-regulating mechanisms such as the renin–angiotensin–aldosterone system. Water restriction is the mainstay of therapy in asymptomatic hyponatremia of chronic SIADH. The associated negative water balance raises the plasma sodium concentration toward normal.

Severe, symptomatic, or resistant hyponatremia often requires the administration of salt. If the plasma sodium concentration is to be elevated, the osmolality of the fluid given must exceed that of the urine. This can be illustrated by a simple example (Table 199.3). Suppose a patient with SIADH and hyponatremia has a U_{Osm} that cannot be reduced below 616 mOsm per kg. If 1,000 mL of isotonic saline is given (containing 154 mEq each of Na and Cl or 308 mOsm), all of the salt is excreted (because sodium handling is intact), but in only 500 mL of water (308 mOsm in 500 mL of water equals 616 mOsm per kg). The retention of half of the administered water leads to a further reduction in the plasma sodium concentration. As a result, correction of the hyponatremia for these cases requires the administration of hypertonic 3% saline intravenously or salt tablets orally, preferably in combination with a drug that lowers the U_{Osm} and increases water excretion by impairing the renal responsiveness to ADH. A loop diuretic is most often used for this purpose.

Demeclocycline and lithium act on the collecting tubule cell to diminish its responsiveness to ADH, thereby increasing water excretion. Demeclocyline may reduce aquaporin-2 expression in the renal inner medulla via cAMP generation [18]. These drugs tend to be too toxic (lithium) or ineffective (demeclocycline) in most patients. By comparison, specific antagonists to the ADH-V_2 (collecting tubule) receptor in the cortical collecting tubule have shown effectiveness, and two of these have been approved by the Food and Drug Administration (FDA) at the time of this writing.

Conivaptan, an antagonist to both the V_1 (vascular) and V_2 (ADH) receptors, was first approved. It must be given intravenously in the hospital and has the propensity to cause phlebitis. Recent data suggest that a single 20 mg bolus intravenously over 30 minutes results in a sustained water diuresis and may avoid vascular injury. It is not suitable for chronic use. Tolvaptan is an oral ADH antagonist which is specific for the V_2 receptor. It must also be initiated in the hospital but can be administered in the outpatient setting after that.

The choice of initial therapy in symptomatic patients is usually 3% saline, and this is the preferred treatment with severe neuropathology (such as seizures). Because there are no controlled prospective studies comparing hypertonic saline with the vaptans, it is difficult to recommend the latter in the SIADH as first-line agents, particularly when cost is considered. Recently, a European Consortium of three medical societies did not recommend the use of vaptans for acute symptomatic hyponatremia in the setting of SIADH or volume overload [19]. When they are administered, it is important to relax fluid restriction during the initial titration with these agents to avoid an excessive rise in the serum sodium concentration. Given the higher cost, liver function test abnormalities, and lack of proven benefit over conventional therapies (hypertonic saline), the role of vaptans is not well defined.

Urea. Oral urea has been used to treat hyponatremia and brain swelling since the 1980s. It is a hydrophilic compound that does not readily cross the blood–brain barrier and creates an osmotic gradient, thereby allowing water to flow out of the brain in a slower fashion that hypertonic saline. With normal kidney function, administered urea is excreted within 12 hours, which promotes the excretion of free water. Although not approved in the United States, its use has been recommended in Europe for the treatment of SIADH [20]. Correction of chronic hyponatremia in rats with the use of urea may be associated with fewer neurologic complication compared with hypertonic saline or lixvaptan [21].

Identification of a reset osmostat is important because the therapeutic recommendations for SIADH discussed here do not apply in this setting. These patients generally have mild, asymptomatic hyponatremia because of downward resetting of the threshold for both ADH release and thirst. Because osmoregulatory function is normal around the new baseline, attempting to raise the plasma sodium concentration increases ADH levels and makes the patient very thirsty, a response that is similar to that seen with water restriction in healthy subjects. Thus, efforts to raise the plasma sodium concentration are both unnecessary and likely to be ineffective. Treatment should be primarily directed at the underlying disease.

Treatment of Hyponatremia in Edematous States. Raising the plasma sodium concentration in patients with edema may be more difficult than in those conditions described earlier. Most of these individuals have advanced CHF or liver disease. Consequently, sodium administration is generally contraindicated.

Congestive Heart Failure. Restricting water intake is the mainstay of therapy in hyponatremic patients with heart failure, although this is often not tolerable because of the intense stimulation of thirst. The combination of an angiotensin-converting enzyme (ACE) inhibitor (or angiotensin receptor blocker [ARB]) and a loop diuretic may induce an elevation in the plasma sodium concentration [22,23]. Tolvaptan may be useful in some patients (see above), but must be initiated in the hospital. Tolvaptan has been approved for the treatment of hyponatremia in the setting of CHF as well as cirrhosis. However, there are no data on improvement in mortality versus conventional therapy [24]. In addition, the FDA in 2013 issued a warning about liver function abnormalities with the use of tolvaptan [25].

Liver Disease. Hyponatremia of patients with hepatic cirrhosis usually develops slowly and produces no cerebral edema or symptoms. It is possible, however, that a low plasma sodium

TABLE 199.3

Mechanism of Normal Saline-Induced Worsening of Hyponatremia in the Syndrome of Inappropriate Antidiuretic Hormone Secretion

	Solute (mOsm)	Water (mL)
Input	308	1,000
Output	308	500
Net gain	0	+500

This calculation assumes that the individual cannot dilute the urine below a urine osmolality of 616 mOsm/kg and that all the administered solute is excreted in the urine.

concentration can exacerbate hepatic encephalopathy. In view of the marked sodium and water retention, the mainstay of therapy in this setting is restricting water intake to a level sufficient to induce negative water balance and partial correction of the hyponatremia. Hypertonic saline or salt tablets are indicated only in patients with symptomatic hyponatremia. Diuretics can be given concurrently to prevent worsening of the edema, but overly rapid correction must be avoided to minimize the risk of central demyelinating lesions. As is the case with hyponatremic CHF patients, demeclocycline has been evaluated in this setting, but its use has been limited because of its nephrotoxicity [26].

Hypernatremia

Hypernatremia can be produced by the administration of hypertonic sodium solutions. However, in almost all cases, there is loss of free water. Persistent hypernatremia does not occur in healthy subjects because the ensuing rise in P_{Osm} stimulates both thirst and the release of ADH, which minimizes further water loss. The associated increase in water intake then lowers the plasma sodium concentration to normal. This regulatory system is so efficient that the P_{Osm} is maintained within a range of 1% to 2% despite wide variations in sodium and water intake. Even patients with diabetes insipidus, who often have marked polyuria because of diminished ADH effect, maintain a near-normal plasma sodium concentration by appropriately increasing water intake.

The result is that hypernatremia occurs primarily in those patients who cannot express thirst normally; most often, these patients are infants and adults with impaired mental status, and the elderly, who also appear to have diminished osmotic stimulation of thirst via an unknown mechanism. A patient with a plasma sodium concentration of 150 mEq per L or more who is alert but not thirsty has, by definition, a *hypothalamic lesion* (either structural or functional) affecting the thirst center.

Etiology of Hypernatremia

The major causes of hypernatremia are listed in Table 199.4.

Free Water Loss. The unreplaced loss of solute-free water leads to an elevation in the plasma sodium concentration. Because the plasma sodium concentration and P_{Osm} are determined by the ratio of total body solutes (i.e., *effective osmoles*, chiefly sodium and potassium salts) to TBW, the amounts of sodium and potassium in a fluid determine how loss of that fluid affects body osmolality [2]. The composition of diarrheal fluid can be used to illustrate this point. Many viral and osmotic diarrheas are associated with an isosmotic diarrheal fluid that has a sodium plus potassium concentration between 40 and 100 mEq per L; organic solutes, which do not affect the plasma sodium concentration, make up the remaining osmoles. Loss of this fluid tends to induce hypernatremia because water is being lost in excess of sodium plus potassium. Similar considerations apply to urinary losses during an osmotic diuresis induced by glucose, mannitol, or urea. Patients with secretory diarrheas such as cholera excrete a diarrheal fluid with a sodium and potassium concentration similar to that of plasma. Loss of this fluid causes volume and potassium depletion but does not directly affect the plasma sodium concentration.

With these considerations in mind, the sources of free water loss that can lead to hypernatremia if intake is not increased include the following:

- *Insensible and sweat losses.* Insensible water losses from the skin by evaporation and sweat are relatively dilute. The loss of this fluid is increased by fever, exercise, and exposure to high temperatures.
- *Gastrointestinal losses.* As mentioned previously, most gastrointestinal losses promote the development of hypernatremia because the sodium plus potassium concentration is less than that in the plasma. An elevation in the plasma sodium concentration with a diarrheal illness is particularly common in infants.
- *Central or nephrogenic diabetes insipidus.* Decreased release of ADH or renal resistance to its effect causes the excretion of relatively dilute urine. Most affected patients have a normal thirst mechanism and, therefore, typically present with polyuria and polydipsia and a high-normal plasma sodium concentration. However, marked and symptomatic hypernatremia occurs if there is inadequate replacement (either oral or intravenous) of the urinary water losses.
  Central diabetes insipidus (CDI) is associated with deficient secretion of ADH. This condition is most often idiopathic (possibly as a result of autoimmune injury to the ADH-producing cells) or induced by trauma, pituitary surgery or infiltration, or hypoxic or ischemic encephalopathy. When CDI develops following trauma or surgery, a triphasic response may be observed [27]. In this condition, initial inhibition of ADH results in polyuria, followed by uncontrolled release of ADH from injured cells, and, subsequently, by permanent CDI.
  Nephrogenic diabetes insipidus (NDI) is characterized by normal ADH secretion but varying degrees of renal resistance to its water-retaining effect. In its mild form, NDI is relatively common because most patients who are elderly or who have underlying renal disease have a reduction in maximum concentrating ability. This defect, however, is not severe enough to produce a symptomatic increase in urine output. True polyuria owing to ADH resistance occurs primarily in four settings: X-linked hereditary NDI in children in which there is an abnormality in the renal V_2 receptors for ADH or in the ADH-sensitive water channel (*aquaporin 2*) [27], chronic lithium use, hypercalcemia, and severe hypokalemia.
- *Osmotic diuresis.* An osmotic diuresis owing to glucose, mannitol, or urea causes an increase in urine output in which the sodium plus potassium concentration is well below that in the plasma because of the presence of the excreted organic solute. Patients with diabetic ketoacidosis or nonketotic hyperglycemia typically present with hyperosmolality, although the plasma sodium concentration may be kept normal or low by the hyperglycemia-induced water movement out of cells.
- *Hypothalamic lesions affecting thirst or osmoreceptor function.* Hypernatremia can occur in the absence of increased water losses if there is a primary hypothalamic disease impairing thirst (called *hypodipsia*). In patients with this problem, forced water intake is usually sufficient to maintain a normal plasma sodium concentration, although CDI, if present, should be treated.

TABLE 199.4

Major Causes of Hypernatremia

Unreplaced water loss
Insensible and sweat losses
Gastrointestinal losses
Central or nephrogenic diabetes insipidus
Hypothalamic lesions affecting thirst or osmoreceptor function
Primary hypodipsia
Essential hypernatremia
Reset osmostat in mineralocorticoid excess
Water loss into cells
Severe exercise or seizures
Sodium overload
Intake of hypertonic sodium solutions

Other hypodipsic patients do not respond to water loading, because the excess water is excreted in the urine with little change in the plasma sodium concentration. These patients have selective injury to the hypothalamic osmoreceptors, with ADH secretion being primarily governed by changes in blood volume (volume receptors remain intact). Thus, the suppression of ADH release by water loading in such patients is caused by the associated mild volume expansion rather than to a fall in P_{Osm} [28]. This disorder was termed *essential hypernatremia*, but is now called adipsic diabetes insipidus. Correction is difficult, because ADH release and suppression is driven by volume and not by the serum osmolality.

True upward resetting of the osmostat has been described only in patients with primary mineralocorticoid excess (such as in primary hyperaldosteronism). Presumably, the suppressive effect of chronic mild volume expansion on ADH release is responsible for this phenomenon. The plasma sodium concentration in these patients is frequently between 141 and 145 mEq per L and may be a clue to the diagnosis.

Water Loss into Cells. Transient hypernatremia, in which the plasma sodium concentration can rise by 10 to 15 mEq per L within a few minutes, can be induced by intense exercise or seizures, activities that are also associated with lactic acidosis. In this setting, the intracellular breakdown of glycogen into smaller, more osmotically active molecules, such as lactate, can increase water uptake into cells. The plasma sodium concentration returns to normal within 5 to 15 minutes after the cessation of exertion.

Sodium Overload. Acute and often marked hypernatremia, with plasma sodium concentrations even higher than 175 mEq per L, can be induced by administration of hypertonic sodium-containing solutions. Examples include salt poisoning in infants and young children, infusion of hypertonic sodium bicarbonate to treat metabolic acidosis, and massive salt ingestion, such as can occur when a highly concentrated saline emetic or gargle is swallowed. This type of hypernatremia corrects spontaneously if renal function is normal, because the excess sodium is rapidly excreted in the urine. Even with optimal therapy, however, the mortality rate is extremely high in adults with a plasma sodium concentration that has suddenly risen to more than 180 mEq per L [29]; for reasons that are poorly understood, severe hypernatremia is often better tolerated in young children.

Symptoms of Hypernatremia

Hypernatremia is basically a mirror image of hyponatremia. The rise in the plasma sodium concentration and osmolality causes rapid water movement out of the brain; this decrease in brain volume can cause tension, thereby leading to rupture of the cerebral veins with focal intracerebral and subarachnoid hemorrhages and possible irreversible neurologic damage. The clinical manifestations of this disorder begin with lethargy, weakness, and irritability and can progress to twitching, seizures, and coma. Severe symptoms usually require an acute elevation in the plasma sodium concentration to more than 158 mEq per L.

Despite the generalized reduction in cell volume with hypernatremia, brain volume is gradually restored because of both water movement from the cerebrospinal fluid into the brain (thereby increasing the interstitial volume) and to the uptake of solutes by the brain cells (thereby pulling water into the cells). The latter response involves an initial uptake of sodium and potassium salts, followed by the later accumulation of osmolytes such as inositol and the amino acids glutamine and glutamate [30]. The effect is that these osmolytes, which do not interfere with cell function, account for approximately 35% of the new cell solute.

As in hyponatremia, the cerebral adaptation in hypernatremia has two important clinical consequences:

1. Chronic hypernatremia is much less likely to induce neurologic symptoms. Assessment of symptoms attributable to hypernatremia is often difficult because most affected adults have underlying neurologic disease, which diminishes the protective thirst mechanism that normally prevents the development of hypernatremia, even in patients with diabetes insipidus.
2. Correction of chronic hypernatremia must occur slowly to prevent rapid fluid movement into the brain leading to cerebral edema, which can cause seizures and coma. Although the brain cells can rapidly lose potassium and sodium in response to this cell swelling, the loss of accumulated osmolytes occurs more slowly, a phenomenon that acts to hold water within the cells. The loss of inositol, for example, requires both a reduction in synthesis of new sodium–inositol cotransporters and the activation of a specific inositol efflux mechanism in the cell membrane. The delayed clearance of osmolytes from the cell can predispose to cerebral edema if the plasma sodium concentration is corrected too rapidly.

Diagnosis of Hypernatremia and Polyuric Disorders

The cause of the hypernatremia is usually evident from the history. When the cause is unclear, the correct diagnosis can usually be established by evaluation of the integrity of the ADH-renal axis via measurement of the U_{Osm}. A rise in the plasma sodium concentration is a potent stimulus to ADH release as well as to thirst; furthermore, a P_{Osm} of more than 295 mOsm per kg (representing a plasma sodium concentration of approximately 145 to 147 mEq per L) generally leads to sufficient ADH secretion to maximally stimulate urinary concentration.

Thus, if both hypothalamic and renal functions are intact, the U_{Osm} of a person with hypernatremia should exceed 700 to 800 mOsm per kg. In this setting, unreplaced insensible or gastrointestinal losses, sodium overload, or, rarely, a primary defect in thirst is likely to be responsible for the hypernatremia. Exogenous ADH does not produce a further rise in the U_{Osm}.

The chemical composition of the urine is diagnostically useful. The urinary sodium concentration should be less than 20 mEq per L when water loss and volume depletion are the primary problems, but it is typically well above 100 mEq per L in a salt-overload state. If the U_{Osm} is significantly lower than that of the hyperosmolar plasma, then either central (ADH-deficient) or nephrogenic (ADH-resistant) diabetes insipidus is present.

Diagnosis of Polyuric States and Diabetes Insipidus. *Polyuria* can be arbitrarily defined as urine output exceeding 3 L per day. It must be differentiated from the more common complaints of frequency and nocturia, which are usually not associated with an increase in the total urine output. Excluding osmotic diuresis from uncontrolled diabetes mellitus, polyuria in the outpatient setting is typically caused by primary polydipsia, CDI, or NDI.

These conditions are all associated with an increase in urine output and the excretion of relatively dilute urine. With primary polydipsia, the polyuria is an appropriate response to excessive water intake and is not associated with hypernatremia. In comparison, the water loss is inappropriate with either form of diabetes insipidus. Thus, a low plasma sodium concentration at presentation (<137 mEq per L) owing to water overload is usually indicative of primary polydipsia, whereas a high-normal plasma sodium concentration (>142 mEq per L) points toward diabetes insipidus. Marked hypernatremia is uncommon in diabetes insipidus because loss of water stimulates the thirst mechanism, resulting in an increase in intake to match the urinary losses. An exception to this general rule is the patient with a central lesion impairing both ADH release and thirst.

The correct diagnosis is often inferred from the plasma sodium concentration and from the history. The patient should be questioned about the causes of CDI or NDI and about the rate of onset of the polyuria; the polyuria is usually abrupt in CDI ("I suddenly began urinating excessively 2 days ago") but gradual in NDI or primary polydipsia. Testing the kidneys' ability to concentrate the urine in response to a high P_{Osm} can confirm the diagnosis. The P_{Osm} can be raised either by water restriction or, less commonly, by the administration of hypertonic saline (0.05 mL/kg/min for no more than 2 hours). These maneuvers are unnecessary if the patient's P_{Osm} is already at or above 295 mOsm per kg because endogenous ADH effect on the kidneys should be maximal.

The water restriction test for the evaluation of polyuria involves measurement of the urine volume and osmolality every hour and plasma sodium concentration and P_{Osm} every 2 hours. The patient should stop drinking 2 to 3 hours before beginning the test; overnight fluid restriction should be avoided because potentially severe volume depletion and hypernatremia can occur in patients with marked polyuria.

The water restriction test is continued until the U_{Osm} reaches a clearly appropriate level of concentration (approximately 600 mOsm per kg, indicating that both ADH release and effect are intact), the U_{Osm} is stable on two or three successive measurements despite a rising P_{Osm}, more than 3% to 5% of body weight is lost, or the P_{Osm} exceeds 295 to 300 mOsm per kg. If urinary concentration is inadequate, exogenous ADH is then given, usually in the form of 10 μg of deamino-8-D-arginine vasopressin [DDAVP; also called desmopressin] by nasal insufflation, and the U_{Osm} and volume are monitored over every 30 minutes for 90 minutes. Measuring the serum ADH level at the start of the test and immediately before DDAVP is administered may be useful.

Each of the causes of polyuria produces a distinct pattern as depicted in Figure 199.3:

1. CDI is usually partial and, therefore, associated with a rise in the U_{Osm} as the P_{Osm} increases. The degree of urinary concentration is clearly submaximal, however; and because ADH release is inadequate, exogenous ADH leads to a rise in the U_{Osm} of 15% to 50% and a corresponding fall in urine output.
2. NDI is also associated with a submaximal rise in U_{Osm}, but there is no urinary response to exogenous ADH. It must be emphasized that NDI is a rare cause of true polyuria in adults in the absence of lithium use, hypercalcemia, hypokalemia, or, rarely, renal tubular disease.
3. Primary polydipsia is associated with a rise in U_{Osm}, usually to more than 500 mOsm per kg, and no response to exogenous ADH because endogenous release is intact. The chronic polyuria in this disorder can partially wash out the medullary interstitial solute gradient; as a result, maximal concentrating ability is impaired, and the U_{Osm} may only reach 500 to 600 mOsm per kg, as compared with 800 mOsm per kg or more in healthy subjects.

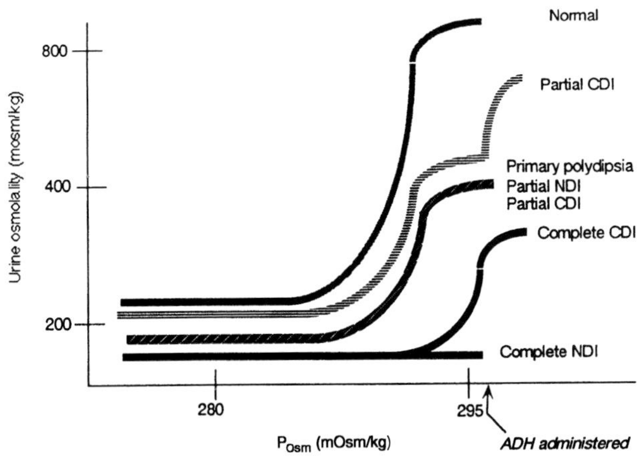

FIGURE 199.3 Response to antidiuretic hormone (ADH) after a water restriction test. ADH is given when the osmolality of plasma (P_{osm}) reaches 295 mOsm per kg, the level at which maximal ADH release and response should be present. This test identifies the cause of polyuria in approximately 80% of patients. Confusion may arise, however, with partial diabetes insipidus (CDI). In this disorder, some individuals have lower than normal ADH levels at a normal P_{osm}, but the increase in ADH (although still subnormal) generates a maximum urine response, presumably because of increased sensitivity. Consequently, these patients exhibit polyuria at a normal P_{osm}, but the curve during the water restriction test may mimic partial nephrogenic diabetes insipidus (NDI) or primary polydipsia. Measurement of plasma ADH levels may be needed to distinguish these possibilities. (From Zerbe R, Robertson G: A comparison of plasma vasopressin measurements with a standard indirect test in the differential diagnosis of polyuria. *N Engl J Med* 305:1539, 1981, with permission.)

There is, however, one major potential source of error. Patients with partial CDI may be hyperresponsive to the submaximal rise in ADH induced by water restriction, perhaps because of receptor upregulation. As a result, they may be polyuric at the normal P_{Osm} of 285 to 290 mOsm per kg when ADH levels are very low, but they may have a maximally concentrated urine at a P_{Osm} of more than 295 mOsm per kg when ADH levels are somewhat higher. In such patients, exogenous ADH is without effect, resulting in a pattern suggestive of primary polydipsia or NDI. Therefore, measurement of plasma ADH levels may be useful.

In some polyuric patients, the increase in urine output is because of a solute or an osmotic diuresis in which decreased solute reabsorption is the primary abnormality. Although glucosuria is the most common cause of osmotic diuresis in outpatients, other conditions may account for some cases. These include high-protein feedings (in which urea acts as the osmotic agent) and volume expansion owing to saline loading or the administration of mannitol. The U_{Osm} in these disorders is usually greater than 300 mOsm per kg, in contrast to the dilute urine typically found with a water diuresis. Total solute excretion, which is calculated from the product of the U_{Osm} and volume of a 24-hour urine sample, is normal with a water diuresis (600 to 900 mOsm per day) but markedly increased with an osmotic diuresis.

Although renal disease can impair sodium conservation in the presence of volume depletion, it rarely causes sufficient sodium wasting to induce true polyuria. For example, the polyuria of postobstructive diuresis is caused by renal excretion of excess fluid and solute, not water and solute wasting. Although urine output may initially exceed 1,000 mL per hour, optimal therapy consists of fluid infusion at a maintenance level, such as 75 mL of one-half isotonic saline per hour. The development of volume depletion, as evidenced by hypotension or a rise in the BUN, is unusual with this regimen.

Treatment of Hypernatremia

The water deficit of a hypernatremic patient can be estimated from the following calculation. The quantity of osmoles in the body is equal to the osmolal space (the TBW) times the osmolality of the body fluids:

$$\text{Total body osmoles} = \text{TBW} \times P_{Osm}$$

$$\text{Water deficit} = \text{current body water (plasma Na}^+/140 - 1)$$

where current (observed) body water = 60% body mass.

This formula estimates the amount of positive water balance required to return the plasma sodium concentration to 140 mEq per L. It does not account for electrolyte losses that may occur conjointly with water losses in such settings as osmotic diuresis or diarrhea.

Rate of Correction. As in hyponatremia, overly rapid correction is potentially dangerous in chronic hypernatremia (present for >48 hours). Rapidly lowering the plasma sodium concentration once osmotic adaptation has occurred may cause cerebral edema and lead to seizures, permanent neurologic damage, or death. This adverse sequence has been described in children in whom hypernatremia was corrected at a rate exceeding 0.7 mEq/L/h. In comparison, no neurologic sequelae were induced when the plasma sodium concentration was lowered at 0.5 mEq/L/h [31]. However, in elderly patients, slow correction (<0.25 mEq/L/h) is associated with increased mortality [32]. Similar to treatment of hyponatremia, the plasma sodium concentration should not be corrected by more than 8 to 10 mEq per L over 24 hours. In contrast, acute hypernatremia should be rapidly corrected over 24 to 48 hours.

The water deficit represents the existing amount of water loss that must be offset; ongoing free water losses, including insensible losses (approximately 40 mL per hour), must also be replaced. The replacement fluid can be administered orally or intravenously as dextrose in water. Sodium or potassium can be added if there are concurrent losses of these cations, but the addition of these solutes decreases the amount of free water that is being given. It should be emphasized that an isotonic saline solution should be used as initial therapy in the volume-depleted, hypotensive patient because restoration of tissue perfusion is of primary importance.

Treatment of Diabetes Insipidus. The major symptoms of both forms of diabetes insipidus are polyuria and polydipsia. Treatment for these disorders is aimed at decreasing the urine output.

Central Diabetes Insipidus. Because the primary problem is deficient secretion of ADH, control of the polyuria can be achieved by hormone replacement using DDAVP (desmopressin), a two–amino acid synthetic analogue of ADH. DDAVP is administered by nasal spray in a usual dose starting at 5 μg once a day. Because nocturia is often the most troubling symptom, the initial dose is usually given at night. Tablets of desmopressin are also available although their absorption may vary in different patients. Therefore, switching from the intranasal form to a tablet may require retitration and close monitoring. The starting dose of the tablet is 0.05 mg per day. The size and necessity for a daytime dose can be determined by the effectiveness of the evening dose. If, for example, polyuria does not recur until noon, then one-half of the evening doses may be sufficient at that time.

One important potential risk inherent in treating CDI with DDAVP is that of water retention leading to the development of hyponatremia. There are several reasons why this may occur. Patients are no longer polyuric once on therapy. Because they are on a fixed dose of DDAVP, their ADH activity is constant and not regulated. V_2 receptors may be upregulated as a result of prolonged deprivation of vasopressin. Finally, some patients may retain their habitually large consumption of water even after their polyuria ceases. Hyponatremia in this context can be avoided by giving the minimum dose that is required to control the polyuria.

Nephrogenic Diabetes Insipidus. NDI results from partial or complete resistance of the kidney to the effects of ADH. As a result, patients with this disorder are not likely to respond to DDAVP.

In adults, a concentrating defect severe enough to produce polyuria as a result of NDI is most often because of chronic lithium use or hypercalcemia. Less frequently, it is caused by other conditions that impair tubular function, such as Sjögren's syndrome. Therapy targets correction of the underlying disorder or discontinuing a causative drug. In hypercalcemic patients, for example, normalization of the plasma calcium concentration usually leads to amelioration of polyuria. In contrast, lithium-induced NDI may be irreversible if the patient already has severe tubular injury and a marked concentrating defect.

Thiazide diuretics can diminish the degree of polyuria in patients with persistent and symptomatic NDI. The combination of a low-sodium diet with a thiazide diuretic (such as hydrochlorothiazide, 25 mg once or twice daily) acts by inducing mild volume depletion. As little as a 1.0- to 1.5-kg weight loss can reduce the urine output by more than 50%, presumably mediated by a hypovolemia-induced increase in proximal sodium and water reabsorption, with diminished water delivery to the ADH-sensitive sites in the collecting tubule.

Thiazide diuretics also limit the ability to dilute the urine. As a result, the concentration of urine in a thiazide-treated individual with NDI typically increases, even in the absence of ADH. This contributes to the decrease in urine volume. As an example, in a patient with a normal solute excretion rate of 900 mOsm/kg/day and a maximum U_{Osm} of 150 mOsm per kg as a result of NDI, a urine output of at least 6 L per day is expected (900 ÷ 150). In contrast, if a thiazide diuretic limits the minimum U_{Osm} to 300 mOsm per day, daily urine output decreases to approximately 3 L each day (900/300).

Thiazide-induced natriuresis can be enhanced by combination therapy with amiloride (or another potassium-sparing diuretic). This regimen has an additional benefit in that amiloride partially blocks the potassium wasting induced by the thiazide. The efficacy of amiloride in patients with reversible lithium nephrotoxicity is directly related to its site and mechanism of action [33]. This drug closes the sodium channels in the luminal membrane of the collecting tubule cells. These channels constitute the mechanism by which filtered lithium normally enters these cells and then interferes with their response to ADH. In contrast to amiloride, thiazide diuretics should be used cautiously, if at all, in patients with lithium-induced NDI *who are still taking lithium* because volume depletion can lead to increased proximal lithium reabsorption and potentially toxic plasma lithium levels.

Nonsteroidal anti-inflammatory drugs (NSAIDs) cause inhibition of renal prostaglandin synthesis. This has the effect of increasing concentrating ability because prostaglandins normally antagonize the urinary concentrating action of ADH. If, for example, healthy subjects are given a submaximal dose of ADH, the ensuing rise in U_{Osm} can be increased by more than 200 mOsm per kg if the patient has been pretreated with an NSAID. The result in patients with NDI may be a 25% to 50% reduction in urine output, a response that is partially additive to that of a thiazide diuretic. Not all NSAIDs are equally effective in a given patient. For example, some patients may have a good response to indomethacin but derive little, if any, benefit from ibuprofen. The impact of cyclooxygenase-2 inhibitors remains to be determined. However, these agents can exacerbate CHF and have been associated with fluid overload, in a manner similar to that of nonselective NSAIDS [34].

Dietary modification via the use of a low-sodium, low-protein diet can diminish the urine output in patients with NDI. The resultant decrease in net solute excretion (as sodium salts and urea) at any given U_{Osm} reduces the urine output.

Most patients with NDI have partial, rather than complete, resistance to ADH. It is, therefore, possible that administering exogenous ADH in doses sufficient to achieve supraphysiologic hormone levels can increase the renal effect of ADH.

DISORDERS OF PLASMA POTASSIUM

Potassium is the major intracellular cation. Only approximately 2% of body potassium is located in the extracellular space, where the concentration (3.5 to 5.0 mEq per L) is much lower than inside cells (125 to 140 mEq per L). This concentration difference is preserved by the Na^+/K^+-adenosine triphosphatase (ATPase) pump that actively transports sodium out of, and potassium into, most cells. Because such a small proportion of K^+ is extracellular, even a slight change in plasma potassium concentration can engender dramatic effects on myoneural cell physiology.

Normal Potassium Homeostasis

Daily potassium intake in the United States varies between 40 and 120 mEq. Most of this (approximately 90%) is eliminated by the kidney; the rest is excreted in stool. In chronic kidney disease, gastrointestinal potassium excretion increases, a process that depends, in part, on aldosterone.

Only approximately 50% of potassium ingested in the diet or administered parenterally appears in the urine during the first 4 hours. Consequently, more than half of an acute potassium load must be rapidly translocated into cells if life-threatening hyperkalemia to be averted.

Transcellular Potassium Shifts

The most important factors involved in transporting K^+ intracellularly are insulin and β-adrenergic stimulation. Insulin stimulates the Na^+/K^+-ATPase pump present in most cell membranes, accelerating the transfer process.

Activation of β-adrenergic receptors (specifically the β_2-receptor) also stimulates K^+ movement from the plasma into cells. The pathophysiology is, in part, owing to direct stimulation of the Na^+/K^+-ATPase pump. The observation that the hypokalemic effect of terbutaline (a β-adrenergic agonist) can be blunted by somatostatin suggests that insulin may have a mediatory role in the hypokalemic response to β-adrenergic stimulation.

Aldosterone is the principal hormone stimulating K^+ secretion by the renal tubule. This effect is important in all epithelial cell surfaces.

Renal Regulation of Potassium Excretion

Potassium is freely filtered at the glomerulus so that the concentration of K^+ entering the early proximal tubule is approximately 4 mEq per L. Ninety percent of the filtered potassium load has been reabsorbed by the time the glomerular filtrate reaches the distal tubule. Most renal K^+ excretion normally occurs as a result of secretion by the distal nephron. Potassium secretion occurs in the principal cells of the cortical collecting tubule (Fig. 199.4). Movement of potassium from the tubular cell into the lumen is controlled by the existing state of potassium balance, the rate of sodium reabsorption (a process driven by aldosterone) that generates a lumen-negative electrical gradient down which K^+ can move, and the rate of distal urine flow that maintains a high tubular cell-to-lumen potassium gradient by washing away secreted K^+.

Aldosterone enters the principal cell from the basolateral (antiluminal) side. Once inside, it binds to receptors, which increase the number of open luminal sodium channels and increase the number and activity of the Na^+/K^+-ATPase pumps in the basolateral membrane. The ensuing increase in cell potassium favors the secretion of K^+ into the lumen, down the electrochemical gradient provided by Na^+ reabsorption.

In states of potassium depletion, potassium secretion in the cortical collecting tubule is reduced, and potassium reabsorption stimulated. Reabsorption takes place in the intercalated (acid-secreting) cells of this nephron segment (Fig. 199.5).

Hypokalemia

Potassium entering the body is largely stored in the cells and then excreted in the urine. Thus, a reduction in the plasma potassium concentration can result from decreased intake, increased cellular uptake, or increased losses. These losses, which are the most common contributors to hypokalemia, can occur via the urine, the gastrointestinal tract, or, less commonly, through the skin (Table 199.5).

Causes of Hypokalemia

Decreased Potassium Intake. Because the kidney can lower potassium excretion to less than 25 mEq per day in response to potassium depletion, decreased intake alone rarely causes hypokalemia, but it can enhance the severity of other causes of potassium depletion such as diuretic therapy.

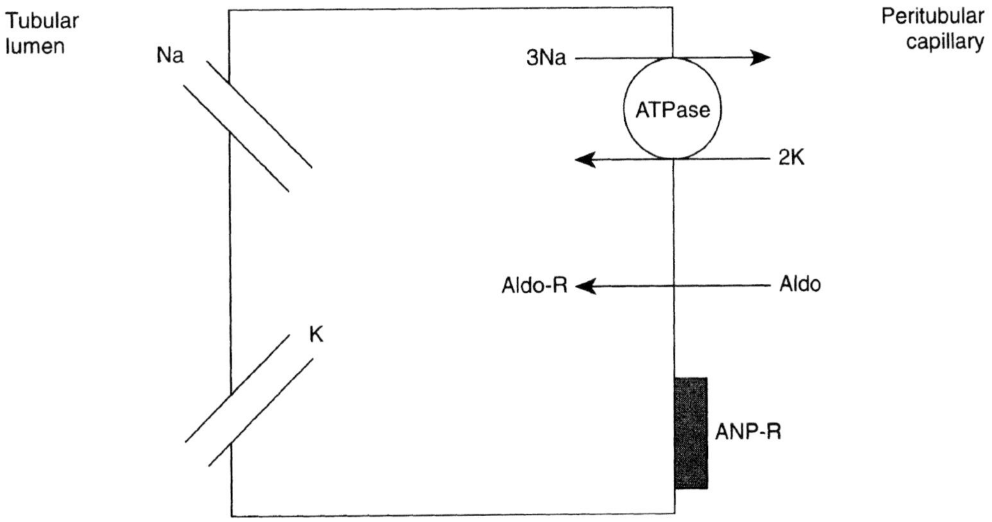

FIGURE 199.4 Schematic representation of sodium and potassium transport mechanisms in the sodium-reabsorbing cells in the collecting tubules. The entry of filtered sodium into the cells is mediated by selective sodium channels in the apical (luminal) membrane; the energy for this process is provided by the favorable electrochemical gradient for sodium (cell interior electronegative and low cell sodium concentration). Reabsorbed sodium is pumped out of the cell by the Na^+/K^+–adenosine triphosphatase (ATPase) pump in the basolateral (peritubular) membrane. The reabsorption of cationic sodium makes the lumen electronegative, thereby creating a favorable gradient for the secretion of potassium into the lumen via potassium channels in the apical membrane. Aldosterone (Aldo), after combining with the cytosolic mineralocorticoid receptor (Aldo-R), leads to enhanced sodium reabsorption and potassium secretion in the cortical collecting tubule by increasing both the number of open sodium channels and the number of Na^+/K^+–ATPase pumps. Atrial natriuretic peptide (ANP), on the contrary, acts primarily in the inner medullary collecting duct by combining with its basolateral membrane receptor (ANP-R) and activating guanylate cyclase. ANP inhibits sodium reabsorption by closing the sodium channels. The potassium-sparing diuretics amiloride and triamterene act by closing the sodium channels directly, and spironolactone acts by competing with aldosterone for binding to the mineralocorticoid receptor.

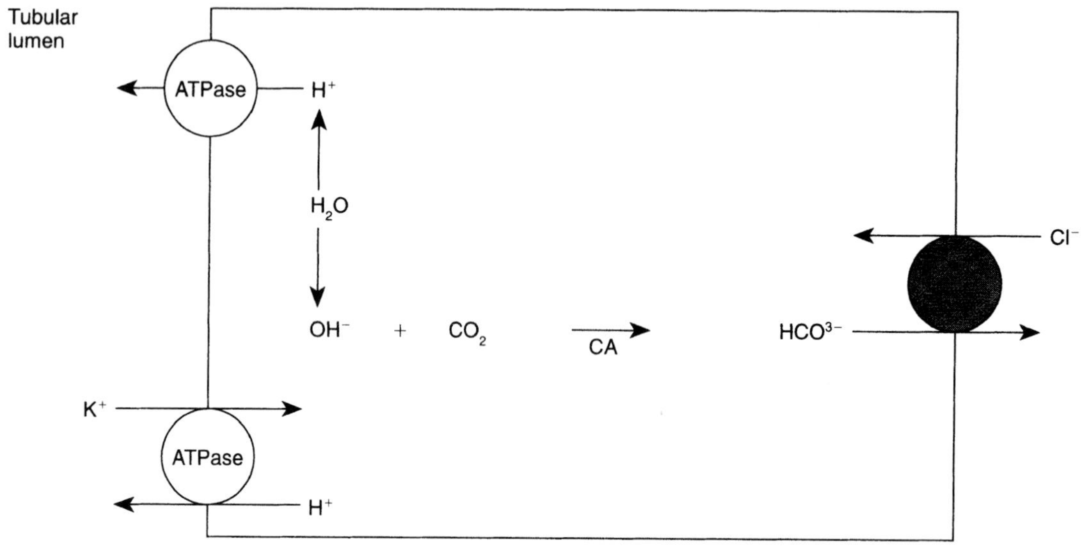

FIGURE 199.5 Transport mechanisms involved in hydrogen secretion and bicarbonate and potassium reabsorption in type-A intercalated cells in the cortical collecting tubule and in the outer medullary collecting tubule cells. Water (H_2O) within the cell dissociates into hydrogen and hydroxyl anions. The former are secreted into the lumen by H–adenosine triphosphatase (ATPase) pumps in the luminal membrane; chloride may be cosecreted with hydrogen to maintain electroneutrality. The hydroxyl anions in the cell combine with carbon dioxide to form bicarbonate in a reaction catalyzed by carbonic anhydrase (CA). Bicarbonate is then returned to the systemic circulation via chloride–bicarbonate exchangers in the basolateral membrane. The favorable inward concentration gradient for chloride (plasma and interstitial concentration greater than that in the cell) provides the energy for bicarbonate reabsorption. H/K-ATPase pumps, which lead to both hydrogen secretion and potassium reabsorption, may also be present in the luminal membrane. The number of these pumps increases with potassium depletion, suggesting that their main function is to promote potassium conservation.

TABLE 199.5

Major Causes of Hypokalemia

- Decreased potassium intake
- Increased entry into cells
  - Elevation in extracellular pH
  - Increased availability of insulin
  - Elevated β-adrenergic activity
  - Hypokalemic periodic paralysis
  - Marked increase in blood cell production
- Increased gastrointestinal losses
- Increased urinary losses
  - Diuretics
  - Primary mineralocorticoid excess
  - Loss of gastric secretions
  - Nonreabsorbable anions
  - Renal tubular acidosis
  - Hypomagnesemia
  - Amphotericin B
  - Aminoglycosides
  - Salt-wasting nephropathies, including Bartter's syndrome
  - Polyuria
- Increased sweat losses
- Dialysis

Increased Entry into Cells. The markedly inequitable distribution of potassium between the cells and the extracellular fluid is maintained by the Na^+/K^+-ATPase pump in the cell membrane. Occasionally, increased potassium entry into cells may result in transient hypokalemia.

Elevation in Extracellular pH. The transcellular hydrogen ion shifts accompanying metabolic and respiratory alkalosis obligate increased sequestration of potassium in cells. In general, this direct effect is relatively small because the plasma potassium concentration falls to less than 0.4 mEq per L for every 0.1-unit rise in pH. This phenomenon provides the rationale for the administration of sodium bicarbonate to treat the hyperkalemia of metabolic acidosis.

Despite the fact that the direct effect of alkalemia is relatively small, hypokalemia is common in metabolic alkalosis. The major reason for this association is that the underlying cause (diuretics, vomiting, or hyperaldosteronism) leads to losses of both hydrogen and potassium ions.

Increased Availability of Insulin. Insulin promotes the entry of potassium into skeletal muscle and hepatic cells by increasing the activity of the Na^+/K^+-ATPase pump in the cell membrane. This effect is most prominent after the administration of insulin to patients with diabetic ketoacidosis or severe nonketotic hyperglycemia.

The plasma potassium concentration can also be reduced in nondiabetic patients by a carbohydrate load. Thus, intravenous administration of potassium chloride in a dextrose-containing solution in an effort to correct hypokalemia can transiently further reduce the plasma potassium concentration and, possibly, lead to cardiac arrhythmias.

Elevated β-Adrenergic Activity. Catecholamines, acting via β_2-adrenergic receptors, promote potassium entry into the cells by increasing Na^+/K^+-ATPase activity. As a result, transient hypokalemia can occur with stress-induced release of epinephrine, as in acute illness, coronary ischemia, theophylline intoxication, or alcohol withdrawal. A similar effect, in which the plasma potassium concentration can fall acutely by more than 0.5 to 1.0 mEq per L, can be achieved by the administration of a β-adrenergic agonist (such as albuterol, terbutaline, or epinephrine). This effect must be considered when diuretic therapy is used for the treatment of hypertension in patients receiving β-agonists for asthma or chronic lung disease. The hypokalemic response to epinephrine can be blocked by a nonselective β-blocker (such as propranolol), but a β_1-selective agent (such as atenolol) offers no protection, at least at lower doses (<100 mg per day).

Hypokalemic Periodic Paralysis. Hypokalemic periodic paralysis is a rare disorder of uncertain cause characterized by potentially fatal episodes of muscle weakness or paralysis that can affect the respiratory muscles. Acute attacks—in which the sudden movement of potassium into the cells can lower the plasma potassium concentration to as low as 1.5 to 2.5 mEq per L—are often precipitated by rest after exercise, stress, or a carbohydrate meal, events that are often associated with increased release of epinephrine or insulin. Hypokalemic periodic paralysis may be familial with autosomal dominant inheritance, or it may be acquired in patients (often, but not exclusively, Asian men) with thyrotoxicosis.

Oral administration of 60 to 120 mEq of potassium chloride usually aborts acute attacks within 15 to 20 minutes. Another 60 mEq can be given if no improvement is noted. The presence of hypokalemia must be confirmed before therapy because potassium can worsen episodes caused by the normokalemic or hyperkalemic forms of periodic paralysis. Furthermore, excess potassium administration during an acute episode may lead to posttreatment hyperkalemia as potassium moves back out of the cells.

Marked Increase in Blood Cell Production. An acute increase in hematopoietic cell production is associated with potassium uptake by the new cells and possible hypokalemia. This most often occurs after the administration of vitamin B_{12} or folic acid to treat a megaloblastic anemia or of granulocyte-macrophage colony-stimulating factor to treat neutropenia.

Metabolically active blood cells may continue to absorb potassium after blood has been drawn. This phenomenon has been described in patients with acute myeloid leukemia and a high white blood cell count. In these patients, the measured plasma potassium concentration may be less than 1 mEq per L (without symptoms) if the blood is allowed to stand at room temperature for a prolonged period before separation of the plasma from the cells.

Hypothermia. Accidental or induced hypothermia (as occurs during cardiac bypass) can accelerate potassium movement into the cells and lower the plasma potassium concentration to less than 3.0 mEq per L. In contrast, hyperkalemia in an individual with severe hypothermia usually signifies irreversible tissue necrosis.

Medications/Toxins. Barium sulfide, used in pesticides, radiologic imaging, and depilatory agents, has been reported to cause severe transient hypokalemia when ingested [35].

Hypokalemia is a complication of severe chloroquine overdose [36].

Increased Gastrointestinal Losses. Loss of gastric or intestinal secretions from any cause (vomiting, diarrhea, laxatives, or tube drainage) is associated with potassium wasting and, possibly, hypokalemia. However, it should be emphasized that the concentration of potassium in gastric secretions is relatively low (5 to 10 mEq per L) and that the potassium depletion is primarily because of increased urinary losses. The metabolic alkalosis that results from loss of gastric secretions raises the plasma bicarbonate concentration and, therefore, the filtered bicarbonate load above its proximal tubular reabsorptive threshold. More sodium bicarbonate and water are thus delivered to the distal potassium secretory site in the presence of hypovolemia-induced aldosterone release. Secreted potassium combines with the negatively charged bicarbonate and is excreted in the final urine, leading to hypokalemia.

The urinary potassium wasting seen with loss of gastric secretions is typically most prominent in the first few days; thereafter, proximal bicarbonate reabsorptive capacity increases, leading to a marked reduction in urinary sodium, bicarbonate, and potassium excretion. At this time, the urine pH falls from more than 7.0 to less than 5.5.

Increased Urinary Losses. Urinary potassium excretion is mostly derived from potassium secretion in the distal nephron, particularly by the principal cells in the cortical collecting tubule. This process is primarily influenced by two factors: aldosterone and the distal delivery of sodium and water. Urinary potassium wasting generally requires increases in aldosterone or in distal flow. Aldosterone acts partly by stimulating sodium reabsorption. The removal of cationic sodium makes the lumen relatively electronegative, thereby promoting passive potassium secretion from the tubular cell into the lumen through specific potassium channels in the luminal membrane.

Diuretics. Any diuretic that acts proximal to the potassium secretory site, including carbonic anhydrase inhibitors and loop and thiazide diuretics, increases distal delivery and, via the induction of volume depletion, activates the renin–angiotensin–aldosterone system. As a result, urinary potassium excretion increases, potentially leading to hypokalemia.

Primary Mineralocorticoid Excess. Urinary potassium wasting is characteristic of any condition associated with primary hypersecretion of a mineralocorticoid, as occurs with an aldosterone-producing adrenal adenoma. Affected patients are usually hypertensive, and the differential diagnosis includes diuretic therapy (which may be surreptitious) in a patient with underlying hypertension and renovascular disease, in which increased secretion of renin leads to enhanced aldosterone release. By comparison, plasma renin activity is suppressed in primary states of mineralocorticoid excess.

Nonreabsorbable Anions. The presence of nonreabsorbable anions in the filtrate draws increased amounts of sodium to the distal nephron where it is reabsorbed at the expense of potassium. Examples of nonreabsorbable anions include bicarbonate in vomiting-induced metabolic alkalosis, β-hydroxybutyrate in diabetic ketoacidosis, hippurate in toluene exposure (glue sniffing), and penicillin in patients receiving high-dose penicillin therapy. The effect of nonreabsorbable anions is augmented when there is concurrent volume depletion. Both the resulting decrease in distal chloride delivery (limiting the ability of chloride reabsorption to dissipate the lumen-negative gradient) and the enhanced secretion of aldosterone promote potassium secretion.

Metabolic Acidosis. Increased urinary potassium losses can occur in several forms of metabolic acidosis by mechanisms similar to those already described. In diabetic ketoacidosis, for example, increased distal sodium and water delivery (because of the glucose-induced osmotic diuresis), hypovolemia-induced hyperaldosteronism, and β-hydroxybutyrate acting as a nonreabsorbable anion all can contribute to potassium wasting. Potassium wasting can also occur in both type-1 (distal) and type-2 (proximal) renal tubular acidosis (RTA) (see Chapter 198).

Hypomagnesemia. Hypomagnesemia is present in up to 40% of patients with hypokalemia. In many cases, such as with diuretic therapy, vomiting, or diarrhea, there are concurrent potassium and magnesium losses. Hypomagnesemia of any cause can lead to increased urinary potassium losses. A direct effect of magnesium on tubular potassium transport is likely the mechanism by which hypomagnesemia promotes kaliuresis [37]. Diagnosis of concomitant hypomagnesemia is particularly important because the hypokalemia often cannot be corrected until the magnesium deficit is repaired.

Salt-Wasting Nephropathies. Occasionally, renal diseases associated with decreased proximal, loop, or distal sodium reabsorption can lead to hypokalemia via a mechanism similar to that induced by diuretics. This problem may arise in patients with Bartter's syndrome or Gitelman's syndrome, tubulointerstitial diseases, such as interstitial nephritis as a result of Sjögren's syndrome or lupus, hypercalcemia, and tubular injury induced by lysozyme in patients with acute monocytic or myelomonocytic leukemia. Increased potassium uptake by the leukemic cells may also contribute to the fall in the plasma potassium concentration.

Polyuria. In the presence of potassium depletion, healthy subjects can lower their urinary potassium concentration to 5 to 10 mEq per L. If, however, the urine output is greater than 5 to 10 L per day, obligatory potassium losses can exceed to 50 to 100 mEq in this period. This problem is most likely to occur in primary polydipsia, in which the urine output may be elevated during a prolonged period. An equivalent degree of polyuria can also occur in CDI, but patients with this disorder typically seek medical care soon after the polyuria has begun.

Transcutaneous Losses. Daily potassium loss through the skin is normally negligible because the volume of perspiration is low and the potassium concentration is only 5 to 10 mEq per L. However, subjects exercising in a hot climate can produce 10 L or more of sweat per day, leading to potassium depletion if these losses are not replaced. Urinary potassium excretion may also contribute because aldosterone release is enhanced by both exercise (via catecholamine-induced renin secretion) and volume loss.

Extensive burns are another situation in which potassium losses through the skin may cause hypokalemia. Although the concentration of potassium in sweat is low, the potassium concentration of fluid lost through the skin after burns may greatly exceed the plasma level because of local tissue breakdown, which leads to the release of potassium from cells.

Dialysis. Although patients with end-stage renal disease typically retain potassium and tend to be mildly hyperkalemic, hypokalemia can be induced in some patients by maintenance dialysis. This is more likely to occur in patients on chronic peritoneal dialysis, in whom dialysis is performed every day. By comparison, hemodialysis treatments are typically administered only three times per week. Nevertheless, transient hypokalemia often follows a hemodialysis treatment.

Clinical Manifestations

Most individuals with mild hypokalemia exhibit no symptoms referable to the low plasma K^+ concentration. The major disturbances seen with more severe K^+ deficiency are changes in cardiovascular, neuromuscular, and renal function. Cardiac toxicity may be manifested by serious arrhythmias because of hyperpolarization of the myocardial cell membrane, leading to a prolonged refractory period and increased susceptibility to reentrant arrhythmias. Earlier electrocardiographic (ECG) changes of hypokalemia include T-wave depression with prominent U waves (Fig. 199.6).

Hyperpolarization also slows down nerve conduction and muscle contractions, which may contribute to symptoms such as muscle weakness, cramps, and paresthesias, although these are usually not observed until the plasma K^+ concentration is less than 2.5 mEq per L. Severe hypokalemia may promote rhabdomyolysis. Profound hypokalemia can also impair respiratory muscle function, leading to hypoventilation.

Polyuria caused by stimulation of thirst and resistance to the action of ADH are the primary renal manifestations of hypokalemia. Increased thirst results from direct stimulation of the hypothalamic thirst center as well as from an appropriate response to polyuria. The mechanism of resistance to ADH appears to be because of reduced expression of the water channel (aquaporin-2).

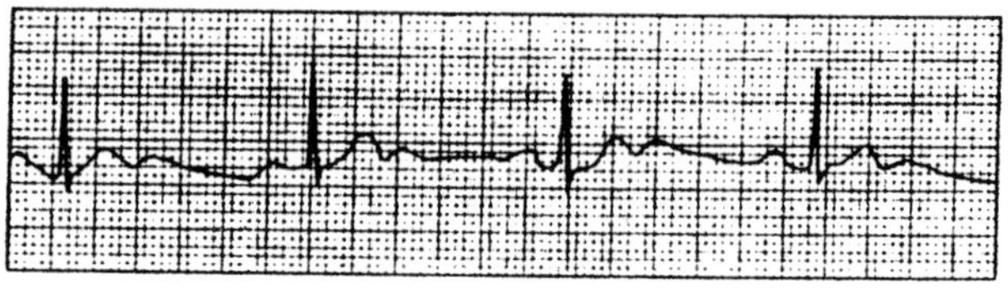

FIGURE 199.6 Both hypokalemia and hyperkalemia can cause changes in the patient's electrocardiogram. The electrocardiogram from a patient with moderate hypokalemia shows prominent U waves.

Diagnosis

The cause of hypokalemia can usually be determined from the history. In some cases, the diagnosis is not readily apparent. The surreptitious vomiting of bulimia or the diarrhea of laxative abuse may be omitted from the patient's history. Measurement of blood pressure and urinary potassium excretion and assessment of acid–base balance are often helpful in such cases.

Urinary Potassium. In the presence of potassium depletion, a healthy subject should lower urinary potassium excretion to less than 30 mEq per day; values above this level reflect at least a contribution from urinary potassium wasting. Random measurement of the urine potassium concentration can be used but is less accurate than a 24-hour collection. Extrarenal losses probably are present if the urine potassium concentration is less than 15 mEq per L, unless the patient is markedly polyuric. Higher values do not necessarily indicate potassium wasting if the urine volume is reduced. The response to potassium depletion is twofold: decreased potassium secretion by the collecting tubule principal cells and increased active potassium reabsorption by H/K-ATPase pumps in the luminal membrane of the adjacent type-A intercalated cells (Fig. 199.5). These pumps, which are activated by hypokalemia, reabsorb potassium and secrete hydrogen.

Once urinary potassium excretion is measured, the following diagnostic possibilities should be considered in the patient with hypokalemia of uncertain origin:

- Metabolic acidosis with a low rate of renal potassium excretion is suggestive of lower gastrointestinal losses as a result of diarrhea, laxative abuse, or a villous adenoma.
- Metabolic acidosis with renal potassium wasting is most often caused by diabetic ketoacidosis or by type-1 (distal) or type-2 (proximal) RTA. A salt-wasting nephropathy can produce similar findings, with the associated renal insufficiency responsible for the acidemia.
- Metabolic alkalosis with a low rate of urinary potassium excretion may be as a result of surreptitious vomiting or diuretic use if the urinary collection is obtained several days after the vomiting or diuretic use has been halted.
- Metabolic alkalosis with renal potassium wasting and a normal blood pressure most often results from ongoing vomiting, diuretic use, or, far less commonly, from Bartter's syndrome or Gitelman's syndrome. A low urine chloride concentration helps to distinguish the hypokalemia of vomiting from that of diuretics or Bartter's syndrome and Gitelman's syndrome.
- Metabolic alkalosis with potassium wasting and hypertension suggests surreptitious diuretic therapy in patients with underlying hypertension, renovascular disease, or one of the causes of primary mineralocorticoid excess.

The possible presence of primary mineralocorticoid excess (with aldosterone and, to a lesser degree, deoxycorticosterone being the major endogenous mineralocorticoids) should be suspected in any patient with hypertension and unexplained hypokalemia and metabolic alkalosis.

The ingestion of licorice can produce a similar clinical and metabolic picture. The active compound in licorice, glycyrrhizic acid, inhibits renal 11*β*-hydroxysteroid dehydrogenase activity. This enzyme normally inactivates cortisol. The result is cortisol-induced stimulation of the mineralocorticoid receptor, leading to renal sodium retention and potassium loss.

The other major cause of hypertension and hypokalemia is renovascular disease, in which the hypersecretion of renin leads sequentially to increased secretion of angiotensin II and then aldosterone. It is important to be aware that hypokalemia is characteristic of malignant hypertension, which is a high renin, high aldosterone state, regardless of the underlying cause.

Treatment

Although hypokalemia can be transiently induced by the entry of potassium into the cells, most cases are caused by gastrointestinal or urinary losses. Optimal therapy depends on the severity of the potassium deficit; somewhat different considerations are required to minimize continued urinary losses caused by diuretic therapy or, less often, to one of the causes of primary hyperaldosteronism.

Potassium Deficit. The total potassium deficit can only be approximated because there is no strict correlation between the plasma potassium concentration and total body potassium stores. In general, the loss of 200 to 400 mEq of potassium is required to lower the plasma potassium concentration from 4 to 3 mEq per L; the loss of an additional 200 to 400 mEq lowers the plasma potassium concentration to approximately 2 mEq per L. Continued potassium losses do not as readily worsen the degree of hypokalemia because of the release of potassium from the intracellular pool.

These estimates assume a normal distribution of potassium between the cells and the extracellular fluid. The most common setting in which this does not apply is diabetic ketoacidosis, a disorder in which hyperosmolality and insulin deficiency favor the movement of potassium out of the cells. As a result, patients with this disorder may have a normal or even elevated plasma potassium concentration at presentation, despite having incurred a marked potassium deficit owing to urinary or gastrointestinal losses, or both. Potassium supplementation for these patients should begin once the plasma potassium concentration is 4.5 mEq per L or less, provided that the patient is producing urine, because the administration of insulin and fluids may cause a precipitous drop in the plasma potassium concentration.

Potassium Preparations. Intravenous or oral potassium chloride generally is the preferred treatment for hypokalemia. Use of the chloride salt has two important advantages. First, potassium chloride more rapidly raises the plasma potassium concentration than does potassium bicarbonate or potassium citrate, the citrate being rapidly metabolized to bicarbonate. Bicarbonate enters cells more readily than does chloride. The retention of chloride in the extracellular fluid, obligated by the need to maintain electroneutrality, limits the initial entry of potassium into the cells, thereby maximizing the rise in the plasma potassium concentration. Second, most patients with hypokalemia also have metabolic alkalosis. For example, with diuretic therapy, vomiting, and hyperaldosteronism, hydrogen loss accompanies that of potassium. Potassium must be given with chloride to such patients if both the hypokalemia and the alkalosis are to be corrected optimally (see Chapter 198). In comparison, potassium bicarbonate or potassium citrate can be given to patients with hypokalemia and metabolic acidosis, such as occurs in RTA and chronic diarrheal states.

Oral potassium chloride can be given in crystalline form (salt substitutes), as a liquid, or in a slow-release tablet or capsule. Salt substitutes contain 50 to 65 mEq per level teaspoon; they may be the ideal form of oral therapy, because they are safe, well tolerated, and much cheaper than the other preparations. Potassium chloride solutions, on the other hand, are often unpalatable, and the slow-release preparations can, in rare cases, cause ulcerative or stenotic lesions in the gastrointestinal tract as a result of the local accumulation of high concentrations of potassium.

Merely increasing the intake of potassium-rich foods such as oranges and bananas is generally less effective in the absence of renal insufficiency. These foods contain phosphate and citrate rather than chloride and are, therefore, less likely to correct the hypokalemia and metabolic alkalosis.

Potassium chloride can be given intravenously to patients who are unable to eat or who have severe hypokalemia. It is usually added to a solution in which the concentration should generally not exceed 40 mEq of potassium per L because higher concentrations can lead to pain and sclerosis of a peripheral vein. A saline solution is preferred to a dextrose solution for initial therapy because the administration of dextrose can lead to a transient 0.2 to 1.4 mEq per L reduction in the plasma potassium concentration because of glucose-induced insulin release.

Mild-to-Moderate Potassium Depletion. The majority of patients have a plasma potassium concentration between 3.0 and 3.5 mEq per L; this degree of potassium depletion usually produces no symptoms, except in patients with advanced liver disease or in patients with heart disease, particularly if they are taking digoxin. Treatment in this setting is directed toward replacing the lost potassium, usually beginning with 40 to 80 mEq of potassium chloride per day, and toward treating the disorder responsible for the loss of potassium.

Potassium replacement alone may be insufficient to treat patients with ongoing urinary losses caused by chronic diuretic therapy, tubular dysfunction, or primary hyperaldosteronism. Potassium-sparing diuretics such as amiloride, triamterene, the aldosterone antagonists, spironolactone, and eplerenone are generally more effective than other agents, because they limit further urinary losses of both potassium and magnesium. It is frequently underappreciated, however, that, in the presence of high levels of aldosterone, greater-than-usual doses (up to 20 to 40 mg of amiloride and 150 to 300 mg of spironolactone) may be required to block potassium secretion. The combination of a potassium-sparing diuretic with potassium supplements should be used only with careful monitoring to prevent possible overcorrection with development of hyperkalemia and should be avoided in most patients with renal insufficiency.

Severe Hypokalemia. Potassium repletion is more urgent for patients with profound or symptomatic hypokalemia (i.e., arrhythmias, marked muscle weakness). This is most easily done orally. The plasma potassium concentration transiently rises by as much as 1.0 to 1.5 mEq per L after 40 to 60 mEq and by 2.5 to 3.5 mEq per L after 135 to 160 mEq. The level then falls because most of the exogenous potassium is taken up by the cells. In light of these fluxes, careful monitoring is required, and more potassium should be given as necessary. A patient with a plasma potassium concentration of 2.0 mEq per L, for example, *may* have a 400 to 800 mEq potassium deficit.

Some patients with severe hypokalemia must be treated intravenously because of medical instability or an inability to take medication orally. There are two potential limitations to intravenous therapy: A *maximum* concentration of 50 to 60 mEq per L can be administered via a peripheral vein without irritation, and, because saline solutions are preferable, volume overload is a potential risk in susceptible subjects.

The necessity for aggressive intravenous therapy occurs primarily in patients with diabetic ketoacidosis or nonketotic hyperglycemia with hypokalemia caused by marked urinary potassium losses. As described previously, treatment with insulin and fluids exacerbates the hypokalemia. Because these patients are also quite volume depleted, the addition of 40 to 60 mEq of potassium chloride to each liter of half-isotonic saline can supply large quantities of potassium with less risk of pulmonary congestion.

In general, the maximum rate of intravenous potassium administration is 10 to 20 mEq per hour, although as much as 40 to 100 mEq per hour has been given to selected patients with paralysis or life-threatening arrhythmias [38]. In these cases, solutions containing as much as 200 mEq of potassium per L (20 mEq in 100 mL of isotonic saline) have been used. They should be infused into a large vein, such as the femoral vein; a central venous line has also been used, but a local increase in the potassium concentration could have a deleterious effect on cardiac conduction.

It must be emphasized that rapid intravenous administration of potassium is potentially dangerous, even in potassium-depleted patients. Thus, careful monitoring of the physiologic effects of hypokalemia (ECG abnormalities, muscle weakness, or paralysis) is essential. Once these problems are no longer severe, the rate of potassium repletion should be slowed down to 10 to 20 mEq per hour, even though there may be persistent hypokalemia.

Hyperkalemia

Hyperkalemia is a relatively common laboratory abnormality in critically ill patients, particularly in those with oliguric acute or chronic kidney disease.

Etiology

Hyperkalemia is rare in healthy subjects because the transcellular and renal disposal adaptations prevent significant potassium accumulation in the extracellular fluid. Furthermore, the efficiency of potassium handling is increased if potassium intake is slowly enhanced, thereby allowing what might otherwise be a fatal potassium load to be tolerated. This phenomenon, called *potassium adaptation*, is mostly because of more rapid potassium excretion in the urine.

Therefore, increasing potassium intake is not commonly a cause of hyperkalemia, unless the patient has an impaired capacity for potassium excretion or the potassium loading occurs too rapidly for such adaptation to occur. As examples, acute hyperkalemia can be induced (primarily in infants because of their small size) by the administration of intravenous potassium penicillin as an intravenous bolus or by the ingestion of a potassium-containing salt substitute.

The net release of potassium from the cells, either because of enhanced release or decreased entry, can also cause hyperkalemia. As with exogenous potassium loading, the elevation is typically transient because the excess potassium is excreted in the urine. Because persistent hyperkalemia requires impairment in urinary potassium excretion, it may be inferred that this problem is generally associated with a reduction in either aldosterone effect or in the delivery of sodium and water to the distal secretory site. The causes of hyperkalemia are listed in Table 199.6.

Increased Potassium Release from Cells

Pseudohyperkalemia. *Pseudohyperkalemia* refers to conditions in which the elevation in the measured plasma potassium concentration is caused by potassium movement out of the cells during or after the blood specimen has been drawn. The major cause of this problem is mechanical trauma during venipuncture, resulting in hemolysis. Because this is an in vitro phenomenon, the patient demonstrates no clinical signs and symptoms of hyperkalemia.

Potassium also moves out of white cells and platelets after clotting has occurred. Thus, the serum potassium concentration normally exceeds the true value in the plasma by as much as 0.5 mEq per L. This difference in normal levels is not clinically important. In contrast, a patient with marked leukocytosis or thrombocytosis (white cell or platelet count >100,000 per μL or 1,000,000 per μL, respectively) may have a measured serum potassium concentration as high as 9 mEq per L. This phenomenon is most often observed in patients with myeloproliferative diseases. With essential thrombocytosis, for example, the measured serum potassium concentration rises by approximately 0.15 mEq per L for every 100,000 per μL elevation in the platelet count.

Pseudohyperkalemia should be suspected whenever there is no apparent cause for an elevated plasma potassium concentration in an asymptomatic patient and particularly in patients with persistent hyperkalemia despite normal renal function. Comparing the serum potassium concentration with that in plasma (collected using a heparinized specimen tube) often establishes the diagnosis. Comparing the serum potassium levels drawn with and without a tourniquet also may be useful diagnostically if a significant difference is observed.

Metabolic Acidosis. The buffering of excess hydrogen ions in the cells can lead to potassium movement into the extracellular fluid; this transcellular shift is necessitated, in part, by the need to maintain electroneutrality. This phenomenon is less likely to occur in the organic acidoses, ketoacidosis, and lactic acidosis. Although the potassium level may be elevated in both of these conditions, hyperkalemia appears to result from insulin deficiency and tissue breakdown, with potassium leakage from cells rather than from the acidosis itself.

Insulin Deficiency, Hyperglycemia, and Hyperosmolality. Insulin promotes potassium entry into cells; thus, the ingestion of glucose (which stimulates endogenous insulin secretion) minimizes the rise in the plasma potassium concentration induced by concurrent potassium intake. On the contrary, in patients with uncontrolled diabetes mellitus, the combination of insulin deficiency and the hyperosmolality induced by hyperglycemia frequently leads to hyperkalemia, even though a patient may be markedly potassium depleted from previously incurred urinary potassium losses.

An elevation in P_{Osm} results in osmotic water movement from cells into the extracellular fluid. This is accompanied by potassium movement out of the cells. A similar rise in plasma potassium can occur with any solute that increases the effective P_{Osm}, such as mannitol, particularly in patients with renal failure.

Somatostatin, by inhibiting insulin release, can raise the plasma potassium concentration by an average of 0.6 mEq per L in healthy subjects but by more than 1.5 mEq per L to potentially dangerous levels in selected patients with end-stage renal disease [39].

Increased Tissue Breakdown. Any cause of increased tissue breakdown can result in the release of potassium into the extracellular fluid. Hyperkalemia is particularly likely to develop in this setting if renal impairment is also present. Clinical examples include breakdown of a large hematoma, as might occur in the wake of a gastrointestinal hemorrhage; rhabdomyolysis from any cause; cell breakdown in patients receiving cytotoxic or radiation therapy for lymphoma or leukemia (the tumor-lysis syndrome); and in patients with severe hypothermia.

***β*-Adrenergic Blockade.** *β*-Adrenergic blockers interfere with the β_2-adrenergic facilitation of potassium uptake by the cells (Fig. 199.4). This effect is associated with only a minor elevation in the plasma potassium concentration in healthy subjects (<0.5 mEq per L) because the excess potassium can be easily excreted in

TABLE 199.6

Major Causes of Hyperkalemia

- Increased potassium release from cells
  - Pseudohyperkalemia
  - Metabolic acidosis
  - Insulin deficiency
  - Hyperglycemia and hyperosmolal states
  - Increased tissue catabolism
  - β-Adrenergic blockade
  - Exercise
  - Other
    - Digitalis overdose
    - Hyperkalemic periodic paralysis
    - Succinylcholine
    - Arginine hydrochloride
- Reduced urinary potassium excretion
  - Hypoaldosteronism
  - Renal disease
  - Reduced effective circulatory volume
  - Selective impairment of potassium excretion
  - Medications
    - Dapsone
    - Trimethoprim
    - Nonsteroidal anti-inflammatory drugs
    - Angiotensin-converting enzyme inhibitors
    - Angiotensin receptor blockers
    - Heparin
    - Potassium-sparing diuretics

the urine. True hyperkalemia is rare, except in conjunction with an additional defect in potassium handling, such as a large potassium load, marked exercise, hypoaldosteronism, or renal failure.

Exercise. Potassium is normally released from muscle cells during exercise. The release of potassium may have a physiologic function, because the local increase in the plasma potassium concentration has a vasodilatory effect, increasing blood flow and energy delivery to the exercising muscle [40].

The increment in the systemic plasma potassium concentration is less pronounced and is related to the degree of exercise: 0.3 to 0.4 mEq per L with slow walking; 0.7 to 1.2 mEq per L with moderate exertion (including prolonged aerobic exercise such as marathon running); and as much as 2.0 mEq per L after exercise to exhaustion [41].

The rise in the plasma potassium concentration is reversed after several minutes of rest and is typically associated with mild-rebound hypokalemia (averaging 0.4 to 0.5 mEq per L below the baseline level) that may be arrhythmogenic in susceptible individuals. The degree of potassium release is attenuated by prior physical conditioning (perhaps owing to increased Na^+/K^+–ATPase activity) but may be exacerbated by the administration of β-blockers.

Exercise can interfere with accurate measurement of the plasma potassium concentration. Repeated fist clenching during blood drawing can acutely raise the plasma potassium concentration by more than 1 mEq per L in that forearm, thereby representing another form of pseudohyperkalemia. Careful drawing of the blood and comparison of the plasma to the serum potassium value should identify most cases [42].

Other. Rarer causes of hyperkalemia because of translocation of potassium from the cells into the extracellular fluid include (a) digitalis overdose from dose-dependent inhibition of membrane Na^+/K^+–ATPase and (b) the hyperkalemic form of periodic paralysis, an autosomal dominant disorder in which episodes of weakness or paralysis are usually precipitated by cold exposure, rest after exercise, or the ingestion of small amounts of potassium. Hyperkalemic periodic paralysis appears related to abnormalities of the skeletal muscle cell sodium channel [43].

Administration of succinylcholine to patients with burns, extensive trauma, or neuromuscular disease can also cause hyperkalemia.

Reduced Urinary Potassium Excretion

Impaired urinary potassium excretion generally requires an abnormality in one or both of the two major factors required for adequate renal potassium handling: aldosterone and distal nephron sodium and water delivery.

Hypoaldosteronism. Any cause of decreased aldosterone release or effect diminishes the efficiency of potassium secretion and can lead to hyperkalemia (Table 199.7). The resulting rise in the plasma potassium concentration directly stimulates potassium secretion, partially overcoming the relative absence of aldosterone. As a consequence, the rise in the plasma potassium concentration is small in patients with normal renal function, but it can be clinically important in the presence of underlying renal insufficiency or a high potassium intake.

Hyperkalemia in hypoaldosteronism is usually associated with a mild metabolic acidosis. This condition has been called *type-4 RTA* and appears to be primarily caused by decreased urinary ammonium excretion.

Although aldosterone also promotes sodium retention, decreased availability of aldosterone is not typically associated with prominent sodium wasting with type-4 RTA in adults because of the ability of other antinatriuretic factors such as angiotensin II and norepinephrine to compensate. Hyponatremia is also uncommon because there is no hypovolemic stimulation for ADH release. If hyponatremia is present, primary adrenal insufficiency should be suspected. In this disorder, the concurrent lack of cortisol is a potent stimulus to ADH secretion, leading to water retention and a fall in the plasma sodium concentration.

The causes of hypoaldosteronism include disorders that affect adrenal aldosterone synthesis, the renal response to aldosterone, or renal (and perhaps adrenal) renin release (Table 199.7).

Hyporeninemic Hypoaldosteronism. The syndrome of hyporeninemic hypoaldosteronism, a form of type-4 RTA, is characterized by coexisting defects in the release of renin by the kidney and aldosterone by the adrenal cortex. This relatively common disorder most often occurs in patients with mild-to-moderate renal insufficiency as a result of diabetic nephropathy or chronic interstitial nephritis. Low plasma renin levels are common in diabetic patients, partly because of a defect in the conversion of the precursor prorenin into active renin. Volume expansion induced by diabetes and other chronic kidney diseases may play a contributory role; the increase in atrial natriuretic peptide release in this setting can suppress both the release of renin and the hyperkalemia-induced secretion of aldosterone. Similar hemodynamic and humoral changes occur in the acute nephritic syndrome of postinfectious glomerulonephritis. For some patients, these changes can lead to hyperkalemia that responds to mineralocorticoid replacement. Recovery of renal function within 1 to 2 weeks is associated with restoration of normal potassium balance.

Low renin and aldosterone levels may also occur in several other settings:

- *NSAIDs.* NSAIDs lower renal renin secretion, which is normally partially mediated by locally produced prostaglandins. The result is that the plasma potassium concentration rises approximately 0.2 mEq per L in subjects with normal renal

TABLE 199.7

Major Causes of Hypoaldosteronism

Hyporeninemic hypoaldosteronism
Renal disease, most often diabetic nephropathy
Nonsteroidal anti-inflammatory drugs
Angiotensin-converting enzyme inhibitors
Cyclosporine
Human immunodeficiency virus infection, including trimethoprim administration
Primary adrenal insufficiency
Potassium-sparing diuretics (trimethoprim may act similarly)
Heparin
Congenital adrenal hyperplasia, with 21-hydroxylase deficiency being most common
Isolated impairment in aldosterone synthesis
Pseudohypoaldosteronism (end-organ resistance)
Severe illness

function but can rise by more than 1.0 mEq per L in the setting of renal insufficiency. This can occur with specific cyclooxygenase-2 inhibitors as well as nonselective NSAIDs.

- *ACE inhibitors, ARBs, and direct renin inhibitors.* Similar considerations apply to agents that block the production or action of angiotensin II, because angiotensin II is necessary for normal aldosterone release in response to volume depletion or hyperkalemia.
- *Other.* Other causes of hyporeninemic hypoaldosteronism include the use of cyclosporine and tacrolimus, which can lead to hyperkalemia in renal transplant recipients, likely from diminished secretion of and responsiveness to aldosterone [44]. The administrations of the antibiotics trimethoprim and pentamidine are other causes of hyperkalemia. Both agents appear to close sodium channels in the distal nephron in a manner similar to that of the potassium-sparing diuretic amiloride.

Primary Adrenal Insufficiency. Primary adrenal cortical failure (also called *Addison's disease*) is associated with lack of cortisol and aldosterone. Pituitary disease, in comparison, does not lead to hypoaldosteronism because ACTH does not have a major role in the regulation of aldosterone release. Primary adrenal insufficiency is frequently because of autoimmune destruction of the steroid-producing cells in the adrenal cortex.

Potassium-Sparing Diuretics. Potassium-sparing diuretics are probably the most common cause of hyperkalemia because of impairment of aldosterone function. These drugs antagonize the action of aldosterone on the collecting tubule cells. Spironolactone and eplerenone compete for the aldosterone receptor, whereas amiloride and triamterene close the sodium channels in the luminal membrane.

Heparin. Commercial heparin preparations exert a direct toxic effect on the zona glomerulosa cells of the adrenal cortex [45]. Even low-dose heparin can lead to a 75% reduction in plasma aldosterone levels. The mechanism appears to involve a reduction in the number and affinity of adrenal angiotensin II receptors involved in aldosterone synthesis and release.

Adrenal Enzyme Deficiency. In children, hypoaldosteronism can result from a deficiency of enzymes required for aldosterone synthesis, which may be associated with concurrent abnormalities in cortisol and androgen production.

Pseudohypoaldosteronism. Decreased aldosterone activity also occurs in the syndrome of pseudohypoaldosteronism. This disorder is associated with generalized resistance to the actions of aldosterone owing to a marked reduction in the number of mineralocorticoid receptors in the kidney and in other target organs such as the colon and sweat glands.

Severe Illness. Hypoaldosteronism caused by decreased adrenal production is common in critically ill patients. The stress-induced hypersecretion of ACTH in these patients may be responsible for this defect by inducing activity of 17α-hydroxylase in the zona glomerulosa. This enzyme enhances the synthesis of cortisol at the expense of aldosterone.

Chronic Kidney Disease. The ability to maintain potassium excretion at near-normal levels is generally maintained in patients with renal disease as long as both aldosterone secretion and distal tubular urine flow are maintained. Patients who are oliguric or who have an additional problem such as a high potassium intake, increased tissue breakdown, or hypoaldosteronism are predisposed to hyperkalemia.

Effective Circulating Volume Depletion. Decreased distal tubular urine flow owing to marked effective volume depletion, as might occur in heart failure or hepatic cirrhosis, can lead to hyperkalemia. In this setting, there is also a fall in the quantity of sodium presented to the potassium secretory site in the collecting tubule. Hyperkalemia may occur even though aldosterone activity is high.

Hyperkalemic Type-1 Renal Tubular Acidosis. In some patients with type-1 (distal) RTA, the primary defect is impaired sodium reabsorption in the cortical collecting tubule. The movement of sodium from the lumen into the cell at this site makes the lumen electronegative, thereby promoting both hydrogen and potassium secretion. Inhibiting the transport of sodium, therefore, reduces both hydrogen and potassium secretion, leading to metabolic acidosis and hyperkalemia. This form of type-1 RTA is most often seen in patients with urinary tract obstruction or sickle cell disease. Patients with type-1 RTA have normal or even high aldosterone levels and are unable to acidify the urine normally (urine pH $\leq$5.0), in contrast to individuals with hypoaldosteronism and other forms of type-4 RTA who frequently exhibit a urine pH of less than 5.3.

Clinical Manifestations

The symptoms induced by hyperkalemia are related to impaired neuromuscular transmission. The ease of generating an action potential, called *membrane excitability*, is related both to the magnitude of the resting membrane potential and to the activation state of membrane sodium channels. Opening of these sodium channels, leading to the passive diffusion of extracellular sodium into the cells, is the primary step in this process. According to the Nernst equation, the resting membrane potential is related to the ratio of the intracellular and the extracellular potassium concentration. An elevation in the extracellular potassium concentration decreases this ratio and, therefore, partially depolarizes the cell membrane, thereby making the resting potential less electronegative. This change initially increases membrane excitability because less of a depolarizing stimulus is required to generate an action potential. However, persistent depolarization inactivates sodium channels in the cell membrane, thereby producing a net decrease in membrane excitability that may be manifested clinically by impaired cardiac conduction or muscle weakness, or both, or by paralysis.

In general, severe symptoms of hyperkalemia do not occur until the plasma potassium concentration is more than 7.5 mEq per L. There is, however, substantial interpatient variability because factors such as hypocalcemia and metabolic acidosis can increase the toxicity of excess potassium. Thus, careful monitoring of the ECG and muscle strength is indicated to assess the functional consequences of the hyperkalemia. A

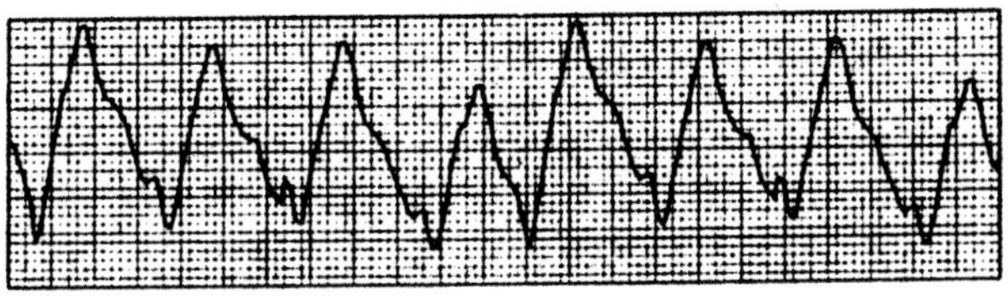

FIGURE 199.7 Marked hyperkalemia results in peaked T waves and widened QRS complexes in this electrocardiogram.

plasma potassium concentration of more than 7.5 to 8.0 mEq per L, severe muscle weakness, or marked ECG changes are potentially life threatening and require immediate treatment using the modalities described here [46].

The earliest ECG abnormality is symmetric peaking of T waves, followed by reduced P-wave voltage and widening of QRS complexes (Fig. 199.7). If untreated, severe hyperkalemia can cause the normal QRS morphology to be lost altogether so that the ECG pattern deteriorates into a sinusoidal ECG form, with one oscillation representing a wide QRS complex and the complementary oscillation representing an abnormal T wave. ECG changes usually do not appear until the plasma K^+ concentration exceeds 6.5 mEq per L, and are more likely to develop when the rise in K^+ occurs rapidly.

The neuromuscular manifestations of hyperkalemia are nonspecific. The earliest findings are paresthesias and weakness, which can progress to paralysis affecting the respiratory muscles. These symptoms are similar to those seen with hypokalemia; cranial nerve function remains unaffected.

Treatment

An asymptomatic patient with a plasma potassium concentration of 6.5 mEq per L and no ECG changes can be treated with a cation exchange resin (Kayexalate) alone, and patients with a level below 6.0 mEq per L can often be treated just with a low-potassium diet and diuretics. Any extra source of potassium intake (salt substitutes, potassium supplements, and foods with a high potassium content) should be eliminated, and any potentiating drugs (e.g., NSAIDs or ACE inhibitors) should be discontinued.

Specific treatment of severe or symptomatic hyperkalemia is directed at antagonizing the membrane effects of potassium, driving extracellular potassium into the cells, or removing excess potassium from the body. The following modalities, which are listed according to their rapidity of action, all may be beneficial.

Calcium. Calcium directly antagonizes the membrane actions of hyperkalemia. As mentioned previously, hyperkalemia-induced depolarization of the resting membrane potential leads to inactivation of sodium channels and decreased membrane excitability. Calcium antagonizes this membrane effect of hyperkalemia, although how this is achieved is not well understood.

The protective effect of calcium begins within minutes but is relatively short lived. As a result, calcium infusions are indicated only for severe hyperkalemia, when it is potentially dangerous to wait the 30 to 60 minutes required for insulin and glucose or sodium bicarbonate to act. The usual dose is 10 mL (1 ampule) of a 10% calcium gluconate solution infused slowly during 2 to 3 minutes with constant cardiac monitoring. This dose can be repeated after 5 minutes if the ECG changes persist.

Calcium should not be given in bicarbonate-containing solutions because this can lead to its precipitation as calcium carbonate. Because hypercalcemia can induce digitalis toxicity, calcium should be administered only when absolutely necessary to patients taking digoxin.

Insulin and Glucose. Increasing the availability of insulin lowers the plasma potassium concentration by driving potassium into the cells by enhancing the activity of the Na^+/K^+–ATPase pump in skeletal muscle. Hyperinsulinemia can be induced either by giving insulin with glucose to prevent hypoglycemia or by the intravenous administration of glucose (50 mL of a 50% glucose solution), which rapidly enhances endogenous insulin secretion in a nondiabetic patient. Glucose alone may produce a smaller rise in the plasma insulin concentration and a lesser reduction in plasma potassium concentration than does the insulin plus glucose regimen. Effective therapy usually produces a 0.5 to 1.5 mEq per L fall in the plasma potassium concentration. This effect begins in 15 minutes, peaks at 60 minutes, and lasts for several hours.

Exogenous insulin can induce symptomatic hypoglycemia unless adequate glucose is given concurrently. If, for example, 10 units of regular insulin are given with 25 g of glucose, the plasma glucose concentration may fall to less than 55 mg per dL in as many as 75% of initially normoglycemic patients. Increasing the initial glucose dose to 40 g, followed by a continuous dextrose infusion, generally prevents this problem.

Proper therapy in diabetic patients varies with the plasma glucose concentration. Both insulin and glucose should be given when the plasma glucose concentration is normal or mildly elevated because endogenous insulin release is impaired. Insulin in this case reduces the plasma potassium concentration directly by preventing a rise in the plasma glucose concentration that can exacerbate the hyperkalemia. The osmotic force generated by the high extracellular glucose concentration pulls water and, secondarily, potassium out of the cells. In comparison, insulin alone is sufficient if the patient is already hyperglycemic.

Sodium Bicarbonate. Raising the systemic pH with sodium bicarbonate promotes hydrogen ion release from the cells and a reciprocal movement of potassium into the cells. The elevation in the plasma bicarbonate concentration appears to have another direct, albeit not delineated, effect on lowering the plasma potassium concentration that is independent of pH.

The potassium-lowering action of sodium bicarbonate is most prominent for patients with metabolic acidosis, beginning within 30 to 60 minutes and persisting for several hours. Sodium bicarbonate appears to be less effective in correcting hyperkalemia for patients with renal failure. Insulin plus glucose or a β_2-agonist is more predictably effective in this setting.

The usual dose is 45 mEq (1 ampule of a 7.5% sodium bicarbonate solution) infused slowly during 5 minutes; this dose can be repeated in 30 minutes if necessary. Alternatively, sodium bicarbonate can be added to a glucose and saline solution. This regimen may have an additional advantage in hyponatremic patients because raising the plasma sodium concentration with this hypertonic solution can also reverse the ECG effects of hyperkalemia. Both an increase in the rate of membrane depolarization and a fall in the plasma potassium concentration by dilution may contribute to this effect. These sodium-containing solutions should be used with extreme caution in edematous patients with advanced heart failure or renal failure. Despite the physiologic rationale, bicarbonate administration appears to be less effective in lowering the serum potassium concentration in patients with end-stage renal disease who are receiving dialysis.

β2-Adrenergic Agonists. Like insulin, β_2-adrenergic agonists drive potassium into the cells by increasing Na^+/K^+–ATPase activity. Albuterol (20.0 mg in 4 mL of saline by nasal inhalation for 10 minutes or 0.5 mg by intravenous infusion) can lower the plasma potassium concentration by 0.5 to 1.5 mEq per L within 30 to 60 minutes. Furthermore, the effect of these agents is additive to that of insulin plus glucose. The only common side effects of the β_2-agonists are mild tachycardia and the possible induction of angina in susceptible individuals. Thus, these agents should probably be avoided in patients with known active coronary disease.

Loop or Thiazide Diuretics. Loop and thiazide diuretics can be used when hyperkalemia is present in an individual with hypertension or volume overload. However, the effectiveness of diuretic therapy is frequently limited by moderate-to-severe renal insufficiency.

Cation Exchange Resin. The most readily available cation exchange resin is sodium polystyrene sulfonate (SPS). In the gut, this resin takes up potassium, and calcium and magnesium to lesser degrees, and releases sodium. Each gram of resin may bind as much as 1 mEq of potassium and release 1 to 2 mEq of sodium. Thus, a potential side effect is exacerbation of any preexisting degree of sodium overload.

The resin can be given either orally or as a retention enema. The oral dose is usually 15 to 30 g. This can be repeated every 4 to 6 hours as necessary. Lower doses (5 to 10 g with meals) are generally well tolerated (no nausea or constipation) and can be used to control chronic mild hyperkalemia in patients with renal insufficiency. Historically, SPS was given with sorbitol to prevent constipation. Intestinal necrosis is a rare complication and has been associated with the use of concomitant sorbitol [47]. After issuance of an FDA black-box warning on the combination of sorbitol and SPS, preparations of SPS containing 70% sorbitol were removed from the market, and the combination is generally not recommended [47].

Recently, there have been reports questioning the effectiveness of SPS. This issue remains unresolved at this time, but anecdotal experience supports its effectiveness in lowering the serum potassium levels for many patients. Still, with the possible, although uncommon, risk of bowel injury, other measures should be tried first.

Two novel agents have recently been studied for the treatment of hyperkalemia in placebo controlled trials. Patiromer is a powder comprised of spherical beads that binds potassium in the colon in exchange for calcium. Sodium zirconium cyclosilicate has a lattice structure and acts as a cation exchanger which entraps potassium in exchange for hydrogen and sodium. Neither of these compounds are approved by the FDA [48].

Dialysis. Dialysis can be used if the conservative measures listed in the preceding sections are ineffective, if the hyperkalemia is severe, if the patient has marked tissue breakdown and is releasing large amounts of potassium from the injured cells, or, of course, if the patient has hyperkalemia in the setting of renal failure. The rate of potassium removal with hemodialysis is preferred in the last two settings because it is many times faster than with peritoneal dialysis.

References

1. Mortiz ML, Kalantar-Zadeh K, Ayus JC, et al: Ecstacy-associated hyponatremia: why are women at risk? *Nephrol Dial Transplant* 28:2206, 2013.
2. Sterns RH: Disorders of plasma sodium—causes, consequences, and correction. *N Engl J Med* 372:55, 2015.
3. Clark BA, Shannon RP, Rosa RM, et al: Increased susceptibility to thiazide-induced hyponatremia in the elderly. *J Am Soc Nephrol* 5:1106, 1994.
4. Iwasaki Y, Oiso Y, Yamauchi K, et al: Osmoregulation of plasma vasopressin in myxedema. *J Clin Endocrinol Metab* 70:534, 1990.
5. Kalogeral KT, Nieman LK, Friedman TC, et al: Inferior petrosal sampling in healthy human subjects reveals a unilateral corticotropin-releasing hormone-mediated arginine vasopressin release associated with ipsilateral adrenocorticotropin secretion. *J Clin Invest* 97:2045, 1996.
6. Fabian TJ, Amico AA, Kroboth PD, et al: Paroxetine-induced hyponatremia in older adults. *Arch Intern Med* 164:327, 2004.
7. Almond CS, Shin AY, Fortescue EB, et al: Hyponatremia among runners in the Boston marathon. *N Engl J Med* 352:1550, 2005.
8. Rosner MH, Kirven J: Exercise-associated hyponatremia. *Clin J Am Soc Nephrol* 2:151, 2007.
9. Issa MM: Technological advances in transurethral resection of the prostate: bipolar versus monopolar TURP. *J Endourol* 22(8):1587–1595, 2008.
10. Aydeniz B, Gruber IV, Schauf B, et al: A multicenter survey of complications associated with 21,676 operative hysteroscopies. *Eur J Obstet Gynecol Reprod Biol* 104(2):160, 2002.
11. Atici S, Zeren S, Ariboğan A: Hormonal and hemodynamic changes during percutaneous nephrolithotomy. *Int Urol Nephrol* 32(3):311, 2001.
12. Ayus J, Wheeler J, Arieff A: Postoperative hyponatremic encephalopathy in menstruant women. *Ann Intern Med* 117:891, 1992.
13. Bichet DG: Vasopressin receptor mutations in nephrogenic diabetes insipidus. *Semin Nephrol* 28(3):245, 2008.
14. Brunner J, Redmond J, Haggar A, et al: Central pontine myelinolysis and pontine lesions after rapid correction of hyponatremia: a prospective magnetic resonance imaging study. *Ann Neurol* 27:61, 1990.
15. Abbot R, Silber E, Felber J, et al: Osmotic demyelination syndrome. *BMJ* 331:829, 2005.
16. Soupart A, Penninckx R, Stenuit A, et al: Treatment of chronic hyponatremia in rats by intravenous saline: comparison of rate versus magnitude of correction. *Kidney Int* 41:1662, 1992.
17. Soupart A, Penninckx R, Stenuit A, et al: Prevention of brain demyelination after excessive correction of chronic hyponatremia in rats by excessive serum sodium lowering [abstract]. *J Am Soc Nephrol* 3:329, 1992.
18. Kortenoeven ML, Sinke AP, Hadrup N, et al: Demeclocycline attenuates hyponatremia by reducing aquaporin-2 expression in the renal inner medulla. *Am J Physiol Renal Physiol* 305:F1705, 2013.
19. Berl T: Vasopressin antagonists. *N Engl J Med* 372:2207, 2015.
20. Sterns RH, Silver SM, Hix JK, et al: Urea for hyponatremia? *Kidney Int* 87:268, 2015.
21. Kengne FG, Couturier BS, Soupart A, et al: Urea minimizes brain complications following rapid correction of chronic hyponatremia compared with vasopressin antagonist or hypertonic saline. *Kidney Int* 87:323, 2014.
22. Oster J, Materson B: Renal and electrolyte complications of congestive heart failure and effects of treatment with angiotensin-converting enzyme inhibitors. *Arch Intern Med* 152:704, 1992.
23. Leier CV, Dei Cas L, Metra M: Clinical relevance and management of the major electrolyte abnormalities in congestive heart failure: hyponatremia, hypokalemia, and hypomagnesemia. *Am Heart J* 128:562, 1994.
24. Habib S, Boyer TD: Vasopressin V2-receptor antagonists in patient with cirrhosis, ascites, and hyponatremia. *Ther Adv Gastroenterol* 5:189, 2012.
25. U.S. Food and Drug Administration: *Samsca (tolvaptan): Drug Warning-potential Risk of Liver Injury*. Washington, DC, U.S. Food and Drug Administration, 2013.
26. Papadakis M, Fraser C, Arieff A: Hyponatraemia in patients with cirrhosis. *Q J Med* 76:675, 1990.
27. Hoorn EJ, Zietse R: Water balance disorders after neurosurgery: the triphasic response revisited. *NDT Plus* 3:42, 2010.
28. DeRubertis F, Michelis M, Davis B: Essential hypernatremia. *Arch Intern Med* 134:889, 1974.
29. Moder K, Hurley D: Fatal hypernatremia from exogenous salt intake: report of a case and review of the literature. *Mayo Clin Proc* 65:1587, 1990.
30. Lien Y, Shapiro J, Chan L: Effect of hypernatremia on organic brain osmoles. *J Clin Invest* 85:1427, 1990.
31. Fang C, Mao J, Dai Y, et al: Fluid management of hypernatraemic dehydration to prevent cerebral oedema: a retrospective case control study of 97 children in China. *J Paediatr Child Health* 46(6):301, 2010.
32. Alshayeb HM, Showkat A, Babar F, et al: Severe hypernatremia correction rate and mortality in hospitalized patients. *Am J Med Sci* 341(5):356–360, 2011.
33. Bedford JJ, Weggery S, Ellis G, et al: Lithium-induced nephrogenic diabetes insipidus: renal effects of amiloride. *Clin J Am Soc Nephrol* 3(5):1324, 2008.
34. Noroian G, Clive D: Cyclo-oxygenase-2 inhibitors and the kidney. *Drug Saf* 25:165, 2002.
35. Sigue G, Gamble L, Pelitre M, et al: From profound hypokalemia to life-threatening hyperkalemia: a case of barium sulfide poisoning. *Arch Intern Med* 160:548, 2000.
36. Clemessy JL, Favier C, Borron SW, et al: Hypokalemia related to acute chloroquine ingestion. *Lancet* 346:877, 1995.
37. Huang CL, Kuo E: Mechanism of hypokalemia in magnesium deficiency. *J Am Soc Nephrol* 18(10):2649, 2007.
38. Kruse J, Carlson R: Rapid correction of hypokalemia using concentration intravenous potassium chloride infusions. *Arch Intern Med* 150:613, 1990.
39. Sharma A, Thiede H, Keller F: Somatostatin-induced hyperkalemia in a patient on maintenance hemodialysis. *Nephron* 59:445, 1991.
40. Daut J, Maiser-Rudolph W, von Beckerath N, et al: Hypoxic dilation of coronary arteries is mediated by ATP-sensitive potassium channels. *Science* 247:1341, 1990.
41. Lindinger M, Heigenhauser G, McKelvie R: Blood ion regulation during repeated maximal exercise and recovery in humans. *Am J Physiol* 262:R126, 1992.
42. Wiederkehr MR, Moe OW: Factitious hyperkalemia. *Am J Kidney Dis* 36:1049, 2000.
43. Jurkat-Rott K, Lehmann-Horn F: Genotype-phenotype correlation and therapeutic rationale in hyperkalemic periodic paralysis. *Neurotherapeutics* 4(2):216, 2007.
44. Naesens M, Kuypers DR, Sarwal M, et al: Calicneurin inhibitor nephrotoxicity. *Clin J Am Soc Nephrol* 4: 481, 2009.
45. Oster JR, Singer I, Fishman LM: Heparin-induced aldosterone suppression and hyperkalemia. *Am J Med* 98:575, 1995.
46. Wilson NS, Hudson JQ, Cox Z, et al: Hyperkalemia-induced paralysis. *Pharmacotherapy* 29:1270, 2009.
47. Harel Z, Harel S, et al: Gastrointestinal adverse events with sodium polystyrene sulfonate (kaexylate) use: a systematic review. *Am J Med* 126:e9, 2013.
48. Inglefinger JR: A new era for the treatment of hyperkalemia? *N Engl J Med* 372:275, 2015.

Chapter 200 ■ Acute Kidney Injury in the Intensive Care Unit

KONSTANTIN ABRAMOV • JAHAN MONTAGUE

OVERVIEW OF ACUTE KIDNEY INJURY

Sudden disruption of previously normal or stable kidney function, usually occurring over hours or days, is termed *acute kidney injury (AKI)*, formerly referred to as *acute renal failure.* AKI occurs in diverse clinical contexts with varied presentations and etiologies. The course of AKI differs from that of chronic kidney disease (CKD), in which renal function declines more slowly.

AKI is often diagnosed when a patient develops an elevation in the blood urea nitrogen (BUN) and serum creatinine. This change typically results from a decline in glomerular filtration rate (GFR), but in certain cases may reflect increased urea and/or creatinine production without any reduction in GFR (Table 200.1). *Oliguria*, a reduction in urine output to less than 20 mL per hour, may be present, although many forms of AKI are nonoliguric. When tubular reabsorption of glomerular filtrate is reduced as a result of either tubular dysfunction or diuretic administration, patients may be polyuric even though GFR is markedly reduced.

Even a small rise in serum creatinine correlates with increased mortality [1,2]. However, AKI can occur prior to a significant increase in creatinine. This is especially true in the ICU setting, where frequent administration of large volume of intravenous fluids can dilute serum creatinine. Therefore, the Acute Dialysis Quality Initiative Group has proposed a classification of AKI based not only on serum creatinine, but also on the degree of urinary output reduction and the requirement for renal replacement therapy [3]. This classification is reflected in the RIFLE criteria (Table 200.2), which have been shown to predict renal outcome and mortality in a variety of critically ill and hospitalized patients [4,5]. Acute Kidney Injury Network and, recently, Kidney Disease Improving Global Outcomes initiative (KDIGO) developed a simplified, three-stage system, which is similarly based on changes in serum creatinine and urinary output (Table 200.3).

AKI may stem from any of three general conditions: impaired renal perfusion without parenchymal injury, damage to the renal parenchyma, or obstruction of the urinary tract. These etiologies are referred to as *prerenal*, *renal*, or *postrenal* causes of AKI, respectively, and are summarized in Table 200.4. Although it is helpful to consider the complete array of renal diseases when evaluating AKI, in the inpatient setting two-thirds of cases will be due to either acute tubular necrosis (ATN) or prerenal azotemia. Hence, an extensive search for other forms of renal disease is indicated in the intensive care unit (ICU) setting only when suggested by clinical signs or laboratory findings such as urinary abnormalities indicative of glomerular disease.

TABLE 200.1

Causes of Blood Urea Nitrogen or Serum Creatinine Elevation Without Reduction of Glomerular Filtration Rate

- Increased biosynthesis of urea
  - Gastrointestinal bleeding
  - Medications
    - Corticosteroids
    - Tetracycline
  - Increased protein intake
  - Amino acid administration
  - Hypercatabolism and febrile illness
- Increased biosynthesis of creatinine
  - Increased release of creatine from muscle (rhabdomyolysis)
- Drug interference with tubular creatinine secretion
  - Cimetidine
  - Trimethoprim
- Spuriously elevated creatinine colorimetric assay
  - Ketoacids (diabetic ketoacidosis)
  - Cephalosporins

Prerenal Azotemia and Autoregulatory Failure

Prerenal azotemia develops when renal perfusion pressure decreases to a point at which GFR falls. This is a functional condition without associated renal parenchymal injury, although it may be superimposed on pre-existing CKD. The causes of prerenal azotemia are listed in Table 200.5. Normalization of renal blood flow, if possible, promptly restores renal function.

Hypovolemia from gastrointestinal losses, hemorrhage, venous pooling, sequestering of fluid in "third spaces," or excessive

TABLE 200.2

RIFLE Criteria of Acute Kidney Injury

	Serum creatinine (Cr)/glomerular filtration rate (GFR) criteria	Urinary output criteria
Risk	Cr increase × 1.5 above baseline or GFR decline >25%	<0.5 mL/kg/h × 6 h
Injury	Cr increase × 2 above baseline or GFR decline >50%	<0.3 mL/kg/h × 24 h
Failure	Cr increase × 3 above baseline or Cr ≥4 mg/dL or GFR decline >75%	<0.3 mL/kg/h 24 h or anuria × 12 h
Loss	Persistent AKI >4 wk	
End stage	End-stage renal disease (AKI >3 mo)	

Summary of RIFLE criteria of AKI. Sensitivity for AKI increases toward the top of the chart, while specificity increases toward the bottom of the chart. [Bellomo R, Ronco C, Kellum JA, et al; Acute Dialysis Quality Initiative Workgroup: acute renal failure—definition, outcome measures, animal models, fluid therapy and information technology needs: the Second International Consensus Conference of the Acute Dialysis Quality Initiative (ADQI) Group. *Crit Care* 8:R204–R210, 2004.]

TABLE 200.3

KDIGO Criteria of Acute Kidney Injury

Stage	Serum creatinine (Cr) criteria	Urine output criteria
1	Cr increase 1.5–1.9× above baseline within 7 d OR at least 0.3 mg/dL increase in 48 hr period	<0.5 mL/kg/h for at least 6 h
2	Cr increase 2–2.9× above baseline	<0.5 mL/kg/h for at least 12 h
3	Cr increase 3× above baseline OR Cr of at least 4 mg/dL OR initiation of dialysis	<0.3 mL/kg/h for at least 24 h OR anuria for at least 24 h

The Kidney Disease Improving Global Outcomes (KDIGO) Acute Kidney Injury criteria are based on based on RIFLE criteria above and Acute Kidney Injury (AKIN) criteria. (Acute Kidney Injury Network: report of an initiative to initiative to improve outcomes of Acute Kidney Injury. *Crit Care* 11:R31, 2007.) Stage 3 in pediatric population (<18 years old) is also defined as estimated glomerular filtration rate (GFR) of <35 mL/min/1.73 m^2. (KDIGO Acute Kidney Injury Workgroup: KDIGO Clinical Practice Guidelines for Acute Kidney Injury. *Kidney Int Suppl* 2:8, 2012.)

TABLE 200.4

Causes of Acute Kidney Injury

- Prerenal azotemia
  - Hypovolemia
  - Reduced effective circulating volume
  - Autoregulatory failure
- Intrinsic renal disease
  - Glomerular diseases
  - Vascular diseases (main renal artery and microcirculation)
  - Tubulointerstitial disease
  - Acute tubular necrosis
  - Acute cortical necrosis
- Postrenal failure
  - Ureteric obstruction (bilateral or solitary kidney)
  - Lower tract obstruction (bladder neck or urethra)

urinary or skin losses of sodium and water may cause prerenal azotemia. Patients will usually exhibit signs of volume depletion, including thirst, diminished skin turgor and dry mucous membranes, and postural hypotension. Patients whose vascular volume is functionally reduced by the hemodynamic alterations of congestive heart failure, cirrhosis, or hypoalbuminemia may develop prerenal azotemia despite having a normal or even expanded extracellular fluid (ECF) volume. Because the *effective circulatory volume* is reduced, renal perfusion is impaired just as in true hypovolemia.

When glomerular perfusion is threatened, autoregulatory mechanisms help maintain glomerular capillary pressure. If autoregulatory mechanisms are inoperative, a given reduction in renal blood flow provokes a sharper decline in GFR. The mechanisms of these processes are shown in Figure 200.1. Use of nonsteroidal anti-inflammatory drugs (NSAIDs) in patients with renal hypoperfusion, for example, can lead to severe AKI. Likewise, administration of angiotensin-converting enzyme (ACE) inhibitors in patients whose renal blood flow is obstructed by bilateral renovascular renal artery stenosis can cause severe azotemia.

Reduced renal perfusion slows down the flow of filtrate through the renal tubules, enhancing the reabsorption of urea. Because creatinine is not reabsorbed in the renal tubules, its clearance is unaffected by these nephronal factors. Thus, the clearance of urea is reduced disproportionately to that of creatinine, explaining the unusually high BUN–creatinine ratio that is often seen in prerenal states. In such situations, the BUN–creatinine ratio typically exceeds 20 to 1.

TABLE 200.5

Causes of Prerenal Azotemia

- Hypovolemia
  - Gastrointestinal losses
    - Vomiting
    - Diarrhea
    - Surgical drainage
  - Renal losses
    - Osmotic agents
    - Diuretics
    - Renal salt-wasting disease
    - Adrenal insufficiency
  - Skin losses
    - Burns
    - Excessive sweating
  - Hemorrhage
  - Translocation of fluid (third spacing)
    - Postoperative
    - Pancreatitis
- Reduced effective circulating volume
  - Hypoalbuminemia
  - Hepatic cirrhosis
  - Left ventricular cardiac failure
  - Peripheral blood pooling (vasodilator therapy, anesthetics, anaphylaxis, sepsis, and toxic shock syndrome)
  - Renal artery occlusion
  - Small vessel disease (malignant hypertension, toxemia, and scleroderma)
  - Renal vasoconstriction (hypercalcemia, hepatorenal syndrome, cyclosporine, and pressor agents)
- Autoregulatory failure
  - Nonsteroidal anti-inflammatory drugs (preglomerular vasoconstriction)
  - Angiotensin-converting enzyme inhibitors (postglomerular vasodilation)

A high urea–creatinine ratio, however, is not pathognomonic of prerenal azotemia. When urea production is accelerated in catabolic states (as is seen with tetracycline or corticosteroid therapy) or by resorption of a large hematoma or with gastrointestinal bleeding, BUN levels rise unless renal urea clearance can increase to meet the augmented urea burden. To establish whether a high BUN–creatinine ratio is due to increased urea production or reduced excretion, calculation of the fractional urea clearance may be useful.

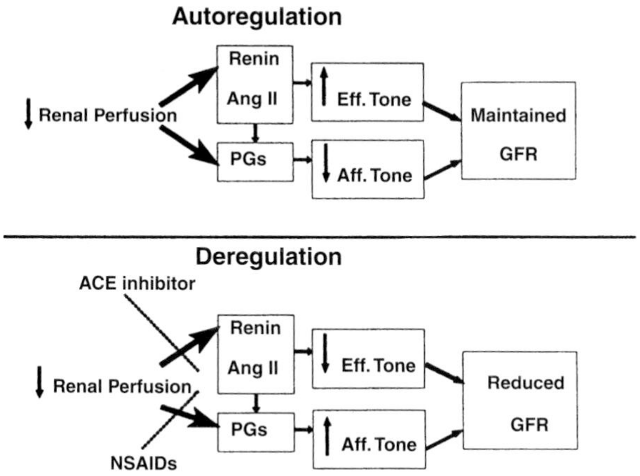

FIGURE 200.1 Diagrammatic representation of autoregulation and deregulation caused by use of either nonsteroidal anti-inflammatory drugs (NSAIDs), which lead to afferent (Aff.) vasoconstriction, or angiotensin-converting enzyme (ACE) inhibitors, which produce efferent (Eff.) vasodilation. Angiotensin II, angiotensin II; GFR, glomerular filtration rate; PGs, prostaglandins.

The hallmark of prerenal conditions is the intense renal conservation of salt and water as reflected in the urine composition, which generally shows a low sodium concentration (U_{Na} <10 mEq per L; fractional excretion of sodium [FE_{Na}] <1%) and a high osmolality (U_{Osm} >500 mOsm per kg). Renal conservation of sodium involves both proximal and distal tubular mechanisms. A low urinary sodium concentration is expected in these states, whereas high urinary sodium in prerenal cases signifies a coexisting abnormality of tubular function, the effect of diuretics, or the presence of nonreabsorbable anionic substances in the urine, such as bicarbonate in patients with metabolic alkalosis, or certain penicillins, that obligate the excretion of cations like sodium. Impaired sodium reabsorption is also seen during osmotic diuresis and in certain forms of chronic renal disease.

Intrinsic Renal Disease

Reduced renal function may also result from renal parenchymal injury. Such injury may arise from glomerular, vascular, and tubulointerstitial disorders (Table 200.4) and may represent either primary kidney disease or the renal effects of an underlying systemic illness (e.g., systemic lupus erythematosus).

Glomerular and Vascular Diseases

The GFR may be abruptly reduced in acute glomerulonephritis. Patients may present with the constellation of hypertension, edema, azotemia, and hematuria, known as the *acute nephritic syndrome*. Hypertension and edema result from impaired excretion of salt and water. Although the history of a previous sore throat or streptococcal infection may provide diagnostic clues, the urinalysis is particularly valuable. The urine may be grossly bloody or tea colored. The urinary sediment contains red blood cells (RBCs) and often RBC casts (Fig. 200.2).

Poststreptococcal glomerulonephritis, the prototypic nephritic disorder, often presents with AKI and oliguria. The crescentic glomerulonephritides (rapidly progressive glomerulonephritis [RPGN]), such as antiglomerular basement membrane disease and ANCA-associated glomerulonephritis, can also cause AKI. Similar findings are frequent in patients with other primary nephritic disorders as well as in secondary nephritides, such as systemic lupus erythematosis and bacterial endocarditis.

Diseases affecting either the main renal arteries or their branches may precipitate AKI. Renal artery occlusion by *acute thrombosis* or *thromboembolism* typically only causes AKI, if it is bilateral or involves a solitary functioning kidney. These processes may be silent or may produce flank pain and hematuria, particularly if abrupt enough to cause renal infarction. Fever, moderate leukocytosis, and an elevated serum level of lactate dehydrogenase should raise the suspicion of infarction. With rare exceptions, renal arterial thromboembolism occurs only in the settings of acute myocardial infarction, atrial fibrillation, bacterial endocarditis, cardiac valvular disease, or hypercoagulable disorders.

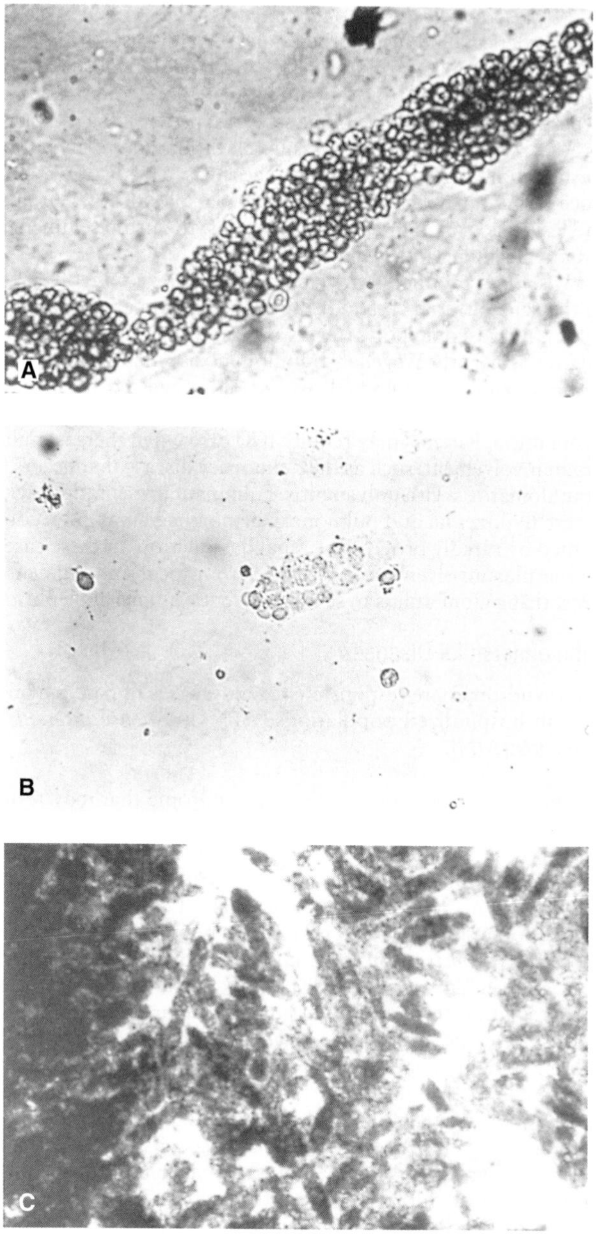

FIGURE 200.2 Typical urinary sediments from patients with parenchymal renal diseases. A: Sediment from patient with acute glomerulonephritis showing free red blood cells and red blood cell casts. B: Sediment from patient with acute interstitial nephritis demonstrating pyuria and white blood cell cast. C: Typical muddy brown, coarse, granular casts in a patient with acute tubular necrosis.

Acute renal vein thrombosis (RVT) seldom causes renal failure unless both kidneys are simultaneously occluded. Acute flank pain and hematuria are the clinical hallmarks. Renal venous obstruction may occur as a complication of nephrotic syndrome and renal cell carcinoma.

Microscopic occlusion of smaller vessels occurs in a variety of disorders, including atheroembolic renal disease, thrombotic thrombocytopenic purpura (TTP) and hemolytic–uremic syndrome, scleroderma, postpartum kidney injury, and malignant hypertension. Scleroderma or malignant hypertension may appear as AKI, with severe blood pressure elevation due to activation of the renin–angiotensin system. These vascular disorders produce renal injury by reducing glomerular blood flow. Because the lesion is proximal to the glomerulus, the urine sediment is usually acellular and bland.

Vasculitis produces AKI either through direct involvement of the renal arterial system or by inducing glomerulonephritis. Often, microscopic polyarteritis or granulomatosis with polyangiitis (formerly Wegener granulomatosis) may present with evident renal parenchymal disease, as suggested by urinary abnormalities such as microscopic hematuria, RBC casts, and proteinuria. Patients may require ICU care when there is multiorgan involvement, such as the pulmonary disease that occurs in granulomatosis with polyangiitis. Fulminant presentations with severe hypoxemia and pulmonary hemorrhage may be accompanied by rapidly progressive renal dysfunction. In these cases, glomerular involvement may range from focal and segmental necrotizing glomerulitis to severe crescentic glomerulonephritis.

Tubulointerstitial Diseases

Two syndromes are responsible for most cases of parenchymal AKI in hospitalized populations: *ATN* and *acute interstitial nephritis (AIN)*.

Acute Tubular Necrosis. ATN is a syndrome that may result from renal ischemia or exposure to nephrotoxins such as aminoglycoside antibiotics, radiocontrast agents, heavy metals, and myoglobin. Despite the term *acute tubular necrosis*, frank tubular cell necrosis does not appear in all cases. Historically, the pathophysiology of AKI in ATN has been attributed to three processes: (a) *obstruction of tubular lumens* by sloughed epithelial cells and cellular debris, (b) *back-leak* of filtered wastes into the circulation through the disrupted tubular epithelium, and (c) *sustained reduction in glomerular blood flow* following the inciting stimulus. For instance, severe cortical vasoconstriction has been noted early in the course of ATN, which is likely mediated by endothelial cell injury and locally acting vasoconstrictors, such as endothelin. Afferent arteriolar vasoconstriction has also been described. In ATN, impaired proximal solute reabsorption increases distal chloride delivery to macular densa, which, in turn, mediates afferent constriction via the secretion of adenosine. This process is termed *tubuloglomerular feedback*. However, it remains unclear whether renal vasoconstriction has a central role in the pathogenesis of ATN, because restoring renal blood flow with vasodilators does not always preserve the GFR. Nonetheless, this process may be important in the initiation of certain forms of ATN such as radiocontrast toxicity.

As already noted, relatively modest hypoperfusion leads to prerenal azotemia, characterized by a modest reduction in urine output and GFR, and preservation of tubular function, which is rapidly reversible. However, a more critical decrease in renal perfusion leads to medullary hypoperfusion and ischemic ATN with greater reductions in GFR, abnormalities of tubular function, and often histologic evidence of tissue injury. Because recovery depends on cellular regeneration, reversal of ATN is much slower than for prerenal azotemia. The most extreme form of hypoperfusion injury is cortical ischemia associated with either patchy or diffuse *cortical necrosis*, typically manifesting the most severe reduction in GFR and a much less certain prognosis for recovery of renal function. The medullary thick ascending limb segment of the loop of Henle is particularly vulnerable to ischemic and nephrotoxic insults because of a combination of low ambient partial pressure of oxygen and intense, transport-driven oxygen consumption. Other factors, such as adenosine triphosphate depletion activation of phospholipases, cytosolic and mitochondrial calcium overload, and release of free radicals, may contribute to cellular damage.

The immune system plays a critical role in pathogenesis of ATN through recruitment of various inflammatory cells, cytokine release, complement activation, and induction of tubular cell apoptosis [6,7]. Adhesion molecules, such as intracellular adhesion molecule 1 (ICAM-1), appear to play a role in the development of postischemic ATN in experimental animal models. However, anti-ICAM antibody failed to protect against ischemic AKI in a clinical trial of kidney transplant patients [8]. Another regulatory molecule expressed in the kidney, the protein neutrophil gelatinase-associated lipocalin (NGAL), is released early in the course of ischemic ATN and appears to attenuate tubular cell injury and apoptosis [9]. There is considerable interest in using NGAL and other molecules as biomarkers of early kidney injury (Table 200.6) with the hope that timely diagnosis of AKI will allow clinicians to make therapeutic interventions that will ultimately improve outcomes (discussed further in "Diagnosis" section).

History of exposure to a predisposing factor, such as prolonged ischemia or toxin, can be elicited in approximately 80% of patients with ATN. Most individuals with this syndrome have the classic findings of sloughed renal tubular epithelial cells, epithelial cell casts, or muddy brown granular casts in the urinary sediment (Fig. 200.2). These findings are not seen in prerenal azotemia. In addition, calculating the fractional excretion of filtered sodium (FE_{Na}) may enable the clinician to differentiate between ATN and prerenal azotemia. The FE_{Na} expresses urinary sodium excretion as a percentage of filtered load. It provides a more precise representation of tubular sodium avidity than the urinary sodium concentration, because it is not influenced by changes in urine concentration or flow

TABLE 200.6

Protein Biomarkers for the Early Detection of Acute Kidney Injury

Biomarker	Associated injury
Cystatin C	Proximal tubule injury
KIM-1	Ischemia and nephrotoxins
NGAL	
L-FABP	
Netrin-1	Sepsis, ischemia, nephrotoxins I
NHE3	Prerenal, ischemia, and postrenal
α-GST	Acute rejection, proximal tubule injury
π-GST	Acute rejection, distal tubule injury
Cytokines (IL-6, IL-8, IL-18)	Delayed graft function
Actin–actin depolymerizing F Keratin-derived chemokine	Tubular cell cycle arrest in early AKI
IGFBP7	
TIMP-2	

GST, glutathione *S*-transferase; IL, interleukin; KIM, kidney injury molecule; L-FABP, L-type fatty acid–binding protein; NGAL, neutrophil gelatinase-associated lipocalin; NHE, sodium–hydrogen exchanger; IGFBP7, insulin-like growth factor–binding protein 7; TIMP-2, tissue inhibitor of metalloproteinases-2.

From Ronco C, Haapio M, House AA, et al: Cardiorenal syndrome. *J Am Coll Cardiol* 52:1527, 2008 and Kashani K, Al-Khafaji A, Ardiles T, et al: Discovery and validation of cell cycle arrest biomarkers in human acute kidney injury. *Crit Care* 17:R25, 2013.

rate. The FE_{Na} is very low in prerenal azotemia as a result of active sodium reabsorption by the renal tubules. When frank tubular damage has occurred, as in ATN, the tubules can no longer reclaim sodium efficiently, and the FE_{Na} is generally high (Fig. 200.3). See "Diagnosis" section for more detail on the FE_{Na}. Urinary concentration is also impaired in tubular necrosis; as a result, urinary osmolality approximates that of plasma, and the ratio of BUN to creatinine is less than 20.

Acute Interstitial Nephritis. The term *acute interstitial* (or *tubulointerstitial*) *nephritis* encompasses a collection of disorders characterized by acute inflammation of the renal interstitium and tubules. Depending on the specific nature of the condition, the inflammatory infiltrate may consist of a combination of neutrophils, eosinophils, and lymphocytes or plasma cells. Most cases of AIN represent an allergic reaction with eosinophilia and skin eruptions, usually induced by medication. Interstitial disease can also occur as a result of infectious agents, including brucellosis, leptospirosis, legionella, toxoplasmosis, and Epstein–Barr virus.

These disorders are to be distinguished from the familiar entity *acute pyelonephritis*. Acute pyelonephritis is a suppurative disease of the tubulointerstitium, usually caused by bacterial infection ascending from the urinary bladder. Acute pyelonephritis rarely causes renal dysfunction. AIN, however, is an important cause of AKI and is discussed in detail later.

Postrenal Azotemia

The term *postrenal azotemia*, or *obstructive uropathy*, refers to azotemia caused by obstruction of urine flow from the kidneys. Renal outflow obstruction has many causes, but the most common causes are prostatic enlargement, nephrolithiasis, and genitourinary tumors. For obstruction to produce azotemia, both kidneys must be involved because one normally functioning kidney is sufficient to maintain a near-normal GFR. AKI may occur with unilateral obstruction in a patient who has one functioning kidney or in whom unilateral obstruction is superimposed on underlying CKD.

The clinical history often helps with the diagnosis of obstructive uropathy. Prior kidney stones should raise the index of suspicion for obstruction, particularly in the setting of symptoms of renal colic. AKI in an elderly man who has been experiencing urinary hesitancy most likely represents obstruction of the bladder outlet by an enlarged prostate. A history of genitourinary malignancy in an azotemic patient also makes obstruction the most likely diagnosis. AKI in the setting of painless gross hematuria and a history of NSAID use should prompt a suspicion of papillary necrosis, a condition in which sloughed-off renal papilla can cause bilateral ureteral obstruction. Finally, renal failure in a newborn infant is likely to be due to congenital anatomic ureteral obstruction.

When urine output declines precipitously or ceases entirely (anuria), complete obstruction of the urinary tract must be ruled out. Such an obstruction is likely to be located at the bladder outlet because the probability of simultaneous obstruction in both ureters from any cause is remote. If the patient has only one kidney (e.g., due to previous nephrectomy, unilateral renal disease, or congenital solitary kidney), however, anuria may occur with unilateral ureteral obstruction. Even though complete obstruction is a common cause of anuria, partial obstruction is not always associated with a decline in urine output. With partial obstruction, damage to the kidney may impair the ability to concentrate urine, resulting in a polyuric state (acquired nephrogenic diabetes insipidus). In patients with complete unilateral obstruction of a ureter, the contralateral kidney often sustains a normal urine output.

Obstructive uropathy is associated with other defects of the distal nephron, including hydrogen ion and potassium secretion, as well as urinary concentration. Consequently, the patient, particularly if there is prolonged high-grade obstruction, may present with hyperkalemia, hyperchloremic metabolic acidosis, hypernatremia, or a combination of all three.

As discussed later, urologic causes of AKI are best diagnosed by renal imaging techniques. The urine chemistry is generally of little help in diagnosing obstructive uropathy. Likewise, the urinalysis provides only indirect evidence of a possible cause of AKI. Hematuria reflects trauma to the urinary epithelium caused by the obstructing lesion. Crystals (calcium oxalate or uric acid) in the urine sediment may suggest a kidney stone.

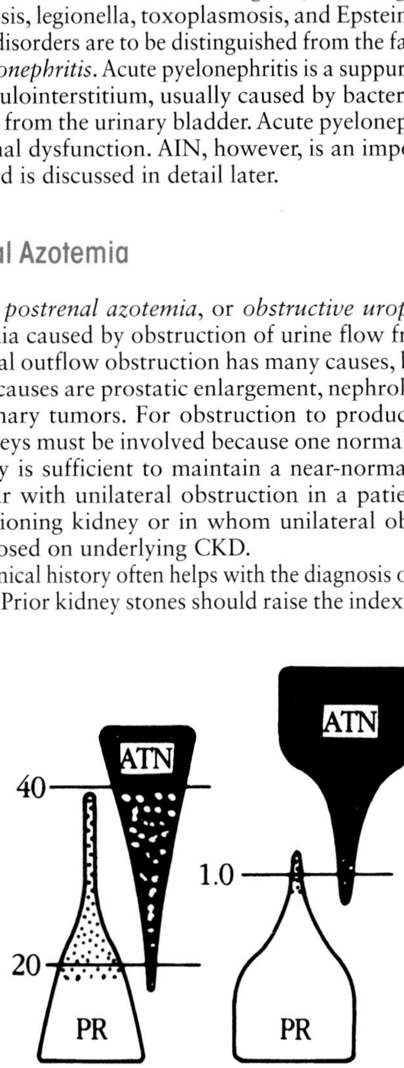

FIGURE 200.3 Diagnostic parameters in acute renal failure. Two laboratory tests used to distinguish prerenal (PR) azotemia from acute tubular necrosis (ATN) are shown. **Left:** Urinary sodium concentration (U_{Na}, mEq per L). **Right:** Fractional excretion of sodium (FE_{Na}, %). Area within each symbol denotes the proportion of patients with each condition correlated with the laboratory parameter. Note that although considerable numbers of patients with PR and ATN fall in an intermediate zone of U_{Na} (20 to 40 mEq per L), the FE_{Na} almost completely differentiates the two groups. (Adapted from Rudnick MR, Bastl CP, Elfinbein IB, et al: The differential diagnosis of acute renal failure, in Brenner BM, Lazarus JM (eds): *Acute Renal Failure*. New York, Churchill Livingstone, 1988, p 177.)

CLINICAL SYNDROMES ASSOCIATED WITH AKI IN THE INTENSIVE CARE SETTING

With the higher level of acuity of illness, and more radical approaches to surgical and pharmacologic therapeutics, the incidence of AKI is increasing. As with other areas of clinical medicine, patterns of presentation often can be recognized and can lead the physician to the most likely diagnoses. The following section explores in greater detail the specific AKI syndromes most commonly encountered in the ICU (listed in Table 200.7).

Ischemic Acute Kidney Injury

The most common forms of AKI in the ICU result from renal hypoperfusion. Because frank hypotension is documented in fewer than half of these cases, the causal events may often be overlooked or obscured by multiple factors. Frequently, more than one causal factor is necessary to provoke AKI. For example, the presence of hypovolemia enhances the risk for AKI due to nephrotoxic insults.

Extracellular Volume Depletion

Extracellular volume depletion accounted for approximately 15% to 20% of cases of AKI. In most instances, urinary losses are the cause of hypovolemia. Injudicious use of diuretics and the osmotic diuresis that accompanies diabetic hyperglycemia

TABLE 200.7

Intensive Care Syndromes Associated with Acute Kidney Injury (AKI)

Ischemic AKI
Extracellular volume depletion
Postoperative (particularly cardiac surgery)
Severe ventricular dysfunction or cardiogenic shock
Sepsis
Pancreatitis
Trauma
Burns
Acute bilateral cortical necrosis
Nephrotoxicity and drug-induced AKI
Myoglobinuric AKI
Radiocontrast nephropathy
Drugs (see Table 200.13)
Renal vascular disease
Major vessel disease
Renal artery embolism or thrombosis
Renal vein thrombosis
Microvascular disease
Atheroembolism
Vasculitis
Scleroderma
Cancer related
Obstructive uropathy
Hypercalcemia
Tumor-lysis syndrome
ATN secondary to chemotherapy
Renal dysfunction with liver disease
Prerenal azotemia
ATN
Hepatorenal syndrome

ATN, acute tubular necrosis.

are the most common etiologies. Cessation of diuretic therapy and volume repletion lead to rapid recovery; consequently, the mortality is quite low.

In rare instances, gastrointestinal losses of substantial magnitude may lead to AKI. (In the developing world, however, this is one of the most common causes of AKI and the major cause of morbidity and mortality where cholera is endemic.) In such cases, the source of the gastrointestinal losses, either gastric or intestinal, may lead to distinctive electrolyte abnormalities. In the former, metabolic alkalosis mandates repletion with chloride-rich replacement solutions (normal saline, usually with potassium chloride, as most patients are also hypokalemic). With intestinal losses of fluid, metabolic acidosis often ensues, and appropriate replacement may consist of a buffer solution of either isotonic bicarbonate or lactate-containing (Ringer) solution in combination with saline. (This is more fully discussed later in this chapter and in Chapter 198.)

Transdermal fluid losses usually occur in the setting of major burns, with the degree of hypovolemia and the severity of AKI corresponding to the extent of thermal injury (body surface-area involvement). Significant burns can lead to severe hypovolemia as a result of massive evaporative and exudative fluid loss across the damaged epidermis as well from redistribution of fluid due to edema in the injured tissues. This hypovolemia can stimulate a sympathetic nerve-mediated response with resultant renal vasoconstriction. In some instances, the severity of renal vasoconstriction, superimposed on hypovolemia, culminates in ATN. In addition, deeper thermal injury with skeletal muscle involvement may induce myoglobinuric AKI (see following discussion). Dermal losses of fluid are also seen in the setting of hyperthermia and heat stroke. The evaporative loss of sweat, which is hypotonic, leads to a hypertonic dehydration for most cases. Replacement with half-normal saline corrects free water and sodium deficits.

Postoperative

Postoperative AKI has long been recognized as a common complication of major vascular, abdominal, and open-heart surgery. The pathogenesis of postoperative renal dysfunction varies with the type of the surgery and the preoperative condition of the patient. AKI following abdominal surgery is often the result of translocation of fluid into the peritoneal cavity. In this phenomenon, third space losses cause intravascular hypovolemia and subsequent renal hypoperfusion. AKI is uncommon in patients undergoing routine abdominal surgery, but the risk is substantial in surgery for obstructive jaundice; this complication may develop in approximately 10% of patients. Major vascular surgery, particularly aortic repairs, is also frequently complicated by AKI, especially in the setting of a ruptured aortic aneurysm. Elective repair of an aortic aneurysm is seldom associated with AKI unless cross clamping is placed above the renal arteries. Although the definition of AKI and its incidence varies among studies, cardiac surgery appears to generate most of the cases in the acute care hospital. Cardiac surgery accounts for nearly two-thirds of the postoperative AKI. Repeated episodes of AKI and sepsis complicating AKI are associated with substantially higher mortality after surgery.

Several predisposing factors for the development of postoperative AKI have been identified, which can be used to stratify risk (Table 200.8). These include emergent surgery, an elevated preoperative serum creatinine, the use of an intra-aortic balloon pump, and combined coronary artery bypass graft and valvular surgery [10]. Still, it is often difficult to prospectively identify those patients at heightened risk for perioperative AKI, especially since 40% of patients who develop AKI do not have frank perioperative hypotension or evidence of shock. Other

TABLE 200.8

A Clinical Score to Predict AKI Requiring Dialysis after Cardiac Surgery

Risk factor	Points
Female gender	1
Congestive heart failure	1
Left ventricular ejection fraction <35%	1
Preoperative use of intra-aortic balloon pump	2
Chronic obstructive pulmonary disease	1
Diabetes requiring insulin	1
Previous cardiac surgery	1
Emergency surgery	2
Valvular surgery only	1
Coronary artery bypass graft surgery plus valvular surgery	2
Other cardiac surgeries	2
Preoperative serum creatinine 1.2 to <2.1 mg/dL	2
Preoperative serum creatinine ≥2.1 mg/dL	5

Minimum score, 0; maximum score, 17. Risk of development of AKI requiring dialysis increases with higher score. Frequency of AKI requiring dialysis for score of 0–2 point is 0.5%, 3–5 points is 2%, 6–8 points is 8%, 9–13 points is 22%.
From Thakar CV, Arrigain S, Worley S, et al: A clinical score to predict acute renal failure after cardiac surgery. *J Am Soc Nephrol* 6:162, 2005.

factors appear to be important for the development of AKI. For example, aprotinin, an antifibrinolytic agent used until recently to decrease perioperative blood loss in cardiac surgery patients, tends to increase AKI and postoperative mortality [11]. Prolonged cardiopulmonary bypass appears to induce oxidative stress, embolism, and systemic inflammation, thus contributing to AKI [12]. Improved mortality and reduced incidence of AKI were observed with the use of "off-pump" technology in one large observational study [13]. Another randomized trial of 2,300 non-CKD patients failed to demonstrate a reduction in mortality or AKI requiring dialysis in the "off-pump" arm. However, the incidence of AKI was low in both arms of this trial [14]. Although a small, randomized trial of CKD patients showed improved renal outcomes in those undergoing "off-pump" surgery [15], more studies are needed to prove the benefit of this technology.

A number of methods have been used unsuccessfully to try to protect kidney function in patients undergoing surgery. Administration of "low-dose" dopamine has long been advocated for the prevention of AKI but has fallen out of favor due to the lack of efficacy. A large, randomized, prospective trial of preventive role of fenoldopam, a selective dopamine receptor agonist, was terminated early due to lack of effect on progression to dialysis or mortality and increase in hypotensive episodes in cardiac surgery patients [16]. Nesiritide, a recombinant human B-type natriuretic peptide, which increases diuresis, natriuresis, and afterload reduction, was studied in a double-blind, randomized trial of 300 patients with mostly preserved renal function undergoing coronary artery bypass graft surgery [17]. The use of nesiritide was associated with improved postoperative serum creatinine and reduced length of hospital stay as compared with the placebo. Nevertheless, a large, randomized trial in nonsurgery patients with acute decompensated heart failure (ADHF) showed little clinical benefit and worsening hypotension [18]. Several other strategies, including perioperative *N*-acetylcysteine (NAC) and mannitol administration, have not been shown to be effective for the prevention of postoperative AKI [19,20]. The use of calcium channel blockers, ACE inhibitors, or diuretics has been disappointing in this context as well [21]. In fact, perioperative furosemide use has been associated with detrimental effect on renal function after cardiac surgery [22]. Loop diuretics should be used only in patients with definite volume overload.

Prevention of postoperative renal failure still hinges on withdrawal of vasopressors as early as safely possible and maintenance of adequate perioperative intravascular volume. To date there is no definitive answer to what type of fluid is preferable for volume expansion. However, in the absence of hemorrhagic shock, the use of colloid hydroxyethyl starch is controversial and not recommended for volume expansion by KDIGO [23]. Identification of modifiable risk factors for the prevention of postoperative AKI is paramount. A retrospective study of 3,500 patients identified three potentially modifiable risk factors associated with AKI after cardiac surgery, such as preoperative anemia, perioperative RBC transfusions, and the need for surgical reexploration [24].

Cardiogenic Shock and Acute Decompensated Heart Failure

Our understanding of "cardiorenal syndrome" is evolving beyond the concept of low cardiac output causing renal dysfunction. We know that approximately half of patients with ADHF have preserved left ventricular function [25]. In the Evaluation Study of Congestive Heart Failure and Pulmonary Artery Catheterization Effectiveness (ESCAPE), optimization of hemodynamics did not prevent AKI, further suggesting that reduction in cardiac output does not fully explain the development of impaired renal function [25].

A complex bidirectional relationship emerges, whereby heart failure and associated renal dysfunction affect each other. In addition to the traditional hemodynamically mediated AKI due to low cardiac output, the heart and the kidney are simultaneously affected by activation of the sympathetic nervous and renin–angiotensin–aldosterone systems. Such activation results in systemic vasoconstriction, salt and water retention, and volume overload, further exacerbating kidney dysfunction and heart failure. In addition, the immune system affects renal and cardiac function through monocyte-mediated endothelial activation, cytokine release, and apoptosis induction [26]. Furthermore, CKD, a risk factor for coronary artery disease, contributes to volume overload, diuretic resistance, and poor prognosis in CHF and ADHF [25]. Here, we will focus on acute ADHF with AKI as a common clinical problem in the ICU setting.

ADHF is frequently complicated by AKI. The Acute Decompensated Heart Failure Registry (ADHERE) of more than 30,000 patients with ADHF suggests that AKI has poor prognostic implications and predicts mortality in this patient group [27]. In one study, more than a quarter of patients with ADHF developed AKI as defined by a rise in serum creatinine of 0.3 mg per dL. However, even this relatively small rise was associated with 7.5-fold increase in hospital mortality [28].

Management of ADHF will be discussed in detail in Chapter 194. However, these patients are frequently diuretic resistant and hypotensive. The optimal diuretic dosing regimen remains undefined as a randomized, placebo-controlled trial did not show any difference between furosemide administered by bolus or continuous infusion [29]. Randomized trials of nesiritide, a recombinant B-type natriuretic peptide, failed to demonstrate a benefit of nesiritide for diuresis or preservation of renal function [18,30]. Tolvaptan, a vasopressin antagonist, has been studied in a large international randomized trial of more than 4,000 heart failure patients [31]. Tolvaptan was statistically better then placebo at improving dyspnea, edema, and weight loss but did not significantly improve the rate of death and rehospitalization for heart failure. The use of ACE inhibitors is often limited by AKI and hyperkalemia.

Other strategies for diuretic-resistant patients with ADHF include mechanical fluid removal with ultrafiltration (UF) or paracentesis. The use of UF in the ICU setting is discussed in detail in Chapter 201. Although early studies suggested benefit from mechanical UF, a randomized trial comparing diuretics and UF in patients with ADHF and worsening renal function demonstrated no difference in diuresis but reduced renal function and more adverse events in those treated with UF [32–34]. Finally, elevated intra-abdominal pressures in ADHF may play a role in the pathogenesis of renal dysfunction [35]. The reduction of intra-abdominal pressure from approximately 13 to 7 mm Hg by paracentesis was associated with a reduction in serum creatinine from 3.4 to 2.4 mg per dL in diuretic-resistant patients.

Severe Sepsis

Sepsis is among the most common causes of AKI. The association between septicemia and AKI is confounded by the experience that renal dysfunction due to other causes is often complicated by infection. Although the incidence of sepsis in patients with AKI has been reported to be as high as 75%, only one-third of patients have clinically apparent sepsis at the onset of renal dysfunction.

AKI may develop in a setting of sepsis through multiple mechanisms. As discussed previously, inflammation appears to play a significant role. In animal models, sepsis can cause renal impairment even in the absence of hypotension [36]. Clinically, it is likely that endotoxin causes a reduction in GFR through hemodynamic mechanisms, including vascular pooling and renal vasoconstriction, which are mediated by local vasoconstrictors such as thromboxane and endothelin. Although cardiac output is often elevated in patients with sepsis, systemic vasodilation coupled with renal vasoconstriction can shunt perfusion away from the kidneys. Vascular pooling and third spacing generally necessitate volume expansion with isotonic saline. Because myocardial suppression, oliguria, and capillary leakage may accompany sepsis, it is essential to monitor the administration of fluids closely. A randomized trial of protocolized early resuscitation efforts in septic patients prevented incidence of AKI when the following goals were achieved within 6 hours of recognition of septic shock: mean arterial blood pressure ≥65 mm Hg, central venous pressure between 8 and 12 mm Hg, reduction of serum lactate levels, and urinary output ≥0.5 mL/kg/h [37]. Although mortality and renal outcomes were not improved by protocolized early sepsis management in recent, large, multicenter trials [38–40], they do support timely antibiotic administration and adequate intravenous fluid administration as cornerstones of septic shock treatment.

Pancreatitis

Pancreatitis may occur in association with various causes of AKI but can itself induce ATN and renal function predicts survival from acute pancreatitis. This is a rare phenomenon and is generally seen in patients with severe or hemorrhagic pancreatitis with serum amylase values of more than 1,000 units per L. Mortality may approach 70% to 80% in this setting, especially in those with multiorgan failure.

Trauma

AKI associated with severe trauma generally reflects the combination of acute volume depletion, hemorrhage, and myoglobinuria (see following discussion). Survival after trauma is markedly reduced when complicated by AKI.

Abdominal Compartment Syndrome

A variety of critical illness can lead to the intra-abdominal hypertension (IAH) and abdominal compartment syndrome (ACS), such as intra-abdominal hemorrhage, peritonitis, third-spacing of fluid into the abdominal cavity associated with abdominal surgery, ileus, or pancreatitis, as well as overdistention with gas following laparoscopy. IAH is defined as an intra-abdominal pressure over 12 mm Hg measured by a bladder transducer on three separate occasions at least 4 hours apart. ACS is defined as an intra-abdominal pressure over 20 mm Hg, associated with one or more organ system failure [41]. The increase in intra-abdominal pressure leads to visceral ischemia, including AKI. The precise incidence of AKI resulting from ACS is unknown, but appears underreported [42]. Treatment usually requires urgent surgical decompression of the abdomen.

Acute Bilateral Cortical Necrosis

Acute bilateral cortical necrosis is rare. Unlike ATN, in which only tubular elements are involved, in acute cortical necrosis, glomeruli and tubules are destroyed by a process in which cortical vessels may be occluded with fibrin thrombi. Cortical necrosis usually occurs after profound hypotension. Approximately two-thirds of cases are related to obstetric complications, including abruptio placentae, pre-eclampsia and eclampsia, septic abortion, and amniotic fluid embolism. Nonobstetric cortical necrosis is most common in shock, sepsis, and disseminated intravascular coagulopathy, but isolated cases have been reported with snakebites, arsenic ingestion, and hyperacute renal allograft rejection. The pathogenesis of AKI in these conditions involves the hemodynamic insults of hypoperfusion and renal vasoconstriction and formation of fibrin thrombi in the renal microvasculature.

Typically, patients with bilateral cortical necrosis have anuric AKI. Although the diagnosis may be suspected early in the course of renal injury, ATN remains far more likely. When renal function fails to recover after several weeks, cortical necrosis may be confirmed by a renal biopsy. Other diagnostic tests are less specific. Renal scintigraphy most often demonstrates complete absence of isotope in the region of the kidneys. Computed tomography (CT) with contrast enhancement may demonstrate similar findings, indicating absence of perfusion to the renal cortex. Renal angiography shows patency of the main renal arteries and either a complete absence of cortical filling or a mottled nephrogram. Given the severity of the inciting disorder, mortality is high in acute cortical necrosis, with fewer than 20% of patients surviving.

Nephrotoxicity and Drug-Induced Acute Kidney Injury

Many cases of AKI in the ICU can be linked to the effects of endogenous and exogenous nephrotoxins.

Myoglobinuria and Hemoglobinuria

Rhabdomyolysis is often associated with leakage of myocyte contents, particularly the pigment protein myoglobin, into the plasma. Myoglobin, with a molecular weight of approximately 17,000 Da, is freely filtered by the glomerulus. In the distal nephron, myoglobin forms proteinaceous casts that obstruct urine flow. Myoglobin may also exert direct cytotoxic effects on tubular epithelium through the generation of reactive oxygen species.

Myoglobinuric AKI is a consequence of massive skeletal muscle injury of diverse causes. Traumatic rhabdomyolysis occurs in the setting of direct mechanical injury (crush syndrome), burns, or prolonged pressure. Myoglobinuric renal failure is an important cause of morbidity in virtually all wide-scale human catastrophes. Indeed, much of what is known about the syndrome derives from experiences with victims of wars and natural disasters. Crush injuries during the Armenian earthquake of 1988, followed by similar disasters in Japan, Turkey, Iran, and Pakistan, necessitated emergent mobilization of dialysis resources on a massive scale [43].

Nontraumatic rhabdomyolysis can occur with toxic, metabolic, and inflammatory myopathies, vigorous exercise, severe potassium and phosphate depletion, and hyperthermic states such as the neuroleptic malignant syndrome and malignant hyperthermia. Lipid-lowering drugs currently represent one of the most common causes of rhabdomyolysis. The use of heroin and amphetamines has also been reported in association with rhabdomyolysis.

As with other forms of AKI, the prognosis depends largely on the gravity of the predisposing condition; AKI following massive trauma can be expected to run a longer course than that associated with nontraumatic causes. In particularly severe cases, oliguria and dialysis dependence may persist for weeks.

Clinical signs and symptoms of muscle injury, such as muscle tenderness, are absent in at least half of cases of significant nontraumatic rhabdomyolysis. The diagnosis is suggested by markedly elevated serum levels of muscle enzymes with serum creatine kinase levels usually higher than 5,000. The serum levels of phosphate and potassium are also typically elevated in rhabdomyolysis because lysis of muscle cells causes release of intracellular contents into the blood. A fall in the serum calcium is quite common. Rebound hypercalcemia often occurs during the recovery phase.

The therapy of myoglobinuria is similar to that of other forms of AKI, but there are several particular considerations. The tubular toxicity of myoglobin is enhanced when urine flow rates are low, urine is concentrated, and urinary acidification is maximal. It is therefore important in the early phases of the illness to ensure that the patient is in a volume-replete state and maintaining a rapid diuresis (i.e., urine output of at least 150 mL per hour). To this end, isotonic fluids may be administered.

Most experts recommend the administration of bicarbonate-rich fluids to alkalinize the urine above a pH of 6.5 so as to improve the solubility of myoglobin. Diuresis may be enhanced with concurrent administration of loop diuretics. Some have argued that loop diuretics may introduce the potentially adverse effect of increasing urinary acid excretion and have advocated the use of osmotic diuretic agents such as mannitol. Mannitol, however, has the potential drawback of causing intravascular volume overload in patients whose kidneys may already have impaired urine output.

Hemoglobinuria can also result in AKI. The pathophysiologic mechanisms are similar to those involved in myoglobinuric AKI. Hemoglobinuric renal failure is relatively rare. Hemoglobin, with a molecular weight almost four times that of myoglobin, is less readily filtered. Furthermore, when hemoglobin is released into the plasma, it binds to haptoglobin, forming a bulky, nonfilterable molecular complex. Only when the haptoglobin-binding capacity is saturated (at plasma hemoglobin concentrations >100 mg per dL) does hemoglobin appear in the tubular fluid. Thus, only massive intravascular hemolysis, as may occur with fulminant transfusion reactions, autoimmune hemolytic crises, and mechanical hemolysis from a dysfunctional prosthetic heart valve (Waring blender syndrome), can induce AKI.

Radiocontrast-Induced Nephropathy

The administration of intravascular radiocontrast agents leads to a syndrome of rapidly developing AKI. Contrast-induced nephropathy (CIN) is commonly defined as an absolute increase in serum creatinine of 0.5 mg per dL or a relative increase of 25% from the baseline within 48 to 72 hours of contrast exposure. The serum creatinine level begins to rise 12 to 24 hours and peaks approximately 4 days after the procedure. Some patients develop a transient increase in urine output as a result of contrast-induced osmotic diuresis, followed by oliguria. The majority of patients are nonoliguric and do not require dialysis. In patients who have undergone endovascular procedures, CIN must be differentiated from atheroembolic disease, which has a significantly worse prognosis.

Prospective studies report that the incidence of radiocontrast-induced kidney injury ranges from 1% to more than 50%. Much of this variance can be attributed to disparities in the definitions of AKI, the number of associated risk factors (particularly CKD), and the type of procedure performed. The incidence appears to be minimal in patients with normal renal function and without risk factors (see Table 200.9). Pre-existing CKD, however, particularly in patients with diabetes, confers a 6- to 10-fold increased likelihood of radiocontrast-induced AKI. Contrast-enhanced CT is associated with a lower risk of CIN as compared with coronary angiography. Noncoronary angiography had the highest incidence of CIN in a study of 660 military veterans, reaching 15% in patients with GFR less than 60 mL per minute per 1.73 m^2 [44]. In the ICU, the risk of contrast-induced AKI is likely much higher as patients often have concomitant nephrotoxic insults such as hypotension or sepsis.

There are several mechanisms by which radiocontrast-induced renal injury may develop. Hemodynamic factors are believed important, as contrast exposure causes initial vasodilation followed by prolonged vasoconstriction of the renal circulation. The finding of a low FE_{Na} in some patients with contrast-induced AKI and the tendency toward rapid recovery suggest a role for reversible vasoconstriction. The intensity and duration of the vasoconstriction may be influenced by the underlying characteristics of the renal microcirculation. Endothelial factors that promote vasoconstriction, such as endothelin and adenosine, may participate in the pathogenesis of radiocontrast-induced nephropathy [45]. Other postulated mechanisms of radiocontrast-induced nephropathy include the generation of reactive oxygen species and the direct cytotoxic effect of the contrast media, especially with highly osmolar agents [46].

Since there is no specific treatment for radiocontrast-induced nephropathy, attention has focused on methods of prevention. Table 200.10 lists a number of preventative measures with possible benefit. However, the best preventive measure remains avoidance of radiocontrast and use of an alternative noncontrast imaging procedure if possible.

Since radiocontrast injury is augmented by hypovolemia, particularly in the presence of prostaglandin inhibitors, modest volume expansion and avoidance of NSAIDs are justifiable. Although isotonic bicarbonate, rather than saline, may reduce the risk of free radical injury, multiple randomized trials have yielded conflicting data [47–49]. Thus, there is no consensus on optimal type, rate, or duration of infusion of fluid for prevention of CIN. For patients at risk (those with renal dysfunction or other risk factors), we use either 0.9% saline or isotonic bicarbonate bolus, 3 mL per kg over 1 hour before administration of contrast agent, followed by 1 mL per kg per hour infusion for 6 hours after procedure. The use of diuretics to augment urine output and manage intravascular volume may provide additional benefit [50,51].

NAC may ameliorate radiocontrast nephrotoxicity, possibly through an antioxidant effect. However, studies have produced conflicting results [52,53]. Though the benefit remains controversial, NAC appears to be a low risk intervention and is still frequently used. We typically give NAC 1,200 mg orally for two doses before and two doses after the contrast exposure.

Low-osmolality contrast formulations (600 to 800 mOsm per kg) have been shown to be less nephrotoxic then high-osmolar agents (>1,400 mOsm per kg) and are now commonly used in all patients. However, iso-osmolar agents, such as iodixanol, have not been shown to have a clear additional benefit as compared with low-osmolar agents [54,55] of patients undergoing contrast enhanced CT and coronary angiography.

TABLE 200.9

Risk Factors Associated with Radiocontrast Nephropathy

Pre-existing renal insufficiency
Diabetic nephropathy, with renal insufficiency
Volume depletion
Diuretic use
Large contrast dose (>2 mL/kg)
Age >60 y
CHF
Hepatic failure
Multiple myeloma (with high-osmolar contrast agent)
Use of intra-aortic balloon pump

TABLE 200.10

Preventive Measures for Radiocontrast Nephropathy

Volume expansion with normal saline or isotonic bicarbonate (3 mL/kg bolus over 1 h prior to the procedure, followed by 1 mL/kg/h for 6 h postexposure)
Limit radiocontrast load to ≤1 mL/kg in high-risk patients
Avoid high-osmolar contrast agents
Discontinue diuretics, ACE inhibitors, and nonsteroidal anti-inflammatory drugs for 24 h postprocedure
N-Acetylcysteine (4 doses of 600–1,200 mg PO every 12 h with 2 doses before and 2 doses after procedure)

Removal of contrast media by hemodialysis or hemofiltration to prevent CIN was studied in several small trials. A meta-analysis of these trials revealed no benefit and even suggested an increase in CIN with hemodialysis [56]. Similarly, there is no clear evidence to support hemodialysis or hemofiltration immediately after contrast exposure to preserve residual renal function in ESRD patients [57]. Therefore, the timing of dialysis after radiocontrast should be based on clinical judgment.

Studies of therapies directed against vasoconstriction have yielded disappointing results. A meta-analysis of theophylline and aminophylline, antagonists of adenosine receptors, showed no benefit in CIN prevention [58]. Fenoldopam, a vasodilatory analog of dopamine, and an endothelin receptor antagonist have been shown minimal or even deleterious effects on renal function after contrast exposure [59,60].

Acute Phosphate Nephropathy

Sodium phosphate, a hyperosmolar laxative, can cause AKI when administered orally or by enema [61]. Risk factors include CKD, volume depletion, and increased dosage. AKI typically occurs days to weeks after exposure and is likely caused by calcium phosphate precipitation with tubular obstruction and injury. Kidney biopsy reveals calcium phosphate deposition in the tubules and interstitium, as well as interstitial inflammation and ATN [62]. The prognosis of APN is poor as kidney function rarely recovers completely and most patients are left with CKD or progress to ESRD.

With growing recognition of acute phosphate nephropathy, the FDA issued warnings regarding the risks of oral sodium phosphate preparations and many products were withdrawn, though some generic preparations remain on the market. However, these agents should be avoided as safer alternatives are widely available.

Drug-Induced Syndromes

Hospitalized patients, particularly those in ICUs, are exposed to numerous pharmacologic agents. Since many drugs are capable of inducing abnormalities in renal function, the appearance of AKI in any patient should prompt the clinician to investigate a possible drug-related cause. Drug-induced AKI has four major syndromes (see Table 200.11).

TABLE 200.11

Syndromes of Drug-Induced Kidney Injury

Acute tubular injury
Aminoglycoside antibiotics
Antifungal agents (amphotericin)
Antiviral agents (tenofovir, foscarnet)
Intravenous immunoglobulin
Heavy metals (cisplatin)
Intratubular micro-obstruction
Methotrexate
Acyclovir
Sulfamethoxazole
Indinavir
Acute interstitial nephritis (see list in Table 200.11)
Autoregulatory failure
Angiotensin-converting enzyme inhibitors
Nonsteroidal anti-inflammatory drugs

Acute Tubular Injury

Nephrotoxic medications often injure the renal tubular epithelium. Tubular damage occurs with variable incidence through a variety of mechanisms including direct toxicity (aminoglycosides, tenofovir), osmotic injury (mannitol, intravenous immunoglobulin), and vasoconstriction (radiocontrast, NSAIDs). Tubular injury is typically reversible after withdrawal of the inciting agent, although recovery may take several days to weeks. Occasionally, specific renal tubular functional abnormalities, such as magnesium and potassium wasting, renal tubular acidosis, and impaired urinary concentration, may persist.

Volume contraction, pre-existing CKD, and liver disease enhance the risk of drug-induced tubular injury. The risk of nephrotoxicity is reduced by ensuring that patients are well hydrated before therapy. If possible, nonnephrotoxic therapeutic alternatives should be used in patients with underlying renal disease.

Intratubular Micro-obstruction

A second form of acute nephrotoxicity is caused by drugs that precipitate in the renal tubules and urinary collecting system and obstruct the nephrons. Such agents are generally poorly soluble at low pH, as characterizes the distal tubular fluid. This syndrome has been reported in patients receiving relatively high-dose intravenous methotrexate and acyclovir, indinavir, low-molecular-weight dextran, and sulfamethoxazole. Prevention of micro-obstructive AKI necessitates optimal hydration of the patient and maintenance of a high urine flow rate. Urinary alkalinization may be of benefit, depending on the nature of the obstructing agent. The syndrome is usually readily reversible and short lived.

Acute Interstitial Nephritis

Many medications can induce AIN, the syndrome of AKI with an inflammatory infiltrate in the renal parenchyma on biopsy (see Table 200.12). Originally associated with allergic manifestations such as skin rash, fever, and eosinophilia, more

TABLE 200.12

Drugs Most Often Implicated in Acute Interstitial Nephritis

Antibiotics
Penicillins
Cephalosporins
Ampicillin
Amoxicillin
Ciprofloxacin
Sulfonamides
Rifampin
Tetracycline
Indinavir
Proton pump inhibitors
Diuretics
Furosemide
Thiazides and related compounds
Nonsteroidal anti-inflammatory drugs
Miscellaneous drugs
Diphenylhydantoin
Cimetidine
Methyldopa
Allopurinol
Captopril
Mesalamine

recent data suggests this clinical triad is relatively uncommon [63], especially in cases caused by NSAIDs. The risk of AIN is not dependent on medication dosage. AIN has a more variable course than syndromes of direct drug nephrotoxicity and cases may vary widely in the time of onset following exposure to the inciting agent (days to years), the severity of the renal injury, and the time required for reversal following withdrawal of the drug (days to months). In addition to hematuria and pyuria, the urine sediment may show a preponderance of eosinophils while heavy proteinuria is rare. White blood cell casts are a common finding (Fig. 200.2). The pathogenesis of AKI in this disorder is poorly understood. The renal histopathology early in the course of the disease shows mainly interstitial infiltration with inflammatory cells, often (but not always) eosinophils.

Although steroids have never been shown to reduce morbidity in a controlled trial, most experts use them in severe cases of AIN (i.e., those in which supportive dialysis may become necessary). See the "Treatment" section for more details on management of AIN.

A variant form of AIN is occasionally encountered in patients who take NSAIDs, particularly fenoprofen, meclofenamate, tolmetin, and indomethacin. The hallmarks of allergy, drug rash, eosinophilia, and eosinophiluria are absent. The urinalysis is nonspecific; some cases are marked by nephrotic range proteinuria. The renal pathology shows interstitial inflammation and normal-appearing glomeruli. As with classic allergic interstitial nephritis, this disorder regresses after cessation of therapy with the offending agent. Patients who have had this disorder should probably be considered at risk for recurrence with other NSAIDs.

Hemodynamic or Autoregulatory Failure

The final form of drug-related AKI pertains to drugs that cause abnormalities of glomerular blood flow. Two pathophysiologic subsets of hemodynamically mediated AKI may be identified, depending on whether the main action of the drug is on the afferent or efferent glomerular arteriole. When the medication increases afferent vasoconstriction, autoregulation of renal blood flow is impaired, and prerenal azotemia develops. This effect may be seen in association with NSAIDs, which reduce the synthesis of vasodilatory prostaglandins, or drugs that directly constrict the preglomerular vessels (i.e., vasopressors and possibly radiocontrast agents). When preglomerular vasoconstriction is severe and prolonged, frank ischemic tubular necrosis may result. More often, a rapidly reversible, prerenal form of AKI occurs.

The other subset of hemodynamically mediated, drug-induced renal failure is seen in association with ACE inhibitors, which block the formation of angiotensin II from angiotensin I. In addition to their role as antihypertensives, these are commonly used as afterload reducers for the treatment of congestive heart failure. When used in this setting, they may engender an improvement of renal perfusion, as reduced peripheral vascular resistance leads to reduced left ventricular impedance. Under conditions of attenuated and fixed renal blood flow, however (as would occur with bilateral renal artery stenosis), ACE inhibitors may cause a sharp reduction in GFR.

These syndromes are encountered almost exclusively in patients with significant underlying impairment of renal perfusion or function. Unless severe renal ischemia has occurred, renal function should rapidly return to baseline levels after withdrawal of the responsible drug.

Renal Vascular Disease

Major Renal Vascular Disease

Renal vascular disease is divisible into major vascular and microvascular syndromes. Major renal vascular disease is an unusual cause of AKI. Renal artery occlusion does not produce AKI unless it is bilateral or occurs in a solitary functioning kidney. The sudden appearance of flank pain and a rising serum creatinine should lead the physician to consider acute renal artery embolism or thrombosis. The differential diagnoses in this scenario include nephrolithiasis, pyelonephritis (with or without urinary obstruction), and RVT.

Renal artery emboli occur most frequently in the setting of cardiac disease, particularly in patients with arrhythmias or mural cardiac thrombi. Frequently, multiple organs are involved, including brain, lung, and spleen. AKI is more likely to occur with a distribution of emboli to both kidneys, although azotemia may occur with a unilateral embolus.

If the thrombus or embolus involves a solitary functioning kidney, oligoanuria and a rising level of azotemia can be expected. In addition to flank pain and diminished urine volume, 50% of patients develop uncontrolled hypertension and 20% experience nausea, fever, or both in a large case series of patients with acute renal infarction [64]. The urinalysis is not specific. Leukocyturia, hematuria, and low-grade proteinuria have been found, as have a bland urine sediment. Radionuclide scanning often demonstrates patchy uptake of isotope or, in the case of total occlusion, no isotopic uptake. CT may demonstrate similar findings of diminished contrast uptake either by the whole kidney or localized wedge-shaped areas of nonperfusion.

Accurate diagnosis of renal arterial disease requires radiologic imaging. Renal artery duplex scan may reveal the absence of Doppler signal if total occlusion occurs, but provides only limited anatomical information if stenosis is present. The renal artery duplex is not as sensitive or specific for the diagnosis of stenosis as compared with angiography or magnetic resonance arteriography. Angiography provides the most accurate anatomic information, but it is also the most invasive test.

Occlusion of the renal artery does not inevitably lead to infarction. Particularly in patients with slowly developing atherosclerotic disease, collateral circulation via capsular or ureteric vessels may protect the kidney from infarction even though renal arterial blood flow is inadequate to maintain function. Surgery may be preferable in patients with renal artery thrombosis, although supportive care with anticoagulation has been the preferred treatment for renal arterial embolism. Reports of successful treatment with fibrinolytic agents (either urokinase or streptokinase) have led some to consider this the preferred treatment for renal artery occlusive disease, particularly in patients for whom surgery represents too great a risk.

Renal Vein Thrombosis

RVT is an uncommon cause of AKI. Bilateral renal vein occlusion occurs most commonly in severely volume-depleted children. In adults, it usually develops in the setting of nephrotic syndrome or renal cell carcinoma, but can also occur with hypercoagulable conditions, sickle cell disease, pregnancy, use of oral contraceptives, or trauma. RVT generally does not cause AKI unless it is acute and bilateral or occurs in a solitary kidney. Flank pain and microscopic hematuria are the usual clinical manifestations in acute RVT. Duplex venography and CT scan can often establish the diagnosis and are less invasive than radiocontrast renal venography. Treatment usually consists of anticoagulation, although fibrinolytic therapy should be considered in patients with AKI and RVT.

Atheroembolic Renal Disease (Cholesterol Emboli)

Atheroembolic renal disease is increasingly recognized as a cause of AKI, but is probably still underdiagnosed. Atheroembolic disease is often found on postmortem examination. It is important to distinguish this syndrome from renal arterial thromboembolism.

Cholesterol embolization occurs only in patients with severe aortic atherosclerosis, usually after trauma to the wall of the aorta such as with aortography, major vascular surgery, or blunt trauma to the abdomen. Atheroemboli may also occur spontaneously, particularly in patients with diabetic macrovascular disease and those receiving anticoagulant therapy. Diffuse occlusion of the microvasculature by atheroemboli leads to tissue damage in either a subacute or an acute fashion. Patients may experience relatively minor abnormalities such as infarction of the tip of a single toe. Renal involvement is particularly common when diffuse embolization accompanies major arteriography or aortic surgery. Involvement of other visceral organs, including the pancreas, bowel, spleen, retina, and brain, may also occur. Typically, the cholesterol emboli form needlelike occlusions in small vessels, which then develop a chronic inflammatory response that can include the formation of a granulomatous reaction. Extensive infarction of bowel or sudden neurologic abnormalities may bring the patient to the ICU, where, in addition to the presenting findings, AKI is noted. In the kidney, occlusion of a sufficient proportion of the microvasculature results in varying degrees of azotemia. The azotemia may be sudden, after the precipitating event, or may develop more slowly and may follow a stuttering course marked by acute deterioration with intervening periods of incomplete recovery. The latter course helps to distinguish this diagnosis from that of radiocontrast nephropathy, which typically occurs within 24 to 48 hours after arteriography.

The diagnosis is often missed unless there are peripheral signs of involvement such as blue distal digits or livedo reticularis of the lower extremities. A more subtle and less frequently observed physical manifestation is the finding of visible cholesterol emboli in the retinal vessels (Hollenhorst plaques). Less specific manifestations include peripheral eosinophilia and hypocomplementemia. The urine sediment is nonspecific.

Patients with atheroembolic renal disease experience the full spectrum of renal dysfunction, from minor degrees of azotemia to full-blown, irreversible renal failure. After an initial rise in serum creatinine, there may be an improvement in GFR over several weeks, probably attributable to nephron adaptation with hyperfiltration in remnant glomeruli. No specific management is available for atheroembolic renal disease. Management of renal failure, including dialytic therapy, may be indicated. Use of anticoagulants may worsen this condition.

Thrombotic Microangiopathies

Thrombotic microangiopathies (TMAs) are a group of disorders characterized by microangiopathic hemolytic anemia and thrombocytopenia often associated with multisystem dysfunction including AKI. TMA can occur as a hereditary or acquired hematologic disorder such as TTP and hemolytic uremic syndrome (HUS). It may also complicate systemic conditions including malignant and pregnancy-related hypertension, rheumatologic diseases such as systemic lupus erythematosis, scleroderma, and antiphospholipid antibody syndrome, various infections, malignancy, and disseminated intravascular coagulation. In primary TMAs, occlusion of the preglomerular and glomerular microvasculature by platelet microthrombi with reactive changes in the endothelium accounts for the rapid deterioration in renal function. Clinical and histopathologic features of malignant hypertension may also be seen.

TTP and HUS, which were previously thought of as the same entity with different clinical presentation, are now considered separate diseases based on different pathogenesis and are discussed in more detail in Chapter 109. TTP often presents with a pentad of fever, thrombocytopenia, microangiopathic hemolytic anemia, AKI, and neurologic abnormalities. In contrast to other forms of TMA, the AKI is often relatively mild. In TTP, diminished activity of a von Willebrand Factor (vWF) cleaving protein called ADAMTS13 generates abnormally enlarged vWF which leads to platelet activation and aggregation, microthrombi formation, and ischemia. Decreased activity or mutations of ADAMTS13 protein are observed in recurrent and familial forms of TTP. TTP can also be seen with certain infections, such as HIV. Several medications are associated with TTP, including clopidogrel, cyclosporine, and chemotherapeutic agents, such as cisplatinum, bleomycin, and others.

In HUS, hematologic and renal features predominate, and ADAMTS13 activity is normal. HUS is associated with a variety of infectious diseases, such as enteric infections, particularly with *Escherichia coli* 0157:H7, Mycoplasma, Legionella, and Coxsackie A and B viruses. Clinical presentation of HUS has a diarrheal and a nondiarrheal form. In the diarrheal form, a Shiga-like toxin is postulated to cause AKI by entering the circulation, binding to the proximal tubular cells as well as arteriolar and glomerular capillary endothelium and causing inflammation and platelet activation. The pathogenesis of the nondiarrheal form appears related to abnormal activation of the alternative complement pathway leading to injury to the renal endothelium.

Treatment of thrombotic angiopathies varies greatly and will be discussed in detail in Chapters 91 and 92. TTP is a medical emergency and without treatment, mortality exceeds 90%. Prompt plasmapheresis and plasma exchange to provide the missing enzyme and to remove vWF cleaving protein inhibitor are essential and are often combined with glucocorticoids. Treatment of HUS is largely supportive. Renal management includes maintenance of adequate intravascular volume, avoidance of nephrotoxins, and dialytic support as needed. There is no proven benefit to plasmapheresis, but eculizumab, a monoclonal antibody directed against C5 has yielded excellent results in HUS related to complement activation [65]. Systemic diseases associated with TMAs are discussed in detail elsewhere in the text.

Acute Kidney Injury in the Cancer Patient

AKI is a relatively common complication in patients with neoplastic diseases. Many malignancies cause hypercalcemia which can induce AKI through alterations in renal hemodynamics (afferent arteriolar vasoconstriction and diminished GFR) and by causing volume depletion. In addition, long-standing hypercalcemia can cause nephrocalcinosis and CKD. The pathogenesis and therapy of hypercalcemia of malignancy are described in detail in Chapters 95 and 140. From a nephrologic perspective, the mainstays of therapy are volume expansion with saline supplemented with loop diuretics to enhance urinary calcium excretion, combined with measures to lower the serum calcium. In cases of severe AKI, dialysis may be needed to lower the calcium level. Of note, bisphosphonates used to treat hypercalcemia can also cause AKI through direct nephrotoxicity leading to ATN as well by inducing collapsing focal glomerulosclerosis [66].

The term *tumor lysis syndrome* refers to the sudden release of tumor cell contents often in response to induction chemotherapy. These intracellular products include phosphate, potassium, uric acid, and other purine metabolites. They may cause diffuse tubular micro-obstruction once they enter the nephron, which results in sudden onset of AKI. The syndrome occurs almost exclusively in patients with hematologic malignancies, especially in the setting of large tumor burden and high cell turnover. Preventive measures include aggressive intravenous hydration to enhance urine flow and minimize precipitation of uric acid and calcium phosphate in the tubules as well as treatment with medications to prevent hyperuricemia. Allopurinol, which decreases the formation of uric acid, and rasburicase, which promotes the degradation of uric acid should be considered [67]. Febuxostat, which also lowers uric acid formation, may be more effective than allopurinol, but carries a greater risk of hepatotoxicity and is much more costly [68]. Alkalinizing the urine enhances uric acid solubility, but also may promote the precipitation of calcium and phosphate in various soft tissues including the kidney. To date, there are no studies showing improved outcomes with urinary alkalinization. A reasonable approach would be to limit hydration with bicarbonate-based solutions to patients with tumor lysis syndrome who also have a significant metabolic acidosis [69]. Of note, once the tumor lysis syndrome becomes established, the resulting oliguria and AKI may further complicate therapy. This requires a delicate balance between continued hydration and intermittent diuretics to maintain urine output and to avoid volume overload.

A number of commonly used antineoplastic agents have renal side effects and can cause AKI. Principal among these is cisplatin, which, like other heavy metals, can induce ATN. The incidence of this complication is less with the newer analog carboplatin. Saline loading of patients who are about to receive platinum-containing chemotherapeutic agents helps reduce the risk of AKI. High-dose (>2 g per day) methotrexate therapy can also cause AKI. The drug is primarily renally excreted and can result in tubular micro-obstruction from intraluminal crystallization of methotrexate metabolites. Raising the urine pH, substantially increases the solubility of methotrexate in the renal tubules. Thus, the cornerstone for prophylaxis relies on volume expansion with a bicarbonate based solution [70].

Many neoplasms involve the ureteric bed or periureteric lymph nodes. Obstructive uropathy must be considered in any case of unexplained AKI in an oncologic patient, particularly one with lymphoma, prostatic, colorectal, or cervical carcinoma. Such obstructions are usually readily detectable by ultrasonographic examination. If the sonogram fails to detect hydronephrosis but obstruction is strongly suspected, further imaging should be done to determine the patency of the ureters. These tests may include CT Urogram, MR Urogram, and retrograde cystoureterography. One must carefully consider the patient's GFR and their ability to receive various contrast solutions before selecting a test. In cases in which ureteral obstruction is confirmed, nephrostomy drainage is often required. Ureteral stents can be considered but may fail if extrinsic compression remains present. Regardless, such drainage measures may only be needed temporarily in tumors that respond sufficiently to radiation or chemotherapy.

Multiple myeloma is a neoplasm that is especially frequently complicated by AKI. Patients with this disease may develop renal injury from several mechanisms. Hypercalcemia is very common in myeloma. In addition, the paraproteins, particularly light chains (Bence–Jones proteins), can be directly nephrotoxic. Finally, filtered paraproteins can form occlusive casts within the urinary space (cast nephropathy).

Tumor infiltration of the renal parenchyma is an unusual cause of AKI, despite the frequency of metastases to the kidneys. Imaging studies should reveal kidney enlargement. Successful reversal with radiation or chemotherapy is unusual. Decisions regarding the use of dialysis in patients with widespread metastatic disease must be based on a realistic appraisal of the prognosis of the underlying disease and on the patient's wishes.

Renal Dysfunction in Patients with Liver Disease

AKI frequently develops in the setting of advanced liver disease with prerenal azotemia being the most common form. Despite obvious fluid retention, these patients have decreased renal perfusion from reduced effective circulating volume due to splanchnic vasodilation, hypoalbuminemia, and various neurohumoral influences. The balance between controlling ascites and peripheral edema while avoiding prerenal azotemia is often difficult. Diuretic dose adjustments, judicious use of crystalloids, colloids, and blood transfusions may not be sufficient to prevent progressive loss of renal function. Patients with liver disease and AKI who do not respond to volume expansion are diagnosed with hepatorenal syndrome (HRS). Table 200.13 details a more specific definition of HRS [71]. HRS is usually seen in advanced

TABLE 200.13

Definition of Hepatorenal Syndrome [71]

- Cirrhosis with ascites
- Serum creatinine >1.5 mg/dL
- No improvement of serum creatinine after 2 d with diuretic withdrawal and volume expansion with albumin. The recommended dose of albumin is 1 g/kg of body weight per day up to a maximum of 100 g/d
- Absence of shock, ongoing bacterial infection, current or recent treatment with nephrotoxic drugs, gastrointestinal or renal fluid loss
- Absence of parenchymal disease as indicated by proteinuria <0.5 g/d, microhematuria (>50 red blood cells per high power field) no abnormalities on renal ultrasound.

cirrhosis, but it has also been reported in patients with acute hepatitis or hepatic neoplasm. Onset of the syndrome may be sudden or insidious.

HRS can be considered a form of prerenal azotemia in patients with severe hepatic dysfunction that is refractory to volume expansion. The pathogenesis of the HRS is principally related to vascular changes induced by portal hypertension. Increased portal pressures cause the release of local vasodilators and splanchnic arterial vasodilation. This results in a drop in systemic perfusion pressure and compensatory activation of the sympathetic nervous system and the renin–angiotensin system which causes severe intrarenal vasoconstriction as depicted in Figure 200.4. HRS is initially a functional condition as evidenced by extreme renal avidity for sodium and water, suggesting AKI from hemodynamic changes rather than parenchymal injury. Furthermore, the process can reverse as involved kidneys function normally when transplanted into a recipient with intact liver function.

The vasodilatation in the splanchnic vascular beds that initiates HRS has been the target of several therapies. Albumin in combination with the vasoconstrictor terlipressin has been shown to be effective in randomized studies reversing HRS in the majority of cases [72,73]. However, terlipressin is currently not available in the United States. In patients under continues hemodynamic monitoring, norepinephrine infusion combined with albumin has been shown to have similar outcomes to terlipressin with fewer ischemic complications [74]. In patients not in the ICU and where terlipressin is not available, treatment with midodrine and octreotide is recommended. Midodrine (7.5 to 15 mg orally three times a day) and octreotide (100 to 200 μg subcutaneously three times a day) is combined with albumin with the goal of increasing mean arterial blood pressure by 15 mm Hg [74–76].

Transjugular intrahepatic portosystemic shunts (TIPS) have not been well studied in cases of HRS. The limited data does show some improvement in renal function but this needs to be weighed against the increased risk of encephalopathy and procedural complication [77]. Finally, in patients with HRS with progressive loss of renal function, dialysis should be considered on a case by case basis [78]. In general, this modality is reserved for patients that are liver transplant candidates or who have reversible forms of hepatic failure.

Hepatic disease predisposes patients to ATN of the other causes (i.e., nephrotoxic drug exposure, radiocontrast exposure, hypotension, and sepsis). Patients with severe hepatic disease often have one or more of these risk factors. Furthermore, hyperbilirubinemia may predispose to AKI through the toxic actions of bile on renal tubules. Although the urinary sediment in most cases of ATN is distinctive with muddy brown granular casts, jaundiced patients without tubular necrosis may

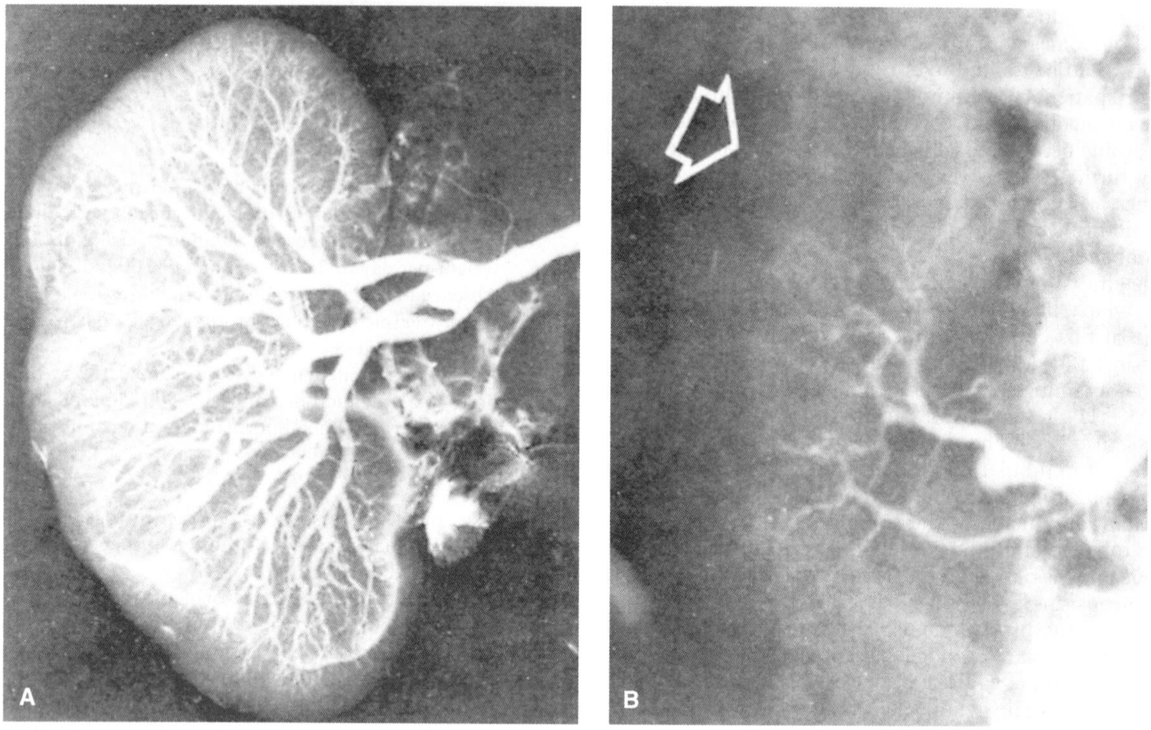

FIGURE 200.4 Angiographic pattern in hepatorenal syndrome with severe renal cortical vasoconstriction. Premortem (**A**) and postmortem (**B**) angiograms of a representative patient are shown. The arrow points to severe cortical vasoconstriction; it is a process that appears to reverse when the involved kidney is transplanted into a hepatically intact host. (Reprinted from Battle DC, Arruda JA, Kurtzman NA: Hyperkalemic distal renal tubular acidosis associated with obstructive uropathy. *N Engl J Med* 304:373, 1981, with permission).

manifest pigmented granular casts simply as a direct result of the interaction of bilirubin with tubular cells. The diagnosis of ATN can be further complicated by the finding of a low FE_{Na}. Patients with ATN typically have a FE_{Na} of greater than 2% as a result of tubular injury impairing sodium reabsorption. Because of the extreme nature of sodium avidity in the setting of cirrhosis, patients may have a FE_{Na} of less than 1% despite renal tubular injury.

Management of cirrhotic patients with sodium and volume overload is extremely challenging. Cirrhotic patients are in a tenuous physiologic state; they have little tolerance for small deviations, either positive or negative, from their optimal state of fluid balance. Sodium balance must be regulated with dietary restriction or diuretics, or both, if ascites and edema are to be controlled. When oliguria develops in patients with advanced cirrhosis, conventional therapy may fail to achieve adequate diuresis. High doses of intravenous diuretics, in combination or as continuous infusions, can be used. Since aldosterone appears to play a significant role in the sodium retention of cirrhosis, spironolactone may be a useful adjunct in diuretic therapy. Although patients with significant peripheral edema can often tolerate as much as a net diuresis of 3 L per day, those with ascites but no edema should be managed more cautiously to avoid AKI.

In patients with significant ascites that is refractory to diet and diuretic therapy, large volume paracentesis (LVP) can help alleviate abdominal pressure and reduce respiratory symptoms. Patients can have up to 5 L of peritoneal fluid removed safely with paracentesis, but simultaneous albumin infusions (8 g of albumin per L removed) should be administered in patients undergoing larger volume removal to avoid hypotension and possible AKI [79]. Although LVP does offer the convenience of rapid resolution of ascites, it does lead to protein loss and carries the risk of procedural complications. Peritoneovenous shunts, such as the Denver and LeVeen shunts, have been used to infuse ascitic fluid into the central circulation. In light of the high perioperative complication rate and the lack of data showing increased survival, the procedure is rarely used. Repetitive paracentesis remains the standard procedure to manage diuretic-resistant ascites.

The biochemical abnormalities that characterize AKI in the patient with hepatic disease are the same as those found in other settings, with a few special considerations. Owing to impaired hepatic synthesis of urea, these patients may have lower BUN levels than expected. In addition, these patients often have dramatically reduced muscle mass; thus, the creatinine level may be deceptively low despite advanced renal dysfunction due to decreased endogenous creatinine production. Azotemic patients with hepatic failure have increased metabolic substrate for ammonia production and therefore are at heightened risk for encephalopathy. Potassium depletion, a common electrolyte imbalance in cirrhosis, further enhances ammonia synthesis. Since cirrhosis is often associated with diminished perfusion pressure, hyponatremia may develop in response to increased antidiuretic hormone (ADH) levels and decreased capacity to excrete free water. Patients with significant hyponatremia should have their water intake restricted to less than 1,500 mL per day.

Acid–base disturbances are common and varied in patients with advanced hepatocellular disease. Respiratory alkalosis can occur as a result of increased progesterone levels stimulating hyperventilation. The use of diuretics as well as the presence of secondary hyperaldosteronism can cause a metabolic alkalosis that can aggravate hepatic encephalopathy. As plasma pH rises, ammonium ions lose protons to the plasma; the resulting ammonia penetrates the blood–brain barrier more readily and can worsen encephalopathy.

Although the finding of metabolic alkalosis is common, acid–base disturbances can rapidly change in the cirrhotic patient. Patients with diarrhea may develop a nonanion gap acidosis. Or in patients with severe hypotension, a high anion gap metabolic acidosis related to lactic acid may develop.

Lactic acidosis may be particularly severe in patients with liver disease because extraction and metabolism of lactic acid from the blood depend largely on hepatic function. In patients with a metabolic alkalosis, the subsequent development of a metabolic acidosis may be missed, as the bicarbonate may be in the normal range. This is a particularly treacherous combined acid–base disturbance because a near-normal serum pH may believe the true extent of the acidosis. As the acidosis worsens, the pH may plummet because of depletion of the bicarbonate buffer system, deficiencies of protein buffers, and inability to maintain adequate respiratory compensation.

DIAGNOSIS OF ACUTE KIDNEY INJURY

History and Physical Examination

In patients with no prior medical data, the history may be useful in establishing whether renal dysfunction is chronic or acute. For example, a patient with long-standing loss of appetite and pruritus is more likely to have CKD than AKI. In these cases, the background information often elicits evidence of previous renal or urinary abnormalities such as hypertension, proteinuria, or a history of diabetes mellitus. A thirsty patient, or one in whom daily weight loss has been documented, may have volume depletion causing prerenal azotemia. The avenues of fluid loss are usually identifiable. Exposure to nephrotoxic agents or a recent episode of sustained hypotension suggests the possibility of ATN. Symptoms of renal colic, abnormal voiding pattern, or a history of genitourinary malignancy point toward an obstructive cause.

The physical examination often furnishes some diagnostic information, particularly regarding volume status. Diminished skin turgor, sunken eyes, dry mucous membranes, the absence of axillary sweat, or orthostatic hypotension supports a diagnosis of prerenal azotemia. In disorders characterized by reduced effective circulatory volume, such as congestive heart failure and nephrotic syndrome, prerenal azotemia may exist in the setting of an expanded extracellular volume. Hypertension in patients with AKI should raise suspicion of intrinsic renal disease. The clinician must be alert for signs of systemic diseases that can cause acute renal injury, including vasculitis, endocarditis, and sepsis. Bladder distention and prostatic enlargement point to an obstructive cause. A full discussion of relevant history and physical findings for the different causes of AKI is beyond the scope of this chapter.

Urine Tests

The laboratory workup should commence with a urinalysis. The measurements of urine osmolality, electrolytes, and creatinine concentration are simple and useful, particularly in differentiating between ATN and prerenal azotemia. Urine specific gravity can be measured at the bedside while the results of the urine chemistry tests are pending. A high urine specific gravity generally correlates with a concentrated urine and is expected in prerenal azotemia, except in the presence of diuretics.

The familiar dipstick tests provide a readily available method for determining whether the urine contains protein or heme pigments. When positive, they should raise the suspicion of intrinsic renal pathology. As the dipstick test for protein measures only albuminuria, Bence–Jones proteins will not be detected. Light chains can be detected by urine protein electrophoresis or immunofixation. Daily urinary protein excretion can be quantified by a 24 hour urine collection. Although influenced by a number of potential confounding variables, the urine protein to creatinine ratio from a random urine specimen rapidly provides a gross estimate of the degree of proteinuria.

Formed elements in the urine sediment yield invaluable information about the nature of AKI, particularly in intrinsic renal disease. The significance of hematuria, pyuria, renal tubular epithelial cells, and casts in the urine has already been discussed. The presence of RBC casts distinguishes the hematuria associated with glomerulonephritis from that of postrenal or urologic causes. Broad and waxy casts suggest that renal disease is chronic. Virtually any lesion that can cause obstruction in the genitourinary tract can produce hematuria. Crystalluria often occurs in association with obstruction due to renal calculi or medications

The FE_{Na} can indicate the degree of renal sodium avidity, which generally reflects renal perfusion. A value of less than 1% typically indicates prerenal azotemia. However, this test can be confounded by concomitant diuretic therapy which will enhance urinary salt losses. In these situations, the FEUrea can be used instead, since urea clearance is unaffected by diuretics. The FEUrea is calculated via the same formula, but substituting urea for sodium and a value of less than 35% is suggestive of renal hypoperfusion (see Table 200.14 for additional details [80]).

Blood Tests

The measurement of the BUN and creatinine is essential to identifying and monitoring AKI. As noted, the ratio of BUN to creatinine carries some diagnostic value, as a high value (>20:1) may indicate prerenal azotemia. Serial blood chemistries will help identify acid–base and electrolyte disturbances common with AKI. Anemia may suggest a more chronic form of kidney disease. Eosinophilia frequently accompanies AIN.

Specialized serologic tests may help answer specific diagnostic questions. The presence of antinuclear antibodies may suggest autoimmune nephropathy such as lupus nephritis or scleroderma, both of which may cause AKI. The serum protein electrophoresis or immunoelectrophoresis may aid in the diagnosis of multiple myeloma, which often presents as AKI of uncertain cause.

Estimates of GFR may be helpful in assessing the severity of AKI as well as for adjusting medication dosages. However, these formulas have limited utility in the early phases of AKI, since the calculations are based on the assumption that serum creatinine reflects a steady state. For example, the creatinine of a patient with AKI from complete loss of renal blood flow will take many days to rise to steady state even though the GFR is negligible from the outset. Estimates of GFR in the first few days will grossly overestimate the patient's residual renal function. See Table 200.14 for equations used to estimate GFR.

Radiographic Studies

Various radiographic techniques may contribute to the evaluation of AKI. The abdominal flat plate (kidneys and urinary bladder) is an easily obtained study that can help establish the presence and size of both kidneys. If both kidneys are small, azotemia may be of a chronic nature. Radiopaque stones may be identified on abdominal plain films.

Renal ultrasonography, a safe, quick, high-yield procedure, is probably the first radiologic test that should be ordered in the evaluation of any azotemic patient. It permits the identification and measurement of both kidneys and is very sensitive for detecting obstructive uropathy (Fig. 200.5). (The specifics on performing point of care ultrasound examination can be found below.) Helical CT, with or without contrast, is a versatile and high-yield technique for establishing the size of the kidneys and recognizing hydronephrosis (Fig. 200.6), but contrast administered during the test can result in AKI in patients at increased risk such as those with renal insufficiency, hypovolemia, or multiple myeloma. Magnetic resonance imaging (MRI) offers

TABLE 200.14

Formulas for Estimating Renal Function

Fractional excretion of sodium (FE_{Na})

The FE_{Na} is the proportion of the filtered load of sodium excreted:

$FE_{Na} = U_{Na}/P_{Na} \times P_{cr}/U_{cr} \times 100$

Urine sodium (U_{Na}) and plasma sodium (P_{Na}) are expressed as millimoles and urine creatinine (U_{cr}) and plasma creatinine (P_{cr}) are expressed as milligrams per deciliter.

Cockcroft-Gault equation

Creatinine clearance (CrCl) can be estimated by using the Cockcroft and Gault formula which uses the patient's age and body weight, where weight is expressed in kilograms and plasma creatinine (P_{cr}) is expressed as milligrams per deciliter:

$C_{cr} = (140 - \text{age}) \times \text{weight}/(P_{cr} \times 72)$

Abbreviated MDRD equation [80]

A series of derivations based on data from the MDRD study have yielded several equations that more accurately represent GFR serum creatinine concentration (SCr) measured in milligrams per deciliter.

GFR, in mL/min/1.73 $m^2 = 186.3 \times \text{SCr} (\exp[-1.154]) \times \text{age} (\exp[-0.203]) \times (0.742 \text{ if female}) \times (1.21 \text{ if black})$

CrCl determined by 24-h urine collection

CrCl can be estimated by collecting a urine sample for 24 h. This formula tends to overestimate the true GFR by at least 10% and some cases significantly more, as some of the creatinine in the urine is derived from tubular secretion.

Urine creatinine (U_{cr}) and plasma creatinine (P_{cr}) are expressed as milligrams per deciliter. U_v is 24-h urine volume in mL.

CrCl, mL/min $= (U_{cr} \times U_v)/(P_{cr} \times 1{,}440)$

GFR, glomerular filtration rate; MDRD, Modification of Diet in Renal Disease.

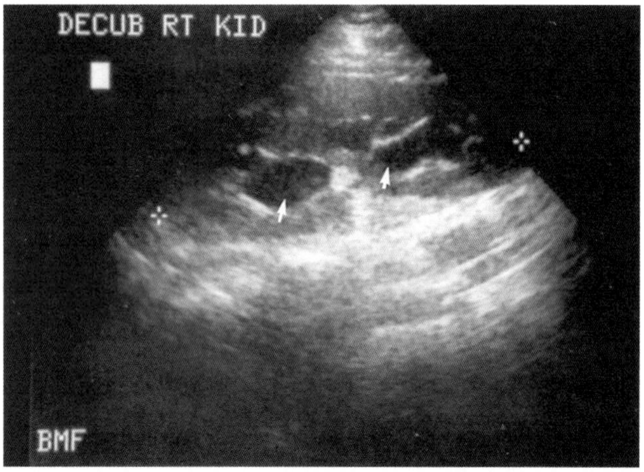

FIGURE 200.5 Sonogram with right hydronephrosis. Kidney poles are marked by crosses. Dark, echolucent areas (*arrows*) in the center represent dilated collecting system.

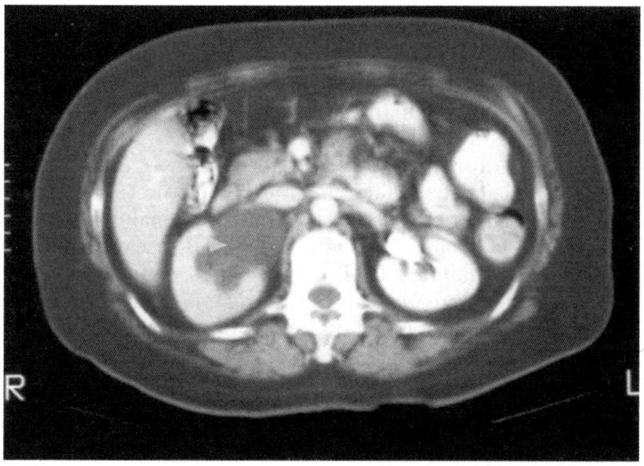

FIGURE 200.6 Computed tomographic scan with right hydronephrosis. **Left:** Unobstructed kidney is shown for comparison. **Right:** Note enlarged pelvocalyceal system on right

similar data as helical CT but is less commonly used because of cost and availability. The use of gadolinium contrast should be avoided, if possible, in the setting of AKI due to the risk of nephrogenic systemic fibrosis.

Retrograde pyelography is reserved for patients in whom urinary tract obstruction is strongly suspected despite the inability to confirm this finding on other imaging techniques. It is generally performed in anticipation of relieving such obstructions as soon as they are identified, usually by placement of ureteral stents.

Isotopic renal scanning provides a safe means for locating the kidneys and allows estimation of their functional capacity. Radionuclide flow studies can be used to assess the rapidity of uptake of tracer by the kidneys. A delay in uptake helps to establish the diagnosis of impaired renal perfusion, whether due to structural renovascular disease or functionally impaired renal blood flow. Prolonged retention of radioisotope by the kidneys is suggestive of outflow obstruction. Radioisotopic scanning may be particularly helpful in assessing patients with prolonged AKI for the absence of blood flow and the possible diagnosis of cortical necrosis or renal infarction (Fig. 200.7).

Renal artery duplex scanning offers an alternative method of assessing renal arterial flow. Although noninvasive, the test requires significant operator expertise. In cases in which a higher degree of sensitivity and specificity is required, CT or MRI angiogram or even full renal arteriography may be necessary. Arteriography is more invasive but offers the opportunity for immediate therapeutic intervention such as angioplasty or vascular stenting.

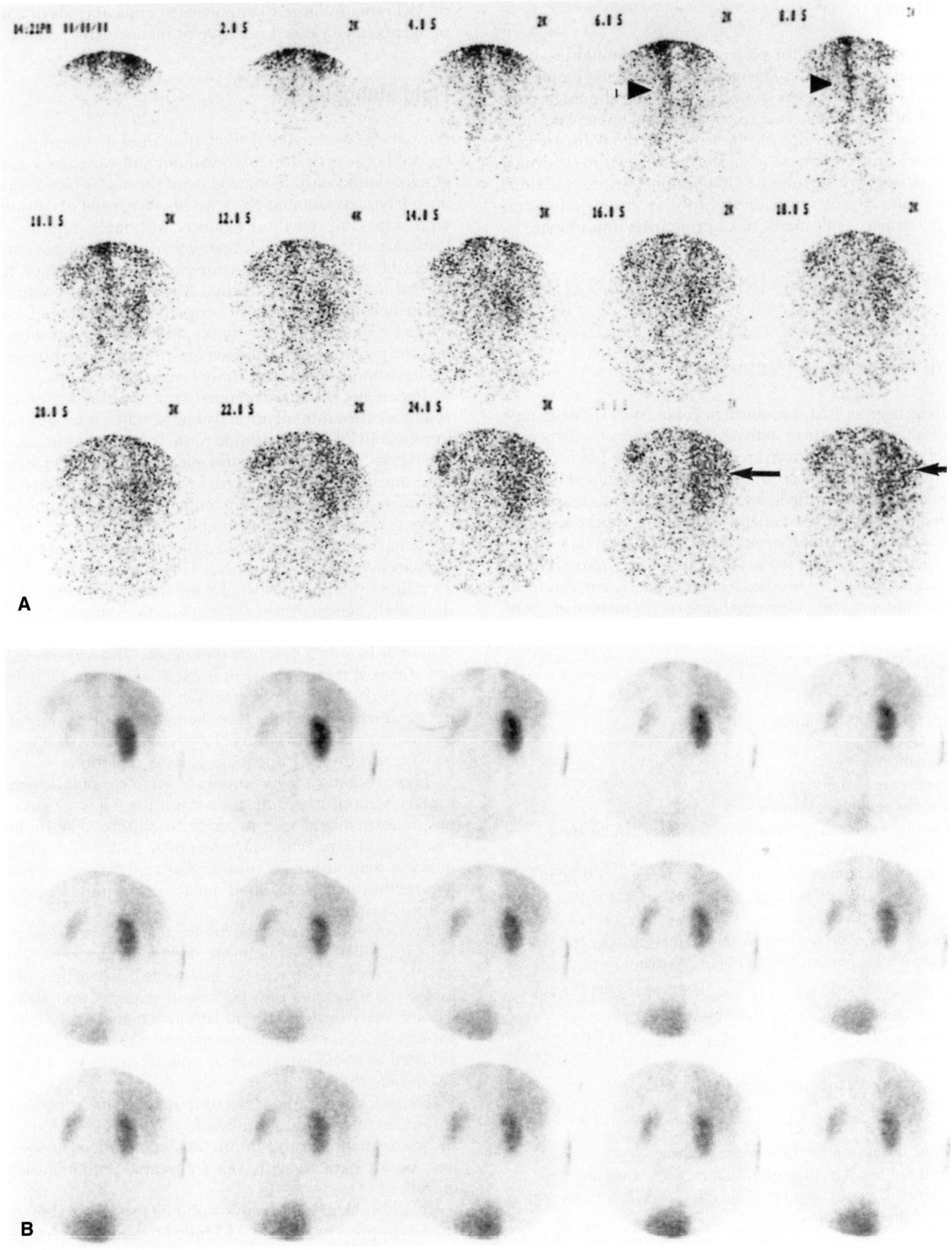

FIGURE 200.7 Renal radioisotopic scan demonstrating poor uptake of tracer in a patient with left renal artery occlusion. **A:** Early flow phase in which each panel represents a 2-second interval. Scintigraphic activity is seen in the proximal aorta (*arrowheads*) and the right kidney (*arrows*). Note the absence of tracer activity over the area of the left kidney. **B:** Functional scan with each panel representing 1-second intervals. Note the marked diminution of scintigraphic activity over the left kidney.

Renal Biopsy

Renal biopsy is reserved for patients who are thought to have parenchymal renal disease. The indications for renal biopsy are a matter of some controversy, but the procedure should be considered when (a) azotemia is of recent onset and unknown cause; (b) there is a possibility that the patient has a renal disease that may require drug treatment (e.g., steroids or cytotoxic drugs) as with patients with probable glomerulonephritis, vasculitis, or AIN; (c) heavy proteinuria or nephrotic syndrome is present; or (d) the biopsy result might be of prognostic importance.

COMPLICATIONS AND TREATMENT OF ACUTE KIDNEY INJURY

General Principles of Treatment

The management of AKI is outlined in Table 200.15. These steps are applicable to any patient with AKI and are quite fundamental. Fluid balance should be measured during each 8-hour nursing shift with input/output recordings, and body weight should be recorded daily. Serum electrolytes and/or arterial blood gases may be needed daily or more frequently depending on the patient's status. One of the most important principles is treatment of the underlying condition that led to AKI. Since renal injury is most often a consequence of another primary illness, correction of that condition is essential for renal recovery. The management of AKI remains largely supportive as clinical trials of a number of agents have yielded negative or inconclusive results.

TABLE 200.15

Management of Acute Kidney Injury

- Fluid balance
  - Weigh patient daily
  - Monitor input and output
  - In volume-depleted patients, replace extracellular fluid with isotonic saline (or bicarbonate)
  - In normovolemic or edematous patients, restrict fluid intake (~1,500 mL/d) and sodium intake (≤2 g/d)
- Acid–base and electrolyte
  - Avoid water overload and hyponatremia (restrict free water intake, particularly in oliguric patients)
  - Restrict potassium intake (≤2 g/d) and treat hyperkalemia
  - Supplement serum bicarbonate to maintain pH >7.1
  - Use phosphate binders (CaCO3) to maintain PO4 ≤5.0 mg/dL
  - Treat symptomatic hypocalcemia (see text)
- Drugs
  - Avoid nephrotoxins when possible
  - Adjust doses of all renally excreted drugs
  - Withhold nonsteroidal anti-inflammatory drugs and angiotensin-converting enzyme inhibitors in patients with prerenal conditions
  - Avoid magnesium-containing drugs (e.g., antacids and milk of magnesia)
- Nutrition
  - Restrict protein intake to ≤0.5 g/kg/d
  - Caloric (carbohydrate) intake of ≥400 kcal/d
- Reduction of infectious risks
  - Remove indwelling urinary catheter in oliguric, nonobstructed patients
  - Strict aseptic technique and rapid removal, when feasible, of vascular catheters

Fluid Management

For patients with renal dysfunction, fluid management is often crucial because of decreased sodium and water excretion. The determination of fluid management should be based on a thorough physical examination as well as evaluation of daily weights, vital signs and net fluid balance. Although respiratory fluid losses are often minimal for patients on mechanical ventilation, insensible losses are significantly increased with high fever or dermal injury. Gastrointestinal fluid losses can be difficult to quantify. Daily weights are often the best means of assessing the net balance between intake and output. Additional data may be provided by measurement of central venous pressures or ultrasound assessment of intravascular volume.

In patients with pure prerenal azotemia attributable to hypovolemia, restoration of normal volume status is usually sufficient to return BUN and creatinine to their normal levels. A normotensive, volume-depleted, azotemic patient can receive up to 1 L of saline during a 4-hour period with the expectation that renal perfusion and urine flow will improve rapidly. Volume-depleted patients with hypotension should receive more aggressive fluid resuscitation, at least until their blood pressure normalizes and signs of hypoperfusion resolve. This maneuver is of diagnostic as well as therapeutic benefit because rapid response to the fluid challenge establishes that azotemia is due, at least in part, to prerenal factors. The estimate of isotonic fluid replacement should be based on the clinical findings. With orthostasis, it may be estimated that the patient is experiencing an ECF deficit of at least 10%. Fluid replacement in these circumstances should be administered regardless of the patient's urine output or the presumptive diagnosis of ATN as recovery of renal function can be hastened by early adequate volume repletion.

Hypovolemia may complicate intrinsic renal disease and urinary tract obstruction, superimposing a low perfusion state on the azotemia caused by these conditions. The finding of a low FE_{Na} in a patient who previously had a high FE_{Na} might indicate that, although tubular function has recovered, renal hypoperfusion persists. Fluid replacement should be given using isotonic saline.

In euvolemic patients, the following formula can be applied to estimate daily fluid requirement: daily fluid replacement (mL per day) = urinary + extrarenal + insensible losses, where insensible losses = 250 mL per day. For febrile patients, add 500 mL per day for every degree Fahrenheit more than 101. In edematous patients requiring volume removal, the rate of diuresis should be adjusted to avoid intravascular volume depletion which could exacerbate the AKI.

Diuretics are a mainstay of management in patients with volume overload and nonoliguric AKI. However, studies have shown no demonstrable improvement in patient survival when nonoliguric patients with AKI are treated with high-dose loop diuretics [81].

In addition, a meta-analysis of nine randomized furosemide studies to prevent or treat AKI failed to show a decreased need for dialysis or improved survival [82].

Despite the paucity of data regarding beneficial effects on renal recovery or survival, diuretics are essential for the maintenance of fluid balance in responsive patients. Loop diuretics are the principal agents and are given as intravenous bolus or through continuous infusion. Dose adjustments may be required to avoid decreased renal perfusion which could impair renal recovery or high dosages which have been associated with hearing loss and tinnitus [83]. Concomitant use of other diuretic agents that act at different segments of the nephron may enhance urine output. Patients with diuretic-resistant oliguria often require renal replacement therapy. This will be discussed in detail in Chapter 75.

Parenchymal Renal Disease

Although AIN usually responds to discontinuation of the culpable drug (see Table 200.12), the recovery may be protracted. The data on steroids in allergic drug-induced acute interstitial nephritis (DI-AIN) is mixed [84]. There are no randomized controlled trials and recommendations rely on case reports and retrospective data. Nevertheless, the use of steroids appears to hasten recovery and reduce the likelihood of developing CKD [85]. Certainly, steroids should be considered for patients with DI-AIN associated with a significant reduction in GFR or for patients who do not promptly respond to withdrawal of the offending agent. These patients often require a renal biopsy to confirm the diagnosis. If steroids are used, the initial dose of prednisone is 1 mg/kg/d for 1 to 2 weeks followed by a slow taper over 1 to 3 months, depending on the response.

The treatment of various forms of glomerulonephritis is beyond the scope of this text. Briefly, in patients with AKI associated with proteinuria and hematuria, the diagnosis of glomerulonephritis should be considered. A renal biopsy may be helpful not only to aid in diagnosis but also as a means of predicting response to therapy. Patients with a sudden loss of renal function associated with nephritis may have "rapidly progressive glomerulonephritis" (RPGN). RPGN is broken down into three categories: pauci-immune glomerulonephritis, anti-GBM disease (Goodpasture), and immune complex mediated disease. The majority of these diseases require immunosuppressive therapy with steroids (high-dose intravenous corticosteroids consisting of 250 to 1,000 mg of methylprednisolone per day for 3 days or oral prednisone)in combination with a steroid sparing agent (cyclophosphamide, mycophenolate, or rituximab), and occasionally plasmapheresis. For example, the pauci-immune nephridities include Granulomatosis with polyangiitis and Microscopic polyangiitis both of which are initially treated with pulse steroids combined with either cyclophosphamide or rituximab [86]. In anti-GBM disease, pulse steroids, oral cytoxan and plasmapherisis are combined for maximal effectiveness. Plasmapherisis is employed to clear the plasma of formed antibodies (e.g., antiglomerular basement membrane antibodies) while the immunosuppressive drugs prevent the formation of new pathogenic antibodies [87]. Immune complex glomerulonephritides include a host of different diseases which require a variety of different approaches. Some of these diseases do not require renal-specific therapies, such as for postinfectious glomerulonephritis or glomerulonephritis associated with bacterial endocarditis. In the former case, spontaneous remission usually occurs; in the latter, antibiotic treatment of the underlying condition may result in clearing of the immune complex–induced renal lesion.

A number of different therapies have been proposed for the treatment of ATN. Dopamine at low doses dilates the interlobular arteries, afferent and efferent arterioles resulting in increased renal blood flow. However, clinical trials have not supported the efficacy low-dose dopamine infusion in the treatment of established ATN, and it is no longer recommended by nephrologists [88].

Fenoldopam, a selective dopamine-1 receptor antagonist which lacks other α- and β-adrenergic effects, has also been proposed as treatment for AKI. A meta-analysis of 16 randomized trials of fenoldopam versus placebo or dopamine for prevention or treatment of AKI found that fenoldopam decreased the need for renal replacement and hospital death [89]. However, a recent, large randomized trial in cardiac surgery patients showed no renal protective effect [16]. Although fenoldopam is not currently recommended [88], further study will be required to fully clarify its role in AKI.

Clinical trials of atrial natriuretic peptide have shown modest improvements in outcomes for patients with AKI [90]. However, given the limitations of design and size of available studies, further investigation is needed to confirm the benefit of this agent in established ATN.

Treatment of Postrenal Failure

Timely relief of urinary obstruction is the goal of therapy for postrenal AKI. Acute intervention is mandatory in the presence of complete or bilateral urinary tract obstruction or severe metabolic or hemodynamic complications of AKI. Coexisting fever or any other evidence of urinary infection proximal to the obstruction requires a rapid decompression procedure to avoid bacteremic shock.

When bladder outlet obstruction is suspected, insertion of a bladder catheter should be attempted. If this is not possible, as is occasionally the case in patients with prostatic enlargement or urethral stricture, urethral dilation or percutaneous cystostomy should be performed. AKI due to upper urinary tract obstruction can be relieved by either the retrograde insertion of a ureteral catheter or by the percutaneous placement (under ultrasonic, fluoroscopic, or CT scan guidance) of a catheter into the renal pelvis.

Because of the defects in distal nephron function associated with high-grade obstruction, patients may develop hyperkalemia, hyperchloremic metabolic acidosis, and hypernatremia. Water and bicarbonate replacement are often required and can be administered as a solution of 5% glucose and water to which sodium bicarbonate has been added. The patient's plasma volume and serum sodium should determine the tonicity of the administered fluid. If the patient is hypovolemic, an isotonic solution should be used. If the patient is hypernatremic, a hypotonic solution is needed. Hyperkalemia may respond to the institution of a diuresis that accompanies the relief of the obstruction and as well as correction of the acidosis.

A dramatic postobstructive diuresis often ensues after relief of urinary obstruction. This usually reflects mobilization of urine sequestered within the dilated ureterovesicular system as well as excess ECF retained during the period of obstruction. As such, this postobstructive diuresis is considered appropriate to the pre-existing volume expansion. In some patients with correction of bilateral obstruction, a large diuresis and natriuresis may ensue, which result in hypovolemia and, sometimes, frank shock. The mechanism for this inappropriate diuresis is poorly understood but may involve release of a natriuretic substance. These patients require fluid replacement, usually with hypotonic saline, to repair the deficit and match urinary losses. A useful technique is to measure the urinary sodium and potassium concentrations periodically to determine the composition of the replacement fluid. However, care must be taken to avoid excessive fluid replacement as this will simply prolong the diuresis.

Abnormal Drug Metabolism

A complete survey of all of the patient's medications should be made. Drugs such as NSAIDs or ACE inhibitors that may interfere with renal blood flow or GFR autoregulation should be discontinued. When possible, aminoglycoside antibiotics or other nephrotoxic drugs should be replaced with nonnephrotoxic agents. Contrast procedures should be avoided so as not to compound renal dysfunction in patients with acute or CKD. If this is not feasible, the risk should be minimized by taking prophylactic measures (see previous discussion). In addition, the dosage of drugs dependent on renal metabolism and excretion should be adjusted appropriately. Some drugs (e.g., aminoglycoside antibiotics and digoxin) are excreted almost entirely by the kidneys. If the dose or dosing interval is unchanged, reduced renal function leads to accumulation of the drug in body fluids and eventual drug toxicity. Other agents are hepatically metabolized, but the active metabolites are renally excreted (e.g., benzodiazepines). Phenytoin, independent of its excretion, may reach toxic concentrations because a larger proportion of the administered drug is displaced from albumin-binding sites in uremia. Drug doses need to be altered in most instances to account for residual renal function and the effect of dialysis on drug removal. It is important to remember that as the patient recovers renal function, upward adjustment of the dosage of renally excreted drugs is necessary. This subject is covered in detail in Chapter 202.

Nutritional Therapy

The management of nutritional therapy in the ICU is discussed in detail in Section 20 (Metabolism/Nutrition). The guidelines for nutritional therapy in AKI are similar to those in other ICU patients. Patients with AKI are often catabolic and increase their production of nitrogenous products that require excretion. The degree of catabolism reflects the level of the patient's metabolic stress and is, in turn, a function of the severity of the underlying illness. Protein and caloric requirements are much higher for patients with catastrophic illness and multiple organ system failure than for those with mild or moderate illness. Although caloric replacement needs to be adequate to reduce tissue catabolism, prevent ketosis, and meet the patient's basal nutritional needs, the clinician must avoid providing excessive substrate for generation of metabolic waste products. This is particularly challenging for patients who are not yet being dialyzed; once patients are on dialysis, they are allowed more liberal fluid intake and can receive a greater intake of carbohydrates, protein, and fat, limited only by the rate of dialytic fluid and solute removal. As discussed in Chapters 212 and 214, the need for nutritional support is becoming an indication for renal replacement therapy [91].

Hyperkalemia

Hyperkalemia is the most immediately life-threatening electrolyte imbalance encountered in patients with renal disease (see Chapter 199). In AKI, hyperkalemia arises from the inability of the kidneys to handle the excretory burden of potassium. Sources of potassium should be identified and regulated appropriately. Potassium loads may be endogenous (e.g., tissue breakdown and hematoma reabsorption) or exogenous (e.g., diet, intravenous fluids, and medications). Even when the GFR is substantially reduced, the kidneys can excrete large amounts of potassium, provided that tubular secretion is intact. For this reason, hyperkalemia more often occurs in patients with parenchymal or postrenal AKI. Urine flow rate is an important determinant of tubular potassium secretion; therefore, oliguric patients are more prone to potassium imbalance than are nonoliguric patients. Many commonly used medications, including heparin, NSAIDs, and ACE inhibitors, can also inhibit tubular potassium secretion. These should be discontinued in hyperkalemic patients.

Metabolic Acidosis

The kidneys' ability to excrete metabolically produced acids may be reduced, particularly in parenchymal and obstructive disease. Because acid excretion is primarily a tubular function, the degree of acidosis may not always correlate with the degree of GFR impairment. Indeed, pure tubular acid excretion abnormalities may exist independently of azotemia (renal tubular acidosis). Metabolic acidosis that results from failure of the tubules to excrete hydrogen ions or conserve bicarbonate normally produces a hyperchloremic or low anion gap acidosis (see Chapter 198). When the GFR is severely impaired, retention of acid wastes may produce a high anion gap acidosis.

Bicarbonate supplementation in the setting of metabolic acidosis remains controversial as there are no studies demonstrating a beneficial effect of this approach. In addition, bicarbonate supplementation may cause volume overload and hypernatremia and may exacerbate hypocalcemia by lowering the ionized calcium level. However, systemic pH <7.1 is associated with a number of adverse hemodynamic effects including decreased myocardial contractility and impaired response to catecholamine pressor agents. Many clinicians empirically administer bicarbonate to maintain pH >7.1 [92].

Abnormal Salt and Water Metabolism

Although most fluids administered to patients are hypotonic, plasma osmolality normally remains within tightly fixed limits. The process by which plasma tonicity is preserved depends on the suppression of vasopressin release and the movement of free water in the ascending limb of the loop of Henle. This latter function is impeded whenever GFR is reduced, which results in water retention and hyponatremia. Conversely, some renal disorders are characterized by failure to conserve water. This situation, referred to as *nephrogenic diabetes insipidus*, is most common in tubulointerstitial disease and in partial obstruction of the urinary tract. Patients with these disorders are prone to dehydration and hypernatremia. The subject is covered in more detail in Chapter 199.

Abnormal Calcium and Phosphorus Metabolism

The ability of the kidney to excrete phosphorus normally is impaired when the GFR falls to approximately one-third of normal. High serum phosphorus levels lead to formation of insoluble calcium phosphate salts, which may precipitate in soft tissue. If the product of the serum calcium and phosphorus concentrations exceeds 70, precipitation in soft tissues becomes more likely. For this reason, administration of calcium to patients with AKI should be reserved for emergent situations, such as the appearance of tetany, seizures, or refractory hypotension. The tendency toward hypocalcemia with AKI may be additionally aggravated by the injured kidneys' failure to form 1,25-dihydroxycholecalciferol, although vitamin D therapy is rarely required in cases of AKI.

Hyperphosphatemia is common in patients with AKI, particularly in patients with rhabdomyolysis or tumor lysis syndrome. Although there is no published data correlating the treatment of hyperphosphatemia with improved outcomes, phosphate binders are typically initiated when phosphate levels rise to more than 6.0 mg per dL. The main phosphate binders available include calcium salts (calcium acetate and calcium carbonate), sevelamer, and lanthanum hydroxide. Unless the patient is hypercalcemic, calcium carbonate can be administered (1.0 to 1.5 g with meals) as the phosphate-binding agent. Although potent, aluminum-based binders are generally avoided because of concerns with aluminum toxicity.

Uremia

Accumulation of endogenous toxins in the body eventually results in uremia. The uremic syndrome is a multisystemic symptom complex. The exact identities of the so-called uremic toxins are not known, although many possibilities have been suggested. Urea and creatinine are not uremic toxins but rather are markers of renal excretory capacity. One cannot deduce on the basis of urea nitrogen and creatinine levels exactly when a patient will become uremic. In general, the syndrome manifests itself at a GFR of less than 10 mL per minute.

Although uremia is considered an indication to initiate dialytic therapy, the syndrome may be insidious in onset and produce only vague symptoms. Lethargy, anorexia, nausea, and malaise, all of which may herald uremia, may well be attributed to extrarenal disease in the patient with AKI. Other, less subjective uremic manifestations constitute stronger indications for prompt initiation of dialysis, including bleeding diathesis, seizures, coma, and the appearance of a pericardial friction rub.

Dialysis

The use of renal replacement therapy in AKI is discussed in depth in Chapter 201. Briefly, the decision of when to initiate dialysis is historically controversial. Patients with intractable volume overload, hyperkalemia, metabolic acidosis, or frank uremia clearly meet criteria for dialysis. However, many patients with significant AKI do not meet one of these criteria. This has led to a discussion regarding the merits of early or even "prophylactic" dialysis. The rationale for forestalling dialysis includes the invasive nature of the procedure as well as concern that renal replacement therapy can exacerbate hemodynamic instability that might prolong the course of AKI. There is also significant labor and cost associated with performing the procedure in the ICU. Nevertheless, several observational studies appear to show decreased morbidity and mortality for patients initiated on early dialysis. It has been argued that early dialysis results in improved volume control as well as the clearance of a variety of cytokines and/or toxins that may be harmful. Unfortunately, at this time, there is still not adequate data to establish the optimal time to initiate dialysis. This issue is discussed in detail in Chapter 75.

Prognosis and Outcome of Acute Kidney Injury

AKI is associated with a substantial increase in hospital mortality, particularly for ICU patients whose mortality with ranges from 40% to 70% [93–96]. The large range in mortality reflects the varied acuity of illness and case mixes in the reports. Patients with prerenal azotemia tend to have an excellent prognosis while critically ill patients with dialysis dependent ATN have had mortality rates that approach 70%. Despite medical advances, mortality in AKI has not improved significantly during the past 50 years [97] though may be due in part to increased acuity of illness of the patient population.

Patients with AKI clearly have increased mortality, but the degree to which this heightened risk is attributable to AKI as opposed to other comorbid conditions remains unclear. A number of published trials show that AKI is an independent risk factor for mortality [93,95,98]. The extent of the risk appears to correlate with the severity of the AKI with dialysis dependent patient being at the highest risk for death. It is not entirely clear how AKI impacts the risk of death, but it is known that patients with significant AKI have compromised immune systems and platelet function placing them at higher risk for complications.

At least half of all cases of AKI are nonoliguric. Nonoliguric renal failure is associated with improved odds of renal recovery and approximately half the mortality of oliguric AKI [99]. Most of these individuals do not have multiorgan failure, and their improved survival may be the result of a less severe primary illness.

The long-term renal prognosis of patients with AKI is impacted by several factors including the severity of the initial injury as well as baseline patient characteristics. Patients with brief ischemic events typically develop a mild form of AKI that often resolves within 72 hours with no long term sequela. Patients with prolonged episodes of ischemia or injury may have variable degrees of recovery [100–102]. A recent study compared 1,610 hospitalized patients with reversible AKI to a control group. At a medium follow-up of 3.3 years, the patients with a history of AKI had almost a twofold increased of CKD (hazard ratio 1.91) compared to controls [100]. For patients with severe initial renal injuries requiring dialysis, the risk of CKD may be as much as 20 times higher than those with less severe injury [103]. In other studies, elderly individuals as well as patients with baseline CKD have been found to have a lower probability of full recovery [101,104,105]. Nevertheless, more than 80% of the patients who survive AKI will recover renal function and remain dialysis free [106].

Utility of Ultrasonography for Evaluation of Acute Kidney Injury

Ultrasonography is a primary imaging modality for evaluation of AKI, so it is an important component of competence in critical care ultrasonography.

Equipment

If available, a curvilinear probe designed for abdominal imaging is used (3.5 to 5.0 MHz). Alternatively, a phased array cardiac probe gives serviceable images when configured with abdominal presets.

Scanning Technique

With the patient in the supine position, the probe is placed in the posterior axillary line over the lower lateral chest wall in order to obtain a transcostal coronal plane view of the left right or left kidney in their longitudinal axis (Video 200.1). Useful landmarks for locating the kidneys are the liver or spleen, as the kidneys are adjacent and caudal to these organs. The inexperienced scanner often scans in too anterior a plane to locate the kidney. A useful rule to locate the kidney is to place the "knuckles on the bed" when the operator is positioned ipsilaterally and scanning the contralateral kidney. This results in an appropriately posterior scanning plane. Once identified, the probe is angled through the kidney in order to obtain multiple tomographic sections of its structure. The operator may rotate the probe counterclockwise by 90 degrees to obtain a transverse view of the kidney while angling through it to obtain multiple tomographic views.

The bladder is imaged by placing the probe just above the pubic bone in the midline. Using a transverse scanning plane, the scanning plane is angled in caudal direction in order to identify the bladder. Once identified, the probe is angled through the bladder in order to obtain multiple tomographic views of its structure. The operator may rotate the probe clockwise by 90 degrees to obtain a longitudinal view of the bladder while angling through it to obtain multiple tomographic views. Doppler analysis of renal blood flow has some applications for assessment of AKI, but requires training above the level typically needed by the frontline intensivist. If indicated, it is obtained on a consultative basis from the radiology service.

Ultrasonography Anatomy

See Video 200.1.

Kidney Size. The normal kidney size is 9 to 12 cm in length. Chronic renal disease results in reduction of kidney size. AKI may result in enlargement of the kidney size.

Kidney Parenchyma. The kidney parenchyma is formed by the outer renal cortex and centrally located medulla with contains the renal pyramids. The renal calyces may be prominently interposed between the pyramids; this is a normal variant. Normal parenchymal thickness is 1.0 to 1.8 cm, and is diminished in CKD. Normally, the renal parenchyma is hypoechoic when compared to the adjacent liver or spleen, and the cortex is slightly hyperechoic relative to the underlying medulla. Both AKI and chronic renal disease result in a hyperechoic parenchyma when compared to the adjacent liver of spleen. When comparing the echogenicity of the kidney parenchyma to the liver and spleen, the operator considers whether there is a disease process that may alter the echogenicity of the liver or spleen.

Kidney Margins. The outer boundary of the kidney is defined by Gerota fascia and perinephric fat. Normally, it is smooth. Persistent fetal lobulations result in distinct V-shaped indentations that are a normal variant.

Pelvocalyceal Area. The central pelvocalyceal area contains the collecting system, sinus fat, and the renal vasculature. It is hyperechoic and demarcated from the surrounding renal parenchyma. Chronic renal failure is associated with loss of demarcation between the pelvocalyceal area and the parenchyma. The normal collecting system is not visible. Obstructive uropathy results in dilation of the collecting system.

Bladder. The bladder is well imaged when filled with urine. The normal bladder is in midline location and is a symmetric organ with thin smooth walls. When nondistended, wall thickness is increased. The empty bladder may be difficult to locate unless a catheter balloon is inflated inside it. It may be difficult to distinguish a distended bladder with co-existing ascites. The operator searches for bowel structures within the fluid filled structure; their presence indicates ascites. If uncertainty persists, injection of agitated saline into the bladder catheter with real-time imaging will generally resolve the issue.

Clinical Applications

Obstructive uropathy is a potentially reversible cause of AKI, so it is important to rule out this entity in the patient who has renal failure in the ICU. The examination can be performed in a short period of time, and is an essential part of competence in critical care ultrasonography (Video 200.2). It includes examination of both kidneys for hydronephrosis and bladder anatomy. The findings of hydronephrosis include dilation of the renal pelvis and calyces by urine with through transmission artifact. It can be classified as mild, moderate, or severe acute obstruction results in calyceal dilation that results in a dilation that ends with an acute angle point. In chronic obstruction, the calyceal dilation ends in curvilinear manner. In long-standing hydronephrosis, the renal parenchyma is thinned and the dilated collecting system comes to occupy most of the kidney profile. The presence of hydronephrosis is not necessarily associated with a reduction in urine flow. The obstruction may be unilateral, so one kidney continues to function; or it may partial, with sufficient pressure backup to harm the kidney but with continued urine flow.

Ultrasonography may identify the source of the obstruction, if it is in the collecting system of the kidney (e.g., kidney stones and malignancy). However, the ureter is difficult to reliably identify with ultrasonography even if dilated; CT scan of the retroperitoneum is the definitive imaging modality for this area. If the obstruction is at the level of the bladder, ultrasonography is useful to identify bladder tumors, blood clots, or prostatic enlargement as the cause for the hydronephrosis (Video 200.3). An occasional cause of anuria is a blocked bladder catheter. The presence of a catheter tip and balloon within the distended bladder indicates a blocked catheter that can be flushed clear. The presence of the inflated balloon within an empty bladder indicates a patent catheter if there is urine output, or an anuric patient if there is none.

The findings on ultrasonography of the kidney in patients with medical causes of renal failure are nonspecific (Video 200.4). The kidney may be enlarged with loss of the medullary cortical interface, and the cortex is typically hyperechoic in comparison to the adjacent liver or spleen. The examination is not useful in categorizing the etiology of the AKI. Chronic renal failure results in small hyperechoic kidneys with reduced parenchymal thickness, and loss of differentiation between the parenchyma and the pelvocalyceal area. In end-stage renal disease requiring dialysis support, the kidney may become so small and hyperechoic that is difficult to locate with ultrasonography.

Limitations of Ultrasonography for Evaluation of AKI

1. **Identification of hydronephrosis:** Obstructive uropathy may take up to 24 hours to manifest with hydronephrosis; so it is appropriate to repeat the examination, if the clinical situation remains ambiguous. The patient with severe medical renal injury may have no urine production by the kidneys. This will obscure the presence of urinary tract obstruction because, with absent kidney function, there can be no hydronephrosis in the unlikely situation where there is a dual diagnosis of severe medical renal failure and obstructive uropathy. Rarely, an infiltrative disease of the kidney (e.g., renal lymphoma) restricts enlargement of the collecting ducts in the presence of downstream obstruction.
2. Without advanced training in renal ultrasonography, the intensivist will regularly encounter abnormalities that are incidental to the main purpose of the ultrasonography examination, which is to determine whether there is evidence of obstructive uropathy. Where the operator identifies an abnormality of uncertain implication, they call for expert consultation with the radiology service. These include the following examples (Video 200.4).
   a. *Renal cyst*: Renal cysts are a common incidental finding that may be unilateral or bilateral. They are often located in the renal parenchymal at the poles of the kidney and occur in wide variety of sizes. Occasionally, they are in the pelvocalyceal area, and may be confused with hydronephrosis.
   A simple renal cyst is anechoic with through transmission artifact, has no wall thickness, and is completely absent of internal echoes. Any other pattern requires radiology consultation.
   b. *Renal mass*: A renal mass is an occasional incidental finding. Regardless of size or location, this requires radiology consultation.
   c. *Renal stone*: Renal stones, if composed of echogenic material, appear as hyperechoic structures within the collecting system of the kidney. They may be single or multiple in number, and characteristically exhibit acoustic shadowing artifact. Ureteral stones are difficult to identify with ultrasonography. Renal stones in association with ipsilateral hydronephrosis raise concern that there is a stone impacted in the ureter.
   d. *Renal abscess and pyelonephritis*: An intraparenchymal or perinephric abscess appears as complex hypoechoic mass with irregular walls. Pyelonephritis does not have specific features on ultrasonography examination, with the exception of emphysematous pyelonephritis where there is a characteristic pattern of air collection within the kidneyIf there is suspicion of renal infection on ultrasonography examination, radiology consultation is indicated.
   e. *Bladder pathology* (Video 200.3): Bladder mass is an occasional incidental finding that requires radiology consultation. Bleeding from the kidney or bladder may result in a thrombus that can obstruct drainage of the bladder. These may be difficult to differentiate from a bladder tumor. Bladder irrigation with removal of the thrombus is diagnostic. Bladder irrigation may be performed with real-time ultrasonography imaging to aid in clearing the

thrombus. A large prostate may protrude into the bladder. Radiology consultation is required to further characterize any bladder mass.

f. *Difficulty with bladder catheter insertion*: If the insertion of a bladder catheter is difficult, it is useful to guide the insertion with real-time scanning. The site of the obstruction is usually an enlarged prostate. Ultrasonography allows the operator to avoid the complication of inadvertent inflation of the balloon within the prostate. This occurs when the tip of the catheter is in the bladder, but the deflated balloon has not been passed into the bladder. Urine flow is noted in the tubing, and the balloon is assumed to be in the bladder. The balloon is inflated thereby causing injury to the proximal urethra and prostate gland. With difficult bladder catheterization, the catheter and its balloon can be seen with real-time scanning within the lumen of the distended bladder before the balloon is inflated.

References

1. Lassnigg A, Schmidlin D, Mouhieddine M, et al: Minimal changes of serum creatinine predict prognosis in patients after cardiothoracic surgery: a prospective cohort study. *J Am Soc Nephrol* 15:1597–1605, 2004.
2. Levy MM, Macias WL, Vincent JL, et al: Early changes in organ function predict eventual survival in severe sepsis. *Crit Care Med* 33(10):2194–2201, 2005.
3. Bellomo R, Ronco C, Kellum JA, et al: Acute renal failure—definition, outcome measures, animal models, fluid therapy and information technology needs: the Second International Consensus Conference of the Acute Dialysis Quality Initiative (ADQI) Group. *Crit Care* 8:R204–R210, 2004.
4. Hoste EA, Clermont G, Kersten A, et al: RIFLE criteria for acute kidney injury are associated with hospital mortality in critically ill patients: a cohort analysis. *Crit Care* 10:R73–R83, 2006.
5. Uchino S, Bellomo R, Goldsmith D, et al: An assessment of the RIFLE criteria for acute renal failure in hospitalized patients. *Crit Care Med* 34:1913–1917, 2006.
6. Ascon M, Ascon DB, Liu M, et al: Renal ischemia-reperfusion leads to long term infiltration of activated and effector-memory T lymphocytes. *Kidney Int.* 75(5):526–535, 2009.
7. Li L, Okusa MD: Blocking the immune response in ischemic acute kidney injury: the role ofadenosine 2A agonists. *Nat Clin Pract Nephrol* 2(8):432, 2006.
8. Salmela K, Wramner L, Ekberg H, et al: A randomized multicenter trial of the anti-ICAM-1 monoclonal antibody (enlimomab) for the prevention of acute rejection and delayed onset of graft function in cadaveric renal transplantation: a report of the European Anti-ICAM-1 Renal Transplant Study Group. *Transplantation* 67(5):729–736, 1999.
9. Mishra J, Dent C, Tarabishi R, et al: Neutrophil gelatinase-associated lipocalin (NGAL) as a biomarker for acute renal injury after cardiac surgery. *Lancet* 365:1241, 2005.
10. Thakar CV, Arrigain S, Worley S, et al: A clinical score to predict acute renal failure after cardiac surgery. *J Am Soc Nephrol* 16(1):162–168, 2005.
11. Fergusson DA, Hebert PC, Mazer CD, et al: A comparison of aprotinin and lysine analogues after a high-risk cardiac surgery. *N Engl J Med* 358:2319–2331, 2008.
12. Rosner MH, Okusa MD: Acute kidney injury associated with cardiac surgery. *Clin J Am Soc Nephrol* 1:19–32, 2006.
13. Chawla LS, Zhao Y, Lough FC, et al: Off-pump versus on-pump coronary artery bypass grafting outcomes stratified by preoperative renal function. *J Am Soc Nephrol* 23: 1389–1397, 2012
14. Shroyer AL, Grover FL, Hattler B: On-pump versus off-pump coronaryartery bypass surgery. *N Engl J Med* 361:1827–1837, 2009
15. Sajja LR, Mannam G, Chakravarthi RM, et al: Coronary artery bypass grafting with or without cardiopulmonary bypass in patients with preoperative nondialysis dependent renal insufficiency: a randomized study. *J Thorac Cardiovasc Surg* 133:378–388, 2007.
16. Bovi T, Zangrillo A, Guarracino F, et al: Effect of fenoldopam on use of renal replacement therapy among patients with acute kidney injury after cardiac surgery: a randomized clinical trial. *JAMA* 312(21):2244–2245, 2014.
17. Mentzer RM, Oz MC, Sladen RN, et al: Effects of perioperative nesiritide in patients with left ventricular dysfunction undergoing cardiac surgery: the NAPA trial. *J Am Coll Cardiol* 49(6):716–726, 2007.
18. O'Connor CM, Starling RC, Hernandez AF, et al. Effect of nesiritide in patients with acute decompensated heart failure. *N Engl J Med* 65:32–43, 2011
19. Haase M, Haase-Fielitz A, Bagshaw SM, et al: Phase II, randomized, controlled trial of high-dose N-acetylcysteine in high-risk cardiac surgery patients. *Crit Care Med* 35:1324–1331, 2007.
20. Yallop KG, Sheppard SV, Smith DC: The effect of mannitol on renal function following cardiopulmonary bypass in patients with normal pre-operative creatinine. *Anaesthesia* 63:576–582, 2008.
21. Zacharias M, Conlon NP, Herbison GP, et al: Interventions for protecting renal function in the perioperative period. *Cochrane Database Syst Rev* (4):CD003590, 2008.
22. Lassnigg A, Donner E, Grubhofer G, et al: Lack of renoprotective effects of dopamine and furosemide during cardiac surgery. *J Am Soc Nephrol* 11(1):97–104, 2000.
23. Kidney Disease: Improving Global Outcomes (KDIGO) Acute Kidney Injury Workgroup: KDIGO Clinical Practice Guidelines for Acute Kidney Injury. *Kidney Int Suppl* 2:37–39, 2012
24. Karkouti K, Wijeysundera DN, Yau TM, et al: Acute kidney injury after cardiac surgery: focus on modifiable risk factors. *Circulation* 119(4):495–502, 2009.
25. Nohria A, Hasselblad V, Stebbins A, et al: Cardiorenal interaction: insights from the ESCAPE trial. *J Am Coll Cardiol* 51:1268–1274, 2008.
26. Ronco C, Haapio M, House AA, et al: Cardiorenal syndrome. *J Am Coll Cardiol* 52(19):1527–1539, 2008.
27. Abraham WT, Adams K, Fonarow GC, et al: In-hospital mortality in patients with acute decompensated heart failure requiring intravenous vasoactive medications. Analysis from the Acute Decompensated Heart Failure Registry (ADHERE). *J Am Coll Cardiol* 46:57–64, 2005.
28. Forman DF, Butler J, Wang Y, et al: Incidence, predictors at admission, and impact of worsening renal function among patients hospitalized with heart failure. *J Am Coll Cardiol* 43:61–67, 2004.
29. Salvador DR, Rey NR, Ramos GC, et al: Continuous infusion versus bolus injection of loop diuretics in congestive heart failure. *Cochrane Database Syst Rev* (3):CD003178, 2005
30. Chen HH, Anstrom KJ, Givertz MM, et al: NHLBI Heart Failure Clinical Research Network: Low-dose dopamine or low-dose nesiritide in acute heart failure with renal dysfunction: The ROSE acute heart failure randomized trial. *JAMA* 310:2533–2543, 2013
31. Gheorghiade M, Konstam MA, Burnett JC Jr, et al: Short-term clinical effects of tolvaptan, an oral vasopressin antagonist, in patients hospitalized for heart failure: the EVEREST Clinical Status Trials. *JAMA* 297(12):1332–1343, 2007.
32. Costanzo MR, Saltzberg MT, Jessup M, et al: Ultrafiltration Versus Intravenous Diuretics forPatients Hospitalized for Acute Decompensated Heart Failure (UNLOAD) Investigators: Ultrafiltration is associated with fewer rehospitalizations than continuous diuretic infusion in patients with decompensated heart failure: Results from UNLOAD. *J Card Fail* 16: 277–284, 2010.
33. Antman EM, Anbe DT, Armstrong PW, et al: ACC/AHA guidelines for the management of patients with ST-elevation myocardial infarction—executive summary: a report of the American College of Cardiology/American Heart Association Task Force on Practice Guidelines (Writing Committee to Revise the 1999 Guidelines for the Management of Patients With Acute Myocardial Infarction). *Circulation* 110(5):588–636, 2004.
34. Cuffe MS, Califf RM, Adams KF Jr, et al: Short-term intravenous milrinone for acute exacerbation of chronic heart failure: a randomized controlled trial. *JAMA* 287(12):1541–1547, 2002.
35. Mullens W, Abrahams Z, Skouri HN, et al: Elevated intra-abdominal pressure in acute decompensated heart failure: a potential contributor to worsening renal function? *J Am Coll Cardiol* 51:300–306, 2008.
36. Wang W, Falk S, Jittikanont S, et al: Protective effect of renal denervation on normotensive endotoxemia-induced acute renal failure in mice. *Am J Physiol Renal Physiol* 283:F583–F587, 2002.
37. Lin SM, Huang CD, Lin HC, et al. A modified goal-directed protocol improves clinical outcomes in intensive care unit patients with septic shock: a randomized controlled trial. *Shock* 26: 551–557, 2006
38. Yealy DM, Kellum JA, Huang DT, et al. ProCESS Investigators: a randomized trial of protocol based care for early septic shock. *N Engl J Med* 370: 1683–1693, 2014.
39. Peake SL, Delaney A, Bailey M, et al. ARISE Investigators; Goal-directed resuscitationfor patients with early septic shock. *N Engl J Med* 371: 1496–1506, 2014.
40. Mouncey PR, Osborne TM, Power GC, et al: trial of early, goal-directed resuscitation for septic shock. *N Engl J Med* 372:1301–1311, 2015.
41. Malbrain ML, Cheatham ML, Kirkpatrick A, et al: Results from the International Conference of Experts on intra-abdominal hypertension and abdominal compartment syndrome: I. Definitions. *Intensive Care Med* 32:1722–1732, 2006.
42. Shibagaki Y, Tai C, Nayak A, et al: Intra-abdominal hypertension is an under-appreciated cause of acute renal failure. *Nephrol Dial Transplant* 21:3567–3570, 2006.
43. Sever MS, Vanholder R, Lameire N: Management of crush-related injuries after disasters. *N Engl J Med* 354:1052–1063, 2006
44. Weisbord SD, Mor MK, Resnick AL, et al: Prevention, incidence, and outcomes of contrast-induced acute kidney injury. *Arch Intern Med* 168:1325–1332, 2008.
45. Lee HT, Jan M, Bae SC, et al: A1 adenosine receptor knockout mice are protected against acute radiocontrast nephropathy in vivo. *Am J Renal Physiol* 290(6):F1367–F1375, 2006.
46. Detrenis S, Meschi M, Musini S, et al: Lights and shadows on the pathogenesis of contrast-induced nephropathy: state of the art. *Nephrol Dial Transplant* 20(8):1542–1550, 2005.
47. Hoste EA, De Waele JJ, Gevaert SA, et al: Sodium bicarbonate for prevention of contrast-induced acute kidney injury: a systematic review and meta-analysis. *Nephrol Dial Transplant* 25(3):747, 2010.
48. Klima T, Christ A, Marana I, et al: Sodium chloride vs. sodium bicarbonate for the prevention of contrast medium-induced nephropathy: a randomized controlled trial. *Eur Heart J* 33(16):2071, 2012.
49. Solomon R, Gordon P, Manoukian SV, et al: Randomized trial of bicarbonate or saline study for the prevention of contrast-induced nephropathy in patients with CKD. *Clin J Am Soc Nephrol* 10(9):1519–1524, 2015.

50. Briguori C, Visconti G, Focaccio A, et al: Renal insufficiency after contrast media administration trial II (REMEDIAL II): renal guard system in high-risk patients for contrast-induced acute kidney injury. *Circulation* 124(11):1260–1269, 2011.
51. Marenzi G, Ferrari C, Marana I, et al: Prevention of contrast nephropathy by furosemide with matched hydration: the MYTHOS (Induced Diuresis With Matched Hydration Compared to Standard Hydration for Contrast Induced Nephropathy Prevention) trial. *JACC Cardiovasc Interv* 5(1):90, 2012.
52. Fishbane S: N-acetylcysteine in the prevention of contrast-induced nephropathy. *Clin J Am Soc Nephrol* 3(1):281, 2008.
53. ACT Investigators: Acetylcysteine for prevention of renal outcomes in patients undergoing coronary and peripheral vascular angiography. *Circulation* 124:1250–1259, 2011
54. Laskey W, Aspelin P, Davidson C, et al: Nephrotoxicity of iodixanol versus iopamidol in patients with chronic kidney disease and diabetes mellitus undergoing coronary angiographic procedures. *Heart J* 158(5):822, 2009.
55. Reed M, Meier P, Tamhane UU, et al: The relative renal safety of iodixanol compared with low-osmolar contrast media: a meta-analysis of randomized controlled trials. *JACC Cardiovasc Interv* 2(7):645, 2009.
56. Cruz DN, Goh CY, Marenzi G, et al: Renal replacement therapies for prevention of radiocontrast-induced nephropathy: a systematic review. *Am J Med* 125(1):66–78, 2012.
57. Rodby RA: Preventing complications of radiographic contrast media: is there a role for dialysis? *Semin Dial* 20(1):19–23, 2007.
58. McCullough PA, Larsen T, Brown JR: Theophylline or aminophylline for the prevention ofcontrast-induced acute kidney injury. *Am J Kidney Dis* 60(3):338, 2012.
59. Stone GW, McCullough PA, Tumlin JA, et al: CONTRAST Investigators: Fenoldopam mesylate for the prevention of contrast-induced nephropathy: a randomized controlled trial. *JAMA* 290:2284–2291, 2003.
60. Wang A, Holcslaw T, Bashore TM, et al: Exacerbation of radiocontrast nephrotoxicity byendothelin receptor antagonism. *Kidney Int* 57(4):1675, 2000.
61. Ori Y, Rozen-Zvi B, Chagnac A, et al: Fatalities and severe metabolic disorders associated with the use of sodium phosphate enemas: a single center's experience. *Arch Intern Med* 172(3):263, 2012.
62. Markowitz GS, Perazella MA: Acute phosphate nephropathy. *Kidney Int* 76(10):1027, 2009.
63. Praga M, González E: Acute interstitial nephritis. *Kidney Int* 77(11):956, 2010.
64. Bourgault M, Grimbert P, Verret C, et al. Acute renal infarction: a case series. *Clin J Am Soc Nephrol*. 3:392–398, 2013
65. Legendre CM, Licht C, Muus P, et al: Terminal complement inhibitor eculizumab in atypical hemolytic-uremic syndrome. *N Engl J Med* 368(23):2169–2181, 2013.
66. Perazella MA, Markowitz GS: Bisphosphonate nephrotoxicity. *Kidney Int* 74(11):1385, 2008.
67. Lopez-Olivo MA, Pratt G, Palla SL, et al. Rasburicase in tumor lysis syndrome of the adult: a systemic review and meta-analysis. *Am J Kidney Dis* 62:481, 2013.
68. Spina M, Nagy Z, Ribera JM, et al: FLORENCE: a randomized, double-blind, phase III pivotal study of febuxostat versus allopurinol for the prevention of tumor lysis syndrome (TLS) in patients with hematologic malignancies at intermediate to high TLS risk. *Ann Oncol*. 26(10):2155–2161, 2015.
69. Coiffier B, Altman A, Pui CH, et al: Guidelines for the management of pediatric and adult tumor lysis syndrome: an evidence-based review. *J Clin Oncol* 26:2767, 2008.
70. Widemann BC, Adamson PC: Understanding and managing methotrexate nephrotoxicity. *Oncologist 11*:694, 2006.
71. Salerno F, Gerbes A, Gines P, et al: Diagnosis, prevention and treatment of hepatorenal syndrome in cirrhosis. *Gut* 56:1310, 2007.
72. Gludd LL, Christensen K, Christensen E, et al: Terlipressin for hepatorenal syndrome. *Cochrane Database Syst Rev* 9:CD005162, 2012
73. Nadim MK, Kellum JA, Davenport A, et al: ADQI Workgroup: hepatorenal-syndrome: the 8th international consensus conference of the Acute Dialysis Quality Initiative (ADQI) Group. *Crit Care* 16: R23, 2012
74. Nassar Junior AP, Farias AQ, D'Albuquerque LA: Terlipressin versus norepinephrine in the treatment of hepatorenal syndrome: a systemic review and meta-analysis. *Plos One* 9:107466, 2014.
75. Esrailian E, Pantangco ER, Kyulo NL, et al: Octreotide/midodrine therapy significantly improves renal function and 30-day survival in patients with type 1 hepatorenal syndrome. *Dig Dis Sci* 52:742–748, 2007.
76. Esrailian E, Runyon BA: Alcoholic cirrhosis-associated hepatorenal syndrome treated with vasoactive agents. *Nat Clin Pract Nephrol* 2:169–172, 2006.
77. Rössle M, Gerbes AL: TIPS for the treatment of refractory ascites, hepatorenal syndrome and hepatic hydrothorax: a critical update. *Gut* 59(7):988, 2010.
78. Witzke O, Baumann M, Patschan D, et al. Which patients benefit from hemodialysis therapy in hepatorenal syndrome? *J Gastroenterol Hepatol* 19:1369, 2004.
79. Runyon BA: Management of adult patients with ascites due to cirrhosis: an update. *Hepatology* 49:2087, 2009.
80. Levey AS, Greene T, Kusek JW, et al. A simplified equation to predict glomerular filtration rate from serum creatinine. *J Am Soc Nephrol*. 11:A0828, 2000.
81. Cantarovich F, Rangoonwala B, Lorenz H, et al: High-dose furosemide for established ARF: a prospective, randomized, double-blind, placebo-controlled, multicenter trial. *Am J Kidney Dis* 44:402, 2004.
82. Ho KM, Sheridan DJ: Meta-analysis of frusemide to prevent or treat acute renal failure. *BMJ* 333:420, 2006.
83. Mehta RL, Pascual MT, Soroko S, et al: Diuretics, mortality, and nonrecovery of renal function in acute renal failure. *JAMA* 288:2547, 2002.
84. Clarkson MR, Giblin L, O'Connell FP, et al: Acute interstitial nephritis: clinical features and response to corticosteroid therapy. *Nephrol Dial Transplant* 19:2778, 2004.
85. Gonzalez E, Gutierrez E, Galeano C, et al: Early steroid treatment improves the recovery of renal function in patients with drug-induced acute interstitial nephritis. *Kidney Int* 73:940, 2008.
86. Stone JH, Merkal PA, Spiera R, et al: Rituximab versus cyclophosphamide for ANCA-associated vasculitis. *N Engl J Med* 363(3):221, 2010.
87. Levy JB, Turner AN, Rees AJ, et al. Long-term outcome of anti-glomerular basement membrane antibody disease treated with plasma exchange and immunosuppression. *Ann Intern Med* 134(11):1033, 2001.
88. KDIGO: KDIGO Clinical Practice Guideline for Acute Kidney Injury. *Kidney Int Suppl* (Suppl 1):8, 2012
89. Landoni G, Biondi-Zoccai GG, Tumlin JA, et al: Beneficial impact of fenoldopam in critically ill patients with or at risk for acute renal failure: a meta-analysis of randomized clinical trials. *Am J Kidney Dis* 49:56, 2007.
90. Nigwekar SU, Navaneethan SD, Parikh CR, et al: Atrial natriuretic peptide for management of acute kidney injury: a systematic review and meta-analysis. *Clin J Am Soc Nephrol* 4(2):261, 2009.
91. Fiaccadori E, Cremaschi E. Nutritional assessment and support in acute kidney injury. *Curr Opin Crit Care* 15:474, 2009.
92. Kraut JA, Madias NE: Treatment of acute metabolic acidosis: a pathophysiologic approach. *Nat Rev Nephrol* 8(10):589–601, 2012.
93. Bagshaw SM, Laupland KB, Doig CJ, et al: Prognosis for long-term survival and renal recovery in critically patients with severe acute renal failure: a population-based study. *Crit Care* 9:R700–R709, 2005.
94. Uchino S, Kellum JA, Bellomo R, et al: Acute renal failure in critically ill patients: a multinational, multicenter study. *JAMA* 294(7):813, 2005.
95. Laingos O, Wald R, O'Bell JW, et al: Epidemiology and outcomes of acute renal failure in hospitalized patients: a national survey. *Clin J Am Soc Nephrol* 1(1):43–51, 2006.
96. Xue JL, Daniels F, Star RA, et al. Incidence and mortality of acute renal failure in hospitalized patients: a national survey. *J Am Soc Nephrol* 17:1135–1142, 2006.
97. Ympa YP, Sakr Y, Reinhart K, et al: Has mortality from acute renal failure decreased? A systematic review of the literature. *Am J Med* 118:827, 2005.
98. Abosaif NY, Tolba YA, Heap M, et al. The outcomes of acute renal failure in the intensive care unit according to RIFLE: Model application, sensitivity, and predictability *Am J Kidney Dis* 46:1038, 2005.
99. Avilo MO, Zanetta DM, Addulkader RC, et al. Urine volume in acute kidney injury: how much is enough? *Renal Fail* 31: 884–890, 2009.
100. Bucaloiu ID, Kirchner HL, Norfolk ER, et al: Increased risk of death and de novo chronic kidney disease following reversible acute kidney injury. *Kidney Int* 81:477–485, 2012.
101. Schmitt R, Coca S, Kanbay M, et al: Recovery of kidney function after acute kidney injury in the elderly: A systematic review and meta-analysis. *Am J Kidney Dis* 52:262–271, 2008.
102. Schiffl H: Renal recovery from acute tubular necrosis requiring renal replacement therapy: a prospective study in critically ill patients. *Nephrol Dial Transplant* 21:1248–1252, 2006
103. Lo LJ, Go AS, Chertow GM, et al. Dialysis-requiring acute renal failure increases the risk of progressive chronic kidney disease. *Kidney Int* 76:893–899, 2009.
104. Hsu CY, Chertow GM, McCulloch CE, et al: Nonrecovery of kidney function and death after acute on chronic renal failure. *Clin J Am Soc Nephrol* 4: 891–898, 2009.
105. Ishani A, Xue JL, Himmelfarb J, et al: Acute kidney injury increases risk of ESRD among elderly. *J Am Soc Nephrol* 20:223, 2009.
106. Liano F, Felipe C, Tenorio MT, et al: Long term outcome of acute tubular necrosis: a contribution to its natural history. *Kidney Int* 71:679, 2007.

Chapter 201 ▪ Renal Replacement Therapy in the Intensive Care Unit

MATTHEW J. TRAINOR • MATTHEW A. NIEMI • PANG-YEN FAN

INTRODUCTION

Rapid deterioration of kidney function in acutely ill patients is common and potentially catastrophic. Acute kidney injury (AKI) occurs in up to 70% of patients admitted to the intensive care unit (ICU) and is associated with a twofold increase in the already high mortality rate for this population. Medical therapy is often inadequate for the management of the metabolic disturbances and fluid overload that complicate AKI. In this setting, renal replacement therapy (RRT) is essential for the survival of the patient. In addition, patients with end-stage renal disease (ESRD) have high rates of hospitalization, particularly for cardiovascular disease and infections. These patients often require ICU care, including RRT.

Despite many technical advances over several decades of dialysis support experience, mortality remains alarmingly high (40% to 60%) for ICU patients with AKI. The high death rate is largely owing to the severity and the array of nonrenal organ system dysfunction, because mortality for patients with AKI is now primarily because of multiorgan system failure (MOSF). Accumulating evidence suggests that the consequences of AKI may in turn contribute to the injury of distant organs and that some forms of RRT may prevent MOSF [1].

The objectives of modern-day RRT now extend beyond correction of metabolic disturbances and volume overload to include facilitation of nutritional support and drug therapies, and even promotion of nonrenal organ system recovery. More proactive treatment strategies have resulted in a trend toward earlier initiation of dialysis. For example, with recognition that fluid overload increases mortality and that volume control can improve outcomes [2–4], RRT is applied more aggressively to prevent volume overload.

An important principle of renal support strategies is that of "capacity (supply) and demand mismatch." Critically ill patients have increased "demand" for renal function. Such patients often generate increased solute from their hypercatabolic metabolism and intensive nutritional support. In addition, they receive enormous amounts of fluid via medications, blood products, enteral and parenteral nutrition, and volume resuscitation. The stress of high solute and fluid loads may overwhelm the excretory capacity of even minimally injured kidneys. Furthermore, the limited "supply" of renal function from kidneys already compromised by AKI is further reduced by tenuous hemodynamics and endogenous/exogenous renal vasoconstrictor activity. RRT supplements the impaired ability of the injured kidney to match the high fluid and solute demand, thereby restoring balance [5].

PRINCIPLES OF SOLUTE CLEARANCE AND FLUID REMOVAL BY DIALYTIC TECHNIQUES

Dialysis therapies involve the movement of solute and plasma water across a semipermeable membrane separating a blood compartment and a dialysate compartment. For intermittent hemodialysis (IHD) and continuous renal replacement therapies (CRRTs), this process occurs within a cartridge called a hemofilter or hemodialyzer, as shown in Figure 201.1. For peritoneal dialysis (PD), the peritoneum serves as the semipermeable membrane separating blood in the mesenteric vasculature from the dialysate in the peritoneal cavity. Characteristics such as membrane thickness and pore dimensions determine the size and transfer rate of molecules that move between the blood and dialysate.

Removal of solute and water using RRT may occur by diffusion or convection. Diffusion (dialysis) involves movement of solute from areas of high concentration to low concentration. Solute molecules have kinetic energy and move in solution. They collide with one another and with water molecules, resulting in an even dispersion throughout the solution. When solute in motion encounters a membrane pore of sufficient dimensions, it moves through the membrane into the adjacent compartment. Small molecules with greater molecular velocity are more readily cleared than are larger molecules even if both fit through the membrane pore. A high concentration of a solute in a given compartment favors a high frequency of membrane collisions and its passage through the pore. Water molecules will also pass easily through the membrane to the compartment with higher

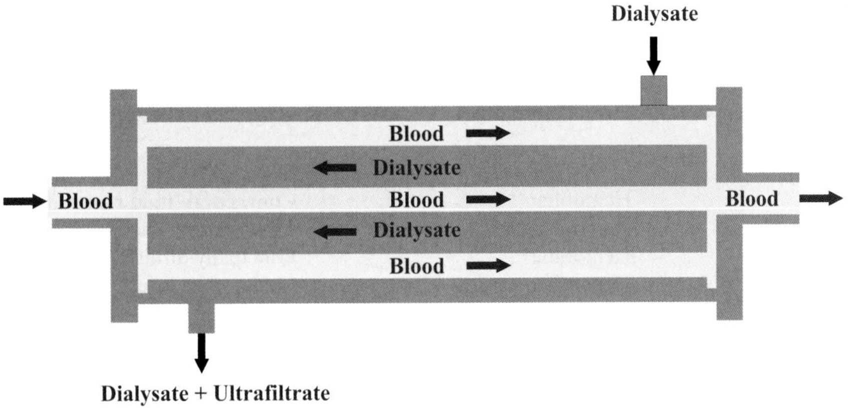

FIGURE 201.1 Schematic diagram of a hollow fiber dialyzer. Blood enters the hemofilter, passes through hollow fibers, and exits at the opposite end. Dialysate enters through the side port, flows around the blood-filled fibers in the opposite direction as the blood, combines with ultrafiltrate, and exits via the side port near the blood entry port.

osmolality. In a static system, net transfer (dialysis) ceases when solute concentrations equilibrate in the compartments. For RRT, blood and dialysate are repeatedly replenished to maintain the high concentration gradients favoring efficient transfer of solute and water.

Convection involves the transfer of solute across a semipermeable membrane driven by a hydrostatic pressure gradient. Those solutes small enough to pass through pores are swept along with water by solvent drag. The membrane acts as a sieve, retaining molecules that exceed the pore size. All filtered solutes below the membrane pore size are removed at rates proportionate to their concentration. The convective removal of fluid in this manner is termed *hemofiltration* or sometimes *ultrafiltration*. This technique does not change the plasma concentration of small solutes (blood urea nitrogen [BUN], creatinine, electrolytes, and glucose), because water is removed in proportion to solute. In contrast, the concentration of larger molecules (albumin) and formed elements (hematocrit) increase as they are sieved off by the smaller membrane pores. Thus, the chemical composition of the filtrate (often referred to as ultrafiltrate) is almost identical to that of the plasma except for the absence of large molecules such as albumin.

OVERVIEW OF DIALYSIS MODALITIES

The general features of different dialysis modalities are summarized in Table 201.1.

Intermittent Hemodialysis

IHD is the standard form of RRT for the majority of stable patients with ESRD in the United States. In IHD, blood is circulated through a dialysis machine and hemodialysis cartridge and then returned to the patient. Utilizing diffusion (principally for solute clearance) and convection (principally for ultrafiltration), this highly efficient modality provides rapid solute and volume removal but requires both specialized equipment and trained staff. Both blood and dialysate are pumped through the hemofilter at high-flow rates. The dialysate flow is countercurrent to blood flow to maximize concentration gradients throughout the course of the filter (Fig. 201.1). Diffusion of solute across the filter is bidirectional. Urea, creatinine, and potassium move from plasma to dialysate, whereas bicarbonate and usually calcium diffuse in an opposite direction (Fig. 201.2).

Standard dialysis machines can also perform isolated ultrafiltration that results in fluid removal but does not significantly alter the chemical composition of plasma. During ultrafiltration, the dialysis machine pumps only blood, but not dialysate through the hemofilter. This process generates a hydrostatic pressure gradient across the hemofilter membrane, resulting in convective fluid removal. However, no dialysate is used, so there is no diffusive solute clearance. Isolated ultrafiltration is typically used when volume overload is the sole concern.

Solute clearance can be adjusted by changing the dialyzer size and membrane; blood and dialysate flow; and dialysis time, as detailed later in this chapter. Fluid removal can be adjusted by changing the hydrostatic pressure gradient between the blood and dialysate compartments within the hemofilter, an automated process performed by the dialysis machine. Although this technique is commonly used in the ICU setting, the rapid shifts in solute and fluid can precipitate hemodynamic instability and may, therefore, be less suitable for critically ill patients. IHD treatments are typically performed for several hours three to four times per week. However, because the technique is labor and resource intensive, more frequent treatments may be limited by staffing and cost.

Peritoneal Dialysis

PD is the main form of RRT for approximately 5% to 10% of patients with ESRD in the United States. In PD, dialysate is instilled into the peritoneal cavity. Through diffusion, solute and volume enter the dialysate, which is periodically drained and replaced with fresh dialysate. Solute clearance is adjusted by altering the volume of dialysate or varying the duration of each “dwell” (the interval between dialysate exchanges). More frequent exchanges will enhance solute removal, provided there is sufficient time between dialysate instillation and drainage to permit diffusion across the peritoneum. Volume is removed by maintaining a high dialysate osmolality through a high concentration of dextrose. This osmolar gradient results in the movement

TABLE 201.1

Dialysis Modalities

Technique	Dialyzer	Physical principle
Hemodialysis		
IHD	Hemodialyzer	Concurrent diffusion (solute clearance) and convection (fluid removal)
SLED	Hemodialyzer	SLED
UF	Hemodialyzer	Convection (fluid removal, limited solute clearance)
CRRT		
SCUF	Hemofilter	Convection (fluid removal, limited solute clearance)
CVVH	Hemofilter	Convection (solute clearance and fluid removal)
CVVHD	Hemofilter	Principally diffusion with some convection
CVVHDF	Hemofilter	Concurrent diffusion and convection
Peritoneal dialysis		
CAPD	None	Principally diffusion with some convection
CCPD	None	Principally diffusion with some convection

CAPD, continuous ambulatory peritoneal dialysis; CCPD, continuous cycling peritoneal dialysis; CRRT, continuous renal replacement therapies; CVVH, continuous venovenous hemofiltration; CVVHD, continuous venovenous hemodialysis; CVVHDF, continuous venovenous hemodiafiltration; IHD, intermittent hemodialysis; SCUF, slow continuous ultrafiltration; SLED, sustained low-efficiency dialysis; UF, ultrafiltration.

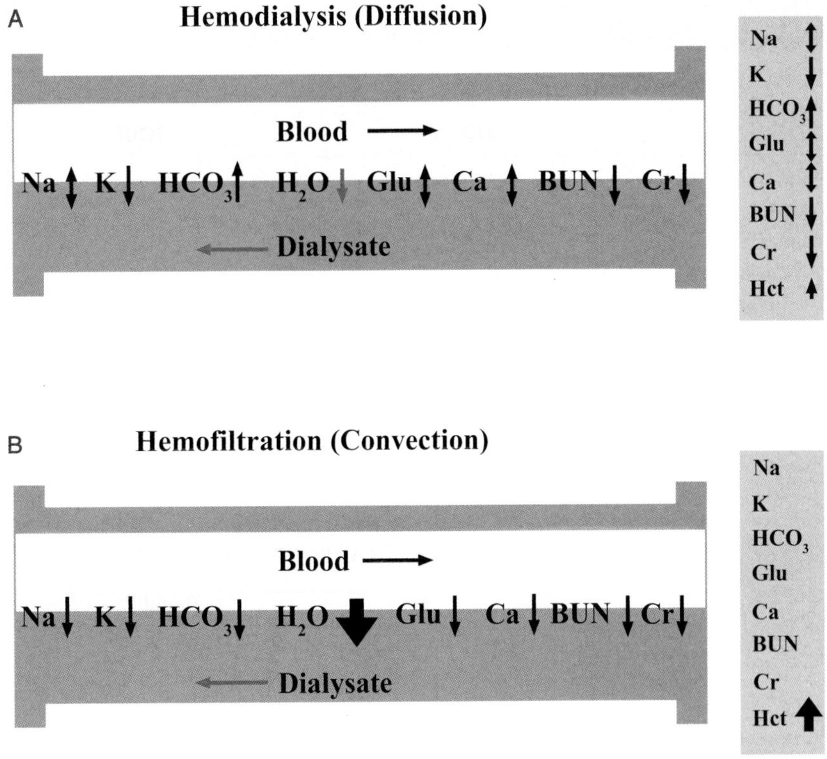

FIGURE 201.2 Solute and water movement across the dialyzer membrane in hemodialysis and hemofiltration. Net effect on serum chemistries and hematocrit shown in box at right. **A:** Significant flux in solute with relatively small shift in water in hemodialysis. Postdialyzer chemistries significantly altered with small increase in hematocrit. **B:** Significant removal of water with concomitant removal of solute in hemofiltration. Posthemofilter chemistries unchanged, because solute is removed in proportion to plasma concentration; however, hematocrit is significantly increased because of high filtration fraction (see text for more detail).

of water into the peritoneal cavity and also contributes to solute clearance through solvent drag. Fluid removal is adjusted by altering the dialysate dextrose content.

PD can be performed as a series of manual dialysate exchanges done during the day (chronic ambulatory peritoneal dialysis or CAPD) or through automated exchanges utilizing a PD machine (cycler) typically done at night (continuous cycled peritoneal dialysis or CCPD). For CAPD, dialysate is changed every 4 to 6 hours with a longer overnight "dwell." For CCPD, the exchanges are typically done every 2 to 3 hours through the night, and the abdomen is often left empty or with only a small volume of dialysate during the day. PD is much less efficient than IHD but is better tolerated hemodynamically, because solute and fluid shifts occur gradually. In the ICU setting, PD is generally reserved for patients with ESRD who are already maintained by this modality. PD is generally not used for AKI because of technical difficulty in establishing dialysis access (discussed later in this chapter) as well as the low efficiency of solute clearance. Furthermore, instillation of 1 to 2 L of dialysate into the peritoneal cavity can impair respiratory mechanics, particularly in the setting of abdominal distention or ileus.

Continuous Renal Replacement Therapies

CRRT denotes several hemodialytic modalities that vary in their mode of solute removal and duration of treatment, but share the characteristic of slow solute and volume removal maintained over an extended period of time rather than high clearances over 3 to 4 hours as with IHD. Although less efficient than IHD, CRRT provides much higher clearances than PD. Like PD, these techniques are better tolerated hemodynamically than IHD, because solute and volume are removed gradually. These modalities are widely used for critical care patients, although they require intensive monitoring and necessitate ICU admission at a hospital with adequate resources and expertise. CRRT can be performed by a number of methods detailed later in the chapter. The operating parameters of different CRRT systems are summarized in Table 201.2. A schematic of the circuitry of the different techniques is presented in Figure 201.3.

Continuous Arteriovenous Hemofiltration, Hemodialysis, and Hemodiafiltration

Early forms of CRRT utilized arteriovenous (AV) systems that relied on the pressure gradient between the arterial and venous circulation to drive ultrafiltration across the hemofilter membrane. However, variations in arterial pressure led to inconsistent rates of ultrafiltration and solute clearance. AV systems also required the placement and long-term maintenance of large-bore arterial catheters at the femoral site. With modern double-lumen venous catheters and advanced pump-driven venovenous systems, these modalities have largely fallen out of favor.

Continuous Venovenous Hemofiltration, Hemodialysis, and Hemodiafiltration

In CRRT, solute removal is achieved by convection or diffusion or a combination of both. Continuous venovenous hemofiltration (CVVH) is a purely convective technique in which a pump system drives blood through the hemofilter and generates ultrafiltration rates of 1 to 4 L per hour. Blood flow rate is generally lower than with IHD, and dialysate is not used. Solute clearance is achieved by replacing these large volumes of ultrafiltrate with fluid that does not contain the solutes targeted for removal (e.g., urea and potassium). Solute clearance and volume removal are adjusted by altering the ultrafiltration rate and the rate of infusion of replacement fluid (RF). The administration of RF maintains fluid balance and lowers the plasma concentration of solute by dilution. RF can be infused before or after the filter along the course of the dialyzer circuit (Fig. 201.3).

In diffusion-based techniques such as continuous venovenous hemodialysis (CVVHD), a dual pump system drives both blood and dialysate through the hemofilter. Dialysate flow and blood flow rates are typically much lower than with IHD. The technique creates less ultrafiltrate (2 to 5 L per day) than CVVH, because

TABLE 201.2

Comparison of RRT Modalities

	IHD	SLED	SCUF	CVVH	CVVHD	CVVHDF
Blood flow (mL/min)	250–400	100–200	<100	200–400	100–200	100–200
Dialysate flow (mL/min)	500–800	100	0	0	17–34	17–34
Filtrate (L/d)	0–4	0–4	0–4	48–96	0	24–48
Replacement fluid (L/d)	0	0	0	46–94	0	23–44
Effluent saturation (%)	15–40	60–70	100	100	85–100	85–100
Solute clearance	Diffusion	Diffusion	Convection	Convection	Diffusion	Both
Duration (h)	3–5	8–12	Variable	>24	>24	>24

IHD, intermittent hemodialysis; CVVH, continuous venovenous hemofiltration; CVVHD, continuous venovenous hemodialysis; CVVHDF, continuous venovenous hemodiafiltration; RRT, renal replacement therapy; SCUF, slow continuous ultrafiltration; SLED, sustained low-efficiency dialysis.

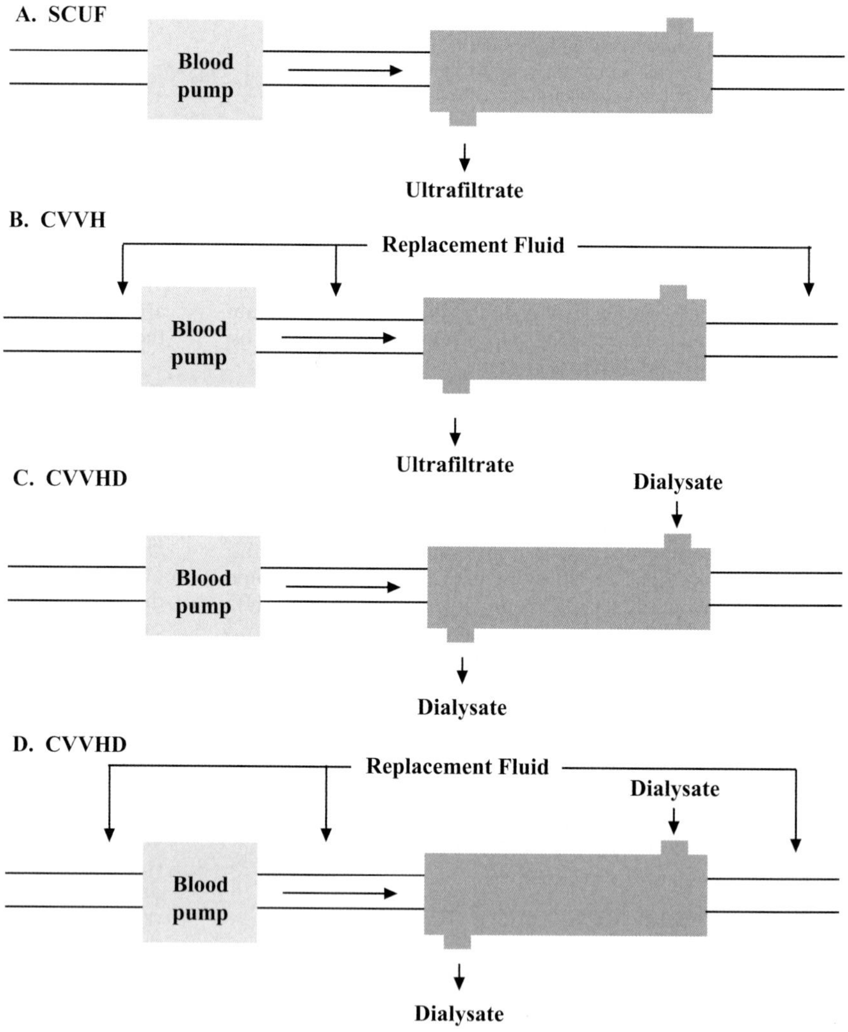

FIGURE 201.3 Schematic diagram of various CRRT configurations. **A:** SCUF. Ultrafiltrate is generated by the transmembrane pressure gradient produced by the blood pump. **B:** CVVH. Large volume ultrafiltrate is generated and replacement fluid is infused preblood pump, prehemofilter, or posthemofilter. **C:** CVVHD. Dialysate is pumped through the filter to generate diffusive solute clearance. **D:** CVVHD. The system utilizes high ultrafiltration with replacement fluid as well as dialysate. CRRT, continuous renal replacement therapy; CVVH, continuous venovenous hemofiltration; CVVHD, continuous venovenous hemodialysis; CVVHDF, continuous venovenous hemodiafiltration; SCUF, slow continuous ultrafiltration.

the infusion pressure of the dialysate lowers the pressure gradient across the hemofilter membrane. As with IHD, diffusion of solute across the filter is bidirectional (Fig. 201.2). No RF is administered. In CVVHD, the flow of dialysate through the filter is countercurrent to the flow of blood, but the dialysate flow rate is significantly slower (1 to 2 L per hour = 17 to 34 mL per minute) than the blood flow rate (100 to 200 mL per minute). This disparity permits full equilibration of plasma urea across the membrane and complete saturation of dialysate.

For all forms of CRRT, solute clearance is directly proportional to the effluent volume (Vef). Thus, Vef is a therapeutic target to ensure dosing adequacy, with effluent targets typically measured in mL/kg/h. The Vef is the product of the filtration process. It comprises the ultrafiltrate in CVVH, the "spent" (equilibrated) dialysate in CVVHD, and the combination of ultrafiltrate and spent dialysate in continuous venovenous hemodiafiltration (CVVHDF). Because urea is freely filtered in CVVH, its concentration in the ultrafiltrate is identical to that of plasma. Thus, 48 L of ultrafiltrate (effluent) represents 48 L of plasma fully cleared of urea. Similarly, in CVVHD, the effluent (spent dialysate) is fully saturated with urea. Each liter of spent dialysate reflects a liter of plasma fully cleared of urea. In diffusive systems, blood flow has little impact on clearance at low dialysate flow (1 to 2 L per hour) but increasing impact as dialysate flow increases.

CVVHDF combines diffusion and convection into a single procedure. Dialysate is infused at 1 to 2 L per hour to boost the convective clearance generated by high (1 to 2 L per hour) ultrafiltration rates. RF is needed to offset the high rate of ultrafiltration. Historically, CVVHDF was developed to overcome clearance limitations posed by the older generation of CRRT equipment, which limited both dialyzer blood and dialysate flow. However, current CRRT equipment delivers blood flow at 400 mL per minute and dialysate flow at up to 10 L per hour. Large bore (13 French [Fr]) catheters are increasingly used to support high-flow systems. These advances allow high-volume ultrafiltrate generation with less complex CVVH or CVVHD systems and have called the role of CVVHDF into question.

Slow Continuous Ultrafiltration

In slow continuous ultrafiltration (SCUF), a pump system maintains low blood flow (usually no more than 100 mL per minute) through a hemofilter and generates low rates of ultrafiltration (typically 100 to 300 mL per hour). This modality provides volume removal but does not alter the chemistry of plasma, because water is removed in proportion to solute. Compared with other CRRT modalities, SCUF is a low-intensity nursing procedure. The procedure is often used in settings of severe volume overload with acceptable chemistries.

TECHNICAL CONSIDERATIONS FOR RENAL REPLACEMENT THERAPY

Anticoagulation

Hemofilter fibers are prone to thrombosis, because removal of fluid through ultrafiltration leads to hemoconcentration at the distal end of the dialyzer. As the filtration fraction (FF), that is, the proportion of plasma flow that is filtered, increases, the risk of filter thrombosis also rises. The FF can be calculated as follows:

$$\begin{aligned} \text{FF} &= \text{ultrafiltration rate/plasma flow rate} \\ &= \text{ultrafiltration rate/(blood flow rate} \times [100 - \text{Hct}]) \end{aligned}$$

Thus, higher rates of ultrafiltration, especially when coupled with low blood flows, predispose to hemofilter thrombosis. Poor filter performance and filter clotting increases sharply at FF greater than 20%. Higher blood flow rates permit greater rates of fluid removal, because hemoconcentration within the filter is limited by the short transit time of blood through the dialysis cartridge.

IHD can generally be performed without anticoagulation. The high blood flows used with this technique permit adequate solute clearance and ultrafiltration with limited risk of dialyzer thrombosis. However, IHD without anticoagulation also necessitates frequent saline flushes through the hemodialyzer to help maintain fiber patency and, therefore, is more labor intensive than standard IHD. In addition, packed red blood cell transfusions cannot be infused through the arterial line of the dialyzer circuit, because the resulting increase in hematocrit will lead to hemofilter clotting.

However, with CRRT, blood flow rates are typically low and ultrafiltration rates high, especially for CVVH, and filter thrombosis is a significant barrier to effective implementation of these therapies, while also increasing nursing and equipment utilization and need for blood transfusions. One approach called *predilutional hemofiltration* involves infusion of RF into the CRRT circuit at a point before the filter, thus lowering the hematocrit through dilution. As a result, a higher ultrafiltration rate may be achieved without compromising filter life. However, prefilter RF also dilutes the solute concentration of blood entering the filter and reduces effective clearance. With this approach, the target Vef should be increased by 25% to compensate for the dilutional effect. Other CRRT parameters such as blood and ultrafiltration rate must be adjusted to compensate for this inefficiency.

Anticoagulation is generally necessary to maintain hemofilter patency with CRRT, especially for principally convective modalities such as CVVH. When heparin is used for anticoagulation, an initial bolus of 1,000 to 2,000 units is typically followed by a continuous infusion of approximately 10 units/kg/h, adjusted to maintain the partial thromboplastin time in the venous line of the blood circuit at 1.5 to 2 times control. However, heparin infusions do result in some systemic anticoagulation and may be contraindicated in patients with active hemorrhage or heparin-induced thrombocytopenia (HIT).

Despite theoretical advantages, low molecular weight heparins do not appear to offer any significant advantages in efficacy or safety over unfractionated heparin for RRT [6]. In addition, these agents are more costly and their anticoagulant effects more difficult to monitor.

For patients with active hemorrhage or high risk of bleeding, regional citrate anticoagulation limited to the CRRT blood circuit offers several advantages [7–9], and is the recommended anticoagulant for CRRT in patients without contraindications to citrate, according to the 2012 kidney disease improving global outcomes (KDIGO) AKI guideline [10]. Citrate infused in the arterial limb of the CRRT circuit prevents hemofilter thrombosis by chelating calcium, a critical component of the clotting cascade. Calcium chloride or calcium gluconate infused into the venous line of the system restores normal systemic calcium levels. This approach appears to reduce the risk of hemorrhage and extend hemofilter patency [11]. In addition, citrate can be used for patient with HIT.

Serum and ionized calcium levels must be carefully monitored when using citrate, especially in patients with significant liver dysfunction, and the calcium infusion appropriately adjusted. Citrate is hepatically metabolized into bicarbonate and can cause metabolic alkalosis. In the setting of hepatic failure, citrate accumulation results in elevated total serum calcium but low ionized calcium levels, reflecting increased circulating calcium bound to citrate. Trisodium citrate solution, typically used in this form of anticoagulation, may also cause hypernatremia.

Other methods of regional anticoagulation such as prostacyclin infusion or heparin reversal with protamine have been less successful. Prostacyclin, an arachidonic acid metabolite, has a half-life of only 3 to 5 minutes and inhibits platelet aggregation. However, it induces vasodilatation, is associated with hypotension, and is costly. Protamine binds and neutralizes heparin, but infusions are technically complex and may be associated with rebound bleeding.

Anticoagulation is unnecessary for PD. However, intraperitoneal fibrin can occlude the dialysis catheter. If fibrin clots are noted in the dialysate, heparin (1,000 units) should be added to each PD exchange for several days. Intraperitoneal heparin is not absorbed and will not cause systemic anticoagulation.

Blood and Dialysate Flow Rates

Maximal urea clearances with standard dialyzers require blood flows of approximately 400 mL per minute. However, when dialysis is initiated for ESRD, blood flow rates begin at 200 to 250 mL per minute and are increased incrementally over several sessions. The low blood flow limits the efficiency of the dialysis and prevents rapid solute and water shifts that can precipitate complications, including delirium, seizures, and dyspnea, collectively known as the dysequilibrium syndrome. With AKI, high blood flow rates (400 mL per minute) may be used immediately, unless the BUN has been markedly elevated for a prolonged period. Blood flow rates for CRRT can vary from 100 to 400 mL per minute, but dysequilibrium syndrome is not a concern because solute and fluid removal occur slowly compared to IHD. The dialysate flow rate typically ranges between 500 to 800 mL per minute in IHD. These rates are sufficiently high so that changes in dialysate flow have relatively little impact on IHD clearances. However, because dialysate flow rates are much lower with CRRT, increases in dialysate flow can significantly enhance solute removal.

Dialyzer Membrane

Most hemofilters are constructed as cylinders containing hollow fibers composed of semipermeable membranes with varying surface areas and pore sizes (Fig. 201.1). Pore diameters are sufficiently small to preclude movement of cellular material or albumin, while allowing movement of smaller and middle-sized molecules. The surface area of the membrane depends on the number and length of these fibers. In the case of a patient with an ingestion of a dialyzable substance, the use of a hemofilter with a larger surface area will enhance clearance. The initial hemofilter membranes, composed of cellulose, have been replaced by synthetic, more biocompatible materials, which cause less complement activation and leukocyte adherence.

Dialysate Composition

The production of dialysate begins with obtaining "ultrapure" water, which is necessary given the potential for backflow of endotoxin or bacteria into the patient. The standard composition of dialysates for both IHD and PD is summarized in Table 201.3.

TABLE 201.3

Dialysate Formulation for Hemodialysis and Peritoneal Dialysis

Solute	Range (usual concentration)
Intermittent hemodialysis	
Na^+	138–145 mEq/L (140)
K^+	0–4 mEq/L (2)
Cl^-	100–110 mEq/L (106)
HCO_3^-	35–45 mEq/L (35)
Ca^+	1.0–3.5 mEq/L (2.5)
Mg^+	1.5 mEq/L (1.5)
Glucose	0–200 mg/dL (200)
Peritoneal dialysis	
Na^+	132 mEq/L
K^+	0
Cl^-	96 mEq/L
Lactate	35 mEq/L
Ca^+	2.5 or 3.5 mEq/L
Mg^+	0.5 or 1.5 mEq/L
Dextrose	1.5%, 2.5%, or 4.25% g/dL

For IHD, chloride, glucose, and magnesium concentrations are generally fixed, whereas sodium, potassium, calcium, and bicarbonate compositions are customizable. Sodium modeling, a strategy employed to prevent hypotension, consists of higher sodium concentrations at the start of dialysis, followed by a gradual reduction, to prevent hypernatremia. The higher sodium concentration helps to prevent rapid fluid shifts when urea is being rapidly cleared.

The dialysate potassium concentration generally ranges from 1.0 to 4.0 mEq per L, with 1.0 mEq per L dialysate generally reserved for cases of severe hyperkalemia. Use of 1.0 mEq per L dialysate is limited by its potential to cause arrhythmias owing to rapid potassium clearance.

The buffer used in dialysate is now uniformly bicarbonate. The concentration of bicarbonate in dialysate usually varies from 33 to 35 mEq per L. Higher bicarbonate concentrations (40 mEq per L) are used in severe acidosis or to offset elevations of carbon dioxide resulting from the permissive hypercapnia that attends low tidal volume ventilation.

Dialysate calcium concentration in maintenance hemodialysis is 2.5 mEq per L of diffusible calcium. Because hypocalcemia is common in AKI and correction of acidosis may further depress ionized calcium, some experts advocate higher dialysate calcium concentration (3.0 to 3.5 mEq per L) in patients with AKI. High-calcium dialysate may be used to correct hypocalcemia but should be used with caution; animal models suggest calcium loading worsens organ dysfunction and mortality from sepsis [12].

For CRRT, a wide variety of dialysate and RFs may be used. The composition of dialysate employed in CVVHD may be identical to that of RF employed in CVVH. Potassium and calcium concentrations are selected to meet patient needs. Base composition may be bicarbonate or lactate or citrate. The latter two buffers are metabolized to bicarbonate and effectively address acidosis in most patients with adequate hepatic function.

The composition of peritoneal dialysate is relatively constant. These commercially produced solutions are available in 2- and 5-L bags and vary only in dextrose content (1.5%, 2.5%, and 4.25% concentrations). Icodextrin, a glucose polymer which is absorbed more slowly than dextrose, has been used for selected patients with severe hyperglycemia or poor ultrafiltration. If necessary, potassium, insulin, heparin, or certain antibiotics can be added to the dialysate.

Dialysis Access

Establishing and maintaining adequate access is paramount to the delivery of all types of RRT. Access is best considered in two distinct settings: the patient with ESRD with permanent access and the patient with AKI requiring temporary access.

Arteriovenous Fistula and Arteriovenous Graft

For the patient with ESRD maintained with IHD, permanent dialysis access options include an arteriovenous fistula (AVF), arteriovenous graft (AVG), or a tunneled central venous catheter (discussed later in this chapter). Created by connecting an artery to a vein, an AVF must "mature," a process during which high blood flow causes gradual dilatation and thickening or "arterialization" of the veins proximal to the AV anastomosis. Once mature, the AVF can be repetitively cannulated several times a week for IHD. Considered the optimal access for IHD, an AVF provides high blood flow (>500 mL per minute), relatively low thrombosis rates, and low infection rates. However, AVFs require long maturation time (typically several months), making them unsuitable for patients with AKI. In addition, AVFs cannot withstand continuous cannulation, precluding their use for CRRT.

For an AVG, a synthetic material is used to connect the artery and vein. Like AVFs, AVGs cannot be used to manage

AKI, because they require several weeks to mature, and they cannot be used for CRRT. Compared with AVFs, AVGs are not as durable, have much higher rates of thrombosis and infection.

To preserve the patency of AVFs and AVGs, measurement of blood pressure, venipuncture, and constricting dressings or tourniquets should be avoided in the access extremity. Acute thrombosis may also occur in the setting of hypotension or severe volume depletion, two conditions common among critically ill patients.

Peritoneal Dialysis Catheters

Unlike IHD and CRRT, patients on PD do not require vascular access. Instead, PD catheters allow for infusion and drainage of dialysate from the peritoneal cavity. Most are made of silicone and have two synthetic cuffs, one placed beneath the skin and one beneath the abdominal fascia, which prevent displacement and infection of the catheter. Use of PD catheters is delayed for 1 or 2 weeks after placement to permit healing of the insertion site and catheter tunnel. In urgent situations, early use of permanent catheters can be attempted with low-volume exchanges and the patient supine, although this may increase the risk of dialysate leak or infection. Although very rarely used, when access is required for AKI, a noncuffed PD catheter can be placed at the bedside and used immediately. This procedure should be reserved for unique situations and be performed by a skilled operator because of the risks of bowel perforation or organ puncture.

Hemodialysis Catheters

For most patients with AKI, dialysis access is achieved by placement of a temporary central venous catheter. These devices fall into two different categories: acute noncuffed, nontunneled lines and long-term cuffed, tunneled catheters. All are of large diameter (12 to 15 Fr) and dual-lumen design. For patients with urgent or emergent need of dialysis, acute catheters provide rapid access for IHD and CRRT and are typically inserted at the bedside into the internal jugular or femoral veins. Complications of these catheters include infection, thrombosis, and vascular perforation, as discussed below.

Cuffed, tunneled catheters are placed when the expected duration of dialytic support exceeds 2 weeks. Composed of soft material such as silicone, they are usually inserted under fluoroscopic guidance into the internal jugular, or femoral vein and exit through a subcutaneous tunnel. These dual-lumen devices are available in different configurations. For appropriate function, the catheters are placed so that the tips extend into the right atrium, thus permitting higher blood flows. Unlike the stiffer acute noncuffed dialysis lines, the softer cuffed catheters do not pose a significant risk of perforation. The subcutaneous cuff and insertion tunnel serve to anchor the catheter and also inhibit infection such that these lines may remain in place for several months or longer. Complications are similar to those with uncuffed catheters and are also discussed below.

INDICATIONS FOR AND TIMING OF INITIATION OF RENAL REPLACEMENT THERAPY

Remarkably, there is no consensus regarding the absolute indications for initiation of RRT in AKI. The absence of objective clinical or biochemical findings that universally warrant dialytic support have resulted in wide variation in clinical practice. A patient's perceived mortality risk may carry as much weight as laboratory-based measures of kidney function [13]. Conventional indications for RRT include:

- Volume overload refractory to or with diuretic therapy
- Hyperkalemia or metabolic acidosis refractory to medical management
- Intoxication with a dialyzable drug or toxin
- Overt uremic signs or symptoms
  - encephalopathy
  - pericarditis
  - uremic bleeding diathesis
- Progressive and advanced asymptomatic azotemia

Reserving RRT for patients who meet one of these criteria may have little impact on the high mortality of AKI, particularly in the setting of MOSF. A treatment strategy that merely prevents uremic complications follows the old paradigm for AKI: these patients die *with*, but not *of*, their renal dysfunction. Despite recognition that AKI carries high mortality risk [14] and that aggressive management of RRT may affect outcomes and reduce mortality, no consensus guideline defines the optimal time to initiate RRT in AKI.

Early versus Late Initiation of RRT

The evidence for early initiation of RRT in AKI is summarized in Table 201.4. Studies are often difficult to interpret, because both timing of RRT initiation and intensity of RRT vary.

A recent retrospective study of Finnish ICU patients with AKI who were treated with RRT compared those who had conventional indications for RRT ("classic RRT") versus those who did not ("preemptive RRT"), and further divided those with classic indications into "classic-delayed" or "classic-urgent," depending on whether RRT was commenced within 12 hours of manifesting indications [15]. Nearly 44% of subjects received "preemptive" RRT, as defined by the authors. Ninety day–adjusted mortality was higher (odds ratio 2.05, $p = 0.04$) among the classic group. Within the classic group, a delay in RRT greater than 12 hours was also associated with a 3.85 odds ratio for mortality ($p = 0.01$). These observational data, therefore, suggest a survival benefit for earlier RRT.

A prospective study of over 1,200 ICU patients with AKI highlighted the nuances of the definition of "early" and "late" RRT initiation [16]. In this study, adjusted patient survival was superior when RRT was started at creatinine levels greater than 3.5 mg per dL, compared with lower levels. However, mortality increased with longer duration of time between ICU admission and RRT initiation. These results suggest the outcomes are not solely dependent on laboratory defined indications for RRT.

A recent single-center randomized trial of "earlier start" (BUN or creatinine of 70 or 7 mg per dL, respectively) versus "usual start" (determined by clinical judgment of treating nephrologist) dialysis for AKI demonstrated a trend toward significantly greater in-hospital mortality among the early-start subjects (20.5% vs. 12.2%). This difference, however, did not reach statistical significance for this outcome or for dialysis dependence at 3 months among survivors [17]. Contrary to the Finnish study cited above, these findings argue against a benefit from starting dialysis in an "early" or "preemptive" fashion in the absence of more conventional indications. Of note, a larger, multicenter study is currently underway to evaluate mortality among critically ill patients who start RRT immediately upon meeting laboratory and urine output-based criteria AKI, versus those who are monitored for additional "severity criteria" [18].

Multiple recent meta-analyses have summarized the evidence the timing of initiation of RRT. A 2008 publication analyzed 18 cohort studies involving more than 2,000 patients [19], for which a pooled 28% risk reduction in mortality was observed with early dialysis. A more recent systematic review and meta-analysis reported an odds ratio of 0.45 (95% confidence interval 0.28 to 0.72) for 28-day mortality with early RRT, in critically ill patients with AKI. In the latter review, early RRT may have also been associated with reduced RRT duration

TABLE 201.4

Summary of Studies Evaluating Timing of Initiation of Renal Replacement Therapy

Study	RRT modality	Study design	Patients	Criteria for early RRT	Criteria for late RRT	Survival (%), early RRT	Survival (%), late RRT	Comment
Gettings et al. [47]	CRRT	Retrospective	100	BUN < 60	BUN > 60	39	20	More MOSF/sepsis in late group
Bouman et al. [48]	CRRT	RCT	106	<12 h after AKI criteria met: UOP < 30 mL/h C^{creat} < 20 mL/min	Standard criteria: BUN > 112, K > 6.5 Pulmonary edema	LV: 69	LV: 75	Low mortality (27%) Underpowered No CRRT in 6/36 late starts
Demirkiliç et al. [49]	CRRT	Retrospective	61	UOP < 100 mL/8 h despite furosemide	Creat > 5 or K > 6.5	77	45	Postcardiac surgery TTI (d) 0.9 vs. 2.6
Elahi et al. [50]	CRRT	Retrospective	64	UOP < 100 mL/8 h despite furosemide	BUN > 84, K > 6.0	78	57	Postcardiac surgery TTI (d) 0.8 vs. 2.6
Liu et al. [51]	CRRT	Retrospective	80	<12 h after ICU admission	Conventional indications	55	28	Sepsis + oliguria Historical controls Early hemofiltration
Seabra et al. [19]	IHD and CRRT	Observational	243	BUN < 76	BUN > 76	65	59	Adjusted RR (death) 1.85 for high BUN
Palevsky [21]	IHD and CRRT	Meta-analysis RCT, cohort	2,378	Variable	Variable			Early-start risk reduction Cohort: 28% RR RCTs: 36% RR
Vaara et al. [15]	IHD and CRRT	Prospective observational	239	Non-conventional	Conventional	70.5	51.5	Mixed critical care population
Bagshaw et al. [16]	IHD and CRRT	Prospective observational	1,238	Urea < 24.2 mmol/L S^{Creat} < 309 mmol/L <2 d from ICU admission to RRT 2–5 d from ICU admission to RRT >5 days from ICU admission to RRT	Urea > 24.2 mmol/L S^{Creat} > 309 mmol/L	36.6 28.6 41.1 37.9 27.2	38.6 46.6	54 ICUs, 23 countries
Jamale [17]	IHD and CRRT	Prospective RCT	208	BUN > 70 or SCreat > 7.0	Traditional	79.5	87.8	Single-center; in-hospital mortality only

BUN, blood urea nitrogen; Ccreat, creatinine clearance; CRRT, continuous renal replacement therapy; HV, high-volume hemofiltration; IHD, intermittent hemodialysis; LV, low-volume hemofiltration; MOSF, multiorgan system failure; RCT, randomized controlled trial; TTI, time to initiation; UOP, urine output.

and ICU length of stay, and higher rates of renal recovery [20]. Both meta-analyses cite significant methodologic limitations that preclude definitive conclusions, including publication bias, variations in technology over the decades-long span of cited studies, heterogeneous definitions of early and late therapy, and a paucity of randomized trials.

Another major methodologic limitation of all observational studies is the omission of patients who never receive RRT from the analysis. Less than 15% of patients who meet RIFLE criteria (threefold increase in creatinine) receive RRT during their hospitalization. Some patients with AKI recover renal function and survive, whereas others may expire before initiating RRT. Yet, neither outcome is integrated into a retrospective analysis. Among AKI patients managed with RRT, patients destined to recover and survive may enrich the early-start groups, whereas patients destined to die of MOSF after an extended ICU course may be overrepresented in late start groups. Future studies on early RRT versus late RRT, whether prospective or observational, must integrate a "No RRT" arm into the study design [21].

The best current guidelines for RRT initiation were formulated by the Acute Kidney Injury Network [22]. We summarize a similar list of indications in Table 201.5. Parameters for starting RRT should be considered within the context of the patient's entire clinical condition. A specific indication may be absolute or relative. An absolute indication represents a stand-alone condition that makes RRT mandatory. A relative indication requires a concomitant condition without which RRT is not mandatory but could be recommended. The presence of an indication in a relatively stable patient with oliguric AKI as single-organ system failure would be viewed differently from the same parameter existing in a critically ill patient with MOSF. The course of illness may be more important than absolute parameters. The strength of an indication for RRT depends on whether the patient's clinical condition is improving or deteriorating or static.

Dialysis Dose

There is no benchmark for the dose or intensity of RRT used to treat AKI. Many experts suggest that IHD in this setting should at least achieve the urea clearance recommended for patients with ESRD, although there are no data validating this approach. Urea clearance can be quantitated through the *Kt*/*V* or urea reduction ratio (URR). The *Kt*/*V* is a dimensionless index of dialysis dose for which *K* is the urea clearance of the dialyzer, *t* is the duration of dialysis, and *V* is the volume of distribution of urea; the *Kt*/*V* is thought to be a measure of time-averaged urea clearance and is determined by applying predialysis and postdialysis urea and volume data to a published formula. The *Kt*/*V* for each IHD should exceed 1.2, assuming single pool urea kinetics. Alternatively, some programs target a URR of more than 65% or 70%. The URR is calculated using the following formula:

$$\text{URR} = (\text{predialysis BUN} - \text{postdialysis BUN}) / \text{predialysis BUN}$$

RRT can also be used simply to maintain the BUN below a target level such as less than 80 to 100 mg per dL.

Methods of increasing urea clearance include maintaining high dialysis blood flows, often necessitating the use of large-bore catheters and high gauge needles, using larger dialyzers, and extending dialysis time or frequency. It is important to note that adequate urea clearance does not ensure that ultrafiltration needs are met and additional RRT may be required to address volume overload.

There is little data regarding the target dosage or intensity of PD for patients with AKI. Guidelines for patients with stable ESRD on this form of RRT remain incompletely validated, even for commonly used techniques such as CCPD. When employed in the ICU setting, the patient's maintenance outpatient regimen is typically continued. However, adjustments such as increased exchange frequency, altered dialysate dextrose concentration, and, rarely, increased dialysate volume can be used to enhance solute and volume removal as clinically indicated.

Guidelines for the intensity of renal support in critically ill patients with AKI, particularly those on CRRT, were previously based on several single-center studies suggesting that more dialysis leads to better outcomes [23–25].

Today's guidelines have been strongly influenced by a large multicenter US trial, the Acute Renal Failure (ATN) trial, which tested the hypothesis that more intensive RRT in critically ill patients would decrease mortality and promote recovery of renal function [26]. A total of 1,124 patients at 27 centers were randomized to intensive therapy (IT) and less intensive therapy (LIT). An integrated treatment strategy was used. Hemodynamically stable patients were managed by IHD, whereas unstable patients were managed with CVVHD or sustained low-efficiency dialysis (SLED). Patients were permitted to move from one modality to another as their hemodynamic status changed. For the IT group, IHD and SLED were performed six times per week, and CVVHDF provided an effluent flow rate of 35 mL/kg/h. For the LIT group, IHD and SLED were performed three times per week, and CVVHDF provided an effluent flow of 20 mL/kg/h. The 60-day mortality was no different (53.6% for IT and 51.5% for LIT). There was no difference between the two groups regarding duration of RRT, rate of recovery of renal function, or recovery from nonrenal organ failure. Another multicenter, randomized trial conducted in Australia and New Zealand compared the effect of CRRT at two levels of intensity [27]. Higher intensity therapy did not reduce mortality at 90 days. Most recently, a multinational European trial revealed no differences in 28-day survival or several other pertinent endpoints, among patients with septic shock and AKI treated with high-volume or standard volume continuous hemofiltration at prescribed doses of 70 or 35 mL/kg/h [28].

Collectively, these studies do not imply that the dose of RRT is unimportant in managing AKI. Patients in the LIT group in the ATN study were better dialyzed than patients receiving usual care in typical clinical practice. Dialysis

TABLE 201.5

General Indications for Renal Replacement Therapy in Patients with Acute Kidney Injury

Indication	Characteristics
Metabolic abnormality	BUN > 100 mg/dL
	Hyperkalemia >6 mEq/L with ECG changes
	Dysnatremia
Acidosis	pH < 7.00
	Lactic acidosis related to metformin use
Anuria/oliguria	<0.5 mL/kg/h × 6 h
	<0.5 mL/kg/h × 12 h
	<0.3 mL/kg/h × 24 h or anuria × 12 h
Fluid overload	Diuretic sensitive
	Diuretic resistant

BUN, blood urea nitrogen; ECG, electrocardiogram.

TABLE 201.6

Major Trials Comparing IHD and CRRT

Study	Design	*N*	Mortality (IHD)	Mortality (CRRT)	Odds of death in IHD (95% CI)	RR[a], CRRT vs. IHD	Comments
Mehta et al. [52]	RCT	166	48	66	0.63 (0.30–1.10)	35% vs. 33%	More liver failure, more MOSF in CRRT group
Augustine et al. [53]	RCT	80	70	68	1.12 (0.40–3.20)	No difference	More fluid removal, less hypotension in CRRT
Uehlinger et al. [54]	RCT	125	51	47	1.16 (0.50–2.50)	50% vs. 42%	
Vinsonneau et al. [38]	RCT	359	68	67	1.05 (0.60–1.7)	90% vs. 93%	5–6 h IHD 4 × per wk Rigorous IHD protocol
Uchino et al. [37]	Observational study	1,218	48	64		85% vs. 66%	CRRT predicted independence from dialysis
Bell et al. [44]	Observational study	2,202	46	51		92% vs. 83%	32 ICUs in Sweden Dialysis dependence at 90 d: 8% vs. 16%
Cho et al. [35]	Multicenter, observational study	398	42	55	RR of death for CRRT, 1.82 (1.26–2.62)	Not reported	Mortality risk of CRRT persists after adjustment for sepsis/liver failure
Schwenger et al. [39]	Prospective randomized	232	49.6	55.6	Not reported	Not reported	SLED treatments were 12 h

[a]Independence from dialysis.
CI, confidence interval; CRRT, continuous renal replacement therapy; ICU, intensive care unit; IHD, intermittent hemodialysis; RCT, randomized controlled trial; RR, renal recovery.

treatment (IHD or SLED) in the LIT group delivered a mean single pool Kt/V_{urea} of 1.30 that generated a mean predialysis BUN of 70. Among patients managed CVVHDF, the median time for treatment was 21 hours per day, substantially longer than times achieved in clinical practice. We support the dosing recommendation of the ATN investigators, which are generally in line with recommendations put forth in the 2012 KDIGO AKI guidelines [10]:

- IHD or SLED
  - Provide hemodialysis three times per week (alternate days).
  - Monitor the delivered dose to ensure delivery of a single pool Kt/V of 1.20 or more.
- CRRT
  - Employ large caliber catheters and systems of anticoagulation to maximize filter life.
  - Ensure effluent flow rate (hemofiltration rate + dialysate flow rate) of 20 mL/kg/h or more.
  - In convective systems which employ RF, add 25% to the prescribed effluent flow rate (RF rate) to adjust for dilutional effects if prefilter RF is used.

MODALITY SELECTION

In the United States, the hemodynamically stable patient with AKI is generally managed with IHD. The technique provides rapid solute clearance and volume removal, but it is of limited utility in the setting of hypotension. Unstable patients are more often managed by one of the CRRTs. Patients may move from one modality to another with changes in hemodynamic status. Dialysis sessions are delivered at a minimum of three times per week. More frequent sessions are often required to achieve specific volume and metabolic targets. The average ICU patient with AKI receives 3.5 L of fluid daily. It is challenging, if not impossible, to mobilize this volume (24 L per week) over three IHD sessions alone. IHD may be supplemented with additional ultrafiltration sessions to meet volume needs.

The principal RRT options are IHD and CRRTs. PD management of AKI has declined markedly over the past 30 years, although it remains an important ICU modality in developing countries [29]; furthermore, a recent meta-analysis reported no differences of pooled mortality between patients with AKI treated with PD versus IHD or CRRT [30]. SLED is used by a minority of programs, often in response to resource considerations.

IHD versus CRRT

Modality selection in AKI is highly variable and appears to be changing in favor of CRRT. Historically, most patients in the United States were treated with IHD. However, a recent survey of VA and US Academic Medical Centers reported a mix of IHD and CRRT modalities [31]. Internationally, CRRT is often the preferred modality for managing AKI [32,33]. The shift toward CRRT is driven by a number of important practical as well as some theoretical advantages for CRRT over IHD:

- CRRT induces less hypotension and is better tolerated by the patient with unstable hemodynamics.
- CRRT permits removal of large fluid volumes without inducing or exacerbating hypotension.
- Because CRRT induces less hypotension, it may promote renal recovery from AKI by avoiding repeated episodes of renal hypoperfusion.
- CRRT provides greater solute clearance than alternate day IHD.
- Because CRRT minimizes/limits hypotension and disequilibrium, it may better preserve cerebral perfusion in acute brain injury and in hepatic failure.
- The convective clearance of CRRT, particularly CVVH, may remove harmful immunomodulatory substances in sepsis.

The major studies comparing IHD with CRRT are summarized in Table 201.6. Retrospective studies show no survival advantage of modality selection in AKI [34,35], and some report higher mortality among the CRRT–treated patients. Prospective randomized trials of different RRT modalities have reported variable results. Some studies suggest improved hemodynamic stability with CCRT [36,37], although none have demonstrated a difference in patient survival or recovery of renal function between CRRT and IHD.

In the largest and most rigorous prospective multicenter trial to date [38], 359 patients from 21 medical centers were randomized to IHD or CVVHDF. Severity of illness was similar among the groups. Pressor support was common at randomization (86% for IHD and 89% for CVVHD) as was sepsis (69% and 56%). Crossover from the IHD group to CVVHDF was low (3.3%), and both groups used the same dialyzer membranes. Sixty-day survival and recovery of renal function were identical among the groups. Unlike other prospective studies, this trial reported similar rates of hypotension. Hemodynamic stability among IHD patients was meticulously promoted by routine use of cool dialysate (35°C), very high dialysate sodium concentration (150 mmol), isovolemic connections, progressive ultrafiltration, and extended dialysis time (>5 hours). This study stands as evidence that most patients could be managed with IHD irrespective of hemodynamics, though it is worth noting that the mean IHD treatment time in this study was 5.2 hours.

A recent study of critically ill patients in a surgical ICU from Germany found no difference in mortality or intradialytic hypotension, between patients treated with CVVH and those treated managed with SLED, consisting of 12-hour dialysis treatments with blood flows of 100 to 120 mL per minute [39]. The SLED group had shorter duration of ICU stay and mechanical ventilation, as well as fewer blood transfusions. In addition, a cost analysis indicated that SLED required significantly less nursing time than CVVH.

Though several previous meta-analyses and systematic reviews concluded that no specific modality of renal support provides a survival advantage or increased freedom from long-term dialysis for patients with AKI [40–42], a recent meta-analysis did report higher rates of dialysis dependence among AKI survivors initially treated with IHD [43]. Included with this analysis were two large studies [37,44] that demonstrated significantly higher dialysis dependence among survivors initially treated with IHD, although mortality was higher for patients managed with CRRT.

In summary, no evidence exists to support a survival advantage of a specific RRT modality in AKI. Some prospective trials suggest improved hemodynamic stability with CRRT, and some retrospective analyses suggest enhanced recovery of renal function. In many circumstances, modality selection is guided by medical and nursing expertise and by availability of equipment or nursing support. When both modalities are available, selection should be individualized according to clinical status. Most US tertiary care centers opt for CRRT in settings of hemodynamic instability. IHD can be used successfully in hemodynamically unstable patients, provided ultrafiltration rates are reduced by increasing the frequency and duration of treatment. Acute hemodialysis programs may be insufficiently staffed to perform high-frequency (five to six times per week) and/or extended (>5 hours) dialysis. The same staffing limitations have lead many US programs to extend the indications for CRRT to the patient with stable hemodynamics, but with severe volume overload and large obligate fluid intake.

Recommendations

We support the practice of most US centers and recommend CRRT over IHD for the management of AKI in the following clinical settings:

- Hypotension requiring pressor support
- Massive volume overload with high obligate fluid intake
- Highly catabolic patients who have failed to reduce BUN less than 80 mg per dL over three IHD sessions
- AKI in the setting of severe liver failure

Technical recommendations:

- We favor CVVH because of its simplicity. There is no evidence that CVVH is associated with better outcomes than CVVHD or CVVHDF [45].
- Regardless of the CRRT modality, the prescribed Vef should be 20 to 25 mL/kg/h.

Discontinuation of Therapy

Recovery of renal function is traditionally defined by the reversal of oliguria and progressive decline in serum creatinine. Increased urine volume may not be apparent in the nonoliguric patient. If the CRRT patient is intensively treated, the serum creatinine may be normal, making it impossible to detect a spontaneous decline. We define recovery of renal function according to the criteria used in the ATN study [26]:

- Urine volume exceeding 30 mL per hour (720 mL per day)
- 6-hour timed urine collection to compute creatinine clearance:

$$C_{creat} = U_{creat} \times \text{volume}/P_{creat} \div 360$$

<12 mL per minute	continue CRRT
12–20 mL per minute	individualize ongoing CRRT
20 mL per minute	discontinue CRRT

COMPLICATIONS OF RENAL REPLACEMENT THERAPY

A comprehensive discussion of RRT complications is beyond the scope of this chapter. For example, complications of central venous catheter placement are discussed in Chapter 6. However, we review selected complications of dialytic support that are common in the ICU setting.

Infection

Infection is a common complication of all RRT modalities. For IHD and CRRT, infection is usually associated with hemodialysis catheter use and may result in interruption of RRT and increased mortality. The largest prospective randomized study comparing internal jugular and femoral catheters showed no difference of the risk for infection after 5 days [46]. This trial randomly assigned 750 patients to receive either jugular or femoral vein catheterization. The rate of catheter-related sepsis was the same for both groups (1.5 vs. 2.3 per 1,000 catheter days for femoral and jugular venous catheterization, respectively). Hematomas were significantly more common for jugular compared with femoral cannulation (3.6% vs. 1.1%). Thus, femoral catheters may be acceptable for short-term use.

Peritonitis is a common infectious complication of PD and is the leading cause of catheter removal and modality conversion. It typically results from bacterial contamination during the exchange procedure or migration along the catheter tunnel. Symptoms and signs include fever, abdominal pain and tenderness, and cloudy dialysate effluent. The peritoneal fluid white blood cell count of greater than 100 cells per mL with at least 50% neutrophils indicates bacterial infection; however, a lymphocyte-predominate cell count may accompany fungal or mycobacterial infections. When peritonitis is suspected, PD fluid cultures should be done prior to antibiotic therapy. *Staphylococcus aureus* and *Staphylococcus epidermidis* are common causes, however; polymicrobial and fungal infections should receive special consideration in the ICU. Patients with suspected peritonitis should receive empiric antibiotics to cover both Gram-positive and Gram-negative organisms, pending culture results.

Electrolyte and Acid–Base Disorders

All forms of RRT can cause a variety of electrolyte and acid–base disturbances. These are most common with CVVH, because convective losses of large volumes of plasma can easily lead to hypocalcemia, hypomagnesemia, hypophosphatemia, hypokalemia, and metabolic acidosis if RF and solute supplementation are not carefully adjusted. Measurements of serum electrolytes are needed at least daily and may be required more frequently in many clinical situations. With IHD and CVVHD, metabolic disturbances are less frequent, because the dialysate composition is adjusted to avoid excessive potassium removal and usually maintains calcium and magnesium levels while supplementing bicarbonate. Hypophosphatemia frequently complicates convective modalities such as CVVH, although it is less common with diffusive RRT.

Access Thrombosis

Thrombosis of vascular access is a frequent complication of RRT. AVF or AVG thrombosis often occurs in the setting of hypotension or severe volume depletion, particularly if there is stenosis of the venous system proximal to the access. AVGs are much more prone to thrombosis than AVFs. The diagnosis is usually obvious, because the access will no longer have a palpable thrill or an audible bruit. In cases of incomplete or impending thrombosis, cannulation of the access may reveal the presence of clots. Rarely, duplex ultrasound of the access is needed to confirm thrombosis. If possible, the access patency should be reestablished by either surgical thrombectomy or mechanical or chemical thrombolysis. The decision to repair or revise the AVF or AVG, as well as the approach used, will depend on the patient's clinical status and the expertise and equipment available.

Less commonly, hemodialysis catheters can develop thrombus, typically manifesting as impaired blood flow through the catheter. A thrombolytic can be instilled into the catheter and allowed to dwell; if this fails to restore blood flow after multiple attempts, the catheter likely needs to be replaced.

Hypotension

Hypotension often complicates volume removal by IHD. Severe reductions in blood pressure during dialysis limit ultrafiltration, perpetuate renal injury, and compromise perfusion to other vital organs. The pathophysiology of intradialytic hypotension involves left ventricular (LV) underfilling and inadequate reactive (pressor) response to decreasing volume. The rate of ultrafiltration, the magnitude of fluid shifts between the extracellular and intracellular compartments, and the plasma refill rate (as fluid moves from the interstitium to plasma) determine LV filling pressure. The risk of hypotension during IHD can be reduced by several methods:

- Reduce ultrafiltration rate by extending the duration of treatment
- Reduce ultrafiltration volume by increasing frequency of treatment
- Minimize intracellular fluid shifts by employing sodium modeling
- Potentiate vasoconstrictor tone by cooling the dialysate as low as 35°C
- Enhance plasma refill rate by infusions of albumin
- Promote vasoconstrictor tone with high dialysate calcium
- Promote vasoconstrictor tone with midodrine prior to dialysis
- Promote vasoconstrictor tone with norepinephrine or vasopressin

References

1. Scheel PJ, Liu M, Rabb H: Uremic lung: new insights into a forgotten condition. *Kidney Int* 74(7):849–851, 2008. doi: 10.1038/ki.2008.390.
2. Bagshaw SM, Brophy PD, Cruz D, et al: Fluid balance as a biomarker: impact of fluid overload on outcome in critically ill patients with acute kidney injury. *Crit Care* 12(4):169, 2008. doi: 10.1186/cc6948.
3. Sutherland SM, Zappitelli M, Alexander SR, et al: Fluid overload and mortality in children receiving continuous renal replacement therapy: the prospective pediatric continuous renal replacement therapy registry. *Am J Kidney Dis* 55(2):316–325, 2010. doi: 10.1053/j.ajkd.2009.10.048.
4. Boyd JH, Forbes J, Nakada T, et al: Fluid resuscitation in septic shock: a positive fluid balance and elevated central venous pressure are associated with increased mortality. *Crit Care Med* 39(2):259–265, 2011. doi: 10.1097/CCM.0b013e3181feeb15.
5. Mehta R: Indications for dialysis in the ICU: renal replacement vs. renal support. *Blood Purif* 19:227–232, 2001.
6. Lim W, Cook DJ, Crowther MA: Safety and efficacy of low molecular weight heparins for hemodialysis in patients with end-stage renal failure: a meta-analysis of randomized trials. *J Am Soc Nephrol* 15(12):3192–3206, 2004. doi:10.1097/01.ASN.0000145014.80714.35.
7. Wu MY, Hsu YH, Bai CH, et al: Regional citrate versus heparin anticoagulation for continuous renal replacement therapy: A meta-analysis of randomized controlled trials. *Am J Kidney Dis* 59(6):810–818, 2012. doi: 10.1053/j.ajkd.2011.11.030.
8. Morabito S, Pistolesi V, Tritapepe L, et al: In-depth review regional citrate anticoagulation for rrts in critically ill patients with AKI. *Clin J Am Soc Nephrol* 9(30):2173–2188, 2014. doi: 10.2215/CJN.01280214.
9. Oudemans-van Straaten HM, Ostermann M: Bench-to-bedside review: citrate for continuous renal replacement therapy, from science to practice. *Crit Care* 16(6):249, 2012. doi: 10.1186/cc11645.
10. KDIGO Clinical Practice Guideline for Acute Kidney Injury. *Kidney Int* 2(1):i–iv; 1–138, 2012. doi: 10.1159/000339789.
11. Kutsogiannis DJ, Gibney RTN, Stollery D, et al: Regional citrate versus systemic heparin anticoagulation for continuous renal replacement in critically ill patients. *Kidney Int* 67(6):2361–2367, 2005. doi: 10.1111/j.1523-1755.2005.00342.x.
12. Collage RD, Howell GM, Zhang X, et al: Calcium supplementation during sepsis exacerbates organ failure and mortality via calcium/calmodulin-dependent protein kinase kinase signaling. *Crit Care Med* 41(11):e352–e360, 2013. doi: 10.1097/CCM.0b013e31828cf436.
13. Thakar CV, Rousseau J, Leonard AC: Timing of dialysis initiation in AKI in ICU: international survey. *Crit Care* 16(6):R237, 2012. doi: 10.1186/cc11906.
14. Uchino S, Kellum JA, Bellomo R, et al: Acute renal failure in critically ill patients—a multinational, multicenter study. *JAMA J Am Med Assoc* 294(7):813–818, 2005.
15. Vaara S, Reinikainen M, Wald R, et al; The FINNAKI Study Group: Timing of RRT based on the presence of conventional indications. *Clin J Am Soc Nephrol* 9:1577–1585, 2014. doi: 10.2215/CJN.12691213.
16. Bagshaw SM, Uchino S, Bellomo R, et al: Timing of renal replacement therapy and clinical outcomes in critically ill patients with severe acute kidney injury. *J Crit Care* 24(1):129–140, 2009. doi: 10.1016/j.jcrc.2007.12.017.
17. Jamale TE, Hase N, Kulkarni M, et al: Earlier-start versus usual-start dialysis in patients with community-acquired acute kidney injury: a randomized controlled trial. *Am J Kidney Dis* 62(6):1116–1121, 2013. doi: 10.1053/j.ajkd.2013.06.012.
18. Gaudry S, Hajage D, Schortgen F, et al: Comparison of two strategies for initiating renal replacement therapy in the intensive care unit: study protocol for a randomized controlled trial (AKIKI). *Trials* 16(1):1–9, 2015. doi: 10.1186/s13063-015-0718-x.
19. Seabra VF, Balk EM, Liangos O, et al: Timing of renal replacement therapy initiation in acute renal failure: a meta-analysis. *Am J Kidney Dis* 52(2):272–284, 2008. doi: 10.1053/j.ajkd.2008.02.371.
20. Karvellas CJ, Farhat MR, Sajjad I, et al: A comparison of early versus late initiation of renal replacement therapy in critically ill patients with acute kidney injury: a systematic review and meta-analysis. *Crit Care* 15(1):R72, 2011. doi: 10.1186/cc10061.
21. Palevsky PM: Indications and timing of renal replacement therapy in acute kidney injury. *Crit Care Med* 36[4 Suppl]:S224–S228, 2008. doi: 10.1097/CCM.0b013e318168e3fb.
22. Gibney N, Hoste E, Burdmann EA, et al: Timing of initiation and discontinuation of renal replacement therapy in AKI: unanswered key questions. *Clin J Am Soc Nephrol* 3(3):876–880, 2008. doi: 10.2215/CJN.04871107.

23. Schiffl H, Lang SM, Fischer R: Daily hemodialysis and the outcome of acute renal failure. *N Engl J Med* 346(5):305–310, 2002.
24. Ronco C, Bellomo R, Homel P, et al: Effects of different doses in continuous veno-venous haemofiltration on outcomes of acute renal failure: a prospective randomised trial. *Lancet* 356(9223):26–30, 2000. doi: 10.1016/S0140-6736(00)02430-2.
25. Saudan P, Niederberger M, De Seigneux S, et al: Adding a dialysis dose to continuous hemofiltration increases survival in patients with acute renal failure. *Kidney Int* 70(7):1312–1317, 2006. doi: 10.1038/sj.ki.5001705.
26. The VA/NIH Acute Renal Failure Trial Network: Intensity of renal support in critically ill patients with acute kidney injury: the VA/NIH acute renal failure trial network. *N Engl J Med* 359(1):7–20, 2008. doi: 10.1056/NEJMoa1404304.
27. Bellomo R, Cass A, Cole L, et al: Intensity of continuous renal-replacementt herapy in critically ill patients. *N Engl J Med* 361(17):1627–1638, 2009. doi: 10.1056/NEJMoa1404595.
28. Joannes-Boyau O, Honoré PM, Perez P, et al: High-volume versus standard-volume haemofiltration for septic shock patients with acute kidney injury (IVOIRE study): a multicentre randomized controlled trial. *Intensive Care Med* 39(9):1535–1546, 2013. doi: 10.1007/s00134-013-2967-z.
29. Ponce D, Caramori JT, Barretti P, et al: Peritoneal dialysis in acute kidney injury: Brazilian experience. *Perit Dial Int* 32(3):242–246, 2012. doi: 10.3747/pdi.2012.00089.
30. Chionh CY, Soni SS, Finkelstein FO, et al: Use of peritoneal dialysis in AKI: a systematic review. *Clin J Am Soc Nephrol* 8(10):1649–1660, 2013. doi:10.2215/CJN.01540213.
31. Overberger P, Pesacreta M, Palevsky PM: Management of renal replacement therapy in acute kidney injury: a survey of practitioner prescribing practices. *Clin J Am Soc Nephrol* 2(4):623–630, 2007. doi: 10.2215/CJN.00780207.
32. Gatward JJ, Gibbon GJ, Wrathall G, et al: Renal replacement therapy for acute renal failure: a survey of practice in adult intensive care units in the United Kingdom. *Anaesthesia* 63(9):959–966, 2008. doi: 10.1111/j.1365-2044.2008.05514.x.
33. Legrand M, Darmon M, Joannidis M, et al: Management of renal replacement therapy in ICU patients: an international survey. *Intensive Care Med* 39(1):101–108, 2013. doi: 10.1007/s00134-012-2706-x.
34. Guérin C, Girard R, Selli JM, et al: Intermittent versus continuous renal replacement therapy for acute renal failure in intensive care units: results from a multicenter prospective epidemiological survey. *Intensive Care Med* 28(10):1411–1418, 2002. doi: 10.1007/s00134-002-1433-0.
35. Cho KC, Himmelfarb J, Paganini E, et al: Survival by dialysis modality in critically ill patients with acute kidney injury. *J Am Soc Nephrol* 17(11):3132–3138, 2006. doi: 10.1681/ASN.2006030268.
36. John S: Effects of continuous haemofiltration vs intermittent haemodialysis on systemic haemodynamics and splanchnic regional perfusion in septic shock patients: a prospective, randomized clinical trial. *Nephrol Dial Transpl* 16:320–327, 2001. doi: 10.1093/ndt/16.2.320.
37. Uchino S, Bellomo R, Kellum J: Patient and kidney survival by dialysis modality in criticall ill patients with acute kidney injury. *Int J Artif Organs* 30:281–292, 2007.
38. Vinsonneau C, Camus C, Combes A, et al: Continuous venovenous haemodiafiltration versus intermittent haemodialysis for acute renal failure in patients with multiple-organ dysfunction syndrome: a multicentre randomised trial. *Lancet* 368(9533):379–385, 2006. doi: 10.1016/S0140-6736(06)69111-3.
39. Schwenger V, Weigand MA, Hoffmann O, et al: Sustained low efficiency dialysis using a single-pass batch system in acute kidney injury—a randomized interventional trial: the REnal Replacement Therapy Study in Intensive Care Unit PatiEnts. *Crit Care* 16(5):451, 2012. doi: 10.1186/cc11815.
40. Rabindranath K, Adams J, Macleod AM, et al: Intermittent versus continuous renal replacement therapy for acute renal failure in adults. *Cochrane Database Syst Rev* (3):CD003773, 2007. doi: 10.1002/14651858.CD003773.pub3.
41. Pannu N, Klarenbach S, Wiebe N, et al: Renal replacement therapy in patients with acute renal failure. *JAMA J Am Med Assoc* 299(7):793–805, 2008.
42. Bagshaw SM, Berthiaume LR, Delaney A, et al: Continuous versus intermittent renal replacement therapy for critically ill patients with acute kidney injury: a meta-analysis. *Crit Care Med* 36(2):610–617, 2008. doi: 10.1097/01.CCM.0B013E3181611F552.
43. Schneider AG, Bellomo R, Bagshaw SM, et al: Choice of renal replacement therapy modality and dialysis dependence after acute kidney injury: A systematic review and meta-analysis. *Intensive Care Med* 39(6):987–997, 2013. doi: 10.1007/s00134-013-2864-5.ww
44. Bell M, Granath F, Schön S, et al: Continuous renal replacement therapy is associated with less chronic renal failure than intermittent haemodialysis after acute renal failure. *Intensive Care Med* 33(5):773–780, 2007. doi: 10.1007/s00134-007-0590-6.
45. Friedrich JO, Wald R, Bagshaw SM, et al: Hemofiltration compared to hemodialysis for acute kidney injury: systematic review and meta-analysis. *Crit Care* 16(4):R146, 2012. doi: 10.1186/cc11458.
46. Parienti J, Thirion M: Femoral vs jugular venous catheterization and risk of nosocomial events in adults. *JAMA J Am Med Assoc* 299(20):2413–2422, 2008. doi: 10.1001/jama.299.20.2413.
47. Gettings LG, Reynolds HN, Scalea T: Outcome in post-traumatic acute renal failure when continuous renal replacement therapy is applied early vs. late. *Intensive Care Med* 25(8):805–813, 1999. doi: 10.1007/s001340050956.
48. Bouman CS, Oudemans-Van Straaten HM, Tijssen JG, et al: Effects of early high-volume continuous venovenous hemofiltration on survival and recovery of renal function in intensive care patients with acute renal failure: a prospective, randomized trial. *Crit Care Med* 30(10):2205–2211, 2002. doi: 10.1097/01.CCM.0000030444.21921.EF.
49. Demirkiliç U, Kuralay E, Yenicesu M, et al: Timing of replacement therapy for acute renal failure after cardiac surgery. *J Card Surg* 19(1):17–20, 2004.
50. Elahi MM, Yann Lim M, Joseph RN, et al: Early hemofiltration improves survival in post-cardiotomy patients with acute renal failure. *Eur J Cardio Thoracic Surg* 26(5):1027–1031, 2004. doi: 10.1016/j.ejcts.2004.07.039.
51. Liu KD, Himmelfarb J, Paganini E, et al: Timing of initiation of dialysis in critically ill patients with acute kidney injury. *Clin J Am Soc Nephrol* 1(5):915–919, 2006. doi: 10.2215/CJN.01430406.
52. Mehta RL, McDonald B, Gabbai FB, et al: A randomized clinical trial of continuous versus intermittent dialysis for acute renal failure. *Kidney Int* 60(3):1154–1163, 2001. doi: 10.1046/j.1523-1755.2001.0600031154.x.
53. Augustine JJ, Sandy D, Seifert TH, et al: A randomized controlled trial comparing intermittent with continuous dialysis in patients with ARF. *Am J Kidney Dis* 44(6):1000–1007, 2004. doi: 10.1053/j.ajkd.2004.08.022.
54. Uehlinger DE, Jakob SM, Ferrari P, et al: Comparison of continuous and intermittent renal replacement therapy for acute renal failure. *Nephrol Dial Transplant* 20(8):1630–1637, 2005. doi: 10.1093/ndt/gfh880.

Chapter 202 ▪ Drug Dosing in Renal and Hepatic Failure: A Pharmacokinetic Approach to the Critically Ill Patient

BRIAN S. SMITH • SHUSEN SUN • KYLE FRAIELLI • REENU NATHAN

Estimates of the incidence of preventable adverse drug events in the intensive care unit (ICU) range from 10 up to 40 per 1,000 patient-days [1,2]. Patients in an ICU are approximately twice as likely to experience an adverse drug event when compared with patients on a general medicine unit. This increased risk is likely a result of the greater number of medical problems faced by patients in the ICU plus their wider range of drug exposures. Critically ill patients are also at increased risk for developing renal dysfunction, because acute kidney injury (AKI) occurs in 7% to 50% of all adults admitted to an ICU and is associated with a several-fold increase in mortality risk [3–5]. Renal injury is also a risk factor for adverse drug events. As many as 45% of patients with an estimated creatinine clearance less than 40 mL per minute receive medications that are dosed as much as 2.5 times higher than the maximum recommended dosage [6]. In addition, adverse drug reactions occur in approximately 9% of patients with blood urea nitrogen less than 20 mg per dL versus 24% of patients with blood urea nitrogen greater than 40 mg per dL [7]. Adverse drug events not only place patients at increased risk for morbidity and mortality but also have a tremendous impact financially. It has been estimated that each adverse drug event increases hospital costs by $2,000 to $4,600 [8–10]. For all of these reasons, appropriate drug dosing for critically ill patients with kidney or liver injury is essential. The following review uses pharmacokinetic principles to discuss key concepts of drug dosing in critically ill patients with renal and hepatic dysfunction.

PHARMACOKINETIC AND PHARMACODYNAMIC PRINCIPLES

To design an effective and safe medication regimen, a clinician must have a general understanding of a drug's pharmacokinetic and pharmacodynamic characteristics and be able to adjust for changes in the drug's disposition that occur with critical illness, AKI, and hepatic failure. *Pharmacokinetics* relates to the principles of drug absorption, distribution, metabolism, and excretion, whereas *pharmacodynamics* describes the pharmacologic response resulting from the drug at the site of action (receptor). Clinical pharmacokinetics is the application of knowledge of drug absorption, distribution, metabolism, and excretion to design patient-specific drug regimens with the goal of maximizing therapeutic outcomes and minimizing toxicity (Fig. 202.1).

Most drugs used for critically ill patients can be modeled using linear, or first-order, pharmacokinetics. This means that the drug is eliminated from plasma at a constant rate. As the plasma concentration increases or decreases, the amount of drug eliminated increases or decreases in a directly proportional relationship. Clinically, if a drug dose is increased, the plasma concentration increases proportionally, as does the amount eliminated (Fig. 202.2). If a drug's plasma concentration is plotted versus time using a logarithmic scale, two different slopes are evident (Fig. 202.3): The upper portion is known as the α (or *distribution*) *phase*, which represents the process of achieving equilibrium between the central and peripheral compartments. When monitoring serum drug concentrations, it is important to sample after the distribution phase is complete to avoid making decisions based on falsely elevated drug levels. The *β* (or *elimination*) *phase* describes the section of the graph once distribution is completed. This phase represents drug elimination from the central compartment. The elimination rate constant (K_{el}) is obtained by calculating the slope of the line during the elimination phase, and it can be used to calculate a drug's half-life ($t_{1/2}$).

Some drugs, such as phenytoin, follow zero-order or nonlinear kinetics. *Zero-order*, or *Michaelis–Menten pharmacokinetics*, refers to removal of a constant quantity of drug per unit of time. As the plasma concentration of the drug decreases or increases, the amount eliminated remains the same. This is the result of metabolism by a saturated enzyme system capable of eliminating drug only at a constant rate, regardless of the serum concentration. Clinically, this means small increases in the drug's dose can lead to large increases in the plasma concentration; hence, the term *nonlinear pharmacokinetics* (Fig. 202.2).

PHARMACOKINETIC TERMINOLOGY

The half-life of a medication is defined as the amount of time required for the concentration of the drug to decrease by 50% and is a function of drug metabolism and elimination. The half-life of a specific drug remains constant provided that the metabolizing and eliminating processes remain constant. If a patient's renal or hepatic function declines, the half-life of the drug can be significantly prolonged.

The half-life of a medication can be used to determine the time required for a drug to reach steady state. Steady state is achieved when the amount of drug entering the body equals the amount eliminated, so plasma drug levels no longer increase. Steady-state conditions are achieved at a time approximately equal to four or five half-lives. A clinician should generally wait for steady state to be achieved before obtaining a drug serum concentration or changing medication dose. Knowledge of a drug's half-life may help estimate how long it should take for a pharmacologic or toxic effect to clear. It is also important to be aware, however, that certain drugs (e.g., azithromycin) may be pharmacologically active longer than would be predicted from serum concentrations.

The rate of drug elimination from the body is described as the K_{el}. With first-order elimination, a constant percentage of drug is removed from the plasma per unit of time and is often expressed as minutes^{-1} or hours^{-1}. The K_{el} is also inversely proportional to the drug's half-life. A drug's K_{el} and half-life are constants and do not change unless the metabolizing or eliminating processes (or both) change.

Volume of distribution is not a physiologic volume but rather a theoretical volume that relates the plasma concentration to the administered dose. It is easiest to explain the concept of volume of distribution by providing an example. If a 700-mg dose of a drug administered as an intravenous bolus to a 70-kg patient results in a calculated maximum plasma concentration of 7 mg per L, it appears as if the drug is dissolved in 100 L of fluid. The volume of distribution would be 100 L or 1.429 L per kg. Under normal physiologic conditions, however, a 70-kg adult does not have 100 L of body fluid. A large volume of distribution means that the amount of drug available to be measured in the plasma is reduced owing to distribution among peripheral compartments

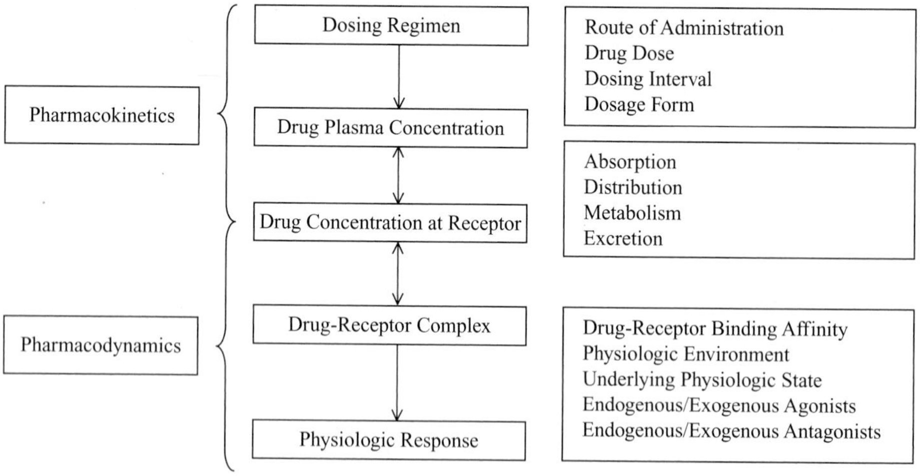

FIGURE 202.1 The relationship between pharmacokinetics and pharmacodynamics. (Adapted from Chernow B (ed): *Critical Care Pharmacotherapy*. Baltimore, MD, Williams & Wilkins, 1995, p 4.)

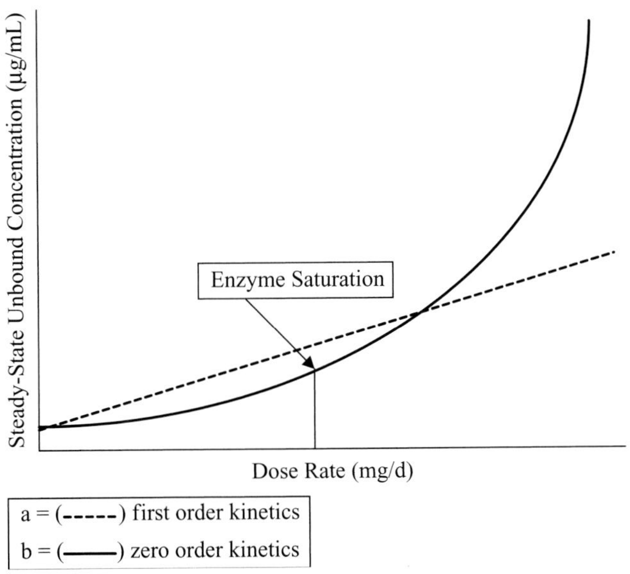

FIGURE 202.2 The effect of increasing daily dose on average steady-state drug concentrations for drugs undergoing nonlinear or zero-order pharmacokinetic modeling (*solid line*). The effect of increasing daily dose on average steady-state drug concentrations for drugs undergoing linear or first-order pharmacokinetic modeling (*dotted line*).

or binding to plasma proteins. Medications that are hydrophilic and remain in the central (vascular) compartment, and without high affinity for plasma protein binding, tend to have a lower volume of distribution with a value that is closer to the intravascular volume. Drugs that are highly lipophilic and distribute to peripheral tissues, or are highly plasma protein bound, tend to have a very large volume of distribution.

Clearance describes the volume of fluid cleared of drug over time. Clearance through an organ is determined by the product of blood flow to the organ and the extraction ratio for the organ. The *extraction ratio* is the percentage of medication removed from the blood as it passes through the eliminating organ: It depends not only on the blood flow rate but also on the free fraction of drug and the intrinsic ability of the organ to eliminate drug.

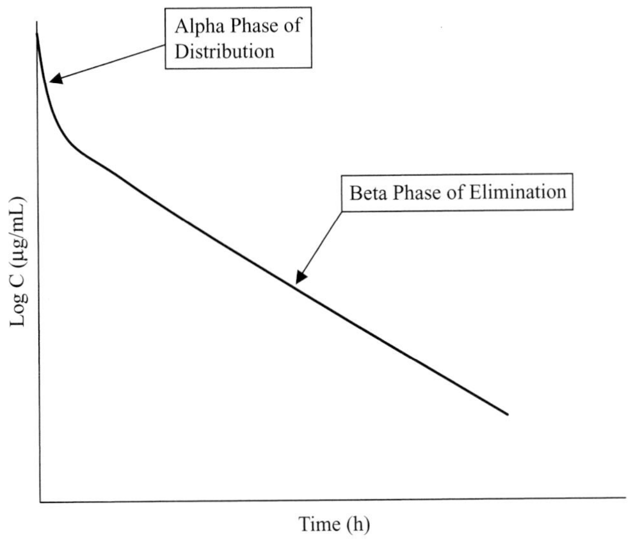

FIGURE 202.3 Logarithm of plasma concentration (Cp) versus time plot for a drug after rapid intravenous injection, delineating the α distribution and β elimination phases.

Changes in blood flow to the organ responsible for clearing the drug or any factor altering the extraction ratio of a drug can alter a drug's clearance. For example, a patient experiencing septic or cardiogenic shock may have impaired blood flow to the liver or the kidneys, hampering the clearance of a particular drug. In addition, if a pharmacologic vasopressor is added to the therapy, blood flow to the gastrointestinal tract may be compromised, resulting in a decreased absorption and transport of drug to the site of action.

RENAL DRUG EXCRETION

The primary organ of drug and drug metabolite clearance for most drugs is the kidney. There are three major processes involved in renal drug clearance: glomerular filtration, tubular secretion, and tubular reabsorption. Both critical illness and renal dysfunction can alter any of these pathways individually or in combination. Studies evaluating the effect of renal impairment on drug elimination typically examine changes in total body clearance or serum concentration, because it is difficult to determine the specific impact on each pathway individually if multiple clearance routes are affected simultaneously.

Glomerular filtration is the most common pathway of renal medication excretion. The glomerular filtration rate (GFR) for an average healthy adult is between 100 and 125 mL per minute and represents approximately 20% of total plasma flow to the kidneys. Many physiologic factors affect glomerular filtration, including hydrostatic pressure and osmotic gradients. For drugs whose primary route of elimination is glomerular filtration, excretion occurs at a rate that is directly proportional to GFR (first-order process). The degree of plasma protein binding also affects filtration because only unbound drug is sufficiently small in size to be filtered across the glomerular capillaries. To estimate the possible impact of decreased filtration, it is important for the clinician to be aware of the fraction of renal drug elimination, in addition to the excretion method for any active or toxic metabolite.

Tubular secretion refers to the active process of drug transport from the interstitial fluid surrounding the proximal tubule into the tubule's lumen. The secretion rate depends on the intrinsic activity of the transporter, proximal tubule blood flow, and the percent of free or unbound drug. Tubular secretion can be an extremely efficient process with drug clearance rates exceeding filtration clearance [11]. Impaired renal function impacts tubular secretion because endogenous and exogenous organic acids and bases accumulate and compete for the transporters required for active secretion. It is difficult to predict whether secretion will be increased or diminished, which may ultimately lead to drug toxicity or reduced efficacy [12].

Tubular reabsorption of drugs can be active or passive. Most of the ultrafiltrate passing through the nephron is reabsorbed. As the volume of fluid in the tubule decreases with this massive reabsorption, there can be a dramatic increase in drug concentration in the tubule, which promotes passive diffusion from inside the tubule into the plasma. Manipulation of urine pH can be used to decrease drug reabsorption and, therefore, increase excretion. Urine alkalization enhances the elimination of weak acids (e.g., barbiturates) by increasing the fraction of ionized drug.

PHARMACOKINETIC CHANGES IN CRITICALLY ILL PATIENTS WITH RENAL DYSFUNCTION

The pharmacokinetics of drugs used in critically ill patients can be altered as a function of the many dynamic physiologic changes that occur. Studies examining the pharmacokinetics of drugs used in the critically ill patient population are limited;

most are performed in healthy volunteers or in relatively stable patients with a specific disease state. Patients with chronic kidney disease take multiple medications, and thus have an inherently increased risk of drug interactions, particularly in the context of altered pharmacokinetics associated with worsening renal dysfunction and critical illness. The next section of this chapter addresses some of the known pharmacokinetic changes and drug interactions that may occur in critically ill patients with renal impairment.

Absorption

Drug absorption in patients with renal dysfunction may be altered for many reasons. Gastrointestinal edema, nausea and vomiting as a result of uremia, and delayed gastric emptying all affect drug absorption in this patient population. In addition, patients may have comorbidities that contribute to changes in drug absorption, such as diabetic gastroparesis, diarrhea, and cardiovascular failure. Patients with chronic kidney disease and diabetic gastroparesis often are prescribed prokinetic agents (e.g., metoclopramide or erythromycin). The use of these agents may decrease enteral absorption of medications owing to decreased gastric transit time, leading to decreased therapeutic effects or delayed onset of action [13]. Patients requiring phosphate binding medications or antacids (aluminum or calcium salts) are at risk for having these medications chelate or bind to other medications and decrease their absorption. To minimize chelation, certain medications administered enterally, such as ciprofloxacin, need to be spaced around the dosing of antacid/phosphate binders by at least 2 hours [14]. Changes in gastric pH from antacids or other acid-suppressing medications may impair the dissolution process of other enteral medications, leading to incomplete drug absorption. Bioavailability studies are often lacking for critically ill patients, because most are conducted in healthy adults. For a majority of medications, however, the bioavailability for patients with impaired renal function is unchanged or increased [15]. To avoid issues relative to uncertain bioavailability among critically ill patients, the intravenous route of administration is often preferred.

Distribution

The distribution of drugs with high binding affinity for plasma proteins can be significantly altered among critically ill patients with renal failure. Highly protein-bound drugs exist in a state of equilibrium between unbound (free) and bound drug (not free). Only the unbound drug is pharmacologically active. This means that if binding decreases, the amount of free drug available to exert a pharmacologic and toxic effect increases. Drug–drug interactions can occur when two highly plasma protein–bound drugs (>90% bound to plasma proteins) compete for the same plasma protein. If drugs such as warfarin, phenytoin, valproic acid, and salicylates (all highly bound to albumin) are administered together, displacement-mediated drug interactions may occur [16]. Drug binding interactions also occur among patients with poor renal function because of changes in the configuration of albumin. For example, the pharmacodynamic effects of phenytoin and warfarin are increased in patients with renal failure because of changes of albumin structure [17,18].

Critically ill patients often have reduced albumin levels because of malnutrition or the metabolic stress of acute illness (or both), and this can lead to higher free fractions of drugs and potentially increase the risk of toxicity. If a patient taking warfarin rapidly develops hypoalbuminemia as a result of critical illness, the result is an increased availability of free drug, resulting in an elevated international normalized ratio and potential risk for bleeding.

The volume of distribution for drugs administered to critically ill patients with renal failure can fluctuate considerably as fluid status changes. This can affect the clearance of drugs, and also protein binding, by altering the amount of free drug available to be metabolized or eliminated or both. Although it is very difficult, if not impossible, to predict these changes in drug distribution, it is important for the clinician to be aware of the risks and monitor for the signs of efficacy and toxicity so that the interactions are recognized and corrected.

Metabolism

The kidneys also actively metabolize medications, and impaired renal function can affect both renal and hepatic drug metabolism. Therefore, clinicians may adjust drug dosages to account for diminished renal metabolism as well as decreased renal elimination [19,20]. Drugs that are oxidized by the cytochrome P450 2D6 isoenzyme are more likely affected than those metabolized by other isoenzymes [21]. The clinical significance of these effects in critically ill patients with renal disease remains to be determined, and the true relevance is difficult to define, because critically ill patients often have impaired metabolic function from nonrenal causes, including hepatic damage, diminished hepatic blood flow, and use of medications that act as enzyme inhibitors or inducers.

Elimination

The kidney is an important organ for drug and metabolite elimination; however, determining drug elimination for the critically ill patient population is challenging. Critically ill patients each have a unique combination of factors that can affect renal drug clearance.

AKI is often accompanied by metabolic acidosis and respiratory alkalosis, which may affect the ionization of drug molecules and, therefore, affect tissue redistribution and clearance. A low serum albumin is often associated with AKI and can lead to an increase in filtration of free drug and increased clearance of drugs that are normally highly plasma protein bound.

Dysfunction of other organ systems can significantly alter renal drug clearance through various mechanisms. For example, renal perfusion may be reduced by low cardiac output from a cardiomyopathy or acute myocardial infarction or by shunting of blood away from the kidney to the heart, brain, and muscle secondary to increased sympathetic nerve activity. Both of these mechanisms decrease drug delivery to the glomeruli, thus reducing the clearance of drugs that are eliminated primarily by glomerular filtration. Retention of fluid may increase a drug's volume of distribution and further reduce drug clearance. States of profound vasodilation, such as sepsis, systemic inflammatory response syndrome, pancreatitis, and liver failure, may impair renal drug elimination by decreasing GFR. Patients with mechanical ventilation may have reduced cardiac output (owing to increased mean intrathoracic pressure), volume of distribution changes, and acid–base imbalance, which can also affect renal drug disposition.

ASSESSING RENAL FUNCTION

Assessment of kidney function of a critically ill patient is challenging but essential for appropriately dosing renally eliminated medications. GFR can be estimated from serum creatinine by equations that use age, gender, race, and body size as surrogates for creatinine generation [22]. However, GFR estimates remain imprecise, despite substantial advances in the accuracy of estimating equations based on creatinine during the past several years. The Cockroft–Gault equation is the most commonly used in the clinical and research settings. It estimates creatinine clearance rather than GFR and thus is expected to overestimate GFR. Appropriate clinical judgment should be exercised. The Modification of Diet in Renal Disease (MDRD) study equation is an alternative method and is the preferred equation for patients with chronic kidney disease [23]. It was derived from a study population with chronic kidney disease and underestimates the measured GFR in populations with higher levels of GFR. The MDRD study equation had greater precision and greater overall accuracy than the Cockcroft–Gault formula. The differences in calculated GFR between MDRD and Cockcroft–Gault equations will yield discordant dose adjustments in 12% to 36% of cases [24–26]. The clinician should be aware of the potential limitations of the currently available methods of GFR estimation and use clinical judgment to assess the level of renal function [27]. A more detailed discussion regarding the assessment of renal function can be found in Chapter 200. See Table 202.1 for drug dosing recommendations based upon renal function.

DIALYSIS

The clinician must often make decisions on medication dose adjustments for patients on renal replacement therapy despite a paucity of available information. It is, therefore, important to consider the dialysis system and drug characteristics that affect drug clearance, in addition to the degree, if any, of residual renal function. Failure to consider dialysis drug clearance may significantly reduce drug efficacy or result in toxicity. Detailed information regarding the many individual factors that must be considered to estimate dialysis drug clearance is discussed elsewhere [28,29]. Postdialysis replacement doses are usually necessary if clearance is particularly efficient, or residual renal function is significant. When drugs are given in multiple daily doses, at least one of the daily doses should be administered soon after the completion of dialysis. Drug dosing in peritoneal dialysis is not discussed here because it is not commonly used in critically ill patients.

Patients may benefit from therapeutic drug monitoring during medication therapy. Drug level monitoring is most useful for medications with established correlation between serum levels and drug efficacy or toxicity. Trough levels are generally drawn 0 to 30 minutes before the next dose is due for administration. Peak levels are usually drawn 1 to 2 hours after oral drug administration and approximately 30 to 60 minutes after parenteral administration to allow an appropriate period of time for tissue distribution (α phase). Peak levels are usually monitored 4 hours postdialysis for drugs with a high volume of distribution (e.g., digoxin) because tissue penetration of these medications is more extensive and, therefore, less of these drugs are available in the blood to be cleared by dialysis. As a result, the intercompartmental reequilibration postdialysis takes longer, so measurement of the level must be delayed to ensure an accurate result. Additional information regarding dialysis can be found in Chapter 201.

PHARMACOKINETIC CHANGES IN CRITICALLY ILL PATIENTS WITH HEPATIC FAILURE

The primary organ responsible for drug metabolism is the liver. Similar to renal disease, liver failure has the potential to significantly alter the pharmacokinetics of many drugs used in critically ill patients. Again, like renal dysfunction, liver failure may alter the absorption, distribution, metabolism, and elimination of a drug. There are limited data to help clinicians assess the impact of liver failure on drug metabolism and facilitate appropriate dose adjustments. Consequently, it is imperative for ICU clinicians to understand the pharmacokinetic and pharmacodynamic profiles of a drug in order to discern the potential effects hepatic failure and critical illness may have on the drug.

Absorption

Drugs administered via the enteral route are absorbed through the gastrointestinal lining, enter the portal circulation, and pass through the liver before entering systemic circulation. Some drugs are metabolized during this initial transit through the liver, a phenomenon known as *first-pass metabolism* or the *first-pass effect*. Critically ill patients with hepatic failure may have a reduced capacity to metabolize drugs, limiting the extent of first-pass metabolism. Patients with cirrhosis may have developed portosystemic shunts, further reducing first-pass metabolism effectively increasing the bioavailability of an enterally administered medication. Medications such as morphine, midazolam, and labetalol undergo significant first-pass metabolism and may have increased bioavailability when given enterally in this setting [30–32].

Distribution

Liver failure may alter a medication's volume of distribution via a reduction in plasma protein synthesis (namely albumin and α-1 acid glycoprotein), development of ascites, edema, or a combination of these factors. The effects of reduced plasma protein binding on volume of distribution in critical illness have been discussed earlier in this chapter. The role of plasma protein binding on hepatic metabolism and elimination is discussed later in this chapter.

Metabolism and Elimination

Liver failure primarily alters the pharmacokinetics of a drug by a reduction in metabolism and elimination. Three major factors that influence the hepatic metabolism and elimination of drugs are enzyme activity, hepatic blood flow, and protein binding.

The two primary pathways responsible for the enzymatic metabolism of medications are phase I metabolism and phase II metabolism. Phase I metabolism involves oxidation, reduction, and hydrolysis reactions via the cytochrome P450 (CYP450) enzyme system to convert a drug's parent compound to a metabolite. Phase II metabolism involves conjugation reactions to increase the water solubility of a parent compound or metabolite to facilitate renal elimination. In chronic liver disease, a reduction of hepatic cell number and activity may lead to a reduced ability to metabolize drugs. It is important to note that liver failure tends to reduce phase I metabolic pathways more than phase II metabolic pathways, although both can be reduced in advanced liver failure [33,34]. An example of this effect can be seen with midazolam and lorazepam. Midazolam undergoes phase I metabolism via CYP450 3A4, and lorazepam undergoes phase II metabolism via glucuronidation. Liver failure significantly reduces the metabolic clearance (phase I) of midazolam, but does not have a significant effect on the clearance (phase II) of lorazepam [35].

Critical illness has the potential to further alter both phase I and phase II metabolism depending on the disease state. For example, there is some evidence to suggest that hepatic metabolism of phenytoin may be increased after severe head injury [36]. Other conditions, such as burn injury, renal dysfunction, cholestasis, hypothermia, and some inflammatory states, have been shown to decrease hepatic enzyme activity [37]. Clinicians must also be aware of other factors that may influence CYP450 activity, such as genetic polymorphisms or drug interactions with the CYP450 system. Detailed discussion

TABLE 202.1

Guidelines for Drug Dosing in Critically Ill Patients with Renal Failure

Drug	Normal dose	Creatinine clearance: 30–50 mL/min	Creatinine clearance: 10–30 mL/min	Creatinine clearance: <10 mL/min	Extracorporeal drug removal: HD	Extracorporeal drug removal: CVVHD and CVVHDF	Notes
Acyclovir [40,41]	5–10 mg/kg IV q8h (higher doses are used in CNS infections and immunocompromised patients) [42]	5–10 mg/kg IV q12h	5–10 mg/kg IV q24h	2.5–5.0 mg/kg IV q24h	2.5–5.0 mg/kg IV q24h; administer after HD	5–10 mg/kg IV q24h	To help avoid nephrotoxicity after IV acyclovir, it is recommended to maintain urine output at >1 mL of urine/d for each 1.3 mg of acyclovir administered [43]
Amikacin [41,44]	7.5 mg/kg IV q12h	7.5 mg/kg IV q18–24h	7.5 mg/kg IV q24–48h	7.5 mg/kg IV q48h	7.5 mg/kg IV based on serum levels, re-dose with levels <5 μg/mL	7.5 mg/kg IV q24–48h	Trough levels should be <10 μg/mL
Amphotericin B (conventional) [44]	0.3–1.0 mg/kg IV q24h (maximum dose: 1.5 mg/kg)	0.3–1.0 mg/kg IV q24h	0.3–1.0 mg/kg IV q24h	0.3–1.0 mg/kg IV q48h	0.3–1.0 mg/kg IV q48h	0.3–1.0 mg/kg IV q24h	—
Amphotericin B (liposomal) [41,45]	3–5 mg/kg IV q24h (higher doses of 15 mg/kg/d have been used) [46]	3–5 mg/kg IV q24h	3–5 mg/kg IV q24h	3–5 mg/kg IV q48h	3–5 mg/kg IV q48h	3–5 mg/kg IV q24h	—
Ampicillin [47]	1–2 g IV q4–6h	1–2 g IV q6–8h	1–2 g IV q8–12h	1–2 g IV q12h	1–2 g IV q12h; supplemental doses are not needed if maintenance doses are scheduled after HD	1–2 g IV q8–12h	—
Ampicillin/sulbactam [41,47,48]	1.5–3.0 g IV q6h	1.5–3.0 g IV q8h	1.5–3.0 g IV q12h	1.5–3.0 g IV q24h	1.5–3.0 g IV q12–24h administered at the end of HD	CVVH: 1.5–3.0 g IV q8–12h CVVHD, CVVHDF: 1.5–3.0 g IV q6–8h	—
Apixaban	Nonvalvular AF: 5 mg PO q12h; VTE: 10 mg PO q12h × 7 D, then 5 mg PO q12h	Nonvalvular AF: see notes; VTE: no change[a]	Nonvalvular AF: see notes; VTE: no change[a]	Nonvalvular AF: see notes; VTE: no change[a]	Nonvalvular AF: 5 mg PO q12h (reduce to 2.5 mg if age ≥80 or weight ≤60 kg)	No dose adjustments available	Reduce nonvalvular AF dosing to 2.5 mg PO q12h if patient meets two of the three following criteria: age ≥80, weight ≤60 kg, or SCr ≥1.5 mg/dL. In patients with severe or ESRD, warfarin remains anticoagulant of choice. [a]Patients with SCr >2.5 mg/dL or CrCl <25 mL/min were excluded from trials.

Aztreonam [47]	1–2 g IV q6–8h	1–2 g IV q6–8h	Loading dose 1–2 g, then 1 g IV q6–8h	Loading dose 1–2 g, then 0.5 g IV q6–8h	Loading dose 1–2 g, then 0.5 g IV q6–8h; administer dose after HD	Loading dose 1–2 g, then 1–2 g IV q8–12h	Note that the dosing interval remains constant, and there is a reduction in dose with worsening renal function
Bivalirudin	Coronary angioplasty: 0.75 mg/kg bolus, then 1.75 mg/kg/h × 4 h [49]; myocardial infarction undergoing PCI: 0.75 mg/kg/h, then 1.75 mg/kg/h during procedure [50]	No change	1 mg/kg/h; no bolus adjustment needed	1 mg/kg/h; no bolus adjustment needed	0.25 mg/kg/h, no bolus adjustment needed	—	Metabolic clearance may be the predominant route of elimination [51]
Cefazolin [41]	1–2 g IV q8h	1–2 g IV q8h	1–2 g IV q12h	1–2 g IV q24h	1–2 g IV q24h administered at the end of HD	CCVHD: 1–2 g IV q12h CVVHDF: 2 g IV q12h	—
Cefepime [41,52,53]	1–2 g IV q8–12h	1–2 g IV q12–24h	1–2 g IV q24h	0.5–1.0 g IV q24h	0.5–1.0 g IV q24h administered at the end of HD	CCVHD: 1–2 g IV q12h CVVHDF: 2 g IV q12h	Covers *Pseudomonas aeruginosa* as well as some Gram-positive organisms
Cefotaxime [41]	1–2 g IV q8h	1–2 g IV q8h	1–2 g IV q12h	1–2 g IV q24h	1–2 g IV q24h administered at the end of HD	CCVHD: 1–2 g IV q12h CVVHDF: 2 g IV q12h	—
Cefotetan [54]	1–2 g IV q12h	1–2 g IV q12h	1–2 g IV q24h	1–2 g IV q48h	1–2 g IV q48h administered at the end of HD	1–2 g IV q12h	—
Cefoxitin	1–2 g IV q6–8h	1–2 g IV q8h	1–2 g IV q12h	1–2 g IV q24h	1–2 g IV q24h administered after HD	1–2 g IV q12h	—
Ceftaroline	600 mg IV q12h	400 mg IV q12h	300 mg IV q12h (15–30 mL/min)	200 mg IV q12h (<15 mL/min)	200 mg IV q12h, dose after HD on HD days	No dose adjustments available	Covers *Staphylococcus aureus* (including methicillin-resistant strains)
Ceftazidime [41,55,56]	2 g IV q8h	2 g IV q12h	Loading dose 2 g IV, then 0.5–1.0 g IV q24h	Loading dose 2 g IV, then 1 g IV q48h	Loading dose 2 g IV, then 1 g IV q48h administered at the end of HD	Loading dose 2 g IV, then 1–2 g IV q12h	Covers *P. aeruginosa*; has limited, if any, Gram-positive coverage
Ceftobiprole [57]	500 mg q8–12h	500 mg q12h	250 mg q12h	—	—	—	—
Ceftolozane/Tazobactam	1.5 g IV q8h	750 mg IV q8h	375 mg IV q8h	No adjustments provided	750 mg for one dose, followed by 150 mg q8h. Administer dose immediately after dialysis on dialysis days.	No dose adjustments available	—
Cefuroxime [40]	0.75–1.5 g IV q8h	0.75–1.5 g IV q8h	0.75–1.5 g IV q12h	0.75–1.5 g IV q24h	0.75–1.5 g IV q24h administered at the end of HD	0.75–1.5 g IV q12h	—

(*continued*)

TABLE 202.1

Guidelines for Drug Dosing in Critically Ill Patients with Renal Failure (*continued*)

		Creatinine clearance			Extracorporeal drug removal		
Drug	**Normal dose**	**30–50 mL/min**	**10–30 mL/min**	**<10 mL/min**	**HD**	**CVVHD and CVVHDF**	**Notes**
Cidofovir [58]	Induction: 5 mg/kg IV once weekly; maintenance: 5 mg/kg q2 wk	Contraindicated	Contraindicated	Contraindicated	Contraindicated	Contraindicated	Administer probenecid and IV hydration with normal saline with each dose; if SCr increases by 0.3–0.4 mg/dL, decrease dose to 3 mg/kg; discontinue if SCr increases by >0.5 mg/dL
Ciprofloxacin [41,47,59,60]	400 mg IV q12h	400 mg IV q8-12h	400 mg IV q24h	250–500 mg PO q24h or 400 mg IV q24h	400 mg IV q24h administered at the end of HD	200–400 mg IV q12–24h	—
Clarithromycin [61]	250–500 mg PO q12h	No change	250–500 mg PO q24h	250–500 mg PO q24h	—	—	—
Colistimethate [41]	2.5–5 mg/kg/d in 2–4 divided doses; 3–8 mg/kg/d in 3 divided doses for cystic fibrosis	SCr 1.3–1.5 mg/dL 2.5–3.8 mg/kg/d divided q12h	SCr 1.6–2.5 mg/d: 2.5 mg/kg/d divided q12–24h	SCr 2.6–4.0 mg/dL: 1.5 mg/kg/d divided q36h	1.5 mg/kg IV q24–48h	2.5 mg/kg IV q48h	CRRT dosing may be as frequent as q12h. [62]
Dabigatran	Nonvalvular AF/VTE: 150 mg PO q12h	AF: no change (75 mg PO q12h if on concomitant dronedarone or ketoconazole) VTE: no change (avoid if on concomitant P-gp inhibitor)	AF: 75 mg PO q12h if CrCl ≥15 mL/min[a] (Avoid if on concomitant P-gp inhibitor) VTE: no recommendations provided	Not recommended	Not included in clinical trials. Approximately 57% removed over 4 h.	—	[a]Dose based on pharmacokinetic data (not recommended in CrCl ≤30 mL/min)
Dalbavancin	1,000 mg IV × 1, followed by 500 mg IV 1 wk later	No change	750 mg IV × 1, followed by 375 mg IV 1 wk later	750 mg IV × 1, followed by 375 mg IV 1 wk later	No adjustment necessary (maybe administered without regard to the timing of HD)	No dose adjustments available	—
Daptomycin [41]	4–6 mg/kg IV q24h	4–6 mg/kg IV q24h	4–6 mg/kg IV q48h	4–6 mg/kg IV q48h	4–6 mg/kg IV q48h administered after HD	4–6 mg/kg IV q48h	—
Demeclocycline [63]	150 mg PO q6h	Not recommended	Not recommended	Not recommended	Not recommended	Not recommended	—
Diazepam	2–10 mg IV/IM q2–4h prn.; 2–10 mg PO q6–12h prn	No change	No change	No change	No change	No change	Active metabolites may accumulate in RF; doses should be titrated to patient response

Digoxin	IV 0.4–1.0 mg/d loading dose, 0.125–0.375 mg/d maintenance dose; PO 0.75–1.25 mg/d loading dose, 0.125–0.375 mg/d maintenance dose	Same loading dose IV/PO; maintenance dose 0.125–0.375 mg q24h	0.625 mg loading dose; IV/PO maintenance dose 0.125–0.375 mg q24–48h	0.625 mg loading dose; IV/PO maintenance dose 0.125–0.375 mg q48h	No supplement for HD	Normal loading dose, IV/PO maintenance dose 0.125–0.375 mg q36h	The volume of distribution of digoxin can decrease by up to 50% in patients with RF, necessitating dose adjustment
Dofetilide [64,65]	500 µg PO bid; IV dose for atrial fibrillation/flutter: 2.5–4.0 µg/kg bolus, repeat doses given 15 min later if conversion did not occur [64]	250 µg PO bid with CrCl 40–60 mL/min	125 µg PO bid with CrCl 20–40 mL/min	Contraindicated when CrCl <20 mL/min	Contraindicated when CrCl <20 mL/min	Contraindicated when CrCl <20 mL/min	Patients should be off amiodarone for at least 3 mo before using dofetilide; >50% of dose is excreted in urine, leading to an increased half-life in RF [65]
Doripenem [66]	500 mg IV q8h	250 mg IV q8h	250 mg IV 12 h	–	—	—	—
Edoxaban	Nonvalvular AF/VTE: 60 mg PO q24h[a]	AF/VTE: 30 mg PO q24h	AF/VTE: 30 mg PO q24h if CrCl ≥15 mL/min	Not recommended	—	—	[a]Do not use if CrCl >95 mL/min owing to increased risk of ischemic stroke. Reduce dose to 30 mg PO q24h if body weight ≤60 kg or on concomitant P-gp inhibitors.
Enoxaparin [67]	Prophylaxis: 30 mg SC q12h or 40 mg SC q24h; treatment: 1 mg/kg SC q12h or 1.5 mg/kg SC q24h	No change, use caution	Prophylaxis: 30 mg SC q24h; treatment: 1 mg/kg SC q24h	Prophylaxis: 30 mg SC q24h; treatment: 1 mg/kg SC q24h	No guidelines determined	No guidelines determined	Patients with renal failure are at increased risk for bleeding
Ertapenem	1 g IV q24h	1 g IV q24h	500 mg IV q24h	500 mg IV q24h	500 mg IV q24h		—
Erythromycin	0.5–1 g IV q6h	No change	No change	0.25–0.5 g IV q6h	0.25–0.5 g IV q6h		—
Famotidine [68]	20–40 mg IV q12h	20 mg IV q12h	20 mg IV q12h	20 mg IV q24h or 40 mg IV q48h	20 mg IV q24h at the end of HD	20 mg IV q12h	—
Fluconazole [41,47,69,70]	400–800 mg IV/PO q24h	Loading dose 400–800 mg IV/PO, then 200–400 mg IV/PO q24h	Loading dose 400–800 mg IV/PO, then 100–200 mg IV/PO q24h	Loading dose 400–800 mg IV/PO, then 100–200 mg IV/PO q24h	100–400 mg IV/PO after each HD only	Loading dose 400–800 mg IV/PO, then 400–800 mg IV/PO q24h	—
Fondaparinux	DVT prophylaxis: 2.5 mg SC q24h	No change, use caution (clearance estimated to be reduced by 40%)	Contraindicated (clearance estimated to be reduced by 55%)	Contraindicated	No guidelines determined	No guidelines determined	Treatment dose not recommended for use in patients with CrCl <30 mL/min. Use of 2.5 mg SC after HD on dialysis days, with anti-Xa monitoring has been reported [71]

(*continued*)

TABLE 202.1

Guidelines for Drug Dosing in Critically Ill Patients with Renal Failure (*Continued*)

		Creatinine clearance			Extracorporeal drug removal		
Drug	**Normal dose**	**30–50 mL/min**	**10–30 mL/min**	**<10 mL/min**	**HD**	**CVVHD and CVVHDF**	**Notes**
Foscarnet [72]	40–80 mg/kg/dose IV q8h	CrCL (mL/min/kg): >1–1.4: 30–45 mg/kg IV q8h >0.8–1: 35–50 mg/kg IV q12h >0.6–0.8: 25–40 mg/kg IV q12h >0.5–0.6: 40–60 mg/kg IV q24h >0.4–0.5: 35–50 mg/kg IV q24h	Not recommended	Not recommended	45–60 mg/kg after each HD session	—	—
Ganciclovir [73]	Induction: 5 mg/kg IV q12h; maintenance: 5 mg/kg IV q24h	Induction: 2.5 mg/kg IV q24h; maintenance: 1.25 mg/kg IV q24h	Induction: 1.25 mg/kg IV q24h; maintenance: 0.625 mg/kg IV q24h	Induction: 1.25 mg IV 3 × wk; maintenance: 0.625 mg/kg IV 3 × wk	Induction: 1.25 mg IV 3 × wk; maintenance: 0.625 mg/kg IV 3 × wk	Induction: 1.25 mg/kg IV q24h; maintenance: 0.625 mg/kg IV q24h	Accumulation of ganciclovir occurs in renal tissue [74]
Gentamicin	Varied, depends on traditional vs. high dose-extended interval dosing regimens; consult institution-specific guidelines	—	—	2 mg/kg based on lean body weight; follow levels once daily and re-dose when trough level is <2.0 μg/mL	2 mg/kg after each HD treatment	Dose based on CrCl of 25 mL/min	Trough aminoglycoside levels post-HD should be drawn 4 h after HD has stopped to allow for equilibrium
Imipenem and cilastatin [41,47,75]	500 mg IV q6h for ≥70 kg; subsequent dose adjustments are based on a total of 2 g/d (considered to be an average ICU dose); 500 mg IV q8h, 60–70 kg; 250 mg IV q6h, 50–60 kg; 250 mg IV q6h, 40–50 kg	500 mg IV q8h for ≥70 kg; 250 mg IV q6h, 60–70 kg; 250 mg IV q6h, 50–60 kg; 250 mg IV q8h, 40–50 kg	250 mg IV q6h for ≥70 kg; 250 mg IV q8h, 60–70 kg; 250 mg IV q8h, 50–60 kg; 250 mg IV q12h, 40–50 kg	250 mg IV q12h for all weights from 40 to ≥70 kg	500 mg IV q12h; administer dose after HD	500 mg IV q6–8h	Use cautiously in patients with renal impairment; adjusting dose may not be adequate to prevent seizure [76]; average time to seizure is 7 d
Levofloxacin [47,60]	500–750 mg IV/PO q24h	Loading dose 500–750 mg IV/PO × 1, then 250–500 mg IV/PO q24h	Loading dose 500–750 mg IV/PO × 1, then 250–500 mg IV/PO q48h	Loading dose 500–750 mg IV/PO × 1, then 250–500 mg IV/PO q48h	Loading dose 500–750 mg IV/PO × 1, then 250–500 mg IV/PO q48h administered at end of HD	Loading dose 500–750 mg IV/PO × 1, then 250–750 mg IV/PO q24–48h	—
Linezolid [41,47,77]	600 mg IV/PO q12h	No change	No change	No change	No change, time dose to occur after HD	No change	Metabolites may accumulate in renal failure but clinical significance is unknown [78,79]

Lorazepam	1–10 mg IV/IM q2–4h prn; 0.5–10 mg PO q4–6h prn	No change	No change	No change	No change	No change	Doses should be titrated to patient response. Use IV lorazepam with caution in patients with RF owing to propylene glycol toxicity [80]
Mannitol	0.25–2 g/kg IV q4–6h	0.25 g/kg IV q6–12h	0.25 g/kg IV q8–12h	Avoid use	Avoid use	Avoid use	Maintain serum osmolarity of 290–310
Meperidine [81]	50–100 mg IV q3–4h, titrate for pain control	37.5–75 mg IV q3–4h, titrate for pain control	37.5–75 mg IV q3–4h, titrate for pain control	25–50 mg IV q3–4h, titrate for pain control	Avoid	37.5–75 mg IV q3–4h, titrate for pain control	Normeperidine, a toxic metabolite, affects the central nervous system and can lead to seizure when meperidine is used in patients with RF
Meropenem [41,47,82,83]	1 g IV q8h	1 g IV q12h	500 mg IV q12h	500 mg IV q24h	500 mg IV q24h; administer dose after HD	0.5–1 g IV q8–12h	Seizures have occurred only in patients with preexisting seizure disorder
Metoclopramide	10–20 mg IV q6h	7.5–15 mg IV q6h	7.5–15 mg IV q6h	5–10 mg IV q6h	5–10 mg IV q6h, administered at the end of HD	7.5–15 mg IV q6h	—
Metronidazole [84]	250–500 mg IV/PO q8h	No change	No change	250 mg IV/PO q8h	Administer dose after HD	No change	Treatment for *Clostridium difficile* diarrhea; causes dark urine
Midazolam [44]	0.01–0.05 mg/kg (0.5–4 mg) IV load over 2–5 min, then 0.02–0.1 mg/kg/h titrated to response	No change	No change	0.5–4 mg/kg load over 2–5 min, then 0.01–0.05 mg/kg/h titrated to response	Guidelines not determined	Guidelines not determined	Prolonged infusions, especially in patients with RF, may result in prolonged sedation because of the accumulation of metabolites; doses should be titrated to patient response [85]
Milrinone [86]	50–75 µg/kg load over 10 min; 0.375–0.75 µg/kg/min infusion based on clinical response	Same load, 0.38–0.43 µg/kg/min infusion based on clinical response	Same load, 0.28–0.33 µg/kg/min infusion based on clinical response	25–50 µg/kg load over 10 min; 0.2–0.23 µg/kg/min infusion based on clinical response	No data	Use normal dose	85% of dose eliminated unchanged in urine within 24 h
Morphine [87]	2–15 mg IV q2–4h, titrate for pain control	1.5–12 mg IV q2–4h, titrate for pain control	1.5–12 mg IV q2–4h, titrate for pain control	1–8 mg IV q2–4h, titrate for pain control	1–8 mg IV q2–4h, titrate for pain control	1.5–12 mg IV q2–4h, titrate for pain control	Although morphine is hepatically metabolized, dose adjustment in renal insufficiency is recommended to avoid accumulation of morphine-6-glucuronide, which may have narcotic activity [88,89]

(continued)

TABLE 202.1

Guidelines for Drug Dosing in Critically Ill Patients with Renal Failure (*Continued*)

Drug	Normal dose	Creatinine clearance 30–50 mL/min	Creatinine clearance 10–30 mL/min	Creatinine clearance <10 mL/min	Extracorporeal drug removal HD	Extracorporeal drug removal CVVHD and CVVHDF	Notes
Nadolol	40–320 mg PO qd in single or divided doses	20–160 mg PO daily in single or divided doses, or use normal dose and change interval to q24–36h	20–160 mg PO daily in single or divided doses, or use normal dose and change interval to q24–48h	10–80 mg PO daily in single or divided doses, or use normal dose and change interval to q48h	Supplement 40 mg after HD	20–160 mg q24h in single or divided doses, or use normal dose and change interval to q24–48h	Alteration of the interval instead of dose is an option
Nesiritide	IV bolus of 2 μg/kg followed by a continuous infusion at a dose of 0.01 μg/kg/min; maximum dose 0.03 μg/kg/min	No change	No change	No change	No guidelines established	No guidelines established	Use of nesiritide in patients with renal insufficiency has been associated with elevations of SCr [90]
Nitroprusside [44]	0.25–10 μg/kg/min; titrate for BP control	No change	No change	No change	No change	No change	Thiocyanate, a toxic metabolite, accumulates in RF, causing seizure and coma; thiocyanate is removed via HD [91]
Norfloxacin [44]	400 mg PO q12h	No change	400 mg PO q24h	400 mg PO q24h	400 mg PO q24h	—	—
Ofloxacin [92]	300 mg PO q12h	300 mg PO q24h	150–300 mg PO q24h	150 mg PO q24h		300 mg PO q24h	—
Oseltamivir [93]	75–150 mg PO q12h	No change	75–150 mg PO q24h	—	30 mg after every other HD	—	Higher doses are recommended for treatment of H1N1 influenza infection [94]
Pancuronium	0.04–0.10 mg/kg load, then 0.01–0.06 mg/kg prn to maintain paralysis	0.02–0.05 mg/kg load, then 0.01–0.03 mg/kg prn to maintain paralysis	0.02–0.05 mg/kg load, then 0.01–0.03 mg/kg prn to maintain paralysis	Avoid use	Guidelines not determined	Guidelines not determined	—
Penicillin G [44,47]	1–4 million units IV q4–6h; 1–2 million units for most uses, 4 million units in meningitis	0.75–3 million units IV q4–6h	0.75–3 million units IV q4–6h	0.5–2 million units IV q4–6h	0.5–2 million units IV q4–6h; supplemental doses are not needed if maintenance doses are scheduled after HD	2–4 million U IV q4–6h	—
Pentamidine [40,42,95]	3–4 mg/kg IV q24h	No change	No change	3–4 mg/kg IV q24–36h	3–4 mg IV q24–36h	—	No adjustment in renal failure has been reported
Peramivir [96]	600 mg IV × 1 dose	150 mg IV × 1 dose	100 mg IV × 1 dose[a]	No recommendation	100 mg IV × 1 dose administered after dialysis	—	—
Pentostatin [97]	4 mg/m^2 q2wk	2–3 mg/m^2 q2wk	2 mg/m^2 q2wk	Not recommended	—	—	—

Phenobarbital	Status epilepticus: 10–20 mg/kg IV; 60–250 mg PO q24h	No change	No change	60–100 mg PO q24h	No change, dose after dialysis	—	Monitor levels closely; therapeutic range: 10–40 μg/mL
Phenytoin	15 mg/kg IV load, then 200–400 mg PO/IV daily divided q8–12h	No change	No change	No change	No change	No change	Monitor levels closely. Phenytoin binding is altered in uremic patients and patients with low albumin; serum levels should be monitored accordingly
Piperacillin [98]	3–4 g IV q4–6h	3–4 g IV q6–8h	3–4 g IV q6–8h	3–4 g IV q8h	3–4 g IV q8h administered at the end of HD	3–4 g IV q6–8h	—
Piperacillin/tazobactam [41,47,98,99]	Nosocomial pneumonia: 4.5 g IV q6h; moderate-to-severe infections: 3.375 g IV q6h	CrCl 20–40 mL/min: nosocomial pneumonia: 3.375 g IV q6h; moderate-to-severe infections: 2.25 g IV q6h	CrCl <20 mL/min: nosocomial pneumonia: 2.25 g IV q6h; moderate-to-severe infections: 2.25 g IV q8h	See CrCl <20 mL/min	Nosocomial pneumonia: 2.25 g IV q8h; moderate-to-severe infections: 2.25 g IV q12h	2.25–3.375 g IV q6–8h	Because HD removes 30%–40% of piperacillin/tazobactam, give a supplementary dose of 0.75 g intravenously after dialysis
Polymyxin B [100]	15,000–25,000 units/kg/d IV divided q12h	11,250–18,750 units/kg/d IV divided q12h	7,500–12,500 units/kg/d IV divided q12h	2,250–3,750 units/kg/d divided q12h	2,250–3,750 units/kg/d divided q12h	—	—
Posaconazole [101,102]	200–400 mg PO q12h	No change	No change	No change	No change	—	Monitor breakthrough fungal infections caused by variability in drug exposure
Procainamide [44,103]	50–100 mg/min IV until arrhythmia is suppressed or dose reaches 500–1,000 mg, then infuse at 2–6 mg/min; oral: 500–1,000 mg PO q4–6h	500 mg PO q6h	500 mg PO q12h	500 mg PO q12–24h	500 mg PO q24h after dialysis	—	Monitor electrocardiogram, procainamide, and NAPA levels closely in renal dysfunction. Procainamide: 4–12 μg/mL; NAPA: 5–15 μg/mL[104]
Ranitidine	50 mg IV q8h or 6.25 mg/h continuous infusion	50 mg IV q12–24h	50 mg IV q12–24h	50 mg IV q24h	50 mg IV q24h, administered at end of HD	50 mg IV q12h	—
Rivaroxaban	Nonvalvular AF: 20 mg PO daily; VTE: 15 mg PO q12h for 21 d, then 20 mg PO daily	Nonvalvular AF: 15 mg PO daily; VTE: No adjustments provided	Nonvalvular AF: 15 mg PO daily if CrCl ≥15 mL/min; VTE: avoid use	Not recommended	Not recommended	—	—
Sotalol	80–320 mg PO q12h; start with 80 mg PO q12h	Lengthen dosing interval to q24h	Lengthen dosing interval to q36–48h, based on clinical response	Dose according to clinical response	Supplement 80 mg after HD	Lengthen dosing interval to q36–48h based on clinical response	Data suggest that HD patients need a decrease in dose and increase in interval [105]
Spironolactone [88]	25–200 mg PO q24h	12.5–100 mg PO q24h	12.5–100 mg PO q24h	Not effective	Not effective	Not effective	Use should be avoided in patients with GFRs <10 mL/min; monitor for hyperkalemia

(continued)

TABLE 202.1

Guidelines for Drug Dosing in Critically Ill Patients with Renal Failure (*Continued*)

		Creatinine clearance			Extracorporeal drug removal		
Drug	**Normal dose**	**30–50 mL/min**	**10–30 mL/min**	**<10 mL/min**	**HD**	**CVVHD and CVVHDF**	**Notes**
Sulfamethoxazole and trimethoprim [106,107]	8–20 mg/kg/d; when IV, divided into q6h; when PO, divided q6–12h	No change	4–10 mg/kg/d; when IV or PO, divided q12h	4–10 mg/kg/d; when IV or PO, divided q12h	4–10 mg/kg/d; when IV or PO, divided q12h, administer dose after HD	4–10 mg/kg/d when IV or PO, divided q12h	Dosing values are based on the trimethoprim component
Ticarcillin/clavulanate potassium [41,47]	3.1 g IV q4–6h	2 g IV q4h	2 g IV q8h	2 g IV q12h	2 g IV q12h, administered at the end of HD	2–3.1 g IV q6–8h	Patients with CrCl <10 mL/min with hepatic dysfunction should receive 2 g IV q24h
Tobramycin	See gentamicin	—	—	—	—	—	—
Valacyclovir [108]	1 g PO q8h	1 g PO q12h	1 g PO q24h	500 mg PO q24h	500 mg PO q24h, administered after HD	—	—
Valganciclovir [42,73]	Induction: 900 mg PO q12;	I: 450 mg PO q12–24h	I: 450 mg PO q24–48h	Not recommended	Not recommended	Maintenance: 450 mg PO q48h [109]	—
	Maintenance: 900 mg PO q24h	Maintenance: 450 mg PO q24–48h	Maintenance: 450 mg PO q48h to 2×/wk	—	—	—	—
Valproic acid	10–15 mg/kg/d	No change	No change	May requite dosage adjustment; see comments	No change	No change	Do not infuse faster than 20 mg/min. With renal impairment, may see increase in free levels. Measurement of total concentration can, therefore, be misleading
Vancomycin [41,110,111]	Refer to institution-specific guidelines	—	—	—	1 g IV every wk, measure random vancomycin level on day 4 after dose to ensure blood levels, dose for level <10 µg/mL	7.5–15 mg/kg q12–48h	—
Voriconazole	6 mg/kg IV q12h × 2 doses; follow with 4 mg/kg IV q12h	IV not recommended	IV not recommended	IV not recommended	IV not recommended	IV not recommended	IV formulation not recommended in CrCL <50 mL/min; accumulation of the intravenous vehicle (cyclodextrin) can occur
Ziprasidone	40–80 mg PO q12h; 10 mg IM q24h	No change for PO. Caution with IM use	No change for PO. Caution with IM use	No change for PO. Caution with IM use	—	—	Injection form contains cyclodextrin sodium that is renally eliminated. Caution recommended with IM use in renal impairment

AF, Atrial fibrillation; bid, twice daily; BP, blood pressure; CNS, central nervous system; CrCl, creatine clearance; CVVDH, continuous venovenous hemodialysis; CVVHDF, continuous venovenous hemodiafiltration; DVT, deep vein thrombosis; ESRD, end-stage renal disease; GFR, glomerular filtration rate; HD, hemodialysis; IM, intramuscularly; IV, intravenous; PCI, percutaneous coronary intervention; P-gp, P-glycoprotein; PO, by mouth; prn; as needed; q; every; RF, renal failure; SC, subcutaneously; VTE, venous thromboembolism.

TABLE 202.2

Guidelines for Drug Dosing in Critically Ill Patients with Hepatic Failure

Drug	Normal dose	Child-Pugh score A (mild)	Child-Pugh score B (moderate)	Child-Pugh score C (severe)	Special circumstances/ notes
Abacavir	300 mg PO q12h OR 6`00 mg PO q24h	200 mg PO q12h	Use is contraindicated	Use is contraindicated	—
Alprazolam	0.25–1 mg PO 2–3 times a d Max: 4 mg/d	—	—	—	Hepatic impairment: reduce dose by 50%–60%; avoid in cirrhosis
Argatroban	HIT/HITTS: initial dose: 2 μg/kg/min; PCI: initial dose: 25 μg/kg/min and administer bolus dose of 350 μg/kg; Cerebral thrombus: 60 mg/d by continuous infusion for 2 d, followed by 10 mg IV twice daily for 5 d. Myocardial infarction: 100 μg/kg IV bolus followed by 2–3 μg/kg/min infusion for 6–72 h.	—	HIT/HITTS: initial dose: 0.5 μg/kg/min	—	During PCI, avoid use in patients with elevations of ALT/AST (>3 times ULN); the use of argatroban in these patients has not been evaluated.
Aspirin [112]	81–325 mg PO q24h	—	—	Avoid use	—
Carvedilol [113]	Hypertension: 6.25–25 mg PO q12h; heart failure: 3.125–50 mg PO q12h	—	—	Use is contraindicated	Extended release is contraindicated in hepatic impairment; liver impairment with cirrhosis: reduce dose by 20%
Caspofungin	Candidiasis, Aspergillosis (invasive): initial dose: 70 mg IV on day 1; subsequent dosing: 50 mg IV q24h	No adjustment necessary	Initial: 70 mg IV loading dose, then 35 mg IV q24h	No clinical experience	—
Colchicine	Acute attacks: PO: 0.5–1.2 mg, followed by 0.6 mg PO q1–2h to a max of 6 mg; IV: 1–2 mg then 0.5 mg q6h to a max of 4 mg	—	—	—	Dosage adjustment should be considered in severe hepatic impairment. Treatment course should not be repeated more than once in a 2-wk period.
Diazepam [114]	2.5–10 mg PO 2–4 times a day ICU sedation: 0.05–0.1 mg/kg IV q30min to q6h; Status epilepticus: IV 5–10 mg q5–10min, max of 30 mg	—	—	—	Patients with cirrhosis: reduce dose by 50%
Esomeprazole [115]	20–40 mg PO/IV 1–2 times a day	No adjustment necessary	No adjustment necessary	Do not exceed 20 mg IV/PO q24h	
Lamotrigine	25–375 mg PO daily in 2 divided doses	No adjustment necessaryv	Without ascites: initial, escalation and maintenance: decrease by 25%; With ascites: initial, escalation and maintenance: decrease by 50%	—	—

(*continued*)

TABLE 202.2

Guidelines for Drug Dosing in Critically Ill Patients with Hepatic Failure (*Continued*)

Drug	Normal dose	Child-Pugh score A (mild)	Child-Pugh score B (moderate)	Child-Pugh score C (severe)	Special circumstances/ notes
Methadone	2.5–40 mg PO/IV q24h	No adjustment necessary	No adjustment necessary	Avoid use	—
Naltrexone	25–50 mg PO q24h	No adjustment necessary	No adjustment necessary	Use with caution	—
Nicardipine	*IV:* initial: 5 mg/h increased by 2.5 mg/h q15min to a maximum of 15 mg/h; consider reduction to 3 mg/h after response is achieved; *immediate release*: 20–40 PO q8h; *sustained release*: 30–60 mg PO q12h	—	—	—	*Immediate release:* starting dose: 20 mg PO q12h with titration; *sustained release:* no initial dose adjustment necessary
Nimodipine [116]	60 mg PO q4h	—	—	—	Liver failure: reduce dosage to 30 mg PO q4h.
Procainamide	*Immediate-release formulation:* 250–500 mg/dose PO q3–6h; *extended-release formulation:* 500 mg–1 g PO q6h; *Procanbid:* 1,000–2,500 mg PO q12h; *IV*: loading dose: 15–18 mg/kg administered as slow infusion over 25–30 min or 100–200 mg/dose repeated q5min as needed to a total dose of 1 g. Maintenance dose: 1–4 mg/min by continuous infusion	—	—	—	Liver impairment: reduce dose by 50%
Quetiapine [117]	*Immediate release:* 25–50 mg PO 2–3 times a day. Max dose of 800 mg/d; *extended release*: 50–300 mg PO q24h. Max dose 800 mg/d	—	—	—	*Immediate release*: initial: 25 mg PO q24h; *extended release:* initial: 50 mg PO q24h
Risperidone	1–6 mg PO q24h; 12.5–50 mg IM q2wk	—	—	—	Initial dose of 0.5 mg PO q12h; initial dose of 12.5 mg IM
Sirolimus [118]	Low-to-moderate immunologic risk renal transplant patients: *Oral:* <40 kg: loading dose: 3 mg/m^2 on day 1, followed by maintenance dosing of 1 mg/m^2 once daily ≥40 kg: loading dose: 6 mg on day 1; maintenance: 2 mg once daily; high immunologic risk renal transplant patients: *Oral:* loading dose: up to 15 mg on day 1; maintenance: 5 mg/d; obtain trough concentration between days 5 and 7 and adjust accordingly	Reduce dose by 33%	Reduce dose by 33%	Reduce dose by 50%	—

Tigecycline	Load: 100 mg IV followed by 50 mg IV q12h	No adjustment necessary	No adjustment necessary	Load: 100 mg IV followed by 25 mg IV q12h	—
Tramadol	*Immediate release formulation:* 50–100 mg PO q4–6h (not to exceed 400 mg/d) *Ultram ER:* patients not currently on immediate release: 100 mg PO q24h (maximum: 300 mg/d)	—	—	*Extended release:* should not be administered	Hepatic impairment with cirrhosis: *Immediate release:* Recommended dose: 50 mg PO q12h; *Ryzolt* should not be used in any degree of hepatic impairment
Triazolam	0.125–0.5 mg PO at bedtime	No adjustment necessary	No adjustment necessary	0.125 mg PO at bedtime	Avoid use in cirrhosis
Voriconazole	100–200 mg PO q12h IV: Load: 6 mg/kg q12h for 2 doses followed by 3–4 mg/kg q12h	Reduce dose by 50%	Reduce dose by 50%	Should only use if benefits outweighs risks	—
Zolpidem [119]	*Ambien:* 10 mg PO immediately before bedtime; maximum dose: 10 mg; *Ambien CR:* 12.5 mg PO immediately before bedtime	—	—	—	Hepatic impairment: Ambien: 5 mg PO at bedtime; Ambien CR: 6.25 mg PO at bedtime

HIT, heparin-induced thrombocytopenia; HITTS, heparin-induced thrombotic thrombocytopenia syndrome; IM, intramuscularly; IV, intravenous; PCI, percutaneous coronary intervention; PO, by mouth; q, every; SC, subcutaneously; TBili, total bilirubin; ULN, upper limits of normal.

of the CYP450 system and drug–drug interactions is beyond the scope of this chapter.

The clearance of drugs by the liver is primarily determined by the extraction ratio and hepatic blood flow. The hepatic extraction ratio is the fraction of drug removed from the blood after one pass through the liver. The rate of hepatic metabolism of drugs with high extraction ratios (>0.7 or 70%) depends more on hepatic blood flow than cellular metabolism. Drugs with high extraction ratios include morphine and fentanyl. For example, if a critically ill patient is receiving intravenous morphine and has a reduction in hepatic blood flow from septic shock, a reduction in morphine metabolism secondary to the reduction in hepatic blood flow is anticipated. Conversely, the rate of hepatic metabolism of drugs with low extraction ratios (<0.3 or 30%) depends more on cellular metabolism than hepatic blood flow. Medications with low extraction ratios include lorazepam, diazepam, and methadone [38,39].

Protein binding also has an important role for hepatic metabolism and the extraction ratio of a drug because only unbound drug is able to be metabolized. Plasma protein binding can be classified as nonrestrictive or restrictive. Medications that bind in a nonrestrictive fashion are easily dissociated from plasma proteins so that free drug is available for hepatic metabolism. Changes in protein binding for drugs exhibiting nonrestrictive binding have minimal impact on hepatic metabolism. Medications that display restrictive binding have a high affinity for plasma proteins, meaning less free drug is available for metabolism. If there is a reduction of plasma proteins during critical illness, there will be an increase in free drug available for metabolism, potentially resulting in an increased extraction ratio. This phenomenon is clinically relevant only for drugs with high extraction ratios.

Estimating Hepatic Drug Metabolism

Although creatinine clearance can be a useful estimate for renal function for critically ill patients, there is currently no readily available, accurate, inexpensive method to quantify hepatic drug metabolism. Some studies have used scoring systems such as the Child's Score or Child's Score with Pugh Modification. While these scoring systems have been useful for assessing the severity of hepatic disease and predicting mortality, they do not accurately quantify the ability of the liver to metabolize medications and should be used cautiously in critically ill patients. In order to appropriately assess hepatic function as it relates to drug metabolism, a clinician must consider many factors, including laboratory data (bilirubin, albumin, and prothrombin time), clinical features (hepatic blood flow, protein binding, and ascites), other medications (drug–drug interactions), a medication's pharmacokinetic profile (absorption, distribution, metabolism, and elimination), the pharmacologic properties of the medication (efficacy and toxicity), and available monitoring parameters (drug concentration and clinical responses). It is important for the clinician to use judgment when applying these dosing recommendations in clinical practice so that drug efficacy and patient safety is optimized. See Table 202.2 for drug dosing recommendations based upon hepatic function.

References

1. Leape LL, Cullen DJ, Clapp MD, et al: Pharmacist participation on physician rounds and adverse drug events in the intensive care unit. *JAMA* 282(3):267–270, 1999.
2. Rothschild JM, Landrigan CP, Cronin JW, et al: The Critical Care Safety Study: the incidence and nature of adverse events and serious medical errors in intensive care. *Crit Care Med* 33(8):1694–1700, 2005.
3. Thakar CV, Christianson A, Freyberg R, et al: Incidence and outcomes of acute kidney injury in intensive care units: a Veterans Administration study. *Crit Care Med* 37(9):2552–2558, 2009.
4. Barrantes F, Tian J, Vazquez R, et al: Acute kidney injury criteria predict outcomes of critically ill patients. *Crit Care Med* 36(5):1397–1403, 2008.
5. Mandelbaum T, Scott DJ, Lee J, et al: Outcome of critically ill patients with acute kidney injury using the Acute Kidney Injury Network criteria. *Crit Care Med* 39(12):2659–2664, 2011.
6. Cantu TG, Ellerbeck EF, Yun SW, et al: Drug prescribing for patients with changing renal function. *Am J Hosp Pharm* 49(12):2944–2948, 1992.
7. Smith JW, Seidl LG, Cluff LE: Studies on the epidemiology of adverse drug reactions. V. Clinical factors influencing susceptibility. *Ann Intern Med* 65(4):629–640, 1966.
8. Bates DW, Spell N, Cullen DJ, et al: The costs of adverse drug events in hospitalized patients. Adverse Drug Events Prevention Study Group. *JAMA* 277(4):307–311, 1997.
9. Classen DC, Pestotnik SL, Evans RS, et al: Adverse drug events in hospitalized patients. Excess length of stay, extra costs, and attributable mortality. *JAMA* 277(4):301–306, 1997.
10. Bates DW, Leape LL, Cullen DJ, et al: Effect of computerized physician order entry and a team intervention on prevention of serious medication errors. *JAMA* 280(15):1311–1316, 1998.
11. Bendayan R: Renal drug transport: A review. *Pharmacotherapy* 16(6):971–985, 1996.
12. Reed WE Jr, Sabatini S: The use of drugs in renal failure. *Semin Nephrol* 6(3):259–295, 1986.
13. Manninen V, Apajalahti A, Melin J, et al: Altered absorption of digoxin in patients given propantheline and metoclopramide. *Lancet* 1(7800):398–400, 1973.
14. Plaisance KI, Drusano GL, Forrest A, et al: Effect of renal function on the bioavailability of ciprofloxacin. *Antimicrob Agents Chemother* 34(6):1031–1034, 1990.
15. Matzke GR, Millikin SP: Influence of renal function and dialysis on drug disposition In: Evans WE, Schentag JJ, Jusko WJ, (eds): *Applied Pharmacokinetics: Principles of Therapeutic Drug Monitoring*. 3rd ed. Vancouver, BC, Canada, Applied Therapeutics, 1992, p 91.
16. Doucet J, Fresel J, Hue G, et al: Protein binding of digitoxin, valproate and phenytoin in sera from diabetics. *Eur J Clin Pharmacol* 45(6):577–579, 1993.
17. MacKichan JJ: Influence of protein binding and the use of unbound (free) drug concentrations. In: Evans WE, Schentag JJ, Jusko WJ, (eds). *Applied Pharmacokinetics: Principles of Therapeutic Drug Monitoring*. 3rd ed. Vancouver, BC, Canada, Applied Therapeutics, 1992, p 192.
18. Swan SK, Bennett WM: Drug dosing guidelines in patients with renal failure. *West J Med* 156(6):633–638, 1992.
19. Pichette V, Leblond FA: Drug metabolism in chronic renal failure. *Curr Drug Metab* 4(2):91–103, 2003.
20. Dreisbach AW: The influence of chronic renal failure on drug metabolism and transport. *Clin Pharmacol Ther* 86(5):553–556, 2009.
21. Touchette MA, Slaughter RL: The effect of renal failure on hepatic drug clearance. *DICP* 25(11):1214–1224, 1991.
22. Stevens LA, Levey AS: Measured GFR as a confirmatory test for estimated GFR. *J Am Soc Nephrol* 20(11):2305–2313, 2009.
23. National Kidney Foundation: K/DOQI clinical practice guidelines for chronic kidney disease: Evaluation, classification, and stratification. *Am J Kidney Dis* 39(2 Suppl 1):S1–S266, 2002.
24. Stevens LA, Nolin TD, Richardson MM, et al: Comparison of drug dosing recommendations based on measured GFR and kidney function estimating equations. *Am J Kidney Dis* 54(1):33–42, 2009.
25. Golik MV, Lawrence KR: Comparison of dosing recommendations for antimicrobial drugs based on two methods for assessing kidney function: cockcroft–gault and modification of diet in renal disease. *Pharmacotherapy* 28(9):1125–1132, 2008.
26. Hermsen ED, Maiefski M, Florescu MC, et al: Comparison of the Modification of Diet in Renal Disease and Cockcroft-Gault equations for dosing antimicrobials. *Pharmacotherapy* 29(6):649–655, 2009.
27. Carlier M, Dumoulin A, Janssen A, et al: Comparison of different equations to assess glomerular filtration in critically ill patients. *Intensive Care Med* 41(3):427–435, 2015.
28. Mohammad RA, Matzke GR: Drug therapy individualization for patients with chronic kidney disease. In: DiPiro JT, Talbert RL, Yee GC, et al, (eds): *Pharmacotherapy: A Pathophysiologic Approach*. 9th ed. New York, NY, McGraw-Hill, 2014.
29. Choi G, Gomersall CD, Tian Q, et al: Principles of antibacterial dosing in continuous renal replacement therapy. *Crit Care Med* 37(7):2268–2282, 2009.
30. Hasselstrom J, Eriksson S, Persson A, et al: The metabolism and bioavailability of morphine in patients with severe liver cirrhosis. *Br J Clin Pharmacol* 29(3):289–297, 1990.
31. Pentikainen PJ, Valisalmi L, Himberg JJ, et al: Pharmacokinetics of midazolam following intravenous and oral administration in patients with chronic liver disease and in healthy subjects. *J Clin Pharmacol* 29(3):272–277, 1989.
32. Homeida M, Jackson L, Roberts CJ: Decreased first-pass metabolism of labetalol in chronic liver disease. *Br Med J* 2(6144):1048–1050, 1978.
33. Paintaud G, Bechtel Y, Brientini MP, et al: Effects of liver diseases on drug metabolism. *Therapie* 51(4):384–389, 1996.

34. Murray M: P450 enzymes. Inhibition mechanisms, genetic regulation and effects of liver disease. *Clin Pharmacokinet* 23(2):132–146, 1992.
35. Greenblatt DJ: Clinical pharmacokinetics of oxazepam and lorazepam. *Clin Pharmacokinet* 6(2):89–105, 1981.
36. McKindley DS, Boucher BA, Hess MM, et al: Effect of acute phase response on phenytoin metabolism in neurotrauma patients. *J Clin Pharmacol* 37(2):129–139, 1997.
37. Smith BS, Yogaratnam D, Levasseur-Franklin KE, et al: Introduction to drug pharmacokinetics in the critically ill patient. *Chest* 141(5):1327–1336, 2012.
38. Rodighiero V: Effects of liver disease on pharmacokinetics. An update. *Clin Pharmacokinet* 37(5):399–431, 1999.
39. Tegeder I, Lotsch J, Geisslinger G: Pharmacokinetics of opioids in liver disease. *Clin Pharmacokinet* 37(1):17–40, 1999.
40. Aronoff GR, Bennett WM, Berns JS, et al: *Drug Prescribing in Renal Failure: Dosing Guidelines for Adults and Children.* 5th ed. Philadelphia, PA, American College of Physicians, 2007.
41. Trotman RL, Williamson JC, Shoemaker DM, et al: Antibiotic dosing in critically ill adult patients receiving continuous renal replacement therapy. *Clin Infect Dis* 41(8):1159–1166, 2005.
42. Gupta SK, Eustace JA, Winston JA, et al: Guidelines for the management of chronic kidney disease in HIV-infected patients: recommendations of the HIV Medicine Association of the Infectious Diseases Society of America. *Clin Infect Dis* 40(11):1559–1585, 2005.
43. Balfour HH Jr, McMonigal KA, Bean B: Acyclovir therapy of varicella-zoster virus infections in immunocompromised patients. *J Antimicrob Chemother* 12[Suppl B]:169–179, 1983.
44. Bennett WM, Aronoff GR, Golper TA, et al: *Drug Prescribing in Renal Failure.* Philadelphia, PA, American College of Physicians, 1994.
45. Lyman CA, Walsh TJ: Systemically administered antifungal agents. A review of their clinical pharmacology and therapeutic applications. *Drugs* 44(1):9–35, 1992.
46. Walsh TJ, Goodman JL, Pappas P, et al: Safety, tolerance, and pharmacokinetics of high-dose liposomal amphotericin B (AmBisome) in patients infected with Aspergillus species and other filamentous fungi: maximum tolerated dose study. *Antimicrob Agents Chemother* 45(12):3487–3496, 2001.
47. Heintz BH, Matzke GR, Dager WE: Antimicrobial dosing concepts and recommendations for critically ill adult patients receiving continuous renal replacement therapy or intermittent hemodialysis. *Pharmacotherapy* 29(5):562–577, 2009.
48. Blum RA, Kohli RK, Harrison NJ, et al: Pharmacokinetics of ampicillin (2.0 grams) and sulbactam (1.0 gram) coadministered to subjects with normal and abnormal renal function and with end-stage renal disease on hemodialysis. *Antimicrob Agents Chemother* 33(9):1470–1476, 1989.
49. Bittl JA, Strony J, Brinker JA, et al: Treatment with bivalirudin (Hirulog) as compared with heparin during coronary angioplasty for unstable or post-infarction angina. Hirulog Angioplasty Study Investigators. *N Engl J Med* 333(12):764–769, 1995.
50. Kushner FG, Hand M, Smith SC Jr, et al: 2009 focused updates: ACC/AHA guidelines for the management of patients with ST-elevation myocardial infarction (updating the 2004 guideline and 2007 focused update) and ACC/AHA/SCAI guidelines on percutaneous coronary intervention (updating the 2005 guideline and 2007 focused update) a report of the American College of Cardiology Foundation/American Heart Association Task Force on Practice Guidelines. *J Am Coll Cardiol* 54(23):2205–2241, 2009.
51. Fox I, Dawson A, Loynds P, et al: Anticoagulant activity of Hirulog, a direct thrombin inhibitor, in humans. *Thromb Haemost* 69(2):157–163, 1993.
52. Allaouchiche B, Breilh D, Jaumain H, et al: Pharmacokinetics of cefepime during continuous venovenous hemodiafiltration. *Antimicrob Agents Chemother* 41(11):2424–2427, 1997.
53. Malone RS, Fish DN, Abraham E, et al: Pharmacokinetics of cefepime during continuous renal replacement therapy in critically ill patients. *Antimicrob Agents Chemother* 45(11):3148–3155, 2001.
54. Martin C, Thomachot L, Albanese J: Clinical pharmacokinetics of cefotetan. *Clin Pharmacokinet* 26(4):248–258, 1994.
55. Davies SP, Lacey LF, Kox WJ, et al: Pharmacokinetics of cefuroxime and ceftazidime in patients with acute renal failure treated by continuous arteriovenous haemodialysis. *Nephrol Dial Transplant* 6(12):971–976, 1991.
56. Slaker RA, Danielson B: Neurotoxicity associated with ceftazidime therapy in geriatric patients with renal dysfunction. *Pharmacotherapy* 11(4):351–352, 1991.
57. Murthy B, Schmitt-Hoffmann A: Pharmacokinetics and pharmacodynamics of ceftobiprole, an anti-MRSA cephalosporin with broad-spectrum activity. *Clin Pharmacokinet* 47(1):21–33, 2008.
58. Hitchcock MJM, Jaffe HS, Martin JC, et al: Cidofovir, a new agent with potent anti-herpesvirus activity. *Antivir Chem Chemother* 7(3):115–127, 1996.
59. Davies SP, Azadian BS, Kox WJ, et al: Pharmacokinetics of ciprofloxacin and vancomycin in patients with acute renal failure treated by continuous haemodialysis. *Nephrol Dial Transplant* 7(8):848–854, 1992.
60. Malone RS, Fish DN, Abraham E, et al: Pharmacokinetics of levofloxacin and ciprofloxacin during continuous renal replacement therapy in critically ill patients. *Antimicrob Agents Chemother* 45(10):2949–2954, 2001.
61. Peters DH, Clissold SP: Clarithromycin. A review of its antimicrobial activity, pharmacokinetic properties and therapeutic potential. *Drugs* 44(1):117–164, 1992.
62. Li J, Rayner CR, Nation RL, et al: Pharmacokinetics of colistin methanesulfonate and colistin in a critically ill patient receiving continuous venovenous hemodiafiltration. *Antimicrob Agents Chemother* 49(11):4814–4815, 2005.
63. Smilack JD, Wilson WR, Cockerill FR 3rd: Tetracyclines, chloramphenicol, erythromycin, clindamycin, and metronidazole. *Mayo Clin Proc* 66(12):1270–1280, 1991.
64. Suttorp MJ, Polak PE, van 't Hof A, et al: Efficacy and safety of a new selective class III antiarrhythmic agent dofetilide in paroxysmal atrial fibrillation or atrial flutter. *Am J Cardiol* 69(4):417–419, 1992.
65. Tham TC, MacLennan BA, Burke MT, et al: Pharmacodynamics and pharmacokinetics of the class III antiarrhythmic agent dofetilide (UK-68,798) in humans. *J Cardiovasc Pharmacol* 21(3):507–512, 1993.
66. Keam SJ: Doripenem: a review of its use in the treatment of bacterial infections. *Drugs* 68(14):2021–2057, 2008.
67. Hirsh J, Bauer KA, Donati MB, et al: Parenteral anticoagulants: American College of Chest Physicians Evidence-Based Clinical Practice Guidelines (8th Edition). *Chest* 133(6 Suppl):141s–159s, 2008.
68. Lin JH, Chremos AN, Yeh KC, et al: Effects of age and chronic renal failure on the urinary excretion kinetics of famotidine in man. *Eur J Clin Pharmacol* 34(1):41–46, 1988.
69. Toon S, Ross CE, Gokal R, et al: An assessment of the effects of impaired renal function and haemodialysis on the pharmacokinetics of fluconazole. *Br J Clin Pharmacol* 29(2):221–226, 1990.
70. Dudley MN: Clinical pharmacology of fluconazole. *Pharmacotherapy* 10(6, Pt 3):141s–145s, 1990.
71. Haase M, Bellomo R, Rocktaeschel J, et al: Use of fondaparinux (ARIXTRA) in a dialysis patient with symptomatic heparin-induced thrombocytopaenia type II. *Nephrol Dial Transplant* 20(2):444–446, 2005.
72. Aweeka FT, Jacobson MA, Martin-Munley S, et al: Effect of renal disease and hemodialysis on foscarnet pharmacokinetics and dosing recommendations. *J Acquir Immune Defic Syndr Hum Retrovirol* 20(4):350–357, 1999.
73. Czock D, Scholle C, Rasche FM, et al: Pharmacokinetics of valganciclovir and ganciclovir in renal impairment. *Clin Pharmacol Ther* 72(2):142–150, 2002.
74. Shepp DH, Dandliker PS, de Miranda P, et al: Activity of 9-[2-hydroxy-1-(hydroxymethyl)ethoxymethyl]guanine in the treatment of cytomegalovirus pneumonia. *Ann Intern Med* 103(3):368–373, 1985.
75. Fish DN, Teitelbaum I, Abraham E: Pharmacokinetics and pharmacodynamics of imipenem during continuous renal replacement therapy in critically ill patients. *Antimicrob Agents Chemother* 49(6):2421–2428, 2005.
76. Leo RJ, Ballow CH: Seizure activity associated with imipenem use: clinical case reports and review of the literature. *DICP* 25(4):351–354, 1991.
77. Mauro LS, Peloquin CA, Schmude K, et al: Clearance of linezolid via continuous venovenous hemodiafiltration. *Am J Kidney Dis* 47(6):e83–e86, 2006.
78. Brier ME, Stalker DJ, Aronoff GR, et al: Pharmacokinetics of linezolid in subjects with renal dysfunction. *Antimicrob Agents Chemother* 47(9):2775–2780, 2003.
79. Tsuji Y, Hiraki Y, Mizoguchi A, et al: Pharmacokinetics of repeated dosing of linezolid in a hemodialysis patient with chronic renal failure. *J Infect Chemother* 14(2):156–160, 2008.
80. Arroliga AC, Shehab N, McCarthy K, et al: Relationship of continuous infusion lorazepam to serum propylene glycol concentration in critically ill adults. *Crit Care Med* 32(8):1709–1714, 2004.
81. American Pain Society: *Principles of Analgesic Use in the Treatment of Acute Pain and Cancer Pain.* 5th ed. Glenview, IL, American Pain Society, 2003.
82. Leroy A, Fillastre JP, Etienne I, et al: Pharmacokinetics of meropenem in subjects with renal insufficiency. *Eur J Clin Pharmacol* 42(5):535–538, 1992.
83. Ververs TF, van Dijk A, Vinks SA, et al: Pharmacokinetics and dosing regimen of meropenem in critically ill patients receiving continuous venovenous hemofiltration. *Crit Care Med* 28(10):3412–3416, 2000.
84. Lau AH, Chang CW, Sabatini S: Hemodialysis clearance of metronidazole and its metabolites. *Antimicrob Agents Chemother* 29(2):235–238, 1986.
85. Bauer TM, Ritz R, Haberthur C, et al: Prolonged sedation due to accumulation of conjugated metabolites of midazolam. *Lancet* 346(8968):145–147, 1995.
86. Woolfrey SG, Hegbrant J, Thysell H, et al: Dose regimen adjustment for milrinone in congestive heart failure patients with moderate and severe renal failure. *J Pharm Pharmacol* 47(8):651–655, 1995.
87. Aronoff GR, Berns JS, Brier ME, et al: *Drug Prescribing in Renal Failure.* 4th ed. Philadelphia, PA, American College of Physicians, 1999.
88. Mazoit JX, Butscher K, Samii K: Morphine in postoperative patients: pharmacokinetics and pharmacodynamics of metabolites. *Anesth Analg* 105(1):70–78, 2007.
89. Portenoy RK, Foley KM, Stulman J, et al: Plasma morphine and morphine-6-glucuronide during chronic morphine therapy for cancer pain: plasma profiles, steady-state concentrations and the consequences of renal failure. *Pain* 47(1):13–19, 1991.
90. Sackner-Bernstein JD, Skopicki HA, Aaronson KD: Risk of worsening renal function with nesiritide in patients with acutely decompensated heart failure. *Circulation* 111(12):1487–1491, 2005.
91. Rindone JP, Sloane EP: Cyanide toxicity from sodium nitroprusside: risks and management. *Ann Pharmacother* 26(4):515–519, 1992.
92. Thalhammer F, Kletzmayr J, El Menyawi I, et al: Ofloxacin clearance during hemodialysis: a comparison of polysulfone and cellulose acetate hemodialyzers. *Am J Kidney Dis* 32(4):642–645, 1998.

93. Robson R, Buttimore A, Lynn K, et al: The pharmacokinetics and tolerability of oseltamivir suspension in patients on haemodialysis and continuous ambulatory peritoneal dialysis. *Nephrol Dial Transplant* 21(9):2556–2562, 2006.
94. Centers for Disease Control and Prevention (CDC): Antiviral treatment options, including intravenous peramivir, for treatment of influenza in hospitalized patients for the 2001–2010 season. Available at http://www.cdc.gov/h1n1flu/EUA/peramivir_recommendations.htm. Accessed January 26, 2010.
95. Conte JE Jr: Pharmacokinetics of intravenous pentamidine in patients with normal renal function or receiving hemodialysis. *J Infect Dis* 163(1):169–175, 1991.
96. Mancuso CE, Gabay MP, Steinke LM, et al: Peramivir: an intravenous neuraminidase inhibitor for the treatment of 2009 H1N1 influenza. *Ann Pharmacother* 44(7/8):1240–1249, 2010.
97. Lathia C, Fleming GF, Meyer M, et al: Pentostatin pharmacokinetics and dosing recommendations in patients with mild renal impairment. *Cancer Chemother Pharmacol* 50(2):121–126, 2002.
98. Dowell JA, Korth-Bradley J, Milisci M, et al: Evaluating possible pharmacokinetic interactions between tobramycin, piperacillin, and a combination of piperacillin and tazobactam in patients with various degrees of renal impairment. *J Clin Pharmacol* 41(9):979–986, 2001.
99. Valtonen M, Tiula E, Takkunen O, et al: Elimination of the piperacillin/tazobactam combination during continuous venovenous haemofiltration and haemodiafiltration in patients with acute renal failure. *J Antimicrob Chemother* 48(6):881–885, 2001.
100. Zavascki AP, Goldani LZ, Cao G, et al: Pharmacokinetics of intravenous polymyxin B in critically ill patients. *Clin Infect Dis* 47(10):1298–1304, 2008.
101. Herbrecht R: Posaconazole: a potent, extended-spectrum triazole anti-fungal for the treatment of serious fungal infections. *Int J Clin Pract* 58(6):612–624, 2004.
102. Courtney R, Sansone A, Smith W, et al: Posaconazole pharmacokinetics, safety, and tolerability in subjects with varying degrees of chronic renal disease. *J Clin Pharmacol* 45(2):185–192, 2005.
103. Gibson TP, Atkinson AJ Jr, Matusik E, et al: Kinetics of procainamide and N-acetylprocainamide in renal failure. *Kidney Int* 12(6):422–429, 1977.
104. Campbell TJ, Williams KM: Therapeutic drug monitoring: antiarrhythmic drugs. *Br J Clin Pharmacol* 46(4):307–319, 1998.
105. Dumas M, d'Athis P, Besancenot JF, et al: Variations of sotalol kinetics in renal insufficiency. *Int J Clin Pharmacol Ther Toxicol* 27(10):486–489, 1989.
106. Varoquaux O, Lajoie D, Gobert C, et al: Pharmacokinetics of the trimethoprim-sulphamethoxazole combination in the elderly. *Br J Clin Pharmacol* 20(6):575–581, 1985.
107. Mofenson LM, Oleske J, Serchuck L, et al: Treating opportunistic infections among HIV-exposed and infected children: recommendations from CDC, the National Institutes of Health, and the Infectious Diseases Society of America. *MMWR Recomm Rep* 53(Rr-14):1–92, 2004.
108. Perry CM, Faulds D: Valaciclovir. A review of its antiviral activity, pharmacokinetic properties and therapeutic efficacy in herpesvirus infections. *Drugs* 52(5):754–772, 1996.
109. Perrottet N, Robatel C, Meylan P, et al: Disposition of valganciclovir during continuous renal replacement therapy in two lung transplant recipients. *J Antimicrob Chemother* 61(6):1332–1335, 2008.
110. Rodvold KA, Blum RA, Fischer JH, et al: Vancomycin pharmacokinetics in patients with various degrees of renal function. *Antimicrob Agents Chemother* 32(6):848–852, 1988.
111. Joy MS, Matzke GR, Frye RF, et al: Determinants of vancomycin clearance by continuous venovenous hemofiltration and continuous venovenous hemodialysis. *Am J Kidney Dis* 31(6):1019–1027, 1998.
112. Tainter ML: *Aspirin in Modern Therapy: A Review.* New York, NY, Bayer Co of Sterling Drugs, 1969, p. 85.
113. Neugebauer G, Gabor M, Reiff K: Pharmacokinetics and bioavailability of carvedilol in patients with liver cirrhosis. *Drugs* 36[Suppl 6]:148–154, 1988.
114. Ochs HR, Greenblatt DJ, Eckardt B, et al: Repeated diazepam dosing in cirrhotic patients: cumulation and sedation. *Clin Pharmacol Ther* 33(4):471–476, 1983.
115. Sjovall H, Hagman I, Holmberg J, et al: Pharmacokinetics of esomeprazole in patients with liver cirrhosis (abstract 346). *Gastroenterology* 118(4):A21, 2000.
116. Gengo FM, Fagan SC, Krol G, et al: Nimodipine disposition and haemodynamic effects in patients with cirrhosis and age-matched controls. *Br J Clin Pharmacol* 23(1):47–53, 1987.
117. Green B: Focus on quetiapine. *Curr Med Res Opin* 15(3):145–151, 1999.
118. Bumgardner GL, Roberts JP: New immunosuppressive agents. *Gastroenterol Clin North Am* 22(2):421–449, 1993.
119. Langtry HD, Benfield P: Zolpidem. A review of its pharmacodynamic and pharmacokinetic properties and therapeutic potential. *Drugs* 40(2):291–313, 1990.

Section 19 GASTROINTESTINAL DISEASE PROBLEMS IN THE INTENSIVE CARE UNIT

DOMINIC J. NOMPLEGGI

Chapter 203 ■ Upper and Lower Gastrointestinal Bleeding

MICHAEL C. BENNETT • C. PRAKASH GYAWALI

Acute gastrointestinal (GI) bleeding is a common emergency that often necessitates admission to the intensive care unit (ICU). There are compelling differences in incidence, clinical presentation, severity, and mortality between lower and upper GI hemorrhage. The annual incidence rate of lower intestinal bleeding is estimated at 20.5 to 33 cases per 100,000 adult populations [1,2], whereas that of upper GI bleeding is estimated between 60 and 125 cases per 100,000 [3,4]. The incidence of upper GI bleeding has declined in those younger than age 70 years to as low as 47 per 100,000 [2,5]. *Helicobacter pylori* eradication efforts and widespread use of proton pump inhibitor (PPI) therapy may account for this decline [6]. The incidence in older populations, however, remains stable possibly from more frequent use of aspirin and nonsteroidal anti-inflammatory drugs (NSAIDs) [4,7]. The majority of upper GI bleeding are nonvariceal (80% to 90%), of which 28% to 59% are attributable to peptic ulcer bleeding [3,4]. Patients with lower GI bleeding are half as likely to present with hemodynamic compromise or require blood transfusion and have significantly higher hemoglobin concentrations at presentation compared to patients with upper GI bleeding [8]. The mortality rate from upper GI bleeding has remained largely stable at 5% to 12%, whereas mortality rate for lower intestinal bleeding remains below 5% [4,8]. Newer surgical, endoscopic, and medical therapies in conjunction with improved ICU care have improved survival [9], and this trend will likely continue in the coming years.

INITIAL EVALUATION AND RESUSCITATION

Resuscitating the actively bleeding patient takes priority over localizing the bleeding source. The immediate goals are to replete intravascular volume and prevent irreversible shock. However, even in situations of exsanguinating hemorrhage, limited attempts to localize bleeding while resuscitation continues may be required to help direct a surgical or angiographic approach.

An initial brief history and physical examination that includes serial measurement of vital signs and evaluation of the volume and character of bleeding helps determine the urgency and degree of resuscitation necessary. Tachycardia (pulse $>$ 100 beat per minute), hypotension (systolic blood pressure $<$ 100 mm Hg), or orthostatic hypotension (an increase in the pulse of $\geq$20 beats per minute or a drop in systolic blood pressure of $\geq$20 mm Hg on standing) indicates significant intravascular volume depletion [4]. Insight into volume status can also be gained from evaluation of mucous membranes and neck veins and measurement of urine output [4]. Bleeding patients need large-bore intravenous (IV)-access catheters (e.g., peripheral catheters 16 or 18 gauge or central venous access), supplemental oxygen, correction of coagulopathies, and prompt packed red blood cell transfusion to patients with tachycardia, hypotension, or hemoglobin less than 7 g per dL in most settings.

Older patients with hemodynamic compromise or shock have a higher risk of mortality; therefore, they need urgent resuscitation and close monitoring. In situations of massive hematemesis, endotracheal intubation provides airway protection and facilitates endoscopic evaluation and therapy. Chest pain may imply a superimposed myocardial infarction or dissecting aneurysm, whereas a history of abdominal vascular surgery adds aortoenteric fistula to the differential diagnoses. GI bleeding is generally not associated with significant abdominal pain, and its presence could signify hemobilia, intestinal infarction, or intestinal perforation.

Although initial aggressive resuscitation is crucial, care must be taken to avoid over-resuscitation. Recent evidence and guidelines support a more restrictive approach to transfusion, with a hemoglobin target of 7 g per dL in most cases [10,11]. Restrictive transfusion goals have been associated with improved outcomes and lower mortality, particularly for patients with cirrhosis and portal hypertension, wherein aggressive resuscitation can increase portal pressure and lead to recurrence of bleeding [10]. However, appropriate target hemoglobin for transfusion depends on the clinical context, with higher goals reasonable in patients with active cardiac ischemia or massive bleeding.

Correction of coagulopathy, when possible, is another important consideration in the initial management of acute GI bleeding. Risk of GI bleeding appears to be similar in patients taking novel anticoagulants such as dabigatran or rivaroxaban, when compared with patients on warfarin [12]. Fresh frozen plasma or prothrombin complex can be administered to rapidly reverse the effect of warfarin. Although the lack of available reversal agents for the newer anticoagulants has been problematic, this concern may soon be alleviated with the development of effective reversal agents [13].

FURTHER EVALUATION AND MANAGEMENT

Resuscitation may need to be continued even after the initial volume deficit has been corrected if there is evidence of ongoing or renewed bleeding. Because of the laxative properties of fresh blood in the GI tract, repeated passage of liquid blood per rectum implies ongoing or recurrent bleeding. As bleeding stops, the stool becomes formed and converts from red or maroon blood to darker stool and eventually to brown stool that contains occult blood, which may persist for as long as 2 weeks after GI bleeding has ceased.

In patients without hematemesis, a nasogastric (NG) tube aspirate of red blood may be a poor prognostic sign [3,4], but the lack of red blood or coffee ground material does not exclude an upper GI bleeding source [4]. NG lavage does not appear to affect clinical outcomes, although it may help predict the presence of high-risk lesions [14].Clinical variables at presentation in combination with endoscopic findings have been used to triage and risk-stratify patients, assess risk of poor outcomes, and aid in guiding management [3,4]. The Glasgow–Blatchford score is a validated tool based solely on pre-endoscopic clinical variables scored from 0 to 23 (Table 203.1), with higher values

TABLE 203.1

Glasgow–Blatchford Score for Clinical Risk Stratification of Gastrointestinal Bleeding

Variable	Score
Blood urea nitrogen (mg/dL)	
<18.2	0
18.2–22.3	2
22.4–27.9	3
28.0–70.0	4
>70.0	6
Hemoglobin in men (g/dL)	
≥13	0
12–12.9	1
10–11.9	3
<10	6
Hemoglobin in women (g/dL)	
≥12	0
10–11.9	1
<10	6
Systolic blood pressure (mm Hg)	
≥110	0
100–109	1
90–99	2
<90	3
Other markers	
Pulse > 100/min	1
Presentation with melena	1
Presentation with syncope	2
Hepatic disease	2
Cardiac failure	2

Adapted from Stanley AJ, Ashley D, Dalton HR, et al: Outpatient management of patients with low-risk upper-gastrointestinal haemorrhage: multicentre validation and prospective evaluation. *The Lancet* 373(9657):42–47, 2009.

TABLE 203.2

Complete Rockall Score for Risk Stratification of Acute Upper GI Bleeding

Variable	Points
Clinical Rockall score	
Age	
<60 y	0
60–79 y	1
≥80 y	2
Shock	
Heart rate > 100 beats/min	1
Systolic blood pressure < 100 mm Hg	2
Coexisting illness	
Coronary artery disease, congestive heart failure, other major illness	2
Renal failure, hepatic failure, metastatic cancer	3
Endoscopic diagnosis	
No finding, Mallory–Weiss tear	0
Peptic ulcer, erosive disease, esophagitis	1
Cancer of the upper GI tract	2
Endoscopic stigmata of recent bleeding	
Clean based ulcer, flat pigmented spot	0
Blood in upper GI tract, active bleeding visible vessel, clot	2

Patients with a clinical Rockall score of 0 or a complete Rockall score of <2 are considered to be at low risk for rebleeding or mortality. Higher scores indicate higher risks.
GI, gastrointestinal.
Adapted from Gralnek IM, Barkun AN, Bardou M: Management of acute bleeding from a peptic ulcer. *N Engl J Med* 359(9):928–937, 2008.

predictive of higher risk. Patients with scores of 0 are at low risk of rebleeding and mortality and can be considered for outpatient management [4,15,16]. The Rockall score can be calculated prior to and after endoscopy (Table 203.2), with higher scores predictive of higher risk of a poor outcome [16,17]. The Glasgow–Blatchford score may be superior to pre-endoscopic Rockall score in predicting need for endoscopic intervention, whereas the full (postendoscopic) Rockall is superior in predicting risk of death [18]. A newer simple pre-endoscopic risk score, AIMS65, includes five clinical measures (albumin < 3 g per dL, international normalized ratio > 1.5, mental status change, systolic blood pressure < 90 mm Hg, and age > 65 years) [19]. Recent evidence suggests that this score performs as well or better than the Glasgow–Blatchford score in predicting mortality, length of stay in hospital, and rebleeding [20]. Although their exact role in clinical management continues to be evaluated, these scores will likely continue to have an increasing role in patient care, particularly in triage of patients at the time of presentation to ICU, inpatient, or outpatient settings [16].

DIAGNOSTIC EVALUATION

Bedside Diagnosis

Although hematemesis is clearly a symptom of upper GI bleeding, black tarry melenic stool predicts an upper GI bleeding source, and brighter colors of red in the stool are more often associated with a distal colonic bleeding source. However, color of bloody stool may not always be helpful in predicting the level of GI bleeding and is subject to interpretation variability by both patients and physicians. Stool color identified by the patient on a color card may be more reliable than physician history in suggesting the level of bleeding in the GI tract [21]. When bright blood in the stool (implying a lower GI bleed) is associated with hemodynamic compromise, as many as 11% of patients may have an upper GI bleeding source, even if the NG aspirate is negative [3,4]. In this setting, an upper endoscopy may be the first endoscopic evaluation even though the presenting symptom is hematochezia.

Upper Endoscopy

When bleeding is suspected to originate proximal to the jejunum, esophagogastroduodenoscopy (EGD; upper endoscopy) is the diagnostic procedure of choice. This identifies the bleeding source in 80% to 90% of cases with a high degree of accuracy, provides therapeutic options, and carries low morbidity [3,4]. Endoscopy has the added advantage of detecting prognostic signs (Table 203.2) and classifies bleeding stigmata as high or low risk for rebleeding based on the Forrest grade (Table 203.3).

Even when an exact diagnosis cannot be made, localizing the bleeding to a specific region within the upper GI tract can be helpful to the surgeon (if resection is indicated) or interventional radiologist (if embolization of the bleeding vessel is recommended). Erythromycin or metoclopramide can be administered

TABLE 203.3

Risk Factors for Further Bleeding and Mortality from Peptic Ulcer

Endoscopic finding	Forrest grade	Further bleeding (%)	Mortality (%)
Active bleeding	IA, IB[a]	55	11
Nonbleeding visible vessel	IIA	43	11
Adherent clot	IIB	22	7
Flat pigmented spot	IIC	10	3
Clean ulcer base	III	5	2

[a]Forrest grade IA indicates spurting or arterial bleeding and IB indicates oozing bleeding.
Adapted from Laine L, Jensen DM: Management of patients with ulcer bleeding. *Am J Gastroenterol* 107(3):345–360, 2012.

IV to induce gastric emptying and clear the stomach of blood and clots prior to endoscopy [22]; repeated lavage with saline through a wide-bore orogastric tube may also be used for this purpose. However, routine gastric lavage may not be necessary. Complications related to endoscopy are higher when the procedure is performed on an emergency basis.

The timing of endoscopy for upper GI bleeding continues to be evaluated. Endoscopy within 12 hours of presentation increased the use of endoscopic therapy but did not reduce rebleeding rates or improve survival rates [23]. However, endoscopy within 24 hours did demonstrate a reduction in the length of hospital stay and need for surgical intervention [24]. Patients with bloody NG aspirate did benefit from endoscopy within 12 hours to reduce the blood transfusion requirements and length of hospital stay [23]. Reduction of the window for endoscopy to 6 hours did not demonstrate benefit in mortality, need for surgery, or transfusion requirements [25]. Current guidelines recommend urgent endoscopy (within 24 hours) for patients with malignancy or cirrhosis, hematemesis, signs of hypovolemia, or hemoglobin less than 8 g per dL [26].

The benefit of a repeat "second-look" endoscopy is an area of investigation, especially in the presence of factors associated with an increased risk of rebleeding (history of peptic ulcer disease, previous ulcer bleeding, presence of shock at presentation, ulcers >2 cm, large underlying bleeding vessel ≥2 mm diameter, and ulcers located in lesser curve of stomach or posterior/superior duodenal bulb) [27,28]. A meta-analysis concluded that second-look endoscopy was associated with a decreased risk of recurrent bleeding but did not alter subsequent surgery rates or mortality [29]. A recent decision-effectiveness and cost-effectiveness analysis suggested that routine second-look endoscopy is not warranted, but for cases with a rebleeding risk of 31% or higher, cost–benefit analysis of second look is favorable [30]. Scheduled repeat endoscopy therefore is not routinely recommended, but can be considered on an individual case basis if clinical signs of recurrent bleeding are present or if there are questions about adequate hemostasis [26,31].

Enteroscopy

If a small bowel lesion is suspected after a negative upper endoscopy, a longer endoscope can be used to evaluate the proximal small bowel (push enteroscopy), which allows visual inspection and endoscopic hemostasis of bleeding lesions as far distal as the proximal jejunum [32]. Bleeding lesions beyond the reach of a push enteroscope can potentially be approached using single- and double-balloon enteroscopy, techniques that allow for visualization of most of the small bowel. Balloons at the endoscope tip and an overtube can be consecutively inflated and deflated while inserting and pulling out the endoscope to allow the bowel to pleat over the overtube, thus allowing deep endoscope insertion into the small bowel, either through the mouth or the anus [32]. Diagnostic yield for push enteroscopy in evaluation of obscure bleeding is 24% to 56%, compared with 43% to 81% for balloon-assisted enteroscopy [33]. Single- and double-balloon enteroscopy also have utility in determining the source of obscure GI bleeding in patients with surgically altered anatomy such as Roux-en-Y gastric bypass [34].

Sigmoidoscopy/Colonoscopy

When a distal lower GI bleeding source is suspected, early sigmoidoscopy may be helpful if the bleeding is not of a magnitude that would prevent adequate visualization. For most situations, however, colonoscopy replaces sigmoidoscopy as the diagnostic approach. Early colonoscopy provides a higher yield of the bleeding source compared to radiologic studies, especially when performed within 24 hours of presentation [35]. In patients with severe hematochezia and diverticulosis, urgent colonoscopy (within 6 to 12 hours of hospitalization or diagnosis of hematochezia) after rapid bowel purge can provide endoscopic treatment of diverticular hemorrhage and may prevent recurrent bleeding and decrease the need for surgery [36]. Only 20% of patients with lower GI bleeding, however, have a lesion amenable to endoscopic intervention [37]. In a community practice setting, a recent retrospective database analysis found that less than 5% of patients received endoscopic hemostasis [38]. Even when the exact cause of bleeding cannot be determined, colonoscopy may localize fresh blood to a segment of colon and direct further therapies such as angiotherapy or surgery. Patients with subacute bleeding or hemorrhage that has ceased can undergo adequate bowel preparation followed by semiurgent colonoscopy.

Video Capsule Endoscopy

Video capsule endoscopy (VCE) has emerged as a useful tool for evaluation of obscure GI bleeding, detecting culprit lesions with rates of 35% to 77% [39]. Diagnostic yield and effect on patient management are improved with early deployment (within 3 days of admission) [40]. VCE is useful for localizing small bowel bleeding sites to guide management with deep enteroscopy or other approaches [33]. Capsule endoscopy has most often been used after both upper and lower endoscopies have been performed. Recent studies have examined the use of VCE earlier in the diagnostic algorithm, either as the initial step in evaluation [41] or immediately following negative EGD [42] in patients with acute GI bleeding, with encouraging results. Larger, randomized studies are needed to clarify the optimal use of VCE in acute bleeding.

Radionuclide Bleeding Scan

The technetium-99m-labeled red blood cell scan (scintigraphy) performed at the bedside offers a noninvasive diagnostic approach to patients suspected of having GI bleeding originating beyond the reach of an endoscope, especially in unstable patients where bowel preparation or endoscopy cannot be safely performed. Although bleeding rates as low as 0.1 mL per minute can be detected by this method, the patient should have evidence of ongoing bleeding during the study [8]. Scintigraphy may help to identify patients needing interventional treatment from those who can be managed conservatively [43]. Combination with CT imaging provides higher precision in localizing bleeding site as well as additional anatomic information that may be useful for management [43]. If the test localizes bleeding, angiography or endoscopy (push enteroscopy, colonoscopy, double-balloon enteroscopy, capsule endoscopy) is needed to confirm the site, to further define the cause, and to offer therapy for ongoing bleeding [8]. If the test is negative, colonoscopy followed by capsule endoscopy is usually performed to evaluate potential small bowel and colonic bleeding sources [32].

Mesenteric Arteriography

Because a more rapid bleeding rate is necessary for a positive arteriogram (0.5 mL per minute), this procedure is typically performed after active bleeding is documented on a radionuclide bleeding scan [8,43]. However, because of the intermittent nature of bleeding and the variable timing of mesenteric arteriography, a positive red blood cell scan does not always result in a diagnostic arteriogram [8]. Arteriography is also useful for upper GI bleeding sources not visualized on upper endoscopy because of rapid bleeding or a blood-filled stomach.

THERAPEUTIC PROCEDURES FOR HEMOSTASIS

Evidence-based recommendations for the therapy of GI bleeding are summarized in Table 203.4.

TABLE 203.4

Summary of Evidence-based Findings for Therapy of GI Bleeding

- Octreotide infusion is an effective adjunct to endoscopic therapy for variceal bleeding [66,71].
- Endoscopic variceal band ligation is the therapy of choice for esophageal variceal bleeding [79].
- TIPS and BRTO are effective nonendoscopic modalities of treating variceal hemorrhage [88,91].
- Identification of patients at high risk for rebleeding and mortality, and early diagnostic endoscopy with hemostatic therapy in patients with high-risk stigmata of rebleeding improve outcome in acute nonvariceal upper GI bleeding [16,19,26,52].
- Intravenous proton pump inhibitors, administered either as intermittent bolus doses or continuous infusion, decrease risk of rebleeding, need for surgery, and death in peptic ulcer bleeding [108–110,112].
- Early colonoscopy for acute lower GI bleeding may identify a bleeding source more often compared to radiologic studies, but the choice of diagnostic test may not affect patient outcomes [35].

GI, gastrointestinal; TIPS, transjugular intrahepatic portosystemic shunt; BRTO, balloon-occluded transvenous obliteration.

Endoscopic Therapy (Endotherapy)

Endotherapy offers a convenient and expedient method for treatment of GI bleeding. Although endotherapy was primarily used for the treatment of upper GI and peptic ulcer bleeding, these modalities can also be applied to patients with lower GI bleeding [4,44,45]. Endotherapy is indicated for all patients with high-risk lesions because of the significant risk of persistent or recurrent bleeding (22% to 55%) and even death if left untreated [3,4,46]. Randomized trials have demonstrated that endotherapy for upper GI bleeding decreases further bleeding, shortens hospital stay, decreases transfusions, decreases emergency surgery, decreases mortality, and lowers costs [47]. Optimal therapy for adherent clots remains controversial; a meta-analysis demonstrated reduced rebleeding rates (RR 0.35, 95% confidence interval [CI] 0.14 to 0.82) with endoscopic removal of clot and treating of the uncovered lesion, but no change in length of hospitalization, need for surgery, transfusion requirements, and mortality compared to only medical therapy [48–50]. However, vigorous lavage of adherent clot can uncover stigmata requiring endoscopic treatment in nearly half of patients and can be performed at the discretion of the endoscopist [11].

The most common modalities of endoscopic therapy used are thermal therapy (heater probe, bipolar probe, argon plasma coagulation), injection therapy (epinephrine, hypertonic saline, sclerosing solutions), and mechanical therapy (hemoclips, endoloops, and band ligation). Newer endoscopic techniques, including over-the-scope clips, endoscopic suturing, mucosal ablation devices, fibrin glue injection, hemostatic spray, and endoscopic ultrasound-guided angiotherapy, may improve success rates in treatment of high-risk lesions [51]. The treatment modalities are generally comparable with respect to efficacy and safety even when used in combination [3]. In a Cochrane database systemic review, addition of an alternative modality of endotherapy to epinephrine injection alone reduced further bleeding (odds ratio [OR] 0.53), need for emergency surgery (OR 0.68), and mortality (OR 0.50) in high-risk ulcers, although no particular form of treatment appeared to be superior to others [52]. These findings are similar to prior meta-analysis and mirror published guidelines [26,53]. However, despite successful endotherapy, rebleeding can occur in up to 30% of patients. The Baylor bleeding score, using patient age, number of illnesses, illness severity, site of bleeding, and stigmata of bleeding, has been proposed to predict the likelihood of rebleeding [54] and may be useful in determining which patients may benefit from second-look endoscopy [30].

Angiotherapy

Intra-arterial vasopressin and/or embolization are used for angiographic control of various bleeding lesions [8,55]. A recent randomized study comparing urgent colonoscopy to radionuclide scanning followed by angiography demonstrated no differences in hospital stay and transfusion requirements despite the fact that colonoscopy identified a definitive bleeding source more often. However, this study used only vasopressin infusion and did not use embolization as a mode of angiotherapy [56]. Vasopressin has potential to cause cardiovascular complications. Gelfoam and metal coils used for embolic therapy after superselective cannulation of the bleeding artery are effective because they can be delivered close to the terminal bleeding vessel and result in localized thrombosis with vessel occlusion. Embolization successfully controls bleeding in 52% to 94% of patients, with approximately 10% of these patients requiring repeat embolization for recurrent bleeding [57]. There is a risk of bowel ischemia following embolization, but this is usually minor and self-limited [55].

Angiotherapy may be a first-line treatment for uncontrolled lower GI bleeding from lesions such as diverticula and angiodysplasia, but its use in the upper gut is reserved for peptic ulcer bleeding that is not localized or controlled by endotherapy. Angiotherapy can be comparable to surgical intervention when endoscopic therapy fails for bleeding peptic ulcers. A retrospective analysis demonstrated no difference between embolization and surgery in recurrent bleeding (29.0% and 23.1%), additional surgery required (16.1% and 30.8%), and mortality (25.8% and 20.5%) despite an older population and higher prevalence of heart disease within embolization group [58]. The timing for the use of angiography and angiotherapy must be individualized and usually is a consensus decision by the involved physicians.

Surgical Therapy

The appropriate timing of when a surgeon should be involved in the care of a bleeding patient is physician and institution dependent, and ranges from an early team approach at presentation to involvement once the risk of significant morbidity and mortality are established after a poor response to medical and endoscopic therapy. Surgical intervention is an effective and safe alternative for patients with uncontrollable bleeding or those unable to tolerate additional bleeding [59]. Prior to surgical intervention, a repeat endoscopy for a patient with persistent or recurrent bleeding can be considered owing to lower risks of side effects from endoscopy compared to surgery [60,61]. A possible exception may be ulcers >2 cm in hypotensive patients where the risk of rebleeding is extremely high with repeat endoscopic therapy [26,61]. Patients with massive hemorrhage that overwhelms the resuscitation effort may need to proceed directly to the surgical suite during ongoing resuscitation. If these patients are high-risk surgical candidates, angiotherapy or a percutaneously or surgically placed portal-hepatic shunt for variceal bleeding may be alternatives.

SPECIFIC BLEEDING LESIONS

Variceal Upper Gastrointestinal Bleeding

Portal hypertension, most frequently a consequence of cirrhosis, leads to portosystemic collateral circulations at the squamocolumnar junctions in the gut (i.e., gastroesophageal, anal, and peristomal), which progressively enlarge to form varices. Bleeding from gastroesophageal varices characteristically is brisk and typically presents as hematemesis, melena, or hematochezia in association with hemodynamic instability. The presentation may be less dramatic because acute blood loss can be self-limited in 50% to 60% of cases [62]. One-half to two-thirds of patients with cirrhosis and acute upper GI bleeding have nonvariceal sources of hemorrhage documented by endoscopy [63]. Upper GI variceal bleeding occurs in at least 20% of all patients with cirrhosis who develop varices, with bleeding episodes carrying a mortality rate of at least 20% at 6 weeks [64,65]. Once active bleeding stops, the likelihood of recurrent variceal hemorrhage is 40% within 72 hours and 60% within 10 days if no definitive treatment is pursued [48]. Risk factors associated with variceal rupture include a portal pressure gradient greater than 12 mm Hg, large variceal size (greater than 5 mm), and progressive hepatic dysfunction [66]. Endoscopic findings that implicate esophageal or gastric varices as the bleeding source include the red sign, where one varix is brighter red than the others from microtelangiectasia (red-sign variants include red-wale marks, cherry-red spots, hematocystic spots, and diffuse redness of varix), and the white-nipple sign, in which a fresh fibrin clot may be seen protruding from a varix [66,67]. Endotracheal intubation protects the airway from aspiration of blood in obtunded patients, especially in the setting of massive bleeding [68]. Additional complications that must be addressed include alcohol withdrawal, aspiration, infection, and electrolyte imbalances.

Octreotide is a somatostatin analog that decreases splanchnic blood flow and portal pressure, controlling variceal bleeding in as many as 85% of patients [69,70] with an efficacy approaching that of endoscopic therapy and providing improved visibility during subsequent endoscopy [70–72]. Octreotide is typically administered IV as a bolus dose of 50 to 100 μg followed by continuous infusion of 25 to 50 μg per hour continued 3 to 5 days after diagnosis, but tachyphylaxis may limit efficacy of repeated bolus administrations [66,71–75]. Aside from transient nausea and abdominal pain with bolus doses, significant adverse effects from octreotide are rare. Vasopressin, once widely used in this setting, has a significant cardiovascular side effect profile and for this reason has been replaced by octreotide.

Infection (specifically spontaneous bacterial peritonitis) occurs in patients with cirrhosis and GI bleeding of any type in 25% to 50% of cases, leading to increased bleeding and mortality [76]. Antibiotic prophylaxis with a fluoroquinolone (norfloxacin or ciprofloxacin) in all cirrhotics with GI hemorrhage reduces the rate of bacterial infections and improves survival [77,78]. IV ceftriaxone is an alternative for patients with advanced cirrhosis or when quinolone-resistant organisms are suspected [78].

Endoscopic evaluation should be performed urgently (within 12 hours) in patients in whom variceal bleeding is suspected [79]. Endoscopic band ligation has gained acceptance as the preferred endoscopic treatment for patients with bleeding esophageal varices, with rapid obliteration of varices, and low rates of complications and rebleeding (Table 203.4) [66,80]. Endoscopic variceal sclerotherapy (injecting a sclerosing solution into the variceal lumen or into the adjacent submucosa), although successful in controlling variceal bleeding, is associated with a 20% to 40% incidence of complications, and has largely been relegated to a second-line therapeutic modality, reserved for patients in whom band ligation is technically difficult [66,81]. Complications of band ligation include recurrent bleeding from treatment-induced esophageal ulcers, stricture formation, esophageal perforation, and acceleration of portal hypertensive gastropathy [82]. Repeat variceal band ligation is performed until varices are obliterated because this approach reduces the incidence of rebleeding [66]. Appropriate interval for repeat band ligation is controversial, with recommendations ranging from 1 to 8 weeks [79].

Gastric varices are detected in approximately 20% of patients with portal hypertension, but can also occur from splenic vein thrombosis. Gastric varices bleed less often, but blood loss can be more substantial compared to esophageal varices [83]. When available, endoscopic injection of a tissue adhesive such as butyl cyanoacrylate is effective, with hemostasis rates approaching that of transjugular intrahepatic portosystemic shunt (TIPS) with fewer recurrences [66,84]. Complications include a propensity for embolic phenomenon posttreatment, including massive pulmonary embolism [85]. Gastric variceal hemorrhage dictates earlier consideration of nonendoscopic therapeutic approaches such as TIPS placement. Embolization of the short gastric veins and varices is a potential management option for isolated gastric varices. In the setting of splenic vein thrombosis, splenectomy may be an appropriate therapy.

A TIPS (an iatrogenic fistula between the hepatic vein and portal vein) decreases portal pressure gradient to less than the 10 mm Hg necessary for the formation of esophagogastric varices [86]. TIPS is commonly recommended if esophageal variceal bleeding recurs after two or more endoscopic attempts at therapy [87], if active bleeding is not responsive to variceal ligation or sclerotherapy, or as first-line treatment for gastric variceal bleeding [66]. Complications include transient deterioration of liver function, new or worsened hepatic encephalopathy (25%), and shunt insufficiency from thrombosis or stenosis [86]. When placed in an emergency setting to control active bleeding, a

10% in-hospital mortality and 40% 30-day mortality have been reported [86,88,89].

Balloon-occluded retrograde transvenous obliteration (BRTO) is an endovascular approach used for managing gastric varices. This technique requires a natural gastrorenal or gastrophrenic shunt, which occur in 95% of cases of gastric varices [90]. A balloon catheter is used to occlude the shunt, following which a sclerosant, for example, ethanolamine is injected into the varix [90]. A recent meta-analysis found a pooled clinical success rate of 97% with a major complication rate of 2.6% [91]. Complications of BRTO include venous thrombosis and pulmonary embolism, renal failure, and infection [90,91]. A significant concern is recurrence or exacerbation of esophageal varices after BRTO because of flow and pressure redistribution [91].

Surgically created shunts reliably control acute bleeding (>90%) and prevent rebleeding (<10%) [92,93] but are limited by high operative mortality and postprocedure encephalopathy. Therefore, surgical shunts are only considered in well-compensated cirrhotic patients with good long-term prognoses [93].

Esophageal or gastric balloon devices may be used for direct tamponade of the bleeding source when definitive therapy is not immediately available. There are two basic types of balloon tubes: those with gastric and esophageal balloons (Sengstaken–Blakemore and Minnesota tubes) and those with a large gastric balloon alone (Linton–Nachlas). The incidence of rebleeding is expectedly high. Other complications (aspiration, balloon migration, airway occlusion, perforation, pressure necrosis) occur in 15% to 30% of patients, including death in 6% [94]. Instructions for correctly placing and maintaining a specific balloon device are included as a product insert and should be reviewed before balloon use.

Peptic Ulcer Bleeding

The most important etiologic factors for peptic ulcer disease are *H. pylori* infection and NSAID use. Although the role of *H. pylori* infection in ulcer formation is established, its exact role in precipitating ulcer bleeding is controversial [95]. With long-term NSAID use, there is a greater risk of gastric ulceration compared to duodenal ulceration. Bleeding risk varies depending on NSAID dose and the agent used. Other cofactors, including older age, a history of past peptic ulcers (especially with ulcer bleeding), and a history of coronary disease, may be independent risk factors for ulcer bleeding [96,97]. Population-based studies have suggested that ulcer formation and bleeding occur even with cyclooxygenase 2 (COX-2) inhibitors, albeit at a lower rate [98]. Both COX-2 inhibitors and their nonselective analogs are associated with increased risk of ulcer bleeding when taken in conjunction with anticoagulants such as warfarin [99]. This risk with nonselective NSAIDs and anticoagulation taken together may be as high as 13 times that of patients taking neither NSAIDs nor anticoagulants [100]. Less than 1% of peptic ulcers result from hypersecretory states such as Zollinger–Ellison syndrome. In a proportion of patients, the disorder remains idiopathic, because of either an inability to demonstrate *H. pylori* or lack of a history of obvious NSAID use.

Although 80% or more patients with acute GI bleeding eventually stop bleeding spontaneously [101], it is important to recognize factors associated with higher risk for morbidity and mortality, including older age, large ulcer size (more than 2 cm), large-volume bleeding, and onset of bleeding while hospitalized. A recent meta-analysis demonstrated a clear relationship between presence of comorbid conditions and risk of death from peptic ulcer bleed [102]. Other prognostic information can be obtained from endoscopy findings, which should detail whether stigmata of recent bleeding (active bleeding, nonbleeding visible vessel, adherent clot, flat pigment spots) or no stigmata (clean ulcer base) were found in association with the ulcer (Table 203.3). These criteria can be used to predict rebleeding and the need for therapeutic intervention [46,101,103]. Patient age, hemodynamic parameters, comorbidities, and endoscopic findings have been compiled into scoring system by Rockall et al. [104] and Blatchford [4]. The Rockall score (Table 203.2) has been validated as a predictor of short-term mortality, but not recurrent bleeding [17].

In vitro data suggest that gastric acid plays an important role in impairing platelet aggregation, clot lysis, and increased fibrinolytic activity that is reversible at pH values above 6 to 6.5 [105,106]. PPIs can effectively raise gastric pH >4.0, but their ability to elevate pH to >6.0 is unclear [105]. However, these differences in gastric pH may not translate into clinical benefit. In contrast to histamine-2 receptor antagonists, PPIs have been established as beneficial in acute nonvariceal upper GI bleeding, with a rapid increase in gastric pH, especially with IV PPI, when a mean pH of 6 is reached approximately 1 hour sooner than oral PPI [107]. A Cochrane meta-analysis reaffirmed the established understanding that IV PPI therapy in the setting of peptic ulcer disease decreased rebleeding rates (OR 0.40, 95% CI 0.24 to 0.67), need for urgent surgery (OR 0.50, 95% CI 0.33 to 0.76), and risk of death (OR 0.53, 95% CI 0.31 to 0.91) [108]. IV PPI therapy upon presentation (when compared to IV PPI therapy initiated after endoscopic therapy) decreases the need for endoscopic therapy but not rebleeding rates, blood transfusion requirements, or mortality, a result supported by meta-analysis [109,110]. This approach has been demonstrated to be cost effective, reducing the need for endoscopic therapy by 7.4% [111]. A recent meta-analysis demonstrates no difference in efficacy between IV PPI therapy when delivered as intermittent bolus dosing compared with continuous infusion in patients with endoscopically treated high-risk bleeding ulcers [112].

Mallory–Weiss Tear

A Mallory–Weiss tear represents bleeding from a mucosal disruption at the area of the esophagogastric junction and is found in approximately 5% to 15% of cases of upper GI bleeding. The classic history is a patient with vomiting of nonbloody gastric contents followed by hematemesis, although this presentation is variable (29% to 86%) [113]. Blood with the initial emesis does not exclude the diagnosis. The great majority of patients (80% to 90%) bleeding from a Mallory–Weiss tear stop bleeding without therapeutic intervention, and rebleeding rates are low (less than 5%). Endoscopy offers diagnosis and the option for endotherapy; rarely nonendoscopic measures such as angiography and embolic therapy are required.

Angiodysplasia

Angiodysplasia lesions are small (3 to 15 mm) vascular mucosal abnormalities that can cause GI bleeding from the stomach, small bowel, or colon. Bleeding upper GI lesions frequently occur in patients with chronic renal failure [114,115], whereas vascular heart disease is associated with colonic lesions [116]. The character of the bleeding usually is subacute and recurrent rather than massive. Angiodysplasia typically is diagnosed at endoscopy; bleeding colonic angiodysplasia lesions can also be detected with angiography. Angiodysplasia lesions are the most frequent finding in the small bowel on wireless capsule endoscopy performed for evaluation of obscure GI bleeding. Endoscopic thermal therapy typically is successful in obliterating the lesions [117]. When large lesions are encountered, the periphery is cauterized first to obliterate the feeder vessels, and the center of the lesion is treated last [118]. Angiotherapy and surgery can be used to treat bleeding vascular lesions.

An iatrogenic risk factor for the development of GI angiodysplasia is implantation of a left ventricular assist device (LVAD), an increasingly common intervention for congestive heart failure. The prevalence of GI bleeding in patients with LVADs is 23% according to a recent meta-analysis, with the most common cause being angiodysplasia in the upper GI tract [119]. Formation of angiodysplasia is thought to be promoted by high shear forces in continuous flow LVADs, decreased activity of von Willebrand factor multimers, gut hypoperfusion caused by low pulse pressure, and changes in vascular smooth muscle tone [119]. Long-term use of anticoagulation in this population also leads to increased rates of bleeding. Endoscopic evaluation has been shown to be safe and effective in this population, detecting a bleeding source in 70% of patients [120].

Dieulafoy Lesion

Dieulafoy lesion, an unusual cause of massive bleeding, represents a mucosal defect, not an ulcer, that exposes an end artery of the same caliber as its feeding submucosal artery [121]. The lesions are typically located in the gastric cardia/proximal stomach but are rarely found in the duodenum and other parts of the GI tract including the colon and rectum [122]. Bleeding is often massive and recurrent yet difficult to diagnose. The site is minute, innocent looking, and frequently not appreciated at endoscopy once bleeding has stopped. Upper endoscopy can offer diagnosis and treat a lesion that was previously considered amenable only to surgical resection [123]. Endoscopic band ligation is one method that has been successful for hemostasis [124].

Colonic Diverticular Bleeding

Bleeding colonic diverticula are the most frequent cause of lower GI bleeding, but a definitive diagnosis (e.g., finding stigmata of recent bleeding) is established in only 20% of patients with hematochezia and colonic diverticula [125]. Diverticular bleeding demonstrated by angiography usually is localized to the right colon, whereas the left colon is the more common location when colonoscopy is performed as the diagnostic study (descending colon, 21%; rectosigmoid, 35%) [126]. The character of diverticular bleeding invariably is bright red or maroon blood per rectum, sometimes associated with orthostasis or hypotension. The majority of patients stop bleeding spontaneously, but approximately 20% to 30% rebleed.

Urgent colonoscopy after a rapid colonic purge (more than 4 to 6 hours) is recommended as an option in patients with ongoing bleeding, once the patient is resuscitated and hemodynamically stable [45]. However, a recent randomized controlled study failed to demonstrate an outcome benefit between urgent colonoscopy and radiologic studies for localization of bleeding, despite a higher likelihood of finding the bleeding source in the urgent colonoscopy group [56]. When a bleeding diverticulum is identified by the finding of a visible vessel or a pigmented protuberance [126], epinephrine injection, thermal contact therapy, or hemoclip application can be considered [44,45,127]. One study demonstrated that visualized diverticular bleeding treated with endoscopic therapy had no recurrent bleeding during a 30-month follow-up compared to 53% of patients with medical therapy alone [45]. Surgical intervention, either segmental or subtotal colectomy, is required in 18% to 25% of patients requiring blood transfusion [128]. Angiotherapy with vasopressin infusion or embolization after superselective cannulation of the bleeding vessel is an alternative approach in patients unstable for surgery.

There is limited evidence that endoscopic therapy can prevent recurrent bleeding and the need for surgery [45]. Alternatively, in patients who have stopped bleeding, elective colonoscopy can be performed during the same hospital stay, after adequate bowel preparation.

Aortoenteric Fistula

The key to recognizing an aortoenteric fistula is inclusion within the differential diagnosis of every patient with bleeding and a history of aortic graft surgery. Although fistulas can occur rarely between a native aortic aneurysm and the intestinal lumen, they more commonly occur in patients who have undergone abdominal aortic graft surgery (0.5% to 2.4%) [129]. This communication with resultant bleeding presents, on average, 4 years after the surgery. The point of intestinal breach can be anywhere from the esophagus to the colon, but occurs most often in the third part of the duodenum (75%). A massive bleeding episode may be preceded by a small "herald bleed" that stops spontaneously. The interval between the first event and the exsanguinating hemorrhage can be hours, weeks, or months (average, 1 to 3 weeks). Making the diagnosis is difficult, but upper endoscopy is useful in excluding the diagnosis by identifying another lesion that is actively bleeding or has stigmata of recent bleeding. Endoscopic visualization of the graft eroding through the intestinal wall is diagnostic but uncommon. In some cases, computed tomography of the abdomen can identify graft abnormalities such as air–fluid levels that may indicate an enteric communication [130]. Angiography has not usually been helpful in the diagnosis unless bleeding is ongoing. If available, a vascular surgeon and an interventional radiologist should be part of the evaluating team. Graft repair surgery or an endovascular approach may be required for a confirmed diagnosis, and exploratory surgery is likely necessary for a presumed diagnosis of a fistulized or infected graft site.

References

1. Longstreth GF: Epidemiology and outcome of patients hospitalized with acute lower gastrointestinal hemorrhage: a population-based study. *Am J Gastroenterol* 92:419–424, 1997.
2. Lanas A, García-Rodríguez LA, Polo-Tomβs M, et al: Time trends and impact of upper and lower gastrointestinal bleeding and perforation in clinical practice. *Am J Gastroenterol* 104:1633–1641, 2009.
3. Peter S, Wilcox CM: Modern endoscopic therapy of peptic ulcer bleeding. *Dig Dis* 26:291–299, 2008.
4. Gralnek IM, Barkun AN, Bardou M: Management of acute bleeding from a peptic ulcer. *N Engl J Med* 359:928–937, 2008.
5. Loperfido S, Baldo V, Piovesana E, et al: Changing trends in acute upper-GI bleeding: a population-based study. *Gastrointest Endosc* 70:212–224, 2009.
6. Hermansson M, Ekedahl A, Ranstam J, et al: Decreasing incidence of peptic ulcer complications after the introduction of the proton pump inhibitors, a study of the Swedish population from 1974–2002. *BMC Gastroenterol* 9:25, 2009.
7. Higham J: Recent trends in admissions and mortality due to peptic ulcer in England: increasing frequency of haemorrhage among older subjects. *Gut* 50:460–464, 2002.
8. Zuckerman GR, Prakash C: Acute lower intestinal bleeding Part I: Clinical presentation and diagnosis. *Gastrointest Endosc* 48:606–616, 1998.
9. Crooks C, Card T, West J: Reductions in 28-day mortality following hospital admission for upper gastrointestinal hemorrhage. *Gastroenterology* 141:62–70, 2011.
10. Villanueva C, Colomo A, Bosch A, et al: Transfusion strategies for acute upper gastrointestinal bleeding. *N Engl J Med* 368:11–21, 2013.
11. Laine L, Jensen DM: Management of patients with ulcer bleeding. *Am J Gastroenterol* 107:345–360, 2012; quiz 361.
12. Abraham NS, Singh S, Alexander GC, et al: Comparative risk of gastrointestinal bleeding with dabigatran, rivaroxaban, and warfarin: population based cohort study. *BMJ* 350:h1857, 2015.
13. Lythgoe M: Effective antidotes for new anticoagulants. *BMJ* 350:h2775, 2015.
14. Huang ES, Karsan S, Kanwal F, et al: Impact of nasogastric lavage on outcomes in acute GI bleeding. *Gastrointest Endosc* 74:971–980, 2011.
15. Stanley AJ, Ashley D, Dalton HR, et al: Outpatient management of patients with low-risk upper-gastrointestinal haemorrhage: multicentre validation and prospective evaluation. *Lancet* 373:42–47, 2009.
16. Stanley AJ: Update on risk scoring systems for patients with upper gastrointestinal haemorrhage. *World J Gastroenterol* 18:2739–2744, 2012.

17. Church NI, Dallal HJ, Masson J, et al: Validity of the Rockall scoring system after endoscopic therapy for bleeding peptic ulcer: a prospective cohort study. *Gastrointest Endosc* 63:606–612, 2006.
18. Yang HM, Jeon SW, Jung JT, et al: Comparison of scoring systems for non-variceal upper gastrointestinal bleeding: a multicenter prospective cohort study. *J Gastroenterol Hepatol* 31:119–125, 2016.
19. Saltzman JR, Tabak YP, Hyett BH, et al: A simple risk score accurately predicts in-hospital mortality, length of stay, and cost in acute upper GI bleeding. *Gastrointest Endosc* 74:1215–1224, 2011.
20. Abougergi MS, Charpentier JP, Bethea E, et al: A prospective, multicenter study of the AIMS65 score compared with the Glasgow-Blatchford score in predicting upper gastrointestinal hemorrhage outcomes. *J Clin Gastroenterol* 50:464–469, 2016.
21. Zuckerman GR, Trellis DR, Sherman TM, et al: An objective measure of stool color for differentiating upper from lower gastrointestinal bleeding. *Digest Dis Sci* 40:1614–1621, 1995.
22. Carbonell N, Pauwels A, Serfaty L, et al: Erythromycin infusion prior to endoscopy for acute upper gastrointestinal bleeding: a randomized, controlled, double-blind trial. *Am J Gastroenterol* 101:1211–1215, 2006.
23. Lin H-J, Wang K, Perng C-L, et al: Early or delayed endoscopy for patients with peptic ulcer bleeding. *J Clin Gastroenterol* 22:267–271, 1996.
24. Cooper GS, Chak A, Way LE, et al: Early endoscopy in upper gastrointestinal hemorrhage: associations with recurrent bleeding, surgery, and length of hospital stay. *Gastrointest Endosc* 49:145–152, 1999.
25. Sarin N, Monga N, Adams PC: Time to endoscopy and outcomes in upper gastrointestinal bleeding. *Can J Gastroenterol* 23:489–493, 2009.
26. Hwang JH, Fisher DA, Ben-Menachem T, et al: The role of endoscopy in the management of acute non-variceal upper GI bleeding. *Gastrointest Endosc* 75:1132–1138, 2012.
27. Chung IK, Kim EJ, Lee MS, et al: Endoscopic factors predisposing to rebleeding following endoscopic hemostasis in bleeding peptic ulcers. *Endoscopy* 33:969–975, 2001.
28. Thomopoulos KC, Theocharis GJ, Vagenas KA, et al: Predictors of hemostatic failure after adrenaline injection in patients with peptic ulcers with non⊠bleeding visible vessel. *Scand J Gastroenterol* 39:600–604, 2004.
29. Marmo R, Rotondano G, Bianco MA, et al: Outcome of endoscopic treatment for peptic ulcer bleeding: is a second look necessary? A meta-analysis. *Gastrointest Endosc* 57:62–67, 2003.
30. Imperiale TF, Kong N: Second-look endoscopy for bleeding peptic ulcer disease: a decision-effectiveness and cost-effectiveness analysis. *J Clin Gastroenterol* 46:e71–e75, 2012.
31. Das A, Wong RCK: Prediction of outcome of acute GI hemorrhage: a review of risk scores and predictive models. *Gastrointest Endosc* 60:85–93, 2004.
32. Raju GS, Gerson L, Das A, et al: American Gastroenterological Association (AGA) institute medical position statement on obscure gastrointestinal bleeding. *Gastroenterology* 133:1694–1696, 2007.
33. Fisher L, Lee Krinsky M, Anderson MA, et al: The role of endoscopy in the management of obscure GI bleeding. *Gastrointest Endosc* 72:471–479, 2010.
34. Skinner M, Peter S, Wilcox CM, et al: Diagnostic and therapeutic utility of double-balloon enteroscopy for obscure GI bleeding in patients with surgically altered upper GI anatomy. *Gastrointest Endosc* 80:181–186, 2014.
35. Green BT, Rockey DC, Portwood G, et al: Urgent colonoscopy for evaluation and management of acute lower gastrointestinal hemorrhage: a randomized controlled trial. *Am J Gastroenterol* 100:2395–2402, 2005.
36. Jensen DM, Machicado GA: Diagnosis and treatment of severe hematochezia. The role of urgent colonoscopy after purge. *Gastroenterology* 95:1569–1574, 1988.
37. Zuckerman GR, Prakash C: Acute lower intestinal bleeding Part II: Etiology, therapy, and outcomes. *Gastrointest Endosc* 49:228–238, 1999.
38. Ron-Tal Fisher O, Gralnek IM, Eisen GM, et al: Endoscopic hemostasis is rarely used for hematochezia: a population-based study from the Clinical Outcomes Research Initiative National Endoscopic Database. *Gastrointest Endosc* 79:317–325, 2014.
39. Wang A, Banerjee S, Barth BA, et al: Wireless capsule endoscopy. *Gastrointest Endosc* 78:805–815, 2013.
40. Singh A, Marshall C, Chaudhuri B, et al: Timing of video capsule endoscopy relative to overt obscure GI bleeding: implications from a retrospective study. *Gastrointest Endosc* 77:761–766, 2013.
41. Gralnek IM, Ching JY, Maza I, et al: Capsule endoscopy in acute upper gastrointestinal hemorrhage: a prospective cohort study. *Endoscopy* 45:12–19, 2013.
42. Schlag C, Menzel C, Nennstiel S, et al: Emergency video capsule endoscopy in patients with acute severe GI bleeding and negative upper endoscopy results. *Gastrointest Endosc* 81:889–895, 2015.
43. Allen TW, Tulchinsky M: Nuclear medicine tests for acute gastrointestinal conditions. *Semin Nucl Med* 43:88–101, 2013.
44. Prakash C, Chokshi H, Walden DT, et al: Endoscopic hemostasis in acute diverticular bleeding. *Endoscopy* 31:460–463, 1999.
45. Jensen DM, Machicado GA, Jutabha R, et al: Urgent colonoscopy for the diagnosis and treatment of severe diverticular hemorrhage. *N Engl J Med* 342:78–82, 2000.
46. Lin H-J, Lo W-C, Lee F-Y, et al: A prospective randomized comparative trial showing that omeprazole prevents rebleeding in patients with bleeding peptic ulcer after successful endoscopic therapy. *Arch Intern Med* 158:54, 1998.
47. Tsoi KKF, Ma TKW, Sung JJY: Endoscopy for upper gastrointestinal bleeding: how urgent is it? *Nat Rev Gastroenterol Hepatol* 6:463–469, 2009.
48. Kahi CJ, Jensen DM, Sung JJY, et al: Endoscopic therapy versus medical therapy for bleeding peptic ulcer with adherent clot: a meta-analysis. *Gastroenterology* 129:855–862, 2005.
49. Laine L: Systematic review of endoscopic therapy for ulcers with clots: can a meta-analysis be misleading? *Gastroenterology* 129:2127, 2005.
50. Sung JJY: The effect of endoscopic therapy in patients receiving omeprazole for bleeding ulcers with nonbleeding visible vessels or adherent clots. *Ann Intern Med* 139:237, 2003.
51. Fujii-Lau LL, Wong Kee Song LM, Levy MJ: New technologies and approaches to endoscopic control of gastrointestinal bleeding. *Gastrointest Endosc Clin N Am* 25:553–567, 2015.
52. Vergara M, Bennett C, Calvet X, et al: Epinephrine injection versus epinephrine injection and a second endoscopic method in high-risk bleeding ulcers. *Cochrane Database Syst Rev* 10:CD005584, 2014.
53. Calvet X, Vergara M, Brullet E, et al: Addition of a second endoscopic treatment following epinephrine injection improves outcome in high-risk bleeding ulcers. *Gastroenterology* 126:441–450, 2004.
54. Saeed ZA, Ramirez FC, Hepps KS, et al: Prospective validation of the Baylor bleeding score for predicting the likelihood of rebleeding after endoscopic hemostasis of peptic ulcers. *Gastrointest Endosc* 41:561–565, 1995.
55. Walker TG, Salazar GM, Waltman AC: Angiographic evaluation and management of acute gastrointestinal hemorrhage. *World J Gastroenterol* 18:1191–1201, 2012.
56. Jensen DM: Management of patients with severe hematochezia-with all current evidence available. *Am J Gastroenterol* 100:2403–2406, 2005.
57. Ljungdahl M, Eriksson L-G, Nyman R, et al: Arterial embolisation in management of massive bleeding from gastric and duodenal ulcers. *Eur J Surg* 168:384–390, 2002.
58. Ripoll C, Bañares R, Beceiro I, et al: Comparison of transcatheter arterial embolization and surgery for treatment of bleeding peptic ulcer after endoscopic treatment failure. *J Vasc Interv Radiol* 15:447–450, 2004.
59. Imhof M, Ohmann C, Roher HD, et al: Endoscopic versus operative treatment in high-risk ulcer bleeding patients—results of a randomised study. *Langenbecks Arch Surg* 387:327–336, 2003.
60. Barkun A, Sabbah S, Enns R, et al: The Canadian Registry on Nonvariceal Upper Gastrointestinal Bleeding and Endoscopy (RUGBE): endoscopic hemostasis and proton pump inhibition are associated with improved outcomes in a real-life setting. *Am J Gastroenterol* 99:1238–1246, 2004.
61. Lau JYW, Sung JJY, Lam Y-H, et al: Endoscopic retreatment compared with surgery in patients with recurrent bleeding after initial endoscopic control of bleeding ulcers. *N Engl J Med* 340:751–756, 1999.
62. Sanyal A, Purdum P, Luketic V, et al: Bleeding gastroesophageal varices. *Semin Liver Dis* 9:328–342, 1993.
63. Peifer KJ, Zuckerman GR, Lisker-Melman M, et al: Frequency of Variceal Upper Gastrointestinal Bleeding (UGIB) in patients with established varices. *Gastrointest Endosc* 59:P163, 2004.
64. El-Serag HB, Everhart JE: Improved survival after variceal hemorrhage over an 11-year period in the Department of Veterans Affairs. *Am J Gastroenterol* 95:3566–3573, 2000.
65. D'Amico G" Upper digestive bleeding in cirrhosis. Post-therapeutic outcome and prognostic indicators. *Hepatology* 38:599–612, 2003.
66. Garcia-Tsao G, Sanyal AJ, Grace ND, et al: Prevention and management of gastroesophageal varices and variceal hemorrhage in cirrhosis. *Hepatology* 46:922–938, 2007.
67. Hirata M, Ishihama S, Sanjo K, et al: Study of new prognostic factors of esophageal variceal rupture by use of image processing with a video endoscope. *Surgery* 116:8–16, 1994.
68. Bornman PC, Terblanche J, Krige JEJ: Management of oesophageal varices. *Lancet* 343:1079–1084, 1994.
69. Avgerinos A, Armonis A, Raptis S: Somatostatin and octreotide in the management of acute variceal hemorrhage. *Hepatogastroenterology* 42:145–150, 1995.
70. Bildozola M: Efficacy of octreotide and sclerotherapy in the treatment of acute variceal bleeding in cirrhotic patients: a prospective, multicentric, and randomized clinical trial. *Scand J Gastroenterol* 35:419–425, 2000.
71. Imperiale TF, Carlos Teran J, McCullough AJ: A meta-analysis of somatostatin versus vasopressin in the management of acute esophageal variceal hemorrhage. *Gastroenterology* 109:1289–1294, 1995.
72. Hwang S-J, Lin H-C, Chang C-F, et al: A randomized controlled trial comparing octreotide and vasopressin in the control of acute esophageal variceal bleeding. *J Hepatol* 16:320–325, 1992.
73. Sung JJY, Lai CW, Lee YT, et al: Prospective randomised study of effect of octreotide on rebleeding from oesophageal varices after endoscopic ligation. *Lancet* 346:1666–1669, 1995.
74. Besson I, Ingrand P, Person B, et al: Sclerotherapy with or without octreotide for acute variceal bleeding. *N Engl J Med* 333:555–560, 1995.
75. Escorsell À, Bandi JC, Andreu V, et al: Desensitization to the effects of intravenous octreotide in cirrhotic patients with portal hypertension. *Gastroenterology* 120:161–169, 2001.
76. Goulis J, Armonis A, Patch D, et al: Bacterial infection is independently associated with failure to control bleeding in cirrhotic patients with gastrointestinal hemorrhage. *Hepatology* 27:1207–1212, 1998.
77. Bernard B, Grang J-D, Khac EN, et al: Antibiotic prophylaxis for the prevention of bacterial infections in cirrhotic patients with gastrointestinal bleeding: a meta-analysis. *Hepatology* 29:1655–1661, 1999.

78. Soares-Weiser K, Brezis M, Tur-Kaspa R, et al: Antibiotic prophylaxis for cirrhotic patients with gastrointestinal bleeding. *Cochrane Database Syst Rev* (2):CD002907, 2002.
79. Hwang JH, Shergill AK, Acosta RD, et al: The role of endoscopy in the management of variceal hemorrhage. *Gastrointest Endosc* 80:221–227, 2014.
80. Masci E, Stigliano R, Mariani A, et al: Prospective multicenter randomized trial comparing banding ligation with sclerotherapy of esophageal varices. *Hepatogastroenterology* 46:1769–1773, 1999.
81. Schuman BM, Beckman JW, Tedesco FJ, et al: Complications of endoscopic injection sclerotherapy: a review. *Am J Gastroenterol* 82:823–830, 1987.
82. Lo G-H, Lai K-H, Cheng J-S, et al: The effects of endoscopic variceal ligation and propranolol on portal hypertensive gastropathy: a prospective, controlled trial. *Gastrointest Endosc* 53:579–584, 2001.
83. Sarin SK, Lahoti D, Saxena SP, et al: Prevalence, classification and natural history of gastric varices: a long-term follow-up study in 568 portal hypertension patients. *Hepatology* 16:1343–1349, 1992.
84. Tan P-C, Hou M-C, Lin H-C, et al: A randomized trial of endoscopic treatment of acute gastric variceal hemorrhage: N-Butyl-2-Cyanoacrylate injection versus band ligation. *Hepatology* 43:690–697, 2006.
85. Hwang SS, Kim HH, Park SH, et al: N-Butyl-2-Cyanoacrylate pulmonary embolism after endoscopic injection sclerotherapy for gastric variceal bleeding. *J Comput Assist Tomogr* 25:16–22, 2001.
86. Jalan R, Redhead DN, Hayes PC: Transjugular intrahepatic portasystemic stent—shunt in the treatment of variceal haemorrhage. *Br J Surg* 82:1158–1164, 1995.
87. Paquet K-J, Feussner H: Endoscopic sclerosis and esophageal balloon tamponade in acute hemorrhage from esophagogastric varices: a prospective controlled randomized trial. *Hepatology* 5:580–583, 1985.
88. Sanyal AJ, Freedman AM, Luketic VA, et al: Transjugular intrahepatic portosystemic shunts for patients with active variceal hemorrhage unresponsive to sclerotherapy. *Gastroenterology* 111:138–146, 1996.
89. McCormick PA, Dick R, Panagou EB, et al: Emergency transjugular intrahepatic portasystemic stent shunting as salvage treatment for uncontrolled variceal bleeding. *Br J Surg* 81:1324–1327, 1994.
90. Kirby JM, Cho KJ, Midia M: Image-guided intervention in management of complications of portal hypertension: more than TIPS for success. *Radiographics* 33:1473–1496, 2013.
91. Park JK, Saab S, Kee ST, et al: Balloon-Occluded Retrograde Transvenous Obliteration (BRTO) for treatment of gastric varices: review and meta-analysis. *Dig Dis Sci* 60:1543–1553, 2015.
92. Orozco Hc, Mercado MA, Chan C, et al: A comparative study of the elective treatment of variceal hemorrhage with beta-blockers, transendoscopic sclerotherapy, and surgery. *Ann Surg* 232:216–219, 2000.
93. Henderson JM, Nagle A, Curtas S, et al: Surgical shunts and tips for variceal decompression in the 1990s. *Surgery* 128:540–547, 2000.
94. Haddock G, Garden OJ, McKee RF, et al: Esophageal tamponade in the management of acute variceal hemorrhage. *Digest Dis Sci* 34:913–918, 1989.
95. Hawkey CJ: Risk of ulcer bleeding in patients infected with *Helicobacter pylori* taking non-steroidal anti-inflammatory drugs. *Gut* 46:310–311, 2000.
96. Soll AH: Nonsteroidal anti-inflammatory drugs and peptic ulcer disease. *Ann Intern Med* 114:307, 1991.
97. Silverstein FE: Misoprostol reduces serious gastrointestinal complications in patients with rheumatoid arthritis receiving nonsteroidal anti-inflammatory drugs. *Ann Intern Med* 123:241, 1995.
98. Mamdani M: Gastrointestinal bleeding after the introduction of COX 2 inhibitors: ecological study. *BMJ* 328:1415–1416, 2004.
99. Battistella M: Risk of upper gastrointestinal hemorrhage in warfarin users treated with nonselective NSAIDs or COX-2 inhibitors. *Arch Intern Med* 165:189, 2005.
100. Shorr RI: Concurrent use of nonsteroidal anti-inflammatory drugs and oral anticoagulants places elderly persons at high risk for hemorrhagic peptic ulcer disease. *Arch Intern Med* 153:1665, 1993.
101. De Muckadell OBS, Havelund T, Harling H, et al: Effect of omeprazole on the outcome of endoscopically treated bleeding peptic ulcers randomized double-blind placebo-controlled multicentre study. *Scand J Gastroenterol* 32:320–327, 1997.
102. Leontiadis GI, Molloy-Bland M, Moayyedi P, et al: Effect of comorbidity on mortality in patients with peptic ulcer bleeding: systematic review and meta-analysis. *Am J Gastroenterol* 108:331–345, 2013; quiz 346.
103. Lau JYW, Sung JJY, Lee KKC, et al: Effect of intravenous omeprazole on recurrent bleeding after endoscopic treatment of bleeding peptic ulcers. *N Engl J Med* 343:310–316, 2000.
104. Rockall TA, Logan RF, Devlin HB, et al: Risk assessment after acute upper gastrointestinal haemorrhage. *Gut* 38:316–321, 1996.
105. Metz DC, Amer F, Hunt B, et al: Lansoprazole regimens that sustain intragastric pH >6.0: an evaluation of intermittent oral and continuous intravenous infusion dosages. *Aliment Pharmacol Ther* 23:985–995, 2006.
106. Patchett SE, Enright H, Afdhal N, et al: Clot lysis by gastric juice: an in vitro study. *Gut* 30:1704–1707, 1989.
107. Laine L, Shah A, Bemanian S: Intragastric pH with oral vs intravenous bolus plus infusion proton-pump inhibitor therapy in patients with bleeding ulcers. *Gastroenterology* 134:1836–1841, 2008.
108. Leontiadis GI, Sharma VK, Howden CW: Proton pump inhibitor treatment for acute peptic ulcer bleeding. *Cochrane Database Syst Rev* (1):CD002094, 2006.
109. Lau JY, Leung WK, Wu JCY, et al: Omeprazole before endoscopy in patients with gastrointestinal bleeding. *N Engl J Med* 356:1631–1640, 2007.
110. Dorward S, Sreedharan A, Leontiadis GI, et al: Proton pump inhibitor treatment initiated prior to endoscopic diagnosis in upper gastrointestinal bleeding. *Cochrane Database Syst Rev* (4):CD005415, 2006.
111. Tsoi KKF, Lau JYW, Sung JJY: Cost-effectiveness analysis of high-dose omeprazole infusion before endoscopy for patients with upper-GI bleeding. *Gastrointest Endosc* 67:1056–1063, 2008.
112. Sachar H, Vaidya K, Laine L: Intermittent vs continuous proton pump inhibitor therapy for high-risk bleeding ulcers: a systematic review and meta-analysis. *JAMA Intern Med* 174:1755–1762, 2014.
113. Graham DY, Schwartz JT: The spectrum of the Mallory-Weiss Tear. *Medicine* 57:307–318, 1978.
114. Zuckerman GR: Upper gastrointestinal bleeding in patients with chronic renal failure. *Ann Intern Med* 102:588, 1985.
115. Clouse RE: Angiodysplasia as a cause of upper gastrointestinal bleeding. *Arch Intern Med* 145:458, 1985.
116. Boley SJ, Sammartano R, Adams A, et al: On the nature and etiology of vascular ectasias of the colon. Degenerative lesions of aging. *Gastroenterology* 72:650–660, 1977.
117. Santos JCM, Aprilli F, Guimarães AS, et al: Angiodysplasia of the colon: endoscopic diagnosis and treatment. *Br J Surg* 75:256–258, 1988.
118. Krevsky B: Detection and treatment of angiodysplasia. *Gastrointest Endosc Clin N Am* 7:509–524, 1997.
119. Draper KV, Huang RJ, Gerson LB: GI bleeding in patients with continuous-flow left ventricular assist devices: a systematic review and meta-analysis. *Gastrointest Endosc* 80:435.e1–446.e1, 2014.
120. Kushnir VM, Sharma S, Ewald GA, et al: Evaluation of GI bleeding after implantation of left ventricular assist device. *Gastrointest Endosc* 75:973–979, 2012.
121. Eidus LB, Rasuli P, Manion D, et al: Caliber-persistent artery of the stomach (Dieulafoy's vascular malformation). *Gastroenterology* 99:1507–1510, 1990.
122. McClave SA, Goldschmid S, Cunningham JT, et al: Dieulafoy's cirsoid aneurysm of the duodenum. *Digest Dis Sci* 33:801–805, 1988.
123. Lin H-J, Lee F-Y, Tsai Y-T, et al: Therapeutic endoscopy for Dieulafoy�s disease. *J Clin Gastroenterol* 11:507–510, 1989.
124. Nikolaidis N, Zezos P, Giouleme O, et al: Endoscopic band ligation of dieulafoy-like lesions in the upper gastrointestinal tract. *Endoscopy* 33:754–760, 2001.
125. Casarella WJ, Kanter IE, Seaman WB: Right-sided colonic diverticula as a cause of acute rectal hemorrhage. *N Engl J Med* 286:450–453, 1972.
126. Foutch PG, Zimmerman K: Diverticular bleeding and the pigmented protuberance (sentinel clot): clinical implications, histopathological correlation, and results of endoscopic intervention. *Am J Gastroenterol* 91:2589–2593, 1996.
127. Binmoeller KF, Thonke F, Soehendra N: Endoscopic hemoclip treatment for gastrointestinal bleeding. *Endoscopy* 25:167–170, 1993.
128. Bounds BC, Friedman LS: Lower gastrointestinal bleeding. *Gastroenterol Clin North Am* 32:1107–1125, 2003.
129. Champion MC, Sullivan SN, Coles JC, et al: Aortoenteric fistula. *Ann Surg* 195:314–317, 1982.
130. Low RN, Wall SD, Jeffrey RB, et al: Aortoenteric fistula and perigraft infection: evaluation with CT. *Radiology* 175:157–162, 1990.

Chapter 204 ■ Stress Ulcer Disease

BENJAMIN E. CASSELL • C. PRAKASH GYAWALI

Stress-related mucosal disease (SRMD) is a term that refers to the broad spectrum of pathologic changes in the gastric mucosa of critically ill patients as a result of physiologic stress [1]. The development of erosive disease in the setting of physiologic stress is not a new concept. In fact, descriptions of acute ulcerations of the intestines in the setting of acute burns date back more than 150 years [2].

Gastric mucosal erosions have been found at protocol endoscopy within hours of intensive care unit (ICU) admission. As many as 90% of ICU patients can have evidence of mucosal erosive disease after 3 days in the ICU [3–7]. Stress-related changes have been related temporally to a number of acute disorders including burns [5,8], cerebral lesions, stroke [6], surgical procedures [3,9,10], and other acute medical illnesses found in an ICU [4]. Fortunately, only a small proportion of these patients will have clinically evident bleeding. Management has largely focused on prevention of erosive disease through acid suppression, although this has been the subject of recent controversy because the risks of the medicines themselves must be balanced with their beneficial effects.

CLINICAL CHARACTERISTICS AND PRESENTATION

Despite the high prevalence of mucosal changes in critically ill patients, only a few will manifest clinically evident bleeding. Gastrointestinal (GI) bleeding from stress ulcers can be classified into the following: (a) occult bleeding, where blood is only detected by hemoccult testing and not by visual inspection of gastric content or stool; (b) overt bleeding, where gross or altered blood is visually evident in gastric aspirate, emesis, or stool; and (c) clinically significant bleeding, for which blood loss is complicated by hypotension, tachycardia, orthostasis, or drop in hemoglobin more than 2 g per dL [11]. Using these definitions, occult bleeding can occur in 15% to 50% of ICU patients, overt bleeding in approximately 5%, and clinically significant bleeding occurs in 1% to 4% of critically ill patients [1,11,12].

The incidence of bleeding from stress ulcers appears to be decreasing over the past several decades. A pooled analysis of studies performed between 1980 and 1998 revealed an incidence of 17%, whereas a similar analysis done for studies published between 1993 and 2010 showed an incidence less than 1% [13]. This improvement has been largely attributed to advances in general ICU care over this time period, including but not limited to routine use of prophylactic medications and earlier initiation of enteral feeding.

When bleeding does occur, it has profound implications. A study done in 2001 showed significant increases in mortality and length of ICU stays when patients with GI bleeding were compared to those who did not bleed [14]. In absolute numbers, mortality rates can be as high as 45% to 55% for patients with clinically significant bleeding [12,14]. This is significantly higher (relative risk 2.2 to 3.7) when compared to patients without bleeding. However, this relationship loses significance when controlled for comorbid medical conditions and other intercurrent factors. This suggests that bleeding is more a barometer of severity of critical illness rather than a direct contributor to death [12,14].

RISK FACTORS

Although by definition, stress ulcer disease is associated with physiologic stress, certain specific disease conditions seem to have a more profound impact on development of SRMD. In a landmark trial in 1994, Cook et al. retrospectively analyzed 2,252 patients for development of ulcer disease. Respiratory failure (need for mechanical ventilation >48 hours) and coagulopathy (platelet count <50,000/μL, international normalized ratio >1.5, or partial thromboplastin time >2 times the upper limit of normal) were significant risk factors by multivariate analysis with odds ratios (ORs) of 15.6 and 4.3, respectively [15]. A more recent analysis of 1,034 patients found chronic liver disease, coagulopathy, need for vasopressors, renal replacement therapy, and use of acid suppression in the first 24 hours of ICU admission to be significant predictors of clinically significant bleeding [12]. Additional risk factors are outlined in Table 204.1.

PATHOPHYSIOLOGY

SRMD occurs when, in the setting of critical illness, the elaborate protection mechanisms of the stomach lining are broken down. Gastric epithelial cells secrete a thick mucus layer that acts as physical barrier against stomach acid and the enzyme pepsin. In addition, bicarbonate ions diffusing across the mucosa and trapped in the mucus layer act as a chemical barrier buffering acidic gastric contents [11,13]. Finally, any injury that does occur is rapidly repaired by moving new epithelial cells through the gastric unit to the mucosal surface of injury, an energy-intensive process [1,13]. Gastric regulatory factors control these processes, of which the most important are prostaglandins [13].

In the setting of critical illness, several factors work to disrupt this intricate system (Fig. 204.1). The key inciting event for SRMD is splanchnic hypoperfusion, specifically gastric hypoperfusion, partly from systemic hypotension and selective shunting of blood

TABLE 204.1

Risk Factors for Stress-related Bleeding [1,12,13,15]

- Prolonged mechanical ventilation (>48 h)
- Coagulopathy
- Shock
- Severe sepsis
- CNS injury/surgery
- Severe burns (>30%)
- Multiple organ failure
- Renal failure
- Need for renal replacement therapy
- Acute and chronic hepatic injury
- Multiple trauma
- Post-organ transplant
- Acute respiratory failure

CNS, central nervous system.

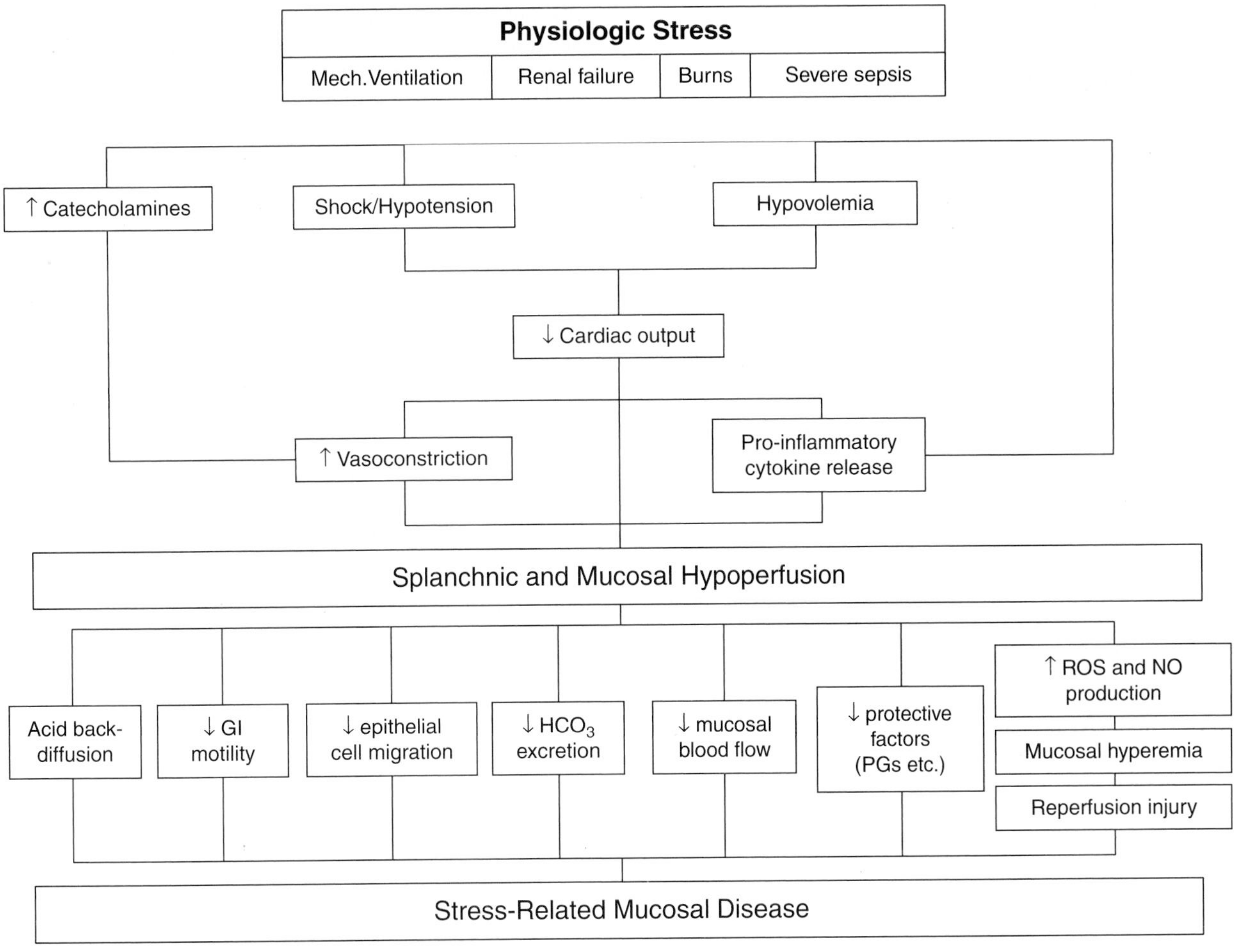

FIGURE 204.1 Pathophysiology of stress-related mucosal disease. In the presence of physiologic stress, hemodynamic and endocrine and paracrine mechanisms lead to decreased blood flow in the splanchnic and specifically gastric circulation. This, in turn, leads to the breakdown of the gastric mucosal defense mechanism, which allows gastric acid and pepsin to erode the gastric mucosa [1,11,13]. HCO_3, bicarbonate; PGs, prostaglandins; ROS, reactive oxygen species; NO, nitric oxide.

away from the splanchnic circulation to essential organs like the kidneys, liver, and brain. This results in gastric mucosal hypoxia, with a decrease in prostaglandin production and an increase in nitric oxide and free oxygen radicals in the mucosa. Nitric oxide leads to vasodilation, with resultant mucosal hyperemia and reperfusion injury, whereas free oxygen radicals are directly toxic to cells. With cell death, pro-inflammatory cytokines are released, which further propagate the injury [11]. In the setting of hypoxia, the mucous bicarbonate barrier breaks down, exposing the gastric epithelium to damage from back diffusion of hydrogen ions as well as direct injury from the protease pepsin. Given the lack of oxygenated blood, the gastric unit is not able to produce the energy needed to replace these damaged epithelial cells [13]. Gastric acid plays a key role in pathogenesis despite the fact that secretion is usually normal or decreased in the setting of critical illness [3,16]. This is illustrated by a number of studies that have shown that raising the gastric pH above 3.5 to 5 can prevent mucosal injury, an effect at least partially explained by optimized mucosal healing and clot formation at higher pH levels [17]. Additional factors such as elevated gastrin and pepsin levels, increased intraluminal bile and urea concentrations, and decreased gastric motility also contribute to the pathogenesis of SRMD [11,18,19].

PROPHYLAXIS

Management of SRMD has largely focused on prophylaxis. By identifying patients at risk of mucosal disease and intervening with pharmacologic therapy before damage occurs, the thought is that bleeding and further morbidity can be prevented. Despite this seemingly simple concept, and despite the fact that stress ulcer prophylaxis has been standard of care for nearly two decades, this remains an area of considerable controversy [20,21].

Some of the controversy stems from the fact that agents used for prophylaxis do not reverse the underlying pathophysiology. Instead, acid suppressive medications prevent damage to the mucosa from the physiologic acidic gastric environment in the setting of the breakdown of the protective measures. This is not without merit because the acid environment also inhibits clot formation and promotes the damaging effects of pepsin [11]. Acid suppression as a means of preventing stress-related bleeding has been proven effective in multiple studies [17] and has become standard of practice, used in ICU patients [22,23] and as part of the sepsis management guidelines [24]. Navigating these standards of practice to provide the best care for patients requires an understanding of the literature and limitations of published outcomes data.

REGIMENS FOR PROPHYLAXIS

Histamine-2 Receptor Antagonists

Histamine-2 receptor antagonists (H2RAs) are an older class of acid suppressants that exert their effects by blocking the action of histamine on the histamine-2 (H2) receptor on the basolateral membrane of parietal cells, thus reducing acid secretion. They are effective in reducing clinically significant GI bleeding in SRMD by over 50% when compared to placebo [17,25]. H2RAs are typically administered intravenously either as bolus dosing or as a continuous infusion. Although continuous infusion has a greater effect on suppressing gastric acid, whether this offers a clinical advantage over bolus dosing is unclear, and bolus dosing is likely satisfactory to achieve the desired endpoint of reducing GI bleeding [26–28].

Proton Pump Inhibitors

Proton pump inhibitors (PPIs) block the final pathway for acid secretion by irreversibly inhibiting H+/K+-ATPase in gastric parietal cells. Like H2RAs, they are often administered intravenously, usually as bolus dosing; oral therapy can be used as well. Over the past several years, PPIs have overtaken H2RAs as the most frequently used agents for stress ulcer prophylaxis [22,23,29] and have been recommended for use over H2RAs in the Surviving Sepsis guidelines [24]. This shift to PPIs over time is based on their potential superiority over H2RAs in the degree of acid suppression, durability of acid suppression, and clinical outcomes in studies evaluating peptic ulcer disease, nonsteroidal anti-inflammatory drug (NSAID)-induced erosive disease, peptic esophagitis, and gastroesophageal reflux disease [30–34].

Despite these potential advantages, data supporting the use of PPIs for stress ulcer prophylaxis are equivocal at best. The majority of available clinical trials over the past decade have compared PPIs to H2RAs, with conflicting results. Some show no difference between the two agents [35,36], others show that PPIs are superior to H2RAs [37,38], and yet others show that PPIs may be worse at preventing bleeding than H2RAs [29,39]. Trials comparing PPI to placebo have shown no significant differences in rates of bleeding [25,35].

Some of the conflicting data can be explained by the fact that the PPI era coincided with a marked decrease in incidence of SRMD-related bleeding [38]. As a result, many of these studies are plagued by low event rates and are largely underpowered to detect true differences in their comparator groups [21]. In addition, many of these studies have methodologic issues making them subject to various forms of bias [21,36–38]. Further, gastric acid plays only a peripheral role in the pathophysiology of SRMD; hence, more acid suppression may not necessarily lead to a better outcome. In contrast, H2RAs have the additional advantage in that they may limit reperfusion injury, a phenomenon that has been observed in animal models [29]. Regardless, based on their method of action and magnitude of acid suppression, PPIs are likely effective for stress ulcer prophylaxis, but they cannot be definitively recommended over H2RAs based on currently available studies.

Sucralfate

Sucralfate is the aluminum salt of sulfated sucrose and does not affect gastric acidity. In contrast to the mechanism of action of acid suppressants, this agent lines denuded gastric mucosa and provides an additional layer of protection against acidic gastric contents. Sucralfate is usually given as a slurry prepared by dissolving 1 g of sucralfate in 5 to 15 mL of water, administered through a nasogastric tube. In terms of efficacy, available data suggest that sucralfate is better than placebo and antacids in preventing stress ulcer bleeding; however, it may be no better and potentially worse than H2RAs in this regard, although data and expert opinion vary [17,40]. Despite this, sucralfate is an agent that remains in the conversation owing to the potential benefit of reducing infectious pulmonary complications for critically ill patients.

Enteral Nutrition

Enteral nutrition has been proposed as another means of prophylaxis of SRMD. The theoretical basis for this is multifaceted. First, most enteral feeding solutions are alkaline and have the potential to raise intragastric pH, although studies indicate a variable effect on gastric pH in actual practice [41]. Further, enteral tube feeds increase mucosal blood flow in animal models [41], which could be attractive if applicable to humans, because this could potentially counteract pathophysiologic events hypothesized to initiate SRMD.

Despite these theoretical advantages, studies evaluating enteral nutrition for SRMD prophylaxis have had mixed results [42]. A meta-analysis of studies assessing stress ulcer prophylaxis showed no additional benefit with an H2RA in patients receiving enteral nutrition, suggesting the feeding itself was protective and that further acid suppression did not have additional impact [43]. However, this study has been criticized for methodologic issues in identifying which patients received parenteral nutrition [13].

COMPLICATIONS OF PROPHYLAXIS

Although some form of stress ulcer prophylaxis has been shown to prevent clinically significant GI bleeding, medications used for prophylaxis are not without side effects. With much lower incidence of stress ulcer bleeding in the present day, universal use of prophylactic agents may shift the risk to benefit ratio toward risk rather than benefit; however, these concepts remain controversial and need further discussion [20].

The major cause for concern with stress ulcer prophylaxis is nosocomial infection, especially nosocomial pneumonia and *Clostridium difficile*–associated diarrhea (CDAD). The acid environment in the stomach acts as an effective barrier to pathogens. Acid suppression, both with H2RAs and PPIs, has been shown to increase bacterial colonization in the stomach and duodenum, with a more profound effect seen with PPIs [44]. Subsequent aspiration of these pathogenic bacteria into the lungs could potentially lead to pneumonia in critically ill patients. With no impact on gastric acidity, sucralfate is not believed to increase rates of nosocomial pneumonia, making this agent a potentially attractive alternative in this setting. However, studies examining the incidence of nosocomial pneumonia with stress ulcer prophylaxis using some form of acid suppression have presented mixed results. A large review by Cook et al. showed no statistically significant increase in pneumonia with the use of H2RA as prophylaxis, when compared to placebo, antacids, or sucralfate [17]. Three of four meta-analyses evaluating PPIs as stress ulcer prophylaxis found no significant increase in rates of pneumonia compared to patients on H2RA [36–38], with only one meta-analysis showing an increase in risk [29]. Another study evaluating PPI versus H2RA in over 20,000 cardiac surgery patients found a slight increase in risk of pneumonia with PPI over H2RA [45]. Finally, a recent meta-analysis including over 1,000 patients showed no increase in rates of nosocomial pneumonia in patients receiving stress ulcer prophylaxis [25].

Acid suppression therapy, particularly PPI therapy, has been linked to CDAD. Incidence of CDAD has been reported to be higher with PPI therapy compared to H2RA with an OR of 3.0, which was higher in that study than the risk attributed to various classes of antibiotics. Another study suggested that the duration of PPI therapy is an independent predictor of CDAD [23,29,46].

IMPACT ON MORTALITY AND RISK TO BENEFIT ANALYSES

Weighing the beneficial effects of stress ulcer prophylaxis against potential adverse events attributed to prophylaxis can be a difficult balancing act. A crude but effective measure is to evaluate the impact that stress ulcer prophylaxis has on all-cause mortality. Studies evaluating this endpoint almost universally reveal no differences in mortality between the various stress ulcer prophylaxis agents or against no prophylaxis [17,25,36–38]. A single study by McLaren et al. showed an increase in mortality with PPIs compared to H2RAs, although the design of this study makes causation difficult to determine [13,29]. Although the lack of mortality benefit appears disheartening, this must be interpreted in light of the knowledge that bleeding from SRMD by itself is not associated with an increase in mortality when controlled for comorbid factors; in contrast, this impacts morbidity and length of hospital stay. Therefore, intervention only intended to prevent bleeding will not necessarily impact the comorbid severe disease processes leading to death.

INAPPROPRIATE USE OF STRESS ULCER PROPHYLAXIS

A consequence of the widespread acceptance of acid suppression for stress ulcer prophylaxis is the fact that acid suppression is used in situations where it is not indicated. In order to shift the risk to benefit ratio toward benefit, use of acid suppression should be restricted to patients with established risk factors for SRMD (Table 204.1). Despite this, inappropriate use of acid suppression occurs frequently in the ICU setting, continuing after transfer out of the ICU and after discharge from the hospital. In the ICU, inappropriate use of acid suppression (defined as use without significant risk factors for SRMD) has been shown to occur in 32% to 68% of patients [22,47,48]. When acid suppression is initiated, a majority remain on these agents after discharge from the ICU, largely when risk factors for their use (if ever present) have resolved [48,49]. Finally, approximately 20% to 50% of patients started on acid suppression in this setting are discharged with instructions to continue on this regimen without an appropriate indication [47–50]. Beyond increasing risk for adverse events, inappropriate use of acid suppressants and stress ulcer prophylaxis can be associated with a significant financial burden [47,50,51].

Based on this data, it is evident that further education of health care personnel regarding appropriate use of stress ulcer prophylaxis is warranted. Indeed, such educational interventions of varying methodology have proven successful in individual medical centers in reducing inappropriate use and controlling costs [52–55]. However, a multicenter survey of stress ulcer prophylaxis usage found no difference in inappropriate use of prophylaxis in those that had institutional stress ulcer prophylaxis guidelines compared to those that did not, suggesting that guidelines alone may not be sufficient [22].

Determination of appropriateness of stress ulcer prophylaxis necessitates in-depth understanding of risks, benefits, and limitations, with special attention to restricting use to active disease conditions where prophylaxis has been shown to be beneficial (Table 204.1). Appropriate use is also dependent on knowing when to stop prophylaxis when risk factors have resolved. Given the multiple factors involved in decision-making, it is not surprising that the guideline-based approach has led to overuse of prophylaxis. On the contrary, appropriate use relies on critical thinking, discretion, and vigilance on the part of the prescriber, which must occur on a case-by-case basis.

MANAGEMENT OF STRESS-RELATED GI BLEEDING

When bleeding does occur, management should follow algorithms laid out for non-variceal upper GI bleeding [56]. Three basic principles are followed: adequate resuscitation, timely endoscopy, and appropriate monitoring postendoscopy. Resuscitation consists of administration of intravenous fluids and appropriate use of red blood cell transfusions. A substantial body of literature exists in supporting a restrictive transfusion strategy of limiting transfusion to settings where hemoglobin levels drop below 7 g per dL [57,58]. PPI therapy is indicated in this setting because it decreases high-risk stigmata (active bleeding, nonbleeding visible vessel, adherent clot) on upper endoscopy and reduces need for endoscopic hemostasis; however, mortality, risk of rebleeding, or need for surgery are not impacted [59]. Timing of endoscopy is dependent on the overall status of the patient; scoring systems such as the Rockall and Blatchford scores can guide decision-making [60,61]. Current guidelines recommend performing upper endoscopy within 24 hours of onset of GI bleeding, except in the case of a high-risk patient (defined as Blatchford score >12), when endoscopy within 13 hours may improve mortality [56,62]. Following endoscopy, PPI should be administered intravenously, with either bolus dosing or continuous infusion for 72 hours if high-risk stigmata are present [56]. If there is evidence of recurrent bleeding, repeat endoscopy should be performed because this has shown to be effective up to 73% of the time [63]. Transcatheter embolization of bleeding vessels is an additional measure that can be useful for peptic ulcer bleeding, but this approach cannot be recommended for stress ulcer bleeding because bleeding tends to be diffuse rather than focal. Surgery can be considered; however, rates of rebleeding and mortality are extremely high in critically ill patients undergoing total or partial gastrectomy [64,65].

CONCLUSIONS

SRMD results from the breakdown of the gastric mucosal barrier in the setting of critical illness. Multiple factors contribute to the pathophysiology, including impaired blood flow to the stomach, presence of inflammatory cytokines, and reperfusion injury. The end result is damage to the intricate gastric mucosal defense mechanisms and exposure of the mucosal cells of the stomach to the caustic effects of gastric acid and pepsin. Over time, this leads to erosions, ulceration, and eventually, to bleeding. Prophylaxis focused on reducing acidity of gastric secretions and as a whole is successful; existing evidence supports the use of H2RAs. Despite a more profound effect on gastric acid secretion, PPIs have not been definitively shown to be better than H2RAs in preventing stress ulcer bleeding. Regardless of the agent used, stress ulcer prophylaxis should only be used for those conditions shown to increase the risk of bleeding (Table 204.1) and should be discontinued once these conditions have resolved. When bleeding occurs, proper therapy consists of adequate resuscitation, timely endoscopic intervention, and close monitoring following endoscopy. A summary of evidence-based guidelines for SRMD is provided in Table 204.2. These therapies and interventions, complemented by other advances in ICU care, have decreased incidence of stress ulcer bleeding and SRMD. Because our understanding of the pathophysiology and treatment of this condition continues to progress, better forms of prophylaxis and therapy could further reduce the incidence and morbidity of this condition.

TABLE 204.2

Summary of Recommendations Based on Clinical Trials

Recommendation	Representative studies
GI bleeding is associated with increased length of stay and mortality in ICU patients	• Cook et al. [14]
H2RAs are effective in reducing clinically significant GI bleeding	• Cook et al. [17] • Krag et al. [25]
PPIs are likely equivalent to H2RAs although some controversy exists	• Lin et al. [36] • Alhazzani et al. [37] • Barletta et al. [39]
Sucralfate and enteral feeding may provide some degree of protection from bleeding	• Cook et al. [17] • Marik et al. [43]
Acid suppression, especially with PPIs, is associated with an increased risk of *Clostridium difficile*–associated diarrhea and potentially, nosocomial pneumonia	• Barletta [46] • MacLaren [29]
Stress ulcer prophylaxis likely has no impact on all-cause mortality	• Krag et al. [25]
Inappropriate use of stress ulcer prophylaxis is common and is associated with increased costs	• Barletta et al. [22]

GI, gastrointestinal; H2RAs, histamine-2 receptor antagonists; ICU, intensive care unit; PPIs, proton pump inhibitors.

References

1. Duerksen DR: Stress-related mucosal disease in critically ill patients. *Best Pract Res Clin Gastroenterol* 17(3):327–344, 2003.
2. Curling TB: On acute ulceration of the duodenum, in cases of burn. *Med Chir Trans* 25:260–281, 1842.
3. Lucas CE, Sugawa C, Riddle J, et al: Natural history and surgical dilemma of "stress" gastric bleeding. *Arch Surg* 102(4):266–273, 1971.
4. Peura DA, Johnson LF: Cimetidine for prevention and treatment of gastroduodenal mucosal lesions in patients in an intensive care unit. *Ann Intern Med* 103(2):173–177, 1985.
5. Czaja AJ, McAlhany JC, Pruitt BA Jr: Acute gastroduodenal disease after thermal injury. An endoscopic evaluation of incidence and natural history. *N Engl J Med* 291(18):925–929, 1974.
6. Kitamura T, Ito K: Acute gastric changes in patients with acute stroke. Part 1: with reference to gastroendoscopic findings. *Stroke* 7(5):460–463, 1976.
7. Eddleston JM, Pearson RC, Holland J, et al: Prospective endoscopic study of stress erosions and ulcers in critically ill adult patients treated with either sucralfate or placebo. *Crit Care Med* 22(12):1949–1954, 1994.
8. Czaja AJ, McAlhany JC, Andes WA, et al: Acute gastric disease after cutaneous thermal injury. *Arch Surg* 110(5):600–605, 1975.
9. Beil AR Jr, Mannix H Jr, Beal JM: Massive upper gastrointestinal hemorrhage after operation. *Am J Surg* 108:324–330, 1964.
10. Goodman AA, Frey CF: Massive upper gastrointestinal hemorrhage following surgical operations. *Ann Surg* 167(2):180–184, 1968.
11. Fennerty MB: Pathophysiology of the upper gastrointestinal tract in the critically ill patient: rationale for the therapeutic benefits of acid suppression. *Crit Care Med* 30[6 Suppl]:S351–S355, 2002.
12. Krag M, Perner A, Wetterslev J, et al: Prevalence and outcome of gastrointestinal bleeding and use of acid suppressants in acutely ill adult intensive care patients. *Intensive Care Med* 41(5):833–845, 2015.
13. Bardou M, Quenot JP, Barkun A: Stress-related mucosal disease in the critically ill patient. *Nat Rev Gastroenterol Hepatol* 12(2):98–107, 2015.
14. Cook DJ, Griffith LE, Walter SD, et al: The attributable mortality and length of intensive care unit stay of clinically important gastrointestinal bleeding in critically ill patients. *Crit Care* 5(6):368–375, 2001.
15. Cook DJ, Fuller HD, Guyatt GH, et al: Risk factors for gastrointestinal bleeding in critically ill patients. Canadian Critical Care Trials Group. *N Engl J Med* 330(6):377–381, 1994.
16. Stannard VA, Hutchinson A, Morris DL, et al: Gastric exocrine "failure" in critically ill patients: incidence and associated features. *Br Med J* 296(6616):155–156, 1988.
17. Cook DJ, Reeve BK, Guyatt GH, et al: Stress ulcer prophylaxis in critically ill patients. Resolving discordant meta-analyses. *JAMA* 275(4):308–314, 1996.
18. Bresalier RS: The clinical significance and pathophysiology of stress-related gastric mucosal hemorrhage. *J Clin Gastroenterol* 13 [Suppl 2]:S35–S43, 1991.
19. Marrone GC, Silen W: Pathogenesis, diagnosis and treatment of acute gastric mucosal lesions. *Clin Gastroenterol* 13(2):635–650, 1984.
20. Alaniz C, Hyzy RC: Time to declare a moratorium on stress ulcer prophylaxis in critically ill. *Crit Care Med* 42(9):e636–e637, 2014.
21. Krag M, Perner A, Wetterslev J, et al: Stress ulcer prophylaxis in the intensive care unit: is it indicated? A topical systematic review. *Acta Anaesthesiol Scand* 57(7):835–847, 2013.
22. Barletta JF, Kanji S, MacLaren R, et al; American-Canadian consortium for Intensive care Drug utilization Investigators: Pharmacoepidemiology of stress ulcer prophylaxis in the United States and Canada. *J Crit Care* 29(6):955–960, 2014.
23. Buendgens L, Bruensing J, Matthes M, et al: Administration of proton pump inhibitors in critically ill medical patients is associated with increased risk of developing *Clostridium difficile*-associated diarrhea. *J Crit Care* 29(4):696.e11–696.e15, 2014.
24. Dellinger RP, Levy MM, Rhodes A, et al: Surviving sepsis campaign: international guidelines for management of severe sepsis and septic shock: 2012. *Crit Care Med* 41(2):580–637, 2013.
25. Krag M, Perner A, Wetterslev J, et al: Stress ulcer prophylaxis versus placebo or no prophylaxis in critically ill patients. A systematic review of randomised clinical trials with meta-analysis and trial sequential analysis. *Intensive Care Med* 40(1):11–22, 2014.
26. Heiselman DE, Hulisz DT, Fricker R, et al: Randomized comparison of gastric pH control with intermittent and continuous intravenous infusion of famotidine in ICU patients. *Am J Gastroenterol* 90(2):277–279, 1995.
27. Ostro MJ, Russell JA, Soldin SJ, et al: Control of gastric pH with cimetidine: boluses versus primed infusions. *Gastroenterology* 89(3):532–537, 1985.
28. Zuckerman GR, Shuman R: Therapeutic goals and treatment options for prevention of stress ulcer syndrome. *Am J Med* 83(6A):29–35, 1987.
29. MacLaren R, Reynolds PM, Allen RR: Histamine-2 receptor antagonists vs proton pump inhibitors on gastrointestinal tract hemorrhage and infectious complications in the intensive care unit. *JAMA Intern Med* 174(4):564–574, 2014.
30. Netzer P, Gaia C, Sandoz M, et al: Effect of repeated injection and continuous infusion of omeprazole and ranitidine on intragastric pH over 72 hours. *Am J Gastroenterol* 94(2):351–357, 1999.
31. Agrawal NM, Campbell DR, Safdi MA, et al: Superiority of lansoprazole vs ranitidine in healing nonsteroidal anti-inflammatory drug-associated gastric ulcers: results of a double-blind, randomized, multicenter study. NSAID-Associated Gastric Ulcer Study Group. *Arch Intern Med* 160(10):1455–1461, 2000.
32. Meneghelli UG, Zaterka S, de Paula Castro L, et al: Pantoprazole versus ranitidine in the treatment of duodenal ulcer: a multicenter study in Brazil. *Am J Gastroenterol* 95(1):62–66, 2000.
33. Jansen JB, Van Oene JC: Standard-dose lansoprazole is more effective than high-dose ranitidine in achieving endoscopic healing and symptom relief in patients with moderately severe reflux oesophagitis. The Dutch Lansoprazole Study Group. *Aliment Pharmacol Ther* 13(12):1611–1620, 1999.
34. Richter JE, Campbell DR, Kahrilas PJ, et al: Lansoprazole compared with ranitidine for the treatment of nonerosive gastroesophageal reflux disease. *Arch Intern Med* 160(12):1803–1809, 2000.
35. Kantorova I, Svoboda P, Scheer P, et al: Stress ulcer prophylaxis in critically ill patients: a randomized controlled trial. *Hepatogastroenterology* 51(57):757–761, 2004.
36. Lin PC, Chang CH, Hsu PI, et al: The efficacy and safety of proton pump inhibitors vs histamine-2 receptor antagonists for stress ulcer bleeding prophylaxis among critical care patients: a meta-analysis. *Crit Care Med* 38(4):1197–1205, 2010.
37. Alhazzani W, Alenezi F, Jaeschke RZ, et al: Proton pump inhibitors versus histamine 2 receptor antagonists for stress ulcer prophylaxis in critically ill patients: a systematic review and meta-analysis. *Crit Care Med* 41(3):693–705, 2013.
38. Barkun AN, Bardou M, Pham CQ, et al: Proton pump inhibitors vs. histamine 2 receptor antagonists for stress-related mucosal bleeding prophylaxis in critically ill patients: a meta-analysis. *Am J Gastroenterol* 107(4):507–520, 2012; quiz 21.

39. Barletta JF: Histamine-2-receptor antagonist administration and gastrointestinal bleeding when used for stress ulcer prophylaxis in patients with severe sepsis or septic shock. *Ann Pharmacother* 48(10):1276–1281, 2014.
40. Huang J, Cao Y, Liao C, et al: Effect of histamine-2-receptor antagonists versus sucralfate on stress ulcer prophylaxis in mechanically ventilated patients: a meta-analysis of 10 randomized controlled trials. *Crit Care* 14(5):R194, 2010.
41. MacLaren R, Jarvis CL, Fish DN: Use of enteral nutrition for stress ulcer prophylaxis. *Ann Pharmacother* 35(12):1614–1623, 2001.
42. Hurt RT, Frazier TH, McClave SA, et al: Stress prophylaxis in intensive care unit patients and the role of enteral nutrition. *JPEN J Parenter Enteral Nutr* 36(6):721–731, 2012.
43. Marik PE, Vasu T, Hirani A, et al: Stress ulcer prophylaxis in the new millennium: a systematic review and meta-analysis. *Crit Care Med* 38(11):2222–2228, 2010.
44. Thorens J, Froehlich F, Schwizer W, et al: Bacterial overgrowth during treatment with omeprazole compared with cimetidine: a prospective randomised double blind study. *Gut* 39(1):54–59, 1996.
45. Bateman BT, Bykov K, Choudhry NK, et al: Type of stress ulcer prophylaxis and risk of nosocomial pneumonia in cardiac surgical patients: cohort study. *BMJ* 347:f5416, 2013.
46. Barletta JF, El-Ibiary SY, Davis LE, et al: Proton pump inhibitors and the risk for hospital-acquired *Clostridium difficile* infection. *Mayo Clin Proc* 88(10):1085–1090, 2013.
47. Perwaiz MK, Posner G, Hammoudeh F, et al: Inappropriate use of intravenous ppi for stress ulcer prophylaxis in an inner city community hospital. *J Clin Med Res* 2(5):215–219, 2010.
48. Farrell CP, Mercogliano G, Kuntz CL: Overuse of stress ulcer prophylaxis in the critical care setting and beyond. *J Crit Care* 25(2):214–220, 2010.
49. Murphy CE, Stevens AM, Ferrentino N, et al: Frequency of inappropriate continuation of acid suppressive therapy after discharge in patients who began therapy in the surgical intensive care unit. *Pharmacotherapy* 28(8):968–976, 2008.
50. Shin S: Evaluation of costs accrued through inadvertent continuation of hospital-initiated proton pump inhibitor therapy for stress ulcer prophylaxis beyond hospital discharge: a retrospective chart review. *Ther Clin Risk Manag* 11:649–657, 2015.
51. Issa IA, Soubra O, Nakkash H, et al: Variables associated with stress ulcer prophylaxis misuse: a retrospective analysis. *Dig Dis Sci* 57(10):2633–2641, 2012.
52. Pitimana-aree S, Forrest D, Brown G, et al: Implementation of a clinical practice guideline for stress ulcer prophylaxis increases appropriateness and decreases cost of care. *Intensive Care Med* 24(3):217–223, 1998.
53. Herzig SJ, Guess JR, Feinbloom DB, et al: Improving appropriateness of acid-suppressive medication use via computerized clinical decision support. *J Hosp Med* 10(1):41–45, 2015.
54. Agee C, Coulter L, Hudson J: Effects of pharmacy resident led education on resident physician prescribing habits associated with stress ulcer prophylaxis in non-intensive care unit patients. *Am J Health Syst Pharm* 72[11 Suppl 1]:S48–S52, 2015.
55. Erstad BL, Camamo JM, Miller MJ, et al: Impacting cost and appropriateness of stress ulcer prophylaxis at a university medical center. *Crit Care Med* 25(10):1678–1684, 1997.
56. Laine L, Jensen DM: Management of patients with ulcer bleeding. *Am J Gastroenterol* 107(3):345–360, 2012; quiz 61.
57. Jairath V, Hearnshaw S, Brunskill SJ, et al: Red cell transfusion for the management of upper gastrointestinal haemorrhage. *Cochrane Database Syst Rev* (9):CD006613, 2010.
58. Villanueva C, Colomo A, Bosch A, et al: Transfusion strategies for acute upper gastrointestinal bleeding. *N Engl J Med* 368(1):11–21, 2013.
59. Sreedharan A, Martin J, Leontiadis GI, et al: Proton pump inhibitor treatment initiated prior to endoscopic diagnosis in upper gastrointestinal bleeding. *Cochrane Database Syst Rev* (7):CD005415, 2010.
60. Rockall TA, Logan RF, Devlin HB, et al: Risk assessment after acute upper gastrointestinal haemorrhage. *Gut* 38(3):316–321, 1996.
61. Blatchford O, Murray WR, Blatchford M: A risk score to predict need for treatment for upper-gastrointestinal haemorrhage. *Lancet* 356(9238):1318–1321, 2000.
62. Lim LG, Ho KY, Chan YH, et al: Urgent endoscopy is associated with lower mortality in high-risk but not low-risk nonvariceal upper gastrointestinal bleeding. *Endoscopy* 43(4):300–306, 2011.
63. Lau JY, Sung JJ, Lam YH, et al: Endoscopic retreatment compared with surgery in patients with recurrent bleeding after initial endoscopic control of bleeding ulcers. *N Engl J Med* 340(10):751–756, 1999.
64. Ritchie W: Stress ulceration, in Nyhus LM, Wastell C (eds): *Surgery of the Stomach and Duodenum*. 4th ed. Boston, MA, Little, Brown and Company, 1986, p 663.
65. Hubert JP Jr, Kiernan PD, Welch JS, et al: The surgical management of bleeding stress ulcers. *Ann Surg* 191(6):672–679, 1980.

Chapter 205 ■ Gastrointestinal Motility for the Critically Ill Patient

FILIPPO CREMONINI • ANTHONY J. LEMBO

The motility of the gastrointestinal tract is a series of coordinated functions that propels its contents through the precise regulation of neural, chemical, and endocrine signals. Although a detailed review of the physiology of motility is beyond the scope of this chapter, it is important for the critical care provider to understand that the closely coordinated movements of the gastrointestinal tract, from mouth to rectum, can frequently be disrupted and deranged in the setting of severe illness.

When systemic illness strikes, such as severe sepsis, the bowels are not a teleologic priority. Rather, physiologic reserve shifts away from the gastrointestinal tract to critical organs such as the lungs, brain, and cardiovascular system, resulting in significant dysfunction and possibly damage of the gastrointestinal tract. This presents most often as delayed transit, or ileus, which may occur at any level of the gastrointestinal tract leading to a number of clinically significant consequences such as gastroesophageal reflux, gastroparesis, abdominal pain and distention, obstipation, and even bowel ischemia and perforation.

Because derangements of gastrointestinal motility are extremely prevalent in the critically ill, providers must be prepared to identify and treat these morbid, and sometimes fatal disorders. Although there has been surprisingly little research dedicated to understanding the pathophysiologic basis of motility abnormalities in the critically ill patient [1], there have nonetheless been several advances in the prevention and treatment of these disorders. This chapter focuses on the clinical presentations of the common motility disorders of the critically ill patient, including gastroesophageal reflux disease (GERD), gastroparesis, ileus, and colonic pseudo-obstruction, and review the current evidence supporting diagnostic and therapeutic approaches for these conditions.

GASTROESOPHAGEAL REFLUX DISEASE

Critically ill patients are especially prone to developing gastroesophageal reflux and related complications, particularly aspiration and erosive esophagitis, which is one of the leading causes of inpatient upper gastrointestinal tract hemorrhage in mechanically ventilated patients, after stress-related mucosal disease [2,3]. GERD is particularly prevalent among the critically ill for several reasons (Fig. 205.1). First, critically ill patients are often in the recumbent position, which promotes acid reflux [4–6] and reduces acid clearance from the esophagus. Second, many critically ill patients are intubated, sedated, or too ill to report symptoms of acid reflux, which can thus go unrecognized until complications occur. Third, critically ill patients are more likely to have increased transient relaxation of the lower esophageal sphincter (LES), due to use of drugs (e.g., morphine, atropine, theophylline, and barbiturates) and to the frequent use

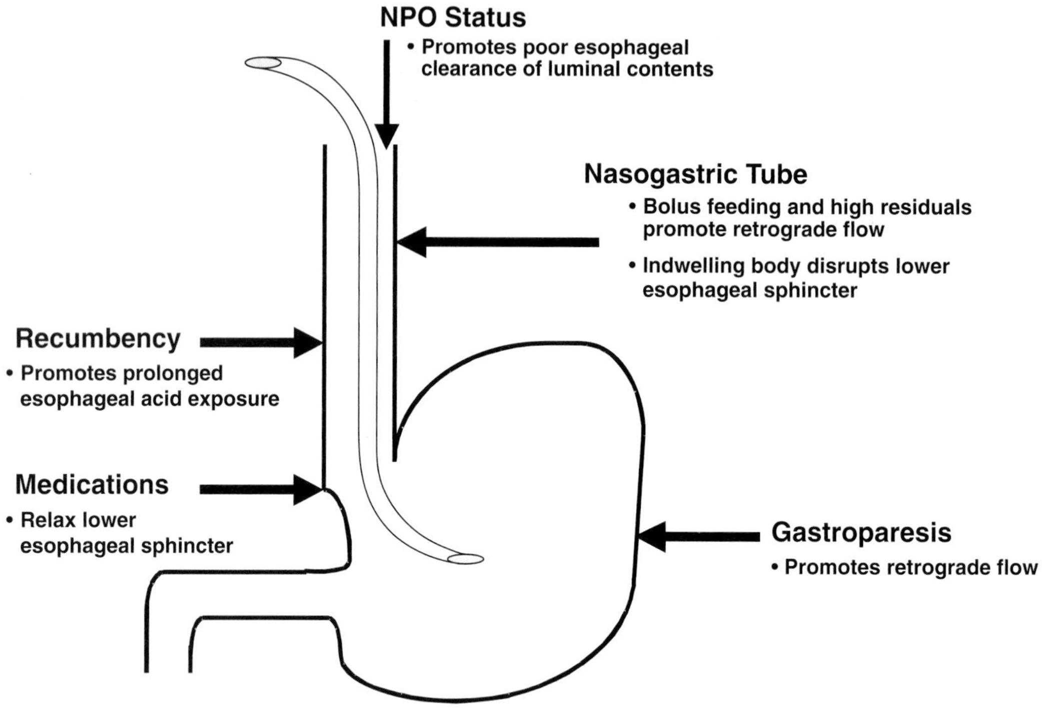
NPO Status
• Promotes poor esophageal clearance of luminal contents
Nasogastric Tube
• Bolus feeding and high residuals promote retrograde flow
• Indwelling body disrupts lower esophageal sphincter
Recumbency
• Promotes prolonged esophageal acid exposure
Medications
• Relax lower esophageal sphincter
Gastroparesis
• Promotes retrograde flow

FIGURE 205.1 The combination of factors contributing to gastroesophageal reflux disease (GERD) in the critically ill patient. Patients in the intensive care unit setting are highly susceptible to each of these factors making GERD a prevalent problem. NPO, nothing by mouth.

of indwelling nasogastric tubes [7–9]. Critically ill patients have reduced propulsive motility in the body of the esophagus [10] and extremely low or absent LES pressures, along with superimposed cough or strain, as a main contributor to GERD [11]. Fourth, critically ill patients often develop concomitant gastroparesis (see following discussion) from a host of factors, which, in turn, favors retrograde flow of gastric contents toward the distal esophagus. Taken together, these multiple mechanisms concur to clinically significant acid reflux and to its related complications.

Several nonpharmacologic steps should be taken in the critical care setting to minimize complications of acid reflux in the critically ill patient. First, patients should be kept in the semi-recumbent or upright position. This maneuver can minimize acid stasis in the distal esophagus and improve emptying of stomach contents, thereby reducing complications of acid reflux [4,5]. The effectiveness of this maneuver alone for patients who are mechanically ventilated remains controversial [5,6]. Another step is to minimize the use of nasogastric tubes. Data indicate that indwelling nasogastric tubes promote GERD and subsequent microaspiration of bacterially contaminated contents into the lower airways [7–9]. Thus, gastroesophageal reflux also can lead to nosocomial pneumonia [12,13]. Results from a small ($n = 17$) randomized trial suggest that the nasogastric tube size (i.e., 2.85 mm vs. 6.0 mm) does not appear to reduce GERD [9], although clearly this study was not powered to demonstrate statistically significant differences in clinically relevant outcomes (such as bleeding or pneumonia). Although placement of a gastrostomy tube in patients undergoing prolonged mechanical ventilation may reduce GERD and its complications, this intervention is not without its own risks and side effects [14].

A key step is to minimize the use of medications known to relax the LES. Many of these agents (Table 205.1) are commonly used in the intensive care setting. It should be noted that while these agents are known to decrease LES resting pressure, their specific impact on the development of GERD complications, including erosive esophagitis or upper gastrointestinal hemorrhage is unknown. Thus, the agents listed in Table 205.1 should not be avoided on the basis of theoretical concerns alone, if their use is otherwise medically justified.

TABLE 205.1

Classes of Medications Commonly Used in the Intensive Care Unit Setting That Relax the Lower Esophageal Sphincter

Anticholinergic agents
Aminophylline
Benzodiazepines
β-Adrenergic agonists
Calcium channel blockers
Nitrates

Pharmacologic therapy is often necessary in the critically ill patient to reduce the potential complications of GERD. Treatment relies primarily on acid suppression. Traditionally, intravenous (IV) histamine-2 receptor antagonists (H2RAs) have served as the mainstay antisecretory therapy in the critical care setting particularly for prophylaxis against stress-related mucosal disease [15] (as opposed to GERD prophylaxis) (see Chapter 204). However, IV proton pump inhibitors (PPIs) (pantoprazole and esomeprazole) have since replaced H2RAs as the antisecretory of choice for active mucosal bleeding. IV PPIs have excellent effectiveness in reducing recurrent hemorrhage following endoscopic hemostasis for bleeding peptic ulcer [16]. Although there are limited clinical data regarding their use for erosive esophagitis, IV PPIs produce potent and longer-lasting acid inhibition [17], making them the preferred antisecretory medication in patients at risk for GERD-related complications [18].

GASTROPARESIS

Gastroparesis, or delayed gastric emptying (GE) in the absence of mechanical obstruction, may lead to several complications among critically ill patients, including malnutrition, erosive esophagitis (as previously noted), and aspiration of gastric contents with resulting nosocomial pneumonia.

As with GERD, gastroparesis arises from a confluence of several common factors (Table 205.2) in the critically ill patient, including medications (especially narcotics and anticholinergic agents), autonomic dysfunction, postsurgical states, and endocrine abnormalities, among others.

Patients with gastroparesis typically present with nausea, vomiting, abdominal pain, early satiety, and postprandial bloating. These symptoms can be blunted or overlooked during critical illness, given the severity of the overall clinical picture and the concomitant treatments. In patients receiving tube feeding, high gastric residuals are a common sign of delayed GE. Because the symptoms of gastroparesis are often nonspecific, the clinician should maintain a low threshold for considering the diagnosis. A combination of physical examination findings and imaging studies confirm gastroparesis and exclude competing diagnoses, including mechanical obstruction and mucosal diseases. On examination, patients with gastroparesis may demonstrate epigastric distention with tenderness but typically lack abdominal rigidity or guarding, signs of a potentially more serious acute diagnosis. The examiner should evaluate for a succussion splash by placing the stethoscope over the left upper quadrant while gently shaking the abdomen laterally by holding either side of the pelvis. A positive test occurs when a splash is heard over the stomach and favors the diagnosis of mechanical gastric outlet obstruction over gastroparesis. Of note, the maneuver is only valid if the patient has not received solids or liquids within the previous 3 hours.

Laboratory testing may help determine the underlying cause of the decreased motility. Serum electrolyte levels, serum glucose level, hemoglobin A1C level, serum cortisol level, thyroid-stimulating hormone level, amylase, and white blood cell count (screen for infection) should be measured. A host of other tests can be used in the outpatient setting to investigate chronic gastroparesis (e.g., erythrocyte sedimentation rate [scleroderma, myopathies, lupus], urinary protein [amyloidosis], chest radiography [lung cancer with gastroparesis as a paraneoplastic syndrome], and antineuronal or anti-Hu antibodies [paraneoplastic gastroparesis]), but these are rarely indicated for the critically ill patient.

Plain films of the abdomen should be obtained to evaluate for evidence of gastric distention and to screen for overt evidence of gastric obstruction. Upper endoscopy should be considered if there is suggestion of gastric outlet obstruction, because significant amounts of retained food, feedings, and secretions can be found in the stomach even in the absence of an obstruction to the pyloric outlet. Additional imaging tests for the investigation of gastroparesis in the intensive care unit (ICU) setting are infrequently indicated. If the problem is suspected by the presentation, becomes a primary issue, and is not easily linked to other disorders, and then confirming the diagnosis by other methods may be merited once the patient leaves the ICU. Formal measurement of gastric motor function is impractical and not routine in the critical care setting. The most accepted diagnostic test, usually performed in the outpatient setting, is a scintigraphic emptying study. Most centers use a 4-hour GE test, with a ^{99}Tc-labeled-egg meal. In health, gastric retention of more than 10% at 4 hours suggests delayed GE [19]. Alternative diagnostic tests include newly approved stable isotope-labeled breath test ([^{13}C]-Spirulina platensis GE breath test), and the wireless motility capsule. Still, the simple finding of persistent high gastric tube residuals should be sufficient to formulate a presumptive diagnosis in the critically ill patient.

Once diagnosed, a search for possible reversible causes of gastroparesis (including mechanical obstruction and medications) should be undertaken. Treatment should begin by with nutritional and dietary modifications including smaller volume, low-fat, and low-fiber meals or tube feeds [20]. Consultation with the nutrition or metabolic support services is often warranted to help select between available liquid caloric supplements. In general, parenteral nutrition should be avoided if possible. Rather, patients who need long-term nutrition support due to gastroparesis should be considered for a jejunostomy tube [21], often placed in conjunction with a gastrostomy tube for venting of the stomach [22].

Metoclopramide and erythromycin are the only currently available prokinetic medications in the United States. Other prokinetics available outside the United States include domperidone, prucalopride, and mosapride. Metoclopramide has multiple actions, including coordination of antral, duodenal, and pyloric muscle function, while simultaneously serving as a centrally acting antiemetic [23,24]. Metoclopramide can be administered orally, intravenously, rectally, and subcutaneously. In the critically ill patient, metoclopramide typically is dosed at 10 to 20 mg IV every 6 hours. The major disadvantage of IV bolus dosing is that plasma levels are often erratic, largely

TABLE 205.2

Common Causes of Gastroparesis in the Critically Ill Patient

- Endocrinopathies
    - Adrenal insufficiency
    - Diabetes
    - Hypoparathyroidism or hyperparathyroidism
    - Hypothyroidism or hyperthyroidism
- Infections
    - Pneumonia
    - Abdominal or pelvic infections
    - Urinary tract infections
    - Sepsis
- Medications
    - Anticholinergic agents
    - Aluminum-hydroxide–containing products
    - *β*-Adrenergic agonists
    - Calcium channel blockers
    - Diphenhydramine
    - Levodopa
    - Narcotics
    - Octreotide
    - Tricyclics
- Neurologic disorders
    - Multiple sclerosis
    - Parkinson disease
    - Stroke
- Postsurgical settings
    - Esophagectomy with gastric pull-through
    - Fundoplication
    - Gastroplasty
    - Gastric bypass surgery
    - Roux-en-Y gastrojejunostomy
    - Vagotomy
    - Whipple procedure
- Vascular disorders
    - Mesenteric ischemia
    - Superior mesenteric artery syndrome
    - Median arcuate ligament syndrome

This list is not comprehensive but is specifically relevant to the critically ill patient.

because levels peak rapidly and the half-life is short. Subcutaneous dosing (two to four times per day in 2-mL aliquots) has been promoted as an alternative route, as it is associated with more stable plasma levels [25]. Although the tardive dyskinesia side effects have been known for decades, the Food and Drug Administration (FDA) recently issued a warning in reference to metoclopramide. Other neurologic side effects include akathisia, sedation, and depression, can impact up to 30% of patients [26]. Reducing the dose and rate of IV infusion may reduce frequency of neurologic side effects.

Erythromycin prokinetic effects are due to its binding to the motilin receptor in the stomach, inducing high-amplitude gastric contractions [27,28]. The preferred route of administration is IV at low doses (e.g., 100 to 200 mg every 6 hours). Erythromycin may be used in combination with metoclopramide for patients with an incomplete response to either agent alone. A randomized-crossover study using ^{13}C breath testing to assess response in ventilated, critically ill patients, showed combination of metoclopramide IV 10 mg every 6 hours and continuous erythromycin infusion 10 mg per hour was most effective at improving GE rate [29]. Oral dosing of erythromycin (125 to 250 mg twice daily) is effective in diabetic patients and has also shown benefits in reducing high tube feed residuals [30]. Unfortunately, long-term use of erythromycin leads to tachyphylaxis from downregulation of motilin receptors [28] and also is associated with antimicrobial resistance.

Another therapy sometimes used for gastroparesis is neuroenteric stimulation (i.e., gastric pacing). However, this treatment is available at only limited centers and is rarely used in critically ill patients. Pyloric botulin toxin injection has not been shown to be effective in gastroparesis and its role in the critically ill patient is unknown [31]. Manipulation of gastrointestinal hormones responsible for delayed GE, such as cholecystokinin, peptide YY, and glucagon-like peptide 1, has been proposed. However, pharmacologic agents with adequate selectivity and bioavailability are currently not available and still under investigation [32].

ILEUS

Any disease state affecting neurohormonal mediators, vascular perfusion, electrolyte balance, and muscular contraction has the potential to affect the coordinated propulsive small and large intestinal motility, resulting in ileus. The postoperative state, inflammation, metabolic derangement, neurogenic impairment, and drug-induced aperistalsis are all common occurrences in the ICU. Patients typically present with abdominal distention, obstipation, nausea, vomiting, abdominal pain, and high tube feed residuals.

Distinguishing ileus from small bowel obstruction is critical, as prolonged mechanical obstruction can lead to bowel ischemia and peritonitis. Table 205.3 compares classical physical examination and radiographic findings of adynamic ileus and small bowel obstruction. These conditions share many clinical manifestations. Peritoneal signs and auscultation of high-pitched bowel sounds favor small bowel obstruction, whereas a silent bowel suggests ileus. Although the skilled clinician often can reliably distinguish small bowel obstruction from ileus on the basis of history and physical examination alone, plain abdominal radiographs may serve to confirm the clinical impression. Ileus typically is characterized by the presence of both small and large bowel dilatation, the presence of gas throughout the bowel and into the rectum, lack of a luminal radiographs may serve to confirm high pitched bowel sounds, small bowel obstruction typically presents with small bowel distention in the absence of colonic gas, a paucity of gas in the rectum, air fluid levels on upright positioning, and with evidence of a luminal transition point. Despite the stereotypical features of small bowel obstruction and ileus, plain film imaging does not always provide a definitive diagnosis, as long-standing ileus or partial small bowel obstruction may appear similar on abdominal imaging. In addition, late-stage mechanical obstruction may lead to exhaustion of intestinal propulsive activity, resembling adynamic ileus without high-pitched bowel sounds and a similar air distribution pattern on plain abdominal X-rays. In cases in which the plain films are inadequate, contrast-enhanced computed tomography (CT) should be considered [33]. A CT scan may provide additional information to complement the clinical picture, such as the presence or absence of intra-abdominal inflammation (e.g., pancreatitis, abdominal abscess) or retroperitoneal pathology.

Once small bowel obstruction has been excluded, the next step is to identify and treat reversible causes of ileus. Common causes in the critically ill patient include electrolyte abnormalities, sepsis, inflammation, postoperative hypomotility, and medications (Table 205.4), initial laboratory studies should include serum potassium, magnesium, calcium, bicarbonate, lipase, blood urea nitrogen, creatinine, and white blood cell count. Medications should be carefully reviewed, and potentially causative agents discontinued or limited if otherwise warranted. There are no specific rules about how and when to discontinue medications in the setting of ileus, especially when necessary pain medications (e.g., narcotics) are involved. Ultimately, the decision rests on a careful balance of clinical factors and meticulous attention to the progress and clinical sequelae of the ileus. In particular, if there is concomitant evidence of significant cecal or large bowel distention to suggest colonic pseudo-obstruction and impending perforation, and then all the medications potentially contributing to aperistalsis should be discontinued.

In contrast, if there are no clinical signs of deterioration and no worsening on serial abdominal X-rays, the ileus is nonprogressive and stable, and a supportive, conservative treatment is preferred, the treatment plan should include adequate IV hydration, electrolyte replacement, and treatment of the underlying condition(s), with close clinical and radiologic follow-up. There is little evidence [34–44] to support insertion of a nasogastric

TABLE 205.3

Differentiation of Ileus and Small Bowel Obstruction

Clinical feature	Ileus	Small bowel obstruction
Bowel sounds	Generally absent	High-pitched and active
Peritoneal signs	Less common	More common, although inconsistent
Involved bowel on radiograph	Small and large bowel dilated	Small bowel dilated
Rectal gas	Present	Absent
Air fluid levels	Absent	Present, although inconsistent
Luminal “cut point”	Absent	Present, although inconsistent

TABLE 205.4

Common Causes of Ileus in Intensive Care Unit Patients

Electrolyte disorders
Medications
Peritoneal inflammation
Postsurgical setting
Mesenteric ischemia
Sepsis
Retroperitoneal disease
Myocardial infarction

tube for decompression of prolonged ileus and worsening abdominal distention; however, when vomiting is present, this is routinely performed. One caveat to this widespread approach is the trend in favor of more atelectasis and pneumonia in patients receiving nasogastric decompression in randomized controlled trials [34–44]. Data from postoperative patients do not support the need for nasogastric tube decompression [37,45].

Unfortunately, pharmacologic treatments for ileus remain limited. Promotility agents are generally ineffective for most cases of ileus.

Patients with an ileus who are receiving narcotics may be experiencing dysmotility from the narcotics. Opioid-induced bowel dysfunction can occur after the initial dose of opioids and not resolve for some time after therapy is discontinued. Unlike many of the other side effects from narcotics, the constipating effect and other bowel dysfunctions do not decrease with prolonged use [46]. Although stool softeners, stimulant, and osmotic laxative are traditionally used, a subset of critically ill patients will not respond to traditional measures and will go on to develop inability to tolerate enteral feedings and laxatives [47]. Opioid reversing agents, with limited systemic bioavailability, have been traditionally used, such as naloxone, naltrexone, and nalmefene. However, early transit across the blood–brain barrier by these agents caused concomitant analgesia reversal and the onset of opioid withdrawal, without consistent restoration of peristalsis [48]. Newer peripherally acting mu opioid receptor antagonists (PAMORAs) do not substantially cross the blood–brain barrier. Methylnaltrexone and naloxegol are efficacious in treating opioid-induced constipation [49]. Methylnaltrexone is available subcutaneously, which is advantageous in critically ill patients. Naloxegol is an oral PAMORA approved by the FDA for opioid-induced constipation. There are no systematic data on the use of naloxegol in the intensive care or postoperative setting. Its oral administration, favorable tolerability and pharmacokinetic profiles support potential clinical utility in opioid-induced ileus [50].

Postoperative ileus has multiple pathophysiologic causes including surgical stress hormones, activation of the endogenous opioid system, exogenous opioids given for pain, and inflammation compounding imbalances in fluid and electrolytes.

Traditional prokinetics have been used for reversal of postoperative ileus. Although metoclopramide has proven efficacy in the foregut, it provides little or no benefit for postoperative ileus [51–55]. There have been few studies of metoclopramide in postoperative ileus, so it is difficult to conclude whether its ineffectiveness in postoperative ileus extends to other forms of ileus. Similarly, randomized controlled trials of erythromycin in postoperative ileus demonstrated minimal, if any, benefit [56]. The somatostatin analog, octreotide, has been used empirically, although no good randomized controlled data exist for its use in humans with postoperative ileus, and there are potential detrimental effects on GE with octreotide that need to be considered before administering in severe whole gut dysmotility.

One trial of 65 postcolectomy patients demonstrated efficacy of methylnaltrexone (see earlier) 0.3 mg given intravenously every 6 hours to achieve a first bowel movement and to hasten discharge from the hospital [57]. These observations support a role for opioid reversal even in the absence of a previous effect of exogenous opioids on gut motor function. Larger trials on methylnaltrexone are needed.

Another opioid antagonist, the selective μ-opioid receptor antagonist, alvimopan, is approved by the FDA for the treatment of postoperative ileus [58,59]. Oral alvimopan is administered preoperatively and postoperatively. In one randomized, controlled, blinded clinical trial of postoperative ileus, alvimopan, 6 mg twice daily, led to a faster passage of flatus (by 21 hours), earlier initiation of bowel movements (by 41 hours), and faster time to discharge (by 23 hours) than placebo [58]. A subsequent larger trial in 510 patients demonstrated similar results [59]. These dramatic effects in postoperative ileus set the stage for the use of alvimopan in other forms of ileus. In a study of 522 patients with noncancer pain requiring an equivalent dose of narcotics more than 30 mg of oral morphine daily, alvimopan was superior to placebo in increasing bowel movement frequency and other endpoints correlated to severe opioid-induced constipation. Although alvimopam has been shown to be effective for opioid-induced constipation it is not FDA approved for this indication due to concerns of cardiovascular side effects demonstrated in one study [60].

ACUTE COLONIC PSEUDO-OBSTRUCTION (OGILVIE SYNDROME)

Acute colonic pseudo-obstruction, or Ogilvie's syndrome, is characterized by marked dilatation of the cecum and ascending colon in the absence of mechanical obstruction (Fig. 205.2). Similar to ileus, colonic pseudo-obstruction generally occurs in critically ill patients with sepsis, recent surgery, electrolyte abnormalities, and trauma, among other conditions. The diagnosis rests on radiographic evaluation of the cecum, where a diameter of more than 9 cm suggests evidence of pseudo-obstruction in the absence of a mechanical obstruction. This threshold is somewhat arbitrary and is based on an early series from 1956 that linked this diameter with clinically significant sequelae, namely colonic perforation [61]. More recent case series suggest that a cecal diameter exceeding 12 cm correlates most highly with bowel perforation and should serve as a critical threshold to track in patients with suspected pseudo-obstruction [62,63].

The exact mechanism by which cecal dilatation occurs remains unclear. There are two competing theories [64]. The first theory, originally postulated by Dr. Ogilvie in 1948 [65], suggests that sympathetic drive to the enteric nervous system is interrupted, thereby promoting unopposed parasympathetic stimulation. This, in turn, could promote unabated distal colonic luminal contractions and a potential source of obstruction. The second theory, espoused by Hutchinson and Griffiths [66], contends that colonic pseudo-obstruction arises from a combination of sympathetic overdrive and parasympathetic suppression, both described in the setting of physiologic stress, thereby leading to colonic hypomotility and eventual paralysis. The proven effectiveness of neostigmine for colonic pseudo-obstruction (see following discussion) supports the validity of the latter theory. In contrast, there are few physiological data to support Ogilvies' original concept of sympathetic interruption. It should be noted that the autonomic nervous system is not the only player in colonic motility. Other factors including neurohormones and gut peptides play a significant role in regulating motility in the gastrointestinal tract.

The clinical presentation of acute colonic pseudo-obstruction is typical of obstructive colonic processes, with the patient

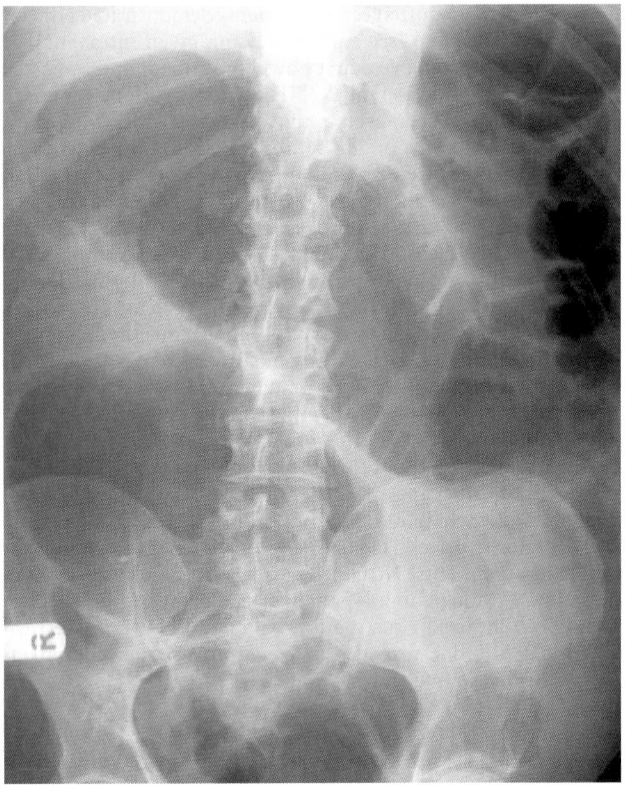

FIGURE 205.2 Marked dilatation of the cecum and other colonic regions in colonic pseudo-obstruction. When the cecal diameter exceeds 12 cm, the risk for perforation rises substantially. (From the Scottish Radiological Society [SRS-X: www.radiology.co.uk/srs-x], with permission.)

demonstrating marked abdominal distention, nausea, vomiting, and abdominal pain. If left untreated, colonic pseudo-obstruction can lead to ischemia, perforation (in approximately 3% of cases overall), peritonitis, and death [67–70]. Thus, the clinician must keep a high index of suspicion for colonic pseudo-obstruction in patients with risk factors, as the consequences of late diagnosis can be grave.

Fortunately, conservative measures are sufficient in most cases, and the cecal dilatation resolves spontaneously. Conservative measures consist of ceasing oral intake, frequent repositioning of the patient, and treating potential underlying causes of dysmotility (as with ileus). Although nasogastric tubes are often employed in cases of colonic pseudo-obstruction, there are no data from randomized controlled studies to support its effectiveness in reducing clinically significant endpoints. Because nasogastric decompression has limited, if any, role in ileus [44–49,51–54], there is little a priori reason to believe that the maneuver would be of benefit in colonic pseudo-obstruction, a condition that is even more distal to the tip of a nasogastric tube than ileus. In contrast, case series do support the effectiveness of colonoscopic decompression, which reduces the cecal diameter in nearly 70% of patients [67,70]. Unfortunately, colonoscopic decompression alone is often short lived, and recurrent distention occurs in approximately half of patients [64,67]. Thus, colonoscopic decompression usually is accompanied by placement of a rectal tube or stent with its proximal tip in the ascending colon. Data from a small controlled clinical trial suggest the efficacy of colonic decompression can be maintained after initial success by administration of polyethylene glycol (PEG) balanced solutions, resulting in increased stool output and flatus, and in reduction of visceral dilation [71]. However, while colonoscopic decompression and tube placement is conceptually attractive, the procedure is challenging and often unsuccessful and it must be conducted in an unprepared bowel without the benefit of full air insufflation.

In patients failing to respond to conservative measures after 24 to 48 hours, including correction of electrolyte abnormalities, IV hydration, correction of underlying medical causes, and minimization of culprit medications, pharmacologic therapy is generally warranted. Moreover, if at any time the cecal diameter exceeds 12 cm, or if there is evidence of worsening clinical status, and then aggressive treatment should be pursued immediately, because these findings constitute a gastroenterologic emergency, which mandates early consultative involvement of a surgeon. In patients with markedly dilated large bowel, some specialists would defer even an initial attempt at colonoscopic decompression to a trial of medical therapy. The acetylcholinesterase inhibitor neostigmine increases the postsynaptic concentration of acetylcholine, thereby favoring a boost in the deranged colonic motor function. Neostigmine is effective in colonic pseudo-obstruction, and its IV administration has been accepted as initial therapy. This recommendation is largely based on a pivotal controlled trial in which 10 of 11 patients randomized to receive neostigmine had prompt evacuation of their colonic contents and normalization of their cecal diameter, whereas none of 10 patients randomized to placebo had these outcomes [68]. Moreover, all of the patients in the placebo arm achieved a response when crossed over to neostigmine in an open-label fashion. The dosage used was 2 mg IV in one infusion followed by an additional 2 mg infusion 3 hours later if there was no initial response or adverse event. Being an anticholinesterase inhibitor, neostigmine has an array of well-defined cholinergic side effects, including bronchoconstriction, abdominal cramping, hypersalivation, diaphoresis, and bradycardia. Hemodynamically relevant side effects, including cardiac arrest and cardiovascular collapse, can occur, requiring neostigmine to be administered in a monitored setting. It is contraindicated in patients with bradycardia, active bronchospasm, and mechanical bowel obstruction. Existing electrolyte imbalances and use of antimotility agents were predictors of poor response to neostigmine. Patients with postoperative colonic ileus had the best response rate [69]. According to a retrospective review of 151 patients, additional predictors of response to neostigmine after failure of conservative management were female gender and older age [72]. The combined administration of 2 mg neostigmine with glycopyrrolate, an anticholinergic agent that has limited activity on the muscarinic receptors of the colon and has the potential of reducing the incidence of cholinergic side effects of neostigmine, has been evaluated in a randomized, controlled study of 13 patients with neurogenic bowel using video fluorographic assessment of evacuation [70]. The neostigmine Korsombination resulted in bowel evacuation with significantly less bradycardia and increase in airways resistance than with neostigmine alone, suggesting that the coadministration would make treatment with neostigmine safer in clinical settings where cardiorespiratory function is compromised.

When severe colonic pseudo-obstruction fails to respond to conservative measures, neostigmine, and colonic decompression, surgery must be considered. In these settings, surgery has a high morbidity and may lead to poor outcomes in patients who are already critically ill. Indeed, case series indicate that one quarter of patients with colonic pseudo-obstruction die in the perioperative period, even in the absence of bowel perforation [65], although the presence of underlying critical illness is arguably the strongest predictor of such a guarded prognosis. Alternatively, endoscopic cecostomy with placement of a percutaneous tube using a modified Seldinger technique similar to percutaneous gastrostomy has been described [73].

SUMMARY

Gastrointestinal motility requires coordinated neural, chemical, and endocrine signals. Systemic illness often deranges motility, leading to syndromes such as GERD, gastroparesis, ileus, and

TABLE 205.5

Summary of Evidence-Based Management Recommendations

- Treatment and prevention of complications from gastroesophageal reflux should include encouraging the semirecumbent or upright position, avoidance of nasogastric tubes, and use of potent antisecretory therapy, such as intravenous proton pump inhibitors.
- Medical therapy for gastroparesis often is ineffective, although modest benefits are seen with metoclopramide (especially subcutaneous administration) and erythromycin.
- Evidence for placement of a nasogastric tube for decompression in postoperative ileus is weak, as indicated by meta-analyses.
- Data indicate that there is little or no benefit of metoclopramide or erythromycin in the setting of ileus.
- Methylnaltrexone is an opioid reversal agent that does not cross the blood–brain barrier and achieves sustained laxation in opioid-induced bowel dysfunction.
- Alvimopan, a highly selective opioid receptor antagonist, has demonstrated excellent results in postoperative ileus in randomized controlled trials.
- Neostigmine was shown in effective medical therapy for the treatment of acute colonic pseudo-obstruction in the presence of colonic diameter >12 cm as determined by direct abdominal X-ray. Endoscopic bowel decompression with insertion of a decompression tube is an effective alternative management option.

colonic pseudo-obstruction. Although there are no randomized trials to support IV PPI therapy versus IV H2RA therapy in the critically ill patient, there is a biologic rationale to consider using IV PPI therapy.

In general, the critical care provider should aim to maintain the appropriate physiologic environment (e.g., normalize electrolytes imbalances and maximize blood flow) and limit known causes of dysmotility (e.g., narcotics and anticholinergics) to ensure at least some level of gastrointestinal motor function. When these measures fail, providers should employ therapies that are supported by the highest level of evidence, namely randomized controlled trials, when available (Table 205.5). Among the therapies described in this chapter, there is high level of evidence to support neostigmine in colonic pseudo-obstruction, alvimopan in postoperative ileus, methylnaltrexone in opioid-induced bowel dysfunction, and good evidence supporting the use of metoclopramide and possibly erythromycin in gastroparesis. Future research for critically ill and injured patients should focus on the effects of novel medications under development on endpoints of motor function, morbidity, and mortality, with fewer systemic side effects and an excellent risk profile.

References

1. Quigley EM: Critical care dysmotility: abnormal foregut motor function in the ICU/ITU patient. *Gut* 54:1351–1352, 2005; discussion 1384-90.
2. Mutlu GM, Mutlu EA, Factor P: Prevention and treatment of gastrointestinal complications in patients on mechanical ventilation. *Am J Respir Med* 2:395–411, 2003.
3. Newton M, Burnham WR, Kamm MA: Morbidity, mortality, and risk factors for esophagitis in hospital inpatients. *J Clin Gastroenterol* 30:264–269, 2000.
4. Torres A, Serra-Batlles J, Ros E, et al: Pulmonary aspiration of gastric contents in patients receiving mechanical ventilation: the effect of body position. *Ann Intern Med* 116:540–543, 1992.
5. Ibanez J, Penafiel A, Raurich JM, et al: Gastroesophageal reflux in intubated patients receiving enteral nutrition: effect of supine and semirecumbent positions. *JPEN J Parenter Enteral Nutr* 16:419–422, 1992.
6. Orozco-Levi M, Torres A, Ferrer M, et al: Semirecumbent position protects from pulmonary aspiration but not completely from gastroesophageal reflux in mechanically ventilated patients. *Am J Respir Crit Care Med* 152:1387–1390, 1995.
7. Nagler R, Spiro HM: Persistent gastroesophageal reflux induced during prolonged gastric intubation. *N Engl J Med* 269:495–500, 1963.
8. Ibanez J, Penafiel A, Marse P, et al: Incidence of gastroesophageal reflux and aspiration in mechanically ventilated patients using small-bore nasogastric tubes. *JPEN J Parenter Enteral Nutr* 24:103–106, 2000.
9. Ferrer M, Bauer TT, Torres A, et al: Effect of nasogastric tube size on gastroesophageal reflux and microaspiration in intubated patients. *Ann Intern Med* 130:991–994, 1999.
10. Kolbel CB, Rippel K, Klar H, et al: Esophageal motility disorders in critically ill patients: a 24-hour manometric study. *Intensive Care Med* 26:1421–1427, 2000.
11. Nind G, Chen WH, Protheroe R, et al: Mechanisms of gastroesophageal reflux in critically ill mechanically ventilated patients. *Gastroenterology* 128:600–606, 2005.
12. DeVault KR: Gastroesophageal reflux disease: extraesophageal manifestations and therapy. *Semin Gastrointest Dis* 12:46–51, 2001.
13. Torres A, El-Ebiary M, Soler N, et al: Stomach as a source of colonization of the respiratory tract during mechanical ventilation: association with ventilator-associated pneumonia. *Eur Respir J* 9:1729–1735, 1996.
14. Douzinas EE, Tsapalos A, Dimitrakopoulos A, et al: Effect of percutaneous endoscopic gastrostomy on gastro-esophageal reflux in mechanically-ventilated patients. *World J Gastroenterol* 12:114–118, 2006.
15. Cook D, Guyatt G, Marshall J, et al: A comparison of sucralfate and ranitidine for the prevention of upper gastrointestinal bleeding in patients requiring mechanical ventilation. Canadian Critical Care Trials Group. *N Engl J Med* 338:791–797, 1998.
16. Lau JY, Sung JJ, Lee KK, et al: Effect of intravenous omeprazole on recurrent bleeding after endoscopic treatment of bleeding peptic ulcers. *N Engl J Med* 343:310–316, 2000.
17. Pisegna JR: Pharmacology of acid suppression in the hospital setting: focus on proton pump inhibition. *Crit Care Med* 30:S356–S361, 2002.
18. Fennerty MB: Pathophysiology of the upper gastrointestinal tract in the critically ill patient: rationale for the therapeutic benefits of acid suppression. *Crit Care Med* 30:S351–S355, 2002.
19. Abell TL, Camilleri M, Donohoe K, et al: Consensus recommendations for gastric emptying scintigraphy: a joint report of the American Neurogastroenterology and Motility Society and the Society of Nuclear Medicine. *Am J Gastroenterol* 103:753–763, 2008.
20. McCallum RW, George SJ: Gastric dysmotility and gastroparesis. *Curr Treat Options Gastroenterol* 4:179–191, 2001.
21. Koretz RL, Lipman TO, Klein S, et al: AGA technical review on parenteral nutrition. *Gastroenterology* 121:970–1001, 2001.
22. Devendra D, Millward BA, Travis SP: Diabetic gastroparesis improved by percutaneous endoscopic jejunostomy. *Diabetes Care* 23:426–427, 2000.
23. Chen JD, Pan J, McCallum RW: Clinical significance of gastric myoelectrical dysrhythmias. *Dig Dis* 13:275–290, 1995.
24. Ricci DA, Saltzman MB, Meyer C, et al: Effect of metoclopramide in diabetic gastroparesis. *J Clin Gastroenterol* 7:25–32, 1985.
25. McCallum RW, Valenzuela G, Polepalle S, et al: Subcutaneous metoclopramide in the treatment of symptomatic gastroparesis: clinical efficacy and pharmacokinetics. *J Pharmacol Exp Ther* 258:136–142, 1991.
26. Ganzini L, Casey DE, Hoffman WF, et al: The prevalence of metoclopramide-induced tardive dyskinesia and acute extrapyramidal movement disorders. *Arch Intern Med* 153:1469–1475, 1993.
27. Kendall BJ, Chakravarti A, Kendall E, et al: The effect of intravenous erythromycin on solid meal gastric emptying in patients with chronic symptomatic post-vagotomy-antrectomy gastroparesis. *Aliment Pharmacol Ther* 11:381–385, 1997.
28. Richards RD, Davenport K, McCallum RW: The treatment of idiopathic and diabetic gastroparesis with acute intravenous and chronic oral erythromycin. *Am J Gastroenterol* 88:203–207, 1993.
29. Hersch M, Krasilnikov V, Helviz Y, et al: Prokinetic drugs for gastric emptying in critically ill ventilated patients: analysis through breath testing. *J Crit Care* 30:655.e7–655.13, 2015.
30. Keshavarzian A, Isaac RM: Erythromycin accelerates gastric emptying of indigestible solids and transpyloric migration of the tip of an enteral feeding tube in fasting and fed states. *Am J Gastroenterol* 88:193–197, 1993.
31. Rayner CK, Horowitz M: New management approaches for gastroparesis. *Nat Clin Pract Gastroenterol Hepatol* 2:454–462, 2005; quiz 493.
32. Luttikhold J, de Ruijter FM, van Norren K, et al: Review article: the role of gastrointestinal hormones in the treatment of delayed gastric emptying in critically ill patients. *Aliment Pharmacol Ther* 38:573–583, 2013.
33. Peck JJ, Milleson T, Phelan J: The role of computed tomography with contrast and small bowel follow-through in management of small bowel obstruction. *Am J Surg* 177:375–378, 1999.
34. Bauer JJ, Gelernt IM, Salky BA, et al: Is routine postoperative nasogastric decompression really necessary? *Ann Surg* 201:233–236, 1985.
35. Cheadle WG, Vitale GC, Mackie CR, et al: Prophylactic postoperative nasogastric decompression. A prospective study of its requirement and the influence of cimetidine in 200 patients. *Ann Surg* 202:361–366, 1985.

36. Cunningham J, Temple WJ, Langevin JM, et al: A prospective randomized trial of routine postoperative nasogastric decompression in patients with bowel anastomosis. *Can J Surg* 35:629–632, 1992.
37. Cheatham ML, Chapman WC, Key SP, et al: A meta-analysis of selective versus routine nasogastric decompression after elective laparotomy. *Ann Surg* 221:469–476, 1995; discussion 476-8.
38. Wolff BG, Pembeton JH, van Heerden JA, et al: Elective colon and rectal surgery without nasogastric decompression. A prospective, randomized trial. *Ann Surg* 209:670–673, 1989; discussion 673-5.
39. Petrelli NJ, Stulc JP, Rodriguez-Bigas M, et al: Nasogastric decompression following elective colorectal surgery: a prospective randomized study. *Am Surg* 59:632–635, 1993.
40. Otchy DP, Wolff BG, van Heerden JA, et al: Does the avoidance of nasogastric decompression following elective abdominal colorectal surgery affect the incidence of incisional hernia? Results of a prospective, randomized trial. *Dis Colon Rectum* 38:604–608, 1995.
41. Pearl ML, Valea FA, Fischer M, et al: A randomized controlled trial of post-operative nasogastric tube decompression in gynecologic oncology patients undergoing intra-abdominal surgery. *Obstet Gynecol* 88:399–402, 1996.
42. Huerta S, Arteaga JR, Sawicki MP, et al: Assessment of routine elimination of postoperative nasogastric decompression after Roux-en-Y gastric bypass. *Surgery* 132:844–848, 2002.
43. Akbaba S, Kayaalp C, Savkilioglu M: Nasogastric decompression after total gastrectomy. *Hepatogastroenterology* 51:1881–1885, 2004.
44. Yoo CH, Son BH, Han WK, et al: Nasogastric decompression is not necessary in operations for gastric cancer: prospective randomised trial. *Eur J Surg* 168:379–383, 2002.
45. Nelson R, Edwards S, Tse B: Prophylactic nasogastric decompression after abdominal surgery. *Cochrane Database Syst Rev* CD004929, 2005.
46. McNicol E, Horowicz-Mehler N, Fisk RA, et al: Management of opioid side effects in cancer-related and chronic noncancer pain: a systematic review. *J Pain* 4:231–256, 2003.
47. De Schepper HU, Cremonini F, Park MI, et al: Opioids and the gut: pharmacology and current clinical experience. *Neurogastroenterol Motil* 16:383–394, 2004.
48. Becker G, Galandi D, Blum HE: Peripherally acting opioid antagonists in the treatment of opiate-related constipation: a systematic review. *J Pain Symptom Manage* 34:547–565, 2007.
49. Thomas J, Karver S, Cooney GA, et al: Methylnaltrexone for opioid-induced constipation in advanced illness. *N Engl J Med* 358:2332–2343, 2008.
50. Corsetti M, Tack J: Naloxegol, a new drug for the treatment of opioid-induced constipation. *Expert Opin Pharmacother* 16:399–406, 2015.
51. Davidson ED, Hersh T, Brinner RA, et al: The effects of metoclopramide on postoperative ileus. A randomized double-blind study. *Ann Surg* 190:27–30, 1979.
52. Jepsen S, Klaerke A, Nielsen PH, et al: Negative effect of Metoclopramide in postoperative adynamic ileus. A prospective, randomized, double blind study. *Br J Surg* 73:290–291, 1986.
53. Tollesson PO, Cassuto J, Faxen A, et al: Lack of effect of metoclopramide on colonic motility after cholecystectomy. *Eur J Surg* 157:355–358, 1991.
54. Seta ML, Kale-Pradhan PB: Efficacy of metoclopramide in postoperative ileus after exploratory laparotomy. *Pharmacotherapy* 21:1181–1186, 2001.
55. Cheape JD, Wexner SD, James K, et al: Does metoclopramide reduce the length of ileus after colorectal surgery? A prospective randomized trial. *Dis Colon Rectum* 34:437–441, 1991.
56. Smith AJ, Nissan A, Lanouette NM, et al: Prokinetic effect of erythromycin after colorectal surgery: randomized, placebo-controlled, double-blind study. *Dis Colon Rectum* 43:333–337, 2000.
57. Viscusi E, Rathmell J, Fichera A, et al: A double-blind, randomized, placebo-controlled trial of Methylnaltrexone (MNTX) for post-operative bowel dysfunction in segmental colectomy patients. *Anesthesiology* 103:A893, 2005.
58. Taguchi A, Sharma N, Saleem RM, et al: Selective postoperative inhibition of gastrointestinal opioid receptors. *N Engl J Med* 345:935–940, 2001.
59. Wolff BG, Michelassi F, Gerkin TM, et al: Alvimopan, a novel, peripherally acting mu opioid antagonist: results of a multicenter, randomized, double-blind, placebo-controlled, phase III trial of major abdominal surgery and postoperative ileus. *Ann Surg* 240:728–734, 2004; discussion 734-5.
60. Webster L, Jansen JP, Peppin J, et al: Alvimopan, a peripherally acting mu-opioid receptor (PAM-OR) antagonist for the treatment of opioid-induced bowel dysfunction: results from a randomized, double-blind, placebo-controlled, dose-finding study in subjects taking opioids for chronic non-cancer pain. *Pain* 137:428–440, 2008.
61. Davis L, Lowman RM: An evaluation of cecal size in impending perforation of the cecum. *Surg Gynecol Obstet* 103:711–718, 1956.
62. Vanek VW, Al-Salti M: Acute pseudo-obstruction of the colon (Ogilvie's syndrome). An analysis of 400 cases. *Dis Colon Rectum* 29:203–210, 1986.
63. Gierson ED, Storm FK, Shaw W, et al: Caecal rupture due to colonic ileus. *Br J Surg* 62:383–386, 1975.
64. Laine L: Management of acute colonic pseudo-obstruction. *N Engl J Med* 341:192–193, 1999.
65. Ogilvie H: Large-intestine colic due to sympathetic deprivation; a new clinical syndrome. *Br Med J* 2:671–673, 1948.
66. Hutchinson R, Griffiths C: Acute colonic pseudo-obstruction: a pharmacological approach. *Ann R Coll Surg Engl* 74:364–367, 1992.
67. Rex DK: Colonoscopy and acute colonic pseudo-obstruction. *Gastrointest Endosc Clin N Am* 7:499–508, 1997.
68. Ponec RJ, Saunders MD, Kimmey MB: Neostigmine for the treatment of acute colonic pseudo-obstruction. *N Engl J Med* 341:137–141, 1999.
69. Mehta R, John A, Nair P, et al: Factors predicting successful outcome following neostigmine therapy in acute colonic pseudo-obstruction: a prospective study. *J Gastroenterol Hepatol* 21:459–461, 2006.
70. Korsten MA, Rosman AS, Ng A, et al: Infusion of neostigmine-glycopyrrolate for bowel evacuation in persons with spinal cord injury. *Am J Gastroenterol* 100:1560–1565, 2005.
71. Sgouros SN, Vlachogiannakos J, Vassiliadis K, et al: Effect of polyethylene glycol electrolyte balanced solution on patients with acute colonic pseudo obstruction after resolution of colonic dilation: a prospective, randomised, placebo controlled trial. *Gut* 55:638–642, 2006.
72. Loftus CG, Harewood GC, Baron TH: Assessment of predictors of response to neostigmine for acute colonic pseudo-obstruction. *Am J Gastroenterol* 97:3118–3122, 2002.
73. Ramage JI Jr, Baron TH: Percutaneous endoscopic cecostomy: a case series. *Gastrointest Endosc* 57:752–755, 2003.

Chapter 206 ■ Hepatic Dysfunction

AVEGAIL G. FLORES • RAJEEV RAMGOPAL • MAURICIO LISKER-MELMAN

Liver function abnormalities are detected among up to 60% of intensive care unit (ICU) patients, often leading to hepatology consultation [1], and early hepatic dysfunction (serum bilirubin > 2 mg per dL within 48 hours of admission) is a specific and independent risk factor for poor prognosis [2]. The presentation of hepatic dysfunction ranges from simple abnormalities in biochemical tests with little impact on a patient's clinical course to complex manifestations of liver failure that require prompt intervention because of high morbidity and mortality. Etiologies of hepatic dysfunction are many and varied. Sometimes, a detailed clinical history is sufficient to establish the cause of the derangement; however, a combination of clinical experience and judicious use of supplemental testing is required to establish a specific diagnosis and suggest a therapeutic course of action. Understanding the anatomic interactions between the liver and other organs and the physiologic principles that determine hepatic function is essential for establishing a rational therapeutic approach for each disorder. In this chapter, we outline aspects of liver physiology that are altered among critically ill patients and review common disorders of hepatic dysfunction seen in this setting. We also discuss complications of chronic hepatic dysfunction and appropriate management of critically ill patients with cirrhosis.

PHYSIOLOGIC CONSIDERATIONS

Blood Flow

In resting conditions, the liver receives 25% of the cardiac output and 10% to 15% of the total body blood volume. About 25% of the liver volume consists of blood (capacitance function). The human liver has dual blood supply. Approximately one-third of the hepatic blood flow is supplied by the hepatic artery (low-flow, high-pressure system, well-oxygenated blood) and two-thirds by the portal vein (high-flow, low-pressure system, poorly oxygenated blood). The hepatic artery supplies the capsule of the liver and bile ducts. The portal vein is formed by the splenic vein, superior mesenteric vein, and inferior mesenteric vein (it drains into the splenic vein). The left gastric vein branches from the portal vein and plays a fundamental role in the formation of esophageal varices for patients with portal hypertension. The portal vein provides venous drainage for several abdominal organs: pancreas, stomach, intestine, and spleen. Once within the liver, arterial and venous bloods mix in the hepatic sinusoids [3]. The sinusoids are involved in the exchange between the blood, space of Disse, and the hepatocytes. The blood flowing through the sinusoids is collected in the central veins and then into the hepatic veins and inferior vena cava.

The sinusoids are composed of fenestrated endothelial cells, Kupffer cells, stellate cells, and natural killer (NK) cells. Endothelial cells represent 50% of the sinusoidal cells. They contain numerous fenestrae (not uniform in size or distribution) with dynamic structure and function. Endothelial cells have several functions including endocytosis, secretion (interleukins, interferon, eicosanoids, endothelin, and nitric oxide), and expression of adhesion molecules. Kupffer cells are phagocytic and remove infective, toxic, and foreign substances from the portal blood. They also release substances involved in the immune response by the liver. Stellate cells, also known as lipocytes, fat storing cells, or Ito cells, store fat vacuoles (major storage sites of retinoids). They have contractile activity regulating the blood flow through the sinusoids. The NK cells, also known as Pit cells, are liver-associated lymphocytes with azurophilic granules having lysosomal activity [4,5].

Blood flow through the liver varies considerably under different physiologic conditions. In the normal state, the liver extracts less than half of its supplied oxygen (4.6 mg/min/100 g liver). Thus, in most conditions of increased oxygen demand, the liver can increase oxygen extraction without an alteration in blood flow [6]. Regulation of total hepatic blood flow occurs primarily at the level of the hepatic artery. If portal venous inflow decreases, compensation is accomplished through vasodilatation of the hepatic artery. However, reductions in mean arterial pressure below 50 mm Hg exceed the capacity of the autoregulatory mechanisms to maintain adequate liver perfusion [7].

Bilirubin Metabolism

The majority of bilirubin (80%) is generated from the breakdown of heme released by senescent red blood cells. Unconjugated bilirubin (indirect bilirubin) circulates bound to albumin before entering the hepatocyte through an active process mediated by transporter proteins. Once inside the hepatocyte, unconjugated bilirubin is transferred to the smooth endoplasmic reticulum, where it is conjugated with glucuronic acid (conjugated or direct bilirubin) and, in turn, secreted into the biliary canaliculi by a pump called multidrug resistance protein 2. Once in the gastrointestinal (GI) tract, bilirubin is deconjugated by gut bacteria enzymes and oxidized to stercobilin and eliminated in the stool. Stercobilin is also reabsorbed in the small intestine, passes the liver, and is reexcreted through the kidney (urobilirubin) in the so-called enterohepatic circulation [8].

Unconjugated hyperbilirubinemia results from increased bilirubin production (e.g., ineffective erythropoiesis, hemolytic disorders), impaired uptake (e.g., Gilbert syndrome, use of certain drugs such as rifampin), or defective conjugation (e.g., Gilbert syndrome, Crigler–Najjar syndrome types I and II). Conjugated hyperbilirubinemia results from a wide spectrum of familial (Dubin–Johnson syndrome and Rotor syndrome), hepatocytic, and biliary disorders that are associated with a benign course, acute or chronic liver cell damage, cholestatic injury, or biliary tree obstruction (intrahepatic or extrahepatic). Cholestasis of an ICU patient may be seen with sepsis, postoperatively after multiple blood transfusions, with severe alcoholic hepatitis, as a result of idiosyncratic reaction to medication (often antibiotics) or drug-induced liver injury (DILI) or while receiving total parenteral nutrition (TPN). Among adults, primary biliary cirrhosis (PBC) and primary sclerosing cholangitis (PSC) are the most common causes of chronic cholestatic liver disease. Patients with decompensated cirrhosis are often jaundiced. Less commonly observed cholestatic chronic liver conditions such as intrahepatic cholestasis of pregnancy, progressive familial intrahepatic cholestasis, and benign recurrent intrahepatic cholestasis may require expert consultation for diagnosis [9,10].

Drug Metabolism

The liver is positioned strategically between the digestive tract and the systemic circulation. Only those substances absorbed by the oral mucosa and the rectum bypass the liver, reaching the systemic circulation directly. Several diverse pathways participate in the metabolism of drugs and toxins by the liver. Three main enzymatic pathways participate in drug metabolism: oxidation, hydrolysis, and reduction, catalyzed by oxidoreductases, hydrolases, and transferases. The oxidoreductases and hydrolases catalyze phase I reactions that increase polarity (or water solubility) of substances and potentially generate toxic metabolites. The transferases catalyze phase II reactions through conjugation and produce less toxic and biologically less active products when compared to the parent compound. The most important drug oxidation system is the P450 system (the electron transport chain associated with the microsomal system). The central protein in this system is cytochrome P450, a hemoprotein [11]. The primary reactions, biochemical or physiologic changes, and toxic consequences to the liver of drug and toxin exposure may be variable and in part dependent on the interaction with the host [12–14].

Hemostatic Function

The liver is the primary site of synthesis of most of the coagulation factors and the major inhibitors of the activated coagulation cascade. The synthesis of procoagulant factors II, VII, IX, and X and anticoagulant factor proteins C and S depends on the presence of vitamin K. The adequacy of hepatic synthetic function can be estimated by the prothrombin time (PT) or international normalized ratio (INR). In the presence of liver disease, there is reduced synthesis of clotting factors and inhibitors of coagulation. The synthesis of abnormal clotting proteins with anticoagulant activity leads to disseminated intravascular coagulation (DIC) and enhanced fibrinolytic activity. In addition, thrombocytopenia, associated with portal hypertension and hypersplenism, and thrombocytopathy are usually identified in patients with end-stage liver disease. Consequently, most patients with liver disease have some measurable defect in hemostasis involving the coagulation system, fibrinolytic system, platelets, and reticuloendothelial system (Kupffer cells). The resultant clinical impact of this bleeding diathesis, however, is of variable importance. When and how the physician institutes therapeutic or prophylactic hemostatic interventions is debated and must be tailored for each patient [15,16].

CLINICAL DISORDERS

Ischemic Hepatitis

Liver ischemia is the consequence of hypoxic liver insult and presents in the setting of reduced liver blood flow, persistent systemic hypotension, or severe hypoxemia. Common synonyms for ischemic hepatitis include acute hepatic infarction, shock liver, and hypoxic hepatitis. The hepatic insult is diffuse, noninflammatory in nature, and results in variable degrees of central vein (zone 3) necrosis and collapse. The syndrome is typically recognized through detailed clinical history and biochemical evaluation because the precipitating factor may not be apparent. Dehydration, heat stroke, hemorrhage, cardiogenic shock, acute decline in cardiac output in the absence of hypotension, traumatic shock, respiratory failure, aortic dissection, pulmonary embolus, and extensive burns have been associated with ischemic hepatitis. For patients with congestive heart failure (left ventricular failure) and chronic passive liver congestion (right ventricular failure), even minor, additional insults may precipitate liver ischemia. The incidence of ischemic hepatitis in the ICU has been reported to be approximately 2.5%, with only half with identifiable hypotensive episode, and yet the in-hospital mortality associated with ischemic hepatitis approaches 50%, highlighting the importance of clinical suspicion and recognition [17,18].

The clinical presentation is highly variable. Biochemically, there is a characteristic rapid rise in serum aminotransferases, reaching 10 to 40 times the upper limits of normal. The lactate dehydrogenase also increases dramatically, whereas abnormalities in serum bilirubin, alkaline phosphatase, and PT are less striking. Peak elevations occur in the first 72 hours. In situations in which the triggering factor resolves, normalization of laboratory tests may occur over 7 to 10 days. Other chemistry abnormalities include renal failure with increased blood urea nitrogen and serum creatinine. Patients may present with hepatic encephalopathy, mild jaundice, weakness, or general malaise. More typically, the dominant clinical features are those of the disorder that triggered the ischemic insult. The differential diagnosis includes other disorders associated with significant, rapid increases in liver enzymes, such as acute viral hepatitis, alcoholic hepatitis, and drug-induced hepatotoxicity. In only rare instances, a liver biopsy is necessary for diagnosis.

Treatment of ischemic hepatitis is directed at correction of the underlying disease or factor that initiated the liver damage. The aim of treatment is to improve cardiac output, optimize liver and peripheral organ perfusion, and improve tissue oxygenation. The specific intervention depends on the precipitating factor and varies from case to case. Ischemic hepatitis is frequently self-limiting, and recovery is associated with normalization of the hepatic architecture. From the liver standpoint, the prognosis depends on the presence of a normal or previously damaged liver and on the etiology of the underlying disorder.

Congestive Hepatopathy

Congestive hepatopathy and passive hepatic congestion are interchangeable terms used to refer to the outcome of increased hepatic vein pressure from a variety of causes. The increased pressure is transmitted through the hepatic veins and venules to the hepatocytes resulting in initial damage to cells in zone 3 [19]. Additional liver damage is thought to occur from decreased hepatic flow and decreased arterial oxygen saturation [20]. The most common causes are ischemic cardiomyopathy, heart failure, valvular heart disease, restrictive lung disease, pulmonary arterial hypertension, and pericardial disease. Right-sided heart failure of any etiology (constrictive pericarditis, tricuspid regurgitation, mitral valve stenosis, or cardiomyopathy) increases the pressure of the inferior vena cava and the hepatic veins and ultimately produces liver congestion [21–23]. Although the clinical presentation of hepatic vein thrombosis (Budd–Chiari syndrome), primary thrombosis limited to hepatic venules, sinusoidal obstructive syndrome (formerly known as veno-occlusive disease), and inferior vena cava thrombosis at its hepatic portion (obliterative hepatocavopathy) may be clinically similar to congestive hepatopathy, accurate differential diagnosis is imperative. The workup of these conditions includes various imaging modalities, such as ultrasound with Doppler flow, fluoroscopic cavography, and magnetic resonance venography; at times, liver biopsy is needed for a definitive diagnosis. These medical conditions have different etiologic factors and treatment approaches [22,24–26].

The patient with liver congestion may present with signs and symptoms of right-sided heart failure and only subtle abnormalities in liver chemistries. The aminotransferases may be mildly elevated, reflecting limited degree of liver cell necrosis. Mild elevations of the alkaline phosphatase and total bilirubin are also common. In more severe presentations, the patient may be jaundiced, suggesting extrahepatic biliary obstruction. Congestive hepatopathy can eventually lead to development of hepatocellular necrosis, broad fibrous septa deposition, regenerative nodule formation, architectural derangement, and frank cirrhosis, previously termed cardiac cirrhosis. Congestion produces tender hepatomegaly, and a pulsatile liver can occur with tricuspid regurgitation. Hepatojugular reflux may be elicited, and ascites is a frequent finding. For these patients, the ascitic fluid albumin is high (>2 g per dL); in contrast, among noncardiac cirrhosis, the ascitic fluid albumin is typically lower (<2 g per dL) [27]. The serum albumin-to-ascites albumin gradient (SAAG) is more than 1.1 g per dL for both conditions. Diagnosis rests on a combination of a high index of suspicion and studies that confirm the presence of cardiopulmonary disease. Pressure measurements through cardiac catheterization, transjugular hepatic venous pressure gradients, and cardiac imaging studies are diagnostic.

A transjugular liver biopsy, ideally obtained at the time of pressure measurements, can be helpful for difficult cases. Classical biopsy findings include centrilobular parenchymal atrophy; sinusoidal and terminal hepatic venular distention; and red blood cell congestion and extravasation into the space of Disse. In addition, perisinusoidal collagen deposition is seen with chronic congestion. Treatment is focused on management of the underlying pulmonary, cardiac, or pericardial disease and removal of precipitating causes such as medications that are negatively inotropic or nephrotoxic. In select cases, advanced heart failure therapies including ventricular assist devices (VAD) and heart transplantation can be considered. Hepatic dysfunction often improves with these therapies when cardiac in origin. Both hepatic and renal dysfunction are predictive of outcomes after VAD and heart transplantation. Cirrhosis is a contraindication to isolated heart transplantation [28–31].

Ascites is managed with diuretics, low-salt diet, or large-volume paracentesis (LVP). Transjugular intrahepatic portosystemic shunt (TIPS) is contraindicated for severe cases of congestive heart failure, tricuspid regurgitation, or pulmonary hypertension, because the marked increase in systemic venous return may precipitate an acute exacerbation of heart failure [32].

Total Parenteral Nutrition

TPN remains a vital medical intervention, and its use has become routine to provide nutrition to those who are unable to eat or tolerate enteral nutrition (short gut syndrome, Crohn disease, radiation enteritis, severe pancreatitis, post-op periods, etc.). Hepatobiliary dysfunction is recognized as a major adverse effect of short-term and long-term TPN use [33–35]. Variable degrees of liver dysfunction, ranging from subtle laboratory abnormalities to clinically apparent liver disease, develop among 40% to 60% of infants and 15% to 40% of adults who require long-term TPN [36,37]. The wide prevalence ranges reflect the difficulty in ascribing liver dysfunction to TPN, particularly in the ICU where the etiology of liver abnormalities may be multifactorial, including infectious, drug-induced, or endocrine disorders. The spectrum of hepatobiliary complications attributable to TPN includes hepatic steatosis, intrahepatic cholestasis, biliary sludge, and cholelithiasis [38]. TPN-related complications are more commonly seen after prolonged periods of parenteral nutrition. Cholestasis is more commonly seen among infants than adults, whereas biliary sludge and cholelithiasis affect both the groups. Progression to cirrhosis and portal hypertension is rare and occurs more frequently among infants and neonates than adults [39].

Most patients with hepatic steatosis are asymptomatic, and liver enzyme levels usually peak within 1 to 4 weeks of TPN initiation. The elevation is often transient, and complete resolution may occur spontaneously despite continued use of TPN. With the development of currently accepted protocols for caloric intake, including lipids as an alternative calorie source, the prevalence of liver steatosis has declined significantly [40–42].

Cholestasis is uncommon among adults on short-term TPN (<3 weeks) [38]. In contrast, among adults on long-term TPN, cholestasis has been reported in up to 65% [36]. Large doses of lipid emulsion (>1 g/kg/d), short bowel syndrome (small bowel remnant < 50 cm), bacterial translocation, hypoxia, and sepsis have been associated with the development of chronic cholestasis [39]. The major concern with cholestasis in those receiving long-term TPN is the risk of progression to chronic liver disease and liver failure. In this setting, TPN may need to be discontinued. TPN-dependent individuals with intestinal failure, who have persistent liver enzyme abnormalities or evidence of impending liver failure, should be considered for isolated intestine transplantation. In the presence of end-stage liver disease, however, combined intestine and liver transplantation (LT) may become necessary. Survival postisolated intestine or combined intestine–liver transplantation is 50% at 5 years, making this a viable therapeutic option [42]. Ursodeoxycholic acid (10 to 30 mg/kg/d) has shown variable success for preterm infants and adults with TPN-induced cholestasis by improving bile flow and reducing gallbladder stasis [43].

Biliary sludge develops in 50% to 100% of individuals after more than 6 weeks on TPN [38,44]. Again, clinical manifestations vary significantly. Some patients may be asymptomatic, whereas others develop striking gallbladder distention, acalculous cholecystitis, or gallstone cholecystitis. Decreased release of cholecystokinin (biliary stasis), use of narcotics (increase in bile duct pressure), and increased bile lithogenicity are contributing factors. Early introduction of oral feeding decreases the incidence of biliary complications. Changes in the rate or composition of the TPN infusion to stimulate gallbladder contraction are impractical and not universally successful [45,46]. Acute acalculous cholecystitis is a serious condition that requires the use of broad-spectrum antibiotics, a percutaneous drainage procedure, or a surgical intervention (i.e., cholecystectomy).

Timing of initiation of parenteral nutrition in the ICU remains controversial. Although prior observational data supported early enteral and/or parenteral feeding, recent data suggests no mortality difference when earlier initiation (within 48 hours) was compared with a late initiation (after day 8). Furthermore, the late initiation group had a lower incidence of cholestasis and ICU-related infections, providing further support for a delayed strategy [47,48].

Management of TPN-related hepatobiliary dysfunction should start with ruling out other causes such as infection or drug induced liver injury (DILI), seeking consultation with nutritionists to optimize parenteral prescriptions, and advancing to enteral feeding when possible [42].

Sepsis and Multiorgan System Failure

The liver often sustains injury and develops dysfunction with sepsis and the systemic inflammatory response syndrome. The injury that occurs in the first hours is most often a consequence of liver hypoperfusion, usually in the setting of shock. This can lead to alterations in liver function including disseminated intravascular coagulation (DIC) and bleeding complications. Progressive liver injury then accompanies systemic effects with the release of bacterial and inflammatory mediators [49]. The liver also contributes to the host immune response through a variety of mechanisms. The portal circulation, which arises from the splanchnic vasculature, is susceptible to vasoconstriction and bacterial translocation during sepsis [50]. The liver is composed of several types of cells, including hepatocytes, Kupffer, endothelial sinusoidal, stellate, NK cells, and others. All these cells contribute to the hepatic response in sepsis through a series of intercellular interactions as well as through circulating or secreted factors. Kupffer cells are responsible for production and clearance of inflammatory mediators, bacterial scavenging, and toxin inactivation [51]. The hepatocytes respond by altering their basic metabolic pathways toward gluconeogenesis and increased production of cytokines and coagulant proteins. Lactate clearance and protein synthesis are reduced. Endothelial cells are responsible for the production of cytokines in response to endotoxins. They further contribute to antimicrobial activity and host defense through production of nitric oxide. Activated neutrophils are also recruited to the liver and respond by release of oxygen-free radicals and destructive enzymes, such as protease and elastase.

The acute-phase reactants produced in this setting promote a procoagulant state and induce activation of other cells involved in the immune response. However, the liver can be damaged by cytokines released by Kupffer cells as well as by factors released from activated neutrophils. The subsequent fibrin deposition and hepatocyte damage can adversely affect the microcirculation of the liver, thereby leading to progressive liver damage and systemic toxicity [52]. The role that the liver plays in the immune and metabolic responses to infection can lead to significant clinical sequelae. The majority of patients with bacteremia have abnormal liver tests. Aminotransferase elevation is characteristic in this setting and is reflective of cellular and mitochondrial injury. Abnormal liver enzymes and jaundice can occur 2 to 3 days after the onset of bacteremia. It is common to see liver enzyme elevations reaching two to three times the upper limit of normal. The serum bilirubin level also may reach 5 to 10 times normal in the setting of sepsis [53].

Prompt treatment of sepsis with supportive care and antibiotic therapy can result in normalization of enzymes and reversal of the associated hepatic dysfunction. There is no current evidence to support the use of antibodies directed toward endotoxins or cytokines for management [54]. The use of a stress dose of steroids has been found to favorably affect host defenses and reduce bacterial colonization of the liver during endotoxemia, but its use in sepsis without shock is controversial and does not appear to be beneficial [55,56].

Multisystem organ failure is an ominous sign of progressive critical illness. Hepatic dysfunction in this setting is a poor prognostic indicator. Sepsis, hemorrhage, severe trauma, or tissue injury such as pancreatitis can precipitate this clinical picture. Hepatic hypermetabolism leads to relative systemic hypoperfusion, and multiple organ injury develops because tissue perfusion is continually compromised. In these conditions, the liver reduces protein synthesis, increases protein catabolism, and decreases detoxification potential. Disproportionately high bilirubin levels compared with aminotransferase levels develop among patients with hepatic dysfunction. Patients with elevations in serum bilirubin greater than 8 mg per dL, without the presence of hemolysis or biliary obstruction, have a mortality rate greater than 90% [56]. Prompt reversal of hypotension can greatly reduce hepatic necrosis, bacterial translocation, and impaired Kupffer cell activity seen in patients with shock.

Drug-induced Liver Injury

Although DILI is suspected to be a common clinical problem, its true incidence is difficult to determine. This is most likely owing to underdiagnosis and underreporting because the abnormalities range from asymptomatic liver chemistry abnormalities with a small potential impact to life or function to fulminant hepatic failure with high morbidity and mortality. The culprit drug or medication may be difficult to identify especially in the setting of polypharmacy. A thorough medication history obtained from the patient, relatives, friends, caregivers, and pharmacy records is essential to identify the most likely precipitating agent. Factors to be considered when assessing patients with suspected DILI include clinical presentation and timeline of symptoms, timeline of drug ingestion, concurrent liver disease and other potential etiologies of liver injury, concomitant medications, herbal and substance abuse, biochemical pattern of liver injury, histologic findings, and response to rechallenge [14].

Overall, the combined rate of death and need for transplantation is estimated to be approximately 10%. Although the incidence of DILI increases with age and individuals older than 65 were more likely to have a cholestatic pattern, mortality and need for transplantation were similar in patients older than 65 years of age as compared to individuals younger than 65 [57,58]. A DILI network has been established as the first broad registry in the United States to understand and assess this problem [14], and an online database is available at livertox.nih.gov. According to the DILI network (apart from acetaminophen), antimicrobials and herbal and dietary supplements (45.5% and 16%, respectively) are the most common drug classes causing liver damage. The most common antibiotics found related to DILI were amoxicillin–clavulanate, trimethoprim–sulfamethoxazole, isoniazid, and nitrofurantoin [57].

DILI occurs through a multistep process that is initiated through drug injury and subsequent immune-mediated injury culminating in cellular apoptosis or necrosis. Injury develops from the direct effect of the drugs or their metabolites during hepatic detoxification process through cell stress, mitochondrial inhibition, and/or immune activation. Toxic by-products produced by the cytochrome P450 system or through conjugation can alter cell plasma membranes, cellular enzyme activity, or mitochondria. Drugs and their metabolites can also induce a host immune defense response with inflammatory cytokines, complement system activation, and nitric oxide, playing integral roles in the development of hepatocyte damage. In the final step, apoptosis occurs via an adenosine triphosphate (ATP)-dependent pathway, and necrosis occurs as a result of mitochondrial dysfunction and ATP depletion [59,60].

With the inception of the Drug Induced Liver Injury Network, the pace of research in the field has grown exponentially. Although categorization was historically presented as either intrinsic (dose dependent and predictable) and idiosyncratic (unpredictable), our current understanding has evolved to consider multiple factors including host metabolism, drug exposure, environmental factors, immune responses, hepatic repair, and genetic polymorphisms [60].

DILI can be classified by patterns of injury and/or clinical phenotype. Injury patterns are described as hepatocellular, cholestatic, or mixed hepatocellular-cholestatic based on liver biochemical parameters. Recognizing these patterns can be helpful for narrowing the differential diagnosis, although different patterns can be caused by the same medication (e.g., anabolic steroids causing cholestatic or mixed pattern) [61]. Isolated serum enzyme abnormalities can be simply related to induction of cytochrome P450 enzymes and are not necessarily indicative of hepatotoxicity. Medications such as phenytoin and rifampicin induce the microsomal oxidase systems and can cause elevated γ-glutamyl transpeptidase (GGT) levels. These elevations are usually present in asymptomatic patients and do not represent cholestasis. Drug-induced cholestasis manifests as elevations in serum alkaline phosphatase, total bilirubin, and GGT. Cholestasis can occur with hepatocellular inflammation and necrosis, with associated systemic symptoms such as fever, myalgias, arthropathy, and rash. Toxicity from erythromycin, chlorpromazine, or oral hypoglycemic agents can present with this clinical picture. Cholestasis with minimal or no systemic symptoms can also occur and is the presentation typically associated with anabolic steroid or estrogen use [62]. Because the presentation of drug-induced cholestasis can resemble biliary obstruction, hepatobiliary imaging is often necessary to exclude biliary ductal dilation or a hepatic or pancreatic mass. Complete recovery after cessation of the offending agent may take several months.

Approximately 50% of cases of fulminant hepatic failure are attributed to acetaminophen and 11% are attributed to non-acetaminophen drugs. Continuous and/or repeated exposures to various drugs (such as amiodarone or methotrexate) can also result in chronic liver injury resembling other causes of chronic liver disease, such as autoimmune hepatitis or alcoholic liver disease [59,63]. Drug discontinuation and supportive care remain paramount in the treatment of DILI. Evidence is mixed on specific therapies for DILI, with the exceptions of N-acetylcysteine for acetaminophen toxicity (see Chapter 98) and L-carnitine for valproic acid [64].

Sinusoidal Obstruction Syndrome

Sinusoidal obstruction syndrome (SOS), previously referred to as hepatic veno-occlusive disease, is a well-recognized complication of high-dose chemotherapy and total body irradiation in stem cell transplantation (SCT) recipients [65]. SOS has also been reported in patients who ingested food contaminated with pyrrolizidine alkaloids (bush tea), following liver transplantation (LT), and after long-term use of azathioprine and other chemotherapeutic agents [66,67]. Although the incidence of SOS varies considerably, there is a perception of a declining occurrence owing to newer nonmyeloablative conditioning regimens, avoidance of cyclophosphamide, and better patient selection.

Initially, the syndrome was thought to occur primarily as a result of injury directed toward the hepatic venules, with progressive venular obliteration, hepatocyte necrosis, and fibrosis. More recent studies indicate that venular involvement is not essential to pathogenesis and that sinusoidal obstruction is the primary mechanism behind disease development [68,69]. In SOS, damage to hepatocytes and sinusoidal endothelial cells is a central pathogenic event.

Classically, 3 to 4 weeks after the triggering event, the affected patient develops weight gain (fluid retention and ascites), right upper quadrant pain (tender hepatomegaly), and jaundice. Laboratory abnormalities begin with isolated hyperbilirubinemia (mostly conjugated or direct), followed by elevations in alkaline phosphatase and aminotransferases [70,71]. A high index of clinical suspicion must be maintained for a successful diagnosis because several other conditions have similar presentations. Clinical presentation may be similar to Budd–Chiari syndrome, congestive hepatopathy (i.e., right-sided heart failure, constrictive pericarditis, tricuspid regurgitation, pulmonary hypertension), graft-versus-host disease (GVHD), or a disseminated fungal infection [72,73].

The initial diagnosis of SOS is often made on clinical grounds, but the gold standard for diagnosis is liver histology. The major histologic features are sinusoidal congestion and fibrosis, necrosis of pericentral hepatocytes, narrowing and eventually fibrosis, and obliteration of sublobular and central venules [74]. In early stages, the histologic changes may be patchy, which may lead to erroneous interpretation. A transjugular approach to measure the hepatic venous pressure gradient (>10 mm Hg) may have diagnostic and prognostic implications and facilitates obtaining a liver biopsy. Numerous biochemical markers, including plasminogen activator inhibitor 1 (PAI-1), serum procollagen type III, and antithrombin, have been investigated as diagnostic markers for SOS, but further investigation is needed prior to clinical application [74–76]. Imaging is useful for excluding other causes of liver dysfunction, such as biliary obstruction or malignancy, than in establishing the diagnosis of SOS.

Prognosis depends on the extent of hepatic injury and is classified into three stages: mild, moderate, and severe. The degree and rate of bilirubin elevation appear to be the best biochemical markers of prognosis. Mild to moderate disease is characterized by eventual resolution of liver dysfunction, whereas severe disease is associated with multiorgan failure and a mortality rate approaching 100%. Death is a consequence of renal, pulmonary, or cardiac failure other than liver failure [77].

Current guidelines recommend various preventive strategies after risk assessment. Risk factors include underlying hepatic disease, age, source of stem cells, conditioning regimen, age, sex, and metastatic malignancy. The strongest evidence exists for the use of defibrotide and ursodeoxycholic acid for prophylaxis, whereas agents such as pentoxifylline, prostaglandin E1, heparin, and antithrombin are not recommended because if mixed data and lack of randomized controlled trials [78–80].

Supportive care is paramount to management of SOS in all stages of disease and includes minimizing sodium load, administration of diuretics, and therapeutic paracentesis. Spontaneous resolution has been reported in 70% to 85% of patients in mild cases [71,81]. There is a paucity of evidence for therapeutic interventions for severe SOS, the strongest of which supports the investigational use of defibrotide.

Defibrotide, a single-stranded oligonucleotide with antithrombotic, thrombolytic, and anti-ischemic effects, has been shown to improve survival in recent phase II and phase III trials and is currently available on an investigational basis for severe SOS. Optimal dosage and route of administration have yet to be determined [78,79,82].

Other therapeutic options for SOS such as TIPS, methylprednisolone, and liver transplantation may be considered, but extensive experience is still lacking [80,82].

GRAFT-VERSUS-HOST DISEASE

GVHD is a major cause of morbidity and mortality affecting up to 60% of patients after allogeneic stem cell transplant (SCT) and is thought to be a reaction between the donor's immune system and the recipient's tissues [83]. Acute GVHD generally presents before day 100 after transplant and commonly affects the skin, the gastrointetsinal tract, and the liver [84]. Chronic GVHD was initially described as occurring after the first 100 days, but recent increases in reduced-intensity conditioning and prophylactic measures have blurred these lines and led to new descriptions of late-onset acute GVHD and overlap syndromes both occurring after 100 days [85]. Discussions within this text will be limited to acute GVHD.

Hepatic involvement of acute GVHD manifests most commonly with elevated bilirubin and alkaline phosphatase with or without hepatitis and rarely occurs without GI or cutaneous manifestations [86,87]. Diagnosis is generally clinical and should be considered in any patient who presents with abdominal pain with diarrhea, classic rash, and/or rising bilirubin within 100 days following transplantation [88]. It is imperative to investigate other causes of hepatic dysfunction, such as sepsis, viral hepatitis, SOS, and drug toxicity. In some cases, a biopsy may be required for histologic confirmation. When hepatic GVHD presents in conjunction with cutaneous and/or GI manifestations, tissue can be obtained from the skin or GI tract. In rare cases of isolated hepatic GVHD, liver biopsy may be needed to confirm the diagnosis. Because many SCT patients present with thrombocytopenia, percutaneous liver biopsy carries significant bleeding risk and a transjugular approach may be preferable.

Grading of disease has prognostic implications and depends on the extent (stage) of dermal, GI, and hepatic involvement as well as performance status. Severe GVHD, grade III and grade IV, carry the worst prognosis with long-term survival being 25% and 5%, respectively, and persistent jaundice is an independent predictor of mortality [89,90].

Prevention and management of GVHD is complex and must be approached in conjunction with a bone marrow transplant center. Treatment of GVHD is nonstandardized and institution specific, but most utilize corticosteroids as first line which is continued for several weeks in responders followed by a slow taper. Patients who do not respond or progress within the first 5 to 7 days are considered steroid refractory and carry a poor prognosis [91]. There is no standard treatment for steroid refractory acute GVHD, but second and third line therapies include mycophenolate mofetil, etanercept, pentostatin, extracorporeal photopheresis, antithymocyte globulin, antitumor necrosis factor-α antibodies, interleukin-2 antibodies, alemtuzumab, and mesenchymal stem cells. In severe refractory hepatic GVHD, several case reports and series have reported LT as an effective therapeutic option [92].

CHRONIC LIVER DISEASE

Chronic liver disease is a result of continuous, long-term hepatic injury. Chronic viral hepatitis is arbitrarily defined as the presence of persistent liver inflammation, liver chemistry abnormalities, and positive serologic and molecular markers for more than 6 months. The persistent nature of the hepatic insult leads to a sequence of damage and repair processes that may ultimately progress to the development of fibrosis, cirrhosis, and hepatocellular carcinoma (HCC). Damage to the hepatic parenchyma, with or without fibrosis, is a common outcome of chronic liver disease. Regardless of whether the insult to the hepatocytes, the biliary ducts, or the hepatic vasculature is toxic, viral, metabolic, autoimmune, or ischemic, the reparative process often leads to similar outcomes.

Cirrhosis is a chronic diffuse condition characterized by replacement of liver cells by fibrotic tissue, which creates a nodular-appearing distortion of the normal liver architecture. Chronic liver disease and cirrhosis affects nearly 5.5 million Americans; cirrhosis is the 12th leading cause of death in the United States [93], but this mortality figures associated with liver disease may be an underestimation because it failed to capture deaths related to specific conditions of chronic liver diseases such as viral hepatitis and HCC [94].

Etiologies

Chronic hepatitis C virus (HCV) disease, alcoholic liver disease, and nonalcoholic fatty liver disease (NAFLD) are the most common causes of chronic liver disease in the United States. HCV infection is the most common chronic blood-borne infection in the United States, with 30,000 new cases reported in 2013 [95]. Recent estimates of HCV infection at 2.2 to 3.2 million cases did not include incarcerated, homeless persons and persons in active military duty, which were not accounted for by national surveys [96]. Recent guidelines from US national health agencies such as the Center for Disease Control [97] and US Preventative Task Force [98] recommend screening HCV in persons born between 1945 and 1965, the so-called baby boomers owing to high prevalence (75%) of HCV in this population [96]. Highly potent direct acting antivirals with cure rates >90% in most cases are creating a significant impact on patients with chronic hepatitis C [99,100].

Worldwide about 240 million people are chronically infected with the hepatitis B virus (HBV), and more than 780,000 die every year of complications such as cirrhosis and liver cancer [101]. It is the most common cause of liver cancer worldwide; and it is unevenly distributed throughout the world. In endemic areas (East Asia and sub-Saharan Africa), the infection is predominantly vertically transmitted from the mother to the infant. In contrast, in Western countries where HBV is relatively uncommon, the infection is acquired in adulthood. In 2013, there were 20,000 new cases of HBV in the United States with an estimated prevalence of 1.4 million [95], but it may be higher at around 2.2 million if adjusted for foreign-born infected persons [102]. Immigration of persons from endemic countries has contributed to the prevalence of chronic HBV in the United States [103].

Alcoholic liver disease is a significant medical and socioeconomic problem worldwide. Although alcohol exerts a direct toxic effect on the liver, significant liver damage develops among only 10% to 20% of those patients with chronic alcohol abuse. The spectrum of alcoholic liver disease is broad, and a single patient may be affected by more than one of the following conditions: fatty liver, alcoholic hepatitis, or alcoholic cirrhosis (common cause of end-stage liver disease and HCC). Severe alcoholic hepatitis is a form of alcoholic liver disease associated with jaundice and coagulopathy, with a 30% to 50% 1-month mortality [104]. Alcoholic hepatitis–related hospitalization increased from 2002 to 2010, and inpatient mortality decreased during this period [105]. Alcoholic liver disease alone or in combination with other liver-related disease is one of the most common indications for liver transplant in the United States [106].

NALFD and its more severe form nonalcoholic steatohepatitis (NASH), is a clinicopathologic syndrome that encompasses several clinical entities that range from simple steatosis, steatohepatitis, fibrosis, and end-stage liver disease in the absence of significant alcohol consumption. It is now recognized as the most common liver disease in the Western world [107]. The worldwide prevalence of NAFLD is estimated at 20% to 30% in Western countries and 5% to 18% in Asia [108]. A meta-analysis estimated a 24% global prevalence of NAFLD correlated with economic status [109]. It affects both children and adults, and the incidence increases with age. NAFLD is associated with an increasing prevalence of type 2 diabetes, obesity, and metabolic syndrome (including abdominal obesity, dyslipidemia, hypertension, and insulin resistance) in the US population. NALFD-induced cirrhosis may progress to HCC and in the Veteran's Affairs population; it is the third most common risk factor for HCC [110]. NASH is predicted to become the leading cause of liver and liver–kidney transplantation in the United States by 2020 [101,111].

Other causes of chronic liver disease include autoimmune liver disease, PSC, PBC, hemochromatosis, Wilson disease, α1-antitrypsin deficiency, and Budd–Chiari syndrome. It is important to recognize acute decompensation in Wilson disease because this condition is universally fatal without a liver transplant.

Clinical Manifestations and Diagnosis

Clinical manifestations of chronic liver disease vary according to the functional and histologic stage of the liver disease. Patients may be asymptomatic or have one or several manifestations of liver dysfunction. Physical findings described in patients with cirrhosis include temporal wasting, jaundice, telangiectasia, gynecomastia, ascites, splenomegaly, caput medusae, palmar erythema, and testicular atrophy. Some laboratory abnormalities are suggestive of cirrhosis. Serum albumin, bilirubin, and PT/INR, which are good indicators of hepatic synthetic function, are frequently abnormal. Thrombocytopenia should raise the suspicion for portal hypertension and cirrhosis. These markers may reflect the degree and progression of chronic liver disease and play an important role in determining patient prognosis.

The severity of chronic liver disease is often scored by the Child–Turcotte–Pugh classification, which considers variables such as serum albumin, serum bilirubin, PT, and the degree of ascites and encephalopathy (Table 206.1). The model for end-stage liver disease (MELD), calculated from the INR, total bilirubin, and creatinine, predicts survival in patients with chronic liver disease awaiting transplant. It was initially envisioned as a tool to evaluate patients undergoing transjugular intrahepatic portosystemic shunt (TIPS); it is now primarily used to prioritize liver allocation for LT in patients with end-stage liver disease [112].

Noninvasive imaging techniques, including ultrasonography, computerized tomography, and magnetic resonance imaging, can identify hepatic steatosis, cirrhosis, and liver cancer but will miss advanced fibrosis and early cirrhosis. There is significant progress in noninvasive fibrosis staging and diagnosis of cirrhosis with the use of serum markers and tools such as elastography. Among the noninvasive techniques, transient elastography is the most validated [113]. Transient elastography that uses the propagation of shear waves to measure liver stiffness is an accepted method of assessing liver fibrosis in patients with HCV

TABLE 206.1

Child–Turcotte–Pugh Scoring System

	Points scored for increasing abnormality		
Clinical and biochemical measurements	**1**	**2**	**3**
Albumin (g/dL)	>3.5	2.8–3.5	<2.8
Bilirubin (mg/dL)	1–2	2–3	>3
For cholestatic disease: bilirubin (mg/dL)	<4	4–10	>10
PT	1–4	4–6	>6
or INR	<1.7	1.7–2.3	>2.3
Ascites	Absent	Slight	Moderate
Encephalopathy (grade)	None	1 and 2	3 and 4

Child A represents 5 and 6 points; Child B, 7–9 points; and Child C, 10–15 points.
PT or INR may be used for scoring.
PT, prothrombin time; INR, international normalized ratio.
From Pugh RNH, Murray-Lyon IM, Dawson JL, et al: Transection of the esophagus for bleeding esophageal varices. *Br J Surg* 60:646–649, 1983, with permission.

by the European guidelines [114]. Transient elastography, as approved by the Food and Drug Administration in 2013, has entered clinical practice in the United States [115]. However, liver biopsy remains the gold standard to establish the severity of liver inflammation and fibrosis.

Complications and Management

The four hallmark complications of cirrhosis are ascites, hepatic encephalopathy, variceal bleeding, and jaundice. The important distinction between compensated cirrhosis and decompensated cirrhosis is the appearance of one of these complications. Hospitalization at diagnosis or at any time with liver disease signals a worse prognosis independent of the cirrhosis stage [116]. Hepatic encephalopathy that ranges from subtle cerebral dysfunction to deep coma is a complication of end-stage liver disease that can result in multiple hospitalizations and decrease life quality. Portal hypertension from cirrhosis has significant consequences. Clinical manifestations of portal hypertension include splenomegaly, esophageal and gastric varices, portal hypertensive gastropathy, colopathy, and ascites. Spontaneous bacterial peritonitis (SBP) occurs in the setting of ascites, and patients with recent upper GI bleeding or Child–Pugh B/C score with low protein ascites are particularly at risk. Hepatorenal syndrome (HRS), a functional renal dysfunction as a result of severe cirrhosis, is associated with poor prognosis and should prompt an urgent evaluation for liver transplant. Complications of chronic liver disease may result in frequent admissions to the ICU.

Hepatic Encephalopathy

Hepatic encephalopathy is a syndrome of disordered consciousness, psychiatric, neurologic, and neuromuscular abnormalities, as a result of chronic liver disease and/or portosystemic shunts [117]. Pathogenesis of this disorder is complex and incompletely understood. In-hospital mortality remains around 15% [118]. Clinical features range in severity from subclinical encephalopathy, manifested by disturbances in psychometric testing to coma (see Chapters 145 and 146). Symptoms may wax and wane over the clinical course of decompensated liver disease. Cerebral edema and elevated intracranial pressure seen with acute liver failure are not present in patients with hepatic encephalopathy and cirrhosis. Serum ammonia is a popular marker for encephalopathy in chronic liver disease. However, there is poor correlation between ammonia levels and clinical disease [119], and, in many cases, results are of uncertain utility [120]. No single test is available to accurately assess the presence or degree of encephalopathy.

Encephalopathy is usually precipitated by an acute event such as increased nitrogen load (GI bleeding, excess dietary protein intake, azotemia, and constipation), the use of certain medications (sedatives, narcotics, and diuretics), infection (SBP, pneumonia, and urinary tract infection), electrolyte abnormalities (hypokalemia and hyponatremia), TIPS, or surgical shunting, or superimposed acute liver disease. Noncompliance to lactulose is a common precipitant. Progression of the underlying liver disease can eventually lead to worsening encephalopathy.

Evaluation of patients with encephalopathy should start with identification of the precipitating event. Metabolic abnormalities such as abnormal serum sodium, potassium, and glucose as well as hypoxemia should be corrected. Hyponatremia is common, and rapid correction may be deleterious. Hypovolemia should be corrected with fluid resuscitation. Infection should be investigated with cultures obtained from urine, blood, sputum, and ascites. Given the coagulopathy associated with chronic liver disease, a lumbar puncture should be pursued only if clinically imperative and after correction of blood clotting abnormalities. The presence of GI bleeding should be investigated. Prior history of medications or toxic ingestions should be reviewed.

Medications that decrease endogenous nitrogen production and nitrogen delivery to the liver play an important role in treating encephalopathy. Lactulose is a nonabsorbable disaccharide that reduces the intestinal production and absorption of ammonia [121]. The dose of lactulose should be titrated to achieve three to five soft stools a day, starting at 30 mL orally or via nasogastric tube every 2 to 4 hours. Lactulose can also be given as an enema in patients with an ileus or in those at increased risk of aspiration (300 mL lactulose in 700 mL distilled water). Rifaximin is a nonabsorbable rifamycin antibiotic that should be added to lactulose if symptoms persist; it has been shown to maintain remission from hepatic encephalopathy and reduce hospitalization related to hepatic encephalopathy [122]. Before rifaximin became available, neomycin and metronidazole have been used in addition to lactulose and may be used as an adjunct in resource-limited setting or where rifaximin is not available. However, side effects such as ototoxicity and nephrotoxicity (neomycin) and peripheral neuropathy and dysgeusia (metronidazole) limit their widespread and long-term use. Oral branched chain amino acids improve manifestations of hepatic encephalopathy without any effects on survival [123]. Glycerol phenylbuterate (GPB) which lowers ammonia by an alternative pathway where it is metabolized and excreted in urine may have additional benefits of reducing episodes of hepatic encephalopathy and hospitalization in patients already on rifaximin [124]. Polyethylene glycol (PEG) 3350-electrolyte solution resulting in rapid gut catharsis was shown to lead to more rapid hepatic encephalopathy resolution compared to lactulose, suggesting possible superiority to lactulose which is the standard of care [115]. However, PEG administration would require an enteral tube, rapid administration of a large volume of the solution over a short period of time, and the potential for electrolyte abnormalities and dehydration. More studies are needed on GPB and PEG before these agents can be recommended. Refractory hepatic encephalopathy can occur in 8% of patients with TIPS and can be successfully managed by downsizing the TIPS [125]. Large spontaneous portosystemic shunts may occur in patients with refractory hepatic encephalopathy, and embolization of these shunts may be safe and effective [126].

Variceal Bleeding

Portal hypertension is characterized by increased resistance to portal flow and increased portal venous inflow owing to splanchnic dilatation. Portal hypertension is defined by measuring the pressure difference between the hepatic vein and the portal vein (normal pressure gradient 3 mm Hg) through transjugular approach. Clinically significant portal hypertension is >10 mm Hg and has a prognostic significance [127]. Portal pressure gradient >12 mm Hg increases the risk of variceal bleeding [128,129].

Portal hypertension induces hemodynamic changes in the hepatic and splanchnic blood flow, with the development of portosystemic collateral circulation (esophagus, stomach, rectum, umbilicus, and retroperitoneum) and splenomegaly. Varices are present in about 50% of patients with cirrhosis [127]. Primary prophylaxis is recommended for patients with small varices with red wale signs or in patients with large varices. Unfortunately, at least 10% of patients are intolerant to nonselective β-blockers [130]. Bleeding from gastric and esophageal varices is a common indication for ICU admission in patients with cirrhosis. Variceal bleeding presents with hematemesis, melena, or hematochezia. The bleeding event is often dramatic and associated with severe hemodynamic instability and frequently followed by hepatic encephalopathy.

Initial management involves airway protection for active hematemesis or advanced encephalopathy and volume resuscitation. Caution against over transfusion is warranted, with recent evidence showing higher mortality in patients who were liberally transfused (hemoglobin > 9 mg per dL) compared to the patients who were judiciously transfused (hemoglobin > 7 mg per dL) [131]. Comprehensive management of patients with GI bleeding related to portal hypertension must include the following considerations: primary prophylaxis (banding of esophageal varices or use of nonselective β-blockers), treatment of the active hemorrhage (blood/volume resuscitation, banding of esophageal varices, octreotide infusion, and antibiotic prophylaxis), and prevention of rebleeding (secondary prophylaxis with nonselective β-blockers). In esophageal bleeding refractory to endoscopic treatment or in the case of bleeding gastric varices, consideration has to be given to salvage therapy with transjugular intrahepatic portosystemic shunt (TIPS) [127]. Balloon retrograde transvenous obliteration (BRTO) of gastric varices is an established technique for the management of bleeding varices. This technique was initially used in Japan and Korea but is becoming increasingly available in the United States. There is insufficient data to compare TIPS and BRTO. Additionally, there are no randomized controlled trials on BRTO [132].

Coagulopathy with markedly elevated PT, INR, and partial thromboplastin time is common in chronic liver disease. The coagulation profile of a patient with chronic liver disease is significantly different from a normal patient because there are deficiencies in the synthesis of coagulation factors in both procoagulant and anticoagulant pathways [133]. Transfusion-related lung injury is a dangerous consequence of overtransfusion and can progress to acute lung injury and acute respiratory distress syndrome. Thrombocytopenia is common among patients with splenomegaly secondary to cirrhosis, and it is a consequence of hypersplenism. In our experience, transfusion of platelets should be limited to those patients who are actively bleeding or undergoing an invasive procedure.

Ascites, Hydrothorax, and Hyponatremia

Mechanisms responsible for the formation of ascites are complicated, multifactorial, and result in sodium and water retention. Circulatory dysfunction characterized by arterial vasodilation and low peripheral vascular resistance with hypotension, high cardiac output, and hypervolemia is seen in patients with portal hypertension and ascites. Levels of nitric oxide, a potent vasodilator, are elevated in the splanchnic circulation of patients with ascites. The ensuing arterial vasodilation triggers activation of baroreceptor-mediated systems, the renin–angiotensin–aldosterone system, and the sympathetic nervous system, inducing sodium retention. Regulation of water balance is also disrupted in patients with cirrhosis. As a result of the reduced effective intravascular volume, arginine vasopressin levels are elevated. The major clinical consequence of this elevation is dilutional hyponatremia, which occurs despite an avid sodium state [134].

Patients with large volume ascites present with abdominal distension with a fluid wave or shifting dullness on examination. Respiratory compromise from associated pleural effusion (hepatic hydrothorax) or increase intra-abdominal pressure may result. Large volume ascites may also induce the development of ventral and umbilical hernias, with increased risk of intestinal strangulation or hernia rupture.

Analysis of the ascitic fluid is essential for the appropriate management of patients with decompensated liver disease. Small volume (60 mL) diagnostic paracentesis should be performed in patients hospitalized with ascites. Even in the presence of severe coagulopathy, it is safe to remove fluid [135]. Infection and bleeding are rare complications (<1%) [136]. The ascitic fluid should be sent for cell count and differential, culture, albumin, and total protein. Additional tests such as triglycerides (chylous ascites), amylase (pancreatic ascites), adenosine deaminase (peritoneal tuberculosis), and cytology (malignant ascites) should only be sent as clinically indicated. An SAAG more than 1.1 g per dL indicates portal hypertension with 97% specificity. An SAAG less than 1.1 g per dL is found in nephrotic syndrome, peritoneal carcinomatosis, serositis, tuberculosis, and biliary and pancreatic ascites. Ascitic fluid total protein is helpful and expectedly low (<2.5 g per L) in portal hypertension. A high SAAG, high-protein ascitic fluid should prompt evaluation for posthepatic etiologies such as heart failure and constrictive pericarditis. Restriction of sodium intake to 2,000 mg per day and minimizing intravenous (IV) sodium load (fluids, antibiotics, TPN, and blood transfusions) play an important therapeutic role.

Most patients will require combination of a potassium-sparing diuretic and a loop diuretic to achieve a more rapid natriuresis and to maintain normal potassium levels. Starting dose of spironolactone is 100 mg daily and furosemide 40 mg daily. Titration every 3 to 5 days (maintaining a 5 to 2 mg ratio) to maximum daily doses of 400 mg of spironolactone and 160 mg of furosemide is the recommended approach [137]. About 10% of patients will fail diuretic therapy and develop refractory ascites. LVP can safely remove 8 to 10 L as a therapeutic measure for patients with tense ascites. The administration of albumin (6 to 8 g per L of ascites removed) during LVP has been associated with a lower incidence of hemodynamic disturbances without affecting survival [138,139]. Refractory ascites is a condition that develops in patients who do not respond adequately to maximum doses of diuretics. Progressive intravascular volume depletion, renal failure, and electrolyte abnormalities may limit the use of high-dose diuretics. Among these patients, the use of angiotensin converting enzyme inhibitor (ACEI) and angiotensin receptor blockers (ARBs) should be avoided. Nonselective β-blocker should be discontinued if there is systemic hypotension. A reasonable alternative in patients with refractory ascites requiring frequent LVPs with preserved liver function is TIPS. Complications associated with TIPS include hepatic encephalopathy, cardiopulmonary compromise, pulmonary edema, transient pulmonary hypertension, infection, bleeding, ischemic hepatitis, and shunt occlusion. Peritoneovenous shunt may be considered for patients who are not TIPS candidate as a palliative measure; unfortunately, occlusion and infection are frequently associated complications that limit their generalized use. Patients with cirrhosis and ascites should be considered for LT. An expedited referral for patients with refractory ascites is recommended [137].

Hepatic hydrothorax is a transudative pleural effusion of patients with portal hypertension in the absence of an underlying cardiopulmonary or pleural process. It occurs in 5% to 10% of cases. Although frequently occurring in the right pleural space caused by direct passage of peritoneal fluids through diaphragmatic defects, left-sided and bilateral hydrothorax occur 13% and 2% of the time, respectively [140]. The medical management is similar to that of ascites with dietary sodium restriction and diuretics. Some of these patients will be considered refractory, and regular thoracentesis will be necessary to alleviate symptoms. Consideration for TIPS in patients with low MELD is a reasonable alternative to regular thoracentesis. A small collection of noncontrolled trials of 198 patients who underwent TIPS reported response rates (both complete and partial) ranging from 59% to 82% is reported [141]. Among selected patients with severe liver disease wherein placement of a TIPS is potentially hazardous such as in cases with MELD score >15, there are some reports of success with implantation of indwelling pleural catheters [142].

Spontaneous bacterial empyema (SBEM) is an important and underdiagnosed complication of hydrothorax, with an observed mortality of 20% to 35% [143]. The name is misleading because there is no pus in the thoracic cavity; and the etiology, pathogenesis, and treatment are different from empyema. The diagnosis is established after pneumonia or parapneumonic effusion is excluded on imaging by pleural fluid analysis showing either (1) a neutrophil count > 250 cells per μL and a positive pleural fluid culture or (2) >500 neutrophils per μL in the absence of a positive culture [144,145]. The typical organisms mirror that of SBP [143]. Treatment with a third-generation cephalosporin for 7 to 10 days is recommended. The concurrent treatment with albumin, as practiced in spontaneous bacterial peritonitis, has not been studied in SBEM. Chest tube placement should be avoided because it is associated with infection, high output, dehydration, and increased mortality [146].

With cirrhosis, hyponatremia develops in the setting of ascites in a state of avid renal sodium retention and increased extracellular fluid volume (hypervolemic hyponatremia) or from excessive losses of sodium and extracellular fluid (hypovolemic hyponatremia). Hyponatremia correlates with the severity of liver disease and is associated with poor outcomes [147]. The patient's volume status determines the treatment. Volume expansion is necessary for hypovolemic hyponatremia. Hypervolemic hyponatremia is common in cirrhosis and is usually tolerated, so rapid correction (>8 mmol per L in a day) should be avoided because of neurologic complications of osmotic demyelination syndrome. There is a lack of data on when treatment for hyponatremia should be initiated. In general, fluid restriction to 1 L per day is recommended for patients with serum sodium <125 mEq per L. Hypertonic saline is only recommended if hyponatremia is associated with neurologic symptoms because of associated problems with infusion [137]. Vaptans are vasopressin receptor 2 antagonists that block the action of arginine vasopressin in the distal tubule of the kidneys. These agents result in solute-free diuresis and have been used in patients with cirrhosis, dilutional hyponatremia, and ascites. There are two approved agents in the United States. Conivaptan is a combined V1a- and V2 receptor antagonist that carries the theoretical risk of hypotension, variceal bleeding, and worsening kidney function. The other approved agent is tolvaptan. A previous long-term study on tolvaptan for the treatment of hyponatremia showed that tolvaptan is safe, resulting in a modest response among cirrhotics with no liver injury reported [148]. However, after a randomized controlled trial that used tolvaptan in adult polycystic kidney disease to inhibit cyst growth and preserve kidney function showed high discontinuation rates owing to hepatic adverse events [149], tolvaptan is no longer approved by the Food and Drug Administration for patients with cirrhosis because of a reported higher frequency of elevation of liver enzymes. It is important to note that the doses used in this trial in adult polycystic kidney disease were much higher than in the previous studies of cirrhosis [150]. In our experience, small doses of vaptans over a short period of time were generally safe, but the small improvement in hyponatremia vanished with discontinuation of the vaptans. A meta-analysis of 12 trials on the safety and efficacy of vaptans showed small benefit in hyponatremia and ascites with no beneficial effect on mortality [151]. Thus, the routine use of vaptans is not recommended [137], but there may be a role in the short-term use of tolvaptan in patients awaiting LT [147].

Spontaneous Bacterial Peritonitis

SBP is an infectious complication resulting from intestinal bacterial translocation that occurs through altered gut permeability and bacterial overgrowth. The intestinal microbiome and genetic and acquired immune defects are linked to the development of infection [152]. SBP develops in the setting of reticuloendothelial system depression and leukocyte dysfunction along with decreased opsonic activity in the ascitic fluid [153,154]. Twelve percent of patients with ascites admitted to the hospital for any reason have SBP, and it is associated with high in-hospital mortality (16% to 23%) [155]. Acute kidney injury (AKI) often complicates SBP and prevention of AKI is associated with reduced mortality [156].

A polymorphonuclear cell count of more than 250 per μL or the presence of a positive bacterial culture in the ascitic fluid establishes the diagnosis of SBP. Inoculation of culture bottles at bedside improves bacterial culture yield [157]. Identification of more than one organism raises the possibility of secondary bacterial peritonitis usually related to another intra-abdominal process. The most common organisms responsible for SBP are the gram-negative enteric bacteria, *Escherichia coli*, *Klebsiella pneumoniae,* and *Streptococcus pneumoniae* [157]. Because the identification of organisms is not immediately available, treatment should be targeted at the most likely culprits. The ideal antibiotic should have both gram-negative and enteric organism coverage without nephrotoxicity. A third- or fourth-generation cephalosporin (cefotaxime and ceftriaxone) and ampicillin/sulbactam are the recommended first-line agents. Repeat paracentesis should be performed in patients who are not responding to therapy after 48 hours. If a 50% decrease in polymorphonuclear cell count is not seen after 72 hours of antibiotic use, antibiotic coverage should be broadened. Antibiotics resistance is increasingly recognized [158], and failure of first-line treatment caused by increasing rates of bacterial resistance is associated with poor prognosis [159]. Nosocomial SBP is very problematic because it is often caused by multidrug-resistant bacteria. Piperacillin/tazobactam or meropenem with and without a glycopeptide is the recommended approach in Europe for nosocomial SBP [158]. A randomized trial showed superior outcomes in nosocomial SBP treated empirically with meropenem and daptomycin compared to ceftazidime (a third generation cephalosporin) [160].

Administration of IV albumin in addition to antibiotics in the setting of SBP results in a lower incidence of renal impairment, improving short-term survival [161,162]. Owing to the high recurrence rate of infection (70%) [163], prophylactic long-term oral antibiotic therapy is recommended after recovery. Secondary prophylaxis can be achieved with daily norfloxacin, ciprofloxacin, or trimethoprim/sulfamethoxazole. Daily dosing is the preferred frequency to avoid the emergence of antibiotic-resistant strains [157]. Primary antibiotic prophylaxis for SBP is indicated in the setting of acute GI bleeding [164], patients with ascitic fluid protein <1.5 g per dL, more advanced cirrhosis (Child B or C), jaundice (bilirubin > 3 mg per dL), and renal impairment (creatinine 1.2 mg per dL, blood urea nitrogen 25, serum sodium 130 mmol per L) [157,158]. Nonselective β-blocker use after an episode of SBP may be associated with increased hospitalization, hepatorenal syndrome, and mortality by exacerbating hemodynamic compromise in patients with already low systolic arterial pressures (<100 mm Hg) [165]. Finally, the association of the development of SBP with proton pump inhibitor (PPI) use should prompt discontinuation of the PPI in patients who do not have a clear indication [166,167].

Hepatorenal Syndrome

HRS develops during the terminal stages of liver failure as a result of intense splanchnic vasodilatation leading to intravascular hypovolemia and severe renal hypoperfusion. It is a feared consequence of end-stage liver disease and is seen in up to 10% of patients hospitalized with cirrhosis and ascites [168]. In HRS, functional renal failure occurs in the absence of obvious abnormalities in kidney structure. Conceptually, the kidneys are structurally normal, and the syndrome is reversible with LT in majority of the patients. The primary mechanism in the pathogenesis of HRS involves intense renal vasoconstriction in response to activation of neurohumoral factors including the renin–angiotensin–aldosterone system and the sympathetic nervous system leading to low renal perfusion and glomerular filtration rate [169].

HRS is a form of AKI. An increase in serum creatinine to 1.5 mg per dL had been the threshold to diagnose AKI in cirrhosis [170]. This creatinine cutoff is problematic in patients with sarcopenia or diminished muscle mass and may not reflect the glomerular filtration rate. In addition, the initial small increase in serum creatinine corresponds to a dramatic drop in glomerular filtration rate. The most recent definition of HRS by the International Ascites Club recognized the diagnostic challenges of AKI in cirrhosis. HRS can now be diagnosed in patients with ascites who meet the criteria given in Table 206.2, where the first stage of AKI is defined as an increase in serum creatinine >0.3 mg per dL within 48 hours or a >50% increase in serum creatinine from a known baseline or presumed to have occurred within the prior 7 days [171].

There are two clinically distinct types in HRS. Type I HRS progresses rapidly and has a close temporal association with a precipitating event that results in progressive loss of kidney function in 2 weeks. Type II HRS progresses in a slower but relentless fashion as a form of expression of circulatory dysfunction and clinically manifests as diuretic-resistant ascites. In contrast to patients with type II HRS that present with better preserved liver function, patients with type I HRS have a very poor prognosis. They are usually severely ill with marked edema, ascites, sodium retention, hyponatremia, and hypotension. In both cases, the presence of ascites is necessary to make the diagnosis of HRS. Precipitants of HRS include SBP, infection, large volume paracentesis without plasma expansion, and GI bleeding.

Although diagnostic criteria for HRS have been established (Table 206.2), the distinction between type I HRS and prerenal azotemia may be extremely difficult. In recent studies, both biomarkers, urinary neutrophil gelatinase–associated lipocalin and interleukin-18, have shown the ability to distinguish hepatorenal syndrome from prerenal azotemia and acute tubular necrosis. However, HRS may not be always an entirely functional condition; it may also involve some degree of parenchymal injury which will limit the utility of these biomarkers where there is an overlap [172]. Pharmacologic therapy with splanchnic vasoconstrictor drugs and IV albumin are usually initiated when HRS is suspected. Splanchnic vasoconstrictors used in the treatment of HRS include terlipressin, norepinephrine, or octreotide in combination with the α-agonist midodrine. Among the vasoconstrictors, terlipressin is the most extensively studied but is not available in the United States. Combination of midodrine (15 mg three times a day), octreotide (200 μg subcutaneously three times a day), and albumin infusion had shown benefit in small studies; this regimen can be given outside the ICU [137]. Terlipressin with albumin has been shown to be more effective than midodrine, octreotide, and albumin [173]. Norepinephrine is a reasonable alternative to terlipressin as it has been shown equivalent with less adverse events [174]. Renal replacement therapy (RRT) is usually required in a majority of these patients as a bridge to LT.

HRS may occasionally be prevented by timely administration of albumin and antibiotics in the treatment of SBP [175]. There had been reports of TIPS as a treatment of types I and II HRS with some success [176–179]; however, the risk of mortality is high because these patients usually have high MELD scores and so TIPS cannot always be advocated. Routine use of RRT may not be beneficial for patients with type 1 HRS already receiving combination treatment of vasoconstrictor plus albumin [180]. Urgent referral for LT is recommended once HRS is suspected. In type I HRS, LT offers better survival. Among patients who do not receive LT, RRT does not provide an improved survival benefit [181]. Although LT is the only curative option, reversal was only seen in 76% of cases of HRS type 1. Duration of pretransplant dialysis was the only observed predictor of reversibility [182].

Hepatopulmonary Syndrome and Portopulmonary Hypertension

Hepatopulmonary syndrome (HPS) is a clinical disorder of impaired oxygenation caused by intrapulmonary vascular dilatation in the setting of portal hypertension and absence of

TABLE 206.2

Diagnostic Criteria for Hepatorenal Syndrome (HRS) [171]

HRS-AKI
Diagnosis of cirrhosis and ascites

Diagnosis of AKI according to ICA-AKI criteria[a]

No response after 2 consecutive days of diuretic withdrawal and plasma volume expansion with albumin 1 g/kg of body weight
Absence of shock
No current or recent use of nephrotoxic drugs
No macroscopic signs of structural kidney injury[a]
Defined as:
- Absence of proteinuria (>500 mg/d)
- Absence of microhematuria (>50 red blood cells per high-power field)
- Normal findings on renal ultrasonography

[a]AKI defined as:

Increase in serum creatinine ≥0.3 mg/dL (≥26.5 μmol/L) within 48 hours, or a percentage increase in serum creatinine ≥50% from baseline which is known, or presumed to have occurred within the prior 7 days

Staging of AKI

Stage 1: increase in sCr ≥0.3 mg/dL (26.5 μmol/L) or an increase in sCr ≥1.5-fold to 2-fold from baseline
Stage 2: increase in sCr > twofold to threefold from baseline
Stage 3: increase in sCr > threefold from baseline or sCr ≥4.0 mg/dL (353.6 μmol/L) with an acute increase ≥0.3 mg/dL (26.5 μmol/L) or initiation of renal replacement therapy

[a]Patients who fulfill this criteria may still have structural damage such as tubular damage.
AKI, acute kidney injury; HRS, hepatorenal syndrome; ICA, International Club of Ascites; sCr, serum creatinine.

primary cardiopulmonary disease [183]. The clinical features platypnea (shortness of breath improved when supine) and orthodeoxia (fall in the arterial PO_2 in the upright position) are unique to this syndrome. Isolated hypoxia should be further investigated with contrast-enhanced echocardiogram or a transthoracic echocardiogram with agitated saline (bubble study). The presence of delayed microbubbles in addition to PaO_2 < 80 mm Hg with an A-a gradient is consistent with HPS [184]. HPS is associated with significant increased risk of death and worse quality of life [185,186]. There is no approved therapy, and LT is the only curative treatment. For this reason, MELD exception points are allocated to patients with HPS with $PaO_2 < 60$ mm Hg to facilitate transplantation. Poor outcomes are seen in patients transplanted with $PaO_2 < 50$ mm Hg [185,187].

Portopulmonary hypertension is pulmonary hypertension (pulmonary artery pressure > 25 mm Hg and pulmonary vascular resistance > 240 dynes/s/cm^5) in the setting of portal hypertension and absence of other primary lung disease [188]. Typical symptoms are dyspnea or nonspecific chest discomfort. Diagnosis usually starts with transthoracic echocardiogram where right ventricle systolic pressure is >40 mm Hg and pulmonary artery pressure is >25 mm Hg. Other etiologies of pulmonary hypertension should be investigated and excluded. A right heart catheterization is required to confirm pulmonary artery pressure and resistance and exclude volume overload or left heart failure. Portopulmonary hypertension is associated with significant morbidity and mortality with an estimated 1-year survival without treatment of 60% [184]. MELD exception points are given to patients with pulmonary artery pressure > 35 mm Hg. Medical treatment for portopulmonary hypertension is similar to that of pulmonary hypertension. LT, although still offered, may not confer a significant survival advantage [189].

Liver Transplantation

LT can be lifesaving in patients with end-stage liver disease. The 1-year survival rate for LT in the setting of chronic liver disease is currently 85% to 90% [190]. With increasing numbers of patients listed for transplantation and the relatively static number of cadaveric organs available, death is not uncommon while awaiting an organ offer. Medical contraindications to LT include uncontrolled sepsis, advanced cardiac or pulmonary disease, multiorgan failure, and advanced malignancies. Psychosocial factors are just as important in transplant listing, and these include unresolved alcoholism, drug addiction, uncontrolled psychiatric disease, compliance issues, and lack of social support or medical insurance coverage. Transplant evaluation should be initiated when there is decompensated liver disease as manifested by the syndromes described in this chapter. In addition, transplant evaluation involves recognizing those patients who are too sick and will not benefit from transplantation. Identification of these patients becomes more difficult because the regional organ allocation for liver prioritizes the sickest patient or the highest MELD score in the list. MELD is an accurate predictor of short-term survival (3 months) in patients with cirrhosis awaiting LT [112,191]. It is a poor predictor of survival posttransplantation [192]. Currently, there are no widely utilized criteria that will accurately predict whether a critically ill patient will survive transplantation.

References

1. Thomson SJ, Cowan ML, Johnston I, et al: 'Liver function tests' on the intensive care unit: a prospective, observational study. *Intensive Care Med* 35(8):1406–1411, 2009.
2. Kramer L, Jordan B, Druml W, et al: Incidence and prognosis of early hepatic dysfunction in critically ill patients—a prospective multicenter study. *Crit Care Med* 35(4):1099–1104, 2007.
3. Bioulac-Sage P, Saric J, Balabaud C: Microscopic anatomy of the intrahepatic circulatory system, in Okuda K, Benhamou J-P (eds): *Portal Hypertension. Clinical and Physiologic Aspects*. Tokyo, Springer-Verlag, 1991, p 13.
4. McCuskey RS: The hepatic microvascular system in health and its response to toxicants. *Anat Rec (Hoboken)* 291(6):661–671, 2008.
5. Sorensen KK, Simon-Santamaria J, McCuskey RS, et al: Liver sinusoidal endothelial cells. *Compr Physiol* 5(4):1751–1774, 2015.
6. Greenway CV, Stark RD: Hepatic vascular bed. *Physiol Rev* 51(1):23–65, 1971.
7. Lautt WW: Hepatic vasculature: a conceptual review. *Gastroenterology* 73(5):1163–1169, 1977.
8. Fabris L, Cadamuro M, Okolicsanyi L: The patient presenting with isolated hyperbilirubinemia. *Dig Liver Dis* 41(6):375–381, 2009.
9. Nguyen KD, Sundaram V, Ayoub WS: Atypical causes of cholestasis. *World J Gastroenterol* 20(28):9418–9426, 2014.
10. Pathobiology of bilirubin and jaundice. *Semin Liver Dis* 8(2):103–199, 1988.
11. Lewis JH: Drug-induced liver disease. *Med Clin North Am* 84(5):1275–1311, x, 2000.
12. Porter TD, Coon MJ: Cytochrome P-450. Multiplicity of isoforms, substrates, and catalytic and regulatory mechanisms. *J Biol Chem* 266(21):13469–13472, 1991.
13. Assis DN, Navarro VJ: Human drug hepatotoxicity: a contemporary clinical perspective. *Expert Opin Drug Metab Toxicol* 5(5):463–473, 2009.
14. Chalasani N, Fontana RJ, Bonkovsky HL, et al: Causes, clinical features, and outcomes from a prospective study of drug-induced liver injury in the United States. *Gastroenterology* 135(6):1924–1934, 1934.e1–1934.e4, 2008.
15. Amitrano L, Guardascione MA, Brancaccio V, et al: Coagulation disorders in liver disease. *Semin Liver Dis* 22(1):83–96, 2002.
16. Northup PG, Caldwell SH: Coagulation in liver disease: a guide for the clinician. *Clin Gastroenterol Hepatol* 11(9):1064–1074, 2013.
17. Tapper EB, Sengupta N, Bonder A: The incidence and outcomes of ischemic hepatitis: a systematic review with meta-analysis. *Am J Med* 128(12):1314–1321, 2015.
18. Merx MW, Weber C: Sepsis and the heart. *Circulation* 116(7):793–802, 2007.
19. Safran AP, Schaffner F: Chronic passive congestion of the liver in man. Electron microscopic study of cell atrophy and intralobular fibrosis. *Am J Pathol* 50(3):447–463, 1967.
20. Giallourakis CC, Rosenberg PM, Friedman LS: The liver in heart failure. *Clin Liver Dis* 6(4):947–967, viii–ix, 2002.
21. Kavoliuniene A, Vaitiekiene A, Cesnaite G: Congestive hepatopathy and hypoxic hepatitis in heart failure: a cardiologist's point of view. *Int J Cardiol* 166(3):554–558, 2013.
22. Moller S, Bernardi M: Interactions of the heart and the liver. *Eur Heart J* 34(36):2804–2811, 2013.
23. Sheth AA, Lim JK: Liver disease from asymptomatic constrictive pericarditis. *J Clin Gastroenterol* 42(8):956–958, 2008.
24. Valla DC: Hepatic vein thrombosis (Budd-Chiari syndrome). *Semin Liver Dis* 22(1):5–14, 2002.
25. Okuda K: Inferior vena cava thrombosis at its hepatic portion (obliterative hepatocavopathy). *Semin Liver Dis* 22(1):15–26, 2002.
26. Sarin SK, Agarwal SR: Extrahepatic portal vein obstruction. *Semin Liver Dis* 22(1):43–58, 2002.
27. Runyon BA: Cardiac ascites: a characterization. *J Clin Gastroenterol* 10(4):410–412, 1988.
28. Lindenfeld J, Albert NM, Boehmer JP, Heart Failure Society of America; et al: HFSA 2010 comprehensive heart failure practice guideline. *J Card Fail* 16(6):e1–e194, 2010.
29. Deo SV, Al-Kindi SG, Altarabsheh SE, et al: Model for end-stage liver disease excluding international normalized ratio (MELD-XI) score predicts heart transplant outcomes: evidence from the registry of the united network for organ sharing. *J Heart Lung Transplant* 35:222–227, 2016.
30. Tsiouris A, Paone G, Nemeh HW, et al: Short and long term outcomes of 200 patients supported by continuous-flow left ventricular assist devices. *World J Cardiol* 7(11):792–800, 2015.
31. Kim B, Tan A, Limketkai BN, et al: Comparison of outcome in patients with versus without ascites referred for either cardiac transplantation or ventricular assist device placement. *Am J Cardiol* 116(10):1596–1600, 2015.
32. Copelan A, Kapoor B, Sands M: Transjugular intrahepatic portosystemic shunt: indications, contraindications, and patient work-up. *Semin Intervent Radiol* 31(3):235–242, 2014.
33. Lindor KD, Fleming CR, Abrams A, et al: Liver function values in adults receiving total parenteral nutrition. *JAMA* 241(22):2398–2400, 1979.
34. Baker AL, Rosenberg IH: Hepatic complications of total parenteral nutrition. *Am J Med* 82(3):489–497, 1987.
35. Delany HM: The interrelationship of the liver and gut. *Nutrition* 12(1):54–55, 1996.
36. Cavicchi M, Beau P, Crenn P, et al: Prevalence of liver disease and contributing factors in patients receiving home parenteral nutrition for permanent intestinal failure. *Ann Intern Med* 132(7):525–532, 2000.
37. Buchman A: Total parenteral nutrition-associated liver disease. *JPEN J Parenter Enteral Nutr* 26[5 Suppl]:S43–S48, 2002.
38. Buchman AL, Iyer K, Fryer J: Parenteral nutrition-associated liver disease and the role for isolated intestine and intestine/liver transplantation. *Hepatology* 43(1):9–19, 2006.
39. Kelly DA: Intestinal failure-associated liver disease: what do we know today? *Gastroenterology* 130[2 Suppl 1]:S70–S77, 2006.
40. Meguid MM, Akahoshi MP, Jeffers S, et al: Amelioration of metabolic complications of conventional total parenteral nutrition. A prospective randomized study. *Arch Surg* 119(11):1294–1298, 1984.

41. Nandivada P, Carlson SJ, Chang MI, et al: Treatment of parenteral nutrition-associated liver disease: the role of lipid emulsions. *Adv Nutr* 4(6):711–717, 2013.
42. Beath SV, Kelly DA: Total parenteral nutrition-induced cholestasis: prevention and management. *Clin Liver Dis* 20(1):159–176, 2016.
43. Kowdley KV: Ursodeoxycholic acid therapy in hepatobiliary disease. *Am J Med* 108(6):481–486, 2000.
44. Messing B, Bories C, Kunstlinger F, et al: Does total parenteral nutrition induce gallbladder sludge formation and lithiasis? *Gastroenterology* 84[5 Pt 1]:1012–1019, 1983.
45. Doty JE, Pitt HA, Porter-Fink V, et al: The effect of intravenous fat and total parenteral nutrition on biliary physiology. *JPEN J Parenter Enteral Nutr* 8(3):263–268, 1984.
46. Priori P, Pezzilli R, Panuccio D, et al: Stimulation of gallbladder emptying by intravenous lipids. *JPEN J Parenter Enteral Nutr* 21(6):350–352, 1997.
47. Alberda C, Gramlich L, Jones N, et al: The relationship between nutritional intake and clinical outcomes in critically ill patients: results of an international multicenter observational study. *Intensive Care Med* 35(10):1728–1737, 2009.
48. Casaer MP, Mesotten D, Hermans G, et al: Early versus late parenteral nutrition in critically ill adults. *N Engl J Med* 365(6):506–517, 2011.
49. Cerra FB, Siegel JH, Border JR, et al: The hepatic failure of sepsis: cellular versus substrate. *Surgery* 86(3):409–422, 1979.
50. Nesseler N, Launey Y, Aninat C, et al: Clinical review: the liver in sepsis. *Crit Care* 16(5):235, 2012.
51. Spapen H: Liver perfusion in sepsis, septic shock, and multiorgan failure. *Anat Rec (Hoboken)* 291(6):714–720, 2008.
52. Allen KS, Sawheny E, Kinasewitz GT: Anticoagulant modulation of inflammation in severe sepsis. *World J Crit Care Med* 4(2):105–115, 2015.
53. Sikuler E, Guetta V, Keynan A, et al: Abnormalities in bilirubin and liver enzyme levels in adult patients with bacteremia. A prospective study. *Arch Intern Med* 149(10):2246–2248, 1989.
54. Arenas J: The role of bacterial lipopolysaccharides as immune modulator in vaccine and drug development. *Endocr Metab Immune Disord Drug Targets* 12(3):221–235, 2012.
55. Annane D, Bellissant E, Bollaert PE, et al: Corticosteroids in the treatment of severe sepsis and septic shock in adults: a systematic review. *JAMA* 301(22):2362–2375, 2009.
56. Barton R, Cerra FB: The hypermetabolism. Multiple organ failure syndrome. *Chest* 96(5):1153–1160, 1989.
57. Chalasani N, Bonkovsky HL, Fontana R, et al: Features and outcomes of 899 patients with drug-induced liver injury: the DILIN prospective study. *Gastroenterology* 148(7):1340.e7–1352.e7, 2015.
58. Marti L, Del Olmo JA, Tosca J, et al: Clinical evaluation of drug-induced hepatitis. *Rev Esp Enferm Dig* 97(4):258–265, 2005.
59. Kaplowitz N: Idiosyncratic drug hepatotoxicity. *Nat Rev Drug Discov* 4(6):489–499, 2005.
60. Au JS, Navarro VJ, Rossi S: Review article: drug-induced liver injury—its pathophysiology and evolving diagnostic tools. *Aliment Pharmacol Ther* 34(1):11–20, 2011.
61. Fontana RJ, Seeff LB, Andrade RJ, et al: Standardization of nomenclature and causality assessment in drug-induced liver injury: summary of a clinical research workshop. *Hepatology* 52(2):730–742, 2010.
62. Chitturi S, Farrell GC: Drug-induced liver disease, in Sorrell MF, Schiff ER, Maddrey WC (eds): *Schiff's Diseases of the Liver*. Philadelphia, PA, Lippincott–Raven Publishers, 2012, p 703.
63. Reuben A, Koch DG, Lee WM: Drug-induced acute liver failure: results of a U.S. multicenter, prospective study. *Hepatology* 52(6):2065–2076, 2010.
64. Bohan TP, Helton E, McDonald I, et al: Effect of L-carnitine treatment for valproate-induced hepatotoxicity. *Neurology* 56(10):1405–1409, 2001.
65. Coppell JA, Richardson PG, Soiffer R, et al: Hepatic veno-occlusive disease following stem cell transplantation: incidence, clinical course, and outcome. *Biol Blood Marrow Transplant* 16(2):157–168, 2010.
66. Sebagh M, Debette M, Samuel D, et al: "Silent" presentation of veno-occlusive disease after liver transplantation as part of the process of cellular rejection with endothelial predilection. *Hepatology* 30(5):1144–1150, 1999.
67. Chojkier M: Hepatic sinusoidal-obstruction syndrome: toxicity of pyrrolizidine alkaloids. *J Hepatol* 39(3):437–446, 2003.
68. Kumar S, DeLeve LD, Kamath PS, et al: Hepatic veno-occlusive disease (sinusoidal obstruction syndrome) after hematopoietic stem cell transplantation. *Mayo Clin Proc* 78(5):589–598, 2003.
69. Poreddy V, DeLeve LD: Hepatic circulatory diseases associated with chronic myeloid disorders. *Clin Liver Dis* 6(4):909–931, 2002.
70. DeLeve LD, Shulman HM, McDonald GB: Toxic injury to hepatic sinusoids: sinusoidal obstruction syndrome (veno-occlusive disease). *Semin Liver Dis* 22(1):27–42, 2002.
71. Wadleigh M, Ho V, Momtaz P, et al: Hepatic veno-occlusive disease: pathogenesis, diagnosis and treatment. *Curr Opin Hematol* 10(6):451–462, 2003.
72. Carreras E, Grañena A, Navasa M, et al: On the reliability of clinical criteria for the diagnosis of hepatic veno-occlusive disease. *Ann Hematol* 66(2):77–80, 1993.
73. Bayraktar UD, Seren S, Bayraktar Y: Hepatic venous outflow obstruction: three similar syndromes. *World J Gastroenterol* 13(13):1912–1927, 2007.
74. Khan AZ, Morris-Stiff G, Makuuchi M: Patterns of chemotherapy-induced hepatic injury and their implications for patients undergoing liver resection for colorectal liver metastases. *J Hepatobiliary Pancreat Surg* 16(2):137–144, 2009.
75. Salat C, Holler E, Kolb HJ, et al: Plasminogen activator inhibitor-1 confirms the diagnosis of hepatic veno-occlusive disease in patients with hyperbilirubinemia after bone marrow transplantation. *Blood* 89(6):2184–2188, 1997.
76. Pihusch M, Wegner H, Goehring P, et al: Diagnosis of hepatic veno-occlusive disease by plasminogen activator inhibitor-1 plasma antigen levels: a prospective analysis in 350 allogeneic hematopoietic stem cell recipients. *Transplantation* 80(10):1376–1382, 2005.
77. Yakushijin K, Atsuta Y, Doki N, et al: Sinusoidal obstruction syndrome after allogeneic hematopoietic stem cell transplantation: incidence, risk factors and outcomes. *Bone Marrow Transplant* 51:403–409, 2015.
78. Ho VT, Revta C, Richardson PG: Hepatic veno-occlusive disease after hematopoietic stem cell transplantation: update on defibrotide and other current investigational therapies. *Bone Marrow Transplant* 41(3):229–237, 2008.
79. Dignan FL, Wynn RF, Hadzic N, et al: BCSH/BSBMT guideline: diagnosis and management of veno-occlusive disease (sinusoidal obstruction syndrome) following haematopoietic stem cell transplantation. *Br J Haematol* 163(4):444–457, 2013.
80. Fan CQ, Crawford JM: Sinusoidal obstruction syndrome (hepatic veno-occlusive disease). *J Clin Exp Hepatol* 4(4):332–346, 2014.
81. Wingard JR, Nichols WG, McDonald GB: Supportive care. *Hematology Am Soc Hematol Educ Program* 372–389, 2004.
82. Richardson PG, Ho VT, Giralt S, et al: Safety and efficacy of defibrotide for the treatment of severe hepatic veno-occlusive disease. *Ther Adv Hematol* 3(4):253–265, 2012.
83. Jagasia M, Arora M, Flowers ME, et al: Risk factors for acute GVHD and survival after hematopoietic cell transplantation. *Blood* 119(1):296–307, 2012.
84. Martin PJ, Schoch G, Fisher L, et al: A retrospective analysis of therapy for acute graft-versus-host disease: initial treatment. *Blood* 76(8):1464–1472, 1990.
85. Filipovich AH, Weisdorf D, Pavletic S, et al: National Institutes of Health consensus development project on criteria for clinical trials in chronic graft-versus-host disease: I. Diagnosis and staging working group report. *Biol Blood Marrow Transplant* 11(12):945–956, 2005.
86. Akpek G, Boitnott JK, Lee LA, et al: Hepatitic variant of graft-versus-host disease after donor lymphocyte infusion. *Blood* 100(12):3903–3907, 2002.
87. Ratanatharathorn V, Nash RA, Przepiorka D, et al: Phase III study comparing methotrexate and tacrolimus (prograf, FK506) with methotrexate and cyclosporine for graft-versus-host disease prophylaxis after HLA-identical sibling bone marrow transplantation. *Blood* 92(7):2303–2314, 1998.
88. Firoz BF, Lee SJ, Nghiem P, et al: Role of skin biopsy to confirm suspected acute graft-vs-host disease: results of decision analysis. *Arch Dermatol* 142(2):175–182, 2006.
89. Cahn JY, Klein JP, Lee SJ, et al: Prospective evaluation of 2 acute graft-versus-host (GVHD) grading systems: a joint Societe Francaise de Greffe de Moelle et Therapie Cellulaire (SFGM-TC), Dana Farber Cancer Institute (DFCI), and International Bone Marrow Transplant Registry (IBMTR) prospective study. *Blood* 106(4):1495–1500, 2005.
90. Leisenring WM, Martin PJ, Petersdorf EW, et al: An acute graft-versus-host disease activity index to predict survival after hematopoietic cell transplantation with myeloablative conditioning regimens. *Blood* 108(2):749–755, 2006.
91. MacMillan ML, Weisdorf DJ, Wagner JE, et al: Response of 443 patients to steroids as primary therapy for acute graft-versus-host disease: comparison of grading systems. *Biol Blood Marrow Transplant* 8(7):387–394, 2002.
92. Zeidan AM, Wozney JL, Torbenson M, et al: Successful treatment of severe refractory hepatic graft-versus-host disease by cadaveric liver transplant. *Leuk Lymphoma* 54(12):2756–2759, 2013.
93. Murphy SL, Xu J, Kochanek KD: Deaths: final data for 2010. *Natl Vital Stat Rep* 61(4):1–117, 2013.
94. Asrani SK, Larson JJ, Yawn B, et al: Underestimation of liver-related mortality in the United States. *Gastroenterology* 145(2):375–382.e1-e2, 2013.
95. Olson JC, Wendon JA, Kramer DJ, et al: Intensive care of the patient with cirrhosis. *Hepatology* 54(5):1864–1872, 2011.
96. Denniston MM, Jiles RB, Drobeniuc J, et al: Chronic hepatitis C virus infection in the United States, National Health and Nutrition Examination Survey 2003 to 2010. *Ann Intern Med* 160(5):293–300, 2014.
97. Smith BD, Morgan RL, Beckett GA, et al: Recommendations for the identification of chronic hepatitis C virus infection among persons born during 1945–1965. *MMWR Recomm Rep* 61(RR-4):1–32, 2012.
98. Moyer VA: Screening for hepatitis C virus infection in adults: U.S. Preventive Services Task Force recommendation statement. *Ann Intern Med* 159(5):349–357, 2013.
99. Liang TJ, Ghany MG: Current and future therapies for hepatitis C virus infection. *N Engl J Med* 368(20):1907–1917, 2013.
100. Muir AJ, Naggie S: Hepatitis C virus treatment: is it possible to cure all hepatitis C virus patients? *Clin Gastroenterol Hepatol* 13(12):2166–2172, 2015.
101. Wree A, Broderick L, Canbay A, et al: From NAFLD to NASH to cirrhosis-new insights into disease mechanisms. *Nat Rev Gastroenterol Hepatol* 10(11):627–636, 2013.
102. Kowdley KV, Wang CC, Welch S, et al: Prevalence of chronic hepatitis B among foreign-born persons living in the United States by country of origin. *Hepatology* 56(2):422–433, 2012.
103. Roberts H, Kruszon-Moran D, Ly KN, et al: Prevalence of chronic hepatitis B virus (HBV) infection in U.S. households: National Health and Nutrition Examination Survey (NHANES), 1988–2012. *Hepatology* 63:388–397, 2016.
104. Mathurin P, Duchatelle V, Ramond MJ, et al: Survival and prognostic factors in patients with severe alcoholic hepatitis treated with prednisolone. *Gastroenterology* 110(6):1847–1853, 1996.

105. Jinjuvadia R, Liangpunsakul S: Trends in alcoholic hepatitis-related hospitalizations, financial burden, and mortality in the United States. *J Clin Gastroenterol* 49(6):506–511, 2015.
106. Kim WR, Lake JR, Smith JM, et al: OPTN/SRTR 2013 Annual data report: liver. *Am J Transplant* 15 Suppl 2:1–28, 2015.
107. Adams LA, Lindor KD: Nonalcoholic fatty liver disease. *Ann Epidemiol* 17(11):863–869, 2007.
108. Masarone M, Federico A, Abenavoli L, et al: Non alcoholic fatty liver: epidemiology and natural history. *Rev Recent Clin Trials* 9(3):126–133, 2014.
109. Zhu JZ, Dai YN, Wang YM, et al: Prevalence of nonalcoholic fatty liver disease and economy. *Dig Dis Sci* 60(11):3194–3202, 2015.
110. Mittal S, Sada YH, El-Serag HB, et al: Temporal trends of nonalcoholic fatty liver disease-related hepatocellular carcinoma in the veteran affairs population. *Clin Gastroenterol Hepatol* 13(3):594.e1–601.e1, 2015.
111. Singal AK, Hasanin M, Kaif M, et al: Nonalcoholic steatohepatitis is the most rapidly growing indication for simultaneous liver kidney transplantation in the United States. *Transplantation* 100:607–612, 2016.
112. Kamath PS, Wiesner RH, Malinchoc M, et al: A model to predict survival in patients with end-stage liver disease. *Hepatology* 33(2):464–470, 2001.
113. Soresi M, Giannitrapani L, Cervello M, et al: Non invasive tools for the diagnosis of liver cirrhosis. *World J Gastroenterol* 20(48):18131–18150, 2014.
114. European Association for the Study of the Liver: EASL Clinical Practice Guidelines: management of hepatitis C virus infection. *J Hepatol* 55(2):245–264, 2011.
115. Rahimi RS, Singal AG, Cuthbert JA, et al: Lactulose vs polyethylene glycol 3350—electrolyte solution for treatment of overt hepatic encephalopathy: the HELP randomized clinical trial. *JAMA Intern Med* 174(11):1727–1733, 2014.
116. Ratib S, Fleming KM, Crooks CJ, et al: 1 and 5 year survival estimates for people with cirrhosis of the liver in England, 1998–2009: a large population study. *J Hepatol* 60(2):282–289, 2014.
117. Vilstrup H, Amodio P, Bajaj J, et al: Hepatic encephalopathy in chronic liver disease: 2014 Practice Guideline by the American Association for the Study of Liver Diseases and the European Association for the Study of the Liver. *Hepatology* 60(2):715–735, 2014.
118. Stepanova M, Mishra A, Venkatesan C, et al: In-hospital mortality and economic burden associated with hepatic encephalopathy in the United States from 2005 to 2009. *Clin Gastroenterol Hepatol* 10(9):1034.e1–1041.e1, 2012.
119. Lockwood AH: Blood ammonia levels and hepatic encephalopathy. *Metab Brain Dis* 19(3–4):345–349, 2004.
120. Ong JP, Aggarwal A, Krieger D, et al: Correlation between ammonia levels and the severity of hepatic encephalopathy. *Am J Med* 114(3):188–193, 2003.
121. van Leeuwen PA, van Berlo CL, Soeters PB: New mode of action for lactulose. *Lancet* 1(8575-6):55–56, 1988.
122. Bass NM, Mullen KD, Sanyal A, et al: Rifaximin treatment in hepatic encephalopathy. *N Engl J Med* 362(12):1071–1081, 2010.
123. Gluud LL, Dam G, Borre M, et al: Oral branched-chain amino acids have a beneficial effect on manifestations of hepatic encephalopathy in a systematic review with meta-analyses of randomized controlled trials. *J Nutr* 143(8):1263–1268, 2013.
124. Rockey DC, Vierling JM, Mantry P, et al: Randomized, double-blind, controlled study of glycerol phenylbutyrate in hepatic encephalopathy. *Hepatology* 59(3):1073–1083, 2014.
125. Riggio O, Angeloni S, Salvatori FM, et al: Incidence, natural history, and risk factors of hepatic encephalopathy after transjugular intrahepatic portosystemic shunt with polytetrafluoroethylene-covered stent grafts. *Am J Gastroenterol* 103(11):2738–2746, 2008.
126. Laleman W, Simon-Talero M, Maleux G, et al: Embolization of large spontaneous portosystemic shunts for refractory hepatic encephalopathy: a multicenter survey on safety and efficacy. *Hepatology* 57(6):2448–2457, 2013.
127. Garcia-Tsao G, Sanyal AJ, Grace ND, et al: Prevention and management of gastroesophageal varices and variceal hemorrhage in cirrhosis. *Hepatology* 46(3):922–938, 2007.
128. Groszmann RJ, Bosch J, Grace ND, et al: Hemodynamic events in a prospective randomized trial of propranolol versus placebo in the prevention of a first variceal hemorrhage. *Gastroenterology* 99(5):1401–1407, 1990.
129. Casado M, Bosch J, Garcia-Pagán JC, et al: Clinical events after transjugular intrahepatic portosystemic shunt: correlation with hemodynamic findings. *Gastroenterology* 114(6):1296–1303, 1998.
130. Merkel C, Marin R, Angeli P, et al: A placebo-controlled clinical trial of nadolol in the prophylaxis of growth of small esophageal varices in cirrhosis. *Gastroenterology* 127(2):476–484, 2004.
131. Villanueva C, Colomo A, Bosch A, et al: Transfusion strategies for acute upper gastrointestinal bleeding. *N Engl J Med* 368(1):11–21, 2013.
132. Saad WE: Endovascular management of gastric varices. *Clin Liver Dis* 18(4):829–851, 2014.
133. Weeder PD, Porte RJ, Lisman T: Hemostasis in liver disease: implications of new concepts for perioperative management. *Transfus Med Rev* 28(3):107–113, 2014.
134. Sola E, Gines P: Renal and circulatory dysfunction in cirrhosis: current management and future perspectives. *J Hepatol* 53(6):1135–1145, 2010.
135. Runyon BA: Paracentesis of ascitic fluid. A safe procedure. *Arch Intern Med* 146(11):2259–2261, 1986.
136. Hoefs JC: Diagnostic paracentesis. A potent clinical tool. *Gastroenterology* 98(1):230–236, 1990.
137. Runyon BA: Management of adult patients with ascites due to cirrhosis: an update. *Hepatology* 49(6):2087–2107, 2009.
138. Gines P, Tító L, Arroyo V, et al: Randomized comparative study of therapeutic paracentesis with and without intravenous albumin in cirrhosis. *Gastroenterology* 94(6):1493–1502, 1988.
139. Gines A, Fernandez-Esparrach G, Monescillo A, et al: Randomized trial comparing albumin, dextran 70, and polygeline in cirrhotic patients with ascites treated by paracentesis. *Gastroenterology* 111(4):1002–1010, 1996.
140. Strauss RM, Boyer TD: Hepatic hydrothorax. *Semin Liver Dis* 17(3):227–232, 1997.
141. Patidar KR, Sydnor M, Sanyal AJ: Transjugular intrahepatic portosystemic shunt. *Clin Liver Dis* 18(4):853–876, 2014.
142. Bhatnagar R, Reid ED, Corcoran JP, et al: Indwelling pleural catheters for non-malignant effusions: a multicentre review of practice. *Thorax* 69(10):959–961, 2014.
143. Chen CH, Shih CM, Chou JW, et al: Outcome predictors of cirrhotic patients with spontaneous bacterial empyema. *Liver Int* 31(3):417–424, 2011.
144. Xiol X, Castellote J, Baliellas C, et al: Spontaneous bacterial empyema in cirrhotic patients: analysis of eleven cases. *Hepatology* 11(3):365–370, 1990.
145. Tu CY, Chen CH: Spontaneous bacterial empyema. *Curr Opin Pulm Med* 18(4):355–358, 2012.
146. Norvell JP, Spivey JR: Hepatic hydrothorax. *Clin Liver Dis* 18(2):439–449, 2014.
147. Sinha VK, Ko B: Hyponatremia in cirrhosis—pathogenesis, treatment, and prognostic significance. *Adv Chronic Kidney Dis* 22(5):361–367, 2015.
148. Berl T, Quittnat-Pelletier F, Verbalis JG, et al: Oral tolvaptan is safe and effective in chronic hyponatremia. *J Am Soc Nephrol* 21(4):705–712, 2010.
149. Torres VE, Devuyst O, Chapman AB, et al: Tolvaptan in patients with autosomal dominant polycystic kidney disease. *N Engl J Med* 367(25):2407–2418, 2012.
150. Cardenas A, Ginès P, Marotta P, et al: Tolvaptan, an oral vasopressin antagonist, in the treatment of hyponatremia in cirrhosis. *J Hepatol* 56(3):571–578, 2012.
151. Dahl E, Gluud LL, Kimer N, et al: Meta-analysis: the safety and efficacy of vaptans (tolvaptan, satavaptan and lixivaptan) in cirrhosis with ascites or hyponatraemia. *Aliment Pharmacol Ther* 36(7):619–626, 2012.
152. Lutz P, Nischalke HD, Strassburg CP, et al: Spontaneous bacterial peritonitis: the clinical challenge of a leaky gut and a cirrhotic liver. *World J Hepatol* 7(3):304–314, 2015.
153. Runyon BA: Low-protein-concentration ascitic fluid is predisposed to spontaneous bacterial peritonitis. *Gastroenterology* 91(6):1343–1346, 1986.
154. Parsi MA, Atreja A, Zein NN: Spontaneous bacterial peritonitis: recent data on incidence and treatment. *Cleve Clin J Med* 71(7):569–576, 2004.
155. Singal AK, Salameh H, Kamath PS: Prevalence and in-hospital mortality trends of infections among patients with cirrhosis: a nationwide study of hospitalised patients in the United States. *Aliment Pharmacol Ther* 40(1):105–112, 2014.
156. Tandon P, Garcia-Tsao G: Renal dysfunction is the most important independent predictor of mortality in cirrhotic patients with spontaneous bacterial peritonitis. *Clin Gastroenterol Hepatol* 9(3):260–265, 2011.
157. Runyon BA: Introduction to the revised American Association for the Study of Liver Diseases Practice Guideline management of adult patients with ascites due to cirrhosis 2012. *Hepatology* 57(4):1651–1653, 2013.
158. Jalan R, Fernandez J, Wiest R, et al: Bacterial infections in cirrhosis: a position statement based on the EASL Special Conference 2013. *J Hepatol* 60(6):1310–1324, 2014.
159. Ariza X, Castellote J, Lora-Tamayo J, et al: Risk factors for resistance to ceftriaxone and its impact on mortality in community, healthcare and nosocomial spontaneous bacterial peritonitis. *J Hepatol* 56(4):825–832, 2012.
160. Piano S, Fasolato S, Salinas F, et al: The empirical antibiotic treatment of nosocomial spontaneous bacterial peritonitis: results of a randomized, controlled clinical trial. *Hepatology* 63:1299–1309, 2016.
161. Sort P, Navasa M, Arroyo V, et al: Effect of intravenous albumin on renal impairment and mortality in patients with cirrhosis and spontaneous bacterial peritonitis. *N Engl J Med* 341(6):403–409, 1999.
162. Fernandez J, Monteaqudo J, Barqallo X, et al: A randomized unblinded pilot study comparing albumin versus hydroxyethyl starch in spontaneous bacterial peritonitis. *Hepatology* 42(3):627–634, 2005.
163. Tito L, Rimola A, Ginès P, et al: Recurrence of spontaneous bacterial peritonitis in cirrhosis: frequency and predictive factors. *Hepatology* 8(1):27–31, 1988.
164. Bernard B, Cadranel JF, Valla D, et al: Prognostic significance of bacterial infection in bleeding cirrhotic patients: a prospective study. *Gastroenterology* 108(6):1828–1834, 1995.
165. Mandorfer M, Bota S, Schwabl P, et al: Nonselective beta blockers increase risk for hepatorenal syndrome and death in patients with cirrhosis and spontaneous bacterial peritonitis. *Gastroenterology* 146(7):1680.e1–1690.e1, 2014.
166. Bajaj JS, Zadvornova Y, Heuman DM, et al: Association of proton pump inhibitor therapy with spontaneous bacterial peritonitis in cirrhotic patients with ascites. *Am J Gastroenterol* 104(5):1130–1134, 2009.
167. Kwon JH, Koh SJ, Kim W, et al: Mortality associated with proton pump inhibitors in cirrhotic patients with spontaneous bacterial peritonitis. *J Gastroenterol Hepatol* 29(4):775–781, 2014.
168. Cardenas A: Hepatorenal syndrome: a dreaded complication of end-stage liver disease. *Am J Gastroenterol* 100(2):460–467, 2005.
169. Arroyo V, Ginès P, Gerbes AL, et al: Definition and diagnostic criteria of refractory ascites and hepatorenal syndrome in cirrhosis. International Ascites Club. *Hepatology* 23(1):164–176, 1996.
170. Salerno F, Gerbes A, Ginès P, et al: Diagnosis, prevention and treatment of hepatorenal syndrome in cirrhosis. *Gut* 56(9):1310–1318, 2007.
171. Angeli P, Ginès P, Wong F, et al: Diagnosis and management of acute kidney injury in patients with cirrhosis: revised consensus recommendations of the International Club of Ascites. *J Hepatol* 62(4):968–974, 2015.

172. Belcher JM: Acute kidney injury in liver disease: role of biomarkers. *Adv Chronic Kidney Dis* 22(5):368–375, 2015.
173. Cavallin M, Kamath PS, Merli M, et al: Terlipressin plus albumin versus midodrine and octreotide plus albumin in the treatment of hepatorenal syndrome: a randomized trial. *Hepatology* 62(2):567–574, 2015.
174. Nassar Junior AP, Farias AQ, D'Albuquerque LA, et al: Terlipressin versus norepinephrine in the treatment of hepatorenal syndrome: a systematic review and meta-analysis. *PLoS One* 9(9):e107466, 2014.
175. Salerno F, Navickis RJ, Wilkes MM: Albumin infusion improves outcomes of patients with spontaneous bacterial peritonitis: a meta-analysis of randomized trials. *Clin Gastroenterol Hepatol* 11(2):123.e1–130.e1, 2013.
176. Guevara M, Ginès P, Bandi JC, et al: Transjugular intrahepatic portosystemic shunt in hepatorenal syndrome: effects on renal function and vasoactive systems. *Hepatology* 28(2):416–422, 1998.
177. Brensing KA, Textor J, Perz J, et al: Long term outcome after transjugular intrahepatic portosystemic stent-shunt in non-transplant cirrhotics with hepatorenal syndrome: a phase II study. *Gut* 47(2):288–295, 2000.
178. Wong F, Pantea L, Sniderman K: Midodrine, octreotide, albumin, and TIPS in selected patients with cirrhosis and type 1 hepatorenal syndrome. *Hepatology* 40(1):55–64, 2004.
179. Ochs A, Rössle M, Haaq K, et al: The transjugular intrahepatic portosystemic stent-shunt procedure for refractory ascites. *N Engl J Med* 332(18):1192–1197, 1995.
180. Zhang Z, Maddukuri G, Jaipaul N, et al: Role of renal replacement therapy in patients with type 1 hepatorenal syndrome receiving combination treatment of vasoconstrictor plus albumin. *J Crit Care* 30:969–974, 2015.
181. Sourianarayanane A, Raina R, Garg G, et al: Management and outcome in hepatorenal syndrome: need for renal replacement therapy in non-transplanted patients. *Int Urol Nephrol* 46(4):793–800, 2014.
182. Wong F, Leung W, Al Beshir M, et al: Outcomes of patients with cirrhosis and hepatorenal syndrome type 1 treated with liver transplantation. *Liver Transpl* 21(3):300–307, 2015.
183. Rodriguez-Roisin R, Krowka MJ: Hepatopulmonary syndrome—a liver-induced lung vascular disorder. *N Engl J Med* 358(22):2378–2387, 2008.
184. Goldberg DS, Fallon MB: The art and science of diagnosing and treating lung and heart disease secondary to liver disease. *Clin Gastroenterol Hepatol* 13(12):2118–2127, 2015.
185. Schenk P, Schöniger-Hekele M, Fuhrmann V, et al: Prognostic significance of the hepatopulmonary syndrome in patients with cirrhosis. *Gastroenterology* 125(4):1042–1052, 2003.
186. Fallon MB, Krowka MJ, Brown RS, et al: Impact of hepatopulmonary syndrome on quality of life and survival in liver transplant candidates. *Gastroenterology* 135(4):1168–1175, 2008.
187. Arguedas MR, Abrams GA, Krowka MJ, et al: Prospective evaluation of outcomes and predictors of mortality in patients with hepatopulmonary syndrome undergoing liver transplantation. *Hepatology* 37(1):192–197, 2003.
188. Krowka MJ, Swanson KL, Frantz RP, et al: Portopulmonary hypertension: results from a 10-year screening algorithm. *Hepatology* 44(6):1502–1510, 2006.
189. Goldberg DS, Batra S, Sahay S, et al: MELD exceptions for portopulmonary hypertension: current policy and future implementation. *Am J Transplant* 14(9):2081–2087, 2014.
190. Busuttil RW, Farmer DG, Yersiz H, et al: Analysis of long-term outcomes of 3200 liver transplantations over two decades: a single-center experience. *Ann Surg* 241(6):905–916, 2005; discussion 916-8.
191. Botta F, Giannini E, Romagnoli P, et al: MELD scoring system is useful for predicting prognosis in patients with liver cirrhosis and is correlated with residual liver function: a European study. *Gut* 52(1):134–139, 2003.
192. Dutkowski P, Oberkofler CE, Slankamenac K, et al: Are there better guidelines for allocation in liver transplantation? A novel score targeting justice and utility in the model for end-stage liver disease era. *Ann Surg* 254(5):745–753, 2011; discussion 753.

Chapter 207 ■ Evaluation and Management of Liver Failure

AVEGAIL G. FLORES • BRITNEY M. RAMGOPAL • MAURICIO LISKER-MELMAN

INTRODUCTION

Acute liver failure (ALF) is a sudden catastrophic deterioration in liver function over a short period of time usually in the absence of preexisting liver disease. The defining feature of ALF is the presence of alterations both in mentation and in coagulopathy. A number of terms have been used for this condition, including fulminant hepatic failure (FHF) and fulminant hepatitis. ALF is the preferred umbrella term [1]. ALF is an uncommon entity, estimated to affect approximately 2,000 to 3,000 patients annually in the United States [2]. Prompt evaluation and aggressive management, including possible liver transplantation (LT), play an integral part in successfully treating patients with ALF in the intensive care unit (ICU). Acute-on-chronic liver failure (ACLF) is the deterioration of liver function in a patient who already has chronic liver dysfunction. It represents a newly recognized, but important, aspect of liver dysfunction among ICU patients. The definition, etiology, clinical features, complications, and management of ALF and ACLF are reviewed in this chapter.

ACUTE LIVER FAILURE

Definition

ALF is an uncommon condition that includes evidence of coagulation abnormalities (international normalized ratio [INR] >1.5) and mental alterations (encephalopathy) of a patient without preexisting cirrhosis and <26 weeks of illness duration [1]. Acute Wilson disease and acute autoimmune hepatitis, when diagnosed within the last 6 months, are widely accepted exceptions that are treated as ALF because of poor outcomes without LT. FHF, although used interchangeably with ALF, has a strict definition when applied to patients under evaluation for LT and is discussed later on in this chapter.

Etiologies

Numerous causes of ALF are recognized, and their relative importance differs around the world. In the United States, acetaminophen accounts for nearly 40% of cases followed by unknown causes (18%) and idiosyncratic drug reactions (13%) [3,4] (see Table 207.1). Acute viral hepatitis has become an infrequent cause of ALF over the last few decades because of effective immunization programs; but in the developing world, it remains the dominant etiology of ALF [5]. The identification of the cause of ALF is important because it can provide prognostic information as well as dictate treatments. Initial laboratory testing to delineate etiology and assess degree of injury is obligatory (Table 207.2). The etiology of ALF may also have prognostic significance in determining outcomes in patients listed for LT [6].

Acetaminophen

Acetaminophen is the most common cause of ALF in the United States and the United Kingdom. This drug is a constituent of numerous over-the-counter preparations and is also commonly combined with prescription analgesics. Although the recommended doses of acetaminophen (up to 4 g per day) are safe in healthy individuals, dose-dependent hepatotoxicity can occur. Hepatotoxicity occurs through intentional or unintentional overdose.

TABLE 207.1

Etiologies of Acute Liver Failure in the United States

Etiology	Percent
Acetaminophen induced	39
Unknown	18
Non-acetaminophen drug induced	13
Hepatitis B	7
Hepatitis A	4
Autoimmune hepatitis	4
Wilson disease	3
Budd–Chiari	2
Pregnancy related	2

Approximately one-third to one-half of cases occur because of efforts at pain relief; these "therapeutic misadventures" occur with lower cumulative doses of ingested acetaminophen, but often times co-ingestion of multiple acetaminophen containing preparations has taken place [7]. These patients may seek late medical attention resulting in delayed physician recognition and worse patient outcomes.

Acetaminophen is 95% eliminated by hepatic conjugation. Approximately 5% of acetaminophen is converted to *N*-acetyl-p-benzoquinone imine (NAPQI), which is inactivated after reaction with cellular glutathione and excreted rapidly. The glutathione stores become progressively depleted in the setting of acetaminophen overdose because the liver produces more NAPQI. When unable to be excreted, NAPQI becomes highly toxic and produces massive liver necrosis. NAPQI accumulates at a higher rate in the setting of increased cytochrome PCY2E1 activity, as seen with chronic alcohol ingestion, and with medications that induce the P450 system.

TABLE 207.2

Initial Laboratory Testing for FHF

- Complete blood count
- Basic metabolic panel
- International normalized ratio (INR)
- Liver chemistry panel
- Lactate
- Blood gas
- Human immunodeficiency virus (HIV) rapid antibody test
- Pregnancy testing
- Blood and urine cultures
- Viral markers
  - Hepatitis A IgM antibody
  - Hepatitis B markers
  - Hepatitis C antibody
  - HSV PCR
- Autoimmune markers
  - Antinuclear antibody
  - Anti-smooth muscle antibody
- Toxicology screen and drug panel
- Imaging and other testing
  - CXR/ECG
  - RUQ US with Dopplers

Liver chemistry panel: aspartate aminotransferase, alanine aminotransferase, alkaline phosphatase, total and direct bilirubin, albumin, total protein.
Hepatitis B markers: hepatitis B surface antigen, hepatitis B surface antibody, hepatitis B core antibodies (IgG and IgM).
FHF, fulminant hepatic failure; HSV PCR, Herpes simplex virus polymerase chain reaction; HIV, human immunodeficiency virus; CXR, chest X-ray; ECG, electrocardiogram; RUQ US, right upper quadrant ultrasound.

Patients with acetaminophen toxicity present in three phases [8]. The first phase involves acute gastrointestinal (GI) symptoms of nausea, vomiting, and abdominal pain within the first few hours after ingestion and aspartate aminotransferase (AST) and alanine aminotransferase (ALT) may begin to rise as early as 8 hours after a massive dose. During the second phase (24 to 72 hours), asymptomatic liver test abnormalities typically occur, with marked elevation of liver enzymes and a high AST to ALT ratio. In severe cases, tender hepatomegaly, jaundice and prolonged prothrombin time may be seen. Nephrotoxicity may also become evident. The third phase (72 to 96 hours) presents with manifestations of hepatic failure, including jaundice and encephalopathy. The mortality of acetaminophen toxicity is higher when associated with severe acidosis, coagulopathy, renal failure, mental status changes, and cerebral edema (CE) [9]. These markers are useful to determine when a patient should be considered for LT.

The effective antidote, *N*-acetylcysteine (NAC), is potentially lifesaving especially when administered within 24 hours of ingestion. Thus, suspicion and early identification of acetaminophen toxicity are of vital importance in treating patients presenting with ALF. Although the therapeutic benefit of NAC is best when given within 10 hours, its effects can still be of value within 72 hours of ingestion [10]. When administered early, NAC leads to greater than 95% survival.

NAC replenishes glutathione stores, preventing depletion and subsequent tissue hypoxia and ischemic damage. Both the oral and intravenous (IV) forms can be used with similar efficacy [8]. Oral NAC is given over 72 hours with a loading dose of 140 mg per kg and subsequent doses of 70 mg per kg every 4 hours for a total of 17 doses. It is not uncommon for oral NAC to induce nausea and vomiting, necessitating nasogastric or nasoduodenal feeding tube placement for administration. If the patient develops significant nausea or vomiting, and has a polysubstance overdose requiring gastric decontamination, GI bleeding, or intestinal obstruction, IV NAC is the preferable administration route. IV NAC is given as a 150 mg per kg loading dose, then 50 mg per kg over 4 hours, followed by 100 mg per kg over 16 hours. However, many practitioners extend NAC treatment until there is improvement in liver chemistry parameters. This extended dosing of NAC is seen most often in severe cases of ALF because the benefits often outweigh any adverse effects from the medication. Anaphylactoid reactions are seen in 10% to 20% of patients, typically occurring after the IV loading dose [8]. Because this reaction may be rate dependent, the loading dose has to be administered over 15 to 60 minutes.

Non-acetaminophen Drugs

Non-acetaminophen agents are second to acetaminophen in known causes of ALF. This group largely comprises antibiotics, antiepileptics, and nonsteroidal anti-inflammatory drugs (NSAIDs). Multiple other agents have also been implicated, including neuropsychiatrics, cardioprotectives, chemotherapeutics, and immunosuppressives, but a complete list is too expansive and beyond the scope of this chapter. Up to 10% of cases may be because of more than one medication [11]. The presentation is often idiosyncratic and may present with a cholestatic, hepatocellular, or mixed pattern of liver enzyme elevations.

Initial management includes prompt identification and cessation of the offending agent. Further management guidelines are variable because this group comprises a wide range of medications and clinical scenarios. NAC is one therapy that has been tried in these patients. NAC was reported to improve transplant-free survival in non-acetaminophen ALF when given in the early stages, that is, before progression to advanced or severe encephalopathy [12]. Analyses of the available data do not demonstrate an overall mortality benefit for patients who received NAC, but mortality benefit was seen in transplant-free survival and posttransplant survival [13]. Overall, NAC can be safely used and may be advocated while awaiting transplantation or even when transplantation is not an option [14].

Hepatotrophic Viruses

The recognized hepatotrophic viruses are hepatitis A, B, C, D, and E. Although relatively rare in the United States and United Kingdom, fulminant viral hepatitis is the leading cause of ALF in developing countries.

Hepatitis A is typically a self-limiting infection, causing ALF in less than 1% of cases in nonendemic areas. The clinical patterns and manifestations may depend on the age of the host: (1) asymptomatic without jaundice, (2) jaundice and self-limiting symptoms for 8 weeks, (3) prolonged jaundice lasting for more than 10 weeks, (4) relapsing cholestasis or jaundice occurring over 6 to 10 weeks, and (5) fulminant hepatitis [15]. Neither cholestatic nor relapsing variant is associated with increased mortality. Fulminant hepatitis leading to ALF manifest in the first week in over 50% of patients and during the first 4 weeks in 90% [16]. The US Acute Liver Failure Study group identified four predictors (creatinine > 2.0 mg per dL on day 1, ALT > 2,600 IU per mL, intubation, and need for pressor support), which in a prognostic model performed better than the King's College criteria and model for end-stage liver disease (MELD) scores [17]. Independently, creatinine > 2 mg per dL still had the best sensitivity and specificity for predicting ALF and mortality [18].

Hepatitis B can cause ALF through acute infection or reactivation. Acute infection causes hepatic damage through immune-mediated lysis of infected hepatocytes. Reactivation typically occurs in the setting of immunosuppression and is generally more severe than acute infection with a higher propensity for ALF and death. Nucleoside/nucleotide analogues are the mainstay of treatment and were found safe and efficacious in reducing short-term mortality in acute on chronic liver failure patients [19]. However, these medications may have no benefit in transplant-free survival in ALF because of the rapid disease progression and short duration of treatment [20]. Nevertheless, nucleoside/nucleotide analogues should still be used because these prevent viral recurrence after transplant.

Hepatitis E virus (HEV) usually causes acute, self-limited infection and most often occur in developing countries. However, two distinct epidemiologic patterns of infection are now observed: (1) acute hepatitis via fecal–oral route in endemic areas or developing countries and (2) chronic hepatitis through ingestion of contaminated meat (zoonotic reservoirs) with rapidly progressive cirrhosis in nonendemic areas or developed countries usually of immunosuppressed patients or recipients of organ transplants. HEV infection can be made by detecting serum immunoglobulin (IgM) (may last up to 4 to 5 months) and IgG antibodies to HEV or HEV ribonucleic acid in stool and serum (not commercially available). The presence of IgM anti-HEV strongly suggests acute infection [21]. Clinical course of HEV infection among pregnant women is known to be more severe and often lead to FHF and death in up to 20% to 25%, specifically among those living in developing countries [22].

Hepatitis C, well known for its role in chronic hepatic failure, is a rare cause of ALF [23].

Non-hepatotrophic Viruses

Herpes simplex virus (HSV) is a rare cause of ALF, but when untreated is associated with a mortality of up to 90%. It is more likely to occur in immunosuppressed or pregnant patients. Liver biopsy is the gold standard for diagnosis, but serum HSV polymerase chain reaction has both a high sensitivity and specificity [24]. Practitioners should have a high index of suspicion because patients may present without mucocutaneous lesions in up to 30% of cases and prompt initiation of acyclovir improves transplant-free survival [10,25].

Epstein–Barr Virus (EBV) is another important but exceedingly rare cause of ALF, accounting for a mere 0.2% of cases. Consistent with its more common disease, infectious mononucleosis, it is mostly seen in young patients [26]. Diagnosis is difficult to make; but if available, monospot testing, EBV serologies, and EBV DNA testing of serum or liver tissue can be useful. There are no current treatment guidelines, but anecdotal evidence suggests antivirals and corticosteroids may be of benefit [26].

Cytomegalovirus (CMV) infection should also be considered in those with ALF. Diagnosis is confirmed by CMV DNA, anti-CMV IgM antibody, or fourfold increase in anti-CMV IgG antibodies [27]. Ganciclovir is the treatment of choice.

Pregnancy

ALF in pregnancy can be divided into acute fatty liver of pregnancy (AFLP) and hypertension-related liver diseases (preeclampsia, hemolysis/elevated liver enzymes/low platelet [HELLP] syndrome). Quick delivery of the fetus can be both lifesaving for the mother and child for both AFLP and HELLP syndrome. Acute hepatic rupture occurs in about 1% of patients with HELLP syndrome with marked mortality risks to the fetus and mother, in addition to inherent risks of ALF in the mother [28]. AFLP is a rare condition caused by microvesicular fatty infiltration of the hepatocytes owing to defects in the long-chain 3-hydroxyacyl coenzyme A dehydrogenase (LCHAD) in the fetal mitochondria. This occurs in the third trimester or within a few days postpartum and is associated with high fetal and maternal mortality [29]. Markers to help identify women at risk of death or LT include elevated lactate despite adequate resuscitation and encephalopathy [30].

Autoimmune Hepatitis

Autoimmune hepatitis can cause ALF in the setting of newly developed disease, exacerbation of chronic disease, or superimposed injury on chronic disease. The histologic features, elevated autoantibodies, and γ-globulins typical of chronic disease may be variably seen in this setting [31]. Current recommendations advise a trial of corticosteroids because this may prevent the need for LT in some patients [32]. Immediate listing for LT may be appropriate in those with ALF because improvement with corticosteroids alone is unsuccessful in 60% of the cases.

Unusual Etiologies

There are multiple rare and important etiologies of ALF. One such entity is *Amanita phalloides* or mushroom poisoning. An accurate history of mushroom ingestion is crucial to recognize and treat this disease. Treatment with gastric lavage or activated charcoal administration is controversial because no evidence exists that this improves clinical outcomes. However, it is a typical practice if patients present early after ingestion. Silibinin, at a dose of 20 to 50 mg/kg/h IV, is recommended for patients who present within 48 hours of ingestion because this has been shown to prevent amanitin uptake into hepatocytes [33]. Penicillin G also prevents amanitin uptake by hepatocytes by displacing it from binding plasma protein. NAC has also been proposed as a treatment strategy in these patients, although data is limited [33]. Mortality from *A. phalloides* poisoning ranges from 10% to 20%.

Another rare but important entity of ALF is Wilson disease. It comprises 3% of those presenting with ALF and can have a mortality up to 95% [34]. Diagnosing Wilson disease as the cause for ALF can be a challenge because serum ceruloplasmin may be falsely elevated because of this acute inflammatory state. Associated clinical data that suggest Wilson disease include Coomb negative hemolytic anemia, coagulopathy that cannot be corrected with vitamin K, modest elevations in aminotransferases, elevated serum copper, and elevated 24-hour urine copper [34]. Treatment of these patients is ultimately LT; however, it is important to note that other sequelae of Wilson disease (i.e., neurologic disease) may not improve after transplantation.

Budd–Chiari syndrome is an important cause of ALF. In mild forms of liver injury, treatment with anticoagulation and diuretics may be of benefit, but in patients who present with ALF, LT is the ultimate therapy [35]. Transjugular intrahepatic portosystemic shunts can be used as a bridge to transplant for some patients.

Case reports have also implicated malignancy as a rare cause of ALF. The majority of these cases are secondary to lymphoma and breast cancer [36]. Mortality in this group is high, and LT is contraindicated.

SYSTEMIC MANIFESTATIONS AND MANAGEMENT

Despite timely intervention, multisystem organ failure can develop among patients with ALF. Hepatic encephalopathy (HE) is the defining clinical feature of ALF, and the development of Cerebral edema (CE) presents a unique set of challenges. Cardiorespiratory failure, renal failure, and infectious complications require aggressive management best done by a multidisciplinary team approach. Supportive management is crucial until the liver recovers or is replaced by transplant. Owing to the rare nature of ALF, evidence-based approaches often rely on analysis of retrospective data from a prospective database such as the US Acute Liver Failure Study group.

Hepatic Encephalopathy

HE is a spectrum of neurologic or psychiatric abnormalities resulting from liver insufficiency and/or portosystemic shunting [37]. It is differentiated into three subtypes according to the underlying diseases: ALF, portosystemic shunting, and cirrhosis. HE from ALF is distinguished from the other two causes by its association with CE with increased intracranial pressure (ICP) and risk of cerebral herniation. The presence of HE is required to establish the diagnosis of ALF. Bedside assessment often relies on clinical assessment scores (Table 207.3), which grade HE from minimal changes in behavior (grade 1) to coma (grade 4). Grades 1 and 2 have mild to moderate confusion with or without asterixis. Grade 3 patients are markedly confused and hypersomnolent but arousable. Grade 4 is defined by a comatose state. Distinguishing patients with low grade (grades 1 and 2) from high grade (grades 3 and 4), HE is important in the early management and triage of patients with ALF. Immediate transfer to a transplant center is recommended when the earliest symptoms of HE are recognized in a patient with acute liver injury. The severity of HE may predict the outcome. Three-week survival without transplantation is 33% and 56% in grades 3 and 4 HE [4].

TABLE 207.3

Clinical Stages of Hepatic Encephalopathy

Grade	Symptoms
1	Lack of awareness, short attention span, altered sleep pattern
2	Agitation, lethargy, seizures
3	Asleep, arousable by pain, confused when aroused
4	Unarousable

From Conn HP: Quantifying the severity of hepatic encephalopathy, in Conn HO, Bircher J (eds): *Hepatic Encephalopathy: Syndromes and Therapies*. Medi-Ed Press, 1994.

Patients with early or low-grade HE can be managed by a skilled nursing staff in a quiet medical ward, with minimal stimulation to the patient. Regular neurologic assessments should be performed because HE may progress rapidly to grade 3 or 4 with severe CE and potential irreversible consequences. It is important to evaluate and treat factors such as electrolyte abnormalities, bleeding, and infection. Head imaging with computerized tomography is only useful if intracranial hemorrhage is suspected. Magnetic resonance imaging of the brain should be avoided because of prolonged scanning time in a confused or agitated patient. Avoidance of sedatives and narcotics is recommended to accurately follow the patient's mental status. However, treatment with short-acting benzodiazepines or propofol may be necessary for cases with extreme agitation. If high-grade HE is suspected, an arterial ammonia level may be useful. Ammonia is an independent risk factor for the development of intracranial hypertension. A level >100 μmol per L predicts severe encephalopathy with 70% accuracy, and a level of 200 μmol per L is associated with intracranial hypertension in half of the ALF patients [38]. Patients with persistent arterial hyperammonemia (>122 μmol per L) for 3 days were more likely to progress and maintain high-grade HE with lower rates of survival (23% vs. 72%), higher incidence of CE (71% vs. 37%), and seizures (41% vs. 7.7%) [39]. Intubation should be performed for airway protection and support with mechanical ventilation when the patient becomes somnolent or develops respiratory distress as a result of metabolic acidosis. Standard therapy for HE of chronic liver disease, such as lactulose, neomycin, or rifaximin, have no proven benefits in ALF and can induce deleterious side effects such as bloating, abdominal pain, nausea, and electrolyte disturbances from diarrheal losses [3].

CE is a devastating complication of ALF. Improvements allowing early recognition, critical care, and the use of emergency LT positively affect the incidence and outcomes of CE. The proportion of patients with intracranial hypertension fell from 76% in 1984 to 1988 to 20% in 2004 to 2008. More importantly, mortality declined from 95% to 55% [40]. The pathophysiology of CE is multifactorial, but ammonia is recognized to play a central role in the development of HE and CE. The liver metabolizes ammonia to urea during homeostasis. Liver failure results in hyperammonemia and ammonia easily crosses the blood–brain barrier. Astrocytes are the only cells in the brain that can metabolize ammonia. Glutamine synthetase in astrocytes converts glutamate and ammonia to glutamine. Glutamine accumulates and acts as an osmolyte and increases astrocyte volume which then contributes to CE [41]. Alternatively, inflammatory cytokines and toxic products from the necrotic liver are proposed to mediate neuroinflammation in ALF. Proinflammatory cytokines have the capacity to alter blood–brain barrier integrity, activate microglia, and act synergistically with ammonia to further cause vasogenic brain edema [41,42].

The most accurate method of diagnosing intracranial hypertension is with the insertion of an ICP monitor. Some centers use ICP monitoring when patients develop grades 3 and 4 HE to help guide management. The normal ICP is 5 to 10 mm Hg and clinically relevant intracranial hypertension exceeds 20 mm Hg. Monitoring mean arterial pressures (MAPs) and maintaining cerebral perfusion pressures (MAP minus ICP) are important. Ideally, ICP should be maintained around 15 mm Hg, with cerebral perfusion pressures greater than 40 to 50 mm Hg. Recovery of neurologic function is optimized by maintaining cerebral perfusion pressures >40 mm Hg. Noninvasive or indirect ICP monitoring such as transcranial Doppler [43–45], transcranial near-infrared spectroscopy [46], jugular venous oximetry [47], and ultrasonic measures of optic nerve sheath diameter [44] had been reported in ALF, but their availability and clinical experience with these monitors are limited.

The use of intracranial pressure monitoring devices in patients with ALF is controversial because of a small but potentially life-threatening risk of intracranial hemorrhage. Practices vary widely based on local transplant center expertise. A review of ICP monitoring in 24 US centers reported ICP monitoring in only 28% of patients with ALF, but the frequency of monitoring significantly differed among centers. Complications of intracranial hemorrhage occurred in 10.3% and may have contributed to the death of two patients. The 30-day survival post-liver transplant was similar in both monitored and nonmonitored groups [48]. A recent retrospective cohort study from the US Acute Liver Failure Study group reported absence of 21-day survival benefit in acetaminophen-ALF and worse outcomes for non-acetaminophen ALF. These results occurred in ICP-monitored patients despite increased intracranial hypertension-directed therapies and more patients receiving liver transplant (41% vs. 18%). Hemorrhagic complications were rare and do not account for the outcomes [49]. Seizures can increase intracranial pressure and should be promptly controlled with phenytoin; however, routine seizure prophylactic treatment is not recommended. In the absence of ICP monitoring, bedside assessment with frequent neurologic evaluation cannot be overstated. The early clinical manifestations of CE often overlap with advanced encephalopathy (grades 3 and 4). The most feared complications are brain herniation and death. Frequent evaluation of mental status (avoiding sedation and neuromuscular blockade if possible), assessment for hyperreflexia, pupillary changes, and sudden systemic hypertension play an important role in monitoring these very ill patients. Prolonged low cerebral perfusion or intracranial hypertension leading to cerebral ischemia and death or a large intracranial bleeding from an underlying coagulopathy eliminates the possibility of transplantation.

Simple recognized strategies to control CE include elevation of the head of the bed to 30° to improve venous drainage, minimization of external stimuli, control of fever and maintaining serum sodium between 145 and 155 mmol per L. IV hypertonic saline continuous infusion rather than boluses (5 to 20 mL 30% saline) should be used [50]. If intracranial hypertension develops despite these prophylactic methods, IV administration of mannitol (100 mL of 20% solution given IV at 0.25 to 0.5 g per kg) can be used as a first-line treatment when ICP is persistently >20 mm Hg for over 10 minutes [51]. Mannitol draws water osmotically from swollen astrocytes back into the intravascular space. It should be avoided in patients with renal failure because of the potential for intravascular volume overload and pulmonary edema. This can be obviated by starting continuous veno-venous hemofiltration. Additional doses of mannitol may be given again as long as the serum osmolality is <320 mOsm per L. The minor survival benefit of mannitol has been shown only in a small series and there are no benefits for cases of severe intracranial hypertension, i.e., >60 mm Hg [52].

Administration of corticosteroids such as dexamethasone has failed to show any benefit in treating elevated ICP [52]. Hypothermia (32°C to 35°C) reduces the production of inflammatory mediators, decreases arterial and cerebrospinal spinal fluid ammonia levels, and attenuates ICP. An earlier small series showed that moderate hypothermia may be effective and safe in patients awaiting liver transplant with intracranial hypertension refractory to standard medical therapy [53]. This result was not duplicated when a retrospective controlled study on moderate hypothermia looked at the impact on survival in ALF patients with high risk of CE. Although no increase in bleeding or infection was seen for therapeutic hypothermia, no effect on 21-day survival was demonstrated [54].

Definitive treatment of CE or intracranial hypertension is achieved with emergency LT. Despite the most appropriate care and stringent inclusion criteria, residual neurologic deficits may persist after transplantation.

Respiratory Complications

Acute lung injury or acute respiratory distress syndrome may be seen in 40% of patients with ALF, and a significant proportion of patients with CE may develop pulmonary edema [55]. Although ALF may have a direct effect in inducing neurogenic pulmonary edema, other etiologies could potentially include aspiration pneumonia, nosocomial pneumonia, transfusion-related lung injury, and intra-alveolar hemorrhage. These patients should be treated with supplemental oxygen or endotracheal intubation as clinically indicated. Intubation, however, is used more frequently for airway protection rather than for respiratory failure. Rapid sequence intubation technique should be used to avoid worsening intracranial hypertension, and nondepolarizing agent cisatracurium is preferable to succinylcholine to avoid muscle contraction which can increase ICP. For sedation, the preferred agent is propofol at 30 to 50 μg/kg/min because of the purported benefits in reducing ICP [56]. Positive pressure ventilation should be used to optimize compliance with caution because the resulting decreased vascular return can lead to increased ICP and cardiac output. The combination of rising ICP and metabolic acidosis in patients with ALF leads to a compensatory hyperventilation and hypocapnia. Forced hyperventilation to $PaCO_2$ of 25 to 30 mm Hg to restore cerebrovascular autoregulation, induce cerebral vasoconstriction, and reduce ICP is not recommended because it showed no impact on reducing the incidence of CE or a survival benefit [57]. Potential worsening of CE caused by cerebral hypoxia secondary to vasoconstriction further limits its utility.

Acute Kidney Injury

The development of acute kidney injury (AKI) is a common complication of ALF and deemed a poor prognostic indicator in ALF. Overall, as many as 70% of patients with ALF developed AKI and 30% received renal replacement therapy (RRT) [58].

AKI etiologies include hepatorenal syndrome, acute tubular necrosis either from sepsis or drug toxicity, and prerenal azotemia. For acetaminophen-induced ALF, a significant proportion of patients develop acute renal failure from direct renal toxicity of NAPQI. Diagnosis of the etiology of AKI requires close monitoring of urine output, volume status, and measurement of urinary sodium and creatinine. Urinary sodium and creatinine can help identify the presence of acute tubular necrosis (high or normal urine sodium) but cannot differentiate between prerenal azotemia and hepatorenal syndrome type 1 (low urine sodium < 10 mmol). Nephrotoxic agents should be avoided in renal failure, and careful renal dosing of medications is vital.

RRT is often initiated early for patients with oliguric renal failure and ALF to prevent complications of volume overload and the risk of intracranial hypertension. The risks of RRT include line sepsis, bleeding, and medication under dosing [59]. Placement of a line under ultrasound guidance may avoid the Trendelenburg position for patients at risk of CE [60]. Citrate anticoagulation is recommended because of high risk of bleeding in ALF, and patients should be monitored for citrate lock wherein hypocalcemia occurs as a result of the formation of calcium citrate complexes in the blood. ALF patients are particularly vulnerable because the liver is unable to metabolize citrate to bicarbonate and patients receive citrate from blood products. It is important to consider adjustments in the dose of NAC (dose increase) in patients on RRT because NAC is dialyzable [61]. As expected, survival was decreased in patients receiving RRT compared to patients without AKI (57% vs. 93%). However, even though AKI is common, it rarely results in chronic kidney disease among patients who survive. Only 4% of patients requiring RRT became dependent on dialysis [58].

Metabolic Disorders

Multiple metabolic derangements occur in ALF. Hyponatremia may occur with volume depletion and as a result of severe splanchnic vasodilation and activation of the renin–angiotensin system. Rapid correction of the serum sodium should be avoided because of the risk of osmotic demyelination syndrome. Metabolic acidosis and alkalosis can occur concurrently. Lactic acidosis is a severe metabolic complication and is widely associated with poor outcomes [62]. Sepsis is an important cause of lactic acidosis that needs proper evaluation. Serum lactate accumulates as a result of tissue hypoxia from hypotension as well as impaired hepatic uptake and metabolism of lactate. Renal dysfunction can further exacerbate metabolic acidosis. Initial treatment involves fluid resuscitation. For metabolic acidosis, half-normal saline with bicarbonate may be required while awaiting RRT [63]. Caution should be taken to avoid volume overload. Hypoglycemia also frequently complicates ALF, given the primary metabolic role of the liver for glycogen storage and gluconeogenesis. Massive hepatic damage is required before serum glucose drops to levels that impair neurologic and cellular function. Frequent glucose monitoring and infusion of concentrated dextrose solutions may be required. Close monitoring of potassium, magnesium, and phosphate levels is likewise necessary. Hypophosphatemia is frequent in ALF and requires aggressive replacement.

Coagulopathy

Coagulopathy is a feature of ALF. The liver synthesizes nearly all circulating coagulation factors and inhibitors, including protein C and protein S, and thrombopoietin, which are essential for platelet production. Laboratory tests such as the prothrombin time (PT), INR, and activated partial thromboplastin time (aPTT) are all prolonged. These parameters are typically followed to monitor hepatic function recovery (in the absence of fresh frozen plasma administration). Clinically significant spontaneous bleeding in ALF is rare [64]. Because of concomitant changes in both procoagulant and anticoagulant pathways, in acute and chronic liver failure, there is a paradoxical state of bleeding and thrombosis in these patients [65]. There is growing evidence of preserved hemostasis in acute liver injury/ALF despite elevated coagulation parameters [66]. Recombinant activated factor VII (rFVIIa) has emerged as a potential treatment and prophylaxis option for bleeding in patients with liver disease. However, prophylactic use of rFVIIa is not the current standard of care. The high cost of rFVIIa as well as the risk of thromboembolic events limits its effectiveness for prophylaxis. The use of rFVIIa in ALF for the rapid correction of INR before an invasive procedure such as placement of an ICP monitor can be advocated in patients who may have CE [67].

GI and oropharyngeal bleeding can result from stress-related mucosal injury. Protection of the gastric mucosa with proton pump inhibitors or H_2 receptor antagonists to prevent mucosal bleeding should be initiated at the onset of coagulopathy. The skin, lungs, and urogenital tract are also potential sites of significant blood loss. Transfusion of blood and blood products are only indicated in patients before invasive procedures or when clinically significant bleeding occurs. Because of the risk of worsening CE and fluid overload with transfusion-related lung injury, use of blood products must be judicious. The effects of fresh frozen plasma on INR are modest and short-lived. In our practice, fresh frozen plasma is infused immediately prior and during procedures to attenuate the risks of bleeding. A single slow infusion of vitamin K 10 mg IV rather than oral form should be given in ALF because vitamin K deficiency has been reported in these patients and intestinal absorption can be unreliable [68]. There are no guidelines for platelet and coagulation transfusion parameters. In the absence of bleeding, a platelet threshold of 10,000 per μL has been recommended and 50,000 per μL or higher when invasive procedures are anticipated. PT, INR, and aPTT cannot adequately predict the bleeding risk in liver disease because of the insensitivity of these tests to the protein C pathway, antithrombin, and tissue factor pathway inhibitor [69,70].

Hemodynamic and Cardiac Complications

Elevated cardiac output (hyperdynamic circulation), decreased peripheral oxygen extraction (tissue hypoxia), and low systemic vascular resistance are present in patients with liver failure. These hemodynamic parameters, possibly because of the release of vasoactive mediators from dying hepatocytes, are similar to those found in patients with sepsis. Splanchnic and peripheral vasodilatation leading to systemic hypotension should be treated with volume replacement. Central venous pressure may be useful in assessing and correcting fluid status in these patients. MAP should be maintained above 65 mm Hg [51]. Norepinephrine is the preferred primary vasopressor because it minimizes tachycardia and preserves splanchnic blood flow. Vasopressin at a fixed rate may be added in refractory cases of hypotension but with caution if CE is suspected. A progressive rise in systolic blood pressure (hypertension) accompanied by bradycardia and widening pulse pressure (Cushing triad), within minutes or hours, can be indicative of intracranial hypertension and impending uncal herniation. Persistent hypotension despite adequate volume resuscitation or empiric broad-spectrum antibiotics should raise concern for adrenal insufficiency. Adrenal insufficiency is common in ALF and correlates with disease severity and should be treated with hydrocortisone 200 to 300 mg per day [71].

Sepsis

Infection commonly occurs in ALF; however, the diagnosis is often difficult as a result of the overlapping hemodynamic changes induced by the liver failure; at times, patients may not demonstrate leukocytosis or fever. The progression of AKI and the worsening of HE should raise the suspicion for infection, and adequate evaluation should be undertaken. The urinary tract and pulmonary system are the most frequent sources of infection. Skin wounds, indwelling vascular access catheters, and ICP monitors are also potential sources of infection. The most common organisms identified are *Staphylococcus*, *Streptococcus*, Gram-negative organisms, and *Candida* species. Fungal infections occur late in the course of illness and are associated with high mortality. Because the hemodynamic, metabolic, and hematologic parameters of ALF are often indistinguishable from sepsis, hospital staff must maintain a high level of suspicion for infectious complications. Because sepsis may be easily overlooked, periodic surveillance cultures (chest radiography, sputum, and urine and blood cultures for fungal and bacterial organisms) can be helpful. However, the routine use of prophylactic antibiotics is controversial and was not shown to reduce the incidence of bloodstream infection or improve 21-day mortality; although, more patients who received prophylactic antibiotics received liver transplants. Multivariable analysis after controlling for confounding showed that antimicrobial prophylaxis did not confer a significant effect on 21-day mortality [72]. Empiric antibiotic and antifungal treatment should be initiated if progression of HE or elements of systemic inflammatory response system (SIRS) is observed. Systemic fungal infection is widely viewed as a contraindication to LT. Transplantation eligibility for patients with evidence of infection and receiving antibiotic treatment is generally reviewed on a case-by-case basis.

Prognosis

Prognostic factors in patients with ALF had been investigated to determine patient survival. Improper selection of a liver transplant recipient who nonetheless will survive with supportive care because of liver regeneration will unnecessarily subject the patient to the morbidity and mortality of transplantation, commit an individual to lifelong immunosuppression, and preclude another medically deserving patient from receiving a LT. Even more crucial is identifying the ALF patient who would die without emergency LT. As a result, several predictive models had been proposed to solve this dilemma.

Among the many predictive models, King's College criteria remain widely used because of the readily available parameters and high specificity for selecting the appropriate patient who will need emergency LT. The King's College criteria produced the first prognosis model in 1989 for both acetaminophen-induced and non-acetaminophen liver failure (Table 207.4). The addition of elevated lactate levels (>3.5 mmol per L) on admission further improved the sensitivity of the model to predict mortality in acetaminophen-induced liver failure [73]. Two recent meta-analyses evaluated the performance of King's College Criteria and found specificity of 82% and 95% but sensitivity of 68% and 58%, respectively [74,75]. Although the King's College criteria are useful wherein a patient meeting its criteria will most assuredly require a liver transplant for survival because of its high specificity, the low sensitivity (58% to 68%) observed implies that a proportion of patients who do not meet the King's College criteria may actually have poor prognosis, may be missed, and not offered emergency LT. Other prognostic models had been proposed for ALF, and they are often reevaluated and modified: MELD [76], sequential organ failure assessment (SOFA) [77], Clichy criteria [78,79], and acute physiology and chronic health evaluation (APACHE) 2 [80]. Although these models overall are useful for identifying patients who will likely need a LT because of poor prognosis (high specificities), the sensitivities of these models are low and reliance on these models alone is not recommended [81].

TABLE 207.4

Indicators of Poor Prognosis in Acute Liver Failure

Etiology	Parameter
Acetaminophen-induced liver failure	Arterial pH < 7.30[a]
	PT > 100 s
	INR > 6.5
	Creatinine > 300 µmol/L (2.3 mg/dL)
	Encephalopathy grades 3 and 4
Nonacetaminophen liver failure	PT > 100 s[b]
	INR > 6.7[b]
	Age <10 or >40
	Serum bilirubin > 300 µmol/L (2.3 mg/dL)
	Seronegative hepatitis or drug reaction

[a]Highest sensitivity (49%), specificity (99%), and positive predictive value (81%).
[b]Highest specificity (100%) but lower sensitivity (34%) and positive predictive value (46%).
INR, international normalized ratio; PT, prothrombin time; s, seconds.
Modified from the King's College Criteria indicating a poor prognosis in acute liver failure.

ACUTE-ON-CHRONIC LIVER FAILURE

Definition and Features

ACLF is defined as an acute deterioration of preexisting chronic liver disease, usually related to a precipitating event and associated with increased 3-month mortality caused by multisystem organ failure [82]. Precipitating events may be viral hepatitis, such as reactivation hepatitis B (typically in Asia) and drug- or alcohol-associated hepatitis or variceal hemorrhage in the West. A multidisciplinary approach involving both the critical care and hepatology teams is recommended. [83]. Hyperbilirubinemia and coagulopathy are chief among the sign/symptoms of ACLF. Bilirubin ≥ 19.9 mg per dL and INR > 2.5 are independent predictors of mortality for this population, as is prior liver decompensation within 6 months [84]. Organ failure is a cardinal feature that often involves the kidneys, brain, heart, lungs, and circulatory and hematologic systems. Development of each new organ failure, renal failure, and the need for inotropic support is associated with increased mortality [84]. SIRS is commonly present and is predictive of mortality especially when associated with renal failure [85].

Treatment and Management Options

There is no single treatment for ACLF. Identification of the precipitating event, directed treatment, prevention of further injury, and supportive care is the standard approach. Integral components to supportive care, when indicated, include mechanical ventilation, vasopressor support, RRT, empiric antibiotics, albumin, and blood products.

Liver support devices have attracted much publicity as a possible treatment option for these patients. The best studied devices are the Prometheus and molecular adsorbents recirculating system (MARS). Unfortunately, studies of these devices have failed to detect mortality benefit of their use. A study of the Prometheus device showed that it was well tolerated and successful at decreasing serum bilirubin level, but with unchanged survival at 28 and 90 days when compared to those who did not undergo this therapy [86]. It was demonstrated that the subgroup of patients with a MELD >30 had improved survival benefit; no further studies have been specifically designed to address this question, and the validity of this results remains unclear [86]. A study of the MARS device showed that it was a well-tolerated procedure, with no increase in adverse events and improvement in serum bilirubin and creatinine; but similarly, no improvement in mortality was seen at 28 or 90 days [87]. The benefits in the subgroup with higher MELD scores were not seen.

Granulocyte colony-stimulating factor (GCSF) is an immunomodulator glycoprotein that was observed in animal models to promote hepatic repair [88], ameliorates hepatic damage, and accelerates regeneration [89]. A study has reported mortality benefits with GCSF compared to placebo at 60 days, as well as improvements in Child–Turcotte–Pugh (CPT), MELD, and SOFA scores [90]. Importantly, a statistically significant decreased risk for development of hepatorenal syndrome, encephalopathy, and sepsis was reported for those treated with GCSF [90]. Moreover, it continues to show promise for the treatment of ACLF owing to reactivation hepatitis B [91] and severe alcoholic hepatitis [92] with some short-term survival benefits.

LT remains controversial for this group of patients because many of the patients have comorbid substance abuse or psychiatric conditions. However, in a retrospective study, there was no increase in mortality posttransplantation among those with ACLF compared to those with chronic liver failure alone [93]. Thus, transplantation for this group may be appropriate with proper identification of candidates.

LIVER TRANSPLANTATION

Patients with ALF and a life expectancy of less than 7 days are deemed to have FHF and granted MELD exception status 1A and priority for LT over patients with chronic liver disease. Criteria for listing include the absence of underlying liver disease, encephalopathy within 8 weeks of the onset of liver disease, an INR > 2, or requirement for RRT or ventilator dependence [94]. A patient with acute decompensated Wilson disease is also granted status 1A as a result of poor survival without a liver transplant. Selection also must discriminate the appropriate patient who would die without a transplant from the patient who is too sick for transplant and the patient who would likely recover only with supportive care. Psychosocial factors are likewise important for determining eligibility and are necessary components of transplant evaluation. Medical contraindications to liver transplant include evidence of uncal herniation, uncontrolled infection despite antibiotic therapy, multiple pressor requirement and multiorgan failure. Failure to recover neurologic function after LT is extremely worrisome but fortunately uncommon. There are reports of regrafting these livers to second recipients with success. In Asia, where living donors are the main source of organs, long-term outcomes of living donor LT for ALF are excellent, regardless of the etiology or classification [95]. In the United States where there is an established system of nonliving donation, the ethical dilemma of donor safety, coercion for donation, and informed consent are debated questions. Auxiliary LT wherein a whole, partial, or hemiliver is transplanted in ALF patients whereas the native liver remains in situ as a bridge to survival, is a technically demanding method that is only practiced in a handful of centers, mostly in Europe (only performed in 2% of cases) [96]. The concept is based on the liver's ability to regenerate completely after ALF, circumventing the need for lifelong immunosuppression.

Significant improvements of outcomes for patients who received liver transplant for ALF had been reported. In the United Kingdom, 1-year survival improved from 63% in 1994 to 1999 to 79% in 2000 to 2004 [97]. In the US ALF study group (patients 1998 to 2010), the longer term survival in ALF liver transplant recipients was excellent (92.4%) and significantly better than that of those patients who did not require a transplant (89.5%) for acetaminophen and 75.5% non-acetaminophen ALF [98].

References

1. Polson J, Lee WM: AASLD position paper: the management of acute liver failure. *Hepatology* 41(5):1179–1197, 2005.
2. Khashab M, Tector AJ, Kwo PY: Epidemiology of acute liver failure. *Curr Gastroenterol Rep* 9(1):66–73, 2007.
3. Bernal W, Wendon J: Acute liver failure. *N Engl J Med* 369(26):2525–2534, 2013.
4. Ostapowicz G, Fontana RJ, Schiødt FV, et al: Results of a prospective study of acute liver failure at 17 tertiary care centers in the United States. *Ann Intern Med* 137(12):947–954, 2002.
5. Blackmore L, Bernal W: Acute liver failure. *Clin Med (Lond)* 15(5):468–472, 2015.
6. Bacak SJ, Callaghan WM, Dietz PM, et al: Pregnancy-associated hospitalizations in the United States, 1999–2000. *Am J Obstet Gynecol* 192(2):592–597, 2005.
7. Lee WM: Acute liver failure. *Semin Respir Crit Care Med* 33(1):36–45, 2012.
8. Bunchorntavakul C, Reddy KR: Acetaminophen-related hepatotoxicity. *Clin Liver Dis* 17(4):587–607, viii, 2013.
9. Chun LJ, Tong MJ, Busuttil RW, et al: Acetaminophen hepatotoxicity and acute liver failure. *J Clin Gastroenterol* 43(4):342–349, 2009.
10. Punzalan CS, Barry CT: Acute liver failure: diagnosis and management. *J Intensive Care Med* 2015.
11. Giordano C, Rivas J, Zervos X: An update on treatment of drug-induced liver injury. *J Clin Transl Hepatol* 2(2):74–79, 2014.
12. Lee WM, Hynan LS, Rossaro L, et al: Intravenous N-acetylcysteine improves transplant-free survival in early stage non-acetaminophen acute liver failure. *Gastroenterology* 137(3):856–864, 864.e1, 2009.
13. Hu J, Zhang Q, Ren X, et al: Efficacy and safety of acetylcysteine in "non-acetaminophen" acute liver failure: a meta-analysis of prospective clinical trials. *Clin Res Hepatol Gastroenterol* 39(5):594–599, 2015.
14. Sales I, Dzierba AL, Smithburger PL, et al: Use of acetylcysteine for non-acetaminophen-induced acute liver failure. *Ann Hepatol* 12(1):6–10, 2013.
15. Jeong SH, Lee HS: Hepatitis A: clinical manifestations and management. *Intervirology* 53(1):15–19, 2010.
16. Williams R: Classification, etiology, and considerations of outcome in acute liver failure. *Semin Liver Dis* 16(4):343–348, 1996.
17. Taylor RM, Davern T, Munoz S, et al: Fulminant hepatitis A virus infection in the United States: incidence, prognosis, and outcomes. *Hepatology* 44(6):1589–1597, 2006.
18. Mackinney-Novelo I, Barahona-Garrido J, Castillo-Albarran F, et al: Clinical course and management of acute hepatitis A infection in adults. *Ann Hepatol* 11(5):652–657, 2012.
19. Yu S, Jianqin H, Wei W, et al: The efficacy and safety of nucleos(t)ide analogues in the treatment of HBV-related acute-on-chronic liver failure: a meta-analysis. *Ann Hepatol* 12(3):364–372, 2013.
20. Dao DY, Seremba E, Ajmera V, et al: Use of nucleoside (tide) analogues in patients with hepatitis B-related acute liver failure. *Dig Dis Sci* 57(5):1349–1357, 2012.
21. Kamar N, Dalton HR, Abravanel F, et al: Hepatitis E virus infection. *Clin Microbiol Rev* 27(1):116–138, 2014.
22. Perez-Gracia MT, García M, Suay B, et al: Current knowledge on hepatitis E. *J Clin Transl Hepatol* 3(2):117–126, 2015.
23. Jayakumar S, Chowdhury R, Ye C, et al: Fulminant viral hepatitis. *Crit Care Clin* 29(3):677–697, 2013.
24. Beersma MF, Verjans GM, Metselaar HJ, et al: Quantification of viral DNA and liver enzymes in plasma improves early diagnosis and management of herpes simplex virus hepatitis. *J Viral Hepat* 18(4):e160–e166, 2011.
25. Navaneethan U, Lancaster E, Venkatesh PG, et al: Herpes simplex virus hepatitis—it's high time we consider empiric treatment. *J Gastrointestin Liver Dis* 20(1):93–96, 2011.
26. Mellinger JL, Rossaro L, Naugler WE, et al: Epstein-Barr virus (EBV) related acute liver failure: a case series from the US Acute Liver Failure Study Group. *Dig Dis Sci* 59(7):1630–1637, 2014.
27. Rosi S, Poretto V, Cavallin M, et al: Hepatic decompensation in the absence of obvious precipitants: the potential role of cytomegalovirus infection/reactivation. *BMJ Open Gastroenterol* 2(1):e000050, 2015.
28. Bacak SJ, Thornburg LL: Liver failure in pregnancy. *Crit Care Clin* 32(1):61–72, 2016.
29. Fesenmeier MF, Coppage KH, Lambers DS, et al: Acute fatty liver of pregnancy in 3 tertiary care centers. *Am J Obstet Gynecol* 192(5):1416–1419, 2005.
30. Westbrook RH, Yeoman AD, Joshi D, et al: Outcomes of severe pregnancy-related liver disease: refining the role of transplantation. *Am J Transplant* 10(11):2520–2526, 2010.
31. Czaja AJ: Acute and acute severe (fulminant) autoimmune hepatitis. *Dig Dis Sci* 58(4):897–914, 2013.
32. Yeoman AD, Westbrook RH, Zen Y, et al: Prognosis of acute severe autoimmune hepatitis (AS-AIH): the role of corticosteroids in modifying outcome. *J Hepatol* 61(4):876–882, 2014.
33. Santi L, Maggioli C, Mastroroberto M, et al: Acute liver failure caused by amanita phalloides poisoning. *Int J Hepatol* 2012:487480, 2012.
34. Patil M, Sheth KA, Krishnamurthy AC, et al: A review and current perspective on Wilson disease. *J Clin Exp Hepatol* 3(4):321–336, 2013.
35. Mackiewicz A, Kotulski M, Zieniewicz K, et al: Results of liver transplantation in the treatment of Budd-Chiari syndrome. *Ann Transplant* 17(1):5–10, 2012.
36. Rich NE, Sanders C, Hughes RS, et al: Malignant infiltration of the liver presenting as acute liver failure. *Clin Gastroenterol Hepatol* 13(5):1025–1028, 2015.
37. Vilstrup H, Amodio P, Bajaj J, et al: Hepatic encephalopathy in chronic liver disease: 2014 Practice Guideline by the American Association for the Study of Liver Diseases and the European Association for the Study of the Liver. *Hepatology* 60(2):715–735, 2014.
38. Bernal W, Hall C, Karvellas CJ, et al: Arterial ammonia and clinical risk factors for encephalopathy and intracranial hypertension in acute liver failure. *Hepatology* 46(6):1844–1852, 2007.
39. Kumar R, Shalimar, Sharma H, et al: Persistent hyperammonemia is associated with complications and poor outcomes in patients with acute liver failure. *Clin Gastroenterol Hepatol* 10(8):925–931, 2012.

40. Bernal W, Hyyrylainen A, Gera A, et al: Lessons from look-back in acute liver failure? A single centre experience of 3300 patients. *J Hepatol* 59(1):74–80, 2013.
41. Bemeur C, Butterworth RF: Liver-brain proinflammatory signalling in acute liver failure: role in the pathogenesis of hepatic encephalopathy and brain edema. *Metab Brain Dis* 28(2):145–150, 2013.
42. Butterworth RF: The concept of "the inflamed brain" in acute liver failure: mechanisms and new therapeutic opportunities. *Metab Brain Dis* 31:1283–1287, 2016.
43. Aggarwal S, Brooks DM, Kang Y, et al: Noninvasive monitoring of cerebral perfusion pressure in patients with acute liver failure using transcranial Doppler ultrasonography. *Liver Transpl* 14(7):1048–1057, 2008.
44. Kim YK, Seo H, Yu J, et al: Noninvasive estimation of raised intracranial pressure using ocular ultrasonography in liver transplant recipients with acute liver failure—A report of two cases. *Korean J Anesthesiol* 64(5):451–455, 2013.
45. Ragauskas A, Bartusis L, Piper I, et al: Improved diagnostic value of a TCD-based non-invasive ICP measurement method compared with the sonographic ONSD method for detecting elevated intracranial pressure. *Neurol Res* 36(7):607–614, 2014.
46. Nielsen HB, Tofteng F, Wang LP, et al: Cerebral oxygenation determined by near-infrared spectrophotometry in patients with fulminant hepatic failure. *J Hepatol* 38(2):188–192, 2003.
47. Rosenberg JB, Shiloh AL, Savel RH, et al: Non-invasive methods of estimating intracranial pressure. *Neurocrit Care* 15(3):599–608, 2011.
48. Vaquero J, Fontana RJ, Larson AM, et al: Complications and use of intracranial pressure monitoring in patients with acute liver failure and severe encephalopathy. *Liver Transpl* 11(12):1581–1589, 2005.
49. Karvellas CJ, Fix OK, Battenhouse H, et al: Outcomes and complications of intracranial pressure monitoring in acute liver failure: a retrospective cohort study. *Crit Care Med* 42(5):1157–1167, 2014.
50. Murphy N, Auzinger G, Bernel W, et al: The effect of hypertonic sodium chloride on intracranial pressure in patients with acute liver failure. *Hepatology* 39(2):464–470, 2004.
51. Siddiqui MS, Stravitz RT: Intensive care unit management of patients with liver failure. *Clin Liver Dis* 18(4):957–978, 2014.
52. Canalese J, Gimson AE, Davis C, et al: Controlled trial of dexamethasone and mannitol for the cerebral oedema of fulminant hepatic failure. *Gut* 23(7):625–629, 1982.
53. Jalan R, Olde Damink SW, Deutz NE, et al: Moderate hypothermia in patients with acute liver failure and uncontrolled intracranial hypertension. *Gastroenterology* 127(5):1338–1346, 2004.
54. Karvellas CJ, Todd Stravitz R, Battenhouse H, et al: Therapeutic hypothermia in acute liver failure: a multicenter retrospective cohort analysis. *Liver Transpl* 21(1):4–12, 2015.
55. Trewby PN, Warren R, Contini S, et al: Incidence and pathophysiology of pulmonary edema in fulminant hepatic failure. *Gastroenterology* 74[5 Pt 1]:859–865, 1978.
56. Wijdicks EF, Nyberg SL: Propofol to control intracranial pressure in fulminant hepatic failure. *Transplant Proc* 34(4):1220–1222, 2002.
57. Ede RJ, Gimson AE, Bihari D, et al: Controlled hyperventilation in the prevention of cerebral oedema in fulminant hepatic failure. *J Hepatol* 2(1):43–51, 1986.
58. Tujios SR, Hynan LS, Vazquez MA, et al: Risk factors and outcomes of acute kidney injury in patients with acute liver failure. *Clin Gastroenterol Hepatol* 13(2):352–359, 2015.
59. Leventhal TM, Liu KD: What a nephrologist needs to know about acute liver failure. *Adv Chronic Kidney Dis* 22(5):376–381, 2015.
60. Ziai WC, Chandolu S, Geocadin RG: Cerebral herniation associated with central venous catheter insertion: risk assessment. *J Crit Care* 28(2):189–195, 2013.
61. Sivilotti ML, Juurlink DN, Garland JS, et al: Antidote removal during haemodialysis for massive acetaminophen overdose. *Clin Toxicol (Phila)* 51(9):855–863, 2013.
62. Bernal W: Lactate is important in determining prognosis in acute liver failure. *J Hepatol* 53(1):209–210, 2010.
63. Stravitz RT, Kramer DJ: Management of acute liver failure. *Nat Rev Gastroenterol Hepatol* 6(9):542–553, 2009.
64. Munoz SJ, Stravitz RT, Gabriel DA: Coagulopathy of acute liver failure. *Clin Liver Dis* 13(1):95–107, 2009.
65. Lisman T, Porte RJ: Rebalanced hemostasis in patients with liver disease: evidence and clinical consequences. *Blood* 116(6):878–885, 2010.
66. Stravitz RT, Lisman T, Luketic VA, et al: Minimal effects of acute liver injury/acute liver failure on hemostasis as assessed by thromboelastography. *J Hepatol* 56(1):129–136, 2012.
67. Le TV, Rumbak MJ, Liu SS, et al: Insertion of intracranial pressure monitors in fulminant hepatic failure patients: early experience using recombinant factor VII. *Neurosurgery* 66(3):455–458, 2010; discussion 458.
68. Pereira SP, Rowbotham D, Fitt S, et al: Pharmacokinetics and efficacy of oral versus intravenous mixed-micellar phylloquinone (vitamin K1) in severe acute liver disease. *J Hepatol* 42(3):365–370, 2005.
69. Caldwell S, Shah N: The prothrombin time-derived international normalized ratio: great for Warfarin, fair for prognosis and bad for liver-bleeding risk. *Liver Int* 28(10):1325–1327, 2008.
70. Weeder PD, Porte RJ, Lisman T: Hemostasis in liver disease: implications of new concepts for perioperative management. *Transfus Med Rev* 28(3):107–113, 2014.
71. Harry R, Auzinger G, Wendon J: The clinical importance of adrenal insufficiency in acute hepatic dysfunction. *Hepatology* 36(2):395–402, 2002.
72. Karvellas CJ, Cavazos J, Battenhouse H, et al: Effects of antimicrobial prophylaxis and blood stream infections in patients with acute liver failure: a retrospective cohort study. *Clin Gastroenterol Hepatol* 12(11):1942.e1–1949.e1, 2014.
73. Macquillan GC, Seyam MS, Nightingale P, et al: Blood lactate but not serum phosphate levels can predict patient outcome in fulminant hepatic failure. *Liver Transpl* 11(9):1073–1079, 2005.
74. McPhail MJ, Wendon JA, Bernal W: Meta-analysis of performance of Kings's College Hospital Criteria in prediction of outcome in non-paracetamol-induced acute liver failure. *J Hepatol* 53(3):492–499, 2010.
75. Craig DG, Ford AC, Hayes PC, et al: Systematic review: prognostic tests of paracetamol-induced acute liver failure. *Aliment Pharmacol Ther* 31(10):1064–1076, 2010.
76. Kamath PS, Wiesner RH, Malinchoc M, et al: A model to predict survival in patients with end-stage liver disease. *Hepatology* 33(2):464–470, 2001.
77. Craig DG, Zafar S, Reid TW, et al: The sequential organ failure assessment (SOFA) score is an effective triage marker following staggered paracetamol (acetaminophen) overdose. *Aliment Pharmacol Ther* 35(12):1408–1415, 2012.
78. Bernuau J, Benhamou JP: Fulminant and subfulminant liver failure, in McIntyre N, Bircher J, Rizzeto M, et al (eds): *Oxford Textbook of Clinical Hepatology*. Oxford, Oxford Medical Publications. 1991, pp 923–942.
79. Ichai P, Legeai C, Francoz C, et al: Patients with acute liver failure listed for superurgent liver transplantation in France: reevaluation of the Clichy-Villejuif criteria. *Liver Transpl* 21(4):512–523, 2015.
80. Mitchell I, Bihari D, Chang R, et al: Earlier identification of patients at risk from acetaminophen-induced acute liver failure. *Crit Care Med* 26(2):279–284, 1998.
81. Lee WM, Stravitz RT, Larson AM: Introduction to the revised American Association for the Study of Liver Diseases Position Paper on acute liver failure 2011. *Hepatology* 55(3):965–967, 2012.
82. Bernal W, Jalan R, Quaglia A, et al: Acute-on-chronic liver failure. *Lancet* 386(10003):1576–1587, 2015.
83. Olson JC, Wendon JA, Kramer DJ, et al: Intensive care of the patient with cirrhosis. *Hepatology* 54(5):1864–1872, 2011.
84. Jalan R, Stadlbauer V, Sen S, et al: Role of predisposition, injury, response and organ failure in the prognosis of patients with acute-on-chronic liver failure: a prospective cohort study. *Crit Care* 16(6):R227, 2012.
85. Jalan R, Gines P, Olson JC, et al: Acute-on chronic liver failure. *J Hepatol* 57(6):1336–1348, 2012.
86. Kribben A, Gerken G, Haag S, et al: Effects of fractionated plasma separation and adsorption on survival in patients with acute-on-chronic liver failure. *Gastroenterology* 142(4):782.e3–789.e3, 2012.
87. Banares R, Nevens F, Larsen FS, et al: Extracorporeal albumin dialysis with the molecular adsorbent recirculating system in acute-on-chronic liver failure: the RELIEF trial. *Hepatology* 57(3):1153–1162, 2013.
88. Piscaglia AC, Shupe TD, Oh SH, et al: Granulocyte-colony stimulating factor promotes liver repair and induces oval cell migration and proliferation in rats. *Gastroenterology* 133(2):619–631, 2007.
89. Yannaki E, Athanasiou E, Xagorari A, et al: G-CSF-primed hematopoietic stem cells or G-CSF per se accelerate recovery and improve survival after liver injury, predominantly by promoting endogenous repair programs. *Exp Hematol* 33(1):108–119, 2005.
90. Garg V, Garg H, Khan A, et al: Granulocyte colony-stimulating factor mobilizes CD34(+) cells and improves survival of patients with acute-on-chronic liver failure. *Gastroenterology* 142(3):505.e1–512.e1, 2012.
91. Duan XZ, Liu FF, Tong JJ, et al: Granulocyte-colony stimulating factor therapy improves survival in patients with hepatitis B virus-associated acute-on-chronic liver failure. *World J Gastroenterol* 19(7):1104–1110, 2013.
92. Singh V, Sharma AK, Narasimhan RL, et al: Granulocyte colony-stimulating factor in severe alcoholic hepatitis: a randomized pilot study. *Am J Gastroenterol* 109(9):1417–1423, 2014.
93. Bahirwani R, Shaked O, Bewtra M, et al: Acute-on-chronic liver failure before liver transplantation: impact on posttransplant outcomes. *Transplantation* 92(8):952–957, 2011.
94. Available from: https://optn.transplant.hrsa.gov/media/1923/liver_adult_meld_exception_guidance_20160815.pdf. Accessed January 12, 2015.
95. Yamashiki N, Sugawara Y, Tamura S, et al: Outcomes after living donor liver transplantation for acute liver failure in Japan: results of a nationwide survey. *Liver Transpl* 18(9):1069–1077, 2012.
96. Germani G, Theocharidou E, Adam R, et al: Liver transplantation for acute liver failure in Europe: outcomes over 20 years from the ELTR database. *J Hepatol* 57(2):288–296, 2012.
97. Bernal W, Cross TJ, Auzinger G, et al: Outcome after wait-listing for emergency liver transplantation in acute liver failure: a single centre experience. *J Hepatol* 50(2):306–313, 2009.
98. Fontana RJ, Ellerbe C, Durkalski VE, et al: Two-year outcomes in initial survivors with acute liver failure: results from a prospective, multicentre study. *Liver Int* 35(2):370–380, 2015.

Chapter 208 ■ Severe and Complicated Biliary Tract Disease

TAREK ABOU HAMDAN • RIAD AZAR

A wide spectrum of acute biliary tract diseases may be seen in the intensive care unit (ICU). Presentations vary from mildly abnormal blood chemistries to life-threatening septic shock. Unrecognized biliary disease can lead to significant morbidity. A practical approach to evaluate and treat biliary disorders using a wide array of noninvasive and invasive diagnostic and therapeutic aids is of paramount importance.

The anatomy of the biliary tract is depicted in Figure 208.1. Approximately 500 mL of bile is secreted at the level of the canaliculus each day. Bile flows through progressively larger ductules until reaching the main bile ducts. The bile duct courses through or immediately adjacent to the head of the pancreas in more than 90% of patients. Hence, any pathology in the head of the pancreas can result in biliary obstruction. Bile flow into the duodenum is regulated by the sphincter of Oddi, which consists of muscle fibers that surround the distal bile duct in the wall of the duodenum at the major ampulla. Tonic contraction of the sphincter increases pressure in the common bile duct (CBD) and allows the gallbladder to fill in a retrograde fashion through the cystic duct. A gallstone passing from the gallbladder to the duodenum would typically encounter resistance to passage in the region of the cystic duct and at the sphincter of Oddi. Biliary tree pathology can be diagnosed by transabdominal ultrasonography, computed tomography (CT), magnetic resonance cholangiopancreatography (MRCP), endoscopic retrograde cholangiopancreatography (ERCP), or endoscopic ultrasonography (EUS). Access to the biliary tree for therapeutic purposes may be obtained through ERCP, EUS, percutaneously, or open surgery.

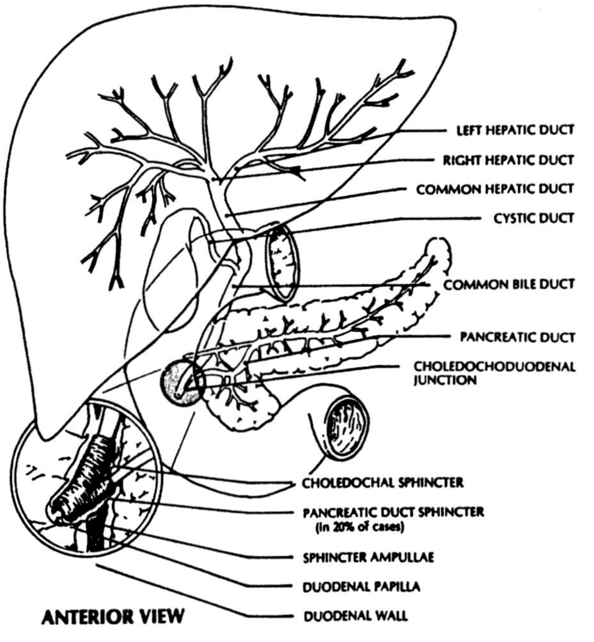

FIGURE 208.1 Normal anatomy of the biliary tract. (From Turner MA, Cho S-R, Messmer JM: Pitfalls in cholangiographic interpretation. *Radiographics* 7:1067, 1987, with permission.)

DIAGNOSTIC EVALUATION

Physical Examination

Physical signs of patients with biliary tract disease may encompass a spectrum from the acute abdomen to nonspecific findings including ileus, fever, or sepsis with hemodynamic instability. Physical exam may reveal icterus, hepatomegaly, ascites, or focal right upper quadrant tenderness.

Laboratory Evaluation

For the obtunded or otherwise compromised ICU patient, abnormal laboratory values often are the first clue to biliary tract disease. All ICU patients should have appropriate laboratory testing on admission, including serum bilirubin, alkaline phosphatase, and transaminases (aspartate aminotransferase or alanine aminotransferase). Bilirubin elevation may indicate an obstructive biliary process, but other processes such as sepsis, drug effects, hemolysis, or other nonbiliary etiologies should be considered for an acutely ill patient. Alkaline phosphatase elevation is not specific for biliary disease; concomitant elevation of γ-glutamyltransferase helps to confirm its hepatobiliary origin. Serum transaminase elevations are the hallmark of hepatocellular injury. However, an elevation in transaminases can also be seen in patients with bile duct obstruction and may precede bilirubin and alkaline phosphatase elevation in the acute setting. Occasionally, laboratory evaluation can be normal as in cholecystitis, without involvement of the CBD and without substantial pericholecystitic hepatitis.

Noninvasive Imaging Studies

Noninvasive radiologic imaging is essential for the evaluation of patients with suspected biliary tract disease.

Plain Abdominal Radiograph

The plain radiographic features of biliary tract disease are usually nonspecific [1]. The most common bowel gas finding seen among patients with acute biliary disease is a generalized ileus. Gallstones are rarely detected on plain radiographs because only 20% of stones are radiopaque. Air in the biliary tree may result from a biliary-enteric fistula or surgical anastomosis, prior sphincterotomy, or infection with gas-producing organisms.

Ultrasonography

Ultrasonography is the initial diagnostic test of choice in the ICU setting and can be performed at the bedside with good results [2]. It is a sensitive test for determining biliary ductal dilatation, acute cholecystitis, and >95% accuracy in detecting cholelithiasis. However, it has low sensitivity (25% to 60%) for detecting choledocholithiasis [3] because gas in the duodenum can obscure visualization of the distal bile duct. In the presence of cholelithiasis or gallbladder sludge, the findings of ductal dilatation, elevated liver enzymes, abdominal pain, and fever are strongly suggestive of cholangitis. Findings on ultrasonography that may indicate acute gallbladder disease include focal tenderness over the gallbladder, thickening of the gallbladder wall, and pericholecystitic fluid collections, but none is specific for cholecystitis. The technique may also detect other abnormalities, including liver lesions, pancreatic masses, abscesses, or ascites.

Radionuclide Scanning

Technetium-99m-labeled hepatic iminodiacetic acid (HIDA) scan yields physiologic and structural information regarding the biliary tract. Filling the gallbladder with radionuclide confirms cystic duct patency, virtually excluding the diagnosis of acute cholecystitis. False-positive examinations can be seen in patients with chronic cholecystitis, on long-term parenteral nutrition, or after prolonged fasting. Delayed views and routine pretreatment with cholecystokinin increase the accuracy of technetium-99m-labeled HIDA scanning for acute cholecystitis to greater than 93% [4]. Radionuclide scanning is also useful in identifying structural abnormalities of the biliary tree, such as significant bile duct leaks; evidence of radiotracer in the abdominal cavity is diagnostic of bile leak. It has a limited role in patients with poor hepatocellular function, complete biliary obstruction, or cholangitis, each of which prevents adequate uptake or excretion of the radiopharmaceutical into the biliary tree.

Computed Tomography

CT scanning has low sensitivity for the detection of choledocholithiasis and is used primarily to document biliary dilation, to exclude other causes of biliary obstruction (e.g., a mass lesion), and to detect local complications such as liver abscess. Unlike ultrasonography or radionuclide scanning, CT cannot be used portably in the ICU. Findings on CT for gallbladder disease include thickening of the gallbladder wall, pericholecystitic fluid, and adjacent abscesses. In addition, CT may reveal a biloma or free fluid in the abdomen. It also allows detailed visualization of the pancreas for grading the severity of pancreatitis and assessing its complications, such as necrosis or pseudocyst formation.

Magnetic Resonance Imaging

The use of magnetic resonance cholangiopancreatogram images can be manipulated to display highly accurate representations of the pancreatobiliary system with high sensitivity (88% to 96%) and specificity (93% to 100%) for the diagnosis of choledocholithiasis [5], strictures, and tumors. It has limited value for detecting stones <6 mm, impacted stone at the ampulla, and dilated bile duct >10 mm [6]. Its use is limited when patients are too sick for transport to the radiology suite.

Summary

When evaluating the ICU patient with suspected biliary tract disease, ultrasonography should be the initial procedure of choice, followed by hepatobiliary scanning if cystic duct obstruction or bile leakage is suspected. Both are portable and noninvasive. Ultrasonography is highly accurate for the detection of gallstones and structural pathology. Hepatobiliary scanning, on the contrary, provides physiologic information, primarily regarding patency of the cystic duct. Functional information can be especially important for patients with suspected calculous or acalculous cholecystitis. CT or MRI should be reserved for those patients in whom sonographic or radionuclide findings are equivocal, if other intra-abdominal pathology needs to be excluded, or if ductal dilatation is seen on ultrasonography without a clearly defined etiology.

Invasive Diagnostic Testing

Endoscopic Retrograde Cholangiopancreatography

The technique of ERCP is used for both diagnostic and therapeutic purposes as described in Chapter 20. In brief, a side-viewing endoscope is passed through the mouth into the second duodenum, where the major ampulla is identified and cannulated. The biliary tree is then opacified with contrast injected through a catheter, allowing a retrograde cholangiogram to be obtained. Fluoroscopy and standard radiographs are used to examine the biliary tree and define abnormalities including stones, strictures, leaks, and obstruction. Endoscopic therapy, including stone removal, biliary drainage, or stricture dilatation, can be accomplished in the same setting. ERCP can be used for the evaluation and therapy of the ICU patient, especially if the patient can be stabilized for endoscopy and transported to a fluoroscopy room. Rarely is it necessary to perform emergent biliary decompression at the bedside using portable fluoroscopy. Coagulopathies should be corrected before the procedure, especially if an endoscopic sphincterotomy (electrocautery incision of the sphincter of Oddi in the duodenal wall for stone removal or drainage) is anticipated. If coagulopathies cannot be satisfactorily corrected, a stent can be placed into the bile duct to allow drainage without performing a sphincterotomy. Major morbidity from the diagnostic procedure includes pancreatitis, cholangitis, perforation, and hemorrhage. The complication rates of ERCP in a recent review noted reduced rates, compared with prior reporting, of pancreatitis at 3.5%, infection at 1.4%, and perforation at 0.6% under standard conditions [7]. The value of ERCP is largely operator-dependent and can be highly successful in the delineation and treatment of biliary disease in the ICU patient [8].

Endoscopic Ultrasonography

EUS involves the transoral passage of an endoscope with an ultrasonic transducer at the tip. The limitations of transabdominal ultrasonography are overcome with this modality because all areas of the biliary tree, including the intrapancreatic portion of the bile duct as well as the pancreas, can be imaged without interference from gas in the intestines. EUS can reliably identify cholelithiasis and is more sensitive than transabdominal ultrasonography in detecting choledocholithiasis with a sensitivity of 95%, specificity of 98%, and an accuracy of 96%. Compared to MRCP, EUS has the additional benefit of being able to detect smaller (<5 mm) stones in small caliber bile ducts [9]. Although EUS is typically an elective procedure and uncommonly used in the ICU, the test may be useful for identifying those patients who would benefit from endoscopic stone extraction by ERCP [10], in particular when clinical predictors of biliary obstruction such as cholestatic liver enzymes and dilated CBD by ultrasonography or CT are unreliable for predicting the presence of CBD stones in the early stages of acute gallstone pancreatitis [11].

Percutaneous Transhepatic Cholangiography

Percutaneous transhepatic cholangiography (PTC) requires fluoroscopy to guide passage of a needle into the intrahepatic bile ducts. The biliary tree is then filled with contrast, and images are obtained. The use of PTC as a diagnostic test has been supplanted by ERCP and noninvasive examinations discussed previously. Currently, PTC is used primarily as an initial step of percutaneous transhepatic biliary drainage. Decompression of the biliary tree via a percutaneous catheter is a highly effective method for rapid nonoperative and nonendoscopic biliary decompression. This procedure is indicated when a patient requires emergent biliary drainage but is not stable enough to undergo ERCP under conscious sedation, if the major papilla cannot be reached endoscopically because of postsurgical anatomy or a technical failure in cannulating the bile duct. The technique involves an initial PTC to delineate the biliary anatomy, followed by selective cannulation of an appropriate intrahepatic bile duct with an 18-gauge needle. A guidewire is then passed into the biliary tree, the tract is dilated, and a drainage catheter is placed. Successful drainage can be established in almost all patients. Percutaneous biliary drainage is an invasive procedure, and acute complications, including hemorrhage, sepsis, and bile leakage, occur in 1% to 5% of patients [12].

Percutaneous Liver Biopsy

Liver biopsy is an important technique for the evaluation of selected patients with hepatobiliary abnormalities who do not have obvious biliary ductal dilatation. Liver biopsy may lead to a rapid pathologic diagnosis in patients with intrinsic liver disease. In cases of infection, tissue can also be cultured. In patients with a coagulopathy, a liver biopsy may be obtained by way of the hepatic vein using a transjugular approach or percutaneously using a sheath, embolizing the tract after completion of the biopsy [13].

BILIARY TRACT DISORDERS ENCOUNTERED IN THE INTENSIVE CARE UNIT

Acute Cholangitis

Acute cholangitis is a life-threatening illness. The presentation of patients with cholangitis may range from intermittent low-grade fever to fulminant septic shock. This diagnosis must be considered and excluded in all patients who present to the ICU with shock and sepsis of unknown origin because of the high mortality if urgent biliary decompression is not accomplished. It occurs as a consequence of partial or complete biliary tract obstruction, typically in patients with biliary stasis in the presence of bacterobilia secondary to stones, strictures, or recent manipulations of the biliary tree [6]. Bacteremia or endotoxemia is correlated directly with the elevated intrabiliary pressure that allows reflux of bacteria into the bloodstream.

Acute cholangitis is a clinical syndrome characterized by fever, jaundice, and abdominal pain (Charcot triad) present in 15% to 72% of patients [14]. Reynold pentad (Charcot triad with the addition of hypotension and altered mental status) may be seen in only 4% to 8% of patients with cholangitis. Liver enzymes are invariably elevated, with a widely variable range. Blood cultures are positive in 21% to 71% [15,16], and gram-negative isolates of *Escherichia coli*, *Klebsiella*, and *Enterococcus* are found most commonly. Anaerobic bacteria are isolated more commonly in polymicrobial infections in patients who have had prior biliary-enteric surgery, are elderly, or have severe disease [6]. Patients who have had recent biliary surgery or who have indwelling stents are more likely to harbor *Enterococcus*, hospital-acquired organisms, or fungi [17].

Because most patients with cholangitis will demonstrate gallstones or a dilated biliary tree, an abdominal ultrasound is the best initial evaluation. This, in association with elevated liver enzymes, fever, or sepsis, is strongly indicative of this diagnosis and should prompt early consultation for decompression.

Treatment

Once cholangitis is suspected, the patient should be treated empirically with broad-spectrum antibiotics with adequate biliary excretion such as ampicillin/sulbactam, piperacillin/tazobactam, third- or fourth-generation cephalosporins, a quinolone, or a carbapenem. Patients who have mild disease usually respond promptly to medical therapy and should undergo biliary decompression and/or definitive therapy for bile duct stones as early as possible, preferably within 24 to 48 hours. Patients who have severe or progressive obstructive biliary disease require urgent biliary drainage in addition to medical therapy. Delay in securing biliary drainage in this subgroup may produce a fatal outcome. This can be accomplished by endoscopic, percutaneous, or surgical means. Selection of a particular approach should be tailored to the patient's condition, local expertise, and the rapid availability of the procedure. Initial efforts for decompensated patients should concentrate on decompression of the biliary tree through ERCP or percutaneous drainage. Definitive therapy may be accomplished at a later time, even if this requires a second procedure. It must be recognized that even with modern support, biliary decompression techniques, and broad-spectrum antibiotics, the mortality from acute fulminant cholangitis ranges from 10% to 50%.

Biliary Obstruction

Biliary obstruction may present without cholangitis. The multiple causes of biliary obstruction are listed in Table 208.1, the most common being stone disease, benign stricture, and malignancy. The patient with physical findings and laboratory studies suggesting obstruction should initially be evaluated with noninvasive imaging or EUS to define the level of obstruction and determine the etiology for definitive therapy planning.

Biliary obstruction without cholangitis is seen more often with malignancy than with stone disease or inflammatory strictures. Definitive therapy for stone disease and benign strictures as well as palliative therapy for malignant strictures may be accomplished utilizing ERCP or PTC. Surgical approaches are preferred for patients who are good operative candidates and who may have resectable malignancy. Bile duct stenting often serves as a bridge to surgery for these patients.

TABLE 208.1

Causes of Biliary Obstruction

- Intrinsic lesions
  - Stones
  - Cholangiocarcinoma
  - Benign stricture
  - Sclerosing cholangitis
  - Periarteritis nodosa
  - Ampullary stenosis
  - Parasites
- Extrinsic lesions
  - Pancreatic carcinoma
  - Metastatic carcinoma
  - Pancreatitis
  - Pancreatic pseudocyst
  - Visceral artery aneurysm
  - Lymphadenopathy
  - Choledochal cyst
  - Hepatic cyst(s)
  - Duodenal diverticulum
- Iatrogenic lesions
  - Postoperative stricture
  - Hepatic artery infusion chemotherapy

Bile Leak

A bile leak may be seen after open or laparoscopic cholecystectomy, hepatic resection, liver transplantation, liver biopsy, PTC, or liver laceration owing to blunt or penetrating trauma. In the postcholecystectomy setting, the most common site of leak is the cystic duct stump; however, leak from the accessory ducts of Luschka, CBD, common hepatic duct, or the liver bed also occurs [18]. The extravasated bile may accumulate focally to form a biloma or freely flow within the peritoneal cavity. The resultant bile peritonitis is usually associated with abdominal pain, ascites, leukocytosis, and fever. Occasionally, collections of bile become infected, resulting in an abscess if untreated. Seldom, patients may present solely with new-onset ascites and an elevated serum bilirubin level. Diagnosis of a biliary leak can usually be made with hepatobiliary scanning. Ultrasonography and CT may reveal a biloma or free fluid in the abdominal cavity. This can be followed by ERCP to determine the exact location of the leak and provide definitive therapy.

Patients with suspected bile leak should be placed on broad-spectrum antibiotics, and the presence of a bile leak should be confirmed with hepatobiliary scanning followed by ERCP. ERCP with therapeutic intent should be performed as soon as possible after diagnosis to limit the degree of bile leakage and patient symptoms. The aim of endoscopic therapy is to decrease or abolish the tone of the sphincter of Oddi, which diverts bile flow away from the leak site. This can be achieved with ERCP and stent placement, with or without sphincterotomy. Stent placement alone is preferred for patients at high risk of post-ES bleeding [19]. Rarely, if endoscopic therapy is unsuccessful for healing a bile leak, surgical repair may be required.

Acute Cholecystitis

Acute cholecystitis is a frequent and important event that occurs in the ICU. The signs and symptoms of acute cholecystitis are often not readily apparent in the compromised ICU patient. A high degree of suspicion and prompt use of noninvasive testing, including ultrasonography and hepatobiliary scanning, are essential to arrive at a timely and correct diagnosis of this entity. *Acalculous cholecystitis* deserves special mention because it can result in significant morbidity and mortality for the ICU patient [20]. Although the signs and symptoms may be similar to those seen with calculous cholecystitis, the presentation in the postoperative or acutely ill ICU patient may be masked by the complicated underlying situation. In this setting, an aggressive diagnostic and therapeutic approach is essential because significant morbidity and even mortality continues to occur from complicated acalculous cholecystitis.

Supportive measures should be undertaken while the patient is being evaluated with noninvasive testing. Antibiotic therapy with broad-spectrum coverage should be initiated for patients with clinical evidence of sepsis, leukocytosis, or fever. Percutaneous cholecystostomy has become the therapy of choice for patients with acute calculous or acalculous cholecystitis who do not respond to conservative therapy and are too unstable for operative cholecystectomy. Percutaneous cholecystostomy is performed at the bedside using ultrasound guidance. A 22-gauge needle is inserted transhepatically into the gallbladder, and bile is aspirated. A guidewire is passed through this needle and the tract is dilated, allowing placement of a drainage catheter, with success rates exceeding 95%. Complications are few and include local wound infection, bleeding, and, rarely, bile peritonitis. The primary advantage of percutaneous cholecystostomy is that it can be done at the bedside without general anesthesia. Percutaneous cholecystostomy is often helpful for patients with suspected gallbladder disease, even if cholecystitis is not found, by excluding the diagnosis. Therefore, percutaneous cholecystostomy should be performed early if gallbladder disease is suspected. The cholecystostomy drainage catheter is left in place until acute symptoms resolve, at which time an elective surgical cholecystectomy or, in the setting of a patent cystic duct and functioning gallbladder, simple tube removal may be performed. For patients with acute calculous cholecystitis and severe underlying medical problems, the gallstones can be removed through the percutaneous tract using various techniques [21]. Such percutaneous gallstone removal is an effective alternate therapy to cholecystectomy for patients with other significant medical conditions. Transpapillary drainage of the gallbladder at ERCP by nasocystic catheter or stent placement and EUS-guided gallbladder drainage via the transluminal route are two endoscopic options to treat patients with acute cholecystitis when standard treatment options fail or is contraindicated. It should be reserved for critically ill patients with severe comorbidities that preclude surgical cholecystectomy and/or patients with contraindications to placement of a percutaneous cholecystostomy tube in case of large-volume ascites, coagulopathy, or the presence of an intervening loop of bowel between the diaphragm and the liver that precludes percutaneous access [11].

Gallstone Pancreatitis

Gallstones are the most common cause of acute pancreatitis. Although most of the cases have an indolent course, about 25% of patients will develop clinically severe acute pancreatitis, usually because of necrotizing pancreatitis. There are several theories regarding the pathogenesis of gallstone pancreatitis, the most accepted being that stone passage or impaction in the ampulla is responsible for this entity. Gallstone pancreatitis should be considered and excluded during the evaluation of all patients with acute pancreatitis because it is a recurrent and treatable cause of this presentation. Standard abdominal ultrasound in combination with laboratory screening for biliary obstruction can be used to exclude gallstones as the cause for the pancreatitis for most patients [22]. Patients with acute pancreatitis should be classified into risk groups based on one of the accepted prognostic scales [23]. These scales include the Ranson criteria, the Glasgow criteria, the Acute Physiology and Chronic Health Evaluation IVa scoring system, and CT criteria for grading severity of pancreatitis. Grading by CT is based on the degree of inflammation, the presence of fluid collections, and the area of pancreatic necrosis seen during bolus infusion of intravenous contrast while scanning. These prognostic scales allow physicians to identify patients who are at risk of developing severe pancreatitis and a complicated hospital course.

Patients with acute pancreatitis from biliary stone disease should be managed initially as detailed in Chapter 209. Although most patients improve with conservative therapy alone, in patients who develop signs of worsening disease or biliary sepsis or coexisting cholangitis, early ERCP is strongly recommended, given the observed benefits in morbidity and mortality [11,24]. Early ERCP may also be beneficial for patients with persistent biliary obstruction (serum bilirubin > 2.5 mg per dL). Data are conflicting as to the benefit of early ERCP for patients with predicted severe disease in the absence of acute cholangitis. Early ERCP [25] allows the removal of impacted or retained CBD stones, limiting further pancreatic inflammation and preventing cholangitis. Consultation with a skilled biliary endoscopist should be obtained early in the course for all patients with severe gallstone pancreatitis. The usual endoscopic approach at ERCP treatment is biliary sphincterotomy, even in the absence of overt stones on cholangiography. This is because small stones and sludge can be missed. In addition, sphincterotomy prevents recurrent pancreatitis in the interim to cholecystectomy, especially if cholecystectomy is not planned within the index admission because of advanced age or severe comorbid medical illnesses. An alternative to sphincterotomy

TABLE 208.2

Evidence-based Management Approaches for Biliary Tract Disorders Encountered in the Intensive Care Unit

- Early ERCP is beneficial in the management of biliary pancreatitis with obstructive jaundice or cholangitis [25].
- ERCP is highly effective in the management of postoperative bile leaks [27].
- In patients with cholangitis, empiric antibiotic therapy should be directed against gram-negative bacteria [17].
- Percutaneous cholecystostomy offers an important therapeutic alternative for critically ill patients with acute cholecystitis [28].

ERCP, endoscopic retrograde cholangiopancreatography.

for patients with coagulopathy is placement of a biliary stent to relieve jaundice and prevent stone impaction. Definitive therapy to prevent recurrent bouts may be accomplished by cholecystectomy or endoscopic sphincterotomy with stone extraction in nonoperative candidates. Although debate continues regarding the timing of surgery, it is generally accepted that all patients who are operative candidates should undergo cholecystectomy during the initial hospital admission after the pancreatitis has subsided [26]. Early operative intervention for patients with active severe gallstone pancreatitis has been associated with unacceptably high morbidity.

Summary

The management of biliary tract disorders encountered in the ICU varies with the specific disorder. Several of the evidence-based treatment approaches are listed in Table 208.2.

References

1. Roszler MH: Plain film radiologic examination of the abdomen. *Crit Care Clin* 10:277, 1994.
2. Romano WM, Platt JF: Ultrasound of the abdomen. *Crit Care Clin* 10:297, 1994.
3. Sugiyama M, Atomi Y: Endoscopic ultrasonography for diagnosing choledocholithiasis: a prospective comparative study with ultrasonography and computed tomography. *Gastrointest Endosc* 45:143–146, 1997.
4. Davis LP, Fink-Bennett D: Nuclear medicine in the acutely ill patient. I. *Crit Care Clin* 10:365, 1994.
5. Verma D, Kapadia A, Eisen GM, et al: EUS vs MRCP for detection of choledocholithiasis. *Gastrointest Endosc* 64:248–54, 2006.
6. Attasaranya S, Fogel E, Lehman G: Choledocholithiasis, ascending cholangitis, and gallstone pancreatitis. *Med Clin N Am* 92:925–960, 2008.
7. Andriulli A, Loperfido S, Napolitano G, et al: Incidence rates of post-ERCP complications: a systematic survey of prospective studies. *Am J Gastroenterol* 102(8):1781–1788, 2007.
8. Cohen SA, Siegel JH: Biliary tract emergencies endoscopic and medical management. *Crit Care Clin* 11:273, 1995.
9. Tse F, Barkun JS, Romagnuolo J, et al: Nonoperative imaging techniques in suspected biliary tract obstruction. *HPB (Oxford)* 8:409–425, 2006.
10. Chak A, Hawes RH, Cooper GS, et al: Prospective assessment of the utility of EUS in the evaluation of gallstone pancreatitis. *Gastrointest Endosc* 49:599, 1999.
11. Ferreira L, Baron T: Acute biliary conditions. *Best Pract Res Clin Gastroenterol* 27:745–756, 2013.
12. Zparchez Z: Percutaneous biliary drainage. Indications, performances, and complications. *J Gastrointestin Liver Dis* 13(2):139–146, 2004.
13. Sawyer AM, McCormick PA, Tennyson GS, et al: A comparison of transjugular and plugged-percutaneous liver biopsy in patients with impaired coagulation. *J Hepatol* 17:81, 1993.
14. Kimura Y, Takada T, Kawarada Y, et al: Definitions, pathophysiology, and epidemiology of acute cholangitis and cholecystitis: Tokyo guidelines. *J Hepatobiliary Pancreat Surg* 14:15–26, 2007.
15. Van Erpecum KJ: Complications of bile-duct stones: acute cholangitis and pancreatitis. *Best Pract Res Clin Gastroenterol* 20:1139–1152, 2006
16. Tanaka A, Takada T, Kawarada Y, et al: Antimicrobial therapy for acute cholangitis: Tokyo guidelines. *J Hepatobiliary Pancreat Surg* 14:59–67, 2007.
17. Rerknimitr R, Fogel EL, Kalayci C, et al: Microbiology of bile in patients with cholangitis or cholestasis with and without plastic biliary endoprosthesis. *Gastrointest Endosc* 56:885–889, 2002.
18. Massoumi H, Kiyici N, Hertan H: Bile leak after laparoscopic cholecystectomy. *J Clin Gastroenterol* 41:301–305, 2007.
19. Sandha GS, Bourke MJ, Haber GB, et al: Endoscopic therapy for bile leak based on a new classification: results in 207 patients. *Gastrointest Endosc* 60:567–574, 2004.
20. Barie P, Eachempati S: Acute acalculous cholecystitis. *Gastroenterol Clin N Am* 39:343–357, 2010.
21. Picus D, Hicks ME, Darcy MD, et al: Percutaneous cholecystolithotomy: analysis of results and complications in 58 consecutive patients. *Radiology* 183:799, 1992.
22. Wang SS, Lin XZ, Tsai YT, et al: Clinical significance of ultrasonography, computed tomography, and biochemical tests in the rapid diagnosis of gallstone-related pancreatitis: a prospective study. *Pancreas* 3:153, 1988.
23. Ranson JH: The current management of acute pancreatitis. *Adv Surg* 28:93, 1995.
24. Tse F, Yuan Y: Early routine endoscopic retrograde cholangiopancreatography strategy versus early conservative management strategy in acute gallstone pancreatitis. *Cochrane Database Syst Rev* (5):CD009779, 2012.
25. Fogel E, Sherman S: ERCP for gallstone pancreatitis. *N Engl J Med* 370:150–157, 2014.
26. Wilson C, de Moya M: Cholecystectomy for acute gallstone pancreatitis: early vs delayed approach. *Scand J Surg* 99: 81–85, 2010.
27. Barkun AN, Rezieg M, Mehta SN, et al: Postcholecystectomy biliary leaks in the laparoscopic era: risk factors, presentation, and management. McGill Gallstone Treatment Group. *Gastrointest Endoscopy* 45:277, 1997.
28. Melin MM, Sarr MG, Bender CE, et al: Percutaneous cholecystostomy: a valuable technique in high-risk patients with presumed acute cholecystitis. *Br J Surg* 82:1274, 1995.

Chapter 209 ■ Acute Pancreatitis

KRUNAL PATEL • WAHID Y. WASSEF

DEFINITION, CLASSIFICATION, AND PATHOLOGY

Pancreatitis is an inflammatory disease of the pancreas. It can be classified as *acute* or *chronic* based on clinical, morphologic, and functional criteria. The focus of this review is acute pancreatitis. *Acute pancreatitis* is defined as an inflammatory process that occurs in a gland that was morphologically and functionally normal before the attack and can return to that state after resolution of the attack.

The pathologic changes associated with acute pancreatitis vary to a great extent with the severity of the attack [1]. Nonsevere acute pancreatitis is associated with interstitial edema, a mild infiltration of inflammatory cells, and evidence of intrapancreatic or peripancreatic fat necrosis, or both. In contrast, severe acute pancreatitis is usually associated with acinar cell necrosis that may be either focal or diffuse. In addition, thrombosis of intrapancreatic vessels, vascular disruption with intraparenchymal hemorrhage, and abscess formation may be noted [2–5].

ETIOLOGY

Acute pancreatitis can be triggered by a number of *etiologies* [6–8]. In developed countries, acute pancreatitis is caused by ethanol abuse or biliary tract disease in 70% to 80% of patients. No etiology can be identified in another 10% to 20% of patients, a condition referred to as idiopathic pancreatitis. And a minority can be related to one of various etiologies listed in Table 209.1. In the less well-developed countries, particularly those in Africa and Asia, acute pancreatitis can develop as a result of malnutrition, ingestion of potentially toxic agents, or both; this type of acute pancreatitis has been called *nutritional* or *tropical* pancreatitis [9–12].

Biliary Tract Stone Disease

Biliary tract stone disease is an especially frequent cause of acute pancreatitis among American Indians of the Southwest, who are prone to development of stones, and among many Asian groups, who have a high incidence of stone formation as a consequence of chronic infection.

Reports by Acosta and Ledesma [13] and Acosta et al. [14] indicated that the onset of pancreatitis associated with biliary tract stones was related to the passage of stones through the terminal biliopancreatic duct and into the duodenum. The mechanism by which stone passage triggers this gallstone pancreatitis has been the subject of considerable speculation and experimental investigation. Three theories have been proposed. The first was the "common channel" theory proposed by Opie [15] in 1901 after he noted gallstones impacted the ampulla of Vater when patients dying of gallstone pancreatitis underwent autopsy examination. He suggested that such stones might create a common biliopancreatic channel proximal to the stone-induced obstruction and that, as a consequence, bile could reflux into the pancreatic ductal system. He reasoned that bile reflux would be injurious to the pancreas and trigger pancreatitis. Subsequent investigations by many groups, however, have challenged the validity of this theory pointing out that pancreatic duct pressure normally exceeds biliary duct pressure, and therefore pancreatic juice reflux into the biliary tract rather than bile reflux into the pancreas would be expected if an obstruction were to create a common channel [16]. Furthermore, many patients develop pancreatitis but lack a common channel that could permit reflux [17], and bile perfused into the pancreatic duct at normal pressure does not induce pancreatitis [18].

Another theory suggested that the stone passing through the sphincter of Oddi could render that sphincter incompetent and, as a result, permit reflux of duodenal juice containing activated digestive enzymes into the pancreas [19]. This "duodenal reflux" would seem to be an unlikely explanation for the development of pancreatitis because it is now clear that neither endoscopic nor surgical procedures that make the sphincter of Oddi incompetent lead to subsequent attacks of acute pancreatitis.

The third theory suggests that either the stone or edema and inflammation resulting from stone passage cause pancreatic duct obstruction and that pancreatic duct obstruction is the event that triggers acute pancreatitis. Studies using a model of acute necrotizing biliary pancreatitis induced in opossums support this theory [20], but in virtually all other species (dog, cat, mouse, rat, rabbit, etc.), pancreatic duct obstruction leads to atrophy of the pancreas with little or no evidence of pancreatitis. This observation has cast considerable doubt on the duct obstruction theory.

Uncertainty regarding mechanisms responsible for gallstone-induced pancreatitis persists. It is generally believed that acute pancreatitis results from an autodigestive injury to the pancreas by enzymes that it normally synthesizes and secretes. Normally, those digestive enzymes are synthesized, intracellularly transported, and secreted from acinar cells as inactive zymogens. Activation normally occurs within the duodenum where the brush border enzyme enterokinase activates trypsinogen and trypsin activates the other zymogens. During pancreatitis, however, zymogen activation appears to occur inside acinar cells, perhaps as a result of pathologic changes in cytoplasmic calcium levels and colocalization of digestive zymogens with lysosomal hydrolases such as cathepsin B. Subsequently, zymogen activation leads to the acinar cell injury/death which is the hallmark of severe pancreatitis [21–25].

TABLE 209.1

Miscellaneous Etiologies of Acute Pancreatitis

- Trauma
- Postoperative setting
  - Common duct exploration
  - Sphincteroplasty
  - Distal gastrectomy
  - Cardiopulmonary bypass
  - Cardiac or renal transplantation
- Endoscopic retrograde cholangiopancreatography
- Translumbar aortography
- Metabolic disorders
  - Hyperparathyroidism
  - Hyperlipoproteinemias types I, IV, and V
- Penetrating ulcer
- Connective tissue disorders
- Scorpion bite
- Renal failure
- Hereditary pancreatitis
- Pancreatic duct obstruction from duodenal diverticulum, ampullary tumor, sphincter of Oddi dysfunction, duodenal Crohn disease, pancreatic tumor
- Drugs
- Bacterial, viral, fungal infections, and parasites
- Pancreatic trauma
- Ischemia or acidosis
- Autoimmune

Ethanol Abuse

For most patients with ethanol-associated pancreatitis, their first clinical attack of pancreatitis develops after many years of ethanol abuse. The incidence of pancreatitis is related to the logarithm of alcohol consumption, but there is no threshold below which alcohol ingestion is not associated with an increased incidence of pancreatitis. The mean consumption of ethanol among patients with ethanol-associated pancreatitis is 150 to 175 g per day. The mean duration of consumption before the first attack is 18 ± 11 years for men and 11 ± 8 years for women [26]. Ethanol-associated pancreatitis, like ethanol abuse itself, is more common among men than among women. Epidemiologic studies suggested that ethanol-associated pancreatitis is most common among those ingesting a high-protein diet with either high or low fat content [26].

The mechanism by which ethanol might cause acute injury to the pancreas is not clear [27–29]. Direct toxic drug-like effect on acinar cells or induction of ductal hypertension as a result of stimulating exocrine secretion and sphincteric contraction are alternating theories [30,31]. Direct cellular injury may be mediated by ethanol metabolites [30–35], and circulating levels of bacterial endotoxin, perhaps released by the intestinal effects of ethanol, may be an important contributing event [34].

Genetic factors certainly predispose to pancreatitis in alcoholics [36,37]. One mechanism is via polymorphisms that may make the above processes more likely (such as increased permeability to endotoxins) and the other as independent pathways that increase susceptibility to mechanisms leading to pancreatic damage in alcoholics. A number of genes have been implicated (SPINK1 [N34S], trypsinogen gene, CFTR); however, genetic testing is not necessarily clinically practical or available.

Drugs

Exposure to certain drugs represents perhaps the third most common cause of acute pancreatitis [38–41] (Table 209.2). The relationship between drug exposure and the development of pancreatitis can be categorized as definite, probable, or equivocal on the strength of the data that indicate that the drug actually causes pancreatitis. The former category includes those drugs whose use is associated with an increased incidence of pancreatitis and that, on specific rechallenge, have been found to induce the disease. On the contrary, drugs in the equivocal category include those that are anecdotally associated with the disease but never demonstrated in prospective studies to be capable of inducing pancreatitis. Historically, diuretic agents such as the thiazides, ethacrynic acid, and furosemide were considered the most likely drugs to cause pancreatitis. More recently, however, drug-related pancreatitis has been reported to be the most common among individuals with acquired immunodeficiency syndrome or acquired immunodeficiency syndrome–related complex receiving dideoxyinosine [42], pentamidine, or related compounds and among transplant patients receiving immunosuppressant agents such as azathioprine. Although previously considered to cause pancreatitis, histamine-2 (H_2)-blockers and steroids are not currently believed to be capable of causing acute pancreatitis.

Pancreatic Duct Obstruction

Obstruction of the pancreatic duct may be caused by duodenal, ampullary, biliary duct, or pancreatic tumors or by inflammatory lesions (e.g., peptic ulcer, duodenal Crohn disease, periampullary diverticulitis) that interfere with pancreatic duct drainage [6]. Pancreatic cysts and pseudocysts and periampullary diverticula filled with food and debris can interfere with duct drainage and as a consequence precipitate pancreatitis. Ductal strictures, frequently the result of traumatic duct injury or previous pancreatitis, can be a cause for obstructive pancreatitis. Finally, certain parasites, such as *Ascaris* and *Clonorchis*, can trigger pancreatitis by physically obstructing the pancreatic duct [6,43]. An association between pancreas divisum and pancreatitis has been claimed, presumably reflecting relative obstruction to pancreatic juice flow at the lesser papilla [44], but this is quite controversial [45,46].

TABLE 209.2

Drugs Associated with Acute Pancreatitis

Definite	
Thiazide diuretics	Valproic acid
Ethacrynic acid	Estrogens
Furosemide	Tetracycline
Azathioprine	Sulfonamides
Asparaginase	Mercaptopurine
Mesalamine	Pentamidine
Dideoxyinosine	
Probable	
Methyldopa	Iatrogenic hypercalcemia
Enalapril	Procainamide
Octreotide	Erythromycin
Chlorthalidone	Phenformin
Equivocal	
Isoniazid	Rifampin
Acetaminophen	Steroids
Histamine-2-blockers	Propoxyphene

Other Miscellaneous Causes of Acute Pancreatitis

Many of the remaining miscellaneous causes of pancreatitis are listed in Table 209.1. Traumatic pancreatitis usually follows blunt abdominal trauma, during which the body of the pancreas is compressed against the vertebral column. As a result, the gland is "cracked," and the duct is either partially or completely transected [47]. Lesser degrees of blunt trauma may be associated with pancreatic contusion, whereas penetrating injury can affect any portion of the pancreas. Traumatic injury to the pancreas can also be associated with surgical procedures performed on or near the pancreas [48–50]. Postoperative pancreatitis is also frequently associated with procedures performed on or near the sphincter of Oddi (duct exploration, sphincteroplasty, and distal gastrectomy), procedures associated with hypoperfusion or atheroembolism of the pancreatic circulation (cardiopulmonary bypass, cardiac transplantation, renal transplantation, and translumbar aortography) [51,52], or procedures involving pancreatic duct injection (endoscopic retrograde cholangiopancreatography [ERCP]) [53].

Hereditary pancreatitis, a familial disease transmitted by a mutation on chromosome 7 that is transmitted as autosomal dominant with incomplete penetrance, can also cause acute pancreatitis among a minority of patients [54]. Reports indicate that the mutation results in the synthesis of a cationic trypsinogen that is resistant to autoinactivation after activation has occurred [55]. Patients with classic cystic fibrosis mutations can present with pancreatitis even in the absence of pulmonary disease. Studies indicate that a substantial number of patients with the so-called idiopathic pancreatitis may have nonclassical cystic fibrosis mutations or polymorphisms of CFTR [56]. The significance of hereditary pancreatitis is the high incidence of pancreatic cancer among this group of patients, which warrants surveillance.

A number of recent reports, particularly from Japan, have drawn attention to a form of autoimmune pancreatitis characterized by extensive lymphoplasmacytic infiltration into the pancreas and sclerosis of the pancreatic and bile ducts. Patients with this form of pancreatitis frequently present with both bile and pancreatic duct obstruction and a mass in the head of the pancreas. They can easily be thought to have neoplastic disease of the pancreas but, if placed on steroid treatment, the changes of autoimmune pancreatitis rapidly resolve. Many, but not all, of these patients have elevated circulating levels of immunoglobulin G (IgG4), and this may permit their identification [57].

Idiopathic Pancreatitis

Approximately 5% to 10% of patients with acute pancreatitis have the disease in the absence of any identifiable etiology. Reports suggest that many of these patients have biliary sludge, that their attacks can be prevented by cholecystectomy, and that they actually have biliary rather than idiopathic pancreatitis [58,59].

CLINICAL PRESENTATION

Symptoms

The symptoms of acute pancreatitis include abdominal pain, nausea, and vomiting [6,7,43,60,61] (Table 209.3). The pain typically is localized to the epigastrium but frequently involves one or both upper quadrants. On occasion, it may be felt in the lower abdomen, one or both shoulders, or the lower chest. The pain is usually described as being of rapid onset, slowly increasing to a maximal severity, and then remaining constant. It usually lacks the waxing and waning character of intestinal or ureteral colic, but it may be diminished by assuming an upright position, leaning forward, or lying on the side with the knees drawn upward. The pain may have a pleuritic component and may be associated with rapid but shallow respirations. Frequently, the pain is described as being a boring or knifelike sensation that passes straight through to the midcentral back from the epigastrium.

Nausea and vomiting commonly are noted among patients with acute pancreatitis. The vomiting typically persists even after the stomach has been emptied and may result in gastroesophageal tears with bleeding (i.e., Mallory–Weiss syndrome). The vomiting and retching may be relieved by passage of a nasogastric tube, but neither the vomiting nor gastric decompression results in reduction of the abdominal pain.

Physical Examination

Patients with acute pancreatitis typically appear anxious and ill. They may be diaphoretic and hyperthermic. Tachycardia, tachypnea, and hypotension are common. Patients often roll or move around in search of a more comfortable position. In this respect, they are quite unlike those with peritonitis caused by a perforated viscus, which remain motionless because movement exacerbates their pain. Most patients with acute pancreatitis have a clear sensorium, but some have mild or even severe alterations in their mental status as a result of drug or ethanol exposure, hypoxemia, hypotension, or release of circulating toxic agents from the inflamed pancreas. Jaundice is common, even in patients with nonbiliary pancreatitis, among whom the hyperbilirubinemia may reflect nonobstructive cholestasis.

The abdominal examination of patients with acute pancreatitis usually reveals abdominal tenderness and voluntary and involuntary guarding. These findings may be limited to the epigastrium or diffusely present throughout the abdomen. A mass, located in the epigastrium or left upper quadrant of the abdomen, or both, may be felt. Direct, percussion, and rebound tenderness usually can be elicited. Abdominal distention also can be seen. Hypovolemia and dehydration are commonly present and can be detected by the presence of hypotension, tachycardia, collapsed neck veins, dry skin, dry mucous membranes, and decreased turgor. Bowel sounds are often diminished or absent. Flank ecchymoses (Grey Turner sign) or other evidence of retroperitoneal bleeding (Cullen sign) may be noted. Examination of the chest may reveal evidence of pleural effusion that may be on either or both sides but is most commonly present on the left. Because of pleuritic and abdominal pain, deep breathing is difficult, and atelectasis, particularly at the bases, is common. Examination of the skin may reveal areas of tender subcutaneous induration and erythema that resemble erythema nodosum; these lesions are believed to result from fat digestion by circulating pancreatic lipases.

TABLE 209.3

Signs and Symptoms of Acute Pancreatitis

Observation	Incidence (%)
Pain	95
Nausea/vomiting	80
Distention	75
Guarding	50
Pain radiating to back	50
Jaundice	20
Abdominal mass	15
Melena	4
Hematemesis	3

LABORATORY TESTS AND RADIOLOGIC EXAMINATIONS

Routine Blood Tests

Acute pancreatitis is associated with significant losses of intravascular fluid. A substantial amount of fluid is lost as a result of the anorexia, nausea, and vomiting that accompanies the disease. In addition to these fluid losses, large volumes of fluid can be sequestered in the retroperitoneum as a result of the pancreatic inflammatory process. In addition, a systemic "capillary leak" process may result in additional fluid sequestration. Taken together, these losses of fluid from the intravascular compartment can cause the hemoglobin, hematocrit, blood urea nitrogen, and serum creatinine to rise. Hypoalbuminemia is common, but the serum electrolytes may remain normal unless vomiting has been significant. Because of the pancreatic inflammatory process, the white blood cell count usually is elevated and the differential may show a "left shift" (neutrophilic predominance). Hyperglycemia, which commonly is noted, may result from the combined effects of elevated circulating catecholamines, decreased insulin release, and hyperglucagonemia [62,63]. A mild rise in serum bilirubin from nonobstructive cholestasis frequently is seen even with nonbiliary acute pancreatitis. When the disease is induced by the passage of gallstones, the hyperbilirubinemia is even more marked, and superimposed cholangitis with bacteremia and positive blood cultures can occur [64]. Markedly elevated circulating triglyceride levels always are seen in individuals whose pancreatitis is caused by hyperlipoproteinemia [65], but hypertriglyceridemia with lactescent serum also can be seen in alcohol-induced acute pancreatitis [66].

Hypocalcemia is relatively common among individuals with acute pancreatitis [67]. For the most part, the hypocalcemia is caused by hypoalbuminemia, and as a result, the ionized calcium level is actually normal. For some patients, however, hypocalcemia can develop that is out of proportion to the degree of hypoalbuminemia and that reflects a true decrease in circulating ionized calcium levels. Tetany and carpopedal spasm and other complications of their hypocalcemia may develop among these patients. Marked hypocalcemia has been considered to be a sign of a poor prognosis. In patients with severe pancreatitis, disseminated intravascular coagulation may develop [68], and as a result, they may have thrombocytopenia, elevated levels of fibrin degradation products, decreased fibrinogen levels, and prolongations of the partial thromboplastin and prothrombin times.

Pancreatic Enzymes and Other Assays

The serum amylase concentration is usually, but not always, elevated during an attack of pancreatitis [7]. The magnitude of that rise does not depend on the severity of pancreatitis, and some reports indicate that as many as 10% of patients with lethal pancreatitis have normal or near-normal serum amylase levels [69]. To a great extent, this may reflect the fact that amylase elevations during pancreatitis typically are transient, with an increase 2 to 12 hours after the onset of an attack and a decline in serum amylase values to near-normal levels 3 to 6 days after the attack has begun. Thus, patients presenting long after the onset of an attack may have normal or only slightly increased serum amylase levels.

Serum amylase activity also may be increased in a number of diseases other than pancreatitis [7,61,70]. Amylase may be synthesized at extrapancreatic sites (e.g., salivary glands, fallopian tube, and lung) or produced by nonpancreatic tumors (e.g., lung, prostate, and ovary), and release of the nonpancreatic amylase into the circulation may result in hyperamylasemia (Table 209.4). Patients with these nonpancreatic extra-abdominal causes for hyperamylasemia rarely are confused with those who have pancreatitis because the clinical features of pancreatitis are usually absent in the former group. On the contrary, some patients with disorders that might be clinically confused with acute pancreatitis may also have hyperamylasemia. This is particularly true for patients with acute cholecystitis, perforated gastric or duodenal ulcers, small bowel obstruction, intestinal ischemia, and intestinal infarction. It may also be true for some patients passing common bile duct stones into the duodenum who do not have pancreatitis.

The overall sensitivity and specificity of amylase determination for the diagnosis of pancreatitis depends on the value chosen as the cutoff level [71] and the presence or absence of clinical features of pancreatitis. Patients with hyperamylasemia but not pancreatitis usually have mild elevations of the circulating amylase level (approximately 200 IU per L) or lack clinical features of pancreatitis, or both, whereas those with pancreatitis usually manifest profound hyperamylasemia (>1,000 IU per L) in association with clinical features of the disease.

Approximately 0.5% of individuals have a condition referred to as macroamylasemia in which amylase is bound to an abnormal circulating protein and, as a result, the amylase is not cleared by the kidney [61,72,73]. Some of these individuals may develop abdominal pain and may be incorrectly suspected of having pancreatitis. In this setting, measurement of urinary amylase activity may be particularly helpful because, in macroamylasemia, urinary amylase levels are usually very low. On the other hand, urinary amylase activity may be particularly helpful for patients who are first seen several days after an attack of pancreatitis and who are found to have normal or near-normal serum amylase activity [63], because urinary amylase level may remain elevated long after serum levels have normalized. Renal clearance of amylase also may be reduced as a result of renal failure, and this reduced clearance can lead to mild hyperamylasemia. On the contrary, enhanced renal clearance of amylase can occur in pancreatitis, and this phenomenon can result in an increase in the clearance ratio for amylase compared with creatinine [73,74]. However, measurement of the so-called amylase to creatinine clearance ratio has not been helpful for the diagnosis of pancreatitis. Alterations of this ratio appear to represent a nonspecific response to an acute illness. Thus, the clearance ratio may be elevated for many patients who lack pancreatitis but may be normal in many who have pancreatitis [72–78].

TABLE 209.4

Causes of Hyperamylasemia

- Pancreatic causes
  - Pancreatitis, pseudocyst, and ascites
  - Pancreatic cancer
  - Pancreatic duct obstruction
  - Pancreatic trauma
  - Endoscopic retrograde cholangiopancreatography
- Nonpancreatic intra-abdominal causes
  - Perforated hollow viscus
  - Bowel obstruction
  - Cholangitis, cholecystitis
  - Mesenteric infarction
  - Ovarian cyst
  - Renal failure
  - Ruptured ectopic pregnancy
- Extra-abdominal causes
  - Salivary gland tumors, trauma, infection, and obstruction
  - Lung tumors
  - Burns
  - Diabetic acidosis
  - Pneumonia

Serum lipase level is commonly checked as part of the assessment for acute pancreatitis. In an acute attack, levels can rise within 4 to 8 hours, peak by 24 hours, and remain elevated for up to 14 days (prolonged elevation of serum lipase may be suggestive of a cyst formation); and for this reason, serum lipase may be the more useful test than serum amylase when evaluating a patient for pancreatitis more than 24 hours after onset of symptoms. Similar to amylase levels, hyperlipasemia may be seen in a number of other diseases, including renal disease, liver cirrhosis, alcohol abuse, small bowel obstruction, acute cholecystitis, peptic ulcer disease, and intestinal infarction. Based on the assays used by different studies, specificity and sensitivity can vary, 42% to 100% and 56% to 100%, respectively. Studies using a higher cutoff to correlate with a diagnosis of acute pancreatitis report a higher specificity at the cost of sensitivity [79]. Although measurements of both enzymes have been used for diagnosing pancreatitis, because of issues involving costs and other factors, most practices will often utilize one of these as the primary assay (studies show that measurements of both enzymes do not increase the accuracy of the diagnosis). Studies using receiver operator characteristics curves show that serum lipase levels gave the greater diagnostic accuracy compared to amylase [80]. The American College of Gastroenterology Guidelines on management of acute pancreatitis recommend clinical correlation with symptoms and presentation when evaluating elevated levels or either enzyme [81].

Circulating levels of other pancreatic enzymes (trypsinogen, chymotrypsinogen, phospholipase, and elastase) or urinary levels of the activation peptide released when trypsinogen is activated (i.e., trypsinogen activation peptide) can also be measured, but there is little or no evidence to suggest that these determinations are more helpful in the diagnosis of pancreatitis than the simpler measurement of serum amylase activity [69,82,83]. Acute pancreatitis also can be associated with methemalbuminemia [84] and with increased circulating levels of several cytokines (e.g., interleukin-1 [IL-1], IL-6, and tumor necrosis factor-α) [85] and acute-phase reactants (e.g., C-reactive protein) [86,87]. The magnitude and duration of these changes may have some prognostic value in pancreatitis, but these changes are not specific to pancreatitis and are therefore of little diagnostic value.

Ultrasonography

Ultrasonography for patients with acute pancreatitis is helpful for detecting gallbladder stones, bile duct dilatation, or both [88]. Endoscopic ultrasound (EUS) can help with investigation of the biliary tree for evaluation of gallstone pancreatitis, especially if a magnetic resonance imaging (MRI) is not feasible. EUS is especially helpful for the investigation of initial or recurrent episodes of idiopathic pancreatitis, in which the endoscopist can assess for smaller stones (including microlithiasis) not previously seen on other imaging modalities, and even for masses, cysts, or tumors as causative agents [36].

Computed Tomography

For acute pancreatitis, particularly during the early stages of the disease, computed tomography (CT) is the most useful imaging modality because it can define the gross features of the pancreas and peripancreatic organs without being limited by the presence of distended gas-filled loops of bowel in the upper abdomen [89]. It is not needed for the diagnosis of the condition, but it should be used if the diagnosis is not clear. The pancreas may be normal or slightly swollen in appearance on CT in mild cases of pancreatitis. Evidence of peripancreatic inflammation, including streaking in the retroperitoneal and transverse mesocolic fat, may also be seen. With more severe attacks, peripancreatic and intrapancreatic fluid collections can be detected. Dynamic CT, performed by rapidly imaging the pancreas during bolus injection of contrast material, can define areas of pancreatic necrosis because those areas do not enhance as a result of contrast administration [90–92]. Detection of these changes may be of prognostic value in acute pancreatitis [93] (see "Prognosis" section), but their major value in the early stages of the disease lies in the fact that their presence confirms the diagnosis of acute pancreatitis. Conversely, the finding of a normal pancreas without signs of peripancreatic inflammation on the CT of a patient suspected of having severe pancreatitis, particularly if that patient's condition is deteriorating, should suggest that the patient does not have pancreatitis.

MRI can also be of great value in the diagnosis of acute pancreatitis. It can reveal the presence of an inciting stone in the distal bile duct. In addition, MRI may be more accurate than CT in defining the extent of pancreatitis-associated necrosis [94].

DIFFERENTIAL DIAGNOSIS

The differential diagnosis of acute pancreatitis includes other processes that may cause upper abdominal pain, nausea, vomiting, and abdominal tenderness. The serum amylase or lipase, or both, is usually elevated in acute pancreatitis and normal or near normal in many other processes that may cause similar symptoms. On the contrary, serum levels of pancreatic enzymes may be elevated with some states that can mimic acute pancreatitis (Table 209.5). On occasion, however, the diagnosis may be uncertain, and CT scan may be helpful.

PROGNOSIS

The management of patients with acute pancreatitis will depend on the severity of their condition. A number of clinical features have been identified that are associated with a poor prognosis. These include age older than 60 years, a "first attack" of pancreatitis, obesity, postoperative pancreatitis, hypocalcemia, methemalbuminemia, and the presence of either Grey Turner or Cullen sign [95]. However, the most common methods for evaluating the severity of acute pancreatitis are *Ranson* criteria [96] and *Imrie criteria* [97] as listed in Tables 209.6 and 209.7, respectively. The presence of fewer than three of the Ranson criteria is associated with mild pancreatitis, little morbidity, and a mortality of less than 1%. In contrast, many patients with three or more of these prognostic signs have severe pancreatitis, with a 34% incidence of septic complications and a mortality that, with seven to eight prognostic signs, may reach 90%. Using the Imrie criteria, severe pancreatitis has been found when three or more of the criteria are present, whereas mild pancreatitis is associated with fewer of the prognostic signs.

Although the criteria developed by the New York and Glasgow groups have proved to be of considerable value in allowing prospective trials in the evaluation of new therapies and interventions for acute pancreatitis, these prognostic criteria are not particularly helpful for the management of an individual patient and should never be used as criteria for the diagnosis of pancreatitis. The Acute Physiology and Chronic Health Evaluation-IV (APACHE-IV) system [98] has been well studied and validated for its ability to predict mortality in patients with acute pancreatitis, with most guidelines recommending a cutoff score of 8 (at admission) above which severe disease is predicted. A newer scoring system, Bedside Index of Severity in Acute Pancreatitis, has been shown to have similar accuracy to the APACHE-2 system with the benefit of being easier to

TABLE 209.5

Differential Diagnosis of Acute Pancreatitis

- Perforated hollow viscus
- Cholecystitis/cholangitis
- Bowel obstruction
- Mesenteric ischemia/infarction

TABLE 209.6

Ranson Prognostic Signs

On admission
- Age > 55 y
- White blood cell count > 16,000/μL
- Blood glucose > 200 mg/dL
- Lactate dehydrogenase > 350 IU/L
- Glutamic oxaloacetic transaminase > 250 Sigma–Frankel units/dL

During initial 48 h
- Hematocrit decrease >10%
- Blood urea nitrogen rise >5 mg/dL
- Serum Ca^{2+} < 8 mg/dL
- Partial pressure of oxygen < 60 mm Hg
- Base deficit > 4 mEq/L
- Fluid sequestration > 6 L

TABLE 209.7

Imrie Prognostic Signs

- Age > 55 y
- White blood cell count > 15,000/μL
- Blood glucose > 10 mmol/L
- Serum urea > 16 mmol/L
- Partial pressure of oxygen < 60 mm Hg
- Serum Ca^{2+} < 2.0 mmol/L
- Lactic dehydrogenase > 600 μg/L
- Aspartate aminotransferase/alanine aminotransferase > 100 μg/L
- Serum albumin < 32 g/L

calculate. A cutoff score of 3 during the earlier phase of the disease identifies patients with an increased risk of death [99].

If a CT scan is obtained, the severity of the pancreatitis can be evaluated based on the Balthazar score [100], in a prospective study involving 83 patients with acute pancreatitis, noted that those with two or more peripancreatic fluid collections seen on CT had a 61% incidence of late pancreatic abscess, those with only one fluid collection or inflammation confined to the pancreas and peripancreatic fat had a 12% to 17% incidence of pancreatic abscess, and those with either no CT changes of pancreatitis or with only pancreatic enlargement on CT had a zero incidence of pancreatic abscess. The morbidity, incidence of abscess formation, and mortality for an attack of pancreatitis also have been shown to be related to the amount of pancreatic tissue that is not enhanced on CT after bolus administration of contrast material during dynamic CT. In addition to these scoring systems, other factors characterizing acute pancreatitis may be helpful for predicting the severity and, thus, the outcome after an attack. Most notable in this regard are the presence or onset, shortly after presentation, of evidence suggesting organ failure and/or evidence of extravascular extravasation of normally intravascular fluid [7,101,102]. This fluid loss can result in renal failure, respiratory failure, or both as well as hemoconcentration, and each of these changes is predictive of a poor outcome. In contrast, the absence of hemoconcentration on admission usually suggests that pancreatic necrosis is unlikely [103,104]. Elevated circulating levels of other factors (e.g., C-reactive protein, certain cytokines, phospholipase A2, trypsinogen activation peptide, and trypsinogen-2) are also suggestive of a severe attack and predictive of poor outcomes [7].

TREATMENT OF ACUTE PANCREATITIS

Initial Management

During the early stages of an acute attack of pancreatitis, efforts should be made to confirm the diagnosis, control pain, and support fluid and electrolyte needs [105].

Treatment of Pain

The pain of pancreatitis is often severe and difficult to control. Most patients require narcotic medications. In clinical practice, narcotics available on inpatient pharmacy formulary plans are used often via a patient controlled administration pump [37].

Fluid and Electrolyte Replacement

The early stage of severe acute pancreatitis is characterized by major fluid and electrolyte losses. External losses, caused by repeated episodes of vomiting and exacerbated by nausea and diminished fluid intake, can lead to hypochloremic alkalosis. Internal losses caused by leakage of intravascular fluid into the inflamed retroperitoneum, pulmonary parenchyma, and soft tissues elsewhere in the body contribute to hypovolemia.

Aggressive and adequate fluid resuscitation, instituted during the early stages of acute pancreatitis, is essential. A growing body of evidence indicates that inadequate fluid resuscitation may promote progression of otherwise mild pancreatitis into severe pancreatitis, with its associated major morbidity and high mortality. Recently, studies have suggested the use of ringer's lactate solution rather than saline to neutralize the development of metabolic acidosis.

Nutrition

Nutrition is the other most important arm of therapy for patients with severe acute pancreatitis. If provided enterally, it can feed the gut and decrease ischemia and transmigration of organisms into areas of necrosis with improved patient outcomes. A number of studies have demonstrated the benefits of nasojejunal tube feedings that support these contentions [106,107]. Furthermore, recent reports suggest that enteral nutrition can be successfully administered by either the nasogastric or the nasojejunal route and that the benefits of using either route are comparable [108,109].

Other Treatments

Recommendations for the use of antimicrobial agents have changed over time. Current guidelines published by the American College of Gastroenterology, based on a number of studies, recommend against prophylactic antibiotics or antifungals, even in cases of severe pancreatitis (strong recommendation with moderate level of evidence quoted). Concomitant infections (such as cholangitis or pneumonia) should be treated appropriately [81]. A summary of treatments of little or unproven value is presented in Table 209.8 and management recommendations for acute pancreatitis are presented in Table 209.9.

Role of Surgery and Endoscopy for Gallstone Pancreatitis

Most patients with biliary tract stone-induced pancreatitis recover quickly and uneventfully because the offending stone is either passed into the duodenum or disimpacts itself from the ampulla of Vater by moving proximally in the duct. The role of early ERCP is well established in cases of severe gallstone pancreatitis. Three prospectively randomized controlled trials and a recent observational, prospective, multicenter trial have evaluated the benefit of early endoscopic sphincterotomy and stone extraction in the management of patients with gallstone pancreatitis [64,110–112]. Each study concluded that early intervention did not alter the course of mild pancreatitis, but they suggested [64,110,112] that the morbidity of severe pancreatitis, particularly if it was associated with cholestasis, was reduced by early stone removal. Therefore, on the basis of currently available data, it seems most appropriate that patients with mild pancreatitis need not undergo either early surgical or endoscopic

TABLE 209.8

Treatments of Limited or Unproven Value

Nasogastric suction
Histamine-2-receptor antagonists
Antacids
Atropine
Glucagon
Calcitonin
Somatostatin
Indomethacin
Steroids
Hypothermia
Thoracic duct drainage
Plasmapheresis
Prostaglandins
Procainamide
Gabexate mesilate
Aprotinin
Isoproterenol
Heparin
Dextran
Vasopressin
Propylthiouracil
Epsilon-aminocaproic acid
Peritoneal lavage

TABLE 209.9

Complications of Acute Pancreatitis

Systemic complications
- Cardiovascular collapse
- Respiratory failure
- Renal failure
- Metabolic encephalopathy
- Disseminated intravascular coagulation
- Gastrointestinal bleeding

Local complications
- Acute fluid collection
- Pancreatic necrosis ± infection
- Pancreatic pseudocyst
- Pancreatic abscess
- Pancreatic ascites
- Pancreatic-pleural fistula
- Duodenal obstruction
- Bile duct obstruction
- Splenic vein thrombosis
- Pseudoaneurysm + hemorrhage

intervention. On the contrary, early intervention by ERCP seems warranted for patients with severe gallstone pancreatitis.

Recurrent attacks of gallstone pancreatitis may develop if stones either in the gallbladder or biliary ducts remain after resolution of the index attack. For that reason, most clinicians recommend that some form of treatment designed to prevent recurrent attacks should be administered before discharge of the patient from the hospital [106]. That might be accomplished by laparoscopic or open cholecystectomy combined with surgical or endoscopic duct clearance if choledocholithiasis is discovered by preoperative magnetic resonance cholangiopancreatography. Alternatively, for patients whose only symptoms are those of ductal disease and who lack symptoms of cholecystolithiasis, endoscopic sphincterotomy and duct clearance may be sufficient, particularly if those patients have high surgical risks.

Treatment of Systemic Complications

Systemic complications of acute pancreatitis include cardiovascular collapse, respiratory failure, renal failure, metabolic encephalopathy, disseminated intravascular coagulation, and gastrointestinal bleeding (Table 209.10). For the most part, the pathogenesis and management of these manifestations of acute pancreatitis are identical to those involved when these processes are superimposed on other diseases that result in severe peritonitis and hypovolemic shock. In other words, there may be nothing specific about these systemic complications of pancreatitis, although they may be worsened by circulating vasoactive agents, activated digestive enzymes, and protein breakdown fragments absorbed from the inflamed pancreas. Please refer to the chapters on peritonitis in chapter 51 and management of shock in chapter 37 for the detailed management of these problems.

LOCAL COMPLICATIONS OF PANCREATITIS

Definitions

Considerable confusion has surrounded the terminology used to describe the local complications of an acute attack of pancreatitis. At a symposium in Atlanta, an international group of

TABLE 209.10

Summary of Management of Acute Pancreatitis

- Early, aggressive fluid resuscitation is beneficial in cases of severe acute pancreatitis associated with shock [114].
- In contrast to morphine, meperidine relaxes the sphincter of Oddi and is thus a favored analgesic in cases of pancreatitis [115,116].
- Use of enteral nutrition has shown benefit over parenteral nutrition in terms of duration of hospital stay, infectious morbidity, and need for surgery in meta-analysis [117–119]. Enteral nutrition, because it is associated with fewer complications, may be the better of these two treatment modalities.
- Antibiotic use remains controversial; meta-analyses have shown utility in preventing infection of pancreatic necrosis [120,121], although a large, randomized, controlled trial failed to demonstrate benefit [122].
- In cases of severe necrotizing pancreatitis, conservative management in an intensive care setting trends toward a survival benefit when compared with early surgical intervention [123].
- Early endoscopic sphincterotomy and stone extraction are beneficial in preventing sepsis in cases of severe gallstone pancreatitis in patients with jaundice [64,110,124].

clinicians and scientists attempted to resolve this confusion by proposing the use of the following definitions [113]:

1. *Acute pancreatic and peripancreatic fluid collections*: Fluid collections in or near the pancreas that occur early in the course of acute pancreatitis and that lack a wall of granulation or fibrous tissue.
2. *Pancreatic necrosis*: An area of nonviable pancreatic tissue that may be diffuse or focal and that typically is associated with peripancreatic fat necrosis. Pancreatic necrosis may be either *sterile* or *infected.*
3. *Pancreatic pseudocyst*: A collection of pancreatic juice that usually is rich in digestive enzymes and that is enclosed by a nonepithelialized wall of fibrous or granulation tissue (Figs. 209.1 and 209.2). It is usually round or ovoid in shape and not present until 4 to 6 weeks have elapsed from the onset of acute pancreatitis. Before this time, the fluid collection

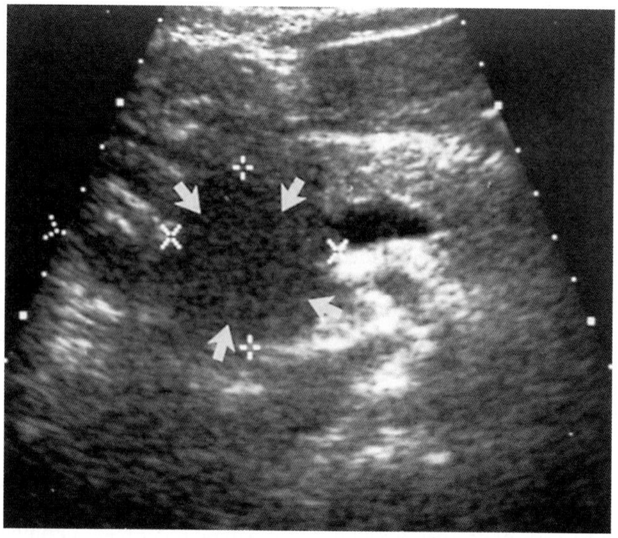

FIGURE 209.1 Ultrasound showing pancreatic pseudocyst (*arrows*).

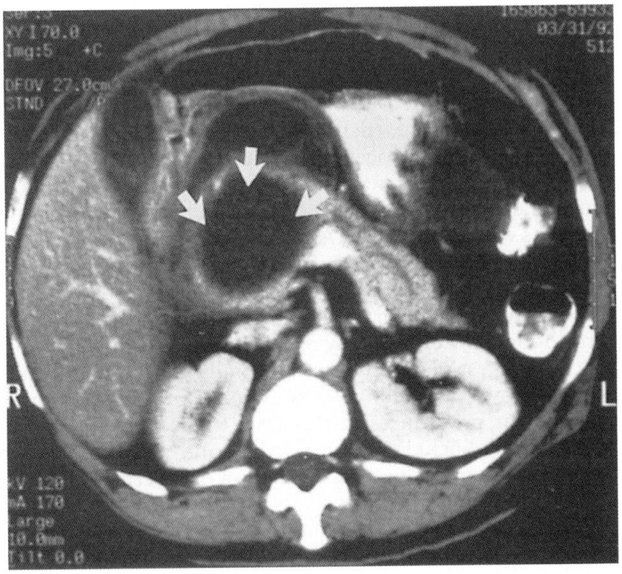

FIGURE 209.2 Computed tomography showing pseudocyst (*arrows*) in the head of the pancreas.

usually lacks a defined wall and may be either an *acute fluid collection* or a localized area of *pancreatic necrosis*. Bacteria may be present in a pseudocyst as a result of contamination; but in this setting, clinical signs of infection usually are absent. When pus is present, however, the lesion should be referred to as a *pancreatic abscess*. Leakage of pseudocysts into the peritoneal cavity or chest leads to the development of *pancreatic ascites* or *pancreatic-pleural fistula*, respectively.

4. *Pancreatic abscess*: A circumscribed intra-abdominal collection of pus, usually in proximity to the pancreas, which contains little or no pancreatic necrosis that arises as a consequence of either acute pancreatitis or pancreatic trauma (Fig. 209.3). The relative absence of necrosis distinguishes *pancreatic abscess* from *infected pancreatic necrosis*.
5. *Walled-off Pancreatic Necrosis (WOPN):* Also called organized pancreatic necrosis, the term walled-off pancreatic necrosis was first introduced in 2005. It is characterized by granulation tissue forming around a collection of enzymes and debris and even bacteria (which can in fact secondarily seed the collection).

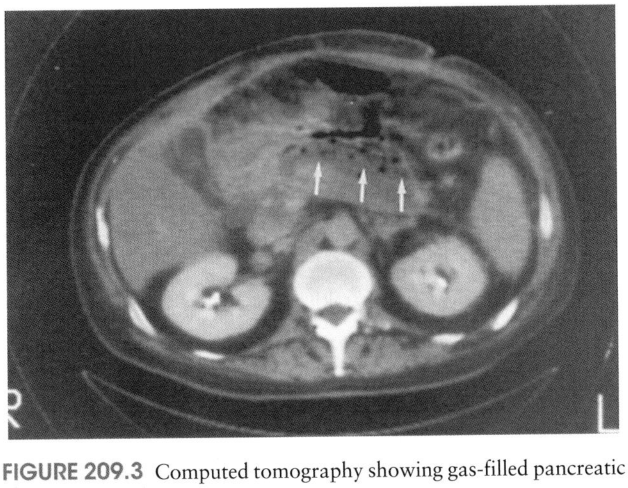

FIGURE 209.3 Computed tomography showing gas-filled pancreatic abscess (*arrows*).

Diagnosis

These types of fluid collections are usually found as a complication of severe acute pancreatitis 7 to 10 days following the onset of symptoms. Usually, patients seem to develop recurrence of their pain in association with fever and leukocytosis.

Dynamic contrast-enhanced CT and MRI are the most accurate means of identifying these complications of acute pancreatitis. The presence of extra-intestinal gas on CT is diagnostic of either infected necrosis or abscess, but this finding is only occasionally noted. More often, patients with either infected necrosis or abscess are found to have poorly enhanced areas on dynamic CT in a clinical setting of suspected sepsis. When doubt about the presence or absence of infection persists, fine-needle aspiration of these areas, under CT or EUS guidance, may yield material that, on Gram stain, reveals the presence of a pathogenic microorganism [125,126].

Management

Acute Fluid Collections

Acute fluid collections generally require no specific treatment. They usually resolve spontaneously within several weeks of an attack. Attempts to drain these collections either by percutaneously placed catheters or by early surgical intervention should be discouraged.

Sterile Necrosis

Patients with sterile necrosis, even if extensive, should be managed nonoperatively during the initial few weeks of their illness [127]. Surgical intervention in such patients may be associated with considerable morbidity and may even result in secondary infection of the inflamed, but previously sterile, pancreas.

Although the consensus view is that patients with sterile necrosis do not need intervention during the early phases of their disease, the potential value of intervention at later times is not entirely clear. Some of these patients experience a very prolonged illness, and full recovery may only be possible after the devitalized pancreatic and peripancreatic tissue has been removed. This can be accomplished surgically by exposing the involved area and removing the necrotic tissue—a procedure that may require repeated operations and can lead to considerable morbidity. Alternatives to this approach have been proposed. They involve transpapillary or transcutaneous placement of irrigating catheters into the involved area followed by debridement achieved by continuous lavage [128–130]. In another approach, debridement is achieved using a percutaneously placed operating nephroscope or laparoscope [131,132]. A more common approach is an endoscopic necrosectomy [133]. Often, unless there is evidence of infected necrosis, an endoscopic necrosectomy is planned for a 4 to 6 weeks after the resolution of the acute episode, allowing for the necrosis to wall off. Even at this time, necrosectomy is often indicated based on symptoms and after further radiologic assessment. It is not uncommon for multiple procedures to be performed over several weeks in order to achieve resolution of the necrosis. Although there have been no randomized controlled trials comparing endoscopic necrosectomy with surgical necrosectomy, the benefits of the former outweigh the morbidity associated with open necrosectomy, and often is the preferred approach for addressing persistent pancreatic necrosis.

Infected Necrosis

Infected necrosis is usually an indication for surgical intervention in symptomatic patients, whether it is detected by the presence of extra-intestinal gas on CT examination or by fine-needle aspiration of an area of pancreatic necrosis. However, more recently endoscopic necrosectomy seems to have also been useful as a less invasive approach. Organisms recovered in areas of infected pancreatic necrosis usually are those that are present in the gastrointestinal tract (*Klebsiella* spp, *Pseudomonas* spp, *Escherichia coli*, *Enterococcus*, *Proteus* spp) [134]. In addition, yeast such as *Candida albicans* may be encountered. It is believed that most of these organisms reach the inflamed pancreas via transmigration from adjacent segments of the intestine. Antibiotic therapy, although indicated, by itself usually represents an inadequate approach to the management of infected pancreatic necrosis. If the endoscopic approach is unsuccessful, surgical debridement and drainage should be considered. This is especially true for the unstable or septic patient who is doing poorly with nonoperative management.

Recent reports have suggested that stable patients with infected necrosis can be managed more electively and conservatively, particularly those stable patients who are asymptomatic; delay in performing surgical debridement may actually be beneficial because it appears to improve survival, decrease surgical complications, and decrease the need for repeated operations when compared with early operation for this group [135]. Furthermore, although most of these patients will eventually need debridement, recent anecdotal reports have indicated that some may be definitively treated with either antibiotics alone or with antibiotics combined with percutaneous drainage [136].

Pseudocyst

Pseudocysts may cause symptoms either because they are themselves tender or because they result in obstruction of adjacent organs such as the stomach, duodenum, and bile duct. On the other hand, many pseudocysts do not cause symptoms. Only symptomatic pseudocysts need to be treated [137–139].

Several methods of treating pseudocysts have been proposed, including either open or laparoscopic internal surgical drainage (cystogastrostomy, cystoduodenostomy, and Roux-en-Y cystojejunostomy), endoscopic drainage (cystogastrostomy, cystoduodenostomy), and percutaneous drainage (aspiration, aspiration followed by administration of somatostatin, and catheter drainage, with or without administration of somatostatin) [140]. Percutaneous drainage has a considerable incidence of either recurrence after aspiration or infection after catheter drainage. On the other hand, endoscopic drainage, via endoscopic cystoduodenostomy or cystogastrostomy, is a highly effective way of managing cysts located in the pancreatic head or body, particularly if they are pressing inward on the duodenum or stomach and there is little in the way of tissue or blood vessels interposed between the cyst and the duodenal or gastric lumen [141]. Surgical internal drainage (i.e., cystojejunostomy, cystogastrostomy) would seem most appropriate for management of cysts in the pancreatic tail or the head/body cysts that cannot be safely accessed endoscopically.

Pancreatic Ascites and Pancreatic Duct Fistulas

Patients with pancreatic ascites or pancreatic-pleural fistulas may respond to nonoperative therapy with bowel rest, parenteral nutrition, and administration of somatostatin or other agents designed to inhibit pancreatic secretion [142–149]. Most, however, fail this method of treatment, and some form of intervention is needed. An ERCP should be performed to identify the site of ductal disruption [150–152] that, if in the pancreatic tail, can be treated easily by distal pancreatectomy. Alternatively, anastomosis of a Roux-en-Y loop of jejunum to the site of rupture, particularly if it is in the head or neck of the gland, may be preferable. Endoscopically placed stents also can be used to prevent leakage of juice from the duct, and this nonoperative approach can be useful in the management of these complications [153].

WOPN

Historically, the curative and first-line treatment for WOPN has been surgical debridement. Alternatively, laparoscopic drainage has been used for patients in whom surgery is deemed too risky a procedure. Both approaches have drawbacks. Often, patients may need more than one operation for complete debridement and can develop abdominal wall hernia as well as external fistulae. And laparoscopic drainage often yields less than complete drainage of the necrotic material. Recent advancements with endoscopic interventions however support EUS-guided or direct endoscopic, transgastric, or transduodenal necrosectomy as an equally effective therapy. Reports suggest that cure rates are similar to those with surgical therapy, approaching 91% at approximately 5 months (with repeat procedures in this time frame). Serious major complications include major bleeding and perforation, and other adverse events may be a function of severity of disease and comorbidities [154].

CONCLUSIONS

The knowledge base for acute pancreatitis has changed dramatically in the past decade. Understanding of the genetic basis of the disease, approaching its management, and the use of less invasive methods of management is currently accepted practice. However, a number of questions still remain: rate of fluid resuscitation, types of fluids to use, and role of oral feedings. It is not until these issues are clearly addressed through clinical trials that we can identify the best way to care of these complicated patients and to develop an acute pancreatitis quality index for the proper care and management of these patients.

ACKNOWLEDGMENT

We thank Dr. Michael Steer for his many contributions to this chapter.

References

1. Kloppel G, Maillet B: Histopathology of acute pancreatitis, in Beger HG, Warshaw AL, Buchler MW, et al (eds): *The Pancreas*. Oxford, Blackwell, 1998, pp 404–409.
2. Sarles H: Introduction and proposal adopted unanimously by the participants of the symposium, in Sarles H (ed): *Pancreatitis-Symposium*. Basel, Switzerland, Verlag S. Karger, 1965, p VI.
3. Sarner M, Cotton PB: Classification of pancreatitis. *Gut* 25:756, 1984.
4. Singer MV, Gyr K: Revised classification of pancreatitis—Marseilles 1984. *Gastroenterology* 89:683, 1985.
5. Dervenis C, Johnson CD, Bassi C, et al: Diagnosis, objective assessment of severity, and management of acute pancreatitis. Santorini consensus conference. *Int J Pancreatol* 25:195, 1999.
6. Steer ML: Acute pancreatitis, in Wolfe MM, Davis G, Farraye FA, et al (eds): *Therapy of Digestive Disorders*. 2nd ed. New York, NY, Elsevier, 2006, pp 417–426.
7. Frossard JL, Steer ML, Pastor CM: Acute pancreatitis. *Lancet* 371:143–152, 2008.
8. Turi S, Kraft M, Lerch MM: Acute pancreatitis associated with metabolic, infectious, and drug-related diseases, in Beger H, Warshaw A, Buchler M, et al (eds): *The Pancreas*. 2nd ed. Oxford, Blackwell, 2008, pp 172–183.
9. Pitchumoni CS: Special problems of tropical pancreatitis. *Clin Gastroenterol* 13:541, 1984.
10. Narendranathan M: Chronic calcific pancreatitis of the tropics. *Trop Gastroenterol* 2:40, 1981.
11. Pitchumoni CS, Jain NK, Lowenfels AF, et al: Chronic cyanide poisoning. Unifying concept for alcoholic and tropical pancreatitis. *Pancreas* 3:220, 1988.
12. Sidu SS, Nundy S, Tandon RK: The effect of the modified Puestow procedure on diabetes in patients with tropical chronic pancreatitis—a prospective study. *Am J Gastroenterol* 96:107, 2001.
13. Acosta JL, Ledesma CL: Gallstone migration as a cause for acute pancreatitis. *N Engl J Med* 290:484, 1974.

14. Acosta JL, Ross R, Ledesma CL: The usefulness of stool screening for diagnosing cholelithiasis in acute pancreatitis: a description of the technique. *Am J Dig Dis* 22:168, 1977.
15. Opie EL: The relationship of cholelithiasis to disease of the pancreas and fat necrosis. *Am J Med Surg* 12:27, 1901.
16. Menguy RB, Hallenbeck GA, Bollman JL, et al: Intraductal pressures and sphincteric resistance in canine pancreatic and biliary ducts after various stimuli. *Surg Gynecol Obstet* 106:306, 1958.
17. Mann FC, Giordano AS: The bile factor in pancreatitis. *Arch Surg* 6:1, 1923.
18. Robinson TM, Dunphy JE: Continuous perfusion of bile protease activators through the pancreas. *JAMA* 183:530, 1963.
19. McCutheon AD: Reflux of duodenal contents in the pathogenesis of pancreatitis. *Gut* 5:260, 1964.
20. Lerch MM, Saluja AK, Runzi M, et al: Pancreatic duct obstruction triggers acute necrotizing pancreatitis in the opossum. *Gastroenterology* 104:853, 1993.
21. Steer ML, Meldolesi J, Figarella C: Pancreatitis: the role of lysosomes. *Dig Dis Sci* 29:934, 1984.
22. Steer ML: The early intraacinar cell events which occur during acute pancreatitis. The Frank Brooks Memorial Lecture. *Pancreas* 17:31, 1998.
23. Steer ML, Sharma A, Tao XH, et al: Where and how does pancreatitis begin? in Amman RW, Buchler MW, Adler G, et al (eds): *Pancreatitis: Advances in Pathobiology, Diagnosis, and Treatment. Falk Symposium 143*. New York, NY, Springer, 2005, pp 3–12.
24. Perides G, Laukkarinen JM, Vassileva G, et al: Biliary acute pancreatitis in mice is mediated by the G protein-coupled cell surface bile acid receptor Gpbar1. *Gastroenterology* 138(2):715–725, 2010.
25. Saluja AK, Donovan EA, Yamaguchi Y, et al: Caerulein-induced in vitro activation of trypsinogen in rat pancreatic acini is mediated by cathepsin B. *Gastroenterology* 113:304, 1997.
26. Sarles H: Chronic pancreatitis: etiology and pathophysiology, in Go VLW, Gardner JD, Brooks EP, et al (eds): *The Exocrine Pancreas: Biology, Pathobiology, and Diseases*. New York, NY, Raven Press, 1986, p 37.
27. Steer ML, Glazer G, Manabe T: Direct effects of ethanol on exocrine secretion from the in-vitro rabbit pancreas. *Dig Dis Sci* 24:769, 1979.
28. Rinderknecht H, Renner IG, Koyama HH: Lysosomal enzymes in pure pancreatic juice from normal healthy volunteers and chronic alcoholics. *Dig Dis Sci* 24:180, 1979.
29. Apte MV, Pirola RC, Wilson JS: Molecular mechanisms of alcoholic pancreatitis. *Dig Dis* 23:232, 2005.
30. Pandol SJ, Raraty M: Pathobiology of alcoholic pancreatitis. *Pancreatology* 7:105, 2007.
31. Vonlaufen A, Wilson JS, Apte MV: Molecular mechanisms of pancreatitis: current opinion. *J Gastroenterol Hepatol* 23:1339, 2008.
32. Criddle DN, Murphy J, Fistetto G, et al: Fatty acid ethyl esters cause pancreatic calcium toxicity via inositol trisphosphate receptors and loss of ATP synthesis. *Gastroenterology* 130:781, 2006.
33. Criddle DN, Raraty MG, Neoptolemos JP, et al: Ethanol toxicity in pancreatic acinar cells: mediation by nonoxidative fatty acid metabolites. *Proc Natl Acad Sci USA* 101:10738, 2004.
34. Vonlaufen A, Xu Z, Kumar DB, et al: Bacterial endotoxin: a trigger factor for alcoholic pancreatitis? Evidence from a novel, physiologically relevant animal model. *Gastroenterology* 134:640, 2008.
35. Renner IG, Savage WE III, Pantoja H, et al: Death due to acute pancreatitis. A retrospective analysis of 405 autopsy cases. *Dig Dis Sci* 30:1005, 1985.
36. Wilcox CM, Varadarajulu S, Eloubeidi M: Role of endoscopic evaluation in idiopathic pancreatitis: a systematic review. *Gastrointest Endosc* 63(7):1037–1045, 2006.
37. Toouli J, Brooke-Smith M, Bassi C, et al: Guidelines for the management of acute pancreatitis. *J Gastroenterol Hepatol* 17 Suppl:15–39, 2002.
38. Thomas FB: Drug-induced pancreatitis: facts vs fiction. *Drug Ther Hosp* 7:60, 1982.
39. Greenberger NJ, Toskes P, Isselbacher KJ: Diseases of the pancreas, in Braunwald E (ed): *Harrison's Principles of Internal Medicine*. New York, NY, McGraw-Hill, 1988, p 1372.
40. McArthur K: Drug induced pancreatitis. *Aliment Pharmacol Ther* 10:238, 1996.
41. Trivedi CD, Pitchumoni CS: Drug-induced pancreatitis: an update. *J Clin Gastroenterol* 39:709, 2005.
42. Lambert JS, Seidlin M, Reichman RC, et al: 2′, 3′-Dideoxyinosine (ddI) in patients with the acquired immunodeficiency syndrome of AIDS-related complex. A phase I trial. *N Engl J Med* 322:1333, 1990.
43. Durr GH: Acute pancreatitis, in Howatt HT, Sarles H (eds): *The Exocrine Pancreas*. London, WB Saunders, 1979, p 352.
44. Warshaw AL, Simeone JF, Schapiro RH, et al: Evaluation and treatment of the dominant dorsal duct syndrome (pancreas divisum redefined). *Am J Surg* 159:59, 1990.
45. Delhaye M, Cremer M: Clinical significance of pancreas divisum. *Acta Gastroenterol Belg* 55:306, 1992.
46. Fogel EL, Toth TG, Lehman GA, et al: Does endoscopic therapy favorably affect the outcome of patients who have recurrent acute pancreatitis and pancreas divisum? *Pancreas* 34:21, 2007.
47. Wilson RH, Moorehead RJ: Current management of trauma to the pancreas. *Br J Surg* 78:1196, 1991.
48. Bardenheier JA, Kaminski DL, William VL: Pancreatitis after biliary tract surgery. *Am J Surg* 16:773, 1968.
49. Peterson LM, Collins JJ, Wilson RE: Acute pancreatitis occurring after operation. *Surg Gynecol Obstet* 127:23, 1968.
50. White TT, Morgan A, Hopton D: Postoperative pancreatitis: a study of seventy cases. *Am J Surg* 120:132, 1970.
51. Adiseshia M: Acute pancreatitis after cardiac transplantation. *World J Surg* 7:519, 1983.
52. Feiner H: Pancreatitis after cardiac surgery. *Am J Surg* 131:684, 1976.
53. Sherman S, Lehman GA: Endoscopic retrograde cholangiopancreatography- and endoscopic sphincterotomy-induced pancreatitis, in Beger HG, Warshaw AL, Buchler MW, et al (eds): *The Pancreas*. Oxford, Blackwell, 1998, pp 291–310.
54. Whitcomb DC, Preston RA, Aston CE, et al: A gene for hereditary pancreatitis maps to chromosome 7g35. *Gastroenterology* 110:1975, 1996.
55. Whitcomb DC, Gorry MC, Preston RA, et al: Hereditary pancreatitis is caused by a mutation in the cationic trypsinogen gene. *Nat Genet* 14:141, 1996.
56. Cohn JA, Friedman KJ, Noone PG, et al: Relation between mutations of the cystic fibrosis gene and idiopathic pancreatitis. *N Engl J Med* 339:653, 1998.
57. Hamano H, Kawa S, Horiuchi A, et al: High serum IgG4 concentrations in patients with sclerosing pancreatitis. *N Engl J Med* 344:732, 2001.
58. Ros E, Navarro S, Bru C, et al: Occult microlithiasis in "idiopathic" acute pancreatitis: prevention of relapses by cholecystectomy or ursodeoxycholic acid therapy. *Gastroenterology* 101:1701, 1991.
59. Lee SP, Nicholls JF, Park HZ: Biliary sludge as a cause of acute pancreatitis. *N Engl J Med* 326:589, 1992.
60. Silen W: *Cope's Early Diagnosis of the Acute Abdomen*. 15th ed. New York, NY, Oxford University Press, 1979.
61. Leavitt MD, Edkfeldt JH: Diagnosis of acute pancreatitis, in Go VLW, Gardner JD, Brooks EP, et al (eds): *The Exocrine Pancreas: Biology, Pathobiology, and Diseases*. New York, NY, Raven Press, 1986, p 481.
62. Solomon SS, Duckworth WC, Jallepalli P, et al: The glucose intolerance of acute pancreatitis. *Diabetes* 29:22, 1980.
63. Drew SI, Joffe B, Vinik A, et al: The first 24 hours of acute pancreatitis. *Am J Med* 64:795, 1978.
64. Fan ST, Lai ECS, Mok FPT, et al: Early treatment of acute biliary pancreatitis by endoscopic papillotomy. *N Engl J Med* 328:228, 1993.
65. Toskes P: Hyperlipidemic pancreatitis. *Gastroenterol Clin North Am* 19:783, 1990.
66. Cameron JL, Crisler C, Margolis S, et al: Acute pancreatitis with hyperlipemia. *Surgery* 70:53, 1971.
67. Imric CW, Beastall GH, Allam BF, et al: Parathyroid hormone and calcium homeostasis in acute pancreatitis. *Br J Surg* 65:717, 1978.
68. Ranson JHC, Lackner H: Coagulopathies, in Bradley EL (ed): *Complications of Pancreatitis*. Philadelphia, PA, WB Saunders, 1982, p 154.
69. Steer ML: Acute pancreatitis, in Yamada T, Owyang C, Powell DW, et al (eds): *Textbook of Gastroenterology*. Philadelphia, PA, JB Lippincott Co, 1991, p 1859.
70. Salt WB, Schenker S: Amylase—its clinical significance: a review of the literature. *Medicine* 55:269, 1976.
71. Steinberg WM, Goldstein SS, Davis ND, et al: Diagnostic assays in acute pancreatitis. A study of sensitivity and specificity. *Ann Intern Med* 102:576, 1985.
72. Berk JE, Kizu H, Wilding P: A newly recognized cause for elevated serum amylase activity. *N Engl J Med* 277:941, 1967.
73. Levitt MD, Rapoport M, Cooperband SR: The renal clearance of amylase in renal insufficiency, acute pancreatitis, and macroamylasemia. *Ann Intern Med* 71:919, 1969.
74. Warshaw AL, Fuller AF: Specificity of increased renal clearance of amylase in diagnosis of acute pancreatitis. *N Engl J Med* 292:325, 1975.
75. McMahon MJ, Playforth MJ, Rashid SA, et al: The amylase-to-creatinine clearance—a nonspecific response to acute illness? *Br J Surg* 69:29, 1982.
76. Levitt MD, Gross JB Jr: Postoperative elevation of amylase/creatinine clearance ratio in patients without pancreatitis. *Gastroenterology* 77:497, 1979.
77. Levin RJ, Galuser FL, Berk JE: Enhancement of the amylase-creatinine clearance ratio in disorders other than acute pancreatitis. *N Engl J Med* 292:329, 1975.
78. Morton WJ, Tedesco FJ, Harter H, et al: Serum amylase determinations and amylase to creatinine clearance ratios in patients with chronic renal insufficiency. *Gastroenterology* 71:594, 1976.
79. Tietz NW, Shuey DF: Denise: lipase in serum—the elusive enzyme: an overview. *Clin Chem* 39(5):746–756, 1993.
80. Treacy J, Williams A, Bais R, et al: Evaluation of amylase and lipase in the diagnosis of acute pancreatitis. *ANZ J Surg* 71(10):577–582, 2001.
81. Tenner S, Baillie J, DeWitt J, et al: American College of Gastroenterology guideline: management of acute pancreatitis. *Am J Gastroenterol* 108:1400–1415, 2013.
82. Banks PA: Acute pancreatitis: clinical presentation, in Go VLW, Gardner JD, Brooks EP, et al (eds): *The Exocrine Pancreas: Biology, Pathobiology, and Diseases*. New York, NY, Raven Press, 1986, p 475.
83. Tenner S, Fernandez-del Castillo C, Warshaw A, et al: Urinary trypsinogen activation peptide (TAP) predicts severity in patients with acute pancreatitis. *Int J Pancreatol* 21:105, 1997.
84. Bank S, Barbezat GO, Marks IN, et al: Methemalbuminaemia in acute abdominal emergencies. *BMJ* 2:86, 1968.
85. Kusske AM, Rungione AJ, Reber HA: Cytokines and acute pancreatitis. *Gastroenterology* 110:639, 1996.

86. Buchler M, Malfertheiner P, Beger HG: Correlation of imaging procedures, biochemical parameters and clinical stage in acute pancreatitis, in Malfertheiner P, Ditschuneit H (eds): *Diagnostic Procedures in Pancreatic Disease*. Berlin, Springer-Verlag, 1986, p 123.
87. Mayer AD, McMahon MJ, Bowen M, et al: C-reactive protein: an aid to assessment and monitoring of acute pancreatitis. *J Clin Pathol* 37:207, 1984.
88. Lees WR: Pancreatic ultrasonography. *Clin Gastroenterol* 13:763, 1984.
89. Freeny PC: Radiology of acute pancreatitis: diagnosis, detection of complications, and interventional therapy, in Glazer G, Ranson JHC (eds): *Acute Pancreatitis*. London, Bailliere Tindall, 1988, p 275.
90. Kivisarri L, Somer K, Standertskjold-Nordenstam C-G, et al: A new method for the diagnosis of acute hemorrhagic-necrotizing pancreatitis using contrast-enhanced CT. *Gastrointest Radiol* 9:27, 1984.
91. Beger HG, Krautzberger W, Bittner R, et al: Results of surgical treatment of necrotizing pancreatitis. *World J Surg* 9:972, 1985.
92. Runzi M, Raptopoulos V, Saluja AK, et al: Evaluation of necrotizing pancreatitis in the opossum by dynamic contrast-enhanced computed tomography: correlation between radiographic and morphologic changes. *J Am Coll Surg* 180:673, 1995.
93. Balthazar EJ: Acute pancreatitis: assessment of severity with clinical and CT evaluation. *Radiology* 223:603, 2002.
94. Matos C, Bali MA, Delhaye M, et al: Magnetic resonance imaging in the detection of pancreatitis and pancrea neoplasms. *Best Pract Res Clin Gastroenterol* 20:157, 2006.
95. Ranson JHC: Prognostication in acute pancreatitis, in Glazer G, Ranson JHC (eds): *Acute Pancreatitis*. London, Bailliere Tindall, 1988, p 303.
96. Ranson JHC, Rifkind KM, Roses DF, et al: Prognostic signs and the role of operative management in acute pancreatitis. *Surg Gynecol Obstet* 139:69, 1974.
97. Imrie CW, Benjamin IS, Ferguson JC, et al: A single-centre double-blind trial of Trasylol therapy in primary acute pancreatitis. *Br J Surg* 65:337, 1978.
98. Larvin M, McMahon MJ: APACHE-2 score for assessment and monitoring of acute pancreatitis. *Lancet* 2:201, 1989.
99. Wu BU: Prognosis in acute pancreatitis. *CMAJ* 183(6):673–677, 2011.
100. Ranson JHC, Balthazar E, Caccavale R, et al: Computed tomography and the prediction of pancreatic abscess in acute pancreatitis. *Ann Surg* 201:656, 1985.
101. Halonen KJ, Pettila V, Leppaniemi AK, et al: Multiple organ dysfunction associated with severe acute pancreatitis. *Crit Care Med* 30:1274, 2002.
102. Vincent JL, de Mendoca A, Cantraine F, et al: Use of the SOFA score to assess the incidence of organ dysfunction/failure in intensive care units: results of a multicenter, prospective study. *Crit Care Med* 26:1793, 1998.
103. Brown A, Orav J, Banks PA: Hemoconcentration is an early marker for organ failure and necrotizing pancreatitis. *Pancreas* 20:367, 2000.
104. Lankisch PG, Mahike R, Blum T, et al: Hemoconcentration: an early marker of severe and/or necrotizing pancreatitis? A critical appraisal. *Am J Gastroenterol* 96:2081, 2001.
105. UK Working Party on Acute Pancreatitis: UK guidelines for the management of acute pancreatitis. *Gut* 54:1, 2001.
106. Heinrich S, Schafer M, Rousson V, et al: Evidence-based treatment of acute pancreatitis: a look at established paradigms, *Ann Surg* 243:154, 2006.
107. Marik PE, Zaloga GP: Meta-analysis of parenteral nutrition versus enteral nutrition in patients with acute pancreatitis. *BMJ* 328:1407, 2004.
108. Whitcomb DG: Acute pancreatitis. *N Engl J Med* 354:2142, 2006.
109. Estock FC, Chong P, Menezes N, et al: A randomized study of early nasogastric versus nasojejunal feeding in severe acute pancreatitis. *Am J Gastroenterol* 100:432, 2005.
110. Neoptolemos JP, Carr-Locke DL, London NJ, et al: Controlled trial of urgent endoscopic retrograde cholangiopancreatography and endoscopic sphincterotomy versus conservative treatment for acute pancreatitis due to gallstones. *Lancet* 2:979, 1988.
111. Folsch UR, Nitsche R, Ludtke R, et al: Early ERCP and papillotomy compared with conservative treatment for acute biliary pancreatitis. The German Study Group on Acute Biliary Pancreatitis. *N Engl J Med* 336:237, 1997.
112. Van Santvoort HC, Besselink MG, de Vries AC, et al: Early endoscopic retrograde cholangiopancreatography in predicted severe acute biliary pancreatitis: a prospective multicenter study. *Ann Surg* 250:68, 2009.
113. Bradley EL: A clinically based classification system for acute pancreatitis. Summary of the International Symposium on Acute Pancreatitis, Atlanta, GA, September 11 through 13, 1992. *Arch Surg* 128:586, 1993.
114. Rivers E, Nguyen B, Havstad S, et al: Early goal-directed therapy in the treatment of severe sepsis and septic shock. *N Engl J Med* 345:1368, 2001.
115. Thune A, Baker RA, Saccone GT, et al: Differing effects of pethidine and morphine on human sphincter of Oddi motility. *Br J Surg* 77:992, 1990.
116. Helm JF, Venu RP, Geenen JE, et al: Effects of morphine on the human sphincter of Oddi. *Gut* 29:1402, 1988.
117. McClave SA, Chang WK, Dhaliwal R, et al: Nutrition support in acute pancreatitis: a systematic review of the literature. *JPEN J Parenter Enteral Nutr* 30:143, 2006.
118. Marik PE, Zaloga GP: Meta-analysis of parenteral nutrition versus enteral nutrition in patients with acute pancreatitis. *BMJ* 328:1407, 2004.
119. Al-Omran M, Groof A, Wilke D: Enteral versus parenteral nutrition for acute pancreatitis. *Cochrane Database Syst Rev* CD002837, 2003.
120. Bassi C, Larvin M, Villatoro E: Antibiotic therapy for prophylaxis against infection of pancreatic necrosis in acute pancreatitis. *Cochrane Database Syst Rev* CD002941, 2003.
121. Golub R, Siddiqi F, Pohl D: Role of antibiotics in acute pancreatitis: a meta-analysis. *J Gastrointest Surg* 2:496, 1998.
122. Isenmann R, Runzi M, Kron M, et al: Prophylactic antibiotic treatment in patients with predicted severe acute pancreatitis: a placebo-controlled double-blind trial. *Gastroenterology* 126:997, 2004.
123. Mier J, Leon EL, Castillo A, et al: Early versus late necrosectomy in severe necrotizing pancreatitis. *Am J Surg* 173:71, 1997.
124. Folsch UR, Nitsche R, Ludtke R, et al: Early ERCP and papillotomy compared with conservative treatment for acute biliary pancreatitis. The German Study Group on Acute Biliary Pancreatitis. *N Engl J Med* 336:237, 1997.
125. Gerzoff SG, Banks PA, Robbins AH, et al: Early diagnosis of pancreatic infection by computed tomography-guided aspiration. *Gastroenterology* 93:1315, 1987.
126. Banks PA, Gerzoff SG: Indications and results of fine needle aspiration of pancreatic exudate, in Beger HG, Buchler M (eds): *Acute Pancreatitis*. Berlin, Springer-Verlag, 1987, p 171.
127. Bradley EL, Allen K: A prospective longitudinal study of observation versus surgical intervention in the management of necrotizing pancreatitis. *Am J Surg* 161:19, 1991.
128. Baron TH, Morgan DE: Endoscopic transgastric irrigation tube placement via PEG for debridement of organized pancreatic necrosis. *Gastrointest Endosc* 50:574, 1999.
129. Freeney PC, Hauptmann E, Althaus AJ, et al: Percutaneous CT-guided catheter drainage of infected acute necrotizing pancreatitis: techniques and results. *Am J Roentgenol* 170:969, 1998.
130. Kozarek RA, Ball TJ, Patterson DJ, et al: Endoscopic transpapillary therapy for disrupted pancreatic duct and peripancreatic fluid collections. *Gastroenterology* 100:1362, 1991.
131. Carter CR, McKay CJ, Imrie CW: Percutaneous necrosectomy and sinus tract endoscopy in the management of infected pancreatic necrosis: an initial experience. *Ann Surg* 232:175, 2000.
132. Horvath KD, Kao LS, Wherry KL, et al: A technique for laparoscopic-assisted percutaneous drainage of infected pancreatic necrosis and pancreatic abscess. *Surg Endosc* 15:1221, 2001.
133. Baron TH: Endoscopic pancreatic necrosectomy. *Gastroenterol Hepatol* 4(9):617–620, 2008.
134. Pemberton JH, Nagorney DM, Dozois RR: Pancreatic abscess, in Go VLW, Gardner JD, Brooks EP, et al (eds): *The Exocrine Pancreas: Biology, Pathobiology, and Diseases*. New York, NY, Raven Press, 1986, p 513.
135. Hartwig W, Maksan SM, Foitzik T, et al: Reduction in mortality with delayed surgical therapy of severe pancreatitis. *J Gastrointest Surg* 30:195, 2002.
136. Runzi M, Niebel W, Goebell H, et al: Severe acute pancreatitis: nonsurgical treatment of infected necroses. *Pancreas* 30:195, 2005.
137. Bradley EL, Clements JL, Gonzales AC: The natural history of pancreatic pseudocysts: a unified concept of management. *Am J Surg* 137:135, 1979.
138. Yeo CJ, Bastidas JA, Lynch-Nyhan A, et al: The natural history of pancreatic pseudocysts documented by computed tomography. *Surg Gynecol Obstet* 170:411, 1990.
139. Vitas GJ, Sarr MG: Selected management of pancreatic pseudocysts: operative versus expectant management. *Surgery* 111:123, 1992.
140. Morali GA, Braverman DZ, Shemesh D, et al: Successful treatment of pancreatic pseudocysts with a somatostatin analogue and catheter drainage. *Am J Gastroenterol* 86:515, 1991.
141. Beckingham IJ, Crige EJ, Bornman PC, et al: Long-term outcome of endoscopic drainage of pancreatic pseudocysts. *Am J Gastroenterol* 94:71, 1999.
142. Sankaran S, Walt AJ: Pancreatic ascites: recognition and management. *Arch Surg* 111:430, 1976.
143. Cameron JL, Kieffer RS, Anderson WJ, et al: Internal pancreatic fistulas: pancreatic ascites and pleural effusions. *Ann Surg* 184:587, 1976.
144. Kavin H, Sobel JD, Dembo AJ: Pancreatic ascites treated by irradiation of pancreas. *BMJ* 2:503, 1971.
145. DeWale B, Van der Spek P, Devis G: Peritoneovenous shunt for pancreatic ascites. *Dig Dis Sci* 32:550, 1987.
146. Variyam EP: Central vein hyperalimentation in pancreatic ascites. *Am J Gastroenterol* 78:178, 1983.
147. Ward PA, Raju S, Suzuki H: Preoperative demonstration of pancreatic fistula by endoscopic pancreatography in a patient with pancreatic ascites. *Ann Surg* 185:232, 1977.
148. Cameron JL, Brawley RK, Bender HW, et al: The treatment of pancreatic ascites. *Ann Surg* 170:668, 1969.
149. Gislason H, Growbech JE, Soreide O: Pancreatic ascites: treatment by continuous somatostatin infusion. *Am J Gastroenterol* 86:519, 1991.
150. Sankaran S, Sugawa C, Walt AJ: Value of endoscopic retrograde pancreatography in pancreatic ascites. *Surg Gynecol Obstet* 148:185, 1979.
151. Rawlings W, Bynum TE, Pasternak G: Pancreatic ascites: diagnosis of leakage site by endoscopic pancreatography. *Surgery* 81:363, 1977.
152. Levine JB, Warshaw AL, Falchuk KR, et al: The value of endoscopic retrograde pancreatography in the management of pancreatic ascites. *Surgery* 81:360, 1977.
153. Kozarek RA, Ball TJ, Paterson DJ, et al: Endoscopic transpapillary therapy for disrupted pancreatic duct and peripancreatic fluid collections. *Gastroenterology* 100:1362, 1991.
154. Gardner TB, Coelho-Prabhu N, Gordon SR, et al: Direct endoscopic necrosectomy for the treatment of walled off pancreatic necrosis: results from a multicenter U.S. series. *Gastrointest Endosc* 73(4):718–726, 2011.

Chapter 210 ■ Diarrhea

JULIEN FAHED • BENJAMIN HYATT • COLIN T. SWALES • LAURA HARRELL RAFFALS

Diarrhea frequently complicates the course of the critically ill patient, occurring in 40% to 50% of patients in the intensive care unit (ICU). Diarrhea is the most common nonhemorrhagic gastrointestinal (GI) complication in this patient population [1–3]. Despite its high prevalence among the ICU patient population, diarrhea is frequently overlooked by physicians and the ICU team, especially when more emergent cardiovascular, respiratory, and infectious issues are present. Inattention to excessive stool output, however, can often result in serious perturbations of fluid and electrolyte balance, promote skin breakdown and infection, and create difficulty in the administration of proper nutritional support. In these instances, proper and immediate evaluation and management are essential to prevent further complications in a critically ill patient. The evaluation of diarrhea is often limited by the patient's status and practical limitations in performing diagnostic studies in the ICU setting.

The term diarrhea often carries a different meaning for patients and health care providers. Increases in stool frequency or fluidity do not necessarily indicate the presence of diarrhea. In a general patient population, an increase in daily stool weight or volume (exceeding 200 g per day) has been used as an objective-defining criterion [4]. In the critically ill patient, however, accurate measurement of stool output may be difficult, if not impossible. Physicians, therefore, must use their best judgment to decide whether diarrhea is present and to determine whether it represents a clinical problem requiring attention. This chapter provides helpful insights for making these decisions, presents guidelines for rapid and directed evaluation, and suggests effective approaches for the management of diarrhea in this setting.

ETIOLOGY

The causative factors of diarrhea in the ICU patient differ considerably from those in the general population. Numerous causes of diarrhea in the ICU setting exist and can be broadly divided into three categories: (a) diarrhea secondary to iatrogenic causes, (b) diarrhea secondary to underlying diseases, and (c) diarrhea resulting as a primary manifestation of specific diseases. Careful review of clinical information will allow physicians to narrow the diagnostic possibilities and avoid overlooking simple and common causes of diarrhea (Table 210.1). In some patients, diarrhea is the result of a combination of factors. Thus, it is incumbent on the physician to carefully review available data to identify the cause(s) of diarrhea.

Iatrogenic Causes

Iatrogenic factors are the most commonly and frequently overlooked cause of diarrhea in the critically ill patient. Furthermore, rapid and successful treatment of iatrogenic diarrhea can often be achieved by eliminating the offending agent or process.

Medications

Medications are a frequent cause of iatrogenic diarrhea in the ICU setting. Many of the drugs commonly used in the ICU can cause diarrhea (Table 210.2). Therefore, any medication or combination of medications should be suspected, and uncertainty on the part of the physician warrants consultation with a pharmaceutical reference. Antibiotic-associated diarrhea occurs among 3% to 29% of hospitalized patients [5]. The frequency of diarrhea varies considerably depending on the antibiotic administered. The rate of diarrhea associated with parenterally administered antibiotics is comparable to orally administered antibiotics, especially antibiotics excreted into the enterohepatic circulation. Antibiotics most commonly associated with diarrhea include ampicillin, tetracycline, clindamycin, azithromycin, clarithromycin, fluoroquinolones, and many of the cephalosporins [6]. Antibiotic agents often cause a nonspecific, noninflammatory diarrhea associated with nausea, abdominal cramping, and bloating. In these instances, diagnostic studies are generally negative. Fluid and electrolyte losses are minimal, and symptoms often abate after withdrawal or change of the medication. Alterations in intestinal flora, breakdown of dietary carbohydrate products, and prokinetic effects (e.g., from erythromycin) are all postulated mechanisms of diarrhea [7].

Clostridium difficile infection (CDI) is the most common cause of infectious diarrhea in the ICU [8]. In fact, residence in the ICU has been identified as a risk factor for developing CDI [9], and some authors believe that *C. difficile* toxins are responsible for 50% of the cases of diarrhea in the ICU setting. CDI in the ICU is increasing not only in incidence but also in

TABLE 210.1

Differential Diagnosis of Diarrhea in the Intensive Care Unit Setting

- Iatrogenic causes
  - Medications
  - Enteral feeding
  - Pseudomembranous colitis
- Diarrhea secondarily related to underlying disease
  - Infections in immunosuppressed patients
  - Neoplastic disease in immunosuppressed patients
  - Gastrointestinal bleeding
  - Neutropenic enteropathy
  - Ischemic bowel disease
  - Postsurgical diarrhea (postcholecystectomy, following gastric surgery)
  - Surgically induced short bowel syndrome or pancreatic insufficiency
  - Fecal impaction
  - Opiate withdrawal
- Diarrhea as a primary manifestation of disease
  - Diabetic diarrhea
  - Renal failure
  - Sepsis
  - Adrenal insufficiency
  - Graft-versus-host disease
  - Vasculitis
  - Diarrhea-causing pathogens
  - Inflammatory bowel disease
  - Celiac sprue

TABLE 210.2

Medications Associated with Diarrhea

Antibiotics (especially erythromycin, ampicillin, clindamycin, azithromycin, and cephalosporins)
Antacids (magnesium containing)
Magnesium and phosphorus supplements
Proton pump inhibitors
Lactulose
Colchicine
Digitalis
Quinidine
Theophylline
Levothyroxine
Aspirin
Nonsteroidal anti-inflammatory agents
Cimetidine
Misoprostol
Diuretics
β-Blocking agents
Chemotherapeutic agents
Immunosuppressants (tacrolimus, sirolimus, mycophenolate mofetil, cyclosporine, and azathioprine)
HIV medications (especially protease inhibitors, e.g., nelfinavir)
Oral hypoglycemics (e.g., metformin)

Additives in the physical formulation of medications (e.g., sorbitol, lactose) may produce diarrhea independently of the primary medication.

severity [10]. CDI must always be considered for ICU patients with diarrhea who are commonly exposed to various mediations, particularly antibiotics that predispose to the development of CDI. Classically, clindamycin, penicillin, and broad-spectrum cephalosporins have been implicated. However, CDI may be caused by any antibiotic, including metronidazole and vancomycin, the agents typically used to treat CDI. Besides antibiotic exposure and environmental factors, the risk factors associated with CDI, include age greater than 60, severe underlying disease, gastric acid suppression, and immunologic susceptibility [7].

C. difficile produces multiple toxins, two of which have been well characterized. Toxin-induced changes in colonocyte function, cytokine release, and alterations in intestinal motility result in the signs and symptoms characteristic of CDI [11]. It is considered complicated and severe when patients are admitted to the ICU, hypotensive requiring pressors, febrile (greater than 38.5°C), have ileus or significant abdominal distention, mental status changes, leukocytosis (more than 35,000 white blood cells [WBC] per μL), leucopenia (less than 2,000 WBC per μL), elevated serum lactate levels (more than 2.2 mmol per L), or end-organ failure (mechanical ventilation, renal failure, etc.). Prompt recognition and treatment of CDI are essential because severe cases of CDI can progress to fulminant colitis and toxic megacolon requiring urgent surgical intervention [12].

Agents that increase the osmotic load in the gut lumen are also frequent causes of diarrhea in the ICU patient. Magnesium-containing antacids (e.g., Maalox and Mylanta) are common examples of such agents. The gut lumen osmotic load can also be increased as a result of aggressive enteral repletion of nutrients, such as magnesium and phosphorus. Lactulose, a useful agent in the treatment of hepatic encephalopathy, provides an osmotic gradient, resulting in increased fluid secretion and stool output. Many medications contain inert additives, sorbitol or lactose, which may also cause an osmotic diarrhea. In one study including 29 tube-fed patients with diarrhea, 48% of the cases were attributed to sorbitol-containing elixirs [13].

Proton pump inhibitors (PPIs), another commonly used class of medication in the ICU setting, frequently cause diarrhea, particularly when administered in higher doses. In fact, in a large study of more than 40,000 patients treated with omeprazole, lansoprazole, or pantoprazole, the most common adverse event was diarrhea [14].

Immunosuppressants used in transplantation (e.g., tacrolimus, sirolimus, mycophenolate mofetil, cyclosporine, and azathioprine) are associated with diarrhea. However, these agents may not be causative. As an example, an alternative explanation was found in 50% of kidney transplant patients who developed diarrhea while receiving mycophenolate [15]. In patients with HIV who are treated with highly active antiretroviral therapy, drug-induced diarrhea occurs in up to 75% of patients, and the protease inhibitors as well as integrase inhibitors are the most common drug-related cause of diarrhea in this population [16]. Symptoms are decreased by dose reduction or eliminated by discontinuation of therapy.

Withdrawal from medications (e.g., long-term sedatives, analgesics) may also be associated with diarrhea [17].

Other medications associated with diarrhea include colchicine, quinidine, digitalis, metoclopramide, theophylline, levothyroxine, aspirin, nonsteroidal anti-inflammatory drugs, misoprostol, cimetidine, diuretics, cholinergic agents (e.g., bethanechol), and β-blockers.

Enteral Feedings

Enteral feedings are the most common cause of diarrhea in the ICU setting, occurring in up to 63% of the ICU patients [1,18]. Numerous studies have investigated the role of enteral feedings in causing diarrhea in the critically ill patient. Certain aspects, such as concurrent administration of antibiotics, osmolality of solution, type of solution, and serum albumin, have been assessed to determine their contributing roles in the occurrence and severity of diarrhea for these patients [19]. In most instances, diarrhea in enterally fed patients is associated with concurrent antibiotic administration [18,20]. However, enteral feeds also cause changes in gut function that can result in diarrhea. The osmolarity of the enteral solution may play a role when elemental-type diets are used, and especially when feedings are rapidly administered directly into the small intestine. Bolus feeding may be more physiologic, especially with regard to glucose homeostasis; however, feedings administered in this manner distal to the pylorus introduce high-osmolar contents rapidly into the small bowel, resulting in a higher incidence of diarrhea [21]. The impact of enteral nutrition-related complications, including diarrhea, was illustrated in a prospective, multicenter cohort study of 400 patients [22]. In this study, 62.8% (251 of 400) patients suffered GI complication with 14.7% of the studied patients experiencing enteral nutrition-related diarrhea. These authors found that patients with GI complications had a reduction in their tube feed volumes, longer length of stay in the ICU, and higher mortality.

Enteral formulas high in lactose or fat content may also be a factor in susceptible patients. Starved or chronically parenterally fed patients who have developed small bowel villus atrophy and a decrease in mucosal disaccharidase enzyme activity may experience diarrhea when enteral feedings are initiated.

The relationship between hypoalbuminemia and diarrhea is controversial. Hwang et al. [2] compared ICU patients with and without diarrhea and found that the albumin level was statistically different between groups (1.90 vs. 3.40 g per dL in the groups with or without diarrhea, respectively). Hypoalbuminemia with resulting lowered oncotic pressure may cause diarrhea by inducing changes in the Starling forces sufficient to inhibit intestinal fluid absorption. Some authors claim that concurrent nutritional intake and correction of the albumin deficit with intravenous salt-poor albumin may result in normalization and maintenance of albumin levels with an improved tolerance to enteral feedings and resolution of diarrhea [23]. Conversely, patients with severe hypoalbuminemia secondary to cirrhosis or nephrotic syndrome do not uniformly have diarrhea. Until further studies show efficacy, routine use of intravenous albumin repletion cannot be recommended.

Studies investigating the role of the intestinal response to tube feedings have revealed that intraduodenal infusion resulted in a normal postprandial pattern of small intestinal motility and an increase in the volume of fluid entering the colon, but did not result in diarrhea [24]. Intragastric infusion, on the contrary, resulted in small intestinal motility and colonic flow similar to fasting, and the majority of subjects developed diarrhea [25]. This has led to the conclusion that enteral feeding–related diarrhea may be secondary to a disorder of colonic function. Further supporting this hypothesis are studies that have shown that the ascending colon, normally the site of maximal absorption of water and electrolytes, actually secretes water, sodium, and chloride during intragastric and intraduodenal infusion [26]. Up to 3.2 L per day was secreted by the ascending colon in these studies. Although this is well within the estimated 5.7 L per day maximal absorptive capacity of the colon, diarrhea still occurred, suggesting that this reversal of normal colonic physiology seriously impairs the absorptive capacity of the colon [27].

Diarrhea Secondarily Related to Underlying Disease

Diarrhea may result from various processes or pathogens associated with disease states commonly seen in the critically ill patient. Diarrhea may occur more frequently in patients who are immunosuppressed, have alterations in cardiac output and blood flow, or have various primary GI diseases.

In immunosuppressed patients, multiple infectious agents may be responsible for the development of diarrhea. Cytomegalovirus (CMV), herpes simplex virus, *Giardia*, *Salmonella*, *Shigella*, *Cryptosporidium*, *Isospora*, *Campylobacter*, and *Mycobacteria* are among the most common identifiable pathogens. Postchemotherapy patients can also experience diarrhea as a result of direct injury to the bowel, ranging from bowel edema to frank infarction. The cause of these changes is unclear; however, infections, direct toxic effects of chemotherapeutic agents, neutropenia, and primary intestinal injury have been postulated as initiating factors [28]. Strongyloides stercoralis should be remembered as a cause of diarrhea in patients who lived or traveled to endemic areas. Untreated immunosuppressed patients may develop hyperinfection with pulmonary infiltrates and infection of the cerebrospinal fluid and blood with enteric gram-negative bacilli [29].

In patients with acquired immunodeficiency syndrome (AIDS), diarrhea is perhaps the most commonly experienced symptom. Aside from iatrogenic causes, these patients can develop diarrhea from a single or multiple pathogens. CMV, *Mycobacterium* spp, *Cryptosporidium*, and *Microsporidium* are the most common agents. *Cryptosporidium* typically results in a severe large-volume secretory diarrhea (often in excess of 1 L per day) [30]. Other pathogens such as *Entamoeba histolytica*, *Isospora belli*, *Giardia lamblia*, *Microsporidium*, adenoviruses, and other species described above are capable of causing diarrhea in patients with AIDS [31]. Bacillary dysentery may become chronic and relapsing, posing challenges with treatment. The herpes simplex virus may cause perianal ulceration, urgency, and frequent mucopurulent discharge, which may be interpreted as diarrhea [32]. The CD4 count (cluster of differentiation four count) indicates the degree of immunocompromise in these patients, and a lower count broadens the differential diagnosis of the etiology of diarrhea. *Cryptosporidium parvum*, *Enterocytozoon bieneusi*, *Encephalitozoon intestinalis*, *Mycobacterium avium* complex (MAC), and enteroaggregative *Escherichia coli* cause self-limited disease in normal and mildly immunosuppressed individuals, but may cause persistent, severe diarrhea in patients with CD4 counts less than 200 cells per μL [3,33–37]. CMV rarely causes diarrhea in patients with CD4 counts greater than 50 cells per mm [3,38]. Patients with AIDS may also develop high-grade intestinal lymphomas predominantly of B-cell origin, which may present as diarrhea. Kaposi sarcoma may cause GI bleeding but rarely causes diarrhea [39].

Intestinal ischemia, especially involving the colon, may result in abdominal pain and diarrhea in the ICU patient. Postsurgical patients, especially those who have undergone repair of an abdominal aortic aneurysm, may have as high as a 6% incidence of colonoscopically documented ischemia [40]. Patients who have undergone an abdominoperineal resection or therapeutic angiography are also at risk. Compromise of the inferior mesenteric artery with left-sided colonic involvement is the primary etiologic factor. Symptoms may occur within hours to a few days following the procedure and may even be delayed for weeks. Patients in shock with depressed cardiac output may be more likely to present with right-sided colonic involvement, which is associated with a worse prognosis [41]. Severity can range from mild, transient ischemic changes to mucosal ulceration or bowel necrosis. Sympathomimetic drugs, vasopressin, ergot preparations, migraine therapies, alosetron, bevacizumab, and digoxin may further place susceptible patients at risk [42]. Likewise, small intestinal ischemia, especially venous ischemia, may present with bloody or nonbloody diarrhea. Bleeding of either the upper or lower GI tract is a frequent cause of bloody diarrhea in the ICU setting. Blood acts as both an irritant and osmotic agent, resulting in diarrhea. Common causes of upper GI bleeding include esophagitis, gastric and duodenal ulcer disease, and hemorrhagic gastropathy; whereas infectious colitis, diverticulosis, and ischemia may result in lower GI bleeding.

Fecal impaction in both medical and surgical patients may cause diarrhea and should be considered in the ICU patient with diarrhea. Drugs such as analgesics, sedatives, aluminum-containing antacids, and sucralfate may decrease intestinal motility and fecal fluidity, resulting in formation of a partially obstructing fecal mass and diarrhea. Diverticulitis may also be present with an accompanying diarrhea.

Diarrhea as a Primary Manifestation of Disease

Several common diseases are occasionally characterized by diarrhea during their courses. For instance, patients with diabetes can experience severe bouts of diarrhea. Diabetic diarrhea is considered to result from an autonomic neuropathy and its subsequent effect on intestinal fluid absorption [43]. These patients invariably have other signs of autonomic neuropathy, including orthostatic hypotension, gastroparesis, anhidrosis, abnormalities in RR wave variation on electrocardiogram, and neurogenic bladder [44]. Abnormalities in motility with intestinal stasis and bacterial overgrowth may also play a role in the development of diarrhea in diabetic patients.

Other endocrine disorders such as adrenal insufficiency and hyperthyroidism should also be considered in the critically ill patient with diarrhea. Adrenal insufficiency, either primary adrenal failure as a result of bilateral adrenal hemorrhage or infarction, or relative deficiency induced by stress in patients chronically exposed to corticosteroids, may present with secretory diarrhea. The symptoms and signs of an adrenal crisis include shock, nausea, vomiting, diarrhea, abdominal pain, fever, fatigue, and sometimes confusion or coma. Patients with hyperthyroidism have increased fecal output largely owing to increased intestinal motility [45].

Graft-versus-host disease (GVHD) may complicate both the short- and long-term course of patients who have undergone transplant (most commonly following allogeneic hematopoietic stem cell transplantation) [46,47]. Acute GVHD, occurring less than 100 days after transplant, typically is characterized by dermatitis, hepatitis, and gastroenteritis usually manifesting with nausea, abdominal pain, and diarrhea. Chronic GVHD (occurring more than 100 days after transplantation) may mimic autoimmune diseases, such as systemic lupus erythematosus, systemic sclerosis, or Sjogren syndrome [48] and often is characterized by a less severe form of diarrhea.

Vasculitic diseases such as systemic lupus erythematosus, dermatomyositis, polyarteritis, and granulomatosis with polyangiitis can involve medium- and small-sized vessels supplying the GI tract. Abdominal pain, fever, bleeding, and diarrhea are common resulting symptoms.

Finally, one must always consider the causes of diarrheal disease that are not unique to the critically ill patient. Infectious causes of diarrhea for immunocompetent hospitalized patients are possible, but are unusual in clinical practice unless the onset of the diarrhea is within the first few days of hospitalization or a nosocomial outbreak of infection is present [49]. Infectious causes that should be considered include *Salmonella*, *Shigella*, *Campylobacter*, *Giardia*, or *E. histolytica*, although other pathogens have also been implicated [50]. Nonenteric infectious causes of diarrhea include toxic shock syndrome and Legionnaires disease. Other causes to be considered include lactose intolerance, inflammatory bowel disease, and celiac sprue.

DIAGNOSIS

History and Physical Examination

The history is important in establishing the diagnosis and etiology of diarrhea in the ICU patient; however, depressed neurological function as the result of the disease state or iatrogenic sedation and intubation may make obtaining a history impossible. Attention to onset, duration, character, relation to enteral intake, and associated symptoms of diarrhea may be helpful etiologic clues. Information on prior episodes of diarrhea, the patient's underlying medical conditions (which may be associated with diarrhea), or prior use of antibiotics is also important to elucidate. Next, a careful review of the patient's current medications and their administration relative to the onset of diarrhea should be performed. Any suspected agent should be discontinued if at all possible or changed to an alternative medication. Every effort should be made at decreasing the number of medications and continuing only those that are absolutely necessary. The physician should also determine whether the initiation of enteral feedings has correlated with the onset of symptoms.

A history of abdominal pain may suggest ischemia, infection, or various inflammatory conditions such as vasculitis or GVHD. Bloody diarrhea may suggest primary GI bleeding, ischemia, or occasionally pseudomembranous colitis secondary to CDI. Passage of frequent small-volume stools with urgency and tenesmus suggests distal, left-sided colonic involvement, whereas passage of less frequent, large-volume stools suggests more proximal involvement (small intestine or right colon). These historic clues, however, are not mutually exclusive, and, in disease states with extensive bowel involvement, the distinction may not be appreciable.

Physical examination may provide further clues to the etiology of diarrhea, but findings are usually nonspecific. More important, the physical examination is essential in assessing the clinical severity of diarrhea. Orthostasis suggests severe volume loss, adrenal insufficiency, or autonomic neuropathy (e.g., from diabetes). Fever may occur in individuals with infection, vasculitis, adrenal insufficiency, or hyperthyroidism. Abdominal tenderness may suggest infectious, ischemic, or vasculitic causes. Skin rashes or mucosal ulcerations in appropriate patients may suggest inflammatory bowel disease, vasculitis, or GVHD. Clinical manifestations of AIDS may be apparent. Abdominal distention, palpable bowel loops, or abnormal rectal examination may suggest a partially obstructing fecal impaction.

Laboratory Studies

Serum electrolytes especially sodium, potassium, magnesium, and phosphorus should be obtained and carefully monitored in patients with diarrhea. Severe diarrhea may result in a hyperchloremic metabolic acidosis and prerenal azotemia. The serum sodium may be normal, elevated, or depressed depending on the severity of diarrhea, oral/parenteral water intake, type of intravenous fluid administered, and other disease states (e.g., hepatic or renal dysfunction). The serum potassium, magnesium, and phosphorus may be normal or depressed, whereas elevations (e.g., in potassium) may suggest adrenal insufficiency or uremia. Leukocytosis may suggest infection or ischemia, whereas neutropenia may suggest an immunosuppressed state or sepsis. Low serum protein levels may be a clue to the presence of a protein-losing gastroenteropathy.

Examination of the stool may be the single most important and most overlooked laboratory investigation in the ICU patient with diarrhea. The presence of fecal leukocytes should be determined, and when present may suggest infection, ischemia, or mucosal inflammation. Newer assays for fecal calprotectin and lactoferrin have been validated for use in dysentery and inflammatory bowel disease, but its usefulness in the ICU setting requires study [51]. Because of the high false-positive rate, *C. difficile* should only be tested in patients with current symptoms of diarrhea. The nucleic acid amplification tests for *C. difficile* toxin gene such as polymerase chain reaction is a standard diagnostic test for CDI and is superior to toxins A + B enzyme immunoassay testing. Once the diagnosis is made, repeat testing is discouraged. Several studies have shown that repeat testing after a negative test is positive in <5% of specimens, thereby increasing the likelihood of false positives [52–54]. On the other hand, when the test comes back negative, empiric treatment for CDI should not be discontinued or withheld in patients with a high pretest suspicion for CDI. That meant, the treatment is monitored by clinical symptoms and not with repeat testing because the stool can remain positive for at least 30 days after the diagnosis is made.

Fresh stool specimens for culture and ova and parasite examination should be requested in patients where there is a clinical suspicion, for example, in dysenteric presentations or when either fecal leukocytes or an elevated fecal calprotectin is found. Indiscriminate ordering of stool culture and ova and parasite test is not warranted. Immunosuppressed patients, however, require more extensive examination of the stool. Often, opportunistic pathogens are not detected readily through stool studies, and endoscopic examination with biopsies is required. Some pathogens such as CMV or MAC isolated from stool do not necessarily represent infection and require evidence of tissue invasion on biopsy for diagnosis.

Qualitative examination of the stool for fat using a Sudan III stain is the best screening test if a malabsorptive state is suspected. Determination of the stool osmolar gap, which is $290 - ([\text{stool } \{Na^+\} + \text{stool } \{K^+\}] \times 2)$, helps to distinguish osmotic and secretory causes of watery diarrhea. A gap greater than 125 mOsm per L is conventional for an osmotic diarrhea. High-volume stool output that persists with fasting suggests a secretory etiology. A low stool pH may suggest bacterial overgrowth or carbohydrate malabsorption [4].

Special Diagnostic Investigations

Plain abdominal radiographs are sometimes helpful and may show signs of ischemia, obstruction, perforation, or a megacolon associated with colitis. Contrast studies better define GI pathology that may result in diarrhea but often cannot be performed in a critically ill patient. Both these studies have been, in practice, supplanted by computed tomography (CT); newer imaging modalities, such as CT enterography and magnetic resonance enterography, have replaced the more cumbersome enteroclysis and may be useful in selected cases.

Flexible sigmoidoscopy, colonoscopy, and upper endoscopy can be extremely useful in diagnosing various causes of diarrhea. Colitides, including infectious, ischemic/vasculitic, and pseudomembranous colitis, will often have a characteristic endoscopic appearance. The classic findings in *C. difficile* colitis include distinct, adherent, raised plaques (pseudomembranes) 2 to 5 mm in size that may be confluent. More commonly, the mucosa is normal; a normal appearance should not exclude the diagnosis of CDI, because mucosal biopsies may reveal pseudomembranes histologically. CMV or herpes colitis are best diagnosed endoscopically. CMV colitis may manifest as discrete ulcerations or widespread mucosal edema, erythema, and erosion. The characteristic vesicles of herpes may or may not be present and can be replaced by extensive ulceration. MAC (aforementioned) is usually diagnosed histologically; small bowel or colonic biopsies reveal abundant acid-fast bacilli. *Cryptosporidium* and *Giardia* can be made by histologic evaluation of small bowel biopsies, whereas identification of *Microsporidium* is more difficult and requires the use of electron microscopy. GVHD is confirmed most commonly by histopathologic findings seen in biopsies obtained during flexible sigmoidoscopy.

Video capsule endoscopy, where a 12-mm capsule is either swallowed or placed in the small bowel endoscopically, captures via telemetry images of the entire small bowel. The mucosal detail provided is excellent, and so small bowel ulcerations, villus abnormalities, strictures, and other mucosal lesions are now more readily detected. In addition, small bowel ulcerations, villus abnormalities, strictures, and other mucosal lesions are now more readily detected. For example, capsule endoscopy allows for a more precise gauge of the extent of Crohn disease and celiac disease, and eosinophilic gastroenteritis has a characteristic capsule endoscopic appearance [55]. Although this technology permits detection of occult small bowel pathology not previously appreciated, its possible role and value in the diagnosis of persisting diarrhea in the ICU patient is unknown.

MANAGEMENT

Initial Management

The first and most important step in management of patients with diarrhea regardless of the etiology is correction of fluid and electrolyte imbalances (Fig. 210.1). Careful monitoring of the patient's physical and laboratory parameters will help guide replacement therapy. Most often, free water, sodium, potassium, phosphorus, or magnesium repletion will be required. If fluid losses are particularly severe or the patient's circulatory status is tenuous or compromised, central venous access and monitoring are essential. Physicians and nursing staff should ensure that proper patient hygiene and skin care are maintained. Suspected infectious causes of diarrhea warrant patient isolation and enteric precautions until a diagnosis is made and proper treatment instituted. Infection control is essential to prevent spread of the disease in the unit. Hospital-based infection control programs are needed to help decrease the incidence of CDI. Intensivists should work on reducing the risk of CDI by antibiotic stewardship as much as possible.

Therapy of Iatrogenic Causes

Iatrogenic causes of diarrhea are among the most readily diagnosed and easily treated etiologies. Suspect medications, especially antibiotics, should be withdrawn or changed to those that are less likely to cause diarrhea.

If a diagnosis of *C. difficile* colitis is suspected or made, the offending antibiotic should be discontinued, or if necessary, replaced by agents that are less likely to cause CDI (Table 210.3). By definition, *C. difficile* colitis that is diagnosed in the ICU is considered complicated and should be treated as such. Management of mild-to-moderate disease will not be treated in the current chapter. That meant, if a patient, who is in the ICU, has a strong pretest suspicion for CDI, empiric therapy should be considered regardless of the laboratory testing result, because the negative predictive values are insufficiently high to exclude disease in these patients. The treatment regimen depends on the patients' condition. If they do not have significant abdominal

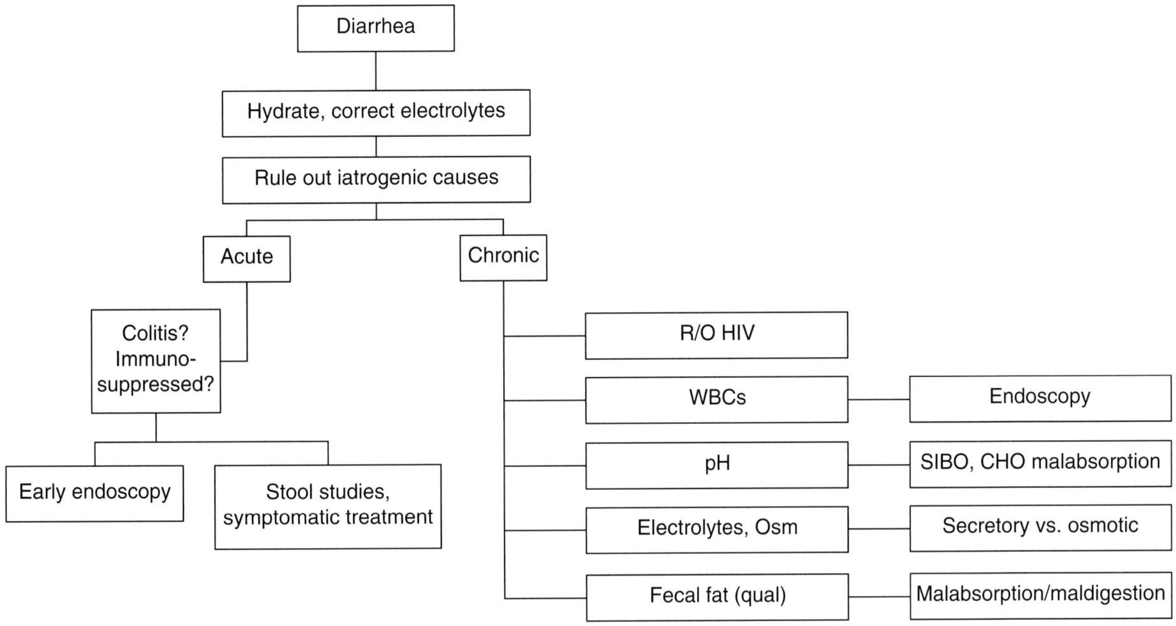

FIGURE 210.1 Algorithm for management of diarrhea in the intensive care unit.

TABLE 210.3

Treatment of *Clostridium difficile* Colitis

General	
	Discontinue offending antibiotic if possible
	Avoid antimotility agents
	Isolation with enteric precautions
Antimicrobial	
	Metronidazole 500 mg PO/IV t.i.d. for 10–14 d
	Vancomycin 125–500 mg PO q.i.d. for 7–14 d

PO, orally; IV, intravenous; t.i.d., three times a day.

distention, they should be treated with vancomycin 125 mg orally four times a day plus metronidazole 500 mg intravenously three times a day. If they have ileus or toxic colon and/or significant abdominal distention, they should be treated with vancomycin 500 mg orally and per rectum four times a day plus metronidazole 500 mg intravenously three times a day. Treatment with PO vancomycin has been a time-honored and highly efficacious therapy, resulting in improvement in more than 95% of patients [56]. Oral route for vancomycin is the preferred route, but in patients in whom oral antibiotics cannot reach a segment of the colon, such as with Hartman pouch, ileostomy, or colon diversion, vancomycin therapy delivered via enema should be added to the oral treatment until the patient improves. Intravenous vancomycin should not be used to treat CDI, because it is not excreted in the stool [57,58]. All patients with complicated CDI should get a CT scan of the abdomen/pelvis and a surgical consult. Surgical therapy should be considered in patients who have a complicated and severe CDI or failed to improve on medical therapy after 5 days. Antiperistaltic agents should be limited or avoided in patients with confirmed or even suspected CDI. Oral or enteral feeding should be continued in the absence of ileus or abdominal distention. Relapse rates may be high, occurring in as many as 24% of patients [59]. There is moderate evidence that two probiotics (*Lactobacillus rhamnosus* GG and *Saccharomyces boulardii*) can decrease the incidence of antibiotic-associated diarrhea, but there is insufficient evidence that they prevent CDI [12].

Data are now emerging that exposure to PPIs is associated with increased odds of CDI in hospitalized patients. The postulate that acid suppression causes enteric infections seems reasonable but remains controversial. These data are observational and, thus, may be subject to uncontrolled confounding. Nonetheless, it is prudent to review the indication for PPI prescription in all patients and restrict use of these drugs appropriately [60].

Antimotility agents should not be used in colitis, because they may lengthen the course of illness and may precipitate toxic megacolon [61]. If the patient with *C. difficile* colitis develops peritoneal signs, bacteremia unresponsive to antibiotics, progressive fever, rigors, or radiologic evidence of significant pericolonic inflammation with increasing bowel wall edema, then surgical intervention is indicated [62]. The recommended procedure is subtotal colectomy with ileostomy, with possible ileorectal anastomosis after the inflammation has subsided.

There are several controlled trials now available which demonstrate the effectiveness of octreotide in chemotherapy and radiation-associated acute diarrhea. In these studies, doses range of 100 to 500 μg is given subcutaneously twice or three times daily. Budesonide is not helpful in these settings [63].

Enteral feedings suspected of causing diarrhea should be reduced in volume, given by continuous infusion or temporarily discontinued. Lactose-free feeds should be used, because the high incidence of stress-induced GI mucosal injury in the ICU population affects loss of disaccharidase activity. Fiber-containing formulas or fiber added to standard formulas may benefit ICU patients with tube feeding-associated diarrhea [64,65]. Elemental diet supplements may also be considered in patients with short bowel syndrome, pancreatic insufficiency, radiation enteritis, fistula, and inflammatory bowel disease. Their major disadvantages are high cost and increased osmolarity [66].

Treatment of Diarrhea Related to Disease

Efforts should always be made to treat the underlying disease-causing diarrhea for the critically ill patient, although such efforts may or may not improve the diarrhea. Diarrhea secondary to sepsis will typically resolve, because the source of sepsis is treated, whereas diarrhea secondary to diabetes or uremia may not improve despite treatment of the primary disease.

Diarrhea-causing pathogens should, in general, be treated. The detection of *Blastocystis hominis* by parasite exams may indicate coinfection with other pathogens, and empiric nitazoxanide or metronidazole may be beneficial [67]. Infections in patients with AIDS and other immunocompromised settings are treatable with currently available therapy [68,69].

Patients with ischemic colitis without transmural necrosis may be managed with supportive care. Drugs that exacerbate ischemia should be discontinued if possible. Aggressive efforts at maintaining circulatory blood volume and maximizing oxygen delivery should be emphasized. Signs of infarction or perforation warrant operative management.

Fistulas should be managed by bowel rest or surgery depending on the clinical circumstances. Postcholecystectomy diarrhea may respond to bile acid sequestrants, such as cholestyramine. Surgically induced cases of short bowel syndrome or malabsorption may be aided by enteral nutrition in the form of elemental diets or, if unsuccessful, parenteral nutrition. Fecal impactions should be removed by manual disimpaction followed by cleansing enemas consisting of tap water, sodium phosphate, or diatrizoate (water-soluble contrast) enemas. More proximal and firm impactions can be broken up using a sigmoidoscope and an irrigating device by directing a water jet into the fecal mass under direct vision. Prevention following treatment with appropriate laxatives or enemas is paramount.

Treatment of Diarrhea as a Primary Manifestation of Disease

Every effort should be made to treat the disease responsible for the diarrheal syndrome. General supportive measures previously discussed should also be employed in all patients. Diseases such as vasculitis should be managed with corticosteroid or immunosuppressive therapy. Adrenal insufficiency will respond promptly to the administration of corticosteroids. Hyperthyroid patients should receive appropriate therapies. GVHD should be managed with corticosteroids and immunosuppressive agents. The chronic form of the disease may be more effectively treated, whereas the acute variety may be less responsive, with a substantial mortality rate. Treatment of the inflammatory bowel diseases is addressed in Chapter 211, but generally includes aminosalicylates, corticosteroids, immunomodulating agents, biologics, and surgery. Celiac sprue will respond to supportive measures and a gluten-free diet.

Palliative Measures

The aforementioned diagnostic and therapeutic approaches will result in proper diagnosis and directed treatment in a majority of patients with diarrhea in the critical care setting. In a modest number of patients, however, a cause for diarrhea will not be

TABLE 210.4

Antidiarrheal Agents and Dosages

Loperamide (Imodium)
- Available forms: capsules (2 mg) and liquid (5 mL [1 tsp] = 1 mg)
- Dosage: 4 mg initially, followed by 2 mg after each diarrheal stool
- Maximum daily recommended dose: 16 mg/d

Diphenoxylate with atropine (Lomotil)
- Available forms: 1 tablet or 5 mL liquid = 2.5 mg diphenoxylate and 0.025 atropine
- Dosage: 2 tablets or 10 mL four times a day (20 mg of diphenoxylate) initially, then decrease and titrate to symptoms
- Maximum daily recommended dose: 20 mg/d (based on diphenoxylate)

Deodorized opium tincture
- Available form: 10 mg morphine per mL
- Dosage: 0.6 mL four times a day (range: 0.3–1 mL 4–6 times a day)
- Maximum daily recommended dose: 6 mL/d

Camphorated opium tincture (paregoric)
- Available form: 0.4 mg morphine per mL
- Dosage: 5–10 mL 1–4 times a day
- Maximum daily recommended dose: 40 mL/d

tsp, teaspoon.

found or a specific treatment will not be readily available. For this category of patients, palliative therapies are available with the goal to decrease fluid losses, patient discomfort, and morbidity (Table 210.4). Antimotility agents such as loperamide, diphenoxylate with atropine, and deodorized tincture of opium (DTO) may decrease frequency and severity of diarrhea in patients with diarrhea of unclear etiology or diarrhea because of enteral feeding or other noninfectious causes. Advantages of loperamide include the absence of central nervous system activity and resultant side effects, whereas DTO is administered in drop form, enhancing dosing flexibility. Octreotide can be used for palliation of diarrhea in patients with AIDS, GVHD, hormone-producing tumors, radiation- and chemotherapy-induced diarrhea, and other causes of secretory diarrhea [70].

CONCLUSION

Diarrhea is a frequently occurring complication in the ICU setting. It is a symptom that tends to be overshadowed by other processes in the ICU, but in and of itself may result in significant morbidity. In most instances, it can be managed following institution of proper diagnostic, therapeutic, or palliative measures.

References

1. Kelly T, Patrick M, Hillman K, et al: Study of diarrhea in critically ill patients. *Crit Care Med* 11:7, 1983.
2. Hwang TL, Lue MC, Nee YJ, et al: The incidence of diarrhea in patients with hypoalbuminemia due to acute or chronic malnutrition during enteral feeding. *Am J Gastroenterol* 89:376, 1994.
3. Dark D, Pingleton S: Nonhemorrhagic gastrointestinal complications in acute respiratory failure. *Crit Care Med* 17:755, 1989.
4. Fine KD, Schiller L: AGA technical review on the evaluation and management of chronic diarrhea. *Gastroenterology* 116:1464, 1999.
5. McFarland LV: Diarrhea acquired in the hospital. *Gastroenterol Clin North Am* 22:563, 1993.
6. Gilbert DN: Aspects of the safety profile of oral antimicrobial agents. *Infect Dis Clin Pract* 4[Suppl 2]:S103, 1995.
7. Dublerke ER, Reshe KA, Yan Y, et al: *Clostridium difficile* associated disease in a setting of endemicity: identification of novel risk factors. *Clin Infect Disease* 45:1543–1549, 2007.
8. Lialios A, Oropello JM, Benjamin E: Gastrointestinal complications in the intensive care unit. *Clin Chest Med* 20:329–345, 1999.
9. Brown E, Talbot G, Axelrod P, et al: Risk factors for *Clostridium difficile* toxin-associated diarrhea. *Infect Control Hosp Epidemiol* 11:283, 1990.
10. Zilberberg MD: *Clostridium difficile*–related hospitalization among US adults, 2006. *Emerg Infect Dis* 15:122–124, 2009.
11. Voth DE, Ballard JD: *Clostridium difficile* toxins: mechanism of action and role in disease. *Clin Microbiol Rev* 18:247–263, 2005.
12. Surawicz C, Brandt L, Binion DG, et al: Guidelines for diagnosis, treatment, and prevention of *Clostridium difficile* infections. *Am J Gastroenterol* 108:478–498, 2013.
13. Edes T, Walk B, Austin J: Diarrhea in tube fed patients: feeding formula not necessarily the cause. *Am J Med* 88:91, 1990.
14. Martin R, Dunn N, Freemantle S, et al: The rates of common adverse events reported during treatment with proton pump inhibitors used in general practice in England. *Br J Clin Pharmacol* 50:366, 2000.
15. Maes B, Hadaya K, de Moor B, et al: Severe diarrhea in renal transplant patients: results of the DIDACT study. *Am J Transplant* 6:1466, 2006.
16. Reijers M, Weigel H, Hart A, et al: Toxicity and drug exposure in a quadruple drug regimen in HIV-1 infected patients participating in the ADAM study. *AIDS* 14:59, 2000.
17. Isto E, VanDyke M, Gimble C, et al: Withdrawal symptoms in critically ill children after long-term administration of sedatives and/or analgesics: a first evaluation. *Crit Care Med* 36:2427–2432, 2008.
18. Keohane P, Attrill H, Love M, et al: Relation between osmolality of diet and gastrointestinal side effects in enteral nutrition. *Br Med J* 288:678, 1984.
19. Cataldi-Betcher E, Seltzer M, Slocum B, et al: Complications occurring during enteral nutritional support: a prospective study. *JPEN J Parenter Enteral Nutr* 7:546, 1983.
20. Keohane P, Attrill H, Jones B, et al: Roles of lactose and *Clostridium difficile* in the pathogenesis of enteral feeding associated diarrhoea. *Clin Nutr* 1:259, 1983.
21. McHugh P, Moran T: Calories and gastric emptying: a regulatory capacity with implications for feeding. *Am J Physiol* 236:254, 1979.
22. Montejo J: Enteral nutrition-relation gastrointestinal complications in critically ill patients: a multicenter study. *Crit Care Med* 27:1447, 1999.
23. Ford E, Jennings L, Andrassy RJ: Serum albumin (oncotic pressure) correlates with enteral feeding tolerance in the pediatric surgical patient. *J Pediatr Surg* 22:7, 1987.
24. Raimundo A, Rogers J, Grimble G, et al: Colonic inflow and small bowel motility during intraduodenal enteral nutrition. *Gut* 29:A1469, 1988.
25. Raimundo A, Rogers J, Silk D: Is enteral feeding related to diarrhoea initiated by an abnormal colonic response to intragastric diet infusion? [abstract] *Gut* 31:A1195, 1990.
26. Bowling T, Raimundo A, Grimble G, et al: Colonic secretory effect in response to enteral feeding in man. *Gut* 35:1734, 1994.
27. Bowling T, Silk D: Colonic responses to enteral tube feeding. *Gut* 42:147, 1998.
28. Starnes H, Moore F, Mentzer S, et al: Abdominal pain in neutropenic cancer patients. *Cancer* 57:616, 1986.
29. Longworth DL, Weller PF: Hyperinfection syndrome with strongyloidiasis. *Curr Clin Top Infect Dis* 7:1–26, 1986.
30. Rodgers V, Kagnoff M: Gastrointestinal manifestations of the acquired immunodeficiency syndrome. *West J Med* 146:57, 1987.
31. Santangelo W, Krejs G: Southwestern Internal Medicine Conference. The gastrointestinal manifestations of the acquired immunodeficiency syndrome. *Am J Med Sci* 292:328, 1986.
32. Baker R, Peppercorn M: Gastrointestinal ailments of homosexual men. *Medicine (Baltimore)* 61:390, 1982.
33. Flanigan T, Whalen C, Turner J, et al: Cryptosporidium infection and CD4 counts. *Ann Intern Med* 116:840, 1992.
34. Asmuth D, DeGirolami P, Federman M, et al: Clinical features of microsporidiosis in patients with AIDS. *Clin Infect Dis* 18:819, 1994.

35. Horsburgh CJ: *Mycobacterium avium* complex infection in the acquired immunodeficiency syndrome. *N Engl J Med* 324:1332, 1991.
36. Durrer P, Zbinden R, Fleisch F, et al: Intestinal infection due to enteroaggregative *Escherichia coli* among human immunodeficiency virus-infected persons. *J Infect Dis* 182:1540, 2000.
37. Wanke C, Mayer H, Weber R, et al: Enteroaggregative *Escherichia coli* as a potential cause of diarrheal disease in adults infected with human immunodeficiency virus. *J Infect Dis* 178:185, 1998.
38. Gallant J, Moore R, Richman D, et al: Incidence and natural history of cytomegalovirus disease in patients with advanced human immunodeficiency virus disease treated with zidovudine. *J Infect Dis* 166:1223, 1992.
39. Weber J, Carmichael D, Boylston A, et al: Kaposi's sarcoma of the bowel presenting as apparent ulcerative colitis. *Gut* 26:295, 1985.
40. Ernst C, Hagihara P, Daugherty M, et al: Ischemic colitis incidence following aortic reconstruction: a prospective study. *Surgery* 80:417, 1976.
41. Sotiriadis J, Brandt LJ: Ischemic colitis has a worse prognosis when isolated to the right side of the colon. *Am J Gastroenterol* 102:2247, 2007.
42. Mueller P, Benowitz N: Toxicologic causes of acute abdominal disorders. *Emerg Med Clin North Am* 7:667, 1989.
43. Chang E, Bergenstal R, Field M: Diarrhea in streptozocin treated rats. *J Clin Invest* 75:1666, 1985.
44. Whalen G, Soergel K, Geenen J: Diabetic diarrhea. *Gastroenterology* 56:1021, 1969.
45. Ryan J, Sleisenger M: Effects of systemic and extraintestinal disease on the gut, in Slesenger M, Fordtran J (eds): *Gastrointestinal Disease*. Philadelphia, PA, WB Saunders, 1993, p 193.
46. McDonald G, Shulman H, Sullivan K, et al: Intestinal and hepatic complications of human bone marrow transplantation. Part I. *Gastroenterology* 90:460, 1986.
47. McDonald G, Shulman H, Sullivan K, et al: Intestinal and hepatic complications of human bone marrow transplantation. Part II. *Gastroenterology* 90:770, 1986.
48. Flowers ME, Kansu E, Sullivan KM: Pathophysiology and treatment of graft-versus-host disease. *Hematol Oncol Clin North Am* 13:1091, 1999.
49. Siegel D, Edelstein P, Nachamkin I: Inappropriate testing of diarrheal diseases in the hospital. *JAMA* 263:979, 1990.
50. Fine K, Krejs G, Fordtran J: Infectious diarrhea, in Sleisenger M, Fordtran J (eds): *Gastrointestinal Disease*. Philadelphia, PA, WB Saunders, 1993, p 1128.
51. Shastri YM, Bergis D, Povse N, et al: Prospective multicenter study evaluating fecal calprotectin in adult acute bacterial diarrhea. *Am J Med* 121:1099, 2008.
52. Debast SB, van Kregten E, Oskam KM, et al: Effect on diagnostic yield of repeated stool testing during outbreaks of *Clostridium difficile*—associated disease. *Clin Microbiol Infect* 14:622–624, 2008.
53. Deshpande A, Pasupuleti V, Pant C, et al: Potential value of repeat stool testing for *Clostridium difficile* stool toxin using enzyme immunoassay? *Curr Med Res Opin* 26: 2635–2641, 2010.
54. Luo RF, Banaei N: Is repeat PCR needed for diagnosis of *Clostridium difficile* infection? *J Clin Microbiol* 48:3738–3741, 2010.
55. May A, Manner H, Schneider M, et al: Prospective multicenter trial of capsule endoscopy in patients with chronic abdominal pain, diarrhea and other signs and symptoms (CEDAP-Plus Study). *Endoscopy* 39:606, 2007.
56. Bartlett J: Treatment of *Clostridium difficile* colitis. *Gastroenterology* 89:1192, 1985.
57. Bolton R, Culshaw M: Faecal metronidazole concentrations during oral and intravenous therapy for antibiotic associated colitis due to *Clostridium difficile*. *Gut* 27:1169, 1986.
58. Friedenberg F, Fernandez A, Kaul V, et al: Intravenous metronidazole for the treatment of *Clostridium difficile* colitis. *Dis Colon Rectum* 44:1176, 2001.
59. Bartlett J, Tedesco F, Schull S, et al: Relapse following oral vancomycin therapy of antibiotic-associated pseudomembranous colitis. *Gastroenterology* 78:431, 1979.
60. Dial MS: Proton pump inhibitor use and enteric infections. *Am J Gastroenterol* 104:S10, 2007.
61. Rubin M, Bodenstein L, Kent C: Severe *Clostridium difficile* colitis. *Dis Colon Rectum* 38:350, 1995.
62. Lipsett P, Samantaray D, Tam M, et al: Pseudomembranous colitis: a surgical disease. *Surgery* 116:491, 1994.
63. Karthaus M, Ballo H, Abenhardt W, et al: Prospective, double-blind, placebo-controlled, multicenter, randomized phase III study with orally administered budesonide for prevention of irinotecan (CPT-11)-induced diarrhea in patients with advanced colorectal cancer. *Oncology* 68:326, 2005.
64. Shimoni Z, Averbuch Y: The addition of fiber and the use of continuous infusion decrease the incidence of diarrhea in elderly tube-fed patients in medical wards of a general regional hospital: a controlled clinical trial. *J Clin Gastroenterol* 41:901, 2007.
65. Rushdi TA, Pichard C, Khater YH: Control of diarrhea by fiber-enriched diet in ICU patients on enteral nutrition: a prospective randomized controlled trial. *Clin Nutr* 23:1344, 2004.
66. Randall H: Enteral nutrition: tube feeding in acute and chronic illness. *J Parenter Enteral Nutr* 8:113, 1984.
67. Rossignol JF, Kabil SM, Said M, et al: Effect of nitazoxanide in persistent diarrhea and enteritis associated with *Blastocystis hominis*. *Clin Gastroenterol Hepatol* 3:987, 2005.
68. Gilbert DN, Moellering RC, Eliopoulos G, et al: *The Sanford Guide to Antimicrobial Therapy 2009*. Sperryville, VA, Antimicrobial Therapy, 2009.
69. Bartlett J: *The Johns Hopkins Hospital 2004 Guide to Medical Care of Patients with HIV Infection*. Philadelphia, PA, Williams & Wilkins, 2004.
70. Gorden P, Comi R, Maton P, et al: Somatostatin and somatostatin analogue (SMS201995) in treatment of hormone-secreting tumors of the pituitary and gastrointestinal tract and non-neoplastic diseases of the gut. *Ann Intern Med* 110:35, 1989.

Chapter 211 ■ Fulminant Colitis and Toxic Megacolon

EMANUELLE A. BELLAGUARDA • STEPHEN B. HANAUER

Ulcerative colitis is characterized by a diffuse, continuous inflammatory process usually limited to the superficial mucosa of the colon. *Fulminant colitis* implies progression of mucosal inflammation into deeper (muscular) layers of the colon wall. It generally is associated with severe bloody diarrhea, fever, tachycardia, and abdominal tenderness. Systemic manifestations result from transmural colitis, which may also produce circular muscle paralysis precipitating dilatation. *Toxic megacolon* refers to acute dilatation of the colon, generally as a complication of ulcerative colitis, but it may occur with any severe inflammatory colitis. Toxic megacolon has been described with inflammatory bowel disease (Crohn disease and ulcerative colitis), and infectious colitis, including amebic colitis, pseudomembranous colitis, and other infections [1]. Two to 8% of patients with *Clostridium difficile* infection will progress to fulminant colitis carrying a mortality rate ranging between 13% and 80% [2]. Toxic megacolon has been reported to complicate from 1% to 10% of all ulcerative colitis cases and from 2% to 3% of Crohn colitis cases [1]. Although mortality from early series was as high as 25% (reaching 50% if colonic perforation occurred), early recognition and management of toxic megacolon have substantially lowered mortality to below 15% [3] and usually below 2% at experienced centers [4]. Factors associated with increased mortality include age older than 40 years, the presence of colonic perforation, and delay of surgery [3,4]. Colonic perforation, whether free or localized, is the greatest risk factor leading to increased morbidity or death.

PREDISPOSING FACTORS

The severity of disease activity is the most important predictor of toxic megacolon, which is more common for extensive colitis than for proctitis or proctosigmoiditis [5]. Limited right- or left-sided segmental colitis also has been associated with toxic megacolon. Concomitant *C. difficile* infection often occurs in hospitalized patients with inflammatory bowel disease and can be associated with refractory disease [6,7]. Similarly, cytomegalovirus (CMV) infections frequently complicate severe colitis with a reported prevalence rate of 4.5% to 16.6% in the setting of immune suppression with corticosteroids or cyclosporine, with a prevalence rate as high as 25% in patients requiring colectomy [8,9]. Treatment of CMV with ganciclovir is controversial; however recent data have shown improved surgery-free outcomes after CMV therapy particularly in patients with a high-grade CMV density on colonic biopsies, defined as 5 or more CMV nuclear inclusions [10].

Toxic megacolon typically occurs early in the course of ulcerative colitis, usually within the first 5 years of disease, and 30% of cases present within 3 months of diagnosis of the initial attack [11]. The onset of toxic megacolon has also been linked to patients who have recently undergone diagnostic examinations, such as barium enemas or colonoscopy, suggesting that manipulation of the inflamed bowel or vigorous laxative preparation may exacerbate the process, possibly through electrolyte imbalance (Table 211.1) [3,12].

Certain drug therapies have been implicated for the development of toxic megacolon. Diphenoxylate hydrochloride/atropine sulfate (Lomotil), loperamide, and other inhibitors of colonic motility such as narcotics may contribute to the development of toxic megacolon by inhibiting colon muscle function for severe transmural disease [11].

Despite early speculations on the role of corticosteroids in inducing toxic megacolon, most experienced clinicians do not accept the implication that corticosteroids or adrenocorticotropic hormone are precipitating factors [1,13]. Concern remains, however, that corticosteroids may suppress signs of perforation, thereby delaying surgical therapy [11].

C. difficile infection can progress to fulminant colitis in and of itself, and a WBC > 20,000 μL or <2,000 μL, elderly >70 years, cardiorespiratory failure, or diffuse abdominal tenderness are predictors of worse outcomes and progression to fulminant colitis [2].

CLINICAL FEATURES

Toxic megacolon usually occurs on the background of chronic inflammatory bowel disease [1,11,13]. The presentation typically evolves with progressive diarrhea, bloody stool, and cramping abdominal pain. Occasionally, patients treated for inflammatory bowel disease over long periods of time have a paradoxical decrease in stool frequency with passage of only bloody discharge or bloody membranes; this can be an ominous sign (Table 211.2). Thereafter, clinical signs of toxemia, including pyrexia (temperature > 101.5°F), tachycardia (heart rate > 120 beats per minute), leukocytosis (total white blood cell count > 10,500 cells per μL), and anemia develop. The abdominal pain and distention become progressive and bowel sounds diminish or cease. Signs of peritoneal irritation, including rebound tenderness and abdominal guarding represent transmural inflammation to the serosa, even in the absence of free perforation. Conversely, peritoneal signs may be minimal or absent in elderly patients or those receiving high-dose prolonged corticosteroid therapy or narcotics for pain control. In such patients, loss of hepatic dullness may be the first clinical indication of colonic perforation.

TABLE 211.1

Potential Precipitants of Toxic Megacolon

- Concurrent pathogens (*Clostridium difficile*, CMV)
- Narcotics
- Anticholinergics
- Antidiarrheal agents (diphenoxylate with atropine, loperamide, opiates)
- Barium enema
- Colonoscopy

CMV, cytomegalovirus.

TABLE 211.2

Clinical Features of Toxic Megacolon

Symptoms and signs
- Increased diarrhea and bleeding
- Fever > 101.5°F
- Abdominal distention
- Decreased or absent bowel sounds
- Peritoneal signs (potentially masked by corticosteroids)
- Hemodynamic instability
- Mental status changes

Imaging findings
- X-ray:
  - Progressive segmental or pancolonic dilatation (may not correlate with physical findings)
  - Pneumocystoides intestinalis
- Abdominal CT:
  - Segmental thinning of the colonic wall
  - Nodular pseudopolyposis
- Endoscopic findings:
  - Extensive ulceration with friable and bleeding mucosa
  - Deep ulcerations

Laboratory test findings
- White blood cell count > 10,000/μL, with pronounced left shift
- Anemia (may not be reflected in initial measurement if dehydrated)
- Hypernatremia (if dehydrated)
- Hypokalemia
- Metabolic alkalosis (diarrhea)/acidosis (sepsis)
- Hypomagnesemia
- Hypophosphatemia
- Hypoalbuminemia

Mental status changes, including confusion, agitation, and apathy, occasionally are noted. Leukocytosis with a left shift generally is present. Anemia, hypokalemia, and hypoalbuminemia are common. The presence of anemia, requirement for transfusion, hypoalbuminemia, malnutrition, and prolonged hospitalization are poor prognostic factors [14–17].

Plain films of the abdomen usually are sufficient radiographic studies, revealing loss of haustration with segmental or total colonic dilatation. Clinical studies have demonstrated a strong correlation between colonic dilatation and deep ulceration involving the muscle layers [18]. The magnitude of dilatation may not be severe, averaging 8 to 9 cm (normal is <5 to 6 cm), although colonic diameter may reach 15 cm before rupture. Maximal dilatation can occur in any part of the colon. Accompanying mucosal thumbprinting or pneumatosis cystoides coli reflect severe transmural disease. Free peritoneal air should serve as an immediate indication for surgery [3]. Infrequently, retroperitoneal tracking of air from a colonic perforation may produce subcutaneous emphysema and pneumomediastinum without pneumoperitoneum. In patients with severe colitis, small bowel ileus may herald toxic megacolon and is a bad prognostic sign for successful medical management. Discrepancies may exist between physical and radiographic findings. Abdominal distention by physical examination can be minimal despite massive colonic dilatation. Conversely, physical findings may dominate the presentation, and peritoneal signs in the absence of free air or dilatation should not be ignored. Computed tomography scans can demonstrate segmental thinning of the colonic wall, nodular pseudopolyposis and air-filled colonic distention over 6 cm or evidence of perforation or abscess [1,19].

Early flexible sigmoidoscopy within the first 48 hours should be performed by an experienced endoscopist to assess severity of disease and obtain biopsies for CMV infection [11,13]. Endoscopic examination generally shows extensive ulceration with friable, bleeding mucosa. In rare instances, however, such as with rectal enema therapy or Crohn disease, the rectum may be normal [20]. More extensive endoscopic examinations, although controversial, generally are contraindicated. If performed, the presence of severe colitis (deep penetrating ulcers) in conjunction with clinical features of severe disease is a poor prognostic sign [18]. Similarly, the presence of extensive and deep ulcerations is a poor prognostic marker of Crohn disease [20].

MANAGEMENT

Few medical emergencies require as close cooperation between medical and surgical personnel as fulminant colitis and toxic megacolon [1,13]. A team approach with early management and continuous assessment is vital not only to determine whether surgery is indicated, but also to support the critically ill patient preoperatively and postoperatively. Early recognition and institution of therapy by an experienced team can alter the outcome of this life-threatening illness (Table 211.3).

Medical Treatment

Despite the fact that "bowel rest" is ineffective as primary therapy for severe colitis, oral intake of fluids should be discontinued in fulminant colitis or once colonic dilatation is recognized due to a possible imminent surgical procedure [1,11,13]. Total parenteral nutrition should be considered for patients at risk for malnutrition. A nasogastric tube is indicated for patients with associated small bowel ileus; however, it is not helpful for colonic decompression [11,13]. Rolling the less toxic patient from front to back may redistribute colonic air and assist in decompression. Rarely, patients who have been made "nothing by mouth" with colonic dilatation *in the absence of toxic signs or symptoms* may benefit from resumption of oral feeding. Anticholinergic and narcotic agents should be discontinued [11,13]. Venous thromboembolism prophylaxis, preferably heparin or low-molecular weight heparin, should also be initiated in all patients hospitalized with severe or fulminant colitis. In ulcerative colitis, studies have shown a sixfold increased risk for thromboembolic events in hospitalized patients when compared to patients treated in the outpatient setting [21–23]. Resuscitative measures, including vigorous fluid, electrolyte, and blood replacement, are paramount. Extracellular fluid loss may be severe and, when combined with a low oncotic pressure from hypoalbuminemia, the hemodynamic state often is unstable. The goal of fluid replacement should be to restore previous losses and continue replenishing ongoing losses from diarrhea, fever, and third spacing of fluids. Transfusion of packed red blood cells should be instituted to maintain the serum hematocrit above 30%. Although severe hypokalemia may not be present, total body potassium depletion is common, and resuscitative measures should include adequate potassium replacement. Phosphate, calcium, and magnesium depletion should be corrected parenterally.

Aminosalicylates, a mainstay of maintenance therapy and the treatment of mild-to-moderate disease, have no role in the treatment of fulminant colitis or toxic megacolon. Their activity, limited to superficial inflammation, is insufficient to abort or control the transmural disease, while the potential adverse effects (e.g., nausea, vomiting, or worsening colitis) may confuse the clinical picture [24]. They should be withheld until the patient has recovered and resumed a normal diet.

Despite the absence of data, most experienced centers continue to administer broad-spectrum antibiotics in the setting of toxic megacolon. Antibiotics with adequate Gram-negative and anaerobic coverage are usually administered without delay once transmural inflammation or toxic megacolon is suspected [11,24]. Antibiotics are continued until the patient stabilizes over several days to a week, or through the initial postoperative period. Nonetheless, the ultimate benefits (or risks) have not been adequately determined.

Corticosteroids have long been used for the management of ulcerative colitis as well as in Crohn colitis. In general, parenteral corticosteroids are essential for patients with toxic megacolon, and most patients are likely to be receiving the drugs before toxic megacolon develops [13]. Augmented doses of corticosteroids should be administered in view of the additional stress of the toxic state. There is no general agreement regarding which corticosteroid preparation or dose should be given. Hydrocortisone, 100 mg every 6 hours, and methylprednisolone, 20 to 30 mg every 12 hours, also are available for intravenous (IV) administration. A continuous infusion of corticosteroids may be beneficial to maintain steady plasma levels; however, a study comparing bolus regimen to continuous steroid infusion found similar rates of clinical remission and colectomy at 1 year [13]. Patients who fail to respond with a reduction in bowel movements, cessation of transfusion requirements, and improvement of C-reactive protein by day 3 are unlikely to respond and rescue therapies should be considered [13,25,26]. Additional tests in anticipation of rescue therapies should be performed early during hospitalization. Tuberculosis exposure should be assessed with a tuberculin skin test or interferon-γ release assay and a chest X-ray. Testing for hepatitis B should be done with hepatitis B surface antigen, hepatitis B core antibody, and surface antibody to screen for immunity in case anti-TNF biologic agents are considered.

Cyclosporine, a calcineurin inhibitor, was the first rescue therapy used to treated severe refractory ulcerative colitis [13]. A small randomized pilot trial showed that cyclosporine given at a dose of 4 mg/kg/d is also an effective single therapy (without steroids) to induce clinical remission for severe ulcerative colitis patients [27]. A trial comparing 2 mg/kg/d with 4 mg/kg/d of cyclosporine in conjunction with corticosteroids for severe colitis demonstrated that the lower dose was equally efficacious with less adverse effects [28]. Our center routinely adjusts the cyclosporine dose based upon serum levels checked 48 hours after initiation of therapy. Total daily dose should be adjusted to achieve a therapeutic level within the range of 250 to 400 mcg per L. Patients who are started on cyclosporine

TABLE 211.3

Management of Toxic Megacolon

Team approach toward management, including medical and surgical personnel
Resuscitation and stabilization—electrolyte and fluid repletion, central venous pressure measurements, blood transfusions to maintain hematocrit greater than 30%, broad-spectrum antibiotics, administration of intravenous corticosteroids (e.g., methylprednisolone, 40–60 mg/d, and hydrocortisone, 400 mg/d)
Evaluate status—abdominal examination every 6 h, radiographs of abdomen every 12–24 h
Surgical intervention required for clinical deterioration at any time, failure of medical management to improve status within 48 h, evidence of perforation, shock, persistent hemorrhage
Consider cyclosporine or infliximab for nontoxic patients without response to intravenous corticosteroids by day 3

should be closely monitored for hypertension, tremors, seizures, opportunistic infections, nephrotoxicity, hypocalcemia, and hypomagnesemia. Individuals with hypocholesterolemia (total <120 mg per dL) or hypomagnesemia (<1.5 mg per dL) have a higher risk of seizures, and the initial cyclosporine dose should be reduced [13]. The role of cyclosporine for toxic megacolon remains controversial [29]. Patients who respond to IV cyclosporine should be transitioned to oral cyclosporine at 5 mg/kg/d and azathioprine should be started concomitantly. Patients will undergo a cyclosporine taper over 3 to 6 months, and should be maintained on trimethoprim–sulfamethoxazole for opportunistic infections prophylaxis during this time periods. There are scant data regarding the long-term outlook after cyclosporine therapy for fulminant or severe colitis, however patients who respond and are maintained on azathioprine have improved long-term outcomes [30].

The biologic chimeric antitumor necrosis factor monoclonal antibody, infliximab, has been used to treat moderate to severely active UC [13]. Formal studies have not been performed in the setting of fulminant colitis or toxic megacolon, although, in the setting of *severe* colitis in hospitalized patients, infliximab may have acute benefits [13]. Recent data has suggested that an accelerated infliximab loading dose regimen with 3 doses given within 24 days significantly decreases the colectomy rate at 3 months when compared to standard loading dose schedule in severe UC patients [31]. This improved response is likely attributed to increased serum levels counter balancing the higher infliximab fecal loss in patients with severe disease [32].

Two recent studies have compared infliximab to cyclosporine in inducing clinical remission in patients with severe ulcerative colitis refractory to IV steroids. Cyclosporine was not more effective than infliximab in inducing clinical remission in this patient population [33,34]. Therefore, both are reasonable first-line options, and the rescue therapy choice should be based on patient's prior medication response, physician's experience and patient's compliance. Current data are reassuring regarding the lack of increased postoperative complications and delay in colectomy for patients on rescue therapies [35]. There is paucity of data regarding the number of rescue therapies one should use in refractory patients, however most tertiary centers agree that surgery should be the treatment of choice should patients fail one rescue therapy by day 7. A summary of the evidence-based medical management approaches for fulminant colitis and toxic megacolon is provided in Table 211.4 and a recently proposed algorithm by Narula et al. is presented in Fig. 211.1.

Resuscitative measures for fulminant infectious colitis resulting in toxic megacolon should be initiated in the same manner as for idiopathic ulcerative colitis. Broad-spectrum antibiotic coverage should be followed by pathogen-specific therapy after the causative organism has been identified. In the setting of severe or fulminant *C. difficile* colitis, oral vancomycin 125 mg four times a day in combination with IV metronidazole 500 mg three times a day is considered the treatment of choice. For patients with an associated ileus or toxic megacolon, the American College of Gastroenterology recommend a higher oral vancomycin dose of 500 mg four times a day in combination with per rectum vancomycin 500 mg in a volume of 500 mL four times a day plus IV metronidazole as described above [7,23]. More recently, fecalmicrobiota transplant has been considered for patients with severe *C. difficile* infection, and some centers have used it with caution in fulminant colitis nonresponsive to standard therapy for 48 hours [36].

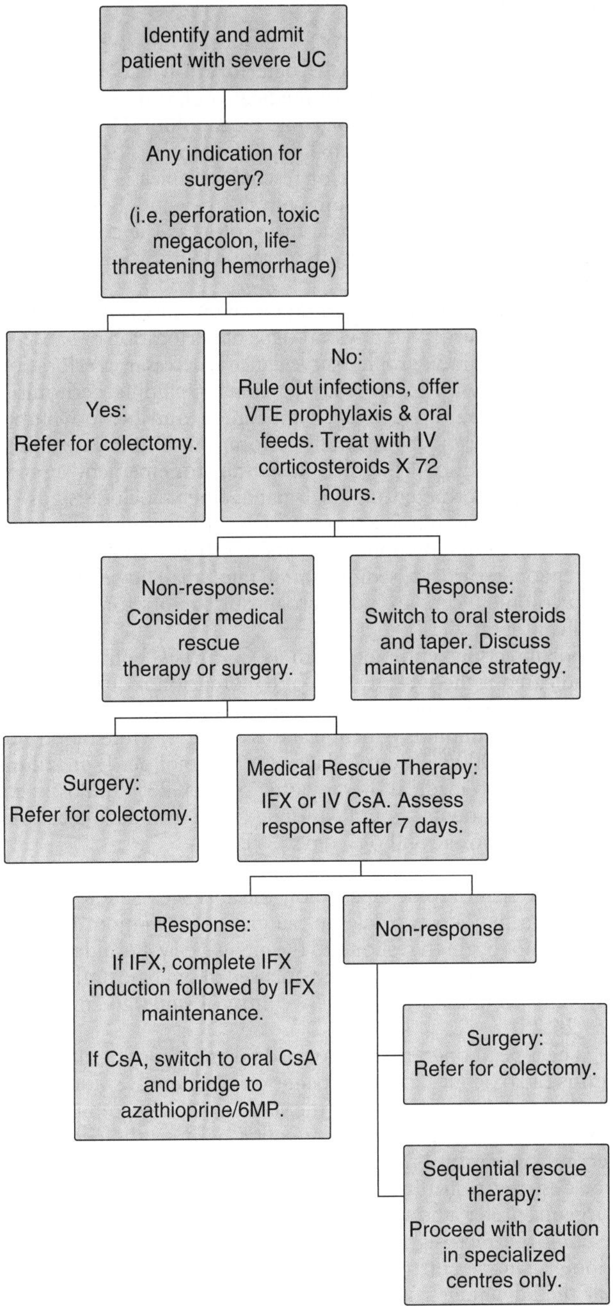

FIGURE 211.1 Proposed algorithm for the treatment of hospitalized patients with severe ulcerative colitis. (From Narula N, Jharap B, Colombel JF: Management of severe ulcerative colitis. *Curr Treat Options Gastroenterol* 13(1):59–76, 2015.)

TABLE 211.4

Evidence-based Therapy of Fulminant Colitis and Toxic Megacolon

Cyclosporine at 4 mg/kg is effective either alone or with corticosteroids to treat severe fulminant ulcerative colitis (toxic megacolon excluded from trials) [27].

Cyclosporine at 2 mg/kg is equally effective as 4 mg/kg in conjunction with corticosteroids in severe ulcerative colitis (toxic megacolon excluded) [28].

Infliximab is effective in moderate-to-severe, refractory ulcerative colitis in the outpatient setting [14]; the role in severe-to-fulminant colitis is less established.

Cyclosporine is not more effective than infliximab in patients with severe ulcerative colitis refractory to intravenous steroids [36].

Surgical Intervention

When no improvement or if deterioration occurs, despite 12 to 24 hours of intensive medical management, surgical intervention is required for toxic megacolon [1]. Failure to substantially improve within 3 days of intensive corticosteroid therapy and within 7 days of rescue therapies is indications for surgery [1,13,25,26]. Some physicians actually view early surgical management of toxic megacolon as the conservative approach, noting that delay of operative therapy may promote higher mortality [15,37].

Evidence of colonic perforation is an unequivocal indication for emergent surgery. If physical signs of perforation are absent, 12- to 24-hour radiographic surveillance is necessary. Perforation is associated with severe complications, including peritonitis, extreme fluid and electrolyte imbalance, and hemodynamic instability. Early recognition of perforation should lessen morbidity or mortality [1]. Other indications for emergent surgery precluding protracted medical management include signs of septic shock and imminent transverse colon rupture (diameter > 12 cm). Hypoalbuminemia, persistently elevated C-reactive protein or erythrocyte sedimentation rate, small bowel ileus, and deep colonic ulcers are poor prognostic factors for successful medical therapy [17].

For infectious etiologies such as *C. difficile* colitis, surgery is indicated if there is any sign of hypotension requiring vasopressor therapy, clinical signs of sepsis and organ dysfunction (renal and pulmonary), mental status changes, white blood cell count > 50,000 cells per L, lactate > 5 mmol per L or failure to improve on medical therapy after 5 days [23,38]. Postoperatively, the patients should continue IV metronidazole or oral vancomycin for a total of 7 days [39].

Although the surgical management of fulminant colitis is similar to that of toxic megacolon, the absence of acute colonic dilatation may permit delay of surgical intervention. Patients who do not begin to respond to the intensive IV steroid regimen should be referred to centers experienced in biologic (infliximab) or cyclosporin therapy in severe colitis, or undergo colectomy [13,24,25].

The type of operation performed for treatment of fulminant colitis or toxic megacolon depends on the clinical status of the patient and the experience of the surgeon [3,4,16]. A one-stage procedure that cures ulcerative colitis without the need for a second operation is appropriate for older patients or those not desiring restorative ileal pouch-anal anastomosis. Most surgeons prefer a limited abdominal colectomy with ileostomy, leaving the rectosigmoid as a mucous fistula or the rectum alone, using a Hartmann procedure [3,13]. This approach has the advantages of limiting the lengthy pelvic dissection in acutely ill patients while allowing for the option of a subsequent restorative, sphincter-saving procedure (ileoanal anastomosis) [40]. In patients with indeterminate colitis or Crohn disease, preservation of the rectum may provide the opportunity for an eventual ileorectal or ileoanal anastomosis to preserve anal continence after temporary diversion and pathologic review of the colectomy specimen.

The surgical management of toxic megacolon must be individualized for each patient. The type of operation selected depends on the clinical condition of the patient and the experience of the surgeon [3,37,41].

References

1. Autenrieth DM, Baumgart DC: Toxic megacolon. *Inflamm Bowel Dis* 18(3):584–591, 2012.
2. van der Wilden GM, Chang Y, Cropano C, et al: Fulminant Clostridium difficile colitis: prospective development of a risk scoring system. *J Trauma Acute Care Surg* 76(2):424–430, 2014.
3. Ausch C, Madoff RD, Gnant M, et al: Aetiology and surgical management of toxic megacolon. *Colorectal Dis* 8(3):195–201, 2006.
4. Jakobovits SL, Travis SP: Management of acute severe colitis. *Br Med Bull* 75–76:131–144, 2005.
5. Farmer RG, Easley KA, Rankin GB: Clinical patterns, natural history, and progression of ulcerative colitis. A long-term follow-up of 1116 patients. *Dig Dis Sci* 38(6):1137–1146, 1993.
6. Regnault H, Bourrier A, Lalande V, et al: Prevalence and risk factors of Clostridium difficile infection in patients hospitalized for flare of inflammatory bowel disease: a retrospective assessment. *Dig Liver Dis* 46(12):1086–1092, 2014.
7. Ananthakrishnan AN, Issa M, Binion DG: Clostridium difficile and inflammatory bowel disease. *Med Clin North Am* 94(1):135–153, 2010.
8. Sager K, Alam S, Bond A, et al: Review article: cytomegalovirus and inflammatory bowel disease. *Aliment Pharmacol Ther* 41(8):725–733, 2015.
9. Kim JJ, Simpson N, Klipfel N, et al: Cytomegalovirus infection in patients with active inflammatory bowel disease. *Dig Dis Sci* 55(4):1059–1065, 2010.
10. Jones A, McCurdy JD, Loftus EV Jr, et al: Effects of antiviral therapy for patients with inflammatory bowel disease and a positive intestinal biopsy for cytomegalovirus. *Clin Gastroenterol Hepatol* 13(5):949–955, 2015.
11. Pola S, Patel D, Ramamoorthy S, et al: Strategies for the care of adults hospitalized for active ulcerative colitis. *Clin Gastroenterol Hepatol* 10(12):1315.e4–1325.e4, 2012.
12. Kumar S, Ghoshal UC, Aggarwal R, et al: Severe ulcerative colitis: prospective study of parameters determining outcome. *J Gastroenterol Hepatol* 19(11):1247–1252, 2004.
13. Narula N, Jharap B, Colombel JF: Management of severe ulcerative colitis. *Curr Treat Options Gastroenterol* 13(1):59–76, 2015.
14. Ananthakrishnan AN, McGinley EL, Binion DG, et al: Simple score to identify colectomy risk in ulcerative colitis hospitalizations. *Inflamm Bowel Dis* 16(9):1532–1540, 2010.
15. Coakley BA, Telem D, Nguyen S, et al: Prolonged preoperative hospitalization correlates with worse outcomes after colectomy for acute fulminant ulcerative colitis. *Surgery* 153(2):242–248, 2013.
16. Ho GT, Mowat C, Goddard CJ, et al: Predicting the outcome of severe ulcerative colitis: development of a novel risk score to aid early selection of patients for second-line medical therapy or surgery. *Aliment Pharmacol Ther* 19(10):1079–1087, 2004.
17. Travis SP: Predicting outcome in severe ulcerative colitis. *Dig Liver Dis* 36(7):448–449, 2004.
18. Carbonnel F, Lavergne A, Lemann M, et al: Colonoscopy of acute colitis. A safe and reliable tool for assessment of severity. *Dig Dis Sci* 39(7):1550–1557, 1994.
19. Moulin V, Dellon P, Laurent O, et al: Toxic megacolon in patients with severe acute colitis: computed tomographic features. *Clin Imaging* 35(6):431–436, 2011.
20. Allez M, Lemann M, Bonnet J, et al: Long term outcome of patients with active Crohn's disease exhibiting extensive and deep ulcerations at colonoscopy. *Am J Gastroenterol* 97(4):947–953, 2002.
21. Grainge MJ, West J, Card TR: Venous thromboembolism during active disease and remission in inflammatory bowel disease: a cohort study. *Lancet* 375(9715):657–663, 2010.
22. Ra G, Thanabalan R, Ratneswaran S, et al: Predictors and safety of venous thromboembolism prophylaxis among hospitalized inflammatory bowel disease patients. *J Crohns Colitis* 7(10):e479–e485, 2013.
23. Surawicz CM, Brandt LJ, Binion DG, et al: Guidelines for diagnosis, treatment, and prevention of Clostridium difficile infections. *Am J Gastroenterol* 108(4):478–498, 2013; quiz 99.
24. Kornbluth A, Sachar DB, Practice Parameters Committee of the American College of Gastroenterology. Ulcerative colitis practice guidelines in adults: American College Of Gastroenterology, Practice Parameters Committee. *Am J Gastroenterol* 105(3):501–523, 2010; quiz 24.
25. Travis SP: Review article: the management of mild to severe acute ulcerative colitis. *Aliment Pharmacol Ther* 20 Suppl 4:88–92, 2004.
26. Travis SP, Farrant JM, Ricketts C, et al: Predicting outcome in severe ulcerative colitis. *Gut* 38(6):905–910, 1996.
27. D'Haens G, Lemmens L, Geboes K, et al: Intravenous cyclosporine versus intravenous corticosteroids as single therapy for severe attacks of ulcerative colitis. *Gastroenterology* 120(6):1323–1329, 2001.
28. Van Assche G, D'Haens G, Noman M, et al: Randomized, double-blind comparison of 4 mg/kg versus 2 mg/kg intravenous cyclosporine in severe ulcerative colitis. *Gastroenterology* 125(4):1025–1031, 2003.
29. Garcia-Lopez S, Gomollon-Garcia F, Perez-Gisbert J: Cyclosporine in the treatment of severe attack of ulcerative colitis: a systematic review. *Gastroenterol Hepatol* 28(10):607–614, 2005.
30. Cohen RD, Stein R, Hanauer SB: Intravenous cyclosporin in ulcerative colitis: a five-year experience. *Am J Gastroenterol* 94(6):1587–1592, 1999.
31. Gibson DJ, Heetun ZS, Redmond CE, et al: An accelerated infliximab induction regimen reduces the need for early colectomy in patients with acute severe ulcerative colitis. *Clin Gastroenterol Hepatol* 13(2):330.e1–335.e1, 2015.
32. Brandse J, Wildenberg M, de Bruyn J, et al: Fecal loss of infliximab as a cause of lack of response in severe inflammatory bowel disease. *Gastroenterology* 144[5 Suppl 1]:S36, 2013.
33. Laharie D, Bourreille A, Branche J, et al: Ciclosporin versus infliximab in patients with severe ulcerative colitis refractory to intravenous steroids: a parallel, open-label randomised controlled trial. *Lancet* 380(9857):1909–1915, 2012.

34. Williams J, Fasihul A, Alrubaiy L, et al: Comparative clinical effectiveness of infliximab and ciclosporin for acute severe ulcerative colitis: early results from the CONSTRUCT trial. Presented at UEGW, Vienna, Austria. October 20, 2014.
35. Powar MP, Martin P, Croft AR, et al: Surgical outcomes in steroid refractory acute severe ulcerative colitis: the impact of rescue therapy. *Colorectal Dis* 15(3):374–379, 2013.
36. Kelly CR, Kahn S, Kashyap P, et al: Update on fecal microbiota transplantation 2015: indications, methodologies, mechanisms, and outlook. *Gastroenterology* 149(1):223–237, 2015.
37. Randall J, Singh B, Warren BF, et al: Delayed surgery for acute severe colitis is associated with increased risk of postoperative complications. *Br J Surg* 97(3):404–409, 2010.
38. Kaiser AM, Hogen R, Bordeianou L, et al: Clostridium difficile infection from a surgical perspective. *J Gastrointest Surg* 19(7):1363–1377, 2015.
39. van der Wilden GM, Subramanian MP, Chang Y, et al: Antibiotic regimen after a total abdominal colectomy with ileostomy for fulminant Clostridium difficile colitis: a multi-institutional study. *Surg Infect (Larchmt)* 16(4):455–460, 2015.
40. Fasen GS, Pandian TK, Pavey ES, et al: Long-term outcome of IPAA in patients presenting with fulminant ulcerative colitis: a matched cohort study. *World J Surg* 39(10):2590–2594, 2015.
41. Berg DF, Bahadursingh AM, Kaminski DL, et al: Acute surgical emergencies in inflammatory bowel disease. *Am J Surg* 184(1):45–51, 2002.

Section 20
METABOLISM/NUTRITION

DOMINIC J. NOMPLEGGI

Chapter 212 ■ Nutritional Therapy in the Critically Ill Patient

DOMINIC J. NOMPLEGGI

The nutritional management of critically ill patients has changed dramatically over the years. The rationale for nutrition support comes from the knowledge that critically ill patients are prone to developing malnutrition, which is known to be associated with serious complications such as sepsis and pneumonia, leading to poor outcomes and even death [1]. In 2009, the Society of Critical Medicine (SCCM) and the American Society for Parenteral and Enteral Nutrition (ASPEN) published guidelines offering basic recommendations supported by the review and analysis of the then current literature [2]. At that time, these joint societies recommended that the guidelines be updated every 3 to 5 years. The target of the 2016 guidelines is intended to be adult patients, who are critically ill and are expected to require a length of stay, in a medical intensive care unit (ICU) of greater than 2 to 3 days. The current guidelines were expanded to include specific populations including organ failure, acute pancreatitis, and surgical subsets including trauma, traumatic brain injury (TBI), and patients with an open abdomen [3]. Based on an expert consensus, the societies recommended that determination of nutritional risk be performed for all patients admitted to the ICU who were not able to consume sufficient calories to meet their caloric requirements. Early enteral nutrition, within 24 to 48 hours, was recommended for all patients determined to be at risk [3]. Traditional nutritional indicators or surrogate markers are no longer recommended because they have not been validated in critical care. Indirect calorimetry (IC) should be used to determine energy requirements when available. When IC is not available, the expert consensus of the panel is that a simplistic weight-based equation (25 to 30 kcal/kg/d) be used to determine daily energy requirements [3].

Although guidelines continue to evolve, there are sufficient data on clinically proven principles and methods of nutrition support to permit practical and useful recommendations for the specific problems and questions confronted by the intensivist.

The SCCM and the ASPEN once again conclude that now after more than 30 years of investigation, nutrition *support* for critically ill patients, once regarded as adjunctive care designed to preserve lean body mass, maintain immune function, and avoid metabolic complications, should now be considered nutrition *therapy* specifically aimed at attenuating the metabolic responses to stress, prevent oxidative injury, and improve the immune response [3]. Table 212.1 does not list all of the recommendations of the panel but summarizes all the recommendations supported by randomized trials.

WHAT IS MALNUTRITION AND HOW DO WE RECOGNIZE IT?

Malnutrition among ICU patients is common and can be present on admission or develop as a result of the metabolic response to injury. This response to injury can lead to changes in substrate metabolism, causing alterations in body composition and nutrient deficiencies that become clinically evident [4]. During starvation, the body uses fat and muscle protein as a source of energy in order to preserve visceral protein [5]. Mobilization of fat for fuel is an important adaptive response for survival because glucose stores, in the form of glycogen, provide only 1,200 kcal in the first 24 hours of starvation. The body attempts to use muscle protein rather than visceral protein because visceral protein is essential for vital functions of the body. Skeletal muscle mass decreases steadily, and its rate of loss exceeds that of weight loss [6]. Because these changes are difficult to assess, intensivists have traditionally used a variety of tools such as clinical, anthropometric, chemical, and immunologic parameters that reflect altered body composition [7].

Nutritional Assessment

It is not known how long a critically ill patient can tolerate lack of nutrient intake without adverse consequences, but because

TABLE 212.1

Summary of Evidence-based Guidelines for Nutrition Support

- EN is preferred over PN for critically ill patients who require nutrition support.
- Bowel sounds are not required for the initiation of enteral feeding.
- Immune modulating enteral formulations should not be used routinely for critically ill patients but may be appropriate for postoperative patients.
- Patients with ARDS and severe acute lung injury should not receive enteral feeding containing anti-inflammatory lipids (i.e., omega-3 fish oil, borage oil) and antioxidants because of conflicting data.
- Antioxidant vitamins and trace minerals, specifically containing selenium, should be given to all critically ill patients receiving nutrition therapy.
- EN regimens not containing glutamine should be reserved for patients with TBI and perioperative patients in the SICU.
- Protocols to promote moderately strict control of serum glucose levels (150–180 mg/dL) when providing nutrition support are recommended.

ARDS, acute respiratory distress syndrome; EN, enteral nutrition; PN, parenteral nutrition; SICU, surgical intensive care unit; TBI, traumatic brain injury. Adapted from McClave SA, Taylor BE, Martindale RG, et al: Guidelines for the provision and assessment of nutrition support therapy in the adult critically ill patient: Society of Critical Care Medicine (SCCM) and American Society for Parenteral and Enteral Nutrition (A.S.P.E.N.) *J Parent Enteral Nutr* 40:159–211, 2016.

critical depletion of lean tissue can occur after 14 days of starvation among severely catabolic patients, it is recommended that nutrition support be instituted for patients who are not expected to resume oral feeding for 7 to 10 days [8]. A study conducted by the European Society of Intensive Care Medicine (ESICM) surveyed intensivists from 35 countries using a 49-item questionnaire to determine how they cope with these issues and to assess the current practice of nutritional management in ICUs [9]. In the ESICM study, 45% of the patients were fed within 24 hours and 47% between 24 and 48 hours of admission to the ICU [9].

The need for nutritional support is determined by the balance between endogenous energy reserves of the body and the severity of stress. The best clinical markers of stress are fever, leukocytosis, hypoalbuminemia, and a negative nitrogen balance.

The purpose of nutritional assessment is to identify the type and degree of malnutrition to devise a rational approach to treatment. Percentage weight loss during the past 6 months, serum albumin level, and total lymphocyte count are readily available, commonly used measures to assess nutritional status. A 10% or 10-lb weight loss over the previous 12 months is an indicator of protein calorie malnutrition. This results from inadequate caloric intake. Hypoalbuminemic malnutrition or kwashiorkor is owing to severe stress or profound malnutrition. Albumin is not a very sensitive indicator of malnutrition among ICU patients because its synthesis is influenced by numerous factors other than nutritional status such as protein-losing states, hepatic function, and acute infection or inflammation [10]. Normal concentrations of albumin are unattainable for many critically ill patients because of large fluid shifts and inadequate synthesis to meet demands. Hypoalbuminemia should be viewed as a marker of injury and not as an indicator of impaired nutrition. Most critically ill patents have a combination of the two. Malnutrition is most effectively treated by nutrition support and treatment of the stresses that led to this severe catabolic condition.

Weight loss of 10 lb or 10% of usual weight is considered clinically important, whereas weight loss of 20% to 30% suggests moderate protein calorie malnutrition and weight loss of greater than 30% suggests severe protein calorie malnutrition. Unfortunately, for many critically ill patients, total body weight is often an insensitive parameter because of progressive total body salt and water retention. The Nutritional Risk Screening 2002 and the nutrition risk in critically ill (NUTRIC) score are the preferred screening and assessment tools because they determine both nutrition status and disease severity [3]. Malnutrition is closely correlated with alterations of immune response as measured by skin test reactivity and total lymphocyte count. A total lymphocyte count less than 1,000 per mm^3 is indicative of altered immune function and is associated with decreased skin test reactivity. Loss of delayed cutaneous hypersensitivity to common antigens is a measure of impaired cellular immunity, which has been consistently found to be associated with malnutrition [10].

Subjective global assessment (SGA) is a method for evaluating nutritional status that uses clinical parameters like history, physical findings, and symptoms [11,12]. The SGA determines whether (a) nutritional assimilation has been restricted because of decreased food intake, maldigestion, or malabsorption; (b) any effects of malnutrition on organ function and body composition have occurred; and (c) the patient's disease process has influenced nutrient requirements. According to the ESICM questionnaire, the critical care community appears to most commonly assess nutritional status using the SGA and laboratory parameters [9]. Current recommendations suggest that these indicators are inaccurate for critically ill patients [3].

HOW MUCH SHOULD YOU FEED?

Macronutrients

Body cell mass is the major determinant of the total caloric requirement. Energy needs can be estimated or measured directly using IC. Although estimated energy requirements have been shown to be adequate in most patients, direct measurement is recommended for patients even when estimating energy needs appears appropriate. Direct measurement is particularly useful in patients who do not appear to respond to therapy (e.g., worsening respiratory function, continued weight loss, or a decrease in prealbumin levels, a more sensitive marker of protein synthesis than albumin).

The general principle of macronutrient support is to provide enough energy to promote anabolic functions and avoid caloric overload. Caloric requirements of 25 to 30 kcal per kg should be based on the usual body weight and are adequate for most patients [3,10]. If patients are not responding to therapy as indicated by the parameters listed previously, or if they are in a severe catabolic state as occurs among multiple trauma or burns patients, the current recommendation is to increase caloric support to up to 35 kcal per kg [3]. However, these recommendations may be changing. A recent meta-analysis of six studies that enrolled 2,517 patients concluded there was no difference in the risk of acquired infection, hospital mortality, length of stay in the ICU, or ventilator-free days among patients receiving an intentional hypocaloric diet as compared to a normocaloric diet [13].

Protein

The usual protein requirement has been estimated to be 1.2 to 1.5 g/kg/d for actual body weight. Another current recommendation by the joint societies is that an ongoing assessment of the adequacy of protein provision be performed. When nitrogen balance studies are not available, weight-based equations (e.g., 1.2 to 2.0 g/kg/d) may be used to monitor adequacy of protein provision by comparing total daily protein calories delivered with that prescribed [3].

Carbohydrates

Generally, patients will need about 25 to 30 kcal/kg/d to meet their energy requirements. Approximately 20 kcal/kg/d of the actual body weight can be provided as carbohydrate. Levels of carbohydrate above 30 kcal/kg/d increase the risk of hyperglycemia. Hyperglycemia should be avoided because it is associated with abnormalities in granulocyte adhesion, chemotaxis, phagocytosis, intracellular killing of pathogens, and poor clinical outcomes.

Hyperglycemia is a major contributing factor to postoperative infections. Blood sugars greater than 220 mg per dL on postoperative day 1 have been associated with a fivefold increased risk of serious infection [14]. A study of patients requiring total parenteral nutrition (TPN) to determine whether the frequency of hyperglycemia and infectious complications can be reduced by an underfeeding strategy (1,000 kcal with 70 g per kg as protein) provision of 1.5 g per kg of protein in conjunction with 25 kcal per kg was not associated with more hyperglycemia or infections than deliberate underfeeding. However, a regimen of 25 kcal per kg in conjunction with 1.5 g per kg of protein did provide significant nutritional benefit in terms of nitrogen balance as compared with hypocaloric TPN [15]. This suggests that it is not a hypocaloric low carbohydrate formula that protects against infection but rather the avoidance of hyperglycemia. Alternatively, TPN can be adjusted and regular insulin can be given, as needed, to maintain a blood glucose level from 150 to 180 mg per dL [3].

Fat

Usually, no more than 15% to 20% of total calories per day should be provided as fat. This will avoid infectious complications that may be caused by the dysfunction of the reticuloendothelial system, which has been associated with the administration of excess lipids [16]. Omega-6 polyunsaturated fatty acids should be provided in doses adequate to prevent essential fatty acid deficiency (at least 7% of total calories). Medium-chain triglycerides (MCTs) can be administered with long-chain triglycerides (LCTs). MCTs are more water soluble and require less lipase activity and bile salts for absorption. Patients with malabsorption, pancreatic insufficiency, and chronic liver disease can absorb them more easily. The ratio of MCT to LCT depends on the route of administration and product availability [10].

Electrolytes, Micronutrients, and Fluid

Potassium, magnesium, phosphate, and zinc should be provided in amounts necessary to maintain normal serum levels. The absolute requirements for vitamins, minerals, and trace elements have not yet been determined. Normal serum and blood levels of vitamins have been established but may vary with the laboratory in which the measurement is obtained [10]. In general, patients should receive 25 mL of fluid per kg actual dry body weight to avoid dehydration. Three milliliters of trace elements injection 5 (Multitrace-5) and 10 mL of multiple vitamin infusion (Infuvite Adult) will provide adequate vitamins, trace elements, and minerals and should be added to TPN daily. The required daily allowance for all vitamins and minerals is usually provided in 1,000 to 1,500 mL of most enteral formulas. If the patient is receiving less than a liter of enteral feeding, vitamin supplementation may be necessary. Spot electrolyte measurements (aliquots of urine, ostomy, nasogastric, or fistulous output) may be very helpful in determining proper replacement. If the total daily volume of the lost fluid is measured, the daily loss of any electrolyte in that fluid can be estimated using the following equation: mmol per L × volume output per 24 hours (in liters) = mmol per 24 hours (e.g., 20 mL of urine contains 100 mmol per L, the daily urine output is 2 L; therefore, the 24-hour urine sodium output is 200 mmol).

WHICH ROUTE OF ADMINISTRATION?

Enteral Feeding

Enteral feeding has been shown in clinical studies to reduce infection and preserve gut integrity, barrier, and immune functions. It is the preferred route of nutrient administration because it is more physiologic, safer, and less expensive than parenteral feeding. Current recommendations support initiation of enteral nutrition as soon as the patient is hemodynamically stable [3]. The only contraindication is a nonfunctioning gut. For example, intragastric feeding requires adequate gastric motility. Gastric residuals should be checked hourly and a volume greater than 500 mL necessitates modification of the infusion rate to minimize reflux and aspiration. Supplemental parenteral nutrition to meet caloric requirements or small bowel feeding to potentially decrease the risk of aspiration will be necessary until normal gastric function returns. Gastric atony and colonic ileus do not preclude enteral feeding but may require gastric decompression or small bowel feeding.

Initiation of enteral feeding does not require active bowel sounds or the passage of flatus or stool. Small bowel feedings can be given in the presence of mild or resolving pancreatitis and low output enterocutaneous fistulas (less than 500 mL per day) [3]. Even patients with severe acute pancreatitis (acute physiology and chronic health evaluation [APACHE II scores 12 to 13] receiving enteral nutrition) have significantly fewer total complications and septic complications than patients receiving parenteral nutrition [17]. A recent study looking at patients with acute pancreatitis (APACHE score of 8 or higher or a modified Glasgow score of 3 or higher) showed no significant differences of rates of major infection, for up to 6 months, among patients fed a nasoenteric diet within 24 hours versus an oral diet initiated at 72 hours [18]. Worsening abdominal distention or diarrhea in excess of 1,000 mL per day requires a medical evaluation. If distention is present, enteral feedings should be discontinued. If no infectious cause for the diarrhea is found, antidiarrheals can be administered and feedings continued [10]. Nasogastric feeding is appropriate for most patients except those with a history of aspiration pneumonia associated with reflux. Those patients should be fed postpylorically or via a G-tube to minimize nasogastric tube-associated reflux of gastric contents and aspiration. In contrast to prior recommendations, the ASPEN/SCCM guidelines now recommend that patients with severe acute pancreatitis can be fed by either the gastric or the jejunal route because there is no difference in tolerance or clinical outcomes [3]. A study of four university-based ICUs at two hospitals found that physicians ordered a daily volume of enteral feeding that was 66% of the requirement; but because only 78% of the ordered volume was infused, patients received only 52% of target calories. Sixty-six percent of the time the reasons given for stopping the infusion were determined to be avoidable. Half the patients whose tube feedings were checked every 4 hours had their feedings held for residual volumes less than 200 mL, when the guideline for stopping the tube feeding was a residual of greater than 200 mL [19]. Protocols for delivery of enteral feeding can avoid this.

Standard isotonic polymeric formulations can meet most patients' nutritional needs. The use of elemental formulas should be reserved for patients with severe small bowel absorptive dysfunction. The "American Gastroenterological Association Medical Position Statement: Guidelines for the use of enteral nutrition" and the current ASPEN/SCCM have concluded that disease- or organ-specific specialty formulations are generally more expensive and have a limited clinical role, and they will require more data to justify their practicality and effectiveness. Immune modulating formulations containing arginine and fish oils can be considered for patients with severe trauma [3,20].

There are numerous issues that arise when providing enteral nutrition to critically ill patients. We provide guidelines to help the readers of this chapter overcome the problems that often arise when administering enteral tube feedings.

In general, most complications associated with the use of feeding tubes relate to placement, displacement, or malfunction of the tubes. It is important to remember that these tubes require frequent maintenance to avoid complications. The position of nasogastric or nasoenteric feeding tubes placed at the bedside should be confirmed endoscopically or radiographically before use because clinical assessment is unreliable. The routine use of promotility drugs has not been shown to be consistently beneficial and although they can increase the volume of feeding, the overall impact is small except for patients at high risk of aspiration [3]. Excessive force during insertion, which can result in malposition, should be avoided. Tubes need to be flushed regularly to avoid clogging with medications or tube feeding. Cycled tube feeding is recommended, if possible, to facilitate this. Little is known about the compatibility of most medications with tube feeding and, therefore, medications should not be mixed with tube feedings because this can lead to precipitation of the medication with blockage of the tube and decreased absorption of the medication.

Placement of tubes across the gastroesophageal junction or pylorus can lead to incompetence of the sphincter, reflux, and aspiration. In patients at risk for or with a history of aspiration associated with reflux, we recommend percutaneously placed gastric or jejunal feeding tubes. Gastric tubes are preferred because the smaller caliber of the jejunal tubes makes them likely to obstruct with administration of anything except liquid medications. Percutaneously placed tubes that fall or are pulled out should be replaced cautiously. Unlike noncritically ill patients who usually have had their feeding tubes in place long term, critically ill patients are likely to have had their tube placed recently or may have impaired healing and, therefore, may not have a fully developed cutaneous fistula. For these reasons, we recommend confirming placement with a contrast-enhanced radiograph before use when replacing these tubes at the bedside.

Elevating the head of the bed 30° and checking for gastric residuals to avoid increases in the volume of the gastric contents, which can lead to hypersecretion and reflux of gastric contents, are also recommended.

Stress gastritis, also known as stress-related erosive syndrome, is a term used to describe gastrointestinal mucosal injury associated with serious systemic disease. Most patients at risk cannot have oral feedings. Histamine H_2 receptor antagonists (H2RAs) have been shown to protect against significant gastrointestinal hemorrhage. There are less data on the efficacy of proton pump inhibitors (PPIs). A reasonable suggestion has been to wait for 6 to 12 hours between stopping parenteral H2RAs before starting to feed and initiating therapy with a PPI [21].

Parenteral Feeding

Parenteral nutrient administration is recommended when the gastrointestinal tract is nonfunctional or inaccessible or enteral feeding is insufficient. Although parenteral nutrient admixtures are not as nutritionally complete as enteral formulations, nutritional goals are achieved more often with the former than the latter. This is usually attributable to a variety of barriers. In patients determined to be at high nutritional risk or severely malnourished, when enteral nutrition is not feasible parenteral nutrition should be initiated as soon as possible. In addition, if patients at high risk do not meet greater than 60% of energy and protein requirements by the enteral route, supplemental parenteral nutrition should be initiated [3].

Parenteral nutrition is associated with an increased risk of infectious complications, especially line infections, and increased costs. Strict adherence to protocols emphasizing aseptic techniques and limiting central line interruption can decrease complications. Peripheral indwelling central catheters or central subclavian or internal jugular lines should be considered, and implanted permanent lines should be avoided [10]. Management of infected temporary lines is easier and has fewer complications.

HOW DO YOU PREVENT COMPLICATIONS AND MAXIMIZE BENEFITS?

Anticipating potential complications leads to early recognition, minimizes the impact of the complications, and improves outcomes. Adherence to general guidelines for energy requirements, as mentioned earlier, should help avoid overfeeding. Overfeeding can lead to a number of problems, such as cholestatic liver disease, hyperglycemia, increased infection risk, and worsening hypercapnic respiratory failure. When there is doubt, expired gas analysis can be used to assess caloric requirements. A respiratory quotient (R/Q) greater than 1 generally indicates overfeeding. R/Q is the quotient of mL of CO_2 produced per mL of O_2 consumed. Increased CO_2 production will cause a rise in the R/Q from 0.80, a normal, average steady state. Reducing total calories (glucose and fat) may benefit patients with chronic lung disease fed parenterally who develop worsening hypercapnia. Assessment of nitrogen balance (the difference between nitrogen produced and nitrogen eliminated in urine and stool) every 5 to 7 days may be useful for assessing the response to adjustments of the protein dose. Prerenal azotemia from excessive protein administration is an indication to decrease nitrogen intake. Patient outcome following acute renal failure (creatinine greater than twice normal) does not improve with the administration of specialized formulations.

Monitoring triglycerides and adjusting continuous fat infusion to keep triglycerides less than 500 mg per dL will avoid hypertriglyceridemia. Monitoring of prealbumin because of its short half-life (i.e., 2 days) can be used to assess response to feeding in the ICU setting. Monitoring of fluid and electrolytes is essential particularly in patients receiving TPN to avoid volume overload. Deficiencies of potassium or calcium can lead to cardiac arrhythmias. Hypophosphatemia can precipitate rhabdomyolysis, severe muscle weakness, and respiratory failure. Hypomagnesemia can cause muscle weakness and even seizures. Zinc deficiency can lead to impaired wound healing, diarrhea, and cutaneous anergy. Routine monitoring of vitamins and minerals for patients on short-term parenteral nutrition support is not useful because deficiencies are usually only associated with long-term therapy. Monitoring on a selected case basis when there are clinical signs or symptoms of a vitamin deficiency (e.g., hyperkeratosis [vitamin A], megaloblastic anemia [folate/vitamin B_{12}]) is more practical. Liver enzymes should be monitored weekly to determine if biliary or liver disease has developed [10].

WHAT IS THE IMPORTANCE OF PROVIDING SPECIAL KEY NUTRIENTS?

Effects of special nutrients on regulation of the processes of inflammation and repair and immune function have been the object of many studies. Although specialized nutrients added to parenteral or enteral formulas have been shown to modulate a variety of cellular responses, their precise clinical utility is still unresolved. For example, arginine is an amino acid that participates in a variety of metabolic processes, including synthesis of nitrous and nitric oxide, compounds known to protect the liver from damage in a murine model of endotoxin-induced hepatic necrosis [22], urea synthesis, lymphocyte proliferation, and wound healing. Other studies have shown that diets rich in fish oils increased the survival of guinea pigs challenged with endotoxin [23,24].

The branched chain amino acids leucine, isoleucine, and valine are essential amino acids required for protein synthesis. Although improvement in nitrogen balance can be observed when these are given in combination with other essential amino acids in doses of 0.5 to 1.2 g/kg/d, their efficacy in improving patient outcomes remains to be defined and their use is not recommended [3,25].

The importance of glutamine to normal cellular function and its unique function in amino acid metabolism, in both health and disease, has been recognized for many years [26]. The skeletal muscle-free amino acid pool is 61% glutamine, and accelerated mobilization of glutamine occurs during catabolic states. In such states, glutamine depletion occurs despite administration of standard parenteral amino acids, which do not contain glutamine because of their instability in aqueous solution. In rats, decline of the intracellular pool of glutamine in the skeletal muscle has been shown to correlate with skeletal muscle protein degradation. The majority of glutamine released from skeletal muscle is taken up by intestinal cells. Rat studies have shown that glutamine-supplemented parenteral nutrition improves gut mucosal metabolism and nitrogen balance during sepsis and also increases villus height and mucosal thickness in starved rats, suggesting that mucosal barrier defense is improved [27,28]. However, in humans, a randomized trial of glutamine supplementation of parenteral nutrition detected no difference in infectious complications or median length of hospital stay between groups and their routine use is not recommended [3,29].

Addition of specialized key nutrients to enteral formulas to enhance immune function has been suggested for the reasons outlined earlier. A meta-analysis of 12 studies that used either of the two most common commercially available enteral feeding preparations enriched with the "immunonutrients" arginine and omega-3 fatty acids concluded that they had no effect on mortality [30]. However, significant reductions in infection rates, ventilator days, and length of stay in hospitals in patients fed these formulas were most pronounced among surgical patients [30]. Although the relative efficacy of any single immune-enhancing component versus its combination with another is impossible to state on the basis of the presently available evidence [31], commercially available formulas fortified with "immunonutrients" may be beneficial, but their routine use in medical ICUs is not recommended [3]. Rather, these formulations should be reserved for patients with TBI and in postoperative patients in surgical ICUs [3].

Although the administration of growth hormone can attenuate the severe catabolic state induced by the metabolic response to injury, surgery, and sepsis, two randomized placebo-controlled clinical trials found that in-hospital mortality, length of stay in the ICU, and duration of mechanical ventilation were greater among patients receiving growth hormone [32].

In summary, nutritional support should be considered essential for the treatment of prolonged critical illness. We have provided some useful guidelines for nutritional assessment, estimation of energy requirement, route of nutrient delivery, estimations of the effectiveness of nutrition provided to critically ill patients, and also suggested some practical points to simplify delivery and avoid associated complications related to parenteral and enteral feeding.

References

1. Giner M, Laviano A, Meguid MM, et al: In 1995 a correlation between malnutrition and poor outcome in critically ill still exists. *Nutrition* 12:23–29, 1996.
2. McClave SA, Martindale RG, Vanek VW, et al: Guidelines for the provision and assessment of nutrition support therapy in the adult critically ill patient: Society of Critical Care Medicine (SCCM) and American Society for Parenteral and Enteral Nutrition (A.S.P.E.N.) *J Parent Enteral Nutr* 33:277–318, 2009.
3. McClave SA, Taylor BE, Martindale RG, et al: Guidelines for the provision and assessment of nutrition support therapy in the adult critically ill patient: Society of Critical Care Medicine (SCCM) and American Society for Parenteral and Enteral Nutrition (A.S.P.E.N.) *J Parent Enteral Nutr* 40:159–211, 2016.
4. Wolfe RR, Durkot MJ, Allsop JR, et al: Glucose metabolism in severely burned patients. *Metabolism* 28:1031–1039, 1979.
5. McMahon M, Bistrian BR: The physiology of nutritional assessment and therapy in protein-calorie malnutrition. *Dis Mon* 36:378–417, 1990.
6. Heymsfield SB, McManus C, Stevens C, et al: Muscle mass: reliable indicator of protein-energy malnutrition severity and outcome. *Am J Clin Nutr* 35:1192–1199, 1982.
7. Jahoor F, Shangraw RE, Miyoshi H, et al: Role of insulin and glucose oxidation in mediating the protein catabolism of burns and sepsis. *Am J Physiol* 257:E323–E331, 1989.
8. Klein S, Kinney J, Jeejeebhoy K, et al: Nutrition support in clinical practice: review of published data and recommendations for future research direction. *J Parenter Enteral Nutr* 21:133–156, 1997.
9. Preiser JC, Berre J, Carpentier Y, et al: Management of nutrition in European intensive care units: results of a questionnaire. *Intensive Care Med* 25:95–101, 1999.
10. Cerra FB, Benitez MR, Blackburn GL, et al: Applied nutrition in ICU patients: a consensus statement of the American College of Chest Physicians. *Chest* 111:769–778, 1997.
11. Marik PE, Hooper MH: Normocaloric versus hypocaloric feeding on outcomes of ICU patients: a systematic review and meta-analysis. *Intensive Care Med* 42:316–323, 2016.
12. Baker JP, Detsky AS, Wesson DE, et al: Nutritional assessment: a comparison of clinical judgment and objective measures. *N Engl J Med* 306:969–972, 1982.
13. Detsky AS, McLaughlin JR, Baker JP, et al: What is subjective global assessment of nutritional status? *J Parenter Enteral Nutr* 11:8–13, 1987.
14. Pomposelli JJ, Baxter JK III, Babineau TJ: Early postoperative glucose control predicts nosocomial infection rate in diabetic patients. *J Parenter Enteral Nutr* 22:77–81, 1998.
15. McCowen KC, Friel C, Sternberg J, et al: Hypocaloric total parenteral nutrition: effectiveness in prevention of hypoglycemia and infectious complications—a randomized clinical trial. *Crit Care Med* 28:3606–3611, 2000.
16. Seidner DL, Mascioli EA, Istfan NW, et al: Effects of long-chain triglyceride emulsions on reticuloendothelial system function in humans. *J Parenter Enteral Nutr* 13:614–619, 1989.
17. Kalfarentzos F, Kehagias J, Mead N, et al: Enteral nutrition is superior to parenteral nutrition in severe acute pancreatitis: results of a randomized prospective trial. *Br J Surg* 84:1665–1669, 1997.
18. Bakker OJ, van Brunschot HC, van Santvoort MG, et al: Early versus on-demand nasoenteric tube feeding in acute pancreatitis. *N Engl J Med* 371:1983–1993, 2014.
19. McClave SA, Sexton LK, Spain DA, et al: Enteral tube feeding in the intensive care unit: factors impeding adequate delivery. *Crit Care Med* 27:1252–1256, 1999.
20. Kirby DF, Delegge MH, Fleming CR: American Gastroenterological Association Medical Position Statement: Guidelines for the use of enteral nutrition. *Gastroenterology* 108:1280–1301, 1995.
21. Wolfe MM, Sachs G: Acid suppression: optimizing therapy for gastroduodenal ulcer healing, gastroesophageal reflux disease, and stress-related erosive syndrome. *Gastroenterology* 118:S9–S31, 2000.
22. Billiar TR, Curren RD, Stueh DJ, et al: Inducible cytosolic enzyme activity for the production of nitric oxides from L-arginine. *Biochem Biophys Res Commun* 168:1034–1040, 1990.
23. Mascioli EA, Leader L, Flores E, et al: Enhanced survival to endotoxin in guinea pigs fed IV fish oil. *Lipids* 23:623–625, 1988.
24. Mascioli EA, Iwasa Y, Trimbo S, et al: Endotoxin challenge after menhaden oil to diet: effects on survival of guinea pigs. *Am J Clin Nutr* 49:277–282, 1989.
25. Nompleggi DJ, Bonkovsky HL: Nutritional supplementation in chronic liver disease: an analytical review. *Hepatology* 19:518–533, 1994.
26. Lacey JM, Wilmore DW: Is glutamine a conditionally essential amino acid? *Nutr Rev* 48:297–309, 1990.
27. Chen K, Okuma T, Okuma K, et al: Glutamine-supplemented parenteral nutrition improves gut mucosal metabolism and nitrogen balance in septic rats. *J Parenter Enteral Nutr* 18:167–171, 1994.
28. Inoue Y, Grant JP, Synder PJ: Effect of glutamine-supplemented total parenteral nutrition on recovery of small intestine after starvation atrophy. *J Parenter Enteral Nutr* 17:165–170, 1993.
29. Powell-Tuck J, Jamieson CP, Bettany EA, et al: A double blind randomized controlled trial of glutamine supplementation in parenteral nutrition. *Gut* 45:82–88, 1999.
30. Beale RJ, Bryg DJ, Bihari DJ: Immunonutrition in the critically ill: a systematic review of clinical outcome. *Crit Care Med* 27:2799–2805, 1999.
31. Bistrian BR: Enteral nutrition: just a fuel or an immunity enhancer? *Minerva Anestesiol* 65:471–474, 1999.
32. Takala J, Ruokonen E, Webster N, et al: Increased mortality associated with growth hormone treatment in critically ill adults. *N Engl J Med* 341:785–792, 1999.

Chapter 213 ■ Parenteral and Enteral Nutrition in the Intensive Care Unit

DAVID F. DRISCOLL • BRUCE R. BISTRIAN

Nutritional and metabolic support during acute illness is an integral part of the clinical care of critically ill patients. The significance of such interventions is predicated on three main factors: (a) degree of metabolic stress; (b) dysfunction of major organ systems; and/or (c) presence of protein-calorie malnutrition (PCM). In the first case, metabolic stress can arise from a variety of sources, including, for example, severe injuries sustained by major trauma such as closed head injury, multiple long-bone fractures, third-degree burns of greater than 25% of body surface area, or severe sepsis and stress of lesser intensity such as thoracoabdominal surgery, pulmonary infection, systemic infection, or any source of active systemic inflammation. Often, more than one form of metabolic stress may be present that can accentuate and/or dysregulate the injury response. Concerning the second factor, metabolically stressed patients may develop acute failure of vital organs during the critical care period or have underlying chronic end-organ dysfunction. Acute or chronic disease, particularly of the cardiopulmonary, renal, or hepatic system, often further complicates the clinical course and requires modification of nutritional support during critical illness, especially among the elderly [1]. Finally, the presence of preexisting or the likely early development of PCM is the key to identifying patients who will derive the greatest clinical benefits from nutritional and metabolic support therapies.

Approximately 35 years ago, the prevalence of PCM among hospitalized general medical and surgical patients was reported to be as high as 50% of all adult admissions to a large teaching hospital [2,3]. More recent reports continue to document high rates of malnutrition among hospitalized patients [4–9]. When moderate to severe PCM accompanies severe metabolic stress, an increase in nutrition-related complications can be expected to occur, including wound dehiscence, nosocomial infections, and severe fluid, electrolyte, and acid–base disturbances. During stress, substantial catabolism of both endogenous and exogenous protein and energy occurs coincident with the injury response. For support of the metabolic response to injury, the breakdown of body protein, principally from muscle and connective tissue stores, supports amino acid and energy needs to mount various beneficial components of the systemic inflammatory response by the release of amino acids for accelerated synthesis of proteins and cells, including leukocytes, hepatic acute phase and cellular proteins for wound repair, and gluconeogenesis. The goal is to optimize energy requirements for metabolically active tissues, including cardiac myocytes, leukocytes, and fibroblasts. An assessment of the degree of this response can be estimated by application of the catabolic index (CI) [10]. However, if PCM complicates injury or infection, the systemic inflammatory response is less intense than that found in normally nourished individuals with a similar degree of injury. Consequently, the degree and duration of the metabolic response, with respect to nitrogen breakdown, may be greatly diminished. In terms of the degree of catabolism, for example, a malnourished elderly patient with significant catabolic injury could manifest nitrogen losses that may be as a much as 50% less than normally nourished younger counterparts with the same injury [1]. Although this might imply a less severe catabolic response sparing lean tissue, the pathologic consequences are more severe as a result of the muting of the beneficial aspects of the systemic inflammatory response, and these adverse effects tend to occur sooner. Moreover, the time course to intervene with nutritional and metabolic support to limit the likelihood of nutrition-related complications is also shortened by as a much as 50% (i.e., 5 to 7 days) in the moderately to severely malnourished versus normally nourished individuals (i.e., 7 to 10 days) with the same metabolic stress. Ultimately, the consequences of ongoing depletion of the metabolically active body cell mass of the malnourished reduce the ability to recover from acute illness, can be associated with severe deficiencies of minerals that are typically found in muscle (potassium, magnesium, and phosphorus), and often lead to severe impairments in immunocompetence, wound healing, and recovery of organ function.

Once the decision to provide nutrition support is made, parenteral nutritional (PN) or enteral nutritional (EN) therapies are available options. In nearly every case, if the gastrointestinal (GI) tract is functional and the patient is hemodynamically stable, EN should be instituted. However, if significant malnutrition also exists and a prolonged recovery is anticipated, it should be recognized that the time frame to achieve eucaloric intakes for EN often takes much longer because of the associated GI intolerance, compared with PN. Because central venous access is generally necessary during critical illness, EN support can often be supplemented with PN [11] so as to avoid the prolongation of caloric deficits during acute illness, which are particularly of concern for initially malnourished patients or for the most severe critically ill with closed head injury, multiple trauma, major burns, and severe sepsis. For such patients, it appears that early feeding within the first 72 hours, whether by enteral, parenteral, or the combination, has the greatest impact on mortality outcomes. Although mild decrements in energy balance in the critical care setting may well be tolerated and, in certain circumstances, appropriate, at least 1 g of protein per kg and 15 kcal per kg advancing to 1.5 g protein per kg and 20 to 25 kcal per kg in the second week of injury should be the goal to avoid adverse, nutrition-related outcomes. Moreover, intensive metabolic support (i.e., the provision of electrolytes and acid–base therapy) can also be accomplished efficiently through the PN admixture. The amount of PNs can be gradually reduced because the patient is transitioned to EN coincident with remission of the stress response and return of full GI tolerance to tube feeding. Thus, in the intensive care unit (ICU), nutrition support is often provided to patients using both enteral and parenteral means, especially during the acute care period. The purpose of supplying both EN and PN where appropriate should not be motivated by attempts to meet protein and energy needs as soon as possible, but rather as a means of providing trophic stimulation to enterocytes and hopefully a quicker transition to full enteral feedings, while PN is used to treat severe metabolic disorders such as hypokalemia, hypophosphatemia, and metabolic alkalosis, that can only be safely and effectively addressed by the intravenous route of administration. The greatest challenge facing the critical care clinician is to appropriately identify those patients who are in greatest need of nutrition support therapy and to provide it in a manner that is both effective and does not produce iatrogenic complications.

CLINICAL CONSEQUENCES OF DELAYING NUTRITIONAL SUPPORT

Although, at times, it is difficult to pinpoint the cause and effect of nutrition-related complications during critical illness, it should be intuitively obvious that withholding nutrition will ultimately lead to death from starvation. This message was poignantly illustrated in the deaths of Maze prisoners in Belfast, Ireland, as detailed in a report from Leiter and Marliss [12] in 1982. Ten Irish Republican Army prisoners went on a hunger strike that led to their deaths over a period of 45 to 73 days of fasting. All were young lean males, and the critical weight loss that resulted in death was approximately 35% calculated from the first day of the fast. It is also generally acknowledged that patients who approach 35% to 40% losses from their ideal or usual body weight through inadequate nutritional intake are at greatest risk of malnutrition-related death. Presumably, at these extreme levels of body mass depletion, both the size and function of vital organs of the viscera are considerably diminished. At some critical point, presumed to be when fat stores become limited, protein catabolism now coming from both skeletal and visceral organs accelerates. If one discontinues providing life-sustaining needs for energy, the loss of a critical mass of body protein is ultimately reached and death from organ failure is imminent.

The effects on the vital organ function can be catastrophic, because oxygen consumption of the visceral organs is much higher than that of resting skeletal muscle. The imbalance between loss of skeletal muscle and visceral organ mass initially favoring visceral organs has also been suggested to explain the higher energy expenditures per body weight seen in severely depleted hospitalized patients (average of approximately 70% of ideal body weight [IBW]) as a result of an approximate 10-fold difference in resting oxygen consumption between skeletal muscle compared to visceral tissues such as the liver [13]. During starvation (with adequate water intake), and in the absence of metabolic stress, a normally nourished, thin individual can survive for periods of approximately 6 to 10 weeks. In terms of total body nitrogen, it is estimated that the loss of 350 to 500 g of nitrogen is potentially lethal. In terms of body mass index (BMI), which is weight in kilogram per height in meters squared, it is generally considered that a BMI less than 13 kg per m^2 in males and less than 11 kg per m^2 in females is incompatible with life [14]. However, the rapidity of weight loss is also a factor, because lesser degrees of semistarvation (i.e., smaller energy deficits) are better tolerated. Table 213.1 depicts the relationship of BMI with nutritional status.

By way of comparison, the metabolically stressed patient experiences greater catabolism coincident with acute illness and can lose as much as 30 g of nitrogen per day, representing about 1 kg of lean tissue from the breakdown of lean body mass. Generally, the majority of these losses can be measured in a 24-hour urine collection as urea nitrogen and used for nitrogen balance estimation. Nitrogen balance studies assess the difference between dietary protein (nitrogen) intake and nitrogen excretion. Healthy individuals consuming an adequate diet in terms of essential nutrients, including protein (0.8 g protein/kg/d) and sufficient energy to provide energy balance, will be in zero nitrogen balance. That is, the nitrogen in is equaled by the nitrogen out in urine (mostly) and feces, reflecting no net change in lean body mass. Net nitrogen losses for patients receiving parenteral or enteral feeding can vary from 0 to 30 g per day, depending on the extent of the injury response and the level of feeding. With the systemic inflammatory response, the utilization of protein to maintain lean body mass is impaired, making the daily requirement increase to about 1.5 g protein/kg/d. Similarly, energy requirements increase, which are offset to some degree by the reduction of physical activity characteristic of the hospitalized patient. With the development of renal dysfunction, the proportionate amounts of nitrogen found in the urine become substantially less, with a concomitant rise in blood urea nitrogen (BUN). In general, in a 70-kg male, every 5 mg% change in BUN represents 2 g of nitrogen catabolized and not excreted, and 1.5 g of nitrogen for a 60-kg female, based on average total body water (TBW) of 60% and 50% for males and females, respectively. Protein intakes must be adjusted to limit the rise in BUN, but nutrition efficacy should not be sacrificed to renal function beyond a reduction to the 1 g protein per kg for other than very brief periods. Renal replacement therapy such as dialysis or hemofiltration should be considered in those circumstances. Once the BUN becomes stable, even if elevated by impaired renal function, a 24-hour urine urea nitrogen excretion represents the amount catabolized over that period. The CI (CI = 24-hour urine urea nitrogen − [0.5 × dietary nitrogen + 3]), adjusts for the effects of dietary intake and obligatory nitrogen loss on urinary urea nitrogen excretion. The CI is the difference between measured and predicted urine urea nitrogen excretion. For example, the major catabolic stresses that produce the highest nitrogen losses and CIs include burns, head injury, severe sepsis, and multiple trauma. The clinical application of nitrogen balance and CI assessments are illustrated in Table 213.2.

There are potential clinical scenarios that may affect the accuracy of nitrogen balance studies. This is especially true for patients with renal dysfunction that may reduce nitrogen output and could erroneously suggest an improvement in nitrogen balance. A correction of the nitrogen balance study can be applied

TABLE 213.1

Body Mass Index and Nutritional Status

Body mass index	= weight in kg ÷ (height in m)^2
Assumptions:	weight: 75 kg; height: 1.84 m
BMI	= 75/(1.84)^2
	= 22.2

Body mass index	Nutritional status
≥30	Obese
≥25–<30	Overweight
20–<25	Normal
<18.5	Moderate malnutrition
<16	Severe malnutrition
<13	Lethal in males
<11	Lethal in females

TABLE 213.2

Clinical Application of the Nitrogen Balance and Catabolic Index Assessments

Nitrogen balance	$= \dfrac{\text{protien intake (g)}}{6.25} - (24\text{ h UUN} + 4)$
	$= \dfrac{105\text{ (g)}}{6.25} - (20 + 4)$
	= −7.2 g
Catabolic index (<0 no significant stress; 0–5 significant stress; >5 severe stress)	= UUN (g) − (½ × dietary nitrogen + 3)
	= 20 g − (0.5 × 16.8 g + 3)
	= 8.6 (severe stress)

Assumptions: 70-kg male; 105 g protein intake; 20 g UUN over 24 hours.
UUN, urine urea nitrogen.

TABLE 213.3

Nitrogen Balance Correction in Renal Dysfunction

Prenitrogen balance data	
BUN = 31 mg/dL; weight = 70 kg; 105 g protein intake	
Prestudy	
Total body water @ 70 kg	= 42 L
Total BUN @ 31 mg/dL	= 42 L × 310 mg/L (or 310 mg/L)
	= **13,020 mg or 13 g**
Postnitrogen balance data	
BUN = 51 mg/dL; weight = 74 kg; 105 g protein intake; 24 h UUN = 20 g	
Poststudy	
Total body water @ 74 kg	= 42 L + 4 L
	= 46 L
Total BUN @ 51 mg/dL (or 510 mg/L)	= 46 L × 510 mg/L
	= **23,460 mg or 23.5 g**
Nitrogen balance	$= \frac{\text{protein intake (g)}}{6.25} - (24\text{ h UUN} + 4)$
	$= \frac{105\text{ (g)}}{6.25} - (20 + 4)$
	= −7.2 g
Corrected N-balance	= 13.02 g − 23.5 g urea nitrogen (blood)
	= −10.5 g not excreted in urine
	= −10.5 g (BUN) + (−7.2 g UUN)
	= **−17.7 g**

Assumptions: total body water = 60% (for males).
BUN, blood urea nitrogen; UUN, urine urea nitrogen.

to account for the nitrogen losses that do not appear in the urine, but result in an increase in the BUN concentration. Assuming nitrogen intake remains constant, two important pieces of data are required to correct for the nitrogen losses not appearing in the urine and include the patient's BUN and body weight at the beginning and end of the 24-hour collection period. These are important because most of the urea is distributed in TBW. A clinical example that applies to this method of correction appears in Table 213.3.

In terms of lean body mass, each gram of nitrogen lost represents approximately 30 g of (hydrated) lean tissue (hydration ratio: approximately 4:1 or 5:1). For patients with daily nitrogen losses of 30 g, which represents the highest catabolic nitrogen loss in the absence of dietary protein intake, approximately 1 kg of lean tissue would be lost each day. Such losses cannot be sustained for protracted periods, and, under these circumstances, nutrition support is clearly indicated within the first 24 to 36 hours even in the previously well-nourished patient to address this extraordinary rate of loss. Using cumulative nitrogen deficits of 350 to 500 g, a sustained loss of this magnitude could theoretically result in death in approximately 2 to 3 weeks, although catabolic rates usually diminish in the later weeks of injury. For the severely malnourished patient of 75% of IBW, one can estimate the critical survival period to be in the range of 1.5 to 2 weeks under the same circumstances. Finally, a cumulative caloric deficit of 10,000 kcal or more during acute illness has been associated with significant morbidity and mortality among surgical ICU patients [15]. However, it is likely that the associated protein deficit played the larger role, because normal individuals have more than 150,000 stored calories as fat, which always makes up the greater proportion of the caloric deficit. A study in the medical ICU has shown that intakes of less than 25% of requirements were associated with a higher rate of bloodstream infections [16].

Of course, projections of survival or complications are estimates and may be highly variable depending on other factors, including nutritional status, metabolic stress, and end-organ function. Moreover, in the clinical setting, such high outputs of nitrogen over long periods will not likely be sustained, because medical and surgical therapies will usually successfully reduce the stress response. Furthermore, both the rate of reduction of lean body mass and the intensity of the systemic inflammatory response diminish as PCM develops. Such patients will invariably receive calories (dextrose) and electrolytes from various parenteral infusions, so that some form of supplementation is given, which also slows the loss of lean tissue. Consequently, the outcome of death from the total lack of nutritional support is rare. However, nutrition-related complications, such as impaired wound healing and immunocompetence leading to nosocomial infections, are the common proximate causes of increased morbidity and mortality under such circumstances.

IDENTIFYING PATIENTS IN NEED OF NUTRITIONAL SUPPORT

In the ICU setting, it is often difficult to identify those patients who are at greatest risk of developing nutrition-related complications because of preexisting malnutrition. Such patients are often volume overloaded because of massive administration of parenteral fluids from multiple drug therapies and often acute volume resuscitation, as well as maintenance intravenous therapy to support intravascular volume. This fluid retention and weight gain is often compounded by the hormonal consequences of the systemic inflammatory response such as enhanced insulin, aldosterone, and antidiuretic hormone secretion, which favor salt and water retention. Consequently, the weight of the patient is artificially high, and major efforts of the ICU team are often directed at reducing volume intake in order to mobilize third-space fluids. A weight history may be difficult to obtain or overlooked entirely because of more acute clinical issues. Moreover, an accurate patient weight is also important to optimize drug therapy. Under these circumstances, a moderately to severely malnourished patient may escape detection by the primary care team, and only be recognized as malnourished after fluid homeostasis is achieved, or worse, a potentially preventable nutrition-related complication, such as wound breakdown, occurs. Clearly, at this point, the opportunity to minimize such complications from expert nutrition support has passed, and the course toward rehabilitation may be long and costly.

To avoid this scenario, a more substantial effort must be undertaken to identify the patients who are at greatest risk. Nutrition screening programs on admission, especially by dieticians, can greatly assist in identifying these patients, but some patients, especially admissions for emergent care, may escape this surveillance process. In these cases, the premorbid weight is very important and should be obtained if at all possible. It will at least provide a baseline prior to the numerous medical and surgical maneuvers that may take place over the ensuing 24 to 48 hours that could dramatically change the patient's weight in the critical care setting.

If the admission weight is not obtained, then the clinician may need to estimate the patient's body weight from available hospital data. Estimations may be made based on the most recent weight recorded and then backtracked through the medical chart using the intake and output records to reconstruct the original weight history. For critically ill patients, such records are usually reliable, and a reasonable estimate may be made. This estimate may be confirmed by subsequent discussions with the patient or family. When confirmed, the body weight can then be compared to standard measures for population-based body weight for height tables, such as the IBW or the BMI. A patient weight less than 85% of IBW or BMI less than 18.5 indicates moderate malnutrition. Severe malnutrition would be considered likely if weight is less than 75% of IBW or BMI is less than 16 kg per m^2. Thus, a greater sense of urgency to intervene with nutrition support is present under these conditions and should be undertaken within several days of the acute injury. If the patient is deemed well nourished, then intervention may be delayed unless the systemic inflammatory response is severe (i.e., major third-degree burns, closed head injury with a Glasgow Coma Score less than 8, multiple trauma with very high acute physiology and chronic health evaluation [APACHE] or injury severity scores, or severe pancreatitis with a positive computed tomography scan and more than three Ranson criteria. Then, because the systemic inflammatory response is likely to endure beyond 1 week, very early nutritional support is indicated. The serum albumin level, which reflects the presence of a recent systemic inflammatory response, is not often helpful in this setting because the invariable systemic inflammatory response and common disturbances in volume status make hypoalbuminemia universal. However, severe hypoalbuminemia (less than 2.4 g per dL) usually reflecting a greater degree and/or longer duration of systemic inflammation identifies a population at much greater nutritional risk. Finally, if the weight-based data are not reliable, a formal nutrition support consult or indirect calorimetry may be indicated.

NUTRITIONAL REQUIREMENTS

Protein

The amount and type of protein administered to the critically ill depends on the clinical circumstances of each patient. Nevertheless, there is an upper limit to the quantity of protein that can be given based on net protein utilization during metabolic stress. In general, providing protein in amounts above 1.75 g/kg/d exceeds the capacity of the body to use the administered protein to increase synthesis [17,18]. Amounts above this level of intake are essentially completely converted to urea and serve no nutritional purpose. At intakes ranging between 0.6 to 1.75 g/kg/d, each increment of intake increases net protein synthesis at a cost of increasing the proportion going to ureagenesis. In patients with nitrogen accumulation disorders (of either renal or hepatic origin), a compromise must often be made between greatest rates of net protein synthesis and lowest rates of urea or ammoniagenesis. For example, as the BUN increases, especially above 100 mg%, the risk of uremic complications increases, including bleeding, or, increasing the production of ammonia in encephalopathic patients. Generally, the optimal protein intake in critically ill patients is given at twice the recommended daily amount (approximately 0.8 g/kg/d) of normal adults, at approximately 1.5 g/kg/d. With renal impairment, at least 1 g per kg should be provided and greater amounts given if tolerated or dialysis is initiated. For patients with liver failure, at least 1 g per kg of standard protein should be provided and up to 1.5 g per kg if tolerated. This is done recognizing the overall impairments in protein utilization that accompanies metabolic stress, as well as the heightened needs during catabolism.

The type of protein administered varies with the patient's condition and the route of administration. For PN support, standard protein mixtures are given in their monomeric form as individual crystalline amino acids and levorotatory isomers, which comprise the essential amino acids (histidine, isoleucine, leucine, lysine, methionine, phenylalanine, threonine, tryptophan, and valine) and the nonessential amino acids (alanine, aminoacetic acid, arginine, cysteine, proline, serine, and tyrosine). In standard amino acid formulations, the branched-chain amino acids (leucine, isoleucine, and valine) comprise approximately 18% to 25% of the amino acid profile. Collectively, they are available in commercial intravenous solutions in concentrations ranging from 3% to 15%. On average, for every 6.25 g of the amino acids in the mixture, 1 g of nitrogen is available, although this number is lower with a number of the specialized amino acid formulas. The caloric value of protein is 4.1 kcal per g, and such calories should be counted in critically ill patients when tracking energy intakes.

Specialized amino acid mixtures have evolved that include selected profiles. For example, renal formulations have been devised that principally provide the essential amino acids (histidine, isoleucine, leucine, lysine, methionine, phenylalanine, threonine, tryptophan, and valine), whereas hepatic formulations have eliminated or reduced aromatic amino acids (phenylalanine, tryptophan, and tyrosine) and the sulfur-containing amino acid methionine and increased the proportion of branched-chain amino acids (isoleucine, leucine, and valine). However, the routine use of these expensive formulations for these conditions over conventional or standard amino acid mixtures has not been convincingly demonstrated and, in certain cases when used to meet full protein needs, may be harmful [19]. For patients with nitrogen accumulation disorders, the use of branched-chain–enriched amino acid formulas in the range of 45% to 50% of the total amino acid profile has been shown to improve protein utilization when total amino acid intakes are given in the 40- to 70-g range and may reduce the risk of encephalopathy when compared to a standard formula. Finally, other attempts at modifying the profiles of amino acid mixtures, such as the extemporaneous preparation by the hospital pharmacy of sterile glutamine in total parenteral nutrition (TPN), have shown some benefits in selected settings, but they require a considerable level of parenteral compounding expertise. In addition, in order to safely provide this compounded sterile preparation, ongoing quality assurance measures as outlined by the *United States Pharmacopeia* (USP) must be performed and, therefore, such practices are subject to the Federal Drug Administration oversight [20]. A glutamine-containing dipeptide formulation, which is commercially available in Europe, has been the subject of some positive trials, but its ultimate place in the care of the critically ill is not yet established. In a recent review of the evidence, however, the safety of glutamine supplementation, when given in pharmacologic doses, has been raised, and caution is advised at this time with respect to its indiscriminant use in the ICU [21]

For EN support, protein is typically provided in either an oligomeric form as protein hydrolysates containing various peptides ranging from di- and tripeptides to polymers of eight or more, or as whole protein usually provided as casein or in its polymeric form as, for example, casein hydrolysates. Less commonly, they can even be provided as the individual amino acids. Most formulations contain a fixed amount of protein in the range of 30 to 40 g per L and thus for fluid-restricted patients in the ICU cannot meet the protein needs of most patients. Alternatively, more concentrated enteral formulas exist that may be used, or the clinician may opt to add protein modules to conventional products to increase protein density. However, in either case, both approaches result in higher osmolarities that may affect GI tolerance.

Carbohydrate

The amount and type of energy provided to improve the utilization of the prescribed protein intake also varies with the individual patient. As well, there are physiologic limits to the amounts given, beyond which significant complications are more likely. For most patients, providing 25 kcal/kg/d is sufficient to support the protein synthetic response to metabolic stress. This is the total energy expenditure of most critically ill, postoperative patients. Amounts above 30 kcal/kg/d exceed the energy expenditure of most hospitalized patients except those with severe burns, closed head injury, and multiple trauma where measured caloric expenditures are usually 30 to 40 kcal per kg. However, providing nutritional support in amounts greater than 30 kcal per kg leads to higher rates of hyperglycemia in both types of patients: in the postoperative setting, because of overfeeding, and in the trauma unit, because of the severity of systemic inflammatory response. Although better glycemic control through the use of insulin would be one way to reduce the infectious risk in the latter instance, it is interesting to note that in several trials of immune-enhancing diets that improved outcomes and reduced infection rates have been seen at energy intakes at 30 kcal per kg or less, in diets that are likely to have been hypocaloric [22]. For carbohydrates, the physiologic limits are linked to the normal endogenous hepatic production rates for glucose, which approximate 2 mg/kg/min or about 200 g per day for a 70-kg healthy adult [23]. This is the amount of glucose needed by the body to meet the obligate needs of tissues dependent on glucose (i.e., brain, renal medulla, red blood cells), and it is derived from body stores of glycogen (glycogenolysis) or made from noncarbohydrate sources such as from protein breakdown to gluconeogenic amino acid precursors (gluconeogenesis). Glycogen stores are limited and, therefore, can be rapidly depleted during acute metabolic stress (i.e., within 24 hours) [24]. Thus, the major source of glucose in the hypocaloric state following stress comes from gluconeogenesis, and higher-than-usual amounts are produced to support the metabolic response to injury, accelerated by the hormonal milieu produced by the increased secretion of catecholamines, glucagon, cortisol, and growth hormone [25]. The judicious provision of nutritional support is designed to attenuate the extent of protein breakdown without exacerbating significant changes in nutritional and metabolic homeostasis. Similar to the case with protein, as carbohydrate intake increases, net oxidation occurs, but with an increasing proportion going to nonoxidative pathways (glycogen synthesis and particularly de novo lipogenesis). However, glycogen synthesis is limited by available storage capacity of about 500 g in normal adults and perhaps 1,000 g in a critically ill patient receiving TPN, with its resultant very high insulin levels. There is effectively no limit for fat storage. The optimal balance is at intakes at about 400 g per day, with maximal glucose oxidized of 700 g per day. Thus, in a 70-kg adult, glucose to amino acid ratio of 2:1 TPN formula providing 400 g per day of glucose and 1.5 g of protein/kg/d represents about 25 kcal/kg/d.

For PN, glucose is the only reasonable carbohydrate fuel or energy source that is widely available for intravenous administration. Generally, it is provided as a monohydrate, and its caloric equivalent is, therefore, 3.4 kcal per g rather than 4 kcal per g for its anhydrous form. It is commercially available in a variety of concentrations ranging from 2.5% to 70% in sterile water for injection. Glucose is the primary energy source of any PN admixture prescribed for central venous alimentation and typically is given in final admixture concentrations from 10% to 25%. Higher concentrations can be given, but are associated with an increase in the number of dextrose-associated complications if the amounts given are too large.

For EN, carbohydrates may be given in a number of chemical forms. For example, they can be given as the monosaccharide, glucose, frequently found in monomeric or elemental formulas. Alternatively, in less refined formulas, carbohydrates may be provided as oligosaccharides, such as hydrolyzed cornstarch, or more complex polysaccharides, such as corn syrup, are frequently used. The selection of a particular enteral formula is largely based on a number of clinical factors, such as GI function, fluid status, and end-organ function.

Fat

Lipids serve as an alternative energy source that is used to substitute for a portion of the carbohydrate calories. PN support prescribed in this fashion, it is referred to as a total nutrient admixture, all-in-one or three-in-one mixed-fuel system [26]. As with protein and carbohydrates, the amount and type of lipids used will vary depending on the clinical condition of the patient. For the most part, long-chain triglycerides (LCTs) derived from vegetable oils have been the principal source of lipid calories used in the clinical setting. Specifically, soybean oil, which is rich in polyunsaturated ω-6 fatty acids, has been extensively used, especially for intravenous nutrition. It is a major source of the proximate essential fatty acids, linoleic, and α-linolenic acids. However, ill-considered prescribing habits, where either excessive quantities or infusion rates have been used, have led to clinically significant adverse effects such as immune dysfunction and pulmonary gas diffusion abnormalities among critically ill patients. The excessive administration of intravenous lipid emulsions (IVLEs) can accumulate in the liver and impair Kupffer cell function, thus interfering with a major component of the reticuloendothelial system [27,28]. In addition, lipid injectable emulsions are composed of various oils that serve as prostaglandin precursors that are immunosuppressive, especially those of the n6 series such as PGE_2, which suppresses lymphocyte proliferation and natural killer cell activity [29], and can reverse hypoxic vasoconstriction in patients with adult respiratory distress syndrome [30]. In contrast, the oxidation and subsequent plasma clearance of lipids are significantly improved when IVLEs are given over 24 hours versus briefer intervals [30]. Impaired plasma clearance of lipids can result in fat overload syndrome and is a particularly significant clinical issue in children [31–42]. Fat overload syndrome can result from the administration of a stable fat emulsion over brief intervals [30,43–48] or from more modest doses of lipid that might be physicochemically unstable [49]. In fact, a review of the literature regarding *stable* fat emulsions has concluded that virtually all of the adverse effects associated with LCTs have occurred when the infusion rate exceeds 0.11 g/kg/h [50]. For a 70-kg adult, this limit would be approximately 13 hours for 500 mL of 20%, which makes three-in-one admixture infusions safer and easier to administer as a continuous infusion over 24 hours rather than as a separate "IV piggyback" over a brief period, which would require an infusion rate almost twice as fast. In addition, piggyback infusion of lipids is not recommended beyond 12 hours [51].

Recent reports regarding the clinical significance of unstable fat emulsions have emerged. On December 1, 2007, the USP, which is recognized by the Food and Drug Administration (FDA) as the official compendium for drug standards, was the first pharmacopeia worldwide to establish globule size limits for IVLEs [52]. This is notable because IVLEs had been used clinically in the United States for more than 30 years (and Europe for more than 45 years), when most drugs have official USP specifications within 5 years of FDA approval [53]. The USP limits specified two size limits: (i) mean droplet size <0.5 µm and (ii) large-diameter tail, expressed as the percent of fat globules >5 µm ($PFAT_5$ $<0.05\%$). The primary motivation for these limits was to avoid the development of microvascular pulmonary embolism from an excessive population of large-diameter fat globules indicating instability of the emulsion.

Around the time the USP announced its intentions to adopt these limits in 2004 [54], a major lipid emulsion product also changed its conventional packaging from glass to plastic containers. With this change in packaging, the lipid emulsion product now failed the large-diameter globule limits of the USP [55]. Lipid emulsions failing USP limits were also shown to produce less stable emulsions when packaged in syringes for neonates [56], when mixed in TPN admixtures [57], and when used in a multichamber bag premixed for TPN therapy [58]. Moreover, lipid emulsions not meeting pharmacopeial limits were also shown to be associated with significant hypertriglyceridemia in premature neonates when compared to lipid emulsions meeting USP limits [59], although this has not been confirmed in a randomized clinical trial. Finally, in animal studies, lipid emulsions failing USP limits were shown to be hepatotoxic [60]. A recent study intended to explore the extent of physiologic damage from the infusion of unstable lipid emulsions produced evidence of hepatic accumulation of fat associated with oxidative stress, liver injury, and a low-level systemic inflammatory response [61].

Triglyceride clearance is maximal at serum triglyceride levels of up to about 400 mg per dL, and patients who initially have serum triglycerides at this level will tolerate even lesser amounts of fat without adverse consequences. Among patients who have normal serum triglyceride levels at initiation of TPN, serum triglyceride levels are usually not monitored. For those with levels greater than 200 mg per dL it is reasonable to check the triglyceride again after a stable regimen has been attained with lipids below 0.11 g/kg/h. Stable levels below 400 mg per dL are acceptable while receiving lipid emulsions.

For PN therapy, soybean oil emulsions continue to dominate the US market, but recently, an 80:20 olive oil to soybean oil physical has been introduced. A 100% fish oil-in-water emulsion has been available on a compassionate use basis for several years, but is primarily directed at the pediatric population as therapy for PN-related liver disease. However, there are a number of different lipid compositions presently available in Europe and under investigation in the United States [62]. They include various mixtures of soybean oil with medium-chain triglycerides (MCTs), olive oil, and fish oil. In nearly every case, soybean oil is included in sufficient proportions to provide adequate amounts of the essential fatty acids [63,64].

For EN therapy, a number of the lipid types available for parenteral use in Europe are widely available in the United States for enteral administration in complete nutritional diets. Typically, they contain 30% to 40% of the total calories as fat and often contain blends of corn and soy oil. However, in the more specialized enteral formulas, MCTs, fish oil, and even structured lipids are available. Moreover, in some of these products, the fat content is either severely restricted (i.e., 3% to 10% of total calories for the fat-intolerant patient) or may be as high as 55% for the patient with pulmonary compromise.

Volume

The maintenance of fluid homeostasis is an important goal in critical care. At times, many patients in the ICU become severely volume overloaded as a consequence of parenteral fluid administration and the fluid-retentive state characteristic of critical illness [65–67]. For this reason, when assessing fluid status, it is important to bear in mind the usual contribution of water to body weight or TBW of the patient under normal, unstressed conditions. In normal adults, TBW comprises approximately 50% to 60% of body weight. Because lean body mass is hydrated in a ratio of approximately 4 parts water to 1 part protein, lean tissue is a significant component of TBW. In the clinical setting, acute changes in weight over short intervals primarily reflect net changes in TBW which almost never reflect lean tissue gains in the hospital setting. For example, a 10% increase in weight over 24 to 48 hours represents a proportional increase in TBW and may be associated with adverse clinical consequences, such as greater ventilator dependence, impaired cardiovascular function, and disturbances of electrolyte homeostasis. Even when the patient is considered euvolemic, the contributions to volume from nutritional support are generally limited to approximately 25 mL/kg/d, because other reasons for fluid administration are usually indicated.

Depending on the volume assessments by the primary care team, the amount of nutrition support that may be provided by either PN or EN may be affected. The most significant effect occurs when volume restrictions are imposed. When this happens, hypocaloric nutrition is usually provided owing to the limitations associated with caloric density. Caloric or macronutrient density is the sum total of calories from protein, carbohydrates, and fat, expressed in kilocalories per milliliter (kcal per mL). Generally, the caloric density of typical formulations routinely prescribed for either PN or EN support is approximately 1 kcal per mL, but special forms of each therapy are available that reasonably allow up to 1.5 kcal per mL to be formulated. However, most enteral formulations are commercially available in fixed concentrations and, therefore, are less easily manipulated to the specific needs of the critically ill patient than with the PN admixture. For example, with a 1,000 mL fluid restriction allotted for PN support, the increased macronutrient density could be achieved to attain eucaloric nutrition for adult patients weighing up to 60 kg (25 kcal per kg). Of course, these special dosage forms are generally more expensive than conventional products, and the cost to benefit ratio has not been fully demonstrated. The usual parenteral formula provided when fluid restriction is necessary is a more standard PN admixture [68], providing 70 g of amino acids and 210 g of glucose (A7D21) approximating 1,000 kcal in a 1 L final volume when compounded from the standard 10% amino acid (700 mL) and 70% dextrose (300 mL) stock solutions, and is usually given for short periods of up to 10 days. Such a formula offers a compromise of the usual desired protein and caloric goals and may provide for a clinical outcome not distinguishable from higher protein, eucaloric regimens [69]. Tables 213.4 and 213.5 provide examples of PN formulations that may be used in the acute critical care setting in adult patients who are fluid restricted (i.e., 1,000 mL for TPN), whose regimens are often hypocaloric for clinical and practical reasons (see Table 213.4), as well as for goal amounts of nutrients in TPN in the absence of fluid restrictions [70]. A recent analysis of highly concentrated TPN admixtures, using a 16% crystalline amino acid solution–containing lipid injectable emulsions in eucaloric amounts, showed them to be stable for up to 30 hours with a net fluid savings of approximately 20% compared with conventional 10% amino acid formulations [71]. Patient-specific PN therapy for pediatric patients (premature, neonate, infant, and adolescent) may be devised using specific practice guidelines [72].

Electrolytes

There are seven key electrolytes that must be monitored and provided as necessary in nutritional admixtures. In some cases, certain electrolytes must be given in *standard* quantities as part of the recommend dietary allowance, whereas others are given in *variable* amounts and replaced according to the clinical needs of the patient. However, in both cases, the daily requirements can be highly variable especially during acute illness for a variety of reasons, including drug therapy [73,74]. As well, in all cases, certain electrolytes may be deliberately omitted because of retention disorders associated with certain disease states. This, of course, is more difficult to accomplish with enteral formulas that contain fixed amounts of nutrients and electrolytes. Nevertheless, avoiding the consequences of wide fluctuations in serum electrolyte concentrations that may assume clinical significance in the critical care setting is an important and necessary goal.

Standard Additives

Calcium. Approximately 98% of total body calcium is present in the skeleton. Thus, the extracellular concentration in plasma is but a fraction of total calcium stores and is tightly regulated by parathyroid hormone. As absorption of calcium from the GI

TABLE 213.4

Hypocaloric 1,000 mL Total Parenteral Nutrition Regimens as a Single-versus Mixed-fuel System in intensive Care Unit Patient

		Single-fuel		Mixed-fuel		
Weight (kg)	Total kcal/d[a]	Amino acids[b] (%)	Glucose[c] (%)	Amino acids (%)	Glucose (%)	Lipids[d] (%)
40	600	40 g or 266 mL (4)[e]	128 g or 183 mL (12.8)[e]	40 g or 266 mL (4)[e]	75 g or 107 mL (7.5)[e]	20 g or 100 mL (2)[e]
50	750	50 g or 333 mL (5)[e]	160 g or 228 mL (16)[e]	50 g or 333 mL (5)[e]	96 g or 137 mL (9.6)[e]	24 g or 120 mL (2.4)[e]
60	900	60 g or 400 mL (6)[e]	192 g or 275 mL (19.2)[e]	60 g or 400 mL (6)[e]	115 g or 164 mL (11.5)[e]	29 g or 145 mL (2.9)[e]
70	1,050	70 g or 466 mL (7)[e]	224 g or 320 mL (22.4)[e]	70 g or 466 mL (7)[e]	135 g or 192 mL (13.5)[e]	34 g or 170 mL (3.4)[e]
80	1,200	80 g or 533 mL (8)[e]	256 g or 366 mL (25.6)[e]	80 g or 533 mL (8)[e]	154 g or 220 mL (15.4)[e]	39 g or 195 mL (3.9)[e]

[a]Calories from the hypocaloric regimen consists of 1 g/kg/d of protein and 15 kcal/kg/d total or approximately 50% to 60% of needs. Hypocaloric regimens that are intended as permissive underfeeding are often intended for patients whose present weight is within 10% of ideal body weight.
[b]Assumes a stock bottle of 15% amino acids at 4.1 kcal/g.
[c]Assumes a stock bottle of 70% hydrated dextrose at 3.4 kcal/g.
[d]Assumes a stock bottle of 20% lipid emulsion at 9 kcal/g and providing approximately 20% of total calories.
[e]Final concentration of nutrient in 1,000 mL of total parenteral nutrition fluid.
From Driscoll DF: Formulation of enteral and parenteral mixtures, in Pichard C, Kudsk KA (eds): *Update in Intensive Care Medicine*. Brussels, Springer-Verlag, 2000, pp 138–150, with permission.

tract diminishes because of impaired absorption or decreased or absent intake, and serum levels begin to fall, the parathyroid glands sense these changes and secrete parathormone that promotes calcium mobilization from bone to restore normal serum concentrations. However, critical illness disturbs normal calcium homeostasis, and mild depressions of total and free calcium concentrations are common [75]. The parenteral equivalent of the recommended dietary allowance (pRDA) for adults is about 25% of the oral RDA or 200 mg (10 mEq or 5 mmol) of elemental calcium daily. Higher amounts may be used if needed when seeking to maintain calcium at the lower limit of normal, but this does increase the risk of incompatibility with phosphate salts that could produce fatal pulmonary emboli [76–78]. Therefore, if higher amounts are needed, it may be necessary to use fat emulsion-free formulas that allow greater amounts of calcium and phosphate to be infused safely. The other alternative, separate infusions of calcium should be done with great care especially if given through peripheral vein, because extravasation injury can be severe [79–81]. In addition, the separate administration of parenteral calcium may be incompatible as a coinfusion with other common infusions applied in the critical care setting, such as sodium bicarbonate. Moreover, if parenteral calcium is given intermittently and the same intravenous line is to be used for other medications, it should be flushed with saline or other suitable parenteral fluid (i.e., D5W) immediately following termination of the calcium infusion. Parenteral forms of calcium are commercially available in three forms, including the gluconate, acetate, and chloride salts. Of these, the gluconate form is preferred in PN admixtures, because it is least capable of forming insoluble products. However, for immediate delivery of calcium in emergency situations such as severe hypocalcemia, the chloride form is the best form for bioavailability reasons,

TABLE 213.5

Eucaloric, Euvolemic Total Parenteral Nutrition Regimens as a Single-versus Mixed-Fuel System in Intensive Care Unit patients

		Single-fuel		Mixed-fuel		
Weight (kg)	Total kcal/d[a]	Amino acids[b]	Glucose[c]	Amino acids	Glucose	Lipids[d]
40	1,000	60 g or 400 mL	222 g or 317 mL	60 g or 400 mL	166 g or 237 mL	21 g or 105 mL
50	1,250	75 g or 500 mL	277 g or 396 mL	75 g or 500 mL	208 g or 297 mL	26 g or 130 mL
60	1,500	90 g or 600 mL	333 g or 476 mL	90 g or 600 mL	250 g or 357 mL	31 g or 155 mL
70	1,750	105 g or 700 mL	388 g or 554 mL	105 g or 700 mL	290 g or 414 mL	37 g or 185 mL
80	2,000	120 g or 800 mL	444 g or 634 mL	120 g or 800 mL	333 g or 476 mL	42 g or 210 mL

[a]Calories from the eucaloric and euvolemic regimen consists of 1.5 g/kg/d of protein and 25 mL/kg/day, respectively. Eucaloric and euvolemic regimens are in conformance with the ASPEN Guidelines for safe total parenteral nutrition formulations and intended for patients whose present weight is within 10% of ideal body weight.
[b]Assumes a stock bottle of 15% amino acids at 4.1 kcal/g.
[c]Assumes a stock bottle of 70% hydrated dextrose at 3.4 kcal/g.
[d]Assumes a stock bottle of 20% lipid emulsion at 9 kcal/g and providing approximately 25% of total calories.
From Driscoll DF: Formulation of enteral and parenteral mixtures, in Pichard C, Kudsk KA (eds): *Update in Intensive Care Medicine*. Brussels, Springer-Verlag, 2000, pp 138–150, with permission.

although it is the most reactive salts with respect to compatibility with nutrient formulas and, therefore, should not be employed when compounding TPN formulas.

Magnesium. Another predominant intracellular cation, magnesium, plays a pivotal role in calcium metabolism. For parathyroid hormone to be secreted in response to hypocalcemia, magnesium is required [82]. In certain instances, corrections of serum magnesium concentrations have been sufficient to normalize hypocalcemia [83]. Such responses have been viewed as an indication of the extent of magnesium deficiency [84]. Furthermore, similar to calcium, hypomagnesemia is commonly seen in critical illness, and the goal is similar (i.e., to maintain levels at about the lower limit of normal). The pRDA is about 33% of the oral RDA or 120 mg (10 mEq or 5 mmol) for elemental magnesium per day. The only parenteral form of magnesium available is as the sulfate salt.

Phosphorus. Phosphorus is an essential element involved in numerous life-sustaining metabolic processes. For example, if omitted from a PN admixture, a life-threatening hypophosphatemia may ensue within days of initiating therapy. Like magnesium and calcium, it too is predominantly found in the intracellular compartment. However, because its GI absorption is highly efficient, the pRDA for phosphorus is the same as its oral RDA at 1,000 mg (30 mmol) daily. The use of milliequivalent units to describe phosphorus concentrations in a solution is often mistakenly applied. At this time, the only parenteral form of phosphorus commercially available in the United States is a mixture of inorganic salts of monobasic ($H_2PO_4^-$) and dibasic (HPO_4^-) phosphate ions. Milliequivalents are defined as the molecular weight (in mg) divided by the valence of a single ion, which is determined by the pH of the final solution. Because the pharmaceutic dosage form is a mixture of two ions and has a finite yet variable pH range, the dosage form cannot be accurately described in mEq units. However, because sodium and potassium are the accompanying anions, it has become traditional to order them in terms of mEq units where, for example, 30 mmol of phosphorus is found in about 40 mEq of the commonly available formulations.

Variable Additives

Sodium. Sodium is often prescribed in daily amounts ranging from 60 to 100 mEq each day. However, certain clinical conditions preclude the use of sodium beyond minute quantities (i.e., 0 to 20 mEq per day) such as found with florid congestive heart failure, end-stage liver disease, and during attempts to reduce massive volume overload characterized by extensive third-spacing of fluids by volume restriction and active diuresis. In contrast, patients with severe sodium deficits can require daily amounts that may be as much as three to four times higher than typical quantities given to those without sodium restrictions. There is limited to no impact of sodium amounts on nutritional efficacy. Parenteral forms of sodium are available as chloride, acetate, and phosphate salts.

Potassium. Potassium is often prescribed in daily amounts ranging from 40 to 80 mEq each day. As described earlier, there are extreme clinical conditions that may require either severe restriction or expansion of the daily dose so that ranges of potassium intake may be from 0 to 400 or more mEq per day. For instance, a severe amphotericin-induced renal loss of potassium of 100 mEq per L with a 4-L urine output can be managed by placing an equivalent amount in the parenteral formula so long as close monitoring of potassium in the serum and urine output is provided. In all cases, serum potassium concentrations should be closely monitored, because the safe clinical range is narrow and levels outside may produce severe and even life-threatening cardiovascular complications. Like sodium, parenteral forms of potassium are available as chloride, acetate, and phosphate salts.

Chloride. Chloride salts are widely used for nutrition support. Most often, they are provided as sodium and potassium salts and quantitatively constitute the majority of anions present in nutritional formulations. In the past, an emphasis on chloride salts with parenteral crystalline amino acid formulations had tended to produce an iatrogenic metabolic acidosis. However, these formulations have since been revised and balanced with an appropriate amount of acetate ions. Thus, it is not necessary to include the inherent concentrations of chloride and acetate present in amino acid products in the additive calculation for the final PN admixture.

Acetate. Acetate salts are primarily used when clinically indicated for the treatment of metabolic acidemia. They are the only suitable alkalinizing salt for use in nutritional formulations. With respect to alkalinizing power, acetate is equivalent to bicarbonate, but this requires cellular metabolism to be effective. Bicarbonate salts should never be used in PN admixtures because they can form insoluble carbonates with calcium ions that are present in most nutritional admixtures and, as such, could result in the formation of fatal pulmonary emboli [85].

Trace Minerals

To provide a balanced nutritional formulation, trace minerals are generally included in most nutritional formulations. These include chromium, copper, manganese, selenium, and zinc. In addition, iodine, and molybdenum may be present in certain formulations. However, for most acute situations, the absence of trace minerals for brief periods (days to weeks) will not produce clinically significant adverse effects. In contrast, the absence of trace minerals in the patient receiving long-term PN support may lead to significant deficiency [86]. However, because manganese is excreted in bile, there is some concern about manganese overload when chronically provided to patients receiving long-term home TPN. Iron is a special case, because hypoferremia is an invariable consequence of the systemic inflammatory response. Furthermore, large amounts of parenteral iron supplementation may worsen septic states. For this reason, iron is not usually provided in TPN formulas during critical illness and when provided to nonseptic patients in home, PN should only be provided when clinically necessary, because iron overload can result in patients with short gut syndromes who have substantial enteral intake. Iron is incompatible in fat emulsion-containing formulas.

Vitamins

Multivitamins are an essential component of all nutritional formulations. This is particularly true for PN formulations. During the national vitamin shortage that occurred in the summer of 1988, three patients died as a result of receiving vitamin-free PN in a matter of 3 to 5 weeks [87]. Ultimately, the cause of death was related to acute thiamine deficiency producing a refractory lactic acidosis. As a water-soluble vitamin, thiamine is an important cofactor in the entry of pyruvate into the Krebs cycle as well as facilitating the processing of glucose within the Krebs cycle. In the absence of thiamine, pyruvate cannot enter the Krebs cycle and is, therefore, converted to lactic acid. The administration of hypertonic dextrose, the major energy component of PN therapy, accelerates the consumption of thiamine and thus accentuates the clinical course of the condition. Therefore, multivitamins are an essential part of any nutrition support regimen.

The FDA has mandated a change in the composition of adult parenteral multivitamins after nearly 30 years of clinical use [88]. The concentrations of four vitamins (thiamine, pyridoxine, ascorbic acid, and folate) were increased by 50% to 100% of previous amounts and, for the first time, vitamin K has been added at 150 mcg per vial. This latter addition may well have some impact on therapeutic doses of warfarin for full anticoagulation as well as for low-dose warfarin therapy for home TPN patients. Lastly, with respect to enteral feeding formulas, the RDA for vitamins is generally met when caloric intakes are between 1,500 to 2,000 kcal per day.

Immunonutrients

There have been a number of nutritional additives that have been alternatively given in supraphysiologic amounts in an effort to improve outcomes. The main ones would include lipids composed of high concentrations of the unsaturated long-chain fatty acids containing n3 or n9 fatty acids, medium-chain saturated fatty acids (MCFAs), and certain "conditionally essential" amino acids. Historically, soybean oil, containing polyunsaturated fatty acids (PUFAs), rich in the 18-carbon essential (cannot be synthesized endogenously) n6 fatty acid linoleic acid and n3 fatty acid α-linolenic acid, has been the main source of fat used in lipid injectable emulsions. These fatty acids are the precursors to the true "necessary" fatty acids, arachidonic and eicosapentaenoic acids from the n6 and n3 families, respectively, whereas the n9 fatty acid, oleic acid is nonessential (i.e., can be synthesized endogenously) [89].

Unfortunately, however, the n6 fatty acids from soybean oil can be proinflammatory and potentially detrimental when provided in large amounts to the critically ill, especially in patients with adult respiratory distress syndrome [30,45–46,90–94]. Therefore, substitution of a portion of the conventional n6 fatty acids with alternative lipid fuels such as the n3 fatty acids (20- and 22-carbon PUFAs) from fish oil, or 18-carbon monounsaturated n9 fatty acids from olive oil, or saturated MCFAs from coconut oil (mostly comprises 8- to 10-carbons), may modulate the proinflammatory response. Thus, one benefit of these alternative lipid sources is a reduction in the intake of the highly vasoactive n6 PUFA precursors to ones with less pronounced effects on eicosanoid metabolism by changing the fatty acid composition of cell membranes [64]. The n6 PUFAs produce proinflammatory eicosanoids (i.e., prostaglandins, prostacyclins, thromboxanes, leukotrienes) and increase the responsiveness of cytokines (i.e., interleukin [IL]-1, IL-6, and tumor necrosis factor) which subsequently lead to an increased systemic inflammatory response. Meanwhile, the n3 and n9 lipids lead to eicosanoids that are less proinflammatory and even anti-inflammatory. Another benefit is related to a unique metabolic action of the substituted lipid(s) that may have favorable clinical implications. In the case of MCFAs, their metabolism is independent of carnitine transport into the mitochondria with rapid oxidation and less interference with the reticuloendothelial system, whereas olive oil may be better tolerated with respect to liver function in certain patients receiving conventional soybean oil–based formulations [95].

Of the amino acids used in clinical nutrition, arginine and glutamine have purportedly been shown to exert favorable immune effects in patients receiving nutrition support. Arginine has been shown to stimulate T-cell function and wound healing, but may be harmful in certain patients under certain conditions depending on dose [96,97]. Thus, its role in immune enhancement has not been clearly defined, and it is most often given as part of a complex nutritional formula containing other potential immunonutrients. Nonetheless, there appears to be a correlation of demonstrable benefits at doses exceeding 4% of the total energy intake [97]. Glutamine is the most abundant amino acid in the human body, a precursor to glutathione, and an important nutrient for rapidly dividing immune cells such as lymphocytes and macrophages. Despite its abundance, serum and tissue glutamine concentrations fall during critical illness, which largely reflects its diverse needs during acute metabolic stress. Its role in clinical nutrition is also not well defined, and, in a large clinical trial in ICU patients, no differences in outcomes were noted between groups receiving 20 g per L versus a conventional enteral formula that was isonitrogenous and isocaloric [98]. Data with parenteral glutamine tend to be more positive in the critically ill, which may reflect the prominent first-pass clearance of enteral glutamine limiting systemic appearance of the amino acid.

Two recent clinical trials have greatly altered the conventional viewpoint that immunonutrients have a net beneficial effect, that is, the so-called "REDOXS" [99] and "METAPLUS" [100] trials. In a recent commentary that included the lead authors of these studies, they point out the "signal of benefit" that has been widely acknowledged comes from older studies from single-center trials, whereas evidence of a "signal of harm", as they have recently reported, is much stronger because the data comes from two large, adequately powered, multicenter trials [101]. They, and others [102,103], have concluded that these diets should not be routinely administered to critically ill patients.

DIFFERENCES BETWEEN ENTERAL AND PARENTERAL NUTRITIONS

Nutrition support may be provided in a variety of ways ranging from noninvasive approaches such as dietary counseling for food and oral supplements to invasive forms of therapy. Of the interventional approaches to nutrition support, these can be accomplished by aseptic placement of intravascular catheters (i.e., PN), or by extravascular devices placed into the GI tract (i.e., EN). Each invasive form of nutrition support has its advantages and disadvantages, and the selection of either approach must be individualized.

Routes of Administration

Enteral Nutrition Options

Like PN therapy, EN can be delivered in a variety of ways with some potential advantages of one access route over the other. The options include gastric, duodenal, and jejunal placement of various enteral feeding catheters. The simplest technique is the nasogastric placement of a feeding tube into the stomach. However, this approach is often associated with the greatest degree of GI intolerance and thus reduced delivery of protein and energy compared to feeding tubes placed in the intestine. A higher degree of successful feeding is likely with nasoenteric tubes or those placed via fluoroscopic, endoscopic, or surgical placement of the feeding catheter beyond the ligament of Treitz. Furthermore, enteral feeding catheters placed in the upper jejunum may allow feeding of patients with severe pancreatitis [104]. However, placement of feeding tubes in the jejunum postinjury rarely occurs spontaneously and generally requires fluoroscopic or endoscopic assistance, which is expensive and can delay feeding. A recent study of mechanically ventilated patients who were fed via a nasogastric or nasojejunal feeding tube for 10 days showed no differences of energy delivery, 71% versus 72% of target, nor rates of ventilator-associated pneumonia, 20% versus 21% [105]. Of note, there was higher incidence of "minor" episodes of GI bleeding in the nasojejunal-fed group, but of the two promotility agents used in this study (metoclopramide and erthyromycin), they received erythromycin more frequently than in the nasogastric-fed group (87% vs. 62%, $p = 0.001$). Erythromycin is known to cause epigastric distress which may be responsible for the GI bleeding observed. Finally, a recent Cochrane meta-analysis of the differences between postpyloric versus gastric tube feeding for preventing pneumonia and improving nutritional outcomes in ICU patients found "moderate-quality" evidence of a 30% reduction in the rate of pneumonia associated with postpyloric feeding, as well as "low-quality" evidence showing an increase in the amount of nutrition delivered [106]. The use of a postpyloric feeding tube was recommended, when feasible.

Parenteral Nutrition Options

PN may be provided by either peripheral or central venous access. Peripheral venous access is clearly less invasive and has minimal complications. The most significant complications are related to maintenance of the patency of the venous catheter and thrombophlebitis and the limited use of each venipuncture site for a relatively short duration. Most peripheral vein catheters will last between 48 and 72 hours from the time of the initial insertion, and, therefore, a systematic rotation of other infusion sites must be performed. Ultimately, however, the number of viable peripheral venipuncture sites is limited and generally of little practical value in the ICU setting. Moreover, owing to the osmolarity limits of these low-flow blood vessels, very large fluid volumes are required to approach protein and energy requirements for most patients, which is not practical in the ICU setting. Peripherally inserted central (venous) catheters (PICCs) generally last longer and can even be used to provide hypertonic PN admixtures. However, the inability to change catheters over guidewires for PICCs, and a greater likelihood of mechanical complications, makes this a less desirable alternative to a central venous catheter.

By far, central venous catheterization is most commonly used to deliver PN therapy. Invariably, central venous access is necessary for virtually all patients requiring ICU care, so the delivery of PN therapy does not introduce unique clinical risks associated with catheter placement (i.e., pneumothorax, catheter malposition, catheter infections, and so forth). In addition to supplying nutrition support, the PN admixture can also be used as a vehicle to provide intensive metabolic support such as replacement of large amounts of electrolytes and correction of acid–base balance, which otherwise could not be accomplished by peripheral vein or EN therapy, largely because of osmolarity limitations. Moreover, it has also been used as a vehicle for selected pharmacotherapies [107].

Parenteral versus Enteral Nutrition and Complications

Approximately 25 years ago, there was a significant push toward the use of EN over PN as being a safer mode of nutrient supplementation. The principal benefit purportedly associated with the use of EN is reduced infectious complications compared with PN support in the critically ill. Three key investigations conducted in trauma patients were largely responsible for promoting EN over PN, showing that patients receiving the latter mode of nutritional support had significantly higher rates of infectious complications [108–110]. In addition, this association appeared to be subsequently confirmed by meta-analysis [111]. However, as eloquently pointed out by Jeejeebhoy [112] in 2001, studies such as these are significantly flawed in that the groups receiving PN have significantly higher energy intakes that are associated with significantly higher blood glucose levels, which predispose them to nosocomial infections. Higher energy intakes are easily obtainable via PN, whereas they are more difficult to achieve with EN during acute illness as a result of GI intolerance [113].

Subsequently, Simpson and Doig [114] conducted a more sensitive approach to meta-analysis comparing studies of PN versus EN only in the critically ill. Previous systematic reviews of the risks and benefits of nutrition support have relied on a composite scales technique that combines certain dimensions of the quality of the selected trial used in the meta-analysis into a combined summary score. Consequently, important differences in methodologic quality (i.e., concealment of allocation, appropriate blinding, and analysis according to the intention-to-treat principle) may be overlooked, making well-conducted studies appear poorly conducted [115]. In contrast, the approach by Simpson and Doig in assessing PN versus EN, using the intent-to-treat principle, applied a component scale technique and demonstrated increased infectious complications with PN, but more importantly, reduced mortality by 50% compared with enteral feeding. This impressive benefit was also shown to be largely the effect of early feeding, because a post hoc analysis of TPN versus early enteral feeding showed no difference in mortality [114]. The latter finding was in contradistinction to previous analyses applying the composite scales approach in assessing the benefits and risks of PN [111,116]. Subsequently, in a large multicenter, randomized clinical trial (1,372 patients), Doig et al. have shown that the use of early PN (ready-to-mix, three-chamber bag containing standard amounts amino acids, glucose, lipids, and electrolytes, but at different infusion rates for energy targets of up to 35 kcal/kg/d) versus "standard care" (which was defined pragmatically outside the PN protocol) did not result in significant differences in 60-day mortality or infection rates, and, thus, there was no associated harm from early PN therapy [117].

The seminal publication by Van den Berghe et al. [118] in 2001 showed a significant morbidity and mortality benefit for surgical ICU patients receiving adequate nutrition either enterally or parenterally or by combination when blood glucose levels were aggressively managed with the intravenous infusion of insulin, and the clinical significance of hyperglycemia in nutritional support was clearly established. Two groups of patients were studied ($n = 1{,}548$) to receive either "intensive" or "conventional" insulin therapy concurrent with PN. Blood glucose management assigned to the "intensive" insulin therapy group was treated with an insulin infusion if levels were above 110 mg%, whereas, in the "conventional" insulin therapy group, insulin was initiated at levels above 215 mg%. The standard infusion consisted of 50 units of insulin in 50 mL of 0.9% sodium chloride solution (1 units per mL), and the maximum insulin dose was arbitrarily set at 50 units per hour for all groups. Hypoglycemia was defined as a blood glucose determination of 40 mg% or less. Within 24 hours, on average, all patients received approximately 1 g of protein and 19 kcal/kg/24 hours, respectively. Significant reductions in in-hospital morbidity (e.g., renal and hepatic function, bloodstream infections, polyneuropathy) and mortality were observed in the "intensive" versus "conventional" insulin therapy group, where, for example, control of the morning blood glucose levels for all patients was significantly different between groups (103 ± 33 mg% vs. 153 ± 19 mg%, respectively). Additional significant clinical benefits (e.g., days on ventilator, lower Simplified Therapeutic Intervention Scoring System-28 scores) were also noted for those patients with ICU stays exceeding 5 days.

A follow-up study by Van den Berghe et al. [119] in 2006 was conducted, but this time it was performed in medical ICU patients receiving EN. Unfortunately, the nutrition support data were not as clearly presented as in the 2001 study, but inferences are made as to how it was supplied. The nutritional goals stated from the outset was 22 to 30 kcal/kg/24 h (with approximately 20% to 40% of energy as fat calories) and protein at between 0.5 and 1.5 g/kg/24 h, with EN beginning as early as possible, once the patient was hemodynamically stable. Subsequently, in the results, two figures are shown that give more details about the success of achieving the stated nutritional goals during this study. One depicts the "total intake of nonprotein calories (kcal per 24 hours)" versus "day" showing that a steady amount of calories (between approximately 1,500 and 1,600 calories per day) were achieved by days 3 and 4 of the 14-day profile. The other depicts the "fraction of kilocalories administered by enteral route" versus "day" showing achievement of 50% of total calories via EN at day 7 and roughly 70% by day 12 of the 14-day profile. The slow progression of EN support is expected in critically ill patients, as contrasted from their previous PN study showing rapid advancement of protein and calories [118]. No significant improvements of mortality were noted, but morbidity (e.g., acute renal failure, days on ventilator) was reduced for patients receiving "intensive" insulin therapy. Of note, for the patients staying in the ICU for less than 3 days (n = 433) ("and for whom data were censored after randomization") [119], 56 deaths occurred in the "intensive" versus 42 deaths in the "conventional" insulin infusion group. Moreover, although the severity of hypoglycemia was similar between groups, hypoglycemia was more common in the "intensive" insulin treatment group. A subsequent logistic regression analysis revealed hypoglycemia to be an independent risk factor for death, prompting the investigators to speculate "that the benefit from intensive insulin therapy requires time to be realized" [119]. For patients staying 3 days or more, the mortality benefits seen in the previous study [118] were similarly observed and may support their theory of a time-dependent benefit of aggressive blood glucose management. From a nutritional perspective, the slow progression of protein and calories via the enteral route suggests significant caution in applying aggressive insulin therapy in medical ICU patients receiving EN support only, because parenteral glucose may make hypoglycemia less likely.

A closer evaluation of the manuscript and the table provided in a supplemental appendix reveals that rather marginal amounts of protein and adequate calories were given to the "intention-to-treat group (n = 1,200)" at approximately 40 g of protein and 1,200 kcal daily, whereas in the "long stayers (in ICU 3 days or more)," approximately 50 g of protein and 1,500 kcal daily were given. It is also obvious from this table that the parenteral infusions were glucose only and not TPN, and that the protein intake in the first 72 hours was about 10 g protein per day. Thus, these critically ill patients did not receive early, adequate feeding, which should be the goal in the critically ill. Furthermore, this less than optimal nutritional therapy was provided at a rather high cost in terms of hypoglycemia with an incidence of 25.1% versus 3.9% in the intensive versus conventional treatment in the long stayers in the ICU. More recently, the risk of significant hypoglycemia in patients receiving EN versus PN has been observed in the so-called "CALORIES" trial. In a randomized trial comparing the route of administration in early nutrition support in critically ill adults, there were no differences between groups in 30-day mortality; however, the EN group experienced significantly higher rates of vomiting and hypoglycemia [120]. GI intolerance would be expected to be higher via EN, but of note, caloric intake was similar in the two groups even though the target delivery of 25 kcal/kg/d was not achieved in a majority of the patients in each study group. Nonetheless, as pointed out by the investigators, the focus of the evaluation of the delivery route was uncomplicated by the dose of nutrients. Importantly, despite the same amounts of calorie intake over 5 days, hypoglycemic episodes occurred in 74 of 1,197 patients in the EN groups versus 44 of 1,191 in the PN group (p = 0.006). Whether this effect was the result of less "absorbable" calories as a result of vomiting and/or the difficulty in managing EN patients with more precise doses of insulin, was not addressed in this study.

A series of recent randomized clinical trials have further clarified the role of nutritional support in the broader group of critically ill patients in general ICUs. A recent large pragmatic trial by Harvey et al. [120] of TPN compared to EN where both groups received 15 to 20 kcal per kg with a goal of 25 kcal per kg, that is, were effectively permissively underfed, demonstrated no morbidity or mortality differences. This study along with the Heidegger et al.'s trial [121], where supplemental TPN at 103% of energy versus 77% of energy (goal 25 kcal per kg for women and 30 kcal per kg for men) with better protein intake (0.8 vs. 1.2 g per kg) in the former, reduced infection rates, strongly support the contention that in modern clinical practice where feeding is with more modest goal intakes of <30 kcal per kg approximating energy expenditure or at lower levels of permissive underfeeding in conjunction with control of blood glucose to <180 mg per dL have made TPN as safe as EN. Permissive underfeeding which is providing a fraction of between 50% and 75% of the caloric expenditure, usually estimated in most studies to be approximately 25 kcal per kg for the majority of critically ill patients in the ICU, certainly makes blood glucose control easier. Whether it improves morbidity or mortality compared to full feeding at 25 kcal per kg is uncertain when the control group receives about 100% of this estimate rather than some larger multiple as was common in earlier studies, and when blood glucose is well controlled. One trial that did compare supplemental TPN feeding in the first week of critical illness that provided 25 kcal per kg in the control group versus <10 kcal per kg in the first week and 15 to 20 kcal per kg over the entire study period had increased infections and ventilator and renal replacement requirements, suggesting a disadvantage to early TPN compared to inadequate feeding [122]. However, the unusual use of hypertonic dextrose, which can be immunosuppressive, for 48 hours before initiation of TPN make this a difficult study to evaluate particularly in light of the more recent evidence of the relative safety of TPN. In a trial of early TPN with a goal of approximately 35 kcal per kg in critically ill patients with short-term relative contraindications to early EN, the treatment group received about 18 kcal per kg in the first week and the control group 8 kcal per kg with protein intakes of about 50 g per day and 25 g per day, respectively [117]. There was a modest improvement in ventilator days and less muscle wasting in the better fed group. In the two trials [123,124] of planned permissive underfeeding conducted by Arabi's group, both the treatment and the permissive underfeeding groups were underfed (59% vs. 71.4% and 46% vs. 71%, respectively) with equal protein intakes in both groups and in both studies by design. The earlier Arabi's study [123] found an improved hospital mortality as a post hoc finding which was not confirmed in the larger trial [124] (i.e., the so-called "PERMIT" trial) with a greater difference in caloric intakes and a longer duration of feeding in this later study despite similar control intakes in both studies. The only disadvantage with the higher calorie intake for the more recent study is that this led to a greater volume intake with a more positive fluid balance and the need for more renal replacement therapy. Thus, whether permissive underfeeding improves outcome over full feeding at 25 kcal per kg has not been definitively determined, but smaller volumes are required with permissive underfeeding. This may be an important factor when the underlying clinical problem is acute respiratory failure. In another recent trial [125] of acute lung injury, adverse mortality experience was found in the intensively fed group receiving nearly adequate energy (84.7% vs. 55.4%) where presumably greater volume was provided. This trial was stopped early because of the higher mortality occurring principally in the first week of therapy in the group with higher energy intake where a positive fluid balance might be particularly harmful. Two other trials [126,127] in acute respiratory failure failed to show an outcome difference between trophic feeding enterally of <5 kcal per kg versus approximately 15 kcal per kg for the first week, but no protein supplementation was provided in the better fed group. Thus, permissive underfeeding was not beneficial in this instance compared to grossly inadequate feeding. In conclusion, recent work has not only better defined the energy goal optimal for the general ICU patient as probably between 50% and 100% of 25 kcal per kg while holding protein constant but has also reinforced the point that a goal is different from what is actually provided, and it is the latter that is of cardinal importance. Although it is possible to achieve these modest goals by feeding enterally or by supplemental feeding parenterally, in practice, underfeeding in relation to goals is the usual outcome for both PN and EN of the critically ill. In such circumstances, permissive underfeeding if protein intakes are maintained at 0.8 to 1 g per kg or even higher should lead to outcomes as good as full feeding at 25 kcal per kg and, probably, better than those found with caloric intakes substantially greater than 25 kcal per kg as was the previous norm. Given the difficulties of assessing caloric needs in the heterogeneous clinical states found in the critically ill without direct measurement of energy expenditure, permissive underfeeding using simple estimates of caloric expenditure like 25 kcal per kg or those derived by use of various other predictive formulas also limits the likelihood of overfeeding in some patients.

In conclusion, much of the increase in morbidity related to PN and EN is as a result of hyperglycemia, which can be significantly reduced by intensive insulin therapy. The level of glycemia necessary to accomplish this goal, whether <110 mg per dL or only <150 mg per dL, is not yet defined. Surgical patients being adequately fed may benefit from the lower range, but a recent large study of intensive insulin therapy alone without full feeding in mixed populations of medical and surgical patients have significantly lower mortality with looser control of <180 mg per dL versus tighter control (81 to 108 mg per dL) [128]. A possible interpretation is that to accomplish early, adequate feeding requires some parenteral feeding in many critically ill patients who may also serve to minimize the risks of hypoglycemia when employing tighter glucose control.

Tolerance

Enteral Nutrition

Tolerance to nutrition support interventions is highly variable and principally depends on the clinical condition of the patient and the mode of administration. In general, critically ill patients are least able to tolerate all forms of nutritional support. This is particularly true with EN and often limits the amount of protein and calories that can be provided, because GI intolerance to feeding is common. As well, a number of other factors associated with ICU care can also interfere with its efficacious delivery [129]. The use of specialized formulations that provide elemental forms of the macronutrients, or are of reduced osmolarity, or of low fat content, may reduce the degree of GI intolerance. Moreover, the use of prokinetic agents, such as metoclopramide and erythromycin, may benefit some patients as well, whether used alone or in combination, but tachyphylaxis limits its use beyond 5 to 7 days [130]. Nevertheless, despite these preventive measures, GI intolerance cannot be successfully managed for all patients. A recent Cochrane meta-analysis assessed the efficacy of metoclopramide for the postpyloric placement of nasoenteric tubes [131]. Although admittedly, the four trials identified for the analysis provided very–low-quality evidence, the authors reported that at doses of 10 and 20 mg, they were equally ineffective when compared to placebo or no intervention. Despite this, they reported it is unlikely that a randomized clinical trial would be performed given the lack of efficacy in this review, and because the available trials for this analysis were all performed before 1995.

Other maneuvers, such as diluting the enteral feeding formula, rarely alleviate the problem and generally should not be undertaken. Providing monomeric or oligomeric formulations with reduced fat content at full strength, given at low rates (i.e., 20 mL per hour) and slowly advanced (i.e., 10 mL per hour every 6 to 12 hours as tolerated) can be applied, but likely of little benefit as well. Three relevant clinical studies in the ICU have focused on additional methods of EN delivery: (1) very low feeding rates or "trophic feeding"; (2) increasing caloric density; and (3) volume-based EN delivery. In the "trophic feeding" study, patients who were expected to require mechanical ventilation for at least 72 hours were randomized to receive "full-energy" EN (25 mL per hour and increased by 25 mL per hour until full feeding is accomplished, 25 to 30 kcal/kg/d) or "initial trophic" EN (10 mL per hour) for 6 days [126]. There were no differences in clinical outcomes, and, as expected, fewer episodes of GI intolerance were observed in the patients receiving the "trophic" regimen.

Increasing the caloric density has also been shown to be possible without increasing adverse effects in the ICU. In a recent multicenter study of mechanically ventilated patients, a standard 1 kcal per mL enteral formula was tested against a concentrated one at 1.5 kcal per mL (maximum rate: 100 mL per hour) for up to 10 days [132]. Daily caloric intakes were estimated to average 1,832 versus 1,125 kcal per day for 1.5- versus 1.0-kcal per day diets, respectively (~EN dose range: 25 to 35 kcal/kg/d, based on IBW). The main difference in the nutritional composition was from the additional calories from fat and carbohydrate in the commercial enteral products used in this study. The two groups received similar volumes of EN (1,221 vs. 1,225 mL per day), but obviously nearly 50% more calories. Of note, the concentrated EN formula was not associated with an increase of GI intolerance (higher gastric residual volumes, diarrhea).

Typical delivery of EN is based on a fixed hourly rate-based feeding (RBF) method, and, according to a recent report, it is shown why EN therapy in the critically ill leads to underfeeding (~50% of caloric requirements) is largely because of delays in initiation, underordering by the physicians, and reduced delivery through frequent interruptions or periods of cessation [133]. Consequently, the patient receives less volume and fewer calories. By adjusting the EN infusion rate upwards to make up for the "interruptions" in delivery, that is, a "volume-based feeding" (VBF) protocol ensures that the intended 24-hour supply of nutrients is achieved. In a small study to evaluate the efficacy of this feeding method, McClave and colleagues found that VBF: (1) allowed more calories than RBF (78% vs. 62%, respectively, of goal: 25 to 30 kcal/kg/d); (2) significantly lowered cumulative caloric deficits during the study, up to 7 days (−776 kcal vs. −1,934 kcal, respectively); and (3) was no better than RBF with regard to incidence of "uninterrupted" EN periods during the study (52% vs. 55%, respectively). A summary of the important clinical issues affecting the delivery of EN therapy appears in Table 213.6.

As a general rule, patients who suffer multiple trauma excluding head injury are usually more tolerant of enteral feeding and allow quicker advancement than those critically ill patients who have closed head injury, sepsis, or are postoperative. Consequently, the time course to achieve eucaloric nutrition is usually longer than with PN.

Parenteral Nutrition

In contrast, patients receiving PN will physically tolerate large amounts of nutrients when given by intravenous administration. The "physiologic brake" that obviously limits EN is not readily apparent. Metabolic abnormalities, such as hyperglycemia and electrolyte and acid–base disturbances, can be easily ascribed to the consequences of the metabolic response to injury, rather than recognizing the contribution of overly aggressive PN support. Furthermore, these iatrogenic metabolic abnormalities are often addressed independently from the PN admixture, such as by separate infusions of insulin, fluid, electrolytes, and so forth, without modifying the PN regimen. The net effect of parenteral overfeeding can unnecessarily complicate the critical care of such patients and lead to significant increases in morbidity and even mortality. However, once metabolic homeostasis is achieved, the

TABLE 213.6

Advances in the Delivery of Enteral Nutrition

Issue	Outcome
Route: nasogastric vs. nasoenteral	No difference in energy delivery [105]; 30% reduction inpneumonia with postpyloric feeding [106]
Blood Glucose: hypoglycemia	Significantly increased risk with EN vs. PN [120]
Prokinetic Agents: metoclopramide, erythromycin	Increased tachyphylaxis after 5–7 d [130]; metoclopramide equally ineffective at 10 and 20 mg doses [131]; erythromycin associated with increased risk of minor episodes of GI bleeding [105]
Nutrient Delivery: rate, caloric density, volume	No difference between very-low/"trophic" vs. full-energy feeding [126]; Increased caloric delivery with high-caloric density vs. low-caloric density, but no difference in clinical outcomes [132]; Volume-based/day vs. rate-based received more calories with reduced cumulative caloric deficits, but no differences in feeding interruptions [133]

EN, enteral nutrition; GI, gastrointestinal; PN, parenteral nutrition.

time course to reach eucaloric nutrition support is usually brief compared with EN therapy.

Fixed Versus Variable Amounts of Nutrients

Enteral Nutrition

There is limited opportunity to manipulate the contents of EN formulations because these products are premade as "complete" commercial products. Of course, they may be modified by the addition of various nutrient modules, but cannot easily be specifically tailored to the patient, especially during acute illness. For example, a number of electrolyte additives may precipitate the complex feeding formulas and cause clogging of the feeding tube. The addition of other components to the enteral formulation increases the osmolarity, which is an important consideration for enteral feeding, as well as increasing the risk of incompatibilities [70]. Thus, the flexibility of enteral therapy is limited, which may make it difficult to achieve the proper balance of nutrients during severe metabolic stress. Once the stress response remits and major organ function improves, this becomes a less pressing concern.

Parenteral Nutrition

Major stability issues associated with PN admixtures preclude the manufacture of ready-to-use commercial products. Of these, the interaction between certain amino acids with dextrose forming oxidized end products, known as the Maillard reaction, is generally acknowledged [72]. The use of multicompartment bags offer a possible alternative to these reactions, but as with enteral products, they too become clinically limiting in the unstable patient in the acute care setting. Thus, PN admixtures are most often made extemporaneously from individual commercial ingredients (i.e., amino acids, dextrose, lipids, electrolytes, and so forth) by qualified pharmacy personnel. The introduction of automated compounding devices and their subsequent widespread use has made the practice of patient-specific admixtures a relatively easy task [134]. Thus, even the sickest of ICU patients can receive some form of nutrition support by the prescribing of unique and specifically designed formulations to support the protein synthetic response to injury.

Costs

Enteral Nutrition

Historically, EN formulations have been a fraction of the cost of PN admixtures because they are ready-to-use and largely comprised of polymeric forms of macronutrients. However, with refinements in these products to construct oligomeric or monomeric forms of protein and carbohydrates, the so-called elemental formulas, the costs have increased substantially. Moreover, the addition of novel nutrients, such as ω-3 fatty acids, glutamine, arginine, and others to produce nutritional supplements that may have pharmacologic effects, particularly with respect to immune function, has increased costs that now exceed most PN formulations per kilocalories. Although the data are promising for these innovative formulations in terms of their potential to reduce length of stay and, possibly, infectious complications, the full extent of these claims have not been fully substantiated.

Parenteral Nutrition

By historical comparison, PN was always more expensive than EN therapy. There were many good reasons for this [135], considering the product had to be specially compounded under aseptic conditions to be suitable and safe for intravenous administration. Because the methods of commercial production improved and became more efficient and competition increased, the costs of PN therapy have significantly declined. Compared with specialized formulas that contain immunonutrients or certain concentrated enteral products, the present costs of PN therapy are equal or, in many cases, less expensive. In contrast, for conventional, polymeric EN supplements, the cost of the formulations is still substantially less than PN formula costs. However, the placement of an enteral feeding tube and components (pumps, sets, and so forth) is dedicated to the provision of nutrition support, whereas central venous lines are already being used for the provision of intravenous fluids, medications, and blood tests. Therefore, additional costs of even conventional EN therapy must be considered.

Complications

The complications or adverse patient events associated with PN and EN include mechanical, septic, and metabolic misadventures [136]. For example, mechanical complications of invasive nutrition support are often associated with the misplacement of various types of feeding access devices (i.e., vascular injury or pneumothorax). With experienced clinicians, the incidence of such complications is substantially reduced and clinically acceptable at about 1% to 2%.

Metabolic and associated septic complications are more common and can have a significant impact on patient outcomes. Severe disturbances in fluid, electrolyte, and acid–base homeostasis are commonly associated with high rates of morbidity and mortality in the ICU. This is especially true for patients with significant heart disease [137]. As well, septic complications in association with hyperglycemia and infections in critically ill patients receiving PN or EN are at least equally significant, if not even more so [138]. Therefore, a more modest provision of energy intake (i.e., approximately 25 total kcal/kg/d) should be the overall goal of therapy by whatever route of delivery and is most likely to succeed, and, with this, fewer nutrition-related complications are likely. However, in the first 3 to 7 days of EN and PN, providing at least 50% of the estimated energy requirement along with protein intake of at least 1 g per kg may be a reasonable compromise meeting the definition or early, adequate feeding while lowering the risk of metabolic and infectious complications. Of note, in the recent permissive underfeeding trial, Arabi et al. showed no differences of clinical outcomes (90-day mortality, feeding intolerance, infections, or hospital length of stay) between groups fed EN for up to 14 days [124]. Not surprisingly, significant increases were observed in the "standard feeding" group versus those in the "permissive underfeeding" group in terms of (1) insulin dose and requirements ($p = 0.02$); (2) blood glucose concentrations ($p = 0.04$); (3) fluid balance ($p = 0.001$); and (4) renal replacement therapy ($p = 0.04$). Also, protein intakes were similar between groups, but daily intake was <1 g/kg/d. Of course, permissive underfeeding should not be applied to high-risk patients, and indirect calorimetry can be helpful for patients with preexisting moderate-to-severe malnutrition.

Appropriate Application of Nutritional Support

Nutritional support does not improve outcomes for operative patients who are well nourished, no matter what route of administration it is given. A number of examples appear in the medical literature supporting this contention. For example, a randomized clinical trial of perioperative nutrition support only found significant improvement in the malnourished group irrespective of feeding mode [139]. Heslin et al. [140] reported no benefit with enteral tube feeding for patients with GI cancer without significant weight loss. In fact, the routine provision of EN in well-nourished patients may cause significant impairments in ventilatory function and mobility [141]. Finally, an extensive review of the literature has corroborated the lack of benefits in the standard prescription of nutrition support for patients who initially are well nourished and undergoing moderate stress following major thoracoabdominal surgery [142]. There is reasonable support for early and adequate feeding for the most critically stressed even when initially well nourished such as those with closed head injury, severe multiple trauma, major third-degree burns, and severe sepsis, not to prevent the development of malnutrition but presumably to limit the severity of the systemic inflammatory response.

In contrast, invasive feeding of the malnourished patient is likely to be effective in a variety of clinical scenarios. This is particularly true during acute metabolic stress, where ongoing catabolism results in significant daily losses of body protein. Patients with weight loss classified as moderate (i.e., 10% or more) or severe (i.e., 20% or more) from usual or IBW are most susceptible to nutrition-related complications, such as infection or wound dehiscence. The absence of nutritional intervention in this vulnerable population for protracted periods of time (i.e., greater than 7 to 10 days) may have a significant impact on outcome. Moreover, even the initially well-nourished patient cannot sustain the protein synthetic response to injury for long periods. For example, in a randomized study of the effects on outcome of postoperative feeding with TPN, those who were inadequately fed for 14 days had a significantly higher morbidity and mortality [143]. Patients who suffer multiple traumas, major burns, or closed head injury are a unique group. Although generally well nourished at the outset, the severity of catabolic response and the likely duration of substantially longer than 7 days make early nutritional intervention within the first few days beneficial.

MONITORING PARAMETERS FOR NUTRITIONAL SUPPORT

Electrolytes

During critical illness, severe electrolyte disorders are common and are primarily the result of various concomitant etiologies, including changes in (a) the function of major organ systems, especially the kidneys; (b) fluid balance affecting intravascular volume and the hormonal milieu produced as a result of the metabolic response to severe stress(es); (c) intracellular or extracellular shifts of ions associated with acid–base disturbances; and (d) multiple drug therapies. Renal dysfunction has profound effects on electrolyte balance by influencing the absorption and excretion of, most notably, sodium, potassium, magnesium, phosphorus, and titratable acids. As renal function declines, the excretion of these electrolytes decreases, and, therefore, the PN admixture must be adjusted accordingly. For example, in some cases, electrolytes are significantly reduced, whereas, in other circumstances, they are entirely omitted from the daily admixture. As well, chloride ions are often substituted with alkalinizing anions such as acetate to combat the metabolic acidosis associated with renal failure.

Fluid overload is a common finding among critically ill patients related to intraoperative support of renal blood flow and function, acute volume resuscitation with crystalloids in the ICU, and the administration of multiple intravenous medications that may produce its own set of complications. For example, acute increases of 10% or greater above usual body weight over short intervals clearly reflect a significant expansion of TBW that may impede the weaning of the patient from mechanical ventilation. Thus, clinical efforts to return to the patient's premorbid weight, such as by aggressive diuretic therapy and concentrating intravenous medications in the least diluent volume possible, are often used. More recently, the use of hemofiltration procedures to accomplish this goal has proven quite effective. Despite "third-spacing" of fluids, the consequences of the antidiuretic and antinatriuretic responses of stress often present as a hyponatremia and can be mistakenly treated by the parenteral administration of sodium salts in an effort to correct the serum sodium concentration. However, given that sodium essentially distributes in TBW, one can easily calculate that, in fact, the patient is both fluid and total body sodium overloaded. Hence, clinical maneuvers to address the problem should be directed at increasing both sodium and free water losses, with gradual restoration of serum sodium concentrations. A clinical example of this estimation appears in Table 213.7.

The acute intracellular or extracellular shifting of electrolytes is primarily the result of the effects of changes in acid–base homeostasis and serum insulin concentrations. In the former case, serum potassium concentrations are most affected by changes in acid–base status. Potassium is predominantly an intracellular ion whose concentration in the intracellular compartment is much higher than its extracellular concentration. When arterial pH falls below normal, potassium shifts to the extracellular compartment and hyperkalemia occurs, and, conversely, metabolic alkalosis produces hypokalemia.

Insulin has also a profound effect on the shifting of potassium, magnesium, and phosphorus between the intracellular and extracellular environments. In fact, the life-threatening refeeding syndrome that occurs in severely malnourished patients is associated with the shifting of these electrolytes from the extracellular to the intracellular compartments [144]. In the atrophic heart muscle characteristic of severe malnutrition (i.e., greater than 30% below IBW), severe reductions of serum potassium (i.e., less than 3 mEq per L) and serum phosphorus (i.e., less

TABLE 213.7

Estimating Total Body Sodium in the Acute Care Setting

Premorbid total body sodium	
Total body water @ 70 kg	= 42 L
Total body sodium	= 42 L × 140 mEq/L
	=5,880 mEq
Present total body sodium	
Total body water @ 91 kg	= 42 L + (91 kg – 70 kg)
	= 63 L
Total body sodium	= 63 L × 130 mEq/L
	= 8,190 mEq
Excess total body sodium	= 8,190 – 5,880
	= 2,310 mEq

Assumptions: premorbid weight = 70 kg male; presently = 91 kg; serum sodium = 140 mEq/L (normal); presently = 130 mEq/L; total body water = 60% (for males).

than 0.2 mg per L) related to feeding may have life-threatening electrophysiologic consequences [145].

Finally, critically ill patients commonly receive multiple drug therapies intravenously for a variety of clinical reasons and include, for example, cardiovascular agents, vasopressors, diuretics, anesthesia/sedation therapy, crystalloids, colloids, antibiotics, anticoagulants, and so forth. These can cause clinically significant effects by altering intended drug actions (i.e., toxic synergism, reduced drug effects) or by addition of substantial diluent volumes (i.e., greater than 500 mL), worsening a fluid-overloaded state. The clinical care of acutely ill patients with severe fluid and electrolyte disorders can be optimally managed through intensive metabolic monitoring and selective manipulations of PN admixture components [73,74,145].

Insulin and Glucose Homeostasis

Notwithstanding its regulatory role in glucose homeostasis in terms of glucose production and breakdown in the liver, as well as its facilitated transport of glucose into muscle and other obligatory tissues, insulin is a complex hormone that exhibits numerous metabolic effects that may be of significant clinical consequences for the critically ill. The mechanisms by which abnormally elevated blood glucose concentrations of critically ill patients produce metabolic dysfunction have been described [146]. With respect to infectious risk, the ability of mononuclear (macrophages and monocytes) and polymorphonuclear neutrophils to exert phagocytic, oxidative bursts, and killing functions is significantly impaired. Thus, infections of the bloodstream, lungs, and superficial wounds (i.e., any surgical incision site, intravascular and extravascular catheter sites, or other topical sites of injury) are significantly increased following periods of hyperglycemia.

Glucose homeostasis is best achieved when parenteral insulin is given in an effective manner. A review of the methods of administration employed emphasize that the route of insulin delivery should be commensurate with the means of administration of carbohydrate calories [147]. In the acute phases of critical illness, patients receiving PN should receive intensive insulin therapy [118]. Once, stabilized (i.e., patients receiving the largest source of glucose as parenteral calories), insulin should be given in the TPN admixture in amounts sufficient to cover the caloric intake from this source over 24 hours. When exclusive PN therapy is given, 24-hour glucose intake may account for as much as 150 to 300 g per L daily (510 to 1,020 kcal), requiring substantial amounts of insulin in the admixture, and can be effectively accomplished [147]. As well, in some cases, supplemental "low-volume, full-strength" EN may provide 50 to 150 g per 24 hours (170 to 510 kcal), which should be managed with subcutaneous or intravenous insulin provided based on blood glucose determinations taken on a regular basis and algorithm-based insulin doses. It should be emphasized that, the insulin administered subcutaneously, either as a continuous intravenous infusion or as a bolus intravenous dose, has a serum half-life of approximately 5 to 7 minutes. The same principles may be applied to patients receiving substantial amounts of glucose in the peritoneal dialytic regimens, where insulin is often best provided in the dialysis solution. Thus, for some cases, such as a patient undergoing both peritoneal dialysis and PN or EN, insulin is given via multiple routes to cover the administration of glucose from various sources to link the insulin administration to the source of exogenous glucose. When hyperglycemia is severe because of severity of the stress response or severity of insulin deficiency (type 1) or insulin resistance (type 2), it is reasonable to employ continuous intravenous insulin and close blood glucose monitoring to quickly establish glucose homeostasis, whatever the source of exogenous glucose.

Goals of Nitrogen Balance

Achieving positive nitrogen balance is an unrealistic goal in the critically ill early in the clinical course. Rather, the principal aim of nutritional intervention is to support the protein synthetic response to injury and, therefore, narrow the negative nitrogen gap (where output exceeds input) that occurs during severe metabolic stress. Even when the metabolic stress has subsided, it should be recognized that nutritional rehabilitation of the moderate-to-severe malnourished patient occurs at a limited rate equivalent to approximately 1 kg of body weight per week, and generally much of this repletion will occur outside the hospital after discharge. This estimation is based on a maximum rate of repletion of a positive nitrogen balance (i.e., approximately +5 g per day) that represents 150 g of lean tissue (hydrated protein) and a calorically equivalent amount of fat (13 g) per day. Weight increases above this rate of repletion can only reflect increases in TBW.

Finally, it should be mentioned that when expending the effort to obtain a 24-hour urine collection, additional laboratory measurements should be performed on this specimen, such as for the determination of creatinine excretion and certain electrolytes (sodium, potassium, and chloride). In this way, important additional clinical information may be provided, including creatinine clearance, urea clearance, fractional excretion of sodium, and quantification of electrolyte losses, among other possible data that may be used in the clinical and nutritional/metabolic care of critically ill patients.

EVIDENCE-BASED GUIDELINES FOR NUTRITIONAL SUPPORT THERAPIES

In 2009, the Society of Critical Care Medicine (SCCM) and the American Society for Parenteral and Enteral Nutrition (ASPEN) developed and copublished "Guidelines for the provision and assessment of nutrition support therapy in the adult critically ill patient" [148,149]. The last statement of the introduction of this document is noteworthy: "Delivering early nutrition support therapy, primarily using the enteral route, is seen as a proactive therapeutic strategy that may reduce disease severity, diminish complications, decrease length of stay in the ICU, and favorably impact patient outcome." Of the 12 categories or conditions (sections A through L), 9 sections related to EN, 2 sections on PN, and 1 section (L) relating to end-of-life situations. It is the authors' opinion that this document is unfortunately biased against the potential utility of PN in many circumstances. The assessment system applied in the guidelines consisted of "Levels of Evidence" and "Grades of Recommendation." "Levels of Evidence" were from I to V, with "Level I" being the strongest evidence and "Level V" being the weakest evidence. The "Grades of Recommendation" were from A to E, with "A" being the highest and "E" being the lowest. If, for example, one scores the grades according to a quality point average (QPA) as applied in education with A = 4.0, B = 3.0 . . . E = 0.0, the evidence is poor for both EN and PN. For example, in the SCCM/ASPEN 2009 guidelines, the QPA for all EN sections was 1.21 and the QPA for all PN sections was 1.25. We selected three controversial statements in the guideline:

A3. "EN is the preferred route of feeding over parenteral nutrition (PN) for the critically ill patient who requires nutrition support therapy. Grade B"

The statement is correct, and fits Dr. Dudrick original thesis "if the guts works, use it," but the principal rationale for its preference, that is, reduced infectious morbidity is misidentified. Although previous studies have shown this association to be true, the premise overlooks the importance of blood glucose control and caloric intake in these studies. Invariably, the PN group in many of the supporting studies received significantly more calories than the EN group and, consequently, had higher blood glucose values that clearly increase infectious complications. This is not surprising because EN is often not well tolerated in eucaloric amounts as PN, and is frequently interrupted for various clinical maneuvers or diagnostic tests in the critical care setting. As well, the insulin required to maintain glucose homeostasis is greater for parenteral compared to enteral glucose. Furthermore, the data supporting this statement was essentially derived before the subsequent eras of reduced energy provision and tight glucose control in the critically ill.

G1. "If the patient is deemed to be a candidate for PN, steps to maximize efficacy (regarding dose, content, monitoring, and choice of additives) should be used. Grade C"

In accordance with the thesis of "do no harm," it would seem intuitively obvious that the safety and efficacy of PN would be accomplished by optimizing the formulation. A "Grade C" recommendation diminishes the importance of dosing nutrients, which unfortunately, is associated with a long history of overfeeding and its attendant complications. In the same section (G6), the use of extemporaneously prepared parenteral glutamine is given the same "Grade C," despite the fact that such an additive is classified as a "HIGH RISK" compounded sterile preparation by the USP [20].

H3. "Serum phosphate levels should be monitored closely and replaced appropriately when needed. Grade E"

The literature is replete with data on the importance of serum phosphate levels is the critically ill, especially with respect to the risks associated with hypophosphatemia on myocardial performance and respiratory function [149]. Moreover, the provision of hypertonic glucose in a PN admixture produces a supraphysiologic increase in serum insulin levels that will cause significant intracellular shifts that may produce life-threatening hypophosphatemia in susceptible patients. A "Grade E" recommendation is inappropriate in this circumstance. Also, in 2009, the European Society of Parenteral and Enteral Nutrition produced "Guidelines on parenteral nutrition: intensive care" [150]. Seventeen statements (categories or conditions) are included, and there are three Grades of Recommendation (A, B, and C) with the strongest evidence being "Grade A" versus the weakest evidence with a "Grade C." Only two statements received "Grade A." We selected three controversial statements in this guideline.

Under "Requirements"

"During acute illness, the aim should be to provide energy as close as possible to the measured energy expenditure in order to decrease negative energy balance. Grade B"

In the ICU setting, particularly during the early phases of critical illness, hypocaloric regimens often seem to be most prudent. Maintenance of normal blood glucose values should take precedence over energy balance in most critical care settings, and then once achieved, judicious increases in calories can commence.

"In the absence of indirect calorimetry, ICU patients should receive 25 kcal/kg/day increasing to target over the next 2–3 days. Grade C"

As already stated, caloric intakes in the ICU should be advanced slowly after the initial provision of 50% of energy and 1.0 to 1.2 g protein per kg to avoid hyperglycemia and infectious morbidity. As stated earlier, for most patients, providing 25 kcal/kg/d is sufficient to support the protein synthetic response to metabolic stress. The guideline, as stated earlier, implies that 25 kcal/kg/d is the starting point, when in fact, for most adult patients, it is the target range [151], and is gradually reached after initiating lesser amounts of calories from the outset.

Under "Amino Acids"

"When PN is indicated in ICU patients the amino acid solution should contain 0.2–0.4 g/kg/day of L-glutamine (e.g., 0.3–0.6 g/kg/day alanyl-glutamine dipeptide). Grade A"

Although there is a commercial product in Europe that is available to provide glutamine supplementation, a recommendation of Grade A seems to be overly optimistic. This is especially true given the recent assessment of L-glutamine in the ICU of an "area of uncertainty" from one of the leading investigators in the field [151]. Thus, such a recommendation seemed premature at the time, and, subsequently, more recent studies have shown this not to be the case [99–103].

At this time, the data is unclear for several reasons. First, the guidelines and methods of assessment must be standardized between organizations. Second, "mining of data" from past studies, many of which are significantly flawed with respect to design and endpoints, cannot yield meaningful guidelines, despite the use of statistical tools, such as meta-analyses. Third, critically ill patients are not homogeneous. As recently pointed out, EN is contraindicated in 10% to 15% of ICU patients; there are very few well-designed, randomized controlled studies of PN efficacy, and preexisting malnutrition, combined with numerous pathophysiologic factors in ICU patients which greatly complicate the role of nutrition support [151, 152].

Thus, it seems that to definitively address the evidence for nutrition support therapy in the ICU setting will require designing better studies in the future rather than the current methods to rehash old data from a previous era using statistical tools. A major emphasis should clearly be on the design (randomized controlled trial, sufficient power, APACHE score, etc.) and specific endpoints for future studies to answer the question of the impact of nutritional therapy in the critically ill on morbidity and mortality and clinical outcome. For example, we now have a series of multicenter studies that have focused on the potential role of early (within 72 hours of ICU admission) and adequate energy (>50%, but <110% of energy requirements) and protein (at least 1.2 g/kg/d), immunonutrients, PN versus EN, and so on. Great progress has been made in the quality of such studies, but to have a truer understanding of the role of nutrition support therapy in the critically ill, more work needs to be done to ensure that nutrition support is provided to those patients most likely to derive clinical benefits, with more precise doses of nutrients and means of delivery, and done so in a timely manner.

CONCLUSIONS

Nutritional and metabolic support is an essential component of the clinical care of critically ill patients. However, if applied in an overly aggressive manner without considering the nutritional status, amounts of nutrients, route of administration, and the clinical condition of the patient, significant iatrogenic complications may occur and little clinical benefit can be expected. Thus, nutritional support of the critically ill must be carefully integrated into the overall clinical care of the patient, with specific and measurable outcome measures in order to obtain the maximum benefits of this important therapy.

References

1. Driscoll DF, Bistrian BR: Special considerations required for the formulation and administration of total parenteral nutrition in the older patient. *Drugs Aging* 2:395–405, 1992.
2. Bistrian BR, Blackburn GL, Hallowell E, et al: Protein nutritional status of general surgical patients. *JAMA* 230:858–860, 1974.
3. Bistrian BR, Blackburn GL, Vitale J, et al: Prevalence of malnutrition in general medical patients. *JAMA* 235:1567–1570, 1976.
4. Reilly JJ, Hull SF, Albert N, et al: Economic impact of malnutrition: a model system for hospitalized patients. *J Parenter Enteral Nutr* 12:371–376, 1988.
5. McWhirter JP, Pennington CR: Incidence and recognition of malnutrition in hospital. *BMJ* 308:945–948, 1994.
6. Shahar A, Feiglin L, Sharar DR, et al: High prevalence and impact of subnormal serum vitamin B_{12} levels in Israeli elders admitted to a geriatric hospital. *J Nutr Health Aging* 5:124–127, 2001.
7. Kyle UG, Genton L, Pichard C: Hospital length of stay and nutritional status. *Curr Opin Clin Nutr Metab Care* 8:397–402, 2005.
8. Singh H, Watt K, Veitch R, et al: Malnutrition is prevalent in hospitalized medical patients: are housestaff identifying the malnourished patient? *Nutrition* 22:350–354, 2006.
9. Kuzu MA, Terzioglu H, Genc V, et al: Preoperative nutritional risk assessment in predicting postoperative outcome in patients undergoing major surgery. *World J Surg* 30:378–390, 2006.
10. Bistrian BR: A simple technique to estimate severity of stress. *Surg Gynecol Obstet* 148:675–678, 1979.
11. Driscoll DF, Blackburn GL: Total parenteral nutrition 1990: a review of its current status in hospitalized patients. The need for patient-specific feeding. *Drugs* 40:346–363, 1990.
12. Leiter LA, Marliss EB: Survival during fasting may depend on fat as well as protein stores. *JAMA* 248:2306–2307, 1982.
13. Ahmad A, Duerksen DR, Munroe S, et al: An evaluation of resting energy expenditure in hospitalized, severely underweight patients. *Nutrition* 15:384–388, 1999.
14. Henry CJ: Body mass index and the limits of human survival. *Eur J Clin Nutr* 44:329–335, 1990.
15. Bartlett RH, Dechert RE, Mault JR, et al: Measurement of metabolism in multiple organ failure. *Surgery* 92:771–779, 1982.
16. Rubinson L, Diette GB, Song X, et al: Low caloric intake is associated with nosocomial blood stream infections in patients in the medical intensive care unit. *Crit Care Med* 32:350–357, 2004.
17. Shaw JHF, Widmore M, Wolfe RR: Whole body protein kinetics in severely septic patients: the response to glucose infusion in total parenteral nutrition. *Ann Surg* 205:66–72, 1987.
18. Shaw JHF, Wolfe RR: Whole body protein kinetics in patients with early and advanced gastrointestinal cancer: the response to glucose infusion and total parenteral nutrition. *Surgery* 103:148–155, 1988.
19. Lamiell JJ, Ducey JP, Freese-Kepczyk BJ, et al: Essential amino acid-induced hyperammonemic encephalopathy and hypophosphatemia. *Crit Care Med* 18:451–452, 1990.
20. *Pharmaceutical Compounding—Sterile Preparations. Physical Tests.* United States Pharmacopeia 34/National Formulary 29. Rockville, MD, United States Pharmacopeia Convention, Inc, 2011, pp. 336–373.
21. Preiser JC, Wernerman J. REDOXs: important answers, many more questions as well. *J Parenter Enteral Nutr* 2013;37:566–567.
22. Bistrian BR: Hyperglycemia and infection: which is the chicken and which is the egg? [Editorial]. *J Parenter Enteral Nutr* 25:180–181, 2001.
23. Cahill GF: Starvation in man. *N Engl J Med* 282:668–675, 1970.
24. Wolfe RR: Carbohydrate metabolism in critically ill patients. *Crit Care Clin* 3:11–24, 1987.
25. Douglas RG, Shaw JHF: Metabolic response to trauma and sepsis. *Br J Surg* 76:115–122, 1989.
26. Driscoll DF: Clinical issues regarding the use of total nutrient admixtures. *Ann Pharmacother* 24:296–303, 1990.
27. Seidner DL, Mascioli EA, Istfan NW, et al: Effects of long-chain triglyceride emulsions on reticuloendothelial system function in humans. *J Parenter Enteral Nutr* 13:614–619, 1989.
28. Jensen GL, Mascioli EA, Seidner DL, et al: Parenteral infusion of long and medium-chain triglycerides and reticuloendothelial system function in man. *J Parenter Enteral Nutr* 14:467–471, 1990.
29. Hwang D: Essential fatty acids and the immune response. *FASEB J* 3:2052–2061, 1989.
30. Mathru M, Dries DJ, Zecca A, et al: Effect of fast vs. slow intralipid infusion on gas exchange, pulmonary hemodynamics, and prostaglandins metabolism. *Chest* 99:426–429, 1991.
31. Belin RP, Bivins BA, Jona JZ, et al: Fat overload with a 10% soybean oil emulsion. *Arch Surg* 111:1391–1393, 1976.
32. Periera GR, Fox WW, Stanley CA, et al: Decreased oxygenation and hyperlipemia during intravenous fat infusions in premature infants. *Pediatrics* 66:26–30, 1980.
33. Heyman MB, Storch S, Ament ME: The fat overload syndrome. Report of a case and literature. *Am J Dis Child* 135:628–630, 1981.
34. Haber LM, Hawkin EP, Seilheimer DK, et al: Fat overload syndrome. An autopsy study with evaluation of the coagulopathy. *Am J Clin Pathol* 90:223–227, 1988.
35. Puntis JW, Rushton DI: Pulmonary intravascular lipid in neonatal necropsy specimens. *Arch Dis Child* 66:26–28, 1991.
36. Schulz PE, Weiner SP, Haber LM, et al: Neurological complications from fat emulsion therapy. *Ann Neurol* 35:628–630, 1994.
37. Toce SS, Keenan WJ: Lipid intolerance in newborns is associated with hepatic dysfunction but not infection. *Arch Pediatr Adolesc Med* 149:1249–1253, 1995.
38. Jasnosz KM, Pickeral JJ, Graner S: Fat deposits in the placenta following maternal total parenteral nutrition with intravenous lipid emulsion. *Arch Pathol Lab Med* 119:555–557, 1995.
39. Gohlke BC, Fahnenstich H, Kowalewski S: Serum lipids during parenteral nutrition with a 10% lipid emulsion with reduced phospholipid emulsifier content in premature infants. *J Pediatr Endocrinol Metab* 10:505–509, 1997.
40. Colomb V, Jobert-Giraud A, Lacaille F, et al: Role of lipid emulsions in cholestasis associated with long-term parenteral nutrition in children. *J Parenter Enteral Nutr* 24:345–350, 2000.
41. Kadowitz PJ, Spannhake EW, Levin JL, et al: Differential effects of prostaglandins on the pulmonary vascular bed. *Prostaglandin Thromboxane Res* 7:731–744, 1980.
42. Driscoll DF, Bistrian BR, Demmelmair H, et al: Pharmaceutical and clinical aspects of lipid emulsions in neonatology. *Clin Nutr* 27:495–503, 2008.
43. Abbott WC, Grakauskas AM, Bistrian BR, et al: Metabolic and respiratory effects of continuous and discontinuous lipid infusions. *Arch Surg* 119:1367–1371, 1984.
44. Hwang TL, Huang SL, Chen MF: Effects of intravenous fat emulsion on respiratory failure. *Chest* 97:934–938, 1990.
45. Smyrniotis VE, Kostopanagiotou GG, Arkadopoulos NF, et al: Long-chain versus medium-chain lipids in acute pancreatitis complicated by acute respiratory distress syndrome: effects on pulmonary hemodynamics and gas exchange. *Clin Nutr* 20:139–143, 2001.
46. Suchner U, Katz DP, Furst P, et al: Effects of intravenous fat emulsions on lung function in patients with acute respiratory distress syndrome or sepsis. *Crit Care Med* 29:1569–1574, 2001.
47. Venus B, Prager R, Patel CB, et al: Hemodynamic and gas exchange alterations during Intralipid infusion in patients with adult respiratory distress syndrome. *Chest* 95:1278–1281, 1989.
48. Skeie B, Askanazi J, Rothkopf MM, et al: Intravenous fat emulsions and lung function: a review. *Crit Care Med* 16:183–194, 1988.
49. Hulman G: The pathogenesis of fat embolism. *J Pathol* 176:3–9, 1995.
50. Klein S, Miles JM: Metabolic effects of long-chain and medium-chain triglycerides in humans. *J Parenter Enteral Nutr* 18:396–397, 1994.
51. Sacks GS, Driscoll DF: Does lipid hang time make a difference? Time is of the essence. *Nutr Clin Pract* 2002;17:284–290.
52. *Globule Size Distribution in Lipid Injectable Emulsions. Physical Tests.* United States Pharmacopeia 32/National Formulary 27. Rockville, MD, United States Pharmacopeia Convention, 2009, pp 283–285.
53. Driscoll DF: Lipid injectable emulsions: pharmacopeial and safety issues. *Pharm Res* 23:1959–1969, 2006.
54. *Globule Size Distribution in Lipid Injectable Emulsions. Pharm Forum* 30:2235–2240, 2004.
55. Driscoll DF: The pharmacopeial evolution of Intralipid injectable emulsions in plastic containers: From a coarse to a fine dispersion. *Int J Pharm* 368:193–198, 2009.
56. Driscoll DF, Ling PR, Bistrian BR: Physical stability of 20% lipid injectable emulsions via simulated syringe infusion: Effects of glass vs. plastic product packaging. *J Parenter Enteral Nutr* 31:148–153, 2007.
57. Driscoll DF, Silvestri AP, Mikrut BA, et al: Stability of adult-based Total nutrient admixtures with soybean oil-based lipid injectable emulsions: The effect of glass versus plastic packaging. *Am J Health-Syst Pharm* 64:396–403, 2007.
58. Driscoll DF, Thoma A, Franke R, et al: Fine vs. Coarse All-In-One (AIOs) as 3-chamber plastic (3-C-P) bags over 48 hours. *Am J Health-Syst Pharm* 66:649–656, 2009.

59. Martin CR, Dumas GJ, Zheng Z, et al: Incidence of hypertriglyceridemia in critically ill neonates receiving lipid injectable emulsions in glass vs. plastic containers: A retrospective analysis. *J Pediatr* 152:232–236, 2008.
60. Driscoll DF, Ling PR, Silvestri AP, et al: Fine vs. coarse total nutrient admixture infusions over 96 hours in rats: Fat globule size and hepatic function. *Clin Nutr* 27:889–894, 2008.
61. Driscoll DF, Ling PR, Andersson C, et al: Hepatic indicators of oxidative stress and tissue damage accompanied by systemic inflammation in rats following a 24-hour infusion of an unstable lipid emulsion admixture. *J Parenter Enteral Nutr* 33:327–335, 2009.
62. Driscoll DF, Adolph M, Bistrian BR: Lipid emulsions in parenteral nutrition, in Rombeau JL, Rolandelli R (eds): *Parenteral Nutrition*. Philadelphia, PA, WB Saunders, 2001, pp 35–59.
63. Driscoll DF: Lipid injectable emulsions: 2006. *Nutr Clin Pract* 21:381–386, 2006.
64. ASPEN Position paper: Clinical role for alternative lipid emulsions. *Nutr Clin Pract* 2012;27:150–192.
65. Simmons RS, Berdine GG, Seidenfeld JJ, et al: Fluid balance and adult respiratory distress syndrome. *Am Rev Respir Dis* 135:924–929, 1987.
66. Lowell JA, Schifferdecker C, Driscoll DF, et al: Postoperative fluid overload: not a benign problem. *Crit Care Med* 18:728–733, 1990.
67. Nahtomi-Shick O, Kostuik JP, Winters BD, et al: Does intraoperative fluid management in spine surgery predict intensive care unit length of stay? *J Clin Anesth* 13:208–212, 2001.
68. Echenique MM, Bistrian BR, Blackburn GL: Theory and techniques of nutritional support in the ICU. *Crit Care Med* 10:546–559, 1982.
69. McCowen KC, Friel C, Sternberg J, et al: Hypocaloric total parenteral nutrition: effectiveness in prevention of hyperglycemia and infectious complications. *Crit Care Med* 28:3606–3611, 2000.
70. Driscoll DF: Formulation of enteral and parenteral mixtures, in Pichard C, Kudsk KA (eds): *Update in Intensive Care Medicine*. Brussels, Springer-Verlag, 2000, pp 138–150.
71. Driscoll DF, Silvestri AP, Nehne J, et al: The physicochemical stability of highly concentrated total nutrient admixtures (TNAs) intended for fluid-restricted patients. *Am J Health Syst Pharm* 63:79–85, 2006.
72. National Advisory Group on Standards and Practice Guidelines for Parenteral Nutrition: Safe practices for parenteral nutrition formulations. *J Parenter Enteral Nutr* 22:49–66, 1998.
73. Driscoll DF: Drug-induced metabolic disorders and parenteral nutrition in the intensive care unit: a pharmaceutical and metabolic perspective. *Ann Pharmacother* 23:363–371, 1989.
74. Driscoll DF: Drug-induced electrolyte disorders in a patient receiving parenteral nutrition [Editorial]. *J Parenter Enteral Nutr* 24:174–175, 2000.
75. Zivin JR, Gooley T, Zager RA, et al: Hypocalcemia: a pervasive metabolic abnormality in the critically ill. *Am J Kidney Dis* 37:689–698, 2001.
76. Flurkey H: A case presentation: precipitate in the central venous line: what went wrong? *Neonatal Netw* 13:51–55, 1994.
77. Hill SE, Heldman LS, Goo EDH, et al: Fatal microvascular pulmonary emboli from precipitation of a total nutrient admixture solution. *J Parenter Enteral Nutr* 20:81–87, 1996.
78. Shay DK, Fann LM, Jarvis WR: Respiratory distress and sudden death associated with receipt of a peripheral parenteral nutrition admixture. *Infect Control Hosp Epidemiol* 18:814–817, 1997.
79. Yoscowitz P, Ekland DA, Shaw RC, et al: Peripheral intravenous infiltration necrosis. *Ann Surg* 182:553–556, 1975.
80. Goldminz D, Barnhill R, McGuire J, et al: Calcinosis cutis following extravasation of calcium chloride. *Arch Dermatol* 124:922–925, 1988.
81. Kagen MH, Bansal MG, Grossman M: Calcinosis cutis following the administration of intravenous calcium therapy. *Cutis* 65:193–194, 2006.
82. Anast CS, Mohs JM, Kaplan SL, et al: Evidence for parathyroid failure in magnesium deficiency. *Science* 177:606–607, 1972.
83. Hermans C, Lefebvre C, Devogelaer JP, et al: Hypocalcemia and chronic alcohol intoxication: transient hypoparathyroidism secondary to magnesium deficiency. *Clin Rheumatol* 15:193–196, 1996.
84. Rude RK, Oldham SB, Sharp CF Jr, et al: Parathyroid hormone secretion in magnesium deficiency. *J Clin Endocrin Metab* 47:800–806, 1978.
85. Food and Drug Administration: Safety alert: hazards of precipitation associated with parenteral nutrition. *Am J Hosp Pharmacol* 51:1427–1428, 1994.
86. Baptista RJ, Bistrian BR, Blackburn GL, et al: Utilizing selenious acid to reverse selenium deficiency in total parenteral nutrition patients. *Am J Clin Nutr* 39:816–820, 1984.
87. Anonymous: Deaths associated with thiamine-deficient total parenteral nutrition. *Morb Mortal Wkly Rep* 38:43–46, 1989.
88. Food and Drug Administration: Parenteral multivitamin products; drugs for human use; drug efficacy implementation; amendment. *Fed Regist* 65:21200–21201, 2000.
89. Bistrian BR: Clinical aspects of essential fatty acid metabolism: Jonathan Rhoads lecture. *J Parenter Enteral Nutr* 27:168–175, 2003.
90. Masclans JR, Iglesia R, Bermejo B, et al: Gas exchange and pulmonary haemodynamic responses to fat emulsions in acute respiratory distress syndrome. *Intensive Care Med* 24:918–923, 1998.
91. Moore FA: Caution: use fat emulsions judiciously in intensive care patients. *Crit Care Med* 29:1569–1574, 2001.
92. Suchner U, Katz DP, Furst P, et al: Impact of sepsis, lung injury, and the role of lipid infusion on circulating prostacyclin and thromboxane A(2). *Intensive Care Med* 28:122–129, 2002.
93. Faucher M, Bregeon F, Gainnier M, et al: Cardiopulmonary effects of lipid emulsions in patients with ARDS. *Chest* 124:285–291, 2003.
94. Lekka ME, Liokatis S, Nathanail C, et al: The impact of intravenous fat emulsion administration in acute lung injury. *Am J Respir Crit Care Med* 169:638–644, 2004.
95. Reimund JM, Arondel Y, Joly F, et al: Potential usefulness of olive oil-based lipid emulsions in selected situations of home parenteral nutrition-associated liver disease. *Clin Nutr* 23:1418–1425, 2004.
96. Grimble RF: Immunonutrition. *Curr Opin Gastroenterol* 21:216–222, 2005.
97. Bistrian BR, McCowen KC: Nutritional and metabolic support in the adult intensive care unit: key controversies. *Crit Care Med* 34:1525–1531, 2006.
98. Hall JC, Dobb G, Hall J, et al: A prospective randomized trial of enteral glutamine in critical illness. *Intensive Care Med* 29:1710–1716, 2003.
99. Heyland DK, Muscedere J, Wischmeyer PE, et al: Canadian Trials Group. Randomized trial of glutamine and antioxidants in critically ill patients. *N Engl J Med* 368:1489–1497, 2013.
100. van Zanten AR, Szark F, Kaisers UX, et al: High-protein enteral nutrition enriched with immune-modulating nutrients vs. standard high protein enteral nutrition and nosocomial infections in the ICU: a randomized clinical trial. *JAMA* 312:514–524, 2014.
101. van Zanten ARH, Hofman Z, Heyland DK: Consequences of the REDOXS and METAPLUS trials: the end of an era of glutamine and antioxidant supplementation for critically ill patients? *J Parenter Enteral Nutr* 39(8):890–892, 2015. doi:10.1177/0148607114567201.
102. Annetta MG, Pittiruti M, Vecchiarelli P, et al: Immunonutrients in critically ill patients: An analysis of the most recent literature. *Minerva Anestesiol* 82(3):320–331, 2015.
103. Evans DC, Hegazi RA: Immunonutrition in critically ill patients: Does one size fit all? *J Parenter Enteral Nutr* 39:500–501, 2015.
104. Fushiki T, Iwai K: Two hypotheses on the feedback regulation of pancreatic enzyme stimulation. *FASEB J* 3:121–128, 1989.
105. Davies AR, Morrison SS, Bailey MJ, et al: A multicentre, randomized controlled clinical trial comparing early nasojejunal with nasogastric nutrition in critical illness. *Crit Care Med* 40:2342–2348, 2012.
106. Alkhawaja S, Martin C, Butler RJ, et al: Post=pyloric vs. gastric tube feeding for preventing pneumonia and improving clinical outcomes in critically ill adults. *Cochrane database Syst Rev* 4:8:CD008875; 2015.
107. Driscoll DF, Baptista RJ, Mitrano FP, et al: Parenteral nutrient admixtures as drug vehicles: theory and practice in the critical care setting. *Ann Pharmacother* 25:276–283, 1991.
108. Moore FA, Moore EE, Jones TN, et al: TEN versus TPN following major abdominal trauma-reduced septic morbidity. *J Trauma* 29:916–923, 1989.
109. Kudsk KA, Croce MA, Fabian TC, et al: Enteral versus parenteral feeding. *Ann Surg* 215:503–513, 1992.
110. Moore F, Feliciano D, Andrassy R, et al: Early enteral feeding compared with parenteral, reduces postoperative septic complications. *Ann Surg* 216:172–183, 1992.
111. Heyland D: Parenteral nutrition in the critically-ill patient: more harm than good? *Proc Nutr Soc* 59:457–466, 2000.
112. Jeejeebhoy KN: Total parenteral nutrition: potion or poison? *Am J Clin Nutr* 74:160–163, 2001.
113. Bistrian BR: Update on total parenteral nutrition [Editorial]. *Am J Clin Nutr* 74:153–154, 2001.
114. Simpson F, Doig GS: Parenteral versus enteral nutrition in the critically ill: a meta-analysis of trials using the intent to treat principle. *Intensive Care Med* 31:12–23, 2005.
115. Huwiler-Muntener K, Juni P, Junker C, et al: Quality of reporting of randomized trials as a measure of methodologic quality. *JAMA* 287:2801–2804, 2002.
116. Heyland DK, MacDonald S, Keefe L, et al: Total parenteral nutrition in the critically ill patient: a meta-analysis. *JAMA* 280:2013–2019, 1998.
117. Doig GS, Simpson F, Sweetman EA, et al: Early parenteral nutrition in critically ill patients with short-term relative contraindications to early enteral nutrition: a randomized controlled trial. *JAMA* 309:2130–2138, 2013.
118. Van den Berghe G, Wouters P, Weekers F, et al: Intensive insulin therapy in critically ill patients. *N Engl J Med* 345:139–167, 2001.
119. Van den Berghe G, Wilmer A, Hermans G, et al: Intensive insulin therapy in medical ICU. *N Engl J Med* 354:449–461, 2006.
120. Harvey SE, Parrott F, Harrison DA, et al: Trial of the route of early nutrition support in critically ill patients. *N Engl J Med* 371:1673–1684, 2014.
121. Heidegger CP, Berger MMN, Graf S, et al: Optimization of energy provision with supplemental parenteral nutrition in critically ill patients: a randomized controlled trial. *Lancet* 381:385–393, 2013.
122. Casaer MP, Mesotten D, Hermans G, et al: Early vs. late parenteral nutrition in critically ill adults. *N Engl J Med* 365:506–517, 2011.
123. Arabi YM, Tamim HM, Dhar GS, et al: Permissive underfeeding and intensive insulin therapy in critically ill patients: a randomized controlled trial. *Am J Clin Nutr* 93:569–577, 2011.
124. Arabi YM, Aldawood AS, Haddad SH, et al: Permissive underfeeding or standard enteral feeding in critically ill adults. *N Engl J Med* 374:2398–2408, 2015.
125. Braunschweig CA, Sheehan PM, Peterson SJ, et al: Intensive nutrition in lung injury: A clinical trial (INTACT). *J Parenter Enteral Nutr* 39:13–20, 2015.
126. Rice TW, Mogan S, Hays WA, et al: Randomized trial of initial trophic vs. full-energy enteral nutrition in mechanically ventilated patients with acute respiratory failure. *Crit Care Med* 39:967–974, 2011.

127. The National Heart, Lung and Blood Institute Acute Respiratory Distress Syndrome (ARDS) Clinical Trials Network: Initial trophic vs. full enteral feeding in patients with acute lung injury. *JAMA* 307:795–803, 2012.
128. The NICE-SUGAR Study Investigators: Intensive versus conventional glucose control in critically ill patients. *N Engl J Med* 360:1283–1297, 2009.
129. McClave SA, Sexton LA, Spain DA, et al: Enteral tube feeding in the intensive care unit: factors impeding adequate delivery. *Crit Care Med* 27:1252–1256, 1999.
130. Nguyen NQ, Chapman N, Fraser RJ, et al: Prokinetic therapy for feed intolerance in critical illness: One drug or two? *Crit Care Med* 35:2561–2567: 2007.
131. Silva CC, Bennett C, Saconato H, et al: Metoclopramide for post-pyloric placement of naso-enteral feeding tubes. *Cochrane Database Syst Rev* (1):CD003353, 2015. doi:10.1002/14651858.CD003353.pub2.
132. Peake SL, Davies AR, Deane AM, et al: Use of a concentrated enteral nutrition solution to increase caloric delivery to critically ill patients: a randomized, double-blind, clinical trial. *Am J Clin Nutr* 100:616–625, 2014.
133. McClave SA, Saad MA, Esterle M, et al: Volume-based feeding in the critically ill patient. *J Parenter Enteral Nutr* 39:707–712, 2015.
134. Driscoll DF, Sanborn MD, Giampietro K: ASHP guidelines on the safe use of automated compounding devices for the preparation of parenteral nutrition admixtures. *Am J Health Syst Pharm* 57:1343–1348, 2000.
135. Anonymous: Follow-up on septicemias associated with contaminated Abbott intravenous fluids. *Morb Mortal Wkly Rep* 20:91–92, 1971.
136. Nehme AE: Nutrition support of the hospitalized patient: the team concept. *JAMA* 243:1906–1908, 1980.
137. Cohen MC, Driscoll DF, Bistrian BR: Parenteral nutrition in patients with cardiac diseases, in Rombeau JL, Caldwell MD (eds): *Parenteral Nutrition*. Philadelphia, PA, WB Saunders, 1993, pp 617–630.
138. Khaodhiar L, McCowen K, Bistrian BR: Perioperative hyperglycemia, infection or risk? *Curr Opin Clin Nutr Metab Care* 7:79–82, 1999.
139. Von Meyenfeldt M, Meijerink W, Rouflart M, et al: Perioperative nutritional support: a randomized clinical trial. *Clin Nutr* 11:180–186, 1992.
140. Heslin M, Lattany L, Leung D, et al: A prospective randomized trial of early enteral feeding after resection of upper gastrointestinal malignancies. *Ann Surg* 226:567–577, 1997.
141. Watters J, Krikpatrick S, Norris S, et al: Immediate postoperative enteral feeding results in impaired respiratory mechanics and decreased mobility. *Ann Surg* 226:369–377, 1997.
142. Klein S, Kinney J, Jeejeebhoy KN, et al: Nutrition support in clinical practice: review of published data and recommendations for future research directions. *Am J Clin Nutr* 66:683–706, 1997.
143. Sandstrom R, Drott C, Hyltander A, et al: The effect of postoperative intravenous feeding (TPN) on outcome following major surgery evaluated in a randomized study. *Ann Surg* 217:185–195, 1993.
144. Apovian C, McMahon MM, Bistrian BR: Guidelines for refeeding the marasmic patient. *Crit Care Med* 18:1030–1033, 1990.
145. Matarese LE, Speerhas R, Seidner DL, et al: Foscarnet-induced electrolyte abnormalities in a bone marrow transplant patient receiving parenteral nutrition. *J Parenter Enteral Nutr* 24:170–173, 2000.
146. Van den Berghe G, Wouters PJ, Bouillon R, et al: Outcome benefit of intensive insulin therapy in the critically ill: insulin dose versus glycemic control. *Crit Care Med* 31:359–366, 2003.
147. McMahon MM, Manji N, Driscoll DF, et al: Parenteral nutrition in patients with diabetes mellitus. Theoretical and practical considerations. *J Parenter Enteral Nutr* 13:545–553, 1989.
148. Martindale RG, McClave SA, Vanek VW, et al: Guidelines for the provision and assessment of nutrition support therapy in the adult critically ill patient. *Crit Care Med* 37:2679–2709, 2009.
149. McClave SA, Martindale RG, Vanek VW, et al: Guidelines for the provision and assessment of nutrition support therapy in the adult critically ill patient. *J Parenter Enteral Nutr* 33:277–316, 2009.
150. Knochel JP: The clinical status of hypophosphatemia. *N Engl J Med* 313:447–449, 1985.
151. Singer P, Berger MM, Van den Burghe G, et al: ESPEN Guidelines on parenteral nutrition: Intensive care. *Clin Nutr* 28:387–400, 2009.
152. Ziegler TR: Parenteral nutrition in the critically ill patient. *N Engl J Med* 361:1088–1097, 2009.

Chapter 214 ■ Disease-Specific Nutrition

DIANA WELLS MULHERIN • ALEXIS P. CALLOWAY • GAY GRAVES • DOUGLAS L. SEIDNER

INTRODUCTION

For the critically ill patient, the constant barrage of multiple physiologic derangements quickly leads to malnutrition. The hypermetabolic response to stress changes the nutritional requirements of these individuals, but failure of the various organ systems complicates the issue. Renal, hepatic, and pulmonary function must be considered when prescribing nutritional therapies in the intensive care unit (ICU). This chapter discusses the metabolic abnormalities associated with these disease processes, the nutritional assessment of the patient in organ failure, and proposes evidence-based guidelines for nutritional support in these disease-specific populations.

RENAL FAILURE

Despite many recent advances of medical therapy, management of the critically ill patient with renal failure remains challenging. Acute kidney injury (AKI) is associated with an overall mortality rate of 50% to 60%, depending on its derivations and comorbid conditions [1]. Hypotension and hypovolemia, secondary to excessive fluid losses, inadequate fluid replacement, or decreased cardiac output are common causes of renal failure among the critically ill. Factors such as shock or sepsis and exposure to nephrotoxic drugs can also predispose patients to renal dysfunction [2]. Early diagnosis and restoration of circulating blood volume to the kidneys may decrease the risk of permanent damage; however, the course to renal recovery is often a complicated one. The patient with chronic kidney disease (CKD) is also at increased risk for morbidity, because these patients often have protein–calorie malnutrition (PCM) at baseline. Moreover, the nutritional support of the patient on renal replacement therapy will offer a unique challenge to the critical care practitioner.

Malnutrition and Metabolic Abnormalities of Renal Disease

In general, renal failure is characterized by altered nutrient metabolism, defective metabolic waste excretion, inadequate nutrient intake, and excessive nutrient losses. Inflammatory cytokine levels are increased in patients with advanced CKD, and this can result in decreased serum albumin concentrations, decreased appetite, and weight loss [1]. In fact, malnutrition and inflammation may occur in approximately 30% to 70% of patients with CKD [3]. For these patients, PCM is most often the result of hypercatabolism, poor dietary intake secondary to uremia-induced gastroparesis, poor-tasting highly restrictive diet prescriptions, and medications with gastrointestinal side effects. The overall effect of these derangements results in protein-energy wasting and cachexia, which is closely associated with morbidity and mortality, particularly among patients with advanced CKD [4]. In addition, 10% to 30% of critically ill patients experience AKI, and therefore, represent a significant portion of critically ill patients who require nutrition support [5].

Common metabolic abnormalities associated with AKI include glucose intolerance, impaired lipolysis, increased protein catabolism, decreased protein synthesis, fluid and electrolyte imbalances, and metabolic acidosis. Catabolic hormones increase glycogenolysis and gluconeogenesis of acutely ill patients, while renal gluconeogenesis and glucagon clearance is decreased in the setting of AKI [5]. This combination of derangements renders patients with AKI particularly prone to hyperglycemia and insulin resistance during critical illness. This is coupled with decreased renal insulin clearance that necessitates close monitoring of blood glucose to avoid hyper- or hypoglycemia. Decreased activity of lipolytic enzymes, such as hepatic triglyceride lipase and lipoprotein lipase, may reduce clearance of parenterally infused lipid emulsion by as much as 60% in patients with AKI compared to subjects with normal renal function [6]. Adequate energy provision may thus be hindered by altered carbohydrate and fat metabolism. Energy requirements of patients with AKI are best met with formulas providing mixed substrates with 10% to 15% of total calories from protein, 55% to 70% from carbohydrates, and 20% to 30% from fat [7].

Several factors contribute to increased protein catabolism and overall negative nitrogen balance of patients with AKI. One aspect of the metabolic response to injury is the breakdown of skeletal muscle proteins for use as an energy source, via an increase of hepatic gluconeogenesis, and for synthesis of acute-phase proteins. Metabolic acidosis, which commonly occurs during renal failure, can trigger skeletal muscle protein breakdown as well. Reduction of muscle protein synthesis among this population has been linked to diminished cellular uptake of glucose and amino acids secondary to insulin resistance, altered cellular ion transport mechanisms, and defective intracellular synthesis [5].

Energy and Protein Requirements of Patients with Renal Disease

Although AKI alone does not result in hypermetabolism, energy requirements are affected by other comorbidities during acute illness and by prior nutritional status. Evidence using indirect calorimetry suggests that energy expenditure of critically ill patients with AKI only increases up to 130% of normal. Thus, the recommended energy delivery for critically ill patients with AKI is similar to those without AKI at 25 to 30 kcal/kg/d [5,8]. Establishing appropriate goals for protein delivery requires consideration of degree of illness, degree of renal insufficiency, and mode of renal replacement therapy. Patients with CKD with modest renal function who are not on intermittent hemodialysis (HD) only require 0.6 to 0.8 g/kg/d of protein. Patients with AKI on intermittent HD can achieve a positive nitrogen balance with 1.5 g/kg/d, while those with CKD receiving maintenance HD require protein of doses at 1.2 g/kg/d. For critically ill patients with AKI the recommended protein doses is 1.2 to 2 g/kg/d of actual body weight be provided [9]. Protein requirements during continuous renal replacement therapy (CRRT) are greatly increased to 1.8 to 2.5 g/kg/d due to the associated level of stress in addition to protein losses in the effluent [1,5]. These protein requirements illustrate the significant role that the mode and dose of renal replacement play on the nutritional status of critically ill patients. Recommendations for energy and protein intake are summarized in Table 214.1.

TABLE 214.1

Recommended Energy and Protein Requirements in Renal Failure

	Per kg dosing weight
Energy requirements in AKI	25–30 kcal/d
Protein requirements without stress	
CKD with residual renal function not on HD	0.6–0.8 g/d
CKD on intermittent HD	1.2 g/d
AKI on HD	1.5 g/d
Protein requirements with stress	
AKI on HD	1.2–2.0 g/d
AKI on CRRT	1.8–2.5 g/d

Comments:
Protein dose should not be restricted to avoid initiation of HD or CRRT.
Protein and amino acid loss during CRRT ranges from 5 to 10 g and 10 to 15 g/d.
Protein loss during HD ranges from 10 to 13 g/session.
Data and comments compiled from Refs. [1,5,8,9–12].
AKI, acute kidney injury; CKD, chronic kidney disease; HD, hemodialysis; CRRT, continuous renal replacement therapy.

Metabolic Abnormalities and Renal Replacement Therapy

Provision of protein can be complex in the setting of AKI and critical illness as protein needs are significantly increased while clearance of urea may be decreased. Although lowering the amount of protein delivered may avoid the development of azotemia, current recommendations suggest that protein doses should not be restricted in an attempt to avoid initiation of HD or CRRT [10]. The protein requirements as previously discussed are in part due to nitrogen loss associated with dialysis. In CRRT, there is a loss of at least 0.2 g amino acids per L of ultrafiltrate (up to 10 to 15 g amino acids per day), and of 5 to 10 g per day of proteins. In contrast, protein losses range from 10 to 13 g per HD session [11,12]. In addition, these patients tend to be severely volume overloaded with fluid shifting to the extravascular space because of capillary leak and hypoalbuminemia. Under these circumstances, it is advised that the clinically appropriate protein dose be met, even if giving extra fluid seems to be counterintuitive, as attaining nitrogen balance for the repletion and reversal of the effects of low serum albumin is of paramount importance in the care of these patients.

While preparing a nutrient prescription, consideration should be given to typical glucose content of the dialysate, as this may make a significant contribution to the caloric load of patients already exhibiting some degree of glucose intolerance. Dextrose-containing CRRT dialysate containing 1.5% dextrose can contribute up to 600 glucose calories during a 10-L per day dialysis infusion [13].

Close monitoring of fluid status is crucial for the maintenance of adequate intravascular volume and renal perfusion. Fluid is typically restricted to 1 to 1.5 L per day in nondialysis anuric or oliguric patients. Sodium often needs to be restricted for these patients as well. In this situation concentrated enteral or parenteral formulas are often used to meet daily nutrient requirements. Renal replacement therapy, particularly CRRT, allows for a liberalization of fluid provisions and often makes it easier to deliver full protein and energy requirements. Finally, sodium intake can be liberalized in the setting of CRRT to help correct acid-base or electrolyte abnormalities.

Serum electrolyte levels often fall outside of the normal range depending on renal excretion, extent of catabolism, and type and duration of dialysis [14]. Increased catabolism of skeletal muscle protein releases phosphorus, potassium, and magnesium and may elevate serum electrolyte concentrations. Therefore, patients with AKI or CKD who are not receiving any form of renal replacement therapy typically need their intake of these electrolytes to be limited [5]. For patients on dialysis, it is important to account for the timing of blood draws in relationship to dialysis as this can have a remarkable effect on the measured serum levels of electrolytes. For example, serum potassium can be significantly decreased during HD, depending on the potassium concentration of the dialysate, duration and modality of HD, and baseline serum potassium concentrations. Conversely, there is a rapid shift of potassium from the intracellular to extracellular compartments following HD that can result in up to a 70% increase of serum potassium within 6 hours [15]. In general, patients receiving HD usually require much lower amounts of electrolyte supplementation, especially between treatments, compared to patients receiving CRRT who often require repletion of sodium, potassium, calcium, magnesium, or phosphorus as these are filtered through this modality. Phosphorus in particular is likely to require repletion, because it is much more efficiently cleared by CRRT compared to HD [8]. This is illustrated in a recent report where nearly 69% of 760 critically ill patients undergoing CRRT for AKI experienced hypophosphatemia. Further, they found that the occurrence of hypophosphatemia during CRRT therapy was independently associated with a 1.5-fold higher 28-day mortality [16]. Patients on CRRT therefore may require the addition of a phosphate source to their dialysate as well as daily monitoring of serum phosphorus so that adequate repletion can be provided. Conversely, depressed serum ionized calcium levels are a common result of uremia that is accompanied by hyperphosphatemia. In this situation supplementation of calcium can be used to prevent the release of calcium from the bone.

The dangers of undershooting electrolyte needs for a malnourished CKD population cannot be overstated. Introducing a carbohydrate load by the parenteral or enteral route to a malnourished patient stimulates insulin production, cellular anabolism, and shifts potassium, magnesium, and phosphorus into the intracellular space [17]. The severe decline of serum electrolyte levels with resultant clinical complications is referred to as *refeeding syndrome*. A series of four patients with CKD who developed significant hypophosphatemia after starting PN due to inadequate electrolyte provisions demonstrates that this problem can even occur when renal function is significantly impaired [18]. It is therefore recommended that dextrose infusions be started gradually, serum electrolyte monitoring be done at least once daily, and abnormalities be corrected appropriately.

It is our practice to provide multivitamin preparations standard to enteral and parenteral formulas for most patients in the ICU with AKI and CKD who are receiving CRRT. However, since vitamins and trace elements may be lost in significant amounts during dialysis [14], it has been suggested that supplementation of folic acid, thiamine, and selenium be provided to patients with AKI undergoing CRRT [5]. We generally do not measure blood levels of vitamins or trace elements unless the patient is at risk for deficiency or excess as interpretation of results is often difficult as concentrations may be affected by the acute-phase response. An exception to this approach is for patients with AKI who are not on dialysis. For these patients supplementation with vitamins C and A should be reduced or eliminated, if possible, as evidence suggests that vitamin C in amounts greater than 100 mg per day can lead to oxalate accumulation with renal injury. Likewise, if signs of vitamin A toxicity are observed, daily provision may need to be withheld.

Nutrition Assessment during Renal Disease

Along with other disease states associated with critical illness, early initiation of nutritional support (i.e., within 24 to 48 hours) is recommended [9]. Unfortunately, common measures of nutritional status, such as serum albumin, prealbumin, serum transferrin, weight changes, and anthropometrics are not reliable for this patient population who is typically volume overloaded with metabolic derangements associated with the inflammatory processes of critical illness. Despite this, serum albumin is considered the strongest laboratory predictor of mortality for hospitalized patients with renal failure and should be considered as an important biomarker in the identification of patients who may benefit from nutritional support [19]. Daily monitoring of weight and intake and output records can help to assess fluid balance in these individuals. It is essential to use a dry weight (i.e., free of edema or ascites) when examining alterations in weight status. The dry or adjusted body weight of a renal patient may then be used to more closely estimate daily nutrient needs.

Enteral and Parenteral Formulations for Renal Disease

A wide array of enteral nutrition (EN) products has been designed for patients in varying stages of renal disease (Table 214.2). Standard enteral formulas are recommended for most critically ill patients with renal failure. The formula should be changed to a specialty formulation if severe electrolyte abnormalities are present [9]. Formula selection may also depend largely on the individual's fluid allowance, as a more concentrated enteral formula is usually preferred in the setting of hypervolemia (i.e., 2 kcal per mL). For patients with AKI in whom CRRT has not been initiated, a formula containing only essential amino acids and histidine with little or no vitamins, minerals, and electrolytes may be appropriate. Products with reduced levels of protein, phosphorus, potassium, magnesium, and vitamin A are useful for patients with chronic renal insufficiency who are not on dialysis. Moderate protein formulas with low electrolyte content are often indicated for patients receiving intermittent dialysis treatments. It is best to initiate tube feedings at a slow rate in this population and advance the feeding rate gradually to prevent osmotic diarrhea. Because patients on CRRT demonstrate improved clearance of nitrogenous wastes, fluid, and electrolytes, standard enteral formulas may be used in addition to protein supplements in order to meet protein requirements. In this case, selection likely depends more on accompanying clinical conditions than on renal status. For example, a low-carbohydrate formula may be more appropriate for the CRRT patient with glucose intolerance than the typical calorically dense renal formulas.

Delayed gastric emptying related to dialysis treatment, diabetes, high blood urea nitrogen levels, hyperglycemia, or postoperative gastrointestinal complications can lead to enteral feeding intolerance in patients with renal failure. Parenteral nutrition (PN) is indicated only when the enteral route cannot safely be used to fully meet daily nutritional requirements. For patients who are normal or mildly malnourished, this should occur 7 to 10 days following ICU admission, while earlier initiation should be considered for those who are severely malnourished [9]. In most cases a standard 10% amino acid solution can be used to prepare PN; however, when fluid volume restriction is necessary a 15% amino acid solution should be considered to provide a maximally concentrated parenteral formula.

Summary of Nutritional Recommendations for Patients with Renal Disease

Primary efforts of the caregiver should be directed toward management of the various nutritional and metabolic disorders commonly associated with renal failure. Adequate nutrient provision may optimize renal function, improve nutritional status, and increase the chances of survival for critically ill patients with AKI. Protein and energy requirements of critically ill patients

TABLE 214.2

Specialty Enteral Products for Use in Renal (1–4), Liver (5), and Pulmonary (6–7) Failure

Indication/ product	Caloric density (kcal/mL)	NPC:N	Pro (g/L)	Carb[c] (%)	Fat[c] (%)	PO_4 (mg/L)	K (mg/L)	Na (mg/L)	Manufacturer recommendation
1. Nepro[a]	1.8	121:1	81	34	48	720	1,060	1,060	CKD 5
2. Suplena[a]	1.8	239:1	45	42	48	717	1,139	802	CKD 3,4
3. Novasource Renal[b]	2.0	113.1	90.7	37	45	819	945	945	AKI, CKD, FR, ER
4. Renalcal[b]	2.0	300:1	34	57	36	100	80	60	AKI, SER
5. NutriHep[b,d,e]	1.5	209:1	40	77	12	1,000	1,320	160	Refractory HE
6. Pulmocare[a,f]	1.5	125:1	62.6	28	55	1,060	1,970	1,310	COPD, CF, RF
7. Oxepa[a,g]	1.5	125:1	62.5	28	55	1,060	1,970	1,310	MV-SIRS, ARDS

[a]Abbott Nutrition (Columbus, OH).
[b]Nestle Healthcare Nutrition (Minnetonka, MN).
[c]As a percentage of total energy.
[d]50% of protein is branched-chain amino acids.
[e]70% of fat is medium-chain triglyceride.
[f]20% of fat is medium-chain triglyceride.
[g]Supplemented with antioxidants, fish and borage oil, and medium-chain triglyceride.
NPC: N, nonprotein calorie to nitrogen ratio; Pro, protein; Carb, carbohydrate; PO_4, phosphorus; K, potassium; Na, sodium; CKD, chronic kidney disease; AKI, acute kidney disease; FR, fluid restriction; ER, electrolyte restriction; SER, severe electrolyte restriction, HE, hepatic encephalopathy; COPD, chronic obstructive pulmonary disease; CF, cystic fibrosis; RF, respiratory failure; MV-SIRS, mechanical ventilation-systemic inflammatory response syndrome; ARDS, acute respiratory distress syndrome.

with renal failure are similar to those without renal failure, with the exception of protein needs which are dictated by the mode of renal replacement [9]. Predictive equations, indirect calorimetry, or simple dry weight-based equations (25 to 30 kcal/kg/d) may be used to determine energy needs for critically ill patients with renal failure [5,8]. Serum electrolytes should be monitored daily with additives adjusted on an individual basis. Standard vitamins and trace minerals can safely be provided to most patients with renal failure in the ICU. Fluid allowances for nondialyzed or HD patients are based on 24-hour urine output with an additional 500 mL for insensible losses. Those undergoing CRRT should be permitted sufficient fluid for provision of full nutritional support.

LIVER FAILURE

As the central regulatory organ of the body, the liver is responsible for the metabolism, storage, activation, transport, and synthesis of many vital nutrients. Biochemical reactions fundamental to carbohydrate metabolism such as glycogenesis and gluconeogenesis are carried out in the liver. Albumin, transferrin, prealbumin, and prothrombin are a few of the major serum proteins generated by the liver. Fatty acid oxidation as well as the production of bile salts, triglycerides, and cholesterol for lipid absorption and transport is part of the normal hepatic function. The liver is also responsible for the catabolism of various potentially toxic substances including ammonia, alcohol, and acetaminophen. Liver damage can lead to the disruption of many of these processes; however, due to hepatic reserve functional capacity, dysfunction is not usually seen until 80% to 90% of the liver cells have been injured [20].

A number of insults can initiate the cellular degeneration of acute or chronic liver disease. Viral infection, alcohol use, medications or other hepatotoxic agents, cardiac shock, chronic cholestasis, metabolic disorders, and autoimmune diseases are all potential instigators of liver injury. The damage can be so sudden and severe that it results in fulminant hepatic failure (FHF), a rare disease involving extensive liver necrosis and often culminating in death. Complications of FHF include metabolic abnormalities such as hypoglycemia or acidosis, hemodynamic instability, cerebral edema, sepsis, immunosuppression, and the hepatorenal syndrome. Treatment of FHF often involves nutritional intervention and while there are no randomized controlled studies to assess the benefits of these therapies for this population, the 2009 ESPEN Clinical Guidelines on Parenteral Nutrition state that PN is a safe second-line option to adequately feed these patients in whom EN is insufficient or impossible [21].

Patients with acute hepatitis tend to be highly catabolic in the setting of severe gastrointestinal distress. Nausea, vomiting, and anorexia with occasionally concurrent acute pancreatitis may preclude adequate oral intake. Short-term nutrition support is often necessary until causes of the acute injury to the liver have been identified and treated.

Chronic liver diseases are characterized by repeated episodes of necrosis, followed by hepatocyte regrowth, formation of connective scar tissue and in severe cases the development of cirrhosis. The resulting disruption of normal hepatic structure increases resistance of blood flow through the liver and leads to portal hypertension, which can be characterized by esophageal varices with gastrointestinal bleeding, splenomegaly, ascites, hypoalbuminemia and hepatic encephalopathy (HE). Malnutrition has been documented for most hospitalized patients with alcoholic liver cirrhosis [22]. Because of the association between PCM and poor clinical outcome these patients are often given PN, EN, or oral nutritional supplements [23,24]. It is important to note that the presence of esophageal varices or ascites does not preclude the use of small bowel nasoenteric tube feeding for malnourished cirrhotic patients [25]. Several controlled trials using EN in this population have demonstrated improvements of liver function tests, nutritional status, nitrogen balance, length of hospitalization, and overall prognosis [26–28]. The achievement of positive nitrogen balance did not have a negative impact on HE, azotemia, edema, or ascites among the study groups.

Malnutrition and Metabolic Abnormalities of Liver Disease

Malnutrition during acute or chronic liver disease is the result of a combination of factors. Inadequate provision of nutrients, the hypermetabolic state of cirrhosis, the diminished synthetic capacity of the liver, and the impaired absorption of nutrients are the main factors that disrupt the metabolic balance of cirrhotic patients [29]. Specifically, a decrease of oral intake is common in the patient with prolonged gastrointestinal distress, early satiety secondary to ascites, or excessive alcohol consumption. Maldigestion and malabsorption leading to steatorrhea is often seen with cholestasis or chronic pancreatitis. Impaired glycogen synthesis and storage as well as decreased hepatic degradation of stress hormones lead to the preferential use of lipid and protein reserves for gluconeogenesis [30]. Insulin resistance and glucose intolerance are usual complications of early liver failure. Hypoglycemia can occur during decompensated cirrhosis or FHF as a result of hepatic glycogen depletion and impaired gluconeogenesis.

Hepatic steatosis with concurrent depletion of adipose tissue stores is a frequent consequence of the imbalance between lipid uptake, fatty acid oxidation, and the release of lipoproteins by the damaged liver. It is important to note that hepatic steatosis is often preventable by avoiding overfeeding. Lipids are a moderate source of energy in EN supplement designed for use in liver failure patients. IV lipids are also metabolized well by critically ill patients with hepatic failure when given in amounts that do not exceed their energy requirements. This was demonstrated by Druml et al. who found no significant differences of uptake, hydrolysis, or oxidation of a 20% IV lipid emulsion in septic patients with hepatic failure compared to healthy controls [31].

Altered protein metabolism is by far the most challenging aspect of providing nutrition therapy to the critically ill patient with liver disease. Cirrhosis has long been established as a catabolic disease, with unremitting protein degradation and inadequate resynthesis leading to depletion of visceral protein stores and muscle wasting [32]. Skeletal muscle autophagic proteolysis and myostatin expression (an inhibitor of protein synthesis) are increased with cirrhosis and believed to contribute to anabolic resistance. A recent prospective study performed to determine the mechanisms of sarcopenia with alcoholic cirrhosis found that impaired mTOR1 signaling increased autophagy of skeletal muscle and that this process is acutely reversed by an oral mixture of branched-chain amino acids (BCAAs) enriched with leucine [33].

Under ordinary circumstances, the skeletal muscle takes up circulating BCAAs for the synthesis of glutamine and alanine, amino acids that are released into the bloodstream and taken up by the liver for use in hepatic gluconeogenesis. Glutamine is also a carrier for ammonia, a potentially toxic by-product of protein metabolism. Ammonia is normally converted into urea by the liver and excreted by the kidneys. As liver function declines, uptake of serum glutamine is diminished and the degradation of ammonia into urea is impaired. In this case, excess serum glutamine and ammonia is diverted to renal pathways for direct excretion by the kidneys.

Adequate protein intake is therefore essential for the liver patient not only for the provision of energy by gluconeogenesis, but also for the preservation of skeletal muscle mass and the prevention of HE. The clinical practice of protein restriction for patients with liver damage is common, for fear of precipitating or worsening central nervous system changes associated with HE. Several protein-related theories have been proposed regarding the development of HE, although it is of significance that the occurrence of encephalopathy has not been observed to directly correlate with protein intake of cirrhotic patients [34]. Intravenous protein solutions with higher concentrations of BCAAs have been developed for use in liver disease based on the following hypothesis. As the use of BCAAs by skeletal muscle increases, serum levels decrease. An imbalance in plasma levels of aromatic amino acids (AAA) phenylalanine, tyrosine, and tryptophan and BCAAs and their BCAA/AAA ratio enhances brain AAA uptake and subsequently disturbs neurotransmission. These alternative neurotransmitters compete with actual neurotransmitters for binding sites and disrupt normal central nervous system function to cause symptoms of HE [35].

Elevated serum ammonia concentrations have also been implicated in the pathogenesis of HE. Ammonia metabolites such as glutamine in cerebrospinal fluid have been correlated with the severity of encephalopathy [36]. Plauth et al. evaluated differences of serum ammonia levels between enterally and parenterally fed cirrhotic patients' status post-transjugular intrahepatic portosystemic shunt placement [37]. The small intestinal metabolism of enterally fed glutamine was found to produce significantly greater serum ammonia levels than the direct systemic infusion of parenterally fed glutamine. This suggests that PN may allow for a safer way to provide protein to encephalopathic patients. Enteral or parenteral administration of glutamine, however, is not recommended for patients with moderate to severe liver disease [38].

Energy and Protein Requirements during Liver Disease

Recently published clinical guidelines for critical illness suggest that, when available, indirect calorimetry should be used to determine energy requirements in all critically ill adults [9]. Guidelines that specifically address nutrition support in liver disease recommend that resting energy expenditure (REE) should be increased by a factor of 1.3 in patients with alcoholic steatohepatitis, cirrhosis, and acute liver failure [21]. If measurement of REE is not available, the target for energy intake in critically ill adults should be 25 to 30 kcal/kg/d [9]. A dry or usual weight should be used instead of actual weight in predictive equations to determine energy and protein goals in patients with cirrhosis and hepatic failure as fluid overload, due to complications of ascites, intravascular volume depletion, edema, portal hypertension, and hypoalbuminemia, can result in the overestimation of needs [9]. Nutrient formulas are generally prepared with mixed substrates to provide 10% to 15% of total calories from protein, 55% to 70% from carbohydrates, and 20% to 30% from fat. Greater proportions of fat should be considered for patients with glucose intolerance as long as the fat is not entirely from oils that are high in n-6 polyunsaturated fatty acids [21].

Recommended protein goals for alcoholic steatohepatitis and cirrhosis range from 1.2 to 1.5 g/kg/d [21]. In acute or subacute liver failure protein dosing should be lowered slightly to 0.8 to 1.2 g/kg/d. For cirrhotic patients with HE, protein should be given at the lower end of this range only until the causes of encephalopathy have been identified and treated. In these instances, once patients show signs of improvement, protein should be advanced as tolerated to goals of 1.2 to 1.5 g/kg/d to help maintain nitrogen balance [39]. In nearly all cases the standard protein or amino acid formula is advised [9]. Recommendations for energy and protein intake are summarized in Table 214.3.

A Cochrane review from 2015 looked at 16 randomized clinical trials that enrolled 827 patients with either overt (12 trials) or minimal (four trials) HE. These studies were performed with oral (eight trials) or intravenous (seven trials) BCAA products as the protein source [40]. BCAA had a beneficial effect on HE (RR 0.76, 95% CI 0.63 to 0.92), though sensitivity analyses found no difference between BCAA compared to lactulose and neomycin (RR 0.66, 95% CI 0.34 to 1.30). It is unclear if these results are applicable to the critically ill and it is because of this

TABLE 214.3

Nutrient Requirements in Various Stages of Liver Disease

	Per kg dosing weight
Energy requirements in liver disease	25–30 kcal/d
Protein requirements without HE	
Alcoholic steatohepatitis and cirrhosis, unstressed	0.8–1.2 g/d
Acute and subacute liver failure	
Alcoholic steatohepatitis and cirrhosis, stressed	1.2–1.5 g/d
Protein requirements with HE	
Alcoholic steatohepatitis and cirrhosis	0.8 g/d
Fulminant hepatic failure	

Comments:
If indirect calorimetry is available, provide REE × 1.3 for energy requirements.
Use standard protein and amino acid formulations when other measures to treat HE are initiated.
Use branched-chain amino acids if HE does not resolve with treatment.
Increase protein dose once HE resolves to promote a positive nitrogen balance.
Data and comments compiled from Refs. [9,21,39].
HE, hepatic encephalopathy.

that the aforementioned guidelines for critically ill patients state that there is no evidence of further benefit of BCAA formulations on coma grade for the ICU patient with encephalopathy who is already receiving first-line therapy with luminal-acting antibiotics and lactulose [9]. In addition, few published studies exist to date, comparing BCAA-enriched PN to parenteral solutions containing standard amino acids [41–43]. No differences in outcomes were noted in each of these studies. This is opposed to the guidelines for liver disease that recommend BCAA formulations for patients with stage III and IV HE [21]. Our approach is to use these special formulations when patients do not improve after instituting measures to reverse and treat HE and following the reduction of the protein dose to 0.8 g/kg/d for 24 to 48 hours.

As is the case in most patients with critical illness, EN is the preferred route of nonvolitional feeding in those with liver disease [9]. IV glucose at a dose of 2 to 3 g/kg/d should be given when EN cannot be given for 12 or more hours because of the risk of hypoglycemia from hepatic glycogen depletion and impaired gluconeogenesis [21]. For patients with FHF, IV glucose at this dose should be given prophylactically to prevent hypoglycemia. PN should be considered when enteral feeding cannot be started within 72 hours for patients with cirrhosis or HE with an unprotected airway [21]. It should be started immediately for patients with alcoholic steatohepatitis or cirrhosis who have moderate to severe malnutrition. It should be started for patients with acute liver failure when it is anticipated that EN cannot be started within 5 to 7 days.

Nutrition Assessment during Liver Disease

Traditional parameters of nutritional status such as weight loss and depletion of visceral protein stores are frequently masked among liver failure patients by the presence of ascites or edema. Serum albumin, prealbumin, and transferrin levels are more reflective of disease-related intravascular volume expansion and increased protein catabolic rate than the severity of nutritional deficit. Despite this, albumin remains an important marker of PCM among liver patients. Because the upper extremities tend to escape the fluid retention often seen in liver patients, midarm muscle circumference and triceps skinfold measurement is considered to be the most accurate tools for nutrition assessment in this population. Severe reduction of midarm muscle circumference and triceps skinfold measurement, suggestive of muscle mass and body fat depletion were found to be independent predictors of survival in a study of 212 hospitalized cirrhotic patients. In this study, Alberino et al. also advised the inclusion of upper-arm anthropometry to improve prognostic accuracy of the Child-Pugh score, a commonly used classification of the severity of liver disease [44]. Recent investigations have focused on the detection of those nutritional parameters most indicative of PCM and predictive of survival of liver failure patients. Computer tomography can be to used quantify skeletal muscle mass at the third lumbar spine and standards using this technique have been developed to define sarcopenia, the age-related decrease of muscle mass. Using this method, 112 patients with cirrhosis who were consecutively evaluated for liver transplantation by investigators who found that muscle wasting was associated with mortality independently of the degree of liver dysfunction as determined the by Child Pugh and MELD scores [45]. Similar findings have been confirmed by others [46]. Until this technique becomes readily available, a comprehensive analysis of all available data, including physical examination, anthropometric measurements, and laboratory values, may therefore be the best determinant of nutritional status during liver disease.

Liver Transplantation

Currently, the best therapy for unsalvageable liver failure is orthotopic liver transplant (OLT). It is of the utmost importance to assess the nutritional status of patients who are candidates for OLT as malnutrition has been shown to contribute to an increase of postoperative infection rates, ventilator dependence, hospital length of stay, and a decrease of 1-year survival [47]. In a survey of 248 patients who had undergone OLT, 45% were found to have sarcopenia by CT and its presence was associated with a longer hospital stay (40 vs. 25 days), and more frequent postoperative bacterial infections (26% vs. 15%) [48]. Although these investigators did not find a relationship between sarcopenia and postoperative mortality, Masuda et al. did find that sarcopenia, which was noted for 47% of the 204 patients who underwent living donor liver transplantation, led to a twofold increase of mortality and a fivefold increase of the risk of developing sepsis following transplantation [49].

Perioperative nutritional support appears to reduce the risk of infection following OLT. A retrospective study comparing a historic cohort of patients who all received EN following living donor liver transplantation was compared to a group that only occasionally received tube feedings, found that the incidence of sepsis of 28.2% for the intermittently fed group was significantly higher than the 10.5% rate of those receiving regular nutritional support ($p = 0.03$) [49]. A randomized controlled trial of 36 patients undergoing living donor liver transplant compared early EN to an oral diet as tolerated and found a significant decrease of postoperative bacterial infections with the intervention (63.2% vs. 29.4%) [50]. A meta-analysis of seven randomized controlled trials involving 501 patients who received perioperative immunonutrition demonstrated a 49% lower risk of infectious and a 4-day shorter length of stay for those receiving immunonutrition [51]. Six trials used fish oil, glutamine, or arginine via the parenteral route while one trial used an enteral product combining all of these nutrients. Although this meta-analysis suggests immunonutrition may be of benefit, a moderately large randomized controlled trial of 101 patients comparing EN supplemented with fish oil, ribonucleic acid and arginine to standard tube feeding for at least

5 days following OLT did not demonstrate a difference of the incidence of postoperative infection (60% vs. 57%) [52]. None of these studies found nutritional support to affect postoperative mortality or hospital length of stay.

Repletion of lean body mass can be difficult following OLT. In a cohort of 53 patients where 33 (66.2%) were found to have sarcopenia prior to OLT, an additional 14 patients developed sarcopenia when followed for up to 19 months after transplantation [53]. No significant change of total-body protein, as measured by neutron activation, was seen after 1 year among the patients who participated in the trial of perioperative immunonutrition versus standard enteral feeding [52]. On the other hand, fat mass increases following OLT and likely contributes to the development of hyperglycemia and hyperlipidemia for some patients. Factors that appeared to contribute to the difficulty in attaining positive nitrogen balance include the postoperative elevation of REE that may occur for up to 1 month following transplantation [54] and an increase in the expression of myostatin that has been attributed to calcineurin inhibitors [53]. These observations illustrate some of the challenges that clinicians face when trying to improve the nutritional status of patients following OLT.

Enteral and Parenteral Formulations for Liver Disease

Enteral and parenteral formulas for use during liver failure are designed to normalize plasma amino acid concentrations and improve encephalopathic symptoms. There is currently one hepatic EN product that is calorically dense, has an increased ratio of BCAA/AAA, and has a low fat content (Table 214.2). Intravenous solutions for use during hepatic failure consist of 8% amino acids with 36% of total amino acids provided as BCAA (e.g., valine, isoleucine, and leucine) and only 2% as AAA (e.g., tryptophan, phenylalanine, and tyrosine). These include Aminosyn-HF (Hospira, Inc., Lake Forest, IL), Hepatasol (Clintec Nutrition, Deerfield, IL), and HepatAmine (B. Braun Medical, Inc., Irvine, CA).

A primary focus of the management of HE should be on treatment of its underlying causes. Dehydration, infection, electrolyte abnormalities, gastrointestinal bleeding, acid–base imbalances, and medications have been implicated as causing or contributing to the occurrence of encephalopathy among critically ill patients. Lactulose is the first-line therapy for hepatic HE. Lactulose may be supplemented with neomycin or rifaximin and intraluminal antimicrobials that work by reducing the burden of enteric flora that contribute to the metabolic by-products that lead to HE. In most acute cases, mental status improves with these interventions. When patients are refractory to these measures, protein intake should be reduced to the lower end of the therapeutic range. Nutrition formulations with modified BCAA/AAA ratios should be considered when HE does not improve following these steps.

Summary of Nutritional Recommendations for Liver Disease

In devising a plan for nutritional management of the critically ill patient with liver disease, one must consider the nutritional status, etiology of the disease, and associated complications and metabolic abnormalities. Although direct measurement of lean body mass holds promise for accurately identifying patients at greatest nutritional risk, physical examination, upper arm and other anthropometric measurements, and laboratory values are currently the best determinants of nutritional status for patients with liver disease. Measurement of REE increased by a factor of 1.3 is the best method to determine energy requirements in alcoholic steatohepatitis, cirrhosis, and acute liver failure, but when this is unavailable a goal of 25 to 30 kcal/kg/d using dry body weight may be used [9,21]. Recommended protein goals are 1.2 to 1.5 g/kg/d for patients with alcoholic steatohepatitis and cirrhosis and 0.8 to 1.2 g/kg/d for those with acute or subacute liver failure [21]. For patients with HE, protein dosing should be reduced to 0.8 g/kg/d only until there is clinical improvement and BCAA-enriched formula should be considered when treatment of HE and reduction of protein dosing of standard formulations does not lead to clinical improvement [39]. Transition to standard formulations with protein goals of 1.2 to 1.5 g/kg/d should be done once HE resolves. EN is the preferred mode of nutrition support and may be administered via a gastric tube in the presence of esophageal varices. Nutrient formulas are generally prepared with mixed substrates to provide 10% to 15% of total calories from protein, 55% to 70% from carbohydrates, and 20% to 30% from fat. Sodium and fluid restriction are indicated with ascites or edema. Recommended daily allowances of vitamins, minerals, and trace elements are usually sufficient for this population, although additional supplementation of thiamine and folate is customary for patients with alcoholic cirrhosis. Although some reports have found that zinc supplementation may improve HE, a recent meta-analysis has questioned the efficacy of zinc as a routine therapy for this condition [55]. Intravenous glucose (2 to 3 g/kg/d) should be given when EN cannot be given for 12 or more hours as depletion of glycogen stores in this population quickly leads to protein breakdown for gluconeogenesis. Infusion of 10% dextrose solutions should be given prophylactically to patients with FHF to prevent hypoglycemia until full feeding by EN or PN, which can provide a more concentrated source of glucose and avoid fluid overload, is firmly established. PN should be considered within 72 hours when EN cannot be started in critically ill patients with liver disease or those were at high risk for aspiration pneumonia. PN should be started immediately for patients with alcoholic steatohepatitis or cirrhosis with moderate to severe malnutrition and for those with acute liver failure who may not be able to start EN within 5 to 7 days. Table 214.4 outlines the summary of randomized controlled trials and clinical guidelines in liver disease.

PULMONARY FAILURE

Optimal pulmonary function is essential to the maintenance of adequate nutritional status. Through the process of gas exchange, the lungs and supporting respiratory structures provide oxygen to vital tissues for nutrient metabolism. The respiratory system also plays a major role for the regulation of acid–base balance. Pulmonary injury or insufficiency can lead to malnutrition and dependence on mechanical ventilation of the critically ill patient. Acute respiratory distress syndrome (ARDS), characterized by severe progressive hypoxemia and mechanical ventilation, is a frequent result of trauma, sepsis, or surgery in the critical care setting. The patient with chronic obstructive pulmonary disease (COPD) may also undergo periods of acute exacerbation requiring intensive care. These two forms of the lung injury illustrates the spectrum of nutritional status encountered in the critical care setting with patient suffering from ARDS often being normal prior to hospitalization and those with COPD being at risk of having chronic disease related malnutrition [56]. Numerous randomized controlled trials have been published over the last several years that have helped clarify the utilization of nutrition support for these patients and will be discussed in this section.

TABLE 214.4

Nutrition Support in Liver Disease: Summary of Controlled Trials and Clinical Guidelines

- Protein restriction is not advised to reduce the risk of hepatic encephalopathy (HE) as it may paradoxically exacerbate this condition and may worsen nutritional status [9].
- Standard protein and amino acid preparations are indicated in most patients [9,21].
- Branched-chain amino acid preparations for liver disease are therapeutically equivalent to lactulose or neomycin for HE [40]. The latter are recommended as first-line therapy [9].
- Branched-chain amino acid preparations for liver disease may be considered in grade III or IV HE [21].
- Enteral nutrition (EN) is the preferred feeding route [9].
- Start PN within 72 h of ICU admission if EN cannot be started in unstressed, mildly malnourished patients or immediately in moderately or severely malnourished patients who cannot be fed enough by mouth or by EN [21].
- IV glucose (2–3 g/kg/d) should be given if EN cannot be given for 12 or more hours as depletion of glycogen stores quickly leads to protein breakdown with loss of lean tissue for gluconeogenesis [21].
- Infusion of 10% dextrose solutions should be given prophylactically to patients with fulminant hepatic failure to prevent hypoglycemia until full feeding by EN or PN can be started [21].
- Perioperative nutrition support reduces the risk of postoperative bacterial infections following orthotopic liver transplantation [50]. Parenteral immunonutrition reduces infectious complications and length of stay [51]. Enteral immunonutrition appears to be equivalent to standard formulas [52].

Malnutrition and Metabolic Abnormalities of Pulmonary Disease

Malnutrition with COPD is the result of an imbalance between energy intake and utilization [57]. Hyperinflation of the lung with an associated decrease in abdominal volume can lead to anorexia, early satiety, and tube feed intolerance. Oral intake may be hampered by dyspnea and fatigue during meal times and impaired leptin regulation, a hormone that reduces food intake. An increase in energy consumption from COPD has been attributed to an increase in the work of breathing, tobacco use and medication (theophylline and β-blockers). Loss of lean body mass may occur as a result of disuse atrophy, tissue hypoxia from arterial hypoxemia, anabolic hormonal insufficiency or systemic inflammation as a result of recurrent infections and an imbalance of inflammatory cytokines. Currently interleukin (IL)-1β is felt to play a more important role than IL-6 or tumor necrosis factor (TNF)-α, as recent studies have not found elevated levels of these latter two cytokines that were previously thought to participate in this process.

Just as pulmonary disease influences the onset of malnutrition, poor nutritional status may significantly impair several structural and functional components of the respiratory system. Respiratory muscles display reduced efficiency and endurance during nutrition deprivation due to loss of muscle mass and depletion of energy reserves. Impaired respiratory muscle function may result in decreased ventilatory drive and inefficient gas exchange with hypercapnia and hypoxemia [58]. Hypophosphatemia is present in up to 30% of critically ill patients and may be more common for those with refeeding syndrome [59]. Phosphate deficiency diminishes diaphragmatic muscle function and adversely affects the hemoglobin–oxygen dissociation curve by limiting the production of adenosine triphosphate and 2,3-diphosphoglycerate. Hypoalbuminemia, associated with critical illness and malnutrition, leads to an expansion of extracellular fluid and increased interstitial lung fluid or pulmonary edema. These factors negatively affect the efficiency of the pulmonary system and place patients with lung disease at risk for respiratory failure. Malnutrition also adversely influences the production of secretory IgA, alveolar macrophage recruitment and function and clearance of bacteria from the upper respiratory tract placing patients at risk for nosocomial pneumonia, the most common fatal infection among hospitalized individuals [60].

Energy and Protein Requirements during Pulmonary Disease

Indirect calorimetry is a clinical tool by which measurements of respiratory gas exchange are used to determine energy requirements and substrate utilization for a given subject. It continues to be the gold standard for establishing nutritional goals. Substrate utilization is the ratio of oxygen consumed to carbon dioxide produced for a given macronutrients and is referred to as the respiratory quotient (*R/Q*). The oxidation of fat, protein, and carbohydrate produces an *R/Q* of 0.7, 0.8, and 1.0, respectively. Ideally, the *R/Q* of a given patient should approximate 0.85 to reflect metabolism of mixed substrates. When carbohydrate or total calorie provisions exceed energy requirements, *R/Q* levels rise above 1.0 to suggest fat synthesis. An *R/Q* of less than 0.7 is indicative of inadequate nutritional support with breakdown body fat and protein stores from adipose and lean tissue. This information is useful for the adjustment of fuel mixtures within the nutrient prescription to avoid potentially harmful effects of under or over feeding the ventilator-dependent patient. Underfeeding energy may increase risk of infection, prolong ventilator dependence, delay wound healing, and increase overall hospital morbidity and mortality, whereas overfeeding energy needs is associated with several metabolic, hepatic, and respiratory complications, including increased carbon dioxide production with inability to wean from mechanical ventilation. Studies comparing estimates of energy requirements by predictive formulas have found a poor correlation with measured energy expenditure; only 25% of hospitalized patients received calories within 10% of energy requirements [61,62]. Although many investigators have recommended using indirect calorimetry to feed critically ill patients, few studies have been able to demonstrate an improvement of clinical outcomes or meaningful endpoints. In one such study, 130 mechanically ventilated patients who were expected to stay in the ICU for at least 3 days were randomized to receive energy as measured by indirect calorimetry or 25 kcal/kg/d [63]. Nutrition support was provided as enteral tube feeding with additional calories being given as PN when the daily energy goal was not met. The group fed based on indirect calorimetry had a trend toward lower hospital mortality (32.3% vs. 47.7%, $p = 0.058$); however, this group was also found to have fewer ventilator free days and required a longer stay in the ICU compared to controls. As previously discussed, current clinical guidelines, that are endorsed by the Society of Critical Care Medicine and the American Society for Parenteral and Enteral Nutrition (SCCM/ASPEN), suggest that indirect calorimetry be used to determine energy requirements when available and in the absence of variables that effect the accuracy of these measurements (such as $FiO_2 > 60\%$) or when these measures cannot be made, published predictive equations or simplistic weight-based equations (25 to 30 kcal/kg/d) should be used to determine energy needs [9].

The provision of IV carbohydrate in excess of 5 mg per kg per minute to severely stressed patients increases carbon dioxide production ($\dot{V}CO_2$) and may delay weaning from mechanical ventilation. Jih et al. reported the case of a septic ARDS patient who developed increased respiratory distress and hypercapnic acidosis in response to hypercaloric carbohydrate infusion [64]. Hypercapnia resolved as carbohydrate and total calories were decreased to levels consistent with indirect calorimetry measurements of REE. Others have shown that total caloric intake has more of an impact on respiratory function for mechanically ventilated patients than excessive carbohydrate calories [65]. No differences of ($\dot{V}CO_2$) was observed upon variation of carbohydrate provisions with consistent total caloric intake (1.3 × REE). In contrast, increasing total caloric provisions (1.5 to 2.0 × REE) with fixed carbohydrate content led to a significant and progressive increase of ($\dot{V}CO_2$).

The substitution of fat for carbohydrate calories may lower *R/Q* and decrease ($\dot{V}CO_2$) to ease weaning from the ventilator [66]. The use of IV fat emulsions (IVFE) is not without its drawbacks, however. Rapid infusion of IVFE may adversely affect gas exchange by decreased rate of clearance, deposition of lipid particles within the reticuloendothelial system, and subsequent reduction of pulmonary diffusion capacity. This effect is most often seen among patients with existing pulmonary dysfunction and with rates of lipid administration more than 0.11 g/kg/hr [67]. There is also concern that higher infusion rates of IVFE may result in immune dysfunction since the products available in the US are manufactured using soybean oil, which is rich in the omega-6 polyunsaturated fatty acids linoleic acid (LA). Large amounts of LA lead to the production of prostaglandins and eicosanoids that favor vasoconstriction and increased inflammation that decreases bacterial clearance from systemic circulation and increases uptake of bacteria by the lungs [68]. Given these concerns, Battistella et al. randomized 57 trauma patients requiring total PN to receive a formula with or without IVFE for 10 days [69]. They found that patients who received IVFE had a significantly greater length of ICU and hospital stay, longer duration of mechanical ventilation, and higher incidence of infection. The results however were criticized because the two groups did not receive isocaloric feeding (21 vs. 28 kcal per day) and it is possible that the excess calories were responsible for the adverse outcomes rather than exposure to IVFE. A meta-analysis of 12 RCT that compared soybean oil based IVFE to soybean oil sparing formulas in 806 patients found a nonstatistical trend toward a reduction of mortality and an increase in the length of mechanical ventilation and ICU length of stay [70] for soybean sparing formulas. There were no significant effects on infectious complications. As a result of these studies, the intersociety clinical guidelines for critical care suggest withholding or limiting soybean oil IVFE during the first week following initiation of PN to a maximum of 100 g per week (often divided into 2 doses per week if there is concern for essential fatty acid deficiency) [9].

Protein requirements of critically ill patients with pulmonary failure are elevated in accordance with the hypercatabolism of stressed states. A prospective observational study of mechanically ventilated patients demonstrated a 50% decrease in 28-day mortality for nonseptic patients when >1.2 g per kg protein was received in conjunction with energy targets [71]. In a similar study a stepwise decrease of 28-day mortality was demonstrated with increased protein provision (group 1: 0.79 g per kg, 27% mortality; group 2: 1.06 g per kg, 24% mortality; group 3: 1.46 g per kg, 16% mortality) [72]. Guideline recommendations suggest that protein intake range from 1.2 to 2.0 g/kg/d of actual body weight [9]. Unfortunately, an increase in ventilatory drive and minute ventilation may be seen with protein infusion. It is therefore recommended that protein provisions be advanced slowly with close attention to ventilatory drive for mechanically ventilated patients. Serum protein markers, such as albumin, prealbumin, transferrin, and CRP, are not reliable for determining adequacy of protein provision in the critical care setting for patients with ongoing inflammation [9].

Nutritional Assessment during Pulmonary Disease

Malnutrition, which is typically defined for COPD patients as a BMI of less than 20 kg per m^2, is an important co-morbidity with an incidence of approximately 20% to 40% [58,73]. The evidence for using this cutoff-point to identify patients at nutritional risk is supported by a multicenter study of hospitalized patients with COPD that found underweight patients with a BMI < 20 kg per m^2 have a significantly lower FEV(1) when compared to patients who were overweight or obese [74]. To determine the impact of nutritional status on mortality, the investigators followed patients for 2 years after initial discharge and found that there were fewer deaths in overweight (BMI 25 to 30 kg per m^2) subjects compared to those who were underweight. For the 49 of 261 subjects that died (19%), this result remained significant after adjustment for FEV(1) with a hazard risk ratio 2.6 (95% CI 1.3 to 5.2). The importance of nutritional status is also supported by its inclusion in the BODE (BMI, airflow obstruction, dyspnoea and exercise capacity) index, a grading system that has been shown to be better than the FEV1 for predicting the risk of death from any cause in patients with COPD [75]. The impact of nutritional intervention has been demonstrated in two meta-analyses of long-term trials of ambulatory malnourished patients with COPD. These reports have demonstrated that when given for two or more weeks, oral and enteral supplements lead to significant gain of weight, lean body mass, fat mass, respiratory muscle strength, physical endurance, and quality of life [76,77].

In regard to defining nutritional status in the ICU, Faisy et al. compared changes of bioelectrical impedance analysis (BIA) with various anthropometric and biologic parameters among patients with COPD and acute respiratory failure [78]. BIA more accurately detected alterations of nutritional status for patients requiring mechanical ventilation, whereas anthropometric data were inconclusive. Low serum albumin levels were also significantly associated with increased mortality among patients in this study. Others have found that weight loss and low percentage of ideal body weight can significantly predict the need for mechanical ventilation among hospitalized COPD patients [79]. Weight changes, serum albumin levels, and BIA, when available, are thus valuable tools in assessment of nutritional status and prediction of outcomes for patients with severe respiratory insufficiency. BIA more accurately identified COPD patients at risk for respiratory failure because low fat free mass, measured with this technique, more accurately identified patients who have a low body weight with low lean body mass (60%), low body weight with a normal lean body mass (20%) and a stable body weight with low lean body mass (20%) [80].

It has been suggested that all patients admitted to the ICU undergo nutritional assessment utilizing a scoring system that examines both nutritional status and disease severity [9]. The Nutrition Risk Screening (NRS) 2002 and NUTRIC score fulfill both of these criteria and have been clinically validated [81,82]. NRS 2002 assigns points for nutritional status (0 to 3) and severity of illness (0 to 3), where 0 = absent, 1 = mild,

2 = moderate, and 3 = severe, and an additional point for age of 70 years or more. NUTRIC score assigns a range of points for age, APACHE II, SOFA, number of comorbidities, and length of stay in the hospital prior to ICU admission. Patients at high nutrition risk are identified by values of ≥5.

Enteral and Parenteral Nutrition for Patients with Pulmonary Disease

Nutritional support is an important component of the care of patients with respiratory failure and acute lung injury (ALI). Several recently performed studies in this cohort of patients serves as the basis for the current version of the SCCM/ASPEN clinical guidelines for critical care [9]. New findings have helped to clarify when nutritional support should be initiated, when trophic versus full enteral feeding should be used, and when PN should supplement enteral tube feeding or be given as a sole source of feeding. The decision on when and how to provide nutrition support requires assessment of the patient's nutritional status and disease severity, functional integrity of the gastrointestinal tract, and the anticipated duration of mechanical ventilation.

EN is the preferred route for feeding patients with respiratory failure because it maintains the mass and function of the intestinal tract, reduces bacterial translocation and the risk of sepsis, reduces the systemic immune response, is lower in cost compared with PN, and is associated with better clinical outcomes [83]. Severe complications are fairly uncommon and include aspiration pneumonia, GI intolerance, electrolyte abnormalities, and intestinal ischemia. An update of the SCCM/ASPEN guidelines meta-analysis of 21 randomized control trials comparing early versus delayed EN found significant reduction of mortality (RR = 0.70; 95% CI 0.49 to 1.0; $p = 0.05$) and infectious morbidity (RR = 0.74; 95% CI 0.58 to 0.93; $p = 0.01$). Based on these results it is recommended that EN be started in 24 to 48 hours for critically ill patients with ARDS/ALI and for those expected to need mechanical ventilation for ≥72 hours [9].

Trophic feeding is defined as EN that provides 10 to 20 kcal per hour and is believed to be of a sufficient amount to prevent mucosal atrophy and maintain gut integrity. It is primarily given for up to 7 to 10 days to patients who are expected to require mechanical ventilation for ≥72 hours and whose nutrition risk stratification is from low to moderate [9]. This recommendation is in part based on two open label, randomized controlled trials which hypothesized that initial trophic feeding for up to 6 days would be as effective as full EN and would have fewer gastrointestinal complications [84,85]. These studies include a single-center trial that enrolled a heterogeneous population of 200 patients with acute respiratory failure [84] and a multicenter trial that enrolled 1,000 patients with ARDS/ALI [85]. Patients given trophic feeding received 300 to 400 kcal per day while the full feeding group received 1,400 kcal per day, which approximated 15% and 75% of the calculated energy requirements, respectively. It was found that both groups had a similar number of ventilator-free days, 60-day mortality, and incidence of nosocomial infections, while the group receiving trophic feeding had a lower incidence of elevated gastric residual volumes and diarrhea. The larger multicenter trial has been criticized for underdelivery of protein (0.6 to 0.8 g/kg/d) and that study patients were moderately critically ill and had a shorter LOS in the ICU, potentially indicating lower nutritional risk [9]. Supplemental PN should not be given to ICU patients at low to moderate nutrition risk during the first week of nutrition support. A large multicenter randomized controlled trial of 4,640 patients, comparing initiation of PN at 48 hours versus PN started after 8 days, demonstrated that the late-initiation group had a significantly lower requirement for mechanical ventilation and renal replacement therapy, fewer infections and incidence of cholestasis, and greater likelihood of being discharged from the ICU and hospital alive [86]. A small randomized controlled trial that specifically investigated the benefit of early PN initiation during ALI was stopped after enrolling 78 subjects because of a significant greater hospital mortality in the early PN group [87].

One should endeavor to provide the full caloric goal within 2 to 3 days of admission to the ICU for patients at high nutrition risk or with severe malnutrition [9]. Though there are no randomized controlled trials to support this recommendation, a large observational study of critically ill patients found significantly lower mortality for high risk patients who received >80% of their goal energy [88] compared to those that did not. EN is most appropriate for reasons that have been discussed; however, for patients with poor tolerance to tube feeding or in those requiring significant vasopressor support the balance of protein and energy requirements should be delivered through the use of PN. The benefits and safety of PN for this group of patients has been demonstrated by studies where protocols provided appropriate doses of energy and protein, achieved good glycemic control, and in some instances, allowed cautious feeding of patients at risk for refeeding syndrome. A randomized multicenter controlled trial of early PN in 1,372 critically ill patients with a relative contraindication to EN compared PN, as the sole source of nutrition support, to standard of care where subjects received EN as tolerated [89]. The study found no differences of ICU and hospital length of stay or 60-day mortality but did note a significant decrease of the duration of mechanical ventilation for the PN group. In a similarly designed study comparing early PN (without EN) to early EN for patients without a contraindication to tube feeding, a similar incidence of 30-day all-cause mortality was noted for all subjects (primary outcome), a significantly lower incidence of hypoglycemia and vomiting was seen in the early PN group, and no difference was noted for infectious complications, 90-day mortality, and other secondary outcome measures [90]. Finally, a randomized controlled trial of 305 critically ill patients comparing EN supplemented with PN to standard EN, found that patient supplemented with PN had a significantly lower number of nosocomial infections (27% vs. 38% with a hazard ratio of 0.65, 95% CI 0.43 to 0.97; $p = 0.03$) [91]. PN should also be used for patients with low to moderate nutritional risk if nutrient requirements cannot be met because of enteral intolerance after 7 to 10 days and for patients with severe malabsorption.

Standard enteral formulas are recommended for most patients with pulmonary dysfunction, even those who are critically ill [9]. Fluid restricted energy-dense formulations that provide 1.5 to 2 kcal per mL should be used for patients with acute respiratory failure who require volume restriction. This includes patients with fluid overload, pulmonary edema, and renal failure. As previously discussed, specialty formulations that have a high ratio of fat to carbohydrate designed to manipulate the respiratory quotient and reduce CO_2 production are not of benefit when energy goals range from 25 to 30 kcal/kg/d. We reserve the use of these products for patients with existing COPD and increasing difficulty weaning off the ventilator. A meta-analysis of six randomized controlled trials that investigated the effect of immune modulating nutrition, which contained fish oil, borage oil, and antioxidants and included reports of mortality, 28-day ICU length of stay and ventilator free days, found no significant effects of this therapy for subjects with ALI/ARDS [92]. The SCCM/ASPEN task force noted significant heterogeneity of these trials based on the method of infusion (continuous versus bolus), the type of oils used and in some instances controls that may have received formulas that had an adverse clinical effect and therefore do

TABLE 214.5

Nutrition Support in Pulmonary Disease: Summary of Controlled Trials and Clinical Guidelines

Early enteral nutrition (EN) reduces mortality and infectious complications [9].
Trophic feeding (10–20 kcals/h) for up to 6 d is as effective as full enteral nutrition and has fewer gastrointestinal complications [84,85] and is recommended in patients with low to moderate nutrition risk.
Early PN is safe if it provides appropriate doses of energy and protein, good glycemic control, and avoids the refeeding syndrome. It has been shown to reduce the duration of mechanical ventilation [89] or be equivalent to EN as tolerated [90]. Early PN supplemented EN reduces the risk of nosocomial infection [91]. It is recommended in patients with severe nutrition risk or malabsorption. It should be delayed for 7–10 d in patients with low to moderate nutrition risk [9].
Energy requirements are best determined by indirect calorimetry. If unavailable, feeding goals are 25–30 kcal/kg/d. Protein goals ranged from 1.2–2.0 g/kg/d. Standard enteral formulas are recommended in most patients with acute respiratory failure. Energy-dense formulations should be used if fluid restriction is needed.
Enteral feeding protocols are recommended to help achieve protein and energy goals [9]. If gastric feeding is not tolerated, then postpyloric delivery reduces the risk of aspiration pneumonia [93,94]. It is not advised to routinely measure gastric residual volume, but when it is termination of feeding should not be done for volumes less than 500 mL [9].
Immunonutrition has not been recommended because of the heterogeneity of the clinical trials [9].

not endorse the use of these products [9]. These products are listed in Table 214.2.

Enteral feeding protocols should be used to increase the likelihood of reaching protein and energy feeding targets [9]. Feeding can be delivered to the stomach for most critically ill patients. Prokinetics, such as metoclopramide and erythromycin, may be considered for patients at high risk for aspiration. Those who are at high risk for aspiration or who have demonstrated intolerance to gastric feeding should be fed beyond the pylorus. These recommendations are based on two meta-analyses of nasogastric versus postpyloric feeding in 1,496 and 1,109 critically ill patients [93,94]. Patients who received feeding distal to the stomach were 30% to 40% less likely to develop aspiration pneumonia, received a greater proportion of prescribed calories, and had lower gastric residual volumes. Mortality, length of ICU stay, and gastrointestinal complications were no different between the groups. Measurement of gastric residual volumes should not be used as part of routine care as results do not correlate with the incidence of regurgitation, aspiration, and aspiration pneumonia [9]. Pitfalls of measuring gastric residual volume include little correlation between large measurements and the development of aspiration pneumonia, lack of standardization between method used to measure its presence, and inconsistent effective prokinetic agents [95]. It is currently advised that volumes of less than 500 mL should not result in termination of enteral feeding potentially leading to greater delivery of enteral feeding to critically ill patients.

Summary of Nutritional Recommendations for Patients with Pulmonary Disease

Malnutrition adversely affects clinical outcomes of patients requiring prolonged mechanical ventilation. Early EN reduces the risk of nosocomial infection and mortality. Trophic feeding provides the same benefits as full EN in patients with a low to moderate nutrition risk with better gastrointestinal tolerance. Full protein and energy requirements should be given in the first 48 to 72 hours after admission to the ICU for patients with severe malnutrition or high nutritional risk scores and to others after 7 to 10 days. If goals cannot be reached with EN then supplemental PN should be provided. Nutritional risk is best determined by using a scoring system that combines assessment of nutritional status and disease severity. Energy requirements are best determined by indirect calorimetry, but when unavailable a simple weight-based equation (25 to 30 kcal/kg/d) may be used. Careful monitoring of intake and output, weight changes, and respiratory status is required when indirect calorimetry is not available. Protein needs to promote recovery from illness range from 1.2 to 2.0 g/kg/d and should be advanced with caution to avoid worsening respiratory function. Maintenance of fluid balance is also of primary importance for the critically ill patient with pulmonary insufficiency. Concentrated parenteral solutions and enteral formulas should be used as necessary. Sodium restriction is indicated for patients with pulmonary edema or congestive heart failure. Hypophosphatemia may be avoided by supplementation and gradual advancement of nutritional support for severely malnourished patients. Serum phosphorus, potassium, and magnesium levels should be monitored routinely and deficiencies should be corrected aggressively in this setting. Table 214.5 outlines the summary of randomized controlled trials and clinical guidelines in pulmonary disease.

References

1. Brown RO, Compher C: A.S.P.E.N. clinical guidelines: nutrition support in adult acute and chronic renal failure. *JPEN J Parenter Enteral Nutr* 34(4):366–377, 2010.
2. McCarthy MS, Phipps SC: Special nutrition challenges: current approach to acute kidney injury. *Nutr Clin Pract* 29(1):56–62, 2014.
3. Peev V, Nayer A, Contreras G: Dyslipidemia, malnutrition, inflammation, cardiovascular disease and mortality in chronic kidney disease. *Curr Opin Lipidol* 25(1):54–60, 2014.
4. Obi Y, Qader H, Kovesdy CP, et al: Latest consensus and update on protein-energy wasting in chronic kidney disease. *Curr Opin Clin Nutr Metab Care* 18(3):254–262, 2015.
5. Gervasio JM, Garmon WP, Holowatyj M: Nutrition support in acute kidney injury. *Nutr Clin Pract* 26(4):374–381, 2011.
6. Druml W, Fischer M, Sertl S, et al: Fat elimination in acute renal failure: long-chain vs medium-chain triglycerides. *Am J Clin Nutr* 55:468–472, 1992.
7. Wolk R, Foulks C: Renal disease, in The A.S.P.E.N: *Adult Nutrition Support Core Curriculum*. 2nd ed. American Society for Parenteral and EN, 2012.
8. Fiaccadori E, Regolisti G, Maggiore U: Specialized nutritional support interventions in critically ill patients on renal replacement therapy. *Curr Opin Clin Nutr Metab Care* 16(2):217–224, 2013.
9. McClave SA, Taylor BE, Martindale RG, et al: Guidelines for the provision and assessment of nutrition support therapy in the adult critically ill patient: Society of Critical Care Medicine (SCCM) and American Society for Parenteral and EN (A.S.P.E.N.). *JPEN J Parenter Enteral Nutr* 40(2):159–211, 2016.
10. Lindsay RM, Spanner E: A hypothesis: the protein catabolic rate is dependent upon the type and amount of treatment in dialyzed uremic patients. *Am J Kidney Dis* 13:382–389, 1989.
11. Davenport A, Roberts NB: Amino acid losses during continuous high-flux hemofiltration in the critically ill patient. *Crit Care Med* 17:1010–1014, 1989.
12. Seidner DL, Matarese LE, Steiger E: Nutritional care of the critically ill patient with renal failure. *Semin Nephrol* 14:53–63, 1994.
13. Wooley JA, Btaiche IF, Good KL: Metabolic and nutritional aspects of acute renal failure in critically ill patients requiring continuous renal replacement therapy. *Nutr Clin Pract* 20(2):176–191, 2005.

14. Maursetter L, Kight CE, Mennig J, et al: Review of the mechanism and nutrition recommendations for patients undergoing continuous renal replacement therapy. *Nutr Clin Pract* 26(4):382–390, 2011.
15. Hung AM, Hakim RM: Dialysate and serum potassium in hemodialysis. *Am J Kidney Dis* 66(1):125–132, 2015.
16. Yang Y, Zhang P, Cui Y, et al: Hypophosphatemia during continuous veno-venous hemofiltration is associated with mortality in critically ill patients with acute kidney injury. *Crit Care* 17:R205, 2013.
17. Walmsley RS: Refeeding syndrome: screening, incidence, and treatment during parenteral nutrition. *J Gastroenteral Hepatol* 28(S4):113–117, 2013.
18. Duerksen DR, Papineau N: Electrolyte abnormalities in patients with chronic renal failure receiving parenteral nutrition. *JPEN J Parenter Enteral Nutr* 22(2):102–104, 1998.
19. Lowrie EG, Lew NL: Death risk in hemodialysis patients: the predictive value of commonly measured variables and an evaluation of death rate differences between facilities. *Am J Kidney Dis* 15(5):458–482, 1990.
20. Delich PC, Siepler JK, Parker P: *Liver Disease. The ASPEN Nutrition Support Core Curriculum: A Case-Based Approach—The Adult Patient*. American Society for Parenteral and Enteral Nutrition, 2007.
21. Plauth M, Cabre E, Campillo B, et al: ESPEN Guidelines on Parenteral Nutrition: hepatology. *Clin Nutr* 28(4):436–344, 2009.
22. Marsano L, McClain CJ: Nutrition and alcoholic liver disease. *JPEN J Parenter Enteral Nutr* 15:337–344, 1991.
23. Koretz RL: The evidence for the use of nutritional support in liver disease. *Curr Opin Gastroenterol* 30(2):208–214, 2014.
24. Koretz RL, Avenell A, Lipman TO: Nutritional support for liver disease. *Cochrane Database Syst Rev* 5:CD008344, 2012.
25. deLedinghen V, Beau P, Mannant PR, et al: Early feeding or enteral nutrition in patients with cirrhosis after bleeding from esophagealvarices? A randomized controlled study. *Dig Dis Sci* 42(3):536–541, 1997.
26. Cabre E, Gonzalez-Huix F, bad-Lacruz A, et al: Effect of total enteral nutrition on the short-term outcome of severely malnourished cirrhotics. A randomized controlled trial. *Gastroenterology* 98:715–720, 1990.
27. Kearns PJ, Young H, Garcia G, et al: Accelerated improvement of alcoholic liver disease with enteral nutrition. *Gastroenterology* 102:200–205, 1992.
28. Mendenhall CL, Tosch T, Weesner RE, et al: VA cooperative study on alcoholic hepatitis. II: prognostic significance of protein-calorie malnutrition. *Am J Clin Nutr* 43:213–218, 1986.
29. Tsiaousi ET, Hatzitolios AI, Trygonis SK, et al: Malnutrition in end stage liver disease: recommendations and nutritional support. *J Gastroenterol Hepatol* 23(4):527–533, 2008.
30. Bugianesi E, Kalhan S, Burkett E, et al: Quantification of gluconeogenesis in cirrhosis: response to glucagon. *Gastroenterology* 115:1530–1540, 1998.
31. Druml W, Fischer M, Ratheiser K: Use of intravenous lipids in critically ill patients with sepsis without and with hepatic failure. *JPEN J Parenter Enteral Nutr* 22:217–223, 1998.
32. McCullough AJ, Tavill AS: Disordered energy and protein metabolism in liver disease. *Semin Liver Dis* 11:265–277, 1991.
33. Tsien C, Davuluri G, Singh D, et al: Metabolic and molecular responses to leucine-enriched branched chain amino acid supplementation in the skeletal muscle of alcoholic cirrhosis. *Hepatology* 61(6):2018–2029, 2015.
34. Mendenhall CL, Moritz TE, Roselle GA, et al: Protein energy malnutrition in severe alcoholic hepatitis: diagnosis and response to treatment. The VA Cooperative Study Group #275. *JPEN J Parenter Enteral Nutr* 19:258–265, 1995.
35. Dejong CH, van de Poll MC, Soeters PB, et al: Aromatic amino acid metabolism during liver failure. *J Nutr* 137[6 Suppl 1]:1579S–1585S, 2007.
36. Latifi R, Killam RW, Dudrick SJ: Nutritional support in liver failure. *Surg Clin North Am* 71:567–578, 1991.
37. Plauth M, Roske A-E, Romaniuk P, et al: Post-feeding hyperammonaemia in patients with transjugular intrahepatic portosystemic shunt and liver cirrhosis: role of small intestinal ammonia release and route of nutrient administration. *Gut* 46(6):849–855, 2000.
38. Li SD, Lue W, Mobarhan S, et al: Nutrition support for individuals with liver failure. *Nutr Rev* 58:242–247, 2000.
39. Amodio P, Bemeur C, Butterworth R, et al: The nutritional management of hepatic encephalopathy in patients with cirrhosis: International Society for Hepatic Encephalopathy and Nitrogen Metabolism Consensus. *Hepatology* 58(1):325–336, 2013.
40. Gluud LL, Dam G, Les I, et al: Branched-chain amino acids for people with hepatic encephalopathy. *Cochrane Database Syst Rev* 9: CD001939, 2015.
41. Kanematsu T, Koyanagi N, Matsumata T, et al: Lack of preventive effect of branched-chain amino acid solution on postoperative hepatic encephalopathy in patients with cirrhosis: a randomized, prospective trial. *Surgery* 104:482–488, 1988.
42. Michel H, Bories P, Aubin JP, et al: Treatment of acute hepatic encephalopathy in cirrhotics with a branched-chain amino acids enriched versus a conventional amino acids mixture. A controlled study of 70 patients. *Liver* 5:282–289, 1985.
43. Rocchi E, Cassanelli M, Gibertini P, et al: Standard or branched-chain amino acid infusions as short-term nutritional support in liver cirrhosis? *JPEN J Parenter Enteral Nutr* 9:447–451, 1985.
44. Alberino F, Gatta A, Amodio P, et al: Nutrition and survival in patients with liver cirrhosis. *Nutrition* 17:445–450, 2001.
45. Montano-Loza AJ, Meza-Junco J, Prado CM, et al: Muscle wasting is associated with mortality in patients with cirrhosis. *Clin Gastroenterol Hepatol* 10:166–173, 2011.
46. Durand F, Buyse S, Francoz C, et al: Prognostic value of muscle atrophy in cirrhosis using psoas muscle thickness on computed tomography. *J Hepatol* 60:1151–1157, 2014.
47. Giusto M, Lattanzi B, Di Gregorio V, et al: Changes in nutritional status after liver transplantation *World J Gastroenterol* 20(31):10682–10690, 2014.
48. Montano-Loza AJ, Meza-Junco J, Baracos VE, et al: Severe muscle depletion predicts postoperative length of stay but is not associated with survival after liver transplantation. *Liver Transpl* 20:640–648, 2014.
49. Masuda T, Shirabe K, Ikegami T, et al: Sarcopenia is a prognostic factor in living donor liver transplantation. *Liver Transplant* 20:401–407, 2014.
50. Kim JM, Joh J-W, Kim HJ, et al: Early enteral feeding after living donor liver transplantation prevents infectious complications: a prospective pilot study. *Medicine* 94(44):1–6, 2015.
51. Lei Q, Wang X, Zheng H, et al. Peri-operative immunonutrition in patients undergoing liver transplantation: a meta-analysis of randomized controlled trials. *Asia Pac J Clin Nutr* 24(4):583–590, 2015.
52. Plank LD, Mathur S, Gane EJ, et al: Perioperative immunonutrition in patients undergoing liver transplantation: a randomized double-blind trial. *Hepatology* 61:639–647, 2015.
53. Tsien C, Garber A, Narayanan A, et al: Post-liver transplantation sarcopenia in cirrhosis: a prospective evaluation. *J Gastroenterol Hepatol* 29(6):1250–1257, 2014.
54. Ferreira LG, Santos LF, Anastácio LR, et al: Resting energy expenditure, body composition, and dietary intake: a longitudinal study before and after liver transplantation. *Transplantation* 96(6):579–585, 2013.
55. Chavez-Tapia NC, Cesar-Arce A, Barrientos-Gutierrez T, et al: A systematic review and meta-analysis of the use of oral zinc in the treatment of hepatic encephalopathy. *Nutr J* 12:74, 2013.
56. Jensen GL, Compher C, Sullivan DH, et al: Recognizing malnutrition in adults: definitions and characteristics, screening, assessment, and team approach. *JPEN J Parenter Enteral Nutr* 37(6):802–807, 2013.
57. Wagner PD: Possible mechanisms underlying the development of cachexia in COPD. *Eur Respir J* 31:492–501, 2008.
58. Itoh M, Tsuji T, Nemoto K, et al: Undernutrition in patients with COPD and its treatment. *Nutrients* 5(4):1316–1335, 2013.
59. Suzuki S, Egi M, Schneider AG, et al: Hypophosphatemia in critically ill patients. *J Crit Care* 28(4):536.e9–536.e19, 2013.
60. Schwartz DB, DiMaria RA: *Pulmonary and Cardiac Failure. The ASPEN Nutrition Support Core Curriculum: A Case-Based Approach—The Adult Patient*. American Society for Parenteral and Enteral Nutrition, 2007.
61. McClave SA, Lowen CC, Kleber MJ, et al: Are patients fed appropriately according to their caloric requirements? *JPEN J Parenter Enteral Nutr* 22:375–381, 1998.
62. Flancbaum L, Choban PS, Sambucco S, et al: Comparison of indirect calorimetry, the Fick method, and prediction equations in estimating the energy requirements of critically ill patients. *Am J Clin Nutr* 69:461–466, 1999.
63. Singer P, Anbar R, Cohen J, et al: The tight calorie control study (TICACOS): a prospective, randomized, controlled pilot study of nutritional support in critically ill patients. *Intensive Care Med* 37(4):601–609, 2011.
64. Jih KS, Wang MF, Chow JH, et al: Hypercapnic respiratory acidosis precipitated by hypercaloric carbohydrate infusion in resolving septic acute respiratory distress syndrome: a case report. *Zhonghua Yi XueZaZhi (Taipei)* 58:359–365, 1996.
65. Talpers SS, Romberger DJ, Bunce SB, et al: Nutritionally associated increased carbon dioxide production. Excess total calories vs high proportion of carbohydrate calories. *Chest* 102(2):551–555, 1992.
66. Kuo CD, Shiao GM, Lee JD: The effects of high-fat and high-carbohydrate diet loads on gas exchange and ventilation in COPD patients and normal subjects. *Chest* 104:189–196, 1993.
67. Klein S, Miles JM: Metabolic effects of long-chain and medium-chain triglyceride emulsions in humans. *JPEN J Parenter Enteral Nutr* 18:396–397, 1994.
68. Grant JP: Nutrition care of patients with acute and chronic respiratory failure. *Nutr Clin Pract* 9:11–17, 1994.
69. Battistella FD, Widergren JT, Anderson JT, et al: A prospective, randomized trial of intravenous fat emulsion administration in trauma victims requiring total parenteral nutrition. *J Trauma* 43:52–58, 1997.
70. Manzanares W, Dhaliwal R, Jurewitsch B, et al: Alternative lipid emulsions in the critically ill: a systematic review of the evidence. *Intensive Care Med* 39(10):1683–1694, 2013.
71. Weijs PJ, Sauerwein HP, Kondrup J: Protein recommendations in the ICU: g protein/kg body weight—which body weight for underweight and obese patients? *Clin Nutr* 31(5):774–775, 2012.
72. Allingstrup MJ, Esmailzadeh N, Wilkens Knudsen A, et al: Provision of protein and energy in relation to measured requirements in intensive care patients. *Clin Nutr* 31(4):462–468, 2012.
73. Cavaillès A, Brinchault-Rabin G, Dixmier A, et al: Comorbidities of COPD. *Eur Respir Rev* 22(130):454–475, 2013.
74. Hallin R, Gudmundsson G, SuppliUlrik C, et al: Nutritional status and long-term mortality in hospitalised patients with chronic obstructive pulmonary disease (COPD). *Respir Med* 101(9):1954–1960, 2007.
75. Celli BR, Cote CG, Marin JM, et al: The body-mass index, airflow obstruction, dyspnea, and exercise capacity index in chronic obstructive pulmonary disease. *N Engl J Med* 350(10):1005–1012, 2004.

76. Collins PF, Elia M, Stratton RJ: Nutritional support and functional capacity in chronic obstructive pulmonary disease: a systematic review and meta-analysis. *Respirology* 18:616–629, 2013.
77. Ferreira IM, Brooks D, White J, et al: Nutritional supplementation for stable chronic obstructive pulmonary disease. *Cochrane Database Syst Rev* 12:CD000998, 2012.
78. Faisy C, Rabbat A, Kouchakji B, et al: Bioelectrical impedance analysis in estimating nutritional status and outcome of patients with chronic obstructive pulmonary disease and acute respiratory failure. *Intensive Care Med* 26:518–525, 2000.
79. Vitacca M, Clini E, Porta R, et al: Acute exacerbations in patients with COPD: predictors of need for mechanical ventilation. *Eur Respir J* 9:1487–1493, 1996.
80. Schols AM, Soeters PB, Dingemans AM, et al: Prevalence and characteristics of nutritional depletion in patients with stable COPD eligible for pulmonary rehabilitation. *Am Rev Respir Dis* 147:1151–1156, 1993.
81. Kondrup J, Rasmussen HH, Hamberg O, et al; Nutritional risk screening (NRS 2002): a new method based on an analysis of controlled clinical trials. *Clin Nutr* 22(3):321–336, 2003.
82. Heyland DK, Dhaliwal R, Jiang X, et al: Identifying critically ill patients who benefit the most from nutrition therapy: the development and initial validation of a novel risk assessment tool. *Crit Care* 15(6):R268, 2011.
83. Fremont RD, Rice TW: Pros and cons of feeding the septic intensive care unit patient. *Nutr Clin Prac* 30(3):344–350, 2015.
84. Rice TW, Mogan S, Hays MA, et al: Randomized trial of initial trophic versus full-energy enteral nutrition in mechanically ventilated patients with acute respiratory failure. *Crit Care Med* 39(5):967–974, 2011.
85. Rice TW, Wheeler AP, Thompson BT, et al; Initial trophic vs full enteral feeding in patients with acute lung injury: the EDEN randomized trial. *JAMA* 307(8):795–803, 2012.
86. Casaer MP, Mesotten D, Hermans G, et al: Early versus late parenteral nutrition in critically ill adults. *N Engl J Med* 365:506–517, 2011.
87. Braunschweig CA, Sheean PM, Peterson SJ, et al: Intensive nutrition and acute lung injury: a clinical trial (INTACT). *JPEN J Parenter Enteral Nutr* 39(1):13–20, 2015.
88. Heyland DK, Stephens KE, Day AG, et al: The success of enteral nutrition and ICU-acquired infections: a multicenter observational study. *Clin Nutr* 30(2):148–155, 2011.
89. Doig GS, Simpson F, Sweetman EA, et al; Early parenteral nutrition in critically ill patients with short-term relative contraindications to early enteral nutrition: a randomized controlled trial. *JAMA* 309:2130–2138, 2013.
90. Harvey SE, Parrott F, Harrison DA, et al: Trial of the route of early nutritional support in critically ill adults. *N Engl J Med* 371(18):1673–1684, 2014.
91. Heidegger CP, Berger MM, Graf S, et al: Optimisation of energy provision with supplemental parenteral nutrition in critically ill patients: a randomised controlled clinical trial. *Lancet* 381:385–393, 2013.
92. Li C, Bo L, Liu W, et al: Enteral immunomodulatory diet (omega-3 fatty acid, γ-linolenic acid and antioxidant supplementation) for acute lung injury and acute respiratory distress syndrome: an updated systematic review and meta-analysis. *Nutrients* 7(7):5572–5585, 2015.
93. Sajid MS, Harper A, Hussain Q, et al: An integrated systematic review and meta-analysis of published randomized controlled trials evaluating nasogastric against postpyloris (nasoduodenal and nasojejunal) feeding in critically ill patients admitted in intensive care unit. *Eur J Clin Nutr* 68(4):424–432, 2014.
94. Alkhawaja S, Martin C, Butler RJ, et al: Post-pyloric versus gastric tube feeding for preventing pneumonia and improving nutritional outcomes in critically ill adults. *Cochrane Database Syst Rev* 8:CD008875, 2015.
95. DeLegge MH: Managing gastric residual volumes in the critically ill patient: an update. *Curr Opin Clin Nutr Metab Care* 14(2):193–196, 2011.

Appendix

CALCULATIONS COMMONLY USED IN CRITICAL CARE

JOSEPH J. FRASSICA

TABLE OF CONTENTS

ABBREVIATIONS USED IN THE APPENDIX

A	Alveolar	atm	Atmosphere
D	Dead	BSA	Body surface area
E	Expiration	cap	Capillary
I	Inspiration	Cr	Creatinine
P	Pressure	dyn	Dynamic
$\dot{Q}$	Net liquid flow	Is	Interstitium
R	Respiratory quotient	St	Static
T	Tidal	ICP	Intracranial pressure
V	Volume	A	Arterial
Δ	Change	D	Distribution
η	Viscosity	L	Length
Π	Oncotic pressure	R	Radius
Σ	Permeability	T	Time
		$\bar{v}$	Mixed venous

FAHRENHEIT AND CELSIUS TEMPERATURE CONVERSIONS

°C	°F	°C	°F
45	113.0	32	89.6
44	111.2	31	87.8
43	109.4	30	86.0
42	107.6	29	84.2
41	105.8	28	82.4
40	104.0	27	80.6
39	102.2	26	78.8
38	100.4	25	77.0
37	98.6	24	75.2
36	96.8	23	73.4
35	95.0	22	71.6
34	93.2	21	69.8
33	91.4	20	68.0

DOSAGE AND ACTION OF COMMON INTRAVENOUS VASOACTIVE DRUGS

	Dosage	α	β_1	β_2
Dopamine	1–2 μg/kg/min	+	+	0
	2–10 μg/kg/min	++	+++	0
	10–30 μg/kg/min	+++	++	0
Dobutamine	2–30 μg/kg/min	+	+++	++
Milrinone	50 μg/kg loading dose, then 0.375–0.75 μg kg/min	0	0	0
Norepinephrine	0.1–3 μg/kg/min	+++	++	+
Epinephrine	0.1–0.5 μg/kg/min	++	+++	+++
Isoproterenol	2–10 μg/min	0	+++	+++
Phenylephrine	100–500 μg bolus, then 0.5–10 μg/kg/min	+++	0	0
Vasopression	0.04 units/min	0	0	0
Labetalol	20 mg, then 40–80 mg boluses, then 2–10 mg/min (300 mg max daily total dose)	–	–	0
Esmolol	500 μg/kg bolus, then 50–200 μg/kg/min	0	–	(–)

Degree of receptor stimulation: 0, none; +, weak; ++, moderate; +++, strong; –, receptor blockade; (–), receptor blockade at high doses.

HEMODYNAMIC CALCULATIONS

MEAN BLOOD PRESSURE (mm Hg)

$$= \overline{BP}$$

$$= \frac{\text{Systolic BP} + (2 \times \text{Diastolic BP})}{3}$$

$$= \text{Diastolic BP} + \frac{1}{3}(\text{Systolic BP} - \text{Diastolic BP})$$

Normal values: 85–95 mm Hg

THE FICK EQUATION FOR CARDIAC INDEX (L/min/m^2)

$$= \text{Cardiac Index (CI)}$$

$$= \frac{\text{Cardiac output (CO)}}{\text{BSA}}$$

$$= \frac{\text{Oxygen consumption}}{\text{O}_2 \text{ content} - \text{Venous O}_2 \text{ content}}$$

$$= \frac{10 \times \dot{V}O_2(\text{mL/min/m}^2)}{\text{Hgb(g/dL)} \times 1.39 \times (\text{Arterial \% saturation} - \text{Venous \% saturation})}$$

Normal values: 2.5–4.2 L/min/m^2

STROKE INDEX (mL/beat/m²)

$$= \frac{\text{CI(L/min/m}^2) \times 1{,}000}{\text{Heartrate (beats/min)}}$$

Normal values: 33–47 mL/beat/m²

SYSTEMIC VASCULAR RESISTANCE (dyne/sec/cm⁵)

$$= \text{SVR}$$

$$= \frac{80 \times (\text{Arterial } \overline{\text{BP}} - \text{Right atrial } \overline{\text{BP}})}{\text{CO(L/min)}}$$

Normal values: 770–1,500 dyne/sec/cm⁵

PULMONARY VASCULAR RESISTANCE (dyne/sec/cm⁵)

$$= \text{PVR}$$

$$= \frac{80 \times (\text{Pulmonary artery } \overline{\text{BP}} - \text{Pulmonary capillary wedge pressure})}{\text{CO (L/min)}}$$

Normal values: 20–120 dyne/sec/cm⁵

TOTAL PULMONARY RESISTANCE (dyne/sec/cm⁵)

$$= \text{TPR}$$

$$= \frac{80 \times \text{Pulmonary artery } \overline{\text{BP}}}{\text{CO (L/min)}}$$

CAPILLARY FLUID FILTRATION

$$= \dot{Q}_f$$

$$= k(P_{cap} - P_{is}) - k\sigma(\pi_{cap} - \pi_{is})$$

NUTRITIONAL CALCULATIONS

BODY MASS INDEX

$$= \text{BMI}$$

$$= \frac{\text{Weight (kg)}}{(\text{Height [cm]})^2}$$

CALORIC CONTENT OF FOODS

Food type	kcal/g	Range
Carbohydrate	3.4	3.4–4.1
Protein	4.0	3.3–4.7
Fat	9.1	9.1–9.5

RESPIRATORY QUOTIENT

$$= \frac{CO_2 \text{ production (mL / min)}}{O_2 \text{ consumption (mL / min)}}$$

$$= \frac{\dot{V}_{CO_2}}{\dot{V}_{O_2}}$$

RELATIONSHIP OF FUEL BURNED TO RESPIRATORY QUOTIENT

Fuel	*R*
Ketones	<0.6
Fat	0.7
Carbohydrate	1.0
Lipogenesis	>1.0

NITROGEN BALANCE

$$= \text{Nitrogen consumed} - \text{Nitrogen excreted}$$

$$= \frac{\text{Proteincalories (kcal/day)}}{25}$$

$$-\text{Urinenitrogen (g/day)} - 5 \text{ (g/day)}$$

HARRIS–BENEDICT EQUATION OF RESTING ENERGY EXPENDITURE (kcal/day)

$$\text{Males} = 66 + (13.7 \times \text{Weight [kg]}) + (5 \times \text{Height [cm]}) - (6.8 \times \text{Age})$$

$$\text{Females} = 655 + (9.6 \times \text{Weight [kg]}) + (1.8 \times \text{Height [cm]}) - (4.7 \times \text{Age})$$

WEIR EQUATION (MODIFIED) OF ENERGY EXPENDITURE (kcal/day)

$$= (3.94 \times \dot{V}_{O_2} \text{ [mL/min]}) + (1.11 \times \dot{V}_{CO_2} \text{ [mL/min]})$$

TYPICAL DRUG DOSAGES FOR RAPID SEQUENCE INTUBATION

Muscle relaxants	
Rocuronium	0.6–1.2 mg/kg
Succinylcholine	1 mg/kg
Vecuronium	0.1–0.20 mg/kg
Sedatives	
Etomidate	0.3–0.4 mg/kg
Ketamine	1–2 mg/kg
Propofol	1–2 mg/kg
Thiopental	3–4 mg/kg

PULMONARY CALCULATIONS

TIDAL VOLUME

$$= V_T$$

$$= \text{Dead space} + \text{Alveolar space}$$

$$= V_D + V_A$$

ALVEOLAR GAS EQUATION

$$PAO_2 = PIO_2 - \frac{PaCO_2}{R}$$

$$= FIO_2(P_{atm} - P_{H_2O}) - \frac{PaCO_2}{R}$$

$$= 150 - \frac{PaCO_2}{R} \text{(room air, sea level)}$$

ALVEOLAR ARTERIOLAR GRADIENT

$= A - a$ gradient

$= PAO_2 - PaO_2$

Normal values (upright): $2.5 + (0.21 \times \text{age})$

ALVEOLAR VENTILATION (L/min)

$= \dot{V}_E$

$= k \dfrac{\dot{V}CO_2}{PaCO_2}$

$= \dfrac{0.863 \times \dot{V}_{CO_2} (\text{mL / min})}{PaCO_2 (1 - V_D / V_T)}$

Normal values: 4–6 L/min

BOHR EQUATION OF DEAD SPACE

Normal values: 0.2–0.3

PHYSIOLOGICAL DEAD SPACE

$$V_D / V_T = \frac{PaCO_2 - PECO_2}{PaCO_2}$$

Normal values: 0.2–0.3

OXYGEN DISSOLVED IN BLOOD (mL/dL)

$= DO_2$

$= 0.003$ (mL, O_2/dL) $\times$ PaO_2 (mm Hg)

OXYGEN CAPACITY OF HEMOGLOBIN (mL O_2/dL)

$= 1.39$ (mL O_2) $\times$ Hgb (g/dL)

Normal values: 17–24 mL/dL

OXYGEN CONTENT OF THE BLOOD (mL/dL)

$= CO_2$

$= DO_2 + (1.39 \times \text{Hgb [g/dL]} \times [\text{\%Hgb saturated with } O_2])$

$= DO_2 + (1.39 \times \text{Hgb [g/dL]} \times S_{O_2})$

Normal values: 17.5–23.5 mL/dL

PERCENTAGE OF SATURATION OF HEMOGLOBIN WITH OXYGEN

$= SO_2$

$= 100 \times \dfrac{CO_2 - DO_2}{1.39 \times \text{Hgb(g/dL)}}$

Normal values: >95%

PHYSIOLOGICAL SHUNT

$= \dot{Q}_S / \dot{Q}_T$

$= \dfrac{C_{capO_2} - C_{O_2}}{C_{capO_2} - C_{\bar{v}O_2}}$

$= \dfrac{1.39 \times \text{Hgb (g/dL)} + 0.003 \times PaO_2 - CaO_2}{1.39 \times \text{Hgb (g/dL)} + 0.003 \times PaO_2 - C\bar{v}O_2}$

Normal values: <5%

COMPLIANCE

$= \Delta V / \Delta P$ (mL/cm H_2O)

On Mechanical Ventilation

Static compliance $= C_{st} = \dfrac{V_T}{P_{plateau} - P_{endexp}}$

Dynamic effective complicance $= C_{dyn} = \dfrac{V_T}{P_{peak} - P_{endexp}}$

During Spontaneous Breathing

Compliance of the lung $= C_L = \dfrac{V_T}{P_{alveolus} - P_{pleura}}$

Compliance of the chest wall $= CW_{cw} = \dfrac{V_T}{P_{pleura} - P_{atm}}$

Compliance of the respiratory system $= C_{rs} = \dfrac{V_T}{P_{alveolus} - P_{atm}}$

Normal values: $C_{st} > 60$ mL/cm H_2O; $C_{dyn} > 60$ mL/cm H_2O

$C_L > 200$ mL/cm H_2O; $C_{rs} > 100$ mL/cm H_2O

RESISTANCE—OHM'S LAW

$= \Delta P/\text{flow} = \Delta P/\dot{Q}$

Normal values: airway resistance of the lung at functional residual capacity = 2 cm H_2O/L/sec

WORK-OF-BREATHING

$$W_{Thorax} = \int_{t_1}^{t_2} (P_{aw} - P_{atm})\dot{V}\,dt$$

$$W_{Lung} = \int_{t_1}^{t_2} (P_{aw} - P_{es})\dot{V}\,dt$$

$$W_{Chest\ wall} = \int_{t_1}^{t_2} (P_{es} - P_{atm})\dot{V}\,dt$$

Normal values: $W_{thorax} = 0.5$ kg M/min

LAPLACE'S LAW OF SURFACE TENSION OF A SPHERE

$P = 2T/r$

POISEUILLE'S LAW OF LAMINAR FLOW

$$\dot{V} = \frac{P\pi r^4}{8\eta l}$$

OXYGENATION INDEX

$FIO_2 \times$ Mean Airway Pressure $\times 100/PaO_2$ [6,7]

(>8.1 Adult Respiratory Distress Syndrome [ARDS])

P/F ratio

PaO_2/FIO_2

COMPOSITION AND PROPERTIES OF COMMON INTRAVENOUS SOLUTIONS

Solution	Na+	Cl⁻	K+	Ca+	Lactate	Kcal/L	mOsm/L
D5W	0	0	0	0	0	170	252
D10W	0	0	0	0	0	240	505
D50W	0	0	0	0	0	1,700	2,530
½ NS	77	77	0	0	0	0	154
NS	154	154	0	0	0	0	308
3% NaCl	513	513	0	0	0	0	1,026
Ringer's lactate	130	109	4	3		0	308
20% mannitol	0	0	0	0	0	0	1,098

ELECTROLYTE AND RENAL CALCULATIONS

ANION GAP

$$= [Na^+] - [Cl^-] - [HCO_3^-]$$

Normal values: 9–13 mEq/L

EXPECTED ANION GAP IN HYPOALBUMINEMIA

= 3 × (albumin [g/dL])

CALCULATED SERUM OSMOLALITY

$$= 2[Na^+] + \frac{[Glucose]}{18} + \frac{[BUN]}{2.8}$$

Normal values: 275–290 mOsm/kg

OSMOLAR GAP

= Serum osmolality measured – Serum osmolality calculated

Normal values: 0–5 mOsm/kg

Na^+ AND GLUCOSE

$[Na^+]$ decreases 1.6 mEq/L for each 100 mg/dL increase in [glucose].

TOTAL CALCIUM AND ALBUMIN

Corrected calcium (mg/dL) = Measured total calcium (mg/dL) + 0.8(4.0 – serum albumin)

GLOMERULAR FILTRATION RATE = GFR

$$\text{Measured} = \text{Creatinine clearance} = \frac{U_{Creat}V}{P_{Creat}}$$

$$= \frac{[\text{Creatinine}]_{urine}\ (g/dL) \times \dfrac{\text{Urine volume (mL/day)}}{1{,}440\ (\text{min/day})}}{[\text{Creatinine}]_{plasma}\ (mg/dL)}$$

$$\text{Estimated for males} = \frac{(140-\text{Age})\times(\text{Lean body weight [kg]})}{P_{Creat} \times 72}$$

Estimated for females = 0.85 × male estimate

Normal values: 74–160 mL/min

WATER DEFICIT IN HYPERNATREMIA (L)

$$= 0.6 \times (\text{Body weight [kg]}) \times \left(\frac{[Na^+]}{140} - 1\right)$$

WATER EXCESS IN HYPONATREMIA (L)

$$= 0.6 \times (\text{Body weight [kg]}) \times \left(1 - \frac{[Na^+]}{140}\right)$$

FRACTIONAL EXCRETION OF SODIUM

$$= F_E\ Na$$

$$= \frac{\text{Excreted } Na^+}{\text{Filtered } Na^+} \times 100$$

$$= \frac{U_{Na^+} \times V}{GFR} \times [Na^+] \times 100$$

$$= \frac{U_{Na^+} / [Na^+]}{U_{Creat} / [Creat]}$$

ACID–BASE FORMULAS

HENDERSON–HASSELBALCH EQUATION

$$pH = pK + \log \frac{[HCO_3^-]}{0.03 \times PaCO_2}$$

HENDERSON'S EQUATION FOR CONCENTRATION OF H^+

$$[H^+](nM / L) = 24 \times \frac{PaCO_2}{[HCO_3^-]}$$

METABOLIC ACIDOSIS

$$\text{Bicarbonate deficit (mEq/L)} = 0.5 \times (\text{Body weight [kg]}) \times (24 - [HCO_3^-])$$

$$\text{Expected } PCO_2 = 1.5 \times [HCO_3^-] + 8 \pm 2$$

METABOLIC ALKALOSIS

$$\text{Bicarbonate excess} = 0.4 \times (\text{Body weight [kg]}) \times ([HCO_3^-] - 24)$$

RESPIRATORY ACIDOSIS

$$\text{Acute: } \frac{\Delta H^+}{\Delta PaCO_2} = 0.8$$

$$\text{Chronic: } \frac{\Delta H^+}{\Delta PaCO_2} = 0.3$$

NEUROLOGICAL CALCULATIONS

GLASGOW COMA SCALE (3–15)

= Eyes (1–4) + Motor (1–6) + Verbal (1–5)

Normal value: 15

CEREBRAL PERFUSION PRESSURE (mm Hg)

$$= \overline{BP} - ICP$$

BODY SURFACE AREA FORMULA AND NOMOGRAM

BODY SURFACE AREA (BSA)

$$= (\text{Height [cm]})^{0.718} \times (\text{Weight [kg]})^{0.427} \times 74.49$$

See Figure A.1 for the nomogram for calculating BSA.

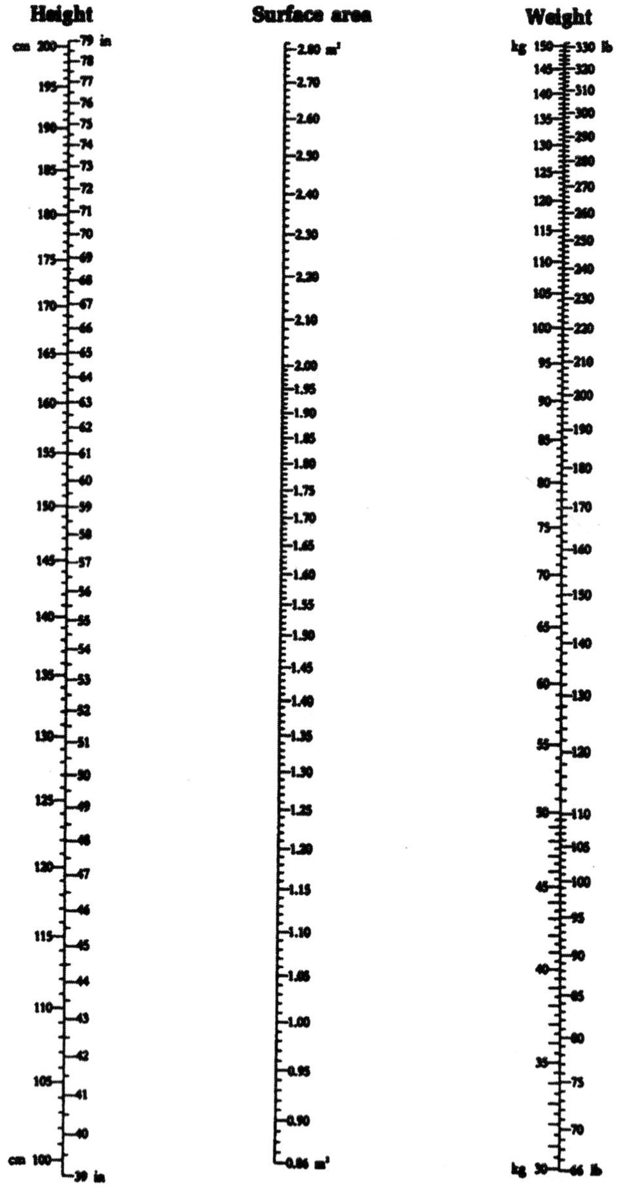

FIGURE A.1 Nomogram for calculation of body surface area (BSA) in square meters by height and weight.

PHARMACOLOGIC CALCULATIONS

DRUG CLEARANCE

$$= V_d \times K_{el}$$

DRUG HALF-LIFE

$$= t_{1/2}$$

$$= \frac{0.693}{K_{el}}$$

DRUG ELIMINATION CONSTANT

$$= K_{el}$$

$$= \frac{\ln\left(\frac{[\text{Peak}]}{[\text{Trough}]}\right)}{t_{peak} - t_{trough}}$$

DRUG LOADING DOSE

$$= V_d\ [\text{Target peak}]$$

DRUG DOSING INTERVAL

$$= \frac{-1}{K_{el}} \times \ln\left(\frac{\text{Desired trough}}{\text{Desired peak}}\right) + \text{Infusion time (hours)}$$

ICU ACUITY SCORING

Type of Admission		Points
	Scheduled surgery	0
	Unscheduled surgery	8
	Medical	6
Chronic diseases	None	0
	Metastatic carcinoma	9
	Hematologic malignancy	10
	AIDS	17
Age (years)	<40	0
	40–59	7
	60–69	12
	70–74	15
	75–79	16
	≥80	18
Temperature	<39°C	0
	>39°C	3
Heart rate	<40	11
	40–69	2
	70–119	0
	120–159	4
	≥160	7
Systolic blood pressure (mm Hg)	<70	13
	70–99	5
	100–199	0
	≥200	2
Urine output	<500 cc/24 h	11
	500–999 cc/24 h	4

Type of Admission		Points
	>1,000 cc/24 h	0
Glasgow Coma Score	<6	26
	6–8	13
	9–10	7
	11–13	5
	14–15	0
Serum urea or Blood Urea Nitrogen (BUN)	<10	0
	10–29.9	6
	≥30	10
Serum sodium (mEq/L)	>146	1
	125–144	0
	<125	5
Serum potassium (mEq/L)	<3	3
	3–4.9	0
	>5	3
WBC	<1,000/mm^3	12
	1,000–19,000/mm^3	0
	>20,000/mm^3	3
HCO_3^- (mEq/L)	<15	6
	15–19	3
	≥20	0
Bilirubin (mg/dL)	<4	0
	4–5.9	4
	≥6	9
PaO_2/FIO_2	<100	11
(if ventilated or CPAP)	100–199	9
	≥200	6

SAPS II, simplified acute physiology score II. [1,2]

APACHE IV VARIABLES (NON-CABG PATIENTS) [3] (TABLES A.1–A.3)

Age

Acute Physiology and Chronic Health Evalution Score from the day of ICU Admission	**Points**
Use the one with the highest point value that is present	
Nonoperative and emergency surgery patients only otherwise = 0	
AIDS	23
Hepatic failure	16
Lymphoma	13
Metastatic cancer	11
Leukemia/multiple myeloma	10
Immunosuppression	10
Cirrhosis	4
None/not available	0
Acute Physiology Score	
PO_2/FIO_2 ratio (or $P(A–a)O_2$) for intubated patients with FIO_2 ≥ 0.5	
Ventilated anytime during day 1	Y/N
ICU admission information	
Admit to ICU from floor	
Transfer to ICU from other hospital	
Admit to ICU from OR/Post Anesthesia Care Unit (PACU)	
Emergency surgery	Y/N
Pre-ICU length of stay (No. of days between ICU and hospital admission)	
Admitting diagnosis	
If Diagnosis is acute Myocardial infarction (MI) is the patient on thrombolytic therapy?	Y/N
Unable to obtain Glascow Coma Scale (GCS) (due to meds, anesthesia, or sedation)	Y/N
GCS	
Acute Physiology Score (APS)	
Pulse (beats/min)	
Select heart rate furthest from 75	
≤39	8
40–49	5
50–99	0
100–109	1
110–119	5
120–139	7
140–154	13
≥155	17
Mean arterial pressure (MAP)	
Select MAP furthest from 90	
≤39	23
40–59	15
60–69	7
70–79	6
80–99	0
100–119	4
120–129	7
130–139	9
≥140	10
Temperature (°C)	
Select core temperature furthest from 38	
Add 1°C to axillary temps prior to selecting worst value	
≤32.9	20
33–33.4	16
33.5–33.9	13
34–34.9	8
35–35.9	2
36–39.9	0
≥40	4
Respiratory rate (breaths/min)	
Select respiratory rate furthest from 19	
For patients on mechanical ventilation no points are given for respiratory rates of 6–12	
≤5	17
6–11	8
12–13	7
14–24	0
25–34	6
35–39	9
40–49	11
≥50	18
PaO_2 (mm Hg)	
Use only for nonintubated patients or intubated patients with FIO_2 <0.5 (50%)	
≤49	15
50–69	5
70–79	2
≥80	0
OR	
$A\text{-}aDO_2$	
Only use $A\text{-}aDO_2$ for intubated patients with FIO_2 ≥0.5 (50%)	

Do not use PaO_2 weights for these patients	
<100	0
100–249	7
250–349	9
350–499	11
≤500	14
Hematocrit (%)	
Select hematocrit furthest from 45.5	
≤40.9	3
41–49	0
≥50	3
WBC (cu/mm)	
Select WBC furthest from 11.5	
<1.0	19
1.0–2.9	5
3.0–19.9	0
20–24.9	1
≥25	5
Creatinine without *Acute Renal Failure* (ARF) (mg/dL)	
Select creatinine furthest from 1	
≤0.4	3
0.5–1.4	0
1.5–1.94	4
≥1.95	7
OR	
Creatinine with ARF (mg/dL)	
ARF is defined as creatinine ≥1.5 mg/dL	
as creatinine ≥1.5 mg/dL and urine output <410 cc/d and no chronic dialysis	
0–1.4	0
≥1.5	10
Urine Output (cc/d)	
Total for day	
≤399	15
400–599	8
600–899	7
900–1,499	5
1,500–1,999	4
2,000–3,999	0
≥4,000	1
BUN (mg/dL)	
Select highest BUN	
≤16.9	0
17–19	2
20–39	7
40–79	11
≥80	12
Sodium (mEq/L)	
Select sodium furthest from 145.5	
≤119	3
120–134	2
135–154	0
≥155	4
Albumin (g/dL)	
Select albumin furthest from 3.5	
≤1.9	11
2–2.4	6
2.5–4.4	0
≥4.5	4

Bilirubin (mg/dL)	
Select highest bilirubin furthest from 0	
≤1.9	0
2–2.9	5
3–4.9	6
5–7.9	8
≥8	16
Glucose (mg/dL)	
Select glucose furthest from 130	
Glucose ≤39 mg/dL is lower weight than 40–59	
≤39	8
40–59	9
60–199	0
200–349	3
≥350	5
Neurological Abnormalities Score	
Acid–Base Abnormalities Score	

Adapted from Cerner Apache. *Apache IV Calculations.xls* with permission.
Note: Mortality prediction calculations based on the APACHE IV are different for the day of ICU admission and subsequent days.

MPM_0-III Scoring System

Category	Variable
Physiology	
	Coma or deep stupor at admission not due to drug overdose
	Heart rate >150 beats/min
	Systolic blood pressure ≤90 mm Hg
Chronic diagnoses	
	Chronic renal compromise or insufficiency
	Cirrhosis
	Metastatic malignant neoplasm
Acute diagnoses	
	Acute renal failure
	Cardiac dysrhythmia
	Cerebrovascular accident
	Gastrointestinal (GI) bleeding
	Intracranial mass effect
Other variables	
	Cardiopulmonary resuscitation within 24 hours before admission
	Mechanical ventilation within one hour of admission
	Medical or unscheduled surgery admission
	Full code status
	Age (years)

Mortality Probability Model 0 - III variables are collected at the time of ICU admission or within 1 hour of admission [4].
Adapted from White Paper Report. Available at: http://www.cerner.com/filedownload.asp?LibraryID = 34399. Accessed July 26, 2010. Cerner Corp © 2005.

TABLE A.1

Specific Components of the Glasgow Coma Scale

Eye opening	
Spontaneous	4
To speech	3
To pain	2
Nil	1
Motor response	
Obeys commands	6
Localizes	5
Withdraws	4
Exhibits abnormal flexion	3
Exhibits abnormal extension	2
Nil	1
Verbal response	
Oriented	5
Confused, conversant	4
Uses inappropriate words	3
Uses incomprehensible sounds	2
Nil	1

TABLE A.2

APACHE IV Nonoperative Diagnoses [3]

Diagnostic group
Cardiovascular diagnoses
Acute Myocardial Infarction
Anterior
Inferior/lateral
Non-Q
Other
Cardiac arrest
Cardiogenic shock
Cardiomyopathy
Congestive heart failure
Chest pain, rule out AMI
Hypertension
Hypovolemia/dehydration (not shock)
Hemorrhage (not related to GI bleeding)
Aortic aneurysm
Peripheral vascular disease
Rhythm disturbance
Sepsis (by infection site)
Cutaneous
Gastrointestinal (GI)
Pulmonary
Urinary tract
Other location
Unknown location
Cardiac drug toxicity
Unstable angina
Cardiovascular, other

TABLE A.2

(continued)

Respiratory diagnoses
Airway obstruction
Asthma
Aspiration pneumonia
Bacterial pneumonia
Viral pneumonia
Parasitic/fungal pneumonia
Chronic obstructive pulmonary disease (emphysema/bronchitis)
Pleural effusion
Pulmonary edema (noncardiac)
Pulmonary embolism
Respiratory arrest
Respiratory cancer (oral, larynx, lung, trachea)
Restrictive lung disease (fibrosis, sarcoidosis)
Respiratory disease, other
GI diagnoses
GI bleeding, upper
GI bleeding lower/diverticulitis
GI bleeding, varices
GI inflammatory disease
Neoplasm
Obstruction
Perforation
Vascular insufficiency
Hepatic failure
Intra/retroperitoneal hemorrhage
Pancreatitis
GI, other
Neurological diagnoses
Intracerebral hemorrhage
Neurologic neoplasm
Neurologic infection
Neuromuscular disease
Drug overdose
Subdural/epidural hematoma
Subarachnoid hemorrhage, intracranial aneurysm
Seizures (no structural disease)
Stroke
Neurologic, other
Trauma diagnoses
Trauma involving the head
Head trauma with either chest, abdomen, pelvis, or spine injury
Head trauma with extremity or facial trauma
Head trauma only
Head trauma with multiple other injuries
Trauma, chest and spine trauma
Trauma, spine only
Multiple trauma (excluding head trauma)
Metabolic/endocrine diagnoses
Acid–base, electrolyte disorder
Diabetic ketoacidosis
Hyperglycemic hyperosmolar nonketotic coma
Metabolic/endocrine, other
Hematologic diagnoses
Coagulopathy, neutropenia, thrombocytopenia, pancytopenia
Hematologic, other%
Genitourinary diagnoses
Renal, other
Miscellaneous diagnoses
General, other

TABLE A.3

APACHE IV Surgical Diagnoses [3]

Diagnostic group

Cardiovascular surgery
- Valvular heart surgery
- Coronary artery bypass grafting (CABG) with double or redo valve surgery
- CABG with single valve surgery
- Aortic aneurysm, elective repair
- Aortic aneurysm, rupture
- Aortic aneurysm, dissection
- Femoral–popliteal bypass graft
- Aortoiliac, aortofemoral bypass graft
- Peripheral ischemia (embolectomy, thrombectomy, dilation)
- Carotid endarterectomy
- Cardiovascular surgery, other

Respiratory surgery
- Thoracotomy, malignancy
- Neoplasm, mouth, larynx
- Thoracotomy, lung biopsy, pleural disease
- Thoracotomy, respiratory infection
- Respiratory surgery, other

GI surgery
- GI malignancy
- GI bleeding
- Fistula, abscess
- Cholecystitis, cholangitis
- GI inflammation
- GI obstruction
- GI perforation
- GI, vascular ischemia
- Liver transplant
- GI surgery, other

Neurologic surgery
- Craniotomy or transsphenoidal procedure for neoplasm
- Intracranial hemorrhage
- Subarachnoid hemorrhage (aneurysm, arteriovenous malformation)
- Subdural/epidural hematoma
- Laminectomy, fusion, spinal cord surgery
- Neurologic surgery, other

Trauma surgery
- Head trauma only
- Multiple trauma sites including the head
- Surgery for extremity trauma
- Multiple trauma (excluding the head)

Genitourinary surgery
- Renal/bladder/prostate neoplasm
- Renal transplant
- Hysterectomy
- Genitourinary surgery, other

Miscellaneous surgery
- Amputation (nontraumatic)

TABLE A.4

The SOFA Score

SOFA score	1	2	3	4
Respiration PaO_2/FiO_2, mmHg	<400	<300	<200 with respiratory support	<100 with respiratory support
Coagulation Platelets × $10^3/mm^3$	<150	<100	<50	<20
Liver Bilirubin, mg/dL (μmol/L)	1.2–1.9 (20–32)	2.0–5.9 (33–101)	6.0–11.9 (102–204)	>12.0 (<204)
Cardiovascular Hypotension	MAP < 70 mmHg	Dopamine ≤ 5 or dobutamine (any dose)[a]	Dopamine > 5 or epinephrine ≤ 0.1 or norepinephrine ≤ 0.1	Dopamine > 15 or epinephrine > 0.1 or norepinephrine > 0.1
Central nervous system Glasgow Coma Score	13–14	10–12	6–9	<6
Renal Creatinine, mg/dL (μmol/L) or urine output	1.2–1.9 (110–170)	2.0–3.4 (171–299)	3.5–4.9 (300–440) or <500 mL/d	>5.0 (>440) or <200 mL/d

[a]Adrenergic agents administered for at least 1 hour (doses given are in μg/kg·min).
Adapted with permission from Vincent JL, Moreno R, Takala J, et al. The SOFA (Sepsis-related Organ Failure Assessment) score to describe organ dysfunction/failure. On behalf of the Working Group on Sepsis-Related Problems of the European Society of Intensive Care Medicine. *Intensive Care Med* 1996;22:707–710.
SOFA, Sequential Organ Failure Assessment.

TABLE A.5

Quick SOFA Score

qSOFA (Quick SOFA) Criteria	Points
Respiratory rate ≥22/min	1
Change in mental status	1
Systolic blood pressure ≤100 mmHg	1

Adapted with permission from Marik PE, Taeb AM. SIRS, qSOFA and new sepsis definition. *J Thoracic Dis* 2017;9:943–945. AME Publishing Company.
SOFA, Sequential Organ Failure Assessment.

NORMAL VALUES OF EXPIRATORY PEAK FLOW [5] (TABLES A.6–A.7)

There is a wide variability in peak expiratory flows because of individual differences. Values also vary slightly depending on the peak flow meter used.

TABLE A.6

Normal Values of Expiratory Peak Flow for Men

	Height				
Age (y)	**60 Inches**	**65 Inches**	**70 Inches**	**75 Inches**	**80 Inches**
20	554	602	649	693	740
25	543	590	636	679	725
30	532	577	622	664	710
35	521	565	609	651	695
40	509	552	596	636	680
45	498	540	583	622	665
50	486	527	569	607	649
55	475	515	556	593	634
60	463	502	542	578	618
65	452	490	529	564	603
70	440	477	515	550	587

TABLE A.7

Normal Values of Expiratory Peak Flow for Women

	Height				
Age (y)	**60 Inches**	**65 Inches**	**70 Inches**	**75 Inches**	**80 Inches**
20	390	423	460	496	529
25	385	418	454	490	523
30	380	413	448	483	516
35	375	408	442	476	509
40	370	402	436	470	502
45	365	397	430	464	495
50	360	391	424	457	488
55	355	386	418	451	482
60	350	380	412	445	475
65	345	375	406	439	468
70	340	369	400	432	461

From Higgins TL, Teres D, Copes WS, et al: Assessing contemporary intensive care unit outcome: an updated Mortality Probability Admission Model (MPM0-III). *Crit Care Med* 35(3):827–835, 2007, with permission.

References

1. Le Gall J, Lemeshow S, Saulnier F: A new simplified acute physiology score (SAPS II) based on a European/North American multicenter study. *JAMA* 270:24, 1993.
2. French Society of Anesthesia and Intensive Care: SAPS II calculator. Available at: http://www.sfar.org/scores2/saps2.html. Accessed August 2, 2006.
3. Zimmerman JE, Kramer AA, McNair DS, et al: Acute Physiology and Chronic Health Evaluation (APACHE) IV: hospital mortality assessment for today's critically ill patients. *Crit Care Med* 34(5):1297–1310, 2006.
4. Higgins TL, Teres D, Copes WS, et al: Assessing contemporary intensive care unit outcome: An updated Mortality Probability Admission Model (MPM0-III). *Crit Care Med* 35(3):827–835, 2007.
5. Leiner GC, Abramowitz S, Small MJ, et al: Expiratory peak flow. Standards for normal subjects. Use as a clinical test of ventilatory function. *Am Rev Respir Dis* 86:644, 1963.
6. Seeley E, McAuley DF, Eisner M, et al: Predictors of mortality in acute lung injury during the era of lung protective ventilation. *Thorax* 63(11): 994–998, 2008. doi: 10.1136/thx.2007.093658
7. Dechert RE, Park PK, Bartlett RH: Evaluation of the oxygenation index in adult respiratory failure. J Trauma Acute Care Surg 76(2): 469–473, 2014. doi:10.1097/TA.0b013e3182ab0d27

Index

Note: Page numbers followed by *f* and *t* indicates figure and table respectively.